Premiering with this edition: A Web site dedicated to the very best in oncology

LWWoncology.com

KEY FEATURES

UNPARALLELED CONTENT

Beginning with the sixth edition of **Cancer: Principles & Practice of Oncology** and branching out to well-known subspecialty texts, LWWoncology.com is your complete resource for both classic and up-to-date clinical information unavailable elsewhere. Additional titles available on the Web site in 2001 include: *Manual of Oncologic Therapeutics, The American Joint Committee on Cancer's Cancer Staging Manual, The Chemotherapy Source Book*, and *Cancer Chemotherapy and Biotherapy.*

PPO UPDATES

LWWoncology.com brings you the popular monthly updates to **Cancer: Principles & Practice of Oncology** so that you can browse or search the latest developments in oncology. PPO Updates published in 2000 are also archived on the site for browsing and searching.

FAST, FOCUSED SEARCHING

The search engine is customized to retrieve exact results to your specific requests for information. Oncology-specific modifiers help refine your search, resulting in focused, high-relevance answers. No more scrolling through scores of "hits" to find the answer you need.

CUSTOM ORGANIZATIONAL TOOLS

Personal Bookmarks. Select chapters or sections from one or multiple books and create your own individual reference, based on your practice and your patients.

Saved Searches. Capture often-used search requests, saving valuable time and allowing fast access to the information most critical to your needs.

Personal Profile. Save links to related sites, key meetings, and other professional information.

MEDLINE LINKING

All references within a resource are linked to PubMed abstracts, so you can easily explore your in-depth interests.

VIDEO

LWWoncology.com enhances your experience with videos that provide a "you-are-there" perspective on surgical procedures.

RELATED TEXTS

LWWoncology.com provides cross-references to other LWW oncology texts and offers you the chance to expand your personal oncology library.

CANCER

Principles & Practice of Oncology

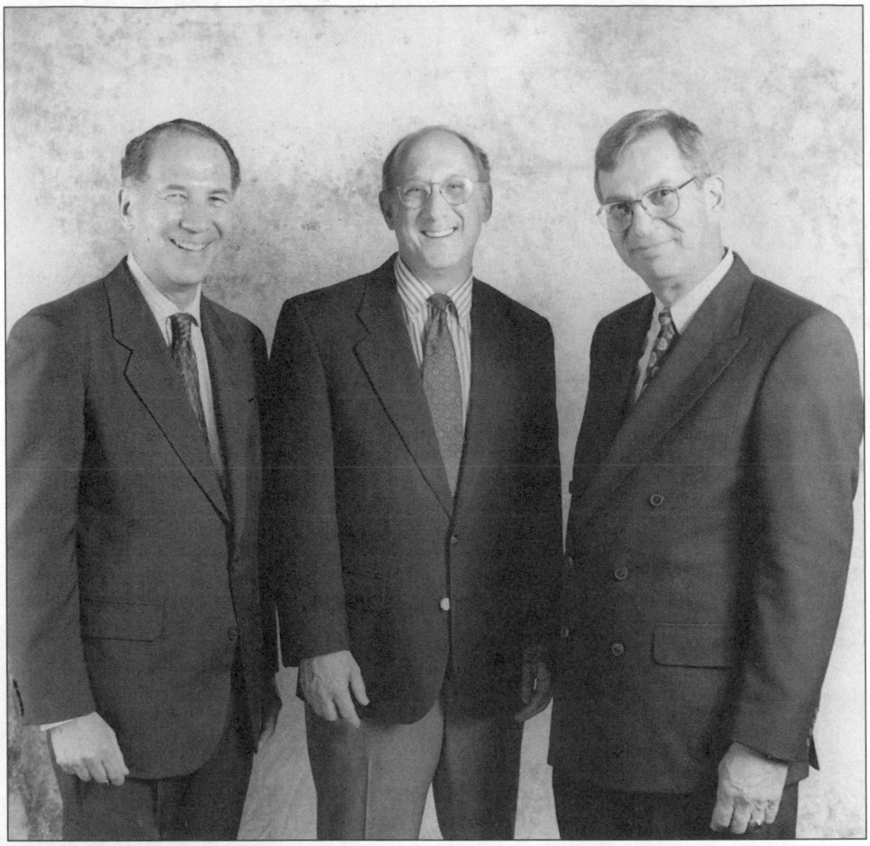

EDITED BY

Vincent T. DeVita, Jr., MD

Director, Yale Cancer Center; Professor of Medicine, Professor of Epidemiology and Public Health, Yale University School of Medicine, New Haven, Connecticut

Samuel Hellman, MD

A. N. Pritzker Distinguished Service Professor, Department of Radiation and Cellular Oncology, University of Chicago, Chicago, Illinois

Steven A. Rosenberg, MD, PhD

Chief of Surgery, National Cancer Institute, National Institutes of Health; Professor of Surgery, Uniformed Services University of the Health Sciences School of Medicine, Bethesda, Maryland; Professor of Surgery, George Washington University School of Medicine, Washington, DC

319 Contributing Authors

CANCER

Principles & Practice of Oncology

6th Edition

www.LWWoncology.com

LIPPINCOTT WILLIAMS & WILKINS
A **Wolters Kluwer** Company
Philadelphia • Baltimore • New York • London
Buenos Aires • Hong Kong • Sydney • Tokyo

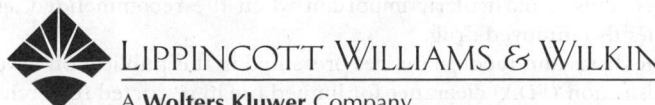

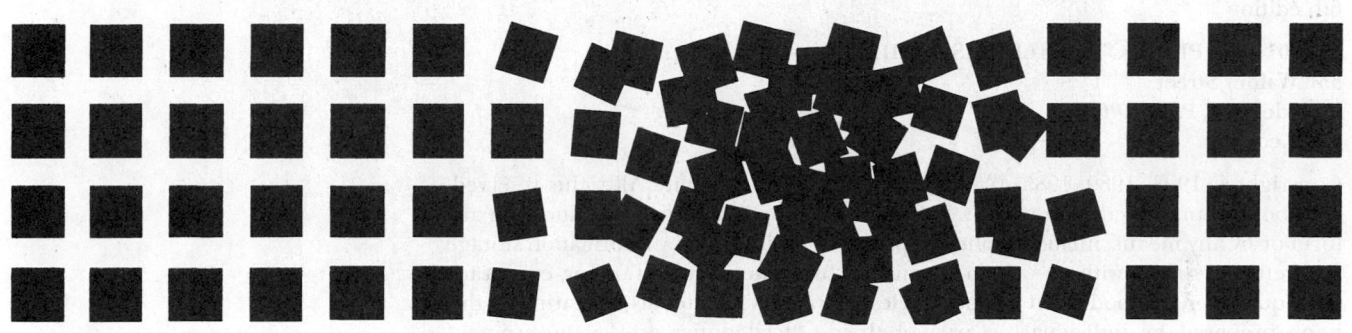

Acquisitions Editor: Stuart Freeman
Developmental Editors: Susan Rhyner, Managing Editor; Anne Snyder, Senior Developmental Editor; and Stephanie Harris, Associate Developmental Editor
Supervising Editor: Toni Ann Scaramuzzo
Production Editors: Kim Langford and Shannon Garza, Silverchair Science + Communications
Manufacturing Manager: Tim Reynolds
Compositor: Silverchair Science + Communications
Printer: Quebecor World, Taunton, MA

6th edition

530 Walnut Street
Philadelphia, PA 19106 USA
LWW.com

Printed in the USA

Library of Congress Cataloging-in-Publication Data
Library of Congress Control Number: 89-649-721
Cancer: principles and practice of oncology [edited by] Vincent T. DeVita, Jr., Samuel Hellman, Steven A. Rosenberg; 319 contributors.—6th
ISSN 0892-0567
ISBN 0-781-72229-2

Care has been taken to confirm the accuracy of the information presented and to describe generally accepted practices. However, the authors, editors, and publisher are not responsible for errors or omissions or for any consequences from application of the information in this book and make no warranty, expressed or implied, with respect to the currency, completeness, or accuracy of the contents of the publication. Application of this information in a particular situation remains the professional responsibility of the practitioner.

The authors, editors, and publisher have exerted every effort to ensure that drug selection and dosage set forth in this text are in accordance with current recommendations and practice at the time of publication. However, in view of ongoing research, changes in government regulations, and the constant flow of information relating to drug therapy and drug reactions, the reader is urged to check the package insert for each drug for any change in indications and dosage and for added warnings and precautions. This is particularly important when the recommended agent is a new or infrequently employed drug.

Some drugs and medical devices presented in this publication have Food and Drug Administration (FDA) clearance for limited use in restricted research settings. It is the responsibility of health care providers to ascertain the FDA status of each drug or device planned for use in their clinical practice.

10 9 8 7 6 5 4 3 2 1

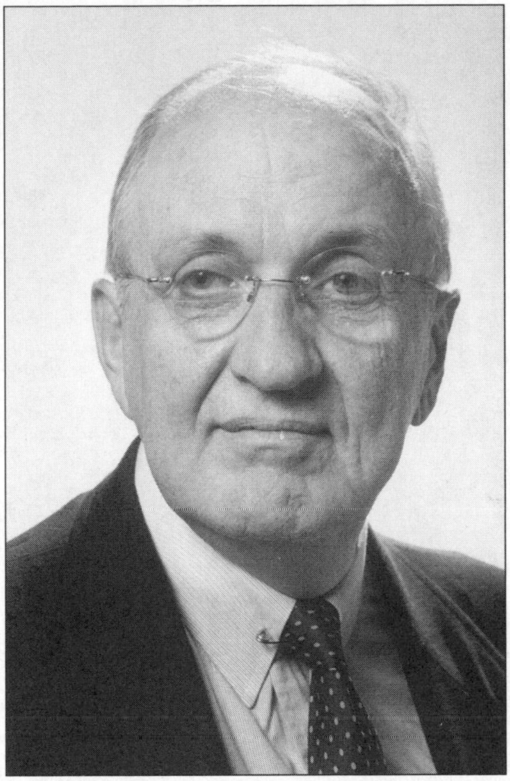

To

Stuart Freeman

whose wisdom and extraordinary skills have guided this text from its inception through all six editions.

His vision for the dissemination of information among all treatment modalities and his commitment to excellence have helped improve the lives of cancer patients.

CONTRIBUTING AUTHORS

James L. Abbruzzese, MD
Annie Laurie Howard Research Distinguished Professor
Department of Gastrointestinal Medical Oncology
The University of Texas M. D. Anderson Cancer Center
Houston, Texas

Gregory P. Adams, PhD
Assistant Member
Department of Medical Oncology
Fox Chase Cancer Center
Philadelphia, Pennsylvania

Daniel M. Albert, MD, MS
F. A. Davis Professor and Chair; Lorenz E. Zimmerman Professor
Department of Ophthalmology and Visual Sciences
University of Wisconsin Center for Health Sciences
Madison, Wisconsin

Kaled M. Alektiar, MD
Assistant Attending
Department of Radiation Oncology
Memorial Sloan-Kettering Cancer Center
New York, New York

H. Richard Alexander, MD
Head, Surgical Metabolism Section
Surgery Branch
National Cancer Institute, National Institutes of Health
Bethesda, Maryland

Carmen J. Allegra, MD
Chief, Medicine Branch
National Cancer Institute, National Institutes of Health
Bethesda, Maryland

Nasser K. Altorki, BCh, MB
Professor of Cardiothoracic Surgery
Weill Medical College of Cornell University
New York, New York

Howard Ira Amols, PhD
Professor of Physics in Radiology
Weill Medical College of Cornell University
Memorial Sloan-Kettering Cancer Center
New York, New York

Susan Anderson, BSN, MFA
Director, Clinical Trials Office
Yale Cancer Center
Yale University School of Medicine
New Haven, Connecticut

Karen H. Antman, MD
Wu Professor of Medicine and Pharmacology
Herbert Irving Comprehensive Cancer Center
Columbia University College of Physicians and Surgeons
New York, New York

James O. Armitage, MD
Professor of Medicine
Dean of the College of Medicine
University of Nebraska Medical Center
Omaha, Nebraska

Susanne M. Arnold, MD
Assistant Professor of Medicine
Department of Hematology and Oncology
Lucille P. Markey Cancer Center
University of Kentucky Chandler Medical Center
Lexington, Kentucky

Michael B. Atkins, MD
Associate Professor of Medicine
Department of Hematology/Oncology
Harvard Medical School
Beth Israel Deaconess Medical Center
Boston, Massachusetts

Richard M. Auchter, MD
Clinical Assistant Professor of Human Oncology
University of Wisconsin Medical School
Madison, Wisconsin

David J. Austin, PhD
Assistant Professor of Chemistry
Yale University School of Medicine
New Haven, Connecticut

Dean F. Bajorin, MD
Professor of Medicine
Weill Medical College of Cornell University
Attending Physician
Memorial Sloan-Kettering Cancer Center
New York, New York

Allen E. Bale, MD
Associate Professor of Genetics
Yale University School of Medicine
New Haven, Connecticut

Bart Barlogie, MD, PhD
Professor of Medicine and Pathology
Director, Arkansas Cancer Research Center
University of Arkansas for Medical Sciences
Little Rock, Arkansas

David L. Bartlett, MD
Surgery Branch
National Cancer Institute, National Institutes of Health
Bethesda, Maryland

Susan E. Bates, MD
Head, Molecular Therapeutics Section, Medicine Branch
National Cancer Institute, National Institutes of Health
Bethesda, Maryland

Jonathan S. Berek, MD
Professor and Chair of Applied Anatomy
Vice Chair and Chief, Division of Gynecologic Oncology
University of California, Los Angeles, UCLA School of Medicine
Los Angeles, California

Ann M. Berger, RN, MSN, MD
Chief of Pain and Palliative Care Service
National Institutes of Health
Bethesda, Maryland

Philip Bierman, MD
Associate Professor of Medicine
Department of Internal Medicine
Section of Oncology/Hematology
University of Nebraska Medical Center
Omaha, Nebraska

Peter McLaren Black, MD, PhD
Franc D. Ingraham Professor of Neurosurgery
Harvard Medical School
Brigham and Women's Hospital
Children's Hospital
Boston, Massachusetts

Clara D. Bloomfield, MD
Professor of Medicine
Ohio State University College of Medicine and Public Health
Department of Internal Medicine
Division of Hematology/Oncology
The Comprehensive Cancer Center
Columbus, Ohio

David A. Bluemke, MD, PhD, MSB
Associate Professor of Radiology
Johns Hopkins University School of Medicine
Baltimore, Maryland

George J. Bosl, MD
Chair, Department of Medicine
Memorial Sloan-Kettering Cancer Center
New York, New York

Douglas E. Brash, PhD
Professor of Therapeutic Radiology and Genetics
Yale University School of Medicine
New Haven, Connecticut

Murray F. Brennan, MD
Chair, Department of Surgery
Memorial Sloan-Kettering Cancer Center
New York, New York

Holly K. Brown, MD
Instructor of Orthopaedic Surgery
Memorial Sloan-Kettering Cancer Center
New York, New York

Suzanne J. Brown, MD
Fellow in Oncology
Yale Comprehensive Cancer Center
Yale University School of Medicine
New Haven, Connecticut

Nick Bryan, MD, PhD
Professor of Radiology
University of Pennsylvania School of Medicine
Philadelphia, Pennsylvania

Gary L. Buchschacher, Jr., MD, PhD
Department of Medicine
Division of Hematology/Oncology
University of California, San Diego, School of Medicine
La Jolla, California

Thomas W. Burke, MD
Professor of Gynecologic Oncology
The University of Texas M. D. Anderson Cancer Center
Houston, Texas

Chandra Burman, PhD
Associate Attending Physicist
Department of Medical Physics
Memorial Sloan-Kettering Cancer Center
New York, New York

Michael A. Caligiuri, MD
Professor of Medicine
Ohio State University College of Medicine and Public Health
Arthur James Cancer Hospital and Research Institute
Columbus, Ohio

Robert B. Cameron, MD
Assistant Professor of Surgery
University of California, Los Angeles, UCLA School of Medicine
Los Angeles, California

Lewis C. Cantley, PhD
Professor of Cell Biology
Harvard Medical School
Beth Israel Deaconess Medical Center
Boston, Massachusetts

Michele Carbone, MD, PhD
Associate Professor of Pathology
Department of Pathology/Cancer Immunology
Loyola University Medical Center
Maywood, Illinois

Christopher L. Carpenter, MD, PhD
Assistant Professor of Medicine
Harvard Medical School
Beth Israel Deaconess Medical Center
Boston, Massachusetts

Peter R. Carroll, MD
Professor and Chair, Department of Urology
University of California, San Francisco, School of Medicine
San Francisco, California

John A. Carucci, MD, PhD
Clinical Instructor of Dermatology
Yale University School of Medicine
New Haven, Connecticut

Webster K. Cavenee, PhD
Professor of Medicine
University of California, San Diego, School of Medicine
Director, Ludwig Institute for Cancer Research
Center for Molecular Genetics; University of California Laboratory of Tumor Biology
La Jolla, California

Bruce A. Chabner, MD
Professor of Medicine
Harvard Medical School
Department of Hematology/Oncology
Massachusetts General Hospital
Boston, Massachusetts

R. S. K. Chaganti, PhD
Member and William E. Snee Chair
Human Genetics
Memorial Sloan-Kettering Cancer Center
New York, New York

Setsuko Kuki Chambers, MD
Professor of Obstetrics and Gynecology
Division of Gynecologic Oncology
Yale University School of Medicine
New Haven, Connecticut

Lisa Chertkov, MD
Fellow in Psychiatry and Behavioral Sciences
Memorial Sloan-Kettering Cancer Center
New York, New York

Bruce D. Cheson, MD
Clinical Professor of Medicine
Georgetown University School of Medicine
Vincent T. Lombardi Cancer Research Center
Washington, DC
Head, Medicine Section
Cancer Therapy Evaluation Program
National Cancer Institute, National Institutes of Health
Bethesda, Maryland

Richard W. Childs, MD
Senior Investigator
Hematology Branch
National Heart, Lung, and Blood Institute, National Institutes of Health
Bethesda, Maryland

Edward Chu, MD
Associate Professor of Medicine and Pharmacology
Yale Cancer Center
Yale University School of Medicine
Director, Veterans Administration Connecticut Cancer Center
New Haven, Connecticut

Chen Chui, PhD
Associate Professor of Medical Physics
Memorial Sloan-Kettering Cancer Center
New York, New York

Rebecca A. Clark-Snow, RN, BSN, OCN
Director of Clinical Services
Oncology and Hematology Associates of Kansas City
Kansas City, Missouri

Daniel G. Coit, MD
Chief of Gastric and Mixed Tumor Service
Department of Surgery
Memorial Sloan-Kettering Cancer Center
New York, New York

Graham A. Colditz, MD, DrPH
Professor of Medicine
Harvard Medical School
Brigham and Women's Hospital
Boston, Massachusetts

Philip Cole, MD, PhD
Professor Emeritus
Department of Epidemiology
University of Alabama School of Medicine
Birmingham, Alabama

Oliver Michael Colvin, MD
Professor of Hematology/Oncology
Director, Duke Comprehensive Cancer Center
Duke University Medical Center
Durham, North Carolina

Dennis L. Cooper, MD
Associate Professor of Medicine
Yale University School of Medicine
Department of Medical Oncology
Yale-New Haven Hospital
New Haven, Connecticut

Carlos Cordon-Cardo, MD, PhD
Member and Director, Division of Molecular Pathology
Department of Pathology
Memorial Sloan-Kettering Cancer Center
New York, New York

José Costa, MD
Professor of Pathology
Yale University School of Medicine
Yale-New Haven Hospital
New Haven, Connecticut

Guido Dalbagni, MD, FACS
Assistant Professor of Urology
Weill Medical College of Cornell University
Memorial Sloan-Kettering Cancer Center
New York, New York

Riccardo Dalla-Favera, MD
Uris Professor of Pathology and Genetics
Director, Institute of Cancer Genetics
Columbia University College of Physicians and Surgeons
New York, New York

Ramsey M. Dallal, MD
Resident of Surgery
University of Pittsburgh Medical Center
Pittsburgh, Pennsylvania

Christopher Daugherty, MD
Assistant Professor of Medicine
University of Chicago Pritzker School of Medicine
Chicago, Illinois

Lisa M. DeAngelis, MD
Chair, Department of Neurology
Memorial Sloan-Kettering Cancer Center
New York, New York

Albert B. Deisseroth, MD, PhD
Ensign Professor of Medicine
Department of Internal Medicine
Yale University School of Medicine
New Haven, Connecticut

Vincent T. DeVita, Jr., MD
Director, Yale Cancer Center
Professor of Medicine
Professor of Epidemiology and Public Health
Yale University School of Medicine
New Haven, Connecticut

Robert B. Dickson, PhD
Professor of Oncology
Georgetown University School of Medicine
Vincent T. Lombardi Cancer Research Center
Washington, DC

Volker Diehl, MD PhD
Professor of Medicine
Department of Internal Medicine I
University Hospital Cologne
Köln, Germany

Joseph J. Disa, MD
Assistant Attending Surgeon
Department of Surgery/Plastic Surgery
Memorial Sloan-Kettering Cancer Center
New York, New York

Gerard M. Doherty, MD
Associate Professor of Surgery
Washington University School of Medicine
St. Louis, Missouri

Sarah S. Donaldson, MD, FACR
Professor of Radiation Oncology
Stanford University School of Medicine
Stanford, California

David H. Ebb, MD
Assistant Professor of Pediatrics
Harvard Medical School
MassGeneral Hospital for Children
Boston, Massachusetts

Richard L. Edelson, MD
Professor and Chair, Dermatology
Yale University School of Medicine
New Haven, Connecticut

Patricia J. Eifel, MD
Professor of Radiation Oncology
The University of Texas M. D. Anderson Cancer Center
Houston, Texas

Lee M. Ellis, MD
Associate Professor of Surgery and Cancer Biology
Department of Surgical Oncology and Cancer Biology
The University of Texas M. D. Anderson Cancer Center
Houston, Texas

Charles Erlichman, MD, FRCP(C)
Professor of Oncology
Department of Medical Oncology
Mayo Medical School
Mayo Clinic
Rochester, Minnesota

Elihu Estey, MD
Professor of Medicine
Department of Leukemia
The University of Texas M. D. Anderson Cancer Center
Houston, Texas

Douglas B. Evans, MD
Professor of Surgery
Department of Surgical Oncology
The University of Texas M. D. Anderson Cancer Center
Houston, Texas

Stefan Faderl, MD
Assistant Professor of Medicine
Department of Leukemia
The University of Texas M. D. Anderson Cancer Center
Houston, Texas

Eric R. Fearon, MD, PhD
Associate Professor of Internal Medicine, Human Genetics, and Pathology
Department of Internal Medicine, Division of Medical Genetics
University of Michigan Medical School
Ann Arbor, Michigan

Isaiah J. Fidler, DVM, PhD
Professor of Cancer Biology and Urology
The University of Texas M. D. Anderson Cancer Center
Houston, Texas

Elliot K. Fishman, MD
Professor of Radiology and Oncology
Johns Hopkins University School of Medicine
Johns Hopkins Hospital
Baltimore, Maryland

Frederick A. Flatow, MD, FACP
Assistant Clinical Professor of Medicine
Department of Oncology
Yale University School of Medicine
New Haven, Connecticut
Medical Director, The Connecticut Hospice
Branford, Connecticut

John C. Flickinger, MD
Professor of Radiation Oncology and Neurological Surgery
Department of Radiation Oncology
University of Pittsburgh Medical Center—Presbyterian Hospital
Pittsburgh, Pennsylvania

Miklos C. Fogarasi, MD
Senior Fellow in Medicine, Section of Medical Oncology
Yale University School of Medicine
Yale Cancer Center
New Haven, Connecticut

Kathleen M. Foley, MD
Professor of Neurology, Neuroscience, and Clinical Pharmacology
Weill Medical College of Cornell University
Attending Neurologist
Memorial Sloan-Kettering Cancer Center
New York, New York

Judah Folkman, MD
Andrus Professor of Pediatric Surgery
Professor of Cell Biology
Harvard Medical School
Children's Hospital
Boston, Massachusetts

Yuman Fong, MD
Attending Surgeon
Memorial Hospital
Member, Memorial Sloan-Kettering Cancer Center
New York, New York

Kwun M. Fong, MD
Hamon Center for Therapeutic Oncology Research
University of Texas Southwestern Medical Center at Dallas
Dallas, Texas

Kenneth A. Foon, MD
Professor of Medicine
Department of Internal Medicine
University of Cincinnati College of Medicine
Director, Barrett Cancer Center
Cincinnati, Ohio

Arlene A. Forastiere, MD
Professor of Oncology
Johns Hopkins University School of Medicine
Baltimore, Maryland

Douglas L. Fraker, MD
Jonathon Rhoads Associate Professor of Surgery
Chief, Division of Surgical Oncology
University of Pennsylvania School of Medicine
Philadelphia, Pennsylvania

Zvi Y. Fuks, MD
Department of Radiation Oncology
Memorial Sloan-Kettering Cancer Center
New York, New York

Brian G. Fuller, MD
Senior Investigator
Radiation Oncology Branch
National Cancer Institute, Radiation Oncology Sciences Program
National Institutes of Health
Bethesda, Maryland

Gianluca Gaidano, MD, PhD
Department of Medical Sciences
Division of Internal Medicine
Amedeo Avogadro University of Eastern Piedmont
Novara, Italy

Don Ganem, MD
Professor of Microbiology and Medicine
Howard Hughes Medical Institute
University of California, San Francisco, School of Medicine
San Francisco, California

Patricia A. Ganz, MD
Professor, School of Medicine and Public Health
Department of Medicine (Hematology-Oncology) and Health Services
University of California, Los Angeles, UCLA School of Medicine
University of California, Los Angeles, Jonsson Comprehensive Cancer Center
Los Angeles, California

Alan C. Geller, MPH, RN
Research Assistant Professor of Dermatology
Boston University School of Medicine
Boston, Massachusetts

Lynn Gerber, MD
Clinical Professor of Medicine
Georgetown University School of Medicine
Chief, Rehabilitation Medicine Department
Clinical Center, National Institutes of Health
Bethesda, Maryland

Jean-Francois H. Geschwind, MD
Assistant Professor of Radiology and Surgery
Johns Hopkins University School of Medicine
Director, Interventional Radiology Research
Department of Radiology and Surgery
Johns Hopkins Hospital
Baltimore, Maryland

Robert J. Ginsberg, MD, FRCS(C)
Professor of Surgery
Weill Medical College of Cornell University
Memorial Sloan-Kettering Cancer Center
New York, New York

Eli Glatstein, MD
Professor of Radiation Oncology
University of Pennsylvania School of Medicine
Hospital of the University of Pennsylvania
Philadelphia, Pennsylvania

Frank A. Greco, MD
Director, Sarah Cannon Cancer Center
Centennial Medical Center
Nashville, Tennessee

Daniel M. Green, MD
Professor of Pediatrics
Roswell Park Cancer Institute
University at Buffalo School of Medicine and Biomedical Sciences
Buffalo, New York

Peter Greenwald, MD, DrPH
Director, Division of Cancer Prevention
National Cancer Institute, National Institutes of Health
Bethesda, Maryland

Michael R. Grever, MD
Professor of Internal Medicine and Hematology and Oncology
Chairman, Department of Internal Medicine
Program Leader for the Experimental Therapeutics Program
James Comprehensive Cancer Center
The Ohio State University
Columbus, Ohio

James D. Griffin, MD
Professor of Medicine
Harvard Medical School
Brigham and Women's Hospital
Department of Adult Oncology
Dana-Farber Cancer Institute
Boston, Massachusetts

Philip H. Gutin, MD
Chief of Neurosurgery; Fred Lebow Chair of Neurooncology
Division of Surgery
Memorial Sloan-Kettering Cancer Center
New York, New York

Douglas Hageman, MPA
Chief, Office of Clinical Informatics
Division of Clinical Sciences
National Cancer Institute, National Institutes of Health
Bethesda, Maryland

John D. Hainsworth, MD
Director, Clinical Research
Sarah Cannon Cancer Center
Centennial Medical Center
Nashville, Tennessee

Ulrike M. Hamper, MD, MBA
Associate Professor of Radiology and Oncology
Johns Hopkins University School of Medicine
Baltimore, Maryland

Jay R. Harris, MD
Professor of Radiation Oncology
Harvard Medical School
Chief of Radiation Oncology
Brigham and Women's Hospital,
Children's Hospital
Dana-Farber Cancer Institute
Boston, Massachusetts

Nancy Lee Harris, MD
Professor of Pathology
Massachusetts General Hospital
Boston, Massachusetts

Louis B. Harrison, MD
Professor of Radiation Oncology
Albert Einstein College of Medicine of
Yeshiva University
Chair, Radiation Oncology
Beth Israel Medical Center
St. Luke's-Roosevelt Hospital Center
New York, New York

Peter W. Heald, MD
Associate Professor of Dermatology
Yale University School of Medicine
New Haven, Connecticut

John H. Healey, MD
Chief, Orthopaedic Surgery Service
Department of Surgery
Memorial Sloan-Kettering Cancer Center
New York, New York

John D. Heiss, MD
Staff Physician
Surgical Neurology Branch
National Institute of Neurological Disorders and Stroke
National Institutes of Health
Bethesda, Maryland

Samuel Hellman, MD
A. N. Pritzker Distinguished Service Professor
Department of Radiation and Cellular Oncology
University of Chicago
Chicago, Illinois

Lee J. Helman, MD
Chief
Pediatric Oncology Branch
Division of Clinical Sciences
National Cancer Institute, National Institutes of Health
Bethesda, Maryland

Charles H. Hennekens, MD, DrPH
Visiting Professor
Department of Medicine and Epidemiology
and Public Health
University of Miami School of Medicine
Miami, Florida

Meenhard Herlyn, DVM, DSc
The Wistar Institute
Philadelphia, Pennsylvania

Harry W. Herr, MD
Attending Surgeon
Department of Urology
Weill Medical College of Cornell University
Memorial Sloan-Kettering Cancer Center
New York, New York

Robert A. Hiatt, MD, PhD
Deputy Director, Division of Cancer Control and Population Sciences
National Cancer Institute, National Institutes of Health
Rockville, Maryland

Jeanne Hicks, MD
Associate Professor of Internal Medicine
George Washington University School of Medicine and Health Sciences
Associate Professor of Rehabilitation Medicine
Department of Orthopedic Surgery
Georgetown University School of Medicine
Washington, DC
Deputy Chief, Department of Rehabilitation Medicines
National Institutes of Health
Bethesda, Maryland

Paulo M. Hoff, MD
Assistant Professor
Department of Gastrointestinal Medical Oncology
The University of Texas M. D. Anderson Cancer Center
Houston, Texas

John P. Hoffman, MD
Professor of Surgery
Temple University School of Medicine
Senior Member, Fox Chase Cancer Center
Philadelphia, Pennsylvania

Steven M. Holland, MD
Senior Clinical Investigator, Laboratory of Host Defenses
National Institute for Allergies and Infectious Diseases and Warren Grant Magnuson Clinical Center
National Institutes of Health
Bethesda, Maryland

McDonald K. Horne III, MD
Senior Clinical Investigator, Clinical Pathology Department
Warren Grant Magnuson Clinical Center, National Institutes of Health
Bethesda, Maryland

Peter M. Howley, MD
George Fabyan Professor of Comparative Pathology
Department of Pathology
Harvard Medical School
Boston, Massachusetts

Susan Molloy Hubbard, RN, MPA
National Cancer Institute, National Institutes of Health
Bethesda, Maryland

Margie Hunt, MS
Assistant Attending
Department of Medical Physics
Memorial Sloan-Kettering Cancer Center
New York, New York

Patrick Hwu, MD
Senior Investigator, Division of Clinical Sciences
National Cancer Institute, National Institutes of Health
Bethesda, Maryland

Bonnie A. Indeck, MSW
Clinical Instructor of Medicine
Department of Social Work/Oncology
Yale University School of Medicine
Yale-New Haven Hospital
New Haven, Connecticut

William Isaacs, PhD
Professor of Urology and Oncology
Johns Hopkins University School of Medicine
Baltimore, Maryland

Robert T. Jensen, MD
Chief, Digestive Diseases Branch
National Institute of Diabetes and Digestive and Kidney Diseases, National Institutes of Health
Bethesda, Maryland

Steven W. Johnson, PhD
Research Assistant Professor of Pharmacology
University of Pennsylvania School of Medicine
Philadelphia, Pennsylvania

Glenn W. Jones, MD, FRCPC, MSc
Associate Professor of Medicine
Department of Radiation Oncology
McMaster University Undergraduate Medical Programme School of Medicine
Hamilton, Ontario, Canada

Barry M. Kacinski, MD, PhD
Professor of Therapeutic Radiology, Obstetrics/Gynecology, and Dermatology
Yale University School of Medicine
New Haven, Connecticut

Robert J. Kaner, MD
Associate Professor of Clinical Medicine
Department of Medicine, Division of Pulmonary and Critical Care Medicine
Weill Medical College of Cornell University
New York Presbyterian Hospital
New York, New York

Christine Kannler, MD, MPH
Medical Resident, Internal Medicine Program
Boston University School of Medicine
Boston, Massachusetts

Hagop M. Kantarjian, MD
Professor of Medicine
Chair, Department of Leukemia
The University of Texas M. D. Anderson Cancer Center
Houston, Texas

Philip W. Kantoff, MD
Associate Professor of Medicine
Harvard Medical School
Director, Lauk Center for Genitourinary Oncology, Adult Oncology
Dana-Farber Cancer Institute
Boston, Massachusetts

Martin S. Karpeh, MD
Assistant Attending
Department of Surgery, Gastric and Mixed Tumor Service
Memorial Sloan-Kettering Cancer Center
New York, New York

Michael B. Kastan, MD, PhD
Member and Chair, Department of Hematology/Oncology
St. Jude Children's Research Hospital
Memphis, Tennessee

David P. Kelsen, MD
Professor of Medicine
Weill Medical College of Cornell University
Chief, Gastrointestinal Oncology Service
Memorial Sloan-Kettering Cancer Center
New York, New York

Nancy Kemeny, MD
Professor of Medicine
Weill Medical College of Cornell University
Attending Physician
Department of of Medicine, Solid Tumor Division, Gastrointestinal Oncology Service
Memorial Sloan-Kettering Cancer Center
New York, New York

Robert S. Kerbel, PhD
Professor and Director
Department of Medical Biophysics
Division of Cancer Biology Research
University of Toronto Faculty of Medicine
Sunnybrook and Women's College Health Sciences Centre
Toronto, Ontario, Canada

Elliott Kieff, MD, PhD
Albee Professor
Department of Medicine and Microbiology and Molecular Genetics
Harvard Medical School
Brigham and Women's Hospital
Boston, Massachusetts

Thomas J. Kilroy, MD
Director of Dental Oncology
Porter Care Hospital
Denver, Colorado

E. Edmund Kim, MD, MS
Professor of Radiology and Medicine
Department of Nuclear Medicine and Diagnostic Radiology
The University of Texas M. D. Anderson Cancer Center
Houston, Texas

John M. Kirkwood, MD
Professor of Medicine, Division of Hematology/Oncology
University of Pittsburgh School of Medicine
Vice Chair for Clinical Research
Director Melanoma Center
University of Pittsburgh Cancer Institute
Pittsburgh, Pennsylvania

David E. Kleiner, Jr., MD, PhD
Director, Clinical Operations
Laboratory of Pathology
National Cancer Institute, National Institutes of Health
Bethesda, Maryland

M. Tish Knobf, RN, PhD
Associate Professor
American Cancer Society Professor of Oncology Nursing
Adult Advanced Practice Program
Yale University School of Nursing
New Haven, Connecticut

Howard K. Koh, MD, MPH
Adjunct Professor
Boston University School of Medicine, School of Public Health
Commissioner of Public Health, Commonwealth of Massachusetts
Boston, Massachusetts

Stanley J. Korsmeyer, MD
Sidney Farber Professor of Pathology
Professor of Medicine
Harvard Medical School
Investigator, Howard Hughes Medical Institute
Director, Program in Molecular Oncology
Department of Cancer Immunology and AIDS
Dana-Farber Cancer Institute
Boston, Massachusetts

Robert C. Kurtz, MD
Professor of Clinical Medicine
Department of Medicine
Weill Medical College of Cornell University
Attending Physician
Memorial Sloan-Kettering Cancer Center
New York, New York

Terry C. Lairmore, MD
Associate Professor of Endocrine and Oncologic Surgery
Washington University School of Medicine
St. Louis, Missouri

Theodore S. Lawrence, MD, PhD
Isadore Lampe Professor and Chair
Department of Radiation Oncology
University of Michigan Medical School
Ann Arbor, Michigan

Hop N. Le, MD
Fellow in Surgery
University of California, San Francisco, School of Medicine
San Francisco, California

Fredrick Leach, MD, PhD
Urologic Oncology Branch
National Cancer Institute, National Institutes of Health
Bethesda, Maryland

Keith L. Lee, MD
Research Fellow in Prostate Cancer
Department of Urology
University of California, San Francisco, School of Medicine
San Francisco, California

David J. Leffell, MD
Professor of Dermatology and Surgery
Yale University School of Medicine
New Haven, Connecticut

Alan T. Lefor, MD, MPH
Associate Professor of Clinical Surgery
University of California, Los Angeles, UCLA School of Medicine
Director, Division of Surgical Oncology
Cedars-Sinai Medical Center
Los Angeles, California

Steven A. Leibel, MD
Chair, Department of Radiation Oncology
Memorial Sloan-Kettering Cancer Center
New York, New York

Victor A. Levin, MD
Professor of Neurooncology
The University of Texas M. D. Anderson Cancer Center
Houston, Texas

Arthur E. Li, MD
Post-Doctoral Fellow in Radiology
Johns Hopkins Hospital
Baltimore, Maryland

Peining Li, PhD
Assistant Director, Cytogenetics Laboratory
Department of Genetics
Yale University School of Medicine
New Haven, Connecticut

Steven K. Libutti, MD
Senior Investigator
Surgery Branch
National Cancer Institute, National Institutes of Health
Bethesda, Maryland

W. Marston Linehan, MD
Chief, Urologic Surgery
Urologic Oncology Branch
National Cancer Institute, National Institutes of Health
Bethesda, Maryland

C. Clifton Ling, PhD
Enid Haupt Chair
Department of Medical Physics
Memorial Sloan-Kettering Cancer Center
New York, New York

Michael P. Link, MD
Professor of Pediatrics
Chief, Division of Hematology, Oncology and Bone Marrow Transplantation
Stanford University School of Medicine
Stanford, California

Lance A. Liotta, MD, PhD
Chief, Laboratory of Pathology
National Cancer Institute, National Institutes of Health
Bethesda, Maryland

Marc E. Lippman, MD
Professor of Oncology and Medicine
Georgetown University School of Medicine
Director, Vincent T. Lombardi Cancer Research Center
Georgetown University Hospital
Washington, DC

Scott M. Lippman, MD
Professor of Medicine and Cancer Prevention
Department of Thoracic/Head and Neck Medical Oncology; Department of Clinical Cancer Prevention
The University of Texas M. D. Anderson Cancer Center
Houston, Texas

Larry I. Lipshultz, MD
Professor of Urology
Chief, Division of Male Reproductive Medicine and Surgery
Baylor College of Medicine
Houston, Texas

Richard F. Little, MD, MPH
Senior Clinical Investigator
HIV and AIDS Malignancy Branch
Division of Clinical Sciences
National Cancer Institute, National Institutes of Health
Bethesda, Maryland

Mark S. Litwin, MD, MPH
Associate Professor of Urology and Health Services
University of California, Los Angeles, UCLA School of Medicine
Los Angeles, California

Edison T. Liu, MD
Director, Division of Clinical Sciences
National Cancer Institute, National Institutes of Health
Bethesda, Maryland

Virginia Livolsi, MD
Professor of Pathology and Laboratory Medicine
University of Pennsylvania School of Medicine
Philadelphia, Pennsylvania

Jay S. Loeffler, MD
Director, Northeast Proton Therapy Center
Department of Radiation Oncology
Massachusetts General Hospital
Boston, Massachusetts

Patrick J. Loehrer, MD
Professor of Medicine
Section of Hematology Oncology
Indiana University School of Medicine
Indianapolis, Indiana

Anthony Lomax, MSc, PhD
Doctor of Radiation Medicine
Paul Scherrer Institut
Villigen, Switzerland

Scott Long, MD, PhD
Assistant Clinical Professor of Medicine
Yale University School of Medicine
New Haven, Connecticut
Physician, The Connecticut Hospice
Branford, Connecticut

Charles L. Loprinzi, MD
Professor and Chair
Department of Medical Oncology
Mayo Medical School
Mayo Clinic
Rochester, Minnesota

Thomas LoSasso, MD
Memorial Sloan-Kettering Cancer Center
New York, New York

Michael T. Lotze, MD
Professor of Surgery, Molecular Genetics, and Biochemistry
University of Pittsburgh School of Medicine
Pittsburgh, Pennsylvania

David N. Louis, MD
Associate Professor of Pathology
Department of Pathology and Neurosurgical Service
Harvard Medical School
Massachusetts General Hospital
Boston, Massachusetts

Andrew M. Lowy, MD
Chief of Surgical Oncology
Associate Medical Director
Barrett Cancer Center
University of Cincinnati Medical Center
Cincinnati, Ohio

Douglas R. Lowy, MD
Chief, Laboratory of Cellular Oncology
Division of Basic Sciences
National Cancer Institute, National Institutes of Health
Bethesda, Maryland

Gigas Mageras, PhD
Associate Attending Physicist
Department of Medical Physics
Memorial Sloan-Kettering Cancer Center
New York, New York

Robert G. Maki, MD, PhD
Clinical Assistant Physician
Department of Medicine
Memorial Sloan-Kettering Cancer Center
New York, New York

Martin M. Malawer, MD, FACS
Professor of Orthopedic Surgery
George Washington University School of Medicine and Health Sciences
Washington Hospital Center, Washington Cancer Institute
Washington, DC
Consultant, Surgery Branch
National Cancer Institute, National Institutes of Health
Bethesda, Maryland

David Malkin, MD
Associate Professor of Pediatrics
Division of Hematology/Oncology
University of Toronto Faculty of Medicine
The Hospital for Sick Children
Toronto, Ontario, Canada

Francesco M. Marincola, MD
Senior Investigator
Surgery Branch
National Cancer Institute, National Institutes of Health
Bethesda, Maryland

Peter Maslak, MD
Assistant Professor
Medicine and Clinical Laboratories
Memorial Sloan-Kettering Cancer Center
New York, New York

Mary Jane Massie, MD
Professor of Clinical Psychiatry
Weill Medical College of Cornell University
Attending Psychiatrist
Department of Psychiatry and Behavioral Science
Memorial Sloan-Kettering Cancer Center
New York, New York

Ellen T. Matloff, MS
Associate Research Scientist
Department of Genetics
Yale University School of Medicine
Yale Cancer Center
New Haven, Connecticut

Peter M. Mauch, MD
Professor of Radiation Oncology
Harvard Medical School
Brigham and Women's Hospital
Boston, Massachusetts

Susan Taylor Mayne, PhD, FACE
Associate Professor of Epidemiology and Public Health
Yale University School of Medicine
Yale Cancer Center
New Haven, Connecticut

Minesh P. Mehta, MD
Associate Professor
Interim Chair
Department of Human Oncology
University of Wisconsin Medical School
Madison, Wisconsin

Marvin L. Meistrich, PhD
Professor of Experimental Radiation Oncology
The University of Texas M. D. Anderson Cancer Center
Houston, Texas

Beth E. Meyerowitz, PhD
Professor of Psychology
University of Southern California School of Medicine
Los Angeles, California

James W. Mier, MD
Associate Professor of Medicine
Harvard Medical School
Beth Israel Deaconess Medical Center
Boston, Massachusetts

Susan D. Miller, PhD
Assistant Professor of Otolaryngology
Georgetown University School of Medicine
Washington, DC

John D. Minna, MD
Professor of Internal Medicine and Pharmacology
Director, Hamon Center for Therapeutic Oncology Research
University of Texas Southwestern Medical Center at Dallas
Dallas, Texas

Bruce D. Minsky, MD
Professor and Vice Chair
Department of Radiation Oncology
Memorial Sloan-Kettering Cancer Center
New York, New York

Jeffrey F. Moley, MD
Associate Professor of Surgery
Washington University School of Medicine
St. Louis, Missouri

Monica Morrow, MD
Professor of Surgery
Northwestern University Medical School
Director, Cancer Department of the American College of Surgeons
Chicago, Illinois

Augusto C. Mota, MD
Senior Fellow in Medicine
Section of Medical Oncology
Yale University School of Medicine
Yale Cancer Center
New Haven, Connecticut

Robert J. Motzer, MD
Associate Attending Physician
Department of Medicine
Memorial Sloan-Kettering Cancer Center
New York, New York

Franco M. Muggia, MD
The Anne Marnick and David H. Cogan Professor of Oncology
New York University School of Medicine
New York, New York

Nikhil C. Munshi, MD
Professor of Medicine
University of Arkansas for Medical Sciences
Myeloma and Transplantation Research Center
Little Rock, Arkansas

John Murren, MD
Associate Professor of Medicine
Yale University School of Medicine
New Haven, Connecticut

Dao M. Nguyen, MD
Senior Investigator
Department of Surgery
National Cancer Institute, National Institutes of Health
Bethesda, Maryland

Jeffrey A. Norton, MD
Professor of Surgery
University of California, San Francisco, School of Medicine
Chief of Surgery, San Francisco Veterans Affairs Medical Center
San Francisco, California

Peter J. O'Dwyer, MB, BCh
Professor of Medicine
Division of Hematology-Oncology
University of Pennsylvania School of Medicine
Philadelphia, Pennsylvania

Edward H. Oldfield, MD
Chief, Surgical Neurology Branch
National Institute for Allergies and Infectious Diseases, National Institutes of Health
Bethesda, Maryland

C. Kent Osborne, MD
Professor of Medicine and Molecular and Cellular Biology
Director, Breast Center
Baylor College of Medicine
Houston, Texas

Willem W. Overwijk, MS
Surgery Branch
National Cancer Institute
Bethesda, Maryland

Robert F. Ozols, MD, PhD
Senior Vice President
Division of Medical Science
Fox Chase Cancer Center
Philadelphia, Pennsylvania

Harvey I. Pass, MD
Professor of Surgery and Oncology
Department of Cardiothoracic Surgery
Wayne State University School of Medicine
Karmanos Cancer Institute
Detroit, Michigan

Roy Patchell, MD
Associate Professor of Surgery (Neurosurgery)
University of Kentucky College of Medicine
Chief of Neuro-Oncology
Division of Neurosurgery
University of Kentucky Medical Center
Lexington, Kentucky

Peter L. Perrotta, MD
Assistant Professor of Pathology
SUNY at Stony Brook School of Medicine
University Hospital
Stony Brook, New York

Jeanne A. Petrek, MD
Attending Surgeon
Memorial Sloan-Kettering Cancer Center
New York, New York

Eric M. Poeschla, MD
Molecular Medicine Program and Division of Infectious Diseases
Mayo Medical School
Mayo Clinic
Rochester, Minnesota

Arthur S. Polans, PhD
Jules and Doris Stein RPB Professor
Department of Ophthalmology and Visual Sciences
University of Wisconsin Medical School
Madison, Wisconsin

Martin G. Pomper, MD, PhD
Assistant Professor of Radiology
Division of Neuroradiology
Johns Hopkins University School of Medicine
Baltimore, Maryland

Amanda Psyrri, MD
Postdoctoral Fellow in Medical Oncology
Yale University School of Medicine
Yale-New Haven Hospital
New Haven, Connecticut

Joe B. Putnam, Jr., MD
Professor of Surgery
Department of Thoracic and Cardiovascular Surgery
The University of Texas M. D. Anderson Cancer Center
Houston, Texas

Mazin B. Qumsiyeh, PhD, FABMG
Associate Professor of Genetics
Yale University School of Medicine
New Haven, Connecticut

Mark J. Ratain, MD
Professor of Medicine
Chair, Committee on Clinical Pharmacology
University of Chicago Pritzker School of Medicine
Chicago, Illinois

Dianne M. Reeves, RN
Senior Research Nurse
Medicine Branch, Division of Clinical Sciences
National Cancer Institute, National Institutes of Health
Bethesda, Maryland

Nicholas P. Restifo, MD
Surgery Branch
National Cancer Institute, National Institutes of Health
Bethesda, Maryland

Stanley R. Riddell, MD
Professor of Medicine
University of Washington School of Medicine
Member, Fred Hutchinson Cancer Research Center
Program in Immunology
Seattle, Washington

Barbara K. Rimer, DrPH
Director, Division of Cancer Control and Population Sciences
National Cancer Institute, National Institutes of Health
Rockville, Maryland

Brad Rodu, DDS
Professor of Pathology
University of Alabama School of Medicine
Birmingham, Alabama

Steven A. Rosenberg, MD, PhD
Chief of Surgery
National Cancer Institute, National Institutes of Health
Professor of Surgery
Uniformed Services University of the Health Sciences School of Medicine
Bethesda, Maryland
Professor of Surgery
George Washington University School of Medicine
Washington, DC

Kenneth Rosenzweig, MD
Assistant Member
Department of Radiation Oncology
Memorial Sloan-Kettering Cancer Center
New York, New York

Andrew J. Roth, MD
Assistant Attending
Department of Psychiatry and Behavioral Sciences
Memorial Sloan-Kettering Cancer Center
New York, New York

Eric K. Rowinsky, MD, FACP
Director, Clinical Research
Institute for Drug Development
Cancer Therapy and Research Center
San Antonio, Texas

José A. Sahel, MD
Professor of Ophthalmology
Clinique Ophthalmologique
Hôpitaux Universitaires de Strasbourg
Strausbourg, France

Kapaettu Satyamoorthy, PhD
Senior Scientist
Department of Molecular and Cellular Oncology
The Wistar Institute
Philadelphia, Pennsylvania

Stimson P. Schantz, MD
Professor of Otolaryngology
The New York Eye and Ear Infirmary
New York, New York

David A. Scheinberg, MD, PhD
Professor of Medicine
Member
Department of Medical Oncology
Memorial Sloan-Kettering Cancer Center
New York, New York

Peter B. Schiff, MD, PhD
Professor and Chair of Radiation Oncology
Columbia University College of Physicians and Surgeons
New York-Presbyterian Hospital
New York, New York

Joellen Schildkraut, PhD
Associate Professor of Community and Family Medicine
Duke University Medical Center
Durham, North Carolina

John T. Schiller, MD
Division of Basic Sciences
National Cancer Institute, National Institutes of Health
Bethesda, Maryland

David S. Schrump, MD
Head, Thoracic Oncology
Department of Surgery
National Cancer Institute, National Institute of Health
Bethesda, Maryland

Peter E. Schwartz, MD
Professor of Obstetrics and Gynecology
Yale University School of Medicine
New Haven, Connecticut

Douglas J. Schwartzentruber, MD
Senior Investigator
Surgery Branch
National Cancer Institute, National Institutes of Health
Bethesda, Maryland

Brahm H. Segal, MD
Assistant Professor of Medicine
Department of Infectious Diseases and Allergy, Immunology, and Rheumatology
University at Buffalo School of Medicine and Biomedical Sciences
Buffalo, New York

Claudia A. Seipp, RN, OCN
Oncology Nurse Clinician
Surgery Branch
National Cancer Institute, National Institutes of Health
Bethesda, Maryland

Yoshitaka Sekido, MD, PhD
Assistant Professor of Clinical Preventive Medicine
Nagoya University School of Medicine
Nagoya, Aichi, Japan

Stuart Seropian, MD
Assistant Professor of Medicine
Department of Internal Medicine, Section of Medical Oncology
Yale University School of Medicine
New Haven, Connecticut

Roy B. Sessions, MD, FACS
Professor of Otolaryngology/Head and Neck Surgery
Albert Einstein College of Medicine of Yeshiva University
Beth Israel Medical Center
New York, New York

Jay Shah, MD
Rehabilitation Medicine Department
National Institutes of Health
Bethesda, Maryland

Robert C. Shamberger, MD
Professor of Surgery
Department of Pediatric Surgery
Harvard Medical School
Children's Hospital
Boston, Massachusetts

Joel Sheinfeld, MD
Associate Member
Department of Urology
Memorial Sloan-Kettering Cancer Center
New York, New York

Richard M. Sherry, MD
Senior Investigator
Surgery Branch
National Cancer Institute, National Institutes of Health
Bethesda, Maryland

Peter G. Shields, MD
Professor of Medicine and Oncology
Cancer Genetics and Epidemiology Program
Georgetown University School of Medicine
Vincent T. Lombardi Cancer Research Center
Washington, DC

William U. Shipley, MD, FACR
Professor of Radiation Oncology
Harvard Medical School
Chair Genitourinary Oncology
Department of Radiation Oncology
Massachusetts General Hospital
Boston, Massachusetts

David Sidransky, BS, MD
Professor of Otolaryngology, Head and Neck Surgery
Johns Hopkins University School of Medicine
Baltimore, Maryland

Mark Siegler, MD
Lindy Bergman Distinguished Service Professor of Medicine
Director, MacLean Center for Clinical Medical Ethics
University of Chicago Pritzker School of Medicine
Chicago, Illinois

Richard Simon, DSc
Chief, Biometric Research Branch
National Cancer Institute, National Institutes of Health
Bethesda, Maryland

Stephen X. Skapek, MD
Assistant Member
Department of Hematology-Oncology (Molecular Therapeutics)
St. Jude Children's Research Hospital
Memphis, Tennessee

Monica Skarulis, MD
Senior Clinical Investigator
National Institute of Diabetes and Digestive and Kidney Diseases, National Institutes of Health
Bethesda, Maryland

John M. Skibber, MD
Associate Professor of Surgery
Department of Surgical Oncology
The University of Texas M. D. Anderson Cancer Center
Houston, Texas

Alfred R. Smith, PhD
Professor of Radiation Oncology
Harvard Medical School
Massachusetts General Hospital
Boston, Massachusetts

J. Stanley Smith, MD
Professor of Surgery
Pennsylvania State University College of Medicine
Milton S. Hershey Medical Center
Hershey, Pennsylvania

Phyllis M. Smith, MS, LCSW
Senior Clinical Social Worker
Department of Social Work
Yale-New Haven Medical Center
New Haven, Connecticut

Edward L. Snyder, MD
Professor of Laboratory Medicine
Yale University School of Medicine
Director, Blood Bank
Yale-New Haven Hospital
New Haven, Connecticut

Wiley W. Souba, MD, ScD, MBA
Waldhausen Professor and Chair
Department of Surgery
Pennsylvania State University College of Medicine
Hershey, Pennsylvania

Ira J. Spiro, MD, PhD
Department of Radiation Oncology
Harvard Medical School
Massachusetts General Hospital
Boston, Massachusetts

Laurel J. Steinherz, MD
Associate Professor of Clinical Pediatrics
Weill Medical College of Cornell University
Associate Member
Memorial Sloan-Kettering Cancer Center
Director of Pediatric Cardiology
Memorial Hospital for Cancer and Allied Diseases
New York, New York

William G. Stetler-Stevenson, MD, PhD
Senior Investigator, Chief, Extracellular Matrix Pathology Section
Laboratory of Pathology
Division of Clinical Sciences
National Cancer Institute, National Institutes of Health
Bethesda, Maryland

James P. Stevenson, MD
Assistant Professor of Medicine
Department of Medical Oncology
University of Pennsylvania School of Medicine
Philadelphia, Pennsylvania

Clinton F. Stewart, PharmD
Associate Member
Department of Pharmaceutical Sciences
St. Jude Children's Research Hospital
Memphis, Tennessee

Diane E. Stover, MD
Professor of Clinical Medicine
Weill Medical College of Cornell University
Chief, Pulmonary Medicine
Head, General Medicine
Memorial Sloan-Kettering Cancer Center
New York, New York

Mario Sznol, MD
Vice President
Department of Clinical Affairs
Vion Pharmaceuticals
New Haven, Connecticut

Moshe Talpaz, MD
Professor of Medicine
Department of Bioimmunotherapy
The University of Texas M. D. Anderson Cancer Center
Houston, Texas

Nancy J. Tarbell, MD
Professor of Radiation Oncology
Harvard Medical School
Massachusetts General Hospital
Boston, Massachusetts

Joel E. Tepper, MD
Professor and Chair
Department of Radiation Oncology
University of North Carolina at Chapel Hill School of Medicine
Chapel Hill, North Carolina

Joseph R. Testa, PhD
Senior Member
Director, Human Genetics Program
Fox Chase Cancer Center
Philadelphia, Pennsylvania

James T. Thigpen, MD
Professor of Medicine
University of Mississippi School of Medicine
University of Mississippi Medical Center
Jackson, Mississippi

Charles R. Thomas, Jr., MD
Associate Professor and Vice Chair
Department of Radiation Oncology
Adjunct Associate Professor of Medical Oncology
University of Texas Health Science Center at San Antonio
San Antonio Cancer Institute
San Antonio, Texas

Michael J. Thun, MD, MS
Vice President
Department of Epidemiology and Surveillance Research
American Cancer Society
Atlanta, Georgia

Anthony W. Tolcher, MD, FRCP(C)
Assistant Clinical Professor of Medicine
University of Texas Health Science Center at San Antonio
San Antonio, Texas

Lois B. Travis, MD, ScD
Senior Investigator
Division of Cancer Epidemiology and Genetics
National Cancer Institute, National Institutes of Health
Bethesda, Maryland

Guido Tricot, MD, PhD
Director, Myeloma Treatment and Transplantation Research Center
University of Arkansas for Medical Sciences
Little Rock, Arkansas

Margaret A. Tucker, MD
Chief, Genetic Epidemiology Branch
Division of Cancer Epidemiology and Genetics
National Cancer Institute, National Institutes of Health
Rockville, Maryland

Robert L. Ullrich, PhD
Professor of Radiation Oncology
University of Texas Medical School at Galveston
Galveston, Texas

Bruce A. Urban, MD
Assistant Professor of Radiology
Johns Hopkins University School of Medicine
Johns Hopkins Hospital
Baltimore, Maryland

Flora E. van Leeuwen, PhD
Professor of Cancer Epidemiology
Department of Epidemiology
The Netherlands Cancer Institute
Amsterdam, The Netherlands

Rena Vassilopoulou-Sellin, MD, FACP, FACE
Professor of Medicine
Internist
Department of Internal Medicine Specialties/Endocrinology
The University of Texas M. D. Anderson Cancer Center
Houston, Texas

Everett E. Vokes, MD
Duchossois Professor of Medicine and Radiation Oncology
Director, Section of Hematology/Oncology
University of Chicago Pritzker School of Medicine
Chicago, Illinois

Margaret von Mehren, MD
Associate Member
Department of Medical Oncology
Fox Chase Cancer Center
Philadelphia, Pennsylvania

Thomas J. Walsh, MD
Senior Investigator
Pediatric Oncology Branch
National Cancer Institute, National Institutes of Health
Bethesda, Maryland

McClellan M. Walther, MD
Department of Urology Oncology
National Cancer Institute, National Institutes of Health
Bethesda, Maryland

Raymond P. Warrell, Jr., MD
President and Chief Executive Officer
Genta Incorporated
Berkeley Heights, New Jersey

Louis M. Weiner, MD
Chair and Professor of Medicine
Department of Medical Oncology
Fox Chase Cancer Center
Philadelphia, Pennsylvania

Howard J. Weinstein, MD
Professor of Pediatrics
Pediatric Hematology-Oncology
Harvard Medical School
MassGeneral Hospital for Children
Boston, Massachusetts

Mark Weiss, MD
Assistant Professor of Medicine
Memorial Sloan-Kettering Cancer Center
New York, New York

Raymond B. Weiss, MD
Clinical Professor of Medicine
Georgetown University School of Medicine
Washington, D.C.

Samuel A. Wells, Jr., MD
Professor of Surgery
Washington University School of Medicine
St. Louis, Missouri

Patrick Y. Wen, MD
Associate Professor of Neurology
Harvard Medical School
Center for Neuro-Oncology
Dana-Farber Cancer Institute
Division of Neuro-Oncology
Brigham and Women's Hospital
Boston, Massachusetts

Jeffrey D. White, MD
Director
Office of Cancer Complementary and Alternative Medicine
National Cancer Institute, National Institutes of Health
Bethesda, Maryland

Christopher G. Willett, MD
Professor of Radiation Oncology
Harvard Medical School
Massachusetts General Hospital
Boston, Massachusetts

Walter C. Willett, MD
Department of Nutrition
Harvard School of Public Health
Boston, Massachusetts

Lynn D. Wilson, MD, MPH
Associate Professor of Therapeutic Radiology
Yale University School of Medicine
New Haven, Connecticut

Eric P. Winer, MD
Associate Professor of Medicine
Department of Adult Oncology
Dana-Farber Cancer Institute
Boston, Massachusetts

Flossie Wong-Staal, PhD
Florence Seeley Riford Professor in AIDS Research
Department of Medicine and Biology
University of California, San Diego, School of Medicine
La Jolla, California

John R. Wunderlich, MD
Surgery Branch
National Cancer Institute, National Institutes of Health
Bethesda, Maryland

Joachim Yahalom, MD
Professor of Radiation Oncology in Medicine
Weill Medical College of Cornell University
Attending and Member
Memorial Sloan-Kettering Cancer Center
New York, New York

James C. Yang, MD
Senior Investigator
Surgery Branch
National Cancer Institute, National Institutes of Health
Bethesda, Maryland

Robert Yarchoan, MD
Chief, HIV and AIDS Malignancy Branch
Division of Clinical Sciences
National Cancer Institute, National Institutes of Health
Bethesda, Maryland

Stuart H. Yuspa, MD
Laboratory Chief
Laboratory of Cellular Carcinogenesis and Tumor Promotion
National Cancer Institute, National Institutes of Health
Bethesda, Maryland

Berton Zbar
Chief, Laboratory of Immunology
Division of Basic Sciences
National Cancer Institute, National Institutes of Health
Bethesda, Maryland

Michael J. Zelefsky, MD
Associate Professor of Radiation Oncology
Director of Brachytherapy
Memorial Sloan-Kettering Cancer Center
New York, New York

Sandra S. Zinkel, MD, PhD
Research Fellow in Cancer Immunology and AIDS
Dana-Farber Cancer Institute
Boston, Massachusetts

PREFACE

The rapid pace of change in knowledge of the scientific basis and clinical practice of oncology presents a daunting challenge to the oncologist. The extraordinary increase in understanding of the molecular basis of cellular processes, the rise of biotechnology, and the steady refinement of each of the major treatment approaches have impacted every phase of the care of the cancer patient. In addition, an increased appreciation of the coordinated role of each of the main treatment modalities in the care of an individual cancer patient has emphasized the need for oncologists to be familiar with developments in all treatment modalities. Each edition of this text, first published in 1982, has attempted to help the oncologist keep pace with these changes.

In this sixth edition of *CANCER: Principles and Practice of Oncology,* we have again attempted to provide a comprehensive resource describing the science underlying recent clinical developments as well as complete information to aid the clinician in the panorama of clinical care ranging from cancer prevention to the care of the terminally ill patient. To accomplish this, the book has been divided into four parts.

PART 1: **Essentials of Modern Oncologic Science** presents a summary of the major areas of modern bioscience carefully distilled to provide the background necessary for an understanding of recent developments in oncology. Thus chapters on molecular biology, genomics, proteomics, signal transduction, and immunology present a primer for the oncologist in these important areas.

Part 2: **Principles of Oncology** has been reorganized to present in further detail the specific scientific areas of greatest relevance to the oncologist, including new chapters on cytogenetics, the cell cycle, apoptosis, and angiogenesis, as well as chapters on the etiology of cancer, and a clear description of modern epidemiologic methods and the incidence of and mortality from cancer.

Chapters on the principles underlying the four modalities of cancer treatment—surgery, radiotherapy, chemotherapy, and biologic therapy—present the basis for continuing changes in the development and application of these treatments. The pharmacology of cancer chemotherapeutics is presented, and a new section is introduced on the rapidly changing area of cancer biotherapeutics as these agents have entered into the practice of oncology.

The final chapter in PART 2 deals with the design and analysis of clinical trials as well as research data and management. As more and more patients are entering clinical trials, knowledge of these areas by the practicing oncologist is of special importance.

PART 3: **Practice of Oncology** provides the practicing clinician with the specific, practical information needed for the management of each cancer patient. Increased emphasis on cancer prevention relating to diet, tobacco, chemopreventive agents, fat, exercise, retinoids, naturally occurring dietary anticarcinogens, and many other areas are covered in detail. A new chapter on the role of surgery in cancer prevention details the emerging use of surgery in preventing cancer in high-risk individuals. Modern techniques of cancer screening, molecular pathology, imaging, and endoscopy are detailed in this section as well.

The hallmark of this book from its inception to the present and a major reason it has gained worldwide acceptance as a definitive source of cancer information has been the description of the treatment of cancer patients by stage of presentation with a tightly coordinated description of the role of each of the treatment modalities in the care of individual patients. To ensure a balanced multidisciplinary approach, each of the major treatment chapters is co-authored by a surgeon, a medical oncologist, and a radiation oncologist. Each of the major treatment sections is preceded by an updated, brief chapter describing the molecular biology of that cancer and the prospects this new information holds for the improved management of cancer patients.

Increased emphasis on supportive care, palliative care, and the quality of life of the cancer patient has led to an enlargement of sections dealing with these areas, including increased information on pain control and the nutritional, sexual, and psychosocial management of the cancer patient as well as issues related to the specialized care of the terminally ill.

PART 4: **Newer Approaches in Cancer Treatment** looks to the future of developments in oncology with special sections on gene therapy, molecular therapy, preventive and therapeutic cancer vaccines, image-guided surgery, and proton beam radiation therapy. In this section, we have attempted to identify those areas that we think will be of increasing value in the several years after the appearance of this text.

As we enter the twenty-first century, both the incidence and mortality of many of the major cancers are beginning to decline. We believe that the dissemination of carefully coordinated information of the scientific foundation and practice of oncology has played and will continue to play an important role in decreasing the devastating impact of cancer on modern society. We present the sixth edition of *CANCER: Principles and Practice of Oncology* to provide the practicing oncologist with the practical as well as cutting-edge information needed to provide the best possible care for each individual patient.

Vincent T. DeVita, Jr., MD
Samuel Hellman, MD
Steven A. Rosenberg, MD, PhD

ACKNOWLEDGMENTS

The editors are grateful to Zia Raven for her excellent help and energy in coordinating all of the contributions to this book and the many organizational details involved in its assembly. We are also grateful to Ruth Crawford, who played an important role in the compilation of many of the manuscripts.

We especially thank Stuart Freeman, Senior Editor, Oncology Program, Lippincott Williams & Wilkins, whose efforts and exceptional talents have been an important part of the preparation of this book through six editions.

VTD
SH
SAR

CONTENTS

PART 1

ESSENTIALS OF MODERN ONCOLOGIC SCIENCE

9

10

11

19

29

51

52

55
Adverse Effects of Treatment 2869

CANCER
Principles & Practice of Oncology

PART 1

ESSENTIALS OF MODERN ONCOLOGIC SCIENCE

Lance A. Liotta
Edison T. Liu

CHAPTER 1

Essentials of Molecular Biology: Basic Principles

STORAGE AND TRANSMISSION OF GENETIC INFORMATION

NUCLEIC ACIDS

The genetic material of all known organisms is nucleic acid: deoxyribonucleic acid (DNA) and ribonucleic acid (RNA). Nucleic acids act as an information storehouse. They also actively participate in the reading and transmission of stored information within the cell and from one cell generation to the next. The usual flow of genetic information is from DNA to RNA to protein. The transition from DNA to RNA is called *transcription*, and the transition from RNA to protein is called *translation*. The direction of flow from DNA to RNA to protein was considered the "central dogma" in biologic sciences because most organisms exhibit this directionality in the expression of genetic information. However, it was found that some viruses, including retroviruses and the virus that causes autoimmune deficiency syndrome, transmit information from RNA to DNA using an enzyme called *reverse transcriptase*. Nucleic acids are polymers comprised of nucleotides (generally four different types) chemically linked together in chains that can be many millions of units long. The number of possible nucleic acid combinations *n* units long is thus 4^n. A nucleic acid only 10 units in length therefore has 4^{10} possible sequences.

Each nucleotide in the chain contains a nitrogenous base, a five-carbon sugar, and a phosphate group. The sequence of bases is the form in which the genetic information is coded.

There are two types of bases: pyrimidines and purines. Pyrimidines are six-membered rings and include cytosine (C), thymine (T), and uracil (U). Purines are fused five- and six-membered rings and include adenine (A) and guanine (G). The chemical structures of the bases is shown in Figure 1-1. Bases C, A, and G are found in both DNA and RNA. T is specific to DNA, and U is specific to RNA.

Nucleosides are constituted by a nitrogenous base linked to a five-carbon sugar (pentose). The linkage is from the N1 position of the pyrimidines or from the N9 position of the purines to the carbon at position 1 on the pentose. DNA and RNA use different pentose sugars. The sugar in DNA is deoxyribose, and the pentose in RNA is ribose. The difference in the two sugars is a hydroxyl group at the 2' position on the sugar.

Nucleotides are nucleoside phosphates. A nucleotide is formed when a phosphate group is added to the 5' position on the pentose. The nucleotides that form the nucleic acid chain are connected in a very specific way: The 5' position of one pentose ring is connected to the 3' position of the next pentose ring by a phosphate group. The connection is called a *phosphodiester bond.*

DNA

The DNA backbone is made up of bonded sugar and phosphate groups in which a phosphate group connects the 5' carbon of one sugar to the 3' carbon of the next sugar in the chain by a phosphodiester bond. As shown in Figure 1-2, the beginning of the DNA chain has a phosphate group attached to the 5' carbon of deoxyribose, whereas the end of the chain has an OH group on the 3' carbon of deoxyribose.

DNA is a double helix. It is a double-stranded polymer. The bases of each chain face inward, with the restriction that a purine is always paired opposite to a pyrimidine; thus, a G on one strand

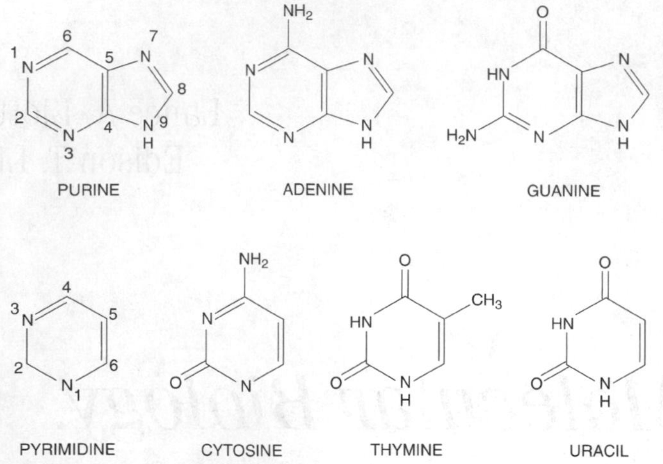

FIGURE 1-1. Purines and pyrimidines.

is paired with a C on the other, and an A is paired with a T. The sugar phosphates are on the backbone of the helix. The resulting negative charge on the outside of the helix is neutralized in the chromosome by metal ions or positively charged proteins.

The two polynucleotide chains in the double helix are connected by hydrogen bonds between the bases. As noted earlier, G hydrogen-bonds specifically with a C, whereas an A can only hydrogen-bond with a T. The resulting base pairs are said to be *complementary.* As shown in Figure 1-3, the GC base pair has three hydrogen bonds, and the AT base pair has only two hydrogen bonds. Each strand can serve as the template for the synthesis of the other, enabling faithful reproduction of the genetic code.

The two polynucleotide chains of the DNA double helix run in opposite directions (antiparallel). Thus, as one strand runs in the 5' to the 3' direction, the partner strand runs in the 3' to 5' direction, as in the following example:

5' P A G T C T G C C A OH 3'
3' HO T C A G A C G G T P 5'

DNA can be methylated in the carbon-5 position of cytosine to form 5-methylcytosine. This occurs in animals in DNA locations where the cytosine is followed on the same strand by guanine. The pattern of methylation is passed on when the DNA replicates.

RNA

In RNA, the pyrimidine uracil replaces the DNA base thymine, and the pentose ribose is used instead of deoxyribose in DNA. During the synthesis of RNA from a DNA template, adenine in DNA is transcribed into uracil in RNA.

Because the pentose ribose is used in RNA instead of deoxyribose, this produces a ribonucleotide having a 2' OH group on the sugar, whereas the 2' OH group is not present in DNA. The important consequence is that RNA is much less stable than DNA. RNA is highly base labile. Although RNA can have a complex secondary structure, it is single stranded, not double stranded like DNA.

RNA is *transcribed* from a DNA template and is the first step by which the genetic information of DNA is converted into the synthesis of specific proteins. A single strand of RNA is generated that is identical in its sequence to one of the strands of the DNA. The DNA strand that has the same sequence (with T instead of U) as the messenger RNA (mRNA) is the coding, or positive, strand; the opposite antiparallel strand is the anticoding, or negative, strand. The RNA itself then becomes the template (mRNA) for translation into the sequence of amino acids that comprise the protein polypeptide.

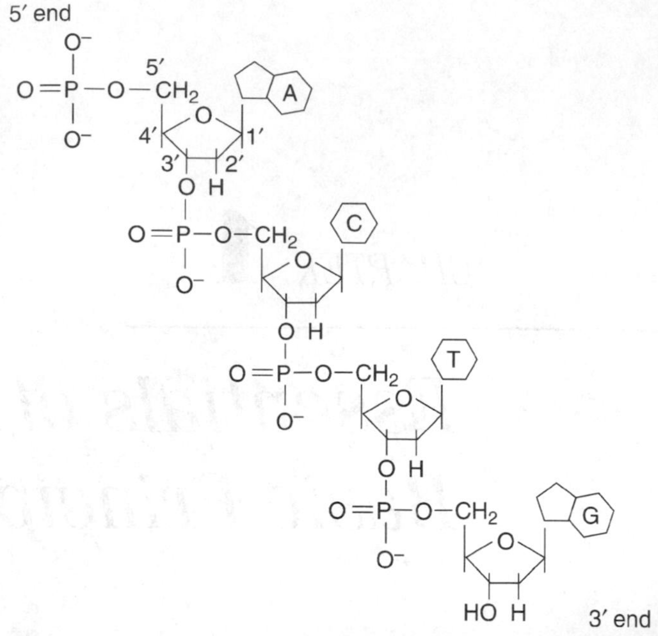

FIGURE 1-2. The backbone of DNA is made of bonded sugar and phosphate groups in which a phosphate group connects the 5' carbon of one sugar to the 3' carbon of the next sugar in the chain. The beginning of the chain has a phosphate group attached to the 5' carbon of deoxyribose.

Three main types of RNA are present in the cell: mRNA, ribosomal RNA (rRNA), and transfer RNA (tRNA). mRNA encodes the sequence for all cellular proteins; however, most

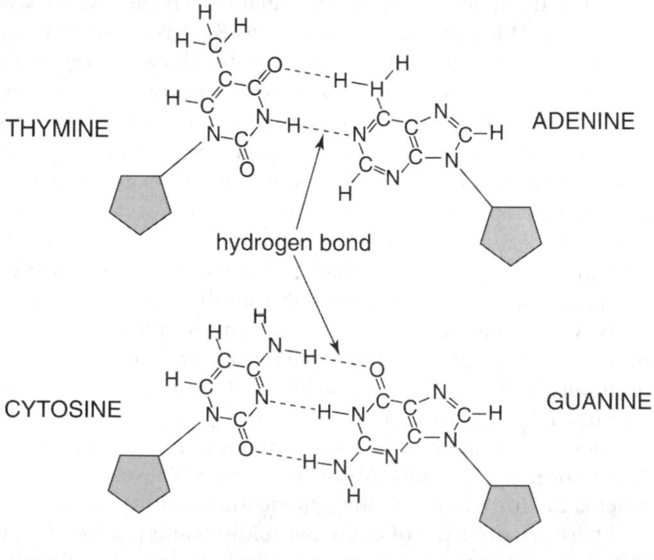

FIGURE 1-3. Base pairs are formed by hydrogen bonds. T=A; G≡C.

		T		C		A		G	
T	T	TTT	phe	TCT	ser	TAT	tyr	TGT	cys
	C	TTC	phe	TCC	ser	TAC	tyr	TGC	cys
	A	TTA	leu	TCA	ser	TAA	ochre	TGA	umber
	G	TTG	leu	TCG	ser	TAG	amber	TGG	trp
C	T	CTT	leu	CCT	pro	CAT	his	CGT	arg
	C	CTC	leu	CCC	pro	CAC	his	CGC	arg
	A	CTA	leu	CCA	pro	CAA	gln	CGA	arg
	G	CTG	leu	CCG	pro	CAG	gln	CGG	arg
A	T	ATT	ile	ACT	thr	AAT	asn	AGT	ser
	C	ATC	ile	ACC	thr	AAC	asn	AGC	ser
	A	ATA	ile	ACA	thr	AAA	lys	AGA	arg
	G	ATG	met	ACG	thr	AAG	lys	AGG	arg
G	T	GTT	val	GCT	ala	GAT	asp	GGT	gly
	C	GTC	val	GCC	ala	GAC	asp	GGC	gly
	A	GTA	val	GCA	ala	GAA	glu	GGA	gly
	G	GTG	val	GCG	ala	GAG	glu	GGG	gly
		T		C		A		G	

FIGURE 1-4. Genetic code. The first base of each codon is presented vertically outside the left margin. The second base of each codon is presented horizontally above and below the chart. The third (wobble) position of each codon is presented just within the left margin.

initial transcripts of mRNA contain large pieces of intervening sequences, or introns, that must be spliced out to leave the coding sequences, or exons. At the 3' end of most mRNA molecules is a poly(A) tail of 150 to 250 adenine nucleotides. The mRNA also has an untranslated leader and tailer sequence at both ends. rRNA does not code for protein. Instead, it comprises part of the machinery that decodes the information in the mRNA. tRNA also does not code for protein. It reads off the mRNA triplet code and matches it with the correct amino acid. tRNA contains specific bases not found in other RNAs: inosine, pseudouridine, and dihydrouridine. At the end of each tRNA is an acceptor arm whose free end is aminoacetylated, or carries the specific amino acid. Another arm on the tRNA contains the anticodon, which recognizes the complementary mRNA codon. Thus, mRNA functions as a transportable copy of the blueprint for the synthesis of protein, and tRNA functions as part of the protein synthetic assembly line.

NUCLEASES AND POLYMERASES

Endonucleases are enzymes that cleave bonds within a nucleic acid chain. They may be specific for RNA, DNA, or hybrids of RNA-DNA or DNA-DNA. Restriction enzymes are a special class of endonucleases that recognize specific short sequences of DNA and cleave the DNA at or next to the recognition sequence. These enzymes are isolated from bacteria and are named after the genus (first letter) and species (second two letters) of the bacteria they are derived from. Because a bacteria can make more than one restriction enzyme, the specific member is designated by a roman numeral (e.g., EcoRI: *Escherichia coli*, strain R, first enzyme from that strain). Restriction enzymes cut DNA at palindromes. The palindrome is a sequence of DNA that is the same when one strand is read left to right (5' to 3') or the other is read right to left (still 5' to 3' because of the antiparallel rule). An example for EcoRI is

5' GAATTC 3'
3' CTTAAG 5'

Restriction endonucleases are now standard tools in molecular biology and permit the cutting of large stretches of DNA at very precise points. They allow fragments of DNA to be "fingerprinted" by the size of the cleaved fragments. Moreover, a restriction enzyme can cleave the DNA so as to leave blunt ends, or staggered "sticky" ends with 5' or 3' overhangs. Because of this property, restriction enzymes are powerful tools to analyze DNA sequences and to create cleaved pieces of DNA that can be shuffled, recombined, and reannealed in the process of DNA cloning.

Polymerases are enzymes that synthesize nucleic acid chains. RNA polymerases synthesize RNA, and DNA polymerases synthesize DNA. All polymerases require a template (nucleic acid strand to be synthesized), which is complementary to the strand being synthesized. They also need a primer, which is a short sequence (oligonucleotide) that is complementary to the 3' end of the template. This provides a free 3' OH end at which the polymerase starts to build a new chain.

Reverse transcriptase is a special polymerase that has, as its primary function, the ability to use RNA as a template to generate a copy in the form of DNA. It is an important enzyme in the life cycle of the human immunodeficiency viruses that cause autoimmune deficiency syndrome and other disorders, and as such, is a prime target for anti–human immunodeficiency virus therapeutics. Reverse transcriptase is also a unique reagent that can be used to create complementary DNA (copy) from mRNA extracted from cells, and therefore it is used in complementary DNA cloning.

The genetic code is a series of three mRNA nucleotides; each is a codon that encodes one amino acid (Fig. 1-4). Three codons are nonsense or termination codons. The genetic code is degenerate, with more than one codon for most amino acids.

GENES AND THEIR EXPRESSION

A gene is a unit of inheritance that carries the information representing a polypeptide or a structural RNA molecule. Genes are stable information packets transmitted from one generation to the next.

A gene includes "control" regions that precede and follow a central coding region and that include the sequences encoding the protein product. The coding region is preceded by a leader sequence and followed by a trailer. The leader and trailer are not translated into protein and represent the 5' and 3' untranslated regions of the mRNA that often function in regulating the half-life of the mRNA or in controlling translation.

The coding region is divided into alternating exons and introns. The exons, which are represented in the mature spliced RNA product, are interrupted or intervened by the introns. The introns are spliced out and do not encode amino acids. The reason for the introns is not obvious, but it is a hallmark of all higher order species in evolution. A gene family is a set of genes whose exons are related. A gene cluster is a group of genes related to each other that are adjacent.

Transcription is the process by which a single-stranded RNA is generated that is identical in sequence with the coding strand of the DNA. A transcription unit is a sequence of DNA that can be transcribed by RNA polymerase into a single RNA, beginning at an initiation start point and ending at a terminator.

Three types of genes are found in eukaryotes that are differentiated from each other by the type of RNA polymerase that transcribes the gene: RNA polymerase I, II, and III. RNA polymerase II produces heterogeneous nuclear RNA, which becomes mRNA after processing and splicing.

Proteins are encoded by mRNA. In the vast majority of cases, therefore, it is the protein product of a polymerase II gene that finally determines gene activity. The genetic code that transfers nucleotide sequences into amino acid sequences is organized as triplets of nucleotides forming a codon. Each codon is recognized by the translational machinery as representing an amino acid. Some codons are used as traffic signals that tell the machinery to start and stop translation (therefore their designation as *start* and *stop codons*). Mutations in important tumor suppressor genes, such as the breast cancer gene BRCA1 and the colon cancer gene APC, are frequently mutations that convert a codon that normally encodes an amino acid to a stop codon. This results in a prematurely truncated and, therefore, inactive protein.

A series of potential points for control of gene expression and functional protein production exist. These include activation of the gene chromatin complex, initiation of transcription, processing and capping of the RNA transcript, splicing of the RNA, polyadenylation of the RNA transcript, transport of the RNA to the cytoplasm, degradation of the RNA, translation of the mRNA into protein, correct folding and posttranslational modifications of the protein, transport and secretion of the protein, cleavage of the protein, or combination with inhibitors or activators.

In the nucleus, DNA exists in a complex with proteins to form chromatin. Structural changes occur to the chromatin to activate the regions of the DNA and unwind regions of the DNA. The eukaryotic chromatin is made from nucleosomes. A nucleosome contains approximately 200 base pairs (bp) of DNA that is wrapped around an octomer of histone proteins. In between the nucleosomes are linker regions that can be digested by DNAases. Transcribable active DNA is particularly sensitive to DNAases.

Between 2% and 7% of cytosines in animal DNA are modified by methylation, most often in sites where a C is followed by a G (CpG doublets). Methylation most often appears in genes that are not being expressed. DNA that is actively transcribed is often undermethylated. CpG-rich islands are often found upstream of constitutively transcribed genes near or at the promoters. This fact has been used by molecular geneticists to identify potential transcription units in large stretches of sequenced genomic DNA.

TRANSCRIPTION CONTROL: PROMOTERS AND ENHANCERS

A promoter is a region of DNA that is involved in binding of RNA polymerase (and associated factors) to initiate transcription and are therefore *cis*-acting sites. Promoters for polymerase I and II are usually located upstream of the transcription unit (initiation start point). Promoters for polymerase III are located downstream.

Transcription factors are *trans*-acting elements that recognize specific *cis*-acting sites in the promoter. *Cis*-acting sites can be spread over regions of DNA that are greater than 100 bp. In general, they can be tentatively identified by footprinting experiments that localize sequences covered by transcription factors. In this type of experiment, a putative promoter DNA binding sequence is allowed to bind to the transcription factor. The DNA is radioactively labeled, digested with nucleases, and then electrophoresed on a sequencing gel. In the region of the binding site, access to nuclease digestion is blocked because of the "footprint" of the transcription factor. Once a candidate promoter sequence is mapped, it is possible to directly test its ability to regulate expression of a reporter gene that is positioned downstream.

Promoters are characterized by short consensus sequences called *boxes*. The TATA box is usually located approximately 25 bp upstream from the start point of transcription. This consensus sequence of AT base pairs (e.g., TATAAAA) is important in the correct positioning of the RNA polymerase II (in concert with a series of transcription factors) at the beginning of the initiation site. The CAAT box (often GGCCAATCT) is located approximately 80 bp upstream of the transcription start point. A large number of different transacting factors recognize the CAAT box. Its role is to determine the strength (frequency or rate of initiation events) of the promoter. The GC box comprises the sequence GGGCGG. It is found in multiple copies in either orientation. The GC box, usually upstream of the TATA box, is the binding site for the Sp1 transcription factor, which regulates the strength of the promoter.

Enhancers are sequences that enhance initiation but may be located at a considerable distance from the start point upstream or downstream. Some enhancers have even been found within introns. Some transcription factors can bind to both promoters and enhancers. In retroviruses, enhancers are located in the viral long terminal repeats and are important for pathogenesis. Papillomaviruses contain enhancer elements that are specific for keratinocytes and thereby contribute to the specific tropism of the virus to these cells. Another example is the immunoglobulin cellular enhancer, which stimulates transcription in specific immune cell types.

Response elements are consensus sequences that allow specific transcription factors to coordinate the transcription of a whole group of genes that all have the consensus sequences. Examples are the heat shock response element, which responds to heat; the glucocorticoid response element, which responds to glucocorticoids; the metal response element; and the tumor promoting element (TRE). The TRE is a response element to TPA the carcinogenic promoting agent. It has the sequence TGACTCA. In response to TPA or phorbol ester, AP-1 transcription factors (a plurifunctional family including Jun and Fos) bind to the TRE.

PROCESSING OF THE RNA TRANSCRIPT

A cap is a complex methylated structure at the 5' end of mRNA that is essential for translation. The first base of a gene that is transcribed into an mRNA molecule is usually a purine (A or G). Almost immediately after transcription starts, a nuclear enzyme guanylyl transferase catalyzes the addition of a 5' G to the first transcribed base of the mRNA. This step is followed by a series of methylation events. The final cap structure maintains the stability of the mRNA transcript as it is forming.

Processing of RNA includes termination and polyadenylation. All eukaryotic mRNAs (except histone genes) contain a poly(A) tail at their 3' end, which is added by poly(A) polymerase. A consensus sequence called the *polyadenylation signal AAUAAA* is located 10 to 30 bases upstream of the poly(A) tail. The polymerase transcribes through the polyadenylation signal, and after termination, an endonuclease cleaves the transcribed RNA at a site 10 to 30 bases downstream of the polyadenylation signal. The site of this event involves small nuclear ribonuclear particles. Once the cleavage occurs, the poly(A) polymerase adds A residues one by one to the 3' free end of the RNA. The poly(A) tail added to the end of the cleaved mRNA may assist the mRNA export out of the nucleus and may also be involved in the stability and lifespan of the mRNA molecule.

Processing of the transcribed RNA is required to remove the introns and produce a continuous linear sequence as a template for translation into the protein polypeptide. The coding region of a gene consists of exons and introns. Splicing is the mechanism by which the introns are removed from the precursor RNA to form a mature mRNA.

Splicing mechanisms differ depending on the type of RNA being spliced. Splicing of heterogeneous nuclear RNA requires a cap structure and is not complete until a poly(A) tail is added. The ends of the intron conform to the GT-AG rule, meaning that each intron in the gene begins with GT and ends with AG. The left 5' site is the donor site, and the right 3' site is the acceptor site. *Alternative splicing* refers to the possibility that there are variations in which exons are spliced together. A large complicated gene with many exons and introns can use alternative splicing to encode different proteins that are generated by different combinations of exons. Cellular genes for structural proteins, such as collagen, fibronectin, and myelin basic proteins, use alternative splicing to produce different proteins with different biologic functions. In this manner, a single gene can produce a number of protein isoforms using sequences within its "start" and "stop" borders.

Translation is the process by which the nucleotide sequence of mRNA is converted into a sequence of amino acids to make a protein. As mentioned, the genetic information of the RNA is organized into triplets of bases called *codons.* Translation requires ribosomal RNA that combines with ribosomal protein to form ribosomes. The ribosomes are docking sites for adaptor molecules, such as tRNA, that can recognize specific codons and the correct amino acid specified by that codon. Thus, the tRNA translates the base sequence of the mRNA into the different language of the amino acid sequence of the protein.

REPAIR OF DNA

Correction of DNA sequence errors is critical to survival. Environmental factors, including radiation, mutagenic chemicals, and thermal energy, can induce errors in the DNA sequence. In addition, errors are occasionally introduced by DNA polymerases during replication. A certain low level of random DNA errors may be required to generate genotype variation to fuel Darwinian evolution. Nevertheless, if most errors were left uncorrected, then both proliferating and nonproliferating cells would accumulate so much genetic damage that they would no longer be viable. Moreover, damage of DNA in germ cells can prevent normal offspring from developing.

Although a significant body of knowledge has been accumulated about DNA polymerase proofreading and excision repair in *E coli,* many of the enzymes required for repairing DNA damage in eukaryotic cells are now being characterized. DNA repair mechanisms have significant roles in carcinogenesis (see Chapter 2).

READING THE GENETIC CODE AND PRODUCTION OF ENCODED PROTEINS

GENETIC CODE

The genetic code refers to triplets of DNA or RNA and the amino acids they specify. A triplet code specifies 4^3 words; thus, there are 4^3 codons. The code is redundant because more than one codon can specify the same amino acid.

An open reading frame is a string of codons that are flanked on the 5' side by an initiation codon and on the 3' side by a termination codon. All proteins start with methionine. The codon AUG specifies methionine and is therefore the initiation codon. Termination or nonsense codons are stop signals for the end of a protein chain. They include the codons UAA, UAG, and UGA. Protein synthesis proceeds from the amino-terminus (N-terminus) to the carboxy-terminus (C-terminus).

Because of the triplet codon, each stretch of mRNA contains three potential open reading frames. The reading frame can be shifted by moving the starting point one or two bases to the right or left. Mutations in which a base is deleted or inserted within an exon are called *frameshift mutations,* because they would alter the reading frame of the sequence.

RIBOSOMES

Ribosomes are the protein synthesizing machinery that brings together the mRNA template and the charged tRNAs. The ribosomes contain two subunits. The small subunit is 40s; it contains an 18s rRNA and 40 proteins and is responsible for binding the tRNAs and the mRNAs. The large subunit, which catalyzes peptide bonds between amino acids on the growing

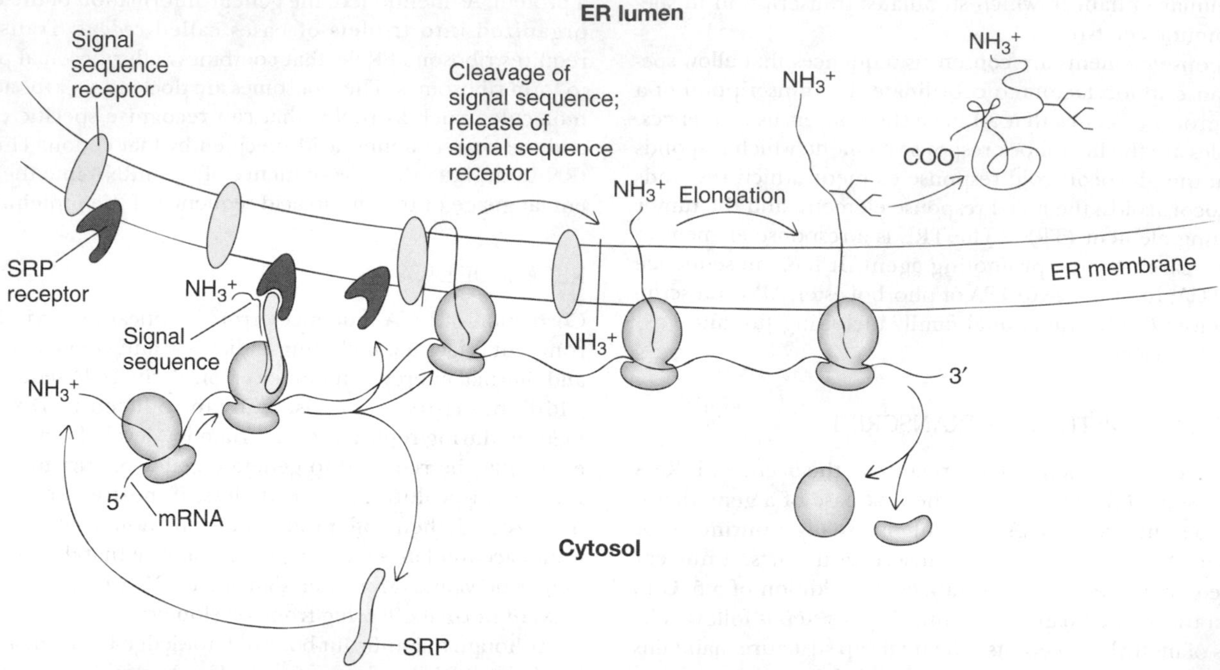

FIGURE 1-5. Synthesis of secretory proteins on the endoplasmic reticulum (ER). An elongated signal recognition particle (SRP) binds to the signal sequence, and then the SRP, nascent polypeptide, and ribosome bind to the ER membrane through the SRP receptor. The signal sequence inserts into the ER membrane and is elongated. The signal sequence is cleaved in the ER lumen by signal peptidase. Carbohydrates are added to asparagine residues by enzymes on the luminal surface. After synthesis is complete, the ribosomes are released and the remaining C-terminus is transferred to the ER lumen. mRNA, messenger RNA.

polypeptide chain, has three rRNAs of 28S, 5.8S and 5S, as well as 50 proteins.

Every tRNA has two properties: It can covalently link to the amino acid it recognizes to form a charged aminoacyl-tRNA, and it contains an anticodon that is complementary to the codon recognizing its amino acid. The anticodon recognizes the codon by complementary base pairing. Some of the base pairs in the third position can be nonstandard or can wobble. This permits one tRNA to recognize more than one codon.

PROTEIN SYNTHESIS: INITIATION, ELONGATION, AND TERMINATION

There are three general steps of protein synthesis: initiation, elongation, and termination. Initiation is the recognition by a specific initiating tRNA for the small ribosome subunit, along with guanosine triphosphate (GTP), and the initiating codon of the mRNA. A special $tRNA^{met}$ binds to the small ribosome subunit, and a molecule of GTP correctly positions the initiating AUG codon of the mRNA on the ribosomal subunit. In concert with several initiating factors, the large ribosomal subunit now binds to the small subunit, met ferrying-$tRNA^{met}$ becomes localized to the ribosome at the P site (peptidyl-tRNA).

Elongation is the extension of the amino acid chain by introducing a second aminoacyl-tRNA to the proper site on the ribosome called the *A site.* With the help of elongation factors, the growing polypeptide chain is attached to the tRNA that brought in the previous amino acid. A peptide bond is formed between the carboxyl group of the methionine and the amino group of the incoming amino acid to make a dipeptide that is attached to the new tRNA. Peptide bond formation requires GTP hydrolysis, which furnishes energy for the reaction. Thus, each elongation step requires two GTPs. Elongation is continued with each new charged tRNA binding to the A site, peptide bond formation, and translocation of the peptidyl-tRNA to the P site (with displacement of the now uncharged tRNA from the P site). In each translocation, the ribosome moves three nucleotides downstream of the mRNA; therefore, more than one polypeptide chain can be produced from one mRNA simultaneously (Fig. 1-5).

Termination occurs when the ribosome reaches the termination codon of the mRNA. A termination factor supports the recognition of the nonsense codon, the release of the last tRNA, and the dissociation of the subunits. This final step also requires GTP hydrolysis.

Once mRNA is transcribed and translated, several factors affect its stability. Degradation of mRNA is a regulated process. Several sequence elements have been detected on mRNAs that regulate decay. An example is the ARE (AU-rich elements) that contain the consensus sequence AUUUA repeated once or several times within the 3' untranslated region.

PROTEIN STRUCTURE AND FUNCTION

AMINO ACIDS

The result of the transcription-translation process is the generation of a protein polypeptide. Proteins, the working molecules of the cell, catalyze a diverse range of chemical reactions, act as information sensors, provide structural scaffolding for cells and extracellular tissue components, control membrane permeability, transduce signals, recognize and covalently bind other molecules, cause motion, and control gene function.

This breadth of tasks are performed by biomolecules constructed from 20 different amino acids. A 100–amino acid protein has 20^{100} possible structures. This enormous potential for variation means that cells and organisms can differ greatly in structure and function even though they are built from a limited number of biopolymer subunits using similar biochemical reactions.

Nineteen of the 20 amino acids contain an amino group (-NH2) and an acidic carboxyl group (-COOH). Proline has an imino group (-NH-) instead of an amino group. All amino acids have a central carbon atom, called an *alpha carbon*, which is bonded to an amino (or imino) group, to the carboxyl group, to a hydrogen atom, and to one variable group called a *side chain* or *R group*. The side chains give the amino acids their individual characteristics. Amino acids with polar but uncharged R groups are serine, threonine, asparagine, and glutamine. Amino acids with positively charged R groups are lysine, arginine, and histidine. Those with negatively charged R groups are glutamic acid and aspartic acid. Amino acids with hydrophobic R groups include alanine, isoleucine, leucine, methionine, phenylalanine, tryptophan, valine, and tyrosine. Special amino acids are cysteine, glycine, and proline.

PROTEIN FOLDING INTO A COLLECTION OF FUNCTIONAL MOTIFS

Peptides are polymers composed of amino acids connected by peptide bonds. The peptide bond joins the carboxyl group of one amino acid to the amino group of the next amino acid. The nature of the peptide bond limits rotation around the alpha carbon and contributes to the three-dimensional spacing and folding of the protein. The newly synthesized protein adopts a three-dimensional conformation through noncovalent (ionic, hydrogen, van der Waals, and hydrophobic) interactions among the amino acids. The final conformation is stabilized by covalent disulfide bonds between cysteines in different parts of the chain, or between two different chains. Multiple different polypeptide chains can interact with each other by noncovalent forces or by covalent bonds, but polypeptide chains are never branched.

Thus, remarkably, the complete three-dimensional shape of a protein is determined by its primary structure, which is the linear sequence of amino acids. The secondary structure of a protein pertains to the folding of parts of the protein into regular structures, such as α helices and β pleated sheets. The tertiary structure describes the interaction of these regular structures into compact domains. The quaternary structure is the final organization of several polypeptide chains (originally encoded by separate genes) into a single protein molecule. The final protein can fold to form a long structural support rod, such as collagen, or a compact ball (globular protein), as in many proteins that catalyze chemical reactions.

Large polypeptides often fold into several globular units rather than one huge unit. Most domains contain between 50 and 300 amino acids. In a water fluid environment, the domains of proteins usually contain a hydrophobic interior and a hydrophilic surface. A regular substructure that occurs in different domains is a motif. Specific motifs are associated with specific functions.

A good example is transcription factor proteins, which have characteristic DNA binding motifs in the protein primary and secondary structure. The helix-turn-helix structure exhibits an α helix, a turn, and a second α helix. An example is the homeodomain in homeobox proteins that regulate development and differentiation. Zinc finger proteins contain tandem repeats of a 30-residue motif that contains cysteine and histidine residues that bind zinc. The zinc finger binds to a consensus sequence GCGTGGGCG on the DNA. Steroid receptors display a zinc binding domain different from the zinc finger and respond to steroid hormones (e.g., estrogen), retinoids, thyroid hormones, and vitamin D. The leucine zippers protein domain appears in many general transcription factors, including Jun and Fos. The zipper itself is a leucine-rich stretch of amino acids in a 30– to 40–amino acid region. The leucines are separated at regular intervals by six amino acids. A conserved repeat of hydrophobic residues is present three residues to the N-terminal side of the leucines (valine or isoleucine). In addition, the leucine zipper proteins have a basic region that is rich in arginines and lysines. The basic region binds to the DNA, and the leucine zipper region forms two parallel α helices in a coiled-coil arrangement. In addition to DNA binding, the leucine zipper plays a role in protein dimerization. Molecules that bind with themselves form homodimers, and those that couple with other proteins form heterodimers. Examples are the homodimers Jun-Jun and the heterodimers Jun-Fos, members of the AP-1 binding proteins involved in transcriptional control.

PROTEIN POSTTRANSLATIONAL MODIFICATIONS

Proteins undergo several types of covalent and noncovalent modifications. These include the cleavage of the N-terminal methionine, the formation of disulfide bridges between two cysteine residues, or cleavage of a precursor polypeptide region. A large number of stable protein modifications can be made, including hydroxylation of proline and lysine in collagen, acetylation of lysine, methylation of histidine, attachment of carbohydrated groups to asparagine, presence of serine or threonine side chains, linkage to lipids, and addition of various groups to the N-terminus.

Protein functions during cell signaling are also controlled by reversible side-chain modifications. A key modification is phosphorylation, which is the substitution of phosphate groups for hydroxyl groups on serine, threonine, or tyrosine. The activity of many critical enzymes in cancer biology is regulated by their state of phosphorylation (e.g., src, HER2/neu, RET, and the retinoblastoma gene product). In fact, phosphatase and kinase enzymes themselves can be regulated by phosphorylation. The phosphorylation is mediated by enzymes called *kinases* and removed by enzymes called *phosphatases*. Thus, the phosphorylation cascade provides a simultaneous means of information exchange, amplification, pathway channeling, and regulation. Its importance in cancer is the fact that many oncogenes are themselves mutated kinases that are rendered constitutively active [e.g., epidermal growth factor receptor (EGFR), bcr-abl] (Fig. 1-6). Moreover, some tumor suppressor genes are strong regulators of kinases (e.g., p16, p27).

SUBCELLULAR MOLECULAR STRUCTURE

PLASMA MEMBRANE

Both prokaryotic and eukaryotic cells are enclosed in a plasma membrane. In addition, most eukaryotic cells contain extensive

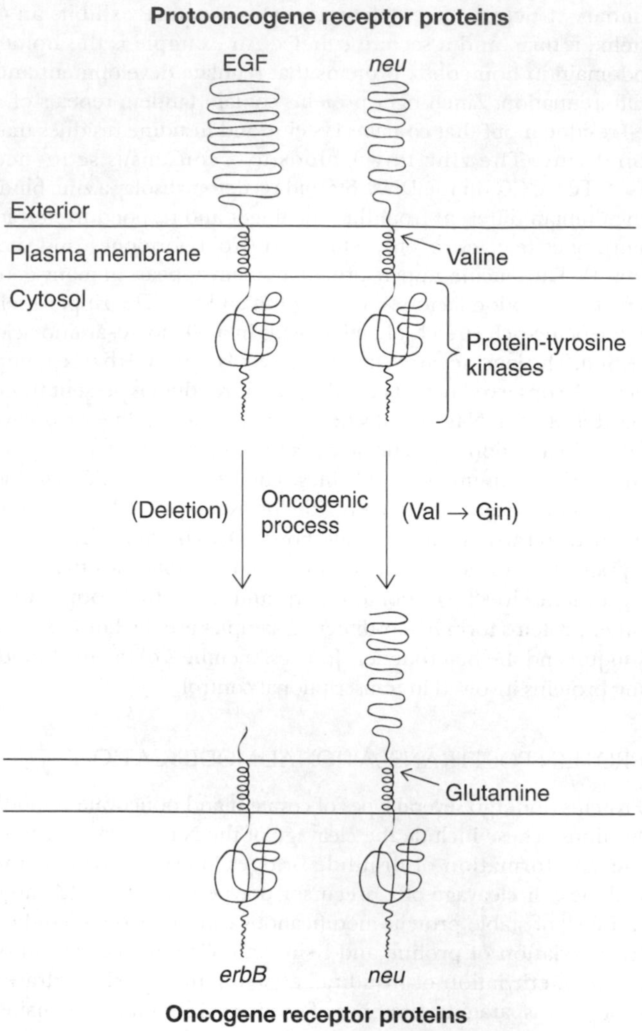

FIGURE 1-6. Oncogenes can arise from protooncogenes that encode cell-surface receptors. On the left, the epidermal growth factor (EGF) receptor becomes oncogenic by loss of the coding region for the extracellular domain. On the right, the *neu* ERB-2 oncogene encodes a protein with a single amino acid substitution in the transmembrane domain.

internal membranes interconnected to the plasma membrane. These internal pockets and sacs define a collection of subcellular organelles. The largest organelle is the nucleus. Examples of other organelles are mitochondria (oxidation of small molecules to generate adenosine triphosphate); rough and smooth endoplasmic reticula, a network of membranes in which glycoproteins and lipids are synthesized; Golgi vesicles, which channel membrane constituents to correct locations in the cell; and lysosomes, which degrade proteins. The organelles maintain a specific, demarcated, confined chemical environment (such as an acid pH in the case of lysosomes) and contain a host of bound enzymes that catalyze requisite chemical reactions.

NUCLEUS

Chromosomal DNA in eukaryotic cells is wrapped in a set of five different positively charged proteins called *histones.* Histone-DNA interactions occur at regular intervals. Every sequence of 150 to 180 bp of DNA is bound to one molecule of histone H1 and to two molecules each of histones H2A, H2B, H3, and H4.

The eukaryotic nucleus is surrounded by two membranes containing phospholipids. The outer membrane is continuous with the cytoplasmic membrane system. The space between the inner and outer membrane communicates with the lumenal cavity of the rough endoplasmic reticulum. The inner membrane defines the nucleus proper. Fibrous proteins called *lamins* form a two-dimensional network on the inner surface of the inner membrane. Ring-like nuclear membrane pores, formed from a special set of membrane proteins, are regulated channels for the movement of material between the nucleus and the cytoplasm.

The nucleolar organizer, a region of one or more chromosomes in the nucleolus, is a focal point for synthesis of ribosomal RNA. Generated ribosomal subunits pass through the nuclear pores into the cytoplasm.

CYTOPLASM

The cytoplasm is the region outside the nucleus of eukaryotic cells, and it contains an array of fibrous proteins collectively constituting the cytoskeleton. The most abundant cytoskeleton components are microfilaments, which are built of actin; slightly wider microtubules, made of tubulin; and intermediate filaments, built of a set of rod-shaped protein subunits. The cytoskeleton is not just a structural scaffolding. It plays critical roles in cell movement, differentiation, intracellular trafficking, cell division (microtubules mediate chromosome movement), and signal transduction. Some of the most active chemotherapeutic agents, such as the taxanes and the vinca alkaloids, directly affect microtubular assembly as their primary mode of action.

The plasma membrane surface is highly specialized to interact with the environment according to the functional requirements of the individual differentiated cell. Protuberances and extensions of the plasma membrane, such as cilia, pseudopods, and villi, contain cores of specialized cytoskeletal extensions and have broad functions in locomotion and macromolecule uptake. The plasma membrane contains embedded receptors and anchor points that bind to the extracellular matrix, surrounding cells, or soluble cytokines.

MEMBRANE PROTEINS

Proteins interact with membranes using a variety of mechanisms. Integral membrane proteins contain amino acid residues with hydrophobic side chains that interact with the fatty acyl groups of the membrane phospholipids. Other integral proteins contain covalently bound fatty acids that function as anchors in the hydrophobic lipid bilayer. An important example is the farnesyl residue of the oncogene p21 ras (the mutant of the normal cellular small g protein) and the myristate residue of the v-src tyrosine kinase oncogene (the mutant of the normal cellular protein c-src). The farnesyl residue is linked by a thioester bond to a cysteine residue four amino acids from the C-terminus of the protein, and then the three C-terminal residues are cleaved off. Myristate is bound by an amide linkage to the glycine residue found at the N-terminus. Cancerous transformation by such oncogenes requires the membrane-attachment function of these covalently attached lipids.

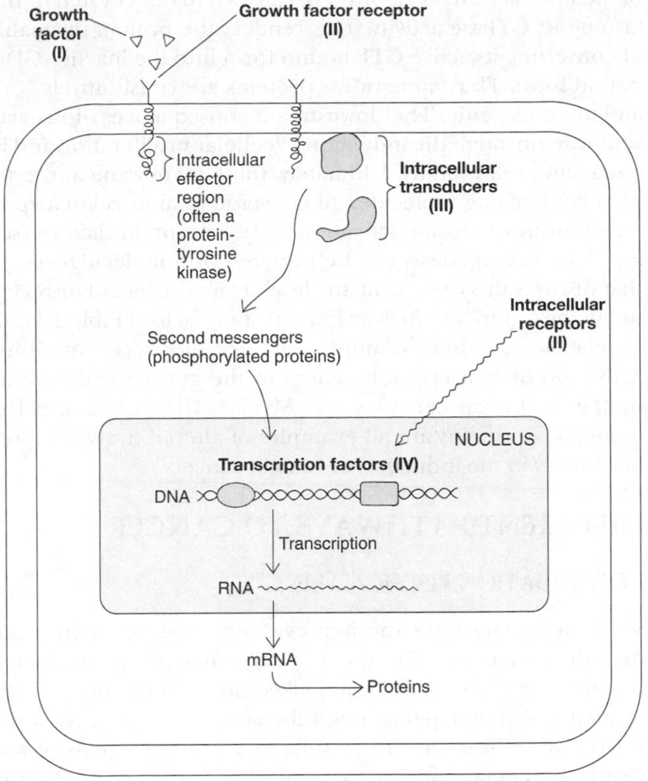

FIGURE 1-7. Control points in cellular regulation that can be targets for carcinogenic events. The following classes can become oncogenes: growth factors (I), receptors (II), transducers (III), and gene regulation factors (IV). mRNA, messenger RNA.

MOLECULAR ONCOGENESIS: CELLULAR SIGNAL TRANSDUCTION

Mutations that cause cancer are mainly those that alter the ability of the cell to maintain genetic stability, such as mutations in repair genes, or those that alter the transmission of signals that control the machinery of cell growth and survival (Fig. 1-7). The transmission of signals within the cell and from inside and outside the cell is called *signal transduction.* Surface receptors are the sensors providing the cell's window to the outside environment. Most receptors fall into one of three general types depending on the signal transduction mechanism used. Channel–linked receptors are ligand gated ion channels involved in rapid synaptic signaling. These receptors belong to a family of homologous multipass transmembrane proteins. Catalytic receptors are activated by a ligand to operate directly as enzymes. Most of the known catalytic receptors are transmembrane proteins with a cytoplasmic domain that normally accepts controlled signals from outside the cell and transmits signals to the inside of the cell. Many of these proteins function as a tyrosine-specific protein kinase. An important example is the receptor for the EGF-related ligands (EGFR). Included in the EGFR family is the ERB2/Neu receptor, which plays a major role in the biology of human breast cancers. When mutated, the RET oncogene is activated and associated with both hereditary and sporadic thyroid cancers, and overexpression of the MET protooncogene leads to increased cell motility and metastatic potential. Conversely, the normal function of the transforming growth factor-β pathway is to suppress growth and oncogenesis. When mutated, the inactivation of the ligand or receptor renders the cell susceptible to transformation. Intracellular kinases that do not transmit signals across the cell membrane but potentially within the cell are also important in oncogenesis. The ABL kinase is activated when participating in the bcr-abl translocation. The majority of these transmembrane receptors normally transduce signals through the controlled phosphorylation of intracellular substrates, usually on tyrosine, serine, or threonine residues that function as signaling nodes in a complex intracellular communications network. The control of phosphorylation and dephosphorylation events are used by cells to relay signals, amplify signals, and regulate pathways and to act by changing the conformation and, therefore, the function of the phosphorylated protein. Any member of a signaling cascade can be a potential target for oncogenic mutation.

A third class of receptors is the G protein–linked receptors. These sensors indirectly activate or inactivate a separate membrane-bound enzyme or ion channel. The interaction takes place through an intermediary protein, the GTP-binding regulatory protein (G protein). The G protein–linked receptors activate a cascade of downstream intracellular messengers. The messengers in turn activate or regulate other target proteins in the cell. Important intracellular messengers are calcium ions, cyclic adenosine monophosphate, and phospholipids.

The Gs protein functions as a shuttle between two membrane proteins: the receptor for the stimulus and the downstream effort enzyme (adenyl cyclase), which generates the second messenger. Thus, Gs is a signal transducer, relaying to the recipient enzyme the conformational change in the receptor triggered by the ligand binding to the receptor (Fig. 1-8). The Gs protein cycles between active and resting forms, which are determined by the state of its subunits. Gs is composed of three polypeptides: an α chain Gsa, which binds and hydrolyzes GTP and activates adenyl cyclase, and a tight complex of a β chain and a γ chain GBg, which anchors Gs to the cytoplasmic face of the plasma membrane. In the resting state, Gsa contains bound guanosine diphosphate (GDP) and is coupled to Gbg. When GTP binds to Gsa, it is hydrolyzed to GDP by the reaction: Gsa + GTP → Gsa + GDP + inorganic phosphate. The change in the receptor conformation is passed on through the Gag to the Gsa and causes GDP to be replaces by GTP. When GTP is bound to Gsa, the Gsa dissociates from the Gbg subunits. The Gsa, with its bound GTP, undergoes a conformational change that enables it to bind and activate adenyl cyclase. In a resting cell, most Gs molecules contain GDP. Binding to a hormone or agonist changes the conformation of the receptor protruding on the inner surface of the membrane. The altered receptor can now bind Gs, causing GDP to be displaced and GTP to be bound. The GTP-bound form of Gsa then acts as a shuttle that translocates to bind adenyl cyclase and activate it to hydrolyze adenosine triphosphate to cyclic adenosine monophosphate and inorganic phosphate. Immediately after activation of adenyl cyclase, Gsa hydrolyzes bound GTP to GDP and returns to its coupled state with Gbg.

All receptors that interact with a G protein share a common stretch of 22 to 24 hydrophobic amino acids that generate seven back and forth *trans* membrane α helixes. A large loop between helixes 5 and 6 protrudes into the cytosol and interacts with the G protein.

In cancer, the most important G proteins are found in the ras family of oncogenes: N-ras, K-ras, and H-ras. Specific mutations

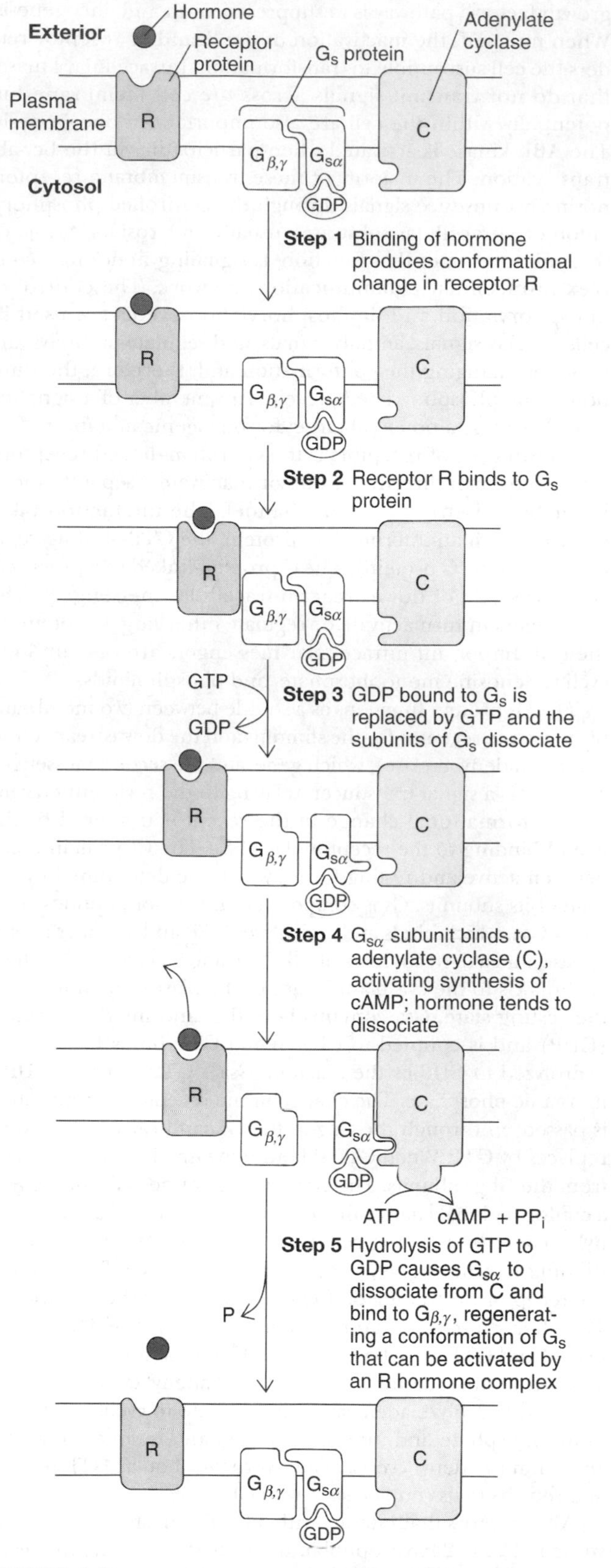

FIGURE 1-8. Cascade of molecular exchange events involved in the transduction of a signal through G protein–linked receptors. ATP, adenosine triphosphate; cAMP, cyclic adenosine monophosphate; GDP, guanosine diphosphate; GTP, guanosine triphosphate; PPi, inorganic pyrophosphate.

of the normal cellular ras protein causes it to be activated by disarming its GTPase activity. This renders the protein incapable of converting its active GTP-bound form into the inactive GDP-bound form. Thus, mutant ras proteins are constitutively "on" and are oncogenic. The downstream consequences of ras activation are through the induction of cellular proliferation and in enhancing cell motility. Ultimately, these membrane and cytoplasmic signaling molecules all converge to alter cellular transcription through the activation of transcription factors (see Fig. 1-7). Oncogenesis can be initiated by a molecular lesion that disrupts this cascade at any level, from the ligand or receptor all the way to the nuclear transcription factor (Table 1-1). In cancer biology, there is ample evidence of direct mutational activation of transcription factors in the genesis and maintenance of the cancerous state. Myc, AML1, MLL, and the homeobox proteins are all examples of altered transcriptional machinery in the induction of human cancers.

DIFFERENT PATHWAYS TO CANCER

PERTURBATIONS IN SIGNALING

Viral oncogenes were the first evidence that host genes can directly cause cancer. Normal cellular genes (protooncogenes, identified by the *c* prefix) are "picked up" or transduced by the retrovirus and mutated through the error-prone process of the retroviral replication. This results in a viral oncogene (v-*onc*) that is functionally arrested in a biochemically activated form. Early studies revealed that the oncogene precursors, the protooncogenes, act as biochemical switches in the command and control processes of a cell, specifically transmitting signals from the outside of the cell to the nucleus. The normal and controlled transfer of extracellular signals is bypassed when one of the relay members is mutated and is made constitutively activated, resulting in the characteristic of a cancer cell—unmanaged growth.

In nature, one finds oncogenic mutations in members of signaling pathways. For example, the receptor tyrosine kinase (EGFR; mutated or overexpressed in brain and epithelial cancers; related retroviral oncogene, v-*erbB*), when stimulated with one of its ligands, transforming growth factor-α (overexpressed in some human cancers), interacts with *ras* (retroviral homologue, v-H-*ras* or v-K-*ras*; mutated in 10% to 20% of human cancers) through bridging proteins. *Ras* is controlled by GTPase-activating proteins (oncogenic homologue is NF1, the gene involved in neurofibromatosis) and transmits signals by activating *raf* (retroviral homologue, v-*raf*). Stimulation of the *ras/raf* pathway results in increased expression of the nuclear proteins *jun, fos,* and *myc* (retroviral homologues, v-*jun*, v-*fos*, v-*myc*; myc is mutated and rearranged in lymphoid malignancies and amplified in breast cancers), which are proteins that can induce the expression of other genes (called *transcription factors*). Thus, every relay node in this signal transduction pathway is a potential site for oncogenic conversion. The complexity of the transformation process is reflected in the multiple parallel signaling pathways that are promiscuous in their selection of biochemical partners. For example, the receptor tyrosine kinase HER-2 physically associates with itself or with related receptor tyrosine kinases, such as EGFR, HER-3, and HER-4; *ras* can be regulated by either *ras*–GTPase-activating proteins or

TABLE 1-1. Selected Oncogenes and Their Proteins

Type/name	*Oncogene found in* Animal retrovirus	*Oncogene found in* Nonviral tumor	*Subcellular location of protein*	*Nature of encoded protein*
Class I: growth factors				
sis	Simian sarcoma		Secreted	A form of platelet-derived growth factor
Class II: receptors				
Cell-surface receptors with protein-tyrosine kinase activity				
fms	McDonough feline sarcoma		Plasma membrane	CSF-1 receptor
erbB	Avian erythroblastosis		Plasma membrane	Epidermal growth factor receptor
neu (or *erbB-2*)		Neuroblastoma	Plasma membrane	Related to epidermal growth factor receptor
ros	UR II avian sarcoma		Plasma membrane	Related to insulin receptor
Intracellular receptors				
erbA	Avian erythroblastosis		Nuclear	Thyroid hormone receptor
Class III: intracellular transducers				
Protein-tyrosine kinase				
src	Rous avian sarcoma		Cytoplasm	
yes	Yamaguchi avian sarcoma		Cytoplasm	
fps (fes)	Fujinami avian sarcoma (and feline sarcoma)		Cytoplasm	Protein kinases that phosphorylate tyrosine residues
abl	Abelson murine leukemia	Chronic myelogenous leukemia	Cytoplasm and nucleus	
met		Murine osteosarcoma		
Protein-serine/threonine kinases				
mos	Moloney murine sarcoma		Cytoplasm	Protein kinases specific for serine or threonine
raf (mil)	3611 murine sarcoma			
Ras proteins				
Ha-*ras*	Harvey murine sarcoma	Bladder, mammary, and skin carcinomas	Plasma membrane inner face	
Ki-*ras*	Kirsten murine sarcoma	Lung and colon carcinomas	Plasma membrane inner face	Guanine nucleotide-binding proteins with GTPase activity
N-*ras*		Neuroblastoma and leukemias	Plasma membrane inner face	
Phospholipase C–related				
crk	Avian sarcoma virus		Cytoplasm	Contains *src*-related regions also homologous with a phospholipase C
Class IV: nuclear transcription factors				
jun	Avian sarcoma virus 17		Nucleus	Transcription factor AP-1
fos	Osteosarcoma		Nucleus	
myc	Avian MC29 myelocytomatosis		Nuclear matrix	
N-*myc*		Neuroblastoma	Nuclear matrix	
myb	Avian myeloblastosis	Leukemia	Nuclear matrix	Proteins possibly involved in regulating transcription
ski	Avian SKV770		Nucleus	
p53		(Demonstrated by cell transformation)	Nucleus	
rel	Avian reticuloendotheliosis		Nucleus and cytoplasm	
RB		Retinoblastoma	Nucleus	Antioncogene that binds to nuclear oncogene proteins of DNA viruses

AP-1, transcription factor; CSF, colony-stimulating factor; GTP, guanosine triphosphate.

NF1; and stimulation of the *ras* pathway activates a number of mitogen-activated protein kinases.

THE WRONG PLACE AT THE WRONG TIME

In human cancers, mutations in protooncogenes result in altered function. However, inappropriate expression of structurally normal proteins that have no role in the biology of a specific tissue can also lead to cancer. Several transcription factors are in this category: *myc*, *tal-1*/SCL, *lyl-1*, *Ttg-1*, and *Ttg-2*. These oncoproteins are structurally identical to their normal forms but are either inappropriately expressed in the cell cycle or in inappropriate tissues. *myc* is expressed in all cells and plays a role in cell division and differentiation. Activation of *myc* due to the t(8;14)(q24;q32) seen in Burkitt's lymphomas and B-cell acute lymphocytic leukemias deregulates *myc* expression, and the exquisite control of *myc* transcription is lost. In lymphoid tissues, this leads to the expansion of pre–B cells in transgenic mice inappropriately expressing *myc*, which ultimately results in the emergence of a lymphoid malignancy. Other members on this list (*tal-1*/SCL, *lyl-1*, *Ttg-1*, and *Ttg-2*) are linked to T-cell acute lymphocytic leukemia. In this group, oncogenic activation is through expression in an inappropriate cell type: *tal-1* is normally expressed in erythroid and myeloid precursors and not in T cells; *lyl-1* is expressed only in myeloid and B-lymphoid cells; and *Ttg-2* transcripts are found in liver, spleen, and kidney but not in activated T cells. In these examples, the inappropriate expression of a transcription factor serves as a molecular switch to induce a malignancy.

RELEASE OF SUPPRESSION

Whereas protooncogenes are identified by a gain of function after mutational damage, another class of cancer genes, tumor suppressor genes, contribute to cancer induction by a loss of function. To this end, tumor suppressor genes, such as the retinoblastoma gene (*Rb-1*) and p53, block cellular proliferation, and each appears to function through distinct pathways. *Rb-1* negatively regulates the important transcription factor E2F, and the deletion of the *Rb* gene (seen in congenital retinoblastoma) releases the suppression of E2F. p53 enhances the expression of p21/CIP1, which is a suppressor of cell-cycle regulatory kinases [cyclin-dependent kinases (CDKs)]. Activation of these CDKs is necessary for progression through the cell cycle, and CDK inhibitors, such as p21/CIP1, block this process. Thus, the loss of p53 and the attenuation of p21/CIP1 expression result in unmanaged progression through the cell cycle.

That both *Rb* and p53 are involved in the genesis of cancer is evidenced by the identification of germline mutations of these genes in individuals with cancer predisposition syndromes, such as congenital retinoblastoma (*Rb*) and the Li-Fraumeni multicancer syndrome (p53). As with oncogenes, the presence of a single abnormal tumor suppressor allele alone is insufficient for cancer to develop; lesions at other genetic lesions are necessary. For example, both *Rb* and p53 may need to be inactivated for some normal cells to be rendered immortal. The DNA tumor virus, the human papillomavirus (HPV) that is the causative agent in many cervical, anal, and penile carcinomas, inhibits both these critical proteins through binding with and inactivation by the HPV viral proteins E6 and E7. In this manner, HPV biochemically achieves the same outcome that carcinogens accomplish through inactivating genetic mutations. In colon cancers, mutations in p53 are frequently associated with other genetic lesions, including those involved in cytoskeletal organization (APC), signal transduction (*ras*), and cell motility (DCC) in the progress toward an invasive cancer.

A tumor suppressor gene can be defined as any gene whose loss of function contributes to cancer progression. One category of suppressor genes are the inhibitors of the CDKs, which are enzymes that control the progression through the cell cycle. They, in turn, are controlled by protein activators (called *cyclins*) and inhibitors (called *CDK inhibitors*). The attenuation of expression of CDK inhibitors, such as p16, p27, and p57, has been associated with a diverse range of cancers, from lung to head and neck, breast, and pancreas cancers, as well as melanoma. In malignant melanoma, the loss of both p16 alleles is found in most primary tumors, and inactivating germline mutations in p16 segregate with familial melanoma syndromes. Therefore, CDK inhibitors, such as p16, maintain the normal cellular state by regulating cell proliferation, and disruption of its inhibitor function leads to cancer.

CELL DEATH

Earlier on, the study of molecular oncogenesis concentrated on processes that stimulated growth. However, the accumulation of cancer cells can also be accomplished by a decrease in cell loss as well as by an increase in cell proliferation. Current evidence suggests that the abrogation of programmed cell death (apoptosis) is an important mechanism for neoplastic transformation. Certain cellular processes, such as cytokine signaling (e.g., tumor necrosis factor, interleukin-3 withdrawal) or DNA damage, can trigger a cascade of events culminating in activation of intracellular proteases. These activated proteases then lead to the regulated cleavage of cellular components, including proteins and DNA, and ultimately to cell death. The cell exerts exquisite control of this process using redundant systems to induce or block apoptosis, and some of these control switches are involved in cancer and cancer treatment.

The clearest example of an oncogene modulating the apoptotic process is *bcl-2*, found to be the oncogene involved in the t(14q;18q) translocation frequently found in follicular lymphomas. *bcl-2* blocks apoptosis when overexpressed or inappropriately expressed, and in lymphomas, translation involving *bcl-2* may be among the earliest oncogene abnormalities that act to prolong the lifespan of cells that are prone to accumulate genetic mutations. In experimental lymphomas, *bcl-2* does not cause cancer directly but is followed by rearrangements at other oncogenes, such as the c-*myc*, which result in accelerated progression of the lymphoma. This *bcl-2*/*myc* interaction highlights another principle of oncogene action—that is, more than one cancer gene must be perturbed for a malignancy to arise. Other bcl-2–related proteins have been identified, all of which are capable of physically interacting with each other as homo- or heterodimers. *bcl-*X_l, like *bcl-2*, is antiapoptotic; overexpression of *bax*, *bak*, *bcl-*X_s, and BAD, however, actually induces apoptosis. Thus, the ratio of antiapoptotic to proapoptotic factors determine the cell's "set point" triggering apoptosis. Significantly, this set point can modulate a cell's responsiveness to radiation and chemotherapy.

More recently, growth factor receptors and other surface signaling molecules have been shown to directly affect the apoptotic process. Many receptor kinases, such as platelet-derived growth factor receptor and *Met*, recruit and activate the phosphatidylinositol 3 kinase (PI3-kinase). PI3-kinase activates the *Akt* protein kinase, which supports cell survival through its phosphorylation and inactivation of BAD, one of the *bcl*-2–related proteins that promotes cell death. Therefore, augmented *Akt* function induced by ligand receptor interactions is predicted to have an antiapoptotic effect. It is not clear why certain tumors genetically alter *bcl*-2 to alter apoptotic potential whereas others use alternative biochemical pathways to accomplish the same ends. Nevertheless, it is clear that normal cells have self-policing mechanisms that activate suicide programs. When the mutational load of a cell exceeds a critical level, self-destruct processes are activated. Cancer, however, may result when genetically abnormal cells are not cleared but are allowed to proliferate, thus accumulating mutations potentially in important cancer genes.

GENETIC INSTABILITY

A characteristic of a cancer cell is its ability to generate and to sustain genetic mutations. Normal cells not only have the ability to identify and repair DNA damage, but also to prevent the expansion of mutation-laden daughter cells by suicide mechanisms such as apoptosis. Defects in DNA repair found in rare disorders such as xeroderma pigmentosum and ataxia-telangiectasia are associated with cancer risk. More recently, however, common human cancers have been linked to abnormalities in repair processes. One example is the hereditary nonpolyposis colon cancer (HNPCC) syndrome. HNPCC is an inherited syndrome characterized by increased risk for colon cancer without the associated polyposis seen in carriers of another hereditable cancer syndrome, adenomatous polyposis coli. Affected individuals with HNPCC show signs of a defect in the repair of DNA mismatches. Additions or reductions in the number of two nucleotide repeats found in human DNA (called *microsatellite instability*) were clonally detected in their tumors. This type of DNA abnormality is a signature for a form of repair defect previously studied in bacteria and yeast. When incorrectly paired nucleotides occur in a DNA duplex, either through misincorporations or nucleotide damage, cells use a mismatch repair system to identify and remove the mismatch. This recognition and cleavage is mediated by the protein products of the MSH2, MSH3, MSH6, MLH1, PMS1, and PMS2 genes. HNPCC patients have primarily mutations in MSH2 and MLH1, although mutations in the other mismatch repair genes also are found. The clinical consequence of this molecular defect in humans is the emergence of colon cancers that differ from the sporadic variety and that are characterized by fewer ras and p53 mutations, as well as fewer allelic losses. Moreover, colon cancer in HNPCC patients appear to have a better prognosis than their sporadic counterparts.

Advances in molecular biology and their application to cancer research have yielded a wealth of new knowledge uncovering molecular mechanisms that can trigger and sustain uncontrolled growth. From the clinical perspective, it is astonishing that the molecular pathways that lead to cancer can be different in different types of neoplasms, in different tissues, and even in the same type of pathology. Nevertheless, elucidating each new molecular pathway involved in cancer provides strategies for diagnosis, intervention, and treatment. Thus, a molecular understanding of cancer clarifies why curing this disease is so difficult, while at the same time, this knowledge provides more precise targets for treatments in the future.

SUGGESTED READINGS

1. Lodish H, Baltimore D, Berk A, et al. *Molecular cell biology.* New York: Scientific American Books, 1995.
2. Hunter T. Signaling—2000 and Beyond. *Cell* 2000;100:113.
3. Sobel ME. Introduction to molecular biology approaches to the study of cancer. In: Cossman J, ed. *Molecular genetics in cancer diagnosis.* New York: Elsevier Scientific Publ. Co., 1990:7.
4. Lewin B. *Genes VII.* New York: Oxford University Press, 1999.
5. Zou X, Calame K. Signaling pathways activated by oncogenic forms of Abl tyrosine kinase. Minireview. *J Biol Chem* 1999;274:18141.
6. Hurtley S. Frontiers in cell biology: quality control. *Science* 1999;286:1881.

Lance A. Liotta
Edison T. Liu

CHAPTER 2

Essentials of Molecular Biology: Genomics and Cancer

UNDERSTANDING CANCER AT THE MOLECULAR LEVEL: THE NEW FRONTIER

Genomic and proteome research is a new frontier for the molecular characterization of cancer. The ongoing revolution in molecular medicine can be divided into three phases. The first phase is gene discovery, in which the tools of molecular biology are applied to identify and sequence previously unknown genes. Identification of most of the expressed human genes will be accomplished before 2002. The second phase is molecular fingerprinting, which correlates the genomic state, the cDNA expression pattern, and the protein repertoire with the functional status of the cells or tissue. The promise of this phase is that expression profiles can uncover clues to functionally important molecules and will generate information to tailor a treatment to the individual patient. The third phase is the synthesis of proteomic information into functional pathways and circuits in cells and tissues. This must take into account the dynamic state of protein posttranslational modifications and protein–protein or protein–DNA interactions. Through an integrated genomic and proteomic analysis, the ultimate outcome will be an actual functional understanding of the molecular events underlying normal development and disease pathophysiology. This higher level of functional understanding will be the basis for true rational therapeutic design.

Progress in these three phases of molecular medicine is largely driven by new technologies. The development of polymerase chain reaction (PCR), high throughput sequencing, and bioinformatics has been a driving force in the first phase. In the second phase, microhybridization arrays applied to genetic analysis and gene expression are a powerful new tool that has entered the commercial sector and is becoming widely available to researchers. As more genes are identified, it is likely that specialized arrays will be offered that are specific for a tissue type (e.g., mammary gland chip), physiologic process (e.g., apoptosis chip, angiogenesis chip, invasion chip), or class of genes (e.g., suppressor gene chip, oncogene chip).

GENETIC MECHANISMS OF CANCER PROGRESSION: CANCER IS A GENETIC DISEASE

Cancer is a genetic disease. Progression from normal tissue to invasive cancer takes place over 5 to 20 years and is influenced by hereditary genetic factors as well as somatic genetic changes (Fig. 2-1). Cancer progression is driven by a series of accumulating genetic changes. Some genetic oncogenic changes contribute to uncontrolled growth or loss of senescence. Some oncogenes cause uncontrolled growth by activating persistent growth stimulatory signal transduction pathways. Some oncogenes cause uncontrolled growth by altering critical nodes in the cell cycle. Uncontrolled growth can be caused by deregulation at the level of DNA transcription factors.

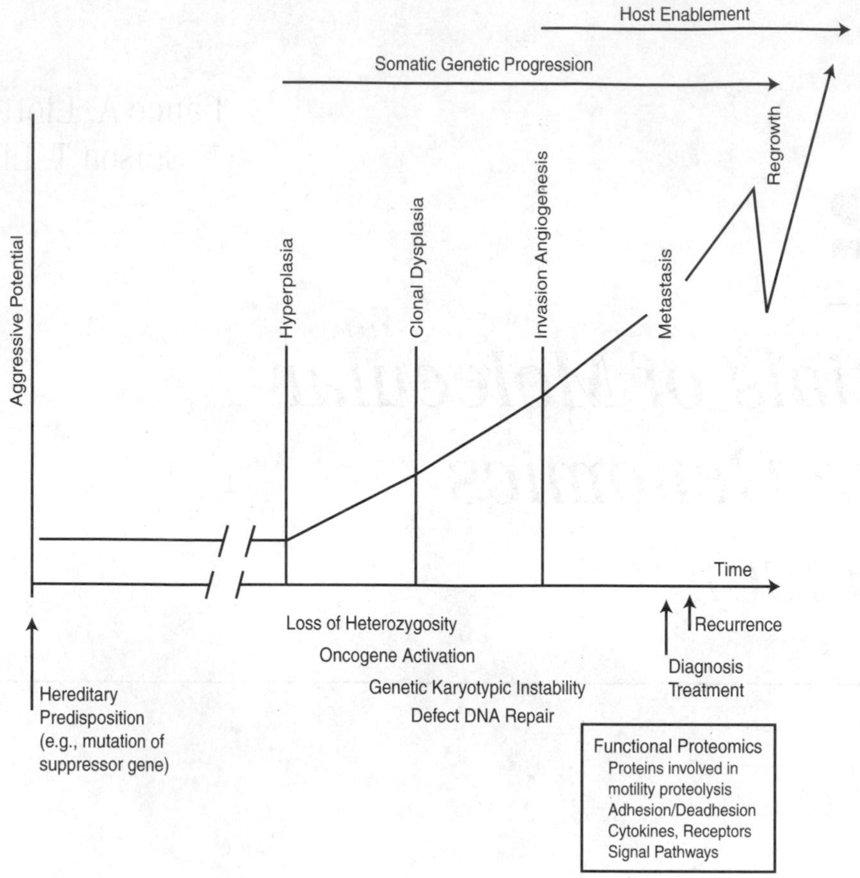

FIGURE 2-1. Molecular progression of cancer. Microscopic premalignant lesions originate within a background of hereditary predisposition. Genetic instability leads to molecular derangements that drive somatic genetic progression. Host interactions enable the cancer lesions to expand, vascularize, and metastasize. Diagnosis usually takes place at a late stage when there is a high probability of metastasis.

Separate genetic changes (beyond those causing uncontrolled growth) are required for tumor invasion and metastasis. Invasion and metastasis form a multistep cascade involving positive and negative regulatory pathways. Cancer invasion and angiogenesis are an uncontrolled version of physiologic invasion.

Genetic instability may predispose the premalignant cell to generate malignant offspring. Instability can take place at the macro level (chromosome karyotype), as well as the micro level (DNA sequence copy fidelity repair). Chromosomal rearrangement can activate silent oncogenes or delete regions containing suppressor genes. Loss of heterozygosity is a hallmark of suppressor gene inactivation in cancer progression. Telomerase defects may affect growth control as well as genetic instability. Mutations in cellular DNA can activate oncogenes or inactivate suppressor genes. Defects in DNA repair mechanisms contribute to the accumulation of genetic defects fueling cancer progression. Genetic defects causing an inhibition of cell death pathways are an important mechanism in tumorigenesis.

CANCER GENES: MODELS OF ACTION

Genetic alterations involved in cancer can activate inductive processes (oncogenes) or block negative pathways (suppressor genes). Early models of cancer genetics categorized cancer genes into oncogenes, which are growth inducing, and tumor suppressor genes, which are growth suppressing. Thus, mutations in oncogenes activate a promoting function, but lesions in tumor suppressors inactivate an inhibitory function. Examples of these models were the ras oncogene and the retinoblastoma (rb) tumor suppressor gene. Mutations in codons 12, 13, and 61 in the ras gene result in biochemical activation of the protein product and an induction of its transforming activity. Deletions or inactivating mutations in the rb gene lead to a compromised suppressor protein that is incapable of inhibiting cell growth. Aberrations in both genes are found as somatic mutations in human cancers and, in the case of rb, also in the germline of individuals at risk for cancer.

Dominant oncogenes play a significant role in human cancers. Ras mutations are found in 10% of cancers and appear frequently in colon and lung adenocarcinomas. Ret is a receptor tyrosine kinase in which activating single nucleotide mutations are associated with hereditary thyroid carcinomas. Myc, encoding a nuclear oncoprotein, is involved in the t(8;14) translocation, which is etiologic for Burkitt's lymphoma. Inappropriate overexpression of myc is sufficient for transformation of lymphocytes in transgenic models. Similarly, amplification and overexpression of the HER2/neu receptor tyrosine kinase not only causes mammary malignancies, but is prognostic in human breast cancers. Although originally these oncogene abnormalities were thought to induce cancer primarily through unregulated growth, other cellular phenotypes such as enhanced survival and motility may be equally important contributors to the cancer state.

It was also originally thought that tumor suppressor genes function mainly by inhibiting cell growth. Later, this was expanded to genes that block the emergence of a tumor, but not growth in culture. More recent studies, however, have uncovered other mechanisms unrelated to growth by which *tumor suppressor* genes act to inhibit cancer formation. In fact, it now seems that the inhibition of growth may not be the most important function of these genetic suppressors. Wild-type (or the normal) p53 is able to slow the proliferation of cancer cells in culture, and naturally occurring mutants of p53 lose this capability. However, many cell lines grow well with both normal p53 and rb genes, suggesting that they are not necessary for cellular proliferation (reviewed in Chapter 1). In the case of p53, one of its major roles is in DNA repair. As it appears, the regulation of growth is coupled with the regulation of DNA repair. When cells suffer DNA damage, cellular *hibernation* manifested by an arrest at the G_1 or G_2 checkpoints permits repair to take place and prevents the accumulation of mutant sequences.[1] Cells harboring mutant p53 genes lose the ability to arrest in G_1 after exposure to gamma irradiation or other genotoxins.[2] Mice with p53 gene disruptions are completely viable, but exhibit an enhanced rate of tumor formation, and the abrogation of the G_1 checkpoint after exposure to DNA-damaging agents.[3,4] In addition, p53 appeared to be involved in two other critical functions: genomic stability and apoptosis. Cells without a functional p53 show an increased ability to amplify their DNA. This measure of genetic plasticity is characteristic of cancer.[5] In addition, a mutant p53 renders cells less likely to undergo apoptosis after cellular stress including gamma irradiation and chemotherapeutic agents. Normal cells that experience a high level of DNA damage, overwhelming their repair capabilities, trigger cell death. This appears to be a mechanism to prevent the accumulation of cells harboring mutant genes. Taken together, these data suggested that the primary role of p53 is not to regulate growth, but to maintain the genetic integrity of a cell.

We know that other important tumor suppressors have similar policing functions. BRCA1 and BRCA2 are structurally unrelated genes with converging clinical effects: Disabling mutations in either gene render an individual more susceptible to breast and ovarian cancers. Although both genes carry the hallmarks of a tumor suppressor gene, their main function is not growth regulation. In gene transfection experiments, BRCA1 is able to inhibit cellular growth only under limited conditions, possibly in cells with an intact retinoblastoma gene product.[6,7] In other experiments, however, BRCA1 and BRCA2 paradoxically appear to be associated with signs of growth promotion. Both are increased at S phase, and mouse embryos that have either gene disrupted die *in utero* exhibiting an increase in the cell-cycle inhibitor p21, a decrease in cyclin E, and a reduction in proliferating cells.[8] These data suggest that BRCA1 and BRCA2 serve to support rather than to suppress proliferation. More important, however, is the finding that BRCA1 and BRCA2 are both associated with each other and with DNA repair proteins RAD51 and PCNA, especially after DNA damage.[9] The functional consequences of this association are exemplified by the experimental data. Cells from a BRCA1 null mouse are defective in transcription-coupled DNA repair.[10] BRCA2 null cells are exquisitely sensitive to gamma irradiation[11] and to chemotherapeutic agents.[12] It is remarkable that two structurally dissimilar proteins interact with the same biochemical entities and lead to similar disease phenotypes. Thus, the fundamental lesson learned from BRCA1 and BRCA2 is that the primary causes of breast cancer may be related to DNA damage and repair and not to excessive growth.

The primacy of repair over growth regulation is also seen in the MLH1 and MSH2 genes that are responsible for the syndrome of hereditary nonpolyposis colorectal cancer. The respective gene products are involved in the recognition and repair of mismatches between complementary DNA strands: When these mismatch repair (MMR) genes are mutated, the mechanism for the correction of nucleotide mismatches is defective. This defect leads to an increased risk of gastrointestinal (especially colorectal) and endometrial cancers.[13]

Oncoproteins such as p53 not only act to induce a cell-cycle arrest in order for DNA repair to complete, but also promotes apoptosis to eliminate damaged cells with a high cancer potential. Therefore, an attenuation of the apoptosis mechanism is therefore likely to support transformation. The cancer susceptibility gene, PTEN/MMAC, is an example of a genetic *guardian* whose primary function is to regulate cell death and survival. PTEN, localized to 10q23, was identified through position cloning as the gene responsible for Cowden's syndrome. Cowden's is a syndrome characterized by gastrointestinal hamartomas, cutaneous trichilemmomas, and increased rates of breast (25% to 50%) and thyroid cancers (3% to 10%), as well as uterine leiomyomas. Although germline PTEN mutations are distinctive for a relatively rare disorder, somatic mutations leading to the loss of PTEN function are detected in a large number of sporadic cancers including high-grade gliomas, thyroid cancers, and endometrial cancers.[14] Transfection of the wild-type PTEN cDNA inhibits growth in established cell lines, and mice with one disrupted PTEN allele exhibit high rates of tumor formation, especially lymphomas, teratocarcinomas, and liver and prostatic cancer.[15] Thus, PTEN fulfills the classic criteria of a tumor suppressor.

Functionally, PTEN is as a multifunctional phosphatase that removes phospho groups from tyrosine and serine residues as well as from phospholipids such as phosphatidylinositol second messengers. The most important biochemical consequence of PTEN is to disarm the PI3'-kinase/AKT pathway.[16] AKT is a pivotal member of a pathway that induces cell survival and motility and was originally found as a retroviral oncogene, v-akt, causing lymphomas in infected mice. More recently, the AKT protooncogene was also found to be amplified in human ovarian cancers. It is thought that AKT phosphorylates BCL2 proapoptotic homologue BAD, resulting in a block to apoptosis.[17] Mutations in PTEN result in an increase in AKT activity, rendering cells more resistant to cell death signals. This mode of cancer induction is similar to the antiapoptotic effects of the bcl2 oncogene. Augmented levels of bcl2 expression associated with the t(14;18) translocation render affected B cells less sensitive to apoptotic signals and more susceptible to be transformed. Thus, activation of the PI3'-kinase/AKT pathway, either through crippling the tumor suppressing phosphatase, PTEN, or augmenting the activity of the AKT kinase, can lead to cancer. This is but one example of the biochemical intersect between classic tumor suppressor and oncogenes that blur the taxonomic distinctions.

Our current state of knowledge of tumor suppressors shows a picture of complex interactions between multiple suppressor genes with oncogenes to generate the malignant state. A dramatic example of the convergence of oncogenic processes is seen in the analysis of the transforming growth factor-β (TGF-β) pathway in gastrointestinal carcinogenesis. It has been long understood that the peptide factor TGF-β can inhibit tumor formation, and that tumor progression is associated with loss of response to TGF-β. This loss of response now appears to be due to the disruption of the type II TGF-β receptor. TGF-β functions by inducing heterodimers between the cognate type I and II receptors (TGF-βRI and TGF-βRII), resulting in the phosphorylation of the type I receptor and activation of downstream pathways. Markowitz and colleagues found that many tumors, especially colorectal cancers, harbor frameshift mutations in a short polyadenine tract within the gene that generates a truncated TGF-β protein bearing defective kinase activity.[18] Interestingly, this frameshift mutation occurs most commonly in cancers with concomitant aberrations in mismatch repair (MMR) as is seen in patients with hereditary nonpolyposis colorectal cancer. Moreover, this mutational *switch* occurs during the conversion from colonic adenoma to malignant carcinoma.[19] Further downstream, the TGF-β signaling pathway requires engagement by the activated receptors and phosphorylation of cytoplasmic SMAD proteins. Activated SMADs form heterodimers between SMAD1 or SMAD2 with SMAD4 and are transported to the nucleus where they interact with DNA-binding proteins to induce transcription of TGF-β–responsive genes.[20] The importance of this pathway is that SMAD4, which is an essential component in the TGF-β signaling pathway, has been found to be disrupted in 50% of human pancreatic cancers and to a lesser extent in gastric, breast, ovarian, and prostatic cancers.[21,22] Thus, the TGF-β pathway alone engages three functional nodes with significant roles in human cancers: mismatch repair, TGF-βRII, and SMAD4. The complexity lies in the fact that these elements are connected not only by biochemistry, but genetics and peculiarities in DNA sequence. It is, therefore, with the use of many of the analytical tools described previously that these relationships can be uncovered.

MOLECULAR PROFILING: PROGNOSIS AND TREATMENT TAILORED TO THE INDIVIDUAL PATIENT

The concept of employing tumor characteristics such as histologic features as a predictor of best treatments has long been part of the practice of oncology. For example, not only are the natural histories of the lymphomas different, but the requirements for optimal therapy are distinct: Burkitt's lymphomas require high-dose alkylator chemotherapy to achieve optimal cure rates, whereas doxorubicin-based therapies are optimal for large cell lymphomas.[23]

A significant refinement of this histology-based approach to selection of therapeutics has been the application of molecular markers and is best exemplified in the use of markers in the treatment of human leukemias. With the availability of effective chemotherapy, it was observed that cytogenetic profiles could discern those who are likely to respond. In acute myeloid leukemia (AML), patients with t(8;21), inv(16), and t(15;17) show the best overall survivals, whereas patients with del(5q)/5q-, del(7q)/7q-, and inv(3) show the lowest complete response rates. Patients with 11q23/+11 abnormalities exhibit average remission rates, but a high probability of relapse and low overall survival.[24]

Many of the genes involved in these leukemia translocations have now been cloned and biochemically characterized. The t(9;22), characterizing common chronic myelogenous leukemia, involves the translocation between bcr on chromosome 22 and the tyrosine kinase abl on chromosome 9. The chimeric bcr-abl oncoprotein activates the abl kinase and the ras pathway and blocks apoptotic processes in hematopoietic precursors.[25] In acute lymphoid leukemias, one of the major discerning factors also appears to be the presence of the bcr-abl rearrangement as exemplified by the t(9;22) translocation. The Philadelphia chromosome (Ph1) and the resultant bcr-abl fusion gene is the single most common abnormality in adult ALL, accounting for up to 50% of the B-lineage disease.[26] Although bcr-abl–positive ALL cases easily achieve complete remissions, relapse is uniform and the potential for cure using standard forms of chemotherapy is low. By contrast, bcr-abl translocations occur only in 5% of pediatric ALL cases, and the low frequency of this adverse prognostic marker may explain some of the differences in survival rates between pediatric and adult ALL.

In AML, the key gene involved in the t(8;21)(q22;q22) translocation found in AML-M2 through positional cloning is AML1, which is related to the *Drosophila* pair rule gene, *runt*. *Runt* is a transcription factor that regulates the expression of specific patterns of the homeobox genes.[27] The human homologues of these homeobox genes have been implicated in hematopoietic differentiation.[28] The normal AML1 binds to a protein partner called CBFβ to exert its physiologic function as a transcription factor. Coincidentally, translocations of CBFβ are also involved in leukemias harboring inv(16) that generates the fusion protein CBFβ-MYHII. This biochemical interaction between the principal gene products of the t(8;21) and the inv(16) rearrangements is even more remarkable in that both translocations are associated with favorable clinical outcomes, although the exact mechanism explaining this association remains unclear. Rearrangements involving chromosome 11q23, however, are uniformly associated with poor outcome and with short durations of remission. Initially described in the uncommon translocation t(4q21;11q23) observed in both AML and ALL, this rearrangement creates a fusion oncogene mutating the ALL1/MLL gene (residing on 11q23). ALL1 is the human homologue of another *Drosophila* gene, *trithorax*, a transcription factor that maintains specific expression patterns of the homeobox genes. Once the exact genetic mutation for the chromosomal rearrangement was identified, other abnormalities at chromosome 11q such as trisomy 11 were found to contain perturbations in ALL1.[29] Moreover, the importance of 11q aberrations in leukemias was further raised when a syndrome characterized by 11q23 translocations in secondary leukemias resulting from etoposide treatment was recognized.[30] In every case, the clinical syndrome linked with 11q abnormalities and its associated ALL1 lesion is characterized by poor clinical outcome.

For solid tumors, the development of tumor markers for the prediction of therapeutic response has been much slower. One impressive positive example, however, has been the HER2/neu gene. HER2 gene encodes a 185-kD protein, which belongs to transmembrane type I tyrosine kinase receptor family including the EGF receptor, HER3, and HER4. Clear evidence from clinical studies demonstrates that HER2 amplification or overexpression is a marker for poor prognosis for node-positive patients. A major question, however, has been whether this poor prognosis is irrevocable or can be bypassed by some intervention. In 1994, the national cooperative group, Cancer and Leukemia Group B (CALGB) published a preliminary study on 442 patients suggesting that the poor clinical outcome of node-positive breast cancer patients with HER2 overexpression can be overcome by adequately dose-intensive regimens of cyclophosphamide, doxorubicin (Adriamycin), and 5-fluorouracil. The HER2-negative group, however, experienced no benefit from the cyclophosphamide, Adriamycin, and 5-fluorouracil dose escalation. Thus, the beneficial effect of dose intensification was present only for the HER2-positive cohort but absent for the HER2-negative patients. In a parallel study, in which node-positive patients were treated with cyclophosphamide, methotrexate, fluorouracil, vincristine, and prednisone (CMFVP) for four cycles, then randomized to completing CMFVP or to vinblastine (Velban), Adriamycin, thiotepa, and fluoxymesterone (Halotestin), patients treated only with CMFVP showed worse survival if their tumors overexpressed HER2. By contrast, patients given Velban, Adriamycin, thiotepa, and Halotestin showed no differential survival between the HER2-positive and -negative groups. These data raised the possibility that the adverse effects of HER2 overexpression can be specifically overcome by effective doses of Adriamycin.

The most definitive test of the HER2–doxorubicin interaction was seen in two studies: the reanalysis of the National Surgical Adjuvant Breast Project trial B-11, and the 10-year follow-up of the analysis of the complete cohort in CALGB 8541.[31] In B-11, node-positive breast cancer patients were randomized between L-PAM and fluorouracil versus L-PAM, Adriamycin, and fluorouracil so that the only treatment variable was doxorubicin. Of the 638 patient tumors, 37.5% were scored as positive for HER2 protein overexpression. After a mean time of study of 13.5 years, clinical benefit from the addition of doxorubicin to L-PAM and fluorouracil was apparent only for HER2-positive patients. The *completion* study of CALGB 8869/8541 conducted by the CALGB looked at over 900 cases from the original CALGB 8869/8541 study with a median follow-up of 9.5 years.[32] Important in the analysis was that the HER2 determination was rigorously validated by concurrent analysis by immunohistochemistry, differential PCR, and fluorescent *in situ* hybridization. Patients with HER2-positive tumors responded with improved overall survival when treated with dose-intensive cyclophosphamide, Adriamycin, and 5-fluorouracil chemotherapy, whereas HER2-negative patients showed no benefit with dose escalation. Although the mechanism of this interaction and putative resistance is unclear, there is evidence that inhibition of HER2 signaling is associated with a decreased ability of the cell to repair DNA damage such is seen after chemotherapeutic exposure.[33]

Thus far, we have centered on examples of how the molecular profile of a cancer may give information pertinent to response to standard chemotherapeutic agents. In most cases, however, the mechanism for this oncogene-associated relative resistance or sensitivity is uncertain. However, many of the markers that define the profile may themselves be suitable targets for molecularly based therapeutics. Given the surface location of HER2 on cells, and the overexpression that occurs mainly in cancerous states, the HER2 oncoprotein represented one such attractive target for antibody-directed therapeutics. One such antibody, 4D5, suppressed cancer cell growth both in *in vitro* and *in vivo* animal studies.[34] When coupled with standard chemotherapeutic agents, 4D5 showed additive and potentially synergistic antiproliferative effects. The humanized form of the murine 4D5 antibody (Herceptin) was developed for clinical applications, and the initial phase II data showed promise: As a single agent in pretreated individuals, Herceptin showed a 16% response rate with 4% complete responders, and a median time to relapse of 9.1 months.[35] The subsequent phase III study was also significant. The study randomized individuals with metastatic breast cancer to chemotherapy alone or chemotherapy plus weekly Herceptin. The results showed that patients treated with chemotherapy alone had a response rate of 32%, a duration of response at 5.9 months, and time to disease progression of 4.6 months. Those treated with chemotherapy and Herceptin exhibited an improvement in all measures: response rate of 49% (vs. 32% with chemotherapy alone), median duration of response of 9.3 months (vs. 5.9 months with chemotherapy alone), and time to progression at 7.6 months (vs. 4.6 months with chemotherapy alone).[36] Thus, as predicted in the *in vitro* investigations, the combination of chemotherapy and Herceptin led to a more favorable outcome.

Since oncogenes are signaling molecules that rely on protein–protein interactions to conduct their signals, interruption of these interactions was predicted to disrupt critical pathways that maintain the cancerous state. Inhibition of the enzymatic activity of certain oncogenes, such as ras proteins and kinases, with small chemically derived molecules has been both an attractive and ultimately successful approach. Some of the most notable clinical successes have been in the treatment of leukemias. Acute promyelocytic leukemia is characterized by the uniform presence of a cytogenetic signature, the reciprocal translocation of chromosomes 15 and 17 [t(15;17)], which generates a fusion between the PML gene and the retinoic acid receptor-α gene (PML/RARA). The resultant fusion protein places the DNA-binding domain of a nuclear protein PML adjacent to a truncated RARA that retains its ligand-binding domain. This observation immediately suggested a molecular explanation for why acute promyelocytic leukemia occasionally responded to available retinoids.[37] This hypothesis was supported by dramatic reports showing clinical remissions to an isomer of retinoic acid, all-*trans*-retinoic acid. In patients with newly diagnosed or relapsing acute promyelocytic leukemia, a 90% complete response rate was seen with single-agent all-*trans*-retinoic acid.[38,39] This response is highly specific: all-*trans*-retinoic acid is ineffective in the absence of the PML-RARA fusion protein. Another significant development has been the Novartis compound, the 2-phenylaminopyrimidine derivative STI571. Derived to inhibit the activity of the activated BCR-ABL tyrosine kinase, STI571 was found to render remissions in the majority of patients with chronic myelogenous leukemia. In both leukemic conditions, other standard chemotherapeutic agents are equally effective. However, the specificity of the drugs significantly avoided the side effects of chemotherapy and underscored the potential of inhibiting a single molecular target to control extensive cancer conditions.

There is currently a rich developmental pipeline for these kinase inhibitors with many potential agents that will be ready for or have been in clinical testing. The targets include the ras proteins PDGF and EGF and the VEGF receptors. The number and diversity of targets, however, make molecular profiling a necessary adjunct to therapeutic decision making. Thus, a comprehensive approach for target detection will no longer remain solely of academic interest, but is predicted to become a clinical necessity.

POSTGENOME CHALLENGE FOR MOLECULAR MEDICINE

Sequencing the human genome will provide new tools and insights that will enhance our understanding of the genetic mechanisms underlying cancer.[40,41] A major objective of the Human Genome Project is the identification of the complete set of human genes. A leading method for rapid gene discovery is single-pass partial sequencing of cDNA clones from one or both ends to generate expressed sequence tags. This strategy has been widely and successfully applied to humans and other species. Before 1991 and the development of the expressed sequence tag method, sequence data existed for fewer than 3000 human genes.[40,41] Now that the entire human genome sequence has been completed, the effect on science and society will be incalculable.[42,43] The combination of data on gene expression and putative gene functions inferred from sequence similarities and motif analysis will provide a powerful means of assessing the transcriptional activity of the genome in the cells and tissue before, during, and after disease. For the next generation of scientists and clinicians, identification of a new gene will be as rare as finding a new species of mammal.

Completion of the human genome sequence is just the beginning. The current challenge is to generate a comprehensive understanding of the *software and the hardware* of the cell and the organism.[44] Less than 2% of the noninfectious human disease burden is monogenic in nature. The rest (98%) is polygenic (caused by multiple genes at once) or is epigenetic (caused by nongenetic or postgenetic alterations in cellular molecules). Consequently, elucidating disease mechanisms and full penetration of the causal mechanisms driving carcinogenesis and cancer progression will require analysis tools ranging from direct DNA sequencing, mRNA expression monitoring, protein sequencing, protein localization studies, and finally to metabolic or physiologic profiling.

A further essential phase will be a description of the normal range of human polymorphisms (base variations in the genome), which may provide a starting point for correlating genetic variance with disease states. The final physiologic state is further complicated because biologic diversity causally associated with disease may be due to posttranslational processes regulated by the cellular environment. These changes cannot be inferred from known DNA variance. Thus, a complete understanding of the molecular basis of cancer depends on a multidisciplinary approach combining genetics, pathology, protein structure and function, cell biology, and clinical medicine.

Finding all the expressed human genes is a different task from sequencing the genome itself. This is because only a small proportion of the genome actually makes up the actual expressed genes and their regulatory elements. The actual number of expressed human genes may be 100,000. However, at any point in time, for any individual cell in any given tissue, the amount of genes *in use* may be as few as 10,000. Of this 10,000, only a proportion may be susceptible to the influence of carcinogenic events. Thus, an important goal for molecular profiling of cancer is to identify a subset of expressed genes that is correlated with, or causally related to, the development and progression of cancer. Setting aside hereditary susceptibility, it is likely that the majority of cancers may originate in tissue that starts with a completely normal genome. Carcinogenic events produce heritable genetic alterations that expand in microscopic premalignant states such as hyperplasia and dysplasia, before frank malignant cancer ensues. Identification of the important genetic derangements and the causally important genes and proteins will depend on direct analysis of actual human cancer tissues, combined with insights gained using animal and cell culture methods. The massive profiling of genes associated with cancer progression is now possible using new technology for microdissection and array hybridization.

cDNA MICROARRAYS ARE A NEW TOOL TO ANALYZE GENE EXPRESSION PATTERNS IN HUMAN CANCER

Every oncologist is daily faced with the biologic heterogeneity of cancer emergence, aggressiveness, and treatment response in individual patients. Every pathologist is daily faced with the enormous histologic diversity of human neoplasms. We assume that the morphologic microscopic appearance (e.g., staining pattern, nuclear shape and contour, cellular configuration and pleomorphism) of a particular neoplastic lesion that spells cancer is the outward manifestation of molecular changes that are occurring inside the interacting tissue cell populations. Scores of molecules and genes can be involved in the behavior of an individual patient's tumor. The clinical heterogeneity of cancer mirrors the underlying molecular heterogeneity of the cancer cell. This is evident in the variable presence of chromosomal translocations, deletions of suppressor genes, and numbers of chromosomes. Consequently, it is critical for molecular oncology of the future to adopt high-throughput technology to survey panels of genes, ranging from hundreds to even the whole human expressed gene set, and apply this technology to the classification of tumor pathologic entities in individual patients.

In response to this challenge, investigators in both the public and private sectors have been perfecting gene-chip arrays that can be used to survey great patterns of gene expression.[45–50] The change in the pattern can then be correlated with histomorphology, clinical behavior, or response to treatment. Typically, the analysis takes the form of rows and rows of oligonucleotide strands lined up in dots on a miniature silicon chip or glass slide or sheet of nitrocellulose. The microarrays work as follows. First, the RNA is extracted from the tumor tissue, amplified, and labeled with a fluorescent or radioactive probe. This of course assumes that the highly labile RNA is preserved when the tissue is extracted. The labeled total RNA, containing the mRNA of the expressed genes, is applied to the surface of the chip or sheet. After appropriate hybridization, the relative intensity of the signal for each spot on the chip corresponds to the abundance of its matching mRNA species and hence reflects the expression level for its gene. With appropriate pattern recognition software it is then possible to assemble a global score for the gene study set represented on the substratum.

Tremendous progress has been made in the use of DNA arrays to analyze gene expression patterns in human cancer cell lines and human cancer tissue. Perou et al. used cDNA microarrays to study 60 cancer cell lines used by the National Cancer Institute to screen anticancer drugs.[48] When they classified the cell lines based on the gene expression subclasses, they obtained a correspondence to the ostensible cell type origin of the cancer cell line (i.e., epithelial or fibroblast or hematopoietic). Specific features of the cell line expression pattern appeared to correlate with the growth rate in culture or drug metabolism. These investigators then went on to use the cultured cell gene expression pattern as a template for comparison with RNA extracted from actual pieces of cancer tissue. They found that the gene pattern

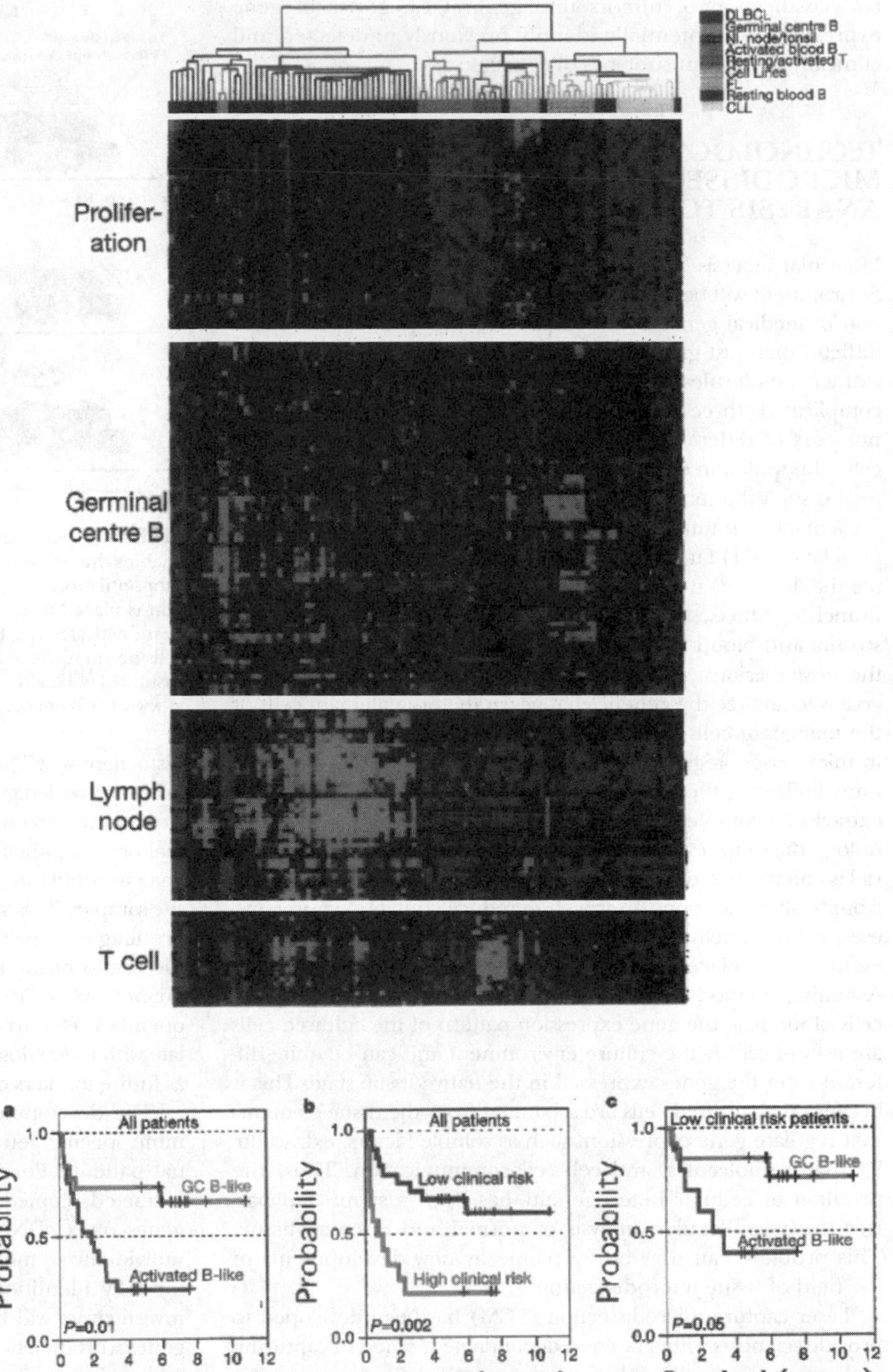

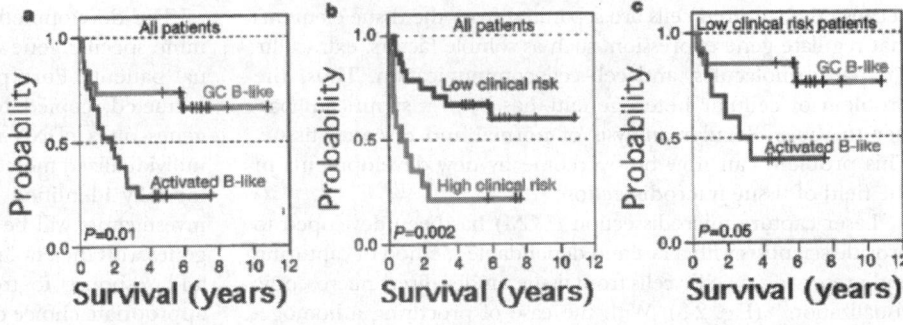

FIGURE 2-2. Diffuse large B-cell lymphoma (DLBCL) clinical subtypes elucidated by DNA chip profiling. Hierarchical clustering of data from the chip profiling of thousands of lymphocyte-relevant genes reveals gene patterns associated with lymph node germinal center B cells (GC B) and activated B cells. The patients with activated B-like profiles underwent a much poorer overall survival. CLL, chronic lymphocytic leukemia; FL, follicular lymphoma. (See Color Fig. 2-2 in the CD-ROM and on the Web at www.LWWoncology.com.)

of the cancer tissue varied greatly from one cancer type to the next. Moreover, the pattern of a carcinoma gene expression appeared to correspond with the cell lines that had an epithelial origin. This study provided direct evidence that tissue pathology was heterogeneous at the level of gene expression patterns and offered hope that this information could potentially be applied to predict patient outcome.

The first major clinical correlation of gene expression patterns with disease outcome was provided by Alizadeh et al.[45] Diffuse large B-cell lymphoma, the most common subtype of non-Hodgkin's lymphoma, is clinically heterogeneous. Sixty percent of the patients succumb to the disease, whereas the remainder respond well to the current therapy and have prolonged survival. This variability in natural history correlated with a distinct pattern of gene expression revealed by DNA arrays. The group identified two molecularly distinct forms of diffuse large B-cell lymphoma (Fig. 2-2): One had a gene expression pattern indicative of a B-cell differentiation pattern. The second type expressed genes induced during *in vitro* activation of peripheral B cells. Patients with the germinal B-like diffuse large B-cell lymphoma had a significantly better overall survival (see Fig. 2-2). This provides evidence that the molecular classification of tumors into general categories of gene expression can potentially identify previously undetected and clinically significant subtypes of cancer.

TECHNOLOGY FOR TISSUE MICRODISSECTION BRINGS MOLECULAR ANALYSIS TO THE TISSUE CELL LEVEL

Molecular analysis of pure cell populations in their native tissue environment will be an important component of the next generation of medical genetics. Accomplishing this goal is much more difficult than just grinding up a piece of tissue and applying the extracted molecules to a panel of assays. This is because tissues are complicated three-dimensional structures composed of large numbers of different types of interacting cell populations. The cell subpopulation of interest may constitute a tiny fraction of the total tissue volume. For example, a biopsy of breast tissue harboring a malignant tumor usually contains the following types of cell populations: (1) fat cells in the abundant adipose tissue surrounding the ducts, (2) normal epithelium and myoepithelium in the branching ducts, (3) fibroblasts and endothelial cells in the stroma and blood vessels, (4) premalignant carcinoma cells in the *in situ* lesions, and (5) clusters of invasive carcinoma. If the goal is to analyze the genetic changes in the premalignant cells or the malignant cells, these subpopulations are frequently located in microscopic regions occupying less than 5% of the tissue volume. Following the computer adage *garbage in, garbage out,* if the extract of a complex tissue is analyzed using a sophisticated technology, the output will be severely compromised if the input material is contaminated by the wrong cells. Culturing cell populations from fresh tissue is one approach to reduce contamination. However, cultured cells may not accurately represent the molecular events taking place in the actual tissue they were derived from. Assuming methods are successful to isolate and grow the tissue cells of interest, the gene expression pattern of the cultured cells are influenced by the culture environment and can be quite different from the genes expressed in the native tissue state. This is because the cultured cells are separated from the tissue elements that regulate gene expression, such as soluble factors, extracellular matrix molecules, and cell–cell communication. Thus, the problem of cellular heterogeneity has been a significant barrier to the molecular analysis of normal and diseased tissue. This problem can now be overcome by new developments in the field of tissue microdissection.

Laser capture microdissection (LCM) has been developed to provide scientists with a fast and dependable method of capturing and preserving specific cells from tissue, under direct microscopic visualization[50] (Fig. 2-3). With the ease of procuring a homogeneous population of cells from a complex tissue using the LCM, the approaches to molecular analysis of pathologic processes are significantly enhanced. The mRNA from microdissected cancer lesions has been used as the starting material to produce cDNA libraries, microchip microarrays, differential display, and other techniques to find new genes or mutations (Fig. 2-4).

Sgroi et al.[51] have combined LCM of breast cancer tissue with cDNA arrays, as an approach to the identification of genes that change their expression during the progression of breast cancer. The group monitored gene expression in LCM-procured pure normal epithelium, invasive cancer, and metastatic tissue cell populations. Differences in the *in vivo* gene expression profile were verified and validated by real-time quantitative PCR and immuno-

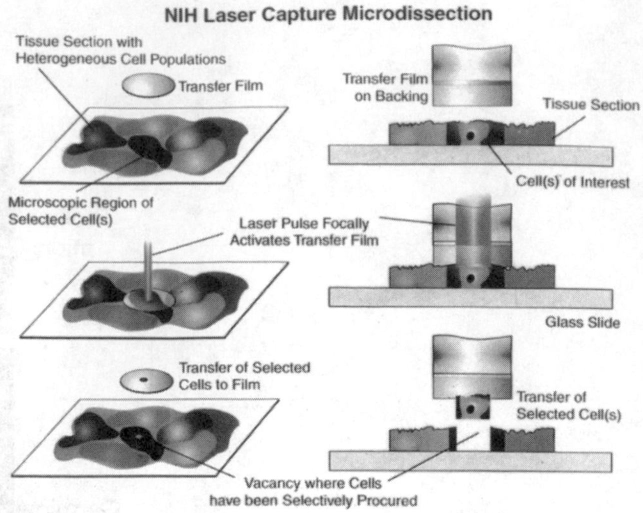

FIGURE 2-3. Laser capture microdissection. This new technology enables the investigator or clinician to directly procure pure tissue cell subpopulations under microscopic visualization. A transparent polymer film is placed in contact with the surface of the tissue section. A laser beam activates the film over the selected cells to actively capture the cells of interest and leave all the unwanted cells behind. NIH, National Institutes of Health. (See Color Fig. 2-3 in the CD-ROM and on the Web at www.LWWoncology.com.)

histochemistry. The combined use of LCM and cDNA microarray analysis revealed genes specifically associated with the progression from normal to metastatic breast cancer cells (Fig. 2-5). Since normal breast epithelium is a minor component of breast tissue, this analysis could not be done with simple ground-up whole breast tissue samples. This study demonstrated that *in vivo* gene expression profiling can be done on specific tissue cell populations, and that the results of the cDNA arrays correlated well with the real-time quantitative PCR analysis and immunohistochemistry. Consequently, cDNA arrays can be used to uncover patterns that correlate with the biology and find lead candidate genes that may serve as future markers or drug targets.

The development of the LCM allows investigators to determine specific gene expression patterns from tissues of individual patients. Pure populations of cells can be obtained, RNA extracted, copied to cDNA, and hybridized to thousands of genes on a cDNA microchip microarray. In this manner, an individualized molecular profile can be obtained for each histologically identified pathology. Using such multiplex analysis, investigators will be able to correlate the pattern of expressed genes with the etiology, premalignant progression (see Fig. 2-5), and response to treatment. A patient's risk for disease and appropriate choice of treatment could, in the future, be personalized based on the profile. A growing clinical database of such results could be used to develop a minimal subset of key markers that will lead to a revolutionary approach for early detection and accurate diagnosis of disease.

Efficient coupling of LCM of serial tissue sections with multiplex molecular analysis techniques[52–57] should lead to sensitive and quantitative methods to visualize three-dimensional interactions between morphologic elements of the tissue. For example, it will be possible to trace the gene expression pattern along the length of a prostate gland or breast duct in order to examine the progression of neoplastic development. The end result will be a new era in the integration of molecular biology with tissue morphogenesis and pathology.

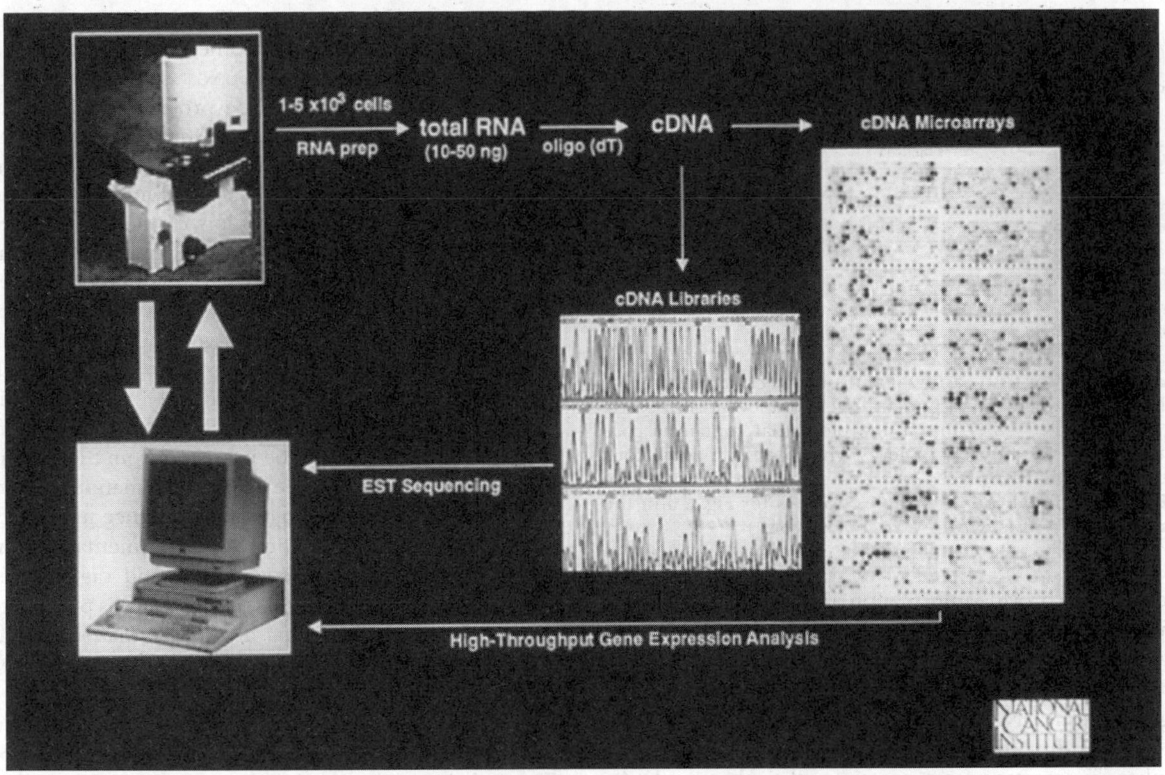

FIGURE 2-4. RNA isolated from tissue is reverse transcribed to cDNA. The sample cDNA is used to prepare cDNA libraries of the expressed genes *in use* by the tissue cells or to probe cDNA arrays of known pathways. EST, expressed sequence tags. (See Color Fig. 2-4 in the CD-ROM and on the Web at www.LWWoncology.com.)

TUMOR TISSUE ARRAYS

Once a putative marker (or set of markers) is identified by cDNA array analysis of cancer tissue samples, the next step is to validate these markers in a large population of human tumors. In the past, immunohistochemistry or *in situ* hybridization has been the method of choice to evaluate an individual patient's tissue sections *one slide at a time.* Consequently, in order to screen hundreds of patient specimens, it was necessary to laboriously stain hundreds of microscopic glass slides. This exhaustive process has now been telescoped into a high-throughput miniaturized tissue array.[52] The array consists of 1000 cylindrical tissue biopsies, each from a different patient, all distributed on a single glass slide. Thus, each tumor is represented by a minute disk-shaped tissue section 0.6 mm in diameter and 4 to 8 μm in thickness (Fig. 2-6). Tumor arrays are ideal for comparing large numbers of solid tumor samples. Full automation of tumor array creation and screening is envisioned as a means to expeditiously correlate marker levels over large study sets of tumors.

BEYOND FUNCTIONAL GENOMICS TO CANCER PROTEOMICS

While DNA is an information archive, proteins do all the work of the cell. The existence of a given DNA sequence does not guarantee the synthesis of a corresponding protein. The DNA sequence is also not sufficient to describe protein structure, function, and cellular location.[53] This is because protein complexity and versatility stems from context-dependent posttranslational processes such as phosphorylation, sulfation, or glycosylation. Moreover, the

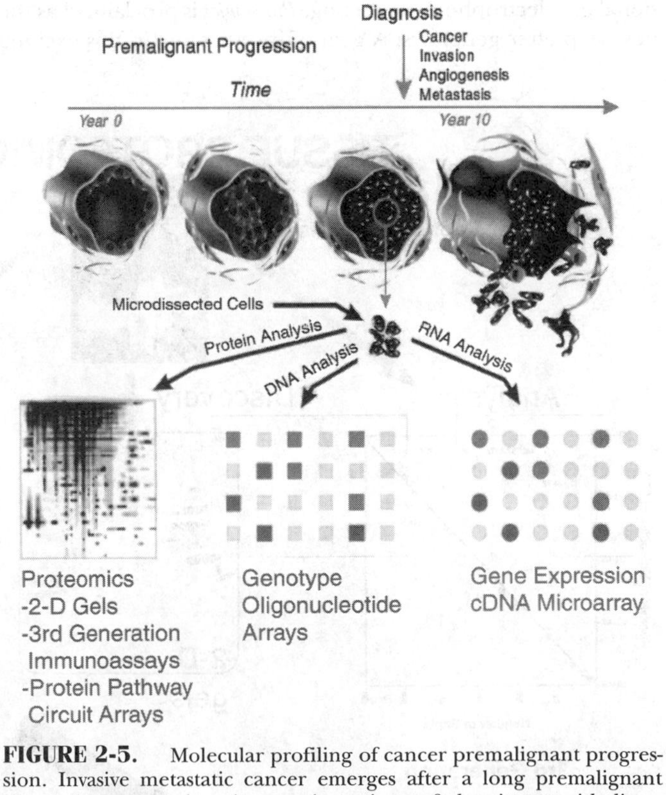

FIGURE 2-5. Molecular profiling of cancer premalignant progression. Invasive metastatic cancer emerges after a long premalignant phase that occurs in microscopic regions of the tissue epithelium. Microdissection makes it possible to profile the molecular patterns that track all the way through from normal epithelium to metastatic cancer in the same patient. (See Color Fig. 2-5 in the CD-ROM and on the Web at www.LWWoncology.com.)

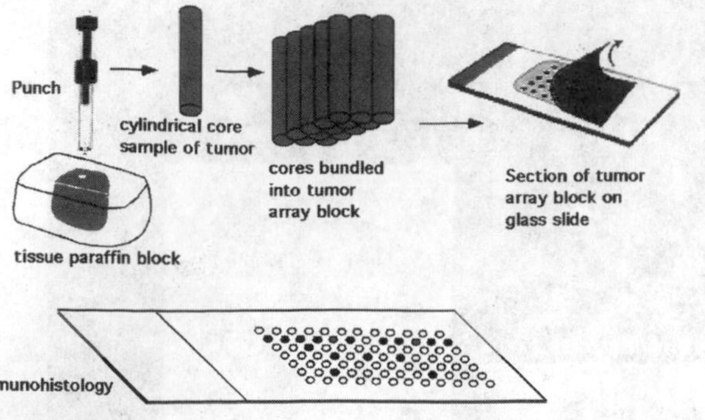

FIGURE 2-6. Tumor tissue arrays. Paraffin-embedded fixed tumor tissue in blocks is sampled with a punch to generate cylindrical cores. The cores are packed together into a new block that contains a core from one of hundreds of different patients. The composite array block is sliced into sections that are placed on a glass slide. The slide now contains hundreds of different tumor samples. (See Color Fig. 2-6 in the CD-ROM and on the Web at www.LWWoncology.com.)

DNA code does not provide information about how proteins link together into networks and functional machines in the cell. In fact, the activation of a protein signal pathway causing a cell to migrate, die, or initiate division can immediately take place before any changes occur in DNA/RNA gene expression. Consequently, the technology to drive the molecular medicine revolution into the third phase is emerging from protein analytical methods. An important goal will be to apply this knowledge at the level of human tissue itself (Fig. 2-7).

The term *proteome*, which denotes all the proteins expressed by a genome, was first coined in late 1994 at the Siena two-dimensional gel electrophoresis meeting. *Proteomics* is proclaimed as the next step after genomics. A goal of investigators in this exciting field is to assemble a complete library of all the proteins. Only a small percentage of the proteome has been cataloged in 2000. Since PCR for proteins does not exist, sequencing the order of 20 possible amino acids in a given protein remains relatively slow and labor intensive, compared with nucleotide sequencing. Although a number of new technologies are being introduced for high-throughput protein characterization and discovery,[54] the mainstay of protein identification continues to be two-dimensional gel electrophoresis.[53–56] Two-dimensional electrophoresis can separate proteins by molecular weight in one dimension and charge in second dimension. When a mixture of proteins is applied to the two-dimensional gel, individual proteins in the mixture are separated out into signature locations on the display, depending on their individual size and charge. Each signature is a *spot* on the gel that can constitute a unique single protein species. The protein spot can be procured from the gel and a partial amino acid sequence can be read. In this manner, known proteins can be monitored for changes in abundance under treatment or new proteins can be identified. An experimental two-dimensional gel image can be captured and overlaid digitally with known archived two-dimensional gels. In this way it is possible to immediately highlight proteins that are differentially abundant in one state versus another (e.g., tumor vs. normal or before and after hormone treatment).

Two-dimensional gels have traditionally required large amounts of protein starting material equivalent to millions of cells. Thus, their application has been limited to cultured cells or ground-up heterogeneous tissue. Not unexpectedly, this approach does not provide an accurate picture of the proteins that are in use by cells in real tissue. Tissues are complicated structures composed of hundreds of interacting cell populations in specialized spatial configurations. The fluctuating proteins expressed by cells in tissues may bear little resemblance to the proteins made by cultured

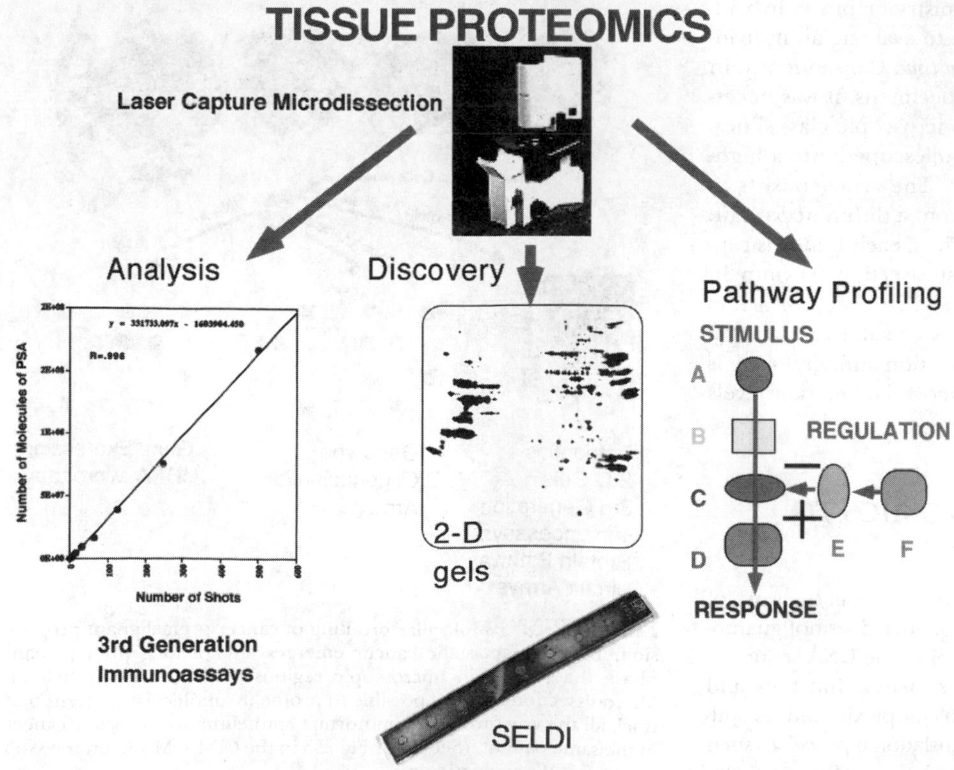

FIGURE 2-7. Tissue proteomics. Proteins extracted from microdissected tissue subpopulations can be applied to quantify known proteins, to discover new proteins, and ultimately to reconstruct signal pathways. PSA, prostate-specific antigen; SELDI, surface-enhanced laser desorption and ionization. (See Color Fig. 2-7 in the CD-ROM and on the Web at www.LWWoncology.com.)

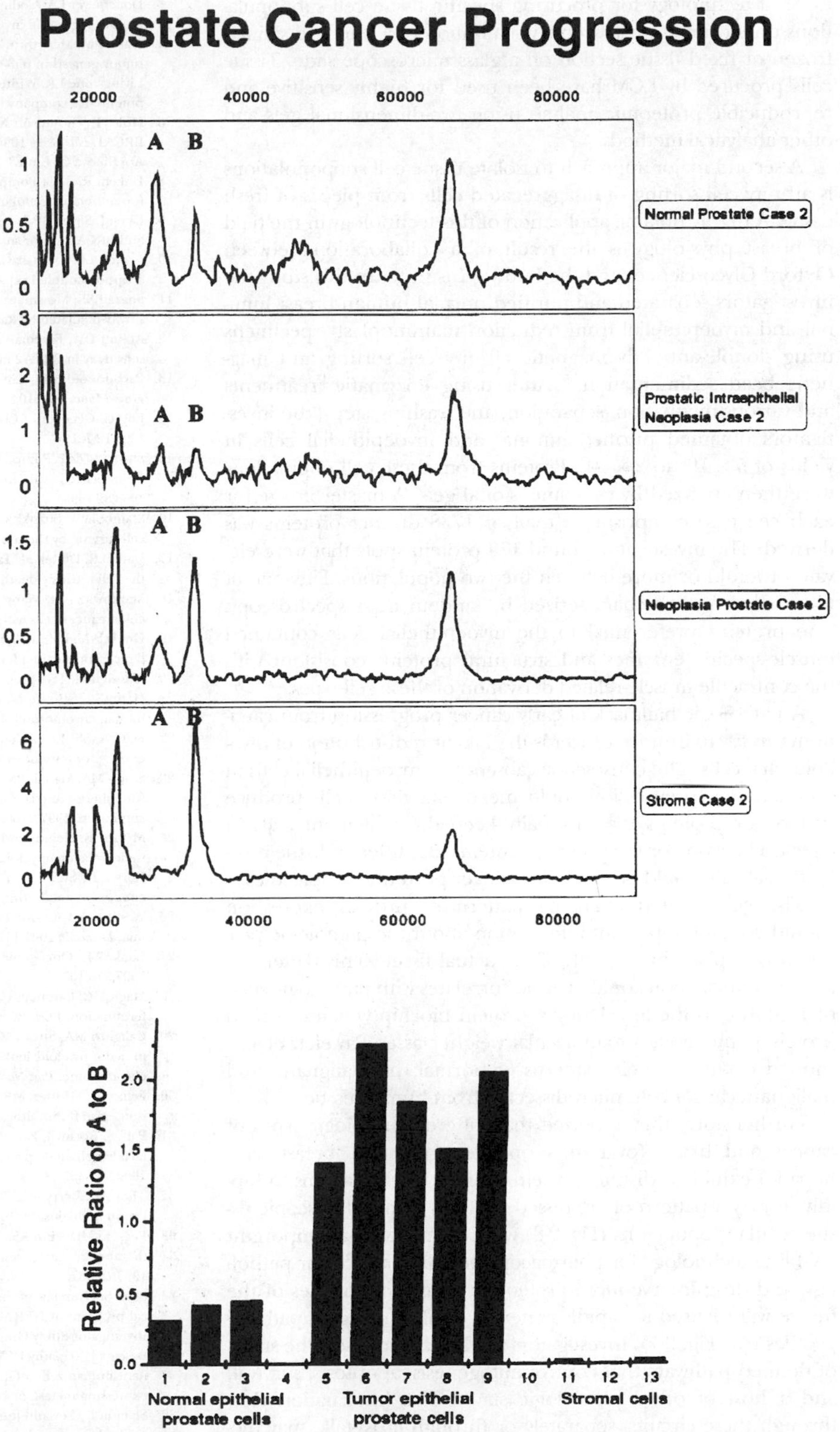

FIGURE 2-8. Surface-enhanced laser desorption and ionization (SELDI) analysis of laser capture microdissection microdissected microscopic stages of human prostate cancer. This technology generates a protein fingerprint consisting of the distribution of molecular weights. In the example study set, the ratios of specific protein peaks change specifically in the invasive carcinoma compared with the normal epithelium.

cells, which are torn from their tissue context and are reacting to a new culture environment. Proteins extracted from ground-up tissue represent an averaging of proteins from all the heterogeneous tissue subpopulations. For example, in the case of breast tissue, the glandular epithelium constitutes a small proportion of the tissue: The vast majority is stroma and adipose. Thus, it has previously been impossible to obtain a clear snapshot of gene or protein expression within normal or diseased tissue cell subpopulations.

To address the tissue-context problem, new technology is again coming to the rescue; *tissue proteomics* is an exciting expanding discipline (see Fig. 2-7). Two major technologic approaches have been successfully used to sample macromolecules directly from subpopulations of human tissue cells. The first technology is

LCM, a technology for procuring specific tissue cell subpopulations under direct microscopic visualization of a standard stained frozen or fixed tissue section on a glass microscope slide. Tissue cells procured by LCM have been used for highly sensitive and reproducible proteomic analysis using two-dimensional gels and other analytical methods.

A second major approach to isolate tissue cell subpopulations is affinity cell sorting of disaggregated cells from pieces of fresh tissue. A highly notable application of this technology in the field of breast physiology is the result of a collaboration between Oxford Glycosciences and the Ludwig Institute. In this study the investigators separated and purified normal human breast luminal and myoepithelial from reduction mammoplasty specimens using double-antibody magnetic affinity cell sorting and magnetic bead sedimentation.[55] After using enzymatic treatments and various incubation, separation, and washing steps, the investigators obtained purified luminal and myoepithelial cells in yields of 5×10^6 to 2×10^7. Proteins from these cell populations were then analyzed by two-dimensional gels. A master image for each cell type comprising a total of 1738 distinct proteins was derived. The investigators found 170 protein spots that were elevated twofold or more between the two populations. Fifty-one of these were further characterized by tandem mass spectroscopy. The proteins preferential to the myoepithelial cells contained muscle-specific enzymes and structural proteins consistent with the contractile muscle-related derivation of these cell types.

A pathologic hallmark of early cancer progression from carcinoma *in situ* to invasive cancer is the loss or redistribution of myoepithelial cells. The conspicuous absence of myoepithelial cells in breast cancer progression could mean that these cells produce suppressor proteins that normally keep the malignant cells in check. Thus, one or more of the proteins identified in tissue myoepithelial cells could be candidate cancer prevention molecules.

The complicated changing pattern of protein expression should contain important information about the pathologic process taking place in the cells of the actual tissue. This pattern of protein information could provide correlates with pathologic state or response to therapy. Using a protein biochip which classified protein populations into molecular weight classes, Paweletz et al.[58] showed distinct protein patterns of normal, premalignant, and malignant cancer cells microdissected from human tissue.

Furthermore, they reported that different histologic types of cancer and tissue (ovarian, esophageal, prostate, breast, and hepatic) exhibited distinct protein profiles. Such a means to rapidly display a pattern of expressed proteins from microscopic tissue cellular populations (Fig. 2-8) will potentially be an important enabling technology for pharmacoproteomics, molecular pathology, and drug intervention. Proteomic array technologies of the future will be used to rapidly generate displays of signal pathway profiles (see Fig. 2-7). Investigators will be able to assess the status of defined pathways that control mitogenesis, apoptosis, survival, and a host of other physiologic states. The information flow through these circuits, separately or through cross-talk, may dictate clinical behavior and susceptibility to therapy.

REFERENCES

1. O'Connor PM. Mammalian G1 and G2 phase checkpoints. *Cancer Surv* 1997;29:151.
2. O'Connor PM, Jackman J, Bae I, et al. Characterization of the p53 tumor suppressor pathway in cell lines of the National Cancer Institute Anticancer Drug Screen and correlations with the growth-inhibitory potency of 123 anticancer agents. *Cancer Res* 1997;57:4285.
3. Donehower LA, Godley LA, Aldaz CM, et al. The role of p53 loss in genomic instability and tumor progression in a murine mammary cancer model. *Prog Clin Biol Res* 1996;395:1.
4. Harvey M, McArthur MJ, Montgomery CA Jr, et al. Spontaneous and carcinogen-induced tumorigenesis in p53-deficient mice. *Nat Genet* 1993;5:225.
5. Livingstone LR, White A, Sprouse J, et al. Altered cell cycle arrest and gene amplification potential accompany loss of wild-type p53. *Cell* 1992;70:923.
6. Holt JT, Thompson ME, Szabo C, et al. Growth retardation and tumour inhibition by BRCA1. *Nat Genet* 1996;12:298.
7. Aprelikova O, Liu ET (*submitted*).
8. Hakem R, de la Pompa JL, Sirard C, et al. The tumor suppressor gene Brcal is required for embryonic cellular proliferation in the mouse. *Cell* 1996;85:1009.
9. Chen J, Silver DP, Walpita D, et al. Stable interaction between the products of the BRCA1 and BRCA2 tumor suppressor genes in mitotic and meiotic cells. *Mol Cell* 1998;2:317.
10. Gowen LC, Avrutskaya AV, Latour AM, Koller BH, Leadon SA. BRCA1 required for transcription-coupled repair of oxidative DNA damage. *Science* 1998;281:1009.
11. Sharan SK, Morimatsu M, Albrecht U, et al. Embryonic lethality and radiation hypersensitivity mediated by RadS1 in mice lacking Brca2. *Nature* 1997;386:804.
12. Abbott DW, Freeman ML, Holt JT. Double-strand break repair deficiency and radiation sensitivity in BRCA2 mutant cancer cells. *J Natl Cancer Inst* 1998;90:978.
13. Papadopoulos N, Lindblom A. Molecular basis of HNPCC: mutations of MMR genes. *Hum Mutat* 1997;10:89.
14. Eng C. Genetics of Cowden syndrome: through the looking glass of oncology. *Int J Oncol* 1998;12:701.
15. Suzuki A, de la Pompa JL, Stambolic V, et al. High cancer susceptibility and embryonic lethality associated with mutation of the PTEN tumor suppressor gene in mice. *Curr Biol* 1998;8:1169.
16. Stambolic V, Suzuki A, de la Pompa JL, et al. Negative regulation of PKB/Akt-dependent cell survival by the tumor suppressor PTEN. *Cell* 1998;95:29.
17. Datta SR, Dudek H, Tao X, et al. Akt phosphorylation of BAD couples survival signals to the cell-intrinsic death machinery. *Cell* 1997;91:231.
18. Markowitz AM, Wang J, Myeroff L, et al. Inactivation of the type II TGF-β receptor in colon cancer cells with microsatellite instability. *Science* 1995;268:1336.
19. Grady WM, Rajput A, Myeroff L, et al. Mutation of the type II transforming growth factor-β receptor is coincident with the transformation. *Cancer Res* 1998;58:3101.
20. Massague J. TGF-β signal transduction. *Annu Rev Biochem* 1998;67:753.
21. Hahn SA, Schutte M, Hoque ATMS, et al. DPC4, a candidate tumor-suppressor gene at human chromosome 18q21.1. *Science* 1996;271:350.
22. Hata A, Shi Y, Massague J. TGFb signaling and cancer: structural and functional consequences of mutations in Smads. *Mol Med Today* 1998;4:257.
23. Shipp MA, Mauch PM, Harris NY. Non-Hodgkin's lymphomas. In: DeVita VT, Hellman A, Rosenberg SA, eds. *Cancer: principles and practice of oncology*, 5th ed. Philadelphia: Lippincott-Raven, 1997:2165.
24. Mrozek K, Heinonen K, de la Chapelle A, Bloomfield CD. Clinical significance of cytogenetics in acute myeloid leukemia. *Semin Oncol* 1997;24:17.
25. Cortez D, Stoica G, Pierce JH, Pendergast AM. The BCR-ABL tyrosine kinase inhibits apoptosis by activating a Ras-dependent signaling pathway. *Oncogene* 1996;13:2589.
26. Westbrook CA. Molecular subsets and prognostic factors in acute lymphoblastic leukemia. *Leukemia* 1997;11(Suppl 4):S8.
27. Look AT. Oncogenic transcription factors in the human acute leukemias. *Science* 1997;278:1059.
28. Magli MC, Largman C, Lawrence HJ. Effects of HOX homeobox genes in blood cell differentiation. *J Cell Physiol* 1997;173:168.
29. Caligiuri MA, Strout MP, Oberkircher AR, et al. The partial tandem duplication of ALL1 in acute myeloid leukemia with normal cytogenetics or trisomy 11 is restricted to one chromosome. *Proc Natl Acad Sci U S A* 1997;94:3899.
30. Felix CA, Hosler MR, Winick NJ, et al. ALL-1 gene rearrangements in DNA topoisomerase II inhibitor-related leukemia in children. *Blood* 1995;85:3250.
31. Paik S, Bryant J, Park C, et al. erbB-2 and response to doxorubicin in patients with axillary lymph node-positive, hormone receptor-negative breast cancer. *J Natl Cancer Inst* 1998;90:1361.
32. Thor AD, Berry DA, Budman DR, et al. erbB-2, p53, and efficacy of adjuvant therapy in lymph node-positive breast cancer. *J Natl Cancer Inst* 1998;90:1346.
33. Pegram MD, Finn RS, Arzoo K, et al. The effect of HER-2/neu overexpression on chemotherapeutic drug sensitivity in human breast and ovarian cancer cells. *Oncogene* 1997;15:537.
34. Shak S. Overview of the trastuzumab (Herceptin) anti-HER2 monoclonal antibody clinical program in HER2-overexpressing metastatic breast cancer. Herceptin Multinational Investigator Study Group. *Semin Oncol* 1999;26:71.
35. Baselga J, Tripathy D, Mendelsohn J, et al. Phase II study of weekly intravenous recombinant humanized anti-p185HER2 monoclonal antibody in patients with HER2/neu-overexpressing metastatic breast cancer. *J Clin Oncol* 1996;14:737.
36. Slamon D, Leyland-Jones B, Shak S, et al. Addition of Herceptin (humanized antiHER-2 antibody) to first line chemotherapy for HER2 overexpressing metastatic breast cancer markedly increases anticancer activity: a randomized, multinational controlled phase III trial. *Proc Am Soc Clin Oncol* 1998;17;98.
37. Flynn PJ, Miller WJ, Weisdorf DJ, et al. Retinoic acid treatment of acute promyelocytic leukemia: in vitro and in vivo observations. *Blood* 1983;62:1211.
38. Huang ME, Ye YC, Chen SR C, et al. Use of all-transretinoic acid in the treatment of acute promyelocytic leukemia. *Blood* 1988;72:567.
39. Degos L, Chomienne C, Daniel MT, et al. Treatment of first relapse in acute promyelocytic leukemia with all-trans retinoic acid. *Lancet* 1990;336:1440.
40. GenBank release 68, June 1991.
41. Adams MD. Initial assessment of human gene diversity and expression patterns based upon 83 million nucleotides of cDNA sequence. *Nature* 1999;377:3.

42. Murray RW. The Human Genome Project—and beyond. *Analytical Chemistry News and Features* 1999, May 1:292.
43. Genes and justice; the growing impact of the new genetics on the courts. *Judicature* 1999;83, entire issue.
44. Hancock W, Apffel A, Chakel J, et al. Integrated genomic/proteomic analysis. *Analytical Chemistry* 1999;71:743.
45. Alizadeh AA. Distinct types of diffuse large B-cell lymphoma identified by gene expression profiling. *Nature* 2000;403:503.
46. Golub TR, Slonim DK, Tamayo P, et al. Molecular classification of cancer: class discovery and class prediction by gene expression monitoring. *Science* 1999;286:531.
47. DeRisi J, Penland L, Brown PO, et al. Use of a cDNA microarray to analyze gene expression patterns in human cancer. *Nat Genet* 1996;14:457.
48. Perou CM, Jeffrey SS, van de Rijn M, et al. Distinctive gene expression patterns in human mammary epithelial cells and breast cancers. *Proc Natl Acad Sci U S A* 1999;96:9212.
49. Ross DT, Scherf U, Eisen MB, et al. Systematic variation in gene expression patterns in human cancer cell lines. *Nat Genet* 2000;24:227.
50. Emmert-Buck MR, Bonner RF, Smith PD, et al. Laser capture microdissection. *Science* 1996;274:998.
51. Sgroi DC, Teng S, Robinson G, et al. In vivo gene expression profile analysis of human breast cancer progression. *Cancer Res* 1999;59:5656.
52. Kononen J, Bubendorf L, Kallioniemi A, et al. Tissue microarrays for high throughput molecular profiling of tumor specimens. *Nat Med* 1998;4:844.
53. Banks RE, Dunn MJ, Forbes MA, et al. The potential use of laser capture microdissection to selectively obtain distinct populations of cells for proteomic analysis. *Electrophoresis* 1999;20:689.
54. Emmert-Buck MR, Gillespie JW, Paweletz CP, et al. An approach to proteomic analysis of human tumors. *Mol Carcinog* 2000;27:158.
55. Humphery-Smith I, Cordwell SJ, Blackstock WP. Proteome research: complementarity and limitations with respect to the RNA and DNA worlds. *Electrophoresis* 1997;18:1217.
56. Gygi SP, Rist B, Gerber SA, et al. Quantitative analysis of complex protein mixtures using isotope-coded affinity tags. *Nat Biotechnol* 1999;17:994.
57. Page MJ, Amess B, Townsend RR, et al. Proteomic definition of normal human luminal and myoepithelial breast cells purified from reduction mammoplasties. *Proc Natl Acad Sci U S A* 1999;96:12589.
58. Paweletz CP, et al. Rapid protein display profiling of cancer progression directly from human tissue using a protein biochip. *Drug Dev Res* 2000;49:34.

Christopher L. Carpenter
Lewis C. Cantley

CHAPTER 3

Essentials of Signal Transduction

Signal transduction is the chemistry that allows communication at the cellular level. Cells sense signals from both the outside environment and other cells and, in response, they regulate protein expression and function. Protein expression is controlled by rates of transcription, translation, and proteolysis, whereas protein activities are affected by location, covalent modifications, and noncovalent interactions. Signal transduction pathways regulate all aspects of cell function, but most pathways target five primary processes: metabolism, cell division, death, differentiation, and movement.

In single-celled organisms, signal transduction pathways determine chemotaxis, mating, and adaptation to varying food sources. In multicellular organisms, signal transduction pathways are necessary for embryonic development, and they regulate differentiation, division, and death in both the mature and developing organism. Signal transduction pathways also control the particular functions of specialized cells (e.g., synthesis and secretion of insulin by the pancreas, migration and phagocytosis by neutrophils) and the abnormal behavior of diseased cells (e.g., invasion and growth of cancer cells).

To emphasize the essentials of signal transduction, we have focused on the variety of solutions to the two common problems faced by cells and organisms in signal transduction: (1) How is a signal sensed and (2) how are the levels and activities of proteins modified in response to the signal? Most signals are transmitted by ligands and are sensed by the receptors to which they bind. Binding of a ligand to a receptor stimulates the activities of proteins necessary to continue the transmission of the signal. Often, this involves the formation of multiprotein complexes and the generation of small-molecule second messengers. Integration of signals from multiple pathways determines the cell's responses to competing and complementary signals.

THE SENSORY MACHINERY: LIGANDS AND RECEPTORS

SIGNALS

Signal transduction pathways have evolved to respond to an enormous variety of stimuli and to generate an equally extensive number of signals. Molecules that initiate signaling cascades include proteins, peptides, amino acids, lipids, nucleotides, gases, and light (Table 3-1). Most extracellular signals, such as growth factors, bind to receptors on the plasma membrane, but others, such as cortisol, diffuse into the cell and bind to receptors in the cytoplasm and nucleus. Single-celled organisms respond primarily to signals that arise from the environment rather than the organism, but they are capable of generating signals, as illustrated by the mating pathway in yeast.[1] Multicellular organisms respond to diverse signals produced from within. Signals can be a direct reaction to a stimulus, such as the secretion of insulin by pancreatic β cells in response to increases in blood glucose. Signal release can be triggered by the nervous system in response to either external or internal cues, as in the release of epinephrine by the adrenal glands in response to stress. Signals also can be continuous, such as those sent by the extracellular matrix. Usually, signaling molecules are stored in the cell and are released to provide communication with other cells under specific conditions. Some ligands are stored outside the cell (e.g., in the extracellular matrix) and become accessible in response to tissue damage or remodeling. Cells also respond to signals that arise from within. Important examples include the checkpoint pathways that ensure the orderly progression of the cell cycle and the pathways that sense and repair damaged DNA.[2,3] When activated, these pathways lead either to cell-cycle arrest, so the damage can be repaired, or to cell death. Exactly how DNA damage and cell-cycle abnormalities are

TABLE 3-1. Ligands That Stimulate Signal Transduction Pathways

Types of Ligands	*Examples*
PROTEINS	
Soluble	Insulin
Matrix	Fibronectin
Bound to other cells	Ephrins
AMINO ACIDS	Glutamate
NUCLEOTIDES	
Soluble	Adenosine triphosphate
DNA	Double-strand breaks
LIPIDS	Prostaglandins
GASES	Nitric oxide
LIGHT	Rhodopsin, visual system

sensed is not yet known, but many components of the pathways that transmit the signals are understood.

RECEPTORS

Usually, signaling pathways begin with binding of a ligand to a receptor (Table 3-2). Receptors can be located either on the cell surface or intracellularly. Ligands that are on the cell surface or cannot transverse the membrane bind to receptors on the plasma membrane, whereas some ligands (e.g., retinoids or nitric oxide) that are membrane-permeable bind to receptors inside the cell. Usually, cells are exquisitely sensitive to ligand-receptor binding. The affinity of receptors for ligands generally is found to be in the p*M* to n*M* range, and very few receptors have to be occupied to transmit a signal. Many cytokine-responsive cells express only a few hundred receptors on the cell surface. (Signal amplification, which allows signals to propagate to the entire cell, is discussed later in Efficiency and Specificity: Formation of Multiprotein Signaling Complexes.)

Both receptors and ligands are multifunctional. Often, ligands can activate more than one receptor, and receptors can bind more than one ligand. The stimulation of most receptors leads to the activation of several downstream pathways that either function cooperatively to activate a common target or stimulate distinct targets. Generally, some of the pathways activated are counter-regulatory and serve to attenuate the signal.

Binding of ligands to receptors leads to a conformational change in the receptor that initiates signaling or oligomerization (or both). As a result of ligand binding, the intrinsic activity of the receptor or of associated proteins is stimulated. Receptors can have intrinsic enzymatic activity or can associate with protein kinases, guanine nucleotide exchange factors, and transcription factors. The receptor families used by eukaryotic cells in signal transduction illustrate both the diversity of receptor type and how signaling is initiated.

Receptor Tyrosine Kinases

Receptor tyrosine kinases are transmembrane proteins that have an extracellular ligand-binding domain, a transmembrane domain, and a cytoplasmic tyrosine kinase domain.[4] The ligands for these receptors are proteins or peptides. Most receptor tyrosine kinases are monomeric, but the insulin receptor family are heterotetramers in which the subunits are linked by disulfide bonds. Receptor tyrosine kinases have been divided into six classes, primarily on the basis of the sequence of extracytoplasmic domain. Examples of tyrosine kinase receptors include the insulin receptor, platelet-derived growth factor receptor, the epidermal growth factor receptor family, and the fibroblast growth factor receptor family.

Activation of receptor tyrosine kinases requires tyrosine phosphorylation of the receptor. Receptor tyrosine kinases transmit signals both by autophosphorylation of the receptor and by phosphorylation of other substrates. Receptor phosphorylation occurs on multiple sites, some of which stimulate the kinase activity of the receptor and others of which allow binding of downstream-signaling molecules. Ligand-dependent oligomerization of receptors brings the kinase domains into close proximity so that they cross-phosphorylate. Often, this transphosphorylation locks the kinase into a high-activity conformation.

Ligands stimulate receptor oligomerization in a variety of ways (Fig. 3-1). Some ligands, such as platelet-derived growth

TABLE 3-2. Receptors in Signal Transduction

Types of Receptors	*Examples*	*Types of Ligands*
Tyrosine kinase	PDGF, EGF, FGF, insulin	Peptide growth factors
Serine kinase	TGF-β	Activin
Heterotrimeric G protein–coupled	Thrombin, smell receptors	Thrombin
Receptors bound to tyrosine kinases	IL-2, interferon	IL-2
TNF family	Fas receptor	Fas
Notch	Notch	Delta-Serrate-LAG-2
Guanylate cyclase		Atrial natriuretic factor, NO
Tyrosine phosphatase	CD45, LAR	Contactin
Nuclear receptors	Estrogen, prostaglandins	Estrogen
Adhesion receptors	Integrins, CD44	Fibronectin, hyaluronic acid

EGF, epidermal growth factor; FGF, fibroblast growth factor; IL-2, interleukin-2; PDGF, platelet-derived growth factor; TGF-β, transforming growth factor-β; TNF, tumor necrosis factor.

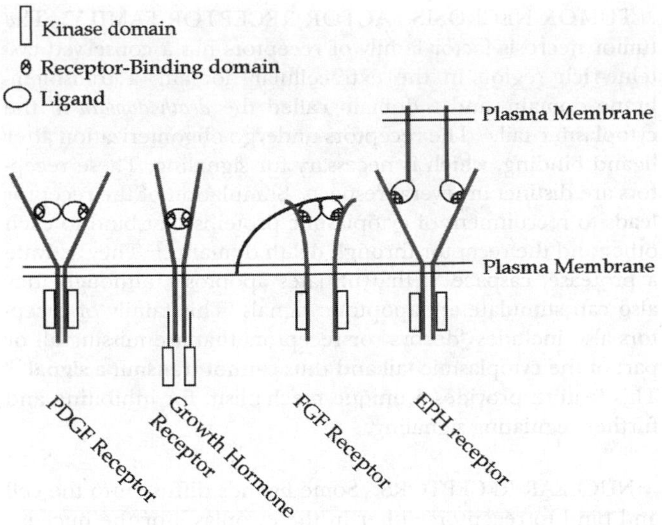

FIGURE 3-1. Dimerization of tyrosine kinase receptors. Most tyrosine kinase receptors are activated by ligand-induced dimerization. Some ligands, such as platelet-derived growth factor (PDGF), are dimeric and induce dimerization using the two receptor-binding domains. Other ligands, such as growth hormone, contain two receptor-binding domains in the same molecule. The fibroblast growth factors (FGF) rely on proteoglycans to aid the formation of ligand dimers. Some ligands, such as the ephrins (EPH), are present on nearby cells and, when the cells come into contact, bind to the receptors and promote clustering.

factor, are dimeric, so that the ligand is able to bind two receptors simultaneously.[5] Other ligands, such as growth hormone, are monomeric but have two receptor-binding sites that allow them to induce receptor dimerization.[6] Fibroblast growth factors (FGF) also are monomeric but have only a single receptor-binding site. FGF molecules bind to heparin sulfate proteoglycans, which promotes dimerization of FGF and the FGF receptor.[7] Epidermal growth factor (EGF) also is monomeric, but it may have a second low-affinity receptor-binding site, or receptor-ligand dimers may bind to a second receptor to allow receptor-receptor interaction and transphosphorylation.[8,9] Ligands not only stimulate receptor-dependent signaling; some ligand-receptor interactions result in signaling by the ligand. Ephrins are ligands for the protein tyrosine kinase EPH receptors. Ephrins are expressed on the surface of adjacent cells, and interaction of EPH receptors and ephrins both activates the tyrosine kinase activity of the receptor and leads to stimulation of signaling by the ligand in the adjacent cell.[10,11] The insulin receptor is an exception to the idea of dimerization leading to activation. The insulin receptor is a heterotetramer before ligand binding, and likely a conformational change brings the cytoplasmic tails in proximity or stimulates kinase activity (or does both).

Studies of the EGF receptor family illustrate some important concepts in signal transduction. The EGF-signaling pathways involve four known receptors (EGF receptor, erbB2, erbB3, and erbB4) and many ligands.[12] EGF can stimulate homodimerization of the EGF receptor but, under certain conditions, heterodimerization with other family members also occurs. The same ligand can activate different signaling pathways, depending on the subgroups of EGF receptor family members expressed in a cell. For example, heparin-binding EGF-like growth factor stimulates mitogenesis but not chemotaxis when it activates the EGF receptor but is both a mitogen and chemotactic factor when it activates Erb4.[13] Recent work also suggests that different ligands binding to the same receptors can activate distinct downstream-signaling pathways.[14] These findings suggest that different ligands may cause distinct conformational changes that lead to the phosphorylation of different sets of tyrosine residues on the receptor and could lead also to phosphorylation of distinct sets of substrates.

RECEPTORS THAT ACTIVATE TYROSINE KINASES. A number of receptors do not have intrinsic enzymatic activity but stimulate associated tyrosine kinases. The cytokine and interferon receptors associate constitutively with members of the Jak family of tyrosine kinases.[15] The kinases appear to be inactive in the absence of ligand but, as happens in receptors with intrinsic tyrosine kinase activity, signaling is initiated by ligand-stimulated heterodimerization of the receptors.[16] Dimerization of the receptors brings the Jak kinases in proximity to each other or to other tyrosine kinases, and transphosphorylation leads to their activation. Downstream signaling is dependent on the active Jak kinases phosphorylating the receptors and other substrates.

SERINE-THREONINE KINASE RECEPTORS. The transforming growth factor-β (TGF-β) family of receptors are serine-threonine kinases.[17] These receptors are transmembrane proteins that have an extracellular ligand-binding domain, a transmembrane domain, and an intracellular serine kinase domain. TGF-β ligands are dimers that lead to oligomerization of type I and type II receptors. The type I and type II receptors are homologous but distinctly regulated. The type II receptors seem to be constitutively active but do not normally phosphorylate substrates, whereas the type I receptors are normally inactive. On ligand-mediated dimerization of the type I and type II receptors, the active type II receptor phosphorylates the type I receptor and converts it to an active kinase. Subsequent signal propagation is dependent on the kinase activity of the type I receptor and the phosphorylation of downstream substrates.

Receptor Phosphotyrosine Phosphatases

Like kinases, receptor protein tyrosine phosphatases (RPTPs) have an extracellular domain, a single transmembrane-spanning domain, and cytoplasmic catalytic domains.[18] The extracellular domains of many receptor tyrosine phosphatases contain fibronectin and immunoglobulin repeats, suggesting that some of these receptors may recognize adhesion molecules as ligands. Several RPTPs are capable of homotypic interaction, but no true ligands are yet known for RPTPs. Most receptor tyrosine phosphatases have two catalytic domains, and both are active in at least some receptors. Both functional and structural evidence suggests that the phosphatase activity of some of these receptors is inhibited by dimerization. Normally, these receptors might be active as tyrosine phosphatases but lose that activity after ligand binding. In this way, constitutive or stimulated tyrosine kinase activity becomes enhanced. Signaling by RPTPs is complicated because they do not always function in opposition to tyrosine kinases. For example, CD45 is necessary for signaling by the B-cell receptor, which also requires tyrosine kinase activity.[19]

G PROTEIN–COUPLED RECEPTORS. G protein–coupled receptors (GPCRs) are by far the most numerous receptors. Of the 19,000 genes in *Caenorhabditis elegans*, approximately 800 (or nearly 5% of the genome) are GPCRs, and nearly 2000 mammalian GPCRs are known.[20,21] The number of GPCRs is so high because they encode the light, smell, and taste receptors, all of which require great diversity. These receptors have seven membrane-spanning domains: The N-terminus, and three of the loops are extracellular, whereas the other three loops and the C-terminus are cytoplasmic. A wide variety of ligands bind GPCRs, including proteins and peptides, lipids, amino acids, and nucleotides. No common binding domain exists for all ligands, and interactions of ligands with GPCRs are fairly distinct.[22] In the case of the thrombin receptor, thrombin cleaves the N-terminus of the receptor, freeing a new N-terminus that self-associates with the ligand pocket, leading to activation. Amines and eicosanoids bind to the transmembrane domains of their GPCRs, whereas peptide ligands bind to both the transmembrane domains and the extracellular loops of their GPCRs. Neurotransmitters and some peptide hormones require the N-terminus for binding and activation.

The receptor appears to be kept in an inactive conformation by intramolecular bonds involving residues in the transmembrane or juxtamembrane regions.[23] In the inactive state, the receptor is bound to a heterotrimeric G protein, which also is inactive. Agonist binding results in a conformational change that activates the guanine nucleotide exchange activity of the receptor. Exchange of guanosine triphosphate (GTP) for guanosine diphosphate (GDP) on the α subunit of heterotrimeric G proteins initiates signaling. Though GPCRs all activate heterotrimeric G proteins, this action ultimately results in the stimulation of other signaling pathways, including protein tyrosine and serine kinases, phospholipases (PLCs A, C, and D) and ion channels.[24] Important recent work has shown that certain GPCRs activate receptor tyrosine kinases. Often, stimulation of GPCRs leads to activation of the EGF receptor, which is necessary for the GPCR to activate the mitogen-activated kinase (MAP kinase) pathway.

NOTCH FAMILY OF RECEPTORS. The Notch receptor has a large extracellular domain, a single transmembrane domain, and a cytoplasmic domain. Ligands for the Notch receptor are proteins expressed on the surface of adjacent cells, and the primary target of notch signaling is activation of the transcription factor SuH in *Drosophila* species or CBF-1 in mammals. Though the mechanisms by which Notch transmits signals have not been worked out definitively, it appears to be fairly different from other receptors.[25] Current evidence suggests that the cytoplasmic domain of the Notch is proteolytically cleaved and translocated to the nucleus, where it interacts directly with transcription factors.

GUANYLATE CYCLASES. Cyclic nucleotides are important second messengers and allosteric regulators of enzyme activities. The synthesis of cAMP by adenylate cyclase is regulated principally by heterotrimeric G proteins, but the synthesis of cGMP is regulated directly by ligands. Plasma membrane guanylate cyclases are receptors for atrial natriuretic hormone, and nitrous oxide binds to soluble guanylate cyclases in the cytoplasm.[26] Both stimuli increase cGMP levels.

TUMOR NECROSIS FACTOR RECEPTOR FAMILY. The tumor necrosis factor family of receptors has a conserved cysteine-rich region in the extracellular domain, a transmembrane domain, and a domain called the *death domain* in the cytoplasmic tail.[27] The receptors undergo oligomerization after ligand binding, which is necessary for signaling. These receptors are distinct in several respects. Stimulation of the receptor leads to recruitment of cytoplasmic proteins that bind to each other and the receptor through death domains.[28] They activate a protease, caspace 8, that initiates apoptosis, although they also can stimulate antiapoptotic signals. This family of receptors also includes "decoys" or receptors that are missing all or part of the cytoplasmic tail and thus cannot transmit a signal.[29] This feature provides a unique mechanism for inhibiting and further regulating signaling.

NUCLEAR RECEPTORS. Some ligands diffuse into the cell and bind to receptors either in the cytoplasm or the nucleus. These ligands include steroids, eicosanoids, retinoids, and thyroid hormone.[30] The receptors for these ligands are transcription factors that have both DNA and ligand-binding domains. The unliganded receptor is bound to heat-shock proteins, from which they release after ligand binding. Release from the chaperone complex and ligand binding allow the DNA-binding domain to contact DNA and the receptors to regulate transcription directly.

ADHESION RECEPTORS. Cell adherence via integrins either to the extracellular matrix or to other cells is mediated by receptors that function mechanically and stimulate intracellular signaling pathways, primarily through tyrosine kinases.[31] Integrins are composed of heterodimers of α and β subunits and bind to an argenine, glycine, aspartate (RGD) motif found in matrix molecules. Activation of integrin signaling involves both binding to ligand and clustering of integrins. Ligand binding can be stimulated also by intracellular signals, presumably by a change in conformation of the integrin. Integrin signaling is necessary for cell movement but, in contrast to many other pathways, adherence provides a continuous signal to cells. This signal appears to be necessary for survival of many cell types. The ability to circumvent the requirement for adherence-dependent survival plays a major role in the development of human cancers by allowing tumor survival in inappropriate locations.

PROPAGATION OF SIGNALS TO THE CELL INTERIOR

Eukaryotic cells use a varied collection of receptors and ligands to initiate cell signaling. Binding of ligands to receptors may stimulate an intrinsic enzymatic activity of the receptor-like protein tyrosine or serine kinases or the guanine nucleotide exchange activity of GPCR. Other receptors do not have intrinsic enzymatic activity, but ligand binding results in activation of downstream enzymes (e.g., proteases by the tumor necrosis factor receptor family or protein tyrosine kinases by the cytokine receptors). Signals are transmitted by all receptors by affecting the function of downstream proteins (Table 3-3). The function of intracellular signaling proteins is regulated by covalent modi-

TABLE 3-3. Enzyme Classes Stimulated by Active Receptors

Enzyme Classes	*Examples*
PROTEIN KINASES	
Tyrosine	Jak
Serine, threonine	ERKs
PROTEIN PHOSPHATASES	
Tyrosine	SHP-2
Serine, threonine	Calcineurin
LIPID KINASES	
Phosphatidylinositol	PI3-kinase
LIPID PHOSPHATASES	
Phosphatidylinositol	SHIP, PTEN
PHOSPHOLIPASES	
A	cPLA2
C	PLC γ
D	—
G PROTEINS	
Heterotrimeric	Gs, Gi
Ras-like	Ras, Rac
NUCLEOTIDE CYCLASES	
Adenylate	—
Guanylate	—

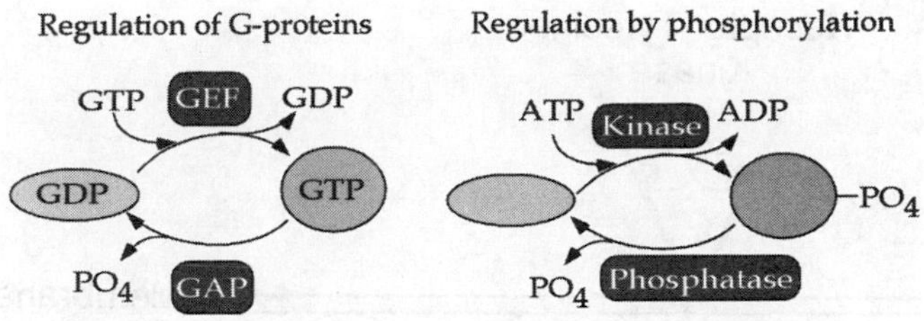

FIGURE 3-2. Regulation of protein activity by phosphate. The activity of many proteins is regulated by phosphate. The exchange of guanosine triphosphate (GTP) for guanosine diphosphate (GDP) bound to G proteins induces an activating conformational change dependent on the additional γ phosphate of GTP. This reaction is catalyzed by guanine nucleotide exchange factors. GTPase-activating proteins (GAP) accelerate the hydrolysis of GTP to GDP to remove the γ phosphate and attenuate G protein signaling. Protein kinases add phosphate to proteins that can result in conformational changes and changes in enzymatic activity. The phosphate can be removed by protein phosphatases to inhibit the signal. Both G proteins and protein kinase substrates undergo a similar cycle of phosphate addition and removal to regulate their activity. ADP, adenosine diphosphate; ATP, adenosine triphosphate; GEF, guanine nucleotide exchange factor.

fications, by noncovalent binding of other proteins and small molecules, and by the level of protein expression.

REGULATION OF PROTEIN KINASES

Proteins undergo many covalent modifications, but phosphorylation is the most common covalent modification involved in the regulation of protein function. Both phosphorylation by kinases and addition of a phosphate moiety in the form of GTP exchange for GDP result in conformational changes that regulate protein activity (Fig. 3-2). Proteolysis is less common in the activation of signaling pathways but is necessary for some pathways (e.g., apoptosis) and also is an important pathway by which signals are attenuated.

The balance between kinase and phosphatase activity controls protein phosphorylation.[32] Protein kinases themselves, transcription factors, and cytoskeletal components are a few examples of proteins regulated by phosphorylation. Most protein kinases in eukaryotic cells are divided into three classes on the basis of residues they phosphorylate: protein tyrosine kinases, protein serine-threonine kinases, and dual-specificity kinases that phosphorylate serine, threonine and tyrosine residues. Important issues in understanding the role and regulation of protein phosphorylation are how specificities of kinases and phosphatases are determined and how phosphorylation alters the function of proteins. Recent work at both the structural and functional levels provides preliminary answers to these questions.

Most signal transduction pathways activate tyrosine kinases, either directly (as in the case of receptor tyrosine kinases) or indirectly. Phosphorylation of proteins on tyrosine can result in either the stimulation or inhibition of enzymatic activity or can provide sites for protein-protein interaction. An example of how tyrosine phosphorylation regulates enzymatic activity is the Src family of protein tyrosine kinases, which are regulated both positively and negatively by tyrosine phosphorylation.[33] Phosphorylation of a tyrosine residue in the C-terminus leads to an intramolecular bond involving this phosphotyrosine and the Src homology 2 (SH2) domain that blocks access of substrate to the catalytic domain. In contrast, phosphorylation of a tyrosine in the T loop of the catalytic domain stimulates the kinase activity by stabilizing the catalytic pocket in an active conformation.

A common theme in the regulation of the activity of both tyrosine and serine-threonine protein kinases is phosphorylation of the T loop as a mechanism of activation. The T loop forms a lip of the catalytic pocket and may occlude the active site, preventing access of the substrate. In the case of the insulin receptor, the unphosphorylated T loop also appears to interfere with adenosine triphosphate (ATP) binding.[34] Crystallographic studies indicate that the T loop is mobile and thus probably is not always in an inhibitory confirmation; hence, a kinase has some constitutive activity. This low level of activity is sufficient to phosphorylate a nearby kinase (e.g., autophosphorylation of a partner in a dimeric receptor). After phosphorylation, the T loop undergoes a conformational change that allows substrate access to the catalytic site.

Once a protein kinase is active, only specific substrates are phosphorylated. This specificity rests on two properties: colocalization of the kinase with the substrate (discussed later in Efficiency and Specificity: Formation of Multiprotein Signaling Complexes) and the presence of sequences in a potential substrate that can be phosphorylated by the kinase. Though protein kinases appear to phosphorylate many substrates *in vitro*, particular motifs have been identified that in some cases govern absolutely whether a protein will be a substrate, such as a proline following a serine or threonine for substrates of MAP kinases.[35,36] In other cases, particular motifs are favored as phosphorylation sites.[37,38] Likely these motifs fit best into the catalytic cleft of the kinase. In some cases, sequences distant from the site of phosphorylation can mediate low-affinity association of a kinase with a substrate and thus can enhance phosphorylation.

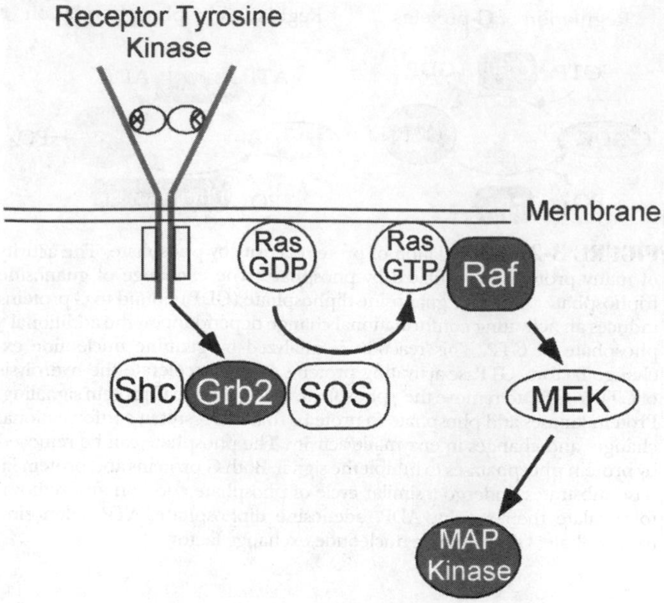

FIGURE 3-3. Activation of the MAP kinase pathway. Many receptors activate the mitogen-activated protein kinases (MAP kinases). Most receptor tyrosine kinases stimulate the activity of the Ras guanine nucleotide exchange factor son of sevenless (SOS), which associates with the linker proteins Shc and Grb2. The activation of Ras by SOS stimulates a protein serine kinase cascade initiated by Raf, which stimulates MEK. MEK then activates the MAP kinases. MAP kinases phosphorylate transcription factors to regulate gene expression. GDP, guanosine diphosphate; GTP, guanosine triphosphate.

Most signaling pathways also activate serine kinases, but a higher level of constitutive phosphorylation of proteins occurs on serine and threonine. Still unclear is how much of this basal phosphorylation is involved in regulation of the activity or location of proteins and how much might be irrelevant. Myriad cellular functions are regulated by serine phosphorylation ranging from the activity of transcription factors and enzymes to the polymerization of actin. Serine kinases themselves are regulated in a variety of ways. Mammalian serine-threonine kinases have been subdivided into 11 subfamilies, on the basis of primary sequence homology, which has been predictive also of related function.[39] Location, phosphorylation, and ligand binding regulate serine kinases. Activation by ligand binding separates some classes of serine protein kinases. For example, cyclic nucleotides (e.g., cAMP) activate the protein kinase A (PKA) superfamily.[40] Calcium and diacylglycerol activate members of the protein kinase C family.[41] The akt family is activated by phosphatidylinositol phosphate products of phosphoinositide 3-kinases (PI3-kinase), which allows phosphoinositide-dependent kinase 1 (PDK1) to phosphorylate the activation, or T loop.[42] Association with cyclins activates the cyclin-dependent kinase family, and the calcium-calmodulin-dependent kinases are activated by calcium.[43,44] Kinase cascades also are important in allowing multiple levels of regulation and amplification of serine kinase activity. For example, MAP kinases are activated by phosphorylation of the T loop after activation of upstream kinases: Activation of Raf leads to phosphorylation and activation of MEK1, which phosphorylates and activates the ERKs (Fig. 3-3).[45]

REGULATION OF PROTEIN PHOSPHATASES

Protein phosphatases remove the phosphate residues from proteins and can either activate or inactivate signaling pathways, depending on the sites that are dephosphorylated. Protein phosphatases can be divided into the same three groups as are the kinases, on the basis of their substrates: tyrosine phosphatases, serine-threonine phosphatases, and dual-specificity phosphatases. Tyrosine phosphatases and dual-specificity phosphatases use a cysteinylphosphate intermediate, whereas the serine-threonine phosphatases are metal-requiring enzymes that dephosphorylate in a single step.[46,47]

Recent structural work has revealed how the activity of some nonreceptor tyrosine phosphatases is regulated. The SHP-2 phosphatase has, in addition to the catalytic domain, two SH2 domains. These domains (discussed in more detail in Domains That Mediate Protein-Protein Binding) mediate binding to other proteins by direct association with phosphorylated tyrosine residues. In the inactive state, the catalytic cleft of SHP-2 is blocked by the N-terminal SH2 domain.[48] Binding of the N-terminal SH2 domain to a phosphotyrosine residue of a target protein induces a conformational change that allows substrate access to the catalytic domain. Tyrosine phosphatases act both to attenuate signals that require tyrosine phosphorylation and to activate pathways inhibited by tyrosine phosphorylation. An example of the negative regulatory function of tyrosine phosphatases is the role of SHP-1 (a homolog of SHP-2) in inhibiting cytokine and B-cell receptor signaling. In contrast, SHP-2 is necessary for cytokine stimulation of cells. On the basis of the ability of phosphatase inhibitors (e.g., vanadate) to activate tyrosine kinase-dependent signaling in the absence of ligands, acute inactivation of specific tyrosine phosphatases may play a more important role than previously appreciated in regulating the balance of tyrosine phosphorylation and dephosphorylation that controls signaling pathways.

Protein phosphatase 1 (PP1), PP2A, PP2B, and PP2C are the major serine-threonine phosphatase activities *in vivo*.[49] Both PP1 and PP2A are composed of catalytic and regulatory subunits. PP1 is involved in regulating many pathways, from glycogen metabolism to the cell cycle. PP2B binds to calmodulin and is regulated by calcium. Phosphorylation of either the regulatory or catalytic subunit regulates the activity of many serine phosphatases. More than 100 PP1 regulatory subunits function to target the catalytic domain to different cellular locations and mediate activation or inhibition. This action provides an example of how a single catalytic activity can perform multiple specific functions as a result of targeting by a regulatory subunit.

GUANOSINE TRIPHOSPHATE–BINDING PROTEINS

Just as covalent modification as a mechanism of protein activity regulation is important, so is noncovalent binding to proteins. A number of small molecules regulate protein function, as does protein-protein interaction. G proteins are the best-studied protein mediators that regulate other proteins.

GTP-binding proteins function as digital switches. They are inactive when bound to GDP, but GTP binding results in a conformational change that allows binding to effector molecules and transmission of a signal (see Fig. 3-2). GTP-binding proteins regulate the same molecules activated by receptors: protein and lipid kinases, phosphatases, and phospholipases. GTP-binding proteins are categorized into two large classes: the heterotrimeric GTP-binding proteins and the Ras-like GTP-binding proteins. Activation of GTP-binding proteins is regulated by guanine nucleotide exchange factors that catalyze the release of GDP and allow GTP to bind to and activate the protein. GTPase-activating proteins (GAPs) accelerate GTP hydrolysis and regulate inactivation of GTP-binding proteins. All GTP-binding proteins have lipid modifications that promote membrane association.

Heterotrimeric GTP-binding proteins have three subunits and are activated by GPCR.[23] In the inactive state, the α, β, and γ subunits are associated as a heterotrimer. In mammalian cells, 20 α subunits, 6 β subunits, and 12 γ subunits are known. The heterotrimeric forms are divided into four classes on the basis of function. Gs stimulates adenylate cyclase, Gi inhibits adenylate cyclase, Gq activates phospholipase C β, and G12 and G13 form a group whose function is not yet known. Activation of GPCR allows them to catalyze GDP/GTP exchange of the α subunit of heterotrimeric G proteins. In response to GTP loading of the α subunit, the α and β/γ subunits dissociate. The β and γ subunits do not dissociate *in vivo*. Both the α subunit and the β/γ complex send signals. The α subunit undergoes a conformational change in response to GTP that allows it to bind to effectors.[50] The β/γ dimer does not undergo a conformational change, but release from the α subunit exposes surfaces that allows it to bind to effectors.[51,52] Both the α and β/γ subunits affect the activity of a wide range of downstream effectors, including ion channels, protein kinases, and phospholipases. Domains termed *regulators of G protein signaling* act as GAPs toward the α subunit and attenuate the signal by catalyzing hydrolysis of GTP to GDP.[53]

Ras-like GTP-binding proteins are monomeric and of lower molecular weight than are the heterotrimeric GTP-binding proteins. Ras-like GTP-binding proteins are classified into five families: the Ras, Rho, Rab, Arf, and Ran families.[54] The Ras and Rho families regulate cell growth, transcription, and the actin cytoskeleton; the Arf family regulates phospholipase D and vesicle trafficking; the Rab family regulates vesicle trafficking; and the Ran family regulates nuclear import.[55–59] Ras-like GTP-binding proteins are activated in a manner similar to that of the α subunit of heterotrimeric G proteins.[60] Exchange of GTP for GDP results in a conformational change that promotes binding to effector molecules.[61] In contrast to heterotrimeric G proteins, nucleotide exchange for Ras-like GTP-binding proteins is not catalyzed by receptors. Specific exchange factors are activated downstream of receptors or in response to specific cellular events. Signals are attenuated by the action of GAPs, analogous to regulators of the G protein–signaling domain-containing proteins that catalyze GTP hydrolysis.

GTP-binding proteins affect the activity of their targets by causing conformational changes and perhaps by serving to localize the target. Recent crystal structures of the catalytic domain of adenylate cyclase bound to G proteins illustrate the conformational change.[62] Gsα binds to the C2a domain of adenylate cyclase, causing rotation of the C1a domain, which likely positions the catalytic residues more favorably for conversion of ATP to cAMP. Though crystal structures of small G proteins bound to portions of their targets also have been solved, the effect on the activity of target molecules as a result of binding has not yet been explained. Studies of the role of Ras in the interaction of Raf suggest that an important role of Ras is localization of Raf to the membrane, but Ras also may help to activate Raf directly.[63]

SMALL-MOLECULE SECOND MESSENGERS

Many small molecules transmit signals by binding noncovalently to protein targets and affecting their function. Many of these molecules are called *second messengers* because they are generated within the cell in response to a first messenger, such as a growth factor, binding to a cell surface receptor. Both the generation and attenuation of small-molecule signals is regulated. Our review of the role of several small molecules in signal transduction pathways is not meant to be comprehensive.

cAMP was the first second messenger discovered.[64] Adenylate cyclase, activated by heterotrimeric G proteins, catalyzes the synthesis of cAMP from ATP.[65] The primary target of cAMP is protein kinase A, and the activation of protein kinase A by cAMP demonstrates how second messengers function.[40] The inactive form of protein kinase A is a tetramer of two catalytic and two regulatory subunits; the regulatory subunit inhibits the activity of the catalytic subunit. The regulatory subunit contains two cAMP-binding sites. Binding of cAMP to the first site causes a conformational change that exposes the second site. Binding of cAMP to the second site causes dissociation of the regulatory and catalytic subunits. The free catalytic subunits are then active.

Many activated receptors stimulate phospholipases C.[66] All three families of phospholipases C (PLC)—β, γ, and δ—are activated by calcium. PLC β is activated by both the α and the β/γ subunits of heterotrimeric G proteins, and PLC γ is activated by tyrosine phosphorylation. The regulation of PLC δ is not as well understood. Phospholipases C cleave PtdIns-4,5-P_2 to produce diacylglycerol and inositol-1,4,5-trisphosphate, resulting in a bipartite signal. Diacylglycerol interacts with the C1 domain of protein kinases C to mediate their membrane localization and activation. Inositol-1,4,5-trisphosphate binds to a calcium channel in the endoplasmic reticulum (ER) and stimulates the release of calcium from intracellular stores.[67] The initial increase in cytoplasmic calcium is followed by an influx of extracellular calcium via capacitive calcium channels at the plasma membrane.[68] Still unclear is how the capacitive calcium channels are activated. In unstimulated cells, cytosolic calcium is much lower than in the extracellular space or ER (100 n*M* versus 1 m*M*), so opening channels in the endoplasmic reticulum or plasma membrane allows calcium to flood into the cytoplasm, temporarily raising the cytoplasmic calcium to micromolar concentrations. Ultimately, calcium returns to basal levels as a result of closing the channels, which increases extracellular transport and pumping calcium into intracellular sites in the ER and mitochondria. Calcium has a multitude of cellular effects, including directly regulating enzymatic activities, ion channels, and transcription. Several calcium-binding domains are known, including the C2 domain and EF hands. Calcium binds directly to enzymes and regulates their activity or it can bind to regulatory subunits, such as calmodulin.

Eicosanoids are ubiquitous signaling molecules that bind to both GPCR and transcription factors. Eicosanoid synthesis occurs in response to a number of stimuli and is an example of rapid cell-to-cell signaling. Unlike most second messengers, eicosanoids produced in one cell can escape that cell and diffuse to nearby cells and either bind to receptors or be metabolized further. Eicosanoid synthesis is regulated by the production of arachidonic acid, which can be produced from diacylglycerol (DAG) via diglyceride lipases or from phospholipids by phospholipases A.[69] Phospholipases A2 cleave the sn-2 acyl group of phospholipids to produce a free fatty acid and a lysophospholipid. The calcium-regulated form of PLA2 shows a preference for substrates containing arachidonic acid. The further metabolism of arachidonic acid results in the synthesis of prostaglandins and leukotrienes.

EFFICIENCY AND SPECIFICITY: FORMATION OF MULTIPROTEIN SIGNALING COMPLEXES

COMPARTMENTATION

The ability of a signal transduction pathway to transmit a signal or to stimulate flux through a pathway is dependent on the probability that a protein finds its target. The likelihood of any two proteins coming into contact is proportional to their concentrations. Recruiting a protein to a specific compartment of a cell allows the local concentration of that protein to be increased markedly, thereby increasing the probability that it will interact with other proteins or small molecules that are recruited to or generated in the same compartment. Colocalization of proteins in a signaling pathway is achieved by recruitment to the same membrane surface or organelle (e.g., plasma membrane versus ER) and ultimately by protein-protein interactions. Conversely, separating proteins or second messengers (or both) into distinct compartments turns off signaling pathways.

The regulation of transport of signaling proteins into the nucleus is important in a number of signal transduction pathways and illustrates the concept of colocalization in the same organelle.[70] Nuclear transport proceeds through nuclear pores that can be transversed by diffusion of proteins of less than 40 kD. Transport of larger molecules requires a nuclear localization signal to which the importin proteins bind. The importins target the protein to the nuclear pore, and the complex is transported into the nucleus. The Ran G protein dissociates the importins from their cargo once they are in the nucleus. Regulated export of proteins from the nucleus is similar to import. A nuclear export signal (NES) is recognized by the protein exportin which then transports the cargo out of the nucleus.

Regulation of nuclear localization of the transcription factor nuclear factor of activated T cells (NFAT), required for its transcriptional activity, is an example of the importance of nuclear localization in signal transduction.[71] In response to T-cell activation and a rise in intracellular calcium, NFAT is dephosphorylated by the calcium-responsive phosphatase calcineurin. Dephosphorylation allows the nuclear localization signal in NFAT to bind to the importins, and NFAT, along with calcineurin, is imported into the nucleus. NFAT also contains a NES, and phosphorylation appears to allow the NES to bind to exportin, resulting in transport to the cytoplasm.

Protein compartmentation can also occur on a smaller scale. Proteins in a signal transduction cascade can exist in a preformed but inactive complex, such as the yeast MAP kinase module composed of the Ste11, Ste7, and MAP kinases bound to the scaffolding protein Ste5.[72] Pheromone signaling activates a G protein, which in turn activates the Ste20 kinase. Ste20 phosphorylates and activates the Ste11, which activates the kinase cascade on Ste5. Once the first kinase in the cascade is activated, the other kinases are phosphorylated quickly and are activated because of their proximity.

A similar scaffolding probably functions in the activation of the Jnk kinase pathway in mammalian cells. The enzymes in the mammalian MAP kinase cascades are homologues of the yeast proteins. A protein originally thought to inhibit Jnk kinase (JIP-1, jnk inhibitory protein) binds to MLK1, MKK7, and Jnk and facilitates the activation of Jnk, presumably by localizing the components in the cascade.[73] Other examples of scaffolding proteins are the A kinase-anchoring proteins.[74] This family of proteins binds the regulatory subunit of protein kinase A and localizes it to such diverse intracellular locations as ion channels, centrosomes, and mitochondria. This activity results in the preferential activation of PKA at specific intracellular locations where the relevant substrates are.

TABLE 3-4. Protein-Protein Interaction Domains and Motifs

Motifs	*Domains That Bind Motif*	*Examples of Proteins That Contain the Domain*
Phosphotyrosine	SH2	Src, PI3-kinase, SHP-2
	PTB	IRS family, SHC
Phosphoserine	WD40	Telomerase, APAF-1, coatamer
	14-3-3	—
	WW	Pin1
	FHA	Rad53
Proline-rich	SH3	Src, PI3-kinase
	WW	YAP, dystrophin
	EVH1	VASP, ENA, WASp
C-terminal sequences	PDZ	ZO-1, lim kinase

DOMAINS THAT MEDIATE PROTEIN-PROTEIN BINDING

Another way in which signal transduction pathways commonly are stimulated is through regulated assembly of protein-protein complexes. Most often, these interactions are mediated by conserved domains found in many signal transduction proteins that recognize phosphorylated tyrosine or serine residues or proline-rich sequences (Table 3-4).

Both SH2 domains and phosphotyrosine-binding (PTB) domains bind to motifs containing phosphorylated tyrosine residues.[75] Tyrosine kinases and phosphatases regulate the formation of complexes involving these domains. Tyrosine kinases themselves can serve as docking sites for other proteins, which is most evident with tyrosine kinase receptors that recruit such proteins as PI3-kinase, p120 Ras GAP, PLC γ, and SHP-2 through SH2 domain-dependent interactions. Tyrosine kinases also phosphorylate other proteins. Tyrosine phosphorylation of the insulin receptor substrate 1 protein by the insulin receptor leads to recruitment of SH2 domain-containing proteins to insulin receptor substrate-1.[76] In addition to mediating protein-protein interactions, binding of SH2 domains to phosphotyrosine residues stimulates the enzymatic activities of such proteins as PI3-kinase and Src kinases.[77,78] In some cases, such as Src kinases, the SH2 domain binds to an intramolecular phosphotyrosine to regulate catalytic activity. Usually, this type of regulation is inhibitory. The crystal structures of several SH2 domains have been determined and reveal a pocket that binds the phosphotyrosine and a groove that determines binding specificity based on the fit of the residues C-terminal (or, in a few cases, N-terminal) to the phosphotyrosine.[79]

PTB domains are functionally analogous to SH2 domains in that they bind phosphotyrosine residues to assemble multiprotein complexes, but they have no sequence or structural similarity to SH2 domains.[80] Thus, they represent an independent evolutionary solution to phosphotyrosine-dependent assembly of protein complexes. A few PTB domains bind to a tyrosine-containing motif in the absence of phosphorylation.

In the last few years, it has become evident that recognition of phosphoserine motifs is also an important means of protein-protein interaction. Forkhead-associated domains, 14-3-3 proteins, and some WD40 and WW domains bind to regions of proteins containing phosphoserine.[81–84] WD40 domains in proteins that are members of the F-box and WD40 repeat family are important in regulating ubiquitination and subsequent proteolysis of proteins, such as the inhibitor of κB (IκB), which regulates the activity of the transcription factor nuclear factor κB (NFκB). 14-3-3 proteins are a family of small proteins whose primary function appears to be binding to phosphoserine motifs. An example of the importance of this interaction is the role of 14-3-3 in regulating the nuclear location of the phosphatase Cdc25 that regulates the cell cycle.[85] Binding of 14-3-3 to phosphorylated Cdc25 leads to its export from the nucleus and a block in the cell cycle.

Src homology 3 (SH3), WW, and ena-vasp homology domains are structurally distinct, but all bind to proline-rich sequences.[86–88] Still not clear is how the interaction of these domains with proline-rich regions in other proteins is regulated. Many proteins that contain SH3 domains also have proline-rich regions that could be involved in intramolecular binding, suggesting that a conformational change in the protein could disrupt intramolecular binding and allow the SH3 domain to interact with other proteins. Similarly, the accessibility of proline-rich regions to SH3 domains may be regulated by conformational changes that expose the proline-rich region or disrupt an intramolecular interaction.

PDZ domains recognize motifs in the C-termini of proteins.[89,90] These domains are found in cytoplasmic proteins, and many contain multiple PDZ domains. PDZ domain–containing proteins often function to aggregate transmembrane proteins, such as the glutamate receptor. Group I PDZ domains bind to a consensus sequence, T/S-X-V/I, where V/I is the C-terminus of the protein.[91] Phosphorylation of the S or T in this motif can disrupt PDZ binding in some cases. For example, phosphorylation of this serine in the β_2-adrenergic receptor was shown to lead to a loss of PDZ domain–mediated binding to EBP50, which regulates endocytic sorting of the receptor.[92]

DOMAINS THAT MEDIATE PROTEIN BINDING TO MEMBRANE LIPIDS

Localization of proteins to membranes greatly limits the space in which proteins can diffuse and increases the probability that enzymes and substrates will contact each other. C1 domains present in protein kinases C (PKC) bind to DAG and thereby recruit PKC to the membrane.[41] Membrane recruitment of PKC is aided also by the C2 domain, which binds to anionic phospholipids in the presence of calcium. This pathway is controlled by DAG production, and the primary source is DAG produced by PLC hydrolysis of PtdIns-4,5-P_2.

Domains homologous to a region in pleckstrin (PH) are present in a number of proteins and bind to phosphoinositides, thereby targeting proteins to the plasma membrane.[93] Both the accessibility of the PH domain and availability of phosphatidylinositol (PtdIns) phosphates likely regulate this interaction. Phosphoinositide kinases regulate the production of phosphoinositides.[94] PtdIns 4-kinases synthesize PtdIns-4-P from PtdIns. Type I phosphatidylinositol phosphate kinases (PIPKs) phosphorylate PtdIns-4-P at the 5 position to make PtdIns-4,5-P_2. PtdIns 3-kinases phosphorylate PtdIns, PtdIns-4-P, and PtdIns-4,5-P_2 at the 3-position of the inositol ring to make PtdIns-3-P, PtdIns-3,4-P_2, and PtdIns-3,4,5-P_3, respectively. Phosphoinositide levels also are regulated by phosphatases. The recessive oncogene PTEN has significant homology to tyrosine phosphatases but recently was shown to remove the phosphate from the 3 position of PtdIns-3,4-5-P_3 and less well from PtdIns-3,4-P_2 and PtdIns-3-P.[95] PTEN thus counteracts PI3-kinase signals, and cells from which PTEN is absent have increased signaling through PI3-kinase-dependent pathways.[96] A family of phosphatases that removes the phosphate from the 5 position of PtdIns-3,4-5-P_3, the SH2 inositol phosphatases, also regulates phosphoinositide signaling pathways.[97]

Some PH domains bind best to PtdIns-4,5-P_2, and others bind best to PtdIns-3,4-P_2 or PtdIns-3,4,5-P_3.[98] Thus, acute production of specific phosphoinositides in a membrane compartment results in the recruitment of proteins containing a PH domain that recognizes the phosphoinositide. Colocalization of a subset of proteins allows them to interact more efficiently. A recent example of the role of PH domains in such a pathway is the activation of akt by PDK1. PDK1 and akt are protein serine-threonine kinases that contain PH domains that bind PtdIns-3,4-P_2 or PtdIns-3,4,5-P_3. Activation of PI3-kinase leads to local synthesis of PtdIns-3,4-P_2 and PtdIns-3,4,5-P_3 recruitment of akt and PDK1 to the same membrane location. This activity facilitates phosphorylation and activation of akt by PDK1.[99] Other domains unrelated to PH domains also bind phosphoinositides. For example, FYVE domains are present in several proteins involved in vesicle trafficking, and they bind to PtdIns-3-P.

Cellular membranes are not uniform and appear to be highly organized. One of the principal structures in the plasma membrane is lipid rafts.[100] They are composed of regions of the membrane that are rich in sphingolipids and cholesterol on the extracellular side of the plasma membrane. The lipid component of the cytoplasmic face of lipid rafts is not known, but some evidence suggests that PtdIns-4,5-P_2 is enriched. Glycophosphatidylinositol-linked proteins, transmembrane proteins, and src family members have been found to localize to lipid rafts. Both the Fcε receptor and the T-cell receptor cluster in lipid rafts, which is necessary for their signaling. The basis of protein recruitment to rafts is not yet known.

REGULATION OF PROTEIN LEVELS: TRANSCRIPTION, TRANSLATION, AND PROTEOLYSIS

In addition to influencing the activity of proteins in the cell, signal transduction pathways also regulate the type and levels of proteins expressed in cells. This sort of regulation is necessary for differentiation and the specific function of distinct cell types. Whether a protein is expressed at all in a cell is regulated at the transcriptional level, whereas transcription, translation, and proteolysis have a role in determining the amount of an expressed protein present in a cell.

Ultimately, many signal transduction pathways regulate gene transcription and, thus, the level and type of proteins expressed in the cell. The magnitude of the effect of a signaling pathway on the transcriptional output of a cell is illustrated by the effects of serum on levels of particular mRNAs in fibroblasts.[101] Of 8600 genes analyzed in this study, more than 500 underwent substantial changes in response to serum stimulation. The ability to transcribe a gene is regulated at many levels, including the structure of chromatin in the region of the gene, modifications of the promoter regions, and the activity of transcription factors and coactivators. Signal transduction pathways regulate histone acetylases and deactylases that determine the accessibility of chromatin to the transcriptional apparatus. Recent work has shown that a number of signals lead to histone hyperacetylation that disrupts the nucleosome to allow transcription. For example, the Rho family small G protein Cdc42 and one of its effectors, Jnk, lead to histone hyperacetylation.[102] Likely these pathways cooperate with the activation of transcription factor to induce transcription.

Signal transduction pathways activate transcription factors by many different means. The binding of ligands to the nuclear receptor family of transcription factors causes dissociation of the receptor from a complex with heat-shock proteins and allows the receptor to bind to DNA. Tyrosine phosphorylation of the STAT family of transcription factors by Jak kinases in response to stimulation of cytokine receptors allows them to dimerize through their SH2 domains and enter the nucleus to bind DNA.[15] TGF-β receptors activate transcription by phosphorylating SMAD proteins on serine residues.[17] Phosphorylation of SMAD proteins promotes heterodimerization with SMAD4 and exposes the DNA-binding domain. Activated SMADs translocate to the nucleus, complex with a protein called *Fast1*, and bind to DNA to regulate transcription.

Activation of transcription factors also can occur much further downstream from the receptor. Stimulation of the transcriptional activity of Elk-1 by EGF requires activation of a Ras exchange factor, which leads to activation of Ras. Active Ras promotes the stimulation of Raf activity. Raf in turn phosphorylates and activates MEK1, which phosphorylates and activates ERK. Active ERK translocates to the nucleus and phosphorylates and stimulates the activity of the transcription factor elk-1.

Translation also is controlled at many levels.[103] The sequence of the RNA can result in stable tertiary structures that bind proteins to regulate location or translation. Often, the ability of these types of RNAs to be translated is regulated by protein kinase cascades. A common target of signal transduction pathways is phosphorylation of initiation factor eIF-4E and availability of eIF-4E. $p70^{S6}$ kinase regulates the translation of specific RNAs containing a 5' terminal oligopyrimidine tract by phosphorylation of thc ribosomal S6 protein.[104] This increases the ability of the ribosome to process such messages.

The levels of proteins also are regulated by proteolysis, which can occur via either the proteosome or the lysosome. Ubiquitination targets proteins to the proteosome.[105] An example of the role of ubiquitination is the regulation of inhibitor of κB (IκB) levels. Phosphorylation of IκB is stimulated by a number of receptor-mediated signaling pathways. This action leads to its dissociation from the transcription factor nuclear factor κB (NFκB) and allows NFκB to enter the nucleus and bind DNA. After phosphorylation, the β transducin repeat–containing protein binds to IκB, recruiting ubiquitin ligase that catalyzes the ubiquitination of IκB and leads to its recognition and degradation by the proteosome.[106]

The second major pathway of protein degradation is the lysosomal pathway, which is important also in signal transduction. An early response to the stimulation of receptors is their internalization into endosomes; some evidence suggests that signaling persists at this location after endocytosis.[107] In the case of receptor tyrosine kinases, ligand-dependent kinase activity is necessary for endocytosis, mediated by clathrin-coated pits. After endocytosis, either receptors may recycle to the plasma membrane or the endosomes may fuse with lysosomes, leading to degradation of the receptor.

REFERENCES

1. Bardwell L, Cook JG, Inouye CJ, Thorner J. Signal propagation and regulation in the mating pheromone response pathway of the yeast *Saccharomyces cerevisiae*. *Dev Biol* 1994;166:363.
2. Skibbens RV, Hieter P. Kinetochores and the checkpoint mechanism that monitors for defects in the chromosome segregation machinery. *Annu Rev Genet* 1998;32:307.
3. Weinert T. DNA damage and checkpoint pathways: molecular anatomy and interactions with repair. *Cell* 1998;94:555.
4. Fantl WJ, Johnson DE, Williams LT. Signaling by receptor tyrosine kinases. *Annu Rev Biochem* 1993;62:453.
5. Fretto LJ, Snape AJ, Tomlinson JE, et al. Mechanism of platelet-derived growth factor (PDGF) AA, AB, and BB binding to alpha and beta PDGF receptor. *J Biol Chem* 1993;268:3625.
6. de Vos AM, Ultsch M, Kossiakoff AA. Human growth hormone and extracellular domain of its receptor: crystal structure of the complex. *Science* 1992;255:306.
7. Spivak-Kroizman T, Lemmon MA, Dikic I, et al. Heparin-induced oligomerization of FGF molecules is responsible for FGF receptor dimerization, activation, and cell proliferation. *Cell* 1994;79:1015.
8. Tzahar E, Pinkas-Kramarski R, Moyer JD, et al. Bivalence of EGF-like ligands drives the ErbB signaling network. *Embo J* 1997;16:4938.
9. Lemmon MA, Bu Z, Ladbury JE, et al. Two EGF molecules contribute additively to stabilization of the EGFR dimer. *Embo J* 1997;16:281.
10. Bruckner K, Pasquale EB, Klein R. Tyrosine phosphorylation of transmembrane ligands for Eph receptors. *Science* 1997;275:1640.
11. Holland SJ, Gale NW, Mbamalu G, et al. Bidirectional signaling through the EPH-family receptor Nuk and its transmembrane ligands. *Nature* 1996;383:722.
12. Hackel PO, Zwick E, Prenzel N, et al. Epidermal growth factor receptors: critical mediators of multiple receptor pathways. *Curr Opin Cell Biol* 1999;11:184.
13. Elenius K, Paul S, Allison G, et al. Activation of HER4 by heparin-binding EGF-like growth factor stimulates chemotaxis but not proliferation. *Embo J* 1997;16:1268.
14. Crovello CS, Lai C, Cantley LC, et al. Differential signaling by the epidermal growth factor-like growth factors neuregulin-1 and neuregulin-2. *J Biol Chem* 1998;273:26954.
15. Leonard WJ, O'Shea JJ. Jaks and STATs: biological implications. *Annu Rev Immunol* 1998;16:293.
16. Moutoussamy S, Kelly PA, Finidori J. Growth-hormone-receptor and cytokine-receptor-family signaling. *Eur J Biochem* 1998;255:1.
17. Massague J. TGF-beta signal transduction. *Annu Rev Biochem* 1998;67:753.
18. Neel BG, Tonks NK. Protein tyrosine phosphatases in signal transduction. *Curr Opin Cell Biol* 1997;9:193.
19. Siminovitch KA, Neel BG. Regulation of B cell signal transduction by SH2-containing protein-tyrosine phosphatases. *Semin Immunol* 1998;10:329.
20. Bockaert J, Pin JP. Molecular tinkering of G protein–coupled receptors: an evolutionary success. *Embo J* 1999;18:1723.
21. The *C. elegans* Sequencing Consortium. Genome sequence of the nematode *C. elegans*: a platform for investigating biology. *Science* 1998;282:2012.
22. Ji TH, Grossmann M, Ji I. G protein–coupled receptors: I. Diversity of receptor-ligand interactions. *J Biol Chem* 1998;273:17299.
23. Hamm HE. The many faces of G protein signaling. *J Biol Chem* 1998;273:669.
24. Hall RA, Premont RT, Lefkowitz RJ. Heptahelical receptor signaling: beyond the G protein paradigm. *J Cell Biol* 1999;145:927.
25. Artavanis-Tsakonas S, Rand MD, Lake RJ. Notch signaling: cell fate control and signal integration in development. *Science* 1999;284:770.
26. Schulz S, Waldman SA. The guanylyl cyclase family of natriuretic peptide receptors. *Vitam Horm* 1999;57:123.
27. Ashkenazi A, Dixit VM. Death receptors: signaling and modulation. *Science* 1998;281:1305.

28. Arch RH, Gedrich RW, Thompson CB. Tumor necrosis factor receptor–associated factors (TRAFs)—a family of adapter proteins that regulates life and death. *Genes Dev* 1998;12:2821.
29. Ashkenazi A, Dixit VM. Apoptosis control by death and decoy receptors. *Curr Opin Cell Biol* 1999;11:255.
30. Kliewer SA, Lehmann JM, Willson TM. Orphan nuclear receptors: shifting endocrinology into reverse. *Science* 1999;284:757.
31. Giancotti FG, Ruoslahti E. Integrin signaling. *Science* 1999;285:1028.
32. Hunter T. Protein kinases and phosphatases: the yin and yang of protein phosphorylation and signaling. *Cell* 1995;80:225.
33. Thomas SM, Brugge JS. Cellular functions regulated by Src family kinases. *Annu Rev Cell Dev Biol* 1997;13:513.
34. Hubbard SR. Crystal structure of the activated insulin receptor tyrosine kinase in complex with peptide substrate and ATP analog. *Embo J* 1997;16:5572.
35. Mukhopadhyay NK, Price DJ, Kyriakis JM, et al. An array of insulin-activated, proline-directed serine/threonine protein kinases phosphorylate the p70 S6 kinase. *J Biol Chem* 1992;267:3325.
36. Vulliet PR, Hall FL, Mitchell JP, et al. Identification of a novel proline-directed serine/threonine protein kinase in rat pheochromocytoma. *J Biol Chem* 1989;264:16292.
37. Songyang Z, Lu KP, Kwon YT, et al. A structural basis for substrate specificities of protein Ser/Thr kinases: primary sequence preference of casein kinases I and II, NIMA, phosphorylase kinase, calmodulin-dependent kinase II, CDK5, and Erk1. *Mol Cell Biol* 1996;16:6486.
38. Kemp BE, Parker MW, Hu S, et al. Substrate and pseudosubstrate interactions with protein kinases: determinants of specificity. *Trends Biochem Sci* 1994;19:440.
39. Hanks SK, Hunter T. Protein kinases 6. The eukaryotic protein kinase superfamily: kinase (catalytic) domain structure and classification. *Faseb J* 1995;9:576.
40. Francis SH, Corbin JD. Cyclic nucleotide-dependent protein kinases: intracellular receptors for cAMP and cGMP action. *Crit Rev Clin Lab Sci* 1999;36:275.
41. Newton AC, Johnson JE. Protein kinase C: a paradigm for regulation of protein function by two membrane-targeting modules. *Biochim Biophys Acta* 1998;1376:155.
42. Alessi DR, James SR, Downes CP, et al. Characterization of a 3-phosphoinositide-dependent protein kinase which phosphorylates and activates protein kinase B alpha. *Curr Biol* 1997;7:261.
43. Roberts JM. Evolving ideas about cyclins. *Cell* 1999;98:129.
44. Soderling TR. The Ca-calmodulin-dependent protein kinase cascade. *Trends Biochem Sci* 1999;24:232.
45. Cobb MH. MAP kinase pathways. *Prog Biophys Mol Biol* 1999;71:479.
46. Barford D. Molecular mechanisms of the protein serine/threonine phosphatases. *Trends Biochem Sci* 1996;21:407.
47. Denu JM, Dixon JE. Protein tyrosine phosphatases: mechanisms of catalysis and regulation. *Curr Opin Chem Biol* 1998;2:633.
48. Hof P, Pluskey S, Dhe-Paganon S, et al. Crystal structure of the tyrosine phosphatase SHP-2. *Cell* 1998;92:441.
49. Barford D, Das AK, Egloff MP. The structure and mechanism of protein phosphatases: insights into catalysis and regulation. *Annu Rev Biophys Biomol Struct* 1998;27:133.
50. Lambright DG, Noel JP, Hamm HE, et al. Structural determinants for activation of the alpha-subunit of a heterotrimeric G protein. *Nature* 1994;369:621.
51. Lambright DG, Sondek J, Bohm A, et al. The 2.0 A crystal structure of a heterotrimeric G protein. *Nature* 1996;379:311.
52. Sondek J, Bohm A, Lambright DG, et al. Crystal structure of a G-protein beta gamma dimer at 2.1A resolution. *Nature* 1996;379:369.
53. Hepler JR. Emerging roles for RGS proteins in cell signaling. *Trends Pharmacol Sci* 1999;20:376.
54. Hall A. Ras-related proteins. *Curr Opin Cell Biol* 1993;5:265.
55. Mackay DJ, Hall A. Rho GTPases. *J Biol Chem* 1998;273:20685.
56. Moore MS. Ran and nuclear transport. *J Biol Chem* 1998;273:22857.
57. Moss J, Vaughan M. Molecules in the ARF orbit. *J Biol Chem* 1998;273:21431.
58. Schimmoller F, Simon I, Pfeffer SR. Rab GTPases, directors of vesicle docking. *J Biol Chem* 1998;273:22161.
59. Vojtek AB, Der CJ. Increasing complexity of the Ras signaling pathway. *J Biol Chem* 1998;273:19925.
60. Boguski MS, McCormick F. Proteins regulating Ras and its relatives. *Nature* 1993;366:643.
61. Schlichting I, Almo SC, Rapp G, et al. Time-resolved X-ray crystallographic study of the conformational change in Ha-Ras p21 protein on GTP hydrolysis. *Nature* 1990;345:309.
62. Simonds WF. G protein regulation of adenylate cyclase. *Trends Pharmacol Sci* 1999;20:66.
63. Campbell SL, Khosravi-Far R, Rossman KL, et al. Increasing complexity of Ras signaling. *Oncogene* 1998;17:1395.
64. Hardman JG, Robison GA, Sutherland EW. Cyclic nucleotides. *Annu Rev Physiol* 1971;33:311.
65. Tesmer JJ, Sprang SR. The structure, catalytic mechanism and regulation of adenylyl cyclase. *Curr Opin Struct Biol* 1998;8:713.
66. Rhee SG, Bae YS. Regulation of phosphoinositide-specific phospholipase C isozymes. *J Biol Chem* 1997;272:15045.
67. Dawson AP. Calcium signaling: how do IP3 receptors work? *Curr Biol* 1997;7:R544.
68. Putney JW Jr. "Kissin' cousins": intimate plasma membrane-ER interactions underlie capacitative calcium entry. *Cell* 1999;99:5.
69. Balsinde J, Balboa MA, Insel PA, et al. Regulation and inhibition of phospholipase A2. *Annu Rev Pharmacol Toxicol* 1999;39:175.
70. Kaffman A, O'Shea EK. Regulation of nuclear localization: a key to the door. *Annu Rev Cell Dev Biol* 1999;15:291.
71. Rao A, Luo C, Hogan PG. Transcription factors of the NFAT family: regulation and function. *Annu Rev Immunol* 1997;15:707.
72. Garrington TP, Johnson GL. Organization and regulation of mitogen-activated protein kinase signaling pathways. *Curr Opin Cell Biol* 1999;11:211.
73. Yasuda J, Whitmarsh AJ, Cavanagh J, et al. The JIP group of mitogen-activated protein kinase scaffold proteins. *Mol Cell Biol* 1999;19:7245.
74. Schillace RV, Scott JD. Organization of kinases, phosphatases, and receptor signaling complexes. *J Clin Invest* 1999;103:761.
75. Pawson T, Scott JD. Signaling through scaffold, anchoring, and adaptor proteins. *Science* 1997;278:2075.
76. White MF. The IRS-signaling system: a network of docking proteins that mediate insulin action. *Mol Cell Biochem* 1998;182:3.
77. Carpenter CL, Auger KR, Chanudhuri M, et al. Phosphoinositide 3-kinase is activated by phosphopeptides that bind to the SH2 domains of the 85-kDa subunit. *J Biol Chem* 1993;268:9478.
78. Liu X, Brodeur SR, Gish G, et al. Regulation of c-Src tyrosine kinase activity by the Src SH2 domain. *Oncogene* 1993;8:1119.
79. Waksman G, Shoelson SE, Pant N, et al. Binding of a high affinity phosphotyrosyl peptide to the Src SH2 domain: crystal structures of the complexed and peptide-free forms. *Cell* 1993;72:779.
80. Zhou MM, Ravichandran KS, Olejniczak EF, et al. Structure and ligand recognition of the phosphotyrosine binding domain of Shc. *Nature* 1995;378:584.
81. Yaffe MB, Cantley LC. Signal transduction. Grabbing phosphoproteins. *Nature* 1999;402:30.
82. Durocher D, Henckel J, Fersht AR, et al. The FHA domain is a modular phosphopeptide recognition motif. *Mol Cell* 1999;4:387.
83. Hart M, Concordet JP, Lassot I, et al. The F-box protein beta-TrCP associates with phosphorylated beta-catenin and regulates its activity in the cell. *Curr Biol* 1999;9:207.
84. Muslin AJ, Tanner JW, Allen PM, et al. Interaction of 14-3-3 with signaling proteins is mediated by the recognition of phosphoserine. *Cell* 1996;84:889.
85. Zeng Y, Forbes KC, Wu Z, et al. Replication checkpoint requires phosphorylation of the phosphatase Cdc25 by Cds1 or Chk1. *Nature* 1998;395:507.
86. Niebuhr K, Ebel F, Frank R, et al. A novel proline-rich motif present in ActA of *Listeria monocytogenes* and cytoskeletal proteins is the ligand for the EVH1 domain, a protein module present in the Ena/VASP family. *Embo J* 1997;16:5433.
87. Ren R, Mayer BJ, Cicchetti P, et al. Identification of a ten-amino acid proline-rich SH3 binding site. *Science* 1993;259:1157.
88. Sudol M, Chen HI, Bougeret C, et al. Characterization of a novel protein-binding module—the WW domain. *FEBS Lett* 1995;369:67.
89. Kim E, Niethammer M, Rothschild A, et al. Clustering of Shaker-type K+ channels by interaction with a family of membrane-associated guanylate kinases. *Nature* 1995;378:85.
90. Kornau HC, Schenker LT, Kennedy MB, et al. Domain interaction between NMDA receptor subunits and the postsynaptic density protein PSD-95. *Science* 1995;269:1737.
91. Songyang Z, Fanning AS, Fu C, et al. Recognition of unique carboxyl-terminal motifs by distinct PDZ domains. *Science* 1997;275:73.
92. Cao TT, Deacon HW, Reczek D, et al. A kinase-regulated PDZ-domain interaction controls endocytic sorting of the beta2-adrenergic receptor. *Nature* 1999;401:286.
93. Rebecchi MJ, Scarlata S. Pleckstrin homology domains: a common fold with diverse functions. *Annu Rev Biophys Biomol Struct* 1998;27:503.
94. Fruman DA, Meyers RE, Cantley LC. Phosphoinositide kinases. *Annu Rev Biochem* 1998;67:481.
95. Maehama T, Dixon JE. The tumor suppressor, PTEN/MMAC1, dephosphorylates the lipid second messenger, phosphatidylinositol 3,4,5-trisphosphate. *J Biol Chem* 1998;273:13375.
96. Stambolic V, Suzuki A, de la Pompa JL, et al. Negative regulation of PKB/Akt-dependent cell survival by the tumor suppressor PTEN. *Cell* 1998;95:29.
97. Huber M, Helgason CD, Damen JE, et al. The role of SHIP in growth factor induced signaling. *Prog Biophys Mol Biol* 1999;71:423.
98. Rameh LE, Arvidsson A, Carraway KL 3rd, et al. A comparative analysis of the phosphoinositide binding specificity of pleckstrin homology domains. *J Biol Chem* 1997;272:22059.
99. Cohen P. The Croonian Lecture 1998. Identification of a protein kinase cascade of major importance in insulin signal transduction. *Philos Trans R Soc Lond B Biol Sci* 1999;354:485.
100. Brown DA, London E. Functions of lipid rafts in biological membranes. *Annu Rev Cell Dev Biol* 1998;14:111.
101. Iyer VR, Eisen MB, Ross DT, et al. The transcriptional program in the response of human fibroblasts to serum. *Science* 1999;283:83.
102. Alberts AS, Geneste O, Treisman R. Activation of SRF-regulated chromosomal templates by Rho-family GTPases requires a signal that also induces H4 hyperacetylation. *Cell* 1998;92:475.
103. Gray NK, Wickens M. Control of translation initiation in animals. *Annu Rev Cell Dev Biol* 1998;14:399.
104. Dufner A, Thomas G. Ribosomal S6 kinase signaling and the control of translation. *Exp Cell Res* 1999;253:100.
105. DeMartino GN, Slaughter CA. The proteasome, a novel protease regulated by multiple mechanisms. *J Biol Chem* 1999;274:22123.
106. Wu C, Ghosh S. Beta-TrCP mediates the signal-induced ubiquitination of Ikb. *J Biol Chem* 1999;274:29591.
107. Fiore PP, Gill GN. Endocytosis and mitogenic signaling. *Curr Opin Cell Biol* 1999;11:483.

Nicholas P. Restifo
John R. Wunderlich

CHAPTER 4

Essentials of Immunology

Potentially harmful challenges to the body include viruses, bacteria, unicellular and multicellular pathogens, and cancer cells. In response to these challenges, the body has evolved active defenses that compose the immune system. While the immune system is composed of a wide range of distinct cell types, lymphocytes play a central role by providing the specificity of immune recognition. Through its various appendages, the immune system is capable of interacting, directly or indirectly, with nearly every cell in the body.

There is a central division in the immune system between the humoral branch, which is largely composed of B lymphocytes and their products, and the cellular branch, many functions of which are performed by T lymphocytes. The humoral (from the Latin word *umor* meaning "fluid") branch of the immune system is involved with the production of antibodies that are capable of neutralizing or destroying harmful challenges to the body. Immune functions classically regarded as cellular immune responses include delayed-type hypersensitivity[1] and rejection of foreign grafts[2] or tumors.[3] As techniques for isolating and identifying cells associated with immune responses developed, it became clear that T cells, or thymus-derived lymphocytes, are the cells essential for cellular immune responses. Thus, understanding the principles of cellular immunity has largely come to mean understanding the development, function, and regulation of T cells.

There are fundamental differences in the ways that the cellular and humoral immune systems recognize antigens (Table 4-1). B cells can recognize antigens not presented in the context of other molecules. T cells, on the other hand, generally recognize antigens in the context of a "self" (major) histocompatibility complex (MHC) molecule on the surface of a cell. T cells use structures on their surfaces called *T-cell receptors* (TCRs) to recognize antigen-MHC molecule complexes; B cells use immunoglobulin (Ig) molecules to react specifically to antigenic stimuli. Whereas Ig is secreted, sometimes in extremely large quantities, few, if any, TCRs are shed by T cells. Underlying the difference in the molecules used for recognition is an important difference in the types of antigens recognized: While B cells can recognize antigen in its native conformation, T cells generally recognize antigen that has been "processed" by another cell and then presented on the surface of the cell by MHC molecules. More specifically, antigen is denatured, cleaved within the cell, and transported into specific subcellular compartments where it is bound by MHC molecules. After a complex of antigen and MHC completes its journey to the cell surface, it is potentially recognizable by a T cell.

We use *antigen* in this chapter for a substance that binds specifically to the combining site of an antibody or a TCR. Some of these substances elicit immune responses (immunogens), whereas others do not. There are exceptions to this terminology, such as *superantigens*, which are discussed later in the section Stimulation of T-Cell Receptors by Superantigens. Also, T cells commonly recognize MHC-peptide complexes, but both the peptide and its parent protein often are termed *antigens* in the literature.

T CELLS AND CELLULAR IMMUNITY

T lymphocytes were first identified as a functional subset of lymphocytes, the development of which depends on the existence of a thymus.[4–6] In conditions of congenital absence of the thymus or following neonatal thymectomy in animal models, a number of immune responses were found to be impaired, including cell-mediated killing and transplantation reactions such as graft-versus-host disease and allograft rejection. Subse-

TABLE 4-1. Toward a Molecular Understanding of Immune Recognition of Antigen

	Humoral	*Cellular*[a]
Recognizing cell	B lymphocyte	T lymphocyte
Recognizing molecule	Immunoglobulin	T-cell receptor
Self-molecules required?	No	Yes
Chemical identity of antigen	Protein, nucleic acid, polysaccharide, other	Protein
Phase of antigen	Fluid or solid	Solid
State of antigen	Native or denatured	"Processed"

[a]Various exceptions are presented in the text.

quent to this functional definition of T lymphocytes, differentiation antigens on T cells were identified using antibodies. The ability to identify T cells and thus to isolate T cells and their subsets, and the ability to grow these cells selectively in culture, has resulted in a body of experimental evidence concerning the mechanisms of maturation, activation, and effector function of this population.

Early experiments showed that the growth of a syngeneic tumor in a mouse could be prevented by prior immunization with that same tumor.[7–11] Since then, the mechanisms involved in the antitumor immune response have been partially elucidated,[12,13] and T cells have been shown to play a critical role.[14–16] Guided by results from animal model studies, human T cells have been shown to be capable of specifically lysing autologous tumor cells *in vitro*.[17,18] T cells can also specifically secrete cytokines, such as interleukin-2 (IL-2), interferon-γ (IFN-γ), granulocyte-macrophage colony-stimulating factor (GM-CSF), and tumor necrosis factor-α (TNF-α), and proliferate in response to stimulation with autologous tumor cells.[19,20] Antitumor T cells can be grown to large numbers *in vitro* and transferred adoptively to treat even substantial tumor burdens in both humans and mice.[21] Finally, tumor antigens recognized by autologous human T cells have been identified by the use of molecular cloning techniques.[22–26] Taken together, these findings provide nearly incontrovertible evidence that a T-cell immune response can occur against an autologous tumor.

ANTIGEN PRESENTATION TO T CELLS

The relative importance of how antigens are recognized by T cells (i.e., what T cells "see") to the biologic therapy of cancer is linked largely to the establishment of new immunotherapies based on T cells. These new therapies have ushered in an entirely new set of challenges having to do with how T cells recognize, or may fail to recognize, tumor antigens.

T-cell responses were found by early investigators to be controlled by the presence of particular genes encoded in the MHC. Polymorphisms at this genetic region were observed to control the ability of an animal to mount a T-cell response. Early attempts to demonstrate direct binding of antigen to T cells failed, while attempts succeeded in the case of B cells. Although a straightforward and still useful model of the recognition of antigen by humoral factors was promulgated before the 1900s, it took nearly another hundred years for a similar event to occur for T cells.

T cells express on their cell surfaces molecules of exquisite sensitivity, very much like the antibody molecules found on the surfaces of B cells. These molecules, called *TCRs*, recognize peptide fragments of antigens, called *epitopes*, that are noncovalently complexed with MHC molecules. The two major types of MHC molecules, class I and class II, are integral membrane glycoproteins that are noncovalently complexed with antigenic peptides. Class I molecules present antigenic peptides to CD8+ lymphocytes; class II molecules perform the same function for CD4+ lymphocytes. CD8+ effector cells sometimes are termed *cytotoxic T lymphocytes* (CTLs), because they can lyse target cells directly through the release of lytic granules as well as through triggering "death" receptors, such as Fas, on target cells. CD4+ T cells, while also capable of cytotoxic activity in some cases, are called *helper T cells*, because they enhance antibody responses by activating B cells, promote other T-cell responses, and activate other important cells in the immune system, such as dendritic cells and macrophages.

A model of how the two major types of T lymphocytes may interact with target cells is depicted in Figure 4-1. A CD8+ T cell is shown interacting directly with a tumor cell, while a CD4+ T cell is shown interacting with an antigen-presenting cell (APC) express-

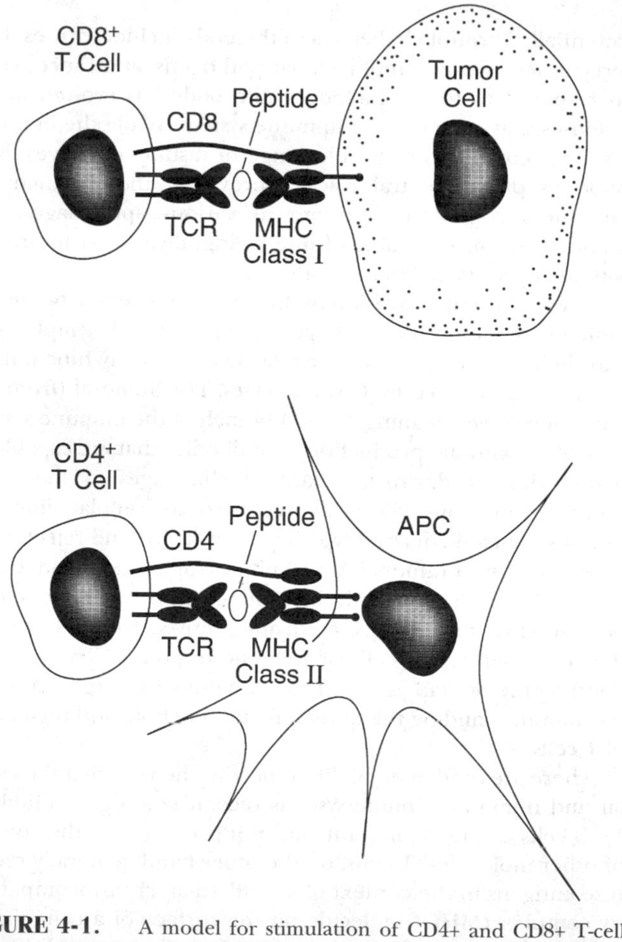

FIGURE 4-1. A model for stimulation of CD4+ and CD8+ T-cell antitumor immunity, based on CD8+ T cells interacting with tumor cells and CD4+ T cells interacting with host antigen-presenting cells (APCs). MHC, major histocompatibility complex; TCR, T-cell receptor.

ing class II molecules. While class I molecules are found on most tumor cells and somatic cells, class II molecules are found in high concentrations on only a subset of tumor cells and on B-cell, bone marrow–derived phagocytic cells (e.g., macrophages), Langerhans'-dendritic cells, follicular dendritic cells and, in lesser quantities, on other cells including subpopulations of thymocytes, activated peripheral T cells, and certain epithelial cells.

MAJOR HISTOCOMPATIBILITY COMPLEX MOLECULES AS ANTIGEN RECEPTORS

A molecular understanding of the structure of MHC molecules has made clear their function with respect to antigen recognition by T cells: MHC molecules are *receptors* for peptide antigens.[27–29] The major locations, or loci, for class I genes are named *A, B,* and *C* in the human and *K, D,* and *L* in the mouse (Fig. 4-2). Class II molecules originate from three major subregions in the human, designated *DP, DQ,* and *DR,* and two in the mouse designated *I-A* and *I-E.* MHC molecules from these major subregions are codominantly expressed. The extent of MHC polymorphism present in the gene pool usually results in heterozygosity for most individuals at every major class I and class II locus. Because there are three different major class I loci and three different major class II loci in the human, most individuals express six different class I alleles and six different class II alleles. Codominant expression in a single individual of MHC molecules originating from multiple loci enhances that individual's ability to present a variety of antigens.

MHC class I molecules can also act as inhibitors of lysis by natural killer (NK) cells and at least some T cells, a function described later in this chapter in the section Natural Killer Cells and in recent reviews.[30,31]

Structure of Major Histocompatibility Complex Molecules

X-ray crystallographic data have indicated that MHC molecules have peptide-binding domains consisting of a deep groove that runs between two long α helices found on the outward-facing surface of the MHC molecule.[27,28,32] X-ray crystallographic findings have since been refined and extended to include x-ray images of particular peptides lying in the clefts of MHC molecules in an extended conformation.[33–40] An ever-clearer crystallographic picture of the interaction of the TCR with the peptide-MHC complex has become available with the solution of the diffraction pattern of this trimolecular structure.[41,42]

While the general architecture of the peptide-binding grooves of MHC class I and class II molecules are almost identical, critical differences fundamentally change the way peptides are bound. Class I molecules bind shorter peptides of defined lengths (generally 8 to 10 residues), whereas class II molecules bind peptides that appear to be arbitrary in length (often 12 to 20 amino acids, but occasionally longer). In fact, class II molecules often bind a core motif of an antigen that can extend in either direction by different lengths (also referred to as *nested sets* of peptides). The binding cleft of class I molecules is closed at both ends, enabling the molecule to make hydrogen bonds with the bound peptides at both the N-terminal and C-terminal. Class II molecules, on the other hand, have a peptide-binding cleft that is open on both ends. In both the class I and class II molecules, peptides are bound by pockets in the binding site.

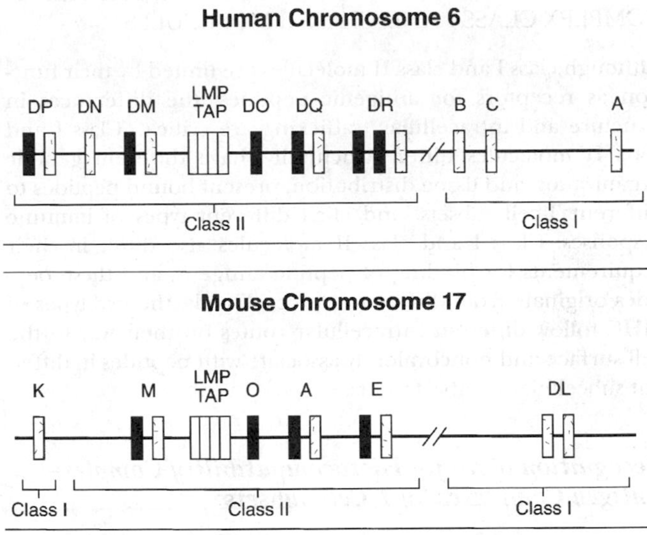

FIGURE 4-2. Highly schematic map of the genomic arrangement of the major histocompatibility complex in humans and mice. For simplicity, class Ib genes and the class III regions are not shown.

The affinity of the TCR for the peptide-MHC complex is far weaker than that of most antibody-antigen interactions, a property consistent with an important role for other antigen-independent T-cell surface receptors acting as cofactors in the triggering process.[43,44] TCR-peptide-MHC complex interactions have low affinities and rapid off-rates, thus allowing for a rapid scanning-type interaction.[45,46]

Polymorphism of Major Histocompatibility Complex Molecules

Sequence studies indicate that MHC class I and class II molecules are among the most highly polymorphic molecules in the genome. The polymorphism of MHC molecules is concentrated in the peptide-binding grooves.[47,48] Specifically, the polymorphism of MHC molecules is concentrated in the pockets along grooves of MHC molecules where amino acid side chains fit into the molecule. The polymorphisms form the molecular basis for the preference of different MHC alleles for different peptide sequence motifs, and they enable each MHC molecule to bind a different set of peptides. It has been demonstrated that MHC polymorphism causes differences in levels of human resistance to specific infections and ensures that, within a species, a broad ability to bind peptides derived from a pathogenic challenge exists.[49,50]

MHC diversity is, of course, what makes the job of the transplantation surgeon so difficult and must be taken into account by the cancer immunotherapist. For example, tyrosinase, which is a tumor antigen associated with normal melanocytes and with melanoma cells, has an epitope that is presented to lytic CD8+ T lymphocytes in the context of the human leukocyte antigen HLA-A24.[51] Use of this peptide in a patient not expressing this class I molecule is likely to be ineffective, because that particular peptide would be unlikely to bind efficiently to other class I alleles and because the appropriate presenting molecule would not be found in that patient.

DIFFERENCES BETWEEN MAJOR HISTOCOMPATIBILITY COMPLEX CLASS I AND CLASS II MOLECULES

Although class I and class II molecules are united by their function as receptors for antigenic peptides, the differences in structure and intracellular trafficking are critical. Class I and class II molecules differ structurally, have different genetic organization and tissue distribution, present bound peptides to different T-cell subsets, and elicit different types of immune responses. Class I and class II molecules also differ in their requirements for binding of peptide antigens, and these peptides originate from different sources. Finally, the two types of MHC follow different intracellular routes on their way to the cell surface and noncovalently associate with peptides in different subcellular compartments.

Recognition of Major Histocompatibility Complex–Antigen Complexes by T-Cell Subsets

There are many interactions involved in T-cell activation, but the specificity of T-cell recognition of a cognate partner cell occurs via the interaction of the TCR with an MHC molecule to which is bound a peptide. The TCR, which is a heterodimer associated on the cell surface with the CD3 complex,[52] is discussed in greater detail later, under Antigen-Specific T-cell Receptors. Although no clear structural or sequence differences between TCRs' detecting class I and detecting class II molecules have been found, a clear difference between the two sets of T cells is found in the ligands for the cell surface markers CD4 and CD8, from which the T-cell sets derive their names. CD8 molecules bind to the α_3 domain of the class I molecules on the target cell,[53–55] and CD4 molecules bind to the β_2 domain of the class II heterodimer on the target cell.[56–59]

Some peptide-MHC complexes, designated *antigenic*, trigger a T-cell response that can consist of proliferation, up-regulation of surface molecules, activation of lytic machinery, secretion of cytokines, or even death by apoptosis. The minimum number of MHC molecules that must be occupied by a particular peptide to activate a very responsive T cell is thought to be extremely low: on the order of 0.03% of the total MHC or fewer than several hundred peptide-MHC complexes.[60,61]

Sources of Antigens Bound by Major Histocompatibility Complex Class I and Class II Molecules

Antigens complexed with MHC class I and class II molecules originate from two different sources (Fig. 4-3). Class I molecules generally present antigens derived from intracellular sources, whereas class II molecules usually present antigens derived from extracellular sources, although clear examples exist that contradict this distinction, especially in "professional" APCs.[62] A more precise understanding of the difference in the sources of antigens can result from an understanding of patterns of intracellular trafficking of these two sets of molecules: Class II molecules intersect endocytosed antigen, whereas class I molecules efficiently bind to intracellular antigens in the endoplasmic reticulum.[63,64] Thus, antigens or antigenic fragments intersecting with the endoplasmic reticulum can be presented by class I molecules; those that intersect with the endosomal subcellular compartment can be presented by class II molecules.

As a result of the differences in the cell biology of MHC molecules, peptides binding to class I molecules are derived mainly from intracellular-cytosolic proteins such as histones and stress proteins, whereas class II peptides are derived primarily from membrane glycoproteins or serum proteins known to enter the acidic vacuolar compartment in large quantities.[65,66] Naturally processed peptides bound to class I molecules are of a very specific size (8 to 10 amino acids) and are smaller than those bound to class II molecules (12 to 20 amino acids), which are much more variable and often nested.[65,66] These peptides bind to MHC molecules with affinities that can range from the picomolar to micromolar range. Despite a restricted length of peptides presented by MHC class II molecules and the even more restricted length of those presented by class I, a tremendous amount of specificity can still occur. (Note that it is possible to make at least 5×10^{11} different peptides of nine amino acids.)

It is now possible to forecast which epitopes within a protein will bind to particular MHC molecules. Allele-specific epitope forecasting has now been done with a large number of human and murine MHC molecules,[67–71] which are characterized by strong preferences for particular amino acid side chains at some positions in the bound peptides and a wide tolerance for amino acid side chains at other positions. Although the anchor positions are critically important in the prediction of which peptides will bind to particular MHC molecules, the amino acid side chains at other positions can play a role and cannot be disregarded.[72]

MAJOR HISTOCOMPATIBILITY COMPLEX CLASS I PATHWAY FOR ANTIGEN PROCESSING

CD8+ T lymphocytes are able to monitor the contents of cells by interacting with class I molecules, presenting a display of peptides carried from the endoplasmic reticulum (ER) to the cell surface.[73–75] Antigen processing is generally necessary for the expression of class I molecules at the cell surface, because class I α chains do not efficiently exit the ER in large quantities unless they are fully assembled with peptide and β_2-microglobulin. Furthermore, they need to bind a peptide to be thermodynamically stable. "Empty" class I molecules appear to be unstable at 37°C but somewhat more stable at lower temperatures.[76] Such empty class I molecules are short-lived and subject to proteolysis but nevertheless are expressed at relatively low levels by certain cells, especially those deficient in antigen processing. Because most nucleated cells express stable class I molecules on their cell surfaces, antigen processing is probably a universal characteristic of normal cells. Thus, the molecules involved in the processing of antigen are likely to be expressed ubiquitously as well.

Structure of Major Histocompatibility Complex Class I Molecules

Class I molecules are heterodimers composed of an extremely polymorphic 45-kD α chain and β_2-microglobulin. Class I molecules are considered by some to be true heterotrimers, as a peptide eight to ten amino acids long having a molecular weight of approximately 1 kD is required for stability and proper expression. Highly schematic structures of class I and class II molecules are shown in Figure 4-4. A bound peptide is presented by the class I molecule.

The α chains of class I molecules (also called *heavy chains*) are encoded in the genome in an eight-exon form. The first

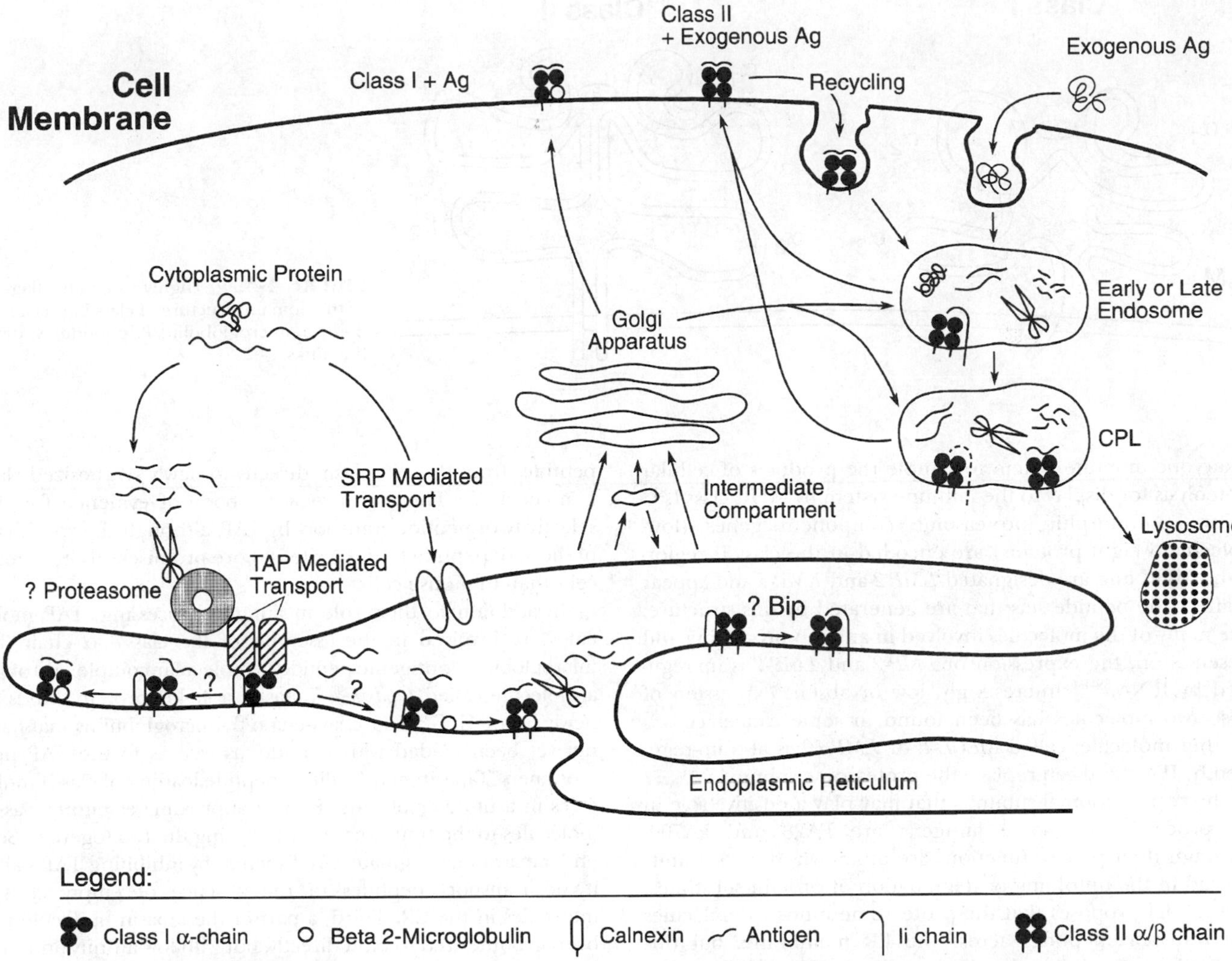

FIGURE 4-3. Intracellular trafficking pathways in the presentation of endogenous and exogenous antigen (Ag). CPL, compartment for peptide loading; SRP, signal recognition particle; TAP, transporter associated with antigen processing.

exon encodes a signal peptide or leader sequence that directs insertion of the rest of the nascent class I molecule into the ER during translation. The next three exons encode the three large extracellular domains (see Fig. 4-4). The α_1 and α_2 domains are directly involved in the binding of peptides. The α_3 domain (exon 4) contains the nonpolymorphic region that is the ligand for the CD8 molecule and shares close homology with the constant region of Igs. Note that β_2-microglobulin also shares structural homology with the Ig constant regions. Exon five encodes a 25–amino acid transmembrane region that forms a hydrophobic α helix that anchors class I into the cell membrane. A short intracytoplasmic segment (30 amino acids long encoded by exons 6, 7, and 8) is involved in the intracellular trafficking of class I molecules and contains regions that interact with the cytoskeleton as well as residues that can be phosphorylated by cyclic adenosine monophosphate–dependent protein kinase A and pp60 src kinase.

β_2-microglobulin is a structural component of the MHC class I molecule presented on the cell surface and plays an indispensable role in the proper folding of the 45-kD class I α chain. The β_2-microglobulin molecule is noncovalently associated with the α chain. Its gene is not encoded within the MHC and has minimal polymorphism, even among mammalian species. A number of human cell lines, including melanomas, renal cell cancers, and a cell line named *Daudi,* express virtually no class I on their cell surfaces as a result of absent or mutated β_2-microglobulin.[77,78] Thus, in these cell lines, the class I α chain molecules do not fold properly, never leave the ER, and are degraded rapidly. β_2-microglobulin-deficient mice have been found to express little, if any, functional class I antigen and have no mature CD8+ T cells.[79]

Origin and Generation of Peptides: The Proteasome

The task of generating peptide fragments from intracellular proteins for presentation by class I molecules is achieved, in part, by a molecular complex known as the *proteasome.*[80] This bulky complex has a remarkable ring-like appearance when visualized through the electron microscope and is composed of at least 16 subunits. Highly conserved through evolution, the proteasome is thought to be involved in the protein economy of cells. This primitive structure was likely adapted by the

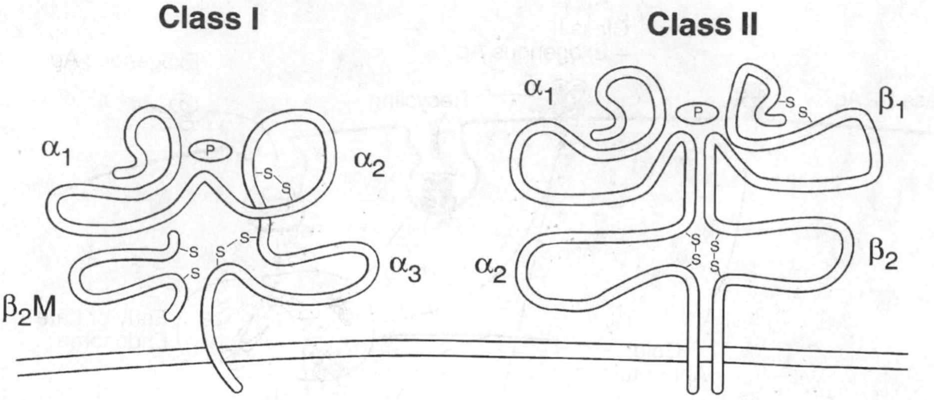

FIGURE 4-4. Highly schematic diagram of the domain structure of class I and class II. β_2-M, β_2-microglobulin; P, peptide; S, disulfide links.

eukaryotic immune system to sample the products of cellular proteolysis for display to the immune system by MHC class I.[81]

Two polymorphic proteasome component genes (low-molecular-weight proteins) are encoded in the class II region of the MHC and are designated *LMP-2* and *LMP-7* and appear to affect the peptide sets that are generated by this structure. Like many of the molecules involved in antigen processing and presentation, the expression of *LMP-2* and *LMP-7* is up-regulated by IFN-γ.[82–84] Interestingly, low or absent expression of these two molecules has been found in some cancer cells.[85] Another molecule, called *MECL-1*, or *LMP-10*, is also up-regulated by IFN-γ and can replace the proteasome subunit Z.[86]

Other proteasomal subunits that may play a positive role in the processing of some antigens are PA28 and PA700. Although their precise functions are unknown, these subunits may aid in the unfolding or degradation of protein substrates. One model proposes that the proteasome binds to molecules that transport peptides across the ER membrane, but this mechanism remains to be demonstrated. IFN-γ changes the proteolytic activity of proteasomes, perhaps to favor the production of peptides capable of binding to MHC class I.[87]

Many cytosolic proteins, the peptide fragments of which eventually find their way onto MHC class I molecules, are first ubiquitinated. Ubiquitin, a protein so named because it seemed to exist everywhere inside the cell at the same time, is attached to proteins that have been targeted for degradation. This attachment is covalent and is mediated by a clustered triad of enzymes called *E1*, *E2*, and *E3*. Ubiquitinated proteins generally are proteolytically degraded by the proteasome.[88]

Translocation of Peptides by TAP and the Role of Tapasin

Once peptide fragments are generated in the cytosol, they must be transported into the ER, a task largely carried out by another product of the MHC region, the transporter associated with antigen processing, called *TAP*. The genes encoding TAP are located in the MHC class II region in both the human and mouse genomes and are interdigitated with the genes encoding the two LMP components of the proteasome. The TAP heterodimer is an adenosine triphosphate–dependent peptide pump, is a member of the ABC (ATP-binding cassette) superfamily of transmembrane transporters, and is related to the products of the multidrug resistance gene.[89–93] TAP transfers peptides from the cytoplasm directly to newly synthesized class I molecules.[94] There is a growing body of evidence for the selectivity of peptide transport by TAP, although the specificity of the TAP peptide-binding site is more promiscuous in human cells than in mouse cells.

In addition to their role in antigen processing, TAP molecules are involved in the assembly of the class I α chain/β_2-microglobulin/antigenic peptide trimolecular complex through a molecule called *tapasin*.[95] Tapasin, a 48-kD protein, binds to newly born MHC class I heavy-chain β_2-microglobulins that have not yet been loaded with peptide, as well as to the TAP heterodimers. Tapasin may facilitate peptide loading of class I molecules in a number of ways. First, it approximates empty class I molecules to the transporters by tethering the two together. Second, tapasin may regulate TAP function by inhibiting TAP's ability to transport peptides in the absence of empty class I molecules in the ER. Third, a part of the tapasin molecule has been hypothesized to bind directly, but with low affinity and with a fast off-rate, to the peptide-binding cleft of the class I heavy chain. This interaction might be similar to the way the peptide-binding grooves of "empty" MHC class II molecules are occupied by a piece of the invariant chain known as *CLIP* [described later in the section Role of Invariant Chain (Ii) in the Folding, Trafficking, and Protection of Class II]. ER-60 is part of the late assembly complexes consisting of MHC class I, tapasin, TAP, calreticulin, and calnexin.

Classical class I molecules assemble in the ER with peptides mostly generated from cytosolic proteins by the proteasome. The activity of the proteasome can be modulated by a variety of accessory protein complexes. A subset of the proteasome β subunits (LMP-2, LMP-7, and MECL-1) and one of the accessory complexes, PA28, are up-regulated by IFN-γ and affect the generation of peptides to promote more efficient antigen recognition. The peptides are translocated into the ER by TAP. A transient complex containing a class I heavy-chain β_2-microglobulin dimer is assembled onto the TAP molecule by successive interactions with the ER chaperones calnexin and calreticulin and a specialized molecule, tapasin. Peptide binding releases the class I β_2-microglobulin dimer for transport to the cell surface, while lack of binding results in proteasome-mediated degradation. The products of certain nonclassical MHC-linked class I genes bind peptides in a similar way. A homologous set of β_2-microglobulin-associated membrane glycoproteins, the CD1 molecules, appears to bind lipid-based ligands within the endocytic pathway.

Chaperones in the Class I Pathway

Although the class I pathway generally presents peptides of cytoplasmic origin, exogenous antigens that are chaperoned by a heat-shock protein (HSP) can gain access to the class I processing pathway of certain cells, such as particular subsets of macrophages.[96,97] HSPs derived from tumor cells may be useful in stimulating antitumor CTLs *in vitro*.[98,99] Furthermore, inoculation of purified HSPs derived from tumor cells can induce protective immune responses against subsequent tumor challenge in experimental animal systems.[100]

Chaperone proteins are involved in the folding of nascent or incompletely folded proteins and are thought to aid proteins in gaining their proper conformation. Two important chaperones that help glycoproteins in the ER to fold are calnexin and calreticulin. Immature class I molecules have been shown to associate transiently with an 88-kD protein called *calnexin*.[101] Calnexin (also called *P88* or *IP90*) probably is involved in the folding of class I molecules. Association of class I α chains with β_2-microglobulin and peptide is likely to cause dissociation of the chaperone molecules.[102] In addition to its possible functions in protein folding, calnexin may be considered a quality-control molecule, because it prevents unfolded, misfolded, or incompletely assembled α chain molecules from exiting the ER.[101,103–107] Calnexin plays a similar role for other proteins, among them such immunologically important proteins as MHC class II[108–110] and the α/β chains of the T-cell receptor, which do not leave the ER until they are fully assembled with the CD3 complex. *Calreticulin*, another ER-resident molecule, is a lectin-like chaperone that may replace calnexin after the MHC class I heavy chain binds with β_2-microglobulin.[111] Calreticulin clearly differs from calnexin in the way that it associates with class I. Another molecule known to associate with immature Ig molecules, called *BiP*, also may associate with a subset of class I molecules or may associate with class I molecules in some not-yet-understood sequence with calnexin.

Role of Interferon-γ

There is genetic evidence for the related functions of many of the various molecules described in the class I pathway: TAP and proteasome component molecules appear to be very closely associated with the MHC region encoding class I α chains and class II on chromosome 17 in the mouse or chromosome 6 in the human. Many of these groups of molecules appear to be regulated in concert, with IFN-γ as the conductor. Molecules known to be up-regulated by IFN-γ include at least two, but probably three, proteasome component and regulatory molecules,[112] the peptide transporters, class I heavy chain, and β_2-microglobulin. Note also that some HSPs also are inducible with IFN-γ.[113] Thus, these groups of molecules appear to share regulatory elements that allow them to be regulated in concert.

Nonclassical Major Histocompatibility Complex and Non-Major Histocompatibility Complex–Encoded Class I Molecules

Nonclassical MHC molecules often are labeled as *MHC class Ib molecules* in the literature. It is now clear that this group of molecules includes members that are not encoded with the MHC region of the genome. As a group, nonclassical MHC molecules generally are expressed at low levels. They are characterized by limited polymorphism, in stark contrast to MHC class I or class II molecules, which are among the most polymorphic genes to be described. Here, we summarize only briefly some examples of nonclassical MHC molecules. A number of excellent reviews of the topic have recently been published.[114–116]

One important class Ib molecule is designated *HLA-E*. Its homologue in the mouse is likely to be *Qa-1*. These molecules have limited sequence polymorphism and are expressed on many different tissues. An important function appears to be modulation of NK-cell activity through binding with NK cell surface CD94/NKG2A (inhibition) or CD94/NKG2C (activation).[117]

HLA-G molecules are expressed by the placenta at the maternal-fetal interface. Mice appear to lack any homologue. Although HLA-G is nonpolymorphic, it behaves in many ways like classical class I molecules in that its loading in the ER is TAP-dependent and it binds to β_2-microglobulin. HLA-G binds to peripheral blood myelomonocytic cells.[118] Like HLA-E, it may contribute to the inhibition of NK cells.[119]

Two other MHC class Ib molecules warrant mention. The first is the mouse *H2-M3* molecule, which appears to have a specialized capacity to bind to N-formylated peptides. Formylated peptides are characteristic of some peptides derived from microorganisms, as well as from "self" mitochondrial proteins. Finally, *CD1* is a molecule encoded outside the MHC that is capable of interacting with both αβ and γδ T cells.[120] CD1 appears to be able to bind and present hydrophobic lipid- and lipoglycan-containing molecules.[121,122] At least two different forms of CD1 exist—CD1a and CD1b—which exhibit different intracellular trafficking patterns and some differences in function.[123,124]

MAJOR HISTOCOMPATIBILITY COMPLEX CLASS II PATHWAY FOR ANTIGEN PROCESSING

The ability of a cell to process antigens via the class II pathway (see Fig. 4-3) is more specialized than the almost ubiquitous ability of nucleated cells to process antigen via the class I pathway. Class II–producing cells include macrophages, dendritic cells, Langerhans cells, and B lymphocytes. These cells not only bear class II heterodimers but also possess the invariant chain monomer, the requisite enzymatic machinery, an important subcellular compartment, and molecules called *HLA-DM*, whose essential function in the class II pathway was discovered more recently. As in the class I system, the interaction of class II–peptide complexes with T cells can now be studied with class II tetramers.[125]

Structure and Assembly of Major Histocompatibility Complex Class II Molecules

The class II molecule is very similar to the class I molecule in its general shape, but it is composed of an α chain of 34 kD and a β chain of 28 kD, both of which are integral membrane glycoproteins (see Fig. 4-4 for a highly schematic representation). α and β chains have transmembrane regions as well as short intracytoplasmic regions. The α_1 and β_1 domains of the class II molecule correspond to the α_1 and α_2 domains of the class I molecule and thus are directly involved in the binding of the presented peptide. The α_2 domain of class II corresponds with the β_2-microglobulin light chain of class I. Finally, the β_2 domain of class II corresponds with the α_3 domain of class I and is involved in the binding of CD4.

Newly synthesized MHC class II molecules assemble in the ER. Three α/β dimers assemble together with an invariant chain trimer to form a nine-chain structure.[126] Such a conglomeration is thought to stabilize these molecules during their transport through the Golgi apparatus and into the endosomal system (sometimes via the cell surface), where they intersect with peptides in a specialized subcellular compartment called the *compartment for peptide loading (CPL)* by some workers.

Compartment for Peptide Loading

The peptides ultimately presented by class II are derived from protein molecules that generally are acquired from outside the cell (i.e., exogenous) by endocytic vesicles. These vesicles change in composition as they move away from the periphery of the cell toward the nucleus, become acidified, and acquire high concentrations of proteolytic enzymes. Pharmacologic agents, such as chloroquine, that disrupt intracellular pH gradients inhibit antigen processing. Furthermore, mutant cell lines, defective in endosomal acidification, diminish antigen-processing abilities. In B cells, surface-bound Ig molecules may be involved in the acquisition of antigens for presentation. Protein molecules to be presented by the class II pathway are processed by denaturation and proteolysis to short linear segments, some of which fit into the antigen-binding groove of class II molecules. These peptides play a role in determining the structure of class II heterodimers.

A unique endosome-related subcellular compartment has been identified in specialized APCs that naturally express class II. Class II molecules are loaded with antigen in this specialized compartment known as the *CPL*.[127–130] Morphologically, CPLs are somewhat heterogeneous in structure. They are spherical or tubular and contain internal membrane vesicles or infoldings, covered with class II α/β. These infoldings presumably increase the surface area for class II and help optimize exposure to potentially antigenic peptides. The invariant chain, Ii, likely targets the class II α/β/Ii complex to the CPL, probably by a dileucine motif in the cytoplasmic tail of the Ii.[127] Because the FcRII-B2 receptor also contains a dileucine motif, such a motif could be implicated in the specific delivery of antigen complexed with antibody to the CPL.

Role of Invariant Chain (Ii) in the Folding, Trafficking, and Protection of Class II

Class II heterodimers associate with the Ii in the ER soon after synthesis. Dissociation occurs before expression on the cell surface (see Fig. 4-3). The invariant chain (Ii) has a single transmembrane domain and an amino-terminal cytoplasmic tail. It is coded for on human chromosome 5 and mouse chromosome 18, and it therefore is not genetically linked with the MHC. Human Ii has been found in at least four forms: p33, p35, p41, and p43. These variations result from combinations of alternative splicing and alternative points of the initiation of translation; their different functions are incompletely understood.[131]

Ii is known to have at least three important functions. First, it facilitates the folding of class II molecules in a chaperone-like fashion. Second, a specialized portion of the Ii called *CLIP* binds to and protects the peptide-binding site from binding by peptides before the designated physiologic site, the CPL.[132] Finally, the cytoplasmic tail of Ii contains an endosomal targeting sequence that directs cellular routing of associated class II heterodimers.

Facilitating Peptide Loading with HLA-DM

Efficient processing of extracellularly derived protein antigens for presentation on class II molecules does not occur in the absence of HLA-DM. The human and the murine (designated *H-2M*) versions of this molecule are heterodimers, the counterparts of which are called *DMA* and *DMB* in the human and *H-2DMa* and *H-2DMb* in the mouse.[133]

These molecules are similar in structure to classical MHC class II molecules, but they are functionally distinct. They do not present peptide antigens to CD4+ lymphocytes but instead reside in the CPL. HLA-DM is likely to induce the dissociation of a nested set of Ii-derived peptides (CLIP) from MHC class II α/β dimers and facilitates peptide loading.[134] This is likely to be a direct enzyme-like interaction that is optimized at an acidic pH.

ANTIGEN PROCESSING AND PRESENTATION IN MALIGNANCY

Most cells in the body express class I peptide complexes, which are the ligands for the TCR on CD8+ T cells. Some tumor cells clearly present antigenic peptides in the context of class I, because specific recognition of tumor cells by cytolytic CD8+ T cells results in their destruction *in vitro* and *in vivo.* Tumor cells that fail to process or present antigen recognizable by T cells may enjoy a selective advantage, because they are not susceptible to antigen-specific T cells.[135]

Tumor cells escape antigen-specific T-cell recognition by a number of mechanisms. For example, some tumor cells derived from epithelium express either greatly reduced or absent levels of class I molecules on their surfaces. These histologies include embryonal carcinomas, choriocarcinomas, cervical carcinomas, mammary carcinomas, small cell carcinomas of the lung, neuroblastomas, some colorectal carcinomas, and some melanomas. Other tumors, including melanoma and renal cell carcinoma, have been shown to loose β_2-microglobulin.[77,78] Other tumors can down-regulate the expression of particular class I loci,[136] or loose the genes for particular class I α chains.[137] Still other tumors, including small cell carcinoma of the lung, can down-regulate the proteasome component molecules LMP-2 and LMP-7 and TAP1 and TAP2.[85]

SPECIALIZED ANTIGEN-PRESENTING CELLS

How are antigens, and tumor antigens in particular, presented to the immune system *in vivo*? Although most tumor cells express class I molecules and some tumor cells express class II molecules, they generally do not express an important set of products called *costimulatory molecules* (discussed in detail in the next section, Dendritic Cells), which are believed to be critical for the activation of many T cells resting from prior stimulation and for the activation of all naive T cells. Naive T cells are those that have not been stimulated by antigen outside the thymus. Specialized cells designated as *accessory cells* can help lymphocytes to respond to antigens. These cells include, first and foremost, dendritic cells (DCs), but they also include mononuclear phagocytes (monocytes and macrophages), activated B lymphocytes, and follicular dendritic cells (FDCs). They are distinguished functionally from the vast majority of somatic cells that can present antigens in the context of MHC only for recognition as target cells by effector T cells. Antigen stimulation by "professional" APCs, exemplified by activated DCs, can stimulate responses not only by resting T cells but also by naive T cells.

DENDRITIC CELLS

DCs were so named because of their distinctive cell shapes. They continually extend and retract processes that are reminiscent of dendrites in neural tissue. These processes presumably increase the DCs' surface area and its ability to sample surrounding tissues. DCs can be differentiated from macrophages by their lack of Fc receptors and their poor endocytic capacity. While macrophages are persistently adherent to plastic *ex vivo,* DCs are transiently adherent. They abundantly express MHC class II molecules as well as a number of costimulatory molecules.[138,139]

DCs are far more potent initiators of T-cell–dependent immune responses than any other APC that has been tested.[140] They have a remarkably high density of both class I and class II molecules on their surfaces,[141] which are loaded with processed antigen acquired in large part from exogenous sources.[142] DCs are of hematopoietic origin, but they lack B, T, and NK markers, and no specific or unique differentiation antigen has been found on their surfaces. They can be derived from mononuclear phagocytes under the influence of immunomodulatory molecules *in vivo.*[143] DCs express large quantities of the costimulatory molecules B7-1/CD80 and B7-2/CD86 as well as other T-cell–activating ligands, including intracellular adhesion molecule-1/CD54 (ICAM-1/CD54). They are likely to play an important role in the activation of antitumor T cells *in vivo.*

DCs are mobile, traveling from the epidermis to the afferent lymphatics as part of a process of maturation. They can be found in peripheral blood or in bone marrow, but in extremely low numbers, and generally are isolated from spleen or blood by a combination of their buoyant density and their adhesive properties. Although dendritic cells are a rare fraction of the total leukocyte population, they can present antigens efficiently for several days after activation. They acquire this antigen through a process called *cross-priming* or *cross-presentation* in which T-cell responses are activated, by DCs, to cellular antigens that originate outside of the DCs.[144–146] DCs can be activated by a number of stimuli including lipopolysaccharide (LPS), the interaction of CD40 and CD40 ligand, and double-stranded RNA.[147–149]

FOLLICULAR DENDRITIC CELLS

FDCs differ from the DCs in many ways. FDCs are likely to be stromal or fibroblast in origin and, unlike DCs, are not from bone marrow stem cells. Although their name may be confusing, suggesting some relationship to DCs, FDCs are, in fact, functionally unrelated to DCs. Their role in the activation of antitumor responses is unclear, but they may have an immunologic role in the activation of B lymphocytes.

B LYMPHOCYTES

B cells can concentrate antigen using membrane-bound Ig. Activated B cells can also express large quantities of the costimulatory molecules B7-1 and B7-2. Finally, B cells clearly present exogenous antigens to CD4+ T cells via their class II molecules, and this is a mechanism for B-cell stimulation of antigen-specific T-cell help.

MONOCYTES AND MACROPHAGES

Mononuclear phagocytes consist mainly of macrophages and monocytes. Monocytes are more differentiated and have more endocytic activity than do macrophages. Macrophages are found in virtually all tissues, especially surrounding blood vessels and near epithelial cells. They generally have what is called a *stellar* morphology. Once they are differentiated, monocytes and macrophages do not divide under normal circumstances. Macrophages in different tissues have different morphologies and different functions. For example, liver macrophages (generally designated *Kupffer cells*) are located in the sinusoids. The Kupffer cells are the major cellular system responsible for the clearance of particulate material or microbes from the circulation. Kupffer cells play a central role in the acute-phase response, releasing IL-1, IL-6, and TNF on phagocytosing bacteria and their products. Macrophages in the peritoneum are a heterogeneous group of cells and can be microbicidal and tumoricidal. Alveolar macrophages efficiently remove particulate materials from the alveolar spaces. They also secrete proteases and bactericidal molecules. Macrophages in bone (osteoclasts) are specialized multinucleated giant cells that are involved in bone resorption and turnover.

Immunologically, macrophages participate as APCs. They can express high quantities of adhesion molecules and, importantly, they express on their surfaces the costimulatory molecules in the B7 family. As noted later, macrophages can participate as major effector cells in antitumor responses and in resisting infectious agents. Finally, macrophages can serve to dampen the immune response by secreting inhibitory cytokines such as IL-10; transforming growth factor-β1 (TGF-β1), -β2, and -β3; and an IL-1 receptor antagonist. They also ameliorate the cellular immune response by promoting connective tissue repair via such factors as fibroblast growth factor.

T-CELL RECOGNITION OF ANTIGENS

Immune activities of T cells commonly are stimulated after they bind to certain types of other cells. The activities are not stimulated simply because of the binding, however. A variety of receptor-ligand interactions occur between the two cell surfaces that initiate T-cell activation. One of these interactions, that between TCRs and MHC-antigen complexes on the opposing cell surface, is critical for normal antigen-specific activation of most T cells.

ANTIGEN-SPECIFIC T-CELL RECEPTOR

Like other cells, T cells express a wide array of cell surface receptors for different ligands. However, that which is distinctively designated *T-cell receptor* reacts with specific antigens, albeit generally only after proper processing and presentation by MHC on a target cell surface. The TCR consists of two paired proteins that form a transmembrane, nonsecreted heterodimer unique for each clone of T cells and determining the antigen specificity of the TCR.[150] Two types of TCR have been identified, the αβ heterodimer and the γδ heterodimer. The crystal structures, determined for four TCRs complexed with peptide-MHC class I and for one TCR complexed with peptide-MHC class II, demonstrate the structural basis for a TCR recognizing both peptide and MHC.[151,152] In addition, recently developed, soluble, fluorescent peptide-MHC complexes permit identification of individual T cells with a particular antigen specificity, including human tumor antigens.[153–155]

T-Cell Receptor Genetics

TCR genetics provide the primary source of TCR diversity and antigen specificity. The α, β, γ, and δ genes encode the TCR by rearrangement from their germline configuration, as do Ig heavy- and light-chain antibody genes. Families of TCR variable (V) genes exist for each receptor chain. During T-cell differentiation, one of the V genes rearranges its position among other gene segments by connecting with one of several alternative joining (J) genes, as a result of losing intervening DNA. A diversity (D) gene between the V and J genes is represented in some but not all classes of chains. This rearranged V(D)J segment encodes the variable region of each TCR chain. After combination with a constant (C) gene, generation of RNA, and RNA splicing to remove unused intervening sequences between V(D)J and C regions, the final protein chain is expressed.

The extracellular, amino-terminal portion of the molecule contains the antigen-binding variable segment, whereas the carboxyl-terminal portion contains the constant region. In contrast to antibodies, the constant region of the T-cell receptor does not contain different subregions that relate to differences in function, such as binding complement or binding to receptors on the surfaces of other cells. The major functions of the constant region appear to be to provide membrane attachment for the TCR and to participate in signal transduction.

The overall diversity in each TCR chain is the result of independent selection of any one of the multiple variable V, D, and J segments and of the combinatorial diversity inherent in the large number of permutations among these choices. Different possible αβ or γδ pairings also contribute to the TCR diversity. Both molecular and serologic probes allow the determination of specific V-, D-, and J-region usage for the antigen receptor chains of a given TCR. Although somatic mutation does not appear to be a source of diversity in TCRs, non–germline-encoded (N) regions at the junctional sites between V-, D-, and J-encoded segments add to overall receptor diversity.

T-Cell Receptor Structure

Through a process of differentiation, a mature receptor-bearing T cell will express either an αβ or a γδ heterodimeric TCR. Nearly all T cells that have been characterized as recognizing specific antigens in an MHC-restricted fashion express αβ receptors.[150] On the cell surface, α and β chains, each approximately 40 to 45 kD in molecular weight, are disulfide-linked. Each mature T cell expresses only one β chain gene, because productive rearrangement of a TCR β gene prevents subsequent full rearrangements of other β genes (allelic exclusion), with rare exceptions.[156,157] The TCR α gene is not subject to allelic exclusion, and T cells have the potential to express two different α chain genes, one from each allele.[158] Most individual T cells, however, appear to be limited to the functional expression of antigen receptors with the same α chains.[159]

A high frequency of T-cell clones react not only with the foreign antigens that stimulated their response but also with allo-MHC determinants.[160] This dual reactivity may represent cross-reactivity of a single TCR with different antigens, which would maintain the rule of one cell, one receptor. Nevertheless, the possibility of significant numbers of T cells expressing two TCR αβ receptors has not been excluded.[161,162]

The second class of T cells are those expressing γδ heterodimers in place of αβ heterodimers.[150,163–165] The γ and δ chains are also the products of rearranged genes. The family of V-region genes in the germline is smaller than that for α and β chains; however, additional mechanisms of diversification exist that expand the mature TCR γδ repertoire. Antigen processing and presentation commonly are not needed, and the antigen specificity mediated by γδ receptors is predominantly MHC-unrestricted. Indeed, many TCR γδ receptors may recognize intact proteins in their native configuration, as Igs do, rather than as MHC-restricted peptides. TCR γδ receptors are not much involved in most of the classical T-cell responses; however, they appear to serve important roles in the immune system. They can react with a variety of different antigens, particularly certain HSPs and phosphate-containing nonpeptidic bacterial antigens that have been highly conserved during evolution. TCR γδ cells are in the epithelia of the skin, lung, female reproductive tract, and intestine, where they may contribute to an early line of host defense.

T-Cell Receptor CD3 Complex

Expression of TCRs at the cell surface and also triggering of T cells after the cross-linking of TCRs through binding with antigen depend on the close but noncovalent association of TCRs with the CD3 complex, which consists of several invariant proteins.[166] Cytoplasmic portions of this complex are critical to TCR-initiated signal transduction, and particular extracellular portions provide serologic markers commonly used to define mature T cells with anti-CD3 antisera.

Stimulation of T-Cell Receptors by Superantigens

Superantigens involve a very different type of interaction between the TCR, MHC, and antigen that results in linking TCR and MHC.[167–170] Superantigens (SAgs) bind in varying degrees to many MHC class II molecules on the target cells and to selected TCR β chain variable (Vβ) regions on T cells, away from the classic antigen-binding regions of these molecules. Crystal structures have been determined for the complex of staphylococcal enterotoxin B (SEB), a bacterial superantigen, with TCR and also for SEB with MHC class II.[171,172] T-cell specificity for SAgs is determined by whether the T cell expresses the relevant TCR Vβ region. SAgs do not require antigen processing and are not MHC-restricted in the classic sense, as they bind to sites on the MHC class II molecule away from the antigen-binding groove. They may be soluble or bound to cells, and they may arise from endogenous cellular genes. SAgs studied thus far are primarily viral and bacterial products, including streptococcal pyrogenic toxins and staphylococcal enterotoxins, notably connected with toxic shock syndrome and selected types of food poisoning. SAgs also appear to be associated with the human immunodeficiency and rabies viruses. Because of SAgs' binding properties, they can interact with a far higher proportion of T cells than do standard T-cell antigens. Both CD4+ and CD8+ T cells, and possibly T cells expressing selected TCR γδ receptors, can be stimulated by SAgs. Like T-cell responses to standard antigens, the potential results of SAg stimulation include T-cell proliferation, cytokine production, enhanced expression of particular cell surface molecules, cytotoxic activity, and anergy or cell death.

Major Histocompatibility Complex–Independent Stimulation of T-Cell Receptors

Cross-linking of TCR/CD3 complexes with subsequent cluster formation appears to be a basic requirement for antigen-specific signal transduction in T cells.[173] Antibodies against extracellular domains of the TCR/CD3 complex will substitute for the MHC-antigen complex if the antibodies are anchored to a surface, such as to other cells through the Fc portion of the antibody or to an artificial surface such as plastic. If the antibody specificity is against a nonpolymorphic determinant, T cells are nonspecifically stimulated. On the other hand, if the antibody specificity is against a determinant unique to the TCR, then T-cell stimulation is highly specific.

T-cell mitogens, such as concanavalin A, bind to a variety of cell surface glycoproteins and stimulate T cells in a nonspecific fashion. The stimulation may depend on cross-linking of the TCR/CD3 complex by the mitogens.

Some antigens that are not SAgs may be recognized by T cells in a fashion that is not MHC-restricted and does not require antigen processing.[163,164,174] Described as being among these antigens are selected polyvalent haptens, myelin basic protein, the heme component of hemoglobin, and underglycosylated mucins produced by particular adenocarcinomas of the breast, pancreas, colon, and ovary. A common feature of these particular antigens is tandem repeats of an epitope, such as a particular amino acid sequence for tumor mucins. One model envisioned for this reactivity is based on an antigenic molecule with a polyvalent epitope that mediates cross-linking of the TCR. These antigens, unlike SAgs, may attach through their epitopes to the classic antigen-binding site of the TCR. However, T-cell activation by the MUC1 mucin tumor antigen requires target cell binding to both the TCR and accessory molecules on the T-cell surface.[175]

In contrast to types of ligands that stimulate T cells independent of MHC, at least two particular types of T cells can recognize antigen in the absence of classical MHC, namely those expressing TCR γδ receptors and also NKT cells, discussed later in the section Natural Killer Cells.

T-CELL MATURATION

During ontogeny and in T-cell development in mature organisms, precursors of T cells migrate from the bone marrow to the thymus, where most T-cell development occurs.[176,177] A series of important maturation events, which define specific functions of mature T cells, occur in the thymus. Here, among a considerable amount of cell proliferation and cell death, T cells first express antigen specificity, develop MHC restriction for antigen recognition, and express the cell surface CD4 or CD8 molecules that relate closely to whether the T cell will recognize MHC class I– or class II–restricted antigens. It is here that individual T cells are limited to the expression of a single functional TCR specificity. It is also here that the first round of selection occurs against maturing T cells that react against the body's normal tissue antigens.

Much of the current understanding of T-cell maturation is based on models that involve genetic changes related specifically to T-cell function, such as transgenic or knockout mice with added or deleted germline genes, respectively, and natural mutants that affect the immune system.[178–180] In addition, mouse models involving T-cell activation by SAgs have served important roles, because they allow one to monitor the maturation of relatively large numbers of T cells with a known antigen specificity.

MARKERS AND PHENOTYPES

Cell surface markers based on antibody reactivity have been identified that permit associating individual T cells with a particular stage of maturation.[181,182] The markers are cell surface molecules, which present a characteristic identifying *phenotype* of the cell when expressed individually or in a certain combination. For example, the TCR/CD3 complex now is commonly used as a marker for mature T cells. Thy-1 (mouse) and CD2 are expressed rather ubiquitously but not exclusively on T cells. CD4 and CD8 are expressed differently by distinct T-cell subpopulations, and mature T cells generally express one but not both.

DEVELOPMENT OF THE T-CELL ANTIGEN REPERTOIRE: ROLE OF THE THYMUS

The antigen repertoire comprises the antigens that a group of T cells can recognize when the T cells are considered as a whole. The limits of the repertoire of all T cells in the body are set by the combined specificities of TCRs that can be generated. The TCRs that are expressed initially by immature T cells in the thymus represent random specificities that include binding affinities not only for determinants foreign to the host but also for determinants produced by the host's cells, including tumor cells. However, as described later in this section and in T-Cell Death in the Thymus, T cells expressing some specificities are favored, whereas many others are deleted in the thymus.

The TCRs that mediate MHC-restricted recognition of foreign antigens are encoded by germline genes that, with the few exceptions of extrathymic maturation, are first expressed in the thymus. The TCR repertoire that is expressed by mature T cells as a whole in an individual, however, is molded during at least two points in T-cell development. The first point occurs in the thymus. The second occurs with mature T cells that have left the thymus, and it is discussed later in the section Peripheral T-Cell Tolerance.

In mouse models, cells with the general phenotype of Thy-1+CD4–CD8– contain the precursors of the T-cell lineage and are located primarily under the capsule in the outer cortex of the thymus. Here, they proliferate rapidly. At this stage, rearrangement of the structural gene for the TCR β chain occurs, which suppresses further rearrangements of the gene and allows assembly of a TCR β chain/surrogate TCR α chain/CD3 complex. This primitive TCR/CD3 complex promotes T-cell maturation to the expression of CD4, CD8, a mature TCR α chain, and cell surface expression of a functional TCR/CD3 complex. The CD4+CD8+ cells are in the thymic cortex, are relatively immature with respect to their functional capacity to respond to a variety of stimuli, and constitute by far the most thymocytes. For the most part, they are destined to die in the thymus.

The CD4+CD8+ double-positive T cells in the thymic cortex undergo selection that results in their deletion or continued maturation (Fig. 4-5). *Positive selection* favors the survival of T cells that, outside the thymus (commonly called the *periphery*), will react with foreign antigens presented by the same MHC determinants that are expressed in the thymic environment. Positive selection and termination of TCR α chain rearrangement follows the interaction of the TCR with MHC-peptide ligands, primarily on the radiation-resistant cortical epithelial cells in the thymus. MHC-bound peptides that promote positive selection are derived primarily from the endogenous pool of normal proteins within the thymus rather than from foreign proteins. Positive selection may depend on an appropriate level of signaling, triggered by the TCR/CD3 complex and determined by the avidity that represents the concentrations of MHC, peptide, TCR, and their affinities. However, the nature of the MHC-peptide ligands driving positive selection in the thymus and their relationship to the MHC-peptide ligands activating T cells in the periphery have not been established; the relationship may include a TCR's cross-reactivity between one or more MHC-restricted self-peptides in the thymus and an MHC-restricted foreign peptide in the periphery.

Expression of the CD4 and CD8 molecules, as well as CD45, has an important role in positive selection and T-cell conversion to CD4 or CD8 single-positive cells.[183–187] TCR and CD45, combined with either CD4 or CD8, frequently are considered as a unit with respect to early signals from the TCR/CD3 complex and their regulation. The mechanism by which the irrelevant coreceptor, CD4 or CD8, is lost as selected double-positive cells mature into *single-positive* CD8+CD4– or CD8–CD4+ T cells and T-cell lineage commitment is not clear.

Self–Major Histocompatibility Complex Defined in the Thymus

Under normal developmental circumstances, the MHC type of the T-cell maturation environment is identical to the genotype of the maturing T cell; that is, the MHC that is functionally recognized as self by the T cell is also genotypically self. However, under certain experimental or clinical circumstances, functional self and genotypic self need not be identical. For example, in bone marrow–transplanted patients or experimental animals, hematopoietic stem cells, including the precursors of T cells, can develop in an MHC environment different from that of the stem cells. In this circumstance, T cells are selected that preferentially recognize foreign antigen in association with MHC determinants of the host type, even when these are different from the genotypically self-MHC determinants of bone marrow–derived cells.[188,189] This situation may present important constraints on the ability of hematopoietically derived cells to function effectively in an MHC-restricted fashion.

T-Cell Death in the Thymus

There appear to be three paths that end in the disappearance of T cells in the thymus (see Fig. 4-5). First, immature T cells die if they fail to express a functional TCR. Second, they

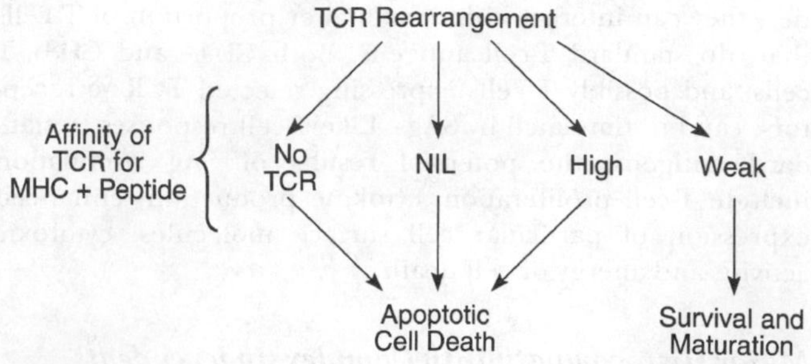

FIGURE 4-5. The fate of T cells maturing in the thymus, based on a model of T-cell receptor (TCR) affinity for the major histocompatibility–antigen complex on antigen-presenting cells. MHC, major histocompatibility complex; NIL, no affinity.

die if the TCR fails to react with MHC-antigen complexes. Third, *negative selection* deletes many of the T cells in the thymus that would otherwise be reactive against normal tissues. These T cells—primarily CD4+CD8+ but also single positive cells, depending on the experimental system—are deleted or sometimes rendered unresponsive in a clonal fashion, based on the ability of the TCR to react with MHC-antigen complexes expressed by cells in the thymic stroma. In contrast to ambiguity about the nature of the TCR ligands (MHC-antigen complexes) that induce positive selection, investigators have identified a variety of ligands that can cause negative selection. In mouse models involving SAgs or transgenic animals in which many T cells express a selected self-antigen specificity, the antigens that activate mature T cells can also trigger antigen-specific deletion of immature T cells in the thymus. Both bone marrow–derived and thymic epithelial cells are effective as APCs for negative selection, although the former appear to be more involved *in vivo*. CD4 and CD8 coreceptors appear to contribute to the triggering of negative selection, as does the lymphocyte function–associated antigen-1/intracellular adhesion molecule (LFA-1/ICAM) interaction. Evidence suggests that clonal T-cell deletion in the thymus has a lower activation threshold than that required for the activation of mature peripheral T cells. This balance would reduce the likelihood of mature peripheral T cells that can react against normal tissues.

T cells in the thymus that are not selected for further maturation die by *apoptosis*, a process resulting in programmed cell death.[190–194] As many as 99% of thymocytes in young rodents may be affected. The process is associated with engagement of the TCR and, possibly, costimulatory determinants that result in the expression of genes connected with apoptosis. Immature T cells whose TCRs fail to bind to other cells in the thymus appear to be preprogrammed for death by apoptosis. Apoptosis is characterized by cytoplasmic blebbing, shrinkage of the cell (including the nucleus), collapsing of the chromatin into patches, DNA fragmentation, breakup of the nucleus and, finally, fragmentation of the cell. Apoptosis in thymocytes appears to involve the activation of "suicide" genes, among which is an endogenous endonuclease. Early in the process, cells undergoing apoptosis *in vivo* are recognized by particular cell surface changes and are ingested by phagocytes, so that the end-stages of the process are not reached and local tissue injury from the release of inflammatory agents by dying cells is minimized.[195]

The differences in events between positive and negative selection that result in T-cell survival or apoptosis are not clear, but apoptosis may be initiated simply by a strong signal or set of signals delivered to the immature thymic T cells by a combination of the TCRs and other receptors. The possibility also exists that different MHC-positive cells in the thymic stroma, and perhaps differences in their MHC-restricted peptides, may contribute to whether the outcome is positive or negative selection. It appears unlikely that Fas, a cell surface molecule belonging to the family of TNF receptors with cytoplasmic segment "death domains," which, if triggered, can initiate apoptosis, is required for thymocyte deletion; however, the issue of Fas involvement is controversial. By contrast, products of the Bcl-2–like family of genes can promote cell survival and contribute to the regulation of apoptosis.[196] Their function appears to be important for maintaining thymocyte viability in older animals, but alone their function or lack thereof does not account for positive or negative selection.

Thymic Maturation of γδ T Cells

T cells that express the TCR γδ receptors for antigen (T γδ) can also arise in the thymus, but they are primarily CD4–CD8–, with a minority being CD4–CD8+. They are the product of a T-cell lineage that shares with T αβ cells a common precursor committed to the T-cell lineage.[163,164,197,198] The lineage of T γδ cells parts from that of T αβ cells early during T-cell maturation in the thymus.[199–202] Studies carried out with mice whose T cells express TCR γδ transgenes indicate that positive and negative selection of these cells, too, occurs in the thymus.

T-Cell Development through Extrathymic Pathways

Extrathymic pathways for T-cell development in the intestinal epithelium have been studied extensively in thymus-deficient mice.[203–205] Several unusual features of these cells have been identified. T cells expressing either TCR αβ or γδ that have developed extrathymically in the intestinal epithelium are predominantly CD4– and commonly express an abnormal form of CD8 consisting of αα homodimers rather than the customary αβ heterodimers. Also, the use of Vβ genes is more restricted than in their thymus-derived counterparts. Selection of at least some developing T cells may also occur in the intestinal epithelium, but this is an unsettled issue. T cells generated in the intestinal epithelium usually do not recirculate to other tissues, which reduces their potential for causing autoimmune reactions. Although their function is not well understood, at least some γ δ T cells have cytotoxic activity. Recently described NKT cells, described later in the section Natural Killer Cells, also develop through extrathymic pathways.

ACTIVATION OF MATURE T CELLS

SIGNAL REQUIREMENTS FOR T-CELL ACTIVATION

The responses of mature T cells to activation commonly include combinations of cell proliferation, cytokine production and release, cytotoxic activity, and even death. The initiation of antigen-specific T-cell activation requires cross-linking and clustering of the TCR/CD3 complex with an antigenic ligand, which generally consists of an antigenic peptide in association with a self-MHC product on the surface of another cell. The antigen that initiates an immune response does not need to be the same as that which triggers effector cell functions by the differentiated T cells. Thus, a foreign antigen, or perhaps a SAg, may trigger a response by T cells not capable of being triggered by self-antigen; however, the resulting effector T cells expressing the same TCRs may also react with self-antigen, albeit at a lower affinity than with the original stimulating antigen. TCR/CD3 signaling is closely involved with two additional cell surface molecules: CD8 or CD4, and CD45.

CD8 and CD4 Molecules as Coreceptors

CD8 and CD4, which are cell surface glycoproteins expressed by mutually exclusive subsets of mature T cells, serve as coreceptors for delivering the TCR/CD3 signals.[152,184,185,206,207] Their role as coreceptors is required for most immune responses by naive T cells and by some activated effector T cells. Acting as coreceptors during antigen recognition, CD8 or CD4 binds to nonpolymorphic regions of the same MHC molecule that presents antigen to the TCR, thus joining with a complex of the TCR/CD3. CD8 and CD4 molecules stabilize the TCR/MHC-peptide complex and contribute to both the binding avidity of TCR to the MHC-antigen complex and to the generation of cytoplasmic signals.

CD45 and T-Cell Activation

CD45, a transmembrane protein tyrosine phosphatase on T cells and other hematopoietic cells, also contributes in a critical fashion to TCR signaling.[208–210] CD45, generally known as the *leukocyte common antigen*, is expressed as multiple isoforms resulting from alternative splicing of three exons encoded by a single gene. It has an essential role in linking antigen-stimulated TCR/CD3 complexes to their cytoplasmic signaling pathways. Although blocking antibodies have not had a notable effect on T-cell function, T-cell lines lacking CD45 are markedly defective in TCR signaling by MHC-antigen complexes; responsiveness of the cells is restored by introducing normal CD45 genes. In CD45-deficient mice, thymocyte maturation is largely blocked, and responses of the few peripheral T cells to MHC-restricted antigens are defective.

Following activation of normal naive T cells, their expression of CD45 changes to a lower-molecular-weight form. The different isoforms of CD45 that are expressed on naive as compared with activated or memory T cells may contribute to the different triggering responses of these cells.[184]

T-Cell Receptor Signal Transduction

The cascades of biochemical reactions that transmit the TCR/CD3 activation signals from the cell surface to nuclear DNA have been partially established.[211,212] Phosphorylation of numerous cytoplasmic and membrane proteins is an essential part of the process. Inositol trisphosphate and diacylglycerol, referred to as *second messengers*, are generated by the hydrolysis of phosphatidylinositol(4,5)bisphosphate, which is initiated through several biochemical intermediates by triggering the TCR/CD3 complex. *Second messenger* is a generic term for molecules produced in response to transduction of a signal initiated by an extracellular ligand, which is the first messenger. The signal cascade is commonly referred to as the *phosphatidylinositol* (PI) *second messenger pathway*. The second messengers are at the beginning of two major intracellular signaling routes. Inositol trisphosphate and diacylglycerol release free calcium from intracellular stores and activate protein kinase C, respectively. The mobilization of calcium and activation of protein kinase C by other means, such as calcium ionophores and phorbol esters, respectively, can also stimulate T-cell division and cytokine production, independent of TCR/CD3 triggering. The two TCR/CD3 signaling routes finally join in a synergistic fashion within the nucleus to initiate gene transcription. TCR/CD3 complexes that have triggered signaling may be internalized, degraded, and replaced. This process permits sequential receptor stimulation by individual MHC-peptide complexes on the target cells, and it improves the opportunity for target cells expressing low densities of antigen to activate T-cell responses.

Some forms of TCR/CD3 triggering may be sufficient to contribute only to partial responses—for example, lymphokine production but not the expression of growth factor receptors or proliferation. Indeed, the type of T-cell response is sensitive even to single amino acid substitutions in the peptide antigen that are sufficiently subtle to preserve TCR/CD3 triggering yet different enough to vary the nature of the TCR/CD3 signal and the T-cell functional response.[213] The ultimate T-cell response depends on the balance of a variety of factors, including the state of differentiation of the responding cell, the nature of the TCR/CD3 signal, and the different modulating signals from its other cell surface receptors, which, in part, reflect the action of cytokines in the environment and the nature of the APC.

Functional Consequences of T-Cell Receptor Triggering

TCR triggering of T cells commonly induces expression of the high-affinity IL-2 receptor, rouses cells to move from the G_0 resting stage of the cell cycle into the G_1 stage, initiates gene transcription for selected cytokines such as IL-2, and activates effector cell functions of cytotoxic T cells. The IL-2 receptor has a major role in the proliferation of T cells after activation by antigen.[214–216] The high-affinity cell surface receptor for IL-2 consists of three transmembrane chains—α, β, and γ—and is expressed only by activated T cells owing to the lack of α chain expression by resting T cells. The high-affinity receptor promotes T-cell proliferation with relatively low concentrations of IL-2. The β chain, which is expressed constitutively by CD8+ but not by CD4+ T cells, combines with the γ chain to form an IL-2 receptor with an intermediate affinity that is approximately $^1/_{100}$ that of the high-affinity receptor and is expressed on naive T cells. Expression of the β chain is also up-regulated following T-cell activation. Thus, signals from triggered TCRs generally leave naive and many memory T cells poised to generate the T-cell growth factor, IL-2, among other cytokines. The cells also are poised to proliferate after IL-2 binding to and triggering of IL-2 receptors. The result of TCR signaling, however, is not necessarily the staging of an antigen-specific immune response. As described later in the section Deletion of Mature T Cells, it may precipitate cell death by apoptosis.

Adhesion and Accessory Molecules

Relatively weak interactions between the TCR and antigen can be reinforced. Binding of accessory molecules to ligands on APCs, such as LFA-1 to ICAMs, CD2 to LFA-3, and CD5 to CD72, enhances conjugation of the two cells and thereby raises the likelihood of interactions between the TCR and the MHC-peptide complexes (Fig. 4-6).[217,218]

Molecules that facilitate the binding of a lymphocyte to its target cell have been referred to as *adhesion* molecules. However, an increasing number of these molecules also appear to provide signaling activity after engagement with their ligands, either by enhancing the signal generated by the TCR or by contributing independent stimulatory signals.[182,219–222] CD28, CD2, CD5, LFA-1, CD44, CD69, CD4, and CD8 are examples of cell surface receptors that contribute to the signaling events. Optimal activation of T cells with weak avidity for an antigen is thus dependent on receptor-ligand interactions that promote the binding of T cells to APCs and that contribute to the T-cell–activating signals.

CD28 SIGNALING IN T-CELL ACTIVATION

Triggering the TCR/CD3 complex is often referred to as the *first signal* for T-cell activation. With naive CD4+ and CD8+ T cells and many memory cells as well, the first signal alone is commonly insufficient for stimulating IL-2 production, proliferation, and differentiation. CD28 molecules on the T-cell surface can provide a critical *second* or *costimulatory signal* by engaging the B7 family of ligands on the APCs, particularly in

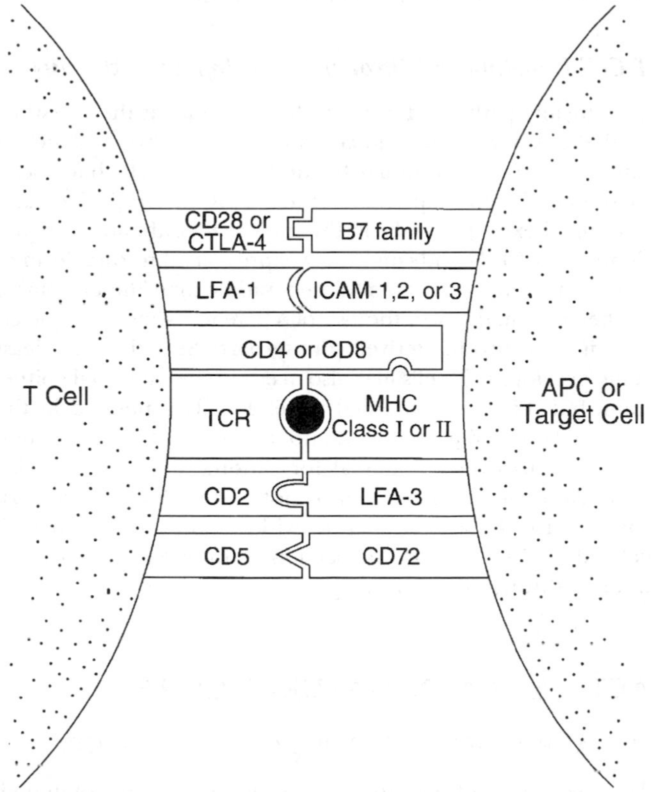

FIGURE 4-6. Some of the cell surface molecules associated with receptor-ligand pairing during T-cell recognition of antigens on antigen-presenting cells (APCs). ICAM, intracellular adhesion molecule; LFA-1, lymphocyte function–associated antigen-1; MHC, major histocompatibility complex; TCR, T-cell receptor.

inflamed sites where APCs are optimally activated.[223,224] Mice that lack CD28 appear unable to generate T-cell responses to certain viruses or to generate T-cell–dependent antibody responses. CD28 is a homodimeric transmembrane glycoprotein found on the majority of human peripheral T cells and, in the mouse, on almost all T cells in lymphoid organs or the peripheral blood. Activation of T cells enhances the expression of CD28 and also induces the expression of CTLA-4, a structural homologue of CD28 with a lower level of surface expression than CD28 but a far higher avidity for ligands in the B7 family.[225–227] CD28 and CTLA-4 signals can have opposite effects. Cross-linking CTLA-4 by B7 ligand can inhibit T-cell activation, IL-2 production, and subsequent cell proliferation. Mice lacking CTLA-4 experience severe, generalized T-cell lymphoproliferation and die within several weeks after birth. Consequently, CTLA-4 may provide a mechanism for down-regulating a T-cell response.

B7 Family of Ligands

The B7 family of ligands for CD28 and CTLA-4 has two key members: B7-1 (CD80), originally called *B7* or *BB1*, and B7-2 (CD86), each of which can trigger second signals.[228–231] They are both expressed by APCs: the DCs, monocyte-macrophages, and activated B cells described earlier in the section Specialized Antigen-Presenting Cells. They have also been detected on activated T and NK cells. Encoded by separate genes, B7-1 and B7-2 each react with CD28 and CTLA-4 with similar binding affinities, and they have, in part, overlapping and redundant functions. However, there are significant differences in their rates of enhanced expression on activated cells and in their contributions to the development of autoimmune disease in several animal models.

Functional Consequences of the Second Signal

For naive and many memory T cells, the signaling pathway associated with triggering CD28 completes the pathway for T-cell activation that was initiated by TCR/CD3.[211] Triggering CD28, among other activities, appears to stimulate prolonged IL-2 production by increasing the half-life of its messenger RNA (mRNA) and by increasing the rate of gene transcription.

IL-2, a single 15-kD polypeptide, is the major growth factor for T cells.[232–234] Although not produced by resting T cells, IL-2 is generated after cell activation, particularly by the Th1 subset of CD4+ helper T cells. Extracellular levels of IL-2 are tightly regulated by the requirement for continuous activation signaling for transcription of its gene, by the controlled half-life of its mRNA, by its serum half-life of minutes, and by the short life span of the activated T cells producing IL-2. IL-2 stimulates both cell proliferation and survival. Activated T cells commonly die without IL-2, as described later in the section Deletion of Mature T Cells.

Mice that are unable to produce IL-2 are only modestly immunodeficient, although they are more prone to autoimmune diseases and die at a young age. The explanation may represent imperfect redundancy among subsets of cytokines. For example, partial compensation for IL-2 may be provided by IL-15, which can stimulate proliferation and differentiation of T cells.[235,236] The second signal also increases the production of other cytokines (e.g., IFN-γ and GM-CSF) likely by the same mechanisms as associated with IL-2. In addition, the second signal activates genes whose products, particularly Bcl-xl, protect against apoptosis, as described later in the section Deletion of Mature T Cells.

In some mouse models, CD28/B7 interactions induce sufficiently high IL-2 production by CD8+ cells that CD8+ CTLs can be generated in the absence of CD4+ T-cell help.[237] Indeed, a major function of helper T cells for CD8+ T-cell responses may be to activate APCs and their expression of costimulatory ligands, such as B7, rather than simply to provide such cytokines as IL-2 directly to the responding CD8+ T cells. Thus, TCR engagement initiates the response in an antigen-specific fashion, while the requirement for a second signal tends to restrict the response of naive T cells to APCs that provide both antigen and second signals.[238]

Normal cells that express a TCR-reactive antigen but lack a second signal ligand will generally not activate naive T cells; indeed, these cells may induce anergy by apoptosis, as described later in the section T-Cell Clonal Anergy. Of note, T cells can respond even if the ligands for first and second signals are on separate cells, as might be the case for activating CD8+ CTL precursors, with a first signal stimulated by tumor cells and a second signal by APCs. Having the two signals initiated by the same cell is far more efficient, however.

The stimulation requirements of one T-cell population can differ substantially from those of another. For example, naive CD8+ and CD4+ T cells require both TCR triggering and second signals to proliferate and generate activated effector cells. Activated effector cells, however, do not require second signals to engage and kill target cells or release cytokines.[239–242] The effector cells also do not need to produce IL-2 or to proliferate.

Costimulatory molecules on APCs that can provide critical second signals in the absence of the B7 family have been reported, such as ICAM-1 (the ligand for LFA-1), heat-stable antigen, and selected members of the TNF family.[222,243,244] They apparently are not, however, the usual primary source of second signals, and the T-cell response is commonly partial and suboptimal. Alternative sources of costimulation are most effective when combined with a strong primary signal from the TCR.

ENDING THE NORMAL IMMUNE RESPONSE OF ACTIVATED T CELLS

Eliminating most of the activating antigen generally results in death by apoptosis for the responding lymphocytes, except for those remaining as memory cells.[177,193,245] After antigen clearance, the priorities of the antigen repertoire of a body's T cells return toward their baseline levels, with emphasis represented by memory cells. Studies of this subject, which are at a relatively early stage, indicate that many factors can contribute to the death or suppression of T cells activated in an immune response and that no factor acting alone is generally responsible. Perhaps the foremost factor is that in the absence of antigen, the stimulation for producing supportive cytokines—particularly IL-2—disappears, resulting in death of the activated T cells. Also, antiapoptosis factors in the Bcl-2 family, which raise the threshold for death from IL-2 withdrawal, diminish without the T-cell activation signals. In addition, activated T cells express CTLA-4 at the cell surface, and triggered CTLA-4 can interfere with CD28-induced activation signals, as described earlier in the section CD28 Signaling in T-cell Activation. Activated T cells also express members of the TNF receptor family with death domains, such as Fas, which can trigger apoptosis when cross-linked. Thus, activated T cells are more at risk for apoptotic death than are resting cells. There are other factors too. Antiinflammatory cytokines, TGF-β and IL-10 in particular, are produced by activated lymphocytes and macrophages or by tumor cells (TGF-β). These cytokines inhibit T-cell expansion, which contributes to the weakening of a response. Recent studies have identified the liver as the key site where circulating, activated CD8+ T cells are trapped, after which they die by apoptosis.[246] Suppressor T cells may interfere with activated T cells or their generation, as described later in the section Supressor T Cells. T-cell responses may also be ended prematurely by mechanisms associated with peripheral T-cell tolerance.

PERIPHERAL T-CELL TOLERANCE

In contrast to immune responses running a normal course, they can be avoided or aborted very early in the face of naive T cells capable of recognizing the antigen of interest. These events contribute to *tolerance*, which can be considered, in the broad sense, as failure of the host to generate a normal T-cell response against the antigen of interest and, consequently, failure of the host to clear away cells expressing the antigen. From the broad view, immunoregulatory factors that contribute to ending a normal T-cell response, discussed in the previous section, may contribute to tolerance too, if they help to abort the response. Of note, mechanisms not addressed here can account for a host's failure to reject cells against which a normal, sustained T-cell response has been generated.

The potential for mature T-cell responses to self-antigens is reduced in the thymus in an antigen-specific fashion by negative selection, a condition referred to as *central tolerance*. However, some T cells leaving the thymus have the potential to react against self-antigens in the periphery. Escape of self-reactive T cells from the thymus is particularly likely for cells that can react in the periphery with tissue-specific antigens unlikely to be presented adequately or imitated in the thymus in a fashion sufficient to induce clonal deletion. The escaped T cells may encounter more potent immunizing conditions in the periphery, which are sufficient to stimulate T-cell activity against MHC/self-peptide complexes on normal host cells that otherwise would be ignored. For example, an inflamed environment occurring naturally or as part of intentional immunization might reach the threshold necessary for triggering otherwise unresponsive, self-reactive T cells by activating APCs and up-regulating cell surface ligands and receptors that promote immune responses. The lack of a reaction between these potential antigen-responsive T cells and relevant antigens that are present in the body has been referred to as a state of *immunologic ignorance* that, when overcome, may result in autoimmunity.

Tolerance among mature T cells can also be induced in the periphery in an antigen-specific fashion by causing cellular anergy, in which the T cells are unresponsive to the antigen, or by deleting the cells.

T-CELL CLONAL ANERGY

In a variety of mouse models, primarily *in vitro* ones, naive T cells and some memory T cells become anergic in an antigen-specific or clonal fashion after TCR triggering (signal 1) in the absence of costimulation (signal 2).[223,247,248] The anergic cells are not deleted; they produce cytokines other than IL-2, albeit at subnormal levels, and they generate increased amounts of high-affinity IL-2 receptor. They do not, however, produce IL-2 or proliferate, even under optimal conditions for normal activation. The antiproliferative state can develop within a day of antigen exposure and presumably can last as long as the anergic cells are exposed to antigen. The anergy results from a block in IL-2 gene transcription.

CD4+ Th1 and many CD8+ naive T cells are susceptible.[249] Anergy appears to be inducible only in cells that secrete IL-2, and it can be reversed in at least some cases with IL-2 or by removing the source of antigen.

The opportunities for delivery of signal 1 alone for antigens associated with autologous cells are numerous. Most nucleated cells express MHC class I with endogenous antigens, but relatively few can also provide signal 2. Signal 1 for antigens complexed with MHC class II may be provided without signal 2 by resting B cells and by selected cell types in areas of inflammation, such as vascular endothelial cells. DCs that express MHC class I–restricted antigens by cross-priming, as discussed earlier in the section Dendritic Cells, but are not well activated may be a common source in draining lymph nodes of tolerance-inducing cells for self-antigens.[250–252] Whether anergy is a prelude to cell death is an unsettled issue.

Other mechanisms or events that have been associated with a reversible, functional inactivation in various models include down-regulation of expression of the TCR/CD3 complex and CD8[253,254] and exposure to structurally suboptimal ligands.[255] Future studies will determine the extent to which the existing observations of anergy and ways of reversing it can be generalized to both CD4+ and CD8+ T cells in various states of activation or differentiation and to *in vivo* situations.

DELETION OF MATURE T CELLS

After activation, mature peripheral T cells can be deleted by repetitive restimulation with high concentrations of antigen.[256–260] Conventional antigens, SAgs, T-cell mitogens, and antibodies against the TCR/CD3 complex have all been associated with the outcome. The process, referred to as *activation-induced cell death* (AICD), can affect Th1 and Th2 CD4+, CD8+, and TCR γδ+ T cells. In most cases, T-cell deletion is preceded by IL-2 release from the activated cells, rapid proliferation, and enhanced expression of Fas and Fas ligand for several days, followed by an apoptotic death. When activated, proliferating T cells pass through the late G_1 or S phase of the cell cycle, where they appear to be far more susceptible to apoptosis than in the resting stage.

The roles of factors contributing to AICD, such as the strength of the TCR stimulation, the presence of various cytokines, and cosignals delivered by accessory cells, are unsettled. However, the deletion appears to be caused by apoptosis triggered primarily by Fas but also by the receptor for TNF, both of which are up-regulated on activated T cells and subject to triggering by their respective ligands, which are also expressed by activated T cells. Studies of Fas-mediated AICD indicate that apoptosis affects primarily the activated T cells with TCRs bound to antigen at the time that Fas is triggered. Activated T cells from mice with a defect in the Fas gene are less susceptible to AICD than normal T cells.[261] These mice exhibit lymphoproliferative and autoimmune disorders. AICD may also serve a normal physiologic function by limiting the height and duration of a T-cell response. Products of the Bcl-2–like family of genes appear to protect against peripheral T-cell apoptosis, particularly Bcl-xl, which can be induced by costimulation from CD28 and can resist either death associated with IL-2 withdrawal or, in some cases, death from activation of Fas.[193,262,263]

A high and persistent load of antigen can induce clonal deletion of CTLs and result in a state designated as *high-zone tolerance*.[264–266] High-zone tolerance may develop through clonal anergy, clonal deletion, or both, and it appears particularly relevant to the tumor-bearing situation where high levels of antigen prevail.

Withdrawal of IL-2 can also result in the death of activated T cells.[193,260,267] The mechanism differs significantly from that associated with the triggering of receptors in the TNF receptor family, such as Fas. IL-2 withdrawal and Fas stimulation probably involve two at least partially different apoptosis pathways. For example, apoptosis associated with IL-2 withdrawal is better inhibited by selected members of the Bcl-2 family than apoptosis associated with Fas. Unlike Fas-mediated apoptosis, IL-2 withdrawal may destabilize mitochondria, resulting in leakage of cytochrome c and subsequent initiation of apoptosis. Moreover, apoptosis from IL-2 withdrawal may be prevented by other T-cell growth cytokines, such as IL-4, IL-7, and IL-15.

STATES OF MATURE T CELLS

NAIVE, EFFECTOR, AND MEMORY T CELLS

Three populations of T cells—naive T cells, effector T cells, and memory T cells—constitute the antigen repertoire of the pool of mature T cells.[268–271] They differ by their state of activation and by prior exposure to antigen. The T cells commonly referred to as *naive* or *virgin* are immunocompetent T cells that have not encountered antigen in the periphery, such as those that have just emerged from the thymus, the primary lymphoid organ for generating mature T cells from nonfunctional precursors. After activation, these cells may develop specific functions associated with cytotoxic activity or the release of particular cytokines. In this activated state, they are referred to as *effector* cells. After a short period in the activated state, most of the cells die, but some appear to become *memory* cells. The extent of T-cell death depends, in part, on the dose of antigen, with lower doses resulting in less death. Products of the Bcl-2–like family of genes provide a level of protection against Fas-mediated apoptosis of activated mature T cells, and this may contribute to the survival of memory T cells after a T-cell response.

Naive T cells are long-lived and circulate through the blood stream and lymphatics between the *secondary lymphoid organs*, such as lymph nodes, where they may encounter APCs presenting their specific antigens and be activated. The long life span of naive T cells appears to depend on their TCRs interacting with normal cells expressing complexes of MHC/self-peptide; otherwise, the naive cells die by apoptosis.[272,273] The interaction does not trigger cell activation and the generation of effector functions,[273] perhaps because TCR triggering is relatively weak, as with positive selection in the thymus. Naive T cells are uncommon in nonlymphoid tissues. They are primarily resting cells that do not proliferate rapidly without antigen stimulation, which would change them to the activated or effector category. Consequently, little of the antigen repertoire represented by naive T cells is against a particular pathogen, unless a SAg is involved, as discussed earlier in the section Stimulation of T-Cell Receptors by Superantigens. As a whole, naive T cells form the bulk of the body's antigen repertoire and, in response to general T-cell depletion, the body's naive T-cell population commonly will expand back to its baseline numbers.[177]

Effector T cells generally are activated, can proliferate rapidly, act immediately after target cell contact (e.g., cytolysis or cytokine release), and are short-lived. Exhibiting homing properties different from those of naive T cells, they are commonly found in nonlymphoid, extravascular tissues.

Memory T cells are characterized by their ability to generate an immune response that is earlier, more intense, and longer-lasting than that of naive cells, after reexposure of the host to the same antigen or a cross-reacting antigen. Unlike effector cells, however, they do not carry out effector cell functions immediately after antigen stimulation, in the context of cytolysis or cytokine release. Their presence in both lymphoid and nonlymphoid peripheral tissues, including areas of inflammation, may reflect the homing patterns of different subsets of memory cells.[274] They appear to be descended from naive T cells that have been activated, although the nature of the progenitors has not been settled, such as naive cells versus effector cells. The memory response probably is associated with a higher frequency of precursors to the effector cells and higher levels of cell surface signaling and adhesion molecules on the memory cells.[275,276] T-cell memory appears to involve a chronic proliferation of T cells responding to persisting antigen, at least for relatively short-term memory. In at least some cases, long-term memory may persist in the absence of the immunizing foreign antigen and even cross-reacting foreign or self-antigen.[177] Some of the memory T cells, probably those not encountering foreign antigen, may be in a resting (nonproliferative) state. As discussed earlier in the sections T-Cell Clonal Anergy and Deletion of Mature T Cells, T cells specifically reactive with the antigen may be deleted or functionally inactivated. In response to general T-cell depletion, the body's memory T cells expand back to their baseline numbers, independent of that for naive T cells and that for B lymphocytes.[177]

PHENOTYPES OF ANTIGEN-STIMULATED T CELLS

Characteristic cell surface markers have greatly facilitated tracking antigen-activated effector T cells and distinguishing them from naive T cells. The activated mature peripheral T cells express CD45RO, a low-molecular-weight isoform of CD45, and relatively little of the higher-molecular-weight form (CD45RA) associated with naive cells. They may also express a variety of cell surface molecules at higher levels than are found on naive T cells, including CD2, LFA-1, LFA-3, CD27, CD29, CD44, CD69, adhesion molecules in the very late activation antigen (VLA) series that react with extracellular matrix proteins, the IL-2R α chain associated with high-affinity IL-2 receptor activity, and MHC class II molecules. CD44 is commonly used as a marker for memory cells, because of persistent expression by the cells. As the activated cells revert to a resting stage, many of the activation markers are lost. An unsettled issue is how well cell surface markers can distinguish between activated cells and memory cells; consequently, the two types of cells are grouped together here.

T-CELL MIGRATION

The antigen repertoire of peripheral T cells can be partitioned, to an extent, in the body through the selected migration of T cells out of the circulation. Naive T cells exit the circulation directly into lymphoid tissues through a specialized type of venule designated *high endothelial venules.*[277–279] The movement of the T cells through the endothelium occurs in several sequential steps that involve progressively tighter binding of the lymphocytes to the endothelial wall and, finally, migration through the endothelium into the extravascular space. Specialized adhesion molecules on naive T cells (e.g., L-selectin), binding to particular mucin-like molecules on the high endothelial venule, provide specificity for the exit site. The process of cell migration into particular tissues and microenvironments is also called *homing.*

Effector and most memory cells do not bear receptors (e.g., L-selectin) associated with migration directly into normal secondary lymphoid tissues. Instead, they migrate to other selected sites, such as the gastrointestinal wall, the skin, and sites of inflammation. Other receptors not expressed by naive cells have been identified (e.g., VLA-4 for inflamed sites and cutaneous lymphocyte antigen for skin) that contribute to the selective exit sites for memory and effector T cells.

Chemotactic cytokines, or *chemokines,* contribute to the exit sites for cells by binding to specific determinants on the endothelial wall, such as macrophage inflammatory protein-1β (MIP-1β), which binds to selected proteoglycans on the endothelium and promotes T-cell adhesion, particularly of CD8+ T cells.[280] Inflammation and associated cytokines also up-regulate lymphocyte-binding ligands expressed by the endothelial cells.

The tissue migration of lymphocytes, and of leukocytes in general, is largely influenced by chemokines.[176,281–283] These small proteins belong to a family of at least 40 members in humans. On the basis of a cysteine motif, most of the chemokines and their receptors are classified as in the CXC (α) or CC (β) subfamilies. At least 15 cell surface, G protein–coupled receptors for chemokines have been identified. Chemokines in the CXC subfamily act primarily on neutrophils and other selected leukocytes, whereas those in the CC subfamily generally act on a different spectrum of leukocytes and not on neutrophils. Within a subfamily, there is redundancy in receptor-ligand pairing in that most receptors bind more than one chemokine and several chemokines can bind to more than one receptor. A single cell can express different chemokine receptors; thus, cell migration may respond to combinatorial patterns and gradients of chemokines. Cells activated by chemokines may change in other ways, too, such as modulating the expression of cell surface adhesion molecules. Although the conditions have not been resolved under which several types of cells do or do not express particular chemokine receptors, a general pattern is emerging in which chemokine receptor expression, and thus responsiveness to chemokines, may vary with the subtype of cell, such as Th1 versus Th2 T cells, with resting or immature versus activated or mature cells, and with the source of activation. For example, immature DCs express receptors for chemokines commonly produced at sites of inflammation by resident cells and infiltrating leukocytes and, hence, may home to these sites, where they gather antigens, are activated by cytokines associated with inflammation, and appear to alter their expression of receptors to ones associated with chemokines produced constitutively in normal lymphoid tissues, with subsequent homing to these sites. Consequently, the recruitment of particular combinations of cells to selected sites, such as naive CD8+ T cells, CD4+ Th1 helper cells, and APCs, is strongly influenced by an integrated combination of cytokines and chemokines. By regulating lymphocyte migration to particular anatomic sites, chemokines affect not only the activation of lymphocytes by antigens but the development and maturation of normal lymphoid tissues.

FUNCTIONS OF MATURE T CELLS

T cells carry out direct and final effector functions. They can also regulate the effector functions of distinct cell populations. This multiplicity of functions confers a potentially pivotal role for the T cell in immune responses.

The CD4+ and CD8+ subsets of T cells differ from one another in important functional parameters.[249,284,285] CD4+ T cells frequently express a "helper" phenotype, as measured by their ability to help B-cell responses (antibody secretion) or the responses of other T-cell populations. CD8+ T cells frequently are cytotoxic or are capable of suppressing the immune response of other lymphoid populations. However, these correlations of CD4/8 phenotype with function are by no means absolute.

The bias toward helper function in CD4+ T cells appears to be the indirect consequence of the fact that most helper cells are MHC class II–restricted, and the bias toward cytotoxic function in CD8+ T cells results from the fact that most cytotoxic T cells are MHC class I–restricted. The restrictions are a consequence of CD4 and CD8 molecules binding to conserved determinants expressed by MHC class II and class I molecules, respectively.

The relationship works out well conceptually in that cells other than APCs, expressing antigenic peptides complexed with MHC class I molecules, generally express endogenously produced antigens, such as virus-infected cells and tumor cells that are targets of the host immune response. In contrast, cells expressing antigenic peptides complexed with MHC class II molecules generally have acquired the antigens from exogenous sources, and these cells stimulate the immune response rather than serve as targets of the response.

HELPER T CELLS

In a variety of immune responses, one T-cell population facilitates or helps the development of effector functions of other T or B lymphocytes. The best-studied example is T-cell help for particular antibody responses by B cells.[286–288] This function may involve specific signals transmitted by direct interaction of helper T cells and B cells as well as signals delivered by T-cell lymphokines.

The generation of CTLs *in situ* also generally requires help from other T cells.[287,288] The helper T cells, activated on APCs, may provide IL-2 and other cytokines for nearby CTL precursor cells attached to the same APCs. The predominant activity of helper T cells, however, may be to promote progressive self-activation and APC activation through TCR/MHC-peptide coupling and CD40/CD40L coupling between conjugated helper T cells and APCs, followed by the activated APCs instigating the critical first (TCR-triggering) and second (e.g., CD28-triggering) signals for activating attached naive CTL precursors.[289–291] In addition, the activated APCs may provide important cytokines, such as IL-12, for CTL activation. The latter pathway allows for the stimulation of CTL precursors by APCs activated in the absence of helper T cells, which occurs with some types of microbial infections.

CD4+ T-CELL SUBSETS

CD4+ helper T cells have been further subdivided into two groups of cells, Th1 and Th2, on the basis of the patterns of cytokines that they secrete after being stimulated.[249,292–298] In contrast to the T-cell receptor, which determines the specificity of the T cell, the secreted cytokines determine the function of the T cell. One group promotes primarily cellular immune responses and the other group humoral immune responses. Thus, in mouse models, Th1 cells secrete primarily IL-2, IFN-γ, and TNF-β (lymphotoxin), but not IL-4, IL-5, IL-6, or IL-10, and they promote delayed-type hypersensitivity responses, cytotoxic cell responses, and macrophage activation. Responses by Th1 cells promote cellular immune inflammatory reactions and appear to provide the primary host immune defenses against intracellular pathogens. By contrast, Th2 cells secrete IL-4, IL-5, IL-6, and IL-10, but not IL-2 or IFN-γ, and they promote B-lymphocyte responses and the synthesis of IgG, IgE, and IgA antibodies. Responses by Th2 cells promote humoral immunity, allergic reactions, and immediate hypersensitivity reactions, which provide defenses against extracellular pathogens. Th1 and Th2 cells appear to represent a later stage of differentiation from Th0 cells, which display an intermediate cytokine profile. Naive T cells generate primarily IL-2 after stimulation, and the pattern of cytokines surrounding these stimulated T cells strongly influences whether a Th1 or Th2 type of response develops.

The responses of the two classes of helper T cells are influenced differently by many factors, including the nature of the antigen and its dose, the type of APC and its membrane-bound costimulatory signals, and various pharmacologic agents. As with humoral and cellular immunity, the responses of the two classes of helper T cells often are regulated in a reciprocal fashion, and here the influence of cytokines is critical. For example, in mouse models, the presence of IFN-γ and IL-12 and the absence of IL-4 tend to promote the activation of Th1 cells, whereas IL-4 and IL-10 tend to promote the activation of Th2 cells. Reciprocal roles for individual cytokines have been observed, in that IFN-γ can directly inhibit the proliferation of Th2 cells, and IL-10 can inhibit cytokine production by Th1 cells indirectly by inhibiting macrophage activation of the Th1 cells.

Patterns of secreted cytokine profiles have been extended to subgroups of CD8+ cytotoxic cells and to T γδ cells as well, which are referred to as *type 1 cells* if they secrete Th1-like cytokines (the major subgroup), or as *type 2 cells* if they secrete Th2-like cytokines.[299–301] Cytotoxic CD8+ T cells in these categories are also referred to as *Tc1* or *Tc2 cells.*

Cytokine patterns themselves have been identified as type 1 or type 2, analogous to those typically produced by Th1 or Th2 mouse cells, to refer to their functions rather than their cellular source.[302] This frame of reference has been useful when cells other than CD4+ T cells contributed to the cytokine pool, such as NK cells (e.g., IFN-γ) and macrophages or B cells (e.g. IL-10).

SUPPRESSOR T CELLS

T-cell suppression of other T cells can be mediated by a variety of mechanisms.[287,303–305] Suppressor cell activity has been associated with both CD4+ and CD8+ T cells.

In some instances, suppression appears to be antigen-nonspecific. Possible mechanisms include an effect of cytokines that nonspecifically interfere with proliferation or differentiation of immune cells. For example, CD4+ Th1 and Th2 helper T cells can each release cytokines that nonspecifically suppress the other, promoting "immune deviation" toward a Th1-propelled cellular response or a Th2-propelled humoral response. Alternatively, bystander T cells, activated against other antigens, may consume the cytokines essential for T-cell responses against the antigen of interest. States of increased nonspecific suppression have been observed in several pathologic conditions, including some tumor-bearing hosts.

In other cases, suppression may be highly antigen-specific.[304,306–308] Suppressor T cells may also act directly on the T cells being suppressed, by exerting veto activity. Veto cells destroy T cells that recognize antigens on the surface of the veto cell.[309–311] In addition, cytotoxic CD4+ Th1 cells may suppress a response by damaging APCs expressing antigens restricted by MHC class II. Cytotoxic CD8+ T cells may act in a similar fashion, as at least some APCs appear able to process exogenous antigens and present them as MHC class I–restricted, as described earlier in the section Dendritic Cells.

Suppressive influences can exist in any immune response. The absence of a strong immune response does not necessarily reflect the absence of antigen recognition by the immune system but rather may reflect suppression.

CYTOTOXIC EFFECTOR CELL MECHANISMS

Different host mechanisms for destroying target cells have evolved, resulting in a diverse collection of cytotoxic cells capable of reacting against a wide variety of foreign cells and organisms. A common feature among them, however, is that cytotoxicity is a regulated process. They are generally activated as a result of cell surface ligands on the target cells binding and triggering selected cell surface receptor molecules on the effector cells.

Major sources of cytotoxic effector cells that have been studied extensively are CTLs, NK lymphocytes, and activated macrophages.

CYTOTOXIC T LYMPHOCYTES

CTLs result from classic T-cell immune responses: (1) The CTL response is initiated by exposure to antigen, (2) generation and regulation of the response depends on a complex MHC-dependent interaction of antigen-processing cells and T cells, (3) the T-cell antigen receptor (TCR) provides MHC-dependent antigen specificity for the interaction between CTLs and target cells, and (4) memory responses commonly follow reexposure to the antigen, resulting in more rapid, longer, and higher-level responses.

CTLs do not have a characteristic morphology. They may appear as small, resting, agranular lymphocytes or as large, blastic, granular cells or as gradations in between.

All CTLs express the TCR/CD3 complex (described earlier in the section T-Cell Receptor CD3 Complex), which triggers antigen-specific responses. Most CTLs do not express cell surface receptors for Ig (FcR).[312,313] Most CTLs express either CD8 or CD4 molecules (primarily CD8) but rarely both. In mouse models, both CD8+ and CD4+ T cells can mediate tumor rejection.[314] The class of MHC molecule with which the target cell antigen is associated correlates with whether the CTL is CD4+ or CD8+: CD8+ CTLs recognize primarily MHC class I–associated antigens, and CD4+ CTLs recognize primarily MHC class II–associated antigens.

The distinction between T cells with cytotoxic activity and those with helper activity is not absolute. For example, stimulated CD4+ Th1 T cells can be cytotoxic by the Fas ligand pathway described later in this section (probably their most cytotoxic common pathway), by the release of cytotoxic granules, or by the release of a relatively slow-acting cytotoxic product, lymphotoxin.[315] Stimulated CD4+ Th1 T cells also may release cytokines, such as IL-2 and IFN-γ, that can promote CTL generation. Moreover, these cells may release GM-CSF after stimulation, which can promote tumor rejection, perhaps through enhancing the development of DCs and their role as APCs.[316] Thus, Th1 or inflammatory CD4+ T cells have the potential to be either helper cells or cytotoxic cells; however, antigen-specific triggering of these cells will be primarily from MHC class II–restricted antigens on the target cells.

Although CTLs use different pathways to destroy target cells, common features are found. The cytolytic reactions generally are triggered by cross-linking of the TCRs on CTLs after contact with target cell antigens expressed at the cell surface. A variety of costimulatory accessory molecules, mentioned earlier in the section Adhesion and Accessory Molecules, may not only facilitate the binding of CTLs to target cells but may contribute to T-cell triggering by the TCRs. Consequently, the activation of only a few TCRs or TCRs with low affinity for MHC-antigen complexes may be capable of triggering T cells with the support of cosignaling molecules. Death of the target cells usually includes apoptosis, with such distinguishing characteristics as membrane blebbing, chromatin condensation, and DNA fragmentation, followed by lysis. In addition, CTLs are not destroyed during the cytolytic reaction; they can recycle to kill more target cells, although their life span is relatively short. CTLs appear to use two significantly different ways of destroying target cells during rapid cytolytic reactions: granule exocytosis and the triggering of target cell receptors by particular TNF-related molecules expressed by the CTLs, such as Fas ligand (FasL/Apo1L/CD95L)[317] and the recently reported TNF-related apoptosis-inducing ligand (TRAIL/Apo2L).[318,319]

With respect to granule exocytosis, specialized granules are secreted into areas of close contact with target cells after triggering of the TCRs. The granules contain two types of proteins that contribute to the destruction of target cells: perforin (cytolysin), which is related to the terminal component of complement and forms pores in the outer membrane of the target cells, and granzymes, a subfamily of serine proteases that are found in lymphocytes and appear to be necessary for apoptosis of the target cells. The serine proteases may enter the target cells through the perforin-generated pores.

Other rapid cytolytic reactions of CTLs with target cells, however, lack features of the granule secretion mechanism and appear to depend on the triggering of receptors for TNF-like molecules on the target cells. A well-characterized example of these receptors is Fas, also referred to as *APO1* or *CD95*, which is expressed on the surface of a wide variety of cell types.[194,320–325] Cross-linking of Fas molecules commonly triggers apoptosis in cells expressing these molecules. A Fas ligand that is a transmembrane protein belonging to the TNF family has been identified on the surface of activated CTLs, particularly among CD8+ T cells and CD4+ Th1 T cells. The antigen specificity of Fas-mediated cytolysis by CTLs may depend on TCR-mediated stimulation of the CTL for brief expression of the Fas ligand in a functional form at the site of contact with the TCR-triggering target cell.[326,327]

Tests of gene-knockout and gene-reconstitution mouse models have clearly established the importance of granule exocytosis and the Fas-mediated pathways.[326–330] Perforin-deficient mice are impaired in their resistance to at least noncytopathic choriomeningitis virus, *Listeria monocytogenes*, and tumors.[331,332] Whereas the granule exocytosis pathway may be used more against pathogens, the Fas-mediated pathway may be more involved with down-regulating immune responses.[191,194,245,260,333,334] Of note, Fas is markedly up-regulated on activated T cells, B cells, and NK cells. However, not all Fas-expressing lymphocytes are susceptible to apoptosis through this pathway; prolonged stimulation for at least a period of days may be needed. Understanding which cells are susceptible to this mode of down-regulation is at an early stage.

At least some T cells express additional receptors that can down-regulate cytotoxic activity through an interaction with MHC class I determinants on target cells.[335,336] Initially found on NK cells, the inhibitory receptors are not related to the antigen-specific TCR. They contribute to the balance between activation and inhibition of T-cell cytotoxic function.

The release of cytotoxic mediators by CTLs is generally antigen-specific and MHC-restricted, because of the TCR-mediated triggering. The cytotoxic activity of the released mediators, however, is not target cell–specific. Only to the extent that their activity is limited to the immediate vicinity of the triggered parent CTLs is cytotoxicity specific for target cells bound to the CTLs. Local activity probably is facilitated by focused effector molecules at the site of target cell contact, concentration gradients, a short burst of cytotoxic molecules from the parent CTLs, and a short half-life of the mediator.

Several exceptions to the antigen specificity of CTL-mediated lysis of target cells have been described.[317,337–340] For example, the expression of Fas ligand on the CTL surface at sites other than contact with the TCR-triggering target cell may destroy innocent bystander cells that express Fas and are in contact with the CTL. In addition, nonspecificity may result from lymphotoxin/TNF-α–like molecules that are released from CTL on triggering by MHC-restricted antigens but, given an opportunity to accumulate in the intercellular space, are nonspecifically toxic. The TNF-related, apoptosis-inducing ligand, TRAIL, may be an exception, as the soluble form appears to be more toxic for cancer cells than for normal cells; as a result, the soluble form is being evaluated as a possible cancer chemotherapeutic agent.[341]

NONSPECIFIC CYTOTOXIC CELLS

NK cells and activated macrophages are the host's major sources of cell-mediated cytotoxic activity that is not triggered by antigen-specific recognition of foreign cells. They are part of the host's innate or front-line defense mechanisms, because to function they require no antigen-specific adaptation of the host or immunization. Although there is no memory response by these cells, NK cells and macrophages can be activated by T-cell cytokines, such as IFN-γ. After cell contact, both types of effector cells can be triggered to kill sensitive target cells by antibody-independent interactions between surface molecules on effector and target cells. The nature of these molecules is at a relatively early stage of identification. By contrast, Ig receptors on NK cells and activated macrophages can trigger antibody-dependent cellular cytotoxicity, if the bound target cells have reacted with appropriate Ig subclasses. Thus, apart from their independent roles in host defense, these cells are also important accessories to cytotoxic immunity. In addition, their production of cytokines and chemokines as part of the early, innate host defense response can strongly influence subsequent adaptive immune responses. For example, activated NK cells may release large amounts of IFN-γ, which can promote inflammatory, Th1-type T-cell responses and also enhance the expression of a wide array of cell surface molecules.

Natural Killer Cells

NK cells are a relatively small population of lymphocytes distinct from T and B lymphocytes.[342–345] They generally are large, granular lymphocytes that originate in the bone marrow. NK cells share a common progenitor with T cells, and NK cell precursors have been identified in the thymus; however, they do not require the thymus for maturation, and they probably diverge from the T-cell lineage at an early stage of differentiation.[176]

Several markers are particularly helpful in distinguishing between NK cells and CTLs.[343,346] Human NK cells are primarily TCR/CD3–, CD5–, CD56+, FcR+. These cell surface features have been used both for physically separating the cells and for functionally distinguishing between NK cell and CTL activity.

Although the picture is far from complete, the basic cytotoxic mechanisms of NK cells and CTLs appear to be similar.[321,346–350] Granule exocytosis, perforin, and granzymes have well-established roles in cytotoxicity mediated by NK cells. As with CTLs, the bulk of lytic activity from NK cells depends on perforin.[351,352] Like CTLs, NK cells depend on surface accessory molecules for the initial binding to target cells. Also like CTLs, accessory molecules expressed on NK cells, such as CD2 and CD69, can contribute to effector cell function when bound to ligand. Granule exocytosis is followed by target cell lysis with apoptosis and then detachment of the NK cell.

NK cells, as with CTLs, can also express or secrete molecules related to TNF, such as FasL and TRAIL, and destroy target cells by apoptosis.[353–355] As in T cells, activation of NK cells increases the expression of these molecules.

Although NK cells are not target cell–specific, they exhibit target cell selectivity by mechanisms independent of antibody and antibody-dependent cellular cytotoxicity.[335,336,342–344,356,357] For example, they are more toxic for tumor cells and virus-infected cells than for most normal cells. Also, different clones of NK cells show different patterns of cytotoxicity with panels of tumor cells from different sources. Different susceptibilities of target cells to NK cells are, in part, due to families of cell surface receptors that can be expressed by NK cells and that recognize polymorphic MHC class I molecules expressed by target cells.[358–363] One family of inhibitory receptors, the NK cell complex, is controlled by genes clustered on human chromosome 12 that encode glycoproteins of the C-type lectin superfamily. Another family, designated *killer inhibitory receptors*, is controlled by genes clustered on human chromosome 19 that encode particular glycoproteins in the Ig superfamily. When cross-linked, the receptors can deliver a dominant signal that inhibits triggering of cytotoxic activity and cytokine expression. Function of the different families of inhibitory receptors is related to a component of their intracytoplasmic tails, the immunoreceptor tyrosine–based inhibition motif (*ITIM*), which on tyrosine phosphorylation can temporarily inhibit the activation of a variety of cellular activities, such as cytotoxicity and cytokine release.[364] This mechanism appears to explain the tolerance of NK cells for normal cells, as a consequence of the inverse relationship between MHC class I expression and susceptibility to NK-mediated cytotoxicity.[365] Thus, there may be two functionally opposed sets of receptors and ligands associated with triggering cytotoxicity. One set, ill-defined, is not MHC-restricted and triggers cytotoxic activity. The other set, which recognizes an MHC class I ligand, can inhibit cytotoxicity. If tumor cells lose MHC class I expression, they escape CTLs; however, they become more susceptible to a subclass of NK cells.

The distinction between NK cells and NK-like activity is important. For example, CTLs cultured with IL-2 can exhibit NK-like activity, but they are not NK cells. Also, a subset of T cells, *NKT cells*, has recently been described, that expresses some of the cell surface markers usually characteristic of NK cells. NKT cells develop outside the thymus, depend on TCR interaction with MHC class I–like CD1 molecules for development, express a very limited TCR repertoire that reacts particularly with galactosylceramide presented by CD1 molecules, and are CD4–CD8– or CD4+CD8–.[366] The TCRs of NKT cells are composed of an invariant TCR-α chain paired preferentially with particular Vβ chains (Vα24/Vβ11 in humans), and they commonly are able to recognize selected lipid or glycolipid antigens or hydrophobic peptide antigens presented by cell surface CD1 molecules. NKT cells mediate NK-like cytotoxicity after triggering of the TCR; however, their role in regulating early responses of NK cells and T cells also appears important because of their ability to release rapidly large amounts of IFN-γ, IL-4, or both after activation.

Lymphokine-Activated Killer Cells

Both CTLs and NK cells cultured with relatively high doses of IL-2 show enhanced nonspecific cytotoxic activity, as revealed by their ability to lyse selectively a broad spectrum of fresh autologous, syngeneic, or allogeneic tumor cells that are relatively insensitive to normal NK-mediated cytotoxicity.[367–369] They are referred to as *lymphokine-activated killer cells.* The greater cytotoxic activity of these cells appears to result, in part, from their activation-enhanced expression of surface molecules that contribute to target cell binding and to triggering cytotoxic activity.

Macrophages

Activated macrophages, as with NK cells and CTL cultured with relatively high doses of IL-2, can be nonspecifically cytotoxic for tumor cells *in vitro*.[314,370–376] IFN-γ and bacterial products, such as LPS, are among the most potent sources of macrophage activators. Macrophages can be activated by many additional factors, including tumor cell contact.[314,370–375] As with NK cells, the basis for triggering cytotoxicity after contact between activated macrophages and tumor cells has not been established.

Macrophages and monocytes are clearly distinct from CTL and NK cells. In contrast to CTL or NK cells, they may be phagocytic; express CD14, CD36, or CD68; have a relatively abundant cytoplasm lacking large azurophilic granules; and are commonly adherent to culture vessel surfaces *in vitro*. Although they may express CD4, they do not express the TCR, CD3, or CD8.[377]

Mediators of cytotoxicity, triggered by the binding of activated macrophages to tumor cells, include the following products: cytolytic proteases; TNF-α and related factors; IFN-α,γ; IL-1; reactive oxygen intermediates, such as H_2O_2; reactive nitrogen intermediates, such as nitric oxide; arginase; thymidine; and lysosomal enzymes.[372,378,379] A serine protease has also been implicated.[373] Many of the cytotoxic mediators may also act on tumor cells that are not in direct contact with macrophages, but most of the cytotoxic effects on bystander cells can be against both normal and tumor cells. Several mechanisms limit bystander effects, including short half-lives of the cytotoxic factors.

Correlations have been established in several animal models between progressive tumor growth *in vivo* and resistance of tumor cells to macrophage cytotoxicity *in vitro*. However, macrophages can also promote growth of some tumors by effects on the tissue stroma, the blood supply, or the tumor cells themselves.[380] The net effect of macrophages on tumors appears to depend on an array of factors that, with naturally occurring host responses, may balance differently for each tumor.

B CELLS AND HUMORAL IMMUNITY

IMMUNOGLOBULIN HETEROGENEITY AND CLASSES

B cells are antibody-producing cells, in addition to serving as APCs. Driven by antigen binding to cell surface, membrane-anchored Ig, mature B cells proliferate and differentiate into end-stage plasma cells, which produce and release soluble antibodies into extracellular fluids. Antibodies are commonly referred to as *immunoglobulins*, which are highly heterogeneous but have a common basic monomeric structure consisting of four disulfide-linked polypeptide chains (Fig. 4-7).[381–383] The two smaller polypeptides of an antibody molecule are identical, are either kappa (κ) or lambda (λ), and are referred to as *light chains*. The two larger chains of a monomeric Ig, also identical, are referred to as *heavy chains*. The great structural heterogeneity of antibody molecules that accounts for the body's ability to react with a vast variety of antigens results from variability in parts of the molecule near the N-terminals of the heavy and light chains, where the binding sites for antigens are located. A four-chain antibody structure has two antigen-binding sites, because each antigen-binding site is formed by the N-terminal regions of a heavy- and light-chain pair.

A second source of structural heterogeneity of antibodies is in the C-terminal portion of the heavy chains. This heterogeneity, which is much less than that associated with antigen-binding activity, accounts for the structural and biologic differences between the five major Ig classes that have been identified in humans: IgG, IgA, IgM, IgD, and IgE. The Ig classes (isotypes) differ from one another with respect to a variety of properties, such as size, carbohydrate content, the concentration in serum, the serum half-life, the portion that is intravascular, and the ability to cross the placenta (Table 4-2). The circulating Ig classes also are associated with particular biologic activities resulting from interactions of the carboxy-terminal region of

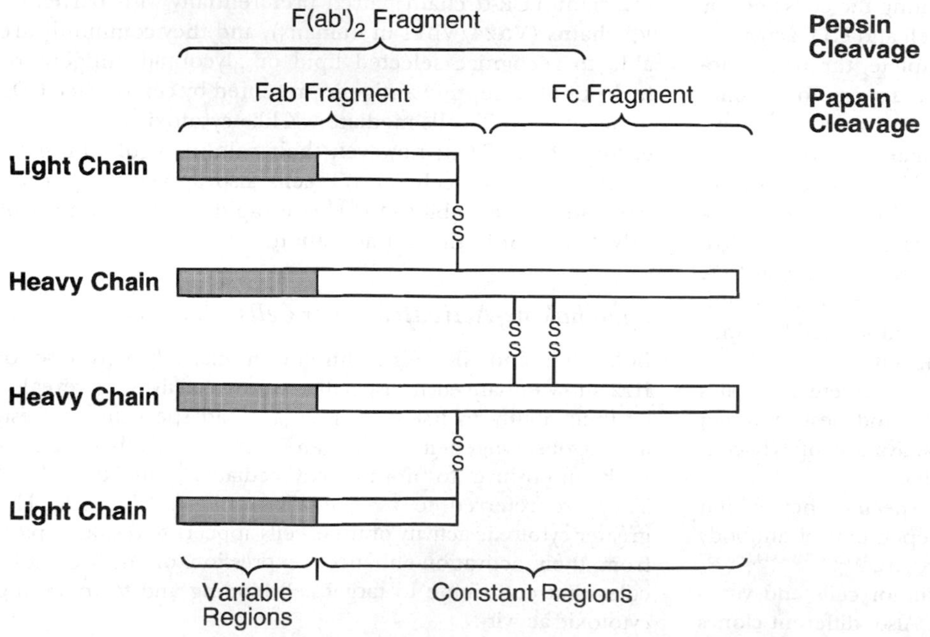

FIGURE 4-7. IgG immunoglobulin molecule with pepsin and papain cleavage sites. SS, disulfide bond.

TABLE 4-2. Some Properties of Human Immunoglobulins

Property	*IgG*				*IgA*				
	IgG1	IgG2	IgG3	IgG4	IgA1	IgA2	*IgM*	*IgD*	*IgE*
Molecular weight ($\times10^{-3}$)[a]	150	150	150	150	160,400	160,400	950,1150	175	190
Antibody valence	2	2	2	2	2,4	2,4	10,12	2	2
% Carbohydrate[a]	3	3	3	3	7	7	12	13	11
Normal serum level (mg/mL)[a]	8	4	1	0.4	3.5	0.4	1	0.03	0.0001
Half-life (days)[a]	23	23	8	23	6	6	5	3	2.5
% Intravascular[b]	40	_	_	_	40	_	80	_	_
Placental transfer	+	+	+	+	0	0	0	0	0
Classic complement activation[c]	+	+	+	0	0	0	+	0	0

[a]Approximate values.
[b]Percentage of immunoglobulin that is intravascular, as determined for the entire IgG and IgA classes rather than subclasses.
[c]Additional classes (IgA, IgD) can activate complement by an alternate pathway.

the heavy chain with Ig receptors on cells or with other soluble molecules. The biologic activities of selected Ig classes bound to antigen include activating the complement cascade (IgG and IgM); triggering cytotoxic activity by macrophages and particular lymphocytes, such as NK cells (IgG); triggering mast and basophil cells to degranulate (IgE); and promoting phagocytosis of antibody-antigen-complement complexes (IgG and IgM). Entering secretions, such as breast milk and on mucosal surfaces, is characteristic of IgA antibodies, and bound antigen is not a prerequisite.

MONOCLONAL ANTIBODIES

Normal humoral immune responses by B lymphocytes are polyclonal and, as a result, the antibodies are heterogeneous. By immortalizing and cloning antibody-producing cells, however, large amounts of homogeneous antibody reacting with a single epitope can be generated.[384–386] Antibody-producing cells, particularly from mice, are commonly immortalized by fusing them with plasma cell tumors that do not produce Ig but nevertheless are capable of supporting antibody synthesis and secretion. The antibody-producing cell contributes the genetic coding for the antibody to the hybridoma brought about by the fusion, and the plasmacytoma provides the ability to replicate indefinitely.

By cloning large numbers of hybridomas and characterizing the antigen specificities of the different monoclonal antibodies, investigators have generated large and renewable quantities of reagents that, as a group, identify an extensive array of biologically important molecules. These include cellular components that stimulate or regulate immune responses, cellular markers that distinguish one class of cell involved with immune responses from another, cellular markers that help to diagnose the nature of a tumor biopsy specimen, and antigens selectively expressed by tumor cells. Monoclonal antibodies are used not only for identifying and purifying molecules or cells but for triggering or blocking activation molecules on cell surfaces and for targeting cytotoxic and diagnostic imaging reagents to tumors *in vivo.* With access to the mRNA coding, mouse monoclonal antibodies have been restructured genetically by recombinant DNA technology to generate new types that may be useful in diagnosing and treating cancer. Examples include humanizing mouse antibodies by introducing human sequences without altering the antigen specificity and reducing the antibody size by coding for variable regions of heavy and light chains connected by a polypeptide spacer.

B-CELL MATURATION IN THE BONE MARROW

Stem cells develop within the adult bone marrow into B cells expressing surface IgM and IgD Igs in a fashion that does not require interaction with foreign antigens.[387–390] These naive or virgin B cells then circulate to lymphoid organs where, stimulated by antigen and appropriate cosignals, they mature further into cells expressing the other Ig classes.

Immunoglobulin Gene Rearrangements as Markers of Maturation Stages

The earliest indication of commitment of a bone marrow stem cell to the B-cell lineage appears to be rearrangement of nonadjacent germline variable V, D, and J genes coding for the variable region of the IgM heavy chain, so that they are next to one another. Successful rearrangement of a V(D)J segment is followed by synthesis of IgM (μ) heavy chains in a fashion similar to that of a T-cell receptor chain, cell surface expression of the μ chain combined with a temporary surrogate light chain, cessation of further rearrangements of H-chain genes, and the start of rearrangements of kappa (κ) light-chain genes. Successful Vκ-Jκ pairing results in κ-chain synthesis; matching of κ and μ heavy chains and expression of monomeric surface IgM molecules; and termination of the gene rearrangements. With a few nonproductive Vκ-Jκ alignments—perhaps only two—rearrangement of κ-chain genes stops and that of lambda (λ) light-chain genes starts, with success resulting in μ heavy chains pairing with λ light chains. The life span appears to be short for cells with nonproductive gene rearrangements. The large diversity among antibody molecules reflects, in part, the different functional gene arrangements and chain pairings that are possible. Developing B cells with light chains and μ heavy chains express surface IgM alone, followed in time by both IgM and IgD, which mark the completion of antigen-independent maturation in the bone marrow.

B-cell tumors and Ig-deficiency disorders often represent arrested stages of normal B-cell development. Characterizing the Ig gene rearrangements in these situations has provided key information about the sequence of events during normal maturation and has helped to identify and classify B-cell tumors.

Igs anchored by transmembrane domains to the cell surface are specific markers for B cells. CD19 and CD20, which are not Igs, are also used for identifying B cells. These cell surface products are expressed by pre–B cells and by mature B cells but not by plasma cells.

In addition to the conventional B-cell lineage, another lineage has been observed in humans and in animal models.[391] Referred to as *B-1 B cells,* in contrast to conventional B-2 B cells, they are bone marrow–derived but differ from the conventional lineage, in part by the general location of mature cells (extra lymphoid sites, such as the peritoneal cavity), cell surface markers (CD5), and the antigen specificity repertoire, which is more restricted, of lower affinity, and of broader specificity than the conventional repertoire. Although not as common as conventional B cells, like Tγδ cells they may contribute to early host reactions against particular pathogens.

B-Cell Antigen Receptor

Igs integrated into the cell surface serve as antigen receptors and cell-signaling molecules.[392,393] These Igs appear to be part of a signaling complex, the B-cell antigen receptor, that includes at least two additional noncovalently bound transmembrane invariant polypeptides, Ig-α and Ig-β, analogous to the TCR/CD3 complex on T cells. Antigen-specific activation of B cells leads to cell proliferation and differentiation through a process of cell signaling that, like T-cell activation, appears to use multiple tyrosine kinases and the phosphatidylinositol second messengers to turn on DNA transcription factors. Analogous to CD4 and CD8 in T-cell activation, the complex of CD19, CD21, and CD81 has been implicated as a coreceptor for B-cell activation by the binding of CD21 (CR2) to fragments of complement CR3 associated with the antigen.

Regulation of B-Cell Maturation in the Bone Marrow

The maturation of B cells is sensitive to a variety of factors in the bone marrow environment, including stromal cells that provide supportive cytokines (e.g., IL-7), chemokines (SDF-1), and direct cell interactions.[388,389,393,394]

Cell surface IgM on developing B cells may have an important role in signaling, similar to the T-cell receptor on thymocytes. B-cell development is arrested in animals genetically unable to express cell surface IgM, which may serve as a source of positive signals for development as a result of relatively low-affinity interactions with self-antigens. However, activation of immature B cells by cross-linking surface IgM molecules with either antigen or anti-IgM antibodies can result in cell deletion, likely by apoptosis, rather than proliferation and differentiation. Fas-dependent mechanisms appear to be associated with the apoptosis. For antigen-mediated deletion of immature B cells, relatively high-affinity binding to the surface IgM may be needed. A pause in cell maturation appears to precede deletion. During this period, a portion of the autoreactive B cells rearrange their light-chain genes by a process referred to as *receptor editing,* and cells with successful rearrangements escape negative selection by expressing new antigen specificities that are not autoreactive.[395]

One Antibody Specificity per Cell

As a consequence of limiting successful gene rearrangements, each B cell generally expresses the heavy chain of only one chromosome, the light chain of only one chromosome (allelic exclusion) and, moreover, only one class of light chain (κ or λ, isotype exclusion).[396] Hence, each B cell generally produces only one antibody specificity.[397] For individual B cells expressing both IgM and IgD molecules, the two classes of antibodies have the same heavy-chain variable region and the same light chains, probably as a result of differential splicing of a single primary RNA transcript that includes the rearranged variable region and both μ and δ constant region genes. Hence, they have the same basic antibody specificity for antigen and preserve the general observation of one specificity per cell. As with T cells, antigen specificity is established before a mature but naive B cell encounters foreign antigen. These B cells, considered as a whole, comprise a host's primary B-cell repertoire. The primary repertoire represents antibodies of lower affinity and broader specificity than what follows with further antigen-driven maturation.

B-CELL MATURATION IN LYMPHOID ORGANS

Mature but naive B cells migrate from the primary lymphoid organ where they are produced—the bone marrow—to secondary lymphoid organs throughout the body, where further maturation is induced by stimulation with antigens and appropriate cosignals. Successfully stimulated B cells differentiate into antibody-secreting plasma cells or into memory cells. Unstimulated cells appear to die by apoptosis after a relatively short life span.

T-Cell–Dependent Antibody Responses

B-cell responses to protein antigens commonly depend on helper (CD4+) T cells.[392,398–402] T-cell–dependent activation of naive B cells starts with antigen binding to Ig cell surface receptors. Antigen processing follows with presentation of MHC class II–restricted peptides. In T-cell–rich areas of lymphoid organs, the B cells act as APCs to helper T cells, with receptors capable of binding to the MHC-restricted peptide. Successful T-cell/B-cell interactions may require previously activated helper T cells. The cognate T-cell/B-cell interaction results in mutually rising levels of activation, including up-regulation of the cell surface B7 family of costimulatory molecules on the B cells. Engagement of the CD40 receptor on B cells by a CD40 ligand (CD40L) on activated helper T cells leads to B-cell activation, enhanced by exposure to T-cell–derived IL-4 and other cytokines and additional B-cell/T-cell receptor-ligand interactions. Establishing germinal centers that include FDCs and helper T cells, the activated B cells undergo class switching, antibody affinity maturation and, finally, differentiation into antibody-secreting plasma cells or memory B cells. The B-cell response to an antigen not previously encountered is, in the early stage, primarily by activated naive cells producing IgM antibodies of relatively low affinity.

Class Switching

Ig class (isotope) switching occurs, in which cells expressing IgM and IgD receptors at the surface differentiate, essentially irreversibly, into cells expressing IgG, IgA, or IgE receptors.[403,404] Antibody molecules resulting from a class switch express a new isotype and new associated biologic functions; however, the antigen specificity remains intact, because the light chains and the variable region of the heavy chain do not change. The switching is controlled by a combination of factors, including B-cell–activating agents (e.g., antigens), contact with helper T cells, and particular cytokines (e.g., IL-4, IFN-γ, and TGF-β). For example, the switch to IgE by B cells previously activated by antigen and T-cell contact is promoted by IL-4 but inhibited by IFN-γ. Class switching involves DNA recombination events between switch regions associated with each heavy-chain constant region. As a result, the V(D)J rearrangement, coding for the variable region of the heavy chain, comes into close approximation to a new constant region gene, probably because of intervening DNA forming a loop and being deleted (e.g., as a circular episome).

Changes in Antibody Affinity for Antigen

Somatic hypermutation in the variable region genes for heavy and light chains of dividing B cells in the germinal centers of secondary lymphoid organs increases the antigen repertoire and the range of antibody-binding affinities for each antigen.[405–407] As a result, B cells expressing high-affinity antibodies preferentially expand in the face of falling levels of antigen associated with the end of the response. If the response is prolonged, such as after immunization with an adjuvant, class switching and affinity maturation may occur later during the initial (primary) response to the antigen.

Memory

Most B cells and plasma cells associated with a primary (IgM) antibody response disappear at the end of the response, which is associated with removal of the antigen and Fas-mediated apoptosis. However, some B cells survive responses to T-dependent antigens as memory cells.[271,392] Memory B cells express surface Ig molecules other than IgM and develop through a T-cell–dependent process. They appear not to be derived from B cells that have generated a primary (IgM) antibody response but rather from a separate differentiation pathway. Expression of Bcl-2 genes in memory cells may protect against apoptosis. Memory cells are not restricted to the site of antigen interaction; they contribute to the pool of recirculating lymphocytes. Long-term memory cells may not need to divide to survive for years. After reexposure to antigen, activated memory cells generate a more rapid response than the primary one. Moreover, the secondary (anamnestic) response is more intense, lasts longer, and exhibits class switching away from IgM antibodies and increased antibody affinity for the antigen.

T-Cell–Independent Antibody Responses

B-cell responses to some antigens, particularly various bacterial products, occur in the absence of MHC class II–restricted T-cell help. These responses are referred to as *T-cell–independent*.[408] They include antigen-specific responses against low doses of haptenated B-cell mitogens (e.g., trinitrophenyl (TNP)-LPS), which can occur in the absence of accessory cells. They also include responses against large nonprotein molecules with repeating, appropriately spaced copies of an antigenic epitope, such as particular bacterial polysaccharides. The multivalent antigens cross-link the B-cell surface Igs capable of binding the epitopes, resulting in a signal that, combined with exposure to particular cytokines (e.g. IL-5), leads to B-cell activation and antibody secretion, particularly IgM. Isotype switching, affinity maturation, and memory do not occur with these responses as they do with T-cell–dependent responses.

Mature B-Cell Tolerance

As with T cells, mature B cells may show tolerance for particular antigens, through deletion, anergy, or ignorance.[409–412] Mature B cells specific for T-dependent antigens are subject to deletion after binding of autoantigen in the absence of successful signaling (e.g., the CD40 ligand) from helper T cells. Apoptosis triggered by Fas on susceptible cells may be involved. B cells can also become unresponsive (anergic) to soluble antigens, probably at a lower antigen concentration or affinity than with deletion, as a result of a failure in signaling from the surface Ig. The life span of anergic B cells is relatively short; hence, the anergy blends into cell deletion. The anergic state may be offset by stimulating the cell surface CD40 molecule and adding IL-4 or by transferring the cells to an antigen-free environment. In addition, B-cell responses that depend on T-cell help can fail as a result of T-cell tolerance. Also, autoreactive B cells may be competitively blocked by other antigen-activated B cells from entering the limited space within the lymphoid follicles of secondary lymphoid organs, where conditions favor optimal stimulation, proliferation, and differentiation. Finally, B cells may simply ignore antigens because of insufficient concentrations or avidity.

SUMMARY

The immune system has evolved as a highly complex and adaptive mechanism for distinguishing between nonself and self and for neutralizing or clearing nonself from the host. Extracellular pathogens are attacked primarily by humoral immune responses, which depend on soluble antibodies produced by B lymphocytes for antigen recognition and for recruitment of effector arms, such as phagocytes and the complement system. Foreign cells, including host cells bearing intracellular pathogens, are recognized and destroyed primarily by cellular immune responses, which depend on the TCR for specific recognition of cell surface antigens and for triggering T-cell activities that kill the foreign cells either directly or through recruitment of other host cells, such as macrophages.

T cells that directly kill foreign cells are commonly CD8+ and generally recognize a cell surface complex of MHC class I molecules and foreign peptides, derived primarily from intracellular proteins processed in the foreign cells through a particular cytoplasmic pathway. Foreign proteins that are shed and picked up by the host's normal APCs, such as macrophages and DCs, are processed mainly by a different cytoplasmic pathway for cell surface presentation if they are expressed as a peptide complex with MHC class II molecules. The peptides bound to MHC class II molecules on APCs are recognized primarily by CD4+ T cells that are not directly cytotoxic but rather function primarily to help immune responses. In this fashion, directly cytotoxic T cells focus on the foreign cells rather than on normal host cells.

Through somatic shuffling of gene components, millions of different gene combinations are efficiently generated by each host to produce antibodies and TCRs that, taken as a whole for the host, can recognize millions of different antigens. Somatic mutations in antibody genes expand the range even further. Generally, each cell in the B-cell lineage expresses only one antibody specificity, and each T cell expresses only one antigen receptor specificity. As a consequence, the immune system can regulate the responses against each antigen by promoting or limiting the expansion and activation of cells that react specifically with the antigen. After immunization, a select portion of lymphocytes may persist as a pool of antigen-specific memory cells, which generate relatively quickly a more intense and longer immune response after reexposure of the host to the antigen.

Stimulating T lymphocytes in an antigen-specific fashion commonly requires two cell surface signals. The first signal selects the cell to respond and provides specificity as a result of triggering the antigen-specific receptor (TCR) on the cell surface. The second is an essential (but by itself insufficient) costimulatory signal from APCs, which adds stringency and reduces the likelihood of careless responses. A first signal without a second signal commonly results in anergy or death. The immune response is promoted or limited by regulatory cells through their secreted cytokines and cell surface ligands, which, as a group, form a network of overlapping activities that reduce the likelihood of general failure of an immune response or of an immune response getting out of hand.

Although far from perfect, immune responses avoid activity against self-antigens generally as a result of processes that remove or inactivate self-reactive cells during the early maturation or adult life of T cells and B cells. Because autologous human tumor antigens recognized by the host's T cells commonly involve unaltered self-proteins, the inactive T cells with potential antitumor activity are of particular interest to tumor immunologists.

REFERENCES

1. Landsteiner K, Chase MW. Experiments on transfer of cutaneous sensitivity to simple compounds. *Proc Soc Exp Biol Med* 1942;49:688.
2. Billingham RE, Brent L, Medawar PB. Quantitative studies on tissue transplantation immunity: II. The origin, strength, and duration of actively and adoptively acquired immunity. *Proc R Soc Lond* 1954;B143:58.
3. Mitchison NA. Passive transfer of transplantation immunity. *Proc R Soc Lond* 1954;B142:72.
4. Miller JF. The thymus and its role in immunity. *Chem Immunol* 1990;49:51.
5. Sprent J. T lymphocytes and the thymus. In: Paul WE, ed. *Fundamental immunology*, 3rd ed. New York: Raven Press, 1993:75.
6. Möller G, ed. Positive T-cell selection in the thymus. *Immunol Rev* 1993;135:5.
7. Gross L. Intradermal immunization of C3H mice against a sarcoma that originated in an animal of the same line. *Cancer Res* 1943;3:326.
8. Foley EJ. Antigenic properties of methylcholanthrene-induced tumors in mice of the strain of origin. *Cancer Res* 1953;13:835.
9. Prehn RT, Main JM. Immunity to methylcholanthrene-induced sarcomas. *JNCI* 1957;18:769.
10. Klein G, Sjögren HO, Klein E, Hellström KE. Demonstration of resistance against methylcholanthrene-induced sarcomas in the primary autochthonous host. *Cancer Res* 1960;20:1561.
11. Klein G, Sjögren HO, Klein E, Hellström KE. Demonstration of resistance against methylcholanthrene-induced sarcomas in the primary autochthonous host. *Cancer Res* 1960;20:1561.
12. Greenberg PD. Adoptive T cell therapy of tumors: mechanisms operative in the recognition and elimination of tumor cells. *Adv Immunol* 1991;49:281.
13. Schreiber H, Ward PL, Rowley DA, Stauss HJ. Unique tumor-specific antigens. *Ann Rev Immunol* 1988;6:465.
14. Greenberg PD, Cheever MA, Fefer A. H-2 restriction of adoptive immunotherapy of advanced tumors. *J Immunol* 1981;126:2100.
15. Rosenberg SA, Spiess P, Lafreniere R. A new approach to the adoptive immunotherapy of cancer with tumor-infiltrating lymphocytes. *Science* 1986;233:1318.
16. Shimizu K, Shen F-W. Role of different T cell sets in the rejection of syngeneic chemically induced tumors. *J Immunol* 1979;122:1162.
17. Itoh K, Platsoucas DC, Balch CM. Autologous tumor-specific cytotoxic T lymphocytes in the infiltrate of human metastatic melanomas: activation by interleukin 2 and autologous tumor cells and involvement of the T cell receptor. *J Exp Med* 1988;168:1419.
18. Topalian SL, Solomon D, Rosenberg SA. Tumor-specific cytolysis by lymphocytes infiltrating human melanomas. *J Immunol* 1989;142:3714.
19. Barth RJ Jr, Mule JJ, Spiess PJ, Rosenberg SA. Interferon gamma and tumor necrosis factor have a role in tumor regressions mediated by murine CD8+ tumor-infiltrating lymphocytes. *J Exp Med* 1991;173:647.
20. Toes RE, Ossendorp F, Offringa R, Melief CJ. CD4 T cells and their role in antitumor immune responses. *J Exp Med* 1999;189:753.
21. Rosenberg SA, Packard BS, Aebersold PM, et al. Use of tumor infiltrating lymphocytes and interleukin-2 in the immunotherapy of patients with metastatic melanoma. Preliminary report. *N Engl J Med* 1988;319:1676.
22. Boon T, Cerottini JC, Van den Eynde B, van der Bruggen P, Van Pel A. Tumor antigens recognized by T lymphocytes. *Annu Rev Immunol* 1994;12:337.
23. Boon T, Gajewski TF, Coulie PG. From defined human tumor antigens to effective immunization? *Immunol Today* 1995;16:334.
24. Rosenberg SA. A new era for cancer immunotherapy based on the genes that encode cancer antigens. *Immunity* 1999;10:281.
25. Boon T, Old LJ. Cancer tumor antigens. *Curr Opin Immunol* 1997;9:681.
26. Boon T, Coulie PG, Van den Eynde B. Tumor antigens recognized by T cells. *Immunol Today* 1997;18:267.
27. Bjorkman PJ, Saper MA, Samraoui B, et al. Structure of the human class I histocompatibility antigen, HLA-A2. *Nature* 1987;329:506.
28. Bjorkman PJ, Saper MA, Samraoui B, et al. The foreign antigen binding site and T cell recognition regions of class I histocompatibility antigens. *Nature* 1987;329:512.
29. Rammensee HG, Falk K, Rotzschke O. MHC molecules as peptide receptors. *Curr Opin Immunol* 1993;5:35.
30. Long EO. Regulation of immune responses by inhibitory receptors. *Adv Exp Med Biol* 1998;452:19.
31. Long EO, Wagtmann N. Natural killer cell receptors. *Curr Opin Immunol* 1997;9:344.
32. Brown JH, Jardetzky TS, Gorga JC, et al. Three-dimensional structure of the human class II histocompatibility antigen HLA-DR1. *Nature* 1993;364:33.
33. Fremont DH, Stura EA, Matsumura M, Peterson PA, Wilson IA. Crystal structure of an H-2Kb-ovalbumin peptide complex reveals the interplay of primary and secondary anchor positions in the major histocompatibility complex binding groove. *Proc Natl Acad Sci U S A* 1995;92:2479.
34. Wilson IA, Fremont DH. Structural analysis of MHC class I molecules with bound peptide antigens. *Semin Immunol* 1993;5:75.
35. Stura EA, Matsumura M, Fremont DH, et al. Crystallization of murine major histocompatibility complex class I H-2Kb with single peptides. *J Mol Biol* 1992;228:975.
36. Matsumura M, Fremont DH, Peterson PA, Wilson IA. Emerging principles for the recognition of peptide antigens by MHC class I molecules. *Science* 1992;257:927.
37. Fremont DH, Matsumura M, Stura EA, Peterson PA, Wilson IA. Crystal structures of two viral peptides in complex with murine MHC class I H-$2K^b$. *Science* 1992;257:919.
38. Stern LJ, Brown JH, Jardetzky TS, et al. Crystal structure of the human class II MHC protein HLA-DR1 complexed with an influenza virus peptide. *Nature* 1994;368:215.
39. Collins EJ, Garboczi DN, Wiley DC. Three-dimensional structure of a peptide extending from one end of a class I MHC binding site. *Nature* 1994;371:626.
40. Smith KJ, Pyrdol J, Gauthier L, Wiley DC, Wucherpfennig KW. Crystal structure of HLA-DR2 (DRA*0101, DRB1*1501) complexed with a peptide from human myelin basic protein. *J Exp Med* 1998;188:1511.
41. Garboczi DN, Ghosh P, Utz U, et al. Structure of the complex between human T-cell receptor, viral peptide and HLA-A2. *Nature* 1996;384:134.
42. Ding YH, Baker BM, Garboczi DN, Biddison WE, Wiley DC. Four A6-TCR/peptide/HLA-A2 structures that generate very different T cell signals are nearly identical. *Immunity* 1999;11:45.
43. Khilko SN, Jelonek MT, Corr M, et al. Measuring interactions of MHC class I molecules using surface plasmon resonance. *J Immunol Methods* 1995;183:77.
44. Corr M, Slanetz AE, Boyd LF, et al. T cell receptor–MHC class I peptide interactions: affinity, kinetics, and specificity. *Science* 1994;265:946.
45. Boniface JJ, Reich Z, Lyons DS, Davis MM. Thermodynamics of T cell receptor binding to peptide-MHC: evidence for a general mechanism of molecular scanning. *Proc Natl Acad Sci U S A* 1999;96:11446.
46. Corr M, Slanetz AE, Boyd LF, et al. T cell receptor–MHC class I peptide interactions: affinity, kinetics, and specificity. *Science* 1994;265:946.
47. Barber LD, Parham P. Peptide binding to major histocompatibility complex molecules. *Annu Rev Cell Biol* 1993;9:163.
48. Parham P. HLA, anthropology, and transplantation. *Transplant Proc* 1993;25:159.
49. Hill AV, Allsopp CE, Kwiatkowski D, et al. Common West African HLA antigens are associated with protection from severe malaria. *Nature* 1991;352:595.
50. Roy S, Scherer MT, Briner TJ, Smith JA, Gefter ML. Murine MHC polymorphism and T cell specificities. *Science* 1989;244:572.

51. Kang X, Kawakami Y, El-Gamil M, et al. Identification of a tyrosinase epitope recognized by HLA-A24-restricted, tumor-infiltrating lymphocytes. *J Immunol* 1995;155:1343.
52. Yagüe J, White J, Coleclough C, et al. The T cell receptor: the α and β chains define idiotype, and antigen and MHC specificity. *Cell* 1985;42:81.
53. Potter TA, Rajan TV, Dick RF II, Bluestone JA. Substitution at residue 227 of H-2 class I molecules abrogates recognition by CD8-dependent, but not CD8-independent, cytotoxic T lymphocytes. *Nature* 1989;337:73.
54. Salter RD, Benjamin RJ, Wesley PK, et al. A binding site for the T- cell co-receptor CD8 on the α_3 domain of HLA-A2. *Nature* 1990;345:41.
55. Connolly JM, Hansen TH, Ingold AL, Potter TA. Recognition by CD8 on cytotoxic T lymphocytes is ablated by several substitutions in the class I alpha 3 domain: CD8 and the T-cell receptor recognize the same class I molecule. *Proc Natl Acad Sci U S A* 1990;87:2137.
56. Konig R, Huang LY, Germain RN. MHC class II interaction with CD4 mediated by a region analogous to the MHC class I binding site for CD8. *Nature* 1992;356:796.
57. Cammarota G, Scheirle A, Takacs B, et al. Identification of a CD4 binding site on the beta 2 domain of HLA-DR molecules. *Nature* 1992;356:799.
58. Ryu SE, Truneh A, Sweet RW, Hendrickson WA. Structures of an HIV and MHC binding fragment from human CD4 as refined in two crystal lattices. *Structure* 1994;2:59.
59. Vignali DA. The interaction between CD4 and MHC class II molecules and its effect on T cell function. *Behring Inst Mitt* 1994;133.
60. Harding CV, Unanue ER. Quantitation of antigen-presenting cell MHC class II/peptide complexes necessary for T-cell stimulation. *Nature* 1990;346:574.
61. Demotz S, Grey HM, Sette A. The minimal number of class II MHC-antigen complexes needed for T cell association. *Science* 1990;249:1028.
62. Kovacsovics-Bankowski M, Rock KL. A phagosome-to-cytosol pathway for exogenous antigens presented on MHC class I molecules. *Science* 1995;267:243.
63. Yewdell JW, Bennink JR. Cell biology of antigen processing and presentation to major histocompatibility complex class I molecule–restricted T lymphocytes. *Adv Immunol* 1992;52:1.
64. Germain RN. MHC-dependent antigen processing and peptide presentation: providing ligands for T lymphocyte activation. *Cell* 1994;76:287.
65. Pichler WJ, Wyss-Coray T. T cells as antigen-presenting cells. *Immunol Today* 1994;15:312.
66. Chicz RM, Urban RG. Analysis of MHC-presented peptides: applications in autoimmunity and vaccine development. *Immunol Today* 1994;15:155.
67. Rammensee HG, Friede T, Stevanoviic S. MHC ligands and peptide motifs: first listing. *Immunogenetics* 1995;41:178.
68. Vogt AB, Kropshofer H, Kalbacher H, et al. Ligand motifs of HLA-DRB5*0101 and DRB1*1501 molecules delineated from self-peptides. *J Immunol* 1994;153:1665.
69. Malcherek G, Gnau V, Stevanovic S, et al. Analysis of allele-specific contact sites of natural HLA-DR17 ligands. *J Immunol* 1994;153:1141.
70. Falk K, Rotzschke O, Stevanovic S, Jung G, Rammensee HG. Pool sequencing of natural HLA-DR, DQ, and DP ligands reveals detailed peptide motifs, constraints of processing, and general rules. *Immunogenetics* 1994;39:230.
71. Rammensee HG. Chemistry of peptides associated with MHC class I and class II molecules. *Curr Opin Immunol* 1995;7:85.
72. Ruppert J, Sidney J, Celis E, et al. Prominent role of secondary anchor residues in peptide binding to HLA-A2.1 molecules. *Cell* 1993;74:929.
73. Benham A, Tulp A, Neefjes J. Synthesis and assembly of MHC-peptide complexes. *Immunol Today* 1995;16:359.
74. Howard JC. Supply and transport of peptides presented by class I MHC molecules. *Curr Opin Immunol* 1995;7:69.
75. Heemels MT, Ploegh H. Generation, translocation, and presentation of MHC class I–restricted peptides. *Annu Rev Biochem* 1995;64:463.
76. Ljunggren HG, Stam NJ, Ohlen C, et al. Empty MHC class I molecules come out in the cold. *Nature* 1990;346:476.
77. Restifo NP, Marincola FM, Kawakami Y, et al. Loss of functional beta 2-microglobulin in metastatic melanomas from five patients receiving immunotherapy. *J Natl Cancer Inst* 1996;88:100.
78. Jakobsen MK, Restifo NP, Cohen PA, et al. Defective major histocompatibility complex class I expression in a sarcomatoid renal cell carcinoma cell line. *J Immunother* 1995;17:222.
79. Zijlstra M, Bix M, Simister NE, et al. β_2-microglobulin deficient mice lack CD4– CD8+ cytolytic T cells. *Nature* 1990;344:742.
80. Rock KL, Goldberg AL. Degradation of cell proteins and the generation of MHC class I–presented peptides. *Annu Rev Immunol* 1999;17:739.
81. York IA, Rock KL. Antigen processing and presentation by the class I major histocompatibility complex. *Annu Rev Immunol* 1996;14:369.
82. Gaczynska M, Goldberg AL, Tanaka K, Hendil KB, Rock KL. Proteasome subunits X and Y alter peptidase activities in opposite ways to the interferon-gamma-induced subunits LMP2 and LMP7. *J Biol Chem* 1996;271:17275.
83. Van Kaer L, Ashton-Rickardt PG, Eichelberger M, et al. Altered peptidase and viral-specific T cell response in LMP2 mutant mice. *Immunity* 1994;1:533.
84. Gaczynska M, Rock KL, Goldberg AL. Gamma-interferon and expression of MHC genes regulate peptide hydrolysis by proteasomes. *Nature* 1993;365:264.
85. Restifo NP, Esquivel F, Kawakami Y, et al. Identification of human cancers deficient in antigen processing. *J Exp Med* 1993;177:265.
86. Rock KL, Goldberg AL. Degradation of cell proteins and the generation of MHC class I–presented peptides. *Annu Rev Immunol* 1999;17:739.
87. Gaczynska M, Rock KL, Goldberg AL. Gamma-interferon and expression of MHC genes regulate peptide hydrolysis by proteasomes. *Nature* 1993;365:264.
88. Michalek MT, Grant EP, Gramm C, Goldberg AL, Rock KL. A role for the ubiquitin-dependent proteolytic pathway in MHC class I–restricted antigen presentation. *Nature* 1993;363:552.
89. Deverson E, Gow IR, Coadwell WJ, et al. MHC class II region encoding proteins related to the multidrug resistance family of transmembrane transporters. *Nature* 1990;348:738.
90. Monaco JJ, Cho S, Attaya M. Transport protein genes in the murine MHC: possible implications for antigen processing. *Science* 1990;250:1723.
91. Parham P. Transporters of delight. *Nature* 1990;348:674.
92. Glynne R, Powis SH, Beck S, et al. A proteasome-related gene between the two ABC transporter loci in the class II region of the human MHC. *Nature* 1991;353:357.
93. Spies T, Bresnhan M, Bahram S, et al. A gene in the human major histocompatibility complex class II region controlling the class I antigen presentation pathway. *Nature* 1990;348:744.
94. Androlewicz MJ, Ortmann B, van Endert PM, Spies T, Cresswell P. Characteristics of peptide and major histocompatibility complex class I/beta 2-microglobulin binding to the transporters associated with antigen processing (TAP1 and TAP2). *Proc Natl Acad Sci U S A* 1994;91:12716.
95. Ortmann B, Androlewicz MJ, Cresswell P. MHC class I/beta 2-microglobulin complexes associate with TAP transporters before peptide binding. *Nature* 1994;368:864.
96. Srivastava PK, Menoret A, Basu S, Binder RJ, McQuade KL. Heat shock proteins come of age: primitive functions acquire new roles in an adaptive world. *Immunity* 1998;8:657.
97. Suto R, Srivastava PK. A mechanism for the specific immunogenicity of heat shock protein-chaperoned peptides. *Science* 1995;269:1585.
98. Chandawarkar RY, Wagh MS, Srivastava PK. The dual nature of specific immunological activity of tumor-derived gp96 preparations. *J Exp Med* 1999;189:1437.
99. Ishii T, Udono H, Yamano T, et al. Isolation of MHC class I–restricted tumor antigen peptide and its precursors associated with heat shock proteins hsp70, hsp90, and gp96. *J Immunol* 1999;162:1303.
100. Tamura Y, Peng P, Liu K, Daou M, Srivastava PK. Immunotherapy of tumors with autologous tumor-derived heat shock protein preparations. *Science* 1997;278:117.
101. Bergeron JJ, Brenner MB, Thomas DY, Williams DB. Calnexin: a membrane-bound chaperone of the endoplasmic reticulum. *Trends Biochem Sci* 1994;19:124.
102. Sugita M, Brenner MB. An unstable beta 2-microglobulin: major histocompatibility complex class I heavy chain intermediate dissociates from calnexin and then is stabilized by binding peptide. *J Exp Med* 1994;180:2163.
103. Hammond C, Braakman I, Helenius A. Role of N-linked oligosaccharide recognition, glucose trimming, and calnexin in glycoprotein folding and quality control. *Proc Natl Acad Sci U S A* 1994;91:913.
104. Rajagopalan S, Xu Y, Brenner MB. Retention of unassembled components of integral membrane proteins by calnexin. *Science* 1994;263:387.
105. David V, Hochstenbach F, Rajagopalan S, Brenner MB. Interaction with newly synthesized and retained proteins in the endoplasmic reticulum suggests a chaperone function for human integral membrane protein IP90 (calnexin). *J Biol Chem* 1993;268:9585.
106. Ou WJ, Cameron PH, Thomas DY, Bergeron JJ. Association of folding intermediates of glycoproteins with calnexin during protein maturation. *Nature* 1993;364:771.
107. Degen E, Cohen-Doyle MF, Williams DB. Efficient dissociation of the p88 chaperone from major histocompatibility complex class I molecules requires both beta 2- microglobulin and peptide. *J Exp Med* 1992;175:1653.
108. Arunachalam B, Cresswell P. Molecular requirements for the interaction of class II major histocompatibility complex molecules and invariant chain with calnexin. *J Biol Chem* 1995;270:2784.
109. Anderson KS, Cresswell P. A role for calnexin (IP90) in the assembly of class II MHC molecules. *EMBO J* 1994;13:675.
110. Schreiber KL, Bell MP, Huntoon CJ, et al. Class II histocompatibility molecules associate with calnexin during assembly in the endoplasmic reticulum. *Int Immunol* 1994;6:101.
111. Basu S, Srivastava PK. Calreticulin, a peptide-binding chaperone of the endoplasmic reticulum, elicits tumor- and peptide-specific immunity. *J Exp Med* 1999;189:797.
112. Realini C, Dubiel W, Pratt G, Ferrell K, Rechsteiner M. Molecular cloning and expression of a gamma-interferon-inducible activator of the multicatalytic protease. *J Biol Chem* 1994;269:20727.
113. Anderson SL, Shen T, Lou J, et al. The endoplasmic reticular heat shock protein gp96 is transcriptionally upregulated in interferon-treated cells. *J Exp Med* 1994;180:1565.
114. Braud VM, Allan DS, McMichael AJ. Functions of nonclassical MHC and non-MHC-encoded class I molecules. *Curr Opin Immunol* 1999;11:100.
115. Burdin N, Kronenberg M. CD1-mediated immune responses to glycolipids. *Curr Opin Immunol* 1999;11:326.
116. O'Callaghan CA, Bell JI. Structure and function of the human MHC class Ib molecules HLA-E, HLA-F and HLA-G. *Immunol Rev* 1998;163:129.
117. Braud VM, McMichael AJ. Regulation of NK cell functions through interaction of the CD94/NKG2 receptors with the nonclassical class I molecule HLA-E. *Curr Top Microbiol Immunol* 1999;244:85.
118. Allan DS, Colonna M, Lanier LL, et al. Tetrameric complexes of human histocompatibility leukocyte antigen (HLA)-G bind to peripheral blood myelomonocytic cells. *J Exp Med* 1999;189:1149.
119. O'Callaghan CA, Tormo J, Willcox BE, et al. Production, crystallization, and preliminary X-ray analysis of the human MHC class Ib molecule HLA-E. *Protein Sci* 1998;7:1264.
120. Brossay L, Chioda M, Burdin N, et al. CD1d-mediated recognition of an alpha-galactosylceramide by natural killer T cells is highly conserved through mammalian evolution. *J Exp Med* 1998;188:1521.
121. Kronenberg M, Brossay L, Kurepa Z, Forman J. Conserved lipid and peptide presentation functions of nonclassical class I molecules. *Immunol Today* 1999;20:515.
122. Ernst WA, Maher J, Cho S, et al. Molecular interaction of CD1b with lipoglycan antigens. *Immunity* 1998;8:331.
123. Sugita M, Grant EP, van Donselaar E, et al. Separate pathways for antigen presentation by CD1 molecules. *Immunity* 1999;11:743.
124. Sugita M, Moody DB, Jackman RM, et al. CD1—a new paradigm for antigen presentation and T cell activation. *Clin Immunol Immunopathol* 1998;87:8.
125. McMichael AJ, Kelleher A. The arrival of HLA class II tetramers. *J Clin Invest* 1999;104:1669.

126. Roche PA, Marks MS, Cresswell P. Formation of a nine-subunit complex by HLA class II glycoproteins and the invariant chain. *Nature* 1991;354:392.
127. Schmid SL, Jackson MR. Making class II presentable. *Nature (London)* 1994;369:103.
128. Amigorena S, Drake JR, Webster P, Mellman I. Transient accumulation of new class II MHC molecules in a novel endocytic compartment in B lymphocytes. *Nature (London)* 1994;369:113.
129. Tulp A, Verwoerd D, Dobberstein B, Ploegh HL, Pieters J. Isolation and characterization of the intracellular MHC class II compartment. *Nature (London)* 1994;369:120.
130. West MA, Lucocq JM, Watts C. Antigen processing and class II MHC peptide-loading compartments in human B-lymphoblastoid cells. *Nature (London)* 1994;369:147.
131. Arunachalam B, Lamb CA, Cresswell P. Transport properties of free and MHC class II–associated oligomers containing different isoforms of human invariant chain. *Int Immunol* 1994;6:439.
132. Roche PA, Cresswell P. Proteolysis of the class II-associated invariant chain generates a peptide binding site in intracellular HLA-DR molecules. *Proc Natl Acad Sci U S A* 1991;88:3150.
133. Russell HI, York IA, Rock KL, Monaco JJ. Class II antigen processing defects in two H2d mouse cell lines are caused by point mutations in the H2-DMa gene. *Eur J Immunol* 1999;29:905.
134. Denzin LK, Cresswell P. HLA-DM induces CLIP dissociation from MHC class II alpha beta dimers and facilitates peptide loading. *Cell* 1995;82:155.
135. Marincola FM, Jaffee EM, Hicklin DJ, Ferrone S. Escape of human solid tumors from T-cell recognition: molecular mechanisms and functional significance. *Adv Immunol* 2000;74:181.
136. Marincola FM, Shamamian P, Simonis TB, et al. Locus-specific analysis of human leukocyte antigen class I expression in melanoma cell lines. *J Immunother* 1994;16:13.
137. Marincola FM, Shamamian P, Alexander RB, et al. Loss of HLA haplotype and B locus down-regulation in melanoma cell lines. *J Immunol* 1994;153:1225.
138. Banchereau J, Steinman RM. Dendritic cells and the control of immunity. *Nature* 1998;392:245.
139. Schuler G, Steinman RM. Dendritic cells as adjuvants for immune-mediated resistance to tumors. *J Exp Med* 1997;186:1183.
140. Steinman RM. The dendritic cell system and its role in immunogenicity. *Annu Rev Immunol* 1991;9:271.
141. Steinman RM, Witmer-Pack M, Inaba K. Dendritic cells: antigen presentation, accessory function and clinical relevance. *Adv Exp Med Biol* 1993;329:1.
142. Pierre P, Turley SJ, Gatti E, et al. Developmental regulation of MHC class II transport in mouse dendritic cells. *Nature* 1997;388:787.
143. Randolph GJ, Inaba K, Robbiani DF, Steinman RM, Muller WA. Differentiation of phagocytic monocytes into lymph node dendritic cells in vivo. *Immunity* 1999;11:753.
144. Heath WR, Carbone FR. Cytotoxic T lymphocyte activation by cross-priming. *Curr Opin Immunol* 1999;11:314.
145. Kurts C, Heath WR, Carbone FR, Kosaka H, Miller JF. Cross-presentation of self antigens to CD8+ T cells: the balance between tolerance and autoimmunity. *Novartis Found Symp* 1998;215:172.
146. Carbone FR, Kurts C, Bennett SR, Miller JF, Heath WR. Cross-presentation: a general mechanism for CTL immunity and tolerance. *Immunol Today* 1998;19:368.
147. Gallucci S, Lolkema M, Matzinger P. Natural adjuvants: endogenous activators of dendritic cells. *Nat Med* 1999;5:1249.
148. Diehl L, den Boer AT, Schoenberger SP, et al. CD40 activation in vivo overcomes peptide-induced peripheral cytotoxic T-lymphocyte tolerance and augments anti-tumor vaccine efficacy. *Nat Med* 1999;5:774.
149. Toes RM, Schoenberger SP, van der Voort EH, Offringa R, Melief CM. CD40-CD40Ligand interactions and their role in cytotoxic T lymphocyte priming and anti-tumor immunity. *Semin Immunol* 1998;10:443.
150. Davis MM, Chien YH. T-cell antigen receptors. In: Paul WE, ed. *Fundamental immunology,* 4th ed. Philadelphia: Lippincott-Raven Publishers, 1999:341.
151. Reinherz EL, Tan K, Tang L, et al. The crystal structure of a T cell receptor in complex with peptide and MHC class II. *Science* 1999;286:1913.
152. Garcia KC, Teyton L, Wilson IA. Structural basis of T cell recognition. *Annu Rev Immunol* 1999;17:369.
153. Yee C, Savage PA, Lee PP, Davis MM, Greenberg PD. Isolation of high avidity melanoma-reactive CTL from heterogeneous populations using peptide-MHC tetramers. *J Immunol* 1999;162:2227.
154. Lee KH, Wang E, Nielsen MB, et al. Increased vaccine-specific T cell frequency after peptide-based vaccination correlates with increased susceptibility to in vitro stimulation but does not lead to tumor regression. *J Immunol* 1999;163:6292.
155. Altman JD, Moss PH, Goulder PR, et al. Phenotypic analysis of antigen-specific T lymphocytes. *Science* 1996;274:94.
156. Padovan E, Giachino C, Cella M, et al. Normal T lymphocytes can express two different T cell receptor beta chains: implications for the mechanism of allelic exclusion. *J Exp Med* 1995;181:1587.
157. Davodeau F, Peyrat MA, Romagne F, et al. Dual T cell receptor beta chain expression on human T lymphocytes. *J Exp Med* 1995;181:1391.
158. Padovan E, Casorati G, Dellabona P, et al. Expression of two T cell receptor alpha chains: dual receptor T cells. *Science* 1993;262:422.
159. Malissen M, Trucy J, Jouvin-Marche E, et al. Regulation of TCR alpha and beta gene allelic exclusion during T-cell development. *Immunol Today* 1992;13:315.
160. Ashwell JD, Chen C, Schwartz RH. High frequency and nonrandom distribution of alloreactivity in T cell clones selected for recognition of foreign antigen in association with self class II molecules. *J Immunol* 1986;136:389.
161. Heath WR, Carbone FR, Bertolino P, et al. Expression of two T cell receptor alpha chains on the surface of normal murine T cells. *Eur J Immunol* 1995;25:1617.
162. Padovan E, Casorati G, Dellabona P, Giachino C, Lanzavecchia A. Dual receptor T-cells. Implications for alloreactivity and autoimmunity. *Ann NY Acad Sci* 1995;756:66.
163. Kabelitz D, Wesch D, Hinz T. gamma delta T cells, their T cell receptor usage and role in human diseases. *Springer Semin Immunopathol* 1999;21:55.
164. Salerno A, Dieli F. Role of gamma delta T lymphocytes in immune response in humans and mice. *Crit Rev Immunol* 1998;18:327.
165. Born W, Cady C, Jones-Carson J, et al. Immunoregulatory functions of gamma delta T cells. *Adv Immunol* 1999;71:77.
166. Malissen B, Ardouin L, Lin SY, Gillet A, Malissen M. Function of the CD3 subunits of the pre-TCR and TCR complexes during T cell development. *Adv Immunol* 1999;72:103.
167. Kotzin BL, Leung DY, Kappler J, Marrack P. Superantigens and their potential role in human disease. *Adv Immunol* 1993;54:99.
168. Möller G. Superantigens. *Immunol Rev* 1993;131:5.
169. Pucillo CE, Palmer LD, Hodes RJ. Superantigenic characteristics of mouse mammary tumor viruses play a critical role in susceptibility to infection in mice. *Immunol Res* 1995;14:58.
170. Lavoie PM, Thibodeau J, Erard F, Sekaly RP. Understanding the mechanism of action of bacterial superantigens from a decade of research. *Immunol Rev* 1999;168:257.
171. Jardetzky TS, Brown JH, Gorga JC, et al. Three-dimensional structure of a human class II histocompatibility molecule complexed with superantigen. *Nature* 1994;368:711.
172. Li H, Llera A, Mariuzza RA. Structure-function studies of T-cell receptor-superantigen interactions. *Immunol Rev* 1998;163:177.
173. Boniface JJ, Rabinowitz JD, Wulfing C, et al. Initiation of signal transduction through the T cell receptor requires the multivalent engagement of peptide/MHC ligands. *Immunity* 1998;9:459.
174. Finn OJ, Jerome KR, Henderson RA, et al. MUC-1 epithelial tumor mucin-based immunity and cancer vaccines. *Immunol Rev* 1995;145:61.
175. Magarian-Blander J, Ciborowski P, Hsia S, Watkins SC, Finn OJ. Intercellular and intracellular events following the MHC-unrestricted TCR recognition of a tumor-specific peptide epitope on the epithelial antigen MUC1. *J Immunol* 1998;160:3111.
176. Spits H, Lanier LL, Phillips JH. Development of human T and natural killer cells. *Blood* 1995;85:2654.
177. Goldrath AW, Bevan MJ. Selecting and maintaining a diverse T-cell repertoire. *Nature* 1999;402:255.
178. von Boehmer H. Thymic selection: a matter of life and death. *Immunol Today* 1992;13:454.
179. Pfeffer K, Mak TW. Lymphocyte ontogeny and activation in gene targeted mutant mice. *Annu Rev Immunol* 1994;12:367.
180. Fischer A, Cavazzana-Calvo M, De Saint B, et al. Naturally occurring primary deficiencies of the immune system. *Annu Rev Immunol* 1997;15:93.
181. Barclay AN, Brown MH, Law SK, et al. *The leucocyte antigen factsbook,* 2nd ed. London: Academic Press, 1997.
182. Shaw S, Turni LA, Katz KS, eds. *Protein Reviews on the Web.* World Wide Web URL: http://www.ncbi.nlm.nih.gov/prow, 1999.
183. Kishihara K, Penninger J, Wallace VA, et al. Normal B lymphocyte development but impaired T cell maturation in CD45-exon6 protein tyrosine phosphatase-deficient mice. *Cell* 1993;74:143.
184. Janeway CA Jr. The T cell receptor as a multicomponent signaling machine: CD4/CD8 coreceptors and CD45 in T cell activation. *Annu Rev Immunol* 1992;10:645.
185. Bosselut R, Zhang W, Ashe JM, et al. Association of the adaptor molecule LAT with CD4 and CD8 coreceptors identifies a new coreceptor function in T cell receptor signal transduction. *J Exp Med* 1999;190:1517.
186. Leitenberg D, Boutin Y, Lu DD, Bottomly K. Biochemical association of CD45 with the T cell receptor complex: regulation by CD45 isoform and during T cell activation. *Immunity* 1999;10:701.
187. Byth KF, Conroy LA, Howlett S, et al. CD45-null transgenic mice reveal a positive regulatory role for CD45 in early thymocyte development, in the selection of CD4+CD8+ thymocytes, and B cell maturation. *J Exp Med* 1996;183:1707.
188. Singer A, Hathcock KS, Hodes RJ. Self recognition in allogeneic radiation bone marrow chimeras. A radiation-resistant host element dictates the self-specificity and immune response gene phenotype of T-helper cells. *J Exp Med* 1981;153:1286.
189. Fink PJ, Bevan MJ. Positive selection of thymocytes. *Adv Immunol* 1995;59:99.
190. King LB, Ashwell JD. Thymocyte and T cell apoptosis: is all death created equal? *Thymus* 1994;23:209.
191. Penninger JM, Kroemer G. Molecular and cellular mechanisms of T lymphocyte apoptosis. *Adv Immunol* 1998;68:51.
192. Moulian N, Berrih-Aknin S. Fas/APO-1/CD95 in health and autoimmune disease: thymic and peripheral aspects. *Semin Immunol* 1998;10:449.
193. Rathmell JC, Thompson CB. The central effectors of cell death in the immune system. *Annu Rev Immunol* 1999;17:781.
194. Nagata S. Apoptosis by death factor. *Cell* 1997;88:355.
195. Savill J, Fadok V, Henson P, Haslett C. Phagocyte recognition of cells undergoing apoptosis. *Immunol Today* 1993;14:131.
196. Chao DT, Korsmeyer SJ. BCL-2 family: regulators of cell death. *Annu Rev Immunol* 1998;16:395.
197. Möller G. Gamma/delta T cells. *Immunol Rev* 1991;120:5.
198. Haas W, Pereira P, Tonegawa S. Gamma/delta cells. *Annu Rev Immunol* 1993;11:637.
199. von Boehmer H, Aifantis I, Azogui O, et al. Crucial function of the pre-T-cell receptor (TCR) in TCR beta selection, TCR beta allelic exclusion and alpha beta versus gamma delta lineage commitment. *Immunol Rev* 1998;165:111.
200. MacDonald HR, Wilson A. The role of the T-cell receptor (TCR) in alpha beta/gamma delta lineage commitment: clues from intracellular TCR staining. *Immunol Rev* 1998;165:87.
201. Robey E, Fowlkes BJ. The alpha beta versus gamma delta T-cell lineage choice. *Curr Opin Immunol* 1998;10:181.

202. Fehling HJ, Gilfillan S, Ceredig R. Alpha beta/gamma delta lineage commitment in the thymus of normal and genetically manipulated mice. *Adv Immunol* 1999;71:1.
203. MacDonald TT. Mucosal T cells. *Chem Immunol* 1998;71:1.
204. Poussier P, Julius M. Speculation on the lineage relationships among CD4(–)8(+) gut-derived T cells and their role(s). *Semin Immunol* 1999;11:293.
205. Beagley KW, Husband AJ. Intraepithelial lymphocytes: origins, distribution, and function. *Crit Rev Immunol* 1998;18:237.
206. Vidal K, Daniel C, Hill M, Littman DR, Allen PM. Differential requirements for CD4 in TCR-ligand interactions. *J Immunol* 1999;163:4811.
207. Devine L, Kavathas PB. Molecular analysis of protein interactions mediating the function of the cell surface protein CD8. *Immunol Res* 1999;19:201.
208. Kong YY, Kishihara K, Yoshida H, Mak TW, Nomoto K. Generation of T cells with differential responses to alloantigens in CD45 exon 6-deficient mice. *J Immunol* 1995;154:5725.
209. Trowbridge IS, Thomas ML. CD45: an emerging role as a protein tyrosine phosphatase required for lymphocyte activation and development. *Annu Rev Immunol* 1994;12:85.
210. Justement LB. The role of CD45 in signal transduction. *Adv Immunol* 1997;66:1.
211. Weiss A. Lymphocyte activation. In: Paul WE, ed. *Fundamental immunology,* 4th ed. Philadelphia: Lippincott-Raven Publishers, 1999:411.
212. Germain RN, Stefanova I. The dynamics of T cell receptor signaling: complex orchestration and the key roles of tempo and cooperation. *Annu Rev Immunol* 1999;17:467.
213. Kersh GJ, Allen PM. Essential flexibility in the T-cell recognition of antigen. *Nature* 1996;380:495.
214. Waldmann TA. The interleukin-2 receptor. *J Biol Chem* 1991;266:2681.
215. Nelson BH, Willerford DM. Biology of the interleukin-2 receptor. *Adv Immunol* 1998;70:1.
216. Karnitz LM, Abraham RT. Interleukin-2 receptor signaling mechanisms. *Adv Immunol* 1996;61:147.
217. Shimizu Y, Shaw S. T lymphocyte adhesion molecules. *Year Immunol* 1990;6:69.
218. Dustin ML, Springer TA. Role of lymphocyte adhesion receptors in transient interactions and cell locomotion. *Annu Rev Immunol* 1991;9:27.
219. Fraser JD, Straus D, Weiss A. Signal transduction events leading to T-cell lymphokine gene expression. *Immunol Today* 1993;14:357.
220. Linsley PS, Ledbetter JA. The role of the CD28 receptor during T cell responses to antigen. *Annu Rev Immunol* 1993;11:191.
221. Schwartz RH. Costimulation of T lymphocytes: the role of CD28, CTLA-4, and B7/BB1 in interleukin-2 production and immunotherapy. *Cell* 1992;71:1065.
222. Watts TH, DeBenedette MA. T cell co-stimulatory molecules other than CD28. *Curr Opin Immunol* 1999;11:286.
223. Powell JD, Ragheb JA, Kitagawa-Sakakida S, Schwartz RH. Molecular regulation of interleukin-2 expression by CD28 co-stimulation and anergy. *Immunol Rev* 1998;165:287.
224. Chambers CA, Allison JP. Co-stimulation in T cell responses. *Curr Opin Immunol* 1997;9:396.
225. Oosterwegel MA, Greenwald RJ, Mandelbrot DA, Lorsbach RB, Sharpe AH. CTLA-4 and T cell activation. *Curr Opin Immunol* 1999;11:294.
226. Thompson CB, Allison JP. The emerging role of CTLA-4 as an immune attenuator. *Immunity* 1997;7:445.
227. Bluestone JA. Is CTLA-4 a master switch for peripheral T cell tolerance? *J Immunol* 1997;158:1989.
228. Robey E, Allison JP. T-cell activation: integration of signals from the antigen receptor and costimulatory molecules. *Immunol Today* 1995;16:306.
229. Azuma M, Lanier LL. The role of CD28 costimulation in the generation of cytotoxic T lymphocytes. *Curr Top Microbiol Immunol* 1995;198:59.
230. June CH, Bluestone JA, Nadler LM, Thompson CB. The B7 and CD28 receptor families. *Immunol Today* 1994;15:321.
231. Hathcock KS, Hodes RJ. Role of the CD28-B7 costimulatory pathways in T cell–dependent B cell responses. *Adv Immunol* 1996;62:131.
232. Morgan DA, Ruscetti FW, Gallo RG. Selective in vitro growth of T-lymphocytes from normal bone marrow. *Science* 1976;193:1007.
233. Rosenberg SA, Grimm EA, McGrogan M, et al. Biological activity of recombinant human interleukin-2 produced in *E. coli. Science* 1984;223:1412.
234. Smith KA. Interleukin-2: inception, impact, and implications. *Science* 1988;240:1169.
235. Waldmann T, Tagaya Y, Bamford R. Interleukin-2, interleukin-15, and their receptors. *Int Rev Immunol* 1998;16:205.
236. Giri JG, Anderson DM, Kumaki S, et al. IL-15, a novel T cell growth factor that shares activities and receptor components with IL-2. *J Leukoc Biol* 1995;57:763.
237. Harding FA, Allison JP. CD28-B7 interactions allow the induction of CD8+ cytotoxic T lymphocytes in the absence of exogenous help. *J Exp Med* 1993;177:1791.
238. Lassila O, Vainio O, Matzinger P. Can B cells turn on virgin T cells? *Nature* 1988;334:253.
239. Chen L, McGowan P, Ashe S, et al. Tumor immunogenicity determines the effect of B7 costimulation on T cell-mediated tumor immunity. *J Exp Med* 1994;179:523.
240. Chen L, Ashe S, Brady WA, et al. Costimulation of antitumor immunity by the B7 counterreceptor for the T lymphocyte molecules CD28 and CTLA-4. *Cell* 1992;71:1093.
241. Townsend SE, Allison JP. Tumor rejection after direct costimulation of CD8+ T cells by B7-transfected melanoma cells. *Science* 1993;259:368.
242. Baskar S, Ostrand-Rosenberg S, Nabavi N, et al. Constitutive expression of B7 restores immunogenicity of tumor cells expressing truncated major histocompatibility complex class II molecules. *Proc Natl Acad Sci U S A* 1993;90:5687.
243. Janeway CA Jr, Bottomly K. Signals and signs for lymphocyte responses. *Cell* 1994;76:275.
244. Sepulveda H, Cerwenka A, Morgan T, Dutton RW. CD28, IL-2-independent costimulatory pathways for CD8 T lymphocyte activation. *J Immunol* 1999;163:1133.
245. Van Parijs L, Abbas AK. Homeostasis and self-tolerance in the immune system: turning lymphocytes off. *Science* 1998;280:243.
246. Mehal WZ, Juedes AE, Crispe IN. Selective retention of activated CD8+ T cells by the normal liver. *J Immunol* 1999;163:3202.
247. Cohn M. The wisdom of hindsight. *Annu Rev Immunol* 1994;12:1.
248. Mueller DL, Jenkins MK. Molecular mechanisms underlying functional T-cell unresponsiveness. *Curr Opin Immunol* 1995;7:375.
249. Fitch FW, McKisic MD, Lancki DW, Gajewski TF. Differential regulation of murine T lymphocyte subsets. *Annu Rev Immunol* 1993;11:29.
250. Sallusto F, Lanzavecchia A. Mobilizing dendritic cells for tolerance, priming, and chronic inflammation. *J Exp Med* 1999;189:611.
251. Miller JF, Kurts C, Allison J, et al. Induction of peripheral CD8+ T-cell tolerance by cross-presentation of self antigens. *Immunol Rev* 1998;165:267.
252. Banchereau J, Steinman RM. Dendritic cells and the control of immunity. *Nature* 1998;392:245.
253. Rocha B, von Boehmer H. Peripheral selection of the T cell repertoire. *Science* 1991;251:1225.
254. Ferber I, Schonrich G, Schenkel J, et al. Levels of peripheral T cell tolerance induced by different doses of tolerogen. *Science* 1994;263:674.
255. Sloan-Lancaster J, Evavold BD, Allen PM. Induction of T-cell anergy by altered T-cell-receptor ligand on live antigen-presenting cells. *Nature* 1993;363:156.
256. Kabelitz D, Pohl T, Pechhold K. Activation-induced cell death (apoptosis) of mature peripheral T lymphocytes. *Immunol Today* 1993;14:338.
257. Green DR, Scott DW. Activation-induced apoptosis in lymphocytes. *Curr Opin Immunol* 1994;6:476.
258. Vacchio MS, Ashwell JD. T cell tolerance. *Chem Immunol* 1994;58:1.
259. Webb DR, Kraig E, Devens BH. Suppressor cells and immunity. *Chem Immunol* 1994;58:146.
260. Lenardo M, Chan KM, Hornung F, et al. Mature T lymphocyte apoptosis—immune regulation in a dynamic and unpredictable antigenic environment. *Annu Rev Immunol* 1999;17:221.
261. Russell JH, Rush B, Weaver C, Wang R. Mature T cells of autoimmune lpr/lpr mice have a defect in antigen-stimulated suicide. *Proc Natl Acad Sci U S A* 1993;90:4409.
262. Cory S. Regulation of lymphocyte survival by the bcl-2 gene family. *Annu Rev Immunol* 1995;13:513.
263. Broome HE, Dargan CM, Krajewski S, Reed JC. Expression of Bcl-2, Bcl-x, and Bax after T cell activation and IL-2 withdrawal. *J Immunol* 1965;155:2311.
264. Mitchison NA. Induction of immunological paralysis in two zones of dosage. *Proc R Soc Lond* 1964;161:275.
265. Moskophidis D, Lechner F, Pircher H, Zinkernagel RM. Virus persistence in acutely infected immunocompetent mice by exhaustion of antiviral cytotoxic effector T cells. *Nature* 1993;362:758.
266. Moskophidis D, Lechner F, Pircher H, Zinkernagel RM. Virus persistence in acutely infected immunocompetent mice by exhaustion of antiviral cytotoxic effector T cells. *Nature* 1993;362:758.
267. Cohen JJ, Duke RC, Fadok VA, Sellins KS. Apoptosis and programmed cell death in immunity. *Annu Rev Immunol* 1992;10:267.
268. Tough DF, Sprent J. Life span of naive and memory T cells. *Stem Cells* 1995;13:242.
269. Sprent J. Immunological memory. *Curr Opin Immunol* 1997;9:371.
270. Dutton RW, Bradley LM, Swain SL. T cell memory. *Annu Rev Immunol* 1998;16:201.
271. Ahmed R, Gray D. Immunological memory and protective immunity: understanding their relation. *Science* 1996;272:54.
272. Freitas AA, Rocha B. Peripheral T cell survival. *Curr Opin Immunol* 1999;11:152.
273. Ernst B, Lee DS, Chang JM, Sprent J, Surh CD. The peptide ligands mediating positive selection in the thymus control T cell survival and homeostatic proliferation in the periphery. *Immunity* 1999;11:173.
274. Sallusto F, Lenig D, Forster R, Lipp M, Lanzavecchia A. Two subsets of memory T lymphocytes with distinct homing potentials and effector functions. *Nature* 1999;401:708.
275. Mackay CR. Immunological memory. *Adv Immunol* 1993;53:217.
276. Gray D. Immunological memory. *Annu Rev Immunol* 1993;11:49.
277. Picker LJ, Butcher EC. Physiological and molecular mechanisms of lymphocyte homing. *Annu Rev Immunol* 1992;10:561.
278. Shimizu Y, Newman W, Tanaka Y, Shaw S. Lymphocyte interactions with endothelial cells. *Immunol Today* 1992;13:106.
279. Springer TA. Traffic signals on endothelium for lymphocyte recirculation and leukocyte emigration. *Annu Rev Physiol* 1995;57:827.
280. Tanaka Y, Adams DH, Shaw S. Proteoglycans on endothelial cells present adhesion-inducing cytokines to leukocytes. *Immunol Today* 1993;14:111.
281. Baggiolini M. Chemokines and leukocyte traffic. *Nature* 1998;392:565.
282. Sallusto F, Lanzavecchia A, Mackay CR. Chemokines and chemokine receptors in T-cell priming and Th1/Th2-mediated responses. *Immunol Today* 1998;19:568.
283. Zlotnik A, Morales J, Hedrick JA. Recent advances in chemokines and chemokine receptors. *Crit Rev Immunol* 1999;19:1.
284. Sprent J, Webb SR. Function and specificity of T cell subsets in the mouse. *Adv Immunol* 1987;41:39.
285. Cantor H. T lymphocytes. In: Paul WE, ed. *Fundamental immunology.* New York: Raven Press, 1984:57.
286. Vitetta ES, Fernandez-Botran R, Myers CD, Sanders VM. Cellular interactions in the humoral immune response. *Adv Immunol* 1989;45:1.
287. Hodes RJ. T-cell-mediated regulation: help and suppression. In: Paul WE, ed. *Fundamental immunology,* 2nd ed. New York: Raven Press, 1989:587.
288. Oxenius A, Zinkernagel RM, Hengartner H. CD4+ T-cell induction and effector functions: a comparison of immunity against soluble antigens and viral infections. *Adv Immunol* 1998;70:313.
289. Lanzavecchia A. Immunology. Licence to kill. *Nature* 1998;393:413.
290. Heath WR, Carbone FR. Cytotoxic T lymphocyte activation by cross-priming. *Curr Opin Immunol* 1999;11:314.

291. Guerder S, Matzinger P. A fail-safe mechanism for maintaining self-tolerance. *J Exp Med* 1992;176:553.
292. Seder RA, Mosmann TM. Differentiation of effector phenotypes of CD4+ and CD8+ T cells. In: Paul WE, ed. *Fundamental immunology,* 4th ed. Philadelphia: Lippincott-Raven Publishers, 1999:879.
293. Romagnani S. The Th1/Th2 paradigm. *Immunol Today* 1997;18:263.
294. Seder RA, Paul WE. Acquisition of lymphokine-producing phenotype by CD4+ T cells. *Annu Rev Immunol* 1994;12:635.
295. Carter LL, Swain SL. Single cell analyses of cytokine production. *Curr Opin Immunol* 1997;9:177.
296. Constant SL, Bottomly K. Induction of Th1 and Th2 CD4+ T cell responses: the alternative approaches. *Annu Rev Immunol* 1997;15:297.
297. O'Garra A. Cytokines induce the development of functionally heterogeneous T helper cell subsets. *Immunity* 1998;8:275.
298. Abbas AK, Murphy KM, Sher A. Functional diversity of helper T lymphocytes. *Nature* 1996;383:787.
299. Sad S, Marcotte R, Mosmann TR. Cytokine-induced differentiation of precursor mouse CD8+ T cells into cytotoxic CD8+ T cells secreting Th1 or Th2 cytokines. *Immunity* 1995;2:271.
300. Mosmann TR, Li L, Sad S. Functions of CD8 T-cell subsets secreting different cytokine patterns. *Semin Immunol* 1997;9:87.
301. Carter LL, Dutton RW. Type 1 and type 2: a fundamental dichotomy for all T-cell subsets. *Curr Opin Immunol* 1996;8:336.
302. Clerici M, Shearer GM. The Th1-Th2 hypothesis of HIV infection: new insights. *Immunol Today* 1994;15:575.
303. Dorf ME, Kuchroo VK, Collins M. Suppressor T cells: some answers but more questions. *Immunol Today* 1992;13:241.
304. Bloom BR, Salgame P, Diamond B. Revisiting and revising suppressor T cells. *Immunol Today* 1992;13:131.
305. North RJ. Down-regulation of the antitumor immune response. *Adv Cancer Res* 1985;45:1.
306. Benacerraf B, Germain RN. A single major pathway of T-lymphocyte interactions in antigen-specific immune suppression. *Scand J Immunol* 1981;13:1.
307. Sambhara SR, Miller RG. Reduction of CTL antipeptide response mediated by CD8+ cells whose class I MHC can bind the peptide. *J Immunol* 1994;152:1103.
308. Hiruma K, Nakamura H, Henkart PA, Gress RE. Clonal deletion of postthymic T cells: veto cells kill precursor cytotoxic T lymphocytes. *J Exp Med* 1992;175:863.
309. Rammensee HG. Veto function in vitro and in vivo. *Int Rev Immunol* 1989;4:175.
310. Miller RG, Muraoka S, Claesson MH, Reimann J, Benveniste P. The veto phenomenon in T-cell regulation. *Ann NY Acad Sci* 1988;532:170.
311. Fink PJ, Shimonkevitz RP, Bevan MJ. Veto cells. *Annu Rev Immunol* 1988;6:115.
312. Lanier LL, Phillips JH, Hackett J Jr, Tutt M, Kumar V. Natural killer cells: definition of a cell type rather than a function. *J Immunol* 1986;137:2735.
313. Trinchieri G, Perussia B. Human natural killer cells: biologic and pathologic aspects. *Lab Invest* 1984;50:489.
314. Greenberg PD. Adoptive T cell therapy of tumors: mechanisms operative in the recognition and elimination of tumor cells. *Adv Immunol* 1991;49:281.
315. Hahn S, Gehri R, Erb P. Mechanism and biological significance of CD4-mediated cytotoxicity. *Immunol Rev* 1995;146:57.
316. Hung K, Hayashi R, Lafond-Walker A, et al. The central role of CD4(+) T cells in the antitumor immune response. *J Exp Med* 1998;188:2357.
317. Henkart PA. Cytotoxic T lymphocytes. In: Paul WE, ed. *Fundamental immunology,* 4th ed. Philadelphia: Lippincott-Raven Publishers, 1999:1021.
318. Ashkenazi A, Dixit VM. Death receptors: signaling and modulation. *Science* 1998;281:1305.
319. Griffith TS, Lynch DH. TRAIL: a molecule with multiple receptors and control mechanisms. *Curr Opin Immunol* 1998;10:559.
320. Rouvier E, Luciani MF, Golstein P. Fas involvement in Ca(2+)–independent T cell–mediated cytotoxicity. *J Exp Med* 1993;177:195.
321. Griffiths GM, Schopp J. *Pathways for cytolysis.* Berlin: Springer-Verlag, 1995.
322. Berke G. The CTL's kiss of death. *Cell* 1995;81:9.
323. Henkart PA. Lymphocyte-mediated cytotoxicity: two pathways and multiple effector molecules. *Immunity* 1994;1:343.
324. Crispe IN. Fatal interactions: Fas-induced apoptosis of mature T cells. *Immunity* 1994;1:347.
325. Nagata S, Golstein P. The Fas death factor. *Science* 1995;267:1449.
326. Kojima H, Shinohara N, Hanaoka S, et al. Two distinct pathways of specific killing revealed by perforin mutant cytotoxic T lymphocytes. *Immunity* 1994;1:357.
327. Walsh CM, Matloubian M, Liu CC, et al. Immune function in mice lacking the perforin gene. *Proc Natl Acad Sci U S A* 1994;91:10854.
328. Lowin B, Hahne M, Mattmann C, Tschopp J. Cytolytic T-cell cytotoxicity is mediated through perforin and Fas lytic pathways. *Nature* 1994;370:650.
329. Kagi D, Vignaux F, Ledermann B, et al. Fas and perforin pathways as major mechanisms of T cell–mediated cytotoxicity. *Science* 1994;265:528.
330. Henkart PA, Williams MS, Nakajima H. Degranulating cytotoxic lymphocytes inflict multiple damage pathways on target cells. *Curr Top Microbiol Immunol* 1995;198:75.
331. Kagi D, Ledermann B, Burki K, Zinkernagel RM, Hengartner H. Molecular mechanisms of lymphocyte-mediated cytotoxicity and their role in immunological protection and pathogenesis in vivo. *Annu Rev Immunol* 1996;14:207.
332. van den Broek ME, Kagi D, Ossendorp F, et al. Decreased tumor surveillance in perforin-deficient mice. *J Exp Med* 1996;184:1781.
333. Crispe IN. Death and destruction of activated T lymphocytes. *Immunol Res* 1999;19:143.
334. Alderson MR, Lynch DH. Receptors and ligands that mediate activation-induced death of T cells. *Springer Semin Immunopathol* 1998;19:289.
335. Lanier LL, Phillips JH. NK cell recognition of major histocompatibility complex class I molecules. *Semin Immunol* 1995;7:75.
336. Bottino C, Vitale M, Pende D, Biassoni R, Moretta A. Receptors for HLA class I molecules in human NK cells. *Semin Immunol* 1995;7:67.
337. Paul NL, Ruddle NH. Lymphotoxin. *Annu Rev Immunol* 1988;6:407.
338. Aggarwal BB, Vilcek J. *Tumor necrosis factors: structure, function, and mechanism of action.* New York: Marcel Dekker Inc, 1992.
339. Beutler B. *Tumor necrosis factors: the molecules and their emerging role in medicine.* New York: Raven Press, 1992.
340. Ratner A, Clark WR. Role of TNF-alpha in CD8+ cytotoxic T lymphocyte–mediated lysis. *J Immunol* 1993;150:4303.
341. Ashkenazi A, Pai RC, Fong S, et al. Safety and antitumor activity of recombinant soluble Apo2 ligand. *J Clin Invest* 1999;104:155.
342. Herberman RB. *NK cells and other natural effector cells.* New York: Academic Press, 1982.
343. Trinchieri G. Biology of natural killer cells. *Adv Immunol* 1989;47:187.
344. Moretta L, Ciccone E, Mingari MC, Biassoni R, Moretta A. Human natural killer cells: origin, clonality, specificity, and receptors. *Adv Immunol* 1994;55:341.
345. Whiteside TL, Herberman RB. The role of natural killer cells in immune surveillance of cancer. *Curr Opin Immunol* 1995;7:704.
346. Lanier LL, Phillips JH. Natural killer cells. *Curr Opin Immunol* 1992;4:38.
347. Berke G. The functions and mechanisms of action of cytolytic lymphocytes. In: Paul WE, ed. *Fundamental immunology,* 3rd ed. New York: Raven Press, 1993:965.
348. Henkart PA, Hayes MP, Shiver JW. The granule exocytosis model for lymphocyte cytotoxicity and its relevance to target cell DNA breakdown. In: Sitkovsky MV, Henkart P, eds. *Cytotoxic cells: recognition, effector function, generation, and methods.* Boston: Birkhauser, 1993:153.
349. Yagita H, Nakata M, Kawasaki A, Shinkai Y, Okumura K. Role of perforin in lymphocyte-mediated cytolysis. *Adv Immunol* 1992;51:215.
350. Shi L, Kraut RP, Aebersold R, Greenberg AH. A natural killer cell granule protein that induces DNA fragmentation and apoptosis. *J Exp Med* 1992;175:553.
351. Doherty PC. Cell-mediated cytotoxicity. *Cell* 1993;75:607.
352. Kagi D, Ledermann B, Burki K, et al. Cytotoxicity mediated by T cells and natural killer cells is greatly impaired in perforin-deficient mice. *Nature* 1994;369:31.
353. Arase H, Arase N, Saito T. Fas-mediated cytotoxicity by freshly isolated natural killer cells. *J Exp Med* 1995;181:1235.
354. Kashii Y, Giorda R, Herberman RB, Whiteside TL, Vujanovic NL. Constitutive expression and role of the TNF family ligands in apoptotic killing of tumor cells by human NK cells. *J Immunol* 1999;163:5358.
355. Zamai L, Ahmad M, Bennett IM, et al. Natural killer (NK) cell–mediated cytotoxicity: differential use of TRAIL and Fas ligand by immature and mature primary human NK cells. *J Exp Med* 1998;188:2375.
356. Yokoyama WM. Natural killer cell receptors specific for major histocompatibility complex class I molecules. *Proc Natl Acad Sci U S A* 1995;92:3081.
357. Gumperz JE, Parham P. The enigma of the natural killer cell. *Nature* 1995;378:245.
358. Long EO. Regulation of immune responses through inhibitory receptors. *Annu Rev Immunol* 1999;17:875.
359. Moretta A, Bottino C, Millo R, Biassoni R. HLA-specific and non-HLA-specific human NK receptors. *Curr Top Microbiol Immunol* 1999;244:69.
360. Yokoyama WM. Natural killer cell receptors. *Curr Opin Immunol* 1998;10:298.
361. Lanier LL. NK cell receptors. *Annu Rev Immunol* 1998;16:359.
362. Parham P. Virtual reality in the MHC. *Immunol Rev* 1999;167:5.
363. Colonna M. Specificity and function of immunoglobulin superfamily NK cell inhibitory and stimulatory receptors. *Immunol Rev* 1997;155:127.
364. Daëron M, Vivier E. Immunoreceptor tyrosine–based inhibition motifs. *Curr Top Microbiol Immunol* 1997;244:1.
365. Karre K. How to recognize a foreign submarine. *Immunol Rev* 1997;155:5.
366. Porcelli SA, Modlin RL. The CD1 system: antigen-presenting molecules for T cell recognition of lipids and glycolipids. *Annu Rev Immunol* 1999;17:297.
367. Grimm EA, Mazumder A, Zhang HZ, Rosenberg SA. The lymphokine activated killer cell phenomenon: lysis of natural killer–resistant fresh solid tumor cells by interleukin 2–activated autologous human peripheral blood lymphocytes. *J Exp Med* 1982;155:1823.
368. Ortaldo JR, Mason A, Overton R. Lymphokine-activated killer cells. Analysis of progenitors and effectors. *J Exp Med* 1986;164:1193.
369. Phillips JH, Lanier LL. Dissection of the lymphokine-activated killer phenomenon: relative contribution of peripheral blood natural killer cells and T lymphocytes to cytolysis. *J Exp Med* 1986;164:814.
370. Fidler IJ, Schroit AJ. Recognition and destruction of neoplastic cells by activated macrophages: discrimination of altered self. *Biochim Biophys Acta* 1988;948:151.
371. Drysdale BE, Agarwal S, Shin HS. Macrophage-mediated tumoricidal activity: mechanisms of activation and cytotoxicity. *Prog Allergy* 1988;40:111.
372. Duerksen-Hughes PJ, Gooding LR. Macrophage-mediated cytotoxicity. In: Sitkovsky MV, Henkart P, ed. *Cytotoxic cells: recognition, effector function, generation, and methods.* Boston: Birkhauser, 1993:439.
373. Adams DO, Hamilton TA. Macrophages as destructive cells in host defense. In: Gallin JI, Golstein IM, Snyderman R, ed. *Inflammation: basic principles and clinical correlates,* 2nd ed. New York: Raven Press, 1992:637.
374. Fauve RM. Fiftieth forum in immunology. Macrophages and cancer. *Ann Inst Pasteur Immunol* 1993;144:265.
375. Bogdan C, Nathan C. Modulation of macrophage function by transforming growth factor beta, interleukin-4, and interleukin-10. *Ann NY Acad Sci* 1993;685:713.
376. Williams MA, Newland AC, Kelsey SM. The potential for monocyte-mediated immunotherapy during infection and malignancy: I. Apoptosis induction and cytotoxic mechanisms. *Leuk Lymphoma* 1999;34:1.

377. Knapp W, Rieber P, Dorken B, et al. Towards a better definition of human leucocyte surface molecules. *Immunol Today* 1989;10:253.
378. Hamilton TA, Adams DO. Mechanisms of macrophage-mediated tumor injury. In: Den Otter W, Ruitenberg EJ, ed. *Tumor immunology: mechanisms, diagnosis, therapy*. Amsterdam: Elsevier, 1987:89.
379. Nathan CF. Secretory products of macrophages. *J Clin Invest* 1987;79:319.
380. Mantovani A. Tumor-associated macrophages in neoplastic progression: a paradigm for the in vivo function of chemokines. *Lab Invest* 1994;71:5.
381. Fahey JL. Antibodies and immunoglobulins: I. Structure and function. *JAMA* 1965;194:183.
382. Fahey JL. Antibodies and immunoglobulins: II. Normal development and changes in disease. *JAMA* 1965;194:255.
383. Frazier JK, Capra JD. Immunoglobulins: structure and function. In: Paul WE, ed. *Fundamental immunology*, 4th ed. Philadelphia: Lippincott-Raven Publishers, 1999:37.
384. Kohler G, Milstein C. Continuous cultures of fused cells secreting antibody of predefined specificity. *Nature* 1975;256:495.
385. Ritter MA, Ladyman HM, eds. *Monoclonal antibodies: production, engineering and clinical application*. Cambridge, UK: Cambridge University Press, 1995.
386. Goding JW. *Monoclonal antibodies: principles and practice*, 3rd ed. London: Academic Press, 1996.
387. Potter M. Neoplastic development in B-lymphocytes. *Carcinogenesis* 1990;11:1.
388. Burrows PD, Cooper MD. B cell development and differentiation. *Curr Opin Immunol* 1997;9:239.
389. Melchers F, Rolink A. B-lymphocyte development and biology. In: Paul WE, ed. *Fundamental immunology*, 4th ed. Philadelphia: Lippincott-Raven Publishers, 1999:183.
390. Küppers R, Klein U, Hansmann ML, Rajewsky K. Cellular origin of human B-cell lymphomas. *N Engl J Med* 1999;341:1520.
391. Kantor AB, Herzenberg LA. Origin of murine B cell lineages. *Annu Rev Immunol* 1993;11:501.
392. DeFranco AL. B-lymphocyte activation. In: Paul WE, ed. *Fundamental immunology*, 4th ed. Philadelphia: Lippincott-Raven Publishers, 1999:225.
393. Benschop RJ, Cambier JC. B cell development: signal transduction by antigen receptors and their surrogates. *Curr Opin Immunol* 1999;11:143.
394. Medina KL, Strasser A, Kincade PW. Estrogen influences the differentiation, proliferation, and survival of early B-lineage precursors. *Blood* 2000;95:2059.
395. Nemazee D. Receptor editing in B cells. *Adv Immunol* 2000;74:89.
396. Melchers F, Rolink A, Grawunder U, et al. Positive and negative selection events during B lymphopoiesis. *Curr Opin Immunol* 1995;7:214.
397. Nossal GJ. The Florey lecture, 1986. The regulatory biology of antibody formation. *Proc R Soc Lond [B] Biol Sci* 1986;228:225.
398. Clark EA, Ledbetter JA. How B and T cells talk to each other. *Nature* 1994;367:425.
399. Bonnefoy JY, Noelle RJ. The CD40.CD40L interaction—all things to all immunologists. *Research in immunology*, vol 145. Paris: Elsevier Science, 1994.
400. Parker DC. T cell–dependent B cell activation. *Annu Rev Immunol* 1993;11:331.
401. Thorbecke GJ, Amin AR, Tsiagbe VK. Biology of germinal centers in lymphoid tissue. *FASEB J* 1994;8:832.
402. Sad S, Marcotte R, Mosmann TR. Cytokine-induced differentiation of precursor mouse CD8+ T cells into cytotoxic CD8+ T cells secreting Th1 or Th2 cytokines. *Immunity* 1995;2:271.
403. Stavnezer J. Antibody class switching. *Adv Immunol* 1996;61:79.
404. Snapper CM, Finkelman FD. Immunoglobulin class switching. Paul WE, ed. *Fundamental immunology*, 4th ed. Philadelphia: Lippincott-Raven Publishers, 1999:831.
405. Neuberger MS, Milstein C. Somatic hypermutation. *Curr Opin Immunol* 1995;7:248.
406. Storb U. Progress in understanding the mechanism and consequences of somatic hypermutation. *Immunol Rev* 1998;162:5.
407. Klein U, Goossens T, Fischer M, et al. Somatic hypermutation in normal and transformed human B cells. *Immunol Rev* 1998;162:261.
408. Mond JJ, Lees A, Snapper CM. T cell-independent antigens type 2. *Annu Rev Immunol* 1995;13:655.
409. Bretscher P, Cohn M. A theory of self-nonself discrimination. *Science* 1970;169:1042.
410. Goodnow CC. Balancing immunity and tolerance: deleting and tuning lymphocyte repertoires. *Proc Natl Acad Sci U S A* 1996;93:2264.
411. Schwartz RH. Immunological tolerance. In: Paul WE, ed. *Fundamental immunology*, 4th ed. Philadelphia: Lippincott-Raven Publishers, 1999:701.
412. Carroll MC. The role of complement in B cell activation and tolerance. *Adv Immunol* 2000;74:61.

PART 2

PRINCIPLES OF ONCOLOGY

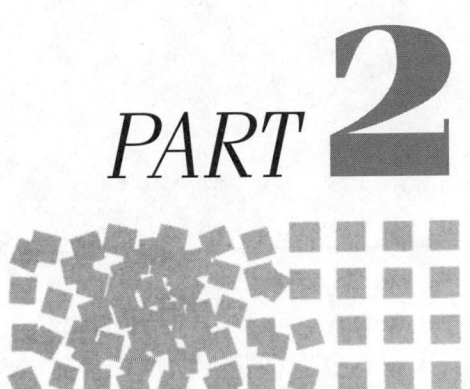

Mazin B. Qumsiyeh
Peining Li

CHAPTER 5

Molecular Biology of Cancer: Cytogenetics

Cytogenetic testing is one of the fastest-growing areas of testing in oncology. In most cytogenetic laboratories, cancer cases have come to constitute more than 50% of cytogenetic testing done. It is difficult to estimate the total testing being done. A recent survey by the Association of Genetic Technologists reported that more than 95,000 cancer studies were performed in the United States in 1998 (reported by 202 responding laboratories from 243 laboratories surveyed). Because large commercial laboratories did not report their numbers, one would estimate that the total number of such tests in the United States is close to 200,000 per year. This number is, however, rapidly rising as clinicians are becoming aware of the prognostic and diagnostic value of chromosome studies. In this chapter, we do not review the molecular cytogenetic knowledge in particular diseases nor discuss the biologic effect of cancer chromosomal abnormalities (e.g., oncogene activation or tumor suppressor genes), because these are covered in detail in separate chapters. We do, however, provide an overview of basic cancer cytogenetics covering terminology, chromosome structure, mechanisms of formation of chromosomal abnormalities, and new technical developments in the field, and cover some genetic topics not covered in other chapters. The continuous advances in techniques of molecular cytogenetics in the last decade are emphasized.

HISTORY OF CANCER CYTOGENETICS

Boveri[1] established the modern paradigm that mutations in somatic cells cause the uncontrolled cell proliferation called *cancer*. The modern era of human cytogenetics confirmed this view. This era was ushered in with the simultaneous publications by Tjio and Levan[2] of good-quality, unbanded human karyotypes showing 46 chromosomes. Technical improvements were the key to the development of clinical cytogenetics. Within a few years (1956 to 1960), researchers identified specific chromosomal abnormalities associated with congenital abnormalities (e.g., Down, Turner's, and Klinefelter's syndromes) and with cancer. The opening salvo in cancer cytogenetics was the demonstration of the Philadelphia chromosome as associated with chronic myelogenous leukemia (CML).[3] The development of banding techniques in 1969 and 1970 allowed further characterization of this aberration as a balanced translocation involving chromosomes 9 and 22.[4] In the last three decades, the knowledge of human cancer cytogenetics has expanded significantly with the addition of new molecular methodologies, such as *in situ* hybridization (discussed later in Fluorescence *In Situ* Hybridization). The field now is best described as *molecular cytogenetics.*

CHROMOSOME STRUCTURE AND FUNCTION

Each normal human somatic cell nucleus has 46 chromosomes, 23 chromosomes being maternal and the other 23 being paternal in origin. This diploid chromosome number is reduced to 23 (haploid) during meiosis, a specialized nuclear division during gametogenesis in the ovaries and testis. At conception, haploid cells from each parent combine to form a new diploid cell (zygote), which then divides via mitosis (somatic nuclear division), ultimately creating the fetus. Errors in mitosis or meiosis can lead to pathogenetic changes (discussed later in Numeric Abnormalities). Genetic instructions are encoded in DNA. DNA replicates during the S phase of the cell cycle and condenses during the prophase of mitosis (somatogenesis) and meiosis (gametogenesis). During metaphase, the characteristic chromosome structures can be observed: Each chromosome represents two chromatids joined at an area of constriction known as the *centromere.*

LOWER-ORDER CHROMATIN STRUCTURE

The human genome consists of approximately 6.8×10^9 base pairs (bp) of DNA in each diploid cell. If stretched end to end, this length of DNA would span 2 meters. In a normal diploid human cell, this DNA is packaged into 44 autosomes and the two sex chromosomes in a compact nucleus. The first level of packaging involves a wrapping of 200 bp in two turns around a histone core, resulting in the complexes called *nucleosomes* with a diameter of 10 nm. This basic DNA fiber then is further condensed in a 30-nm-diameter spiral called a *solenoid fiber.* The solenoid in turn forms larger fibers that are visible with the light microscope as chromatin fibers. Chromatin loops of 60 to 90 kb are anchored at scaffold attachment regions. These loops also appear to represent functional replication domains called *replicons.*

HIGHER-ORDER CHROMATIN STRUCTURE

The development of various banding techniques in the period from 1969 to 1971 revealed that various chromosomal regions respond differently to biochemical and physical treatments. This suggested that there is a higher-order structure for human chromosomes. One of the first recognized divisions of chromatin is into the categories of euchromatin and heterochromatin. Heterochromatin was the material that stained dark (heteropyknotic) with various staining techniques, giving rise to chromocenters in interphase. We now know that this dark staining is a result of the more condensed DNA structure in these regions picking up more DNA dyes.

There are two types of heterochromatin. *Constitutive heterochromatin* is chromatin that is constitutionally condensed in all cells and cell types and is composed of highly repeated sequences that can be detected in cytogenetic preparations using the technique of C-banding. In humans, constitutive heterochromatin is found at the centromeric regions of all chromosomes as well as in the pericentromeric areas of chromosomes 1, 9, and 16 and in the distal long arm of the Y chromosome. *Facultative heterochromatin* can switch from condensed to decondensed and vice versa. An example of the latter type is the inactivation of the X chromosome in female cells for gene dosage compensation. Meiotic pairing has been shown to require heterochromatin homology and to be sensitive to repeat numbers in both male and female *Drosophila.*[5] Banding is produced along the chromosomal length of euchromatin because of both structural and functional differences in light and dark G-bands (Table 5-1).

TELOMERES AND TELOMERASE

A double-strand break in DNA is susceptible to recombination and fusion and also triggers cell-cycle arrest mediated by p53. Further, DNA replication, as it is now understood, would result in shortening of the ends of replicating linear DNA owing to the mechanisms of function of the DNA replication proteins. Thus, there is an obvious need for telomeres to be unique. Examination of human cells as well as cells from other vertebrates showed that the ends of chromosomes are capped by a simple repeat of six nucleotides (TTAGGG). The telomere sequence is synthesized by a specialized DNA polymerase called *telomerase* (reviewed in ref. 6). The telomerase function includes an enzymatic protein component as well as an RNA component acting as a primer. Telomerase is responsible for programmed end healing *in vivo* after breaks and in maintaining telomere length. The telomeres further bind other specific proteins that appear to function in protecting the ends of the chromosomes from recombination, nuclease attack, activation of cell-cycle checkpoints, and end-to-end fusions.

Hayflick and Moorehead[7] recognized that fibroblast cells grown in culture have limited replicative potential (50 to 100 cell divisions). This Hayflick phenomenon is now understood as explained by age-related deterioration of telomeres.[8] In the

TABLE 5-1. Functional Significance of Chromosomal Banding Patterns

	R-Bands (Light G-Bands)	*G-Bands (Dark R-Bands)*
Quinacrine	Dull	Bright
Heteropyknosis in prometaphase	Negative	More condensed
Replication in S phase	Early	Late
Mitotic condensation (to metaphase)	Fast	Slow
Chiasmata and break frequency	High	Low
DNA base composition	GC-rich	AT-rich
Repeats	SINE	LINE
	Alu (humans)	L1
	B1, B2 in mouse	—
Gene regulation	CpG islands	TATA boxes
Common genes	Housekeeping + some TS	TS

L1, a mouse long interspersed element; LINE, long interspersed nuclear element; SINE, short interspersed nuclear element; TS, tissue specific.
(Modified from R Drouin, GP Holmquist, CL Richer. High-resolution replication bands compared with morphologic G- and R-bands. *Adv Hum Genet* 1994;22:47.)

absence of telomerase, the ends of the chromosomes would shorten gradually (by 25 to 200 bp in each replication) owing to the end-replication problem. It is believed that in normal cells, this deterioration of telomeres can eventually lead to cell-cycle arrest and, thus, cellular senescence. The reverse is also true; it was shown that telomerase reactivation is important in immortalization of cell lines and in cancer development and metastasis.[9,10] The technique developed by Kim et al.,[9] called *telomeric repeat amplification protocol*, is used, with several available commercial and other modifications, to detect telomerase activity in cell extracts.

It is now recognized that telomerase activity is found in the majority of primary human tumors.[11] There is the potential for development of novel cancer therapies by regulating telomerase or proteins that in turn regulate telomerase levels in cancer cells. Prognostic value for examining telomerase activity in certain cancers is being discussed. An example of this is a significantly worse prognosis in meningiomas with telomerase activity versus those without it.[12] One complicating factor is that there are other pathways for developing "immortality" besides telomere maintenance or for maintaining telomeres without detectable telomerase activity (e.g., involving recombination). In fact, some human cancer cells even at metastasis have decreased telomeres and are susceptible to end-to-end attachments in metaphase. This phenomenon was recognized very early in human cytogenetics as "sticky" chromosomal ends. This reduction in telomere length is usually attributed to the increased cell division (most cancers start from a single cell with increased proliferative capacity). Further, genetically engineered mice lacking telomerase RNA lose their telomeres but are still capable of developing tumors.[13]

Some human premature aging syndromes result from decreased replicative capacity of the cells. In the example of Hutchison-Gilford progeria, telomeres are markedly reduced, resulting in decreased replicative capacity. Similar findings are reported in Down syndrome, which predisposes to premature senescence of the immune system as well as predisposition to early Alzheimer's disease.[14] Other nuclear and mitochondrial genes seem to influence aging. For example, Werner and Bloom syndromes are characterized by mutations in DNA helicases.[15]

CENTROMERES

The centromeric DNA is vital to the attachment of specialized proteins to form a functioning structure called the *kinetochore.* Kinetochores are responsible for the segregation of the chromatids to the opposite poles of the dividing nucleus during anaphase of mitosis and the segregation of the homologous chromosomes during anaphase of the first meiotic division. The centromere provides a useful landmark along the chromosome axis, dividing each chromosome into two segments or arms: a short arm (known as the *p arm* from the French *petit*) and a long arm (the *q arm*, named after the next letter in the alphabet). By convention, chromosomes are identified by their centromeres. Thus, a derivative chromosome, mostly chromosome 3 material but only one centromere of chromosome 21, is a derivative chromosome 21. Human chromosomes are normally monocentric. Cancer cells occasionally have dicentric and even polycentric chromosomes. Chromosomes are classified by their centromere positions and size into seven groups, A through G (Fig. 5-1). Metacentric chromosomes have equal or almost equal arms (centromere at or almost at the middle of the chromosome). Acrocentrics (chromosomes 13, 14, 15, 20, 21) have a very tiny short arm carrying a satellite of repeat sequences and the nucleolar organizer region and the DNA coding for recombinant RNA (rRNA). A *submetacentric* is a chromosome wherein the short arm is less than one-half the length of the long arm. Centromeres can be detected using antikinetochore antibodies (e.g., from serum of patients with combined calcinosis cutis, Raynaud's phenomenon, esophageal dysfunction, sclerodactyly, and telangiectasia) as well as using alpha satellite DNA probes.

CYTOGENETIC METHODS

SPECIMEN REQUIREMENTS

Most cancer cytogenetic testing involves bone marrow for hematologic malignancies. However, solid-tumor cytogenetics is likely to be the next area of increased clinical relevance, especially with the new techniques of molecular cytogenetics. For hematologic malignancies, a bone marrow aspirate is the preferred sample, although success can also be achieved in some difficult cases using core biopsies. Peripheral blood samples can be submitted if there are circulating blast cells. A lymph node biopsy may also be used in cases with lymph node involvement. Technologies have developed such that even fine-needle aspirates can be tested for cytogenetic abnormalities. Other types of specimens can be studied, including infiltrates, pleural effusion, spinal fluid, and basically any tissue that may contain dividing cancer cells.

It is important to provide clinical information on specimens submitted for testing. This helps to select appropriate culture and analysis procedures and, in some cases, to suggest additional tests. Examples include (1) the need to stimulate cultures with B-cell mitogens (e.g., Epstein-Barr virus, lipopolysaccharide, or 12-O-tetradecanoyl-phorbol-13-acetate) in B-cell malignancies; (2) the importance of longer culture time in some myeloid disorders [e.g., for detection of t(15;17) in acute myelogenous leukemia (AML) M3]; and (3) offering fluorescence *in situ* hybridization (FISH) tests in cases of certain translocations should the routine cytogenetics prove negative [e.g., inv(16) in M4e or t(9;22) in CML]. It is recommended that cytogenetic studies be performed at diagnosis and for follow-up of cancer progression. Occasionally, failure to obtain results can be due to the fact that a patient is under treatment (treatments are intended to block cell division). Because the study requires viable cells, specimen handling is important in cytogenetics. Drawing of a bone marrow or a blood sample should be performed using heparinized (sodium heparin) and sterile collection tools and containers. For bone marrow aspirates, volumes can be from 0.25 to 1.0 mL; for blood, 3 to 5 mL is adequate. However, small specimens can also be processed; the best approach is to check with the laboratory.

BANDING TECHNIQUES (CLASSIC CYTOGENETICS)

Chromosome analysis requires examining cells in the process of mitosis in which the chromosome structure is most clearly defined (most commonly cells in late prophase or early metaphase). Spontaneously dividing tissues, such as occur in hematopoiesis or in cancer, would be expected to provide mitotic cells for analysis even in a direct harvest of the material submitted. In practice, the quality of such preparations is suboptimal, and cell culture may be required in some cases. The time required for culture and analysis varies, depending on the tissue sampled and specific testing requested. Average turnaround time

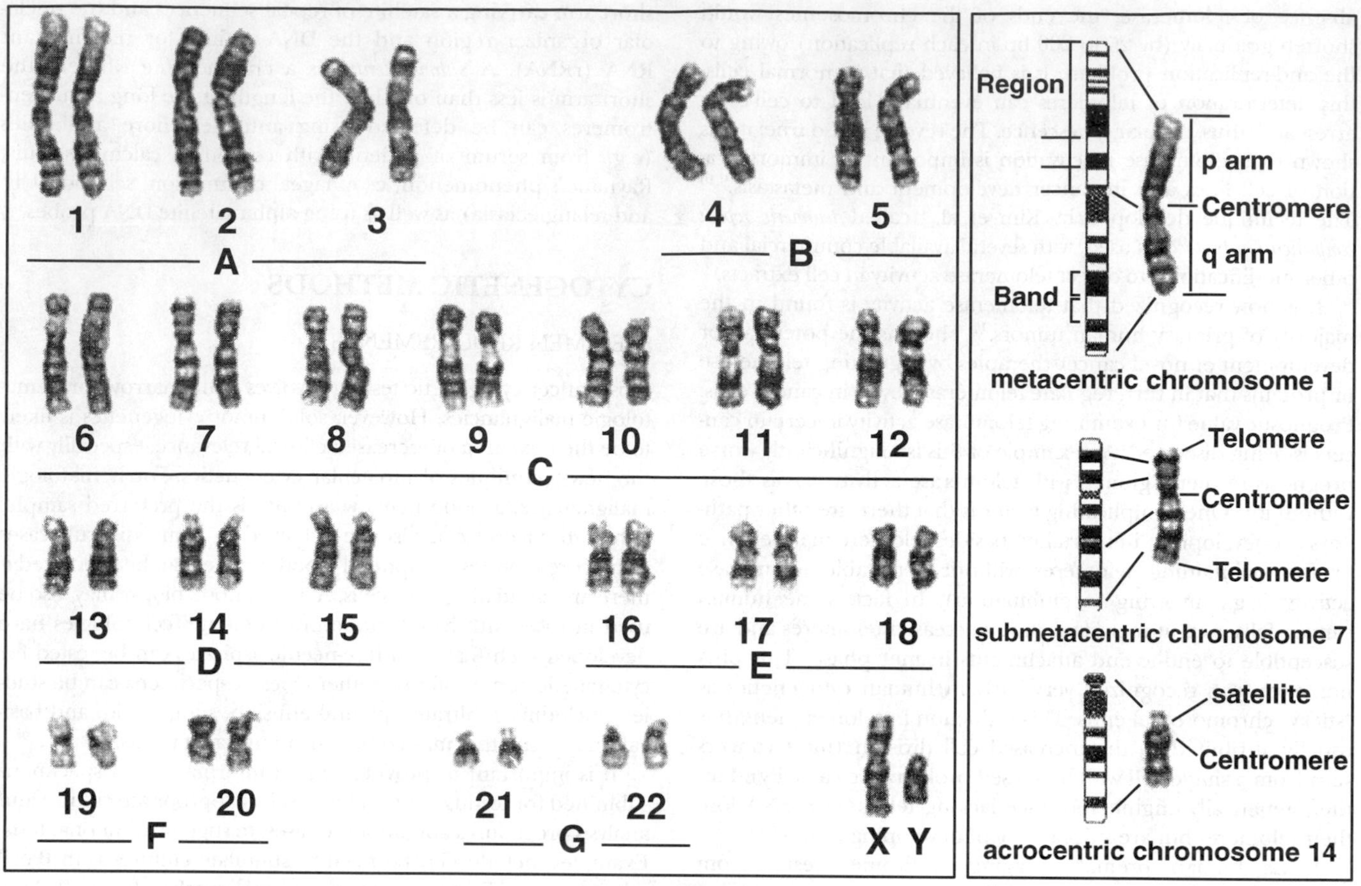

FIGURE 5-1. Chromosome numbering and nomenclature. The figure illustrates a normal male karyotype. Chromosomes are numbered according to size and centromere position (left panel). Chromosomes are classified into groups based on size and centromere position and, within groups, by banding patterns. Groups A (1–3), B (4,5), C (6–12, X), D (13–15), E (16–18), F (19–20), G (21, 22, Y). Examples of a metacentric, a submetacentric, and an acrocentric chromosome (right panel).

for studies can be as short as 2 to 3 days for bone marrow, 4 to 7 days for blood, and up to 3 weeks for some solid-tissue biopsies. Chromosomes are prepared on glass slides and are treated by digestion (e.g., with trypsin) and then stained to produce a banding pattern. The most commonly used staining techniques are G-banding and R-banding, which produce characteristic staining or banding patterns for each human chromosome. These techniques, in combination with the physical chromosomal structure, allow for the identification of individual chromosomes.

FLUORESCENCE *IN SITU* HYBRIDIZATION

Mammalian DNA is a double-stranded helix with a phosphate and sugar backbone and hydrogen bonds linking the nucleotides cytosine (C) to guanine (G) and adenine (A) to thymine (T). Under appropriate conditions, the double-stranded DNA can be resolved to single strands, and the complementary single-stranded DNA can be reannealed to a double-stranded helix. The property of DNA strand complementarity is used in various molecular methods involving DNA hybridization. By merging the nucleic acid hybridization onto metaphase chromosome spreads, FISH has established a solid technical foundation for the field of molecular cytogenetics. The principle of FISH is the hybridization of a DNA probe with incorporated reporter molecule to its complementary chromosomal locus, followed by detection of the hapten using fluorescent microscopy, usually with computer-assisted imaging analysis. A routine FISH protocol involves multistep procedures. The reporter molecule can be a protein, such as biotin or digoxigenin, or a fluorescent molecule, such as rhodamine or fluorosiothiocyanate. Incorporation of the reporter molecule in the probe is performed using nick translation or primer extension with labeled nucleotides. The labeled DNA probe and targeted specimen are treated to denature double-stranded DNA to single strands and then are allowed to hybridize for 2 to 24 hours (depending on specimen and probe).

FISH analysis extends routine cytogenetic banding methods by resolving ambiguous diagnosis and providing a new tool to diagnose submicroscopic abnormalities. FISH is a relatively simple, fast, and reliable procedure. Depending on the sequence complexity of labeled DNA probe and the content of tested specimen, FISH has variable signal sensitivity and spatial resolution. Hybridization probes range from very small DNA fragments (500 bp) to large yeast artificial chromosomes or bacterial artificial chromosomes. The spatial resolution measured by the closest separable signals could range from 5 Mbp on metaphase chromosomes to 100 Kbp on interphase chromatins. The most important features of FISH techniques are its applicability to different specimens and its use for simultaneous detection of several targets using multiple probes. Specimens that can be used for FISH include peripheral blood cells, cultured cell lines, bone

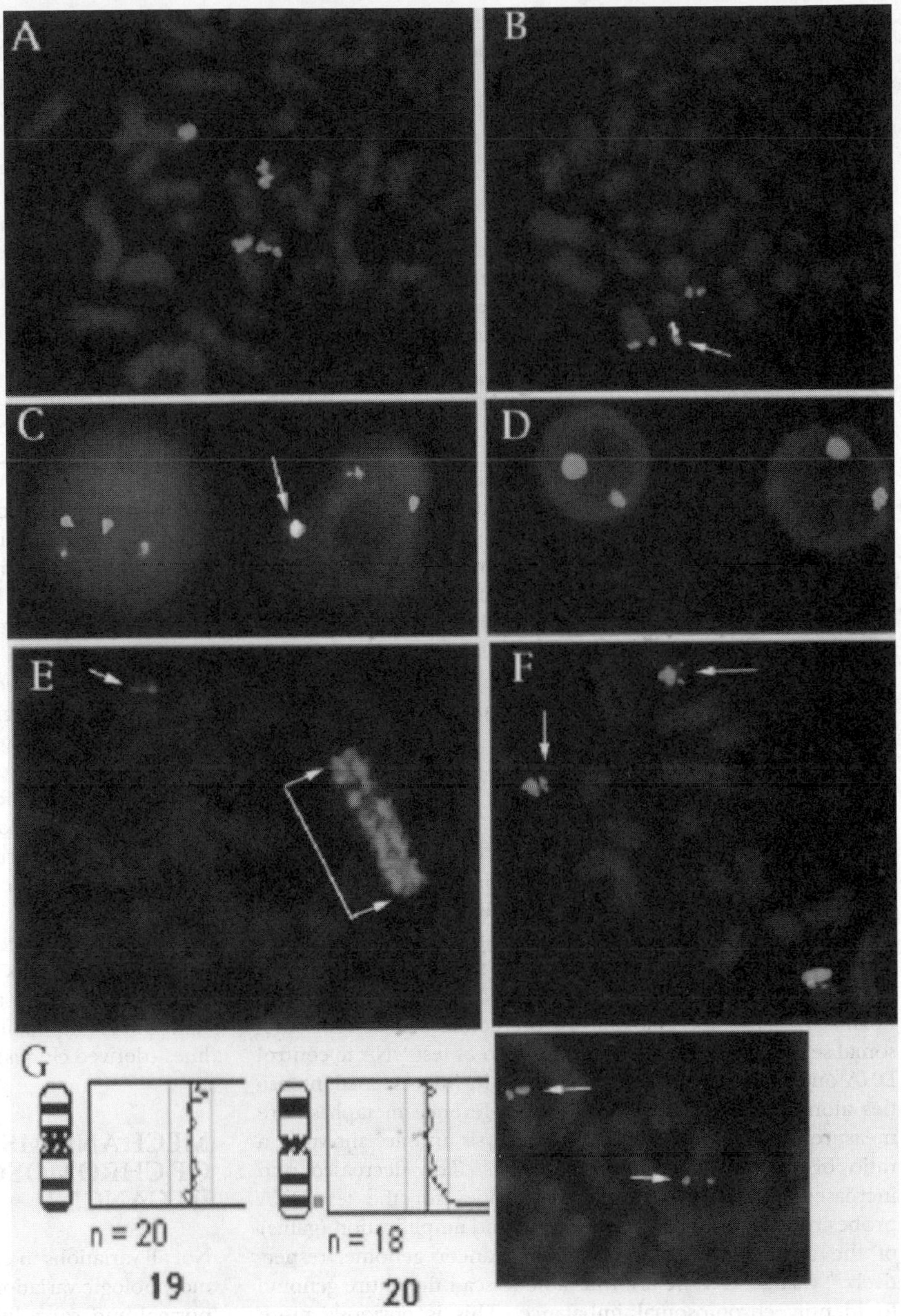

FIGURE 5-2. Examples of application of molecular cytogenetics. **A:** Fluorescence *in situ* hybridization (FISH) using probes for ETV6 gene at 12p13 (*green*) and CBFA2 (AML1) gene at 21q22 (*red*). These are useful probes for the detection of the t(12;21), a very common translocation in childhood acute lymphocytic leukemia. **B:** FISH using probes for BCR at 22q11.2 (*green*) and ABL at 9q34 in a case of chronic myelogenous leukemia. Arrow shows the Philadelphia chromosome with fused signals. **C:** Using same probes as in **B**, showing the ability to detect a fusion in the interphase nucleus on the right (*arrow*). **D:** Use of repetitive probes for X (*red*) and Y (*green*) in sex-mismatched bone marrow transplant. **E:** Illustration of FISH use in gene amplification using a probe for c-myc on 8q24. The probe labels the distal 8q in this case (*arrow*) plus an amplified area on the homologous 8q (*between arrows*). **F:** Use of FISH to identify two marker chromosomes (*arrows*) as derived from chromosome 15 (probes for 15p in green and proximal 15q in red). **G:** Comparative genomic hybridization profile of two chromosomes (19 and 20) from a case of melanoma showing amplification of the distal end of 20q. FISH using BTAK(STK1 5), a gene that hybridizes to 20q and is amplified in a number of cancers showing normal signal on metaphases from normal blood cells. (See Color Fig. 5-2.)

marrow cells, paraffin-embedded tissue sections, and frozen tissues. Specific applications of FISH include:

1. Delineation of chromosomal numeric abnormalities. For example, interphase FISH has been used for detection of trisomy 8 in myeloid disorders, trisomy 7 in prostate cancer,[16] and trisomy 12 in chronic lymphocytic leukemia,[17,18] and ovarian cancers.[19]
2. Detection of specific translocations, such as those involving immunoglobulin genes in lymphomas, and other translocation seen in leukemias (Fig. 5-2; see Color Fig. 5-2)
3. Determining degree of engraftment after sex-mismatched bone marrow and cord blood transplantations (see Fig. 5-2*D*; see Color Fig. 5-2*D*)
4. Determining the origin of specific translocations and marker chromosomes using paint probes in cases where G-banding cannot identify the origin (see Fig. 5-2*F*; see Color Fig. 5-2*F*)
5. Revealing cases with gene amplification (e.g., see Fig. 5-2*E*; see Color Fig. 5-2*E*).

MULTICOLOR FISH AND SPECTRAL KARYOTYPING

In the last few years, new development of FISH allowed for detection of different chromosomes using probes combinatorially labeled with several fluorescent dyes. One method of analysis of this is to image each fluorophore separately and then to allow a computer to translate the different color combinations to values or ratios that are then pseudocolored, resulting in a karyotype with 24 colors for each of the human chromosomes (1 through 22, X, and Y). This multicolor FISH technique can be used to identify derivative and marker chromosomes. A similar technique, named *spectral karyotyping*, also was introduced by using a combination of epifluorescence microscopy, CCD (cooled-coupled device) imaging, and Fourier spectroscopic measurement.[20,21] Multicolor FISH and spectral karyotyping cannot detect intrachromosomal anomalies, such as inversions, still require metaphases from the test specimen of good quality, and are limited in resolution to abnormalities involving one or more bands at a 450-band level.

PRIMED *IN SITU* LABELING

Primed *in situ* labeling is a method combining complementary DNA hybridization and *in situ* primer extension.[22] The method consists of annealing DNA primers to their complementary sequences on fixed chromosomes, followed by a primer extension reaction catalyzed by DNA polymerase to incorporate labeled nucleotides and then visualization of synthesized DNA by image analysis. Primed *in situ* labeling has been used in interphase analysis of aneuploidy in cancer cell lines[23] and in the detection and sizing of telomeric repeat DNA *in situ*.[24]

COMPARATIVE GENOMIC HYBRIDIZATION

Comparative genomic hybridization (CGH) is a molecular cytogenetic approach with potential for detecting chromosomal imbalance without the need for dividing cells. The method entails isolating DNA from a test sample (which can be a few cells from any source, including fixed material and even paraffin sections), labeling this test DNA with one color, and cohybridizing this DNA with a control DNA labeled with another color to normal metaphases. The ratio of the colors on each chromosomal segment will, thus, reflect the ratio of test DNA to control DNA on that segment. The differences in fluorescence intensities along the chromosomes on the reference metaphase are measured through a digital image analysis and are shown as a ratio of the two distinct fluorophores. The decreased and increased ratios of fluorescent intensities for the test DNA probes represent the deletion (losses) and amplification (gains) of the chromosomal regions in the cancer genome, respectively.[25] Using CGH, we are thus able to scan the entire genome to identify chromosomal imbalance. This is obviously more involved than FISH and requires use of specific software to allow calculation of color ratios along each chromosome.

The CGH technique provides a genomic fingerprint at a megabase level of resolution for detecting gains and losses of DNA sequences.[26] Therefore, it is particularly appropriate for cancer studies to identify recurrent chromosomal gains and losses, which serve as starting points for the characterization and isolation of pathogenetically relevant genes, such as oncogene amplifications or the deletion of segments containing a tumor suppressor gene. CGH could also be used to detect chromosomal imbalances for monitoring tumor progression and providing prognostic relevance, to analyze markers of genomic instability, and to identify clonal differences within a specimen.[16,21,27] A recent review by Knuutila et al.[28] showed rapid adoption of these techniques in diverse neoplasms, including detecting abnormalities of 1p32-p36, 1q, and 12q13-q21 in sarcomas; 2p13-p16 and 18q in non-Hodgkin's lymphoma; 2p23-p25 in neuroblastomas and small cell lung cancer; and 3q, 5p, 8q, 12p, 17p11.2-p12, 17q12-q21, 17q22-qter, 20q, and Xp11-q13 in prostate cancer. CGH analysis also reveals unique genomic response toward clinical treatment. Visakorpi et al.,[29] using CGH, demonstrated that an Xp11-q13 amplicon containing the androgen receptor is present in relapsed (but not in primary) prostate cancer. When prostate cancer is treated with androgen depletion therapy, amplification of the androgen receptor gene enables the cell to recover from the depletion therapy. This is a finding with evident therapeutic implications.

INTERNATIONAL SYSTEM OF CYTOGENETIC NOMENCLATURE

As indicated, chromosomes are classified by size and centromere position (see Fig. 5-1). The bands along each chromosome are numbered consecutively, by region, starting at the centromere, and each individual band is given a region and a band number from the centromere toward the telomere (see Fig. 5-1). Bands may also be divided into sub-bands. Thus, in this international nomenclature, a description of 3q22.3 indicates the long arm of chromosome 3, region 2, band 2, sub-band 3. Occasionally, more sophisticated techniques, such as high-resolution banding of late prophase chromosomes or *in situ* hybridization with DNA probes, are called for to identify chromosomal abnormalities beyond the resolution limits of the routine banding methods. An International System of Cytogenetic Nomenclature (ISCN)[30] ensures uniformity of the terminology used to describe cytogenetic results. Table 5-2 lists examples of the karyotype designations based on the ISCN. Note that the order of listing of abnormalities is sex chromosomes first, followed by numeric order (regardless of abnormality). The order of clone presentation is to list the main clonal abnormalities followed by any sidelines (derived clones) and, finally, by the normal cells.

MECHANISMS AND IMPLICATIONS OF CHROMOSOMAL ABNORMALITIES IN CANCER

Not all variations in chromosome structure are pathologic; some morphologic variations in human chromosomes are considered normal and carry little, if any, clinical significance. Increased amounts of repetitive DNA in the heterochromatic regions on chromosomes 1, 9, and 16 and the Y chromosome are seen frequently and are not associated with any clinical manifestations. A large Y chromosome is common in Asian populations and some Bedouin tribes and is entirely due to a large heterochromatic region on the distal long arm. Another common nonpathogenic variant is a pericentric (around the centromere) inversion of the heterochromatic region of chromosome 9. These normal or acceptable variations in chromosome structure are called *polymorphisms*. Other changes may be seen with little or no pathologic significance. In normal individuals of advanced age, the loss of one of the two X chromosomes in lymphocytes of women and of the Y chromosome in men is a common observation.

Beyond the polymorphic and normal variations, structural or numeric abnormalities can be causative of congenital anom-

TABLE 5-2. Examples of the International System of Cytogenetic Nomenclature

Term	*Definition*
47,XY,+21	Male with trisomy 21.
45,X,-X[15]/46,XX[5]	Loss of X chromosome seen in 15 cells (not a constitutional event).
45,Xc[15]/46,XX[5]	A mosaic monosomy X (constitutional) as may be seen in a patient with Turner syndrome (no somatic mutations).
46,XY,t(9;22)(q34;q11.2),i(17)(q10)	Male with the Philadelphia translocation and also an isochromosome for the long arm of chromosome 17 (breakpoint at the centromeric area).
46,XX,-7,t(9;22)(q34;q11.2),+der(22)t(9;22)	Monosomy 7, the Philadelphia translocation, and an extra Philadelphia chromosome (the small deleted 22 occurs in two copies).
46,XX,-7,t(9;22)(q34;q11.2),+der(22)t(9;22)[13]/47,idem,+8[7]	As above, but a secondary clone is noted with an additional abnormality (trisomy 8) in 7 of the 20 cells examined.
46,XX,del(11)(q23)	Deletion of the distal end of the long arm of chromosome 11 with breakpoint at 11q23 (most are likely interstitial deletions; see Deletions, later in the chapter).
46,XY,dup(1)(q22q25)	Duplication of the segment of 1q extending from q22 to q25.
46,X,ins(5;X)(p14;q21q25)	Insertion of material from chromosome X (from Xq21 to Xq25) into chromosome 5 at 5p14.
46,XY,add(19)(p13)	Additional material of unknown origin on the short arm of chromosome 19 (region 1, band 3).
46,XY,+21c,-7	A male patient with a constitutional trisomy 21 (Down syndrome) and a malignancy-related monosomy 7.
46-50,XX,del(3)(p14),+4,+10,+16,+mar[cp24]	cp24 stands for a composite karyotype summarizing the common abnormalities seen in those 24 cells. Mar is a marker chromosome of unknown origin.
47,XX,+mar.ish der(10)(WCP10+)	Marker unidentified by routine banding, but FISH using a whole chromosome paint probe indicates this marker to be derived from 10.
nuc ish 15q22(PMLx2),17q12(RARAx2)(PML con RARAx1)	Nuclear *in situ* hybridization showing evidence for juxtaposition of the PML gene on 15q22 and the RARA gene on 17q12.

FISH, fluorescence *in situ* hybridization.

alies (if constitutional) or malignancy (if somatic or acquired; Fig. 5-3). Somatic or acquired chromosomal abnormalities occur after conception and commonly are present only in specific tissues. Constitutional abnormalities are determined at conception and may be present in all somatic tissues of an individual (rarely as tissue-limited mosaicism).

NUMERIC ABNORMALITIES

During the anaphase of meiosis I in germ cells, the homologous chromosomes separate (disjoin) after accomplishing recombination (crossover). During the anaphase of mitosis and the second meiotic division, chromatids separate (disjoin) and migrate to the opposite poles of the cell. A failure of separation in either of these situations is termed *nondisjunction.* Rather than both daughter cells receiving the expected number of chromosomes, there will be gain of material in one daughter nucleus and loss of genetic material in the other daughter nucleus. For human autosomes, the normal situation is *disomy* (two copies of each chromosome). Thus, *trisomy* refers to having an extra chromosome and *monosomy* to having a missing chromosome.

Another mechanism for producing a chromosome abnormality is anaphase lag, wherein a chromosome lags at anaphase and fails to be included in daughter nuclei and so is lost. This can result only in monosomy. Trisomies and monosomies are common in human cancers. Polyploidy occurs when cells have more than the normal two sets of chromosomes (diploidy). Thus, a triploid cell will have three sets of chromosomes (modal number of chromosomes, 69) and a tetraploid cell four sets (modal number of chromosomes, 92). Polyploidy is noted in both hematologic malignancies and solid tumors and usually is seen duplicating a set of chromosomes that already have abnormal chromosomes (structural or numeric).

Our understanding of the impact of numeric abnormalities on development and progression of cancer has actually lagged

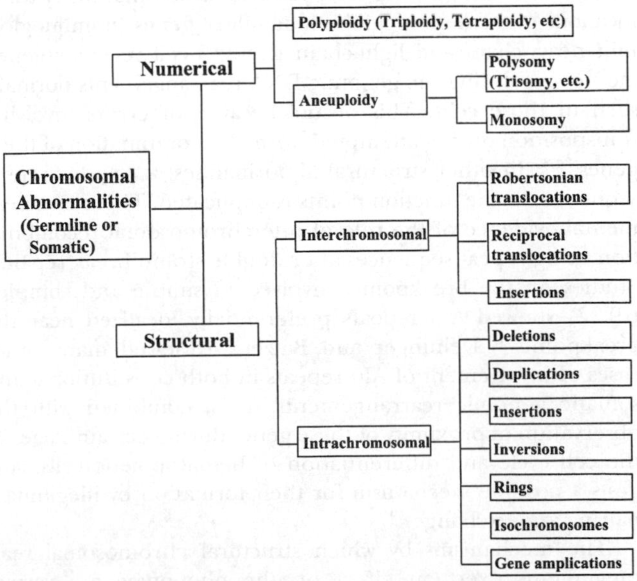

FIGURE 5-3. Various types of chromosomal aberrations seen in cancer.

behind that of structural abnormalities. For monosomy, speculation about loss of tumor suppressor genes on these chromosomes abound but, for the most common monosomies (e.g., monosomy 7 in myeloid disorders), no confirmed tumor suppressor genes have yet been cloned that are proven to be directly related to these monosomies. Trisomies are even more problematic, as it is difficult to show that specific genes on the extra chromosome are responsible for cell proliferation because of a dosage effect (three vs. two copies of the gene). Recently, it was demonstrated that the extra chromosome 7 in papillary renal carcinomas with trisomy 7 includes the mutant MET allele.[31] This indicates that one mechanism for the effect of a trisomy is duplication of mutant oncogenes. Other involved mechanisms include gene interactions, imprinting, or position effects.[32,33]

STRUCTURAL ABNORMALITIES

Numeric chromosomal abnormalities entail loss or gain of whole chromosomes. By contrast, structural abnormalities involve changes in part of one or more chromosomes. By definition, structural chromosomal aberrations require one or more breaks in the DNA sequence. Structural chromosomal rearrangements are expected to be deleterious. Thus, it is not surprising that strong selective forces in evolution resulted in numerous mechanisms to reduce the rate of chromosomal aberrations, including numerous pathways of DNA repair or cell-cycle arrest after DNA breaks (e.g., p53-mediated cell-cycle arrest in response to double-stranded DNA breaks); protective nuclear architecture with chromosome domains; increased nuclear size in the gametocytes; and asynchrony of DNA replication. Despite these mechanisms, a high incidence of chromosomal abnormalities clearly escapes this negative selection, resulting in an estimated 1% of newborns with constitutional chromosomal abnormalities and, of course, the many chromosomal abnormalities seen in cancer.[32,33]

While DNA breaks can occur in any sequence, there are clear preferential sites for DNA rearrangements. Several studies on recurrent cancer translocations are particularly illustrative of possible mechanisms for the origin of these abnormalities. In lymphoid neoplasms, it is now well established that many translocations in the immunoglobulin family of genes (immunoglobulin heavy-chain and light-chain genes, T-cell receptor genes, etc.) occur during the genomic DNA rearrangements normally seen in those cells. This occurs because of errors involving transposition during attempted normal recombination of these genes.[34,35] In other structural abnormalities, a role for repeat sequences at the junction points is implicated. There is experimental evidence of the role of interchromosomal recombination using repeat sequences after double-strand break repair.[36] Studies on the breakpoints involved in simple and complex t(9;22) showed Alu repeats preferentially localized near the breakpoints.[37] Deininger and Batzer[38] reviewed many other cases of involvement of Alu repeats in both constitutional and somatic genomic rearrangements. This, combined with the observation of proximity of these genes during certain stages of the cell cycle and differentiation of hematopoietic cells, suggests a possible mechanism for their formation by illegitimate pairing and exchange.[39]

The mechanisms by which structural chromosomal rearrangements exert an effect on the phenotype are varied. Clearly, balanced translocations in cancer lead to fusion products or gene regulation changes (e.g., overexpression of certain genes) that have a direct impact on cellular proliferation, escape from cell-cycle arrest, or apoptosis. In the case of deletions, duplications, trisomies, and monosomies, a gene dosage effect can also be involved. However, gene regulation at the translocation breakpoint or dosage effects probably do not explain all cases. Accumulated data suggest that structural chromosomal abnormalities can impact gene expression not only of the affected chromosomes but of nearby chromosomal regions. In cancer, the acquisition of "suites" of particular chromosomal rearrangements in cancers after the presumed initial cancer genetic change may be explained by nuclear position effects.[32] Another example is cited for the repeated establishment of isochromosome 17q in certain cancers.[40] However, gene alterations at or near the breakpoints clearly explain the effects of the majority of translocations in cancer cytogenetics. This still provides a veritable gold mine for positional cloning of new cancer related genes.

Reciprocal Translocations

A common type of structural chromosome change is the reciprocal translocation. This involves breakage of two chromosomes, a reciprocal exchange, and resealing of the broken ends (Fig. 5-4*D*). Considering the size of the genome and the small percentage of the DNA that is coding, most random breaks resulting in balanced translocations would not produce a phenotypic effect because no genetic material is lost or gained in the process and no genes are disrupted. A clinically significant abnormality may result when a translocation causes disruption or activation of genes or has a long-range effect on other genes. Although phenotypically normal themselves, carriers of constitutional reciprocal translocations are at increased risk of producing chromosomally unbalanced offspring. Somatic (acquired) translocations in cancer usually result in fusion gene products or in activation of an oncogene function or in both (discussed in Chapters 45.1 and 46.1).

A few examples here are worth commenting on. The t(14;18)(q32;q21) is found in a majority of lymphomas with follicular center cell morphology and in one-third of diffuse large cell lymphoma. The translocation is associated with overexpression of BCL2 gene at 18q21. The BCL-2 protein is localized in mitochondria, the endoplasmic reticulum, and the nuclear envelope and is involved in cell-cycle regulation. Various rearrangements involving 11q23 occur in acute lymphocytic leukemia (ALL) and a subset of cases with AML. The disrupted gene is the MLL gene at 11q23 with more than 30 different partner genes involved (hence, MLL is called a *promiscuous oncogene*). The t(11;22)(q24;q12) is found in more than 90% of cases of Ewing's sarcoma and can be very diagnostic. FISH can be used to detect all these translocations using dual color probes (see Fig. 5-2 and Color Fig. 5-2).

Robertsonian Translocations

Robertsonian translocations specifically involve breakage at or near the centromeres of two acrocentric chromosomes with the long arms joining to form a novel metacentric or submetacentric chromosome. Because the short arms of these acrocentric chromosomes carry only ribosomal genes, these translocations can reduce the chromosome number without

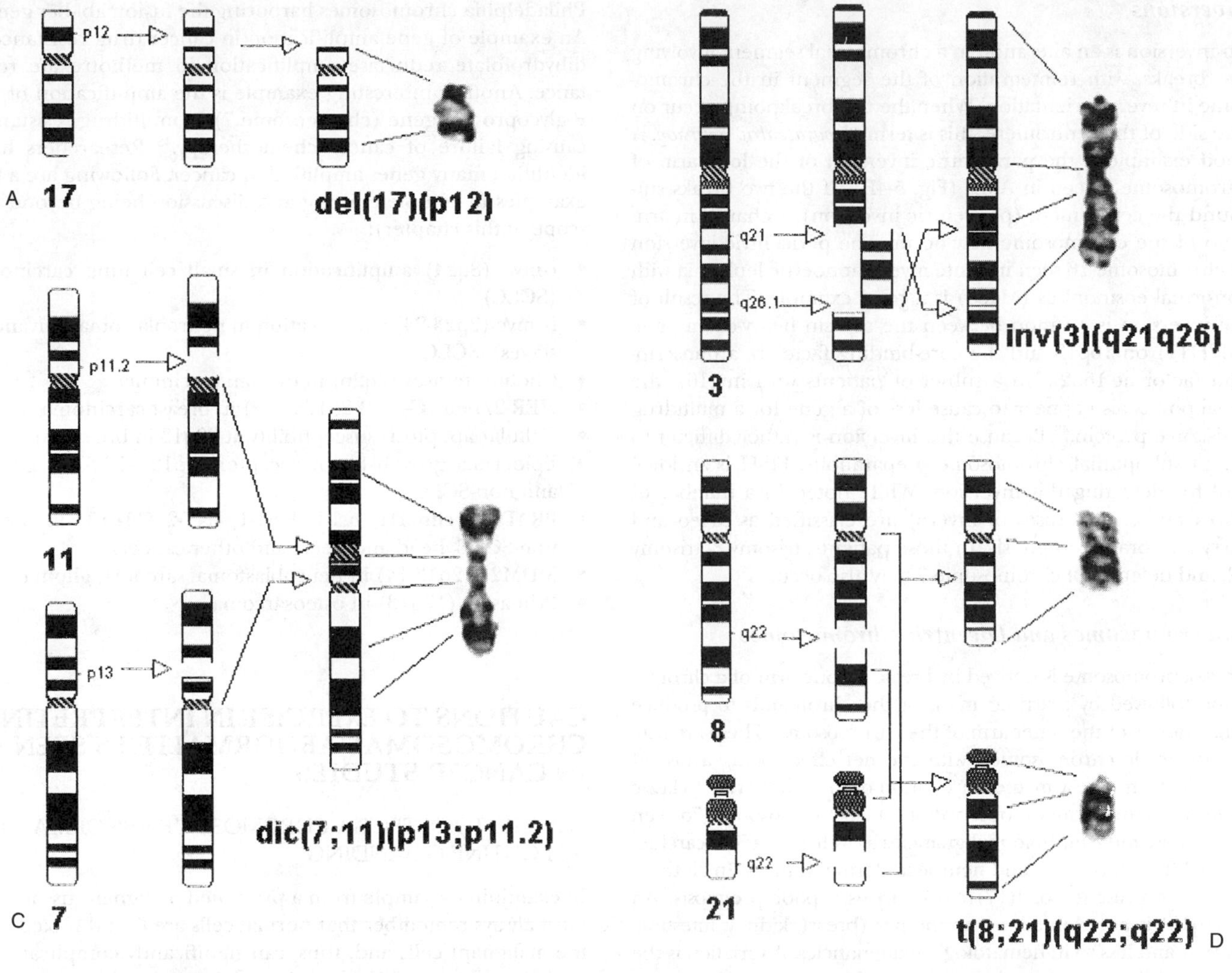

FIGURE 5-4. Some structural chromosomal abnormalities seen in cancer cytogenetics; compare with normal banding pattern in Figure 5-1. **A:** Deletion of the short arm of 17. **B:** Paracentric inversion of the long arm of chromosome 3. **C:** Dicentric chromosome with centromeres from chromosomes 7 and 11 (breakpoints on the short arm). **D:** Common reciprocal translocation of 8q and 21q noted in acute myelogenous leukemia M2.

causing a phenotypic abnormality. While these are the most common constitutional translocations, they are very rare as somatic mutations in cancer. When they have been noted in cancer, they seem to exert an effect by being unbalanced translocations resulting in trisomies for the long arms of the acrocentric chromosomes.

Deletions

Deletions are common in cancer cells. At the G-band level, these may appear as terminal deletions (i.e., one breakpoint with loss of material distal to the breakpoint; Fig. 5-4A). However, most, if not all, are likely not true terminal deletions, and there is no proof that terminal deletions exist in cancer, probably because of cell-cycle arrest due to failure to correct breaks. There are very rare examples of telomere regeneration. The single confirmed recapping by telomeres of a terminally deleted chromosome is the reported chromosome 16 deletion noted in rare cases of patients with mental retardation and hemoglobin abnormalities. Deletions designated as *terminal*, on the basis of G-band examination, are either interstitial deletions or cryptic unbalanced translocations. For example, a molecular study of melanoma cell lines with identified "terminal deletions"[41] showed that there is subtelomeric material from other chromosomes located at the ends of these shortened chromosomes. A specialized deletion that occurs on both ends of the chromosome with joining of the two ends results in ring chromosomes.

Duplication

An intrachromosomal duplication requires at least two breakpoints with the segment between them duplicated either head to tail (direct duplication) or head to head (inverted duplication). One of the most common duplications seen in hematologic malignancies is the duplication of the long arm of chromosome 1 (breakpoints at q12-21 and q31-q44). This duplication is especially noted in lymphoid malignancies (ALL and lymphomas), usually as a secondary abnormality with poor prognosis.

Inversions

An inversion is an alteration in a chromsomal segment involving two breaks, with reintegration of the segment in the chromosome in reverse orientation. When the two breakpoints occur on one side of the centromere, this is termed *paracentric inversion.* A good example is the paracentric inversion of the long arm of chromosome 3 seen in AML (Fig. 5-4B). If the two breaks surround the centromere (pericentric inversion), a change in arm ratio of the chromosome may occur. The pericentric inversion of chromosome 16 seen in acute myelomonocytic leukemia with abnormal eosinophils (M4eo) is a good example. The result of the inversion is a fusion between the myosin heavy-chain gene (MYH11) on 16p13 and the core-binding factor b, a transcription factor at 16q22. In a subset of patients with inv(16), the breakpoints also appear to cause loss of a gene for a multidrug resistance protein.[42] Because this inversion is rather difficult to see in suboptimal chromosome preparations, FISH is an ideal tool for detecting this inversion. While noted in a number of FAB classes, most cases of inv(16) are classified as M4eo and carry a favorable prognosis. In those patients, trisomy 8, trisomy 22, and deletion of chromosome 7 may also occur.

Isochromosomes and Dicentric Chromosomes

An isochromosome is derived by breaks in one arm of a chromosome followed by rearrangement of the chromatids to produce duplications of the other arm of the chromosome. These are usually dicentric chromosomes, with the net effect being a loss of material from one arm and duplication of the other arm. A classic example is the common observation of isochromosome 17q seen in myeloid and lymphoid malignancies as well as in adenocarcinomas (different organs) and neuroectodermal tumors. In all these cases, the presence of i(17)(q10) carries a poor prognosis. An i(1)(q10) is noted in adenocarcinomas (breast, kidney, intestine, uterus) and less so in hematologic malignancies. A variation is the break involving two nonhomologous chromosomes forming a dicentric chromosome (Fig. 5-4*C*).

Gene Amplification

Molecular genetic methods allowed for rigorous study of variations in gene copy number in mammalian cells. This allowed for the understanding of the earlier cytogenetic observation of "double minutes" (DMs) and of homogeneously staining regions (HSRs) in cancer cells and drug-resistant cell lines. HSRs and other forms of chromosomal DNA amplification are notable as unusually banded regions on the chromosomes. DMs are extrachromosomal, acentric (lacking centromeres), circular DNA molecules (lacking telomeres) and can be variable in size. Generally, DMs are less stable than HSRs in culture, which is expected, as DMs lack centromeres and would not segregate properly to daughter nuclei in mitosis. Gene amplification is noted in many biologic phenomena, including amplification of insecticide detoxification genes in insects, induced amplification of certain genes in cultured cells (used to produce certain proteins industrially), amplification of developmental genes in *Xenopus* and other organisms, amplification of drug resistance genes, and amplification of certain oncogenes in cancer.

It is the latter topic that is of interest here. A duplication of a chromosome or a chromosome region is not considered here under amplification (e.g., CML patients can have two or three Philadelphia chromosomes harboring the fusion abl-bcr gene). An example of gene amplification in cancer drug resistance is dihydrofolate reductase amplification in methotrexate resistance. Another interesting example is the amplification of the P glycoprotein gene (chromosome 7) in multidrug resistance, causing failure of cancer chemotherapy.[43] Researchers have identified many genes amplified in cancer. Following are a few examples (a complete listing and discussion being beyond the scope of this chapter):

- c-myc (8q24) amplification in small cell lung carcinoma (SCLC)
- N-myc (2p23-24) amplification in neuroblastoma (advanced stages), SCLC
- Cholinesterases (3q26) in ovarian carcinoma
- HER-2/neu (C-erbB-2, 17q11.2) in breast carcinoma
- Cellular apoptosis susceptibility at 20q13 in breast cancer
- Epidermal growth factor receptor (7p12.1-12.3) in glioma and non-SCLC
- PRAD1/cyclin D1, bcl-1, HST-1, INT-2 (11q13) in breast, non-SCLC, head and neck, and other cancers
- MDM2 (12q13-14) in neuroblastoma, sarcoma, glioma
- Primase 1 (12q13) in osteosarcoma.

CAUTIONS TO EXERCISE IN INTERPRETING CHROMOSOMAL ABNORMALITIES SEEN IN CANCER STUDIES

FAILURE TO DETECT A CHROMOSOME ABNORMALITY BY ROUTINE G-BANDING

In examining a sample from a presumed malignant tissue, one must always remember that normal cells are found mixed with the malignant cells and, thus, can significantly complicate the analysis. A report of 20 normal metaphases should be read with caution, as these metaphases could be those of a cancer that happens to be diploid and to lack visible structural abnormalities or of normal surrounding cells. In some malignancies, normal cells in the submitted sample can give much better chromosome morphology than abnormal cells. This is especially true in acute lymphoblastic leukemia. Experienced cytogenetic technologists learn to analyze fuzzy, poor metaphases and quickly to identify these abnormalities, even in poor cells. Further, there are expected variations between laboratories owing to different referral bases. Physicians differ in their referral patterns, and individual referral may vary, depending on such factors as the patient-specific situation, stage of the disease, and even financial considerations. As more data accumulate, there are now more clear indications for cytogenetic studies that should decrease (but not eliminate) variation in the rate of detection of chromosomal abnormalities by different laboratories.

Failure to note the aberration in routine analysis may also occur because the abnormality involves a small amount of chromosomal material or produces little change in perceived banding patterns. The t(15;17)(q22;q22) in AML M3 and inv(16)(p13q22) seen in AML M4eo are not easily noted in short or poorly banded chromosomes. A more interesting example is the complete failure of detection of t(12;21) by banding methods because the exchange is between segments of these chromosomes that stain similarly (light) by G-banding. The translocation resulting in a fusion of the ETV6 (TEL) gene at 12p13 and the CBFA2 (AML1) gene at 21q22 is variably reported in 16% to 36% of cases of childhood ALL. This t(12;21)(p13;q22) is reported to be associated with B-cell precursor ALL, with presumed favorable prognosis. FISH using probes for ETV6 and CBFA2 is the method of choice for identifying this translocation (see Fig. 5-2A).

CONSTITUTIONAL CHROMOSOMAL ABNORMALITIES

Some chromosomal abnormalities are present at birth and are not related to neoplasia. These include balanced translocations, Robertsonian translocations, inversions, and insertions that are found at some level in normal-appearing individuals (but in most cases affecting their reproductive success or resulting in the birth of children with congenital abnormalities or both). Other constitutional abnormalities can be associated with an abnormal phenotype, and some predispose to cancer development (e.g., Down, Klinefelter's, and chromosome breakage syndromes). Of course, these abnormalities usually are found in all cells in a person and are not limited to a particular tissue type. Thus, when we find such abnormalities in all examined cells, we are suspicious of a potential constitutional translocation. Obvious exceptions to this assumption are translocations classically noted in certain cancers, such as t(9;22) in CML, in which all examined cells may have the translocation, but it is not a constitutional translocation. To distinguish between a constitutional translocation and a novel translocation found in all sampled cells, a cytogeneticist may request a constitutional chromosome study. The simplest is to get a peripheral blood sample cultured for 48 to 96 hours using B- or T-cell stimulants (mitogens) to ensure adequate numbers of actively dividing cells for analysis. Chromosome studies may also be performed using other cells, such as skin fibroblasts.

FRAGILE SITES

Cytogeneticists regularly observe breaks in preparations of human chromosomes. Fragile sites are visible cytogenetically as breaks at consistent sites in the genome. Some of these sites are induced by certain chemicals (e.g., aphidicolin, methotrexate). The sites, which now number more than 100, are heterogeneous in their method of induction (some are constitutively expressed and are not induced) and in their location and the sequences involved. Some are associated with integration sites for oncogenic viruses. Some occur in or near tumor suppressor genes and may be associated with the chromosomal events leading to loss of those genes. The best example of the latter phenomenon is the aphidicolin-induced fragile site at 3p14.2 (FRA3B), which occurs within the tumor suppressor gene FHIT involved in numerous cancers, including the translocation t(3;8)(p14.2;q24) seen in clear cell renal carcinoma.[44] Much more work needs to be done to resolve the relationship between other fragile sites and chromosome translocations and aberrations seen in cancer. When fragile sites are found in one or a few examined metaphases, this is noted in the workup. Such findings may fall into one of three categories: (1) rare events in normal individuals noted as chromatid and chromosome breaks (not clinically significant), (2) breaks at the same site in multiple untreated cells, considered constitutional fragile sites (their relevance to the cancer being unknown now), or (3) multiple breaks in many cells at different sites, possibly suggesting one of the chromosome breakage syndromes (e.g., ataxia-telangiectasia or xeroderma pigmentosum) or other pathologic mechanisms.

SATELLITE ASSOCIATIONS

The human karyotype normally includes five pairs of acrocentric chromosomes (chromosomes 13, 14, 15, 21, and 22). On average, seven to eight of the short arms of these chromosomes carry satellites and a satellite stalk with the nucleolar organizer region. Satellite associations can be seen persisting through metaphase as remnants of the nucleolar associations. These are normal findings. Speculations in the literature that this predisposes to Robertsonian translocations have not been confirmed. Robertsonian translocations are common in animals that lack nucleolar organizer regions or satellites on the short arms of involved chromosomes.

PROBLEMS WITH SOLID TUMORS

A biopsy of a solid tumor usually contains a number of tissue types (e.g., blood vessels, epithelial cells, fibroblast) in addition to the tumor cells. Further, tumor cell growth is usually not very good, and normal cells can grow faster than tumor cells *in vitro*. Various technical tricks can be used to obtain decent results from such specimens, including selecting appropriate media (avoiding media that stimulate growth of normal fibroblasts), treating primary cultures with trypsin to remove fibroblasts, and culturing at lower density. Recent molecular cytogenetic methods can obviate the need for cell culture in assaying for specific chromosomal abnormalities.

CLONAL EVOLUTION AND CHROMOSOME EVOLUTION

Early studies using X-inactivation as a marker for clonality in female cells suggested that most, if not all, cancers originate clonally. Later chromosome studies confirmed the clonal origin of cancer cells with specific chromosomal abnormalities. However, there are published cases of apparently independent clones with distinct chromosomal abnormalities (occurring in approximately 1% of cases of leukemias and lymphomas). The generally accepted explanation for most of these cases is that a unifying submicroscopic event occurred, with further genetic alterations appearing as unique events (i.e., they are an evolution of the original clone). True multiclonal cancers are indeed rare. In testing, we usually examine a minimum of 20 metaphases in an attempt to locate a clone with a chromosomal abnormality. According to the ISCN (1995),[30] a clone is recognized if three or more cells have the same missing chromosome or two or more cells exhibit the same additional chromosome or structural abnormality. The reason for the difference in number of cells needed to define a clone with a missing chromosome (monosomy) versus one with trisomy relates to the possibility in cytogenetic preparation of overspreading of chromosomes and, hence, artifactual "missing" chromosomes. If one of the first 20 cells showed a particular aberration likely related to the cancer, a count of additional cells can be initiated or molecular cytoge-

TABLE. 5-3. Constitutional Chromosomal Abnormalities Predisposing to Cancer Development

Syndrome	*Associated Cancers*
13q14 deletion	Retinoblastoma
45,X/46,XY or 45,X/46,X,der(Y)	Gonadoblastoma
Ataxia-telangiectasia	Leukemia (especially T-cell), lymphoma, breast cancer
Bannayan-Riley-Ruvalcaba syndrome	Multiple lipomas, hemangiomas, hamartomatous gastrointestinal polyps, lymphangiomas
Bloom syndrome	Leukemia, lymphoma, colon, breast, stomach, Wilms' tumor
Cockayne's syndrome	Skin, aging-related cancers
Denys-Drash syndrome	Wilms' tumor
Diamond-Blackfan anemia	Acute myelogenous leukemia primarily, many others
Down syndrome (trisomy 21)	Leukemia
Fanconi's anemia	Leukemia, myelodysplastic syndromes, hepatocellular carcinoma
Flamm syndrome (dysplastic nevus syndrome)	Melanoma
Frasier syndrome	Gonadoblastoma, Wilms' tumor
Gardner's syndrome (familial adenomatous polyposis)	Colorectal cancer, hepatoblastoma, medulloblastoma, thyroid cancer
Gorlin's syndrome (nevoid basal cell carcinoma)	Multiple basal cell carcinoma, medulloblastoma, ovarian cancer
Hemihyperplasia, isolated	Wilms' tumor, hepatoblastoma, neuroblastoma, adrenocortical carcinoma
Immunodeficiency, centromeric instability, facial anomalies	T-cell leukemia
Klinefelter's syndrome (47,XXY)	Germ cell tumors, breast cancer
Multiple endocrine neoplasia type 2B	Thyroid cancer, pheochromocytoma
N syndrome	T-cell leukemia
Neurofibromatosis type 1	Malignant peripheral nerve sheath tumors, leukemia, neural tumors
Neurofibromatosis type 2	Schwannomas, meningiomas
Nijmegen breakage syndrome	Lymphoma (especially B-cell type)
Peutz-Jeghers syndrome	Gastrointestinal and other malignancies (including breast, pancreatic, reproductive tract cancers)
Reifenstein's syndrome	Male breast cancer
Renal cell carcinoma, hereditary papillary	Papillary renal cell carcinoma
Rothmund-Thomson syndrome	Osteosarcoma, skin cancer (squamous and basal cell carcinomas)
Rubinstein-Taybi syndrome	Medulloblastoma
Simpson-Golabi-Behmel syndrome	Wilms' tumor
Tuberous sclerosis	Renal and cardiac rhabdomyomas, brain and retinal cancers
von Hippel-Lindau syndrome	Central nervous system hemangioblastomas, renal, pancreatic cancers
Wilms' tumor, aniridia, genital anomalies, mental retardation (WAGR syndrome)	Wilms' tumor
Werner syndrome	Osteosarcoma, meningioma
Wiedemann-Beckwith syndrome	Wilms' tumor, hepatoblastoma, neuroblastoma, adrenocortical carcinoma
Xeroderma pigmentosum	Skin and corneal cancers
Extra Y syndrome	Myelomonocytic leukemia, refractory anemia with excess blasts
XY gonadal dysgenesis	Gonadoblastoma, dysgerminoma

netic methods used to confirm the presence of a clone. In any case, once a clone is identified, this can provide a baseline for diagnosis, prognosis, and follow-up study of relapse.

Many cancers are seen with only simple aberrations, such as the t(9;22) in CML. Early cytogenetic studies, however, still showed significant complex karyotypes in many cancers, suggesting that these early events can progress to more complex karyotypes. The stepwise progression of cancer by acquiring additional abnormalities is now well established for a number of cancers. A good example of this is colorectal carcinoma, which involves a successive series of genetic alterations. One must caution, though, that simplistic multistage scenarios usually are not the common pattern seen. For many solid tumors, chromosome instability results in massive karyotypic changes that appear totally unrelated to selective advantage. One possible explanation is that a genetic event resulting in cancer or predisposition to cancer removes a cell-cycle checkpoint involved in preventing damaged cells from dividing. An example is that cells missing p53 can accumulate chromosomal abnormalities because of the absence of p53-mediated cell-cycle arrest after double-stranded DNA breaks.

CONSTITUTIONAL CHROMOSOMAL ABNORMALITIES PREDISPOSING TO CANCER DEVELOPMENT

We do not review here hereditary cancer syndromes due to gene mutation (e.g., hereditary breast cancer and Li-Fraumeni syndrome). We are more interested in syndromes with microscopically visible chromosomal abnormalities that predispose to cancer. A partial listing of the latter conditions is shown in

TABLE 5-4. Web Sites of Interest in Cancer Genetics and Cytogenetics

American Cancer Society Web page (informative site for basic cancer material): www.cancer.org
Atlas of Genetics and Cytogenetics in Oncology and Haematology (excellent resource): www.infobiogen.fr/services/chromcancer
Breakpoint map of recurrent chromosomal aberrations in cancer at the National Center for Biotechnology Information (NCBI): www.ncbi.nlm.nih.gov/CCAP/mitelsum.cgi
Cancer Web information from the United Kingdom and National Cancer Institute: www.graylab.ac.uk/cancerweb.html
Chromosome Web (mostly for researchers but also includes protocols and many links): http://infofarm.cc.affrc.go.jp/~shignak/chromosome.net/
Common cytogenetic findings in hematologic disorders from Michigan State University: www.phd.msu.edu/cyto/hemat.htm
DNA Database of Japan: www.ddbj.nig.ac.jp/
European Molecular Biology Laboratory (includes sequence information): www2.ebi.ac.uk/
GenBank: www.ncbi.nlm.nih.gov/Genbank/index.html
Genome Database by the Human Genome Project Organization: www.gdb.org/hugo
Genomics lexicon (terms and definitions): http://www.phrma.org/genomics/lexicon/
Genome Link (a site to allow access to genome databases, genome project sites, and appr000000oximately 24 genetic sites of interest): www-ls.lanl.gov/HGhotlist.html
Glossary of Genetic Terms (by Birgid Schlindwein): www.weihenstephan.de/ schlind/genglosalfa.html
Human Chromsome Launchpad (information on each human chromosome): www.ornl.gov/hgmis/launchpad/
Human chromosome maps, linkage mapping information, tools, and the like: www.genlink.wustl.edu/chrmaps/
Human Genome Chromosome Databases: MRC www.hgmp.mrc.ac.uk/GenomeWeb/human-gen-db-chromosomes.html#0
Karyotypic region-based integrated information resource for mapping and sequencing data: sgiweb.ncbi.nlm.nih.gov:80/Zjing/yac.html
National Cancer Institute (informative sites on various cancers and links to databases for loci, etc.): http://www.ncbi.nlm.nih.gov/disease/Cancer.html
Online Mendelian Inheritance in Man (the ultimate reference for genetic disorders but not cytogenetic; detailed with references and histories): www.ncbi.nlm.nih.gov/omim
U.S. Department of Energy, Oak Ridge National Laboratory, Human Genome Web site: www.ornl.gov/hgmis/

Table 5-3. Many of these syndromes are detailed and continuously updated on the Web via *Online Mendelian Inheritance in Man* (http://www3.ncbi.nlm.nih.gov/Omim/). Specific information about cancer risks for certain syndromes are available at http://www.infobiogen.fr/services/chromcancer/Kprones/Kproneliste.html. Both Bloom syndrome and Werner syndrome genes have been cloned and found to code for putative helices on chromosomes 15 and 8, respectively. Because, in both of these conditions, chromosome breakage is increased, it is suspected that the absence of these helices increases the probability of illegitimate recombination.

DATA MINING IN CANCER CYTOGENETICS

The proliferation of information in the rapidly growing cancer cytogenetics field has been a great asset to both clinicians and researchers. Fortunately, the development of information technology has made it easier to keep abreast of the rapid developments in this field. There are commercial or semicommercial databases for cancer cytogenetics. An example is the software called *Cancer Cytogenetics Lookup* published by Gilbert B. Coté. Further, the large text by Mitelman, titled *Catalogue of Chromosome Aberration in Cancer*,[45] is also available as a compact disk (John Wiley & Sons). However, the proliferation of free Internet resources with online direct access to continuously updated data has mushroomed. Table 5-4 lists some specialized Web pages of interest. Of course, there are many other resources to the student of cancer cytogenetics, including subscribing to bibliographic updates (e.g., *Current Contents*, now available on the Web), running search engines for Web pages (e.g., Yahoo, Infoseek, Excite, etc.), and local and national library search engines (e.g., Medline).

There are also specialized list servers that help to facilitate communications between researchers and clinicians. For example, one could get onto the Molecular Genetics list serve at www.hum-molgen.de and be able to ask and answer questions for various areas of molecular genetics.

GLOSSARY

acrocentric: of chromosome whose centromere is very close to one end

amplicon: a unit of gene amplification, usually containing a large segment of DNA containing many genes

amplification: an increase in the number of copies of a particular DNA sequence

aneuploidy: meaning "not euploid," having missing or additional chromosomes or chromosome material

centromeres (from *kentron* = center, *meros* = part): the site of attachment of chromosomes to the mitotic or meiotic spindle; considered by some to be the kinetochore (the functional centromere) and that centromere should refer only to repetitive DNA sequences (in humans, alphoid repeats) that attract centromere proteins

chromatid: one of the two visibly distinct longitudinal parts of a replicated chromosome seen in late prophase and in metaphase; after separation, becomes a daughter chromosome

chromosome: a nuclear subunit that includes linked genes as well as a centromere structure (found in eukaryotes)

diploidy: having the normal two homologous sets of chromosomes

disjunction: the separation of daughter chromosomes (chromatids) or of homologous chromosomes (in meiosis I)

haploid: having one set of chromosomes (present in gametes)

kinetochore: a specialized structure at the centromere that functions to elongate or digest microtubules to allow disjunction in meiosis and mitosis; a functioning centromere produces the primary constriction of a chromosome

metacentric: of chromosome, the centromere of which is roughly in a median position

monosomic: a condition in which one chromosome is missing; thus, in humans, having 45 chromosomes (2n – 1)

polyploidy: having one or more extra sets of chromosomes (triploidy, tetraploidy, etc.)

telomerase (telomere terminal transferase): a specialized ribonucleoprotein that uses its RNA component as a template to synthesize telomeric repeats

telomeres: repeated DNA sequences (TTAGGG in vertebrates) found at the ends of linear chromosomes; provide protection of the end from degradation and attract proteins that prevent the ends from recombination and from triggering cell-cycle checkpoints

TRAP(Telomeric Repeat Amplification Protocol): a technique using polymerase chain reaction to measure telomerase activity in cell extracts; developed by Kim et al.[9] and now having numerous available modifications

trisomy: a condition in which there is one extra chromosome; thus, in humans, having 47 chromosomes (2n + 1)

REFERENCES

1. Boveri T. *Zur Frage der Entstehung maligner Tumoren.* Jena: Gustav Fischer, 1914.
2. Tjio JH, Levan A. The chromosome number of man. *Hereditas* 1956;42:1.
3. Nowell PC, Hungerford DA. A minute chromosome in human chronic granulocytic leukemia. *Science* 1960;132:1497.
4. Rowley JD. A new consistent chromosomal abnormality in chronic myelogenous leukemia identified by quinacrine fluorescence and Giemsa staining. *Nature* 1973;243:290.
5. Irick H. A new function for heterochromatin. *Chromosoma* 1994;103(1):1.
6. Kipling D. *The telomere.* Oxford: Oxford University Press, 1995:208.
7. Hayflick L, Moorhead PS. The serial cultivation of human diploid strains. *Exp Cell Res* 1961;25:585.
8. Harley CB, Futcher AB, Greider CW. Telomeres shorten during aging of human fibroblasts. *Nature* 1990;345:458.
9. Kim NW, Piatyszek MA, Prowse KR, et al. Specific association of human telomerase activity with immortal cells and cancer. *Science* 1994;266(5193):2011.
10. de Lange T. Activation of telomerase in a human tumor. *Proc Natl Acad Sci U S A* 1994;91:2882.
11. Shay JW, Bacchetti S. A survey of telomerase activity in human cancer. *Eur J Cancer* 1997;33:787.
12. Langford LA, Piatyszek MA, Xu R, et al. Telomerase activity in ordinary meningiomas predicts poor outcome. *Hum Pathol* 1997;28:416.
13. Blasco MA, Lee HW, Hande MP, et al. Telomere shortening and tumor formation by mouse cells lacking telomerase RNA. *Cell* 1997;91:25.
14. Vaziri H, Schachter F, Uchida I, et al. Loss of telomeric DNA during aging of normal and trisomy-21 human lymphocytes. *Am J Hum Genet* 1993;52(4):661.
15. Yu CE, Oshima J, Fu YH, et al. Positional cloning of the Werner's syndrome gene. *Science* 1996;272(5259):258.
16. Fox JL, Hsu PH, Legator MS, Morrison LE, Seelig SA. Fluorescence in situ hybridization: powerful molecular tool for cancer prognosis. *Clin Chem* 1995;41(11):1554.
17. Kwong YL, Pang J, Ching LM, et al. Trisomy 12 in chronic lymphocytic leukemia—an interphase cytogenetic study by fluorescence in situ hybridization. *Cancer Genet Cytogenet* 1994;72(2):83.
18. Qumsiyeh MB, Tharapel SA. Interphase detection of trisomy 12 in B-cell chronic lymphocytic leukemia by fluorescence hybridization in situ. *Leukemia* 1992;6(6):602.
19. Persons DL, Hartmann LC, Herath JF, Keeney GL, Jenkins RB. Fluorescence in situ hybridization analysis of trisomy 12 in ovarian tumors. *Am J Clin Pathol* 1994;102(6):775.
20. Schröck E, du Manoir S, Veldman T, et al. Multicolor spectral karyotyping of human chromosomes. *Science* 1996;273:494.
21. Ried T, Liyanage M, duManoir S, et al. Tumor cytogenetics revisited: comparative genomic hybridization and spectral karyotyping. *J Molec Med Immunol* 1997;75(11–12):801.
22. Gosden J, Hanratty D, Starling J, et al. Oligonucleotide-primed in situ DNA synthesis (PRINS)—a method for chromosome mapping, banding, and investigation of sequence organization. *Cytogenet Cell Genet* 1991;57(2–3):100.
23. Pellestor F, Andreo B, Coullin P. Interphasic analysis of aneuploidy in cancer cell lines using primer in situ labeling. *Cancer Genet Cytogenet* 1999;111:111.
24. Serakinci N, Koch J. Detection and sizing of telomeric repeat DNA in situ. *Nat Biotech* 1999;17:200.
25. Kallioniemi A, Kallioniemi O, Sudar D, et al. Comparative genomic hybridization for molecular cytogenetic analysis of solid tumors. *Science* 1992;258:18.
26. Parentc F, Gaudray P, Carle GF, TurcCarel C. Experimental assessment of the detection limit of genomic amplification by comparative genomic hybridization CGH. *Cytogenet Cell Genet* 1997;78(1):65.
27. Lichter P, Bentz M, Joos S. Detection of chromosomal aberrations by means of molecular cytogenetics: painting of chromosomes and chromosomal subregions and comparative genomic hybridization. *Methods Enzymol* 1995;254:334.
28. Knuutila S, Bjorkqvist A-M, Autio K, et al. DNA copy number amplifications in human neoplasms: review of comparative genomic hybridization studies. *Am J Pathol* 1998;152:1107.
29. Visakorpi T, Kallioniemi AH, Syvanen A-C, et al. Genetic changes in primary and recurrent prostate cancer by comparative genomic hybridization. *Cancer Res* 1995;55:342.
30. Harnden DG, Klingor HP, eds. *ISCN: an international system for human cytogenetic nomenclature.* Basel, Karger, 1995.
31. Zhuang ZP, Park WS, Pack S, et al. Trisomy 7-harbouring non-random duplication of the mutant MET allele in hereditary papillary renal carcinomas. *Nat Genet* 1998;20(1):66.
32. Qumsiyeh MB. Impact of rearrangements on function and position of chromosomes in the interphase nucleus and on human genetic disorders. *Chromosome Res* 1995;3:455.
33. Qumsiyeh MB. Structure and function of the nucleus: anatomy and physiology of chromatin. *Cell Mol Life Sci* 1999;55:1129.
34. Riom K, Melek M, Gellert M. DNA transposition by the RAG1 and RAG2 proteins: a possible source of oncogenic translocations. *Cell* 1998;94:463.
35. Retiere CFH, Peyrat MA, Le Deist F, Bonneville M, Hallet MM. The mechanism of chromosome 7 inversion in human lymphocytes expressing chimeric gamma beta TCR. *J Immunol* 1999;162:903.
36. Richardson C, Moynahan ME, Jasin M. Double-strand break repair by interchromosomal recombination: suppression of chromosomal translocations. *Genes Dev* 1998;12(24):3831.
37. Jeffs AR, Benjes SM, Smith TL, Sowerby SJ, Morris CM. The BCR gene recombines preferentially with Alu elements in complex BCR-ABL translocations of chronic myeloid leukaemia. *Hum Mol Genet* 1998;7(5):767.
38. Deininger PL, Batzer MA. Alu repeats and human disease. *Mol Genet Metab* 1999;67(3):183.
39. Neves H, Ramos C, da Silva M, Parreira A, Parreira L. The nuclear topography of ABL, BCR, PML, and RARalpha genes: evidence for gene proximity in specific phases of the cell cycle and stages of hematopoietic differentiation. *Blood* 1999;93:1197.
40. Matioli GT. On a mechanism for isochromatid 17q in a subset of Ph+ chronic myeloid leukemia patients. *Med Hypotheses* 1998;50(5):375.
41. Meltzer PS, Guan XY, Trent JM. Telomere capture stabilizes chromosome breakage. *Nat Genet* 1993;4(3):252.
42. Kuss BJ, Deeley RG, Cole SPC, et al. The biological significance of the multidrug resistance gene MRP in inversion 16 leukemias. *Leuk Lymphoma* 1996;20(5–6):357.
43. Trambas CM, Muller HK, Woods GM. P-glycoprotein mediated multidrug resistance and its implications for pathology. *Pathology* 1997;29(2):122.
44. Mimori K, Druck T, Inoue H, et al. Cancer-specific chromosome alterations in the constitutive fragile region FRA3B. *Proc Natl Acad Sci U S A* 1999;96(13):7456.
45. Mitelman F, Johansson B, Mertens F. *Catalogue of chromosome aberrations in cancer.* New York: Wiley-Liss, 1994.

Michael B. Kastan
Stephen X. Skapek

CHAPTER 6

Molecular Biology of Cancer: The Cell Cycle

A cell's ability to produce exact replicas of itself is an essential component of life. This process must be performed with great fidelity in order for whole organisms and species to propagate. The molecular machinery used to control the cell division cycle and replicate is highly organized and well conserved through evolution. Although we are only beginning to unravel the mechanisms in this process, it is clear that multiple extracellular and intracellular signals must be integrated in order to accomplish this complex task.

Although evolution and cellular differentiation may rely on some subtle genetic or epigenetic changes in a given cell, these changes must occur in an orderly and controlled fashion to prevent disastrous outcomes. Gross lack of fidelity in the cellular reproduction process leads to genetic instability, which appears to significantly contribute to the development of malignancy. In order to understand how cancers start and to devise optimal strategies to eliminate cancer cells, we must be able to identify the molecular distinctions between normal cells and tumor cells. Aberrations of normal cell-cycle control reflect some of the molecular alterations that are characteristic of cancer cells.

In this chapter, we review (1) the present understanding of mechanisms by which a normal cell controls the ordered progression through its cell cycle, (2) how regulatory mechanisms are integrated with extracellular signals, and (3) how a normal cell monitors its own progress through several *checkpoints* in the cell division cycle. We emphasize how these normal processes may go awry in cancer cells. Finally, we discuss the potential implications of this knowledge for our understanding of cancer biology and the development of novel therapeutic strategies.

MECHANICS OF THE CELL DIVISION CYCLE

BRIEF OVERVIEW

Cell-Cycle Phases

In any proliferating mammalian cell, the replication of the entire genome and the division of the cell into genetically identical daughter cells can be broken down into four distinct cell-cycle phases (Fig. 6-1). In the first phase, known as G_1 (for *gap 1*), the cell undergoes biochemical changes to prepare for entry into S phase in which new DNA is synthesized. As discussed later, in section G_1 to S Transition, a number of these biochemical events are now known; however, cellular factors that drive these changes, such as cell size, protein content, or nutrient environment, are still poorly understood for mammalian cells. In S phase, the cell generates a complete copy of its genetic material and then proceeds into a second preparatory phase, known as G_2 (for *gap 2*), before entry into mitosis (M phase). In M phase, the replicated DNA is carefully condensed into compact chromosomes that are precisely segregated so that two daughter cells each receive a full complement of the genetic material. Following mitosis, a proliferating cell directly reenters G_1 phase as it prepares for further replication.

Because of the complexity and irreversibility of cellular replication, eukaryotic cells have evolved several checkpoints, which are biochemically defined points in the cell cycle that can be activated to prevent the transition across certain cell-cycle phases[1,2] (see Fig. 6-1). In this way, a normal cell can ensure that DNA synthesis is not initiated or is not continued under adverse conditions, and that chromosomes do not condense and segregate

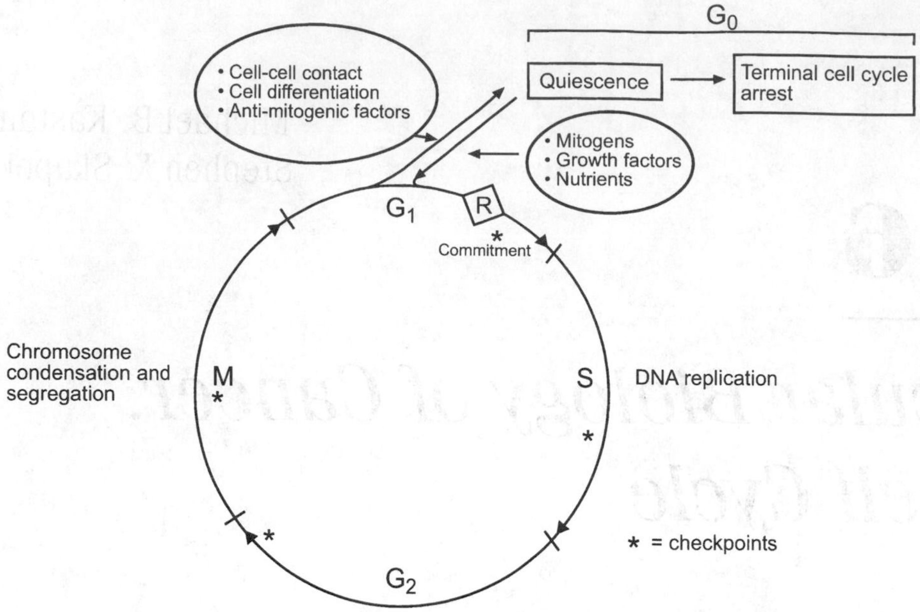

FIGURE 6-1. Schematic representation of cell-cycle phases. Mitogenic growth factors can drive a quiescent cell from G_0 into the cell cycle. Once the cell cycle passes beyond the restriction point (R), mitogens are no longer required for progression into and through S phase. The DNA is replicated in S phase and the chromosomes are condensed and segregated in mitosis. In early G_1 phase, certain signals can drive a cell to exit the cell cycle and enter a quiescent phase. Other signals such as cellular differentiation can make this irreversible. Cell-cycle checkpoints (denoted by asterisks and discussed in the text) in G_1, S, G_2, and M have been identified.

into daughter cells until the entire genome has been accurately replicated and prepared for mitosis. Loss of these checkpoints, which would have disastrous implications by leading to a variety of genetic abnormalities, is commonplace in cancer cells.

As depicted in Figure 6-1, any proliferating cell has an additional option, which is the entry into a quiescent state known as G_0. Entry into G_0 phase from G_1 is an important decision in cellular development (such as in lymphocyte or skeletal muscle cell maturation). *In vitro*, it is largely governed by the presence or absence of growth factors or nutrients that allow the procession through G_1 into S phase. If these growth factors are adequate, the cell traverses a point in G_1 phase after which the growth factors are not required. This point or transition is known as the *restriction point* (see Fig. 6-1).[3] If cellular environmental conditions are not right for a cell to proceed across the restriction point, it enters G_0 phase. Importantly, entry into G_0 may be reversible or it may be irreversible, such as during skeletal muscle or neuronal differentiation. Although the restriction point was described over 20 years ago, the precise biochemical events that define it are still not known.[4]

Regulatory Mechanisms

As described in further detail later in this chapter, research has characterized many of the molecular and biochemical events that control the transition across different cell-cycle phases and into or out of a quiescent phase. Two common regulatory themes have emerged. First, many of the key regulatory proteins are controlled by posttranslational modifications in a cell-cycle–dependent manner. Perhaps the best known example of this is the hyperphosphorylation of the retinoblastoma gene product, RB, which renders it inactive as a cell crosses the restriction point.[5,6] The hyperphosphorylation of RB and many other components of the cell-cycle machinery is mediated by heterodimeric complexes of regulatory proteins known as cyclins and their catalytically active partners known as cyclin-dependent kinases (cdks).[5] Regulation of cyclin/cdk activity is central to all phases of the mammalian cell cycle.

A second important theme that has emerged is that many of the posttranslational modifications of cell-cycle proteins alter their stability and increase their proteolytic degradation.[7,8] Because protein degradation is irreversible, it seems to be a natural mechanism to ensure that the cell cycle progresses in only one direction. This regulatory mechanism is important in every cell-cycle phase and has been conserved in many eukaryotic organisms.

As one might expect, because cancer cells have fundamental abnormalities in cell-cycle control, it is not surprising that they have been found to have abnormalities in many of the components that control each of the cell-cycle phases. These abnormalities are described in greater detail as specific phases of the cell cycle are discussed.

G_1 TO S TRANSITION

In a proliferating cell, molecular events in G_1 phase prepare the cell for the synthesis of new DNA. In different types of mammalian cells grown in culture, there can be great variations in the length of this phase, which may be very short or last for many hours. The length of the G_1 phase is somewhat dependent on extracellular signals (such as nutrients or growth factors in the environment) and may be coupled to a cell's growth in size.[9] Although much is known about events that lead up to the exit from G_1 into S phase, how the length of G_1 is determined for an individual cell is not clear.

Not only is the length of the G_1 phase of the cell cycle variable, but whether a cell completely traverses this phase at all seems to be an active *decision*. As noted previously, when a cell does not traverse G_1, it enters a quiescent phase known as G_0. *In vivo*, there are many examples of different types of mammalian cells, such as epithelial cells or lymphocytes, which are normally arrested in a quiescent phase but may be induced to reenter a proliferative phase by certain physiologic stimuli such as mitogenic growth factors (see Fig. 6-1). This arrest and reentry into the cell cycle can be largely recapitulated in cell culture systems for normal cells. However, the ability to arrest in G_0 phase of the cell cycle (e.g., because

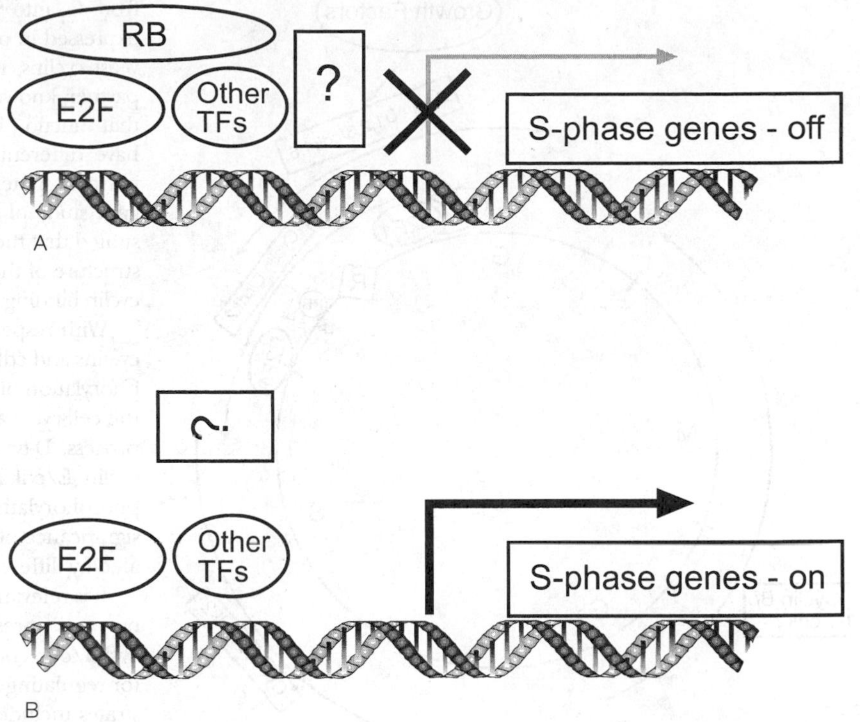

FIGURE 6-2. Schematic model for the control of E2F-dependent genes and S-phase entry by RB. **A:** When active, RB can form a complex with the transcription factor E2F. The localization of RB to this complex by E2F can suppress the transactivation function of E2F as well as other transcription factors (TFs) that may be colocalized. Other proteins (?) have been suggested to be in such a transcription repressor complex such as histone deacetylase-1.[29,30] This complex represses the expression of genes required for S-phase entry. **B:** When RB is inactivated (by phosphorylation of the protein or by mutation of the gene) the repressor complex presumably does not form and genes required for S phase are expressed.

of contact with other cells or lack of external mitogenic growth factors) is fundamentally abnormal in cancer cells.

In addition to entry into a *reversible* G_0 state, under some conditions the entry into such a state can be irreversible (see Fig. 6-1). This occurs during the terminal differentiation of cells such as skeletal muscle or neurons and during cellular senescence, which is largely an *in vitro* phenomenon that may be analogous to cellular aging.[10,11] The molecular mechanisms by which this *irreversible* arrest occurs and is maintained are only now becoming clear in certain settings, such as in skeletal muscle cells, which require the retinoblastoma gene product RB for irreversible cell-cycle arrest.[12,13]

In vitro, it is clear that the complete transit across G_1 phase is governed by the presence of extracellular growth factors that push a cell past the restriction point.[3] This point is functionally defined as a time in late G_1 phase beyond which growth factors are not required for initiation and completion of DNA synthesis and mitosis. Without adequate growth factors, the cell enters a reversible G_0 arrest described previously. Biochemical events that are concurrent with passage through this restriction point include the hyperphosphorylation of RB, the functional activation of a cellular transcription factor known as E2F-1, the accumulation of a certain threshold level of cyclin/cdk activity, and the loss of key cyclin-dependent kinase inhibitors.[5,14] However, whether or not this point can actually be attributed to any single event in mammalian cells is formally unknown.

Of these possible biochemical events that may form the restriction point, most work has focused on the role of the retinoblastoma gene product RB. Disruption of the RB gene was first found in retinoblastoma tissue[15] and subsequently in tumors from patients with sporadic forms of cancer.[16,17] The first clues to RB function came when it was found that its forced expression caused cells to arrest in G_1 phase.[18] Naturally occurring mutations in the RB gene rendered the protein unable to stop cell proliferation.[19] Hence, RB was the first tumor suppressor identified that directly functioned to block cell proliferation.

Further insight into how RB itself was regulated came from studying how it was altered during the cell cycle. Numerous studies have now proven that RB becomes progressively hyperphosphorylated as cells pass from G_1 into S phase.[20,21] This correlation suggested that hyperphosphorylation inactivated RB and allowed cell-cycle progression into S phase. Although this inactivation may be important, it is probably not the sole basis for the restriction point because cells that lack the RB gene still retain certain aspects of restriction point control.[22]

One logical extension of these studies was to determine the mechanism by which RB prevented S phase entry and how RB hyperphosphorylation blocked this function. Insight into this has come from a large body of work focused on identifying cellular proteins that interact with RB. There have been over 20 such proteins identified using a variety of assays.[23] One of the proteins identified, the transcription factor E2F-1, is central to how RB prevents cell proliferation.[24,25]

E2F-1 was the founding member of what is now known to be a family of at least six related transcription factors, which seem to have specific, nonoverlapping functions *in vivo.*[24] Most is known about E2F-1, which may be particularly important for regulating the G_1 to S transition. As a transcription factor E2F-1 activates the expression of a variety of genes, many of which encode either transcription factors that are induced as cells enter S phase or proteins that are involved in DNA synthesis, such as dihydrofolate reductase.[24] In fact, E2F-1–mediated activation of these genes is so critical that the forced expression of E2F-1 alone is sufficient to drive some cells from quiescence into S phase.[26] A number of studies have also shown that when

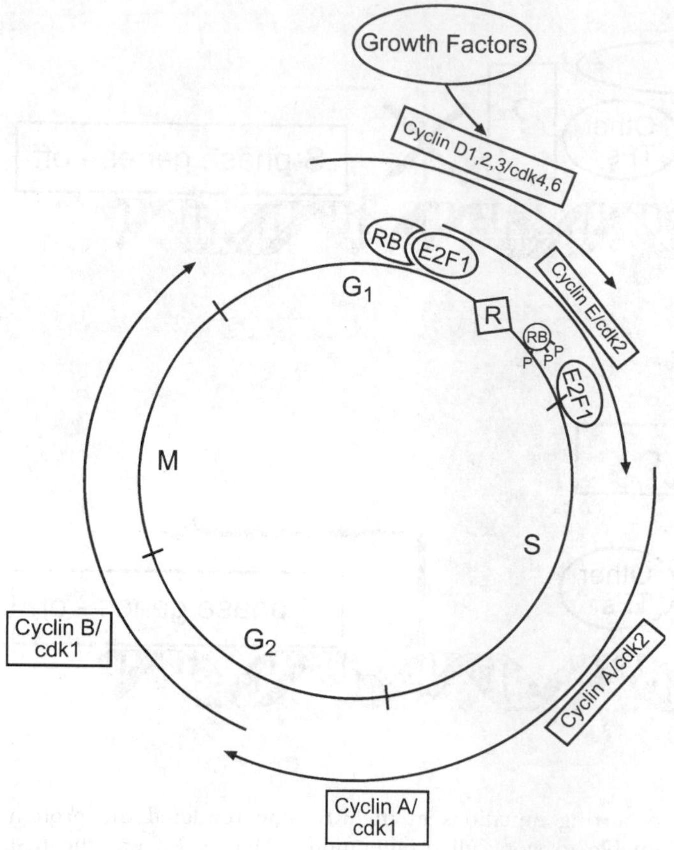

FIGURE 6-3. Schematic representation of changes in cyclins and cdks through the cell cycle. Synthesis of D-type cyclins are stimulated by growth factor signals in the G_1 phase of the cycle and associate primarily with cdks 4 and 6. Cyclin E is synthesized later in G_1 and associates with cdk2. Cyclin A is synthesized late in G_1, throughout S phase, and into early G_2 and associates with cdk2 in early S phase and cdc2 in late S phase and early G_2. Cyclin B is synthesized late in G_2 and M phase and associates with cdk1 (also known as *cdc2*). The loss of cyclin B/cdk1 activity at the end of M phase is required for reentry into the next G_1 phase.

RB physically interacts with E2F-1, it blocks E2F-1–mediated activation of these genes.[27,28] Hence, it has been proposed that the RB suppresses tumor formation by repressing genes normally induced by E2F-1 and the loss of RB would be expected to disrupt this active repressor complex (Fig. 6-2). How RB and E2F-1 form an active repressor complex is not known, but there are provocative data that this complex may alter chromatin structure by modulating histone deacetylase activity.[29,30] Despite these studies, the importance of histone deacetylase as a mediator of RB tumor suppression is not yet known.

Given the proposed model that hypophosphorylated RB and E2F-1 form an active repressor complex that is disrupted by RB hyperphosphorylation, it is important to understand the mechanisms driving RB hyperphosphorylation. The first insight into this came with the discovery of a class of genes known as cyclins in yeast cells. These cyclins are expressed in a cell-cycle–dependent manner and are required for the transition from G_1 into S phase in yeast.[5] It was later discovered that mammalian cells also had cyclins, which were expressed in a cell-cycle–dependent manner and were functionally similar to yeast cyclins. Mammalian cyclins are actually a family of related genes that includes D-type cyclins (D1, D2, and D3) and cyclin E, which are expressed maximally as cells progress from G_1 into S phase, and cyclin A, and B-type cyclins, which are expressed in other phases of the cell cycle[5,14,31] (Fig. 6-3). Like the yeast cyclins, mammalian cyclins form complexes with a catalytic partner, known as a *cdk*. There are at least seven mammalian cdks that function in distinct phases of the cell cycle (see Fig. 6-3) and have different biochemical properties including different cyclin partners, potential substrates, and link to human cancer.[14,31] Elegant study of the crystal structure of cyclin A and cdk2 demonstrated that the binding of the cyclin to the cdk physically alters the structure of the cdk and activates the enzyme.[32] In addition to this, cyclin binding may provide substrate specificity to the cdk.

With respect to the G_1 to S phase control, the key function of cyclins and cdks is to phosphorylate the RB protein.[33,34] The phosphorylation of certain serine or threonine residues in RB reverses the cell-cycle arrest by disrupting the RB-E2F-1 complex.[35] In this process, D-type cyclin/cdk complexes are activated earlier than cyclin E/cdk2, and both cyclins are required for the efficient phosphorylation of RB and entry into S phase (see Fig. 6-3).[36] The significance of potential differences in RB phosphorylation mediated by different cyclin/cdk complexes is not known.

It is relevant to emphasize that many aspects of cyclin/cdk biology are unresolved. First, although RB clearly is a target for cyclin/cdk complexes, whether it is the most important substrate for regulating entry into S phase is not known. Other possible substrates include RB-related proteins p107 and p130[37,38] that seem to have partially redundant roles with RB in cell-cycle control, components of the DNA synthesis machinery (discussed later in S Phase), and even E2F-1 itself.[39] Second, it is not obvious why mammalian cells should require so many different cyclins/cdks to phosphorylate RB. This is especially true when one considers, for example, that cyclin E seems to be able to accomplish everything that cyclin D1 can do in an elegant *knockout/knockin* experiment in mice.[40] It seems likely that as more is understood about possible *in vivo* targets for different cyclin/cdk complexes, the purpose of such a large family of cyclins will also become clearer.

Because cyclin/cdk activity is so important for regulating the G_1-to S-phase transition, their activity can be regulated at numerous levels. At present, it appears that cyclin/cdk activity can be controlled by at least six different mechanisms (Fig. 6-4).[14,41] The first level of regulation is that different cyclins are synthesized at discrete stages of the cell cycle. In this regard, the expression of D-type cyclins is closely coupled to the presence or absence of mitogenic growth factors and may be viewed as growth factor sensors.[42] Second, in addition to the regulation of cyclin synthesis, there is active regulation of cyclin degradation. In yeast cells in G_1, this is mediated by a cellular activity known as the *SCF* (for Skp-1, cullin, and F-box).[43] A similar complex has been identified in mammalian cells as well. This *machine*, which is analogous to the anaphase promoting complex (APC), that regulates mitosis, targets certain cell-cycle proteins for degradation by the ubiquitin-proteosome system. Third, in addition to the regulation of cyclin protein levels, cyclin activity is regulated by the requirement for complex formation with a cdk as discussed previously. Fourth, the cyclin/cdk complex must be activated by a cdk-activating kinase, which phosphorylates a conserved threonine residue on the cdk.[44] Fifth, additional amino acid residues in the cdk must be dephosphorylated. This is accomplished by both inhibiting certain kinases (known as Wee1/Myt1) and activating certain phosphatases (known as cdc25 A, B, and C).[41] Finally, cyclin/cdk activity is controlled by

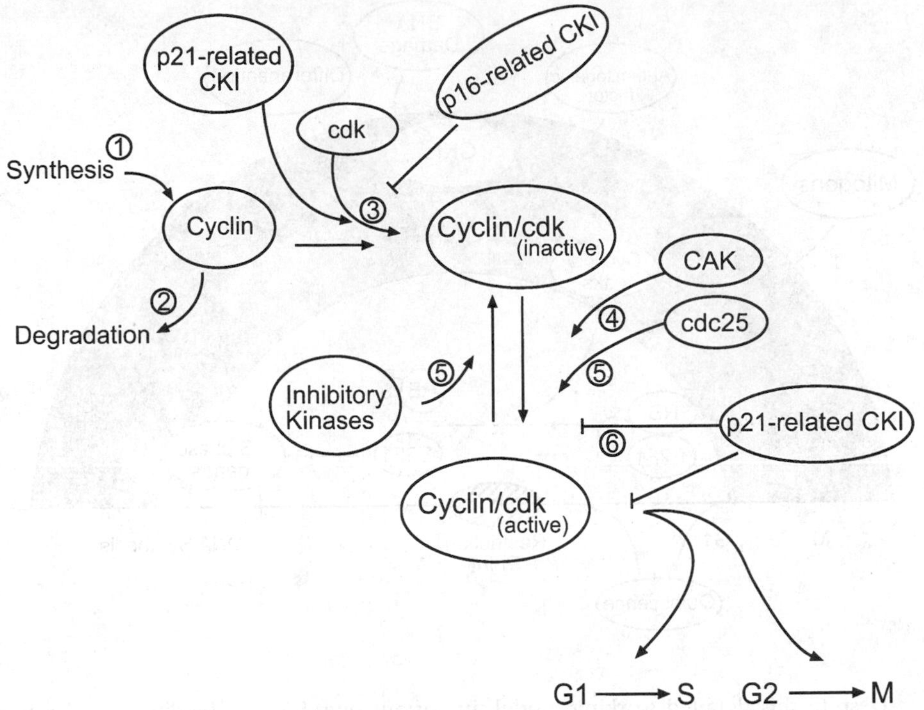

FIGURE 6-4. Multiple levels of regulation of cyclin/cyclin-dependent kinase (cdk) activity. The activity of cdks can be regulated by at least six different mechanisms: (1) and (2) cyclins are synthesized and degraded at specific stages of the cycle; (3) cdks must associate with cyclins in order to be active; p21-related and p16-related cyclin/cdk inhibitors (CKIs) can positively and negatively influence this step, respectively; (4) cdks complexed with cyclins must be activated by a cdk-activating kinase; (5) cdk activity is further controlled by inhibitory phosphorylation at threonine 14 and tyrosine 15, which can be removed (and thereby activate the cyclin/cdk) by cdc25 phosphatases; and (6) p21-related CKIs can further inhibit cyclin/cdk activity by direct complex formation with the cyclin/cdk. The activated cyclin/cdk complex phosphorylates a variety of substrates to facilitate both the G_1- to S-phase and the G_2-to M-phase transitions.

further protein-protein interactions between cdks or cyclin/cdk complexes and other proteins known as *cyclin/cdk inhibitors* (CKIs). Once fully activated, cyclin/cdk complexes phosphorylate a variety of substrates that are involved in both the G_1 to S transition as well as the G_2 to M transition.

CKIs have grown in importance and in number since they were first described. Thus far, two groups of CKIs have been identified (Table 6-1). One group includes $p21^{WAF1/CIP1}$, $p27^{KIP1}$, and $p57^{KIP2}$, which appear to be *universal* inhibitors of cyclin/cdk activity that function by forming a complex with the cyclin/cdk.[45–50] A second group includes $p16^{INK4a}$, $p15^{INK4b}$, $p18^{INK4c}$, and $p19^{INK4d}$.[51–54] These four specifically inhibit cyclin D–associated cdk4 and cdk6 (hence, the name *inhibitors of cdk4*). As was said of cyclins and cdks, why there should be such a large number of CKIs is an interesting question. To be sure, there are clear biologic differences between these two families. First of all, although $p16^{INK4a}$ clearly functions as a tumor suppressor in humans, the full role of other CKIs in human cancer is not yet clear.[55] There are also biochemical differences among different CKIs. For example, p21-like CKIs bind to the cyclin/cdk complex, whereas p16-like CKIs bind to the cdk4 or cdk6 subunit to prevent cyclin D/cdk complex formation[14] (see Fig. 6-4). Intriguingly, p21-related CKIs may function in some capacity as activators of cyclin/cdks.[56] This is based on the observation that p21-like CKIs can bind to cyclin/cdks at greater than 1:1 stoichiometry. The activity of the cyclin/cdk complex is only inhibited at high ratios of p21-like CKI to cyclin/cdk.[57,58] Finally, different CKIs can be regulated in distinct ways. For example, $p21^{WAF1/CIP1}$ was identified because the p53 tumor suppressor gene can induce its expression.[46] As such, it was an obvious candidate effector for p53-mediated cell-cycle arrest after genotoxic stress such as gamma irradiation[59,60] (see Cell-Cycle Checkpoints, later in this chapter). Similarly, both $p27^{KIP1}$ and $p15^{INK4b}$ can be modulated by transforming growth factor-β, and hence may be functional effectors of the antimitogenic effects of transforming growth factor-β.[52,61] It is likely that further understanding of the biochemical differences between different CKIs and *in vivo* studies of their function will help clarify their relevance to human cancer.

In summary, mammalian cells have developed an elegant system in which several layers of regulators control the *decision* to traverse G_1 phase and enter S phase (Fig. 6-5). RB and possibly other RB-related proteins function by actively repressing E2F-1–dependent genes at the working end of this biochemical and genetic pathway. The ability of RB to form a repressor complex with E2F-1 is regulated by multiple members of cyclin/cdk family. Of these, D-type cyclins may be particularly important as an intranuclear *sensor* of extracellular growth factors. The activity of cyclin/cdk complexes is regulated by multiple mechanisms to coordinate the decision to enter S phase with extracellular cues. These mechanisms include positive and negative influences by members of two families of CKIs that respond to both extracellular and intracellular signals. At some critical point that seems to be defined by the activation of a threshold level of cyclin/cdk activity, the RB-E2F repressor activity is turned off and the cell makes the commitment to enter S phase.

TABLE 6-1. Classes of Cyclin-Dependent Kinase (cdk) Inhibitors

Inhibits Multiple Cyclin/cdk Complexes	*Inhibits Cyclin D/cdk4 or 6*
$p21^{WAF1/CIP1}$	$p16^{INK4a}$
$p27^{KIP1}$	$p15^{INK4b}$
$p57^{KIP2}$	$p18^{INK4c}$
	$p19^{INK4d}$

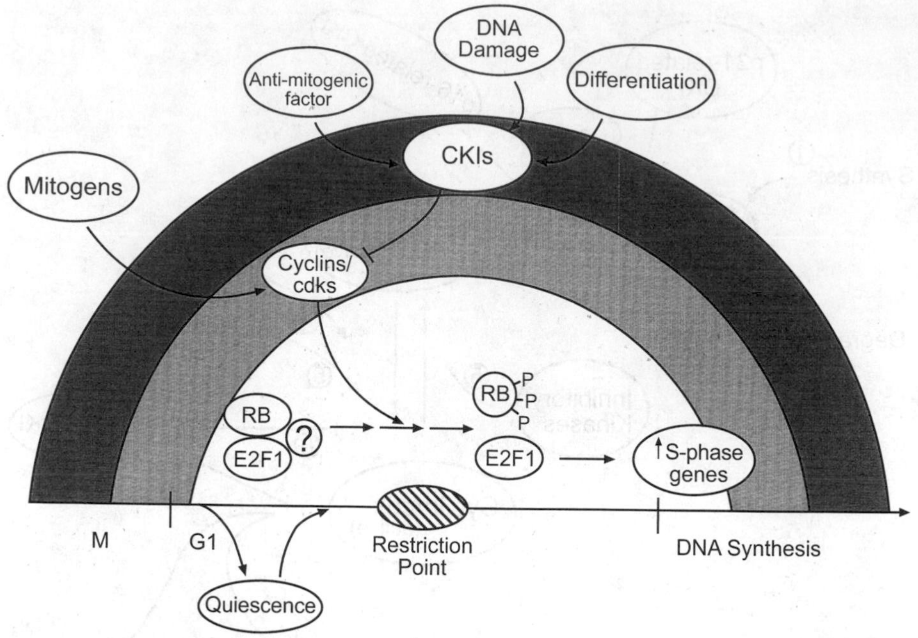

FIGURE 6-5. Schematic diagram showing several layers governing the regulation of G_1-to S-phase transition. At present, the event most closely correlated with the transition across the restriction point seems to be the phosphorylation of RB, which disrupts the RB/E2F-1 repressor complex. This leads to the induction of E2F-1–dependent genes and commitment to enter and progress through S phase. The function of RB in this complex is controlled by a number of cyclin/cdk (cyclin-dependent kinases) complexes that are active in G_1 phase. These cyclin/cdk complexes are, in turn, largely negatively regulated by a number of cyclin/cdk inhibitors (CKIs). The activity of both cyclin/cdk complexes and CKIs are lastly regulated by a number of extracellular signals (such as mitogenic or antimitogenic factors) and intracellular signals (such as DNA damage or differentiation factors).

Despite this detailed working model, important questions remain. For example, clarifying the molecular basis for the restriction point will be an important advance in the basic understanding of cell-cycle control. Determining the importance of different regulatory proteins in different types of human cancer will also be important. Finally, understanding how RB and E2F actually function as an active repressor may open up new therapeutic avenues based on better understanding of the working end of this pathway.

S PHASE

The task of generating an exact copy of more than 3 billion base pairs of DNA in the human genome is quite daunting. As is described here, mammalian cells have had to surmount a number of mechanistic difficulties to accomplish this. The importance of the machinery that accomplishes this task is clear because many of the components have been highly conserved from bacteria to humans. What is perhaps an even more important task, though, is how to regulate this DNA synthesis machinery. Each of these 3 billion base pairs must be copied one time, and only one time, during each cell division cycle. Except in rare circumstances in certain organisms or certain developmental states, the synthesis of DNA more or less than one time per cell cycle would be devastating. Since the last writing of this chapter, much insight has been gained into how DNA synthesis is regulated.

It is now known that DNA synthesis begins at defined sequences in the genome of most organisms. These *origins of replication* contain specific DNA sequences, which have been referred to as *autonomously replicating sequences* or *replicator* elements.[62] A technique known as *DNA footprinting* was used to evaluate proteins that were bound to these DNA elements at different phases of the cell cycle. These studies have shown that there are two different footprint patterns on replicator elements at different phases of the cell cycle, and a change in this pattern occurs as DNA synthesis begins. The multiple proteins that form a DNA-binding complex to generate these footprints are known as the origin of replication complex (ORC).[63] Based on the timing of the two observed ORC footprints, it is thought that these represent a prereplication ORC (pre-RC) and a postreplication ORC (post-RC).[64] The pre-RC is assembled and competent to begin replication in G_1 phase but is held in check by some mechanism to prevent the formal initiation of DNA synthesis (i.e., the conversion of a pre-RC to a post-RC) until S phase. The post-RC represents a complex that is competent to carry out DNA synthesis from the origin of replication to which it is bound.

The molecular components of a pre-RC and post-RC have been studied using biochemical and genetic approaches in different types of eukaryotic cells. There are a large number of proteins of different classes that form these pre-RCs and post-RCs. Some of these proteins, such as ORC proteins 1 through 6 and MCM proteins 2 through 7, have been identified and are beginning to be biochemically characterized.[64] However, mechanistic details for how ORCs function are largely unknown.

In addition to identifying the individual components of the pre-RC and post-RC, work has focused on understanding how a pre-RC is converted to a post-RC and how this is directly linked with DNA synthesis. The changes in footprint pattern as a pre-RC becomes a post-RC coincide with the loss or gain of different molecular components of this complex. Because of the importance of cyclin/cdk activation at the G_1 to S transition, it is likely that cyclin/cdk complexes will be shown to phosphorylate particular substrates that directly affect the pre-RC and post-RC complexes. For example, there is some evidence that MCM proteins, which are components of the ORC, are phosphorylated at the transition to S phase.[65] The phosphorylation of at least one of these (MCM4) can be mediated by a cyclin/cdk.[66] Such a posttranslational modification may be involved in changing a pre-RC to a post-RC and actually driving the formal initiation of DNA synthesis.

The regulation of pre-RC and post-RC is also probably coupled to the mechanism by which a cell prevents *rereplication* of DNA in S phase. The cell cycle can be generally divided into two states: an assembly state and a replication state.[64] The former

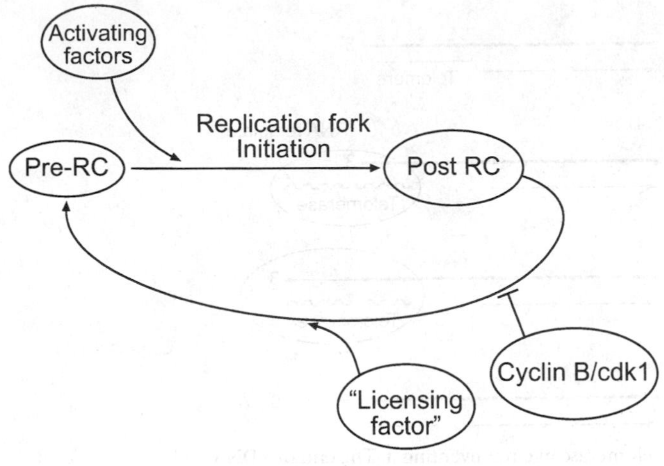

FIGURE 6-6. Schematic model of how the ability to synthesize new DNA may be regulated. After mitosis is complete, a cell becomes competent to initiate new DNA synthesis. This competency correlates with the presence of a prereplication complex (pre-RC) bound to DNA replicator elements. At the formal initiation of DNA synthesis (replication fork initiation), which is driven by certain poorly defined events (activating factors), the pre-RC complex changes to a post-RC complex while DNA is synthesized. This post-RC complex is unable to bind to new DNA replicator elements and, hence, DNA can only be synthesized one time per cell cycle. The transition from a post-RC back to a pre-RC, on completion of the next mitotic phase, is negatively and positively regulated by cyclin B/cdk1 and a poorly defined licensing factor (see text for details).

state allows the assembly of pre-RCs at replicator elements but prevents the formal initiation of DNA synthesis until other critical factors are supplied (such as G_1/S cyclin/cdk activity) (Fig. 6-6). The latter state allows DNA synthesis from preassembled ORCs but does not allow assembly of *new* pre-RCs. The loss of cyclin/cdk activity at the end of mitosis is one factor that probably allows the reformation of the pre-RCs. There may also be other factors, such as *licensing factor*,[67] which seems to be supplied to a cell only *after* completion of mitosis to prevent rereplication of DNA (see Fig. 6-6). As more is learned about the existence of states that are competent and not competent for new DNA synthesis, many more regulatory details will be elucidated.

In addition to the task of allowing DNA synthesis only one time during the cell cycle, the cell faces the task of ensuring that newly synthesized DNA is *accurately* copied. The enzymes that accomplish this are called DNA polymerases, three of which are known to be involved in DNA replication (as opposed to repair) in eukaryotic cells (DNA polymerases a, d, and e). The double-stranded nature of genomic DNA provides a mechanism to ensure accuracy because each existing strand serves as a template for a new strand. Although the DNA polymerases copy it with high fidelity, they are not perfect. Approximately one incorrect nucleotide is incorporated for every 10^5 to 10^6 correct nucleotides. At this rate, 1000 to 10,000 mutations would be generated with each cell division. In order to prevent this, the DNA polymerases are endowed with *proofreading* functions that allow misincorporated nucleotides to be detected and removed by 3' to 5' exonuclease activity of the DNA polymerase. This process reduces the error rate by approximately 1000-fold.[68] In addition to the repair activity that is closely coupled to DNA synthesis, other repair processes detect and replace mismatched DNA bases or other DNA abnormalities to further limit errors associated with DNA replication. Inefficiencies in DNA repair machinery appear to be important in the development of some forms of cancer, such as certain forms of hereditary colon cancer that are linked to abnormalities in DNA mismatch repair enzymes.[69]

In addition to the problem of accuracy, the cell faces a problem due to the sheer magnitude of the task of copying all 3 billion base pairs. A single replication fork traveling at approximately 3000 bases per minute would require approximately 1 month to replicate just one of the 46 human chromosomes.[70] As described previously, the cell addresses this problem by initiating DNA replication at multiple origins of replications. Interestingly, these multiple origins appear to fire in an ordered fashion.[64] The mechanisms by which origins fire early or late in S phase are not understood.

After any individual ORC is activated to begin DNA synthesis, how the polymerase generates an elongating strand of newly synthesized DNA is another mechanistic hurdle. Because DNA is a double-stranded helix, it must be unwound and both strands of the DNA must be copied simultaneously. The synthetic process is started from an RNA primer on each of these strands and makes the new strand in the 5' to 3' direction (Fig. 6-7). Because the double-stranded DNA is arranged in an antiparallel fashion, one new strand is synthesized continuously (*leading strand*) and the other discontinuously (*lagging strand*). As described for the ORCs, much work has focused on identifying the proteins that are required for DNA synthesis at the replication forks of eukaryotic cells. These include PCNA, RPA, RFC, DNA polymerases, DNA primase, and RNAseH.[71] Some of the mechanics of the process are now understood, such as PCNA forming a molecular *sliding clamp* to hold the polymerase on the DNA.[72] After the DNA polymerase complex has proceeded along the length of a strand of DNA to the next replicon, the RNA primer is replaced by DNA and a DNA ligase closes the gap between the two newly synthesized stretches of DNA. With this, DNA synthesis is essentially complete.

One final hurdle, though, for a cell to *completely* copy the entire genome involves the synthesis of new DNA at the end of each chromosome. Because DNA polymerases require an RNA primer to begin this process and because they only assemble a new strand in the 5' to 3' direction, each linear chromosome would fail to copy DNA at the very 3' end of each chromosome with every round of replication (see Fig. 6-7).[73] This would be deleterious because numerous rounds of DNA replication would result in a large amount of DNA being lost from the chromosome ends.

It appears that eukaryotic cells deal with this *end-replication* problem by the use of specialized structures called *telomeres*, which are simple tandemly repeated sequences at the end of each chromosome (see Fig. 6-7). These repeated DNA sequences are recognized by telomerase, a holoenzyme containing a reverse transcriptase (polymerase) and an RNA component that is complementary to the repeated DNA sequences of a telomere. The reverse transcriptase extends the 3' end of the chromosomal DNA by *reading* the RNA component as a template[73,74] (see Fig. 6-7). In this way, telomerase prevents the loss of this 3' end of the DNA to defeat the end-replication problem.

In addition to providing a mechanism to complete the DNA synthesis task, telomerase activity is particularly important for cancer biology because it confers unlimited cell proliferation capacity,[73,74] which is a hallmark of a malignant cancer cell. There is good experimental evidence that most telomerase-

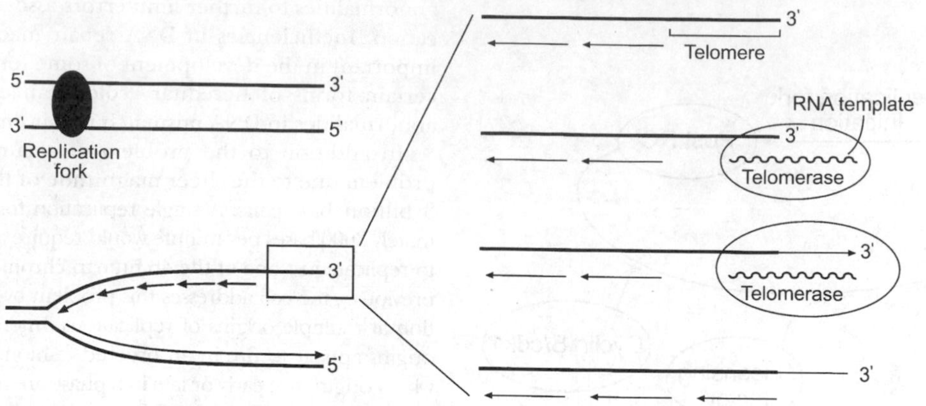

FIGURE 6-7. The end-replication problem and role of telomerase in circumventing it. The end of a DNA molecule is replicated on one strand by continuous replication proceeding to the end of the molecule, whereas the other strand is replicated discontinuously using RNA primers and Okazaki fragments. Removal of the RNA primer and Okazaki fragment ligation leaves a region at the 3' end of one nascent DNA strand unreplicated (*box*). If there were no mechanism to fill the gap, the chromosome end would get shorter with each round of replication. Telomerase solves this problem by binding to the telomere at the 3' end of the nascent DNA strand and extending this end. This provides an elongated template for the DNA polymerase to use, which allows the entire original genomic DNA sequence to be completely replicated. (Adapted from ref. 74, with permission.)

deficient cells can only replicate a finite number of times until the telo–meric ends of the chromosomes become shortened to a critical point that arrests further cell proliferation.[73] Because most normal cells in the body do not have telomerase activity, it has been suggested that the loss of telomeric DNA may be the basis for cellular aging. On the other hand, tumor cells appear to be immortalized by virtue of the increased telomerase activity.[75] Because increased telomerase activity is relatively specific to cancer cells in a human body, the pharmacologic inhibition of telomerase may, indeed, be a new therapy for cancer that is directly based on better understanding of the DNA synthesis process.

M-PHASE ENTRY AND EXIT

Once the cell has copied the entire genome, it enters a second gap phase, known as G_2, to prepare for entry into mitosis, the phase in which the duplicated genome is segregated to two daughter cells. The successful completion of mitosis may be considered the most crucial phase in the cell cycle because errors in this process are irreversible and lead to dramatic alterations in the genetic material such as the loss or gain of entire chromosomes. Much insight has been gained into the regulation of this process since the last writing of this chapter and can be found in excellent, detailed reviews.[8,76,77] Three main features of this regulation are presented here. Because of its complexity, it is helpful to consider mitosis in several distinct phases (Fig. 6-8*A*). In the first place, the actual entry into mitosis is carefully controlled to prevent the segregation of chromosomes that have not completed DNA synthesis. Second, there are many structural changes that occur in a cell during mitosis such as chromosomal condensation, centrosome migration, microtubule polymerization, spindle assembly, nuclear membrane dissolution, microtubule and kinetochore attachment, alignment of all chromosomes on a plane between the centrosomes, and the separation of sister chromatids (see Fig. 6-8*A*). The actual separation of sister chromatids, a process that constitutes the metaphase to anaphase transition, represents an important checkpoint for a cell because chromatid separation is not easily reversed. Finally, after anaphase is complete, the chromosomes lose their highly condensed structure, the nuclear envelope reforms, and the cell undergoes cytoplasmic division (cytokinesis) to complete the cell cycle. At this stage, the cell must formally exit mitosis to reset itself for the next cell division cycle. Most of what is known about mitotic control in mammalian cells relates to how the entry into mitosis, the metaphase to anaphase transition, and the exit from mitosis are governed.

The first regulatory mechanism for mitosis involved the maturation- (or mitosis) promoting factor (MPF), which was identified as a cytoplasmic activity in metaphase-blocked *Xenopus* oocytes that could drive other cells into mitosis.[78] MPF was characterized as a complex of cyclin B and cdk1 (also known as cdc2) (Fig. 6-8*B*).[79] Many studies have demonstrated that the activation of cyclin B/cdk1 is the most crucial step governing whether a cell enters mitosis.[77] Because of this central role, cyclin B/cdk1 is regulated at many levels, including some that are different from the G_1/S cyclin/cdks discussed previously. First, the levels of cyclin B protein are increased during late S and G_2 phase by both increased synthesis and decreased destruction. Second, newly synthesized cyclin B binds to unphosphorylated cdk1, which becomes activated by phosphorylation at threonine 161 by cdk-activating kinase. Approximately concurrent with this, the *cytoplasmic* cyclin B/cdk1 complexes must be relocalized to the nucleus by an as yet unclear mechanism.[80] In addition, the competing kinases (Wee1/Mik1/Myt1) and phosphatases (cdc25 B and C), which govern the phosphorylation of threonine 14 and tyrosine 15 on cdk1, must allow dephosphorylation of these residues to activate the cyclin/kinase activity (see Fig. 6-8*B*).[77] Once activated, a positive feedback loop between cyclin B/cdk1 and cdc25C exists to allow further activation of B/cdk1, which drives the initiation of mitosis by phosphorylating specific nuclear proteins.[77] The identification of the specific proteins that are phosphorylated by cyclin B/cdk1 to drive the initiation of mitosis will be important for our understanding of this phase of the cell cycle. Because the cdc25 phosphatase plays a key role in the initial activation of cyclin B/cdk1, it is not surprising that it also has an important role in a checkpoint pathway that can be activated to prevent the entry into mitosis in response to genotoxic stress (see section G_2- to M-Phase Checkpoint, later in this chapter).

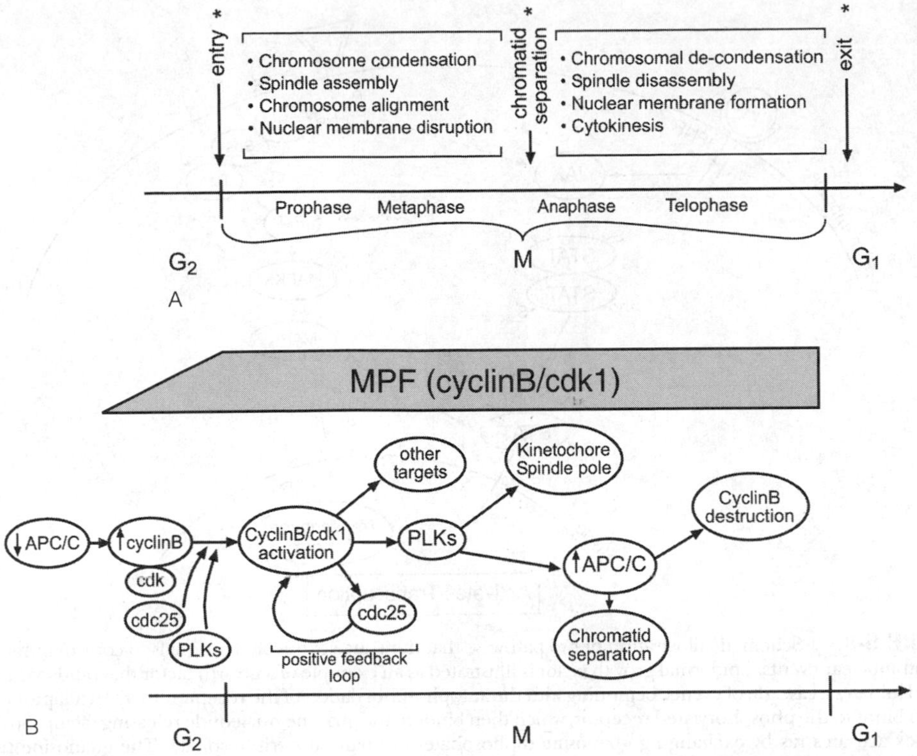

FIGURE 6-8. Schematic diagram of G_2- to M-phase regulation. **A:** The large number of complex structural changes that occur during M phase generally seem to be regulated at three key transition points: the formal entry into mitosis, the metaphase to anaphase transition, and the formal exit from mitosis. **B:** Regulation of the transition across M phase involves multiple events. First, the accumulation of maturation- (or mitosis) promoting factor (MPF) (cyclin B/cdk1) to a critical level seems to mark the formal beginning of M phase. The accumulation of cyclin B is governed by decreased anaphase promoting complex/cyclosome (APC/C) activity, and a number of other cyclin/cdk (cyclin-dependent kinase) activating steps (see Fig. 6-4). Once activated cyclin B/cdk1 phosphorylates a number of targets, including cdc25 phosphatase, which positively feeds back to activate more cyclin B/cdk1. Cyclin B/cdk1 also seems to activate polo-like kinases (PLKs), which are kinases physically localized to (and hence may regulate) certain key mitotic structures such as kinetochores and spindle pole bodies. Finally, PLKs can activate APC/C again during M phase, which leads to the degradation of proteins that may be directly involved in the separation of sister chromatids (metaphase to anaphase transition). APC/C activation also causes the degradation of cyclin B, which both ends the mitotic phase and facilitates the reformation of the pre-RC to set the stage for the next cell-cycle phase (see Fig. 6-6).

A second important regulatory mechanism may help link biochemical changes such as phosphorylation of specific proteins with structural changes such as spindle body assembly. This mechanism involves a family of kinases known as polo-like kinases (PLKs) after polo kinase, the first of this family identified in *Drosophila*.[76] Like cdks, PLKs represent a family of kinases conserved from yeast to humans. Although they may have functions at several stages of the cell cycle, the best-characterized roles are during mitosis.[76] In the first place, they indirectly activate cyclin B/cdk1 by phosphorylating and activating cdc25. Whether PLKs are initial activators of cyclin B/cdk1 or play a role in the positive feedback loop for B/cdk1 activation is not known. Second, at different stages of mitosis PLKs are localized to spindle pole bodies, kinetochores, and the spindle midzone, which suggests that they may play a role in spindle apparatus assembly, sister chromatid pairing and separation, and even cytokinesis. Because cyclin B/cdk1 may activate them, PLKs could directly link the biochemical activity of MPF with structural changes that occur during mitosis. However, the mechanistic details of this are far from understood. Finally, PLKs may also activate the APC/cyclosome (APC/C), which has roles in both the metaphase to anaphase transition as well as the formal exit from mitosis.

Finally, it has become clear that regulated destruction of certain proteins is a central force driving entry into, transition through, and exit from mitosis. At the heart of this is a large complex of proteins known as the APC/C. As with PLKs, the importance of the APC/C is indicated by the fact that it has been conserved in evolution from yeast to humans.[8,81] It functions by *marking* particular proteins with a ubiquitin molecule that leads to the destruction of the ubiquitinated protein by the 26S proteosome degradation machine. Numerous studies have shown that the down-regulation of APC/C activity contributes to the accumulation of cyclin B, which is required for a cell to enter into mitosis (see Fig. 6-8*B*).[82] In addition, the APC/C contributes to the destruction of the *glue* that holds sister chromatids together; hence, it drives the metaphase to anaphase transition.[82] Finally, activation of the APC/C eventually guides the destruction of cyclin B protein to mark the end of mitosis.[82] Importantly, by destroying all mitotic cyclin/cdk activity, the APC/C also allows the entry into the *next* G_1 phase by allowing the formation of new pre-RC (see Fig. 6-6). Moreover, the APC/C remains active to prevent the reaccumulation of cyclin B until the next mitotic entry is scheduled.

CONTROL OF THE CELL DIVISION CYCLE

Obviously, the cell does not use the complex DNA synthesis and cell division machinery in a vacuum. It must continuously integrate extracellular signals from the environment as well as

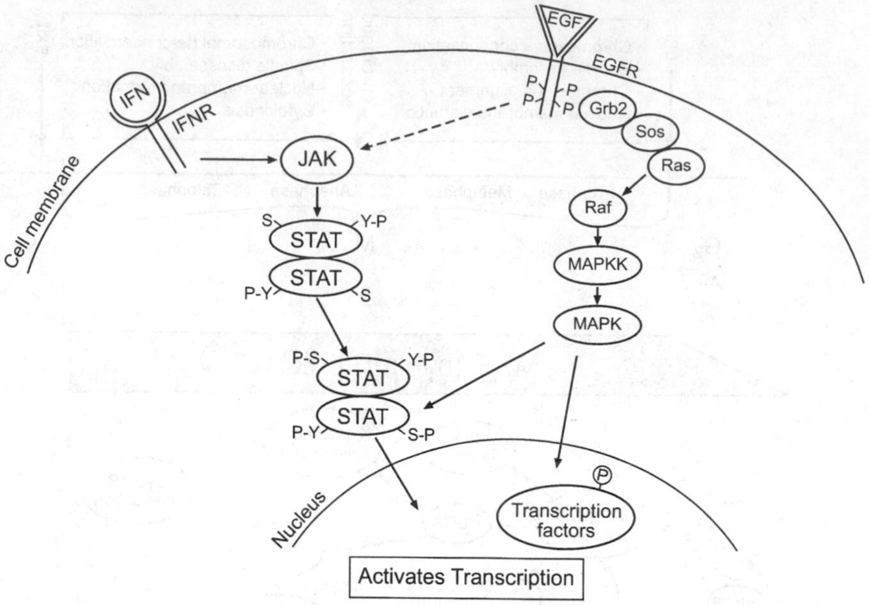

FIGURE 6-9. Schematic illustration of two pathways that transduce extracellular signals to control intracellular and intranuclear events. Epidermal growth factor is illustrated as an example of a growth factor that binds to its receptor and initiates a cascade of events, beginning with the autophosphorylation of the receptor itself. An adaptor protein (Grb2) binds to the phosphorylated receptor, which then binds to the guanine nucleotide releasing factor (Sos). This complex activates ras by exchanging guanosine diphosphate for guanosine triphosphate. The guanosine triphosphate–bound active form of ras binds to and activates the serine/threonine kinase raf. Raf phosphorylates and activates mitogen-activated protein-kinase kinase (MAPKK), which in turn phosphorylates and activates mitogen-activated protein kinase (MAPK). The targets phosphorylated by MAPK appear to be both cytoplasmic and nuclear proteins, at least some of which can activate transcription of certain gene products involved in cell proliferation. The Jak/STAT pathway is illustrated as being initiated by interferon (IFN) binding to its receptor (IFNR), which leads to activation of members of the Jak family of nonreceptor tyrosine kinases. These kinases then phosphorylate members of the STAT family of transcription factors on tyrosine residues, which translocate to the nucleus, bind specific DNA sequences, and promote transcription. There may be significant cross-talk between signaling pathways. In this example, this is illustrated by (1) the activation of the Jak pathway by certain peptide growth factors (*dashed arrow*) and (2) the phosphorylation of serine residues on STAT proteins by MAP kinase.

intracellular signals regarding the status of the genome. These signals contribute to the control of cell division and also constitute formal checkpoints that may be activated in times of cellular stress. How a cell accomplishes the integration of extracellular signals and the mechanisms by which it checks its progress through cell division are reviewed in this section.

EXTRACELLULAR SIGNALS

Nutrient status, cell-cell contact, and extracellular peptides can all influence intracellular events. The significant question that arises is how do these extracellular factors communicate with the intracellular machinery to influence cell-cycle progression? For example, growth factors cause cells in the resting or G_0 phase of the cell cycle to enter and proceed through the cycle. Continued growth factor exposure is required for progression through G_1 until the cell reaches the restriction point (see Fig. 6-3), after which time the cell proceeds through the rest of the cell cycle. How does the presence of an extracellular polypeptide, such as a growth factor, influence the cell cycle in this way? Much progress has been made in understanding the exact details of the many events that occur after any single growth factor stimulates a cell to proliferate. Unfortunately, these events are so complex that it would be impossible to provide adequate detail in this chapter. Therefore, we address general themes that have emerged more recently.

Many growth factors (or cytokines) are soluble proteins that mediate cellular communication. In general, these growth factors bind to specific receptors on the surface of cells and initiate a cascade of biochemical signals that influence intracellular events. Typically, one of the first events is the phosphorylation of the receptor or a protein associated with the receptor.[83] Some cytokine receptors contain intrinsic tyrosine kinase domains, whereas other cytokine receptors have no intrinsic kinase function but are capable of recruiting and activating nonreceptor tyrosine kinases, which can transduce signals *downstream* to other proteins. A common end point for this cascade is the change in activity of certain transcription factors leading to the induction or repression of specific genes involved in cell proliferation, cell differentiation, or cell survival (Fig. 6-9). Examples of such signaling pathways include the activation of the RAS-RAF-MAP kinase pathway in response to epidermal growth factor signaling,[83–85] or the activation of the Janus kinase (Jak) family that then activates the STAT family of transcriptional regulators in response to interleukin signaling.[86–88] With the role that growth factor receptors and signal transduction components have in mediating the cellular decision to proliferate by driving the G_1 to S transition, it is not surprising that many of these components have been found to be abnormal in human cancers. The HER2/neu epidermal growth factor–like growth factor receptor is an elegant example of both the identification of important components of this pathway and how such knowledge has been translated into a novel therapeutic approach that is specifically designed to disrupt this pathway using anti-HER2/neu antibodies.[89]

It must be emphasized that these are only two of a large number of pathways that have been identified. Moreover, these apparently linear pathways are not linear at all, as there is much cross-talk between different components of a pathway, which suggests that the cellular responses to any single factor may depend on the balance of signals from different growth factor pathways.[90]

Despite the complexity of these mitogenic signaling pathways, there is the suggestion that most converge on a common intranuclear event. It has been observed that most, if not all, mitogenic growth factors at some point lead to increased expression of certain D-type cyclins.[5] As noted previously, this is an essential component of the ultimate activation of cyclin D/cdk activity (see Fig. 6-4). However, the induction of cyclin D protein is not sufficient to drive the entire decision for a cell to proliferate. Therefore, it must be integrated with other biochemical events in the nucleus. This observation provides a framework to think about how signaling of cells at the cell membrane by extracellular growth factors can affect the machinery that directly drives cell proliferation across the G_1 to S boundary. As more is learned about mitogenic signal transduction pathways, the knowledge of how growth factors influence the cell-cycle machinery should lead to novel therapeutic strategies to treat cancer.

CELL-CYCLE CHECKPOINTS

The events of the cell cycle appear to be highly ordered into dependent pathways so that the initiation of any event in the cell cycle is dependent on the completion of earlier events. For example, mitosis is dependent on completion of DNA synthesis, chromatid separation is dependent on kinetochore assembly and chromosome alignment, and DNA replication during S phase is *licensed* by the cell having completed a prior mitosis. The control mechanisms that enforce this ordered dependency are called cell-cycle checkpoints.[1,2] It is important to emphasize that a variety of signals, from both extracellular as well as intracellular events, can activate these checkpoints to prevent cell-cycle progression. For example, nutrient deprivation, temperature changes and other forms of environmental stress, nucleotide depletion, or damage to the DNA all can inhibit cell-cycle progression by invoking these cell-cycle checkpoint controls.

It is now clear that cell-cycle checkpoints are actively regulated by components of the cell-cycle machinery. For example, cell-cycle arrest following DNA damage is not simply a by-product of the structural damage to the DNA. Moreover, mutations in the genes that control these checkpoints can disrupt the arrest signals and allow continued cell-cycle progression when it may be inappropriate. Such mutations could result in altered responses to environmental or therapeutic DNA-damaging agents, such as increased or decreased cell death, increased mutation rate, and genetic instability. It is not surprising, then, that mutations in cell-cycle checkpoint genes are now thought to both significantly contribute to cancer development and affect the responses of tumor cells to chemotherapy and radiation therapy.[91]

Damage to the DNA by ionizing radiation is the one stimulus for cell-cycle checkpoint activation that has been the most intensively studied. When nuclear DNA has been damaged by either intrinsic or extrinsic processes, normal cells cease progressing through the cell cycle at one of several points: either before entry into S phase, within S phase, or before entry into mitosis (see Fig. 6-1). Presumably, arrest at these particular points in the cell cycle would limit the propagation of genetic mutations to daughter cells by allowing for DNA repair, and it may also prevent cell death. We briefly review what is known about each of these DNA damage checkpoints as well as two additional checkpoints that are not directly activated by DNA damage but may still be relevant to cancer development.

G_1- to S-Phase Checkpoint

The tumor suppressor gene, p53, appears to be a critical component of the signaling pathway that arrests cells in G_1 after DNA damage (Fig. 6-10). It is mutated in a large proportion of human cancers and the Li-Fraumeni familial cancer syndrome is caused by germline mutations in the p53 gene,[92,93] which supports the importance of p53 function in cancer prevention. There are two potential mechanisms by which the loss of the p53-mediated G_1 to S checkpoint could lead to increased cancer susceptibility. First, DNA damage is known to increase p53 protein level and activity, which secondarily increases the level of the $p21^{WAF1/CIP1}$ CKI. Increased $p21^{WAF1/CIP1}$ inhibits the activity of cyclin/cdk complexes that drive the G_1- to S-phase transition by preventing the hyperphosphorylation of RB (see Fig. 6-10). In cells that lack $p21^{WAF1/CIP1}$, the G_1 to S arrest after DNA damage is defective.[60] In addition to being critical for G_1 to S arrest, p53 also can drive programmed cell death or apoptosis in certain cells in response to DNA damage.[94,95] What governs whether p53 causes cell-cycle arrest or programmed cell death is not well understood. Nonetheless, it is clear that the loss of p53 can result in inappropriate cellular response to DNA damage by two mechanisms: allowing damaged DNA to be replicated and allowing the survival of cells that normally would undergo programmed cell death (see Fig. 6-10). In this regard, it is easy to understand how p53 mutations would be critical to cancer development. In addition, the loss of p53-mediated apoptosis in response to therapies that cause DNA damage could have a significant effect on tumor response. Two new genes, p73 and p63, have been identified as relatives of p53.[96,97] The full importance of these p53-related genes in human cancer and the G_1 to S checkpoint will require further study.

S-Phase Checkpoint

The molecular controls of S-phase arrest after DNA damage in mammalian cells are less well understood, but a number of yeast genes, such as MEC1, MEC2, and HUS1, have been identified that control the S-phase checkpoint.[98] Although clear mammalian counterparts to these genes are just now being identified, the ATM gene, which is *mutated in ataxia-telangiectasia* and is related to MEC1, seems to be particularly important for the S-phase checkpoint. The first insight into this came from the study of patients with ataxia-telangiectasia, who are cancer prone, and from study of these patients' cells, which are defective in all three DNA damage-induced checkpoints, including the S-phase checkpoint.[99] The ATM gene product is a nuclear and cytoplasmic protein kinase that can phosphorylate certain proteins that are known to be involved in DNA damage checkpoints and DNA repair, such as p53.[100] Although studies of ATM-related genes in yeast have suggested potential biochemical and genetic mechanisms,[2] how ATM regulates the S-phase checkpoint is not yet known (see Fig. 6-10).

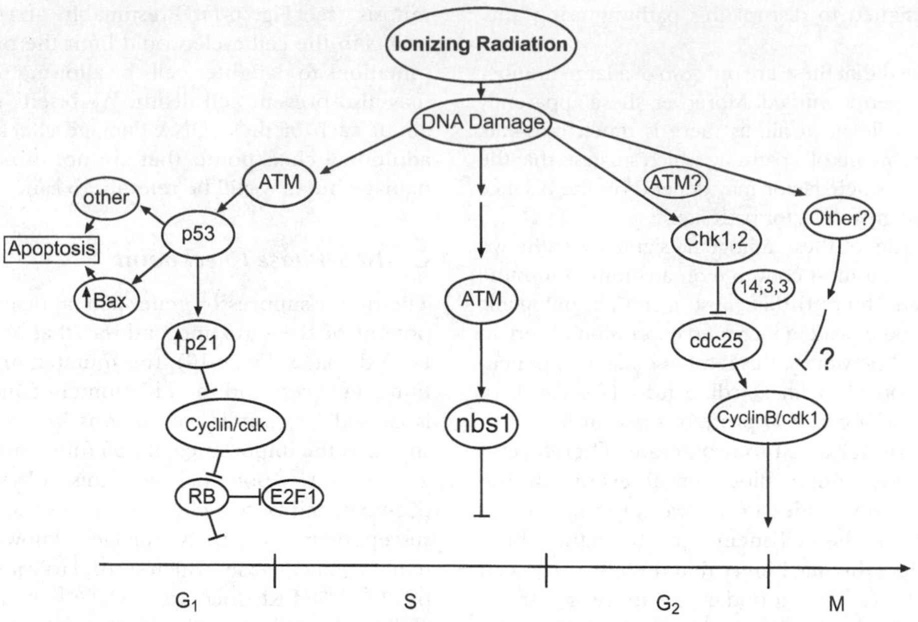

FIGURE 6-10. Schematic diagram of several cell-cycle checkpoints in mammalian cells. Ionizing radiation causes DNA damage in the form of strand breaks. This activates several signal transduction pathways, depending on the phase of the cell cycle. For cells in G_1, DNA damage leads to increased p53 protein, which is dependent on signaling through ATM. Increased p53 protein levels lead to transcriptional activation of certain genes, such as gadd45, mdm2, p21, cyclin G, and Bax, which causes either cell-cycle arrest by induction of $p21^{WAF1/CIP1}$ or apoptosis. For cells in S phase, DNA damage arrests further DNA synthesis in an ATM-dependent and an nbs1-dependent manner.[150] In cells in G_2 and M phase, DNA damage leads to the activation of proteins such as chk1 and chk2, which can phosphorylate cdc25 phosphatase. Phosphorylated cdc25 is then bound by, and hence inactivated by, 14-3-3 proteins, which therefore prevents the activation of cyclin B/cdk1 (MPF). The role of ATM and potentially other proteins in this checkpoint are not yet known. It is important to emphasize that the cell-cycle checkpoints differ in response to different types of DNA damage, such as that induced by gamma irradiation versus various genotoxic drugs or ultraviolet irradiation.

G_2- to M-Phase Checkpoint

The DNA damage-induced arrest of cells in the G_2 phase of the cell cycle is prominent in most mammalian cell types and has been intensively studied by radiobiologists for years because of an apparent link between G_2 arrest and radiosensitivity.[101] In yeast, the RAD9, RAD17, RAD24, MEC1, MEC2, and MEC3 genes all appear to be involved in signaling the cell to arrest in G_2 after DNA damage,[91] and mutations in these genes lead to increased genetic instability and increased radiosensitivity. Work clarifying many details of this pathway in mammalian cells indicates that it controls the activation of cyclin B/cdk1, which is particularly important for regulating entry into mitosis (see Fig. 6-8). Briefly, in yeast it has been shown that DNA damage activates a kinase known as chk1, which can phosphorylate cdc25, the phosphatase that is critical for activating cyclin B/cdk1 at entry into mitosis. Phosphorylated cdc25 can be bound and, hence, inactivated by interaction with 14-3-3 proteins (see Fig. 6-10).[102] Similar themes are emerging from study of mammalian cells. ATM also appears to have a role in this pathway; however, the molecular details are not yet known.

Mitotic Spindle Checkpoint

In addition to the DNA damage-induced checkpoint to prevent entry into mitosis, there is another mitotic checkpoint that involves the mitotic spindle apparatus. This checkpoint functions to prevent the metaphase to anaphase transition until all sister chromatid pairs are aligned and attached to the mitotic spindle apparatus (see M-Phase Entry and Exit, earlier in this chapter) (see Fig. 6-8). Abnormalities in this checkpoint can lead to gross changes in chromosome number, which is a common occurrence in cancer cells. Several yeast genes (MAD1, MAD2, MAD3, BUB1, BUB2, and BUB3) have been found that control mitotic arrests when the microtubule apparatus is poisoned,[91] but mammalian counterparts have not been identified. Interestingly, p53 has been implicated in a spindle checkpoint in mouse cells,[103] which again demonstrates its importance in numerous aspects of cancer cell biology.

Cellular Senescence

Finally, it has been suggested that cellular senescence also represents a type of cell-cycle checkpoint that is activated when chromosomal telomeres become shortened to a critical point.[104] It is thought that critically shortened telomeres may cause DNA strand abnormalities to activate one or more cell-cycle arrest signals and prevent further cell proliferation (hence, senescence). This could be significant for tumorigenesis because tumor cells may have defective checkpoint-signaling pathways. Thus, in addition to expressing telomerase activity (see S Phase, earlier in this chapter), the loss of a growth inhibitory checkpoint signal to induce senescence could also contribute to the development of cellular immortality in tumor cells.

IMPLICATIONS FOR CANCER

CANCER DEVELOPMENT

Cancer cells exhibit a diverse set of phenotypic abnormalities, including loss of differentiation, increased motility or invasive-

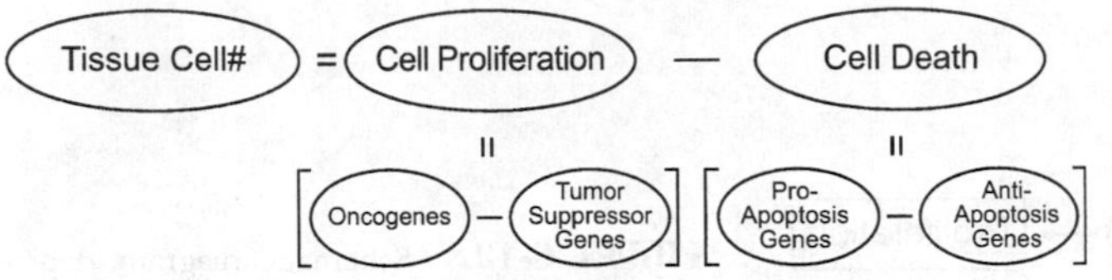

FIGURE 6-11. The steady-state number of cells in a tissue is a function of the relative amount of cell proliferation and cell death. Cell proliferation is influenced by the balance of positive effects of oncogenes and negative effects of tumor suppressor genes. Cell death is influenced by the balance of positive and negative effects of proapoptotic and antiapoptotic gene products. Simplistically, cell number may be increased by increased activity of oncogenes or antiapoptotic genes or by decreased activity of tumor suppressor genes or proapoptotic genes.

ness, and decreased drug sensitivity. However, one phenotypic abnormality that is virtually pathognomonic of all cancer cells is dysregulation of cell-cycle control. A common misconception is that cancer cells replicate faster than normal cells. Rather, the growth abnormality in cancer cells appears to result from two factors: (1) lack of appropriate control responses to the signals that normally cause the cell to stop going through the cell cycle, and (2) lack of a cellular death program in response to appropriate stimuli or stresses. The transformation of a normal cell to a tumor cell appears to be dependent on mutations in gene products important in integrating extracellular and intracellular signals to the cell cycle and cell death machinery and on those gene products involved in directly controlling cell-cycle progression. Loss of either type of function would lead to loss of regulatory cell growth signals.

An evolution has occurred over the past 25 years in our thinking about the nature of the growth abnormalities present in cancer cells. The discovery of oncogenes in the 1970s and their overexpression or increased activity in tumor cells led to the suggestion that the abnormality in tumor cells was the presence of too much of a signal that pushed the cell through the cell cycle. The discovery of tumor suppressor genes in the 1980s added to this model by suggesting that the growth abnormalities of tumor cells resulted from a combination of too few of the cell-cycle *brakes* (tumor suppressors) and too many of the cell-cycle *accelerators* (oncogenes).

This model has been even further revised in the past several years with the recognition of the importance of cell death controls in maintaining appropriate numbers of cells in a given tissue. Changes in tissue cell number are dictated by the number of new cells generated by cellular proliferation and the number of cells lost to the tissue by cell death (Fig. 6-11). The number of proliferating cells is controlled by a combination of the gene products driving the cell through the cycle (can be considered oncogenes in a simplified model) and the gene products that inhibit cell-cycle progression (considered tumor suppressor genes in a simplified model). In a simplified model, the number of cells dying in a tissue is a function of the relative activities of the gene products that block programmed cell death (antiapoptosis genes) and the gene products that enhance programmed cell death (apoptosis-enhancing genes). Thus, tumors may develop and malignant cells may continue to increase their numbers by acquiring mutations in genes that result in combinations of increased drive through the cell cycle (increased *oncogene* activity), decreased inhibition of cell-cycle progression (loss of *tumor suppressor* genes), increased antiapoptosis signals (e.g., overexpressed BCL2) and decreased proapoptosis signals (e.g., decreased BAX or mutated p53). Cell differentiation is also probably associated with slowing or stopping cell proliferation, and some abnormal gene products in malignancies that drive proliferation also appear to inhibit differentiation.

Oncogenes

One formal definition for an oncogene is that the oncogene product contributes to malignant transformation either *in vitro* or *in vivo*. The concept used previously that oncogenes are gene products that enhance cell-cycle progression is not always true, but is useful for the discussion here. Oncogenic mutations in tumor cells will not be discussed in great detail here. However, it is clear that many of the genes that have been classified as oncogenes are positive growth signals. They can fall into categories of abnormally activated growth factors (e.g., c-SIS), growth factor receptors (e.g., HER2/neu and c-FMS), intracellular signaling molecules (e.g., c-SRC, RAS, and c-RAF), and nuclear transcription factors (e.g., c-MYC). Such signaling pathways were discussed previously as influencing the actual cell-cycle machinery, and it is easy to envision how activating mutations in any of these genes could lead to enhanced signals that inappropriately keep the cell going through the cell cycle. Positive signals directly involved in the cell-cycle machinery have been linked to oncogenesis by the observations of abnormally high levels of cyclin expression in certain tumor cells.[105] In addition, the cdk-activating cdc25 phosphatases have been demonstrated to have cooperative oncogenic activity in soft agar and nude mouse tumor assays and appear to be overexpressed in a significant percentage of primary human breast carcinomas.[106]

Tumor Suppressor Genes

The existence of tumor suppressor genes, predicted in the 1970s by the elegant epidemiologic studies of Knudson[107] and by subsequent cell fusion studies,[108] finally became a reality with the discovery of the retinoblastoma (RB) gene and later the role of the p53 gene in the 1980s.[109] Although a number of tumor suppressor genes have been identified to date (including APC, BRCA1, BRCA2, NF1 and NF2, WT1, and VHL), RB and p53 are unusual tumor suppressor genes in that they directly influence the cell-cycle machinery. As discussed previously, RB expression inhibits cell-cycle progression by binding to E2F-1 and blocking transcription of genes necessary for entry into S phase. p53 inhibits cell-cycle progression by inducing the transcriptional activation of the CKI, $p21^{WAF1/CIP1}$, which in turn inhibits activation of the cdk such that it cannot phosphorylate substrates such as RB.

As discussed previously, p53 participates in a cell-cycle checkpoint signal transduction pathway that causes either a G_1 arrest or apoptotic cell death after DNA damage. Loss of p53 function during tumorigenesis thus can result in both inappropriate progression through the cell cycle after DNA damage and survival of a cell that might otherwise have been destined to die. It is easy to conceive how this would cause both increased genetic instability and decreased apoptosis and contribute to malignant transformation. Additionally, roles for p53 in controlling certain aspects of the progression from the G_2 phase of the cell through mitosis and chromosome segregation have been suggested.[110,111] Thus, it is not surprising that p53 is the most commonly mutated gene in human cancers identified to date, with at least 50% of tumors

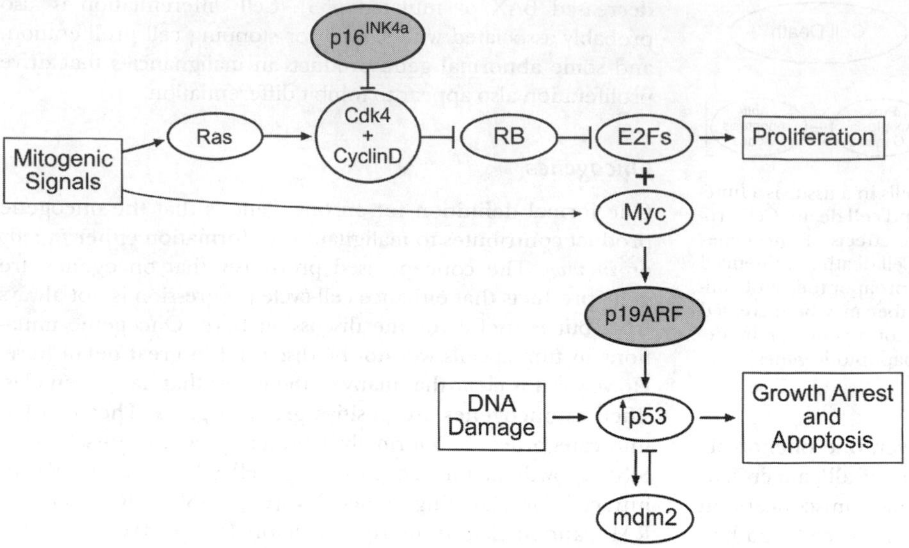

FIGURE 6-12. Schematic diagram depicting the cell-cycle checkpoints mediated by the $p16^{INK4a}/p19^{ARF}$ genetic locus. Mitogenic signals that activate cyclin D/cdk4 to lead to cell proliferation can be blocked by $p16^{INK4a}$. In certain cellular contexts, mitogenic signals that would normally drive cell proliferation can instead activate the $p19^{ARF}$ pathway. Activated $p19^{ARF}$ indirectly activates p53 by a mechanism that involves mdm2. Activated p53 may lead to cell-cycle arrest or apoptosis as noted in Figure 6-10. In this way, $p19^{ARF}$ can act as a checkpoint to "sense" what may be inappropriate oncogenic cell proliferation signals. Of note, the DNA damage response checkpoint, which also involves p53, is independent of $p19^{ARF}$. (Adapted from ref. 122, with permission.)

having abnormal p53 genes.[92] Some tumors also develop other mechanisms of inactivating p53 function by overexpression of the p53-binding protein, mdm2,[112] or by infection with high-risk human papilloma tumor virus (HPV) and expression of the HPV E6 protein, which binds to p53 and enhances its degradation.[113] Inactivation of p53 by overexpression of mdm2 appears to occur primarily in sarcomas and inactivation by HPV infection in cervical carcinomas.[112,114] Thus, many tumors appear to inactivate p53 function by these mechanisms, rather than by mutation of the p53 gene itself, but the end result is the same since p53 function and certain aspects of cell-cycle control are abrogated.

The RB gene is mutated in a number of different tumor types, but others may have mutations elsewhere in the cell-cycle pathways that use RB. For example, cyclin D/cdk4 complexes phosphorylate RB and it appears that $p15^{INK4b}$ and $p16^{INK4a}$, which are inhibitors of cyclin D/cdk4, are mutated in a variety of tumor types. In contrast, the $p21^{WAF1/CIP1}$ and $p27^{KIP1}$ cdk inhibitors are rarely mutated.[115] In principle, any cdk inhibitor might act as a tumor suppressor protein.[14] Loss of RB pathway function could certainly lead to loss of normal inhibitory controls of cell-cycle progression. However, some data also suggest that loss of RB function alone enhances apoptosis tendencies of cells, so by itself might not result in tumor development.[116–119] It has been suggested[119] that loss of RB function, leading to enhanced cell proliferation, coupled with genetic changes that cause loss of apoptosis signals, would be an efficient combination for enhancing malignant transformation (see Apoptosis: Another Step in the Cell Cycle That Goes Awry in Tumor Cells?, later in this chapter).

Characterization of the tumor suppressor locus coding for the cyclin kinase inhibitor $p16^{INK4a}$ revealed a novel tumor suppressor gene and a genomic organization that is unprecedented in mammalian cells and affects both the RB and p53 pathways.[120] The $p19^{ARF}$ gene was found as an alternatively spliced gene encoded within the genetic locus that codes for $p16^{INK4a}$. Interestingly, the $p19^{ARF}$ gene product induces a growth arrest that is dependent on the p53 protein.[121,122] Thus, this single genetic locus codes for two proteins, one of which ($p16^{INK4a}$) inhibits proliferation via the RB pathway by inhibiting activation of cyclin-dependent kinases and a second protein ($p19^{ARF}$) that inhibits proliferation via activation of p53 (Fig. 6-12).[122] The mechanism by which $p19^{ARF}$ affects p53 protein levels has been shown to be via binding to the mdm2 protein and sequestering mdm2 in the nucleolus.[122–127] The sequestration of mdm2 results in increased p53 protein levels because mdm2 normally binds to p53 and enhances its proteolytic degradation. This $p19^{ARF}$-mediated increased level of p53 protein results in growth arrest of a cell.

The genetic locus coding for these two genes is on chromosome 9p in human cells and is a common area of mutation in human tumors.[128] Intriguingly, oncogene activation is one cellular stimulus that has been shown to activate $p19^{ARF}$ and initiate this p53-mediated growth arrest.[129,130] If this pathway were not inactivated during tumor formation, activation of an oncogene would simply cause a p53-mediated growth arrest or apoptosis. Thus, tumor cells can bypass this normal cellular response to oncogene activation by mutating either $p19^{ARF}$ or p53 (see Fig. 6-12). Furthermore, since this same locus also codes for a gene product that limits cellular proliferation by inhibiting the RB pathway, deletion of this locus would eliminate two gene products that limit cellular proliferation through two different critical pathways. Thus, it is not at all surprising that this locus is so commonly mutated in human tumors.

Apoptosis: Another Step in the Cell Cycle That Goes Awry in Tumor Cells?

Apoptosis is a mode of cellular death that is an energy-dependent, programmed event (hence the name *programmed cell death*) that occurs in response to certain stimuli. There are characteristic morphologic (nuclear condensation and fragmentation, cell shrinkage, and relative sparing of the cellular membrane and internal organelles) and biochemical (DNA fragmentation and selected proteolysis) events that occur during apoptotic cell death.[131] In addition, a variety of stimuli, such as irradiation or chemotherapy, viral infection, growth factor or hormone withdrawal, and cytotoxic lymphocyte killing, can initiate this death program. Obviously, some of these stimuli are cell-type specific. Apoptosis is also a critical event in normal development and in normal tissue homeostasis, clearly

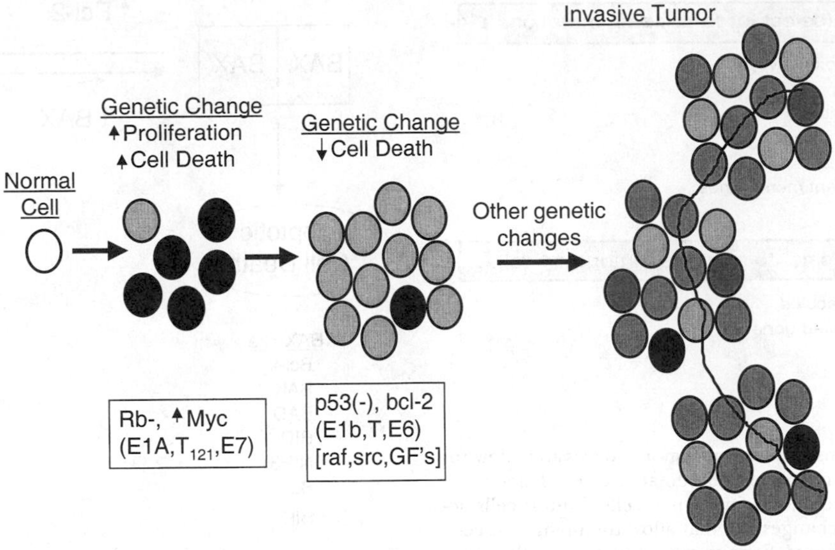

FIGURE 6-13. Model of multistep tumor progression incorporating current concepts of genetic changes occurring during tumorigenesis. Genetic changes such as loss of RB function or overexpressed c-MYC may lead to increased cell proliferation. However, these changes also lead to increased apoptosis (*black ovals*) and thus there is no significant net increase in cell number. The viral gene products, E1A from adenovirus, T antigen from SV40, and E7 from human papilloma virus, appear to have similar effects on the cell by virtue of binding to RB. Subsequent genetic changes that decrease apoptosis (such as loss of $p19^{ARF}$ or p53 or overexpression of bcl-2) would then lead to increases in total cell number. Viral gene products, such as adenovirus E1b, SV40 large T antigen, and human papilloma virus E6, appear to accomplish this by binding to p53 protein. Additional genetic changes further contribute to the malignant cell phenotype by enhancing local invasiveness and metastasis. Although the order of the genetic events may vary in different settings, the concept that both increased proliferation signals and decreased cell death signals contribute to tumorigenesis probably applies to most tumor types. (Concept adapted from ref. 119, with permission.)

playing a role, for example, in nervous system development and in lymphocyte selection processes in the immune system.

Some of the gene products that control the cell cycle also appear to influence apoptosis tendencies (e.g., c-myc, p53, RB). It has been suggested that apoptosis occurs when *conflicting* cell-cycle signals are simultaneously active in the cell or when survival signals coming from extracellular peptides are blocked. Some models also conceive of apoptosis as an integral part of the cell cycle, with apoptotic death being viewed as a type of permanent exit from the cycle, just as the G_0 quiescent phase is an exit from the cycle. It has also been suggested that apoptotic death is the natural *default* outcome for cycling cells unless a survival factor (hormone or growth factor) is present to keep the cell alive as it progresses through the cycle. Since responses to current antineoplastic therapies (chemotherapy and radiation therapy) are also likely to be affected by the apoptosis tendencies of cells, this process has obvious therapeutic implications.

It appears that a decrease in apoptosis tendencies is a key step in tumor development (Fig. 6-13). Experimental tumorigenesis systems using DNA tumor virus models and transgenic animal models led to the suggestion that an initial mutation in a cell may occur in a gene that increases cellular proliferation. Examples of such mutations include loss of function of RB or overexpression of c-MYC. However, these genetic changes, which increase proliferation, also appear to lead to increased apoptotic cell death, thus leading to no net increase in absolute cell number in the tumor.[132] However, if one cell in this proliferating (and apoptotic-prone) population then developed a mutation that abrogated the cell death response, then it is easy to envision how this would lead to a significant increase in cell number in the population. Dysfunction of p53 or overexpression of BCL2 are examples of genetic changes that could inhibit the death response initiated by c-MYC overexpression or RB mutation. Subsequent genetic changes in these cells could then contribute to other phenotypic changes associated with tumors, such as invasiveness and metastasis.

In addition to oncogenic genetic changes providing a selection pressure for loss of apoptotic signals during tumor development, the harsh microenvironment surrounding the tumor mass can similarly favor cellular alterations that oppose death pathways. As the number of cells in a tumor mass grows, significant cellular stresses ensue. For example, the tumor mass is exposed to periods of hypoxia as well as oxidative stress during reperfusion. In addition, suboptimal blood supplies to tumor masses result in periods of time in which the tumor is exposed to acid pH and deprivation of nutrients and glucose. Growth of the tumor mass also results in cellular detachment from normal tissue basement membranes. All of these microenvironmental situations might typically kill the exposed cells. In order for a tumor mass to grow beyond a certain size, it must develop mechanisms to survive in this harsh microenvironment. Similar to the mechanisms a developing tumor uses to survive the oncogenic stresses discussed previously, mutations in death-signaling pathway would allow the developing tumor to survive these microenvironmental stresses. Thus, mutations in survival-signaling molecules or gene products involved the apoptosis machinery, and alterations in growth factor or cytokine exposure favor continued development of a tumor mass (Fig. 6-14).

Significant insights have been gained into the molecular steps involved in cell death-signaling pathways. These insights began

Tumor Cell Stresses (select for "anti-death mutations")

Hypoxia +/- reperfusion (oxidative)
Acid pH
Nutrient/glucose deprivation
Oncogene activation
Viral oncoproteins
Detachment from basement membranes

A

"Anti-Death Mechanisms" to promote tumor survival

Mutation in signaling molecules
Mutation in apoptosis-related genes
Viral oncoproteins
Growth factors/cytokines

B

FIGURE 6-14. Mutations involved in tumor progression allow tumor cells to survive harsh microenvironmental stresses. Tumor cell stresses **(A)** would lead to cell death in normal cells. Tumor cells acquire a number of genetic changes **(B)** that allow the malignant cells to survive these harsh conditions. For any given tumor type, the exact nature of these genetic changes may not be known. Little is known about the sequence of these genetic changes during tumor development *in vivo.*

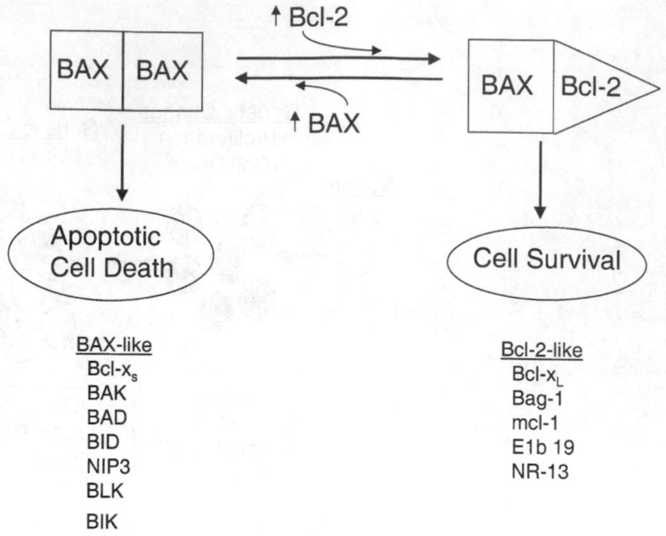

FIGURE 6-15. Overexpression of Bcl-2 inhibits apoptotic cell death following many different stimuli. The current model of how Bcl-2 accomplishes this is based on the observation that Bcl-2 protein binds to BAX protein. It has been proposed that BAX protein binds to itself and drives the cell toward apoptosis. Bcl-2 can bind to BAX and prevent BAX homodimerization. A number of different proteins similar to Bcl-2 and BAX have been identified, some of which are proapoptotic (listed as BAX-like) and some of which are antiapoptotic (listed as Bcl-2–like). The use of these different proapoptotic and antiapoptotic proteins may be cell-type specific. [Model based on the work of Korsmeyer and colleagues (ref. 134), with permission.]

with the molecular characterization of the t(14;18) chromosomal translocation commonly seen in follicular lymphomas resulting in identification of the antiapoptotic gene BCL2.[133] The concept developed in the follicular lymphoma model was that the abnormal lymphoid cells grow initially because of loss of cell death tendencies due to BCL2 overexpression caused by the translocation of the BCL2 gene from chromosome 18 to the actively transcribed immunoglobulin gene on chromosome 14 in B-lymphoid cells. At this point, such lymphomas are rather indolent, but are difficult to cure with chemotherapy. However, at some later stage, they develop other genetic changes and become more aggressive. We now know of a family of related gene products that interact with each other to influence apoptotic tendencies. Korsmeyer and colleagues developed a model in which the bcl-2–like protein, bax, can drive the cell toward apoptosis when it forms complexes with itself[134,135] (Fig. 6-15). When bcl-2 protein is expressed at high levels in cells, it forms complexes with bax, preventing bax homodimerization and inhibiting cell death. Other antiapoptotic proteins with homologies to bcl-2 and bax, such as bcl-x_L and mcl-1, have also been identified.[136,137] The list of antiapoptotic and proapoptotic gene products continues to grow and it appears that some of this apparent redundancy of proteins results from tissue-specific expression and use of the different proteins in different signaling pathways.

Critical details in death-signaling pathways have been elucidated in recent years and incorporate much of what had been known about the bcl-2 family and survival-signaling pathways. One major insight was the identification of a family of specific proteases, now referred to as *caspases,* which are critical for apoptosis signaling.[138] Current models suggest that apoptosis is dependent on a series of highly regulated proteolytic cleavages that result in selected activation or inactivation of certain molecules and eventually result in the highly ordered internal destruction of the cell (Fig. 6-16). The release of cytochrome C from the mitochondria and association of cytochrome C with the apaf-1 protein and caspase 3, is a critical step in death induced by genotoxic damage, as would be induced by many chemotherapeutic agents.[138,139] Predictably, growth factors, such as interleukin-3, which provide survival signals to cells, appear to act via modulation of one or more steps in these pathways.[140,141] One particularly interesting mechanism along these lines is the interleukin-3–induced phosphorylation of the *pro*apoptotic protein, BAD, which causes the release of the *anti*-apoptotic protein, bcl-x_L, promoting cell survival.[142]

It is now clear that a group of extracellular molecules can also act as death-inducing signals by interaction with selected cell surface receptors (called *death receptors*) to initiate cellular suicide via activation of a different caspase-dependent pathway, one that may not involve mitochondria (see Fig. 6-16).[135,143] Fas ligand and Fas receptor are examples of an extracellular molecule and death receptor that initiate programmed cell death in this way, and this pathway appears to be particularly important in the regulation of cell death in lymphoid cells. Tumor necrosis factor and the TRAIL family[143] are additional examples of cytokines that act via this type of pathway. As discussed previously, alterations in these death-signaling pathways can contribute to tumor development by keeping the tumor cells alive in the face of genetic changes or microenvironmental stresses that would normally result in cell death. The potential impact of loss of these death-signaling pathways on tumor responses to therapy is obvious.

CANCER THERAPY

A major limiting factor for cancer cures at this time is the toxicity of chemotherapy and radiation therapy to normal tissues.

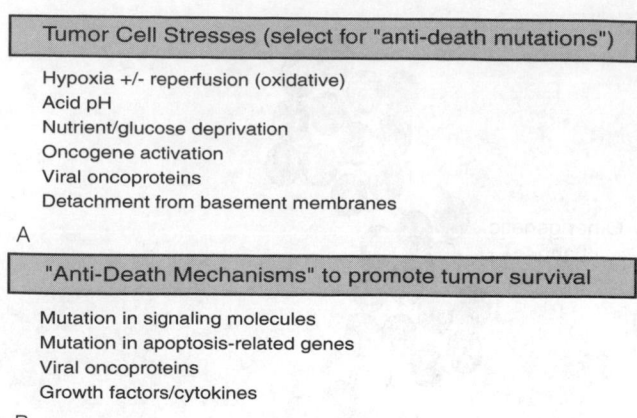

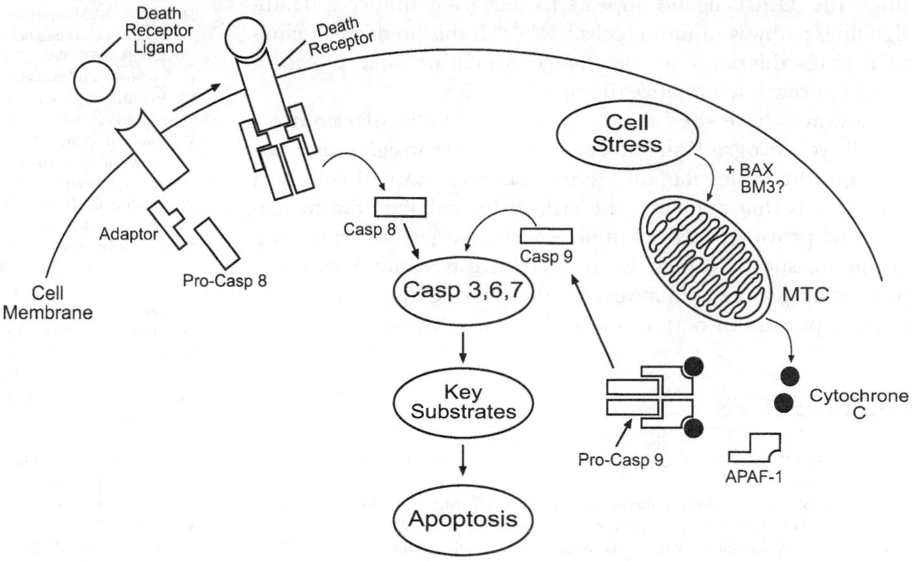

FIGURE 6-16. Schematic diagram depicting mechanisms for activation of caspases that lead to apoptosis in mammalian cells. One pathway that can be activated by a variety of cellular stresses (see text for details) involves the release of cytochrome C from mitochondria (MTC). Cytochrome C and apaf-1 activate procaspase 9, which subsequently activates a series of effector caspases (Casp 3, 6, 7), which mediate proteolytic destruction of cellular proteins resulting in apoptosis. A second apoptotic pathway can be activated by extracellular signaling molecules. Receptor activation leads to activation of procaspase 8, followed by activation of effector caspases. This latter pathway may be independent of mitochondrial activities. (Adapted from Green DR. Apoptotic pathways: the roads to ruin. *Cell* 1998; 94:695, with permission.)

The doses of current antineoplastic agents that would be required to kill resistant tumors would also lead to patient mortality. The selection pressures for loss of apoptotic pathways during tumor development would only make this selective killing of tumor cells with cytotoxic agents more difficult. The more we understand about the molecular and cellular differences between tumor cells and normal cells, the more likely we are to be able to achieve this selectivity by identifying specific targets within tumor cells.

Since alteration in cell-cycle control is one hallmark difference between normal and cancer cells, it is reasonable to consider cell-cycle targets to achieve this desired specificity. Unfortunately, these same cell-cycle alterations may also contribute to making tumor cells more resistant to cytotoxic therapies. For example, genetic instability is a common feature of tumor cells and presumably contributes to the large number of mutations that occur during tumorigenesis. Such genetic instability, arising from mutations in cell-cycle checkpoint or DNA repair genes, could also give the tumor cell an advantage by creating the capability for it to mutate to find ways to become resistant to therapeutic agents. Two ways to address this are to find ways to limit instability or to find ways to kill the cells quickly so that they do not have time to become resistant. Although it is not clear how one might go about reducing genetic instability, taking advantage of new insights into apoptotic signaling pathways could allow us to more effectively induce rapid apoptosis and achieve this second goal.

It has been suggested that we could take advantage of altered cell-cycle checkpoints in tumor cells to make chemotherapy and radiotherapy given in a particular sequence more specifically toxic for tumor cells.[91] For example, although loss of the G_1 checkpoint in tumor cells by itself does not make tumor cells more sensitive to irradiation, selective combinations of therapies could theoretically selectively kill the tumor cells that continued to progress through the cell cycle after treatment with the first cytotoxic agent while the normal cells that arrested are relatively protected. Another scenario arises from the observations that yeast that are defective in the G_2 checkpoint are more sensitive to irradiation[1] and that abrogation of the G_2 checkpoint in mammalian cells (e.g., by caffeine) makes the cells more sensitive to DNA-damaging agents. It has been suggested that tumor cells, particularly those tumor cells that have lost the G_1 checkpoint because of mutations in p53, may be particularly sensitive to inhibition of the G_2 checkpoint.[144–146]

Telomerase provides another potential cell-cycle–related, tumor-specific target. As discussed previously, telomerase activity is expressed in embryonic tissues and is usually turned off in differentiated somatic cells, but appears to be reexpressed in tumor cells, giving them unlimited replication potential.[75] Thus, since telomerase is a relatively tumor-specific gene product and since inhibition of its activity would theoretically lead to eventual cessation of cellular replication, telomerase is an attractive potential novel target for antineoplastic therapies. Potential problems with this as a target are the potential toxicity to stem cells in the gastrointestinal tract or bone marrow and the question of how long it would be necessary to inhibit its activity before the tumor cell stopped growing. It is possible that the latter problem may be circumvented by using telomerase inhibitors in combination with other cytotoxic agents.

Perhaps the most direct way to make tumor cells more sensitive to current therapies is to enhance the apoptosis tendencies of the tumor cells either directly or in conjunction with exposure of the cells to chemotherapy and radiotherapy. It can be argued that the inherent rapid apoptosis tendencies of tumors dictate our observed response rates with current therapies. The tumors in which we have reasonable cure rates (e.g., lymphoid malignancies, germ cell tumors) probably derive from tissues that have greater tendencies to undergo DNA damage-induced apoptosis than the tissues that give rise to relatively resistant tumors (e.g., carcinomas of colon, pancreas, breast). As we continue to elucidate the steps controlling apoptosis responses, then our opportunities to biochemically modulate these responses are enhanced such that a rapid apoptosis response may be initiated on exposure of a resistant carcinoma cell to chemotherapy and radiation therapy. Specificity could also theoretically be achieved by appropriate use of death receptor-ligand interactions or use of cell-type specific survival factors.[147] For example, at least in certain settings, the TRAIL ligand appears to selectively induce a death-signaling pathway in tumor cells.[143,148,149] If this holds up in clinical settings, this particular death-receptor pathway may provide a novel approach to enhance therapeutic index.

Advances have shed much light on the molecular controls of cell-cycle progression and cell death. These insights also suggest specific molecular differences between normal cells and tumor cells that appear to be critical for cellular transformation and provide potential tumor-specific targets for improving antineoplastic therapies. Continued investigations into these molecular processes may eventually provide the answers we need to prevent or better treat malignant processes.

REFERENCES

1. Hartwell LH, Weinert TA. Checkpoints: controls that ensure the order of cell cycle events. *Science* 1989;246:629.
2. Elledge SJ. Cell cycle checkpoints: preventing an identity crisis. *Science* 1996;274:1664.
3. Pardee AB. G_1 events and regulation of cell proliferation. *Science* 1989;246:603.
4. Zetterberg A, Larsson O, Wiman KG. What is the restriction point? *Curr Opin Cell Biol* 1995;7:835.
5. Sherr CJ. G_1 phase progression: cycling on cue. *Cell* 1994;79:551.
6. Weinberg RA. The retinoblastoma protein and cell cycle control. *Cell* 1995;81:323.
7. Krek W. Proteolysis and the G_1-S transition: the SCF connection. *Curr Opin Cell Biol* 1998;8:36.
8. Townsley FM, Ruderman JV. Proteolytic ratchets that control progression through mitosis. *Trends in Cell Biology* 1998;8:238.
9. Neufeld TP, Edgar BA. Connections between growth and the cell cycle. *Curr Opin Cell Biol* 1998;10:784.
10. Hayflick L. The limited in vitro lifetime of human diploid cell strains. *Exp Cell Res* 1965;37:614.
11. Hastie ND, Dempster M, Dunlop MG, et al. Telomere reduction in human colorectal carcinoma and with aging. *Nature* 1990;346:866.
12. Schneider JW, Gu W, Zhu L, Mahdavi V, Nadal-Ginard B. Reversal of terminal differentiation mediated by p107 in RB-/-muscle cells. *Science* 1994;264:1467.
13. Novitch BG, Mulligan GJ, Lassar AB. Skeletal muscle cells lacking the retinoblastoma protein display defects in muscle gene expression and accumulate in S and G_2 phases of the cell cycle. *J Cell Biol* 1996;135:441.
14. Sherr CJ, Roberts JM. Inhibitors of mammalian G_1 cyclin-dependent kinases. *Genes Dev* 1995;9:1149.
15. Lee W-H, Bookstein R, Hong F, et al. Human retinoblastoma susceptibility gene: cloning, identification, and sequence. *Science* 1987;235:1394.
16. Harbour JW, Lai S-H, Whang-Peng J, et al. Abnormalities in structure and expression of the human retinoblastoma gene in SCLC. *Science* 1988;241:353.
17. Lee EYHP, To H, Shew J-Y, et al. Inactivation of the retinoblastoma susceptibility gene in human breast cancers. *Science* 1988;241:218.
18. Goodrich DW, Wang NP, Qian Y, Lee EYHP, Lee W-H. The retinoblastoma gene product regulates progression through G_1 phase of the cell cycle. *Cell* 1991;67:293.
19. Qin X-Q, Chittenden T, Livingston D, Kaelin WG. Identification of a growth suppression domain within the retinoblastoma gene product. *Genes Dev* 1992;6:953.
20. Chen P-L, Scully P, Shew J-Y, Wang JYJ, Lee W-H. Phosphorylation of the retinoblastoma gene product is modulated during the cell cycle and cellular differentiation. *Cell* 1989;58:1193.
21. Buchkovich K, Duffy LA, Harlow E. The retinoblastoma protein is phosphorylated during specific phases of the cell cycle. *Cell* 1989;58:1097.
22. Herrera RE, Sah VP, Williams BO, et al. Altered cell cycle kinetics, gene expression, and G_1 restriction point regulation in Rb-deficient fibroblasts. *Mol Cell Biol* 1996;16:2402.
23. Skapek SX, Qian Y-W, Lee EYHP. The retinoblastoma protein: more than meets the eyes. *Progress in Retinal and Eye Research* 1997;16:591.
24. Dyson N. The regulation of E2F by pRB-family proteins. *Genes Dev* 1998;12:2245.
25. Nevins JR. E2F: A link between the Rb tumor suppressor protein and viral oncoproteins. *Science* 1992;258:424.
26. Johnson DG, Schwarz JK, Cress WD, Nevins JR. Expression of E2F1 induces quiescent cells to enter S phase. *Nature* 1993;23:349.
27. Hiebert SW, Chellappan SP, Horowitz JM, Nevins JR. The interaction of RB with E2F coincides with an inhibition of the transcriptional activity of E2F. *Genes Dev* 1992;6:177.
28. Helin K, Harlow E, Fattaey A. Inhibition of E2F-1 transactivation by direct binding of the retinoblastoma protein. *Mol Cell Biol* 1993;13:6501.
29. Brehm A, Miska EA, McCance DJ, et al. Retinoblastoma protein recruits histone deacetylase to repress transcription. *Nature* 1998;391:597.
30. Magnaghi-Jaulin L, Groisman R, Naguibneva I, et al. Retinoblastoma protein represses transcription by recruiting a histone deacetylase. *Nature* 1998;391:601.
31. Hunter T, Pines J. Cyclins and cancer II: cyclin D and CDK inhibitors come of age. *PMID* 1994;79:573.
32. Jeffrey PD, Russo AA, Polyak K, et al. Mechanism of CDK activation revealed by the structure of a cyclin A-CDK2 complex. *Nature* 1995;376:313.
33. Ewen ME, Sluss HK, Sherr CJ, et al. Functional interactions of the retinoblastoma protein with mammalian D-type cyclins. *Cell* 1993;73:487.
34. Hinds PW, Mittnacht S, Dulic V, et al. Regulation of retinoblastoma protein functions by ectopic expression of human cyclins. *Cell* 1992;70:993.
35. Knudsen ES, Wang JYJ. Dual mechanisms for the inhibition of E2F binding to RB by cyclin-dependent kinase-mediated RB phosphorylation. *Mol Cell Biol* 1997;17:5771.
36. Resnitzky D, Reed SI. Different roles for cyclins D1 and E in the regulation of the G1-S transition. *Mol Cell Biol* 1995;15:3463.
37. Ewen ME, Xing YG, Lawrence JB, Livingston DM. Molecular cloning, chromosomal mapping, and expression of the cDNA for p107, a retinoblastoma gene product-related protein. *Cell* 1991;66:1155.
38. Hannon GJ, Demetrick D, Beach D. Isolation of the Rb-related p130 through its interaction with CDK2 and cyclins. *Genes Dev* 1993;7:2378.
39. Peeper DS, Keblusek P, Helin K, et al. Phosphorylation of a specific cdk site in E2F-1 affects its electrophoretic mobility and promotes pRB-binding in vitro. *Oncogene* 1995;10:39.
40. Geng Y, Whoriskey W, Park MY, et al. Rescue of cyclin D1 deficiency by knockin cyclin E. *Cell* 1999;97:767.
41. Morgan DO. Principles of CDK regulation. *Nature* 1995;374:131.
42. Matsushime H, Roussel MF, Ashmun RA, Sherr CJ. Colony-stimulating factor 1 regulates novel cyclins during the G1 phase of the cell cycle. *Cell* 1991;65:701.
43. Peters J-M. SCF and APC: the yin and yang of cell cycle regulated proteolysis. *Curr Opin Cell Biol* 1998;10:759.
44. Fisher RP, Morgan DO. A novel cyclin associates with MO15/cdk7 to form the cdk-activating kinase. *Cell* 1994;78:713.
45. Harper JW, Adami GR, Wei N, Keyomarsi K, Elledge SJ. The p21 CDK-interacting protein Cip1 is a potent inhibitor of G1 cyclin-dependent kinases. *Cell* 1993;75:805.
46. El-Deiry WS, Tokino T, Velculescu VE, et al. WAF1, a potential mediator of p53 tumor suppression. *Cell* 1993;75:817.
47. Xiong Y, Hannon GH, Zhang H, et al. p21 is a universal inhibitor of cyclin kinases. *Nature* 1993;366:701.
48. Polyak K, Lee M-H, Erdjument-Bromage H, et al. Cloning of $p27^{Kip1}$ a cyclin-cdk inhibitor and a potential mediator of extracellular antimitogenic signals. *Cell* 1994;78:59.
49. Toyoshima H, Hunter T. p27, a novel inhibitor of G_1 cyclin-cdk protein kinase activity, is related to p21. *Cell* 1994;78:67.
50. Matsuoka S, Edwards MC, Bai C, et al. $p57^{(KIP2)}$, a structurally distinct member of the $p21^{(CIP1)}$ CDK inhibitor family, is a candidate tumor suppressor gene. *Genes Dev* 1995;9:650.
51. Serrano M, Hanno GJ, Beach D. A new regulatory motif in cell-cycle control causing specific inhibition of cyclin D/CDK4. *Nature* 1993;366:704.
52. Hannon GJ, Beach D. $p15^{INK4B}$ is a potential effector of TGFβ induced cell cycle arrest. *Nature* 1994;371:257.
53. Guan K, Jenkins Y, Nichols MA, et al. Growth suppression by p18, a $p16^{INK4/MTS1}$- and $p14^{INK4B/MTS2}$-related CDK6 inhibitor, correlates with wild-type pRb function. *Genes Dev* 1994;8:2939.
54. Hirai H, Roussel MF, Kato J-Y, Ashmun RA, Sherr CJ. Novel Ink4 proteins, p19 and p18, are specific inhibitors of the cyclin D-dependent kinases cdk4 and cdk6. *Mol Cell Biol* 1995;15:2672.
55. Sherr CJ. Cancer cell cycles. *Science* 1996;274:1672.
56. Sherr CJ, Roberts JM. CDK inhibitors: positive and negative regulators of G_1-phase progression. *Genes Dev* 1999;13:1501.
57. Zhang H, Hannon GJ, Beach D. p21-containing cyclin kinases exist in both active and inactive states. *Genes Dev* 1994;8:1750.
58. LaBaer J, Garrett MD, Stevenson LF, et al. New functional activities for the p21 family of CDK inhibitors. *Genes Dev* 1997;11:847.
59. El-Deiry WS, Harper JW, O'Conner PM, et al. WAF1/CIP1 Is Induced in p53-mediated G1 arrest and apoptosis. *Cancer Res* 1994;54:1169.
60. Deng C, Zhang P, Harper JW, Elledge SJ, Leder P. Mice lacking $p21^{CIP1/WAF1}$ undergo normal development, but are defective in G1 checkpoint control. *Cell* 1995;82:675.
61. Polyak K, Kato JY, Solomon MJ, et al. $p27^{Kip1}$, a cyclin-Cdk inhibitor, links transforming growth factor-β and contact inhibition to cell cycle arrest. *Genes Dev* 1994;8:9.
62. DePamphilis ML. Origins of DNA replication in metazoan chromosomes. *J Biol Chem* 1993;268:1.
63. Newlon CS. Two jobs for the origin replication complex. *Science* 1993;262:1830.
64. Dutta A, Bell SP. Initiation of DNA replication of eukaryotic cells. *Annu Rev Cell Dev Biol* 1997;13:293.
65. Todorov IT, Attaran A, Kearsey SE. BM28, a human member of the MCM2-3-5 family, is displaced from chromatin during DNA replication. *J Cell Biol* 1995;129:1433.
66. Hendrickson M, Madine M, Dalton S, Gautier J. Phosphorylation of MCM4 by cdc2 protein kinase inhibits the activity of the minichromosome maintenance complex. *Proc Natl Acad Sci U S A* 1996;93:12223.
67. Blow JJ, Laskey RA. A role for the nuclear envelope in controlling DNA replication within the cell cycle. *Nature* 1988;332:546.
68. Kunkel TA. Exonucleolytic proofreading. *Cell* 1988;53:837.
69. Kinzler KW, Vogelstein B. Lessons from hereditary colorectal cancer. *Cell* 1996;87:159.
70. Laskey RA, Rairman MP, Blow JJ. S Phase of the cell cycle. *Science* 1989;246:609.
71. Stillman B. Smart machines at the DNA replication fork. *Cell* 1994;78:725.
72. Krishna TS, Kong XP, Burgers PM, Kuriyan J. Crystal structure of the eukaryotic DNA polymerase processivity factor PCNA. *Cell* 1994;79:1233.
73. Levy MZ, Allsopp RC, Futcher AB, Greider CW, Harley CB. Telomere end-replication problem and cell aging. *J Mol Biol* 1992;225:951.
74. Greider CW. Telomeres, telomerase and senescence. *BioEssays* 1990;12:363.
75. Kim NW, Piatyszek MA, Prowse KR, et al. Specific association of human telomerase activity with immortal cells and cancer. *Science* 1994;266:2011.
76. Glover DM, Hagan IM, Tavares AAM. Polo-like kinases: a team that plays throughout mitosis. *Genes Dev* 1998;12:3777.

77. Ohi R, Gould KL. Regulating the onset of mitosis. *Curr Opin Cell Biol* 1999;11:267.
78. Masui Y, Markert CL. Cytoplasmic control of nuclear behavior during meiotic maturation of frog oocytes. *J Exp Zool* 1971;177:129.
79. King RW, Jackson PK, Kirschner MW. Mitosis in transition. *Cell* 1994;79:563.
80. Nurse P. Ordering S phase and M phase in the cell cycle. *Cell* 1994;79:547.
81. King RW, Deshaies RJ, Peters J-M, Kirschner MW. How proteolysis drives the cell cycle. *Science* 1996;274:1652.
82. Zachariae W, Nasmyth K. Whose end is destruction: cell division and the anaphase-promoting complex. *Genes Dev* 1999;13:2039.
83. Schlessinger J, Bar-Sagi D. Activation of Ras and other signaling pathways by receptor tyrosine kinases. *Cold Spring Harbor Symposia on Quantum Biology* 1994;59:173.
84. Blenis J. Signal transduction via the MAP kinases: proceed at your own RSK. *Proc Natl Acad Sci U S A* 1993;90:5889.
85. Aaronson SA. Growth factors and cancer. *Science* 1991;254:1146.
86. Muller M, Briscoe J, Laxton C, et al. The protein tyrosine kinase JAK1 complements defects in interferon-α/β and γ signal transduction. *Nature* 1993;366:129.
87. Zhong Z, Wen ZL, Darnell JE Jr. STAT3-a STAT family member activated by tyrosine phosphorylation in response to epidermal growth factor and interleukin-6. *Science* 1994;264:95.
88. Taniguchi T. Cytokine signaling through nonreceptor protein tyrosine kinases. *Science* 1995;268:251.
89. Shak S. Overview of the trastuzumab (Herceptin) anti-HER2 monoclonal antibody clinical program in HER2-overexpressing metastatic breast cancer. Herceptin Multinational Investigator Study Group. *Semin Oncol* 1999;26:71.
90. Robinson MJ, Cobb MH. Mitogen-activated protein kinase pathways. *Curr Opin Cell Biol* 1997;9:180.
91. Hartwell LH, Kastan MB. Cell cycle control and cancer. *Science* 1994;266:1821.
92. Hollstein M, Sidransky D, Vogelstein B, Harris CC. p53 mutations in human cancers. *Science* 1991;253:49.
93. Levine AJ, Momand J, Finlay CA. The p53 tumor suppressor gene. *Nature* 1991;351:453.
94. Lowe SW, Schmitt EM, Smith SW, Osborne BA, Jacks T. p53 is required for radiation-induced apoptosis in mouse thymocytes. *Nature* 1993;362:849.
95. Clarke AR, Purdie CA, Harrison DJ, et al. Thymocyte apoptosis induced by p53-dependent and independent pathways. *Nature* 1993;362:849.
96. Jost CA, Marin MC, Kaelin WG Jr. p73 is a human p53-related protein that can induce apoptosis. *Nature* 1997;389:191.
97. Yang A, Kaghad M, Wang Y, et al. p63, a p53 Homolog at 3q27-29, encodes multiple products with transactivating, death-inducing, and dominant-negative activities. *Mol Cell* 1998;2:305.
98. Weinert TA, Kiser GL, Hartwell LH. Mitotic checkpoint genes in budding yeast and the dependence of mitosis on DNA replication and repair. *Genes Dev* 1994;8:9.
99. Morgan SE, Kastan MB. p53 and ATM: cell cycle, cell death and cancer. *Adv Cancer Res* 1997;71:1.
100. Canman CE, Lim D-S, Cimprich KA, et al. Activation of the ATM kinase by ionizing radiation and phosphorylation of p53. *Science* 1998;281:1677.
101. Weinert TA, Hartwell LH. The RAD9 gene controls the cell cycle response to DNA damage in saccharomyces cerevisiae. *Science* 1988;241:317.
102. Weinert T. A DNA damage checkpoint meets the cell cycle engine. *Science* 1997;277:1450.
103. Cross SM, Sanchez CA, Morgan CA, et al. A p53-dependent mouse spindle checkpoint. *Science* 1995;267:1353.
104. de Lange T. Activation of telomerase in a human tumor. *Proc Natl Acad Sci U S A* 1994; 91:2882.
105. Keyomarsi K, Pardee AB. Redundant cyclin overexpression and gene amplification in breast cancer cells. *Proc Natl Acad Sci U S A* 1993;90:1112.
106. Galaktionov K, Lee AK, Eckstein J, et al. CDC25 phosphatases as potential human oncogenes. *Science* 1995;269:1575.
107. Knudson AG. Mutation and cancer: statistical study of retinoblastoma. *Proc Natl Acad Sci U S A* 1971;68:820.
108. Stanbridge EJ. Suppression of malignancy in human cells. *Nature* 1976;260:17.
109. Weinberg RA. Tumor suppressor genes. *Science* 1991;254:1138.
110. Fukasawa K, Choi T, Kuriyama R, Rulong S, Vande Woude GF. Abnormal centrosome amplification in the absence of p53. *Science* 1996;271:1744.
111. Bunz F, Dutriaux A, Lengauer C, et al. Requirement for p53 and p21 to sustain G2 arrest after DNA damage. *Science* 1998;282:1497.
112. Oliner JD, Kinzler KW, Meltzer PS, George DL, Vogelstein B. Amplification of a gene encoding a p53-associated protein in human sarcomas. *Nature* 1992;358:80.
113. Scheffner M, Werness BA, Huibregtse JM, Levine AJ, Howley PM. The E6 oncoprotein encoded by human papillomavirus types 16 and 18 promotes the degradation of p53. *Cell* 1990;63:1129.
114. zur Hausen H, Schneider A. The role of papillomaviruses in human anogenital cancer. In: Howley PM, Salzman NP, eds. *The Papovaviridae*. Vol. 2: Papillomaviruses. New York: Plenum, 1987:245.
115. Hirama T, Koeffler HP. Role of the cyclin-dependent kinase inhibitors in the development of cancer. *Blood* 1995;86:841.
116. Howes KA, Ransom N, Papermaster DS, et al. Apoptosis or retinoblastoma: alternative fates of photoreceptors expressing the HPV-16 E7 gene in the presence or absence of p53. *Genes Dev* 1994;8:1300.
117. Pan H, Griep AE. Altered cell cycle regulation in the lens of HPV-16 E6 or E7 transgenic mice: implications for tumor suppressor gene function in development. *Genes Dev* 1994;8:1285.
118. Morgenbesser SD, Williams BO, Jacks T, DePinho RA. p53-dependent apoptosis produced by Rb-deficiency in the developing mouse lens. *Nature* 1994;371:72.
119. Symonds H, Krall L, Remington L, et al. p53-dependent apoptosis suppresses tumor growth and progression in vivo. *Cell* 1994;78:703.
120. Quelle DE, Zindy F, Ashmun RA, Sherr CJ. Alternative reading frames of the *INK4a* tumor suppressor gene encode two unrelated proteins capable of inducing cell cycle arrest. *Cell* 1995;83:993.
121. Kamijo T, Zindy F, Roussel MF, et al. Tumor suppression at the mouse INK4a locus mediated by the alternative reading frame product $p19^{ARF}$. *Cell* 1997;91:649.
122. Sherr CJ. Tumor surveillance via the ARF-p53 pathway. *Genes Dev* 1998;12:2984.
123. Kamijo T, Weber JD, Zambetti G, et al. Functional and physical interactions of the ARF tumor suppressor with p53 and Mdm2. *Proc Natl Acad Sci U S A* 1998;95:8292.
124. Pomerantz J, Schreiber-Agus N, Liegeois NJ, et al. The INK4a tumor suppressor gene product, $p19^{Arf}$, interacts with MDM2 and neutralizes MDM2's inhibition of p53. *Cell* 1998;92:713.
125. Stott F, Bates SA, James M, et al. The alternative product from the human CDKN2A locus, $p14^{ARF}$, participates in a regulatory feedback loop with p53 and MDM2. *EMBO J* 1998;17:5001.
126. Zhang Y, Xiong Y, Yarbrough WG. ARF promotes MDM2 degradation and stabilizes p53: ARF-INK4a locus deletion impairs both the Rb and p53 tumor suppression pathways. *Cell* 1998;92:725.
127. Weber JS, Taylor LJ, Roussel MF, Sherr CJ, Bar-Sagi D. Nucleolar Arf sequesters Mdm2 and activates p53. *Nature Cell Biol* 1999;1:20.
128. Ruas M, Peters G. The p16INK4a/CDKN2A tumor suppressor and its relatives. *Biochim Biophys Acta* 1998;1378:F115.
129. de Stanchina E, McCurrach ME, Zindy F, et al. E1A signaling to p53 involves the $p19^{ARF}$ tumor suppressor. *Genes Dev* 1998;12:2434.
130. Zindy F, Eischen CM, Randle DH, et al. Myc signaling via the ARF tumor suppressor regulates p53-dependent apoptosis and immortalization. *Genes Dev* 1998;12:2424.
131. Wyllie AH. Apoptosis (The 1992 Frank Rose Memorial Lecture). *Br J Cancer* 1993;67:205.
132. Evan GI, Wyllie AH, Gilbert CS, et al. Induction of apoptosis in fibroblasts by c-myc protein. *Cell* 1992;69:119.
133. Tsujimoto Y, Gorham J, Cossman J, Jaffe E, Croce CM. The t(14;18) chromosome translocations involved in B-cell neoplasms result from mistakes in VDJ joining. *Science* 1985;229:1390.
134. Oltvai ZN, Milliman CL, Korsmeyer SJ. Bcl-2 heterodimerizes in vivo with a conserved homolog, Bax, that accelerates programmed cell death. *Cell* 1993;74:609.
135. Gross A, McDonnell JM, Korsmeyer SJ. BCL-2 family members and the mitchondria in apoptosis. *Genes Dev* 1999;13:1899.
136. Boise LH, Gonzalez-Garcia M, Postema CE, et al. Bcl-x, a Bcl-2-related gene that functions as a dominant regulator of apoptotic cell death. *Cell* 1993;74:597.
137. Kozopas KM, Yang T, Buchan HL, Zhou P, Craig RW. Mcl-1, a gene expressed in programmed myeloid cell differentiation, has sequence similarity to Bcl-2. *Proc Natl Acad Sci U S A* 1993;90:3516.
138. Cryns V, Yuan J. Proteases to die for. *Genes Dev* 1998;12:1551.
139. Zou H, Henzel WJ, Liu X, Lutschg A, Wang X. Apaf-1, a human protein homologous to C. elegans CED-4, participates in cytochrome c-dependent activation of caspase-3. *Cell* 1997;90:405.
140. Vander Heiden MG, Chandel NS, Schumacker PT, Thompson CB. $Bcl\text{-}x_L$ prevents cell-death following growth factor withdrawal by facilitating mitochondrial ATP/ADP exchange. *Mol Cell* 1999;3:159.
141. Packham G, White EL, Eischen CM, et al. Selective regulation of Bcl-XL by a jak kinase-dependent pathway is bypassed in murine hematopoietic malignancies. *Genes Dev* 1998;12:2475.
142. Zha J, Harada H, Yang E, Jockel J, Korsmeyer SJ. Serine phosphorylation of death agonist BAD in response to survival factor results in binding to 14-3-3 not $BCL\text{-}L_L$. *Cell* 1996;87:619.
143. Ashkenazi A, Dixit VM. Death receptors: signaling and modulation. *Science* 1998;281:1305.
144. Fan S, Smith ML, Rivet DJ II, et al. Disruption of p53 function sensitizes breast cancer MCF-7 cells to cisplatin and pentoxifylline. *Cancer Res* 1995;55:1649.
145. Powell SM, DeFrank JS, Connell P, et al. Differential sensitivity of $p53^{(-)}$ and $p53^{(+)}$ cells to caffeine-induced radiosensitization and override of G_2 delay. *Cancer Res* 1995;55:1643.
146. Russell KJ, Wiens LW, Demers GW, et al. Abrogation of the G_2 checkpoint results in differential radiosensitization of G_1 checkpoint-deficient and G_1 checkpoint-competent cells. *Cancer Res* 1995;55:1639.
147. Canman CE, Gilmer T, Coutts S, Kastan MB. Growth factor modulation of p53-mediated growth arrest vs. apoptosis. *Genes Dev* 1995;9:600.
148. Pan G, Ni J, Wei Y-F, et al. An antagonist decoy receptor and a death domain-containing receptor for TRAIL. *Science* 1997;277:815.
149. Sheridan JP, Marsters SA, Pitti RM, et al. Control of TRAIL-induced apoptosis by a family of signaling and decoy receptors. *Science* 1997;277:818.
150. Lim D-S, Kim S-T, Xu B, et al. ATM phosphorylates p^{95}/nbs1 in an S-phase checkpoint pathway. *Nature* 2000;404:613.

Stanley J. Korsmeyer
Sandra S. Zinkel

CHAPTER 7

Molecular Biology of Cancer: Apoptosis

APOPTOSIS

Multicellular organisms have developed a highly organized and carefully regulated mechanism of cell suicide to craft the development of multiple lineages and to maintain cellular homeostasis. Normal development and morphogenesis proceed by the production of excess cells, which are then removed by a genetically programmed, evolutionarily conserved process. This same program of cell death is used by the organism to remove damaged cells, including virally infected cells.

Programmed cell death may have first been recognized in the developing neuronal system of the toad by Vogt.[1] Kerr and colleagues described cell deaths with distinct ultrastructural features, including plasma membrane blebbing, volume contraction, nuclear condensation, and endonucleolytic cleavage of DNA. They noted that these features were consistent with an active, regulated process and coined the term *apoptosis* from the Greek word used to describe "dropping off" or "falling off" of petals from flowers or leaves from trees.[2,3]

Studies of chromosomal translocations in human lymphoid malignancies yielded the *BCL-2* gene, the first component of the cell death pathway to be identified. The most common chromosomal translocation found in these malignancies is the t(14;18):(q32;q21) harbored by 85% of follicular and 20% of diffuse B-cell lymphomas.[4,5] The breakpoint proved to be the result of aberrant immunoglobulin heavy-chain gene rearrangements,[6–8] in which *BCL-2* was introduced from chromosome 18.[9] The consequence of this rearrangement is to place *BCL-2* under the transcriptional control of the immunoglobulin (Ig) heavy-chain locus. B cells harboring this translocation express inappropriately elevated levels of BCL-2 protein.[10]

Clues to the biologic consequence of BCL-2 overexpression reside in the natural history of follicular lymphoma.[11] The disease usually follows an indolent course, with symptoms that wax and wane over years. Transformation to a high-grade lymphoma with diffuse mixed or diffuse large cell morphology often occurs within the first decade.[11] When a *BCL-2-Ig* minigene that recapitulated the t(14:18) breakpoint was inserted into the germline of a mouse, follicular hyperplasia resulted (Fig. 7-1). This polyclonal expansion of small resting B cells was principally in G_0,G_1 phase of the cell cycle.[12,13] Over time, these mice progress to diffuse, large cell immunoblastic lymphoma. Long latency followed by progression to high-grade malignancy is essentially diagnostic for the acquisition of second genetic abnormalities. Indeed, approximately one-half of the high-grade tumors have acquired an additional translocation, placing *c-myc* under the control of the Ig heavy-chain locus, thus combining an inherent survival advantage (*Bcl-2*) with a gene that promotes proliferation (*c-myc*).[14] Further evidence for the potent synergy of such a combination emerged when *Bcl-2* transgenic mice were mated to *myc* transgenic mice, resulting in the rapid appearance of an undifferentiated hematolymphoid leukemia.[15,16] The oncogenic potential of BCL-2 is not restricted to the B-cell lineage; overexpression in T cells results in peripheral T-cell lymphomas.[17,18]

Tumorigenesis reflects the accumulation of excess cells, which formally results from increased cell proliferation and decreased cell death.[10,19,20] The first oncogenes to be discovered were genes involved in signal transduction or regulation of transcription. Gain of function mutations in these genes results in oncogenesis by increased proliferation. A second class of oncogenes was subsequently identified whose normal function is to inhibit growth and proliferation. It is often loss of function

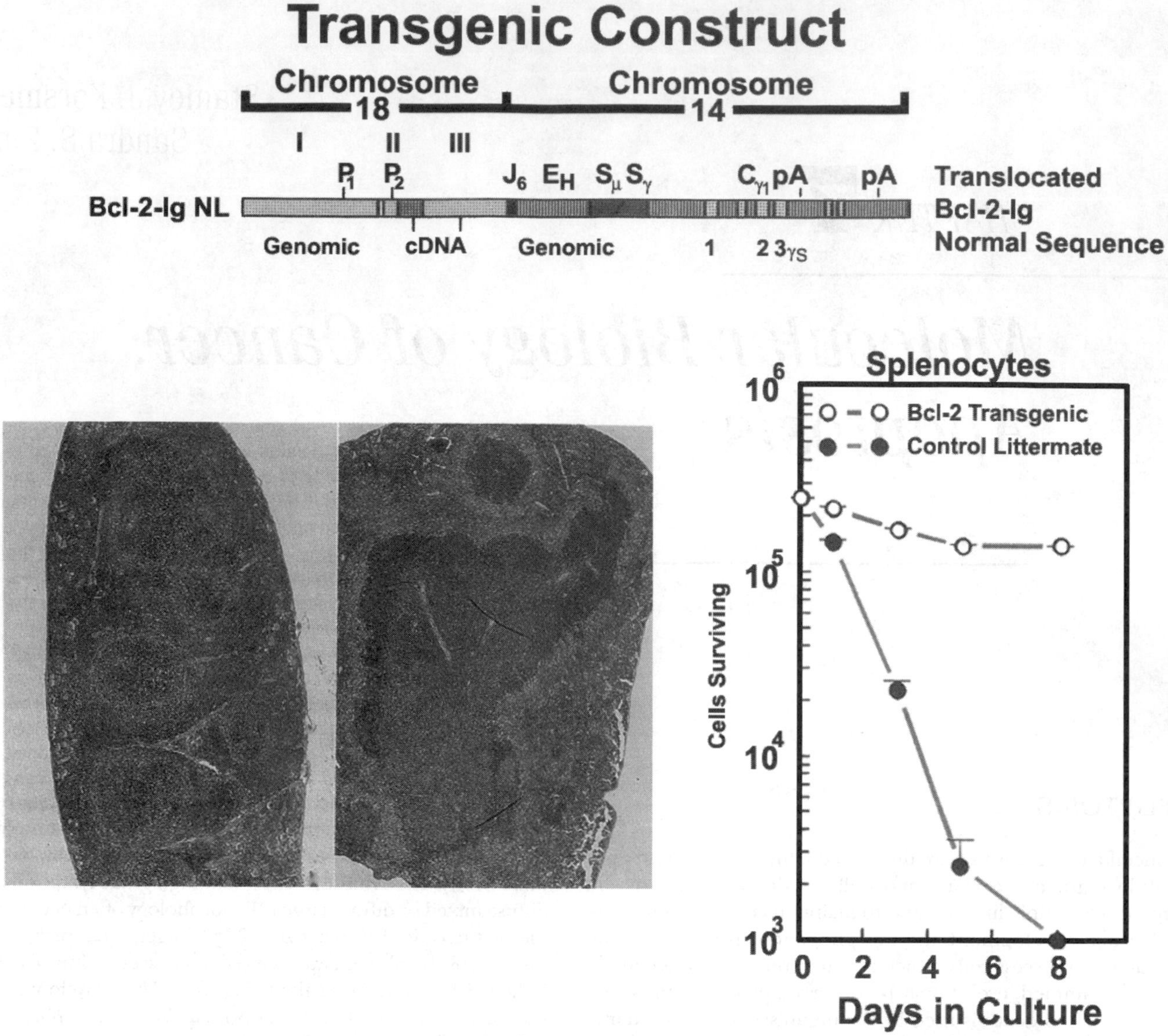

FIGURE 7-1. *Bcl-2-Ig* transgenic mice. The *Bcl-2-Ig* minigene recapitulates the t(14;18) chromosomal translocation of follicular B-cell lymphoma. Gain of function *Bcl-2* leads to B-cell expansion and an enlarged white pulp in the transgenic spleen (*left*) versus control spleen (*right*). B cells accumulate due to extended cell survival (*graph*).[12] (See Color Fig. 7-1 in the CD-ROM and on the Web at www.LWWoncology.com.)

mutations in this class of genes that results in tumors. *BCL-2* represents the cardinal member of a third class of oncogenes, which regulate cell death, resulting in resistance to apoptosis that enables the accumulation of additional genetic aberrations.[12–16,20]

GENETICS OF CELL DEATH

A genetic program of developmental cell death emerged from the study of the nematode *Caenorhabditis elegans*. These worms are particularly well suited to the study of cell fates because they are transparent, allowing visualization of individual cells. During the development of the *C elegans* hermaphrodite, 1090 cells are generated, and 131 of these cells undergo programmed cell death.[21,22] Genes have been identified that reside in a common, core pathway responsible for the regulation of all 131 cell deaths. Moreover, lineage-specific genes that reside in private pathways more upstream are responsible for initiating the cell deaths. Furthermore, two complementary sets of genes have been identified that control the phagocytosis of cell corpses. Functional mammalian counterparts to many of these genes have been identified (Fig. 7-2), indicating that the basic tenets of apoptosis are conserved from nematodes to humans.

The *ced-9* (for cell death abnormal) gene confers resistance to cell death. Loss of function mutations of *ced-9* result in massive cell death leading to death of the worm.[23] Conversely, overexpression of *ced-9* inhibits cell death. Thus, *ced-9* is both a structural and functional homologue of *Bcl-2*.[24,25]

Three additional genes required for apoptosis have been identified, *egl-1* (egg-laying abnormal), *ced-3*, and *ced-4*. Loss of function mutations in either *ced-3* or *ced-4* can rescue cells from death.[22] *Egl-1* functions as an upstream, negative regulator of

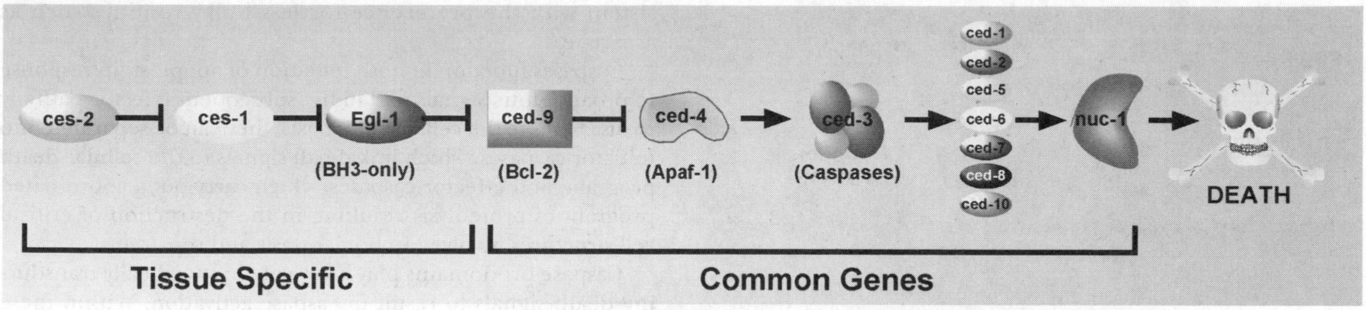

FIGURE 7-2. The genetic pathway regulating cell death in the nematode *Caenorhabditis elegans* has been well characterized and has been conserved in evolution from worms to mammals. Cell death in the nematode transpires by a mechanism in which death is executed by a single protease (CED-3), whose activity is regulated by a single activator (CED-4) and inhibitor (CED-9).[28] Mammalian counterparts for the *C elegans* genes are indicated in parentheses. (See Color Fig. 7-2 in the CD-ROM and on the Web at www.LWWoncology.com.)

the *BCL-2* homologue *ced-9*.[26] Whereas the killing activity of *ced-4* requires functional *ced-3*, the killing activity of *ced-3* is independent of active *ced-4*.[27] *Ced-4* thus appears to function upstream of *ced-3* in this genetic pathway. An overall genetic pathway consistent with all the observations would be *egl-1* → *ced-9* → *ced-4* → *ced-3*.

Ced-3 encodes a cysteine protease homologous to the mammalian interleukin 1 beta-converting enzyme (ICE), or caspase 1, required for the proteolytic activation of pro–interleukin-1β.[28–30] Transient expression of either CED-3 or ICE induces apoptosis in mammalian cells, suggesting that this family of proteases plays a critical role in programmed cell death.[31] The mechanism by which cell death in the nematode transpires is remarkably simple: Death is executed by a protease (CED-3) whose activity is regulated by an activator (CED-4) and an inhibitor (CED-9).[32] Mammalian counterparts for each of the members of the *C elegans* apoptotic pathway exist (see Fig. 7-2).

DEATH RECEPTORS

In mammals, the initiation of programmed cell death occurs through interaction of death ligands such as tumor necrosis factor-α (TNF-α), Fas, or TNF-related apoptosis-inducing ligand (TRAIL), with their respective receptors followed by aggregation of these receptors.[33] Recruitment of adaptor proteins, such as Fas-associated death domain (DD) protein (FADD), TNF receptor-associated DD protein (TRADD), and receptor interacting protein (RIP), to a plasma membrane complex ensues through interactions between yet a third domain, the death domain (DD), present on both the receptor and adaptor proteins.[34–37] Recruitment of the initiator caspase 8 (also called Fas-associated death domain–like interleukin 1 beta-converting enzyme [FLICE]) through interaction of its death effector domain (DED), results in its subsequent activation, evidently by self-proteolytic cleavage (Fig. 7-3). Caspase recruitment can be inhibited by proteins such as FLICE-inhibitory protein (FLIP) whose DED interacts with and ties up adaptor proteins.[38]

In addition to transducing a death signal through caspase activation, engagement of the TNF-α receptor results in a survival signal through nuclear factor κB (NFκB).[39–42] An additional survival signal appears to be mediated by TNF-induced activation of stress-activated protein kinase/c-JUN amino-terminal kinase.[43,44] It is the balance between these opposing signals that ultimately determines whether a cell lives or dies (Fig. 7-4). Accordingly, mice deficient in the RelA subunit of NFκB die between embryonic days 15 and 16 of massive liver apoptosis.[45] Mice deficient in the upstream DD kinase RIP survive this critical stage of development, but die between days 1 and 3 with apoptosis of the thymus and adipose tissue.[46] T-cell death mediated by TNF receptor-2 requires RIP; induction of RIP during T-cell activation promotes a change in TNF receptor-2 signaling from NFκB activation to apoptosis, suggesting a role for this kinase in the switch from survival to apoptosis in some situations.[47]

Evidence that NFκB plays a role in cellular transformation arises from both human and animal tumors.[48] T-cell–specific expression of the avian retroviral oncogene *v-rel* gives rise to T-cell leukemias in transgenic mice. Direct alterations of the NFκB2 locus have been reported in T-cell lymphomas.

Other death stimuli, including DNA-damaging agents and staurosporine, trigger the release of cytochrome *c* from the mitochondrial intermembrane space, resulting in the formation of a caspase 3 activating complex, termed the *apoptosome.* The requisite members of the apoptosome include cytochrome *c*, deoxyadenosine triphosphate (dATP), Apaf-1 (a mammalian homologue of CED-4), and caspase 9.[49–51] In the presence of cytochrome *c* and dATP, Apaf-1 oligomerizes together with procaspase 9 via caspase activation and recruitment domains (CARD).[52] Procaspase 9 is subsequently activated by proteolysis and, in turn, activates caspase 3.[53] Activated effector caspases carry out their role in cell death through the proteolytic cleavage of antiapoptotic proteins and repair proteins, as well as through the degradation of cell structures such as the nuclear lamina.[54]

CASPASES

Caspase 1 is the prototype of a large family of proteases whose members function in inflammation or apoptosis.[54] Caspases are expressed as inactive proenzymes and are activated by proteolytic cleavage after a death stimulus. Members of the caspase family possess a common structural motif consisting of three domains: an amino-terminal domain, a large subunit, and a small subunit. Caspase cleavage consensus sites separate each domain. After cleavage, the large and small subunits associate to form a heterodimer. Crystallographic analyses of both caspase 1 and caspase 3 show association of two heterodimers to form a

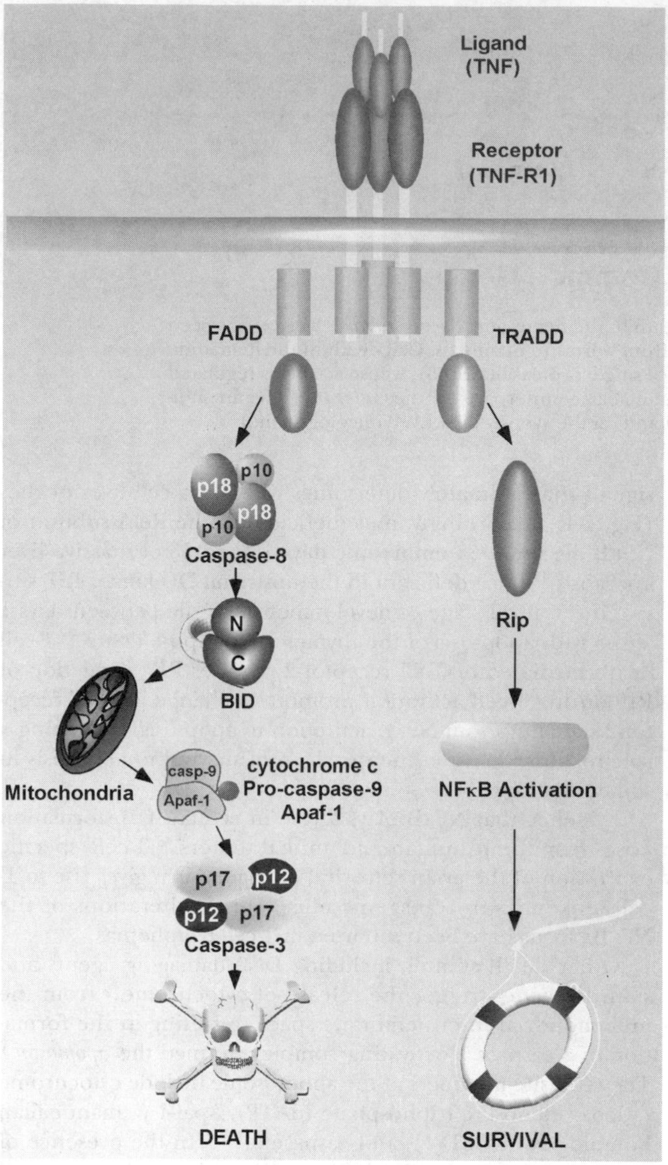

FIGURE 7-3. Cell fate after activation of tumor necrosis factor (TNF) family receptors (TNFR) is determined by the balance between cell survival and cell death signals. Signals through Fas-associated death domain (DD) protein (FADD) result in recruitment and activation of the initiator caspase8 followed by activation of downstream effector caspases, ultimately resulting in cell death. Signals through TNF receptor-associated DD protein (TRADD) result in recruitment of receptor interacting protein (Rip), followed by nuclear factor κB (NFkB) activation and transcription of genes involved in cell survival. The balance between these two opposing pathways determines the ultimate fate of the cell. (See Color Fig. 7-3 in the CD-ROM and on the Web at www.LWWoncology.com.)

tetramer. Both the large and small subunits contribute residues important for substrate binding and specificity. The two catalytic sites of the tetramer appear to function independently.[55–57]

Caspases are cysteine proteases that cleave substrates after an aspartate residue. Substrate specificity of individual caspases is determined by the size of the substrate binding pocket, which dictates the preferred amino acids immediately amino-terminal to this aspartate residue.[55–59] In the case of caspase 1, a relatively large pocket is consistent with the preference for bulky, hydrophobic residues, whereas the smaller pocket of caspase 3 is consistent with the preference for less bulky residues such as aspartate.

Caspases function in both initiation of apoptosis in response to proapoptotic signals and in the subsequent effector pathway to disassemble the cell. On this basis, they can be separated into initiator caspases, which link death signals to the cellular death program, and effector caspases, which carry out a coordinated program of proteolysis resulting in the destruction of critical cell structures involved in homeostasis and repair.

Caspase prodomains play a key role in specifically transducing death signals to result in caspase activation. Within these prodomains, two distinct structural domains have been identified that mediate specific protein-protein interactions: DED and CARD. DEDs are found in initiator caspases, such as caspase 8 and caspase 10. These domains mediate caspase targeting to death receptors via interaction with DEDs on adaptor proteins such as FADD/MORT1.[34,60–64] Activation of upstream caspases initiates a proteolytic cascade that allows rapid transmission and exponential amplification of a death stimulus. Effector caspases such as caspase 3 are activated, culminating in destruction of the cell by apoptosis. Depending on the death signal and the cell type involved, this process appears to proceed through a pathway of mitochondrial dysfunction and the release of cytochrome *c* or, alternatively, a mitochondrial-independent pathway.[65]

THE Bcl-2 FAMILY

The Bcl-2 family of proteins is situated upstream of irreversible cell damage in the apoptotic pathway (see Fig. 7-4),[66] providing a pivotal decisional checkpoint in the fate of a cell after a death stimulus. At least two effector pathways exist downstream for the execution of apoptosis, the caspase pathway and mitochondrial dysfunction. Mitochondrial dysfunction manifests as altered mitochondrial transmembrane potential ($\Delta\psi m$); release of proteins from the mitochondrial intermembrane space, including cytochrome *c*, that triggers the activation of Apaf-1 and caspases; and the production of reactive oxygen species. Thus, the effector caspases may be activated directly following engagement of a surface death receptor or downstream of a mitochondrial amplification loop.

Both pro- and antiapoptotic family members have been identified (Fig. 7-5). Members of the family possess up to four conserved α helical domains, designated *BH1*, *BH2*, *BH3*, and *BH4*.[67–69] Mutagenesis studies of BCL-2 indicate that the conserved domains are necessary for the interaction with proapoptotic proteins such as BAX and for the inhibition of cell death.[70] The proapoptotic and apoptotic family members may also have independent activities.[71,72] An intact amphipathic α helical BH3 domain is required for the proapoptotic proteins BAX or BAK to initiate apoptosis.[73,74] BAX and BAK are more highly conserved prodeath members of the BCL-2 family bearing BH1, BH2, and BH3 domains. A subset of proapoptotic Bcl-2 family members possess sequence homology only within the BH3 domain, further emphasizing the concept that this region forms a critical DD. The recognition that the upstream proapoptotic molecule in *C elegans*, EGL-1, was also a "BH3 only" protein supports the role of these proteins at the intersection with the core apoptotic pathway.[75]

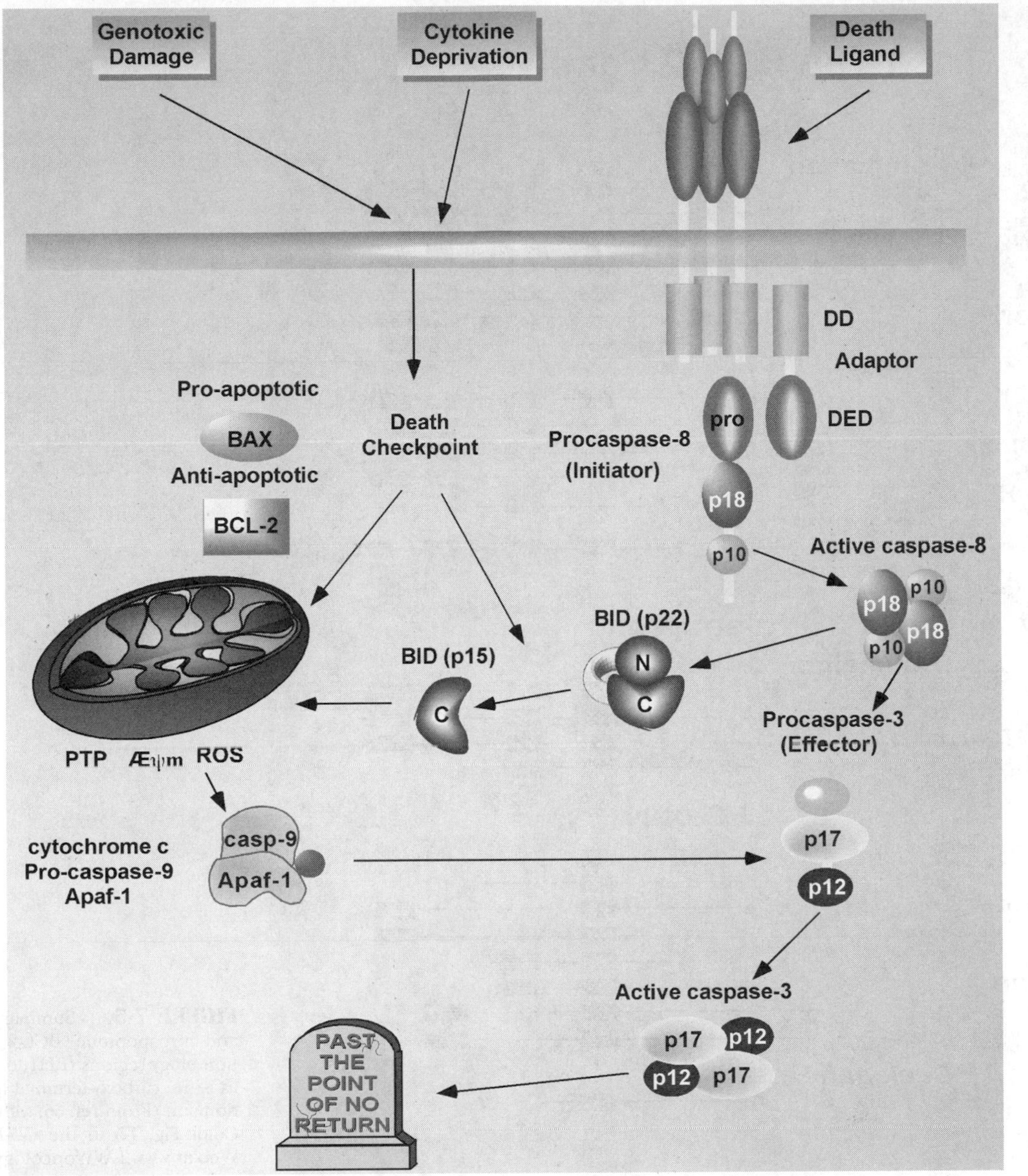

FIGURE 7-4. Model of the mammalian cell death pathway. Left: A major checkpoint in this pathway is the ratio of proapoptotic (BAX) to antiapoptotic (BCL-2) members. Downstream of this checkpoint are two major execution programs: mitochondrial dysfunction and caspase activation. Mitochondrial dysfunction is manifested as altered mitochondrial transmembrane potential (Δψm); disturbed mitochondrial physiology, including ROS production; and, at times, mitochondrial swelling. Cytochrome *c* is released from the mitochondrial membrane space to complex with Apaf-1 and activate caspase 9. Caspase activation may occur following a mitochondrial loop with Apaf-1/cytochrome *c* or directly in cells in which caspase 8 activates effector caspase 3. Caspases are activated by two cleavage events between the prodomain and the large subunit, and subsequently between the large and small subunits. The active caspase consists of a complex with two large and two small subunits. These activated caspases cleave death substrates, such as poly (ADP-ribose) polymerase (PARP) and laminin, culminating in cell death. Right: Activation of a Fas/TNF-α–family cell surface receptor leads to recruitment and activation of caspase 8, which in turn cleaves cytosolic p22 BID. After cleavage, truncated BID (tBID) translocates to the mitochondria, resulting in the release of cytochrome *c*. (See Color Fig. 7-4 in the CD-ROM and on the Web at www.LWWoncology.com.)

The three-dimensional structures for both an antiapoptotic molecule, BCL-X_L, and the proapoptotic molecule BID have been determined.[76–78] The Bcl-X_L α helical structure includes two central hydrophobic cores sandwiched by two amphipathic α helices similar to the membrane translocation domain of the bacterial toxin diphtheria toxin fragment B and the colicins. In fact, electrophysiologic studies have shown that BAX and BCL-2 are capable of forming ion channels in artificial membranes.[79] In their closed, monomeric forms, the α helices comprising domains BH1 to BH3 of the full family members are juxtaposed to form a hydrophobic pocket; this pocket receives the hydrophobic face of a BH3 amphipathic α helix to form hetero- or homodimers.[80,81]

As predicted from their structure, antiapoptotic molecules are principally integral membrane proteins found in the outer

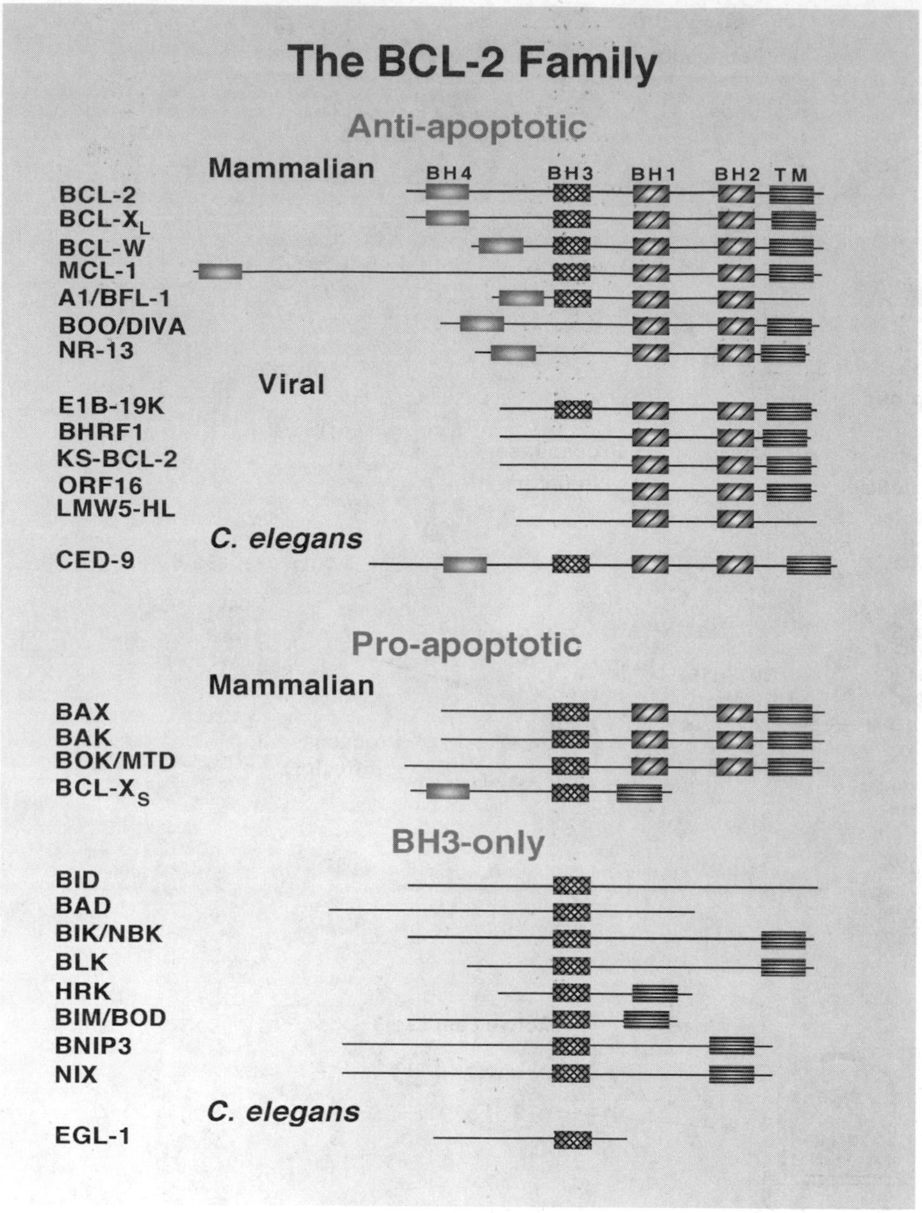

FIGURE 7-5. Summary of antiapoptotic and proapoptotic BCL-2 members. BCL-2 homology regions (BH1 to BH4) are denoted, as is the carboxy-terminal hydrophobic (TM) domain. (From ref. 66, with permission.) (See Color Fig. 7-5 in the CD-ROM and on the Web at www.LWWoncology.com.)

mitochondrial membrane, endoplasmic reticulum, or outer nuclear membrane.[82–85] In contrast, many of the proapoptotic molecules, especially the "BH3 domain only" subset are localized to the cytosol or cytoskeleton and undergo posttranslational modification after a death signal, which allows them to target and integrate into the mitochondrial membrane.[86–89] These modifications in response to death stimuli suggest that these BH3-only molecules are candidates for an upstream link between the BCL-2 checkpoint and proximal signal transduction (Fig. 7-6).

In support of this thesis, the BH3-only protein BAD is modified by phosphorylation on two serine residues in the presence of the survival factor interleukin-3 (IL-3).[90] In its phosphorylated form, BAD is inactive, bound, and sequestered by a cytosolic molecule, 14-3-3. On exposure to a death stimulus, such as IL-3 deprivation, BAD is dephosphorylated, resulting in the interaction of the BH3 domain of active BAD with the hydrophobic pocket of BCL-X$_L$ at the mitochondrial membrane.[91]

Distinct kinases appear to be responsible for the phosphorylation of the two serine sites in BAD. The phosphoinositide 3 kinase pathway regulates the phosphorylation of serine 136 in BAD. AKT, a serine/threonine survival signaling kinase in that pathway, can phosphorylate BAD serine 136.[92–95] AKT can also phosphorylate and inactivate the proapoptotic transcription factor FKHRL1 and caspase 9.[94,95] The phosphorylation and inactivation of serine 112 is mediated at the mitochondrial membrane by cyclic adenosine monophosphate–dependent protein kinase that is tethered to this locale by a mitochondrial-based A kinase anchoring protein (AKAP).[96] Thus, a single proapoptotic molecule BAD has multiple signal transduction pathways that converge to inactivate it. This example indicates how complex the regulation of this pathway is and offers additional steps for therapeutic intervention.

Another BH3-only protein, BID, connects the death signal through TNF-α or Fas to the downstream death effectors. BID exists in the cytoplasm as an inactive 22-kD protein. After TNF-

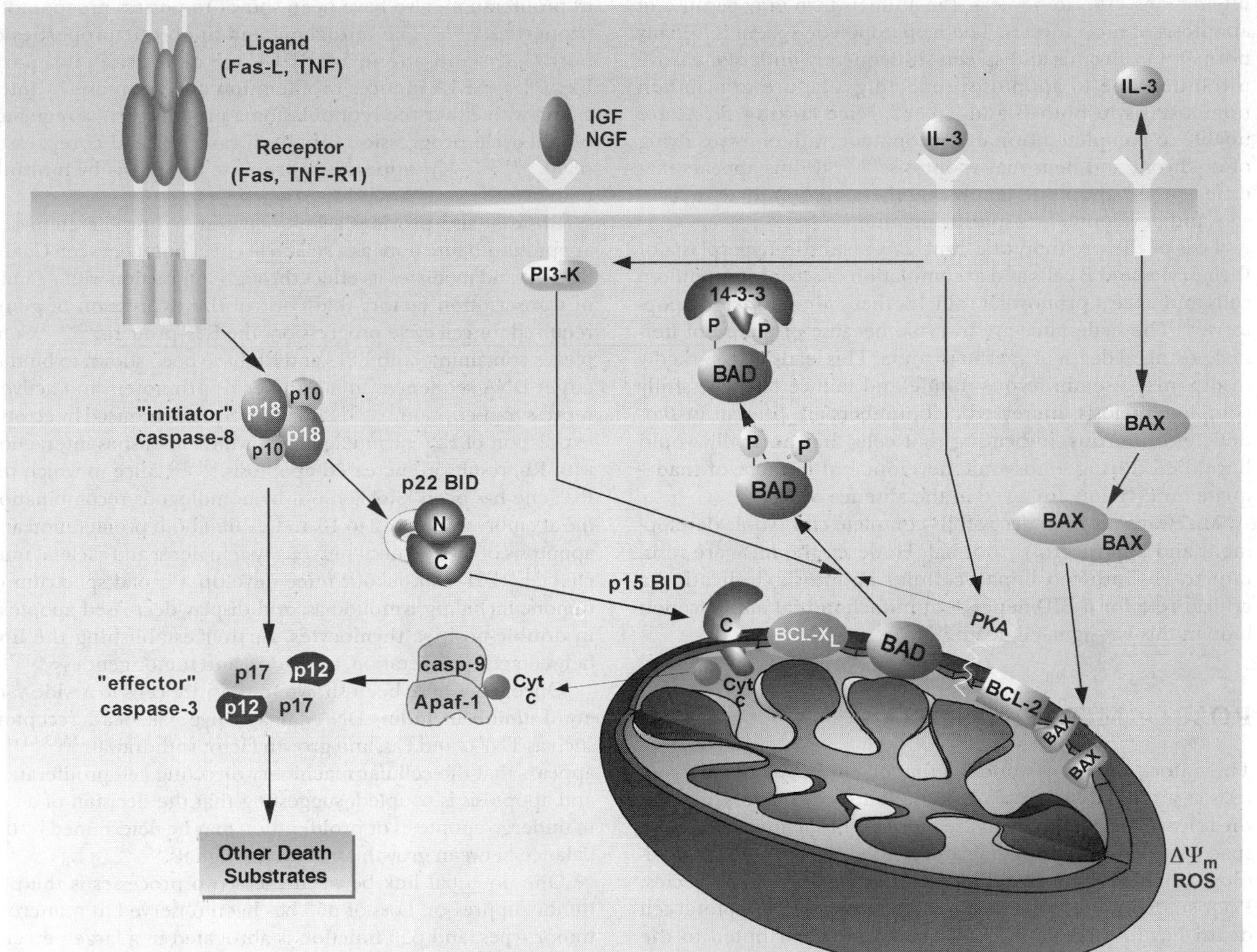

FIGURE 7-6. Model of apoptotic and survival signaling pathways involving the BCL-2 members. Left: Activation of tumor necrosis factor (TNF)/Fas cell surface receptor leads to activation of caspase 8. Caspase 8 cleaves cytosolic p22 BID, generating a p15 carboxy-terminal fragment that translocates to the mitochondria, resulting in the release of cytochrome *c*. Released cytochrome *c* activates Apaf-1, which in turn activates a downstream caspase program. Right: A death stimulus interleukin-3 (IL-3) deprivation induces the translocation of BAX to the mitochondria, where it is an integral membrane homo-oligomerized complex. Center: Activation of the insulin-like growth factor (IGF), nerve growth factor (NGF), or interleukin-3 (IL-3) receptors stimulates phosphoinositide 3 kinase (PI3-K) and Akt, resulting in the phosphorylation of BAD at serine 136. Survival factors, such as IL-3, also activate the mitochondrial-based cyclic adenosine monophosphate–dependent protein kinase (PKA) holoenzyme, resulting in the phosphorylation of BAD at serine 112. Phosphorylated BAD is inactive, sequestered to the cytosol by the phosphoserine-binding protein 14-3-3. Δψm, mitochondrial transmembrane potential. (See Color Fig. 7-6 in the CD-ROM and on the Web at www.LWWoncology.com.)

α or Fas signals, BID is cleaved in an unstructured loop by caspase8 to generate an active 15-kD fragment, truncated BID (tBID) which translocates and inserts into the mitochondrial membrane.[97–100] Cleavage eliminates the amino-terminal inhibitory α_1 helix, exposing the hydrophobic face of the BH3 domain as well as two central hydrophobic cores. Once integrated into the mitochondrial membrane, p15 BID results in the release of cytochrome *c*. The presence of BCL-2 or BCL-X_L ties up tBID, often preventing the release of cytochrome *c*.

The proapoptotic full family members BAX and BAK also demonstrate inactive and active conformations. Inactive BAX exists as a monomer in the cytosol, which translocates to the mitochondrial membrane where it resides as an active homo-oligomerized integral membrane protein. The translocation and oligomerization steps that activate BAX are, interestingly, blocked in cells protected by BCL-2.

Bcl-2 FAMILY MEMBERS PLAY CRITICAL ROLES IN TISSUE HOMEOSTASIS

The most stringent test for the role of a gene in normal development and homeostasis is an animal in which the gene of interest has been disrupted. Newborn *Bcl-2* knockout mice are viable, but the majority die within a few weeks of birth.[101–103] The surviving mice develop renal failure due to severe polycystic kidney disease. BCL-2 functions in the normal fetal kidney to maintain cell survival during inductive epithelial-mesenchymal interactions. At 5 to 6 weeks, the animals turn gray because of apoptosis of melanocytes. The hematopoietic system is initially normal, but thymus and spleen subsequently undergo massive involution due to apoptosis, reflecting a failure to maintain homeostasis in both B and T cells. Mice lacking *Bcl-X*$_L$ are unable to complete normal development, with embryos dying of erythroid and neuronal apoptosis.[104,105] It thus appears that different antiapoptotic family members predominate in a tissue- and developmental-specific manner.

Loss of the proapoptotic gene *Bax* results in hyperplasia of thymocytes and B cells and accumulation of atrophic granulosa cells and excess primordial follicles that fail to undergo apoptosis.[106] The male mice are infertile because of failure of normal postnatal death of spermatogonia. This leads to a markedly disorganized seminiferous tubule and failure to successfully complete meiosis. Increased cell numbers are present in *Bax*-deficient neurons, indicating that cells that normally would have died during embryonic development because of inadequate innervation are saved in the absence of *Bax.*[107]

Mice without BID successfully complete embryonic development and appear grossly normal. However, the mice are resistant to Fas-induced hepatocellular apoptosis, indicating a critical role for a BID-dependent mitochondrial amplification loop in this Fas-signaled death.[108]

ROLE OF MITOCHONDRIA

The mitochondrial dysfunction that occurs in cell death manifests as an initial hyperpolarization, followed by a loss of $\Delta\psi m$; the release of proteins from the mitochondrial intermembrane space, such as cytochrome *c*; and altered mitochondrial physiology, including the production of reactive oxygen species. Prior studies of necrotic death and late stages of apoptotic cell death have noted mitochondrial swelling attributed to the opening of a mitochondrial permeability transition pore that allows the passage of solutes and dissipation of the transmembrane gradient. The localization of antiapoptotic molecules, such as *BCL-2* and *BClX*$_L$, as well as the translocation of proapoptotic BAX and tBID to the mitochondrial membrane, emphasizes the importance of mitochondrial dysfunction in the action of these molecules. The specific mechanisms by which these proteins elicit their mitochondrial effects is an area of intense interest.

The importance of the mitochondria in the execution of apoptosis varies depending on both cell type and death stimulus. In certain cell types, activation of the TNF/Fas death receptor activates robust quantities of caspase 8 and subsequent effector caspase 3 with no requisite role for mitochondria, whereas other cells such as liver require the mitochondrial amplification loop to die. Other death stimuli, such as growth factor deprivation, may proceed in the absence of caspases and depend heavily on mitochondrial dysfunction.[109–111]

CELL PROLIFERATION AND APOPTOSIS

Apoptosis represents a brake on cellular expansion, countering abnormal cell proliferation. Substantial evidence exists for cross-talk between proliferation and apoptosis pathways.[112] The oncoproteins *c-Myc* and adenovirus E1A, both potent inducers of proliferation, also have been shown to possess proapoptotic properties.[113–116] The mitogenic and apoptotic properties of both *c-Myc* and adenovirus E1A are genetically inseparable.[113,117,118] E1A induces proliferation and apoptosis by interacting with either the retinoblastoma protein (Rb), a regulator of cell-cycle progression, or the transcriptional corepressor p300.[119–123] *c-Myc* appears to promote apoptosis by multiple pathways.[112]

Rb itself also provides a link between cell proliferation and apoptosis. Rb functions as a cell-cycle checkpoint between G_1 and S phase and mediates its effect through interaction with a family of transcription factors that control the expression of genes required for cell-cycle progression, the E2F proteins.[124–126] Complexes containing both E2Fs and Rb have been shown to bind to target DNA sequences in a number of promoters and actively repress transcription.[127–130] Entry into S phase induced by ectopic expression of E2F or mutagenesis, which abolishes interaction with Rb, results in increased apoptosis.[131–133] Mice in which the Rb gene has been knocked out by homologous recombination die at embryonic day 12 to 13 and exhibit both proliferation and apoptosis of liver, central nervous system, lens, and skeletal muscle.[134,135] E2F-1 knockout mice develop a broad spectrum of tumors, including lymphomas, and display decreased apoptosis in double-positive thymocytes, further establishing the link between cell proliferation, apoptosis, and tumorigenesis.[136,137]

Oncogenes have been shown to sensitize cells to a wide variety of stimuli, including DNA damage, hypoxia, death receptors such as TNF-α and Fas, and growth factor withdrawal.[113,138–144] It appears that the cellular machinery directing cell proliferation and apoptosis is coupled, suggesting that the decision of a cell to undergo apoptosis or proliferation may be determined by the balance between growth and survival signals.[145]

One potential link between these two processes is the p53 tumor suppressor. Loss of p53 has been observed in numerous tumor types, and p53 function is abrogated in a large percentage of tumors.[146,147] p53 expression is induced in response to a variety of cellular stresses, including DNA damage, hypoxia, and oncogene activation, resulting in cell-cycle arrest or apoptosis. Mice deficient for p53 are developmentally normal, but 75% develop spontaneous tumors by 6 months of age.[148] Germline mutation of p53 in humans results in Li-Fraumeni syndrome, and more than 50% of these individuals develop tumors by 30 years of age.[149]

The majority of p53 mutations in human tumors cluster within the DNA-binding domain, suggesting that p53 exerts its tumor suppressor effects through transcriptional regulation of target genes.[150] The mechanism by which p53 exerts its apoptotic effect appears to be multifactorial. p53 is able to induce the expression of *BAX* and *FAS*, as well as another member of the TNF family of death receptors, DR5.[151–154] In addition, p53 inhibits the expression of *BCL-2*, and BCL-2 can inhibit p53-induced apoptosis in select settings.[155–158] p53 also appears to induce apoptosis by post-translational mechanisms.[159,160]

POSSIBILITIES FOR THERAPEUTIC INTERVENTION

Given the ability to induce apoptosis in lymphoid cells and many types of tumor cells, the death receptors are attractive targets for therapeutic intervention in cancer. However, infusion of TNF-α causes a lethal inflammatory response resembling septic shock, which results from proinflammatory activation of macrophages and endothelial cells,[161,162] and infusion of agonistic anti-Fas antibody causes lethal hepatic apoptosis. The related death ligand TRAIL (APO2L) appears to possess the ability to induce apoptosis in a wide variety of tumor cell lines. *In vivo* administration of a leucine zipper form of TRAIL in which the molecule is stabilized as a trimer suppresses the growth of a mammary adenocarcinoma cell line in SCID (severe combined immunodeficiency) mice.[163] Normal cells treated *in vitro* with TRAIL showed no decreased viability. Similarly, recombinant TRAIL administered shortly after tumor xenograft injection markedly reduces tumor incidence. In addition, treatment of mice bearing solid tumors resulted in tumor cell apoptosis as well as improved survival. A synergistic effect was obtained with TRAIL and 5-fluorouracil or irinotecan (CPT-11). Encouragingly, intravenous injections of TRAIL into nonhuman primates did not result in toxicity to tissues or organs.

The *BCL-2* gene provides another promising target for therapeutic intervention, particularly in the therapy of low-grade lymphoma in which BCL-2 overexpression plays an important role.[164] The strategy of antisense oligonucleotide therapy has been used to "silence" *BCL-2* expression. Antisense oligonucleotides are short stretches of DNA, approximately 16 to 20 bases in length. The oligonucleotides are internalized by cells through a saturable endocytosis pathway. On injection into a host, expression of a specific gene can be blocked by hybridization with the target messenger RNA through Watson-Crick base pairing. The result is either degradation of the RNA-DNA complex by Rnase H or block in translation of the RNA.

An 18-base-pair antisense oligonucleotide, G3139 (Genta, San Diego, CA), was designed against *Bcl-2* for the treatment of follicular lymphoma.[165] Initial studies in a t(14;18) murine xenograft lymphoma model were encouraging, with absence of disease by polymerase chain reaction in 10 of 12 animals tested. A phase I clinical trial of G3139 has been completed on patients with relapsed B-cell non-Hodgkin's lymphoma with evidence of BCL-2 overexpression by immunohistochemistry of lymph node biopsy.[166] The main toxicity was reversible thrombocytopenia. Of the 20 evaluable patients (N = 21), one complete response was achieved in a patient with stage IV follicular lymphoma. Two patients had partial responses, eight patients had stable disease, and nine patients progressed. Current phase II studies are under way to investigate the role of G3139 in combination with conventional chemotherapy.

BCL-2 also has been shown to play a role in solid tumors. In prostate cancer, Bcl-2 overexpression confers both chemoresistance and resistance to apoptotic cell death after androgen withdrawal.[167–172] In an androgen-dependent tumor model, *in vitro* treatment of tumor cells with antisense *BCL-2* enhances cytotoxicity of paclitaxel.[167] *In vivo* administration of antisense *BCL-2* oligonucleotides in combination with paclitaxel to animals with established tumors results in inhibition of tumor growth. In addition, treatment in combination with paclitaxel after castration results in a significant delay in tumor recurrence. BCL-2 is also highly expressed in malignant melanoma.[173,174] In a preclinical xenograft model, *BCL-2* antisense oligonucleotides significantly sensitized the tumor cell response to subsequent dacarbazine.[175] It thus appears that *BCL-2* antisense therapy may have a potential role in combination with other chemotherapeutic drugs as a chemosensitizing agent.

CONCLUSIONS

Apoptosis is an evolutionarily conserved, highly regulated mechanism for maintaining homeostasis in multicellular organisms. Numerous signals are capable of modulating cell death. After a death stimulus, the signal is propagated and amplified through the activation by proteolytic cleavage of caspases, culminating in the ordered disassembly of the cell. The process may transpire through a mitochondrial-dependent or -independent pathway, depending on the death signal and cell type involved. The Bcl-2 family of proteins is situated upstream of irreversible cell damage in the apoptotic pathway, providing a pivotal checkpoint in the fate of a cell after a death stimulus. The proapoptotic molecules BID, BAD, and BAX undergo modification and intracellular translocation on receipt of a death stimulus, connecting distinct upstream signal transduction pathways with the common, core apoptotic pathway. The distribution of inactive conformers of the BH3-only members suggests that they may function as sentinels for recognizing cellular damage.[66] BIM would monitor microtubule function, BID would amplify minimal caspase 8 activation, and BAD would patrol for metabolic stress after loss of critical survival factors. This model would explain how seemingly diverse cellular injuries converge on a final common pathway of cell death.

Finally, the cellular pathway to apoptosis appears to communicate with the pathway for cell proliferation.[112] As a result, activation of cell proliferation by oncogenes also results in sensitization to apoptosis. Reciprocally, the expression of antiapoptotic molecules often retards cell-cycle progression.[176] This interconnection provides a means for limiting the threatening expansion of cells with a lesion in either pathway. These observations fit the evidence that defects are required in both proliferation and cell death pathways, as single defects tend to be self-correcting in their net effect on cell number. The molecules mediating apoptotic pathways provide an exciting opportunity for rational design of new therapeutic agents to specifically promote apoptosis of cancer cells.

REFERENCES

1. Vogt C. Untersuchungen uber die Entwickllungsgeschichte der Geburtshelferkroete (Alytes obsttertricians). Solothurn, Switzerland: Jent and Gassman, 1842.
2. Kerr JF, Wylie AH, Currie AR. Apoptosis: a basic biological phenomenon with wide-ranging implications in tissue kinetics. *Br J Cancer* 1972;26:239.
3. Wylie AH. Apoptosis, cell death in tissue regulation. *J Pathol* 1987;153:313.
4. Fukuhara S, Rowley JD, Varrakojis D, Golumb HM. Chromosomal abnormalities in poorly differentiated lymphocytic lymphoma. *Cancer Res* 1979;39:3119.
5. Yunis JJ, Frizzera G, Oken MM, et al. Multiple recurrent genomic defects in follicular lymphoma. *N Engl J Med* 1987;316:79.
6. Tsujimoto Y, Gorham J, Cossman J, Jaffe E, Croce CM. The t(14;18) chromosome translocations involved in B-cell neoplasms result from mistakes in VDJ joining. *Science* 1985;229:1390.
7. Bakhshi A, Jensen JP, Goldman P, et al. Cloning the chromosomal breakpoint of t(14;18) human lymphomas: clustering around JH on chromosome 14 and near a transcriptional unit on 18. *Cell* 1985;41:889.
8. Cleary ML, Sklar J. Nucleotide sequence of a t(14;18) chromosomal breakpoint in follicular lymphoma and demonstration of a breakpoint cluster region near a transcriptionally active locus on chromosome 18. *Proc Natl Acad Sci U S A* 1985;82:7439.
9. Tsujimoto Y, Croce CM. Analysis of the structure, transcription, and protein products of bcl-2, the gene involved in human follicular lymphoma. *Proc Natl Acad Sci U S A* 1986;83:5214.
10. Korsmeyer SJ. Bcl-2 gene family and the regulation of programmed cell death. *Cancer Res* 1999;59[Suppl]:1693s.
11. Horning SJ. Natural history of and therapy for the indolent non-Hodgkin's lymphomas. *Semin Oncol* 1993;20:75.
12. McDonnell TJ, Dean N, Platt FM, et al. Bcl-2-immunoglobulin transgenic mice demonstrate extended B-cell survival and follicular lymphoproliferation. *Cell* 1989;57:79.

13. McDonnell TJ, Nunez G, Platt FM, et al. Deregulated Bcl-2-immunoglobulin transgene expands a resting but responsive IgM/IgD B-cell population. *Mol Cell Biol* 1990;10:1901.
14. McDonnell TJ, Korsmeyer SJ. Progression from lymphoid hyperplasia to high-grade malignant lymphoma in mice transgenic for the t(14;18). *Nature* 1991;349:6306.
15. Strasser A, Harris AW, Bath ML, Cory S. Novel primitive lymphoid tumors induced in transgenic mice by cooperation between myc and bcl-2. *Nature* 1990;348:331.
16. Vaux DL, Cory S, Adams J. Bcl-2 gene promotes haemopoietic cell survival and cooperates with c-myc to immortalize pre-B cells. *Nature* 1988;335:440.
17. Hockenberry D, Nunez G, Milliman C, Schreiber RD, Korsmeyer SJ. Bcl-2 is an inner mitochondrial membrane protein that blocks programmed cell death. *Nature* 1990;348:334.
18. Nunez G, London L, Hockenberry D, et al. Deregulated c Bcl-2 expression selectively promotes survival of growth factor-deprived hematopoietic cell lines. *J Immunol* 1990;144:3602.
19. Bishop JM. The molecular genetics of cancer. *Science* 1987;235:305.
20. Korsmeyer SJ. Bcl-2 initiates a new category of oncogenes: regulators of cell death. *Blood* 1992;80:879.
21. Sulston JE, Horvitz HR. Post-embryonic cell lineages of the nematode, Caenorhabditis elegans. *Dev Biol* 1977;56:110.
22. Sulston JE, Schierenberg E, White JG, Thomson JN. The embryonic cell lineage of the nematode Caenorhabditis elegans. *Dev Biol* 1983;100:64.
23. Hengartner M, Ellis R, Horvitz HR. C. elegans gene ced-9 protects cells from programmed cell death. *Nature* 1992;356:494.
24. Hengartner MO, Horvitz HR. C. elegans survival gene ced-9 encodes a functional homologue of the mammalian proto-oncogene bcl-2. *Cell* 1994;76:665.
25. Vaux DL, Weissman I, Kim S. Prevention of programmed cell death in Caenorhabditis elegans by human bcl-2. *Science* 1992;258:1955.
26. Conradt B, Horvitz HR. The C. elegans protein EGL-1 is required for programmed cell death and interacts with the Bcl-2-like protein CED-9. *Cell* 1998;93:519.
27. Shaham S, Horvitz HR. Developing Caenorhabditis elegans neurons may contain both cell-death protective and killer activities. *Genes Dev* 1996;10:578.
28. Cerretti DP, Kozlosky CJ, Mosley B, et al. Molecular cloning of the interleukin-1β converting enzyme. *Science* 1992;256:97.
29. Thornberry N, Bull HG, Calaycay JR, et al. A novel heterodimeric cysteine protease is required for interleukin-1β processing in monocytes. *Nature* 1992;356:768.
30. Ledoux S, Ellis HM, Horvitz HR. The C. elegans cell death gene ced-3 encodes a protein similar to mammalian interleukin-1β-converting enzyme. *Cell* 1993;75:641.
31. Miura M, Zhu H, Rotello R, Hartweig EA, Yuan J. Induction of apoptosis in fibroblasts by IL-1β-converting enzyme, a mammalian homologue of the C. elegans cell death gene ced-3. *Cell* 1993;75:653.
32. Cryns V, Yuan J. Proteases to die for. *Genes Dev* 1998;12:1551.
33. Nagata S. Apoptosis by death factor. *Cell* 1997;88:355.
34. Chinnaiyan AM, O'Rourke K, Tewari M, Dixit VM. FADD, a novel death domain–containing protein, interacts with the death domain of Fas and initiates apoptosis. *Cell* 1995;81:505.
35. Chinnaiyan AM, Tepper CG, Seldin MF, et al. FADD/Mort1 is a common mediator of CD95 (Fas/APO-1) and tumor necrosis factor–induced apoptosis. *J Biol Chem* 1996;271:4961.
36. Hsu H, Xiong J, Goeddel DV. The TNF receptor I–associated protein TRADD signals cell death and NF-κB activation. *Cell* 1995;81:495.
37. Stanger BZ, Leder P, Lee TH, Kim E, Seed B. RIP: a novel protein containing a death domain that interacts with Fas/APO-1 (CD95) in yeast and causes cell death. *Cell* 1995;81:513.
38. Irmler M, Thome M, Hahne M, et al. Inhibition of death receptor signals by cellular FLIP. *Nature* 1997;388:190.
39. Baeuerle PA, Baltimore D. NF-κB, ten years after. *Cell* 1996;87:13.
40. Wang CY, Mayo MW, Baldwin AS Jr. TNF and cancer therapy–induced apoptosis: potentiation by inhibition of NF-κB. *Science* 1996;274:784.
41. Van Antwerp DJ, Martin SJ, Kafri T, Green DR, Verma IM. Suppression of TNF-α-induced apoptosis by NF-κB. *Science* 1996;274:787.
42. Beg AA, Baltimore D. An essential role for NF-κB in preventing TNF-α-induced cell death. *Science* 1996;274:782.
43. Liu ZG, Hsu H, Goeddel DV, Karin M. Dissection of TNF receptor 1 effector functions: JNK activation is not linked to apoptosis while NF-κB activation prevents cell death. *Cell* 1996;87:565.
44. Natoli G, Costanzo A, Ianni A, et al. Activation of SAPK/JNK by TNF receptor 1 through a noncytotoxic TRAF2-dependent pathway. *Science* 1997;275:200.
45. Beg AA, Sha WC, Bronson RT, Ghosh S, Baltimore D. Embryonic lethality and liver degeneration in mice lacking the RelA component of NF-κB. *Nature* 1995;376:167.
46. Kelliher MA, Grimm S, Ishida Y, et al. The death domain kinase RIP mediates the TNF-induced NF-κB signal. *Immunity* 1998;8:297.
47. Pimental-Muinos FX, Seed B. Regulated commitment of TNF receptor signaling: a molecular switch for death or activation. *Immunity* 1999;11:783.
48. Gilmore TD, Koedood M, Piffat KA, White DW. Rel/NF-kappaB/IkappaB proteins and cancer. *Oncogene* 1996;13:1367.
49. Liu X, Kim CN, Yang J, Jemmerson R, Wang X. Induction of apoptotic program in cell-free extracts: requirement for dATP and cytochrome c. *Cell* 1996;86:147.
50. Li F, Srinivasan A, Wang Y, et al. Cell-specific induction of apoptosis by microinjection of cytochrome c. Bcl-X_L has activity independent of cytochrome c release. *J Biol Chem* 1997;272:30299.
51. Zou H, Henzel W, Liu X, Lutschg A, Wang X. Apaf-1, a human protein homologous to C. elegans CED-4, participates in cytochrome c–dependent activation of caspase-3. *Cell* 1997;90:405.
52. Zou H, Henzel WJ, Liu X, Wang X. An Apaf-1-cytochrome c multimeric complex is a functional apoptosome that activiates procaspase-9. *J Biol Chem* 1999;274:11549.
53. Zou H, Henzel WJ, Liu X, Wang X. An Apaf-1-cytochrome c multimeric complex is a functional apoptosome that activates procaspase-9. *J Biol Chem* 1999;274:11549.
54. Thornberry NA, Lazebnik Y. Caspases, enemies within. *Science* 1998;281:1312.
55. Walker NPC, Talanian RV, Brady LC, et al. Crystal structure of the cysteine protease interleukin-1β-converting enzyme: a (p20/p20)2 homodimer. *Cell* 1994;78:739.
56. Wilson KP, Black JAF, Thomson JA, et al. Structure and mechanism of interleukin-1β converting enzyme. *Nature* 1994;370:270.
57. Rotonda J, Nicholson DW, Fazil K. The three dimensional structure of apopain/CPP32, a key mediator of apoptosis. *Nature Struct Biol* 1996;3:619.
58. Talanian RV, Quinlan C, Trautz S, et al. Substrate specificities of caspase family proteases. *J Biol Chem* 1997;272:9677.
59. Thornberry N, Rano T, Peterson E, et al. A combinatorial approach defines specificities of members of the caspase family and granzyme B. Functional relationships established for key mediator of apoptosis. *J Biol Chem* 1997;272:17907.
60. Boldin MP, Goncharov TM, Goltsev TV, Wallach D. Involvement of MACH, a novel MORT1/FADD-interacting protease, in Fas/APO-1 and TNF receptor–induced cell death. *Cell* 1996;85:803.
61. Boldin MP, Varfolomeev EE, Pancer Z, et al. A novel protein that interacts with the death domain of Fas/APO-1 contains a sequence motif related to the death domain. *J Biol Chem* 1995;270:7795.
62. Fernandes-Alnemri T, Armstrong RC, Krebs J, et al. In vitro activation of CPP32 and Mch3 by Mch4, a novel apoptotic cysteine protease containing two FADD-like domains. *Proc Natl Acad Sci U S A* 1996;93:7464.
63. Muzio M, Chinnaiyan AM, Kischkel FC, et al. Flice, a novel FADD-homologous ICE/CED-3-like protease, is recruited to the CD95 (Fas/APO-1) death-inducing signaling complex. *Cell* 1996;85:817.
64. Vincenz C, Dixit VM. Fas-associated death domain protein and interleukin-1β-converting enzyme 2 (FLICE2), an ICE/Ced-3 homologue, is proximally involved in CD95- and p55-mediated death signaling. *J Biol Chem* 1997;272:6578.
65. Scaffidi C, Fulda S, Srinivasan A, et al. Two CD95(APO-1/Fas) signaling pathways. *EMBO J* 1998;273:3388.
66. Gross A, McDonnell JM, Korsmeyer SJ. Bcl-2 family members and the mitochondria in apoptosis. *Genes Dev* 1999;13:1899.
67. Adams JM, Cory S. The Bcl-2 protein family: arbiters of cell survival. *Science* 1998;281:1322.
68. Keleker A, Thompson CB. Bcl-2–family proteins: the role of the BH3 domain in apoptosis. *Trends Cell Biol* 1998;8:324.
69. Reed JC. Bcl-2 family proteins. *Oncogene* 1998;17:3225.
70. Yin XM, Oltvai ZN, Korsmeyer SJ. BH1 and BH2 domains of Bcl-2 are required for inhibition of apoptosis and heterodimerization with Bax. *Nature* 1994;369:321.
71. Cheng EHY, Levine B, Boise LH, Thompson CB, Hardwick JM. Bax-independent inhibition of apoptosis by Bcl-X_L. *Nature* 1996;379:554.
72. Perez GI, Robles R, Knudson CM, et al. Prolongation of ovarian lifespan into advanced chronological age by Bax-deficiency. *Nat Genet* 1999;21:200.
73. Chittenden T, Flemington C, Houghton AB, et al. A conserved domain in Bak, distinct from BH1 and BH2, mediates cell death and protein binding functions. *EMBO J* 1995;14:5589.
74. Wang K, Yin XM, Chao DT, Milliman CL, Korsmeyer SJ. BID: a novel BH3 domain-only death agonist. *Genes Dev* 1996;10:2859.
75. Conradt B, Horvitz HR. The C. elegans protein EGL-1 is required for programmed cell death and interacts with the Bcl-2-like protein CED-9. *Cell* 1998;93:519.
76. Muchmore SW, Sattler M, Liamg H, et al. X-ray and NMR structure of human Bcl-X_L, an inhibitor of programmed cell death. *Nature* 1996;381:335.
77. Chou JJ, Li H, Salveson GS, Yuan J, Wagner G. Solution structure of BID, an intracellular amplifier of apoptotic signalling. *Cell* 1999;96:615.
78. McDonnell JM, Fushman CL, Milliman CL, Korsmeyer SJ, Cowburn D. Solution structure of the pro-apoptotic molecule BID: a structural basis for apoptotic agonists and antagonists. *Cell* 1999;96:625.
79. Schlesinger PH, Gross A, Yin XM, et al. Comparison of the ion channel characteristics of proapoptotic BAX and antiapoptotic BCL-2. *Proc Natl Acad Sci U S A* 1997;94:11357.
80. Sattler M, Liang H, Nettesheim D, et al. Structure of Bcl-X_L-Bak peptide complex: recognition between regulators of apoptosis. *Science* 1997;275:983.
81. Zha J, Harada H, Osipov K, et al. BH3 domain of BAD is required for heterodimerization with Bcl-X_L and pro-apoptotic activity. *J Biol Chem* 1997;272:24101.
82. Hockenberry D, Nunez G, Milliman C, Schreiber RD, Korsmeyer SJ. Bcl-2 is an inner mitochondrial membrane protein that blocks programmed cell death. *Nature* 1990;348:334.
83. Krajewski S, Tanaka S, Takayama S, et al. Investigation of the subcellular distribution of the bcl-2 oncoprotein: residence in the nuclear envelope, endoplasmic reticulum, and outer mitochondrial membranes. *Cancer Res* 1993;53:4701.
84. De Jong D, Prins FA, Mason DY, et al. Subcellular localization of the bcl-2 protein in malignant and normal lymphoid cells. *Cancer Res* 1994,54.256.
85. Zhu W, Cowie A, Wasfy GW, et al. Bcl-2 mutants with restricted subcellular location reveal spatially distinct pathways for apoptosis in different cell types. *EMBO J* 1996;15:4130.
86. Hsu YT, Wolter KG, Youle RJ. Cytosol to membrane redistribution of Bax and Bcl-X(L) during apoptosis. *Proc Natl Acad Sci U S A* 1997;94:3668.
87. Gross A, Jockel J, Wei MC, Korsmeyer SJ. Enforced dimerization of BAX results in its translocation, mitochondrial dysfunction, and apoptosis. *EMBO J* 1998;17:3878.
88. Puthalakath H, Huang DC, O'Reilly LA, King SM, Strasser A. The proapoptotic activity of the Bcl-2 family member Bim is regulated by interaction with the dynein motor complex. *Mol Cell* 1999;3:287.

89. Zha JP, Harada H, Yang E, Jockel J, Korsmeyer SJ. Serine phosphorylation of death agonist Bad in response to survival factor results in binding to 14-3-3 not Bcl-X_L. *Cell* 1996;87:619.
90. Zha JP, Harada H, Osipov J, et al. BH3 domain of BAD is required for heterodimerization with BCL-X_L and pro-apoptotic activity. *J Biol Chem* 1997;272:24101.
91. Datta SR, Dudek H, Tao X, et al. Akt phosphorylation of BAD couple survival signal to the cell-intrinsic death machinery. *Cell* 1997;91:231.
92. Del Peso L, Ganzalez-Garcia M, Page C, Herrera R, Nunez G. Interleukin-3-induced phosphorylation of BAD through the protein kinase Akt. *Science* 1997;278:687.
93. Blume-Jensen P, Janknecht R, Hunter T. The kit receptor promotes cell survival via activation of PI3-kinase and subsequent Akt-mediated phosphorylation of Bad on Ser136. *Curr Biol* 1998;8:779.
94. Brunet A, Binni A, Zigmond MJ, et al. Akt promotes cell survival by phosphorylating and inhibiting a Forkhead transcription factor. *Cell* 1999;96:857.
95. Cardone MH, Roy N, Stennicke HR, et al. Regulation of cell death protease caspase-9 by phosphorylation. *Science* 1998;282:1318.
96. Harada H, Becknell B, Wilm M, et al. Phosphorylation and inactivation of BAD by mitochondria-anchored protein kinase A. *Mol Cell* 1999;3:413.
97. Li P, Zhu H, Xu CJ, Yuan J. Cleavage of BID by caspase 8 mediates the mitochondrial damage in the Fas pathway of apoptosis. *Cell* 1998;94:491.
98. Luo X, Budihardjo I, Zou H, Slaughter C, Wang X. Bid, a Bcl2 interacting protein, mediates cytochrome c release from mitochondria in response to activation of cell surface death receptors. *Cell* 1998;94:481.
99. Gross A, Yin XM, Wang K, et al. Caspase cleaved BID targets mitochondria and is required for cytochrome c release, while BCL-X_L prevents this release but not tumor necrosis factor-R1/Fas death. *J Biol Chem* 1999;274:1156.
100. Han Z, Bhalla K, Pantazis P, Hendrickson EA, Wyche JH. Cif (cytochrome c efflux-inducing factor) activity is regulated by Bcl-2 and caspases and correlates with the activity of Bid. *Mol Cell Biol* 1999;19:1381.
101. Veis DJ, Sorenson CM, Shutter JR, Korsmeyer SJ. Bcl-2 deficient mice demonstrate fulminant lymphoid apoptosis, polycystic kidneys, and hypopigmented hair. *Cell* 1993;75:229.
102. Nakayama K, Negisha I, Kuida K, Sawa H, Loh DY. Targeted disruption of Bcl-2 in mice: occurrence of grey hair, polycystic kidney disease, and lymphocytopenia. *Proc Natl Acad Sci U S A* 1994;91:3700.
103. Kamada S, Shimono A, Shinto Y, et al. Bcl-2 deficiency in mice leads to pleitrophic abnormalities: accelerated lymphoid cell death in thymus and spleen, polycystic kidney, hair hypopigmentation, and distorted small intestine. *Cancer Res* 1995;55:354.
104. Motoyama N, Wang F, Roth KA, et al. Massive cell death of immature hematopoietic cells and neurons in Bcl-X_L-deficient mice. *Science* 1995;267:1506.
105. Ma A, Pena JC, Chang B, et al. Bclx regulates the survival of double positive thymocytes. *Proc Natl Acad Sci U S A* 1995;92:4763.
106. Knudson CM, Tung SK, Tourtellotte WG, Brown GAJ, Korsmeyer SJ. Bax-deficient mice with lymphoid hyperplasia and male germ cell death. *Science* 1995;270:96.
107. Deckworth TL, Elliott JL, Knudson CM, et al. Bax is required for neuronal death after trophic factor deprivation and during development. *Neuron* 1996;17:401.
108. Yin XM, Wang K, Gross A, et al. Bid-deficient mice are resistant to Fas-induced hepatocellular apoptosis. *Nature* 1999;400:886.
109. Ashkenazi A, Dixit VM. Death receptors: signaling and modulation. *Science* 1998;281: 1305.
110. Wallach D, Kavalenko AV, Varfolomeev EE, Boldin MP. Death-inducing functions of ligands of the tumor necrosis family: a Sanhedrin verdict. *Curr Opin Immunol* 1998;10:279.
111. Scaffidi C, Schmitz I, Zha J, et al. Differential modulation of apoptosis sensitivity in CD95 type I and type II cells. *J Biol Chem* 1999;274:22532.
112. Evan G, Littlewood T. A matter of life and cell death. *Science* 1998;281:1317.
113. Evan GM, Wylie AH, Gilbert CS, et al. Induction of apoptosis in fibroblasts by c-myc protein. *Cell* 1992;69:119.
114. Sakamuro D, Eviner V, Elliott KJ, et al. c-Myc induces apoptosis in epithelial cells by both p53-dependent and p53-independent mechanisms. *Oncogene* 1995;11:2411.
115. Shi Y, Glynn JM, Guilbert LJ, et al. Role for c-myc in activation-induced cell death in T cell hybridomas. *Science* 1992;257:212.
116. White E, Cipriani R, Sabbatini P, Denton A. Adenovirus E1B 19-kilodalton protein overcomes the cytotoxicity of E1A proteins. *J Virol* 1991;65:2968.
117. Amati B, Littlewood TD, Evan GI, Land H. The c-Myc protein induces cell cycle progression and apoptosis through dimerization with Max. *EMBO J* 1993;12:5083.
118. Raychaudhuri P, Bagchi S, Devoto SH, Kraus VB, Moran E. Domains of the adenovirus E1A protein required for oncogenic activity are also required for dissociation of E2F transcription factor complexes. *Genes Dev* 1991;5:1200.
119. Flint J, Shenk T. Viral transactivating proteins. Annu Rev Genet 1997;31:177.
120. Samuelson AV, Lowe SW. Selective induction of p53 and chemosensitivity in RB-deficient cells by E1A mutants unable to bind the RB-related proteins. *Proc Natl Acad Sci U S A* 1997;94:12094.
121. Shisler J, Duerksen-Hughes P, Hermiston TM, Wold WS, Gooding L. Induction of susceptibility to tumor necrosis factor by E1A is dependent on binding to either p300 or p105-Rb and induction of DNA synthesis. *J Virol* 1996;70:68.
122. Querido E, Teodoro JG, Branton PE. Accumulation of p53 induced by the adenovirus E1A protein requires regions involved in the stimulation of DNA synthesis. *J Virol* 1997;71:3526.
123. Mymryk JS, Shire K, Bayley ST. Induction of apoptosis by adenovirus type 5 E1A in rat cells requires a proliferation block. *Oncogene* 1994;9:1187.
124. Johnson DG, Schneider-Broussard R. Role of E2F in cell cycle control and cancer. *Front Biosci* 1998;3:d447.
125. Weinberg RA. The retinoblastoma protein and cell cycle control. *Cell* 1995;81:323.
126. Nevins JR. E2F: a link between the Rb tumor suppressor protein and viral oncoproteins. *Science* 1992;258:424.
127. LaThangue NB. DRTF/E2F: an expanding family of heterodimeric transcription factors implicated in cell cycle control. *Trends Biochem Sci* 1994;19:108.
128. Weintraub SJ, Prater CA, Dean DC. Retinoblastoma protein switches the E2F site from positive to negative element. *Nature* 1992;358:259.
129. Lam EWF, Watson RJ. An E2F-binding site mediates cell-cycle regulated repression of mouse B-myb transcription. *EMBO J* 1993;12:2705.
130. Dynlacht BD, Flores O, Lees JA, Harlow E. Differential regulation of E2F transactivation by cyclin/cdk2 complexes. *Genes Dev* 1994;8:1772.
131. Qin XQ, Livingston DM, Kaelin WG Jr, Adams PD. Deregulated E2f-1 transcription factor expression leads to S-phase entry and p53-mediated apoptosis. *Proc Natl Acad Sci U S A* 1994;91:10918.
132. Adams PD, Kaelin WG. The cellular effects of E2F overexpression. *Curr Top Microbiol Immunol* 1996;208:79.
133. Shan B, Lee WH. Deregulated expression of E2F-1 induces S-phase entry and leads to apoptosis. *Mol Cell Biol* 1994;14:8166.
134. Jacks T, Fazeli A, Schmitt E, et al. Effects of an RB mutation in the mouse. *Nature* 1992;359:295.
135. Clarke AR, Maandag ER, van Roon M, et al. Requirement for a functional Rb-1 gene in murine development. *Nature* 1992;359:328.
136. Yamasaki L, Jacks T, Bronson R, et al. Tumor induction and tissue atrophy in mice lacking E2F-1. *Cell* 1996;85:537.
137. Field SJ, Tsai FY, Kuo F, et al. E2F-1 functions in mice to promote apoptosis and suppress proliferation. *Cell* 1996;85:549.
138. Packham G, Cleveland JL. The role of ornithine decarboxylase in c-Myc-induced apoptosis. *Curr Top Microbiol Immunol* 1995;194:283.
139. Galaktionov K, Chen X, Beach D. Cdc25 cell-cycle phosphatase as a target of c-myc. *Nature* 1996;382:511.
140. Nip J, Strom DK, Fee BE, et al. E2F-1 cooperates with topoisomerase II inhibition and DNA damage to selectively augment p53-independent apoptosis. *Mol Cell Biol* 1997;17:1049.
141. Lowe SW, Ruley HE, Jacks T, Housman DE. P53-dependent apoptosis modulates the cytotoxicity of anticancer agents. *Cell* 1993;74:957.
142. Alarcon RM, Rupnow BA, Graeber TG, Knox SJ, Giaccia AJ. Modulation of c-myc activity and apoptosis in vivo. *Cancer Res* 1996;56:4315.
143. Klefstrom J, Vastrik I, Saksela E, et al. C-Myc induces susceptibility to the cytotoxic action of TNF-alpha. *EMBO J* 1994;13:5442.
144. Hueber AO, Zornig M, Lyon D, et al. Requirement for the CD95 receptor-ligand pathway in c-Myc-induced apoptosis. *Science* 1997;278:1305.
145. Harrington EA, Fanidi A, Evan GI. Oncogenes and cell death. *Curr Opin Genet Dev* 1994;4:120.
146. Hollstein M, Sidransky D, Vogelstein B, Harris CC. The p53 mutations in human cancers. *Science* 1991;280:1089.
147. Vogelstein B, Kinzler KW. p53 function and dysfunction. *Cell* 1992;70:523.
148. Donehower LA, Harvey M, Slagle BL, et al. Mice deficient for p53 are developmentally normal but susceptible to spontaneous tumors. *Nature* 1992;356:215.
149. Malkin D, Li FP, Strong FC, et al. Germ line p53 mutations in a familial syndrome of breast cancer, sarcomas, and other neoplasms. *Science* 1990;250:1233.
150. Cho Y, Gorina S, Jeffrey PD, Pavletich NP. Crystal structure of a p53 tumor suppressor–DNA complex: understanding tumorigenic mutations. *Science* 1994;265:346.
151. Burn TF, El-Deiry WS. The p53 pathway and apoptosis. *J Cell Physiol* 1999;181:231.
152. Miyashita T, Reed JC. Tumor suppressor p53 is a direct transcriptional activator of the human bax gene. *Cell* 1995;80:293.
153. Owen-Scaub LB, Zhang W, Cusack JC, et al. Wild-type human p53 and a temperature-sensitive mutant induce fas/APO1 expression. *Mol Cell Biol* 1995;15:3032.
154. Wu GS, Burns TF, McDonald ER III, et al. KILLER/DR5 is a DNA damage–inducible p53-regulated death receptor gene. *Nat Genet* 1997;17:141.
155. Wang Y, Szekely L, Okan I, Klein G, Wiman KG. Wild-type p53-triggered apoptosis is inhibited by bcl-2 in a v-myc-induced T-cell lymphoma line. *Oncogene* 1993;12:3427.
156. Marin MC, Hsu B, Meyn RE, et al. Evidence that p53 and bcl-2 are regulators of a common cell death pathway important for in vivo lymphomagenesis. *Oncogene* 1994;9:3107.
157. Chiou SK, Rao L, White E. Bcl-2 blocks p53-dependent apoptosis. *Mol Cell Biol* 1994;4:25560.
158. Froesch BA, Aime-Sempe C, Leber B, Andrews D, Reed JC. Inhibition of p53 transcriptional activity by Bcl-2 requires its membrane-anchoring domain. *J Biol Chem* 1999;274:6469.
159. Brady HJ, Salomons GS, Bobeldijk RC, Berns AJ. T cells from baxalpha transgenic mice show accelerated apoptosis in response to stimuli but do not show restored DNA damage–induced cell death in the absence of p53. *EMBO J* 1996;15:1221.
160. Fuchs EJ, McKenna KA, Bedi A. P53-dependent DNA damage–induced apoptosis requires Fas/APO-1-independent activation of CPP32 beta. *Cancer Res* 1997;57:2550.
161. Ashkenazi A, Pai RC, Fong S, et al. Safety and antitumor activity of recombinant soluble Apo2 ligand. *J Clin Invest* 1999;104:155.
162. Tartaglia L, Goeddel D. Two TNF receptors. *Immunol Today* 1992;13:151.
163. Walczak H, Miller RE, Ariail K, et al. Tumoricidal activity of tumor necrosis factor–related apoptosis-inducing ligand in vivo. *Nat Med* 1999;5:157.
164. Cotter F. Antisense therapy of hematologic malignancies. *Semin Hematol* 1999;36:9.
165. Cotter FE, Johnson P, Hall P, et al. Antisense oligonucleotides suppress B-cell lymphoma growth in a SCID-hu mouse model. *Oncogene* 1994;9:3049.
166. Webb A, Cunningham D, Cotter F, et al. Bcl-2 antisense therapy in patients with non-Hodgkin's lymphoma. *Lancet* 1997;349:1137.
167. Miayake H, Tolcher A, Gleave ME. Chemosensitization and delayed androgen-independent recurrence of prostate cancer with the use of Bcl-2 antisense oligodeoxynucleotides. *J Natl Cancer Inst* 2000;92:34.

168. McDonnell TJ, Troncosco P, Brisby SM, et al. Expression of the proto-oncogene Bcl-2 in the prostate and its association with the emergence of androgen resistance. *Cancer Res* 1992;52:6940.
169. Colombel M, Symmans F, Gil S, et al. Detection of the apoptosis-suppressing oncoprotein Bcl-2 in hormone-refractory prostate cancers. *Am J Pathol* 1993;143:390.
170. Berchem GJ, Bosseler M, Sugars LY, et al. Androgen resistance to bcl-2-mediated apoptosis in LNCaP prostate cancer cells. *Cancer Res* 1995;55:735.
171. Raffo AJ, Perlman H, Chen MW, Streitman JS, Buttyan R. Overexpression of Bcl-2 protects prostate cancer cells from apoptosis in vitro and confers resistance to androgen depletion in vivo. *Cancer Res* 1995;55:4438.
172. Bauer JJ, Sesterhenn IA, Mostofi FK, et al. Elevated levels of apoptosis regulator proteins p53 and bcl-2 are independent prognostic biomarkers in surgically treated clinically localized prostate cancer. *J Urol* 1996;156:1511.
173. Grover R, Wilson GD. Bcl-2 expression in malignant melanoma and its prognostic significance. *Eur J Surg Oncol* 1996;22:347.
174. Tron VA, Krajewski S, Klein-Parder H, et al. Immunohistochemical analysis of Bcl-2 protein regulation in cutaneous melanoma. *Am J Pathol* 1995;146:643.
175. Jansen B, Schlagbauer-Wadl H, Brown BD, et al. Bcl-2 antisense therapy chemosensitizes human melanoma in SCID mice. *Nat Med* 1998;4:232.
176. Linette GP, Li Y, Roth K, Korsmeyer SJ. Cross talk between cell death and cell cycle progression: BCL-2 regulates NFAT-mediated activation. *Proc Natl Acad Sci U S A* 1996;93:9545.

William G. Stetler-Stevenson
David E. Kleiner, Jr.

CHAPTER 8

Molecular Biology of Cancer: Invasion and Metastases

Metastasis is the spread of cancer cells from a primary tumor to vital organs and distant sites in the cancer patient's body. Metastatic disease is the hallmark of malignant cancer. The formation of tumor metastasis is the major cause of treatment failure in cancer patients and is a principal contributing factor to cancer morbidity and mortality. Metastatic disease has significant biologic and prognostic impact on cancer diagnosis and treatment.

The formation of metastatic foci is a continuous process that can begin early in the growth of the primary tumor and increases in frequency with tumor duration and tumor burden. Metastases may also disseminate to form new metastatic lesions in other organs (metastases will metastasize). The variation in size, age, dispersed anatomic location, and heterogeneous composition of metastases makes complete eradication of metastatic disease by currently available therapeutic strategies extremely difficult. The patient with metastatic disease succumbs to organ failure secondary to anatomic compromise caused by multiple metastases or to complications associated with systemic therapy directed against the metastatic disease. The design of more effective therapies to treat metastatic cancer requires better understanding of the molecular events and cellular processes that are involved in the process of metastasis formation.

THE METASTATIC CASCADE

It is well established, from both clinical observations and mechanistic studies, that metastasis formation is an inefficient process. Studies have demonstrated that late events in metastasis formation are largely responsible for the inefficiency of this process. Large numbers of tumor cells and tumor cell clumps are shed into the vascular drainage system of a primary tumor.[1,2] It has been demonstrated experimentally that, after intravenous injection of highly metastatic tumor cells, only approximately 0.01% of these cells form tumor foci. The number of circulating tumor cells and tumor emboli correlate with the size and age of the primary tumor (i.e., larger tumors shed more tumor cells and emboli). However, the number of circulating tumor cells does not correlate with the clinical outcome of metastases.

The inefficiency of tumor cells in completing the metastatic cascade is the result of the fact that successful formation of metastatic foci consists of several highly complex and interdependent steps. Each step is rate limiting in that failure to complete any of these events completely disrupts metastasis formation. The steps involved in metastasis formation are thought to be similar in all tumors and are characterized as follows (Fig. 8-1):

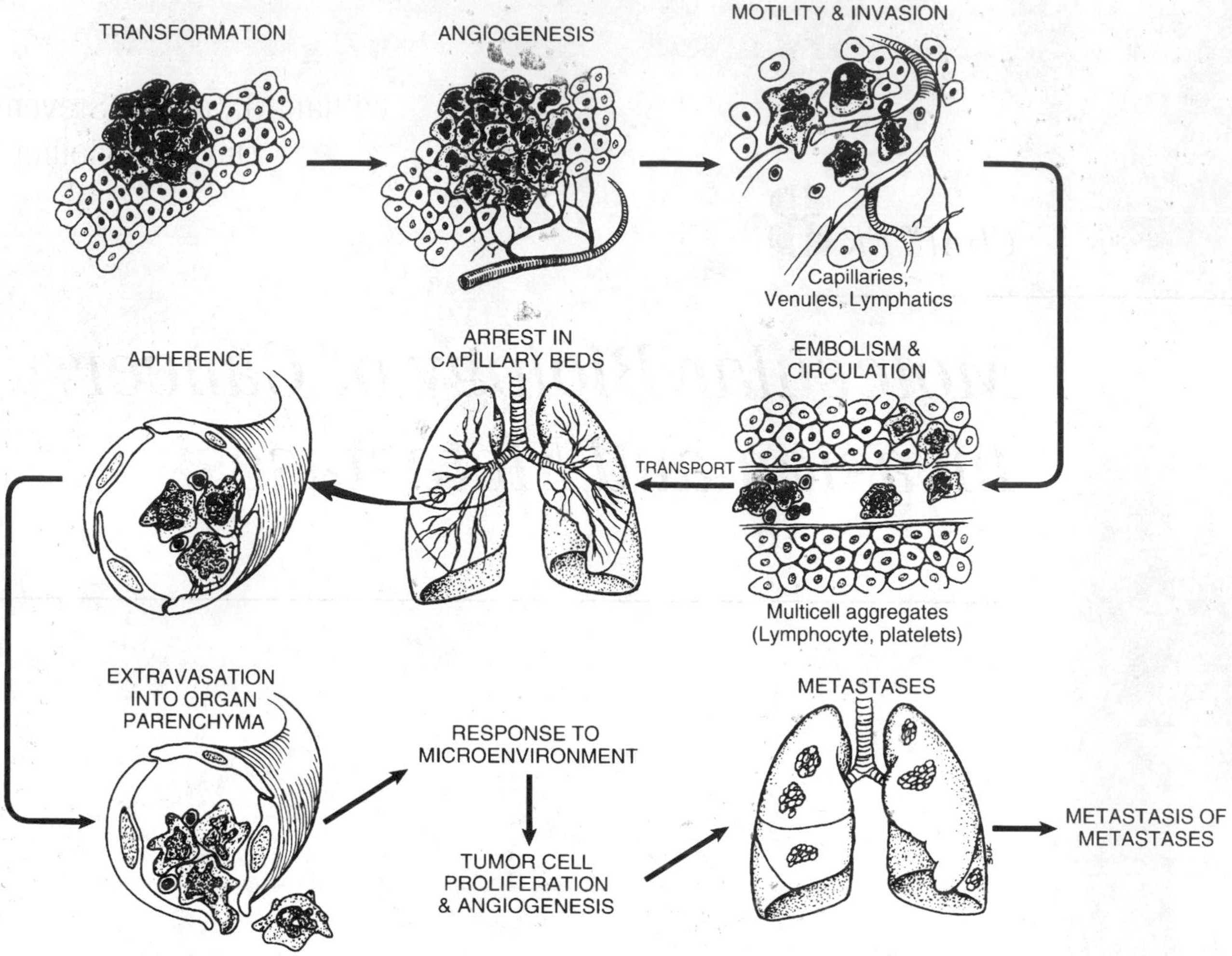

FIGURE 8-1. The pathogenesis of cancer metastasis. To produce metastases, tumor cells must detach from the primary tumor, invade the extracellular membrane and enter the circulation, survive in the circulation to arrest in the capillary bed, adhere to subendothelial basement membrane, gain entrance into the organ parenchyma, respond to paracrine growth factors, proliferate and induce angiogenesis, and evade host defenses. The pathogenesis of metastasis is therefore complex and consists of multiple sequential, selective, and interdependent steps whose outcome depends on the interaction of tumor cells with homeostatic factors.

1. Oncogenesis (tumorigenesis). After the initial neoplastic transformation, the tumor cells undergo progressive proliferation that is accompanied by further genetic changes and development of a heterogeneous tumor cell population with varying degrees of metastatic potential. The initial growth of the primary tumor is supported by the surrounding tissue microenvironment, which eventually becomes rate limiting for further growth.
2. Angiogenic switch. As the tumor grows and central tumor cells become hypoxic, the tumor initiates recruitment of its own blood supply. This process is called the *angiogenic switch* and involves the secretion of various angiogenic factors and the removal or suppression of angiogenesis inhibitors. Vascularization of the tumor is also associated with a dramatic increase in the metastatic potential of these tumors. Studies demonstrate that some tumors and metastases arising in vascularized tissues may first co-opt existing vasculature before initiating recruitment of new vessels.
3. Clonal dominance and invasive phenotype. Continued genetic alterations in the tumor cell population results in selection of tumor cell clones with distinct growth advantage and acquisition of an invasive phenotype. Invasive tumor cells down-regulate cell-cell adhesion, alter their attachment to the extracellular matrix (ECM) by changing integrin expression profiles, and proteolytically alter the matrix. Collectively, these changes result in enhanced cell motility and the ability of these invasive cells to separate from the primary tumor mass. These cells can detach from the primary tumor and create defects in the ECM that define tissue boundaries, such as basement membranes, thus accomplishing stromal invasion. Furthermore, the poorly formed tumor vasculature that forms in response to the angiogenic switch in phenotype of the primary tumor, as well as thin walled lymphatic channels in the surrounding stroma, are readily penetrated by these invasive tumor cells and offer ready conduits to the systemic circulation. Endothelial cells responding to the angiogenic stimulus produced by the primary tumor also express an invasive phenotype.

4. Survival in the circulation. Once the tumor cells and tumor cell clumps (emboli) have reached the vascular or lymphatic compartments, they must survive a variety of hemodynamic and immunologic challenges. Little is known about how these factors may impact on the inefficiency of the metastatic process in human cancers.
5. Tumor cell arrest. After survival in the circulation, tumor cells must arrest in distant organs or lymph nodes. This arrest may occur by size trapping on the inflow side of the microcirculation, or by adherence of tumor cells through specific interactions with capillary or lymphatic endothelial cells, or by binding to exposed basement membrane.
6. Extravasation and growth at the secondary site. In most cases, arrested tumor cells extravasate before proliferating. Studies suggest that extravasation of tumor cells is not dependent on protease activity and is independent of metastatic potential. After exiting the vascular or lymphatic compartments, metastatic tumor cells may proliferate in response to paracrine growth factors or become dormant. After extravasation, tumor cells migrate to a local environment more favorable for their continued growth. Findings using *in vivo* videomicroscopy demonstrate that the poor growth of tumor cells after extravasation from the circulation is a major factor contributing to the inefficiency of the metastatic process.
7. Angiogenesis in metastatic foci. Finally, continued growth of the metastatic foci is also dependent on angiogenesis. The development of this neovascular network at the metastatic site enhances the metastatic potential of these cells just as it does for the primary tumor.
8. Evasion of immune response. Metastatic foci of tumor cells must evade eradication by immune responses that may be either nonspecific or targeted directly against the tumor cells.

As might be expected from the highly complex nature of metastasis formation, no single gene product is responsible for metastasis formation. Successful completion of many of the steps of the metastatic cascade is the result of both the acquisition of positive effectors as well as the loss of negative regulators. Unrestrained growth is not sufficient to result in tumor invasion and metastasis. Tumor invasion is not a passive process secondary to tumor growth, and it may require additional genetic changes other than those associated with the tumorigenic phenotype. Tumorigenicity and metastatic competence have some overlapping features but are clearly under separate genetic control. Research on tumor cells has identified gene products that can facilitate completion of each of the steps outlined above. These are the molecular effectors of tumor invasion and metastasis. In many cases, research also has identified gene products that function to block successful completion of each of the steps in the metastatic cascade. The idea that there is loss of negative effectors, as well as positive phenotypic changes, associated with malignant progression and metastasis formation is now well established. In this chapter, some of the steps in the metastatic cascade are examined with the aim of identifying both the molecular mechanisms and the effector and suppressor genes that may become a target for new and effective cancer therapies. Immune modulation of cancer is discussed elsewhere (see Chapter 4), as is the process of tumor-associated angiogenesis (see Chapter 9). In addition, the angiogenic response at the metastatic foci is conceptually the same as in the primary tumor; therefore, the discussion of these points is limited here.

ONCOGENESIS: METASTASIS AND TUMORIGENESIS ARE UNDER SEPARATE GENETIC CONTROL

Many tumors progress through distinct stages that can be identified by histopathologic examination. Pathologists use the identification of these distinct phases to diagnose and classify tumors into different prognostic categories (e.g., normal tissue, hyperplasia, dysplasia, carcinoma *in situ*, and frankly invasive carcinoma). Genetic analysis of these different stages of tumor progression resulted in the multistep theory of tumorigenesis, which involves activation of oncogenes, inactivation of tumor suppressor genes, and identification of a host of tumor-associated molecules (cancer markers). The progressive alteration in cellular oncogenes and inactivation of tumor suppressor genes that results in uncontrolled growth and loss of contact-dependent cell growth has been well documented in many tumor types, and it is the subject of separate chapters in this text (see Chapters 1 and 2). It also has been demonstrated that transfection of certain of these oncogenes into the correct recipient cell can result in acquisition of invasive and metastatic phenotype. Thorgeirsson et al.[3] were first to demonstrate that transfection of activated Ras oncogene sequences into fetal mouse fibroblasts result in acquisition of a metastatic phenotype when these cells are implanted in the nude mouse. This finding has been confirmed in both fibroblast and epithelial cells of human and rodent origin when transfected with Ras. Similar findings, but with lower efficiency, have been observed with several other oncogenes (Mos, Raf, Src, Fes, and Fms) when transfected into an *appropriate* recipient cell.

At first, these results might suggest that the metastatic phenotype might arise from genetic alterations associated with the acquisition of tumorigenicity. However, cells can be transformed by oncogene transfection, but not all cells acquire a metastatic phenotype after oncogene transfection.[4] In addition, the adenovirus 2E1A gene was shown to suppress Ras induction of the metastatic phenotype without alteration in tumorigenicity or inhibition of soft agar colony formation.[5] These findings demonstrate that a clear separation exists between the genetic changes that drive tumorigenicity and the metastatic phenotype. These findings can be explained by the fact that invasion and metastasis require activation of additional effector genes or suppression of local inhibitors over and above those required for uncontrolled growth alone. The failure to induce metastatic competence by Ras in some cell systems is explained by a deficiency or suppression of these effector molecules in these cell types. These metastasis effector genes or gene products may be downstream of Ras or totally independent pathways that are involved in cell attachment or regulation of protease activity. In studies in which Ras effectively confers a metastatic phenotype, the metastasis effector genes are activated and suppressor genes are inactivated before Ras transfection, and the addition of Ras oncogene allows completion of the metastatic cascade. This finding is demonstrated by the observation that Ras plus E1A reverses the metastatic potential and metalloproteinase expression observed in rat embryo cell lines.[5,6] Candidate effector genes include those associated with cellular adhesion to ECM components, as well as proteases, motility factors, angiogenic factors, and growth regulation. Candidate suppressor genes would include genes associated with enhanced cell-cell attachment; phosphatase activities that regulate focal adhesion assembly; angiogenesis inhibitors; protease inhibitors; and factors that suppress cell migration, invasion, and growth.

ANGIOGENESIS: BALANCE OF POSITIVE AND NEGATIVE EFFECTORS

Classic studies by Folkman and colleagues in the 1970s demonstrated that continued growth of tumors requires persistent new blood vessel growth and that inhibition of this angiogenic response results in tumor dormancy.[7,8] These studies suggested that tumor cells release soluble factors that induce the angiogenic response (i.e., angiogenic factors). This process is now referred to as the *angiogenic switch*—that is, the switch from a nonangiogenic to an angiogenic phenotype.[9]

It has been experimentally demonstrated that shedding of malignant cells into the venous drainage is commensurate with the initiation of a tumor angiogenic response and is quantitatively related to the surface area of new tumor vessel.[10] This process may be facilitated by the immature nature of newly formed tumor vessels. Weidner and colleagues have reported the correlation of angiogenic response with the frequency of metastasis, disease recurrence, and reduced survival in a number of different human tumors.[11–13]

Some reports challenge the presumption that most tumors and metastases originate as small, avascular tumor cell clumps that must recruit new vessels for continued growth. Studies find that tumors arising or metastasizing into vascularized tissues may initially co-opt existing blood vessels.[14] Subsequently, there is regression of the co-opted vessels and increased production of angiogenic factors by the tumor cells that recruit a neoangiogenic response.

Researchers have begun to identify angiogenesis inhibitors that either must be modified or removed during the tumor-induced angiogenic response. Examples of these inhibitors include platelet factor-4, interferon-α, thrombospondin, and protease inhibitors [tissue inhibitors of metalloproteinases (TIMPs)]. The list of inhibitors of angiogenesis continues to grow with the identification of pigment epithelium–derived factor.[15] Inhibitors of angiogenesis can work at many levels by blocking endothelial cell growth, cell attachment, or migration.

A novel direction in angiogenesis inhibitors is the identification of cryptic inhibitors that are revealed by proteolytic modification of ECM components. This finding suggests a class of angiogenesis inhibitors that are contained within other proteins that are not antiangiogenic and must undergo proteolytic processing to uncover the antiangiogenic activity. Examples of these types of inhibitors include a 29-kD fragment of fibronectin[9]; the 16-kD fragment of prolactin; angiostatin released from plasminogen[16,17]; and endostatin, a C-terminal fragment of collagen XVIII.[18] The newest member of this group is the cleaved conformation of the serpin antithrombin.[19] Thus, local regulation of angiogenesis can be achieved by proteolytic release of cryptic angiogenesis inhibitors.

In a study by Bergers et al.,[20] the RIP1-Tag2 model of pancreatic islet β-cell tumors has been useful in examining the effects of angiogenesis inhibitors on multistage carcinogenesis in mice. The findings of this study demonstrate that antiangiogenic drugs can be targeted to selective stages of cancer progression and that combination of agents with different mechanisms of action should be used at different stages of tumor development.

Tumor angiogenesis is the result of a tightly regulated process and a delicate balance of both pro- and antiangiogenic factors. The process of endothelial cell invasion and formation of new blood vessels has many functional similarities to the process of tumor cell invasion.[21] Understanding the mechanisms of cell invasion may allow identification of new strategies to disrupt the invasive process. In addition to therapeutic use of antiangiogenic agents, it should be possible to target molecules that are involved in the process of cellular invasion that is required for both angiogenesis and tumor metastasis.

TUMOR HETEROGENEITY AND CLONAL DOMINANCE

It is now well recognized that most neoplasms consist of several tumor cell populations that vary widely in several important biologic characteristics. These characteristics include growth rates, karyotype, production of growth factors and stimulators of angiogenesis, hormone production, receptor content, and susceptibility to damage by cytotoxic agents, immune response, and hypoxia. Fidler et al.[22–24] first demonstrated the concept of heterogeneity of primary neoplasms in 1977. This concept is important because it suggested that not all tumor cells in the primary tumor population share the same propensity to form metastases and that formation of metastatic foci selects for an aggressive subpopulation of tumor cells out of the primary tumor. It was logical to assume that the size of the aggressive subpopulation in the primary tumor would reflect the propensity of that tumor to metastasize. This assumption would be of prognostic significance if a clinical assay of the primary tumor were able to detect and determine the presence of the highly aggressive subpopulation. However, evidence of a significant difference between the average metastatic propensity of cells comprising a primary tumor compared with those from an established metastasis was not forthcoming. This discrepancy was examined experimentally by Kerbel et al.[25–27] by using genetic markers to tag different subpopulations in the primary tumor. This work demonstrated that the metastatic subpopulation dominates the primary tumor mass early in its development. This dominance arises secondary to a selective growth advantage in the metastatic cells responding to local growth factors. Thus, the measurement of the average level of a molecular marker associated with metastatic propensity in the primary tumor reflects the likelihood of that tumor to form metastases. This finding has subsequently been confirmed in clinical studies by demonstration that the average level of a specific marker or oncogene measured within the primary tumor can be correlated with clinical evidence of metastasis or recurrence.

DEFINING THE INVASIVE PHENOTYPE

During the transition from benign to invasive carcinoma, extensive changes occur in the quantity, organization, and distribution of subepithelial basement membrane. The hallmark of invasive carcinoma is disruption of the epithelial basement membrane and the presence of cancer cells in the stromal compartment.[21,28] Benign proliferative disorders, such as fibrocystic disease, sclerosing adenosis, intraductal hyperplasia, intraductal papilloma, and fibroadenoma, are all characterized by disorganization of the normal epithelial architecture. But no matter how extensive this disorganization may become, these benign lesions are always characterized by a continuous basement membrane that separates the neoplastic epithelium from the stroma.[21,28]

In contrast, invasive carcinoma is characterized by a loss of basement membrane around the invasive tumor cells in the stroma. Once the basement membrane barrier is compromised, it is impossible to determine the quantity or location of tumor cells that may have escaped from the primary tumor. Thus, local invasion is paramount to malignant conversion.

The ability to cross basement membrane barriers is not unique to malignant carcinoma cells. During an inflammatory response, nonneoplastic immune cells regularly cross the subendothelial basement membranes, as do endothelial cells during the angiogenic response. Trophoblasts invade the endometrial stroma and blood vessels to establish contact with the maternal circulation during development of the hemochorial placenta. However, these normal cell types respond to additional signals that result in differentiation and subsequent loss of their invasive phenotype. Indeed, both normal and tumor cell invasion share functional similarities. In tumor cell invasion, however, it is the lack of response to negative signals or regulators and the continued invasion with ongoing tumor cell growth that is unique to cancer metastasis.[21,28]

Tumor cell interaction with the basement membrane is defined as the critical event of tumor invasion that signals the initiation of the metastatic cascade.[21,28] Basement membranes are composed of a dense meshwork of type IV collagen, laminin, and heparin sulfate proteoglycans that is interspersed with entactin and other minor components. Basement membranes do not contain pores that would allow passive tumor cell migration. Early studies on defining the invasive phenotype on malignant tumor cells focused on the interaction of tumor cells with the epithelial basement membrane. These studies defined the three-step hypothesis of tumor cell invasion: tumor cell attachment to the basement membrane, creation of proteolytic defects in the basement membrane, and migration of tumor cells through these defects.[21,28] It is now recognized that these three steps describe tumor cell interaction with all types of ECM and not just basement membrane. Furthermore, nonneoplastic invasive cells, such as trophoblasts, endothelial cells, and inflammatory cells, all use mechanisms for invasion that are functionally similar to tumor cells. The difference between these normal invasive processes and the pathologic nature of tumor cell invasion is therefore one of regulation. An understanding of the factors that control cellular processes essential to the invasive phenotype should allow identification of novel targets for therapeutic intervention to prevent and treat both angiogenesis and metastasis formation.

CELL-CELL ADHESION SUPPRESSES OR FACILITATES METASTASIS FORMATION

The initial events in cellular invasion are changes in cell adhesion. These changes consist of alteration in both cell-cell adhesion and interactions with the ECM. A variety of cell surface receptors that mediate these interactions have been characterized, including the cadherins, integrins, immunoglobulin superfamily, and CD44. Tumor cells must decrease cell and matrix adhesive interactions to escape from the primary tumor. At later stages in the metastatic cascade, however, tumor cells may need to increase adhesive interactions with cells and ECM, such as during arrest and extravasation at a distant site. The apparent contribution of each class of cell adhesion molecules to invasive behavior will in some way be dependent on the tumor cell population and model system used to study these interactions. We review the contribution of changes in cell-cell adhesion to tumor progression before considering alterations in association with the ECM.

The majority of human cancers arise in epithelial cells. Several types of junctional structures, such as desmosomes, tight junctions, and adherens-type junctions tightly interconnect normal epithelial cells. The formation and maintenance of these contacts require Ca^{2+}-dependent homophilic interactions mediated by the cell-adhesion molecules known as *cadherins* (Fig. 8-2). Cadherins are a superfamily of single-pass transmembrane glycoproteins that mediate Ca^{2+}-dependent cell-cell adhesion. The cadherin superfamily now consists of five subfamilies: the classic type I and type II cadherins, desmosomal cadherins, protocadherins, and cadherin-related proteins.[29,30] The classic cadherin, epithelial cadherin (or E-cadherin), mediates homotypic cell adhesion in epithelial cells. E-cadherin is a transmembrane glycoprotein that has five extracellular homologous domains (ectodomains), a single membrane-spanning region, and a cytosolic domain. E-cadherin is physically anchored to the actin cytoskeleton by cytoplasmic proteins termed *catenins.* β-Catenin is also a major component of the WNT signaling pathway.

Any disruption of the intracellular E-cadherin–catenin complex results in loss of cell adhesion. This would include changes in E-cadherin expression or function, as well as genes other than E-cadherin that are required for complex formation and function. Abundant evidence indicates that E-cadherin function is frequently lost during progression of many human cancers, including those arising in the breast, prostate, esophagus, stomach, colon, skin, kidney, lung, and liver.[31,32] This loss of E-cadherin function arises via several different mechanisms. In familial gastric carcinomas, germline mutations in the E-cadherin gene predispose individuals to develop malignant cancer. Mutations in β-catenin are found in many primary tumors, including prostatic cancer, melanoma, and gastric and colon cancer. Another mechanism disrupting E-cadherin function during tumor progression is hypermethylation of the E-cadherin promoter, resulting in decreased gene expression. This has been found to be a major mechanism in papillary thyroid cancer in that 83% of cases of this disease demonstrated hypermethylation of the E-cadherin promoter.[33] Yet another mechanism to alter E-cadherin function is proteolytic modification. Lochter et al.[34] have reported that E-cadherin function can be disrupted by degradation of E-cadherin's extracellular domains by stromelysin-1, a member of the matrix metalloproteinase (MMP) family that has been closely linked with tumor progression. Constitutive expression of active stromelysin in mammary epithelial cells results in cleavage of E-cadherin and progressive phenotypic changes *in vitro,* including loss of catenins from cell-cell contacts, down-regulation of cytokeratins, and up-regulation of vimentin and MMP-9. These changes result in a stable epithelial to mesenchymal transition of

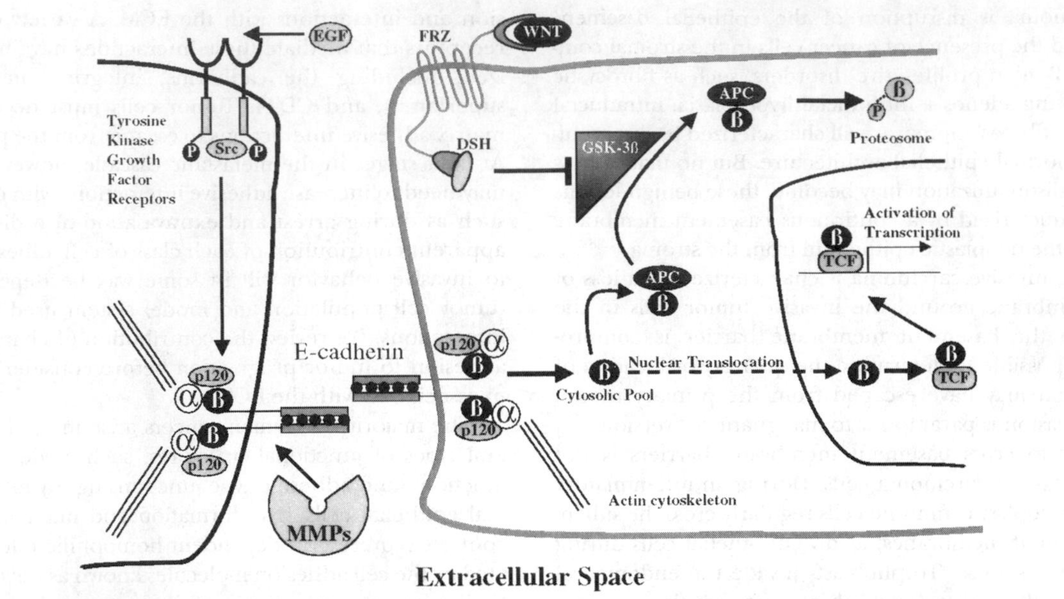

FIGURE 8-2. Disruption of cell-cell adhesion concomitant with tumor progression. E-cadherin is a homotypic cell adhesion molecule containing five homologous, extracellular domains (ectodomains) that bind divalent calcium ions. Calcium binding promotes homophilic cell-cell E-cadherin complexes found in such structures as desmosomes, tight junctions, and adherens-type junctions. The cytoplasmic tail of E-cadherin involved in cell-cell adhesion interacts with β-catenin, α-catenin, and p120^{CAS} (p120). Loss of E-cadherin function, by germline mutation, promoter hypermethylation, or destruction of the ectodomains by matrix metalloproteinase (MMP) activity, results in an increase in free cytosolic β-catenin levels. Increased cytoplasmic β-catenin can be directed to the proteosome complex by glycogen-synthetase kinase 3β (GSK3β) phosphorylation and subsequent interaction with the adenomatous polyposis coli (APC) gene product. The frizzled (FRZ)-disheveled (DSH) pathway for WNT signaling can down-regulate the activity of GSK3β. Activation of the WNT signaling pathway or loss of APC function facilitate the increase in cytosolic β-catenin levels, which are associated with loss of E-cadherin function, or mutations of the β-catenin gene, which result in reduced association with E-cadherin cytoplasmic domain. Translocation of β-catenin to the nucleus results in gene expression associated with cell transformation and tumor growth (i.e., c-Myc, cyclin D1). It is noteworthy that this cascade of cellular transformation can be initiated by expression of an extracellular protease that culminates in enhanced chromosomal instability.[35] EGF, epidermal growth factor; P, phosphorylated amino acid residue(s); TCF, tissue coding factor.

cellular phenotype. *In vivo* stromelysin expression promotes mammary carcinogenesis that includes stereotyped genomic changes distinct from those seen in other mouse breast cancer models.[35] It has been reported that loss of H-cadherin expression occurs during the progression of breast cancer,[36] but little is known about the function of other cadherin family members during tumor progression. In summary, a decrease in cell-cell adhesion is associated with malignant conversion. Forced expression of E-cadherin in tumor cell lines results in reversion from an invasive to a benign tumor cell phenotype.[31,32]

In normal cells, β-catenin is sequestered in the intracellular adhesion complex with the cytoplasmic domain of E-cadherin, α-catenin, γ-catenin, and p120^{CAS} (Crk-associated substrate). Loss of cell-cell adhesion results in disruption of the adhesion complex and free β-catenin. Free β-catenin is bound by the adenomatous polyposis coli (APC) gene product and is rapidly phosphorylated by glycogen-synthetase kinase 3β (GSK3β). Phosphorylated β-catenin is subsequently degraded in the ubiquitin proteosome pathway. In many colon cancer cells, the tumor suppressor gene APC is nonfunctional. This lack of function can lead to accumulation of high levels of cytoplasmic β-catenin that can subsequently be translocated to the nucleus. The WNT-1 protooncogene–initiated signaling pathway, which includes the frizzled (FRZ) and disheveled (DSH) gene products, can block activity of GSK3β, which can also result in accumulation of β-catenin. In the nucleus, free nonphosphorylated β-catenin can bind to members of the TCF (tissue-coding factor)/LEF-1 (lymphoid enhancer-binding factor 1) family of transcription factors. It has been demonstrated that, after inactivation of APC function, the increase in available β-catenin enters the nucleus, complexes with transcription factor Tcf-4, and up-regulates c-Myc expression.[37] It also has been shown that β-catenin activates transcription from the cyclin D1 promoter and contributes to neoplastic transformation by causing accumulation of cyclin D1.[38] These findings link changes in cell-cell adhesion with intracellular signaling, oncogene expression, and tumor cell growth. Thus, loss of cadherin-mediated cell-cell adhesion is an important event that has many far-reaching consequences for acquisition of the invasive phenotype and tumor progression.

Other types of cell-cell adhesive interactions can actually facilitate metastasis formation. These may be particularly important during tumor cell arrest and extravasation. These molecules include members of the immunoglobulin superfamily, such as nerve cell adhesion molecule and vascular cell adhesion molecule-1.[39–43] The immunoglobulin superfamily has a wide variety of members involved in cellular immunity and signal transduction, as well as cell adhesion. Members of the superfamily share the immunoglobulin homology unit that consists of 70 to 110 amino acid residues organized into seven to nine β-sheet structures. The diversity of superfamily members precludes generalization about their role in tumor cell invasion and metastasis. However, the role of one family member seems straightforward. Vascular cell adhesion molecule-1 is an endothelial cell, cytokine-inducible, counterreceptor for VLA-4 (very late antigen-4) integrin, also known as a_4b_1 *integrin receptor.* The role of integrin receptors is discussed separately (see Role of Integrins in Tumor Invasion, later in this chapter). Normally, VLA-4 is expressed on leukocytes and functions in mediating leukocyte attachment to endothelial cells. VLA-4 is also found on tumor cells in malignant melanoma[44] and metastatic sarcoma but not in adenocarcinomas.[45] It is thought that expression of VLA-4 may facilitate interaction of circulating tumor cells with endothelium before tumor cell extravasation. This was demonstrated by intravenous injection of human melanoma cells into nude mice pretreated with VLA-4–inducing cytokines, which resulted in an enhanced number of lung metastases formed compared with no cytokine pretreatment of the mice.[46] Cell-cell adhesive interactions can either suppress or facilitate metastasis formation. Either role is dependent on the specific context and molecular mechanisms of cell-cell interaction.

CELL–EXTRACELLULAR MATRIX INTERACTIONS IN TUMOR PROGRESSION

As already discussed, the interaction of the tumor cell with the ECM, in particular the basement membrane, defines the invasive phenotype, and tumor invasion is paramount to metastasis. It is now recognized that the ECM exerts a profound influence on cell behavior and that cells direct the assembly and disassembly of the matrix. This concept is known as *dynamic reciprocity* and also applies to the interaction of malignant tumor cells with the ECM. During the process of metastasis formation, malignant tumor cells must interact with a variety of different types of ECM. These types include the subepithelial basement membrane of the tissue of origin, stromal elements of the tissue of origin, subendothelial basement membranes during extravasation, and the stromal and basement membranes of the organ(s) at the site of metastasis growth. Attachment of nonneoplastic cells to the ECM is prerequisite for cell survival. A fundamental difference for neoplastic cells is the loss of anchorage requirement for cell survival and growth. The anchorage-independent growth of tumor cells may result from an uncoupling of cell survival signals transduced from the ECM by attachment, coupled with activation of cell-cycle progression that is associated with neoplastic transformation. Tumor cell interactions with the ECM have profound implications for both cell-cycle regulation and migration.

ROLE OF CD44 IN TUMOR INVASION

CD44 is a transmembrane glycoprotein with a large ectodomain and single cytoplasmic domain. CD44 is involved in cell adhesion to hyaluronan (HA). The gene encoding CD44 is on the short arm of human chromosome 11[47] and contains both constant and variable exons.[48] As a result of this gene structure, a number of differentially spliced isoforms of CD44 can be generated. The isoform containing no variant exon sequences is referred to as *standard CD44.* A total of nine variant regions (v2 to v10) can encode protein sequences. Alternatively spliced messenger RNA variants of CD44 (CD44v) can contain one or more variant coding regions. More than 30 different splice variants have been detected by polymerase chain reaction analysis.[49] In addition to these variants, cell type–specific differences in glycosylation of the core protein also exist. The pattern of glycosylation and presence of variant exons influence the ability of CD44 to function in HA binding.[50]

Several lines of evidence suggest that CD44 expression plays a role in metastasis formation. Clinical correlation studies demonstrate that a variety of different types of cancer that express high cell surface levels of CD44 have a poorer clinical outcome when compared with tumors that have low CD44 surface expression.[51–53] Forced expression of CD44v4 to v7 confers metastatic ability to a nonmetastasizing rat pancreatic carcinoma cell line.[54] Metastasis formation could be blocked using antivariant antibodies.[55] However, the exact role of CD44v in metastasis formation remains elusive.

In some tumors, CD44-associated increases in tumor growth and metastatic potential correlate with CD44-mediated cell attachment to HA.[56–58] CD44 also functions in HA uptake and degradation that is also correlated with tumor cell behavior.[56,59,60] It also has been demonstrated that CD44 aggregation on the cell surface creates a binding site for the active MMP-9.[61] It is postulated that bound MMP-9 may liberate ECM-bound HA and facilitates tumor cell HA uptake and degradation. These findings link cell adhesion and ECM turnover. In addition, they suggest that CD44 may function at different stages of tumor cell invasion and metastasis and that the specific CD44 role may depend on the specific stage of metastasis formation that is examined.

ROLE OF INTEGRINS IN TUMOR INVASION

Integrins are heterodimeric transmembrane proteins that are formed by the noncovalent association of α and β subunits.[61–64] Considerable redundancy within cell-ECM interaction mediated by integrins exist, because most integrins bind to several individual matrix proteins, and ECM components, such as laminin, fibronectin, vitronectin, and collagens, bind to several different integrin receptors. This fact suggests that integrins are capable of providing the cell with detailed information about the surrounding ECM environment, which is then integrated at the cellular level to generate a cellular response (Fig. 8-3). It is now well established that integrins can signal across the cell membrane in both directions.[65–67] Binding of ECM ligands to integrins is known to initiate signal transduction pathways that can result in cell proliferation, differentiation, migration, or cell death (apoptosis, anoikis). This is referred to as *outside-in signaling.* It is also known that intracellular events can modulate the binding activity of integrins for their ligands in the ECM, which is referred to as *inside-out signaling.* Both integrin clustering and ligand occupancy are crucial for the initiation of intracellular integrin-mediated signal pathways.[68]

Integrin-mediated signal transduction involves both direct activation of signaling pathways and collaborative signaling (also referred to as *cooperative signaling*), in which integrins modulate signaling events initiated through receptor tyrosine kinases.[67,69] The *cis* association of integrins with other receptors on the same cell surface results in formation of multireceptor complexes. There is little evidence that these multireceptor complexes signal through exclusive, integrin-specific pathways, but instead they cooperate with the other receptors to influence a variety of signaling pathways. Direct integrin signaling starts after engagement of the integrin with their ECM ligands, lateral clustering of the integrin receptors, and interaction of the integrin cytoplas-

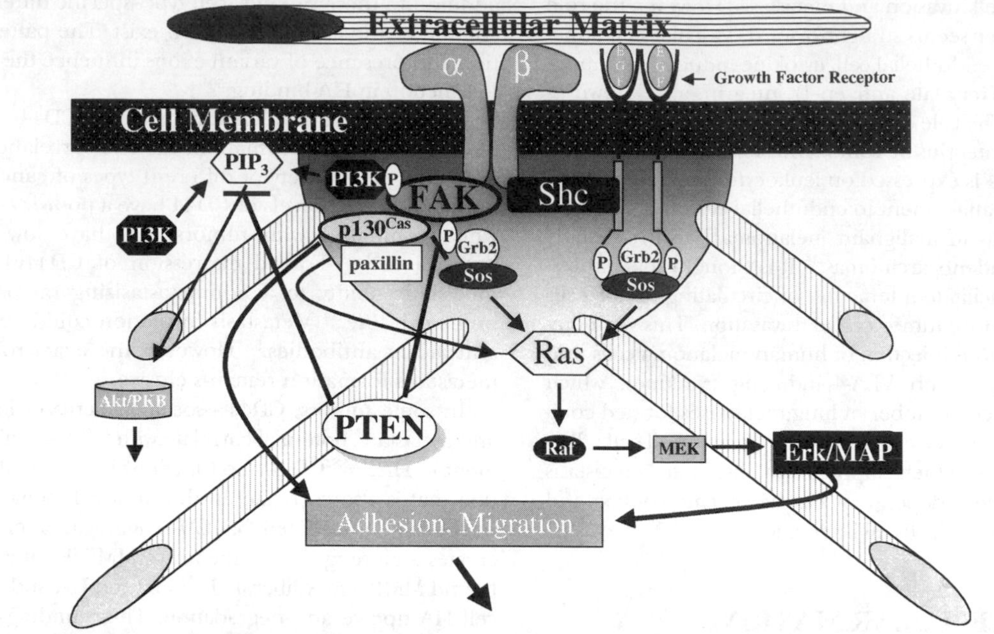

FIGURE 8-3. Role of integrins in tumor cell invasion and metastasis: integration of kinase and phosphatase activities. Binding of extracellular matrix components to integrin receptors initiates an intracellular signaling cascade that results in formation of a focal adhesion complex consisting of cytoskeletal and signal transduction molecules. Ligand binding to the integrin receptor results in integrin clustering and association of signal transduction molecules. Integrin receptor clustering induces autophosphorylation of focal adhesion kinase (FAK) on tyrosine 397. Subsequently, a Src homology 2 (SH2)-containing (Shc) adapter protein of the Src kinase family that binds to specific phosphotyrosine residues (Y397) on FAK is recruited to the integrin-FAK complex. Recruitment of additional proteins, such as α-actinin, talin, and paxillin, to this complex connects the focal adhesion complex to the filamentous actin cytoskeleton. Interaction of Shc with FAK results in additional sites of phosphorylation on the FAK molecule and subsequent recruitment of additional SH2 adapter proteins, such as Grb2 and the nucleotide exchange factor Sos. These interactions lead to activation of the mitogen activated protein (MAP) pathway, which stimulates tumor cell growth, adhesion, and migration. Similarly, receptors for growth factors can transiently associate with the focal adhesion complex to synergistically activate the MAP kinase pathway.

FAK activation also acts upstream of the Akt/protein kinase B (PKB) signaling pathway, which promotes cell survival. Association of the p85 subunit of phosphatidylinositol-3 kinase (PI3K) with tyrosine 397 in FAK mediates this effect. The rapid elevation of the phosphatidylinositol(3,4,5)triphosphate (PIP_3) lipid product of PI3K activity stimulates the Akt/PKB pathway, leading to enhanced cell survival.

Crk-associated substrate ($p130^{CAS}$) is another SH2- and SH3-conatining signal transduction that associates with FAK on integrin binding to the extracellular matrix. Interaction of $p130^{CAS}$ with FAK is mediated by a prolinc-rich region on FAK (residues 712–178) that interacts with the SH3 domain of $p130^{CAS}$. Activation of $p130^{CAS}$ promotes cell migration and invasion that is associated with enhanced metastatic behavior. The tumor suppressor gene PTEN inhibits cell adhesion, migration, and invasion. This inhibition is mediated by direct PTEN dephosphorylation of FAK and Shc, leading to negative regulation of the $p130^{CAS}$ pathway, which affects cell attachment, migration, and invasion. Down-regulation of the MAP kinase pathway by PTEN dephosphorylation of FAK and Shc negatively affects cell growth in addition to attachment and migration. PTEN is also known to directly dephosphorylate PIP_3 and negatively regulate the downstream Akt/PKB cell survival pathway. PTEN may also disrupt this pathway indirectly by dephosphorylation of FAK, which alters P13K activation. Thus, integrin-mediated regulation of cell growth, adhesion, migration, and invasion is a complex network of signal transduction cascades that have both positive (kinase) and negative (phosphatase) regulatory elements. EGF, epidermal growth factor; Erk, extracellular signal–regulated kinase; MEK, MAP kinase or ERK kinase; P, phosphorylated amino acid residual(s).

mic domain to form complexes with proteins that link to the cytoskeleton. This results in organization of cell structures known as *focal adhesions*.

Autophosphorylation of the focal adhesion kinase (FAK) was among the first integrin-mediated signaling events to be identified. This autophosphorylation event on tyrosine 397 results in recruitment of Src-family protein kinases that in turn results in phosphorylation of additional tyrosine residues on FAK. Phosphorylation of FAK can result in activation of the extracellular signal–regulated kinase (ERK)/mitogen-activated protein (MAP) kinase pathway. Activation of the MAP kinase pathway has been linked to induction of cell migration.[70] The activation of MAP kinase can be mediated by Grb-2 recruitment to FAK that then binds Sos, a guanine nucleotide exchange factor for Ras.[67,71] Alternatively, activation of the MAP kinase pathway can result from FAK phosphorylation of paxillin and the Crk-associated substrate ($p130^{Cas}$) that leads to binding of link proteins, such as Nck.[72] In addition, phosphorylation of FAK at tyrosine 397 creates a binding site for the regulatory subunit of phosphoinositol-3 kinase and triggers activation of this signal pathway.[73]

The knowledge that FAK is tyrosine phosphorylated on integrin activation suggests that focal adhesion–associated protein tyrosine phosphatases (PTP) could modulate Fak function. Several PTPs that interact with components of the focal adhesion

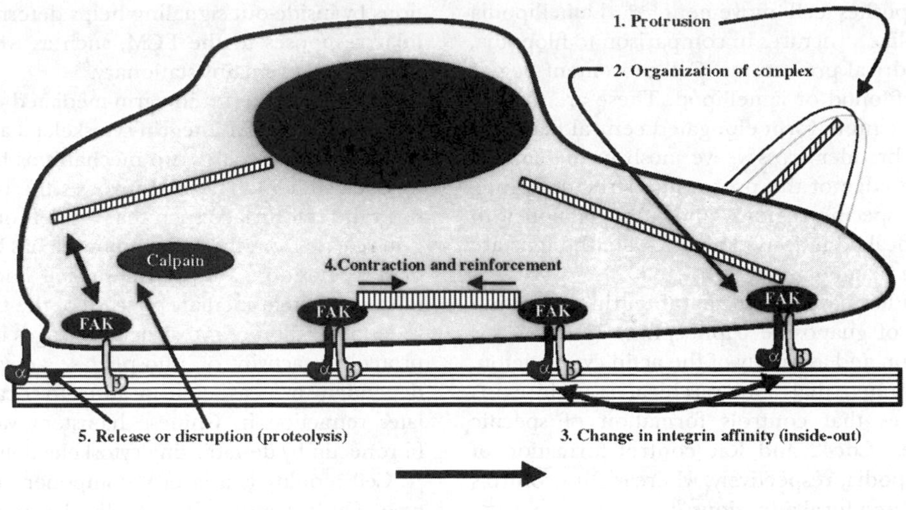

FIGURE 8-4. Cellular migration. Cell migration requires transmission of force from the extracellular matrix to the cytoskeleton. This is accomplished in distinct steps, several of which are illustrated. First, there is protrusion of a cellular projection (filopodia or lamellipodia), which is mediated by actin polymerization. The second step involves organization of the focal adhesion complex and connection with the actin cytoskeleton. This is accomplished via mechanisms described in Figure 8-3. Evidence suggests that if the integrin component of these complexes is not activated, these complexes are continually recycled across the cell surface without cell movement. Step 3 entails engagement of the integrin with the extracellular matrix, which is mediated by a change in integrin affinity. Traction force is generated and transmitted by the contraction and reinforcement of the actin cytoskeleton. The final step in cell locomotion is the release or disruption of the focal adhesion complex at the trailing edge of the migrating cell. Step 5 is accomplished by release of components of the integrin complex or via proteolytic disruption of focal adhesion kinase connections with the filamentous actin cytoskeleton.

complex have been identified. These are PTP-α and PTP-PEST [protein tyrosine phosphatase rich in proline (P), glutamic acid (E), serine (S), and threonine (T)], which negatively regulate Src and paxillin, respectively.[74,75] It has been shown that, in PTP-PEST–deficient cells, a defect in cell motility correlates with an increase in the size and number of focal adhesions.[76] This defect appears to be due in part to the constitutive increase in tyrosine phosphorylation of paxillin, as well as $p130^{CAS}$ and FAK.

A PTP that interacts directly with FAK is referred to as *PTEN*.[77] PTEN was identified as a tumor suppressor gene on human chromosome 10q23, which is frequently mutated or deleted in a wide variety of human cancers, including gliomas and prostate, breast, lung, bladder, endometrial, kidney, and oropharyngeal cancers.[71] The gene encodes both a phosphatase domain and also has extensive sequence homology to the cytoskeletal protein tensin. PTEN functions as a dual-specificity phosphatase in that not only is it a PTP but it also dephosphorylates the lipid phosphoinositol(3,4,5,)triphophaste (PIP_3). The current view is that both phosphatase activities function as tumor suppressor activities. The lipid phosphatase activity regulates levels of PIP_3, which in turn regulates activation of the protein kinase B pathway that is protective against programmed cell death (apoptosis, anoikis). As a PTP, PTEN regulates the phosphorylation status of FAK and Shc that in turn regulate cell adhesion, migration, cytoskeletal organization, and MAP kinase activation. To summarize, loss of PTEN function results in alterations in integrin-mediated signaling via FAK and PIP_3 pathways, which results in achievement of an invasive phenotype.[71] The protein kinase activity just described functions to promote cell invasion. This process is countered by the PTP activities, which act as tumor suppressors.

The roles of specific integrins in tumor progression and metastasis formation are dichotomous. The decreased expression of some integrins is associated with cellular transformation and tumorigenesis. These include $\alpha_5\beta_1$ and $\alpha_2\beta_1$ integrins. HT29 colon carcinoma cells lacking $\alpha_5\beta_1$ expression are either significantly less tumorigenic or completely nontumorigenic when forced to express α_5.[78] Loss of $\alpha_2\beta_1$ expression in breast epithelial cells correlates with the transformed phenotype, and reexpression of this integrin abrogates the malignant phenotype.[79] On the other hand, expression of some integrins directly correlates with tumorigenicity and tumor progression. For example, the $\alpha_v\beta_3$ integrin is expressed in metastatic melanoma but not in benign melanocytic lesions.[80,81] Antibodies against α_v integrins blocked growth of human melanoma xenografts in nude mice.[82] Integrin α_6 expression is increased in oropharyngeal and bladder cancers and in lung tumors.[46,83–87] Tumor progression is associated with expression of $\alpha_3\beta_1$ in 82% of tumors. The molecular events associated with enhanced integrin expression and tumor progression are not well defined. Clearly, in nontransformed cells, integrins are implicated in growth regulation. But tumor cell growth is anchorage-independent. This observation suggests that the role of integrins in tumor invasion and metastasis may only be secondarily related to growth control. Integrins are also directly involved in cell migration.

CELLULAR MIGRATION: NEW INSIGHTS

Cell migration requires transmission of propulsive force from the ECM to the cytoskeleton of the migrating tumor or endothelial cell (Fig. 8-4). Repetitive assembly of cytoskeletal elements to form membrane ruffles, lamellipodia, filopodia, and pseudopodia accomplishes cell movement.[88,89] Lamellipodia are broad, flat, sheet-like structures in comparison to filopodia, which are thin, cylindrical projections. Cell movement begins with protrusion of a filopod or lamellipod. These are formed by polymerization of actin to form elongated central filaments in the filopod and a broader cross-weave mesh in the lamellipod.[90] At the leading edge of the protruding structures, integrins concentrate in specific regions, and after ligation with ECM, ligands form focal adhesions. These focal adhesions are anchored to the actin filaments.

Microinjection studies have shown that integrin association with the Rho family of guanosine triphosphate (GTP)ases is critical for organization and assembly of the actin cytoskeleton. It has been demonstrated that a hierarchical cascade exists among these GTPases that controls formation of specific cytoskeletal structures. Cdc42 and Rac control formation of filopodia and lamellipodia, respectively, whereas Rho controls stress fiber formation and focal adhesions.[91]

The integrin connection to the ECM provides adhesive traction, and contraction of the actin filaments results in forward propulsion of the cell body. As the cell moves, new projections occur at the leading edge and are anchored with new focal adhesions. As the cell moves forward, the focal adhesions appear to move in a retrograde fashion on the cell surface. This apparent movement of the focal adhesions has been observed using fluorescent-tagged beads coated with integrin substrates or antiintegrin antibodies.[92–94] These coated beads can also be used to actually measure the integrin-cytoskeletal traction forces generated, which has led to the demonstration that the strength of the integrin-cytoskeletal interaction can be modulated by the rigidity of the extracellular substrate. When cells are on a rigid substrate, more restraining force is exerted to prevent movement of the focal adhesion. Cells can detect this change in the substrate, and they respond by increasing the force generated by cytoskeletal linkage to the focal adhesion so that the cell pulls harder. This is referred to as *reinforcement of the integrin-cytoskeletal attachments.* Data suggest that Src kinases may be selectively involved in regulating this reinforcement.[94] Researchers have shown that beads binding to the fibronectin receptor in fibroblast containing either wild-type or Src-deficient cells show similar reinforcement of the fibronectin-receptor–actin cytoskeletal linkage. In contrast, when they use vitronectin, there is little reinforcement of the vitronectin receptor in wild-type Src-expressing cells, but a strong reinforcement in the Src-deficient fibroblasts. These authors also show selective association of kinase-defective Src–green fluorescent protein fusion with the α_v integrin subunit of the vitronectin receptor, but not with the fibronectin receptor. Possible interpretations of these results are that either Src is normally a selective inhibitor of reinforcement of force generation through the vitronectin receptor or that Src promotes the turnover of links between cytoskeletal and integrin components of the focal adhesion complex.

Investigators have used a β_1 integrin–green fluorescent protein chimcra to follow focal adhesion cycling over the cell surface.[95] These experiments demonstrate that, in stationary cells, focal adhesions were highly motile and moved in a linear fashion to the cell center. In motile cells, the focal adhesions remained stationary and only moved at the trailing edge of the cell. These authors postulate a cellular "clutch-like mechanism" in which alteration in integrin affinity is seen in response to migratory stimulus. Regulation of integrin-ligand interactions by inside-out signaling helps determine the nature of cellular responses to the ECM, such as whether a cell becomes migratory or remains stationary.[96]

The last step in integrin-mediated cell migration is the release of the ECM integrin-cytoskeletal attachments at the trailing edge of the cell.[88] Two mechanisms have been identified in this detachment. The first involves the release of the integrins from the cell surface such that it is left on the substratum. Integrin release from the cell membrane has been observed in fibroblast migration[97] and by tumor cell lines *in vitro.*[98] A second mechanism that mediates release of the trailing edge of the cell is destabilization of cytoskeletal linkages intracellularly by either proteolytic activity or phosphatase activity. Calpain is a Ca^{2+}-dependent protease that localizes to focal adhesions and regulates retraction in Chinese hamster ovary cells migrating on fibronectin by destabilizing cytoskeletal linkages.[99]

Cell motility is a critical component of the invasive phenotype. Understanding the molecular mechanisms that confer tumor cell motility should allow identification of novel targets for disrupting this process and preventing tumor dissemination. Tumor cell motility can be correlated with metastatic behavior. When parameters such as pseudopod extension, membrane ruffling, or vectorial translation are measured, a quantitative increase in highly invasive and metastatic tumor cells is seen when compared with nonmetastatic counterparts. A variety of stimuli have been shown to stimulate tumor cell motility *in vitro,* including host-derived factors, growth factors, and tumor-secreted factors that function in an autocrine fashion to stimulate tumor cell motility. Autocrine motility factor is a 60-kD glycoprotein produced by human melanoma cells that stimulates tumor cell migration. Autocrine motility factor has been identified as neuroleukin/phosphohexose isomerase.[100,101] Autotaxin (ATX) is a 125-kD glycoprotein that elicits chemotactic and chemokinetic responses at picomolar to nanomolar concentrations in human melanoma cells. ATX contains a peptide sequence identified as the catalytic site in type I alkaline phosphodiesterases (PDEs), and it possesses 5-nucleotide PDE [EC 3.1.4.1 (Enzyme Commission designation for this enzymatic activity)] activity.[102–104] ATX binds adenosine triphosphate (ATP) and is phosphorylated only on threonine. Thr210 at the PDE active site of ATX is required for phosphorylation, 5-nucleotide PDE, and motility-stimulating activities. ATX also has adenosine-5-triphosphatase (ATPase) and ATP pyrophosphatase activities. ATX catalyzes the hydrolysis of GTP to guanosine diphosphate and guanosine monophosphate, of either adenosine monophosphate or inorganic pyrophosphate to inorganic phosphate, and the hydrolysis of nicotinamide adenine dinucleotide to adenosine monophosphate, and each of these substrates can serve as a phosphate donor in the phosphorylation of ATX. ATX possesses no detectable protein kinase activity toward histone, myelin basic protein, or casein. These results have led to the proposal that ATX is capable of at least two alternative reaction mechanisms—threonine (T-type) ATPase and 5-nucleotide PDE/ATP pyrophosphatase—with a common site (Thr210) for the formation of covalently bound reaction intermediates, threonine phosphate and threonine adenylate, respectively.[103]

PROTEASES IN TUMOR CELL INVASION

As has been noted, matrix proteolysis has been recognized as a key part of the mechanism of tumor cell invasion. Tumor cells

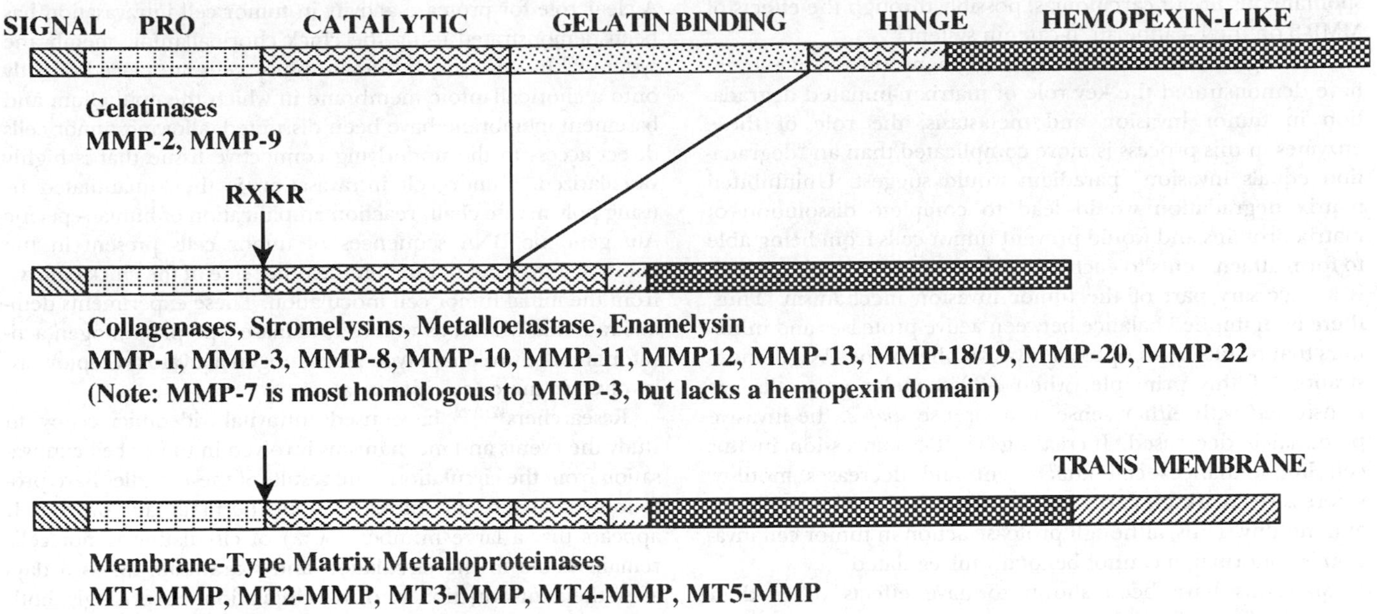

FIGURE 8-5. Simplified schematic domain structure of the matrixin family members. Most matrixins have the same basic domain structure, consisting of signal, pro, catalytic, hinge, and hemopexin-like domains. Matrix metalloproteinase 7 (MMP-7) lacks the hemopexin-like domain, and the gelatinases and membrane-type (MT) matrixins have additional domains. The arrow indicates the location of the furin RXKR cleavage site of MMP-11 and the MT matrixins. The length of each segment is roughly proportional to the number of amino acids that comprise the domain.

must be able to move through connective tissue barriers, such as the basement membrane, to spread from their site of origin. Although a variety of proteases have been implicated in this process, the family of proteases that has received the most attention has been the matrixins or MMPs. Matrixins and their specific inhibitors, the TIMPs, play important roles in normal physiology, because the ECM is a dynamic matrix of structural proteins, growth factors, and latent enzymes that is constantly being remodeled. Approximately 20 matrixins and four TIMPs have been characterized in humans and other animals.[105,106] The matrixins share a common domain structure (Fig. 8-5), although not all domains are represented in all family members. All of the enzymes have a signal peptide sequence; a propeptide domain (prodomain); a catalytic domain, which includes a highly conserved binding site for the catalytic zinc ion; and a hemopexin-like domain. Two family members, MMP-2 and MMP-9, have a gelatin binding domain containing three fibronectin type II repeats inserted into the catalytic domain just on the amino side of the active site sequence. Five family members have a carboxy-terminal transmembrane domain after the hemopexin domain. This subgroup is also known as the *membrane-type MMPs.* They reside on the cell surface, in contrast to the other family members, which are all secreted as proenzymes into the extracellular milieu. The TIMPs also share a high level of homology, including 12 absolutely conserved cysteine residues that are all involved in intramolecular disulfide bonds. TIMPs are divided into two domains by the disulfide-bonding pattern. An amino-terminal domain contains the inhibitory site, and a carboxy-terminal domain has other binding interactions. Because most of the MMP enzymes are secreted in their proenzyme forms, activation is a key regulatory step. Many of the matrixins are activated by an initial protease cleavage within the prodomain by another matrixin or by a serine protease, such as plasmin or urokinase-type plasminogen activator. This cleavage destabilizes the bond between a conserved prodomain cysteine sulfhydryl group and the catalytic zinc in the active site. The bond breaks and the prodomain is released, which frees the active site for catalysis. Unlike the other family members, which are typically activated outside the cell, MMP-13 and the membrane-type MMP subgroup are activated intracellularly by a furin-dependent cleavage of a conserved RXKR sequence that lies between the prodomain and the catalytic domain. The activation mechanisms have been the subject of a review by Murphy et al.[107]

An early indication of the importance of matrixins in tumor biology was the characterization in 1980 of a MMP secreted from a melanoma cell line that was able to degrade basement membrane collagen.[108,109] This finding was followed by numerous studies showing that secretion of matrixins enhanced tumor cell invasion in experimental model systems and that inhibition of protease activity by TIMPs or by synthetic metalloproteinase inhibitors impeded invasion. For example, the invasion of HT-1080 fibrosarcoma cells through Matrigel (a reconstituted basement membrane) is enhanced by addition of activated MMP-2 and inhibited by the addition of TIMP-2 or by zinc chelators.[110] *In vitro* evidence has been supported by the results of *in vivo* experiments using transfected cell lines. For example, when MYU3L bladder carcinoma cells are transfected with *mmp-2,* they have enhanced metastatic potential, whereas transfecting the highly metastatic LMC19 cell line with *timp-2* reduces its metastatic potential.[111,112] Mice genetically engineered to overexpress MMP-3 in breast epithelial cells develop spontaneous breast carcinomas, possibly through the effects of MMP-3 on the E-cadherin/β-catenin system.[35]

Although these experiments and many others like them have demonstrated the key role of matrixin-initiated degradation in tumor invasion and metastasis, the role of these enzymes in this process is more complicated than an "degradation equals invasion" paradigm would suggest. Uninhibited matrix degradation would lead to complete dissolution of matrix proteins and would prevent tumor cells from being able to form attachments to each other or to matrix proteins, which is a necessary part of the tumor invasion mechanism. Thus, there is an implied balance between active proteases and inhibitors that results in an optimal invasive phenotype. As a demonstration of this principle, when A2058 melanoma cells are transfected with either sense or antisense *timp-2*, the invasive potential is decreased. Increasing TIMP-2 expression in this cell line enhances cell attachment and decreases motility, whereas decreasing expression decreases both cell attachment and motility. Thus, although protease action in tumor cell invasion is abnormal, it cannot be totally unregulated.

Matrixins have been shown to have effects other than removal of structural barriers to invasion. As noted above, some matrixins act on other proteins to reveal hidden activity. MMP-2 specifically degrades the γ2 chain of laminin-5, a structural protein in basement membrane, to reveal a site on the α3 chain that has chemotactic properties.[113] The physiologic role of this fragment may be to act as a wound-related chemoattractant; in tumors, however, this peptide may attract tumor cells to breaks in the basement membrane. In an analogous situation, MMPs have been shown to degrade plasminogen into angiostatin, the angiogenesis inhibitor.[114,115]

Research has focused on the interaction between cell surface adhesion molecules and the matrixin family. One obvious interaction is the simple degradation of cell surface adhesion molecules. For example, MMP-3 degrades E-cadherin on mammary epithelial cells, inducing an increased expression of vimentin and decreased expression of keratin.[34] The cell-matrix adhesion molecule CD44 is also cleaved by matrixins, permitting detachment from the matrix.[116] Decreased cell-cell or cell-matrix adhesion can be a proinvasive phenotype. However, beyond mere degradation of adhesion molecules, cells may control the scope of degradative activity by binding the soluble matrixins with cell surface adhesion molecules, thus limiting degradation to a zone in the immediate vicinity of the cell. On endothelial cells, the integrin $\alpha_v\beta_3$ binds MMP-2 through the matrixin's hemopexin domain in response to angiogenic stimuli.[117,118] Similarly, CD44 has been shown to bind MMP-9 to the surface of breast carcinoma and melanoma cells.[60] Interestingly, stimulation of melanoma cells by antibodies to CD44 increased expression of MMP-2,[119] suggesting that binding of matrixins to cell surface receptors might not only provide a mechanism for localizing protease activity but also may serve as an autocrine-stimulating loop mechanism for increased expression of matrixins.

INTRAVASATION, EXTRAVASATION, AND ORTHOTOPIC EFFECT

The mechanisms of tumor cell intravasation have not been investigated as intensively as the other events in the metastatic cascade. This is due in part to the lack of suitable model systems. A clear role for protease activity in tumor cell intravasation has been demonstrated using the chick chorioallantoic membrane system.[120] In this model, human tumor cells are placed directly onto a chorioallantoic membrane in which the epithelium and basement membrane have been disrupted, allowing tumor cells direct access to the underlying connective tissue that is highly vascularized. Tumor cell intravasation is then quantitated by using polymerase chain reaction amplification of human-specific Alu genomic DNA sequences of tumor cells present in the chorioallantoic membrane on the other side of the chick embryo from the initial tumor cell inoculation. These experiments demonstrate that MMPs, as well as urokinase-type plasminogen activator and the urokinase-type plasminogen activator receptor, are involved in tumor cell intravasation.

Researchers[121,122] have used intravital videomicroscopy to study the events and mechanisms involved in tumor cell extravasation from the circulation. The results of these studies have profoundly changed our thinking about the metastatic process. It appears that a large number (80%) of circulating tumor cells remain viable in the circulation and extravasate up to 3 days after their introduction into the circulation. Surprisingly, both metastatic and nonmetastatic cells extravasate, and this process is not protease-dependent. However, only a small subset of cells (1 in 40) grow to form micrometastases, and even fewer (1 in 100) continue to grow, forming macroscopic tumors. Almost 40% of injected tumor cells remained as dormant solitary cancer cells. These findings suggest that the control of postextravasation growth of individual cancer cells is a dominant effect in metastatic inefficiency. More recent data suggest that the local environment of the target organ may profoundly influence the growth potential of extravasated tumor cells. The importance of tissue microenvironment (host) on growth of the primary tumor is well known and is referred to as *orthotopic effect.*[123]

Xenografts of human metastatic tumor cells in nude or SCID (severe combined immunodeficiency) mice infrequently recapitulate the behavior of the parent tumor to show a spontaneously metastatic phenotype. When injected intravenously, however, many of these same human tumor cells are capable of experimental metastasis formation in what are known as *lung colonization assays.* In pioneering experiments,[124–126] it has been demonstrated that this effect is due in part to important tumor-host interactions that are not usually provided by models using subcutaneous injection of tumor xenografts. Using orthotopic implantation of tumor xenografts, these investigators have demonstrated that the host microenvironment has a profound influence on a number of tumor cell parameters,[127] including tumor growth, invasive behavior,[126] response to chemotherapeutic agents,[128,129] growth factor and cytokine production,[130,131] and protease profiles for both urokinase and metalloproteinases.[132–134] An important host contribution to tumor progression is the frequent association of MMP production by stimulated stromal fibroblasts adjacent to invading tumor cells.[135]

During the 1990s, tremendous progress has been made in understanding the process of tumor cell invasion and metastasis formation, which is being revealed as a complex cascade of both promoting agents and suppressors. Loss of function (suppressor inactivation) may occur not only in the tumor cell but also in the host. Such tumor cell-host interactions are complex and difficult to examine in a controlled fashion. However, understanding these complexities is the future of research on cancer metastasis and tumor dissemination. The goal of this research will be the development of new strategies for eradication of established metastases and prevention of new metastatic growth.

REFERENCES

1. Butler TP, Gullino P. Quantitation of cell shedding into efferent blood vessels of mammary adenocarcinoma. *Cancer Res* 1975;35:512.
2. Liotta LA, Kleinerman J, Saidel G. Quantitative relationships of intravascular tumor cells, tumor vessels and pulmonary metastasis. *Cancer Res* 1974;34:977.
3. Thorgeirsson UP, et al. NIH/3T3 cells transfected with human tumor DNA containing activated ras oncogenes express the metastatic phenotype in nude mice. *Mol Cell Biol* 1985;5:259.
4. Tuck AB, Wilson SM, Chambers AF. ras transfection and expression does not induce progression from tumorigenicity to metastatic ability in mouse LTA cells. *Clin Exp Metastasis* 1990;8:417.
5. Pozzatti R, et al. Primary rat embryo cells transformed by one or two oncogenes show different metastatic potentials. *Science* 1986;232:223.
6. Sreenath T, et al. Expression of matrix metalloproteinase genes in transformed rat cell lines of high and low metastatic potential. *Cancer Res* 1992;52:4942.
7. Gimbrone MAJ, et al. Tumor dormancy *in vivo* by prevention of neovascularization. *J Exp Med* 1972;136:261.
8. Brem S, et al. Prolonged tumor dormancy by prevention of neovascularization in the vitreous. *Cancer Res* 1976;36:2807.
9. Hanahan D, Folkman J. Patterns and emerging mechanisms of the angiogenic switch during tumorigenesis. *Cell* 1996;86:353.
10. Liotta LA, Saidel MG, Kleinerman J. The significance of hematogenous tumor cell clumps in the metastatic process. *Cancer Res* 1976;36:889.
11. Vermeulen PB, et al. Quantification of angiogenesis in solid human tumours: an international consensus on the methodology and criteria of evaluation. *Eur J Cancer* 1996;32A:2474.
12. Weidner N. Tumoural vascularity as a prognostic factor in cancer patients: the evidence continues to grow [Editorial]. *J Pathol* 1998;184:119.
13. Weidner N. Intratumoral vascularity as a prognostic factor in cancers of the urogenital tract. *Eur J Cancer* 1996;32A:2506.
14. Holash J, Maisonpierre PC, Compton D, et al. Vessel cooption, regression, and growth in tumors mediated by angiopoietins and VEGF. *Science* 1999;284:1994.
15. Dawson DW, et al. Pigment epithelium-derived factor: a potent inhibitor of angiogenesis. *Science* 1999;285:245.
16. O'Reilly MS, et al. Angiostatin: a novel angiogenesis inhibitor that mediates the suppression of metastases by a Lewis lung carcinoma [see comments]. *Cell* 1994;79:315.
17. O'Reilly MS, et al. Angiostatin induces and sustains dormancy of human primary tumors in mice. *Nat Med* 1996;2:689.
18. O'Reilly MS, et al. Endostatin: an endogenous inhibitor of angiogenesis and tumor growth. *Cell* 1997;88:277.
19. O'Reilly MS, et al. Antiangiogenic activity of the cleaved conformation of the serpin antithrombin [see comments]. *Science* 1999;285:1926.
20. Bergers G, et al. Effects of angiogenesis inhibitors on multistage carcinogenesis in mice. *Science* 1999;284:808.
21. Liotta LA, Steeg PS, Stetler-Stevenson WG. Cancer metastasis and angiogenesis: an imbalance of positive and negative regulation. *Cell* 1991;64:327.
22. Fidler IJ, Kripke ML. Metastasis results from preexisting variant cells within a malignant tumor. *Science* 1977;197:893.
23. Fidler IJ, Gersten DM, Hart IR. The biology of cancer invasion and metastasis. *Adv Cancer Res* 1978;28:149.
24. Fidler IJ, Hart IR. Biological diversity in metastatic neoplasms: origins and implications. *Science* 1982;217:998.
25. Waghorne C, et al. Genetic evidence for progressive selection and overgrowth of primary tumors by metastatic cell subpopulations. *Cancer Res* 1988;48:6109.
26. Kerbel RS, Cornil I, Korezak B. New insights into the evolutionary growth of tumors revealed by Southern gel analysis of tumors genetically tagged with plasmid or proviral DNA insertions. *J Cell Sci* 1989;94(Pt 3):381.
27. Kerbel RS. Growth dominance of the metastatic cancer cell: cellular and molecular aspects. *Adv Cancer Res* 1990;55:87.
28. Stetler-Stevenson WG, Aznavoorian S, Liotta LA. Tumor cell interactions with the extracellular matrix during invasion and metastasis. *Annu Rev Cell Biol*, 1993;9:541.
29. Suzuki ST. Protocadherins and diversity of the cadherin superfamily. *J Cell Sci* 1996;109:2609.
30. Takeichi M. Morphogenic roles of classical cadherins. *Curr Opin Cell Biol* 1995;7:619.
31. Bracke ME, van Roy FM, Mareel MM. The E-cadherin/catenin complex in invasion and metastasis. *Curr Top Microbiol Immunol* 1996;213(Pt 1):123.
32. Birchmeier W, Behrens J. Cadherin expression in carcinomas: role in the formation of cell junctions and the prevention of invasiveness. *Biochem Biophys Acta* 1994;1198:11.
33. Graff JR. Distinct patterns of E-cadherin CpG island methylation in papillary, follicular, Hűrthle's cell, and poorly differentiated human thyroid carcinoma. *Cancer Res* 1998;58:2063.
34. Lochter A, et al. Matrix metalloproteinase stromelysin-1 triggers a cascade of molecular alterations that lead to stable-epithelial-to-mesenchymal conversion and a premalignant phenotype in mammary epithelial cells. *J Cell Biol* 1997;139:1861.
35. Sternlicht MD, et al. The stromal proteinase MMP3/stromelysin-1 promotes mammary carcinogenesis. *Cell* 1999;98:137.
36. Lee SW. H-cadherin, a novel cadherin with growth inhibitory functions and diminished expression in human breast cancer. *Nat Med* 1996;2:776.
37. He TC, et al. Identification of c-MYC as a target of the APC pathway. *Science* 1998;281:1509.
38. Tetsu O, McCormick F. β-Catenin regulated expression of cyclin D1 in colon carcinoma cells. *Nature* 1999;398:422.
39. Johnson JP. Identification of molecules associated with the development of metastasis in human malignant melanoma. *Invasion Metastasis* 1994;14:123.
40. St-Pierre Y, et al. Dissemination of T cell lymphoma to target organs: a post-homing event implicating ICAM-1 and matrix metalloproteinases. *Leuk Lymphoma* 1999;34:53.
41. Umansky V, Schirrmacher V, Rocha M. New insights into tumor-host interactions in lymphoma metastasis. *J Mol Med* 1996;74:353.
42. Johnson JP. Cell adhesion molecules of the immunoglobulin supergene family and their role in malignant transformation and progression to metastatic disease. *Cancer Metastasis Rev* 1991;10:11.
43. Pantel K, et al. Early metastasis of human solid tumours: expression of cell adhesion molecules. *Ciba Found Symp* 1995;189:157; discussion, 170.
44. Albelda SM. Role of integrins and other cell adhesion molecules in tumor progression and metastasis. *Lab Invest* 1993;68:4.
45. Paavonen T, et al. *In vivo* evidence of the roll of α4β1-VCAM interaction in sarcome, but carcinoma extravasation. *Int J Cancer* 1994;58:298.
46. Garofolo A, et al. Involvement of the very late antigen 4-integrin on melanoma in interleukin-1-augmented experimental metastasis. *Cancer Res* 1995;55:414.
47. Goodfellow PN, et al. The gene, MIC4, which controls expression of the antigen defined by monoclonal antibody F10.44.2, is on human chromosome 11. *Eur J Immunol* 1982;12:659.
48. Screaton GR, et al. Genomic structure of DNA encoding the lymphocyte homing receptor CD44 reveals at least 12 alternatively spliced exons. *Proc Natl Acad Sci U S A* 1992;89:12160.
49. van Weering DH, Baas PD, Bos JL. A PCR-based method for the analysis of human CD44 splice products. *PCR Methods Appl* 1993;3:100.
50. Bennett KL, et al. Regulation of CD44 binding to hyaluronan by glycosylation of variably spliced exons. *J Cell Biol* 1995;131(Pt 1):1623.
51. Jalkanen S, et al. Lymphocyte homing and clinical behavior of non-Hodgkin's lymphoma. *J Clin Invest* 1991;87:1835.
52. Pals ST, et al. Expression of lymphocyte homing receptor as a mechanism of dissemination in non-Hodgkin's lymphoma. *Blood* 1989;73:885.
53. Sneath RJ, Mangham DC. The normal structure and function of CD44 and its role in neoplasia. *Mol Pathol* 1998;51:191.
54. Gunthert U, et al. A new variant of glycoprotein CD44 confers metastatic potential to rat carcinoma cells. *Cell* 1991;65:13.
55. Seiter S, et al. Prevention of tumor metastasis formation by anti-variant CD44. *J Exp Med* 1993;177:443.
56. Yu Q, Toole BP, Stamenkovic I. Induction of apoptosis of metastatic mammary carcinoma cells *in vivo* by disruption of tumor cell surface CD44 function. *J Exp Med* 1997;186:1985.
57. Sy MS, Guo YJ, Stamenkovic I. Distinct effects of two CD44 isoforms on tumor growth *in vivo*. *J Exp Med* 1991;174:859.
58. Bartolazzi A, et al. Interaction between CD44 and hyaluronate is directly implicated in the regulation of tumor development. *J Exp Med* 1994;180:53.
59. Culty M, et al. Binding and degradation of hyaluronan by human breast cancer cell lines expressing different forms of CD44: correlation with invasive potential. *J Cell Physiol* 1994;160:275.
60. Yu Q, Stamenkovic I. Localization of matrix metalloproteinase 9 to the cell surface provides a mechanism for CD44-mediated tumor invasion. *Genes Dev* 1999;13:35.
61. Giancotti FG, Ruoslahti E. Integrin signaling. *Science* 1999;285:1028.
62. Hynes RO, Lander AD. Contact and adhesive specificities in the associations, migrations, and targeting of cells and axons. *Cell* 1992;68:303.
63. Clark EA, Brugge JS. Integrins and signal transduction pathways: the road taken. *Science* 1995;268:233.
64. Yamada K. Integrin signaling. *Matrix Biol* 1997;16:137.
65. Zhang Z, et al. Integrin activation by R-ras. *Cell* 1996;85:61.
66. Hughes PE, et al. Suppression of integrin activation: a novel function of a Ras/Raf-initiated MAP kinase pathway. *Cell* 1997;88:521.
67. Howe A, et al. Integrin signaling and cell growth control. *Curr Opin Cell Biol* 1998;10:220.
68. Miyamoto S, Akiyama SK, Yamada KM. Synergistic roles for receptor occupancy and aggregation in integrin transmembrane function. *Science* 1995;267:883.
69. Porter JC, Hogg N. Integrins take partners: cross-talk between integrins and other membrane receptors. *Trends Cell Biol* 1998;8:390.
70. Klernke RL, et al. Regulation of cell motility by mitogen-activated protein kinase. *J Cell Biol* 1997;137:481.
71. Tamura M, et al. PTEN gene and integrin signaling in cancer. *J Natl Cancer Inst* 1999;91:1820.
72. Schlaepfer DD, Broome MA, Hunter T. Fibronectin-stimulated signaling from a focal adhesion kinase-c-Src complex: involvement of the Grb2, p130cas, and Nck adaptor proteins. *Mol Cell Biol* 1997;17:1702.
73. Chen HC, et al. Phosphorylation of tyrosine 397 in focal adhesion kinase is required for binding phosphatidylinositol 3-kinase. *J Biol Chem* 1996;271:26329.
74. Harder KW, et al. Protein-tyrosine phosphatase alpha regulates Src family kinases and alters cell-substratum adhesion. *J Biol Chem* 1998;273:31890.
75. Shen Y, et al. Direct association of protein-tyrosine phosphatase PTP-PEST with paxillin. *J Biol Chem* 1998;273:6474.
76. Angers-Loustau A, et al. Protein tyrosine phosphatase-PEST regulates focal adhesion disassembly, migration, and cytokinesis in fibroblasts. *J Cell Biol* 1999;144:1019.
77. Tamura M, et al. Inhibition of cell migration, spreading, and focal adhesions by tumor suppressor PTEN. *Science* 1998;280:1614.
78. Varner JA, Emerson DA, Juliano RL. Integrin alpha 5 beta 1 expression negatively regulates cell growth: reversal by attachment to fibronectin. *Mol Biol Cell* 1995;6:725.
79. Zutter MM, et al. Re-expression of the alpha 2 beta 1 integrin abrogates the malignant phenotype of breast carcinoma cells. *Proc Natl Acad Sci U S A* 1995;92:7411.

80. Danen EH, et al. Alpha v-integrins in human melanoma: gain of alpha v beta 3 and loss of alpha v beta 5 are related to tumor progression *in situ* but not to metastatic capacity of cell lines in nude mice [published erratum appears in *Int J Cancer* 1995;62:365]. *Int J Cancer* 1995;61:491.
81. Albelda SM, et al. Integrin distribution in malignant melanoma: association of the beta 3 subunit with tumor progression. *Cancer Res* 1990;50:6757.
82. Mitjans F, et al. An anti-alpha v-integrin antibody that blocks integrin function inhibits the development of a human melanoma in nude mice. *J Cell Sci* 1995;108(Pt 8):2825.
83. Costantini RM, et al. Integrin (alpha 6/beta 4) expression in human lung cancer as monitored by specific monoclonal antibodies. *Cancer Res* 1990;50:6107.
84. Gaetano C, et al. Retinoic acid negatively regulates beta 4 integrin expression and suppresses the malignant phenotype in a Lewis lung carcinoma cell line. *Clin Exp Metastasis* 1994;12:63.
85. Liebert M, et al. The monoclonal antibody BQ16 identifies the alpha 6 beta 4 integrin on bladder cancer. *Hybridoma* 1993;12:67.
86. Van Waes C, Carey TE. Overexpression of the A9 antigen/alpha 6 beta 4 integrin in head and neck cancer. *Otolaryngol Clin North Am* 1992;25:1117.
87. Van Waes C, et al. The A9 antigen associated with aggressive human squamous carcinoma is structurally and functionally similar to the newly defined integrin alpha 6 beta 4. *Cancer Res* 1991;51:2395.
88. Lauffenburger DA, Horowitz AF. Cell migration: a physically integrated molecular process. *Cell* 1996;84:359.
89. Gumbiner BM. Cell adhesion: the molecular basis of tissue architecture and morphogenesis. *Cell* 1996;84:345.
90. Mitchison TJ, Cramer LP. Actin-base cell motility and cell locomotion. *Cell* 1996;84:371.
91. Tapon N, Hall A. Rho, Rac and Cdc42 GTPases regulate the organization of the actin cytoskeleton. *Curr Opin Cell Biol* 1997;9:86.
92. Sheetz MP, Felsenfeld DP, Galbraith CG. Cell migration: regulation of force on extracellular-matrix-integrin complexes. *Trends Cell Biol* 1998;8:51.
93. Choquet D, Felsenfeld DP, Sheetz MP. Extracellular matrix rigidity causes strengthening of integrin-cytoskeleton linkages. *Cell* 1997;88:39.
94. Felsenfeld DP, et al. Selective regulation of integrin—cytoskeleton interactions by the tyrosine kinase Src. *Nat Cell Biol* 1999;1:200.
95. Smilenov LB, et al. Focal adhesion motility revealed in stationary fibroblasts. *Science* 1999;286:1172.
96. Palecek SP, et al. Integrin-ligand binding properties govern cell migration speed through cell-substratum adhesiveness [published erratum appears in *Nature* 1997;388:210]. *Nature* 1997;385:537.
97. Palecek SP, et al. Integrin dynamics on the tail region of migrating fibroblasts. *J Cell Sci* 1996;109(Pt 5):941.
98. Niggemann B, et al. Locomotory phenotypes of human tumor cell lines and T lymphocytes in a three-dimensional collagen lattice. *Cancer Lett* 1997;118:173.
99. Huttenlocher A, et al. Regulation of cell migration by the calcium-dependent protease calpain. *J Biol Chem* 1997;272:32719.
100. Niinaka Y, et al. Expression and secretion of neuroleukin/phosphohexose isomerase/maturation factor as autocrine motility factor by tumor cells. *Cancer Res* 1998;58:2667.
101. Watanabe H, et al. Tumor cell autocrine motility factor is the neuroleukin/phosphohexose isomerase polypeptide. *Cancer Res* 1996;56:2960.
102. Murata J, et al. cDNA cloning of the human tumor motility-stimulating protein, autotaxin, reveals a homology with phosphodiesterases. *J Biol Chem* 1994;269:30479.
103. Clair T, et al. Autotaxin is an exoenzyme possessing 5-nucleotide phosphodiesterase/ATP pyrophosphatase and ATPase activities. *J Biol Chem* 1997;272:996.
104. Lee HY, et al. Stimulation of tumor cell motility linked to phosphodiesterase catalytic site of autotaxin. *J Biol Chem* 1996;271:24408.
105. Kleiner DE, Stetler-Stevenson G. Matrix metalloproteinases and metastasis. *Cancer Chemother Pharmacol* 1999;43:S42.
106. Nagase H, Woessner JF. Matrix metalloproteinases. *J Biol Chem* 1999;274:21491.
107. Murphy G, et al. Mechanisms for pro matrix metalloproteinase activation. *APMIS* 1999;107:38.
108. Liotta LA, et al. Metastatic potential correlates with enzymatic degradation of basement membrane collagen. *Nature* 1980;284:67.
109. Salo T, Liotta LA, Tryggvason K. Purification and characterization of a murine basement membrane collagen-degrading enzyme secreted by metastatic tumor cells. *J Biol Chem* 1983;258:3058.
110. Albini A, et al. Tumor cell invasion inhibited by TIMP-2. *J Natl Cancer Inst* 1991;83:775.
111. Kawamata H, et al. Marked acceleration of the metastatic phenotype of a rat bladder carcinoma cell line by the expression of human gelatinase A. *Int J Cancer* 1995;63:568.
112. Kawamata H, et al. Over-expression of tissue inhibitor of matrix metalloproteinases (TIMP1 and TIMP2) suppresses extravasation of pulmonary metastasis of a rat bladder carcinoma. *Int J Cancer* 1995;63:680.
113. Giannelli G, et al. Induction of cell migration by matrix metalloprotease-2 cleavage of laminin-5. *Science* 1997;277:225.
114. O'Reilly MS, et al. Regulation of angiostatin production by matrix metalloproteinase-2 in a model of concomitant resistance. *J Biol Chem* 1999;274:29568.
115. Dong ZY, et al. Macrophage-derived metalloelastase is responsible for the generation of angiostatin in Lewis lung carcinoma. *Cell* 1997;88:801.
116. Okamoto I, et al. CD44 cleavage induced by a membrane-associated metalloprotease plays a critical role in tumor cell migration. *Oncogene* 1999;18:1435.
117. Brooks PC, et al. Disruption of angiogenesis by PEX, a noncatalytic metalloproteinase fragment with integrin binding activity. *Cell* 1998;92:391.
118. Brooks PC, et al. Localization of matrix metalloproteinase MMP-2 to the surface of invasive cells by interaction with integrin alpha v beta 3. *Cell* 1996;85:683.
119. Takahashi K, Eto H, Tanabe KK. Involvement of CD44 in matrix metalloproteinase-2 regulation in human melanoma cells. *Int J Cancer* 1999;80:387.
120. Kim J, et al. Requirement for specific proteases in cancer cell intravasation as revealed by a novel semiquantitative PCR-based assay. *Cell* 1998;94:353.
121. Chambers AF, et al. Steps in tumor metastasis: new concepts from intravital videomicroscopy. *Cancer Metastasis Rev* 1995;14:279.
122. Luzzi KJ, et al. Multistep nature of metastatic inefficiency: dormancy of solitary cells after successful extravasation and limited survival of early micrometastases. *Am J Pathol* 1998;153:865.
123. Naumov GN, et al. Cellular expression of green fluorescent protein, coupled with high-resolution *in vivo* videomicroscopy, to monitor steps in tumor metastasis. *J Cell Sci* 1999;112(Pt 12):1835.
124. Pettaway CA, et al. Selection of highly metastatic variants of different human prostatic carcinomas using orthotopic implantation in nude mice. *Clin Cancer Res* 1996;2:1627.
125. Dinney CP, et al. Isolation and characterization of metastatic variants from human transitional cell carcinoma passaged by orthotopic implantation in athymic nude mice. *J Urol* 1995;154:1532.
126. Fabra A, et al. Modulation of the invasive phenotype of human colon carcinoma cells by organ specific fibroblasts of nude mice. *Differentiation* 1992;52:101.
127. Stephenson RA, et al. Metastatic model for human prostate cancer using orthotopic implantation in nude mice. *J Natl Cancer Inst* 1992;84:951.
128. Wilmanns C, et al. Orthotopic and ectopic organ environments differentially influence the sensitivity of murine colon carcinoma cells to doxorubicin and 5-fluorouracil. *Int J Cancer* 1992;52:98.
129. Fidler IJ, et al. Modulation of tumor cell response to chemotherapy by the organ environment. *Cancer Metastasis Rev* 1994;13:209.
130. Gutman M, et al. Regulation of interleukin-8 expression in human melanoma cells by the organ environment. *Cancer Res* 1995;55:2470.
131. Singh RK, et al. Organ site-dependent expression of basic fibroblast growth factor in human renal cell carcinoma cells. *Am J Pathol* 1994;145:365.
132. Nakajima M, et al. Influence of organ environment on extracellular matrix degradative activity and metastasis of human colon carcinoma cells [see comments]. *J Natl Cancer Inst* 1990;82:1890.
133. Gohji K, et al. Regulation of gelatinase production in metastatic renal cell carcinoma by organ-specific fibroblasts. *Jpn J Cancer Res* 1994;85:152.
134. Gohji K, et al. Organ-site dependence for the production of urokinase-type plasminogen activator and metastasis by human renal cell carcinoma cells. *Am J Pathol* 1997;151:1655.
135. Chambers AF, Matrisian LM. Changing views of the role of matrix metalloproteinases in metastasis. *J Natl Cancer Inst* 1997;89:1260.

Isaiah J. Fidler
Robert S. Kerbel
Lee M. Ellis

CHAPTER 9

Biology of Cancer: Angiogenesis

One crucial step for the continuous growth of tumors and the development of metastasis is the induction of vasculature (i.e., angiogenesis).[1–3] A tumor mass that is less than 0.5 mm in diameter can receive oxygen and nutrients by diffusion, but any increase in tumor mass beyond 0.5 mm requires the proliferation and morphogenesis of vascular endothelial cells.[2] The process of angiogenesis consists of multiple, sequential, and interdependent steps. It begins with local degradation of the basement membrane surrounding capillaries, which is followed by invasion of the surrounding stroma by the underlying endothelial cells in the direction of the angiogenic stimulus. Endothelial cell migration is accompanied by the proliferation of endothelial cells and their organization into three-dimensional structures that join with other similar structures to form a network of new blood vessels (Fig. 9-1).[4]

NEOPLASTIC ANGIOGENESIS: THE BALANCE OF PROANGIOGENIC AND ANTIANGIOGENIC MOLECULES

The onset of angiogenesis involves an alteration in the balance between proangiogenic and antiangiogenic molecules.[1,5] These molecules may mediate multiple steps in the process of angiogenesis and also may affect the function of diverse cell types not involved in angiogenesis. A more refined definition of an angiogenic factor is a factor that selectively alters the characteristics of endothelial cells and associated perivascular structures (i.e., pericytes, vascular smooth muscle cells) but does not affect the function of other cell types. Table 9-1 lists most of the proangiogenic and antiangiogenic factors that have been well characterized to date.

Vascular endothelial growth factor–vascular permeability factor (VEGF/VPF) was initially detected as a factor secreted by tumor cells into tissue culture medium or ascites fluid *in vivo*.[6] The factor was identified as a heparin-binding protein of molecular weight 34 to 42 kD and was termed *VPF*. It was later demonstrated that VPF also stimulated endothelial cell division.[7] Independently, several groups isolated a secreted protein that had selective mitogenic activity for cultured endothelial cells, which they called *VEGF*.[8,9] On the basis of amino acid and complementary DNA sequence analysis, it is now known that VEGF and VPF are the same protein,[10] and *VEGF* is the term more commonly used to describe this angiogenic factor.

VEGF is a homodimeric heparin-binding glycoprotein that exists in at least four isoforms due to alternative splicing of the primary messenger RNA (mRNA) transcript. The isoforms are designated $VEGF_{121}$, $VEGF_{165}$, $VEGF_{189}$, and $VEGF_{205}$, according to the number of amino acids that each protein contains.[10] The vascular permeability induced by VEGF is 50,000 times that induced by histamine, the standard for induction of permeability.[11] Induction of permeability by VEGF allows for the diffusion of proteins into the interstitium on which endothelial cells migrate.

The receptors for VEGF are expressed almost exclusively on endothelial cells. Rarely, expression of the various VEGF receptors has been demonstrated on cells of neural origin, Kaposi's sarcoma cells, hematopoietic precursor cells, and other rare tumor cell types.[12,13] Three VEGF/VPF receptors have been identified. The fms-like tyrosine kinase (Flt-1) and fetal liver kinase 1/kinase insert domain–containing receptor (Flk-1/KDR) are high-affinity VEGF/VPF receptors with an extracellular domain containing seven immunoglobulin-like domains and a split tyrosine kinase intracellular domain.[8] Flk-1 has 85% homology with the human homologue, KDR. Both Flt-1 and Flk-1/KDR have been shown to be important regulatory systems for vasculogenesis and physiologic angiogenesis.[14] However, the interaction of VEGF/VPF with Flk-1/KDR is believed to be the more important interaction for tumor angiogenesis, as it is essential for induction of

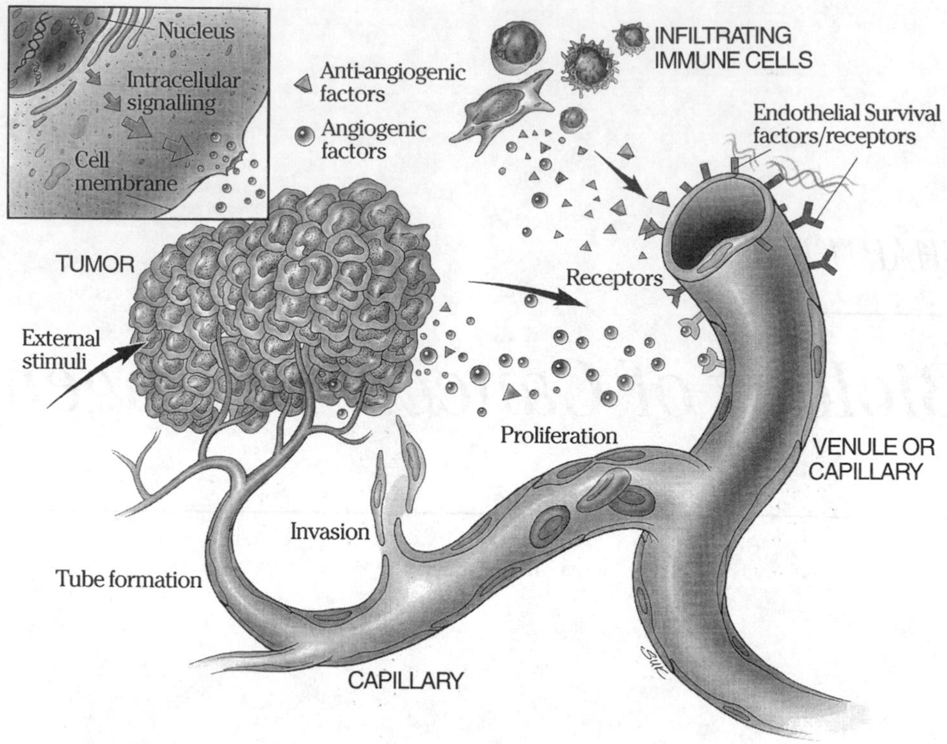

FIGURE 9-1. The angiogenic process. The process of angiogenesis is a series of linked and sequential steps that ultimately lead to the development of a neovascular blood supply to the tumor mass. Different steps in the angiogenic process may be occurring in different parts of the tumor at the same time. Tumor cells or host cells (infiltrating immune cells or adjacent normal tissue) secrete angiogenic growth factors, which then bind to specific receptors on endothelial cells. This ligand-receptor interaction leads to endothelial cell proliferation, migration, invasion and, eventually, capillary tube formation. Factors also affect endothelial cell survival under adverse conditions that occur in tumors. The proangiogenic process is balanced by the activity of antiangiogenic molecules that are necessary for homeostatic processes. When the activity of the proangiogenic molecules exceeds the activity of the antiangiogenic molecules, new blood vessel formation occurs. Proangiogenic factors may be constitutively expressed, but their expression may be increased by certain stimuli, such as hypoxia, low pH, cytokines, growth factors, tumor size, activated oncogenes, signal transduction pathways, or loss of tumor suppressor gene function.

the full spectrum of VEGF/VPF functions.[8] In fact, many compounds and molecules developed to block VEGF/VPF activities mediated by Flk-1/KDR have been shown to have antiangiogenic activity in animal models.[14] Most recently, VEGFR-3 (Flt-4) has been shown to be the receptor for VEGF-C, which is most likely involved with lymph angiogenesis.[14]

There are at least four other members of the VEGF family. The above-referenced VEGF is referred to as *VEGF-A*. *VEGF-B* most likely plays an important role in vasculogenesis but may have other functions such as activation of invasive enzymes on endothelial cells.[14,15] *VEGF-C* is most commonly associated with lymph angiogenesis but, more recently, its expression has been associated with tumor angiogenesis in several systems.[16–19] VEGF-C also binds preferentially to the VEGFR-3. The role of *VEGF-D* is less well defined, but this protein may bind to VEGFR-2 and VEGFR-3 and may induce *in vivo* angiogenesis.[20,21] Little is known about *VEGF-E*, except that it binds to VEGF-R2 and can induce endothelial cell mitosis and angiogenesis.[22,23]

Another family of endothelial cell–specific molecules is the angiopoietin (Ang) family. At present, its members are designated *angiopoietins 1 through 4*. The best characterized of these factors are Ang-1 and Ang-2. Ang-1 and -2 bind to the specific tyrosine kinase receptor Tie-2 on endothelial cells. Ang-1 acts as an agonist and is involved in endothelial cell differentiation and stabilization.[24] In contrast, Ang-2 binds to Tie-2 and blocks the binding of Ang-1 to this receptor.[25] This blockade leads to endothelial cell destabilization and vascular regression.[26] Although the receptor Tie-1 has been identified on endothelial cells, its ligand remains to be identified.

An insightful method for studying the function of various angiogenesis-related molecules is to develop knockout mice for the gene under question. Homozygous knockout of the genes for VEGF or any of the VEGF receptors lead to embryonic death in mice (reviewed in Gale and Yancopoulos[27]). Study of these embryos at the time of death reveals defective vascular development. Similarly, knockout of the genes for Ang-1, Ang-2, Tie-1, and Tie-2 also lead to embryonic lethality and defective vascular development in mice.[28,29] Thus, these factors that are being controlled in such mice are critical for vasculogenesis and likely play an essential role in tumor angiogenesis as well.

Numerous nonspecific angiogenic molecules affect not only the growth of endothelial cells but also the growth of other cell types. These factors include the fibroblast growth factors (FGF), acidic and basic; transforming growth factor-α (TGF-α); and epidermal growth factor (EGF); platelet-derived growth

TABLE 9-1. Proangiogenic Growth Factors

Factor	*Properties*	*Receptor*	*Study*
Vascular endothelial growth factor–vascular permeability factor	Endothelial mitogen, survival factor, and permeability inducer produced by many types of tumor cells	Flk-1/KDR (VEGFR-2), Flt-1 (VEGFR-1) (both present on activated endothelium)	Veikkola et al.[14]
Placental growth factor	Weak endothelial mitogen	Flt-1 (VEGFR-1)	Veikkola et al.[14]
Basic fibroblast growth factor (bFGF/FGF-2)	Endothelial mitogen, angiogenesis inducer, and survival factor; inducer of Flk-1 expression	FGF-R1–4	Baird and Klagsbrun,[149] Gimenez-Gallego and Cuevas[150]
Acidic fibroblast growth factor (aFGF/FGF-1)	Endothelial mitogen and angiogenesis inducer	FGF-R1–4	Baird and Klagsbrun,[149] Gimenez-Gallego and Cuevas[150]
Fibroblast growth factor 3 (FGF-3/*int*-2)	Endothelial mitogen and angiogenesis inducer	FGF-R1–4	Baird and Klagsbrun,[149] Gimenez-Gallego and Cuevas[150]
Fibroblast growth factor 4 (FGF-4/*hst*/K-FGF)	Endothelial mitogen and angiogenesis inducer	FGF-R1–4	Baird and Klagsbrun,[149] Gimenez-Gallego and Cuevas[150]
Transforming growth factor-α (TGF-α)	Endothelial mitogen and angiogenesis inducer; inducer of vascular endothelial growth factor expression	Epidermal growth factor-R	Schmitt and Soares[151]
Epidermal growth factor (EGF)	Weak endothelial mitogen; inducer of vascular endothelial growth factor expression	Epidermal growth factor-R	Mooradian and Diglio[152]
Hepatocyte growth factor/scatter factor (HGF/SF)	Endothelial mitogen, motogen, and angiogenesis inducer	c-Met	Lamszus et al.[153]
Transforming growth factor-β (TGF-β)	*In vivo*–acting angiogenesis inducer; endothelial growth inhibitor; inducer of vascular endothelial growth factor expression	Transforming growth factor-β RI, II, III	Pepper[154]
Tumor necrosis factor-α (TNF-α)	*In vivo*–acting angiogenesis inducer; endothelial mitogen (low concentrations) or inhibitor (at high concentrations); inducer of vascular endothelial growth factor expression	TNF-R55	Yoshida et al.[155]
Platelet-derived growth factor	Mitogen and motility factor for endothelial cells and fibroblasts; *in vivo*–acting angiogenesis inducer	Platelet-derived growth factor-R	Kuwabara et al.[156]
Granulocyte colony-stimulating factor	*In vivo*–acting angiogenesis-inducing factor with some mitogenic and motogenic activity for endothelial cells	Granulocyte colony-stimulating factor	Bussolino et al.[157]
Interleukin-8	*In vivo*–acting, possibly indirect angiogenesis inducer	Interleukin-8R presence on endothelial cells remains uncertain	Desbaillets et al.[48]
Pleiotropin	Angiogenesis-inducing pleiotropic growth factor	Proteoglycan	Choudhuri et al.[158]
Thymidine phosphorylase (TP)–platelet-derived endothelial cell growth factor (PD-ECGF)	*In vivo*–acting angiogenesis factor	Unknown	Takahashi et al.[38]
Angiogenin	*In vivo*–acting angiogenesis inducer with RNAse activity	170-kD angiogenin receptor	Hartmann et al.[47]
Proliferin	35-kD angiogenesis-inducing protein in mouse	Unknown	Jackson et al.[159]

(Modified with permission from ref. 164.)

factor (PDGF); platelet-derived endothelial cell growth factor (PD-ECGF); angiogenin; and the CXC chemokines interleukin-8 (IL-8), macrophage inflammatory protein-1(MIP), platelet factor-4(PF-4), and growth-related oucogene-α(GRO-α).[30]

The process of angiogenesis is dynamic and complex. In fact, the development of a neovascular blood supply is a series of interlinked processes that eventually leads to new blood vessel formation. Studies have demonstrated that different operations in the overall process of angiogenesis may be regulated by different angiogenic factors.[31] For example, basic FGF (bFGF) is the most potent mitogen for endothelial cells, followed by VEGF and PD-ECGF. VEGF and bFGF are also the most potent survival factors for endothelial cells. However, bFGF is the angiogenic factor most associated with increasing activity of degradative enzymes. Hepatocyte growth factor enhances endothelial cell motility more than any other angiogenic factor studied. The more recent recognition of Ang-1 and -2 and their role in endothelial cell stabilization suggests that these molecules are also important in endothelial cell survival.[26]

LYMPHOID CELL–MEDIATED ANGIOGENESIS

Angiogenesis is essential to homeostasis, and its regulation by lymphoid cells, such as T lymphocytes, macrophages, and mast cells, is well recognized.[32–35] A local inflammatory reaction consisting of T lymphocytes and macrophages often is associated with invasive cutaneous melanoma, and an intense inflammatory reaction often is associated with an increased risk of metastasis, suggesting that angiogenesis induced by inflammation may contribute to melanoma progression and metastasis.[35]

Immunologic mechanisms involved in physiologic angiogenesis are activated subsequent to wound healing.[33] Systemic chemotherapy has been shown to retard the process of wound healing, possibly by decreasing the immune response; whether this is mediated by inhibition of angiogenesis is unclear.[36] We have investigated the role of tumor vascularization and its effect on tumor growth in immunosuppressed mice. The growth of weakly immunogenic B16 melanoma was retarded in myelosuppressed mice as compared with control mice.[35] Further evidence implicating myelosuppression in the retardation of tumor growth and vascularity was obtained from doxorubicin-pretreated animals injected with normal spleen cells 1 day before tumor challenge. Tumor growth in these mice was comparable to that in control mice.[35] Similar results were obtained in athymic mice, suggesting that the tumor vascularization observed in doxorubicin-treated mice reconstituted with normal splenocytes was not mediated solely by T lymphocytes. Because reconstitution with spleen cells enhanced vascularization of the B16 tumors, the results suggest that myelosuppressive chemotherapeutic drugs (e.g., doxorubicin) can inhibit host-mediated vascularization and support the concept that developing tumors can usurp homeostatic mechanisms to their advantage.[37]

The role of infiltrating cells in the angiogenesis of human colon cancer has been reported.[38] High expression of PD-ECGF was found in infiltrating cells, mostly macrophages and lymphocytes, though very little PD-ECGF was expressed in the cancer epithelium. The intensity of staining for PD-ECGF in infiltrating cells correlated with vessel counts, suggesting the involvement of these cells in the angiogenesis of human colon cancer.

Macrophages have been recognized for a number of years as important angiogenesis effector cells.[32,33] They may influence new capillary growth by several different mechanisms. First, macrophages produce factors that act directly to influence angiogenesis-linked endothelial cell functions. *In vitro* studies have shown that macrophages produce in excess of 20 molecules that reportedly influence endothelial cell proliferation, migration, and differentiation *in vitro*[32] and that are potentially angiogenic *in vivo*. A second mechanism by which macrophages might modulate angiogenesis is by modifying the extracellular matrix (ECM). The composition of the ECM has been shown to influence endothelial cell shape and morphology dramatically and may profoundly influence new capillary growth.[39] Macrophages can influence the composition of the ECM either through the direct production of ECM components or through the production of proteases, which effectively alter the structure and composition of the ECM.[33] A third mechanism is by producing substances that suppress angiogenesis. Macrophages have been shown to express the angiogenesis inhibitor thrombospondin-1 (TSP-1) when treated with the chemopreventive agent retinoic acid.[39–41]

The generation of angiostatin by subcutaneous Lewis lung carcinoma[42] requires the presence of macrophages and is directly correlated with their metalloelastase activity.[43] For example, the addition of plasminogen to Lewis lung carcinoma (3LL) cells cultured *in vitro* did not result in generation of angiostatin, whereas the addition of plasminogen to cocultures of macrophages and 3LL cells did. Elastase activity in macrophages was up-regulated by the cytokine granulocyte-macrophage colony-stimulating factor (GM-CSF). GM-CSF secreted by Lewis lung carcinoma cells significantly enhanced the production of elastase by macrophages and, hence, the generation of angiostatin from plasminogen.[43] These data suggest that elastase released from tumor-infiltrating macrophages is responsible for the angiostatin production in this tumor model and for the angiogenesis-inhibiting role of macrophages.

REGULATION OF ANGIOGENIC FACTOR EXPRESSION IN TUMORS

Tumor cells may constitutively overexpress angiogenic factors, or they may respond to external stimuli. The most potent external stimulus of angiogenic factor expression is hypoxia.[44,45] Hypoxia is a consequence of tissue that is poorly perfused, and teleologically represents the appropriate response of a cell trying to survive. Hypoxia typically increases angiogenic factor expression by inducing signal cascade pathways that eventually lead to an increase in transcription of VEGF as well as stabilization of the mRNA transcript. The expression of other angiogenic factors such as angiogenin, PD-ECGF, and IL-8 may also be induced by hypoxia.[46–48] Other microenvironmental factors that increase the angiogenic response include various cytokines and growth factors. The cytokines, insulin growth factor-1, insulin growth factor-2, EGF, hepatocyte growth factor, IL-1, and PDGF have all been shown to up-regulate VEGF.[49–51] Thus, antiangiogenic therapy may involve down-regulation of upstream targets of the angiogenic factors rather than targeting of angiogenic factors themselves.[52,53] Furthermore, protein products of tumor suppressor genes such as the von Hippel-Lindau *(VHL)* or *p53* gene also regulate angiogenesis.[54,55]

ENDOGENOUS INHIBITORS OF ANGIOGENESIS

A large, growing, and structurally diverse family of endogenous protein inhibitors of angiogenesis has been discovered (e.g.,

TABLE 9-2. Some Endogenous Inhibitors of Angiogenesis

Name	*Description*	*Study*
Thrombospondin-1 and internal fragments of thrombospondin-1	Large, modular (180-kD) extracellular matrix protein	Tolsma et al.[57]
Angiostatin	38-kD fragment of plasminogen involving either kringle domains 1–3 or smaller kringle 5 fragments	O'Reilly et al.[42]
Endostatin	20-kD zinc-binding fragment of type XVIII collagen	O'Reilly et al.[61]
Vasostatin	NH_2 terminal fragment (amino acids 1–80) of calreticulin	Pike et al.[63]
Vascular endothelial growth factor inhibitor	174–amino acid protein with 20–30% homology to tumor necrosis factor superfamily	Zhai et al.[62]
Fragment of platelet factor-4	N-terminal fragment of platelet factor-4	Gupta et al.[65]
Derivative of prolactin	16-kD fragment of prolactin	Clapp et al.[60]
Restin	NC10 domain of human collagen XV	Ramchandran et al.[160]
Proliferin-related protein	Protein related to the proangiogenic molecule proliferin	Jackson et al.[159]
SPARC cleavage product	Fragments of *s*ecreted *p*rotein, *a*cidic and *r*ich in *c*ysteine	Vasquez[64]
Osteopontin cleavage product	Thrombin-generated fragment containing an RGD sequence	Sage[161]
Interferon-α-β	Well-known antiviral proteins, may down-regulate angiogenic factor expression	Ezekowitz et al.[59]
METH-1 and METH-2	Proteins containing metalloprotease and thrombospondin domains, and disintegrin domains in NH_2 termini	Vasquez,[64] Sage[161]
Angiopoietin-2	Antagonist of angiopoietin-1 that binds to Tie-2 receptor	Davis and Yankopoulos,[25] Maisonpierre et al.[162]
Antithrombin III fragment	A fragment missing the carboxy-terminal loop of antithrombin III (a member of the serpin family)	O'Reilly et al.[66]
Interferon-inducible protein-10	Up-regulated by IFN-γ and whose mechanism of antiangiogenic effect is unknown	Moore et al.[163]

(Modified with permission from RS Kerbel, Tumor angiogenesis: past, present and the near future. *Carcinogenesis* 2000;21:505.)

TSP-1[56,57]; the interferons IFN-α, -β, and -γ[58,59]; the 16-kD fragment of prolactin[60]; angiostatin[42]; endostatin[61]; VEGF or vascular endothelial cell growth inhibitor[62]; vasostatin[63]; METH-1 and METH-2[64]; and cleavage products of platelet factor 4[65] or antithrombin III,[66] among many others (Table 9-2). Some of these are internal fragments of various proteins that normally lack any antiangiogenic activity[67]; for example, the active component of angiostatin comprises one or more fragments of plasminogen,[42] and endostatin is a fragment of type XVIII collagen.[61]

It is now thought that the tumor angiogenic switch is triggered as a result of a shift in the balance of stimulators to inhibitors.[5] When the ratio is low, tumor angiogenesis is blocked or modest in magnitude; in contrast, when the ratio is high, the angiogenic switch is turned to the on position.[5] Of considerable interest is the finding by Dameron et al.[56] that loss of wild-type *p53* gene function resulted in a loss of TSP expression. Not only did this finding establish a possible critical link between the genetic basis of cancer and tumor angiogenesis; it also opened up the now flourishing field of endogenous angiogenesis inhibitors. Furthermore, it is now increasingly recognized that oncogenes, such as mutant ras or src, may also contribute to tumor angiogenesis by influencing (i.e., enhancing) the production of proangiogenic molecules such as VEGF.[52,68,69] Such effects were slow to be uncovered in the oncogene and tumor suppressor gene fields, given the predominant use of pure tumor cell culture systems to study the function of cancer-causing genetic alterations.

CLINICAL UTILITY OF ANGIOGENESIS

THE PROGNOSTIC SIGNIFICANCE OF TUMOR ANGIOGENESIS

With few exceptions, benign neoplasms are sparsely vascularized and tend to grow slowly, whereas malignant neoplasms are highly vascular and fast-growing.[1,2,4] The increase in vasculature also increases the probability that tumor cells will enter the circulation and possibly give rise to metastases.[3] Immunohistochemical staining of breast cancer sections with antibodies against factor VIII, a protein expressed predominantly on the surface of endothelial cells, allowed Weidner et al.[70] to determine the density of the microvasculature. The number of microvessels in microscopic fields selected from the most vascular areas ("hot spots") of the sections correlated directly with metastasis and inversely with survival.

Most recent studies have concluded that increased microvessel density in the areas of most intense neovascularization is a significant and independent prognostic indicator in early-stage breast cancer.[70–80] Studies of other neoplasms such as prostate cancer, melanoma, ovarian carcinoma, gastric carcinoma, and colon carcinoma also support the conclusion that the angiogenesis index is a useful prognostic factor.[81–86] However, the expectation that an angiogenesis index can identify all patients with occult metastatic disease or those with probable distant metastases may be unrealistic for several reasons.[1,87] First, human tumors are heterogeneous and consist of subpopulations of cells having different biologic properties.[88–92] Heterogeneity of angiogenic molecule expression has recently been documented in human renal carcinomas and human colon.[93,94] Second, the process of cancer metastasis is sequential and selective, consisting of a series of interlinked but independent steps.[89,92] To produce clinically relevant metastases, tumor cells must complete all the steps in this process. Tumor cells that can induce intense angiogenesis but cannot survive in the circulation or proliferate in distant organs will not produce metastases.[89,92] Like all other steps in the metastatic cascade, angiogenesis is necessary but not sufficient for the pathogenesis of a metastasis. Third, although not all large angiogenic tumors metastasize, inhibition of angiogenesis prevents the growth of tumor cells at both the primary and secondary sites and thus can prevent the development of clinically relevant metastases.[42,61,67]

To study angiogenesis in tumor specimens using current technology, it is necessary to obtain tissue for histologic evaluation. The criterion standard for evaluation of human tumor specimens is to highlight the tumor endothelium with antibodies that differentiate endothelial cells from other cells within the tumor.[95] The first such antibody used was factor VIII-RA (FVIII-RA), and this is still the antibody used in many studies reported in the literature. Other endothelial cell–specific antibodies that are used in the study of angiogenesis include CD31/PECAM, CD34, CD36, TEC-11, and ulex europaeus(UEA). Currently, the antibodies most commonly used in the study of angiogenesis are FVIII-RA, CD31, and CD34 antibodies. Once histologic preparation of a slide is complete, it is necessary to quantify the level of angiogenesis within the tumor. It is essential that an investigator examine angiogenesis systematically. For example, investigators may choose the five most vascularized areas in a tumor by scanning at low power and then count vessels in these areas under higher magnification. In certain tumors, such as colon cancer and gastric cancer, it is necessary to define the location at which tumor counts are obtained, as counts made close to the invading edge of the tumor may be significantly different from counts made further away from the invading edge.[82,83] The number of blood vessels in individual tumor specimens can be quantified either as the number in a single high-power field or as the average number in several high-power fields.

In addition to counting blood vessels in a high-power field, it also is possible to grade the degree of vasculature on a scale of 0 to 3+, with 3+ being the most vascular. Obviously, this approach is subjective and prone to problems of reproducibility. Another method of analyzing tumor angiogenesis involves highlighting the vessels with an endothelial cell–specific antibody and, with the aid of computer imaging analysis, determining the area within a high-power field that is occupied by positively stained cells. Access to imaging systems and computer software is necessary for this technique. A third method for quantifying the degree of angiogenesis is to count the number of branch points in vessels within a tumor. Finally, a very common method employed in Europe is the Chalkley-Grid method.[96] In this methodology, an eyepiece marked with overlapping crossbars is used to visualize the high-power field of a tumor stained with an endothelial cell–specific antibody. The areas where an endothelial cell intersects a crossbar are counted, and the total sum in a high-power field of these counts is equal to the Chalkley score.

The recognition that tumors with a high angiogenic index may be associated with subsequent metastasis suggests that these patients may be the ones most likely to benefit from adjuvant therapy. In a study evaluating the prognostic role of angiogenesis in late-stage lung carcinoma, adjuvant therapy improved survival in patients with a high vessel count but not in patients with a low vessel count.[97] However, the observation that patients with highly angiogenic tumors benefit from adjuvant therapy is not universal. In several studies of node-positive breast cancer patients treated with adjuvant chemotherapy or hormonal therapy, those whose tumors had a high microvessel density were found to have a *worse* prognosis than those whose tumors had a low microvessel density, despite adjuvant chemotherapy.[98,99] In fact, one recent study suggested that patients with a low VEGF expression have a more favorable outcome secondary to adjuvant therapy.[100] Tumors with a high angiogenic index may represent a biologically more aggressive variant of the disease, against which conventional adjuvant therapies are ineffective. Perhaps antiangiogenic therapy is indicated in these patients. Obviously, well-controlled clinical trials should be designed to determine the efficacy of antiangiogenic therapy as an adjunct in the treatment of patients with highly vascularized solid malignancies.

OVERVIEW OF ANTIANGIOGENIC STRATEGIES

Antiangiogenic agents currently used in the clinic can be categorized into several broad classes based on the biologic activity of the compounds used. The first class of compounds, metalloproteinase inhibitors, blocks degradation of the basement membrane. Most of the studies on these agents reported to date have been phase I studies in which major toxicity was associated with musculoskeletal and joint pain owing to defects in collagen remodeling.

A second class of antiangiogenic agents includes those designed to inhibit endothelial cell function. These include TNP-470, thalidomide, squalamine, combretastatin A-4 prodrug, and endostatin. Less is known about the biologic effects of these drugs as compared to the first class, and most of these drugs are currently in phase I or phase II trials. How these drugs exert their antiangiogenic activities in *in vivo* models is not fully elucidated at this time; perhaps well-designed clinical trials will shed some light on their mechanisms of action.

A third class of antiangiogenic agents specifically targets an angiogenic factor or factors. These agents include tyrosine kinase inhibitors of the receptors of such factors as VEGF, bFGF, and PDGF. In addition, antibodies directed against these receptors or the factors themselves are either in clinical trials or in the process of being developed for clinical trials. In preclinical trials in animal models, most of these agents inhibited tumor growth, but very few have caused tumor regression. This suggests that tumor regression, which is the typical end point for successful cytotoxic chemotherapy, may not be appropriate for antiangiogenic therapies. Thus, it is necessary to redefine the end points for biologic therapy.

Because endothelial cell survival has recently been recognized as an important characteristic of the development of a neovascular blood supply, drugs that target survival factors are beginning to be introduced into clinical trials. These drugs include antagonists to integrins that are present on the endothelial cell surface. In addition, as VEGF currently is thought of as both a survival factor for endothelial cells and an angiogenic factor, anti-VEGF therapy may affect the survival of tumor endothelial cells.

TUMOR ENDOTHELIUM ("ACTIVATED ENDOTHELIUM") AS DISTINCT FROM NORMAL ENDOTHELIUM

The discovery of VEGF receptors and their up-regulation in newly formed blood vessels highlights the fact that there can indeed be major phenotypic differences between mature, quiescent vessels and their newly formed counterparts. Such differences are essential to avoid unwanted toxicity to normal vessels when using antiangiogenic drugs while still achieving a sufficient therapeutic index. A number of such differences in the phenotypes of endothelial cells in normal versus malignant tissues are now known and include a significant elevation of expression of the integrins avb3 and avb5.[101,102] In breast cancer, it has been demonstrated that antibodies to avb3 preferentially stain the tumor vasculature but not the normal vasculature, suggesting that avb3 is a marker for activated endothelium.[103]

An important issue in antiangiogenic strategies is the fact that tumor endothelium at different sites and within different tumors may be phenotypically distinct. Tumor endothelium is heterogeneous in terms of the ability to bind specific peptide sequences.[104] Other markers that are up-regulated in activated endothelial cells include adhesion molecules such as E-selectin,[105] endoglin,[106] glycoproteins such as prostate-specific membrane antigen,[107] the ED-B domain of fibronectin,[108] and various proteases.[109] Many of these unique characteristics of the tumor endothelium can be exploited not only as potential therapeutic targets but also for detection of cancer by various clinical imaging techniques.[108]

ANTIANGIOGENIC ACTIVITY OF INTERFERON

The IFN family consists of three major glycoproteins that exhibit species specificity: leukocyte-derived IFN-α, fibroblast-derived IFN-β, and immune cell–produced IFN-γ. Although IFN-α and IFN-β share a common receptor (the type I IFN receptor) and induce a similar pattern of cellular responses, certain cellular reactions can be stimulated only by IFN-β, probably by the phosphorylation of a receptor-associated protein that is uniquely responsive to IFN-β.[110] In addition to their well-recognized activity as antiviral agents, IFNs regulate multiple biologic activities such as cell growth,[111] differentiation,[112] oncogene expression,[113] host immunity,[114] and tumorigenicity.[115–117] IFNs can also inhibit a number of steps in the angiogenic process. IFN has antiproliferative properties, especially on tumor cells,[118,119] an effect that has been demonstrated also on endothelial cells *in vitro.* IFN-α can inhibit FGF-induced endothelial proliferation[120]; IFN-γ also can inhibit endothelial proliferation.[121] IFN-α and IFN-γ have been shown to be cytostatic to human dermal microvascular endothelial cells[122] and human capillary endothelial cells.[123]

Systemic therapy using recombinant IFNs produces antiangiogenic effects in vascular tumors, including life-threatening infantile hemangioma,[59,124,125] Kaposi's sarcoma,[126] giant cell tumor of the mandible,[127] and bladder carcinoma.[128] These tumors have also been documented as producing the high levels of bFGF often detectable in the urine or serum of these patients.[129,130] IFN-α and IFN-β, but not IFN-γ, down-regulate the expression of bFGF mRNA and protein in human carcinoma cells.[58] Indeed, systemic administration of human IFN-α decreased the *in vivo* expression of bFGF, decreased blood vessel density, and inhibited tumor growth of a human bladder carcinoma implanted orthotopically in nude mice.[131]

ANTIANGIOGENIC THERAPY: ISSUES AND EXPECTATIONS

The understanding that angiogenesis is essential for tumor growth and metastasis formation has led to a large effort to discover effective antiangiogenic compounds. It must be understood that angiogenesis occurs not only in pathologic processes but also in homeostasis. Physiologic angiogenesis is important in reproduction, wound healing, menses, and vascular diseases such as coronary artery and peripheral vascular diseases. Thus, as always, a balance must be maintained between limiting angiogenesis to the tumor and causing significant toxicity to the host.

In addition to the potential toxicity, another issue in antiangiogenic therapy is the chronic nature of this therapy. Because antiangiogenic therapy is designed to inhibit the development of new blood vessels, the end points for success or failure must be redefined. For example, a desired response to standard chemotherapy is one that decreases the cross-sectional area of a tumor by 50% within a few months. However, antiangiogenic therapy is likely to produce stable disease, which early on may be considered a failure. Thus, in evaluating antiangiogenic therapy in the clinic or the laboratory, different criteria for effectiveness must be outlined.

Because antiangiogenic therapy may not decrease tumor growth, it is likely that this therapy will need to be delivered on a chronic basis. Hence, the agent must be easily delivered (i.e., oral) and have few long-term side effects. One must also consider that the effect of antiangiogenic therapy may require a longer interval between evaluations than does chemotherapy, as the stability of disease may be difficult to determine at short intervals.

There have, of course, been reports of complete regression of tumors in experimental models of angiogenesis.[61,132] However, these reports are few, and the vast majority of studies in this field have demonstrated that antiangiogenic therapy leads to an inhibition of tumor growth.[133,134] Thus, it is critical that the reader be able to interpret experimental studies appropriately and avoid creating unrealistic expectations. For example, the sites of tumor injection must be considered when experimental antiangiogenic studies are being conducted. It is clear that endothelia from different organs are phenotypically distinct[104] and that therapy effective at one site may be ineffective at another site. In addition, the growth and patterns of metastases depend on the site of injection.[135] Thus, the most relevant model for evaluating antiangiogenic therapy is an orthotopic model in which the tumor is growing in the appropriate host environment. Moreover, in designing experiments or reading the literature, it is important to determine whether antiangiogenic therapy is being designed as (1) a chemopreventive agent (delivered prior to or at the time of tumor inoculation), (2) adjuvant therapy (delivered when the tumor is at a relatively small volume, such as shortly after tumor injection), or (3) a therapeutic modality (delivered to animals with established tumors).

In evaluating responses to antiangiogenic therapy, one must define the end points prior to initiation of the study. Typically, tumor size or mass is determined at initiation of therapy and at termination of the study. As a surrogate means of assessing drug activity, biopsies of accessible tumors can be obtained for immunohistochemical staining to determine vessel counts, tumor cell proliferation and apoptotic rates, and endothelial cell proliferation and apoptotic rates. More important, survival studies may better assess the effectiveness of antiangiogenic therapy.

Preclinical data suggest that the efficacy of a conventional cytotoxic drug can be improved by combination with an angiogenesis inhibitor.[136] Indeed, a number of antiangiogenic clinical trials currently in progress have been designed to compare the effects of a particular cytotoxic agent alone with the effects of the same agent in combination with an angiogenesis inhibitor. Clearly, the success of Herceptin in improving the effects of cytotoxic chemotherapy in a proportion of advanced-stage breast cancer patients has enhanced the credibility of this strategy of evaluating cytostatic drugs.[137] This could allow conventional end points, such as tumor shrinkage and prolonged survival of very sick patients, to be used, albeit indirectly, as a convenient means of more rapidly assessing the merit of antiangiogenic drugs.

Another possible approach to effect tumor vascular growth could be the increased use of improved antivascular targeting strategies that can cause acute tumor regression, as shown in various preclinical models. For example, certain tubulin-binding agents,[138] such as combretastatin A-4, can cause such an effect,[139,140] as can antibodies that target tissue factor to newly formed blood vessels, thus causing an intravascular thrombogenic response in such vessels.[141] These drugs kill endothelial cells of newly formed blood vessels by different mechanisms[139] that result in vascular collapse and the subsequent death of much larger numbers of tumor cells. Clearly, the problem here will be to develop drugs that have this ability to cause such a dramatic tumor infarction[141] without major, perhaps even life-threatening, toxic side effects. In this regard, a potentially significant development in the near future could be the use of genomics-based technologies to uncover a large number of highly (or even totally) specific molecular markers for the activated endothelial cells of newly formed blood vessels. This could make antibody-based therapeutics safer and more effective.

Cytostatic antiangiogenic agents have the desired biologic (i.e., antiangiogenic) effect *in vivo.* In experimental animal models, tumors can be resected and analyzed for such changes as the extent of vascularization, vascular structure, and endothelial cell viability or apoptosis as well as for markers of angiogenic activity (e.g., expression of VEGF, bFGF, IL-8). Performing serial biopsies of metastatic tumors will not be practical; thus, reliable surrogate markers of tumor angiogenesis found in serum or urine may be necessary. At present, few, if any such markers (at least of a reliable nature) exist. The use of noninvasive medical imaging strategies (e.g., magnetic resonance imaging, Doppler ultrasound) to monitor changes in tumor blood flow, vascular structure, and permeability may be helpful, and considerable research efforts to determine their efficacy are under way.[142–145]

Toxic effects associated with chronic antiangiogenic therapy may not show up in short-term early-phase clinical trials or in animal models but, rather, only after very protracted courses of therapy. The development of spastic diplegia in some infants or children who had been treated previously and successfully over 1 year with antiangiogenic (IFN-α2-B) therapy for their life-threatening hemangiomas[146] is an example of such delayed toxic side effects. This undoubtedly will increase the need for targeting tumor blood vessels. The growing interrelationship between the clotting and fibrinolytic pathways and angiogenesis[66] raises the possibility of inciting bleeding and coagulation disorders in patients who receive certain antiangiogenic drugs, as well as the possibility of causing or exacerbating existing cardiovascular defects in older patients. In addition, there is the obvious concern about affecting physiologic forms of angiogenesis in various situations. Thus, wound healing may be adversely affected in a cancer patient who is receiving antiangiogenic drugs, as reproductive angiogenesis would be (e.g., corpus luteum development in adult women and development of the vasculature in embryos). Growth in neonates may also be compromised by angiogenesis inhibitor therapies.[147] However, given the unique structural features of the tumor vasculature, some angiogenesis inhibitors may selectively block tumor angiogenesis without actually affecting other physiologic forms of angiogenesis. This possibility could turn out to be an important factor in selecting the optimal angiogenesis inhibitors for clinical development and their use in cancer patients.

ANTIANGIOGENIC THERAPY AS A COMPONENT OF OTHER ANTINEOPLASTIC REGIMENS

The combination of an antiangiogenic drug (or drugs), such as TNP-470, with a conventional cytotoxic agent, such as cisplatin, paclitaxel, or cyclophosphamide, can significantly improve the antitumor efficacy of the cytotoxic drug.[136] These effects of combination therapy, which have also been observed for the combination of radiation therapy and angiogenesis inhibitors,[148] could play a significant role in the clinical evaluation and effects of angiogenesis inhibitors.

A more rational, yet futuristic, approach to the treatment of patients with malignancies is to determine the molecular alterations that lead to the various processes involved in tumor growth. Angiogenesis is but one component of the process of tumor growth and metastasis, and overexpression of other genes involved in protection from apoptosis, cell proliferation, and cell invasion (i.e., an individual tumor's malignant fingerprint) must be examined. With the rapid development of gene chip technology, it may be possible in the future to determine the malignant fingerprint of individual tumors and to develop therapies that specifically target the molecular phenotype of an individual tumor. Antiangiogenic therapy may therefore be one component of diverse biologic therapy delivered in combination with anti–growth factor therapy or with agents that induce apoptosis in tumor cells and tumor vessel endothelial cells.

CONCLUSIONS

Angiogenesis is a dynamic process essential for the growth of primary and metastatic malignancies as well as hematopoietic cancers. Understanding of the basic principles of the biology of angiogenesis has led to the development of new prognostic factors, tumor markers, imaging techniques, and therapeutic modalities. The challenge lies in integrating this knowledge into the care of patients with malignant diseases of all types and stages. An understanding of the basic biology of angiogenesis and tumor biology ultimately will lead to the rational implementation of new paradigms for the treatment of patients with cancer.

A comprehensive review of current antiangiogenic clinical trials is not feasible, as this area of clinical research is in constant evolution. However, the U.S. National Cancer Institute maintains an up-to-date Web site at which information on clinical trials can be accessed: http://cancertrials.nci.nih.gov/news/angio/table.html. In addition, an overview of antiangiogenesis can be found at http://cancertrials.nci.nih.gov/news/angio/index.html/.

Acknowledgments

This work was supported in part by Cancer Center Support Core grant CA16672 and grant R35-CA42107 (I.J.F.), grant CA41223 (R.S.K.), grant R01-CA74821 (L.M.E.) from the U.S. National Cancer Institute, National Institutes of Health, and grant MT-5815 from the Medical Research Council of Canada (R.S.K.).

REFERENCES

1. Fidler IJ, Ellis LM. The implications of angiogenesis to the biology and therapy of cancer metastasis. *Cell* 1994;79:185.
2. Folkman J. Angiogenesis in cancer, vascular, rheumatoid and other disease. *Nature Med* 1995;1:27.
3. Liotta LA, Steeg PS, Settler-Stevenson WG. Cancer metastasis and angiogenesis: an imbalance of positive and negative regulation. *Cell* 1991;64:327.
4. Auerbach W, Auerbach R. Angiogenesis inhibition: a review. *Pharmacol Ther* 1994;63:265.
5. Hanahan D, Folkman J. Patterns and emerging mechanisms of the angiogenic switch during tumorigenesis. *Cell* 1996;86:353.
6. Senger DR, Galli SJ, Dvorak AM, et al. Tumor cells secrete a vascular permeability factor that promotes accumulation of ascites fluid. *Science* 1983;219:983.
7. Connolly DT, Heuvelman DM, Nelson R, et al. Tumor vascular permeability factor stimulates endothelial cell growth and angiogenesis. *J Clin Invest* 1989;84:1470.
8. Ferrara N, Henzel WJ. Pituitary follicular cells secrete a novel heparin-binding growth factor specific for vascular endothelial cells. *Biochem Biophys Res Commun* 1989;161:851.
9. Gospodarowicz D, Abraham JA, Schilling J. Isolation and characterization of a vascular endothelial cell mitogen produced by pituitary-derived folliculo stellate cells. *Proc Natl Acad Sci U S A* 1989;86:7311.
10. Thomas KA. Vascular endothelial growth factor, a potent and selective angiogenic agent. *J Biol Chem* 1996;271:603.
11. Dvorak HF, Nagy JA, Berse B, et al. Vascular permeability factor, fibrin, and the pathogenesis of tumor stroma formation. *Ann NY Acad Sci* 1992;667:101.
12. Ziegler BL, Valtieri M, Porada GA, et al. KDR receptor: a key marker defining hematopoietic stem cells. *Science* 1999;285:1553.
13. Ferrer FA, Miller LJ, Lindquist R, et al. Expression of vascular endothelial growth factor receptors in human prostate cancer. *Urology* 1999;53:567.
14. Veikkola T, Karkkainen, M, Claesson-Welsh L, Alitalo K. Regulation of angiogenesis via vascular endothelial growth factor receptors. *Cancer Res* 2000;60:203.
15. Olofsson B, Korpelainen E, Pepper MS, et al. Vascular endothelial growth factor B (VEGF-B) binds to VEGF receptor-1 and regulates plasminogen activator activity in endothelial cells. *Proc Natl Acad Sci U S A* 1998;95:11709.
16. Tsurusaki T, Kanda S, Sakai H, et al. Vascular endothelial growth factor-C expression in human prostatic carcinoma and its relationship to lymph node metastasis. *Br J Cancer* 1999;80:309.
17. Veikkola T, Alitalo K. VEGFs, receptors, and angiogenesis. *Semin Cancer Biol* 1999;9:211.
18. Salven P, Lymboussaki A, Heikkila P, et al. Vascular endothelial growth factors VEGF-B and VEGF-C are expressed in human tumors. *Am J Pathol* 1998;153:103.
19. Lymboussaki A, Partanen TA, Olofsson B, et al. Expression of the vascular endothelial growth factor C receptor VEGFR-3 in lymphatic endothelium of the skin and in vascular tumors. *Am J Pathol* 1998;153:395.
20. Marconcini L, Marchio S, Morbidelli L, et al. c-Fos-induced growth factor/vascular endothelial growth factor D induces angiogenesis *in vivo* and *in vitro*. *Proc Natl Acad Sci U S A* 1999;96:9671.
21. Achen MG, Jeltsch M, Kukk E, et al. Vascular endothelial growth factor D (VEGF-D) is a ligand for the tyrosine kinases VEGF receptor 2 (Flk1) and VEGF receptor 3 (Flt4). *Proc Natl Acad Sci U S A* 1998;95:548.
22. Meyer M, Clauss M, Lepple-Wienhues A, et al. A novel vascular endothelial growth factor encoded by Orf virus, VEGF-E, mediates angiogenesis via signaling through VEGFR-2 (KDR) but not VEGFR-1 (Flt-1) receptor tyrosine kinases. *EMBO J* 1999;18:363.
23. Ogawa S, Oku A, Sawano A, et al. A novel type of vascular endothelial growth factor, VEGF-E (NZ-7 VEGF), preferentially utilizes KDR/Flk-1 receptor and carries a potent mitotic activity without heparin-binding domain. *J Biol Chem* 1998;273:31273.
24. Papapetropoulos A, Garcia-Cardena G, Dengler TJ, et al. Direct actions of angiopoietin-1 on human endothelium: evidence for network stabilization, cell survival, and interaction with other angiogenic growth factors. *Lab Invest* 1999;79:213.
25. Davis S, Yancopoulos GD. The angiopoietins: Yin and Yang in angiogenesis. *Curr Topics Microbiol Immunol* 1999;237:173.
26. Holash J, Maisonpierre PC, Compton D, et al. Vessel cooperation, regression, and growth in tumors mediated by angiopoietins and VEGF. *Science* 1999;284:1994.
27. Gale NW, Yancopoulos GD. Growth factors acting via endothelial cell–specific receptor tyrosine kinases: VEGFs, angiopoietins, and ephrins in vascular development. *Genes Dev* 1999;13:1055.
28. Patan S. TIE1 and TIE2 receptor tyrosine kinases inversely regulate embryonic angiogenesis by the mechanism of intussusceptive microvascular growth. *Microvasc Res* 1998;56:1.
29. Suri C, Jones PF, Patan S, et al. Requisite role of angiopoietin-1, a ligand for the TIE2 receptor, during embryonic angiogenesis. *Cell* 1996;87:1171.
30. Moore BB, Arenberg DA, Addison CL, Keane MP, Strieter RM. Tumor angiogenesis is regulated by CXC chemokines. *J Lab Clin Med* 1998;132:97.
31. Kumar R, Yoneda J, Bucana CD, Fidler IJ. Regulation of distinct steps of angiogenesis by different angiogenic molecules. *Int J Oncol* 1998;12:749.
32. Polverini PJ, Leibovich JS. Induction of neovascularization *in vivo* and endothelial proliferation *in vitro* by tumor-associated macrophages. *Lab Invest* 1984;51:635.
33. Sunderkotter C, Steinbrink K, Goebeler M, et al. Macrophages and angiogenesis. *J Leukoc Biol* 1994;55:410.
34. Leek RD, Harris AL, Lewis CE. Cytokine networks in solid human tumors: regulation of angiogenesis. *J Leukoc Biol* 1994;56:423.
35. Gutman M, Singh RK, Yoon S, et al. Leukocyte-induced angiogenesis and subcutaneous growth of B16 melanoma. *Cancer Biother* 1994;9:163.
36. Noh R, Karp GI, Devereaux DF. The effect of doxorubicin and mitoxanthrone on wound healing. *Cancer Chemother Pharmacol* 1991;29:141.
37. Fidler IJ. Modulation of the organ microenvironment for the treatment of cancer metastasis [Editorial]. *J Natl Cancer Inst* 1995;84:1588.
38. Takahashi Y, Bucana CD, Liu W, et al. Platelet derived endothelial cell growth factor in human colon cancer angiogenesis: role of infiltrating cells. *J Natl Cancer Inst* 1996;88:1146.
39. Polverini PJ. How the extracellular matrix and macrophages contribute to angiogenesis-dependent diseases. *Eur J Cancer* 1996;32A:2430.
40. DiPietro LA, Polverini PJ. Angiogenic macrophages produce the angiogenic inhibitor thrombospondin 1. *Am J Pathol* 1993;143:678.
41. Lingen MW, Polverini PJ, Bouck N. Retinoic acid induces cells cultured from oral squamous cell carcinomas to become antiangiogenic. *Am J Pathol* 1996;149:247.
42. O'Reilly MS, Holmgren L, Shing Y, et al. Angiostatin: a novel angiogenesis inhibitor that mediates the suppression of metastases by a Lewis lung carcinoma. *Cell* 1994;79:315.
43. Dong Z, Kumar R, Yang X, Fidler IJ. Macrophage-derived metalloelastase is responsible for the generation of angiostatin in Lewis lung carcinoma. *Cell* 1997;88:801.
44. Shweiki D, Itin A, Stoffer D, Keshet E. Vascular endothelial growth factor induced by hypoxia may mediate hypoxia-initiated angiogenesis. *Nature* 1992;359:843.
45. Levy AP, Levy NS, Wegner S, Goldberg MA. Transcriptional regulation of the rat vascular endothelial growth factor gene by hypoxia. *J Biol Chem* 1995;270:13333.
46. Griffiths L, Dachs GU, Bicknell R, Harris AL, Stratford IJ. The influence of oxygen tension and pH on the expression of platelet-derived endothelial cell growth factor/thymidine phosphorylase in human breast tumor cells grown *in vitro* and *in vivo*. *Cancer Res* 1997;57:570.
47. Hartmann A, Kunz M, Kostlin S, et al. Hypoxia-induced up-regulation of angiogenin in human malignant melanoma. *Cancer Res* 1999;59:1578.
48. Desbaillets I, Diserens AC, Tribolet N, Hamou MF, Meir EGV. Upregulation of interleukin 8 by oxygen-deprived cells in glioblastoma suggests a role in leukocyte activation, chemotaxis, and angiogenesis. *J Exp Med* 1997;186:1201.
49. Akagi Y, Liu W, Xie K, Zebrowski B, Ellis LM. Regulation of vascular endothelial growth factor expression in human colon cancer by insulin-like growth factor-I. *Cancer Res* 1998;58:4008.
50. Akagi Y, Liu W, Xie K, et al. Regulation of vascular endothelial growth factor expression in human colon cancer by interleukin-1. *Br J Cancer* 1999;80:150b.
51. Tsai JC, Goldman CK, Gillespie GY. Vascular endothelial growth factor in human glioma cell lines: induced secretion by EGF, PDGF-BB, and bFGF. *J Neurosurg* 1995;82:864.
52. Ellis LM, Staley CA, Liu W, et al. Downregulation of vascular endothelial growth factor in a human colon carcinoma cell line transfected with an antisense expression vector specific for c-src. *J Biol Chem* 1998;273:1052.
53. Bouvet M, Ellis LM, Nishizaki M, et al. Adenovirally mediated wild-type p53 gene transfer down-regulates vascular endothelial growth factor expression and inhibits angiogenesis in human colon cancer. *Cancer Res* 1998;58:2288.
54. Pal S, Claffey KP, Dvorak HF, Mukhopadhyay D. The von Hippel-Lindau gene product inhibits vascular permeability factor/vascular endothelial growth factor expression in renal cell carcinoma by blocking protein kinase C pathways. *J Biol Chem* 1997;272:27509.
55. Levy AP, Levy NS, Goldberg MA. Hypoxia-inducible protein binding to vascular endothelial growth factor mRNA and its modulation by the von Hippel-Lindau protein. *J Biol Chem* 1996;271:25492.
56. Dameron KM, Volpert OV, Tainsky MA, Bouk N. Control of angiogenesis in fibroblasts by p53 regulation of thrombospondin-1. *Science* 1994;265:1502.
57. Tolsma SS, Volpert OV, Good DJ, et al. Peptides derived from two separate domains of the matrix protein thrombospondin-1 have anti-angiogenic activity. *J Cell Biol* 1993;122:497.

58. Singh RK, Gutman M, Bucana CD, et al. Interferons alpha and beta downregulate the expression of basic fibroblast growth factor in human carcinoma. *Proc Natl Acad Sci U S A* 1995;92:4562.
59. Ezekowitz RAB, Mulliken JB, Folkman J. Interferon alpha-2a therapy for life-threatening hemangiomas of infancy. *N Engl J Med* 1992;326:1456-1463.
60. Clapp C, Martial JA, Guzman RC, Rentier-Delrue F, Weiner RI. The 16-kilodalton N-terminal fragment of human prolactin is a potent inhibitor of angiogenesis. *Endocrinology* 1993;133:1292.
61. O'Reilly MS, Boehm T, Shing Y, et al. Endostatin: an endogenous inhibitor of angiogenesis and tumor growth. *Cell* 1997;88:277.
62. Zhai Y, Ni J, Jiang GW, et al. VEGI, a novel cytokine of the tumor necrosis factor family, is an angiogenesis inhibitor that suppresses the growth of colon carcinomas *in vivo*. *FASEB J* 1999;13:181.
63. Pike SE, Yao L, Jones KD, et al. Vasostatin, a calretriculin fragment, inhibits angiogenesis and suppresses tumor growth. *J Exp Med* 1998;188:2349.
64. Vasquez F, Hastings G, Ortega MA, et al. METH-1, a human ortholog of ADAMTS-1, and METH-2 are members of a new family of proteins with angioinhibitory activity. *J Biol Chem* 1999;274:23349.
65. Gupta SK, Hassel T, Singh JP. A potent inhibitor of endothelial cell proliferation is generated by proteolytic cleavage of the chemokine platelet factor 4. *Proc Natl Acad Sci U S A* 1995;92:7799.
66. O'Reilly MS, Pirie-Shepherd S, Lane WS, Folkman J. Antiangiogenic activity of the cleaved conformation of the Serpin antithrombin III. *Science* 1999;285:1926.
67. Folkman J. Angiogenesis inhibitors generated by tumors. *Mol Med* 1995;1:120.
68. Rak J, Mitsuhashi Y, Bayko L, et al. Mutant ras oncogenes upregulate VEGF/VPF expression: implications for induction and inhibition of tumor angiogenesis. *Cancer Res* 1995;55:4575.
69. Viloria-Petit AM, Rak J, Hung MC, et al. Neutralizing antibodies against EGF and ErbB-2/neu receptor tyrosine kinases downregulate VEGF production by tumor cells in vitro and in vivo: angiogenic implications for signal transduction therapy of solid tumors. *Am J Pathol* 1997;151:1523.
70. Weidner N, Semple JP, Welch WR, Folkman J. Tumor angiogenesis and metastasis-correlation in invasive breast cancer. *N Engl J Med* 1991;324:1.
71. Gasparini G, Weidner N, Bevilacqua P, et al. Tumor microvessel density, p53 expression, tumor size, and peritumoral lymphatic vessel invasion are relevant prognostic markers in node-negative breast carcinoma. *J Clin Oncol* 1994;12:454.
72. Weidner N, Folkman J, Pozza F, et al. Tumor angiogenesis: a new significant and independent prognostic indicator in early-stage breast carcinoma. *J Natl Cancer Inst* 1992;84:1875.
73. Toi M, Kashitani J, Tominaga T. Tumor angiogenesis is an independent prognostic indicator in primary breast carcinoma. *Int J Cancer* 1993;55:371.
74. Obermair A, Czerwenka K, Kurz C, Kaider A, Sevelda P. Tumoral vascular density in breast tumors and their effect on recurrence-free survival. *Chirurg* 1994;65:611.
75. Visscher DW, Smilanetz S, Drozdowicz S, Wykes SM. Prognostic significance of image morphometric microvessel enumeration in breast carcinoma. *Anal Quant Cytol Histol* 1993;15:88.
76. Horak ER, Leek R, Klenk N, et al. Angiogenesis, assessed by platelet/endothelial cell adhesion molecule antibodies, as an indicator of node metastases and survival in breast cancer. *Lancet* 1992;340:1120.
77. Bosari S, Lee AKC, DeLellis RA, et al. Microvessel quantitation and prognosis in invasive breast carcinoma. *Hum Pathol* 1992;23:755.
78. Axelsson K, Ljung BM, Moore DH 2nd, et al. Tumor angiogenesis as a prognostic assay for invasive ductal breast carcinoma. *J Natl Cancer Inst* 1995;87:997.
79. Hall N, Fish D, Hunt N, et al. Is the relationship between angiogenesis and metastasis in breast cancer real? *Surg Oncol* 1992;1:223.
80. Van Hoef ME, Knox WF, Dhesi SS, Howell A, Schor AM. Assessment of tumour vascularity as a prognostic factor in lymph node negative invasive breast cancer. *Eur J Cancer* 1993;29A:1141.
81. Weidner N, Carroll PR, Flax J, Flumenfeld W, Folkman J. Tumor angiogenesis correlates with metastasis in invasive prostate carcinoma. *Am J Pathol* 1993;143:401.
82. Takahashi Y, Cleary KR, Mai M, et al. Significance of vessel count and vascular endothelial growth factor and its receptor (KDR) in intestinal-type gastric cancer. *Clin Cancer Res* 1996;2:1679.
83. Takahashi Y, Kitadai Y, Bucana CD, Cleary KR, Ellis LM. Expression of vascular endothelial growth factor and its receptor, KDR, correlates with vascularity, metastasis, and proliferation of human colon cancer. *Cancer Res* 1995;55:3964.
84. Maeda K, Chung YS, Takatsuka S, et al. Tumour angiogenesis and tumour cell proliferation as prognostic indicators in gastric carcinoma. *Br J Cancer* 1995;72:319.
85. Hollingsworth HC, Kohn EC, Steinberg SM, Rothenberg ML, Meriono MJ. Tumor angiogenesis in advanced stage ovarian carcinoma. *Am J Pathol* 1995;147:33.
86. Graham CH, Rivers J, Kerbel RS, Stankiewicz KS, White WL. Extent of vascularization as a prognostic indicator in thin (<0.76 mm) malignant melanomas. *Am J Pathol* 1994;145:510.
87. Ellis LM, Fidler IJ. Angiogenesis and breast cancer metastasis. *Lancet* 1995;346:388.
88. Fidler IJ. Tumor heterogeneity and the biology of cancer invasion and metastasis. *Cancer Res* 1978;38:2651.
89. Fidler IJ. Critical factors in the biology of human cancer metastasis: twenty-eighth GHA Clowes Memorial Award Lecture. *Cancer Res* 1990;50:6130.
90. Fidler IJ, Hart IR. Biological diversity in metastatic neoplasms: origins and implications. *Science* 1982;217:998.
91. Liotta LA, Stetler-Stevenson WG. Tumor invasion and metastasis: an imbalance of positive and negative regulation [Review]. *Cancer Res* 1991;51:5054s.
92. Poste G, Fidler IJ. The pathogenesis of cancer metastasis. *Nature* 1979;283:139.
93. Kitadai Y, Ellis LM, Takahashi Y, et al. Multiparametric *in situ* mRNA hybridization analysis to detect metastasis-related genes in surgical specimens of human colon carcinomas. *Clin Cancer Res* 1995;1:1095.
94. Singh RK, Bucana CD, Gutman M, et al. Organ site-dependent expression of basic fibroblast growth factor in human renal cell carcinoma cells. *Am J Pathol* 1994;145:365.
95. Vermeulen PB, Gasparini G, Fox SB, et al. Quantification of angiogenesis in solid human tumours: an international consensus on the methodology and criteria of evaluation. *Eur J Cancer* 1996;32A:2474.
96. Makris A, Powles TJ, Kakolyris S, et al. Reduction in angiogenesis after neoadjuvant chemoendocrine therapy in patients with operable breast carcinoma. *Cancer* 1999;85:1996.
97. Angeletti CA, Lucchi M, Fontanini G, et al. Prognostic significance of tumoral angiogenesis in completely resected late stage lung carcinoma (stage IIIA-N2): impact of adjuvant therapies in a subset of patients at high risk of recurrence. *Cancer* 1996;78:409.
98. Viens P, Jacquemier J, Bardou VJ, et al. Association of angiogenesis and poor prognosis in node-positive patients receiving anthracycline-based adjuvant chemotherapy. *Breast Cancer Res Treat* 1999;54:205.
99. Gasparini G, Harris AL. Clinical importance of the determination of tumor angiogenesis in breast carcinoma: much more than a new prognostic tool. *J Clin Oncol* 1995;13:765.
100. Gasparini G, Toi M, Miceli R, et al. Clinical relevance of vascular endothelial growth factor and thymidine phosphorylase in patients with node-positive breast cancer treated with either adjuvant chemotherapy or hormone therapy. *Cancer J Sci Am* 1999;5:101.
101. Brooks PC, Montgomery AMP, Rosenfeld M, et al. Integrin avb3 antagonists promote tumor regression by inducing apoptosis of angiogenic blood vessels. *Cell* 1994;79:1157.
102. Stromblad S, Cheresh DA. Cell adhesion and angiogenesis. *Trends Cell Biol* 1996;6:462.
103. Gasparini G, Brooks PC, Biganzoli E, et al. Vascular integrin alpha(v)beta3: a new prognostic indicator in breast cancer. *Clin Cancer Res* 1998;4:2625.
104. Pasqualini R, Ruoslahti E. Organ targeting *in vivo* using phage display peptide libraries. *Nature* 1996;380:364.
105. Bischoff J. Approaches to studying cell adhesion molecules in angiogenesis. *Trends Cell Biol* 1995;5:69.
106. Burrows FJ, Derbyshire EJ, Tazzari PL, et al. Upregulation of endoglin vascular endothelial cells in human solid tumors: implications for diagnosis and therapy. *Clin Cancer Res* 1995;1:1623.
107. Chang SS, Reuter VE, Heston WD, et al. Five different anti-prostate-specific membrane antigen (PSMA) antibodies confirm PSMA expression in tumor-associated neovasculature. *Cancer Res* 1999;59:3192.
108. Neri D, Carnemolla B, Nissim A, et al. Targeting by affinity-matured recombinant antibody fragments of an angiogenesis associated fibronectin isoform. *Nat Biotechnol* 1997;15:1271.
109. Hiraoka N, Allen E, Apel IJ, Gyetko MR, Weiss SJ. Matrix metalloproteinases regulate neovascularization by acting as pericellular fibrinolysins. *Cell* 1998;95:365.
110. Uze G, Lutgalla G, Morgensen KE. α and β Interferons and their receptors and their friends and relations. *J Interferon Cytokine Res* 1995;15:3.
111. Tamm I, Lin SL, Pfeffer LM, et al. Interferons alpha and beta as cellular regulatory molecules. In: Gresser I, ed. *Interferon 9*. London: Academic Press, 1987:13.
112. Rossi G. Interferons and cell differentiation. In: Gresser I, ed. *Interferon 6*. London: Academic Press, 1985:31.
113. Reznitzky D, Yarden A, Zipori D, et al. Autocrine β-related interferon controls c-myc suppression and growth arrest during hematopoietic cell differentiation. *Cell* 1986;46:31.
114. Strander H. Interferon treatment of human neoplasia: effects on the immune system. *Adv Cancer Res* 1986;46:36.
115. Ferrantini M, Proietti E, Santodonato L, et al. α1-Interferon gene transfer into metastatic Friend leukemia cells abrogated tumorigenicity in immunocompetent mice: antitumor therapy by means of interferon-producing cells. *Cancer Res* 1993;53:1107.
116. Gresser I, Belardelli F, Maury C, et al. Injection of mice with antibody to interferon enhances the growth of transplantable murine tumors. *J Exp Med* 1983;158:2095.
117. Gutterman JU. Cytokine therapeutics: lessons from interferon α. *Proc Natl Acad Sci U S A* 1994;91:1198.
118. Johns TG, Mackay IR, Callister KA, et al. Antiproliferative potencies of interferons on melanoma cell lines and xenografts: higher efficacy of interferon-β. *J Natl Cancer Inst* 1992;84:1185.
119. Sica G, Fabbroni L, Castagnetta L, et al. Antiproliferative effect of interferons on human prostate carcinoma cell lines. *Urol Res* 1989;17:111.
120. Heyns AP, Eldor A, Vlodavsky I, et al. The antiproliferative effect of interferon and the mitogenic activity of growth factors are independent cell cycle events. *Exp Cell Res* 1985;161:297.
121. Friesel R, Komoriya A, Maciag T. Inhibition of endothelial cell proliferation by gamma-interferon. *J Cell Biol* 1987;104:689.
122. Ruszczak Z, Detmar M, Imcke E, et al. Effects of rIFN-α, -β, -γ on the morphology, proliferation, and cell surface antigen expression of human dermal microvascular endothelial cells *in vitro*. *J Invest Dermatol* 1990;95:693.
123. Hicks C, Breit SN, Penny R. Response of microvascular endothelial cells to biological response modifiers. *Immunol Cell Biol* 1989;67:271.
124. Orchard PJ, Smith CM, Woods WG. Treatment of hemangioendotheliomas with interferon-alpha. *Lancet* 1989;2:565.
125. White CW, Sondheimer HM, Crouch EC, et al. Treatment of pulmonary hemangiomatosis with recombinant interferon-α-2a. *N Engl J Med* 1989;320:1197.
126. Mitsuyasu RT. Interferon alpha in the treatment of AIDS-related Kaposi's sarcoma. *Br J Haematol* 1991;79:69.
127. Kaban LB, Mulliken JB, Ezekowitz RA, et al. Antiangiogenic therapy of a recurrent giant cell tumor of the mandible with interferon alpha-2a. *Pediatrics* 1999;103:1145.
128. Stadler WM, Kuzel TM, Raghavan D, et al. Metastatic bladder cancer: advances in treatment. *Eur J Cancer* 1997;33:23.
129. Nguyen M, Watanabe H, Budson AE, et al. Elevated levels of an angiogenic peptide, basic fibroblast growth factor, in the urine of patients with a wide spectrum of cancers. *J Natl Cancer Inst* 1994;86:356.

130. Nanus DM, Schmitz-Drager BJ, Motzer RJ, et al. Expression of basic fibroblast growth factor in primary human renal tumors: correlation with poor survival. *J Natl Cancer Inst* 1994;85:1597.
131. Dinney CPN, Bielenberg DR, Reich R, et al. Inhibition of basic fibroblast growth factor expression, angiogenesis, and growth of human bladder carcinoma in mice by systemic interferon-alpha administration. *Cancer Res* 1998;58:808.
132. Lode HN, Moehler T, Xiang R, et al. Synergy between an antiangiogenic integrin alpha antagonist and an antibody-cytokine fusion protein eradicates spontaneous tumor metastases. *Proc Natl Acad Sci U S A* 1999;96:1591.
133. Warren RS, Yuan H, Matli MR, Gillett NA, Ferrara N. Regulation by vascular endothelial growth factor of human colon cancer tumorigenesis in a mouse model of experimental liver metastasis. *J Clin Invest* 1995;95:1789.
134. Shaheen RM, Davis DW, Liu W, et al. Antiangiogenic therapy targeting the tyrosine kinase receptor for vascular endothelial growth factor receptor inhibits the growth of colon cancer liver metastasis and induces tumor and endothelial cell apoptosis. *Cancer Res* 1999;59:5412.
135. Takahashi Y, Mai M, Wilson MR, et al. Site-dependent expression of vascular endothelial growth factor, angiogenesis and proliferation in human gastric carcinoma. *Int J Oncol* 1996;8:701.
136. Teicher BA. Potentiation of cytotoxic cancer therapies by antiangiogenic agents. In: Teicher BA, ed. *Antiangiogenic agents in cancer therapy.* Totowa, NJ: Humana Press, 1999:277.
137. Pegram MD, Lipton A, Hayes DF, et al. Phase II study of receptor-enhanced chemosensitivity using recombinant humanized anti-p185HER2/neu monoclonal antibody plus cisplatin in patients with HER2/neu-overexpressing metastatic breast cancer refractory to chemotherapy treatment. *J Clin Oncol* 1998;16:2659.
138. Chaplin DJ, Pettit GR, Parkins CS, Hill SA. Antivascular approaches to solid tumour therapy: evaluation of tubulin binding agents. *Br J Cancer* 1996;74[Suppl 27]:S86.
139. Dark GG, Hill SA, Prise VE, et al. Combretastatin A-4, an agent that displays potent and selective toxicity toward tumor vasculature. *Cancer Res* 1997;57:1829.
140. Iyer S, Chaplin DJ, Rosenthal DS, et al. Induction of apoptosis in proliferating human endothelial cells by the tumor-specific antiangiogenesis agent combretastatin A-4. *Cancer Res* 1998;58:4510.
141. Huang X, Molema G, King S, et al. Tumor infarction in mice by antibody-directed targeting of tissue factor to tumor vasculature. *Science* 1997;275:547.
142. Frouge C, Guinebretiere JM, Contesso G, Di Paola R, Blery M. Correlation between contrast enhancement in dynamic magnetic resonance imaging of the breast and tumor angiogenesis. *Invest Radiol* 1994;29:1043.
143. Cohen FM, Kuwatsuru R, Shames DM, et al. Contrast-enhanced magnetic resonance imaging estimation of altered capillary permeability in experimental mammary carcinomas after X-irradiation. *Invest Radiol* 1994;29:970.
144. Pham CD, Roberts TP, van Bruggen N, et al. Magnetic resonance imaging detects suppression of tumor vascular permeability after administration of antibody to vascular endothelial growth factor. *Cancer Invest* 1998;16:225.
145. Wu CC, Lee CN, Chen TM, et al. Incremental angiogenesis assessed by color Doppler ultrasound in the tumorigenesis of ovarian neoplasms. *Cancer* 1994;73:1251.
146. Barlow CF, Priebe CJ, Mulliken JB, et al. Spastic diplegia as a complication of interferon alfa-2a treatment of hemangiomas of infancy. *J Pediatr* 1998;132:527.
147. Gerber HP, Hillan KJ, Ryan AM, et al. VEGF is required for growth and survival in neonatal mice. *Development* 1999;126:1149.
148. Mauceri HJ, Hanna NN, Beckett MA, et al. Combined effects of angiostatin and ionizing radiation in antitumour therapy. *Nature* 1998;394:287.
149. Baird A, Klagsbrun M. The fibroblast growth factor family. *Cancer Cells* 1991;3:239.
150. Gimenez-Gallego G, Cuevas P. Fibroblast growth factors, proteins with a broad spectrum of biological activities. *Neurol Res* 1994;16:313.
151. Schmitt FC, Soares R. TGF-α and angiogenesis. *Am J Surg Pathol* 1999;23:358.
152. Mooradian DL, Diglio CA. Effects of epidermal growth factor and transforming growth factor-β1 on rat heart endothelial cell anchorage-dependent and -independent growth. *Exp Cell Res* 1990;186:122.
153. Lamszus K, Laterra J, Westphal, M, Rosen EM. Scatter factor/hepatocyte growth factor (SF/HGF) content and function in human gliomas. *Int J Dev Neurosci* 1999;17:517.
154. Pepper MS. Transforming growth factor-beta: vasculogenesis, angiogenesis, and vessel wall integrity. *Cytokine Growth Factor Rev* 1997;8:21.
155. Yoshida S, Ono M, Shono T, et al. Involvement of interleukin-8, vascular endothelial growth factor, and basic fibroblast growth factor in tumor necrosis factor alpha-dependent angiogenesis. *Mol Cell Biol* 1997;17:4015.
156. Kuwabara K, Ogawa S, Matsumoto M, et al. Hypoxia-mediated induction of acidic/basic fibroblast growth factor and platelet-derived growth factor in mononuclear phagocytes stimulates growth of hypoxic endothelial cells. *Proc Natl Acad Sci U S A* 1995;92:4606.
157. Bussolino F, Ziche M, Wang JM, et al. *In vitro* and *in vivo* activation of endothelial cells by colony-stimulating factors. *J Clin Invest* 1991;87:986.
158. Choudhuri R, Zhang HT, Donnini S, Ziche M, Bicknell R. An angiogenic role for the neurokines midkine and pleiotrophin in tumorigenesis. *Cancer Res* 1997;57:1814.
159. Jackson D, Volpert OV, Bouck N, Linzer DI. Stimulation and inhibition of angiogenesis by placental proliferin and proliferin-related protein. *Science* 1994;266:1581.
160. Ramchandran R, Dhanabal M, Volk R, et al. Antiangiogenic activity of restin, NC10 domain of human collagen XV: comparison to endostatin. *Biochem Biophys Res Commun* 1999;255:735.
161. Sage EH. Pieces of eight: bioactive fragments of extracellular proteins as regulators of angiogenesis. *Trends Biol Sci* 1999,7.182.
162. Maisonpierre PC, Suri C, Jones PF, et al. Angiopoietin-2, a natural antagonist for Tie2 that disrupts *in vivo* angiogenesis. *Science* 1997;277:55.
163. Moore BB, Arenberg, DA, Addison CL, Keane MP, Strieter RM. Tumor angiogenesis is regulated by CXC chemokines. *J Lab Clin Med* 1998;132:97.
164. Dedhar S, Hannigan GE, Rak J, Kerbel RS. Extracellular environment and cancer. In: Tannock I, Hill RP (eds). *Basic science of oncology.* New York: McGraw-Hill, 1998:197.

CHAPTER 10

Etiology of Cancer: Viruses

SECTION 1

ERIC M. POESCHLA
GARY L. BUCHSCHACHER, JR.
FLOSSIE WONG-STALL

RNA Viruses

RNA viruses, particularly retroviruses, have been studied as important causes of human cancer and as tools for understanding both viral and nonviral oncogenesis at the molecular level. The retrovirus human T-cell leukemia virus type I (HTLV-I) is the causative agent of adult T-cell leukemia (ATL). Two other RNA viruses, human immunodeficiency virus (HIV) and hepatitis C virus (HCV), are strongly associated with human malignancies. In addition, the discovery and characterization of oncogenes and the subsequent elucidation of protooncogene functions have been closely intertwined with the study of retroviruses.

Retroviruses have been classified on the basis of pathogenic roles into Oncovirinae (tumor viruses), Lentivirinae (genetically complex agents, including HIV), and Spumavirinae (foamy viruses, not known to be associated with human disease). Other classifications based on particle morphology (virus types A–D) and genetic relatedness[1,2] also are used. To illustrate different molecular mechanisms of oncogenesis, this discussion is principally concerned with the Oncovirinae, including the mammalian type C tumor viruses, the avian leukemia/sarcoma viruses, and HTLV-I and -II. The roles played by HIV in the various malignancies associated with acquired immunodeficiency syndrome (AIDS) and by HCV (a flavivirus) in hepatocellular carcinoma (HCC) also are discussed. In all examples, although these virus infections may play key initiating or contributory roles to carcinogenesis, additional, sequential alteration of cellular DNA is generally required to yield the fully malignant phenotype.[3]

RETROVIRAL GENETICS: SELECTIVE ACCESS TO THE GROWTH CONTROL GENES OF THE CELL

Special features of their replication cycle have made retroviruses useful for investigating the molecular basis of neoplasia. Retroviruses are unique among animal viruses in having an RNA genome that replicates through a DNA intermediate. The virally encoded reverse transcriptase converts the single-stranded RNA genome into a double-stranded DNA copy; a subsequent reaction catalyzed by the retroviral integrase covalently and irreversibly integrates this DNA molecule into a host chromosome where it resides as a provirus. This process can result in mutagenesis, translocation, or altered regulation of any locus in the genome.[4,5]

An integrated provirus resembles other multiexon cellular genes in that it is duplicated along with the cell's genome, passed on to daughter cells during mitosis, and subsequently transcribed into full-length and spliced RNAs [messenger RNAs (mRNAs)]. The ends of the provirus are made up of identical genetic control regions called *long terminal repeats* (LTRs), which are composed of U3 (unique 3' region), R (repeat), and U5 (unique 5' region). The promoter and enhancer functions necessary for RNA polymerase II to initiate viral mRNA transcription reside within the LTR, primarily in U3. Transcription initiates just downstream of the TATA box at the 5' U3/R junction and proceeds through to the polyadenylation (polyA) signal usually located in the R region of the 3' LTR (Fig. 10.1-1).

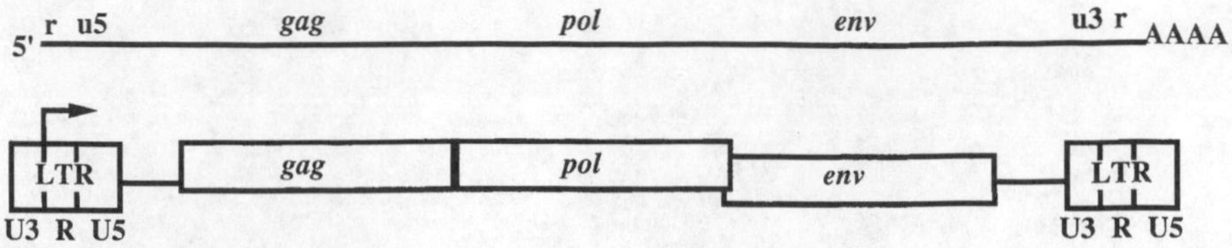

FIGURE 10.1-1. Retrovirus genome organization. General genome structure of a typical replication-competent oncoretrovirus. The structure of the double-stranded DNA copy (provirus) is shown below that of the genomic RNA. In the provirus, *gag* (encoding viral core proteins), *pol* (viral replication enzymes), and *env* (viral envelope glycoproteins) genes are flanked on each end by the long terminal repeats (LTR). The viral promoter is located in the 5' U3 region, with transcription termination and poly A signals located in the 3' LTR. The arrow indicates point and direction of transcription initiation. R, repeat.

The locations of transcription initiation and termination result in virion (genomic) RNA that carries the viral promoter (U3 element) downstream of the genes to be transcribed (in contrast to the structure of the provirus). Because a genomic transcript possesses neither an upstream U3 nor a downstream U5, the essential rearrangements that occur during the RNA template strand switching of reverse transcription are establishment of a 5' promoter and of integration-competent termini. The retention of a duplicate U3 promoter element in the 3' LTR of the provirus, though generally not active, has implications for retroviral oncogenesis.

Retrovirus virions normally encapsidate a dimer of identical plus-sense RNA genomes, both of which are used as templates during reverse transcription. However, it is possible for nonidentical transcripts (heterodimers) to be packaged together. Studies with dual selectable markers show that each infectious virion, even if heterozygous, produces only one provirus. Heterodimer packaging plays an important role in the creation of oncogenic retroviruses because, after recombination and reverse transcription, it can result in the creation of novel proviruses. Even when identical RNAs are packaged, aberrant strand transfers during reverse transcription result in high rates of genetic recombination and rearrangement, including sequence deletions, duplications, and inversions.[1,5–8] Recombination can occur between two viruses infecting the same cell or, less commonly, between viral and cellular sequences.

MECHANISMS OF RETROVIRAL ONCOGENESIS

In the case of acutely transforming retroviruses such as Rous sarcoma virus (RSV), virtually all infected cells are swiftly transformed, whereas for other retroviruses, transformation is an unusual and much delayed outcome that often depends on the cell's accrual of additional alteration of its DNA. The latter group includes agents such as HTLV-I and avian leukosis virus (ALV). Most transforming retroviruses are not cytopathic. Reverse transcription and integration of the viral genome into that of the cell favor the three major mechanisms by which retroviruses may participate in the malignant transformation process (Fig. 10.1-2):

1. Acutely transforming retroviruses (e.g., RSV) incorporate and exert control over cellular growth–related genes (protooncogene capture) and subsequently transfer these deregulated genes into new cells.
2. Slowly transforming viruses (e.g., ALV) alter cellular gene expression by chance insertion of *cis*-acting viral regulatory sequences adjacent to these genes (insertional mutagenesis).
3. *Trans*-acting retroviruses (e.g., HTLV-I) alter cellular gene expression and function through viral regulatory protein(s) that act in *trans.*

ACUTELY TRANSFORMING (TRANSDUCING) RETROVIRUSES AND GENE CAPTURE

Acutely transforming retroviruses provided evidence for viral oncogenesis even before the existence of viruses was recognized. A porcelain filtrate of tumor lysates prepared from chicken sarcomas was shown to cause sarcomas when injected into animals. The causative agent, RSV, is a prototype of the acutely transforming (transducing) retroviruses. It is the only replication-competent oncogene-carrying retrovirus; since oncogene insertions usually supplant essential viral sequences, all other known acutely transforming retroviruses are defective for replication and require a helper virus to supply one or more viral proteins in *trans.* RSV contains the full complement of replicative genes in addition to a transforming gene.

It was not until the 1940s that the first mammalian retrovirus, mouse mammary tumor virus, was isolated; later, a murine leukemia virus was isolated from neonatal mice. Investigation of the actual physical nature of these agents awaited the advent of cell culture, elucidation of the genetic code, and the framework of the "central dogma" (i.e., genetic information flow proceeds unidirectionally from DNA to RNA to protein). The term *retrovirus* was coined when Temin and Mizutani[9] and Baltimore[10] overturned this dogma with their co-discovery of reverse transcriptase in 1970.

RSV mutants defective only for transformation but not for replication were isolated. The mutants were either conditional (temperature-sensitive) or nonconditional. The latter had genomes roughly 20% shorter in length than the oncogenic strain of RSV.[11] Molecular hybridization experiments revealed that the missing "oncogenic" sequences hybridized not only to DNA from infected chicken cells but also to normal chicken, human, and even invertebrate DNA.[11] The inference was that the sequence (*v-src*) was not a native viral gene but rather an altered version of a normal cellular homologue (*c-src*) that had been captured by RSV at some unknown point in evolution. Such cellular genes are designated protooncogenes (or c-oncs). All retroviral v-oncs are dispensable for viral replication, and in

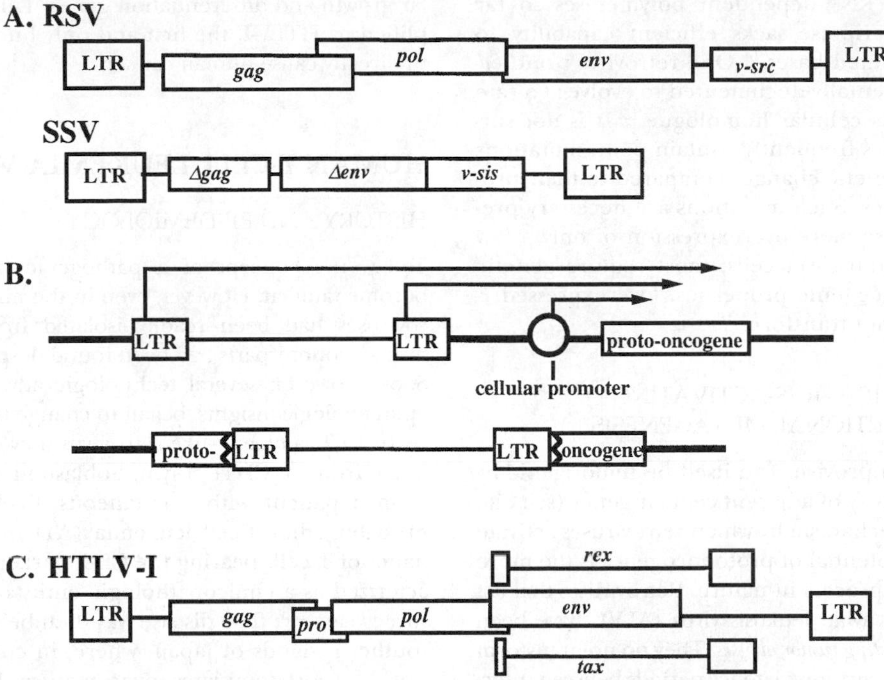

FIGURE 10.1-2. Three types of oncogenic retroviruses. **A:** Acutely transforming retroviruses. Rous sarcoma virus (RSV) and simian sarcoma virus (SSV), retroviruses that contain oncogenes, are shown. RSV is unique in that the oncogene, *v-src,* has been added to the viral genome without concomitant loss of replicative genes. SSV, an example of the more common oncogene-containing retroviruses, is not replication-competent; the recombination that led to *v-sis* insertion resulted in deletion of some viral sequences. **B:** Slowly transforming retroviruses. In the upper example, a provirus has integrated upstream of a cellular protooncogene. The viral promoters may alter protooncogene expression directly [via read-through transcription originating from the 5' long terminal repeat (LTR) or from transcripts aberrantly originating in the 3' LTR] or indirectly via the effect of viral enhancers increasing transcription from cellular promoters (the viral enhancer can also affect expression of cellular genes 5' to, and in the opposite orientation of, the site of provirus integration). In the lower example, insertional mutagenesis is illustrated. This may lead to inactivation of a tumor suppressor or to production of a mutant cellular protein that could lead to oncogenesis. In both cases, aberrant splicing could lead to production of chimeric viral-cellular proteins. Arrows indicate points of initiation and direction of transcription. **C:** *Trans*-acting retroviruses. In addition to *gag, pol,* and *env,* human T-cell leukemia virus type I (HTLV-I) encodes viral regulatory proteins. Tax is implicated in the genesis of adult T-cell leukemia through its interactions with cellular transcription factors, resulting in alteration of expression of many growth-related genes.

all cases homology exists to cellular genes conserved over long evolutionary distances.

The genetic mechanism whereby retroviruses captured and transduced oncogenes remained surprisingly ambiguous for more than a decade after the characterization of RSV and other transforming retroviruses. Two prevailing models postulate that recombination, generally illegitimate (nonhomologous), occurs after a retrovirus integrates in the vicinity of a protooncogene. Both models require co-packaging into one virion of an abnormal viral transcript containing cellular sequences with that of another viral genome. They differ in the level at which the initial rearrangement takes place. The first model proposes two different events, with the first being a presumably rare deletion of the 3' portion of an integrated provirus. The key feature is that deletion of the 3' LTR brings internal retroviral sequences in contiguity with a downstream protooncogene. The hybrid transcript initiated in the 5' LTR is then processed (e.g., by splicing) and packaged into virions along with a wild-type genome from another provirus infecting the same cell. After infection of another cell, illegitimate recombination during reverse transcription then provides the oncogene-containing molecule with a 3' LTR that supports integration and, in some cases, subsequent replication. In the second model, no deletion of chromosomal DNA is required.[12] Transduction of sequences downstream of the provirus is instead accomplished at the posttranscriptional level by packaging of RNA transcripts generated when RNA polymerase II terminates inefficiently at the retroviral polyadenylation signal in the R repeat. The model postulates co-packaging of such read-through transcripts, followed by illegitimate recombination during reverse transcription. Direct evidence has been obtained for such a mechanism by placing a selectable drug marker transcriptional unit downstream of Rous-associated virus, with and without mutations of the viral polyadenylation signal.[12]

Increased mutation is another dramatic consequence that arises from the transfer of cellular sequences from the host genome into the genome of retroviruses. The point mutation rates of RNA viruses (10^{-3} to 10^{-5} per nucleotide per replication cycle) are roughly 1 million–fold in excess of cellular DNA.[13] Like all RNA-dependent polymerases so far studied, reverse transcriptase lacks efficient capability to proofread misincorporated bases.[14] One retroviral v-onc (*v-mos*) has been experimentally documented to evolve at a rate 10^6-fold higher than its cellular homologue.[15] It is not surprising, then, that v-oncs frequently contain point mutations in addition to other genetic changes compared to their protooncogene homologues. Such mutations are necessary preludes to cancer, because mere overexpression of only a few protooncogenes can transform cells; most require genetic alteration for their oncogenic properties. Overexpressed *c-src*, for example, does not transform.[16]

SLOWLY TRANSFORMING (*CIS*-ACTIVATING) RETROVIRUSES: INSERTIONAL MUTAGENESIS

Genomic insertion of a provirus can itself be tumorigenic by leading to aberrant activity of adjacent cellular genes (see Fig. 10.1-2). This second mechanism by which retroviruses activate the latent oncogenic potential of protooncogenes is the more common transforming process in nature. Retroviruses that act in this manner, such as avian leukosis virus (ALV), have been termed *chronic*, or *slow-acting tumor viruses*. They do not transform cells in tissue culture. *In vivo*, long latency periods between infection and tumorigenesis are typical, whereas acutely transforming retroviruses reliably transform cultured cells and cause tumors with high probability shortly after infection. Also in contrast to acutely transforming retroviruses, the tumors are monoclonal for the site of insertion. In general, slowly transforming viruses require a second mutagenic event for their transforming properties to become apparent.

In B-cell lymphomas associated with ALV, tumors arising from independent transformation events invariably have ALV proviruses clonally integrated in the vicinity of the *c-myc* gene.[17] These tumors illustrate two general ways in which insertional mutagenesis may operate: promoter insertion and enhancer insertion. In the former, the ALV provirus integrates upstream of, and in the same orientation as, *c-myc*. 3' LTR-promoted *c-myc* transcripts are produced at up to 100-fold higher than normal levels (the transcripts, however, encode a normal *c-myc* protein). Enhancer insertion, however, can occur if the provirus inserts downstream of *c-myc*, or upstream but in opposite orientation to the gene. In this scenario, enhancer elements within the LTR may abnormally increase gene expression. These two roles of retroviruses in studies of *myc*—gene capture and insertional mutagenesis—elegantly confirm the protooncogene hypothesis: The gene was first identified as a protooncogene not from insertional mutagenesis studies, but from its mutant v-onc homologue in a transforming retrovirus.[2,4]

A related transforming mechanism occurs when insertion of a retrovirus occurs within the c-onc itself or if the 5' LTR-promoted read-through RNAs result in downstream protooncogene transcription.[18] In either case, viral-protooncogene hybrid spliced transcripts encoding novel proteins with transforming potential can then be produced.

TRANS-ACTIVATING RETROVIRUSES

A third mechanism of transformation involves a *trans*-acting viral protein that regulates the expression or function of cellular growth and differentiation genes. This mechanism is exemplified by HTLV-I, the first and only human retrovirus known to directly cause human cancer.

HUMAN T-CELL LEUKEMIA VIRUS TYPE I

HISTORY AND EPIDEMIOLOGY

Today, the concept of a pathogenic human retrovirus has become familiar. However, even in the mid-1970s, although retroviruses had been readily isolated from many species, no human counterparts had been found despite intensive attempts. Soon, however, several technologic advances, combined with epidemiologic insights, began to change the picture.[19,20]

In 1978, a type C–like retrovirus now called *HTLV-I* was isolated from a CD4+ T-lymphoblastoid cell line established from a patient with a cutaneous T-cell lymphoma,[21] most probably adult T-cell leukemia (ATL). An aggressive malignancy of T cells bearing the CD4 marker, ATL had been characterized as a clinicopathologic entity only in the preceding three years.[22,23] The disease was then believed confined to the southern islands of Japan, where, in contrast to most of the world, it predominates over mature B-cell leukemia/lymphoma. The geographic clustering suggested an infectious etiology, and serologic testing of Japanese ATL patients with antigens prepared from the newly discovered HTLV-I revealed nearly 100% seropositivity.[24,25] Other epidemiologic clusters consistent with an etiologic role for endemic HTLV-I infection have since been documented, most notably in the Caribbean basin, the southeastern United States, northeastern South America, Central Africa, and Papua New Guinea. Moreover, transmission of HTLV-I by blood transfusion (but, unlike HIV, not cell-free blood products), needle sharing, breast feeding, and from male to female (rarely the reverse) by sexual intercourse has been well documented.

In addition to seroepidemiologic studies of patients and their close contacts, several lines of evidence support a direct causal role for HTLV-I in ATL. The virus can be isolated reproducibly from ATL patients. Leukemic cells invariably contain an HTLV-I provirus, whereas other cells from these patients do not. Infected individuals born in an endemic region carry their risk of developing ATL with them if they move elsewhere, suggesting that risk is not dependent on environmental cofactors peculiar to endemic areas. Infection clearly precedes transformation, because the tumor cells carry monoclonal or oligoclonal insertions of HTLV-I DNA and have a single T-cell antigen receptor-β gene rearrangement.[26,27] This monoclonality also provides additional evidence that transformation is a rare sequel to infection.

Primary T cells infected with HTLV-I do not senesce after a month in culture, as normal T cells do, but become immortalized, acquiring the ability to divide continually in the presence of interleukin-2 (IL-2). Continued culture of immortalized cells eventually can result in selection of a transformed, IL-2–independent clone of cells. There is evidence that, in addition to CD4+ T cells (the phenotype of the majority of ATLs), HTLV-I can also infect and transform CD8+ T cells, as well as immature CD4– CD8– T-cell precursors in bone marrow.[28]

THE VIRAL REPLICATION CYCLE AND ITS IMPLICATIONS FOR VIRAL SPREAD AND EVOLUTION

Although HTLV-I shares many features with the type C viruses, it is considerably more complex genetically and biologically. In addition to *gag*, *pol*, and *env*, the virus genome contains several additional open reading frames (see Fig. 10.1-2). Of these, the two best characterized genes code the *trans*-regulating proteins Tax and Rex. Both proteins are expressed early in the viral replication cycle and are important for expression of viral genes; as such, they are analogous to the HIV proteins Tat and Rev.[29–32] Rex and Rev, through an interaction with a human nuclear export receptor, CRM-1,[33,34] act as adaptors for the nuclear export of unspliced retroviral mRNA. Additional cellular proteins interfacing with the splicing/export pathways are also involved in mediating Rev/Rex function.[35] Tax is a nuclear protein that activates transcription from the HTLV-I LTR in *trans* by associating with a number of cellular transcription factors.[36–38] A 21-base-pair repeat sequence within the HTLV-I U3 is necessary for Tax activity and confers Tax inducibility to heterologous genes placed downstream.[39,40]

Little, if any, HLTV-I replication or gene expression is detectable *in vivo* by analyzing primary leukemic cells from humans[41,42]; significant viremia is not detected. The molecular mechanisms that maintain viral latency *in vivo* are unclear. The *in vivo* latency and low levels of viremia in HTLV patients has important implications both for virus spread and evolution. Unlike HIV, there is remarkably little genetic variability among HTLV-I isolates,[43] with 97% to 99% sequence identity among strains derived from Japanese patients and generally 96% to 99% identity across widely diverse geographic regions.[41] Again, unlike HIV, cell-free transmission rarely occurs, either in cell culture or *in vivo*. This property is one factor in the less efficient, endemic transmission of HTLV-I compared to the epidemic spread of HIV-1, even though the same routes of infection appear to be operative.

When a cytopathic virus such as HIV rapidly destroys its host cell, continuous viral spread is imperative. The alternative adopted by HTLV-I is to keep virion burden low but promote gradually accelerating amplification of cells harboring transcriptionally quiescent proviral DNA over the course of the host organism's lifetime. Because infection is by cell transfer, spread in the population is thereby promoted and only in some cases does the process ultimately give rise to frank leukemia.

MODELS FOR HTLV-I LEUKEMOGENESIS

The most common outcome of HTLV-I infection is an asymptomatic carrier state; HTLV-I carriers have an estimated lifetime risk of developing ATL of approximately 5%.[44] Therefore, factors other than simple viral infection must be necessary for leukemogenesis. Despite the mono- or oligoclonality of HTLV-I proviral insertions in ATL tumors, the sites of proviral insertion are random from patient to patient, indicating that *cis*-acting insertional mutagenesis does not play a role in tumorigenesis. Nor does the virus appear to encode a host-derived oncogene: No homologies between human cellular genes and nonstructural HTLV-I genes have been observed. A third genetic mechanism for tumorigenesis, which appears to be a multistep process, is thus implicated, with the Tax protein being central to transformation.

Tax promotes viral gene expression by indirectly activating the viral promoter in the LTR via interaction with cellular transcription proteins. However, the interaction of Tax with various transcription factors also transactivates numerous cellular gene promoters. A molecular basis for the pleiotropism of Tax was shown to reside in its interaction with the conserved basic regions of varied basic region–leucine zipper DNA-binding domains within such factors, thus altering both affinity and selectivity of the factors for varied cellular promoters.[45,46] The numerous cellular transcription pathways activated by Tax in this way include activating transcription factor/cyclic AMP-responsive element binding protein(ATF/CREB), nuclear factor (NF)-κB/c-Rel, and serum response factor.[47,48] Tax is able to bind directly to the TATA-binding protein, a component of the transcriptional complex, and to p300 and CREB-binding protein, both of which are transcriptional coactivators.[49]

Among the cellular genes transactivated by Tax, the most relevant are the IL-2 and IL-2 receptor (IL-2R) genes.[36,50–52] Unlike normal resting T cells, ATL cells and T cells transformed *in vitro* by HTLV-I constitutively express the α chain of the IL-2 receptor at high levels that cannot be down-regulated. In this way, an autocrine loop might arise, stimulating continuous proliferation of infected cells. The autocrine mechanism is not sufficient to explain leukemogenesis, however. For example, in contrast to the invariable expression of IL-2R, not all HTLV-I immortalized cells express IL-2.[53] Possible interactions between another HTLV-I protein (p12I) and the gamma subunit of IL-2R may contribute to the ligand-independent activation of this receptor,[54] resulting in stimulation and expansion of the pool of infected cells at risk for further genetic alteration.

In regard to the latter process, Tax also has been shown to down-regulate expression of a cellular DNA repair enzyme, beta-DNA polymerase,[55] a potentially straightforward link to accelerated accumulation of mutation. In addition, expression of a large number of genes involved in cell proliferation is transactivated by Tax. These include granulocyte-macrophage colony-stimulating factor (GM-CSF), the protooncogenes *c-fos* and *c-sis*, HLA class I molecules,[56] vimentin, and tumor necrosis factor.[19,20,41,42]

The IL-2 independence of HTLV-I–infected T cells involves a cell signaling pathway in which receptor-associated protein kinases in the Janus kinase (Jak) family phosphorylate cytoplasmic transcription factors called *STATS* (for signal transducers and activators of transcription).[57] After phosphorylation, STATS translocate to the cell nucleus and bind to specific DNA elements to modulate transcription. The Jak-STAT pathway is triggered by IL-2 in normal T cells; however, transition to IL-2 independence after HTLV-I infection was associated with constitutive activation of the pathway.[58,59]

Tax also has been shown to interact with and presumably inactivate a number of cell-cycle–related proteins, including the cyclin-dependent kinase (cdk) inhibitor $p16^{INK4A}$ and the cell-cycle checkpoint protein MAD1.[47,60,61] Tax activates the promoter of $p21^{waf1/cip1}$, also a cdk inhibitor, and through the activation of the ATF/CREB pathway, suppresses the activity of p53, which can prevent p53-induced apoptosis.[47,54,60] It also has been suggested that constitutive action of the IL-2 receptor pathway allows cells, through an unknown mechanism, to avoid apoptosis.[62]

In summary, although the exact steps in HTLV-I–induced leukemogenesis are unclear, Tax seems to play a critical role by direct interaction with cellular proteins involved in transcription, cell-cycle regulation, cell proliferation, and apoptosis. Whatever the role of the virus, however, it seems that a second mutational event is necessary for the transition from cell immortalization to monoclonality and acute ATL. Immortalization and propagation of cells probably allows alterations in the cell cycle and apoptosis pathways to accumulate, allowing a transformed clone to emerge.

CLINICAL FEATURES OF HTLV-I DISEASE

The clinical presentation, differential diagnosis, and treatment of ATL are discussed elsewhere in this volume, but are described briefly here.[44] In acute ATL, the tumor aggressively infiltrates multiple organs, commonly involving lymph nodes, liver, spleen, skin, and lung. Median survival is measured in months. The age of onset averages 58 years (range, 24 to 85 years), with a male to female ratio of 1.4:1. Either a leukemic or a non–Hodgkin's T-cell lymphoma presentation may predominate. ATL has been classified into four stages: acute, chronic, smoldering, and lymphomatous.[63] Hypercalcemia is commonly seen in the acute and lymphomatous types; death is often the result of opportunistic infection.

The differential diagnosis includes mycosis fungoides, Sézary syndrome, Hodgkin's disease, and T-cell chronic lymphocytic leukemia. HTLV-I seropositivity, negative terminal deoxynucleotidal transferase (TdT) staining, and CD4 positivity are characteristic of ATL. Detection of a mono- or oligoclonally integrated HTLV-I provirus makes the diagnosis definitive.

In addition to ATL, HTLV-I is also associated with tropical spastic paraparesis/HTLV-associated myelopathy (TSP/HAM), a chronic progressive neurologic disorder.[44]

HUMAN T-CELL LEUKEMIA VIRUS TYPE II

HTLV-II is closely related to HTLV-I, sharing the same overall genetic organization and 70% homology at the amino acid level. Although it also infects and transforms T cells *in vitro*, HTLV-II is preferentially tropic *in vitro* for the CD8+ subset.[64] The virus was isolated in 1982 from a patient with atypical T-cell variant hairy cell leukemia and subsequently from two other individuals.[65] Other disease associations have been reported; however, convincing epidemiologic data for an etiologic role for HTLV-II in human disease are lacking. Most patients with either T- or B-cell hairy cell leukemia are not HTLV-II infected, and so far no disease has a demonstrated increased incidence in HTLV-II–infected populations. In contrast to HTLV-I, HTLV-II is able to transform T cells in a manner not dependent on activation of the Jak/STAT pathway,[66] although the exact mechanism of cell transformation by HTLV-II remains unknown.

HTLV-II is transmitted by the same routes as HTLV-I. Like HTLV-I, and unlike HIV, the genome of HTLV-II is quite stable. Again, this is postulated to be due largely to the latent infection and expansion of infected cells within a person and to transmission being mainly via infected cells, as opposed to free virus.[67] HTLV-II is recognized to be endemic in African pygmies and in many indigenous New World populations, including the Navajo, Pueblo, and Seminole Indians in North America, the Guyami Indians in Panama, and various quite widely separated and remote tribes in South America.[68]

HUMAN IMMUNODEFICIENCY VIRUS

Although the annual incidence of HIV infection in the United States declined in the late 1990s, HIV disease remains a formidable global health problem. New infections continue at a significant rate, particularly in parts of the world such as Southeast Asia. In addition, a large number of asymptomatic HIV-infected persons are expected to develop AIDS. Newer pharmacologic therapies have slowed the rate of progression to AIDS, but do not eradicate infection.[69,70] Treatment failures due to noncompliance or drug resistance are common, the drugs themselves have a number of potentially serious side effects, and the cost of lifelong therapy can be prohibitive, particularly in underdeveloped countries.

HIV-1 and HIV-2 are members of the lentivirus subfamily of retroviruses. It is now known that both viruses became human pathogens after zoonotic (cross-species) transmission to humans from primate reservoirs. Sooty mangabeys (*Cercocebus atys*) are the reservoir of simian immunodeficiency virus strain sm (SIVsm) and the probable ancestor of HIV-2.[71] A subspecies of common chimpanzee (*Pan troglodytes troglodytes*) inhabiting west equatorial Africa is the reservoir of SIVcpz and the source of at least three independent transmissions of this virus to humans, resulting in the evolution of HIV-1 groups M, N, and O.[72] The hunting and preparation of chimpanzees for food, a common practice in equatorial Africa, provides the most likely mechanism by which the zoonotic infections occurred. Although HIV-2 can also cause AIDS in humans and monkeys, the majority of AIDS cases worldwide are the result of HIV-1 infection. Therefore, this discussion focuses on HIV-1 disease.

As with HTLV-I, the HIV genome and replication cycle are complex (Fig. 10.1-3). In sharp contrast to HTLV-I, however, HIV replicates actively after initial infection, which results in high levels of viremia.[73–75] This high rate of replication, in concert with a high mutation rate, results in the extreme genetic variability that has been documented for HIV-1. This variability occurs both within individual patients, among patients, and between definable geographic subtypes.[13,74] HIV, unlike HTLV-I, is highly cytopathic for CD4+ T cells.

HIV encodes two *trans*-acting proteins, Tat and Rev, that are analogous in function to the HTLV proteins Tax and Rex.[76] Like HTLV-I Tax, HIV Tat is necessary for efficient expression from the viral promoter in the 5' LTR. At a molecular level, however, Tat and Tax act through different mechanisms. Instead of interacting indirectly with a region of the proviral LTR via interactions with cellular transcription factors, Tat interacts directly with a 5' region of HIV RNA known as the *trans*-activating region (TAR) and promotes processive transcription through further interactions with cellular factors that modify RNA polymerase II function.

In contrast, HTLV Rex and HIV Rev use similar mechanisms to promote expression of viral structural and enzymatic proteins. Rex and Rev bind to their respective RNA response elements, *rxre* and *rre*, to mediate the export of full length and singly spliced viral transcripts from the nucleus to the cytoplasm. In addition to Tat and Rev, HIV encodes a number of accessory proteins not found in other retroviruses.[76] These include Vif, Vpu, and Nef, the functions of which are not yet fully elucidated. The protein Vpr contributes to the ability of HIV to infect nondividing cells, a property unique to lentiviruses.

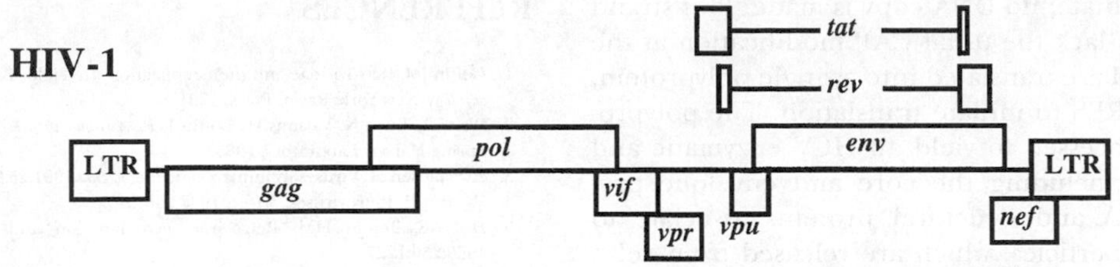

FIGURE 10.1-3. Human immunodeficiency virus (HIV) genome. Overall, the genomic organization of HIV is the same as for the simpler retroviruses, with *gag*, *pol*, and *env* genes flanked on each end by long terminal repeats (LTR). HIV also encodes other proteins involved in the viral replication cycle.

The immunodeficiency resulting from HIV infection can contribute to tumor development and patient prognosis. There is, however, little evidence that HIV is directly oncogenic.[77] Although HIV infection may contribute to the pathogenesis or complicate the treatment of neoplastic diseases, no viral protein has been shown to be directly transforming. Transduction of cellular oncogenes has not been observed. Despite rare reports of insertional mutagenesis resulting in T-cell lymphoma,[78] this disease does not occur disproportionately in HIV infection.

In HIV infected persons, non-Hodgkin's lymphoma, Kaposi's sarcoma (KS), Hodgkin's disease, and cervical cancer are all AIDS-defining illnesses. Many of the neoplasms common to AIDS patients are associated with infection by DNA viruses. These include human herpes virus-8 (HHV-8), Epstein-Barr virus (EBV), and human papillomavirus.[79] These viruses and their associations with oncogenesis are discussed in detail elsewhere in this volume, but are mentioned briefly here.

The tumor biology of KS is not well understood.[80] Unlike most tumors that have readily identifiable neoplastic cells, KS tumors are histologically complex. The predominant cell and the most likely candidate tumor cell of KS is the spindle cell, but other cells, including infiltrating leukocytes, are present in the tumor. It is unclear how much of the tumor is made up of true neoplastic cells versus hyperplastic, secondary inflammatory, or angiogenic cells. Instead of monoclonality, a polyclonal, multicentric proliferative process seems to occur, which is reflected in the frequently observed waxing and waning clinical course of KS. For example, lesions may disappear in one region, only to be supplanted by new lesions elsewhere. Although evidence supports HHV-8 as the etiologic agent of KS, HIV is clearly an important cofactor in KS development.

In addition to immunodeficiency induced by HIV-1 infection, the viral Tat protein also may be involved in the pathogenesis of KS. Tat increases the level of a variety of cytokines, including interferon-γ, tumor necrosis factor-α, IL-1, and IL-6.[81] These factors may promote growth of endothelial cells and production of angiogenic substances, including basic fibroblast growth factor and vascular endothelial growth factor.[82,83] Additionally, Tat protein that is released from HIV-infected cells can be taken up by other cells, thereby widening its potential effects.[84] Thus, a complex interplay between HIV, the cytokines induced by HIV infection, and HHV-8 may provide the microenvironment and stimulus for KS development.[80,85,86]

AIDS patients are also at increased risk for the development of non-Hodgkin's lymphomas.[87–89] The majority of these lymphomas are of B-cell origin, and many are associated with EBV infection or with rearrangements of *c-myc*. In general, these malignancies carry a poor prognosis. An aggressive form of non-Hodgkin's lymphoma seen in AIDS patients is primary central nervous system lymphoma, a malignancy that is rare in the general population. Unlike the systemic lymphomas, primary central nervous system non-Hodgkin's lymphoma is nearly universally associated with EBV infection. In this respect it is similar to the posttransplant lymphoproliferative disorder seen in organ transplant recipients. Another form of systemic non-Hodgkin's lymphoma, primary effusion lymphoma, has been associated with infection by HHV-8; co-infection of cells with EBV also has been observed.[90,91] Multicentric Castleman's disease also is associated with HHV-8 infection.[92] The role that HIV itself might play in the genesis of the AIDS-associated lymphoproliferative disorders is not clear. In addition to the immunosuppression caused by T-cell depletion, it has been theorized that HIV may contribute to lymphomagenesis by affecting cytokine production and by altering B-cell regulation.

Cervical carcinoma and anal squamous cell carcinoma are two other malignancies seen in AIDS patients; both are associated with human papillomavirus infection. These malignancies may present in a more advanced or invasive form than in non-HIV–infected patients. Immune suppression may support development of and complicates treatment of these tumors, but at this time there is no evidence that HIV plays a more direct role in their genesis.

HEPATITIS C VIRUS

HCV infection is a well-established risk factor for the development of hepatocellular carcinoma (HCC), although its role in oncogenesis may not be direct.[93,94] HCV belongs to the *Flaviviridae* family of viruses. Virions consist of a single-stranded plus sense RNA molecule surrounded by a nucleocapsid and envelope.[95] The viral genome is approximately 9500 nucleotides long and has a single, large open reading frame encoding viral proteins. The 5' leader sequence of the viral genome contains stem-loop structures, one of which acts as an internal ribosome entry site (IRES). The 5' end of the large open reading frame encodes the capsid (C) protein and envelope (E1,E2) glycoproteins, whereas the enzymatic proteins are encoded by the 3' end. These enzymatic proteins include a metalloprotease, a serine protease and helicase, and the RNA-dependent RNA polymerase responsible for viral nucleic acid replication. The extreme 3' end of the RNA genome contains a short untranslated region.

After entry into cells, the viral genome is replicated by the viral-encoded RNA-dependent RNA polymerase via a minus-strand RNA intermediate; no DNA copy is made. Plus strand viral RNA molecules lack the usual CAP modification at the 5' end of mRNAs and are translated into a single polyprotein, making use of the IRES to initiate translation. The polyprotein produced is processed to yield all HCV enzymatic and structural proteins, including the core and envelope proteins. Genomic RNA and structural proteins associate to form progeny virus particles, which are released from cells, most likely through the endoplasmic reticulum and host cell secretory pathways.

HCV is transmitted by contaminated blood products, by shared needles of intravenous drug users, perinatally, and via sexual routes, but in approximately 10% of cases known risk factors for transmission are not identified. It is estimated that approximately 3 million people in the United States are chronically infected with HCV.[96] HCV infection is strongly associated with the development of cirrhosis and HCC, although the regional prevalence of HCV infection in HCC varies.[96,97] HCV infection is chronic in 75% to 85% of cases, with a subset of people developing chronic hepatitis and cirrhosis. The rate of HCC development in those with cirrhosis is estimated to be 1% to 4% per year. However, an individual patient's risk for progression to HCC development is difficult to assess because many additional factors affect the likelihood of HCC development. For example, alcohol consumption or co-infection with hepatitis B virus greatly increases the relative risk for developing HCC.[98]

The role of HCV in HCC pathogenesis is not entirely clear. There is a 20- to 30-year period after initial HCV infection before development of HCC. It has been postulated that HCC largely develops indirectly as a result of the inflammatory responses that lead to hepatocyte destruction, regeneration, and fibrosis. Nevertheless, the virus may play a more direct role in neoplastic transformation of hepatocytes. For example, growing evidence suggests that the HCV core protein may contribute to tumor development.[99–101] Infection by different strains of HCV may also pose different levels of risk for HCC development. Many groups have reported that HCV genotype 1b confers an elevated risk for developing HCC. However, the observed effects were variable and not seen in all studies.[102–104]

For those infected with HCV, interferon-α therapy is effective in a minority of cases in stably reducing viral load and improving histologic hepatic changes.[105,106] In this subgroup of patients, the risk of HCC development appears to be decreased but not eliminated.[107–110] It is still not certain if this treatment can decrease permanently the risk of developing HCV-associated HCC. Treatment with both interferon and ribavirin, a synthetic guanosine analogue, can increase the number of sustained responders to treatment to 30% to 40%.[111] Unfortunately, attempts at early detection of HCV-associated HCC by ultrasound or α-fetoprotein levels have not proven effective in reducing HCC-related mortality.

In addition to infecting hepatocytes, HCV can infect hematopoietic cells, including lymphocytes and CD34+ precursor cells. Patients infected with HCV are suggested to be at increased risk for the development of B-cell non-Hodgkin's lymphoma.[112,113] This association, however, has not been observed in all studies. Further studies are needed to resolve fully the potential contribution of HCV infection to the development of some subtypes of B-cell lymphoproliferative disorders.

REFERENCES

1. Coffin JM. Retroviridae and their replication. In: Fields BN, Knipe DM, eds. *Fundamental virology.* New York: Raven Press, 1991.
2. Weiss R, Teich N, Varmus H, Coffin J. *RNA tumor viruses.* Cold Spring Harbor, NY: Cold Spring Harbor Laboratory, 1985.
3. zur Hausen H. Viruses in human cancers. *Science* 1991;254:1167.
4. Varmus H. Retroviruses. *Science* 1988;240:1427.
5. Hu WS, Temin HM. Retroviral recombination and reverse transcription. *Science* 1990;250:1227.
6. Hu WS, Temin HM. Genetic consequences of packaging two RNA genomes in one retroviral particle: pseudodiploidy and high rate of genetic recombination. *Proc Natl Acad Sci U S A* 1990;87:1556.
7. Temin HM. Sex and recombination in retroviruses. *Trends Genet* 1991;7:71.
8. Zhang J, Temin HM. Rate and mechanism of nonhomologous recombination during a single cycle of retroviral replication. *Science* 1993;259:234.
9. Temin HM, Mizutani S. RNA-dependent DNA polymerase in virions of Rous sarcoma virus. *Nature* 1970;226:1211.
10. Baltimore D. RNA-dependent DNA polymerase in virions of RNA tumour viruses. *Nature* 1970;226:1209.
11. Stehelin D, Varmus HE, Bishop JM, Vogt PK. DNA related to the transforming gene(s) of avian sarcoma viruses is present in normal avian DNA. *Nature* 1976;260:170.
12. Swain A, Coffin JM. Mechanism of transduction by retroviruses. *Science* 1992;255:841.
13. Domingo E, Holland J. Mutation rates and rapid evolution of RNA viruses. In: Morse S, ed. *The evolutionary biology of viruses.* New York: Raven Press, 1994:161.
14. Steinhauer DA, Domingo E, Holland JJ. Lack of evidence for proofreading mechanisms associated with an RNA virus polymerase. *Gene* 1992;122:281.
15. Gojobori T, Yokoyama S. Rates of evolution of the retroviral oncogene of Moloney murine sarcoma virus and of its cellular homologues. *Proc Natl Acad Sci U S A* 1985;82:4198.
16. Parker RC, Varmus HE, Bishop JM. Expression of v-src and chicken c-src in rat cells demonstrates qualitative differences between pp60v-src and pp60c-src. *Cell* 1984;37:131.
17. Hayward WS, Neel BG, Astrin SM. Activation of a cellular onc gene by promoter insertion in ALV-induced lymphoid leukosis. *Nature* 1981;290:475.
18. Nilsen TW, Maroney PA, Goodwin RG, et al. c-erbB activation in ALV-induced erythroblastosis: novel RNA processing and promoter insertion result in expression of an amino-truncated EGF receptor. *Cell* 1985;41:719.
19. Wong-Staal F, Gallo RC. Human T-lymphotropic retroviruses. *Nature* 1985;317:395.
20. Gallo RC. Human retroviruses: a decade of discovery and link with human disease. *J Infect Dis* 1991;164:235.
21. Poiesz BJ, Ruscetti FW, Reitz MS, Kalyanaraman VS, Gallo RC. Isolation of a new type C retrovirus (HTLV) in primary uncultured cells of a patient with Sézary T-cell leukaemia. *Nature* 1981;294:268.
22. Yodoi J, Takatsuki K, Masuda T. Two cases of T-cell chronic lymphocytic leukemia in Japan [Letter]. *N Engl J Med* 1974;290:572.
23. Uchiyama T, Yodoi J, Sagawa K, Takatsuki K, Uchino H. Adult T-cell leukemia: clinical and hematologic features of 16 cases. *Blood* 1977;50:481.
24. Robert-Guroff M, Nakao Y, Notake K, et al. Natural antibodies to human retrovirus HTLV in a cluster of Japanese patients with adult T cell leukemia. *Science* 1982;215:975.
25. Kalyanaraman VS, Sarngadharan MG, Nakao Y, et al. Natural antibodies to the structural core protein (p24) of the human T-cell leukemia (lymphoma) retrovirus found in sera of leukemia patients in Japan. *Proc Natl Acad Sci U S A* 1982;79:1653.
26. Jarrett RF, Mitsuya H, Mann DL, et al. Configuration and expression of the T cell receptor beta chain gene in human T-lymphotrophic virus I-infected cells. *J Exp Med* 1986;163:383.
27. Matsuoka M, Hagiya M, Hattori T, et al. Gene rearrangements of T cell receptor beta and gamma chains in HTLV-I infected primary neoplastic T cells. *Leukemia* 1988;2:84.
28. Markham PD, Salahuddin SZ, Macchi B, Robert-Guroff M, Gallo RC. Transformation of different phenotypic types of human bone marrow T-lymphocytes by HTLV-1. *Int J Cancer* 1984;33:13.
29. Chen IS, Slamon DJ, Rosenblatt JD, et al. The x gene is essential for HTLV replication. *Science* 1985;229:54.
30. Felber BK, Paskalis H, Kleinman-Ewing C, Wong-Staal F, Pavlakis GN. The pX protein of HTLV-I is a transcriptional activator of its long terminal repeats. *Science* 1985;229:675.
31. Wachsman W, Cann AJ, Williams JL, et al. HTLV x gene mutants exhibit novel transcriptional regulatory phenotypes. *Science* 1987;235:674.
32. Seiki M, Hikikoshi A, Taniguchi T, Yoshida M. Expression of the pX gene of HTLV-I. general splicing mechanism in the HTLV family. *Science* 1985;228:1532.
33. Fornerod M, Ohno M, Yoshida M, Mattaj IW. CRM1 is an export receptor for leucine-rich nuclear export signals. *Cell* 1997;90:1051.
34. Neville M, Stutz F, Lee L, Davis LI, Rosbash M. The importin-beta family member Crm1p bridges the interaction between Rev and the nuclear pore complex during nuclear export. *Curr Biol* 1997;7:767.
35. Li J, Tang H, Mullen TM, et al. A role for RNA helicase A in post-transcriptional regulation of HIV type 1. *Proc Natl Acad Sci U S A* 1999;96:709.
36. Leung K, Nabel GJ. HTLV-1 transactivator induces interleukin-2 receptor expression through an NF-kappa B–like factor. *Nature* 1988;333:776.
37. Nyborg JK, Dynan WS, Chen IS, Wachsman W. Binding of host-cell factors to DNA sequences in the long terminal repeat of human T-cell leukemia virus type I: implications for viral gene expression. *Proc Natl Acad Sci U S A* 1988;85:1457.
38. Armstrong AP, Franklin AA, Uittenbogaard MN, Giebler HA, Nyborg JK. Pleiotropic effect of the human T-cell leukemia virus Tax protein on the DNA binding activity of eukaryotic transcription factors. *Proc Natl Acad Sci U S A* 1993;90:7303.

39. Brady J, Jeang KT, Duvall J, Khoury G. Identification of p40x-responsive regulatory sequences within the human T-cell leukemia virus type I long terminal repeat. *J Virol* 1987;61:2175.
40. Fujisawa J, Seiki M, Sato M, Yoshida M. A transcriptional enhancer sequence of HTLV-I is responsible for *trans*-activation mediated by p40 chi HTLV-I. *Embo J* 1986;5:713.
41. Cann AJ, Chen ISY. Human T cell leukemia viruses types I and II. In: Fields BN, Knipe DM, eds. *Virology*. New York: Raven Press, 1990.
42. Feuer G, Chen IS. Mechanisms of human T-cell leukemia virus–induced leukemogenesis. *Biochim Biophys Acta* 1992;1114:223.
43. Wattel E, Vartanian JP, Pannetier C, Wain-Hobson S. Clonal expansion of human T-cell leukemia virus type I–infected cells in asymptomatic and symptomatic carriers without malignancy. *J Virol* 1995;69:2863.
44. Manns A, Hisada M, La Grenade L. Human T-lymphotropic virus type I infection. *Lancet* 1999;353:1951.
45. Perini G, Wagner S, Green MR. Recognition of bZIP proteins by the human T-cell leukaemia virus transactivator Tax. *Nature* 1995;376:602.
46. Baranger AM, Palmer CR, Hamm MK, et al. Mechanism of DNA-binding enhancement by the human T-cell leukaemia virus transactivator Tax. *Nature* 1995;376:606.
47. Bex F, Gaynor RB. Regulation of gene expression by HTLV-I Tax protein. *Methods* 1998;16:83.
48. Azimi N, Brown K, Bamford RN, et al. Human T cell lymphotropic virus type I Tax protein *trans*-activates interleukin 15 gene transcription through an NF-kappaB site. *Proc Natl Acad Sci U S A* 1998;95:2452.
49. Kwok RP, Laurance ME, Lundblad JR, et al. Control of cAMP-regulated enhancers by the viral transactivator Tax through CREB and the co-activator CBP. *Nature* 1996;380:642.
50. Inoue J, Seiki M, Taniguchi T, Tsuru S, Yoshida M. Induction of interleukin 2 receptor gene expression by p40x encoded by human T-cell leukemia virus type 1. *Embo J* 1986;5:2883.
51. Maruyama M, Shibuya H, Harada H, et al. Evidence for aberrant activation of the interleukin-2 autocrine loop by HTLV-1-encoded p40x and T3/Ti complex triggering. *Cell* 1987;48:343.
52. Siekevitz M, Feinberg MB, Holbrook N, Wong-Staal F, Greene WC. Activation of interleukin 2 and interleukin 2 receptor (Tac) promoter expression by the *trans*-activator (tat) gene product of human T-cell leukemia virus, type I. *Proc Natl Acad Sci U S A* 1987;84:5389.
53. Arya SK, Wong-Staal F, Gallo RC. T-cell growth factor gene: lack of expression in human T-cell leukemia-lymphoma virus–infected cells. *Science* 1984;223:1086.
54. Mulloy JC, Crownley RW, Fullen J, Leonard WJ, Franchini G. The human T-cell leukemia/lymphotropic virus type 1 p12I proteins bind the interleukin-2 receptor beta and gamma chains and affects their expression on the cell surface. *J Virol* 1996;70:3599.
55. Jeang KT, Widen SG, Semmes OJ, Wilson SH. HTLV-I *trans*-activator protein, tax, is a *trans*-repressor of the human beta-polymerase gene. *Science* 1990;247:1082.
56. Mann DL, Popovic M, Sarin P, et al. Cell lines producing human T-cell lymphoma virus show altered HLA expression. *Nature* 1983;305:58.
57. Darnell JE Jr, Kerr IM, Stark GR. Jak-STAT pathways and transcriptional activation in response to IFNs and other extracellular signaling proteins. *Science* 1994;264:1415.
58. Migone TS, Lin JX, Cereseto A, et al. Constitutively activated Jak-STAT pathway in T cells transformed with HTLV-I. *Science* 1995;269:79.
59. Takemoto S, Mulloy JC, Cereseto A, et al. Proliferation of adult T cell leukemia/lymphoma cells is associated with the constitutive activation of JAK/STAT proteins. *Proc Natl Acad Sci U S A* 1997;94:13897.
60. Hollsberg P. Mechanisms of T-cell activation by human T-cell lymphotropic virus type I. *Microbiol Mol Biol Rev* 1999;63:308.
61. Jin DY, Spencer F, Jeang KT. Human T cell leukemia virus type 1 oncoprotein Tax targets the human mitotic checkpoint protein MAD1. *Cell* 1998;93:81.
62. Cereseto A, Kislyakova T, Washington Parks R, Nicot C, Franchini G. Differential response to genotoxic stress in immortalized or transformed human T-lymphotropic virus type I–infected T-cells. *J Gen Virol* 1999;80:1575.
63. Shimoyama M. Diagnostic criteria and classification of clinical subtypes of adult T-cell leukaemia-lymphoma. A report from the Lymphoma Study Group (1984–87). *Br J Haematol* 1991;79:428.
64. Ijichi S, Ramundo MB, Takahashi H, Hall WW. *In vivo* cellular tropism of human T cell leukemia virus type II (HTLV-II). *J Exp Med* 1992;176:293.
65. Rosenblatt JD, Chen IS, Wachsman W. Infection with HTLV-I and HTLV-II: evolving concepts. *Semin Hematol* 1988;25:230.
66. Mulloy JC, Migone TS, Ross TM, et al. Human and simian T-cell leukemia viruses type 2 (HTLV-2 and STLV-2(pan-p)) transform T cells independently of Jak/STAT activation. *J Virol* 1998;72:4408.
67. Salemi M, Vandamme AM, Desmyter J, Casoli C, Bertazzoni U. The origin and evolution of human T-cell lymphotropic virus type II (HTLV-II) and the relationship with its replication strategy. *Gene* 1999;234:11.
68. Manns A, Blattner WA. The epidemiology of the human T-cell lymphotrophic virus type I and type II: etiologic role in human disease. *Transfusion* 1991;31:67.
69. Flexner C. HIV-protease inhibitors. *N Engl J Med* 1998;338:1281.
70. Palella FJ Jr, Delaney KM, Moorman AC, et al. Declining morbidity and mortality among patients with advanced human immunodeficiency virus infection. HIV Outpatient Study Investigators. *N Engl J Med* 1998;338:853.
71. Gao F, Yue L, White AT, et al. Human infection by genetically diverse SIVSM-related HIV-2 in West Africa. *Nature* 1992;358:495.
72. Gao F, Bailes E, Robertson DL, et al. Origin of HIV-1 in the chimpanzee *Pan troglodytes troglodytes*. *Nature* 1999;397:436.
73. Wei X, Ghosh SK, Taylor ME, et al. Viral dynamics in human immunodeficiency virus type 1 infection. *Nature* 1995;373:117.
74. Coffin JM. HIV population dynamics *in vivo*: implications for genetic variation, pathogenesis, and therapy. *Science* 1995;267:483.
75. Perelson AS, Neumann AU, Markowitz M, Leonard JM, Ho DD. HIV-1 dynamics *in vivo*: virion clearance rate, infected cell life-span, and viral generation time. *Science* 1996;271:1582.
76. Tang H, Kuhen KL, Wong-Staal F. Lentivirus replication and regulation. *Annu Rev Genet* 1999;33:133.
77. Sanguineti-Diaz C, Rodriguez-Tafur J, Patarca R. Primate retroviruses and oncogenesis. *Crit Rev Oncog* 1998;9:209.
78. Shiramizu B, Herndier BG, McGrath MS. Identification of a common clonal human immunodeficiency virus integration site in human immunodeficiency virus–associated lymphomas. *Cancer Res* 1994;54:2069.
79. Feigal EG. AIDS-associated malignancies: research perspectives. *Biochim Biophys Acta* 1999;1423:C1.
80. Gallo RC. The enigmas of Kaposi's sarcoma. *Science* 1998;282:1837.
81. Fiorelli V, Barillari G, Toschi E, et al. IFN-gamma induces endothelial cells to proliferate and to invade the extracellular matrix in response to the HIV-1 Tat protein: implications for AIDS-Kaposi's sarcoma pathogenesis. *J Immunol* 1999;162:1165.
82. Samaniego F, Markham PD, Gendelman R, Gallo RC, Ensoli B. Inflammatory cytokines induce endothelial cells to produce and release basic fibroblast growth factor and to promote Kaposi's sarcoma–like lesions in nude mice. *J Immunol* 1997;158:1887.
83. Barillari G, Sgadari C, Fiorelli V, et al. The Tat protein of human immunodeficiency virus type-1 promotes vascular cell growth and locomotion by engaging the $\alpha 5\beta 1$ and $\alpha v\beta 3$ integrins and by mobilizing sequestered basic fibroblast growth factor. *Blood* 1999;94:663.
84. Chang HC, Samaniego F, Nair BC, Buonaguro L, Ensoli B. HIV-1 Tat protein exits from cells via a leaderless secretory pathway and binds to extracellular matrix–associated heparan sulfate proteoglycans through its basic region. *AIDS* 1997;11:1421.
85. Fiorelli V, Gendelman R, Sirianni MC, et al. γ-Interferon produced by CD8+ T cells infiltrating Kaposi's sarcoma induces spindle cells with angiogenic phenotype and synergy with human immunodeficiency virus-1 Tat protein: an immune response to human herpesvirus-8 infection? *Blood* 1998;91:956.
86. Barillari G, Sgadari C, Palladino C, et al. Inflammatory cytokines synergize with the HIV-1 Tat protein to promote angiogenesis and Kaposi's sarcoma via induction of basic fibroblast growth factor and the $\alpha v\beta 3$ integrin. *J Immunol* 1999;163:1929.
87. DeMario MD, Liebowitz DN. Lymphomas in the immunocompromised patient. *Semin Oncol* 1998;25:492.
88. Lyons SF, Liebowitz DN. The roles of human viruses in the pathogenesis of lymphoma. *Semin Oncol* 1998;25:461.
89. Aboulafia D. Epidemiology and pathogenesis of AIDS-related lymphomas. *Oncology* (Huntingt) 1998;12:1068; discussion 1081.
90. Nador RG, Cesarman E, Chadburn A, et al. Primary effusion lymphoma: a distinct clinicopathologic entity associated with the Kaposi's sarcoma–associated herpes virus. *Blood* 1996;88:645.
91. Horenstein MG, Nador RG, Chadburn A, et al. Epstein-Barr virus latent gene expression in primary effusion lymphomas containing Kaposi's sarcoma–associated herpesvirus/human herpesvirus-8. *Blood* 1997;90:1186.
92. Soulier J, Grollet L, Oksenhendler E, et al. Kaposi's sarcoma–associated herpesvirus-like DNA sequences in multicentric Castleman's disease. *Blood* 1995;86:1276.
93. Di Bisceglie AM. Hepatitis C and hepatocellular carcinoma. *Hepatology* 1997;26:34S.
94. Colombo M. The role of hepatitis C virus in hepatocellular carcinoma. *Recent Results Cancer Res* 1998;154:337.
95. Houghton M. Hepatitis C viruses. In: Fields BN, Knipe DM, Howley PM, et al., eds. *Fields virology*. Philadelphia: Lippincott–Raven Publishers, 1996:1035.
96. El-Serag HB, Mason AC. Rising incidence of hepatocellular carcinoma in the United States. *N Engl J Med* 1999; 340:745.
97. Recommendations for prevention and control of hepatitis C (HCV) infection and HCV-related chronic disease. *MMWR Morb Mortal Wkly Rep* 1998;47:1.
98. Donato F, Tagger A, Chiesa R, et al. Hepatitis B and C virus infection, alcohol drinking, and hepatocellular carcinoma: a case-control study in Italy. Brescia HCC Study. *Hepatology* 1997;26:579.
99. Moriya K, Fujie H, Shintani Y, et al. The core protein of hepatitis C virus induces hepatocellular carcinoma in transgenic mice. *Nat Med* 1998;4:1065.
100. Ray RB, Steele R, Meyer K, Ray R. Hepatitis C virus core protein represses p21WAF1/Cip1/Sid1 promoter activity. *Gene* 1998;208:331.
101. Ray RB, Steele R, Meyer K, Ray R. Transcriptional repression of p53 promoter by hepatitis C virus core protein. *J Biol Chem* 1997;272:10983.
102. Bruno S, Silini E, Crosignani A, et al. Hepatitis C virus genotypes and risk of hepatocellular carcinoma in cirrhosis: a prospective study. *Hepatology* 1997;25:754.
103. Tanaka H, Tsukuma H, Yamano H, et al. Hepatitis C virus 1b(II) infection and development of chronic hepatitis, liver cirrhosis and hepatocellular carcinoma: a case-control study in Japan. *J Epidemiol* 1998;8:244.
104. Reid AE, Koziel MJ, Aiza I, et al. Hepatitis C virus genotypes and viremia and hepatocellular carcinoma in the United States. *Am J Gastroenterol* 1999;94:1619.
105. Ikeda K, Saitoh S, Arase Y, et al. Effect of interferon therapy on hepatocellular carcinogenesis in patients with chronic hepatitis type C: a long-term observation study of 1,643 patients using statistical bias correction with proportional hazard analysis. *Hepatology* 1999;29:1124.
106. International Interferon-alpha Hepatocellular Carcinoma Study Group. Effect of interferon-alpha on progression of cirrhosis to hepatocellular carcinoma: a retrospective cohort study [published erratum appears in *Lancet* 1998:352:1230]. *Lancet* 1998;351:1535.
107. Shindo M, Ken A, Okuno T. Varying incidence of cirrhosis and hepatocellular carcinoma in patients with chronic hepatitis C responding differently to interferon therapy. *Cancer* 1999;85:1943.

108. Yoshida H, Shiratori Y, Moriyama M, et al. Interferon therapy reduces the risk for hepatocellular carcinoma: national surveillance program of cirrhotic and noncirrhotic patients with chronic hepatitis C in Japan. Inhibition of Hepatocarcinogenesis by Interferon Therapy Study Group. *Ann Intern Med* 1999;131:174.
109. Kasahara A, Hayashi N, Mochizuki K, et al. Risk factors for hepatocellular carcinoma and its incidence after interferon treatment in patients with chronic hepatitis C. Osaka Liver Disease Study Group. *Hepatology* 1998;27:1394.
110. Okanoue T, Itoh Y, Minami M, et al. Interferon therapy lowers the rate of progression to hepatocellular carcinoma in chronic hepatitis C but not significantly in an advanced stage: a retrospective study in 1148 patients. Viral Hepatitis Therapy Study Group. *J Hepatol* 1999;30:653.
111. McHutchison JG, Gordon SC, Schiff ER, et al. Interferon alfa-2b alone or in combination with ribavirin as initial treatment for chronic hepatitis C. Hepatitis Interventional Therapy Group. *N Engl J Med* 1998;339:1485.
112. Collier JD, Zanke B, Moore M, et al. No association between hepatitis C and B-cell lymphoma. *Hepatology* 1999;29:1259.
113. Silvestri F, Pipan C, Barillari G, et al. Prevalence of hepatitis C virus infection in patients with lymphoproliferative disorders. *Blood* 1996;87:4296.

PETER M. HOWLEY
DON GANEM
ELLIOTT KIEFF

SECTION 2

DNA Viruses

Viral oncology has its foundations in scientific observations made at the turn of the twentieth century and defining the transmissibility of avian leukemia (in Denmark in 1908) and an avian sarcoma in chickens (in 1911).[1,2] These important discoveries were not appreciated at the time, and their impact on virology and medicine was not recognized for decades. The importance of the work of Peyton Rous[2] demonstrating that cell-free extracts from a sarcoma in chickens could, within a few weeks, induce tumors in injected chickens, even when the extracts were passed through filters that retained bacteria, finally was recognized by a Nobel prize in 1968. Rous's original work pointed out that this infectious agent not only was capable of inducing tumors but also imprinted the phenotypic characteristics of the original tumor on the recipient cell. At the time, this early work was relegated to the rank of avian curiosities, and its importance remained unrecognized for several decades.

In the 1930s, Richard Shope published a series of articles demonstrating cell-free transmission of tumors in rabbits. The first studies involved fibromatous tumors found in the footpads of wild cottontail rabbits that could be transmitted by injecting cell-free extracts in either wild or domestic rabbits.[3] Subsequent studies have shown that this virus, now referred to as the *Shope fibroma virus*, is a pox virus. Additional studies carried out by Shope demonstrated that cutaneous papillomatosis in wild cottontail rabbits could also be transmitted by cell-free extracts. In a number of cases, these benign papillomas would progress spontaneously into squamous cell carcinomas in infected domestic rabbits or in the infected cottontail rabbits.[4,5] In general, however, the field of viral oncology lay dormant until the early 1950s, with the discovery of the murine leukemia viruses by Ludwig Gross[6] and of the mouse polyomavirus by Gross et al.[7,8] Such findings of tumor viruses in mice led many cancer researchers and virologists to the field of viral oncology. These researchers hoped that these initial observations in mammals could be extended to humans and that a fair proportion of human tumors might also be found to have a viral etiology. The Special Viral Cancer Program at the National Cancer Institute grew from this intense interest in viral oncology and the hope that human tumor viruses would be identified.

Many of the most important developments in modern molecular biology derive from studies in viral oncology from the 1960s and 1970s. The discovery of reverse transcriptase, the development of recombinant DNA technology, the discovery of messenger RNA (mRNA) splicing, and the discovery of oncogenes and, more recently, tumor suppressor genes all are developments that derive directly from studies in viral oncology. Oncogenes were first recognized as cellular genes that had been acquired by retroviruses through recombinational processes to convert them into acute transforming RNA tumor viruses. It is now recognized that oncogenes participate in many different types of tumors and can be involved at different stages of tumorigenesis and viral oncology. This has contributed significantly to the concepts of nonviral carcinogenesis. It is likely that the direct, transforming, oncogene-transducing retroviruses do not play a major causative role in naturally occurring cancers in animals or in humans but rather represent laboratory-generated recombinants. A list of human viruses with oncogenic properties is presented in Table 10.2-1. This list includes such viruses as the transforming adenoviruses, which are capable of transforming normal cells into malignant cells in the laboratory but which have not been associated with any known human tumors. The list also includes viruses such as the papillomaviruses, which have been etiologically associated with specific human cancers and which have been shown to encode transforming viral oncogenes. Finally, it includes such viruses as the hepatitis B and C viruses, which have been closely linked with a specific human tumor, hepatocellular carcinoma (HCC), for which the evidence of a *bona fide* viral oncogene remains unclear.

This chapter focuses primarily on the DNA viruses that have been associated with specific human cancers and discusses the biology and pertinent molecular biology of these viruses. Chapter 10.1 deals with the RNA viruses, particularly the human retroviruses. The evidence pertaining to the association of each of these viruses with specific types of human neoplasia is presented, and the mechanisms by which these viruses may contribute to malignant transformation are discussed.

HEPADNAVIRUSES AND HEPATOCELLULAR CARCINOMA

HCC is one of the world's most common malignancies. Though rare in the West, the disease is highly prevalent in Southeast Asia and sub-Saharan Africa. In the 1970s, this distribution was recognized to mirror the distribution of chronic hepatitis B virus (HBV) infection. This fact, and the long-recognized histopathologic association between HCC and chronic hepatitis in the surrounding nontumorous liver, led to the strong presumption that chronic HBV infection predisposes to hepatic cancer.[9] This presumption has been strikingly validated in large prospective epidemiologic studies in Taiwan, in which chronically infected individuals were followed for deaths due to this tumor.[10] These studies showed that chronic

TABLE 10.2-1. Human Viruses with Oncogenic Properties

Virus Family	*Type*	*Human Tumor*	*Cofactors*
Adenovirus	Types 2, 5, 12	None	—
Hepadnavirus	Hepatitis B (HBV)	Hepatocellular carcinoma	Aflatoxin, alcohol, smoking
Hepatotropic viruses (other)	Hepatitis C (HCV)	Hepatocellular carcinoma	—
Herpesviruses	Epstein-Barr (EBV)	Burkitt's lymphoma	Malaria
		Immunoblastic lymphoma	Immunodeficiency
		Nasopharyngeal carcinoma	Nitrosamines, HLA genotype
		Hodgkin's disease	
	KSHV (HHV-8)	Kaposi's sarcoma	HIV infection
		Body cavity–based lymphoma	HIV infection
		Castleman's disease	HIV infection
Papillomaviruses	HPV-16, -18, -33, -39	Anogenital cancers and some upper airway cancers	Smoking, ? other factors
	HPV-5, -8, -17	Skin cancer	Genetic disorders, sunlight exposure, immunosuppression
Polyomavirus	BK, JC	? Neural tumors	—
	SV40	? Insulinomas	—
		? Mesotheliomas	—
Retroviruses	HTLV-I	Adult T-cell leukemia or lymphoma	Uncertain
	HTLV-II	Hairy cell leukemia	Unknown

HHV-8, human herpes virus-8; HIV, human immunodeficiency virus; HLA, human leukocyte antigen; HPV, human papillomavirus; HTLV-I, human T-cell leukemia virus type I; HTLV-II, human T-cell leukemia virus type II; KSHV, Kaposi's sarcoma herpesvirus; SV40, simian virus 40.

HBV infection is associated with a 100-fold increase in HCC risk over that of controls who are not chronically infected.

HBV is a small DNA virus classified as a member of the hepadnavirus family (for *hepatotropic DNA viruses*); for review, see Ganem and Schneider.[11] HBV is the only human virus in this family, which also includes related viruses of woodchucks [woodchuck hepatitis virus (WHV)], ground squirrels [ground squirrel hepatitis virus, (GSHV)], and ducks [duck hepatitis B virus (DHBV)] (Table 10.2-2). Primary infection of susceptible hosts with HBV produces either a subclinical infection or acute hepatitis B, depending on the age of the host and many other poorly understood factors. In adult hosts, 95% of such infections resolve, with clearance of virus from liver and blood and the induction of lasting immunity to reinfection. However, 5% of these infections do not resolve but result in persistent hepatic infection and viremia; most of the demonstrated HCC risk falls within this subgroup of infections. Persistent HBV infections usually last for the life of the host and can have a variety of pathologic consequences. In many hosts thus affected, such infections are subclinical and accompanied by little hepatocellular injury. This asymptomatic carrier state provides evidence that the HBV replication cycle is not directly cytopathic for host cells,

TABLE 10.2-2. The Hepadnavirus Family

	HBV	*WHV*	*GSHV*	*DHBV*
Genome	3.2 kb	3.3 kb	3.3 kb	3.0 kb
ORFs	S, C, P, X	S, C, P, X	S, C, P, X	S, C, P
Hosts	Humans	Woodchucks	Ground squirrels	Ducks
	Chimps	Woodchucks	Geese	Chipmunks
Replication	Liver	Liver	Liver	Liver
	Kidney	Kidney		Kidney
	Pancreas	Pancreas		Pancreas
	WBC	WBC		Spleen
		Other		Other?
Diseases	ACS	ACS	ACS	ACS
	Hepatitis	Hepatitis	Hepatitis	Hepatitis
	Cirrhosis			
	HCC	HCC	HCC	

ACS, asymptomatic carrier state; DHBV, duck hepatitis B virus; GSHV, ground squirrel herpesvirus; HBV, hepatitis B virus; HCC, hepatocellular carcinoma; ORF, open reading frame; WBC, white blood cell; WHV, woodchuck herpesvirus.
(From BN Fields, DM Knipe, PM Howley, eds. *Field's Virology*. Philadelphia: Lippincott-Raven, 1996, with permission.)

an inference that has been strongly sustained by studies of viral replication in cultured cells.[11] Nonetheless, 20% to 25% of persistently infected hosts display hepatocellular injury, in the form of either chronic persistent hepatitis (inflammation limited to the periportal areas, with scant necrosis and no disruption of hepatic architecture) or chronic active hepatitis (necroinflammatory changes extending from portal to central areas). The latter is considered a severe lesion with significant potential to progress to cirrhosis and liver failure.

It is thought that in such hosts, the hepatocyte injury is due to host immune responses triggered by recognition of viral antigens presented on the surface of infected cells.[12] Much has been learned recently about the mechanisms of such injury. Cytotoxic T lymphocytes (CTLs) appear to play a key role in this process. In experiments with transgenic mice expressing viral antigens, transfer of CTLs specific for those antigens leads to a hepatitis, the severity of which depends on the dose of transferred T cells.[13] Importantly, however, direct killing of the cells is only a part of the story.[14] Much of the injury produced in such experiments is due to secondary, antigen-nonspecific responses triggered by the initial CTL activation and cytokine release[15]: release of inflammatory molecules that recruit other inflammatory cell types, production of toxic reactive oxygen radicals, and the like. In addition, infected cells displaying deregulated viral gene expression may display enhanced sensitivity to tumor necrosis factor (TNF) and other inflammatory cytokines.[16]

The induction of hepatocellular injury is believed to be important in HCC pathogenesis because it triggers in the liver a stereotypical proliferative response. Two types of regenerative response are known in the liver, which depend to some extent on the nature of the hepatic insult. (The mechanisms by which these responses occur remain obscure.) In classical liver regeneration (as observed, for example, after a partial liver resection), all mature hepatocytes in the liver—which, under normal circumstances, are nondividing—synchronously reenter the cell cycle, resulting in the prompt restoration of normal hepatic mass.[17] A somewhat different proliferative response is observed after treatment with certain toxic or carcinogenic chemicals. In this response, poorly characterized cells in the periductal areas (termed *oval cells*, largely on the basis of their morphology) undergo expansion. These cells are thought to be precursor cells to both bile duct epithelium and hepatocytes.[18] They also share many of the biochemical properties of cells seen in hepatic cancers (e.g., α-fetoprotein production) and, for this reason, are thought by some to be the target cell for transformation in hepatic carcinogenesis by a variety of agents. Although it is likely that both forms of proliferative response are operative in chronic hepatitis, considerable debate continues to surround this issue.

However, the fact that major liver cell proliferation is operative throughout the prolonged preneoplastic period is undisputed and is believed to be an important precondition for carcinogenesis. Such proliferation increases opportunities for replicative errors (mutations) that, over time, can contribute to the loss of normal cellular growth control; cells harboring such mutations will have a selective advantage that further perpetuates this cycle. Attesting to the importance of cellular injury and turnover in HCC development is the fact that HCC usually is accompanied by pathologic signs of severe liver injury (chronic active hepatitis and cirrhosis) in the nontumorous liver; it is distinctly uncommon to see hepatoma in hosts whose livers contain minimal evidence of injury.

In the preceding formulation, HBV serves as an agent of oncogenesis chiefly by (indirectly) provoking cellular proliferation in response to immune-mediated injury. In this view, no direct genetic contribution is made by viral sequences acting *in cis* or viral gene products acting *in trans*. If this view is correct, then other agents, which similarly provoke chronic liver cell injury and regeneration, should likewise be associated with hepatic cancer. In this connection, it is of interest that chronic infection with hepatitis C virus, a genetically unrelated hepatotropic RNA virus that similarly produces chronic hepatitis, also confers an increased risk for HCC development.[19]

Despite strong experimental support for the pathogenetic scheme just presented, there is reason to believe that hepadnaviruses may also make a more direct genetic contribution to HCC. Phylogenetic analyses of hepadnaviral genome organization reveal that the structure of the oncogenic mammalian viruses differs from that of the nononcogenic avian viruses in an important way.[11] The mammalian viruses all harbor an additional coding region, termed *ORF X* (for *open reading frame X;* Fig. 10.2-1), that encodes a small regulatory protein.[20] This open reading frame is absent in the avian viruses, which fail to induce HCC in their native hosts despite the regular induction of persistent infection. Interestingly, in several lines of transgenic mice displaying constitutive hepatic expression of *ORF X*, HCC arises with increased frequency.[21,22] Tumors in such mice do not begin until midlife, suggesting that additional genetic changes are necessary for loss of normal growth control.

The sequence of *ORF X* reveals no homology to known oncogenes or growth regulatory loci, and little is known of its

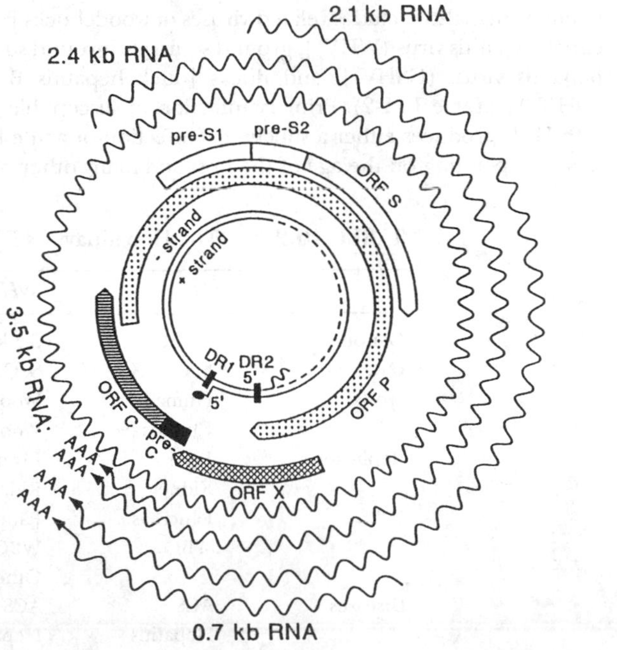

FIGURE 10.2-1. Genomic and transcriptional organization of the human hepatitis B virus. The inner circle represents the partially double-stranded virion DNA, with dashes specifying the single-stranded genomic region. The locations of the direct repeat (DR1 and DR2) regions are indicated. The boxed arcs specify the viral coding regions, and the arrows indicate the direction of translation. The outermost wavy lines depict the viral RNAs identified in infected cells, with the arrows indicating the direction of transcription and the AAAs indicating the polyadenylated 3' tails. ORF, open reading frame.

biochemical function. In transient cotransfection assays, X expression up-regulates a wide variety of viral and cellular promoters, but the mechanism by which this activation is achieved has remained obscure. In some situations, X appears to stimulate cytoplasmic signal transduction pathways (e.g., the ras-raf MAP kinase pathway),[23,24] whereas in other settings, it may function as a nuclear transcriptional activator.[25,26] It has also been suggested that X protein might bind to and inactivate the tumor suppressor gene product p53,[27] but such reports require confirmation. The relationship of all of these activities to the putative oncogenic function of ORF X is unproven.

Another class of more direct genetic contributions that HBV might make to HCC derives from the existence of integrated copies of viral DNA in the tumor cells. Unlike retroviruses, hepadnaviruses do not specify genetic functions directing genomic integration, and such integration is not essential for HBV replication.[11] (HBV replication actually proceeds from episomal DNA via reverse transcription of an RNA intermediate.) In fact, because every nucleotide of the viral genome is in a coding region, integration of HBV DNA generally disrupts essential genes and is incompatible with replication. Yet most hepatoma cells arising in HBV-infected patients harbor multiple integrated HBV genomes, and in general, active viral replication has been extinguished.[28] The tumors are clonal with respect to these viral insertions: All cells of the tumor bear the same pattern of integrated sequences, indicating that integration preceded or accompanied the final transforming event. However, close inspection of these integrated sequences indicates that they usually are highly rearranged, with multiple deletions, inversions, reduplications, or other mutations typically present.[28] Although individual integrated sequences may retain certain coding functions, no one viral coding region is invariably preserved, as are E6 and E7 of the human papillomaviruses (HPVs; see the section Papillomaviruses and Human Cancer).

These facts have led to interest in the model that the viral sequences might be contributing *cis*-acting regulatory signals rather than *trans*-acting proteins to the host cell. Ample precedent for such a model exists in retroviral oncogenesis in animals, wherein insertion of powerful retroviral enhancer sequences into the chromosome can activate the expression of growth-regulatory genes flanking the insert. Strong evidence that hepadnaviruses can mediate such activation events *in cis* has been proffered for WHV. WHV is strikingly oncogenic in its native host: Virtually 100% of animals chronically infected from birth will develop HCC.[29] The oncogenic drive in an infected animal is remarkably strong; many adult animals can be shown to harbor multiple independent HCCs. As in HBV-induced cancer, the tumors display multiple viral insertions, often highly rearranged, and in a clonal pattern. However, here, remarkably, the vast majority of tumors can be shown to harbor at least one viral insertion *in cis* to the protooncogene N-myc.[30–32] This gene, normally silent in adult liver, is strongly up-regulated by this insertion, and such activation can be seen early in the oncogenic sequence, even in premalignant lesions.[33] Many insertions are within a few kilobases of the N-myc locus, but insertions as far away as 250 kb appear to be activating.[31] Clearly, insertional activation of N-myc plays a major role in WHV oncogenesis.

Similar efforts to identify common integration sites for integrated HBV genomes in human HCC have not met with comparable success. Human hepatomas do not harbor N-myc rearrangements and, although isolated examples of dramatic insertion events have been described (e.g., insertions near loci for retinoid receptors or cyclin A homologues), none of these has been identified in more than one tumor, despite extensive searches.[34,35] The practitioner does well to remember that, despite its many similarities to HBV, WHV differs strikingly in its oncogenic potency; it is possible that insertional activation of N-myc loci is responsible for this difference.

PAPILLOMAVIRUSES AND HUMAN CANCER

The viral nature of human warts was first demonstrated at the turn of the century by transmission using a cell-free filtrate.[36] This important group of viruses has remained refractory to standard virologic studies, however, because propagating the papillomaviruses in the laboratory in tissue culture under standard conditions is difficult. Although some advances have been made in propagating the virus using organotypic raft cultures of epithelial cells, most knowledge about the molecular biology and genetics of the papillomaviruses has resulted from advances in basic research and the application of reverse genetics using cloned viral DNAs.

The papillomaviruses are found in many higher vertebrate species ranging from birds to humans. Although originally classified as papovaviruses because of their icosahedral shape and circular, double-stranded DNA genome, the papillomaviruses now are recognized to be separate from the other papovaviruses such as polyoma and simian virus 40 (SV40), on the basis of different biologic and genetic characteristics. The papillomaviruses contain a double-stranded circular DNA genome of 8000 base pairs, which is larger than the polyomaviruses (5000 base pairs), and the virion particles have a correspondingly larger capsid diameter (55 nm vs. 40 nm). The papillomaviruses have not yet been propagated in tissue culture under standard conditions.

More than 80 different HPV types have been described in detail to date,[37] and evidence exists that there may be as many as 30 to 40 additional viruses that have not yet been as well characterized. Unlike some human viruses such as adenoviruses, it has not been possible to type the papillomaviruses by serologic methods, as antisera that can distinguish between the different HPV types are currently not available. Through the 1970s and 1980s, the HPVs were typed by DNA hybridization under stringent annealing conditions, but currently the DNA sequence of a portion of the L1 ORF (in the so-called late region of the HPV genome) is used to define new HPV types. A list of many of the HPV types that have now been categorized, and the clinical syndromes with which they are associated or from which they have been isolated, is presented in Table 10.2-3.

The papillomaviruses are highly species-specific and induce squamous epithelial and fibroepithelial tumors in their natural hosts. These viruses have a specific tropism for squamous epithelial cells, and their full productive cycle is supported only in squamous epithelial cells. The productive infection of cells by papillomaviruses is divided into stages, and these stages are linked to the differentiation state of the epithelial cell. The specific tropism of the papillomaviruses for squamous epithelial cells is evidenced by the restriction of the viral replication functions (vegetative viral DNA synthesis, the production of viral

TABLE 10.2-3. The Human Papillomaviruses

HPV Type	*Location*	*Association*
1	Cutaneous	Plantar warts
2	Cutaneous	Common warts
3	Cutaneous	Flat warts
4	Cutaneous	Common and plantar warts
5	Cutaneous	Macular lesions in EV and cancers
6	Genital tract, other mucosae	Genital warts, laryngeal papillomatosis
7	Genital tract, other mucosae	"Butcher's" warts
8	Cutaneous	Macular lesions (EV) and cancers
9	Cutaneous	Macular lesions (EV)
10	Cutaneous	Flat warts
11	Genital tract, other mucosae	Genital warts, laryngeal papillomas
12	Cutaneous	Macular lesions (EV)
13	Oral	Oral focal epithelial hyperplasia
14	Cutaneous	Macular lesions (EV) and cancers
15	Cutaneous	Macular lesions (EV)
16	Genital tract, other mucosae	Intraepithelial neoplasia and cancers
17	Cutaneous	Macular lesions (EV) and cancers
18	Genital tract, other mucosae	Intraepithelial neoplasia and cancers
19	Cutaneous	Macular lesions (EV)
20	Cutaneous	Macular lesions (EV) and cancers
21	Cutaneous	Macular lesions (EV)
22	Cutaneous	Macular lesions (EV)
23	Cutaneous	Macular lesions (EV)
24	Cutaneous	Macular lesions (EV)
25	Cutaneous	Macular lesions (EV)
26	Cutaneous	Common warts
27	Cutaneous	Common warts
28	Cutaneous	Flat warts
29	Cutaneous	Common warts
30	Genital tract, other mucosae	Intraepithelial neoplasia and cancer
31	Genital tract, other mucosae	Intraepithelial neoplasia and cancers
32	Oral	Oral focal epithelial hyperplasia, oral papillomas
33	Genital tract, other mucosae	Intraepithelial neoplasia and cancers
34	Genital tract, other mucosae	Intraepithelial neoplasia
35	Genital tract, other mucosae	Intraepithelial neoplasia and cancers
36	Cutaneous	Actinic keratosis, EV lesions
37	Cutaneous	Not yet known, isolated from a keratoacanthoma
38	Cutaneous	Not yet known, isolated from a melanoma
39	Genital tract, other mucosae	Intraepithelial neoplasia and cancers
40	Genital tract, other mucosae	Intraepithelial neoplasia
41	Cutaneous	Flat warts
42	Genital tract, other mucosae	Intraepithelial neoplasia
43	Genital tract, other mucosae	Intraepithelial neoplasia
44	Genital tract, other mucosae	Intraepithelial neoplasia
45	Genital tract, other mucosae	Intraepithelial neoplasia and cancers
46[a]	Cutaneous	Macular lesions (EV)
47	Cutaneous	Macular lesions (EV)
48	Cutaneous	Cutaneous squamous cell carcinoma (transplant patient)
49	Cutaneous	Flat wart (immunosuppressed patient)
50	Cutaneous	Macular lesions (EV)
51	Genital tract, other mucosae	Intraepithelial neoplasia and cancers
52	Genital tract, other mucosae	Intraepithelial neoplasia and cancers
53	Genital tract, other mucosae	Intraepithelial neoplasia
54	Genital tract, other mucosae	Intraepithelial neoplasia
55	Genital tract, other mucosae	Intraepithelial neoplasia
56	Genital tract, other mucosae	Intraepithelial neoplasia and cancers
57	Oral, genital tract, other mucosae	Oral papillomas and inverted maxillary sinus papilloma

(continued)

TABLE 10.2-3. (*Continued*)

HPV Type	*Location*	*Association*
58	Genital tract, other mucosae	Intraepithelial neoplasia and cancers
59	Genital tract, other mucosae	Anogenital intraepithelial neoplasia
60	Cutaneous	Epidermoid cysts, plantar warts
61	Genital tract, other mucosae	Intraepithelial neoplasia
62	Genital tract, other mucosae	Intraepithelial neoplasia
63	Cutaneous	Isolated from a plantar wart
64	Genital tract, other mucosae	Intraepithelial neoplasia
65	Cutaneous	Isolated from a pigmented wart
66	Genital tract, other mucosae	Intraepithelial neoplasia and cancers
67	Genital tract, other mucosae	Isolated from an intraepithelial neoplasia
68	Genital tract, other mucosae	Isolated from an intraepithelial neoplasia
69	Genital tract, other mucosae	Intraepithelial neoplasia and cancers
70	Genital tract, other mucosae	Isolated from a vulvar papilloma
71	Genital tract, other mucosae	Isolated from an intraepithelial neoplasia
72	Oral	Isolated from an oral papilloma (HIV patient)
73	Oral	Isolated from an oral papilloma (HIV patient)
74	Genital tract, other mucosae	Isolated from an intraepithelial neoplasia
75	Cutaneous	Isolated from a common wart in organ allograft recipient
76	Cutaneous	Isolated from a common wart in organ allograft recipient
77	Cutaneous	Isolated from a common wart in organ allograft recipient

EV, epidermodysplasia verruciformis; HIV, human immunodeficiency virus; HPV, human papillomavirus.
[a]HPV-46 is now designated *HPV-20b*.
(From refs. 37, 40, and 146, with permission.)

capsid proteins, and the assembly of virions) to the most terminally differentiated keratinocytes.

In a normal squamous epithelium, the basal cell is the only cell normally capable of supporting cellular DNA synthesis and undergoing cellular division. The virus, therefore, must infect the basal cell to establish a persistent lesion. *In situ* hybridization experiments have demonstrated that the papillomavirus DNA is indeed present within the basal cell of a papilloma.[38] In a squamous epithelium, as the cells migrate upward through the stratum spinosum and into the granular layer, they undergo a program of differentiation. The control of papillomavirus late gene expression is tightly linked to the differentiation state of the squamous epithelial cells.[39] Vegetative viral DNA synthesis and expression of the capsid proteins occurs only in the more differentiated squamous epithelial cells.

All HPV types examined to date have a similar genomic organization. The DNA genomes of each of the HPVs sequenced, as well as of the other animal papillomaviruses, are approximately 8000 base pairs in size. All of the ORFs that could serve to encode proteins are located on only one of the two viral DNA strands. RNA studies have indicated that only one strand is transcribed. A more detailed description of the molecular biology of the papillomaviruses can be found in the current edition of *Field's Virology*.[40]

The HPV genome can be divided into two distinct regions: an "early" region, which encodes the viral proteins involved in viral DNA replication, transcriptional regulation, and cellular transformation, and a "late" region, which encodes the viral capsid proteins. This functional division is based largely on genetic studies that were carried out with the bovine papillomavirus.[41] A diagram of the organization of a typical HPV-16 is shown in Figure 10.2-2. The genes located in the early region of the genes are designated as *E1, E2*, and so on, and the genes located in the late region are designated as *L1* and *L2*. Studies with the HPVs indicate that it is likely that *E4* encodes a "late" gene, which is expressed only in productively infected keratinocytes.[42] Thus, although this ORF is located with the early ORFs, its function may be important only in the vegetative replication of the virus. A listing of the functions assigned to the HPV-16 ORFs is provided in Table 10.2-4.

In productively infected tissue (i.e., tissue in which viral particles are made, such as a wart), mRNA is transcribed from the early *and* late regions of the genome.[39] Nonproductive infection of host cells (as seen in the lower cells of the epithelium in a wart) is accompanied by transcription of mRNA from only the early region of the genome. The restricted expression of the genome to only the early region involves regulation of transcription at the levels of the initiation of RNA synthesis, RNA stability, and transcriptional termination.

The molecular biology of the papillomaviruses has been most extensively studied for the bovine papillomavirus (BPV-1), which is capable of transforming a variety of rodent fibroblast cell lines in tissue culture. In these transformed cells, the DNA remains as a stable extrachromosomal plasmid, and this system has served as an excellent model for studying latent infection by papillomavirus (reviewed in Spalholz and Howley[43]). This virus has served as the prototype for unraveling many aspects of the molecular biology of the papillomaviruses over the last 20 years. Two independent transforming activities have been mapped in BPV-1: one to the *E5* gene and the other to the *E6* and *E7* genes. Transformation by the BPV-1 E5 oncoprotein appears to be mediated through activation by binding of the platelet-derived growth factor-β (PDGF-β) receptor.[44] The mechanisms by which the *E6* and *E7* genes of BPV-1 trans-

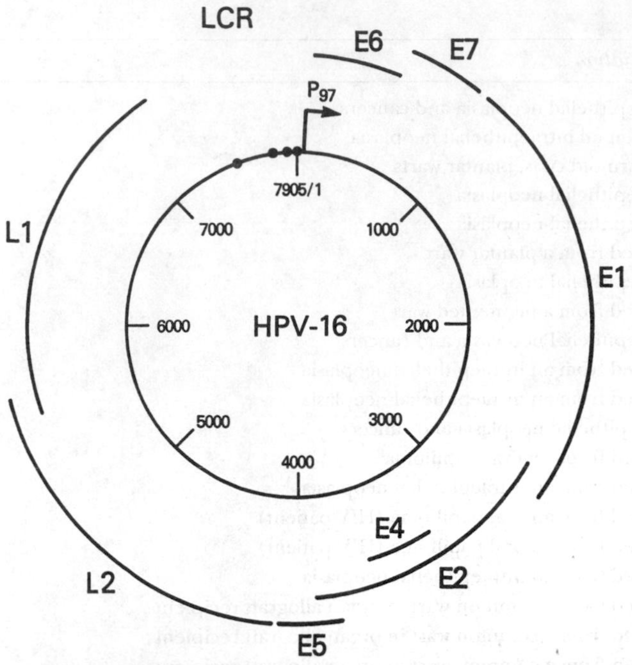

FIGURE 10.2-2. The genomic map of human papillomavirus-16 (HPV-16) deduced from the DNA sequence. The nucleotide numbers are noted within the circular maps, transcription proceeds clockwise, and the major open reading frames (E1 to E7, L1, and L2) are indicated. The only transcriptional promoter mapped to data for HPV-16 is designated P_{97}. The viral long control region (LCR) containing the putative viral transcriptional and replication regulatory elements is noted. The closed circles on the genome represent the four E2 binding sites, which have been noted in the LCR. (From ref. 16, with permission.)

form have not yet been fully elucidated. BPV-1 E6 has been shown to bind the focal adhesion protein paxillin, and the binding of E6 to paxillin has been implicated in the cellular transformation phenotype through the disruption of the actin cytoskeleton.[45,46]

The papillomavirus E2 proteins are regulatory proteins that have roles in viral DNA replication and in viral transcription.[47] E2 is a DNA-binding protein that was first described as a transcriptional activator[48]; however, subsequent studies have shown that it can also function as a transcriptional repressor depending on the context of the E2 binding sites within the promoter.[49] E2 has several roles in viral DNA replication and plasmid maintenance in infected cells.[50] E2 ensures viral DNA partitioning in persistently infected cells by tethering the viral DNA to the mitotic chromosomes during mitosis.[51,52] E2 also binds to the viral E1 protein and cooperatively promotes origin-dependent viral DNA replication.[53,54] The *E1* gene encodes a protein necessary for extrachromosomal replication and has been shown to have DNA-binding, DNA helicase, and adenosine triphosphatase activities.[55,56] No function has yet been found for the E3 or E8 ORFs of BPV-1. The L1 ORF of the papillomaviruses encodes the major capsid protein, and the L2 ORF encodes a minor capsid protein.[57,58] The L1 and L2 ORFs are expressed only in the terminally differentiated keratinocytes.[39]

Although initial papillomavirus transformation studies focused on BPV-1 because it could effectively transform rodent

TABLE 10.2-4. HPV-16 Gene Functions

ORF	*Function*
L1	L1 protein, major capsid protein
L2	L2 protein, minor capsid protein
E1	Initiation of viral DNA replication, helicase, adenosine triphosphatase
E2	Transcriptional regulatory protein, auxiliary role in viral DNA replication, complexes E1
E4	Late protein; disrupts cytokeratins
E5	Membrane transforming protein may interact with growth factor receptors
E6	Transforming protein of HPVs; targets degradation of p53; activates telomerase; other potential targets
E7	Transforming protein of HPVs; binds to the retinoblastoma protein and other "pocket proteins"

HPV, human papillomavirus; ORF, open reading frame.

cells in tissue culture, recent studies have focused more on the high-risk HPVs, in particular HPV-16 and HPV-18, which are associated with human cervical cancer. Although the genomic organization of the HPVs is quite similar to that of BPV-1, there appear to be important differences in the mechanisms by which they transform cells. The principal transforming genes for the cancer-associated HPVs have been mapped to E6 and E7, as will be discussed later in this section. *E7* alone is sufficient for the transformation of primary rodent cells.[59–61] *E7* also is capable of cooperating with an activated *ras* oncogene to transform primary rodent cells.[60] Expression of *E6* and *E7* together is sufficient for the efficient immortalization of primary human cells, most notably primary human keratinocytes, which are the normal host cell for the HPVs.[62,63] Cellular targets for the HPV E6 and E7 proteins have been identified, as discussed later in this section. HPV *E5* may also have transforming activities, but it has not been studied as well as has BPV E5 and does not appear to function through interaction with the PDGF-β receptor.

Only a subgroup of the papillomaviruses is associated with lesions that are at risk for progression to cancer. These viruses and their associated malignancies are listed in Table 10.2-5. The papillomavirus that infects cottontail rabbits in nature (CRPV) was first identified by Shope as the etiologic agent of cutaneous papillomatosis in rabbits.[4] CRPV has been extensively studied as a model for papillomavirus-induced carcinogenesis.[5,64] One of the features of carcinogenic progression with the papillomaviruses is the synergy between the virus and carcinogenic external factors (see Table 10.2-3). In the case of CRPV, carcinomas develop at an increased frequency in virus-induced papillomas that are painted with cool tar or methylcholanthrene.[65,66] These CRPV-associated carcinomas contain copies of the viral DNA that are transcriptionally active, an observation which supports the hypothesis that these viruses play an active role in the cancers that develop. There has been limited study of the molecular mechanisms involved in CRPV-associated carcinogenesis.

In cattle, BPV-4 has been associated with esophageal papillomatosis and also is associated with squamous cell carcinomas of the upper alimentary tract.[67,68] Interestingly, however, only those cattle from the highlands of Scotland that are infected with BPV-4 and that also feed on bracken fern (known to con-

TABLE 10.2-5. Papillomaviruses Associated with Lesions That May Progress to Cancer

Papillomaviruses	*Cancers*	*Other Factors*
CRPV (Shope)	Skin cancer	Methylcholanthrene
Bovine (BPV-4)	Tongue, esophageal, foregut cancers	Bracken fern
Bovine	Ocular cancer	Ultraviolet light
Ovine	Skin cancer	Ultraviolet light
Human (HPV-5, -8; and others)	Skin cancer (in EV patients and immunosuppressed patients)	Ultraviolet light
Human (HPV-16, -18, -31; and other high-risk HPVs)	Anogenital cancer; some upper airway cancers (including tonsillar cancer)	Smoking, ? HSV, ? oral contraceptive use

BPV, bovine papillomavirus; CRPV, cottontail rabbit papillomavirus; EV, epidermodysplasia verruciformis; HPV, human papillomavirus; HSV, herpes simplex virus.

tain a radiomimetic substance) have a high incidence of squamous cell carcinomas of the esophagus and of the foregut.[67] In contrast to the CRPV-associated carcinomas in which the viral DNA can invariably be found, extensive analysis of the squamous cell carcinomas of the upper alimentary tract in these cattle infected with BPV-4 has failed to reveal a consistent pattern of viral DNA sequences within the malignant tumors.[69] In the case of these alimentary tract tumors, possibly the continued presence of BPV-4 DNA sequences is not required for maintenance of the cancer.

The first evidence that HPVs were associated with human cancer came from studies in patients with epidermodysplasia verruciformis (EV), a rare, lifelong disease in humans that usually begins in infancy or childhood (reviewed in Jablonska and Majewski[70]). The disease is characterized by disseminated, polymorphic cutaneous lesions that resemble flat warts and by reddish macules sometimes referred to as *pityriasis-like* lesions.[71] Approximately one-half of the patients with EV develop multiple skin cancers, usually during the third or fourth decade of life. Papillomavirus particles have been detected within the benign lesions and not in the carcinomas. EV is considered an autosomal recessive disorder, and genetic studies of affected families have led to the mapping of a susceptibility gene to 17q, the same region that has been found to contain a dominant locus for the susceptibility to familial psoriasis.[72] It is thus tempting to speculate that distinct defects affecting the same gene may be involved somehow in the pathogenesis of these two hyperproliferative skin conditions. Of interest is that the carcinomas that develop in these patients arise in sun-exposed areas, and it is suspected that ultraviolet radiation plays a cocarcinogenic role with the papillomaviruses in the etiology of these cancers. Although EV is a very rare disease, it has been under intense study by dermatologists and virologists. More than 20 different HPV types have now been demonstrated in individual lesions in patients with this rare disease (see Table 10.2-3). Furthermore, recent studies have shown that these EV HPVs are widespread and point to psoriasis as a potential reservoir for HPV-5, one of the HPVs commonly found in EV.[73] Whether the EV-associated HPVs also are involved in the pathogenesis of psoriasis remains to be determined.

The cutaneous carcinomas in patients with EV can be bowenoid carcinomas, *in situ* carcinomas, or invasive squamous cell carcinomas. Of the HPV types found in patients with EV, only a subset of them is associated with a risk of malignant progression, most notably HPV-5 and HPV-8, although other types occasionally are found in EV cancers. The role of the HPVs in EV cancers is suggested by the presence of viral DNA of specific HPV types in the EV cancers. Although metastasis is uncommon in the cancers in these patients, the presence of HPV-5 in the two metastatic lymph node lesions examined strengthens the agreement for an etiologic role for HPV in these carcinomas.[74,75] Further studies have established that the viral genomes are transcriptionally active within these carcinomas[76] and that HPV-5 and HPV-8 encode cellular transformation functions.[77] Little work has been done yet to establish the mechanisms by which the EV HPVs contribute to cancer.

The role of HPVs in cutaneous cancers in humans extends beyond EV patients to other patients, both immunosuppressed and immunocompetent. New HPV types have been found in squamous and basal cell carcinomas of immunosuppressed patients and in some of the same tumors in immunocompetent patients.[78,79] However, the cutaneous HPVs are very prevalent in the population, and it has not yet been determined whether the virus has a role in promoting these cancers in immunosuppressed patients or whether it merely persists as a passenger.

The epidemiology of genital warts follows a pattern characteristic of a sexually transmitted disease (STD) with a high prevalence in populations of highly promiscuous women.[80,81] Two general types of genital wart viral infections—condylomata acuminata and squamous intraepithelial lesions (SILs)—are now recognized and can be differentiated by their clinical appearance. Condylomata acuminata can be localized to the penis, the vulva, the perineum, the anus and, rarely, the uterine cervix, and are caused by papillomaviruses. Papillomavirus particles have been demonstrated by the electron microscope.[82,83] HPV-6 and HPV-11 DNAs were directly cloned from condylomata acuminata lesions, and the genomes of these HPV types can be demonstrated in more than 90% of the lesions of condylomata acuminata examined.[84,85] Less frequently, other HPV types can be found in condylomata acuminata. Malignant conversion of condylomata acuminata into squamous cell carcinoma is uncommon. A lesion described by Buschke and Löwenstein and designated as a *giant condyloma* has characteristics similar to a locally invasive squamous cell carcinoma. These tumors are also associated with HPV-6 and HPV-11.[84,85] The majority of cervical carcinomas and other genital tract carcinomas, however, are negative for HPV-6 and HPV-11.

In the mid-1970s, zur Hausen[86] suggested an association between papillomaviruses and genital cancers. Compelling evidence linking an HPV infection with cervical carcinoma came from the recognition that the morphologic changes previously interpreted on Papanicolaou smears and tissue sections of the cervix as cervical dysplasia were due to a papillomavirus infection.[87–89] The characteristic cell that is diagnostic for a cervical papillomavirus infection is the koilocyte.[90] Electron microscopy demonstrated papillomavirus particles in the koilocytotic cells supporting the papillomavirus etiology.[91,92] Subsequent studies found papillomavirus-specific capsid antigens and HPV DNA within cervical dysplastic lesions, providing confirmation of the viral etiology of cervical dysplasia.

Epidemiologic studies had long implicated an infectious agent in the etiology of human cervical carcinoma.[93,94] Venereal transmission of a carcinogenic factor with a long latency had been suggested by early epidemiologic studies. Sexual promiscuity, an early age of onset of sexual activity, and poor sexual hygiene are known risk factors for cervical carcinoma. There is a correlation between the incidence rates of cervical cancer and penile carcinoma in various geographic areas, although the incidence rates for penile carcinoma are 20-fold lower when compared to those of cervical carcinoma. The similar ratio of incidence between cervical carcinoma and penile carcinoma is maintained, however, in areas of high, medium, or low prevalence, suggesting that the etiologic factors for penile and cervical carcinoma may be the same. The "male factor" also appears to implicate a sexually transmitted agent. Women who are monogamous are at a higher risk for cervical carcinoma if their spouses have multiple sexual partners.

The suggestion that an infectious agent might be involved in the etiology of cervical carcinoma has prompted many studies over the years, evaluating genital pathogens as potential causative agents. Infections by trichomonads, chlamydiae, and bacteria, such as syphilis and gonorrhea, have not been linked to cervical carcinoma. In the late 1960s and early 1970s, genital infection by herpes simplex virus type 2 (HSV-2) was considered as a possible etiologic candidate.[95,96] Support for the notion that HSV might be a cancer-associated virus came from studies demonstrating the ability of HSV to transform certain rodent cells in the laboratory *in vitro* and from some initial serologic studies that suggested a higher frequency of antibodies to HSV-2 in patients with cervical carcinoma. However, subsequent carefully performed molecular studies, attempting to demonstrate HSV RNA or HSV DNA in cervical cancer tissues, could not provide convincing evidence for a role for HSV in cervical cancer.[97] A large prospective epidemiologic study carried out by Vonka et al.[98,99] also failed to support the involvement of HSV-1 or HSV-2 infections in cervical cancer.

The association of an HPV with cervical dysplasia [also referred to as *cervical intraepithelial neoplasia* (CIN) and *SIL*] sparked an examination of cervical cancers for HPV sequences. The natural history linking CIN to carcinoma *in situ* and to invasive squamous cell carcinoma of the cervix had already been well established.[100–102] Initial experiments from a number of laboratories revealed HPV sequences in occasional cases of cervical carcinoma and anogenital carcinoma, but no consistent pattern of positivity emerged. Using radioactively labeled HPV-11 DNA under conditions of hybridization of low stringency, Durst et al.[103] and Boshart et al.[104] examined human cervical carcinoma DNAs for related HPV DNAs and, in the early 1980s, identified two new papillomavirus DNAs, HPV-16 and HPV-18. Using these HPV DNAs as probes, HPV types 16 and 18 could be demonstrated in approximately 70% of cervical carcinomas.[105] The use of low-stringency hybridization and the polymerase chain reaction with degenerative primers has led to the identification of approximately 20 different HPVs now associated with genital tract lesions (see Table 10.2-3). HPV-31, -33, -39, -42, and other HPVs are each associated with a small percentage of cervical carcinomas. Specific HPVs can be found regularly in 85% to 90% of human cervical carcinoma tissues and in a lower percentage of other human genital carcinomas such as penile carcinomas, vulvar carcinomas, and perianal carcinomas. The availability of HPV DNA probes has permitted the extensive analysis of specific clinical lesions. Bowenoid papulosis of the penis, also referred to as *penile intraepithelial neoplasia*, is associated with HPV-16 and is the male counterpart of CIN in the female.[106,107] Approximately 20 HPVs are associated with anogenital lesions. These can generally be further classified as either high-risk or low-risk on the basis of whether the genital tract lesions with which these HPVs are associated are at significant risk for malignant progression. Such low-risk viruses as HPV-6 and -11 are associated with venereal warts, whereas such high-risk viruses as HPV-16 and -18 are associated with SILs of the genital tract. The other high-risk viruses include HPV-31, -33, -35, -39, -45, -51, -52, and -56. The 85% to 90% of cervical carcinomas that are HPV-positive contain a high-risk DNA.

Studies of cervical cancers and derived cell lines that are HPV-positive have indicated that the DNA often is integrated, although in some cases the DNA is apparently also extrachromosomal. In those cases in which the DNA is integrated, the pattern of integration is clonal, indicating that the association of the HPV preceded the clonal outgrowth of the tumor. Integration of the viral DNA is not at specific sites in the host chromosome, although in some cell lines the integration event has occurred in the vicinity of known oncogenes. For instance, in the HeLa cell line (which is an HPV-18-positive cervical carcinoma cell line), the integration of the viral genome has occurred within approximately 50 kb of the c-myc locus on human chromosome 8.[108] It is not known whether such an integration event provides a selective advantage for the progression of a preneoplastic lesion to a cancer. It does seem plausible that in some individual cancers, the integration of the viral DNA could result in genetic changes such as the activation of a cellular oncogene or the inactivation of a tumor suppressor gene that could contribute to carcinogenic progression.

In HPV-positive cancers, there appears to be a selection for the integrity of the E6–E7 coding region and the upstream regulatory region, which contains the promoter elements that regulate *E6* and *E7* expression. Furthermore, the *E6* and *E7* genes are regularly expressed in HPV-positive cervical cancers.[108–110] Interestingly, integration of the viral genome into the host chromosome in the cancers often is associated with disruption of the viral *E1* or *E2* genes.[108,109] HPV E2 is an important viral regulatory factor that can negatively regulate the transcriptional promoter directing the *E6* and *E7* genes.[49,111] The manner of integration observed is such that it results in an increase in the expression of the *E6* and *E7* viral genes. The disruption of the *E2* gene by integration releases the viral promoter of the *E6* and *E7* genes from the inhibitory activity of *E2*, increasing the expression of these genes. The reexpression of *E2* in HPV-positive cervical cancer cells results in a cell-cycle arrest due to repression of the viral promoter directing expression of the E6 and E7 oncoproteins.[112]

The E6 and E7 proteins encoded by the high-risk HPVs are oncoproteins and contribute to cellular transformation by bind-

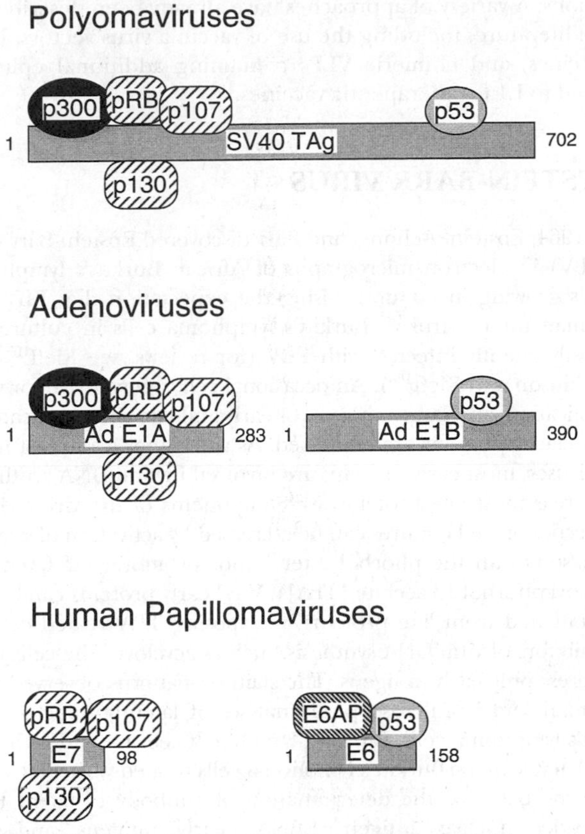

FIGURE 10.2-3. The transforming proteins encoded by three distinct groups of DNA tumor viruses target similar cellular proteins. The binding of human papillomavirus E6 oncoproteins to p53 is mediated by a cellular protein called *E6-AP*.[124] SV40, simian virus 40.

ing to the cell regulatory proteins p53 and RB, respectively (Fig. 10.2-3). The E7 proteins encoded by the high-risk HPVs share sequence similarity to adenovirus E1A and to SV40 large T antigen, and in all three proteins these regions are critical for the transformation properties of the respective viral oncoproteins. The regions of amino acid sequence similarity between E7 and adenovirus E1A that are shared with SV40 large T antigen are regions that have been shown to participate in the binding of a number of important cellular regulatory proteins, including the product of the retinoblastoma tumor suppressor gene (pRB) and the related "pocket" proteins, p107 and p130.[113–116] The E7 proteins may function in carcinogenic progression, at least in part, through interaction with the product of the retinoblastoma susceptibility gene, *pRB.* One consequence of this interaction is the disruption of a complex between pRB and the E2F-1 transcription factor.[117] The E7-mediated release of E2F from these complexes then activates the expression of genes in cell-cycle progression. Genetic studies indicate, however, that there must be other cellular targets of E7 and that complex formation between E7 and the pocket proteins, including pRB, is not sufficient to account for the immortalization and transforming functions of this viral oncoprotein.[118] Studies in several laboratories have identified additional targets, the physiologic significance of which must still be determined. One intriguing E7 target is the cellular cyclin-dependent kinase inhibitor p21[CIP], which appears to have a role in skin differentiation.[119]

The immortalization-transformation properties of the E6 protein were first revealed by studies using primary human genital squamous epithelial cell.[62,63] Efficient immortalization of primary human cells by HPV-16 or HPV-18 requires both the E6 and E7 genes.[62,63,120] The ability of the E6 and E7 proteins to cooperate and efficiently immortalize primary human keratinocytes is a characteristic of the high-risk but not the low-risk HPVs.[121,122] Like SV40 large T antigen and the 55-kD protein encoded by adenovirus E1B, the E6 proteins of the high-risk HPVs can enter into a complex with p53.[123] The interaction of E6 with p53 is not direct but is mediated by a cellular protein, called the *E6-associated protein* (E6AP).[124] E6AP is a ubiquitin protein ligase and, in the presence of E6, directly participates in the ubiquitination of p53.[125,126] Multiubiquitinated p53 then is recognized by the 26S proteasome for proteolysis. Consequently, the half-life and level of p53 are low in E6-immortalized cell lines and in HPV-positive cancers.[127,128] Through its ubiquitination of p53, HPV-16 E6 can abrogate the transcriptional activation and repression properties of p53[129] and disrupt the ability of wild-type p53 to mediate cell-cycle arrest in response to DNA damage.[130] The p53 protein can sense DNA damage and prevent the replication of mutated DNA through its transcriptional activation of the p21 cyclin-dependent kinase inhibitor. Thus, the functional abrogation of p53 by high-risk HPV E6 results in decreased genomic stability and accumulation of DNA abnormalities in high-risk HPV E6–expressing cells. Hence, E6 can be directly implicated in the establishment and propagation of genomic instability, a hallmark in the pathology of malignant progression of cervical lesions.[131]

The high-risk HPV E6 proteins also have other activities that are not linked to their ability to target p53. For instance, it has been shown that expression of the HPV E6 oncoprotein results in the activation of telomerase activity in infected cells.[132] Furthermore, E6 can interact with several additional cellular proteins, including a putative calcium-binding protein referred to as the *E6-binding protein*[133] and a novel GAP protein, E6TP1.[134] The high-risk HPV E6 proteins as well as the oncogenic BPV E6 protein can complex with paxillin, a cellular focal adhesion protein that may serve as an adapter in transmitting signals from integrin molecules to the actin cytoskeleton.[46,135] The high-risk HPV E6 protein has also been reported to bind p300.[136] HPV-16 E6 can also bind and inhibit the transcription activation function of interferon regulatory factor-3, an interaction that may have more to do with the virus-evading host cell defenses than cellular transformation.[137] It should be noted, however, that the significance of the interaction of E6 with these cellular targets and others described in the literature, other than p53 through E6AP, has yet to be fully established.

It is clear that infection by a specific HPV alone is not sufficient for the development of cervical cancer. Only a small fraction of those individuals who are infected by a specific HPV will eventually develop cancer, and the time interval between infection and invasive cancer can be several decades. Thus, the genetic information carried by the virus *per se* is not sufficient for malignant progression. Other factors must be involved in the progression of virus-associated lesions to these genital tract cancers, and clearly additional genetic mutations in the infected cell are required for a cancer to arise. Epidemiologic studies have suggested that smoking is a risk factor for developing cervical carcinoma.[138–140] The recognition that other factors are involved in the progression to cervical carcinomas suggests that papillomavirus infections may work synergistically with these other factors. It has been suggested that tobacco condensate in women who smoke could accumulate in the vaginal fluids, bathing the cervix and acting as a cofactor with the papillomavirus infection.[141] Likewise, it has been postulated that herpesvirus infection might act synergistically with specific papillomaviruses to induce human cervical carcinoma.[142]

The use of restriction fragment–length polymorphisms has revealed that a loss of heterozygosity on the short arm of chromosome 3p implicates a potential tumor suppressor gene seen in cervical cancer,[143] which may be the recently described *FHIT* gene.[144] The somatic cell hybrid work of Stanbridge[145] implicates a potential tumor suppressor gene on human chromosome 11. A gene on human chromosome 11 can suppress the tumorigenicity of HPV-positive cervical carcinoma cells. It has been proposed that the loss of this gene on chromosome 11 in HeLa cells results in loss of expression of the cellular interfering factor, which negatively regulates HPV expression in these cells.[146] Further evidence that a negative regulator of HPV transcription is included on chromosome 11 is that fibroblasts with a deletion in the short arm of chromosome 11 can be more efficiently immortalized by HPV-16 than can normal fibroblasts.[147] The identification of genes on human chromosome 11 involved in tumor suppression in cervical cancer cell lines will obviously be a very important advance. Tumor progression, however, is complex and may involve additional loci. It should be noted that late stages of cervical carcinomas are associated with amplification and overexpression of the cellular oncogene myc.[148]

The availability of specific HPV DNA probes has provided investigators the opportunity to carry out extensive screenings of a variety of human cancers for HPV sequences. Based on the animal models, it seemed likely that any carcinomas of any squamous epithelium or an epithelium that can undergo squamous metaplasia would be a potential candidate for association with an HPV. Studies examining oral, upper airway, and tonsillar carcinomas have revealed some HPV-positive carcinomas.[149–151] HPV DNA has been found in benign oral papillomas,[152–155] and oral focal epithelial hyperplasia has been firmly established as having a papillomavirus etiology.[156,157] In addition, papillomavirus DNA sequences have been found associated with some cases of oral leukoplakia.[153,158] Esophageal carcinomas in humans have not yet been convincingly shown to be associated with an HPV. The esophagus is lined by a squamous epithelium, and squamous cell papillomas of the esophagus have been described in humans.[159,160] Additional studies would seem warranted to investigate a possible role of HPV in human esophageal cancers. In addition, sporadic reports in the literature associate occasional human tumors, including colon cancer, ovarian cancer, prostate cancer, and even melanomas, with the presence of HPV DNA. In general, it seems prudent to be skeptical of such reports until systematic and well-performed studies are confirmed in multiple laboratories.

Significant advances have been made recently in the development of vaccines against papillomavirus infections. The expression in yeast and in insect cells of the major capsid protein L1, either alone or together with L2, leads to the assembly of virus-like particles (VLPs) that are morphologically identical to native virion particles.[161,162] Further, these VLPs present the conformational epitopes necessary for the development of a high-titer neutralizing antisera. Such VLPs now are being used in clinical trials in humans. In addition, there is interest in the development of therapeutic vaccines directed against the E6 and E7 proteins expressed in cancers and preneoplastic lesions. A variety of approaches have already been described in the literature, including the use of vaccinia virus vectors, DNA vaccines, and chimeric VLPs containing additional epitopes fused to L1 for therapeutic vaccines.[163]

EPSTEIN-BARR VIRUS

In 1964, Epstein, Achong, and Barr discovered Epstein-Barr virus (EBV) in electron micrographs of African Burkitt's lymphoma cells growing in culture; raising the expectation that EBV is a human tumor virus.[164] Burkitt's lymphoma cells in culture are mostly latently infected with EBV (for reviews, see Kieff[165] and Rickinson and Kieff[166]). An occasional cell is permissive for virus replication, and large amounts of early and late virus replication–associated proteins are expressed. As with other groups of herpesviruses, most early proteins are involved in viral DNA synthesis, whereas most late proteins are components of the virion. Lytic infection in cell cultures can be increased by activation of protein kinase C with the phorbol ester tumor promoter (12-0-tetradecanoyl-phorbol-13-acetate [TPA]). Viral early proteins can be differentiated from late proteins by exposing TPA-treated cells to inhibitors of viral DNA synthesis, such as acyclovir; the cells then express only early antigens. The staining patterns observed with human sera in microscopical analyses of latently infected Burkitt's lymphoma cells, Burkitt's lymphoma cells treated with TPA and acyclovir, or Burkitt's lymphoma cells treated with TPA alone are the basis for the determination of antibody to latent EBV-encoded nuclear antigen (EBNA), early antigens, and viral capsid antigen, respectively. EBV proteins are serologically distinct from proteins of other human herpesviruses. Early seroepidemiologic studies established that antibody to EBV is prevalent in all human populations and that high titers of antibody correlate with specific malignancies; Burkitt's lymphoma, nasopharyngeal carcinoma, and Hodgkin's disease (Fig. 10.2-4).[167–169]

The host range of EBV, *in vitro*, is limited to primate B lymphocytes. B lymphocytes express large amounts of CD21, a surface glycoprotein for which the major EBV envelope glycoprotein has high affinity. Consistent with the notion that EBV is a human tumor virus, infection of normal B lymphocytes confers an ability to proliferate continuously, *in vitro*,[170] in nude mouse brain after intracerebral inoculation or in the mesentery of severe combined immunodeficiency mice after intravenous inoculation.[171] Infection of some new world primates with EBV reproducibly induces an acutely fatal lymphoproliferative disease.[172] A similar lymphoproliferative disease can occur with primary EBV infection in male children with X-linked lymphoproliferative disease[173] or in profoundly immunosuppressed patients with human immunodeficiency virus (HIV) infection or liver, heart, lung, or bone marrow transplantation.[174,175] Although EBV-transformed B lymphocytes have substantial capacity for continuous proliferation, they remain fully differentiated and exhibit phenotypic markers similar to antigen-activated normal B lymphocytes.

In latently infected transformed B lymphocytes growing *in vitro*, in the peripheral blood of patients with primary EBV infection, or in polyclonal lymphoproliferative disease, EBV encodes six EBNAs, two latent infection–associated membrane proteins (LMPs), and two small nonpolyadenylated RNAs (EBV encoded small RNA [EBERs]). Molecular genetic analyses using specifically mutated EBV recombinants indicate that EBNA3B, LMP2,

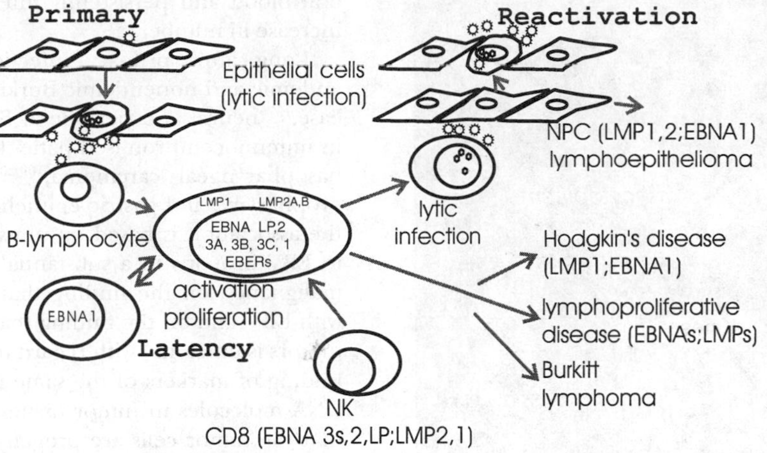

FIGURE 10.2-4. Schematic diagram of the events in Epstein-Barr virus (EBV) infection. Primary EBV infection begins at the oropharyngeal epithelium, where it can produce symptomatic pharyngitis. B lymphocytes are infected as they traffic in close proximity to the oropharyngeal epithelium. EBV BCRF1 is a close homologue of human interleukin-10 and blunts the initial natural killer (NK) CD8 T lymphocyte and gamma interferon responses, enabling EBV better to infect B lymphocytes. In acutely infected B lymphocytes, EBV expresses all EBV-encoded nuclear antigens (EBNAs), latent infection–associated membrane proteins (LMPs), and EBV encoded small RNA (EBERs), causing cell proliferation. In immunosuppressed patients, an acute lymphoproliferative disease may emerge, and the EBNAs, LMPs, and EBERS are expressed in the tumor cells. An EBV-specific CD8+ T-lymphocyte response is demonstrable in normal people shortly after EBV infection and is presumed to account for the fall in peripheral blood EBV-infected B-lymphocyte number from as much as 1 in 10 in acute infection to 1 in 10^5 to 10^6 with convalescence from acute EBV infection. CD8 T lymphocytes recognize determinants from EBNA2, -3A, -3B, -3C or -LP or from LMP1 or LMP2 in the context of specific class 1 major histocompatibility complex (MHC) molecules. B lymphocytes expressing these proteins must continue to be present, as a high level of EBV-immune CD8 T lymphocytes persists for life. EBV persists in some lymphocytes that express only EBNA1. Because CD8 responses to EBNA1 are rare, EBNA1-expressing lymphocytes can escape immune surveillance. Lymphocytes probably carry virus to other organs and to epithelial surfaces, including the oropharynx. LMP2 keeps the virus from reactivating as latently infected B lymphocytes circulate in the peripheral blood and tissues, where they encounter ligands for surface immune globulin or for CD19 or class II MHC. Persistent replication in the oropharynx depends on activation of lytic infection in lymphocytes when they traffic close to oropharyngeal epithelial cells. Years after primary EBV infection, Burkitt's lymphoma, Hodgkin's disease, and nasopharyngeal carcinoma (NPC) tumors occur. These tumors can initiate from a clone of EBV-infected cells. Most African Burkitt's lymphoma, 50% of Hodgkin's disease, and all anaplastic nasopharyngeal carcinomas are composed of EBV-infected cells.

the small RNAs, and most of the viral genome that is expressed in lytic infection can be mutated without a significant effect on the ability of the virus to transform primary B lymphocytes. The other EBNAs and LMP1 are important for lymphocyte transformation. Although not a mediator of cell transformation, LMP2 is important in maintaining latency by preventing lytic infection in response to lymphocyte activation signals.[176]

EBNA1 is an EBV DNA replication origin-binding protein, which is important in latent infection for origin function in episome maintenance and transcriptional activation.[177] The other EBNAs, the functions of which are established, are regulators of transcription of viral or cellular genes. EBNA2 is the best characterized of these virally encoded transactivators and is an acidic type transactivator.[178] EBNA2 lacks DNA sequence–specific binding activity and is dependent on interactions with sequence-specific cell proteins for recognition of enhancer elements. All known EBNA2 response elements have a sequence, which binds the cell protein Jκ that, in turn, recruits EBNA2. This interaction is not entirely sufficient for EBNA2 responsiveness; for example, PU.1 is essential for EBNA2 responsiveness of the LMP1 promoter. EBNA3A and EBNA3C also regulate transcription in lymphocyte transformation. Like EBNA2, EBNA3A and EBNA3C achieve specificity in their interaction with viral and cellular promoters by interacting with the cell protein Jκ.[179] The interaction of three different EBV proteins with Jκ may indicate an importance for Jκ-mediated cell gene regulation in B-lymphocyte growth. This is reinforced by the recent findings that *Notch*, a T-cell leukemia gene, activates transcription through Jκ.[180,181] From a different perspective, EBNA2 and EBNA3s can be viewed as usurpers of the Notch signaling pathway.

LMP1 is a key gene in EBV-mediated cell growth transformation. *LMP1* can transform immortalized rodent fibroblasts to loss of contact inhibition, anchorage independence, or nude mouse tumorigenicity. When expressed in normal resting B lymphocytes or in non–EBV-infected Burkitt's lymphoma cells that have a nonactivated phenotype with regard to markers of normal B-lymphocyte activation, LMP1 induces most B-lymphocyte activation and adhesion markers, activates NFκB, and induces Bcl2 and A20, proteins important in preventing apoptosis. In epithelial cells, LMP1 induces epidermal growth factor receptor expression and inhibits differentiation.[176,182] Specific mutations in the *LMP1* gene in EBV recombinants have provided direct evidence that LMP1 is essential for primary B-lymphocyte growth transformation.[183] LMP1 has multiple transmembrane domains that enable it to aggregate in a patch in the plasma membrane, mimicking an activated growth factor receptor. The first 45 amino acids of the LMP1 C-terminal cytoplas-

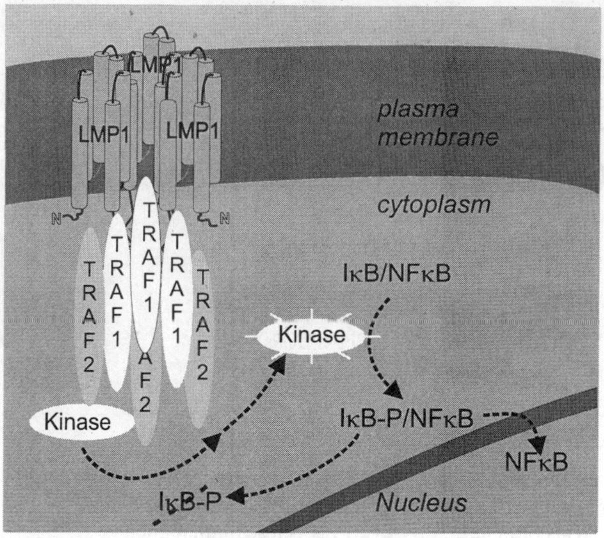

FIGURE 10.2-5. The first 44 amino acids of latent infection–associated membrane protein type 1 (LMP1) engage tumor necrosis factor receptor–associated factors (TRAF) 1, 2, and 3 and activate NFκB through interaction with TRAF1 and TRAF2. Activation is presumed to proceed by constitutive activation of a TRAF2-associated kinase. It is known that phosphorylation of IκB leads to degradation of IκB and release of NFκB to the nucleus.

mic domain are essential for primary B-lymphocyte growth transformation, whereas the N-terminal cytoplasmic domain and the more distal 155 amino acids of the LMP1 C-terminus are not necessary. The essential C-terminal 45–amino acid domain interacts in the cytoplasm with cellular proteins that ordinarily transduce signals from the TNF receptor (TNFR) family.[184,185] TNF signaling is critical in normal lymphoid development, and the B-lymphocyte TNFR family member, CD40, is remarkably similar to LMP1 in its growth-promoting and NFκB-activating effects (Fig. 10.2-5).

Primary EBV infection in most normal people causes clinically apparent or milder forms of acute infectious mononucleosis. Infection initiates in the oropharyngeal epithelium[186] and then spreads to B lymphocytes. As many as 10% of the circulating B lymphocytes may be EBV-infected and express EBNAs and LMPs.[187,188] These infected cells engender a massive natural killer response, followed by a human leukocyte antigen class I and EBV antigen–specific, cytotoxic CD8+ T-cell response.[189,190] The number of responding cells substantially exceeds the number of infected B lymphocytes. As a consequence of the cellular response, the number of infected B lymphocytes falls to 1 in 106 and remains at that level. Somewhat higher levels persist in tonsils. The persisting cells may express only EBNA1, EBNA1 and LMPs, or all of the EBNAs and LMPs.[191] The EBNA1-only type latency appears to be undetectable by T-cell surveillance, whereas the other EBNAs are well recognized by CD8+ T cells.[192–194] In normal people, high-level CD8+ T-cell recognition persists for life, restricting the growth of EBV-infected lymphocytes that progress to expression of all EBNAs and LMPs.[195] The continuous presence of specific CD8+ T cells is unusual and indicates ongoing stimulation of the immune response with EBNA- and LMP-expressing cells. Virus replication also persists in the oropharyngeal epithelium, although this requires reintroduction of virus from the lymphocyte pool. With immunosuppression, latently infected cells in the peripheral blood and persistently infected cells in the oropharynx increase in number.[196]

Long after primary infection, EBV is associated with endemic and nonendemic Burkitt's lymphoma, Hodgkin's disease,[197] neural and peripheral B lymphomas and leiomyomas in immunocompromised patients,[198–201] T-cell malignancies,[202] nasopharyngeal carcinoma,[169,203] squamous tumors of the oropharynx, and gastric epitheliomas.[204,205] In most instances, the association is based on unusually high serologic reactivity to EBV proteins in a substantial number of patients with the malignancy, on the finding that the tumor cells are infected with EBV, and on the finding that the resident EBV genome in tumors is uniclonal with regard to EBV infection events.[206] The finding of markers of the same infection event in all the EBV DNA molecules in tumor tissue and in metastases is evidence that the tumor cells are progeny of a single infected cell and that EBV was present in the cell before the cell became malignant.[207] The EBERs are transcribed in high abundance in latent EBV infection of nonepithelial cells, and *in situ* hybridization to EBERs has been useful in demonstrating the specific association of EBV with Hodgkin's disease tumor cells. Hodgkin's cells express EBNA1 and high levels of LMP1; other EBNAs are not expressed.[208] EBNA1, LMP1, and LMP2 are the only EBV proteins expressed in nasopharyngeal carcinoma and in preneoplastic lesions of the nasopharynx, consistent with a role for these proteins in the latent infection and associated cell growth alteration.[203]

The role of EBV in Burkitt's lymphoma and in other late-onset malignancies is complicated. The presence of EBV in all the tumor cells and the uniclonality of the tumor cells with regard to EBV infection indicate that the tumors arise in an EBV-infected cell.[207] Thus, EBV infection clearly sets the stage at the cellular level for progression to malignancy. At the cellular level, EBV infection may enable further evolution of the malignancy by increasing *NFκB, c-myc,* immune globulin, and *RAG* gene expression and by preventing apoptosis. Increased c-myc, Ig, and *RAG* gene expression may increase the frequency of *c-myc/Ig* translocation, which can result in constitutive c-myc activation.[209,210] On the basis of transgenic models, constitutive c-myc activation can further expand the B-cell pool and predispose to subsequent genetic changes that lead to more malignant phenotypes. EBV genes may initially complement c-myc in promoting cell growth but eventually become redundant. In Africa and New Guinea, the very high-level predisposition of EBV to Burkitt's lymphoma appears to be due to holoendemic malaria; malaria infection stimulates B-cell proliferation and depresses cytotoxic T-cell function.[211,212] In this regard, malarial infection has effects in endemic Burkitt's lymphoma that overlap with the effects of HIV infection or high-level immunosuppressive therapy in EBV-associated lymphoproliferative disease.[213] The significance of the failure of T-cell immune surveillance in the evolution of lymphoproliferative disease in immunosuppressed patients[213] has been experimentally confirmed by the beneficial effects of EBV-specific or nonspecific reconstitutive therapy or prophylaxis.[214] Cytotoxic T-cell failure rarely is complete, and Burkitt's lymphoma or similar uniclonal B lymphomas involving EBV-infected cells that emerge in normal or immunocompromised patients frequently are characterized by the absence of cells that express EBV proteins other than EBNA1. Thus, the current model for EBV-associated B-cell malignancy is that EBV causes B-lymphocyte proliferation.

The number of EBV-infected cells can increase as a result of CD8+ T-cell disorders. Given sufficient immunosuppression, several clones of EBV-infected B cells or the best-growing clone may emerge as a lymphoproliferative disease. EBV infection also predisposes to c-myc translocation, and a more malignant cell clone can eventually emerge as a tumor cell in a host with normal immune function.

EBV also causes oral hairy leukoplakia, a benign proliferation of epithelial cells that occurs in acquired immunodeficiency syndrome (AIDS) patients. The lesions are sites of persistent EBV replication and disappear in response to suppression of EBV replication with acyclovir.[215] As no evidence exists for EBV latency in these lesions, the pathogenesis of oral hairy leukoplakia may involve secretion of a cytokine from lytically infected cells.[216]

KAPOSI'S SARCOMA–ASSOCIATED HERPESVIRUS (HUMAN HERPESVIRUS-8)

Kaposi's sarcoma (KS) is the most common neoplasm associated with AIDS.[217,218] Initially described as a rare and indolent tumor of elderly Mediterranean men, it was later recognized to occur at a higher frequency in Africa.[219] Still later, KS was documented among immunosuppressed organ transplant recipients.[220] In all cases, the histologic picture of the disease is strikingly similar and highly distinctive. Unlike most tumors, which arise from the clonal outgrowth of a single cell, KS lesions contain many cell types.[217] Advanced lesions contain a predominance of spindle-shaped cells (spindle cells), the histogenesis of which remains uncertain but which are believed to arise from endothelial cells (or a more primitive mesenchymal precursor of such cells). In addition, there are infiltrating mononuclear cells (including plasma cells and monocyte-macrophages) and a highly characteristic profusion of slit-like neovascular spaces. The vascularity of the lesion gives KS its distinctive reddish or violaceous appearance.

This complex histology sets KS apart from most other tumors and raises important questions about its pathogenesis. Based on the properties of spindle cells cultivated from AIDS-related KS specimens, many studies have pointed to a key role for growth factors and cytokines in the evolution of a KS lesion.[217,221–223] In general, such cells are not fully tumorigenic: Most do not produce stable, transplantable tumors in nude mice or grow in soft agar. In fact, they are dependent on exogenous growth factors for their proliferation[221,224,225] and, in turn, they produce an array of growth factors and angiogenic factors.[226] When transplanted into nude mice,[223,227] they survive only transiently, then involute. However, during their period of viability, they recruit host inflammatory cells and neovascular structures very reminiscent of KS. When the human spindle cells involute, the entire lesion disappears. This suggests a model for KS in which the proliferating spindle cells drive the rest of the lesion via the elaboration of growth and angiogenic factors. The central question then is: What drives the proliferation of the spindle cells?

One early model attempted to relate spindle cell growth to HIV infection.[217] Certainly, HIV infection is an enormous risk factor for KS development: The prevalence of KS in AIDS patients is 20,000 times that in the general population and 300 times that observed in other immunosuppressed populations.[228] However, both *in vivo* and in cell culture, spindle cells do not appear to carry the HIV genome, ruling out direct infection by HIV as the growth-promoting event. Rather, HIV infection is limited to the smaller lymphoid and mononuclear cell components of KS. Such HIV-infected cells can be shown *in vitro* to release factors that promote cultured spindle cell growth, including both cellular cytokines and the HIV *tat* gene product.[229,230] These observations suggest a plausible mechanism by which HIV infection could drive KS lesion formation without directly infecting the spindle cell.

However, doubts soon arose concerning the ability of HIV infection alone to account for the etiology of KS. First, of course, KS can certainly arise in HIV-negative hosts. More important, even within the HIV-infected population, large differences in KS risk are not accounted for by the preceding formulation.[228–231] KS risk is highest in homosexual men with AIDS: A full 20% to 30% of such individuals will develop KS in the course of their HIV disease. By contrast, fewer than 1% to 2% of AIDS cases related to hemophilia (i.e., blood product administration) will be complicated by KS, and KS is rarer still among pediatric AIDS cases in which HIV infection is acquired vertically from infected mothers. These and other data[231] suggest the possibility of a sexually transmitted cofactor in KS etiology or pathogenesis. In 1994, Chang et al.[232] used a polymerase chain reaction–based method to identify DNA sequences that were present in DNA extracted from an AIDS-KS specimen but absent from normal genomic DNA from the same patient. Two small DNA fragments emerged that were shown to be highly correlated with KS: Virtually all AIDS-KS tumors were positive for these sequences, whereas available tissue specimens from a large number of HIV-negative hosts were negative, as were most non-KS tissues from patients with KS. Interestingly, approximately 10% to 15% of lymphoid tissues from AIDS patients who did not have KS were also positive, indicating that the sequences track with both KS and the risk for KS development. Sequence analysis of these two small DNA fragments reveals homology to two known lymphotropic herpesviruses, human EBV and the simian herpesvirus saimiri (HVS). These seminal findings point to the existence of a novel herpesvirus, termed *KS-associated herpesvirus* (KSHV) or *human herpes virus-8* (HHV-8), and suggest it as a candidate for the exogenous cofactor earlier predicted by epidemiologists.

Subsequent work has confirmed these findings and extended them in important ways, all of which are consistent with a role for this virus in KS development. First, KSHV/HHV-8 sequences are present in virtually all KS specimens from HIV-negative patients with the disease, as well as their HIV-positive counterparts.[233–237] Because most HIV-negative KS patients are not grossly immunodeficient, it is unlikely that KSHV/HHV-8 is simply an opportunistic saprophyte that overruns the profoundly immunodeficient host. In KS tumors, KSHV DNA is found primarily in the spindle cells[238]—the key cell type in KS pathogenesis—and active but restricted viral gene expression consistent with latent infection is demonstrable in the vast majority of these cells.[239,240] In addition, a small subset of the spindle cells appears to harbor viral genomes undergoing lytic replication. Second, KSHV/HHV-8 sequences have been identified in the peripheral blood mononuclear cells (PBMCs) of 30% to 50% of KS patients and a much smaller proportion (10% to 15%) of AIDS patients lacking clinical KS.[241] Importantly, in KS-negative AIDS patients, the risk of subsequent KS development is much greater among patients whose initial PBMC sample harbored KSHV than among those whose PBMCs did not.[241] Thus, viral infection precedes the development of KS, and prior infection appears to be predictive of increased KS risk.

These early inferences have been sustained by more recent seroepidemiologic studies, which have yielded the following important conclusions. First, KSHV infection is not ubiquitous; among screened (low-risk) U.S. and European blood donors, only approximately 5% to 7% are seropositive. (This number probably slightly underestimates the true prevalence of infection in the general population.) However, in HIV-positive populations, seroprevalence tracks very strikingly with KS risk: While 30% to 60% of HIV-infected homosexual men are KSHV-seropositive, fewer than 5% of HIV-positive hemophiliacs or women show serologic evidence of KSHV infection, and KSHV seroreactivity is surprisingly rare among U.S. children with AIDS.[242–245] In large prospective studies, KSHV seroreactivity was shown to antedate the onset of the tumor (often by up to 10 years) and strongly predicted an increased risk of KS development.[246–248] Studies in male homosexuals in the United States produced strong evidence for sexual transmission in this group: KSHV seroprevalence rises sharply with increasing numbers of sexual partners and with histories of other STDs, for example. In a key study, Martin et al.[246] showed that the risk of subsequent KS among KSHV-seropositive individuals was the same even after normalizing for the prevalence of other STDs.[246] This result indicates that it is KSHV infection itself, not some cotransmitted STD, that is responsible for KS risk.

These data clearly indicate that KSHV is the agent predicted by KS epidemiology and strongly implicate KSHV in KS pathogenesis. The epidemiologic case for involvement of KSHV in KS biogenesis now is as compelling as the cases for HBV and hepatoma or HPV and cervical cancer. Given the large number of subjects studied to date, the evidence supports the assertion that KS is virtually never observed in the absence of documented KSHV infection. Accordingly, most experts in the field now accept that KSHV is necessary for KS development. However, there is also strong consensus that it is not sufficient for this process. For example, 5% to 7% of the general population in the United States is infected by KSHV, yet this population has no significant KS risk. Clearly, therefore, one or more cofactors, in addition to KSHV, are required to promote tumorigenesis. In the case of AIDS-KS, of course, that cofactor is HIV, although exactly what HIV contributes to pathogenesis is much debated. Some argue that HIV's link to KS generation is simply the production of an immunodeficient state; others hypothesize that individual HIV proteins released from infected cells (specifically tat or HIV-induced host cytokines) participate directly in spindle cell growth deregulation in a paracrine fashion.[226,249,250] Such notions need not, of course, be mutually exclusive. The nature of the cofactors in the HIV-negative forms of KS remains unknown.

Studies of KSHV seroepidemiology conducted in the developing world have yielded additional new insights. First, the prevalence of KSHV in the general population is remarkably elevated in countries in which classic KS is common. For example, in southern Italy, Sicily, and Sardinia, KSHV antibodies are found in more than 20% of the general population[251,252]; in many populations in sub-Saharan Africa, where classic KS was common even in the pre-AIDS era, 60% to 80% of the population is seropositive.[253–256] Thus, KS seroprevalence tracks with KS risk even outside of HIV-positive cohorts. However, these numbers also reflect major epidemiologic differences between KSHV infection in Africa and the Mediterranean, on the one hand, and KS risk in Western Europe and America, on the other. In the latter countries, homosexual men represent a major reservoir of infection, with much lower rates in women and very little infection in prepubertal children.[257,258] By contrast, in Africa and the Mediterranean, seroconversions begin in childhood, and the seroprevalence rises nearly continuously throughout the first four to five decades of life. Moreover, seroprevalence is equal in both genders, in sharp contrast to the developed world. The basis for this strikingly different epidemiology is not yet understood. The frequent occurrence of infection in young children in the Mediterranean and Africa suggests the existence of nonsexual routes of spread, and the equal infection rates in adult men and women also suggests different routes of spread from those observed in the West.

How does KSHV infection predispose to KS? Understanding of this association at the molecular level is still fragmentary. Because most KS tumor cells are latently infected, efforts to identify and characterize KSHV latency genes have been made, presuming, as in EBV, that these genes will play strong roles in spindle cell growth deregulation. To date, several interesting genes have been identified in this fashion. An important group of latency genes is clustered in one region of the viral genome, where two transcription units have been mapped.[259,260] One expresses a set of three genes, including (1) LANA, an antigen that appears to function in KSHV genomic maintenance in latency,[261] (2) a viral homologue of cellular cyclin D1, and (3) a homologue of cellular inhibitors of caspase activation (Flice-inhibitory protein). The viral cyclin can bind and activate cdk6, indicating that it is a functional cyclin.[262,263] It appears to display reduced sensitivity to the inhibitory effects of certain cdk inhibitors.[264–266] It is easy to imagine how such a gene might figure in growth deregulation, especially given the known links between deregulation of cellular cyclin D1 and several forms of human cancer.[267] The viral Flice-inhibitory protein presumably functions to block apoptosis—a potentially important activity, as overexpression of viral cyclin sensitizes cells to apoptosis.[268] A second transcription unit encodes a family of related proteins, the kaposins, which are generated by a complex translational strategy.[269] Their transcripts are used widely to identify latently infected cells,[270,271] but the functions of their gene products remain unknown. Remote from these genes, at the right-hand terminus of the genome, is a coding region for a multiply spliced transcript encoding a series of transmembrane proteins called *latency-associated membrane proteins* (LAMPs).[272,273] These proteins contain a variety of motifs suggestive of roles in cellular signal transduction and can bind tumor necrosis factor receptor–associated factors (TRAFs) 1, 2, and 3 *in vitro*, but their *in vivo* roles remain to be defined.[272]

As noted, KS tumors also harbor smaller numbers of lytically infected cells.[270,274] The significance of lytic infection in KS tumorigenesis is unknown, but there are reasons to believe that the lytic cycle may play a more profound role in KS than in other herpesvirus-induced malignancies. First, a recent clinical trial has shown that even in patients with advanced AIDS, treatment with ganciclovir, which is active only against lytic herpesvirus infection, profoundly reduced the subsequent development of KS over the ensuing 6 to 12 months.[275] Although this result might mean simply that lytic reactivation from the lymphoid reservoir is necessary for spread to the endothelium to initiate latent infection there, it is also compatible with a requirement for ongoing KSHV replication in KS pathogenesis. The latter is an attractive notion, because the virus contains numerous genes that are potent signaling molecules expressed principally during lytic growth.[276–278] Some of these are secreted factors (e.g., homologues of interleukin-6, chemokines, and other factors), whereas others (e.g., the K1 protein and a virus-specific G protein–coupled receptor) are transmembrane proteins that trigger deregulated signal transduction in the host, often leading to secretory products that can influence surrounding cells.[279–281] For example, virus-specific G protein–coupled receptor expression induces the release of vascular endothelial growth factor,[282] a protein long speculated to play a role in the angiogenic phenotype of KS. Some of the viral chemokines can trigger angiogenesis as well[283]; moreover, these molecules would be expected to contribute to the influx of inflammatory cells in the lesion, another hallmark of KS. Defining the relative contributions of latency and lytic growth to KS pathogenesis will be a major focus of KSHV research in the coming decade.

The homologies to EBV and the simian herpesvirus saimiri place KSHV/HHV-8 within the lymphotropic herpesvirus subfamily, an assignment supported by the finding of viral DNA in the B-cell compartment of the PBMC population.[237] This raises the possibility that the virus might participate in lymphoid neoplasia as well and, in recent years, viral infection has in fact been associated with at least two lymphoproliferative conditions. The first is a rare B-cell lymphoma, termed *body cavity–based lymphoma,* that has thus far been limited to HIV-positive hosts.[284] It presents as ascitic tumors in the pleural and peritoneal cavities, often without clinically evident lymphadenopathy or bone marrow involvement. Body cavity–based lymphoma cells are uniformly latently infected with HHV-8; many (but not all) also bear latent EBV genomes. Cultured B-cells derived from such tumors are latently infected and, in some of these cells, lytic viral replication can be induced *in vitro* with phorbol esters.[285] The other lesion associated with HHV-8 is *multicentric Castleman's disease* (MCD), a complex and poorly understood lymphoproliferative syndrome that can occur in both HIV-positive and HIV-negative individuals. The HIV-positive form appears to be uniformly associated with KSHV/HHV-8, whereas only approximately half of the HIV-negative forms can be shown to harbor this virus.[286] Although the role of the virus in this condition is unclear, it is interesting that an association of Castleman's disease with KS has long been recognized, though little discussed.

Study of viral gene expression in MCD has revealed some provocative surprises. Within the involved tissue, viral DNA is confined to B cells in the mantle zones surrounding the lymphoid follicles. There, both latently and lytically infected cells can be found, with a rather larger proportion of the infected cell population being in the lytic cycle than there are in KS.[287,288] Interestingly, although MCD-involved nodes contain equal numbers of B cells bearing κ and λ light chains, all the infected cells appear to bear λ chains on their surface. Though this might simply indicate clonality of these cells, it is striking that among more than a dozen analyzed cases, no KSHV-infected cells with surface κ chains have yet been described. The meaning of this observation is not yet clear, but it may suggest a particular stage in B-cell ontogeny is targeted by KSHV during MCD pathogenesis. Although the links of KSHV to primary effusion lymphoma and MCD are very strong, it bears noting that formal epidemiologic evidence for causality—of the type that has been so compelling for KS—is lacking for these disorders, owing primarily to their rarity.

REFERENCES

1. Ellermann V, Bang O. Experimentelle leukamie bei huhnern. *Zentralbl Bakteriol Abt I* 1908;46:595.
2. Rous P. A sarcoma of the fowl transmissible by an agent separable from the tumor cells. *J Exp Med* 1911;13:397.
3. Shope RE. A filtrable virus causing a tumor-like condition in rabbits and its relationship to virus myxomatosum. *J Exp Med* 1932;56:803.
4. Shope RE, Hurst EW. Infectious papillomatosis of rabbits; with a note on the histopathology. *J Exp Med* 1933;58:607.
5. Rous P, Beard JW. The progression to carcinoma of virus-induced rabbit papillomas (Shope). *J Exp Med* 1935;62:523.
6. Gross L. Pathogenic properties, and "vertical" transmission of the mouse leukemia agent. *Proc Soc Exp Biol Med* 1951;62:523.
7. Gross L. A filtrable agent, recovered from Akr leukemia extracts, causing salivary gland carcinomas in C3H mice. *Proc Soc Exp Biol Med* 1953;83:414.
8. Steward SE. Leukemia in mice produced by a filterable agent present in AKR leukemic tissues with notes on a sarcoma produced by the same agent. *Anat Rev* 1953;117:532.
9. Szmuness W. Hepatocellular carcinoma and the hepatitis B virus: evidence for a causal association. *Prog Med Virol* 1978;24:40.
10. Beasley RP. Hepatitis B virus—the major etiology of the hepatocellular carcinoma. *Cancer* 1988;61:1942.
11. Ganem D, Schneider RJ. Hepadnaviridae and their replication. In: Knipe DM, Howley PM, eds. *Field's Virology*. Philadelphia: Lippincott Williams & Wilkins, 2000 *(in press)*.
12. Chisari FV, Ferrari C. Hepatitis B virus immunopathogenesis. *Annu Rev Immunol* 1995;13:29.
13. Moriyama T, Guilhot S, Klopchin K, et al. Immunobiology and pathogenesis of hepatocellular injury in hepatitis B virus transgenic mice. *Science* 1990;248:361.
14. Ando K, Moriyama T, Guidotti LG, et al. Class I restricted cytotoxic T lymphocytes are directly cytopathic for their target cells *in vivo*. *J Immunol* 1994;152:3245.
15. Guidotti L, Ishikawa T, Hobbs M, et al. Intracellular inactivation of hepatitis B virus by cytotoxic T lymphocytes. *Immunity* 1996;4:25.
16. Gilles PN, Guerrette DL, Ulevitch RJ, Schreiber RD, Chisari FV. HB_sAg retention sensitizes the hepatocyte to injury by physiological concentrations of interferon-gamma. *Hepatology* 1992;16:655.
17. Michalopoulos G. Liver regeneration: molecular mechanisms of growth control. *FASEB J* 1990;4:176.
18. Sell S, Hunt JM, Knoll B, Dunsford H. Cellular events during hepatocarcinogenesis in rats and the question of premalignancy. *Adv Cancer Res* 1987;48:10.
19. Tsukuma H, Hiyama T, Tanaka S, et al. Risk factors for hepatocellular carcinoma among patients with chronic liver disease. *N Engl J Med* 1993;328:1797.
20. Yen TSB. Hepadnaviral X protein: review of recent progress. *J Biomed Sci* 1996;3:20.
21. Kim C-Y, Koike K, Saito I, Miyamura T, Jay G. HBx gene of hepatitis B virus induces liver cancer in transgenic mice. *Nature* 1991;351:317.
22. Koike K, Moriya K, Iino S, et al. High-level expression of hepatitis B virus HBx gene and hepatocarcinogenisis in transgenic mice. *Hepatology* 1994;19:810.
23. Benn J, Schneider R. Hepatitis B virus HBx protein activates ras-GTP complex formation and establishes a ras, raf, MAP kinase signaling cascade. *Proc Natl Acad Sci U S A* 1994;91:10350.
24. Natoli G, Avantaggiati M, Chirillo P, et al. Ras and raf-dependent activation of cjun transcriptional activity by the hepatitis B virus transactivator pX. *Oncogene* 1994;9:2837.
25. Unger T, Shaul Y. The X protein of the hepatitis B virus acts as a transcription factor when targeted to its responsive element. *EMBO J* 1990;9:1889.
26. Williams J, Andrisani O. The hepatitis B virus X protein targets the basic region-leucine zipperdomain of CREB. *Proc Natl Acad Sci U S A* 1995;92:3819.
27. Wang X, Forrester K, Yeh H, et al. Hepatitis B virus X protein inhibits p53 sequence-specific DNA binding, transcriptional activity and association with transcription factor ERCC3. *Proc Natl Acad Sci U S A* 1994;91:2230.
28. Nagaya T, Nakamura T, Tokino T, et al. The mode of hepatitis B virus DNA integration in chromosomes of human hepatocellular carcinoma. *Genes Dev* 1987;1:773.
29. Popper H, Roth L, Purcell RH, Tennant BC, Gerin JL. Hepatocarcinogenicity of the woodchuck hepatitis virus. *Proc Natl Acad Sci U S A* 1987;84:866.
30. Fourel G, Trepo C, Bougueleret L, et al. Frequent activation of N-myc genes by hepadnavirus insertion in woodchuck liver tumours. *Nature* 1990;347:294.
31. Fourel G, Couturier J, Wei Y, et al. Evidence for long-range oncogene activation by hepadnavirus insertion. *EMBO J* 1994;13:2526.
32. Hansen LJ, Tennant BC, Seeger C, Ganem D. Differential activation of myc gene family members in hepatic carcinogenesis by closely related hepatitis B virus. *Mol Cell Biol* 1993;13:659.
33. Yang D, Alt E, Rogler CE. Coordinate expression of N-myc 2 and insulin-like growth factor II in pre-cancerous altered hepatic foci in woodchuck hepatitis virus carriers. *Cancer Res* 1993;53:2020.
34. de The G, Zeng Y. Population screening for EBV markers: toward improvement of nasopharyngeal carcinoma control. In: Epstein MA, Achog BS, eds. *The Epstein-Barr virus*. New York: John Wiley and Sons, 1986:237.
35. Wang J, Chenivesse X, Henglein B, Brechot C. Hepatitis B virus integration in a cyclin A gene in a hepatocellular carcinoma. *Nature* 1990;343:555.

36. Ciuffo G. Imnfesto positivo con filtrato di verruca volgare. *Giorn Ital Mal Venereol* 1907;48:12.
37. DeVilliers E-M. Human pathogenic papillomaviruses: an update. *Curr Top Microbiol Immunol* 1994;86:1.
38. Schneider A, Oltersdorf T, Schneider V, Gissmann L. Distribution of human papillomavirus 16 genome in cervical neoplasia by molecular *in situ* hybridization of tissue sections. *Int J Cancer* 1987;39:717.
39. Baker CC, Howley PM. Differential promoter utilization by the papillomavirus in transformed cells and productively infected wart tissues. *EMBO J* 1987;6:1027.
40. Howley PM. Papillomavirinae: the viruses and their replication. In: Fields BN, Knipe DM, Howley PM, eds. *Field's Virology*, vol 2. Philadelphia: Lippincott-Raven Publishers, 1996:2045.
41. Lowy DR, Dvoretzky I, Shober R, et al. *In vitro* tumorigenic transformation by a defined subgenomic fragment of bovine papillomavirus DNA. *Nature* 1980;287:72.
42. Doorbar J, Campbell D, Grand RJA, Gallimore PH. Identification of the human papillomavirus-1a E4 gene products. *EMBO J* 1986;5:355.
43. Spalholz BA, Howley PM. Papillomavirus-host cell interactions. *Adv Viral Oncol* 1989;8:27.
44. DiMaio D, Petti L, Hwang E-S. The E5 transforming proteins of the papillomaviruses. *Semin Virol* 1994;5:369.
45. Tong X, Salgia R, Li J-L, Griffin JD, Howley PM. The bovine papillomavirus E6 protein binds to the LD motif repeats of paxillin and blocks its interaction with vinculin and the focal adhesion kinase. *J Biol Chem* 1997;272:33373.
46. Vande Pol SB, Brown MC, Turner CE. Association of bovine papillomavirus type 1 E6 oncoprotein with the focal adhesion protein paxillin through a conserved protein interaction motif. *Oncogene* 1998;16:43.
47. McBride AA, Romanczuk H, Howley PM. The papillomavirus E2 regulatory proteins. *J Biol Chem* 1991;266:18411.
48. Spalholz BA, Yang Y-C, Howley PM. Transactivation of a bovine papillomavirus transcriptional regulatory element by the E2 gene product. *Cell* 1985;42:183.
49. Thierry F, Yaniv M. The BPV1 E2 *trans*-acting protein can be either an activator or a repressor of the HPV18 regulatory region. *EMBO J* 1987;6:3391.
50. Ustav M, Stenlund A. Transient replication of BPV-1 requires two viral polypeptides encoded by the E1 and E2 open reading frames. *EMBO J* 1991;10:449.
51. Skiadopoulos MH, McBride AA. Bovine papillomavirus type 1 genomes and the E2 transactivator protein are closely associated with mitotic chromatin. *J Virol* 1998;72:2079.
52. Lehman CW, Botchan MR. Segregation of viral plasmids depends on tethering to chromosomes and is regulated by phosphorylation. *Proc Natl Acad Sci U S A* 1998;95:4338.
53. Mohr IJ, Clark R, Sun S, et al. Targeting the E1 replication protein to the papillomavirus origin of replication by complex formation with the E2 transactivator. *Science* 1990;250:1694.
54. Yang L, Li R, Mohr IJ, Clark R, Botchan MR. Activation of BPV-1 replication *in vitro* by the transcription factor E2. *Nature* 1991;353:628.
55. MacPherson P, Thorner L, Parker L, Botchan M. The bovine papillomavirus E1 protein has ATPase activity essential to viral DNA replication and efficient transformation in cells. *Virology* 1994;204:403.
56. Seo Y-S, Muller F, Lusky M, et al. Bovine papillomavirus (BPV)-encoded E2 protein enhances binding of E1 protein to the BPV replication origin. *Proc Natl Acad Sci U S A* 1993;90:2865.
57. Pilacinski WP, Glassman DL, Krzyzek RA, Sadowski PL, Robbins AK. Cloning and expression in *Escherichia coli* of the bovine papillomavirus L1 and L2 open reading frames. *Biotechnology* 1984;1:356.
58. Komly CA, Breitburd F, Croissant O, Streeck RE. The L2 open reading frame of human papillomavirus type 1a encodes a minor structural protein carrying type-specific antigens. *J Virol* 1986;60:813.
59. Bedell MA, Jones KH, Laimins LA. The E6-E7 region of human papillomavirus type 18 is sufficient for transformation of NIH 3T3 and rat-1 cells. *J Virol* 1987;61:3635.
60. Phelps WC, Yee CL, Münger K, Howley PM. The human papillomavirus type 16 E7 gene encodes transactivation and transformation functions similar to those of adenovirus E1A. *Cell* 1988;53:539.
61. Matlashewski G, Schneider J, Banks L, et al. Human papillomavirus type 16 DNA cooperates with activated ras in transforming primary cells. *EMBO J* 1987;6:1741.
62. Münger K, Phelps WC, Bubb V, Howley PM, Schlegel R. The E6 and E7 genes of the human papillomavirus type 16 together are necessary and sufficient for transformation of primary human keratinocytes. *J Virol* 1989;63:4417.
63. Hawley-Nelson P, Vousden KH, Hubbert NL, Lowy DR, Schiller JT. HPV16 E6 and E7 proteins cooperate to immortalize human foreskin keratinocytes. *EMBO J* 1989;8:3905.
64. Rous P, Kidd JG, Smith WE. Experiments on the cause of the rabbit carcinomas derived from virus-induced papillomas. *J Exp Med* 1953;96:159.
65. Rous P, Kidd JG. The carcinogenic effect of a virus upon tarred skin. *Science* 1936;83:468.
66. Kidd JG, Rous P. Effect of the papillomavirus (Shope) upon tar warts of rabbits. *Proc Soc Exp Biol Med* 1937;37:518.
67. Jarrett WFH, McNeil PE, Grimshaw WIR, Selman IE, McIntyre WIM. High incidence area of cattle cancer with a possible interaction between an environmental carcinogen and a papillomavirus. *Nature* 1978;274:215.
68. Jarrett WFH, Murphy J, O'Neill BW, Larid HM. Virus-induced papillomas of the alimentary tract of cattle. *Int J Cancer* 1978;22:323.
69. Campo MS, Moar MH, Sartirana ML, Kennedy IM, Jarrett WGF. The presence of bovine papillomavirus type 4 DNA is not required for the progression to, or maintenance of, the malignant state in cancers of the alimentary tract in cattle. *EMBO J* 1985;4:1819.
70. Jablonska S, Majewski S. Epidermoplasia verruciformis: immunological and clinical aspects. *Curr Top Microbiol Immunol* 1994;186:157.
71. Lutzner M, Croissant O, Ducasse MF, et al. A potentially oncogenic human papillomavirus (HPV-5) found in two renal allograft recipients. *J Invest Dermatol* 1980;75:353.
72. Ramoz N, Rueda LA, Bouadjar B, Favre M, Orth G. A susceptibility locus for epidermodysplasia verruciformis, an abnormal predisposition to infection with the oncogenic human papillomavirus type 5, maps to chromosome 17qter in a region containing a psoriasis locus. *J Invest Dermatol* 1999;112:259.
73. Favre M, Orth G, Majewski S, et al. Psoriasis: a possible reservoir for human papillomavirus type 5, the virus associated with skin carcinomas of epidermodysplasia verruciformis [see comments]. *J Invest Dermatol* 1998;110:311.
74. Orth G. Epidermodysplasia verruciformis: a model for understanding the oncogenicity of human papillomaviruses. *Ciba Found Symp* 1986;120:157.
75. Ostrow RS, Bender M, Niimura M, et al. Human papillomavirus DNA in cutaneous primary and metastasized squamous cell carcinomas from patients with epidermodysplasia verruciformis. *Proc Natl Acad Sci U S A* 1982;79:1634.
76. Yutsudo M, Hakura A. Human papillomavirus type 17 transcripts expressed in skin carcinoma tissue of a patient with epidermodysplasia verruciformis. *Int J Cancer* 1987;39:586.
77. Iftner T, Bierfelder S, Csapo Z, Pfister H. Involvement of human papillomavirus type 8 genes E6 and E7 in transformation and replication. *J Virol* 1988;62:3655.
78. Berkhout RJM, Tieben LM, Smits HL, et al. Nested PCR approach for detection and typing of epidermoplasia verruciformis–associated human papillomavirus types in cutaneous cancers from renal transplant recipients. *J Clin Microbiol* 1995;33:690.
79. Shamanin V, Glover M, Rausch C, et al. Specific types of human papillomavirus found in benign proliferations and carcinomas of the skin in immunosuppressed patients. *Cancer Res* 1994;54:4610.
80. Underwood PB, Hester L. Diagnosis and treatment of premalignant lesions of the vulva. *Am J Obstet Gynecol* 1971;110:849.
81. Waugh M. Condylomata acuminata. *Br Med J* 1972;2:527.
82. Dunn AE, Ogilvie MM. Intranuclear virus particles in human genital wart tissue: observation on the ultrastructure of epidermal layer. *J Ultrastruct Res* 1968;22:282.
83. Oriel JD, Almeida JD. Demonstration of virus particles in human genital warts. *Br J Vener Dis* 1970;46:37.
84. Gissmann L, de Villiers EM, zur Hausen H. Analysis of human genital warts (condylomata acuminata) and other genital tumors for human papillomavirus type 6 DNA. *Int J Cancer* 1982;29:143.
85. Gissmann L, Wolnik L, Ikenberg H, et al. Human papillomavirus types 6 and 11 DNA sequences in genital and laryngeal papillomas and in some cervical cancers. *Proc Natl Acad Sci U S A* 1983;80:560.
86. zur Hausen H. Condylomata acuminata and human genital cancer. *Cancer Res* 1976;36:530.
87. Meisels A, Fortin R. Condylomatous lesions of the cervix and vagina: I. Cytologic patterns. *Acta Cytol* 1976;20:505.
88. Purola E, Savia E. Cytology of gynecologic condyloma acuminatum. *Acta Cytol* 1977;21:26.
89. Laverty CR, Russell P, Hills E, Booth N. The significance of noncondylomatous wart virus infection of the cervical transformation zone. *Acta Cytol* 1978;22:195.
90. Koss LG, Durfee GR. Unusual patterns of squamous epithelium of the uterine cervix: cytologic and pathologic study of poilocytotic atypia. *Ann NY Acad Sci* 1956;63:1245.
91. Della Torre G, Pilotti S, De Palo G, Rilke F. Viral particles in cervical condylomatous lesions. *Tumori* 1978;64:549.
92. Hills E, Laverty CR. Electron microscopic detection of papilloma virus particles in selected koilocytotic cells in a routine cervical smear. *Acta Cytol* 1979;23:53.
93. Kessler IL. Human cervical cancer as a venereal disease. *Cancer Res* 1976;36:783.
94. zur Hausen H. Human papillomaviruses and their possible role in squamous cell carcinomas. *Curr Top Microbiol Immunol* 1977;78:1.
95. Rawls WE, Tompkins WAF, Figueroa ME, Melnick JL. Herpes simplex virus type 2: association with carcinoma of the cervix. *Science* 1968;161:1255.
96. Nahmias AJ, Josey WE, Naib ZM, Luce CF, Guest BA. Antibodies to herpes virus hominus types 1 and 2 in humans: II. Women with cervical cancer. *Am J Epidemiol* 1970;91:547.
97. zur Hausen H. Herpes simplex virus in human genital cancer. *Int Rev Exp Pathol* 1983;25:307.
98. Vonka V, Kanda J, Hirsch I, et al. Prospective study on the relationship between cervical neoplasia and herpes simplex type-2 virus: II. Herpes simplex type-2 antibody presence in sera taken at enrollment. *Int J Cancer* 1984;33:61.
99. Vonka V, Kanda J, Jelinek J, et al. Prospective study on the relationship between cervical neoplasia and herpes simplex type-2 virus: I. Epidemiological characteristics. *Int J Cancer* 1984;33:49.
100. Peterson O. Spontaneous course of cervical precancerous conditions. *Am J Obstet Gynecol* 1956;72:1063.
101. Kinlen LJ, Spriggs AI. Women with positive cervical smears but without surgical intervention: a follow-up study. *Lancet* 1978;2:463.
102. Richart RM, Barrow BA. A follow-up study of patients with cervical dysplasia. *Am J Obstet Gynecol* 1969;105:386.
103. Durst M, Gissmann L, Idenburg H, zur Hausen H. A papillomavirus DNA from a cervical carcinoma and its prevalence in cancer biopsy samples from different geographic regions. *Proc Natl Acad Sci U S A* 1983;80:3812.
104. Boshart M, Gissmann L, Ikenberg H, et al. A new type of papillomavirus DNA, its presence in genital cancer biopsies and in cell lines derived from cervical cancer. *EMBO J* 1984;3:1151.
105. Gissmann L, Schwarz E. Persistence and expression of human papillomavirus DNA in genital cancer. In: Evered D, Clark S, eds. *Papillomaviruses.* Chichester: John Wiley and Sons, 1986:190.
106. Ikenberg H, Gissmann L, Gross G, et al. Human papillomavirus type-16-related DNA in genital Bowen's disease and in Bowenoid papulosis. *Int J Cancer* 1983;32:563.
107. Gross G, Hagedorn M, Ikenberg H, et al. Bowenoid papulosis. Presence of human papillomavirus (HPV) structural antigens and of HPV-16 related DNA sequences. *Arch Dermatol* 1985;121:858.
108. Durst M, Croce C, Gissmann L, Schwarz E, Huebner K. Papillomavirus sequences integrate near cellular oncogenes in some cervical carcinomas. *Proc Natl Acad Sci U S A* 1987;84:1070.
109. Schwarz E, Freese UK, Gissmann L, et al. Structure and transcription of human papillomavirus sequences in cervical carcinoma cells. *Nature* 1985;314:111.
110. Yee CL, Krishnan-Hewlett I, Baker CC, Schlegel R, Howley PM. Presence and expression of human papillomavirus sequences in human cervical carcinoma cell lines. *Am J Pathol* 1985;119:361.

111. Dowhanick JJ, McBride AA, Howley PM. Suppression of cellular proliferation by the papillomavirus E2 protein. *J Virol* 1995;69:7791.
112. Francis DA, Schmid SI, Howley PM. Repression of the integrated papillomavirus E6/E7 promoter is required for growth suppression of cervical cancer cells. *J Virol* 2000;74:2679.
113. DeCaprio JA, Ludlow JW, Figge J, et al. SV40 large tumor antigen forms a specific complex with the product of the retinoblastoma susceptibility gene. *Cell* 1988;54:275.
114. Whyte P, Williamson NM, Harlow E. Cellular targets for transformation by the adenovirus E1A proteins. *Cell* 1989;56:67.
115. Ewen MB, Ludlow JW, Marsilio E, et al. An N-terminal transformation-governing sequence of SV40 large T antigen contributes to the binding of both p110 RB and a second cellular protein, p120. *Cell* 1989;58:257.
116. Münger K, Werness BA, Dyson N, Phelps WC, Howley PM. Complex formation of human papillomavirus E7 proteins with the retinoblastoma tumor suppressor gene product. *EMBO J* 1989;8:4099.
117. Chellappan S, Kraus VB, Kroger B, et al. Adenovirus E1A, simian virus 40 tumor antigen and human papillomavirus E7 protein share the capacity to disrupt the interaction between transcription factor E2F and the retinoblastoma gene product. *Proc Natl Acad Sci U S A* 1992;89:4549.
118. Jewers RJ, Hildebrandt P, Ludlow JW, Kell B, McCance DJ. Regions of human papillomavirus type 16 E7 oncoprotein required for immortalization of human keratinocytes. *J Virol* 1992;66:1329.
119. Jones DL, Alani RM, Münger K. The human papillomavirus E7 oncoprotein can uncouple cellular differentiation and proliferation in human keratinocytes by abrogating p21cip1-mediated inhibition of cdk2. *Genes Dev* 1997;11:2101.
120. Hudson JB, Bedell MA, McCance DJ, Laimins LA. Immortalization and altered differentiation of human keratinocytes *in vitro* by the E6 and E7 open reading frames of human papillomavirus type 18. *J Virol* 1990;64:519.
121. Barbosa MS, Vass WC, Lowy DR, Schiller JT. *In vitro* biological activities of the E6 and E7 genes vary among HPVs of different oncogenic potential. *J Virol* 1991;65:292.
122. Schlegel R, Phelps WC, Zhang YL, Barbosa M. Quantitative keratinocyte assay detects two biological activities of human papillomavirus DNA and identifies viral types associated with cervical carcinoma. *EMBO J* 1988;7:3181.
123. Werness BA, Levine AJ, Howley PM. Association of human papillomavirus types 16 and 18 E6 proteins with p53. *Science* 1990;248:76.
124. Huibregtse JM, Scheffner M, Howley PM. A cellular protein mediates association of p53 with the E6 oncoprotein of human papillomavirus types 16 or 18. *EMBO J* 1991;10:4129.
125. Scheffner M, Huibregtse JM, Vierstra RD, Howley PM. The HPV-16 E6 and E6-AP complex functions as a ubiquitin-protein ligase in the ubiquitination of p53. *Cell* 1993;75:495.
126. Talis AL, Huibregtse JM, Howley PM. The role of E6AP in the regulation of p53 protein levels in human papillomavirus (HPV) positive and HPV negative cells. *J Biol Chem* 1998;273:6439.
127. Hubbert NL, Sedman SA, Schiller JT. Human papillomavirus type 16 E6 increases the degradation rate of p53 in human keratinocytes. *J Virol* 1992;66:6237.
128. Scheffner M, Munger K, Byrne JC, Howley PM. The state of the p53 and retinoblastoma genes in human cervical carcinoma cell lines. *Proc Natl Acad Sci U S A* 1991;88:5523.
129. Mietz JA, Unger T, Huibregtse JM, Howley PM. The transcriptional transactivation function of wild-type p53 is inhibited by SV40 large T-antigen and by HPV-16 oncoprotein. *EMBO J* 1992;11:5013.
130. Kessis TD, Slebos RJ, Nelson WG, et al. Human papillomavirus 16 E6 expression disrupts the p53-mediated cellular response to DNA damage. *Proc Natl Acad Sci U S A* 1993;90:3988.
131. White A, Livanos EM, Tlsty TD. Differential disruption of genomic integrity and cell cycle regulation in normal human fibroblasts by the HPV oncoproteins. *Genes Dev* 1994;8:666.
132. Klingelhutz AJ, Foster SA, McDougall JK. Telomerase activation by the E6 gene product of human papillomavirus type 16. *Nature* 1996;380:79.
133. Chen JJ, Reid CE, Band V, Androphy EJ. Interaction of papillomavirus E6 oncoproteins with a putative calcium-binding protein. *Science* 1995;269:529.
134. Gao Q, Srinivasan S, Boyer SN, Wazer DE, Band V. The E6 oncoproteins of high-risk papillomaviruses bind to a novel putative GAP protein, E6TP1, and target it for degradation. *Mol Cell Biol* 1999;19:733.
135. Tong X, Howley PM. The bovine papillomavirus E6 oncoprotein interacts with paxillin and disrupts the actin cytoskeleton. *Proc Natl Acad Sci U S A* 1997;94:4412.
136. Patel D, Huang SM, Baglia LA, McCance DJ. The E6 protein of human papillomavirus type 16 binds to and inhibits co-activation by CBP and p300. *EMBO J* 1999;18:5061.
137. Ronco LV, Karpova AY, Vidal M, Howley PM. The human papillomavirus 16 E6 oncoprotein binds to interferon regulatory factor-3 and inhibits its transcriptional activity. *Genes Dev* 1998;12:2061.
138. Clarke EA, Morgan RW, Newman AM. Smoking as a risk factor in cancer of the cervix: additional evidence from a case control study. *Am J Epidemiol* 1982;115:59.
139. Wigle DT. Smoking and cancer of the cervix: hypothesis. *Am J Epidemiol* 1980;111:125.
140. Winkelstein WJ. Smoking and cancer of the uterine cervix. *Am J Epidemiol* 1977;106:257.
141. Hoffmann D, Hecht SS, Haley NJ, et al. Tumorigenic agents in tobacco products and their uptake by chewers, smokers and nonsmokers. *J Cell Biochem* 1985;9C:33.
142. zur Hausen H. Human genital cancer: synergism between two virus infections or synergism between a virus infection and initiating events. *Lancet* 1982;2:1370.
143. Yokota J, Tsukada Y, Najajima T, et al. Loss of heterozygosity on the short arm of chromosome 3 in carcinoma of the uterine cervix. *Cancer Res* 1989;49:3598.
144. Ohta M, Inoue H, Cotticelli MG, et al. The FHIT gene, spanning the chromosome 3p14.2 fragile site and renal carcinoma-associated t(3;8) breakpoint, is abnormal in digestive tract cancers. *Cell* 1996;84:587.
145. Stanbridge EJ. Suppression of malignancy in human cells. *Nature* 1976;260:17.
146. zur Hausen H. Papillomavirus infections—a major cause of human cancers. *Biochim Biophys Acta* 1996;1288:55.
147. Smits HL, Raadsmeer E, Rood I, et al. Induction of anchorage independent growth of human fibroblasts with a deletion in the short arm of chromosome 11 by human papillomavirus 16 DNA. *J Virol* 1988;62:4538.
148. Riou G, Barrois M, Le MG, et al. C-myc proto-oncogene expression and prognosis in early carcinoma of the uterine cervix. *Lancet* 1987;1:761.
149. Kahn T, Schwarz E, zur Hausen H. Molecular cloning and characterization of the DNA of a new human papillomavirus from a laryngeal carcinoma. *Int J Cancer* 1986;37:61.
150. Loning T, Ikenberg H, Becker J, et al. Analysis of oral papillomas, leukoplakias, and invasive carcinomas for human papillomavirus type related DNA. *J Invest Dermatol* 1985;84:417.
151. Brandsma JL, Steinberg BM, Abromson AL, Winkler B. Presence of human papillomavirus type 16 related sequences in verrucous carcinoma of the larynx. *Cancer Res* 1986;46:2185.
152. Jenson AB, Lancaster WD, Hartmann DP, Shaffer EL. Frequency and distribution of papillomavirus structural antigens in verrucae, multiple papillomas, and condylomata of the oral cavity. *Am J Pathol* 1982;107:212.
153. Lind PO, Syrjanen SM, Syrjanen KJ, Koppang HS, Aas E. Local immunoreactivity and human papillomavirus (HPV) in oral precancer and cancer lesions. *Scand J Dent Res* 1986;94:419.
154. DeVilliers E-M, Neumann C, Le JY, Weidauer H, zur Hausen H. Infection of the oral mucosa with defined types of human papillomaviruses. *Med Microbiol Immunol (Berl)* 1986;174:287.
155. Naghasfar Z, Sawada E, Kutcher MK, et al. Identification of genital tract papillomaviruses HPV-6 and HPV-16 in warts of the oral cavity. *J Virol* 1985;62:660.
156. Pfister H, Hettich I, Runne U, Gissmann L, Chilf GN. Characterization of human papillomavirus type 13 from lesions of focal epithelial hyperplasia Heck lesions. *J Virol* 1983;47:363.
157. Beaudenon S, Praetorius F, Kremsdorf D, et al. A new type of human papillomavirus associated with oral focal epithelial hyperplasia. *J Invest Dermatol* 1987;88:130.
158. Syrjanen S, Syrjanen K, Lambert MA. Detection of human papillomavirus DNA in oral mucosal lesions using *in situ* DNA hybridization applied on paraffin sections. *Oral Surg Oral Med Oral Pathol* 1986;62:660.
159. Syrjanen K, Pyrhonen S, Aukee S, Koskela E. A tumor probably caused by human papillomavirus (HPV). *Diagn Histopathol* 1982;5:291.
160. Winkler B, Capo V, Reumann W, et al. Human papillomavirus infection of the esophagus. *Cancer* 1985;55:149.
161. Zhou J, Stenzel DJ, Sun XY, Frazer IH. Synthesis and assembly of infectious bovine papillomavirus particles *in vitro*. *J Gen Virol* 1993;74:763.
162. Kirnbauer R, Booy F, Cheng N, Lowy DR, Schiller JT. Papillomavirus L1 major capsid protein self-assembles into virus-like particles that are highly immunogenic. *Proc Natl Acad Sci U S A* 1992;89:12180.
163. Jochmus I, Schafer K, Faath S, Muller M, Gissmann L. Chimeric virus-like particles of the human papillomavirus type 16 (HPV 16) as a prophylactic and therapeutic vaccine. *Arch Med Res* 1999;30:269.
164. Epstein MA, Barr YM. Cultivation *in vitro* of human lymphoblasts from Burkitt's malignant lymphoma. *Lancet* 1964;1:252.
165. Kieff E. Epstein-Barr virus and its replication. In: Fields BN, Knipe DM, Howley PM, eds. *Field's Virology*. Philadelphia: Lippincott-Raven Publishers, 1996:2343.
166. Rickinson A, Kieff E. Epstein-Barr virus. In: Fields BN, Knipe DM, Howley PM, eds. *Field's Virology*. Philadelphia: Lippincott-Raven Publishers, 1996:2397.
167. Henle W, Henle G. Seroepidemiology of the virus. In: Epstein MA, Achong BG, eds. *The Epstein-Barr Virus*. Berlin: Springer-Verlag, 1979:61.
168. de The G, Geser A, Day NE, et al. Epidemiological evidence for causal relationship between Epstein-Barr virus and Burkitt's lymphoma from Ugandan prospective study. *Nature* 1978;274:756.
169. Zeng Y. Seroepidemiological studies on nasopharyngeal carcinoma in China. *Adv Cancer Res* 1985;44:121.
170. Henle W, Diehl V, Kohn G, zur Hausen H, Henle G. Herpes-type virus and chromosome marker in normal leukocytes after growth with irradiated Burkitt cells. *Science* 1967;157:1064.
171. Rowe M, Young LS, Crocker J, et al. Epstein-Barr virus (EBV)-associated lymphoproliferative disease in the SCID mouse model: implications for the pathogenesis of EBV-positive lymphomas in man. *J Exp Med* 1991;173:147.
172. Shope TC, Dechairo D, Miller G. Malignant lymphoma in cotton-top marmosets after inoculation with Epstein-Barr virus. *Proc Natl Acad Sci U S A* 1973;70:2487.
173. Harrington DS, Weisenburger DD, Purtilo DT. Malignant lymphomas in the X-linked lymphoproliferative syndrome. *Cancer* 1987;59:1419.
174. Shapiro RS, McClain K, Frizzera G, et al. Epstein-Barr virus-associated B cell lymphoproliferative disorders following bone marrow transplantation. *Blood* 1988;71:1234.
175. Young LS, Alfieri C, Hennessy K, et al. Expression of Epstein-Barr virus transformation-associated genes in tissues of patients with EBV lymphoproliferative disease. *N Engl J Med* 1989;321:1080.
176. Miller C, Burkhardt A, Lee J, et al. Integral membrane protein 2 (LMP2) of Epstein-Barr virus regulates reactivation from latency through dominant negative effects on protein tyrosine kinases. *Immunity* 1995;2:155.
177. Reisman D, Sugden B. Trans-activation of an Epstein-Barr viral (EBV) transcriptional enhancer by the EBV nuclear antigen 1. *Mol Cell Biol* 1986;6:3838.
178. Tong X, Drabkin R, Yalamanchili R, Mosialos G, Kieff E. The Epstein-Barr virus nuclear protein 2 acidic domain interacts with a novel cellular coactivator that can associate with TFIIE. *Mol Cell Biol* 1995;15:4735.
179. Robertson E, Grossman S, Johannsen E, et al. Epstein-Barr virus nuclear protein 3C modulates transcription through interaction with the sequence specific DNA binding protein J kappa. *J Virol* 1995;69:3108.
180. Ellisen LW, Bird J, West DC, et al. Tan-1, the human homolog of the *Drosophila* notch gene, is broken by chromosomal translocations in T lymphoblastic neoplasms. *Cell* 1991;66:649.
181. Fortini ME, Artavanis-Tsakonas S. The suppressor of hairless protein participates in notch receptor signaling. *Cell* 1994;79:273.
182. Wilson JB, Weinberg W, Johnson R, Yuspa S, Levine AJ. Expression of the BNLF-1 oncogene of Epstein-Barr virus in the skin of transgenic mice induces hyperplasia and aberrant expression of keratin 6. *Cell* 1990;61:1315.

183. Kaye K, Izumi K, Mosialos G, Kieff E. The Epstein-Barr virus LMP1 cytoplasmic carboxy-terminus is essential for B lymphocyte transformation; fibroblast co-cultivation complements a critical function within the terminal 155 residues. *J Virol* 1995;69:675.
184. Mosialos G, Birkenbach M, Yalamanchili R, et al. The Epstein-Barr virus transforming protein LMP1 engages signaling proteins for the tumor necrosis factor receptor family. *Cell* 1995;80:389.
185. Izumi KM, McFarland EC, Ting AT, et al. The Epstein-Barr virus oncoprotein latent membrane protein 1 engages the tumor necrosis factor receptor–associated proteins TRADD and receptor-interacting protein (RIP) but does not induce apoptosis or require RIP for NF-κB activation. *Mol Cell Biol* 1999;19:5759.
186. Sixbey JW, Nedrud JG, Raab-Traub N, Hanes RA, Pagano JS. Epstein-Barr virus replication in oropharyngeal epithelial cells. *N Engl J Med* 1984;310:1225.
187. Robinson J, Smith D, Niederman J. Mitotic EBNA-positive lymphocytes in peripheral blood during infectious mononucleosis. *Nature* 1980;287:334.
188. Tierney RJ, Steven N, Young LS, Rickinson AB. Epstein-Barr virus latency in blood mononculear cells: analysis of viral gene transcription during primary infection and in the carrier state. *J Virol* 1994;68:7374.
189. Tomkinson BE, Maziarz R, Sullivan JL. Characterisation of the T cell–mediated cellular cytotoxicity during acute infectious mononucleosis. *J Immunol* 1989;143:660.
190. Tosato G, Magrath I, Koski I, Dooley N, Blaese M. Activation of suppressor T cells during Epstein-Barr virus–induced infectious mononucleosis. *N Engl J Med* 1979;301:1133.
191. Babcock GJ, Decker LL, Volk M, Thorley-Lawson DA. EBV persistence in memory B cells *in vivo*. *Immunity* 1998;9:395.
192. Khanna R, Burrows SR, Kurilla MG, et al. Localization of Epstein-Barr virus cytotoxic T cell epitopes using recombinant vaccinia: implications for vaccine development. *J Exp Med* 1992;176:169.
193. Murray RJ, Kurilla MG, Brooks JM, et al. Identification of target antigens for the human cytotoxic T cell response to Epstein-Barr virus (EBV): implication for the immune control of EBV-positive malignancies. *J Exp Med* 1992;176:157.
194. Shapiro A, Imreh M, Leonchiks A, Imreh S, Masucci MG. A minimal glycine-alanine repeat prevents the interaction of ubiquitinated IκB alpha with the proteasome: a new mechanism for selective inhibition of proteolysis. *Nature Med* 1998;4:939.
195. Tan LC, Gudgeon N, Annels NE, et al. A re-evaluation of the frequency of CD8+ T cells specific for EBV in healthy virus carriers. *J Immunol* 1999;162:1827.
196. Preiksaitis JK, Diaz-Mitoma F, Mirzayons F, Roberts S, Tyrrell DLJ. Quantitative oropharyngeal Epstein-Barr virus shedding in renal and cardiac transplant recipients: relationship to immunosuppressive therapy, serologic responses, and the risk of post-transplant lymphoproliferative disorder. *J Infect Dis* 1992;166:989.
197. Anagnostopoulos I, Herbst H, Niedobitek G, Stein H. Demonstration of monoclonal EBV genomes in Hodgkin's disease and Ki-1-positive anaplastic large cell lymphoma by combined Southern blot and *in situ* hybridisation. *Blood* 1989;74:810.
198. Hamilton-Dutoit S, Rea D, Raphael M, et al. Epstein-Barr virus–latent gene expression and tumour cell phenotype in acquired immunodeficiency syndrome–related non-Hodgkin's lymphoma. Correlation of lymphoma phenotype with three distinct patterns of viral latency. *Am J Pathol* 1993;143:1072.
199. Pelicci PG, Knowles DM, Arlin ZA, et al. Multiple monoclonal B-cell expansions and c-myc oncogene rearrangements in acquired immunodeficiency syndrome–related lymphoproliferative disorders. *J Exp Med* 1986;164:2049.
200. McGrath MS, Shiramizu B, Meeker TC, Kaplan LD, Herndier B. AIDS-associated polyclonal lymphoma: identification of a new HIV-associated disease process. *J AIDS* 1991;4:408.
201. MacMahon EME, Glass JD, Hayward SD, et al. Epstein-Barr virus in AIDS-related primary central nervous system lymphoma. *Lancet* 1991;338:969.
202. Leyvraz S, Henle W, Chahinian AP, et al. Association of Epstein-Barr virus with thymic carcinoma. *N Engl J Med* 1985;312:1296.
203. Brooks L, Yao QY, Rickinson AB, Young LS. Epstein-Barr virus latent gene transcription in nasopharyngeal carcinoma cells: coexpression of EBNA1, LMP1, and LMP2 transcripts. *J Virol* 1992;66:2689.
204. Nicholls JM, Pittaluga S, Chung LP, So KC. The association between carcinoma of the tonsil and Epstein-Barr virus: a study using radiolabelled *in situ* hybridisation. *Pathology* 1994;26:94.
205. Shibata D, Weiss LM. Epstein-Barr virus–associated gastric adenocarcinoma. *Am J Pathol* 1992;140:769.
206. Raab-Traub N, Flynn K. The structure of the terminal of the Epstein-Barr virus as a marker of clonal cellular proliferation. *Cell* 1986;47:883.
207. Cleary ML, Nalesnik MA, Shearer WT, Sklar J. Clonal analysis of transplant-associated lymphoproliferations based on the structure of genomic termini of the Epstein-Barr virus. *Blood* 1988;72:349.
208. Herbst H, Dallenbach F, Hummel M, et al. Epstein-Barr virus latent membrane protein expression in Hodgkin and Reed-Sternberg cells. *Proc Natl Acad Sci U S A* 1991;88:4766.
209. Altiok E, Klien G, Zech L, et al. Epstein-Barr virus transformed pro-B cells are prone to illegitimate recombination between the switch region of the μ chain gene and other chromosomes. *Proc Natl Acad Sci U S A* 1989;86:6333.
210. Dalla-Favera R, Bregni M, Erikson J, et al. Human C-myc oncogene is located on the region of chromosome 8 that is translocated in Burkitt lymphoma cells. *Proc Natl Acad Sci U S A* 1982;79:7824.
211. Kafuko GW, Burkitt DP. Burkitt's lymphoma and malaria. *Int J Cancer* 1970;6:1.
212. Whittle HC, Brown J, Marsh K, et al. T-cell control of Epstein-Barr virus–infected B-cells is lost during *P. falciparum* malaria. *Nature* 1984;312:449.
213. Savoie A, Perpete C, Carpentier L, Jonas J, Alfieri C. Direct correlation between the load of Epstein-Barr virus–infected lymphocytes in the peripheral blood of pediatric transplant patients and risk of lymphoproliferative disease. *Blood* 1994;83:2715.
214. Papadopoulos EB, Ladanyi M, Emanuel D, et al. Infusions of donor leukocytes to treat Epstein-Barr virus–associated lymphoproliferative disorders after allogeneic bone marrow transplantation. *N Engl J Med* 1994;330:1185.
215. Greenspan D, De Souza YG, Conant MA, et al. Efficacy of desciclovir in the treatment of Epstein-Barr virus infection in oral hairy leukoplakia. *J AIDS* 1990;3:571.
216. Niedobitek G, Young LS, Lau R, et al. Epstein-Barr virus infection in oral hairy leukoplakia: virus replication in the absence of a detectable latent phase. *J Gen Virol* 1991;72:3035.
217. Ensoli B, Barillari G, Gallo RC. Pathogenesis of AIDS-associated Kaposi's sarcoma. *Hematol Oncol Clin North Am* 1991;5:281.
218. Ganem D. AIDS. Viruses, cytokines and Kaposi's sarcoma. *Curr Biol* 1995;5:469.
219. Ziegler J, Templeton AC, Voegel GL. KS: a comparison of classical, endemic and epidemic forms. *Semin Oncol* 1984;11:47.
220. Penn I. Kaposi's sarcoma in organ transplant recipients. *Transplantation* 1979;27:8.
221. Nakamura S, Salahuddin SZ, Bieberfeld P, et al. Kaposi's sarcoma cells: long term culture with growth factor from retrovirus-infected CD4+ T cells. *Science* 1988;242:426.
222. Ensoli B, Nakamura S, Salahuddin SZ, et al. AIDS–Kaposi's sarcoma–derived cells express cytokines with autocrine and paracrine growth effects. *Science* 1989;243:223.
223. Salahuddin SZ, Nakamura S, Biberfeld P, et al. Angiogenic properties of Kaposi's sarcoma–derived cells after long-term culture *in vitro*. *Science* 1988;242:430.
224. Miles SA, Rezai AR, Salazar-Gonzalez JF, et al. AIDS–Kaposi sarcoma–derived cells produce and respond to interleukin 6. *Proc Natl Acad Sci U S A* 1990;87:4068.
225. Nair BC, DeVico AL, Nakamura S, et al. Identification of a major growth factor for AIDS–Kaposi's sarcoma cells as oncostatin M. *Science* 1992;255:1430.
226. Ensoli B, Gendelman R, Markham P, et al. Synergy between basic fibroblast growth factor and HIV-1 tat protein in induction of Kaposi's sarcoma. *Nature* 1994;371:674.
227. Nakamura S, Sakaurada S, Salahuddin SZ, et al. Inhibition of development of Kaposi's sarcoma–related lesions by a bacterial cell wall complex. *Science* 1992;255:1437.
228. Beral V. Epidemiology of Kaposi's sarcoma. In: Beral V, Jaffe HW, Weiss R, eds. *Cancer Surveys: 10. Cancer, HIV and AIDS.* Cold Spring Harbor, NY: Cold Spring Harbor Press, 1991:5.
229. Buonaguro L, Barillari G, Chang H, et al. Effects of HIV-1 tat protein on the expression of inflammatory cytokines. *J Virol* 1992;66:7159.
230. Barillari G, Gendelman R, Gallo RC, Ensoli B. The tat protein of HIV1, a growth factor for AIDS Kaposi's sarcoma and cytokine-activated vascular cells, induces adhesion of the same cell types by using integrin receptors recognizing the RGD amino acid sequence. *Proc Natl Acad Sci U S A* 1993;90:7941.
231. Beral V, Peterman T, Berkelman R, Jaffe HW. Kaposi's sarcoma among persons with AIDS: a sexually transmitted infection? *Lancet* 1990;335:123.
232. Chang Y, Cesarman E, Pessin MS, et al. Identification of herpesvirus-like DNA sequences in AIDS-associated Kaposi's sarcoma. *Science* 1994;266:1865.
233. Moore P, Chang Y. Detection of herpesvirus-like DNA sequences in Kaposi's sarcoma patients with and those without HIV infection. *N Engl J Med* 1995;332:118.
234. Huang Y, Li JJ, Kaplan M, Friedman-Kien A. Human herpesvirus-like DNA sequence in various forms of Kaposi's sarcoma. *Lancet* 1995;345:759.
235. Schalling M, Eukman M, Kaaya E, Linde A, Biberfeld P. A role for a new herpesvirus (KSAV) in different forms of Kaposi's sarcoma. *Nature Med* 1995;1:707.
236. Chuck S, Grant RM, Katongole-Mbidde E, Conant M, Ganem D. Frequent presence of herpesviral-like DNA sequences in lesions of HIV-negative Kaposi's sarcoma. *J Infect Dis* 1996;173:248.
237. Ambroziak J, Blackbourn D, Herndier B, et al. Herpesvirus-like sequences in HIV-infected and uninfected Kaposi's sarcoma patients [technical comment]. *Science* 1995;268:582.
238. Boshoff C, Schulz TF, Kennedy MM, et al. Kaposi's sarcoma–associated herpesvirus infects endothelial and spindle cells. *Nature Med* 1995;1:1274.
239. Zhong W, Wang H, Herndier B, Ganem D. Restricted expression of Kaposi's sarcoma–associated herpesvirus genes in Kaposi's sarcoma. *Proc Natl Acad Sci U S A* 1996 *(in press).*
240. Staskus K, Zhong W, Gebhardt K, et al. Kaposi's sarcoma–associated herpesvirus genes are expressed predominantly in the endothelial (spindle) tumor cells of Kaposi's sarcoma. Manuscript submitted 1996.
241. Whitby D, Howard MR, Tenant-Flowers M, et al. Detection of Kaposi sarcoma associated herpesvirus in peripheral blood of HIV-infected individuals and progression to Kaposi's sarcoma. *Lancet* 1995;346:799.
242. Kedes DH, Operskalski E, Busch M, et al. The seroepidemiology of human herpesvirus 8 (Kaposi's sarcoma–associated herpesvirus): distribution of infection in KS risk groups and evidence for sexual transmission. *Nature Med* 1996;2:918.
243. Gao SJ, Kingsley L, Hoover DR, et al. Seroconversion to antibodies against Kaposi's sarcoma–associated herpesvirus-related latent nuclear antigens before the development of Kaposi's sarcoma. *N Engl J Med* 1996;335:233.
244. Simpson GR, Schulz TF, Whitby D, et al. Prevalence of Kaposi's sarcoma associated herpesvirus infection measured by antibodies to recombinant capsid protein and latent immunofluorescence antigen. *Lancet* 1996;348:1133.
245. Zhu L, Wang R, Sweat A, et al. Comparison of human sera reactivities in immunoblots with recombinant human herpesvirus (HHV)-8 proteins associated with the latent (ORF73) and lytic (ORFs 65, K8.1A, and K8.1B) replicative cycles and in immunofluorescence assays with HHV-8-infected BCBL-1 cells. *Virology* 1999;256:381.
246. Martin JN, Ganem DE, Osmond DH, et al. Sexual transmission and the natural history of human herpesvirus 8 infection. *N Engl J Med* 1998;338:948.
247. Moore PS, Kingsley LA, Holmberg SD, et al. Kaposi's sarcoma–associated herpesvirus infection prior to onset of Kaposi's sarcoma. *AIDS* 1996;10.175.
248. Renwick N, Halaby T, Weverling GJ, et al. Seroconversion for human herpesvirus 8 during HIV infection is highly predictive of Kaposi's sarcoma. *AIDS* 1998;12:2481.
249. Gallo RC. The enigmas of Kaposi's sarcoma. *Science* 1998;282:1837.
250. Ensoli B, Sirianni MC. Kaposi's sarcoma pathogenesis: a link between immunology and tumor biology. *Crit Rev Oncog* 1998;9:107.
251. Whitby D, Luppi M, Barozzi P, et al. Human herpesvirus 8 seroprevalence in blood donors and lymphoma patients from different regions of Italy. *J Natl Cancer Inst* 1998;90:395.
252. Calabro ML, Sheldon J, Favero A, et al. Seroprevalence of Kaposi's sarcoma–associated herpesvirus/human herpesvirus 8 in several regions of Italy. *J Hum Virol* 1998;1:207.

253. Ariyoshi K, Schim van der Loeff M, Cook P, et al. Kaposi's sarcoma in the Gambia, West Africa is less frequent in human immunodeficiency virus type 2 than in human immunodeficiency virus type 1 infection despite a high prevalence of human herpesvirus 8. *J Hum Virol* 1998;1:193.
254. Gessain A, Mauclere P, van Beveren M, et al. Human herpesvirus 8 primary infection occurs during childhood in Cameroon, Central Africa. *Int J Cancer* 1999;81:189.
255. Mayama S, Cuevas LE, Sheldon J, et al. Prevalence and transmission of Kaposi's sarcoma–associated herpesvirus (human herpesvirus 8) in Ugandan children and adolescents. *Int J Cancer* 1998;77:817.
256. Sitas F, Carrara H, Beral V, et al. Antibodies against human herpesvirus 8 in black South African patients with cancer. *N Engl J Med* 1999;340:1863.
257. Blauvelt A, Sei S, Cook PM, Schulz TF, Jeang KT. Human herpesvirus 8 infection occurs following adolescence in the United States. *J Infect Dis* 1997;176:771.
258. Goedert JJ, Kedes DH, Ganem D. Antibodies to human herpesvirus 8 in women and infants born in Haiti and the USA. *Lancet* 1997;349:1368.
259. Dittmer D, Lagunoff M, Renne R, et al. A cluster of latently expressed genes in Kaposi's sarcoma–associated herpesvirus. *J Virol* 1998;72:8309.
260. Sarid R, Wiezorek JS, Moore PS, Chang Y. Characterization and cell cycle regulation of the major Kaposi's sarcoma–associated herpesvirus (human herpesvirus 8) latent genes and their promoter. *J Virol* 1999;73:1438.
261. Ballestas ME, Chatis PA, Kaye KM. Efficient persistence of extrachromosomal KSHV DNA mediated by latency-associated nuclear antigen. *Science* 1999;284:641.
262. Godden-Kent D, Talbot SJ, Boshoff C, et al. The cyclin encoded by Kaposi's sarcoma–associated herpesvirus stimulates cdk6 to phosphorylate the retinoblastoma protein and histone H1. *J Virol* 1997;71:4193.
263. Chang Y, Moore PS, Talbot SJ, et al. Cyclin encoded by KS herpesvirus. *Nature* 1996;382:410.
264. Swanton C, Mann DJ, Fleckenstein B, et al. Herpes viral cyclin/Cdk6 complexes evade inhibition by CDK inhibitory proteins. *Nature* 1997;390:184.
265. Ellis M, Chew YP, Fallis L, et al. Degradation of p27(Kip) cdk inhibitor triggered by Kaposi's sarcoma virus cyclin-cdk6 complex. *EMBO J* 1999;18:644.
266. Mann DJ, Child ES, Swanton C, Laman H, Jones N. Modulation of p27(Kip1) levels by the cyclin encoded by Kaposi's sarcoma–associated herpesvirus. *EMBO J* 1999;18:654.
267. Motokura T, Bloom T, Kim HG, et al. A novel cyclin encoded by a bcl1-linked candidate oncogene. *Nature* 1991;350:512.
268. Schulz TF. Kaposi's sarcoma–associated herpesvirus (human herpesvirus-8). *J Gen Virol* 1998;79:1573.
269. Sadler R, Wu L, Forghani B, et al. A complex translational program generates multiple novel proteins from the latently expressed kaposin (K12) locus of Kaposi's sarcoma–associated herpesvirus. *J Virol* 1999;73:5722.
270. Staskus KA, Zhong W, Gebhard K, et al. Kaposi's sarcoma–associated herpesvirus gene expression in endothelial (spindle) tumor cells. *J Virol* 1997;71:715.
271. Sturzl M, Wunderlich A, Ascherl G, et al. Human herpesvirus-8 (HHV-8) gene expression in Kaposi's sarcoma (KS) primary lesions: an *in situ* hybridization study. *Leukemia* 1999;13:S110.
272. Glenn M, Rainbow L, Aurad F, Davison A, Schulz TF. Identification of a spliced gene from Kaposi's sarcoma–associated herpesvirus encoding a protein with similarities to latent membrane proteins 1 and 2A of Epstein-Barr virus. *J Virol* 1999;73:6953.
273. Poole LJ, Zong JC, Ciufo DM, et al. Comparison of genetic variability at multiple loci across the genomes of the major subtypes of Kaposi's sarcoma–associated herpesvirus reveals evidence for recombination and for two distinct types of open reading frame K15 alleles at the right-hand end. *J Virol* 1999;73:6646.
274. Orenstein JM, Alkan S, Blauvelt A, et al. Visualization of human herpesvirus type 8 in Kaposi's sarcoma by light and transmission electron microscopy. *AIDS* 1997;11:35.
275. Martin DF, Kuppermann BD, Wolitz RA, et al. Oral ganciclovir for patients with cytomegalovirus retinitis treated with a ganciclovir implant. Roche Ganciclovir Study Group. *N Engl J Med* 1999;340:1063.
276. Nicholas J, Zong JC, Alcendor DJ, et al. Novel organizational features, captured cellular genes, and strain variability within the genome of KSHV/HHV8. *J Natl Cancer Inst Monogr* 1998;23:79.
277. Nicholas J, Ruvolo V, Zong J, et al. A single 13-kilobase divergent locus in the Kaposi sarcoma–associated herpesvirus (human herpesvirus 8) genome contains nine open reading frames that are homologous to or related to cellular proteins. *J Virol* 1997;71:1963.
278. Neipel F, Albrecht JC, Fleckenstein B. Cell-homologous genes in the Kaposi's sarcoma associated rhadinovirus human herpesvirus 8: determinants of its pathogenicity? *J Virol* 1997;71:4187.
279. Lee H, Guo J, Li M, et al. Identification of an immunoreceptor tyrosine-based activation motif of K1 transforming protein of Kaposi's sarcoma–associated herpesvirus. *Mol Cell Biol* 1998;18:5219.
280. Lee H, Veazey R, Williams K, et al. Deregulation of cell growth by the K1 gene of Kaposi's sarcoma–associated herpesvirus. *Nature Med* 1998;4:435.
281. Lagunoff M, Majeti R, Weiss A, Ganem D. Deregulated signal transduction by the K1 gene product of Kaposi's sarcoma–associated herpesvirus. *Proc Natl Acad Sci U S A* 1999;96:5704.
282. Bais C, Santomasso B, Coso O, et al. G-protein-coupled receptor of Kaposi's sarcoma–associated herpesvirus is a viral oncogene and angiogenesis activator. *Nature* 1998;391:86.
283. Boshoff C, Endo Y, Collins PD, et al. Angiogenic and HIV inhibitory functions of KSHV-encoded chemokines. *Science* 1997;278:290.
284. Cesarman E, Chang Y, Moore PS, Said JW, Knowles D. Kaposi's sarcoma associated herpesvirus-like DNA sequences in AIDS-related body cavity based lymphomas. *N Engl J Med* 1995;332:1186.
285. Renne R, Zhong W, Herndier B, et al. Lytic growth of Kaposi's sarcoma–associated herpesvirus (human herpesvirus 8) in a cultured B cell lymphoma line. *Nature Med* 1996;2:342.
286. Soulier J, Grollet L, Oksenhendler E, et al. Kaposi's sarcoma–associated herpesvirus-like DNA sequences in multicentric Castleman's disease. *Blood* 1995;86:1276.
287. Dupin N, Fisher C, Kellam P, et al. Distribution of human herpesvirus-8 latently infected cells in Kaposi's sarcoma, multicentric Castleman's disease, and primary effusion lymphoma. *Proc Natl Acad Sci U S A* 1999;96:4546.
288. Parravicini C, Chandran B, Corbellino M, et al. Differential viral protein expression in KSVH-associated diseases: Kaposi's sarcoma, primary effusion lymphoma, and multicentric Castleman's disease. *American Journal of Pathology* 2000;156:743.

Stuart H. Yuspa
Peter G. Shields

CHAPTER 11

Etiology of Cancer: Chemical Factors

The chemical origin of human malignancies was recognized by observations of unusual cancer incidences in persons in certain occupational groups. The capacity for chemicals to cause cancer was subsequently confirmed in numerous experimental animal studies. The extent to which chemical exposures contribute to cancer incidence was not appreciated fully until population-based studies documented differing organ-specific cancer rates among geographically distinct populations. Changes in cancer frequency among migrating ethnic groups, high cancer rates associated with specific occupations, and the high risk of smoking-associated cancers confirmed that environmental and lifestyle exposures were major determinants of human cancer risk. Current data indicate that changing lifestyles and exposures can modify cancer risk.[1] Individual genetic factors also can influence cancer risk in several ways. In hereditary cancer syndromes, genetic factors dictate a very high cancer risk for a small group of individuals. However, the general population carries hereditary susceptibility genes that increase cancer risk for particular exposures. Thus, most human cancer is not simply a genetically determined sequela of aging but rather the manifestation of personal and cultural behavior superimposed on individually determined hereditary susceptibility.

The experimental induction of tumors in animals, neoplastic transformation of cultured cells by chemicals, and analysis of environmentally induced human tumors have revealed important concepts regarding the pathogenesis of cancer.[2–5] Often, chemical carcinogens are organ-specific, target epithelial cells, and cause genetic damage (i.e., are genotoxic). Chemically related DNA damage can occur either directly from environmental exposures or indirectly by activation of endogenous mutagenic pathways (e.g., nitric oxide and oxy radicals).[6] Most chemically induced tumors are clonal in origin and require an accumulation of genetic changes in a multistage progression from normal to premalignant to carcinoma. The risk of developing a chemically induced tumor may be modified by nongenotoxic exogenous and endogenous exposures and factors and by accumulated exposure to the same or different genotoxic carcinogens. Somatic mutations relevant to cancer pathogenesis have been documented after carcinogen exposures in experimental animals and humans, and pathways for carcinogen metabolism have defined a set of genetic variables that contribute to human cancer risk. Studies with cultured rodent and human cells[7] confirm the remarkable qualitative similarities among mammalian species for responses to carcinogens but also have revealed some important quantitative differences that have enhanced our understanding of chemical carcinogenesis in human populations.

Analysis of the chemical induction of cancer in animal models and human populations has had a major impact on human health. Experimental studies have been instrumental in validating hypotheses generated from human studies. Animal experiments confirmed the carcinogenic and tumor-promoting properties of cigarette smoke and identified the active chemical and gaseous components.[8] The transplacental carcinogenicity of diethylstilbestrol and the hazards of specific occupational carcinogens [e.g., vinyl chloride, benzene, aromatic amines, and bis (chloromethyl) ether] led to the removal of the suspected human carcinogens from the environment and reduction of the cancer rate. Dietary factors that enhance or inhibit cancer development have been identified in models of chemical carcinogenesis,[9] resulting in a reduction of cancer incidence through nutritional alterations. The application of cancer chemoprevention strategies, particularly retinoids, antiestrogens, and inhibitors of the arachidonic acid cascade, are the direct result of studies conducted in models of chemical carcinogenesis[10] and are reducing the tumor incidence in high-risk populations.

THE NATURE OF CHEMICAL CARCINOGENS: CHEMISTRY AND METABOLISM

A wide variety of chemicals and chemical classes can cause cancer in animals and humans,[11] yet the process is very specific. Most chemicals are not known to be carcinogenic. Within chemical classes, stereoisomers may vary widely in carcinogenicity. Carcinogens can be genotoxic, nongenotoxic, or both. Sometimes, the distinction is arbitrary.[12,13] Genotoxic carcinogens have high chemical reactivity (such as alkylating agents) or can be metabolized to reactive intermediates by the host. They form covalent adducts with macromolecules and target DNA in the nucleus and mitochondria.[5,14] Because a good correlation exists between the ability to form DNA adducts and the potency to induce tumors in laboratory animals, DNA is considered the ultimate target for most carcinogens. Genotoxic carcinogens may transfer simple alkyl or complexed (aryl) alkyl groups to specific sites on DNA bases (Fig. 11-1)[5,14] These alkylating and arylalkyating agents include (but are not limited to) N-nitroso compounds, aliphatic epoxides, aflatoxins, mustards, polycyclic aromatic hydrocarbons, and other combustion products of fossil fuels and vegetable matter. Others transfer arylamine residues to DNA (see Fig. 11-1) as exemplified by aryl aromatic amines, aminoazodyes, and heterocyclic aromatic amines; the latter are produced by overcooking meat, poultry, or fish at high temperatures.[15] For genotoxic carcinogens, the interaction with DNA is not random, and each class of agents reacts selectively with purine and pyrimidine targets (see Fig. 11-1).[14,16] Furthermore, targeting of carcinogens to particular sites in DNA is determined by nucleotide sequence,[17] by host cell,[18] and by selective DNA repair processes, rendering some genetic material at risk over others. As expected from this chemistry, genotoxic carcinogens are potent mutagens, particularly adept at causing base mispairing or small deletions and leading to missense or nonsense mutations.[16] Others may cause macrogenetic damage, such as chromosome breaks and large deletions.[19] In all cases, mutations detected in tumors represent a combination of the effect of the mutagenic change on the function of the protein product and the effect of the functional alteration on the behavior of the specific host cell type.

A number of chemicals that cause cancers in laboratory rodents are not demonstrably genotoxic.[12,13,20] Synthetic pesticides and herbicides fall within this group, as do a number of natural products that are ingested.[21] In general, these agents are carcinogenic at high doses in laboratory animals and require prolonged exposure. The mechanism of action by nongenotoxic carcinogens is controversial and may be related in some cases to toxic cell death and regenerative hyperplasia.[20,22]

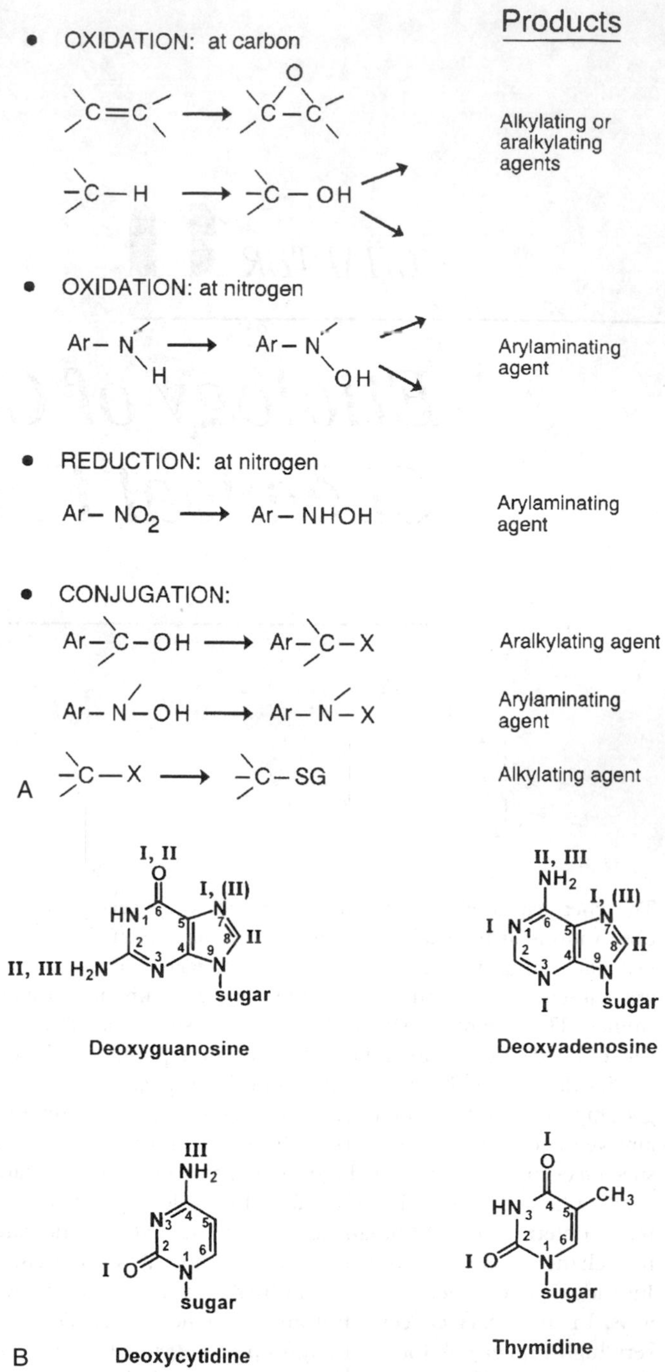

FIGURE 11-1. **A:** Metabolic activation to yield DNA-reactive alkylating, arylaminating, and aralkylating agents. Ar is an aromatic residue, X is a leaving group, and SG represents a glutathione residue. **B:** Sites of substitution of DNA bases by genotoxic carcinogens. Sites modified by alkylating agents are marked by the numeral *I*, those modified by arylaminating agents are marked by a *II*, and those modified by polycyclic aralkylating agents are marked by a *III*. Because C8-substituted arylamino adducts have been suggested to have arisen from N7-substituted precursors, the arylaminating agents are listed parenthetically at the 7-position of the purines. (Reproduced by permission of the author, Dr. Anthony Dipple, and the publisher, Oxford University Press, from *Carcinogenesis* 1995;16:437.)

TABLE 11-1. Enzymatic Pathways of Carcinogen Metabolism in Experimental Animals and Humans

Enzyme	*Mammalian Isoforms*	*Major Reaction (Minor)*	*Major Activity (Minor)*	*Typical Substrates*	*Inducible*	*Polymorphic*
Cytochrome P-450	>40	N- or C-oxidation (reduction)	Activation (detoxication)	PAH, nitrosamines, aromatic amines, benzene, aflatoxin, heterocyclic amines	Yes	Yes
Microsomal flavin-containing monoxygenase	5	N- or S-oxidation	N-detoxication, S-detoxication	2-Naphthylamine	Yes	Yes
Peroxidases	Multiple	Oxidation	Activation	Aromatic amines	Yes	Yes
NADPH/P-450 reductase, other reductases	1	Reduction	Detoxication (activation)	Dinitropyrene, chromium	Yes	Yes
Glutathione S-transferase	>10	Glutathione conjugation	Detoxication (activation)	Oxygenated carcinogens	Yes	Yes
N-acetyltransferase	>2	N- or O-acetylation	Activation Detoxication	4-Aminobiphenyl, 2-aminofluorene, heterocyclic amines	Yes	Yes
Sulfotransferase	>4	O-sulfation	Activation (detoxication)	4-Aminobiphenyl, 2-aminofluorene, heterocyclic amines	Yes	Yes
UDP-glucuronosyl transferase	>10	N- or O-glucuronidation	Detoxication	4-Aminobiphenyl, 2-naphthylamine, heterocyclic amines	Yes	Yes
Epoxide hydrolases	3	Reduction	Detoxication	PAH epoxides	Yes	Yes

PAH, polycyclic aromatic hydrocarbons.

Induction of endogenous mutagenic mechanisms, such as DNA oxy radical damage,[23] depurination, and deamination of 5-methylcytosine by exposure to nongenotoxic carcinogens, may contribute to carcinogenicity of these agents. In other cases, nongenotoxic carcinogens may have hormonal effects, influencing hormone-dependent tissues directly.[24,25] Though the contribution of nongenotoxic carcinogens to human cancer causation is not certain, they may serve also as modifiers in concert with genotoxic agents.

A number of metabolic pathways activate or detoxify carcinogens and procarcinogens (chemicals that can be transformed into active carcinogens).[5,26,27] These pathways are complex and interactive (Table 11-1), and genetic polymorphisms in animal models and humans are thought to be major determinants of cancer susceptibility.[28] In general, metabolic activation of carcinogens involves oxidation at carbon-carbon double bonds or saturated carbon atoms, in the latter case often requiring a further esterification (see Fig. 11-1). Oxidation at nitrogen on aromatic amines or reduction at nitrogen of aromatic nitro compounds yields reactive intermediates that transfer an arylamine residue to DNA. An esterified intermediate may be required, as in the case of heterocyclic amine carcinogens.[29] Conjugations are also frequent intermediates of metabolism of many carcinogens and can be both activating and detoxifying pathways (see Fig. 11-1 and Table 11-1).[14,27] The importance of metabolic activation to carcinogenesis and the polymorphic nature of metabolic activity among individuals provides an approach to estimate individual risk profiles for particular exposures.[30] Furthermore, a number of metabolic pathways are inducible (see Table 11-1) and modified by diet, hormones, and additional exposures, adding further complexity to the process of carcinogenesis.

ANIMAL MODEL SYSTEMS AND MULTISTAGE CARCINOGENESIS

Virtually every major form of human cancer can be reproduced in experimental animals by exposure to specific chemical carcinogens. In many cases, the cell of origin, morphogenesis, phenotypic markers, and genetic alterations are qualitatively identical to corresponding human cancers (Table 11-2).[2] Animal models have demonstrated the modifying effect of tumor promoters and hormones or cofactors, such as asbestos or viral infections. Furthermore, animal models have revealed the constancy of carcinogen-host interaction among mammalian species by reproducing organ-specific cancers in animals with chemicals identified as human carcinogens, such as coal tar and squamous cell carcinomas; vinyl chloride and hepatic angiosarcomas; aflatoxin and hepatocarcinoma; and aromatic amines and bladder cancer. These results validate the qualitative value of animal models in carcinogenesis research and support the extrapolation of data from experimental studies to human applications with specific limitations. The introduction of genetically modified mice designed to reproduce specific human cancer syndromes has accelerated both the understanding of the contributions of chemicals to cancer causation and the identification of potential exogenous carcinogens.[31,32]

From analyses of both human cancer pathogenesis and experimental animal tumor induction by chemical carcinogens, specific stages that have been identified have typical phenotypic, genetic, and biochemical characteristics (Fig. 11-2). However, in reality, these stages are not distinct, and steps to cancer do not follow a straight line. Mutations in single cells frequently "initiate" carcinogenesis. On clonal expansion, initiated cells form a premalignant lesion, often a benign tumor (e.g., an adenoma)

TABLE 11-2. Animal Models for Chemical Carcinogenesis

Target	*Species*	*Agents*	*Tumor Type*	*Modifiers*	*Associated Genetic Changes*	*References*
Skin	Mouse, rat	Nitrosamines, alkylating agents, aromatic amines, PAH, ultraviolet light, cigarette smoke condensate	Squamous papillomas, squamous cell and basal cell carcinomas	Phorbol ester, cigarette smoke condensate, benzoyl peroxide, anthralin, ultraviolet light, wounding, TGF-β, TGF-α	H-*ras* mutations, trisomy chromosome 6, 7, LOH chromosome 11, *P53* mutations	175–177
Skin	Hamster, guinea pig	7,12-dimethylbenz[a]anthracene	Melanoma	Phorbol ester	None identified	178
Liver	Mouse, rat, hamster, nonhuman primate	Nitrosamines, aromatic amines, vinyl chloride, PAH, heterocyclic amines, aflatoxin, tamoxifen	Hepatocellular adenoma and carcinoma, angiosarcoma, cholangiocarcinoma	Phenobarbital, dioxin, PCB, hepatitis B virus envelope protein, TGF-α, liver fluke	H-*ras* mutations (mice), K-*ras* mutations (rats)	179,180
Lung	Mouse, rat, hamster, dog	Nitrosamines, asbestos, PAH, urethane, cigarette smoke	Adenocarcinoma and squamous cell carcinoma, mesothelioma	Asbestos, silica dust, BHT	K-*ras* mutations	40,181
Breast	Mouse, rat, dog	Methylnitrosourea, aromatic amines, heterocyclic amines, butadiene, 7,12-dimethylbenz[a]anthracene	Adenocarcinoma, ductal hyperplasias, hyperplastic alveolar nodules	Pregnancy, prolactin, estrogen, diet, apoptosis, N-*ras* overexpression, TGF-α, TGF-β, selenium	H-*ras* mutations, LOH at 1q22 (rat), *P53* mutations (mouse), LOH chromosome 11 (mouse)	45,182, 183
Colon	Mouse, rat	Heterocyclic amines, nitrosamines, dimethyhydrazine	Acinar cell carcinoma, adenomatous polyps, adenocarcinoma	High-fat diet, bile salts, calcium, aspirin, vitamin D_3, COX-2 inhibitors	K-*ras* mutations, Apc mutations	67,184, 185
Pancreas	Rat, hamster, guinea pig	Azaserine, nitrosamines	Adenocarcinoma, ductal carcinoma	High-fat diet, soybean protein, cholecystokinin	K-*ras* mutations, inactivation of DCC and Rb-1	186,187
Bladder	Mouse, rat, hamster, dog	Aromatic amines, nitrosamines, cyclophosphamide, nitrofurans	Transitional cell and squamous cell carcinoma	Infection, urinary precipitates, urinary EGF, arsenic	H-*ras* mutations, *P53* mutations	187–189
Prostate	Rat	Methylnitrosourea, nitrosamines, testosterone, cadmium, 3,2'-dimethy-4-aminobiphenyl	Adenocarcinoma	Testosterone, antiandrogens, 5α reductase inhibitors, estrogens, cadmium	K-*ras* mutations	190,191
Nervous system	Rat	Ethyl and methylnitrosourea	Glioma, neurinoma	Age, transplacental exposure	*Neu* mutations	192

BHT, butylated hydroxytoluene; EGF, epidermal growth factor; PAH, polycyclic aromatic hydrocarbons; PCB, polychlorinated biphenyl; TGF, transforming growth factor.

but also recognized as hyperplastic or dysplastic foci in some tissue sites. Agents that cause clonal expansion of initiated cells are called *tumor promoters.* Tumor promotion may occur as a consequence of exogenous exposures, such as cigarette smoke or viral infections. Promotion may be an endogenous process, such as hormonal stimulation in breast and prostate cancer or bile salts in colon cancer. Premalignant lesions undergo further phenotypic changes, often in a predictable sequence and commonly multifocal within a single lesion. Some foci progress at a faster rate than others, and these are at highest risk for malignant conversion. Premalignant progression encompasses the majority of the tumor latency period prior to malignant conversion, when the lesion shows invasive properties.

Usually, initiation is a low-frequency genetic event and is directly dependent on carcinogen dose. The phenotype of initiated cells varies according to tissue site and includes a defect in maturation, resistance to cytotoxicity, escape from senescence, and altered dependence on growth factors and hormones.[2] At the molecular level, initiation involves an alteration in signal transduction pathways that regulate cellular responses to extracellular signals, and these are internally regulated by protooncogenes and tumor suppressor genes.[33–35] Mutational activation of protooncogenes to oncogenes and inactivation of tumor suppressor genes contribute to initiation in most tissue sites.

Usually, experimental tumor promoters are nongenotoxic and frequently are tissue-specific and have multiple mechanisms of action, generally resulting in a disturbance of tissue homeostasis.[36,37] The mechanisms of tumor promotion include activation of cell-surface receptors; activation or inhibition of cytosolic enzymes and nuclear transcription factors; stimulation of proliferation;

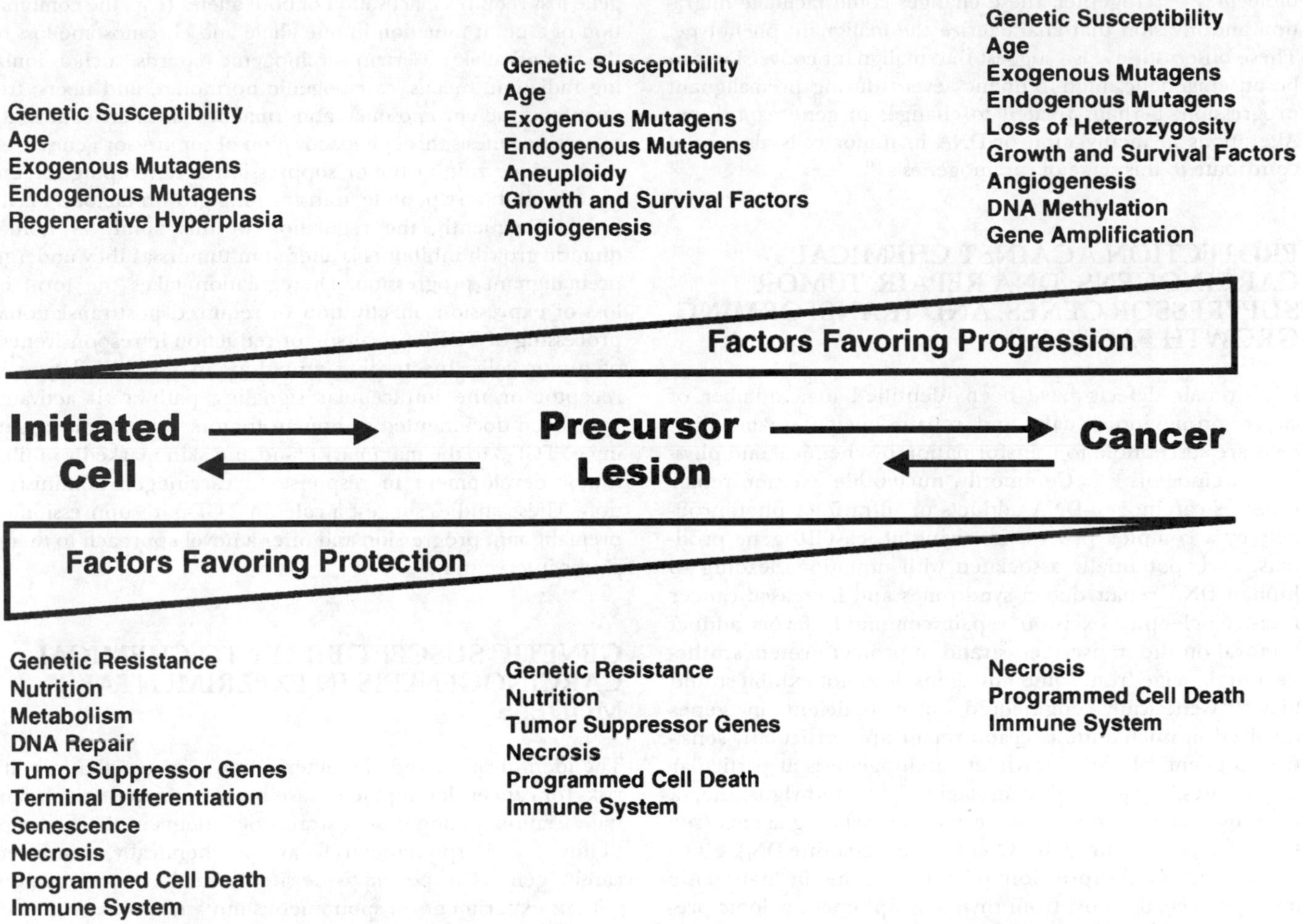

FIGURE 11-2. Factors influencing multistage carcinogenesis from environmental exposures. Early events reflect a balance of protective and initiating factors that determine the long premalignant latency period. As the process proceeds, protective factors are superseded by phenotypic alterations in the emerging neoplasm, whereas genetic instability accelerates selection of more deviant clones, even in the absence of exogenous exposures. The emerging cancerous clones are resistant to most of the endogenous protective mechanisms.

inhibition of apoptotic cell death; and direct cytotoxicity.[2,38] Genotoxic carcinogens also can have promoting properties, and repeated exposures to low concentrations of genotoxic carcinogens can induce tumors more effectively than do fewer exposures to the same total dose in experimental carcinogenesis.[39] Exogenous tumor promoters can determine the target site for tumor formation when experimental animals are initiated systemically with widely acting carcinogenic agents.[2,37] Thus, tumor promoters may contribute to target organ specificity when germline mutations produce an initiated state in multiple cell types. In general, initiated cells respond differently than do normal cells to promoters, and this is the basis for a clonal selection of an initiated population.[2,37] The contribution of exogenous tumor promoters to human cancer risk is clear only in a few cases, such as cigarette smoke and asbestos,[40] although other experimental promoting agents are found in the human environment (see Table 11-2).[37] Any change that causes a selective outgrowth of a preneoplastic cell, including additional genetic changes that selectively enhance growth of initiated cells, can be considered a promoting stimulus.

Premalignant progression in an initiated cell clone can occur spontaneously without further exposures, but this stage is accelerated by additional exposures to genotoxic agents, including some cancer chemotherapeutic drugs.[41] Spontaneous premalignant progression has been attributed to genomic instability that is constitutive in the premalignant phenotype.[42] Premalignant progression in most tumor models and in humans is associated with nonrandom, sequential chromosomal aberrations, including duplications, deletions, and loss of heterozygosity,[43] suggesting repeated episodes of cell selection and producing modally dominant chromosomal aberrations. Thus, at least one function of the relevant genetic events in premalignant progression must result in a growth advantage for the affected cell. In rodent populations, the genetic background of specific strains is determinant for the rate of premalignant progression, suggesting that constitutional factors influence both early and late events in cancer progression.

Frequently, malignant conversion is a multifocal change in premalignant lesions. Experimentally, malignant conversion has been linked to up-regulation of AP-1 transcriptional activity, gene amplification, and alterations in cell-cycle regulatory genes and secreted proteases.[44–47] Other studies have revealed gene splicing changes with expression of modified cell-surface molecules.[48,49] Together, these changes could facilitate migration and invasion that characterize the malignant phenotype. These observations also suggest that malignant conversion can be an epigenetic, high-frequency event during premalignant progression, perhaps related to changes in gene expression. Alterations in methylation of DNA in tumor cells also could contribute to this stage of carcinogenesis.[50,51]

PROTECTION AGAINST CHEMICAL CARCINOGENS: DNA REPAIR, TUMOR SUPPRESSOR GENES, AND TRANSFORMING GROWTH FACTOR-β

DNA repair defects have been identified in a number of cancer-prone individuals, and repair-deficient mammalian cells are susceptible to transformation by chemical and physical carcinogens.[52–55] Commonly, nucleotide excision repair removes carcinogen-DNA adducts or ultraviolet photoproducts by a complex process involving at least 10 gene products, each potentially associated with mutations leading to human DNA repair defect syndromes and increased cancer rates. Nucleotide excision repair commonly favors adduct removal on the transcribed strand to protect protein synthesis, but damage from some mutagens does not exhibit strand bias.[56] Genetically engineered mice deficient in genes involved in nucleotide excision repair are particularly sensitive to chemical and ultraviolet carcinogenesis at particular organ sites.[54] The highly mutagenic O^6-methylguanine, a consequence of exposure to certain methylating agents (see Fig. 11-1), is repaired by O^6-alkyldeoxyguanine-DNA alkyltransferase. Overexpression of this enzyme in transgenic mice protects the host from thymic lymphomas, colonic preneoplastic lesions, and colonic K-*ras* mutations after exposure to methylating agents.[57] O^6-alkyldeoxyguanine-DNA alkyltransferase activity varies in different tissues and cell types, and the enzyme can be inhibited by exogenous exposures that may act as cofactors in carcinogenesis.[58,59] Recently, interest has focused on a multigenic nucleotide mismatch repair system designed to repair mismatched bases after replication.[60] Mutations in components of this pathway increase risk for colon cancer in humans, and engineered mice that are null for a gene in this pathway are predisposed to develop tumors.[61]

Tumor suppressor genes represent a growing family of regulators of the cell cycle, genomic stability, cell senescence, cell death, or cell-cell communication that are inactivated during carcinogenesis.[4] Some may be direct targets of carcinogens, such as the *P53* gene in liver and the K-*ras* gene in lung cancer,[8,18] whereas others may become spontaneously altered during premalignant progression or may be suppressed by promoter methylation.[51] Suppressor genes can be inactivated by structural gene changes, but genomic imprinting, reduction in stability of the protein product, or mutations with a dominant-negative effect that suppresses the function of the product of the normal allele variously have been reported.[18,62] Inactivation of a single allele of a tumor suppressor gene (in which mutations at multiple sites may cause inactivation) occurs commonly, because it is a higher-probability event than is activation of an oncogene (in which specific changes at a few selected sites are required). However, a dominant effect of a tumor suppressor gene loss requires inactivation of both alleles (e.g., the combination of a point mutation in one allele and chromosome loss of the second allele). Certain carcinogenic hazards, such as ionizing radiation, metals, carcinogenic hormones, and fibers, frequently cause chromosomal abnormalities and may contribute to carcinogenesis through inactivation of suppressor genes.

A unique role in tumor suppression is developing for the growth inhibitory peptide, transforming growth factor-β (TGF-β).[63,64] Frequently, the regulation of this family of homodimeric growth inhibitors is altered in tumors as they undergo premalignant progression. Dysregulation takes the form of loss of expression, inactivation of required posttranslational processing of TGF-β precursor, or reduction in responsiveness of tumor cells. Inactivating mutations in the TGF-β type II receptor or the intracellular signaling pathway it activates have been documented in human tumors. Transgenic targeting of TGF-β to the mammary gland and skin markedly inhibit tumor development in response to carcinogen administration. These studies suggest a role for TGF-β in suppression of premalignant progression and offer a novel approach to therapeutic intervention.

GENETIC SUSCEPTIBILITY TO CHEMICAL CARCINOGENESIS IN EXPERIMENTAL MODELS

The identification and characterization of genes that modify risks for cancer development have been facilitated by substantial variation among inbred strains of rodents in their susceptibility to spontaneous and chemically induced carcinogenesis at specific tissue sites.[65] Furthermore, carcinogenesis experiments in spontaneous mutant strains or genetically modified mice created by transgenic or knockout technology have identified specific loci that modify cancer risk. For a variety of tissue sites, including lung, liver, breast, and skin, pairs of inbred mice that differ by 100-fold in risk for tumor development have been characterized. Detailed analyses of these differences using backcross, recombinant inbred, and recombinant congenic breeding protocols have shown specific determinants for initiation, promotion, premalignant progression, and metastatic stages.[66] In most cases, susceptibility or resistance is a property of the target tissue, not the host. Genetically determined differences in the affinity for the aryl hydrocarbon hydroxylase (Ah) receptor or other differences in metabolic processing of carcinogens is one modifier that has a major impact on experimental cancer risk.[28,30] Other loci regulate the growth of premalignant foci, the response to tumor promoters, the immune response to metastatic cells, and the basal proliferation rate of target cells.[65] In mice susceptible to colon cancer due to a constitutive mutation in the *apc* gene,[67] a locus on mouse chromosome 4 confers resistance to colon cancer.[68] Similarly, an autosomal dominant locus in the rat genome protects susceptible rats from chemically induced mammary gland neoplasia.[69] Recent advances in mapping of the mouse and rat genome[70] now promise to provide precise localization and identification of the loci involved in experimental genetic susceptibility, and translation of this information to syntenic loci of the human genome[71] should provide important insights into human susceptibility traits.

TABLE 11-3. Testing for Carcinogenicity

Method	*Examples*	*Advantages*	*Limitations*
In vitro testing	*Salmonella typhimurium* (Ames') mutation assay; HGPRT forward mutation assays; chromosomal aberrations; unscheduled DNA synthesis; cell transformation assays	Rapid results; human cells can be used; economical	Uncertain *in vitro*-to-*in vivo* extrapolations; frequent false-positives and -negatives; mutagenicity is not the same as carcinogenicity; substantial interlaboratory variation
Animal bioassay	National Toxicology Program rodent bioassays	More predictive of human experience than short-term tests; elucidates species differences	Expensive; doses are higher than those experienced by humans; uncertain animal-to-human extrapolation
Epidemiology	Prospective cohort studies; case-control studies	Direct measurement of human experience; covariants examined; dose-response data; now incorporating genetic and other biomarkers	Insensitive; does not prove causation; unknown confounding variables; biomarker data studies in early stage of development and validation

DETERMINATION OF CHEMICAL CARCINOGENS FOR HUMANS AND POPULATION-BASED RISK ASSESSMENT

Current understanding of carcinogenesis and risk to human health comes from a variety of models and methods, including mutagenesis assays, mammalian cell-culture experiments, animal studies, and both classic and molecular epidemiology. The goal of these studies is to elucidate cancer etiologies, to define cancer risks in humans (population and individual), and to identify more rational cancer prevention methods. Physicians are challenged when they attempt to determine what causes a cancer in a particular individual. The determination process requires an accurate history and physical examination and interpretation of research data. Often, the latter are beyond the scope of the practitioner and, in many cases, beyond the current state of knowledge. Nevertheless, methods for cancer risk assessment have been proposed and resources are available.[72] Several types of study models are used to assist in elucidating carcinogenic mechanisms and identifying potential human carcinogens. The usefulness of each method for identifying carcinogenic mechanisms and for identifying cancer risk can be contrasted with its limitations (Table 11-3). A direct relationship of *in vitro* experimental studies (i.e., metabolic activation of chemicals by cytochrome P-450s), *in vitro* mutagenicity tests, experimental animal studies, and human epidemiology has not been proved, but most chemicals that are positive in one method generally are positive with other methods. Nevertheless, 100% concordance does not exist; though sensitivity is high, specificity is low. It may be that consideration of multiple assays yields greater productivity, but this is not yet proved, and the concordance from animal to human experience is variable, although carcinogens that are more potent in one species tend to be more potent in others, including humans.

Human investigations provide the most relevant data regarding human risk. Classic epidemiology measures the incidence or prevalence of disease in human populations. Epidemiologic studies have identified such previously unknown risks as asbestos-related pleural mesothelioma, benzene-induced leukemia, and bladder cancer in dye workers. Study design and controlling for confounding variables are important determinants of a true association. It must be realized that epidemiologic methods, by themselves, do not demonstrate causation, and specific guidelines for assessing causation are available (Table 11-4).[73] The concordance between different scientific methods for inferring human cancer risk is variable.

Physicians can look to various regulatory, governmental, or review organizations for extensive evaluation of the scientific literature. Some organizations generate documents that report findings of experts who critically review the scientific literature, whereas others simply summarize data from other organizations. Several lists of carcinogens also have been published, but the evaluations of the literature and the definitions can vary greatly among organizations. Physicians should be aware of the purposes and goals of an organization when requesting its information. For example, the National Institute for Occupational Safety and Health and the American Council of Governmental Industrial Hygienists are concerned primarily with occupational exposures. The Environmental Protection Agency is concerned primarily with environmental exposures, quantitative risk assessments, and regulations relating to health hazard prevention for the entire population. The International Agency for Research on Cancer and the National Toxicology Program do not limit themselves to occupational or environmental exposures. The Agency for Toxic Substances and Disease Registry was created to study persons exposed to environmental toxins and to evaluate the adequacy of scientific literature. The known and potential

TABLE 11-4. Evaluating Cancer Etiology: Bradford-Hill Criteria[73]

Criteria	*Explanation*
Strength of association	What is magnitude of risk?
Consistency	Are there repeated observations by multiple investigators in different populations?
Specificity	Is the effect specific or are there other known causes?
Temporality	Does exposure precede effect?
Biologic gradient	Is there a dose-response relation?
Biologic plausibility	Is the effect predictable?
Coherence	Is the effect consistent with other scientific data?
Analogy	Do other similar agents act similarly?

TABLE 11-5. Known or Suspected Chemical Carcinogens in Humans

Target Organ	*Agents*	*Industries*	*Tumor Type*
Lung	Tobacco smoke, arsenic, asbestos, crystalline silica, benzo[a]pyrene, beryllium, *bis*(chloro)methyl ether, 1,3-butadiene, chromium VI compounds, coal tar and pitch, nickel compounds, soots, mustard gas	Aluminum production, coal gasification, coke production, hematite mining, painters	Squamous, large cell and small cell cancer and adenocarcinoma
Pleura	Asbestos, erionite		Mesothelioma
Oral cavity	Tobacco smoke, alcoholic beverages, nickel compounds	Boot and shoe production, furniture manufacturer, isopropyl alcohol production	Squamous cell cancer
Esophagus	Tobacco smoke, alcoholic beverages		Squamous cell cancer
Gastric system	Smoked, salted, and pickled foods	Rubber industry	Adenocarcinoma
Colon	Heterocyclic amines, asbestos	Pattern makers	Adenocarcinoma
Liver	Aflatoxin, vinyl chloride, tobacco smoke, alcoholic beverages, thorium dioxide		Hepatocellular carcinoma, hemangiosarcoma
Kidney	Tobacco smoke, phenacetin		Renal cell cancer
Bladder	Tobacco smoke, 4-aminobiphenyl, benzidine, 2-naphthylamine, phenacetin	Magenta manufacture, auramine manufacture	Transitional cell cancer
Prostate	Cadmium		Adenocarcinoma
Skin	Arsenic, benzo[a]pyrene, coal tar and pitch, mineral oils, soots, cyclosporin A, PUVA	Coal gasification, coke production	Squamous cell cancer, basal cell cancer
Bone marrow	Benzene, tobacco smoke, ethylene oxide, antineoplastic agents, cyclosporin A	Rubber workers	Leukemia, lymphoma

Note: These carcinogen designations are determined by regulatory or review agencies based on public health needs. They do not imply proof of carcinogenicity in individuals. This table is not all-inclusive. For additional information, the reader is referred to agency documents and publications.[11,72,193–197]

human carcinogens, as reported by various regulatory and research organizations, are listed in Table 11-5.

A formal quantitative risk assessment is used by regulatory agencies to estimate the risk to a population exposed to a particular carcinogen at a specific dose. Risk assessments serve public health interests as they attempt to predict the frequency of cancer in a population before epidemiologic investigations can be performed (i.e., before significant exposure and adverse outcomes occur). Risk estimates are formulated for potential dietary, airborne, and workplace carcinogens. Several mathematical models are used by various regulatory bodies to predict risks and to regulate allowable exposures. Risk assessments include four general steps: (1) hazard assessment, which qualitatively reviews scientific literature to decide whether a hazard might exist; (2) dose-response assessment, which evaluates the doses used in scientific studies and relates them to human exposures; (3) exposure assessment, which examines a population thought to be at risk regarding the quantity, duration, and routes of exposure; and (4) risk characterization, which incorporates the foregoing information and evaluates the assumptions used and the uncertainties to estimate risk. The modeling process requires many assumptions that are open to debate, and safety factors are incorporated to compensate for the uncertainties. At the conclusion, an incidence of cancer will be predicted, such as one additional case in 1 million persons. Owing to methodological limitations and uncertainties, wide confidence limits often prevail for the prediction.

MOLECULAR EPIDEMIOLOGY OF CANCER RISK FROM CHEMICALS

The field of molecular epidemiology seeks to identify cancer risk on the basis of individual exposures and genetically determined susceptibilities to cancer. Cancer epidemiology differs from traditional epidemiology because of its complexity. Traditional epidemiology paradigms implicate single causative agents that cause specific diseases (i.e., demonstrated through Koch's postulates). However, cancer is caused by multiple agents, and different combinations of agents can cause the same cancer. Conversely, the same agents might contribute to the development of different cancers. Molecular approaches to epidemiology use *a priori* hypotheses and biomarkers, rather than simply seeking associations between an exposure and disease (Fig. 11-3). Two fundamental principles underlie current studies of molecular epidemiology. First, carcinogenesis is a multistage process, and behind each stage are genetic events and complex pathways that may be responsible for these events. Thus, characterizing a specific risk factor against a background of many risk factors is difficult for scientists and can limit statistical power. Second, wide interindividual variation in response to carcinogen exposure and carcinogenic processes indicate that the human response to carcinogens is not homogeneous; hence, other studies (e.g., the use of a single-cell clone to study a gene's effect experimentally or the assumption that the population responds similarly to the mean in epidemiology studies) might not be representative of susceptible and resistant groups within a population.

The carcinogenic process is driven by genetic events (mutations or epigenetic changes), and in most people they are triggered by environmental exposures modified by host susceptibility. These are so-called gene-environment interactions.[74] Cancer-causing genes can be categorized into caretaker and gatekeeper genes.[75] Caretaker genes are involved in maintaining genomic integrity, such as those of DNA repair and carcinogen detoxification. Gatekeeper genes are involved in normal cellular function, such as those that are involved in cell-

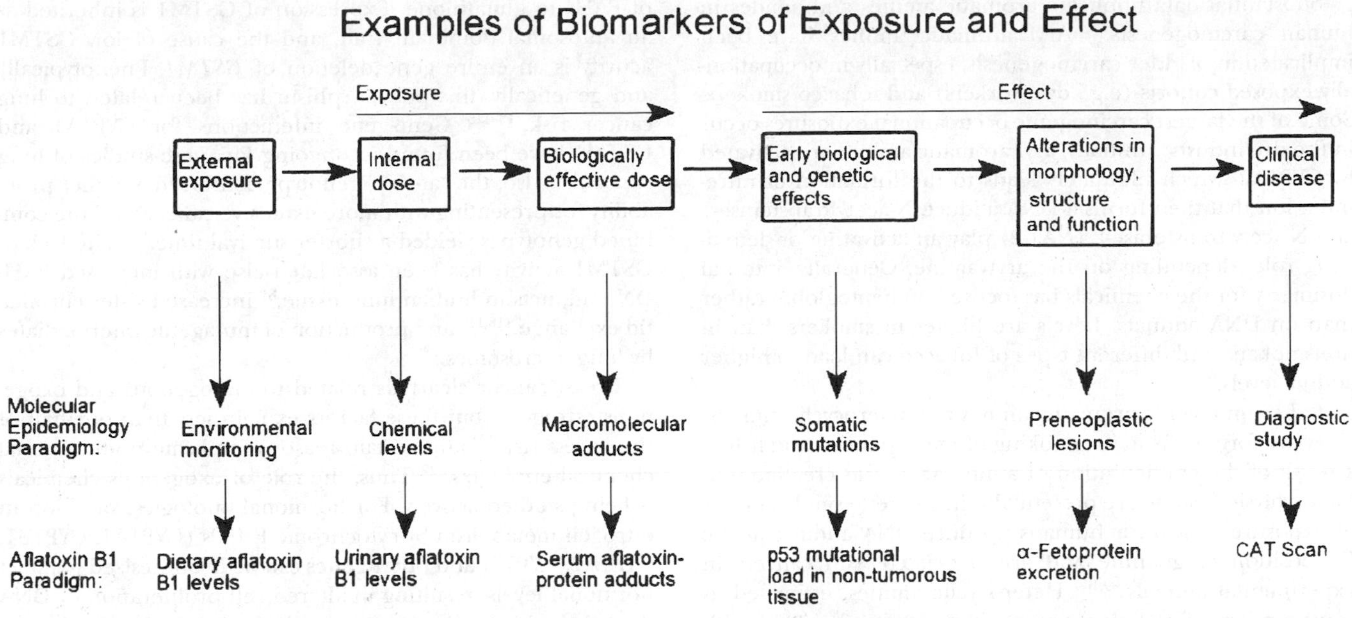

FIGURE 11-3. Schematic model depicting the range (from exposure to effect) and types of biomarkers that might be used for cancer risk assessments. Aflatoxin-B_1 is shown as a paradigm for the range of biomarkers. CAT, computer-aided tomography.

cycle control or apoptosis. Also, given that cancers are caused by multiple exposures causing damage in different genes, now the carcinogenic process is being considered as $gene^N$-$environment^N$ interactions. This new paradigm will lead to different perspectives of cancer genetics and cancer risk factors, wherein some genetic effects will be modeled differently (see Fig. 11-2).

EXPOSURE ASSESSMENT AND INTERNAL DOSIMETRY

Chemicals cause genetic damage in different ways: formation of carcinogen-DNA adducts leading to base mutations or bringing about gross chromosomal changes. Carcinogen-macromolecular adducts are formed when a mutagen, or part of it, irreversibly binds to DNA so that it can cause a base substitution, insertion, or deletion during DNA replication. Gross chromosomal mutations are chromosome breaks, gaps, or translocations. The level of DNA damage is the biologically effective dose in a target organ,[76] and reflects the net result of carcinogen exposure, activation, lack of detoxification, lack of DNA repair, and lack of programmed cell death or necrosis.

A variety of assays are available to identify carcinogen-macromolecular adducts in human tissues. These assays include the ^{32}P-postlabeling assay-nucleotide chromatography, immunoassays that include immunohistochemistry, fluorescence spectroscopy, gas chromatography–mass spectroscopy, and electrical chemical detection. Each has its usefulness and limitations, and all are challenged by sensitivity or specificity (or both). The effect of an individual's metabolism on carcinogen-DNA adduct formation might be different at different levels of exposure—where adduct levels formed from lower exposures are relatively higher—and similar to that of persons with decreased metabolic capacity but higher exposures.[77] The relationship of such surrogate markers as carcinogen-DNA adducts in blood to the target organ has been studied partially[78,79] but is not yet well established, and the use of target organs[80,81] can provide specific information about potentially carcinogenic effects.

The detection of gross chromosomal changes in normal-appearing cells is technically difficult. Presumed surrogate measures of chromosomal damage include the estimate of sister chromatid exchanges or baseline gross chromosomal changes. The latter has been associated with increased cancer risk, but these studies have significant limitations.[82,83]

The effect of some potential carcinogens has been studied extensively using molecular epidemiological tools.[8,84,85] These carcinogens tend to be present in tobacco smoke and, in some cases, diet and workplace.

Commonly, people are exposed to N-nitrosamine and other N-nitroso compounds from dietary[86] and tobacco exposures,[8] which are associated with DNA adduct formation and cancer in laboratory animals.[87] Exposure can occur through endogenous formation of N-nitrosamines from nitrates in food[88] or directly from dietary sources, cosmetics, drugs, household commodities, and tobacco smoke. The greatest source of exposure in the United States is from processed meats and (until recently) beer. Endogenous formation occurs in the stomach from the reaction of nitrosatable amines and nitrate, used as a preservative, which is converted to nitrites by bacteria. Host capacity to form N-nitrosamines is associated with risk of stomach[89] and esophageal cancer.[90,91] It has been shown also that coadministration of vitamin C can reduce the rate of endogenous nitrosation. N-nitrosamines undergo metabolic activation by cytochrome P-450s (*CYP2E1*, *CYP2A6*, and *CYP2D6*) and form DNA-adducts that have been identified in target tissues or have been associated with specific cancers.[92–94]

Exposures to polycyclic aromatic hydrocarbon (PAH) compounds are associated with an increased risk of lung and skin cancer. Industrial pollution, fossil fuels, and tobacco smoke account for the major environmental sources, although diet is considered the major source.[95] DNA damage in white blood cells has been documented for a variety of exposures.[85] PAH-adducts can be formed from the consumption of charcoal-broiled foods, where adduct levels exceed those from smoking.[96]

Substantial data implicate aromatic amines and amides in human carcinogenesis.[77] Aryl aromatic amines have been implicated in bladder carcinogenesis, especially in occupationally exposed cohorts (e.g., dye workers) and tobacco smokers. Some of the largest carcinogenic occupational exposures occur in the dye industry. Initially, aryl aromatic amines are activated by CYP1A2, which ultimately leads to the formation of nitrenium ion that then forms a DNA adduct. N-acetyltransferase-1 and N-acetyltransferase-2 (NAT-2) play an activating or detoxifying role, depending on the aryl amine. Generally, internal dosimetry for the chemicals has focused on hemoglobin rather than on DNA adducts. Levels are higher in smokers than in nonsmokers, and different types of tobacco can lead to higher adduct levels.[97]

Other mutagenic aromatic amines are heterocyclic amines. They are formed from the cooking of meat, poultry, and fish as a result of the condensation of amino acids and creatine during pyrolysis.[98] Some are present also in cigarette smoke. Levels of exposure typical for humans produce DNA adducts at the C8 position of guanine and are associated with cancers in experimental animals.[99,100] Heterocyclic amines, estimated as consumption of well-done meat, have been associated with breast and colon cancer.[101]

Aflatoxins are suspected human liver carcinogens and are considered to be a major contributor to liver cancer in China and parts of Africa. Aflatoxin remains one of the best examples of the range and use of biomarkers for cancer risk (see Fig. 11-3). The primary adduct formed from aflatoxin exposure is to the N7 position of guanine.[102] The metabolic activation in humans is similar to that of sensitive laboratory animals.[103] Urinary aflatoxin adduct levels vary among regions of the world, depending on dietary exposures.[104] Serum albumin adducts correlate with dietary intake and urinary excretion of the M1 metabolite.[105] Important is that urinary aflatoxin adduct levels correlate with the incidence of hepatocellular carcinomas, and an interaction is seen with hepatitis B infection.[84]

GENETIC SUSCEPTIBILITY

The cancer risk from genetic variation can range from small to large, depending on its penetrance. Highly penetrant cancer susceptibility genes cause familial cancers and account for fewer than 1% of all cancers.[106] Low-penetrant genes cause common sporadic cancers, which have large public health consequences. Table 11-6 lists several investigated genetic polymorphisms and their association with cancer risk. A genetic polymorphism is defined as a genetic variant present in at least 1% of the population.

Lung cancer has been studied most extensively for gene-environment interactions. Among the low-penetrant genes studied most commonly are cytochrome P-450 (CYP)1A1 and glutathione S-transferase M1 (*GSTM1*). The CYP1A1 enzyme is the first step in the metabolic activation of polycyclic aromatic hydrocarbons, which are known human lung and skin carcinogens. Studies of Japanese subjects indicated an interaction between a CYP1A1 polymorphism and smoking for lung cancer risk,[107] wherein the combination of the homozygous minor allele and smoking yielded odds ratios similar to having one of the other genotypes and a greater smoking history.[108] Western studies, however, do not show the same association.[109–112] GSTM1 is a detoxifying enzyme that catalyzes the conjugation of PAHs to glutathione. Expression of GSTM1 is inherited as an autosomal dominant trait, and the cause of low GSTM1 activity is an entire gene deletion of *GSTM1*. Phenotypically and genetically, this polymorphism has been related to lung cancer risk.[113–115] Gene-gene interactions for CYP1A1 and GSTM1 have been found in ongoing Japanese studies of lung cancer.[116] Also, the "at-risk" genotype conferred a higher probability for presenting with more extensive cancer, and the combined genotypes yielded a shorter survival time.[117] The lack of GSTM1 activity has been associated also with increased PAH-DNA adducts in human lung tissue,[81] increased sister chromatid exchange,[118,119] and production of mutagenic intermediates by lung microsomes.[120]

Breast cancer clearly is related to endogenous and exogenous estrogens, but these factors explain less than one-half of the excess risk,[121] and certain reasons implicate nonhormonal chemical etiologies.[122] Thus, the role of exogenous chemicals is being studied actively. For hormonal etiologies, variation in estrogen metabolism by cytochrome P-450s (CYP1A1, CYP1B1, CYP1A2, CYP17) and other genes can be hypothesized to affect hormonal levels, resulting in altered cell proliferation or DNA damage and subsequent cancer risk. One study has implicated cytochrome 17,[123] whereas others have provided conflicting evidence for catechol-methyltransferase that detoxifies estradiol.[124,125] For chemical etiologies, aromatic amines have been implicated as potential human breast carcinogens.[122] These chemicals are detoxified by NAT-2, in which a genetic polymorphism governs the metabolism of isoniazid for tuberculosis treatments.[126] One study indicated that tobacco smoking is associated with breast cancer in white postmenopausal women who have a decreased capacity to detoxify aromatic amines, because they are NAT-2 slow acetylators.[127] Although a prospective study of nurses[128] seemingly provided conflicting data, differences were found in data analysis and study size. Considering a specific role for polycyclic aromatic hydrocarbons in breast cancer, some suggestions posit that one polymorphic variant of CYP1A1 might be a risk factor for breast cancer in subsets of smokers,[129,130] whereas another polymorphism might be a risk factor in African Americans.[131] A nested case-control study from a prospective cohort of women in Maryland found a 2.1-fold increased risk for women who lacked GSTM1,[132] although two studies have not found similar results.[129]

The role for genetic determinants of carcinogen metabolism in cancer risk is established for other cancers, although this area of study is newer.[113] Several studies have implicated deficient GSTM1 and NAT-2 detoxification of smoke-related or occupational carcinogens in bladder cancer.[77,133] For colon cancer, studies have demonstrated that risk increases for NAT-2 rapid acetylators,[134,135] wherein, in contrast to its detoxification role in bladder and breast cancer, evidence suggests that NAT-2 works to activate heterocyclic amines formed from the overcooking of meats.[136]

Genetic polymorphisms for housekeeping genes controlling such cellular functions as cell-cycle control and DNA repair logically may affect cancer risk.[106] In the general population, DNA repair capacity in humans decreases with aging,[137,138] which would make this decrease an acquired risk factor for cancer and might explain a portion of the increased cancer risk in the elderly.[139] However, inherited susceptibilities via specific genetic polymorphisms that affect the efficiency of DNA repair,

TABLE 11-6. Selected Examples of Inherited Susceptibilities for Cancer

Gene	*Examples of Substrate*	*Associated Cancer*	*Comments*
METABOLIC ACTIVATION			
CYP2D6	Debrisoquine, dextromethorphan	Lung	Phenotyping method available; more than 13 polymorphisms have been identified, and families have been shown to inherit multiple copies; wide racial variation exists.
CYP1A1	Polycyclic aromatic hydrocarbons	Lung, breast, oral cavity	Different polymorphisms exist in different racial populations; several studies relate a functionally active polymorphism to lung cancer in Japanese; wide racial variation and crossover occurred in some races.
CYP2E1	N-nitrosamines, benzene, urethane, 1,3-butadiene	Lung	Phenotyping methods available; different polymorphisms exist in different racial groups; one has been associated with lung cancer in Japanese.
CYP2A6	N-nitrosamines	Lung	Genotyping method available but technically difficult and may not be accurate.
CYP1A2	Aromatic amines, aflatoxin	Colon	Phenotyping methods available; racial variation exists.
CYP3A4	Polycyclic aromatic hydrocarbons, aflatoxin	Unknown	Phenotyping methods available; racial variation exists.
CYP1B1	Polycyclic aromatic hydrocarbons, estrogens	Unknown	Several polymorphisms identified.
N-acetyltransferase-1	Aryl and heterocyclic aromatic amines	Bladder, oral cavity, colon	Phenotyping methods available; genotype may not correlate with phenotype; multiple variants exist with different and complex pathways for different substrates.
N-acetyltransferase-2	Aryl and heterocyclic aromatic amines	Bladder, colon	Phenotyping methods available; multiple polymorphisms known; wide racial variation; polymorphisms can alter activity in both directions.
Epoxide hydrolase	Polycyclic aromatic hydrocarbons, aflatoxin	Liver, oral cavity, lung	Two variants known, each can affect activity; also considered a detoxification enzyme (aflatoxin).
AHH receptor	AHH receptor–binding sites	Lung	Wide interindividual variation but not determined at the genetic level.
CYP17	Estrogens	Breast	Related to age at menarche; might increase transcription.
CYP19	Estrogens	Breast	Two polymorphisms known, but no functional effect.
Catechol-methyltransferase	Estrogens	Breast	Opposite results reported in literature.
Nitroquinone oxoreductase	Benzene	Leukemia	Functional polymorphism.
DETOXICATION ENZYMES			
Glutathione S-transferase M1	Polycyclic aromatic hydrocarbons, aromatic amines, others	Lung, breast	The polymorphism results in the deletion of the entire gene; other GSTs also are important but are not polymorphic.
Glutathione S-transferase Pi	Polycyclic aromatic hydrocarbons	Lung, oral cavity	Phenotype questionably associated with genotype.
Alcohol dehydrogenase	Ethanol	Oral cavity, breast, liver	Two polymorphisms are known that determine detoxication of alcoholic beverages.
Aldehyde dehydrogenase	Acetaldehyde	Liver	Two separate polymorphisms are known that determine detoxication of alcoholic beverages.
UDP-glucuronosyl transferases	Aromatic amines, polycyclic aromatic hydrocarbons, phenols, steroids	Unknown	Interindividual variation known but appears to be unimodal.
Sulfotransferases	Phenols, aromatic amines	Unknown	Very little information is known about this enzyme; phenotyping methods are not easily available; a liver biopsy is required.
PROTOONCOGENES			
L-myc	Not applicable	Lung, sarcoma, gastric	A functional effect of this polymorphism has not been determined; it is a risk factor in Japanese only.
H-ras	Not applicable	Lung, breast, colon, bladder	A functional effect of this polymorphism has not been demonstrated.
erb-b2	Not applicable	Unknown	There is a single base substitution in an intron of unknown significance.
TUMOR SUPPRESSOR GENE			
p53	Not applicable	Lung	Variants have no functional importance; polymorphism is associated with lung cancer in Japanese.
REPLICATION/REPAIR			
Poly(ADP-ribose) polymerase	DNA-binding protein	Myeloma, prostate	The polymorphism is a 193 bp duplicated conserved region in the pseudogene.
O^6-alkyl-deoxyguanine-DNA-alkyltransferase	N-nitrosamine-related damage	Unknown	Wide interindividual variation exists.
XRCC1	Not applicable	Unknown	Three polymorphic sites, one with phenotypic relationship.

such as for nucleotide excision repair, are largely unknown. A nonspecific DNA repair assay that measures chromosomal aberrations in human cultured lymphocytes after an *in vitro* challenge with a mutagen has shown initial promise. An increased mutagen-related aberration rate has been observed in persons with primary and secondary upper aerodigestive tract cancers,[140] multiple primary cancers,[141] and lung cancer.[142]

MUTATIONAL SPECTRUM OF HUMAN CANCERS

The study of mutations in human tumors and experimental models is elucidating important carcinogenic mechanisms.[143] *In vitro* studies using prokaryotic and simple eukaryotic assays, including human cells (e.g., site-specific mutagenesis assays), indicate that human exposure to mutagens might result in a narrow spectrum of mutations that are nonrandom.[18] Some carcinogenic agents produce a "fingerprint" of mutations. In eukaryotic studies, for example, examining the mutational spectra in endogenous genes[144] or exogenous genes transfected into cell systems[145,146] have identified different phenotypes, depending on the exposures. These assays, however, may underestimate the induced mutational frequency due to deletions, chromosomal nondysjunction, and frameshift mutations that cause loss of other genes essential for cell survival and result in cytotoxicity or apoptosis. The data also show that the fingerprint hypothesis is likely the exception rather than the rule, because most mutagens actually can form several types of mutations, depending in part on the conformation of DNA and the type and the location of the adduct.[143] Nonetheless, a comparison of the mutational spectrum at the *aprt* locus in Chinese hamster ovary cells induced by ionizing radiation, ultraviolet radiation, or benzo[a]pyrene-diol-epoxide is consistent with the mutagenesis models for these exposures.[144] Promutagenic cyclobutane and pyrimidine-pyrimidone(6-4) photoproducts are induced by ultraviolet light, whereas ionizing radiation frequently causes deletions, and benzo[a]pyrene-diol-epoxide causes the predicted G:C→T:A transversion.

The study of mutations in the *P53* tumor suppressor gene is suited uniquely for the study of cancer etiology, exposure, and susceptibility, because *P53* is involved in many cellular processes, including maintenance of genomic stability, programmed cell death, DNA repair, and others.[147] The *P53* mutation frequency varies by organ site and histological subtype,[18] indicating that cancers occur through different pathways and different exposures at the cellular level. Several examples of particular carcinogenic exposures are linked to cancers via a *P53* mutational mechanism, especially the demonstration that ultraviolet light exposure and skin cancer are associated with cytosine-cytosine to thymine-thymine tandem transitions.[148] Another example is dietary aflatoxin B1 exposure and a consistent finding of mutations in the third nucleotide pair of codon 249 of liver cancers in regions with endemic exposure to aflatoxin B1.[149,150] Combinations of exposures can lead also to different outcomes in the same organ site. An interactive effect of alcohol drinking and cigarette use in oral cavity cancers yields different types of *P53* mutations.[151]

Showing that the *P53* mutation frequency is modulated by gene-environment interactions has been difficult because of the technical difficulties in determining the mutational spectra in large numbers of cancer patients, but preliminary evidence exists. The mutational spectra of lung[18] and breast cancers[152] are different among whites, African Americans, and Japanese, consistent with the hypothesis that differences exist in both exposure and the frequency of genetically determined carcinogen metabolism and DNA repair. More specific evidence for a relationship of gene-environment interactions and mutations in the *P53* gene can be found from Japanese studies of *CYP1A1, GSTM1,* and lung cancer.[153]

Among the most exciting areas in molecular epidemiology is the potential ability to identify mutations and preneoplastic lesions prior to the development of cancer or as a diagnostic test for early cancer. Analyses of stool from cancer patients have found cells with the same K-*ras* mutations present in the cancer.[154] Similar findings have been reported in sputum samples from patients with head and neck cancers.[155] Analysis of codon 12 mutations in the K-*ras* gene of bronchoalveolar cells has shown a 33% rate of detection in cancer patients, with an acceptable specificity; many of the positive samples were cytologically negative for cancer.[156] Archived sputum samples also have revealed, in K-*ras,* mutations that were matched later to a confirmed diagnosis of lung cancer.[157]

TOBACCO SMOKING AND CANCER RISK

Tobacco smoking is the major cause of cancer and accounts for almost 96% of all male lung cancers in whites. Though the risk of lung cancer decreases after smoking cessation, the risk never returns to that for nonsmokers. According to 1990 estimates, persons who died of smoking-related diseases would have lived an additional 15 years if they had never smoked. Tobacco smoke contains more than 3500 chemicals, of which more than 20 are carcinogens.[8] Specific chemicals in tobacco smoke include PAHs and N-nitrosamines, aromatic amines, ethylene oxide, 1,3-butadiene, and agents that cause oxy radical damage. For example, tobacco-specific nitrosamines (TSN)—that is, 4-(methyl-nitrosamino)-1-(3-pyridyl)-1-butanone (NNK) and N'-nitrosonornicotine (NNN), which are potent carcinogens in laboratory animals[158]—result in the formation of hemoglobin adducts.[159] PAHs and TSNs are considered to be the most potent carcinogens in tobacco smoke.[8] During the last 40 years, the approximate threefold decrease in tar (containing PAHs) and nicotine content has been accompanied by an increase of other carcinogens, including TSNs.[160]

Convincing laboratory animal and human studies demonstrate a relationship between tobacco smoke constituents, carcinogen-DNA adduct formation, and cancer.[161] In humans, case-control studies find a positive relationship for lung and bladder cancer.[162,163] Also, studies of tobacco smoke exposure have shown increased adduct formation in the lung,[78,164,165] blood,[78,163,166] and larynx.[167–169] However, wide interindividual variation for adduct levels is common, so several studies have failed to show a direct relationship between smoking and adducts.[81,162,170,171]

The *P53* gene, in particular, has a unique spectrum of mutations in tobacco-associated lung cancers.[172] Also, an increased frequency of *P53* tumor suppressor gene mutations has been reported at non-CpG sites in smokers with head and neck cancers, especially in conjunction with alcohol consumption.[151] The decrease in nicotine content in cigarettes has led to a paradoxical increase in smoking, owing to the drive for maintaining higher blood nicotine levels.

Several determinants of tobacco carcinogen exposure and cancer risk exist, including the number of cigarettes smoked per day, years smoked, cigarette type (e.g., tar content, which is the total dry particulate component of smoke), and smoking topography (e.g., how much smoke entering the lung is measured by puff volume, number of puffs per cigarette, puff duration, and interpuff interval).[173]

Also important is that not all smokers experience the same carcinogenic risks; only 1 in 10 heavy smokers develop lung cancer, and some heavy smokers live to their 90s. Thus, interindividual variation in host susceptibility likely is important for cancer risk (e.g., those related to carcinogen metabolism, DNA repair, or behavior).[174] Overall risk is related to dose, which is directly affected by nicotine addiction; more cigarettes are consumed to maintain nicotine blood levels, and cigarettes with lower nicotine levels result in the need to smoke more, thereby increasing the exposure to tobacco carcinogens.

REFERENCES

1. Wingo PA, Ries LA, Giovino GA, et al. Annual report to the nation on the status of cancer, 1973–1996, with a special section on lung cancer and tobacco smoking. *J Natl Cancer Inst* 1999;91:675.
2. Yuspa SH, Poirier MC. Chemical carcinogenesis: from animal models to molecular models in one decade. *Adv Cancer Res* 1988;50:25.
3. Harris CC. Chemical and physical carcinogenesis: advances and perspectives for the 1990s. *Cancer Res* 1991;51:5023s.
4. Stanley LA. Molecular aspects of chemical carcinogenesis: the roles of oncogenes and tumour suppressor genes. *Toxicology* 1995;96:173.
5. Lawley PD. Historical origins of current concepts of carcinogenesis. *Adv Cancer Res* 1994;65:17.
6. Wink DA, Vodovotz Y, Laval J, et al. The multifaceted roles of nitric oxide in cancer. *Carcinogenesis* 1998;19:711.
7. Harris CC. Human tissues and cells in carcinogenesis research. *Cancer Res* 1987;47:1.
8. Hecht SS. Tobacco smoke carcinogens and lung cancer. *J Natl Cancer Inst* 1999;91:1194.
9. Kohlmeier L, Simonsen N, Mottus K. Dietary modifiers of carcinogenesis. *Environ Health Perspect* 1995;103[Suppl 8]:177.
10. Wattenberg LW. Inhibition of tumorigenesis in animals. *IARC Sci Publ* 1996;139:151.
11. *Report on carcinogens,* 8th ed. Washington, DC: US Department of Health and Human Services, Public Health Service, National Toxicology Program, Integrated Laboratory Systems, Inc, 1998.
12. Jackson MA, Stack HF, Waters MD. The genetic toxicology of putative nongenotoxic carcinogens. *Mutat Res* 1993;296:241.
13. Ashby J, Paton D. The influence of chemical structure on the extent and sites of carcinogenesis for 522 rodent carcinogens and 55 different human carcinogen exposures. *Mutat Res* 1993;286:3.
14. Dipple A. DNA adducts of chemical carcinogens. *Carcinogenesis* 1995;16:437.
15. Felton JS, Knize MG. Occurrence, identification, and bacterial mutagenicity of heterocyclic amines in cooked food. *Mutat Res* 1991;259:205.
16. Essigmann JM, Wood ML. The relationship between the chemical structures and mutagenic specificities of the DNA lesions formed by chemical and physical mutagens. *Toxicol Lett* 1993;67:29.
17. Levy DD, Groopman JD, Lim SE, et al. Sequence specificity of aflatoxin B_1-induced mutations in a plasmid replicated in xeroderma pigmentosum and DNA repair proficient human cells. *Cancer Res* 1992;52:5668.
18. Greenblatt MS, Bennett WP, Hollstein M, et al. Mutations in the *p53* tumor suppressor gene: clues to cancer etiology and molecular pathogenesis. *Cancer Res* 1994;54:4855.
19. Barrett JC. Mechanisms of multistep carcinogenesis and carcinogen risk assessment. *Environ Health Perspect* 1993;100:9.
20. Tennant RW. A perspective on nonmutagenic mechanisms in carcinogenesis. *Environ Health Perspect* 1993;101[Suppl 3]:231.
21. Ames BN, Gold LS. The causes and prevention of cancer: the role of environment. *Biotherapy* 1998;11:205.
22. Tennant RW. The genetic toxicity database of the National Toxicology Program: evaluation of the relationships between genetic toxicity and carcinogenicity. *Environ Health Perspect* 1991;96:47.
23. Guyton KZ, Kensler TW. Oxidative mechanisms in carcinogenesis. *Br Med Bull* 1993;49:523.
24. Davis DD, Bradlow HL, Wolff M, et al. Medical hypothesis: xenoestrogens as preventable causes of breast cancer. *Environ Health Perspect* 1993;101:372.
25. Dunnick JK, Elwell MR, Huff J, et al. Chemically induced mammary gland cancer in the National Toxicology Program's carcinogenesis bioassay. *Carcinogenesis* 1995;16:173.
26. Gonzalez FJ, Gelboin HV. Role of human cytochromes p450 in the metabolic activation of chemical carcinogens and toxins. *Drug Metab Rev* 1994;26:165.
27. Guengerich FP. Metabolic activation of carcinogens. *Pharmacol Ther* 1992;54:17.
28. Gonzalez F. Genetic polymorphism and cancer susceptibility: fourteenth Sapporo cancer seminar. *Cancer Res* 1995;55:710.
29. Ames BN, Gold LS, Willett WC. The causes and prevention of cancer. *Proc Natl Acad Sci U S A* 1995;92:5258.
30. Poulsen HE, Loft S, Wassermann K. Cancer risk related to genetic polymorphisms in carcinogen metabolism and DNA repair. *Pharmacol Toxicol* 1993;72[Suppl 1]:93.
31. Tennant RW, Spalding J, French JE. Evaluation of transgenic mouse bioassays for identifying carcinogens and noncarcinogens. *Mutat Res* 1996;365:119.
32. Macleod KF, Jacks T. Insights into cancer from transgenic mouse models. *J Pathol* 1999;187:43.
33. Cantley LC, Auger KR, Carpenter C, et al. Oncogenes and signal transduction. *Cell* 1991;64:281.
34. Hunter T. Cooperation between oncogenes. *Cell* 1991;64:249.
35. Weinberg RA. The molecular basis of oncogenes and tumor suppressor genes. *Ann NY Acad Sci* 1995;758:331.
36. Slaga TJ. *Mechanisms of tumor promotion,* vols 1–3. Boca Raton, FL: CRC Press, 1983.
37. Yuspa SH. Tumor promotion. In: Fortner JF, Rhoads JE, eds. *Accomplishments in cancer research, 1986.* Philadelphia: JB Lippincott Co, 1987:169–182.
38. Marsman DS, Barrett JC. Apoptosis and chemical *Carcinogenesis Risk Anal* 1994;14:321.
39. Iversen OH. The skin tumorigenic and carcinogenic effects of different doses, numbers of dose fractions and concentrations of 7,12-dimethylbenz[a]anthracene in acetone applied on hairless mouse epidermis. Possible implications for human carcinogenesis. *Carcinogenesis* 1991;12:493.
40. Willey JC, Harris CC. Cellular and molecular biological aspects of human bronchogenic carcinogenesis. *Crit Rev Oncol Hematol* 1990;10: 181.
41. Hennings H, Shores RA, Poirier MC, et al. Enhanced malignant conversion of benign mouse skin tumors by cisplatin. *J Natl Cancer Inst* 1990;82:836.
42. Loeb LA. Microsatellite instability: marker of a mutator phenotype in cancer. *Cancer Res* 1994;54:5059.
43. Fearon ER, Vogelstein B. A genetic model for colorectal tumorigenesis. *Cell* 1990;61:759.
44. Dong Z, Birrer MJ, Watts RG, et al. Blocking of tumor promoter-induced AP-1 activity inhibits induced transformation in JB6 mouse epidermal cells. *Proc Natl Acad Sci U S A* 1994;91:609.
45. Gould MN. Cellular and molecular aspects of the multistage progression of mammary carcinogenesis in humans and rats. *Semin Cancer Biol* 1993;4:161.
46. Bianchi AB, Fischer SM, Robles AI, et al. Overexpression of cyclin D1 in mouse skin carcinogenesis. *Oncogene* 1993;8:1127.
47. Aznavoorian S, Murphy AN, Stetler-Stevenson WG, et al. Molecular aspects of tumor cell invasion and metastasis. *Cancer* 1993;71:1368.
48. Gunthert U, Hofman M, Rudy S, et al. A new variant of glycoprotein CD44 confers metastatic potential to rat carcinoma cells. *Cell* 1991;65:13.
49. Tennenbaum T, Belanger AJ, Glick AB, et al. A splice variant of a6 integrin is associated with malignant conversion in mouse skin tumorigenesis. *Proc Natl Acad Sci U S A* 1995;92:7041.
50. Jones PA, Laird PW. Cancer epigenetics comes of age. *Nat Genet* 1999;21:163.
51. Baylin SB, Herman JG, Graff JR, et al. Alterations in DNA methylation: a fundamental aspect of neoplasia. *Adv Cancer Res* 1998;72:141.
52. Rajewsky MF, Engelbergs J, Thomale J, et al. Relevance of DNA repair to carcinogenesis and cancer therapy. *Recent Results Cancer Res* 1998;154:127.
53. Yu Z, Chen J, Ford BN, et al. Human DNA repair systems: an overview. *Environ Mol Mutagen* 1999;33:3.
54. de Boer J, Hoeijmakers JH. Cancer from the outside, aging from the inside: mouse models to study the consequences of defective nucleotide excision repair. *Biochimie* 1999; 81:127.
55. Weeda G, de Boer J, Donker I, et al. Molecular basis of DNA repair mechanisms and syndromes. *Recent Results Cancer Res* 1998;154:147.
56. Leadon SA. Transcription-coupled repair of DNA damage: unanticipated players, unexpected complexities. *Am J Hum Genet* 1999;64:1259.
57. Zaidi NH, Pretlow TP, O'Riordan MA, et al. Transgenic expression of human *MGMT* protects against azoxymethane-induced aberrant crypt foci and G to A mutations in the K-*ras* oncogene of mouse colon. *Carcinogenesis* 1995;16:451.
58. Grafstrom RC, Pegg AE, Trump BF, Harris CC. O^6-alkylguanine-DNA alkyltransferase activity in normal human tissues and cells. *Cancer Res* 1984;44:2855.
59. Krokan H, Grafstrom RC, Sundqvist K, et al. Cytotoxicity, thiol depletion and inhibition of O^6-methylguanine-DNA methyltransferase by various aldehydes in cultured human bronchial fibroblasts. *Carcinogenesis* 1985;6:1755.
60. Kolodner RD, Marsischky GT. Euxaryotic DNA mismatch repair. *Curr Opin Genet Dev* 1999;9:89.
61. Edelmann W, Yang K, Umar A, et al. Mutation in the mismatch repair gene Msh6 causes cancer susceptibility. *Cell* 1997;91:467.
62. Lane DP. *P53* and human cancers. *Br Med Bull* 1994;50:582.
63. Akhurst RJ, Balmain A. Genetic events and the role of TGF-b in epithelial tumour progression. *J Pathol* 1999;187:82.
64. Reiss, M. Transforming growth factor-b and cancer: a love-hate relationship? *Oncol Res* 1997;9:447.
65. Drinkwater NR. Effect of genetic susceptibility on tumor induction. In: Arcos JC, Argus M, Woo Y, eds. *Chemical induction of cancer: modulation and combination effects.* Boston: Birkhauser, 1995:451-472.
66. Balmain A, Nagase H. Cancer resistance genes in mice: models for the study of tumour modifiers. *Trends Genet* 1998;14:139.
67. Moser AR, Pitot HC, Dove WF. A dominant mutation that predisposes to multiple intestinal neoplasia in the mouse. *Science* 1990;247:322.

68. Dietrich WF, Lander ES, Smith JS, et al. Genetic identification of *Mom-1*, a major modifier locus affecting *Min*-induced intestinal neoplasia in the mouse. *Cell* 1993;75:631.
69. Fernandez-Salguero P, Pineau T, Hilbert DM, et al. Immune system impairment and hepatic fibrosis in mice lacking the dioxin-binding Ah receptor. *Science* 1995;268:722.
70. Kelloff GJ, Crowell JA, Hawk ET, et al. Clinical development plan: 13-*cis*-retinoic acid. *J Cell Biochem Suppl* 1996;26:168.
71. Kelloff GJ, Crowell JA, Hawk ET, et al. Clinical development plan: vitamin A. *J Cell Biochem Suppl* 1996;26:269.
72. Shields PG, Harris CC. Environmental causes of cancer. *Med Clin North Am* 1990;74:263.
73. Hill AB. The environment and disease: association or causation. *Proc R Soc Med* 1965;58:295.
74. Khoury MJ. Genetic epidemiology and the future of disease prevention and public health. *Epidemiol Rev* 1997;19:175.
75. Kinzler KW, Vogelstein B. Cancer-susceptibility genes. Gatekeepers and caretakers [news; comment]. *Nature* 1997;386:761.
76. Perera FP. Molecular cancer epidemiology: a new tool in cancer prevention. *J Natl Cancer Inst* 1987;78:887.
77. Vineis P, Pirastu R. Aromatic amines and cancer. *Cancer Causes Control* 1997;8:346.
78. Wiencke JK, Kelsey KT, Varkonyi A, et al. Correlation of DNA adducts in blood mononuclear cells with tobacco carcinogen-induced damage in human lung. *Cancer Res* 1995;55:4910.
79. Stone JG, Jones NJ, McGregor AD, et al. Development of a human biomonitoring assay using buccal mucosa: comparison of smoking-related DNA adducts in mucosa versus biopsies. *Cancer Res* 1995;55:1267.
80. Dunn BP, Vedal S, San RH, et al. DNA adducts in bronchial biopsies. *Int J Cancer* 1991; 48:485.
81. Kato S, Bowman ED, Harrington AM, et al. Human lung carcinogen–DNA adduct levels mediated by genetic polymorphisms in vivo. *J Natl Cancer Inst* 1995;87:902.
82. Bonassi S, Abbondandolo A, Camurri L, et al. Are chromosome aberrations in circulating lymphocytes predictive of future cancer onset in humans? Preliminary results of an Italian cohort study. *Cancer Genet Cytogenet* 1995;79:133.
83. Hagmar L, Brogger A, Hansteen IL, et al.Cancer risk in humans predicted by increased levels of chromosomal aberrations in lymphocytes: Nordic study group on the health risk of chromosome damage. *Cancer Res* 1994;54:2919.
84. Groopman JD, Kensler TW. The light at the end of the tunnel for chemical-specific biomarkers: daylight or headlight? *Carcinogenesis* 1999;20:1.
85. Schoket, B. DNA damage in humans exposed to environmental and dietary polycyclic aromatic hydrocarbons. *Mutat Res 424*: 143-153, 1999.
86. Bartsch H, Ohshima H, Pignatelli B, et al. Endogenously formed N-nitroso compounds and nitrosating agents in human cancer etiology. *Pharmacogenetics* 1992;2:272.
87. Hecht SS. Approaches to cancer prevention based on an understanding of N-nitrosamine carcinogenesis. *Proc Soc Exp Biol Med* 1997;216:181.
88. Lijinsky W. N-nitroso compounds in the diet. *Mutat Res* 1999;443:129.
89. Kamiyama S, Ohshima H, Shimada A, et al. Urinary excretion of N-nitrosamino acids and nitrate by inhabitants in high- and low-risk areas for stomach cancer in northern Japan. *IARC Sci Publ* 1987;84:497.
90. Lu SH, Ohshima H, Fu HM, et al. Urinary excretion of N-nitrosamino acids and nitrate by inhabitants of high- and low-risk areas for esophageal cancer in Northern China: endogenous formation of nitrosoproline and its inhibition by vitamin C. *Cancer Res* 1986;46:1485.
91. Wu Y, Chen J, Ohshima H, et al. Geographic association between urinary excretion of N-nitroso compounds and oesophageal cancer mortality in China. *Int J Cancer* 1993;54:713.
92. Shields PG, Povey AC, Wilson VL, et al. Combined high-performance liquid chromatography/^{32}P-postlabeling assay of N^7-methyldeoxyguanosine. *Cancer Res* 1990;50:6580.
93. Wilson VL, Weston A, Manchester DK, et al. Alkyl and aryl carcinogen adducts detected in human peripheral lung. *Carcinogenesis* 1989;10:2149.
94. Umbenhauer D, Wild CP, Montesano R, et al. O^6-methyldeoxyguanosine in oesophageal DNA among individuals at high risk of oesophageal cancer. *Int J Cancer* 1985;36:661.
95. Phillips DH. Polycyclic aromatic hydrocarbons in the diet. *Mutat Res* 1999;443:139.
96. Rothman N, Poirier MC, Baser ME, et al. Formation of polycyclic aromatic hydrocarbon-DNA adducts in peripheral white blood cells during consumption of charcoal-broiled beef. *Carcinogenesis* 1990;11:1241.
97. Bryant MS, Vineis P, Skipper PL, et al. Hemoglobin adducts of aromatic amines: associations with smoking status and type of tobacco. *Proc Natl Acad Sci U S A* 1988;85:9788-9791.
98. Keating GA, Layton DW, Felton JS. Factors determining dietary intakes of heterocyclic amines in cooked foods. *Mutat Res* 1999;443:149.
99. Turteltaub KW, Frantz CE, Creek MR, et al. DNA adducts in model systems and humans. *J Cell Biochem Suppl* 1993;17F:138.
100. Schut HA, Snyderwine EG. DNA adducts of heterocyclic amine food mutagens: implications for mutagenesis and carcinogenesis. *Carcinogenesis* 1999;20:353.
101. Zheng W, Gustafson DR, Sinha R, et al. Well-done meat intake and the risk of breast cancer. *J Natl Cancer Inst* 1998;90:1724.
102. Scholl P, Musser SM, Kensler TW, et al. Molecular biomarkers for aflatoxins and their application to human liver cancer. *Pharmacogenetics* 1995;5:S171.
103. Wild CP, Hasegawa R, Barraud L, et al. Aflatoxin-albumin adducts: a basis for comparative carcinogenesis between animals and humans. *Cancer Epidemiol Biomarkers Prev* 1996;5:179.
104. Wild CP, Jiang YZ, Allen SJ, et al. Aflatoxin-albumin adducts in human sera from different regions of the world. *Carcinogenesis* 1990;11:2271.
105. Gan LS, Skipper PL, Peng XC, et al. Serum albumin adducts in the molecular epidemiology of aflatoxin carcinogenesis: correlation with aflatoxin B1 intake and urinary excretion of aflatoxin M1. *Carcinogenesis* 1988;9:1323.
106. Fearon ER. Human cancer syndromes: clues to the origin and nature of cancer. *Science* 1997;278:1043.
107. Nakachi K, Imai K, Hayashi S, et al. Genetic susceptibility to squamous cell carcinoma of the lung in relation to cigarette smoking dose. *Cancer Res* 1991;51:5177.
108. Okada T, Kawashima K, Fukushi S, et al. Association between a cytochrome P-450 CYPIA1 genotype and incidence of lung cancer. *Pharmacogenetics* 1995;4:333.
109. Alexandrie A, Sundberg MI, Seidegard J, et al. Genetic susceptibility to lung cancer with special emphasis on CYP1A1 and GSTM1: a study on host factors in relation to age at onset, gender and histological cancer types. *Carcinogenesis* 1994;15:1785.
110. Hirvonen A, Husgafvel-Pursiainen K, Karjalainen A, et al. Point-mutational MspI and Ile-Val polymorphisms closely linked in the CYP1A1 gene: lack of association with susceptibility to lung cancer in a Finnish study population. *Cancer Epidemiol Biomarkers Prev* 1992;1:485.
111. Shields PG, Caporaso NE, Falk RT, et al. Lung cancer, race, and a CYP1A1 genetic polymorphism. *Cancer Epidemiol Biomarkers Prev* 1993;2:481.
112. Tefre T, Ryberg D, Haugen A, et al. Human CYP1A1 (cytochrome P(1)450) gene: lack of association between the Msp I restriction fragment length polymorphism and incidence of lung cancer in a Norwegian population. *Pharmacogenetics* 1991;1:20.
113. Brockmoller J, Cascorbi I, Kerb R, et al. Polymorphisms in xenobiotic conjugation and disease predisposition. *Toxicol Lett* 1998;102–103:173.
114. Kihara M, Noda K. Lung cancer risk of GSTM1 null genotype is dependent on the extent of tobacco smoke exposure. *Carcinogenesis* 1994;15:415.
115. Rebbeck TR. Molecular epidemiology of the human glutathione S-transferase genotypes GSTM1 and GSTT1 in cancer susceptibility. *Cancer Epidemiol Biomarkers Prev* 1997;6:733.
116. Nakachi K, Imai K, Hayashi S, et al. Polymorphisms of the CYP1A1 and glutathione S-transferase genes associated with susceptibility to lung cancer in relation to cigarette dose in a Japanese population. *Cancer Res* 1993;53:2994.
117. Goto I, Yoneda S, Yamamoto M, et al. Prognostic significance of germ line polymorphisms of the CYP1A1 and glutathione S-transferase genes in patients with non-small cell lung cancer. *Cancer Res* 1996;56:3725.
118. Norppa H, Hirvonen A, Jarventaus H, et al. Role of GSTT1 and GSTM1 genotypes in determining individual sensitivity to sister chromatid exchange induction by diepoxybutane in cultured human lymphocytes. *Carcinogenesis* 1995;16:1261.
119. Wiencke JK, Kelsey KT, Lamela RA, et al. Human glutathione S-transferase deficiency as a marker of susceptibility to epoxide-induced cytogenetic damage. *Cancer Res* 1990;50: 1585.
120. Bartsch H, Petruzzelli S, De Flora S, et al. Carcinogen metabolism and DNA adducts in human lung tissues as affected by tobacco smoking or metabolic phenotype: a case-control study on lung cancer patients. *Mutat Res* 1991;250:103.
121. Madigan MP, Ziegler RG, Benichou J, et al. Proportion of breast cancer cases in the United States explained by well-established risk factors. *J Natl Cancer Inst* 1996;87:1681.
122. Ambrosone CB, Shields PG. Molecular epidemiology of breast cancer. In: Aldaz CM, Gould MN, McLachlan J, et al., eds. *Etiology of breast and gynecological cancers.* New York: Wiley-Liss, 1997:83.
123. Feigelson HS, Coetzee GA, Kolonel LN, et al. A polymorphism in the CYP17 gene increases the risk of breast cancer. *Cancer Res* 1997;57:1063.
124. Lavigne JA, Helzlsouer KJ, Huang HY, et al. An association between the allele coding for a low activity variant of catechol-O-methyltransferase and the risk for breast cancer. *Cancer Res* 1997;57:5493.
125. Thompson PA, Shields PG, Freudenheim JL, et al. Genetic polymorphisms in catechol-O-methyltransferase (COMT), menopausal status and breast cancer risk. *Cancer Res* 1998;58:2107.
126. Evans DAP, Manley FA, McKusick VA. Genetic control of isoniazid metabolism in man. *Br Med J* 1960;2:485.
127. Ambrosone CB, Freudenheim JL, Graham S, et al. Cigarette smoking, N-acetyltransferase 2 genetic polymorphisms, and breast cancer risk. *JAMA* 1996;276:1494.
128. Hunter DJ, Hankinson SE, Hough H, et al. A prospective study of NAT2 acetylation genotype, cigarette smoking, and risk of breast cancer. *Carcinogenesis* 1997;18:2127.
129. Ambrosone CB, Freudenheim JL, Graham S, et al. Cytochrome P4501A1 and glutathione S-transferase (M1) genetic polymorphisms and postmenopausal breast cancer risk. *Cancer Res* 1995;55:3483.
130. Ishibe N, Hankinson SE, Colditz GA, et al. Cigarette smoking, cytochrome P450 1A1 polymorphisms, and breast cancer risk in the Nurses' Health Study. *Cancer Res* 1998;58:667.
131. Taioli E, Trachman J, Chen X, et al. A CYP1A1 restriction fragment length polymorphism is associated with breast cancer in African-American women. *Cancer Res* 1995;55:3757.
132. Helzlsouer KJ, Selmin O, Huang HY, et al. Association between glutathione S-transferase M1, P1, and T1 genetic polymorphisms and development of breast cancer. *J Natl Cancer Inst* 1998;90:512.
133. Ross RK, Jones PA, Yu MC. Bladder cancer epidemiology and pathogenesis. *Semin Oncol* 1996;23:536.
134. Lang NP, Butler MA, Massengill J, et al. Rapid metabolic phenotypes for acetyltransferase and cytochrome P4501A2 and putative exposure to food-borne heterocyclic amines increase the risk for colorectal cancer or polyps. *Cancer Epidemiol Biomarkers Prev* 1994;3:675.
135. Vineis P, McMichael A. Interplay between heterocyclic amines in cooked meat and metabolic phenotype in the etiology of colon cancer. *Cancer Causes Control* 1996;7:479.
136. Sinha R, Rothman N. Exposure assessment of heterocyclic amines (HCAs) in epidemiologic studies. *Mutat Res* 1997;376:195.
137. Liu Y, Hernandez AM, Shibata D, et al. BCL2 translocation frequency rises with age in humans. *Proc Natl Acad Sci U S A* 1994;91:8910.
138. Wei Q, Matanoski GM, Farmer ER, et al. DNA repair and aging in basal cell carcinoma: a molecular epidemiology study. *Proc Natl Acad Sci U S A* 1993;90:1614.
139. Simpson AJ. The natural somatic mutation frequency and human carcinogenesis. *Adv Cancer Res* 1997;71:209.
140. Cloos J, Spitz MR, Schantz SP, et al. Genetic susceptibility to head and neck squamous cell carcinoma. *J Natl Cancer Inst* 1996;88:530.

141. Cloos J, Braakhuis BJ, Steen I, et al. Increased mutagen sensitivity in head-and-neck squamous-cell carcinoma patients, particularly those with multiple primary tumors. *Int J Cancer* 1994;56:816.
142. Spitz MR, Hsu TC, Wu X, et al. Mutagen sensitivity as a biological marker of lung cancer risk in African Americans. *Cancer Epidemiol Biomarkers Prev* 1995;4:99.
143. Dogliotti E, Hainaut P, Hernandez T, et al. Mutation spectra resulting from carcinogenic exposure: from model systems to cancer-related genes. *Recent Results Cancer Res* 1998;154:97.
144. Skandalis A, Glickman BW. Endogenous gene systems for the study of mutational specificity in mammalian cells. *Cancer Cells* 1990;2:79.
145. Sarasin A. Shuttle vectors for studying mutagenesis in mammalian cells. *J Photochem Photobiol [B]* 1989;3:143.
146. Basu AK, Essigmann JM. Site-specifically alkylated oligodeoxynucleotides: probes for mutagenesis, DNA repair and the structural effects of DNA damage. *Mutat Res* 1990;233:189.
147. Levine AJ. *P53*, the cellular gatekeeper for growth and division. *Cell* 1997;88:323.
148. Brash DE, Rudolph JA, Simon JA, et al. A role for sunlight in skin cancer: UV-induced *P53* mutations in squamous cell carcinoma. *Proc Natl Acad Sci U S A* 1991;88:10124.
149. Bressac B, Kew M, Wands J, et al. Selective G to T mutations of *p53* gene in hepatocellular carcinoma from southern Africa. *Nature* 1991;350:429.
150. Hsu IC, Metcalf RA, Sun T, et al. Mutational hotspot in the *p53* gene in human hepatocellular carcinomas. *Nature* 1991;350:427.
151. Brennan JA, Boyle JO, Koch WM, et al. Association between cigarette smoking and mutation of the *p53* gene in squamous-cell carcinoma of the head and neck. *N Engl J Med* 1995;332:712.
152. Hartmann A, Baszyk H, Kovach JS, et al. The molecular epidemiology of *p53* gene mutations in human breast cancer. *Trends Genet* 1997;13:27.
153. Kawajiri K, Eguchi H, Nakachi K, et al. Association of CYP1A1 germ line polymorphisms with mutations of the *p53* gene in lung cancer. *Cancer Res* 1996;56:72.
154. Sidransky D, Tokino T, Hamilton SR, et al. Identification of ras oncogene mutations in the stool of patients with curable colorectal tumors. *Science* 1992;256:102.
155. Boyle JO, Mao L, Brennan JA, et al. Gene mutations in saliva as molecular markers for head and neck squamous cell carcinomas. *Am J Surg* 1994;168:429.
156. Mills NE, Fishman CL, Scholes J, et al. Detection of K-ras oncogene mutations in bronchoalveolar lavage fluid for lung cancer diagnosis. *J Natl Cancer Inst* 1995;87:1056.
157. Mao L, Hruban RH, Boyle JO, et al. Detection of oncogene mutations in sputum precedes diagnosis of lung cancer. *Cancer Res* 1994;54:1634.
158. Hecht SS, Hoffmann D. Tobacco-specific nitrosamines, an important group of carcinogens in tobacco and tobacco smoke. *Carcinogenesis* 1988;9:875.
159. Hecht SS, Haley NJ, Hoffman D. Monitoring exposure to tobacco products by measurement of nicotine metabolites and derived carcinogens. In: Groopman JD, ed. *Molecular dosimetry and human cancer.* Boca Raton, FL: CRC Press, 1991:325.
160. Hoffmann D, Hoffmann I. The changing cigarette, 1950–1995. *J Toxicol Environ Health* 1997;50:307.
161. Nakayama J, Yuspa SH, Poirier MC. Benzo(a)pyrene-DNA adduct formation and removal in mouse epidermis in vivo and in vitro: relationship of DNA binding to initiation of skin carcinogenesis. *Cancer Res* 1984;44:4087.
162. Peluso M, Airoldi L, Armelle M, et al. White blood cell DNA adducts, smoking, and NAT2 and GSTM1 genotypes in bladder cancer: a case-control study. *Cancer Epidemiol Biomarkers Prev* 1998;7:341.
163. Tang D, Santella RM, Blackwood AM, et al. A molecular epidemiological case-control study of lung cancer. *Cancer Epidemiol Biomarkers Prev* 1995;4:341.
164. Cuzick J, Routledge MN, Jenkins D, et al. DNA adducts in different tissues of smokers and non-smokers. *Int J Cancer* 1990;45:673.
165. Schoket B, Phillips DH, Kostic S, et al. Smoking-associated bulky DNA adducts in bronchial tissue related to CYP1A1 MspI and GSTM1 genotypes in lung patients. *Carcinogenesis* 1998;19:841.
166. Vineis P, Bartsch H, Caporaso N, et al. Genetically based N-acetyltransferase metabolic polymorphism and low-level environmental exposure to carcinogens. *Nature* 1994;369:154.
167. Degawa M, Stern SJ, Martin MV, et al. Metabolic activation and carcinogen-DNA adduct detection in human larynx. *Cancer Res* 1994;54:4915.
168. Flamini G, Romano G, Curigliano G, et al. 4-Aminobiphenyl-DNA adducts in laryngeal tissue and smoking habits: an immunohistochemical study. *Carcinogenesis* 1998;19:353.
169. Romano G, Sgambato A, Boninsegna A, et al. Evaluation of polycyclic aromatic hydrocarbon-DNA adducts in exfoliated oral cells by an immunohistochemical assay. *Cancer Epidemiol Biomarkers Prev* 1999;8:91.
170. Grinberg-Funes RA, Singh VN, Perera FP, et al. Polycyclic aromatic hydrocarbon-DNA adducts in smokers and their relationship to micronutrient levels and the glutathione-S-transferase M1 genotype. *Carcinogenesis* 1994;15:2449.
171. van Schooten FJ, Hillebrand MJ, van Leeuwen FE, et al. Polycyclic aromatic hydrocarbon-DNA adducts in lung tissue from lung cancer patients. *Carcinogenesis* 1990;11:1677.
172. Bennett WP, Hussain SP, Vahakangas KH, et al. Molecular epidemiology of human cancer risk: gene-environment interactions and p53 mutation spectrum in human lung cancer. *J Pathol* 1999;187:8.
173. Hofer I, Nil R, Wyss F, et al. The contributions of cigarette yield, consumption, inhalation and puffing behaviour to the prediction of smoke exposure. *Clin Invest* 1992;70:343.
174. Harris CC. Interindividual variation among humans in carcinogen metabolism, DNA adduct formation and DNA repair. *Carcinogenesis* 1989;10:1563.
175. Yuspa SH. The pathogenesis of squamous cell cancer: lessons learned from studies of skin carcinogenesis—Thirty-third G.H.A. Clowes Memorial Award Lecture. *Cancer Res* 1994;54:1178.
176. DiGiovanni J. Multistage carcinogenesis in mouse skin. *Pharmacol Ther* 1992;54:63.
177. Dooley TP. Recent advances in cutaneous melanoma oncogenesis research. *Oncol Res* 1999;6:1.
178. Montesano R, Kirby GM. Chemical carcinogens in human liver cancer. In: Brechot C, ed. *Primary liver cancer: etiological and progression factors.* Boca Raton, FL: CRC Press, 1995:57.
179. Dragan YP, Pitot HC. The role of the stages of initiation and promotion in phenotypic diversity during hepatocarcinogenesis in the rat. *Carcinogenesis* 1992;13:739.
180. Witschi H. Modulation of lung tumor development in rats, hamsters and mice. In: Homburger F, ed. *Progress in experimental tumor research.* Basel: Karger, 1991:132.
181. McKenzie K, Sukumar S. Molecular mechanisms of chemical carcinogenesis in rodent models. *Cancer Treat Res* 1994;71:313.
182. Russo J, Gusterson BA, Rogers AE, et al. Comparative study of human and rat mammary tumorigenesis. *Lab Invest* 1990;62:244.
183. Galloway DJ. Animal models in the study of colorectal cancer. *Cancer Surv* 1989;8:169.
184. Pories SE, Ramchurren N, Summerhayes I, et al. Animal models for colon carcinogenesis. *Arch Surg* 1993;128:647.
185. Reddy J, Rao MS. Progress in pancreatic cancer: implications of phenotypic and molecular plasticity. *Lab Invest* 1995;72:383.
186. Chang KW, Laconi S, Mangold KA, et al. Multiple genetic alterations in hamster pancreatic ductal adenocarcinomas. *Cancer Res* 1995;55:2560.
187. Cohen SM, Johansson SL. Epidemiology and etiology of bladder cancer. *Urol Clin North Am* 1992;19:421.
188. Yamamoto S, Konishi Y, Matsuda T, et al. Cancer induction by an organic arsenic compound, dimethylarsinic acid (cacodylic acid), in F344/DuCrj rats after pretreatment with five carcinogens. *Cancer Res* 1995;55:1271.
189. Bosland MC. Animal models for the study of prostate carcinogenesis. *J Cell Biochem Suppl* 1992;16H:89.
190. Masui T, Shirai T, Imaida K, et al. Ki-ras mutations with frequent normal allele loss versus absence of *p53* mutations in rat prostate and seminal vesicle carcinomas induced with 3,2'-dimethyl-4-aminobiphenyl. *Mol Carcinog* 1995;13:21.
191. Koestner A. Characterization of N-nitrosourea-induced tumors of the nervous system: their prospective value for studies of neurocarcinogenesis and brain tumor therapy. *Toxicol Pathol* 1990;18:186.
192. *American Conference of Government Industrial Hygienists' threshold limit values for chemical substances and physical agents and biological exposure indices.* Cincinnati: American Conference of Government Industrial Hygienists, 1993.
193. *IARC monographs on the evaluation of carcinogenic risks to humans. Overall evaluations of carcinogenicity: an updating of IARC monographs,* vols 1–42. Lyon: International Agency for Research on Cancer, 1987.
194. National Toxicology Program fifth annual report on carcinogens. Rockville, MD: US Department of Health and Human Services, 1989.
195. US Department of Health and Human Services, Public Health Service, Centers for Disease Control. *NIOSH pocket guide to chemical hazards.* Cincinnati: National Institute for Occupational Safety and Health, 1990.
196. World Health Organization, International Agency for Research on Cancer. *IARC monographs on the evaluation of carcinogenic risks to humans.* Lyon: International Agency for Research on Cancer, 1995.
197. Theriault G, Infante-Rivard C, Armstrong B, et al. Occupational neoplasia. In: Zenz C, Dickerson OB, Horvath EP Jr, eds. *Occupational medicine,* 3rd ed. Baltimore: Mosby, 1994:813.

Robert L. Ullrich

CHAPTER 12

Etiology of Cancer: Physical Factors

This chapter discusses the induction of cancer by three physical agents that are known to cause cancer in humans: radiation, UV light, and asbestos. Exposures to ionizing radiation can come from both natural and man-made sources. We are continually exposed to naturally occurring radioisotopes contained in soil and rocks, and, as a result, in building materials and even in our own bodies. In addition, we are exposed to cosmic rays from the sun and radon. The levels of this naturally occurring environmental radiation, often referred to as *background radiation*, varies with altitude, geology, and types of building materials used to construct homes and other buildings. One of the most important man-made sources of exposure is from imaging and therapy procedures in medicine. It is also one of the largest sources of exposure. On average, the dose to the general population from medical exposures is similar to that received from background radiation.

UV light from the sun is responsible for an increasing number of skin cancers throughout the world. Risks for skin cancer vary with altitude, latitude, and pigmentation, all of which modify exposure to UV light. UV light and certain types of ionizing radiation, such as x-rays and gamma rays, are all part of the electromagnetic spectrum, which also includes static magnetic fields, fields generated by 50 or 60 cycle alternating current, radiowaves, microwaves, infrared light, and visible light. UV light and electromagnetic forms of ionizing radiation have the highest frequencies and energies.

Asbestos is a third physical agent that is a well-known human carcinogen. Asbestos is a naturally occurring mineral silicone that results from fibrous crystallization. Health effects, including lung cancer, arise from its commercial uses that lead to high occupational exposures. Health effects from low-level exposures, such as those to the general population, are more controversial. The concern over the effects from occupational exposures and potential health risks in the general population has markedly reduced the mining and use of asbestos worldwide.

Because their carcinogenic potential is well known, questions about these physical agents focus on the degree of risk to humans as a function of level of exposure and on mechanisms of cancer development. These mechanistic studies can provide insight into potential risks at very low levels of exposure, for which effects cannot be directly measured by epidemiologic studies. These studies also provide information about potential sensitive subpopulations, suggest ways to reduce risks, and provide insight into fundamental mechanisms of cancer development.

INTERACTIONS OF RADIATION WITH CELLS AND TISSUES

Gamma rays, x-rays, and UV light are all part of the electromagnetic spectrum, which is shown in Figure 12-1.[1] Their interactions with biologic material depend on the frequency or wavelength of the radiation. At the short wavelengths of x-rays, electromagnetic radiation has sufficient energy to produce ionizations as a result of the removal of electrons from atoms. At the longer wavelengths of the other forms of electromagnetic radiation, from UV light to low-level electric and magnetic fields, the energy deposition is insufficient to produce ionizations, and these forms are often generally referred to as *nonionizing radiations*.

IONIZING RADIATION

In addition to the electromagnetic forms of ionizing radiation (such as x-rays and gamma rays), electrons, protons, alpha particles, and neutrons are particulate forms of ionizing radiation. The spatial distribution of the ionizations produced by these different forms of ionizing radiation provide a means of classification based on their interactions in matter, including their

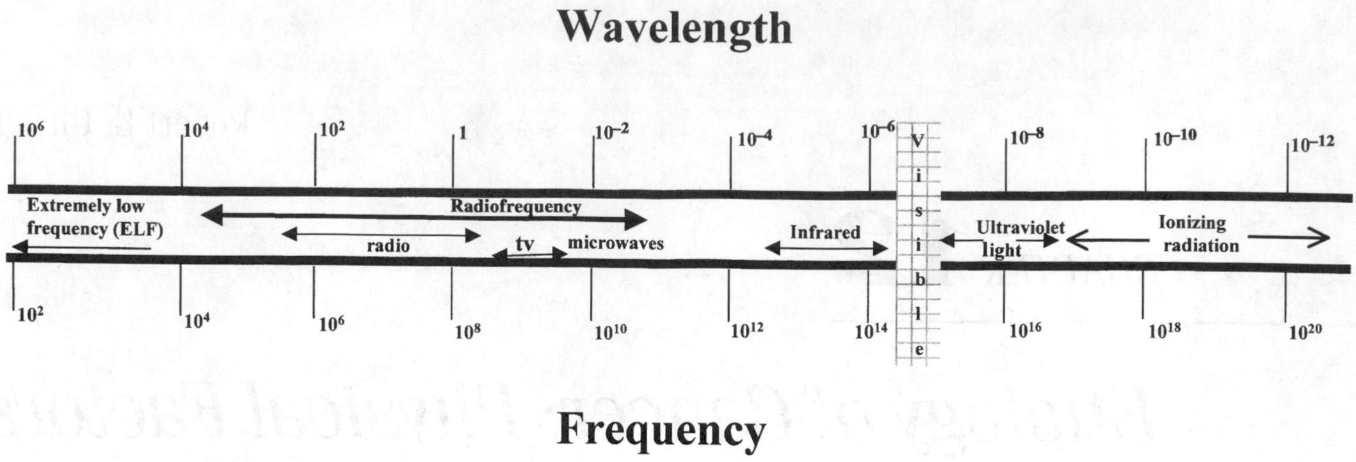

FIGURE 12-1. Electromagnetic spectrum.

interaction with biologic material. This spatial distribution of ionization is measured as the energy transferred per unit track length [linear energy transfer (LET)] in units of keV/mm.[2] On this basis, x-rays, gamma rays, and electrons are classified as *sparsely ionizing*, whereas alpha particles (such as those associated with radon) and neutrons are *densely ionizing*. The density of the ionization tracks can have a substantial impact on the biologic effects of the radiation. These influences can be qualitative as well as quantitative. The quantitative differences in the effectiveness of different ionizing radiations are measured by comparing the dose of the test radiation (e.g., neutrons) to produce a specific level of effect against the dose of x-rays (or sometimes gamma rays) to produce that same level of effect. That ratio is the relative biologic effectiveness (RBE). For cell killing effects, RBEs for neutrons and alpha particles are often approximately 3 to 5; for cancer induction in animals, the RBE values can be 20 or higher (RBEs of 50 or more have been reported).[3] The RBE increases with increasing LET to a maximum at approximately 100 keV/mm. At this LET, the average separation of ionizing events is approximately the diameter of the double helix. This results in a high probability that a single track of radiation of this LET can produce a double-strand break. Qualitative differences between high and low LET radiation are suggested by the fact that, for all effects observed, including cell killing, chromosome aberrations, mutations, and cancer induction, the radiation damage that induces these effects appears to be less easily repaired by the cell or organism after exposure to high LET radiation.[2]

Energy deposited in biologic material can produce ionizations in target molecules, such as DNA, directly or indirectly by interactions with water molecules that result in the formation of free radicals. These free radicals can then produce damage to DNA. Because ionizing events from low LET radiation exposures are sparsely distributed, damage to DNA and other targets from such radiation is principally a result of indirect mechanisms mediated by free radicals. High LET effects are more generally mediated via direct effects on the target molecules.[2]

Whether the effects are directly or indirectly produced, ionizing radiation results predominantly in base damage, and single- and double-strand breaks in DNA. As already mentioned, for low LET radiations, these effects are mediated via reactive oxygen species much like those produced by normal cellular processes. The reason that ionizing radiations are able to cause the degree of damage that they do is because of the different spatial distribution of energy that results in a markedly different distribution of these reactive oxygen species than occurs during normal cellular processes. Ionizations from the deposition of ionizing radiation are highly clustered, which results in localized areas of sites in DNA molecules with multiple and complex lesions consisting of a combination of base damage and single- and double-strand breaks.[2,4] These more complex lesions are less easily repaired with fidelity than are the more simple forms of DNA damage.[4,5] For high LET radiations, because of the density of the ionization clusters, the molecular damage can be particularly complex and difficult to repair.

ULTRAVIOLET LIGHT

UV radiation does not have sufficient energy to produce ionizations. Rather, its effects are the result of molecular excitation after absorption of energy by the molecule. UV light can be categorized into three types, based on wavelength: UVC with wavelengths ranging from 240 to 290 nm, UVB ranging from 290 to 320 nm, and UVA ranging from 320 to 400 nm. UVC is not in sunlight that reaches earth because it is readily absorbed by the atmosphere. It has proven to be useful, however, for other reasons. It is produced by low-pressure mercury lamps commonly used for sterilization. In addition, because the peak wavelength of these lamps (254 nm) is very close to the peak for absorption in DNA molecules (260 nm), it has been an important experimental tool for studies of UV light effects on DNA. UVB appears to be primarily responsible for skin cancer induction after sunlight exposure via direct damage to DNA. The amount to which the population is exposed depends on many factors, including the ozone layer. Effects of UVB and UVC appear to be mediated via effects on DNA. Interactions of UVB and UVC with DNA result in a number of molecular changes, the most prevalent of which are dimers between adjacent pyrimidines.[6] The most biologically important of these are the cyclobutane dimer and the 6-4 photoproduct. Other products are less frequent, but these two, especially the cyclobutane dimers, appear to play a major role in the mutagenic and carcinogenic effects of UVB. UVA is not absorbed by the atmosphere and penetrates deeper into the skin than UVB. Because of its wavelength, DNA and proteins only weakly absorb UVA, but it has been shown to be carcinogenic. This carcinogenic effect appears to be due to the production of reactive oxygen species and free radicals through its interactions with target chromophores. As a result, such products induce indirect damage to DNA.[7]

For UVC and UVB, the distribution of specific changes in the genome depends on base sequence and secondary and tertiary genomic structure. For example, cytosine absorbs higher wavelengths of UV radiation than thymine, resulting in dimers containing cytosine being more readily formed after UVB radiation. Data have shown that methylation at specific sequences in the p53 molecule enhance formation of dimers in specific regions, resulting in mutations that are relatively specific for UV damage.[8] These specific mutations have been found quite early in skin tumors.[9,10]

IONIZING RADIATION AND CANCER

HISTORY AND SOURCES OF INFORMATION

The benefits of ionizing radiation in the diagnosis and treatment of disease were recognized by the medical community very soon after the discovery of x-rays and radioactivity.[11] Almost as quickly, the risks of exposure began to be recognized as well. The first cancers, detected a few years after the discovery of x-rays, were skin cancers that developed after high skin doses received by early workers who often used their hands to test the output of x-ray tubes. These cases were followed by cases of radiation-induced leukemias among radiologists and radioisotope workers. These early studies established that radiation could cause cancer in humans, but the extent of the risk as a function of dose was not known. This began to change in the 1950s and 1960s with the study of the Japanese survivors of the atomic bombs, the study of patient populations exposed to radiation for therapeutic and diagnostic procedures, and occupationally exposed populations, such as radiologists, uranium miners, and nuclear industry workers. A partial list of the principal sources of information is shown in Table 12-1. These studies, which began in the 1950s and continue today, have provided and continue to provide extensive quantitative information about radiation dose and cancer risk. In addition, such studies provide information on tissue and organ sensitivity and risk-modifying factors, such as age and genetic background.

The largest population studied and the one that has served as the primary source for risk estimates are the populations in Hiroshima and Nagasaki, Japan, who survived the atomic bombings of these two cities.[12–15] The doses received were single acute exposures of a mixture of gamma rays and neutrons to the entire body. The doses ranged from lethal to very small, depending on the location of the individuals at the time. The average dose received by the survivors was less than 0.3 Sv. The study of this group, which began a few years after the exposures, has provided extensive information on risk as a function of dose and provided insight into variations in tissue and organ sensitivity. Because the age distribution of the population was wide, including the old and the very young (as well as children exposed *in utero*), this study is also an important source of information about the effects of age on risk and on the time between radiation exposure and the appearance of leukemias and solid cancers (latent period). This study is still ongoing, and a large fraction of the population exposed as children, adolescents, and young adults are still living. Because of this fact, we are continuing to learn about the risks from radiation exposure, and this population will continue to provide new information for many years to come.

TABLE 12-1. Studies of Radiation-Exposed Populations

Atomic bomb
Japanese survivors
Occupational exposures
Radiologists
Underground miners
Radium dial painters
Nuclear workers
Radiation technologists
Medical exposures
Ankylosing spondylitis patients
Tinea capitis
Thymic enlargement
Benign breast disease
Benign gynecologic disease
Fluoroscopy during treatment for tuberculosis
Cervical cancer
Hodgkin's disease
Breast cancer
Childhood cancer

Another major source of information is patient populations exposed to ionizing radiation as a result of therapeutic or diagnostic procedures. The numbers of patients in each individual study are smaller than in the atomic bomb survivors, but the number of such studies is relatively large.[16] In spite of the large numbers of studies, only a few have been useful for the quantification of risk as a function of dose. Because such populations generally receive localized exposures, these groups generally provide information on cancer risks in specific organs and tissues. Such populations also have provided insight into modifying factors, such as age and genetic background. Studies of second cancers after radiation therapy has become an increasingly important source of information.[17] This group is discussed in more detail later in the section Second Cancers. In the past, radiation was used to treat a number of benign disorders, including enlarged thymus glands and tonsils, tinea capitis, ankylosing spondylitis, and peptic ulcers.[16] Epidemiologic studies of such treated populations have provided information on radiation-induced leukemia, as well as thyroid, breast, and stomach cancers. In general, diagnostic procedures result in very low radiation exposures; however, a few studies have provided evidence for increased cancer risks. One of the most intensively studied of these is a group of tuberculosis patients who were subjected to multiple diagnostic fluoroscopies during their treatment.[18,19] In these studies, female patients have been shown to be at an increased risk for breast cancer. Although individual doses were low, the number of exposures resulted in the accumulation of relatively large doses.

As is the case for other carcinogenic agents, occupational exposures also have been a valuable source of information. Studies of uranium miners and other underground miners have been a particularly valuable source of information on risks of lung cancer after exposure to radon.[20]

RADIATION AND CANCER RISKS

Tissue Sensitivity and Latent Period

Although radiation can induce many different types of cancer, certain organs, tissues, and cell types are more sensitive than others. Chronic myelocytic leukemia and acute leukemia are very sensitive to induction, whereas no evidence indicates that chronic lymphocytic leukemia, Hodgkin's disease, or non-Hodgkin's lymphoma can be induced by radiation exposure.[14] Among solid cancers, cancers of the thyroid gland, female breast, and lung appear to be the most sensitive.[13] Evidence also suggests increased risk for salivary gland tumors; colon cancer; stomach cancer; and cancers of the liver, ovary, bladder, esophagus, skin, and central nervous system; however, these sites are not as sensitive. Most skin cancers are basal cell and squamous cell carcinomas, whereas there is little evidence for the induction of melanomas. In general, bone sarcoma and cancer of connective tissues require relatively high doses before a significant increased risk can be detected. No clear evidence exists for the induction of cancers of the pancreas, prostate, uterine cervix, small intestine, or most childhood cancers (except for acute leukemia).

Radiation-induced leukemias are the first to appear after radiation exposure.[21,22] Depending on dose, these leukemias can begin to appear as early as 2 years after exposure, with peak incidence occurring between 4 and 8 years after irradiation. After this peak, the incidence begins to drop toward baseline levels. In general, solid cancers do not appear until 10 or more years after the radiation exposure, and it is not unusual for the latent period to exceed 20 years.[16] The time between irradiation can depend on the age at exposure, the dose, and a variety of host factors. For example, the appearance of breast cancer is greatly influenced by age at the time of irradiation. The time between radiation exposure and the appearance of breast cancer is quite long for a prepubertal or adolescent girl, whereas for a woman in her late twenties or early thirties, the latent period is generally shorter. A close look at the relationship between age at exposure and time of appearance for breast cancer indicates that these radiation-induced cancers appear at a time when the natural incidence of these cancers is also rising. This is likely a result of host factors that play an important role in breast cancer development and that also appear to strongly influence the expression of radiation-initiated cells. These data have important implications for potential mechanisms of radiation carcinogenesis. These very long latent periods, particularly for younger individuals, are also important to remember when assessing risks associated with specific treatment protocols.

Dose-Response Relationships

Understanding the relationship between cancer frequency, or risk, and radiation dose is important for providing insight into mechanisms underlying radiation carcinogenesis. It is also important for estimating risks at low doses for which effects cannot be directly determined from experimental or epidemiologic studies. Accurate risk estimates at low doses are essential in regulating environmental and occupational exposures.[21] It is also essential in decisions about medical uses of radiation when weighing the benefits of the procedure versus its risks.[2] One of the most prominent examples of this issue has been the debate over mammography, both with respect to its general use to screen women for breast cancer and with respect to the age at which such screening should be initiated and practiced routinely. The question of whether the benefits of this screening outweigh the risks for inducing new breast cancers depends on many complex issues, but central to these issues is the risk of breast cancer from the doses received. It is virtually impossible

TABLE 12-2. Approximate Doses from Common Diagnostic Procedures

Procedure	*Dose (mGy)*
Chest x-ray (single PA film) (air kerma[a])	0.16
Dental bitewing (air kerma)	1.0
Mammography (mean glandular dose)	1.6

PA, posterior to anterior beam projection
[a] Air kerma is dose in air in units of joules/kg of air.

low doses received as a result of a single mammographic procedure (or for that matter any diagnostic procedure) (Table 12-2), so estimates must be based on models of dose-response relationships that allow estimates to be derived. Mainly because of these low-dose risk issues, a substantial amount of effort in epidemiologic studies and in experimental studies of radiation carcinogenesis has been to define dose-response relationships and test predictions of dose-response models.

From theoretical models of radiation interactions at the cellular and molecular level, and from experimental and epidemiologic studies, two dose-response models are most prominent: the linear model and the linear-quadratic model.[21,23] As suggested by its name, with the linear model cancer risk (or I, incidence) is linearly related to dose ($I = \alpha D$). With the linear-quadratic model, risk at low doses is linearly related to dose, whereas at higher doses, the risk increases more rapidly as a function of dose. In this region, risk increases as a function of the square of the dose. As a result, the dose response takes the form $I = \alpha D + \beta D^2$. The linear-quadratic model is based on biophysical theories of radiation interactions. The βD^2 component represents effects produced by the interaction of multiple ionization tracks, whereas the αD component represents effects produced by single ionization tracks. For sparsely ionizing low LET radiation at low doses, the probability is that only a few ionization tracks will traverse a cell (at very low doses perhaps only one such ionization track might traverse a cell). Therefore, any effects observed, such as a double-strand break or a chromosome aberration, must have been a result of effects produced by such single tracks. At higher doses, in which multiple tracks would be traversing a cell, such effects would be expected to be a result of interactions of damage produced by these multiple tracks. Because the probability of inducing a complex type of damage, such as a double-strand break, is greater with multiple events occurring in close proximity, the dose response would be expected to rise more rapidly than at low doses. For densely ionizing radiation, ionization tracks through a cell are few, but the density of the ionization is sufficient to produce complex effects with single tracks with a high probability. As a result, the dose response is expected to be linear over a wide range of doses.

Irrespective of the model, the prediction at low doses is that the dose response is linear. This prediction implies that any dose of radiation received has a probability of inducing damage and, therefore, results in some increased risk for cancer development. Although there is some argument about this assumption at very low doses because of the repair and damage response capabilities of cells, current information about underlying mechanisms of cancer induction by ionizing radiation would tend to support the view that any dose of radiation confers some degree of risk.

At high dose, the linear quadratic and linear models differ not only in form but also in predictions about risks at low dose rates and fractionated exposures.[24] Such predictions impact lifetime risks for those exposed occupationally at low dose rates over many years and also impact estimates of risks from multiple medical procedures, such as mammography, computed tomographic scans, fluoroscopies, or even dental x-rays over a lifetime. The linear model in its most simple form predicts that lowering the dose rate or giving many small fractions confers the same cancer risk as the same dose delivered as a single, high dose-rate exposure. The linear-quadratic model predicts that, at high total doses, reducing the rate at which the total dose is received or giving the dose in multiple small fractions reduces the risk. This makes sense when considering acute effects of radiation. A dose of 4 Gy delivered instantaneously would have the chance of being lethal in a short time, whereas that same dose accumulated over a lifetime would not produce such acutely lethal effects. But whether this same concept holds for the damage that results in increased cancer risk is not certain. Theoretically, because effects are likely to be a result of the interaction of damages produced by independent tracks, lowering the dose rate or fractionating the exposure reduces the probability of the interaction of damage because of cellular repair processes that rapidly respond to such damage. If this theory applies to the damage responsible for radiation-induced cancers, the cancer risk at low dose rates and after low dose fractions would be lower than that predicted from high dose, high dose-rate exposures. At very low dose rates and very low doses per fraction, this results in a predicted dose response that simply is a continuation of the slope of the dose-response curve at low doses [i.e., the dose response would be linear ($I = \alpha D$)].[23] Because most epidemiologic studies involve populations irradiated at high dose rates, the applicability of this model potentially impacts the accuracy of estimates of risk for low dose, low dose-rate, and fractionated exposures derived from such studies. Whether this model is appropriate and the degree of the so-called dose-rate effect is a matter of debate and study. Epidemiologic and experimental data are not adequate to resolve the issue at the present time.

Analyses of results from epidemiologic studies of the atomic bomb survivors suggest a linear quadratic dose response for the induction of all leukemia, although a simple linear model also fits the data.[21,25] For all solid cancers combined, a linear dose response is suggested based on the data at hand.[21,25] Except for a few tumor types, such as breast cancer, data for individual cancers are insufficient to address the issue of dose response. It must be remembered that the solid tumor data are incomplete at present because of the late onset of these cancers and because a significant fraction of the population who were children and young adults at the time of the bombing are still alive. Studies of radiation-induced breast cancer in the atomic bomb survivors support a linear dose response over a wide range of doses.[13,21] This linear response is supported by studies of other populations as well.[18,21,26]

For breast cancer, limited data on fractionation effects are available from studies of tuberculosis patients who received multiple diagnostic fluoroscopies during their course of treatment. Although the doses from the individual fluoroscopies were small, relatively large total doses were accumulated. Analysis of these data suggest similar risks for radiation-induced breast cancer in this group compared with those derived from the atomic bomb survivors and other groups who received radiation at a high dose rate.[18,19,21,23,26] The lack of an apparent fractionation effect is in contrast to results of analyses of the same tuberculosis patients for lung cancer. Comparing the risk for lung cancer in the groups receiving fractionated exposures from fluoroscopy to the risk in the atomic bomb survivors indicates that fractionation resulted in a markedly decreased risk for radiation-induced lung cancer.[27] Information on dose-response relationships for high LET radiation–induced cancer in human populations is relatively limited but suggest linear dose-response relationships.[20] Some of the most extensive dose-response data are for lung cancer in underground miners exposed to radon (see Radon, later in this chapter).

Experimental studies examining dose-response relationships for leukemia and a variety of solid cancers generally support the linear-quadratic model.[23,24,28–30] In addition, most of these studies have found that reducing the dose rate or fractionating the dose into small fractions reduces the risk for development of radiation-induced cancer in the manner predicted by the linear-quadratic model. The degree of the dose-rate effect appears to vary with tumor type. Interestingly, in mice the dose-rate effect for the induction of lung cancer is greater than that for breast cancer.[24] Dose-response relationships for cancer induction after exposure to high LET radiation are limited mainly to studies of neutrons and only a few tumor types, but the data available clearly demonstrate linear dose-response relationships.[3,31,32] Fractionating the exposure or delivering the exposure at low dose rates has little effect on the dose response in most instances. However, data for mammary tumors in mice, and for transformation *in vitro*, have shown a so-called inverse dose-rate effect in which doses delivered at low dose rates were seen to be more effective with respect to cancer induction than single acute exposures.[32–34]

MODIFIERS OF RISK

Age

Age has a significant impact on susceptibility to radiation-induced cancer. Increased risks for thyroid cancer are primarily found after exposure of children to radiation, whereas the risk in adults after exposure to radiation is small.[13] For breast cancer, young children and adolescents are at the highest risk.[13,17,21,35–38] Risks, although still increased, are lower for young adults in their twenties and thirties compared with younger individuals. For women older than 45 to 50 years of age, radiation appears to have little influence on breast cancer risk.[17,39,40] Although not as dramatic, risks for acute leukemia, colon cancer, cancer of the central nervous system, and skin cancer are all greater if the exposure occurs early in life.[13,17,22]

Reports in the mid-1950s suggested for the first time an increased risk of childhood leukemia and all childhood solid cancers as a result of *in utero* radiation exposure from diagnostic procedures.[41,42] Initial concerns of a selection bias that might have resulted in more *in utero* exposures because of an underlying medical problem that was the actual risk factor were essentially dispelled by confirmation of these results in a study of twins in which such a selection bias could be minimized.[43,44] Similar studies of effects from *in utero* exposure in atomic bomb survivors have not observed such an increased risk. However, it is generally accepted that an increased risk exists for childhood cancers, including leukemia, from *in utero* exposure, which should be avoided.[45] Studies to date on risks of adult cancers after *in utero* exposure are inconclusive.[46]

Genetic Susceptibility

It has been recognized for many years that there are individuals within the population who have a higher risk for spontaneous cancer. Studies of these individuals and their families have led to the discovery of several genes involved in heritable susceptibility to specific cancer. A number of these genes have now been cloned. In individuals with such susceptibility, the probability of developing a tumor during their lifetime can exceed 50%, and in some instances the probability is higher.[47–49] However, such mutations are relatively rare in the population. The prevalence of currently known, high penetrance genes account for approximately 5% of the total cancers in the population, and the prevalence of such genes in the total population is less than 1%. Because of this incidence, it is difficult to obtain adequate data to assess the impact of such genes on susceptibility to radiation-induced cancer.

Most information has come from studies of second cancers after radiation therapy. Studies to date have demonstrated increased risks for radiation-induced osteosarcoma and soft tissue sarcoma in patients with the hereditary form of retinoblastoma.[50] Studies of patients with basal cell nevus carcinoma syndrome have been found to be at an increased risk for basal cell carcinoma and ovarian tumors in the irradiated field.[51] In addition, patients with Li-Fraumeni syndrome appear to be at an increased risk for radiation-induced cancer.[52,53] In each instance, these patients have defects in genes that are known to act as tumor suppressor genes, the retinoblastoma gene (RB), the human homologue of the patched gene PTCH, and the p53 gene, respectively. It has also been proposed that the gene involved in ataxia-telangiectasia (AT) may also influence susceptibility to radiation-induced cancer.[54] AT is a recessive inherited syndrome that results in hypersensitivity to acute radiation effects, such as cell killing, because of mutations in the ATM gene, which is involved in DNA damage signaling and response pathways.[55,56] Patients homozygous for mutated ATM are extremely sensitive to acute radiation effects and are at a high risk for the development of certain forms of cancer. It has been suggested that individuals heterozygous for mutated ATM are also at an increased risk for radiation-induced cancer, in particular breast cancer.[54] The sensitivity of these individuals to acute effects of radiation is generally within the normal range. This hypothesis has been difficult to definitively test, and the question of enhanced susceptibility remains unresolved. Also unknown at the present time is the impact of the breast cancer genes BRCA1 and BRCA2 on susceptibility to radiation-induced cancer.

A major area of uncertainty and increasing interest is the potential impact of low-penetrance mutations that are likely to be relatively common in the population.[48] Such genes are difficult to identify in epidemiologic studies. Experimental studies in animal models and in human cells have provided evidence for such mutations and provided data implicating such mutations in susceptibility to radiation-induced cancer. It is also likely that such low-penetrance mutations could be involved in other delayed effects, such as radiation-induced fibrosis. The identification of such susceptible subpopulations is now a major research activity in radiation oncology.

SECOND CANCERS

As the treatment of cancer has improved, long-term survivors have begun to develop second cancers as a result of treatment. Studies of such populations can provide information on the nature of potential risks and suggest new approaches to treatment that may reduce risks. Several studies have now been reported on risks of second cancers from radiation therapy. The most extensive data are available from studies of second cancers arising after treatment for childhood cancer, cervical cancer, Hodgkin's disease, and breast cancer. Data also are becoming available regarding risks of second cancers after whole body irradiation for bone marrow transplantations.

Relatively little information has been reported on radiation-induced second cancers in long-term survivors of childhood cancer.[17] Interpretation of results are complicated by the fact that many of these cancers are associated with germinal mutations that can influence susceptibility to the development of second cancers independent of the radiation or perhaps enhance susceptibility to radiation exposure. Another complicating factor is that many of these patients received chemotherapeutic agents as well. Furthermore, in many cases insufficient time has passed for risks for adult solid tumors to be properly assessed. The most common second cancers appear after treatment of childhood cancers appears to be bone and soft tissue sarcomas. By far the largest source of information on these sarcomas come from study of retinoblastoma patients, many of whom have an elevated risk for such cancers independent of the radiation exposure because of heritable mutations in the RB gene.[17,50,57] In these children, risk after radiation therapy can be as high as 50%. Although genetic susceptibility of these children to the familial form of these cancers can complicate interpretation, studies of retinoblastoma patients who do not have the familial form and studies of patients with other forms of childhood cancer also show increased risks for these sarcomas. Not unexpectedly, based on the earlier discussion about age susceptibility (see Age, earlier in this chapter), the risk for thyroid, breast, and skin cancers also are elevated after radiation therapy for a variety of childhood cancers, as are tumors of the central nervous system and leukemias.[17] It appears, however, that the effects of radiation are primarily on the induction of solid cancers. The relative increase in risk for leukemia development after radiation therapy is lower than that for the development of a subsequent solid cancer.

A series of large studies have examined the development of second cancers in cervical cancer patients treated with high doses of ionizing radiation.[58,59] Increased risks for second cancers have been difficult to detect, although a small (twofold) increased risk of leukemia was detected when the sample size was increased to include several hundred thousand women. The reason for such a small increase in leukemia risk is likely a result of a number of factors. First, the high doses delivered to a small volume likely resulted in cell killing in nearby target cells, and the dose outside the field was relatively low so that the fraction of target cell irradiated may have been small. Second, the doses were protracted (brachytherapy), fractionated, or both. In spite of the small numbers of leukemias, a dose-response curve was constructed that showed a rise in leukemia risk up to approximately 4 Gy, followed by a decline from the peak at higher doses. This decline at higher doses was suggested to be a result of cell killing that could have reduced the number of transformed cells. With respect to time of occurrence, a minimum latent period of approximately 2 years was seen, and the risk remained elevated for approximately 15 years before declining to normal levels. Within the field of irradiation, cancers of the bladder and bone, as well as soft tissue sarcomas, were observed. Outside of this field, cancers of the stomach were seen, probably as a result of scatter radiation of approximately 1 Gy.

In long-term survivors of Hodgkin's disease, the risk of leukemia appears to be mainly associated with the use of alkylating agents. Radiation in combination with chemotherapeutic agents does not seem to markedly enhance the risk of leukemia over that associated with chemotherapy alone.[17,60–62] Although these data would suggest that radiation is not a particularly effective leukemogenic agent, studies of second solid cancers indicate radiation is capable of increasing the risks of a number of solid cancers, including cancers of the breast, thyroid, stomach, bone, and skin.[35,36,39] Second cancers of the breast are particularly pronounced in women treated at young ages.[35] It has been reported that the relative risk for women treated when they were younger than 15 years is 136. For those treated between the ages of 15 and 24, the relative risk was 19; for ages 25 to 29 years, a relative risk of 7.3 was reported. Women treated at older ages did not appear to be at an increased risk. It is also important to note that the time between radiation exposure and the onset of breast cancer was long. The risk was higher at times beyond 15 years after treatment than before 15 years. Clearly, such patients should be identified as high risk and monitored carefully on a long-term basis.

In addition to breast cancer, an excess of lung cancer has been reported.[63,64] Unlike breast cancer, lung cancer has been reported to appear as early as 5 years after treatment. As might be expected, a strong interaction between smoking and radiation with respect to lung cancer risk has been reported. An increased risk for thyroid cancer has been found in patients treated at very young ages but not in adults, and an increased risk for bone cancer has been reported mainly in patients treated as adolescents.[65,66] Concerns over these second cancer risks, particularly breast cancer, has led to treatment modifications but not to elimination of radiation as an important tool in the treatment of Hodgkin's disease.[17] In spite of the risk, radiation is very effective, and the potential benefits of its continued use (a high probability of long-term survival) is thought to outweigh the risks of a second cancer many years later.

On the basis of epidemiologic studies of breast cancer risks in other populations, the dose to the contralateral breast during radiation therapy for breast cancer is sufficient to result in an increased risk for a second breast cancer. This potential risk has been shown to be the case in several studies.[39,40] An increase in risk has been found in women irradiated before age 45 who survive longer than 10 years. For women older than 45 at the time of treatment, the risk does not appear to be increased. In addition to breast cancer in the contralateral breast, an increased risk of lung cancer also has been reported.[67]

Studies have been reported on patients receiving whole body irradiation for bone marrow transplantations who received radiation doses in the range of 10 to 15 Gy. It was found that, in those patients who survived 10 or more years, the risk was 8.3 times higher than expected. Risks were elevated for cancer of the buccal cavity, liver, brain and central nervous system, thyroid, bone, and connective tissue, as well as for malignant melanoma. Those treated at younger ages were at higher risk than those treated at older ages.[68]

RADON

Radon is a gas that comes from the naturally occurring uranium in rocks and soil. As a gas, it is able to flow from rocks and soil into the air, and because of this, underground mines, especially uranium mines, often contain high levels of radon. Homes in many areas also contain measurable levels of radon because of the makeup of the rocks and soil in the area. Radon, although radioactive, is chemically inert and uncharged. The spontaneous decay of radon results in radon progeny that are also radioactive but are electrically charged. These charged particles can attach to dust particles and, when inhaled, can deposit in the lung, where decay of these progeny results in irradiation of lung tissue with alpha particles.

Studies of underground miners exposed to high levels of radon have clearly demonstrated that radon and its progeny are responsible for an increased risk of lung cancer.[20] The risk is specific for lung cancer, and an increased risk for leukemia and other cancers is not observed. Based on extensive studies of such miners, an exposure-response relationship has been constructed that indicates a linear relationship between exposure and lung cancer risk, as would be expected for high LET radiations, such as alpha particles. It has been more difficult to detect risks due to radon in homes, but newer analyses have provided evidence of such risks and appear to confirm that the exposure-response relationship derived from the underground miner studies adequately projects risks at low radon levels as well. All of these estimates are complicated because of the overwhelming risk associated with smoking that must be taken into account in many study groups. On the basis of estimates from the uranium miners and studies of risks of radon in homes, it is currently estimated that approximately 10% to 15% of lung cancers in the U.S. population each year could be attributed to radon exposure.[20]

MECHANISMS

It is clear from the discussion in the previous section that a single dose of ionizing radiation can result in an increased risk of cancer from years to decades later. Although it is generally assumed that these carcinogenic effects are somehow related to its mutagenic and clastogenic potential, the precise mechanisms through which radiation results in this increased frequency of cancer is unknown. The long period between radiation exposure and cancer development and the multistage nature of carcinogenesis make it particularly difficult to sort out radiation-induced changes from other alterations that occur once the process has been initiated. Radiation-induced cancers do not appear to be unique or specifically identifiable. The mutations and the growth characteristics of tumors likely caused by radiation are the same as those spontaneously occurring tumors of the same site. Attempts to identify radiation-specific changes have not been successful, despite fairly extensive investigation. However, there are clues to possible underlying mechanisms that emerge from epidemiologic and experimental investigations.

Based on experimental studies, it is generally thought that the induction of complex forms of double-strand breaks is the most biologically important type of lesion induced by ionizing radiation. That is, this type of double-strand break is likely to be responsible for subsequent molecular and cellular effects.[4] Attempts to repair these complex lesions are likely to be error-prone, and it is thought that this error-prone repair process can lead to gross chromosomal effects and mutagenesis. Molecular analyses of radiation-induced mutations have found a full range of mutations, including base pair substitutions, frameshift mutations, and deletions. Importantly, the most common alterations are deletions rather than point mutations. Because mutations predominate, theories of radiation-induced cancer have focused mainly on effects in oncogenes and tumor suppressor genes that would be expected to occur through this mode of action rather than through the induction of point mutations. Thus, mechanisms involving gene and chromosome rearrangements, loss of heterozygosity, and gene deletion are considered the most likely radiation-induced events to initiate the process of cancer development. Some support for this view comes from the molecular analysis of radiation-induced cancers. In the papillary form of thyroid cancer, rearrangements in the RET protooncogene are a common feature,[69] and it has been demonstrated that such rearrangements can occur in thyroid cells after irradiation.[70–72] Radiation-induced myeloid leukemia in mice appears to be associated with specific deletions in chromosome 2 that occur very early after irradiation.[73–75] In a murine model of p53 deficiency containing mice with one normal and one mutant allele of the p53 gene, it has been shown that these mice are highly sensitive to radiation tumorigenesis.[76] Analysis of these tumors has demonstrated loss of the wild-type allele and duplication of the mutant p53 allele. In patients with familial forms of RB, basal cell nevus carcinoma syndrome, and Li-Fraumeni syndrome, the pathogenesis of second cancers after radiation therapy appears to involve a similar mechanism. In each case, the patient has a germline mutation in one allele at birth, and radiation appears to facilitate the loss of the normal allele.

More recently, experimental studies have questioned whether the initiating events produced by radiation are direct effects on specific genes or whether the mutations and chromosomal rearrangements result indirectly as a consequence of genomic instability induced by the radiation exposure.[77–80] The observation of genomic instability is relatively recent. It had been generally believed that all the mutagenic and cytogenetic effects of radiation occurred in the first, or at least the first few, cell divisions. It has now been shown that increased mutation rates and new cytogenetic damage can occur in a large proportion of the progeny of irradiated cells many generations later (Fig. 12-2). This has led to the hypothesis that this radiation-induced instability, which appears to be broadly based, is the initiating event responsible for subsequent mutations and chromosomal rearrangements that ultimately lead to cancer. Interestingly, analyses of mutations arising in genomically unstable cells indicate that they are more frequently point mutations rather than deletions. According to this hypothesis, this instability puts all genes at an increased risk for mutations, and it is this increased mutation rate that ultimately results in cancer development (Fig. 12-3).

The mechanism for induction of radiation-induced instability is not known, but it does not appear to be a result of the induction of a mutation in a specific gene or set of genes. The argument against a specific gene mutation is based on the high frequency of radiation-induced instability after relatively small doses. The probability of a specific gene mutation after 1 Gy of ionizing radiation ranges from 1 in 10,000 to 1 in 100,000, whereas approximately one in five cells or more will express radiation-induced instability. The strongest evidence to date in support of this hypothesis comes from mouse studies that have found a genetic association between susceptibility to radiation-induced chromosomal instability and susceptibility to breast cancer.[81]

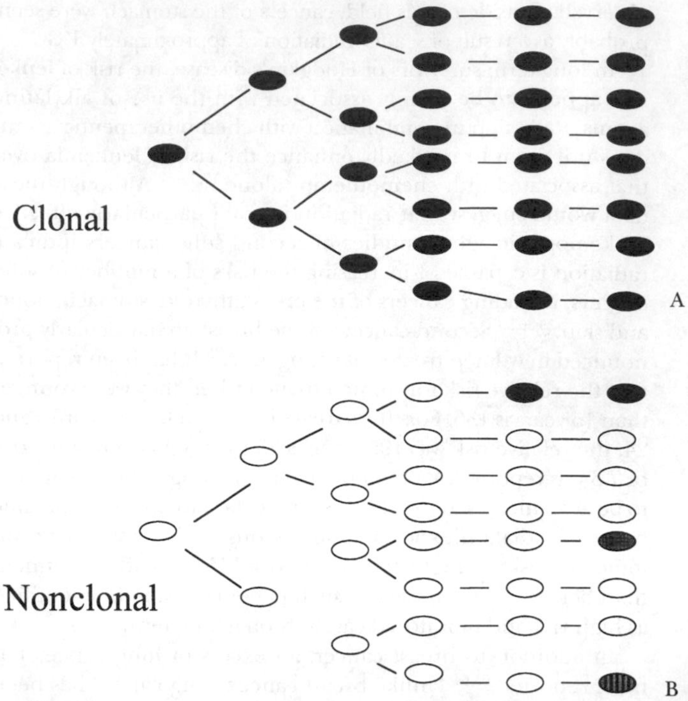

FIGURE 12-2. Comparison of mutations and cytogenetic damage as a result of direct radiation damage or as a result of radiation-induced genomic instability. **A:** Directly induced mutations or chromosome aberrations are passed to all progeny (i.e., the alterations are clonal). **B:** In contrast, mutations or aberrations arising as a result of radiation-induced instability arise in the progeny of irradiated cells that have not been directly irradiated. This leads to a nonclonal, or mosaic, pattern. Because the alterations arise in the progeny of the cells, another characteristic of instability is that the mutational or clastogenic effects are delayed with respect to the radiation exposure.

ULTRAVIOLET LIGHT

Skin cancer is one of the most common forms of cancer, and its incidence is rising.[82–84] Although it is difficult to estimate overall incidence rates for nonmelanoma skin cancer, it is estimated that the annual incidence in 1996 was on the order of 800,000 new cases. Approximately 80% of all nonmelanoma skin cancers are basal cell carcinomas. Squamous cell carcinoma comprises the other 20%. Mortality rates for these nonmelanoma cancers are low. However, this is not the case for melanoma, which has been increasing at a rate of approximately 3% per year in the United States. In 1998, an estimated 41,600 new cases of melanoma were diagnosed, an estimated 7300 of which ultimately will be fatal.[85] A major cause of all forms of skin cancer is UV light from the sun.

SUNLIGHT AND SKIN CANCER

The evidence that UV light is responsible for a large proportion of skin cancer is considerable. Skin cancer is more frequent in populations in regions with high ambient solar radiation and in individuals exposed to sunlight as a result of their occupations (e.g., farmers). Nonmelanoma skin cancer is most frequent in sites that are the most exposed to sunlight, such as the head, neck, and arms. Pigmented skin is less susceptible to nonmelanoma skin cancer, and lack of pigmentation increases the risk. A high incidence of skin tumors is seen in young individuals associated with sunlight exposure who have xeroderma pigmentosum, a disease that is

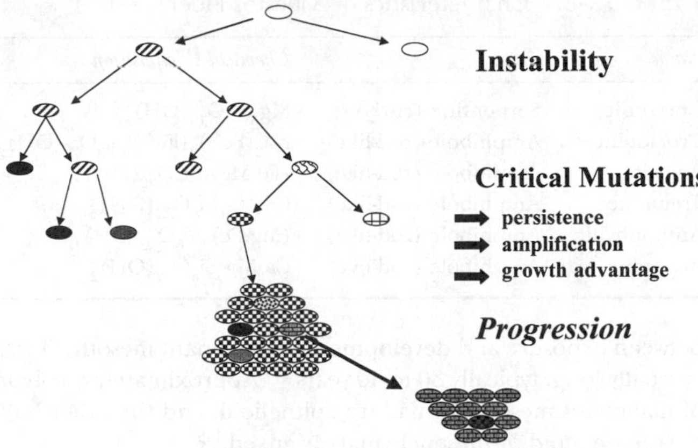

FIGURE 12-3. Proposed role of radiation-induced cytogenetic instability in radiation-induced cancer. Radiation exposure induces instability in a high percentage of the progeny of the irradiated cells (*striped* cells represent unstable progeny). As a result of this instability, the rate of chromosome aberrations and mutations is increased. Some mutations result in cell death (*black*) or slow-growing cells (*gray*), whereas some occur in critical genes involved in the regulation of cell growth and differentiation, or in the maintenance of the stability of the genome. These mutations result in the persistence and amplification of genomic instability or in cells with a growth advantage. As these cells continue to develop into a clonal outgrowth, further mutations result in additional cellular changes, which lead to death or progression toward neoplasia. Cells with other patterns represent cells with specific mutations or sets of mutations that arose subsequent to radiation exposure.

caused by a deficiency in the ability to repair UV light–induced DNA damage. In the United States, the incidence of basal cell carcinoma and squamous cell carcinoma increase by approximately 2% to 3% for every 1% increase in ambient UV light, and melanoma incidence increases by approximately 0.5% to 1.0%.[86] On a worldwide level, the incidence of skin cancer is extremely dependent on latitude, which equates with level of exposure to UV light; the closer to the equator, the greater the risk. This is particularly true for countries in which a large proportion of the population is lightly pigmented, such as Australia.[87]

Melanoma is also associated with sunlight exposure but is less dependent on total exposure, and it is not correlated with chronically exposed anatomic sites. Rather, increased risk for melanoma appears to be related more to acute burns rather than accumulated dose.[82] Additional evidence for a role for sunlight in melanoma development comes from the observation that children who move to countries with high ambient sunlight are at an increased risk of melanoma.[87] The same does not appear to be true when individuals move at older ages. These finding suggest that both exposure factors and factors involved in age-dependent susceptibility are involved. A greater risk for nonmelanoma skin cancer is seen in children and adolescents as well.

GENETICS AND RISK

One of the major discoveries that established a direct link between UV light to DNA damage and skin cancer was that patients with xeroderma pigmentosum are defective in nucleotide excision repair.[89] Nucleotide excision repair is the repair pathway that removes the cyclobutane pyrimidine dimers produced in DNA by UV light, as well as other large adducts, and replaces the damaged site.[90,91] This pathway is complex and involves a number of sequential steps, including recognition of the lesion; assembly of the enzymes that make up the excision complex, which excises a 27- to 29-nucleotide region containing the photoproduct; removal of this oligonucleotide containing the damage; and, finally, replacement and filling of the resulting gap by polymerization and ligation. Another pathway, base excision repair, removes less complex base damage. Both pathways are complex processes that are influenced by many factors, including transcriptional activity, the sequence of nucleotides surrounding the damaged site, and DNA conformation.

In addition to xeroderma pigmentosum, a number of other disorders result in increased acute sensitivity to UVC or UVB.[92] These include Cockayne's syndrome and trichothiodystrophy. Both are related to disorders in genes involved in DNA damage repair, but neither has an increased sensitivity to UV-induced skin cancer. Studies of these disorders are providing additional insights into details of underlying mechanisms of UV-induced skin cancer. For example, it has been found that cells from Cockayne's syndrome patients are able to repair only transcriptionally inactive genes.[93] Perhaps repair of transcriptionally active genes is more important for the prevention of mutagenesis and carcinogenesis.

MECHANISMS

Squamous Cell Carcinoma and Basal Cell Carcinoma

The development of squamous cell carcinoma and basal cell carcinoma is associated with chronic exposure to sunlight. In other words, multiple exposures of UV light from the sun are necessary for the induction of these cancers. This finding is consistent with experimental evidence indicating that UV radiation (UVB and UVC) acts both as an initiator and a promoter for squamous cell cancers.[85] UV-induced mutations in p53 appear to be an early event in this process.[94,95] Further exposures may lead to additional mutations in oncogenes and tumor suppressor genes, but, in addition, these further exposures facilitate clonal expansion of initiated cells through killing effects on normal but not p53 mutant cells. Exposure to UV light also has been shown to suppress the immune system's ability to suppress tumor growth.[96,97] High doses of UV radiation apparently affect the ability of Langerhans' cells to efficiently transfer antigenic signals to T cells in local lymph nodes.

Studies of patients with basal cell nevus carcinoma syndrome have provided insight into mechanisms of development of basal cell carcinomas. These patients are highly susceptible to basal cell carcinoma as a result of exposure to both ionizing and UV radiation, but keratinocytes from these patients show no difference in sensitivity to cell killing effects.[98] It has been shown that the gene associated with this syndrome is PTC, which is the human homologue of the *Drosophila* patched gene (ptc).[99] In *Drosophila*, this gene plays a role in cell-cell communication and transforming growth factor-β signaling. The most common genetic alteration in nonfamilial basal cell carcinoma is loss of heterozygosity at chromosome 9q22, which contains the PTC locus. This loss of heterozygosity has been observed even in very small tumors, suggesting that alteration of PTC is an early event.[100]

Melanoma

Epidemiologic evidence has established a causal relationship between sunlight exposure and melanoma that appears to be primarily a function of acute sunburn rather than chronic exposure, as is the case for squamous cell and basal cell carcinoma. A history of five or more sunburns as an adolescent has been found to double the risk for melanoma.[88] Experimental studies with a fish model suggest that the majority of melanomas are induced by UVA.[101] If this is the case, DNA damage would be predicted to be a result of damage mediated through reactive oxygen species rather than the cyclobutane dimers and 6-4 photoproducts that are associated with exposure to UVB and UVC. In the familial form of melanoma, susceptibility is associated with chromosome 9p21, which contains CDKN2A, the gene encoding p16 and p19.[102] This gene is involved in cell-cycle regulation. In both sporadic and familial forms of melanoma, loss of heterozygosity is found in several chromosomes, including 9p, 6, 8, and 10.[103,104] As yet, no evidence indicates that these changes are a direct result of damage produced by UV light.

ASBESTOS

Asbestos use has spanned many centuries. Major industrial use began in the late 1800s and became widespread during World War II. Use peaked in the 1970s, and recognition of its health effects has led to major reductions in mining and use of asbestos, as well as programs aimed at removal of asbestos from existing structures. The carcinogenic effects of asbestos have been clearly demonstrated in studies of individuals exposed in the mining and industrial use of asbestos.[105]

FIBER QUALITY AND DISEASE

Asbestos is actually a group of fibers, with each type having a unique structure and chemical composition (Table 12-3).[106] Each type also appears to differ in its chemical reactivity. Not unexpectedly, each type also appears to have differing biologic properties as well. There are two main subgroups. Chrysotile fibers are long, curly snake-like fibers. Amphibole fibers are shorter and rod-like in structure. The most common amphibole types include crocidolite, amosite, and tremolite. Few malignant mesotheliomas are associated with occupational exposure to chrysotile fibers, probably because they do not tend to persist in lung. The persistence of amphibole fibers, which are more commonly linked with mesothelioma, is significantly greater.

CANCER RISK AND ASBESTOS EXPOSURE

The most common form of cancer associated with asbestos exposure is malignant mesothelioma, but the risk of bronchogenic cancer is also significantly elevated. Although lung cancer is generally associated with asbestos exposure, other cancers that have been reported to occur at an increased frequency include cancers of the larynx, oropharynx, kidney, esophagus, and gallbladder/bile duct.[107,108]

Because it is very rare, it has been relatively easy to link the risk of mesothelioma to asbestos exposure. Occupational exposure can be linked to 50% to 80% of all patients with malignant mesotheliomas.[107,109] In a study of tile workers exposed to asbestos over a 50-year period, it was found that the incidence of mesothelioma was as high as 2%.[110] A study of a large group of asbestos insulation workers found that mesothelioma was responsible for approximately 8% of all deaths.[111] The latent period

TABLE 12-3. Characteristics of Asbestos Fibers

Name	*Type*	*Chemical Composition*
Chrysotile	Serpentine (curly)	$Mg_6Si_4O_{10}(OH)_8$
Crocidolite	Amphibole (rod-like)	$Na_2(Fe^{3+})_2(Fe^{2+})_3Si_8O_{22}(OH)_2$
Amosite	Amphibole (rod-like)	$(Fe,Mg)_7Si_8O_{22}(OH)_2$
Tremolite	Amphibole (rod-like)	$Ca_2Mg_5Si_8O_{22}(OH)_2$
Anthophyllite	Amphibole (rod-like)	$(Mg,Fe)_7Si_8O_{22}(OH)_2$
Actinolite	Amphibole (rod-like)	$Ca_2Mg_5Si_8O_{22}(OH)_2$

between exposure and development of malignant mesothelioma is usually long, typically 30 to 40 years.[107] Approximately one-half of malignant mesotheliomas are epithelioid, and the other half are sarcomatoid or mesenchymal, or mixed.[112]

A link between asbestos and bronchogenic carcinomas was first reported in the 1930s and has been subsequently confirmed in several investigations.[113] Although the vast majority of bronchogenic carcinomas are related to smoking, it has been estimated that from 3% to 17% of such cancers are from occupational exposures, including asbestos.[114] Asbestos and smoking appear to interact in a multiplicative manner, and risk is decreased when exposure to either agent is stopped. Whereas the majority of smoking-related tumors are squamous cell carcinomas originating in the upper lobes of the lung, those associated with asbestos are more often adenocarcinomas located in the lower lobes.[115–117] The asbestos-related tumors are also often associated with areas of fibrosis.[118]

MECHANISMS

Asbestos fibers are cytotoxic and genotoxic. They have been shown to induce DNA damage, including double-strand breaks, mutations, and chromosomal damage.[119,120] Evidence also indicates that asbestos fibers can impair mitosis and chromosomal segregation, which can result in aneuploidy. The majority of these effects are believed to be due to oxidoreductive processes that result in the formation of reactive oxygen species.[121,122] Support for this view comes from studies showing that the amount of damage induced is increased if iron is present in the chemical structure of the fibers. Besides the direct induction of reactive oxygen species, these effects may also be induced indirectly as a result of phagocytosis of the asbestos fibers. Fibers also tend to induce inflammatory responses, resulting in the release of cytokines.[106] Such cytokines may facilitate the growth, selection, and expansion of initiated cells.

Loss of one copy of chromosome 22 is one of the most common chromosomal alteration in malignant melanoma. A wide range of other changes also are seen, including deletions in chromosomes 1p, 3p, 6q, 9p, 13q, 15q, and 22q. Analysis of tumors with these chromosomal alterations have found deletions of CDKN2A, located on chromosome 9p, and mutations in NF2 (the neurofibromatosis type 2 gene that is located on chromosome 22q), coupled with the loss of the normal NF2 allele associated with loss of one of an entire chromosome 22, as common features.[123]

REFERENCES

1. Johns HE, Cunningham JR. *The physics of radiology.* Springfield, IL: Charles C Thomas Publisher, 1983.

2. Hall EJ. *Radiobiology for the radiologist.* New York: JB Lippincott Co, 1994.
3. National Council on Radiation Protection and Measurements. Influences of radiation quality (LET) on relative biological effectiveness. NCRP report of Scientific Committee 40. Bethesda, MD. National Council on Radiation Protection and Measurements, 1989.
4. Ward JF. Damage produced by ionizing radiation in mammalian cells: identities, mechanisms of formation and reparability. *Prog Nucleic Acid Res Mol Biol* 1988;35:95.
5. Jeggo PA. Identification of genes involved in repair of DNA double strand breaks in mammalian cells. *Radiat Res* 1998;150:S80.
6. Niggli HJ, Cerutti PA. Cyclobutane-type pyrimidine photodimer formation and excision in human skin fibroblasts after irradiation with 313-nm ultraviolet light. *Biochemistry* 1983;22:1390.
7. Tyrrell RM, Pidoux M. Action spectra for human skin cells: estimates of the relative cytotoxicity of the middle ultraviolet, near ultraviolet, and violet regions of sunlight on epidermal keratinocytes. *Cancer Res* 1987;47:1825.
8. Tommasi S, Denissenko MF, Pfeifer GP. Sunlight induces pyrimidine dimers preferentially at 5-mehylcytosine bases. *Cancer Res* 1997;57:4727.
9. Brash DE, Rudolph JA, Simon JA, et al. A role for sunlight in skin cancer: UV-induced p53 mutations in squamous cell carcinoma. *Proc Natl Acad Sci U S A* 1991;88:10124.
10. Ziegler A, Jonason AS, Leffell DJ, et al. Sunburn and p53 in the onset of skin cancer. *Nature* 1994;372:773.
11. Miller RW. Delayed efforts of external radiation exposure: a brief history. *Radiat Res* 1995;144:160.
12. Mabuchi K, Soda M, Ron E, et al. Cancer incidence in atomic bomb survivors. Part I: Use of the tumor registries in Hiroshima and Nagasaki for incidence studies in the atomic bomb survivors. *Radiat Res* 1994;137:S1.
13. Thompson DE, Mabuchi K, Ron E, et al. Cancer incidence in atomic bomb survivors. Part II: Solid tumors, 1958–1987. *Radiat Res* 1994;137:S17.
14. Preston DL, Kusumi S, Tomonaga M, et al. Cancer incidence in atomic bomb survivors. Part III: Leukemia, lymphoma and multiple myeloma, 1950–1987. *Radiat Res* 1994;137:S68.
15. Ron E, Preston DL, Mabuchi K, Thompson DE, Soda M. Cancer incidence in atomic bomb survivors. Part IV: Comparison of cancer incidence and mortality. *Radiat Res* 1994;137:S98.
16. Boice JD. *Radiation epidemiology: past and present.* In: Proceedings of the Thirty-Second Meeting of the National Council on Radiation Protection and Measurements, Washington, DC, 1997:7.
17. Inskip PD. Second cancers following radiotherapy. In: Neugut AI, Meadows AT, Robinson E, eds. *Multiple primary cancers.* Philadelphia: Lippincott Williams & Wilkins, 1999:91.
18. Little MP, Boice JD Jr. Comparison of breast cancer incidence in the Massachusetts tuberculosis fluoroscopy cohort and in the Japanese atomic bomb survivors. *Radiat Res* 1999;151:218.
19. Howe GR, McLaughlin J. Breast cancer mortality between 1950 and 1987 after exposure to fractionated moderate-dose-rate ionizing radiation in the Canadian fluoroscopy cohort study and a comparison with breast cancer mortality in the atomic bomb survivors study. *Radiat Res* 1996;145:694.
20. National Research Council, Committee on Health Effects of Exposure to Radon. *B E I R VI report.* Washington, DC: National Academy Press, 1999.
21. National Research Council, Committee on the Biological Effects of Ionizing Radiations. *Health effects of exposure to low levels of ionizing radiation: BEIR V report.* Washington, DC: National Academy Press, 1990.
22. Boice JD Jr, Land CE, Preston DL. Ionizing radiation. In: Schottenfeld D, Fraumeni JF Jr, eds. *Cancer epidemiology and prevention.* New York: Oxford University Press, 1996:319.
23. National Council on Radiation Protection and Measurements. *Influence of dose and its distribution in time on dose-response relationships for low LET radiations.* Report no. 64. Washington, DC: National Council on Radiation Protection and Measurements, 1980.
24. Ullrich RL, Jernigan MC, Satterfield LC, Bowles ND. Radiation carcinogenesis: time-dose relationships. *Radiat Res* 1987;111:179.
25. UNSCEAR (United Nations Scientific Committee on the Effects of Atomic Radiation). *Sources and effects of ionizing radiation.* Publ. no. E.94.IX.11. New York: United Nations, 1994.
26. Land CE, Boice JD Jr, Shore RE, Norman JE, Tokunaga M. Breast cancer risk from low-dose exposures to ionizing radiation: results of parallel analysis of three exposed populations of women. *J Natl Cancer Inst* 1980;65:353.
27. Howe GR. Lung cancer mortality between 1950 and 1987 after exposure to fractionated moderate-dose-rate ionizing radiation in the Canadian fluoroscopy cohort study and a comparison with lung cancer mortality in the atomic bomb survivors study. *Radiat Res* 1995;142:295.
28. Upton AC, Randolph ML, Conklin JW. Late effects of fast neutrons and gamma rays in mice as influenced by the dose rate of irradiation: induction of neoplasia. *Radiat Res* 1970;41:467.
29. Ullrich RL, Storer JB. Influence of gamma ray irradiation on the development of neoplastic disease in mice. I. Reticular tissue tumors. *Radiat Res* 1979;80:303.
30. Ullrich RL, Storer JB. Influence of gamma ray irradiation on the development of neoplastic disease in mice. II. Solid tumors. *Radiat Res* 1979;80:317.
31. Ullrich RL, Jernigan MC, Cosgrove GE, et al. The influence of dose and dose rate on the incidence of neoplastic disease in RFM mice after neutron irradiation. *Radiat Res* 1976;68:115.
32. Ullrich RL, Jernigan MC, Storer JB. Neutron carcinogenesis: dose and dose rate effects in BALB/c mice. *Radiat Res* 1977;72:487.
33. Hill CK, Zhu L. Energy and dose-rate dependence of neoplastic transformation and mutations induced in mammalian cells by fast neutrons. *Radiat Res* 1991;128:S53.
34. Miller RC, Brenner DJ, Randers-Person G, Marino SA, Hall EJ. The effects of temporal distribution of dose on oncogenic transformation by neutrons and charged particles of intermediate LET. *Radiat Res* 1990;124:S62.
35. Hancock SL, Tucker MA, Hoppe RT. Breast cancer after treatment of Hodgkin's disease. *J Natl Cancer Inst* 1993;85:25.
36. Bhatia S, Robinson LL, Oberlin O, et al. Breast cancer and other second neoplasms after childhood Hodgkin's disease. *N Engl J Med* 1996;334:745.
37. Hildreth NG, Shore RE, Dvoretsky PM. The risk of breast cancer after irradiation of the thymus in infancy. *N Engl J Med* 1989;321:1281.
38. Aisenberg AC, Finkelstein DM, Doppke KP, et al. High risk of breast carcinoma after irradiation of young women with Hodgkin's disease. *Cancer* 1997;79:1203.
39. Boice JD Jr, Harvey E, Blettner M, Stovall M, Flannery JT. Cancer in the contralateral breast after radiotherapy for breast cancer. *N Engl J Med* 1992;326:781.
40. Storm HH, Andersson M, Boice JD Jr, et al. Adjuvant radiotherapy and risk of contralateral breast cancer. *J Natl Cancer Inst* 1992;84:1245.
41. Stewart A, Web J, Giles D, Hewitt D. Malignant disease in childhood and diagnostic irradiation *in utero. Lancet* 1956;2:447.
42. Stewart A, Webb J, Hewitt D. A survey of childhood malignancies. *BMJ* 1958;1:1495.
43. Mole RH. Antenatal irradiation and childhood cancer: causation or coincidence? *Br J Cancer* 1974;30:199.
44. Harvery EB, Boice JD Jr, Honeyman M, Fannery JT. Prenatal x-ray exposure and childhood cancer in twins. *N Engl J Med* 1985;312:541.
45. Doll R, Wakeford R. Risk of childhood cancer from fetal irradiation. *Br J Radiology* 1997;70:130.
46. Boice JD Jr, Miller RW. Childhood and adult cancer following intrauterine exposure to ionizing radiation. *Teratology* 1999;59:227.
47. Harvard Report on Cancer Prevention. Causes of human cancer. *Cancer Causes Control* 1996;7[Suppl 1]:S3.
48. Sharp C, Cox R. Genetic susceptibility to radiation effects: possible implication for medical ionizing radiation exposures. *Eur J Nucl Med* 1999;26:425.
49. Sankaranarayanan K, Chakraborty R. Cancer predisposition, radiosensitivity and the risk of radiation induced cancers. I: Background [Review]. *Radiat Res* 1995;143:121.
50. Wong FL, Boice JD Jr, Abramson DH, et al. Cancer incidence after retinoblastoma: radiation dose and sarcoma risk. *JAMA* 1997;278:1262.
51. Strong LC. Theories of pathogenesis: mutation and cancer. In: Mulvihill JJ, Miller RW, Fraumeni JF Jr, eds. *Genetics of human cancer.* New York: Raven Press, 1977:401.
52. Li FP, Fraumeni JF Jr, Mulvihill JJ, et al. A cancer family syndrome in twenty-four kindreds. *Cancer Res* 1988;48:5358.
53. Srivastava S, Zou Z, Pirollo K, Blattner W, Chong EH. Germ-line transmission of a mutated p53 gene in a cancer prone family with Li-Fraumeni syndrome. *Nature (Lond)* 1990;348:747.
54. Swift M, Morrell D, Massey RB, Chase CL. Incidence of cancer in 161 families affected by ataxia-telangiectasia. *N Engl J Med* 1999;325:1831.
55. Lavin JF, Shiloh Y. The genetic defect in ataxia-telangiectasia. *Ann Rev Immunol* 1997;15:177.
56. Morgan SE, Kastan MB. P53 and ATM: cell cycle, death and cancer. *Adv Cancer Res* 1997;71:125.
57. Eng C, Li FP, Abramson DH, et al. Mortality from second tumors among long-term survivors of retinoblastoma. *J Natl Cancer Inst* 1993;85:1121.
58. Boice JD Jr, Engholm G, Kleinerman RA, et al. Radiation dose and second cancer risk in patients treated for cancer of the cervix. *Radiat Res* 1988;116:3.
59. Boice JD Jr, Blettner M, Kleinerman RA, et al. Radiation dose and leukemia risk in patients treated for cancer of the cervix. *J Natl Cancer Inst* 1987;79:1295.
60. Van Leeuwen FE, Klokman WJ, Hagenbeek A, et al. Second cancer risk following Hodgkin's disease: a 20-year follow-up study. *J Clin Oncol* 1994;12:312.
61. Boivin JF, Hutchison GB, Zauber AG, et al. Incidence of second cancers in patients treated for Hodgkin's disease. *J Natl Cancer Inst* 1995;87:732.
62. Swerdlow AJ, Barber JA, Horwich A, et al. Second malignancy in patients with Hodgkin's disease treated at the Royal Marsden Hospital. *Br J Cancer* 1997;75:116.
63. Van Leeuwen FE, Klokman WJ, Stovall M, et al. Roles of radiotherapy and smoking in lung cancer following Hodgkin's disease. *J Natl Cancer Inst* 1995;87:1530.
64. Kaldor JM, Day NE, Bell J, et al. Lung cancer following Hodgkin's disease: a case-control study. *Int J Cancer* 1992;52:677.
65. Tucker MA, Morris Jones PH, Bice JD Jr, et al. Therapeutic irradiation at a young age is linked to secondary thyroid cancer. *Cancer Res* 1991;51:2885.
66. Tucker MA, Meadows AT, Boice JD Jr, Hoover RN, Fraumeni JF Jr. Late Effects Study Group. Cancer risk following treatment of childhood cancer. In: Boice JD Jr, Fraumeni JF Jr, eds. *Radiation carcinogenesis: epidemilogy and biological significance.* New York: Raven Press, 1984:211.
67. Inskip PD, Stovall M, Flannery JT. Lung cancer and radiation dose among women treated for breast cancer. *J Natl Cancer Inst* 1994;86:983.
68. Curtis RE, Rowlings PA, Deeg HJ, et al. Solid cancers after bone marrow transplantation. *N Engl J Med* 1997;336:897.
69. Zimmerman D. Thyroid neoplasia in children. *Curr Opin Pediatr* 1997;9:413.
70. Bongarzone I, Butti MG, Fugazzola L, et al. Comparison of the breakpoint regions of ELEI and RET genes involved in the generation of RET/PTC3 oncogene in sporadic and in radiation-associated papillary thyroid carcinomas. *Genomics* 1997;42:252.
71. Klugbauer S, Lengerfelder E, Demidchik EP, et al. High prevalence of ret rearrangements in thyroid tumours of children from Belarus after the Chernobyl reactor accident. *Oncogene* 1995;11:2459.
72. Mizuno T, Kyoizumi S, Suzuki T, et al. Continued expression of a tissue specific activated oncogene in the early steps of radiation-induced human thyroid carcinogenesis. *Oncogene* 1997;15:1455.
73. Breckon G, Papworth D, Cox R. Murine radiation myeloid leukamogenesis: a possible role for radiation sensitive sites on chromosome 2. *Genes Chromosomes Cancer* 1991;3:367.
74. Bouffler SD, Meijne EIM, Morris DJ, et al. Chromosome 2 hypersensitivity and clonal development in murine radiation acute myeloid leukemia. *Int J Radiat Biol* 1997;72:181.
75. Hayata I, Seki M, Yoshida K, et al. Chromosomal aberrations observed in 52 mouse myeloid leukemias. *Cancer Res* 1983;43:367.

76. Kemp CJ, Wheldon T, Balmain A. p53-deficient mice are extremely susceptible to radiation-induced tumorigenesis. *Nat Genet* 1994;8:66.
77. Selvanayagam CS, Cornforth MN, Ullrich RL. Latent expression of p53 mutations and radiation-induced mammary cancer. *Cancer Res* 1995;55:3310.
78. Little JB, Nagasawa H, Pfenning T, Vetrovs H. Radiation-induced genomic instability: delayed mutagenic and cytogenetic effects of x-rays and alpha particles. *Radiat Res* 1997;148:299.
79. Morgan WF, Day JP, Kaplan MI, McGhee EM, Limoli CL. Genomic instability induced by ionizing radiation. *Radiat Res* 1996;146:247.
80. Kadhim MA, MacDonald DA, Goodhead DT, et al. Transmission of chromosomal instability after plutonium alpha particle irradiation. *Nature* 1992;355:738.
81. Ponnaiya B, Corforth MN, Ullrich RL. Radiation-induced chromosomal instability in BALB/c and C57BL/6 mice: the difference is as clear as black and white. *Radiat Res* 1997;147:121.
82. Urbach F. Photocarcinogenesis: from the widow's coif to the p53 gene. *Photochem Photobiol* 1997;655:1295.
83. Leigh IM, Bishop JAN, Kripke ML, eds. Skin cancer. *Cancer Surv* 1996;26:1.
84. Marks R. An overview of skin cancers: incidence and causation. *Cancer* 1995;75[Suppl]:607.
85. International Commission on Radiological Protection. The biological basis for dose limitation in the skin. ICRP report 59. *Ann ICRP* 1999;22:1.
86. Landis SH, Murray T, Bolden S, Wingo PA. Cancer statistics, 1998. *CA Cancer J Clin* 1998;48:6.
87. Armstrong BK, Kricker A. Epidemilogy of sun exposure and skin cancer. *Cancer Surv* 1996;26:133.
88. Weinstock MA. Controversies in the role of sunlight in the pathogenesis of cutaneous melanoma. *Photochem Photobiol* 1996;63:406.
89. Cleaver JE. Defective repair replication in xeroderma pigmentosum. *Nature* 1968;218:652.
90. Sancar A. Mechanisms of DNA excision repair. *Science* 1994;266:1954.
91. Sancar A, Sancar GB. DNA repair enzymes. *Ann Rev Biochem* 1988;57:29.
92. Bootsma D, Kraemer KH, Cleaver JE, Hoeijmakers JHJ. Nucleotide excision repair syndromes: xeroderma pigmentosum, Cockayne syndrome, and trichothiodystrophy. In: Vogelstein B, Kinzler KW, eds. *The genetic basis of human cancer.* New York: McGraw-Hill, 1998:245.
93. Venema J, Mullenders JH, Natarajan AT, Zeeland AAV, Mayne LY. The genetic defect in Cockayne syndrome is associated with a defect in repair of UV-induced DNA damage in transcriptionally active DNA. *Proc Natl Acad Sci U S A* 1990;87:4707.
94. Brash D. Sunlight and onset of skin cancer. *Trends Genetics* 1997;13:410.
95. Berg JW, van Krauen H J, Rebel HG, et al. Early p53 alterations in mouse skin carcinogenesis by UVB radiation: immunohistochemical detection of mutant p53 protein in clusters of preneoplastic epidermal cells. *Proc Natl Acad Sci U S A* 1996;93:274.
96. Daynes RA, Bernhard EJ, Gurish MF, Lynch DH. Experimental photoimmunology: immunologic ramifications of UV-induced carcinogenesis. *J Invest Dermatol* 1981;77:77.
97. Kripke ML. Immunobiology of photocarcinogenesis. In: Parish JA, ed. *Effect of ultraviolet radiation on the immune system.* New Brunswick, NJ: Johnson and Johnson, 1983:87.
98. Stacey M, Thacker S, Taylor AMR. Cultured skin keratinocytes from both normal individuals and basal cell naevus syndrome patients are more resistant to gamma-rays and UV light compared with cultured skin fibroblasts. *Int J Radiat Biol* 1989;56:45.
99. Gailani MR, Bale AE. Developmental genes and cancer: role of patched in basal cell carcinoma of the skin. *J Natl Cancer Inst* 1997;89:1103.
100. Gailani MR, Leffell DJ, Ziegler AM, et al. Relationship between sunlight exposure and a key genetic alteration in basal cell carcinoma. *J Natl Cancer Inst* 1996;88-349.
101. Setlow RB. Spectral regions contributing to melanoma: a personal view. *J Investig Dermatol Symp Proc* 1999;4:46.
102. Monzon J, Liu L, Brill H, et al. CDKN2A mutations in multiple primary melanomas. *N Engl J Med* 1998;338:879.
103. Bastian BC, LeBoit PE, Hamm H, Brocker EB, Pinkel D. Chromosomal gains and losses in primary cutaneous melanomas detected by comparative genome hybridization. *Cancer Res* 1998;58:2170.
104. Trent JM, Stanbridge EJ, McBride HL, et al. Tumorigenicity in human melanoma cell lines controlled by introduction of human chromosome 6. *Science* 1990;247:568.
105. Albin M, Magnani C, Krstev S, Rapiti E, Shefer I. Asbestos and cancer: an overview of current trends in Europe. *Environ Health Perspect* 1999;107[Suppl 2]:289.
106. Mossman BT, Kamp DW, Weitzman SA. Mechanisms of carcinogenesis and clinical features of asbestos-associated cancers. *Cancer Invest* 1996;14:466.
107. Mossman BT, Gee JBL. Asbestos-related diseases. *N Engl J Med* 1989;320:1721.
108. Selikoff KJ. Historical developments and perspectives in inorganic fiber toxicity in man. *Environ Health Perspect* 1990;88:269.
109. Light RW. Tumors of the pleura. In: Murray JF, Nadel JA, eds. *Textbook of Respiratory Medicine,* vol 2. New York: WB Saunders, 1994:2222.
110. Peto J, Doll R, Hermon C, et al. Relationship of mortality to measures of environmental asbestos pollution in an asbestos textile factory. *Ann Occup Hyg* 1985;29:305.
111. Selikoff I. Latency of asbestos disease among insulation workers in the United States and Canada. *Cancer* 1980;46:2736.
112. Hillerdal G. Malignant mesothelioma 1982: review of 4710 published cases. *Br J Dis Chest* 1983;77:321.
113. Enterline PE. Changing attitudes and opinions regarding asbestos and cancer. *Am J Indust Med* 1997;20:685.
114. Ernster VL, Mustacchi P, Osann K, Osann KE. Epidemiology of lung cancer. In: Murray JF, Nadel JA, eds. *Textbook of respiratory medicine,* vol 2. New York: WB Saunders, 1994:1504.
115. Byers TE, Vena JE, Rzepka TF. Predilection of lung cancers for the upper lobes: an epidemiologic inquiry. *J Natl Cancer Inst* 1984;72:1271.
116. Craighead JE, Abraham JL, Churg A, et al. The pathology of asbestos-associated diseases of the lungs and pleural cavities: diagnostic criteria and proposed grading schema. *Arch Pathol Lab Med* 1982;106:540.
117. Raffin E, Lynge E, Korsgaard B. Incidence of lung cancer by histological type among asbestos cement workers in Denmark. *Br J Indust Med* 1993;50:85.
118. Kipen HM, Lilis R, Suzuki Y, et al. Pulmonary fibrosis in asbestos insulation workers with lung cancer: a radiological and histopathological evaluation. *Br J Indust Med* 1987;44:96.
119. Okayasu R, Takahashi S, Yamada S, Hei T, Ullrich RL. Asbestos and DNA double strand breaks. *Cancer Res* 1999;59:298.
120. Jaurand MC. Mechanisms of fiber-induced genotoxicity. *Environ Health Perspect* 1997;105[Suppl 5]:1073.
121. Walker C, Everitt J, Barrett JC. Possible cellular and molecular mechanisms for asbestos carcinogenicity. *Am J Ind Med* 1992;21:253.
122. Kamp DW, Graceffa P, Pryor WA, Weitzman, SA. The role of free radicals in asbestos-induced diseases. *Free Radic Biol Med* 1992;12:293.
123. Murthy SS, Testa JR. Asbestos, chromosomal deletions, and tumor suppressor gene alterations in human malignant mesothelioma. *J Cell Phys* 1999;180:150.

Allen E. Bale
Suzanne J. Brown

CHAPTER 13

Etiology of Cancer: Cancer Genetics

Hundreds of genetic traits are associated with an increased risk of neoplasia.[1] The extent to which cancer risk is attributable to genetic factors varies among tumor types. For rare childhood cancers up to 30% occur in genetically predisposed individuals,[2] whereas not more than 5% to 10% of common adult cancers arise in an hereditary setting.[3] For those malignant tumors most closely associated with environmental carcinogens, the risk attributable to genetic factors is low; but genetic variation may still influence the effect of environmental agents on the host (e.g., sun exposure is a major risk factor for skin cancer, but dark-skinned individuals are virtually immune).[4]

Many of the genes underlying hereditary cancer predisposition are fundamentally involved in the control of cell growth and differentiation or in DNA repair and maintenance of genomic integrity. Analysis of the molecular basis for cancer predisposition has contributed a great deal to our understanding of the biology of tumor cells.

CANCER AS A GENETIC DISEASE

Cancer is a clonal disorder. All cells in a tumor arise from a single cell in which regulatory mechanisms for proliferation have been disrupted. Malignant cells have several qualities that distinguish them from their normal counterparts. They are immortal, often grow more rapidly than normal cells of the same origin, and fail to exhibit normal cell-cell interactions. This latter quality results in their ability to invade and to metastasize and grow in an abnormal cellular environment.[5] The transition from completely normal to frankly malignant occurs through a series of steps or *hits* (e.g., a cell may first acquire one abnormal property, such as immortality, and then become truly malignant when additional abnormal qualities develop) (Fig. 13-1).[6]

Hits are mutations or other alterations of genes involved in regulation of cell growth and cell interactions. They may occur by random chance during DNA synthesis and cell replication, as the result of exposure to environmental carcinogens (chemical mutagens, ultraviolet or ionizing radiation, oncogenic viruses), or they may be inherited as germline mutations. Regardless of the source of the genetic alterations, a cell must acquire two or more hits before becoming malignant, a process that usually takes years to decades in humans.

Several types of genes are involved in carcinogenesis.[5] Normal cell regulation results from a balance between the function of growth-promoting genes and growth-suppressing genes. When the former type of gene is *activated* through amplification or mutation to a hyperfunctioning form, it exerts a positive effect of cell growth. Such genes are known as *oncogenes.* The latter type of gene is known as a *tumor suppressor.* Loss of function of both homologous copies of a tumor suppressor gene has a powerful growth-promoting effect. Loss of just one copy typically has little effect. DNA repair genes are another class that may be mutated in cancer cells and do not clearly fit into the categories of oncogene or tumor suppressor gene.

MECHANISMS OF CANCER PREDISPOSITION

Molecular analysis of inherited cancer susceptibility has elucidated a number of mechanisms by which germline mutations can lead to cancer predisposition. Several categories can be distinguished based on the functional characteristics of the genes

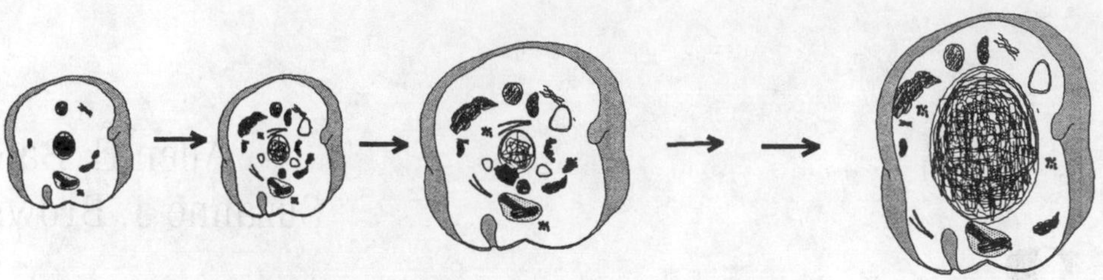

FIGURE 13-1. Carcinogenesis is a multistep process. The transition from completely normal to frankly malignant occurs through a series of mutations in genes that control cell growth and differentiation. Epigenetic phenomena, such as methylation, also play a role. Early hits may have little apparent phenotypic effect, but ultimately growth patterns and cellular morphology are altered.

involved, and additional mechanisms may yet be discovered. The examples that follow use rare genetics defects with a very high risk for cancer to illustrate mechanisms of cancer predisposition. Milder and more common defects in genes belonging to any of these categories may account for a significant portion of cancer risk attributable to hereditary factors.

GERMLINE TUMOR SUPPRESSOR GENE INACTIVATION

Tumor suppressor genes were identified through their role in familial predisposition to cancer. However, these genes are now known to be critically important in growth control of both sporadic and hereditary tumors. It appears that the majority of hereditary cancer predisposition is attributable to germline mutations in tumor suppressor genes. The retinoblastoma gene (RB1) was the first of this class to be isolated.

Retinoblastomas are eye tumors occurring in young children. Most are sporadic, occurring in one eye of children between the ages of 2 and 4 years. In 30% of patients, multiple retinoblastomas arise in one or both eyes and occur before the age of 2 years. Such children often come from families in which retinoblastoma is segregating as an autosomal dominant trait. Based on these observations Knudson[7] proposed that children with hereditary retinoblastoma have inherited a *first genetic hit* that affects every cell in their bodies. Tumors arise from retinoblasts in which a somatic *second hit* has occurred. Given the large number of retinoblasts in a child's eye, it is not surprising that retinoblastomas would arise from multiple cells of predisposed children at an early age. In sporadic retinoblastoma, both hits must occur in a single somatic cell. Because of the much lower probability of two somatic hits, sporadic retinoblastomas are uncommon, occur later in childhood, and are solitary. Knudson did not know the nature of the first and second hits. Mapping and cloning of the retinoblastoma gene proved the two-hit hypothesis and elucidated the nature of tumor suppressor genes.

Clues to the location of the retinoblastoma gene came from studies of the constitutional karyotype of a group of patients with multifocal retinoblastoma plus other physical abnormalities. It was hypothesized that such patients might have an abnormality of one copy of the retinoblastoma gene, but had other genetic defects as well. The simplest explanation for this complex phenotype was an underlying deletion involving the retinoblastoma gene and surrounding genes. A variety of deletions of chromosome 13 were found in such patients, the smallest region of overlap being 13q14 (the cytogenetic study of retinoblastoma tumors might have yielded the same information, but as with many types of cancer, retinoblastoma cells show a great variety of chromosomal defects including but not limited to chromosome 13).

This putative location for the retinoblastoma gene was confirmed by linkage studies in heredity retinoblastoma families.[8] A polymorphic maker, esterase D (ESD), on chromosome 13q14 was shown to map very close to the retinoblastoma locus. In a related study, a patient with bilateral retinoblastoma was described who had half the normal levels of ESD in constitutional tissues but no visible deletion.[9] Presumably, a submicroscopic deletion in one copy of chromosome 13 had eliminated the retinoblastoma gene and the ESD gene. Cytogenetic studies of tumor cells from this patient showed that one copy of chromosome 13 was consistently absent. Biochemical studies of tumors found no ESD activity. Therefore, the first hit in this patient was a constitution deletion involving the retinoblastoma as well as ESD genes. The second hit in tumor cells was loss of the copy of chromosome 13 containing the normal retinoblastoma and ESD homologue. This study indicated that retinoblastomas arise only when both copies of the gene are defective or absent. Several mechanisms for first and second hits have been described.[10] Often the first hit is a point mutation or tiny deletion. The second hit may be loss of the entire homologous chromosome by nondisjunction in mitosis, loss of a portion of the homologous chromosome by deletion, point mutation of the second copy of the gene, or gene conversion through mitotic recombination (Fig. 13-2). An epigenetic mechanism involving methylation of one copy has been shown to play a role in inactivation of other tumor suppressor genes.[11]

The retinoblastoma gene (RB1) was one of the first to be positionally cloned[12] (i.e., the gene was isolated based on its location with no prior knowledge of its sequence). RB1 extends over more than 100 kb of genomic DNA and encodes a nuclear phosphoprotein (pRb),[13] which is constitutively expressed in a large variety of cell types during all phases of the cell cycle. However, its growth-suppressing activity seems to be modulated through varying levels of phosphorylation. It is relatively dephosphorylated during the G_1 phase and phosphorylated during the remainder of the cell cycle. It appears that pRb normally maintains cells in a resting state but can be overcome by signals from the cell-cycle machinery, particularly phosphorylation by cyclin-dependent kinases. The effect of pRb is probably mediated through its ability to bind and sequester several transcription factors. The oncogene products of several DNA tumor viruses function by binding and inactivating the pRb protein. Notably, reintroduction of wild-type RB1 into tumors lacking a functional copy of the gene results in reversion of the tumor cells to a less malignant phenotype.

Homozygous inactivation of RB1 may be sufficient to transform a cell from completely normal to frankly malignant. However, additional genetic changes may enhance the growth and invasiveness of retinoblastoma cells.[2] There is compelling evidence that homozygous inactivation of other tumor suppressors is not sufficient for tumorigenesis (e.g., germline homozygous mutation of the CDKN2 gene[14] does not produce a more severe

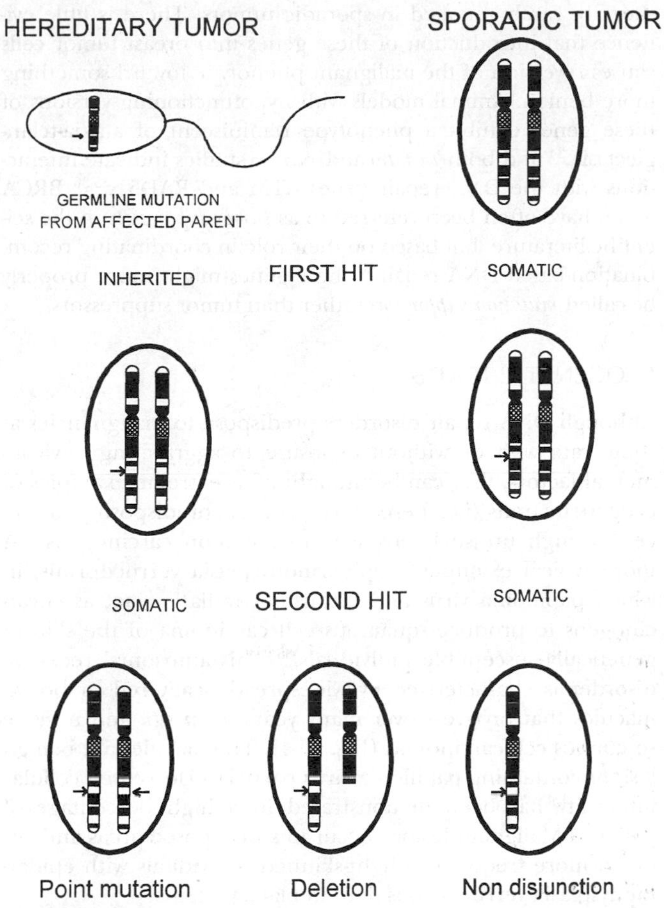

FIGURE 13-2. Germline mutation in a tumor suppressor gene gives cells a head start in multistep carcinogenesis. Homozygous inactivation of the gene in an individual with an inherited mutation requires a single somatic hit. In a normal individual two hits in the same cell are required. In addition to point mutations, gross chromosomal mechanisms such as deletion or nondisjunction may be involved in somatic hits.

phenotype than heterozygous germline mutation). Other alterations must be required for development of tumors or else tumors would be present in every cell of the relevant organs almost from the time of birth.

The RB1 gene is often inactivated in tumors other than retinoblastoma, such as breast cancer, lung cancer, and genitourinary cancer, but it may not play an essential role in regulation of cell growth in many tissue types. Patients with germline mutation of RB1 are prone to osteosarcoma, soft tissue sarcoma, and perhaps melanoma and brain tumors, but not breast, lung, and genitourinary cancers.[15] In the latter group of neoplasms, loss of RB1 may contribute to malignant characteristics, but apparently is not essential to growth control in these tissues.

There is increasing evidence that inactivation of just one homologue of a tumor suppressor gene may have an effect on cell growth and differentiation. In the heterozygous state, mutations in the FAP gene (familial adenomatous polyposis) may promote excessive proliferation of the colon epithelium. A more dramatic effect is seen with heterozygous mutations in the WT1 (Wilms' tumor gene), which lead to congenital anomalies of the genitourinary system.[16,17]

GERMLINE ONCOGENE ACTIVATION

Expression of protooncogenes in normal cells appears to be carefully regulated.[18] Different oncogenes are turned on and off at different steps of the cell cycle, at different stages of embryologic development, and in different cell types. The biochemistry and molecular biology of oncogene function is a rapidly evolving field. In general, protooncogenes function as messengers in the pathway by which external stimuli received at the cell surface lead to DNA synthesis, cell growth, and division. It follows that activating mutations of such genes could lead to abnormal, unrestrained stimulation of cell proliferation in the absence of appropriate signals.

Although activating mutations of oncogenes have for many years been considered as a possible cause of hereditary cancer predisposition, extensive investigations of a wide variety of disorders have until relatively recently yielded no positive results.

The first evidence for *constitutional* (but not germline) activation of an oncogene came from studies of McCune-Albright syndrome,[19] a sporadic disorder characterized by precocious puberty, adenomas of several endocrine tissues, areas of bone dysplasia, and café au lait spots. Many of the endocrine tumors that can be seen in this syndrome were known to arise with activating mutations of the gene encoding a G protein. G proteins resemble ras very closely and are known to function as oncogenes. Analysis of a variety of normal and neoplastic tissues from patients with the syndrome showed that they are all mosaic for activating mutations in the α subunit of the G(s) gene. These mutations are not inherited, but arise somatically at an early stage in embryogenesis.

The first disorders shown to be caused by true germline activation of an oncogene were multiple endocrine neoplasia (MEN) type 2a and MEN 2b.[20–23] These autosomal dominant syndromes are characterized by medullary thyroid carcinoma and pheochromocytoma. MEN 2b has additional features including mucosal neuromas, blubbery lips, and marfanoid habitus; and MEN 2a can be complicated by hyperparathyroidism. The genes for both syndromes were mapped to the centromeric region of chromosome 10, but the related tumors did not show allelic loss at this site, suggesting that a tumor suppressor mechanism did not underlie the cancer predisposition. The ret protooncogene had previously been mapped to the same region as the MEN 2 genes, and analysis of RET revealed mutations in both MEN 2a and MEN 2b kindreds. Ret encodes a transmembrane receptor tyrosine kinase. All MEN 2b cases have the same single base alteration in exon 16, a region responsible for the tyrosine kinase activity of the protein product. Most MEN 2a patients have a mutation in codon 634 in exon 11, but mutations in exon 10 have been identified as well.[24] All of the exon 10 and 11 alterations lead to substitution of another amino acid for the normal cysteine residue in an extracellular region immediately adjacent to the transmembrane domain. There is a strong correlation between hyperparathyroidism and a cysteine to arginine change in codon 634.

That the spectrum of ret mutations is extremely limited and none is a stop signal suggests that they have a specific and probably activating effect on the gene product. Transfection studies show that MEN 2a and MEN 2b mutations can indeed induce transformation of NIH3T3 cells.[25,26] Curiously, inactivating mutations of ret have been shown to cause a completely different disorder, Hirschsprung disease.[27] The main clinical feature is pseudo-obstruction of the colon caused by lack of intestinal parasympathetic ganglia. Apparently ret is required for the proper migration of ganglion precursors during embryogenesis.

Other disorders caused by germline activation of growth-promoting genes include hereditary papillary renal carcinoma (met oncogene)[28] and rare cases of familial melanoma (CDK4).[29]

DNA REPAIR DEFECTS

In the context of cancer as a genetic disease, it is easy to see how disorders involving DNA repair defects would lead to malignancy because failure to repair DNA damage would increase the risk of mutations in cancer-related genes.

A typical disorder of this type is xeroderma pigmentosum, an autosomal recessive disease characterized by extreme photosensitivity, premature aging of skin, and neoplasia of skin and, to a lesser extent, other organs (Fig. 13-3). The molecular basis for this disease is inability to repair the types of DNA damage caused by ultraviolet light. Complementation studies performed by fusing cells from different individuals with xeroderma pigmentosum suggest that there are at least eight different genes for this phenotype (genetic heterogeneity). The genes for several types of xeroderma pigmentosum have been cloned, and their activities include photoproduct binding, helicase, and endonuclease.[30]

Other disorders with faulty DNA repair or replication include ataxia-telangiectasia (x-ray hypersensitivity; defect in a signal transduction protein that mediates multiple responses to DNA damage such as cell-cycle checkpoint control, activation of DNA repair enzymes, and control of programmed cell death),[31,32] Fanconi pancytopenia (sensitivity to DNA cross-linking agents, several genes of unknown function),[1] and Bloom's syndrome (high frequency of spontaneous chromosome breaks, helicase defect).[33] All of these syndromes are rare autosomal recessive disorders associated with an increased risk of cancer.

BRCA1 and BRCA2, which are responsible for approximately 5% of all breast cancers, are important members of this class. Germline mutations in these genes lead to an autosomal dominant syndrome of breast and other cancers. The genes are homozygously inactivated in tumor tissue from patients with germline mutations, but in contrast to typical tumor suppressors they are rarely mutated in sporadic tumors. There is little evidence that introduction of these genes into breast tumor cells causes reversion of the malignant phenotype toward something more benign. Animal models with hypofunctioning versions of these genes exhibit a phenotype reminiscent of ataxia-telangiectasia,[34] and both *in vitro* and *in vivo* studies indicate interactions with the DNA repair genes ATM and RAD51.[35,36] BRCA genes have often been referred to as *tumor suppressors* in the scientific literature, but based on their role in coordinating recombination-based DNA repair,[37] these genes might more properly be called *mutation suppressors* rather than tumor suppressors.

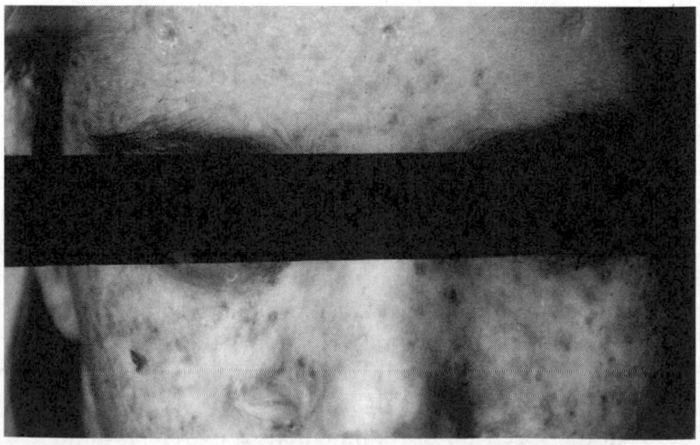

FIGURE 13-3. DNA repair defects accelerate the process of multistep carcinogenesis because alterations in tumor suppressors and oncogenes are not corrected. This 13-year-old girl with xeroderma pigmentosum and severe actinic changes (lentigines, atrophy, and ectropion) has had more than 10 epidermal malignancies. Patients with xeroderma pigmentosum are prone to internal malignancies as well as skin cancer. (Courtesy of Drs. J. DiGiovanna and G. Peck.)

ECOGENETIC TRAITS

Although DNA repair disorders predispose to malignancies at some rate with or without exposure to aggravating environmental factors, they can be thought of as extreme examples of ecogenetic traits (i.e., hereditary disorders predisposing to cancer through unusual sensitivity to common carcinogens). A more typical example is epidermodysplasia verruciformis, in which papilloma virus and ultraviolet radiation act as cocarcinogens to produce squamous cell carcinoma of the skin in genetically susceptible individuals.[38] This autosomal recessive disorder is characterized by widespread, scaly, red or brown macules that progress over many years to *in situ* and invasive squamous cell carcinomas (Fig. 13-4). The macules are benign lesions containing papilloma virus particles. Decreased cellular immunity has been demonstrated in a high percentage of patients. Malignant lesions occur in sun-exposed areas and are much more frequent in light-skinned individuals with epidermodysplasia verruciformis than in black patients.

Genetic factors influencing host responses to environmental carcinogens may contribute to susceptibility to several common cancer types. Lung cancer has a strong association with cigarette smoking, and the risk attributable to hereditary factors is small. Nevertheless, metabolism of the carcinogens in tobacco smoke may be influenced by genetic variation in detoxifying enzymes. Numerous studies have related polymorphisms in CYP1A1, CYP2D6, and CYP2E1 to lung cancer susceptibility.[39] Likewise aflatoxin B_1 exposure contributes to the risk of hepatocellular carcinoma, and genetic variation in epoxide hydrolase (EPHX) may have an important influence on susceptibility to this agent.[40]

ABNORMAL TISSUE ARCHITECTURE

Juvenile polyposis (JPS) is an autosomal dominant disease characterized by hamartomatous polyps and predisposition to colorectal malignancy. JPS can be caused by germline mutations in the PTEN gene on chromosome 10 or the SMAD4 gene on chromosome 18.[41–43] The polyps in JPS are composed primarily of stromal cells among which nests of epithelial cells become trapped. The growth of these epithelial cells in an abnormal environment is probably responsible for dysplasia and eventual neoplasia. Presumably, the genetic alterations that contribute to malignant transformation of epithelial cells are similar to those that occur in any colon tumor. Allelic loss of PTEN has been seen in the nonmalignant, stromal component of juvenile polyps[44] but not in the epithelial component of malignancies that arise in JPS patients. The best interpretation of these data is that the JPS gene sets the stage for accumulation of other genetic alterations.

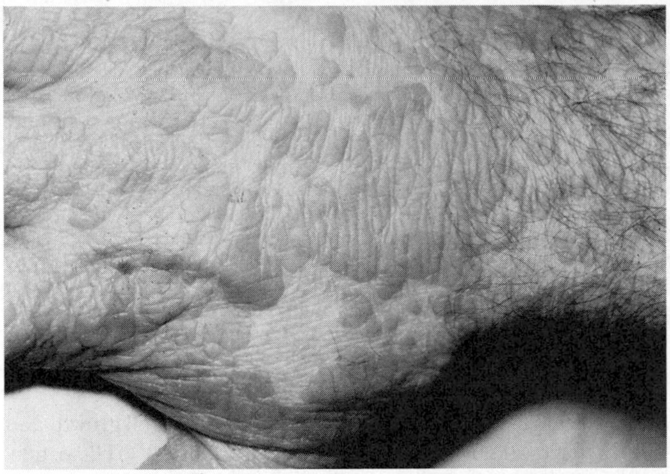

FIGURE 13-4. Benign skin lesions of epidermodysplasia verruciformis. Papilloma virus and ultraviolet light act as cocarcinogens in producing skin cancer in patients with this ecogenetic trait. In the absence of these environmental agents, affected individuals are not predisposed to cancer. (Courtesy of Dr. D. Lowy.)

Another disorder that may follow this model is epidermolysis bullosa dystrophica, a genetically heterogeneous disease characterized by subdermal blistering that results in chronic inflammation and scarring.[45] Aggressive squamous cell carcinoma of the skin is a well-known complication of this disease[46] and probably arises through increased turnover of epidermal cells leading to a risk of genetic alterations during DNA replication. This mechanism is reminiscent of the carcinogenesis that occurs in chronic, nonhealing burn wounds.

HUMORAL TUMOR PROMOTORS AND REPRESSORS

Circulating factors, such as hormones and components of the immune system, may play a role in tumor promotion or progression. Genetic disorders causing immune deficiency or an abnormal hormonal milieu can lead to an increased risk of cancer. Polycystic ovary syndrome, for example, is a common disorder characterized by hyperandrogenism and chronic anovulation. Associated malignancies, related to an abnormal balance between estrogen and androgen and possibly excess luteinizing hormone, include endometrial and ovarian cancer.[47] The etiology of polycystic ovary syndrome is heterogeneous, but several studies support a strong hereditary component.[48,49] Genetic alterations in three genes have been implicated in this disorder including luteinizing hormone, CYP11a (involved in the synthesis of androgens), and the 21-hydroxylase gene (involved in synthesis of many steroids).[50–52]

GATEKEEPERS, CARETAKERS, AND LANDSCAPERS

The term *gatekeepers* has been proposed to describe genes whose function is essential in control of growth and differentiation.[53] Gatekeepers directly prevent the development of tumors by inhibiting growth or promoting terminal differentiation and cell death. In the original gatekeeper concept, it was proposed that each tissue type had one key gene of this type, and mutation of the gatekeeper gene was necessary for the development of tumors. Hence, both sporadic and hereditary tumors would be expected to bear mutations in gatekeepers. RB1 is a gatekeeper gene with tissue specificity primarily for the developing retina, and this gene is mutated in all or nearly all retinoblastomas. Other genes serve this gatekeeper function in other tissue types. For some tissues, either inactivation of a gatekeeper or activation of another member of the same biochemical pathway can lead to malignant transformation. Melanomas, for example, often arise with inactivating mutations in CDKN2A, a negative regulator of cyclin-dependent kinases. An alternate route to melanoma is mutation of cyclin-dependent kinase 4 to an activated form that is resistant to negative regulation by CDKN2A. Both inactivating mutations in CDKN2A and activating mutations in CDK4 can cause hereditary melanoma.[29,54,55] Other examples of tissues that may arise with mutation in a gatekeeper or another member of the same pathway include colon carcinoma[56] and basal cell carcinoma of the skin.[57] Germline mutation of a gatekeeper leads to a risk of cancer at least 100 times greater than that in the general population.

Caretaker genes are involved in DNA repair and maintenance of genomic integrity. Inactivation of a caretaker does not directly promote tumor formation, but facilitates the development of mutations in gatekeeper genes and other cancer-related genes. Caretakers, like gatekeepers, may be tissue specific, but mutation in a caretaker is neither necessary nor sufficient for the development of cancer. The risk of cancer is modestly elevated in syndromes caused by germline caretaker mutations, and sporadic tumors rarely have mutations in these genes. BRCA1 is an example of a gene in this class.

Landscaper genes,[58] such as the genes for JPS, also act indirectly to cause cancer. Mutations in these genes lead to tissue dysplasia, but are not necessary for the development of cancer and are rarely seen in sporadic tumors.

CLINICAL CHARACTERISTICS OF CANCER FAMILIES

The hallmarks of hereditary cancer are relatively early age of onset compared with similar sporadic tumors, multiple and bilateral tumors, and a family history of cancer. Some cancer predisposition syndromes also include birth defects or other distinctive physical features. An underlying hereditary disorder should be considered when rare tumor types are encountered because a significant percentage of certain rare cancers are attributable to genetic factors (e.g., retinoblastoma). The same applies to cancers that are common in one gender occurring in the other gender (e.g., male breast cancer).[59]

Because the genes that underlie hereditary cancer predisposition may be important in a variety of tissues, germline mutation may lead to multisystem disease. The production of multiple phenotypic effects by a single mutant gene is called *pleiotropy*.[60] Often different members of a single kindred have different manifestations of the same genetic defect, a phenomenon known as *variable expressivity* (Fig. 13-5). Development of cancer is a multistep process involving two or more independent events. There is always some probability that no cell in a genetically cancer-prone individual will suffer sufficient somatic hits to become neoplastic. In this event a gene carrier could escape all manifestations of disease and be a *nonpenetrant* carrier. Virtually all adult-onset cancer predisposition syndromes have age-dependent penetrance

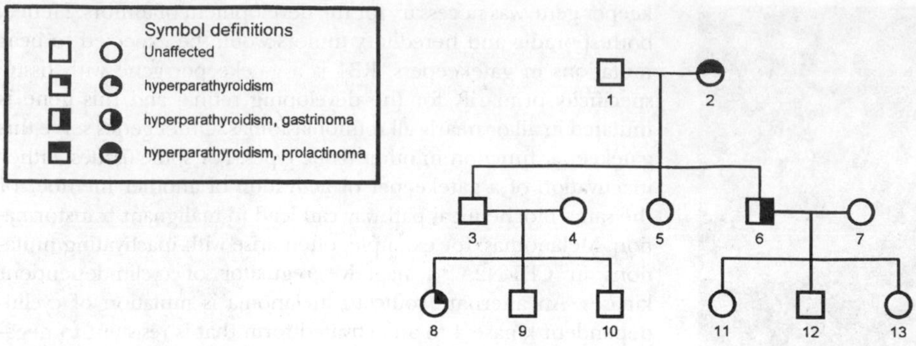

FIGURE 13-5. Multiple endocrine neoplasia type 1 is an autosomal dominant disorder characterized by parathyroid, pancreatic islet, and pituitary tumors. This kindred demonstrates nonpenetrance (individual 3 is an obligate gene carrier because his mother and daughter are affected, yet he has no signs of the disease) and variable expressivity (the three affected individuals have different constellations of neoplasia). Typically, few individuals in the younger generations have signs of the disorder because multistep carcinogenesis may take years to decades even with one inherited hit.

because the probability of accumulating sufficient hits to develop cancer increases with age. Presumably nonpenetrant carriers would develop cancer if they lived long enough.

In addition to the effects of random chance, perhaps coupled with environmental exposures, penetrance may be influenced by modifying genes. For example, women who carry a mutation in the BRCA1 gene have a risk of ovarian cancer in the range of 30%. Why do some BRCA1 carriers get ovarian cancer whereas others do not? Common variants in the HRAS gene appear to influence susceptibility to this malignancy. Women with both a BRCA1 mutation and an unfavorable HRAS variant are twice as likely to get ovarian cancer as those without the variant. Susceptibility to breast cancer is not affected by the presence of these unfavorable variants.[61]

MULTISYSTEM GENETIC SYNDROMES WITH A HIGH RISK OF CANCER

Many disorders involving cancer predisposition are characterized by a distinctive pattern of neoplasia involving several different organs or neoplasia plus unusual physical features. These genetic *syndromes* often can be definitively diagnosed on the basis of medical and family history plus astute physical examination. Hereditary retinoblastoma/osteosarcoma, MEN 2, and xeroderma pigmentosum fall into this group. Several other syndromes are worth mentioning because they are fairly frequent or are responsible for a significant proportion of certain rare tumors.

NEUROFIBROMATOSIS TYPE 1

Neurofibromatosis type 1 (NF1) is an autosomal dominant disorder affecting approximately 1 in 3000 individuals. The defining clinical features are café au lait spots of the skin, benign Schwann cell tumors known as *neurofibromas,* and hamartomas of the iris known as *Lisch nodules.* Other manifestations include macrocephaly, segmental hypertrophy, bone dysplasia leading to pseudoarthrosis, learning disability, and seizures. A variety of CNS tumors occur to excess including optic gliomas, astrocytomas, and meningiomas. Malignant tumors such as neurofibrosarcomas, pheochromocytomas, and leukemia are also part of this syndrome.[62]

The gene for this disease was mapped to chromosome 17 in 1987[63,64] and was cloned in 1990.[65,66] Its function involves interaction with the ras oncogene product.[67–69] Ras proteins have a role in growth regulation through adenylate cyclase activation. They are homologous to G proteins and like G proteins they bind guanosine triphosphate (GTP) in response to signals from cell surface. The GTP-bound form is active in promoting cell growth and slowly inactivates itself by hydrolyzing the bound GTP to guanosine diphosphate. The latter function is influenced by another protein known as the GTPase-activating protein. It follows that homozygous inactivation of the GTPase-activating protein would result in unrestrained stimulation of adenylate cyclase by the activated ras protein. Portions of the NF gene are highly homologous to GTPase-activating protein. Presumably the normal function of this gene is to negatively regulate cell stimulation by the ras gene product or similar growth-promoting proteins. In both benign and malignant tumors related to neurofibromatosis, the NF1 gene is homozygously inactivated.[70,71] Other features of the syndrome could be due to haploinsufficiency (i.e., loss of just one copy of the gene may produce abnormalities in some tissues).

No single clinical feature is sufficient for diagnosis of NF1; in particular, many individuals without NF1 have one or more café au lait spots. Until a valid, gene-based test becomes available, the clinical criteria proposed by the 1988 National Institutes of Health Consensus Development Conference[72] should be used. The life expectancy of patients with NF1 is reduced due to malignant complications,[73] and suggested clinical management includes annual evaluation of blood pressure, skin examination, neurologic evaluation, and ophthalmologic examination.[74] In addition, children should be checked for growth and development, with particular attention to learning disability, sexual maturation, skeletal abnormalities, and speech.

NEUROFIBROMATOSIS TYPE 2

Neurofibromatosis type 2 (NF2) shares with NF1 several characteristics including café au lait spots, skin neurofibromas, and an autosomal dominant mode of inheritance. The defining feature of this syndrome, however, is bilateral vestibular schwannomas (previously called *acoustic neuromas*). Schwannomas of other cranial nerves and spinal nerve roots, meningiomas, and retinal hamartomas are also seen. Cataracts, particularly the posterior capsular type, are common. NF2 is far less common than NF1, with a prevalence of approximately 1 in 35,000.[75] The gene for NF2 is related to the ezrin family of proteins that link the cell cytoskeleton to cell membrane proteins, and its mode of action is not fully understood.[76]

The diagnosis of NF2 should be considered in patients with bilateral vestibular schwannomas, unilateral schwannoma before the age of 40, or meningioma and any other feature of the syndrome. In the setting of a family history of NF2, DNA-based testing of at-risk individuals is recommended.[77] Recommended follow-up studies in gene carriers include gadolinium-enhanced magnetic resonance imaging to detect early spine and CNS tumors. In the case of vestibular schwannomas, surgical removal of small tumors can preserve some useful hearing.[78]

HEREDITARY WILMS' TUMOR AND RELATED SYNDROMES

On the order of 1% of Wilms' tumor cases occur in a familial setting, following an autosomal dominant inheritance pattern with incomplete penetrance.[79] Twenty percent of familial cases and 3% of sporadic cases are bilateral, consistent with a two-hit model for development of this neoplasm.[80] Rare cases have, in addition to Wilms' tumor, aniridia, hemihypertrophy, genitourinary anomalies, and mental retardation (WAGR syndrome)[81]; and cytogenetic analysis has revealed deletions of chromosome 11p13 in such patients.[82,83] The WAGR complex qualifies as a *contiguous gene syndrome* (i.e., the multiple features are caused by loss of more than one gene). Denys-Drash syndrome involves Wilms' tumor, genitourinary abnormalities similar to those in WAGR, pseudohermaphroditism, and nephropathy[84,85] without aniridia or mental retardation; and no chromosome abnormality has been identified.

The Wilms' tumor gene on chromosome 11p13 was isolated by positional cloning, and encodes a zinc finger protein[86,87] possibly involved in transcriptional regulation of insulin-like growth factor-2 (IGF-2) and a variety of other growth factors. Additional motifs in the gene may have a role in RNA processing.[88] During development WT1 is expressed specifically in the developing kidney and the genital ridge and fetal gonad, and point mutations in WT1 are capable of causing the genitourinary abnormalities seen in the WAGR syndrome and Denys-Drash syndrome.[16,17] It seems clear that there is not a separate gene for the *G* part of the WAGR syndrome, although there is a separate gene for aniridia and almost certainly for mental retardation.

WT1 mutations are not the only cause of genetic predisposition to Wilms' tumor.[79] Beckwith-Wiedemann syndrome, which maps to chromosome 11p15, is characterized by a high frequency of Wilms' tumor. Other features of this disorder are large size at birth, disproportionately large tongue, omphalocele, and linear creases in the earlobe. Several families have been described in which the gene causing predisposition to Wilms' tumor maps to neither chromosome 11p13 nor 11p15.

There is no clear consensus on appropriate screening studies in children at risk for Wilms' tumor.[89–91] Computed tomographic scanning is superior to ultrasound in detecting early tumors. However, the low cost and lack of radiation exposure make ultrasound an attractive option for serial studies. Magnetic resonance imaging may prove useful as a high-quality imaging tool that does not involve radiation exposure. In practice, abdominal ultrasound at 3- to 6-month intervals is the most common screening method. The exact duration of screening is variable, but most tumors in genetically predisposed individuals occur between birth and the age of 5.

LI-FRAUMENI SYNDROME

In 1968, Miller[92] analyzed 21,659 death certificates of U.S. children who died of cancer and found an excess mortality from sarcomas and brain tumors in siblings. To pursue the observation, Li and Fraumeni[93] reviewed several hundred hospital charts of children with rhabdomyosarcoma. There were four families with multiple childhood sarcomas occurring in association with other childhood cancers and early-onset breast cancer. Subsequent studies established an autosomal dominant pattern of occurrence of at least six tumors: premenopausal breast cancer and childhood soft tissue sarcomas, osteosarcoma, brain tumors, adrenal cortical carcinomas, and acute leukemia.[94] Similar familial aggregates were identified by Strong[95,96] and Birch and colleagues[97] through studies of hospital-based and population-based series of childhood sarcomas, respectively. Segregation analyses suggested that 50% of carriers in affected families would develop cancer by 35 years of age and 90% by age 70.[97] Penetrance appears to be higher in female subjects, who are at risk of breast cancer in adulthood. Patients who survive cancer are prone to develop second primary neoplasms, often within the field of prior radiotherapy.[94]

In 1990, germline mutations in the p53 tumor suppressor gene were identified in five families with Li-Fraumeni syndrome, and the observation was soon confirmed by several groups.[98] In addition, germline p53 mutations have been identified in a small fraction of unselected patients with early-onset multiple primary cancers, multifocal brain tumors, childhood sarcoma, and childhood adrenal cortical carcinoma.[99–101] However, less than 1% of breast cancer patients have germline p53 mutations. The germline p53 mutational spectrum is similar to that for somatic p53 mutations in sporadic cancers and tends to occur in exons 5 through 9.[102] Germline p53 mutations have not been detected in a substantial minority of Li-Fraumeni families, suggesting that other genes might produce the syndrome.[103] Genetic heterogeneity is also indicated by exclusion of linkage to p53 for at least one affected family.[104]

When germline p53 mutations were identified, the possibility of predictive testing to identify unaffected carriers became feasible. However, the risks and benefits of predictive testing for a syndrome of multiple cancers are unknown. In particular, early detection at a curable stage is problematic for the component cancers of this syndrome.[105] Several small research programs of predictive genetic testing for p53 mutations have been offered to adults in families with a known alteration. Lessons from p53 testing may be useful in developing testing programs for more common inherited susceptibility genes for breast and colon cancer.[106,107]

NEVOID BASAL CELL CARCINOMA SYNDROME

The nevoid basal cell carcinoma syndrome (NBCC), also known as *Gorlin syndrome* and the *basal cell nevus syndrome,* is an autosomal dominant disorder that predisposes to basal cell carcinomas of the skin, medulloblastomas, and ovarian fibromas.[108] Its prevalence has been estimated at 1 per 56,000, and 1% to 2% of medulloblastomas and 0.5% of basal cell carcinomas are attributable to the syndrome.[109,110] Other neoplasms that probably occur to excess include fibrosarcomas, meningiomas, rhabdomyosarcomas, and cardiac fibromas.

In addition to benign and malignant tumors, malformations are a striking component. The syndrome is associated with pits of the palms and soles, keratocysts of the jaw and other dental malformations, cleft palate, characteristic coarse facies, strabismus, dysgenesis of the corpus callosum, calcification of the falx cerebri, spina bifida occulta and other spine anomalies, bifid ribs and other rib anomalies, ectopic calcification, mesenteric cysts, macrocephaly, and generalized overgrowth.[111–113]

The NBCC gene was mapped to chromosome 9[114–116] and the demonstration that the exact same region is deleted in a high percentage of sporadic basal cell carcinomas and other tumors related to the disorder provided strong evidence that the gene functions as a tumor suppressor. Positional cloning identified a human homologue of Drosophila patched as the gene for this syndrome,[117] and subsequent studies showed that patched is mutated in a high percentage of sporadic basal cell carcinomas.[118] Patched is a negative regulator of the hedgehog pathway, several members of which are known to function as oncogenes in skin and brain tumors. Mutation of patched may be a necessary if not sufficient step in basal cell carcinoma development. Minute basal cell carcinomas are as likely as large tumors to have patched mutations, and all histologic subtypes, whether primary or recurrent, have a high frequency of loss of patched. Tumors with allelic loss on chromosome 9 sometimes show additional areas of loss on other chromosomes, but no tumors have loss on other chromosomes without involvement of chromosome 9.[114] Patched appears to function as a gatekeeper gene in the epidermal cell type from which basal cell carcinomas arise.[119]

In contrast to many other disorders caused by tumor suppressors congenital anomalies are a prominent feature of NBCC. One hypothesis to explain at least some of these anomalies is a two-hit mechanism in which a single fetal or embryonic cell that has lost the normal copy of the gene gives rise to a developmentally abnormal clone.[120] However, other symmetric generalized features of the syndrome (e.g., overgrowth, corpus callosum defects) suggest that loss of just one copy of the NBCC gene exerts an effect on growth and differentiation.

The diagnosis of NBCC should be considered in anyone below the age of 30 with a single basal cell carcinoma and in older individuals with multiple basal cell carcinomas. Medulloblastoma, keratocysts of the jaw, and typical skeletal anomalies should raise the suspicion of NBCC regardless of the presence or absence of basal cell carcinomas. Palmar and plantar pits are pathognomonic. DNA-based testing is available for individuals at risk with a family history of NBCC and for sporadic patients as well. The most important follow-up study in affected individuals is dermatologic examination for basal cell carcinomas at intervals of 6 months to 1 year. Yearly dental examinations, with particular attention to the possibility of jaw cysts, are also recommended. Because the frequency of medulloblastoma in this syndrome probably does not exceed 5% and may be as low as 1%, screening studies for this tumor type in children are controversial.[111,113]

TWO MECHANISMS LEADING TO FAMILIAL COLON CANCER

Familial aggregation of carcinomas of the colon and rectum have been reported in multiple studies in the literature.[121] Close relatives of an affected individual have approximately twofold increased risk of the disease.[122] Risk increases with the number of affected members in the kindred. Some families develop colo rectal carcinoma in an autosomal dominant pattern, strongly suggesting the influence of highly penetrant gene(s).

Familial adenomatous polyposis (FAP) was the first hereditary colorectal cancer syndrome to be clinically recognized. The inheritance pattern is autosomal dominant, and the disorder accounts for approximately 1% of colorectal carcinoma. Affected individuals develop hundreds to thousands of colonic adenomas by the second decade, and almost all develop colorectal carcinomas by age 45.[123] FAP carries a substantial risk for small intestine and gastric adenomas with a 5% lifetime risk of small bowel or gastric carcinoma.[124] Although most families develop only polyposis and cancer of the colon and rectum, others have associated osteomas of the jaw and skull, fibromas of the skin, and benign and malignant tumors of the ampulla of Vater and stomach (Gardner's syndrome). In addition, polyposis coli has been reported in association with brain tumors, a condition called *Turcot's syndrome.* The association of brain tumors and colon cancer without polyps has also been termed *Turcot's syndrome* but is genetically distinct.[125]

Early efforts to identify the gene for adenomatous polyposis coli (APC) were unrevealing. Eventually, a case report of a patient with mental retardation, multiple congenital anomalies, adenomatous polyposis of the colon, and a chromosome 5 deletion localized the APC gene to the long arm of chromosome 5(5q).[126] In 1991, the APC gene was cloned and shown to have the characteristics of a tumor suppressor gene.[127,128] APC promotes the degradation of the β-catenin, which can function as an oncoprotein in colon carcinoma.[57] Most APC germline mutations yield a truncated protein product, and correlations have been found between size of the APC protein and phenotype.[129] Mutations in the 5'(proximal) end of the gene result in small protein products and attenuated manifestations of polyposis coli. Pigmented lesions in the eye (congenital hypertrophy of retinal pigment epithelium) in polyposis cases are associated with APC mutations clustering around exons 10 through 14.[130] An APC mutational *hot spot* is at codon 1309 (exon 15), and mutations in this region are associated with larger numbers of polyps of early onset.[131] These patients have poor prognoses for survival when compared with those with mutations at other APC sites. I1307K, a common variant among Ashkenazi Jews, causes genetic instability in the APC gene and a tendency toward somatic mutations.[132] This variant is associated with a small increase in the risk of colorectal cancer and possibly an increased risk of other types of cancer as well,[133] but not with large numbers of colon polyps. A role for clinical testing for this mutation is not established.

The other major form of hereditary colorectal cancer is hereditary nonpolyposis colorectal cancer (HNPCC). In this autosomal dominant disorder, the colon is not carpeted with polyps, but the lifetime risk of colon cancer is still very high. Other tumor types that occur in this syndrome include carcinomas of the endometrium, stomach, ovary, small bowel, pancreas, hepatobiliary tract, ureter, and renal pelvis.[134] Muir-Torre syndrome is a variant of HNPCC with sebaceous adenomas, carcinomas, and keratoacanthomas.[135] Because colorectal carcinoma is common in the general population, familial aggregates of two or three cases might be caused by chance association or shared environmental influences. The International Collaborative Group on HNPCC has proposed that the diagnosis be based on the following findings (called the *Amsterdam criteria*): three or more relatives with histologically diagnosed colorectal cancer, of whom one is a first-degree relative to the other two; cancers involve at least two generations; at least one case diagnosed before age 50; and exclusion of FAP.[136]

In 1993, an HNPCC gene was mapped to the short arm of chromosome 2 (2p16).[137] Simultaneously, two studies described widespread genetic instability in short repeated DNA markers (microsatellites) in cancers of the proximal colon, particularly within tumors of familial cases.[138,139] The widespread genetic instability raised the possibility that the inherited defect in HNPCC might involve mutations in mismatch repair genes that had been well characterized in yeast and *Escherichia coli.* Fishel and associates cloned several human homologues of yeast mismatch repair genes, and found that MSH2 is mapped to human chromosome 2p.[140] They then demonstrated inherited MSH2 mutations in several families with HNPCC. Using a second approach, positional cloning, Leach and colleagues independently demonstrated MSH2 as the colon cancer gene on chromosome 2.[141] Within months, a second HNPCC gene, MLH1, was mapped to the short arm of chromosome 3 and cloned.[142,143] MSH2 and MLH1 account for the large percentage of HNPCC families including cases of Muir-Torre syndrome. Other genes that can cause HNPCC include MSH6 and PMS1 and PMS2, which are homologous to *E coli* MUTL and yeast PMS1.[144,145] Mutations in mismatch repair genes are found in a high percentage of families that conform to the Amsterdam criteria, particularly if endometrial cancer is present in the family as well as colon cancer.[136]

Management of hereditary colon cancer involves surveillance and preventive treatment of affected patients for colonic and extracolonic cancers, counseling of patients and their families, and presymptomatic diagnostic testing of at-risk family members.[146–148] In FAP, prophylactic colectomy is recommended in all affected patients during the second or third decade. Regular endoscopic checkup of the upper gastrointestinal tract is necessary to detect malignant transformation of duodenal and gastric polyps. For HNPCC patients, only preventive measures such as regular colonoscopic and gynecologic examinations are recommended. Prophylactic colectomy or hysterectomy are not considered to be routine procedures at present. On a research basis, trials of chemopreventive agents are under way. Substances being explored in colorectal cancer prevention include (1) the nonsteroidal antiinflammatory drugs, which inhibit the formation and evolution of adenomas in animal models presumably by their inhibition of cyclooxygenase and prostaglandin synthesis; and (2) antioxidants, such as vitamin E or C, which may modulate carcinogenic substances and correlate with lower colon cancer risk in epidemiologic studies. Dietary intervention with decreased fat intake and increased fiber consumption has also been linked to a lower incidence of colon cancer in epidemiologic studies.[149]

NONSYNDROMIC HEREDITARY CANCER

In the absence of a characteristic pattern of neoplasia or neoplasia plus developmental defects, diagnosis of hereditary cancer predisposition is far more difficult than in the case of a distinctive genetic syndrome. Nevertheless, a family history of cancer, early age of onset, and multiple primaries strongly suggests an underlying genetic disorder, particularly in the absence of known carcinogen exposure. Laboratory testing for mutations in cancer predisposition genes will become increasingly important for diagnosis of site-specific, nonsyndromic cancer. Evaluation of patients with isolated, site-specific cancer predisposition is discussed elsewhere in this book.

REFERENCES

1. *Online Mendelian Inheritance in Man,* OMIM(TM). The Human Genome Data Base Project, Johns Hopkins University, Baltimore, MD. World Wide Web URL: http://gdb-www.gdb.org/omim/docs/omimtop.html, 1995.
2. Haber DA, Housman DE. Rate-limiting steps: the genetics of pediatric cancers [Review]. *Cell* 1991;64:5.
3. Marx J. New colon cancer gene discovered. *Science* 1993; 260:751.
4. Scotto J, Fraumeni JF. Skin (other than melanoma). In: Schottenfeld D, Fraumeni JF, eds. *Cancer epidemiology and prevention.* Philadelphia: WB Saunders, 1982:254.
5. Bishop JM. Molecular themes in oncogenesis. *Cell* 1991;64:235.
6. Vogelstein B, Kinzler KW. The multistep nature of cancer. *Trends Genet* 1993;9:138.
7. Knudson AG. Mutation and cancer: statistical study of retinoblastoma. *Proc Natl Acad Sci U S A* 1971;68:820.
8. Sparkes RS, Murphree AL, Lingua RW, et al. Gene for hereditary retinoblastoma assigned to human chromosome 13 by linkage to esterase D. *Science* 1983;219:971.
9. Benedict WF, Murphree AL, Banerjee A, et al. Patient with 13 chromosome deletion: evidence that the retinoblastoma gene is a recessive cancer gene. *Science* 1983;219:973.
10. Cavenee WK, Dryja TP, Phillips RA. Expression of recessive alleles by chromosomal mechanisms in retinoblastoma. *Nature* 1983;305:779.
11. Laird PW, Jackson-Grusby L, Fazeli A, et al. Suppression of intestinal neoplasia by DNA hypomethylation. *Cell* 1995;81:197.
12. Friend SH, Bernards R, Rogel S, et al. A human DNA segment with properties of the gene that predisposes to retinoblastoma and osteosarcoma. *Nature* 1986;323:643.
13. Weinberg RA. The retinoblastoma protein and cell cycle control [Review]. *Cell* 1995; 81:323.
14. Gruis NA, Vandervelden PA, Sandkuijl LA, et al. Homozygotes for CDKN2 (P16) germline mutation in Dutch familial melanoma kindreds. *Nat Genet* 1995;10:351.
15. Eng C, Li FP, Abramson DH, et al. Mortality from second tumors among long-term survivors of retinoblastoma. *J Natl Cancer Inst* 1993;85:1121.
16. Pelletier J, Bruening W, Kashtan CE, et al. Germline mutations in the Wilms' tumor suppressor gene are associated with abnormal urogenital development in Denys-Drash syndrome. *Cell* 1991;67:437.
17. Pelletier J, Bruening W, Li FP, et al. WT1 mutations contribute to abnormal genital system development and hereditary Wilms' tumour. *Nature* 1991;353:431.
18. Cantley LC, Auger KR, Carpenter C, et al. Oncogenes and signal transduction. *Cell* 1991;64:281.
19. Weinstein LS, Shenker A, Gejman PV, et al. Activating mutations of the stimulatory G protein in the McCune-Albright syndrome. *N Engl J Med* 1991;325:1688.
20. Mulligan LM, Kwok JB, Healey CS, et al. Germ-line mutations of the RET proto-oncogene in multiple endocrine neoplasia type 2A. *Nature* 1993;363:458.
21. Donis-Keller H, Sou S, Chi D, et al. Mutations in the RET proto-oncogene are associated with MEN 2A and FMTC. *Hum Mol Genet* 1993;2:851.
22. Hofstra RMW, Landsvater RM, Ceccherini I, et al. A mutation in the RET proto-oncogene associated with multiple endocrine neoplasia type 2B and sporadic medullary thyroid carcinoma. *Nature* 1994;367:375.
23. Carlson KM, Dou S, Chi D, et al. Single missense mutation in the tyrosine kinase catalytic domain of the RET protooncogene is associated with multiple endocrine neoplasia type 2B. *Proc Natl Accad Sci U S A* 1994;91:1579.
24. Mulligan LM, Eng C, Healey CS, et al. Specific mutations of the RET proto-oncogene are related to disease phenotype in MEN 2A and FMTC. *Nat Genet* 1994;6:70.
25. Santoro M, Carlomagno F, Romano A, et al. Activation of RET as a dominant transforming gene by germline mutations of MEN2A and MEN2B. *Science* 1995;267:381.
26. Asai N, Iwashita T, Matsuyama M, Takahashi M. Mechanism of activation of the ret proto-oncogene by multiple endocrine neoplasia 2A mutations. *Mol Cell Biol* 1995;15:1613.
27. van Heyningen V. One gene—four syndromes. *Nature* 1994;367:319.
28. Schmidt L, Duh FM, Chen F, et al. Germline and somatic mutations in the tyrosine kinase domain of the MET proto-oncogene in papillary renal carcinomas. *Nat Genet* 1997;16:68.
29. Zuo L, Weger J, Yang Q, et al. Germline mutations in the p16INK4a binding domain of CDK4 in familial melanoma. *Nat Genet* 1996;12:97.
30. Cleaver JE. It was a very good year for DNA repair [Review]. *Cell* 1994;76:1.
31. Savitsky K, Bar-Shira A, Gilad S, et al. A single ataxia telangiectasia gene with a product similar to Pl-3 kinase. *Science* 1995;268:1749.
32. Meyn MS. Ataxia-telangiectasia and cellular responses to DNA damage. *Cancer Res* 1995;55:5991.
33. Ellis NA, Groden J, Ye TZ, et al. The Bloom's syndrome gene product is homologous to RecQ helicases. *Cell* 1995;83:1.
34. Shen SX, Weaver Z, Xu X, et al. A targeted disruption of the murine Brca1 gene causes gamma-irradiation hypersensitivity and genetic instability. *Oncogene* 1998;17:3115.
35. Scully R, Chen J, Plug A, et al. Association of BRCA1 with RAD51 in mitotic and meiotic cells. *Cell* 1997;88:265.
36. Gowen LC, Avrutskaya AV, Latour AM, et al. BRCA1 required for transcription-coupled repair of oxidative DNA damage. *Science* 1998;281:1009.
37. Moynahan ME, Chiu JW, Koller BH, et al. Brca1 controls homology-directed DNA repair. *Mol Cell* 1999;4:511.
38. Jablonska S, Orth G, Jarzabek-Chorzelska M, et al. Twenty-one years of follow-up studies of familial epidermodysplasia verruciformis. *Dermatologica* 1979;158:309.
39. Rannug A, Alexandrie AK, Persson I, et al. Genetic polymorphism of cytochromes P450 1A1, 2D6, and 2E1: regulation and toxicological signficance. *J Occup Environ Med* 1995;37:25.
40. McGlynn KA, Rosvold EA, Lustbader ED, et al. Susceptibility to hepatocellular carcinoma is associated with genetic variation in the enzymatic detoxification of aflatoxin B1. *Proc Natl Acad Sci U S A* 1995;92:2384.
41. Olschwang S, Serova-Sinilnikova M, Lenoir GM, et al. *PTEN* germline mutations in juvenile polyposis coli. *Nat Genet* 1998;18:12.
42. Howe JR, Roth S, Ringold JC, et al. Mutations in the *SMAD4/DPC4* gene in juvenile polyposis. *Science* 1998;280:1086.
43. Lynch ED, Ostemeyer EA, Lee MK, et al. Inherited mutations in PTEN that are associated with breast cancer, Cowden disease, and juvenile polyps. *Am J Hum Genet* 1997;61:1254.
44. Jacoby RF, Schlack S, Cole CE, et al. A juvenile polyposis tumor suppressor locus at 10q22 is deleted from nonepithelial cells in the lamina propria. *Gastroenterology* 1997;112:1398.

45. Uitto J, Pulkkinen L, McLean WH. Epidermolysis bullosa: a spectrum of clinical phenotypes explained molecular heterogeneity. *Mol Med Today* 1997;3:457.
46. Reed WB, College J, Francis MJO, et al. Epidermolysis bullosa dystrophica with epidermal neoplasms. *Arch Dermatol* 1974;110:894.
47. Schildkraut JM, Schwingl PJ, Bastos E, et al. Epithelial ovarian cancer risk among women with polycystic ovary syndrome. *Obstet Gynecol* 1996;88:554.
48. Legro RS, Driscoll D, Strauss JF 3rd, et al. Evidence for a genetic basis for hyperandrogenemia in polycystic ovary syndrome. *Proc Natl Acad Sci U S A* 1998;95:14956.
49. Govind A, Obhrai MS, Clayton RN. Polycystic ovaries are inherited as an autosomal dominant trait: analysis of 20 polycystic ovary syndrome and 10 control families. *J Clin Endocrinol Metab* 1999;84:38.
50. Azziz R, Slayden SM. The 21-hydroxylase-deficient adrenal hyperplasias: more than ACTH oversecretion. *J Soc Gynecol Invest* 1996;3:297.
51. Gharani N, Waterworth DM, Batty S, et al. Association of the steroid synthesis gene CYP11a with polycystic ovary syndrome and hyperandrogenism. *Hum Mol Genet* 1997;6:397.
52. Tapanainen JS, Koivunen R, Fauser BC, et al. A new contributing factor to polycystic ovary syndrome: the genetic variant of luteinizing hormone. *J Clin Endocrinol Metab* 1999;84:1711.
53. Kinzler KW, Vogelstein B. Gatekeepers and caretakers. *Nature* 1997;386:761.
54. Hussussian CJ, Struewing JP, Goldstein AM, et al. Germline p16 mutations in familial melanoma. *Nat Genet* 1994;8:15.
55. Kamb A, Gruis NA, Weaver-Feldhaus J, et al. A cell cycle regulator potentially involved in genesis of many tumor types. *Science* 1994;264:436.
56. Morin PJ, Sparks AB, Korinek V, et al. Activation of beta-catenin-tcf signaling in colon cancer by mutations in beta-catenin or APC. *Science* 1997;275:1787.
57. Xie J, Murone M, Luoh SM, et al. Activating Smoothened mutations in sporadic basal-cell carcinoma. *Nature* 1998;391:90.
58. Kinzler KW, Vogelstein B. Landscaping the cancer terrain. *Science* 1998;280:1036.
59. Everson RB, Fraumeni JF Jr, Wilson RE, et al. Familial male breast cancer. *Lancet* 1976;1:9.
60. Thompson MW, McInnes RR, Willard HF, eds. *Genetics in medicine.* 5th ed. Philadelphia: WB Saunders, 1991.
61. Phelan CM, Rebbeck TR, Weber BL, et al. Ovarian cancer risk in BRCA1 carriers is modified by the HRAS1 variable number of tandem repeat (VNTR) locus. *Nat Genet* 1996; 12:309.
62. Riccardi VM. Von Recklinghausen neurofibromatosis. *N Engl J Med* 1981;305:1617.
63. Seizinger BR, Rouleau GA, Ozelius LJ, et al. Genetic linkage of von Recklinghausen neurofibromatosis to the nerve growth factor receptor gene. *Cell* 1987;49:589.
64. Barker D, Wright E, Nguyen K, et al. Gene for von Recklinghausen neurofibromatosis is in the pericentromeric region of chromosome 17. *Science* 1987;236:1100.
65. Wallace MR, Marchuk DA, Andersen LB, et al. Type 1 neurofibromatosis gene: identification of a large transcript disrupted in three NF1 patients. *Science* 1990;249:181.
66. Cawthon RM, Weiss R, Xu GF, et al. A major segment of the neurofibromatosis type 1 gene: cDNA sequence, genomic structure, and point mutations. *Cell* 1990;62:193.
67. Xu GF, Lin B, Tanaka K, et al. The catalytic domain of the neurofibromatosis type 1 gene product stimulates ras GTPase and complements ira mutants of S. cerevisiae. *Cell* 1990;63:835.
68. Buchberg AM, Cleveland LS, Jenkins NA, et al. Sequence homology shared by neurofibromatosis type-1 gene and IRA-1 and IRA-2 negative regulators of the RAS cyclic AMP pathway. *Nature* 1990;347:291.
69. Ballester R, Marchuk D, Boguski M, et al. The NF1 locus encodes a protein functionally related to mammalian GAP and yeast IRA proteins. *Cell* 1990;63:851.
70. Colman SD, Williams CA, Wallace MR. Benign neurofibromas in type 1 neurofibromatosis (NF1) show somatic deletions of the NF1 gene. *Nat Genet* 1995;11:90.
71. Glover TW, Stein CK, Legius E, et al. Molecular and cytogenetic analysis of tumors in von Recklinghausen neurofibromatosis. *Genes Chromosomes Cancer* 1991;3:62.
72. National Institutes of Health (NIH) Consensus Development Conference Statement: neurofibromatosis. *Neurofibromatosis* 1988;1:172.
73. Sorensen SA, Mulvihill JJ, Nielsen A. Long-term follow-up of von Recklinghausen neurofibromatosis: survival and malignant neoplasms. *N Engl J Med* 1986;314:1010.
74. Committee on Genetics. Health supervision for children with neurofibromatosis. *Pediatrics* 1995;96:368.
75. Parry DM, Eldridge R, Kaiser-Kupfer MI, et al. Neurofibromatosis 2 (NF2): clinical characteristics of 63 individuals and clinical evidence for heterogeneity. *Am J Med Genet* 1994;52:450.
76. Trofatter JA, MacCollin MM, Rutter JL, et al. A novel moesin-, ezrin-, radaixin-like gene is a candidate for the neurofibromatosis 2 tumor suppressor [published erratum appears in *Cell* 1993 19;75:826]. *Cell* 1993;72:791.
77. National Institutes of Health Consensus Development Conference Statement on Acoustic Neuroma, December 11–13, 1991. The Consensus Development Panel [Review]. *Arch Neurol* 1994;51:201.
78. Briggs RJ, Brackmann DE, Baser ME, et al. Comprehensive management of bilateral acoustic neuromas. Current perspectives [Review]. *Arch Otolaryngol Head Neck Surg* 1994;120:1307.
79. van Heyningen V, Hastie ND. Wilms' tumour: reconciling genetics and biology. *Trends Genet* 1992;8:16.
80. Knudson AG, Strong LC. Mutation and cancer: a model for Wilms' tumor of the kidney. *J Natl Cancer Inst* 1972;48:313.
81. Miller RW, Fraumeni JF, Manning MD. Association of Wilms' tumor with aniridia, hemihypertrophy and other congenital malformations. *N Engl J Med* 1964;270:922.
82. Riccardi VM, Sujansky E, Smith AC, et al. Chromosomal imbalance in the aniridia—Wilms' tumor association: 11p interstitial deletion. *Pediatrics* 1978;61:604.
83. Francke U, Riccardi VM, Hittner HM, et al. Interstitial del(11p) as a cause of the aniridia-Wilms tumor association: band localization and a heritable basis. *Am J Hum Genet* 1978;30: 81A(abst).
84. Denys P, Malvaux P, van den Berghe H, et al. Association d'un syndrome anatomo-pathologique de pseudohermaphrodisme masculin, d'une tumeur de Wilms, d'une nephropathie parenchymateuse et d'un mosaicisme XX/XY. *Arch Franc Pediatr* 1967;24:729.
85. Drash A, Sherman F, Hartmann WH, et al. A syndrome of pseudohermaphroditism, Wilms' tumor, hypertension, and degenerative renal disease. *J Pediatr* 1970;76:585.
86. Call KM, Glaser T, Ito CY, et al. Isolation and characterization of a zinc finger polypeptide gene at the human chromosome 11 Wilms' tumor locus. *Cell* 1990;60:509.
87. Gessler M, Poustka A, Cavenee W, et al. Homozygous deletion in Wilms tumours of a zinc-finger gene identified by chromosome jumping. *Nature* 1990;343:774.
88. Larsson SH, Charlieu JP, Miyagawa K, et al. Subnuclear localization of WT1 in splicing or transcription factor domains is regulated by alternative splicing. *Cell* 1995;81:391.
89. Craft AW, Parker L, Stiller C, et al. Screening for Wilms' tumour in patients with aniridia, Beckwith syndrome, or hemihypertrophy. *Med Pediatr Oncol* 1995;24:231.
90. Green DM, Breslow NE, Beckwith JB, et al. Screening of children with hemihypertrophy, aniridia, and Beckwith-Wiedemann syndrome in patients with Wilms tumour: a report from the National Wilms Tumour Study. *Med Pediatr Oncol* 1993;21:188.
91. White KS, Kirks DR, Bove KE. Imaging of nephroblastomatosis: an overview [Review]. *Radiology* 1992;182:1.
92. Miller RW. Deaths from childhood cancer in sibs. *N Engl J Med* 1968;279:122.
93. Li FP, Fraumeni JF Jr. Familial breast cancer, soft-tissue sarcomas, and other neoplasms. *Ann Intern Med* 1975;83:833.
94. Garber JE, Goldstein AM, Kantor AF. Follow-up study of twenty-four families with Li-Fraumeni syndrome. *Cancer Res* 1991;51:6094.
95. Strong LC. Cancer in survivors of childhood soft tissue sarcoma and their relatives. *J Natl Cancer Inst* 1987;79:1213.
96. Strong LC, Williams WR, Tainsky MA. The Li-Fraumeni syndrome: from clinical epidemiology to molecular genetics. *Am J Epidemiol* 1992;135:190.
97. Birch JM, Hartley AL, Marsden HB. Excess risk of breast cancer in the mothers of children with soft tissue sarcomas. *Br J Cancer* 1984;49:325.
98. Malkin D, Li FP, Strong LC, et al. Germline p53 mutations in a familial syndrome of breast cancer, sarcomas, and other neoplasms. *Science* 1990;250:1233.
99. Malkin D, Jolly KW, Barbier N, et al. Germline mutations of the p53 tumor-suppressor gene in children and young adults with second malignant neoplasms. *N Engl J Med* 1992;326:1309.
100. Anton-Culver H, Lee-Feldstein A, Taylor T. The association of bladder cancer risk with ethnicity, gender, and smoking. *AEP* 1993;3:429.
101. Sameshima Y, Tsunematsu Y, Watanabe S, et al. Detection of novel germ-line p53 mutations in diverse-cancer-prone families identified by selecting patients with childhood adrenocortical carcinoma. *J Natl Cancer Inst* 1992;9:703.
102. Caron de Fromentel C, Soussi T. TP53 tumor suppressor gene: a model for investigating human mutagenesis. *Genes Chromosomes Cancer* 1992;4:1.
103. Frebourg T, Barbier N, Yan Y, et al. Germline p53 mutations in 15 families with Li-Fraumeni syndrome. *Am J Hum Genet* 1995;56:9.
104. Birch JM, Heighway J, Teare MD, et al. Linkage studies in a Li-Fraumeni family with increased expression of p53 protein but no germline mutation in p53. *Br J Cancer* 1994;70:1176.
105. Li FP, Garber JG, Friend SH, et al. Recommendations on predictive testing for germ line p53 mutations among cancer prone individuals. *J Natl Cancer Inst* 1992;84:1156.
106. Li FP, Fraumeni JF Jr. Meeting report: collaborative interdisciplinary studies of p53 and other predisposing genes in Li-Fraumeni syndrome. *Cancer Epidemiol Biomarkers Prev* 1994;3:1.
107. Birch JM, Hartley AL, Tricker KJ, et al. Prevalence and diversity of constitutional mutations in the p53 gene among 21 Li-Fraumeni families. *Cancer Res* 1994;54;1298.
108. Gorlin RJ, Goltz RW. Multiple nevoid basal-cell epithelioma, jaw cysts and bifid rib. A syndrome. *N Engl J Med* 1962;262:908.
109. Evans DGR, Farndon PA, Burnell LD, et al. The incidence of Gorlin syndrome in 173 consecutive cases of medulloblastoma. *Br J Cancer* 1991;64:959.
110. Springate JE. The nevoid basal cell nevoid basal cell carcinoma syndrome. *J Pediatr Surg* 1986;21:908.
111. Gorlin RJ. Nevoid basal-cell carcinoma syndrome. *Medicine* 1987;66:98.
112. Bale SJ, Amos CI, Parry DM, et al. The relationship between head circumference and height in normal adults and in the nevoid basal cell carcinoma syndrome and neurofibromatosis type 1. *Am J Med Genet* 1991;40:206.
113. Kimonis VE, Goldstein AM, Pastakia B, et al. Clinical manifestations in 105 persons with nevoid basal cell carcinoma syndrome. *Am J Med Genet* 1997;69:299.
114. Gailani MR, Bale SJ, Leffell DJ, et al. Developmental defects in Gorlin syndrome related to a putative tumor suppressor gene on chromosome 9. *Cell* 1992;69:111.
115. Farndon PA, Del Mastro RG, Evans DGR, et al. Location of gene for Gorlin syndrome. *Lancet* 1992;339:581.
116. Reis A, Kuster W, Linss G, et al. Localization of gene for the nevoid basal cell carcinoma syndrome. *Lancet* 1992;339:617.
117. Hahn H, Wicking C, Zaphiropoulos PG, et al. Mutations of the human homologue of *Drosophila patched* in the nevoid basal cell carcinoma syndrome. *Cell* 1996;85:841.
118. Gailani MR, Stahle-Bäckdahl M, Leffell DJ, et al. The role of the human homologue of *Drosophila patched* in sporadic basal cell carcinomas. *Nat Genet* 1996;13:78.
119. Sidransky D. Is human patched the gatekeeper of common skin cancers? *Nat Genet* 1996;14:7.
120. Levanat S, Gorlin RJ, Fallet S, et al. A two-hit model for developmental defects in Gorlin syndrome. *Nat Genet* 1996;12:85.
121. Li FP. Familial cancer syndromes and clusters. *Curr Probl Cancer* 1990,14.75.
122. Fuchs CS, Giovannucci EL, Colditz GA, et al. A prospective study of family history and the risk of colorectal cancer. *N Engl J Med* 1994;331:1669.
123. O'Sullivan MJ, McCarthy TV, Doyle CT. Familial adenomatous polyposis: from bedside to benchside. *Am J Clin Pathol* 1998;109:521.
124. Wallace MH, Phillips RK. Upper gastrointestinal disease in patients with familial adenomatous polyposis. *Br J Surg* 1998;85:742.
125. Paraf F, Jothy S, Van Meir EG. Brain tumor-polyposis syndrome: two genetic diseases? *J Clin Oncol* 1997;15:2744.
126. Herrera L, Kakati S, Gibas L, et al. Gardner syndrome in a man with an interstitial deletion of 5q. *Am J Med Genet* 1986;25:473.

127. Kinzler KW, Nilbert MC, Su LK, et al. Identification of FAP locus genes from chromosome 5q21. *Science* 1991;253:661.
128. Groden J, Thliveris A, Samowitz W, et al. Identification and characterization of the familial adenomatous polyposis coli gene. *Cell* 1991;66:589.
129. Olschwang S, Laurent-Puig P, Groden J, et al. Germ-line mutations in the first 14 exons of the adenomatous polyposis coli (APC) gene. *Am J Hum Genet* 1993;52:273.
130. Olschwang S, Tiret A, Laurent-Puig P, et al. Restriction of ocular fundus lesions to a specific subgroup of APC mutations in adenomatous polyposis coli patients. *Cell* 1993;75:959.
131. Caspari R, Friedl W, Mandl M, et al. Familial adenomatous polyposis: mutation at codon 1309 and early onset of colon cancer. *Lancet* 1994;343:629.
132. Laken SJ, Petersen GM, Gruber SB, et al. Familial colorectal cancer in Ashkenazim due to a hypermutable tract in APC. *Nat Genet* 1997;17:79.
133. Woodage T, King SM, Wacholder S, et al. The APC I1307K allele and cancer risk in a community-based study of Ashkenazi Jews. *Nat Genet* 1998;20:62.
134. Lynch HT, Smyrk T. Hereditary nonpolyposis colorectal cancer (Lynch syndrome). An updated review. *Cancer* 1996;78:1149.
135. Lynch HT, Fusaro RM. Muir-Torre syndrome: heterogeneity, natural history, diagnosis, and management. *Probl Gen Surg* 1993;10:1.
136. Wijnen JT, Vasen HF, Khan PM, et al. Clinical findings with implications for genetic testing in families with clustering of colorectal cancer. *N Engl J Med* 1998;339:511.
137. Peltomaki P, Aaltonen L, Sistonen P, et al. Genetic mapping of a locus predisposing to human colorectal cancer. *Science* 1993;5:279.
138. Aaltonen LA, Peltomaki P, Leach FS, et al. Clues to the pathogenesis of familial colorectal cancer. *Science* 1993;260:812.
139. Thibodeau SN, Bren G, Schaid D. Microsatellite instability in cancer of the proximal colon. *Science* 1993;260:816.
140. Fishel R, Lescoe MK, Rao MRS, et al. The human mutator gene homolog MSH2 and its association with hereditary nonpolyposis colon cancer. *Cell* 1993;75:1027.
141. Leach FS, Nicolaides NC, Papadopoulos N, et al. Mutations of a mutS homolog in hereditary nonpolyposis colorectal cancer. *Cell* 1993;75:1215.
142. Bronner CE, Baker SM, Morrison PT, et al. Mutation in the DNA mismatch repair gene homologue hMLH1 is associated with hereditary nonpolyposis colon cancer. *Nature* 1994;368:258.
143. Papadopouls N, Nicolaids NC, Wei YF, et al. Mutation of a mutL homolog in hereditary colon cancer. *Science* 1994;263:1625.
144. Miyaki M, Konishi M, Tanaka K, et al. Germline mutation of MSH6 as the cause of hereditary nonpolyposis colon cancer. *Nat Genet* 1997;17:271.
145. Nicolaides NC, Papdopoulos N, Liu B, et al. Mutations of two PMS homologues in hereditary nonpolyposis colon cancer. *Nature* 1994;371:75.
146. Debinski HS, Spigelman AD, Hatfield A, et al. Upper intestinal surveillance in familial adenomatous polyposis. *Eur J Cancer* 1995;31A:1149.
147. Luk GD. Diagnosis and therapy of hereditary polyposis syndromes. *Gastroenterologist* 1995;3:153.
148. Lynch HT, Lemon SJ, Karr B, et al. Etiology, natural history, management and molecular genetics of hereditary nonpolyposis colorectal cancer (Lynch syndromes): genetic counseling implications. *Cancer Epidemiol Biomarkers Prev* 1997;6:987.
149. Garay CA, Engstrom PF. Chemoprevention of colorectal cancer: dietary and pharmacologic approaches. *Oncology* 1999;13:89.

CHAPTER 14

Epidemiology of Cancer

SECTION 1

MARGARET A. TUCKER

Epidemiologic Methods

Cancer epidemiology is the study of cancer patterns in populations and cancer causation. Through epidemiologic studies, we have learned about changing patterns of cancer incidence and mortality worldwide, risk factors for specific cancers, potential prevention strategies, and the role of genetic variation in cancer etiology. Leads from these studies have formed the basis of many laboratory investigations that have revealed biologic mechanisms for the associations first described in epidemiologic studies. It is beyond the scope of this chapter to detail the complex methodology of epidemiologic studies. A number of excellent texts elucidate the nuances of study design and conduct.[1–5] The object of this chapter is to provide clinicians with information about epidemiologic approaches and the strengths and shortcomings of various study designs so that they may evaluate the literature more critically.

Similar to clinical trials, epidemiologic studies are of human populations and, therefore, are frequently multiple years in duration and subject to certain limitations. Epidemiologic studies are usually observational and sometimes opportunistic, to learn as much as possible when humans are unexpectedly exposed to potentially harmful substances. An example is the long-term study of the population of Seveso, Italy, after the 1976 explosion that exposed the local population to high levels of 2,3,7,8-tetrachlorodibenzo-para-dioxin.[6] Another example involves the study of long-term toxicities of therapeutic irradiation and chemotherapy for cancer treatment (one of the few instances in which humans are deliberately exposed to well-documented doses of carcinogens; see Chapter 55.7). These studies have greatly enhanced our understanding of cancer biology and have affected treatment (e.g., less radiation therapy for heritable retinoblastoma).[7,8] The central distinction in epidemiologic studies is between the observational and experimental approaches (Fig. 14.1-1).[2] The experimental approach controls exposures to some extent and, therefore, presents different issues in design, conduct, and analyses of studies. This chapter focuses predominantly on observational studies, since the experimental approach is covered in other chapters on prevention and clinical trials.

OBSERVATIONAL STUDIES

Observational epidemiologic studies can be divided into two broad categories: descriptive studies and analytic studies. Descriptive studies are usually large, population-level studies of patterns of disease based on demographic data, such as age, gender, race, geographic residence, calendar year, type of cancer, and possibly other attributes. Descriptive studies provide important information for public health decisions and are often hypothesis-generating. Examples of these studies are the comparison of cancer rates among migrants to a different country, such as the evaluation of breast and colon cancer in Asians after migration to Western countries[9,10] and the evaluation of melanoma among individuals of British origin in Australia.[11] Analytic studies are designed to test hypotheses by obtaining individual information about potential risk factors for specific types of cancer. Examples would be the resultant investigation of the role of Western diet and lifestyle among Asian migrants to the United States[12,13] and the role of sun exposure in the development of melanoma among migrants to Australia.[11]

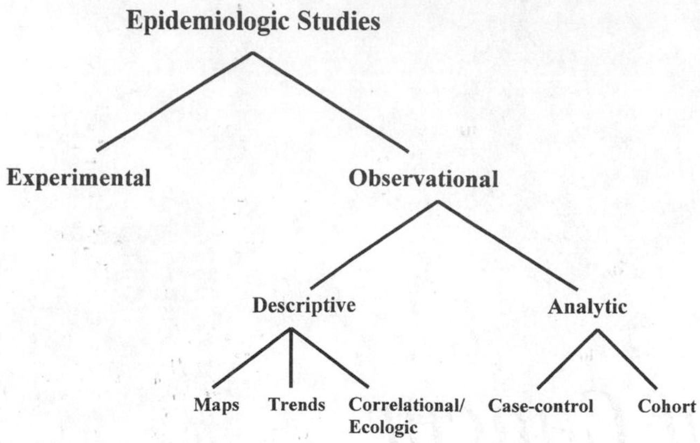

FIGURE 14.1-1. Schematic of types of epidemiologic studies.

Certain general concepts are important to the evaluation and interpretation of all epidemiologic studies. The inference of causation from epidemiologic studies is quite complex; there are no fixed and agreed-on criteria to establish causation.[2,3] Most formulations, however, derive from the criteria originally proposed at the time of the controversy about cigarette smoking and lung cancer.[14,15] Descriptive studies in general will not lead to causal inferences. No one analytic study, however large and methodologically robust, is likely to "prove" a causal association. Because epidemiologic studies are largely observational, it is important to replicate findings from one study in other groups or populations to evaluate the consistency of the results. The consistency of results should be interpreted taking into account the relative rigor of both the study designs and the conduct of the investigations and the size and statistical power of the studies. Within appropriately designed and conducted studies, the magnitude of the risks demonstrated and the statistical significance of the risks are important. The greater the magnitude of the risk, the stronger the evidence for causation. Evidence of increasing risk of cancer with increasing exposure to a risk factor strengthens a postulated association. Data from studies must be interpreted within the current body of knowledge of that exposure and that cancer. There needs to be sufficient time between the exposure and the development of cancer as well as biologic plausibility of the exposure. Animal studies demonstrating carcinogenicity of an exposure lend credence to the hypothesis.

In trying to determine whether an association found in an investigation is plausible and valid, it is important to consider the possibility of bias in the data, confounding factors, and chance associations. Bias can result from a flaw in the design of the study or in the collection of the data. For instance, the study could be designed such that individuals with cancer are identified several months after the cancer is diagnosed. For individuals with a cancer for which there is high survival, this may not be a problem. For individuals with a cancer for which the survival is poor and mortality is rapid, only a subset of better-prognosis individuals would be alive to participate. This subset of individuals may fundamentally differ from those with more aggressive disease in host susceptibility or in risk factor exposures, if either is related to more aggressive disease. Another type of problem could be in long-term follow-up of groups under study. If there is differential effort in locating individuals with specific exposures or differential effort in locating individuals who may have become ill, there could be profound effects on the data. If interviewers know who has cancer and who does not, they may be (even unconsciously) more persistent in prompting individuals with cancer for answers to specific questions. This could lead to a systematic bias in data collection. These types of difficulties cannot be accommodated well in the data analyses and affect how one can interpret the results.

Confounders are variables associated with disease risk and with an exposure under investigation.[2] If confounder variables are not appropriately recognized and dealt with in analyses, the risks associated with the exposure of interest may be altered, either increased or decreased. Confounder variables must demonstrate three characteristics: (1) The confounder must be related to disease risk in individuals with and without the exposure of interest; (2) the confounder variable must be associated with the exposure of interest in the group from which the study participants come; and (3) a confounding variable cannot be an intermediate end point in the development of disease.[16] These relationships can be complex to disentangle but can frequently be handled by specific analytic techniques. An example of a confounder would be cigarette smoking in participants in a case-control study that is investigating the role of alcohol consumption in the etiology of oral cancer.[17,18] Cigarette smoking is related to alcohol consumption and is a risk factor for oral cancer. If the level of cigarette smoking is not accounted for in the analysis, the risk shown for alcohol consumption would be altered.

In interpreting results of epidemiologic studies, one must always also consider that a finding occurs by chance alone. These spurious associations are more likely in large, complex analyses with multiple comparisons. Chance associations usually do not show evidence of a dose response and may or may not have biologic plausibility. Evaluating the level of statistical significance of a finding is usually helpful also. Most risk estimates are accompanied either by a test of statistical significance or by confidence intervals. Ninety-five percent confidence intervals that do not include 1.0 indicate significance of at least the 0.05 level. This can be interpreted as a 1 in 20 likelihood of the observation occurring by chance alone. The more comparisons that are done, the more likely it is that a chance association will occur.

In descriptive studies, most demographic data are collected from institutions, not individuals. In those data, the completeness of ascertainment of data and quality of data from the relevant sources are important to evaluate. In analytic studies, response rates indicate the percentage of people approached who actually complete components of an investigation. Especially in analytic studies, epidemiologists are dependent on the generosity of study participants to spend time, provide sensitive or confidential information (or both), and donate biologic specimens. This is becoming an increasing problem. In the late 1970s and early 1980s, response rates in excess of 90% were not uncommon. As individuals have become more concerned about privacy issues and as studies have become more demanding of time, biologic specimens, and other impositions, response rates have dropped substantially. It is now common to have response rates of 50% or lower if biologic specimens are requested. Lower response rates are of concern because it often is not clear that respondents are identical to nonrespondents in terms of risk factor exposures or genetic susceptibility factors. Inferences about the entire group are quite limited if only a minority of individuals provide information. In addition, low response rates affect the statistical power of the study to detect associations.

DESCRIPTIVE STUDIES

Descriptive studies are important for noting differences in patterns of cancer among different populations or over time.[19] Evaluating changes in cancer incidence has been essential in determining public health priorities. To have equivalent data to compare across populations or time, crude data are adjusted to standard age distributions. Crude incidence is the number of new cancer cases in a selected group that occur over a specified time period, divided by the total number of people in that selected group (usually the number at the midpoint of the specified time period). Similarly, crude mortality is the total number of deaths from cancer in a selected group that occur over a specified time period, divided by the total number of people in that selected group. For international comparisons, these crude rates usually are adjusted to an age-standardized population, as the age structure of populations varies widely and cancer rates are age-dependent. In an equivalent manner, to compare rates in the same population over different calendar periods, the crude rates need to be adjusted to a similar population structure.

Descriptive studies are highly dependent on the quality of data collected. The quality of incidence data varies substantially, depending on the medical care systems, the thoroughness with which a diagnosis of a specific type of cancer is pursued, the completeness of reporting a new diagnosis of cancer to whatever institution is collecting the data, and the accuracy of the population numbers. The percentage of histologic confirmation of new cancer diagnoses also varies widely among health care systems and among tumor registries.[20,21] In some areas, where there is better reporting of causes of death than of new cases of cancer, mortality may be a more reliable estimate of rates, particularly if the type of cancer is associated with poor survival. The ideal population for evaluating cancer rates would be a large, diverse one in which there is little in or out migration, one health care system provides high-quality care from birth to death, and each individual has a unique identifier for life.

Maintaining the infrastructure for these descriptive studies is essential for monitoring trends in cancer incidence and mortality over time, which is necessary for monitoring the health of the population. For instance, through evaluating data from the Surveillance, Epidemiology, and End Results (SEER) program, it is clear that lung cancer incidence has leveled overall for men.[21] For women, however, the rates are still increasing, and lung cancer now is the leading cause of cancer-related deaths in women. The SEER data are now available on the National Cancer Institute (NCI) Web site http://www-seer.ims.nci.nih.gov/. These data provide population-based incidence rates, survival, and mortality for the United States, based on information from 11 population-based registries and three supplemental registries. These registries cover approximately 14% of the U.S. population, with measures of poverty and education similar to the U.S. population. The SEER population tends to be more urban, with a higher percentage of foreign-born persons than the general U.S. population.[21] For international comparisons, the World Health Organization's International Agency for Research on Cancer and the International Association of Cancer Registries publishes *Cancer Incidence in Five Continents*.[22] This volume is extremely useful in comparing the wide variation in cancer incidence. The Scandinavian countries have long-standing active cancer registries.[23] Several years ago, the NCI and the Danish Tumor Registry collaborated on analyzing data regarding multiple primary tumors occurring in Connecticut and Denmark over approximately a 50-year period.[24]

The NCI has also published *Atlas of Cancer Mortality in the United States 1950–94*, which is available at Web site http://www.nci.nih.gov/atlas/.[25] Two components comprise this atlas: a static version and a dynamic version. These maps were used to show a substantial change in geographic patterns of lung cancer mortality over time that correlates with changes in smoking patterns.[26] The mortality is higher for white male individuals in the Southeast (Fig. 14.1-2), for white female subjects in the West, and for African Americans in the urban North.[25] This is also an example of another variant in descriptive studies, a correlational or ecologic study, in which statistics gathered for another purpose are correlated with cancer incidence. An earlier version of the mortality maps showed an excess of lung cancer in white men along the southern seaboard.[25] A number of analytic studies were undertaken to evaluate potential risk factors that revealed that the excess was largely due to asbestos exposure in shipyards during World War II.[27–29] In the recent maps, this coastal excess has essentially disappeared for white men (see Fig. 14.1-2). These mortality maps can be used to generate many new hypotheses related to the geographic clustering. Newer technologies, such as satellite mapping that provides data for geographic information systems, will likely become increasingly important in the future for ecologic or correlational studies.

ANALYTIC STUDIES

In contrast to descriptive studies, in which only demographic information is available, analytic studies obtain information on specific risk factors from individuals. Each of the two broad categories of analytic studies—cohort studies[30] and case-control studies[31]—has specific advantages and limitations.

COHORT STUDIES

Cohort studies are frequently prospective and longitudinal. A group is identified and defined and then followed prospectively for outcomes of interest. There are multiple advantages of this type of design. Information on specific risk factors can be obtained before onset of disease. This is particularly important for risk factors that may be altered in individuals who have become symptomatic from their disease. For example, the diet of a patient who has just had a colectomy for colon cancer or a gastrectomy for stomach cancer will be quite different from that patient's diet before diagnosis. There may be recall bias in remembering previous dietary intakes. Usually, updated information is collected at regular intervals, so that longitudinal patterns of exposure can be obtained (variations in smoking patterns, alcohol consumption, etc.). Because information is collected on a large number of people at regular intervals, information is best collected on relatively common exposures. It is impractical to expect participants to complete extensive questionnaires every year or two. Biologic samples can also be obtained, so that sequential patterns of exposure (micronutrients, viral titers, nicotine metabolites) can be quantified and

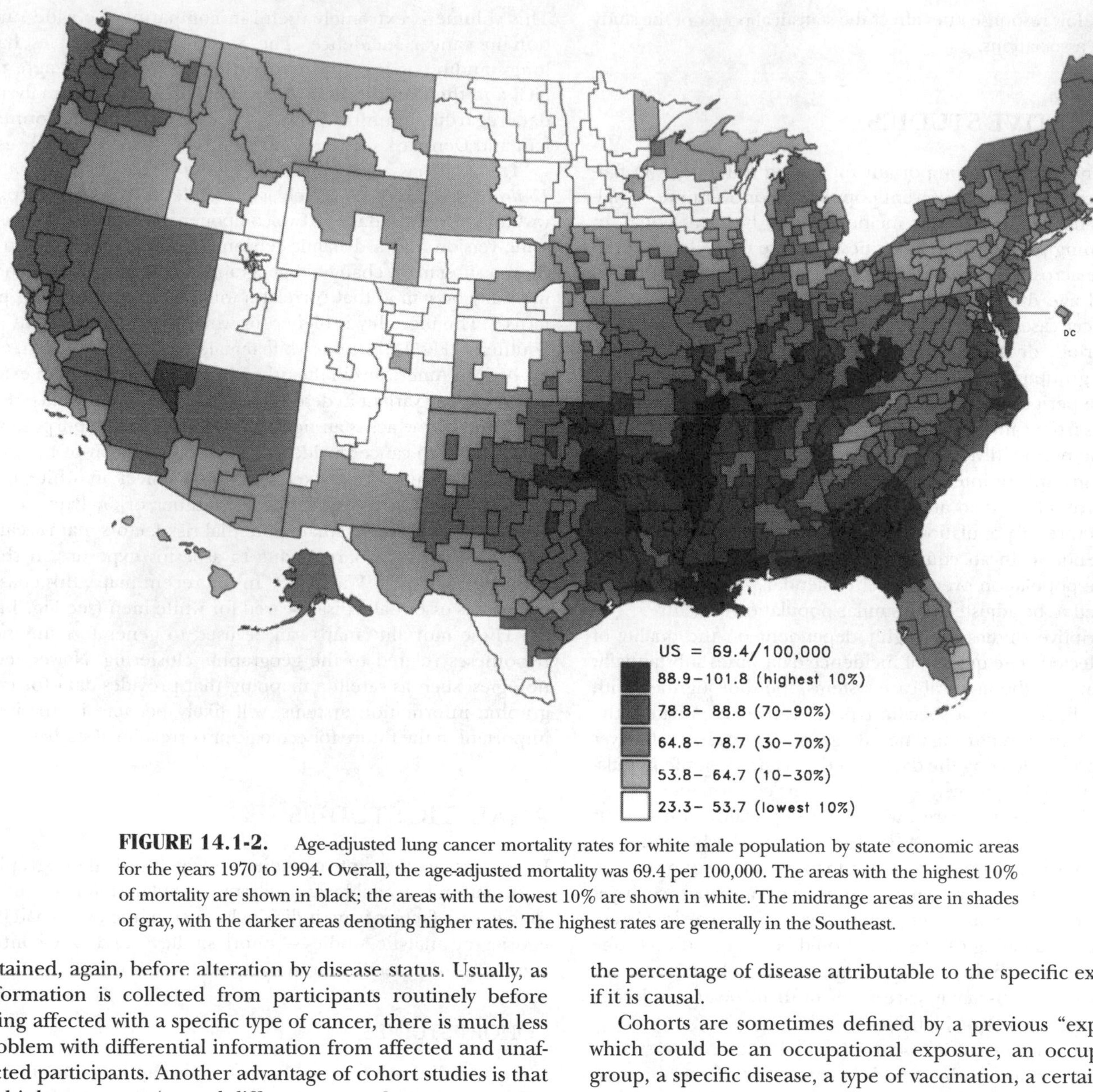

FIGURE 14.1-2. Age-adjusted lung cancer mortality rates for white male population by state economic areas for the years 1970 to 1994. Overall, the age-adjusted mortality was 69.4 per 100,000. The areas with the highest 10% of mortality are shown in black; the areas with the lowest 10% are shown in white. The midrange areas are in shades of gray, with the darker areas denoting higher rates. The highest rates are generally in the Southeast.

obtained, again, before alteration by disease status. Usually, as information is collected from participants routinely before being affected with a specific type of cancer, there is much less problem with differential information from affected and unaffected participants. Another advantage of cohort studies is that multiple outcomes (several different types of cancer, mortality from other causes, morbidity if data are collected, etc.) can be evaluated.

In a prospective cohort, when part of the cohort has a specific exposure (e.g., cigarette smoking) and part does not, the relative risk of developing disease is calculated by the ratio of the proportion of exposed individuals who develop cancer to the proportion of unexposed individuals who develop cancer.[2] This is a direct comparison of the rate of cancers (or for mortality rate of death) in the exposed and unexposed groups. A relative risk of 2 means that the exposed group is twice as likely to develop the cancer as the unexposed group; a relative risk of 0.5 means that the exposed group is half as likely to develop the cancer. The terms in these calculations usually include the time interval over which the event occurred, usually person-years of observation. Relative risks are usually reported with 95% confidence intervals. If the 95% confidence intervals do not include 1.0, the relative risk is considered statistically significant. One can also calculate other measures of risk that reflect the percentage of disease attributable to the specific exposure, if it is causal.

Cohorts are sometimes defined by a previous "exposure," which could be an occupational exposure, an occupational group, a specific disease, a type of vaccination, a certain medication, and the like. In these retrospective studies, individuals are followed up from a specific time of exposure in the past to onset of disease, death, or time of study. The rates of cancers (or death, if evaluating mortality) over the time period frequently are compared to the general population rates rather than to an unexposed group (which may not be available). This comparison assumes that the group under study would have the same baseline rate of cancer as the general population, absent the exposure under study.

In both the prospective and retrospective cohort designs, careful definition of study participants and exposition of follow up procedures are crucial for interpreting data. This includes how potential participants are identified (and contacted), initial and continuing participation rate, loss to follow-up, and refusal rate (which may change over time). In evaluating the relationship of exposure to disease, methods and precision of quantification of exposure are important. Exposure measures can range from industrial hygiene estimations of occupational exposures, to dietary histories (or diaries), smoking history, medication records, and biologic measures, such as DNA adducts or metabolites of specific substances in specimens. The potential error in these measures must be considered in interpreting the data. An advantage of cohort investigations is that when onset of exposures is well documented, one can evaluate latency of the exposure to disease diagnosis and the duration of an effect after exposure. For instance, 20 years after the explosion in Seveso, detectable levels of dioxin persisted in the blood of heavily exposed individuals.[32] As with all epidemiologic studies, confounding variables should be identified when possible.

A relative disadvantage of cohort studies is that they are usually large, long-term, complex, and very expensive endeavors. Outcomes in prospective cohorts may not be apparent for decades, and it is extremely difficult to motivate study participants to continue. With increasing concerns about privacy and confidentiality of data, fewer participants are willing to undertake the commitment. If a substantial part of the proposed cohort does not participate or if there is continuous loss of participants due to refusal or withdrawal from the study, the results may become difficult to interpret. The participant group may no longer reflect the entire group from which they were derived. Even with very large cohorts, it is difficult to study relatively rare diseases or uncommon exposures (unless the cohort was chosen because of the exposure). Because of the limitations of imposition on cohort participants, detailed information on other exposures of interest may be lacking. This lack of focused exposure information can be a problem when specific cancers are evaluated. To overcome these constraints, within larger cohort investigations, additional information on other exposures of interest (including confounders) may be collected from smaller substudies of identified individuals with a specific cancer and a subgroup of the cohort (either matched controls or a selected sample of the cohort).[2] These are called either *nested case-control* or *case-cohort analyses.* These approaches may be cost-effective mechanisms for evaluating specific cancers of interest free of selection bias if the participants with the cancer are still alive to provide the information. Another approach within the cohort design for evaluating rare cancers is to combine data from several cohorts.

CASE-CONTROL STUDIES

Case-control studies, also called *case-referent studies,* usually obtain data within a limited time frame on previous exposures of interest. They are, therefore, considered retrospective. Cases (individuals with the cancer of interest) and controls (individuals similar to the cases but who do not have the cancer) are identified in a systematic manner, and data are collected. These data are frequently collected using questionnaires, abstracting occupational or medical records, or examining participants. Usually, there is not longitudinal follow-up. Several advantages accompany this design. The studies are much shorter in duration than cohort studies and, therefore, are less costly. The amount of data collected at one time can be greater than in a cohort study because the investigators will not be imposing on the participants repeatedly over many years. Questionnaires can be longer, with detailed information about more risk factors specific to the type of cancer being studied. This may allow evaluation of interaction of risk factors. Because the cancers have already occurred, it is more feasible to identify a larger number of individuals with relatively rarer tumors to include in the study than to wait to accrue a sufficient number in a large cohort. It is, therefore, more efficient and cost-effective to try to study a rare tumor in a case-control study than in a cohort study.

Biologic specimens can also be collected relatively efficiently, often in close temporal proximity to extensive information about recent exposures. In contrast to cohort studies, however, for the cases, this will be after the onset of disease. If the disease process directly or indirectly affects the exposure measure, there will be difficulty in interpreting the results. (Biospecimen collection as part of case-control studies is discussed later in Molecular Epidemiologic Studies.) Other limitations in case-control studies include recall bias, as individuals with cancer may have spent time already pondering the causes of their illness. In contrast to cohort studies, in which multiple types of cancers can be evaluated as outcomes, in case-control studies, usually only one cancer type or a small number of closely related cancer types is evaluated in one study.

The identification of cases and the selection of controls are crucial to the validity of the investigation. Two general approaches are used to identify cases. The first is through population-based registries. Theoretically, this should lead to the least biased ascertainment of cases and should identify cases representative of the group from which they are identified. For cancers associated with high survival, this technique can be highly successful. There is frequently a several-month delay between the time the cancer is diagnosed and the time that the case is identified from the registry, however, which can cause a selection bias for cancers with high mortality. This delay can also cause problems if biologic specimens to measure exposure or host characteristics are to be collected. Many of the bioassays would be profoundly altered by interval treatment with radiation therapy or chemotherapy. In some instances, special efforts are made to identify cases rapidly. Although this is necessary for some types of cancer, it is frequently very costly.

The second general approach is to identify the cases from a hospital or clinic setting. If essentially all cases from a defined area are treated in the hospital from which the cases are identified, the cases may be essentially as representative of the population as the true population-based ascertainment. An advantage of hospital ascertainment is that the cases may be more cooperative, and it is logistically easier to enroll them and to collect the data, including biospecimens. Again, if biologic samples are collected, which could be affected by being in the hospital (dietary factors, smoking, occupational exposures, etc.), the results may be difficult to interpret. For both of these methods of identification, it is important to evaluate closely how scrupulously the cases were identified.

Equally important to the validity of the study is the selection of the controls. The controls should be from the same population group as the cases. Controls are frequently matched to the cases on characteristics that are important in determining risk of disease, such as gender, age, and ethnicity, or on potential confounder variables (e.g., socioeconomic status or, possibly, smoking status). Controls may be population-based (i.e., identified from the same population by use of population registries or lists, random-digit dialing if telephones are common in the population, neighborhood canvassing, or other methods). Although theoretically these methods should yield controls that are most representative of the population from which the cases come, if only a small proportion of individuals approached agree to participate in the study, this may not happen. The participants may differ from the nonparticipants in manners that are difficult to quantify and may not be representative. True population-based controls are becoming increasingly difficult to enroll in studies, at least partially because of privacy concerns.

If the cases are identified from hospitals or clinics, an alternative control selection could be patients from the same hospital or clinic. Care must be taken to select individuals who have the same likelihood of coming to that hospital or clinic if they developed the same disease as the cases (a surrogate may be the same catchment area for the control disease as for the type of cancer the case has). Selecting individuals as possible controls who have a variety of diagnoses that do not include conditions related to the development of the type of cancer of interest is also important to minimize bias. For instance, considering individuals being evaluated for skin conditions in a dermatology clinic as controls for a melanoma case-control study would often be inappropriate, because the reason they were being seen may be related to melanoma risk factors.[33] If there is a clinical component to the study, such as a structured physical examination, this is often best performed in a clinical setting. Obtaining biologic specimens can also be facilitated in a clinical facility, but similar difficulties in interpreting results can occur as with cases. Cooperation and participation are frequently higher among hospital- or clinic-based controls.

The measure of association in case-control studies is the odds ratio, which is an estimate of the relative risk. Unlike cohort studies, case-control studies cannot directly evaluate the actual rate or risk associated with a specific exposure, because the rates in the unexposed and exposed populations are not known. This estimate is the ratio of the odds of exposure among cases (number of exposed cases divided by number of unexposed cases) to the odds of exposure among controls.[3] The odds ratio is a good approximation of the relative risk when cancer is uncommon in the population. Estimates can also be made for the attributable risk, which also cannot be directly measured as in cohort studies. Similar to cohort studies, the odds ratio shows a positive association between exposure and disease when it is greater than 1.0 and a negative association (or protective effect) when it is less than 1.0. Odds ratios usually are reported with 95% confidence intervals, which are considered statistically significant when they do not include 1.0. In case-control studies, detailed exposure information may have been collected on several exposures and potential confounders identified. The other risk factors and confounders should be considered in the analyses and dealt with appropriately. In large studies, with sufficient numbers of participants exposed to two risk factors, interactions between two exposures, such as asbestos and smoking in lung cancer, can be examined.[26–28]

In limited situations, a variant of a case-control design or analysis, a case-case design, may be appropriate. This type of analysis can be useful when attributes or risk factors are not available or present in controls or when controls are not available. This design cannot evaluate main effects of specific genes or exposures but can evaluate the interaction between a genotype and an environmental exposure.[34] Case-only or case-case studies are more efficient than case-control studies for detecting interaction. These analyses require that the genotype and the exposure be independent. The inferences from this type of analysis are often difficult to interpret and somewhat limited, because the risks do not reflect comparisons between affected and unaffected individuals but between affected individuals. An example might be comparing cases with a specific genotype to cases without the genotype, when the genotype is rare in the control population. Another example could be a study comparing somatic mutations in tumors to risk factors.

MOLECULAR EPIDEMIOLOGIC STUDIES

Two other variations of both cohort and case-control studies must be considered: molecular and genetic epidemiologic studies. Molecular epidemiologic studies have been developed over the last decade or so to enhance exposure measurement methods. These have generally ranged in three large categories: (1) studies that directly assay exposure to specific substances; (2) those that evaluate phenotype or genotype information about metabolic pathways that may alter effective dose of an exposure or other host susceptibility factors; and (3) those that use markers of a specific effect to refine disease categories for analyses (of heterogeneity, prognosis, etiology, etc.). The type of specimen collected is determined by the exposure of interest and the methods available to quantify that exposure. Some investigations focus on directly measuring exposure, such as blood levels of substances (e.g., toxins, carcinogens, nutrients, micronutrients, viral titers), DNA adducts, levels of metabolites in urine, and the like. These data are then correlated with measures of exposure from occupation records, questionnaire responses, medical records, and other sources of data. If the metabolic pathways of the exposure of interest are known, often genes with variations (polymorphisms) are evaluated and correlated with either biologic measurements of dose or historic measures or both. Other host susceptibility factors (e.g., immune response determinants) may be related to time to progression, disease severity, or other parameters.[35,36]

Molecular epidemiologic studies have all of the logistic and methodologic characteristics of conventional epidemiologic studies. They also have the added constraints of laboratory components.[37,38] Molecular epidemiologic studies are, by definition, interdisciplinary and require investigators from highly divergent fields to collaborate closely from study design to completion. The complexity of these investigations manifests in both the epidemiologic and the laboratory components.

Many of the early molecular epidemiologic investigations were relatively small, exploratory studies to determine the feasibility of this approach, to validate biologic markers, and to estimate level of risk.[37] Even when assessing polymorphisms present in one-half of the population, these relatively small studies do not have power to evaluate modest risks, especially in subgroup analyses.[39–41] With the advances in laboratory techniques and the identification of many genetic variations that alter effective dose of exposure, much larger studies now are necessary to test adequately hypotheses involving complex exposures.[42,43] Careful estimates of sample size to detect the level of risk expected, given the frequency of exposure expected and the variation in biologic measures, must be accomplished as part of the early planning. The epidemiologic study design is directly affected by the sample size necessary for molecular studies. These investigations typically need to include hundreds or thousands of study subjects to detect a significant difference in, for instance, the effect of a genetic polymorphism that occurs in one-third of the population or a difference in adduct levels when one-half of the population is exposed. Even larger numbers are necessary to try to evaluate gene-exposure or gene-gene interactions. The appropriate controls for these molecular epidemiologic studies have also been under extensive discussion.[37,44] The type and quantity of biologic specimens to be collected has to be selected with the laboratory investigators. The specimens requested will have an effect not only on the study design and cost but on the response rate of the potential participants.[45] Adequate consent procedures are complex and essential. Because many of the exact laboratory assays may not have been selected (or developed) at the time the participant is enrolled in the study, specifying exactly what will be done with the specimen may be somewhat problematic. Many investigators are now using a consent that allows for different levels of use of the specimen (e.g., for only the specified assays or for other assays related to the disease of interest) or for any future use. Analytic methods to incorporate laboratory information as well as more standard epidemiologic information must be carefully developed.

The additional complexity of the laboratory components begins with establishing appropriate collection, processing, and transportation of biologic specimens with necessary quality control measures. Because many of the specimens must be stored for various lengths of time before being assayed, some type of repository system is needed to locate and track specimens. As laboratory assays are completed for the samples, each sample becomes more valuable because of the laboratory information in combination with the epidemiologic information connected to each sample. Repository functions, including proper identification and tracking of each sample, remain essential. All the routine difficulties of validity and reproducibility of the laboratory techniques being used on the specimens must be resolved before analysis of the samples. Many of the assays of particular interest may be technically challenging or quite complex. The laboratory collaborators often have to develop the methods to conduct the assays or genotyping on large numbers of samples (hundreds or thousands). Despite the risk of these complex studies, they hold the promise of more closely integrating biologic measures of exposure to the more traditional questionnaire and record abstraction of exposure information.

Many investigators conducting cohort studies try to collect biologic specimens for future use. One major advantage of these collections is that specimen collection occurs before disease onset. Because, in large cohorts, a majority of individuals will not develop the diseases of interest, many specimens will not be informative about the diseases the study was designed to investigate. With the sequential information gathered over time, new hypotheses and different outcomes can be evaluated in these cohorts, however. Collection and storage of large numbers of specimens for decades is costly, especially because relatively few of the samples will actually be assayed (in nested case-control or case-cohort analyses). Storage costs are proportional to volume of material and number of specimens collected. For cohort studies with large numbers and continuing contact with the study participants, the type of specimen collected is a trade-off between imposition costs for the participants, the storage needs and costs of the specimen, and the potential uses of those specimens. For low-cost blood storage for DNA, limited quantities of blood (100 to 150 μL) can be stored on collection cards.[46] For noninvasive collection of genetic materials, buccal cell collection is a reasonable option with limitations.[47] Because, for most cohort studies, specimen collections will be relatively limited with finite quantities, extremely careful selective use of samples for assays is essential. As new laboratory techniques develop that consume less of the total sample, these invaluable resources can be increasingly informative.

Case-control studies may offer more efficient collection and storage of specimens but, as noted earlier under Case-Control Studies, these samples may be altered by the presence of disease in the cases or by hospital-related exposures or lack of exposures in cases and controls. A relative advantage is that the specimens will be quickly informative. In contrast to cohort studies, there is not a long latency before cases occur and samples are potentially useful for proposed laboratory tests. Greater volumes of specimens (e.g., blood) can possibly be collected and stored, because the participants are not being sequentially contacted and long-term storage (for decades) before use is not anticipated. Storage issues for thousands of samples accrued over a several-year period are not trivial, however. Consent issues may still be problematic, as with cohort studies, because new hypotheses or laboratory tests may be developed that were not originally anticipated when participants were accrued. Case-control studies may be a more efficient design to investigate interactions between host susceptibility factors and exposures (gene-exposure and gene-gene interactions), especially when the type of cancer being studied is relatively rare.[37]

GENETIC EPIDEMIOLOGIC STUDIES

Genetic epidemiologic studies overlap substantially with molecular epidemiologic studies, particularly when the "molecular" component is evaluating variations in genes. The field of genetic epidemiology has rapidly increased with the advent of gene identification and large-scale genotyping. Genetic epidemiology in its broad context, however, includes family studies, molecular epidemiologic studies with genetic components, and more traditional cohort and case-control studies with family history components. Similar to the molecular epidemiologic studies, genetic epidemiologic studies are multidisciplinary from the outset and involve clinicians, geneticists, epidemiologists, and laboratory investigators. These studies include all the complications of molecular epidemiologic studies, often with the additional complexity of having to deal with family dynamics.[48]

Family studies have been essential for mapping and identifying the more than 20 major cancer susceptibility genes found in the late 1990s.[49] (The methods for identifying and evaluating these genes are discussed in Chapter 13.) Once the contribution of genetic variation to disease within the families has been established, however, these variations should be evaluated in relation to known exposure factors for the specific cancers of interest (parity, reproductive factors for breast cancer; sun for melanoma, etc.). Complex analytic techniques that incorporate both genotype information and environmental risk factors into a regressive model have been developed.[50] Again, large numbers of families are necessary for these gene-environment and, potentially, gene-gene interactions. Care must be taken in these analyses to account for familial relationships, as the observations within families are not necessarily independent. Families share not only genes but environmental exposures and lifestyles. Within high-risk families, selected because there are many living members, penetrance (risk of developing disease associated with carrying an altered gene) estimates will be high but useful for determining an upper limit on the risk associated with alteration of a specific gene.

Larger population studies are important for estimating the effect of an altered gene outside of high-risk families selected for linkage analyses. Because most cancers are adult-onset, complex diseases, even when a major susceptibility gene is mutated, other factors may be important. Large epidemiologic studies are needed to identify these additional risk factors so that the complex chain of events that results in a cancer development can be interrupted. One approach is to conduct a large case-control study in which usual risk factors are obtained and large genes, such as *BRCA1* or *BRCA2* (each having hundreds of mutations throughout the gene), are analyzed.[51] This is logistically challenging, laboratory time-intensive, and costly. Even though mutations in such genes as *BRCA1* and *BRCA2* account for a percentage of familial breast cancer and are important for understanding the biology of breast cancer development, they account for only a small fraction of breast cancer in the general population.[51] Sample sizes for these studies must, therefore, be large and, even then, the limitation is the number of mutation carriers in the referent (control) population.

Another approach to understanding the role of mutations in the development of cancers is to take advantage of the opportunity afforded by relatively isolated populations with so-called founder mutations, recurrent mutations prevalent in a specific group. Unlike other populations in which an entire gene needs to be sequenced, these founder mutations can be more easily genotyped because the laboratory searches for one or a limited number of specific mutations.[52] It is thus feasible to screen thousands of samples for the specific mutation. Founder mutations have been identified in a number of populations worldwide. For example, breast, ovarian, and prostate cancer risk associated with prevalent mutations in *BRCA1* and *BRCA2* were estimated in volunteers from the Jewish community of Washington, DC.[46] To estimate risk of cancer among mutation carriers, a novel analytic technique was devised, called the *kin-cohort method*.[53] The risk of breast and ovarian cancers could not be directly estimated among the genotyped participants because of the potential survival bias. Information on cancer history of first-degree relatives of genotyped individuals was used to estimate penetrance of breast, ovarian, and prostate cancers. The cumulative risk of each type of cancer in relatives of carriers was compared to that of noncarriers and found to be much lower than that in high-risk families.[46,53,54] Other novel analytic techniques will need to be developed for other types of data sets to maximize the information gleaned from both genetic and environmental risk factors.

Family history data from case-control or cohort studies can be used to evaluate clustering of cancers in families. Information on first-degree relatives is usually accurate among well-educated Americans,[55,56] but this type of information is culture-specific. In cultures where notification of cancer diagnoses is not routine, obviously information on cancer diagnoses in relatives will not be accurate. One approach to identifying families with known ascertainment for clustering studies or linkage analyses is to identify individuals from case-control or cohort studies with a family history of interest, contact the individual to ask for permission to contact other family members, and then evaluate the family members who are willing to participate. Another approach to systematically identifying families at increased risk of specific cancers is through population registries,[48] where genetic findings can be extrapolated to the population from which the cases are derived.[48,57] Individuals with a disease of interest are identified at the time of registration, and family history is obtained. If the family meets the criteria, family members are invited to participate in a family registry study. This approach is being developed to provide resources for the research community.[49]

Genetic epidemiologic studies that investigate other genes not considered among the major susceptibility genes are similar to those described in molecular epidemiology. There are some special issues for genetic epidemiologic studies, however.[48] Informed consent is complex. (The issues of consent in families are discussed in Chapter 56.4.) A growing concern among potential participants in any type of genetic epidemiologic study is the implementation of confidentiality practices to protect the privacy of genetic information. Another concern is notifying participants of results and the approach of this notification. If all identifiers are removed, individual notification becomes impossible. In most large studies, it is not feasible to counsel participants individually about their genotype status, even if it were possible to interpret the meaning of such variation. One approach is to notify participants about aggregate results, so that they can then pursue clinical, rather than research, genetic testing with their physicians.

INTERVENTION STUDIES

In some senses, intervention studies represent the culmination of descriptive studies that reveal patterns of cancer and analytic studies that discover risk factors for developing the cancers. The ultimate goal of both approaches is to identify individuals at high risk of developing cancer, to establish risk factors for the cancer, and to develop rational approaches to interrupting the causal pathway in cancer development. Intervention studies are designed to test ways of disrupting the chain of events that may lead to cancer causation. As such, some investigations are designed to evaluate intermediates in tumor development. The hypotheses in general are developed from case-control and cohort studies. Intervention studies randomize individuals to a group receiving some type of prevention intervention and those not receiving the intervention. The risk of cancer is compared in the two groups using similar analytic techniques as in the cohort studies. These intervention trials may be dietary (e.g., giving supplementary micronutrients to individuals at risk of esophageal or stomach cancer)[58]; chemopreventive (e.g., the tamoxifen trial for women at increased risk of breast cancer)[59]; vaccine trials (e.g., hepatitis B[60] or the papilloma virus[61] vaccination trials); medical screening (e.g., the NCI's Prostate, Lung, Colon, and Ovary screening trial); or lifestyle-altering (e.g., sun exposure) programs.[62] When individuals are randomized, confounding factors should be equivalently distributed between the groups. The baseline characteristics should also be equivalent among the randomized groups. Most of these trials are conducted with participants who are considered to be at high risk for disease. An important consideration is that because participants are healthy individuals, prevention strategies should not have substantial side effects: That is, toxicity should not outweigh potential benefit.

In the design of these trials, sample size estimates are crucial. Even among selected high-risk participants, cancer outcomes may be relatively rare, and a large number of participants may have to be enrolled and followed up for decades. Oversight committees are not uncommon; they are quite useful in monitoring data and helping with the ethical decision to stop a trial if a substantial benefit is shown in one group.

FUTURE DIRECTIONS

Epidemiologic studies have pointed to the direction of many fruitful avenues of cancer research in the basic sciences and have established the causes and major risk factors for many cancers. Much needs to be done, however. The major progress in the next few years will likely emerge from large, interdisciplinary, highly collaborative research programs with improved measures of host susceptibility and environmental exposure. A new era of chemopreventive studies, based on identifying high-risk individuals and the biologic mechanisms of tumor progression, hold great promise for altering the natural history of disease. The identification of genetic factors that may influence addiction to tobacco[63–65] could, in time, reduce the number of individuals who smoke.

Acknowledgments

I am deeply grateful to my husband, Dr. David Schlafer, for his support and help; to my colleagues, Drs. Neil Caporaso, Alisa Goldstein, and Patricia Hartge, for their insightful comments; and to Dan Grauman for providing the mortality maps.

REFERENCES

1. Gordis L. *Epidemiology.* Philadelphia: WB Saunders, 1996.
2. Rothman KJ, Greenland S, eds. *Modern epidemiology,* 2nd ed. Philadelphia: Lippincott Williams & Wilkins, 1998.
3. MacMahon B, Trichopoulos D. *Epidemiology: principles and methods,* 2nd ed. Boston: Little, Brown and Company, 1996.
4. Mausner JS, Kramer S. *Mausner and Bahn epidemiology: an introductory text,* 2nd ed. Philadelphia: WB Saunders, 1985.
5. Schottenfeld D, Fraumeni JF Jr, eds. *Cancer epidemiology and prevention,* 2nd ed. New York: Oxford University Press, 1996.
6. Bertazzi PA, di Domenico A. Chemical, environmental, and health aspects of the Seveso, Italy, accident. In: Schecter A, ed. *Dioxins and health.* New York: Plenum Publishing, 1994:587.
7. Wong FL, Boice JD Jr, Abramson DM, et al. Cancer incidence after retinoblastoma: radiation dose and sarcoma risk. *JAMA* 1997;278:1262.
8. National Cancer Institute. PDQ. *Curr Clin Trials Oncol* 1999;6:158.
9. Shimizu H, Mack TM, Ross RK, Henderson BE. Cancer of the gastrointestinal tract among Japanese and white immigrants in Los Angeles County. *J Natl Cancer Inst* 1987;78:223.
10. Shimizu H, Ross RK, Bernstein L, et al. Cancers of the prostate and breast among Japanese and white immigrants in Los Angeles County. *Br J Cancer* 1991;63:963.
11. Elwood JM, Gallagher RP. Sun exposure and the epidemiology of melanoma. In: Gallagher RP, Elwood JM, eds. *Epidemiologic aspects of cutaneous malignant melanoma.* Boston: Kluwer Academic Publishers, 1994:15.
12. Ursin G, Wu AH, Hoover RN, et al. Breast cancer and oral contraceptive use in Asian-American women. *Am J Epidemiol* 1999;150:561.
13. Le Marchand L. Combined influence of genetic and dietary factors in colorectal cancer incidence in Japanese Americans. *Monogr Natl Cancer Inst* 1999;26:101.
14. Hill AB. The environment and disease: association or causation? *Proc R Soc Med* 1965;58:295.
15. Advisory Committee to the Surgeon General. Smoking and health. Public Health Service publication no. 1103. Washington, DC: U.S. Government Printing Office, 1964.
16. Rothman KJ. *Modern epidemiology.* Boston: Little, Brown and Company, 1986:92.
17. Jensen OM, Paine SL, McMichael AJ, Ewertz M. Alcohol. In: Schottenfeld D, Fraumeni JF Jr, eds. *Cancer epidemiology and prevention,* 2nd ed. New York: Oxford University Press, 1996:290.
18. Saracci R. The interactions of tobacco smoking and other agents in cancer etiology. *Epidemiol Rev* 1987;9:175.
19. Esteve J, Benhamou E, Raymond L. Statistical methods in cancer research. Descriptive epidemiology. *IARC Sci Publ* 1994;4(128):1.
20. Sobue T, Ajiki W, Tsukuma H, et al. Trends of lung cancer incidence by histologic type: a population-based study in Osaka, Japan. *Jpn J Cancer Res* 1999;90:6.
21. Ries LAG, Kossary CL, Mankey BF, eds. *SEER cancer statistics review, 1973–1996.* Bethesda, MD: National Cancer Institute, 1999.
22. Parkin DM, Wheland SL, Ferlay J, et al. Cancer incidence in five continents. *IARC Sci Publ* 1997;143.
23. Jensen OM, Carstensen B, Glattre E, et al. *Atlas of cancer incidence in the Nordic countries.* Nordic Cancer Union. Helsinki: Puna Musta, 1988.
24. Boice JD Jr, Storm HH, Curtis RE, eds. *Multiple primary cancers in Connecticut and Denmark.* National Cancer Institute monograph 68. Washington, DC: U.S. Government Printing Office, 1985.
25. Devesa SS, Grauman DJ, Blot WJ, et al. *Atlas of cancer mortality in the United States, 1950–1994.* NIH publication no. 99-4564. Bethesda, MD: National Institutes of Health, 1999.
26. Devesa SS, Grauman DJ, Blot WJ, Fraumeni JF Jr. Cancer surveillance series: changing geographic patterns of lung cancer mortality in the United States, 1950 through 1994. *J Natl Cancer Inst* 1999;91:1040.
27. Blot WJ, Morris LE, Stroube R, et al. Lung and laryngeal cancers in relation to shipyard employment in coastal Virginia. *J Natl Cancer Inst* 1980;65:571.
28. Blot WJ, Harrington JM, Toledo A, et al. Lung cancer after employment in shipyards during World War II. *N Engl J Med* 1978;299:620.
29. Blot WJ, Davies JE, Morris LE, et al. Occupation and the high risk of lung cancer among men in northeast Florida. *Cancer* 1982;50:364.
30. Breslow NE, Day NE. Statistical methods in cancer research. The design and analysis of cohort studies. *IARC Sci Publ* 1987;2(82):1.
31. Breslow NE, Day NE. Statistical methods in cancer research. The analysis of case-control studies. *IARC Sci Publ* 1980;1(32):5.
32. Landi MT, Needham LL, Lucier G, et al. Concentrations of dioxin 20 years after Seveso. *Lancet* 1997;349:1811.
33. Tucker MA, Halpern A, Holly EA, et al. Clinically recognized dysplastic nevi: a central risk factor for cutaneous melanoma. *JAMA* 1997;277:1439.
34. Goldstein AM, Andrieu N. Detection of interaction involving identified genes: available study designs. *Monogr Natl Cancer Inst* 1999;26:49.
35. Hildesheim A, Schiffman M, Scott DR, et al. Human leukocyte antigen class I/II alleles and development of human papilloma virus-related cervical neoplasia: results from a case-control study conducted in the United States. *Cancer Epidemiol Biomarkers Prev* 1998;7:1035.
36. Ung A, Kramer TR, Schiffman M, et al. Soluble interleukin 2 receptor levels and cervical neoplasia: results from a population-based case-control study in Costa Rica. *Cancer Epidemiol Biomarkers Prev* 1999;8:249.
37. Caporaso N, Rothman N, Wacholder S. Case-control studies of common alleles and environmental factors. *Monogr Natl Cancer Inst* 1999;26:25.
38. Schaid DJ, Buetow K, Weeks DE, et al. Discovery of cancer susceptibility genes: study designs, analytic approaches, and trends in technology. *Monogr Natl Cancer Inst* 1999;26:1.
39. London SJ, Daly AK, Cooper J, et al. Polymorphism of glutathione S-transferase M1 and lung cancer risk among African-Americans and Caucasians in Los Angeles County, California. *J Natl Cancer Inst* 1995;87:1246.
40. Jourenkova N, Reinikanen M, Bouchardy C, et al. Effects of glutathione S-transferases GSTM1 and GSTT1 genotypes on lung cancer risk in smokers. *Pharmacogenetics* 1997;7:515.
41. Le Marchand L, Sivaram L, Pierce L, et al. Associations of CYP1A1, GSTM1 and CYP2E1 polymorphisms with lung cancer suggest cell type specificities to tobacco carcinogens. *Cancer Res* 1998;58:4858.
42. Garcia-Closas M, Rothman N, Lubin J. Misclassification in case-control studies of gene-environment interactions: assessment of bias and sample size. *Cancer Epidemiol Biomarkers Prev* 1999;8:1043.
43. Garcia-Closas M, Lubin J. Power and sample size calculations in case-control studies of gene-environment interactions: comments on different approaches. *Am J Epidemiol* 1999;149:689.
44. Thomas DC. Design of gene characterization studies: an overview. *Monogr Natl Cancer Inst* 1999;26:17.
45. Hunter DJ. Methodological issues in the use of biological markers in cancer epidemiology: cohort studies. *IARC Sci Publ* 1997;142:39.
46. Struewing JP, Hartge P, Wacholder S, et al. The risk of cancer associated with specific mutations of BRCA1 and BRCA2 among Ashkenazi Jews. *N Engl J Med* 1997;336:1401.
47. Lum A, Le Marchand L. A simple mouthwash method for obtaining genomic DNA in molecular epidemiologic studies. *Cancer Epidemiol Biomarkers Prev* 1998;7:719.
48. Whittemore AS, Nelson LM. Study design in genetic epidemiology: theoretical and practical considerations. *Monogr Natl Cancer Inst* 1999;26:61.
49. Klausner RD. *The nation's investment in cancer research: a budget proposal for fiscal year 2000.* NIH publication no. 98-4373. Bethesda, MD: National Institutes of Health, 1998:40.
50. Demenais F, Lathrop M. REGRESS: a computer program including the regressive approach into the LINKAGE programs. *Genet Epidemiol* 1994;11:291.
51. Newman B, Mu H, Butler LM, et al. Frequency of breast cancer attributable to BRCA1 in a population-based series of American women. *JAMA* 1998;279:915.
52. Struewing JP, Abeliovich D, Peretz T, et al. The carrier frequency of the BRCA1 185delAG mutation is approximately 1 percent in Ashkenazi Jewish individuals. *Nat Genet* 1995;11:198.
53. Wacholder S, Hartge P, Struewing JP, et al. The kin-cohort study for estimating penetrance. *Am J Epidemiol* 1998;148:623.
54. Gail MH, Pee D, Carroll R. Kin-cohort designs for gene characterization. *Monogr Natl Cancer Inst* 1999;26:55.
55. Bondy ML, Strom SS, Colopy MN, et al. Accuracy of family history of cancer obtained through interviews with relatives of patients with childhood sarcoma. *J Clin Epidemiol* 1994;47:89.
56. Novakovic B, Goldstein AM, Tucker MA. Validation of family history of cancer in deceased family members. *J Natl Cancer Inst* 1996;88:1492.
57. Hopper JL, Chenevix-Trench G, Jolley DJ, et al. Design and analysis issues in a population-based case-control-family study of the genetic epidemiology of breast cancer and the Co-operative Family Registry for Breast Cancer Studies (CFRBCS). *Monogr Natl Cancer Inst* 1999;26:95.
58. Mark SD, Liu SF, Li JY, et al. The effect of vitamin and mineral supplementation on esophageal cytology: results from the Linxian Dysplasia Trial. *Int J Cancer* 1994;57:162.

59. Dunn BK, Kramer BS, Ford LG. Phase III, large-scale chemoprevention trials. Approach to chemoprevention clinical trials and phase III clinical trial of tamoxifen as a chemopreventive for breast cancer—the U.S. National Cancer Institute experience. *Hematol Oncol Clin North Am* 1998;12:1019.
60. Oda T. Viral hepatitis and hepatocellular carcinoma prevention strategy in Japan. *Jpn J Cancer Res* 1999;90:1051.
61. Murakami M, Gurski KJ, Steller MA. Human papillomavirus vaccines for cervical cancer. *J Immunother* 1999;22:212.
62. Lindholm LH, Isacsson A, Slaug B, Moller TR. Acceptance by Swedish users of a multimedia program for primary and secondary prevention of malignant melanoma. *J Cancer Educ* 1998;13:207.
63. Lerman C, Audrain J, Orleans CT, et al. Investigation of mechanisms linking depressed mood to nicotine dependence. *Addict Behav* 1996;21:9.
64. Lerman C, Shields PG, Audrain J, et al. The role of serotonin transporter gene in cigarette smoking. *Cancer Epidemiol Biomarkers Prev* 1998;7:235.
65. Lerman C, Caporaso N, Main D, et al. Depression and self-medication with nicotine: the modifying influence of the dopamine D4 receptor gene. *Health Psychol* 1998; 17:56.

SECTION **2**

PHILIP COLE
BRAD RODU

Descriptive Epidemiology: Cancer Statistics

The malignant diseases have both a descriptive and an analytic epidemiology. Descriptive epidemiology consists primarily of vital statistics, particularly incidence and mortality rates. These usually relate to large populations divided according to age, gender and race. Differences in these statistics from one place or time to another are part of descriptive epidemiology. Survivorship also is descriptive. The descriptive epidemiology of the malignancies is described in this Section.

Analytic epidemiology consists of the knowledge of suspect and known causes of disease. It is developed from disease-specific or cause-specific investigations. The analytic epidemiology of the malignancies is described in Section 3 of this chapter.

DESCRIPTIVE EPIDEMIOLOGY

USA

Most data presented here pertain to the United States of America (USA). This is not limiting in that cancer patterns vary relatively little over the developed world. Further, differences that occur reflect geographic and cultural variations in the distribution of the causes of cancer, not differences in the causes themselves. However, in the developing world cancer patterns vary from that of the developed world and differ from one region to another. In many developing countries there are high frequencies of cancers of the liver, stomach, cervix and, in parts of Asia, cancer of the nasopharynx. Cancer patterns in many newly industrialized societies are changing rapidly towards those of the West. This reflects their recent large-scale adoption of cigarette smoking.[1] Global variations in the descriptive epidemiology of cancer are reviewed in "Global cancer statistics" by Parkin, Pisani and Ferlay.[2]

CANCER ENTITIES

Depending on the cancers of interest and on their grouping, there could be several dozen groups of malignancies for which statistics are available. This Section describes "all cancer" and 20 specific cancers and groups of cancer that cause the largest numbers of deaths in the USA. These entities accounted for 88% of cancer deaths in 1996. Table 14.2-1 ranks them by number of deaths. The names in the table were chosen for brevity. The cancers included in each group will be specified.

INCIDENCE

The incidence (sometimes called the incident number) of a cancer is the number of cases of the disease diagnosed in a specified population, or group of people, over a specified time, usually one year. The more commonly used measure, the incidence rate (***I***), relates the incident number to the size of the population and to the interval in which the cases were diagnosed. ***I*** is expressed as cases per 100,000 persons per year or, usually, as cases per 100,000 person-years (py). An ***I*** may relate to an entire population (the ***I*** of lung cancer in the USA is 54 cases per 100,000 py), may be specific, e.g., as to gender (the ***I*** of lung cancer among males in the USA is 70 per 100,000 py) or may be ever more specific, e.g., as to males of one race and of a narrow age range. Whether or not they are specific, ***I's*** that span a broad age range usually are age-adjusted to facilitate comparison with one another. Age-adjustment nearly eliminates age as the explanation for any differences seen among a group of ***I's***. All ***I's*** and mortality rates in the remainder of this chapter are adjusted to the age distribution of the total USA population in 1970.

Cancer ***I*** data in the USA are provided mainly by population-based cancer registries. These vary in size and somewhat in the quality and completeness of their data. Most of the incidence data come from a national system of cancer registries that has existed since 1973. This Surveillance, Epidemiology and End Results (SEER) Program now includes 11 registries. The incidence data reported for 1973 and later are from SEER's nine original registries which include about 10.5% of the USA population.[3]

Data from a cancer registry less than 20 years old are viewed cautiously. As a registry matures its coverage will improve, possibly giving the false impression of a rise in ***I's***. There are other potential sources of distortion in ***I's***, even those from established registries.[4,5] These include a population's increased use of cancer screening services and improvements in access to medical care. Improvements in diagnostic capabilities and, rarely, changes in diagnostic categories also affect ***I's***. All of these advances may convey the false impression of a rise in cancer ***I's***.

MORTALITY

Cancer mortality or the number of deaths, and the cancer mortality rate (***M***) are analogous to the corresponding measures of incidence. Of course these measures relate to deaths certified as due to cancer not to diagnosed cases of cancer. ***M*** usually is expressed as deaths per 100,000 py and may be made specific for population subgroups just as is ***I***.

TABLE 14.2-1. Incidence and Mortality Data for Major Forms of Cancer. USA, Total Population 1996

Mortality Rank	Form of Cancer	Incidence						Mortality				
		Number	*I**	Rank	%	Cum. %	B/W**	Number	*M**	%	Cum. %	B/W
	All cancer	1154328	389	-	-	-	1.1	539533	167	-	-	1.3
01	Lung, bronchus	161301	54.2	03	13.0	13	1.3	152015	48.8	28.2	28	1.2
02	Colon	100160	30.3	04	7.0	20	1.2	48587	14.4	9.0	37	1.4
03	Breast (female)	176757	111	02	13.6	34	1.1	43091	24.3	8.0	45	1.6
04	Prostate gland	171423	136	01	23.3	57	1.7	34123	24.1	6.3	52	2.5
05	Pancreas	26066	8.6	14	1.9	59	1.6	27260	8.3	5.1	57	1.5
06	Non-Hodg. lymph.	46883	15.5	06	3.9	63	0.8	22934	6.9	4.2	61	0.7
07	Leukemia	28613	9.7	12	2.0	65	0.8	20340	6.3	3.8	65	1.0
08	Stomach	20917	6.6	15	1.7	66	2.1	13336	4.0	2.5	67	2.2
09	Ovary	22533	14.1	13	2.0	68	0.6	13161	7.4	2.4	70	0.8
10	Nervous system	16181	5.8	17	1.3	70	0.6	12376	4.2	2.3	72	0.5
11	Liver, biliary tract	18502	4.2	16	1.5	71	1.7	11584	3.6	2.1	74	1.5
12	Urinary bladder	51835	16.2	05	3.9	75	0.5	11452	3.2	2.1	76	0.9
13	Esophagus	11929	4.0	20	0.9	76	2.3	11231	3.6	2.1	78	2.0
14	Kidney, renal pelvis	29891	9.4	10	2.3	78	1.2	11095	3.5	2.1	80	1.0
15	Multiple myeloma	12811	4.2	19	1.1	79	2.4	10248	3.1	1.9	82	2.2
16	Rectum	43176	12.5	07	2.9	82	0.9	8167	2.4	1.5	84	1.2
17	Oral cavity, pharynx	29809	10.0	11	2.2	85	1.4	7854	2.6	1.5	85	1.8
18	Melanoma of skin	41612	13.8	08	2.8	87	0.1	7279	2.3	1.3	86	0.1
19	Endometrium	33999	21.1	09	2.5	90	0.7	6311	3.3	1.2	88	1.9
20	Uterine cervix	12705	7.7	18	0.1	90	1.5	4542	2.7	0.8	88	2.2

*New cases or deaths per 100,000 person-years. Adjusted to the age-distribution of the total USA population in 1970.
**Black : White. Age-adjusted race ratio: the ratio of the rate for Blacks to the corresponding rate for Whites. The race-specific rates are not shown.

M's are of very high quality in the USA,[6] especially for cancer. Nearly 90% of persons considered to have died from cancer, on the basis of autopsy, will have the disease correctly listed on their death certificate.[7] Numbers of deaths and ***M's*** are available annually in great detail for the entire country. In this Section we usually present mortality data for 1996. This is the latest year for which detailed information is available and it is the same as the year for most incidence data presented. Preliminary mortality data are available for 1997 and 1998. This recent information extends all of the trends described in this Section. All of the mortality data come from publications of the National Center for Health Statistics.[8,9,10]

SEX RATIO

Males and females differ in their rates of most cancers. These male:female differences are expressed as the age-adjusted sex ratio, the ratio of the age-adjusted male ***I*** or ***M*** to the corresponding female rate. Since this ratio is based on age-adjusted rates it accommodates the fact that the female population is larger and older than the male.

RACE RATIO

For brevity ***I's*** and ***M's*** are presented for all races combined. However, we also present the ratio of age-adjusted ***I's*** and ***M's*** of Blacks to those of Whites. The ratio of Black to White ***M's*** is typically higher than the ***I*** ratios and this discrepancy, for each cancer, may be an index, albeit a crude index, of the access to and use of cancer-related services by the two races.

SURVIVORSHIP

Survivorship is described by the five-year ***relative*** survival rate (***RSR-5***). The ***RSR-5*** is the proportion of persons with a particular form (and usually, stage) of cancer who survive to the fifth anniversary of their diagnosis, divided by the proportion of the general population expected to live that long. The expectation is based on mortality rates from all causes among persons with the same age, gender and race composition as the cancer patients. An ***RSR-5*** of, say 75%, indicates that five years after diagnosis the cancer group has 25% fewer survivors than does the comparable population. The ***RSR-5*** is based on all deaths in the cancer group, so it does not describe mortality from the specific cancer in question. Instead, it indicates the incremental mortality imposed by that cancer. Because ***RSR-5's*** are available for specific stages of a cancer, they permit evaluation of long-term gains in patient survival.

AGE PATTERNS, TIME TRENDS

Patterns of ***I's*** and ***M's*** are described by age for men and women for each of the cancers addressed. For cancers of greatest public health importance and for several others of special interest, the age-patterns are also presented graphically. Time trends are presented graphically for ***I's*** and ***M's*** for cancers of

TABLE 14.2-2. Incidence and Mortality Data for Major Forms of Cancer by Gender. USA, Total Population 1996

		Incidence					*Mortality*				
		Male		*Female*			*Male*		*Female*		
Mortality Rank	*Form of Cancer*	Number	*I**	Number	*I*	*SR***	Number	*M**	Number	*M*	*SR*
	All cancer	590373	455	563955	342	1.3	281898	207	257635	139	1.5
01	Lung, bronchus	92001	70.0	69300	42.3	1.7	91620	68.2	60395	34.3	2.0
02	Colon	48594	34.9	51566	26.6	1.3	23770	14.4	24817	14.3	1.0
03	Breast (female)	-	-	176757	111	-	-	-	43091	24.3	-
04	Prostate gland	171423	136	-	-	-	34123	24.1	-	-	-
05	Pancreas	12936	10.0	13670	7.4	1.4	13027	9.6	14233	7.2	1.3
06	Non-Hodgkin's lymphoma	26303	19.2	20580	12.2	1.6	11962	8.6	10972	5.6	1.5
07	Leukemia	15971	12.3	12642	7.7	1.6	11179	8.2	9161	4.8	1.7
08	Stomach	13031	9.8	7886	4.2	2.3	7859	5.7	5477	2.7	2.1
09	Ovary	-	-	22533	14.1	-	-	-	13161	7.4	-
10	Nervous system	9314	7.2	6867	4.5	1.6	6733	5.0	5643	3.4	1.5
11	Liver, biliary tract	11036	6.4	7466	2.4	2.7	7404	5.3	4180	2.3	2.3
12	Urinary bladder	37306	27.7	14259	7.4	3.7	7683	5.5	3769	1.7	3.2
13	Esophagus	8831	6.8	3098	1.7	4.0	8400	6.3	2831	1.5	4.2
14	Kidney, renal pelvis	18438	12.9	11456	6.5	2.0	6757	5.1	4338	2.3	2.2
15	Multiple myeloma	6836	5.3	5975	3.4	1.6	5253	3.8	4995	2.6	1.5
16	Rectum	23972	16.1	19204	9.6	1.7	4515	2.6	3652	2.2	1.2
17	Oral cavity, pharynx	19981	14.8	9828	5.9	2.5	5215	3.9	2639	1.4	2.8
18	Melanoma of skin	23048	17.0	18564	11.4	1.5	4490	3.2	2789	1.5	2.1
19	Endometrium	-	-	33999	21.1	-	-	-	6311	3.3	-
20	Uterine cervix	-	-	12705	7.7	-	-	-	4542	2.7	-

*New cases or deaths per 100,000 person-years. Adjusted to the age-distribution of the total USA population in 1970.
**Age-adjusted sex ratio: the ratio of the male to the corresponding female rate.

the greatest public health significance and for those of interest for some other reason. Finally, ***RSR's*** are presented for 1950-1959, 1974-1976, 1979-1981 and 1989-1991, for all cancer and the 20 cancers of major interest. The data come from the SEER program[3] and its predecessor, the End Results Group.[11]

ALL CANCER

(This category includes all malignant neoplasms except non-melanoma cancers of the skin. It is not limited to the 20 cancer groups that follow.) Variation in the causes and the descriptive patterns of malignancies make statistics for "all cancer" difficult to interpret. Moreover, lung cancer accounts for about 15% of all cancer cases and 30% of deaths. As a result descriptive patterns for "all cancer" reflect those of lung cancer. Yet, an overview of the malignancies as a whole gives perspective to national issues such as time trends, improvements in survivorship, the value of cancer screening, etc. Further, the public has an abiding interest in "cancer" as a group.

Table 14.2-1 shows that the ***I*** of all cancers combined in the USA population in 1996 was 389 cases per 100,000 py. Table 14.2-2 shows that the rate was 455 for males and 342 for females, an age-adjusted incidence sex ratio of 1.3. The Black:White (B/W) incidence ratio of 1.1 indicates that for all cancer combined, Blacks have a slightly higher incidence rate than do Whites. Useful explanations of B/W ratios different from 1.0 are specific to each form of cancer and are beyond our scope.

The ***M*** of all cancer for the total population in 1996 was 167 deaths per 100,000 py, 207 for males and 139 for females. The age-adjusted mortality sex ratio is 1.5, slightly higher than the corresponding ratio of 1.3 for incidence. This discrepancy does not indicate that females survive cancer better than do males since males experience relatively more cases of the more fatal malignancies (lung, stomach, liver, esophagus). Actually, women do survive most cancers better than do men. But this is best inferred from a comparison of the sex-specific ***RSR-5's*** of each form of cancer.

The B/W mortality ratio for all cancer is 1.3, larger than the 1.1 incidence ratio. The discrepancy between the incidence and the mortality ratio may reflect the fact that Blacks have less access to, and use, medical care less than do Whites.

Figure 14.2-1 shows age patterns of ***I's*** and ***M's*** for all cancer for males and females, respectively, averaged for 1992-1996. These five years were combined because age-specific ***I's*** are not available for any individual recent year. The pattern of ***I's*** shows an upward inflection during the late 40's for men. The rates start to rise earlier and increase more gradually for women. The earlier rise of ***I's*** among women reflects the early onset of breast cancer and cervix cancer. For both genders, ***I's*** then increase nearly linearly to about age 75 and peak in the early 80's. The "late-age decline" appearing in these data is common and is usually an artifact due to underdiagnosis of cancer among the elderly and to overestimation of the size of the elderly population. For both genders the pattern of mortality lags that of incidence by about 10 years and there is no late age decline seen for either gender.

Age-specific cancer ***I's*** were used to estimate the risk of developing cancer over a lifetime and over several age spans of

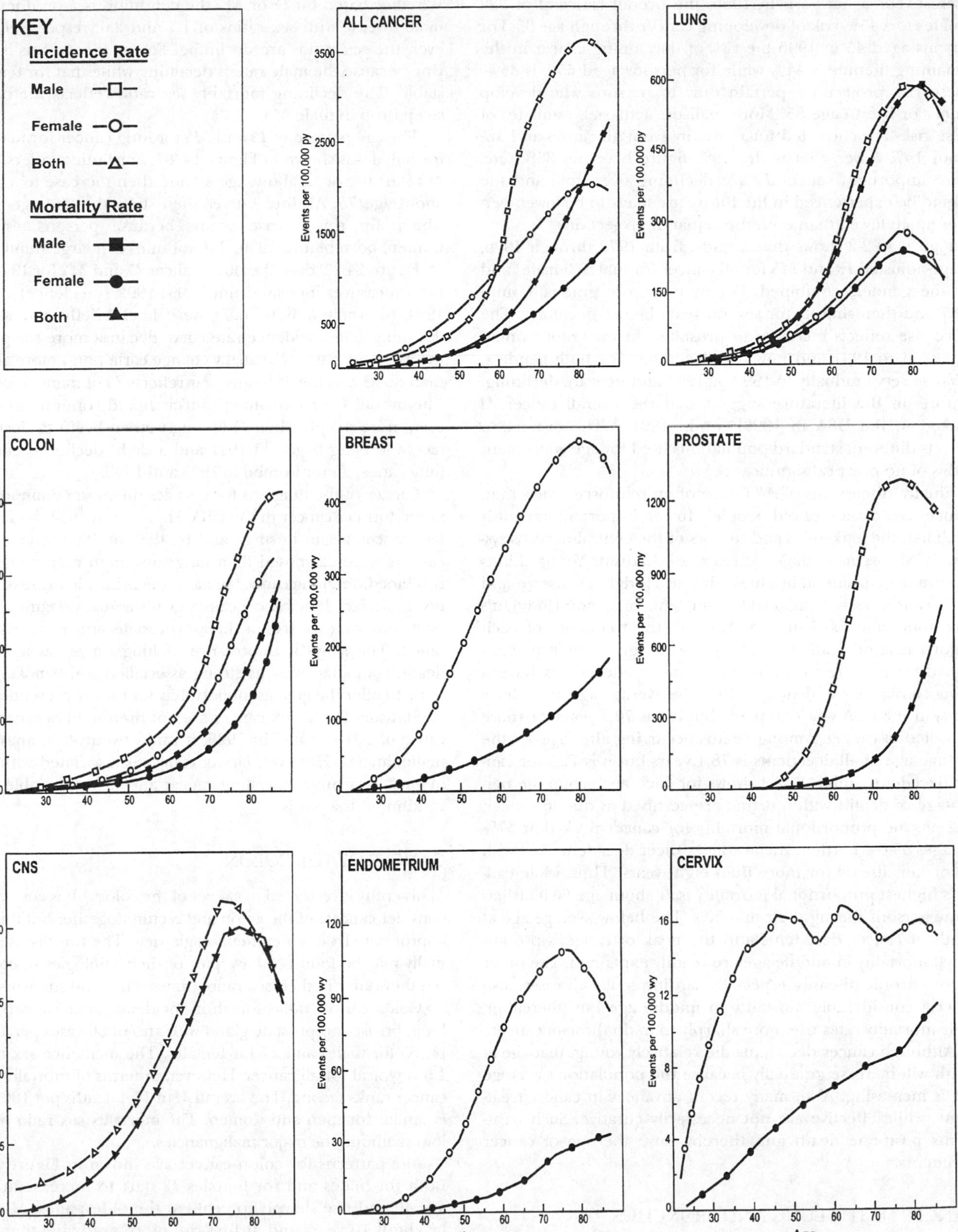

FIGURE 14.2-1. Incidence rates and mortality rates for all cancer and for seven selected cancers. According to age.

interest. For a newborn in 1996, the overall cancer ***I*** of 389 equates to a 45% risk of developing cancer through age 85. For persons aged 45 in 1996 the risk of developing cancer in the remaining lifetime is 44% while for persons aged 65 it is 35%. These risk projections pertain only to persons who develop cancer or live to age 85. More realistic, actuarial, estimates of these risks are corrected for mortality from all causes and are about 15% lower, that is the 45% figure becomes 38%, etc. More important, cancer ***I's*** are declining over time and the risks to be experienced in the future are likely to be lower, perhaps much lower, than even the actuarial projections.

Figure 14.2-2 shows time trends, from 1973 through 1996, of age-adjusted ***I's*** and ***M's*** for all cancer for males, females and for the genders combined. For men ***I's*** rose gradually until 1987 and then sharply for several years before declining. The sharp rise reflects increases in prostate cancer. ***I's*** for women increased to 1991 and now are declining. For both genders, ***M's*** rose very gradually to 1990 or 1991 and now are declining. Reports in the literature suggest that the overall cancer ***M*** peaked in the USA in 1990[12] or in 1991.[13] The distinction reflects different standard populations used for age-adjustment and is of no practical significance.

Finally, discussions of *All Cancer* often reinforce a view that, "cancer is a disease of old people". In two important ways, it is not. First, the leukemias and tumors of the central nervous system (CNS) remain major threats to children. Young adults experience considerable illness due to Hodgkin's disease and testis cancer as well as death from leukemia, non-Hodgkin's lymphoma and CNS tumors. Second, the frequency of each major cause of death rises sharply with age. Among persons who die from the major diseases, cancer decedents have a ***below*** average age at death. In 1996 the average age of all decedents in the USA was 72.0 years, but it was 70.7 years for those who died of cancer. Among deaths occurring after age 45, the average age of all decedents is 78.1 years but it is 72.5 for cancer decedents. Table 14.2-3 shows for each age group the percentage of deaths within it that are certified as due to cancer. In 1996 the proportional mortality for cancer peaked at 37% for ages 55-64. Further, the average cancer decedent lived with his or her disease for more than eight years. Thus, while cancer's highest proportional mortality is at about age 60 it afflicts many persons during their mid-50's. The below average age at death of cancer decedents and the peak of cancer's proportional mortality in middle age are readily explained. The other major chronic diseases, especially cardiovascular diseases, also exact a considerable mortality in middle age but, thereafter, their mortality rates rise more sharply than do those of cancer.

Although cancer decedents die relatively young, that age at death will increase gradually because the population's average age is increasing. Also, many recent advances in cancer treatment, while effective are not necessarily curative. Such treatments postpone death and thereby raise the age of cancer decedents.[5]

CANCER OF THE LUNG AND BRONCHUS

(This category includes cancers of the trachea, lung and bronchus and of the pleura. Less than one percent of cases or deaths in this category are cancers of the pleura.) Lung cancer had an overall *I* of 54 cases per 100,000 py in 1996, 70 for males and 42 for females. The corresponding ***M's*** were 49, 68 and 34. Whether based on ***I's*** or ***M's*** the condition is a predominantly male disease with sex ratios of 1.7 and 2.0, respectively. However, the sex ratios are declining. For incidence this is occurring because the male rate is declining while that for females is stable. The declining mortality sex ratio reflects the ongoing steep drop in male ***M's***.

The age pattern of ***I's*** and ***M's*** for lung cancer for males and for females is shown in Figure 14.2-1. For both genders, ***I's*** and ***M's*** start to rise at about age 40 and then increase to a peak at about age 75. All four curves then show the late age decline which, for this disease occurs because persons, especially women, born before 1930, did not smoke in large numbers.

Figure 14.2-2 describes lung cancer ***I's*** and ***M's*** for 1973-1996. Both measures increased until 1991-1992 (incidence) or 1990-1994 (mortality). Both rates were level briefly and now are declining. The incidence rate curve declines more steeply than the mortality curve. ***I's*** usually change earlier and more abruptly than do ***M's***, as the ***M*** in any year reflects ***I's*** of many prior years. The overall ***I*** curve for lung cancer should continue to decline even more steeply when ***I's*** among women begin to decline. In fact, a leveling began in 1991 and a slight decline occurred in lung cancer ***I's*** for women in 1995 and 1996.

Cancer of the lung was for decades the most commonly diagnosed form of cancer in the USA. However, in 1984 the ***I*** of prostate cancer began to surge and by 1989 or 1990 more prostate cancers were diagnosed than lung cancers in men and women combined. Yet, lung cancer remains the principle cause of cancer deaths. In fact, lung cancer causes nearly as many deaths as do the next four cancers (colon, breast, prostate and pancreas) combined. The singular importance of lung cancer as a cause of death, combined with its strong association with smoking, continue to offer the greatest opportunity for cancer prevention.

Statistics for larynx cancer are not presented because as the cause of 3918 deaths in 1996, it ranks twenty-first among the malignancies. However, larynx cancer is associated with smoking just as strongly as is lung cancer and so is amenable to prevention on that basis.

CANCER OF THE COLON

(This entity is restricted to cancer of the colon.) It is customary to consider cancers of the colon and rectum together but this is not appropriate from an epidemiologic view. The two diseases eventually may be found to have part of their etiologies in common but they differ in their sex ratios, time trends and survivorship.

Colon cancer ranks fourth in incidence after cancers of the lung, breast and prostate gland with an ***I*** of 30 cases per 100,000 py, 35 for males and 27 for females. The incidence sex ratio of 1.3 is typical for all cancer. However, in terms of mortality, colon cancer ranks second. The overall ***M*** of 14.4 deaths per 100,000 py is similar for men and women. The mortality sex ratio of 1.0 is lowest among the major malignancies.

Age patterns for colon cancer are shown in Figure 14.2-1. Both for males and for females ***I's*** start to increase at about age 40 and rise sharply to peaks at the oldest ages. ***M's*** lag ***I's*** by about 10 years and at first rise more gradually than do ***I's*** but then accelerate upward. Colon cancer's time trends appear in Figure 14.2-2. ***I's*** peaked at about 38 cases per 100,000 py in 1987 and then began declining. Mortality has declined since at least 1979, the first year for which data specific to the colon are available.

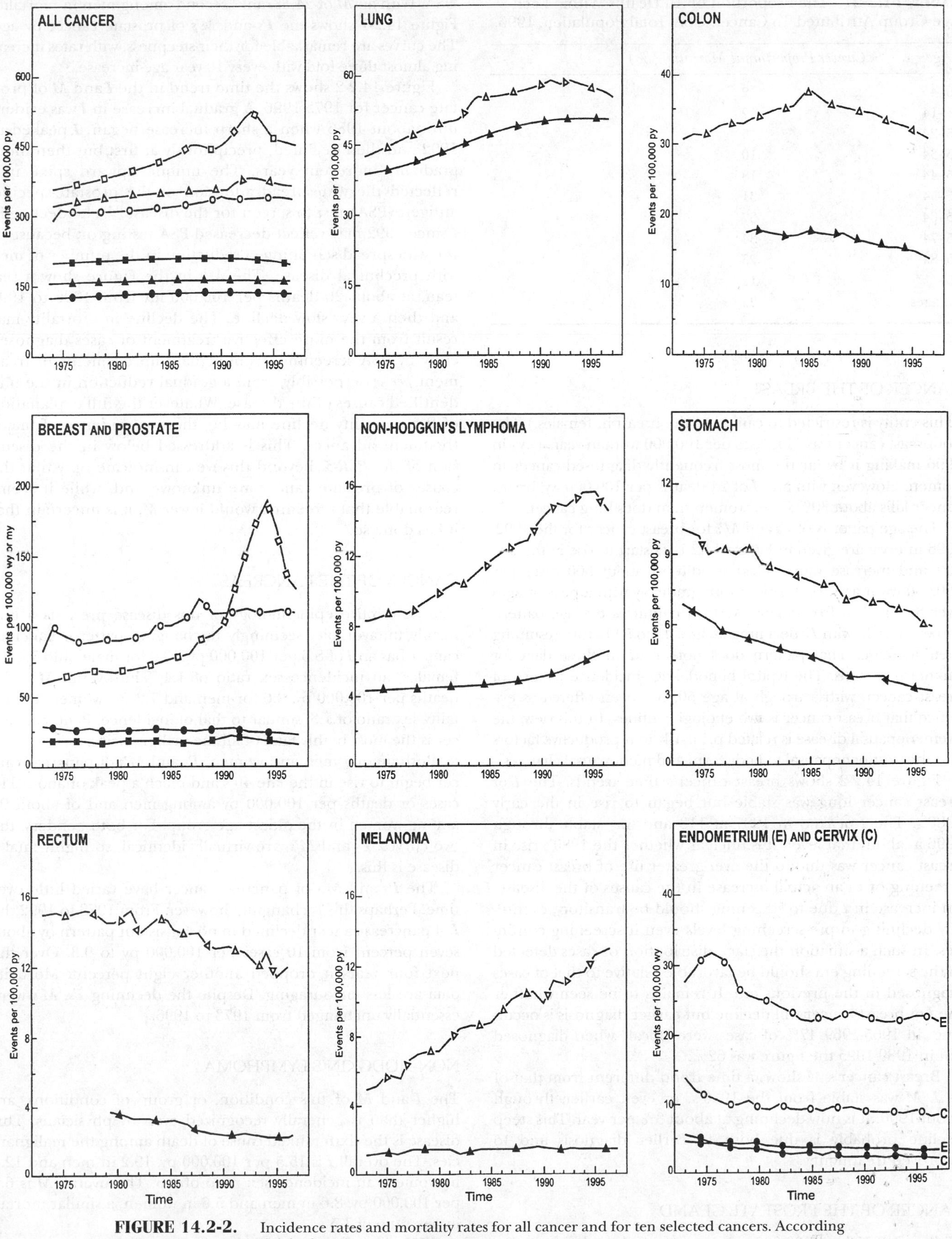

FIGURE 14.2-2. Incidence rates and mortality rates for all cancer and for ten selected cancers. According to time. See Figure 14.2-1 for key.

TABLE 14.2-3. The Proportion of All Deaths Within Each Age Group Attributed To Cancer. USA Total Population, 1996.

Age	*Cancer Proportional Mortality (%)*
0–4	2
5–14	12
15–24	5
25–34	10
35–44	18
45–54	31
55–64	37
65–74	34
75–84	23
85+	12
All ages	23

CANCER OF THE BREAST

(This entity is restricted to cancer of the breast in females.) The ***I*** of breast cancer was 111 cases per 100,000 woman-years (wy) in 1996 making it by far the most frequently diagnosed cancer in women. However, with an ***M*** of 24 deaths per 100,000 wy, breast cancer kills about 30% fewer women than does lung cancer.

The age patterns of ***I's*** and ***M's*** for breast cancer for the 1992-1996 interval are given in Figure 14.2-1. ***I's*** start to rise in the late 20's and increase more-or-less steadily to about 500 cases per 100,000 wy at age 70. ***M's*** rise more gradually with a peak at ages over 85. In data from many Western countries the age pattern shows a notch, with ***I's*** declining at ages 45 to 54 before resuming their increase. That pattern does not occur in these data for unknown reasons. The typical bimodal age-incidence pattern of breast cancer, with a trough at age 50, has been offered as evidence that breast cancer is two etiologic entities. In this view, the premenopausal disease is related primarily to reproductive factors and the postmenopausal to body form and menopausal changes.

Figure 14.2-2 shows breast cancer's time trends. The ***I*** of breast cancer long was stable but began to rise in the early 1980's. The ***I*** peaked in 1987 at 113 and was stable through 1996 at about that level. It is unclear whether the 1980's rise in breast cancer was due to the ever-greater use of breast cancer screening or to an actual increase in the causes of the disease. An increase in ***I*** due to screening should be transitory, eventually declining to pre-screening levels even if screening continues. In such a situation the stage distribution of cases detected in the screening era should be favorable relative to that of cases diagnosed in the previous era. It remains to be seen whether the ***I*** of breast cancer will decline but earlier diagnosis is occurring: in 1965-1969 47% of cases were "local" when diagnosed but in 1989-1995 the figure was 62%.

Breast cancer's ***M*** shows a time trend different from that of its ***I***. ***M*** was stable from the 1930's, or even earlier, through about 1990. It is now declining at about 3% per year. This steep decline probably is due both to earlier diagnosis and to improved treatment.

CANCER OF THE PROSTATE GLAND

With an ***I*** of 136 per 100,000 man-years (my) this cancer is by far the most frequently diagnosed malignancy among men in the USA. With an ***M*** of 24, it ranks second among men in mortality. Figure 14.2-1 shows the ***I's*** and ***M's*** of prostate cancer by age. The curves are remarkable for their steepness, with rates increasing almost three-fold with every 10-year age increase.

Figure 14.2-2 shows the time trend in the ***I*** and ***M*** of prostate cancer for 1973-1996. A gradual increase in ***I*** was evident until about 1986 when a sharp increase began. ***I*** peaked in 1992 and then declined, precipitously at first but then more gradually in recent years. The unique upward spike in ***I*** reflected the widespread adoption of the prostate-specific-antigen (PSA) test to screen for the disease.[14] The decline in ***I*** since 1992 may reflect decreased PSA testing or, because of the widespread screening, a reduction in the number of men with preclinical disease. The ***M's*** in the Figure show a plateau, at about 26 deaths per 100,000 my from 1990 to 1993 and then a very slow decline. The decline in mortality may result from the more effective treatment of cases diagnosed early by PSA screening, from actual improvements in treatment *per se* or, possibly, from a gradual reduction in the unidentified causes of the disease. Whatever the full explanation of the mortality decline may be, there is evidence of major treatment advances. This is addressed below in the discussion of the ***RSR-5***. Beyond this we can indicate only that the causes of prostate cancer are unknown and, while it seems reasonable that screening would lower ***M***, it is uncertain that it has done so.

CANCER OF THE PANCREAS

The descriptive epidemiology of this disease presents a uniformly unfavorable, seemingly unchanging pattern. Pancreas cancer has an ***I*** of 8.6 per 100,000 py, 10.0 for males and 7.4 for females, an incidence sex ratio of 1.4. The overall ***M*** is 8.3 deaths per 100,000 py, 9.6 for men and 7.2 for women, a mortality sex ratio of 1.3, similar to that of incidence. Pancreas cancer is the most highly fatal of all the malignancies.

Both among men and women, ***I's*** and ***M's*** of pancreas cancer begin to rise in the late 40's and reach a peak of about 110 cases or deaths per 100,000 py among men and of about 90 among women in the oldest age group. For both genders, the two curves, ***I's*** and ***M's***, are virtually identical, so highly fatal a disease is this.

The ***I's*** and ***M's*** of pancreas cancer have varied little over time. Perhaps this is changing, however. From 1973 to 1992 the ***I*** of pancreas cancer declined in no consistent pattern by about seven percent from 10 cases per 100,000 py to 9.3. Over the next four years it dropped another eight percent. Mortality data are less encouraging. Despite the declining ***I's***, ***M's*** were essentially unchanged from 1973 to 1996.

NON-HODGKIN'S LYMPHOMA

The ***I*** and ***M*** of this condition, or group of conditions, are higher than is generally recognized even by physicians. This disease is the sixth-ranked cause of death among the malignancies. The overall ***I*** is 15.5 per 100,000 py, 19.2 in men and 12.2 in women, an incidence sex ratio of 1.6. The overall ***M*** is 6.9 per 100,000 py, 8.6 in men and 5.6 in women, a similar mortality sex ratio of 1.5.

NHL shows increased ***I's*** as early as the mid-20's. ***I's*** increase sharply after about age 50 and ***M's*** after about age 60 in men.

For women the upward inflections occur at ages 60 and 70. Figure 14.2-2 shows the time trends in ***I's*** and ***M's***. ***I's*** now are rising sharply, increasing by 80%, from 8.6 cases per 100,000 py to 15.5 from 1973 to 1996. It has been suggested that some of this increase is an artifact due to changes in diagnostic classifications, which are bringing new entities into the lymphoma family.[15] However, such changes are unlikely to explain more than one-fourth of the increase seen. ***M's*** also are increasing but more slowly and may now be stabilizing. The increase from 1973 (4.7 deaths per 100,000 py) to 1994 (6.9 deaths) was 47%. However, there was no further increase in 1995 or 1996.

LEUKEMIA

(Leukemia here refers collectively to the four major forms of the disease, acute lymphocytic leukemia (ALL), acute myelogenous leukemia (AML), chronic lymphocytic leukemia (CLL) and chronic myelogenous leukemia (CML)). This discussion does not specifically address leukemia in children. Ninety percent of all leukemia cases occur after age 20. The statistics presented are inclusive of all ages but the observations pertain to leukemia in adults.

The leukemias are a category of diseases combined under one label both by historical precedent and by practical considerations of contemporary diagnosis and treatment. Nonetheless, while the leukemias eventually may be found to share some etiologic factors, this has been shown only for ionizing radiation and CLL is exempt even from that.

The ***I*** of leukemia was 9.7 cases per 100,000 py, 12.3 in males and 7.7 in females, an incidence sex ratio of 1.6. ***M's*** were 6.3 deaths per 100,000 py overall and 8.2 and 4.8 for males and females, giving a nearly identical mortality sex ratio of 1.7.

The ***I*** of leukemia is relatively high at 6.8 cases per 100,000 under age 5. It is then steady at about 2 to 5 until about age 40 when it begins to rise at a constant rate. The ***I*** of leukemia reaches a peak of 120 cases per 100,000 in men and 71 in women at ages 85 and over.

Leukemia ***M's*** are no longer particularly high in childhood; they remain under 1.3 deaths per 100,000 py through age 20 and then begin a steady increase to ages 85 and over.

Age-adjusted ***I's*** of leukemia were essentially unchanged at about 10.5 cases per 100,000 py from 1973 to 1995. In 1996 the ***I*** was 9.7, perhaps signaling the start of a decline. ***M's*** have declined from 6.7 deaths per 100,000 in 1973 to 6.3 at present. This 6% decline is identical for males and females and largely reflects treatment advances for the leukemias of childhood.

CANCER OF THE STOMACH

Although cancer of the stomach long has been declining, it remains the eighth-ranked cause of cancer death. The overall ***I*** is 6.6 per 100,000 py, 9.8 in men and 4.2 in women, a rather high incidence sex ratio of 2.3. The overall ***M*** is 4.0, with rates of 5.7 in men and 2.7 in women giving a sex ratio of 2.1.

I's of stomach cancer start to rise at about age 40. They rise progressively to age 85 and over, reaching a maximum of 119 cases per 100,000 py in men and 58 in women. The age pattern of ***M's*** closely follows that of ***I's*** but is one-third lower.

The ***I*** of stomach cancer has declined one to two percent per year for as long as data have been available, that is, since the mid-1930's. Mortality data suggest that the disease has been declining, at the same rate, since 1900. Stomach cancer was by far the most common cause of cancer death in men until surpassed by colorectal cancer in the late-1940's. It was also the most common cause of cancer death in women until about 1937 when it declined to fourth place. The "intestinal" type of stomach cancer declined two to three times faster than did the "diffuse" type of disease.[16,17] During the last 25 years or so, the long-term declines in stomach cancer have continued unchanged (Figure 14.2-2). ***I*** was 10.2 cases per 100,000 py in 1973 and declined about 1.5% per year to the 1996 level of 6.6, an overall reduction of 35%. The decline was identical in both sexes. ***M's*** have declined more, the reduction being 43% from 7.0 deaths per 100,000 py in 1973 to 4.0 in 1996. It was the same in both sexes.

The reason for the declining ***I*** of the intestinal type of stomach cancer is unknown. However, the decline extends over 90 years indicating that one or more causes of the disease started downward before 1900. The similarity of the decline in both sexes is remarkable and suggests that the declining cause is closely tied to domestic life or to residential, not occupational, settings. The favored hypothesis relates to the introduction of refrigeration and chemical food additives, several of which have anti-oxidant properties.[18] These twentieth-century methods of food preservation gradually displaced older methods such as the smoking, salting and pickling of foods. This hypothesis is supported by the fact that stomach cancer is strongly, and inversely, associated with economic status as the well-to-do adopted the newer methods first. Some other unidentified aspect of improving living standards also may have played a role in the decline of this disease. For example, *Helicobacter pylori*, a bacillus that colonizes the stomach of about 45% of Americans, was recognized as a cause of stomach cancer in 1994.[19] The prevalence of *H. pylori* infection also is strongly and inversely related to economic well being.

CANCER OF THE OVARY

The ***I*** of cancer of the ovary is 14.1 cases per 100,000 wy while the ***M*** is 7.4. The ***I*** has been stable for 40 years. An apparent rise in ***I*** from 1945 to 1960 probably resulted from improving ability to diagnose the condition. Despite the constancy of the ***I's***, ***M's*** have declined recently from 8.4 in 1973 to 7.4 in 1996, about 0.3% per year.

The age pattern of cancer of the ovary is exceptional in that ***I's*** start to increase in the late teens. Both ***I*** and ***M*** increase slowly until about age 40 or 45 and then rise sharply to peaks at about age 80.

CANCER OF THE NERVOUS SYSTEM

(This entity includes cancers of the brain, spinal cord, other central nervous system and the peripheral nervous system. However, 97% of deaths due to malignancies in this group are from tumors of the brain. We refer to this group as "CNS" cancer.) In 1996 CNS cancer had an overall ***I*** of 5.8 per 100,000 py in the USA, 7.2 in males and 4.5 in females. The corresponding ***M's*** are 4.2 and 5.0 and 3.4 for men and women respectively. With age-adjusted sex ratios of 1.6 for incidence and 1.5 for mortality this disease has a typical male predilection.

The age patterns for CNS cancer are shown in Figure 14.2-1. They are unusual in the long, gradual rise that extends from about age 20 to age 60 followed by a leveling, and then sharp declines. The leveling and decline in the statistics may result from a progressively greater underdiagnosis of cases and under-certification of deaths due to CNS cancer with increasing age. This would occur because of confusion of the cancer's symptoms with those of the much more common condition, stroke.[20]

The ***I's*** of CNS cancer long have been increasing. The rise during the middle of the century was probably due to improving diagnosis. More recently, ***I's*** rose from 5.0 cases per 100,000 py in 1973 to a peak of about 6.4 in 1987-1989. There has since been a gradual reduction to the current ***I*** of 5.8. The pattern of ***M's*** closely follows that of ***I's*** with a short lag. ***M's*** rose from 3.7 deaths per 100,000 py in 1973 to a peak of 4.3 in 1990. ***M*** is now stable at about 4.1 deaths per 100,000 py.

LIVER AND BILIARY TRACT

(This entity includes all primary cancers of the liver, bile ducts and gall bladder. We refer to it as liver cancer.) Liver cancer had an ***I*** of 4.2 cases per 100,000 py in 1996, 6.4 for men and 2.4 for women, a high incidence sex ratio of 2.7. For mortality the corresponding figures are 3.6 deaths per 100,000 py overall, 5.3 and 2.3 for men and women, a mortality sex ratio of 2.3.

Age patterns of liver cancer both among men and women are unremarkable. ***I's*** start to rise by the mid-30's among men and by the mid-40's among women and peak at about age 80. ***M's*** are virtually identical to ***I's*** in every respect.

Since 1973 ***I's*** for liver cancer have been increasing steadily from 2.3 cases per 100,000 py to the 1996 figure of 4.2. This 80% increase in just 23 years is worrisome but has attracted little attention. This is strange, since ***M's*** show a similar pattern, a 50% increase from 2.4 deaths per 100,000 py in 1973 to 3.6 in 1996. Moreover, the increases are occurring both among men and women.

Liver cancer is caused by the carrier state of the hepatitis-B and -C virus and these agents are the overwhelming cause of the disease in much of the developing world. Together, they probably account for about 50% of the disease in the USA.[21] In the USA there is also a clear association between abuse of alcoholic beverages and liver cancer.

URINARY BLADDER

(This entity includes cancer of the urinary bladder and "other urinary organs", essentially the ureter and urethra. Cancers of the kidney and renal pelvis are in a separate category. Ninety-seven percent of cancers in this group are bladder cancers and we refer to the disease that way.) Bladder cancer is the number 12-ranked cancer killer, responsible for 11,452 deaths in the USA in 1996. The overall ***I*** is 16.2 cases per 100,000 py. With ***I's*** of 27.7 for men and 7.4 for women, the incidence sex ratio is a striking 3.7. This reflects men's higher prevalence of smoking and greater exposure to occupational carcinogens. The overall ***M*** is 3.2 deaths per 100,000 py. With ***M's*** of 5.5 and 1.7 for men and women, respectively, the sex ratio is also a remarkably high 3.2.

Bladder cancer ***I's*** begin rising at about age 40 in men and 45 in women. A peak of 297 cases per 100,000 py is reached in men at ages 85 and over. A much lower peak of 75 appears at the same age in women. ***M's*** lag ***I's*** by about 10 years and peak at 139 and 42 deaths per 100,000 py for men and women, respectively.

I's for bladder cancer rose from 14.6 cases per 100,000 py in 1973 to a peak of 17.5 in 1987. A slow decline is now occurring with a rate of 16.2 in 1996. ***M's*** for bladder cancer declined 25%, about 1% per year, from 4.2 deaths per 100,000 py in 1973 to 3.2 in 1996. The decline has been slightly greater for men than for women.

CANCER OF THE ESOPHAGUS

This disease has an overall ***I*** of 4.0 per 100,000 py but for men the ***I*** is 6.8 while for women it is 1.7. The corresponding ***M's*** are 3.6 overall and 6.3 and 1.5 for men and women respectively. With age-adjusted sex ratios of 4.0 for incidence and 4.2 for mortality, this disease is the most strongly male-associated malignancy.

I's start to rise at about age 35 in men and 45 in women. There is then a sharp rise to an ***I*** of 41 cases per 100,000 py in men, 15 in women, at ages over 80. ***M's*** are virtually identical to ***I's***. The ***I*** of esophagus cancer increased gradually from 3.4 cases per 100,000 py in 1973 to 4.0 in 1996. However, there was almost no change in ***I's*** among women while rates among men increased about one percent per year from 5.5 in 1973 to 6.8 in 1996. The patterns of ***M's*** are virtually the same.

Cancer of the esophagus results from smoking, alcoholic beverage abuse and the combination of the two. Poor nutrition, particularly micronutrient deficiency may also be involved in causing this disease, especially in regions of the world where rates are very high.[22] If there is some good news in this it is that the now ongoing long term decline in smoking should bring reductions in ***I's*** of esophagus cancer in developed countries both directly and also by reducing the impact of alcohol abuse. In developing countries the correction of micronutrient deficiencies, which is relatively practical, may produce reductions in the disease.

CANCER OF THE KIDNEY AND RENAL PELVIS

(This group includes cancers of the kidney and of the renal pelvis, an unfortunate combination with a historical basis. Kidney cancer nearly always is a renal cell adenocarcinoma while renal pelvis cancer is a tumor of transitional or squamous cells. The renal pelvis is better seen as an extension of the bladder than of the kidney and both the histology and epidemiology of its cancer reflect that. Ninety-eight percent of tumors in this group are kidney cancers and we will refer to it as such.) The ***I*** of kidney cancer is 9.4 cases per 100,000 py, 12.9 among men and 6.5 among women. The corresponding ***M's*** are 3.5, 5.1 and 2.3. The respective sex ratios are relatively high at 2.0 and 2.2.

Both for men and women the age patterns of cancer of the kidney are unremarkable. ***I's*** start to increase in the 30's and peak at about age 80. ***M's*** show a similar pattern but lag ***I's*** by 5 to 10 years. The ***I*** of kidney cancer has undergone a 40% increase from 6.7 cases per 100,000 py in 1973 to 9.4 in 1996, nearly 1.7% per year. The increase is somewhat higher for women (48%) than for men (38%). The time trend in ***M's*** is similar but less striking. For both genders there was about a 20% increase from 2.9 deaths per 100,000 py in 1973 to 3.5 in 1996.

Kidney cancer and renal pelvis cancer are clearly though not strongly associated with smoking. This may explain why ***I's*** have been rising more sharply among women than among men. The fact that ***I's*** of kidney cancer reached a peak among men of 13.3 cases per 100,000 py in 1994 and may now be declining also supports the idea that long-term smoking patterns influence the disease's descriptive statistics. That is, the gender-specific time trends of ***I's*** for kidney cancer may duplicate, later in time and at a lower level, those of lung cancer.

MULTIPLE MYELOMA

The ***I*** of multiple myeloma was 4.2 cases per 100,000 py in 1996, 5.3 in men and 3.4 in women, an incidence sex ratio of 1.6. The corresponding ***M's*** were 3.1 deaths per 100,000 py, 3.8 for men and 2.6 for women, a mortality sex ratio of 1.5.

The age patterns, both of ***I's*** and ***M's*** for multiple myeloma are unexceptional. ***I's*** begin to rise in the early 40's and increase to a peak in the late 70's. ***M's*** lag ***I's*** by about 5 years and both ***I's*** and ***M's*** rise more sharply among men than among women.

I's of multiple myeloma have changed on a long term basis moving from 3.8 cases per 100,000 py in 1973 to a peak of 4.8 in 1987. There has been some decline since 1987 but the current ***I*** remains at 4.2. In contrast, ***M's*** have been increasing steadily. Both for men and for women the increase was about 35% from 1973 to 1996.

CANCER OF THE RECTUM

(This condition includes cancers of the rectum, rectosigmoid junction and anal canal.) Cancer of the rectum had an ***I*** of 12.5 cases per 100,000 py in 1996, 16.1 for men and 9.6 for women, an incidence sex ratio of 1.7. In the same year, ***M's*** were 2.4 deaths per 100,000 py overall, 2.6 for men and 2.2 for women, a lower mortality sex ratio of 1.2. These statistics are quite different from those of colon cancer which has lower sex ratios of 1.3 and 1.0.

Both for men and women ***I's*** rise in the 30's and rise sharply after age 45 to peaks at ages 75-79. For both genders, ***M's*** lag ***I's*** considerably and peak at 44 deaths per 100,000 py among men and at 34 among women. The time trend for rectum cancer is shown in Figure 14.2-2. The ***I*** of cancer of the rectum peaked at 15.2 cases per 100,000 py in 1981 and then declined slowly to 12.5 in 1996, a reduction of 18% in 15 years. This pattern was similar for males and females. ***M's*** have shown a similar pattern.

CANCER OF THE ORAL CAVITY AND PHARYNX

(This entity includes cancers of the entire oral cavity and of the pharynx. We refer to it as OCC, oral cavity cancer.) In 1996 the ***I*** of OCC was 10.0 cases per 100,000 py, 14.8 for males and 5.9 for females. The corresponding ***M's*** were 2.6, 3.9 and 1.4. The respective sex ratios were 2.5 and 2.8.

I's of OCC rise sharply among men from about 2 cases per 100,000 py at age 30 to a near peak of 65 at ages 60-64 and then rise slowly to a peak of 77 at ages 80-84. The pattern for women is similar although more gradual with a peak ***I*** of 34 at ages 85 and over. For each gender the age pattern of mortality closely follows that of incidence but ***M's*** typically are only about one-fourth of the corresponding ***I's***. ***I's*** of OCC declined over the period 1973-1996, about 15% for men and 10% for women. ***M's*** declined much more, about 30% both for men and women.

OCC shares much of its etiology with cancer of the esophagus, the lower sex ratio notwithstanding. It is not known whether the considerable decline in ***M's*** of OCC is due to increased screening for the disease, especially by dentists, or to treatment advances. However, stage-specific increases in survival have been relatively small, suggesting major benefits from earlier detection.

MALIGNANT MELANOMA OF THE SKIN

In 1996 melanoma had an ***I*** of 13.8 cases per 100,000 py, 17.0 for men and 11.4 for women, an incidence sex ratio of 1.5. For mortality, the corresponding rates were 2.3 deaths per 100,000 py, 3.2 and 1.5 for men and women, a mortality sex ratio of 2.1, much higher than that of incidence. The relatively poor survival of males occurs because a high proportion of their lesions are on the trunk and carry a poorer prognosis than do those on the extremities.[23]

I's of malignant melanoma begin to rise early in life, at about age 15 in both genders. There is a steep increase among men to a plateau of about 45 cases per 100,000 py at ages 70 and over. Among women the increase is more gradual to a lower plateau of about 30 cases per 100,000 py at ages 70 and over. For both genders, ***M's*** lag ***I's*** considerably in age and reach peaks of 27 and 12 deaths per 100,000 py among men and women, respectively, at ages 85 and over. The ***I's*** of melanoma have increased greatly, particularly over the last 25 years. This is shown in Figure 14.2-2. The increase from 1973 to 1996 was 140% overall, 178% and 110% for men and women respectively. However, ***M's*** have increased much less, 44% among men and only 15% among women. The increase in ***I's*** is due in part to an increased awareness of the disease and efforts to find it by physical examination of the skin. Part of the increase is also real and possibly due to increases in leisure time and sun exposure.

CANCER OF THE ENDOMETRIUM

(This entity includes cancer of the endometrium and cancer "of the uterus, not otherwise specified". At least 78% of cancers of the uterus, not otherwise specified, are cancers of the endometrium[24] and we refer to the entity that way.)

As shown in Figure 14.2-1 ***I's*** of endometrial cancer begin to rise at about age 30 and increase sharply to about 84 cases per 100,000 wy at age 64. They then increase more gradually to a peak of 109 at ages 75-79 and then decline slowly. ***M's*** start to increase at age 45 and rise gradually to a peak of 36 deaths per 100,000 wy at ages 85 and over. The ***I*** of cancer of the endometrium is 21.1 cases per 100,000 while the ***M*** is 3.3.

As shown in Figure 14.2-2 the ***I*** of endometrial cancer peaked at 32 cases per 100,000 wy in 1975. This reflected the gradually increasing use of estrogens, particularly conjugated equine estrogens, to manage symptoms of menopause. When that causal relation was recognized,[25] and this use of estrogens diminished, the ***I*** began to drop sharply reaching 21 in 1986 and changing little since. ***M's*** for this condition declined from 4.6 deaths per 100,000 wy in 1973 to 3.4 in 1989 and are now stable.

CANCER OF THE UTERINE CERVIX

This disease has an ***I*** of 7.7 cases per 100,000 wy and an ***M*** of 2.7 deaths per 100,000 wy. The exceptional age pattern of ***I's*** for cervix cancer is shown in Figure 14.2-1. The disease occurs among the young and ***I's*** rise sharply to age 35 and are then more-or-less steady for the remainder of the life span. This pattern strongly suggests that the rate of exposure to the causal agent is constant after about age 30 or that the agent's carcinogenic potency is reduced after that age. The age pattern of ***M's*** is unexceptional. The continued rise, long after ***I's*** have stabilized does, however, indicate that death can occur long after diagnosis.

I's of cervical cancer have declined since at least the 1940's. And, as shown in Figure 14.2-2, the recent decline was from 14.2 in 1973 to 7.9 in 1996, about 2% per year. ***M's*** are also in a long-term downtrend from 5.2 deaths per 100,000 wy in 1973 to 2.8 in 1996, also 2% per year. Some of the decline, both in ***I*** and ***M***, reflects the gradually increasing proportion of women in the population who have had a hysterectomy. Also, this disease is strongly and inversely related to economic well-being and so some general aspect of improving standards of living may play a protective role.

Screening for cervical cancer with the pap smear probably is responsible for some of the decline in ***I's*** and ***M's***. However, the relationship is not straightforward. The use of the pap smear increased greatly during the 1960's, 1970's and 1980's and, while this test is intended to detect dysplasia and *in situ* carcinoma, it also detects invasive disease. Thus, the early effect of the gradually increasing use of the pap smear should have been to ***increase*** the apparent ***I***. Eventually, the identification of large numbers of *in situ* cases presumably would lower the ***I*** of invasive cases and ***M***. Nonetheless, ***I's*** and ***M's*** of cervical cancer were declining long before pap smear programs could have had any major effect. This is not to deny the value of these programs, especially among high-risk women. Whatever may be the full explanation for the long-term declines of cervical cancer it seems likely that causes of the disease have been diminishing since at least the 1930's.

RELATIVE SURVIVAL RATES

Table 14.2-4 shows ***RSR-5's*** for all cancer and for the 20 major forms of cancer. The diagnosis intervals presented are 1950-1959, 1974-1976, 1979-1981 and 1989-1991; hereafter, 1955, 1975, 1980 and 1990. For most of these cancers, information is available for three stages of the disease: local, regional and all. These categories allow reasonably valid comparisons of survival statistics from as long ago as 1975. The 1955 data are of good quality but are not fully comparable with the subsequent data. They are provided for interest but are not discussed.

For all cancer, no improvement is seen in survival for any stage from 1975 to 1980, possibly because of the short interval between the two periods. Substantial gains occurred in each of the three stage groups from 1980 to 1990, a 15% increase (from 78% to 90%) for local disease and 25% for regional. The 16% improvement, from an ***RSR-5*** of 50% to 58% for all stages of all cancer is remarkable. It suggests a reduction in deaths of about 1.5% per year and conveys the ***magnitude*** of the gain that occurred during this 10 to 15 year period.

The data for all 20 forms of cancer allow 104 stage-specific comparisons to be made from one time period to another, e.g., for colon cancer, regional, from 1975 to 1980. Of these 104 comparisons, 82 (79%) show an increase in the ***RSR-5***, 10 show a decline and 12 were unchanged. This indicates the ***breadth*** of the gains that have occurred. This breadth makes it unlikely that the gains over the last 20 years in the all cancer ***RSR-5's*** would be explained by any gradual increase in the proportion of cancers that are inherently more benign.

In 1986 Bailar and Smith[26] indicated that cancer ***M's*** were still increasing and that gains in ***RSR-5's*** probably reflected earlier diagnosis or a "lead time" bias, not a true increase in cures or delay of death. The statement regarding mortality rates was accurate but, if lung cancer had been excluded, ***M's*** for all other cancers combined would have been seen to be declining as early as the mid 1950's.[27] It is more difficult to exclude lead time as the explanation of the small gains in ***RSR-5's*** through 1980 or even of the larger gains thereafter. However, data for breast cancer and prostate cancer may be useful for addressing this. From 1975 to 1990 these cancers became special targets for earlier diagnosis by screening and public education. Most of the lead time bias from screening, in terms of a seeming lengthening of survival, results from advancing the time of diagnosis of local disease and little results from earlier diagnosis of regional disease. Therefore, we may infer that survival gains for regional disease largely reflect actual treatment effects. Both for breast cancer and, especially for prostate cancer, for 1975 to 1990, large gains are seen in the ***RSR-5's*** for regional disease in Table 14.2-4. These gains suggest that there has been real improvement from medical care advances above and beyond any lead time effect. In another approach to this question, Cole and Rodu evaluated survival data for patients diagnosed from 1950-1991 and focussed on particular stages of specific cancers for which lead time gains presumably would be minimal or absent. Even for these conditions they found gains of about 0.5% per year in survival. They suggested that about one-half of the ongoing 1.0% per year decline in the overall cancer ***M*** that they reported for 1990-1995 was due to real advances in medical care.[12] A gain of 0.5% per year due to improvements in all aspects of medical care may seem disappointing. But we should bear in mind that for gains to occur each advance must favorably alter the course of ever more difficult cases, those that were resistant to prevailing diagnosis and treatment.

PERSPECTIVES

The descriptive epidemiology of the malignancies during the last quarter of the twentieth century provides five important observations:

First, the ***I's*** of the four major cancers (lung, colon, breast, prostate), and of all cancer combined are declining.[28] In fact, the ***I's*** of many forms of cancer, including cancers of the stomach, cervix, endometrium, rectum and oral cavity, were declining during the 1980's or before.

Second, ***RSR-5*** is increasing for most stages of many forms of cancer. It is unlikely that lead-time bias explains this because the improvements are occurring even for conditions for which diagnostic advances probably have been minimal.[12] Further, practicing oncologists now report seeing survival gains on a regular basis among patients with all stages of disease. These clinical observations can not be dismissed as anecdotal because they are nearly universal and because they are supported by improved survival figures and by declining cancer ***M's***.

Third, ***M's*** are declining for all cancer combined and for most forms of cancer and this has been true since 1991.[12] We must conclude that by 1996, there had been a decline in mortality for many forms of cancer extending over a period of at least 35 years that was due at least in part to advances in medical care.

TABLE 14.2-4. Five-Year Relative Survival Rate, as Percent, for All Cancer and for Twenty Major Forms of Cancer, by Stage, According to Time Period of Diagnosis

	Time Period of Diagnosis			
Cancer (stage)	1950-1959	1974-1976	1979-1981	1989-1991
All cancer*				
Local		78	78	90
Regional		47	48	60
All		50	50	58
Lung, bronchus				
Local	26	38	33	50
Regional	7	11	14	20
All	8	12	13	14
Colon				
Local	72	84	87	92
Regional	41	55	59	69
All	44	50	55	62
Breast (female)				
Local	83	91	90	97
Regional	51	67	69	77
All	60	75	75	85
Prostate				
Local	61	81	86	101
Regional	46	71	74	96
All	47	67	73	90
Pancreas				
Local	5	6	6	17
Regional	2	3	5	6
All	1	3	3	4
Non-Hodgkin's lymphoma				
All	29	47	50	51
Leukemia				
All	13	34	37	43
Stomach				
Local	40	53	57	62
Regional	13	14	17	21
All	12	15	17	21
Ovary				
Local	69	81	86	95
Regional	31	49	54	78
All	29	37	39	49
Brain, Nervous				
All	25	22	25	31
Liver, bil tract				
Local	5	11	6	16
Regional	0	2	2	5
All	1	4	3	5
Urinary bladder				
Local	68	85	89	93
Regional	21	40	46	51
All	55	73	77	81
Esophagus				
Local	6	8	11	24
Regional	4	4	4	10
All	4	5	6	11
Kidney				
Local	59	83	83	88
Regional	29	52	53	62
All	34	52	52	60

(*continued*)

TABLE 14.2-4. (*Continued*)

Cancer (stage)	*Time Period of Diagnosis* 1950–1959	1974–1976	1979–1981	1989–1991
Multiple myeloma				
All	7	24	27	29
Rectum				
Local	65	78	78	85
Regional	32	43	45	57
All	40	49	51	60
Oral, pharynx**				
Local		77	77	81
Regional		42	42	43
All		53	53	53
Melanoma				
Local	75	90	91	95
Regional	37	57	54	58
All	56	80	82	88
Endometrium				
Local	83	95	91	95
Regional	52	65	68	66
All	71	88	82	84
Uterine cervix				
Local	77	88	85	91
Regional	47	49	52	49
All	59	69	68	71

* Data not available for all cancer for 1950-1959.
** Data for oral cavity and pharynx for 1950-1959 judged not comparable with subsequent information and not presented.

In 1997, Bailar and Gornick[29] repeated the suggestion that declining ***M's*** were unlikely to be due to advances in diagnosis and treatment. This was based primarily on the view that the declines were minimal and that ***M's*** for most cancers were continuing upward. However, the decline in cancer mortality is accelerating downward (from 1996 to 1998 alone, the decline amounted to four percent[8,10]) and most forms of cancer are, in fact, declining.[14]

Fourth, a national pattern of the breadth and depth of the ongoing cancer mortality reductions can neither start nor stop abruptly. The length of cancer induction periods and the likely reduced exposure to carcinogens over the last 25 years make it reasonable to expect ***M's*** to continue down until at least 2010.

Fifth, we are winning but have not won the war on cancer. Bailar and Gornick[29] are correct in their view that more emphasis should be placed on prevention and prevention-related research. Several of the malignancies, notably non-Hodgkin's lymphoma and malignant melanoma, continue to increase in incidence and others, notably cancer of the esophagus and pancreas, remain resistant to diagnostic and treatment advances. Yet, to achieve the greatest overall reduction in cancer deaths, the target remains clear and unchanging; anti-smoking efforts must be reinvigorated and, most especially, heavy smokers must be provided with alternative ways to quit.[30]

Finally, the largest perspective. During the twentieth century cancer emerged from a minor position and became a major public health problem in the developed world. Over the next 30 to 50 years it will resume a minor position.[31] This waxing and waning occurred for virtually all the great scourges of mankind and it will occur for cancer. The descriptive epidemiology tells us that cancer's decline is now well established.

REFERENCES

1. Peto R. Smoking and death: the past 40 years and the next 40. *BMJ* 1994;309:937.
2. Parkin DM, Pisani P, Ferlay J. Global cancer statistics. *CA Cancer J Clin* 1999;49:33.
3. Ries LA, Kosary CL, Hankey BF, et al., eds. *SEER cancer statistics review, 1973–1996.* Bethesda, MD: National Cancer Institute, 1999.
4. The cancer epidemic: fact or misinterpretation? *Lancet* 1992;340:399.
5. Cole P, Sateren W. The evolving picture of cancer in America. *J Natl Cancer Inst* 1995; 87:159.
6. Rosenberg H, Maurer J, Sorlie P, et al. *Quality of death rates by race and Hispanic origin: a summary of current research, 1999. National vital statistics reports, vol 2, no. 128.* Hyattsville, MD: National Center for Health Statistics, 1999.
7. Kircher T, Nelson J, Burdo H. The autopsy as a measure of accuracy of the death certificate. *N Engl J Med* 1985;313:1263.
8. Peters KD, Kochanek KD, Murphy SL. *Deaths: final data for 1996. National vital statistics reports, vol 47, no. 9.* Hyattsville, MD: National Center for Health Statistics, 1998.
9. Hoyert DL, Kochanek KD, Murphy SL. *Deaths: final data for 1997. National vital statistics reports, vol 47, no. 19.* Hyattsville, MD: National Center for Health Statistics, 1999.
10. Martin JA, Smith BL, Mathews TJ, Ventura SJ. *Births and deaths: preliminary data for 1998. National vital statistics reports, vol 47, no. 25.* Hyattsville, MD: National Center for Health Statistics, 1999.
11. Axtell LM, Cutler SJ, Myers MH. *End results in cancer, report No. 4.* Bethesda, MD: U.S. Department of Health, Education, and Welfare, National Cancer Institute, 1972.
12. Cole P, Rodu B. Declining cancer mortality in the United States. *Cancer* 1996; 78:2045.
13. Wingo P, Ries L, Rosenberg H, Miller D, Edwards B. Cancer incidence and mortality: 1973–1995. A report card for the U.S. *Cancer* 1998;82:1197.
14. Devesa S, Blot W, Stone B, et al. Recent cancer trends in the United States. *J Natl Cancer Inst* 1995;87:175.

15. Porcu P, Nichols C. Evaluation and management of the "new" lymphoma entities: mantle cell lymphoma, lymphoma of mucosa-associated lymphoid tissue, anaplastic large-cell lymphoma, and primary mediastinal B-cell lymphoma. *Curr Probl Cancer* 1998;22:283.
16. Muñoz N, Connelly R. Time trends of intestinal and diffuse types of gastric cancer in the United States. *Int J Can* 1979;8:158.
17. Sidoni A, Lancia D, Pietropaoli N, Ferri I. Changing patterns in gastric carcinoma. *Tumori* 1989;75:605.
18. National Academy of Sciences, National Research Council, Commission on Life Sciences, Food and Nutrition Board. *Diet and health: implications for reducing chronic disease risk.* Washington DC: National Academy Press, 1989.
19. Infection with *Helicobacter pylori. IARC Monogr Eval Carcinog Risks Hum* 1994;61:177.
20. Schoenberg BS, Christine BW, Whisnant JP. The resolution of discrepancies in the reported incidence of primary brain tumors. *Neurology* 1978;28:817.
21. Ince N, Wands J. The increasing incidence of hepatocellular carcinoma [Editorial]. *N Engl J Med* 1999;340:798.
22. Chen F, Cole P, Mi Z, Xing L. Dietary trace elements and esophageal cancer mortality in Shanxi, China. *Epidemiology* 1992;3:402.
23. Vossaert K, Silverman M, Kopf A, et al. Influence of gender on survival in patients with stage I malignant melanoma. *J Am Acad Dermatol* 1992;26:429.
24. Percy CL, Horm JW, Young JL, Asire AJ. Uterine cancers of unspecified origin—a reassessment. *Public Health Rep* 1983;98:176.
25. Ziel H, Finkle W. Increased risk of endometrial carcinoma among users of conjugated estrogens. *N Engl J Med* 1975;293:1167.
26. Bailar JC, Smith EM. Progress against cancer? *N Engl J Med* 1986;314:1226.
27. Wingo PA, Ries LA, Giovino GA, et al.. Annual report to the nation on the status of cancer, 1973–1996, with a special section on lung cancer and tobacco smoking. *J Natl Cancer Inst* 1999;91:675.
28. Bailar J, Gornick H. Cancer undefeated. *N Engl J Med* 1997;336:1569.
29. Rodu B, Cole P. Nicotine maintenance for inveterate smokers. *Technology* 1999;6:17.
30. Cole P. Preface. In: Whelan E, ed. *Preventing cancer.* New York: Norton, 1977.

SECTION 3

PHILIP COLE
BRAD RODU

Analytic Epidemiology: Cancer Causes

Most known causes of cancer of human beings became suspect because of observations made by physicians and surgeons treating cancer patients. These "alert practitioners" noted unusual characteristics among several patients with the same disease. Investigations by themselves or others then identified a cause of the cancer. An early example is the observation in 1895 by the German urologist, Rehn, that three men with bladder cancer had worked at a particular chemical facility, a dyestuffs manufacturer.[1]

Cancer causation also is studied in experimental settings. Such studies can be complex and difficult to perform but may permit a straightforward judgement of causation to be made. When several investigators reproduce an experimental finding it is usually accepted as demonstrating causation.

Evaluating causality with epidemiologic research is more problematic. Epidemiology is not an experimental science. The epidemiologist observes heterogeneous, free-living human beings and has no control over their exposures or any other aspect of their lives. Further, the observations may be distorted by the retrospective nature of most epidemiologic research. That is, studies are made of exposures and of illnesses or deaths that occurred in the past, often in the distant past. For these reasons and others epidemiologic studies of cancer causation may produce highly variable results. History shows that studies of true and moderately strong causal associations will be reasonably consistently positive. However, a series of studies of a non-existent association will produce positive findings as well as the correct negative ones.

In 1965 Hill advanced guidelines for evaluating causality in epidemiologic studies of diseases with a long induction period.[2] The "Hill criteria", especially the major ones, the strength, consistency and plausibility/coherence of associations remain useful. A recently-developed set of guidelines[3] are more detailed than Hill's and are specific to the different circumstances in which causality is assessed. Several of these guidelines apply to the results of an individual study while others apply to a general causal hypothesis. Yet others address causality in the exposure-illness experience of a specific person.

EVALUATING CARCINOGENICITY

Many considerations underlie the judgement that a suspect agent is or is not a carcinogen for human beings. An important factor is whether the determination is to serve scientific or public health and regulatory purposes. The scientific focus addresses the question, "Is this agent, virtually certainly, a cause of cancer in man?" An affirmative response could be based on strong, consistent evidence from epidemiologic studies or on overwhelming evidence of carcinogenicity in animals and the absence of meaningful negative findings in human beings. In practice, a positive judgement usually rests on both consistent human and animal evidence.

When public health and regulatory purposes are the focus the question will be, "Is the probability that this agent is a human carcinogen sufficiently high that exposure to it should be eliminated or restricted?" The evidence needed for a positive response is less than that needed for the scientific question. The use of a lower standard means that a positive judgement does not imply that the agent is considered a carcinogen but only that society should act ***as if*** it is.

These different purposes partly explain why available lists of carcinogens are rather different. For example, the National Toxicology Program (NTP) of the USA lists 33 agents as "known to be human carcinogens" and an additional 274 as "reasonably anticipated to be" human carcinogens,[4] the "NTP-A" and "NTP-B" lists, respectively. It is clear that the NTP, in compiling both lists, is addressing the scientific question. At the other extreme, the EPA of California attempts to serve a regulatory purpose. It lists 456 "known" carcinogens, but there is no representation that the agents are known to cause cancer in human beings.[5]

Agencies also produce differing lists of carcinogens because they evaluate different agents or group them differently. For example, while the NTP-A list includes 33 entries the International Agency for Research on Cancer (IARC) has a "Group 1" list of 75 items for which there is "sufficient evidence" of human carcinogenicity.[6] This discrepancy seems surprising, since both agencies have a scientific mission. However, the IARC uses three categories: "agents", "mixtures" and "exposure circumstances". The category "agents" includes 25 items and, considering variations in the way agents are grouped, is virtually identical to the NTP-A list. The NTP recently has begun to evaluate "mixtures" and "exposure circumstances". When we turn from "known" to "suspect" carcinogens, we find that the NTP-B list includes 274 agents while the IARC has a Group 2A ("probably carcinogenic to humans") and a Group 2B ("possibly carcinogenic") which include 59 and 227 listings respectively, a total of 286. While the two lists are not directly comparable their similar lengths suggest correctly that their contents are very much alike.

There are important lessons in the 25-year experience of various agencies in classifying carcinogens. First, once suspicion falls on a true human carcinogen it usually soon is recognized as such. In contrast, despite decades of research on them, hundreds of items languish on lists of suspect carcinogens, especially on those of regulatory agencies. For example, the NTP-B list has included at least 274 agents since 1980. Only two of these ever were "promoted" to the NTP-A list, both in 1998. During the same 18-year interval 12 compounds were added directly to the NTP-A list without appearing on the "B" list. Evidently, the probability that a suspect item will come to be recognized as a human carcinogen is small. Second, the identification of "known" causes of human cancer has slowed. During the 1990's, the NTP added only four agents to its "A" list of known carcinogens, including the two from the "B" list. Ten had been added during the 1980's. This slowdown occurred despite ever more intensive searches for causes of cancer. The public health implication of this slowdown is that the extension of declines in cancer ***I's*** will require more effort against the known causes of cancer. The clinical implication is that improved access to medical care and improved methods for the detection, diagnosis and treatment of cancer will be needed to extend the ongoing increases in patient survival.

CAUSES OF CANCER

The causes of the malignancies are as diverse as the causes of disease in general. They include genetic defects, environmental and lifestyle factors, and chemical, physical and biologic agents. We address primarily the known human carcinogens but will mention a few suspect agents in context. Our list of 72 causes, or groups of causes, (Table 14.3-1) is adapted from the IARC's Group 1 list of 75 agents, mixtures and exposure circumstances for which there was judged to be sufficient evidence of carcinogenicity for human beings. We organized related agents into groups and combined them into five major categories. We added a few lifestyle factors of the type that the IARC does not consider. IARC does not list genetic causes of cancer and this Section does not address them. Finally, we indicate the NTP classification for each agent.

Many items in the table could be listed in more than one of the five categories. For example, solar radiation is an *environmental* factor but excessive sun exposure could be a *lifestyle* choice. It also poses an *occupational* hazard for outdoor workers, especially farmers. We placed each agent in the category where it seemed that most adverse exposure occurs. For each of the five categories, we estimated the attributable risk percent (***AR%***) for the general population. This is the proportion of cancer cases that would be prevented if the agents in the category were virtually entirely controlled. ***AR%'s*** were determined from estimates of the proportion of the USA population exposed to each agent in a category and the relative risks of cancer for such persons. We also considered the related efforts of Doll and Peto,[7] Trichopoulos *et al*[8] and of others. Collectively, a series of ***AR%'s*** provides an overview of the profile of cancer causation in a large population. But ***AR%'s*** are highly variable from one population or time period to another.

Table 14.3-1 includes the major malignancies resulting from each of the causes listed. For cancers for which reasonably reliable data are available, we provide an estimate of the relative risk (***RR***). This is the ***I*** of the cancer among persons with a typical exposure to the listed cause divided by the ***I*** among non-exposed.

We do not review the evidence relating to these established causal relationships but provide one or two references in support of each. In some instances we referenced the IARC discussion itself. We describe some of the causal relationships that are of greatest public health significance and a few others because of some biologic or epidemiologic feature that they exhibit. Reviews of known and suspected cause-effect relationships are available in two widely-used textbooks of cancer epidemiology.[9,10]

ENVIRONMENTAL FACTORS

For decades the mass media represented to the American public that the general environment was becoming polluted and that as a result cancer was increasing. Little attention was given to the underlying issue: Are the carcinogens in the environment or our exposure to them increasing?

From an epidemiologist's view the "environment" includes both the general or shared environment and individual behaviors and lifestyles. Only in this inclusive sense of the word is it correct that more than 90% of cancer is due to environmental, that is to all non-genetic, factors. On the other hand, in lay usage, the word "environment" designates only the shared environment, i.e., the air, water, ground and food supplies. We have adopted this usual meaning of the word, but point out that insofar as is known, individual behaviors are much more important causes of cancer than is the general environment.

All aspects of the long-term environmental deterioration in this country differ from place to place. There is no accurate way to summarize what the major contaminants were, when their inappropriate discharge occurred or when there was human exposure to them. Nevertheless, in much of the country the accumulated contamination had become consequential by about 1940. Most solid tumors of adults have an average induction period of about 20 years so it would be expected that cancers caused by environmental contaminants would have started to occur in about the mid-1950's.

Public awareness of the large scale of America's environmental problems began in 1962 with the publication of *Silent Spring*.[11] When Lake Erie and the Cuyahoga River caught fire in 1969 there was a public outrage that led to the environmental regulations and the broad-based cleanup that continue to this day. But, despite the cleanup the exposure of human beings to environmental contaminants probably continued to increase in much of the country until at least the mid-1970's and more likely until about 1980. Thus, environmental cancers would have increased in frequency until about 2000 or later.

In reality, ***M's*** from all cancer were increasing in this country by the early 1900's. ***I's*** would have begun to increase even

TABLE 14.3-1. Known Causes of Cancer of Human Beings and the Major Cancers that They Cause

*Causes**	*NTP***	*Forms of Cancer (RR)****	*References*
I. Environmental (4 factors, *AR*%: 5%)			
1. aflatoxins	A	hepatocellular	22
2. erionite	A	mesothelioma	19
3. radon	A	lung (2)	72
4. solar radiation	—	malignant melanoma (3), non-melanotic skin cancer	73,74
II. Lifestyle (6 factors, *AR*%: 45%)			
1. tobacco smoke	—	lung (12), larynx (12), oral cavity (5), esophagus (4), kidney (3), bladder (3), pancreas (2)	75, 76, 47, 79, 77, 78, 45
2. smokeless tobacco	—	oral cavity (2)	80
3. betel quid with tobacco	—	oral cavity (9)	81
4. alcoholic beverages	—	oral cavity (5), esophagus (4), larynx (4), liver (3)	82
5. dietary factors, salted fish (Chinese style)	—	nasopharynx (5)	83
6. reproductive factors****	—	breast, endometrium, ovary	84, 49, 57
III. Occupational (35 factors, *AR*%: 4%)			
1. 4-aminobiphenyl	A	bladder (10)	85
2. benzidine	A	bladder (30)	86
3. beta-naphthylamine	A	bladder (30)	87
4. benzene	A	leukemia (3)	88
5. bis-chloromethyl ether	A	lung (10)	89
6. vinyl chloride	A	hemangiosarcoma liver (300), hepatocellular, brain, lung, lymphatic/hematopoietic	90,91
7. ethylene oxide	B	lymphatic/hematopoietic (1.2)	92
8. mustard gas	A	lung (2)	93
9. dioxin	B	lung (1.4)	94
10. arsenic	A	skin (1.4), lung (6)	95,96
11. cadmium	B	lung	97
12. chromium VI	A	lung (2), sinonasal (10)	98
13. nickel	B	lung, nasal	99
14. beryllium	B	lung (2)	100
15. asbestos	A	mesothelioma (6), lung (3), larynx (2)	101,102
16. silica	B	lung (2)	103
17. talc (asbestiform)	—	lung (3)	104
18. ionizing radiation****	—	leukemia (2), lung (1.5), bladder (4), ovary (2), thyroid (10), bone (>2), soft tissue sarcoma (10)	105
19. coal tar, pitches	A	skin (scrotum)	106
20. mineral oils	A	skin (scrotum) (5)	107
21. shale oils	—	skin (scrotum)	108
22. soots	A	skin (scrotum)	109
23. wood dust	—	nasopharynx (5)	110
24. aluminum manufacture	—	lung (2)	111
25. auramine manufacture	—	bladder	112
26. boot/shoe manufacture, repair	—	nose (7)	113
27. coal gasification	—	lung, bladder, skin	114
28. coke production	—	lung (5), kidney (7)	115
29. furniture, cabinet manufacture	—	nose (80)	116
30. iron and steel founding	—	lung (2)	117
31. isopropanol manufacture, strong acid process	—	larynx	118
32. magenta manufacture	—	bladder (2)	119
33. painter	—	lung (1.3)	120
34. rubber industry	—	bladder (2)	121
35. sulfuric acid mist	—	nose, larynx	118
IV. Pharmacologic (18 factors, *AR*%: 2%)			
Alkylating agents			
1. chlorambucil	A	AML (10)	122
2. cyclophosphamide	A	leukemia (5)	123

(continued)

TABLE 14.3-1. (*Continued*)

*Causes**	*NTP***	*Forms of Cancer (**RR**)****	*References*
3. melphalan	A	AML (50)	124
4. methyl-CCNU	A	AML (25)	125
5. MOPP, and others	—	AML (50)	126
6. myleran	A	AML (20)	127
7. thiotepa	A	leukemia (5)	128
8. treosulfan	—	AML (>100)	128
9. chlornaphazine	A	bladder (4)	129
Immunosuppressants			
10. azathioprine	A	NHL (13)	130
11. cyclosporin	A	lymphoma (4), Kaposi's (50)	131
Hormones			
12. nonsteroidal estrogens	A	vagina (200), breast (1.5), testis (2.5)	58,132,133
13. steroidal estrogens	A	endometrium (5)	134
14. oral contraceptives, seq.	B	endometrium (4)	135
15. oral contraceptives, comb.	B	hepatocellular (7)	136
16. tamoxifen	—	endometrium (5)	137
Other			
17. methoxypsoralen + UV-A	A	non-melanotic skin (20)	138
18. analgesic mixtures with phenacetin	A	renal pelvis and bladder (7)	139
V. Biologic (9 factors, *AR*%: 4%)			
1. Epstein-Barr virus	—	Burkitt's lymphoma (30), sinonasal lymph, immunosuppressant-related lymphoma, Hodgkin's disease, nasopharyngeal cancer	140
2. *Helicobacter pylori*	—	stomach (4)	141
3. Hepatitis-B virus	—	liver (100)	142
4. Hepatitis-C virus	—	liver (20)	143
5. HIV-type 1	—	Kaposi's sarcoma (1000), NHL (100)	144
6. Human papilloma virus–types 16, 18	—	cervix (20)	63
7. Human T-cell lympho. virus–type 1		adult T-cell lymphoma (4)	145
8. *Opisthorchis viverrini*	—	cholangiocarcinoma (5)	146
9. *Schistosoma haematobium*	—	bladder (5)	147

*Adapted from IARC's Group 1 list of known carcinogens.
**From NTP; A = "A" list of known carcinogens; B = "B" list of suspect agents; — = not listed.
***Relative risk for persons with a typical exposure, as compared to a risk of 1 for non-exposed persons.
****Not listed by IARC or NTP.

earlier. That is, the overall cancer ***I*** probably had been increasing for fifty years before environmental pollution could have had any discernible effect. The overall ***I*** of cancer began declining in 1991[12] and many forms of cancer began declining in the 1970's. This implies that many causes of cancer had begun to decline by 1970, that is, 30 or more years before an environmental cleanup could have had a beneficial effect.

While our concern with environmental causes of cancer is focused on ***I's***, there is reason to review ***M's*** as well. The principle reason is the superior quality and representativeness of ***M's*** over ***I's*** when evaluating long-term, large-scale patterns of a relatively fatal disease. Excluding lung cancer, ***M's*** for "all other cancer" have been declining continuously since 1950.[13] Mortality from all cancer, even including lung cancer, has been declining since 1991[14] and is now accelerating downward.[15,16] This overall decline reflects reductions in the ***M's*** of many specific forms of cancer, including the four major cancers.[17] In fact, the American cancer experience, never static, is now changing favorably and profoundly: there was no meaningful increase in the ***number*** of cancer deaths from 1996 through 1998.[16] This is impressive because the USA's population is increasing in size and age—two demographic changes that would increase the annual number of cancer deaths substantially even if age-specific ***M's*** were constant.

We can not exclude agents in the environment as causes of some cancer. However, the study of general environments has led to the identification of only one cause of cancer in human beings. In that instance, endemic pleural mesothelioma in three villages in Turkey was found to be due to erionite, a naturally-occurring mineral which shares physical properties, including fiber size and shape, with asbestos.[18,19] Moreover, if an environmental agent were to cause cancer, cases probably would first appear as a "cancer cluster" in a residential or social (e.g., school or house-of-worship) setting. Erionite came to attention in this way. However, none of the other investigations of hundreds of cancer clusters by the Centers for Disease Control and Prevention[20] or by a state health department[21] identified a culpable agent, old or new. There is no way to know how many such investigations have gone unpublished because they provided no useful clue to the identity of a carcinogen. These considerations do not reduce the need to seek environmental carcinogens when their presence is suspected. And, they do not justify the environmental contamination that occurred. But they do indicate that there are more fruitful arenas in which to seek human carcinogens.

Table 14.3-1 lists the four natural environmental agents that are on IARC's list of known carcinogens. Arsenic also could be listed here. Except for the inclusion of radon gas, and occupations involving exposure to radon, IARC makes no mention of ionizing radiation and its sources, natural or man-made. Aflatoxins and erionite cause little or no cancer in this country but aflatoxins are discussed because of scientific interest. Solar radiation is addressed elsewhere in this text. Man-made environmental contaminants are addressed below.

Aflatoxins

Aflatoxins are a group of toxins formed by the fungus *Aspergillus sps.* which lives on peanuts, maize and animal fodder. The aflatoxins kill bacteria which compete with the fungus for the vegetable material as food. Aflatoxin B1, produced by *Aspergillus flavus,* is a potent cause of several forms of cancer in many species. It is considered a cause of hepatocellular carcinoma (HCC) in man on the basis of animal and epidemiologic studies.[22] HCC caused by aflatoxin is a major public health problem in Africa, in China and elsewhere in Asia.[23] In these regions it also may interact with hepatitis viruses to cause a large amount of HCC, probably the most common cancer in the world, among men. The frequency of HCC caused by afla toxin in developed countries probably is very low.[24]

Concern over environmental carcinogens usually is focussed on agents discharged in large amounts into the air or water supplies or dumped inappropriately. Rarely is there concern about naturally occurring geophysical factors or agents, even though the cancer burden imposed by natural agents is likely to exceed greatly that imposed by artificial ones.[25] Only three agents on IARC's Group 1 list of known carcinogens were widely distributed in the environment by man. These are arsenic, asbestos and benzene. These agents were distributed primarily through the application of pesticides (arsenic), use of insulation and automotive brake materials (asbestos) and motor vehicle exhausts (benzene). Other Group 1 agents (e.g., the metals) also were dumped in large amounts but in limited areas.

How much cancer is caused by the three man-made, or man-distributed, agents in IARC's Group 1? That question can not be answered with precision. However, several groups[7,8] have suggested that less than four percent of cancer deaths in America are caused by known carcinogens that pollute the environment. Perhaps the issue of greatest interest is that of general air pollution and lung cancer. Although this is not an established causal relationship, estimates of the ***AR%*** abound. For example, in 1990 the EPA estimated that less than one percent of lung cancer in the USA was caused by all of the "toxic pollutants" in air.[26] However, the estimate related to known, or suspect, carcinogens. Thus, the actual amount of lung cancer caused may be somewhat higher because of the possible additional effects of unidentified agents. On the other hand, the actual percentage may be or soon may become lower if the environmental cleanup of the last 25 years produces benefits.

Benzene can be used to illustrate the effort to estimate the ***AR%*** of a widely-dispersed environmental carcinogen. In this example, we focus on benzene as a cause only of leukemia and not of lymphomas as has been suggested by some persons. Several benzene-leukemia risk assessments[27,28] suggest that a benzene exposure of 50 to 100 part-per-million years is needed to double a person's risk of leukemia. The higher estimate, implying that benzene is weaker, is probably superior but we will use 50 ppm-years as the "first doubling dose" for leukemia. The "years" in the assessments refer to a year's work, that is 240 days at eight hours per day or about 22% of a full year. In highly contaminated public areas, e.g., a congested intersection in a major city, benzene levels in air rarely exceed 0.005 ppm. A person who spent a 75 year lifespan (about 350 work years) in this highly contaminated environment would accumulate a benzene exposure of 1.8 ppm-years (350 years × 0.005 ppm). This is about four percent of the first doubling dose of leukemia. Members of a population living under this condition would have a lifetime probability of death from leukemia of 1.04% instead of the usual 1.0%. This estimate may be too high as there is evidence that the benzene-leukemia relationship is a threshold phenomenon in animals[29] and that benzene does not produce leukemia in human beings at cumulative doses below 50 ppm-yrs.[30]

Benzene was used to illustrate the basis for the existing low estimates of the carcinogenic effects of environmental pollutants. Estimates for arsenic and asbestos are even lower because of their limited dispersal. Thus, the suggestion that environmental pollutants cause an appreciable amount of cancer in the USA usually rests upon conjectures: Unrecognized environmental pollutants are the culprits. Risk assessments such as that described are too general; concern should focus on local areas where exposures are uniquely high. The risk assessments do not consider possible synergistic effects of combinations of carcinogens. Or, finally, the population includes highly susceptible persons who will develop cancer at doses much lower than those experienced by the workers whose experience provides the basis for most risk assessments. It is correct that IARC's Group 2A and 2B together include about two dozen agents and mixtures that are suspected to cause cancer in human beings and are widespread. Trichloroethylene, polychlorinated biphenyls and diesel exhausts are relevant examples. But, whether these agents, alone or combined, do cause cancer is unknown.

LIFESTYLE FACTORS

There are five "mixtures" on IARC's Group 1 list that are included as lifestyle factors in Table 14.3-1. Each except the third, betel quid with tobacco, is discussed. We added reproductive factors. The NTP includes no lifestyle factor on its lists. We consider that about 45% of cancer in the USA is attributable to lifestyle factors but two-thirds of this 45% results from smoking.

Smoking

Smoking was not the first cause of cancer identified in human beings but it is premiere in almost every other way. It was the first lifestyle factor shown to cause cancer and probably the first established by epidemiologic means. Most important, ***smoking causes more cancer in the USA than do all other known causes combined.*** A typical 50 year old smoker has a risk of dying from cancer that is three times as great as that of a nonsmoker. Smoking leads to at least 25% and perhaps 35% of cancer deaths.

Finally, smoking is preventable and its elimination would lower cancer mortality more than would the optimization of all other known preventive and treatment strategies combined.

CANCER OF THE LUNG. Cigarette smoking began in about 1900 and increased among men during World War I and the "roaring" twenties. It continued upward through the 1950's. Large numbers of women began to smoke during World War II and their smoking increased until the mid-1960's.[31] By the 1930's many physicians suspected that the increase in lung cancer seen in their practices resulted from cigarette smoking. But this was contentious because many persons thought that the undoubted rise was due to urban air pollution. The importance of smoking was established in 1950 when the earliest case-control studies[32,33] showed the strength of its association with lung cancer. The association was widely accepted as causal by the public health and medical communities by the mid-1950's.

When the first Surgeon General's Report on Smoking and Health appeared in 1964,[34] smoking was a well-established cause of lung cancer. Interest had shifted to estimating benefits from smoking cessation and from switching to filter-tipped and to "low tar" cigarettes. It is now known that the ***RR*** of lung cancer declines 60% within 10 years of quitting smoking, and more thereafter.[35] However, a switch to filter-tipped and low tar cigarettes only minimally lowers risks.[36] Low tar cigarettes also have a low nicotine level and so "switchers" practice compensatory smoking, largely negating potential benefits.[37] Recent concerns relate to the effects of environmental tobacco smoke or "passive smoking". Although lung cancer remains uncommon among nonsmokers, nonsmoking spouses and associates of smokers have a 25% increased risk of the disease from environmental tobacco smoke.[38]

The persistence of smoking-induced lung cancer requires that conventional public health approaches to smoking control be reconsidered. These 40 year old programs have produced some beneficial effects. For example, the proportion of adults who smoke declined from about 50% in 1960 to 30% in 1990. However, it has not declined further. Moreover, there is something of a puzzle: Anti-smoking campaigns reduced the prevalence of smokers substantially in the mid-1960's. Why, then, did not lung cancer stabilize and begin to decline by the mid- to late 1970's? In fact, lung cancer stabilized (in men) only in the late 1980's and, so far, has declined only about nine percent. The explanation is that it was almost exclusively light smokers who quit first. Yes, light smokers do experience elevated lung cancer risks. However, it is the heavy or "inveterate" smokers, persons who are unable to quit, who suffer the greatest lung cancer mortality.[39] The prevalence of heavy smokers has declined relatively little and only recently.[40] Moreover, this decline is occurring not because the heavy smokers are quitting, but because they are dying. It still may be possible to save many of these heavy smokers, more than one-half of whom otherwise will die of a smoking-related illness,[41] by a harm reduction strategy which switches them *permanently* from cigarettes to an alternative nicotine source. This strategy is distinct from the usual one in which alternative sources (nicotine patch, gum) are employed only temporarily to assist conventional smokers to quit. No nicotine source is ideal for permanent use but, esthetic considerations aside, smokeless tobacco packets come closest.[39]

CANCER OF THE LARYNX. Smoking's association with larynx cancer is as strong as that with lung cancer. However, the risk of the disease among nonsmokers is so low that even the high ***RR*** among smokers produces rather few cases among them. The increased risk of larynx cancer from smoking is magnified by abuse of alcoholic beverages. A similar interaction or synergy is seen for cancer of the oral cavity and of the esophagus.

CANCER OF THE ORAL CAVITY (OCC). This condition, including cancer of the pharynx, is caused by smoking with a ***RR*** of about 5.

CANCER OF THE ESOPHAGUS. The risk of this disease is increased in smokers with a ***RR*** of about 4. It is a strikingly male disease, uncommon even among women who smoke.

URINARY TRACT CANCER. Renal cell cancer has a weak association with cigarette smoking with ***RR's*** rarely exceeding 2. However, the association is consistent and widely accepted as causal. The disease presumably is caused by a urogenous agent(s), possibly the same as that, or those, which cause squamous and transitional cell carcinomas of the lower urinary tract.

Smoking was causally linked to cancer of the bladder by the mid-1950's.[42] Smoking also is a likely cause of carcinomas of the other urinary passages, the renal pelvis, ureter and urethra.[43] These associations are moderate, with ***RR's*** of 2-4 and are consistent. There is some evidence that aromatic amines, especially 4-aminobiphenyl,[44] created from tobacco proteins by the pyrolysis of smoking, explain these causal relationships. One of the largest studies found that persons who quit smoking lowered their ***RR*** of bladder cancer by 20 to 30% within about four years.[45] This suggests that the urogenous carcinogen in cigarette smoke acts as a late-stage carcinogen in producing bladder cancer, whether or not it also acts as an early-stage carcinogen.

OTHER CANCERS. IARC considers smoking a cause of pancreas cancer. Smoking is moderately to strongly suspect as a cause of cancer of the cervix and liver and of leukemia.

Smokeless Tobacco

Use of smokeless tobacco imposes a moderate ***RR*** of 2 for OCC. However, this risk may be declining because the suspect carcinogens in smokeless tobacco, naturally-occurring tobacco-specific nitrosamines (TSNAs), have been reduced over the past two decades. In Sweden, where *per capita* consumption of smokeless tobacco is very high, TSNAs levels are undetectable and recent studies report no OCC attributable to the use of Swedish products.[46]

Alcoholic Beverages

Four forms of cancer are caused by abuse of alcoholic beverages (AB), OCC and cancers of the larynx, esophagus and liver. ***RR's*** averaged over different levels of AB abuse and from different studies are about 4 for these cancers. Thus, 75% of these cancers that occur among AB abusers is attributable to their drinking. In a general population with a six percent prevalence of AB abusers, a typical figure for men and women combined,[31] about 20% of these cancers, and about 3% of all cancers, is attributable to AB abuse. Similar estimates have been made by others.[7,8] However, none of these estimates includes the synergistic effects of smoking with AB in causing OCC and larynx and esophagus cancer.

Smoking and alcohol show a strong synergy in causing OCC and cancers of the larynx and esophagus. For example, among men, the ***RR*** of OCC is 5 for smokers and 5 for AB abusers. However, it is about 25 for men who have both exposures.[47] Each of these three cancers has a distinctly high incidence sex ratio: 4.1, 4.0 and 2.5 for cancers of the larynx, esophagus and OCC, respectively. These high sex ratios probably occur because the combination of heavy smoking and AB abuse is four times as common among men as among women.[47] A practical reality is that all three of the cancers would decline by 40% or so if AB abuse were to cease.

Despite its acceptance as a cause of four forms of cancer, the carcinogenic effect of AB abuse is unexplained. Ethanol is not carcinogenic in animals or *in vitro.*[48] It has been suggested that AB abuse is associated with cancer because of the poor diet, including micronutrient and vegetable deficiencies, that characterize AB abusers. Another suggestion is that alcohol acts as a topical solvent on epithelial tissues and increases the amount of carcinogens in food or cigarette smoke or in the AB themselves that penetrate cells. Both suggestions have existed for decades without becoming established or disproven.

Dietary Factors

Diet is widely seen as a cause of a high proportion of cancer in human beings. This perception has three major bases, the 1981 report by Doll and Peto,[7] a wealth of seemingly incriminating research and an intuitive appeal. Doll and Peto estimated that 35% of cancer deaths in the USA ***might be*** attributable to diet (with a range of 10-70%). They wrote, "It must be emphasized that the figure chosen is highly speculative and chiefly refers to dietary factors which are not yet reliably identified." This qualification of the 35% estimate is as valid today as it was 20 years ago.

If the estimate is restricted to known and strongly suspect dietary causes of cancer it is much lower than 35%. IARC includes only one dietary item, Chinese style salted fish, on its list of known carcinogens. It causes nasopharynx cancer where heavily salted fish is eaten in large amounts by persons of all ages, including children. This item presumably causes almost no cancer in America.

Although not a dietary factor in the usual sense, caloric excess and the resultant obesity may be seen as a cause of cancer. This is virtually certain for cancer of the endometrium[49] and likely for breast cancer.

The items in the American diet often linked to cancer are red meat especially when charred,[50] animal fats[51] and "pesticide residues" ingested on over-treated and under-washed fruits and vegetables. The cancers related to these items are those of the stomach, colon, breast and prostate. None of these associations is established as causal. Similarly, many dietary agents have been suggested as protective against one or another form of cancer. These include, as examples, zinc and cancer of the larynx and esophagus,[52] fruits and vegetables and cancers of the gastrointestinal tract, lung and endometrium.[53] None of these associations is established.

Reproductive Factors

Virtually every aspect of a woman's reproductive life is associated with alterations in her breast cancer risk. These include age at menarche (earlier, increased risk), age at first delivery (later, including nulliparity, increased risk), parity (more children, lowered risk), lactation (longer, lowered risk), age at menopause (earlier, lowered risk) and the use of exogenous estrogens (increased risk). Prolonged use of oral contraceptives (OCs) by younger women may increase breast cancer risk but this relationship remains poorly understood. The observations seem consistent in suggesting that the duration of a woman's reproductive life is the primary risk determinant.[54] But, there also is evidence that much of a woman's breast cancer risk is determined in her youth and young adulthood.[54,55] And yet, there is no accepted mechanism that links these reproductive features to a causal agent or to a means of preventing breast cancer.

Cancer of the endometrium and ovary share descriptive epidemiologic features with breast cancer and their risk is increased by nulliparity. But they share few of the other reproductive correlates of risk. Endometrial cancer is caused by use of sequential but not of combined OCs. This is presumably due to the regimen of sequential agents which involves two weeks per month of exposure to estrogens unmodified by a progestogen. Endometrial cancer also is caused by exogenous estrogens, primarily estrone, that until 1975 were prescribed frequently and in relatively high doses for the control of menopausal symptoms. These observations suggest that endogenous estrone is also a cause of the disease. In any event, some aberration of endogenous hormone production or metabolism is likely to cause endometrial cancer. This is consistent with the correlation of endometrial cancer risk with male pattern (upper body) obesity in which hormonal aberrations commonly are seen.[50] Finally, endometrial cancer is caused by tamoxifen, anti-estrogenic for the breast but estrogenic for the endometrium.[56]

There is no established cause of ovarian cancer except ionizing radiation, although several agents are suspect. These include asbestos, talc and hair dyes. Parity is moderately protective with ***RR's*** declining gradually from 1.0 for nulliparas to about 0.4 for women with four or more children. Lactation may be moderately protective with perhaps a 30% risk reduction from prolonged lactation. Five or more years of use of combined OCs may lower risk by 40%. Weiss et al[57] indicated that major progress will require a massive study which evaluates demographic features and possible causes separately for each of the major types of ovarian tumor (germ cell, sex cord and stromal and epithelial).

OCCUPATIONAL FACTORS

No area of epidemiologic research has identified as many human carcinogens as has occupational epidemiology. One-half of the 75 agents on the IARC Group 1 list of known carcinogens were identified, or confirmed, by occupational investigations. Yet, only about four percent of cancer in the USA is due to occupational factors.

The discovery of new carcinogens in occupational settings has slowed but this research setting remains important for four reasons: 1) There are several strong suspect occupational carcinogens. 2) For many agents thousands of workers are exposed in the USA and several hundred thousand worldwide. Thus, the hazard to workers alone from an occupational carcinogen could pose a major public health problem. 3) Workers typically are exposed to high concentrations of the agents with which they work and so serve as sentinels for the general population. 4) Almost all occupational studies are of the retrospective follow-up (also termed retrospective cohort) type. This design permits all causes of death, or all major illnesses, to be identified. Thus, these studies may identify not only carcinogens but causes of other diseases as well.

Only one occupational carcinogen, creosote, has been added to the NTP "A" list since 1981. More generally, the health of employed groups now is remarkably high and is likely only to improve as advances in industrial hygiene and manufacturing efficiency make the workplace cleaner.

PHARMACOLOGIC/IATROGENIC FACTORS

The use of a carcinogen as a therapeutic agent is justified for treating a life-threatening condition and even for treating severe non-fatal conditions. At least one known carcinogen, tamoxifen, is also a cancer preventative in women at high risk of breast cancer.[56] The need to evaluate carefully the risks from the therapeutic use of a carcinogen in each patient is obvious. This is especially so for children since a child cured of a malignancy has a life expectancy much longer than the induction period of any cancer. It is not so well recognized that the same issue applies to adults. Even a 60 year old person in the USA has a life expectancy of 20 years or more, an adequate induction period for many forms of cancer and especially for the leukemias induced by oncolytic therapy.

IARC's Group 1 list of known carcinogens includes 18 agents and mixtures that are, or were, used in medical practice. There are nine alkylating agents (including as one, MOPP and other combinations that include an alkylating agent), four hormone groups, 1 hormone antagonist, two immunosuppressants, and two additional mixtures. They are listed in Table 14.3-1. Most of the agents are used to treat cancer and a few are used to treat other life-threatening conditions, e.g., transplanted organ rejection. Several, such as the estrogen mixtures are, or were, used to treat relatively benign conditions and OCs are used without a therapeutic indication.

The carcinogenic effects of therapeutic agents can be difficult to recognize and to quantify. The reasons are best described if we consider first the agents used for non-malignant conditions. The carcinogenic effect of these agents is difficult to evaluate because, although they are available only on prescription, the actual amounts prescribed and consumed are uncertain as any patient (or member of the general public) may obtain the drugs. A patient, or another physician may change the drug prescribed to another which has a similar biologic effect but which has a different carcinogenic potential, e.g., substitution of non-steroidal for steroidal estrogens. Finally, if the patient is not under long-term observation at a single medical center a cancer that occurs will not be noted, much less be related to drug use.

Perhaps because of the difficulties just mentioned, as well as the low risk of cancer posed by agents that are not anti-neoplastic, Table 14.3-1 lists few such agents. This dearth does ***not*** reflect a lack of suspicion or of searches for carcinogenic effects of pharmacologic agents. Many agents have been evaluated and not found to be carcinogenic. For example, the IARC's Group 3 ("Unclassifiable as to carcinogenicity to humans") includes, among other medications, chloral, acetaminophen (the major metabolite of phenacetin), reserpine and spironolactone.

The causal relationship between DES exposure *in utero* and clear cell adenocarcinoma (CCA) of the vagina in young women warrants mention. DES is the only non-oncolytic pharmacologic agent that imposes a massive ***RR*** of cancer on exposed persons. Although the association is strong with an ***RR*** >100 the disease is nonetheless rare among exposed women; their lifetime risk of developing CCA is only 1 in 1000.[58]

When we turn to the anti-neoplastic agents, most of the investigative problems mentioned above are reduced. The identity and dosage of the agents prescribed are documented. Outpatient compliance with treatment is presumed to be good. The agents are not used by the general public and so the baseline number of cancers of a particular type to be expected among treated patients can be estimated. However, there are three problems that complicate the study of the carcinogenicity of anti-neoplastic agents: 1) The agents often are used in combinations both simultaneous and sequential or with radiation therapy. This makes it difficult to identify the effect of any one agent and also introduces the possibility of synergistic effects. There is particular concern about synergy between pharmacologic agents and radiation therapy. However, there is as yet no evidence of this synergy.[59] 2) Many cancer patients survive relatively few years after receiving chemotherapy. This makes it difficult to accumulate a substantial number of person-years at risk after the passage of a reasonable minimum induction period for a second cancer. 3) Cancer patients are at increased risk of developing a second primary cancer for reasons unrelated to their treatment. These include the high risk of a second primary of the same type as the first. The causes of one type of cancer also cause others, e.g., patients with lung cancer have an increased risk of bladder cancer, and vice versa, because smoking causes both. Also, causes of cancer often cluster in an individual, e.g., smoking, AB abuse and poor diet. Finally, there is the possibility of a "cancer diathesis", the prospect that, for some constitutional reason, e.g., genetic makeup, a person who developed one cancer has an inherently increased risk of developing another.

The many reasons why a cancer patient might develop a second primary tumor cause us to be skeptical of reports of an excess of second primaries following anti-neoplastic treatment. This is especially so if the excess is minimal or is restricted to cancers of the same type or etiology as the first. However, as Table 14.3-1 indicates, a characteristic of the risk of second primaries following cancer treatment is that almost all of the ***RR's*** are 5 or greater. And, the second cancer commonly is AML, irrespective of the cancer for which treatment was given. The associations in the table are virtually certainly attributable to the agents listed and not to any of the other reasons why a cancer patient might develop a second tumor.

BIOLOGIC FACTORS

Oncogenic biologic agents long have challenged laboratory investigators and epidemiologists. For nearly a century one microbe after another that appeared to cause cancer in man was identified but soon discarded. Few contemporary researchers will remember the "*Bacillus hodgkini*" – the "cause" of Hodgkin's disease discovered in 1915.[60] More memorable, if only because of their recency, are the various "B" and "C" particles that were considered fragments of a virus which was thought to cause breast cancer in women. *Herpesvirus hominis, type 2,* was virtually established in the mid-1970's as the cause of cervix cancer. But, by 1981, in their review of known and suspect causes of cancer, Doll and Peto[7] indicated only that the EBV-Burkitt's lymphoma relationship seemed likely to be causal and they appeared to accept the hepatitis-B virus and HCC association as causal. They suggested as, "a very uncertain best estimate" that 10% of cancer deaths in the USA might prove to be due to infectious agents.

Now, the discovery of causes of cancer has slowed in virtually every area except that of biologic agents. Almost certainly as a direct result of advances in molecular biology, there are nine biologic agents known to cause cancer in human beings (Table 14.3-1). All nine agents are of considerable scientific and clinical interest but only the hepatitis viruses, the human papilloma viruses (HPV) and *H. pylori* cause enough cancer to be considered public health problems in the USA. The hepatitis-B and -C viruses together cause about 50% of the cases of HCC that occur[61] and so cause about 6000 deaths per year. HPV causes about 90% of cervical cancer or 4000 deaths per year.[62] Both categories of agents produce much more disease in the developing world, as does EBV. *H. pylori* is estimated to cause 60% of stomach cancer or about 7000 deaths per year in the USA. The other known infectious agents combined probably cause less than 500 cancer deaths per year. The total for infectious agents is about 18,000 deaths per year or about four percent of cancer deaths. Doll and Peto's "best estimate" of 10% still seems reasonable as a virus etiology may yet be found for several forms of cancer, especially in the leukemia-lymphoma group.

Cervical cancer is the most common cancer in the world, among women. It has a long and rich epidemiologic history. Its long-term declining ***I*** and ***M*** in developed countries, its striking association with poverty, with "reproductive" factors, and the large-scale use of the pap smear all have caused this disease to receive considerable attention from the cancer research community. Cancer of the cervix is the "epidemiologic opposite" of the other major cancers of women. It is associated with early childbearing, high parity and poverty. However, the representation that cervix cancer is associated with "reproductive" factors is a euphemism. The disease actually is associated largely with sexual practices. The more sexual partners a woman has had, especially before age 20, the higher her risk of cervical cancer.[63] We now recognize that this association reflected a woman's probability of becoming infected with HPV. There may be small, independent associations of cervical cancer risk with factors beyond those that are indices of exposure to HPV. These factors are use of OCs and micronutrient, especially vitamin, deficiencies.

A notable feature of the epidemiology of cervical cancer is the recent increase of adenocarcinomas. This condition has an epidemiology like that of cancer of the endometrium and unlike that of the usual squamous cell carcinoma of the cervix.[64]

PERSPECTIVES

The year 2001 is the thirtieth anniversary of the National Cancer Act and of the USA's "War on Cancer". These three decades brought major achievements. Since at least 1972 ***M's*** of most forms of cancer have been declining; in 1991 the overall cancer ***M*** started to decline and is now accelerating downward. This favorable trend probably will continue for many years. Thus, progress may now be described as, at the very least, substantial.

TABLE 14.3-2. Percentage of Cancer Deaths Attributable to Agents in Eleven Categories

Category	*Year* 1981*	2000**
1. Pollution	2%	2%
2. Geophysical	3	3
3. Smoking	30	30
4. Alcohol	3	3
5. Diet	35	5
6. Food additives	1	0
7. Reproductive/Sexual	7	7
8. Occupation	4	4
9. Industrial products	1	1
10. Medicines/Procedures	1	2
11. Biologic	10	4
Total	97%	61%

*From reference 7.
**Present authors.

Cancer ***M's*** started to decline earlier and still decline more sharply than do ***I's***. This is *prima facie* evidence of major improvements in medical care. And yet ***I's*** finally are also declining indicating that prevention efforts are bringing results. This is what we address here. Do we now know, and protect against, the causes of more cancers than we did 20 or 30 years ago?

ARE MORE CANCERS NOW OF KNOWN ETIOLOGY?

At the beginning of this Section we compared the 1998 NTP-A list of known carcinogens with its 1980 counterpart. The list increased from about 20 agents to about 33. However, the added items are almost all pharmacologic agents that, combined, cause less than three percent of cancer deaths.

In 1981 Doll and Peto estimated the percentage of cancer deaths in the USA attributable to each of 11 major causes or groups of causes of cancer.[7] The left column of Table 14.3-2 is an adaptation of their summary estimates of ***AR%'s***. (We made minor alterations in their format, described below.) The 97% figure of Doll and Peto does not imply that they thought they were explaining nearly all cancer. The ***AR%'s*** listed are not mutually exclusive and the totals presented are only general indicators of how much disease might be prevented if the causes listed were controlled. The right column in Table 14.3-2 shows our present estimates of the all-cancer ***AR%'s*** for the same categories of agents. A comparison of the two sets of estimates seems to imply that there has been little progress. The total in the second column is actually moderately ***lower*** than that in the first! Do we know the causes of fewer cancers than we did 20 years ago? No. The explanation of the decline in the ***AR%'s*** lies in the different bases of the two sets of estimates. Doll and Peto addressed what reasonably might be true; we describe what is known or highly probable. To clarify this we address several categories in the table.

We labeled the third category "smoking" but Doll and Peto termed it "tobacco". The distinction is important. During the last 20 years in the USA many anti-smoking campaigns shifted their focus from preventing deaths caused by smoking to preventing tobacco use. If we refocus attention on deaths from smoking we can learn a valuable lesson from Sweden, the only country which has met the World Health Organization's goal of a less than 20% prevalence of smokers. It also has Europe's lowest rates of lung cancer, larynx cancer, OCC and bladder cancer.[65] How were these benchmarks attained? There may be several explanations, but it is certainly relevant that Sweden has the highest *per capita* use in Europe of smokeless tobacco.[66]

Whether we refer to "tobacco" or "smoking", the situation has not changed in 20 years: smoking causes about 30% of cancer deaths. It will now change. Lung cancer and other smoking-related cancers will decline sharply over the next decade. The impending decline in lung cancer deaths will occur because the number occurring among inveterate, that is heavy, smokers at last has started down. These persons are literally a dying breed whose numbers, finally, are not being replaced fully by equally heavy smokers. The misfortune is that the decline in smoking-related morbidity and mortality that is now beginning might have occurred 20 or more years ago if our initial efforts against smoking had focussed on the heavy smokers.

Doll and Peto thought that dietary factors might cause about 35% of cancer. Yet, the evidence that dietary factors are carcinogens is as elusive today as it was 20 years ago. Our present estimate even of just five percent is defensible only as "strongly suspect". Despite limitations and controversy the information on diet and cancer is useful. Virtually all of the dietary alterations recommended today to reduce cancer risk are, at the least, prudent. The specific reason why people choose a healthful diet and whether it is the "prudent" diet,[67] the Asian diet, or the Mediterranean diet[68] may matter little. Each of the diets, adopted not as a temporary regimen, but as a part of one's lifestyle will contribute to weight control, reduce intake of animal fats and increase the intake of fruits and vegetables. This should lower the risks of cardiovascular diseases and, perhaps, of cancer.

Doll and Peto considered only two of the virus-cancer relationships in Table 14.3-1 as "likely". Today, none of the relationships in the table is controversial. However, there is uncertainty over the ***RR's*** and ***AR%'s*** of cancer associated with infectious agents. Our summary estimate of four percent, developed above, is a reasonably firm estimate of the minimum amount of cancer caused by infectious agents.

We consider Doll and Peto's estimate of one percent of cancer due to "medicines, procedures" and our analogous estimate of two percent as identical if only because both are imprecise. The amount of cancer caused by these agents is unlikely to be increasing. In fact, in a carefully developed opinion in 1977 Jick and Smith suggested two percent.[69] Cancer due to pharmacologic and iatrogenic agents probably is declining because of their more guarded use.

No, we do not know the causes of fewer cancers today than we did 20 years ago. But, if we focus on what we know, as distinct from what may be true, we do not know the causes of many more, either.

HAVE WE REDUCED EXPOSURE TO RECOGNIZED CAUSES OF CANCER?

Yes. The population's smoking, both active and passive, is diminishing, albeit slowly. Exposure to workplace carcinogens probably is declining and occupational cancers are in decline.[8] *H. pylori* is treated widely, sunblockers are in common use and carcinogenic agents in medical practice are used carefully. Although obesity unfortunately is increasing,[70] animal fat in the American diet is declining while the amount of fruit and vegetables is increasing.[71] Also, contaminants in the general environment, possibly including carcinogens, are in decline. It is impractical to estimate the cancer reductions that these changes will bring. But, the reductions already are evident and appear certain to increase.

REFERENCES

1. Rehn L. Blasengeschwulste bei fuchsin-arbeitern. *Arch Klin Chir* 1895;50:588.
2. Hill AB. The environment and disease: association or causation? *Proc R Soc Med* 1965;293.
3. Cole P. Causality in epidemiology, health policy, and law. *Environ Law Reporter* 1997;27:10279.
4. US Department of Health and Human Services. National Toxicology Program. *Eighth report on carcinogens 1998 summary.* Also available at: http://ehis.niehs.nih.gov/roc/toc8.html.
5. California Regulatory Notice Register. *Safe drinking water and toxic enforcement act of 1986 (Proposition 65): Notice to interested parties.* August 20, 1999. Also available at: www.oeha.org/prop65/899not.html.
6. IARC current website: http://www.iarc.fr.
7. Doll R, Peto R. *The causes of cancer.* New York: Oxford University Press, 1981.
8. Trichopoulos D, Li F, Hunter D. What causes cancer? *Sci Am* 1996;275:80.
9. Greenwald P, Kramer B, Weed D, eds. *Cancer prevention and control.* New York: Marcel Dekker, 1995.
10. Schottenfeld D, Fraumeni JF Jr, eds. *Cancer epidemiology and prevention.* 2nd ed. New York: Oxford University Press, 1996.
11. Carson R. *Silent spring.* Boston: Houghton Mifflin, 1962.
12. Wingo P, Ries L, Giovino G, et al. Annual report to the nation on the status of cancer, 1973–1996, with a special section on lung cancer and tobacco smoking. *J Natl Cancer Inst* 1999;91:675.
13. Rodu B, Cole P. The fifty year decline of cancer in America. *J Clin Oncol* 2000 (*in press*).
14. Cole P, Rodu B. Declining cancer mortality in the United States. *Cancer* 1996;78:2045.
15. Hoyert DL, Kochanek KD, Murphy SL. Deaths: final data for 1997. *National Vital Statistics Reports.* Vol 47, no. 19. Hyattsville, MD: National Center for Health Statistics, 1999.
16. Martin JA, Smith BL, Mathews TJ, Ventura SJ. Births and deaths: preliminary data for 1998. *National Vital Statistics Reports.* Vol 47, no. 25. Hyattsville, MD: National Center for Health Statistics. 1999.
17. Wingo P, Ries L, Rosenberg H, Miller D, Edwards B. Cancer incidence and mortality: 1973–1995; a report card for the U.S. *Cancer* 1998;82:1197.
18. IARC Monographs on the evaluation of carcinogenic risks to humans: silica and some silicates. Lyon, France: *IARC Monograph* Vol. 42, 1987.
19. Simonato L, Baris R, Saracci R, Skidmore J, Winkelmann R. Relation of environmental exposure to erionite fibres to risk of respiratory cancer. *IARC Scientific Publications* 1989;90:398.
20. Caldwell GG. Twenty-two years of cancer cluster investigations at the Centers for Disease Control. *Am J Epidemiol* 1990;132:S43.
21. Devier JR, Brownson RC, Bagby JR Jr, Carlson GM, Crellin JR. A public health response to cancer clusters in Missouri. *Am J Epidemiol* 1990;132:S23.
22. IARC monographs on the evaluation of carcinogenic risks to humans: some naturally occurring substances: food items and constituents, heterocyclic aromatic amines and mycotoxins. Lyon, France: *IARC Monograph* Vol. 56, 1993.
23. Montesano R, Hainaut P, Wild C. Hepatocellular carcinoma: from gene to public health. *J Natl Cancer Inst* 1997;89:1844.
24. Stoloff F. Aflatoxin as a cause of primary liver-cell cancer in the United States: a probability study. *Nutr Cancer* 1983;5:165.
25. Ames B, Magaw R, Gold L. Ranking possible carcinogenic hazards. *Science* 1987;236:271.
26. U.S. EPA. *Cancer risk from outdoor exposure to air toxics.* Vol. 1: final report. EPA-450/1-90-004a. Washington, DC: U.S. Environmental Protection Agency, 1990.
27. Austin H, Delzell E, Cole P. Benzene and leukemia: a review of the literature and a risk assessment. *Am J Epidemiol* 1988;127:419.
28. Paxton M. Leukemia risk associated with benzene exposure in the pliofilm cohort. *Environ Health Perspect* 1996;104:1461.
29. Cronkite E, Drew R, Inoue T, Hirabayashi Y, Bullis J. Hematotoxicity and carcinogenicity of inhaled benzene. *Environ Health Perspect* 1989;82:97.
30. Paxton M, Chincilli V, Brett S, Rodricks J. Leukemia risk associated with benzene distribution. *Risk Analysis* 1994;14:147.
31. National Center for Health Statistics. *Health, United States, 1995.* Hyattsville, MD: Public Health Service, 1996.
32. Doll R, Hill AB. Smoking and carcinoma of the lung. *BMJ* 1950;2:739.
33. Wynder EL, Graham EA. Tobacco smoking is a possible etiologic factor in bronchiogenic carcinoma. A study of six hundred eighty-four proved cases. *JAMA* 1950;143:329.
34. U.S. Department of Health, Education, and Welfare. *Smoking and health. Report of the Advisory Committee to the Surgeon General of the Public Health Service.* Public Health Service Publication No. 1103. Washington, DC: U.S. Government Printing Office, 1964.
35. Halpern M, Gillespie B, Warner K. Patterns of absolute risk of lung cancer mortality in former smokers. *J Natl Cancer Inst* 1993;85:457.
36. Stellman S, Garfinkel L. Lung cancer risk and cigarette tar yield. *Prev Med* 1989;18:518.

37. Wilcox H, Schoenberg J, Mason T, Bill JS, Stemhagen A. Smoking and lung cancer: risk as a function of cigarette tar content. *Prev Med* 1988;17:262.
38. Fontham E, Correa P, Chen V. Passive smoking and lung cancer. *J LA State Med Soc* 1993;145:132.
39. Rodu B, Cole P. Nicotine maintenance for inveterate smokers. *Technology* 1999;6:17.
40. Surveillance for selected tobacco-use behaviors: United States, 1900–1994. *MMWR* 1994;43:1.
41. Thun MJ, Day-Lally CA, Calle EE, Flanders WD, Heath CW Jr. Excess mortality among cigarette smokers: changes in a 20-year interval. *Am J Public Health* 1995;85:1223.
42. Lilienfeld AM, Levin M, Moore GE. The association of smoking with cancer of the urinary bladder in humans. *Arch Intern Med* 1956;98:129.
43. Schmauz R, Cole P. Epidemiology of cancer of the renal pelvis and ureter. *J Natl Cancer Inst* 1974;52:1431.
44. Vineis P, Caporaso N, Tannenbaum S, Skipper P, et al. Acetylation phenotype, carcinogen-hemoglobin adducts, and cigarette smoking. *Cancer Res* 1990;50:3002.
45. Hartge P, Silverman D, Hoover R, Schairer C, et al. Changing cigarette habits and bladder cancer risk: a case-control study. *J Natl Cancer Inst* 1987;78:1119.
46. Lewin F, Norell S, Johansson H, Gustavsson P, et al. Smoking tobacco, oral snuff, and alcohol in the etiology of squamous cell carcinoma of the head and neck: a population-based case-referent study in Sweden. *Cancer* 1998;82:1367.
47. Blot W, McLaughlin J, Winn D, et al. Smoking and drinking in relation to oral and pharyngeal cancer. *Cancer Res* 1988;48:3282.
48. Rubin E. The questionable link between alcohol intake and cancer. *Clin Chim Acta* 1996;246:143.
49. Swanson C, Potischman N, Wilbanks G, Twiggs L, et al. Relation of endometrial cancer risks to past and contemporary body size and body fat distribution. *Cancer Epidemiol Biomarkers Prev* 1993;2:321.
50. Augustsson K, Skog K, Jagerstad M, Dickman P, Steineck G. Dietary heterocyclic amines and cancer of the colon, rectum, bladder and kidney: a population-based study. *Lancet* 1999;353:703.
51 .Kolonel L. Fat and cancer: the epidemiologic evidence in perspective. *Adv Exper Med Biol* 1997;422:1.
52. Rogers M, Thomas D, Dais S, Vaughan T, Nevissi A. A case-control study of element levels and cancer of the upper aerodigestive tract. *Cancer Epidemiol Biomarkers Prev* 1993;2:305.
53. Steinmetz K, Potter J. Vegetables, fruit, and cancer prevention: a review. *J Am Diet Assoc* 1996;96:1027.
54. Henderson B, Pike M, Bernstein L, Ross R. Breast cancer. In: Schottenfeld D, Fraumeni JF Jr., eds. *Cancer epidemiology and prevention.* 2nd ed. New York: Oxford University Press, 1996.
55. Adami H, Signorello L, Trichopoulos D. Towards an understanding of breast cancer etiology. *Semin Cancer Biol* 1998;8:255.
56. White I. The tamoxifen dilemma. *Carcinogenesis* 1999;20:1153.
57. Weiss N, Cook L, Farrow D, Rosenblatt K. Ovarian Cancer. In: Schottenfeld D, Fraumeni JF Jr., eds. *Cancer epidemiology and prevention.* 2nd ed. New York: Oxford University Press, 1996.
58. Herbst A, Cole P, Colton T, et al. Age-incidence and risk of DES-related clear cell adenocarcinoma of the vagina and cervix. *Am J Obstet Gynecol* 1977;128:43.
59. Little J. Cellular, molecular and carcinogenic effects of radiation. *Hematol Oncol Clin North Am* 1993;7:337.
60. Yates J, Bunting C. The rational treatment of Hodgkin's disease. *JAMA* 1915;64:1953.
61. Ince N, Wands J. The increasing incidence of hepatocellular carcinoma. *N Engl J Med* 1999;340:798.
62. Schiffman M. Recent progress in defining the epidemiology of human papilloma virus infection and cervical neoplasia. *J Natl Cancer Inst* 1992;84:394.
63. Schiffman M, Burk R. Human papilloma viruses. In: Evans A, Kaslow R, eds. *Viral infections of humans.* 4th ed. New York: Plenum, 1997.
64. Kjaer S, Brinton L. Adenocarcinomas of the uterine cervix: the epidemiology of an increasing problem. *Epidemiol Rev* 1993;15:486.
65. LaVecchia C, Lucchini F, Negri E, Boyle P, et al. Trends of cancer mortality in Europe, 1955–1989: II and IV. *Eur J Cancer* 1992;28:514 and 1992;28A:1210.
66. Schildt E, Eriksson M, Hardell L, Magnusson A. Oral snuff, smoking habits and alcohol in relation to oral cancer in a Swedish case-control study. *Intl J Cancer* 1998;77:341.
67. Wynder E. Nutrition and cancer. *Fed Proc* 1976;35:1309.
68. Jenkins N. *The Mediterranean diet cookbook.* New York: Bantam Books, 1994.
69. Jick H, Smith P. Regularly used drugs and cancer. In: Hiatt H, Watson J, Winsten J, eds. *Origins of human cancer.* Cold Spring Harbor, NY: Cold Spring Harbor Laboratory, 1977.
70. National Center for Health Statistics. Health, United States, 1999 with Health and Aging Chartbook. Hyattsville, MD: Public Health Service, 1999.
71. National Center for Health Statistics. Healthy People 2000 Review, 1998–99. Hyattsville, MD: Public Health Service, 1999.
72. Axelson O, Andersson K, Desai G, et al. Indoor radon exposure and active and passive smoking in relation to the occurrence of lung cancer. *Scand J Work Environ Health* 1988;14:286.
73. Elwood J, Jopson J. Melanoma and sun exposure: an overview of published studies. *Int J Cancer* 1997;73:198.
74. Moan J, Dahlback A, Setlow R. Epidemiological support for an hypothesis for melanoma induction indicating a role for UVA radiation. *Photochem Photobiol* 1999;70:243.
75. Doll R, Peto R. Mortality in relation to smoking: 20 years' observations on male British doctors. *BMJ* 1976;2:1525.
76. Falk RT, Pickle LW, Brown LM, Mason TJ, et al. Effect of smoking and alcohol consumption on laryngeal cancer risk in coastal Texas. *Cancer Res* 1989;49:4024.
77. Tuyns AJ, Esteve J. Pipe, commercial and hand-rolled cigarette smoking in oesophageal cancer. *Intl J Epidemiol* 1983;12:110.
78. McLaughlin JK, Mandel JS, Blot WJ, Schuman LM, et al. A populationnbased casencontrol study of renal cell carcinoma. *J Natl Cancer Inst* 1984;72:275.
79. IARC Monographs on the Evaluation of Carcinogenic Risks to Humans: Tobacco smoking. Lyon, France: *IARC Monograph* Vol. 38, 1986.
80. Winn DM, Blot WJ, Shy CM, Pickle LW, et al. Snuff dipping and oral cancer among women in the southern United States. *N Engl J Med* 1981;304:745.
81. Gupta P, Pindborg J, Mehta F. Comparison of carcinogenicity of betel quid with and without tobacco: an epidemiological review. *Ecol Dis* 1982;1:213.
82. Jensen O, Paine S, McMichael A, Ewertz M. Alcohol. In: Schottenfeld D, Fraumeni JF Jr., eds. *Cancer epidemiology and prevention.* 2nd ed. New York: Oxford University Press, 1996.
83. Yu MC, Huang TB, Henderson BE. Diet and nasopharyngeal carcinoma: a case-control study in Guangzhou, China. *Intl J Cancer* 1989;43:1077.
84. Madigan M, Ziegler R, Benichou J, Byrne C, Hoover R. Proportion of breast cancer cases in the United States explained by well-established risk factors. *J Natl Cancer Inst* 1995;87:1681.
85. Melick WF. Bladder carcinoma and xenylamine. *N Engl J Med* 1972;287:1103.
86. Meigs JW, Marrett LD, Ulrich FU, Flannery JT. Bladder tumor incidence among workers exposed to benzidine: a thirty-year follow-up. *J Natl Cancer Inst* 1986;76:1.
87. Schulte PA, Ringen K, Hemstreet GP, et al. Risk assessment of a cohort exposed to aromatic amines. Initial results. *J Occup Med* 1985;27:115.
88. Wong O. An industry wide mortality study of chemical workers occupationally exposed to benzene. I. General results. *Br J Ind Med* 1987;44:365.
89. Weiss W. Epidemic curve of respiratory cancer due to chloromethyl ethers. *J Natl Cancer Inst* 1982;69:1265.
90. Tamburro CH. Relationship of vinyl monomers and liver cancers: angiosarcoma and hepatocellular carcinoma. *Semin Liver Dis* 1984;4:158.
91. Wong O, Whorton MD, Foliart DE, Ragland D. An industry-wide epidemiologic study of vinyl chloride workers, 1942–1982. *Am J Ind Med* 1991;20:317.
92. Bisanti L, Maggini M, Raschetti R, et al. Cancer mortality in ethylene oxide workers. *Br J Ind Med* 1993;50:317.
93. Easton DF, Peto J, Doll R. Cancers of the respiratory tract in mustard gas workers. *Br J Ind Med* 1988;45:652.
94. IARC Monographs on the Evaluation of Carcinogenic Risks to Humans: Polychlorinated dibenzo-*para*-dioxins and polychlorinated dibenzofurans. Lyon, France: *IARC Monograph* Vol. 69, 1997.
95. Brown KG, Boyle KE, Chen CW, Gibb HJ. A dose-response analysis of skin cancer from inorganic arsenic in drinking water. *Risk Anal* 1989;9:519.
96. Lee-Feldstein A. Cumulative exposure to arsenic and its relationship to respiratory cancer among copper smelter employees. *J Occup Med* 1986;28:296.
97. Hayes RB. The carcinogenicity of metals in humans. *Cancer Causes Control* 1997;8:371.
98. Davies JM, Easton DF, Bidstrup PL. Mortality from respiratory cancer and other causes in United Kingdom chromate production workers. *Br J Ind Med* 1991;48:299.
99. Doll R, Mathews JD, Morgan LG. Cancers of the lung and nasal sinuses in nickel workers: a reassessment of the period of risk. *Br J Ind Med* 1977;34:102.
100. Steenland K, Ward E. Lung cancer incidence among patients with beryllium disease: a cohort mortality study. *J Natl Cancer Inst* 1991;83:1380.
101. Seidman H, Selikoff IJ, Gelb SK. Mortality experience of amosite asbestos factory workers: dose-response relationships 5 to 40 years after onset of short-term work exposure. *Am J Ind Med* 1986;10:479.
102. Brown LM, Mason TJ, Pickle LW, et al. Occupational risk factors for laryngeal cancer on the Texas Gulf Coast. *Cancer Res* 1988;48:1960.
103. Amandus H, Costello J. Silicosis and lung cancer in U.S. metal miners. *Arch Environ Hlth* 1991;46:82.
104. Thomas TL, Stewart PA. Mortality from lung cancer and respiratory disease among pottery workers exposed to silica and talc. *Am J Epidemiol* 1987;125:35.
105. Boice J, Land C, Preston D. Ionizing radiation. In: Schottenfeld D, Fraumeni JF Jr., eds. *Cancer epidemiology and prevention.* 2nd ed. New York: Oxford University Press, 1996.
106. Doll R, Vessey MP, Beasley RWR, Buckley AR, et al. Mortality of gasworkers—final report of a prospective study. *Br J Ind Med* 1972;29:394.
107. Jarvholm B, Lavenius B. Mortality and cancer morbidity in workers exposed to cutting fluids. *Arch Environ Health* 1987;42:361.
108. Miller BG, Cowie HA, Middleton WG, Seaton A. Epidemiologic studies of Scottish oil shale workers: III. Causes of death. *Am J Ind Med* 1986;9:433.
109. Hogstedt C, Andersson K, Frenning B, Gustavsson A. A cohort study on mortality among long-time employed Swedish chimney sweeps. *Scand J Work Environ Health* 1982;8(Suppl 1):72.
110. Demers PA, Kogevinas M, Boffetta P, et al. Wood dust and sino-nasal cancer: pooled reanalysis of twelve case-control studies. *Am J Ind Med* 1995;28:151.
111. Spinelli JJ, Band PR, Svirchev LM, Gallagher RP. Mortality and cancer incidence in aluminum reduction plant workers. *J Occup Med* 1991;33:1150.
112. Vineis P, Pirastu R. Aromatic amines and cancer. *Cancer Causes Control* 1997;8:346.
113. Pippard EC, Acheson ED. The mortality of boot and shoe makers, with special reference to cancer. *Scand J Work Environ Health* 1985;11:249.
114. Loeb L, Ernster V, Warner K, et al. Smoking and lung cancer: an overview. *Cancer Res* 1984;44:5940.
115. Redmond CK. Cancer mortality among coke oven workers. *Environ Health Perspect* 1983;52:67.
116. Gerhardsson MR, Norell SE, Kiviranta HJ, Ahlbom A. Respiratory cancers in furniture workers. *Br J Ind Med* 1985;42:403.
117. Sorahan T, Cooke MA. Cancer mortality in a cohort of United Kingdom steel foundry workers: 1946–85. *Br J Ind Med* 1989;46:74.
118. Sathiakumar N, Delzell E, Amoateng-Adjepong Y, et al. Epidemiologic evidence on the relationship between mists containing sulfuric acid and respiratory tract cancer. *Crit Rev Toxicol* 1997;27:233.
119. Boyko RW, Cartwright RA, Glashan RW. Bladder cancer in dye manufacturing workers. *J Occup Med* 1985;27:799.
120. IARC Monographs on the Evaluation of Carcinogenic Risks to Humans. Some organic solvents, resin monomers and related compounds, pigments and occupational exposures in pain manufacture and painting. Lyon, France: *IARC Monograph* Vol. 47, 1989.

121. Delzell E, Monson RR. Mortality among rubber workers. III. Cause-specific mortality, 1940–1978. *J Occup Med* 1981;23:677.
122. Travis LB, Curtis RE, Stovall M, et al. Risk of leukemia following treatment for non-Hodgkin's lymphoma. *J Natl Cancer Inst* 1994;86:1450.
123. Hass JF, Kittelmann B, Mehnert WH, et al. Risk of leukaemia in ovarian tumour and breast cancer patients following treatment by cyclophosphamide. *Br J Cancer* 1987;55:213.
124. Greene MH, Boice JD Jr, Greer BE, Blessing JA, Dembo AJ. Acute nonlymphocytic leukemia after therapy with alkylating agents for ovarian cancer: a study of five randomized clinical trials. *N Engl J Med* 1982;307:1416.
125. Boice JD Jr, Greene MH, Killen JY Jr, et al. Leukemia and preleukemia after adjuvant treatment of gastrointestinal cancer with semustine (methyl-CCNU). *N Engl J Med* 1983;309:1079.
126. Boivin JF, Hutchison GB, Lyden M, Godbold J, et al. Second primary cancers following treatment of Hodgkin's disease. *J Natl Cancer Inst* 1984;72:233.
127. Stott H, Fox W, Girling DJ, Stephens RJ, Galton DA. Acute leukaemia after busulphan. *BMJ* 1977;2:1513.
128. Kaldor JM, Day NE, Pettersson F, et al. Leukemia following chemotherapy for ovarian cancer. *N Engl J Med* 1990;322:1.
129. Thiede T, Christensen BC. Bladder tumours induced by chlornaphazine. A five-year follow-up study of chlornaphazine-treated patients with polycythaemia. *Acta Med Scand* 1969;185:133.
130. Kinlen LJ. Incidence of cancer in rheumatoid arthritis and other disorders after immunosuppressive treatment. *Am J Med* 1985;78:44.
131. Alexander JW, First MR, Hariharan S, et al. Recent contributions to transplantation at the University of Cincinnati. *Clin Transplants* 1991:159.
132. Colton T, Greenberg ER, Noller K, et al. Breast cancer in mothers prescribed diethylstilbestrol in pregnancy. Further follow-up. *JAMA* 1993;269:2096.
133. Depue RH, Pike MC, Henderson BE. Estrogen exposure during gestation and risk of testicular cancer. *J Natl Cancer Inst* 1983;71:1151.
134. Marrett LD, Meigs JW, Flannery JT. Trends in the incidence of cancer of the corpus uteri in Connecticut, 1964–1979, in relation to consumption of exogenous estrogens. *Am J Epidemiol* 1982;116:57.
135. Weiss NS, Sayvetz TA. Incidence of endometrial cancer in relation to the use of oral contraceptives. *N Engl J Med* 1980;302:551.
136. Neuberger J, Forman D, Doll R, Williams R. Oral contraceptives and hepatocellular carcinoma. *BMJ* 1986;292:1355.
137. Fisher B, Costantino JP, Redmond CK, Fisher ER, et al. Endometrial cancer in tamoxifen-treated breast cancer patients: findings from the National Surgical Adjuvant Breast and Bowel Project (NSABP) B-14. *J Natl Cancer Inst* 1994;86:527.
138. Stern RS, Laird N, Melski J, Parrish JA, et al. Cutaneous squamous-cell carcinoma in patients treated with PUVA. *N Engl J Med* 1984;310:1156.
139. Piper JM, Tonascia J, Matanoski GM. Heavy phenacetin use and bladder cancer in women aged 20 to 49 years. *N Engl J Med* 1985;313:292-5.
140. IARC Monographs on the Evaluation of Carcinogenic Risks to Humans. Epstein-Barr virus and kaposi's sarcoma herpesvirus/human herpesvirus 8. Lyon, France: *IARC Monograph* Vol. 70, 1997.
141. Forman D, Newell DG, Fullerton F, et al. Association between infection with *Helicobacter pylori* and risk of gastric cancer: evidence from a prospective investigation. *BMJ* 1991;302:1302.
142. London WT. Primary hepatocellular carcinoma: etiology, pathogenesis, and prevention. *Hum Pathol* 1981;12:1085.
143. Stroffolini T, Chiaramonte M, Tiribelli C, et al. Hepatitis C virus infection, HBsAg carrier state and hepatocellular carcinoma: relative risk and population attributable risk from a case-control study in Italy. *J Hepatol* 1992;16:360.
144. Levine AM. AIDS-related malignancies: the emerging epidemic. *J Natl Cancer Inst* 1993;85:1382.
145. Hinuma Y, Nagata K, Hanaoka M, et al. Adult T-cell leukemia: antigen in an ATL cell line and detection of antibodies to the antigen in human sera. *Proc Natl Acad Sci* 1981;78:6476.
146. Schwartz DA. Cholangiocarcinoma associated with liver fluke infection: a preventable source of morbidity in Asian immigrants. *Am J Gastroenterol* 1986;81:76.
147. Vizcaino AP, Parkin DM, Boffetta P, Skinner ME. Bladder cancer: epidemiology and risk factors in Bulawayo, Zimbabwe. *Cancer Causes Control* 1994;5:517.

Steven A. Rosenberg

CHAPTER 15

Principles of Cancer Management: Surgical Oncology

Surgery is the oldest treatment for cancer and, until recently, was the only treatment that could cure patients with cancer. The surgical treatment of cancer has changed dramatically over the last several decades. Advances in surgical techniques and a better understanding of the patterns of spread of individual cancers have allowed surgeons to perform successful resections for an increased number of patients. The development of alternate treatment strategies that can control microscopic disease has prompted surgeons to reassess the magnitude of surgery necessary.

The surgeon who treats cancer must be familiar with the natural history of individual cancers and with the principles and potentialities of surgery, radiation therapy, chemotherapy, immunotherapy, and other new treatment modalities. The surgeon has a central role in the prevention, diagnosis, and definitive treatment of the disease and in palliation and rehabilitation of the cancer patient. The principles underlying each of these roles of the surgical oncologist are discussed in this chapter.

HISTORICAL PERSPECTIVE

Although the earliest discussions of the surgical treatment of tumors are found in the Edwin Smith papyrus from the Egyptian Middle Kingdom (circa 1600 BC), the modern era of elective surgery for visceral tumors began in frontier America in 1809.[1,2] Ephraim MacDowell removed a 22-pound ovarian tumor from a patient, Mrs. Jane Todd Crawford, who survived for 30 years after the operation. This procedure, the first of 13 ovarian resections performed by MacDowell, was the first elective abdominal operation and provided a great stimulus to the development of elective surgery.

The treatment of most tumors depended on two subsequent developments in surgery. The first of these was the introduction of general anesthesia by two dentists, Dr. William Morton and Dr. Crawford Long. The first major operation using general ether anesthesia was an excision of the submaxillary gland and part of the tongue, performed by Dr. John Collins Warren on October 16, 1846, at the Massachusetts General Hospital. The second major development stimulating the widespread application of surgery resulted from the introduction of the principles of antisepsis by Joseph Lister in 1867. Based on the concepts of Pasteur, Lister introduced carbolic acid in 1867 and described the principles of antisepsis in an article in the *Lancet* in that same year.

These developments freed surgery from pain and sepsis and greatly increased its use for the treatment of tumors. In the decade before the introduction of ether, only 385 operations were performed at the Massachusetts General Hospital. By the last decade of the nineteenth century, more than 20,000 operations per year were performed at that same hospital.[3]

Table 15-1 lists selected milestones in the history of surgical oncology. Although this list does not include all the important developments, it does provide the tempo of the application of surgery to cancer treatment.[4] Major figures in the evolution of surgical oncology included Albert Theodore Billroth who, in addition to developing meticulous surgical techniques, performed the first gastrectomy, laryngectomy, and esophagectomy. In the 1890s, William Stewart Halsted elucidated the principles of *en bloc* resections for cancer, as exemplified by the radical mastectomy. Examples of

TABLE 15-1. Selected Historical Milestones in Surgical Oncology

Year	Surgeon	Event
1809	Ephraim McDowell	Elective abdominal surgery (excised ovarian tumor)
1846	John Collins Warren	Use of ether anesthesia (excised submaxillary gland)
1867	Joseph Lister	Introduction of antisepsis
1860–1890	Albert Theodore Billroth	First gastrectomy, laryngectomy, and esophagectomy
1878	Richard von Volkmann	Excision of cancerous rectum
1880s	Theodore Kocher	Development of thyroid surgery
1890	William Stewart Halsted	Radical mastectomy
1896	G. T. Beatson	Oophorectomy for breast cancer
1904	Hugh H. Young	Radical prostatectomy
1906	Ernest Wertheim	Radical hysterectomy
1908	W. Ernest Miles	Abdomenoperineal resection for rectal cancer
1912	E. Martin	Cordotomy for the treatment of pain
1910–1930	Harvey Cushing	Development of surgery for brain tumors
1913	Franz Torek	Successful resection of cancer of the thoracic esophagus
1927	G. Divis	Successful resection of pulmonary metastases
1933	Evarts Graham	Pneumonectomy
1935	A. O. Whipple	Pancreaticoduodenectomy
1945	Charles B. Huggins	Adrenalectomy for prostate cancer
1958	Bernard Fisher	Organization of NSABP to conduct prospective randomized trials

NSABP, National Surgical Adjuvant Breast and Bowel Project.

radical resections for cancers of individual organs include the radical prostatectomy by Hugh Young in 1904, the radical hysterectomy by Ernest Wertheim in 1906, the abdominoperineal resection for cancer of the rectum by W. Ernest Miles in 1908, and the first successful pneumonectomy performed for cancer by Evarts Graham in 1933. Modern technical innovations continue to extend the surgeon's capabilities. Recent examples include the development of microsurgical techniques that enable the performance of free grafts for reconstruction, automatic stapling devices, sophisticated endoscopic equipment that allows for a wide variety of "incisionless" surgery, and major improvements in postoperative management and critical care of patients that have extended the safety of major surgical therapy.

Critics who believe that the application of surgery has reached a plateau beyond which it will not progress should remember the words of a famous British surgeon, Sir John Erichsen, who, in his introductory address to the medical institutions at University College, said,

> There must be a final limit to the development of manipulative surgery, the knife cannot always have fresh fields for conquest and although methods of practice may be modified and varied and even improved to some extent, it must be within a certain limit. That this limit has nearly, if not quite, been reached will appear evident if we reflect on the great achievements of modern operative surgery. Very little remains for the boldest to devise or the most dextrous to perform.

These comments, published in the *Lancet* in 1873, preceded most important developments in modern surgical oncology.

ANESTHESIA FOR ONCOLOGIC SURGERY

Modern anesthetic techniques have greatly increased the safety of major oncologic surgery. Regional and general anesthesia play important roles in a wide variety of diagnostic techniques, in local therapeutic maneuvers, and in major surgery. These techniques should be understood by all oncologists.

Anesthetic techniques may be divided into those for regional and general anesthesia. Regional anesthesia involves a reversible blockade of pain perception by the application of local anesthetic drugs. These agents generally work by preventing the activation of pain receptors or by blocking nerve conduction. Agents commonly used for local and topical anesthesia for biopsies in cancer patients are shown in Tables 15-2 and 15-3.[5] Topical anesthesia refers to the application of local anesthetics to the skin or mucous membranes. Good surface anesthesia of the conjunctiva and cornea, oropharynx and nasopharynx, esophagus, larynx, trachea, urethra, and anus can result from the application of these agents.

Local anesthesia involves injecting anesthetic agents directly into the operative field. *Field block* refers to injection of local anesthetic by circumscribing the operative field with a continuous wall of anesthetic agent. Lidocaine (Xylocaine) in concentrations from 0.5% to 1% is the most common anesthetic agent used for this purpose. Peripheral nerve block results from the deposition of a local anesthetic surrounding major nerve trunks. It can provide local anesthesia to entire anatomic areas.

Major surgical procedures in the lower portion of the body can be performed using epidural or spinal anesthesia. Epidural anesthesia results from the deposition of a local anesthetic agent into the extradural space within the vertebral canal. Catheters can be left in place in the epidural space, allowing the intermittent injection of local anesthetics for prolonged operations. The major advantage of epidural over spinal anesthesia is that it does not involve puncturing the dura, and the injection of foreign substances directly into the cerebrospinal fluid is avoided.

Spinal anesthesia involves the direct injection of a local anesthetic into the cerebrospinal fluid. Puncture of the dural

TABLE 15-2. Infiltration Anesthesia

		Plain Solution		*Epinephrine-Containing Solution*	
Drug	*Concentration (%)*	Maximum Dose (mg)	Duration (min)	Maximum Dose (mg)	Duration (min)
Short duration					
Procaine					
Chloroprocaine	1.0–2.0	800	15–30	1000	30–90
Moderate duration					
Lidocaine	0.5–1.0	300	30–60	500	120–360
Mepivacaine	0.5–1.0	300	45–90	500	120–360
Prilocaine	0.5–1.0	500	30–90	600	120–360
Long duration					
Bupivacaine	0.25–0.5	175	120–240	225	180–420
Etidocaine	0.5–1.0	300	120–180	400	180–420

(From ref. 5, with permission.)

sac generally is performed between the L-2 and L-4 vertebrae. Spinal anesthesia provides excellent anesthesia for intraabdominal operations, operations on the pelvis, or procedures involving the lower extremities. Because the patient is awake during spinal anesthesia and is breathing spontaneously, it often has been thought that spinal anesthesia is safer than general anesthesia. There is no difference in the incidence of intraoperative hypotension with spinal anesthesia compared with general anesthesia, and there is no clear benefit in using spinal anesthesia for patients with ischemic heart disease.[6] Because patients are awake during spinal anesthesia and can become agitated during the surgical procedure, spinal anesthesia actually can cause more myocardial stress than general anesthesia. The health status of patients with preoperative evidence

TABLE 15-3. Various Preparations Intended for Topical Anesthesia

Anesthetic Ingredient	*Concentration (%)*	*Pharmaceutical Application Form*	*Intended Area of Use*
Benzocaine	1–5	Cream	Skin, mucous membrane
	20	Ointment	Skin, mucous membrane
	20	Aerosol	Skin, mucous membrane
Cocaine	4	Solution	Ear, nose, throat
Dibucaine	0.25–1	Cream	Skin
	0.25–1	Ointment	Skin
	0.25–1	Aerosol	Skin
	0.25	Solution	Ear
	2.5	Suppositories	Rectum
Cyclonine	0.5–1	Solution	Skin, oropharynx, tracheobronchial tree, urethra, rectum
Lidocaine	2–4	Solution	Oropharynx, tracheobronchial tree, nose
	2	Jelly	Urethra
	2.5–5	Ointment	Skin, mucous membrane, rectum
	2	Viscous	Oropharynx
	10	Suppositories	Rectum
	10	Aerosol	Gingival mucosa
Tetracaine	0.5–1	Ointment	Skin, rectum, mucous membrane
	0.5–1	Cream	Skin, rectum, mucous membrane
	0.25–1	Solution	Nose, tracheobronchial tree
EMLA	2.5	Cream	Skin
TAC	Tetracaine, 0.5 Epinephrine, 1:2000 Cocaine, 11.8	Solution	Skin

EMLA, eutectic mixture of lidocaine and prilocaine; TAC, tetracaine, epinephrine, and cocaine.
(From ref. 5, with permission.)

of congestive heart failure is more likely to be worsened by general anesthesia than by spinal anesthesia. In one series, heart failure developed *de novo* in 4% of adults older than age 40 who were undergoing major surgery and worsened in 22% of patients who had a history of heart failure.[6] Spinal anesthesia was not associated with any new or worsened heart failure. Because of local irritating effects of general anesthesia on the lung, it has been suggested that spinal anesthesia may be safer for patients with severe pulmonary disease.

General anesthesia refers to the reversible state of loss of consciousness produced by chemical agents that act directly on the brain. Most major oncologic procedures are performed using general anesthesia, which can be induced using intravenous or inhalational agents. The advantages of intravenous anesthesia are the extremely rapid onset of unconsciousness and improved patient comfort and acceptance. Ultra-short-acting barbiturates, such as sodium thiopental, or tranquilizers, such as the benzodiazepines or droperidol, are the most frequently used intravenous agents for general anesthesia or for sedation during regional anesthesia.

A variety of inhalational anesthetic agents are in clinical use. Nitrous oxide is popular, usually in combination with narcotics and muscle relaxants. This technique provides a safe form of general anesthesia with the use of nonexplosive agents. Two other agents in widespread use are the fluorinated hydrocarbons, halothane (Fluothane) and enflurane (Ethrane). Although they are used frequently, the fluorinated hydrocarbons have a variety of side effects. Halothane depresses myocardial function, reduces cardiac output, causes significant vasodilation, and sensitizes the myocardium to endogenous and administered catecholamines that can lead to life-threatening cardiac arrhythmias. In rare instances, halothane can cause severe hepatotoxicity, which begins 2 to 5 days after surgery. Enflurane also depresses myocardial function but does not appear to sensitize the myocardium to catecholamines and has not been associated with hepatic toxicity. The newest of the halogenated hydrocarbons is isoflurane, which was introduced in 1980. Isoflurane depresses the myocardium less than halothane or enflurane, but it has more potent vasodilatory properties.

Virtually all general anesthetics affect biochemical mechanisms, including depression of bone marrow, alteration of the phagocytic activity of macrophages, and exhibition of immunosuppressive properties. General anesthetic agents, such as cyclopropane and diethyl ether, rarely are used because of their explosive potential.

Intravenous neuromuscular blocking agents, called *muscle relaxants*, are commonly used during general anesthesia. These agents are nondepolarizing (e.g., curare), preventing access of acetylcholine to the receptor site of the myoneural junction, or are depolarizing (e.g., succinylcholine), acting in a manner similar to that of acetylcholine by depolarizing the motor end plate. These agents induce profound muscle relaxation during surgical procedures but have the disadvantage of inhibiting spontaneous respiration because of paralysis of respiratory muscles. Succinylcholine is short-acting (3 to 5 minutes), with a rapid recovery phase. Curare-induced paralysis lasts for 30 to 40 minutes after usual clinical doses of 0.3 to 0.5 mg/kg. Pancuronium has fewer side effects than curare but can induce tachycardia by means of sympathetic stimulation.

DETERMINATION OF OPERATIVE RISK

As with any treatment, the potential benefits of surgical intervention in cancer patients must be weighed against the risks of surgery. The incidence of operative mortality is of major importance in formulating therapeutic decisions and varies greatly in different patient situations (Table 15-4). The incidence of operative mortality is a complex function of the basic disease process that involves surgery, anesthetic technique, operative complications and, most important, the general health status of patients and their ability to withstand operative trauma.

In an attempt to classify the physical status of patients and their surgical risks, the American Society of Anesthesiologists (ASA) has formulated a general classification of physical status that appears to correlate well with operative mortality.[7] Patients are classified into five groups depending on their general health status (as shown in Table 15-5).

Operative mortality usually is defined as mortality that occurs within 30 days of a major operative procedure. In oncologic patients, the basic disease process is a major determinant of operative mortality. Patients undergoing palliative surgery for widely metastatic disease have a high operative mortality rate even if the surgical procedure can alleviate the symptomatic problem. Examples of these situations include surgery for intestinal obstruction in patients with widespread ovarian cancer and surgery for gastric outlet obstruction in patients with cancer of the head of the pancreas. These simple palliative procedures are associated with mortality rates of approximately 20% in most series because of the debilitated state of the patient and the rapid progression of the basic disease.

Mortality caused by anesthetic administration alone is related directly to the physical status of the patient. In a review of 32,223 operations, Dripps et al.[8] determined the mortality thought to be related to anesthetic administration alone (Table 15-6). It is extremely difficult to differentiate the mortality caused by anesthesia from that resulting from other contributors to operative mortality. However, this analysis indicates that operative mortality due to anesthesia in physical status class 1 patients is extremely low, fewer than 1 in every 16,000 operations. The anesthetic mortality increased with worsened physical status.

There is considerable evidence that anesthesia-related mortality has decreased in the last two decades, largely because of the development of rigid practice standards and improved intraoperative monitoring techniques.[9–11] A summary of the specific intraoperative monitoring methods used to achieve improved anesthetic safety is presented in Table 15-7.[12] A study of 485,850 anesthetics administered in 1986 in the United Kingdom revealed the risk of death from anesthesia alone in patients from all ASA classes to be

TABLE 15-4. Determinants of Operative Risk

General health status
Severity of underlying illness
Degree to which surgery disrupts normal physiologic functions
Technical complexity of the procedure (related to incidence of complications)
Type of anesthesia required
Experience of personnel

TABLE 15-5. American Society of Anesthesiologists Classification of Physical Status

CLASS I
A normal healthy patient with no organic, physiologic, biochemical, or psychiatric disturbance. The abnormal process for which operation is to be performed is localized and does not entail a systemic disturbance (i.e., a fit patient with inguinal hernia or a fibroid uterus in an otherwise healthy woman).

CLASS II
A patient with mild to moderate systemic disturbance caused either by the condition to be treated surgically or by other pathophysiologic processes (i.e., nonorganic or only slightly limiting organic heart disease, mild diabetes, essential hypertension, or anemia). Some might list the neonate or the octogenarian, even if no discernible systemic disease is present. Extreme obesity and chronic bronchitis may be included in this category.

CLASS III
A patient with severe systemic disease that limits activity but is not incapacitating, even though it may not be possible to define the degree of disability with finality (i.e., severely limiting organic heart disease; severe diabetes with vascular complications; moderate to severe degrees of pulmonary insufficiency; and angina pectoris or healed myocardial infarction).

CLASS IV
A patient with an incapacitating systemic disease that is a constant threat to life and not always correctable by operation (i.e., patients with organic heart disease showing marked signs of cardiac insufficiency, persistent anginal syndrome, or active myocarditis; and advanced degrees of pulmonary, hepatic, renal, or endocrine insufficiency).

CLASS V
A moribund patient who is not expected to survive 24 hours without operation or who has little chance of survival but is submitted to operation in desperation (i.e., the burst abdominal aneurysm with profound shock, major cerebral trauma with rapidly increasing intracranial pressure, and massive pulmonary embolus). Most of these patients require operation as a resuscitative measure with little, if any, anesthesia.

STATUS E
In the event of emergency operation, precede the number with an E. Any patient in one of the classes listed previously who is operated on as an emergency is considered to be in poorer physical condition. The letter E is placed beside the numeric classification. Thus, the patient with a hitherto uncomplicated hernia now incarcerated and associated with nausea and vomiting is classified as 1E. By definition, class 5 always constitutes an emergency.

(From ref. 7, with permission.)

approximately 1 in 185,000.[9] In a retrospective review encompassing cases from 1976 through 1988, Eichorn[10] estimated anesthetic mortality in ASA class I and II patients to be 1 in 200,200. These are probably underestimates, since underreporting of anesthetic-related deaths is a problem in all studies. Most cancer patients undergoing elective surgery fall between physical status I and II; thus, an anesthetic mortality rate of 0.01% to 0.001% is a realistic estimate for this group.

Anesthesia-related mortality is rare, and factors related to the patient's preexisting general health status and disease are far more important indicators of surgical outcome. A study of the factors contributing to the risk of 7-day operative mortality

TABLE 15-6. Mortality Related to Physical Status

Physical Status Grade	*Spinal Anesthesia (Frequency)*	*General Anesthesia and Relaxants (Frequency)*
Definitely related to anesthesia		
1	1:100,000[a]	1:25,000[a]
2	1:3500	1:1000
3	1:400	1:350
4	1:35	1:46
5	1:16	1:24
Possibly related to anesthesia		
1	0:10,164	0:6028
2	1:2260	1:600
3	1:228	1:150
4	1:19	1:23
5	1:16	1:10

[a]Estimated.
(From ref. 8, with permission.)

after 100,000 surgical procedures is shown in Table 15-8.[13] The 7-day perioperative mortality in this study was 71.4 deaths per 10,000 cases, and the major determinants of death were the physical status of the patient, the emergent nature of the procedure, and the magnitude of the operation.

Several specific health factors can increase the risks of the operative procedure. Using discriminant analysis, Goldman et al.[6] identified nine independent variables that correlated with life-threatening and fatal cardiac complications in patients undergoing noncardiac surgical procedures. By assigning a point value to each variable, a cardiac risk index could be computed (Table 15-9) that separated patients into four categories of risk (Table 15-10). The two risk factors most predictive of life-threatening complications were the presence of a third heart sound (S_3) or jugular vein distention (11 points) or a myocardial infarction in the previous 6 months (10 points).

A recent myocardial infarction significantly increases the incidence of reinfarction and cardiac death associated with surgery (Table 15-11). Significant improvements have occurred as new techniques of anesthetic monitoring and hemodynamic support have been developed.[14–16]

The impact of general health status on operative mortality is seen when operative mortality as a function of age is analyzed. Palmberg Hirsjarvi[17] studied the postoperative mortality of 17,199 patients undergoing general surgical procedures. The overall mortality rate of patients younger than age 70 was 0.25%, as compared with 9.2% for patients older than 70. In these elderly patients, the operative mortality rate for emergency operations was 36.8%, as compared with 7.8% for elective surgical procedures. The four leading causes of operative mortality that accounted for approximately 75% of all postoperative deaths in this age group were pulmonary embolism, pneumonia, cardiovascular collapse, and the primary illness itself.

TABLE 15-7. Summary of Specific Intraoperative Monitoring Methods

Variable	*Monitoring Methods*
Inspired gas	Oxygen analyzer with a low oxygen concentration alarm
Blood oxygenation	A quantitative method, such as pulse oximetry; adequate illumination and exposure to assess color
Endotracheal tube position	Correct positioning in the trachea must be verified by clinical assessment and identification of CO_2 in the expired gas
Ventilation	Clinical assessment; monitoring of CO_2 content and volume of expired gas encouraged
Ventilator disconnect	A device with audible alarm, capable of detecting disconnection of components of the breathing system when a mechanical ventilator is used
Circulation	Continuous electrocardioography; blood pressure and heart rate determined every 5 min; continual evaluation of circulation by pulse palpation, heart auscultation, intraarterial pressure tracing, ultrasonographic pulse monitor, pulse plethysmography, or oximetry
Temperature	Measurement when changes in temperature are intended, anticipated, or suspected

(From ref. 12, with permission.)

More recently, Hoskings et al.[18] reviewed the outcome of surgery performed on 795 patients aged 90 or older. Surgery was generally well tolerated. As with younger patients, the ASA classification was an important predictor of outcome.

Cancer is often a disease of the elderly, and there is sometimes a tendency to avoid even curative major surgery for cancer in patients of advanced age. In the United States and in most Western countries, life expectancies for the elderly have increased substantially. The average life expectancies for 80-year-old men and women in the United States are 7 and 9.1 years, respectively.[19] The 5-year expected survival rates of 90-year-old men and women are 30% and 39.8%, respectively; for 95-year-olds, the rates are 16.5% and 23.2%, respectively. Thus, even in the very old cancer patient, aggressive curative surgery can be warranted.

Reports of most surgical series include an account of operative mortality and operative complications. These results, combined with a consideration of the general health status of the patient, allow a reasonable estimate of the operative mortality for any given surgical intervention in the treatment of cancer.

TABLE 15-8. Risk Factors Associated with 7-Day Operative Mortality

Variable	*Description*	*Relative Odds of Dying*
Patient factors		
Age	>80 y versus <60 y	3.29
Gender	Female versus male	0.77
Physical status	ASA III–V versus ASA I–II	10.65
Surgical factors		
Operation type	Major versus minor	3.82
Length	>2 h versus <2 h	1.08
Urgency	Emergency versus elective	4.44
Anesthesia factors		
Techniques	Inhalation + narcotic versus inhalation alone	0.76
	Narcotic alone versus inhalation alone	1.41
	Narcotic + inhalation versus inhalation alone	0.79
	Spinal versus inhalation alone	0.53
	Number of anesthetic drugs: 1–2 versus >3	2.94
Experience of anesthetist	>600 procedures/y for 8+ y versus <600 procedures/y for <8 y	1.06

ASA, American Society of Anesthesiologists.
(From ref. 13, with permission.)

TABLE 15-9. Computation of the Cardiac Risk Index

Criteria	*Multivariate Discriminant-Function Coefficient*	*Points*
History		
Age older than 70 y	0.191	5
Myocardial infarction in previous 6 mo	0.384	10
Physical examination		
S_3 gallop or jugular vein distention	0.451	11
Important valvular aortic stenosis	0.119	3
Electrocardiogram		
Rhythm other than sinus or premature atrial contractions on last preoperative electrocardiogram	0.283	7
>5 premature ventricular contractions per min documented at any time before operation	0.278	7
General status		
pO_2 <60 or pCO_2 >50 mm Hg; K <3 or HCO_3 <20 mEq/liter; BUN >50 or Cr >3 mg/dL; abnormal SGOT, signs of chronic liver disease or patient bedridden from noncardiac causes	0.132	3
Operation		
Intraperitoneal, intrathoracic, or aortic operation	0.123	3
Emergency operation	0.167	4

BUN, blood urea nitrogen; Cr, creatinine; HCO_3, bicarbonate; K, potassium; pCO_2, partial pressure of carbon dioxide; pO_2, partial pressure of oxygen; SGOT, serum glutamic oxaloacetic transaminase.
(Adapted from ref. 6.)

TABLE 15-10. Cardiac Risk Index

Class	*No. of Patients*	*Point Total*	*No or Only Minor Complications (n = 943)*	*Life-Threatening Complication[a] (n = 39)*	*Cardiac Deaths (n = 19)*
I	537	0–5	532 (99%)	4 (0.7%)	1 (0.2%)
II	316	6–12	295 (93%)	16 (5%)	5 (2%)
III	130	13–25	112 (86%)	15 (11%)	3 (2%)
IV	18	>26	4 (22%)	4 (22%)	10 (56%)

[a]Documented intraoperative or postoperative myocardial infarction, pulmonary edema, or ventricular tachycardia without progression to cardiac death.
(Adapted from ref. 6.)

ROLES FOR SURGERY

PREVENTION OF CANCER

Because surgeons are often the primary providers of medical care, they are responsible for educating patients about carcinogenic hazards and about direct surgical intervention for the prevention of cancer. All surgical oncologists should be aware of the high-risk situations that require surgery to prevent subsequent malignant disease.

Underlying conditions or congenital or genetic traits are associated with an extremely high incidence of subsequent cancer. When these cancers are likely to occur in nonvital organs, it is necessary to remove the offending organ to prevent subsequent malignancy.[20] Examples of diseases associated with a high incidence of cancer that can be prevented by prophylactic surgery are presented in Table 15-12. An excellent example is presented by patients with the genetic trait for multiple polyposis of the colon. If colectomy is not performed in these patients, approximately one-half will develop colon cancer by the age of 40. By age 70, virtually all patients with multiple polyposis will develop colon cancer.[20] It is, therefore, advisable for all patients containing the mutant gene for multiple polyposis to undergo prophylactic colectomy before age 20 to prevent these cancers.

In this situation, as for many of the other familial conditions associated with a high incidence of cancer, the surgeon has a responsibility for alerting the family to the hereditary nature of the disorder and its possible occurrence in other family members. Another disease associated with a high incidence of cancer of the colon is ulcerative colitis. Approximately 40% of patients with total colonic involvement ultimately die of colon cancer if they survive the ulcerative colitis.[21] Three percent of children with ulcerative colitis develop cancer of the colon by the age of 10, and 20% develop cancer during each ensuing decade.[22] Colectomy is indicated for patients with ulcerative colitis if the chronicity of this disease is well established.

Other disorders that require early treatment to prevent subsequent cancers include cryptorchidism and multiple endocrine neoplasia. Cryptorchidism is associated with a high incidence of testicular cancer that probably can be prevented by early prophylactic surgery.

In the past, patients with multiple endocrine neoplasia type 2a (MEN 2a) were screened for the presence of C-cell hyperplasia and calcitonin secretion using pentagastrin stimulation tests to determine the possible need for prophylactic surgery to prevent the occurrence of medullary thyroid cancer. Recent studies using polymerase chain reaction–based direct DNA testing for mutations in the *RET* protooncogene have shown it to be the preferred method for screening MEN 2a kindreds to identify individuals in whom total thyroidectomy is indicated, regardless of the plasma calcitonin levels.[23]

A more complex example of the role of surgery in cancer prevention involves women at high risk for breast cancer. Because the risk of cancer in some women is increased substantially over the normal risk (but does not approach 100%), counseling is required. Women in this situation must carefully balance the benefits and risks of prophylactic mastectomy. A careful understanding of the factors involved in increased breast cancer incidence is essential for the surgical oncologist to provide sound advice in this area. Statistical techniques can provide approximations of the risk for patients, depending on the fre-

TABLE 15-11. Incidence of Perioperative Myocardial Infarction in Patients with a Previous Myocardial Infarction

Time from MI to Operation (mo)	*Incidence of Reinfarction[a]* Topkins and Artusio[14] (1959–1963)	Tarhan et al.[15] (1975–1976)	Rao et al.[16] (1976–1982)
0–3	12/22 (55%) (0–3 and 4–6)	3/8 (37%)	3/52 (6%)
4–6		3/19 (16%)	2/36 (2%)
7–12	9/36 (25%)	2/24 (5%)	1/104 (1%)
>12	—	(5%)	(1%)

MI, myocardial infarction.
[a]The incidence of MI in patients with no previous evidence of an MI is approximately 0.3%.

TABLE 15-12. Conditions in Which Prophylactic Surgery Can Prevent Cancer

Underlying Condition	*Associated Cancer*	*Prophylactic Surgery*
Cryptorchidism	Testicular	Orchiopexy
Polyposis coli	Colon	Colectomy
Familial colon cancer	Colon	Colectomy
Ulcerative colitis	Colon	Colectomy
Multiple endocrine neoplasia types 2 and 3	Medullary cancer of the thyroid	Thyroidectomy
Familial breast cancer	Breast	Mastectomy
Familial ovarian cancer	Ovary	Oophorectomy

quency of disease in the family history, the age at the first pregnancy, and the presence of fibrocystic disease. For example, a woman who has a family history of breast cancer in a sister or mother, has fibrocystic disease, and is nulliparous or had a first pregnancy at a late age has an 18% probability of developing breast cancer over a 5-year period.[20] These estimates can be of value in advising women about prophylactic mastectomy.

DIAGNOSIS OF CANCER

The major role of surgery in the diagnosis of cancer lies in the acquisition of tissue for exact histologic diagnosis. The principles underlying the biopsy of malignant lesions vary, depending on the natural history of the tumor under consideration. Various techniques exist for obtaining tissues suspected of malignancy, including aspiration biopsy, needle biopsy, incisional biopsy, and excisional biopsy.

Aspiration biopsy involves the aspiration of cells and tissue fragments through a needle that has been guided into the suspect tissue. Cytologic analysis of this material can provide a tentative diagnosis of the presence of malignant tissue. However, major surgical resections should not be undertaken solely on the basis of the evidence of aspiration biopsy. Even the most experienced cytologist can mistake inflammatory or benign reparative changes for malignant cells. This error is inherent in the uncertainties of an individual cell analysis and, even in the best of hands, provides an error rate substantially higher than that of standard histologic diagnosis.

Needle biopsy refers to obtaining a core of tissue through a specially designed needle introduced into the suspect tissue. The core of tissue provided by needle biopsies is sufficient for the diagnosis of most tumor types. Soft tissue and bony sarcomas often present major difficulties in differentiating benign and reparative lesions from malignancies and often cannot be diagnosed accurately. If these latter lesions are considered in the diagnosis, attempts should be made to obtain larger amounts of tissue than are possible from a needle biopsy.

Incisional biopsy refers to removal of a small wedge of tissue from a larger tumor mass. Incisional biopsies often are necessary for diagnosing large masses that require major surgical procedures for even local excision. Incisional biopsies are the preferred method of diagnosing soft tissue and bony sarcomas because of the magnitude of the surgical procedures necessary to extirpate these lesions definitively. The treatment of many visceral cancers cannot be undertaken without an incisional biopsy, but be aware of opening new tissue planes contaminated with tumor by performing excisional biopsies for large lesions. An inappropriately performed excisional biopsy can compromise subsequent surgical excision. When this is a possibility, incisional biopsies should be performed.

In excisional biopsy, an excision of the entire suspected tumor tissue with little or no margin of surrounding normal tissue is done. Excisional biopsies are the procedure of choice for most tumors if they can be performed without contaminating new tissue planes or further compromising the ultimate surgical procedure.

The following principles guide the performance of all surgical biopsies:

1. Needle tracks or scars should be placed carefully so that they can be conveniently removed as part of the subsequent definitive surgical procedure. Placement of biopsy incisions is extremely important, and misplacement often can compromise subsequent care. Incisions on the extremity generally should be placed longitudinally so as to make the removal of underlying tissue and subsequent closure easier.
2. Care should be taken not to contaminate new tissue planes during the biopsy. Large hematomas after biopsy can lead to tumor spread and must be scrupulously avoided by securing excellent hemostasis during the biopsy. For biopsies on extremities, the use of a tourniquet may help in controlling bleeding. Instruments used in a biopsy procedure are another potential source of contamination of new tissue planes. It is not uncommon to take biopsy samples from several suspected lesions at one time. Care should be taken not to use instruments that may have come in contact with tumor when obtaining tissue from a potentially uncontaminated area.
3. Choice of biopsy technique should be made carefully to obtain an adequate tissue sample for the needs of the pathologist. For the diagnosis of selected tumors, electron microscopy, tissue culture, or other techniques may be necessary. Sufficient tissue must be obtained for these purposes if diagnostic difficulties are anticipated.
4. Handling of the biopsy tissue by the pathologist is also important. When the orientation of the biopsy specimen is important for subsequent treatment, the surgeon should mark distinctive areas of the tumor carefully to facilitate subsequent orientation of the specimen by the pathologist. Certain fixatives are best suited to specific types or sizes of tissue. If all biopsy specimens are placed in formalin immediately, the opportunity to perform valuable diagnostic tests may be lost. The handling of excised tissue is the surgeon's responsibility. Biopsy tissue obtained from breast cancer lesions, for example, should be saved for estrogen receptor studies and placed in cold storage until ready for processing.

Surgery also has a role in diagnosing pathologic states in cancer patients that do not directly involve the diagnosis of cancer. Cancer patients often are immunosuppressed by their disease or their treatment and are subject to opportunistic infections not commonly seen in most general surgical patients. Open lung or liver biopsies are often important in diagnosing these lesions adequately and in planning suitable therapy.

Oncologists are becoming increasingly aware of the need for precise staging of patients when planning treatment. Lack of proper staging information can lead to poor treatment planning and compromise the ability to cure patients. Staging laparotomy can be important in determining the exact extent of spread of lymphomas.

In performing accurate surgical staging, the surgeon must be familiar with the natural history of the disease under consideration. The development of ovarian cancer treatment is an excellent example. The tendency of ovarian cancer to metastasize to the undersurface of the diaphragm is a good example of the need to obtain a biopsy of an anatomic site that would not normally be subjected to biopsy by most surgeons. Extensive surgical staging may be required before undertaking other major surgical procedures with curative intent. For example, biopsy of the celiac and paraaortic lymph nodes in patients with cancer of the esophagus is often important so that unnecessary esophageal resections can be avoided.

Placement of radioopaque clips during biopsy and staging procedures is important to delineate areas of known tumor and as a guide to the subsequent delivery of radiation therapy to these areas.

TREATMENT OF CANCER

Surgery can be a simple, safe method to cure patients with solid tumors when the tumor is confined to the anatomic site of origin. When patients with solid tumors present to the physician for the first time, approximately 70% already have micrometastases beyond the primary site. The extension of the surgical resection to include areas of regional spread can cure some of these patients, although regional spread often is an indication of undetectable distant micrometastases.

The emergence of effective nonsurgical therapies has had a profound impact on the treatment of cancer patients and on the role and responsibilities of the surgeon treating the cancer patient. John Hunter, a brilliant eighteenth-century surgeon, characterized surgery as being "like an armed savage who attempts to get that by force which a civilized man would get by strategem."

Although surgery continues to be the most important aspect of the treatment of most patients presenting with solid tumors, modern clinical research in oncology has been devoted to applying other adjuvant "strategems" to improve the cure rates of those 70% in whom surgical therapy alone ultimately fails. The role of surgery in the treatment of cancer patients can be divided into six separate areas: (1) definitive surgical treatment for primary cancer, selection of appropriate local therapy, and integration of surgery with other adjuvant modalities; (2) surgery to reduce the bulk of residual disease (e.g., Burkitt's lymphoma, ovarian cancer); (3) surgical resection of metastatic disease with curative intent (e.g., pulmonary metastases in sarcoma patients, hepatic metastases from colorectal cancer); (4) surgery for the treatment of oncologic emergencies; (5) surgery for palliation; and (6) surgery for reconstruction and rehabilitation. In each area, interactions with other treatment modalities can be essential for a successful outcome.

Primary Cancer

There are three major challenges confronting the surgical oncologist in the definitive treatment of solid tumors: accurate identification of patients who can be cured by local treatment alone; development and selection of local treatments that provide the best balance between local cure and the impact of treatment morbidity on the quality of life; and development and application of adjuvant treatments that can improve the control of local and distant invasive and metastatic disease. The selection of the appropriate local therapy to be used in cancer treatment varies with the individual cancer type and the site of involvement. In many instances, definitive surgical therapy that encompasses a sufficient margin of normal tissue is sufficient local therapy. The treatment of many solid tumors falls into this category, including the wide excision of primary melanomas in the skin that can be cured locally by surgery alone in approximately 90% of cases. The resection of colon cancers with a 5-cm margin from the tumor results in anastomotic recurrences in fewer than 5% of cases.

In other instances, surgery is used to obtain histologic confirmation of diagnosis, but primary local therapy is achieved through the use of a nonsurgical modality, such as radiation therapy. Examples include the treatment of Ewing's sarcoma in long bones and the treatment of selected primary malignancies in the head and neck. In each instance, selection of the definitive local treatment involves careful consideration of the likelihood of cure balanced against the morbidity of the treatment modality.

The magnitude of surgical resection is modified in the treatment of many cancers by the use of adjuvant treatment modalities. Rationally integrating surgery with other treatments requires a careful consideration of all effective treatment options. The surgical oncologist must be thoroughly familiar with adjuncts and alternatives to surgical treatment. It is a knowledge of this rapidly changing field that separates the surgical oncologist from the general surgeon most distinctly.

In some instances, effective adjuvant modalities have led to a decrease in the magnitude of surgery. The evolution of childhood rhabdomyosarcoma treatment is a striking example of the successful integration of adjuvant therapies with surgery in the treatment of cancer.[24,25] Childhood rhabdomyosarcoma is the most common soft tissue sarcoma in infants and children. Before 1970, surgery alone was used almost exclusively, and 5-year survival rates of 10% to 20% were commonly reported. Local surgery alone failed in patients with rhabdomyosarcomas of the prostate and extremities because of extensive invasion of surrounding tissues and the early development of metastatic disease. The failure of surgery alone to control local disease in patients with childhood rhabdomyosarcoma led to the introduction of adjuvant radiation therapy. This resulted in a marked improvement in local control rates that was further improved dramatically by the introduction of combination chemotherapy with vincristine, dactinomycin, and cyclophosphamide. Long-term cure rates are in the range of 80%. Many other examples of the integration of surgery with other treatment modalities appear throughout this book.

Residual Disease

The concept of cytoreductive surgery has received much attention in recent years.[26,27] In some instances, the extensive local spread of cancer precludes the removal of all gross disease by surgery. The surgical resection of bulk disease in the treatment of selected cancers may well lead to improvements in the ability to control residual gross disease that has not been resected. Studies that suggest the merit of this approach are discussed in Chapters 45 and 36 (Burkitt's lymphoma and ovarian cancer, respectively).

Enthusiasm for cytoreductive surgery has led to the inappropriate use of surgery for reducing the bulk of tumor in some cases. Clearly, cytoreductive surgery is of benefit only when other effective treatments are available to control the residual disease that is unresectable. Except in rare palliative settings, there is no role for cytoreductive surgery in patients for whom little other effective therapy exists.

Metastatic Disease

The value of surgery in the cure of patients with metastatic disease tends to be overlooked. As a general principle, patients with a single site of metastatic disease that can be resected without major morbidity should undergo resection of that metastatic cancer. Many patients with few metastases to lung or liver or brain can be cured by surgical resection. This approach is especially true for cancers that do not respond well to systemic chemotherapy. The resection of pulmonary metastases of soft tissue and bony sarcomas can cure disease in as many as 30% of patients. As effective systemic therapy is developed for the treatment of these diseases, cure rates may increase. Studies have shown that similar cure rates occur in patients with adenocarcinomas when resected metastatic disease to the lung is the sole clinical site of metastases. Small numbers of pulmonary metastases often are the only clinically apparent metastatic disease in patients with sarcomas. However, this is rare in the natural history of most adenocarcinomas. If solitary metastases to the lung do occur in patients with carcinoma of the colon or other adenocarcinomas, surgical resection is indicated.

Similarly, there is increasing enthusiasm for the resection of hepatic metastases, especially from colorectal cancer, in patients in whom the liver is the only site of known metastatic disease. In patients with solitary hepatic metastases from colorectal cancer, resection can lead to long-term cure in approximately 25%. This far exceeds the cure rates of any other available treatment.

The resection for cure of solitary brain metastases should also be considered when the brain is the only site of known metastatic disease. The exact location and functional sequelae of resection should be considered when making this treatment decision.

Oncologic Emergencies

As in the treatment of all patients, emergencies arise for oncologic patients that require surgical intervention. These generally involve the treatment of exsanguinating hemorrhage, perforation, drainage of abscesses, or impending destruction of vital organs. Each category of surgical emergency is unique and requires an individual approach.

The oncologic patient often is neutropenic and thrombocytopenic and has a high risk of hemorrhage or sepsis. Perforations of an abdominal viscus can result from direct tumor invasion or from tumor lysis resulting from effective systemic treatments. Perforation of the gastrointestinal tract after effective treatment for lymphoma involving the intestine is not uncommon. The ability to identify patients at high risk for perforation may lead to the use of surgery to prevent this problem. Surgery to decompress cancer invading the central nervous system represents another surgical emergency that can lead to preservation of function.

Palliation

Surgical resection often is required for the relief of pain or functional abnormalities. The appropriate use of surgery in these settings can improve the quality of life for cancer patients. Palliative surgery may include the relief of mechanical problems, such as intestinal obstruction, or the removal of masses that are causing severe pain or disfigurement.

Reconstruction and Rehabilitation

Surgical techniques are being refined that aid in the reconstruction and rehabilitation of cancer patients after definitive therapy. The ability to reconstruct anatomic defects can substantially improve function and cosmetic appearance. The development of free flaps using microvascular anastomotic techniques is having a profound impact on the ability to bring fresh tissue to resected or heavily irradiated areas. Lost function (especially of extremities) often can be rehabilitated by surgical approaches. This includes lysis of contractures or muscle transposition to restore muscular function that has been damaged by previous surgery or radiation therapy.

THE SURGICAL ONCOLOGIST

Several factors have led to a recent increase in the development of surgical oncology and to the organization of separate sections of surgical oncology in large hospitals and departments of surgery within universities. This enthusiasm derives from the recognition that modern oncologic management requires levels of expertise in cancer surgery, chemotherapy, and radiation therapy that are not common to most general surgeons and from a desire to use effectively the resources being committed to cancer care and research by hospitals, private foundations, and the federal government. A sense of urgency has existed because some surgical leaders believe that the surgeon is experiencing a declining intellectual role in modern cancer treatment and research and that steps must be taken to reassert the surgeon's role in modern oncology.

Many surgeons have resisted the development of surgical oncology as a specialty area because of the fear of fragmenting the field of general surgery. A survey of 124 university surgery departments in the United States between January and July of 1985 revealed that 38% had formal divisions of surgical oncology, compared with the divisions of medical oncology present in 95%, radiation oncology in 94%, pediatric oncology in 76%, and gynecologic oncology in 79%.[28] Of the 47 divisions of surgical oncology that did exist, only 13 (28%) had formal clinical training programs in surgical oncology.[28] This lack of emphasis on surgical oncology at universities may be a factor in the decreasing success of surgeons in obtaining grant support from the National Cancer Institute. From 1980 to 1985, an analysis of 6407 applications submitted from clinical departments of medical schools for peer-reviewed grants revealed that 44% were submitted from departments of medicine and only 16% from departments of surgery.[29] Thirty-four percent of applications submitted from departments of medicine were awarded, compared with 25% from departments of surgery.[29] The publication of research in major surgical journals appears to be decreasing.[30]

The development of surgical oncology as a specialty area of surgery depends on a clear delineation of its role. There are six major areas in which the modern surgical oncologist can play a valuable role in the care of cancer patients at major treatment centers[31]:

- Organizing surgical oncology teaching programs for staff, residents, and students
- Providing expert consultation for unusual or difficult oncologic patient problems
- Providing unique surgical expertise in surgical cases unfamiliar to general surgeons (e.g., major soft tissue resections, exenterations, head and neck resections, isolation perfusions)
- Organizing clinical research protocols for surgical oncology patients
- Coordinating surgical oncology efforts with medical and radiation oncologists
- Conducting experimental research programs in oncology where possible

The rapid development of new information in surgery, chemotherapy, and medical oncology and of newer disciplines of immunotherapy, hyperthermia, and phototherapy requires the continuing education of all surgical staff. Surgical oncologists maintain close contact with all these areas and should be responsible for teaching programs for general surgical staff, residents, and students.

Because of the unique training and exposure to oncologic problems, the surgical oncologist has expertise in dealing with unusual or difficult oncologic patient problems and can provide expert consultation in these areas. The surgical oncologist is trained to perform many types of surgical procedures not commonly performed by general surgeons. Although most surgeons are able to perform many of the standard cancer resections, some operations are not performed frequently by general surgeons and can be performed better by a specialist in surgical oncology.

In most hospital settings, general surgeons operate on cancer patients. It is often essential, however, that patients receiving care for various cancers enter clinical protocols that help to answer important questions related to the treatment of that cancer. The surgical oncologists can help to organize clinical research protocols for surgical oncology patients treated by all surgeons at that institution. A large surgical group should have a surgical specialist capable of coordinating efforts with medical and radiation oncologists. Successful coordination with these nonsurgical specialists requires expertise in medical oncology and radiation therapy that is not common among most general surgeons.

The surgical oncologist can also be involved in administering and defining the need for adjuvant treatments. Adjuvant chemotherapy commonly is administered by surgeons when the chemotherapy regimens use well-known single or combination agents. The future development of immunotherapies and other new adjuvant treatments can be logically administered by surgical oncologists to their patients after recovery from the surgical procedure.

The surgical oncologist, when the situation allows, is in a position to perform experimental research in oncology that can lead to the introduction of new diagnostic and treatment regimens in clinical care. Laboratory research programs that contribute to basic knowledge of cancer biology also provide an important source of stimulation to residents and students.

The emergence of a subspecialty of surgical oncology within general surgery requires that special attention be given to the training of surgeons interested in pursuing this area of clinical care. Although it is generally agreed that all surgical oncologists should be well-trained general surgeons, attempts have been made to define additional areas of expertise that must be studied. In 1978, a group of surgical oncologists met under the sponsorship of the Society of Surgical Oncology and the Division of Cancer Research, Resources, and Centers of the National Cancer Institute to develop guidelines for the training of surgical oncologists. The guidelines adopted by this meeting include suggestions for such training[32,33]:

- Two-year training program on a surgical oncology service after completion of eligibility for general surgical certification by the American Board of Surgery or other surgical specialty board
- Training at an institution with a cancer program approved by the Commission on Cancer of the American College of Surgeons and whose clinical resources provide a sufficient variety and volume of clinical material to ensure exposure to a broad variety of clinical cancer problems
- Training at a center with sufficient basic science resources to provide education in these areas, with exposure to basic and clinical research
- Training at an institution that provides adequate operative experience, including standard curative and palliative procedures, with broad exposure to surgical procedures unique to the oncologic patient
- A full-time assignment during the training period to radiation oncology and chemotherapy services to allow the trainee to gain confidence and knowledge in these nonsurgical disciplines

These training recommendations are designed to provide general surgeons with the expertise in oncology and nonsurgical disciplines necessary to bring the best aspects of all disciplines of modern oncology to the care of the cancer patient.

REFERENCES

1. Brested JH. *The Edwin Smith surgical papyrus.* Chicago: University of Chicago Press, 1930.
2. Thorwald J. *Science and the secrets of early medicine.* New York: Harcourt, Brace, & World, 1962.
3. Wangensteen OH. Has medical history importance for surgeons? *Surg Gynecol Obstet* 1975;140:434.
4. Hill GJ. Historic milestones in cancer surgery. *Semin Oncol* 1979;6:409.
5. Strichartz GR, Berde CB. Local anesthetics. In: Miller RD, ed. *Anesthesia.* New York: Churchill Livingstone, 1994.
6. Goldman L, Caldera DL, Nussbaum SR, et al. Multifactorial index of cardiac risk in noncardiac surgical procedures. *N Engl J Med* 1977;297:845.
7. Dripps RD, Eckenhoff JE, Vandam LD. *Introduction to anesthesia,* 2nd ed. Philadelphia: WB Saunders, 1988.
8. Dripps RD, Lamont A, Eckenhoff JE. The role of anesthesia in surgical mortality. *JAMA* 1961;178:261.
9. Buck N, Devlin HB, Lunn JN. *Report on the confidential enquiry into perioperative deaths.* London: Nuffield Provincial Hospitals Trust, The Kings Fund Publishing House, 1987.
10. Eichhorn JH. Prevention of intraoperative anesthesia accidents and related severe injury through safety monitoring. *Anesthesiology* 1989;70:572.
11. Eichhorn JH. Documenting improved anesthesia outcome. *J Clin Anesth* 1991;3:351.
12. Ross AF, Tinker JH. Anesthesia risk. In: Miller RD, ed. *Anesthesia.* New York: Churchill Livingstone, 1994.
13. Cohen MM, Duncan PG, Tate RB. Does anaesthesia contribute to operative mortality? *JAMA* 1988;260:2859.

14. Topkins MJ, Artusio JF. Myocardial infarction and surgery: a five year study. *Anesth Analg* 1964;43:715.
15. Tarhan S, Moffitt EA, Taylor WF, et al. Myocardial infarction after general anesthesia. *JAMA* 1972;199:318.
16. Rao TLK, Jacobs KH, El-Etr AA. Reinfarction following anesthesia in patients with myocardial infarction. *Anesthesiology* 1983;59:499.
17. Palmberg S, Hirsjarvi E. Mortality in geriatric surgery. *Gerontology* 1979;25:103.
18. Hoskings MP, Warner MA, Lobdell EM, Offord KP, Melton LJ. Outcomes of surgery in patients 90 years of age and older. *JAMA* 1989;261:1909.
19. Manton KC, Vaupel JW. Survival after the age of 80 in the United States, Sweden, France, England, and Japan. *N Engl J Med* 1995;333:1232.
20. Mulvihill JJ. Cancer control through genetics. In: Arrighi FE, Rao PN, Stubblefield E, eds. *Genes, chromosomes, and neoplasia.* New York: Raven Press, 1980.
21. MacDougall IPM. The cancer risk in ulcerative colitis. *Lancet* 1964;2:655.
22. Devroede GJ, Taylor WF, Sauer WG. Cancer risk and life expectancy of children with ulcerative colitis. *N Engl J Med* 1971;285:17.
23. Wells SA, Chi DD, Toshima K, et al. Predictive DNA testing and prophylactic thyroidectomy in patients at risk for multiple endocrine neoplasia type 2A. *Ann Surg* 1994;220:237.
24. Kilman JW, Clatworthy HW Jr, Newton WA, et al. Reasonable surgery for rhabdomyosarcoma: a study of 67 cases. *Ann Surg* 1973;3:346.
25. Heyn RM, Holland R, Newton WA, et al. The role of combined chemotherapy in the treatment of rhabdomyosarcoma in children. *Cancer* 1974;34:2128.
26. Silberman AW. Surgical debulking of tumors. *Surg Gynecol Obstet* 1982;155:577.
27. Wong RJ, De Cosse JJ. Cytoreductive surgery. *Surg Gynecol Obstet* 1990;170:276.
28. Lawrence W Jr, Wilson RE, Shingleton WW, et al. Surgical oncology in university departments of surgery in the United States. *Arch Surg* 1986;121:1088.
29. Avis FP, Ellenberg S, Friedman MA. Surgical oncology research: a disappointing status report. *Ann Surg* 1988;207:262.
30. Nahrwold DL, Pereira SG, Dupuis J. United States research published in major surgical journals is decreasing. *Ann Surg* 1995;222:263.
31. Rosenberg SA. The organization of surgical oncology in university departments of surgery. *Surgery* 1984;95:632.
32. Leffall LD Jr. Presidential address: surgical oncology—expectations for the future. *Cancer* 1980;42:2925.
33. Schweitzer RJ, Edwards MH, Lawrence W, et al. Training guidelines for surgical oncology. *Cancer* 1981;48:2336.

Samuel Hellman

CHAPTER 16

Principles of Cancer Management: Radiation Therapy

To understand the practice of radiation therapy, one must seek its roots in principles derived from three separate areas. The first is practical radiation physics, which must be understood much as the surgeon understands the use of the equipment available in the operating room and as the internist understands the pharmacologic basis of therapeutics. The basic concepts of physics necessary to consider radiation therapy in the disease-related chapters of this textbook are introduced in this chapter.

The second important discipline to be understood is cell, tissue, and tumor biology. This chapter describes the fundamental principles of radiation biology and cell kinetics. These two discussions provide the rudiments of cell biology necessary to understand the uses of radiation.

A large clinical experience in radiation use has resulted in certain principles of treatment. These are discussed separately and are related to the physical and biologic concepts that may underlie their success.

PHYSICAL CONSIDERATIONS

Only the most important concepts of the physics of ionizing radiation can be discussed in this chapter. If more detailed information is needed, a standard textbook of radiation physics is a more appropriate source of information.[1]

Ionizing radiation is energy that, during absorption, causes the ejection of an orbital electron. A large amount of energy is associated with ionization. Ionizing radiation can be considered as a wave and as a packet of energy (a photon). The packet of energy is large enough to cause ionizations, and these are distributed unevenly through tissue. Examples of particulate radiation are the subatomic particles: electrons, protons, α particles, neutrons, negative pi mesons, and atomic nuclei. All of these have been experimentally considered or are being used in radiation therapy.

ELECTROMAGNETIC RADIATION

Electromagnetic radiation consists of roentgen and gamma radiation. They differ only in the way in which they are produced: Gamma rays are produced intranuclearly, and roentgen rays are produced extranuclearly. In practice, this means that gamma rays used in radiation therapy are produced by the decay of radioactive isotopes and that almost all of the roentgen rays used in radiation therapy are made by electrical machines. Exceptions are roentgen rays produced by orbital electron rearrangements, as in the decay of iodine 125 (^{125}I), which is a radioactive isotope but produces photons by extranuclear processes. ^{125}I also emits a small number of gamma rays from the nucleus.

The intensity of electromagnetic radiation dissipates as the inverse square of the distance from the source. The dose of radiation 2 cm from a point source is 25% of the dose at 1 cm.

The relative prevalence of the three dominant absorption mechanisms of electromagnetic radiation depends on the energy of the radiation. The first is photoelectric absorption, which predominates at lower energies. In this circumstance, the photon interaction results in the ejection of a tightly bound orbital electron. The vacancy left in the atomic shell is then filled by another electron falling from an outer shell of the same atom or from outside the atom. All or most of the photon energy of the transition is lost in this process. Photoelectric absorption varies with the cube of the atomic number (Z^3). This fact has significant practical implications because it explains why materials with high atomic numbers, such as lead, are such effective shielding materials. It also means that bones absorb significantly more radiation than soft tissues at lower photon energies, the basis for conventional diagnostic radiology.

The second type of radiation absorption is the Compton type. In this process, the photon interaction is with a distant orbital electron that has a low binding energy. In this absorptive

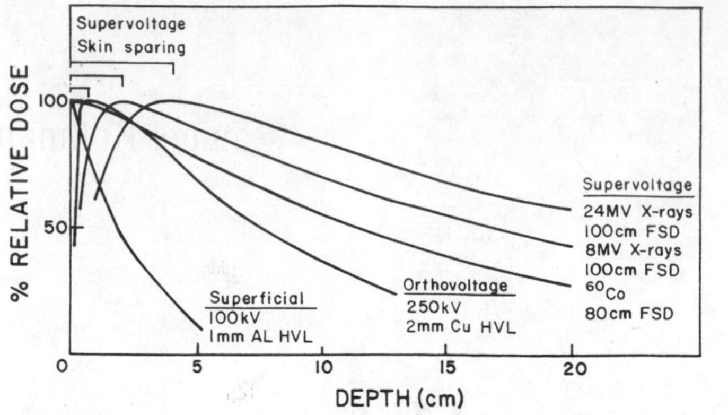

FIGURE 16-1. Relative dose at different depths for various types of ionizing radiation.

process, the photon does not give up all its energy to a single electron; an appreciable portion reappears as a secondary photon, which is created in the interaction. In contrast to the photoelectric effect, the probability of Compton absorption does not depend much on atomic number, but rather on electron density. This explains why films made at supervoltage energy do not show much difference between bone and soft tissue, but air cavities are clearly distinguished.

The third type of absorption is the pair production process. This type of absorption requires an incident photon energy greater than 1.02 MeV. In this process, positive and negative electrons are produced at the same time.

The fundamental quantity necessary to describe the interaction of radiation with matter is the amount of energy absorbed per unit mass. This quantity is called *absorbed dose*, and the rad was the most commonly used unit. Absorbed dose is measured in joules per kilogram; another name for 1 J/kg is the gray (1 Gy = 100 rad), which is now the recommended unit. The roentgen (R) is a unit of roentgen rays, or gamma rays, based on the ability of radiation to ionize air. At the energies used in radiation therapy, 1 R of roentgen rays, or gamma rays, results in a dose of somewhat less than 1 rad (0.01 Gy) in soft tissue.

The different ranges of electromagnetic radiations used in clinical practice are superficial radiation, or roentgen rays from approximately 10 to 125 keV; orthovoltage radiation, or electromagnetic radiation between 125 and 400 keV; and supervoltage, or megavoltage, radiation for energies of more than 400 keV. There are important differences between these classes. As energy increases, the penetration of the roentgen rays increases (Fig. 16-1), and at supervoltage energies, absorption in bone is not higher than that in surrounding soft tissues, as is the case with lower energies. This is because at supervoltage energies, Compton absorption predominates. Compared with orthovoltage, supervoltage radiation is skin sparing, meaning that the maximum dose is not reached in the skin, but instead occurs below the surface. The electrons created in the interaction travel some distance and do not attain full intensity until they reach some depth, resulting in a reduced dose to the skin. With orthovoltage radiation, the skin frequently is the dose-limiting normal tissue.

RADIATION TECHNIQUES

Two general types of radiation techniques are used clinically: brachytherapy and teletherapy. In brachytherapy, the radiation device is placed within or close to the target volume. Examples of this are interstitial and intracavitary radiation used in the treatment of many gynecologic and oral tumors. Teletherapy uses a device located at a distance from the patient, as is the case with supervoltage machines.

Because the radiation source is close to or within the target volume with brachytherapy, the dose is determined largely by inverse-square considerations. This means that the geometry of the implant is important. Spatial arrangements have been determined for different types of applications based on the particular anatomic considerations of the tumor and important normal tissues. An example of isodose distribution around an intracavitary application for carcinoma of the cervix is shown in Figure 16-2. The dose decreases rapidly as the distance from the applicator increases. This emphasizes the importance of proper placement. The applicator pictured is used to treat the cervix, uterus, and important paracervical tissues while limiting excessive irradiation of the bladder and rectum in front of and behind the tumor.

Historically, the removable interstitial and intracavitary sources used were radium and radon, the latter primarily for permanent implants. Marie Curie, the discoverer of radium, recognized its importance early and championed the medical use of these isotopes. They were important tools in early cancer therapy but now have been largely replaced by man-made isotopes, which overcome most of the disadvantages of the naturally occurring ones.

Initially, even removable isotopes were used by directly applying the isotope, thereby exposing the operator to significant radiation doses. This problem has largely been circumvented through the use of cesium 137, iridium 192, and cobalt 60. The iridium and cesium have a lower energy and are much easier to shield. Afterloading techniques are used for removable implants as often as possible. Receptacles for the radioactive material are placed in the patient in the form of needles, tubes, or intracavitary applicators. When they have been satisfactorily placed, they are afterloaded with the radiation sources. Remote afterloading using high-intensity sources whose dwell time is determined for a particular dose distribution is now a common treatment method. Permanent implants are primarily done today with gold 198 and ^{125}I and palladium 109.

Typical teletherapy isodose distributions are shown in Figure 16-3. The dose depends on inverse-square considerations and tissue absorption. The distribution of radiation depends on characteristics of the machine and the patient. The isodose curve depends on the energy of radiation, the distance from the source of radiation, and the density and atomic number of the absorbing material. The beam of radiation produced in typical radiation treatment may be modified to make isodose distributions conform to the specific target volume, and individually designed shields are used to protect vital normal tissues.

Figure 16-4 shows some radiation treatment plans in which the target volumes are depicted. This volume contains the tumor and the normal tissues intimately involved with the tumor. The diagram also contains the transited normal tissues, or transit volume. The purpose of the treatment plan is to maximize the dose to the target volume and minimize the dose to the transit volume. It is important that the tumor dose is relatively homogenous, because the maximum dose in the target volume is often the cause of complications, and the minimum dose in the target volume determines the likelihood of tumor recurrence. The volumes of interest in the patient have been specified as the: gross tumor volume (GTV), clinical tumor volume, and planning target volume.

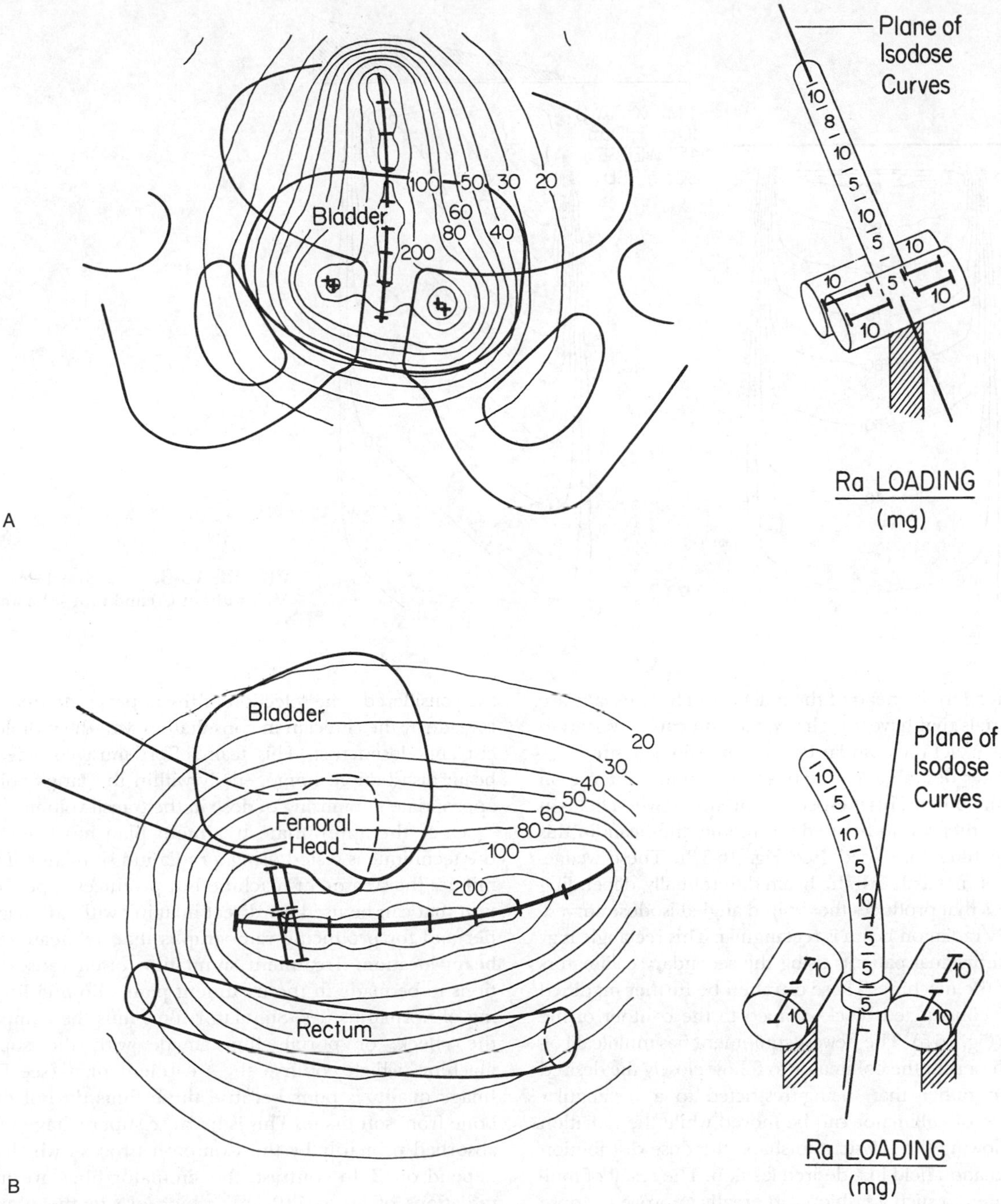

FIGURE 16-2. Isodose distribution around an intrauterine radium (Ra) applicator. **A:** Anteroposterior view. **B:** Lateral view.

The GTV is the clinically evidenced tumor volume, taking into account all diagnostic procedures. The clinical tumor volume is the GTV plus the volume considered at risk for microscopic extensions. The planning target volume includes the GTV and a margin for physiologic organ motion.

BEAM-MODIFYING DEVICES

In modern radiation therapy, teletherapy is given almost exclusively with supervoltage equipment. These radiations are produced by the decay of radioactive cobalt or with the production of roentgen rays in the range of 2 to 35 MeV (the most common are 4 to 8 MeV). High-energy photons and electrons are made by linear accelerators.

Regardless of the radiation source, the beam must be modified for clinical use. With electrical machines, the beam tends to have a much greater intensity in the center than on the sides. Modification to give a uniform dose of radiation across the beam is done with a flattening filter (unnecessary in cobalt units). For the beam to be limited to the designated size, colli-

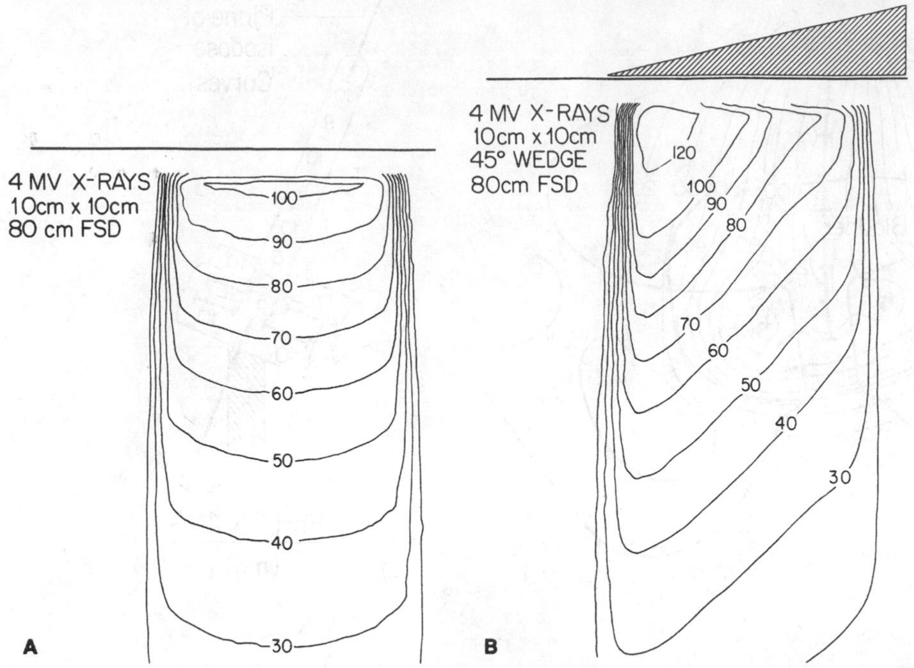

FIGURE 16-3. Isodose distributions for 4 MeV without **(A)** and with **(B)** a wedge filter.

mators are placed in the head of the machine. These usually are made of materials that have a high *Z* value and can be varied to conform to the exact rectangular beam dimensions desired.

It is sometimes desirable for the beam to be more intense on one side than the other. This is especially important when fields at angles to each other are to be used. To modify the beam in this fashion, wedge filters are used (see Fig. 16-3*B*). These wedge-shaped pieces of metal absorb the beam differentially, depending on the thickness that produces the desired angled isodose curves.

The primary radiation beam is rectangular. This rectangle may be varied for individual patients using the secondary collimators in the head of the machine. These can then be further modified by individually constructed blocks shaped to the contour of the normal tissue (Fig. 16-5). The newest equipment has multileaf collimators, which permit the collimator to follow closely the desired portal contour, rather than being restricted to a rectangular shape. This type of collimator can be moved while the radiation beam is on, allowing the physicist to shape the dose distribution within each radiation field in a desired fashion. The result of multiple fields treated in such a fashion can greatly improve the dose distribution so that the transited normal tissue dose is greatly reduced. This is described in Chapter 29.4.

RADIATION TREATMENT

Once the decision has been made to treat a patient with radiation, pretreatment procedures must be performed. First, the target volume must be accurately localized and the dose-limiting, transited normal tissues must be determined. This localization requires physical examination, radiography, ultrasonography, computed tomography (CT), and other diagnostic procedures. Before this step, the clinician must understand the natural history of the disease and its patterns of spread.

Once localization has been completed, the treatment planning process begins, in which alternative techniques of treatment are considered. The selection of the appropriate treatment plan is made by the clinician in consultation with the radiologic physicist and dosimetrist. This team effort must consider the best beam distribution, homogeneity within the target volume, and appropriate minimizing of dose in the transit volume.

Once the appropriate treatment plan has been accepted, the technique is tested using a radiation simulator. This device mimics the treatment machine but produces superficial radiation that can be used for direct imaging with an image intensifier and for producing radiographs that delineate exactly the beam location. Treatment simulation often causes modifications to be made in the treatment plan, allowing further sparing of normal tissues. Simulator films must be compared with the check, or portal, films made with the supervoltage machine, which confirm the treatment plan (see Fig. 16-5). Image quality is poor because these films do not distinguish bone from soft tissue. This is because supervoltage radiation is absorbed primarily by the Compton process, which does not depend on *Z*. In contrast, the simulator films are made with radiations of 80 to 110 keV, which are in the photoelectric range and therefore dependent on Z^3. Treatment planning and simulation are now greatly facilitated using a CT simulator. This single device combines CT image acquisition with treatment planning in the treatment position.

For the treatment to be applied as designed on the radiation simulator, proper immobilization and marking techniques must be used. These also ensure that daily treatments are given to the same volume. Markings on the patient's skin may be temporary or permanent. Usually, temporary marks are used to supplement the permanent small dots, or "tattoos," ensuring that the treatment is given to the same volume each day. Should the patient require further therapy at a later date, these markings accurately indicate the location of previous treatment portals. Within the treatment room, light localizers describe the outline of the field, and small laser dots are used to check whether the patient is in

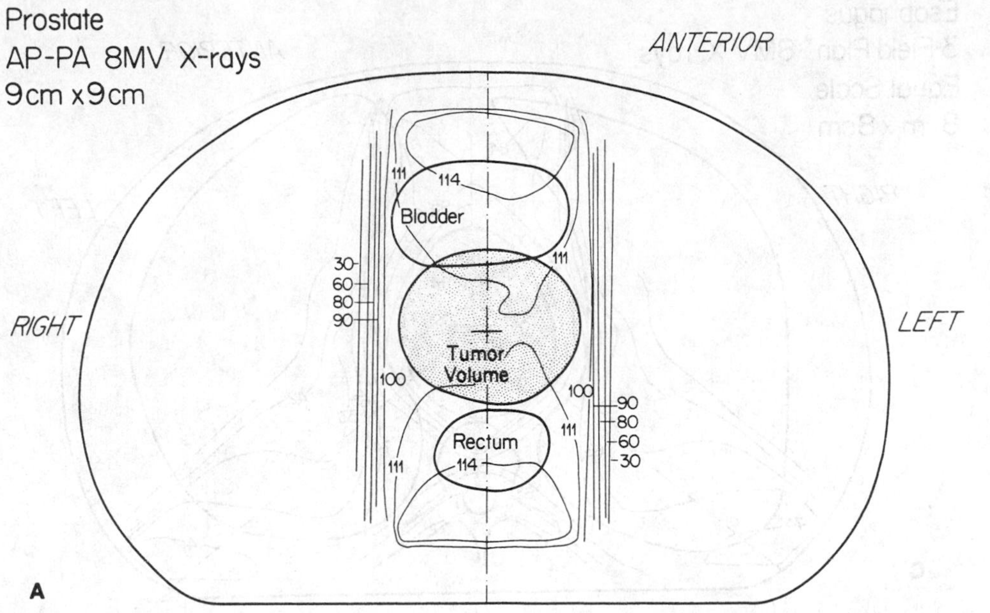

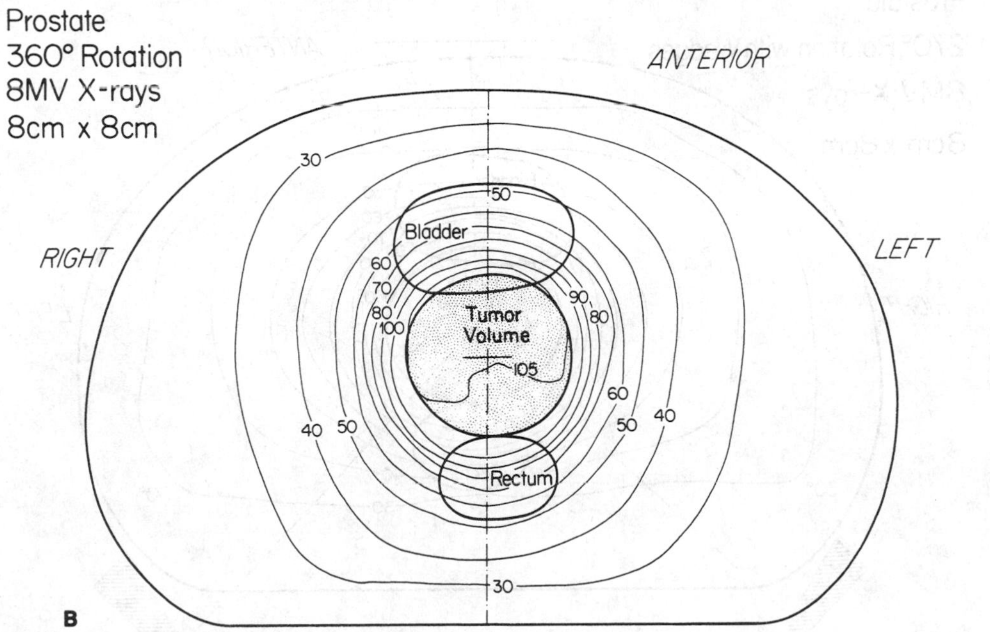

FIGURE 16-4. Typical supervoltage treatment plans for opposing fields (**A**), rotation (**B**), three fields (**C**), and wedge rotation (**D**). (Figure continues on next page.)

the correct position. Immobilization of the patient usually is achieved by devices made of foam, plastic, plaster, and other materials that can be made to conform to each patient's anatomy. It is most important that the patient be put in a position that is comfortable and easily reproduced from day to day.

ELECTRON THERAPY

Electrons differ greatly in their characteristic depth-dose distributions (Fig. 16-6). The maximum dose is reached and followed by a prompt fall. Little skin sparing is possible with electron beam therapy. It is the most useful radiation in the treatment of superficial tumors because the deeper tissue is spared by the prompt fall in the radiation dose. With higher electron energy, the penetration is greater and the fall in depth dose not as steep. A major problem with electrons is that absorption can be modified greatly by bone or air-containing tissues. Bone greatly reduces the depth dose because it absorbs much more of the radiation; the contrary is true for air-containing spaces.

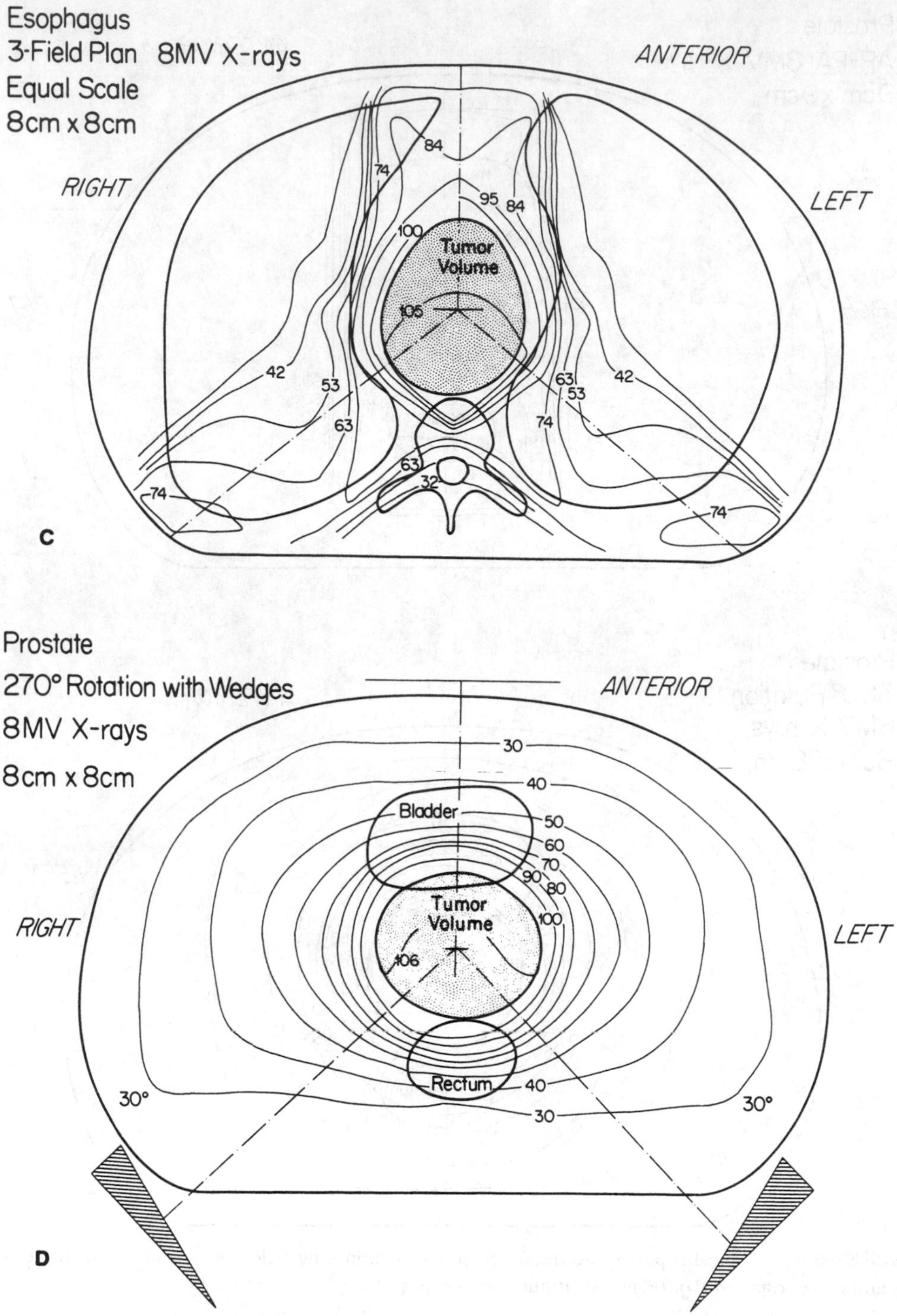

FIGURE 16-4. *(Continued)*

Currently there is a great deal of interest in proton therapy, which is discussed in more detail in Chapter 65.

BIOLOGIC CONSIDERATIONS

RADIATION INTERACTION WITH BIOLOGIC MATERIALS

Because mammalian cells may be considered dilute aqueous solutions, there are two possible mechanisms of interaction with biologically important molecules—the direct effect of radiation on the important target molecule, and the indirect effect produced by intermediary radiation products. For most events, the important target molecule is thought to be the DNA, and when considering the maintenance of reproductive integrity, it is useful to assume that DNA is the target. Whatever the critical target, it can be affected directly by ionizing radiation that causes a change in the molecular structure of the biologically important molecule. This direct effect is most common for high linear energy transfer (LET) radiation. Alternatively, the photon may interact with water, the predominant molecule in these dilute solutions, to produce free radicals. All of these forms of radiation are short-lived; they can interact with biologically important material, caus-

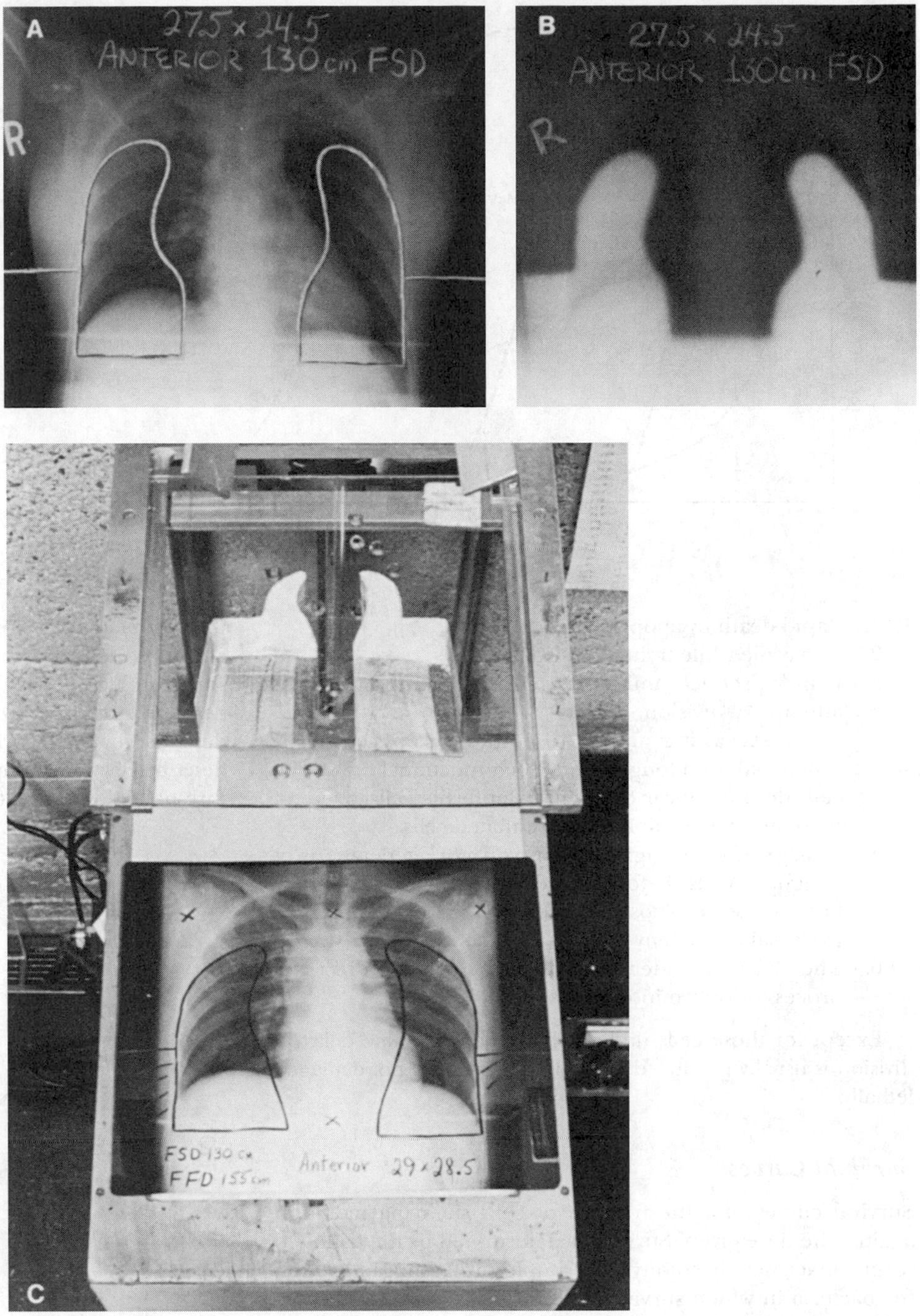

FIGURE 16-5. **A:** A film made on a therapy simulator on which outlines for shielding blocks are drawn. **B:** Supervoltage portal film with blocks in place. **C:** Technique for checking accuracy of the blocks with simulator films.

ing a detrimental effect, or they can react innocently and revert to their former state. The likelihood of interaction or reversion can be modified by reaction with molecular oxygen, which favors prolonging the life of a reactive species, or by reaction with sulfhydryl compounds, which reduces the lifespan of the free radicals by combining with them to return to innocuous substances.

CELL SURVIVAL CONSIDERATIONS

Radiation effects, whether direct or indirect, are random, an important principle in the general nature of cell killing. The biologically important effects of radiation therapy are those concerned with reproductive integrity. It usually is assumed that DNA is the critical target for this radiation effect, although it has not been proved with certainty. Other biologically important effects of radiation (e.g., edema) are far more likely to be caused by its action on membranes.

At least four possible consequences of radiation interaction with cells can affect long-term reproductive viability of the cell or its progeny: necrosis, apoptosis, accelerated senescence, and terminal differentiation. Current research is focused on these different effects of radiation on cells.

A cell that is damaged by radiation and loses its reproductive integrity may divide once or more often before all the progeny are rendered reproductively sterile. Possible consequences to the cell include the following:

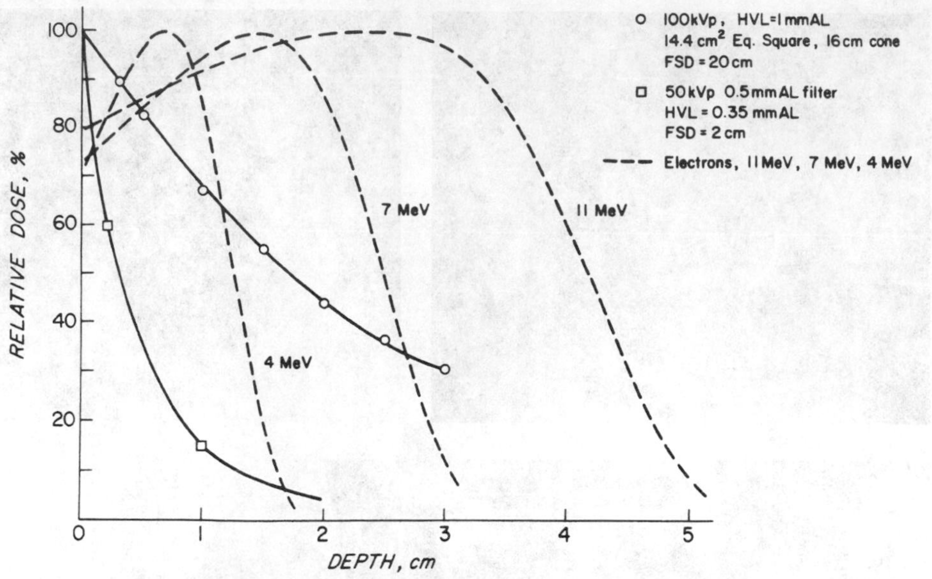

FIGURE 16-6. Electron and superficial roentgen ray depth–dose curves.

1. Rapid death by apoptosis.
2. It may die while trying to divide.
3. It may produce unusual forms as a result of aberrant attempts at division.
4. It may stay as it is, unable to divide, but physiologically functional for a long period. Such functional but sterile cells do not appear different from fertile cells. Some of these may be terminally differentiated cells.
5. It may divide, giving rise to one or more generations of daughter cells before some or all of the progeny become sterile. Those colonies in which some reproductively viable progeny emerge may then regrow.[2]
6. The cell may undergo no alterations in the divisional process or only minor ones.

Except for those cells undergoing apoptosis, some delay in division is usually produced, even in cells that are not damaged lethally.

Survival Curves

Survival curves plot the fraction of cells surviving radiation against the dose given. Survival is determined by the ability to form a macroscopic colony. The simplest relation can be seen for bacteria in which survival is a constant exponential function of dose. The importance of this exponential relation is that, for a given dose increment, a constant proportion (rather than a constant number) of cells is killed. Because of the randomness of radiation damage, if there is, on average, one lethal lesion per cell, some cells have one lesion, some more than one, and some fewer than one. Under such circumstances, the proportion of cells that have fewer than one (i.e., no lethal events) is e^{-1}, or a survival fraction of 0.37. The dose required to reduce the survival fraction to 37% on the exponential curve is known as the D_o. This term is related to the slope of the exponential survival curve. If a smaller dose is required to reduce the survival fraction to 37%, the cells are more sensitive to radiation.

Survival curves of most mammalian cells differ from those of bacterial cells by having a "shoulder" in the low-dose region and the exponential relation at higher doses. This shoulder indicates a reduced efficiency of cell killing. Such an idealized curve is shown in Figure 16-7, with the shorthand terminology used to describe survival curves. The terminal exponential portion is described by the D_o, whereas the initial shoulder region can be described by the extrapolation number n or the D_q, the quasi-threshold dose. The former is the number on the ordinate

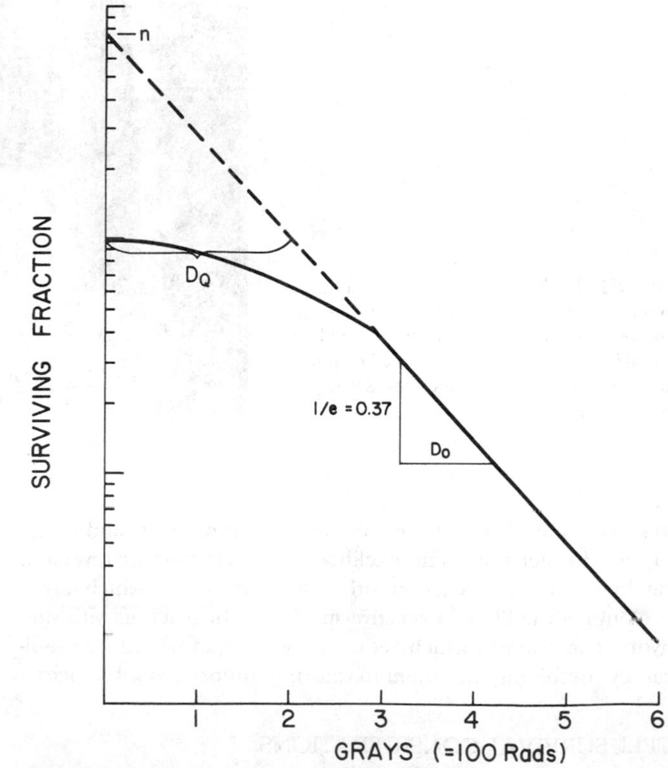

FIGURE 16-7. Idealized radiation survival curve. D_o, dose required to reduce the survival fraction to 37% on the exponential curve, D_q, the quasi-threshold dose, 1/e, dose energy divided by dose loss.

found when the exponential portion is extrapolated to O dose, whereas D_q is the dose at which the straight portion of the survival curve extrapolated backward intersects the line where the survival fraction is unity. If any two of these are known, the third can be calculated. The survival curve is described as follows: log $e^n = D_q/D_o$. This curve is best described by a linear quadratic model with the following formula[3]:

$$S = e^{-(\alpha D + \beta D2)}$$

The α and β terms in this equation and their ratio are used to describe survival curve characteristics and to classify cellular response to radiation. Survival curves have been determined for benign or neoplastic mammalian cells in culture. No general characteristics of tumor cells make them different from normal cells in culture. The survival curves for various human tumors thought to be sensitive and resistant to radiation were studied by Weichselbaum and colleagues,[4] who did not show any survival-curve characteristics that allow these two to be separated. Therefore, the differences in clinical response cannot be explained by simple acute differences in survival curves, although recurrent tumors have the radiobiologic characteristics of the more resistant subclones of the primary tumor.

Normal tissues also have been studied using clonogenic survival as an end point, with survival curves determined analogously to those for cells in tissue culture. The simplest clonal system, as originally described by Till and McCulloch,[5] is that used for murine bone marrow stem cells. When bone marrow cells are injected into lethally irradiated recipient animals, colonies are formed in the animals' spleens. These can be used to assess the reproductive integrity of the injected cells. The viability of the small intestinal clonogenic mucosal cells can be assessed by looking at sections of the small intestine at various times after irradiation and determining the appearance of colonies derived from cells surviving this radiation.[6] Using these and other techniques, the general properties of survival curves of normal and tumor cells are shown in Table 16-1. There are no characteristic differences in survival curves between normal tissues and tumors. Tumors generally resemble their normal tissue of origin in this respect.

Repair of Radiation Damage

When cells are irradiated, lethal damage can occur, or the damage may be modified and not lead irrevocably to cell death. Such amelioration of radiation damage is called *repair.* Repair can be divided into potentially lethal damage repair and sublethal damage repair.

Potentially lethal damage, under certain circumstances, leads to cell death. If postirradiation conditions are modified to allow repair, cells that would have died can be salvaged. In general, postirradiation conditions that suppress cell division are the ones most favorable to repair of potentially lethal damage. The simplest example of this was shown first in bacteria for UV and x-radiation.[7] A similar effect was seen in mammalian cells and persists into the first few postirradiation generations.[8–10] Potentially lethal damage repair may be most important in relating the cell culture studies of human tumors to their clinical response. Weichselbaum and colleagues[11] have shown that osteogenic sarcoma, a tumor characteristically thought to be resistant to radiation, has a great capacity for potentially lethal damage repair compared with tumors that may be much more responsive to radiation. After irradiation in the clinical circumstance, the tumor cell may not be faced with the necessity of rapid cell division, and it may have the opportunity for potentially lethal damage repair.

One explanation for the shoulder of the radiation survival curve is that the cell can repair some of the radiation damage, including a great proportion of the damage incurred with low doses of radiation. This is called *sublethal damage.* Elkind and Sutton[12] have studied the shoulder and its return by using divided doses of radiation. They have shown that if the dose of radiation is divided into two fractions and a few hours elapse between radiation doses, the shoulder will return. Therefore, two doses of radiation separated in time are less effective than the same total dose given as a single dose. Both D_q and the α/β ratio measure similar characteristics of the survival curve. With the exception of the bone marrow stem cells, acutely responding normal tissues have a large D_q and a large α/β ratio. This suggests that multiple small fractions of radiation can preserve these tissues, but not bone marrow.

Varying the dose rate of radiation may be considered a form of radiation fractionation. When the dose rate is low, such as during interstitial or intracavitary irradiation, it can be considered as a large number of small doses on the shoulder of the survival curve.[13] Therefore, differences between the dose-limiting normal tissues and the tumor in their shoulder characteristics and differences in the break point between shoulder and steep exponential have great clinical implications for such continuous radiation.

Apoptosis is an important response to radiation in many cells.[14] The relative proportion of cells undergoing apoptosis rather than pausing in the cell cycle to repair radiation damage may be a very important determinant of the likelihood of the radiation curability of a tumor. Certain normal cells, such as

TABLE 16-1. Survival Curve Parameters for Some Mammalian Cells

Cell Type	*How Determined*	D_o *(Rad)*	*n*	D_q *(Rad)*
Hamster V-79 fibroblast	*In vitro*	~160	~7	250–300
Chang liver	*In vitro*	150	2	150
HeLa	*In vitro*	130	4	180
P388 leukemia	*In vivo*	130	8.5	280
Mouse bone marrow	*In vivo*	90–100	1.5–2.0	~60
Mouse small intestine	*In vivo*	100	50	390
Mouse chondroblast	*In vivo*	160	9	350
Rat endothelium	*In vivo*	170	7	340

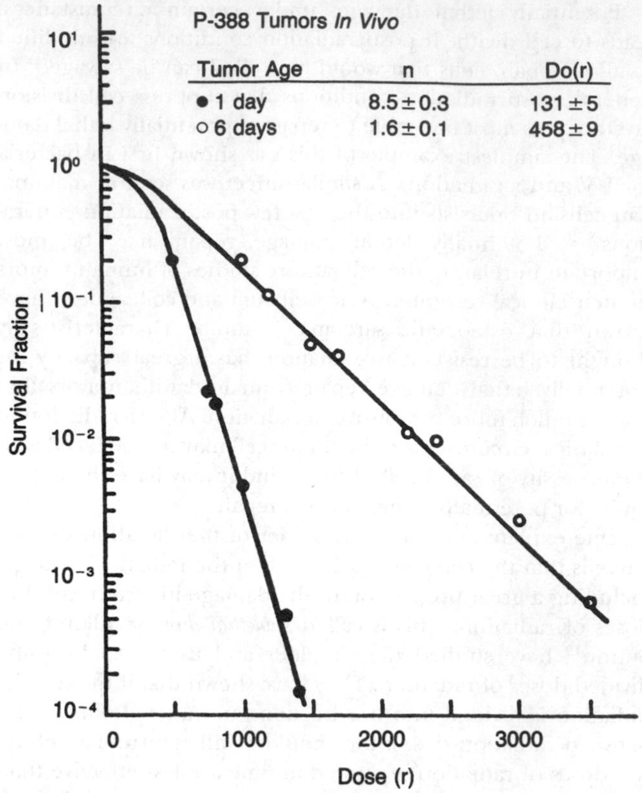

FIGURE 16-8. *In vivo* survival curves for oxic and hypoxic tumor cells. (From ref. 21, with permission.)

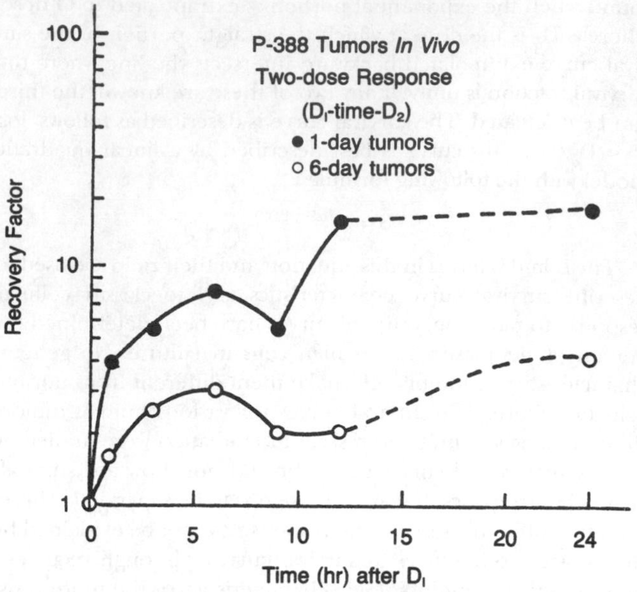

FIGURE 16-9. *In vivo* curves comparing two-dose survival to single-dose survival for oxic and hypoxic tumor cells. (From ref. 21, with permission.)

lymphocytes and germ cells, show apoptosis with very small doses of radiation. The reciprocal nature of radiation repair and apoptosis may explain the correlation between potentially lethal damage repair and radiocurability; cells with a great capacity for potentially lethal damage repair have little apoptotic response to radiation. It may be the latter that is the determining characteristic. The loss of the apoptotic response seems to be correlated to tumor progression. A number of genes associated with oncogenesis affect the likelihood of a cell demonstrating programmed cell death after DNA damage, including Bcl-2, Bcl-x, and P53.[15,16] A variety of factors can induce or stimulate apoptosis,[16] including those stimulated by radiation.[17]

Importance of Oxygen

The most important modifier of the biologic effect of ionizing irradiation is molecular oxygen. First noted in the 1920s, its importance was not realized until Mottram studied it systematically.[18] The general scientific community became aware of this phenomenon with the publications by Read[19] and Gray et al.[20] in the early 1950s. Figure 16-8 shows a survival curve for cells under aerobic and hypoxic conditions.[21] For equivalent cell killing at every level of survival, greater doses are required under hypoxic conditions compared with oxic conditions. There is some disagreement in the literature as to whether the dose ratio is the same throughout the survival curve. Most data suggest a smaller difference when low doses are used. A shorthand term, the *oxygen enhancement ratio* (OER), often is used. OER is the ratio of dose required for equivalent cell killing in the absence of oxygen compared with the dose required in the presence of oxygen. This term has most relevance on the exponential portion of the curve, because there appears to be a reduced shoulder on the survival curve of cells under hypoxic conditions.[21] Tumor cells allowed to grow into physiologic hypoxia have reduced capacity to repair sublethal damage (Fig. 16-9).

The OER range for different cells that have been studied varies from approximately 2.5 to 3.5. This means that, for reduction to a given survival level, three times as much radiation is required under hypoxic conditions as under oxic conditions. Because the curves are exponential, the ratio of survival fractions increases with dose. For example, in Figure 16-8, at 1000 rad the ratio of survival is 30.

Study of the phenomenon reveals that oxygen must be present during irradiation. Figure 16-10 shows the relative radi-

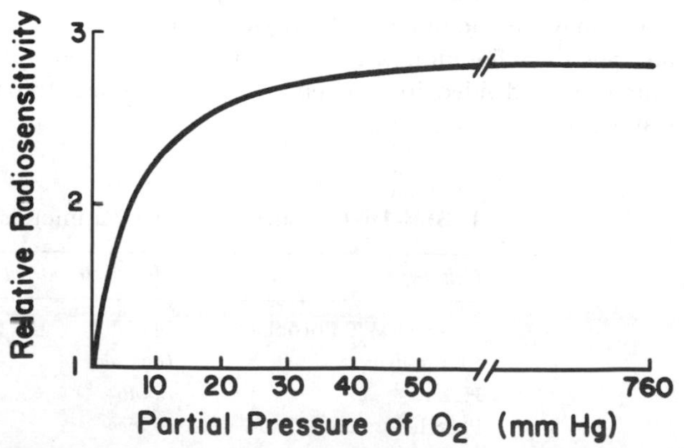

FIGURE 16-10. Radiation sensitivity as a function of ambient oxygen pressure. (Modified from Deschner EE, Gray LH. Influence of oxygen tension of x-ray induced chromosomal damage in Ehrlich ascites tumor cells irradiated *in vitro* and *in vivo*. *Radiat Res* 1959;11:115, with permission.)

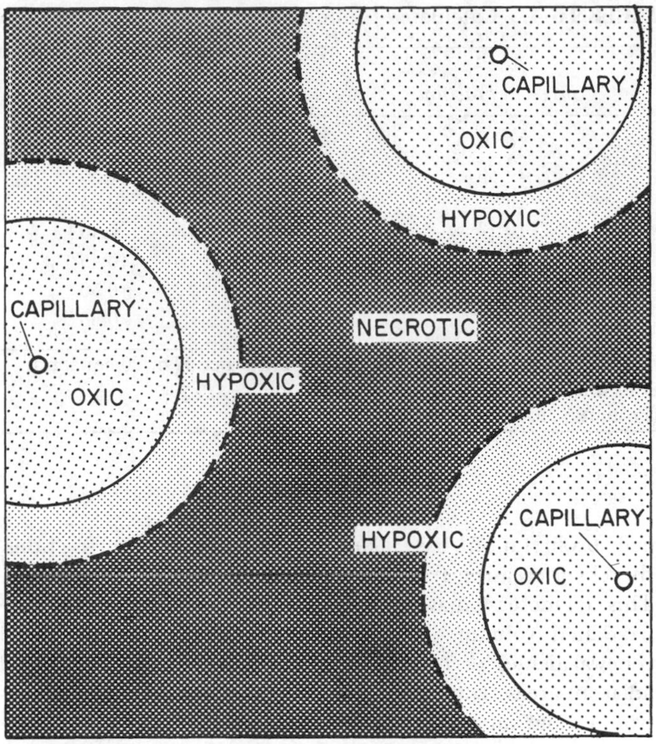

FIGURE 16-11. Diagrammatic representation of a tumor.

osensitivity of cells as a function of the oxygen tension at the time of irradiation. A low oxygen tension must be reached before there is a protective effect of hypoxia. The exact mechanism of the oxygen effect has not been determined definitively. It is believed that oxygen affects the initial chemical products of the interaction of radiation with biologic material. The important free radicals have short half-lives. A useful way to think about them is that they may return to an innocuous state or remain highly reactive molecules. Oxygen appears to favor the latter, whereas the presence of high levels of sulfhydryl compounds favors the former.

Thomlinson and Gray[22] recognized the importance of the oxygen effect in a classic paper in which they showed that tumors from humans frequently had anoxic regions. Calculations of oxygen diffusion from capillaries and metabolism predicted that the oxygen tension would decrease to zero at approximately 150 μm. They measured the width of tumor cords and showed that tumors can be modeled as shown in Figure 16-11. Those cells within approximately 100 μm of the capillary are well oxygenated, those beyond 150 μm are anoxic and necrotic, and those between 100 and 150 μm are hypoxic at an oxygen tension that might protect cells from radiation. This model has had a profound influence on radiobiologic and radiotherapeutic thinking. If all tumors look this way and such hypoxic regions contain cells that ultimately could cause tumor regrowth, then no clinically apparent tumor would be cured by radiation therapy. Because this is not the case, this paradox must be explained.

Laboratory experiments have indicated that immediately after a single dose of radiation, the surviving tumor cells are mainly the original hypoxic cells. After a period, the proportion of hypoxic cells returns to the preradiation level. This process has been called *reoxygenation.*[23] The term can be confusing because these are indirect experiments and do not record the fate of individual cells. The results of these experiments can be explained by suggesting that tumor cells do reoxygenate for several reasons: (1) reduced total tumor cell population relative to the surface area of tumor blood vessels; (2) reduced separation of hypoxic cells from the blood vessels, resulting from preferential cell kill of oxygenated cells; (3) increased oxygen diffusion; and (4) decreased intratumoral pressure, which opens blood vessels.

TABLE 16-2. Results of a Randomized Prospective Trial of Hyperbaric Oxygen in the Radiation Treatment of Head and Neck Cancer

	Local Control (%)	*Survival Rate (%)*
Hyperbaric oxygen	61	56
Conventional treatment	40	27

(From ref. 24, with permission.)

Alternatively, a large number of these hypoxic cells might in fact be doomed because, with proliferation in the oxic regions, they are pushed outward, ultimately forced to reside in the anoxic regions, and therefore die. Hypoxic cells, rather then being determinant in tumors surviving irradiation, may be on the way to anoxia and death, thus having limited clinical importance. It is likely that different mechanisms pertain under different circumstances in the laboratory and in the clinic.

The clinical importance of the oxygen effect has led to clinical and laboratory experiments, including the use of high-pressure oxygen with radiation therapy to improve results. These studies have indicated that, with a small number of radiation fractions, hyperbaric oxygen increases curability. If normal fractionation schemes are used, hyperbaric oxygen often does not show an advantage. However, some reports of tumors of the head, neck, and uterine cervix indicate that hyperbaric oxygen with 10 fractions of radiation results in greater cure than conventional daily fractionation.[24–26] Table 16-2 depicts the results with head and neck cancers. Despite these promising studies, the hyperbaric oxygen technique is cumbersome, difficult for the patient, and prohibits the use of the careful beam definition and beam modification so important in radiation therapy. The technique has been abandoned in most radiotherapy centers.

A more attractive alternative has been the development of hypoxic cell sensitizers. In the 1960s, Adams and colleagues[27,28] began searching for compounds that would mimic oxygen in its effect. They sought agents that would be metabolized slowly and reach all portions of the tumor. This is an important distinction, because high-pressure oxygen increases diffusion only slightly, whereas slowly metabolized sensitizers can reach all areas of the tumor. Although newer methods were based on replacing molecular oxygen, other effects of the nitroimidazoles, the most well-studied class of these agents, have been described. They appear to be cytotoxic to hypoxic cells and may sensitize cells to chemotherapeutic agents.[29,30] How important these last two points are in their use remains to be seen. However, this general class of agents offers a whole new approach to the chemical treatment of tumors based on a known tumor–normal tissue difference (i.e., the presence of hypoxic cells in tumors).

TABLE 16-3. Effects of Anemia on Pelvic Recurrence in Stage IIB or III Cervical Cancer

	Control		*Transfused*
Hemoglobin	<12 g/dL	>12 g/dL	>12 g/dL
Pelvic recurrence	10/20 (50%)	11/48 (23%)	11/67 (16%)

(Adapted from ref. 31, with permission.)

TABLE 16-4. Calculated Cumulative Survival Fraction[a]

Survival Fraction	X^{32} X =	X^{20} X =
10^{-11}	0.45	0.28
10^{-10}	0.49	0.32
10^{-9}	0.52	0.35
10^{-8}	0.56	0.40
10^{-7}	0.60	0.45
10^{-6}	0.65	0.50
10^{-5}	0.70	0.56

[a]Calculated cumulative survival fraction for either 32 or 20 equal fractions when the fractional survival is varied.
(From ref. 39, with permission.)

A practical clinical concern is whether the presence of anemia affects tumor response to radiation. Historic review and a prospective study from the Princess Margaret Hospital (Table 16-3) appear to indicate that anemia results in an adverse effect on tumor curability by radiation, presumably because it increases the hypoxic component of tumor cells.[31]

A review of intercapillary distance and tissue oxygen tension correlates local recurrence with evidence of hypoxia using these parameters in studying carcinoma of the cervix.[32] These studies emphasize the promise of techniques that improve tissue oxygenation in the treatment of epithelial cancers. *In vitro* measurement of hypoxia using radioactively labeled hypoxic sensitizers may alter selection of appropriate tumors for such therapeutic manipulation.[33,34]

Variable Radiation Response during the Division Cycle

The cell cycle can be divided into four phases: G_1, S, G_2, and M. Terasima and Tolmach[35] and Sinclair and Morton[36] studied synchronized populations to determine whether there is a difference in response to radiation as a function of the cell's position in the division cycle. They found that, generally, the mitotic phase (M) is most sensitive and G_2 almost as sensitive. G_1 is relatively sensitive in cells with a short G_1 phase. Cells gradually increase in resistance as they proceed through the late G_1 and S phases, reaching a maximum of resistance in the late S phase. In cells with a long G_1 phase, a peak of resistance is seen early in G_1. These findings *in vitro* also seem to be true *in vivo* for normal and tumor cells.[37,38]

The changes in radiation response are reflected in changes in the shoulder of the survival curve and in the terminal slope. These differences can be large. The difference between the most resistant and the most sensitive can show slope ratios equal to that of the oxygen effect.

The clinical consequences of different fractional survival after 2 Gy can be seen in Table 16-4. Small differences in fractional survival when repeated have profound consequences in the level of cell killing.

A second consequence of differential cell killing and the mitotic delay induced by radiation is a tendency to partially synchronize the cells. The timing of the second dose of a fractionated scheme may be critical. This synchronization is short-lived because cells desynchronize rapidly and redistribute themselves according to the original cell age distribution. This phenomenon, which could pose a clinical problem or a clinical advantage, does not seem to be important unless an incomplete redistribution between fractions exists.

Cell Proliferation

During a course of fractionated radiation, the ultimate response of the tumor and normal tissue depends on whether cell proliferation has taken place between the fractions, thereby increasing the number of cells exposed to radiation. This cell increase may be caused by cell proliferation within the irradiated volume (i.e., within the tumor or normal cell renewal tissue) or by cells that immigrate from unirradiated adjacent areas. The latter situation is seen in the skin, oral gastrointestinal mucosa, or from great distances, as found with bone marrow and lymph node repopulation. The balance between radiation-induced cell killing and repopulation is responsible for most of the clinical findings seen during fractionated radiotherapy treatment.

In addition to spontaneous repopulation, an induced cell proliferation, or recruitment of cells, may take place.[40,41] Physiologically, many tissues of the body respond to trauma by being recruited into rapid proliferation (e.g., after a wound in the skin, a break in bone, or a partial hepatectomy). The reparative process requires proliferation of the undamaged cells. Similarly, when the oral mucosa is irradiated, strong evidence indicates that the cell-cycle time is decreased and that net cell proliferation increases. This also may occur in some tumors but appears to be of less magnitude than that in normal tissues.[42] If cell proliferation is greater in the tumor, then fewer fractions will be desired. Part of the differential effect of fractionated radiation may lie in differential recruitment of normal versus tumor cells.

TRANSCRIPTIONAL ACTIVATION, GENE INDUCTION, AND REGULATION AFTER IONIZING RADIATION

A new class of actions of ionizing radiation may explain a number of perplexing effects. Immediately after exposure to ionizing radiation, expression of genes such as FOS, JUN, and EGR1 appear to take place.[43,44] This seems to occur in the presence of protein synthesis and is thought to be due to transcriptional activation and inhibition of protein degradation. Radiation also induces tumor necrosis factor-α,[45–47] which may produce additive, synergistic, and distant cytotoxic effects of radiation. Platelet-derived growth factor-α and fibroblast growth factor are induced and released from vascular endothelium.[48] It is suggested that this release stimulates proliferation of smooth muscle cells in the smaller arterioles and contributes to the undesirable long-term vascular events associated with radiation exposure.[49]

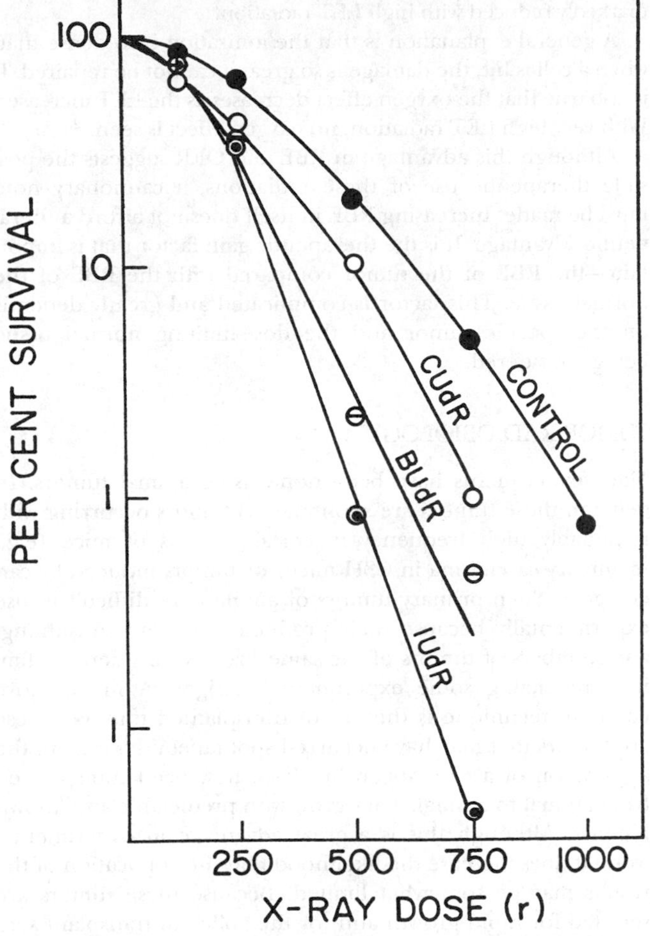

FIGURE 16-12. Radiation survival curve for cells incorporating halogenated pyrimidines. (From ref. 50, with permission.)

PHARMACOLOGIC MODIFICATION OF RADIATION EFFECTS

Pharmacologic agents can modify the basic parameters of radiation response. Figure 16-12 shows a radiation survival curve for cells that have semiconservatively incorporated the halogenated pyrimidine bromodeoxyuridine into their DNA. Under such circumstances, these cells are more sensitive to radiation, their survival curve having the slope and the shoulder modified.[50] This occurs only when the halogenated pyrimidines bromodeoxyuridine or iododeoxyuridine are incorporated into the DNA; their presence at the time of radiation is not sufficient. Sublethal damage repair also is markedly inhibited under these circumstances.

A second class of agents includes those that primarily affect the shoulder and only slightly affect the slope. The two most important of these agents are dactinomycin and doxorubicin. Sublethal damage apparently is inhibited by dactinomycin but not by doxorubicin.[51–57] Strong evidence suggests that these drugs can and do modify radiation effects when given simultaneously. Furthermore, when given after radiation therapy, they can recall the irradiated volumes by erythema on the skin or by producing pulmonary reactions.[52,55,58,59] Chemicals may also interact with radiation by preferentially killing cells that are more resistant to radiation. For example, agents that, along with radiation, preferentially destroy cells in the most resistant phase of the cell cycle (S) increase the cell kill; an example of this is hydroxyurea.[60] Radioprotective agents, such as sulfhydryl-containing compounds, act in the reverse fashion and tend to make cells more resistant.[61] They also reduce the chromosome abnormalities associated with radiation.

Agents with dose-limiting normal tissue toxicities different from radiation may be used effectively with radiation. This is one of the basic principles of multiple-drug chemotherapy—add agents with nonoverlapping toxicities. This strategy also works well with radiation.

The combined effects of drugs and radiation, or of two drugs, can be divided into the following types:

1. Independent. The agents act independently, their mechanisms of action are independent, and their damage is independent.
2. Additivity. The agents act on the same loci, and therefore their sublethal damage and their lethal damage are additive. Because of additive sublethal damage, the lethality of the two together may be greater than the lethality of each alone added together.
3. Synergism. The two agents have a result that is more effective than pure additivity.
4. Antagonism. The cell killing is less than independent action.

The most important parameter for the clinician is the therapeutic index. The sigmoid curve of tumor cure and that of dose-limiting toxicity are portrayed in Figure 16-13. If both curves are moved but their relative place (one to the other) is not changed, then the proportion cured for a given level of toxicity is unchanged. Drug–roentgen ray interaction is useful only when the curves are separated and not merely displaced.

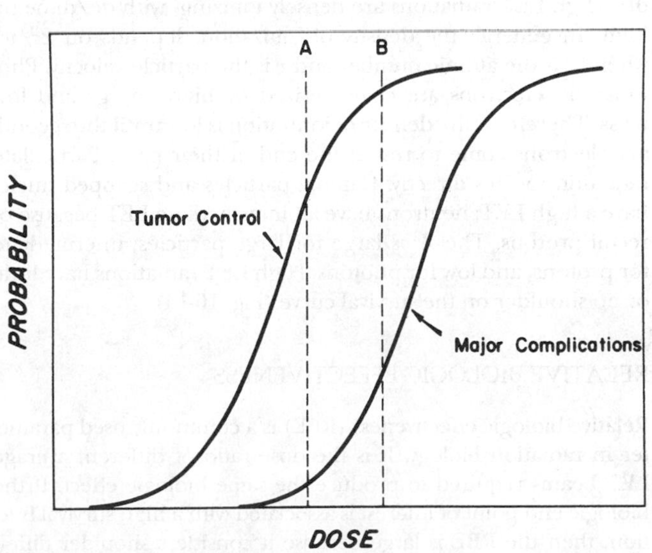

FIGURE 16-13. Sigmoid curves of tumor control and complications. Dose for tumor control with minimum complications (*A*). Maximum tumor dose with significant complications (*B*).

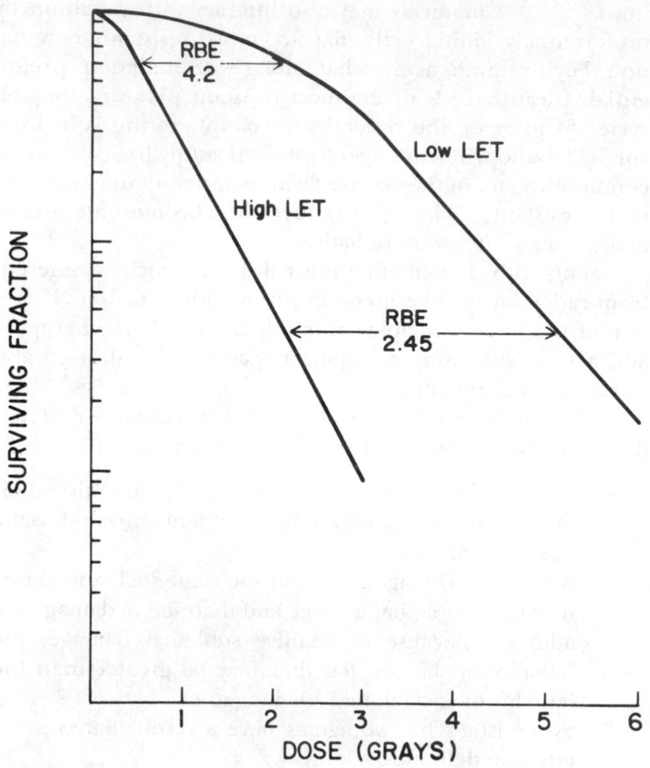

FIGURE 16-14. Survival fractions for high and low linear energy transfer (LET) radiations. RBE, relative biologic effectiveness.

HIGH LINEAR ENERGY TRANSFER RADIATION

Most of the discussion so far has been concerned with sparsely ionizing radiation, such as that produced by photons or high-energy electrons. More densely ionizing radiation is produced by larger atomic particles. The biologic actions of these two types of radiation are different and relate to the density of ionization. LET is the rate of energy loss along the path of the particle (de/dl). High LET radiations are densely ionizing, with de/dl being high. In general, the density of ionization depends on Z^2/v^2, where Z is the atomic number and v is the particle velocity. Photons and electrons are characterized by high energy and low mass. Therefore, the density of ionization is low until the secondary electrons come to rest at the end of their path. Particulate radiation ionizes directly. Gamma particles and stripped nuclei have a high LET; neutrons have an intermediate LET because of recoil protons. The Z^2 is large for large particles, intermediate for protons, and low for photons. High LET radiations have little or no shoulder on the survival curve (Fig. 16-14).

RELATIVE BIOLOGIC EFFECTIVENESS

Relative biologic effectiveness (RBE) is a commonly used parameter in radiation biology. It is the dose ratio of different average LET beams required to produce the same biologic effect. If the biologic end point of interest is associated with a high survival fraction, then the RBE is large because it considers shoulder differences and those of the terminal slope. If the biologic end point involves a low survival fraction, the RBE is less because it primarily considers slope differences. In general, RBE increases as the dose decreases. Not only is the shoulder reduced, but other measures of sublethal damage repair or potentially lethal damage repair are markedly reduced with high LET radiation.

A general explanation is that the ionization is so dense that, when a cell is hit, the damage is so great it cannot be repaired. It is also true that the oxygen effect decreases as the LET increases. With very high LET radiation, no oxygen effect is seen.[62]

Although this advantage in RBE and OER suggests the possible therapeutic use of these radiations, a cautionary note must be made. Increasing RBE in itself does not afford a therapeutic advantage. It is the therapeutic gain factor that is important—the RBE of the tumor compared with the RBE of the normal tissue. This factor is complicated and greatly depends on the specific tumor and the dose-limiting normal tissue being considered.

TUMOR RADIOBIOLOGY

Many experiments have been done using animal tumors. In general, these tumors are spontaneous tumors occurring with reasonably high frequency in certain strains of mice (e.g., mammary carcinoma in C3H mice) or tumors induced by carcinogens. Such primary tumors of animals are difficult to use experimentally because their production is time consuming, and numbers of tumors of the same size and location are limited, restricting some experimental designs. A much more common technique is the use of transplanted tumors. These are tumors that may have occurred spontaneously or from the application of a carcinogen but have now been transplanted from animal to animal. They grow with predictable and known kinetics. Although this is a great advantage in experimental work, it does increase the likelihood that the application of the results may be somewhat limited. Because these tumors are selected for rapid growth and for the ability to transplant serially, they may not represent tumors that occur spontaneously in the host animal. Currently, many laboratories study human tumors transplanted into "nude" mice. These genetically immunosuppressed mice permit the growth of these xenographs, but interpretation of these experiments is limited by the artificiality of the experimental circumstance.

Tumors can be used in radiobiologic experiments and assayed in a number of ways. The simplest is to study the likelihood for cure. A researcher implants a tumor into animals, allows it to grow to palpable size, treats it with a specific regimen, and then determines how many tumors of this type in various host animals are cured. If the dose of radiation is plotted against the likelihood for cure, a sigmoid curve is generated (Fig. 16-15).[64] There is insufficient cell kill to cause tumor cure at very low doses. As the dose is raised (to approximately one lethal event per cell), the statistics of random cell kill become important. Occasionally, tumors have zero viable cells and are cured. The likelihood of cure rises rapidly with dose at this portion of the curve; it starts to plateau when the maximum effect of the particular technique is reached. The dose required to increase a 10% likelihood of tumor control to 90% is approximately three times the D_0 dose. This sigmoid relation is important, because it is true not only for tumors in experimental animals but also for clinical situations. The steepness of the curve in the effective range emphasizes the importance of small increases in dose.

The shape and steepness of the sigmoid dose-response relation for tumors can be affected by many factors. If the D_0 is

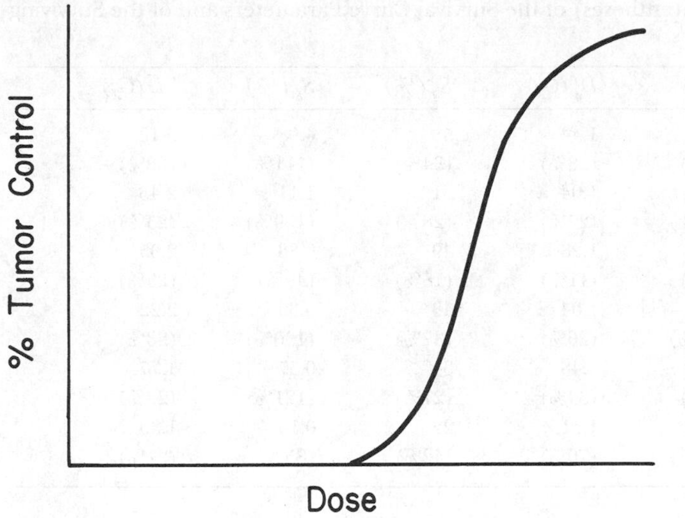

FIGURE 16-15. Sigmoid curve of tumor control.

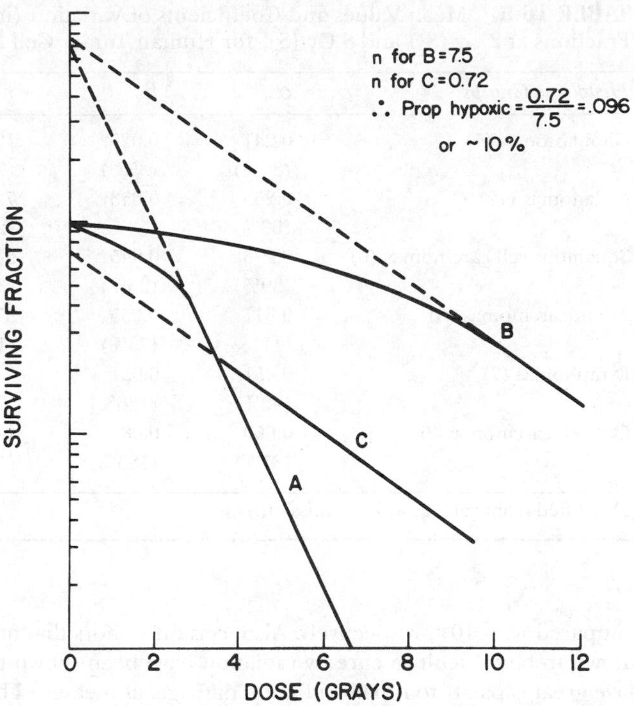

FIGURE 16-16. Idealized survival curves for oxic tumor cells (*A*), hypoxic tumor cells (*B*), and a tumor containing both oxic and hypoxic tumor cells (*C*). Prop, proportion.

large, then the dose-response curve is also shallow. It also is affected by host defense mechanisms. This curve is steep with nonimmunogenic tumors or in hosts with an abrogated immune response, but it is significantly shallower in immunogenic tumors.[65] The shallowness means that occasional cures are found at low doses and occasional failures are noted at very high doses.

A similar sigmoid relation is seen when plotting the likelihood for complications against tumor control. Figure 16-13 shows the two sigmoid curves, one for cure and one for complications. This is presented optimistically—the important complication curve is placed to the right of the tumor cure curve. The difference between these curves is a measure of therapeutic gain. Much of clinical medicine and research in cancer treatment is concerned with separating these curves.[63] After the curves are separated, for a given level of complications, the likelihood of cure can be increased. Or, for a high likelihood of cure, the likelihood of complications can be decreased. Some methods for separating these curves include better restriction of the radiation dose by using techniques such as intensity-modulated radiation therapy (see Chapter 29.4). Combining agents with nonoverlapping toxicity, such as certain chemotherapeutic agents, antiangiogenic agents, or even gene therapy, offer the promise of improved cure without increasing the radiation toxicity. It may also be possible to modify radiation toxicity without decreasing effectiveness.

Tumors, like normal tissues, have certain physiologic characteristics. We associate some of these with the definition of malignancy: continued growth and extension into surrounding tissues, and the ability to metastasize. In addition, growing tumors must induce a blood supply to meet their increasing metabolic needs. The production of these blood vessels appears to result from the release of substances described by Folkman and colleagues[66–68] as "tumor angiogenesis factors" and may have important clinical implications. If tumors can be prevented from producing such substances, they cannot grow beyond a size supported by diffusion alone.[66–68] From the radiobiologic point of view, it means that, when irradiating a tumor, the radiobiology of the tumor and the vascular endothelial cells are important. Complete destruction of the ability of tumor blood vessels to proliferate effectively limits tumor growth.

As tumors grow, they often exceed their blood supply and develop areas of necrosis and hypoxia (see Fig. 16-11). The proportion of hypoxic cells in a tumor can be determined by studying the radiation survival curves. In Figure 16-16, curve A represents a well-oxygenated cell population, curve B describes hypoxic cells, and curve C represents a mixture of oxic and hypoxic cells (as in a tumor). Extrapolation of the curves to the ordinate gives the proportion of hypoxic cells within a tumor, first described by Powers and Tolmach.[69] In most experimental tumors studied, the percentage of hypoxic cells is 10% to 20%.

There has been great interest in trying to determine whether appropriate laboratory correlates exist for clinical radiation treatment.[70,71] Table 16-5 shows important parameters found by *in vitro* survival determinations for six histologic groups of human tumor cells.[72] The first four parameters have already been described. S_2 and S_8 are the survival fractions found with 2 Gy and 8 Gy, respectively. $\bar{D}$ is the mean inactivation dose, a mathematically determined characteristic of the initial portion of the survival curve. It appears that S_2 and $\bar{D}$ correlate directly with clinical radiocurability, whereas α is inversely related. All of these are measures of the initial portion of the radiation survival curve; S_2 is the most closely correlated with clinical practice, because doses between 1.5 and 2.5 Gy are used most often in patient care.

Because in radiation therapy the dose is divided into many fractions, small differences in S_2 can have significant consequences. Table 16-4 shows that, in a typical 32-fraction radiation treatment, the difference between survival fractions of 0.45 and 0.60 results in an ultimate survival fraction of 10^{-11}

TABLE 16-5. Mean Values and Coefficients of Variation (in Parentheses) of the Survival Curve Parameters and of the Surviving Fractions at 2 Gy (S_2) and 8 Gy (S_8) for Human Tumor Cell Lines

Histologic Groups	α	β	*n*	D_o *(Gy)*	S_2 *(%)*	S_8 *(%)*	$\bar{D}$ *(Gy)*
Glioblastomas (5)	0.241	0.029	12	1.44	58	4.98	3.10
	(86%)	(37%)	(71%)	(28%)	(34%)	(111%)	(38%)
Melanomas (19)	0.255	0.053	73	1.04	51	1.11	2.43
	(69%)	(56%)	(265%)	(27%)	(28%)	(109%)	(25%)
Squamous cell carcinomas (6)	0.273	0.045	5	1.28	49	0.88	2.35
	(39%)	(25%)	(38%)	(11%)	(18%)	(49%)	(25%)
Adenocarcinomas (6)	0.311	0.055	37	1.04	48	0.39	2.22
	(117%)	(79%)	(166%)	(26%)	(37%)	(130%)	(28%)
Lymphomas (7)	0.451	0.051	1.8	1.48	34	0.57	1.77
	(42%)	(126%)	(79%)	(34%)	(27%)	(121%)	(22%)
Oat cell carcinomas (6)	0.650	0.081	1.8	1.51	22	0.14	1.33
	(37%)	(183%)	(104%)	(70%)	(42%)	(85%)	(21%)

(Modified from ref. 72, with permission.)

compared with 10^{-7}, respectively. Also, certain tumors that are known to be difficult to cure by radiation have been shown to have great capacity to repair radiation damage, as measured by allowing the cells time for repair before plating them for *in vitro* growth.[73] That these two simple laboratory determinations correlate with clinical results gives hope that *in vitro* techniques can be used to determine mechanisms of modifying clinical parameters. This does not mean that the other biologic parameters, such as oxygenation, position in the cell cycle, and cell proliferation, are not important; no doubt, all of these factors add to the complexity of correlating the clinical response with *in vitro* determinations.

NORMAL TISSUE RADIATION BIOLOGY

To understand normal tissue radiation biology, an appreciation of the cell kinetics of cell renewal tissues is vital. The effects on organ function depend on the reproductive requirements of the irradiated cells. Tissues whose functional activity does not require cell renewal (e.g., muscle and neurologic tissue) are considered resistant to radiation. Both muscle and neurologic tissue also have important vasculoconnective tissue stroma that support them.[74] These stromal cells may be required to divide and, therefore, determine the organ response to radiation. The radiation response of endothelial cells demonstrates a D_q = 340 rad, n = 7, and a D_o = 170 rad, values similar to those of epithelial cells.[75]

Many tissues of the body require continued cellular proliferation for their function, and they promptly demonstrate the effects of radiation. These cell renewal tissues include the skin and its appendages, the gastrointestinal mucosa, bone marrow, reproductive tissues, and many exocrine glands. Clonogenic survival curves for bone marrow stem cells, gastrointestinal epithelial cells, and skin are all available.

Tissues such as the liver and bone require little or no proliferation during the steady state, and normal function can be maintained despite large doses of radiation. However, both of these respond to injury with rapid cell renewal. If trauma (fracture or partial hepatectomy) occurs, then the cells die when they attempt repair. Irradiation of the liver has few consequences in moderate doses, but if this is followed by a partial hepatectomy, hepatic failure can occur. This finding has been of clinical importance in the preoperative irradiation of right-sided Wilms' tumors attached to the liver, in which a significant amount of liver must be removed.[76] Under such circumstances, it is far better to operate, allow the liver to regenerate, and then irradiate.

Patients who have received large amounts of radiation to the bone do perfectly well unless the bone is fractured. The damaged bones fail to be reconstituted or heal slowly, causing a significant deformity and disability to the patient. These examples are included to stress that it is not the different cells that have such great differences in radiation response, but rather that the proliferative requirements of different tissues largely determine the radiation effects. If the proliferative requirements are low, the organ is considered resistant to radiation. If the proliferative requirements are high, it is considered radiosensitive. Some common limitations on all systems may apply, based on the radiosensitivity of the stromal support cells, such as connective tissue and endothelial cells.[74] Stem cells of the cell renewal tissues may have a limited proliferative capacity, and stem cell exhaustion appears to be a cause of late organ failure after irradiation.[77]

Many other effects of radiation that do not depend on reproductive viability may have clear clinical relevance. For example, radiation is damaging to the cell membrane and changes membrane transport. Subsequent radiation-induced edema is seen with moderate doses of radiation. Damage to certain membrane lipids can cause apoptosis without nuclear damage. These nonreproductive effects of radiation are far less well understood but may be important in understanding the effects of radiation on nondividing tissue, especially on the central nervous system.

Large doses of whole body irradiation have obvious clinical consequences, which generally are not relevant to conventional radiation therapy. However, because whole body irradiation has been used in low doses in treating the lymphomas and in high doses in treating metastatic carcinoma, this topic is discussed briefly.

After large doses of radiation, the prodromal syndrome of nausea, vomiting, diarrhea, cramps, fatigue, sweating, fever, and headache occurs. Three distinct modes of death may occur. The first, with very high doses of radiation (more than 10,000 rad), is seen within hours and appears to result from neurologic and cardiovascular damage. Because this occurs so quickly, it probably is not caused by failure of cell proliferation but rather by extranuclear events within these organs. At intermediate doses of radiation (500 to 1000 rad), death occurs within days. It is associated with extensive gastrointestinal mucosal damage, resulting in prolonged, severe, bloody diarrhea; dehydration; and secondary infection occurring as the gastrointestinal mucosa is denuded. At lower doses of radiation (near the LD_{50}), death is caused by hematopoietic failure. This complication has a latency period because the formed blood elements are nondividing, and bone marrow failure does not occur until the progeny of the proliferating cells are required to maintain the patient. The lymphocyte level falls promptly as some of these cells die by apoptosis. The granulocyte level falls on approximately day 5 or 6, and thrombocytopenia occurs later. Anemia does not occur as a direct result of a failure of red blood cell production, because of the long life of the red blood cell, but it may be caused by hemorrhage.

Whole body irradiation appears to have significant antitumor activity exceeding that seen when the same dose is given to the tumor alone.[78,79] Very low doses of whole body radiation in humans (10 to 15 rad, two to three times per week for 6 to 10 fractions) may be effective treatment for lymphomas and may cause marked depression of the formed blood elements. The mechanism of action of this type of treatment is not understood. The effects on tumor and normal tissue are greater than can be explained by the typical survival curve. One possible explanation is the release of TNF-α after radiation.[45,46,48] Perhaps the release of this and other factors may contribute to the general effects of low-dose whole body radiation and the abscopal (distant) effects of regional irradiation. Many of the effects of radiation on both tumors and normal tissues may be mediated or modified by the release of cytokines. Their effect may be tissue specific; for example, basic fibroblast growth factor protects against the apoptotic microvascular component of radiation pneumonitis but has no effect on other mediastinal organs.[49]

ADVERSE EFFECTS OF RADIATION

Some biologic considerations of localized radiation may decrease the likelihood for tumor control. The first and most commonly discussed is the effect of radiation on the immune response. High-dose, whole body irradiation has a well-known and profound effect on the immune response. This generalized treatment rarely is used in clinical therapy, however, except as preparation for bone marrow transplantation.

Shortly after the discovery of roentgen rays, whole body irradiation before the administration of antigens was found to suppress the production of antibodies. After whole body irradiation, a prompt fall in the lymphocyte count is seen. The lymphocytes appear to have two types of radiation response: Approximately 80% apoptose, but some lymphocytes survive the radiation. When assayed on the basis of reproductive capacity by exposure to mitogens after irradiation or other functional end points, their radiation survival curves looked similar to that of hematopoietic cells with a D_o of approximately 70 to 80 rad and an n of approximately 1.[80] Response depends on the classes of lymphocytes involved, the extent of cell proliferation required, cell traffic, and the balance between suppressor and helper systems. The following conclusions concerning the effect of radiation on the immune response can be made[81]:

1. B lymphocytes are radiosensitive and undergo interphase (apoptosis) and mitotic death after irradiation.
2. All functional T-cell subpopulations have sensitive precursor cells. Suppressor T-cell precursors may undergo interphase death.
3. The homing potential of cells is affected by radiation.
4. Resting cells are more sensitive to interphase death than are the same cells when stimulated to divide before irradiation. (In the latter case, they have an n and D_o similar to those of hematopoietic stem cells.)
5. The effects of whole body irradiation are qualitatively and quantitatively different from those caused by localized or regional irradiation.

Whole body irradiation is more effective in preventing response to new antigens than in modifying response to a previously encountered antigen. Survival of second-set skin grafts are affected much less than are initial grafts. Localized radiation, as used in radiation therapy, affects the immune response by decreasing the number of circulating lymphocytes, presumably by irradiating and destroying them as they pass through the irradiated volume and by the release of certain cytokines.

Other adverse effects of radiation on the patient may be seen in addition to those affecting host-defense mechanisms. Radiation-induced mutagenesis is of concern for germline and somatic cells. If the gonads are irradiated, there is an increased likelihood of mutation with increasing doses, without any evidence of a threshold dose or of an ameliorating effect of fractionation. At higher doses, significant cell killing takes place, and the dose-response curve is no longer linear, presumably because the cells that mutated received sufficient radiation to become sterile. Abnormal live births are uncommon after gonadal irradiation because most radiation-induced mutations are recessive. Furthermore, dominant mutations, when they occur, usually are lethal. In the mouse, some evidence indicates that the risk of mutation decreases with time after ovarian irradiation. Whether this is true in humans and how the mechanism occurs in animals are not known. It does not appear to be true for irradiation of the testes.

The mutagenic effects of radiation depend on the type of irradiation. The RBE for high LET radiation can be extremely high for mutations. It is difficult to quantify the risk because experiments with mice indicate a large difference in the mutation rate for different loci, with as much as a 1000-fold variation in the mutation rate.[81] In general, the prudent figure used is that the mutation rate doubles with approximately every 50 rad.

Perhaps of even greater concern are somatic mutations, especially those that may lead to tumors. A great deal of evidence indicates that low doses of radiation increase the incidence of tumors after significant latent periods. This information comes largely from whole body exposures to the atomic bomb and experience with patients irradiated for benign diseases.[82–84] In general, there appears to be a linear increase in tumor incidence with dose until high doses are reached, at which point the incidence reaches a plateau or even falls.[85,86] Presumably, this is true, again, because of cell killing. Figure 16-17 is an example of this biphasic dose-response curve. Such tumor induction is associated with a latent period of 3 to 5 years for leukemia but is much longer for solid tumors. There are different ages at which tumor induction is most likely. For example, the induction of breast cancer by radia-

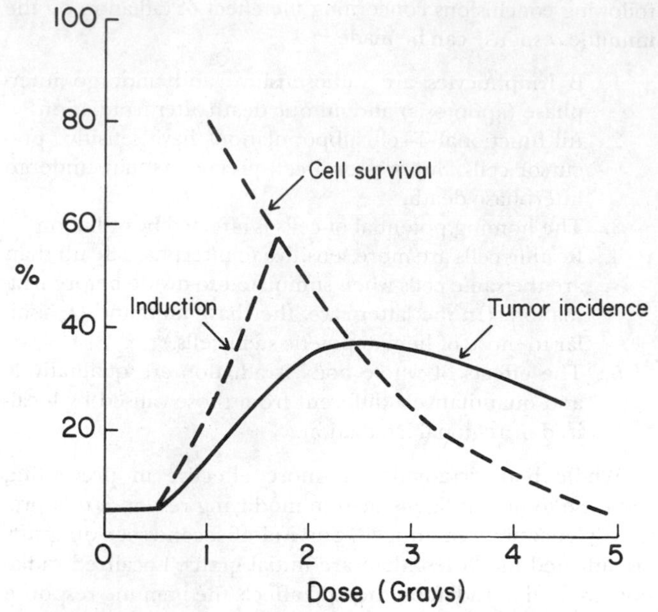

FIGURE 16-17. Biphase curve of tumor incidence. (Adapted from refs. 85 and 86.)

tion appears primarily with exposure in the first and second decades of life and decreases with radiation later in life.

CLINICAL CONSIDERATIONS

It is often suggested that the goal of treatment is the greatest probability of uncomplicated cure. Although this goal is desirable, circumstances actually may dictate a different policy. Consider Figure 16-13, in which the curve for complications is to the right of the sigmoid curve for tumor control. If tumor failure can be salvaged by subsequent surgery but complications are severe, long-lived, and difficult to manage, then line A is the optimal line.[63] An example of this would be the treatment of T2 and T3 glottic cancer. On the other hand, if complications are not severe or are remediable but cancer failure is fatal, then line B would be appropriate. This is the case in stage II and III carcinoma of the uterine cervix. There is no simple answer. Often, the worst complication of treatment is tumor recurrence.

Many clinical examples of sigmoid dose-response curves have been reported. An example for tumors of the head and neck is shown in Figure 16-18 and for Hodgkin's disease in Figure 16-19.[87,88] In Figure 16-18, the ordinate is arranged to convert a sigmoid curve to a straight line. An instructive clinical experience is described by Stewart and Jackson[90] in which a consistent ~10% change in dose was used. Figure 16-20 shows the results in tumor control and complications. The small increase in dose markedly improved the curability of the larger tumors, presumably because this dose is on the steep portion of the sigmoid dose-response curve. It did not change the cure rate for small tumors very much because, presumably, the dose already was large enough to be on the plateau of the dose-response curve, where changes in dose do not affect the cure appreciably. Similarly, complications were not increased significantly. The point indicating complications is to the right, still on the shallow portion of the curve. This is a good example of separation of response between

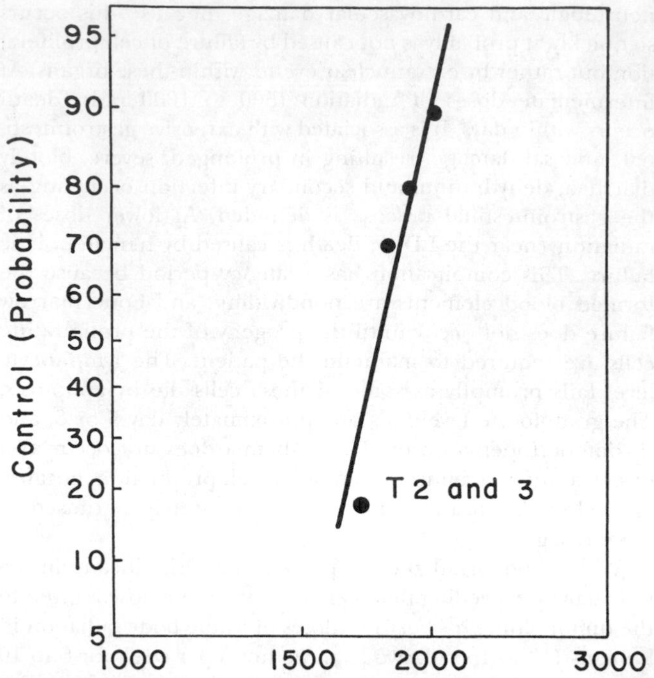

FIGURE 16-18. Tumor control versus dose for supraglottic carcinoma. (From ref. 87, with permission.)

tumor and normal tissues. It also shows displacement of the curve for cure as a function of tumor size.

Even though tumors have a very steep dose-response relationship, significant intertumor heterogeneity may cause great flattening in the radiation dose-control curves.[90] Considerable heterogeneity exists between tumors of the same histologic type and location, and this consideration explains the shallower nature of the clinical dose-response curves compared with those for experimental animals. These analyses further indicate that,

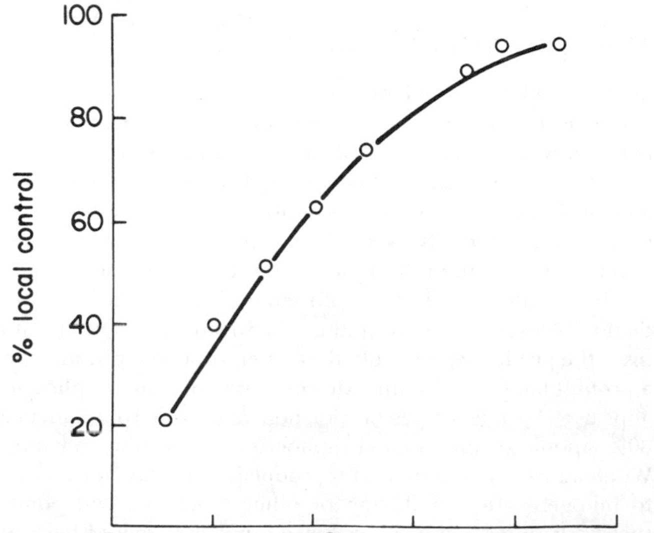

FIGURE 16-19. Tumor control versus dose for Hodgkin's disease. (From ref. 88, with permission.)

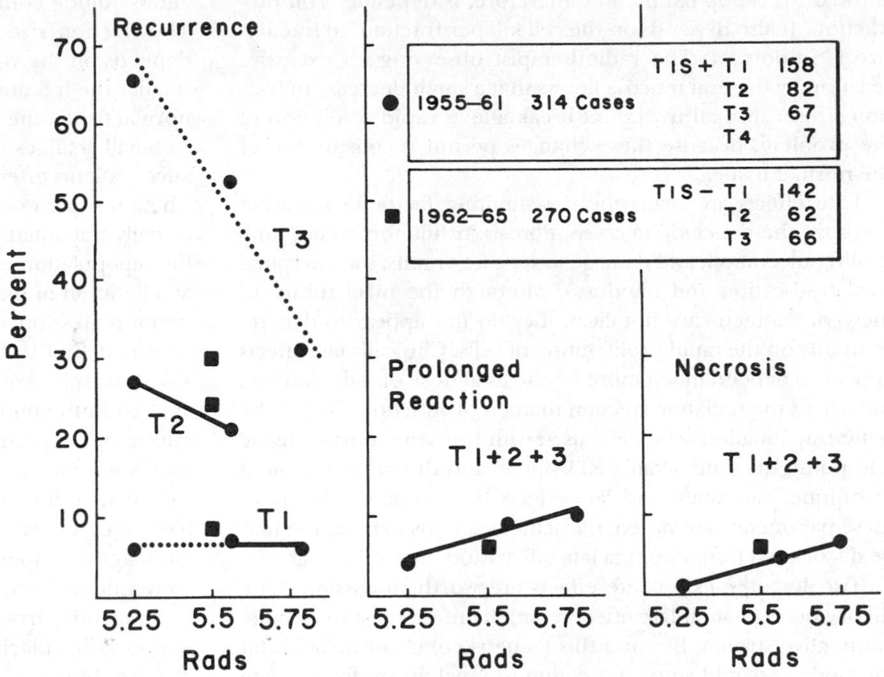

FIGURE 16-20. Tumor control versus dose for cancer of the larynx (4 MeV given over 3 weeks for a treatment period of 5 years). (From ref. 89, with permission.)

when the tumor control probability is low, the major reason is a high S_2. This fact emphasizes the importance of identifying prospectively tumors that have a high S_2. Changes in the likelihood of apoptosis after radiation may have an important effect on S_2.

FRACTIONATION

Early in the twentieth century, as the practice of radiation therapy evolved, the virtues of dividing the radiation into small fractions were noticed. The reasons given were often incorrect, but the clear observation was that fractionation of the dose allowed more effective tumor cure without excessive complications.

Fractionation considers the size and number of radiation increments. Protraction considers the overall time during which the course of radiation therapy is given. Both factors affect all radiation therapy plans. The fashioning of a plan for fractionated radiation therapy for carcinoma of the larynx by Coutard,[91] whose work was based on the principles of Regaud,[92] laid the foundation for the development of radiation therapy. The principles of such treatment were as follows:

1. Fractionation is important.
2. A relation exists between the acute reaction of the skin and oropharyngeal mucosa to cure and to late effects.

The association between acute and late effects has sometimes led radiotherapists astray. This relation depends on the fractionation scheme, the energy of radiation used, and other factors. In general, acute effects are much more dependent on time than late effects. Late effects are influenced primarily by the total dose and fraction size.

CONTINUOUS RADIATION

Another important technique of radiation therapy that evolved in the early part of the twentieth century was the application of continuous radiation by interstitial or intracavitary application.[93] If the dose rate was too high or the volume too large, unacceptable complications occurred. Rules for treatment were developed that resulted in the cure of certain tumors without unacceptable complications. These rules required that the dose rate be kept moderate (less than 100 rad/hour) and an attempt at a good implant geometry be made to avoid unnecessary hot and cold spots.

The whole question of homogeneity of dose is much more difficult with intracavitary and interstitial irradiation than with external-beam techniques. To a great extent, the clinical use of radioactive isotopes, especially by implantation techniques, developed separately from external-beam radiation therapy. Some physicians only practiced one or the other of these techniques. More recently, external-beam and interstitial treatment have been used together to take advantage of the virtues of both modalities. Good examples of this combined treatment are described in the chapters dealing with tumors of the head and neck and uterine cervix (see Chapters 30 and 36). The increase in the use of high-dose-rate afterloading techniques, although having the practical and logistical advantages, eliminate the dose-rate advantage of brachytherapy. It remains to be determined whether this will have significant clinical consequences (see Chapter 36.2).

ACUTE AND LATE NORMAL TISSUE EFFECTS

Acute radiation effects occur largely in renewing tissues, such as skin, oropharyngeal mucosa, small intestine, rectum, bladder mucosa, and vaginal mucosa. These cell-renewing tissues are rapidly proliferating, and as they are confronted with fractionated radiation, the processes of repair, repopulation, and recruitment all obtain. Because the response of rapidly renewing tissues depends on the balance between cell birth and cell death, acute tissue reaction is crucially affected by the time allowed for repopulation and, therefore, is dependent on protraction. It also depends on the cell kill per fraction, so fraction size is important. The radiotherapist observing an excessive reaction by the oral mucosa knows that a small decrease in fraction size or a small treatment break allows rapid resolution of the problem, because these changes permit reconstitution of the normal tissue.

Late effects are really the dose-limiting factor in radiation therapy. These include necrosis, fibrosis, fistula formation, nonhealing ulceration, and damage to specific organs, such as spinal cord transection and blindness. Although the mechanisms of these phenomena are not clear, they do not appear to depend primarily on the rapid proliferation of cells. Clinically late effects appear to depend much more on the total dose of radiation and the size of the radiation fraction than on protraction. Only if the same fractionation scheme is used with the same normal tissue end point, the same irradiated volume, and the same treatment technique, can acute and late effects be correlated. If any of these parameters are varied, the acute reactions to radiation may be dissociated from eventual late effects and are misleading.

Two hypotheses for late effects are worth discussion. One theory holds that all late effects result from damage to vasculoconnective stroma. Because this tissue is common throughout the body, it would suggest a common mechanism for the late effects in any organ.[74] A variation on this hypothesis is that it is damage to the endothelial cells, ubiquitous throughout the body, that determines late effects.[75] An alternative hypothesis suggests that the acute and the late effects of radiation and cytotoxic chemotherapy are caused by cell depletion of the targeted cell-renewal tissues. Acute effects depend on the balance between cell killing and compensatory replication of the stem and proliferative cells. The development of late effects requires that stem cells have only a limited proliferative capacity.[94,95] Compensation for extensive or repeated cell killing may exhaust this capacity, resulting in eventual tissue failure.[73,96]

ALTERING THE THERAPEUTIC INDEX

Goodman and Gilman[98] define the therapeutic index as the relation between desired and undesired effects of therapy. For the oncologist, separation of the sigmoid curve of complications from that of local control (see Fig. 16-13) is the graphic representation of manipulation of the therapeutic index. Some techniques of time-dose relations used by the radiation oncologist to take advantage of this are fractionation, protraction, split-course technique, interstitial treatment, and manipulation of the target volume. Although fractionation has been discussed, the use of multiple small fractions two, three, or more times a day (hyperfractionation), is being explored, with some good results.[98–100]

Another technique to reduce complications is the use of normal-size fractions given more than once a day. This is referred to as *multifraction, multiple daily fractions*, or *accelerated fractionation*.[101]

When tumor cells are proliferating rapidly, accelerated fractionation makes sense. Waiting 24 hours between each fraction may allow significant proliferation. Perhaps the best example of the changing therapeutic index obtained with accelerated fractionation is the enhanced success in treating Burkitt's lymphoma.[102]

In general, most radiotherapists administer conventional radiation in fractions between 180 and 250 rad each day. This allows tumor control without excessive acute or late effects. The fraction size that is tolerated in terms of acute effects depends on the volume irradiated (the larger the volume, the smaller the fraction size), the amount and type of dose-limiting normal tissue, the age of the patient, and other clinical factors.

Small changes in fraction size make a big difference in tolerance. Patients often are given small breaks during the treatment. These rest periods usually are caused by weekend interruptions of daily fractionation. This protraction of the treatment allows for repopulation and recruitment. The days of rest also allow amelioration of many acute effects, and they may allow time for tumor regression, resulting in reoxygenation.

An attempt to formalize and extend treatment breaks is the so-called split course technique.[103–105] Two to 3 weeks are allowed in the middle of treatment for recovery from the acute effects and to permit tumor regression. When the dose of radiation is not increased, accumulating evidence indicates that this treatment (although better tolerated) may be associated with less tumor control.[106] When the split course is administered with an increase in total dose, the results seem to be comparable to conventional fractionation but perhaps with greater late effects.

Interstitial irradiation is administered by permanently or temporarily placing radioactive material into tissues. It requires biologic and physical considerations. Great inhomogeneity is found, even in the most geometrically perfect implant. There is large inhomogeneity of dose and a similar variation in dose rate; the dose rate of radiation is greater in areas of high dose. The half-life of ^{125}I is long (60 days), resulting in a significant amount of the dose being given so slowly that significant cell division may occur in the tumor and some normal cells. Therefore, the important dose may not be the total dose, but rather the dose per cell cycle, which is different for each cell type and different as the isotope decays. Also, ^{125}I irradiates primarily by the emission of very low-energy photons, some of which are absorbed by the seeds themselves, leading to further inhomogeneity.[107]

When implants can be used alone or in combination with external irradiation, the results are often better in terms of the therapeutic index than with external-beam techniques alone. The high local dose, continuous radiation, and even inhomogeneity allowing normal tissue regrowth all contribute to better cosmetic and functional results and cure of the tumor. Examples are breast cancer and tumors of the tongue and other head and neck sites.[108,109] Tumor volume also is important in clinical radiotherapy. Although the gross tumor extent can be determined, most clinicians recognize that a characteristic of tumors is to extend beyond those macroscopically identifiable borders. Determination of the target volume must include this consideration, but if a larger volume must be irradiated, then a smaller dose is tolerated. Conversely, if the volume of the tumor is larger, then a larger dose is required. This dilemma limited the success of early radiotherapy of certain tumors by reducing the target volume, resulting in recurrences at the treatment margins, or by causing significant complications in the treatment of large target volumes. Today, distinctions are made between gross tumor and the subclinical extensions into apparently normal tissues. Subclinical disease means small numbers of cells, perhaps favorable to irradiation (well oxygenated), which can be controlled with modest doses of radiation (Table 16-6). The large number of cells present in the clinically evidenced tumor

TABLE 16-6. Control of Subclinical Disease

	Control Rate (%)	
Dose (Gy)	Adenocarcinoma of the Breast	Carcinoma of Upper Aerodigestive Tract
30–35	60–70	60–70
40	80–90	>90
50	>90	>90

(From Fletcher GH. Clinical dose-response curves of human malignant epithelial tumors. *Br J Radiol* 1973;46:1, with permission.)

requires higher doses (see curves in Figs. 16-20 and 16-21). This difference has led to the development of techniques for administering different doses to microscopic tumor extensions and to the gross tumor. These include shrinking-field techniques, boost treatments, and certain strategies of combined surgery and radiotherapy.

Shrinking-field technique means giving the largest potential tumor bed a moderate dose of radiation, then reducing the target volume to the tumor and its immediate confines and raising the dose. This can be done by reducing the fields; changing the treatment technique and target volume; or using a treatment technique such as intensity-modulated radiation therapy, which gives the desired moderate dose to the larger volume and a higher dose to the smaller volume. Attempts have been made to consider fractionation, protraction, and even implantation used with external beam in some form of mathematical formulae, all of which tend to oversimplify complex clinical circumstances and can be misleading.

The dose-limiting normal tissues are of two kinds: those transited by the radiation as a consequence of irradiating the target volume, and those normal tissues within the target volume (e.g., the urethra in a prostatic target volume). Radiotherapy with detailed treatment planning, CT scanning, and computer-controlled radiation therapy may reduce the dose to the transited volume, possibly changing the therapeutic index.[110] However, it is unlikely that significant physical techniques will be available for reducing the dose to normal tissues in the target volume. This can be done only by some biologic mechanism that distinguishes tumor from normal tissues.

RADIOSENSITIVITY

The term *radiosensitivity* is used in different ways in the literature and can mean what is defined as radiosensitivity, radioresponsiveness, or radiocurability. Each is a somewhat different concept. To the radiation biologist, radiosensitivity means the innate sensitivity of the cells to radiation. For cells that die a reproductive death, this is related to the slope of the survival curve, or the D_0.

Radioresponsiveness means the clinical appearance of tumor regression promptly after moderate doses of radiation. This may be a function of the cell's radiosensitivity, but it also may be a function of the active cell kinetics of a tumor. Bergonie and Tribondeau[114] first established an association between the rate of proliferation and the response of normal tissues, although they considered this to be radiosensitivity. A similar relation was presumed to apply to tumors. Because cells do not undergo a reproductive death until they face mitosis, some tumors that proliferate rapidly regress rapidly,

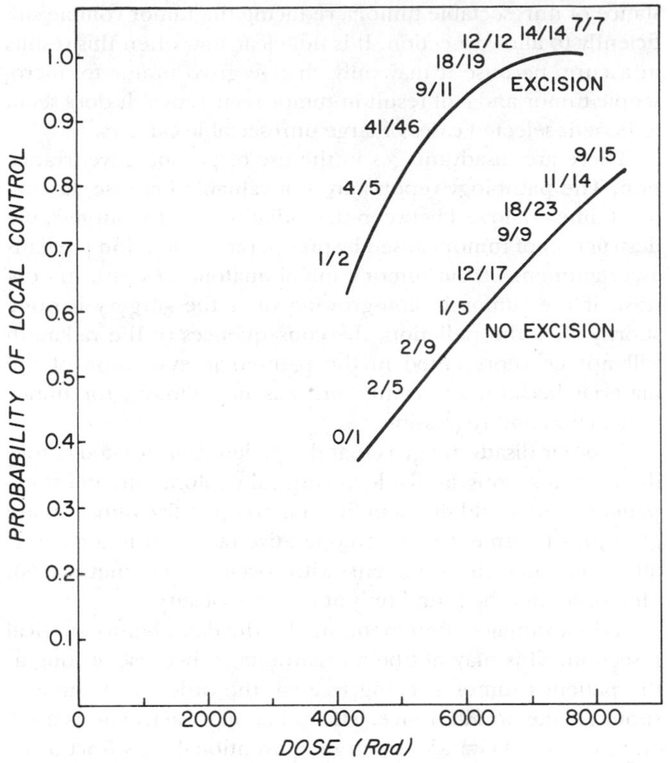

FIGURE 16-21. Tumor control versus dose for stage II and III breast cancer. (From Hellman S. Improving the therapeutic index in breast cancer treatment. *Cancer Res* 1980;40:4335, with permission.)

but they also may regrow rapidly. This is often confused with radiosensitivity.

Radiocurability means that the tumor–normal tissue relations are such that curative doses of radiation can be applied regularly without excessive damage to normal tissues. Examples of such radiocurable tumors are carcinomas of the cervix, larynx, breast, and prostate, in addition to Hodgkin's disease and seminomas. Some of these are radioresponsive, some are radiosensitive, and some are neither.

RADIATION AND SURGERY

Radiation and surgery can be combined in many different ways. The general rationale for combining surgery and radiation is that the mechanism of failure for the two techniques is different. Radiation rarely fails at the periphery of tumors, where cells are small in number and well vascularized. When radiation fails, it usually does so in the center of the tumor where there are large volumes of tumor cells, often under hypoxic conditions. Surgery, in contrast, is limited by the required preservation of vital normal tissues adjacent to the tumor. In resectable cancers, the gross tumor can be removed, but it is these vital normal tissues that limit the anatomic extent of the dissection. When surgery fails under these circumstances, it is usually because of microscopic tumor cells left behind. It seems logical, therefore, to consider combining the two techniques.

Radiation can be given before or after surgery. Preoperative radiation has the advantages of sterilizing cells at the edges of the resection, sterilizing cells that perhaps would be dislodged and seeded at the time of surgery and, in the special circumstance of unresectable tumors, reducing the tumor volume sufficiently to allow resection. It is not clear how often this results in a cure, because it may only change gross tumor to microscopic tumor and still result in tumor recurrence. It does seem to benefit selected cases of large unresectable cancers.[112]

There are disadvantages in the use of preoperative irradiation. The pathology reports are not valuable because, if sufficient time is allowed between the radiation and the surgery, the destruction of tumor caused by preoperative radiation prevents ascertainment of the tumor's initial anatomic extent. In contrast, if the tumor is slow-growing or if the surgery is done shortly after the radiation, the consequences of the radiation will not be represented in the pathologic evaluation of the material because sufficient time was not allowed for tumor destruction and regression.

Another disadvantage is that the patient is irradiated before the careful staging available at surgical exploration, and some patients who would not benefit from preoperative radiation are given this treatment (e.g., preoperative radiation to a colorectal carcinoma in a patient with occult liver metastases). Metastases may be found only at the time of surgery.

A disadvantage often mentioned is the delay before surgical resection. This may not be a disadvantage, because as long as the patient's tumor is being treated, the order of treatments should make no difference. The radiation dose usually is moderate (40 to 50 Gy) and given in conventional 2-Gy fractions 5 days a week or in smaller total doses given more quickly in larger fractions. If the total dose of radiation is kept small (less than or equal to 20 Gy), then the delay between radiation and surgery is small. When the dose reaches approximately 40 Gy, it is valuable to delay the surgery (usually 4 to 6 weeks) to allow the tissues to recover from the radiation. If the total dose is greater than 50 Gy, then the surgery often will be more difficult. However, with moderate doses of radiation and some time allowed between radiation and surgery, the resection can proceed without difficulty.

Postoperative radiation has a number of advantages as well. The subgroup of patients who may be helped by radiation can be defined accurately as a consequence of the surgical exploration and pathologic review. Unnecessary irradiation to patients who are not likely to benefit can be avoided, and the target volumes are tailored to meet what is found at surgery. Time can be allowed for wound healing so that the radiation does not interfere with this process. A disadvantage of such treatment is that it has no effect on seeding at the time of surgery. Surgery also may alter the physiology of the tumor left behind because of reduction of the vascular supply. Cells that were well oxygenated may be rendered physiologically hypoxic and more resistant to radiation. Another disadvantage in the peritoneal cavity is that the surgery causes loops of bowel to be fixed in specific positions and increases the likelihood of small intestinal damage by radiation.

Some uncertainty exists as to which technique is better for particular clinical circumstances. Both preoperative and postoperative radiation appear to be valuable, and the choice of the method, the dose of radiation, and time between radiation and surgery should be considered in terms of the goals planned.

An additional technique for combining surgery with radiation is limited surgical removal of the gross tumor. Because the gross tumor limits the radiotherapeutic treatment, new interest has been raised in using surgery as the boost technique. Full courses of radiation combined with tumorectomy are given. This surgery can be done before or after the irradiation. An example of this strategy is the "lumpectomy" used in the treatment of breast masses before definitive radiation (see Chapter 37).[113,114] In the latter there appears to be evidence to suggest that the removal of gross tumor displaces the sigmoid curve of cure to lower radiation doses and makes it change more steeply with dose (see Fig. 16-21).

RADIATION AND CHEMOTHERAPY

The purpose of combined radiation and chemotherapy treatment is not to decrease the dose of radiation to gain the same effect, but rather to increase the therapeutic index. This may be achieved using techniques that take advantage of the different mechanisms of action of systemic chemotherapy and regional irradiation. Chemotherapeutic agents that directly modify the radiation survival curve may be used. A good example of this is the use of dactinomycin in the treatment of childhood rhabdomyosarcoma or Wilms' tumor. A second way to increase the therapeutic index is to use drugs that specifically affect tumor response to radiation; the most exciting of these are the hypoxic sensitizers, because they affect hypoxic cells that usually are restricted to tumors.

A third mechanism is the combination of drugs and roentgen rays with independent action or additivity. This strategy is just beginning to be explored but appears to be of value in increased local control achieved in head and neck cancer. Because the major advantage of chemotherapy is its wide distribution throughout the body, the combination of radiation and chemotherapy may improve the therapeutic index because, like the combination of surgery and irradiation, the target volumes are different. Adjuvant chemotherapy with radiation for breast cancer, or with surgery and radiation for colon cancer, may improve survival because the chemotherapy is effective against occult micrometastases outside the radiation field. Similarly, radiation may be of value in the treatment of leukemia by chemotherapy because the radiation can be applied to specific sanctuary sites, such as the central nervous system.

REFERENCES

1. Johns HE, Cunningham JR. *The physics of radiology.* Springfield, IL: Charles C Thomas, 1977.
2. Thompson LH, Suit HD. Proliferation kinetics of x-irradiated mouse L cells studied with timelapse photography, part II. *Int J Radiat Biol* 1969;15:347.
3. Elkind MM. The initial part of the survival curve: does it predict the outcome of fractionated radiotherapy? *Radiat Res* 1988;144:425.
4. Weichselbaum RR, Nove J, Little JB. X-ray sensitivity of human tumor cells *in vitro. Int J Radiat Oncol Biol Phys* 1980;6:437.
5. Till JE, McCulloch EA. A direct measurement of the radiation sensitivity of normal mouse bone marrow cells. *Radiat Res* 1961;14:213.
6. Withers HR, Elkind MM. Microcolony survival assay for cells of mouse intestinal mucosa exposed to radiation. *Int J Radiat Biol* 1970;17:261.
7. Alper T, Gillies NE. Restoration of *Escherichia coli* strain B irradiation: its dependence on suboptimal growth conditions. *J Gen Microbiol* 1958;18:461.
8. Phillips RA, Tolmach LJ. Repair of potentially lethal damage in x-irradiated HeLa cells. *Radiat Res* 1966;29:413.
9. Little JB, Hahn GM, Frindel E, et al. Repair of potentially lethal radiation damage *in vitro* and *in vivo. Radiology* 1973;106:689.
10. Belli JA, Shelton M. Potentially lethal radiation damage: repair of mammalian cells in culture. *Science* 1969;165:490.
11. Weichselbaum R, Little JB, Nove J. Response of human osteosarcoma *in vitro* to irradiation: evidence for unusual cellular repair activity. *Int J Radiat Biol* 1977;31:295.
12. Elkind MM, Sutton H. Radiation response of mammalian cells grown in culture: part 1. Repair of x-ray damage in surviving Chinese hamster cells. *Radiat Res* 1960;13:556.

13. Hall EJ. Radiation dose-rate: a factor of importance in radiobiology and radiotherapy. *Br J Radiol* 1972;45:81.
14. Dewey WC, Ling CC, Meyn RE. Radiation-induced apoptosis: relevance to radiotherapy. *Int J Radiat Oncol Biol Phys* 1995:33:781.
15. Boise LH, González-Garcia M, Postema CE, et al. bcl-x, a bcl-2-related gene that functions as a dominant regulator of apoptotic cell death. *Cell* 1993:74:597.
16. Thompson CB. Apoptosis in the pathogenesis and treatment of disease. *Science* 1995:267:1456.
17. Fuks Z, Persaud RS, Alfieri A, et al. Basic fibroblast growth factor protects endothelial cells against radiation-induced programmed cell death *in vitro* and *in vivo*. *Cancer Res* 1994:54:2582.
18. Mottram JC. Factors of importance in radiosensitivity of tumors. *Br J Radiol* 1936;9:606.
19. Read J. The effect of ionizing radiation on the broad beam root: the dependence of the x-ray sensitivity on dissolved oxygen. *Br J Radiol* 1952;25:89.
20. Gray LH, Coger AD, Ebert M, et al. The concentration of oxygen dissolved in tissues at the time of irradiation as a factor in radiotherapy. *Br J Radiol* 1953;26:638.
21. Belli JA, Dicus GJ, Bonte FJ. Radiation response of mammalian tumor cells. I. Repair of sublethal damage *in vivo*. *J Natl Cancer Inst* 1967;38:673.
22. Thomlinson RH, Gray LH. The histological structure of some human lung cancers and possible implications for radiotherapy. *Br J Cancer* 1955;9:539.
23. Kallman RF. The phenomenon of reoxygenation and its implications for fractionated radiotherapy. *Radiology* 1972;105:135.
24. Henk JM, Kindler PB, Smith CW. Radiotherapy and head and neck cancer: final report of the first clinical trial. *Lancet* 1977;2:101.
25. Henk JM, Smith CW. Radiotherapy and head and neck cancer: interim report of second clinical trial. *Lancet* 1977;2:104.
26. Watson ER, Halman KE, Dische S, et al. Hyperbaric oxygen and radiotherapy: a Medical Research Council trial in carcinoma of the cervix. *Br J Radiol* 1978;51:879.
27. Adams GE, Dewez DL. Hydrated electrons and radiobiological sensitization. *Biochem Biophys Res Commun* 1963;12:473.
28. Adams GE, Ahmed L, Fielden EM, et al. The development of some nitroimidazoles as hypoxic cell sensitizers. *Cancer Clin Trials* 1980;3:37.
29. Stratford LJ, Adams GE. Effect of hyperthermia on differential cytotoxicity of a hypoxic cell radiosensitizer RO-07-0582 on mammalian cells *in vitro*. *Br J Cancer* 1977;35:307.
30. Rose CM, Millar JL, Peacock JH, et al. Differential enhancement of toxicity in tumors and normal tissues by misonidazole. In: *Proceedings of the Key Biscayne Conference on Hypoxic Cell Sensitizers and Radioprotectors.* New York: Masson, 1980.
31. Bush RS, Jenkin RP, Allt WE, et al. Definitive evidence for hypoxic cells influencing cure in cancer therapy. *Br J Cancer* 1978;37:302.
32. Kolstad P. Intercapillary distance, oxygen tension, and local recurrence in cervix cancer. *Scan J Clin Lab Invest* 1968;106[suppl]:145.
33. Urtasun RC, Koch CJ, Franko AJ, et al. A novel technique for measuring human tissue PO_2 at the cellular level. *Br J Cancer* 1986;54:453.
34. Urtasun RC, Chapman JD, Raleigh JA, Franko AJ, Koch CJ. Binding of 3H-misonidazole to solid human tumors as a measure of tumor hypoxia. *Int J Radiat Oncol Biol Phys* 1986;12:1263.
35. Terasima R, Tolmach LJ. X-ray sensitivity and DNA synthesis in synchronous populations of HeLa cells. *Science* 1963;140:490.
36. Sinclair WK, Morton RA. X-ray sensitivity during the cell generation cycle of cultured Chinese hamster cells. *Radiat Res* 1966;29:450.
37. Chaffey JT, Hellman S. Differing responses to radiation of murine bone marrow stem cells in relation to the cell cycle. *Cancer Res* 1971;31:1613.
38. Madoc-Jones H, Mauro F. Age response to x-rays vinca alkaloids and hydroxyurea of murine lymphoma cells synchronized *in vivo*. *J Natl Cancer Inst* 1970;45:1131.
39. Hellman S. Cell kinetics, models, and cancer treatment: some principles for the radiation oncologist. *Radiology* 1975;114:219.
40. Chaffey JT, Hellman S. Radiation fractionation as applied to murine colony-forming units in differing proliferative states. *Radiology* 1969;93:1167.
41. Chaffey JT, Hellman S. Studies on dose fractionation as measured by endogenous spleen colonies in the mouse. *Radiology* 1968;90:363.
42. Hermens AF, Barendson GW. Changes in cell proliferation characteristics in a rat rhabdomyosarcoma before and after x-irradiation. *Eur J Cancer Clin Oncol* 1969;5:173.
43. Sherman ML, Datta R, Hallahan DE, et al. Ionizing radiation regulates expression of the *c-jun* proto-oncogene. *Proc Natl Acad Sci U S A* 1990;87:5663.
44. Hallahan DE, Sukhatme VP, Sherman ML, et al. Protein kinase C mediates x-ray inducibility of nuclear signal transducers EGR1 and JUN. *Proc Natl Acad Sci U S A* 1991;88:2156.
45. Hallahan DE, Spriggs DR, Beckett MA, et al. Increased tumor necrosis factor α mRNA after cellular exposure to ionizing radiation. *Proc Natl Acad Sci U S A* 1989;86:10104.
46. Sherman ML, Datta R, Hallahan DE, et al. Tumor necrosis factor gene expression is transcriptionally and post-transcriptionally regulated by ionizing radiation in human myeloid leukemic cells and peripheral blood monocytes. *J Clin Invest* 1991;87:1794.
47. Witte L, Fuks Z, Haimovitz-Friedman A, et al. Effects of radiation on the release of growth factors from cultured bovine, porcine and human endothelial cells. *Cancer Res* 1989;49:5066.
48. Weichselbaum RR, Hallahan DE, Sukhatme V, et al. Biological consequences of gene regulation after ionizing radiation exposure. *J Natl Cancer Inst* 1991;83:480.
49. Fuks Z, Alfieri A, Haimovitz-Friedman A, Seddon A, Cordon-Cardo A. Intravenous basic fibroblast growth factor protects the lung but not mediastinal organs against radiation-induced apoptosis *in vivo*. *Cancer J Sci Am* 1995:1:62.
50. Szybalski W. X-ray sensitization by halopyrimidines. *Cancer Chemother Rep* 1974;58:539.
51. Piro AJ, Taylor CC, Belli JA. Interaction between radiation and drug damage in mammalian cells, part 1. Delayed expression of actinomycin D/x-ray effects in exponential and plateau phase cells. *Radiat Res* 1975;63:346.
52. D'Angio GJ, Farber S, Maddock CL. Potentiation of x-ray effects by actinomycin D. *Radiology* 1959;73:175.
53. Bases RE. Modification of the radiation response determined by single-cell techniques: actinomycin D. *Cancer Res* 1959;19:1223.
54. Elkind MM, Whitmore GF, Alescio T. Actinomycin D: suppression of recovery in x-irradiated mammalian cells. *Science* 1964;143:1454.
55. Pinkel D. Actinomycin D in childhood cancer: a preliminary report. *Pediatrics* 1959;23:342.
56. Hellman S, Hannon E. Effects of Adriamycin on the radiation response of murine hematopoietic stem cells. *Radiat Res* 1976;67:162.
57. Belli JA, Piro AJ. The interaction between radiation and Adriamycin damage in mammalian cells. *Cancer Res* 1977;37:1624.
58. Cassady JR, Richter MP, Piro AJ, et al. Radiation-Adriamycin interactions: preliminary clinical observations. *Cancer* 1975;36:946.
59. Donaldson SC, Glick JM, Wilbur JR. Adriamycin activating a recall phenomenon after radiation therapy. *Ann Intern Med* 1974;81:407.
60. Sinclair WK. Hydroxyurea: effects on Chinese hamster cells grown in culture. *Cancer Res* 1967;27:297.
61. Yuhas JM, Yurconic M, Kligerman MM, et al. Combined use of radioprotective and radiosensitizing drugs in experimental radiotherapy. *Radiat Res* 1977;70:433.
62. Barendsen GW. Response of cultured cells, tumours, and normal tissues to radiations of different linear energy transfer. *Curr Top Radiat Res* 1968;4:293.
63. Bloomer WD, Hellman S. Normal tissue responses to radiation therapy. *N Engl J Med* 1975;293:80.
64. Holthusen H. Erfahrungen über die Vertaglichkeitsgrenze fur Röntgenstrahler und deren Nutzanwendung zur Verhutung von Schaden. *Strahlentherapie* 1936;57:254.
65. Suit HD, Goitein M. Rationale for use of charged-particle and fast-neutron beams in radiation therapy. In: Meyn RE, Withers HR, eds. *Radiation biology in cancer research.* New York: Raven Press, 1980.
66. Folkman J, Tyler K. Tumor angiogenesis: its possible role in metastasis and invasion. In: Day B, Myers WP, Stans Garattini S, et al., eds. *Cancer invasion and metastasis: mechanisms and therapy,* Vol 5. New York: Raven Press, 1977:95.
67. Folkman J. Tumor angiogenesis: a possible control point in tumor growth. *Ann Intern Med* 1975;82:96.
68. Folkman J, Langer R, Linhardt RJ, et al. Angiogenesis inhibition and tumor regression caused by heparin or a heparin fragment in the presence of cortisone. *Science* 1983;221:719.
69. Powers WE, Tolmach LV. A multicomponent x-ray survival curve for mouse lymphosarcoma cells irradiation *in vitro*. *Nature* 1963;197:710.
70. Fertil B, Malaise EP. Inherent cellular radiosensitivity as a basic concept for human tumor radiotherapy. *Int J Radiat Oncol Biol Phys* 1981;7:621.
71. Deacon J, Peckham MJ, Steel GG. The radioresponsiveness of human tumours and the initial slope of the cell survival curve. *Radiother Oncol* 1984;2:317.
72. Malaise EP, Fertil B, Chavaudra N, et al. Distribution of radiation sensitivities for human tumor cells of specific histological types: comparison of *in vitro* to *in vivo* data. *Int J Radiat Oncol Biol Phys* 1986;12:617.
73. Weichselbaum RR, Dahlberg W, Little JB. Inherently radioresistant cells exist in some human tumors. *Proc Natl Acad Sci U S A* 1985;82:4732.
74. Rubin P, Casarett GW. *Clinical radiation pathology.* Philadelphia: WB Saunders, 1968.
75. Reinhold HS, Buisman GH. Radiosensitivity of capillary endothelium. *Br J Radiol* 1973;46:54.
76. Filler RM, Tefft M, Vawter GF, et al. Hepatic lobectomy in childhood: effects of x-ray and chemotherapy. *J Pediatr Surg* 1969;4:31.
77. Reincke U, Hannon EC, Rosenblatt M, Hellman S. Proliferative capacity of murine hematopoietic stem cells *in vitro*. *Science* 1982;215:1619.
78. Medinger FG, Craver LF. Total-body irradiation. *Am J Roentgenol Radium Ther Nucl Med* 1942;48:651.
79. Hellman S, Chaffey JT, Rosenthal DS, et al. Place of radiation therapy in the treatment of non-Hodgkin's lymphomas. *Cancer* 1977;39:843.
80. Anderson RE, Warner NL. Ionizing radiation and the immune response. *Adv Immunol* 1976;24:215.
81. Kohn HI, Melvold RW. Divergent x-ray-induced mutation rates in the mouse for Hand "7 locus" groups of loci. *Nature* 1976;259:209.
82. Folley JH, Borges W, Yamawaki T. Incidence of leukemia in survivors of the atomic bomb in Hiroshima and Nagasaki, Japan. *Am J Med* 1952;13:311.
83. Smith PG, Doll R. Late effects of x-irradiation in patients healed for metropathia hemorrhagica. *Br J Radiol* 1976;49:224.
84. Court Brown WM, Doll R. Mortality from cancer and other causes after radiotherapy for ankylosing spondylitis. *BMJ* 1965;2:1327.
85. Gray LH. Radiation biology and cancer. In: *Cellular radiation biology—the M. D. Anderson Hospital and Tumor Institute 18th Symposium on Fundamental Cancer Research.* Baltimore: Williams & Wilkins, 1965:7.
86. Upton AC, Randolph ML, Conklin JW. Late effects of fast neutrons and gamma rays in mice as influenced by the dose rate of irradiation: induction of neoplasia. *Radiat Res* 1970;41:467.
87. Shukovsky LJ. Dose, time, volume relationships in squamous cell carcinoma of the supraglottic larynx. *Am J Roentgenol Rad Ther Nucl Med* 1970;108:27.
88. Kaplan HS. Evidence for a tumoricidal dose level in the radiotherapy of Hodgkin's disease. *Cancer Res* 1966;26:1221.
89. Stewart JG, Jackson AW. The steepness of the dose-response curve both for tumor and normal tissue injury. *Laryngoscope* 1975;85:1107.
90. Zagars GK, Schultheiss TE, Peters LJ. Inter-tumor heterogeneity and radiation dose-control curves. *Radiother Oncol* 1987;8:353.
91. Coutard H. Roentgen therapy of epitheliomas of the tonsillar region, hypopharynx, and larynx from 1920 to 1926. *AJR Am J Roentgenol* 1932;28:313.

92. Regaud C, Ferroux R. Discordance des effets des rayons X, d'une part dans la peau, d'autre part dans le testicule par le fractionement de la dose: diminution de l'efficacite dans le peau, maintien de l'efficacite dans le testicule. *Compt Rend Soc Biol* 1927;97:431.
93. Danlos H. Quelques considerations sur le traitement des dermatoses par le radium. *J Physiotherapie* (Paris) 1905;3:98.
94. Botnick L, Hannon EC, Hellman S. Multisystem stem cell failure after apparent recovery from alkylating agents. *Cancer Res* 1978;38:1942.
95. Hellman S, Botnick LE. Stem cell depletion: an explanation of the late effects of cytotoxins. *Int J Radiat Oncol Biol Phys* 1977;2:181.
96. Harris JR, Recht A, Almaric R, et al. Time course and prognosis of local recurrence following primary radiation therapy for early breast cancer. *J Clin Oncol* 1984;2:37.
97. Goodman LS, Gilman A. *The pharmacological basis of therapeutics.* London: Macmillan, 1970:21.
98. Withers HR, Peters LJ, Thames HD, et al. Hyperfractionation. *Int J Radiat Oncol Biol Phys* 1982;8:1807.
99. Withers HR, Thames HA, Peters LJ. Dose fractionation and volume effects in normal tissues and tumors. *Cancer Treat Symp* 1984;1:75.
100. Shank B, Chu FCH, Dinsmore R, et al. Hyperfractionated total body irradiation for bone marrow transplantation: results in seventy leukemia patients with allogeneic transplants. *Int J Radiat Oncol Biol Phys* 1983;9:1607.
101. Thames HD Jr, Peters LJ, Withers HR, et al. Accelerated fractionation vs hyperfractionation: rationales for several treatments per day. *Int J Radiat Oncol Biol Phys* 1983;9:127.
102. Norin T, Onyango J. Radiotherapy in Burkitt's lymphoma: conventional or superfractionated regime—early results. *Int J Radiat Oncol Biol Phys* 1977;2:399.
103. Scanlon P. Split-dose radiotherapy: the original premise. *Int J Radiat Oncol Biol Phys* 1980;6:527.
104. Sambrook DK. Split-course radiation therapy in malignant tumors. *AJR Am J Roentgenol* 1964;91:37.
105. Parsons JT, Thar TL, Bova FJ, et al. An evaluation of split-course irradiation for pelvic malignancies. *Int J Radiat Oncol Biol Phys* 1980;6:175.
106. Parsons JT, Bova FJ, Million RR. A re-evaluation of the University of Florida split-course technique for squamous carcinoma of the head and neck. *Int J Radiat Oncol Biol Phys* 1980;6:1645.
107. Ling CC, Anderson LL, Shipley WU. Dose inhomogeneity in interstitial implants using ^{125}I seeds. *Int J Radiat Oncol Biol Phys* 1979;5:419.
108. Pierquin B, Chassagne D, Baillet F, et al. Clinical observations on the time factor in interstitial radiotherapy using iridium-192. *Clin Radiol* 1973;24:506.
109. Beadle GF, Silver B, Botnick L, et al. Cosmetic results following primary radiation therapy for early breast cancer. *Cancer* 1984;54:2911.
110. Levene MB, Kijewski PK, Chin LM, et al. Computer controlled radiation therapy. *Radiology* 1978;129:769.
111. Bergonie J, Tribondeau L. Interpretation of some results of radiotherapy and an attempt at determining a logical technique of treatment. *Radiat Res* 1959;11:587.
112. Kligerman MM. Radiotherapy and rectal cancer. *Cancer* 1977;39:896.
113. Harris JR, Beadle GF, Hellman S. Clinical studies on the use of radiation therapy as primary treatment of early breast cancer. *Cancer* 1984;53:705.
114. Hellman S. Improving the therapeutic index in breast cancer treatment. *Cancer Res* 1980;40:4335.

Edward Chu
Vincent T. DeVita, Jr.

CHAPTER 17

Principles of Cancer Management: Chemotherapy

The introduction of chemotherapy in the fifth and sixth decades of the twentieth century has resulted in the development of curative therapeutic interventions for patients with several types of advanced solid tumors and hematologic neoplasms. These advances provided important proof of the principle that anticancer drugs could cure cancer and subsequently resulted in their integration into treatment programs with surgery and radiation therapy in early stages of disease, with excellent results. The important obstacles encountered in the use of chemotherapy have been toxicity to the normal tissues of the body and the development of cellular resistance to these chemotherapeutic agents. During the 1990s, the application of molecular techniques for analysis of the DNA of normal and neoplastic cells began to identify some of the critical mechanisms through which chemotherapy induces cell death. This modern-day technology has also provided insight into the changes within these cells that can confer either sensitivity or resistance to drug treatment. This new level of understanding of the molecular pathways through which chemotherapy works and by which genetic change can result in resistance to drug therapy has opened the door for novel therapeutic strategies in which molecular, genetic, and biologic therapies can be used in combination to attack directly new and specific targets to increase the chemosensitivity of malignant cells to treatment and to protect the normal tissues of the body from therapy-induced side effects. The implementation of such novel therapeutic approaches may provide an important paradigm shift in the manner in which therapy is delivered as we move into the next millennium. Clearly, the long-term goal is to improve the outcome of cancer patients undergoing treatment, especially in those with neoplasms that currently are resistant to conventional-dose therapy.

HISTORY

The systemic treatment of cancer has its roots in the work of Paul Ehrlich, who coined the word *chemotherapy.* Erlich's use of *in vivo* rodent model systems to develop antibiotics for treatment of infectious diseases led George Clowes, at Roswell Park Memorial Institute in Buffalo, New York, in the early 1900s, to develop inbred rodent lines bearing transplanted tumors that could be used to screen potential anticancer drugs. This *in vivo* system provided the foundation for mass screening of novel compounds.[1] Alkylating agents represent the first class of chemotherapeutic drugs to be used in the clinical setting. Of note, they were a product of the secret gas program of the United States in both world wars. The exposure of military seamen to mustard gas in World War II led to the observation that alkylating agents caused marrow and lymphoid hypoplasia.[2,3] This observation then led to the direct application of such agents in humans with hematologic neoplasms, including Hodgkin's disease and lymphocytic lymphomas, at the Yale Cancer Center in 1943. However, given the secret nature of the gas warfare program, this work was not published until 1946.[1,4] The demonstration of dramatic regressions in advanced lymphomas with chemotherapy generated much excitement. At approximately this same time, Sidney Farber reported that folic acid had a significant proliferative effect on leukemic cell growth in children with lymphoblastic leukemia. These observations led to the development of folic acid analogs as cancer drugs to inhibit folate metabolism; thus, the era of cancer chemotherapy began in earnest.

The cure of childhood leukemias and Hodgkin's disease with combination chemotherapy in the 1960s proved the much-disputed point that a fraction of human cancers, even in their advanced stages, could be cured by drugs. This seminal work laid the foundation for the application of chemotherapy in the treatment of solid tumors. The most disappointing aspect of the work with solid tumors was the failure to cure more patients once it was shown that cancer cells might be more sensitive to cytotoxic drugs than normal cells. This is an especially relevant issue in the adjuvant setting where, because of low tumor burden, cancer cells were thought to be more sensitive to eradication by drug therapy.[5] In addition, a curious and perplexing distribution of responses to chemotherapy has been noted, in that nearly 90% of all drug cures occur in only 10% of cancer types.[6]

Chemotherapy failure was, at first, thought to be due to variations in tumor growth characteristics. Attention then shifted to the role of specific and permanent mechanisms of resistance to individual chemotherapeutic agents that were either acquired after exposure to cancer drugs or were already present as a consequence of intrinsic genetic mutations within the tumor.[7] During the 1980s, a new form of multidrug resistance (mdr gene) to a host of natural-product antitumor agents, including the anthracyclines, the taxanes, the vinca alkaloids, and a few antifolate analogs, was identified. This resistance mechanism was believed to play a significant role in the failure of cancer chemotherapy *in vitro.* The mdr gene encodes a 170-kD membrane glycoprotein that acts to extrude these various anticancer agents from the cell, resulting in decreased intracellular drug accumulation. Recently, the mrp gene, a related family member, has been characterized in pleiotropic drug-resistant cancer cells. This gene encodes a 190-kD protein that functions in a fashion similar to that of the p170 glycoprotein to mediate the rapid efflux of drug from the cell.[8,9] Although mdr and mrp appear to play a key role in the development of drug resistance *in vitro* and *in vivo,* their actual relevance to clinical drug resistance remains unclear.

The therapeutic emphasis in the design of early studies was on maximizing the interaction of the active component of cancer drugs with the cycling cancer cell. The availability of tritiated thymidine, a DNA precursor taken up during the S phase of the cell cycle, made possible the study of the kinetics of cell proliferation. It was quickly determined that cancer cells did not divide faster than normal cells; rather, a larger fraction of the population was dividing.[10] This capacity to enter the cell cycle more frequently was referred to as the *tumor growth fraction,* and it is widely appreciated that cancers, in general, have a significantly higher growth fraction than their normal cell of origin.[11] Though the molecular technology at the time was limited, it was clear even then that the essence of a malignant cell was a critical defect in the ability to control its own growth.

Much of the early clinical work in cancer chemotherapy was based on the kinetic modeling of the drug therapy of the murine leukemia L1210 cell line. Cell kinetic studies revealed this system to be an exponentially growing malignancy with a growth fraction approaching 100%.[12] Except for the rare Burkitt's lymphoma, however, a growth fraction this high has no parallel in human solid tumors. For this reason, the mathematics of cell kill based on the L1210 murine leukemic model could never properly account for the ability to cure some human cancers with a relatively small fraction of cycling cells.[5]

The work with the L1210 model also was the basis for the long-held dogma that rapidity of growth and frequency of cycling in responsive tumors determined sensitivity to chemotherapy. Thus, slowly growing tumors are not kinetically vulnerable, whereas faster-growing tumors are both responsive and curable. Largely because of their good response to treatment, leukemias and lymphomas were considered to be rapidly growing. This observation led to the odd conclusion that solid tumors, such as lung cancer, colon cancer, and other "resistant tumors," were slow-growing, even though there was insufficient evidence for this. It also ran counter to another important clinical observation: Certain human cancers that display a spectrum of growth patterns from indolent to aggressive become significantly more treatable as well as potentially curable as the cell of origin becomes less differentiated and the growth rate, as measured by thymidine-labeling index, increases. When this same tumor transforms, however, to a highly aggressive phenotype, paradoxically it often becomes almost totally incurable.

Non-Hodgkin's lymphoma is an ideal example of this treatment paradox. Diffuse large cell lymphoma (DHL) is a more rapidly growing form of non-Hodgkin's lymphoma that is curable by combination chemotherapy in its advanced stages. Indolent, low-grade lymphomas are more slowly growing tumors than DHL and, while they are highly responsive to treatment, they are generally incurable in their advanced form with conventional-dose chemotherapy. Thus, despite a similar cell of origin, the more rapidly proliferating cells are subject to complete eradication by chemotherapy. However, further increases in growth rates within populations of patients with diffuse aggressive lymphomas, as predicted by the degree of expression of the Ki-67 antigen, a nuclear antigen that closely parallels the labeling index, negatively predict for both response to treatment and curability.[13] This finding suggests that, beyond a certain point, the emergence of drug resistance in some way accompanies an increase in the growth rate of the tumor.

Another important and curious clinical observation not easily explained by the dogma on acquired drug resistance was that normal renewing tissue, such as the bone marrow and gastrointestinal (GI) mucosa, never develop resistance to these drugs. These are the two host tissues that are most commonly affected by most anticancer agents used in the clinic. It is a consistent and disconcerting clinical experience to have a patient's tumor respond to treatment with associated marrow suppression, only to have the tumor grow back in the face of continued treatment while the sensitivity of the marrow to chemotherapy-induced toxicity remains invariant. The same can be said for toxicity to GI mucosa.[6] It is now well-appreciated that the genetic machinery involved in the cell-cycle checkpoint and apoptosis is preserved in normal host tissues. This fact most likely explains why normal host cells are constantly sensitized to the toxic effect of cytotoxic agents.

CHEMOTHERAPY AS PART OF THE INITIAL TREATMENT OF CANCER

Currently, chemotherapy has a role in four different clinical settings[14]: (1) as induction treatment for advanced disease, (2) as an adjunct to local methods of treatment, (3) as the primary treatment for some patients who present with localized disease, in whom local forms of therapy by themselves are inadequate, and (4) by direct instillation into sanctuary sites or by site-directed perfusion of specific regions of the body directly affected by the cancer.

The term *induction chemotherapy* has been used to describe drug therapy given as the primary treatment for patients who present with advanced cancer for which no alternative treatment exists.[15] Adjuvant chemotherapy denotes the use of systemic treatment after the primary tumor has been controlled by an alternative modality, such as surgery and radiation therapy. The selection of an adjuvant treatment program for a particular patient usually is based on response rates in separate groups of patients with advanced cancers of the same histologic type. The determination of a population of patients as suitable for adjuvant treatment is based on available data about their average risk of recurrence after local treatment alone. Currently, adjuvant chemotherapy is considered standard treatment for early-stage breast and colorectal cancer.[16,17] There is also evidence to support the use of chemotherapy after surgical resection of anaplastic astrocytomas.[18]

Primary (neoadjuvant) chemotherapy denotes the use of chemotherapy as the initial treatment for patients who present with localized cancer for which there is an alternative but less than completely effective local treatment.[19,20] For chemotherapy to be used as the initial (primary) treatment of a cancer partially curable by either surgery or radiation therapy, there must be considerable evidence for the effectiveness of the drug program in question against advanced disease of the same type. At this time, neoadjuvant therapy has been effectively used in the treatment of anal cancer, bladder cancer, breast cancer, esophageal cancer, laryngeal cancer, locally advanced non–small cell lung cancer, and osteogenic sarcoma. For some of these tumors, it has now been determined that chemotherapy, when given concurrently with radiation therapy, is superior to sequencing chemotherapy before radiation therapy.

CLINICAL END POINTS IN EVALUATING RESPONSE TO CHEMOTHERAPY

INDUCTION CHEMOTHERAPY

In induction chemotherapy for patients with advanced cancer and measurable disease, it is possible to assess response to drugs on a case-by-case basis. Partial response is usually defined as the fraction of patients who demonstrate at least a 50% reduction in measurable tumor mass. There is growing evidence to suggest that quality-of-life indices are better in patients who show either a response to therapy or a minimal response as compared to supportive care, even if overall survival is not improved. However, partial responses are also useful in the evaluation of new drugs or new drug regimens, to determine whether the particular experimental approach is worthy of further clinical development.

It is clear, however, that the most important indicator of the effectiveness of chemotherapy is the complete response rate. No patient with advanced cancer has ever been cured without first achieving a complete remission. When new programs consistently produce more than an occasional complete remission, they have invariably been proven to be of significant practical value in medical practice. Thus, in clinical trials, complete and partial responses should always be reported separately. The most important indicator of the quality of a complete remission is the relapse-free survival from the time treatment is discontinued. This criterion is the only clinical counterpart of the quantifiable cytoreductive effect of drugs in the *in vivo* rodent system. The use of freedom from progression in patients who have attained a mixture of complete and partial responses can be misleading when evaluating a new treatment.[20] This method of analyzing clinical outcomes is a relatively simple indicator of the practical potential of a new treatment but, for experimental treatments, it obscures the value of a relapse-free survival of complete responders as the major determinant of the quality of remission and the potential for cure. Other end points, such as median response duration and median survival, are also of little practical value until treatment results have been refined so that the complete response rate is higher than 50%.

ADJUVANT CHEMOTHERAPY

There was initially great excitement with the concept of using chemotherapy as an adjunct to local treatment. The rationale for adjuvant chemotherapy was to treat micrometastatic disease at a time when tumor bulk would be at a minimum, thereby enhancing the potential efficacy of drug treatment. It was assumed that drug therapy, at this stage, would result in a much higher cure rate.[21,22]

The major indicator of effectiveness of a chemotherapy program—the complete remission rate—is lost in the adjuvant setting because the primary tumor has already been removed. In the clinic, treatment is selected for individual patients based on response rates in an entirely different population of patients with advanced disease of the same histologic type. In adjuvant programs, relapse-free survival remains the major end point but, in each patient, micrometastases consist of a mixture of tumor cells, some of which could have been expected to be sensitive to chemotherapy and others of which could have been expected to be resistant to chemotherapy. The relapse-free survival in the adjuvant setting, therefore, measures time to regrowth to clinically detectable levels of cells unresponsive, partially responsive, or very sensitive to chemotherapy and is the equivalent of the duration of remission of a combined group of complete responders, partial responders, and nonresponders. In this sense, it is similar to the use of freedom from progression in patients with advanced disease.

PRIMARY (NEOADJUVANT) CHEMOTHERAPY

The unique feature of using chemotherapy in patients with localized tumor before or in place of purely local treatments, such as surgical excision or radiation therapy (or both), is the preservation of the presenting tumor mass as a biologic marker of responsiveness to the drugs. Moreover, this approach has allowed the sparing of vital normal organs, such as the larynx, the anal sphincter, and the bladder, as the primary tumor is reduced in size and rendered easier to deal with by traditional local measures. As with induction chemotherapy for patients with advanced cancer, it is possible to determine, on an individual basis, the potential efficacy of a new treatment program. A good response to chemotherapy identifies a patient who may benefit from further treatment. A poor response of the primary tumor to chemotherapy identifies a patient for whom alternative methods of treatment should be seriously considered. Another feature of primary chemotherapy is the ability to differentiate partial responders with varying degrees of prognosis. Removal of residual tumor masses and histologic examination of the tissue allow determination of the viability and character of the remaining tumor cells. The response duration of complete and partial responders must be catalogued separately. Such an approach could result in briefer, less morbid, and more effective treatment programs.[14] When chemotherapy is administered concurrently with radiation therapy, the determinants of sensitivity to drugs are obviated unless compared to radiation alone in a control arm.

The use of chemotherapy as primary treatment is reviewed in each of the appropriate disease-oriented chapters. Table 17-1 lists the specific malignancies in which primary chemotherapy for localized forms of the cancer in question already have been incorporated into clinical usage (first and second categories) and in which current clinical trials show considerable promise (third category).[23–32]

TABLE 17-1. Primary Chemotherapy

NEOPLASMS IN WHICH CHEMOTHERAPY IS THE PRIMARY THERAPEUTIC MODALITY FOR LOCALIZED TUMORS
Large cell lymphoma
Lymphoblastic lymphoma
Burkitt's and non-Burkitt's, undifferentiated lymphoma
Childhood and some adult stages of Hodgkin's disease
Wilms' tumor
Embryonal rhabdomyosarcoma
Small cell lung cancer
Central nervous system lymphomas
NEOPLASMS IN WHICH PRIMARY CHEMOTHERAPY CAN ALLOW LESS MUTILATING SURGERY
Anal carcinoma
Bladder carcinoma
Breast cancer
Esophageal cancer
Laryngeal cancer
Osteogenic sarcoma
Soft tissue sarcoma
NEOPLASMS IN WHICH CLINICAL TRIALS INDICATE AN EXPANDING ROLE FOR PRIMARY CHEMOTHERAPY IN THE FUTURE
Non–small cell lung cancer
Bladder cancer
Breast cancer
Cervical cancer
Esophageal cancer
Gastric cancer
Nasopharyngeal cancer
Other cancers of the head and neck region
Pancreatic cancer
Prostate cancer

PRINCIPLES GOVERNING THE USE OF COMBINATION CHEMOTHERAPY

With rare exceptions (e.g., choriocarcinoma and Burkitt's lymphoma), standard single drugs at clinically tolerable doses have been unable to cure cancer. In the early years of cancer chemotherapy, drug combinations were developed based on known biochemical actions of available anticancer drugs rather than on their clinical efficacy. These regimens were largely ineffective.[33–37] The era of effective combination chemotherapy began when an array of active drugs from different classes became available for use in combination in the treatment of leukemias and lymphomas. Combination chemotherapy has now been extended to the treatment of most solid tumors, as described throughout this book.

Combination chemotherapy using conventional cytotoxic agents accomplishes several important objectives not possible with single-agent treatment. First, it provides maximal cell kill within the range of toxicity tolerated by the host for each drug as long as dosing is not compromised. Second, it provides a broader range of interaction between drugs and tumor cells with different genetic abnormalities in a heterogeneous tumor population. Finally, it may prevent or slow the subsequent development of drug resistance.

Certain principles have been useful in the selection of drugs in the most effective drug combinations, and they guide the development of new drug therapeutic programs. First, only drugs known to be partially effective against the same tumor when used alone should be selected for use in combination. If available, drugs that produce some fraction of complete remission are preferred to those that produce only partial responses. Second, when several drugs of a class are available and are equally effective, a drug should be selected on the basis of toxicity that does not overlap with the toxicity of other drugs to be used in the combination. Although such selection leads to a wider range of side effects, it minimizes the risk of a lethal effect caused by multiple insults to the same organ system by different drugs and allows dose intensity to be maximized.

Additionally, drugs should be used in their optimal dose and schedule, and drug combinations should be given at consistent intervals. Because long intervals between cycles negatively affect dose intensity (discussed in further detail later in Concept of Dose Intensity), the treatment-free interval between cycles should be the shortest possible time necessary for recovery of the most sensitive normal target tissue, which is usually the bone marrow. Finally, there should be a clear understanding of the biochemical, molecular, and pharmacokinetic mechanisms of interaction between the individual drugs in a given combination, to allow for maximal effect.

Omission of a drug from a combination may allow overgrowth by a cell line sensitive to that drug alone and resistant to other drugs in the combination. In addition, arbitrary reduction in the dose of an effective drug to add other less effective drugs may dramatically reduce the dose of the most effective agent below the threshold of effectiveness and destroy the capacity of the combination to cure disease in a given patient.

Most standard treatment programs were designed around the kinetics of recovery of the bone marrow in response to exposure to a cytotoxic agent. The introduction of the colony-stimulating factors (CSFs) has been a significant advance for cancer therapy, as they help to accelerate bone marrow recovery and prevent the occurrence of severe myelosuppression.[38] They play an instrumental role in decreasing the incidence of infections and the need for hospitalizations and allow for maintenance of optimal dose intensity of chemotherapy. Clearly, these cytokine growth factors have revolutionized the next generation of chemotherapy treatment.

Bone marrow has a storage compartment that supplies mature cells to the peripheral blood for 8 to 10 days after the stem cell pool has been damaged by cytotoxic drugs. Events in the peripheral blood are usually a week behind events occurring in the bone marrow. In previously untreated patients not primed by CSFs, leukopenia and thrombocytopenia are observed on the ninth or tenth day after initial dosing. Nadir blood counts are noted between days 14 and 18, with the onset of recovery beginning by day 21 and usually completed by day 28 in patients who have not had prior treatment with drugs or x-irradiation. This sequence may be altered in patients with previous therapy by depletion of the stem cell pool, shortening the time to the appearance of leukopenia and thrombocytopenia and prolonging the recovery time. The interval of greatest importance in the clinic is the duration of the nadir level of leukocytes and platelets. The highest risk of infection or bleeding occurs with granulocyte counts lower than 500/dL and platelet counts lower than 10,000/dL. If this nadir lasts only 4 to 7 days, it is tolerated by most patients without the need for supplemental support. Increasing doses of most anticancer drugs within the range of the maximally tolerated standard dose does not usually ablate the marrow or even prolong the time to recovery; however, it does usually influence the nadir count levels. Repeated dosing during the phase of early recovery of the marrow (days 16 to 21) may result in more severe toxicity in the second treatment cycle in patients whose marrow is not the source of, or involved with, the tumor.

These clinical observations, coupled with the kinetic studies of bone marrow recovery in mice and humans, led to the now-familiar 2-week interval between cycles of the most effective drug combinations, using standard doses without CSFs (new cycles begin on days 21 or 28 after the first dose) to accommodate the recovery time of human bone marrow. Although this treatment schedule is suitable for some tumors, the rapid regrowth of others, such as DHLs, Burkitt's lymphoma, and leukemia, often permit the tumor volume to return to pretreatment levels in the interval required for bone marrow recovery, and other approaches to cycling drug combinations are being explored.

No rigid schedule can accommodate all the variables assumed to be important for maximum effectiveness of combination chemotherapy and the requirements of the patients in the practice of medical oncology. Physicians must often adjust doses at intervals to allow for the safe administration of drugs. The certainty that the therapeutic effect of a drug or drug combination can be lost if the dose or schedule is altered should temper these judgments. Reductions in dose rates also often result in only minimal decreases in toxicity but major reduction in the capacity to attain a complete remission in patients with drug-responsive tumors.[6] Adherence to the standard sliding scale for dose adjustments, usually published with most new treatments, or the prompt initiation of CSF adjunct therapy is the most appropriate way to optimize the delivery of chemotherapy without compromising long-term outcome. The application of appropriate guidelines for dose reductions preserves the intervals between treatment cycles, preserves the integrity of each drug combination and, finally, provides consistency between patients and various clinical studies.[39]

For many years, clinical trial design has been dominated by the use of alternating cycles of combination chemotherapy. The basis for this study design came from the translation of preclinical experimental data into a model for clinical treatment. In 1943, Luria and Delbruck[40] observed that the bacterium *Escherichia coli* developed resistance to bacterial viruses (bacteriophage) not by surviving exposure but by expanding clones of bacteria that had spontaneously mutated to a type inherently resistant to phage infection. This was a seminal principle in bacterial genetics that laid the framework for the understanding of the development of spontaneous resistance to cancer chemotherapy.[40] In 1979, Goldie and Coldman[41] applied this principle to the development of resistance to anticancer drugs by cancer cells without prior exposure to these drugs. They proposed that the nonrandom cytogenetic changes now known to be associated with most human cancers probably were tightly associated with the development of the capacity to resist the action of certain types of anticancer drugs. They developed a mathematical model that predicted that tumor cells mutate to drug resistance at a rate intrinsic to the genetic instability of a particular tumor. Their model predicted that such events would begin to occur at population sizes between 10^3 and 10^6 tumor cells (1000 to 1 million cells), much lower than the mass of cells considered to be clinically detectable (10^9, or 1 billion cells). The probability that a given tumor will contain resistant clones when a patient's disease is newly diagnosed would be a function of both tumor size and the inherent mutation rate. If the mutation rate is as infrequent as 10^{-6}, a tumor composed of 10^9 cells (a 1-cm mass) would be predicted to have at least one drug-resistant clone; however, the absolute number of resistant cells in a tumor composed of 10^9 cells would be relatively small. Therefore, in the clinic, such tumors should initially respond to treatment with a partial or complete remission but would recur as the resistance clone expands to repopulate the tumor mass. Such a pattern is commonly seen in the clinical setting with the use of chemotherapy in many drug-responsive tumors.

The Goldie-Coldman hypothesis, therefore, predicts that cellular drug resistance should be present even with small tumors and that the maximal chance for cure occurs when all available effective drugs are given simultaneously.[41] Because this would involve using eight to 12 drugs simultaneously, this approach has not generally been tested in the clinic for fear that the use of more than five cytotoxic drugs, at full doses, would not be possible. An alternative approach, using two programs of equally effective, non–cross-resistant drug combinations in alternating cycles, has been under evaluation since the mid-1980s. However, many studies purporting to test the Goldie-Coldman hypothesis have not been properly designed. First, in many instances, inadequate testing has been carried out to determine whether the alternate combination is truly non–cross-resistant and is as effective as the primary treatment. In most instances, these requirements are not met. Second, except in rare instances, dosing is usually not controlled properly. Doses of essential drugs are modified downward, *a priori*, without testing the potential impact of such dose reductions on outcome. Finally, the requirement for symmetry in biologic characteristics of tumors in different patients is unrealistic. The use of alternating cycles of combination chemotherapy has not yet proven to be more effective than full doses of a single effective combination program.

In 1986, Day[42] and Norton and Day[43] reanalyzed the Goldie-Coldman hypothesis and relaxed the requirement for symmetry in the model. Although it verified the basic tenets of the Goldie-Coldman hypothesis, their model suggested a different approach to sequencing combinations: In many instances, the sequential use of combinations should outperform alternating cycles, because no two combinations are likely to be strictly non–cross-resistant or have equal cell-killing capacity, the symmetry assumed by Goldie and Coldman. Day formulated "the worst-drug rule," which refers to any strategy using more or earlier doses of a treatment that is the least effective of two or more available options.[6] The worst-drug rule has interesting implications. First, it is a nonintuitive approach. If two treatments—treatments A and B—are available and B is known to be better, a physician is more likely to use B first. Cells that are resistant to the best treatment, B, must be eliminated by the weaker program, A; however, because it is the weaker program, one cannot wait too long to use it or the overgrowth of the population resistant to B will place the physician and patient in a situation that is difficult to overcome. The model predicts that if six cycles of A and B are planned, use of the weaker program, A, first offers a better outcome. There have been clinical examples in which sequential therapies have outperformed alternating cyclic use of the same programs if the dose intensity of the two regimens is carefully controlled.[44,45]

EFFECT OF THE BIOLOGY OF TUMOR GROWTH ON RESPONSE TO CHEMOTHERAPY

Applying the principles of chemotherapy developed by Skipper et al.[12,46,47] in leukemia L1210 to the drug treatment of human cancers requires a clear understanding of the differences between the growth characteristics of this rodent leukemia and of human cancers as well as an understanding of the differences in growth rates of normal target tissues between mice and humans. For example, L1210 is a rapidly growing leukemia with a high percentage of cells synthesizing DNA, as measured by the uptake of tritiated thymidine (the labeling index). Because L1210 leukemia has a growth fraction of 100% (i.e., all its cells are actively progressing through the cell cycle), its life cycle is consistent and predictable.[48]

The time to death of animals bearing L1210 leukemia is the interval required to achieve a population size of approximately 10^9 (1 billion) cells. With a growth fraction of 100% and a doubling time of 12 hours, 10^9 cells accumulate by 19 days after the injection of a single cell, by 10 days after the injection of 10^5 cells, and by 5 days after the administration of 10^8 cells. Skipper et al.[46,47] postulated that the increase in host life span after cytotoxic chemotherapy of L1210 leukemia was largely due to the cytocidal effect of treatment on the tumor cell population. In these early elegant mouse experiments, they calculated the residual number of cells after treatment by extrapolating back from the duration of prolongation of life after a single treatment. An increase of 2 days in life would be equivalent to a 90% destruction of tumor cells (a 1-log kill), or a reduction in the cell number from 10^6 to 10^5. A 99.999% destruction of tumor cells, a number that seems enormous to most clinicians, represents only a 5-log kill and does not cure disease in animals unless the initial inoculum is small, perhaps 10^4 cells or fewer. If multiple treatments are given, the net tumor cell kill per treatment is the sum of the surviving cells plus the regrowth of the tumor cell population before the next treatment.

The cytotoxic effects of cancer drugs in this tumor model follow log cell-kill kinetics. Thus, if a particular dose of an individual drug kills 3 logs of tumor cells and reduces tumor burden from 10^{10} to 10^7 cells, the same dose used at a tumor burden of 10^5 cells reduces the tumor mass to 10^2. Cell kill, therefore, is proportional, regardless of tumor burden. This model fits the response of L1210 murine leukemia to chemotherapy. When treatment failed in sensitive cell lines, it was because the initial tumor burden was too high to allow the delivery of curative doses of chemotherapy to eradicate the last leukemia cell. The cardinal rule of chemotherapy—the invariable inverse relation between cell number and curability—was established in this model and applies to other model systems. Skipper et al.[12] proceeded to show that this rodent leukemia could be cured by specifically designing doses and schedules of administration that were based on tumor volume and growth characteristics.

Although growth of murine leukemias closely follows exponential cell kinetics, available data suggest that most human solid tumors do not grow in an exponential fashion. For example, the concept of log kill would have predicted that some large tumors in the clinic should have been more sensitive to treatment than has been experienced. *In toto*, the experimental data in human solid cancers support a Gompertzian model of tumor growth and regression. The critical distinction between Gompertzian and exponential growth is that in Gompertzian kinetics, the growth fraction of the tumor is not constant but decreases exponentially with time (exponential growth is matched by exponential retardation of growth). The growth fraction peaks when the tumor is approximately 37% of its maximum size. In a Gompertzian model, when a patient with advanced cancer is treated, the tumor mass is larger, its growth fraction is low, and the fraction of cells killed is, therefore, small. An important feature of Gompertzian growth is that response to chemotherapy in drug-sensitive tumors depends, in large measure, on where the tumor is in its particular growth curve. Sensitive Gompertzian-growing tumors respond to cytotoxic drugs in a Gompertzian fashion.

Therefore, predictions can be made about the behavior of small tumors, such as the microscopic tumor burdens that might be present after primary surgical therapy. When the tumor is clinically undetectable, its growth fraction would be at its largest and, although the numerical reduction in cell number is small, the fractional cell kill from a known-to-be-effective therapeutic dose of chemotherapy would be higher than later in the tumor course. This observation was initially used to justify dose reductions at lower tumor volumes. However, such an unnecessary dose reduction may account for some of the disappointment in the outcome of adjuvant studies in breast cancer. The Gompertzian model for tumor growth is important for another reason: It affects the patterns of regrowth of residual tumor cells. In breast cancer, Norton[43,49] has analyzed the clinical data from multiple adjuvant studies and from available studies of untreated patients with localized disease.[6,50] In each clinical study, the Gompertzian model precisely fit the growth curves of these tumors. In the adjuvant setting, the model showed that relapse-free survival and survival curves are unable to discriminate between residual cell populations of only one cell and a residual population of 1 million cells, because the regrowth of residual cell populations will be faster at smaller volumes than it will be at larger volumes, producing identical results sometimes at 5 years after diagnosis and treatment. These findings suggest that short of total eradication of micrometastases (cure), varying residual volumes produce similar 5-year relapse-free survival and obscure the major differences in tumor reduction by different programs. This information has been especially useful in the design of new adjuvant treatment protocols for early-stage breast cancer.

APOPTOSIS, CELL-CYCLE CONTROL, AND RESISTANCE TO CHEMOTHERAPY

The kinetic models described are realistic only in the context of a tumor that is sensitive to chemotherapy. Only recently have we arrived at a new understanding of the critical determinants of drug sensitivity and resistance. For more than 30 years, the classic view of anticancer drug action has involved the specific interaction between a given drug and its respective target. Cell death arises as a direct consequence of this drug-receptor interaction. However, the critical molecular mechanisms involved in facilitating the initial coupling of the stimulus to the final response of the cell were never clearly elucidated. With an enhanced understanding of the molecular mechanisms underlying the control of the cell cycle and the process of programmed cell death (apoptosis), it is now clear that this very simplistic model must be reevaluated. In contrast to the drug-target interaction directly leading to cell death as was viewed in the classic model, it is now well appreciated that such an interaction acts as a stimulus to initiate a cascade of events eventually resulting in apoptosis. It is doubtful that cell death induced by chemotherapy occurs by any other mechanism. This pathway involves some type of sensor that detects a death-inducing signal, a signal transduction network, and an execution machinery that facilitates the process of cell death. Moreover, this entire process is exceedingly complex as it is highly dependent on the specific cell type under study, the specific anticancer agent being tested, and the cellular context and environment in which the drug-target interaction is being considered.

In addition, it now appears that the capacity of certain cancers to resist the cytotoxic effects of cancer chemotherapy may be more closely connected to either abnormalities in the genetic machinery of cancer cells or to alterations in the critical pathways of cell-cycle checkpoint control and apoptosis than to the specific mechanisms of resistance unique to each agent. This observation is underscored by the general failure to overcome resistance to chemotherapy in the clinic with approaches that attack only the classic biochemical or molecular mechanisms of resistance (or both). Although this section briefly reviews the complex interrelationship between products of cell-cycle checkpoint genes, oncogenic viruses, transcription factors, apoptosis, and chemotherapy as they relate to drug resistance, more detailed discussion of these topics are reviewed elsewhere.[51–59]

As noted earlier in the History section of this chapter, normal tissues never develop resistance to chemotherapy. However, one of the most remarkable features of both radiation therapy and chemotherapy, when used to treat sensitive tumors, is that their cytotoxic effects may be initially greater in neoplastic cells than in normal host tissues, including the bone marrow and the GI tract. Doses that eradicate some sensitive tumors will not ablate the bone marrow or destroy the capacity of the GI mucosa to regenerate. No molecular basis for this therapeutic selectivity was available until just recently. However, this difference in cytotoxic action between normal and malignant cells appears to relate to mechanisms that allow normal renewing cell populations, such as bone marrow and GI precursor cells, to monitor and repair damaged DNA or destroy cells with irreparable DNA, rather than allowing damaged cells to proceed through the cell cycle and potentially replicate their damaged DNA. Because they express an intact genetic machinery, normal cells can almost always recover from exposure to DNA-damaging anticancer agents, except in the case of high-dose chemotherapy, as used in transplantation programs. In this particular setting, the high doses of chemotherapy are able to overwhelm these protective mechanisms or to destroy the DNA of exposed cells by direct necrosis (or both). Initially, sensitive cancer cells can be destroyed by effective chemotherapy but, if not, they develop resistance to further treatment, perhaps in part because of drug-induced mutations in their DNA. This resistance may be linked to the dysregulation of the same genetic and signaling pathways that control entry into the cell cycle and the process of programmed cell death.

p53

p53 (Fig. 17-1) is a tumor suppressor protein and critical transcriptional activator that causes both G_1 and G_2 arrest of the cell cycle when cells are exposed to DNA-damaging agents.[51–54,57,60–62] This function is thought to be critical in preserving the integrity of the cellular genome in response to treatment with a cytotoxic agent. In addition to its role in the cell-cycle checkpoint, p53 is a potent inducer of programmed cell death (apoptosis) within a cell in which DNA damage has occurred.[50] The basis for the cell's decision either to undergo growth arrest and repair DNA damage or to induce apoptosis remains unknown. Significant research efforts are focused on elucidating the critical factors that determine the eventual cellular function of p53. This is undoubtedly a complex issue, however, that must take into account the extent of DNA damage, the stage of the cell cycle at which the DNA damage occurs, the presence of other genetic abnormalities in either the cell-cycle regulatory apparatus or the signaling machinery, or the specific cellular context. It is now clear that some cell types, such as lymphocytes and the tumors derived from them, have a more rapid access to apoptotic mechanisms than the large majority of epithelial cancers.

Mutations in the p53 gene are among the most common genetic alterations observed in human tumor samples and have been estimated to occur in at least 50% of all human tumors.[63] The initial studies showing that loss of p53 function was associated with resistance to radiation therapy as well as chemotherapy came from *in vivo* model systems using p53 knockout mice.[64–67] Subsequent studies have confirmed that various

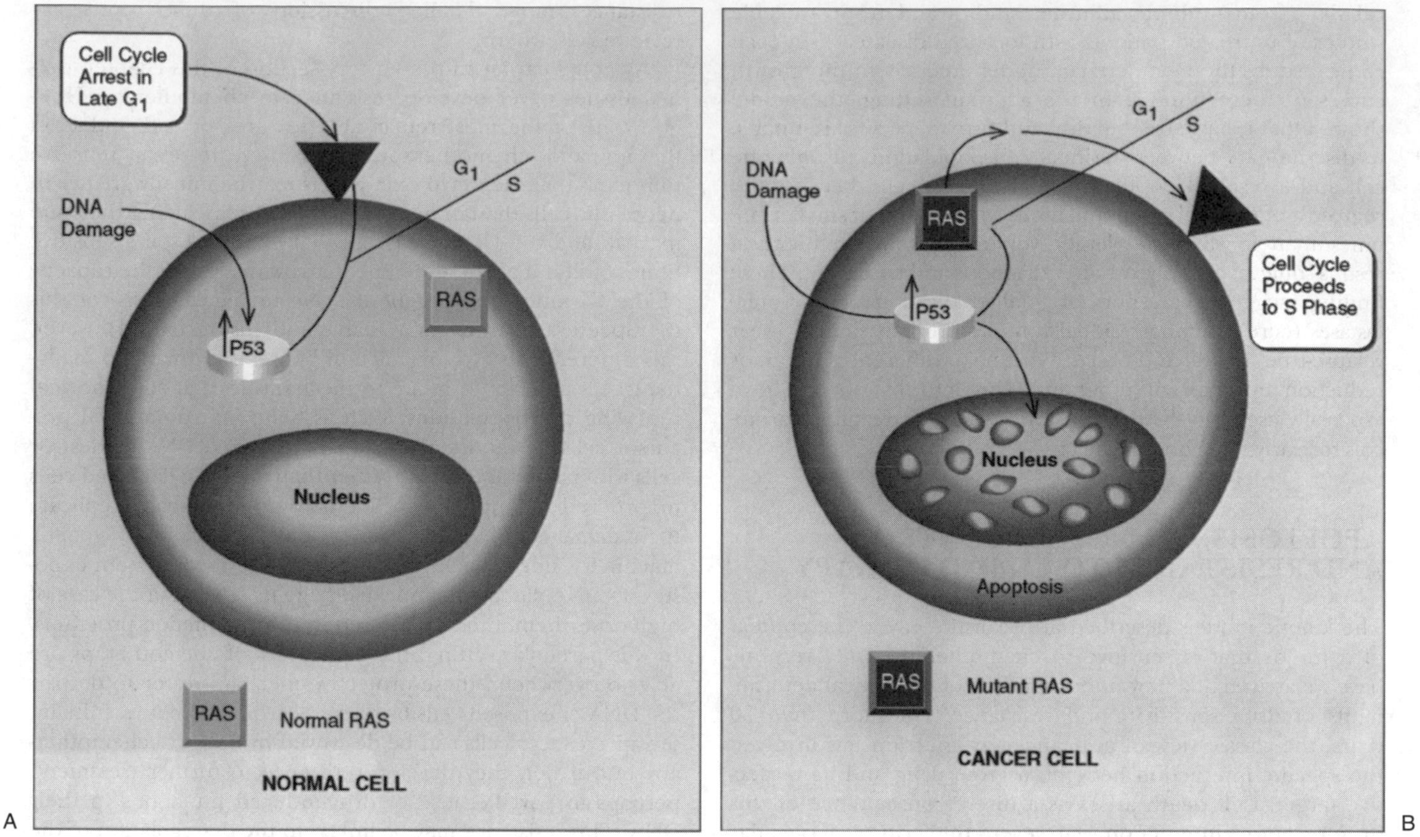

FIGURE 17-1. Role of p53 in chemotherapy sensitivity in normal and neoplastic cells. Exposure of normal cells **(A)** to DNA-damaging agents results in increased levels of p53, which induces an arrest of progression from the G_1 or quiescent phase to the S or DNA synthetic phase of the cell cycle. Exposure of cancer cells **(B)** to DNA-damaging agents increases p53 but does not stop cell-cycle progression to S phase, owing to mutant Ras. This results in apoptosis. (From AB Deisseroth, VT DeVita. The cell cycle: probing new molecular determinants of resistance and sensitivity to cytotoxic agents. *Cancer J Sci Am* 1995;1:15, with permission.)

malignant cell lines and tumors expressing mutant or deleted p53 are chemoresistant to a wide range of anticancer agents.[68] However, loss of p53 function is not always associated with chemoresistance. Some studies suggest that cells with impaired p53 function can become sensitized to various anticancer agents.[69] Thus, the relationship between p53 status and chemosensitivity is complex and is presumably dependent on a number of factors, including the specific cytotoxic stimuli, tissue-specific differences, and the specific cellular context that incorporates the overall genetic machinery and the various intracellular signaling pathways.

The specific cytotoxic treatment, the conditions of treatment, p53 status, and other cell-cycle regulatory elements may all contribute to the outcome of an exposure of a cell to DNA damaging agents. If the dose of the treatment is very high, nonapoptotic cell death (e.g., necrotic cell death due to DNA or other damage) may occur. At an intermediate level of dose intensity, p53-dependent or p53-independent apoptotic cell death can occur. When p53 function is intact, the level of inhibitors of p53 is not high, and the regulatory environment of the cell is such that the cell circumvents the interruption of the cell-cycle progression that occurs after DNA damage, the cell will undergo p53-dependent apoptosis. However, in the setting of abnormal p53 function, whether through the acquisition of point mutations in the p53 gene, posttranslation inactivation of p53 through binding to other protein partners (e.g., MDM2) or enhancement of the degradation (e.g., the E6 protein of the human papilloma virus), or decreased translation of wild-type p53 messenger RNA by the folate-dependent enzyme thymidylate synthase, the cell is unable to undergo cell-cycle arrest or apoptosis in response to DNA damage. In a tumor population, the functional inactivation of p53 through any of these regulatory mechanisms facilitates genomic instability and contributes to the development of cellular resistance. Normal hematopoietic cells tend to be more genetically stable during chemotherapy as a result of an intact p53 mechanism that provides an opportunity to repair DNA damage. In contrast, the malignant cell with functional p53 may be more sensitive to chemotherapy than normal cells because of the fact that common transforming mutations in other proteins, such as ras, which tend to drive cells into S phase, overcome the p53-dependent mechanisms that allow for repair. Because the p53-dependent apoptotic mechanisms, triggered by DNA damage, may remain intact, the tumor cell dies after chemotherapy, whereas the normal cell survives. When the function of p53 is finally lost, the stability of the genome of the tumor cells

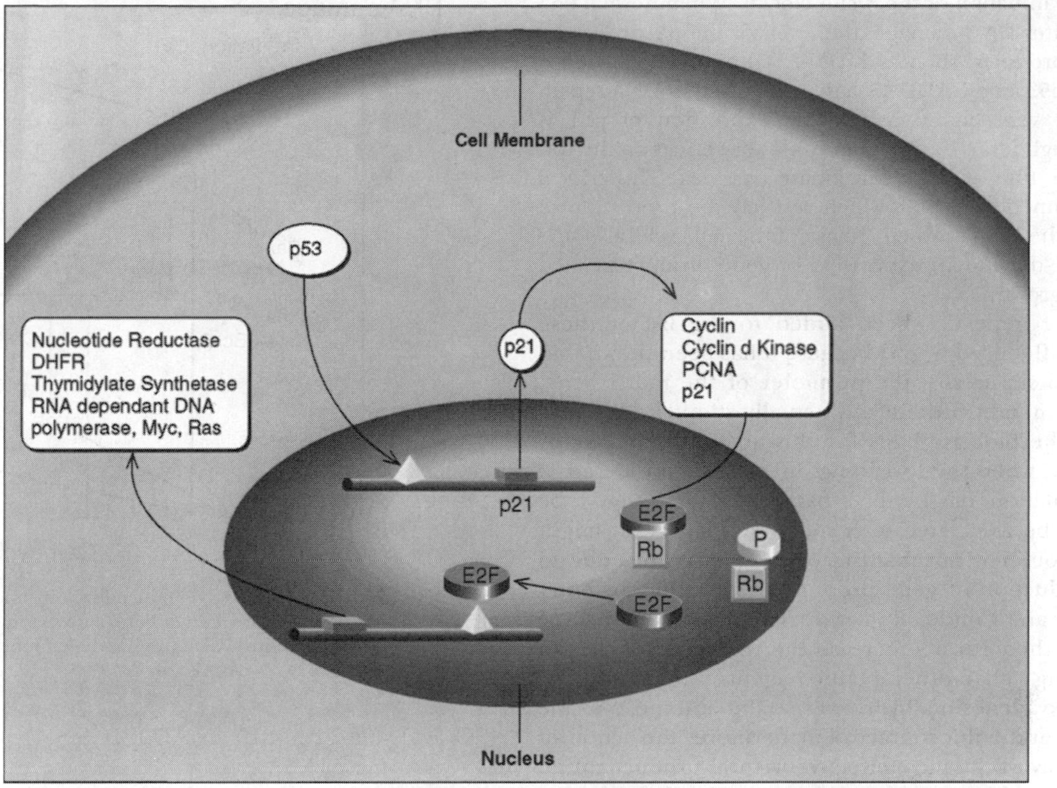

FIGURE 17-2. Once its level is high within the cell, p53 can induce p21 expression to such an extent that the cyclin-dependent kinase activation complex does not occur. The absence of this kinase activity permits the retinoblastoma protein to remain in its unphosphorylated form, in which it binds to the transcription factor E2F. This, in turn, prevents the release of E2F and its binding to the transcriptional enhancers of the genes necessary for DNA synthesis to occur. DHFR, dihydrofolate reductase; PCNA, proliferating cell nuclear antigen. (From AB Deisseroth, VT DeVita. The cell cycle: probing new molecular determinants of resistance and sensitivity to cytotoxic agents. *Cancer J Sci Am* 1995;1:15, with permission.)

decreases, and the disease progresses rapidly to higher and higher levels of resistance to therapy and to a more advanced pattern of dysregulated growth and metastasis.

Although it was initially thought that drug-curable tumors, in general, were less often found to have p53 mutations, this is not always the case. In addition to p53-dependent mechanisms, it is well appreciated that p53-independent mechanisms also exist. In general, the presence of p53 mutations has been correlated with a poor prognosis, even in such treatable tumors as lymphomas.[70] However, the issue of whether mutations determine cure or no cure will be addressed only by reexamination of the tissue specimens of patients cured many years ago, to separate easily the impact of a damaged cell-cycle checkpoint control system on early response to treatment rather than cure.

This is an important question. If drugs can kill only cells with an intact apoptotic mechanism, as expressed by a functioning p53 gene, the chemotherapy of cancer may have gone as far as it can go in its present form, except for the increment of additional cures that may be attained by using high-dose regimens that overwhelm these mechanisms. If cures are possible in tumors with mutant p53, responsiveness to treatment may relate more to the degree of dysregulation of the checkpoint control system, which is downstream from p53 in the growth regulatory pathway, something that possibly can be manipulated as an approach to treatment.

How might dysregulation of this pathway increase drug resistance beyond the failure to induce apoptosis? p53 affects events within the cell by binding to p53 recognition sites located in the transcriptional regulatory regions of genes.[71–76] The acquisition of point mutations in the p53 gene can affect the DNA-binding function and the transcriptional activation functions of p53 at these regulatory sites.[59]

Some of the genes that are transcriptionally activated by p53 belong to a class of proteins known to inhibit the cyclin-dependent kinases (Fig. 17-2). One of these proteins, known as *p21* (Waf-1, Cip-1), can form a complex with proliferating cell nuclear antigen or inhibit the full activation of the cyclin-dependent kinase.[76] When the cyclin kinase is fully active, it acts on another tumor suppressor, the retinoblastoma (RB) gene, to phosphorylate it.[77] This causes the release of the E2F family of transcription factors, which then bind to the regulatory regions of a number of genes that participate in the synthesis of DNA. These genes are shown in Figure 17-2 and include ribonucleotide reductase, dihydrofolate reductase, DNA-dependent RNA polymerase, thymidylate synthase, c-myc, c-fos, and c-myb.

Activation of this family of proteins promotes and supports the entry of the cell into S phase. The activation of cyclin-dependent kinases and the consequent turning on of the DNA synthetic machinery by release of E2F from RB occur in normal cells after growth factor stimulation, which probably provides the signal for the initiation of the cyclin clock.[78] When normal p53 is activated after DNA damage, the levels of the p21, p27, and other gene products, such as MDM-2, an apparent feedback regulator of p53, and GADD 45, a gene involved in DNA repair, may become very high.[79] When the expression of p21 is induced to high levels, it exerts an inhibitory effect on the formation of the fully active cyclin kinase complex. This critical checkpoint function of p53, which restricts the procession of the cell into the DNA synthetic phase of the cell cycle, also prevents the E2F-dependent expression of gene products related to rapid cell growth.

The mdr-1 gene has been added to the list of those potentially influenced by p53 because it has been shown that wild-type p53 suppresses the promoter of the mdr-1 gene, whereas the mutant protein can actually stimulate the promoter.[80,81] The biologic basis for this action is not readily apparent but, when the foregoing effects are considered *in toto*, dysregulation of the p53 pathway, which would be expected to be associated with more rapid growth, might well be a prominent mechanism of drug resistance due to the overproduction of gene products responsible for entry into S phase and rapid cell growth. The activation of these genes could theoretically increase the resistance of cells to the following chemotherapeutic agents: methotrexate, 2-chlorodeoxyadenosine, hydroxyurea, fludarabine, cytosine arabinoside, and 5-fluorouracil. Furthermore, the action of an entire array of the most effective natural product antitumor agents could be suppressed through stimulation of the mdr-1 promoter directly by a mutant form of p53.

Thus, an active p53 in the setting of such DNA-damaging agents as chemotherapy or irradiation increases the levels of key gene products to levels that are sufficient to inhibit the phosphorylation of the RB gene by cyclin-dependent kinase (Fig. 17-3). This, in turn, prevents the expression of the gene products necessary for DNA synthesis to occur.

It is conceivable that increasing growth rates may be associated with increasing levels of drug resistance through the increased transcription of genes involved in rapid cell growth and entry into the cell cycle. The high degree of resistance in more advanced tumors, including the spontaneous development of resistance, which was the basis of the Goldie-Coldman hypothesis, and the development of multidrug resistance, appear more likely to be related to mutations in key genes in the cell-cycle regulatory system than to drug-specific spontaneous mutations, as has been proposed in the past. Cell death in response to exposure to DNA-damaging agents may require an intact p53-dependent apoptotic mechanism under some experimental circumstances. On the other hand, it also may depend on the activation of alternative pathways of apoptosis or some degree of reregulation of the system which would ultimately lead to the reduced release of transcription factors from genes such as RB, or a homologous gene, p107, and the production of lower levels of growth-related gene products, thereby sensitizing cells to chemotherapeutic agents. An enhanced understanding of the complexities surrounding chemotherapy-induced cell death may shed light on critical insights with profound implications for the design of future approaches to therapy that might couple standard cytotoxic agents to new biologic agents that attack specific molecular targets to reregulate the cell-cycle checkpoint.

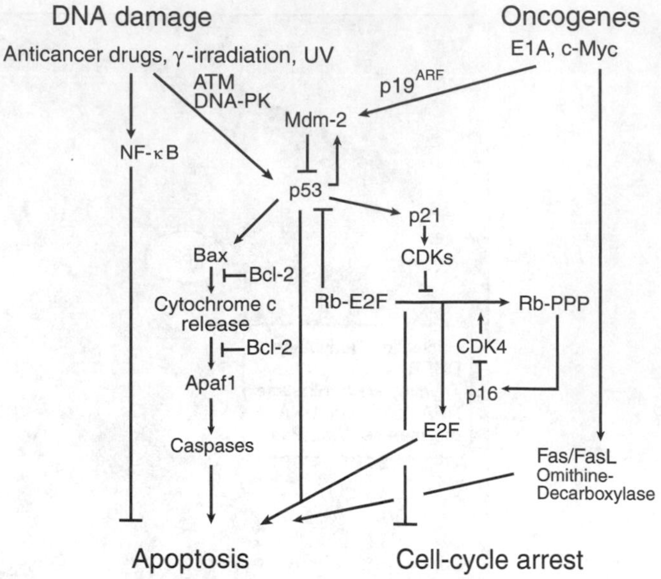

FIGURE 17-3. DNA damage induced by anticancer drugs and irradiation and oncogene expression initiate pathways involved in apoptosis or cell-cycle arrest (or both). CDKs, cyclin-dependent kinases; UV, ultraviolet. (From ref. 56, with permission.)

ROLE OF Bcl-2 FAMILY IN APOPTOSIS

Because apoptosis is a genetically programmed event, inactivation of genes that induce the apoptotic program or activation of antiapoptotic genes can result in the development of cellular drug resistance. Bcl-2 is a potent suppressor of apoptotic cell death, and a number of studies have shown that it is able to repress cell death triggered by either γ-irradiation or a variety of anticancer agents (see Fig. 17-3).[54,56,82] In further support of the role of Bcl-2 as an inhibitor of cell death are studies that show that treatment of certain human leukemia or lymphoma cells with an antisense strategy directed against bcl-2 leads to the reversal of chemoresistance. Lymphoma cells treated with either antisense oligonucleotides or with plasmid constructs that overexpress antisense bcl-2 messenger RNA are sensitized to the cytotoxic effects of methotrexate and cytosine arabinoside.[83] In addition, the phosphorylation status of bcl-2 may play an important role as a determinant of chemosensitivity. It has been suggested that phosphorylated bcl-2 may interact less efficiently with its heterodimer protein partner bax, resulting in cell death. Some work suggests that Bcl-x_l, a functional and structural homologue of Bcl-2, is also able to confer protection against radiation-induced apoptosis as well as against a wide number of anticancer agents, including bleomycin, cisplatin, etoposide, and vincristine. Recently, the antiapoptotic effects of Bcl-2 and Bcl-x_l were compared. Using FL5.12 lymphoid cells, it was shown that these two proteins have a differential ability to protect against chemotherapy-induced cell death.[84] This differential effect depends more on the molecular mechanism targeted as opposed to the cell-cycle specificity of an individual drug. In contrast to Bcl-2 and Bcl-x_l, other family members, including Bax, Bcl-x_s, and Bak, have been shown to promote apoptosis in response to either radiation or various anticancer drugs (or both). The underlying mechanisms through which these Bcl-2 family members control apoptosis remains unknown at this time. However, the mitochondrial pathway with altered release of cytochrome C presumably plays a critical role in this process.

ROLE OF STRESS-ACTIVATED PROTEIN KINASE IN APOPTOSIS

The mitogen-activated protein kinase family of proteins is highly conserved among all eukaryotic species.[85] These kinases play a critical role in mediating signal transduction pathways that are sensitive to extracellular stimuli. Stress-activated protein kinase (SAPK), also known as *c-Jun N-terminal protein kinases,* represents one of the key mitogen-activated protein kinase–signaling pathways. It is now well appreciated that SAPK activation is necessary for cell death in response to exposure to certain forms of cell stress and that defects in SAPK signaling promote cell survival. With regard to chemotherapy, SAPK functions are an important mediator of apoptosis.[86–88] Inhibition of SAPK activation has a protective effect against cancer cells treated with various anticancer agents, including the anthracyclines and etoposide. In addition, SAPK is required for ceramide-induced apoptosis, a key mediator of cytotoxicity induced by various cancer drugs.[89] Thus, the SAPK-signaling pathway plays an essential role in facilitating chemotherapy-induced apoptosis. The precise mechanism by which the SAPK pathway is actually activated remains the focus of much research. However, one potential clue rests with the observation that DNA damage induced by genotoxic stress is sensed by kinases, including the DNA-dependent protein kinase or the ataxia-telangiectasia-mutated gene product (or both).[90,91] These proteins can then phosphorylate p53, resulting in its activation. In addition, DNA-dependent protein kinase can stimulate c-Abl tyrosine kinase, which in turn leads to direct activation of SEK-1, an upstream signal in the SAPK cascade.[92]

DEATH EXECUTIONER PATHWAY

The molecular mechanisms and signal transduction pathways initiated by a given cellular stress may differ significantly. However, the final stage of these various death pathways occurs through the activation and function of the caspases (see Fig. 17-3).[59] The caspases represent a conserved family of cysteine proteases with specificity for aspartic acid residues in their substrates. The cleavage of certain essential substrates then results in cell death. Exogenous inhibition of caspase proteases by CrmA promotes the development of resistance of human leukemia cells to a broad array of anticancer agents.[93] In addition, some knockout mouse models with germline disruptions of Apaf1, caspase-3, or caspase-9 have shown these genetically engineered mice to be resistant to γ-irradiation and a wide number of chemotherapeutic drugs.[59,94,95]

CELL SURVIVAL PATHWAYS

It has been shown that a number of external stimuli, including various cytokines, tumor necrosis factor-α (TNF-α), chemotherapy, and radiation, lead to activation of the transcription factor NF-κB.[96] Paradoxically, activation of NF-κB results in potent suppression of the apoptotic potential of these stimuli.[97] Several studies have demonstrated that inhibition of NF-κB *in vitro* leads to enhanced apoptosis in response to different stimuli.[98] Some *in vivo* work shows that the adenoviral delivery of a modified form of IκBα, an inhibitor of NF-κB, results in inhibition of NF-κB expression. Moreover, the chemoresistant fibrosarcoma tumors derived from HT1080 cells become sensitized to the apoptotic potential of TNF-α and the topoisomerase I compound, CPT-11, leading to significant tumor regression.[99] These findings suggest that activation of NF-κB expression in response to chemotherapy may represent an important mechanism of inducible tumor chemoresistance. Moreover, they suggest that strategies to inhibit NF-κB may lead to enhanced antitumor therapy through increased apoptosis.

DEVELOPMENT OF NOVEL THERAPEUTIC STRATEGIES

Significant efforts continue to be placed on elucidating the critical intracellular signal transduction pathways required for cell-cycle control and the induction of apoptosis and cell death. However, based on current knowledge, attempts are already being made to manipulate these intracellular programs so as to design and develop novel therapeutic approaches to improve the efficacy of chemotherapy. Tumor suppressor genes were originally identified because of the ability of transforming viruses to bind to the protein product of the tumor suppressor gene and induce the growth required for the virus lytic growth cycle. It has been shown that some viral gene products, such as the adenovirus E1A protein, which by itself is nontransforming, can actually sensitize cells to agents that induce apoptosis. E1A is involved in the release of E2F from the RB protein, which could be expected to facilitate entry of cells into S phase. It has been hypothesized that the transmission of conflicting signals, which act both to slow and to stimulate growth simultaneously, may lead to E1A-induced apoptosis.[100] Thus, the identification of analogs of E1A to be used in this setting is an attractive concept.

Clearly, it will be important to identify novel strategies that are selective in their targeting of malignant cells while preserving normal function of host tissues. Along these lines, viral vectors expressing apoptotic genes can now be directly introduced into the tumor. Adenoviral vectors that express p53 have been injected into human tumors, resulting in suppression of tumor growth.[101,102] Moreover, this gene therapy approach shows a synergistic interaction with various cytotoxic agents to produce enhanced antitumor activity with minimal host toxicity. This strategy has been taken into the clinic where a phase I study was performed in patients with non–small cell lung cancer.[103]

TNF-related apoptosis-inducing ligand, or TRAIL, is a type II transmembrane protein that was initially identified based on the homology of its extracellular domain with CD95L. Like TNF and Fas, TRAIL induces apoptosis in a wide range of tumor cells.[104] Walczak et al.[105] evaluated the ability of TRAIL as a therapeutic agent. They created leucine zipper (LZ) forms of human (hu) and murine (mu) TRAIL to promote trimerization and found that these trimers of LZ-TRAIL effectively killed cultured mammary adenocarcinoma cells but not normal, nontransformed mammary epithelial cells, fibroblasts, renal tubule cells, skeletal muscle cells, pulmonary epithelial cells, and melanocytes. Administration of either the hu or mu TRAIL was nontoxic to the normal tissues of mice *in vivo.* Finally, repeated administration of LZ-huTRAIL showed impressive antitumor activity against human mammary adenocarcinoma MDA-231 cells implanted in severe combined immunodeficient mice, and histologic examination of tumors revealed clear areas of apoptosis within 9 to 12 hours of injection. These findings show that TRAIL exerts potent antitumor activity *in vivo* by selectively and directly activating tumor cell death without affecting normal tissues. Studies are ongoing to determine whether TRAIL-based therapy may be used either alone or in combination with other cytotoxic agents and whether these promising results can be effectively translated into the clinic.

It has been suggested that initiation of the cyclic production of cyclins in the cell is due, in part, to the effect of growth factors. Some cyclin classes, such as the D cyclins, may indeed be the essential sensors for multiple growth factor signals.[60] In some experimental systems, a determining factor in the decision of a cell either to undergo cell-cycle arrest and repair damaged DNA or to undergo apoptosis may be the presence of key growth factors within the cellular environment.[106,107] Thus, in the absence of a growth signal, with growth factors serving as a survival factor, the cell becomes committed to the apoptotic pathway. It is presumed that apoptosis is taking place within the context of an intact p53 mechanism. However, one issue is whether, even in the presence of mutations of p53 or other checkpoint genes (or both), deprivation of critical growth factor signals would still result in enhanced sensitivity to chemotherapy.

Experiments using *in vivo* mouse models bearing human tumor xenografts suggest that this may be so. An antiepidermal growth factor receptor, monoclonal antibody C225 targeted to the epidermal growth factor receptor, was used in combination with the anticancer agent doxorubicin against human A431 squamous carcinomas and human MDA468 breast carcinomas. The effects of either the antibody or the drug alone are modest, with no long-term survivors. However, when the antibody is administered before doxorubicin, the effects of the combination are dramatic, often leading to complete tumor regression and long-term survival.[108] Similar results were observed in mice bearing human GEO colon cancer xenografts. Complete tumor regression was noted only in mice treated with the topoisomerase I inhibitor topotecan and the C225 monoclonal antibody.[109] These effects at first seem paradoxical, as the cytotoxic effects of an anticancer drug are being enhanced by a biologic agent that presumably is slowing down growth. However, an alternative explanation is that treatment with the antibody sensitizes the tumor to chemotherapy by depriving it of a vital growth factor signal, thereby facilitating the process of apoptosis. The results are provocative enough that other monoclonal antibodies that block key growth factor receptors have been coupled with chemotherapy and are being tested in the clinic. A similar approach is being taken with the use of the anti-HER2 (Herceptin) antibody for the treatment of advanced breast cancer, in combination with either paclitaxel (Taxol) or with the combination of cyclophosphamide (Cytoxan) and doxorubicin (Adriamycin).[110,111] Based on the promising clinical results, these combination regimens have been approved by the U.S. Food and Drug Administration for women with advanced breast cancer.

CONCEPT OF DOSE INTENSITY

Irrespective of the molecular mechanisms underlying the development of human cancers, a principal factor limiting the capacity to cure is proper dosing. The dose-response curve in biologic systems is usually sigmoidal in shape, with a threshold, a lag phase, a linear phase, and a plateau phase. For radiation therapy and chemotherapy, therapeutic selectivity is dependent on the difference between the dose-response curves of normal and tumor tissue that must be exploited during treatment. In experimental models, the dose-response curve is usually steep in the linear phase. Almost without exception in rodents bearing transplantable tumors, a reduction of dose in the linear phase of the dose-response curve usually results in a loss of the capacity to cure the tumor effectively before a diminution in the response rate is seen. Thus, although complete remissions continue to be observed with a dose reduction as small as 20%, the residual tumor cells may not be eliminated, allowing for eventual relapse to occur. There is an extremely important lesson in these animal data for clinicians who, in their daily practice, judge the adequacy of their therapy by measuring the response rate of visible or palpable tumor masses and only much later are able to evaluate the treatment by survival results. This point is nicely illustrated in Table 17-2, which summarizes data from numerous experiments conducted by Skipper[112] at the Southern Research Institute using the transplantable and palpable Ridgway osteosarcoma tumor model. Reduction in the average dose intensity of the two-drug combination of L-phenylalanine mustard and cyclophosphamide causes a marked decrease in the cure rate before a significant reduction in the complete remission rate occurs. On average, a dose reduction of approximately 20% leads to a loss of 50% of the cure rate. The converse is also true. In tumors with a high growth fraction, a twofold increase in dose often leads to a tenfold increase (1-log) in tumor cell kill. Although *in vivo* systems are not the perfect model for human malignancies, the invariable nature of these data indicates that the general principle may be applied to the clinic. Because anticancer drugs are toxic, it is often appealing to avoid acute but not life-threatening toxicity by either reducing the dose or increasing the time interval between each cycle of treatment. This kind of empiric dose adjustment is a major reason for treatment failure in patients with drug-sensitive tumors who are undergoing induction chemotherapy.

One problem facing clinicians is the difficulty in adequately comparing the impact of different dosing practices on the clin-

TABLE 17-2. Ridgway Osteogenic Sarcoma: Response to Different Dose Intensity of Two-Drug Combination of Cyclophosphamide and L-PAM

Relative Dose Intensity			*Complete Response*	
CPA	L-PAM	Average	*Rate (%)*	*Cure Rate (%)*
0.38	0.82	0.60	100	60
0.75	0.18	0.47	100	44
0.25	0.55	0.44	100	0
0.50	0.12	0.31	10	0
0.17	0.36	0.27	0	0

CPA, cyclophosphamide; L-PAM, L-phenylalanine mustard.
Note: Tumors weighed 2–3 g.
(Modified from HE Skipper, Booklet no. 5. Birmingham, AL: Southern Research Institute, 1986.)

ical efficacy of chemotherapy. To approach this issue, Hryniuk et al.[113–118] analyzed treatment outcomes in various tumor types as a function of dose intensity. Dose intensity is defined as the amount of drug delivered per unit of time, expressed as milligrams per square meter per week, regardless of the schedule or route of administration. Relative dose intensity (RDI) is the amount of drug delivered per unit of time relative to an arbitrarily chosen standard single drug or, for a combination regimen, the decimal fraction of the ratio of the average dose intensity of all drugs of the test regimen compared with the standard regimen. A sample calculation of the RDI for a commonly used regimen, the cyclophosphamide, methotrexate, and 5-fluorouracil (CMF) combination for breast cancer, is provided in Table 17-3.[73] To calculate the average RDI for a regimen containing fewer drugs than the standard regimen, a dose intensity of zero is assigned to the missing drug, and the average RDI of the test regimen is divided by the total number of drugs in the standard.[114] The dose intensity of each drug regimen is then determined based on the time period in which the treatment program is administered. Specific calculations can be made of the intended dose intensity, the dose intensity as described in the treatment protocol, or the actually received dose intensity. However, determination of the received dose intensity would seem to be the most clinically relevant as it reflects the direct impact of dose reductions and treatment delays imposed in actual practice.[118] A positive relation between dose intensity and response rate has, in fact, been demonstrated in several solid tumors, including advanced ovarian, breast, lung, and colon cancers, and in the lymphomas.[113,114,116–118]

Because dose intensity is determined based on the amount of drug given per week, regardless of schedule, treatment delays are given equal weight with dose reductions. Calculations of the dose intensity, therefore, assume that differences in scheduling do not influence treatment outcome. Although this concept may at first appear to be contradictory, close scrutiny of all available data in humans and rodents reveals that the schedule of administration influences outcome mainly by affecting toxicity. In this way, higher doses of drug can be administered over the same time frame. As one example, daily administration of low doses of methotrexate is extremely toxic and severely limits the dose and duration of therapy with this drug. However, a twice-weekly schedule, which is much more effective in rodents and humans, allows much higher doses to be delivered over a longer period. Of note, this particular schedule is associated with significantly less host toxicity. As calculated, the dose intensity of the twice-weekly schedule is much greater than that of the daily oral schedule. In practice, the impact of scheduling on the calculation of dose intensity can be neutralized by comparing programs in which drugs with toxicities affected by scheduling, such as the antimetabolites, are given on similar schedules.

TABLE 17-3. Sample Calculations: Dose Intensity, Relative Dose Intensity, and Average Relative Dose Intensity

CALCULATION OF RELATIVE DOSE INTENSITY (RDI)

Standard: Cyclophosphamide, 80 $mg/m^2/d$ (continuously), 560 $mg/m^2/wk$

Test schedule: Cyclophosphamide, 100 $mg/m^2/d$ (days 1–14, q28d), 350 $mg/m^2/wk$

RDI = 350/560 = 0.62

CALCULATION OF AVERAGE RDI

Standard[a]:

Cyclophosphamide, 2 mg/kg/d, 560 $mg/m^2/wk$

Methotrexate, 0.7 mg/kg/wk, 28 $mg/m^2/wk$

5-Fluorouracil, 12 mg/kg/wk, 480 $mg/m^2/wk$

Test regimen:

Cyclophosphamide, 100 $mg/m^2/d$ (days 1–14), 350 $mg/m^2/wk$; RDI = 350/560 = 0.62

Methotrexate, 40 mg/m^2 on days 1 and 8, 20 $mg/m^2/wk$; RDI = 20/28 = 0.71

5-Fluorouracil, 600 mg/m^2 on days 1 and 8, 300 $mg/m^2/wk$; RDI = 300/480 = 0.62

Repeat cycles q28d

Average RDI = (0.62 + 0.71 + 0.62)/3 = 0.65

[a]Assume standard regimen to be cyclophosphamide, methotrexate, and 5-fluorouracil. To convert milligrams per kilogram (mg/kg) to milligrams per square meter (mg/m^2), multiply by 40.[115]

One of the potential limitations of the dose-intensity concept is that calculations of an average RDI of a drug combination assume that each drug has equal efficacy against the tumor being treated. In most clinical settings, this is usually not the case. However, the impact of a single drug or combinations of two or three drugs in a multidrug combination can be assessed separately. Such an analysis has been performed to show the greater impact of cisplatin in a drug combination for ovarian cancer[113–116] and to show the importance of adequate doses of alkylating agents and vinca alkaloids in lymphoma treatment. The most active drug in a combination regimen can be identified, and this information is important because such data can help to avoid dose adjustments that may radically alter the clinical outcome. Moreover, by identifying the most essential drugs in a given regimen, protocols can focus on administering the optimal dose intensity of those specific agents.

To judge adequately the dosing of a particular protocol, data on total dose of each drug used and cumulative doses of each drug are necessary. However, the collection of such information is not part of the routine practice in medical oncology, and reports are not generally available in the literature. Therefore, for proper assessment of the impact of dosing schedules in clinical trials, it is critical that such data be provided.

Calculations of the impact of dose intensity on outcome are particularly important in estimating the value and exploring some of the pitfalls of adjuvant chemotherapy. The steep dose-response curve for anticancer drugs indicates that dose reductions in adjuvant drug treatment programs are likely to be associated with significantly less therapeutic effect. Dose reduction, however, has been the norm in the design of adjuvant trials. One example is the standard CMF regimen for breast cancer referred to in Table 17-3. The initial reports of this regimen revealed an impressive complete remission rate of approximately 30%, albeit at the expense of considerable host toxicity.[119] When this regimen was advanced for use in the cooperative group setting, initially for advanced disease and later for adjuvant trials by Bonadonna et al.,[120] its doses were arbitrarily reduced without pretesting the potential impact of such reductions on clinical outcome. In addition, further reduction was empirically made for patients older than 60 years, with the assumption that such a dose reduction would be required for age. When the effect of these reductions is correlated with outcome, there is a strong suggestion of a negative impact.[120,121] In premenopausal women, the differences in relapse-free survival at both low and high doses of CMF are statistically significant. The importance of dose effect was further confirmed by a large study in which a survival benefit was observed as a result of increasing dose intensity in the adjuvant chemotherapy for women with stage II, node-positive breast cancer.[122]

An increase in the dose intensity represents one approach to improve on the effect of specific drugs or drug combination, but it may not be useful in all clinical circumstances. In the setting of large tumor burdens, the dose-response curve tends to shift to the right. At the low end of the curability curve (i.e., in the presence of the highest tumor burdens), an increase in dose intensity may not improve treatment outcome, as the dose-response curve is flat, but most often leads to unacceptable host toxicity. In addition, increasing the dose intensity of drug regimens that are already associated with curing nearly 100% of a subset of patients would not be expected to be of clinical benefit. Such a scenario would hold for the treatment of germ cell cancer using the cisplatin, etoposide, bleomycin combination and for Hodgkin's disease, using either the mechlorethamine, vincristine (Oncovin), procarbazine, and prednisone regimen; the doxorubicin, bleomycin, vinblastine, and dacarbazine regimen; or regimens derived from them, such as BEACOPP (see Chapter 45.3). However, for most drugs, there appears to be a threshold dose that produces clinical response. The success of high-dose chemotherapy programs with stem cell support in refractory lymphomas, breast cancer, childhood sarcomas, and neuroblastomas suggests that maximizing dose intensity can improve response rates or cure in drug-responsive tumors.

Frei et al.[123] and Hryniuk et al.[124] have proposed the term *summation dose intensity* to reflect the relationship between dose and combination chemotherapy. As part of this concept, they suggested that the final outcome of either a high-dose or combination treatment must be related in some manner to the sum of the dose intensities of all the agents used in that treatment. The intrinsic chemosensitivity of a given tumor is critical for treatment success. An active agent is defined as one that, when used alone, is associated with at least a 30% response rate for a given tumor. It is now well appreciated that for almost all malignancies, a combination regimen incorporating at least three active drugs is necessary for cure. In the case of childhood leukemia, the cure rate increases linearly when the number of active drugs increases from three to seven. The critical issue for this concept is that all active agents must be used at their full therapeutic doses. However, until the advent of the various cytokine growth factors and autologous or peripheral stem cell transplantation (or both), the effective administration of maximal doses of chemotherapy has not been possible. Although the concept of summation dose intensity is not new, it does offer a unified approach for the careful design and interpretation of clinical trials.

IN VITRO DRUG-RESPONSE ASSAYS

Several methods have been developed since the 1950s to determine the *in vitro* drug sensitivities of human tumor cells to various anticancer agents.[125–139] The advent of reliable *in vitro* drug-response assays has raised the possibility of selecting effective anticancer agents to be used either alone or in combination to treat a patient's individual tumor. In this setting, identification of agents with an extremely low probability of response makes it possible to eliminate the use of such agents and thus their potential for adverse events. A number of methods have been used to investigate the sensitivity of tumors and tumor cell lines, including clonogenic, differential staining cytotoxicity assay; colorimetric, rapid ^{3}H-thymidine incorporation assay; and chemotherapeutic treatment of athymic nude mice with human tumor xenografts. Fruehauf and Bosanquet[140] reviewed the correlation between the results of *in vitro* sensitivity testing and a patient's tumor response to chemotherapy and, in general, they found an overall sensitivity of 85% and an overall specificity of 80%.

In the mid-1950s, Black and Spear[134,135] were the first to report the use of an *in vitro* assay to predict patient response. Their studies compared the *in vitro* activity of aminopterin with its clinical response. Their assay technology was based on the colorimetric detection of viable cells using a substrate for mitochondrial succinate dehydrogenase. Although the predictive accuracy of their results was not particularly strong, the development of the clonogenic stem cell assay in the 1970s brought *in vitro* testing of solid tumors into the mainstream.[137] However, the results of these studies indicated that there were significant technical issues to overcome.[138,139] As illustrated in Table 17-4, further work to improve on the technology led to a variety of techniques and approaches with a pronounced ability to identify drug resistance accurately. The major distinction among the differing assay methods is the end point used to measure cell viability. Assay end points include colony growth from single stem cells, incorporation of tritiated thymidine, microscopic examination of cells with vital dyes, mitochondrial enzyme activity, cytosolic esterase activity, and adenosine triphosphate content. Given the variety of assay types, it is remarkable that the predictive accuracy for the identification of chemosensitivity for most of these approaches appears to be at least 90%. Several issues should be considered when evaluating an assay technology (Table 17-5).[125,127,140]

The clonogenic assay evaluates the ability of chemotherapeutic agents to inhibit tumor stem cell proliferation in agarose, a medium that precludes proliferation of nontransformed cells.[133,134] Most of the *in vitro* drug-response techniques use similar methods for tumor preparation. Solid tumors are disaggregated into suspensions of multicellular clumps with scissors and by passing the fragments through mesh or by stirring tissue fragments with collagenase. Single-cell suspensions then are generated by passing the cellular aggregates through high-gauge needles.[133,138] Cell suspensions are incubated with drug for 1 hour, rinsed, and plated on an agar base with growth media. After a period of 14 to 28 days, the number of colonies that have grown from the treated cells is compared with the number of colonies from untreated control cells. The fraction of control growth provides an index of drug activity. Studies by the National Cancer Institute and the Southwest Oncology Group indicate that the assay is reproducible among multiple laboratories.[138] Problems with assay interpretation arising from the initial plating of small cell clumps were overcome with the use of chromomycin A3.[138,139]

The conventional clonogenic stem cell assay has suffered from a relatively low success rate (<50%) of specimens yielding results, rendering it difficult to accrue adequate numbers of

TABLE 17-4. Correlations of *In Vitro* Test Results with Patient Response

Assay Type	*Patients*	*TP*	*TN*	*FP*	*FN*	*Predictive Accuracy*[a] +	*Predictive Accuracy*[a] –	*Sensitivity (%)*[b]	*Specificity (%)*[c]
Clonogenic	2300	512	1427	226	135	69	91	79	86
5 d thymidine	494	123	432	119	20	51	92	86	66
3 h thymidine	171	90	40	21	20	81	67	82	66
DiSC	510	247	175	72	16	77	92	94	71
MTT	326	187	74	37	28	83	73	87	67
ATP	129	74	37	6	12	93	76	86	86
FCA	333	154	116	52	11	75	91	93	69
Total	4263	1387	2101	533	242	72	90	85	80

ATP, adenosine triphosphate; DiSC, differential staining cytotoxicity; FCA, fluorescent cytoprint assay; FN, patients who are resistant *in vitro* but respond clinically; FP, patients who are sensitive *in vitro* but resistant clinically; MTT, tetrazolium dye; TN, patients who are resistant *in vitro* and do not respond to chemotherapy; TP, patients who are sensitive *in vitro* and respond to therapy.
[a]Predictive accuracy: + indicates TP/(TP – FP), percentage of patients with sensitivity in the test who respond; – indicates TN/(TN + FN), percentage of patients with resistance in the test who do not respond to therapy.
[b]Test's ability to detect clinically responsive patients.
[c]Test's ability to detect clinically unresponsive patients; clinical response is greater than or equal to a 50% reduction in assessable disease.[85]
Note: Summary of clinical correlations is pooled from individual studies referenced in text.

patients into clinical trials.[133] Although this factor initially dampened enthusiasm for this approach, a significant number of clonogenic assays (>2500 cases) have now been performed by various groups, with an overall positive predictive value of 69% and a negative predictive value of 91% (see Table 17-4).[120]

Tritiated thymidine incorporation, as an assay end point, was introduced in part to eliminate the problem of discriminating between true colony growth from a single cell and from a clump of cells plated at the outset. This technique also decreased the assay time from more than 14 days to less than 1 week and was associated with an improved success rate of diagnostic yield to 85%.[125–127,141,142]

Processing and plating of the tumor for the thymidine assay is similar to that for the clonogenic assay. However, in the thymidine assay, small clumps rather than single cells are preferred to maintain cell-cell interactions. In addition, cells are grown in an agar suspension, which allows tumor growth *in vitro* to recapitulate the three-dimensional *in vivo* morphology. Cell-cell interactions resulting from three-dimensional growth may be critical for the detection of acquired drug resistance, which can be missed in monolayer cultures.[143]

In contrast to the clonogenic assay, prolonged drug exposures are utilized in the thymidine-based system. Tumor suspensions are continuously exposed to drug for 5 days, and tritiated thymidine is added during the final 48 hours of the assay to label proliferating cells. Determination of drug action is based on a comparison of the incorporation of labeled thymidine by untreated controls with incorporation by the groups treated with different drugs. Clinical correlations obtained using this assay technique demonstrate a reasonable overall predictive accuracy (72%) and indicate that it is an accurate predictor of drug resistance (99%).[126] The prolonged drug exposure in the thymidine assay results in a five- to 20-fold higher concentration × time factor than that used in the clonogenic assay, biasing assay accuracy toward detection of drug resistance. Tumor growth after drug exposure in the thymidine assay is associated with multifold drug resistance, which led the authors of one article to describe it as the "extreme drug resistance assay."[126] Some paclitaxel-resistant tumors identified with this technique have been found to overexpress P170 glycoprotein, suggesting that this assay can be used to identify the activity of specific mechanisms of drug resistance in different tumor histologies.[144]

Another promising assay is the differential staining cytotoxicity (DiSC) assay.[140,145] The DiSC assay relies on the structural integrity of cells. In the DiSC assay, cells are incubated with drugs for 4 days. Dead cells are stained in suspension with fast green dye in the absence or presence of nigrosin, and duck red blood cells are added as an internal standard for counting. The specimen is cytocentrifuged to deliver discs of cells onto microscope slides. Live cells then are stained with either hematoxylin-eosin or Romanowsky stain. The end point of this test is the morphologic identification of tumor cell cytotoxicity as compared with the internal control of fixed duck erythrocytes. The DiSC assay requires more than 10% tumor cells and measures cell kill in both dividing and nondividing tumor cell populations. Microscopic identification of the cell population renders it possible to determine the differential kill of normal and tumor cells,

TABLE 17-5. Factors Influencing the Utility of the *In Vitro* Assay

Tumor heterogeneity: Is the assay end point selective for malignant cells versus stromal cells?
Is the assessability rate greater than 80%?
Have the assays been correlated with clinical response and survival?
Can the tests evaluate all histologic types, or are they restricted to only certain types of tumors?
Are clinically appropriate drugs evaluated in the test?
Does the turnaround time meet clinical requirements?
Is the test information easily interpreted and applied?
Is the test cost-effective?

and this is the therapeutic index for new agents undergoing *in vitro* screening for activity. The DiSC assay (see Table 17-4) offers an overall predictive accuracy of 83%, with a sensitivity of 94% and a specificity of 71%.[125,132,145]

The potential efficacy of individualized chemotherapy selected by *in vitro* drug sensitivity testing for patients with cancer has been reviewed.[146,147] A number of issues seriously limit the widespread use of this approach in the clinic. First, *in vitro* drug sensitivity testing is relatively expensive and time-consuming. Second, the efficient procurement of tumor tissue remains a serious problem. In fact, only two studies, both from the National Cancer Institute, have evaluated the ability to obtain tumor tissue from patients with limited- and extensive-stage small cell lung cancer.[147,148] Tumor tissue was obtained from 30% of patients with limited-stage disease, in contrast to nearly 70% of patients with extensive-stage disease. Third, even with successful procurement of tumor tissue, a host of technical issues limits the ability for efficient and successful drug testing. In fact, of 12 different trials reviewed, only slightly more than one-half of all tumor samples had sufficient cell numbers for drug testing. Finally, only one-third of all patients entered in prospective trials of *in vitro* drug testing were actually treated with an *in vitro* best regimen. In those patients, the response rates appear to be as good as, and perhaps even slightly better than, those achieved with empiric therapy. It is not surprising, then, that when all the clinical studies are taken together, no potential benefit in survival is observed for this approach. Of note, however, is a survival advantage that has been reported, in a small select series of studies, in patients treated with an individualized *in vitro* best regimen.[148]

The reliability of newer *in vitro* assay technologies to identify drug sensitivity suggests that such assays can help the clinician to avoid exposure of patients to the toxicity of drugs with little clinical benefit. Although the promise of an *in vitro* sensitivity assay has not yet been met, there remains value in identifying inactive agents before their administration and eliminating them from drug combinations. These tests render it possible to tailor drug combinations for the individual cancer patient. They also offer a rational stopping point for both the patient and clinician in situations in which the patient's tumor demonstrates extreme resistance to all conventional anticancer agents. An understanding of when to terminate therapy in hopeless situations is as important as any management issue facing the clinician.[149] Although only a few hundred patients have been enrolled to date to evaluate the impact of *in vitro* assay-directed therapy on survival, it is intuitively obvious that there should be a therapeutic advantage in the activity of agents to which a tumor is highly responsive *in vitro* as compared with agents that demonstrate significant *in vitro* drug resistance.[125] Further prospective, randomized studies are needed to define more properly the true role of *in vitro* drug testing in the selection of chemotherapy for cancer patients in the adjuvant, induction, or salvage setting.

Although *in vitro* tissue culture studies serve as an important guide for selecting chemotherapy, they are inadequate at addressing the issues of tumor cell heterogeneity, drug distribution, drug bioactivation, and host toxicity. *In vivo* model systems overcome some of these obstacles, and several have been developed, including the subrenal capsule assay, a semipermeable membrane in the Millipore diffusion chamber as vessels for tumor implantation into mice, and the tumor xenograft model, which is perhaps the most widely used method for drug testing.[140,150–152] However, each of these experimental systems has its unique drawbacks. Recently, a novel system was developed using a semipermeable polysulfone fiber with a molecular weight cutoff of 30 kD. Human cancer cells derived from tissue culture or from patient tumor specimens are injected directly into semipermeable fibers that are then implanted into immunocompetent rats.[153,154] Animals are treated with the given drug and, after a defined period, they are sacrificed, the fibers are recovered, and the remaining viable cells are counted using the trypan dye exclusion method. There are several advantages to this polysulfone fiber model. First, the entire process of tumor recovery, injection, and implantation of fibers, drug treatment, fiber recovery, and cell analysis can be completed in less than 1 week. This short period minimizes the potential waiting time for selection of the optimal drug, thereby rendering this model feasible for application in the clinical setting in treating a patient. Second, the results from this model system are consistent, reliable, and highly reproducible. As many as six to seven fibers can be implanted into an individual rat; thus, each fiber can be injected with the same cell type and the individual rat treated with the same drug. In addition, this reduces the unnecessary expense of using multiple animals for drug *in vivo* testing. Third, because up to six to seven fibers can be implanted into an individual rat, cancer cells derived from different primary tumors can be tested simultaneously for drug sensitivity, a process that can result in greater cost and time efficiency. Further testing and validation are required to determine whether such a novel *in vivo* system can help to individualize and optimize the clinical therapy of cancer patients.

Finally, studies by Waldman et al.[155] have raised concerns regarding the validity of the *in vitro* colony formation assay as a measure of the cytotoxicity of DNA-damaging agents in tumor cells with altered checkpoint response. Using the human colon cancer HCT116 cell line that expresses wild-type p53 and p21 (p21+/+) and a subline that was rendered p21-deficient (p21−/−) by homologous recombination, these researchers tested the effects of γ-irradiation using the *in vitro* colony formation assay and an *in vivo* xenograft model. Of note, they observed no differences in sensitivity to ionizing radiation, as determined by the *in vitro* colony formation assay. However, using the nude mouse xenograft model, they found that tumors derived from the parent p21+/+ cell line were able to survive exposure to ionizing radiation. In contrast, a significant fraction of the tumors deficient in p21 underwent apoptosis and were thus completely cured. Clearly, the *in vitro* assay was unable to detect this significant difference in sensitivity, as both the processes of cell arrest and apoptosis preclude the outgrowth of colonies. Given the critical role of checkpoint status as a determinant of chemosensitivity, these findings are important as they suggest that *in vivo* assays may represent a more relevant model system to compare the effects of anticancer agents.[156] Moreover, such an *in vivo* model may be ideal for testing novel agents that specifically target cell-cycle control and the pathways associated with the process of apoptosis.

REFERENCES

1. Marchall EK Jr. Historical perspectives in chemotherapy. *Adv Chemother* 1964:1:1.
2. Hersh SM. *Chemical and biological warfare: America's hidden arsenal.* New York: Bobbs Merrill, 1968.
3. Alexander SF. Final report of Bari mustard casualties. Washington, DC: Allied Force Headquarters, Office of the Surgeon. APO 512, June 20, 1944.
4. DeVita VT. The evolution of therapeutic research in cancer. *N Engl J Med* 1978;298:907.

5. DeVita VT. Cell kinetics and the chemotherapy of cancer. *Cancer Chemother Rep* 1971;3:2323.
6. DeVita VT. The influence of information on drug resistance on protocol design: the Harry Kaplan Memorial Lecture given at the Fourth International Conference on Malignant Lymphoma, June 6–9, 1990, Lugano, Switzerland. *Ann Oncol* 1991;2:93.
7. Goldie JH, Coldman AJ. The genetic origin of drug resistance in neoplasms: implication for systemic therapy. *Cancer Res* 1984;44:3643.
8. Endicott JA, Ling V. The biochemistry of P-glycoprotein mediated multidrug resistance. *Annu Rev Biochem* 1989;58:137.
9. Chaudhary PM, Roninson IB. Expression and activity of P-glycoprotein, a multidrug efflux pump, in human hematopoietic stem cells. *Cell* 1992;66:85.
10. Young RC, DeVita VT. Cell cycle characteristics of human solid tumors in vivo. *Cell Tissue Kinet* 1970;3:285.
11. Mendelsohn ML. Autoradiographic analysis of cell proliferation in spontaneous breast cancer in C3H mice: III. The growth fraction. *J Natl Cancer Inst* 1962;28:1015.
12. Skipper HE, Schabel FM, Wilcox WS. Experimental evaluation of potential anti-cancer agents: XII. On the criteria and kinetics associated with "curability" of experimental leukemia. *Cancer Chemother Rep* 1964;35:1.
13. Miller TP, Grogan TM, Dahlberg S, et al. Prognostic significance of the Ki-67-associated proliferative antigen in aggressive non-Hodgkin's lymphoma: a prospective Southwest Oncology Group trial. *Blood* 1994;83:1460.
14. DeVita VT. On the value of response criteria in therapeutic research. *Colloque INSERM* 1988;75:863.
15. Holland JF. Induction chemotherapy: an old term for an old concept. *Colloque INSERM* 1986;137:45.
16. Goldhirsch A, Wood WC, Senn HJ, et al. Meeting highlights: international consensus panel on the treatment of primary breast cancer. *J Natl Cancer Inst* 1995;87:14.
17. Fuchs CS, Mayer RJ. Adjuvant chemotherapy for colon and rectal cancer. *Semin Oncol* 1995;22:472.
18. Cokgor I, Friedman HS, Friedman AH. Chemotherapy for adults with malignant glioma. *Cancer Invest* 1999;17:264.
19. Frei A III, Clark JR, Miller D. The concept of neoadjuvant chemotherapy. In: Salmon SE, ed. *Adjuvant therapy of cancer,* 5th ed. Orlando, FL: Grune & Stratton, 1987:67.
20. Muggia FM. Primary chemotherapy: concepts and issues. In: *Primary chemotherapy in cancer medicine.* New York: Alan R. Liss, 1985:377.
21. DeVita VT. The relationship between tumor mass and resistance to treatment of cancer. *Cancer* 1983;51:1209.
22. Skipper HE. Critical variables in the design of combination chemotherapy regimens to be used alone or in adjuvant setting. *Colloque INSERM* 1986;137:11.
23. Goldie JH. Scientific basis for adjuvant and primary (neoadjuvant) chemotherapy. *Semin Oncol* 1987;14:1.
24. Bonadonna G, Veronesi U, Brambilla C, et al. Primary chemotherapy to avoid mastectomy in tumors with diameters of three centimeters or more. *J Natl Cancer Inst* 1990;82:1539.
25. Jacobs C. Adjuvant and neoadjuvant treatment of head and neck cancers. *Semin Oncol* 1991;18:504.
26. Forastiere AA, Urba SG. Combined modality therapy for cancer of the esophagus. In: DeVita VT, Hellman S, Rosenberg SA, eds. *Principles and practice of oncology,* 5th ed. Philadelphia: Lippincott-Raven Publishers, 1997;10:1.
27. Bosset JF, Gignoux M, Triboulet JP, et al. Chemoradiotherapy followed by surgery compared with surgery alone in squamous-cell cancer of the esophagus. *N Engl J Med* 1997;337:161.
28. Herr HN, Whitmore NF, Morse MJ, et al. Neoadjuvant chemotherapy in invasive bladder cancer: the evolving role of surgery. *J Urol* 1990;144:1083.
29. Jacquillat C, Weil M, Baillet F, et al. Results of neoadjuvant chemotherapy and radiation therapy in the breast conserving treatment of 250 patients with all stages of infiltrative breast cancer. *Cancer* 1990;66:119.
30. DeVita VT. Primary chemotherapy can avoid mastectomy but there is more to it than that [Editorial]. *J Natl Cancer Inst* 1990;82:1522.
31. Green MR. Chemotherapy and radiation in the nonoperative management of stage III non-small cell lung cancer. In: DeVita VT Jr, Rosenberg SA, eds. *Important advances in oncology 1993.* Philadelphia: Lippincott-Raven Publishers, 1993:125.
32. Rusch VW, Albain KS, Crowley JJ, et al. Surgical resection of stage IIIA and stage IIIB non-small cell lung cancer after concurrent induction of chemoradiotherapy. *J Thorac Cardiovasc Surg* 1993;105:97.
33. Nathanson L, Hall TC, Schilling AC, et al. Concurrent combination chemotherapy of human solid tumors: experience with three-drug regimen and review of the literature. *Cancer Res* 1969;29:419.
34. Potter VR. Sequential blocking of metabolic pathways in vivo. *Proc Soc Exp Biol Med* 1951;75:41.
35. Elion GB, Singer S, Hitchings GH. Antagonists of nucleic acid derivatives: VIII. Synergism in combinations of biochemically related antimetabolites. *J Biol Chem* 1954;208:477.
36. Sartorelli AC. Approaches to the combination chemotherapy of transplantable neoplasms. *Prog Exp Tumor Res* 1965;6:228.
37. DeVita VT, Schein PS. The use of drugs in combination for the treatment of cancer: rationale and results. *N Engl J Med* 1973;288:998.
38. Vose JM, Armitage JO. Clinical applications of hematopoietic growth factors. *J Clin Oncol* 1995;13:1023.
39. DeVita VT. Only if you believe in magic. In: Jones SE, Salmon SE, eds. *Adjuvant therapy of cancer,* 4th ed. Orlando, FL: Grune & Stratton, 1984:3.
40. Luria SE, Delbruck M. Mutations of bacteria from virus sensitivity to virus resistance. *Genetics* 1943;28:491.
41. Goldie JH, Coldman AJ. A mathematical model for relating the drug sensitivity of tumors to thc spontancous mutation rate. *Cancer Treat Rep* 1979;63:1727.
42. Day RS. Treatment sequencing, asymmetry and uncertainty: protocol strategies for combination chemotherapy. *Cancer Res* 1986;46:3876.
43. Norton L, Day RS. Potential innovations in scheduling in cancer chemotherapy. In: DeVita VT Jr, Hellman S, Rosenberg SA, eds. *Important advances in oncology 1991.* Philadelphia: Lippincott-Raven Publishers, 1991:57.
44. Buzzoni R, Bonadonna G, Valagussa P, et al. Adjuvant chemotherapy with doxorubicin plus cyclophosphamide, methotrexate, and fluorouracil in the treatment of resectable breast cancer with more than three positive axillary nodes. *J Clin Oncol* 1991;9:2134.
45. Bonadonna G, Zambetti M. Sequential or alternating doxorubicin and CMF regimens in breast cancer with more than three positive nodes. *JAMA* 1995;273:542.
46. Skipper HE. Reasons for success and failure in treatment of murine leukemias with the drugs now employed in treating human leukemias. In: *Cancer chemotherapy.* Ann Arbor, MI: University Microfilms International, 1978:1.
47. Skipper HE, Schabel FM Jr, Mellet LB, et al. Implications of biochemical, cytokinetic, pharmacologic and toxicologic relationships in the design of optimal therapeutic schedules. *Cancer Chemother Rep* 1950;54:431.
48. Yankee RA, DeVita VT, Perry S. The cell cycle of leukemia L1210 cells in vivo. *Cancer Res* 1968;27:2381.
49. Norton LA. A Gompertzian model of human breast cancer growth. *Cancer Res* 1988;48:7067.
50. Bloom H, Richardson M, Harris B. Natural history of untreated breast cancer (1804–1933): comparison of treated and untreated cases according to histologic grade of malignancy. *Med J* 1962;2:213.
51. Hickman JA. Apoptosis induced by anticancer drugs. *Cancer Metastasis Rev* 1992;11:121.
52. Leonard CJ, Canman CE, Kastan MB. The role of p53 in cell-cycle control and apoptosis: implications for cancer. In: DeVita VT, Hellman S, Rosenberg SA, eds. *Important advances in oncology 1995.* Philadelphia: Lippincott-Raven Publishers, 1995:33.
53. Levine AJ. p53, the cellular gatekeeper for growth and division. *Cell* 1997;88:323.
54. Ko LJ, Prives C. p53: puzzle and paradigm. *Genes Dev* 1996;10:1054.
55. El-Deiry WS. Regulation of p53 downstream genes. *Cancer Biol* 1998;8:345.
56. Schmitt CA, Lowe SW. Apoptosis and therapy. *J Pathol* 1999;187:127.
57. Haq R, Zanke B. Inhibition of apoptotic signaling pathways in cancer cells as a mechanism of chemotherapy resistance. *Cancer Metastasis Rev* 1998;17:233.
58. McGill G, Fisher DE. p53 and cancer therapy: a double-edged sword. *J Clin Invest* 1999;104:223.
59. Green DR. Apoptotic pathways: the roads to ruin. *Cell* 1998;94:695.
60. Sherr CJ. Mammalian G1 cyclins. *Cell* 1993;73:1059.
61. Livingstone LR, et al. Altered cell cycle arrest and gene amplification potential accompany loss of wild-type p53. *Cell* 1993;70:923.
62. Keurbitz SJ, Plunkett BS, Walsh WV, Kastan MB. Wild-type p53 is a cell cycle checkpoint determinant following irradiation. *Proc Natl Acad Sci USA* 1992;89:7492.
63. Hollstein M, Sidransky DE, Vogelstein B, Harris CC. p53 mutations in human cancers. *Science* 1991;253:49.
64. Lowe SW, Schmitt EM, Smith SW, et al. p53 is required for radiation-induced apoptosis in mouse thymocytes. *Nature* 1993;362:847.
65. Clarke AR, Purdie CA, Harrison DJ, et al. Thymocyte apoptosis induced by p53-dependent and independent pathways. *Nature* 1993;362:849.
66. Lowe SW, Ruley HE, Jacks T, Housman DE. p53-dependent apoptosis modulates the cytotoxicity of anticancer agents. *Cell* 1993;74:957.
67. Lowe SW, Bodis S, McClatchey A, et al. p53 status and the efficacy of cancer therapy in vivo. *Science* 1994;266:807.
68. Wu GS, El-Deiry WS. p53 and chemosensitivity. *Nature Med* 1996;2:255.
69. Wahl AF, Donaldson KL, Fairchild C, et al. Loss of normal p53 function confers sensitization to taxol by increasing G_2/M arrest and apoptosis. *Nature Med* 1996;2:72.
70. Piris MA, Pezzella F, Martinez-Montero JC, et al. p53 and bcl-2 expression in high-grade B-cell lymphomas: correlation with survival time. *Br J Cancer* 1994;69:337.
71. Kern SE, Kinzler KW, Bruskin A, et al. Identification of p53 as a sequence-specific DNA-binding protein. *Science* 1991;252:1708.
72. El-Deiry WS, Tokino T, Velculescu VE, et al. WAF1, a potential mediator of p53 tumor suppression. *Cell* 1993;75:817.
73. Funk WD, Pak DT, Karas RH, et al. A transcriptionally active DNA-binding site for human p53 protein complexes. *Mol Cell Biol* 1992;12:2866.
74. Zhang W, Funk WD, Wright WE, et al. Novel DNA binding of p53 mutants and their role in transcriptional activation. *Oncogene* 1993;8:2555.
75. Zhang H, Hannon GJ, Beach D. p21 containing cyclin kinases exist in both active and inactive states. *Genes Dev* 1994;8:1750.
76. Polyak K, Xia Y, Zweier JL, et al. A model for p53-induced apoptosis. *Nature* 1997;389:300.
77. Sherr CJ. G1 phase progression: cycling on cue. *Cell* 1994;79:551.
78. Ewen ME. The cell cycle and the retinoblastoma family. *Cancer Metastasis Rev* 1994;13:45.
79. Smith MD, Chen I-T, Zhan Q, et al. Interaction of the p53-regulated protein Gadd 45 with proliferating cell nuclear antigen. *Science* 1994;266:1376.
80. Wang Q, Beck WT. Transcriptional suppression of multidrug resistance-associated protein (MRP) gene expression by wild-type p53. *Cancer Res* 1998;58:5762.
81. Zhou G, Kuo MT. Wild-type p53-mediated induction of rat mdr1b expression by the anticancer drug daunorobucin. *J Biol Chem* 1998;273:15387.
82. Miyashita T, Reed JC. Bcl-2 oncoprotein blocks chemotherapy-induced apoptosis in a human leukemia cell line. *Blood* 1993;81:151.
83. Kitada S, Takayuma S, Dak RK, et al. Reversal of chemoresistance of lymphoma cells by antisense-mediated reduction of bcl-2 gene expression. *Antisense Res Dev* 1994;4:71.
84. Simonian PL, Grillot DAM, Nunez G. Bcl-2 and bcl-xl can differentially block chemotherapy-induced cell death. *Blood* 1997;3:1208.
85. Davis RJ. The mitogen-activated protein kinase signal transduction pathway. *Biol Chem* 1993;268:14553.

86. Seimiya H, Mashima T, Toho M, Tsuruo T. c-Jun NH2-terminal kinase-mediated activation of interleukin-1beta converting enzyme/CED-3-like protease during anticancer drug-induced apoptosis. *J Biol Chem* 1997;272:4631.
87. Osborn MT, Chambers TS. Role of the stress-activated/c-Jun NH2-terminal protein kinase pathway in the cellular response to adriamycin and other chemotherapeutic drugs. *J Biol Chem* 1996;271:30950.
88. Zanke BW, Boudreau K, Rubie E, et al. The stress-activated protein kinase pathway mediates cell death following injury induced by cis-platinum, UV radiation, or heat. *Curr Biol* 1996;6:606.
89. Verheil M, Bose R, Lin XH, et al. Requirement for ceramide-initiated SAPK/JNK signaling in stress-induced apoptosis. *Nature* 1996;380:75.
90. Woo RA, McLure KG, Lees-Miller SP, et al. DNA-dependent protein kinase acts upstream of p53 in response to DNA damage. *Nature* 1998;394:700.
91. Kharbanda S, Pandey P, Ren R, et al. c-Abl activation regulates induction of the SEK1/stress-activated protein kinase pathways in the cellular response to 1-beta-D-arabinofuranosylcytosine. *J Biol Chem* 1995;270:30728.
92. Kharbanda S, Ren R, Pandey P, et al. Activation of the c-Abl tyrosine kinase in the stress response to DNA-damaging agents. *Nature* 1995;376:785.
93. Kuida K, Haydar TF, Kuan CY, et al. Reduced apoptosis and cytochrome c-mediated caspase activation in mice lacking caspase 9. *Cell* 1998;94:325.
94. Antoku K, Liu Z, Johnson DE. Inhibition of caspase proteases by CrmA enhances the resistance of human leukemia cells to multiple chemotherapeutic agents. *Leukemia* 1997;11:1665.
95. Eastman A. Survival factors, intracellular signal transduction, and the activation of endonucleases in apoptosis. *Semin Cancer Biol* 1995;6:45.
96. Wang CY, Mayo MW, Baldwin AS. TNF- and cancer therapy-induced apoptosis: potentiation by inhibition of NF-κB. *Science* 1996;274:784.
97. Van Antwerp D, Martin SJ, Kafri T, et al. Suppression of TNF-a-induced apoptosis by NF-κB. *Science* 1996;274:787.
98. Wang CY, Cusack JC Jr, Liu R, Baldwin AS. Control of inducible chemoresistance: enhanced anti-tumor therapy through increase apoptosis by inhibition of NF-κB. *Nature Med* 1999;5:412.
99. Lowe SW, Ruley HE. Stabilization of the p53 tumor suppressor gene is induced by adenovirus 5 E1A and accompanies apoptosis. *Genes Dev* 1993;7:535.
100. Wu XW, Levine AJ. p53 and E2F-1 cooperate to mediate apoptosis. *Mol Cell Biol* 1994;14:2556.
101. Nielson LL, Maneval DC. p53 tumor suppressor gene therapy for cancer. *Cancer Gene Ther* 1998;5:52.
102. Spitz FR, Nguyen D, Skibber JM, et al. In vitro adenovirus-mediated p53 tumor suppressor gene therapy for colorectal cancer. *Anticancer Res* 1996;16:3415.
103. Roth JA, Swisher SG, Merritt JA, et al. Gene therapy for non-small cell lung cancer: a preliminary report of a phase I trial of adenoviral p53 gene replacement. *Semin Oncol* 1998;25[Suppl 8]:33.
104. French LE, Tschopp J. The TRAIL to selective tumor death. *Nature Med* 1999;5:146.
105. Walczak H, Miller RE, Ariail K, et al. Tumoricidal activity of tumor necrosis factor-related apoptosis-inducing ligand in vivo. *Nature Med* 1999;5:157.
106. Shan B, Chang CY, Jones D, Lee WH. The transcription factor E2F-1 mediates autoregulation of RB expression. *Mol Cell Biol* 1994;12:299.
107. Shan B, Lee WH. Deregulated expression of E2F-1 induces S-phase entry and leads to apoptosis. *Mol Cell Biol* 1994;14:8166.
108. Baselga J, Norton L, Masui H, et al. Antitumor effects of doxorubicin in combination with anti-epidermal growth factor receptor monoclonal antibodies. *J Natl Cancer Inst* 1993;85:1327.
109. Ciardello F, Bianco R, Damiano V, et al. Antitumor activity of sequential treatment with topotecan and anti-epidermal growth factor receptor monoclonal antibody C225. *Clin Cancer Res* 1999;5:909.
110. Baselga J, Norton L, Albanell J, et al. Recombinant anti-HER2 antibody (Herceptin) enhances the antitumor activity of paclitaxel and doxorubicin against HER2/neu overexpressing human breast cancer xenografts. *Cancer Res* 1998;58:2825.
111. Slamon D, Leyland-Jones B, Shak W, et al. Addition of Herceptin (humanized anti-HER2 antibody) to first-line chemotherapy for HER2 overexpressing metastatic breast cancer (HER2+/MBC) markedly increases anticancer activity: a randomized, multinational controlled phase III trial. *Proc Am Soc Clin Oncol* 1998;17:98a.
112. Skipper H. Data and analysis having to do with the influence of dose intensity and duration of treatment (single drugs and combinations) on lethal toxicity and the therapeutic response of experimental neoplasms. Birmingham, AL: Southern Research Institute, Booklets 13, 1986, and 2–13, 1987.
113. Hryniuk WM. The importance of dose intensity in the outcome of chemotherapy. In: DeVita VT, Hellman S, Rosenberg SA, eds. *Important advances in oncology 1988.* Philadelphia: JB Lippincott, 1988:121.
114. Hryniuk W, Levine MN. Analysis of dose intensity for adjuvant chemotherapy trials in stage II breast cancer. *J Clin Oncol* 1986;4:1162.
115. Hryniuk WM. Average relative dose intensity and the impact on design of clinical trials. *Semin Oncol* 1987;14:65.
116. Levin L, Hryniuk W. Dose intensity analysis of chemotherapy regimens in ovarian carcinoma. *J Clin Oncol* 1987;5:756.
117. Hryniuk W, Bush H. The importance of dose intensity in chemotherapy of metastatic breast cancer. *J Clin Oncol* 1984;2:1281.
118. Hryniuk W, Goodyear M. The calculation of received dose intensity. *J Clin Oncol* 1990;8:1935.
119. Canellos GP, DeVita VT, Gold GL, et al. Cyclical combination chemotherapy for advanced breast carcinoma. *Br Med J* 1974;1:218.
120. Bonadonna G, Brusamalino MP, Valagussa R, et al. Combination chemotherapy as an adjuvant treatment in operable breast cancer. *N Engl J Med* 1976;298:405.
121. Bonadonna G, Calagussa R. Dose-response effect of adjuvant chemotherapy in breast cancer. *N Engl J Med* 1981;304:10.
122. Wood W, Korzan AH, Cooper R, et al. Dose and dose intensity of adjuvant chemotherapy for stage II node positive breast cancer. *N Engl J Med* 1994;330:1253.
123. Frei E III, Elias A, Wheeler C, et al. The relationship between high-dose treatment and combination chemotherapy: the concept of summation dose intensity. *Clin Cancer Res* 1998;4:2027.
124. Hryniuk W, Frei E III, Wright FA. A single scale for comparing dose- intensity of all chemotherapy regimens in breast cancer: summation dose-intensity. *J Clin Oncol* 1998;16:3137.
125. Bird MC, Godwin VA, Antrobus JH, Bosanquet AG. Comparison of an in vitro drug sensitivity by the differential staining cytotoxicity (DiSC) and colony-forming assays. Br J Cancer 1987;55:429.
126. Kern DH, Weisenthal LM. Highly specific prediction of antineoplastic drug resistance with an in vitro assay using suprapharmacologic drug exposures. *J Natl Cancer Inst* 1990;82:582.
127. Kochli OR, Sevin BU, Averette HE, Haller U. Overview of currently used chemosensitivity test systems in gynecologic malignancies and breast cancer. *Contrib Gynecol Obstet* 1994;19:12.
128. Andreotti PE, Cree IA, Kurbacher CM, et al. Chemosensitivity testing of human tumors using a microplate adenosine triphosphate luminescence assay: clinical correlation for cisplatin resistance of ovarian carcinoma. *Cancer Res* 1995;55:5276.
129. Schandendorf D, Worm M, Algermissen B, et al. Chemosensitivity testing of human malignant melanoma: a retrospective analysis of clinical response and in vitro drug sensitivity. *Cancer* 1994;73:103.
130. Elledge RM, Clark GM, Thant HM, et al. Rapid in vitro assay for predicting response to fluorouracil in patients with metastatic breast cancer. *J Clin Oncol* 1995;13:419.
131. Silber R, Degar B, Costin D, et al. Chemosensitivity of lymphocytes from patients with B-cell chronic lymphocytic leukemia to chlorambucil, fludarabine, and camptothecin analogs. *Blood* 1994;84:3440.
132. Bosanquet AG. Short-term in vitro drug sensitivity tests for cancer chemotherapy: a summary of correlations of test result with both patient response and survival. *Forum Trends Exp Clin Med* 1994;4:179.
133. Von Hoff DD, Kronmal R, Salmon SE, et al. A Southwest Oncology Group study on the use of human tumor cloning assay for predicting response in patients with ovarian cancer. *Cancer* 1991;67:20.
134. Black MM, Spear FD. Effects of cancer chemotherapeutic agents on dehydrogenase activity of human cancer tissue in vitro. *Am J Clin Pathol* 1953;218.
135. Black MM, Spear FD. Further observations on the effects of cancer chemotherapeutic agents on the in vitro dehydrogenase activity of cancer tissue. *J Natl Cancer Inst* 1954;143:1147.
136. Puck TT, Marcus PI. A rapid method for viable titration and clone production with HeLa cells in tissue culture: the use of X-irradiated cells to supply conditioning factors. *Proc Natl Acad Sci USA* 1955;41:432.
137. Salmon SE, Hamburger AW, Soehnlen B, et al. Quantitation of differential sensitivity of human tumor stem cells to anticancer drugs. *N Engl J Med* 1978;298:1321.
138. Clark GM, Von Hoff DD. Quality control of a multicenter human tumor cloning systems: the Southwest Oncology Group experience. In: Salmon SE, Trent JM, eds. *Human tumor cloning.* Orlando, FL: Grune & Stratton, 1984:255.
139. Selby P, Buick RN, Tannock I. A critical appraisal of the "human tumor stem cell assay." *N Engl J Med* 1983;308:129.
140. Fruehauf JP, Bosanquet AG. In vitro determination of drug response: a discussion of clinical application. In DeVita VT Jr, Hellman S, Rosenberg SA, eds. *Principles and practice of oncology,* 4th ed. Philadelphia: JB Lippincott, 1993;4:1.
141. Tanigawa N, Kern DH, Hikasa Y, Morton DL. Rapid assay for evaluating the chemosensitivity of human tumors in soft agar culture. *Cancer Res* 1982;42:2159.
142. Sondak VK, Bertelsen CA, Tanigawa N, et al. Clinical correlations with chemosensitivities measured in a rapid thymidine incorporation assay. *Cancer Res* 1984;44:1725.
143. Graham CH, Kobayashi H, Strankiewicz KS, et al. Rapid acquisition of multicellular drug resistance after a single exposure of mammary tumor cells to antitumor alkylating agents. *J Natl Cancer Inst* 1994;86:975.
144. Fruehauf JP, Kyshtoobayeva A, Parker R, et al. Quantitative determination of breast cancer MDR-1 expression by image analysis demonstrates a direct relationship between MDR-1 levels and in vitro resistance to taxol and doxorubicin. *Br Cancer Treat Rep* 1996;37[Suppl]:106.
145. Fruehauf JP, Manetta A. Use of the extreme drug resistance assay to evaluate mechanisms of resistance in ovarian cancer: taxol resistance and MDR-1 experience. *Contrib Gynecol Obstet* 1994;19:39.
146. Markman M. Chemosensitivity and chemoresistance assays: Are they clinically relevant? *Cancer* 1996;77:1020.
147. Cortazar P, Gazdar AF, Woods E, et al. Survival of patients with limited-stage small cell lung cancer treated with individualized chemotherapy selected by in vitro drug sensitivity testing. *Clin Cancer Res* 1997;3:741.
148. Cortazar P, Johnson BE. Review of the efficacy of individualized chemotherapy selected by in vitro drug sensitivity testing for patients with cancer. *J Clin Oncol* 1999;17:1625.
149. Benner SE, Fetting JH, Brenner MH. A stopping rule for standard chemotherapy for metastatic breast cancer: lessons from a survey of Maryland medical oncologists. *Cancer Invest* 1994;12:451.
150. Phillip RM, Bibby MC, Double JA. Appraisal of the predictive value of in vitro chemosensitivity assays. *J Natl Cancer Inst* 1990;82:1.
151. Griffin TW, Bogden AE, Reich SD, et al. Initial trials of the subrenal capsule assay as a predictor of tumor response to chemotherapy. *Cancer* 1983;52:2185.
152. Bennett JA, Pilon VA, MacDowell RT. Evaluation of growth and histology of human tumor xenografts implanted under the renal capsule of immunocompetent and immunodeficient mice. *Cancer Res* 1985;45:4963.
153. Lipsky MH, Chu MY, Yee LK, et al. Predictive sensitivity of human cancer cells to anticancer agents in vivo. *Proc Am Assoc Cancer Res* 1994;35:371.
154. Chu MY, Lipsky MH, Epstein J, et al. Predictive sensitivity of human cancer cells in vivo using semipermeable polysulfone fibers. *Pharmacology* 1998;56:318.
155. Waldman T, Zhang Y, Dillehay L, et al. Cell-cycle arrest versus cell death in cancer therapy. *Nat Med* 1997;3:1034.
156. Lamb JR, Friend SH. Which guesstimate is the best guesstimate? Predicting chemotherapeutic outcomes. *Nat Med* 1997;3:962.

Steven A. Rosenberg

CHAPTER 18

Principles of Cancer Management: Biologic Therapy

Biologic therapy is cancer treatment that produces antitumor effects primarily through the action of natural host defense mechanisms or the administration of natural mammalian substances. Biologic therapy has emerged as an important fourth modality for the treatment of cancer.* Its increased application is the result of a better understanding of the basic aspects of host defense mechanisms against cancer and rapid biotechnologic developments that made molecules available in quantities large enough for use in manipulating biologic processes *in vivo.* Although this field is still in its infancy, there are many examples of the successful application of biologic therapy to the treatment of human cancers.

BASIC PRINCIPLES OF TUMOR IMMUNOLOGY

Most applications of biologic therapy for cancer have attempted to stimulate immune defense mechanisms. The immune system evolved as a means to detect and eliminate molecules or pathogens that are recognized as "nonself" but not to react to host (self) tissues. Many immunotherapies attempted to cause the tumor to appear more "foreign" compared with normal tissues or tried to magnify relatively weak host immune reactions to growing tumors.

The immune system differs from most other organ systems because its cells are not in constant contact with each other. They circulate freely throughout the body in and out of the circulatory and lymphatic systems. Immune reactivity involves the integrated action of lymphocytes, monocytes, macrophages, basophils, eosinophils, dendritic cells, endothelial cells, and many other cells throughout the body. Although separate functions have been assigned to these cell types, it is now clear that they interact in many ways and can regulate one another's activities.

Immune cells secrete two major classes of soluble protein. The first of these lymphocyte products to be recognized was the antibody. Antibodies are a group of proteins composed of one or several units, each of which is composed of two pairs of different polypeptide chains (i.e., heavy and light chains). Each unit possesses two recognition sites, which are capable of combining with the immunizing antigen. The unique bond between antigen and antibody is part of the basis for the exquisite specificity that is the hallmark of immunologic reactivity. The existence of circulating antibodies was first demonstrated in 1890, and until recently, scientific studies of antibodies monopolized the study of immune reactions.

Since the 1970s, it has become clear that selected subpopulations of lymphoid cells can secrete a second (nonantibody) class of protein molecules. These molecules are not biochemically similar to antibodies, are produced in tiny amounts, and are not normally detectable in the circulation. Collectively called *cytokines,* they represent a new class of hormones with actions on many different target cells within and outside the immune system. Increasing knowledge of a wide variety of cytokines has dramatically altered the understanding of the functions of the immune system and created new possibilities for cancer immunotherapy.

*For a definitive compendium of information on the biologic therapy of cancer, refer to the companion volume, Rosenberg SA, ed. *Principles and practice of the biologic therapy of cancer.* Philadelphia: Lippincott Williams & Wilkins, 2000.

CELLS OF THE IMMUNE SYSTEM

The central cell in immune function is the lymphocyte. Lymphocytes constitute approximately 20% of blood leukocytes and fall into three major classes—B cells, T cells, and null cells—on the basis of ontogeny and function. Basic aspects of modern cellular immunology are presented in Chapter 4. Analysis of cell surface molecules, usually using monoclonal antibodies, revealed substantial heterogeneity in human leukocytes and lymphocytes. In 1982, the First International Workshop on Human Leukocyte Differentiation Antigens was held in Paris to attempt to codify the proliferating number of cell surface determinants detected on leukocytes and the antibodies used to detect them. As a result of the testing of large numbers of antibodies on target cells of many different leukocyte types, cluster analysis permitted the definition of groups of antigens that are similar and those that are clearly different on each type of target cell. This workshop defined the clusters of differentiation (CD), now used to describe cell surface components on leukocytes. A summary of selected CD classifications, the cells on which they are found, and the principal antibodies that are used to detect them as assigned by the Fourth International Workshop in 1989 are shown in Table 18-1.

The results of the Fifth International Workshop on Human Leukocyte Differentiation Antigens were presented in November 1993 and represented the efforts of more than 500 laboratories that analyzed 1450 antibodies. Based on these findings, 48 new CD clusters and subclusters were adopted and 14 previously established clusters were redefined. These additions and changes are shown in Table 18-2. An updated source of detailed information concerning all CD molecules can be found on the internet at http://www.ncbi.nlm.nih.gov/prow/guide/45277084.htm.

IMMUNE EFFECTOR MECHANISMS RESULTING IN CELL DESTRUCTION

A variety of immune effector mechanisms can cause destruction of vascularized tissue or of circulating tumor cells (see Chapter 4).

Antibodies can mediate cell destruction by the binding of complement or by action as an opsonin to facilitate phagocytosis by macrophages or by other phagocytic cells bearing Fc receptors.

The direct interaction of an immune cell with a target cell can also result in lysis, and a variety of immune cytotoxic cells have been described. The best-characterized lytic immune cell is the cytotoxic T lymphocyte (CTL). These T cells can interact with specific cell surface antigens by an interaction with the T-cell receptor and a class I or II major histocompatibility complex (MHC) molecule. This lysis appears to involve direct cell contact and can occur quickly, with the initial lytic events initiated within minutes of the adhesion of the target cell to the lymphocyte. Although binding of the CTL to the tumor target occurs by means of the T-cell receptor, other means for binding lytic cells to targets also produce lysis. One such mechanism is antibody-dependent cellular cytotoxicity. In this lysis, antibody bound to immune cells serves as a cross-link to a cytolytic cell bearing an Fc receptor. The Fc receptor on the immune effector binds to the free Fc portion of the antibody on the target cell; after this cross-linkage, lysis of the target cell occurs. Similarly, the phenomenon of lectin-dependent cellular cytotoxicity involves the association of a lytic cell with a target using a lectin such as concanavalin A or phytohemagglutinin as the cross-linking agent.

Natural killer (NK) cells can lyse selected cultured target cells without a prior sensitizing stimulus. The most common target for NK cells is the K562 leukemia cell line. NK lymphocytes have little or no ability to kill fresh tumor cells, and their physiologic role as an antitumor effector mechanism is unclear.

Lymphokine-activated killer (LAK) cells are lymphocytes that acquire the ability to lyse a broad array of tumor cells after incubation in interleukin (IL)-2. The precursor of LAK cells is a null lymphocyte, and most mature LAK cells do not bear T- or B-cell markers. However, one subpopulation of LAK cells has been shown to be CD3+, and precursor and effector LAK cells appear to bear the Leu-19 cell surface marker. LAK cells can lyse a broad array of malignant, but not normal, fresh target cells in 4-hour chromium-release assays. LAK cells also can lyse normal and malignant cultured lines. LAK cells are capable of lysing most cells that have their membranes perturbed by malignant transformation, culture, or other activation processes.

Activated macrophages also recognize and lyse tumor cells. Although most lymphocyte-mediated lysis can easily be detected in 4 hours, the measurement of significant macrophage-mediated lysis often requires 48 to 72 hours.

Many of the cytokines secreted by immune cells can mediate toxicity of tissue directly or by the recruitment of other inflammatory processes. For example, tumor necrosis factor (TNF) can interfere with the blood supply of tumors. Interferon (IFN)-γ has an antiproliferative effect on some tumor cells. Many chemotactic and vascular permeability factors that are involved in inflammatory responses also can indirectly mediate tumor destruction and may play a role in tumor immune phenomena.

CYTOKINES

Cytokines are soluble proteins produced by mononuclear cells of the immune system (usually lymphocytes or monocytes) that have regulatory actions on other cells of the immune system or target cells involved in immune reactions. Cytokines produced by lymphocytes are referred to as *lymphokines*, and cytokines produced by monocytes are referred to as *monokines*. Cytokines are true hormones, acting on other cells at a distance from the secreting cells.

It has been known for more than two decades that the soluble substances produced by immune cells are involved in immune function and regulation. These cytokines were first identified by the function they exhibit in *in vitro* assays. Lymphokines that inhibited the migration of macrophages were known as *migration-inhibition factors*, and other factors that activated macrophages were known as *macrophage-activation factors*. This identification of cytokines on the basis of function led to a confusing situation in which the same molecules were often described by various investigators using different assays for their detection.

Substantial progress in this field resulted from the use of molecular biologic techniques to clone the genes for these cytokines, express them in bacteria, purify them to homogeneity, and produce large amounts of homogeneous cytokines for detailed study. A new nomenclature referring to cytokines as *ILs* (meaning "between leukocytes") has been introduced that supplants the acronyms based on functional properties. In 1979, a meeting of the Second International Lymphokine Workshop in Ermatingen, Switzerland, reached a consensus that a variety of lymphokines that had been referred to as *T-cell*

TABLE 18-1. Workshop Antigen Designation by the Nomenclature Committee of the Fourth International Workshop on Human Leukocyte Differentiation Antigens[a]

CD Designation	*Selection of Assigned Monoclonal Antibodies*	*Main Cellular Reactivity*	*Recognized Membrane Component*	*Sequence/ CH-Structure Analyzed*
CD1a	NA1/34, T6, VIT6, Leu-6	Thy, DC, B subset	gp49	Y
CD1b	WM-25, 4A76, NUT2	Thy, DC, B subset	gp45	Y
CD1c	L161, M241, 7C6, PHM3	Thy, DC, B subset	gp43	Y
CD2	9.6, T11, 35.1	T	CD58 (LFA-3) receptor, gp50	Y
CD2R	T11.3, VIT13, D66	Act T	CD2 epitopes restr to act T	Y
CD3	T3, UCHT1, 38.1, Leu-4	T	CD3-complex (five chains), gp/p26, 20, 16	Y
CD4	T4, Leu-3a, 91.D6	T subset	Class II/HIV receptor, gp59	Y
CD5	T1, UCHT2, T101, HH9, AMG4	T, B subset	gp67	Y
CD6	T12, T411	T, B subset	gp100	
CD7	3a1, 4A, CL1.3, G3–7	T	gp40	Y
CD8	α Chain: T8, Leu-2a, M236, UCHT4, T811; β chain: T8/ 2T8-5H7	T subset	Class I receptor, gp32, αα or αβ dimer	Y
CD9	CLB-thromb/8, PHN200	Pre-B, M, plt	p24	
CD10	J5, VILAI, BA-3	Lymph prog, cALL, germ ctr B, G	Neutral endopeptidase, gp100, CALLA	Y
CD11a	MHM24, 2F12, CRIS-3	Leukocytes, broad	LFA-1, gp180/95	Y
CD11b	Mol, 5A4.C5, LPM19C	M, G, NK	C3bi receptor, gp155/95	
CD11c	B-LY6, L29, BL-4H4	M, G, NK, B subset	gp150/95	
CDw12	M67	M, G, plt	(p90–120)	
CD13	MY7, MCS-2, TÜK1, MOU28	M, G	Aminopeptidase N, gp150	Y
CD14	Mo2, UCHM1, VIMI3, MoP15	M, (G), LHC	gp55	Y
CD15	My1, VIM-D5	G, (M)	3-FAL, X-hapten	Y
CD16	BW209/2, HUNK2, VEP13, Leu-11c	NK, G, mac	FcRIII, gp50–65	Y
CDw17	GO35, Huly-m13	G, M, plt	Lactosylceramide	
CD18	MHM23, M232, IIH6, CLB54	Leukocytes broad	β chain to CD11a,b,c	Y
CD19	B4, HD37	B	gp95	Y
CD20	B1, 1F5	B	p37/32, ion channel?	Y
CD21	B2, HB5	B subset	C3d/EBV rec. (CR2), p140	Y
CD22	HD39, S-HCL1, To15	Cytopl B/surface B subset	gp135, homology to myelin assoc. gp (MAG)	Y
CD23	Blast-2, MHM6	B subset, act M, eo	FcεRII, gp45–50	Y
CD24	VIBE3, BA-1	B, G	gp41/38?	Y
CD25	TAC, 7G7/B6, 2A3	Act T, B, M	IL-2R β chain, gp55	Y
CD26	134-2C2, TS145	Act T	Dipeptidylpeptidase IV, gp120	Y
CD27	VIT14, S152, OKT18A, CLB-9F4	T subset	p55 (dimer)	
CD28	9.3, KOLT2	T subset	gp44	Y
CD29	K20, 4B4, A-1A5	Broad, T subset	VLA-β chain, integrin β1 chain, plt GPIIa	Y
CD30	Ki-1, Ber-H2, HSR4	Act T, B; Sternberg-Reed	gp120, Ki-1	Y
CD31	SG134, TM3	Plt, M, G, B, (T)	gp140, plt GPIIa	Y
CDw32	CIKM5, 41H16, IV.3	M, G, B	FcRII, gp40	Y
CD33	My9, H153, L4F3	M, prog, AML	gp67	Y
CD34	My10, B1-3C5, ICH-3	Prog	gp105–120	Y
CD35	TO5, CB04, J3D3	G, M, B	CR1	Y
CD36	5F1, CIMeg1	M, P, (B)	gp90, plt GPIV	Y
CD37	HD28, HH1, G28-1	B, (T, M)	gp40–52	Y
CD38	HB7, T16	Lymph prog, PC, act T	p45	Y
CD39	AC2, G28-2	B subset, (M)	gp70–100	Y
CD40	G28-5	B, carcinomas	gp50, homology to NGF receptor	Y
CD41	LO-PL3b, PBM 6.4, CLB-thromb/7	Plt	Plt GPIIb/IIIa complex	Y
CD42a	FMC25, BL-H6, GR-P	Plt	Plt GPIX, gp23	Y
CD42b	PHN89, PHN103, GN287	Plt	Plt GPIb, gp135/25	Y
CD43	OTH 71C5, G19-1, MEM-59	T, G, brain	Leukosialin, gp95	Y

(*continued*)

TABLE 18-1. (*Continued*)

CD Designation	*Selection of Assigned Monoclonal Antibodies*	*Main Cellular Reactivity*	*Recognized Membrane Component*	*Sequence/ CH-Structure Analyzed*
CD44	GRHL1, F10-44-2, 33-383, BRIC35	T, G, brain, RBC	Pgp-1, gp80–95	Y
CD45	T29/33, BMAC 1, AB187	Leukocytes	LCA, T200	Y
CD45RA	G1–15, FB-11-13, 73.5	T subset, B, G, M	Restricted T200, gp220	Y
CD45RB	PT17/26/16	T subset, B, G, M	Restricted T200	Y
CD45RO	UCHL1	T subset, B, G, M	Restricted T200, gp180	Y
CD46	HULYM5, 122-2, J4B	Leukocytes broad	Membrane cofactor protein, gp66/56	Y
CD47	BRIC 126, CIKM1, BRIC 125	Broad	gp47–52, N-linked glycan, Rh assoc.	
CD48	WM68, LO-MN25, J4–57	Leukocytes	gp41, PI-linked	
CDw49b	CLB-thromb/4, Gi14	Plt, act T, thy	VLA-α2 chain, plt GP1a	Y
CDw49d	B5G10, HP2/1, HP1/3	M, T, B, LHC, thy	VLA-α4 chain, gp150	
CDw49f	GoH3	Plt, (T)	VLA-α6 chain, gp140	
CDw50	101-1D2, 140-11	Leukocytes broad	gp180/108 PI-linked	
CD51	13C2, 23C6, NKI-M7, NKI-M9	Plt, (B)	VNR-α chain	Y
CDw52	097, YTH66.9, Campath-1	Leukocytes	Campath-1, gp21–28	
CD53	H129, H136, MEM-53, HD77	Leukocytes	gp32–40, PI-linked	
CD54	7F7, WEHI-CAMI	Broad	ICAM-1	Y
CD55	143-30, BRIC 110, BRIC 128, F2B-7.2	Broad	Decay accelerating factor	Y
CD56	Leu-19, NKH1, FP2-11.14, L185	NK, act lymph	gp220/135, NKH1, isoform of N-CAM	Y
CD57	Leu-7, L183, L187	NK, T, B sub, brain	gp110, HNK1	
CD58	G26, BRIC 5, TS2/9	Leukocytes, epithel	LFA-3 gp40–65	Y
CD59	Y53.1, MEM-43	Broad	gp18–20	
CDw60	M-T32, M-T21, M-T41, UM4D4	T sub	NeuAc-NeuAc-Gal-	Y
CD61	Y2/51, CLB-thromb/1, VI-PL2, BL-E6	P, (B)	Integrin β3 chain, VNR-β chain, plt GPIIIa	Y
CD62	CLB-thromb/6, CLB-thromb/5, RUU-SP1.18.1	Plt act	GMP-140 (PADGEM), gp140	Y
CD63	RUU-SP2.28, CLB-gran/12	Plt act, M, G, T, B	gp53	
CD64	Mab32.2, Mab22	M	FcRI, gp75	Y
CDw65	VIM2, HE10, CF4, VIM8	G, M	Ceramide-dodecasaccharide 4c	Y
CD66	CLB gran/10, YTH71.3	G	Phosphoprotein pp 180–200	
CD67	B13.9, G10F5, JML-H16	G	p100, PI-linked	
CD68	EBM11, Y2//131, Y-1/82A, Ki-M7, Ki-M6	Macrophages	gp110	
CD69	MLR3, L78, BL-Ac/p26, FN50	Act B, T	gp32/28, AIM	
CDw70	Ki-24, HNE 51, HNC 142	Act B, T, Sternberg-Reed	Ki-24	
CD71	138-18, 120-2A3, MEM-75, VIP-1, Nu-T1R2	Proliferating cells, mac	Transferrin receptor	Y
CD72	S-HCL2, J3-109, BU-40, BU-41	B	gp43/39	
CD73	1E9.28.I, 7G2.2.11, AD2	B subset, T subset	Ecto-5'-nucleotidase, p69	
CD74	LN2, BU-43, BU-45	B, M	Class II assoc. invariant chain, gp41/35/33	
CDw75	LN1, HH2, EBU-141	Mature B, (T subset)	p53?	
CD76	HD66, CRIS-4	Mature B, T subset	gp85/67	
CD77	38.13(BLA), 424/4A11, 424/3D9	Restr B	Globotriaosylceramide (Gb3)	
CDw78	Anti-Ba, LO-panB-a, 1588	B, (M)	?	

act, activated; AML, acute myeloid leukemia; B, B cells; cytopl, cytoplasmic; cALL, common null cell acute lymphocytic leukemia; CALLA, common acute lymphoblastic leukemia antigen; DC, dendritic cells; EBV, Epstein-Barr virus; eo, eosinophil; epithel, epithelial cells; G, granulocytes; germ ctr B, germinal center B cells; GMP, granule membrane protein; ICAM-1, intercellular adhesion molecule 1; IL, interleukin; LCA, leukocyte common antigen; LFA-1, lymphocyte function–associated antigen-1; LHC, epidermal Langerhans cells; lymph, lymphocyte; M, monocytes; mac, macrophages; MAG, myelin-associated glycoprotein; N-CAM, neural cell adhesion molecule; NGF, nerve growth factor; NK, natural killer cells; PADGEM, platelet activation–dependent granule–external membrane protein; PC, plasma cell; plt, platelets; prog, progenitor cells; RBC, red blood cell; Sternberg-Reed, Reed-Sternberg cells; T, T cells; thy, thymocytes; VLA, virus-like antigen.

[a]To be approved by International Union of Immunological Societies/World Health Organization. Members: Workshop Council: Bernard A, Beverley P, Boumsell L, Kishimoto T, Knapp W, McMichael A, Milstein C, Schlossman SF, Reinherz E, Riethmüller G, Springer TA, Winchester R; Workshop Organizers, T-Cell Section: Rieber P, Kurrle R, Meuer S; B-Cell Section: Dörken B, Moldenhauer G, Möller P, Pezzutto A, Schwartz-Albiez R; Myeloid Antigen Section: Knapp W, Bettelheim P, Gadd S, Köller U, Majdic O, Peschel C, Radaszkiewicz T, Stockinger H, Tetteroo PAT, van der Schot E; NK-/NL-Section: Schmidt RE, Feller AC, Hadam MR, Johnson J, Schubert J, Schwinzer R, Stoll M, Uciechowski P, Wonigeit K; Activation Antigen Section: Stein H, Schwarting R. Platelet Section: Kr.v.d. Borne AEG, de Bruijne-Admiraal LG, Modderman PW, Niewenhuis HK; Statistics Section: Gilks WR, Oldfield L, Rutherford A.

(From *J Immunol* 1989;143:758, with permission.)

TABLE 18-2. Modifications and Additions to CD Nomenclature by the Fifth International Workshop on Human Leukocyte Differentiation Antigens

CD Designation	*Common Name*	*Workshop Section*	*MW Reduced*	*CD Designation*	*Common Name*	*Workshop Section*	*MW Reduced*
CD15s	sLe^x, Sialyl Lewis^x	Adhesion	—	CD87	UPA-R	Myeloid	50–65
CD16	FcRIIIA/FcR-IIIB	Myeloid	50–65	CD88	C5aR	Myeloid	42
CD16b	FcRIIIB	Myeloid	48	CD89	FcαR	Myeloid	55–75
CD32	Previously CDw32, FcRII	Myeloid	40	CDw90	Thy-1	Myeloid	25–35
CD42a	GPIX	Platelets	23	CD91	α_2M-R	Myeloid	600
CD42b	GPIB-α	Platelets	135, 23	CDw92	—	Myeloid	70
CD42c	GPIB-β	Platelets	22	CD93	—	Myeloid	120
CD42d	GPV	Platelets	85	CD94	KP43	NK cell	43
CD44	Pgp-1	Adhesion	80–90	CD95	APO-1, FAS	Activation	42
CD44R	Restricted epitope on CD44	Adhesion	—	CD96	TACTILE	Activation	160
CD49a	VLA-1, α1 integrin chain	Adhesion	210	CD97	—	Activation	74, 80, 89
CD49b	VLA-2, α2 integrin chain	Adhesion	160	CD98	4F2, 2F3	T cell	80, 40
CD49c	VLA-3, α3 integrin chain	Adhesion	125	CD99	E2, MIC2	T cell	32
CD49d	VLA-4, α4 integrin chain	Adhesion	150, 80, 70	CD99R	CD99 monoclonal antibody restricted	T cell	32
CD49e	VLA-5, α5 integrin chain	Adhesion	135, 25	CD100	BB18, A8	T cell	150
CD49f	VLA-6, α6 integrin chain	Adhesion	120, 25	CDw101	BB27, BA27	T cell	140
CD50	ICAM-3	Adhesion	124	CD102	ICAM-2	Adhesion	60
CD51/CD61	Complex dependent epitope	Adhesion	—	CD103	HML-1	Adhesion	150, 25
CD52	Campath-1	Blind	21–28	CD104	β4 integrin chain	Adhesion	220
CD62E	E-selectin, ELAM-1	Adhesion	115	CD105	Endoglin	Endothelial	95
CD62L	L-selectin, LAM-I, TQ-1	Adhesion	75–80	CD106	VCAM-1, INCAM-110	Endothelial	100, 110
CD62P	P-selectin, GMP-140, PADGEM	Adhesion	150	CD107a	LAMP-1	Platelet	110
CD66a	BGP	Myeloid	180–200	CD107b	LAMP-2	Platelet	120
CD66b	CD67, p100, CGM6	Myeloid	95–100	CDw108	—	Adhesion	80
CD66c	NCA	Myeloid	90–95	CDw109	8A3, 7D1	Endothelial	170/150
CD66d	CGM1	Myeloid	30	CD115	CSF-1R, M-CSFR	Myeloid	150
CD66e	CEA	Myeloid	180–200	CDw116	HGM-CSFR, GM-CSFR	Cytokine	75–85
CD67	Now CD66b	—	—	CD117	SCFR, cKIT	Cytokine	145
CD70	CD27-ligand	Activation	55, 75, 95, 110, 170	CDw119	IFN-γR	Cytokine	90
CDw76	Previously CD76	B cell	NA	CD120a	TNFR; 55 kD	Cytokine	55
CD79a	mb-1, Igα	B cell	33, 40	CD120b	TNFR; 75 kD	Cytokine	75
CD79b	B29, Igβ	B cell	33, 40	CDw121a	IL-1R; type 1	Cytokine	80
CD80	B7, BB1	B cell	60	CDw121b	IL-1R; type 2	Cytokine	68
CD81	TAPA-1	B cell	22	CD122	IL-2R; 75 kD, IL-2Rβ	Cytokine	75
CD82	R2, IA4, 4F9	B cell	50–53	CDw124	IL-4R	Cytokine	140
CD83	HB15	B cell	43	CD126	IL-6R	Cytokine	80
CDw84	—	B cell	73	CDw127	IL-7R	Cytokine	75
CD85	VMP-55, GH1/75	B cell	120, 83	CDw128	IL-8R	Cytokine	58–67
CD86	FUN-1, BU63	B cell	80	CDw130	IL-GR-gp130SIG	Cytokine	130

BGP, biliary glycoprotein; CEA, carcinoembryonic antigen; HGM-CSFR, human granulocyte-macrophage colony-stimulating factor receptor; HML, human mucosal lymphocyte; ICAM, intercellular adhesion molecule; IFN, interferon; IL, interleukin; INCAM, inducible cell adhesion molecule; LAMP, lysosome-associated membrane protein; NCA, nonspecific cross-reacting antigen; NK, natural killer cell; TNFR, tumor necrosis factor receptor; UPA-R, urokinase plasminogen activator receptor; VCAM, vascular cell adhesion molecule; VLA, virus-like antigen. (From Schlossman SF, Boumsell L, Gills W, et al. CD antigens 1993. *Blood* 1994;83:879, with permission.)

growth factor, thymocyte-stimulating factor, thymocyte mitogenic factor, killer cell helper factor costimulator, and *secondary CTL-inducing factor* were all the same molecule and should be referred to as *IL-2.* The term *IL-1* was adopted to refer to a monocyte product previously called *lymphocyte-activating factor.* Since that time, many cytokines have been described. This list is rapidly expanding as new hormones produced by cells of the immune system are described.

Cytokines are proteins or glycoproteins, mostly with molecular weights in the range of 15,000 to 40,000, and many are glycosylated, although it appears that the glycosylation is often not essential for function. In many cases, the cytokines described in mouse and human are structurally related. For example, IL-1α shows a 61% to 65% amino acid homology among human, rabbit, and mouse. Some lymphokines exhibit species specificity; for example, IL-1, IL-2, IL-5, and IL-6 derived from human are active on cells from mouse and human, but IL-3, IL-4, and IFN-γ derived from humans are active only on human cells and not on mouse cells.

Most research on cytokines has involved *in vitro* studies or animal studies. Many cytokines, such as IFN-α, IFN-β, IFN-γ, IL-2, TNF, and the colony-stimulating factors, have reached clinical application in patients with cancer.

A summary of the major characteristics of IL-1 through IL-18 follows and is taken from S. K. Durum in *Principles and Practice of Biologic Therapy of Cancer*, S. A. Rosenberg, ed. The characteristics of the IFN and colony-stimulating factors are shown in Table 18-3 and are further discussed in Chapters 20.1 and 53.4.

INTERLEUKIN-1

IL-1[1,2] was among the earliest cytokines identified because it has so many potent activities. Many features of the IL-1 system, however, are not particularly representative of cytokines. IL-1 has an unusual mechanism of release from the cells that produce it. The two family members, α and β, are only distantly related but act on the same receptor. It has two dedicated inhibitors that block ligand-receptor interaction. IL-1 is a powerful inducer of inflammatory processes, both local and global, although knockout of the IL-1 system only modestly reduces these processes. Clinically, the main goals have been to block the IL-1 system in inflammatory states, such as rheumatoid arthritis (RA) and septic shock.

Proteins

Three members of the IL-1 family exist: α, β, and the receptor antagonist, encoded by a cluster of genes. IL-1α[3] and -β[4] have little homology to one another, but it is accurate to term them both *IL-1* because they act on the same receptor. Neither α nor β has a typical signal sequence, and both are released from the producing cell by an unusual mechanism. Mature 17-kD IL-1α is produced from a biologically inactive 31-kD precursor by cleavage[5] with caspase 1. Mature 17-kD IL-1α is also produced by cleavage from a different 31-kD precursor, which is biologically active. The receptor antagonist[6] is produced in two forms by alternative message splicing: one

TABLE 18-3. Interferons, Colony-Stimulating Factors, and Tumor Necrosis Factor, with Their Biologic Activities

Cytokine	*Molecular Weight (kD)*[a]	*Biologic Effects*
IFN-α or -β1[b]	16–27	Antiproliferative to certain tumor cells; promotes partial reversal of the malignant phenotype; enhances the expression of surface molecules, including β2-microglobulin, Fc receptors, tumor-associated antigens, and MHC class I antigens; augments NK activity; modulates B-cell function; inhibits suppressor T-cell activity; activates monocytes/macrophages; exerts antiviral activity; interacts with (enhances, inhibits) growth factors, oncogenes, and other cytokines; activates CTL
IFN-γ	15.5–25.0	Exerts antiviral activity; augments NK activity; induces expression of MHC class I and II molecules; activates macrophages; interacts with (enhances, inhibits) other cytokines; induces IL-2 receptors; mediates antimicrobial activity; regulates lipid metabolism; induces B-cell immunoglobulin production; suppresses IL-4 activities on B cells; activates CTL; enhances tumor-associated antigen expression; regulates differentiation
TNF-α[c]	17 (secretory), 26 (membrane form)	Stimulates T-cell proliferation; enhances NK activity; induces macrophage tumoricidal activity; directly cytotoxic to some tumor cells; induces systemic acute phase responses; activates PMNs; costimulates mitogen-activated B cells; enhances expression of MHC class I and class II molecules; stimulates production of other cytokines, including CSFs; affects (reduces or increases) expression of oncogene products; induces cytokine receptor expression; activates endothelial cells (expression of adhesion molecules); mediates catabolic processes, septic shock, and inflammation; induces myeloid differentiation
G-CSF	20–25	Stimulates growth of granulocyte colonies; activates mature granulocytes; increases antibody-dependent, neutrophil-mediated cytotoxicity; stimulates proliferation and differentiation of leukemic cells
GM-CSF	18–30	Stimulates growth of granulocyte, monocyte, and early erythrocyte progenitors; stimulates some megakaryocyte progenitors; enhances ADCC; activates mature granulocytes and monocytes; some stimulation of proliferation of leukemic progenitors; chemotactic for monocytes and PMNs; up-regulates CR3 receptors on PMNs and monocytes; stimulates production of other cytokines (M-CSF and TNF) by monocytes
M-CSF	45–70	Stimulates growth of monocyte colonies; supports survival of macrophages; activates mature monocytes; enhances ADCC by monocytes; stimulates production/secretion of cytokines, plasminogen activator, oxygen reduction products, and acidic isoferritins by macrophages; enhances Fc receptor, CR3 receptor, and MHC class II expression on macrophages; stimulates macrophage pinocytosis; chemotactic

ADCC, antibody-dependent cellular cytotoxicity; CR3, complement receptor-3; CSF, colony-stimulating factor; CTL, cytotoxic T lymphocyte; G, granulocyte; IFN, interferon; IL, interleukin; M, macrophage; MHC, major histocompatibility complex; NK, natural killer cell; PMN, polymorphonuclear leukocyte; TNF, tumor necrosis factor.

[a]Molecular weights vary according to level of glycosylation; G- and GM-CSF are single polypeptide chains; M-CSF is a homodimer.

[b]More than 20 closely related genes for IFN-α exist (subtypes: 80% to 85% amino acid homology to each other; 90% nuclear homology). Only a single gene exists for IFN-γ, and possibly two genes for IFN-β.

[c]TNF-β lymphotoxin. Lymphotoxin is produced by lymphocytes, is approximately 30% homologous with TNF-α, acts at the same receptor, and shares multiple biologic activities with TNF-α. Other members of this cytokine family may exist that have yet to be purified, sequenced, and cloned; these proteins have been implicated in monocyte- and lymphocyte-mediated tumor cell killing and are not neutralized by monoclonal antibodies to TNF-α or TNF-β.

(From Mulé JJ, Rosenberg SA. Catalogue of cytokines. *Biol Ther Cancer Updates* 1992;2:1, with permission.)

secreted form with a signal peptide and a second intracellular form lacking a signal peptide.

Producers

The most prolific IL-1–producing cells are macrophages following stimulation with a variety of microbial products or other agents, including cytokines. Many other cell types, such as keratinocytes, also produce IL-1. The IL-1 promoters are complex, perhaps accounting for the ability of these genes to respond to so many different stimuli in different cell types. In macrophages, the mechanism of IL-1 induction is partly based on the PU-1 transcription factor in cooperation with other nuclear factors.[7,8] IL-1 production is also regulated by message stability, message translation, and the release mechanism. The receptor antagonist is produced concurrently with IL-1α and -β in many cell types, acting as a natural buffer to the action of IL-1.

Receptors and Cellular Response

Two IL-1 binding proteins exist: IL-1RI, which serves all known receptor function,[9] and IL-1RII, which serves as a "decoy" receptor.[10] These genes are also linked to the IL-1 gene cluster in humans, but not in mice. IL-1RI is a member of the "toll" family of receptors. After IL-1 binding, IL-1 receptor accessory proteins,[11] a kinase [IL-2 receptor–associated kinase (IRAK)][12] and TRAF6,[13] are recruited to the complex. IL-18 receptor forms a similar complex (see Interleukin-18, later in this chapter). MyD88 serves as an adaptor protein, linking IRAK to the receptor complex.[14] Intracellular cascades lead to activation of several types of transcription factors, including nuclear factor κB[15] and AP-1.[16] This results in the induction of many genes, including a number of other inflammatory cytokines, such as IL-6. A wide variety of cell types respond to IL-1. IL-18 signaling has many parallels with that of IL-1.

Activities

IL-1 is considered a key mediator of inflammation.[2] It has a broad spectrum of inflammatory activities, including local effects, such as induction of prostaglandins, chemokines, and adhesion molecules. IL-1 also has global effects, such as fever, the acute-phase response, and hypotension. Knockout mice show deficiency in local inflammation and delayed-type hypersensitivity and are resistant to collagen-induced arthritis.[17] The fact that IL-1 deficiency does not eliminate inflammation has been interpreted to mean that other cytokines with overlapping activities, such as TNF and IL-6, are equally important.

Clinical Use

Trials were performed in cancer patients[18] with some benefit in preventing thrombocytopenia induced by chemotherapy, but significant toxic side effects, such as hypotension, arrhythmia, and pulmonary-capillary leakage, occurred. Intratumoral injection in mouse cancers has shown promising responses. Blocking IL-1 activity via receptor antagonist, soluble receptors, or newly tailored drugs shows promise in controlling inflammatory diseases, such as RA and septic shock, probably most effectively if combined with blockade of other inflammatory cytokines, such as TNF and IL-6.

INTERLEUKIN-2

IL-2 was originally discovered as a growth factor for T cells *in vitro* and is one of the most extensively studied cytokines. Knockout of IL-2 in mice suggests complex regulatory roles, perhaps in programming T cells for death. The IL-2 receptor complex shares components with receptors for IL-4, -7, -9, and -15. IL-2 has been used clinically for acquired immunodeficiency syndrome, cancer, and for *ex vivo* expansion of T cells directed against tumors and viruses.

Protein

IL-2[19,20] is a 15-kD protein, contains one internal disulfide bond, and is a member of a family of cytokines (IL-4, -7, -9, and -15) containing α helixes.

Producers

IL-2 is produced by T lymphocytes after activation by antigen-MHCs and costimulators on the surface of antigen-presenting cells. The T helper 1 (Th1) subset of memory T cells retains the capacity to produce IL-2, whereas the Th2 subset loses this capacity, producing IL-4 instead.[21]

Receptor and Cellular Response

The IL-2 receptor comprises three chains: α,[22] β,[23] and γ_c.[24] The β and γ_c chains are members of a cytokine receptor superfamily, whereas the α chain is related to IL-15Rα. The β and γ chains are essential for signaling, whereas the α chain increases affinity of the complex for IL-2 but is not required. After binding of IL-2, the Janus kinase Jak3,[25,26] associated with the γ_c chain, phosphorylates tyrosines on the β chain, which serve as docking sites for signal transducers and activators of transcription protein (STAT)3 and -5. The STATs[22,27] are then phosphorylated and translocate to the nucleus, where they serve as transcription factors. Many other intracellular second messenger pathways are also triggered by IL-2[28] and involve lck, syk, ras, phosphoinositide 3 kinase (PI3-kinase), protein kinase C, and Akt. The γ_c chain of the IL-2 receptor is shared by the receptors for IL-4, -7, -9, and -15. Jak3 is also a component of the signaling complex in these receptors.

Activities

The property that led to the discovery of IL-2 was its induction of activated T-cell proliferation.[19] Thus, IL-2 is widely used for propagating T-cell lines. Knockout of IL-2 in mice,[29] however, resulted in excessive, uncontrolled T-cell proliferation, leading to the concept that IL-2 is not essential for growth *in vivo,* but is essential for programming T cells to die. Other activities of IL-2 include stimulation of cytotoxicity in NK and T cells and acting as a cofactor in activating macrophages and B cells.

Clinical Use

IL-2 has been used clinically in several ways (see Chapter 20.2). Treatment of malignant melanoma renal cell carcinoma has shown efficacy.[30,31] A significant side effect of IL-2 is the vascular leak syndrome.[32] IL-2 has been used for *ex vivo* expansion of

LAK cells, tumor-infiltrating T cells,[33] and antiviral T cells,[34–36] which are then returned to the patient. Anti–IL-2 receptor shows promise in blocking rejection of organ transplantations.[37]

INTERLEUKIN-3

IL-3 is produced by activated T cells and induces hematopoiesis. Its receptor shares components with IL-5 and granulocyte-macrophage colony-stimulating factor (GM-CSF). It is used clinically to sustain explanted hematopoietic stem cells before reinfusion.

Proteins

IL-3[38,39] is linked to IL-4, -5, -9, and -13 in humans.

Producers

Activated T cells are the major producers of IL-3.[40] Activated mast cells are also producers.

Receptors

Two chains that compose the IL-3 receptor exist in humans: IL-3Rα[41] and IL-3Rβ_c,[42] which are shared by the receptors for GM-CSF and IL-5. In the mouse, two different β chains exist. Both α and β are members of the cytokine receptor superfamily. Cross-linking of the α to the β chain triggers receptor activation.[43] The nature of this cross-linking process is thought to resemble that of the IL-2 and IL-4 receptors, in that the ligand directly binds one chain with intermediate affinity. The second receptor chain, which cannot bind ligand on its own, then recognizes some features of the complex formed by the ligand and the other receptor component. Jak2 is associated with the β chain[44] and activates STAT5.[45] A number of other second messenger pathways are also activated.[46] The cellular response includes survival, such as the pathway leading to disposal of BAD, the proapoptotic protein.[46,47]

Activities

IL-3 stimulates production of macrophages, granulocytes, erythrocytes, and megakaryocytes from primitive pluripotential stem cells. Knockouts indicate that IL-3 is not required during normal hematopoiesis, indicating its importance probably lies in the hematopoietic stimulation during immune responses. Mature myelomonocytic-lineage cells also react to IL-3.

Clinical Use

IL-3 has been tested extensively for a variety of potential clinical uses.[48] In individuals with normal hematopoiesis, IL-3 treatment increased platelets, reticulocytes, and leukocytes and showed only mild side effects.[49] To increase hematopoiesis, IL-3 has been tested in myelodysplastic syndrome, aplastic anemia, Diamond-Blackfan anemia, chemotherapy, bone marrow transplantation, and stem cell mobilization. Although responses were observed, it has not been adopted as a therapeutic agent. IL-3 is widely used, however, as part of a cytokine cocktail to sustain hematopoietic stem cells *ex vivo* for treatment after radiation or chemotherapy (i.e., promoting introduction of recombinant constructs for gene therapy).[50,51]

INTERLEUKIN-4

IL-4 is an important cofactor in B-lymphocyte activation, particularly for production of immunoglobulin E (IgE). One type of IL-4 receptor incorporates γ_c, as do IL-2, -7, -9, and -15. IL-4 is closely related to IL-13 and can share receptor components and signaling pathways. IL-4 is critical in directing activated T cells into the Th2 pathway. Overproduction is implicated in atopy.

Proteins

IL-4[52–54] is 20 kD, with six cysteines involved in intrachain disulfide bonds, and forms four α helices. The human IL-4 gene is found in a cluster together with genes for IL-3, -5, -9, and -13.

Producers

Several types of T cells produce IL-4 after activation by antigen-MHC complexes and costimulators on the surface of antigen-presenting cells.[21] IL-4 is a key member of the spectrum of cytokines produced by Th2 T cells. In mice, CD4 T cells that express NK1 are also producers, as are a subset of CD8 T cells. Mast cells and basophils also produce IL-4.[55] The induction of Th2 cell development is dependent on IL-4 produced by T cells themselves.[56] Production of IL-4 requires the transcription factor GATA3[57] and, possibly, c-maf.[58]

Receptors

The primary binding chain, IL-4Rα,[59] forms two types of receptor complexes: IL-4Rα + γ_c and IL-4Rα + IL-13Rα.[60] These receptor chains are members of the cytokine receptor superfamily. IL-4 first binds to IL-4Rα; γ_c is then recruited to the complex. The Janus kinase Jak3, bound to the intracellular domain of γ_c, is required for many, but not all, IL-4 effects.[61] STAT6 is required for IL-4 signaling.[62] IRS-1 is an important adaptor molecule, coupling the receptor to second messenger pathways other than the Jak-STAT pathway.[60,63]

Activities

IL-4 was discovered as a growth factor for preactivated B cells and induces class II MHC expression on B cells. In macrophages, it suppresses production of inflammatory cytokines and it has effects on endothelial cells and fibroblasts. Knockout mice show major defects in Th2 cell generation and in IgE production,[64] suggesting that the selective value of IL-4 may be immunity against parasitic infections.

Clinical Use

An overactive IL-4 pathway appears to be one component of atopy.[65–67] Therefore, IL-4 presents a therapeutic target for allergy. IL-4 itself could be used to divert immunity away from autoimmune or inflammatory directions.

INTERLEUKIN-5

IL-5 induces production of eosinophils during immune responses, which probably contributes to protection against some kinds of parasites. It shares a receptor component with IL-3 and GM-CSF.

Proteins

IL-5[68,69] is a disulfide-linked homodimer, which is unusual among the ILs, and is heavily glycosylated. Its crystal structure resembles that of two IL-4 molecules with two bundles, each with four α helices.[70] It is genetically linked to IL-3, -4, -9, and -13 in humans.[68]

Producers

IL-5 is produced by activated Th2 cells,[21] as well as mast cells and eosinophils.

Receptors

The receptors for IL-5 consist of two chains: IL-5Rα[71] and IL-5Rβ_c,[42] which is shared by the receptors for GM-CSF and IL-3. Both chains are members of the cytokine receptor superfamily. Cross-linking principles are similar to IL-3, as are the ensuing Jak2-STAT5 pathways and other second-messenger pathways.[46]

Activities

IL-5 was initially identified as a T-cell factor that induced production of eosinophils.[72] Knockout of IL-5 eliminated the eosinophilia induced by helminth infection,[73] whereas baseline production of eosinophils was normal. IL-5 also promotes local accumulation[74] and sustains the life span and function of eosinophils in tissues, such as the lung and bowel. Evidence exists that IL-5, presumably via its eosinophil activities, contributes to protection from helminth infections.[75,76]

Clinical Use

IL-5 has long been implicated in allergic asthma.[77] Efforts are therefore being made to develop IL-5 antagonists.[78]

INTERLEUKIN-6

IL-6 is a key inflammatory mediator produced by many cell types. It is the major inducer of the acute-phase response and fever. IL-6 receptor shares the gp130 chain with several other cytokine receptors.

Proteins

IL-6 is a glycoprotein of 21 to 28 kD.

Producers

IL-6 is produced after stimulation by many cell types, including T and B lymphocytes, macrophages, fibroblasts, and endothelial cells.

Receptors

Two components of the IL-6 receptor exist: a ligand-specific α chain[79] and a signal-transducing gp130 chain,[80] which is shared by receptors for leukocyte inhibitory factor (LIF), oncostatin M (OSM), ciliary neurotrophic factor (CNTF), IL-11, and CT-1. The α chain binds IL-6. This complex then cross-links multiple gp130 chains, initiating signal transduction. Unlike many cytokine receptors, the α chain has no intracellular signaling function in this class of receptors. The Janus kinases Jak1, Jak2, and Tyk2 are activated, as are the transcription factors STAT1, -3, and -5, as well as other signal transduction pathways, such as the ras–mitogen-activated protein kinase pathway.[81]

Activities

IL-6[82,83] was originally characterized based on its activity in inducing Ig synthesis by activating B cells. Knockout of IL-6[84,85] showed defects in a number of inflammatory processes, including production of acute-phase reactants and bone loss after estrogen depletion. Fever responses depend on IL-6.[86] Hematopoietic defects were also found in IL-6 knockouts.[87]

Clinical Use

Blocking IL-6 may alleviate RA and may also be effective in other autoimmune, inflammatory, and bone-erosive diseases. In mice, IL-6 is required for development of oil-induced plasmacytomas[88] and is involved in tumor cachexia.[89] In humans, IL-6 is a growth factor for myelomas,[90] suggesting further applications of IL-6 blockers.

INTERLEUKIN-7

IL-7 is produced by stromal cells and is essential for T lymphopoiesis, partly because of a survival or "trophic" effect, a partial role in VDJ recombination. This is the pathway deficient in X-linked, severe combined immunodeficiency in humans. IL-7 also has trophic effects on mature T and B lymphocytes and is therefore potentially useful in the clinic as an adjuvant.

Proteins

IL-7 is a 25-kD protein predicted to contain four α helices and an internal disulfide bond.[91] After secretion, it binds to extracellular matrix via a glycosaminoglycan-binding site,[92] which could be the form encountered by developing thymocytes.

Producers

Unlike most ILs, IL-7 is produced constitutively by nonhematopoietic cells. In the thymus, the IL-7 producer resembles the cortical epithelial cell.[93] In bone marrow, the producer is a reticular stromal cell.[94] Other sources include the intestine,[95] skin,[96] and follicular dendritic cells.[94]

Receptors

The primary binding chain for IL-7 is IL-7Rα.[97] The IL-7–IL-7Rα complex then recruits γ_c,[98,99] bearing Jak3 to the complex. TSLP, a homologue of IL-7, also binds the IL-7Rα chain but does not recruit γ_c and Jak3.[100] Jak1 and a number of other kinases are induced,[101] including PI3-kinase. STAT3 and -5 partly mediate the nuclear effects. Because γ_c is also a component of the receptors for IL-2, -4, -9, and -15, some similarities appear to exist in the signal transduction pathways.

Activities

IL-7 was discovered based on its activity in inducing proliferation of murine pro-B cells.[91] B-cell development depends on IL-7 in mice, but not in humans.[102] Normal T-cell development requires IL-7 based on the knockout phenotypes for IL-7[103] and its receptor,[104] which show a severe block at an early stage in T-cell development. A related block is seen in X-linked, severe combined immunodeficiency in humans, which is in γ_c, a component of the IL-7 receptor. This requirement for IL-7 is partly attributed to its trophic activity on lymphoid progenitors[105] and its promotion of VDJ recombination.[106] In mice, the γσ lineage is particularly dependent on IL-7, perhaps not only during thymic generation, but also for survival in the intestine and skin. Pharmacologic activity of IL-7 has been observed in mice, inducing increases in B and T cells.[107,108] Overexpression of IL-7 in mice can induce lymphomagenesis.[109] In human skin, IL-7 may provide trophic support for the survival of lymphoma cells.[110]

Clinical Use

IL-7 has not been tested clinically. Potential clinical uses of IL-7 include boosting immunity to infectious diseases or prolonging the life of lymphocytes, as in acquired immunodeficiency syndrome. Antagonists to IL-7 might be effective in treating autoimmune diseases, blocking rejection of allografted organs, or treating lymphoma.

INTERLEUKIN-8

IL-8 induces chemotaxis and activation of neutrophils. It is one of the chemokines, a large group of chemotactic cytokines. IL-8 signals through seven transmembrane G protein–coupled receptors that are related to other chemokine receptors.

Proteins

IL-8[111–114] is a 6- to 8-kD glycoprotein containing two intrachain disulfide bonds. At high concentrations, IL-8 homodimerizes via hydrogen bonding. It is presented to neutrophils on endothelial cell surfaces.[115] IL-8 was the first to be discovered of the family of cytokines known as *chemokines.*[116] More than 50 members have been identified; only IL-8 has the IL terminology. IL-8 is one of a subgroup termed *CXC chemokines* and is linked to a group of these genes. Mice lack a close homologue to human IL-8. It is thought that IL-8's inflammatory roles are fulfilled in mice by other chemokines using the same receptor.

Producers

Many cell types produce IL-8 after stimulation with lipopolysaccharide, IL-1, or TNF,[117] including macrophages, endothelial cells, and keratinocytes.

Receptors

Two functional IL-8 receptors exist: CXCR1[118] and CXCR2.[119,120] They are both members of the seven-transmembrane family of receptors that includes rhodopsin. These receptors also respond to other chemokines. The two receptors induce some overlapping and distinct responses.[121] Receptors are coupled to G proteins, including Gi2α,[122] which trigger downstream events involving phospholipase C, diacylglycerol, inositol triphosphate, release of calcium from intracellular stores, RhoA, and the ras pathway.

Activities

IL-8 induces neutrophil chemotaxis, respiratory burst, and degranulation. In rabbits, blocking IL-8 with antibodies has potent inhibitory effects on some inflammatory processes, particularly of the lung.[123–125] Knockouts in mice cannot directly address IL-8 function because no close IL-8 homologue exists in mice. Mice lack CXCR1. Knockout of the receptor CXCR2, however, greatly affects neutrophil attraction to inflamed peritoneum,[126] which establishes that chemokines are involved in neutrophil accumulation *in vivo.* IL-8 also induces angiogenesis.[127]

Clinical Use

Increased IL-8 is detected in a variety of human clinical conditions, ranging from myocardial infarction to RA,[128] and suggests potential applications for IL-8 blockers. In rabbits, a number of studies have shown that anti–IL-8 inhibits inflammation of various tissues. Despite the numerous chemokines that exist, blocking IL-8 alone can be sufficient.

INTERLEUKIN-9

IL-9 is related to IL-2, -4, -7, and -15 and has some overlapping activities based most likely on sharing some receptor components. It is produced by T cells and acts on lymphocytes and mast cells. It may be involved in Hodgkin's disease and lymphoma.

Proteins

IL-9[129,130] is predicted to have an α-helical topology like IL-2, -4, -7, and -15. The human IL-9 gene is found in a cluster together with genes for IL-3, -4, -5, -9, and -13. This does not apply to mice. Ten cysteines exist, implying extensive intrachain disulfide bonding, heavy N-linked glycosylation, and a high isoelectric point (approximately ten).

Producers

Memory helper T cells produce IL-9 after activation.[131] This induction involves a cascade of cytokines, including IL-2, -4, and -10, eventually leading to IL-9 production.[132] Murine Th2 clones are producers.[133]

Receptors

The IL-9 receptor α chain[134] is a member of the hematopoietin superfamily. In humans, the IL-9 receptor α chain is unusual because it is encoded on chromosomes X and Y.[135] Four IL-9Rα pseudogenes also exist. The receptor complex shares the γ_c chain[136] with receptors for IL-2, -4, -7, and -15. After receptor ligation, Jak3 (γ_c-associated) and Jak1 (IL-9Rα–associated) increase their tyrosine kinase activity, phosphorylating the IL-9Rα chain, adaptor protein IRS-1,[137] and transcription factors STAT1, -3, and -5.[138,139]

Activities

IL-9 was discovered as a growth factor for T-cell clones[129] and independently as a growth factor for mast cell lines.[130,140] It is not clear, however, whether a normal T-cell growth role should be ascribed to IL-9, because normal T cells have not been found to proliferate in response to it until after 10 days or so of prior *in vitro* stimulation. Some transformed T cells, however, can respond to IL-9, and human T-cell leukemia–transformed T cells produce it[141]; overexpression of IL-9 as a transgene induced T-cell transformation,[142] suggesting possible autocrine function. This was also suggested for Hodgkin's disease.[143] Mast cells and eosinophils, B lymphocytes,[144] and hematopoietic stem cells[145] also respond to IL-9. Because its receptor is a member of the γ_c family, overlapping activities are expected to be present with other cytokines in this group.

Clinical Use

No extensive preclinical data on IL-9 are available. The possibility that it has autocrine activity in Hodgkin's disease and T lymphomas suggests potential uses for IL-9 antagonists.

INTERLEUKIN-10

IL-10 is a powerful inhibitor of inflammatory and immune responses, partly via its inhibition of some macrophage functions. It is produced by Th2 cells. Its receptor is related to IFN receptors.

Proteins

Human IL-10 is an 18-kD monomer with little glycosylation and two presumed intrachain disulfide bonds.

Producers

Activated Th2 cells were the originally described IL-10 producers. Other cell types, including macrophages and keratinocytes, however, also produce IL-10. Epstein-Barr virus encodes an active IL-10 homologue.[146]

Receptors and Cellular Response

The first identified component of IL-10 receptor[147,148] is related to the IFN receptors. It is expressed by many types of hematopoietic cells. In mice, a second receptor component, CRF2-4, has been identified,[149] which is related and linked to the IFN receptors. Jak1 and Tyk2 are activated by IL-10.[150] STAT3 mediates some downstream effects in macrophages.[151]

Activities

IL-10 was originally discovered and cloned[152] as an inhibitor of the ability of Th1 cells to synthesize IFN. This inhibition occurs largely via effects on antigen-presenting cells, such as macrophages, especially by inhibiting their IL-12 production. Other macrophage functions also are inhibited, such as synthesis of inflammatory cytokines (i.e., IL-1, IL-6, IL-8, and TNF) and phagocytosis. IL-10 knockout mice show extensive pathology, particularly in the gut, which is thought to arise from unattenuated immune responses to gut flora.[153] Receptor knockout mice have similar pathology.[149]

Clinical Use

IL-10 has been shown to inhibit some lipopolysaccharide-induced inflammatory responses in humans.[154] Clinical trials are under way in inflammatory bowel disease, RA, thoracic-abdominal aortic surgery, acute lung injury, multiple sclerosis, psoriasis, and human immunodeficiency virus infection.[155] Evidence exists that the Epstein-Barr virus IL-10 homologue acts as an autocrine in B lymphomas, suggesting benefit in blocking IL-10.[156,157]

INTERLEUKIN-11

IL-11 is a mesenchymal cell product with activity on hematopoietic cells. IL-11 has been used to promote hematopoiesis in patients. IL-11 receptor shares the gp130 component with IL-6, LIF, OSM, CNTF, and CT-1. IL-11 is required for embryonic implantation in the uterus.

Proteins

IL-11[158] is a 19-kD protein with no intrachain disulfide bonds. IL-11 is slightly homologous to IL-6, OSM, and LIF.

Producers

IL-11 is produced by a variety of mesenchymal cells, including keratinocytes, chondrocytes, osteoblasts, fibroblasts, and bone marrow stromal cells.[159]

Receptors and Cellular Response

The IL-11 receptor includes a ligand-specific α chain and gp130, which is common to IL-6, LIF, OSM, CNTF, and CT-1. Two alternative α chains exist in the mouse. The ligand-binding chains of this family do not contribute to signaling, which is wholly performed by gp130. Thus, the intracellular cascades should be the same for all members (gp130 signaling is discussed in Interleukin-6, earlier in this chapter). As in the IL-6 system, soluble IL-11 receptor can capture its ligand and then associate with cell-bound gp130 and signal.[160]

Activities

IL-11 was identified based on promoting growth of a plasmacytoma line.[158,159] It stimulates multilineage hematopoiesis when administered to mice and humans and is particularly effective in stimulating thrombopoiesis by inducing production of megakaryocytes. Knockout of the major receptor did not show a requirement in hematopoiesis[161] but revealed an IL-11 requirement in the uterine response to implantation.[162]

Clinical Use

Trials performed in breast cancer patients show that IL-11 can significantly restore suppressed hematopoiesis and alleviate thrombocytopenia induced by chemotherapy.[163] In mice, IL-11 also protects intestinal cells from damage induced by chemotherapy and radiotherapy.[164]

INTERLEUKIN-12

IL-12 is produced by antigen-presenting cells. IL-12 promotes Th1 cell development and IFN production. It is required for development of some types of autoimmunity in mice.

Proteins

IL-12[165–167] is a heterodimer consisting of disulfide-linked 35-kD and 40-kD subunits encoded by distinct genes. Both subunits are glycosylated and have intrachain disulfide bonds. Homodimers of p40 also are observed[168] and, in mice, have receptor-antagonist activity. This does not apply to humans.

Producers

Macrophages, B lymphocytes, and dendritic cells are major producers of IL-12. In macrophages, this synthesis is stimulated by microbial products and during contact with T cells via CD40L-CD40 interaction.[169] The two IL-12 chains associate intracellularly before secretion. The p35 subunit is expressed by a much wider range of cell types than the p40 subunit.[166,170]

Receptors and Cellular Response

Two components comprise the IL-12 receptor, the β1 and β2 chains.[171,172] Th2 cells fail to respond to IL-12 because they lack the β2 chain.[173] Many protein kinases are triggered by the IL-12 receptor, including the Janus kinases tyk2 and Jak2,[174] which are associated with the β1 and β2 chains, respectively.[175] STAT3, STAT4, and IRF-1 are implicated in gene induction by IL-12.[176,177]

Activities

IL-12 was discovered as one factor promoting CTLs and as an independent factor for promoting NK cells. These activities include proliferation, differentiation, and cytokine secretion, especially of IFN. The IFN-g–inducing activity of IL-12 is as a cofactor, such as with IL-18 (see Interleukin-18, later in this chapter). IL-12 knockout mice[178] showed greatly suppressed IFN production and revealed a requirement for IL-12 in development of Th1 cells in some settings but not in others.[179]

Clinical Use

IL-12 has been tested in cancer patients in phase 1 trials with no major toxicity other than a decrease in circulating lymphocytes, which, nevertheless, showed increased activity.[180] In preclinical studies, antitumor activity of IL-12 was detected,[181] and increased effects were seen in combination with a pulse of IL-2.[182] In mice, IL-12 is a required component of some types of autoimmunity in tissues, including the bowel, joint, eye, pancreas, and central nervous system.[183]

INTERLEUKIN-13

IL-13 is a T-cell product closely related to IL-4 and shares a receptor component. It elicits a subset of IL-4 responses and is implicated in Th2 cell generation and IgE synthesis. IL-13 is antiinflammatory.

Proteins

IL-13[184] is a 12-kD protein, and it is structurally related to IL-4, although the homology is low.[185,186] The gene is clustered together with IL-3, -4, -5, and -9.

Producers

IL-13 is expressed in Th2 cells after activation by antigen-MHC complexes and costimulators on the surface of antigen-presenting cells. Unlike IL-4, IL-13 expression is not strictly repressed in Th1 cells. IL-13 also is produced by dendritic cells.

Receptors and Cellular Response

The IL-13 receptor is comprised of IL-13Rα together with IL-4Rα. The same receptor complex also responds to IL-4. Two homologous IL-13Rα chains exist with different affinities for IL-13 in the absence of IL-4Rα: a high-affinity α2 chain[187] and a low-affinity α1 chain.[188] Receptors are expressed on monocytes, macrophages, eosinophils, basophils, mast cells, keratinocytes, and endothelial cells. Human B cells express the receptor, whereas mouse B cells do not. T cells have not been found to express receptors or respond to IL-13. Jak1 and Tyk2 are activated by receptor ligation. Unlike IL-4, Jak3 is not activated,[189] because it is associated with γ_c, which is not part of this receptor complex. STAT6 is phosphorylated and accounts for one set of responses, whereas IRS-2 is phosphorylated and initiates other second-messenger pathways.

Activities

Knockout of IL-13[190] revealed a requirement in Th2 development, which is perhaps indirect given the lack of receptors on T cells. IL-13 induces a subset of IL-4 effects, including effects on human B cells and macrophages, but not T cells. No apparently unique IL-13 effects have been noted. IL-13 activities include inducing IgE synthesis in human B cells. Whereas an IL-4 requirement for B cells to produce IgE was verified by IL-4 knockout, the same logic cannot be applied to IL-13 because mouse B cells do not express IL-13 receptors and do not respond to IL-13. Although IL-13 knockout did reduce IgE production, this may have occurred indirectly via decreased Th2 and IL-4 production. IL-13[184] is a potent inhibitor of inflammatory product synthesis by macrophages *in vitro* and an effective antiinflammatory *in vivo;* it can also induce monocytes to differentiate into dendritic cells.

Clinical Use

The induction of IgE synthesis implicates blocking the IL-13 pathway as a potential target in atopy. Other applications are suggested by IL-13 inhibiting inflammatory processes in mice.

INTERLEUKIN-14

Difficulties have occurred in reproducing the original observations regarding IL-14 and are therefore not discussed.

INTERLEUKIN-15

IL-15 resembles IL-2 in its activities on T cells and shares some receptor components with IL-2. It is essential for NK cell development. Unlike IL-2, the IL-15 gene is expressed by many cell types, but little protein is produced.

Proteins

IL-15[191–193] is a 15-kD glycoprotein with two internal disulfide bonds. IL-15 is predicted to fold into a four-part α helix structure like IL-2 and IL-4. It is genetically linked to IL-4, -5, and -9.

Producers

Unlike most of the ILs, many cell types constitutively transcribe the IL-15 gene. However, considerable constraints on translation imposed by the 5' and signal peptide region of the message exist.[194]

Receptors and Cellular Response

The IL-15 receptor shares the β and γ_c chains with the IL-2 receptor[195] but uses its own unique α chain that is expressed on more cell types than the IL-2Rα chain.[196] Mast cells appear to have a different receptor.[197] Jak1 and -3, and STAT3 and -5 are activated by the receptor in T cells, whereas Jak2 and STAT5 are activated in mast cells.

Activities

IL-15 was discovered as a T-lymphocyte growth factor activity. NK cell development can be induced by IL-15.[198] The knockout of IL-15Rα verified its requirement for NK development.[199] Mast cells also respond to IL-15, as do mature T and B lymphocytes, which are also deficient in knockouts.

Clinical Use

IL-15 has not been tested clinically. It may find use in boosting innate or T-cell immunity, or in *ex vivo* expansion of NK and T cells before reinfusion. Antagonists could be immunosuppressive.

INTERLEUKIN-16

IL-16 is a product of CD8 T cells that has activities on CD4 cells, including chemotaxis. It is implicated in airway inflammation in asthma.

Proteins

IL-16[200–202] is the C-terminal 17-kD peptide cleaved from a larger nonglycosylated precursor by caspase 3.[203] IL-16 lacks a typical signal peptide and is therefore released from cells by an atypical process. It is not homologous or linked to other cytokines, has an unusual protein structure with a PDZ domain otherwise found in intracellular proteins, and aggregates in solution.[204]

Producers

IL-16 is constitutively transcribed and translated by CD8 T cells. Release of the active form is then induced by stimuli, such as T-cell antigen cross-linking, histamine, and serotonin.[205] Other producers include eosinophils[206] and airway epithelial cells.[207]

Receptors and Cellular Response

IL-16 binds to CD4, which it appears to cross-link, inducing signaling.[208] The second messenger pathway does not require lck, which is associated with CD4. Implications of PI3-kinase and protein kinase C involvement exist.

Activities

IL-16 was discovered based on chemotactic activity for CD4 T cells.[200–202] It is also chemotactic for monocytes and eosinophils. IL-16 induces G_0 to G_1 transition in CD4 T cells, but not entry into S phase, which can be induced by IL-2. IL-16 inhibits the activation of T cells induced by the T-cell receptor, perhaps by sterically inhibiting CD4 interaction with class II MHC.[209] It inhibits human immunodeficiency virus replication, not through competing with entry via CD4, but through the human immunodeficiency virus promoter.[210]

Clinical Use

IL-16 has been implicated as the attractant for CD4 T cells in asthmatic inflammation of airways in humans,[202] suggesting uses for antagonists. It could possibly be used to induce T-cell blast transformation.

INTERLEUKIN-17

IL-17 is a product of memory T cells, with inflammatory, immunologic, and hematopoietic activities. IL-17 and its receptor bear little resemblance to other genes, although they do bear resemblance to the IL-17 homologue in a herpesvirus.

Proteins

IL-17[211–213] is a 17-kD peptide that can dimerize via disulfide bridges.[214]

Producers

IL-17 is produced by activated T cells, particularly the memory CD4 subset.[214] The gene was captured by *Herpesvirus saimiri*, whose product is biologically active.

Receptors and Cellular Response

One IL-17 receptor chain has been identified that bears remarkably little resemblance to other receptor types and results in nuclear factor κB activation.[215] This receptor chain is expressed on many different cell types.

Activities

IL-17 was discovered as a complementary DNA (cDNA) of unknown function, homologous to a sequence in a herpesvirus also of unknown function.[211] It has been shown to trigger several types of responses in cells, including IL-6 and IL-8 induction in fibroblasts.[214,215] It also has induced production of hemopoietic cytokines and neutrophils in bone marrow cultures and *in vivo*.[214] Blocking IL-17 suppresses T-cell proliferative responses.[215] This result may partly be because IL-17 promotes dendritic cell differentiation. This, in turn, may explain how blocking IL-17 prolonged allografts in mice.[216] Preliminary IL-17 receptor knockout data have not shown gross abnormalities.[217]

Clinical Use

IL-17 appears to promote immune and inflammatory responses. Thus, blocking its activity in humans could be immunosuppressive, as it is in mice.

INTERLEUKIN-18

IL-18 was discovered based on its induction of IFN-γ synthesis. Its own structure and that of its receptor system resemble IL-1. It promotes Th1 activities, inhibits Th2 activities, and induces macrophages to produce inflammatory cytokines.

Protein

IL-18[218,219] is a member of the IL-1 family. Like IL-1β, IL-18 is synthesized as a biologically inactive proform, which is cleaved by caspase 1, generating the active mature form.[220,221]

Producers

Kupffer cells were the source that led to the cloning of murine IL-18. Blood and tissue macrophages are avid producers, but unlike most cytokines, IL-18 production and release do not require stimulation of the macrophage.[222] Keratinocytes also produce IL-18 constitutively.

Receptors and Cellular Response

The organization of the cellular receptors for IL-18 is remarkably similar to that of IL-1. IL-18 initially associates with a binding chain,[223,224] which is encoded near IL-1 receptor[225]; this recruits a second signaling chain.[226] As with IL-1, a "decoy" receptor exists.[227] The active IL-18 receptor complex recruits the same kinase (IRAK) and initiates the TRAF6 pathway, as does IL-1.[228] MyD88 serves as an adaptor that links IRAK to the IL-18 and IL-1 receptor complex.[14] The IL-18 receptor is expressed on Th1 cells, but not on Th2 cells. Receptor expression is induced by IL-12 on both T and B cells.[229]

Activities

IL-18 was discovered based on its activity in inducing IFN-γ production. It has been verified in IL-18 knockout mice[230] that IFN-γ production is greatly reduced after inflammatory stimuli, although polyclonal T cell activation induces IFN-γ normally. This is probably explained by the observations that IL-18 primarily participates in IFN-γ induction as a cofactor together with IL-12; this synergy is partly based on IL-12 inducing expression of the IL-18 receptor. IL-18 promotes Th1 activities and inhibits Th2 activities via IFN-γ, such as IgE induction. IL-18 induces macrophages to synthesize secondary inflammatory cytokines, such as IL-1, IL-6, and chemokines.

Clinical Use

Possible clinical uses based on animal studies include giving IL-18 to promote IFN-γ production during viral or mycobacterial infections. IL-18 may combat allergy or asthma. Antagonizing IL-18 (i.e., by using the decoy receptor) could have antiinflammatory uses.

TUMOR ANTIGENS

IMMUNE RESPONSE TO TUMORS IN RODENTS

Early attempts to identify tumor antigens in mouse models by immunizing mice with spontaneous or carcinogen-induced tumors were confused by the immune reactions that arose to normal transplantation antigens present on tumors. The development of inbred mouse strains made it possible to differentiate tumor antigens from normal histocompatibility antigens and led to the first demonstrations that tumors did contain unique tumor-associated antigens on their surface.

In 1943, Gross[231] demonstrated that the intradermal immunization of inbred mice against a methylcholanthrene-induced sarcoma could result in immunization of that mouse against subsequent tumor challenge. These findings encouraged studies of the nature of the immune response to transplantable tumors in inbred mice, which demonstrated that tumor-specific antigens did exist in a variety of murine tumors.[232–237] These tumor antigens could not be detected in the normal tissues of mice, as demonstrated by studies showing that immunization with tumor cells did not immunize mice against normal tissue grafts from the mouse donating the tumor.[234] Immunity to tumor antigens existed in the same mice in which the tumors had originated, demonstrating that the tumor antigens were not the result of minor allogeneic differences between the transplantable tumor and the host.[235] Tumor antigens were found on a variety of tumors induced with chemical or physical carcinogens and on spontaneous tumors.[238–249]

Tumors induced by chemical carcinogens appear to have limited cross-reactivity, as evidenced by immunization-challenge experiments: Even two sarcomas induced in the same mouse do not cross-react.[233,243–245,276] The uniqueness of tumor antigens on chemically induced tumors contrasts with the shared antigens that are often found on virally induced tumors.[246–248] The sharing of antigens on tumors induced by RNA and DNA viruses has facilitated the study of the biologic and molecular nature of these antigens. For example, studies performed with simian virus 40–induced tumors identified the large T antigen, which is expressed primarily in the nucleus and is necessary to maintain the malignant phenotype of these tumor cells.[249,250] Similarly, the polyomavirus has a middle T antigen and small T antigen localized in the nucleus that can be detected by serologic tests. Boon and coworkers[251] isolated the genes that code for murine tumor-associated antigens induced by chemical mutagenesis. The isolated genes from several murine tumors bear little homology with one another or with other known genes.

In most animal studies of tumor immunity, tumor antigens are detected in experiments in which animals are immunized and then challenged with the same transplantable tumor. Lack of growth of a tumor challenge after immunization is taken as evidence for the existence of tumor antigens. *In vitro* assays involving reactivity of the tumor cell with antibodies or immune cells can also provide evidence for the existence of tumor antigens. Although tumors induced by high doses of chemical carcinogens or by viruses often exhibit high levels of immunogenicity in mice, it has been thought that spontaneous murine cancers are far less immunogenic.[252,253] The ability to detect tumor-associated antigens depends on the method used, and as more sensitive methods for detecting tumor antigens are developed, unsuspected antigens are likely to be observed.

A significant difference exists in the nature of the antigens recognized by humoral and cellular detection systems. Humoral antibodies detect specific epitopes on antigenic molecules, and it is the interaction of these molecules with the variable region of the antibody that produces recognition. In contrast, antigens recognized by T-cell receptors recognize processed peptides on the surface of the tumor cell or on an antigen-presenting cell in conjunction with MHC molecules. CD4+ lymphocytes recognize small peptides bound to MHC class II molecules, and CD8+ cells recognize peptides attached to class I molecules. Monoclonal antibodies are not capable of detecting the small processed peptides on MHC molecules on the cell surface, and the nature of the antigens recognized by humoral and cellular immune responses are therefore very different.

Tumor-infiltrating lymphocytes (TILs) provide a valuable reagent for detecting cellular immune responses to tumor antigens, revealing unique tumor antigens on a variety of methylcholanthrene-induced sarcomas in inbred mice.[254-258] TILs can recognize tumor antigens based on direct lysis of tumor cells or by the specific release of cytokines such as IFN-γ, GM-CSF, or TNF-α when the TILs are cocultured with the specific tumor. These TILs are derived from animals bearing established tumors and may differ from the cellular immune responses that are detected in animals that are highly immunized against the tumor as a result of artificial manipulations.

The detection of tumor antigens on human cancers presents unique problems because of the inability to use the immunization-challenge experiments, which have so effectively demonstrated tumor antigens on animal tumors. Attempts to detect human tumor antigens have relied almost exclusively on the availability of *in vitro* assays that could detect humoral or cellular immune responses.

IDENTIFICATION OF HUMAN CANCER ANTIGENS RESTRICTED BY CLASS I MAJOR HISTOCOMPATIBILITY COMPLEX AND RECOGNIZED BY CD8+ T CELLS

Attempts to apply the insights gained from increasing knowledge of cellular immunology to the development of effective immunotherapies for patients with cancer fall into three main areas: (1) The identification of antigens on human cancers that are capable of mediating immune responses, (2) the development of techniques for effective immunization of humans using tumor antigens, (3) and overcoming obstacles that enable the tumor to escape antitumor immune reactions. Significant progress has been made in the identification of human tumor antigens, and extensive efforts to develop effective means of immunizing patients have begun. Although substantial progress has been made, the clinical impact of these advances is still limited.

Much experimental evidence points to the importance of cellular immune reactions in mediating the regression of established tumors. Thus, considerable effort has been devoted to identifying human cancer antigens that elicit cellular immune responses. Both class I and class II restricted antigens, mediated by CD8+ and CD4+ lymphocytes, respectively, appear to be important in mediating immune destruction.

TABLE 18-4. Techniques for Cloning Tumor Antigens Recognized by CD8+ Cells and Presented on Major Histocompatibility Complex (MHC) Class I

Screen complementary DNA libraries from tumor using MHC class I–restricted T cells to identify the appropriate transfectants.
Identify peptides eluted from tumor cells, pulsed onto target cells bearing the appropriate MHC class I, and recognized by MHC class I–restricted T cells.
Raise MHC class I–restricted T cells against candidate antigens by *in vitro* sensitization techniques and then test the ability of these T cells to recognize tumor cells ("reverse immunology").

Several techniques for cloning tumor antigens recognized by CD8+ cells and presented on MHC class I have been developed and are presented in Table 18-4. Most class I–restricted antigens have been identified by screening cDNA libraries from tumor using MHC class I–restricted T cells to identify the relevant transfectants.[259-261] Alternatively, peptides have been eluted from tumor cells, pulsed onto target cells bearing the appropriate MHC class I antigen, and then tested by using the MHC class I–restricted T cells to identify the appropriate peptide fractions.[262] By obtaining partial sequences from cDNA libraries or from eluted peptides, it has been possible to identify a variety of class I–restricted tumor antigens.

Both of these approaches, however, depend on the ability to generate T cells capable of recognizing antigens presented on the surface of tumor cells. It is often difficult to generate these T cells *in vitro,* and thus a third approach, commonly referred to as *reverse immunology*, has been used. This approach attempts to determine whether candidate antigens, presumed to have a high likelihood of being tumor antigens based on their biologic characteristics, are actually presented on tumor cells. Class I–restricted T cells that work against these candidate antigens are raised by *in vitro* sensitization techniques. A variety of techniques have been developed, including the use of protein-pulsed or transfected antigen-presenting cells, or *in vitro* sensitization against synthetic peptides from the candidate antigen. If MHC class I–restricted T cells can be raised by these *in vitro* sensitization techniques, then the T cells are tested for the ability to recognize tumor cells and thus confirm the ability of these putative antigens to act as immunotherapeutic targets.

By making use of these approaches, a variety of cancer antigens restricted by MHC class I and recognized by CD8+ T cells have been derived (Table 18-5). The first cancer antigens to be described were shared cancer-testes antigens.[263] These antigens are present on a subset of patients with a variety of tumor types and appear to be expressed on cells in the testis but not on other normal cells. Several families of these cancer-testes antigens have been described and are presented in Table 18-6.[264]

Another major class of tumor antigens are the shared melanocyte-differentiation antigens (see Table 18-5). These antigens are present on melanomas as well as on normal melanocytes, the cells of origin of melanomas. At least six different shared melanocyte differentiation antigens have been described, including MART-1,[265,266] gp100,[267] tyrosinase,[268,269] TRP1,[270] TRP2,[271] and MC1R.[272]

TABLE 18-5. Cancer Antigens Restricted by Class I Major Histocompatibility Complex and Recognized by CD8+ T Cells

Shared cancer-testis antigens
MAGE-A1 to A12
MAGE-B1 to B4
MAGE-C1 and C2
BAGE
GAGE
NY-ESO-1
Shared melanocyte differentiation antigens
MART-1
gp100
Tyrosinase
TRP-1
TRP-2
MC1R
Unique mutant antigens
β-Catenin
CDK-4
MUM-1
Caspase-8
KIA
Widely expressed antigens with selective expression on cancer cells
p15
PRAME
SART-1
Viral antigens that contain T-cell epitopes
Epstein-Barr virus (EBNA 1–6; LMP1, -2)
Human T-cell leukemia virus type I (tax, gag, envelope)
Hepatitis B virus
Human papillomavirus-16 (E6, E7)
Normal proteins overexpressed on epithelial cancers
MUC-1
HER-2/neu
CEA
PSA
p53
Mutant oncoproteins or fusion proteins
Ras
p53
p16
BCR-ABL fusion (?)
EWS-ATF1 fusion (?)

CEA, carcinoembryonic antigen; PSA, prostate-specific antigen.

TABLE 18-6. Cancer-Testis Antigens

Gene	*HLA Restriction*	*Peptide*	*Position*
MAGE-A1	A1	EADPTGHSY	161–169
	A24	NYKHCFPEI	135–143
MAGE-A2	A2	YLQLVFGIEV	157–166
MAGE-A3	A1	EVDPIGHLY	168–176
	A2	FLWGPRALV	271–279
	A2	KVAELVHFL	112–120
	A24	IMPKAGLLI	195–203
	B44	MEVDPIGHLY	167–176
	DR11	TSYVKVLHHMVKISG	281–295
	DR13	AELVHFLLLKYRAR	114–127
	DR13	LLKYRAREPVTKAE	121–134
MAGE-A6	A34	MVKISGGPR	290–298
MAGE-A10	A2	GLYDGMEHL	254–262
MAGE-A12	A2	FLWGPRALV	271–279
BAGE	Cw16	AARAVFLAL	2–10
GAGE-1, 2, 8	Cw6	YRPRPRRY	9–16
NY-ESO-1	A2	QLSLLMWITQC	155–165
	A31	ASGPGGGAPR	53–62
	A31	LAAQERRVPR	ALT.ORF

(Adapted from Boon T, Van den Eynde BJ. *Principles and practices of the biologic therapy of cancer,* 3rd ed., with permission.)

The identification of these differentiation antigens on melanomas has led to the conjecture that differentiation antigens unique to other tissues might also be expressed on tumors arising from those tissues and thus serve as immunotherapeutic targets. Thus, differentiation antigens present on the epithelial cells of a variety of organs not essential for life, such as testis, ovary, prostate, breast, and thyroid, might also serve as tumor antigens.

Several tumor antigens such as beta-catenin,[273] CDK4,[274] MUM1,[275] caspase 8,[276] and KIA,[277] have been described and result from individual base mutations that give rise to amino acid differences. These mutated proteins thus represent antigens expressed only on cancer cells and not normal cells. Because each of these antigens is unique to the individual patient bearing the mutation, its use in the development of generally applicable cancer vaccines is limited.

Several unusual antigens with selective expression on cancer cells have been identified. Messenger RNA–encoding antigens, such as p15,[278] PRAME,[279] and SART-1,[280] are presented as antigens in a variety of tissues, but the encoded proteins do not appear to be present on cells other than cancers.

Several viral epitopes are known to be expressed on tumors caused by these viruses. Examples in this category include antigens from the Epstein-Barr virus,[281,282] human T-cell leukemia virus type I,[283] the hepatitis B virus,[284] and the E6 and E7 proteins from human papillomavirus-16. Several other normal or mutant proteins that are overexpressed in epithelial cells or represent mutated oncoproteins or fusion proteins have been hypothesized to be capable of acting as tumor antigens, although convincing evidence to support this hypothesis is lacking.

CANCER ANTIGENS RESTRICTED BY CLASS II MAJOR HISTOCOMPATIBILITY COMPLEX AND RECOGNIZED BY CD4+ T CELLS

Three general techniques for identifying MHC class II–restricted antigens recognized by CD4+ T cells are presented in Table 18-7. The testing of known class I–restricted antigens for the presence of class II–presented epitopes resulted in the identification of class II–restricted epitopes on tyrosinase[285] and gp100[286] (Touloukian et al., unpublished data). CD4+ T cells can recognize antigen-presenting cells pulsed with tumor lysates or proteins. It has thus been possible to purify proteins from tumor cell lysates that can elicit CD4 reactivity; the triosephosphate isomerase antigen was identified using this technique.[287] A general technique for the identification of class II antigens present on cancers as well as on cells from a variety of other diseases has been described.[288] This technique involves

TABLE 18-7. Techniques for Cloning Tumor Antigens Recognized by CD4+ Cells and Presented on Major Histocompatibility Complex Class II

Test known class I–restricted antigens
Purification of proteins from tumor cell lysates that elicit CD4 reactivity when incubated with APC
Screening of complementary DNA library transfected into an "engineered" APC containing:
DR α and β
DMA and DMB
Invariant chain

APC, antigen-presenting cell.

the screening of cDNA libraries transfected into antigen-presenting cells engineered to express the appropriate class II α and β molecules, the DMA and DMB molecules required for antigen processing as well as invariant chain. This technique was based on the unique aspects of the presentation of class II antigens and the inability of normal cytoplasmic proteins to be presented in the class II pathway. Using this genetic approach, several antigens, such as the CDC27 protein[30] and a mutated fusion protein, were identified[289] (Table 18-8).

HUMAN CANCER ANTIGENS: GENERAL PRINCIPLES

Tumor antigens can be derived from a variety of sources, including normal differentiation antigens, normal nonmutated antigens expressed on tumors and germ cells, intronic sequences, single base mutations, chromosomal rearrangements, aberrant processing, or alternative open reading frames of normal genes (Table 18-9). Because of the large number of mutations and chromosomal abnormalities present in cancer cells, it appears likely that many, if not all, cancers contain unique sequences capable of being recognized by human immune reactions. In support of this hypothesis are the examples that exist of individual patients who develop immune reactions against multiple different antigens present on their tumor. Two examples of this are shown in Table 18-10. TIL 586 from patient B.C. developed HLA-A31–restricted reactivity against four different epitopes, including one from an alternative open reading frame of TRP1, from the normal open reading frame of TRP2, and from both the normal and alternative open reading frames of the NY-ESO-1 antigen.[271,290,291] Similarly, patient M.G., whose tumors gave rise to TIL 888 and 1290, developed HLA-A24–restricted epitopes from four completely different proteins, including tyrosinase, p15, β-catenin, and gp100.[269,273,278,292]

Of importance for the general application of tumor antigens in human immunization is the ability of individual tumor antigens to present immune epitopes on a variety of HLA antigens (Table 18-11). Thus, the gp100 molecule has peptide epitopes that are presented on HLA A2, A3, A24, CDW8, and DR4.[286,292–295] Similarly, tyrosinase has known epitopes presented on HLA A1, A2, A24,[285,296–298] DRB1*0401, DRB1*1501, and B*4402. Thus, individual antigens can potentially be applicable to the immunization of a majority of patients with different HLA types.

TABLE 18-8. Cancer Antigens Restricted by Class II Major Histocompatibility Complex and Recognized by CD4+ Tumor-Infiltrating Lymphocytes

Antigens	*HLA Restrictions*	*Peptides*
Tyrosine	HLA-DR4	QNILLSNAPLGPQFP (56–70)
	HLA-DR4	SYLQDSDPDSFQD (448–462)
	HLA-DR15	FLLHHAFVDSIFEQWLQRHRP (386–406)
	HLA-DR4	EIWRDIDFAHE (193–203)
gp100	HLA-DR4	WNRQLYPEWTEAQRLD (44–59)
MAGE-3	HLA-DR11	TSYVKVLHHMVKISG (281–295)
	HLA-DR13	AELVHFLLLKYRAR (114–127)
	HLA-DR13	FLLLKYRAREPVTKAE (119–134)
TPI	HLA-DR1	GELIGILNAAKVPAD (23–37)
LDFP	HLA-DR1	PVIWRRAPA (312–323)
	HLA-DR1	WRRAPAPGA (315–323)
CDC27	HLA-DR4	FSWAMDLDPKGA (760–771)

(From Wang RF, Rosenberg SA. Human tumor antigens for cancer vaccine development. *Immunol Rev* 1999;170:85, with permission.)

TABLE 18-9. Sources of Human Tumor Antigens

Normal differentiation antigens
Intronic sequences
Posttranscriptional control of expression
Single base mutations
Chromosomal rearrangement
Aberrant processing
Alternative open reading frames

ANTIBODIES FOR DETECTING TUMOR ANTIGENS

Igs in all species have the same basic structure and consist of two polypeptide chains: the light chain, with a molecular weight of approximately 23,000, and the heavy chain, with a molecular weight of 55,000 to 70,000 (reviewed in Chapter 4).

Five different classes of Igs have been identified based on structural differences within the heavy-chain constant regions: IgM, IgG, IgA, IgD, and IgE. IgG constitutes the predominant

TABLE 18-10. A Single Patient Can Develop Reactivity against Multiple Epitopes on Different Antigens

T Cell	*Antigen*	*MHC Restriction*	*Peptides*
TIL 586 (patient B.C.)	TRP-1	A31	MSLQRQFLR (ORF3)
	TRP-2	A31	LLPGGRPYR
	NY-ESO-1	A31	ASGPGGGAPR
	NY-ESO-1	A31	LAAQERRVPR (ORF2)
TIL 888 and 1290 (patient M.G.)	Tyrosinase	A24	?
	p15	A24	AYGLDFYIL
	β-Catenin	A24	SYLDSGIHF
	gp100	A24	VYFFLPDHL (intron)

MCH, major histocompatibility complex.

TABLE 18-11. A Single Cancer Antigen Can Present Peptides on Multiple Class I and Class II Major Histocompatibility Complex Types

Protein	*HLA Restriction*	*Peptides*
gp100	A2	KTWGQYWQV
	A2	ITDQVPFSV
	A2	YLEPGPVTA
	A2	LLDGTATLRL
	A2	VLYRYGFSV
	A2	RLMKQDFSV
	A2	RLPRIFCSC
	A2	AMLGTHTMEV
	A2	SLADTNSLAV
	A3	SLIYRRRLMK
	A3	ALLAVGATK
	A24	VYFFLPDHL
	Cw8	SNDGPTLI
	DR4	WNRQLYPEWETAQRLD
Tyrosinase	A1	KCDICTDEY
	A1	SSDYVIPIGTY
	A2	MLLAVLYCL
	A2	YMDGTMSQV
	A24	AFLPWHRLF
	DRB1*0401	QNILLSNAPLGPQFP
	DRB1*0401	SYLQDSDPDSFQD
	DRB1*0401	EIWRDIDFAHE
	DRB1*1501	FLLHHAFVDSIFEQWLQRHRP
	B*4402	SEIWRDIDF

Ig fraction in sera, and most antibody activity is associated with IgG antibodies. IgM constitutes approximately 5% to 10% of serum Igs and is the largest of the Ig molecules. IgA is the predominant Ig in exocrine secretions, and IgE Igs are involved in allergic reactions. The exact function of IgD Igs is unknown.

Kohler and Milstein[299] were the first to demonstrate that somatic cells could be fused with murine myelomas and that monoclonal antibodies with unique specificities could be produced. A vast array of monoclonal antibodies have now been produced against a wide variety of human tumor-associated antigens (reviewed in Chapter 20.5). Most hybridoma cell lines can produce between 1 and 10 μg of Ig per 1 mL in culture, and ascites fluids can produce between 1 and 10 mg of Ig per 1 mL. In the generation of most monoclonal antibodies, mice are immunized against a specific antigen, and their cells are fused with the mouse myeloma cell. It is possible, however, to use human lymph node or peripheral blood cells for fusion with human myelomas. These human monoclonal antibodies may be able to identify antigens that are not immunogenic in the mouse and are less immunogenic in humans than murine monoclonal antibodies. It is possible to make recombinant chimeric monoclonal antibodies that contain the variable region of murine origin and the constant region of human origin.

Virtually all monoclonal antibodies have at least some reactivity with normal tissues, although the degree of cross-reactivity can be minimal. The potential clinical applications of monoclonal antibodies are summarized in Table 18-12 and Chapter 20.5.

TABLE 18-12. Clinical Applications of Monoclonal Antibodies (MoAbs)

Diagnosis
- Screening of body fluids (serum, sputum, effusions, urine, cerebrospinal fluid) for the presence of circulating TAA
- Nuclear scanning with radiolabeled MoAb
- Detection of primary or metastatic lesions (intravenous, subcutaneous, or iliopsoas administration of radiolabeled MoAb)
- The use of radiolabeled MoAb and intraoperative γ detecting probe
- Immunopathology
  - The diagnostic dilemma; malignant versus benign
  - Differential diagnosis of tumor type
  - Subclassification of tumor based on TAA expression
  - Metastatic potential
  - Specific favored sites of metastasis
  - Predicted response (or lack thereof) to specific therapeutic regimens
  - Prognosis

Monitoring of disease progression
- Screening of body fluids for circulating TAA
- Nuclear scanning with radiolabeled MoAb to detect or quantitate tumor recurrence
- Immunopathology for detection of occult metastases
  - Aspiration cytology
  - Lymph node or bone marrow biopsy
  - Cytology of body fluids

Therapy
- Direct cytotoxicity of MoAb
  - Complement mediated
  - Cell mediated
- Drug conjugation of MoAb (e.g., doxorubicin)
- Toxin conjugation of MoAb (e.g., ricin)
- Radionuclide conjugation of MoAb (e.g., α or β emitters)
- *Ex vivo* tumor removal from harvested bone marrow
- Inhibition of receptors for growth factors
- Administration of antiidiotype MoAbs to induce specific active immunity to tumor antigens

TAA, tumor-associated antigen.

IMMUNOTHERAPY

Strategies for the immunotherapy of cancer can be divided into active and passive approaches (Table 18-13). *Active immunotherapy* refers to the immunization of the tumor-bearing host with materials designed to elicit an immune reaction capable of eliminating or retarding tumor growth. Active immunotherapy can be subdivided into nonspecific or specific immunization. Most early attempts at the immunotherapy of cancer used nonspecific active approaches to immune stimulation with adjuvants such as bacillus Calmette-Guérin, *Corynebacterium parvum,* and levamisole. These early approaches were almost uniformly unsuccessful in humans and have largely been abandoned.

The advent of recombinant cytokines provided a more selective means for stimulating the immune system. Treatment with the IFNs or with IL-2 is a form of nonspecific active immunotherapy, although the selective action of these purified lymphokines provides a greater ability to manipulate immune responses than was previously possible.

TABLE 18-13. Classification of Cancer Immunotherapies

Classification	*Examples*
Active immunotherapy	
Nonspecific	Immune adjuvants such as bacillus Calmette-Guérin, *Corynebacterium parvum*, levamisole
	Interferon
	Interleukin-2
Specific	Immunization with tumor antigen vaccines
Passive immunotherapy	
Antibodies	Monoclonal or polyclonal antibodies alone or conjugated with toxins or radiolabels
Cells	Tumor-infiltrating lymphocytes
Indirect	Removal or blocking factors; inhibition of growth factors or angiogenic factors

INTERLEUKIN-2

Major progress in immunotherapy has resulted from the identification of the cytokine IL-2 that enabled the *ex vivo* growth of human T lymphocytes.[19] The identification of the gene encoding IL-2,[20] the biologic characterization of recombinant IL-2,[300] increasing information about the dominant role of IL-2 in regulating immune reactions, and extensive studies of IL-2 administration to tumor-bearing mice[301] led to studies of the clinical use of this molecule in patients with advanced cancer (see Chapter 20.2). IL-2 is now in common use for the treatment of patients with metastatic melanoma and renal cancer and has been instrumental for the conduct of *in vitro* studies identifying human cancer antigens. IL-2 also has been used as an adjuvant for *in vivo* immunization protocols.

The best evidence that manipulation of the human immune system can result in the regression of advanced cancer in patients resulted from clinical studies in which high-dose bolus IL-2 was administered to patients with metastatic melanoma and metastatic renal cancer.[5] IL-2 has no direct impact on cancer cells, and all of its effects result from its ability to stimulate *in vivo* immune reactions. In the National Cancer Institute's Surgery Branch, 409 consecutive patients with either advanced melanoma (n = 182) or renal cancer (n = 227) were treated with high-dose bolus IL-2 alone at a dose of 720,000 IU/kg every 8 hours.[30] The results of the treatment are shown in Tables 18-14 and 18-15. Seven percent of patients with melanoma underwent a complete response, and 9% underwent a partial response. In patients with renal cancer the complete and partial response rates were 9% and 10%, respectively. Complete responses were most often durable. Of 12 patients with metastatic melanoma who achieved a complete response, only two have recurred, with the remainder having ongoing complete responses of between 95 and 173 months. Of 21 patients with metastatic renal cell cancer who achieved a complete regression, four have recurred and 17 have ongoing responses between 46 and 159 months. The lack of recurrences after 5 years and the follow-up of several patients beyond 10 years indicate that these patients have probably been cured by the administration of high-dose IL-2 (Fig. 18-1).

TABLE 18-14. Response of Patients with Metastatic Cancer Treated with High-Dose Bolus Interleukin-2

		Number of Patients (%)		
Diagnosis	*Total*	CR	PR	CR + PR
Melanoma	182	12 (7%)	16 (9%)	28 (15%)
Renal cell cancer	227	21 (9%)	22 (10%)	43 (19%)
Total	409	33 (8%)	38 (9%)	71 (17%)

CR, complete response; PR, partial response.
Patients accrued between September 1985 and November 1996.
Follow-up as of April 1, 2000 (median follow-up, 9.2 y).

TABLE 18-15. Duration of Response in Patients with Metastatic Cancer Treated with High-Dose Bolus Interleukin-2

Diagnosis	*CR (mo)*	*PR (mo)*
Melanoma	173+, 122+, 120+, 118+, 116+, 109+, 105+, 96+, 96+, 95+, 16, 12	35, 31, 19, 10, 10, 8, 8, 7, 7, 6, 5, 5, 5, 4, 4, 2
Renal cell cancer	159+, 148+, 140+, 119+, 119+, 115+, 111+, 111+, 104+, 95+, 89+, 88+, 87+, 85+, 74+, 64+, 46+, 35, 23, 19, 19	52, 30, 30, 22, 20, 17, 16, 15, 14, 14, 13, 11, 9, 8, 8, 7, 7, 6, 4, 4, 4, 4

+, ongoing response as of April 1, 2000; CR, complete response; PR, partial response.
Note: Of 33 patients with CR, 27 remain in CR at 46 to 173 mo.

As experience with the use of IL-2 increased, improved methods for managing the side effects of its administration were developed, and the safety of IL-2 administration has improved dramatically.[302] A consecutive series of 1241 metastatic cancer patients who received 720,000 IU/kg IL-2 every 8 hours by intravenous bolus infusion, either alone or in conjunction with other treatments, were evaluated for the incidence of treatment-related toxicities.[303] Significant decreases in the incidence of grade III and IV toxicities were found as experience with the use of IL-2 increased over the 12 years of this study. Although a 1% to 3% treatment-related mortality was seen in the first 4 years of the administration of IL-2, no treatment-related deaths were reported in this series between May 1989 and January 1997, including the treatment of 809 consecutive patients. These trends suggested that high-dose IL-2 could be safety administered to metastatic cancer patients when appropriate treatment guidelines were used and that the administration of IL-2 could

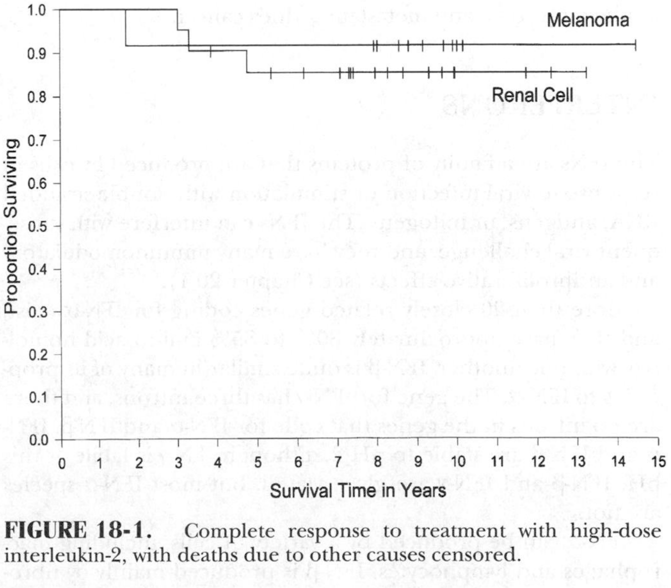

FIGURE 18-1. Complete response to treatment with high-dose interleukin-2, with deaths due to other causes censored.

TABLE 18-16. Response of Various Cancers to Interferon-α

Tumor Type	*Response Rate (%)*
Cervical intraepithelial neoplasia	80–90
Basal cell cancer	90
Superficial bladder cancer	60–70
Malignant neuroendocrine tumors	30–80
Kaposi's sarcoma (acquired immunodeficiency syndrome–related)	35
Ovarian cancer	
Parenteral	10–15
Intraperitoneal	40
Gliomas	30
Renal cell cancer	15–20
Nasopharyngeal cancer	20
Melanoma	10–15
Colorectal cancer	<10
Osteogenic sarcoma	<10
Lung (small and non–small cell)	<10
Breast cancer	<10
Hairy cell leukemia	80–90
Chronic myelogenous leukemia	
Newly diagnosed	70–80
Advanced	10–25
Philadelphia-negative myeloproliferative disorders, essential thrombocythemia and polycythemia vera	75
Cutaneous T-cell lymphomas	
No prior therapy	80
Previously treated	55
Non-Hodgkin's lymphomas (relapsed)	
Low grade	40–50
Intermediate and high grade	15
Hodgkin's disease (relapsed)	20
Multiple myeloma	
No prior therapy	50
Previously treated	15–25
Chronic lymphocytic leukemia	10–15
Acute lymphocytic leukemia	10–20

result in durable responses in a small subset of patients with metastatic melanoma and metastatic kidney cancer.

INTERFERONS

The IFNs are a family of proteins that are produced by cells in response to viral infection or stimulation with double-stranded RNA, antigens, or mitogens. The IFNs can interfere with subsequent viral challenge, and they have many immunomodulatory and antiproliferative effects (see Chapter 20.1).

More than 20 closely related genes coding for IFN α exist, and they have approximately 80% to 85% amino acid homology with one another. IFN-β is quite similar in many of its properties to IFN-α. The gene for IFN-γ has three introns, and there are no introns in the genes that code for IFN-α and IFN-β. IFN-α and IFN-β are stable to pH 2, although IFN-γ is labile at this pH. IFN-β and IFN-γ are glycosylated, but most IFN-α species are not.

IFN-α can be produced by a variety of cells, including macrophages and lymphocytes. IFN-β is produced mainly by fibroblasts and epithelial cells. IFN-γ can be produced by a variety of lymphocyte subtypes, such as CD4+ or CD8+ cells, NK cells, and LAK cells. Secretion of IFN-γ occurs after stimulation by mitogens or antigens. IFNs have a variety of biologic properties, including immunomodulatory activities, antiviral activities, the ability to interfere with cell proliferation, inhibition of angiogenesis, regulation of differentiation, and enhancement of the expression of a variety of cell surface antigens. Although the direct antiproliferative activity of the IFNs is thought to play a major role in the antitumor effects of these compounds, other actions of the IFNs may also be important.

The IFNs have antitumor activity against a variety of tumor types, including hairy cell leukemia, chronic myelogenous leukemia, cutaneous T-cell lymphoma, and Kaposi's sarcoma.

The response rates of various solid tumors and hematologic malignancies to treatment with IFN-α are summarized in Table 18-16. IFN-α and IFN-β, but not IFN-γ, demonstrate direct antitumor activity. The side effects associated with IFN therapy include flu-like symptoms, rashes, gastrointestinal complaints, hepatic dysfunction, neurologic complaints, and chronic fatigue, and they are highly dose and schedule dependent.

TABLE 18-17. Variables Involved in the Immunization of Humans against Cancer Antigens

Choice of antigen
MART-1
gp100
Others
Vector of administration
Peptide
Protein
DNA
Recombinant viruses
Adenovirus
Fowlpox virus
Vaccinia virus
Vehicle of administration
Saline
Adjuvant (IFA, QS-21, Ribi, and others)
Antigen-presenting cells
Route of administration
Intradermal
Subcutaneous
Intramuscular
Intravenous
Immune adjuvants
Interleukin-2
Interleukin-7
Interleukin-10
Interleukin-12

DEVELOPMENT OF APPROACHES TO THE IMMUNIZATION OF HUMANS AGAINST CANCER ANTIGENS

Although many human cancer antigens have now been identified, relatively little is known about the best methods for successful immunization of patients against these antigens. The number of variables involved in determining optimal methods of immunization of humans presents a daunting challenge and are shown in Table 18-17.

TABLE 18-18. General Principles for Human Vaccination against Cancer Antigens Based on Animal Models

Immunizations most effective in generating reactive T cells are the most therapeutically effective.
Therapeutic efficacy of immunization is enhanced by the administration of interleukin-2 and -12.
The more immunogen the better.
Repeated boost immunizations with different vehicles containing the same antigen (i.e., to avoid immunization to the vehicle itself) is optimal.

A variety of cancer antigens are available. Multiple vectors can be used to provide immunization, including peptides, proteins, DNA, and a variety of recombinant viruses such as adenovirus, fowlpox virus, and vaccinia virus. When using these immunizing vectors, the vehicle can be important as well. It is possible to inject these vectors in saline and in a variety of adjuvants, such as incomplete Freund's adjuvant, QS21, or others. Similarly, these antigens can be presented on professional antigen-presenting cells, such as mature dendritic cells. The route of immunization is also a variable that must be considered (e.g., intradermal, subcutaneous, intramuscular, or intravenous injection). Immune adjuvants may increase the immune response to these immunogens, and studies exploring the use of IL-2, IL-7, IL-10, and IL-12 have been performed. Because of the myriad of possibilities for immunization of humans, substantial effort has been placed on elucidation in animal models of the general principles for vaccination against cancer antigens. Four general principles resulting from these murine studies are presented in Table 18-18 and have guided the work in humans. A detailed discussion of cancer vaccines is presented in Chapters 63.1 and 63.2.

It is possible to immunize cancer patients against antigens present on their autologous cancers and raise high levels of circulating immune lymphocytes.[304–306] An example of one such series of experiments in which 11 patients with metastatic melanoma were immunized with a modification of the gp100:209–217 epitope, from the gp100 melanoma antigens, which was modified with a methionine substitution in the 210 position, is shown in Table 18-19.[306] The introduction of this amino acid

TABLE 18-19. Reactivity of Peripheral Blood Mononuclear Cells from Patients Immunized with 209-2M Peptide in IFA

		Assay Stimulator[a] (pg IFN-τ/mL)							
		Before Immunization				*After Immunization[b]*			
Patient	*Experiment*	T2	T2 (280)	T2 (209)	T2 (209-2M)	T2	T2 (280)	T2 (209)	T2 (209-2M)
1	1	21	22	12	20	42	37	6897	57,060
2	1	58	56	66	50	54	48	1851	4012
	2	1	4	2	ND	30	22	>1000	ND
3	1	33	26	33	35	46	53	56	54
	2	145	127	124	ND	49	36	46	ND
4	1	133	123	184	213	40	35	2631	6086
	2	50	36	41	43	45	52	1618	3751
	3	351	299	501	470	86	825	944	1057
5	1	28	30	21	24	41	35	4366	6402
	2	154	156	152	142	128	129	295	323
	3	29	18	37	32	27	22	856	1126
6	1	38	28	24	31	44	47	152	671
	2	154	166	210	153	128	72	662	887
	3	96	61	117	127	22	14	2374	5407
7	1	44	66	72	82	104	81	4424	5411
	2	10	8	13	16	197	224	1293	1583
	3	127	105	ND	120	61	67	1244	ND
8	1	ND	ND	ND	ND	17	25	845	ND
	2	1553	562	719	ND	79	78	2326	ND
	3	ND	ND	ND	ND	43	ND	1768	ND
9	1	345	337	355	ND	209	183	2253	ND
	2	13	13	10	ND	229	262	1550	ND
	3	1434	816	513	ND	495	517	2408	ND
10	1	247	283	413	ND	29	39	1271	ND
	2	135	102	146	ND	86	74	24,150	ND
	3	117	147	150	ND	6	9	39,690	ND
11	1	53	53	56	ND	65	71	154	ND
	2	46	50	47	ND	29	39	63	ND
	3	ND	ND	ND	ND	87	83	205	ND

IFN, interferon; ND, not done.
[a]Day 11 to 13 after culture with 209-2M peptide, peripheral blood mononuclear cells were tested for IFN-τ release after 24-hr incubation with peptide pulsed T2 cells.
[b]Patient 1 after one immunization; all other patients after two immunizations.
(From ref. 306, with permission.)

modification greatly increased the binding of this peptide to the HLA-A2 molecule and thus appeared to increase both its *in vitro* and *in vivo* immunogenicity.[307] Despite the ability to reproducibly generate immune reactions against this tumor epitope, little antitumor effect was seen unless IL-2 was simultaneously injected. In pilot human trials, it appeared that the response rate to immunization with the gp100 209–217 (210M) epitope plus the administration of IL-2 resulted in response rates almost three times greater than that due to IL-2 alone.[308] However, the confirmation of this result will require evaluation in prospective randomized trials in which patients are treated with either IL-2 alone or IL-2 plus the peptide immunogen.

ADOPTIVE IMMUNOTHERAPY

Adoptive immunotherapy—the transfer to the tumor-bearing host of cells with antitumor activity—has substantial therapeutic attractiveness as an approach to treating human cancer.[308–311] Early cell-transfer experiments in animals demonstrated that the cellular arm of the immune response is crucial in mediating the rejection of allogeneic grafts and syngeneic tumors. In most experimental systems, the transfer of immune cells, but not of antibody directed against cellular antigens, produces immunity to tissue transplantations.

The major obstacle to the development of successful adoptive immunotherapies for the treatment of cancer in humans has been the inability to develop immune cells with specific reactivity for human tumors that could be obtained in large enough numbers for transfer to tumor-bearing patients. However, several new approaches have been developed for generating human cells with reactivity to tumor.

Beginning in 1980, Rosenberg and colleagues[312–314] described a technique for generating lymphoid cells from mice and humans that were capable of lysing fresh tumor cells but not normal cells. The incubation of resting murine splenocytes or human peripheral blood lymphocytes with IL-2 for 3 to 4 days generates LAK cells that can lyse fresh tumor cells.

The characteristics of LAK cells have been extensively studied.[314–316] These cells represent a lytic population distinct from NK cells or CTLs, and their phenotypic surface markers are characteristic of non–MHC-restricted killer cells. LAK cells can be CD3+ or CD3–, are nonadherent, and bear NK-like markers such as CD16 and CD56. The nature of the determinants recognized on fresh tumor targets by LAK cells is unknown, although the determinants appear to be broadly expressed on fresh and cultured tumor cells and in cultured normal cells. Fresh normal cells do not appear to bear cell surface determinants recognized by LAK cells.

After the description of the LAK cell phenomenon, animal studies evaluated the use of LAK cells in the adoptive immunotherapy of established tumors. These studies demonstrated that the adoptive transfer of LAK cells in conjunction with IL-2 could mediate the regression of established pulmonary, hepatic, and subdermal metastases in a variety of animal models.[317,318] IL-2 stimulated *in vivo* expansion of LAK cells with maintenance of cellular function.[319]

Based on these *in vitro* studies and animal models, clinical protocols were developed for the systemic administration of LAK cells plus IL-2 to patients with advanced cancer.[309] Results from a prospective randomized trial in the National Cancer Institute's Surgery Branch comparing treatment of patients with metastatic melanoma or renal cancer using either IL-2 or LAK cells plus IL-2 revealed no difference in survival.

TABLE 18-20. Treatment of Patients with Melanoma with Tumor-Infiltrating Lymphocytes

Patient Status	*NR*	*Objective Response (PR + CR)*	*PR + CR (all)*	*Rate (%)*
No previous IL-2				
IL-2 + CY	26	14	14/140	35
IL-2 (no CY)	12	6	6/18	33
Previous IL-2				
IL-2 + CY	11	6	6/17	35
IL-2 (no CY)	8	3	3/11	27

CR, complete response; CY, cyclophosphamide; IL, interleukin; NR, no response; PR, partial response.

TUMOR-INFILTRATING LYMPHOCYTES AND INTERLEUKIN-2

TILs are lymphocytes that infiltrate growing tumors and can be isolated by growing single-cell suspensions from the tumor in IL-2.

In animals, the adoptive transfer of TILs can be from 50 to 100 times as potent as LAK cells in mediating the regression of established micrometastases.[254] TILs have been isolated from virtually all types of human tumors and can recognize tumor-associated antigens.[320–346] Based on these *in vitro* and *in vivo* studies, pilot trials of TILs for the treatment of advanced cancers in humans have been conducted.[290–292] The results of a pilot trial studying patients with metastatic melanoma treated with TILs in the National Cancer Institute's Surgery Branch are presented in Table 18-20.

TILs traffic to and accumulate in tumor deposits. This finding led to attempts to genetically alter TILs to increase their antitumor activity at the tumor site. In an initial phase of this effort, TILs transduced with the gene for neomycin phosphotransferase were infused into patients with advanced melanoma, as were TILs transduced with the gene for TNF.[310,347,348] This study and additional efforts to develop gene therapies for patients with cancer are considered in Chapter 62.1. Improved methods for developing lymphocytes with antitumor activity by *in vitro* sensitization with tumor-specific peptides, as well as the use of cloned cells, are under development and may provide valuable reagents for use in future adoptive immunotherapy studies.[349–352]

REFERENCES

1. Gery I, Gershon RK, Waksman BH. Potentiation of the T-lymphocyte response to mitogens. I. The responding cell. *J Exp Med* 1972;136:128.
2. Dinarello CA. Interleukin-1, interleukin-1 receptors and interleukin-1 receptor antagonist. *Int Rev Immunol* 1990;16:157.
3. Lomedico PT, Gubler U, Hellmann CP, et al. Cloning and expression of murine interleukin-1 cDNA in *Escherichia coli. Nature* 1984;312:458.
4. Auron PE, Webb AC, Rosenwasser LJ, et al. Nucleotide sequence of human monocyte interleukin 1 precursor cDNA. *Proc Natl Acad Sci U S A* 1984;81:7907.
5. Black RA, Kronheim SR, Cantrell M, et al. Generation of biologically active interleukin-1 beta by proteolytic cleavage of the inactive precursor. *J Biol Chem* 1988;263:9437.
6. Eisenberg SP, Evans RJ, Arend WP, et al. Primary structure and functional expression from complementary DNA of a human interleukin-1 receptor antagonist. *Nature* 1990;343:341.
7. Buras JA, Reenstra WR, Fenton MJ. NF beta A, a factor required for maximal interleukin-1 beta gene expression is identical to the ets family member PU.1. Evidence for structural alteration following LPS activation. *Mol Immunol* 1995;32:541.

8. Kominato Y, Galson D, Waterman WR. Monocyte expression of the human prointerleukin 1 beta gene IL-1B is dependent on promoter sequences which bind the hematopoietic transcription factor Spi-1/PU.1. *Mol Cell Biol* 1995;15:59.
9. Sims JE, Gayle MA, Slack JL. Interleukin 1 signaling occurs exclusively via the type I receptor. *Proc Natl Acad Sci U S A* 1993;90:6155.
10. Colotta F, Re F, Muzio M. Interleukin-1 type II receptor: a decoy target for IL-1 that is regulated by IL-4. *Science* 1993;261:472.
11. Greenfeder SA, Nunes P, Kwee L, et al. Molecular cloning and characterization of a second subunit of the interleukin 1 receptor complex. *J Biol Chem* 1995;270:13757.
12. Cao Z, Henzel WJ, Gao X. IRAK: a kinase associated with the interleukin-1 receptor. *Science* 1996;271:1128.
13. Cao Z, Xiong J, Takeuchi M, et al. TRAF6 is a signal transducer for interleukin-1. *Nature* 1996;383:443.
14. Adachi O, Kawai T, Takeda K, et al. Targeted disruption of the MyD88 gene results in loss of IL-1 and IL-18-mediated function. *Immunity* 1998;9:143.
15. Shirakawa F, Chedid M, Suttles J, et al. Interleukin-1 and cyclic AMP induce kappa immunoglobulin light-chain expression via activation of an NF-kappa B–like DNA-binding protein. *Mol Cell Biol* 1989;9:959.
16. Muegge K, Williams TM, Kant J, et al. Interleukin-1 costimulatory activity on the interleukin-2 promoter via AP-1. *Science* 1989;246:249.
17. Shornick LP, De Togni P, Mariathasan S, et al. Mice deficient in IL-1 beta manifest impaired contact hypersensitivity to trinitrochlorobenzone. *J Exp Med* 1996;183:1427.
18. Smith JW, Longo DL, Alvord WG, et al. The effects of treatment with interleukin-1 alpha on platelet recovery after high-dose carboplatin. *N Engl J Med* 1993;328:756.
19. Morgan DA, Ruscetti FW, Gallo R. Selective *in vitro* growth of T lymphocytes from normal human bone marrows. *Science* 1976;193:1007.
20. Taniguchi T, Matsui H, Fujita T, et al. Structure and expression of a cloned cDNA for human interleukin-2. *Nature* 1983;302:305.
21. Mosmann TR, Sad S. The expanding universe of T-cell subsets: Th1, Th2 and more. *Immunol Today* 1996;17:138.
22. Leonard WJ, Depper JM, Crabtree GR, et al. Molecular cloning and expression of cDNAs for the human interleukin-2 receptor. *Nature* 1984;311:626.
23. Hatakeyama M, Tsudo M, Minamoto S, et al. Interleukin-2 receptor beta chain gene: generation of three receptor forms by cloned human alpha and beta chain cDNA's. *Science* 1989;244:551.
24. Takeshita T, Asao H, Ohtani K, et al. Cloning of the gamma chain of the human IL-2 receptor. *Science* 1992;257:379.
25. Johnston JA, Kawamura M, Kirken RA, et al. Phosphorylation and activation of the Jak-3 Janus kinase in response to interleukin-2. *Nature* 1994;370:151.
26. Witthuhn BA, Silvennoinen O, Miura O, et al. Involvement of the Jak-3 Janus kinase in signalling by interleukins 2 and 4 in lymphoid and myeloid cells. *Nature* 1994;370:153.
27. Leonard WJ, O'Shea JJ. Jaks and STATs: biologic implications. *Annu Rev Immunol* 1998;16:293.
28. Gomez J, Gonzalez A, Martinez A, Rebollo A. IL-2-induced cellular events. *Crit Rev Immunol* 1998;18:185.
29. Schorle H, Holtschke T, Hunig T, Schimpl A, Horak I. Development and function of T cells in mice rendered interleukin-2 deficient by gene targeting. *Nature* 1991;352:621.
30. Rosenberg SA, Yang JC, White DE, Steinberg SM. Durability of complete responses in patients with metastatic cancer treated with high-dose interleukin-2: identification of the antigens mediating response. *Ann Surg* 1998;228:307.
31. Davey JR, Chaitt DG, Albert JM, et al. A randomized trial of high- versus low-dose subcutaneous interleukin-2 outpatient therapy for early human immunodeficiency virus type 1 infection. *J Infect Dis* 1999;179:849.
32. Baluna R, Vitetta ES. Vascular leak syndrome: a side effect of immunotherapy. *Immunopharmacology* 1997;37:117.
33. Kawakami Y, Rosenberg SA. Immunobiology of human melanoma antigens MART-1 and gp100 and their use for immuno-gene therapy. *Int Rev Immunol* 1997;14:173.
34. Brodie SJ, Lewinsohn DA, Patterson BK, et al. *In vivo* migration and function of transferred HIV-1-specific cytotoxic T cells. *Nat Med* 1999;5:34.
35. Walter EA, Greenberg PD, Gilbert MJ, et al. Reconstitution of cellular immunity against cytomegalovirus in recipients of allogeneic bone marrow by transfer of T-cell clones from the donor [See comments]. *N Engl J Med* 1995;333:1038.
36. O'Reilly RJ, Small TN, Papadopoulos E, et al. Biology and adoptive cell therapy of Epstein-Barr virus–associated lymphoproliferative disorders in recipients of marrow allografts. *Immunol Rev* 1997;157:195.
37. Waldmann TA, O'Shea J. The use of antibodies against the IL-2 receptor in transplantation. *Curr Opin Immunol* 1998;10:507.
38. Yokota T, Lee F, Rennick D, et al. Isolation and characterization of a mouse cDNA clone that expresses mast-cell growth-factor activity in monkey cells. *Proc Natl Acad Sci U S A* 1984;81:1070.
39. Yang YC, Ciarletta AB, Temple PA, et al. Human IL-3 multi-CSF: identification by expression cloning of a novel hematopoietic growth factor related to murine IL-3. *Cell* 1986;47:3.
40. Schrader JW, Nossal GJ. Strategies for the analysis of accessory-cell function: the *in vitro* cloning and characterization of the P cell. *Immunol Rev* 1980;53:61.
41. Kitamura T, Sato N, Arai K, Miyajima A. Expression cloning of the human IL-3 receptor cDNA reveals a shared beta subunit for the human IL-3 and GM-CSF receptors. *Cell* 1991;66:1165.
42. Hayashida K, Kitamura T, Gorman DM, et al. Molecular cloning of a second subunit of the receptor for human granulocyte-macrophage colony-stimulating factor (GM-CSF): reconstitution of a high-affinity GM-CSF receptor. *Proc Natl Acad Sci U S A* 1990;87:9655.
43. Stomski FC, Sun Q, Bagley CJ, et al. Human interleukin-3 (IL-3) induces disulfide-linked IL-3 receptor alpha- and beta-chain heterodimerization, which is required for receptor activation but not high-affinity binding. *Mol Cell Biol* 1996;16:3035.
44. Quelle FW, Sato N, Witthuhn BA, et al. JAK2 associates with the beta c chain of the receptor for granulocyte-macrophage colony-stimulating factor, and its activation requires the membrane-proximal region. *Mol Cell Biol* 1994;14:4335.
45. Mui AL, Wakao H, O'Farrell AM, Harada N, Miyajima A. Interleukin-3, granulocyte-macrophage colony-stimulating factor and interleukin-5 transduce signals through two STAT5 homologs. *EMBO J* 1995;14:1166.
46. Guthridge MA, Stomski FC, Thomas D, et al. Mechanism of activation of the GM-CSF, IL-3, IL-5 family of receptors. *Stem Cells* 1998;16:301.
47. del Peso L, Gonzalez-Garcia M, Page C, Herrera R, Nunez G. Interleukin-3-induced phosphorylation of BAD through the protein kinase Akt. *Science* 1997;278:687.
48. Eder M, Geissler G, Ganser A. IL-3 in the clinic. *Stem Cells* 1997;15:327.
49. Ganser A, Lindemann A, Seipelt G, et al. Effects of recombinant human interleukin-3 in patients with normal hematopoiesis and in patients with bone marrow failure. *Blood* 1990;76:666.
50. Brugger W, Heimfeld S, Berenson RJ, Mertelsmann R, Kanz L. Reconstitution of hematopoiesis after high-dose chemotherapy by autologous progenitor cells generated *ex vivo*. *N Engl J Med* 1995;333:283.
51. Dzierzak EA, Papayannopoulou T, Mulligan RC. Lineage-specific expression of a human beta-globin gene in murine bone marrow transplant recipients reconstituted with retrovirus-transduced stem cells. *Nature* 1988;331:35.
52. Yokota T, Otsuka T, Mosmann T, et al. Isolation and characterization of a human interleukin cDNA clone, homologous to mouse B-cell stimulatory factor 1, that expresses B-cell- and T-cell-stimulating activities. *Proc Natl Acad Sci U S A* 1986;83:5894.
53. Noma Y, Sideras P, Naito T, et al. Cloning of cDNA encoding the murine IgGl induction factor by a novel strategy using SP6 promoter. *Nature* 1986;319:640.
54. Lee F, Yokota T, Otsuka T, et al. Isolation and characterization of a mouse interleukin cDNA clone that expresses B-cell stimulatory factor 1 activities and T-cell- and mast-cell-stimulating activities. *Proc Natl Acad Sci U S A* 1986;83:2061.
55. Seder RA, Paul WE, Dvorak AM, et al. Mouse splenic and bone marrow cell populations that express high-affinity Fc epsilon receptors and produce interleukin-4 are highly enriched in basophils. *Proc Natl Acad Sci U S A* 1991;88:2835.
56. Schmitz J, Thiel A, Kuhn R, et al. Induction of interleukin 4 (IL-4) expression in T helper (Th) cells is not dependent on IL-4 from non-Th cells. *J Exp Med* 1994;179:1349.
57. Zheng W, Flavell RA. The transcription factor GATA-3 is necessary and sufficient for Th2 cytokine gene expression in CD4 T cells. *Cell* 1997;89:587.
58. Ho IC, Hodge MR, Rooney JW, Glimcher LH. The proto-oncogene c-af is responsible for tissue-specific expression of interleukin-4. *Cell* 1996;85:973.
59. Mosley B, Beckmann MP, March CJ, et al. The murine interleukin-4 receptor: molecular cloning and characterization of secreted and membrane bound forms. *Cell* 1989;59:335.
60. Nelms K, Huang H, Ryan J, Keegan A, Paul WE. Interleukin-4 receptor signalling mechanisms and their biologic significance. *Adv Exp Med Biol* 1998;452:37.
61. Oakes SA, Candotti F, Johnston JA, et al. Signaling via IL-2 and IL-4 in JAK3-deficient severe combined immunodeficiency lymphocytes: JAK3-dependent and independent pathways. *Immunity* 1996;5:605.
62. Kaplan MH, Schindler U, Smiley ST, Grusby MJ. Stat6 is required for mediating responses to IL-4 and for development of Th2 cells. *Immunity* 1996;4:313.
63. Keegan AD, Nelms K, White M, et al. An IL-4 receptor region containing an insulin receptor motif is important for IL-4-mediated IRS-1 phosphorylation and cell growth. *Cell* 1994;76:811.
64. Kuhn R, Rajewsky K, Muller W. Generation and analysis of interleukin-4 deficient mice. *Science* 1991;254:707.
65. Mitsuyasu H, Izuhara K, Mao XQ, et al. Ile50Val variant of IL4R alpha upregulates IgE synthesis and associates with atopic asthma [Letter]. *Nat Genet* 1998;19:119.
66. Song Z, Casolaro V, Chen R, et al. Polymorphic nucleotides within the human IL-4 promoter that mediate overexpression of the gene. *J Immunol* 1996;156:424.
67. Parronchi P, Maggi E, Romagnani S. Redirecting Th2 responses in allergy. *Curr Top Microbiol Immunol* 1999;238:27.
68. Kinashi T, Harada N, Severinson E, et al. Cloning of complementary DNA encoding T-cell replacing factor and identity with B-cell growth factor II. *Nature* 1986;324:70.
69. Azuma C, Tanabe T, Konishi M, et al. Cloning of cDNA for human T-cell replacing factor interleukin-5 and comparison with the murine homologue. *Nucleic Acids Res* 1986; 14:9149.
70. Milburn MV, Hassell AM, Lambert MH, et al. A novel dimer configuration revealed by the crystal structure at 2.4 Å resolution of human interleukin-5. *Nature* 1993;363:172.
71. Tavernier J, Devos R, Cornelis S, et al. A human high affinity interleukin-5 receptor (IL5R) is composed of an IL5-specific alpha chain and a beta chain shared with the receptor for GM-CSF. *Cell* 1991;66:1175.
72. Sanderson CJ, Warren DJ, Strath M. Identification of a lymphokine that stimulates eosinophil differentiation *in vitro*. Its relationship to interleukin-3, functional properties of eosinophils produced in cultures. *J Exp Med* 1985;162:60.
73. Kopf M, Brombacher F, Hodgkin PD, et al. IL-5-deficient mice have a developmental defect in CD5+ B-1 cells and lack eosinophilia but have normal antibody and cytotoxic T cell responses. *Immunity* 1996;4:15.
74. Yamaguchi Y, Hayashi Y, Sugama Y, et al. Highly purified murine interleukin 5 (IL-5) stimulates eosinophil function and prolongs *in vitro* survival. IL-5 as an eosinophil chemotactic factor. *J Exp Med* 1988;167:1737.
75. Matthaei KI, Foster P, Young IG. The role of interleukin-5 (IL-5) *in vivo* studies with IL-5 deficient mice. *Mem Inst Oswaldo Cruz* 1997;92[Suppl 2]:63.
76. Sugaya H, Aoki M, Yoshida T, Takatsu K, Yoshimura K. Eosinophilia and intracranial worm recovery in interleukin-5 transgenic and interleukin-5 receptor alpha chain-knockout mice infected with *Angiostrongylus cantonensis*. *Parasitol Res* 1997;83:583.
77. Okudaira H, Nogami M, Matsuzaki G, et al. T-cell-dependent accumulation of eosinophils in the lung and its inhibition by monoclonal anti-interleukin-5. *Int Arch Allergy Appl Immunol* 1991;94:171.
78. McKinnon M, Page K, Uings IJ, et al. An interleukin 5 mutant distinguishes between two functional responses in human eosinophils. *J Exp Med* 1997;186:121.
79. Yamasaki K, Taga T, Hirata Y, et al. Cloning and expression of the human interleukin-6 BSF-2/IFN beta 2 receptor. *Science* 1988;241:825.

80. Taga T, Hibi M, Hirata Y, et al. Interleukin-6 triggers the association of its receptor with a possible signal transducer, gp130. *Cell* 1989;58:573.
81. Nakashima K, Taga T. gp130 and the IL-6 family of cytokines: signaling mechanisms and thrombopoietic activities. *Semin Hematol* 1998;35:210.
82. Hirano T, Yasukawa K, Harada H, et al. Complementary DNA for a novel human interleukin BSF-2 that induces B lymphocytes to produce immunoglobulin. *Nature* 1986;324:73.
83. May LT, Helfgott DC, Sehgal PB. Anti-beta-interferon antibodies inhibit the increased expression of HLA-B7 mRNA in tumor necrosis factor–treated human fibroblasts: structural studies of the beta 2 interferon involved. *Proc Natl Acad Sci U S A* 1986;83:8957.
84. Kopf M, Baumann H, Freer G, et al. Impaired immune and acute-phase responses in interleukin-6-deficient mice. *Nature* 1994;368:339.
85. Poli V, Balena R, Fattori E, et al. Interleukin-6 deficient mice are protected from bone loss caused by estrogen depletion. *EMBO J* 1994;13:1189.
86. Zetterstrom M, Sundgren-Andersson AK, Ostlund P, Bartfai T. Delineation of the proinflammatory cytokine cascade in fever induction. *Ann N Y Acad Sci* 1998;856:48.
87. Bernad A, Kopf M, Kulbacki R, et al. Interleukin-6 is required *in vivo* for the regulation of stem cells and committed progenitors of the hematopoietic system. *Immunity* 1994;1:725.
88. Hilbert DM, Kopf M, Mock BA, Kohler G, Rudikoff S. Interleukin 6 is essential for *in vivo* development of B lineage neoplasms. *J Exp Med* 1995;182:243.
89. Strassmann G, Kambayashi T. Inhibition of experimental cancer cachexia by anti-cytokine and anti-cytokine-receptor therapy. *Cytokines Mol Ther* 1995;1:107.
90. Hawley RG, Berger LC. Growth control mechanisms in multiple myeloma. *Leuk Lymphoma* 1998;29:465.
91. Namen AE, Lupton S, Hjerrild K, et al. Stimulation of B-cell progenitors by cloned murine interleukin-7. *Nature* 1988;333:571.
92. Kitazawa H, Muegge K, Badolato R, et al. IL-7 activates $\alpha4\beta1$ integrin in murine thymocytes. *J Immunol* 1997;159:2259.
93. Oosterwegel MA, Haks MC, Jeffry U, Murray R, Kruisbeek AM. Induction of TCR gene rearrangements in uncommitted stem cells by a subset of IL-7 producing, MHC class-II-expressing thymic stromal cells. *Immunity* 1997;6:351.
94. Funk PE, Stephan RP, Witte PL. Vascular cell adhesion molecule 1–positive reticular cells express interleukin-7 and stem cell factor in the bone marrow. *Blood* 1995;86:2661.
95. Watanabe M, Ueno Y, Yajima T, et al. Interleukin-7 is produced by human intestinal epithelial cells and regulates the proliferation of intestinal mucosal lymphocytes. *J Clin Invest* 1995; 95:2945.
96. Kroncke R, Loppnow H, Flad HD, Gerdes J. Human follicular dendritic cells and vascular cells produce interleukin-7: a potential role for interleukin-7 in the germinal center reaction. *Eur J Immunol* 1996;26:2541.
97. Goodwin RG, Friend D, Ziegler SF, et al. Cloning of the human and murine interleukin-7 receptors: demonstration of a soluble form and homology to a new receptor superfamily. *Cell* 1990;60:941.
98. Noguchi M, Nakamura Y, Russell SM, et al. Interleukin-2 receptor gamma chain: a functional component of the interleukin-7 receptor. *Science* 1993;262:1877.
99. Kondo M, Takeshita T, Higuchi M, et al. Functional participation of the IL-2 receptor gamma chain in IL-7 receptor complexes. *Science* 1994;263:1453.
100. Levin SD, Koelling RM, Friend SL, et al. Thymic stromal lymphopoietin: a cytokine that promotes the development of IgM+ B cells *in vitro* and signals via a novel mechanism. *J Immunol* 1999;162:677.
101. Foxwell BM, Beadling C, Guschin D, Kerr I, Cantrell D. Interleukin-7 can induce the activation of Jak 1, Jak 3 and STAT 5 proteins in murine T cells. *Eur J Immunol* 1995;25:3041.
102. Prieyl JA, LeBien TW. Interleukin 7 independent development of human B cells. *Proc Natl Acad Sci U S A* 1996;93:10348.
103. von Freeden-Jeffry U, Vieira P, Lucian LA, et al. Lymphopenia in interleukin (IL)-7 gene-deleted mice identifies IL-7 as a nonredundant cytokine. *J Exp Med* 1995;181:1519.
104. Peschon JJ, Morrissey PJ, Grabstein KH, et al. Early lymphocyte expansion is severely impaired in interleukin-7 receptor-deficient mice. *J Exp Med* 1994;180:1955.
105. Kim K, Lee CK, Sayers TJ, Muegge K, Durum SK. The trophic action of IL-7 on pro-T cells: inhibition of apoptosis of pro-T1, -T2, -T3 cells correlates with Bcl-2 and Bax levels and is independent of Fas and p53 pathways. *J Immunol* 1998;160:5735.
106. Muegge K, Vila MP, Durum SK. Interleukin-7: a cofactor for VDJ rearrangement of the T cell receptor beta gene. *Science* 1993;261:93.
107. Morrissey PJ, Conlon P, Charrier K, et al. Administration of IL-7 to normal mice stimulates B-lymphopoiesis and peripheral lymphadenopathy. *J Immunol* 1991;147:561.
108. Komschlies KL, Gregorio TA, Gruys ME, et al. Administration of recombinant human IL-7 to mice alters the composition of B-lineage cells and T cell subsets, enhances T cell function, induces regression of established metastases. *J Immunol* 1994;152:5776.
109. Rich BE, Campos-Torres J, Tepper RI, Moreadith RW, Leder P. Cutaneous lymphoproliferation and lymphomas in interleukin-7 transgenic mice. *J Exp Med* 1993;177:305.
110. Dalloul A, Laroche L, Bagot M, et al. Interleukin-7 is a growth factor for Sézary lymphoma cells. *J Clin Invest* 1992;90:1054.
111. Yoshimura T, Matsushima K, Tanaka S, et al. Purification of a human monocyte-derived neutrophil chemotactic factor that has peptide sequence similarity to other host defense cytokines. *Proc Natl Acad Sci U S A* 1987;84:9233.
112. Walz A, Peveri P, Aschauer H, Baggiolini M. Purification and amino acid sequencing of NAF, a novel neutrophil-activating factor produced by monocytes. *Biochem Biophys Res Commun* 1987;149:755.
113. Schroder JM, Mrowietz U, Morita E, Christophers E. Purification and partial biochemical characterization of a human monocyte-derived, neutrophil-activating peptide that lacks interleukin-1 activity. *J Immunol* 1987;139:3474.
114. Schmid J, Weissmann C. Induction of mRNA for a serine protease and a beta-thromboglobulin-like protein in mitogen-stimulated human leukocytes. *J Immunol* 1987;139:250.
115. Middleton J, Neil S, Wintle J, et al. Transcytosis and surface presentation of IL-8 by venularendothelial cells. *Cell* 1997;91:385.
116. Wang JM, Su S, Gong W, Oppenheim JJ. Chemokines, receptors, and their role in cardiovascular pathology. *Int J Clin Lab Res* 1998;28:83.
117. Baggiolini M, Dewald B, Moser B. Interleukin-8 and related chemotactic cytokines—CXC and CC chemokines. *Adv Immunol* 1994;55:97.
118. Murphy PM, Tiffany HL. Cloning of complementary DNA encoding a functional human interleukin-8 receptor. *Science* 1991;253:1280.
119. Holmes WE, Lee J, Kuang WJ, Rice GC, Wood WI. Structure and functional expression of a human interleukin-8 receptor. *Science* 1991;253:1278.
120. Murphy PM. Neutrophil receptors for interleukin-8 and related CXC chemokines. *Semin Hematol* 1997;34:311.
121. Jones SA, Wolf M, Qin S, Mackay CR, Baggiolini M. Different functions for the interleukin-8 receptors (IL-8R) of human neutrophil leukocytes: NADPH oxidase and phospholipase D are activated through IL-8R1 but not IL-8R2. *Proc Natl Acad Sci U S A* 1996;93:6682.
122. Damaj BB, McColl SR, Mahana W, Crouch MF, Naccache PH. Physical association of Gi2alpha with interleukin-8 receptors. *J Biol Chem* 1996;271:12783.
123. Sekido N, Mukaida N, Harada A, et al. Prevention of lung reperfusion injury in rabbits by a monoclonal antibody against interleukin-8. *Nature* 1993;365:654.
124. Broaddus VC, Boylan AM, Hoeffel JM, et al. Neutralization of IL-8 inhibits neutrophil influx in a rabbit model of endotoxin-induced pleurisy. *J Immunol* 1994;152:2960.
125. Folkesson HG, Matthay MA, Hebert CA, Broaddus VC. Acid aspiration–induced lung injury in rabbits is mediated by interleukin-8-dependent mechanisms. *J Clin Invest* 1995;96:107.
126. Cacalano G, Lee J, Kikly K, et al. Neutrophil and B cell expansion in mice that lack the murine IL-8 receptor homolog. *Science* 1994;265:682.
127. Moore BB, Arenberg DA, Addison CL, Keane MP, Strieter RM. Tumor angiogenesis is regulated by CXC chemokines. *J Lab Clin Med* 1998;132:97.
128. Harada A, Mukaida N, Matsushima K. Interleukin-8 as a novel target for intervention therapy in acute inflammatory diseases. *Mol Med Today* 1996;2:482.
129. Van Snick J, Goethals A, Renauld JC, et al. Cloning and characterization of a cDNA for a new mouse T cell growth factor P40. *J Exp Med* 1989;169:363.
130. Hultner L, Druez C, Moeller J, et al. Mast cell growth-enhancing activity (MEA) is structurally related and functionally identical to the novel mouse T cell growth factor P40/TCGFIII interleukin-9. *Eur J Immunol* 1990;20:1413.
131. Renauld JC, Goethals A, Houssiau F, et al. Human P40/IL-9. Expression in activated CD4+ T cells, genomic organization, and comparison with the mouse gene. *J Immunol* 1990;144:4235.
132. Houssiau FA, Renauld JC, Fibbe WE, Van Snick J. IL-2 dependence of IL-9 expression in human T lymphocytes. *J Immunol* 1992;148:3147.
133. Gessner A, Blum H, Rollinghoff M. Differential regulation of IL-9-expression after infection with *Leishmania major* in susceptible and resistant mice. *Immunobiology* 1993;189:419.
134. Renauld JC, Druez C, Kermouni A, et al. Expression cloning of the murine and human interleukin-9 receptor cDNAs. *Proc Natl Acad Sci U S A* 1992;89:5690.
135. Vermeesch JR, Petit P, Kermouni A, et al. The IL-9 receptor gene, located in the Xq/Yq pseudoautosomal region, has an autosomal origin, escapes X inactivation and is expressed from the Y. *Hum Mol Genet* 1997;6:1.
136. Kimura Y, Takeshita T, Kondo M, et al. Sharing of the IL-2 receptor gamma chain with the functional IL-receptor complex. *Int Immunol* 1995;7:115.
137. Yin T, Tsang ML, Yang YC. JAK1 kinase forms complexes with interleukin-4 receptor and 4PS/insulin receptor substrate-1-like protein and is activated by interleukin-4 and interleukin-9 in T lymphocytes. *J Biol Chem* 1994;269:26614.
138. Demoulin JB, Uyttenhove C, Van Roost E, et al. A single tyrosine of the interleukin-9 (IL-9) receptor is required for STAT activation, antiapoptotic activity, growth regulation by IL-9. *Mol Cell Biol* 1996;16:4710.
139. Bauer JH, Liu KD, You Y, Lai SY, Goldsmith MA. Heteromerization of the gamma c chain with the interleukin-9 receptor alpha subunit leads to STAT activation and prevention of apoptosis. *J Biol Chem* 1998;273:9255.
140. Yang YC, Ricciardi S, Ciarletta A, et al. Expression cloning of cDNA encoding a novel human hematopoietic growth factor: human homologue of murine T-cell growth factor P40. *Blood* 1989;74:1880.
141. Kelleher K, Bean K, Clark SC, et al. Human interleukin-9: genomic sequence, chromosomal location, sequences essential for its expression in human T-cell leukemia virus (HTLV)-I-transformed human T cells. *Blood* 1991;77:1436.
142. Renauld JC, van der Lugt N, Vink A, et al. Thymic lymphomas in interleukin 9 transgenic mice. *Oncogene* 1994;9:1327.
143. Merz H, Houssiau FA, Orscheschek K, et al. Interleukin-9 expression in human malignant lymphomas: unique association with Hodgkin's disease and large cell anaplastic lymphoma. *Blood* 1991;78:1311.
144. Petit-Frere C, Dugas B, Braquet P, Mencia-Huerta JM. Interleukin-9 potentiates the interleukin-4-induced IgE and IgG1 release from murine B lymphocytes. *Immunology* 1993;79:146.
145. Donahue RE, Yang YC, Clark SC. Human P40 T-cell growth factor interleukin-9 supports erythroid colony formation. *Blood* 1990;75:2271.
146. Hsu DH, de Waal M, Fiorentino DF, et al. Expression of interleukin-10 activity by Epstein-Barr virus protein BCRF1. *Science* 1990;250:830.
147. Ho AS, Liu Y, Khan TA, et al. A receptor for interleukin 10 is related to interferon receptors. *Proc Natl Acad Sci U S A* 1993;90:11267.
148. Liu Y, Wei SH, Ho AS, de Waal M, Moore KW. Expression cloning and characterization of a human IL-10 receptor. *J Immunol* 1994;152:1821.
149. Spencer SD, Di Marco F, Hooley J, et al. The orphan receptor CRF2-4 is an essential subunit of the interleukin 10 receptor. *J Exp Med* 1998;187:571.
150. Finbloom DS, Winestock KD. IL-10 induces the tyrosine phosphorylation of tyk2 and Jak1 and the differential assembly of STAT1 alpha and STAT3 complexes in human T cells and monocytes. *J Immunol* 1995;155:1079.
151. O'Farrell AM, Liu Y, Moore KW, Mui AL. IL-10 inhibits macrophage activation and proliferation by distinct signaling mechanisms: evidence for Stat3-dependent and -independent pathways. *EMBO J* 1998;17:1006.

152. Moore KW, Vieira P, Fiorentino DF, et al. Homology of cytokine synthesis inhibitory factor IL-10 to the Epstein-Barr virus gene BCRFI. *Science* 1990;248:1230.
153. Kuhn R, Lohler J, Rennick D, Rajewsky K, Muller W. Interleukin-10-deficient mice develop chronic enterocolitis. *Cell* 1993;75:263.
154. Pajkrt D, Camoglio L, Tiel-van Buul MC, et al. Attenuation of proinflammatory response by recombinant human IL-10 in human endotoxemia: effect of timing of recombinant human IL-10 administration. *J Immunol* 1997;158:3971.
155. Opal SM, Wherry JC, Grint P. Interleukin-10: potential benefits and possible risks in clinical infectious diseases. *Clin Infect Dis* 1998;27:1497.
156. Beatty PR, Krams SM, Martinez OM. Involvement of IL-10 in the autonomous growth of EBV-transformed B cell lines. *J Immunol* 1997;158:4045.
157. Khatri VP, Caligiuri MA. A review of the association between interleukin-10 and human B-cell malignancies. *Cancer Immunol Immunother* 1998;46:239.
158. Paul SR, Bennett F, Calvetti JA, et al. Molecular cloning of a cDNA encoding interleukin 11, a stromal cell-derived lymphopoietic and hematopoietic cytokine. *Proc Natl Acad Sci U S A* 1990;87:7512.
159. Du X, Williams DA. Interleukin-11: review of molecular, cell biology, clinical use. *Blood* 1997;89:3897.
160. Baumann H, Wang Y, Morella KK, et al. Complex of the soluble IL-11 receptor and IL-11 acts as IL-6-type cytokine in hepatic and non-hepatic cells. *J Immunol* 1996;157:284.
161. Nandurkar HH, Robb L, Tarlinton D, et al. Adult mice with targeted mutation of the interleukin-11 receptor IL11Ra display normal hematopoiesis. *Blood* 1997;90:2148.
162. Robb L, Li R, Hartley L, et al. Infertility in female mice lacking the receptor for interleukin-11 is due to a defective uterine response to implantation. *Nat Med* 1998;4:303.
163. Tepler I, Elias L, Smith JW, et al. A randomized placebo-controlled trial of recombinant human interleukin-11 in cancer patients with severe thrombocytopenia due to chemotherapy. *Blood* 1996;87:3607.
164. Du XX, Williams DA. Interleukin-11: a multifunctional growth factor derived from the hematopoietic microenvironment. *Blood* 1994;83:2023.
165. Gubler U, Chua AO, Schoenhaut DS, et al. Coexpression of two distinct genes is required to generate secreted bioactive cytotoxic lymphocyte maturation factor. *Proc Natl Acad Sci U S A* 1991;88:4143.
166. Wolf SF, Temple PA, Kobayashi M, et al. Cloning of cDNA for natural killer cell stimulatory factor, a heterodimeric cytokine with multiple biologic effects on T and natural killer cells. *J Immunol* 1991;146:3074.
167. Trinchieri G. Interleukin-12: a cytokine at the interface of inflammation and immunity. *Adv Immunol* 1998;70:83.
168. Mattner F, Fischer S, Guckes S, et al. The interleukin-12 subunit p40 specifically inhibits effects of the interleukin-12 heterodimer. *Eur J Immunol* 1993;23:2202.
169. Shu U, Kiniwa M, Wu CY, et al. Activated T cells induce interleukin-12 production by monocytes via CD40-CD40 ligand interaction. *Eur J Immunol* 1995;25:1125.
170. Schoenhaut DS, Chua AO, Wolitzky AG, et al. Cloning and expression of murine IL-12. *J Immunol* 1992;148:3433.
171. Chua AO, Chizzonite R, Desai BB, et al. Expression cloning of a human IL-12 receptor component. A new member of the cytokine receptor superfamily with strong homology to gp130. *J Immunol* 1994;153:128.
172. Presky DH, Yang H, Minetti LJ, et al. A functional interleukin 12 receptor complex is composed of two beta-type cytokine receptor subunits. *Proc Natl Acad Sci U S A* 1996;93:14002.
173. Szabo SJ, Dighe AS, Gubler U, Murphy KM. Regulation of the interleukin (IL)-12R beta 2 subunit expression in developing T helper 1 (Th1) and Th2 cells. *J Exp Med* 1997; 185:817.
174. Bacon CM, McVicar DW, Ortaldo JR, et al. Interleukin 12 (IL-12) induces tyrosine phosphorylation of JAK2 and TYK2: differential use of Janus family tyrosine kinases by IL-2 and IL-12. *J Exp Med* 1995;181:399.
175. Zou J, Presky DH, Wu CY, Gubler U. Differential associations between the cytoplasmic regions of the interleukin-12 receptor subunits beta1 and beta2 and JAK kinases. *J Biol Chem* 1997;272:6073.
176. Jacobson NG, Szabo SJ, Weber-Nordt RM, et al. Interleukin 12 signaling in T helper type 1 (Th1) cells involves tyrosine phosphorylation of signal transducer and activator of transcription Stat3 and Stat4. *J Exp Med* 1995;181:1755.
177. Coccia EM, Passini N, Battistini A, et al. Interleukin-12 induces expression of interferon regulatory factor-1 via signal transducer and activator of transcription-4 in human T helper type 1 cells. *J Biol Chem* 1999;274:6698.
178. Magram J, Connaughton SE, Warrier RR, et al. IL-12-deficient mice are defective in IFN gamma production and type 1 cytokine responses. *Immunity* 1996;4:471.
179. Piccotti JR, Li K, Chan SY, et al. Alloantigen-reactive Th1 development in IL-12-deficient mice. *J Immunol* 1998;160:1132.
180. Robertson MJ, Cameron C, Atkins MB, et al. Immunological effects of interleukin 12 administered by bolus intravenous injection to patients with cancer. *Clin Cancer Res* 1999;5:9.
181. Brunda MJ, Luistro L, Warrier RR, et al. Antitumor and antimetastatic activity of interleukin 12 against murine tumors. *J Exp Med* 1993;178:1223.
182. Wigginton JM, Komschlies KL, Back TC, et al. Administration of interleukin-12 with pulse interleukin-2 and the rapid and complete eradication of murine renal carcinoma. *J Natl Cancer Inst* 1996;88:38.
183. Caspi RR. IL-12 in autoimmunity. *Clin Immunol Immunopathol* 1998;88:4.
184. de Vries JE. The role of IL-13 and its receptor in allergy and inflammatory responses. *J Allergy Clin Immunol* 1998;102:1657.
185. Brown KD, Zurawski SM, Mosmann TR, Zurawski G. A family of small inducible proteins secreted by leukocytes are members of a new superfamily that includes leukocyte and fibroblast-derived inflammatory agents, growth factors, indicators of various activation processes. *J Immunol* 1989;142:679.
186. McKenzie AN, Culpepper JA, de Waal M, et al. Interleukin-13, a T-cell-derived cytokine that regulates human monocyte and B-cell function. *Proc Natl Acad Sci U S A* 1993;90:3735.
187. Aman MJ, Tayebi N, Obiri NI, et al. cDNA cloning and characterization of the human interleukin-13 receptor alpha chain. *J Biol Chem* 1996;271:29265.
188. Hilton DJ, Zhang JG, Metcalf D, et al. Cloning and characterization of a binding subunit of the interleukin-13 receptor that is also a component of the interleukin-4 receptor. *Proc Natl Acad Sci U S A* 1996;93:497.
189. Keegan AD, Johnston JA, Tortolani PJ, et al. Similarities and differences in signal transduction by interleukin-4 and interleukin-13: analysis of Janus kinase activation. *Proc Natl Acad Sci U S A* 1995;92:7681.
190. McKenzie GJ, Emson CL, Bell SE, et al. Impaired development of Th2 cells in IL-13-deficient mice. *Immunity* 1998;9:423.
191. Grabstein KH, Eisenman J, Shanebeck K, et al. Cloning of a T cell growth factor that interacts with the beta chain of the interleukin-2 receptor. *Science* 1994;264:965.
192. Burton JD, Bamford RN, Peters C, et al. A lymphokine, provisionally designated interleukin T and produced by a human adult T-cell leukemia line, stimulates T-cell proliferation and the induction of lymphokine-activated killer cells. *Proc Natl Acad Sci U S A* 1994;91:4935.
193. Cosman D, Kumaki S, Anderson D, et al. Interleukin 15. *Biochem Soc Trans* 1997;25:371.
194. Bamford RN, DeFilippis AP, Azimi N, Kurys G, Waldmann TA. The 5' untranslated region, signal peptide, the coding sequence of the carboxyl terminus of IL-15 participate in its multifaceted translational control. *J Immunol* 1998;160:4418.
195. Giri JG, Ahdieh M, Eisenman J, et al. Utilization of the beta and gamma chains of the IL-2 receptor by the novel cytokine IL-15. *EMBO J* 1994;13:2822.
196. Giri JG, Kumaki S, Ahdieh M, et al. Identification and cloning of a novel IL-15 binding protein that is structurally related to the alpha chain of the IL-2 receptor. *EMBO J* 1995;14:3654.
197. Tagaya Y, Burton JD, Miyamoto Y, Waldmann TA. Identification of a novel receptor/signal transduction pathway for IL-15/T in mast cells. *EMBO J* 1996;15:4928.
198. Williams NS, Klem J, Puzanov IJ, et al. Natural killer cell differentiation: insights from knockout and transgenic mouse models and *in vitro* systems. *Immunol Rev* 1998;165:47.
199. Lodolce JP, Boone DL, Chai S, et al. IL-15 receptor maintains lymphoid homeostasis by supporting lymphocyte homing and proliferation. *Immunity* 1998;9:669.
200. Center DM, Cruikshank W. Modulation of lymphocyte migration by human lymphokines. I. Identification and characterization of chemoattractant activity for lymphocytes from mitogen-stimulated mononuclear cells. *J Immunol* 1982;128:2563.
201. Cruikshank W, Center DM. Modulation of lymphocyte migration by human lymphokines. II. Purification of a lymphotactic factor LCF. *J Immunol* 1982;128:2569.
202. Cruikshank WW, Kornfeld H, Center DM. Signaling and functional properties of interleukin-16. *Int Rev Immunol* 1998;16:523.
203. Zhang Y, Center DM, Wu DM, et al. Processing and activation of pro-interleukin-16 by caspase-3. *J Biol Chem* 1998;273:1144.
204. Muhlhahn P, Zweckstetter M, Georgescu J, et al. Structure of interleukin-16 resembles a PDZ domain with an occluded peptide binding site. *Nat Struct Biol* 1998;5:682.
205. Laberge S, Cruikshank WW, Kornfeld H, Center MD. Histamine-induced secretion of lymphocyte chemoattractant factor from CD8+ T cells is independent of transcription and translation. Evidence for constitutive protein synthesis and storage. *J Immunol* 1995;155:2902.
206. Lim KG, Wan HC, Bozza PT, et al. Human eosinophils elaborate the lymphocyte chemoattractants. IL-16 lymphocyte chemoattractant factor and RANTES. *J Immunol* 1996;156:2566.
207. Bellini A, Yoshimura H, Vittori E, Marini M, Mattoli S. Bronchial epithelial cells of patients with asthma release chemoattractant factors for T lymphocytes. *J Allergy Clin Immunol* 1993;92:412.
208. Cruikshank WW, Greenstein JL, Theodore AC, Center DM. Lymphocyte chemoattractant factor induces CD4-dependent intracytoplasmic signaling in lymphocytes. *J Immunol* 1991;146:2928.
209. Theodore AC, Center DM, Nicoll J, et al. CD4 ligand IL-16 inhibits the mixed lymphocyte reaction. *J Immunol* 1996;157:1958.
210. Maciaszek JW, Parada NA, Cruikshank WW, et al. IL-16 represses HIV-1 promoter activity. *J Immunol* 1997;158:5.
211. Rouvier E, Luciani MF, Mattei MG, Denizot F, Golstein P. CTLA-8, cloned from an activated T cell, bearing AU-rich messenger RNA instability sequences, and homologous to a herpesvirus saimiri gene. *J Immunol* 1993;150:5445.
212. Yao Z, Painter SL, Fanslow WC, et al. Human IL-17: a novel cytokine derived from T cells. *J Immunol* 1995;155:5483.
213. Yao Z, Timour M, Painter S, Fanslow W, Spriggs M. Complete nucleotide sequence of the mouse CTLA8 gene. *Gene* 1996;168:223.
214. Fossiez F, Djossou O, Chomarat P, et al. T cell interleukin-17 induces stromal cells to produce proinflammatory and hematopoietic cytokines. *J Exp Med* 1996;183:2593.
215. Yao Z, Fanslow WC, Seldin MF, et al. Herpesvirus Saimiri encodes a new cytokine, IL-17, which binds to a novel cytokine receptor. *Immunity* 1995;3:811.
216. Antonysamy MA, Fanslow WC, Fu F, et al. Evidence for a role of IL-17 in organ allograft rejection: IL-17 promotes the functional differentiation of dendritic cell progenitors. *J Immunol* 1999;162:577.
217. Spriggs MK. Interleukin-17 and its receptor. *J Clin Immunol* 1997;17:366.
218. Okamura H, Tsutsi H, Komatsu T, et al. Cloning of a new cytokine that induces IFN-gamma production by T cells. *Nature* 1995;378:88.
219. Fantuzzi G, Dinarello CA. Interleukin-18 and interleukin-1 beta: two cytokine substrates for ICE caspase-1. *J Clin Immunol* 1999;19:1.
220. Gu Y, Kuida K, Tsutsui H, et al. Activation of interferon-gamma inducing factor mediated by interleukin-1beta converting enzyme. *Science* 1997;275:206.
221. Ghayur T, Banerjee S, Hugunin M, et al. Caspase-1 processes IFN-gamma-inducing factor and regulates Lps-induced IFN-gamma production. *Nature* 1997;386:619.
222. Puren AJ, Fantuzzi G, Dinarello CA. Gene expression, synthesis, secretion of interleukin-18 and interleukin-1 beta are differentially regulated in human blood mononuclear cells and mouse spleen cells. *Proc Natl Acad Sci U S A* 1999;96:2256.

223. Parnet P, Garka KE, Bonnert TP, Dower SK, Sims JE. IL-1Rrp is a novel receptor-like molecule similar to the type I interleukin-1 receptor and its homologues T1/ST2 and IL-1R AcP. *J Biol Chem* 1996;271:3967.
224. Torigoe K, Ushio S, Okura T, et al. Purification and characterization of the human interleukin-18 receptor. *J Biol Chem* 1997;272:25737.
225. Dale M, Nicklin MJ. Interleukin-1 receptor cluster: gene organization of IL-1R2, IL-1R1, IL-1RL2 IL-1Rrp2, IL-1RL1 T1/ST2, IL-18R1 IL-1Rrp on human chromosome 2q. *Genomics* 1999;57:177.
226. Born TL, Thomassen E, Bird TA, Sims JE. Cloning of a novel receptor subunit, AcPL, required for interleukin-18 signaling. *J Biol Chem* 1998;273:29445.
227. Novick D, Kim SH, Fantuzzi G, et al. Interleukin-18 binding protein: a novel modulator of the Th1 cytokine response. *Immunity* 1999;10:127.
228. Kojima H, Takeuchi M, Ohta T, et al. Interleukin-18 activates the IRAK-TRAF6 pathway in mouse EL-4 cells. *Biochem Biophys Res Commun* 1998;244:183.
229. Xu D, Chan WL, Leung BP, et al. Selective expression and functions of interleukin-18 receptor on T helper (Th) type 1 but not Th2 cells. *J Exp Med* 1998;188:1485.
230. Takeda K, Tsutsui H, Yoshimoto T, et al. Defective NK cell activity and Th1 response in IL-18-deficient mice. *Immunity* 1998;8:383.
231. Gross L. Intradermal immunization of C3H mice against a sarcoma that originated in an animal of the same line. *Cancer Res* 1943;3:326.
232. Foley EJ. Antigenic properties of methylcholanthrene-induced tumors in mice of the strain of origin. *Cancer Res* 1953;13:835.
233. Baldwin RW. Immunity to methylcholanthrene-induced tumors in inbred rats following atrophy and regression of implanted tumors. *Br J Cancer* 1955;9:652.
234. Prehn RT, Main JM. Immunity to methylcholanthrene-induced sarcomas. *J Natl Cancer Inst* 1957;18:769.
235. Klein G, Sjögren HO, Klein E, Hellström KE. Demonstration of resistance against methylcholanthrene-induced sarcomas in the primary autochthonous host. *Cancer Res* 1960;20:1561.
236. Old LJ, Boyse EA, Clarke DA, Carswell EA. Antigenic properties of chemically induced tumors. *Ann N Y Acad Sci* 1962;101:80.
237. Globerson A, Feldmann M. Antigenic specificity of benzo[a]pyrene-induced sarcomas. *J Natl Cancer Inst* 1964;32:1229.
238. Vaage J. Nonvirus-associated antigens in virus-induced mouse mammary tumors. *Cancer Res* 1968;28:2477.
239. Morton DL, Miller GF, Wood DA. Demonstration of tumor-specific immunity against antigens unrelated to the mammary tumor virus in spontaneous mammary adenocarcinomas. *J Natl Cancer Inst* 1969;42:289.
240. Carswell EA, Wanebo HJ, Old LJ, Boyse EA. Immunogenic properties of reticulum cell sarcomas of SJL/J mice. *J Natl Cancer Inst* 1970;44:1281.
241. Koch S, Zaleberg JR, McKenzie IFC. Description of a murine B lymphoma tumor-specific antigen. *J Immunol* 1984;133:1070.
242. Baldwin RW. Tumor-specific immunity to spontaneous rat tumors. *Int J Cancer* 1966;1:257.
243. Basombrio MA. Search for common antigenicity among twenty-five sarcomas induced by methylcholanthrene. *Cancer Res* 1970;30:2458.
244. Basombrio MA, Prehn RT. Studies on the basis for diversity and time of appearance of antigens in chemically induced tumors. *Natl Cancer Inst Monogr* 1972;35:117.
245. Baldwin RW, Price MR. Neoantigen expression in chemical carcinogenesis. In: Becker FF, ed. *Cancer: a comprehensive treatise,* vol 1, 2nd ed. New York: Plenum, 1982:507.
246. Defendi V. Effects of SV40 virus immunization on growth of transplantable SV40 and polyoma virus tumors in hamsters. *Proc Soc Exp Biol Med* 1963;113:12.
247. Khera KS, Ashkenazi A, Rapp F, Melnick JL. Immunity in hamsters to cells transformed *in vitro* among the papovaviruses. *J Immunol* 1963;91:604.
248. Sjögren HO, Hellström I, Klein G. Resistance of polyoma virus–immunized mice to transplantation of established polyoma tumors. *Exp Cell Res* 1961;23:204.
249. Chang CR, Martin RG, Livingston DM, et al. Relationship between T-antigen and tumor specific transplantation antigen in simian virus 40-transformed cells. *J Virol* 1979;29:69.
250. Livingston DM, Bradley MK. The simian virus 40 large T antigen. A lot packed into a little. *Mol Biol Med* 1987;4:63.
251. Boon T, Van Pel A, DePlaen E, et al. Genes coding for T-cell-defined tumor transplantation antigens: point mutations, antigenic peptides, and subgenic expression. *Cold Spring Harbor Symp Quant Biol* 1989;1:587.
252. Hewitt HB, Blake ER, Walder AS. A critique of the evidence for active host defense against cancer based on personal studies of 27 murine tumors of spontaneous origin. *Br J Cancer* 1976;33:241.
253. Middle JG, Embleton MJ. Naturally arising tumors of the inbred WAB/Not rat strain. II. Immunogenicity of transplanted tumors. *J Natl Cancer Inst* 1981;67:637.
254. Rosenberg SA, Spiess P, Lafreniere R. A new approach to the adoptive immunotherapy of cancer with tumor-infiltrating lymphocytes. *Science* 1986;233:1318.
255. Topalian SL, Rosenberg SA. Tumor infiltrating lymphocytes (TIL). Evidence for specific immune reactions against growing cancers in mice and humans. In: DeVita VT, Hellman S, Rosenberg SA, eds. *Important advances in oncology.* Philadelphia: JB Lippincott, 1990:19.
256. Barth RJ, Mulé JJ, Asher AL. Identification of unique murine tumor associated antigens by tumor infiltrating lymphocytes using tumor specific secretion of interferon-gamma and tumor necrosis factor. *J Immunol Methods* 1991;140:269.
257. Hellström I, Hellström KE, Sjögren HO, et al. Demonstration of cell-mediated immunity to human neoplasms of various histological types. *Int J Cancer* 1971;7:1.
258. Hellström I, Hellström KE, Shepard TH. Cell-mediated immunity against antigens common to human colonic carcinomas and fetal gut epithelium. *Int J Cancer* 1970;6:346.
259. Boon T, Coulie PG, Van den Eynde B. Tumor antigens recognized by T cells. *Immunol Today* 1997;18:267.
260. Rosenberg SA. A new era for cancer immunotherapy based on the genes that encode cancer antigens. *Immunity* 1999;10:281.
261. Rosenberg SA. Cancer vaccines based on the identification of genes encoding cancer regression antigens. *Immunol Today* 1997;18:175.
262. Cox AL, Skipper J, Chen Y, et al. Identification of a peptide recognized by five melanoma-specific human cytotoxic T cell lines. *Science* 1994;264:716.
263. Van der Bruggen P, Traversari C, Chomez P, et al. A gene encoding an antigen recognized by cytolytic T lymphocytes on a human melanoma. *Science* 1991;254:1643.
264. Van Den Eynde B, Peeters O, De Backer O, et al. A new family of genes coding for an antigen recognized by autologous cytolytic T lymphocytes on a human melanoma. *J Exp Med* 1995;182:689.
265. Kawakami Y, Eliyahu S, Delgado CH, et al. Cloning of the gene coding for a shared human melanoma antigen recognized by autologous T cells infiltrating into tumor. *Proc Natl Acad Sci U S A* 1994;91:3515.
266. Coulie PG, Brichard V, Van Pel A, et al. A new gene coding for a differentiation antigen recognized by autologous cytolytic T lymphocytes on HLA-A2 melanomas. *J Exp Med* 1994;180:35.
267. Kawakami Y, Eliyahu S, Delgado CH, et al. Identification of a human melanoma antigen recognized by tumor infiltrating lymphocytes associated with *in vivo* tumor rejection. *Proc Natl Acad Sci U S A* 1994;91:6458.
268. Brichard V, Van Pel A, Wolfel T, et al. The tyrosinase gene codes for an antigen recognized by autologous cytolytic T lymphocytes on HLA-A2 melanomas. *J Exp Med* 1993;178:489.
269. Robbins PF, El-Gamil M, Kawakami Y, Rosenberg SA. Recognition of tyrosinase by tumor infiltrating lymphocytes from a patient responding to immunotherapy. *Cancer Res* 1994;54:3124.
270. Wang RF, Robbins PF, Kawakami Y, Kang XQ, Rosenberg SA. Identification of a gene encoding a melanoma tumor antigen recognized by HLA-A31-restricted tumor-infiltrating lymphocytes. *J Exp Med* 1995;181:799.
271. Wang RF, Appella E, Kawakami Y. Identification of TRP-2 as a human tumor antigen recognized by cytotoxic T lymphocytes. *J Exp Med* 1996;184:2207.
272. Salazar-Onfray F, Nakazawa T, Chhajlani V, et al. Synthetic peptides derived from the melanocyte-stimulating hormone receptor MC1R can stimulate HLA-A2-restricted cytotoxic T lymphocytes that recognize naturally processed peptides on human melanoma cells. *Cancer Res* 1997;57:4348.
273. Robbins PF, El-Gamil M, Li YF, et al. A mutated B-catenin gene encodes a melanoma-specific antigen recognized by tumor infiltrating lymphocytes. *J Exp Med* 1996;183:1185.
274. Wolfel T, Hauer M, Schneider J, et al. A p16INK4A-insensitive CDK4 mutant targeted by cytolytic T lymphocytes in a human melanoma. *Science* 1995;269:1281.
275. Coulie PG, Lehmann F, Lethe B, et al. A mutated intron sequence codes for an antigenic peptide recognized by cytolytic T lymphocytes on a human melanoma. *Proc Natl Acad Sci U S A* 1995;92:7976.
276. Mandruzzato S, Brasseur F, Andry G. A CASP-8 mutation recognized by cytolytic T lymphocytes on a human head and neck carcinoma. *J Exp Med* 1997;186:785.
277. Gueguen M, Matard JJ, Gaugler B. An antigen recognized by autologous CTLs on a human bladder carcinoma. *J Immunol* 1998;160:6188.
278. Robbins PF, El-Gamil M, Li Y, et al. Cloning of a new gene encoding an antigen recognized by melanoma-specific HLA-A24-restricted tumor-infiltrating lymphocytes. *J Immunol* 1995;154:5944.
279. Ikeda H, Lethe B, Lehmann F. Characterization of an antigen that is recognized on a melanoma showing partial HLA loss by CTL expressing an NK inhibitory receptor. *Immunity* 1999;6:199.
280. Shichijo S, Nakao M, Imai Y. A gene encoding antigenic peptides of human squamous cell carcinoma recognized by cytotoxic T lymphocytes. *J Exp Med* 1998;187:277.
281. Khanna R, Burrows SR, Kurilla MG, et al. Localization of Epstein-Barr virus cytotoxic T cell epitopes using recombinant vaccinia: implications for vaccine development. *J Exp Med* 1992;176:169.
282. Murray RJ, Kurilla MG, Brooks JM, et al. Identification of target antigens for the human cytotoxic T cell response to Epstein-Barr virus (EBV): implications for the immune control of EBV-positive malignancies. *J Exp Med* 1992;176:157.
283. Kannagi M, Matsushita S, Shida HHS. Cytotoxic T cell response and expression of the target antigen in HTLV-1 infection. *Leukemia* 1994;8:S54.
284. Cerny A, Ferrari C, Chisari FV. The class I–restricted cytotoxic T lymphocyte response to predetermined epitopes in the hepatitis B and C viruses. *Curr Top Microbiol Immunol* 1994;189:169.
285. Topalian SL, Rivoltini L, Mancini M, et al. Human CD4+ T cells specifically recognize a shared melanoma-associated antigen encoded by the tyrosinase gene. *Proc Natl Acad Sci U S A* 1994;91:9461.
286. Halder T, Pawelec G, Kirkin AF, et al. Isolation of novel HLA-DR restricted potential tumor-associated antigens from the melanoma cell line FM3. *Cancer Res* 1997;57:3238.
287. Pieper R, Christian RE, Gonzales MI, et al. Biochemical identification of a mutated human melanoma antigen recognized by CD4+ T cells. *J Exp Med* 1999;189:757.
288. Wang RF, Wang X, Atwood AL, Topalian SL, Rosenberg SA. Cloning genes encoding MHC class II–restricted antigens: mutated CDC27 as a tumor antigen. *Science* 1999;284:1351.
289. Wang RF, Wang X, Rosenberg SA. Identification of a novel major histocompatibility complex class II–restricted tumor antigen resulting from a chromosomal rearrangement recognized by CD4+ T cells. *J Exp Med* 1999;189:1659.
290. Wang RF, Parkhurst MR, Kawakami Y, Robbins PF, Rosenberg SA. Utilization of an alternative open reading frame of a normal gene in generating a novel human cancer antigen. *J Exp Med* 1996;183:1131.
291. Wang RF, Johnston SL, Topalian SL, Schwartzentruber DJ, Rosenberg SA. A breast and melanoma-shared tumor antigen: T cell responses to antigenic peptides translated from different open reading frames. *J Immunol* 1998;161:3596.
292. Robbins PF, El-Gamil M, Li YF, et al. The intronic region of an incompletely spliced gp100 transcript encodes an epitope recognized by melanoma-reactive tumor infiltrating lymphocytes. *J Immunol* 1997;159:303.
293. Kawkami Y, Eliyahu S, Jennings C. Recognition of multiple epitopes in the human melanoma antigen gp100 associated with *in vivo* tumor regression. *J Immunol* 1995;154:3961.
294. Kawakami Y, Robbins PF, Wang X, et al. Identification of new melanoma epitopes on melanosomal proteins recognized by tumor infiltrating T lymphocytes restricted by HLA-A1, -A2, and -A3 alleles. *J Immunol* 1998;161:6985.

295. Skipper JC, Kittlesen DJ, Hendrickson RC. Shared epitopes for HLA-A3-restricted melanoma-reactive human CTL include a naturally processed epitope from Pmel-17/gp100. *J Immunol* 1996;157:5027.
296. Kang XQ, Kawakami Y, Sakaguchi K. Identification of a tyrosinase epitope recognized by HLA-A24 restricted tumor-infiltrating lymphocytes. *J Immunol* 1995;155:1343.
297. Kittlesen DJ, Thompson LW, Gulden PH, et al. Human melanoma patients recognize an HLA-A1-restricted CTL epitope from tyrosinase containing two cysteine residues: implications for tumor vaccine development. *J Immunol* 1998;160:2099.
298. Wolfel T, Van Pel A, Brichard V, et al. Two tyrosinase nonapeptides recognized on HLA-A2 melanomas by autologous cytolytic T lymphocytes. *Eur J Immunol* 1994;24:759.
299. Kohler G, Milstein C. Continuous culture of fused cells secreting antibodies of predefined specificity. *Nature* 1975;256:495.
300. Rosenberg SA, Grimm EA, McGrogan M, et al. Biologic activity of recombinant human interleukin-2 produced in *E. coli*. *Science* 1984;223:1412.
301. Rosenberg SA, Mule JJ, Spiess PJ, Reichert CM, Schwarz S. Regression of established pulmonary metastases and subcutanous tumor mediated by the systemic administration of high-dose recombinant IL-2. *J Exp Med* 1985;161:1169.
302. Schwartzentruber DJ. Interleukin-2: clinical applications: principles of administration and management of side effects. In: Rosenberg SA, ed. *Principles and practice of biologic therapy of cancer.* Philadelphia: Lippincott Williams & Wilkins 2000:32.
303. Kammula US, White DE, Rosenberg SA. Trends in the safety high-dose bolus interleukin-2 administration in patients with metastatic cancer. *Cancer* 1998;83:797.
304. Cormier JN, Salgaller ML, Prevette T, et al. Enhancement of cellular immunity in melanoma patients immunized with a peptide from MART-1/Melan A. *Cancer J Sci Am* 1997;3:37.
305. Salgaller ML, Marincola FM, Cormier JN, Rosenberg SA. Immunization against epitopes in the human melanoma antigen gp100 following patient immunization with synthetic peptides. *Cancer Res* 1996;56:4749.
306. Rosenberg SA, Yang JC, Schwartzentruber DJ, et al. Immunologic and therapeutic evaluation of a synthetic vaccine for the treatment of patients with metastatic melanoma. *Nature Med* 1998;4:321.
307. Parkhurst MR, Salgaller ML, Southwood S, et al. Improved induction of melanoma reactive CTL with peptides from the melanoma antigen gp100 modified at HLA-A* 0210 binding residues. *J Immunol* 1996;157:2539.
308. Rosenberg SA, Lotze MT, Muul LM, et al. Observations of the systemic administration of autologous lymphokine-activated killer cells and recombinant interleukin-2 to patients with metastatic cancer. *N Engl J Med* 1985;313:1485.
309. Rosenberg SA, Lotze MT, Muul LM, et al. A progress report on the treatment of 157 patients with advanced cancer using lymphokine activated killer cells and interleukin-2 or high-dose interleukin-2 alone. *N Engl J Med* 1987;316:889.
310. Rosenberg SA. The immunotherapy and gene therapy of cancer. *J Clin Oncol* 1992;180.
311. Rosenberg SA, Terry W. Passive immunotherapy of cancer in animals and man. *Cancer Res* 1977;25:323.
312. Yron I, Wood TA Jr, Spiess PJ, Rosenberg SA. *In vitro* growth of murine T cells. V. The isolation and growth of lymphoid cells infiltrating syngeneic solid tumors. *J Immunol* 1980;125:238.
313. Lotze MT, Grimm E, Mazumder A, et al. *In vitro* growth of cytotoxic human lymphocytes. IV. Lysis of fresh and cultured autologous tumor by lymphocytes cultured in T cell growth factor (TCGF). *Cancer Res* 1981;41:4420.
314. Grimm EA, Ramsey KM, Mazumder A, et al. Lymphokine-activated killer cell phenomenon. II. The precursor phenotype is serologically distinct from peripheral T lymphocytes, memory CTL, and NK cells. *J Exp Med* 1983;157:884.
315. Roberts R, Lotze MT, Rosenberg SA. Separation and functional studies of the human lymphokine-activated killer cell. *Cancer Res* 1987;47:4366.
316. Phillips LL. Dissection of the LAK phenomenon. *J Exp Med* 1986;164:814.
317. Mulé JJ, Shu S, Schwartz SL, Rosenberg SA. Adoptive immunotherapy of established pulmonary metastases with LAK cells and recombinant interleukin-2. *Science* 1984; 225:1487.
318. Lafreniere R, Rosenberg SA. Adoptive immunotherapy of murine hepatic metastases with lymphokine activated killer (LAK) cells and recombinant interleukin-2 (RIL-2) can mediate the regression of both immunogenic and non-immunogenic sarcomas and an adenocarcinoma. *J Immunol* 1985;135:4273.
319. Ettinghausen SE, Lipford EH III, Mulé JJ, et al. Recombinant interleukin-2 stimulates *in vivo* proliferation of adoptively transferred lymphokine activated killer (LAK) cells. *J Immunol* 1985;135:3623.
320. Topalian SL, Rosenberg SA. Adoptive cellular therapy: basic principles. In: DeVita VT, Hellman S, Rosenberg SA, eds. *Biologic therapy of cancer.* Philadelphia: JB Lippincott, 1991:178.
321. Galili U, Vanky F, Rodriguez L, et al. Activated T lymphocytes within human solid tumors. *Cancer Immunol Immunother* 1979;6:129.
322. Whiteside TL, Miescher S, Hurlimann J, et al. Separation, phenotyping, and limiting dilution analysis of T-lymphocytes infiltrating human solid tumors. *Int J Cancer* 1986;38:803.
323. Whiteside TL, Miescher S, Hurlimman J, et al. Clonal analysis and *in situ* characterization of lymphocytes infiltrating human breast carcinomas. *Cancer Immunol Immunother* 1986;23:169.
324. Paine JT, Handa H, Yamasaki T, et al. Immunohistochemical analysis of infiltrating lymphocytes in central nervous system tumors. *Neurosurgery* 1986;18:766.
325. Itoh K, Tilden AB, Balch CM. Interleukin-2 activation of cytotoxic T-lymphocyte infiltrating into human metastatic melanomas. *Cancer Res* 1986;46:3011.
326. Kurnick JT, Kradin RL, Blumberg R, et al. Functional characterization of T lymphocytes propagated from human lung carcinoma. *Clin Immunol Immunopathol* 1986;38:367.
327. Rabinowich H, Cohen R, Bruderman J, et al. Functional analysis of mononuclear cells infiltrating into tumors; lysis of autologous human tumor cells by cultured infiltrating lymphocytes. *Cancer Res* 1987;47:173.
328. Muul LM, Spiess PJ, Director EP, et al. Identification of specific cytolytic immune responses against autologous tumor in humans bearing malignant melanoma. *J Immunol* 1987;138:989.
329. Heo DL, Whiteside TL, Johnson JT, et al. Long-term interleukin-2-dependent growth and cytotoxic activity of tumor-infiltrating lymphocytes from human squamous cell carcinomas of the head and neck. *Cancer Res* 1987;47:6353.
330. Itoh K, Platsooucas CD, Balch CM. Autologous tumor-specific cytotoxic T lymphocytes in the infiltrate of human metastatic melanomas: activation by interleukin-2 and autologous tumor cells and involvement of the T cell receptor. *J Exp Med* 1988;168:1419.
331. Kuppner MC, Hamou MF, de Tribolet N. Immunohistological and functional analyses of lymphoid infiltrates in human glioblastomas. *Cancer Res* 1988;48:6926.
332. Saito T, Tanaka R, Yoshida S, et al. Immunohistochemical analysis of tumor-infiltrating lymphocytes and major histocompatibility antigens in human gliomas and metastatic brain tumors. *Surg Neurol* 1988;29:435.
333. Heo DS, Whiteside TL, Kanbour A, et al. Lymphocytes infiltrating human ovarian tumors. I. Role of Leu-19 (NKH1)-positive recombinant IL-2 activated cultures of lymphocytes infiltrating human ovarian tumors. *J Immunol* 1988;140:4042.
334. Belldegrun A, Muul LM, Rosenberg SA. Interleukin-2 expanded tumor-infiltrating lymphocytes in human renal cell cancer: isolation, characterization, and anti-tumor activity. *Cancer Res* 1988;48:206.
335. Radrizzani M, Gambacorti-Passerini C, Parmiani G, et al. Lysis by interleukin-2 stimulated tumor-infiltrating lymphocytes of autologous and allogeneic tumor target cells. *Cancer Immunol Immunother* 1989;28:67.
336. Topalian SL, Solomon D, Rosenberg SA. Tumor-specific cytolysis by lymphocytes infiltrating human melanomas. *J Immunol* 1989;142:3714.
337. Tagaki S, Chen K, Schwarz R, et al. Functional and phenotypic analysis of tumor-infiltrating lymphocytes isolated from human primary and metastatic liver tumors and cultured in recombinant interleukin-2. *Cancer* 1989;63:102.
338. Balch CM, Riley LB, Bae TJ, et al. Patterns of human tumor infiltrating lymphocytes in 120 human cancers. *Arch Surg* 1990;125:200.
339. Haas GP, Solomon D, Rosenberg SA. Tumor infiltrating lymphocytes from non renal urological malignancies. *Cancer Immunol Immunother* 1990;30:342.
340. Rivoltini L, Avienti F, Orazi A, et al. Phenotypic and functional analysis of lymphocytes infiltrating pediatric tumors, with a characterization of the tumor phenotype. *Cancer Immunol Immunother* 1992;34:241.
341. Schwartzentruber DJ, Topalian SL, Mancini MJ, et al. Specific release of granulocyte-macrophage colony-stimulating factor, tumor necrosis factor-α, and IFN-γ by human tumor-infiltrating lymphocytes after autologous tumor stimulation. *J Immunol* 1991;146:153.
342. Hom SS, Topalian SL, Simoni ST, et al. Common expression of melanoma tumor-associated antigens recognized by human tumor-infiltrating lymphocytes: analysis by HLA restriction. *J Immunother* 1991;10:153.
343. Darrow TL, Slingluff CL, Seigler HF. The role of class 1 antigens in recognition of melanoma cells by tumor-specific cytotoxic T lymphocytes: evidence for shared tumor antigens. *J Immunol* 1989;142:3329.
344. Stotter H, Wiebke EA, Tomita S, et al. Cytokines alter target cell susceptibility to lysis. II. Evaluation of tumor infiltrating lymphocytes. *J Immunol* 1989;142:1767.
345. Kawakami Y, Rosenberg SA, Lotze MT. Interleukin-4 promotes the growth of tumor-infiltrating lymphocytes cytotoxic for human autologous melanoma. *J Exp Med* 1988;168:2183.
346. Kawakami Y, Zakut R, Topalian SL, et al. Shared human melanoma antigens: recognition by tumor infiltrating lymphocytes in HLA-A2.1-transfected melanomas. *J Immunol* 1992;148:638.
347. Rosenberg SA, Aebersold P, Cornetta K, et al. Gene transfer into humans—immunotherapy of patients with advanced melanoma, using tumor-infiltrating lymphocytes modified by retroviral gene transduction. *N Engl J Med* 1990;323:570.
348. Rosenberg SA. Gene therapy for cancer. *JAMA* 1992;268:2416.
349. Riddell SR, Watanabe KS, Goodrich JM, et al. Restoration of viral immunity in immunodeficient humans by the adoptive transfer of T cell clones. *Science* 1992;257:238.
350. Yee C, Gilbert MJ, Riddell SR. Isolation of tyrosinase-specific CD8+ and CD4+ T cell clones from the peripheral blood of melanoma patients following *in vitro* stimulation with recombinant vaccinia virus. *J Immunol* 1996;157:4079.
351. Dudley ME, Nishimura MI, Czopik AK, Rosenberg SA. Anti-tumor immunization with a minimal epitope (G9-209-2M) leads to a functionally heterogeneous CTL response. *J Immunother* 1999 (*in press*).
352. Yee C, Savage PA, Lee PP, Davis MM, Greenberg PD. Isolation of high avidity melanoma-reactive CTL from heterogeneous populations using peptide-MHC tetramers. *J Immunol* 1999;162:2227.

CHAPTER 19

Pharmacology of Cancer Chemotherapy

SECTION 1

MARK J. RATAIN

Pharmacokinetics and Pharmacodynamics

Medical oncologists prescribe and administer those drugs with the narrowest therapeutic index in all of medicine. Thus, understanding variability in toxicity and response is of utmost importance. Such variability can be divided into two components, pharmacokinetics and pharmacodynamics. Pharmacokinetics, the relationship between time and plasma concentration (Fig. 19.1-1), is concerned with understanding issues such as metabolism and excretion. It can be simply described as "what the body does to the drug."

The clinical interpretation of pharmacokinetic results requires another set of information, the relationship between plasma concentrations (or dose as a surrogate) and effect, or pharmacodynamics (Fig. 19.1-2). This can be described as "what the drug does to the body." The understanding of anticancer pharmacodynamics has increased dramatically, although most studies that have successfully correlated concentration with effect have focused on toxicity end points.[1]

It has become fashionable to conduct clinical pharmacology studies in conjunction with early clinical trials of new anticancer agents, even in multiinstitution (i.e., Cooperative Group) studies. Such studies may have as their objectives pharmacokinetic or pharmacodynamic end points, or both. In phase I trials, the primary pharmacologic objective is to define the pharmacokinetics to optimize scheduling and dosing for subsequent studies. Pharmacodynamic end points are generally secondary, unless an adequate number of patients are studied at or near the recommended phase II dose. Phase II trials offer a different opportunity, because generally all patients are treated at the same dose. Thus, variability in toxicity or response may potentially be related to variability in pharmacokinetics.[2] In addition, population pharmacokinetic studies can be conducted at this phase, with a relatively large patient base, sparse sampling (one to four samples per patient), and the implementation of sophisticated modeling programs.

PHARMACOKINETICS: FUNDAMENTAL PRINCIPLES

The study of pharmacokinetics is classically considered to consist of four aspects: absorption, distribution, metabolism, and excretion. Each of these issues is addressed in their general aspects, and specific examples are given as appropriate.

ABSORPTION

Because most anticancer drugs are administered intravenously, most oncologists have only infrequently dealt with those issues specific to the clinical pharmacology of orally administered agents.[3] The term *absorption* has historically implied transport across the intestinal mucosa, although it has been recognized that the intestinal mucosa is important in xenobiotic metabolism.[4,5]

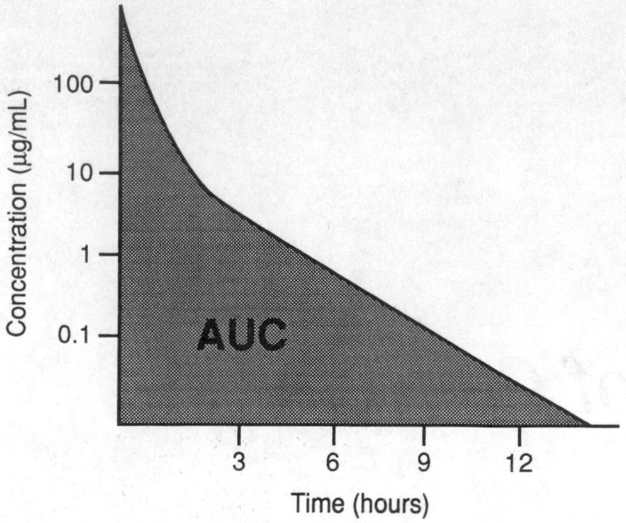

FIGURE 19.1-1. A representative pharmacokinetic profile relating time and concentration. The area under the concentration-time curve (AUC) is shaded.

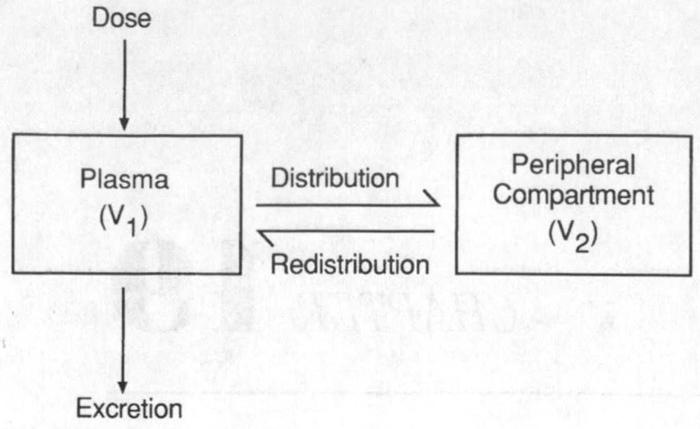

FIGURE 19.1-3. A schematic diagram of a standard two-compartment pharmacokinetic model. V, volume.

The degree of absorption can be expressed as the bioavailability, which in practice is determined by comparing the area under the concentration-time curve (AUC) after oral administration to the AUC after intravenous administration. A low bioavailability can be due to either poor absorption per se, or high first-pass metabolism.[6,7] In addition, the presence of transport proteins in the gut, such as P glycoprotein, also impact on the oral bioavailability of anticancer agents.[8]

Alteration in gastrointestinal absorptive capacity can be due to a variety of factors common in patients with cancer. Recent surgery may influence absorption, as demonstrated in regard to UFT (tegafur, uracil, and 5-fluorouracil) administration in the early postoperative period after partial gastrectomy.[9] Prior chemotherapy can be a major issue, and diminished absorption may be present in the absence of clinical gastrointestinal toxicity.[10] Concomitant medications affecting gastrointestinal motility, such as opiates or metoclopramide, may also be a factor.[11] It also should be recognized that cytotoxic chemotherapy may alter plasma concentrations of other medications given on a chronic basis, such as phenytoin or verapamil.[12,13]

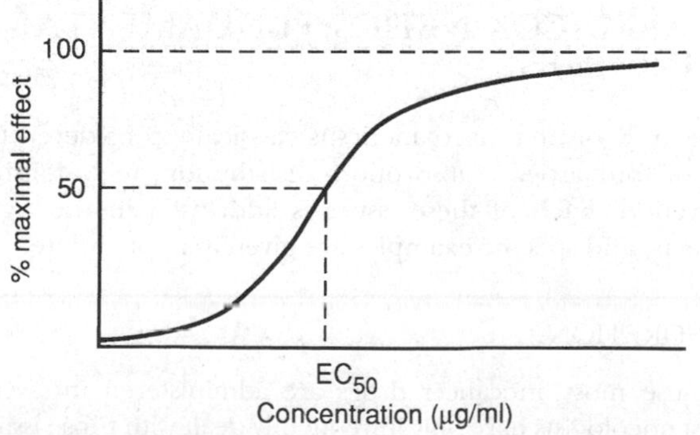

FIGURE 19.1-2. A representative pharmacodynamic profile relating concentration and effect. The concentration at which there is half-maximal effect (EC_{50}) is indicated. Note that the concentration-response curve is steepest around the EC_{50} and is relatively flat at both low and high concentrations.

Absorption also must be considered in regard to subcutaneous or intramuscular dosing. Although bioavailability via these routes is usually close to 100%, there may be decreased bioavailability due to local drug degradation or other factors.[14]

DISTRIBUTION

Drugs usually distribute after administration from the plasma into extracellular and intracellular fluids. If a hypothetical drug were given as a 100-mg instantaneous bolus, the initial concentration would be 100 mg divided by the volume of distribution (the higher the volume, the lower the initial concentration). Subsequent concentrations would then be determined by the drug's rate of elimination. In the simplest pharmacokinetic model, the clearance is equal to the product of the volume of distribution and the elimination rate constant.

In actuality, distribution is much more complex. A drug's pharmacokinetics can be described by one or more interconnected compartments, and distribution is then represented by drug moving from the "central" compartment to a "peripheral" compartment (Fig. 19.1-3). This description is important for several reasons.

Because the central compartment is usually plasma, the site of action is probably more closely related to a peripheral compartment (i.e., intracellular fluid). Thus, plasma concentrations may be falling as the pharmacologic effect increases (Fig. 19.1-4). This inverse relationship may be compounded further for anticancer drugs by the known delay between the cytotoxic event and its clinical manifestations.

In general, drug that distributes to the peripheral compartments eventually redistributes back to the plasma or central compartment. Drugs that are extensively distributed usually have a long terminal half-life, which can be highly dependent on the rate of redistribution. Such drugs are often highly protein-bound. This can have important clinical ramifications for highly schedule-dependent agents such as methotrexate, which distributes to "third spaces" such as pleural effusions or ascites.

METABOLISM

Metabolism is the most critical and complex aspect of pharmacokinetics for most agents. The great majority of xenobiotic metabolism takes place in the liver, although cytochrome P-450

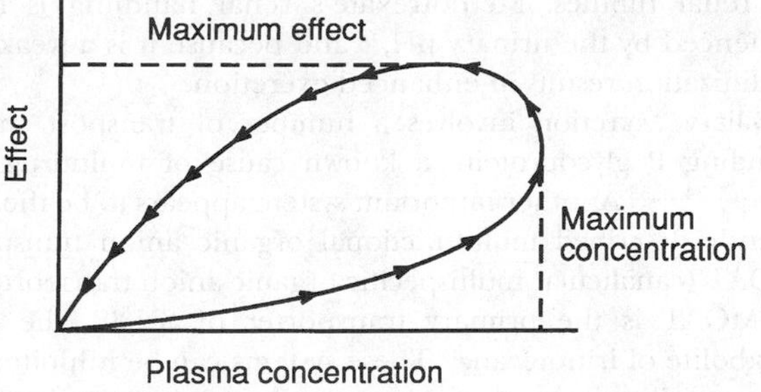

FIGURE 19.1-4. A reverse hysteresis loop representing the relationship between concentration, time, and pharmacologic effect (e.g., DNA damage). The plasma concentration rises during the period of drug administration (i.e., 24-hour infusion). The plasma concentration falls immediately after the infusion ends, but the tumor concentration continues to rise (due to distribution). Thus, the maximal effect occurs later than the end of the infusion (maximal plasma concentrations). Although the same plasma concentration occurs both during infusion and after infusion, the effect is greater when the concentration is falling.

enzymes and uridine diphosphate–glucuronosyltransferases are present in the small bowel,[5,15] and both carboxylesterases[16] and deaminases[17] are present in plasma and other tissues.

Xenobiotic metabolism can be divided into phase I and phase II reactions[18] (Table 19.1-1). Phase I reactions are oxidative, or reductive, reactions and include the P-450 system. Phase II reactions are conjugative reactions, such as acetylation and glucuronidation. Phase I reactions usually make a drug more susceptible to phase II reactions, which generally produce molecules amenable to biliary or renal excretion. These metabolic reactions evolved for the purpose of xenobiotic detoxification, but can also result in drug activation.

An area of rapidly increasing importance is genetically determined variability in drug-metabolizing enzymes.[19] Such genetic variability can result in enhanced toxicity because of impaired detoxification,[20] enhanced activation,[21] or lack of desired effect due to impaired activation.[22] Furthermore, genetically determined variability may also be a risk factor for carcinogenesis.[23] A number of distinct drug-metabolizing enzymes have been conclusively demonstrated to be polymorphic (see Table 19.1-1).

An individual's metabolic capacity can also be affected by a variety of other factors, such as hepatic dysfunction, nutrition, and other medications.[18] These are all factors that are highly variable in patients receiving chemotherapy.[24,25]

Phase I metabolism (i.e., the P-450 system) appears to be more sensitive to hepatic dysfunction than phase II enzymes (i.e., glucuronidation).[26,27] Although oncologists generally monitor liver function tests during chemotherapy, the serum bilirubin (the most commonly used measure) is a very insensitive measure of changes in plasma drug clearance. Malnutrition, like hepatic dysfunction, may result in decreased synthesis of drug-metabolizing enzymes, decreased clearance, and enhanced toxicity.[25,28–30]

One of the most important considerations with regard to the elimination of anticancer drugs is the effect of other medi-

TABLE 19.1-1. Selected Drug-Metabolizing Enzymes of Importance in Oncology

Reaction	*Substrates*	*Polymorphic*
Phase I reactions		
Cytochrome P-450		
CYP1A1	Benzo(a)pyrene	X
CYP1A2	Theophylline, caffeine	X
CYP2B6	Cyclophosphamide	
CYP2C8	Paclitaxel	
CYP2C9	Phenytoin, warfarin	X
CYP2C19	Omeprazole, diazepam	X
CYP2D6	Codeine, granisetron	X
CYP2E1	Ethanol	X
CYP3A4	Etoposide, vinca alkaloids, ifosfamide, docetaxel, irinotecan	X
Ketoreductase	Anthracyclines	
Aldehyde dehydrogenases	Aldoifosfamide	
Carboxylesterases	Irinotecan	
Dihydropyriminidine dehydrogenase	5-Fluorouracil	X
Cytosine deaminase	Cytarabine	
Phase II reactions		
N-acetylation		
NAT2	Isoniazid, amonafide	X
Glucuronidation		
UGT1A1	Bilirubin, SN-38	X
UGT2B7	Morphine, epirubicin	
Methyltransferases		
TPMT	6-Mercaptopurine, azathioprine	X

TABLE 19.1-2. Potential Drug Interactions with Chemotherapy

Inhibition of CYP3A4 by ketoconazole, itraconazole, erythromycin, clarithromycin, or grapefruit juice may result in decreased clearance of etoposide, vinca alkaloids, or irinotecan or decreased activation of ifosfamide
Inhibition of glucuronysyl transferases by valproic acid may result in decreased clearance of SN-38 (active metabolite of irinotecan)
Inhibition of xanthine oxidase by allopurinol may result in decreased clearance of 6-mercaptopurine
Induction of CYP3A4 by corticosteroids, phenytoin, phenobarbital, rifampin, cyclophosphamide, or ifosfamide may result in enhanced clearance of etoposide, vinca alkaloids, or irinotecan or enhanced activation of ifosfamide
Inhibition of biliary excretion by cyclosporine A (and other P-glycoprotein inhibitors) may result in decreased clearance of a wide range of agents
Inhibition of renal tubular secretion by probenecid, salicylates or penicillins may result in decreased clearance of methotrexate, topotecan, or SN-38

cations. Cancer patients receive a large number of medications that can affect metabolism (and excretion) of concomitant chemotherapy (Table 19.1-2). Given the complexity of most treatment regimens (multiple cytotoxic agents, antiemetics, analgesics, anticonvulsants, corticosteroids), relatively few specific data are available in this regard.

EXCRETION

There are two major routes of excretion, renal and biliary. Both are complex processes involving a chain of events, any of which can be modulated by disease processes or other medications.[31–34]

Xenobiotics may undergo filtration, secretion, and reabsorption on their journey from the glomeruli to the ureter. The creatinine clearance, either measured from a timed urine specimen or calculated based on a variety of formulas, is often used as a surrogate for the glomerular filtration rate (GFR), although these formulas have limited accuracy.[35–37] Furthermore, this surrogate may be used to describe an individual's overall renal function. Patients with reduced renal function should be considered for dose reduction if renal excretion is a major component of the agent's clearance.[32]

A great effort has been expended in trying to predict carboplatin pharmacokinetics.[31,38–40] The most accurate approach uses chromium-labeled EDTA (ethylenediamine-tetraacetic acid).[41,42] Simpler techniques, such as using a measured or calculated creatinine clearance, have inconsistently been predictive, because of the poor correlation between creatinine clearance and GFR.[35–37,43,44]

Physicians also commonly use a measured or estimated creatinine clearance to guide cisplatin dosing, primarily as a determinant of dose modifications from a standard body surface area (BSA)–adjusted dose. It is important to recognize that GFR is normally correlated with BSA, so that smaller patients appear to have poorer renal function, unless the GFR is also adjusted for the BSA (mL/min/m^2 or mL/min/1.73 m^2).

Tubular secretion and reabsorption may also be important in drug excretion.[45–47] As an example, it has been suggested that cisplatin's reabsorption is saturable, resulting in enhanced proportional reabsorption when administered by infusion, potentially resulting in enhanced toxicity.[48,49] Methotrexate and topotecan[50] also undergo secretion and reabsorption in the renal tubules. Methotrexate's renal handling is highly influenced by the urinary pH,[51] and because it is a weak acid, alkalinization results in enhanced excretion.

Biliary excretion involves a number of transport systems, including P glycoprotein, a known cause of multidrug resistance.[33,34,52,53] Another important system appears to be the more recently described multifunctional organic anion transporter, cMOAT (canalicular multispecific organic anion transporter).[54]

cMOAT is the primary transporter of SN-38, the active metabolite of irinotecan.[55] These systems can be inhibited by a variety of disease processes, as well as by other drugs (cyclosporine A, PSC-833) or formulants (Cremophor).[56,57]

After biliary excretion, reabsorption may take place in the small intestine, leading to an enterohepatic circulation.[58,59] This is particularly relevant for those drugs whose primary metabolite is a glucuronide, because of the presence of bacterial β-glucuronidases in the gut, which cleave off the glucoronide.[60,61]

The serum bilirubin is often used to determine dose modifications for hepatically cleared drugs. However, this is only a marker of impaired excretion, and it is poorly correlated with impaired metabolism. (Metabolism may be better represented by measures of synthetic function, such as serum albumin.)

PHARMACOKINETICS: WHAT'S IMPORTANT TO THE CLINICIAN?

CLEARANCE

The generation of pharmacokinetic data is easy, but its interpretation can be quite overwhelming, especially to a clinician attempting to apply such data to a particular patient or study. A good starting point is the assessment of total plasma clearance. Clearance can be calculated in one of two ways: either by measurement (or estimation) of the AUC after a single dose (see Fig. 19.1-1), or by determination of the steady-state concentration (C_{ss}) during continuous infusion.

$$\text{Clearance} = \frac{\text{dose}}{\text{AUC}}$$

or

$$\text{Clearance} = \frac{\text{dose rate}}{C_{ss}}$$

Although the absolute value of the clearance may be of some interest to the pharmacologist, the clinician should be primarily concerned with variability in clearance, best represented as the coefficient of variation (CV), the ratio of the standard deviation (not standard error) to the mean. The CV may be as low as 10% to 20% for drugs with low variability, or as high as 75% to 100% for drugs with high variability. Most drugs have a CV in the 20% to 40% range.

After understanding the extent of variability, the next question is to explain it, particularly if the CV is quite large. This becomes even more relevant if patients with a low clearance have an increased risk of toxicity. Drugs with a very high CV should be closely studied for genetically determined polymorphisms of the primary metabolizing system.[62,63]

Another important source of variability is saturation of the major metabolic or excretory site. If saturation occurs at clinically relevant concentrations, the clearance generally decreases dramatically at higher doses, and the drug is considered to have nonlinear pharmacokinetics. Optimal administration of such drugs requires a full understanding of the complexities involved, as well as the potential effects of disease and other medications.

In assessing variability in AUC or clearance, variability in protein binding may be an important issue. The degree of protein binding may range from negligible to more than 99%. Only the free (unbound) drug is active, whereas conventional assays quantitate the total (free plus bound) drug. If significant variability in protein binding is found for a highly bound drug, it may be difficult to interpret plasma concentrations without directly measuring the free drug or extent of protein binding. For some agents, however, such as etoposide, it may be possible to estimate protein binding from simple parameters, such as serum albumin, bilirubin, and age.[64,65]

A potential source of variability that has been greatly exaggerated in oncology practice is variability in body size. Minimal data support the dosing of chemotherapy on the basis of BSA in adults. Because size may have no significant correlation with clearance, this practice may even increase the extent of variability in AUC.[66–69] Further studies of this important issue are needed, if only to decrease the complexity of oncology practice.

HALF-LIFE

For highly schedule-dependent drugs, variability in half-life may be more important than variability in clearance. Although half-life and clearance are generally inversely correlated, an increased half-life may also be a consequence of an increased volume of distribution. This may have significant consequences, as has been well established for methotrexate's distribution into ascites or pleural effusions.[70]

Variability in half-life influences variability in time above any specific plasma concentration. This finding is becoming increasingly well recognized as an important factor in both toxicity and response.[71,72]

Knowledge of the half-life may also be important for protocol designs, because schedule-dependent drugs with short half-lives (e.g., cytarabine, 5-fluorouracil) might be best administered by continuous infusions or frequent dosing. It may also be critical to know the half-life for estimating when plasma cytotoxic activity is negligible in the context of peripheral stem cell reinfusion or colony-stimulating factor administration.[73,74]

ACTIVE METABOLITES

Although metabolism generally results in detoxification, some drugs may have active circulating metabolites (Table 19.1-3). These include drugs that are true prodrugs, having no intrinsic cytotoxic activity, and drugs that have metabolites with comparable or greater cytotoxicity to the parent. It is also important to understand the pathways through which activation occurs. There may be theoretical advantages to enhancing or inhibiting formation of the active metabolites, which may have a different "therapeutic index" (ratio of beneficial to harmful effects) than the parent drug. This alteration of active metabolite formation can potentially be accomplished by the use of inhibitors (e.g., ketoconazole) or inducers (i.e., phenobarbital) of specific drug-metabolizing enzyme systems.[75,76] Finally, an identifiable genetic basis for differences in activation may exist, which leads to different effects in specific patient populations.[22]

TABLE 19.1-3. Oncology Drugs with Active Circulating Metabolites

Chemotherapy drugs
Alkylating agents
Cyclophosphamide
Ifosfamide
Procarbazine
Dacarbazine
Temozolomide
Hexamethylmelamine
Thio-TEPA
Anthracyclines
Doxorubicin
Idarubicin
Epirubicin
Camptothecins
Irinotecan
Antimetabolites
UFT
Methotrexate
6-Mercaptopurine
Antiestrogens
Toremifene
Tamoxifen
Retinoids
All-*trans*-retinoic acid
Other oncology drugs
Analgesics
Morphine
Codeine
Hydrocodone

TEPA, triethylenephosphoramide; UFT, tegafur, uracil, and 5-fluorouracil.

ROUTES OF ELIMINATION

Oncologists are generally well aware of the potential for drug elimination to be impaired in patients with end-organ dysfunction. However, relatively little information is available to guide dose modifications. Even if a physician knew an individual's clearance before dosing, it would be difficult to predict the extent of toxicity because of the risk of prolonged low concentrations (for schedule-dependent drugs) or concomitant pharmacodynamic factors (resulting in enhanced sensitivity, such as malnutrition).

The only generalization that can be made is that variability increases as end-organ dysfunction develops. Formal phase I studies are warranted in patients with end-organ dysfunction.[77–79]

BASIC METHODOLOGY OF PHARMACOKINETIC STUDIES

The first pharmacokinetic studies of a new agent are almost always conducted in conjunction with phase I studies. Proper conduct of such studies requires a great deal of planning, as well as technical and logistical expertise. Data from preclinical studies are critical in the design. These generally include evaluations of *in vitro* cytotoxicity, preclinical pharmacokinetics, *in vitro* metabolism, *in vitro* toxicology (myelosuppression), and whole-animal toxicology.

Pharmacokinetic data can be collected using either intensive or sparse sampling strategies. In the first pharmacokinetic studies, intensive sampling is used to try to model each individual's pharmacokinetics. Data from all patients can be combined in two basic ways: either with a simple descriptive summary (mean ± standard deviation) of the fundamental parameters, or by pooling all data into a single analysis. The latter approach requires a high level of statistical and computational sophistication, but may generate insights not available by other means.[80]

It is also useful to begin to plan subsequent pharmacologic studies in the context of the initial pharmacokinetic analysis. These subsequent studies are often primarily concerned with pharmacodynamic issues, relating toxicity or response to pharmacokinetic variables. Such studies benefit greatly from the use of optimal sampling strategies, in which only a few samples are collected on each patient.[81–87]

PHARMACODYNAMICS

FUNDAMENTAL PRINCIPLES

The fundamental objective of pharmacodynamic studies is understanding variability in effect.[24] In phase I trials, the primary objective is to understand variability in effect (toxicity) as a function of dose. The investigator can also begin to understand the relationship between pharmacokinetic end points (i.e., AUC) and effect.

However, because phase I trials encompass multiple doses, dose is correlated with AUC (and other end points), and relationships between AUC and effect are confounded if the dose range is wide.[88] Thus, phase II trials in which all patients receive a single drug at a fixed dose offer an important opportunity to correlate pharmacokinetic end points (due solely to pharmacokinetic variability) and effect (both toxicity and response).[2]

Since the 1980s, a progressively increasing number of studies have been published that have included pharmacodynamic end points.[1,24,88,89] Such studies primarily have used AUC or C_{ss} as the pharmacokinetic parameter, and blood count nadirs as the pharmacodynamic end point. More recently, several studies have demonstrated that time above a threshold concentration is an important pharmacokinetic parameter, which is consistent with the understanding that schedule is an important determinant of antineoplastic drug action.[71,72,90]

METHODOLOGIC ISSUES

The methodology for pharmacodynamic studies should use generally recognized outcomes. Historically, blood count nadirs have been used, although this approach has several limitations. Nadir blood counts, by definition, measure the lowest observed blood count, which is highly dependent on the number of observations. In addition, nadir blood counts are not useful in the context of high-dose chemotherapy. Thus, it is potentially desirable to incorporate all blood counts and to use a methodology robust enough to properly analyze missing data.[91–94]

Nonhematologic toxicity is an even more difficult problem, as it is often graded rather than continuous, and subjective rather than objective. Statistical methodologies appropriate for such end points are necessary, such as logistic regression and its variants.[88]

The "holy grail" of antineoplastic clinical pharmacologists is to correlate pharmacologic end points with response. Although examples of plasma clearance being correlated with response are available,[95–97] it is likely that variability in response is primarily due to tumor factors (i.e., intrinsic drug resistance) rather than patient factors (i.e., altered clearance).[98,99]

TABLE 19.1-4. Pharmacokinetic and Pharmacodynamic Determinants of Chemotherapy Toxicity

Pharmacokinetic
Metabolism
Genetic
Hepatic synthetic function
Other medications
Diet
Smoking
Alcohol
Age
Performance status
Excretion
Renal function
Biliary function
Other medications
Age
Performance status
Distribution
Pleural effusions or ascites
Obesity
Amputation
Pharmacodynamic
Prior therapy
Bone marrow replacement
Age
Performance status
Genetic
Other medications
Comorbidity

Another major challenge is to expand the knowledge of anticancer pharmacodynamics from single agents to combinations. Such studies are logistically difficult, because plasma samples must be collected at times appropriate for each of the drugs in the regimen. Some work in this area has been done with regard to the effect of a second drug on carboplatin-induced thrombocytopenia.[100–102]

RATIONAL USE OF PHARMACOKINETIC AND PHARMACODYNAMIC DATA IN CLINICAL ONCOLOGY

Although oncologists may have difficulty exactly defining pharmacokinetics and pharmacodynamics, many of the important principles are incorporated into oncology clinical practice. By understanding that the principles are not foreign, the oncologist can better use principles of clinical pharmacology to optimize dosing of these highly toxic agents.

DOSE MODIFICATION FOR TOXICITY

It is common practice to reduce drug dosages for excessive toxicity. But a variety of reasons may be responsible for excessive toxicity, which can generally be categorized as either pharmacokinetic or pharmacodynamic (Table 19.1-4). It is important

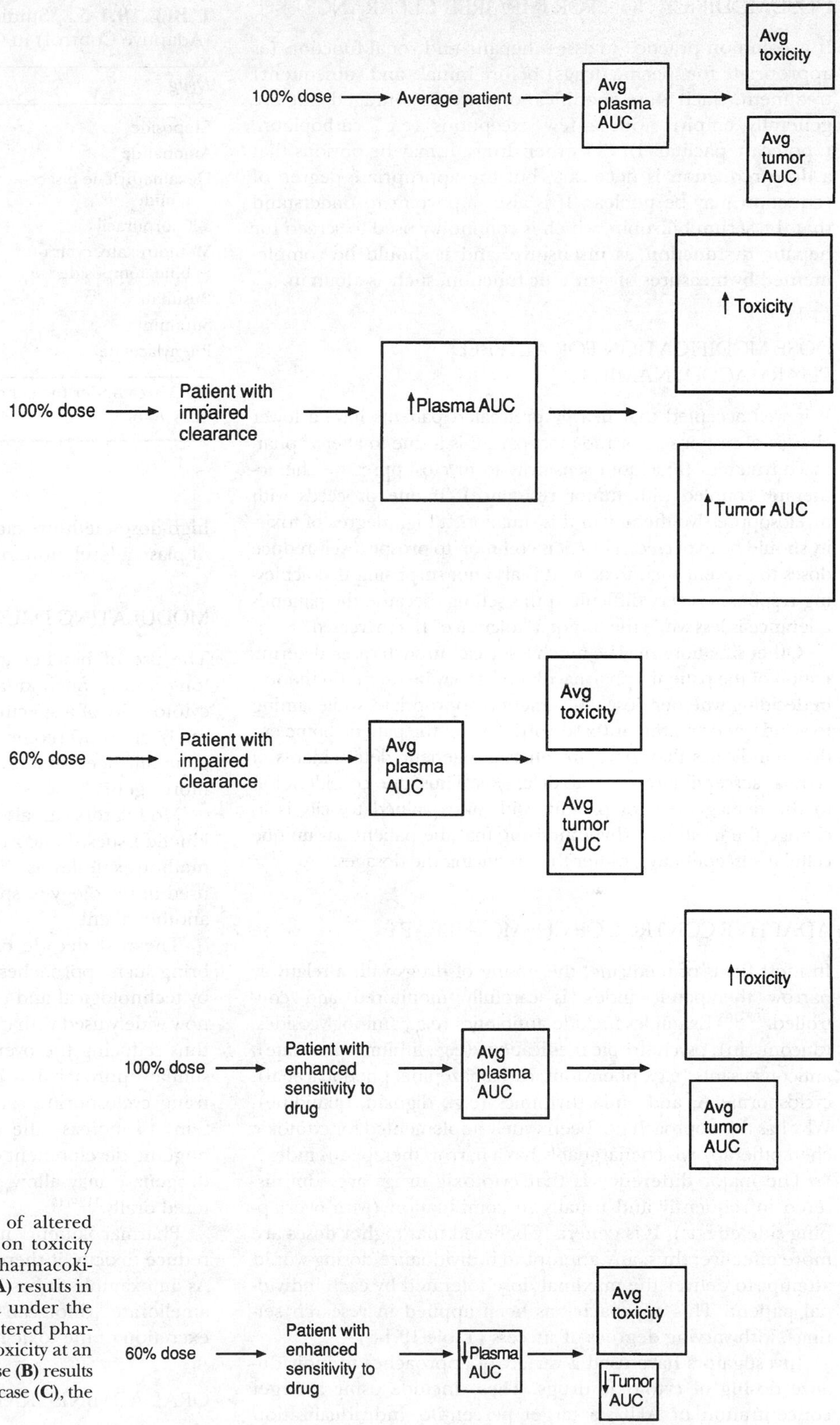

FIGURE 19.1-5. Comparison of effect of altered pharmacokinetics and pharmacodynamics on toxicity and tumor concentrations. Alteration of pharmacokinetics **(B)** compared to an average patient **(A)** results in enhanced toxicity due to an increased area under the concentration-time curve (AUC), whereas altered pharmacodynamics **(C)** may result in enhanced toxicity at an average AUC. Dose reduction in the former case **(B)** results in an average tumor AUC, whereas in the latter case **(C)**, the tumor AUC may be subtherapeutic.

to understand this distinction. If one assumes that decreasing drug exposure (AUC) reduces the likelihood of response, then dose reduction may be inappropriate for patients with increased toxicity on a pharmacodynamic basis, whereas patients with altered clearance can be dose-reduced yet maintain an acceptable AUC (Fig. 19.1-5). Hypothetically, patients with normal clearance but excessive toxicity might be best served by a change in treatment (or discontinuation of treatment if no alternative is available), rather than reduction to what might be a subtherapeutic AUC.

DOSE MODIFICATION FOR IMPAIRED CLEARANCE

It is common practice to assess hepatic and renal function (as appropriate for specific drugs) before initial (and subsequent) treatment. Such dose modifications are encouraged but are generally empiric with a few exceptions (e.g., carboplatin, topotecan, paclitaxel). For other drugs, it may be obvious that a dose reduction is necessary, but the appropriate degree of reduction may be unclear. It is also important to understand that the serum bilirubin, which is commonly used to screen for hepatic dysfunction, is insensitive, and it should be complemented by measures of synthetic function, such as albumin.

DOSE MODIFICATION FOR ALTERED PHARMACODYNAMICS

It is well accepted that heavily pretreated patients have a lower chance of response. For the most part, this is due to altered pharmacodynamics (increased sensitivity to myelosuppressive chemotherapy coupled with tumor resistance). If one proceeds with myelosuppressive therapy in this situation, a high degree of toxicity should be expected. Thus, it is common to prospectively reduce doses to prevent such toxicity. It is also not surprising that achieving responses is very difficult in this setting, because the patient's tolerance is less while the tumor's "tolerance" has increased.

Other situations may be much less clear. In such cases, determination of the patient's pharmacokinetics may be useful (in theory) in deciding whether dose adjustment is appropriate, while aiming to avoid undertreatment (based on AUC) of the patient. Some evidence indicates that there are pharmacogenetic determinants of cellular susceptibility to cytotoxic agents. Thus, one consideration in the management of patients with unexplained toxicity is to change the treatment (hypothesizing that the patient has unique cellular susceptibility), rather than reducing the dosages.

ADAPTIVE CONTROL OF CHEMOTHERAPY

In most fields of medicine, the dosing of drugs with a relatively narrow therapeutic index is carefully monitored and controlled.[103–105] Examples include antibiotics (e.g., aminoglycosides, vancomycin), psychotropic medications (e.g., lithium carbonate), anticonvulsants (e.g., phenytoin, carbamazepine, phenobarbital), cyclosporine A, and antiarrhythmics (e.g., digoxin, quinidine). Why has this approach not been widely implemented for cytotoxic chemotherapy, which inarguably has a narrow therapeutic index?

The major difference is that cytotoxic drugs are administered infrequently and usually in combination (with overlapping side effects). It is generally believed that higher doses are more effective; thus, any attempt to individualize dosing would attempt to deliver the maximal dose tolerated by each individual patient. This approach has been applied in research settings, with varying degrees of success (Table 19.1-5).

Investigators have used a variety of approaches to individualize dosing of cytotoxic drugs. These include using a target concentration or AUC, a target percentile, individualization based on both concentration and pharmacodynamic factors, and individualization based on metabolism of a probe drug. These studies have yielded important insights into the understanding of the potential importance of pharmacokinetic and pharmacodynamic variability. However, adaptive control remains a research tool. Analysis of methotrexate levels after high-dose methotrexate is still the only generally accepted use of plasma level monitoring in clinical oncology.[106]

TABLE 19.1-5. Studies of Therapeutic Drug Monitoring (Adaptive Control) in Oncology

Drug	*End Point*	*References*
Etoposide	Predicted nadir WBC	118, 119
Amonafide	Predicted nadir WBC	120
Hexamethylene bisacetamide	Predicted nadir platelet count	121, 122
5-Fluorouracil	Predicted AUC	123
Methotrexate, cytarabine, teniposide	Target concentration range	97, 124
Busulfan	Target concentration range	125–127
Suramin	Target concentration range	128–132
Phenylacetate	Target concentration range	133

AUC, area under the concentration-time curve; WBC, white blood cell count.

MODULATING DRUGS

The use of biochemical modulators of chemotherapy has a long history. Such an approach has been used to enhance the cytotoxicity of a specific agent (e.g., leucovorin with 5-fluorouracil) or to overcome drug resistance. Such modulators have generally been used to affect the pharmacodynamics of one or more agents.[107]

Modulators can also be administered because of pharmacokinetic issues. Leucovorin is commonly dosed on the basis of methotrexate levels.[108] But drugs have not yet been routinely used in oncology to specifically affect the pharmacokinetics of another agent.

The first decade of the twenty-first century will probably bring such approaches into mainstream oncology, driven both by technological and cost issues. For example, ketoconazole is now widely used with cyclosporine to improve its bioavailability, thus reducing the overall cost of cyclosporine therapy.[109,110] A similar approach has been applied to oral anticancer agents, using cyclosporine (an inhibitor of CYP3A4 and P glycoprotein) to increase the oral bioavailability of paclitaxel.[111] The ongoing development of inhibitors of dihydropyrimidine dehydrogenase may allow 5-fluorouracil to be effectively administered orally.[112–115]

Pharmacokinetic modulators may also be beneficial to reduce toxicity, if there is more than one route of elimination. As an example, it has been suggested that cyclosporine A may ameliorate irinotecan-induced diarrhea by inhibiting biliary excretion of the toxic metabolite SN-38.[116,117]

ORAL ADMINISTRATION

A resurgence of interest has been seen in oral administration of cytotoxic chemotherapy. If successful, this route of administration may be more acceptable to patients and potentially be cost effective as well.[3] Prolonged oral administration will allow a more detailed evaluation of specific drugs, but will introduce new complexities caused by diet, drug interactions, and compliance. Oncologists should become familiar with these issues and master a general understanding of interpatient and intrapatient variability in bioavailability.

REFERENCES

1. Kobayashi K, Jodrell DI, Ratain MJ. Pharmacodynamic-pharmacokinetic relationships and therapeutic drug monitoring. *Cancer Surv* 1993;17:51.
2. Ratain MJ, Rosner G, Allen SL, et al. Population pharmacodynamic study of amonafide: a Cancer and Leukemia Group B study. *J Clin Oncol* 1995;13:741.
3. DeMario MD, Ratain MJ. Oral chemotherapy: rationale and future directions. *J Clin Oncol* 1998;16:2557.
4. Kolars JC, Schmiedlin-Ren P, Schuetz JD, et al. Identification of rifampin-inducible P450IIIA4 (CYP3A4) in human small bowel enterocytes. *J Clin Invest* 1992;90:1871.
5. Watkins PB. Drug metabolism by cytochromes P450 in the liver and small bowel. *Gastroenterol Clin North Am* 1992;21:511.
6. Pond SM, Tozer TN. First-pass elimination. Basic concepts and clinical consequences. *Clin Pharmacokinet* 1984;9:1.
7. Weiss M. Use of metabolite AUC data in bioavailability studies to discriminate between absorption and first-pass extraction. *Clin Pharmacokinet* 1990;18:419.
8. Schinkel AH. The physiological function of drug-transporting P-glycoproteins. *Semin Cancer Biol* 1997;8:161.
9. Maehara Y, Takeuchi H, Oshiro T, et al. Effect of gastrectomy on the pharmacokinetics of tegafur, uracil, and 5- fluorouracil after oral administration of a 1:4 tegafur and uracil combination. *Cancer Chemother Pharmacol* 1994;33:445.
10. Choi KE, Ratain MJ, Williams SF, et al. Plasma pharmacokinetics of high-dose oral melphalan in patients treated with trialkylator chemotherapy and autologous bone marrow reinfusion. *Cancer Res* 1989;49:1318.
11. Quijano RF, Ohnishi N, Umeda K, et al. Effect of atropine on gastrointestinal motility and the bioavailability of cyclosporine A in rats. *Drug Metab Dispos* 1993;21:141.
12. Neef C, de Voogd-van der Straaten I. An interaction between cytostatic and anticonvulsant drugs. *Clin Pharmacol Ther* 1988;43:372.
13. Kuhlmann J, Woodcock B, Wilke J, et al. Verapamil plasma concentrations during treatment with cytostatic drugs [published erratum appears in *J Cardiovasc Pharmacol* 1987;10:247]. *J Cardiovasc Pharmacol* 1985;7:1003.
14. Salmonson T, Danielson BG, Wikstrom B. The pharmacokinetics of recombinant human erythropoietin after intravenous and subcutaneous administration to healthy subjects. *Br J Clin Pharmacol* 1990;29:709.
15. Radominska-Pandya A, Little JM, Pandya JT, et al. UDP-glucuronosyltransferases in human intestinal mucosa. *Biochim Biophys Acta* 1998;1394:199.
16. Leinweber FJ. Possible physiological roles of carboxylic ester hydrolases. *Drug Metab Rev* 1987;18:379.
17. Thompson PW, Jones DD, Currey HL. Cytidine deaminase activity as a measure of acute inflammation in rheumatoid arthritis [see comments]. *Ann Rheum Dis* 1986;45:9.
18. Sitar DS. Human drug metabolism *in vivo*. *Pharmacol Ther* 1989;43:363.
19. Iyer L, Ratain MJ. Pharmacogenetics and cancer chemotherapy. *Eur J Cancer* 1998;34:1493.
20. Diasio RB, Beavers TL, Carpenter JT. Familial deficiency of dihydropyrimidine dehydrogenase. Biochemical basis for familial pyrimidinemia and severe 5-fluorouracil-induced toxicity. *J Clin Invest* 1988;81:47.
21. Dalen P, Frengell C, Dahl ML, Sjoqvist F. Quick onset of severe abdominal pain after codeine in an ultrarapid metabolizer of debrisoquine. *Ther Drug Monit* 1997;19:543.
22. Sindrup SH, Brosen K. The pharmacogenetics of codeine hypoalgesia. *Pharmacogenetics* 1995;5:335.
23. Taningher M, Malacarne D, Izzotti A, et al. Drug metabolism polymorphisms as modulators of cancer susceptibility. *Mutat Res* 1999;436:227.
24. Ratain MJ, Schilsky RL, Conley BA, et al. Pharmacodynamics in cancer therapy. *J Clin Oncol* 1990;8:1739.
25. Murry DJ, Riva L, Poplack DG. Impact of nutrition on pharmacokinetics of anti-neoplastic agents. *Int J Cancer* 1998;11[Suppl]:48.
26. Ghabrial H, Desmond PV, Watson KJ, et al. The effects of age and chronic liver disease on the elimination of temazepam. *Eur J Clin Pharmacol* 1986;30:93.
27. Hoyumpa AM, Schenker S. Is glucuronidation truly preserved in patients with liver disease? *Hepatology* 1991;13:786.
28. Jung D. Pharmacokinetics of theophylline in protein-calorie malnutrition. *Biopharm Drug Dispos* 1985;6:291.
29. Tranvouez JL, Lerebours E, Chretien P, et al. Hepatic antipyrine metabolism in malnourished patients: influence of the type of malnutrition and course after nutritional rehabilitation. *Am J Clin Nutr* 1985;41:1257.
30. Davis LE, Lenkinski RE, Shinkwin MA, et al. The effect of dietary protein depletion on hepatic 5-fluorouracil metabolism. *Cancer* 1993;72:3715.
31. Sorensen BT, Stromgren A, Jakobsen P, et al. Renal handling of carboplatin. *Cancer Chemother Pharmacol* 1992;30:317.
32. Kintzel PE, Dorr RT. Anticancer drug renal toxicity and elimination: dosing guidelines for altered renal function. *Cancer Treat Rev* 1995;21:33.
33. Meijer DK, Mol WE, Muller M, et al. Carrier-mediated transport in the hepatic distribution and elimination of drugs, with special reference to the category of organic cations. *J Pharmacokinet Biopharm* 1990;18:35.
34. LeBlanc GA. Hepatic vectorial transport of xenobiotics. *Chem Biol Interact* 1994;90:101.
35. Van Lente F, Suit P. Assessment of renal function by serum creatinine and creatinine clearance: glomerular filtration rate estimated by four procedures. *Clin Chem* 1989;35:2326.
36. van Acker BA, Koomen GC, Koopman MG, et al. Creatinine clearance during cimetidine administration for measurement of glomerular filtration rate [see comments]. *Lancet* 1992;340:1326.
37. Hellerstein S, Alon U, Warady BA. Creatinine for estimation of glomerular filtration rate [see comments]. *Pediatr Nephrol* 1992;6:507.
38. Calvert AH, Newell DR, Gumbrell LA, et al. Carboplatin dosage: prospective evaluation of a simple formula based on renal function [see comments]. *J Clin Oncol* 1989;7:1748.
39. Newell DR, Pearson AD, Balmanno K, et al. Carboplatin pharmacokinetics in children: the development of a pediatric dosing formula. The United Kingdom Children's Cancer Study Group [see comments]. *J Clin Oncol* 1993;11:2314.
40. Chatelut E, Canal P, Brunner V, et al. Prediction of carboplatin clearance from standard morphological and biological patient characteristics [see comments]. *J Natl Cancer Inst* 1995;87:573.
41. Martensson J, Groth S, Rehling M, et al. Chromium-51-EDTA clearance in adults with a single-plasma sample. *J Nucl Med* 1998;39:2131.
42. Martin L, Chatelut E, Boneu A, et al. Improvement of the Cockcroft-Gault equation for predicting glomerular filtration in cancer patients. *Bull Cancer* 1998;85:631.
43. Okamoto H, Nagatomo A, Kunitoh H, et al. Prediction of carboplatin clearance calculated by patient characteristics or 24-hour creatinine clearance: a comparison of the performance of three formulae. *Cancer Chemother Pharmacol* 1998;42:307.
44. van Warmerdam LJ, Rodenhuis S, ten Bokkel Huinink WW, Maes RA, Beijnen JH. Evaluation of formulas using the serum creatinine level to calculate the optimal dosage of carboplatin. *Cancer Chemother Pharmacol* 1996;37:266.
45. Williams WM, Chen TS, Huang KC. Effect of penicillin on the renal tubular secretion of methotrexate in the monkey. *Cancer Res* 1984;44:1913.
46. Caterson R, Etheredge S, Snitch P, et al. Mechanisms of renal excretion of cisdichlorodiamine platinum. *Res Commun Chem Pathol Pharmacol* 1983;41:255.
47. Klein J, Bentur Y, Cheung D, et al. Renal handling of cisplatin: interactions with organic anions and cations in the dog. *Clin Invest Med* 1991;14:388.
48. Forastiere AA, Belliveau JF, Goren MP, et al. Pharmacokinetic and toxicity evaluation of five-day continuous infusion versus intermittent bolus *cis*-diamminedichloroplatinum(II) in head and neck cancer patients. *Cancer Res* 1988;48:3869.
49. Reece PA, Stafford I, Russell J, et al. Nonlinear renal clearance of ultrafilterable platinum in patients treated with *cis*-dichlorodiammineplatinum (II). *Cancer Chemother Pharmacol* 1985;15:295.
50. Zamboni WC, Houghton PJ, Johnson RK, et al. Probenecid alters topotecan systemic and renal disposition by inhibiting renal tubular secretion. *J Pharmacol Exp Ther* 1998; 284:89.
51. Ferrazzini G, Sohl H, Robieux I, et al. Diurnal variation of methotrexate disposition in children with acute leukaemia. *Eur J Clin Pharmacol* 1991;41:425.
52. Thalhammer T, Stapf V, Gajdzik L, et al. Bile canalicular cationic dye secretion as a model for P-glycoprotein mediated transport. *Eur J Pharmacol* 1994;270:213.
53. Smit JW, Duin E, Steen H, et al. Interactions between P-glycoprotein substrates and other cationic drugs at the hepatic excretory level. *Br J Pharmacol* 1998;123:361.
54. Ito K, Suzuki H, Hirohashi T, et al. Functional analysis of a canalicular multispecific organic anion transporter cloned from rat liver. *J Biol Chem* 1998;273:1684.
55. Chu XY, Kato Y, Sugiyama Y. Multiplicity of biliary excretion mechanisms for irinotecan, CPT-11, and its metabolites in rats. *Cancer Res* 1997;57:1934.
56. Speeg KV, Maldonado AL, Liaci J, et al. Effect of cyclosporine on colchicine secretion by a liver canalicular transporter studied *in vivo*. *Hepatology* 1992;15:899.
57. Song S, Suzuki H, Kawai R, et al. Effect of PSC 833, a P-glycoprotein modulator, on the disposition of vincristine and digoxin in rats. *Drug Metab Dispos* 1999;27:689.
58. Peris-Ribera JE, Torres-Molina F, Garcia-Carbonell MC, et al. General treatment of the enterohepatic recirculation of drugs and its influence on the area under the plasma level curves, bioavailability, and clearance. *Pharm Res* 1992;9:1306.
59. Semmes RL, Shen DD. A reversible clearance model for the enterohepatic circulation of drug and conjugate metabolite pair. *Drug Metab Dispos* 1990;18:80.
60. Slattum PW, Cato AE III, Pollack GM, et al. Age-dependent intestinal hydrolysis of valproate glucuronide in rat. *Xenobiotica* 1995;25:229.
61. Gupta E, Lestingi TM, Mick R, et al. Metabolic fate of irinotecan in humans: correlation of glucuronidation with diarrhea. *Cancer Res* 1994;54:3723.
62. Meyer UA, Zanger UM, Skoda RC, et al. Genetic polymorphisms of drug metabolism. *Prog Liver Dis* 1990;9:307.
63. Boddy AV, Idle JR. The role of pharmacogenetics in chemotherapy: modulation of tumour response and host toxicity. *Cancer Surv* 1993;17:79.
64. Stewart CF, Fleming RA, Arbuck SG, et al. Prospective evaluation of a model for predicting etoposide plasma protein binding in cancer patients. *Cancer Res* 1990;50:6854.
65. Liu B, Earl HM, Poole CJ, et al. Etoposide protein binding in cancer patients. *Cancer Chemother Pharmacol* 1995;36:506.
66. Grochow LB, Baraldi C, Noe D. Is dose normalization to weight or body surface area useful in adults? *J Natl Cancer Inst* 1990;82:323.
67. Gurney H. Dose calculation of anticancer drugs: a review of the current practice and introduction of an alternative. *J Clin Oncol* 1996;14:2590.
68. Gurney HP, Ackland S, Gebski V, et al. Factors affecting epirubicin pharmacokinetics and toxicity: evidence against using body-surface area for dose calculation [see comments]. *J Clin Oncol* 1998;16:2299.
69. Ratain MJ. Body-surface area as a basis for dosing of anticancer agents: science, myth, or habit? [Editorial; see comments]. *J Clin Oncol* 1998;16:2297.
70. Chabner BA, Stoller RG, Hande K, et al. Methotrexate disposition in humans: case studies in ovarian cancer and following high-dose infusion. *Drug Metab Rev* 1978;8:107.
71. Clark PI, Slevin ML, Joel SP, et al. A randomized trial of two etoposide schedules in small-cell lung cancer: the influence of pharmacokinetics on efficacy and toxicity. *J Clin Oncol* 1994;12:1427.
72. Gianni L, Kearns CM, Giani A, et al. Nonlinear pharmacokinetics and metabolism of

paclitaxel and its pharmacokinetic/pharmacodynamic relationships in humans. *J Clin Oncol* 1995;13:180.

73. Kohl P, Koppler H, Schmidt L, et al. Pharmacokinetics of high-dose etoposide after short-term infusion. *Cancer Chemother Pharmacol* 1992;29:316.
74. Mulder PO, de Vries EG, Uges DR, et al. Pharmacokinetics of carboplatin at a dose of 750 mg m-2 divided over three consecutive days. *Br J Cancer* 1990;61:460.
75. Gupta E, Wang X, Ramirez J, et al. Modulation of glucuronidation of SN-38, the active metabolite of irinotecan, by valproic acid and phenobarbital. *Cancer Chemother Pharmacol* 1997;39:440.
76. Yu LJ, Drewes P, Gustafsson K, et al. *In vivo* modulation of alternative pathways of P-450-catalyzed cyclophosphamide metabolism: impact on pharmacokinetics and antitumor activity. *J Pharmacol Exp Ther* 1999;288:928.
77. O'Reilly S, Rowinsky E, Slichenmyer W, et al. Phase I and pharmacologic studies of topotecan in patients with impaired hepatic function. *J Natl Cancer Inst* 1996;88:817.
78. O'Reilly S, Rowinsky EK, Slichenmyer W, et al. Phase I and pharmacologic study of topotecan in patients with impaired renal function [see comments]. *J Clin Oncol* 1996;14:3062.
79. Venook AP, Egorin MJ, Rosner GL, et al. Phase I and pharmacokinetic trial of paclitaxel in patients with hepatic dysfunction: Cancer and Leukemia Group B 9264. *J Clin Oncol* 1998;16:1811.
80. Vozeh S, Steimer JL, Rowland M, et al. The use of population pharmacokinetics in drug development [see comments]. *Clin Pharmacokinet* 1996;30:81.
81. Ratain MJ, Vogelzang NJ. Limited sampling model for vinblastine pharmacokinetics. *Cancer Treat Rep* 1987;71:935.
82. Ratain MJ, Staubus AE, Schilsky RL, et al. Limited sampling models for amonafide (NSC 308847) pharmacokinetics. *Cancer Res* 1988;48:4127.
83. Ratain MJ, Robert J, van der Vijgh WJ. Limited sampling models for doxorubicin pharmacokinetics. *J Clin Oncol* 1991;9:871.
84. Launay MC, Milano G, Iliadis A, et al. A limited sampling procedure for estimating adriamycin pharmacokinetics in cancer patients. *Br J Cancer* 1989;60:89.
85. van Warmerdam LJ, ten Bokkel Huinink WW, Maes RA, et al. Limited-sampling models for anticancer agents. *J Cancer Res Clin Oncol* 1994;120:427.
86. Shaw LM, Bonner HS, Fields L, et al. The use of concentration measurements of parent drug and metabolites during clinical trials. *Ther Drug Monit* 1993;15:483.
87. Jodrell DI, Murray LS, Hawtof J, et al. A comparison of methods for limited-sampling strategy design using data from a phase I trial of the anthrapyrazole DuP-941. *Cancer Chemother Pharmacol* 1996;37:356.
88. Mick R, Ratain MJ. Statistical approaches to pharmacodynamic modeling: motivations, methods, and misperceptions. *Cancer Chemother Pharmacol* 1993;33:1.
89. Canal P, Chatelut E, Guichard S. Practical treatment guide for dose individualisation in cancer chemotherapy. *Drugs* 1998;56:1019.
90. Bruno R, Hille D, Riva A, et al. Population pharmacokinetics/pharmacodynamics of docetaxel in phase II studies in patients with cancer. *J Clin Oncol* 1998;16:187.
91. Karlsson MO, Port RE, Ratain MJ, et al. A population model for the leukopenic effect of etoposide. *Clin Pharmacol Ther* 1995;57:325.
92. Rosner GL, Muller P. Pharmacodynamic analysis of hematologic profiles. *J Pharmacokinet Biopharm* 1994;22:499.
93. Karlsson MO, Molnar V, Bergh J, et al. A general model for time-dissociated pharmacokinetic-pharmacodynamic relationship exemplified by paclitaxel myelosuppression. *Clin Pharmacol Ther* 1998;63:11.
94. Minami H, Sasaki Y, Saijo N, et al. Indirect-response model for the time course of leukopenia with anticancer drugs. *Clin Pharmacol Ther* 1998;64:511.
95. Evans WE, Crom WR, Abromowitch M, et al. Clinical pharmacodynamics of high-dose methotrexate in acute lymphocytic leukemia. Identification of a relation between concentration and effect. *N Engl J Med* 1986;314:471.
96. Lilleyman JS, Lennard L. Mercaptopurine metabolism and risk of relapse in childhood lymphoblastic leukaemia. *Lancet* 1994;343:1188.
97. Evans WE, Relling MV, Rodman JH, et al. Conventional compared with individualized chemotherapy for childhood acute lymphoblastic leukemia. *N Engl J Med* 1998;338:499.
98. Johnston PG, Lenz HJ, Leichman CG, et al. Thymidylate synthase gene and protein expression correlate and are associated with response to 5-fluorouracil in human colorectal and gastric tumors. *Cancer Res* 1995;55:1407.
99. Etienne MC, Cheradame S, Fischel JL, et al. Response to fluorouracil therapy in cancer patients: the role of tumoral dihydropyrimidine dehydrogenase activity. *J Clin Oncol* 1995;13:1663.
100. Belani CP, Egorin MJ, Abrams JS, et al. A novel pharmacodynamically based approach to dose optimization of carboplatin when used in combination with etoposide [see comments]. *J Clin Oncol* 1989;7:1896.
101. Reyno LM, Egorin MJ, Canetta RM, et al. Impact of cyclophosphamide on relationships between carboplatin exposure and response or toxicity when used in the treatment of advanced ovarian cancer. *J Clin Oncol* 1993;11:1156.
102. Belani CP, Kearns CM, Zuhowski EG, et al. Phase I trial, including pharmacokinetic and pharmacodynamic correlations, of combination paclitaxel and carboplatin in patients with metastatic non-small-cell lung cancer. *J Clin Oncol* 1999;17:676.
103. Holt DW, Fashola TO, Johnston A. Monitoring cyclosporin: is it still important? *Immunol Lett* 1991;29:99.
104. McLeod HL, Evans WE. Pediatric pharmacokinetics and therapeutic drug monitoring. *Pediatr Rev* 1992;13:413.
105. Preskorn SH, Burke MJ, Fast GA. Therapeutic drug monitoring. Principles and practice. *Psychiatr Clin North Am* 1993;16:611.
106. Ackland SP, Schilsky RL. High-dose methotrexate: a critical reappraisal. *J Clin Oncol* 1987;5:2017.
107. O'Dwyer PJ. Biochemical modulation as an approach to reversal of antimetabolite resistance. *Cancer Treat Res* 1994;73:201.
108. Abelson HT, Fosburg MT, Beardsley GP, et al. Methotrexate-induced renal impairment: clinical studies and rescue from systemic toxicity with high-dose leucovorin and thymidine. *J Clin Oncol* 1983;1:208.
109. Keogh A, Spratt P, McCosker C, et al. Ketoconazole to reduce the need for cyclosporine after cardiac transplantation [see comments]. *N Engl J Med* 1995;333:628.
110. Gomez DY, Wacher VJ, Tomlanovich SJ, et al. The effects of ketoconazole on the intestinal metabolism and bioavailability of cyclosporine. *Clin Pharmacol Ther* 1995;58:15.
111. Meerum Terwogt JM, Beijnen JH, ten Bokkel Huinink WW, et al. Co-administration of cyclosporin enables oral therapy with paclitaxel [Letter; published erratum appears in *Lancet* 1998;352:824]. *Lancet* 1998;352:285.
112. Baccanari DP, Davis ST, Knick VC, et al. 5-Ethynyluracil (776C85): a potent modulator of the pharmacokinetics and antitumor efficacy of 5-fluorouracil. *Proc Natl Acad Sci U S A* 1993;90:11064.
113. Cao S, Rustum YM, Spector T. 5-Ethynyluracil (776C85): modulation of 5-fluorouracil efficacy and therapeutic index in rats bearing advanced colorectal carcinoma. *Cancer Res* 1994;54:1507.
114. Naguib FN, Hao SN, el Kouni MH. Potentiation of 5-fluorouracil efficacy by the dihydrouracil dehydrogenase inhibitor, 5-benzyloxybenzyluracil. *Cancer Res* 1994;54:5166.
115. Tatsumi K, Yamauchi T, Kiyono K, et al. 3-Cyano-2,6-dihydroxypyridine (CNDP), a new potent inhibitor of dihydrouracil dehydrogenase. *J Biochem* (Tokyo) 1993;114:912.
116. Gupta E, Safa AR, Wang X, et al. Pharmacokinetic modulation of irinotecan and metabolites by cyclosporin A. *Cancer Res* 1996;56:1309.
117. Ratain MJ, Iyer L, Fagbemi S, et al. A phase I study of irinotecan with pharmacokinetic modulation by cyclosporine A and phenobarbital. *Proc Am Soc Clin Oncol* 1999;18:202a.
118. Ratain MJ, Schilsky RL, Choi KE, et al. Adaptive control of etoposide administration: impact of interpatient pharmacodynamic variability. *Clin Pharmacol Ther* 1989;45:226.
119. Ratain MJ, Mick R, Schilsky RL, et al. Pharmacologically based dosing of etoposide: a means of safely increasing dose intensity. *J Clin Oncol* 1991;9:1480.
120. Ratain MJ, Mick R, Janisch L, et al. Individualized dosing of amonafide based on a pharmacodynamic model incorporating acetylator phenotype and gender. *Pharmacogenetics* 1996;6:93.
121. Conley BA, Forrest A, Egorin MJ, et al. Phase I trial using adaptive control dosing of hexamethylene bisacetamide (NSC 95580). *Cancer Res* 1989;49:3436.
122. Conley BA, Egorin MJ, Sinibaldi V, et al. Approaches to optimal dosing of hexamethylene bisacetamide. *Cancer Chemother Pharmacol* 1992;31:37.
123. Santini J, Milano G, Thyss A, et al. 5-FU therapeutic monitoring with dose adjustment leads to an improved therapeutic index in head and neck cancer. *Br J Cancer* 1989;59:287.
124. Evans WE, Rodman J, Relling MV, et al. Individualized dosages of chemotherapy as a strategy to improve response for acute lymphocytic leukemia. *Semin Hematol* 1991;28:15.
125. Grochow LB. Busulfan disposition: the role of therapeutic monitoring in bone marrow transplantation induction regimens. *Semin Oncol* 1993;20:18.
126. Yeager AM, Wagner JE Jr, Graham ML, et al. Optimization of busulfan dosage in children undergoing bone marrow transplantation: a pharmacokinetic study of dose escalation. *Blood* 1992;80:2425.
127. Demirer T, Buckner CD, Appelbaum FR, et al. Busulfan, cyclophosphamide and fractionated total body irradiation for autologous or syngeneic marrow transplantation for acute and chronic myelogenous leukemia: phase I dose escalation of busulfan based on targeted plasma levels. *Bone Marrow Transplant* 1996;17:491.
128. Myers C, Cooper M, Stein C, et al. Suramin: a novel growth factor antagonist with activity in hormone-refractory metastatic prostate cancer [see comments]. *J Clin Oncol* 1992; 10:881.
129. Jodrell DI, Reyno LM, Sridhara R, et al. Suramin: development of a population pharmacokinetic model and its use with intermittent short infusions to control plasma drug concentration in patients with prostate cancer [see comments]. *J Clin Oncol* 1994;12:166.
130. Eisenberger MA, Reyno LM, Jodrell DI, et al. Suramin, an active drug for prostate cancer: interim observations in a phase I trial [see comments; published erratum appears in *J Natl Cancer Inst* 1994;86:639]. *J Natl Cancer Inst* 1993;85:611.
131. Cooper MR, Lieberman R, La Rocca RV, et al. Adaptive control with feedback strategies for suramin dosing. *Clin Pharmacol Ther* 1992;52:11.
132. Scher HI, Jodrell DI, Iversen JM, et al. Use of adaptive control with feedback to individualize suramin dosing. *Cancer Res* 1992;52:64.
133. Thibault A, Cooper MR, Figg WD, et al. A phase I and pharmacokinetic study of intravenous phenylacetate in patients with cancer. *Cancer Res* 1994;54:1690.

SECTION 2

Cancer Drug Development

EDWARD CHU
MICHAEL R. GREVER
BRUCE A. CHABNER

Identification and Screening of New Agents

More than five decades of research effort in cancer drug discovery and development have provided approximately six dozen approved products for the treatment of malignancy.[1,2] Although major advances have been made in the chemotherapeutic management of some patients, particularly in hematologic malignancies, one-half of all cancer patients either do not respond to therapy or relapse from the initial response and ultimately die from their metastatic disease. Thus, the continued commitment to the arduous task of discovering new cancer therapeutic agents remains critically important.[3] Many of the existing antineoplastic agents share a common mechanism of action. Current research efforts are more diverse than ever, being driven by explosive discoveries in molecular biology and related areas to fully elucidate the development of the malignant process (e.g., factors controlling tumor angiogenesis and metastatic potential). The hope for improvement in treatment outcome for most patients with metastatic disease resides in continued research designed to discover novel therapeutic products that exploit differences in molecular targets between normal and tumor cells and to use them in combination with biologic agents and immune therapies to eradicate systemic disease not curable by surgery or irradiation.

Beyond the intellectual challenge of drug discovery, formidable effort, time, and expense are required for the complex development processes that move a new agent from discovery to its ultimate approval for use in the treatment of malignancy. Numerous pitfalls may threaten the progress of a promising agent (e.g., excessive early toxicity, ineffective route or schedule of administration, inappropriate formulation, long-term unpredicted toxicities, and delays in the execution of clinical trials). Although the time to drug approval for the treatment of cancer has varied considerably, depending on the specific agent (e.g., 6 to 12 years from the time of initiation of clinical trials), efforts are being made to expedite both the preclinical and clinical components of investigation. In other areas of medicine, the time to develop specific drugs may be equally long and difficult. However, the potentially fatal consequences of unsuccessful treatment of this disease continue to impart urgency in the discovery and development of novel anticancer agents.

DRUG DISCOVERY

HOW DRUGS ARE DISCOVERED

This section considers strategies for identifying new chemical entities, whether they be synthesized chemicals or compounds extracted or derived from plant, microbial, and marine animal sources. The parallel process for discovery and development of biologic agents is discussed elsewhere in this text. (See Chapter 18.)

In establishing a program for drug discovery, cancer researchers must address two fundamental questions: What screening system should be used to detect a compound of interest? What compounds should be tested in this system? The answers to these questions determine whether the research effort is empiric, with few preconceived notions about where to search for compounds and what to use as the screen, or whether it focuses on a specific biologic target, such as an oncogene, and tests a specific set of materials, such as natural products and rationally synthesized inhibitors of a target enzyme. The history of cancer drug discovery reflects an evolution from highly empiric approaches, based on testing of randomly selected compounds against rapidly proliferating murine leukemia, to the current, more focused testing of natural products, rationally synthesized agents, and biologic products against well-characterized tumor cell lines or molecular targets. Even in its earliest days, however, cancer drug discovery attracted scientists who had a theoretical basis for testing certain types of compounds. Perhaps the two best examples are the antifolates, initially tested by Farber et al.,[4] and the fluoropyrimidines synthesized by Heidelberger and colleagues[5] (see Chapter 19.5).

The story of the discovery of antifolates is particularly instructive because it illustrates the important interplay between cancer biology and drug discovery. The earliest uses of an antifolate as a chemotherapeutic agent resulted from the astute observations of Farber and associates,[4] who observed an acceleration of the leukemic process in patients being treated with folic acid. A series of folic acid antagonists were provided to Farber and colleagues by the medicinal chemists at Lederle Laboratories. Although structure-activity relations of antifolates and the intracellular target of these compounds were unknown at that time, it was clear from laboratory studies that modified folates could inhibit tumor cell growth. The initial clinical trial involved the administration of pteroylaspartic acid (an analogue of folic acid, or pteroylglutamate) to a moribund patient with progressive acute myelogenous leukemia, which resulted in a markedly hypocellular bone marrow without actually producing clinical benefit. The investigators were sufficiently encouraged, however, to administer a more powerful folic acid antagonist, aminopterin (2,4-diaminopteroylglutamate), to children with advanced stages of acute leukemia. Substitution of an amino group at the 4 position of the folate pteridine ring created a tight-binding inhibitor of dihydrofolate reductase and yielded drugs with the potential to induce remissions. Approximately 10 of the first 16 patients treated with aminopterin demonstrated evidence of hematologic and clinical improvement. These early clinical experiences provided the foundation for medicinal chemists to synthesize a number of agents with structural similarities to naturally occurring folates. Moreover, these studies revealed that various substitutions resulted in different sites of action, in addition to inhibition of dihydrofolate reductase (Fig. 19.2-1).

From these relatively primitive beginnings, rational design efforts have progressed to the use of computer modeling of drug-enzyme interactions as the basis for cancer drug discovery. Advances in x-ray crystallographic and nuclear magnetic resonance structural characterization of ligands and their target molecules have significantly enhanced the potential for

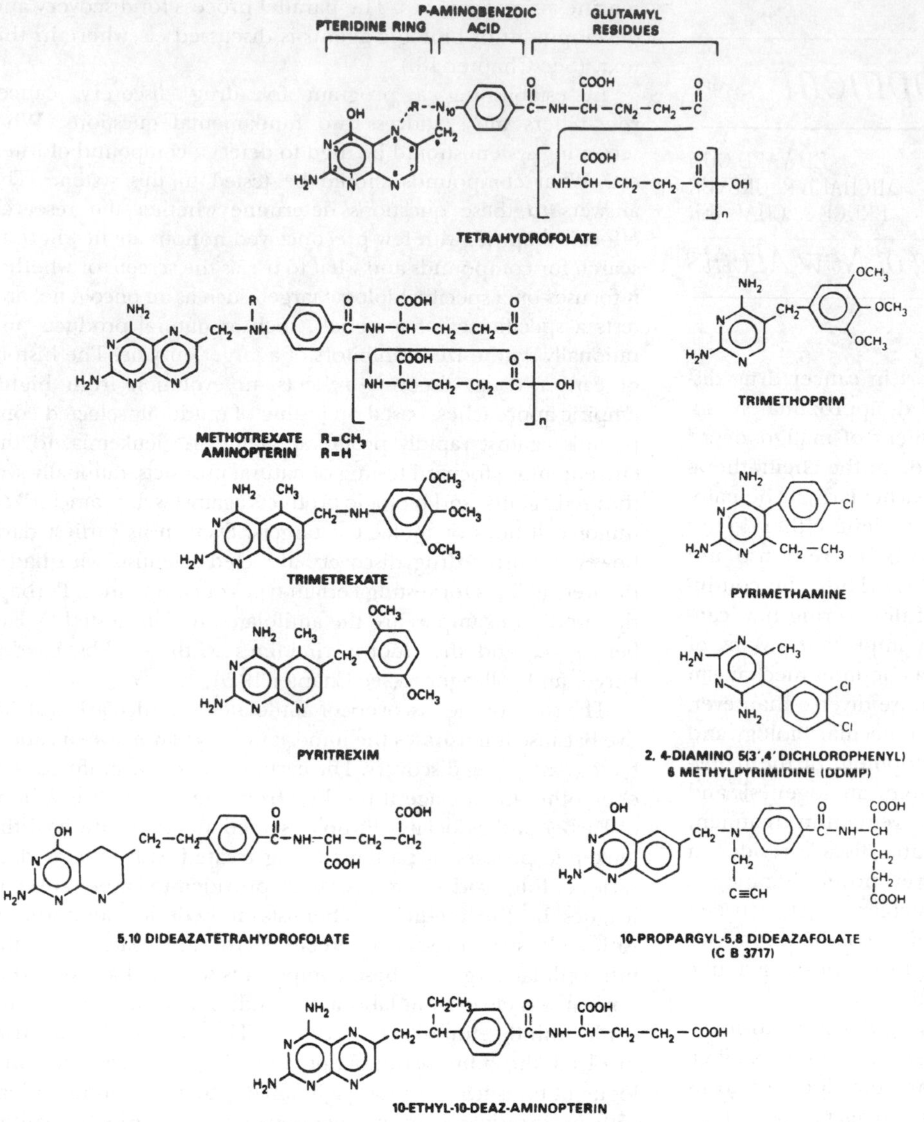

FIGURE 19.2-1. Structure of tetrahydrofolate and clinically useful antifolate compounds. (From Chabner BA, Collins JM, eds. *Cancer chemotherapy and biotherapy: principles and practice.* Philadelphia: Lippincott–Raven, 1996:112, with permission.)

rational design and, as is described later (see the section Molecular-Targeted Screening), such research efforts are now beginning to identify effective small molecules with efficacy against various human malignancies. Symmetric inhibitors of the protease of human immunodeficiency virus type 1 that were designed on the basis of the three-dimensional symmetry of the active enzyme site are currently in clinical use, thus demonstrating the feasibility and merit of such an approach.[6]

In most current drug discovery efforts, the rational and empiric approaches are being combined. Lead compounds are identified as inhibitors for molecular targets through molecular screening.[7] The lead compound can then be modified or enhanced by chemical analogue synthesis based on a variety of considerations, including a detailed study of target-inhibitor interaction. The complete characterization of the target and its interaction with the lead agent provides the basis for enhancing drug-target interaction. A key decision in this approach is the selection of a suitable target that is likely to have an impact on clinical outcome (enzyme, growth factor receptor, or oncogene product). The next challenge is the development of an appropriate and practical assay to identify the actual lead agents.

Although early efforts in cancer drug discovery tested agents either from the broad universe of synthetic chemicals or from a more targeted rational effort, attention increasingly has focused on natural products as an important, untapped source of promising lead compounds with unique sites of action as antineoplastic drugs.[8] The enormous diversity and complexity of chemical entities that have evolved as part of nature's chemical warfare cannot be readily duplicated by compounds synthesized in the laboratory and be made available for screening. However, the technological advances in combinatorial approaches for synthesizing large numbers of complex substances have provided an entire new source for novel antineoplastic agents.[9,10] Combinatorial chemistry can provide two different kinds of libraries that can then be used for further drug development.[11–13] The first is a generic library, which is used to discover a novel structural motif or feature that possesses a certain biologic activity. The goal of such an unbiased library is to identify a completely novel lead compound. The second type is a focused, biased library that serves to fine-tune the properties and biologic activity of an existing lead compound. In this case, the objective is to identify new lead com-

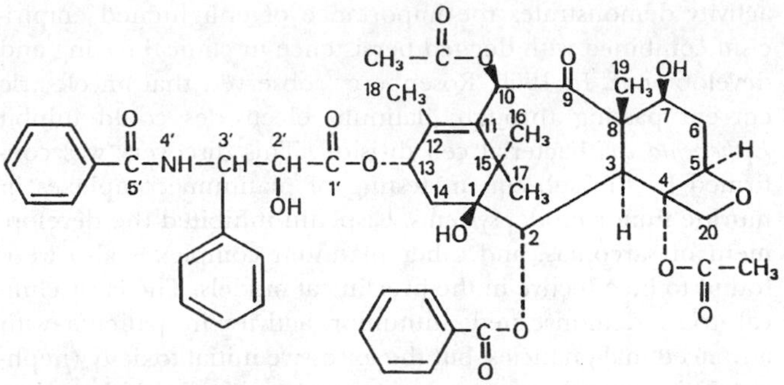

FIGURE 19.2-2. Structure of Taxol. (From Chabner BA, Collins JM, eds. *Cancer chemotherapy and biotherapy: principles and practice.* Philadelphia: Lippincott–Raven, 1996, with permission.)

pounds based on known structures that have already proven to be biologically active.

Approximately 30% of the currently effective antineoplastic agents are from natural sources or are derivatives of a natural product lead.[14] Certain themes run through the efforts to discover and develop natural products. Active compounds often have exceedingly complex structures that complicate efforts at total synthesis. Problems of supply and dependence on a natural resource, therefore, must be anticipated. Structure-activity relations are difficult to elucidate because of the basic problems presented by the unusual chemistry of these compounds and by the multiple chiral centers in these molecules (Fig. 19.2-2). However, the overall contribution of these complex chemical entities to the management of patients has been extremely rewarding.

Among the natural products, microbial antibiotics have been the most important source of cytotoxic agents. As a result of the great advances in the field of microbiology during the 1940s and the dawn of effective antibiotic therapy, potent anticancer drugs were sought in fermentation broths obtained from soil microbes, including bacteria, fungi, and related organisms. The discoveries of the actinomycins, anthracyclines, bleomycin, deoxycoformycin, and other agents have contributed valuable new entities to the repository of effective antineoplastic agents. Natural product drug discovery, however, must be complemented by efforts to improve leads through chemical modification and analogue synthesis. The discovery and subsequent clinical development of anthracyclines highlights the need for the close interplay of chemistry, biology, and clinical pharmacology in producing improved anticancer agents.

Daunorubicin, isolated from a colony of *Streptomyces* in 1957, eventually was demonstrated to have significant antileukemic activity in patients.[15] Additional research to induce mutant strains of the fungus *Streptomyces* resulted in the isolation of doxorubicin. Although the difference between these two anthracyclines is limited chemically to a single hydroxyl group, a marked difference exists in their spectrum of antitumor activity. Doxorubicin has been more effective than daunorubicin in the treatment of metastatic solid tumors and sarcomas. The cardiac toxicity associated with the chronic administration of both these agents, however, has provided impetus to design a new generation of anthracycline analogues. The long-term assessment of clinical outcome for children successfully treated for malignancy further substantiates the concerns regarding anthracycline-induced cardiotoxicity.[16] None of these anthracycline analogues is devoid of cardiac toxicity, but closely related molecules may have significant advantages. For example, the anthraquinones (e.g., mitoxantrone) demonstrate less cardiotoxicity and have remission-inducing activity in acute nonlymphocytic leukemia.[17] Thus, in modifying the chemical structure of a natural product in an attempt to enhance its therapeutic selectivity, the synthetic organic chemist plays a critical role in this process of drug development.

Natural product research has yielded other effective antineoplastic drugs. Although most of these agents have been identified in fermentation broths of microbial organisms, plants also have provided a number of active antineoplastic agents. One of the earliest plant-derived drugs resulted from a chance observation. In the 1950s, Noble and colleagues[18] were investigating interesting plant extracts used by primitive peoples. This attempt to take advantage of tribal medications, primarily natural products, represented an early entree into the discipline known as *ethnopharmacology*.

The leaves of the Jamaican periwinkle plant, *Vinca rosea*, were used to make a tea that was reported to be of benefit in diabetes.[18] During the initial animal investigations, the extract of these leaves was administered orally to both rats and rabbits without any observed effect on blood sugar levels. Subsequent administration of the aqueous extract of the periwinkle plant by injection to rats had a dramatic lethal effect within a week. Postmortem examination of the animals demonstrated that the rats had died of sepsis related to bone marrow suppression. Isolation and chemical characterization of the responsible chemical factors were accomplished using a bioassay-guided approach (i.e., granulocytopenia in the treated animals) for identifying the effective component of this aqueous extract of the plant. The compound was determined to be an organic base and subsequently was called *vincaleukoblastine.* This agent demonstrated carcinostatic activity against both a transplanted murine mammary adenocarcinoma and a rat-transplanted sarcoma.[18] The mechanism of action (i.e., inhibition of microtubule formation) proved to be unique and provided the basis for an entirely new area of research for cancer drug development.

In contrast to using the complicated biologic end point of the peripheral blood granulocyte count from an intact animal, simple and more rapid screens (e.g., molecular target–based or *in vitro* cell cytotoxicity assays) currently are used to guide fractionation of extracts for isolation and characterization of active components. After final chemical identification of the plant-derived chemical antineoplastic entity, validation of antitumor activity in an *in vivo* tumor model is still required. Sufficient supplies of the active agents isolated from natural product sources are needed to conduct adequate *in vivo* confirmatory studies. Adequate supply was a problem with the periwinkle extract in its early development, and it remains problematic for many natural product agents now being isolated.

Several new plant-derived natural products have proven to be of extreme interest in the treatment of cancer. Taxol was isolated from the bark of the Pacific yew tree in 1971,[19] and it has a unique mechanism of antitumor activity that involves stabilization of microtubule assembly with resultant inhibition of the normal dynamics of microtubule formation.[20] This agent has a broad spectrum of antitumor activity, and it is active against a number of human tumor xenografts, including breast cancer, ovarian cancer, and other malignancies. Subsequent clinical studies have confirmed the high degree of activity in patients with a wide range of solid tumors, including breast, ovary, head and neck, esophagus, testes, and lung malignancies.[21] Initially, a major obstacle to defining the role of Taxol in cancer therapy related to the difficulties encountered with drug supply.[14] Semisynthesis from 10-acetyl baccatin III, was eventually accomplished, and new sources of Taxol from nursery species have been identified. The supply issue has now been fully resolved with the successful total synthesis of this complex molecule.[22,23] Moreover, advances in the chemistry of isoserines and taxoid anticancer agents have facilitated the synthesis of second-generation taxoid compounds with activity against drug-resistant cancer cells.[24] The history of the development of Taxol is important because it highlights the complexities involved with development of any cancer drug—namely challenges in supply of drug, difficulties with synthesis of drug, issues of drug formulation, and obstacles associated with the implementation of successful clinical studies.

Another natural product that has been under investigation for many years, but only now found to have broad activity against various human malignancies, is derived from the bark of *Camptotheca accuminata*, a tree prized for its medicinal properties in traditional Chinese medicine.[25] The camptothecin derivatives are unique because they inhibit topoisomerase I, a key enzyme that maintains DNA in a torsionally relaxed state.[26,27] Both topotecan and CPT-11, which are derivatives of camptothecin, have significant activity in patients with advanced malignancies, including colorectal cancer, esophageal cancer, non–small cell and small cell lung cancer, and cervical cancer.[28–30] Significant efforts continue to focus on developing novel analogues of camptothecin with enhanced biophysical and biologic activity. 9-Nitroaminocamptothecin and 9-aminocamptothecin are currently in advanced stages of clinical testing.[31]

Marine organisms represent a largely unexplored and untapped source of unique toxic chemicals. These toxins are elaborated by sponges and other sessile saltwater organisms as defenses against their predators. Several highly potent agents demonstrate interesting antitumor activity against unique molecular targets in preclinical models, and some examples include the bryostatins (which inhibit protein kinase C), the dolastatins and halichondrins (which bind to microtubules), and the tunicate-derived ecteinascidins (which bind in the minor groove of DNA).[8,14,32–36] Although the marine environment represents an untapped potential source for interesting new chemical entities, certain unique problems affect this biosphere. Scale-up procurement of bulk material from marine sources presents a special challenge in biomass collection. The potency of many of these agents may ameliorate this supply problem, but selectivity against the tumor (and not the normal host) must first be demonstrated. In addition, the highly potent natural products present additional challenges for clinical investigators conducting phase I studies. For example, clinical pharmacologic studies may be impossible if the active species is present in such low levels that detection by even very sensitive analytic methods is not feasible at clinically tolerated doses. The rich diversity of chemical structures found in nature provides the impetus for continued research in this area. Moreover, the use of combinatorial chemistry technology may be incorporated into the process once novel therapeutic leads are identified from these natural products.

Cancer drug discovery may also result from a totally fortuitous experimental observation. The discovery of platinum complexes as antiproliferative agents with remarkable clinical activity demonstrates the importance of enlightened empiricism combined with dogged persistence in clinical testing and development. In 1965, Rosenberg[37] observed that an electric current passing through platinum electrodes could inhibit *Escherichia coli* bacterial cell division. This discovery was confirmed by the subsequent testing of platinum complexes in murine tumor model systems. Cisplatin inhibited the development of sarcomas, and other platinum complexes also were found to be effective in the preclinical models. The early clinical trials demonstrated antitumor activity in patients with advanced malignancies, but the excessive initial toxicity (nephrotoxicity) raised serious concern among the clinical investigators. The demonstration that adequate hydration and slow infusion reduce the degree of renal toxicity permitted further evaluation of the agent. The responses observed in testicular cancer and ovarian cancer led to approval of the drug approximately 6 years after the initial clinical trial. This excellent anticancer drug might have been discarded in error without the foresight of both preclinical and clinical investigators who were convinced of the drug's potential, were committed to the systematic testing of the drug, and were clever enough to find ways to deal with its toxicity. Most of the antineoplastic agents have been discovered though empiric screening efforts or represent chemical modifications of lead compounds discovered in cancer screenings.

Screening methods can either be simple, such as a well-characterized cell line or a defined enzymatic target, or complex, such as an *in vivo* animal tumor. In general, current efforts favor simple systems that accommodate high volumes of unknown compounds. The end point of the cancer screen may be a biologic target (e.g., tumor cell cytotoxicity, growth inhibition, differentiation) or a biochemical-molecular target that is known to be important for the survival of cancer cells. The advantages and disadvantages of each of these approaches is presented in Table 19.2-1. Both the cell line and molecular approach may be combined through the use of genetically engineered cell lines that express a specific molecular target.

The evolution of strategies at the National Cancer Institute (NCI) illustrates the changes in screening that have resulted from the advances in cancer biology and cancer genetics. The early NCI cancer screening efforts used murine leukemias (L1210 and P388) as the index tumors in an *in vivo* screening effort.[38] The screen identified agents that had efficacy in humans in the treatment of leukemias and lymphoproliferative malignancies, such as hydroxyurea and the nitrosoureas. However, the failure of this screen to identify active drugs for the major solid tumors resulted in a significant change in 1975 in the approach of the NCI when animal solid tumor and human tumor xenografts were added as a secondary *in vivo* tumor panel.[38] In 1985, a second major change was made.[38,39] The increasing availability of a growing number of cell lines derived from human solid tumors and well characterized with respect to drug response patterns, growth factor dependence, oncogene expression, and other biochemical and molecular features presented an opportunity to focus screening efforts on the unique biology of human solid tumors.

A number of human solid tumor cell lines were selected to provide a disease-oriented approach to drug discovery in contrast with the previous compound-oriented drug discovery methods. A total of 60 human tumor cell lines derived from seven cancer types (e.g., lung, colon, melanoma, kidney, ovary, brain,

TABLE 19.2-1. Comparison of Cancer Screening Devices

Screen	*Advantages*	*Disadvantages*
Tumor cell line–based assays	High-volume assay	Mechanism of action not defined by this approach
	Has identified many current cancer drugs	May define agents that are nonspecifically toxic to cells
	Defines agent with effect on tumor cell and displays the pattern of cellular response	Does not elucidate the cellular target responsible for the observed effect
	Defines agents that cross cell membrane and withstand the intracellular milieu	
Mechanistic or molecular targeted assays	High-volume assay	Despite scientific appeal, approach only more recently implemented
	Has a rational basis for drug discovery	No guarantee that agents will enter the cell or withstand intracellular milieu
	May provide agents specifically aimed at a critical point in the tumor cell	No guarantee that agents will be selective
	Potential selective antitumor activity	
	May provide novel classes of antitumor agents	

leukemia) formed the original cell line panel. Breast cancer cell lines were subsequently added. The initial concept proposed that leads demonstrating disease specificity would be identified, and activity could be further examined by *in vivo* testing in nude mice, using the most sensitive *in vitro* index tumor cell lines.

In the current NCI anticancer screen, each candidate agent is tested over a broad concentration range against every cell line in the panel.[2,3,38–40] Active compounds are selected for further testing based on several different criteria: disease-type specificity in the *in vitro* assay, unique structure, potency, and demonstration of a unique pattern of cellular cytotoxicity or cytostasis, indicating a unique mechanism of action or intracellular target. The agents selected for further investigation are then subjected to additional testing to assess their *in vivo* therapeutic index.[3,41] The current version of the cancer drug screening program of the NCI has been in operation since 1990, and a number of novel chemical entities have been identified for further evaluation. This high-capacity screen was designed to accommodate approximately 10,000 individual chemicals tested annually, with additional capacity for screening natural product extracts. Approximately 5% of the compounds tested in the initial screen show sufficient activity to warrant further evaluation in *in vivo* screens or biochemical-molecular assays. More than 60,000 agents have been screened against a panel of 60 human cancer cell lines. The tumors that are represented in this cell line panel include melanomas; leukemias; and cancers of the breast, prostate, colon, ovary, kidney, and central nervous system. To date, this approach has identified five novel agents (e.g., a tyrosine kinase inhibitor, a protein kinase C inhibitor, and several disease-specific agents) for further testing in clinical trials. It is hoped that an overall assessment of the clinical usefulness of this novel cell line screening approach will be feasible in the near future.

The concept of cancer drug discovery that is based on high-volume screens, whether oriented toward a cell line–based or molecular target, relies on the acquisition of a large source of diverse materials for examination. In the case of the NCI, an extensive program for acquiring both defined chemical entities and diverse natural products has been pursued. Enormous effort was initially invested to standardize the *in vitro* assay, and sufficient time should be provided to fully evaluate the clinical utility of its early findings.

The pharmaceutical industry is also actively engaged in the procurement of large numbers of interesting chemical structures and natural products for testing in their respective cancer screens, many of which focus on specific molecular targets. Difficult decisions must be made to choose among the large number of unknown entities for initial testing and to aid in the prioritization of known active compounds for further development. Computer programs have been developed to assist in this prioritization and to enhance the diversity of potential chemical entries and crude natural products introduced into the screening process.[40,42] For example, there are significant challenges in representing, analyzing, and storing the vast amount of experimental data generated by the substances tested in the *in vitro* screen of the NCI. In Figure 19.2-3, drug testing data are represented as a mean graph presenting growth inhibition in a standard bar graph.[38] The mean graph is constructed by projecting bars to the right or left of the mean, depending on whether an individual cell line is more or less sensitive than the average line in the panel. Furthermore, the length of each bar is proportional to the relative sensitivity of the cell lines. Thus, each agent can be represented by a characteristic fingerprint of cell line responsiveness.

After an agent has been tested in the cancer screen, its unique response pattern can be compared with the results from all other agents within the database. A computer program called *COMPARE* uses a simple algorithm for aligning and contrasting the patterns for each compound with the patterns of other compounds in the database.[43,44] A compound is entered into the program as a seed, and the computer database elicits a list of those agents that have similar patterns of tumor cellular responsiveness. In Table 19.2-2, an example is presented for the introduction of a seed compound and the resulting list of agents that had similar patterns of cellular cytotoxicity. A correlation coefficient is also expressed, relating the closeness of the seed to those agents listed by the computer program. Close correlations between agents appear to have biologic and pharmacologic importance, implying a common intracellular target despite a dissimilarity in structure (e.g., tubulin-binding agents, topoisomerase-interactive agents). The COMPARE program has several important features.[44] It can identify the intracellular target or mechanism of action of a new compound through a comparison of its fingerprint with known agents. It

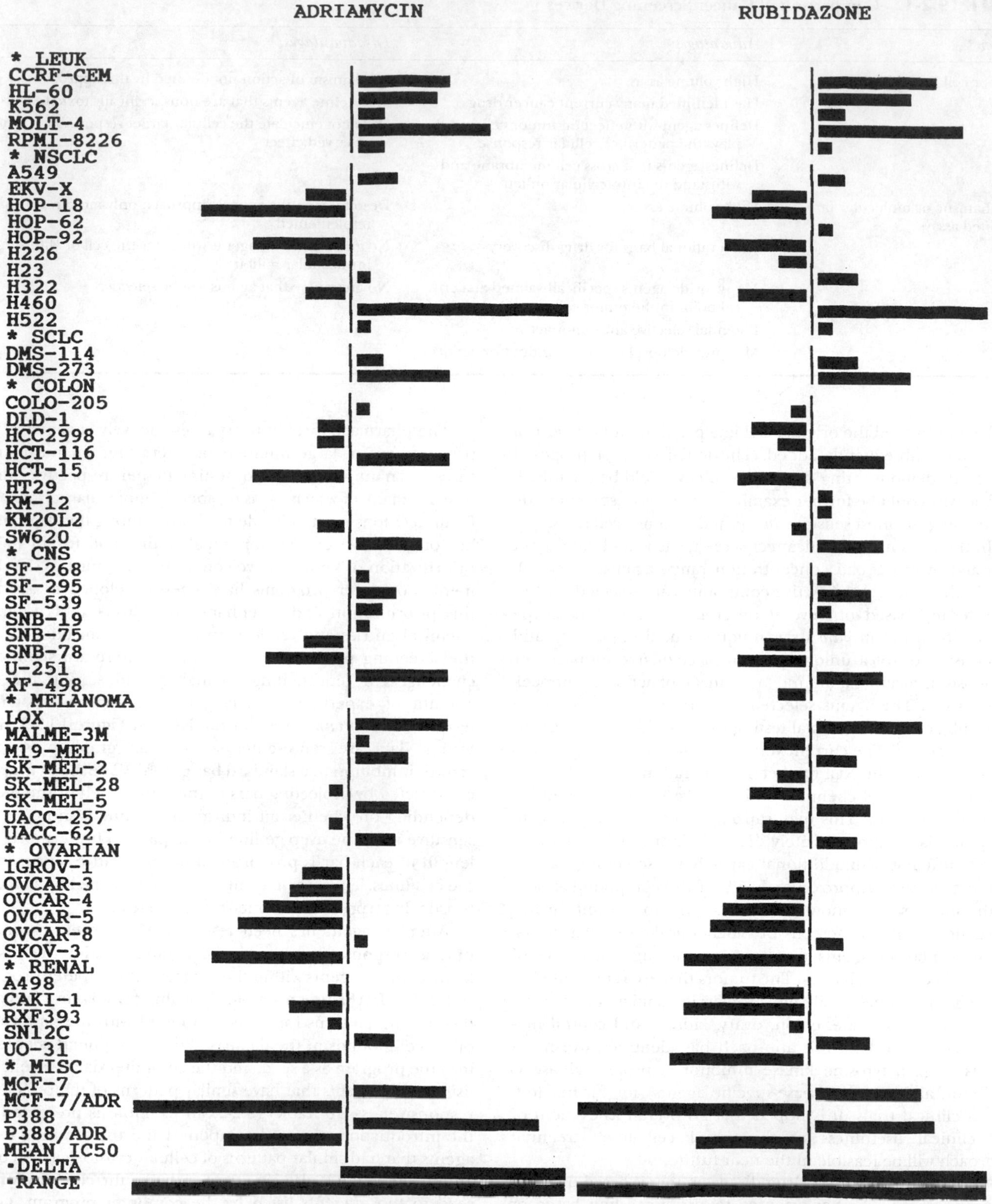

FIGURE 19.2-3. Mean graph representation of antitumor effects in the National Cancer Institute's (NCI) cancer screen. The effects of a specific agent on the tumor cell lines in the NCI cancer screen are shown by the construction of a mean graph presentation of the data. Screening results for two anthracyclines are charted. A mean concentration of the agent that produces the same level of response for all the cell lines in the screen forms an anchor point for this graphic presentation. The individual response of each cell line to the agent is then depicted by a bar graph extending to the right or left of the mean, depending on whether the cell line was either more or less sensitive than the average response, respectively. The length of each bar is proportional to the relative sensitivity when compared with the mean determination. CNS, central nervous system; Leuk, leukemia; NSCLC, non–small cell lung carcinoma; Misc, miscellaneous; SCLC, small cell lung carcinoma.

TABLE 19.2-2. The COMPARE Program[a]

	Parent = Taxol		
NSC Number	High Concentration	Correlation Coefficient	*Chemical Name*
153858	1.00E-09	0.812	Maytansine
49842	2.50E-06	0.767	Vinblastine sulfate
332598	5.00E-06	0.745	Rhizoxin
609395	1.00E-08	0.703	Halichondrin B
757	6.25E-04	0.691	Colchicine
67574	1.00E-03	0.628	Vincristine sulfate
376128	1.00E-08	0.628	Dolastatin

[a]An extensive database has been generated from the many agents tested in the National Cancer Institute's cancer screen. The unique patterns of cellular response can be used to characterize an agent by its "fingerprint" of cytostasis or cytotoxicity. Agents that have common cellular targets can be identified by the use of the computerized database. For example, introduction of a seed or parent compound into the COMPARE program elicits a list of those agents that exhibit similar patterns of tumor cell response. In the example in this table, the agents listed are known to be tubulin-interactive agents. The correlation coefficient for the relation of each agent to the seed or parent compound is provided. *High concentration* refers to the highest concentration of the agent used during the screening experiment. *NSC Number* refers to the individual identification number assigned to each agent submitted to the National Cancer Institute.

can search for compounds previously tested in the cancer screen that have a fingerprint similar to that of a lead compound known to inhibit a unique target. It also has the power to detect inhibition of integrated biochemical and molecular pathways that are not adequately represented by a single molecule or molecular interaction. The comparison also allows recognition of a new agent that does not match with compounds of known mechanisms of action. Given the critical roles of an intact cell-cycle checkpoint and apoptotic pathways in determining chemosensitivity, it is clear that such an algorithmic approach may help identify candidate anticancer drugs that are not dependent on an intact checkpoint and apoptosis function. Finally, this strategy provides the rational basis for future pharmacophore development.

Computer approaches to data analysis similar to that described by the NCI are being developed by industry to search for agents interacting with specific molecular targets. In addition, the NCI has conducted an elaborate characterization of specific molecular targets expressed by the existing tumor cell lines within its screen. For example, because certain cell lines are known to contain a mutated or overexpressed oncogene, such as k-ras or HER-2/neu, it is possible to search the existing database for agents active against only those particular cell lines. This process may ultimately combine the advantages of both cell line–based and molecular screens, but will require separate validation to confirm that identified leads do indeed interact with the purported molecular target in specific assays directed at that entity. Although the NCI cell line screen represents a carefully constructed system for obtaining and analyzing voluminous data on diverse compounds, alternative screening systems in academic centers and industry increasingly rely on high throughput assays based on specific molecular targets, against which combinatorial chemistry inventories are tested. A good example of this approach is the potent antimitotic agent monastrol, isolated by Mayer et al.[45] This agent targets kinesin Eg5, a mitotic protein required for spindle bipolarity and, thus, acts to inhibit the process of mitosis.

MOLECULAR-TARGETED SCREENING

From a scientific perspective, a compelling argument can be made for focusing on a well-defined molecular target and for using computer-based approaches to design small molecules that would specifically interact with this target.

With the rapid advances being made in defining the molecular pathology of neoplastic cells, specific oncogenes have been identified that are expressed uniquely in malignant tissue. The discovery of inappropriately expressed or mutated genes has provided an impetus for the establishment of numerous screens designed to detect specific inhibitors or modulators of the products of these abnormal genes. Intracellular signaling pathways that mediate the actions of growth factors and oncogenes on cell proliferation, such as protein kinases, G proteins, and transcription activators, provide additional novel targets for anticancer drugs. However, given the considerable overlap of access to various growth-factor signaling pathways (many signals use the same distal steps), signal transduction inhibitors may lack specificity for the neoplastic cells.[46]

As an alternative to targeting these intracellular pathways, significant attention has focused on strategies to inhibit the process of angiogenesis.[47] This concept stems from the seminal work of Folkman and colleagues[47a] who proposed that the growth of a tumor mass is dependent on the formation of a vascular network that supplies the tumor with essential nutrients. The targeting of the tumor vasculature has two potential advantages over conventional biochemical and molecular targets. The first is that this approach does not require tailoring of therapy to the unique genetic makeup of the tumor, because it appears that all solid tumors are dependent, to some extent, on angiogenesis for growth. In addition, the target of this approach is the normal vascular endothelial cells that are genetically stable and, thus, less likely to become drug-resistant.

Advocates for the use of mechanistic-based approaches to novel drug discovery have emphasized the potential for selectivity that may result from the use of molecular targeting.[7,48–50] The expression of identical or closely related molecular or biochemical targets in normal tissue must always be considered. Mutant oncogenes and their corresponding protein products appear to be the most attractive targets for drug design. Two examples include the fusion protein that results from the BCR-ABL translocation in chronic myelogenous leukemia (CML) and the interference with tumor suppression resulting from the binding of papillomavirus proteins to the RB (retinoblastoma) gene in cervical carcinoma.

In CML and in approximately 20% of adult patients with acute lymphocytic leukemia (ALL), a characteristic reciprocal translocation between chromosomes 9 and 22 is observed. The protooncogene (ABL) from chromosome 9 is translocated at the breakpoint cluster region (BCR) on chromosome 22. This translocation encodes the Bcr-Abl protein, which expresses constitutively activated tyrosine kinase function. It is a 210-kD oncoprotein, and expression of p210 BCR-Abl induces a disease in mice resembling CML, confirming the critical role of this oncoprotein in the development of CML.[51,52] The p210 Bcr-Abl protein is present in 95% of patients with CML and in 5% to 10% of adults with ALL for whom there is no evidence of CML. A second fusion protein of 185 kD is found in 10% of adult cases and 5% to 10% of pediatric cases of ALL, but not in CML.

It is clear that expression of this genetic rearrangement is essential for maintaining the malignant phenotype.[53] In addition, transfection of the specific DNA for the BCR-ABL–encoded protein kinase into the hematopoietic stem cells of mice results in the induction of a malignant disorder *in vivo* with similarities to the clinical illness in humans.[54] Modification of these murine models could provide a potential opportunity to test promising new therapeutic products *in vivo.* Moreover, the aberrant tyrosine kinase resulting from these abnormal genetic rearrangements (BCR-ABL) within the hematopoietic stem cells does not exist in normal host cells. This abnormal gene provides an ideal molecular target for therapeutic intervention. The crystal structure of several protein kinases has been solved, and a number of compounds have been designed based on the structure of the adenosine triphosphate (ATP) binding site or the active site of the enzyme. In screening against the recombinant BCR-ABL kinase protein, the 2-phenylaminopyrimidine derivative known as *CGP 57148* (STI 571) proved to be a potent and selective inhibitor, targeting the ATP binding pocket.[55] This compound inhibits all ABL tyrosine kinases at submicromolar concentrations *in vitro,* and it has minimal to no inhibitory effect on the colony-forming potential of normal bone marrow cells. CGP 57148 appears to be selectively toxic to cells expressing the BCR-ABL tyrosine kinase.[56,57] A phase I clinical trial has been completed in CML patients who were unsuccessful with interferon therapy.[58,59] CGP 57148 was given orally on a daily basis, and treatment was well tolerated, with the most common toxicities being only mild nausea (grade 1), muscle cramps, and arthralgias. With regard to its clinical activity, significant hematologic responses have been observed, with 100% clinical complete response at daily doses greater than 300 mg and a 40% to 50% cytogenetic response. Clinical investigations are in progress to validate the clinical efficacy of this novel agent. Studies have shown that the drug also has potent activity against the platelet-derived growth factor receptor, and in experimental studies, it inhibits tumors that overexpress this receptor. Thus, this compound may have broader application than just for CML.

Another potential target for therapeutic intervention has evolved from an enhanced understanding of the role of aberrant tumor suppressor protein function in the malignant process. It is appreciated that more than 80% of cervical carcinomas have evidence of integrated DNA sequences from papillomaviruses.[60] Human papillomavirus-16 has been implicated frequently as a causal role of this malignancy. Extensive molecular investigation of the association of human papillomavirus with cervical carcinoma has identified specific nuclear proteins that interact with the tumor suppressor gene RB.[61] In fact, the complex protein-protein interaction between the E7 protein from human papillomavirus-16 and the retinoblastoma suppressor protein (pRB) is believed to be important in the cellular transformation that leads to cervical carcinoma. Expression of the E7 protein apparently occurs both within cells from patients with cervical carcinoma and from cell lines derived from this malignancy. The inactivation of the RB tumor suppressor gene by this protein appears to be reversible. There is significant interest in identifying agents that could selectively interfere with this deleterious E7-RB interaction.

DRUG DEVELOPMENT

There is an urgent need to move promising new therapies into clinical trials. However, important and clinically relevant information may be lost by proceeding immediately from a primary *in vitro* screen to a clinical trial without defining the *in vivo* activity of an agent, its pharmacokinetics and schedule dependency in animals, and its profile of toxicity for normal and malignant cells and tissues. Each of these issues is important and must be addressed in a timely manner to provide safe and reasonable starting doses for implementing phase I trials in patients. The steps required in the development of a cancer agent for clinical practice are complex, and as outlined in Figure 19.2-4, they are both time- and resource-intensive.

Secondary *in vitro* studies to optimize the exposure time to an agent and to define mechanisms of resistance are useful for the investigators planning *in vivo* studies. Examination of the dose-response data for several tumor cell lines should permit a selection of the optimal tumor system for subsequently evaluating *in vivo* efficacy. Furthermore, preliminary pharmacologic studies in non–tumor-bearing animals provide useful information about the plasma concentrations achievable and an estimate of the acute toxicity after systemic administration of a new agent. Success in identifying new therapies relies on the expeditious, yet careful, conduct of those studies pertinent to developing a promising *in vitro* observation (derived from either the cell line screen or the molecular models) into an actual drug candidate.[62–65]

IN VIVO ANTITUMOR ASSAYS CURRENTLY IN USE

In the current NCI development schema, the human tumor cell line most sensitive to an active candidate *in vitro* is selected

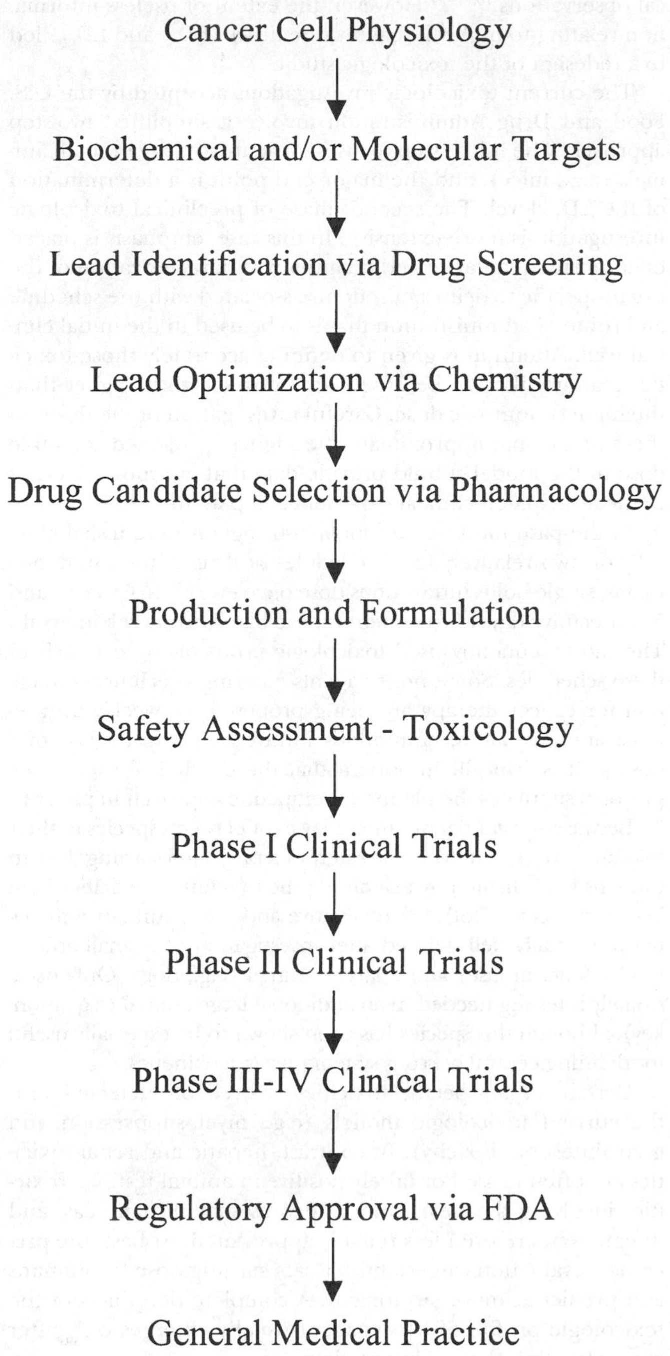

FIGURE 19.2-4. Steps in cancer drug development. FDA, U.S. Food and Drug Administration.

for testing as a xenograft in a subcutaneous implant site in a nude mouse. Compounds identified in molecular screens are usually tested against human or murine tumors engineered to overexpress the specific drug target.

Failure to demonstrate *in vivo* efficacy for agents that display strong *in vitro* evidence of antitumor activity should prompt additional studies to determine whether a pharmacokinetic or metabolic explanation exists for the loss of activity. The initial lead, either discovered by an empiric screen or as a result of rational chemical design, is usually not the optimal chemical entity for clinical investigation. Lead optimization and an iterative process between chemists and tumor biologists may be required to enhance the *in vivo* therapeutic index. Factors such as poor solubility and rapid *in vivo* metabolism may be corrected by analogue development. More potent and less toxic derivatives can often be subsequently developed (i.e., provided the molecule is amenable to modification).

PRECLINICAL PHARMACOLOGY

Preclinical studies in mice, rats, and dogs provide essential information about pharmacokinetics and provide a basis for rational schedule development for the new drugs in humans. Factors such as bioavailability (for agents administered by the oral route), metabolism, renal excretion, and penetration into the central nervous system contribute to the understanding of how best to test a new drug in humans. Although there is no guarantee that human subjects will handle a new drug in the same way as the animal species, in most instances the major pathways for drug metabolism and excretion are qualitatively, if not quantitatively, the same across species.

Pharmacokinetic information in animals can also provide a rational basis for dose escalation in humans. Collins and associates[66] have hypothesized that dose-limiting toxicity in mice and humans is a function of drug exposure, as measured by the area under the drug concentration in plasma × time curve (C × T). They predict that animals and humans encounter dose-limiting toxicity at the same C × T for any given drug and that the experimentally determined dose-limiting C × T can be used as a target for dose escalation in humans. An analysis of experience with phase I drug trials suggested that for most, but not all, drugs, the relationship of C × T to toxicity holds across species. This work potentially allows the clinical investigator to base initial dose escalation steps on measurements of C × T. Dose escalation can proceed in a more rapid fashion than formerly possible using empiric schemes, and wasteful multiple steps in dose escalation can be avoided. This approach, although apparently valid in retrospective studies, still requires broader validation in a prospective manner.

Drugs that demonstrate substantial interspecies variation in patterns of target tissue activation are not good candidates for this approach. For example, drugs activated by deoxycytidine kinase, such as fludarabine phosphate, are much more toxic to human marrow cells than to mouse bone marrow, presumably as a result of the higher levels of this activating enzyme in human cells.[67] In this instance, toxicity in humans would not be accurately predicted by the C × T approach. Furthermore, drug candidates that are excessively potent (e.g., several of the marine natural products) may have biologic effects at plasma concentrations lower than the level of reproducible detection. Consequently, such agents are not acceptable candidates for pharmacologically guided dose escalation.

FORMULATION STUDIES

Although the preliminary pharmacologic and toxicologic studies may begin before a decision on the final formulation of a product, the Investigational New Drug (IND)–directed toxicology should be performed with the final formulation. In addition, other critical studies may be influenced by the formulation (e.g., bioavailability of an oral formulation, insolubility of an agent demonstrating interesting antitumor activity in the cancer screen). Three important factors that have an impact on formulation studies include solubility, stability, and dosage requirements.[68]

Because the route of drug administration for antineoplastic agents has primarily been through the intravenous approach, the issue of solubility has provided a substantial challenge for a number of agents with limited aqueous solubility. Efforts to improve the solubility of an agent have primarily involved physical measures, including the use of various mixed solvent systems. Novel approaches, including the use of micronization, liposomal encapsulation, and other unique delivery systems (e.g., cyclodextrins and coacervate systems), have been investigated in an effort to improve methods of drug delivery to tissues. Major efforts are needed to expand the vehicles that are available for intravenous drug delivery of agents with limited aqueous solubility and stability.

The prodrug approach uses chemical modification to solve the difficulty associated with drug insolubility. The most recent example of a simple prodrug approach is the synthesis of the monophosphate of 2-fluoro-adenine arabinoside (fludarabine).[69] In essence, the halogenated nucleoside was poorly soluble in aqueous solution. In contrast, the monophosphate (fludarabine) was more soluble and readily cleaved enzymatically *in vivo* to the 2-fluoro-adenine arabinoside. The nucleoside is rapidly rephosphorylated after transport to the intracellular compartment and, thus, can be effective as an anticancer agent.

Unique opportunities exist to use monoclonal antibodies to selectively deliver antineoplastic agents to targeted tumor cells. New methods of prodrug administration (e.g., ADEPT) are being evaluated that couple the administration of an anthracycline glucuronide and the use of a human β-glucuronidase conjugated to a monoclonal antibody for selected delivery to a tumor-bearing animal. It is hoped that this novel approach will enhance the selectivity of anticancer agents, and it may have particular utility in the case of highly potent compounds.

TOXICOLOGIC INVESTIGATION

Preclinical toxicology is frequently the final step in the progression of a new chemotherapeutic drug from discovery to initial phase I testing in humans (see Fig. 19.2-4). The major objectives of the preclinical toxicologic studies include (1) the definition of the qualitative and quantitative organ toxicities (including dose and schedule dependencies), (2) the reversibility of these effects, and (3) the initial safe starting dose proposed for humans. In general, the ideal approach is to ensure that the preclinical toxicologic studies accurately reflect the intended clinical investigations in humans (i.e., identical formulation, schedules, and routes of drug administration, and dose levels anticipated to reflect the likely experience in patients).

The protocols for performing the preclinical toxicology at the NCI have changed dramatically since the late 1970s.[70,71] Numerous schedules of drug administration were examined in a variety of animal species in the era before 1980. The emphasis later focused on mouse lethality studies for the initial dose-range–finding studies [i.e., lethal dose in 10% of mice (LD_{10}), LD_{50}, and LD_{90}]. The subsequent toxicologic studies were performed on fixed schedules to refine the doses associated with lethal and nonlethal toxicities. The preclinical toxicities reported correlated reasonably well with the subsequent clinical observations.[70,72–74] However, the extent of useless information relating to highly lethal murine doses (LD_{50} and LD_{90}) led to a redesign of the toxicologic studies.

The current toxicologic investigations accepted by the U.S. Food and Drug Administration involve a simplified two-step approach. The initial step focuses on acute toxicity in small animals (e.g., mice), and the major end point is a determination of the LD_{10} level. The second phase of preclinical toxicologic investigation is more extensive. In this case, emphasis is placed on a careful qualitative and quantitative characterization of the organ-specific toxicities in rodents associated with the schedule and route of administration that is to be used in the initial clinical trial. Attention is given to defining accurately those toxicities that are likely to be observed at doses slightly higher than the highest nontoxic dose. Careful investigation of the doses in the animals that approximate the highest projected tolerable dose in the model should provide data that are more relevant to the anticipated clinical experience in patients.

In the past, most new antineoplastic agents were tested clinically on two relatively fixed schedules of drug administration—that is, single-bolus intravenous dose once every 3 to 4 weeks, and 5 consecutive days of treatment repeated at 3- to 4-week intervals. The most frequently used toxicologic protocols reflect each of these schedules. Some newer agents entering preclinical evaluation for cancer therapy are being proposed for weekly intravenous administration, continuous intravenous infusion, or oral dosing. It is critically important that the preclinical toxicologic protocol simulates the planned therapeutic approach in patients.

Because substantial variation may exist between species in their tolerance to a given drug, the safety of a projected starting dose in humans is confirmed by examining the preclinical toxicities in at least two species. Both the qualitative and the quantitative toxicities are usually well defined after investigation of a small animal model (e.g., mouse) and a larger animal (e.g., dog). Only occasionally is testing needed in an additional large animal (e.g., monkey), although this species has been shown to be especially useful for defining central nervous system pharmacokinetics.

Certain organ-specific toxicities are reliably detected with the current toxicologic models (e.g., myelosuppression and gastrointestinal toxicity). In contrast, hepatic and renal toxicities are often missed or falsely positive in animal testing. Toxicities involving the heart, lung, nervous system, pancreas, and integument are even less reliably appreciated. At best, the preclinical evaluation can establish a safe starting dose for humans and predict acute organ toxicity. A complete definition of the toxicologic profile of a new agent usually emerges only after extensive clinical experimentation.

CONCLUSION

The discovery and development of novel anticancer agents involves substantial time, effort, and resources. The strategies used for drug discovery range from empiric screening (the source of most of the current active drugs) to rational drug design based on an enhanced understanding of the various biochemical and molecular targets. As outlined in this chapter, an extensive series of preclinical investigations are necessary before the decision to enter clinical trials is made. Significant efforts are then required for the successful completion of clinical studies, in which an individual agent is taken from the ini-

TABLE 19.2-3. Stages in Clinical Testing of New Anticancer Agents

Stage of Drug Testing	*Objectives*	*Patient Population Studied*
Phase I	Determine tolerance Maximally tolerable dose Limiting toxicity Reversibility of toxicity Proper schedule Pharmacology Bioavailability Plasma clearance Biotransformation Excretion Therapeutic effect Secondary	Histologically confirmed advanced malignancies; no longer amenable to conventional therapy; physiologically well compensated.
Phase II	Therapeutic effect Determine effectiveness in a panel of human tumors Dose-response relationships Nontherapeutic effects Toxicity in relationship to therapeutic effect	Histologically confirmed advanced malignancy; measurable tumor masses; no longer amenable to conventional therapy; a variety of tumor types in groups of 15 to 30; physiologically well compensated.
Phase III	Therapeutic effectiveness Compare experimental therapy to existing standard therapy Nontherapeutic effects Are toxic effects tolerable in the context of observed therapeutic effect and in comparison with standard therapy?	Histologically confirmed malignancy; patient sample must be of adequate size and uniformity; usually previously untreated; controls usually are selected randomly, but on occasion, historical controls are used.
Phase IV	Therapeutic effectiveness Integration of drug therapy into primary treatment in combination with surgery or radiation therapy (e.g., postoperative drug treatment in breast cancer) Compare to concurrent standard program Nontherapeutic effects Are toxic effects sufficiently minimal to risk giving drug to patients whose tumor might not necessarily recur? Long-term toxic effects require monitoring (second tumors, sterility, marrow aplasia)	Histologically confirmed malignancy; patient sample must be of adequate size and uniformity; controls usually randomized.

tial phase I testing through to the randomized phase III and IV settings (Table 19.2.-3). The effective development of new cancer agents demands the close cooperation of a multidisciplinary team that includes basic research scientists, clinical pharmacologists, clinical research nurses, data managers, and clinical investigators. The combined resources of government, academic centers, and the pharmaceutical industry are needed for successfully dealing with the formidable task of identifying effective new therapeutic agents for cancer patients.

REFERENCES

1. Kaufman D, Chabner BA. Clinical strategies for cancer treatment: the role of drugs. In: Chabner BA, Longo DL, eds. *Cancer chemotherapy and biotherapy*. New York: Lippincott–Raven, 1996:1.
2. Grever MR. Cancer drug screening. In: Schilsky RL, ed. *Principles of antineoplastic drug development and pharmacology*. New York: Marcel Dekker Inc, 1996:1.
3. Grever MR, Schepartz S, Chabner BA. The National Cancer Institute: cancer drug discovery and development program. *Semin Oncol* 1992;19:622.
4. Farber S, Diamond LK, Mercer RD, Sylvester RF, Wolff JA. Temporary remissions in acute leukemia in children produced by folic acid antagonist, 4-aminopteroyl-glutamic acid (aminopterin). *N Engl J Med* 1948;238:787.
5. Heidelberger C, Chaudhari NK, Danneberg P, et al. Fluorinated pyrimidines. A new class of tumor-inhibitory compounds. *Nature* 1957;179:663.
6. Erickson J, Neidhart DJ, VanDrie J, et al. Design, activity, and 2.8 A crystal structure of a C2 symmetric inhibitor complexed to HIV-1 protease. *Science* 1990;249:527.
7. Johnson RK. Screening methods in antineoplastic drug discovery. *J Natl Cancer Inst* 1990;82:1082.
8. Suffness M, Newman DJ, Snader K. Discovery and development of antineoplastic agents from natural sources. *Bioorg Marine Chem* 1989;3:131.
9. Salmon SE, Lam KS, Felder S, et al. One bead, one chemical compound: use of the selectide process for anticancer drug discovery. *Acta Oncol* 1994;33:127.
10. Lam KS, Wu J, Lou Q. Identification and characterization of a novel synthetic peptide substrate specific for Src-family protein kinases. *Int J Pept Protein Res* 1995;45:587.
11. Amzel LM. Structure-based drug design. *Curr Opin Biotechnol* 1998;9:366.
12. Cargill JF, Lebl M. New methods in combinatorial chemistry—robotids and parallel synthesis. *Curr Opin Chem Biol* 1997;1:67.
13. Spaller MR, Burger MT, Fardis M, Bartlett PA. Synthetic strategies in combinatorial chemistry. *Curr Opin Chem Biol* 1997;1:47.
14. Cragg GM, Newman DJ, Weiss RB. Coral reefs, forests, and thermal vents: the worldwide exploration of nature for novel antitumor agents. *Semin Oncol* 1997;24:156.
15. Weiss RB, Sarosy G, Clagett-Carr K, Russo M, Leyland-Jones B. Anthracycline analogs: the past, present, and future. *Cancer Chemother Pharmacol* 1986;18:185.
16. Steinherz LJ, Steinherz PG, Tan C. Cardiac failure and dysrhythmias 6–19 years after anthracycline therapy: a series of 15 patients. *Med Pediatr Oncol* 1995;24:352.
17. Smith IE. Mitoxantrone (Novantrone): a review of experimental and early clinical studies. *Cancer Treat Rev* 1983;10:103.
18. Noble RL, Beer CT, Cutts JH. Role of chance observations in chemotherapy: *Vinca rosea*. *Ann N Y Acad Sci* 1958;76:882.
19. Wani MC, Taylor HL, Wall ME, Coggon P, McPhail AT. Plant antitumor agents. VI. The isolation and structure of Taxol, a novel antileukemic and antitumor agent from *Taxus brevifolia*. *J Am Chem Soc* 1971;93:2325.
20. Schiff PB, Fant J, Horwitz SB. Promotion of microtubule assembly *in vitro* by Taxol. *Nature* 1979;277:665.
21. Rowinsky EK, Donehower RC. Drug therapy: paclitaxel (Taxol). *N Engl J Med* 1995;332:1004.
22. Mann J. Steps to a successful synthesis. *Nature* 1994;367:594.
23. Gordon M. Taxol supply problem? What problem? *Nat Biotechnol* 1996;14:1635.
24. Ojima I, Lin S, Wang T. Recent advances in the medicinal chemistry of taxoids with novel beta-amino acid side chains. *Curr Med Chem* 1999;6:927.
25. Wall ME, Wani MC, Cook CE, et al. Plant antitumor agents. I. The isolation and structure of camptothecin, a novel alkaloidal leukemia and tumor inhibitor from *Camptotheca accuminata*. *J Am Chem Soc* 1966;88:3888.
26. Hsiang YH, Hertzberg R, Hecht S, Liu LF. Camptothecin induces protein-linked DNA breaks via mammalian DNA topoisomerase I. *J Biol Chem* 1985;260:14873.
27. Hsiang YH, Liu LF. Identification of mammalian DNA topoisomerase I as an intracellular target of the anticancer drug camptothecin. *Cancer Res* 1988;48:1722.

28. Rothenberg ML, Blanke CD. Topoisomerase I inhibitors in the treatment of colorectal cancer. *Semin Oncol* 1999;26:632.
29. Cunningham D. Setting a new standard—irinotecan (Campto) in the second-line therapy of colorectal cancer: final results of two phase III studies and implications for clinical practice. *Semin Oncol* 1999;26:1.
30. Ilson DH, Saltz L, Enzinger P, et al. Phase II trial of weekly irinotecan plus cisplatin in advanced esophageal cancer. *J Clin Oncol* 1999;17:3270.
31. Giovanella BC, Stehlin JS, Wall ME, et al. DNA topoisomerase I–targeted chemotherapy of human colon cancer in xenografts. *Science* 1989;246:1046.
32. Pettit GR, Herald CL, Doubek DL, et al. Isolation and structure of bryostatin I. *J Am Chem Soc* 1982;104:6846.
33. Bai R, Pettit GR, Hamel E. Dolastatin 10, a powerful cytostatic peptide derived from a marine animal. Inhibition of tubulin polymerization mediated through the vinca alkaloid binding domain. *Biochem Pharmacol* 1990;39:1941.
34. Bai RL, Paul KD, Herald CL, et al. Halichondrin B and homohalichondrin B, marine natural products binding in the vinca domain of tubulin: discovery of tubulin-based mechanism of action by analysis of differential cytotoxicity data. *J Biol Chem* 1991;266:15882.
35. Bonfanti M, LaValle E, Fernandez JM, et al. Effect of ecteinascidin-743 on the interaction between DNA binding proteins and DNA. *Anticancer Drug Des* 1999;14:179.
36. Rinehart KL. Antitumor compounds from tunicates. *Med Res Rev* 2000;20:1.
37. Rosenberg B. Fundamental studies with cisplatin. *Cancer* 1985;55:2303.
38. Boyd MR. Status of the NCI preclinical antitumor drug discovery screen. *PPO Updates* 1989;3:1.
39. Skehan P, Storeng R, Scudiero D, et al. New colorimetric cytotoxicity assay for anticancer drug screening. *J Natl Cancer Inst* 1990;82:1107.
40. Chabner BA. In defense of cell-line screening. *J Natl Cancer Inst* 1990;82:1083.
41. Double JA, Bibby MC. Therapeutic index: a vital component in selection of anticancer agents for clinical trial. *J Natl Cancer Inst* 1989;81:988.
42. Hodes L. Computer-aided selection of compounds for antitumor screening: validation of a statistical-heuristic method. *J Chem Inf Comput Sci* 1981;21:123.
43. Paull KD, Shoemaker RH, Hodes L, et al. Display and analysis of patterns of differential activity of drugs against human tumor cell lines: development of mean graph and COMPARE algorithm. *J Natl Cancer Inst* 1989;81:1088.
44. Weinstein JN, Myers TG, O'Connor PM, et al. An information-intensive approach to the molecular pharmacology of cancer. *Science* 1997;275:343.
45. Mayer TU, Kapoor TM, Haggerty SJ, et al. Small molecule inhibitor of mitotic spindle bipolarity identified in a phenotype-based screen. *Science* 1999;29:971.
46. Gibbs JB. Anticancer drug targets: growth factors and growth factor signaling. *J Clin Invest* 2000;105:9.
47. Keshet E, Ben-Sasson SA. Anticancer drug targets: approaching angiogenesis. *J Clin Invest* 1999;104:1497.
47a. Hanahan D, Folkman J. Patterns and emerging mechanisms of the angiogenic switch during tumorigenesis. *Cell* 1996;86:353.
48. Kaelin WG. Choosing anticancer drug targets in the postgenomic era. *J Clin Invest* 1999;104:1503.
49. Sellers WR, Fisher DE. Apoptosis and cancer drug targeting. *J Clin Invest* 1999;104:1655.
50. Shapiro GI, Harper JW. Anticancer drug targets: cell cycle and checkpoint control. *J Clin Invest* 1999;104:1645.
51. Kelliher M, Knott A, McLaughlin J, Wittee ON, Rosenberg N. Differences in oncogenic potency but not target cell specificity distinguish the two forms of the bcr/abl oncogene. *Mol Cell Biol* 1991;11:4710.
52. Daley GQ, Van Etten RA, Baltimore D. Induction of chronic myelogenous leukemia by the P210bcr/abl gene of the Philadelphia chromosome. *Science* 1990;247:824.
53. Szczylik C, Skorski T, Nicholaides NC, et al. Selective inhibition of leukemia cell proliferation by BCR-ABL antisense oligodeoxynucleotides. *Science* 1991;253:562.
54. Kelliher MA, McLaughlin J, Wittee ON, Rosenberg N. Induction of a chronic myelogenous leukemia-like syndrome in mice with v-ABL and BCR/ABL. *Proc Natl Acad Sci U S A* 1990;87:6649.
55. Druker BJ, Tamura S, Buchdunger E, et al. Effects of a selective inhibitor of the ABL tyrosine kinase on the growth of BCR-ABL positive cells. *Nature Med* 1996;2:561.
56. Deininger MW, Goldman JM, Lydon N, Melo JV. The tyrosine kinase inhibitor CGP57148B selectively inhibits the growth of BCR-ABL-positive cells. *Blood* 1997;90:3691.
57. LeCoutre P, Mologni L, Cleris L, et al. *In vivo* eradication of human BCR-ABL-positive leukemia cells with an ABL kinase inhibitor. *J Natl Cancer Inst* 1999;91:163.
58. Druker BJ, Sawyers CL, Talpaz M, et al. Phase I trial of a specific abl tyrosine kinase inhibitor, CGP 57148, in interferon refractory chronic myelogenous leukemia patients. *Proc Am Soc Clin Oncol* 1999;18:24(abst).
59. Druker BJ, Lydon NB. Lessons learned from the development of an Abl tyrosine kinase inhibitor for chronic myelogenous leukemia. *J Clin Invest* 2000;105:3.
60. zur Hausen H. Molecular pathogenesis of cancer of the cervix and its causation by specific human papillomavirus types. In: zur Hansen H, ed. *Human pathogenic papillomavirus*. Berlin: Springer-Verlag, 1994:131.
61. Jones RE, Wegrzyn RJ, Patrick DR, et al. Identification of HPV-16 E7 peptides that are potent antagonists of E7 binding to the retinoblastoma suppressor protein. *J Biol Chem* 1990;265:12782.
62. Corbett TH, Wozniak A, Gerpheide S, Hanka L. *In vitro* and *in vivo* models for detection of new antitumor drugs. In: Hanka IJ, Kondo T, White RJ, eds. *Proceedings of a workshop at the 14th International Congress of Chemotherapy at Kyoto*. Tokyo: University of Tokyo Press, 1985:5.
63. Grindey GB. Current status of cancer drug development: failure or limited success? *Cancer Cells* 1990;2:163.
64. Bogden AE. The subrenal capsule assay and its use as a drug screening system. In: Hellman K, Carter SK, eds. *Fundamentals of cancer chemotherapy*. New York: McGraw-Hill, 1987:173.
65. Corbett TH, Valeriote FA, Baker LH. Is the P388 murine tumor no longer adequate as a drug discovery model? *Invest New Drugs* 1987;5:3.
66. Collins JH, Grieshaber CK, Chabner BA. Pharmacologically guided phase I clinical trials based upon preclinical drug development. *J Natl Cancer Inst* 1990;82:1321.
67. DeSouza JJV, Leiby JM, Staubus AE, Grever MR, Malspeis L. Altered pharmacokinetics of fludarabine phosphate by 2'-deoxycoformycin in the dog and analysis of a route of fludarabine activation. *Proc Am Assoc Cancer Res* 1985;26:1413.
68. Davignon JP, Craddock JC. The formulation of anticancer drugs. In: Hellman K, Carter SK, eds. *Fundamentals of cancer chemotherapy*. New York, McGraw-Hill, 1987:212.
69. Brockman RW, Cheng YC, Schabel FM, Montgomery JA. Metabolism and chemotherapeutic activity of 9-B-D-arabinofuranosyl-2-fluoroadenine against murine leukemia L1210 and evidence for its phosphorylation by deoxycytidine kinase. *Cancer Res* 1980;40:3610.
70. Grieshaber CK, Marsoni S. Relation of preclinical toxicology to findings in early clinical trials. *Cancer Treat Rep* 1986;70:65.
71. Lowe MC, Davis RD. The current toxicology protocol of the National Cancer Institute. In: Hellman K, Carter SK, eds. *Fundamentals of cancer chemotherapy*. New York: McGraw-Hill, 1987:228.
72. Schein P, Anderson T. The efficacy of animal studies in predicting clinical toxicity of cancer chemotherapeutic drugs. *Int J Clin Pharmacol* 1973;8:228.
73. Lowe M. Large animal toxicological studies of anticancer drugs. In: Hellman K, Carter SK, eds. *Fundamentals of cancer chemotherapy*. New York: McGraw-Hill, 1987:238.
74. Schurig JE, Bradner WT. Small animal toxicology of cancer drugs. In: Hellman K, Carter SK, eds. *Fundamentals of cancer chemotherapy*. New York: McGraw-Hill, 1987:248.

DAVID J. AUSTIN

Combinatorial Chemistry

PRINCIPLES OF COMBINATORIAL CHEMISTRY

REVOLUTION IN SYNTHETIC AND MEDICINAL CHEMISTRY

The field of combinatorial chemistry represents a revolution in both the concepts and construction of chemical entities. This revolution has not only changed the fields of chemical catalysis, materials science, and methods development, but also has impacted the field of drug development. The impact of combinatorial chemistry is likely to be as significant to drug development as the polymerase chain reaction was in advancing cloning techniques for molecular biology. The postgenomic era is predicted to present us with between 50,000 and 150,000 unique genes, each encoding a protein product that is potentially a therapeutic target.[1] Between 1000 and 3000 unique members are predicted to exist within the protein kinase family, which is an important class of therapeutic targets.[2] Because the average medicinal chemist can synthesize approximately 100 molecules per year, it is difficult to envision the identification of unique inhibitors for thousands of proteins using traditional techniques.

This chapter introduces the field of combinatorial chemistry and describes how it has impacted drug development and how it will likely impact future drug development. The aim of this introduction is to serve as a primer for researchers wishing to incorporate chemical diversity into their research program.

WHAT IS COMBINATORIAL CHEMISTRY AND HOW DOES IT RELATE TO CHEMICAL DIVERSITY?

To properly understand what combinatorial chemistry is, the concept of chemical diversity must first be addressed. If diversity is defined as that which represents all possible permutations of a given set, then chemical diversity can be described as the atomic representation of all possible permutations of molecular structure or functional space. The concept of chemical diversity has been recognized since the early days of drug development, when natural products (biologically active chemical entities found in nature) were the main focus of the pharmaceutical industry. At that point, the methods of achieving chemical diversity—in other words, the techniques required to synthesize 10^3 to 10^6 molecules—were unknown, and researchers depended on nature for diversity. *Combinatorial chemistry* is a collective term referring to those techniques that are used to achieve chemical diversity. A collection of diverse molecules is referred to as a *chemical library* or, often, a *combinatorial library*.

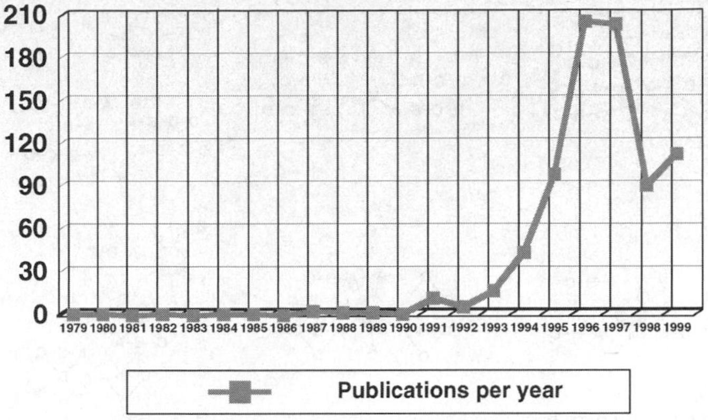

FIGURE 19.2-5. Graphic representation of the number of literature articles containing the keywords *combinatorial chemistry* or *solid-phase organic synthesis*, from 1979 to 1999.

THE HISTORY OF COMBINATORIAL CHEMISTRY

TECHNICAL ADVANCES THAT ENABLED COMBINATORIAL SYNTHESIS

The chemical techniques for generating diversity have their origin in the solid-phase synthesis of peptides and nucleotides, both of which had a major impact on the growing field of molecular biology and biotechnology. These technical developments in combinatorial chemistry can be grouped into three major categories: the development of solid-phase chemical synthesis techniques, the development of deconvolution and encoding strategies for combinatorial library construction, and the development of arrayed technologies and chemical synthesizers for the rapid synthesis of molecules. A search of literature reference databases for the keywords *combinatorial chemistry* or *solid-phase organic synthesis* provides interesting insight into the rapidity of growth in the field of combinatorial chemistry. By plotting the number of literature citations as a function of year, an almost logarithmic growth is seen in the number of references between the years 1993 and 1996. Most of the major technical achievements in combinatorial chemistry were made before 1990 and were largely influenced by the demands of the pharmaceutical industry.

It should also be noted that the decrease in references to combinatorial chemistry that begins in 1997 is most likely not a function of the field slowing down, but rather a function of the acceptance of combinatorial chemistry in science as a whole. This can be thought of as *keyword disappearance*. In an analogous fashion, every paper mentioning the polymerase chain reaction technique shortly after its development would contain the phrase in the title or abstract. After its acceptance as a common technique, however, it was relegated to the experimental section of papers. As the technique of combinatorial chemistry becomes more widespread in the literature, it will cease to be the main focus of papers, becoming merely the technique used to solve much greater research problems. This is likely the trend that is taking place now, as illustrated in Figure 19.2-5.

HIGH-THROUGHPUT SCREENING AND COMBINATORIAL CHEMISTRY

Since its inception, high-throughput screening has become a major source of novel drug leads in the pharmaceutical industry. After the existing pharmaceutical chemical stocks had been processed, however, a need for more screening materials emerged. This need far outweighed the potential efforts of the medicinal and natural product isolation chemists. The initial technical advances required for combinatorial chemistry were already in place (see Figure 19.2-5) and promised to be a potential source for large quantities of new chemical entities. Initial libraries were composed mainly of natural peptides. Later, as newer and more general coupling techniques became available, libraries of peptides with unnatural amino acids became commonplace. In general, peptides and peptide-like molecules are usually not a direct source of drugs because of their susceptibility to proteases, poor pharmacodynamics, and potential for antigenic response; therefore, they require extensive chemical development. This fact prompted a large effort in the development of novel chemistry that would be compatible with solid-phase resins. The growth of solid-phase organic synthesis began with the development of solid-phase protocols of known solution-phase reactions. As solid-phase synthetic efforts became more sophisticated, the emergence of complex, even pharmacologically proven, molecules (such as the benzodiazepine core) became commonplace.[3]

THE BENEFIT OF SOLID-PHASE SYNTHESIS

The development of solid-phase techniques for the manipulation of peptides and nucleotides preceded the development of combinatorial library techniques and thus paved the way for automation by allowing the synthesis of biopolymers in a reproducible format.[4] As mentioned earlier, solid-phase synthesis was an important factor in the development of consistent, high-yielding syntheses of polynucleotides and polypeptides. The concept of solid-phase synthesis is summarized in Figure 19.2-6. A solid-phase resin is a beaded form of polystyrene, or any polymeric material, that is chemically functionalized to allow the synthesis of molecules while they are attached to the bead. As is shown in Figure 19.2-6*A*, each new component can be attached to the previous one in a processive manner, allowing both the automation of the synthesis procedure and a reduced need for chemical purification. Because reagents can be used in large excess, then simply washed away, the only purification step that is required is the last one, after resin cleavage. Developments in solid-phase chemistry involve the development of new resins, more advanced chemistry, and improvement in linking strategies. More advanced approaches to solid-phase synthesis

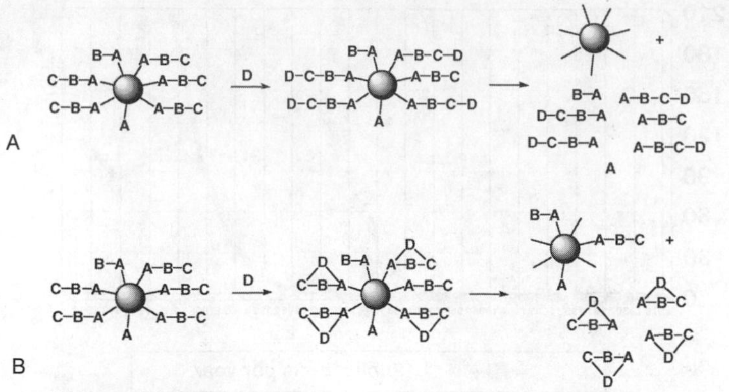

FIGURE 19.2-6. Solid-phase synthesis and selective resin cleavage. **A:** The major benefit of solid-phase synthesis is a reduced need for chromatographic separation, because only the last step requires purification. **B:** Through synthetic design, some solid-phase synthesis techniques eliminate chromatography altogether.

involve improvements in the cleavage step (see Fig. 19.2-6*B*), in which the final transformation in a synthesis alters the nature of the connection to the solid support. In this manner, a selective resin cleavage is achieved, thereby removing the need for purification altogether. This has been demonstrated in many cases, including cyclic peptides,[5,6] metathesis reactions,[7–9] and cycloaddition-cycloreversion reactions.[10,11]

PARALLEL VERSUS COMBINATORIAL SYNTHESIS

It should be pointed out that the term *combinatorial*, which is often used as a general term for the entire field, has a specific meaning in terms of library synthesis. The field is collectively known as *chemical diversity*; however, the term *combinatorial chemistry* is still largely ingrained in the literature. Two types of synthetic procedures are used in chemical diversity: parallel and combinatorial synthesis. Figure 19.2-7*A* shows an example of a combinatorial synthesis. In this method, each reaction takes place in a separate reaction vessel. After the first step, the beads are combined and split apart again. Each mixture is then subjected to a second chemical reaction, pooled, and then split apart again. This process is commonly referred to as the *split-pool technique*. Each bead travels through a different path in the overall scheme, and ultimately, each possible combination is made. In parallel synthesis (Fig. 19.2-7*B*), the pools are never recombined and the syntheses proceed independently. The benefits, drawbacks, and required technical advances for each of these synthetic protocols are discussed in the next two sections, Combinatorial Chemical Libraries and Parallel Chemical Libraries.

Combinatorial Chemical Libraries

The major difficulty with the implementation of a combinatorial synthesis strategy is the identification of active molecules. Because the strategy involves the pooling of beads, all of the molecules are mixed together in solution, and individual library members must somehow be characterized once they are identified as having biologic activity. For this reason, early developments in combinatorial synthesis focused on deconvolution strategies. Later, methods were developed that involved the encoding of individual beads. The combinatorial deconvolution procedure involves a split-pool synthesis, as seen in Figure 19.2-7*A*. However, the last set of mixtures are not pooled together, but rather are tested as a mixture. The active "pool" is then resynthesized, but during the resynthesis, the final mixtures are not pooled. This method is called *serial deconvolution*.[12] A related method, referred to as *recursive deconvolution*, has been developed, in which a fraction of each reaction mixture is saved at each stage of synthesis.[13] In this manner, resynthesis involves only adding the last monomer at each stage of deconvolution. This method works best when evaluating a combinatorial library in cell-based assays, because the mixtures can be cleaved off the resin and tested as a whole.

Another type of combinatorial synthesis is referred to as the *"one bead, one molecule" approach*.[14] This procedure also uses the split-pool technique; however, instead of relying on a deconvolution strategy, each bead is chemically tagged after it has been chemically modified. These tags are chemically orthogonal to the growing chemistry chain and have proven useful for the on-bead analysis of protein affinity[15] and in off-bead strategies using spatial arrays of beads.[16] Once a bead has been identified to contain an active component, the tag is removed and "read" to

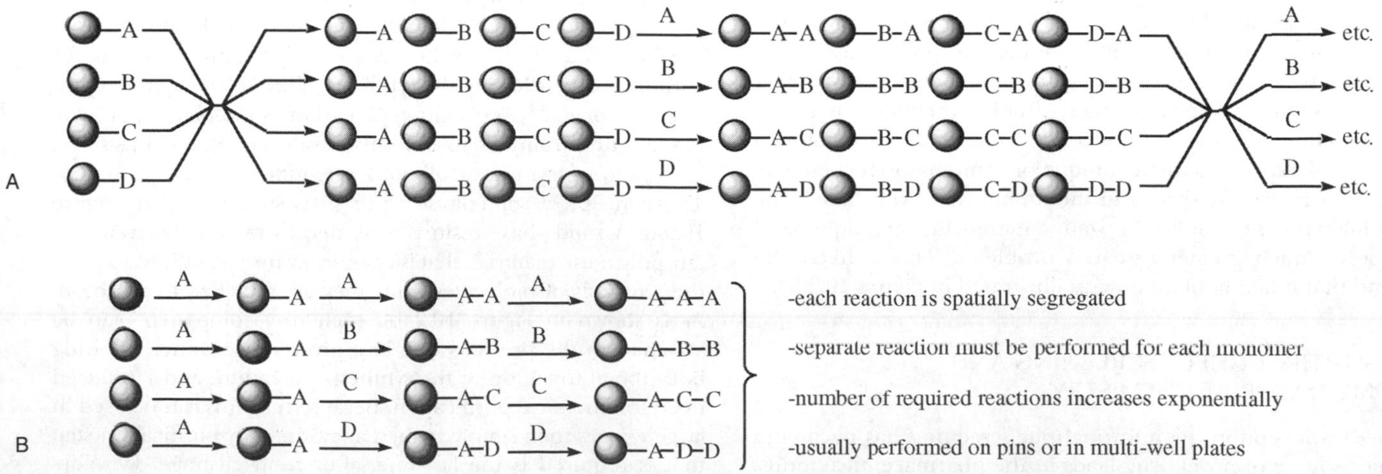

FIGURE 19.2-7. Combinatorial versus parallel library synthesis. **A:** Combinatorial synthesis involves the combination of library components during the synthetic sequence. **B:** Parallel synthesis involves the spatial segregation of library members during each reaction scheme.

determine the identity of the molecule. Some of the tagging strategies that have been used include nucleotides,[16,17] gas-chromatography (GC)–detectable electrophoric molecules,[18] and high pressure liquid chromatography (HPLC)–detectable secondary amines.[19] Modern mass spectrometry methods are becoming powerful enough to allow the direct detection of the molecules attached to the solid-phase resin.[20] The split-mix technology remains the best method for the construction of libraries of more than 10^3 members.[21]

Parallel Chemical Libraries

The need for technical advances in the development of parallel synthetic techniques is much less than for combinatorial approaches, because the major requirement involves the spatial arraying of each molecule. Two early developments in this field involve the pin[22] and teabag methods.[23] In pin-based library synthesis, the molecules are synthesized on the head of functionalized pins, which serve as probes that can be inserted into any number of solvent or reagent wells. The randomization process takes place by the nature of the fact that each pin is exposed to a different set of reagents or monomers. The teabag approach is similar, in that each separate bag is moved from one reagent or reaction mixture to another. In this case, the molecules are spatially arrayed in the individual bags. A popular advance on this technique involves the use of radiolabels to tag each bead, thus allowing a rapid handling of each bag.[24] Microarray chip technology also allows the spatial arraying of a combinatorial library and has proven useful in library synthesis. More recent developments involve synthesis in multiwell plates on automated synthesizers. In general, the pharmaceutical industry has turned to this technique, using discrete molecules in a high-throughput format. This technique has been facilitated by the development of large-scale machine-based organic synthesizers.

THE PRACTICE OF COMBINATORIAL CHEMISTRY

IDENTIFYING AN INHIBITOR FOR A SPECIFIC RECEPTOR

Once a protein is identified as a potential therapeutic target, the major goal is to evaluate a biologic system in the absence of the protein activity. Gene technology has been developed to generate knockout mice that lack a specific protein of interest; however, the mouse must reach development without the aid of this protein and often this gene is required for proper development. Furthermore, it is often more desirable to study the biologic effect in a cell line before proceeding to an animal model.

A number of methods have been developed for identifying inhibitors of receptors. The most common, often used in the pharmaceutical industry, is high-throughput screening. This method often involves an automated assay based on affinity or some related *in vitro* cell-based or cell-free phenotype and a large library of chemical compounds. These chemicals may originate from a natural product isolation, combinatorial synthesis, or an in-house library grown over many years of chemical development. Such a library can be a great place to start to determine whether a molecule or class of molecules with affinity for either the receptor of interest or a closely related receptor from the same family has already been identified.

In the case in which no known inhibitor exists for the class of receptor of study, or for identifying a novel inhibitor for a specific receptor, then access to chemical diversity is essential. There are two ways of obtaining chemical diversity: It can be made or bought. Because this chapter is intended for a nonchemical audience, we discuss methods of buying chemical diversity.

NATURAL PEPTIDES AS A STARTING POINT FOR CHEMICAL DIVERSITY

The presentation of peptides on the surface of bacteriophage particles is known as *phage display.*[25] Phage display of peptide libraries has become a common method for quickly obtaining large libraries of natural peptides.[26] The benefit of a natural peptide is that it can elucidate the type of functionality that binds to the receptor of interest, and many peptide phage display libraries are commercially available. Once a natural peptide inhibitor is identified, peptidomimetic strategies can be used to identify nonpeptide inhibitors. The development of nonpeptide inhibitors is usually performed by the further analysis of molecules that mimic the functional nature of the peptide, yet eliminate the poor drug-like qualities of the peptides. One popular and potentially very powerful modification of peptides to improve function and biologic activity is the cyclization of the peptide, which results in a cyclic peptide with a limited number of ground-state conformations and a reduced susceptibility to proteases. However, the cyclization may result in locking the peptide in an inactive conformation, limiting the success of the method. For this reason, many individuals begin screening with cyclized libraries rather than cyclizing a linear peptide. This can even be achieved in phage display by using a randomized peptide sequence that is flanked by cysteine residues. Once the phage is secreted from the cell, the flanking cysteine residues form a disulfide bond and create a cyclic structure. Peptidomimetics has become one of the most studied areas of molecular recognition.[27] Indeed, many natural products themselves are mimics of biologically active peptides.[28]

NATURAL PRODUCTS AS A STARTING POINT FOR CHEMICAL DIVERSITY

Natural products have a rich history in the elucidation of biologic processes and in drug development.[29] Even in those cases in which the natural product itself is not a potential drug, it can offer a glimpse as to what kinds of molecules will be effective in drug development. It is often found that the product of nature lacks the specificity that is desired for therapeutic activity. Combinatorial chemistry offers the possibility of developing a more specific inhibitor using the chemical nature of the natural product as a good starting point for diversity. However, the modification of a natural product or the construction of a novel library based on a natural product is chemically intensive and usually requires collaboration with a chemistry laboratory or pharmaceutical company.

THE MATHEMATICS OF DIVERSITY

One issue that must be addressed when designing a chemical library or evaluating a combinatorial phage peptide library is the total number of individual molecules in that library. Table 19.2-4 shows the diversity that one might expect from different chemical and biologic libraries. The formula for diversity, in any library, can be described as the number of monomer units raised to the power of the number of variable positions. For example, if we chemically synthesize a heptapeptide library using all 20 natural amino acids, our library will contain 20^7 or 1.28 billion different molecules. If we use phage display to create the same heptapeptide library, we must account for the redundancy of the genetic code and consider each codon as a monomer unit. In this case, the diversity increases to 64^7, or 4.4×10^{12}, library members, which is an unmanageable number of clones. Proper design of the library and use of the wobble position can reduce the required number of codons to 32, reducing the diversity to 32^7, or 3.4×10^{10}, library members. This is still a very large number but is slightly more realistic.

It is important to consider the size and chemical diversity of the library. There is increasing data to suggest that it is more important for a library to be diverse than to be large. Permutational libraries, such as peptides, do not have to cover their diversity. In all likelihood, the epitope is likely to be smaller than the total positions varied. For example, a peptide sequence such as RGD, a common motif in integrin recognition, would come up many times in a heptapeptide library. Some phage display libraries contain 12 randomized amino acids, with no hope of containing that diversity. Yet these libraries are very useful for the identification of discontinuous epitopes within the same peptide. In summary, phage display offers the most accessible first entry into chemical diversity, but often it must be followed up with a synthetic library.

COMBINATORIAL CHEMISTRY IN PHARMACEUTICAL DRUG DEVELOPMENT

"HIT" GENERATION AND "HIT TO LEAD" DEVELOPMENT

Modern drug development often begins with the screening of thousands of molecules to generate chemical "hits" against a therapeutic target or cell line. A *hit* is defined as a molecule that shows activity in an assay below a certain activity level. High-throughput screening of chemical compounds emerged in the early 1990s to aid the rapid evaluation of the large chemical stocks that were being amassed in the pharmaceutical industry. The high-throughput assay is usually an *in vitro* assay, although it is not necessarily cell-free. Once a molecule has been identified as a hit, it is evaluated by a medicinal chemist who begins a synthetic effort to obtain a structure activity relationship for the molecule. If the activity of the initial hit can be optimized for *in vitro* activity, the molecule becomes a "lead" molecule. This process is known as *"hit to lead" development.* Although each pharmaceutical company and, indeed, each therapeutic target has different criteria for the categorization of a lead molecule, the development process is basically the same. Once a lead is identified, a series of *in vivo* tests and further development take place to determine whether the chemical lead has the proper pharmacologic properties and *in vivo* efficacy to become an actual drug.

COMBINATORIAL CHEMISTRY AND LEAD DEVELOPMENT

Although the desire for large numbers of compounds led to the rapid growth of combinatorial chemistry and solid-phase synthetic techniques, it was quickly recognized that a combinatorial approach to lead generation could also be developed. This approach involves the synthesis of secondary libraries, synthesized in a manner that allow the randomization of chemical functionality that was not, or could not be, addressed in the first library. In this manner, an entire library is not synthesized, but rather a small sample of the library is synthesized, and that hit is used as a starting point for a subsequent library generation. This is a convenient method of evaluating a library that has more diversity than can be synthesized. Consider, for example, a library with six potential sites of randomization (see Figure 19.2-6). If twenty monomers were chosen to construct this library, 64 million molecules would have to be synthesized. This diversity is much higher than that which could ever be achieved with a parallel synthesis approach, and it is even outside the limit of a combinatorial synthesis. The premise of this approach is that an actual drug resides within the design of the library and that an activity-driven search of diversity space will pick it out. This is analogous to the needle in the haystack dilemma.

CANCER-RELATED TARGETS

Combinatorial chemistry is still in its adolescent stage with regard to drug development. However, many cancer-related targets have been discovered with combinatorial approaches. Farnesyl transferase, responsible for targeting the oncoprotein p21ras to the cellular membrane, was one of the first targets explored with combinatorial chemistry because of the well-defined CAAX nature of the farnesylation site.[30] Cell surface receptors such as vitronectin, implicated in the complex mechanism of cellular metastasis, have been the target of attempts to inhibit tumor cell adhesion.[31] The receptor tyrosine kinases and cellular kinases have been implicated as therapeutic cancer targets, and the development of kinase inhibitors is a very active area with many combinatorial library approaches.[32] In addition to the active site of kinases, the SH2 recognition and SH3 regulation domains, also involved in kinase activation, are targets of cancer intervention.[33,34] Their peptide nature makes them excellent targets for combinatorial development.

COMBINATORIAL BIOLOGY: NATURE'S BIOLOGIC DIVERSITY

Herceptin,[35] an antibody targeted against the her-2/neu/erb-B2 receptor, is an example of biologic products developed for cancer treatment. Peptide phage display is an efficient and convenient method of obtaining a self-encoded combinatorial library of natural peptides, both linear and cyclic. It is also a convenient method for obtaining combinatorial mixtures of randomized proteins. Although *in vivo* techniques are still the primary source for antibody production, phage display offers the potential for accessing nonantibody proteins for the development of biologic cancer chemotherapeutics. Although this technique has been used mainly for the investigation of basic biology, combinatorial antibodies against a malignant melanoma have been reported.[36] An interesting combination of biologic techniques for the construction of chemical libraries involves polyketide synthase gene swapping. It has been demonstrated that small-molecule diversity can be achieved by randomizing the order of polyketide synthase genes in bacterial systems. This method is unique, because it offers the promise of a biologic synthesis format once an active molecule is identified.

TABLE 19.2-4. The Mathematics of Chemical Diversity[a]

Libraries	*Number of Positions*	*Number of Compounds*
Synthetic libraries		
8^n, where n = number of positions		
	1	8
	2	64
	3	512
	4	4096
	5	32,768
	6	262,144
	7	2,097152
	8	16,777,216
20^n, where n = number of positions		
	1	20
	2	400
	3	8000
	4	160,000
	5	3,200,000
	6	64,000,000
	7	1,280,000,000
$8 \times 12 \times n$, where n = number of plates	*Number of Plates*	*Number of Compounds*
	4	384
	48	4608
	480	46,080
	4800	460,800
	48,000	4,608,000
DNA/RNA libraries		
4^n, where n = number of positions	*Number of Positions*	*Number of Compounds*
	1	4
	2	16
	3	64
	4	256
	5	1024
	6	4096
	7	16,384
	8	65,536
	9	262,144
	10	1,048,576
	20	1.09×10^{12}
	30	1.15×10^{18}
	40	1.21×10^{24}
Phage display libraries		
64^n, where n = number of positions	*Number of Positions*	*Number of Phage*
	1	64
	2	4096
	3	262,144
	4	16,777,216
	5	1,073,741,824
	6	68,719,476,740
	7	4,398,046,511,000
32^n, where n = number of positions	*Number of Positions*	*Number of Phage*
	1	32
	2	1024
	3	32,768
	4	1,048,576
	5	33,554,432
	6	1,073,741,824
	7	34,359,738,370

[a]The way in which the number of molecules in a library relates to Avogadro's number, 6.0221×10^{23}.

THE FUTURE OF CHEMICAL DIVERSITY IN DRUG DEVELOPMENT

The need for a large numbers of molecules for high-throughput screening has led to the rapid growth of combinatorial chemistry; however, only now are scientists recognizing the need for the development of chemical diversity.[37] As the field of combinatorial chemistry matures, it is becoming more apparent that library design is more important than library size. Although large chemical libraries may provide the potential for hit generation, it is not yet established that such libraries will replace the use of natural products for hit generation. At a minimum, it should be expected that natural products, peptides, and signaling molecules will continue to be a source of inspiration for the design of chemical libraries.

In addition to natural product leads, structural biology is continually providing insight into the structural nature of biologic macromolecules. The combination of chemical diversity with structural and molecular biology and computational chemistry will undoubtedly provide the greatest advance in modern drug development.[37]

The use of chemical diversity to address genomic diversity is likely to be the single most important effort for chemical diversity in the postgenomic era.[38] Proteomics has already emerged as a field in need of small-molecule probes. Biologic techniques, such as expression cloning, complementary DNA phage display, and cellular display systems, offer the opportunity to probe protein function with small molecule diversity. Indeed, if the potential of combinatorial diversity can be realized, we envision a small-molecule inhibitor for every protein encoded by the human genome.

REFERENCES

1. Schuler GD, Boguski MS, Stewart EA, et al. A gene map of the human genome. *Science* 1996;274:540.
2. Hunter T. 1001 protein kinases redux—towards 2000. *Semin Cell Biol* 1994;5:367.
3. Bunin BA, Plunkett MJ, Ellman JA. The combinatorial synthesis and chemical and biological evaluation of a 1,4-benzodiazepine library. *Proc Natl Acad Sci U S A* 1994;91:4708.
4. Merrifield RB. Solid phase peptide synthesis. I. The synthesis of a tetrapeptide. *J Am Chem Soc* 1963;85:2149.
5. Mihara H, Yamabe S, Niidome T, Aoyagi H, Kumagai H. Efficient preparation of cyclic peptide mixtures by solid phase synthesis and cyclization cleavage with oxime resin. *Tetrahedron Lett* 1995;36:4837.
6. Lee BH. Solid-phase synthesis of cyclooctadepsipeptide PF1022A analogs using a cyclization-cleavage method with oxime resin. *Tetrahedron Lett* 1997;38:757.
7. vanMaarseveen JH, denHartog JAJ, Engelen V, et al. Solid phase ring-closing metathesis: cyclization/cleavage approach towards a seven membered cycloolefin. *Tetrahedron Lett* 1996;37:8249.
8. Nicolaou KC, Winssinger N, Pastor J, et al. Synthesis of epothilones A and B in solid and solution phase. *Nature* (London) 1997;387(6630):268.
9. Piscopio AD, Miller JF, Koch K. Solid phase heterocyclic synthesis via ring closing metathesis: traceless linking and cyclative cleavage through a carbon-carbon double bond. *Tetrahedron Lett* 1997;38(41):7143.
10. Whitehouse DL, Nelson KH, Savinov SN, Austin DJ. A chemoselective rhodium (II) mediated solid phase 1,3-dipolar cycloaddition and its application to a thermally self-cleaving furan scaffold. *Tetrahedron Lett* 1997;38:7139.
11. Whitehouse DL, Nelson KH Jr, Savinov SN, Lowe RS, Austin DJ. A metathetical cycloaddition-cycloreversion approach to the formation of furan scaffold libraries. *Bioorg Med Chem* 1998;6:1273.
12. Houghten RA, Pinilla C, Blondelle SE, et al. Generation and use of synthetic peptide combinatorial libraries for basic research and drug discovery. *Nature* 1991;354:84.
13. Erb E, Janda KD, Brenner S. Recursive deconvolution of combinatorial chemical libraries. 1994;91:11422.
14. Lam KS, Lebl M, Krchák V. The "one-bead-one-compound" combinatorial library method. *Chemical Reviews* 1997;97(2):411.
15. Lam KS, Salmon SE, Hersh EM, et al. A new type of synthetic peptide library for identifying ligand-binding activity. *Nature* 1991;354:82.
16. Chen CL, Strop P, Lebl M, Lam KS. One bead–one compound combinatorial peptide library: different types of screening. *Methods Enzymol* 1996;267:211.
17. Needels MC, Jones DG, Tate EH, et al. Generation and screening of an oligonucleotide-encoded synthetic peptide library. *Proc Natl Acad Sci U S A* 1993;90:10700.
18. Burbaum JJ, Ohlmeyer MHJ, Reader JC, et al. A paradigm for drug discovery employing encoded combinatorial libraries. *Proc Natl Acad Sci U S A* 1995;92:6027.
19. Ni Z, Maclean D, Holmes C, et al. Versatile approach to encoding combinatorial organic syntheses using chemically robust secondary amine tags. *J Med Chem* 1996;39:1601.
20. Brown BB, Wagner DS, Geysen HM. A single-bead decode strategy using electrospray ionization mass spectrometry and a new photolabile linker: 3-amino-3-(2-nitrophenyl)propionic acid. *Mol Divers* 1995;1:4.
21. Furka A, Bennett WD. Combinatorial libraries by portioning and mixing. *Comb Chem High Throughput Screen* 1999;2:105.
22. Geysen HM, Meloen RH, Barteling SJ. Use of peptide synthesis to probe viral antigens for epitopes to a resolution of a single amino acid. *Proc Natl Acad Sci U S A* 1984;81:3998.
23. Houghten RA. General method for the rapid solid-phase synthesis of large numbers of peptides: specificity of antigen-antibody interaction at the level of individual amino acids. *Proc Natl Acad Sci U S A* 1985;82:5131.
24. Nicolaou KC, Xiao XY, Parandoosh Z, Senyei A, Nova MP. Radiofrequency encoded combinatorial chemistry. *Angew Chem Int Ed Engl* 1995;34:2289.
25. Smith GP. Fimentous fusion phage: novel expression vectors that display cloned antigens on the viron surface. *Science* 1985;228:1315.
26. Scott JK, Smith GP. Searching for peptide ligands with an epitope library. *Science* 1990;249:386.
27. Qabar M, Urban J, Sia C, Klein M, Kahn M. Pharmaceutical applications of peptidomimetics. *Lett Pept Sci* 1996;3:25.
28. Barrow CJ, Thompson PE. Natural product peptidomimetics. *Adv Amino Acid Mimetics Peptidomimetics* 1997;1:251.
29. Rosen MR, Schreiber SL. Natural products as probes of cellular function: studies of immunophilins. *Angew Chem Int Ed Engl* 1992;31:384.
30. Buday L, Downward J. Epidermal growth factor regulates p21ras through the formation of a complex of receptor, Grb2 adapter protein, and Sos nucleotide exchange factor. *Cell* 1993;73:611.
31. Hoekstra WJ, Poulter BL. Combinatorial chemistry techniques applied to nonpeptide integrin antagonists. *Curr Med Chem* 1998;5:195.
32. Lloyd AW. Combinatorial chemistry—hydroxystilbene kinase inhibitor library. *Drug Discov Today* 1997;2:556.
33. Combs AP, Kapoor TM, Feng S, et al. Protein structure-based combinatorial chemistry: discovery of non-peptide binding elements to src SH3 domain. *J Am Chem Soc* 1996;118:287.
34. Feng S, Kapoor TM, Shirai F, Combs AP, Schreiber SL. Molecular basis for the binding of SH3 ligands with non-peptide elements identified by combinatorial synthesis. *Chem Biol* 1996;3:661.
35. Baselga J, Norton L, Albanell J, Kim YM, Mendelsohn J. Recombinant humanized anti-HER2 antibody (Herceptin) enhances the antitumor activity of paclitaxel and doxorubicin against HER2/neu overexpressing human breast cancer xenografts. *Cancer Res* 1998;58:2825.
36. Pereira S, VanBelle P, Elder D, et al. Combinatorial antibodies against human malignant melanoma. *Hybridoma* 1997;16:11.
37. Borman S. Reducing time to drug discovery. *Chem Eng News* 1999;77:33.
38. Veber DF, Drake FH, Gowen M. The new partnership of genomics and chemistry for accelerated drug development. *Curr Opin Chem Biol* 1997;1:151.

SECTION 3 OLIVER MICHAEL COLVIN

Antitumor Alkylating Agents

HISTORY OF THE ALKYLATING AGENTS

A nitrogen mustard alkylating agent was the first nonhormonal chemical that demonstrated significant clinical antitumor activity. The clinical evaluation of nitrogen mustards as antitumor agents evolved from the observed clinical effects of sulfur mustard gas used as a weapon in World War I. This gas was used because of its vesicant effect on the skin and mucous membranes, especially the eyes and respiratory tract.[1] However, in addition to this deadly effect, depression of the hematopoietic and lymphoid systems was observed in victims and experimental animals.[2] These observations led to further studies that used the less volatile nitrogen mustards (Fig. 19.3-1). Studies published in 1946 demonstrated regression of tumors, especially lymphomas[3–5] and led to the introduction of the compound nitrogen mustard (mechlorethamine, Mustargen) into clinical practice. Subsequently, less toxic and more clinically effective nitrogen mustard derivatives and other types of alkylating agents have been developed.

CHEMISTRY AND CYTOTOXICITY OF ALKYLATING AGENTS

The alkylating agents react with (or "alkylate") many electron-rich atoms in cells to form covalent bonds. The most important reactions with regard to their antitumor activities are reactions with DNA bases. Some alkylating agents are monofunctional and react with only one strand of DNA. Others are bifunctional and react with an atom on each of the two strands of DNA to produce a "cross-link" that covalently links the two strands of the DNA double helix. Unless repaired, this lesion will prevent the cell from replicating effectively. The lethality of the monofunctional alkylating agents results from the recognition of the DNA lesion by the cell and the response of the cell to that lesion. Analogous cellular reactions may occur to the interstrand cross-links, but such reactions have not been definitively established.

CLASSES OF ALKYLATING AGENTS AND THEIR PROPERTIES

NITROGEN MUSTARDS

Mustargen

Mustargen is currently used in the MOPP [Mustargen, vincristine (Oncovin), procarbazine, prednisone] regimen for the treatment of Hodgkin's disease[6] but rarely for other purposes. The other nitrogen mustards in significant clinical use are cyclophosphamide, ifosfamide, melphalan, and chlorambucil (Fig. 19.3-2). All these compounds produce cytotoxicity by forming covalent interstrand cross-links in DNA (as shown in Fig. 19.3-3 for Mustargen). The nitrogen mustard cross-link has been demonstrated to occur in the G-X-C/C-Y-G configuration,[7] as opposed to the G-C/C-G cross-link that had previously been predicted.[8] The formation of the G-X-C/C-X-G cross-link has been postulated to occur on the basis of the greater frequency of approximation of the N7 atoms of the two guanylates in the G-X-C/C-X-G configuration, as opposed to the G-C/C-G configuration.[9]

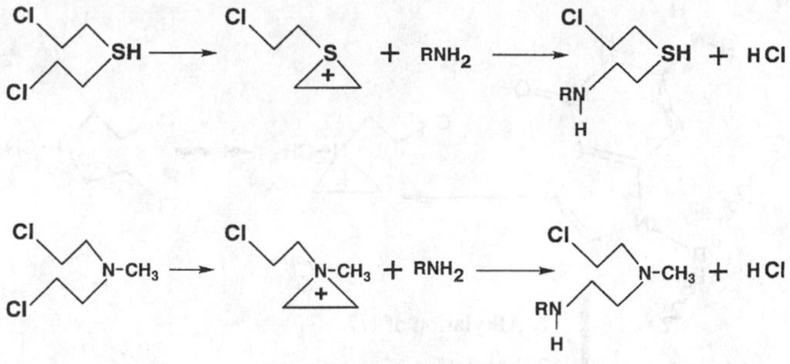

FIGURE 19.3-1. Structures and alkylation mechanisms for sulfur mustard and the nitrogen mustard, Mustargen (mechlorethamine).

Mustargen is available only as an intravenous preparation that can also be used topically for cutaneous malignancies. In the MOPP regimen, Mustargen is used at a dose of 6 mg/m^2 on days 1 and 8 of the monthly schedule. Toxicities unique to the agent are topical irritation and pain on injection if given too rapidly. The clearance of the drug is very rapid, but pharmacokinetics have not been performed with modern techniques.

Cyclophosphamide

The most frequently used alkylating agent, cyclophosphamide, is used for the treatment of breast cancer in combination with doxorubicin (Adriamycin)[10] or with methotrexate and 5-fluorouracil[11] and for the treatment of lymphomas,[12,13] childhood tumors,[14,15] and many solid tumors.[16] High doses of cyclophosphamide are frequently used in conjunction with bone marrow transplantation[17–19] and for the treatment of autoimmune diseases.[20,21]

Cyclophosphamide is inactive *in vitro* and is metabolized by P-450 enzymes in the liver to active species, as shown in Figure 19.3-4. The initial product is 4-hydroxycyclophosphamide (4-HC), which is released from the liver into the circulation.[22] This compound is in equilibrium with an open-ring tautomer, aldophosphamide. Aldophosphamide spontaneously eliminates acrolein to produce phosphoramide mustard,[23] which is an active bifunctional alkylating species.[24] Phosphora-

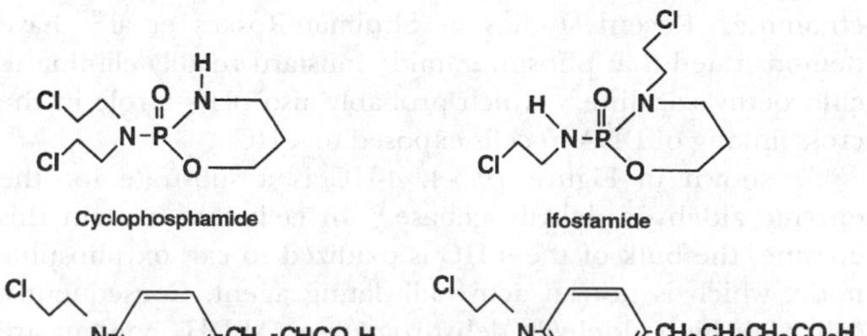

FIGURE 19.3-2. Nitrogen mustards in frequent clinical use.

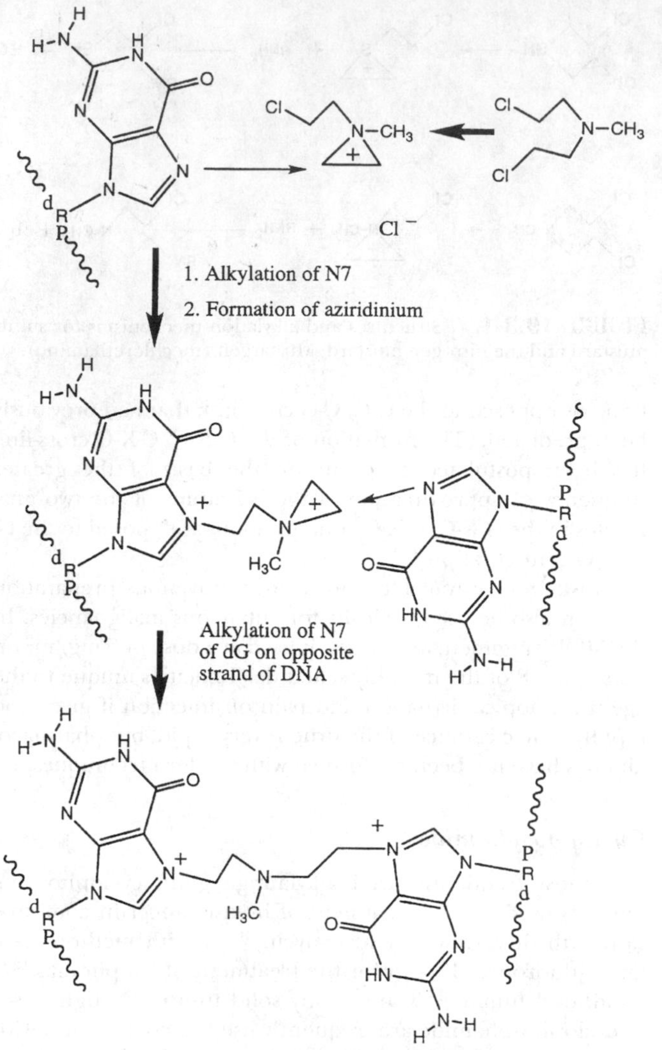

FIGURE 19.3-3. Alkylation of DNA and formation of interstrand cross-link by nitrogen mustard.

mide mustard is zwitterionic at physiologic pH[25] and enters cells poorly. 4-HC-aldophosphamide is not charged and enters cells facilely. While phosphoramide mustard is toxic to cells *in vitro* at concentrations of 100 µM and higher, 4-HC is cytotoxic in the range of 10 µM.[26] Thus, 4-HC-aldophosphamide serves as an efficient delivery system for phosphoramide mustard, which has been demonstrated to produce an interstrand DNA cross-link analogous to the cross-link produced by mechlorethamine.[7] Recent studies by Shulman-Roskes et al.[27] have demonstrated that phosphoramide mustard readily eliminates chloroethylaziridine,[27] which probably also plays a role in the cross-linking of DNA in cells exposed to 4-HC.

As shown in Figure 19.3-4, 4-HC is a substrate for the enzyme aldehyde dehydrogenase.[28] In cells that contain this enzyme, the bulk of the 4-HC is oxidized to carboxyphosphamide, which is not an active alkylating agent. Consequently, cells with high aldehyde dehydrogenase (ALDH) content are resistant to the metabolites of cyclophosphamide.[29,30] Early hematopoietic stem cells and megakaryocytes contain high levels, as do the epithelial stem cells in the small intestine and mucous membranes.[30,31] These observations explain why cyclophosphamide administration produces a shorter period of hematopoietic depression,[32] is relatively sparing of platelets, and is associated with less gastrointestinal toxicity and mucositis than other alkylating agents.[33]

4-HC is too unstable to be used as a reagent, but the compound 4-hydroperoxycyclophosphamide (see Fig. 19.3-4) is spontaneously converted in aqueous solution to 4-HC and can be used for *in vitro* studies of cell sensitivity.[34,35] This compound has also been used for the *in vitro* treatment of autologous bone marrow to reduce the number of tumor cells returned to the patient.[36]

Cyclophosphamide is available as tablets for oral administration or as an intravenous preparation. The drug is used at a variety of doses and schedules. Oral administration is particularly used for autoimmune diseases at a daily dose of approximately 100 mg. Because of its rapid absorption and high bioavailability, even very high doses can be given orally, but high intermittent doses are usually given intravenously. In moderate-dose combination chemotherapy, doses of cyclophosphamide in the range of 750 mg are usually used. For high-dose therapy in conjunction with hematopoietic cell transplantation, doses of up to 50 mg/kg for 2 or 4 days in combination with other agents are used.

The bulk (nearly 70%) of a dose of cyclophosphamide is excreted in the urine as the inactive carboxyphosphamide.[37,38] At high doses (approximately 50 mg/kg), plasma concentrations of up to 400 µM of cyclophosphamide are achieved,[38] and clearance depends on the renal clearance and the rate of microsomal metabolism in the liver. With improved and more facile techniques to measure 4-HC concentrations accurately, the clinical pharmacology of cyclophosphamide and this critical transport intermediate are being more carefully defined. Studies in patients receiving high-dose therapy have demonstrated considerable variation in the rates of clearance of cyclophosphamide between patients, with consequent differences in the peak concentrations (1 to 15 µM) and total exposure of the patient to 4-HC (60 to 140 µM.hours).[39,40] The total exposure to 4-HC is probably the major determinant of therapeutic effect. Currently, several programs are evaluating dose adjustment regimens based on the initial pharmacokinetics of cyclophosphamide and 4-HC. While it is known that substantial concentrations of phosphoramide mustard are present in plasma (up to 10 µM after 60 mg/kg of cyclophosphamide[38]), this concentration is well below the concentrations needed for *in vitro* cytotoxicity of phosphoramide mustard.[26]

A unique toxicity of cyclophosphamide and other oxazophosphorines is a characteristic hemorrhagic cystitis[41,42] due to irritation of the bladder mucosa from urinary metabolites. Acrolein has been identified as the metabolite most responsible for this effect,[43] but phosphoramide mustard and chloracetaldehyde may contribute to this toxicity. Careful hydration and emptying of the bladder are crucial to avoiding this toxicity, which has produced massive and even fatal hemorrhage. Another toxicity that has been associated with cyclophosphamide is an antidiuretic effect, especially at high doses.[44] This effect may produce marked fluid retention and electrolyte abnormalities, particularly low sodium, and seizures and fatalities have been seen.[45] It is important to avoid low-sodium-containing fluids after high-dose cyclophosphamide, and the fluid retention syndrome has been treated with furosemide to promote free water clearance.[46] The most severe dose-limiting toxicity of cyclophosphamide is a fulminant cardiac toxicity,[47] which is often fatal when seen clini-

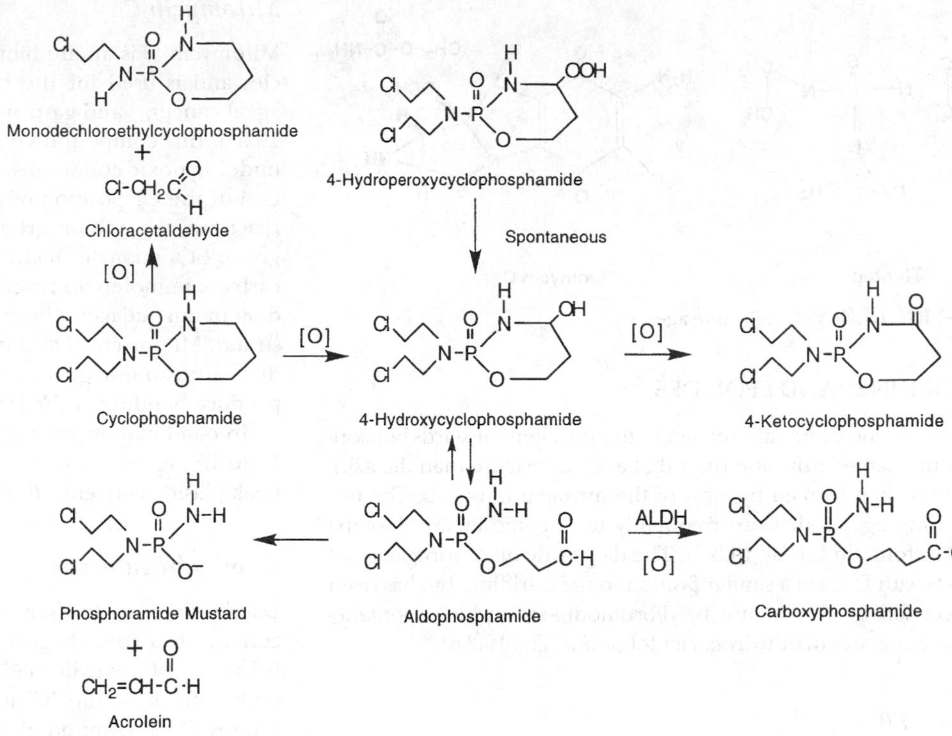

FIGURE 19.3-4. Metabolism of cyclophosphamide.

cally. This toxicity is seen only after the high doses used in bone marrow transplantation. It was initially seen in patients receiving 60 mg/kg/d of cyclophosphamide for 4 days, and the incidence has decreased since lower doses have been used. The syndrome usually presents with severe cardiac failure, beginning approximately 10 days after drug administration, with a dilated heart and low electrocardiogram voltage. There is a characteristic pathologic picture of edema, interstitial hemorrhage, and cardiac necrosis.[47]

Ifosfamide

Ifosfamide is a structural isomer of cyclophosphamide that is often used in the treatment of sarcomas and pediatric tumors (see Fig. 19.3-2). There is more chloroethyl side chain oxidation of ifosfamide (up to 50%) than of cyclophosphamide (<10%), and the degree of such metabolism is more variable than with cyclophosphamide.[48] Oxidation of the chloroethyl groups produces chloroacetaldehyde, which is probably responsible for the neurotoxicity[49] and renal toxicity[50] that have been seen with ifosfamide therapy. Since the oxidation of a chloroethyl side chain produces a much less toxic monofunctional agent, higher doses of ifosfamide than cyclophosphamide must be used clinically. The studies of the clinical pharmacology of ifosfamide have been more limited than those of cyclophosphamide but have demonstrated large intrapatient variability in the pharmacokinetics and metabolism of the agent during repeated administrations.[51,52]

Melphalan

Melphalan is now used principally for the treatment of multiple myeloma,[53] for high-dose myeloablative therapy in conjunction with bone marrow transplantation,[54] and for the isolated limb perfusion of localized tumors,[55] especially malignant melanoma and sarcomas (see Fig. 19.3-2). Melphalan is an amino acid analogue and is actively transported into cells by amino acid transport systems.[56,57] It has been demonstrated that cellular uptake[58] and transport into the central nervous system (CNS)[59] of melphalan can be modulated by the amino acid content in the extracellular fluid.

Melphalan is available both as tablets and as an intravenous preparation. For the treatment of multiple myeloma, melphalan is usually used orally at a dose of 0.25 mg/kg for 4 days, with prednisone on the same schedule every 4 to 6 weeks. At these doses, peak plasma concentrations of 0.625 μM are found, but absorption is variable.[60] For bone marrow transplantation, doses of melphalan of 100 to 140 mg/m² are used.[61] At these doses, peak concentrations of melphalan of 40 to 50 μM are reached.[61,62]

Chlorambucil

Chlorambucil is used for the treatment of B-cell chronic lymphocytic leukemia[63] and lymphomas[64] and for the immunosuppressive therapy of autoimmune diseases.[65] It is administered orally and is well tolerated when given either by daily administration or intermittent high-pulse doses.[64] Chlorambucil is well tolerated by most patients and can be used successfully for patients who have severe nausea and vomiting with cyclophosphamide or melphalan.

Chlorambucil is available only in an oral formulation. For chronic leukemia and immunosuppression, daily doses of 3 to 6 mg are given for a number of weeks, or 12 mg/m² may be given monthly. Pulsed dose pulse chlorambucil for lymphoma is given orally at a dose of 16 mg/m² daily for 5 consecutive days each month.[64] Chlorambucil is metabolized to a less active derivative—phenylacetic acid mustard—and the clinical pharmacology of chlorambucil is very similar to that of melphalan.[66]

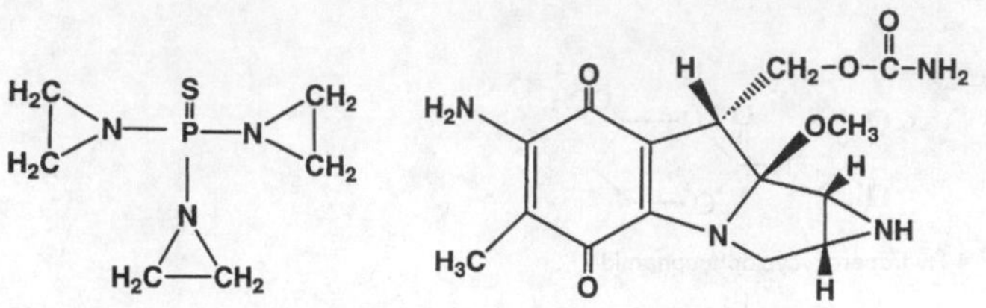

Thiotepa   Mitomycin C

FIGURE 19.3-5. Aziridine agents.

AZIRIDINES AND EPOXIDES

The aziridine agents are related to the nitrogen mustards but contain uncharged aziridine rings that are less reactive than the aziridinium rings formed by most of the nitrogen mustards. The two aziridine agents that are frequently used clinically are thiotepa and mitomycin C (Fig. 19.3-5). The diepoxide dianhydrogalactitol reacts with DNA in a similar fashion to the aziridines but has been succeeded in clinical use by dibromodulcitol, which spontaneously generates dianhydrogalactitol *in situ* (Fig. 19.3-6).

Thiotepa

Thiotepa is now used most frequently in combination with other alkylating agents in high-dose therapy with stem cell support.[39,67] Thiotepa has been demonstrated to react with the N7 position of guanylic acid in DNA[68] and to cross-link DNA,[69] indicating that it is acting similarly to the nitrogen mustards. Thiotepa is desulfurated by cytochrome P-450 enzymes[70] to produce tepa. Tepa is less toxic than thiotepa and has been demonstrated to produce alkali-labile sites in DNA, rather than cross-links.[69] These findings suggest that tepa reacts differently from thiotepa and produces monofunctional alkylation of DNA.

In combination with cyclophosphamide for high-dose therapy, thiotepa has been given as a continuous infusion for 4 days, at a daily dose of 200 mg/m^2. Under these conditions, steady-state levels of 2 to 6 μM of thiotepa are rapidly achieved.[71] Thiotepa is also used at a dose of 900 mg/m^2 in combination with high-dose cyclophosphamide and cisplatin.[72]

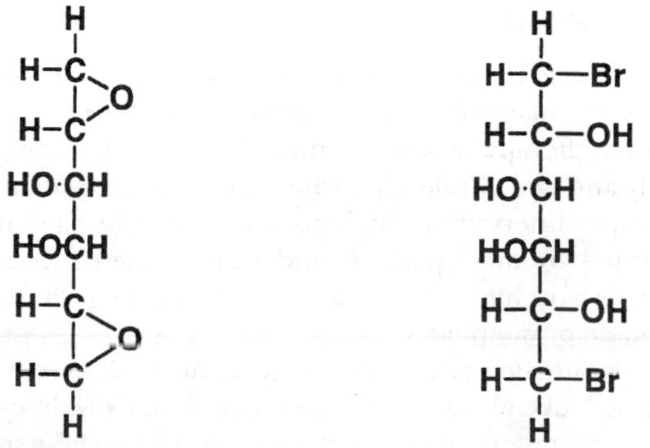

Dianhydrogalactitol   Dibromodulcitol

FIGURE 19.3-6. Structures of dianhydrogalactitol and its prodrug, dibromodulcitol.

Mitomycin C

Mitomycin C is an antibiotic extracted from a *Streptomyces* species and is used for the treatment of breast cancer,[73] esophageal cancer,[74] and gastrointestinal tumors.[75] As seen in Figure 19.3-5, this compound contains an aziridine ring. Particularly under hypoxic conditions, mitomycin C is reduced, with activation of the C1 position of the aziridine ring. This carbon then reacts in the minor groove with the extracyclic N2 amino group of a guanylic acid,[76,77] positioning the 10 carbon of the carbamate moiety to react with the N2 of a guanylic acid residue in an adjacent base pair in the complementary DNA strand. Mitomycin C and its reduced metabolites can also produce intrastrand guanylic acid–guanylic acid cross-links that produce bending of the DNA.[78]

In combination regimens, mitomycin C is given at doses of 10 to 15 mg/m^2 every 4 to 6 weeks. After a dose of 15 mg/m^2, peak plasma concentrations of 3 μM are seen.[79]

Dianhydrogalactitol

Dianhydrogalactitol (see Fig. 19.3-6) is a hexitol derivative that contains two epoxide groups and cross-links DNA through the N7 atoms of guanylic acid,[80] presumably through the nucleophilic attack of the N7 atoms on the strained-ring epoxide groups. This compound was evaluated in clinical trials and demonstrated modest antitumor activity.[81,82] However, the structurally related dibromodulcitol (see Fig. 19.3-6) has demonstrated more antitumor activity[83,84] and is still being used in combination chemotherapy of breast cancer, cervical cancer, and brain tumors. Dibromodulcitol is hydrolyzed to dianhydrogalactitol, and its better antitumor activity is presumably due to more effective localization of the reactive agent in tumor cells.[85] Dibromodulcitol is usually administered at a dose of 1 g/m^2, which produces a maximum plasma concentration of approximately 50 μM.[86]

ALKYL SULFONATES: BUSULFAN

Busulfan (Myeleran), other alkyl sulfonates, and the related sulfamates react with DNA by a direct displacement reaction (as shown in Fig. 19.3-7). Busulfan has been demonstrated to cross-link DNA,[87] but the structure of the cross-link has not been established. A chemically related agent, hepsulfam, with seven methylene units between the reactive groups, has been demonstrated to form a DNA G-X-C/C-X-G interstrand cross-link analogous to those formed by the nitrogen mustards.[88] Haddow and Timmis[89] reported in 1953 that busulfan was active against chronic myelogenous leukemia. Busulfan was for many years the principal agent used to treat this disease, before being replaced by the use of hydroxyurea[90] and interferon-α,[91] both of which have proved to be more effective than busulfan. The most frequent use of busulfan in cancer therapy today is in high-dose therapy for many tumors, including chronic myelogenous leukemia, in conjunction with bone marrow or stem cell transplantation. For this application, high doses of busulfan are combined with cyclophosphamide, total body irradiation, or other agents.[18,92–94] The effectiveness of busulfan for this purpose is undoubtedly related to its marked myeloablative properties,[95] the mechanistic bases of which are not understood.

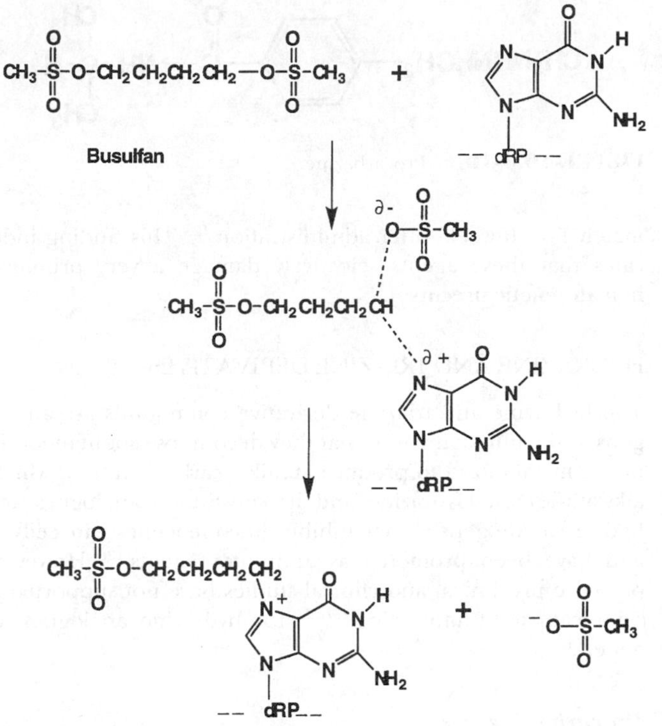

FIGURE 19.3-7. Alkylation of guanylate in DNA by busulfan through S_N2 alkylation. A second displacement reaction with the N7 of a guanylate in the complementary strand creates a G-X-C/C-X-G interstrand cross-link.

Until recently, busulfan was available only as an oral preparation, but intravenous preparations are now available. For hematopoietic transplantation, busulfan is usually given as 1 mg/kg every 6 hours for 4 days, for a total dose of 16 mg/kg. Peak concentrations of busulfan after each dose are approximately 10 µM.[96] High doses of busulfan have been associated with venoocclusive disease of the liver. This syndrome consists of hepatomegaly, jaundice, ascites, and hepatic failure with a high mortality rate.[97] Grochow et al.[96] have demonstrated that pharmacokinetic monitoring and dose adjustment of the busulfan can markedly reduce the incidence of venoocclusive disease.

NITROSOUREAS

The members of the nitrosourea group of therapeutic alkylating agents are related to the alkylnitrosoamines and similar compounds that have long been known to be carcinogenic. Methylnitrosoguanidine and methylnitrosourea are monofunctional alkylating agents and were found to have modest antitumor activity.[98,99] Montgomery[100] and others[101,102] evaluated a number of analogues of these compounds and demonstrated remarkable antitumor effects of bischloroethylnitrosourea (BCNU; Fig. 19.3-8) against mouse tumors, and particularly against intracerebral tumors, which had been refractory to most agents because of the blood–brain barrier.[100–102] BCNU was found to produce interstrand cross-linking of DNA,[103] which has been demonstrated to occur through the spontaneous generation of a chloroethyldiazonium species[104] and the series of reactions illustrated in Figure 19.3-9.[105] As illustrated, this interstrand cross-link occurs between a guanylate in DNA and the base-paired cytidylate in the other strand of the DNA.[106]

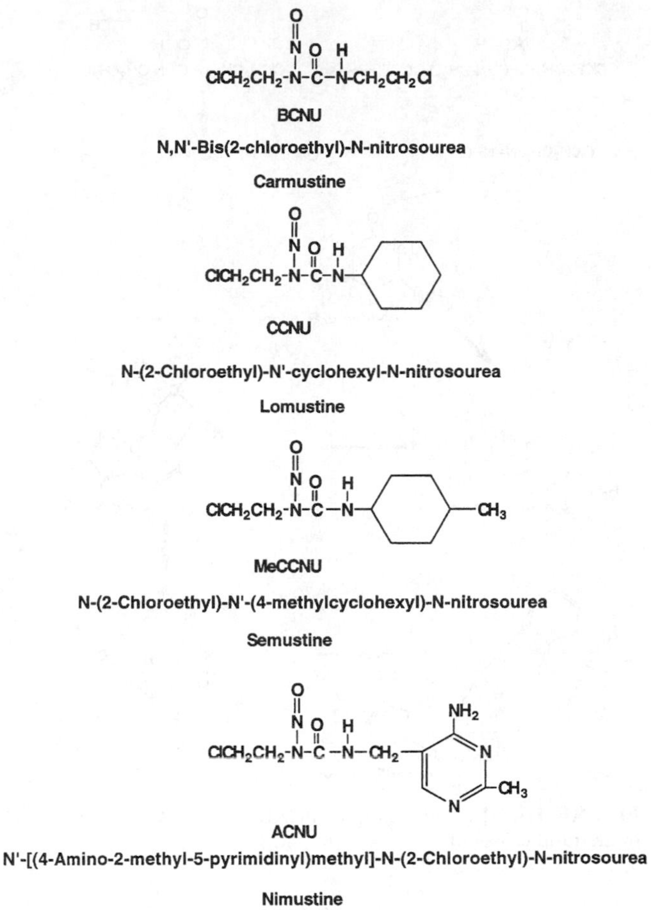

FIGURE 19.3-8. Nitrosoureas.

Bischloroethylnitrosourea

BCNU (carmustine; see Fig. 19.3-8) demonstrated activity against brain tumors clinically[107] and has continued to be used in the treatment of gliomas and other brain tumors. BCNU has also been used in the treatment of multiple myeloma[108] and in high-dose therapy in conjunction with bone marrow and stem cell transplantation.[109] BCNU can also be administered to brain tumors by direct injection[110] and by the implantation of biodegradable polymers containing BCNU into the brain.[111]

Cyclohexylchloroethylnitrosourea

Cyclohexylchloroethylnitrosourea (CCNU, lomustine; see Fig. 19.3-8) is a more lipid-soluble nitrosourea. It is administered orally and is used in the treatment of brain tumors.[112,113]

Methylcyclohexylchloroethylnitrosourea

Methylcyclohexylchloroethylnitrosourea (semustine; see Fig. 19.3-8) is an oral investigational drug that has been used in the treatment of gastrointestinal tumors.[114]

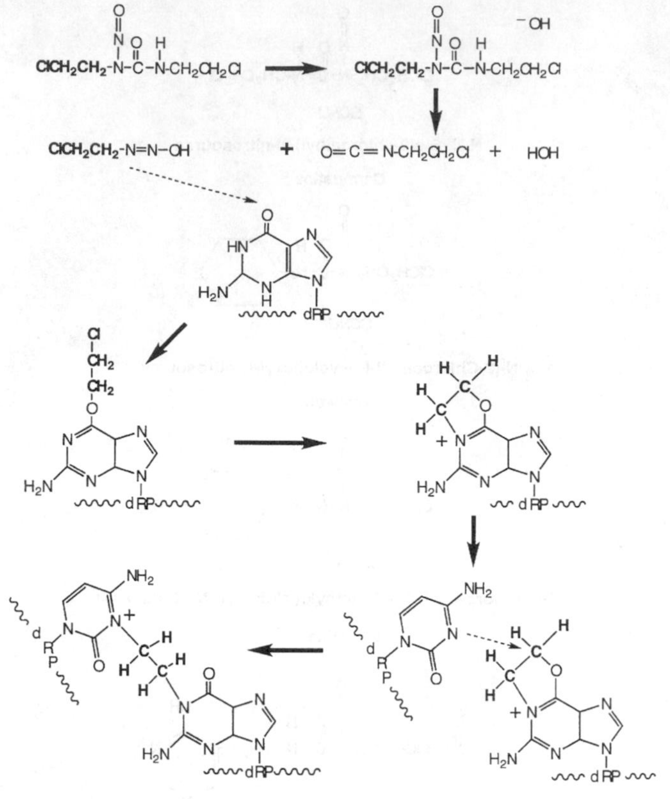

FIGURE 19.3-9. Reaction of BCNU with DNA to produce a G-C interstrand cross-link.

N'-[(4-amino-2-methyl-5-pyrimidinyl)methyl]-N-(2-chloroethyl)-N-nitrosourea

N'-[(4-amino-2-methyl-5-pyrimidinyl)methyl]-N-(2-chloroethyl)-N-nitrosourea (nimustine; see Fig. 19.3-8) is more water-soluble than the other chloroethylnitrosoureas and has been used for the treatment of CNS tumors by the intraarterial[115] and intrathecal routes.[116]

Clinical Pharmacology

As a single agent, BCNU is usually used in a dose of 125 to 200 mg/m^2 every 6 to 8 weeks. In combination with doxorubicin for multiple myeloma, a dose of 30 mg/m^2 every 3 to 4 weeks has been used.[117] After doses in the range of 100 mg/m^2, peak plasma concentrations are in the range of 5 μM.[118] For high-dose therapy of breast cancer, BCNU is given at a dose of 600 mg/m^2 in combination with cyclophosphamide and cisplatin.[119] After this dose of BCNU, the peak plasma levels of BCNU have been shown to be approximately 5 μM.[120] Phenobarbital has been demonstrated to increase the clearance of BCNU[121] and to decrease the toxic and therapeutic effects. CCNU is administered in doses similar to those of BCNU. The parent CCNU has not been detected, but the peak concentrations of the ring hydroxylated metabolites are approximately 3 μM after doses of 130 mg/m^2.[122]

Specific Toxicities

Hematopoietic toxicity of the nitrosoureas is severe and is delayed, with the nadir of the granulocytes occurring approximately 5 to 6 weeks after administration.[123] This finding indicates that these agents selectively damage a very primitive hematopoietic precursor.

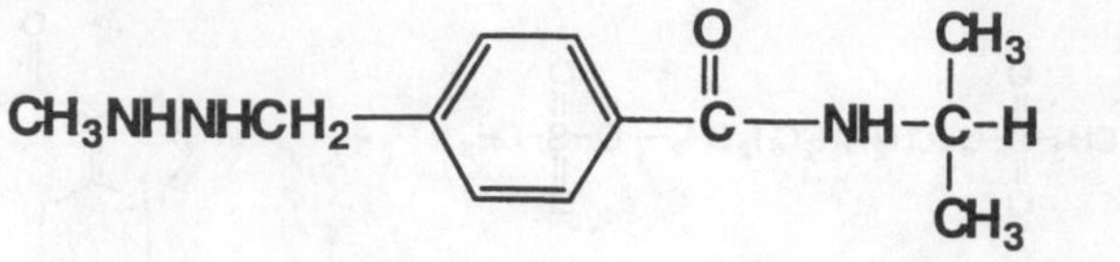

FIGURE 19.3-10. Procarbazine.

HYDRAZINE AND TRIAZINE DERIVATIVES

The hydrazine and triazene derivative compounds are analogous to the nitrosoureas in that they decompose spontaneously or are metabolized to produce an alkyl carbonium ion, which alkylates DNA. Hydrazine and its substituted analogues are known carcinogens[124] that inhibit gluconeogenesis in cells[125] and have been promoted as antitumor agents.[126] However, objective preclinical and clinical studies have not supported a significant antitumor effect[127,128] for hydrazine analogues in general.

Procarbazine

Procarbazine is a phenylhydrazine derivative that was initially developed as an inhibitor of monoamine oxidase but was found to have significant antitumor activity in preclinical models and clinically (Fig. 19.3-10).[129] Procarbazine was one of the components of the first effective combination chemotherapy regimen, MOPP, for Hodgkin's disease.[6] The agent is currently used for the treatment of Hodgkin's disease[6,130] and for the treatment of primary brain tumors.[113,131] Procarbazine has been demonstrated to be metabolized to a DNA-methylating agent,[132–134] which is most likely methylazoxyprocarbazine.[135,136] Since procarbazine is a monoamine oxidase inhibitor, patients can experience CNS depression[137] or stimulation[138] and acute hypertension, especially after the ingestion of tyramine-rich foods.

Dacarbazine

Dacarbazine, or DTIC [(dimethyltriazeno)imidazole-carboxamide], is a triazene derivative that is metabolized by microsomal N-demethylation, predominantly in the liver, to an intermediate that spontaneously decomposes to release a methyldiazonium that methylates DNA (Fig. 19.3-11).[139–141] Dacarbazine is used in the regimen of doxorubicin, bleomycin, vinblastine, and dacarbazine for the treatment of Hodgkin's disease[130,142] and for the treatment of malignant melanoma.[119,143]

Temozolomide

Temozolomide is a triazene analogue that spontaneously decomposes to produce a methyl diazonium ion, as illustrated in Figure 19.3-11.[144,145] This compound may produce a more homogeneous distribution of the short-lived MITC [(methyltriazeno)-imidazole-carboxamide], which is spontaneously generated from temozolomide at all sites, than does dacarbazine, which is metabolized to MITC in the liver. The principal toxicities seen in phase I trials have been neutropenia and thrombocytopenia,

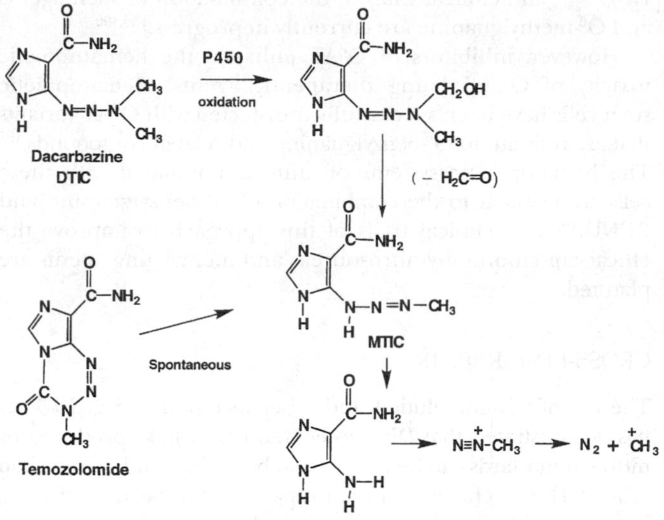

FIGURE 19.3-11. Generation of methyl diazonium from the triazenes dacarbazine and temozolomide.

and tumor responses were seen in those trials[146,147] in patients with glioma and melanoma. Phase II trials in patients with gliomas have shown response rates of 20% to 30%,[148,149] but phase II trials in patients with sarcomas[150] and pancreatic cancer[151] did not demonstrate significant responses.

These agents exert their toxicity predominantly through the methylation of the O^6 position of guanylic acid in DNA. Therefore, cells that contain significant O^6-alkyltransferase or are deficient in mismatch repair will be resistant to them (as discussed in the section Mechanisms of Toxicity and Drug Resistance).

Procarbazine is an oral preparation and used in the MOPP regimen for Hodgkin's disease at a dose of 100 mg/m^2/d for 14 days.[142] Because of its complex metabolism, pharmacokinetic studies have been limited. Dacarbazine is an intravenous preparation and is used in the regimen of doxorubicin, bleomycin, vinblastine, dacarbazine for Hodgkin's disease at a dose of 375 mg/m^2/d for 15 days.[142] For the treatment of malignant melanoma, a dose of 200 to 250 mg/m^2/d for 5 days is used and, at this dose, peak plasma concentrations of dacarbazine are approximately 30 μM.[152] This agent has been used as a single agent with bone marrow transplantation at a dose of 2000 mg/m^2.[153] At this dose, the maximum plasma concentration of dacarbazine was 800 μM.[153] Temozolomide is usually given orally at 150 to 250 mg/m^2/d for 5 days. Reid et al.[154] measured peak concentrations of MTIC of 0.5 to 5 μM after administration of these doses of temozolomide.[154] Baker et al.[155] studied the pharmacokinetics of ^{14}C-labeled temozolomide and found peak concentrations of temozolomide of approximately 30 μM and peak concentrations of MTIC of approximately 1 μM.

MECHANISMS OF TOXICITY AND DRUG RESISTANCE

REACTION WITH CELLULAR MOLECULES

The alkylating agents are potent electrophiles and react with many electron-rich molecules within the cell to be inactivated.

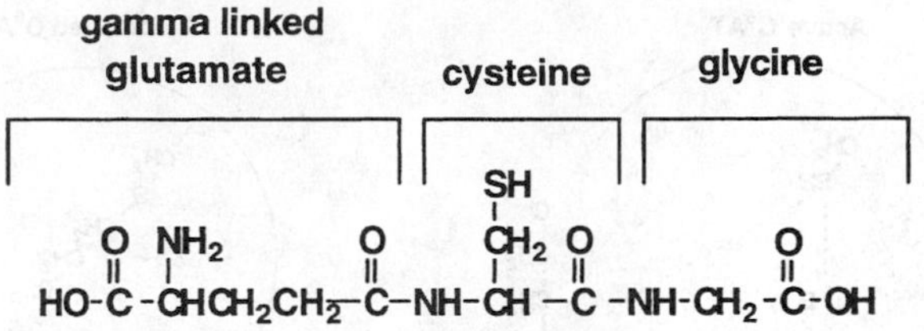

FIGURE 19.3-12. Structure of glutathione.

The principal such molecule is glutathione (GSH), a tripeptide with a free cysteine sulfhydryl that is present at millimolar concentrations in cells (Fig. 19.3-12). This small nucleophile is known to react with and inactivate virtually all the therapeutic alkylating agents, and a correlation between elevated cellular GSH concentrations and resistance to nitrogen mustards has been demonstrated.[156,157] The GSH S-transferase enzymes catalyze the conjugation of GSH with electrophiles, and increased activity of this class of enzymes enhances GSH-mediated resistance.[158–160] The GSH conjugates of specific alkylating agents have been characterized,[161–163] and the specific isoenzymes of GST that catalyze their formation have been characterized.[164–168]

Buthionine sulfoximine is an inhibitor of gamma-glutamylcysteine synthetase, the rate-limiting enzyme in the GSH synthesis pathway, and decreases the GSH concentration in cells.[169] Exposure to this compound sensitizes both normal and tumor cells to alkylating agents.[156,170,171] In a phase I clinical trial, buthionine sulfoxime has been shown to increase the hematologic toxicity of melphalan[172] and is currently in further clinical trials to determine whether this agent can increase the clinical antitumor efficacy of melphalan.

Cells can also be sensitized to alkylating agents by exposure to inhibitors of GSH S-transferases,[173,174] and a clinical trial of the GSH S-transferase inhibitor sulfasalazine with melphalan demonstrated increased nausea and vomiting but no increase in hematopoietic toxicity.[175] The membrane transporter multidrug resistance protein is known to mediate the efflux of GSH conjugates from the cell,[176] and Barnouin et al.[177] have demonstrated that this system can transport the GSH conjugates of chlorambucil and melphalan from cells. The observations suggest that modulation of these systems could enhance the efficacy of alkylating agents.

Kelley et al.[178] demonstrated that transfection of metallothionein into cells produced increased resistance to chlorambucil and melphalan. Subsequently, Yu et al.[179] have demonstrated that the thiol groups of metallothionein will bind melphalan and phosphoramide mustard.[180] It has also been demonstrated that exposure of cells to zinc will increase metallothionein concentration in the cell and increase resistance of the cells to melphalan, doxorubicin, and cisplatin.[181]

ENHANCED DNA REPAIR: O^6 ALKYLATION

Another mechanism of cellular resistance to alkylating agents is repair of the DNA damage that the agents produce. The most defined mechanism of cellular repair of alkylating agent damage is that of the enzyme O^6-alkylguanine-alkyltransferase. As illustrated in Figure 19.3-13, this enzyme can remove an alkyl group from the O^6 position of guanine, and the alkylated enzyme is then rapidly degraded.[182] This mechanism has been shown to be effective in protecting normal and tumor cells

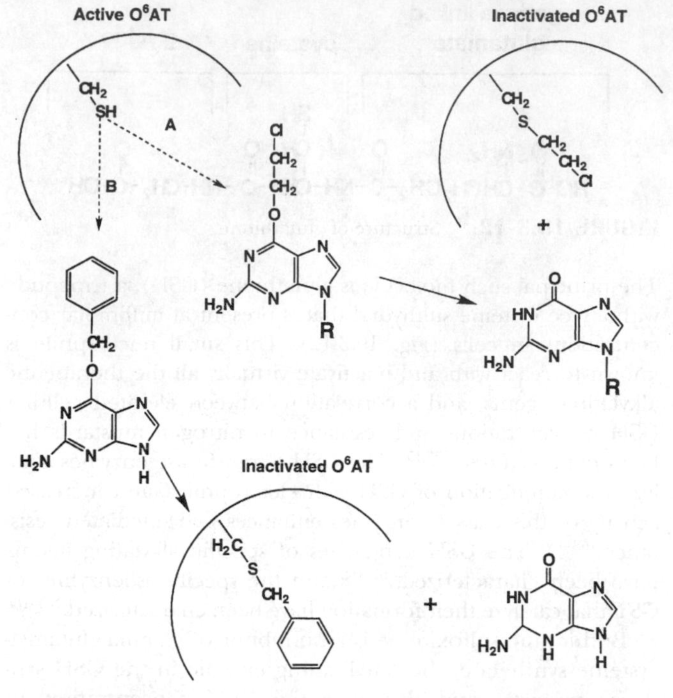

FIGURE 19.3-13. Interactions of O^6-alkylguanine-DNA alkyltransferase. Pathway A: Repair of O^6 alkylation by O^{6}AT. Pathway B: Inactivation of O^{6}AT by benzylguanine.

from the carcinogenic and toxic effects of DNA methylating agents, such as temozolomide and procarbazine.[183] Erickson et al.[184] demonstrated that this enzyme would also remove the 6-chloroethyl lesion produced by the alkylation of guanine by the chloroethylnitrosoureas and produce resistance to these compounds, and this observation has been confirmed and extended.[185]

It has been shown that such compounds as O^6-benzylguanine will be acted on by O^6-alkylguanine-DNA alkyltransferase (see Fig. 19.3-13) to remove the benzyl group[186] and that the enzyme will be rapidly degraded and depleted. Such compounds have been demonstrated to reverse tumor resistance due to O^{6}AT to the O^6 alkylating agents *in vitro* and *in vivo*,[187,188] and clinical trials of the combination of such agents and O^6-methylguanine are currently in progress.[189,190]

However, inhibitors of O^{6}AT enhance the hematopoietic toxicity of O^6 alkylating therapeutic agents. Hematopoietic stem cells have been successfully transfected with O^{6}AT variants that are resistant to O^6-benzylguanine and related compounds.[191] The hematopoietic systems of animals populated with these cells are resistant to the combination of O^6-benzylguanine and BCNU,[192] and clinical trials of this approach to improve the efficacy of chloroethylnitrosoureas and methylating agents are planned.

CROSS-LINK REPAIR

The use of alkaline elution and other techniques (Fig. 19.3-14) has demonstrated that DNA interstrand cross-links produced by nitrogen mustards can be removed in bacteria[193] and mammalian cells.[194] The mechanism of such repair has not been elucidated, but nucleotide excision repair[195] and poly(adenosine diphosphate–ribose) polymerase[196] appear to play a role.

Caffeine and related compounds have been demonstrated to enhance the cytotoxicity of nitrogen mustard.[197] This effect was associated with abrogation of G_2 arrest. O'Connor et al.[198,199] demonstrated that the G_2 arrest associated with nitrogen mustard resistance was associated with decreased activity of cdc2 kinase in the resistant cells. Caffeine has also been shown to inhibit nucleotide excision repair by binding to the subunit that recognizes the damage and helps to mediate this repair activity.[200] Elevated Bcl-2 has also been associated with nitrogen mustard resistance.[201]

A medulloblastoma cell line has been demonstrated to be resistant to activated cyclophosphamide (4-hydroperoxycyclophosphamide) on the basis of increased removal of DNA interstrand cross-links.[34,202] This cell does not appear to repair cross-links produced by BCNU and busulfan, indicating that the recognition of the nitrogen mustard cross-link is fairly specific.

IN VIVO RESISTANCE

Kobayashi et al.[203] and St. Croix et al.[204] have described resistance to alkylating agents and other antitumor agents that is

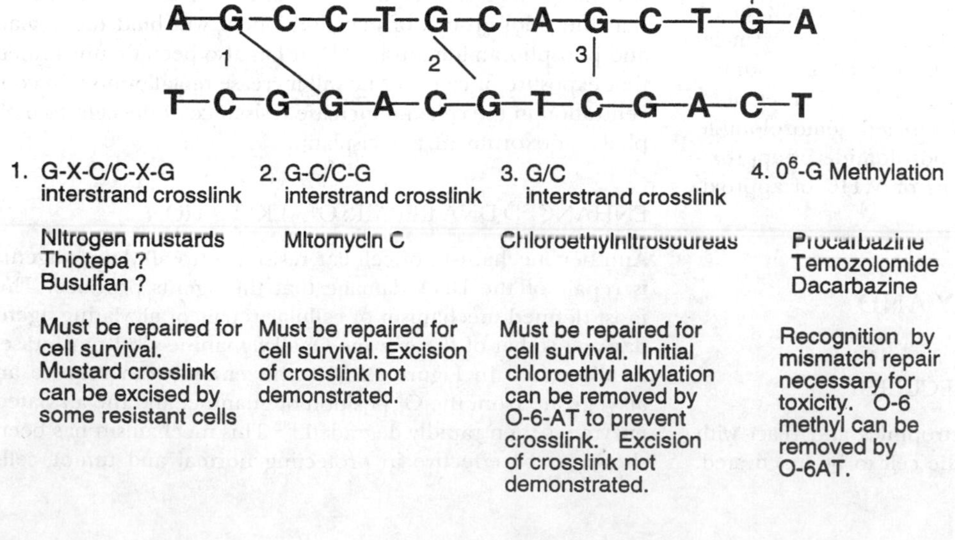

FIGURE 19.3-14. DNA lesions produced by alkylating agents.

associated with aggregation of tumor cells. This resistance is present when the tumor cells are growing *in vivo* or in three-dimensional *in vitro* culture with adherence between the cells but is not present when the cells are dispersed in two-dimensional culture. This type of resistance has also been associated with increased metastatic potential.[205]

COMMON TOXICITIES

Toxicities that are associated with specific alkylating agents are described in the discussions of the individual agents. The toxicities common to the alkylating agents as a class are described here.

HEMATOPOIETIC TOXICITY

The usual dose-limiting toxicity for an alkylating agent is hematopoietic toxicity. As described, cyclophosphamide usually produces a relatively rapid nadir of the granulocytes, with recovery within 3 weeks after a single dose or short course.[32,33,206] Cyclophosphamide is also relatively platelet-sparing. The reason for the relative hematopoietic sparing properties of cyclophosphamide is the high concentrations of the enzyme aldehyde dehydrogenase in hematopoietic stem cells and megakaryocytes.[30,31]

The nitrosoureas produce an unusual delayed hematopoietic toxicity, with nadirs of both granulocytes and platelets at 5 to 6 weeks after administration.[123] Severe granulocytopenia and thrombocytopenia are also characteristic of busulfan.[207] An interesting characteristic of busulfan is its relative sparing of lymphocytes. The different hematopoietic effects of alkylating agents, except for the characteristics of cyclophosphamide, are not explained but suggest significant differences in selectivity of the agents for hematopoietic precursors.

GASTROINTESTINAL TOXICITY

The alkylating agents frequently produce nausea and vomiting, although this effect is usually not as severe as with the platinum agents. Cyclophosphamide produces severe nausea and vomiting in some patients, but these patients usually tolerate chlorambucil, which is clinically less emetogenic. The nausea and vomiting produced by alkylating agents are known to be mediated significantly through the CNS.[208,209] With the higher doses of alkylating agents used in bone marrow transplantation, increased nausea and vomiting are seen but can usually be controlled by corticosteroids and the newer antiserotonin antiemetics.[210–212] The alkylating agents can cause significant toxicity to the gastrointestinal mucosa and produce mucositis, stomatitis, and diarrhea, especially with the high doses of melphalan and thiotepa used in bone marrow transplantation.[213]

GONADAL TOXICITY

The alkylating agents can produce significant gonadal toxicity. The characteristic testicular lesion in men is depletion of germ cells without damage to the Sertoli cells, which was first described with nitrogen mustard in 1948.[214] This lesion is also seen, often in association with oligospermia or aspermia, after treatment with other alkylating agents.[215,216] Spermatogenic dysfunction is reversible in some patients.[217,218]

Women treated with alkylating agents may develop amenorrhea associated with a marked decrease in ovarian follicles.[215,219,220] This complication and its irreversibility increase with the age of the woman.[221]

PULMONARY TOXICITY

Interstitial pneumonitis and fibrosis were initially reported as a consequence of busulfan therapy[222] but have subsequently been reported to occur after therapy with melphalan,[223] chlorambucil,[224] cyclophosphamide,[225,226] mitomycin C,[227] and BCNU.[228,229] The clinical manifestations of this toxicity are dyspnea and a nonproductive cough, which can progress to cyanosis, pulmonary insufficiency, and death. The syndrome has particularly been associated in frequency and severity with high doses of BCNU.[230,231] The greater pulmonary toxicity of BCNU may be due to the spontaneous decomposition of BCNU, which produces chloroethyl isocyanate in addition to the alkylating chloroethyl diazonium moiety described.[232] Chloroethyl isocyanate is an analogue of methyl isocyanate, a known pulmonary toxin that produced many deaths when released in an industrial accident in Bhopal, India.[233]

ALOPECIA

Alopecia from chemotherapy was first described after administration of dimethylmyeleran, an analogue of busulfan.[234] The alkylating agents now most associated with alopecia are cyclophosphamide and ifosfamide. Feil and Lamoureux[235] examined the alopecia-producing effects of metabolites and analogues of cyclophosphamide and proposed that the alopecic effect was due to the facile entry of a lipophilic metabolite (now known to be 4-HC) into the hair follicles. This hypothesis is consistent with the fact that vincristine, doxorubicin, and the taxanes, all associated with alopecia, are fairly lipophilic.

TERATOGENICITY

All the therapeutically used alkylating agents are teratogenic in animal studies.[236–239] A review of the literature in 1968 found that 4 of 25 children born to mothers who received alkylating agents during the first trimester of pregnancy had fetal malformations.[240] On the basis of the limited information available, women treated with an alkylating agent during the first trimester of pregnancy may have a risk as high as 15% of having a malformed infant. Administration of alkylating agents during the second and third trimesters has not been associated with increased fetal malformations.[241,242] More recent reviews support the lack of malformations produced by treatment during the second and third trimesters,[243,244] and one review cites 19 women treated during the first trimester with no infant malformations.[244]

CARCINOGENESIS

In the 1970s, there were reports of acute leukemia occurring in patients who had been treated with alkylating agents,[245–249] and subsequent experience has confirmed the occurrence of this complication. The incidence of leukemia is difficult to estimate because of the variety of agents, doses, and combinations used but is probably approximately 5%. In one group of 12 ovarian cancer patients receiving a high dose of melphalan, 4 developed acute leukemia.[248] In one report, the incidence of leukemia was found to be higher after melphalan treatment than after cyclophosphamide therapy.[250] This observation may be related to the stem cell–sparing properties of cyclophosphamide.[30] An increased frequency of solid tumors also occurs after alkylating agent therapy.[251,252]

IMMUNOSUPPRESSION

In 1921, Hektoen and Corper[253] reported an inhibitory effect of sulfur mustard on antibody production. While all the alkylating agents produce some degree of immunosuppression, cyclophosphamide is the most immunosuppressive.[254] Cyclophosphamide and chlorambucil are the alkylating agents most commonly used for the treatment of autoimmune diseases.[255–259]

Selective inhibition of immunosuppressor cells with low doses of an activated analogue of cyclophosphamide and with melphalan has been demonstrated *in vitro*[260–263] and *in vivo*[263,264] and enhancement of the immune response has been shown *in vivo*.[263] For this reason, low doses of cyclophosphamide have been used in conjunction with immunotherapy.[265,266] Because of its potent immunosuppressive properties, cyclophosphamide has long been used in preparative regimens for allogeneic stem cell transplantation for malignancy[267] and more recently for the autologous transplantation of autoimmune disease.[268,269] The use of high doses of cyclophosphamide without stem cell support has now been reported to produce complete remissions in autoimmune diseases.[21,270,271]

REFERENCES

1. Rhodes R. *The making of the atomic bomb.* New York: Simon & Schuster, 1986.
2. Adair CPJ, Bogg HJ. Experimental and clinical studies of the treatment of cancer by dichloroethylsulfide (mustard gas). *Ann Surg* 1931;93:190.
3. Rhoads C. Nitrogen mustards in treatment of neoplastic disease. *JAMA* 1946;131:6568.
4. Goodman LS, Wintrobe MM, Dameshek W, et al. Use of methyl-bis(beta-chlorethyl)amine hydrochloride for Hodgkin's disease, lymphosarcoma, leukemia. *JAMA* 1946;132:126.
5. Jacobson LP, Spurr C, Barron E, et al. Studies of the effect of methyl-bis(beta-chloroethyl)amine hydrochloride on neoplastic diseases and allied disorders of the hematopoietic system. *JAMA* 1946;132:263.
6. DeVita VT Jr, Serpick AA, Carbone PP. Combination chemotherapy in the treatment of advanced Hodgkin's disease. *Ann Intern Med* 1970;73(6):881.
7. Millard JT, Raucher S, Hopkins PB. Mechlorethamine cross links deoxyguanosine residues at 5´ GNC sequences in duplex DNA sequences in duplex DNA fragments. *J Am Chem Soc* 1990;112:2459.
8. Brookes P, Lawley PD. The reaction of mono- and difunctional alkylating agents with nucleic acids. *Biochem J* 1961;80:486.
9. Dong Q, Barsky D, Colvin ME, et al. A structural basis for a phosphoramide mustard-induced DNA interstrand cross-link at 5´-d(GAC). *Proc Natl Acad Sci U S A* 1995;92(26):12170.
10. Fisher B, Anderson S, Wickerham DL, et al. Increased intensification and total dose of cyclophosphamide in a doxorubicin-cyclophosphamide regimen for the treatment of primary breast cancer: findings from National Surgical Adjuvant Breast and Bowel Project B-22. *J Clin Oncol* 1997;15(5):1858.
11. Falkson G, Tormey DC, Carey P, Witte R, Falkson HC. Long-term survival of patients treated with combination chemotherapy for metastatic breast cancer. *Eur J Cancer* 1991;27(8):973.
12. DeVita VT Jr, Chabner B, Schein P, Hubbard SP, Young RC. Advanced diffuse histiocytic lymphoma, a potentially curable disease. *Lancet* 1975;1:248.
13. Chao NJ, Rosenberg SA, Horning SJ. CEPP(B): an effective and well-tolerated regimen in poor-risk, aggressive non-Hodgkin's lymphoma. *Blood* 1990;76(7):1293.
14. Carpenter PA, White L, McCowage GB, et al. A dose-intensive, cyclophosphamide-based regimen for the treatment of recurrent/progressive or advanced solid tumors of childhood—a report from the Australia and New Zealand Children's Cancer Study Group. *Cancer* 1997;80(3):489.
15. McCowage G, Tien R, McLendon R, et al. Successful treatment of childhood pilocytic astrocytomas metastatic to the leptomeninges with high-dose cyclophosphamide. *Med Pediatr Oncol* 1996;27(1):32.
16. Colvin OM. Drug resistance in the treatment of sarcomas. *Semin Oncol* 1997;24(5):580.
17. Santos GW, Tutschka PJ, Brookmeyer R, et al. Marrow transplantation for acute nonlymphocytic leukemia after treatment with busulfan and cyclophosphamide. *N Engl J Med* 1983;309(22):1347.
18. Blazar BR, Ramsay NK, Kersey JH, et al. Pretransplant conditioning with busulfan (Myleran) and cyclophosphamide for nonmalignant diseases. Assessment of engraftment following histocompatible allogeneic bone marrow transplantation. *Transplantation* 1985;39(6):597.
19. Antman K, Ayash L, Elias A, et al. High-dose cyclophosphamide, thiotepa, and carboplatin with autologous marrow support in women with measurable advanced breast cancer responding to standard dose therapy: analysis by age. *J Natl Cancer Inst Monogr* 1994;16:91.
20. Ferrara F, Copia C, Annunziata M, et al. Complete remission of refractory anemia following a single high dose of cyclophosphamide. *Ann Hematol* 1999;78(2):87.
21. Brodsky RA, Petri M, Smith BD, et al. Immunoablative high-dose cyclophosphamide without stem-cell rescue for refractory, severe autoimmune disease. *Ann Intern Med* 1998;129(12):1031.
22. Colvin M, Hilton J. Pharmacology of cyclophosphamide and metabolites. *Cancer Treat Rep* 1981;3:89.
23. Colvin M, Padgett CA, Fenselau C. A biologically active metabolite of cyclophosphamide. *Cancer Res* 1973;33(4):915.
24. Colvin M, Brundrett RB, Kan MN, Jardine I, Fenselau C. Alkylating properties of phosphoramide mustard. *Cancer Res* 1976;36(3):1121.
25. Gamcsik MP, Ludeman SM, Shulman-Roskes EM, et al. Protonation of phosphoramide mustard and other phosphoramides. *J Med Chem* 1993;36(23):3636.
26. Hilton J. Deoxyribonucleic acid cross-linking by 4-hydroperoxycyclophosphamide in cyclophosphamide-sensitive and -resistant L1210 cells. *Biochem Pharmacol* 1984;33(12):1867.
27. Shulman-Roskes EM, Noe DA, Gamcsik MP, et al. The partitioning of phosphoramide mustard and its aziridinium ions among alkylation and P-N bond hydrolysis reactions. *J Med Chem* 1998;41(4):515.
28. Hilton J. Role of aldehyde dehydrogenase in cyclophosphamide-resistant L1210 leukemia. *Cancer Res* 1984;44(11):5156.
29. Russo JE, Hilton J. Characterization of cytosolic aldehyde dehydrogenase from cyclophosphamide resistant L1210 cells. *Cancer Res* 1988;48(11):2963.
30. Kastan MB, Schlaffer E, Russo JE, et al. Direct demonstration of elevated aldehyde dehydrogenase in human hematopoietic progenitor cells. *Blood* 1990;75(10):1947.
31. Russo JE, Hilton J, Colvin OM. The role of aldehyde dehydrogenase isozymes in cellular resistance to the alkylating agent cyclophosphamide. *Prog Clin Biol Res* 1989;290:65.
32. Nissen-Meyer R, Host H. A comparison between the hematological side effects of cyclophosphamide and nitrogen mustard. *Cancer Chemother Rep* 1960;9:51.
33. Mullins GM, Colvin M. Intensive cyclophosphamide (NSC-26271) therapy for solid tumors. *Cancer Chemother Rep* 1975;59(2):411.
34. Dong Q, Bullock N, Aliosman F, et al. Repair analysis of 4-hydroperoxycyclophosphamide induced DNA interstrand cross-linking in the C-Myc gene in 4-hydroperoxycyclophosphamide-sensitive and -resistant medulloblastoma cell lines. *Cancer Chemother Pharmacol* 1996;37(3):242.
35. Gamcsik MP, Millis KK, Colvin M. Noninvasive detection of elevated glutathione levels in Mcf-7 cells resistant to 4-hydroperoxycyclophosphamide. *Cancer Res* 1995;55(10):2012.
36. Rowley SD, Jones RJ, Piantadosi S, et al. Efficacy of ex vivo purging for autologous bone marrow transplantation in the treatment of acute nonlymphoblastic leukemia. *Blood* 1989;74(1):501.
37. Bakke JE, Feil VJ, Fjelstul CE, Thacker EJ. Metabolism of cyclophosphamide by sheep. *J Agric Food Chem* 1972;20(2):384.
38. Jardine I, Fenselau C, Appler M, et al. Quantitation by gas chromatography–chemical ionization mass spectrometry of cyclophosphamide, phosphoramide mustard, and nornitrogen mustard in the plasma and urine of patients receiving cyclophosphamide therapy. *Cancer Res* 1978;38(2):408.
39. Chen TL, Kennedy MJ, Anderson LW, et al. Nonlinear pharmacokinetics of cyclophosphamide and 4-hydroxycyclophosphamide/aldophosphamide in patients with metastatic breast cancer receiving high-dose chemotherapy followed by autologous bone marrow transplantation. *Drug Metab Dispos* 1997;25(5):544.
40. Ren S, Kalhorn TF, McDonald GB, et al. Pharmacokinetics of cyclophosphamide and its metabolites in bone marrow transplantation patients. *Clin Pharmacol Ther* 1998;64(3):289.
41. Phillips FS, Sternberg SS, Cronin AP, PM V. Cyclophosphamide and urinary bladder toxicity. *Cancer Res* 1961;21:1577.
42. Forni AM, Koss LG, Geller W. Cytological study of the effect of cyclophosphamide on the epithelium of the urinary bladder in man. *Cancer* 1964;17:1348.
43. Cox PJ. Cyclophosphamide cystitis—identification of acrolein as the causative agent. *Biochem Pharmacol* 1979;28(13):2045.
44. DeFronzo RA, Braine H, Colvin M, Davis PJ. Water intoxication in man after cyclophosphamide therapy. Time course and relation to drug activation. *Ann Intern Med* 1973;78(6):861.
45. Harlow PJ, DeClerck YA, Shore NA, et al. A fatal case of inappropriate ADH secretion induced by cyclophosphamide therapy. *Cancer* 1979;44(3):896.
46. Green TP, Mirkin BL. Prevention of cyclophosphamide-induced antidiuresis by furosemide infusion. *Clin Pharmacol Ther* 1981;29(5):634.
47. Slavin RE, Millan JC, Mullins GM. Pathology of high dose intermittent cyclophosphamide therapy. *Hum Pathol* 1975;6(6):693.
48. Colvin M. The comparative pharmacology of cyclophosphamide and ifosfamide. *Semin Oncol* 1982;9(4)[Suppl 1]:2.
49. Pratt CB, Green AA, Horowitz ME, et al. Central nervous system toxicity following the treatment of pediatric patients with ifosfamide/mesna. *J Clin Oncol* 1986;4(8):1253.
50. Pratt CB, Meyer WH, Jenkins JJ, et al. Ifosfamide, Fanconi's syndrome, and rickets. *J Clin Oncol* 1991;9(8):1495.
51. Boddy AV, Yule SM, Wyllie R, et al. Intrasubject variation in children of ifosfamide pharmacokinetics and metabolism during repeated administration. *Cancer Chemother Pharmacol* 1996;38(2):147.

52. Boddy AV, Proctor M, Simmonds D, Lind MJ, Idle JR. Pharmacokinetics, metabolism and clinical effect of ifosfamide in breast cancer patients. *Eur J Cancer* 1995;1:69.
53. Cuttner J, Wasserman LR, Martz G, et al. The use of low-dose prednisone and melphalan in the treatment of poor-risk patients with multiple myeloma. *Med Pediatr Oncol* 1975;1(3):207.
54. Vesole DH, Crowley JJ, Catchatourian R, et al. High-dose melphalan with autotransplantation for refractory multiple myeloma: results of a southwest oncology group phase II trial. *J Clin Oncol* 1999;17(7):2173.
55. Norda A, Loos U, Sastry M, Goehl J, Hohenberger W. Pharmacokinetics of melphalan in isolated limb perfusion. *Cancer Chemother Pharmacol* 1999;43(1):35.
56. Goldenberg GJ, Lee M, Lam HY, Begleiter A. Evidence for carrier-mediated transport of melphalan by L5178Y lymphoblasts in vitro. *Cancer Res* 1977;37(3):755.
57. Begleiter A, Lam HY, Grover J, Froese E, Goldenberg GJ. Evidence for active transport of melphalan by two amino acid carriers in L5178Y lymphoblasts in vitro. *Cancer Res* 1979;39(1):353.
58. Vistica DT, Rabon A, Rabinovitz M. Amino acid conferred protection against melphalan: comparison of amino acids which reduce melphalan toxicity to murine bone marrow precursor cells (CFU-C) and murine L1210 leukemia cells. *Res Commun Chem Pathol Pharmacol* 1979;23(1):171.
59. Groothuis DR, Lippitz BE, Fekete I, et al. The effect of an amino acid–lowering diet on the rate of melphalan entry into brain and xenotransplanted glioma. *Cancer Res* 1992;52(20):5590.
60. Pallante SL, Fenselau C, Mennel RG, et al. Quantitation by gas chromatography–chemical ionization–mass spectrometry of phenylalanine mustard in plasma of patients. *Cancer Res* 1980;40(7):2268.
61. Hersh MR, Ludden TM, Kuhn JG, Knight WA 3rd. Pharmacokinetics of high dose melphalan. *Invest New Drugs* 1983;1(4):331.
62. Pinguet F, Martel P, Fabbro M, et al. Pharmacokinetics of high-dose intravenous melphalan in patients undergoing peripheral blood hematopoietic progenitor-cell transplantation. *Anticancer Res* 1997;17(1B):605.
63. Han T, Rai KR. Management of chronic lymphocytic leukemia. *Hematol Oncol Clin North Am* 1990;4(2):431.
64. Portlock CS, Fischer DS, Cadman E, et al. High-dose pulse chlorambucil in advanced, low-grade non-Hodgkin's lymphoma. *Cancer Treat Rep* 1987;71(11):1029.
65. Branten AJW, Reichert LJM, Koene RAP, Wetzels JFM. Oral cyclophosphamide versus chlorambucil in the treatment of patients with membranous nephropathy and renal insufficiency. *QJM* 1998;91(5):359.
66. Alberts DS, Chang SY, Chen H-SG, Larcom BJ, Evans TL. Comparative pharmacokinetics of chlorambucil and melphalan in man. *Recent Results Cancer Res* 1980;74:124.
67. Przepiorka D, Khouri I, Thall P, et al. Thiotepa, busulfan and cyclophosphamide as a preparative regimen for allogeneic transplantation for advanced chronic myelogenous leukemia. *Bone Marrow Transplant* 1999;23(10):977.
68. Andrievsky GY, Sukhodub LF, Pyatigorskaya TL, et al. Direct observation of the alkylation products of deoxyguanosine and DNA by fast atom bombardment mass spectrometry. *Biol Mass Spectrom* 1991;20(11):665.
69. Cohen NA, Egorin MJ, Snyder SW, et al. Interaction of N,N',N''-triethylenethiophosphoramide and N,N',N''-triethylenephosphoramide with cellular DNA. *Cancer Res* 1991;51(16):4360.
70. Chang TK, Chen G, Waxman DJ. Modulation of thiotepa antitumor activity in vivo by alteration of liver cytochrome P450-catalyzed drug metabolism. *J Pharmacol Exp Ther* 1995;274(1):270.
71. Kennedy MJ, Armstrong DK, Huelskamp AM, et al. Phase I and pharmacologic study of the alkylating agent modulator novobiocin in combination with high-dose chemotherapy for the treatment of metastatic breast cancer. *J Clin Oncol* 1995;13(5):1136.
72. Hussein AM, Petros WP, Ross M, et al. A phase I/II study of high dose cyclophosphamide, cisplatin, and thiotepa followed by autologous bone marrow and granulocyte colony stimulating factor-primed peripheral blood progenitor cells in patients with advanced malignancies. *Cancer Chemother Pharmacol* 1996;37(6):561.
73. Lyss AP, Luedke S, Einhorn L, Luedke DW, Raney M. Vindesine and mitomycin C in metastatic breast cancer. A Southeastern Cancer Study Group Trial. *Oncology* 1989;46(6):357.
74. Hong RL, Sheen TS, Ko JY, et al. Induction with mitomycin C, doxorubicin, cisplatin and maintenance with weekly 5-fluorouracil, leucovorin for treatment of metastatic nasopharyngeal carcinoma: a phase II study. *Br J Cancer* 1999;80(12):1962.
75. Arbuck SG, Silk Y, Douglass HO Jr, et al. A phase II trial of 5-fluorouracil, doxorubicin, mitomycin C, and leucovorin in advanced gastric carcinoma. *Cancer* 1990;65(11):2442.
76. Borowy-Borowski H, Lipman R, Chowdary D, Tomasz M. Duplex oligodeoxyribonucleotides cross-linked by mitomycin C at a single site: synthesis, properties, and cross-link reversibility. *Biochemistry* 1990;29(12):2992.
77. Tomasz M, Lipman R, Chowdary D, et al. Isolation and structure of a covalent cross-link adduct between mitomycin C and DNA. *Science* 1987;235(4793):1204.
78. Rink SM, Lipman R, Alley SC, Hopkins PH, Tomasz M. Bending of DNA by the mitomycin C-induced, GpG intrastrand cross-link. *Chem Res Toxicol* 1996;9(2):382.
79. den Hartigh J, McVie JG, van Oort WJ, Pinedo HM. Pharmacokinetics of mitomycin C in humans. *Cancer Res* 1983;43(10):5017.
80. Institoris E, Tamas J. Alkylation by 1,2:5,6-dianhydrogalactitol of deoxyribonucleic acid and guanosine. *Biochem J* 1980;185(3):659.
81. Haas CD, Baker L, Thigpen T. Phase II evaluation of dianhydrogalactitol in lung cancer: a Southwest Oncology Group Study. *Cancer Treat Rep* 1981;65(1):115.
82. Edmonson JH, Frytak S, Letendre L, Kvols LK, Eagan RT. Phase II evaluation of dianhydrogalactitol in advanced head and neck carcinomas. *Cancer Treat Rep* 1979;63(11):2081.
83. Levin VA, Edwards MS, Gutin PH, et al. Phase II evaluation of dibromodulcitol in the treatment of recurrent medulloblastoma, ependymoma, and malignant astrocytoma. *J Neurosurg* 1984;61(6):1063.
84. Nguyen HN, Nordqvist SR. Chemotherapy of advanced and recurrent cervical carcinoma. *Semin Surg Oncol* 1999;16(3):247.
85. Horvath IP, Csetenyi J, Kerpel-Fronius S, et al. Pharmacokinetics and metabolism of dianhydrogalactitol DAG in patients: a comparison with the human disposition of dibromodulcitol DBD. *Eur J Cancer Clin Oncol* 1986;22(2):163.
86. Kelley SL, Peters WP, Andersen J, et al. Pharmacokinetics of dibromodulcitol in humans: a phase I study. *J Clin Oncol* 1986;4(5):753.
87. Hartley JA, Berardini MD, Souhami RL. An agarose gel method for the determination of DNA interstrand cross-linking applicable to the measurement of the rate of total and "second-arm" cross-link reactions. *Anal Biochem* 1991;193(1):131.
88. Streeper RT, Cotter RJ, Colvin ME, Hilton J, Colvin OM. Molecular pharmacology of hepsulfam, NSC 329680l: identification of alkylated nucleosides, alkylation site, and site of DNA cross-linking. *Cancer Res* 1995;55(7):1491.
89. Haddow A, Timmis GM. Myeleran in chronic myeloid leukemia-chemical constitution and biological action. *Lancet* 1953;1:207.
90. Hehlmann R, Heimpel H, Hasford J, et al. Randomized comparison of busulfan and hydroxyurea in chronic myelogenous leukemia: prolongation of survival by hydroxyurea. The German CML Study Group. *Blood* 1993;82(2):398.
91. Ohnishi K, Tomonaga M, Kamada N, et al. A long term follow-up of a randomized trial comparing interferon-alpha with busulfan for chronic myelogenous leukemia. The Kouseisho Leukemia Study Group. *Leuk Res* 1998;22(9):779.
92. Nevill TJ, Barnett MK, Klingemann HG, et al. Regimen-related toxicity of a busulfan-cyclophosphamide conditioning regimen in 70 patients undergoing allogeneic bone marrow transplantation. *J Clin Oncol* 1991;9(7):1224.
93. Santos GW. Busulfan and cyclophosphamide versus cyclophosphamide and total body irradiation for marrow transplantation in chronic myelogenous leukemia—a review. *Leuk Lymph* 1993;1:201.
94. Chao NJ, Stein AS, Long GD, et al. Busulfan/etoposide—initial experience with a new preparatory regimen for autologous bone marrow transplantation in patients with acute nonlymphoblastic leukemia. *Blood* 1993;81(2):319.
95. Elson LA. Hematologic effects of the alkylating agents. *Ann NY Acad Sci* 1958;68:826.
96. Grochow LB, Jones RJ, Brundrett RB, et al. Pharmacokinetics of busulfan: correlation with veno-occlusive disease in patients undergoing bone marrow transplantation. *Cancer Chemother Pharmacol* 1989;25(1):55.
97. Jones RJ, Lee KS, Beschorner WE, et al. Venoocclusive disease of the liver following bone marrow transplantation. *Transplantation* 1987;44(6):778.
98. Leiter J, Schneiderman MA. Screening data from the Cancer Chemotherapy National Service Center Screening Laboratories. *Cancer Res* 1959;19(2):31.
99. Johnston TP, McCaleb GS, Montgomery JA. The synthesis of antineoplastic agents: XXXII. N-nitrosoureas. *J Med Chem* 1963;6:669.
100. Montgomery JA. Chemistry and structure-activity studies of the nitrosoureas. *Cancer Treat Rep* 1976;60(6):651.
101. Schabel FM Jr. Nitrosoureas: a review of experimental antitumor activity. *Cancer Treat Rep* 1976;60(6):665.
102. Schepartz SA. Early history and development of the nitrosoureas. *Cancer Treat Rep* 1976;60(6):647.
103. Kohn KW. Interstrand cross-linking of DNA by 1,3-bis(2-chloroethyl)-1-nitrosourea and other 1-(2-haloethyl)-1-nitrosoureas. *Cancer Res* 1977;37(5):1450.
104. Colvin M, Brundrett RB, Cowens W, Jardine I, Ludlum DB. A chemical basis for the antitumor activity of chloroethylnitrosoureas. *Biochem Pharmacol* 1976;25(6):695.
105. Tong WP, Kirk MC, Ludlum DB. Mechanism of action of the nitrosoureas: V. Formation of O^6-(2-fluoroethyl)guanine and its probable role in the cross-linking of deoxyribonucleic acid. *Biochem Pharmacol* 1983;32(13):2011.
106. Fischhaber PL, Gall AS, Duncan JA, Hopkins PB. Direct demonstration in synthetic oligonucleotides that N,N'-bis(2-chloroethyl)-nitrosourea cross-links N-1 of deoxyguanosine to N-3 of deoxycytidine on opposite strands of duplex DNA. *Cancer Res* 1999;59(17):4363.
107. Walker MD, Alexander E Jr, Hunt WE, et al. Evaluation of BCNU and/or radiotherapy in the treatment of anaplastic gliomas. A cooperative clinical trial. *J Neurosurg* 1978;49(3):333.
108. Blade J, Rozman C, Montserrat E, et al. Treatment of alkylating resistant multiple myeloma with vincristine, BCNU, doxorubicin and prednisone (VBAP). *Eur J Cancer Clin Oncol* 1986;22(10):1193.
109. Eder JP, Antman K, Peters W, et al. High-dose combination alkylating agent chemotherapy with autologous bone marrow support for metastatic breast cancer. *J Clin Oncol* 1986;4(11):1592.
110. Garfield J, Dayan AD, Weller RO. Postoperative intracavitary chemotherapy of malignant supratentorial astrocytomas using BCNU. *Clin Oncol* 1975;1(3):213.
111. Brem H, Piantadosi S, Burger PC, et al. Placebo-controlled trial of safety and efficacy of intraoperative controlled delivery by biodegradable polymers of chemotherapy for recurrent gliomas. *Lancet* 1995;345(8956):1008.
112. Paleologos NA, Macdonald DR, Vick NA, Cairncross JG. Neoadjuvant procarbazine, CCNU, and vincristine for anaplastic and aggressive oligodendroglioma. *Neurology* 1999;53(5):1141.
113. Prados MD, Scott C, Curran WJ, et al. Procarbazine, lomustine, and vincristine (PCV) chemotherapy for anaplastic astrocytoma: a retrospective review of Radiation Therapy Oncology Group protocols comparing survival with carmustine or PCV adjuvant chemotherapy. *J Clin Oncol* 1999;17(11):3389.
114. Clark JL, Barcewicz P, Nava HR, Goodwin PS, Douglass HO Jr. Adjuvant 5-FU and MeCCNU improves survival following curative gastrectomy for adenocarcinoma. *Am Surg* 1990;56(7):423.
115. Paccapelo A, Piana C, Rychlicki F, et al. Treatment of malignant gliomas: a new approach. *Tumori* 1998;84(5):529.
116. Arita N, Ushio Y, Hayakawa T, et al. Intrathecal ACNU—a new therapeutic approach against malignant leptomeningeal tumors. *J Neurooncol* 1988;6(3):221.
117. Alberts DS, Durie BG, Salmon SE. Doxorubicin/B.C.N.U. chemotherapy for multiple myeloma in relapse. *Lancet* 1976;1(7966):926.

118. Levin VA, Hoffman W, Weinkam RJ. Pharmacokinetics of BCNU in man: a preliminary study of 20 patients. *Cancer Treat Rep* 1305;62(9):1305.
119. Meisenberg BR, Ross M, Vredenburgh JJ, et al. Randomized trial of high-dose chemotherapy with autologous bone marrow support as adjuvant therapy for high-risk, multi-node-positive malignant melanoma. *J Natl Cancer Inst* 1993;85(13):1080.
120. Henner WD, Peters WP, Eder JP, et al. Pharmacokinetics and immediate effects of high-dose carmustine in man. *Cancer Treat Rep* 1986;70(7):877.
121. Levin VA, Stearns J, Byrd A, Finn A, Weinkam RJ. The effect of phenobarbital pretreatment on the antitumor activity of 1,3-bis(2-chloroethyl)-1-nitrosourea (BCNU), 1-(2-chloroethyl)-3-cyclohexyl-1-nitrosourea (CCNU) and 1-(2-chloroethyl)-3-(2,6-dioxo-3-piperidyl-1-nitrosourea (PCNU), and on the plasma pharmacokinetics and biotransformation of BCNU. *J Pharmacol Exp Ther* 1979;208(1):1.
122. Lee FY, Workman P, Roberts JT, Bleehen NM. Clinical pharmacokinetics of oral CCNU (lomustine). *Cancer Chemother Pharmacol* 1985;14(2):125.
123. DeVita VT, Carbone PP, Owens AH Jr, et al. Clinical trials with 1,3-Bis(2-chloroethyl)-1-nitrosourea, NSC-409962. *Cancer Res* 1965;25:1876.
124. Toth B. Synthetic and naturally occurring hydrazines as possible cancer causative agents. *Cancer Res* 1975;35(12):3693.
125. Silverstein R, Bhatia P, Svoboda DJ. Effect of hydrazine sulfate on glucose-regulating enzymes in the normal and cancerous rat. *Immunopharmacology* 1989;17(1):37.
126. Gold J. Use of hydrazine sulfate in terminal and preterminal cancer patients: results of investigational new drug (IND) study in 84 evaluable patients. *Oncology* 1975;32(1):1.
127. Herndon JE, Fleishman S, Kosty MP, Green MR. A longitudinal study of quality of life in advanced non-small cell lung cancer—Cancer and Leukemia Group B 8931. *Control Clin Trials* 1997;18(4):286.
128. Kamradt JM, Pienta KJ. The effect of hydrazine sulfate on prostate cancer growth. *Oncol Rep* 1998;5(4):919.
129. Spies SK, Snyman HW. Procarbazine (Natulan) in the treatment of Hodgkin's disease and other lymphomas. *S Afr Med J* 1966;40(44):1061.
130. Glick JH, Young ML, Harrington D, et al. MOPP/ABV hybrid chemotherapy for advanced Hodgkin's disease significantly improves failure-free and overall survival: the 8-year results of the intergroup trial. *J Clin Oncol* 1998;16(1):19.
131. Brandes AA, Ermani M, Turazzi S, et al. Procarbazine and high-dose tamoxifen as a second-line regimen in recurrent high-grade gliomas: a phase II study. *J Clin Oncol* 1999;17(2):645.
132. Fink D, Aebi S, Howell SB. The role of DNA mismatch repair in drug resistance. *Clin Cancer Res* 1998;4(1):1.
133. Friedman HS, Johnson SP, Dong Q, et al. Methylator resistance mediated by mismatch repair deficiency in a glioblastoma multiforme xenograft. *Cancer Res* 1997;57(14):2933.
134. Bianchini F, Weiderpass E, Kyrtopoulos S, et al. Detection of DNA methylation adducts in Hodgkin's disease patients treated with procarbazine. *Biomarkers* 1996;1(4):226.
135. Erikson JM, Tweedie DJ, Ducore JM, Prough RA. Cytotoxicity and DNA damage caused by the azoxy metabolites of procarbazine in L1210 tumor cells. *Cancer Res* 1989;49(1):127.
136. Swaffar DS, Horstman MG, Jaw JY, et al. Methylazoxyprocarbazine, the active metabolite responsible for the anticancer activity of procarbazine against L1210 leukemia. *Cancer Res* 1989;49(9):2442.
137. Massie MJ, Holland JC. Diagnosis and treatment of depression in the cancer patient. *J Clin Psychiatry* 1984;45(3):25.
138. Pfefferbaum B, Pack R, van Eys J. Monoamine oxidase inhibitor toxicity. *J Am Acad Child Adolesc Psychiatry* 1989;28(6):954.
139. Farina P, Benfenati E, Reginato R, et al. Metabolism of the anticancer agent 1-(4-acetylphenyl)-3,3-dimethyltriazene. *Biomed Mass Spectrom* 1983;10(8):485.
140. Skibba JL, Beal DD, Ramirez G, Bryan GT. N-demethylation the antineoplastic agent4(5)-(3,3-dimethyl-1-triazeno)imidazole-5(4)-carboxamide by rats and man. *Cancer Res* 1970; 30(1):147.
141. Vaughan K, Tang Y, Llanos G, et al. Studies of the mode of action of antitumor triazenes and triazines: 6. 1-Aryl-3-(hydroxymethyl)-3-methyltriazenes: synthesis, chemistry, and antitumor properties. *J Med Chem* 1984;27(3):357.
142. DeVita VT, Mauch PM, Harris NL. Hodgkin's disease. In: DeVita VT Jr, Hellman S, Rosenberg S, eds. *Cancer: principles & practice of oncology*. Philadelphia: Lippincott-Raven Publishers, 1997:2268.
143. Falkson CI, Ibrahim J, Kirkwood JM, et al. Phase III trial of dacarbazine versus dacarbazine with interferon alpha-2b versus dacarbazine with tamoxifen versus dacarbazine with interferon alpha-2b and tamoxifen in patients with metastatic malignant melanoma: an Eastern Cooperative Oncology Group study. *J Clin Oncol* 1998;16(5):1743.
144. Lowe PR, Sansom CE, Schwalbe CH, Stevens MF, Clark AS. Antitumor imidazotetrazines: 25. Crystal structure of 8-carbamoyl-3-methylimidazo[5,1-d]-1,2,3,5-tetrazin-4(3H)-one (temozolomide) and structural comparisons with the related drugs mitozolomide and DTIC. *J Med Chem* 1992;35(18):3377.
145. Denny BJ, Wheelhouse RT, Stevens MF, Tsang LL, Slack JA. NMR and molecular modeling investigation of the mechanism of activation of the antitumor drug temozolomide and its interaction with DNA. *Biochemistry* 1994;33(31):9045.
146. Nicholson HS, Krailo M, Ames MM, et al. Phase I study of temozolomide in children and adolescents with recurrent solid tumors—a report from the Children's Cancer Group. *J Clin Oncol* 1998;16(9):3037.
147. Hammond LA, Eckardt JR, Baker SD, et al. Phase I and pharmacokinetic study of temozolomide on a daily-for-5-days schedule in patients with advanced solid malignancies. *J Clin Oncol* 1999;17(8):2604.
148. Paulsen F, Hoffmann W, Becker G, et al. Chemotherapy in the treatment of recurrent glioblastoma multiforme: ifosfamide versus temozolomide. *J Cancer Res Clin Oncol* 1999;125(7):411.
149. Newlands ES, Oreilly SM, Glaser MG, et al. The Charing Cross Hospital experience with temozolomide in patients with gliomas. *Eur J Cancer* 1996;13:2236.
150. Woll PJ, Judson I, Lee SM, et al. Temozolomide in adult patients with advanced soft tissue sarcoma: a phase II study of the EORTC Soft Tissue and Bone Sarcoma Group. *Eur J Cancer* 1999;35(3):410.
151. Moore MJ, Feld R, Hedley D, Oza A, Siu LL. A Phase II study of temozolomide in advanced untreated pancreatic cancer. *Invest New Drugs* 1998;16(1):77.
152. Breithaupt H, Dammann A, Aigner K. Pharmacokinetics of dacarbazine (DTIC) and its metabolite 5-aminoimidazole-4-carboxamide (AIC) following different dose schedules. *Cancer Chemother Pharmacol* 1982;9(2):103.
153. Adkins DR, Irvin R, Kuhn J, et al. A phase I clinical and pharmacological profile of dacarbazine with autologous bone marrow transplantation in patients with solid tumors. *Invest New Drugs* 1993;11(2):169.
154. Reid JM, Stevens DC, Rubin J, Ames MM. Pharmacokinetics of 3-methyl-(triazen-1-yl)imidazole-4-carboximide following administration of temozolomide to patients with advanced cancer. *Clin Cancer Res* 1997;3(12):2393.
155. Baker SD, Wirth M, Statkevich P, et al. Absorption, metabolism, and excretion of 14C-temozolomide following oral administration to patients with advanced cancer. *Clin Cancer Res* 1999;5(2):309.
156. Friedman HS, Colvin OM, Kaufmann SH, et al. Cyclophosphamide resistance in medulloblastoma. *Cancer Res* 1992;52(19):5373.
157. Suzukake K, Petro BJ, Vistica DT. Reduction in glutathione content of L-PAM resistant L1210 cells confers drug sensitivity. *Biochem Pharmacol* 1982;31(1):121.
158. Buller AL, Clapper ML, Tew KD. Glutathione S-transferases in nitrogen mustard-resistant and -sensitive cell lines. *Mol Pharmacol* 1987;31(6):575.
159. Puchalski RB, Fahl WE. Expression of recombinant glutathione S-transferase pi, Ya, or Yb1 confers resistance to alkylating agents. *Proc Natl Acad Sci U S A* 1990;87(7):2443.
160. Townsend AI, Fields WR, Haynes RL, et al. Chemoprotective functions of glutathione S-transferases in cell lines induced to express specific isozymes by stable transfection. *Chem Biol Interact* 1998;112:389.
161. Dulik DM, Colvin OM, Fenselau C. Characterization of glutathione conjugates of chlorambucil by fast atom bombardment and thermospray liquid chromatography/mass spectrometry. *Biomed Environ Mass Spectrom* 1990;19(4):248.
162. Dulik DM, Fenselau C, Hilton J. Characterization of melphalan-glutathione adducts whose formation is catalyzed by glutathione transferases. *Biochem Pharmacol* 1986;35(19):3405.
163. Yuan ZM, Fenselau C, Dulik DM, et al. Laser desorption electron impact: application to a study of the mechanism of conjugation of glutathione and cyclophosphamide. *Anal Chem* 1990;62(8):868.
164. Bolton MG, Colvin OM, Hilton J. Specificity of isozymes of murine hepatic glutathione S-transferase for the conjugation of glutathione with L-phenylalanine mustard. *Cancer Res* 1991;51(9):2410.
165. Ciaccio PI, Tew KD, LaCreta FP. The spontaneous and glutathione S-transferase-mediated reaction of chlorambucil with glutathione. *Cancer Commun* 1990;2(8):279.
166. Dirven HA, van Ommen B, van Bladeren PI. Involvement of human glutathione S-transferase isoenzymes in the conjugation of cyclophosphamide metabolites with glutathione. *Cancer Res* 1994;54(23):6215.
167. Pallante SL, Lisek CA, Dulik DM, Fenselau C. Glutathione conjugates. Immobilized enzyme synthesis and characterization by fast atom bombardment mass spectrometry. *Drug Metab Dispos* 1986;14(3):313.
168. Horton JK, Roy G, Piper JT, et al. Characterization of a chlorambucil-resistant human ovarian carcinoma cell line overexpressing glutathione S-transferase mu. *Biochem Pharmacol* 1999;58(4):693.
169. Anderson ME. Glutathione: an overview of biosynthesis and modulation. *Chem Biol Interact* 1998;112:1.
170. Smith AC, Liao JT, Page JG, Wientjes MG, Grieshaber CK. Pharmacokinetics of buthionine sulfoximine (NSC 326231) and its effect on melphalan-induced toxicity in mice. *Cancer Res* 1989;49(19):5385.
171. Friedman HS, Colvin OM, Griffith OW, et al. Increased melphalan activity in intracranial human medulloblastoma and glioma xenografts following buthionine sulfoximine-mediated glutathione depletion. *J Natl Cancer Inst* 1989;81(7):524.
172. Bailey HH, Ripple G, Tutsch KD, et al. Phase I study of continuous-infusion L-S,R-buthionine sulfoximine with intravenous melphalan. *J Natl Cancer Inst* 1997;89(23):1789.
173. Morgan AS, Ciaccio PI, Tew KD, Kauvar LN. Isozyme specific glutathione S-transferase inhibitors potentiate drug sensitivity in cultured human tumor cell lines. *Cancer Chemother Pharmacol* 1996;37(4):363.
174. Zhang K, Yang EB, Wong KP, Mack P. GSH, GSH-related enzymes and GS-X pump in relation to sensitivity of human tumor cell lines to chlorambucil and adriamycin. *Int J Oncol* 1999;14(5):861.
175. Gupta V, Jani JP, Jacobs S, et al. Activity of melphalan in combination with the glutathione transferase inhibitor sulfasalazine. *Cancer Chemother Pharmacol* 1995;36(1):13.
176. Keppler D, Leier I, Jedlitschky G, Konig J. Atp-dependent transport of glutathione S-conjugates by the multidrug resistance protein Mrp1 and its apical isoform Mrp2. *Chem Biol Interact* 1998;112:153.
177. Barnouin K, Leier I, Jedlitschky G, et al. Multidrug resistance protein-mediated transport of chlorambucil and melphalan conjugated to glutathione. *Br J Cancer* 1998;77(2):201.
178. Kelley S, Basu A, Teicher BA, et al. Overexpression of metallothionein confers resistance to anticancer drugs. *Science* 1988;241(4874):1813.
179. Yu X, Wu Z, Fenselau C. Covalent sequestration of melphalan by metallothionein and selective alkylation of cysteines. *Biochemistry* 1995;34(10):3377.
180. Wei D, Fabris D, Fenselau C. Covalent sequestration of phosphoramide mustard by metallothionein—an in vitro study. *Drug Metab Dispos* 1999;27(7):786.
181. Satoh M, Cherian MG, Imura N, Shimizu H. Modulation of resistance to anticancer drugs by inhibition of metallothionein synthesis. *Cancer Res* 1994;54(20):5255.
182. Pegg AE, Boosalis M, Samson L, et al. Mechanism of inactivation of human O^6-alkylguanine-DNA alkyltransferase by O^6-benzylguanine. *Biochemistry* 1993;32(45):11998.

183. Pegg AE. Mammalian O^6-alkylguanine-DNA alkyltransferase: regulation and importance in response to alkylating carcinogenic and therapeutic agents. *Cancer Res* 1990;50(19):6119.
184. Erickson LC, Laurent G, Sharkey NA, Kohn KW. DNA cross-linking and monoadduct repair in nitrosourea-treated human tumour cells. *Nature* 1980;288(5792):727.
185. Bodell WJ, Tokuda K, Ludlum DB. Differences in DNA alkylation products formed in sensitive and resistant human glioma cells treated with N-(2-chloroethyl)-N-nitrosourea. *Cancer Res* 1988;48(16):4489.
186. Dolan ME, Moschel RC, Pegg AE. Depletion of mammalian O^6-alkylguanine-DNA alkyltransferase activity by O^6-benzylguanine provides a means to evaluate the role of this protein in protection against carcinogenic and therapeutic alkylating agents. *Proc Natl Acad Sci U S A* 1990;87(14):5368.
187. Gerson SL, Berger SI, Varnes ME, Donovan C. Combined depletion of O^6-alkylguanine-DNA alkyltransferase and glutathione to modulate nitrosourea resistance in breast cancer. *Biochem Pharmacol* 1994;48(3):543.
188. Cussac C, Rapp M, Mounetou E, et al. Enhancement by O^6-benzyl-N-acetylguanosine derivatives of chloroethylnitrosourea antitumor action in chloroethylnitrosourea-resistant human malignant melanocytes. *J Pharmacol Exp Ther* 1994;271(3):1353.
189. Friedman HS, Kokkinakis DM, Pluda J, et al. Phase I trial of O-6-benzylguanine for patients undergoing surgery for malignant glioma. *J Clin Oncol* 1998;16(11):3570.
190. Spiro TP, Gerson SL, Liu LL, et al. O-6-benzylguanine: a clinical trial establishing the biochemical modulatory dose in tumor tissue for alkyltransferase-directed DNA repair. *Cancer Res* 1999;59(10):2402.
191. Allay JA, Dumenco LL, Koc ON, Liu L, Gerson SL. Retroviral transduction and expression of the human alkyltransferase cDNA provides nitrosourea resistance to hematopoietic cells. *Blood* 1995;85(11):3342.
192. Koc ON, Reese JS, Davis BM, et al. Delta MGMT-transduced bone marrow infusion increases tolerance to O-6-benzylguanine and 1,3-bis(2-chloroethyl)-1-nitrosourea and allows intensive therapy of 1,3-bis(2-chloroethyl)-1-nitrosourea-resistant human colon cancer xenografts. *Hum Gene Ther* 1999;10(6):1021.
193. Kohn KW, Steigbigel NH, Spears CL. Cross-linking and repair of DNA in sensitive and resistant strains of *E. coli* treated with nitrogen mustard. *Proc Natl Acad Sci U S A* 1154;53(5):1154.
194. Crathorn AR, Roberts JJ. Mechanism of the cytotoxic action of alkylating agents in mammalian cells and evidence for the removal of alkylated groups from deoxyribonucleic acid. *Nature* 1966;211(45):150.
195. Sancar A. Mechanisms of DNA excision repair. *Science* 1994;266(5193):1954.
196. Stevnsner T, Ding R, Smulson M, Bohr VA. Inhibition of gene-specific repair of alkylation damage in cells depleted of poly(ADP-ribose) polymerase. *Nucleic Acids Res* 1994;22(22):4620.
197. Das SK, Lau CC, Pardee A. Comparative analysis of caffeine and 3-aminobenzamide as DNA repair inhibitors in Syrian baby hamster kidney cells. *Mutat Res* 1984;131(2):71.
198. O'Connor PM, Ferris DK, White GA, et al. Relationships between cdc2 kinase, DNA cross-linking, and cell cycle perturbations induced by nitrogen mustard. *Cell Growth Differ* 1992;3(1):43.
199. O'Connor PM, Ferris DK, Hoffmann I, et al. Role of the cdc25C phosphatase in G2 arrest induced by nitrogen mustard. *Proc Natl Acad Sci U S A* 1994;91(20):9480.
200. Selby CP, Sancar A. Molecular mechanisms of DNA repair inhibition by caffeine. *Proc Natl Acad Sci U S A* 1990;87(9):3522.
201. Walton MI, Whysong D, O'Connor PM, et al. Constitutive expression of human Bcl-2 modulates nitrogen mustard and camptothecin induced apoptosis. *Cancer Res* 1993;53(8):1853.
202. Dong Q, Johnson SP, Colvin OM, et al. Multiple DNA repair mechanisms and alkylator resistance in the human medulloblastoma cell line D-283 Med (4-HCR). *Cancer Chemother Pharmacol* 1999;43(1):73.
203. Kobayashi H, Man S, Graham CH, et al. Acquired multicellular-mediated resistance to alkylating agents in cancer. *Proc Natl Acad Sci U S A* 1993;90(8):3294.
204. St Croix B, Man S, Kerbel RS. Reversal of intrinsic and acquired forms of drug resistance by hyaluronidase treatment of solid tumors. *Cancer Lett* 1998;131(1):35.
205. Kerbel RS, Kobayashi H, Graham CH. Intrinsic or acquired drug resistance and metastasis: are they linked phenotypes? *J Cell Biochem* 1994;56(1):37.
206. Mullins GM, Anderson PN, Santos GW. High dose cyclophosphamide therapy in solid tumors. Therapeutic, toxic, and immunosuppressive effects. *Cancer* 1950;36(6):1950.
207. Fried W, Kedo A, Barone J. Effects of cyclophosphamide and of busulfan on spleen colony-forming units and on hematopoietic stroma. *Cancer Res* 1977;37(4):1205.
208. Borison HL, Brand ED, Orland RK. Emetic action of nitrogen mustard in dogs and cats. *Am J Physiol* 1968;192:410.
209. Fetting JH, McCarthy LE, Borison HL, Colvin M. Vomiting induced by cyclophosphamide and phosphoramide mustard in cats. *Cancer Treat Rep* 1982;66(8):1625.
210. Spitzer TR, Grunberg SM, Dicato MA. Antiemetic strategies for high-dose chemoradiotherapy-induced nausea and vomiting. *Support Care Cancer* 1998;6(3):233.
211. Perez EA. 5-HT3 antiemetic therapy for patients with breast cancer. *Breast Cancer Res Treat* 1999;57(2):207.
212. Bauduer F, Coiffier B, Desablens B. Granisetron plus or minus alprazolam for emesis prevention in chemotherapy of lymphomas: a randomized multicenter trial. *Leuk Lymph* 1999;34(3-4):341.
213. Antman K, Eder JP, Elias A, et al. High-dose thiotepa alone and in combination regimens with bone marrow support. *Semin Oncol* 1990;17[Suppl 3]:33.
214. Spitz S. The histological effects of nitrogen mustards on human tumors and tissues. *Cancer* 1948;1:383.
215. Miller DG. Alkylating agents and human spermatogenesis. *JAMA* 1971;217(12):1662.
216. Sherins RJ, DeVita VT Jr. Effect of drug treatment for lymphoma on male reproductive capacity. Studies of men in remission after therapy. *Ann Intern Med* 1973;79(2):216.
217. Blake DA, Heller RH, Hsu SH, Schacter BZ. Return of fertility in a patient with cyclophosphamide-induced azoospermia. *Johns Hopkins Med J* 1976;139(1):20.
218. Hinkes E, Plotkin D. Reversible drug-induced sterility in a patient with acute leukemia. *JAMA* 1490;223(13):1490.
219. Galton DAG, Till M, Wiltshaw E. Busulfan (1,4-dimethanesulfonyloxybutane, Myeleran): summary of clinical results. *Ann NY Acad Sci* 1958;68:967.
220. Rose DP, Davis TE. Ovarian function in patients receiving adjuvant chemotherapy for breast cancer. *Lancet* 1977;1(8023):1174.
221. Koyama H, Wada T, Nishizawa Y, Iwanaga T, Aoki Y. Cyclophosphamide-induced ovarian failure and its therapeutic significance in patients with breast cancer. *Cancer* 1403;39(4):1403.
222. Oliner H, Schwartz R, Rubio FJ. Interstitial pulmonary fibrosis following busulfan therapy. *Am J Med* 1961;31:134.
223. Codling BW, Chakera TM. Pulmonary fibrosis following therapy with melphalan for multiple myeloma. *J Clin Pathol* 1972;25(8):668.
224. Cole SR, Myers TJ, Klatsky AU. Pulmonary disease with chlorambucil therapy. *Cancer* 1978;41(2):455.
225. Mark GJ, Lehimgar-Zadeh A, Ragsdale BD. Cyclophosphamide pneumonitis. *Thorax* 1978;33(1):89.
226. Patel AR, Shah PC, Rhee HL, Sassoon H, Rao KP. Cyclophosphamide therapy and interstitial pulmonary fibrosis. *Cancer* 1976;38(4):1542.
227. Orwoll ES, Kiessling PJ, Patterson JR. Interstitial pneumonia from mitomycin. *Ann Intern Med* 1978;89(3):352.
228. Bailey CC, Marsden HB, Jones PH. Fatal pulmonary fibrosis following 1,3-bis(2-chloroethyl)-1-nitrosourea (BCNU) therapy. *Cancer* 1978;42(1):74.
229. Holoye PY, Jenkins DE, Greenberg SD. Pulmonary toxicity in long-term administration of BCNU. *Cancer Treat Rep* 1976;60(11):1691.
230. Litam JP, Dail DH, Spitzer G, et al. Early pulmonary toxicity after administration of high-dose BCNU. *Cancer Treat Rep* 1981;65(1):39.
231. Wilczynski SW, Erasmus JJ, Petros WP, Vredenburgh JJ, Folz RJ. Delayed pulmonary toxicity syndrome following high-dose chemotherapy and bone marrow transplantation for breast cancer. *Am J Respir Crit Care Med* 1998;157(2):565.
232. Colvin M, Cowens JW, Brundrett RB, Kramer BS, Ludlum DB. Decomposition of BCNU (1,3-bis(2-chloroethyl)-1-nitrosourea) in aqueous solution. *Biochem Biophys Res Commun* 1974;60(2):515.
233. Vijayan VK, Sankaran K. Relationship between lung inflammation, changes in lung function and severity of exposure in victims of the Bhopal tragedy. *Eur Respir J* 1977;9(10):1977.
234. Bierman HR, Kelly KH, Knudson AG Jr, Maekawa T, Timmis GM. The influence of 1,4-dimethylsulfonoxy-1,4-dimethylbutane (CB 2348, dimethylmyeleran) in neoplastic disease. *Ann NY Acad Sci* 1968;68:1211.
235. Feil VJ, Lamoureux CH. Alopecia activity of cyclophosphamide metabolites and related compounds in sheep. *Cancer Res* 1974;34(10):2596.
236. Bodenstein D, Goldin A. A comparison of the effects of various nitrogen mustard compounds on embryonic cells. *J Exp Zool* 1948;108:75.
237. Murphy ML, Del Moro A, Lacon C. The comparative effects of five polyfunctional alkylating agents on the rat fetus, with additional notes on the chick embryo. *Ann NY Acad Sci* 1958;68:762.
238. Hales BF. Effects of phosphoramide mustard and acrolein, cytotoxic metabolites of cyclophosphamide, on mouse limb development in vitro. *Teratology* 1989;40(1):11.
239. Mirkes PE. Cyclophosphamide teratogenesis: a review. *Teratog Carcinog Mutagen* 1985;5(2):75.
240. Nicholson HO. Cytotoxic drugs in pregnancy. Review of reported cases. *J Obstet Gynaecol Br Comm* 1968;75(3):307.
241. Lergier JE, Jimenez E, Maldonado N, Veray F. Normal pregnancy in multiple myeloma treated with cyclophosphamide. *Cancer* 1974;34(4):1018.
242. Ortega J. Multiple agent chemotherapy including bleomycin of non-Hodgkin's lymphoma during pregnancy. *Cancer* 1977;40(6):2829.
243. Reichman BS, Green KB. Breast cancer in young women: effect of chemotherapy on ovarian function, fertility, and birth defects. *J Natl Cancer Inst Monogr* 1994;16:125.
244. Aviles A, Diaz-Maqueo JC, Talavera A, Guzman R, Garcia EL. Growth and development of children of mothers treated with chemotherapy during pregnancy: current status of 43 children. *Am J Hematol* 1991;36(4):243.
245. Hochberg MC, Shulman LE. Acute leukemia following cyclophosphamide therapy for Sjögren's syndrome. *Johns Hopkins Med J* 1978;142(6):211.
246. Rosner F, Grunwald H. Multiple myeloma terminating in acute leukemia. Report of 12 cases and review of the literature. *Am J Med* 1974;57(6):927.
247. Rosner F, Grunwald H. Hodgkin's disease and acute leukemia. Report of eight cases and review of the literature. *Am J Med* 1975;58(3):339.
248. Einhorn N. Acute leukemia after chemotherapy (melphalan). *Cancer* 1978;41(2):444.
249. Reimer RR, Hoover R, Fraumeni JF Jr, Young RC. Acute leukemia after alkylating-agent therapy of ovarian cancer. *N Engl J Med* 1977;297(4):177.
250. Greene MH, Harris EL, Gershenson DM, et al. Melphalan may be a more potent leukemogen than cyclophosphamide. *Ann Intern Med* 1986;105(3):360.
251. Einhorn N, Eklund G, Lambert B. Solid tumours and chromosome aberrations as late side effects of melphalan therapy in ovarian carcinoma. *Acta Oncol* 1988;27(3):215.
252. Tucker MA, Coleman CN, Cox RS, Varghese A, Rosenberg SA. Risk of second cancers after treatment for Hodgkin's disease. *N Engl J Med* 1988;318(2):76.
253. Hektoen L, Corper HJ. The effect of mustard gas (dichloroethylsulphide) on antibody formation. *J Infect Dis* 1921;28:279.
254. Makinodan T, Santos GW, Quinn RP. Immunosuppressive drugs. *Pharmacol Rev* 1970;22(2):189.
255. Barratt TM, Soothill JF. Controlled trial of cyclophosphamide in steroid-sensitive relapsing nephrotic syndrome of childhood. *Lancet* 1970;2(7671):479.
256. Laros RKJ, Penner JA. "Refractory" thrombocytopenic purpura treated successfully with cyclophosphamide. *JAMA* 1971;215(3):445.
257. Kleta R. Cyclophosphamide and mercaptoethane sulfonate therapy for minimal lesion glomerulonephritis. *Kidney Int* 1999;56(6):2312.

258. Bargman JM. Management of minimal lesion glomerulonephritis: evidence-based recommendations. *Kidney Int* 1999;55[Suppl 70]:S3.
259. Viallard JF, Pellegrin JL, Vergnes C, et al. Three cases of acquired von Willebrand disease associated with systemic lupus erythematosus. *Br J Haematol* 1999;105(2):532.
260. Ozer H, Cowens JW, Colvin M, Nussbaum-Blumenson A, Sheedy D. In vitro effects of 4-hydroperoxycyclophosphamide on human immunoregulatory T subset function: I. Selective effects on lymphocyte function in T-B cell collaboration. *J Exp Med* 1982; 155(1):276.
261. Smith JJ, Mihich E, Ozer H. In vitro effects of 4-hydroxyperoxycyclophosphamide on human immunoregulatory T subset function. *Methods Find Exp Clin Pharmacol* 1987;9(9):555.
262. Mokyr MB, Colvin M, Dray S. Cyclophosphamide-mediated enhancement of antitumor immune potential of immunosuppressed spleen cells from mice bearing a large MOPC-315 tumor. *Int J Immunopharmacol* 1985;7(1):111.
263. Dray S, Mokyr MB. Cyclophosphamide and melphalan as immunopotentiating agents in cancer therapy. *Med Oncol Tumor Pharmacother* 1989;6(1):77.
264. Berd D, Mastrangelo MJ. Effect of low dose cyclophosphamide on the immune system of cancer patients: depletion of CD4+, 2H4+ suppressor-inducer T-cells. *Cancer Res* 1988;48(6):1671.
265. Berd D, Mastrangelo MJ. Active immunotherapy of human melanoma exploiting the immunopotentiating effects of cyclophosphamide. *Cancer Invest* 1988;6(3):337.
266. Mitchell MS, Kempf RA, Harel W, et al. Effectiveness and tolerability of low-dose cyclophosphamide and low-dose intravenous interleukin-2 in disseminated melanoma. *J Clin Oncol* 1988;6(3):409.
267. Santos GW, Sensenbrenner LL, Anderson PN, et al. HL-A-identical marrow transplants in aplastic anemia, acute leukemia, and lymphosarcoma employing cyclophosphamide. *Transplant Proc* 1976;8(4):607.
268. Burt RK, Traynor AE. Hematopoietic stem cell transplantation: a new therapy for autoimmune disease. *Stem Cells* 1999;17(6):366.
269. Wulffraat N, van Royen A, Bierings M, et al. Autologous haemopoietic stem-cell transplantation in four patients with refractory juvenile chronic arthritis. *Lancet* 1999;353(9152):550.
270. Brodsky RA, Sensenbrenner LL, Jones RJ. Complete remission in severe aplastic anemia after high-dose cyclophosphamide without bone marrow transplantation. *Blood* 1996;87(2):491.
271. Nousari HC, Brodsky RA, Jones RJ, Grever MR, Anhalt GJ. Immunoablative high-dose cyclophosphamide without stem cell rescue in paraneoplastic pemphigus: report of a case and review of this new therapy for severe autoimmune disease. *J Am Acad Dermatol* 1999;40(5):750.

SECTION **4**

STEVEN W. JOHNSON
JAMES P. STEVENSON
PETER J. O'DWYER

Cisplatin and Its Analogues

The platinum drugs represent a unique and important class of antitumor compounds. Alone or in combination with other chemotherapeutic drugs, *cis*-diamminedichloroplatinum (II) (cisplatin) and its analogues have made a significant impact on the treatment of a variety of solid tumors. The realization that platinum complexes exhibit antitumor activity arose somewhat serendipitously in a series of experiments carried out by Rosenberg and colleagues beginning in 1961.[1] These studies involved determining the effect of electromagnetic radiation on the growth of bacteria in a chamber equipped with a set of platinum electrodes. Exposure of the bacteria to an electric field resulted in a profound change in their morphology and, in particular, the appearance of long filaments that were several hundred times longer than that of their untreated counterparts. This effect was not due to the electric field directly, but to the electrolysis products produced from the platinum electrodes. An analysis of these products revealed that the predominant species was ammonium chloroplatinate $[NH_4]_2[PtCl_6]$. This compound was inactive at reproducing the filamentous growth originally observed; however, Rosenberg and colleagues[1] soon discovered that the conversion of this complex to a neutral species by UV light resulted in an active species. Attempts to synthesize the active neutral platinum complex failed. They realized, however, that the neutral compound could exist in two isomeric forms, *cis* or *trans*, and that the latter species is the one they had synthesized. Subsequently, the *cis* isomer was synthesized and shown to be the active compound.

The observation that *cis*-diamminedichloroplatinum (II) and *cis*-diamminetetrachloroplatinum (IV) inhibited bacterial growth led to the testing of four neutral platinum compounds for antineoplastic activity in mice bearing the Sarcoma-180 solid tumor and L1210 leukemia cells.[2] All four compounds showed significant antitumor activity, with *cis*-diamminedichloroplatinum (II) exhibiting the most efficacy. Further studies in other tumor models confirmed these results and indicated that cisplatin exhibited a broad spectrum of activity. Although early clinical trials demonstrated significant activity against several tumor types, particularly testicular tumors, the severe renal and gastrointestinal toxicity caused by the drug nearly led to its abandonment. Cvitkovic et al.[3,4] showed that these effects could be ameliorated, in part, by aggressive prehydration, which rekindled interest in its clinical use. Currently, cisplatin is curative in testicular cancer and significantly prolongs survival in combination regimens for ovarian cancer. The drug also has therapeutic benefit in head and neck, bladder, and lung cancer.[5]

The unique activity and toxicity profile observed with cisplatin has fueled the development of platinum analogues that are less toxic and more effective against a variety of tumor types, including those that have developed resistance to cisplatin. Two other platinum drugs are widely used: *cis*-diamminecyclobutanedicarboxylato platinum (II) (carboplatin) and 1,2-diaminocyclohexaneoxalato platinum (II) (oxaliplatin). Several new analogues with unique activities are currently in various stages of clinical development. Continued progress in the development of superior analogues requires a thorough understanding of the chemical, biological, pharmacokinetic, and pharmacodynamic properties of this important class of drugs. A review of these properties is the focus of this chapter.

PLATINUM CHEMISTRY

Platinum exists primarily in either a 2+ or 4+ oxidation state. These oxidation states dictate the stereochemistry of the carrier ligands and leaving groups surrounding the platinum atom. Platinum (II) compounds exhibit a square planar geometry, whereas platinum (IV) compounds exhibit an octahedral geometry. Interconversion of the two oxidation states may readily occur. However, the kinetics of this reaction depend on the nature of the bound ligands. The nature of the ligands also determines the stability of the complex and the rate of substitution. For platinum (II) compounds, the rate of substitution of a ligand is strongly influenced by the type of ligand located opposite to it. Therefore, ligands that are bound more strongly stabilize the moieties that are situated *trans* to it. For *cis*-diamminedichloroplatinum (II), the two chloride ligands are prone to substitution, whereas substitution of the amino groups is thermodynamically unfavorable.[6] The stereochemistry of platinum complexes is critical to their antitumor activity, as evidenced by the significantly reduced efficacy observed with *trans*-diamminedichloroplatinum (II).

In aqueous solution, the chloride leaving groups of cisplatin are subject to mono- and diaqua substitution, particularly at chloride concentrations below 100 mmol, which exist intracellularly. The equilibria may be described by the following two equations:

$$cis\text{-}(NH_3)_2PtCl_2 + H_2O \leftrightharpoons Cl^- + cis\text{-}(NH_3)_2PtCl(H_2O)^+$$

$$cis\text{-}(NH_3)_2PtCl(H_2O)^+ + H_2O \leftrightharpoons Cl^- + cis\text{-}(NH_3)_2Pt(H_2O)_2^{\,2+}$$

where equilibria constants for each reaction may be written

$$K_1 = \frac{[Cl^-][cis-(NH_3)_2PtCl(H_2O)^+]}{[cis-(NH_3)_2PtCl_2]} \text{ and}$$

$$K_2 = \frac{[Cl^-][cis-(NH_3)_2Pt(H_2O)_2^{2+}]}{[cis-(NH_3)_2PtCl(H_2O)^+]}$$

These descriptions illustrate the key role of ambient chloride concentrations in determining aquation rates. In weakly acidic solutions, the monochloromonoaqua and diaqua complexes become deprotonated to form the neutral dihydroxo species. The monohydroxo and dihydroxo complexes are the predominant species present in low chloride-containing environments, such as the nucleus. A detailed analysis of the equations and rate constants that govern these reactions has been published.[7] Based on studies of the reaction of cisplatin metabolites with inosine, the predominant cisplatin species that react with DNA are likely to be the chloroaqua and hydroxoaqua species.[7]

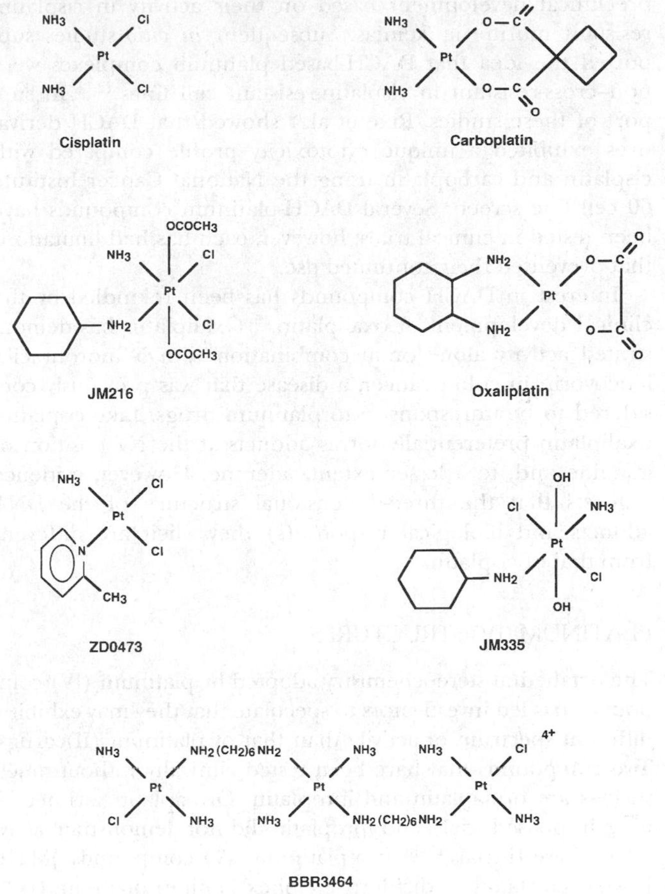

FIGURE 19.4-1. Structures of platinum complexes.

EVOLUTION OF NOVEL PLATINUM COMPLEXES

Cisplatin therapy has two major limitations: an undesirable toxicity profile and the development of resistance by tumor cells. Therefore, substantial effort has gone into developing analogues that are less toxic, with a different spectrum of antitumor activity. Progress in understanding the chemistry and pharmacokinetics of cisplatin has guided the development of new analogues. In general, modification of the chloride leaving groups of cisplatin results in compounds with different pharmacokinetics, whereas modification of the carrier ligands alters the activity of the resulting complex. This section summarizes the features of the more important platinum analogues that have been developed, which are shown in Figure 19.4-1.

CARBOPLATIN

The search for a less toxic platinum drug, pursued at the Institute for Cancer Research in the United Kingdom, led to the development of carboplatin.[8,9] It was hypothesized that modification of cisplatin to contain a more stable leaving group could alter toxicity without necessarily influencing the cytotoxicity profile. Using a murine screen for nephrotoxicity, it was discovered that substituting a cyclobutanedicarboxylate moiety for the two chloride ligands of cisplatin resulted in a complex with reduced renal toxicity. Instead, myelosuppression was dose-limiting, a toxicity that is not associated with cisplatin therapy. At effective doses, carboplatin produces less nausea, vomiting, nephrotoxicity, and neurotoxicity than cisplatin and has demonstrated essentially equivalent survival rates in ovarian cancer patients. Similar findings have been observed in other solid tumors. Therefore, based on its superior therapeutic index, greater ease of administration, and more predictable individualized dosing, carboplatin has replaced cisplatin in many chemotherapeutic regimens.

1,2-DIAMINOCYCLOHEXANE DERIVATIVES

The example of carboplatin provided a paradigm for the development of other platinum coordination compounds with modified leaving groups. However, the antitumor activity of these drugs generally overlap, and they are not considered effective for the treatment of cisplatin-resistant disease. Therefore, the development of platinum analogues that produce responses in cisplatin/carboplatin-resistant tumors became necessary, and it was hypothesized that modifying the carrier ligands might achieve this. The antitumor activity of a series of platinum compounds containing the 1,2-diaminocyclohexane (DACH) carrier ligand was initially described by Connors et al.[10] in 1972. Several of these compounds exhibited a significantly higher therapeutic index compared with cisplatin using a murine ADJ/PC6A tumor model. Kidani et al.[11] also reported significant antitumor activity of DACH platinum complexes. Burchenal and colleagues[12] selected several DACH derivatives for preclinical development based on their activity in cisplatin-resistant murine leukemias. Subsequent *in vitro* studies supported the idea that DACH-based platinum complexes were non–cross-resistant in cisplatin-resistant cell lines.[12,13] In support of these studies, Rixe et al.[14] showed that DACH derivatives exhibited a unique cytotoxicity profile compared with cisplatin and carboplatin using the National Cancer Institute 60 cell line screen. Several DACH-platinum compounds have been tested in clinical trials; however, each has had limitations that prevented their continued use.

Interest in DACH compounds has been rekindled by the clinical development of oxaliplatin.[15] Oxaliplatin has demonstrated activity alone or in combination with 5-fluorouracil/leucovorin in colon cancer, a disease that was previously considered to be unresponsive to platinum drugs. Like cisplatin, oxaliplatin preferentially forms adducts at the N7 position of guanine and, to a lesser extent, adenine. However, evidence suggests that the three-dimensional structure of the DNA adducts and biological response(s) they elicit are different from that of cisplatin.

PLATINUM (IV) STRUCTURES

The octahedral stereochemistry adopted by platinum (IV) compounds has led investigators to speculate that they may exhibit a different spectrum of activity than that of platinum (II) drugs. Two compounds that have been tested clinically without much success are ormaplatin and iproplatin. Ormaplatin was neurotoxic in phase I trials, and iproplatin did not demonstrate activity in phase II trials.[16–18] Two platinum (IV) compounds, JM216 [bis(acetato)amminedichloro(cyclohexylamine) platinum (IV)] and JM335 [*trans*-ammine(cyclohexylamine)dichlorodihydroxo platinum (IV)], have been developed in the United Kingdom and contain several unique features.[19] These compounds may also be classified as mixed amines or ammine/amine platinum (IV) complexes. JM216 is the first orally active platinum compound and is currently undergoing phase II testing. A response rate of 38% was observed in patients with small cell lung cancer[20]; however, no significant antitumor activity was observed in patients with non–small cell lung cancer.[21] Based on the lack of antitumor activity of transplatin [*trans*-diamminedichloroplatinum (II)], it has been generally believed that most, if not all, *trans* platinum compounds were inactive. Renewed interest in *trans* compounds has occurred, however, with the observation that JM335 and a related group of complexes exhibited significant antitumor activity in murine ADJ/PC6 and human ovarian cancer models.[19] Khokhar and colleagues[22] also have produced *trans*-platinum (IV) compounds containing the DACH moiety that they demonstrated to be non–cross-resistant to cisplatin.

MULTINUCLEAR PLATINUM COMPLEXES

The synthesis and preclinical studies of multinuclear platinum compounds was first reported by Farrell et al.[23] These compounds are unique in that their interaction with DNA is considerably different from that of cisplatin, particularly in the abundance of interstrand cross-links formed. Also, the observation that multinuclear platinum complexes containing the *trans* geometry exhibit antitumor activity contradicts the original dogma that platinum drugs containing the *trans* geometry are inactive. Currently, the lead compound in this class of drugs is BBR3464. Its structure is described as two *trans*-$[PtCl(NH_3)_2]^+$ units linked together by a noncovalent tetraamine $[Pt(NH_3)_2[H_2N(CH_2)_6NH_2]_2]^{2+}$ unit. Preclinical testing of BBR3464 shows it to be significantly more potent than cisplatin and to be active in cisplatin-resistant xenografts and p53 mutant tumors. Preliminary data from a phase I clinical trial of BBR3464 have indicated that diarrhea and myelosuppression are dose-limiting (P. Calvert, H. Calvert, C. Sessa, G. Camboni, personal communication, 1999). In this study, a partial response was observed in a patient with metastatic pancreatic cancer.

OTHER PLATINUM COMPLEXES

Another approach for the design of novel platinum analogues is to identify compounds that can circumvent specific cisplatin resistance mechanisms. An example of this is ZD0473 (AMD473) [*cis*-amminedichloro(2-methylpyridine) platinum (II)], which is a sterically hindered platinum complex that was designed to preferentially react with nucleic acids instead of thiol-containing molecules such as glutathione.[19] ZD0473 exhibits activity against acquired cisplatin-resistant cell lines and is active when administered by oral or intraperitoneal routes in human ovarian cancer xenografts.[24,25] The results of a phase I clinical trial have indicated that myelosuppression is dose-limiting and that nephrotoxicity, neuropathy, and ototoxicity are not prominent.[26] Antitumor activity was observed in previously platinum-treated head and neck and ovarian cancer patients.

MECHANISM OF ACTION

DNA ADDUCT FORMATION

The observation by Rosenberg[2] that cisplatin induces filamentous growth in bacteria without affecting RNA and protein synthesis implicated DNA as the cytotoxic target of the drug. Evidence from several subsequent experiments supported this idea.[27–31] The differential cytotoxic effects observed with platinum drugs are determined, in part, by the structure and relative amount of DNA adducts formed. Cisplatin and its analogues react preferentially at the N7 position of guanine and adenine residues to form a variety of monofunctional and bifunctional adducts.[32] The first step of the reaction involves the formation of monoadducts. These monoadducts may then react further to form intrastrand or interstrand cross-links. The predominant bidentate lesions that are formed with DNA *in vitro* or in cultured cells are the d(GpG)Pt, d(ApG)Pt, and d(GpNpG)Pt intrastrand cross-links. In a study of cisplatin-treated Chinese hamster ovary (CHO) cells, these lesions were determined to account for approximately 60%, 15%, and 20% of the total platinum DNA adducts, respectively.[33] Cisplatin also forms interstrand cross-links between guanine residues located on opposite strands that account for less than 5% of the total DNA bound platinum. These adducts may contribute to the drug's cytotoxicity, because they impede certain cellular processes that require the separation of both DNA strands, such as replication and transcription.

The adducts that are formed between the reaction of carboplatin with DNA in cultured cells are essentially the same as that of cisplatin. However, higher concentrations of carboplatin are required (20- to 40-fold for cells) to obtain equivalent total platinum-DNA adduct levels because of cisplatin's slower rate of aquation.[34] The relative amounts of each lesion are different, with the d(GpNpG)Pt intrastrand adduct being the most prevalent (approximately 40%) followed by the d(GpG)Pt (approximately 30%) and d(ApG)Pt (approximately 15%) intrastrand adducts, respectively.[33] As with cisplatin, a relatively low number of monoadducts and interstrand cross-links are observed. The relative amounts and frequencies of the DNA adducts formed in cultured cells by oxaliplatin have also been examined. Oxaliplatin intrastrand adducts form more slowly because of a slower rate of conversion from monoadducts; however, they are formed at similar DNA sequences and regions as cisplatin adducts. Saris et al.[35] reported that oxaliplatin forms predominantly d(GpG)Pt and d(ApG)Pt intrastrand cross-links *in vitro* and in cultured cells. At equitoxic doses, however, oxaliplatin forms fewer DNA adducts compared with cisplatin. This suggests that oxaliplatin lesions are more cytotoxic than those formed by cisplatin.

The differences observed in cytotoxicity between the diamine (e.g., cisplatin, carboplatin) and DACH platinum compounds is not dependent on the type and relative amounts of the adducts formed, but more likely due to the overall three-dimensional structure of the adduct and its recognition by various cellular proteins. Structural analysis of the cisplatin d(GpG)Pt intrastrand cross-link has been accomplished by both x-ray crystallography and nuclear magnetic resonance spectroscopy. These studies revealed that the binding of platinum to DNA causes a variety of perturbations in the double helix, including a roll of 26° to 50°C between the cross-linked guanine bases, displacement of platinum from the planes of the guanine rings, a bend of the helical axis toward the major groove, and an unwinding of the DNA.[36] Scheef et al.[37] used computer modeling to demonstrate that oxaliplatin produces a similar DNA bend, base rotation, and base propeller as cisplatin. The major difference, however, is the protrusion of the DACH moiety of oxaliplatin into the major groove of DNA, thus producing a bulkier adduct than that of cisplatin. This bulkier, more hydrophobic adduct may be recognized differently by a host of cellular proteins involved in sensing DNA damage.[38] The functional consequence of these effects are twofold: Proteins, such as polymerases, that recognize and participate in reactions on DNA under normal circumstances may be perturbed, whereas processes that are controlled by proteins that recognize damaged DNA may become activated. The latter group of proteins may function in the DNA repair process or in the initiation of programmed cell death.

PLATINUM-DNA DAMAGE–RECOGNITION PROTEINS

Several damage-recognition proteins have been identified that preferentially bind to DNA damaged by cisplatin, but not to the inactive transplatin isomer.[39,40] The first of these to be discovered were the HMG1 (high mobility group 1) and HMG2 proteins. These proteins are capable of bending DNA as well as recognizing bent DNA structures, such as that produced by cisplatin binding. The HMG domain, which consists of a highly basic 80 amino acid motif, has been found in other proteins, most of which are involved in gene expression.[41] Although many theories exist as to how HMG proteins may influence cisplatin sensitivity, relationships between HMG protein function and expression have not yet been clearly established. Recognition of platinum-DNA adducts by the mismatch repair (MMR) complex also has been implicated in cisplatin sensitivity.[42] For example, the MSH2 (MutS homologue) and MLH1 (MutL homologue) proteins participate in the recognition of DNA adducts formed by cisplatin.[43,44] The presence of a platinum lesion results in a continuous futile cycle of repair synthesis on the DNA strand opposite the lesion, possibly causing the accumulation of DNA strand breaks that may result in cell death. Interestingly, oxaliplatin adducts are not recognized by this MMR protein complex, which may account for differences in the cytotoxic mechanism of the two platinum compounds.

PLATINUM DRUG–INDUCED CELL DEATH

The sequence of events that lead to cell death after the formation of platinum-DNA adducts have not yet been elucidated. However, cells treated with platinum drugs display the biochemical and morphologic features of apoptosis.[45] These features are common to cells treated with other cytotoxic and biological agents. Therefore, understanding the pathway(s) that are involved in the early stages of programmed cell death, including the detection/initiation and decision/commitment phases, are important for understanding the unique activities of platinum drugs. The sensitivity of a cell to a platinum drug depends, in part, on cell cycle. For example, proliferating cells are relatively sensitive, whereas quiescent cells or cells in G_0/G_1 are relatively insensitive.[46] Thus, it is possible that programmed cell death initiated at various cell-cycle checkpoints is governed by different proteins and signal transduction pathways.

A model for cisplatin-induced cell death in CHO cells has been provided by Sorrenson and Eastman.[47] In this study, cisplatin-treated CHO/AA8 cells experienced slow progression through S phase and accumulated in G_2. At low drug concentrations, the cells recovered and continued to cycle. At high drug concentrations, the cells died after a protracted G_2 arrest. An aberrant mitosis was observed before apoptosis. Further studies with G_2-synchronized cells revealed that passage through S phase is necessary for G_2 arrest and cell death, suggesting that DNA replication on a damaged template may result in the accumulation of further damage, ultimately causing the cells to die. Cisplatin-induced accumulation of human tumor cells in G_2 also has been observed in mice. Abrogating the G_2 checkpoint with pharmacologic agents, such as caffeine or 7-hydroxystaurosporine, have been shown to enhance the cytotoxicity of cisplatin.[48] It is not yet clear how these events specifically transduce a proapoptotic signal. However, the observations provide a valuable framework to begin to elucidate the initial steps.

The decision/commitment phase of apoptosis hinges on the balance between survival and death signals. Each cell contains a damage threshold that, once surpassed, results in the onset of apoptosis. It is not clear what signaling pathways influence the response of cells to platinum drugs. However, it has been shown that activators or inhibitors of known signal transduction pathways can influence platinum drug sensitivity. For example, treatment of various cell lines with tamoxifen, epidermal growth factor, interleukin-1α, tumor necrosis factor-α bombesin, and rapamycin enhance cisplatin cytotoxicity.[49–53] Also, the expression of certain protooncogenes, including *Ha-Ras, v-abl,* and Her2/*neu*, has been shown in some instances to promote cell survival after cisplatin exposure.[54–57] This is an area of investigation that requires further study, and the overall balance of cell survival and cell death signals may be critical in determining the response of tumors to chemotherapy.

In addition to the mounting evidence supporting the existence of programmed cell death pathways, substantial evidence indicates that cell death is influenced by cellular signal transduction pathways such as those that control growth, differentiation, and stress response. These signals are mediated primarily by small guanosine triphosphatases and protein serine-threonine kinases. Members of the extracellular signal-related kinase/mitogen-activated kinase family, as well as their upstream activators, have been implicated in these events. The c-JUN amino-terminal kinase (JNK)/stress-activated protein kinase (SAPK) and p38 kinase pathways have been shown to be activated by a variety of environmental stimuli and inflammatory cytokines.[58] JNK/SAPK and p38 phosphorylate and regulate the activity of the ATF2 (alcohol acetyltransferase II) and Elk-1 transcription factors. JNK/SAPK also phosphorylates c-JUN, a component of the AP-1 (activating protein 1) transcription factor complex, on serine residues 63 and 73. Considerable evidence suggests that these protein kinases are involved in transmitting a drug-induced cell death signal. For example, Zanke et al.[59] demonstrated that, in mouse fibroblasts, the inhibition of JNK phosphorylation by the stable transfection of a dominant-negative complementary DNA encoding SEK1, the protein kinase responsible for activating JNK, resulted in reduced sensitivity to cisplatin. Sanchez-Perez et al.[60] observed a prolonged activation of JNK by cisplatin that was related to cell death. Modulating the activity of kinases upstream of JNK, including c-Abl, MKK3/MKK6, MEKK1, and ASK1, also influences cellular drug sensitivity.[61] For example, Chen et al.[62] demonstrated that overexpression of a dominant-negative ASK1, which inhibits activation of JNK, resulted in an inhibition of cisplatin-induced apoptosis. Clearly, activation of these pathways occurs after drug exposure in some cells, and it is important to understand the contribution of these intracellular signaling events to overall platinum drug sensitivity. Within these pathways may reside the key to understanding the molecular basis for platinum drug–induced cell death.

MECHANISMS OF RESISTANCE

The major limitation to the successful treatment of solid tumors with platinum-based chemotherapy is the emergence of drug-resistant tumor cells.[63] Platinum drug resistance may be intrinsic or acquired and may occur through multiple mechanisms. These mechanisms may be classified into two major groups: (1) those that limit the formation of cytotoxic platinum-DNA adducts and (2) those that prevent cell death from occurring after platinum-DNA adduct formation. The first group of mechanisms includes decreased drug accumulation and increased drug inactivation by cellular protein and nonprotein thiols. The second group of mechanisms includes increased platinum-DNA adduct repair and increased platinum-DNA damage tolerance. These mechanisms have been described previously in *in vitro* resistance models, and their relevance to clinical resistance is unknown (Table 19.4-1).

TABLE 19.4-1. Correlation Coefficients Derived from the Relationships between Cisplatin-Sensitivity and Cisplatin-Resistance Mechanisms in Two Human Ovarian Cancer Model Systems

Resistance Mechanism	In Vitro–*Selected Cisplatin-Resistant Model*[a]	*Unrelated Ovarian Tumor Cell Lines*[b]
Glutathione levels	0.94	0.13
Cellular platinum accumulation	0.85	–0.11
Platinum-DNA adduct formation	0.83	–0.38
Platinum-DNA adduct removal	0.83	0.44
Platinum-DNA adduct tolerance	0.99	0.84

[a]A2780/C series of cell lines derived from the repeated exposure of the A2780 human ovarian cancer cell line to cisplatin. (Data adapted from refs. 71, 91, and 92.)

[b]Panel of human ovarian cancer cell lines derived from patients that were either untreated or treated with platinum-based chemotherapy.[110]

REDUCED ACCUMULATION

The majority of cell lines that have been selected for cisplatin resistance *in vitro* exhibit a decreased platinum accumulation phenotype, and it is generally believed that this is due to decreased drug uptake rather than enhanced drug efflux. Cisplatin and its analogues may accumulate within cells by passive diffusion or facilitated transport.[64] Cisplatin uptake has been shown to be nonsaturable, even up to its solubility limit, and not inhibited by structural analogues. Carrier-mediated transport is supported by the observation that uptake is partially energy-dependent, ouabain-inhibitable, sodium-dependent, and influenced by membrane potential and cyclic adenosine monophosphate levels. Although no specific drug transporters have been implicated in the reduced platinum accumulation phenotype, some insight into a possible pathway has been provided. Using two different acquired cisplatin resistance model systems, Shen et al.[65] reported that the loss of the folate binding protein (FBP) was associated with decreased cellular accumulation of cisplatin, methotrexate, arsenate, and arsenite. Although the loss of FBP was not shown to be directly responsible for reduced cisplatin accumulation, the regulatory mechanism responsible for the reduction in FBP gene expression may be linked to the expression of a transport protein that may influence cisplatin uptake.

The prospect of an active efflux mechanism for platinum drugs has been rekindled by the discovery of a group of multidrug resistance protein (MRP)-related transport proteins. MRP is a member of the adenosine triphosphate–binding cassette family of transport proteins that participates in the extrusion of glutathione-coupled and unmodified anticancer drugs out of cells.[66] Overexpression of MRP confers resistance to a variety of drugs, but not to cisplatin. For platinum complexes, the formation of a glutathione-platinum drug conjugate may be the rate-limiting step for producing an MRP substrate. The MRP homologue cMOAT (canalicular multispecific organic anion transporter) shares 49% amino acid sequence identity and a similar substrate specificity with that of MRP. Taniguchi et al.[67] has shown that cMOAT (MRP2) is overexpressed in some cisplatin-resistant human cancer cell lines exhibiting a decreased platinum accumulation phenotype. These investigators also demonstrated that transfection of an antisense cMOAT complementary DNA into HepG2 cells results in decreased cMOAT protein levels and a fivefold increase in cisplatin sensitivity.[68] Kool et al.[69] examined the expression of MRP, cMOAT, and three other MRP homologues (MRP3, MRP4, MRP5) in a set of cell lines selected for cisplatin resistance *in vitro*. MRP1 and MRP4 messenger RNA levels were not increased in any of the cisplatin-resistant sublines. MRP3 and MRP5 were overexpressed in a few cell lines, but the messenger RNA levels were not associated with cisplatin resistance. In contrast, cMOAT was substantially overexpressed in some of the cisplatin-resistant cell lines. An immunohistochemical analysis of the expression of P glycoprotein, MRP1, and MRP2 revealed that none of these transporters was associated with response to platinum-based chemotherapy in ovarian cancer.[70]

INACTIVATION

As mentioned above, the formation of conjugates between glutathione (GSH) and platinum drugs may be an important step for their inactivation and elimination from the cell. For many years, investigators have attempted to make positive correlations between platinum drug sensitivity, GSH levels, and the relative expression of the enzymes involved in GSH metabolism. There have been many reports showing a strong association between platinum drug sensitivity and GSH levels.[71–74] However, reducing intracellular GSH levels with drugs such as buthionine sulfoximine has resulted in only low to modest potentiation of cisplatin sensitivity.[75,76] Part of the reason for this may be due to the fact that the formation of GSH-platinum conjugates is a slow process.[77] The formation of a GSH-platinum complex, however, has been reported to occur in cultured cells, and GSH has been shown to quench platinum-DNA monoadducts *in vitro*, preventing them from being converted to potentially cytotoxic cross-links.[78–80] These findings raise the question of whether the intracellular reaction is catalyzed by glutathione S-transferases (GSTs). In support of this theory, a threefold increase in cisplatin resistance was reported in CHO cells transfected with the GSTπ isoenzyme.[81] In contrast, transfection of NIH3T3 cells with GSTπ resulted in hypersensitivity to cisplatin.[82] Studies attempting to associate GST activity with cisplatin sensitivity in cell lines and tumor biopsies have not consistently shown a positive correlation between GST expression or activity and cisplatin sensitivity.[72–74,83]

Inactivation of the platinum drugs may also occur through binding to the metallothionein (MT) proteins. The MTs are a family of sulfhydryl-rich, small-molecular-weight proteins that participate in heavy metal binding and detoxication. *In vitro*, cisplatin binds stoichiometrically to metallothionein, and up to ten molecules of cisplatin can be bound to one molecule of metallothionein.[84] Kelley et al.[85] demonstrated that overexpression of the full-length MT-II_A in mouse C127 cells conferred a fourfold resistance to cisplatin. Furthermore, this group showed that embryonic fibroblasts isolated from MT-null mice were hypersensitive to cisplatin.[86] These studies clearly show that modulating MT levels can alter cisplatin sensitivity. However, the contribution of MT to clinical platinum drug resistance is unclear. In some cell lines, elevated MT levels have been shown to be associated with cisplatin resistance, whereas in others, they have not.[72,87] Studies with human tumors have shown that, in some instances, metallothionein expression level is associated with response to chemotherapy. For example, a significant correlation between MT overexpression and response or survival was reported in urothelial transitional cell carcinoma patients.[88] Overexpression of MT also has been observed in bladder tumors from patients that were unsuccessful with cisplatin chemotherapy.[89]

INCREASED DNA REPAIR

Once platinum-DNA adducts are formed, cells must either repair or tolerate the damage to survive. The capacity to rapidly and efficiently repair DNA damage clearly plays a role in determining a tumor cell's sensitivity to platinum drugs and other DNA damaging agents. Evidence suggests that cell lines derived from tumors that are unusually sensitive to cisplatin, such as testicular nonseminomatous germ cell tumors, are deficient in their ability to repair platinum-DNA adducts.[90] Increased repair of platinum-DNA lesions in cisplatin-resistant cell lines as compared with their sensitive counterparts has been shown in several human cancer cell lines, including ovarian,[91,92] breast,[93] glioma,[94] and murine leukemia cell lines.[95] Evidence for increased repair of cisplatin interstrand cross-links in specific gene and nongene regions in cisplatin-resistant cell lines also has been demonstrated. These studies have been done using a variety of *in vivo* methods, including unscheduled DNA synthesis, host cell reactivation of cisplatin-damaged plasmid DNA, atomic absorption spectrometry, quantitative polymerase chain reaction, and renaturing agarose gel electrophoresis.

The repair of platinum-DNA adducts occurs predominantly by nucleotide excision repair (NER). However, the molecular basis for the increased repair activity observed in cisplatin-resistant cells is unknown.[96] Because the rate-limiting step in this process is platinum-adduct recognition/incision, increased expression of the proteins that control this step are likely to enhance nucleotide excision repair activity. Using an *in vitro* assay, Ferry et al.[97] demonstrated that the addition of the ERCC1/XPF (excision repair) protein complex increased the platinum-DNA adduct excision activity of an ovarian cancer cell extract. Circumstantial evidence also implicates *ERCC1* expression with increased NER and cisplatin resistance. For example, expression levels of the *ERCC1* and *XPA* genes have been shown to be higher in malignant tissue from ovarian cancer patients resistant to platinum-based therapy compared with those responsive to treatment.[98] *ERCC1* expression also has been shown to correlate with NER activity and cisplatin resistance in human ovarian cancer cells.[97] Increased levels of XPE, a putative DNA repair protein that recognizes many DNA lesions, including platinum-DNA adducts, has been observed in tumor cell lines resistant to cisplatin.[99] It should be noted, however, that XPE is not a necessary component for the *in vitro* reconstitution of NER.[96,100] Increased expression of DNA polymerases α and β have been observed in cisplatin-resistant cell lines, and increased expression of these polymerases, as well as DNA ligase, has been described in human tumors after cisplatin exposure *in vivo*.[94] The possible significance of these findings is unclear because the primary polymerases involved in NER are thought to be DNA polymerases δ or ε.[96] Although it is probably not involved in NER, DNA polymerase β may be involved in translesion DNA synthesis.[101]

Inhibiting DNA repair activity to enhance platinum drug sensitivity has been an active area of investigation. Agents that have been used include nucleoside analogues, such as gemcitabine, fludarabine, and cytarabine; the ribonucleotide reductase inhibitor hydroxyurea; and the inhibitor of DNA polymerases α and γ, aphidicolin. All of these agents interfere with the repair synthesis stage of various repair processes, including nucleotide excision repair, and it should be noted that these compounds are also likely to affect DNA replication and, as such, should not be strictly characterized as repair inhibitors. The potentiation of cisplatin cytotoxicity by treatment with aphidicolin has been studied extensively in human ovarian cancer cell lines. Although some studies have demonstrated a clear synergism with this drug combination,[102,103] others have not.[104] In an *in vivo* mouse model of human ovarian cancer, the combined treatment of cisplatin and aphidicolin glycinate, a water-soluble form of the drug, was found to be significantly more effective than cisplatin alone.[105] The combination of cytarabine and hydroxyurea was found to demonstrate cytotoxic synergy with cisplatin in a human colon cancer cell line[106] and in rat mammary carcinoma cell lines.[107] Moreover, the modulatory effect of cytarabine and hydroxyurea on cisplatin was associated with an increase in DNA interstrand cross-links in both cellular systems. Similarly, the drugs gemcitabine[108] and fludarabine[109] have both been shown to synergize with cisplatin in causing cell death in *in vitro* systems, and both of these drugs have been shown to interfere with the removal of cisplatin-DNA adducts. The likelihood of a significant improvement in the therapeutic index of cisplatin in refractory patients by the coadministration of a repair inhibitor, however, is limited by the multifactorial nature typical of resistant tumor cells. The combination of an inhibitor of the repair process with other modulators of resistance may be a more viable avenue in treating patients with recurrent disease. Furthermore, a modest change in drug sensitivity may bring some refractory tumors into a range that is treatable with conventional chemotherapy.

INCREASED DNA DAMAGE TOLERANCE

Platinum-DNA damage tolerance is a phenotype that has been observed in both cisplatin-resistant cells derived from chemotherapy-refractory patients and cells selected for primary cisplatin resistance *in vitro*. The contribution of this mechanism to resistance is significant, and it has been shown to correlate strongly with cisplatin resistance as well as to resistance to other drugs in two ovarian cancer model systems (see Table 19.4-1).[92,110] Like other cisplatin resistance mechanisms, this phenotype may result from alterations in a variety of cellular pathways.

One component of DNA damage tolerance that has been observed in cisplatin-resistant cells involves the loss of function of the DNA MMR system. The main function of the MMR system is to scan newly synthesized DNA and to remove mismatches that result from nucleotide incorporation errors made by the DNA polymerases. In addition to causing genomic instability, it has been reported that loss of MMR is associated with low-level cisplatin resistance and that the selection of cells in culture for resistance to this drug often yields cell lines that have lost a functional MMR system.[111] MMR deficiency may create an environment that promotes the accumulation of mutations in drug-sensitivity genes. Another hypothesis is that the MMR system serves as a detector of platinum-DNA adducts. MSH2 alone, and in combination with MSH6, has been shown to bind to cisplatin 1,2-d(GpG)Pt intrastrand adducts with high efficiency.[44,112] Additionally, MSH2- and MLH1-containing protein-DNA complexes have been observed when nuclear extracts of MMR-proficient cell lines were incubated with DNA preincubated with cisplatin, but not with oxaliplatin. These data suggest that MMR recognition of damage may trigger a programmed cell death pathway, rendering cells with intact MMR more sensitive to DNA damage.[43] Another possibility is that the cytotoxicity involves repeated rounds of synthesis past the platinum-DNA lesions followed by recognition and subsequent removal of the newly synthesized strand by the MMR system. This futile cycling may generate DNA strand gaps and breaks that trigger programmed cell death.[113] Loss of MMR thus increases the cell's ability to tolerate platinum-DNA lesions.

Another possible tolerance mechanism related to MMR is enhanced replicative bypass, which is defined as the ability of the replication complex to synthesize DNA past a platinum adduct.[101,114] Increased replicative bypass has been shown to occur in cisplatin-resistant human ovarian cancer cells.[114] These cells are also MMR-deficient, and it has been shown that in steady-state chain elongation assays, a 2.5- to 6.0-fold increase in replicative bypass of cisplatin adducts occurred. Oxaliplatin adducts are not recognized by the MMR complex, and no significant differences in bypass of oxaliplatin adducts in MMR-proficient and -defective cells were observed. DNA polymerase β, the most inaccurate of the DNA polymerases, may also function in this process.[101] The activity of this enzyme was found to be significantly increased in cells derived from a human malignant glioma resistant to cisplatin compared with its drug-sensitive counterpart.[94]

The tolerance mechanisms just mentioned are related primarily to cisplatin resistance. Because the platinum-DNA damage tolerance phenotype is often associated with cross-resistance to other unrelated chemotherapeutic drugs,[110] the existence of a more general resistance mechanism must be considered. One possible explanation is that the platinum-DNA damage tolerance phenotype is the result of decreased expression or inactivation of one or more components of the programmed cell death pathway. As mentioned above in Platinum Drug–Induced Cell Death, a number of pro- and antiapoptotic signaling pathways have been implicated in cisplatin sensitivity. The possibility exists that cells containing defective or constitutively down-regulated stress signaling pathways, such as SAPK/JNK, may exhibit resistance to platinum drugs. A number of other proteins that regulate these pathways may also have the capacity to influence drug sensitivity. In addition, cell death may also be influenced by expression of members of the bcl-2 gene family. This group of pro- and antiapoptotic proteins regulates mitochondrial function, and they serve as a cell survival/cell death rheostat by forming homo- and heterodimers with one another. The antiapoptotic bcl-2 and bcl-X_L proteins are localized in the outer mitochondrial membrane and may be involved in the formation of transmembrane channels. Overexpression of bcl-2 or bcl-X_L has been shown to prevent disruption of the mitochondrial transmembrane potential and to prolong cell survival in some cells after exposure to cisplatin and other anticancer drugs.[115,116] The activity of these proteins is negated, however, in the presence of high levels of the proapoptotic protein BAX, another bcl-2 family member. Therefore, the relative intracellular levels of these proteins may also confer resistance to platinum drugs. An interesting connection between the bcl-2 gene family and SAPK/JNK has been reported by Kharbanda et al.[117] They found that, after genotoxic stress, SAPK/JNK is translocated to the mitochondria, where it phosphorylates bcl-X_L, presumably rendering it inactive.

TABLE 19.4-2. Comparative Pharmacokinetics of Platinum Analogues after Bolus or Short Intravenous Infusion

	Cisplatin	*Carboplatin*	*Oxaliplatin*
$T_{1/2}\alpha$ (min)			
Total platinum	14–49	12–98	26
Ultrafiltrate	9–30	8–87	21
$T_{1/2}\beta$ (h)			
Total platinum	0.7–4.6	1.3–1.7	—
Ultrafiltrate	0.7–0.8	1.7–5.9	—
$T_{1/2}\gamma$ (h)			
Total platinum	24–127	8.2–40.0	38–47
Ultrafiltrate	—	—	24–27
Protein binding	>90%	24–50%	85%
Urinary excretion	23–50%	54–82%	>50%

$T_{1/2}\alpha$, half-life of first phase; $T_{1/2}\beta$, half-life of second phase; $T_{1/2}\gamma$, half-life of terminal phase.
Data adapted from references 120–129.

CLINICAL PHARMACOLOGY

PHARMACOKINETICS

The pharmacokinetic differences observed among platinum drugs may be attributed to the structure of their leaving groups. Platinum complexes containing leaving groups that are less easily displaced exhibit reduced plasma protein binding, longer plasma half-lives, and higher rates of renal clearance. These features are evident in the pharmacokinetic properties of cisplatin, carboplatin, and oxaliplatin, which are summarized in Table 19.4-2. Platinum drug pharmacokinetics also have been reviewed elsewhere.[118–120]

Cisplatin

After intravenous infusion, cisplatin rapidly diffuses into tissues and is covalently bound to plasma protein. More than 90% of platinum is bound to plasma protein at 4 hours postinfusion.[121] The disappearance of ultrafilterable platinum is rapid and occurs in a biphasic fashion. Half-lives of 10 to 30 minutes and 0.7 to 0.8 hours have been reported for the initial ($T_{1/2}\alpha$) and terminal phases ($T_{1/2}\gamma$), respectively.[122,123] Cisplatin excretion is dependent on renal function, which accounts for the majority of its elimination. The percentage of platinum excreted in the urine has been reported to be between 23% and 40% at 24 hours postinfusion.[124,125] Only a small percentage of the total platinum is excreted in the bile.[126]

Carboplatin

The differences in pharmacokinetics observed between cisplatin and carboplatin depend primarily on the slower rate of conversion of carboplatin to a reactive species. Thus, the stability of carboplatin results in a low incidence of nephrotoxicity. Carboplatin diffuses rapidly into tissues after infusion, but it is considerably more stable in plasma. Only 24% of a dose was reported to be bound to plasma protein at 4 hours postinfusion.[127]

The disappearance of platinum from plasma after short intravenous infusions of carboplatin has been reported to occur in a biphasic or triphasic manner. The initial half-lives for total platinum, which vary considerably among several studies, are listed in Table 19.4-2. The $T_{1/2}\alpha$ ranges from 12 to 98 minutes and ranges from 1.3 to 1.7 hours during the second phase ($T_{1/2}\beta$). Half-lives reported for the $T_{1/2}\gamma$ range from 8.2 to 40.0 hours. The disappearance of ultrafilterable platinum is biphasic, with $T_{1/2}\alpha$ and $T_{1/2}\beta$ values ranging from 7.6 to 87.0 minutes and 1.7 to 5.9 hours, respectively. Carboplatin is excreted predominantly by the kidneys, and cumulative urinary excretion of platinum is 54% to 82%, most as unmodified carboplatin. The renal clearance of carboplatin is closely correlated with the glomerular filtration rate (GFR).[127] This observation enabled Calvert et al.[128] to design a carboplatin dosing formula based on an individual patient's GFR.

Oxaliplatin

After oxaliplatin infusion, platinum accumulates into three compartments: plasma-bound platinum, ultrafilterable platinum, and platinum associated with erythrocytes. Approximately 85% of the total platinum is bound to plasma protein at 2 to 5 hours postinfusion.[129] Plasma elimination of total platinum and ultrafiltrates is biphasic. The $T_{1/2}\alpha$ and $T_{1/2}\gamma$ are 26 minutes and 38.7 hours, respectively, for total platinum and 21 minutes and 24.2 hours, respectively, for ultrafilterable platinum (see Table 19.4-2).[120] Thus, as with carboplatin, substantial differences between total and free drug kinetics are not observed. Similar to cisplatin, a prolonged retention of oxaliplatin is observed in red blood cells. Unlike cisplatin, however, oxaliplatin does not accumulate to any significant level after multiple courses of treatment.[129] This may explain why neurotoxicity associated with oxaliplatin is reversible. Oxaliplatin is eliminated predominantly by the kidneys, with more than 50% being excreted in the urine at 48 hours.

PHARMACODYNAMICS

Pharmacodynamics relates pharmacokinetic indices of drug exposure to biological measures of drug effect, which is usually defined by toxicity to normal tissues or by amount of tumor cell kill. Two issues to be addressed in such efforts are whether the effectiveness of the drug can be enhanced or the toxicity attenuated by knowledge of the platinum pharmacokinetics in an individual. These questions are appropriate to the use of cytotoxic agents with relatively narrow therapeutic indices. Toxicity to normal tissues can be quantitated as a continuous variable when the drug causes myelosuppression. Thus, the early studies of carboplatin demonstrated a close relationship of changes in platelet counts to the area under the concentration-time curve (AUC) in the individual. The AUC was itself closely related to renal function, which was determined as creatinine clearance. Based on these observations, Egorin et al.[130] and Calvert et al.[128] derived formulas based on creatinine clearance to predict either the percent change in platelet count or a target AUC. More recently, Chatelut and colleagues[131] have derived a formula that relies on serum creatinine as well as morphometric determinants of renal function. Application of pharmacodynamically guided dosing algorithms for carboplatin has been widely adopted as a means of avoiding overdosage (by producing acceptable nadir platelet counts) and of maximizing dose intensity in the individual. Good evidence suggests that this approach can decrease the risk of unacceptable toxicity. Accordingly, a dosing strategy based on renal function is recommended for the use of carboplatin.

A key question is whether maximizing carboplatin exposure in an individual can measurably increase the probability of tumor regression or survival. In an analysis by Jodrell et al.,[132] carboplatin AUC was a predictor of response, thrombocytopenia, and leukopenia. The likelihood of a tumor response increased with increasing AUC up to a level of 5 to 7 mg × hr/mL, after which a plateau was reached. Similar results were obtained with carboplatin in combination with cyclophosphamide, and neither response nor survival rates were determined by the carboplatin AUC in a cohort of ovarian cancer patients.[133]

The relationship of pharmacokinetics to response may also be explored by investigating the cellular pharmacology of these agents.[134] As discussed above in DNA Adduct Formation, platinum compounds form various types of DNA adducts. The formation and repair of these adducts in human cells are not easily measured. One approach is to measure specific DNA adducts (using antibody-based assays); another is to measure total platinum bound to DNA. The formation and repair of platinum-DNA adducts has been studied in white blood cells obtained from various groups of patients. Ma et al.[135] have reevaluated the pharmacokinetic and pharmacodynamic interactions of cisplatin administered as a single agent. In a series of patients with head and neck cancer, they found that cisplatin exposure (measured as the AUC) closely correlated with both the peak DNA adduct content in leukocytes and the area under the DNA-adduct–time curve.[136] These measures were important predictors of response, both individually and in logistic regression analysis. An adaptive dosing study in which the dose of cisplatin is modified based on DNA-adduct levels is in progress.

Based on the variability of both pharmacokinetics in individuals and of tumor genotype determinants of susceptibility to platinum agents, it seems most likely that direct investigations of these factors will elucidate how best to use these drugs. Single-nucleotide polymorphism associations with toxicity and tumor gene expression profiles determining susceptibility will, it is hoped, further enhance the therapeutic index by prospectively identifying sensitive and resistant populations.

FORMULATION AND ADMINISTRATION

Cisplatin

Cisplatin is administered in a chloride-containing solution intravenously over 0.5 to 2.0 hours. To minimize the risk of nephrotoxicity, patients are prehydrated with at least 500 mL of salt-containing fluid. Immediately before cisplatin administration, mannitol (12.5 to 25.0 g) is given parenterally to maximize urine flow. A diuretic, such as furosemide, may also be used, along with parenteral antiemetics, which currently include dexamethasone together with a 5-hydroxytryptamine$_3$ (5-HT_3) antagonist. A minimum of 1 L of posthydration fluid is usually given.[137] The intensity of hydration varies somewhat with the dose of cisplatin. High-dose cisplatin (up to 200 mg/m^2 per course) may be administered in a formulation containing 3% sodium chloride, but this method is no longer widely used. Cisplatin may also be administered regionally to increase local drug exposure and to diminish side effects. Its intraperitoneal use was defined by Ozols et al.[138] and by Howell and colleagues.[139] Measured drug exposure in the peritoneal cavity is some 50-fold higher than levels achieved with intravenous administration.[139] At standard doses in ovarian cancer patients with low-volume disease, a randomized intergroup trial suggested that intraperitoneal administration is superior to intravenous cisplatin in combination with intravenous cyclophosphamide.[140] The development of combinations of carboplatin with paclitaxel has, however, superseded this technique in ovarian cancer, and the intraperitoneal route is now infrequently used. Regional use also includes intraarterial delivery (as for hepatic tumors, melanoma, and glioblastoma), but none has been adopted as a standard method of treatment. There is growing interest in chemoembolization for the treatment of tumors confined to the liver, and cisplatin is a component of many popular regimens.[141]

Carboplatin

Cisplatin treatment over 3 to 6 hours is burdensome for clinical resources and tiring for cancer patients. Previously given as in-hospital treatment, it is now usually administered in the outpatient setting. The exigencies of the modern health care environment have contributed to the expanding use of carboplatin as an alternative to cisplatin, except in circumstances in which cisplatin is clearly the superior agent. Carboplatin is substantially easier to administer. Extensive hydration is not required because of the lack of nephrotoxicity at standard doses.[142] Carboplatin is reconstituted in chloride-free solutions (unlike cisplatin, because chloride can displace the leaving groups) and administered over 30 minutes as a rapid intravenous infusion. Carboplatin has been incorporated in high-dose chemotherapy regimens at doses more than threefold higher than those of the standard regimens.[143] In some regimens, continuous infusion has been substituted for a rapid intravenous infusion; however, it is doubtful that there is an advantage to this approach. Carboplatin doses up to 20 mg × min/mL may be safely administered in 200 mL of D5W over 2 hours.[144]

Oxaliplatin

Oxaliplatin is also uncomplicated in its clinical administration. For bolus infusion, the required dose is administered in 500 mL of chloride-free diluent over a period of 2 hours. In studies of colorectal cancer, oxaliplatin has been administered as a 5-day continuous infusion, during which the dosage rate has been modified to observe principles of chronopharmacologic administration.[145] Oxaliplatin is more frequently given as a single dose every 2 weeks (85 mg/m^2) or every 3 weeks (130 mg/m^2), alone or with other active agents. It is common to pretreat patients with active antiemetics, such as a 5-HT_3 antagonist, but the nausea is not as severe as with cisplatin. No prehydration is required. The predominant toxicity of oxaliplatin is neurotoxicity. The development of an oropharyngeal dysesthesia, often precipitated by exposure to cold, requires prolongation of the duration of administration to 6 hours.

TOXICITY

A substantial body of literature documents the side effects of platinum compounds. The nephrotoxicity of cisplatin almost led to its abandonment, until Cvitkovic and colleagues[3,4] intro-

TABLE 19.4-3. Toxicity Profiles of Platinum Analogues in Clinical Use

Toxicity	*Cisplatin*	*Carboplatin*	*Oxaliplatin*
Myelosuppression		X	
Nephrotoxicity	X		
Neurotoxicity	X		X
Ototoxicity	X		
Nausea and vomiting	X	X	X

duced aggressive hydration, which prevented the development of acute renal failure. As already noted, the toxicity of cisplatin was a driving force both in the search for less toxic analogues and for more effective treatments for its side effects, especially nausea and vomiting. The toxicities associated with cisplatin, carboplatin, and oxaliplatin are described in detail in the next three sections and are summarized in Table 19.4-3.

Cisplatin

The side effects associated with cisplatin (at single doses of more than 50 mg/m^2) include nausea and vomiting, nephrotoxicity, ototoxicity, neuropathy, and myelosuppression. Rare effects include visual impairment, seizures, arrhythmias, acute ischemic vascular events, glucose intolerance, and pancreatitis.[137] The nausea and vomiting stimulated a search for new antiemetics. These symptoms are currently best managed with 5-HT$_3$ antagonists and usually given with a glucocorticoid, although other combinations of agents are still widely used. In the weeks following treatment, continuous antiemetic therapy may be required. Nephrotoxicity is ameliorated but not completely prevented by hydration. The renal damage to both glomeruli and tubules is cumulative, and after cisplatin treatment, serum creatinine is no longer a reliable guide to the measurement of glomerular filtration rate. An acute elevation of serum creatinine may follow a cisplatin dose, but this index returns to normal with time. Tubule damage may be reflected in a salt-losing syndrome that also resolves with time.

Ototoxicity is a cumulative and irreversible side effect of cisplatin treatment that results from damage to the inner ear. Therefore, audiograms are recommended every 2 to 3 cycles.[137] The initial audiographic manifestation is loss of high-frequency acuity (4000 to 8000 Hz). When acuity is affected in the range of speech, cisplatin should be discontinued under most circumstances and carboplatin substituted where appropriate. Peripheral neuropathy is also cumulative, although less common than with agents such as vinca alkaloids. This neuropathy usually is reversible, although recovery is often slow. A number of agents with the potential for protection from neuropathy have been developed, but none is yet used widely.[146]

Carboplatin

Myelosuppression, which is not usually severe with cisplatin, is the dose-limiting toxicity of carboplatin.[142] The drug is most toxic to the platelet precursors, but neutropenia and anemia are frequently observed. The lowest platelet counts after a single dose of carboplatin are observed 17 to 21 days later, and recovery usually occurs by day 28. The effect is dose-dependent, but individuals vary widely in their susceptibility. As shown by Egorin et al.[130] and Calvert et al.,[128] the severity of platelet toxicity is best accounted for by a measure of the drug exposure in an individual, the AUC. Both groups derived pharmacologically based formulas to predict toxicity and guide carboplatin dosing. That of Calvert and colleagues targets a particular exposure to carboplatin:

$$\text{Dose (mg)} = \text{target AUC} \times \left(\frac{\text{mg} \cdot \text{min}}{\text{mL}}\right) \times \left(\frac{\text{GFR mL}}{\text{min} + 25}\right)$$

This formula has been widely used to individualize carboplatin dosing, and it permits targeting at an acceptable level of toxicity. Patients who are elderly or have a poor performance status or a history of extensive pretreatment have a higher risk of toxicity, even when dose is calculated with these methods,[128,130] but the safety of drug administration has been enhanced. In the combination of carboplatin and paclitaxel, AUC-based dosing has helped to maximize the dose intensity of carboplatin.[147] Doses some 30% higher than a dosing strategy based solely on body surface area may safely be used. A determination of whether this approach to dosing improves outcome requires a randomized trial, which is in progress.

The other toxicities of carboplatin are generally milder and better tolerated than those of cisplatin. Nausea and vomiting, although frequent, are less severe, shorter in duration, and more easily controlled with standard antiemetics (i.e., Compazine, dexamethasone, lorazepam) than those symptoms typical after cisplatin treatment. Renal impairment is infrequent, although alopecia is common, especially with the paclitaxel-containing combinations. Neurotoxicity is also less common than with cisplatin, although it is observed more frequently with the increasing use of high-dose regimens. Ototoxicity is also less common.

Oxaliplatin

The dose-limiting toxicity of oxaliplatin is sensory neuropathy, a characteristic of all DACH-containing platinum derivatives. The severity of the toxicity is dramatically less than that observed with another DACH-containing analogue, ormaplatin. This side effect takes two forms. First, a tingling of the extremities, which may also involve the perioral region, occurs early and usually resolves within a few days. With repeated dosing, symptoms may last longer between cycles but do not appear to be of long duration or cumulative. Laryngopharyngeal spasm and cold dysesthesias also have been reported but are not associated with significant respiratory symptoms; they can be prevented by prolonging the duration of infusion. A second neuropathy, more typical of that seen with cisplatin, affects the extremities and increases with repeated doses. Definitive physiologic characterization of oxaliplatin-induced neuropathy has proven difficult in large studies. Electromyograms performed in six patients treated by Extra et al.[148] revealed an axonal sensory neuropathy, but nerve conduction velocities were unchanged. Peripheral nerve biopsies performed in this study showed decreased myelinization and replacement with collagen pockets. The neurologic effects of oxaliplatin appear to be cumulative in that they become more pronounced and of greater duration with successive cycles. Unlike those with cisplatin, however, they are reversible with drug cessation. In a review of 682 patient experiences, Brienza et al.[149] reported that 82% of patients who experienced grade 2 or higher neurotoxicity had their symptoms regress within 4 to 6 months. Ototoxicity is not observed with oxaliplatin. Nausea and vomiting do occur and generally respond to 5-HT_3 antagonists. Myelosuppression is uncommon and is not severe with oxaliplatin as a single agent, but it is a feature of combinations including this drug. Oxaliplatin therapy is not associated with nephrotoxicity.

REFERENCES

1. Rosenberg B, VanCamp L, Trosko J, Mansour V. Platinum compounds: a new class of potent antitumor agents. *Nature* 1969;222:385.
2. Rosenberg B. Platinum complexes for the treatment of cancer: why the search goes on. In: Lippert B, ed. *Cisplatin: chemistry and biochemistry of a leading anticancer drug.* Zurich, Switzerland: Verlag Helvetica Chimica Acta, 1999:3.
3. Cvitkovic E, Spaulding J, Bethune V, Martin J, Whitmore W. Improvement of *cis*-dichlorodiammineplatinum (NSC 119875): therapeutic index in an animal model. *Cancer* 1977;39:1357.
4. Hayes D, Cvitkovic E, Golbey R, et al. High dose *cis*-platinum diammine dichloride: amelioration of renal toxicity by mannitol diuresis. *Cancer* 1977;39:1372.
5. O'Dwyer P, Stevenson J, Johnson S. Clinical status of cisplatin, carboplatin and other platinum-based antitumor drugs. In: Lippert B, ed. *Cisplatin: chemistry and biochemistry of a leading anticancer drug.* Zurich, Switzerland: Verlag Helvetica Chimica Acta, 1999:31.
6. Roberts J, Thomson A. The mechanism of action of antitumor platinum compounds. *Prog Nucleic Acids Res* 1979;22:71.
7. Martin R. Platinum complexes: hydrolysis and binding to N(7) and N(1) of purines. In: Lippert B, ed. *Cisplatin: chemistry and biochemistry of a leading anticancer drug.* Zurich, Switzerland: Verlag Helvetica Chimica Acta, 1999:183.
8. Harrap K. Preclinical studies identifying carboplatin as a viable cisplatin alternative. *Cancer Treat Rev* 1985;12:A21.
9. Harrap K. Initiatives with platinum- and quinazoline-based antitumor molecules. Fourteenth Bruce F. Cain memorial award lecture. *Cancer Res* 1995;55:2761.
10. Connors T, Jones M, Ross W, et al. New platinum complexes with anti-tumour activity. *Chem Biol Interact* 1972;5:415.
11. Kidani Y, Inagaki K, Tsukagoshi S. Examination of antitumor activities of platinum complexes of 1,2-diaminocyclohexane isomers and their related complexes. *Gann* 1976;67:921.
12. Burchenal J, Kalaker K, Dew K, Lokyst L. Rationale for development of platinum analogs. *Cancer Treat Rep* 1979;63:1493.
13. Burchenal J, Irani G, Kern K, Lokys L, Turkevich J. 1,2-Diaminocyclohexane platinum derivatives of potential clinical value. *Recent Results Cancer Res* 1980;74:146.
14. Rixe O, Ortuzar W, Alvarez M, et al. Oxaliplatin, tetraplatin, cisplatin, and carboplatin: spectrum of activity in drug-resistant cell lines and in the cell lines of the National Cancer Institute's anticancer drug screen panel. *Biochem Pharmacol* 1996;52:1855.
15. Cvitkovic E, Bekradda M. Oxaliplatin: a new therapeutic option in colorectal cancer. *Semin Oncol* 1999;26:647.
16. Hubbard K, Pazdur R, Ajani J, et al. Phase II evaluation of iproplatin in patients with advanced gastric and pancreatic cancer. *Am J Clin Oncol* 1992;15:524.
17. Murphy D, Lind M, Prendiville J, et al. Phase I/II study of intraperitoneal iproplatin in patients with minimal residual disease following platinum-based systemic therapy for epithelial ovarian carcinoma. *Eur J Cancer* 1992;28A:870.
18. Schilder R, LaCreta F, Perez R, et al. Phase I and pharmacokinetic study of ormaplatin (Tetraplatin, NSC 363812) administered on a day 1 and day 8 schedule. *Cancer Res* 1994;54:709.
19. Kelland L. The development of orally active platinum drugs. In: Lippert B, ed. *Cisplatin: chemistry and biochemistry of a leading anticancer drug.* Zurich, Switzerland: Verlag Helvetica Chimica Acta, 1999:497.
20. Fokkema E, Groen HJ, Bauer J, et al. Phase II study of oral platinum drug JM216 as first-line treatment in patients with small-cell lung cancer. *J Clin Oncol* 1999;17:3822.
21. Judson I, Cerny T, Epelbaum R, et al. Phase II trial of the oral platinum complex JM216 in non-small-cell lung cancer: an EORTC early clinical studies group investigation. *Ann Oncol* 1997;8:604.
22. Khokhar A, al-Baker S, Shamsuddin S, Siddik Z. Chemical and biological studies on a series of novel (trans-(1R,2R)-, trans-(1S,2S)-, and cis-1,2-diaminocyclohexane)platinum(IV) carboxylate complexes. *J Med Chem* 1997;40:112.
23. Farrell N, Qu Y, Bierbach U, Valsecchi M, Menta E. Structure-activity relationships within di- and trinuclear platinum phase-I clinical anticancer agents. In: Lippert B, ed. *Cisplatin: chemistry and biochemistry of a leading anticancer drug.* Zurich, Switzerland: Verlag Helvetica Chimica Acta, 1999.
24. Holford J, Sharp S, Murrer B, Abrams M, Kelland L. *In vitro* circumvention of cisplatin resistance by the novel sterically hindered platinum complex AMD473. *Br J Cancer* 1998;77:366.
25. Raynaud F, Boxall F, Goddard P, et al. cis-Amminedichloro(2-methylpyridine) platinum(II) (AMD473), a novel sterically hindered platinum complex: *in vivo* activity, toxicology, and pharmacokinetics in mice. *Clin Cancer Res* 1997;3:2063.
26. Trigo J, Beale P, Judson I, et al. Phase I and pharmacokinetic (PK) study of cis-amminedichloro (2-methylpyridine) platinum (II) (ZD0473), a novel sterically hindered platinum complex, in patients (pts) with advanced solid malignancies. *Proc Am Soc Clin Oncol* 1999;18:169a.
27. Harder H, Rosenberg B. Inhibitory effects of anti-tumor platinum compounds on DNA, RNA and protein syntheses in mammalian cells *in vitro*. *Int J Cancer* 1970;6:207.
28. Howle J, Gale G. Cis-dichlorodiammineplatinum (II). Persistent and selective inhibition of deoxyribonucleic acid synthesis *in vivo*. *Biochem Pharmacol* 1970;19:2757.
29. Reslova S. The induction of lysogenic strains of *Escherichia coli* by *cis*-dichloro-diammineplatinum (II). *Chem Biol Interact* 1971;4:66.
30. Poll EHA, Abrahams PJ, Arwert F, Eriksson AW. Host cell reactivation of *cis*-diamminedichloroplatinum (II)-treated SV40 DNA in normal human, Fanconi anaemia and xeroderma pigmentosum fibroblasts. *Mutat Res* 1984;132:181.
31. Fraval HNA, Rawlings CJ, Roberts JJ. Increased sensitivity of UV-repair deficient human cells to DNA bound platinum products which unlike thymine dimers are not recognized by an endonuclease extracted from *Micrococcus luteus*. *Mutat Res* 1978;51:121.
32. Eastman A. The formation, isolation and characterization of DNA adducts produced by anticancer platinum complexes. *Pharmacol Ther* 1987;34:155.
33. Blommaert F, van Kijk-Knijnenburg H, Dijt F, et al. Formation of DNA adducts by the anticancer drug carboplatin: different nucleotide sequence preferences *in vitro* and in cells. *Biochemistry* 1995;34:8474.
34. Knox R, Friedlos F, Lydall D, Roberts J. Mechanism of cytotoxicity of anticancer platinum drugs: evidence that *cis*-diamminedichloroplatinum(II) and *cis*-diammine-(1,1-cyclobutanedicarboxylato)platinum(II) differ only in the kinetics of their interaction with DNA. *Cancer Res* 1986;46:1972.
35. Saris C, van de Vaart P, Rietbroek R, Blommaert F. *In vitro* formation of DNA adducts by cisplatin, lobaplatin and oxaliplatin in calf thymus DNA in solution and in cultured cells. *Carcinogenesis* 1996;17:2763.
36. Zamble D, Lippard S. The response of cellular proteins to cisplatin-damaged DNA. In: Lippert B, ed. *Cisplatin: chemistry and biochemistry of a leading anticancer drug.* Zurich, Switzerland: Verlag Helvetica Chimica Acta, 1999:73.
37. Scheef E, Briggs J, Howell S. Molecular modeling of the intrastrand guanine-guanine DNA adducts produced by cisplatin and oxaliplatin. *Mol Pharmacol* 1999;56:633.
38. Raymond E, Faivre S, Woynarowski J, Chaney S. Oxaliplatin: mechanism of action and antineoplastic activity. *Semin Oncol* 1998;25:4.
39. Toney J, Donahue B, Kellett P, et al. Isolation of cDNAs encoding a human protein that binds selectively to DNA modified by the anticancer drug *cis*-diamminedichloroplatinum. *Proc Natl Acad Sci U S A* 1989;86:8328.
40. Bruhn S, Pil P, Essigmann J, Housman D, Lippard S. Isolation and characterization of human cDNA clones encoding a high mobility group box protein that recognizes structural distortions to DNA caused by binding of the anticancer agent cisplatin. *Proc Natl Acad Sci U S A* 1989;89:2307.
41. Grosschedl R, Giese K, Pagel J. HMG domain proteins: architectural elements in the assembly of nucleoprotein structures. *Trends Genet* 1994;10:94.
42. Fink D, Zheng H, Nebel S, et al. *In vitro* and *in vivo* resistance to cisplatin in cells that have lost DNA mismatch repair. *Cancer Res* 1997;57:1841.
43. Fink D, Nebel S, Aebi S, et al. The role of DNA mismatch repair in platinum drug resistance. *Cancer Res* 1996;56:4881.
44. Mello J, Acharya S, Fishel R, Essigmann J. The mismatch-repair protein hMSH2 binds selectively to DNA adducts of the anticancer drug cisplatin. *Chem Biol* 1996;3:579.
45. Sorenson C, Barry M, Eastman A. Analysis of events associated with cell cycle arrest at G2 phase and cell death induced by cisplatin. *J Natl Cancer Inst* 1990;82:749.
46. Evans D, Dive C. Effects of cisplatin on the induction of apoptosis in proliferating hepatoma cells and nonproliferating immature thymocytes. *Cancer Res* 1993;53:2133.
47. Sorrenson C, Eastman A. Mechanism of *cis*-diamminedichloroplatinum (II)-induced cytotoxicity: role of G2 arrest and DNA double-strand breaks. *Cancer Res* 1988;48:4484.
48. Bunch R, Eastman A. 7-Hydroxystaurosporine (UCN-01) causes redistribution of proliferating cell nuclear antigen and abrogates cisplatin-induced S-phase arrest in Chinese hamster ovary cells. *Cell Growth Differ* 1997;8:779.
49. McClay EF, Albright KD, Jones JA, et al. Modulation of cisplatin resistance in human malignant melanoma cells. *Cancer Res* 1992;52:6790.
50. Kroning R, Jones JA, Hom DK, et al. Enhancement of drug sensitivity of human malignancies by epidermal growth factor. *Br J Cancer* 1995;72:615.
51. Chang MJ, Yu WD, Reyno LM, et al. Potentiation by interleukin 1 alpha of cisplatin and carboplatin antitumor activity: schedule-dependent and pharmacokinetic effects in the RIF-1 tumor model. *Cancer Res* 1994;54:5380.
52. Isonishi S, Jekunen AP, Hom DK, et al. Modulation of cisplatin sensitivity and growth rate of an ovarian carcinoma cell line by bombesin and tumor necrosis factor-alpha. *J Clin Invest* 1992;90:1436.
53. Shi Y, Frankel A, Radvanyi L, et al. Rapamycin enhances apoptosis and increases sensitivity to cisplatin *in vitro*. *Cancer Res* 1995;55:1982.
54. Sklar M. Increased resistance to *cis*-diamminedichloro platinum (II) in NIH3T3 cells transformed by ras oncogenes. *Cancer Res* 1988;48:793.
55. Isonishi S, Hom DK, Thiebaut FB, et al. Expression of the c-Ha-ras oncogene in mouse NIH 3T3 cells induces resistance to cisplatin. *Cancer Res* 1991;51:5903.
56. Chapman RS, Whetton AD, Chresta CM, Dive C. Characterization of drug resistance mediated via the suppression of apoptosis by Abelson protein tyrosine kinase. *Mol Pharmacol* 1995,48.334.
57. Benz CC, Scott GK, Sarup JC, et al. Estrogen-dependent, tamoxifen-resistant tumorigenic growth of MCF-7 cells transfected with HER2/neu. *Breast Cancer Res Treat* 1993;24:85.
58. Ip YT, Davis RJ. Signal transduction by the c-Jun N-terminal kinase (JNK)—from inflammation to development. *Curr Opin Cell Biol* 1998;10:205.
59. Zanke B, Boudreau K, Rubie E, et al. The stress-activated protein kinase pathway mediates cell death following injury induced by *cis*-platinum, UV irradiation or heat. *Curr Biol* 1996;6:606.
60. Sanchez-Perez I, Murguia J, Perona R. Cisplatin induces a persistent activation of JNK that is related to cell death. *Oncogene* 1998;16:533.

61. Jarpe M, Widmann C, Knall C, et al. Anti-apoptotic versus pro-apoptotic signal transduction: checkpoints and stop signs along the road to death. *Oncogene* 1998;17:1475.
62. Chen Z, Seimiya H, Naito M, et al. ASK1 mediates apoptotic cell death induced by genotoxic stress. *Oncogene* 1999;18:173.
63. Johnson S, Ferry K, Hamilton T. Recent insights into platinum drug resistance in cancer. *Drug Resistance Updates* 1998;1:243.
64. Gately DP, Howell SB. Cellular accumulation of the anticancer agent cisplatin: a review. *Br J Cancer* 1993;67:1171.
65. Shen DW, Pastan I, Gottesman M. Cross-resistance to methotrexate and metals in human cisplatin-resistant cell lines results from a pleiotropic defect in accumulation of these compounds associated with reduced plasma membrane binding proteins. *Cancer Res* 1998;58:268.
66. Borst P, Kool M, Evers R. Do cMOAT (MRP2), other MRP homologues, and LRP play a role in MDR? *Semin Cancer Biol* 1997;8:205.
67. Taniguchi K, Wada M, Kohno K, et al. A human canalicular multispecific organic anion transporter (cMOAT) gene is overexpressed in cisplatin-resistant human cancer cell lines with decreased drug accumulation. *Cancer Res* 1996;56:4124.
68. Koike K, Kawabe T, Tanaka T, et al. A canalicular multispecific organic anion transporter (cMOAT) antisense cDNA enhances drug sensitivity in human hepatic cancer cells. *Cancer Res* 1997;57:5475.
69. Kool M, de Haas M, Scheffer G, et al. Analysis of expression of cMOAT (MRP2), MRP3, MRP4, and MRP5, homologues of the multidrug resistance–associated protein gene (MRP1), in human cancer cell lines. *Cancer Res* 1997;57:3537.
70. Arts H, Katsaros D, Vries ED, et al. Drug resistance–associated markers P-glycoprotein, multidrug resistance–associated protein 1, multidrug resistance–associated protein 2, and lung resistance protein as prognostic factors in ovarian carcinoma. *Clin Cancer Res* 1999;5:2798.
71. Godwin A, Meister A, O'Dwyer P, et al. High resistance to cisplatin in human ovarian cancer cell lines is associated with marked increase in glutathione synthesis. *Proc Natl Acad Sci U S A* 1992;89:3070.
72. Hosking LK, Whelan RDH, Shellard SA, Bedford P, Hill BT. An evaluation of the role of glutathione and its associated enzymes in the expression of differential sensitivities to antitumor agents shown by a range of human tumour cell lines. *Biochem Pharmacol* 1990;40:1833.
73. Mistry P, Kelland L, Abel G, Sidhar S, Harrap K. The relationships between glutathione, glutathione-S-transferase and cytotoxicity of platinum drugs and melphalan in eight human ovarian carcinoma cell lines. *Br J Cancer* 1991;64:215.
74. Britten RA, Green JA, Broughton C, et al. The relationship between nuclear glutathione levels and resistance to melphalan in human ovarian tumour cells. *Biochem Pharmacol* 1991;41:647.
75. Hamilton T, Winker M, Louie K, et al. Augmentation of Adriamycin, melphalan and cisplatin cytotoxicity in drug-resistant and -sensitive human ovarian cancer cell lines by buthionine sulfoximine mediated glutathione depletion. *Biochem Pharmacol* 1985;34:2583.
76. Smith E, Brock AP. An *in vitro* study comparing the cytotoxicity of three platinum complexes with regard to the effect of thiol depletion. *Br J Cancer* 1988;57:548.
77. Dedon P, Borch R. Characterization of the reactions of platinum antitumor agents with biologic and nonbiologic sulfur-containing nucleophiles. *Biochem Pharmacol* 1987;36:1955.
78. Ishikawa T, Ali-Osman F. Glutathione-associated *cis*-diamminedichloroplatinum (II) metabolism and ATP-dependent efflux from leukemia cells. *J Biol Chem* 1993;268:20116.
79. Mistry P, Loh S, Kelland L, Harrap K. Effect of buthionine sulfoximine on PtII and PtIV drug accumulation and the formation of glutathione conjugates in human ovarian carcinoma cell lines. *Int J Cancer* 1993;55:848.
80. Eastman A. Cross-linking of glutathione to DNA by cancer chemotherapeutic platinum coordination complexes. *Chem Biol Interact* 1987;61:241.
81. Miyazaki M, Kohno K, Saburi Y, et al. Drug resistance to *cis*-diamminedichloroplatinum (II) in Chinese hamster ovary cell lines by transfection with glutathione S-transferase pi gene. *Biochem Biophys Res Commun* 1990;166:1358.
82. Nakagawa K, Saijo N, Tsuchida S, et al. Glutathione S-transferase p as a determinant of drug resistance in transfectant cell lines. *J Biol Chem* 1990;265:4296.
83. Hrubisko M, McGown AT, Fox BW. The role of metallothionein, glutathione, glutathione S-transferases and DNA repair in resistance to platinum drugs in a series of L1210 cell lines made resistant to anticancer platinum agents. *Biochem Pharmacol* 1993;45:253.
84. Pattanaik A, Bachowski G, Laib J, et al. Properties of the reaction of *cis*-dichlorodiammineplatinum(II) with metallothionein. *J Biol Chem* 1992;267:16121.
85. Kelley S, Basu A, Teicher B, et al. Overexpression of metallothionein confers resistance to anticancer drugs. *Science* 1988;241:1813.
86. Kondo Y, Woo ES, Michalska AE, Choo KHA, Lazo JS. Metallothionein null cells have increased sensitivity to anticancer drugs. *Cancer Res* 1995;55:2021.
87. Kojima M, Kikkawa F, Oguchi H, et al. Sensitisation of human ovarian carcinoma cells to *cis*-diamminedichloroplatinum (II) by amphotericin B *in vitro* and *in vivo*. *Eur J Cancer* 1994;30A:773.
88. Siu L, Banerjee D, Khurana F, et al. The prognostic role of p53, metallothionein, P-glycoprotein, and MIB-1 in muscle-invasive urothelial transitional cell carcinoma. *Clin Cancer Res* 1998;4:559.
89. Wood D, Klein E, Fair W, Chaganti R. Metallothionein gene expression in bladder cancer exposed to cisplatin. *Mod Pathol* 1993;6:33.
90. Koberle B, Grimaldi K, Sunters A, et al. DNA repair capacity and cisplatin sensitivity of human testis tumour cells. *Int J Cancer* 1997;70:551.
91. Johnson S, Perez R, Godwin A, et al. Role of platinum-DNA adduct formation and removal in cisplatin resistance in human ovarian cancer cell lines. *Biochem Pharmacol* 1994;47:689.
92. Johnson S, Swiggard P, Handel L, et al. Relationship between platinum-DNA adduct formation and removal and cisplatin cytotoxicity in cisplatin-sensitive and -resistant human ovarian cancer cells. *Cancer Res* 1994;54:5911.
93. Yen L, Woo A, Christopoulopoulos G, et al. Enhanced host cell reactivation capacity and expression of DNA repair genes in human breast cancer cells resistant to bi-functional alkylating agents. *Mutat Res* 1995;337:179.
94. Ali-Osman F, Berger M, Rairkar A, Stein D. Enhanced repair of a cisplatin-damaged reporter chloramphenicol-O-acetyltransferase gene and altered activities of DNA polymerases α and β, and DNA ligase in cells of a human malignant glioma following *in vivo* cisplatin therapy. *J Cell Biochem* 1994;54:11.
95. Eastman A, Schulte N. Enhanced DNA repair as a mechanism of resistance to *cis*-diamminedichloroplatinum(II). *Biochemistry* 1988;27:4730.
96. Wood R. Nucleotide excision repair in mammalian cells. *J Biol Chem* 1997;272:23465.
97. Ferry K, Hamilton T, Johnson S. Increased nucleotide excision repair in cisplatin-resistant ovarian cancer cells: role of ERCC1-XPF. *Biochem Pharmacol* 2000;60:1305.
98. Dabholkar M, Vionnet J, Bostick-Bruton F, Yu J, Reed E. Messenger RNA levels of XPAC and ERCC1 in ovarian cancer tissue correlate with response to platinum-based chemotherapy. *J Clin Invest* 1994;94:703.
99. Chu G, Chang E. Cisplatin-resistant cells express increased levels of a factor that recognizes damaged DNA. *Proc Natl Acad Sci U S A* 1990;87:3324.
100. Mu D, Park CH, Matsunaga T, et al. Reconstitution of human DNA repair excision nuclease in a highly defined system. *J Biol Chem* 1995;270:2415.
101. Hoffmann JS, Pillaire MJ, Maga G, et al. DNA polymerase beta bypasses *in vitro* a single d(GpG)-cisplatin adduct placed on codon 13 of the HRAS gene. *Proc Natl Acad Sci U S A* 1995;92:5356.
102. Masuda H, Tanaka T, Matsuda H, Kusaba I. Increased removal of DNA-bound platinum in a human ovarian cancer cell line resistant to *cis*-diamminedichloroplatinum (II). *Cancer Res* 1990;50:1863.
103. Katz E, Andrews P, Howell S. The effect of DNA polymerase inhibitors on the cytotoxicity of cisplatin in human ovarian carcinoma cells. *Cancer Commun* 1990;2:159.
104. Dempke WCM, Shellard SA, Fichtinger-Schepman AMJ, Hill BT. Lack of significant modulation of the formation and removal of platinum-DNA adducts by aphidicolin glycinate in two logarithmically growing ovarian tumour cell lines *in vitro*. *Carcinogenesis* 1991;12:525.
105. O'Dwyer P, Moyer J, Suffness M, et al. Antitumor activity and biochemical effects of aphidicolin glycinate (NSC 303812) alone and in combination with cisplatin *in vivo*. *Cancer Res* 1994;54:724.
106. Albain K, Swinnen L, Erickson L, et al. Cytotoxic synergy of cisplatin with concurrent hydroxyurea and cytarabine: summary of an *in vitro* model and initial clinical pilot experience. *Semin Oncol* 1992;19:102.
107. Alaoui-Jamali M, Loubaba BB, Robyn S, Tapiero H, Batist G. Effect of DNA-repair-enzyme modulators on cytotoxicity of L-phenylalanine mustard and *cis*-diamminedichloroplatinum (II) in mammary carcinoma cells resistant to alkylating agents. *Cancer Chemother Pharmacol* 1994;34:153.
108. Peters GJ, Bergman AM, Ruiz van Haperen VW, Veerman G, Kuiper CM. Interaction between cisplatin and gemcitabine *in vitro* and *in vivo*. *Semin Oncol* 1995;22:72.
109. Li L, Keatin M, Plunkett W, Yang LY. Fludarabine-mediated repair inhibition of cisplatin-induced DNA lesions in human chronic myelogenous leukemia-blast crisis K562 cells: induction of synergistic cytotoxicity independent of reversal of apoptosis resistance. *Mol Pharm* 1997;52:798.
110. Johnson S, Laub P, Beesley J, Ozols R, Hamilton T. Increased platinum-DNA damage tolerance is associated with cisplatin resistance and cross-resistance to various chemotherapeutic agents in unrelated human ovarian cancer cell lines. *Cancer Res* 1997;57:850.
111. Aebi S, Kurdi-Haidar B, Gordon R, et al. Loss of DNA mismatch repair in acquired resistance to cisplatin. *Cancer Res* 1996;56:3087.
112. Duckett D, Drummond J, Murchie A, et al. Human MutSalpha recognizes damaged DNA base pairs containing O6-methylguanine, O4-methylthymine, or the cisplatin-d(GpG)adduct. *Proc Natl Acad Sci U S A* 1996;93:6443.
113. Karran P, Bignami M. DNA damage tolerance, mismatch repair and genome instability. *Bioessays* 1994;16:833.
114. Mamenta E, Poma E, Kaufmann W, et al. Enhanced replicative bypass of platinum-DNA adducts in cisplatin-resistant human ovarian carcinoma cell lines. *Cancer Res* 1994;54:3500.
115. Miyashita T, Reed JC. Bcl-2 oncoprotein blocks chemotherapy-induced apoptosis in a human leukemia cell line. *Blood* 1993;81:151.
116. Minn A, Rudin C, Boise L, Thompson C. Expression of Bcl-x_l can confer a multidrug resistance phenotype. *Blood* 1995;86:1903.
117. Kharbanda S, Saxena S, Yoshida K, et al. Translocation of SAPK/JNK to mitochondria and interaction with Bcl-x(L) in response to DNA damage. *J Biol Chem* 2000;275:322.
118. Duffull S, Robinson B. Clinical pharmacokinetics and dose optimisation of carboplatin. *Clin Pharmacokinet* 1997;33:161.
119. van der Vijgh W. Clinical pharmacokinetics of carboplatin. *Clin Pharmacokinet* 1991;21:242.
120. Extra J, Marty M, Brienza S, Misset J. Pharmacokinetics and safety profile of oxaliplatin. *Semin Oncol* 1998;25:13.
121. DeConti R, Toftness B, Lange R, Creasey W. Clinical and pharmacological studies with *cis*-diamminedichloroplatinum (II). *Cancer Res* 1973;33:1310.
122. Himmelstein K, Patton T, Belt R, et al. Clinical kinetics on intact cisplatin and some related species. *Clin Pharmacol Ther* 1981;29:658.
123. Vermorken J, van der Vijgh WVD, Klein I, et al. Pharmacokinetics of free and total platinum species after short-term infusion of cisplatin. *Cancer Treat Rep* 1984;68:505.
124. Gormley P, Bull J, LeRoy A, Cysyk R. Kinetics of *cis*-dichlorodiammineplatinum. *Clin Pharmacol Ther* 1979;25:351.
125. Belt R, Himmelstein K, Patton T, et al. Pharmacokinetics of non-protein-bound platinum species following administration of *cis*-dichlorodiammineplatinum(II). *Cancer Treat Rep* 1979;63:1515.
126. Casper E, Kelsen D, Alcock N, Young C. Platinum concentrations in bile and plasma following rapid and 6-hour infusions of *cis*-dichlorodiammineplatinum(II). *Cancer Treat Rep* 1979;63:2023.
127. Harland S, Newell D, Siddik Z, et al. Pharmacokinetics of *cis*-diammine-1,1-cyclobutane dicarboxylate platinum(II) in patients with normal and impaired renal function. *Cancer Res* 1984;44:1693.

128. Calvert A, Newell D, Gumbrell L, et al. Carboplatin dosage: prospective evaluation of a simple formula based on renal function. *J Clin Oncol* 1989;7:1748.
129. Gamelin E, Bouil A, Boisdron-Celle M, et al. Cumulative pharmacokinetic study of oxaliplatin, administered every three weeks, combined with 5-fluorouracil in colorectal cancer patients. *Clin Cancer Res* 1997;3:891.
130. Egorin M, Echo DV, Olman E, et al. Prospective validation of a pharmacologically based dosing scheme for the *cis*-diamminedichloroplatinum(II) analogue diamminecyclobutanedicarboxylatoplatinum. *Cancer Res* 1985;45:6502.
131. Chatelut E, Canal P, Brunner V, et al. Prediction of carboplatin clearance from standard morphological and biological patient characteristics. *J Natl Cancer Inst* 1995;87:573.
132. Jodrell D, Egorin M, Canetta R, et al. Relationships between carboplatin exposure and tumor response and toxicity in patients with ovarian cancer. *J Clin Oncol* 1992;10:520.
133. Reyno L, Egorin M, Canetta R, et al. Impact of cyclophosphamide on relationships between carboplatin exposure and response or toxicity when used in the treatment of advanced ovarian cancer. *J Clin Oncol* 1993;11:1156.
134. O'Dwyer P, Hamilton T, Yao K, Ozols R, Gallo J. Cellular pharmacodynamics of anticancer drugs. In: Schilsky R, Milano G, Ratain M, eds. *Cancer pharmacology*. New York: Marcel Dekker Inc, 1996:329.
135. Ma J, Verweij J, Planting A, et al. Current sample handling methods for measurement of platinum-DNA adducts in leucocytes in man lead to discrepant results in DNA adduct levels and DNA repair. *Br J Cancer* 1995;71:512.
136. Schellens J, Ma J, Planting A, et al. Relationship between the exposure to cisplatin, DNA-adduct formation in leucocytes and tumour response in patients with solid tumours. *Br J Cancer* 1996;73:1569.
137. Loehrer P, Einhorn L. Drugs five years later. Cisplatin. *Ann Intern Med* 1984;100:704.
138. Ozols R, Corden B, Jacob J, et al. High-dose cisplatin in hypertonic saline. *Ann Intern Med* 1984;100:19.
139. Howell S, Pfeifle C, Wung W, Olshen R. Intraperitoneal *cis*-diamminedichloroplatinum with systemic thiosulfate protection. *Cancer Res* 1983;43:1426.
140. Alberts D, Liu P, Hannigan E, et al. Intraperitoneal cisplatin plus intravenous cyclophosphamide versus intravenous cisplatin plus intravenous cyclophosphamide for stage III ovarian cancer. *N Engl J Med* 1996;335:1950.
141. Solomon B, Soulen M, Baum R, et al. Chemoembolization of hepatocellular carcinoma with cisplatin, doxorubicin, mitomycin-C, ethiodol, and polyvinyl alcohol: prospective evaluation of response and survival in a U.S. population. *J Vasc Interv Radiol* 1999;10:793.
142. Evans B, Raju K, Calvert A, Harland S, Wiltshaw E. Phase II study of JM8, a new platinum analog, in advanced ovarian carcinoma. *Cancer Treat Rep* 1983;67:997.
143. Ozols R, Behrens B, Ostchega Y, Young R. High dose cisplatin and high dose carboplatin in refractory ovarian cancer. *Cancer Treat Rev* 1985;12:59.
144. Schilder R, Johnson S, Gallo J, et al. Phase I trial of multiple cycles of high-dose chemotherapy supported by autologous peripheral-blood stem cells. *J Clin Oncol* 1999;17:2198.
145. Levi F, Giacchetti S, Adam R, et al. Chronomodulation of chemotherapy against metastatic colorectal cancer. International Organization for Cancer Chronotherapy. *Eur J Cancer* 1995;31A:1264.
146. McMahon S, Priestley J. Peripheral neuropathies and neurotrophic factors: animal models and clinical perspectives. *Curr Opin Neurobiol* 1995;5:616.
147. Langer C, Leighton J, Comis R, et al. Paclitaxel and carboplatin in combination in the treatment of advanced non-small-cell lung cancer: a phase II toxicity, response, and survival analysis. *J Clin Oncol* 1995;13:1860.
148. Extra J, Espie M, Calvo F, et al. Phase I study of oxaliplatin in patients with advanced cancer. *Cancer Chemother Pharmacol* 1990;25:299.
149. Brienza S, Vignoud J, Itzhaki M, Krikorian A. Oxaliplatin (L-OHP): global safety in 682 patients. *Proc Am Soc Clin Oncol* 1995;14:209.

EDWARD CHU
AUGUSTO C. MOTA
MIKLOS C. FOGARASI

SECTION 5

Antimetabolites

METHOTREXATE

Aminopterin was the first antimetabolite to demonstrate clinical activity in the treatment of patients with malignancy. This antifolate analogue was used to induce remissions in children with acute leukemia in the 1940s.[1] Aminopterin has since been replaced by methotrexate (MTX), the 4-amino, 10-methyl analogue of folic acid. MTX remains the most widely used antifolate in cancer chemotherapy, with documented activity against a wide range of human malignancies, including leukemia, breast cancer, colorectal cancer, head and neck cancer, lymphoma, osteogenic sarcoma, urothelial cancer, and choriocarcinoma. Antifolates have also been used to treat a host of nonmalignant disorders, including psoriasis, rheumatoid arthritis, graft-versus-host disease, bacterial and plasmodial infections, and parasitic infections associated with the acquired immunodeficiency syndrome.[2] This class of agents represents the best-characterized and most versatile of all chemotherapeutic drugs in current clinical use.

MECHANISM OF ACTION

MTX is a tight-binding inhibitor of dihydrofolate reductase (DHFR), a critical enzyme in folate metabolism (Fig. 19.5-1).[2] The importance of DHFR stems from its role in maintaining the intracellular folate pool in its fully reduced form as tetrahydrofolates. These compounds serve as one-carbon carriers required for the synthesis of thymidine-5'-monophosphate (thymidylate), purine nucleotides, and certain amino acids. Thymidylate synthase (TS) catalyzes the formation of thymidine-5'-monophosphate from 2'-deoxyuridine 5'monophosphate (deoxyuridylate, dUMP) (Fig.

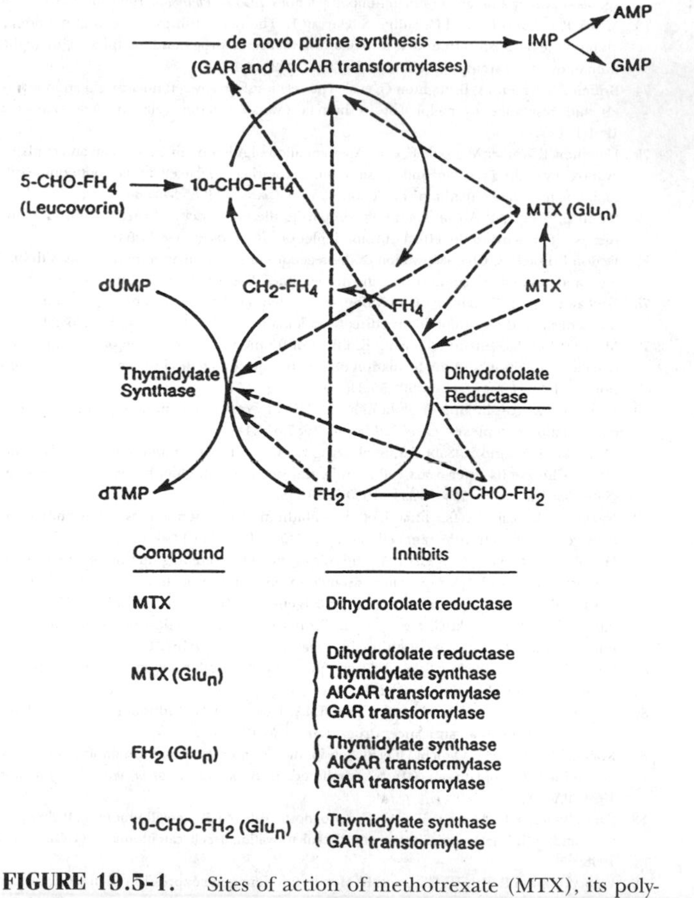

FIGURE 19.5-1. Sites of action of methotrexate (MTX), its polyglutamated metabolites [MTX(Glu_n)], and folate by-products of the inhibition of dihydrofolate reductase, including dihydrofolate (FH_2) and 10-formyl-dihydrofolate (10-CHO-FH_2). Also shown are 5,10-methylenetetrahydrofolate (CH_2FH_4), the folate cofactor required for thymidylate synthesis, and 10-formyltetrahydrofolate (10-CHO-FH_4), the required cofactor for *de novo* purine synthesis. AICAR, aminoimidazole carboxamide ribonucleotide transformylase; AMP, adenosine monophosphate; dTMP, thymidylate; dUMP, deoxyuridylate; GAR, glycinamide ribonucleotide transformylase; GMP, guanine monophosphate; IMP, inosine monophosphate.

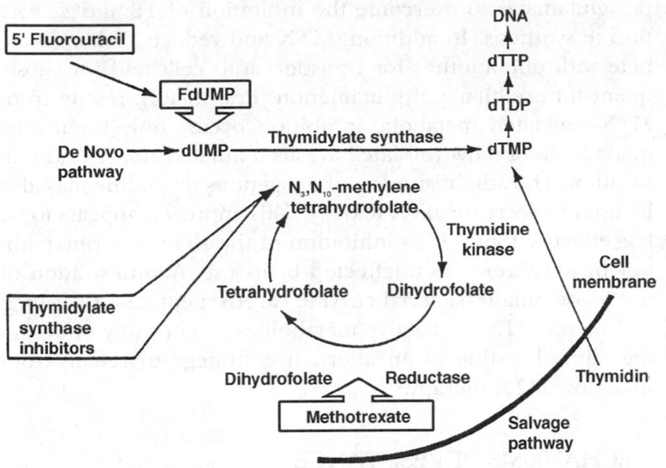

FIGURE 19.5-2. The thymidylate synthase enzyme pathway. dTDP, thymidine diphosphate; dTMP, thymidylate; dTTP, thymidine triphosphate; dUMP, deoxyuridylate; FdUMP, 5-fluoro-2'-deoxyuridine monophosphate.

19.5-2). This reaction uses 5,10-methylenetetrahydrofolate as a methyl donor and results in the oxidation of the reduced folate to dihydrofolate. The activity of the TS reaction thus creates the requirement for DHFR to maintain the intracellular reduced folate pool needed for one-carbon transfer reactions. The reduced folate, 10-formyltetrahydrofolate, serves as a substrate for two folate-dependent enzymes of *de novo* purine synthesis, glycinamide ribonucleotide (GAR) transformylase and aminoimidazole carboxamide ribonucleotide transformylase. An intact DHFR pathway is therefore necessary for continued *de novo* thymidylate and purine nucleotide biosynthesis.

The precise mechanism by which MTX produces metabolic inhibition remains a subject of ongoing debate. The long-held view has been that inhibition of DHFR results in an accumulation of oxidized folates at the expense of reduced folates owing to the continued synthetic function of TS. Ultimate depletion of the required reduced folates would result in cessation of *de novo* thymidylate and purine biosynthesis as well as inhibition of protein synthesis. However, several investigators have demonstrated that after exposure of malignant cells to inhibitory concentrations of MTX, intracellular reduced folates are depleted by only 50% to 70%, a level presumably insufficient to account for the observed inhibition of DNA synthesis.[2,3] Additional metabolic effects of MTX result from its transformation to polyglutamate forms (see Fig. 19.5-1). MTX and physiologic folate polyglutamates are formed by the enzyme folylpolyglutamyl synthetase, which adds up to five to seven glutamyl groups in a γ-peptide linkage. Polyglutamation is a time- and concentration-dependent process that occurs in tumor cells and, to a lesser extent, in normal tissues.[4] These polyglutamate metabolites have a prolonged intracellular half-life and allow for prolonged drug action in malignant cells. The relative difference in polyglutamate formation in normal versus malignant cells may account for the selective activity of the drug. As much as 80% of MTX found in malignant tissues is in the polyglutamated forms, and these metabolites are potent, direct inhibitors of several folate-dependent enzymes, including DHFR, TS, and aminoimidazole carboxamide ribonucleotide and GAR transformylases.[1–3,5,6] Thus, metabolic inhibition resulting from MTX exposure is a multifactorial process and may depend on several factors, including partial depletion of reduced folates and direct inhibition of folate-dependent enzymes by the polyglutamates of both MTX and dihydrofolate that accumulate after inhibition of DHFR.

The precise mechanism by which MTX induces cytotoxicity remains an area of continued investigation. MTX-induced depletion of thymidine triphosphate (dTTP) and purine nucleotides interferes with the cellular capacity to repair DNA, resulting in DNA strand breaks.[7,8] Furthermore, the need for repair is accentuated by an intracellular accumulation of dUMP resulting from the inhibitory effects of MTX on TS. dUMP can be converted to the triphosphate nucleotide form (dUTP), which is then incorporated into DNA, resulting in inhibition of chain elongation and DNA synthesis. Excision repair of the DNA containing these misincorporated dUTP moieties by the enzyme uracil DNA glycosylase results in further DNA fragmentation.

Novel mechanisms by which MTX may exert its cytotoxic action have been described. Treatment with MTX results in a significant dose-dependent reduction in methionine synthase enzyme activity.[9,10] This enzyme catalyzes the folate-dependent reaction in which 5-methyltetrahydrofolate serves as a critical one-carbon carrier methyl donor and mediates the conversion of homocysteine to methionine. Thus, inhibition of methionine synthase leads to inhibition of a number of key downstream pathways, including transmethylation reactions, polyamine biosynthesis, protein synthesis, or all three.[11] Treatment of cultured Ehrlich ascites tumor cells with MTX resulted in up to a 3.5-fold increase in 5'-phosphoribosyl-1-pyrophosphate (PRPP) levels, which was associated with a significant suppression in the rate of glucose transport. Coadministration of MTX and hypoxanthine completely protected against the growth-inhibitory action of MTX and reversed the effect on PRPP production and on the rate of glucose transport.[12] Thus, MTX may exert its anticancer effect, in part, through inhibition of critical glucose transport mechanisms, thereby starving the cancer cell of essential nutrients required to maintain cellular metabolism and growth.

MTX is most active against rapidly proliferating cells, as its cytotoxic effects occur primarily during the S phase of the cell cycle. During longer periods of drug exposure, a higher fraction of cells can enter the S phase of the cell cycle, resulting in greater cell kill. In addition, MTX polyglutamate formation is substantially enhanced with longer periods of drug exposure, thereby increasing cytotoxicity. The cytotoxic effects of MTX are also greater with increasing drug concentrations. Therefore, MTX cytotoxicity is highly dependent on the absolute drug concentration and the duration of drug exposure.

MTX enters cells by the same active transport mechanisms used by physiologic reduced folates. In general, intracellular drug concentrations reach steady state in less than 30 minutes. Folate transport is a complex process with at least two carrier-mediated, energy-dependent mechanisms existing in mammalian cells. The first is the classic reduced folate carrier (RFC) system that has a relatively low affinity for MTX and reduced folates such as leucovorin (LV), with affinity constants in the micromolar range.[2,13–17] The RFC system has a large capacity and is primarily responsible for transport of MTX into cells at pharmacologic concentrations. The human RFC gene has been mapped to the long arm of chromosome 1, and it encodes a protein with a predicted molecular weight of 59 to 68 kD.

A second folate transport system involves a high-affinity, membrane-bound folate receptor-binding protein with affinity constants for reduced folates and folic acid in the nanomolar range.[18,19] MTX is a relatively poor substrate for this folate-binding protein, and its affinity is 10- to 30-fold lower than that of physiologic reduced folates. The human folate receptor protein (FR) is a 38- to 40-kD glycoprotein bound to the cellular membrane via a C-terminal, glycosylphosphatidylinositol tail.[20] It is expressed on the surface of various normal tissues, including human placenta, choroid plexus, renal tubules, and fallopian tubes. Of note, this receptor is also highly expressed on the surface of a number of epithelial tumors, including ovarian cancer, but not on normal ovarian tissue, making it an attractive target for antigen-directed anticancer therapies.[21] Alterations in the tissue expression of FR can be induced by changes in the exogenous folate concentration or by alteration in normal physiology such as in pregnancy. At least three different isoforms of the human FR have been described to date, and they are classified as FR-α, FR-β, and FR-γ.[17,22] These isoforms have unique folate-binding affinities and variable expression in specific tissues. FR-α is highly expressed in human epithelial tissues and in some cancers such as ovarian cancer, whereas FR-β is expressed in human placenta and other nonepithelial tissues. Although the FR-α and FR-β isoforms share 70% to 80% amino acid sequence homology, they differ significantly in their respective affinities and stereospecificities for reduced folates. Human FR-γ lacks a glycosylphosphatidylinositol tail, and this isoform most likely represents a secretory protein.

An additional MTX transport system has been described in murine L1210 leukemic cells that is completely distinct from either the RFC or the FR systems.[23,24] Further studies are under way to characterize the role of this transporter as a determinant of MTX cytotoxicity. It is likely that the relative function of each of these distinct transport systems depends on the extracellular folate concentration, and their expression may vary significantly among different cell lines. Their interrelationship and role in MTX transport remains an active area of research. Nonclassic antifolate compounds, such as trimetrexate and trimethoprim, do not rely on specific transport systems for cellular entry. Such analogues are active against various malignant cell lines resistant to MTX on the basis of decreased transport capacity. In addition to these transport systems, two energy-dependent MTX efflux transport systems have been described in murine leukemic L1210 cells using *inside out* membrane vesicles.[25] These two systems appear to be functionally distinct and sensitive to a different range of chemical inhibitors. The major efflux transporter is identical to a glutathione conjugate membrane pump and accounts for nearly 70% of MTX efflux.

Reduced folates, such as 5-formyltetrahydrofolate (LV), prevent, rescue, or both prevent and rescue cells from the toxic effects of MTX. The predominant species of reduced folate in human plasma, 5-methyltetrahydrofolate, circulates with levels in the range of 5 to 50 n*M*, a concentration inadequate to rescue cells. Administration of appropriate doses of LV after high-dose MTX therapy can prevent toxicity to the bone marrow and gastrointestinal epithelium, the two most rapidly dividing cells in the body. The dose of LV required to rescue normal tissues is dependent on the antifolate concentration at the time of antidote administration.[26] The competitive nature of this rescue suggests that LV does more than simply replete intracellular reduced folate pools. LV is converted to intracellular folates that can compete with both MTX and dihydrofolate polyglutamates to overcome the inhibition of TS and *de novo* purine synthesis. In addition, MTX and reduced folates compete with one another for transport into cells and for subsequent intracellular polyglutamation. Presumably, rescue from MTX-associated metabolic inhibition occurs only when adequate levels of dihydrofolate have accumulated after LV administration. The administration of exogenous thymidine may also be used to decrease MTX toxicity. This approach appears to be less effective than LV, as inhibition of the *de novo* purine pathway by MTX remains unaffected by its use. Administration of the recombinant bacterial enzyme carboxypeptidase G_2, which hydrolyzes MTX to inactive metabolites, is currently undergoing clinical testing as an alternative strategy to rescue from high-dose MTX therapy.[27]

MECHANISMS OF RESISTANCE

The development of cellular resistance to MTX remains a major obstacle to its effective clinical use. In experimental systems, resistance to antifolates may result from several mechanisms, including an alteration in antifolate transport due to either a defect in the RFC or FR systems,[28–31] decreased capacity to polyglutamate MTX through either decreased expression of folylpolyglutamyl synthetase or increased expression of the catabolic enzyme gamma-glutamyl hydrolase,[32–35] and alterations in the target enzyme DHFR through either increased expression of the wild-type protein or overexpression of a mutant protein with reduced binding affinity for MTX.[2,36,37]

Amplification of the DHFR gene is one of the most common forms of MTX resistance observed in experimental systems.[2] The amplified gene may be stably integrated into chromosomal DNA in the form of a homogeneously staining region, or it may exist in extrachromosomal pieces of DNA known as *double-minute chromosomes.*[38] Homogeneously staining region–mediated gene amplification is associated with the development of stable resistance to MTX. In contrast, double-minute chromosomes are unequally distributed during cell division, and, in the absence of continued selective pressure of MTX, cells eventually revert to a sensitive phenotype with wild-type levels of DHFR expression. It was shown that resistant human leukemic HL-60 cells coamplify both DHFR and hMSH3, the human *mutS* homologue 3 gene.[39] Overproduction of hMSH3 results in virtually complete sequestration of the nuclear hMSH2 mismatch repair (MMR) protein. The net effect of this protein-protein interaction is a marked reduction in the efficiency of base-base MMR. As MMR deficiency has been implicated as a potential mechanism of resistance to the platinum analogues cisplatin and carboplatin, DNA methylating agents, and doxorubicin (Adriamycin), it is conceivable that this same resistance phenotype may contribute to the development of resistance to MTX and other antifolate analogues.

An alternative mechanism of resistance has been ascribed to mutations that result in a DHFR protein product with an altered binding affinity for MTX. There is evidence that naturally occurring DHFR alleles with differing affinities to MTX may exist in cells and provide a mechanism for the rapid emergence of MTX resistance.[40] In several *in vitro* experimental model systems, the levels of DHFR enzyme activity acutely increase after exposure to MTX, other antifolate analogue compounds, or both.[41,42] This acute induction of DHFR in response to drug exposure is mediated, in part, by a translational regulatory mechanism.[43] DHFR protein, in its unbound or free state, is capable of specifically repressing the translation of its own messenger RNA (mRNA). However, when DHFR protein is bound to an antifolate inhibitor, it is unable to repress DHFR mRNA translation, and the rate of new DHFR protein synthesis increases.[43,44] Thus, induction of DHFR may represent a clinically relevant mechanism for the acute development of cellular drug resistance.

Apoptosis, the process of programmed cell death, is a critical event during normal development and in the pathogenesis of several disease states, including cancer, autoimmune disorders, viral infection, and neurodegenerative diseases. Bcl-2 can repress cell death triggered by a wide array of stimuli, including chemotherapy and gamma-irradiation. Bcl-XL, a structural homologue of Bcl-2, has also been shown to provide protection against a wide range of anticancer agents. These prosurvival proteins presumably act at some common final step to prevent or overcome the cell death pathway induced by various anticancer agents. It has been shown that murine lymphoid FL5.12 cells transduced with Bcl-XL as compared with another antiapoptotic gene Bcl-2, become resistant to the cytotoxic effects of MTX.[45] Thus, the expression of Bcl-XL may represent an important indicator for predicting chemosensitivity to MTX and other antifolate analogues.

Despite many years of active investigation, the relative contribution of each of these mechanisms as a determinant of MTX resistance remains unclear. However, there is growing evidence to support the concept that the emergence of MTX resistance, in the clinical setting, is a multifactorial process. In fact, DHFR gene amplification, defective transport, and decreased polyglutamate formation have all been observed in clinical specimens taken from MTX-resistant patients.[46–49]

CLINICAL PHARMACOLOGY AND PHARMACOKINETICS

Accurate monitoring of MTX concentrations in plasma is essential for the safe and optimal use of this agent in cancer chemotherapy, particularly with high-dose regimens. At least four methods are presently available for the clinical monitoring of MTX drug levels, including the DHFR enzyme inhibition assay, a competitive protein-binding assay, a fluorescence-polarization radioimmunoassay technique, and an enzyme-multiplied immunoassay system.[2]

The absorption of oral MTX is saturable and erratic at higher doses, such that oral doses should be kept to less than 25 mg/m^2. The drug is usually administered intravenously. The volume of distribution of MTX approaches that of total body water, and approximately 60% of the drug is bound to serum albumin at pharmacologic drug concentrations.[2] Although plasma pharmacokinetics are variable, MTX metabolism generally follows a three-phase pattern. The initial distribution phase, which lasts for only a few minutes, is followed by a second phase lasting 12 to 24 hours, during which time the drug is eliminated with a half-life of 2 to 3 hours. The final phase of drug clearance has a half-life of 8 to 10 hours. The last two phases of drug elimination are considerably lengthened in patients with renal dysfunction. There is substantial evidence that a more rapid systemic clearance of drug is associated with a high risk of relapse in children receiving MTX for maintenance therapy of acute lymphocytic leukemia.

The distribution of MTX into third-space fluid collections, such as pleural effusions and ascitic fluid, can substantially alter MTX pharmacokinetics. The slow release of accumulated MTX from these third spaces over time prolongs the terminal half-life of the drug, leading to potentially increased clinical toxicity.[50] Although no strict guidelines exist for the treatment of patients with ascites or pleural effusions, it is advisable to evacuate these fluid collections before treatment and monitor plasma drug concentrations closely. In addition, patients with bladder cancer who have undergone cystectomy and ileal conduit loop diversion may experience a significant increase in toxicity secondary to MTX treatment.[51] Thus, caution should be given when beginning therapy with MTX in this particular subset of patients.

Elimination of MTX occurs primarily through renal excretion. MTX is filtered by the glomerulus and is actively secreted in the proximal tubule. Renal clearance usually equals or exceeds creatinine clearance. However, rates of drug clearance may vary widely, and they do not precisely parallel renal function. Renal excretion of MTX is inhibited by probenecid, penicillins, cephalosporins, aspirin, and nonsteroidal antiinflammatory drugs.[2] The combination of MTX and nonsteroidal antiinflammatory drugs has been associated with severe toxicity in patients receiving high-dose MTX. Patients with impaired renal function (creatinine clearance less than 60 mL/min) should not be treated with high-dose MTX. Moreover, standard doses of MTX should be reduced in proportion to reductions in creatinine clearance.

The introduction of high-dose MTX regimens led to the identification of at least two MTX metabolites. 7-Hydroxymethotrexate (7-OH-MTX) constitutes 20% to 46% of drug excreted in urine from 12 to 24 hours after the start of a high-dose infusion. It is formed through the action of aldehyde oxidase in the liver and is a weak inhibitor of DHFR. 7-OH-MTX is a substrate for folylpolyglutamyl synthetase, and the resulting polyglutamate metabolites are inhibitors of the folate-dependent enzymes TS and aminoimidazole carboxamide ribonucleotide transformylase, with a potency similar to that of MTX polyglutamates.[52] A second metabolite, 2,4 diamino-N10-methyl pteroic acid (DAMPA), a product of bacterial degradation of MTX in the gut lumen, is inactive and constitutes approximately 25% of the excreted drug at 24 to 48 hours after drug infusion. The exact role of these metabolites in producing MTX toxicity or enhancing therapeutic activity remains uncertain.

Biliary excretion of MTX represents approximately 10% of overall MTX drug clearance.[53] However, in the presence of renal dysfunction, enterohepatic circulation may represent an important pathway of drug elimination. Most MTX excreted in bile is reabsorbed as intact drug, but an undefined fraction is converted by intestinal flora to DAMPA. Intestinal binding of drug with oral charcoal or the anion-exchange resin cholestyramine enhances nonrenal drug excretion. Given the relatively minor role of biliary excretion in drug elimination, no adjustments in MTX dose are necessary for patients with hepatic dysfunction.

SCHEDULES OF ADMINISTRATION

The safe use of high-dose MTX with LV rescue requires a thorough understanding of MTX pharmacokinetics. High-dose MTX therapy is used in the treatment of high-grade lymphomas, osteogenic sarcoma, and acute leukemia. These regimens use otherwise lethal infusions of MTX given over 6 to 42 hours in doses of 500 mg/m^2 or higher. High-dose MTX can be safely administered to patients provided that careful attention is paid to intravenous fluid hydration, urinary alkalinization, plasma drug level monitoring, and adequate administration of LV.

During infusion of high-dose MTX, rapid renal excretion results in high urinary drug concentrations. Urinary MTX concentrations approaching 10 mM exceed solubility, resulting in intratubular precipitation and acute renal failure with potentially disastrous consequences. This complication can be avoided by vigorous hydration (3 L fluid/m^2/24 hours, beginning 12 hours before infusion and continuing for 36 hours), and urinary alkalinization to increase drug solubility. Administration of MTX should not begin until urine flow is 100 mL/h and urine pH is 7 or greater, and these parameters should be carefully monitored during the course of therapy. High-dose MTX therapy should not be used in patients with impaired renal function (creatinine clearance less than 60 mL/min).

Close monitoring of MTX plasma levels is essential for guiding the duration and amount of LV required to prevent severe MTX-associated toxicity. Given the competitive interaction between MTX and LV, the dose of the rescue agent must be increased in proportion to the plasma concentration of MTX. If the MTX level exceeds 0.5 μM 48 hours from the start of the infusion, the LV dose may be adjusted to 15, 100, or 200 mg/m^2 every 6 hours for MTX levels of 0.5, 1.0, and 2.0 μM, respectively. Drug levels should be rechecked every 24 hours and the LV dose adjusted until the drug concentration is less than 50 n*M*. However, clinicians should be aware that overzealous use of LV may counteract the cytotoxic effects of MTX in tumor cells as well as in host cells.[54] For this reason, it is important to use doses of LV that are adequate but not excessive, so that normal but not tumor cells will be rescued. In patients with delayed MTX excretion, LV is usually given intravenously, because its oral bioavailability is decreased at total doses higher than 40 mg.

Despite careful attention to detail, persistent elevations of plasma MTX levels may sometimes occur. Plasma MTX levels higher than 10 μM at 48 hours are poorly rescued even with high doses of LV. Hemodialysis and peritoneal dialysis are ineffective in removing MTX, with clearance rates of only 35 to 40 mL/min. Experimental approaches to reduce toxic levels of MTX include hemoperfusion over a charcoal column, oral administration of activated charcoal or cholestyramine to increase enterohepatic drug loss, and intravenous infusion of the degradative enzyme carboxypeptidase G_2.[27,55]

MTX penetrates poorly into the cerebrospinal fluid (CSF), and CSF levels are 30-fold lower than plasma levels at equilibrium.[56] However, after high-dose MTX therapy, peak CSF levels greater than the therapeutic threshold of 1 μM can be achieved. Systemic high-dose MTX therapy has been used to prevent meningeal leukemia and lymphoma. Intrathecal injection of MTX can also be used for prophylaxis. For treatment of meningeal carcinomatosis, injection of MTX through an indwelling Ommaya reservoir is recommended because drug administered into the CSF via the lumbar space circulates poorly into the ventricles, resulting in inadequate CSF drug levels. A total intrathecal dose of 12 mg is advised for all persons older than 3 years of age. In normal patients, the CSF half-life is approximately 12 hours, but it may be prolonged in patients with active meningeal disease. Delayed clearance from the CSF has been associated with an increased risk of MTX neurotoxicity.

TOXICITY

The primary toxic effects of MTX therapy are myelosuppression and gastrointestinal mucositis. The occurrence of these adverse effects and other toxicities depends on the dose, schedule, and route of drug administration. Mucositis usually appears 3 to 7 days after MTX therapy and precedes the decrease in granulocyte and platelet count by several days. Myelosuppression and mucositis are usually completely reversed within 14 days, unless drug elimination mechanisms are impaired. In patients with compromised renal function, even small doses of MTX may result in serious toxicity.

MTX-induced nephrotoxicity is thought to result from the intratubular precipitation of MTX and its metabolites, 7-OH-MTX and DAMPA, in acidic urine. Antifolates may also exert a direct toxic effect on the renal tubules. Vigorous hydration and urinary alkalinization have greatly reduced the incidence of renal failure in high-dose regimens.[2]

MTX is associated with both acute and chronic hepatotoxicity. Acute elevations in hepatic enzyme levels, as well as hyperbilirubinemia, are often observed during high-dose therapy, but these usually return to normal within 10 days. Chronic administration of daily oral MTX, as has been used in the treatment of psoriasis, is associated with the development of hepatic fibrosis in as many as 25% of patients. Cirrhosis of the liver has also been described in this group. Intermittent, weekly MTX therapy, rather than continuous daily treatment, is associated with a lower incidence of hepatotoxicity. Although the precise mechanism of MTX hepatotoxicity is not known, liver biopsies of patients with drug-induced liver disease reveal increased lipid deposition in the liver.

MTX causes a poorly defined, self-limited pneumonitis characterized by fever, cough, and interstitial pulmonary infiltrates. Lung biopsies have not revealed consistent pathologic findings. Although a hypersensitivity reaction has been proposed as a possible explanation, rechallenge with MTX does not uniformly result in a return of symptoms. With the increasing use of chronic, low-dose MTX therapy for rheumatoid arthritis, there is now a growing number of cases of MTX-associated lung damage. No specific therapy for MTX pneumonitis is recommended other than withholding MTX therapy during the acute episode.

Three distinct neurotoxic syndromes are associated with intrathecal MTX therapy.[57] The most common syndrome is an acute chemical arachnoiditis that arises immediately after intrathecal drug administration. This syndrome is characterized by severe headaches, nuchal rigidity, vomiting, fever, and an inflammatory cell infiltrate in the CSF. A subacute form of neurotoxicity is seen in approximately 10% of patients and usually occurs after the third or fourth course of intrathecal therapy. It is most common in adults with active meningeal leukemia and consists of motor paralysis, cranial nerve palsies, and seizures or coma, or both. A change in therapy is absolutely indicated, because continued intrathecal MTX therapy may result in death. The third syndrome is a chronic, demyelinating encephalopathy, typically occurring in children months to years after receiving intrathecal MTX. Patients present with dementia, limb spasticity, and, in advanced cases, coma. Computed tomography scan reveals ventricular enlargement, cortical thinning, and diffuse intracerebral calcifications.[83]

High-dose systemic MTX therapy is occasionally associated with an acute, transient cerebral dysfunction with symptoms of paresis, aphasia, and behavioral abnormalities, and seizures have also been described in 4% to 15% of patients receiving high-dose MTX.[58] Symptoms occur within 6 days of MTX treatment and usually completely resolve within 48 to 72 hours. In addition, a chronic form of neurotoxicity is manifested as an encephalopathy with dementia and motor paresis developing in the second or third month after treatment. At present, the underlying mechanism of CNS toxicity from MTX remains unknown.

There is no evidence to support the therapeutic use of LV in patients who develop neurotoxic symptoms.

True anaphylactic reactions to MTX are exceedingly rare. There have been a few reported cases of toxic skin erythema and desquamation of the hands after high-dose MTX therapy. In men treated with high-dose MTX, a reversible defect in spermatogenesis may occur. However, no alterations in reproductive function have been reported in women treated with MTX.

NEW ANTIFOLATES

TRIMETREXATE

In the 1990s, several new antifolates were developed in an attempt to circumvent some of the known mechanisms of resistance to MTX, to target folate-dependent enzymes other than DHFR, or both. The more lipid-soluble quinazoline antifolate trimetrexate (TMTX, Neutrexin) differs from MTX by not requiring the RFC system for cellular transport and by lacking the potential for polyglutamation. Like MTX, it is a potent inhibitor of DHFR and produces metabolic inhibition through mechanisms similar to MTX. It was thought that malignant cells that had become resistant to MTX, by virtue of either reduced membrane transport or deficient polyglutamation, would remain sensitive to this antifolate analogue. Because TMTX is not polyglutamated, its intracellular half-life is shorter than MTX, necessitating frequent or continuous dosing schedules. In contrast to MTX, TMTX can serve as a substrate for the P-glycoprotein-associated efflux pump. As a result, cross-resistance to TMTX and a host of natural products, including anthracyclines, taxanes, and vinca alkaloids, can develop in multidrug resistant cancer cells overexpressing the P170 glycoprotein.

TMTX has been tested using a variety of dose schedules. It is highly protein bound (more than 90%) and cleared principally from the body by hepatic metabolism.[59] The terminal plasma half-life of the drug ranges from 12 to 20 hours. TMTX has been tested in the phase II setting for the treatment of a variety of malignancies, principally with a regimen of 8 to 12 mg/m^2 daily for 5 days every 3 weeks.[60,61] The dose-limiting toxicity has been myelosuppression. Other toxicities include rash, mucositis, fever, nausea and vomiting, and reversible transaminasemia. Antitumor responses have ranged from 13% to 26%, with the highest rates in head and neck (26%) and non–small cell lung (19%) cancers. As a single agent, the compound has shown little activity against gastrointestinal cancers. However, when used in combination with 5-fluorouracil (5-FU) and LV, response rates on the order of 30% to 35% have been reported in patients with previously untreated metastatic colorectal cancer.[62]

TOMUDEX

Raltitrexed (ZD1694, Tomudex) is a quinazoline antifolate that is a potent and specific inhibitor of TS. Like MTX, raltitrexed is transported into the cell via the RFC. To exert its cytotoxic activity, this compound needs to be metabolized to its higher polyglutamated forms. The polyglutamates of raltitrexed are approximately 100-fold more potent than the parent compound with regard to their affinity for TS, and they exhibit prolonged intracellular retention.[63] The principal mechanism of action of this compound is inhibition of TS, resulting in depletion of key nucleotide precursors required for DNA repair and synthesis. Mechanisms of resistance to raltitrexed include reduced transport, decreased polyglutamation, and overexpression of the target enzyme, TS.[64,65]

Raltitrexed has undergone phase I testing, and the recommended dosing schedule is 3 mg/m^2 given as a 15-minute intravenous infusion every 3 weeks.[60,61] The drug is cleared from the body principally by renal excretion, and its clearance follows a three-compartment elimination model with a terminal half-life of 10 to 22 hours. The major toxicities include an anorexia and fatigue syndrome, diarrhea, myelosuppression, and reversible transaminasemia. Several phase II clinical trials have investigated the activity of this drug in patients with a wide spectrum of malignancies, including advanced colorectal, breast, hepatocellular, platinum-resistant ovarian, non–small cell lung, gastric, and pancreas cancers.[66] Response rates have ranged from 14% for patients with pancreas cancer to 25% for those with breast cancer. The largest reported experience has been for first-line treatment of patients with advanced colorectal carcinoma. An overall response rate of 26% was observed in a phase II trial involving 176 patients. Randomized, phase III trials to compare the efficacy of raltitrexed versus LV-modulated 5-FU have been completed.[67,68] Raltitrexed has comparable response rates and similar palliative and survival benefits when compared with 5-FU/LV. Reduced toxicity was observed with this novel antifolate analogue, however, and it was associated with a more convenient administration schedule. This drug is approved as first-line therapy for patients with advanced colorectal cancer in Australia, Canada, and several European countries. Further studies are ongoing to determine the role of this antifolate TS inhibitor compound, either alone or in combination with other anticancer agents, in the therapy of colorectal cancer in North America.

OTHER ANTIFOLATES

Several pteroyl glutamate analogues have shown superior preclinical activity compared with MTX, and this enhanced effect is thought to be due to enhanced transport, more avid polyglutamation, or a unique site of action. 10-Ethyl-5-deazaaminopterin (Edatrexate), a potent inhibitor of DHFR with enhanced transport and more efficient polyglutamation relative to MTX, has demonstrated activity against non–small cell lung cancer.[60,61,69] Mucositis is the dose-limiting toxicity. 5,10-Dideazatetrahydrofolate (Lometrexol) is a new antifolate that impairs *de novo* purine synthesis by virtue of its direct inhibitory effects on GAR transformylase. Phase I studies have been performed, and this agent is currently undergoing phase II clinical investigation.

LY231514 was originally developed as a pure antifolate inhibitor of TS. However, preclinical studies suggest that it is not entirely specific for TS and that it inhibits other folate-dependent enzymes, including DHFR and GAR transformylase.[60,61,70] Like raltitrexed, this analogue requires polyglutamation for its potent inhibitory effects on TS, and it uses the RFC for entry into cells. This compound has been investigated in several phase I studies, and the major toxicities include neutropenia, anorexia and fatigue syndrome, gastrointestinal toxicity, and reversible transaminasemia.[71] Promising antitumor activity has been noted in a wide variety of tumor types, and phase II studies have confirmed activity against non–small cell lung cancer and mesothelioma.[72]

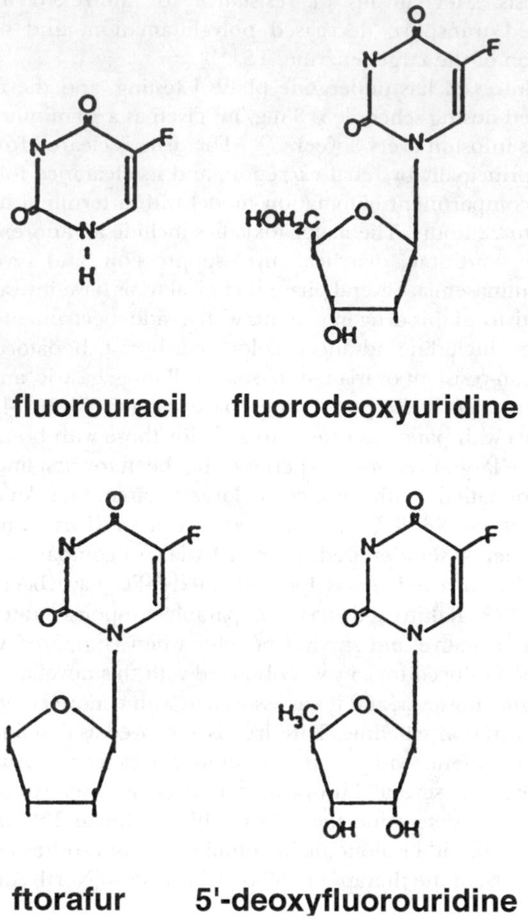

FIGURE 19.5-3. Structures of fluoropyrimidines of clinical interest.

5-FLUOROPYRIMIDINES

The rationale for the synthesis of the fluoropyrimidines stemmed from the observation that rat hepatoma cells use uracil more efficiently than normal rat intestinal mucosa.[73] This finding suggested that uracil metabolism might represent a potential target for cancer chemotherapy.

The chemical structures of the fluoropyrimidines in common clinical practice are shown in Figure 19.5-3. 5-FU has a fluorine atom substituted in place of hydrogen at the carbon-5 position of the pyrimidine ring (see Fig. 19.5-3). The deoxyribonucleoside derivative, 5-fluoro-2'-deoxyuridine (FUdR) is limited in its clinical use because of its rapid degradation in normal and tumor tissues. It has mainly been used for hepatic arterial infusions. Ftorafur and 5'-deoxyfluorouridine represent two fluoropyrimidine analogues that have been incorporated in oral prodrug forms of 5-FU, and they both demonstrate promising clinical activity.

5-FU has antitumor activity against a wide spectrum of solid tumors, including epithelial malignancies arising in the breast, gastrointestinal tract, head and neck, and ovary, with single-agent response rates of 10% to 30%.[74] Significant efforts have focused on identifying agents that can biochemically modulate the cytotoxic effects of 5-FU. Such modulators of 5-FU include other antineoplastic agents such as MTX, cisplatin, and CPT-11, ionizing radiation, cytokines such as the interferons, and agents that by themselves have little to no activity such as LV and 5-ethynyluracil (EU).[74,75] Thus, in the clinical setting, 5-FU is most often incorporated as part of a combination regimen.

Intracellular Metabolism and Mechanism of Action

Intracellular activation is required for the fluoropyrimidines to exert their cytotoxic effects. 5-FU readily enters cells via the facilitated uracil transport mechanism, whereas FUdR is a substrate for the facilitated nucleoside transport system. These compounds are anabolized to cytotoxic forms by several biochemical pathways (Fig. 19.5-4). 5-FU is converted to FUdR by thymidine phosphorylase. Subsequent phosphorylation of FUdR by thymidine kinase results in formation of the active 5-FU metabolite, 5-fluoro-2'-deoxyuridine monophosphate (FdUMP). In the presence of the reduced folate cofactor, 5,10-methylenetetrahydrofolate, FdUMP forms a stable covalent complex with TS.[76] TS catalyzes the sole intracellular *de novo* formation of thymidine-5'-monophosphate from dUMP (see Fig. 19.5-2). Inhibition of TS leads to depletion of dTTP, thus interfering with DNA biosynthesis and repair. 5-FU may be anabolized to fluorouridine monophosphate through the sequential action of uridine phosphorylase and uridine kinase. In the presence of PRPP, orotic acid phosphoribosyltransferase directly converts 5-FU to fluorouridine monophosphate. This metabolite is further metabolized to fluorouridine diphosphate and then to the triphosphate form (FUTP), which is subsequently incorporated into RNA. An alternate pathway for FdUMP synthesis is via conversion of fluorouridine diphosphate to fluorodeoxyuridine diphosphate (FdUDP) by ribonucleotide reductase (RR).

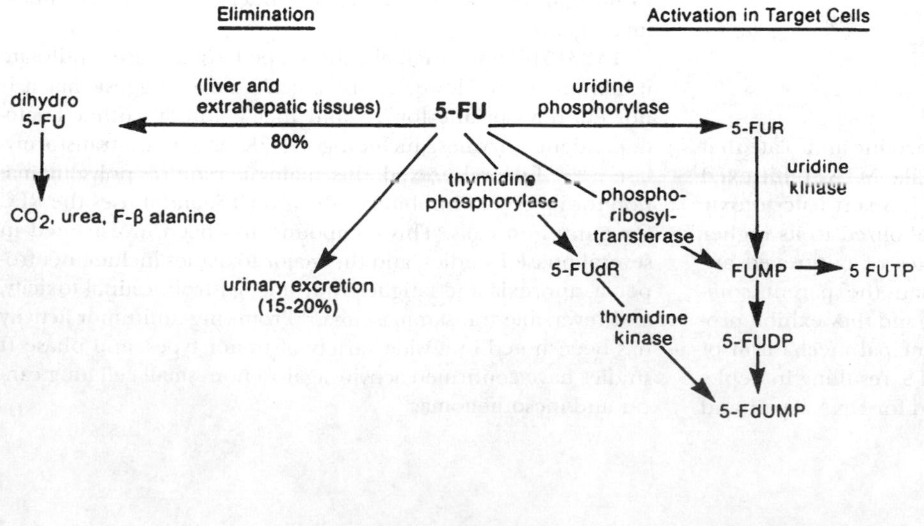

FIGURE 19.5-4. Metabolism of 5-fluorouracil (5-FU). 5-FdUMP, 5-fluoro-2'-deoxyuridine monophosphate; 5-FUDP, fluorouridine diphosphate; 5-FUdR, 5-fluoro-2'-deoxyuridine; FUMP, fluorouridine monophosphate; 5-FUR, fluorouridine; 5 FUTP, fluorouridine triphosphate.

Inhibition of TS by FdUMP is one of the principal mechanisms of 5-FU action. The TS-FdUMP-folate ternary complex is slowly dissociable, and the intracellular level of 5,10-methylenetetrahydrofolate is critical for ternary complex formation as well as for maintaining enzyme inhibition. Depletion of intracellular reduced folate pools prevents ternary complex formation in various tissue culture systems.[74] Pharmacologic concentrations of LV enhance the cytotoxicity of 5-FU by expanding the intracellular pools of 5,10-methylenetetrahydrofolate, thereby increasing the extent and duration of TS inhibition. Randomized clinical trials in advanced colorectal cancer indicate that the addition of LV to bolus 5-FU significantly improves the response rate compared with bolus 5-FU alone.[77,78] However, the actual benefit in patient survival is marginal and on the order of only 2 to 3 months.

5-FU is extensively incorporated into both nuclear and cytoplasmic RNA species, and this process interferes with normal RNA processing and function.[79–84] The extent of 5-FU-RNA incorporation correlates with cytotoxicity in some *in vitro* tissue culture and *in vivo* models. The following effects have been described as a consequence of 5-FU-RNA incorporation: alteration of the secondary structure of RNA; inhibition of mRNA polyadenylation, which decreases mRNA stability; inhibition of the conversion of high-molecular-weight nuclear RNA species to lower molecular-weight ribosomal RNA; quantitative and qualitative changes in protein synthesis; and incorporation into uracil-rich small nuclear RNA species, which interferes with normal splicing. 5-FU–containing transfer RNA forms covalent complexes with enzymes involved in posttranslational modification of uracil residues, thereby inhibiting their function. Despite the significant progress made in this area of research, it remains unclear as to how these 5-FU–mediated RNA effects translate into cytotoxicity.

Inhibition of TS leads not only to depletion of dTTP, but to accumulation of dUMP. Both FdUMP and dUMP may be subsequently metabolized to their respective triphosphate forms. Incorporation of dUTP and FdUTP into cellular DNA, with resultant inhibition of DNA synthesis and function, may represent another mechanism of cytotoxicity. Two enzymatic mechanisms limit the DNA incorporation of (F)dUTP: dUTP nucleotidohydrolase degrades the triphosphate forms, and uracil-DNA glycosylase removes uracil residues from DNA.[85,86] The combined effects of dTTP depletion and (F)dUTP-DNA incorporation are associated with inhibition of nascent DNA chain elongation, altered DNA stability, production of DNA single-strand breaks, and interference with DNA repair. The genotoxic stress resulting from TS inhibition may activate programmed cell death pathways in susceptible cells, resulting in induction of parental DNA fragmentation. Both internucleosomal DNA laddering typical of classic apoptosis and very high-molecular-weight DNA fragmentation (50 kb or greater) have been described.[87] Factors operating downstream from TS (e.g., bcl-2 and p53 status) may influence the cellular response to such genotoxic stress.[88,89] Some studies suggest that in some human colon cancer cells, the process of thymineless death resulting from 5-FU therapy may be mediated via the Fas-signaling pathway.[90]

The relative contribution of each of these mechanisms of action to the cytotoxicity of 5-FU remains unclear and may depend on the specific patterns of intracellular 5-FU metabolism, which vary among different normal tissues and tumor types. The concentration of drug and the duration of exposure play crucial roles in determining the ultimate mechanism of cytotoxicity. However, there is now increasing support for the critical role of TS as a therapeutic target. The specific lines of evidence for this view include the enhanced activity of LV-modulated 5-FU in the therapy of both early stage and advanced colorectal cancer, the strong correlation between low TS content in tumor tissue and response to 5-FU–based therapy, the correlation between level of TS enzyme inhibition in tumors after 5-FU administration and response to 5-FU therapy, and the clinical activity of selective TS inhibitors such as Tomudex.[74,91,92]

Mechanisms of Resistance

Given the multiple sites of cytotoxic action of 5-FU and the various metabolic pathways required for its activation, it is not surprising that several mechanisms of resistance have been identified in experimental and clinical settings.[74,92] However, the relative contribution of each of these mechanisms in the development of cellular resistance to 5-FU in the actual clinical setting remains unclear.

In human and murine tumor cells selected *in vitro* for resistance to 5-FU, a variety of mechanisms have been described. Deletion or diminished activity of thymidine or uridine kinase, thymidine or uridine phosphorylase, and orotate phosphoribosyl transferase interferes with metabolic activation. Decreased accumulation of FUTP, FdUMP, and (F)dUTP may result from increased activity of catabolic enzymes [acid and alkaline phosphatases, dUTP hydrolase, and dihydropyrimidine dehydrogenase (DPD)].[93] Expansion of intracellular cytidine triphosphate (CTP) pools associated with elevated CTP synthase activity results in feedback inhibition of uridine kinase, thus decreasing the metabolism of 5-FU to ribonucleotide forms. Decreased incorporation of 5-FU into both RNA and DNA may result in decreased sensitivity.[92,94] A relative deficiency of the reduced folate substrate 5,10-methylenetetrahydrofolate may also compromise the cytotoxic action of FdUMP on TS. This may result from low extracellular levels of reduced folates, decreased membrane transport of reduced folates, or reduced activity of folylpolyglutamate synthase, thereby preventing its polyglutamation.[95]

Alterations in the target enzyme TS represent the most commonly described mechanism of resistance to 5-FU. A decrease in binding affinity of the 5-FU metabolite FdUMP to the TS target has resulted from point mutations in the protein-coding region of the TS gene.[96] *In vitro, in vivo,* and clinical model systems have shown a strong correlation between the levels of TS enzyme activity and TS protein and chemosensitivity to 5-FU. In this regard, cell lines, tumors with higher levels of TS, or both are relatively more resistant to 5-FU. This increase in TS protein content is usually associated with amplification of the TS gene.[97] In cell lines made resistant to cisplatin or doxorubicin, cross-resistance to 5-FU may develop on the basis of increased TS expression as a consequence of increased transcription of the TS gene.[98] In several *in vitro* and *in vivo* model systems, the levels of TS enzyme activity and TS protein have been shown to acutely increase after exposure to 5-FU, other specific TS inhibitor compounds, or both.[74,99,100] Moreover, acute increases in the expression of TS protein have been identified in the clinical setting in paired tumor tissue biopsies obtained from patients before and during therapy with 5-FU.[101] This acute induction of TS protein in response to drug exposure is mediated by a translational regulatory mechanism.[102] TS protein, in its unbound or free state, is capable of specifically repressing the translation of its own mRNA. However, when TS protein is bound to either nucleotide, antifolate inhibitors, or both, it is unable to repress TS mRNA translation, and the rate of new TS protein synthesis increases.[103] Thus, induction of TS may represent an efficient and clinically relevant mechanism for the acute development of drug resistance.

Clinical Pharmacology

An understanding of 5-FU pharmacokinetics is important given the wide choice of routes and schedules of administration available, each of which has advantages in terms of differing spectrum of host toxicity. The most widely used methods for quantitating 5-FU in biologic fluids are high-pressure liquid chromatography (HPLC) and gas chromatography–mass spectrometry.[104] Nuclear magnetic resonance imaging with ^{19}F offers the potential for noninvasive monitoring of intratumoral accumulation of 5-FU; trapping of 5-FU within tumor tissue has been associated with clinical response.

5-FU is administered by either intravenous bolus or continuous infusion. The volume of distribution is slightly larger than the extracellular space, and 5-FU readily penetrates into tissues, CSF, and extracellular third-space accumulations such as ascites or pleural effusions. After intravenous bolus doses of 370 to 720 mg/m^2, peak plasma concentrations reach 300 μM to 1 mM; thereafter, metabolic elimination is rapid, with a primary half-life of 8 to 14 minutes. Plasma levels of 5-FU fall below 1 μM within 2 hours, an approximate threshold for cytotoxic effects. A prolonged third elimination phase of 5-FU after intravenous bolus (half-life, approximately 5 hours), detected by a sensitive gas chromatography–mass spectrometry method, may reflect release of 5-FU from tissues. Less than 10% of parent drug is excreted in the urine, whereas the balance is cleared through metabolic pathways (catabolism is greater than intracellular anabolism). 5-FU is enzymatically inactivated to dihydrofluorouracil by DPD.[105] Although the liver expresses the highest levels of DPD in the body, this enzyme is widely distributed in other tissues, including gastrointestinal mucosa and peripheral lymphocytes. Dihydropyrimidinase subsequently converts dihydrofluorouracil to α-fluoro-ureidopropionic acid, then β-alanine synthase catalyzes the irreversible formation of α-fluoro-β-alanine with the release of ammonia and CO_2. 5-FU and its catabolites undergo biliary excretion and enterohepatic circulation.

5-FU clearance is saturable; total body clearance decreases with increasing doses and deviates from a linear relationship above a certain dose (depending on schedule of administration). For example, clearance ranges from approximately 350 to 850 mL/min/m^2 with bolus doses of 720 and 370 mg/m^2. It may be difficult to predict plasma concentrations or the risk of severe toxicity at high doses.

Rare patients with inherited DPD deficiency may have life-threatening or fatal toxicity if treated with fluoropyrimidine-based chemotherapy.[106,107] Because affected individuals are otherwise in good health, the first indication of the presence of this inborn error of metabolism usually follows an unexpectedly severe reaction to 5-FU chemotherapy. Careful testing of DPD-deficient patients has revealed an autosomal recessive pattern of inheritance. It is now estimated that as many as 3% to 5% of adult cancer patients may have this pharmacogenetic syndrome. Several molecular defects, including point mutations and deletions due to exon skipping, have been identified in DPD-deficient patients who experience severe toxicity to 5-FU. Further studies are in progress to establish the precise relationship between the level of DPD activity and 5-FU host toxicity.

Frequently used continuous infusion schedules include protracted venous infusion (300 mg/m^2/d when given alone), 96- to 120-hour infusion every 3 weeks (1000 mg/m^2/d), and a weekly 24-hour infusion (2600 mg/m^2/d). 5-FU clearance is faster with constant infusion, varying from approximately 2000 to 3000 mL/min/m^2 depending on the dose rate. The incidence of serious clinical toxicity tends to increase with higher systemic exposure (steady-state plasma concentrations during constant infusion and total area under the concentration time curve with bolus administration). Pharmacologic monitoring with intracycle dose modifications offers the potential to avoid serious toxicity. Variation in 5-FU steady-state plasma levels according to time of day have been reported during constant infusion, although the time of day at which peak and trough plasma values occurred has not been consistent between studies.

Hepatic metastases obtain their blood supply predominantly from the arterial circulation via the hepatic artery. In patients with metastases confined to the liver, hepatic arterial infusion of 5-FU or FUdR provides high local drug concentrations to the tumor. The first-pass extraction of FUdR by the normal hepatic parenchyma approaches 95%, and little drug enters the systemic circulation. In contrast, the first-pass extraction of 5-FU ranges from 20% to 50%.[108] The recommended dosage of FUdR is 0.2 mg/kg/d for up to 14 days (7 mg/m^2/d), whereas 440 to 555 mg/m^2/d of 5-FU may be given for up to 14 days; lower 5-FU doses (total of 300 mg/d) may be tolerated for longer periods. The response rates reported for previously untreated colorectal carcinoma approach 50% in selected series.[109] Although the time to hepatic disease progression is significantly longer compared with systemic therapy with single-agent 5-FU or 14-day intravenous infusion of FUdR, the time to extrahepatic disease progression and overall survival remain unchanged. Approximately 30% of patients with liver-only metastases who have failed to respond to systemic 5-FU may respond to hepatic arterial infusion FUdR. Systemic toxicities are usually dose limiting with hepatic arterial infusion of 5-FU, presumably because a higher concentration of drug reaches the systemic circulation. These side effects include oral mucositis and gastrointestinal symptoms such as nausea, vomiting, and diarrhea. Myelosuppression occurs less often. Local and regional toxicities include peptic ulceration and chemical hepatitis (usually mild). In contrast, systemic toxicities are less common with FUdR, whereas local and regional toxicities predominate. Hepatic toxicity is dose limiting, and gastritis, duodenitis, or frank ulcers occur in 20% to 25% of patients.

5-FU and FUdR may also be given by the intraperitoneal route. Both drugs are absorbed primarily through the portal circulation and are subject to first-pass clearance in the liver before reaching the systemic circulation. In early trials, dialysate concentrations of 5 mM or less 5-FU maintained by intermittent exchanges of fluid for up to 5 days were tolerated, and the ratio of intraperitoneal to plasma 5-FU levels was approximately 300. 5-FU clearance is slower from the peritoneal cavity than from plasma (half-life approximately 1.5 hours). Up to 20 mM 5-FU given intraperitoneally for 4 hours with 90 mg/m^2 cisplatin every 4 weeks is tolerated, except for mild nausea and vomiting and sometimes diarrhea, whereas granulocytopenia occurs with higher dialysate concentrations. FUdR, 3000 mg given in 2 L of dialysate for 4 hours daily for 3 days, is well tolerated. The major systemic toxicity is nausea and vomiting, and this is usually well controlled. The peritoneal to plasma FUdR ratio is approximately 2700, suggesting a potential pharmacologic advantage for the use of intraperitoneal FUdR over 5-FU.

Clinical Toxicity

The primary effects of 5-FU are exerted on rapidly dividing tissues, specifically gastrointestinal mucosa and bone marrow. The spectrum of toxicities associated with 5-FU varies considerably according to the dose, schedule, and route of administration. The most frequently used dose and schedules of single-agent 5-FU given by bolus injection are 600 mg/m^2/week and 425 mg/m^2/d for 5 days every 3 to 4 weeks. The dose of 5-FU generally should be reduced when used in combination with LV, the magnitude of which varies according to the schedule and LV dose. Epithelial ulceration may occur throughout the gastrointestinal tract and may manifest as mucositis, pharyngitis, dysphagia, esophagitis, gastritis, colitis, or proctitis. Diarrhea may be watery or bloody, and the combination of nausea, vomiting, and profuse diarrhea can lead to profound dehydration and hypotension. Disruption of the integrity of the gut lining may permit access of enteric organisms into the blood stream, with the potential for overwhelming sepsis, particularly if the granulocyte nadir coincides with diarrhea. 5-FU should be withheld in the face of ongoing mucositis or diarrhea, even if mild, and subsequent doses should be reduced when the patient has fully recovered. If diarrhea occurs, supportive care and vigorous hydration should be given. Antidiarrheal agents, such as diphenoxylate and loperamide, may help control mild diarrhea, but they are generally ineffective in controlling diarrhea of greater severity.[110] In this setting, the somatostatin analogue octreotide seems to have greater efficacy. Mouth cooling (oral cryotherapy) with oral ice chips for 30 minutes starting immediately before bolus 5-FU substantially reduces the severity of mucositis. Nausea and vomiting may occur but are usually controlled with antiemetics. Myelosuppression may also be observed, with granulocytopenia occurring more than thrombocytopenia. With the schedule of a daily dose for 5 days, the granulocyte and platelet nadirs tend to occur during the second or third week of treatment. In contrast, myelosuppression generally occurs after the fourth weekly dose of the weekly bolus 5-FU schedule.

Continuous intravenous infusion of 5-FU at doses of 1000 mg/m^2/d for 5 days every 3 weeks results in only minor myelosuppression, whereas stomatitis and diarrhea are the principal dose-limiting toxicities. With protracted venous infusion of 5-FU (300 mg/m^2/d), serious myelosuppression is less common. The infusion can be interrupted at the first signs of mouth soreness or diarrhea, thus limiting the severity of toxicity. However, palmar-plantar erythrodysesthesia (hand-foot syndrome) is a more subacute toxicity that may eventually be dose limiting.[111] With a weekly 24-hour infusion of 2600 mg/m^2 5-FU, neurotoxicity and gastrointestinal toxicity are dose limiting.

Other dermatologic toxicities associated with 5-FU therapy include alopecia, changes in the fingernails, and dermatitis that varies from a pruritic erythematous rash followed by scaling to more severe cases with vesicle formation. 5-FU enhances the cutaneous toxicity of radiation, and reactions usually occur within 7 days of radiation. Photosensitivity reactions, increased pigmentation over the veins into which 5-FU has been administered, as well as more generalized hyperpigmentation, and atrophy are possible. Hand-foot syndrome most often occurs with protracted infusion schedules of 5-FU, but may also be seen in patients receiving LV-modulated 5-FU. Ocular toxicity includes blepharitis, epiphora, tear duct stenosis, and acute and chronic conjunctivitis. The acute inflammatory response is reversible when the drug is discontinued early in the treatment course, but progression may require surgical correction of ectropion and tear duct stenosis.

Acute neurologic symptoms, including somnolence, cerebellar ataxia, and upper motor signs, are primarily seen in patients receiving intracarotid infusions for head and neck tumors, but neurologic toxicity may also occur with weekly schedules (24-hour infusion is greater than bolus). The premise that 5-FU catabolites play a role in the neurotoxicity is supported by preclinical models of neurotoxicity. However, patients with DPD deficiency may experience severe neurologic toxicity in the absence of myelosuppression and gastrointestinal toxicity after 5-FU therapy.[112] Thus, the exact 5-FU metabolite responsible for 5-FU neurotoxicity remains unclear.

A syndrome of chest pain, cardiac enzyme elevations, and electrocardiographic changes consistent with myocardial ischemia may be seen in temporal association with 5-FU administration. In some patients, coronary angiography revealed no abnormalities, suggesting vasospasm as a possible mechanism. This toxicity has been attributed to parent drug and to the catabolites, fluoro-β-alanine and fluoroacetate. Concentration-dependent vasoconstriction occurs when isolated vascular smooth muscle rings are exposed *in vitro* to 5-FU, and this can be reversed with nitrates.

Intrahepatic administration of FUdR is complicated mainly by cholestatic jaundice and biliary sclerosis. These adverse side effects are thought to result from direct perfusion of the blood supply to the gallbladder and upper bile duct with high local drug concentrations. Of note, this complication occurs much less frequently with hepatic arterial infusion of 5-FU. Biliary sclerosis typically occurs by the third cycle of treatment. Therapy with FUdR may be reinstituted at a lower dose after normalization of serum hepatic enzyme levels, but most patients become progressively less tolerant. Catheter-related complications include thrombosis of the catheterized vessel, hemorrhage or infection at the site of insertion, and slippage of the catheter into the gastroduodenal artery with resultant necrosis of the intestinal epithelium, hemorrhage, and perforation.

Drug Interactions

A host of drug interactions have been investigated in an attempt to enhance the cytotoxicity and therapeutic selectivity of fluoropyrimidine chemotherapy. The interaction of 5-FU with MTX is of particular interest as both drugs are often used in combination chemotherapy for breast and colorectal cancer. When given before 5-FU, MTX-mediated inhibition of DHFR results in accumulation of PRPP.[74] Increased availability of PRPP promotes formation of fluorouridine monophosphate via the reaction catalyzed by orotic acid phosphoribosyltransferase, with enhanced FUTP incorporation into RNA. In contrast, administration of 5-FU before MTX antagonizes the antipurine effects of MTX by preventing the accumulation of dihydrofolate and maintaining the pool of reduced folates needed for *de novo* purine synthesis. A 24-hour interval is superior to a 1-hour interval in some preclinical and clinical studies.[113] The dose of MTX in clinical trials has varied, but doses of 100 mg/m^2 or more are usually followed by LV rescue. A metaanalysis of randomized trials of MTX and 5-FU revealed a higher response rate compared with single-agent bolus 5-FU.[114]

Synergy between 5-FU and cisplatin has been noted in several preclinical models. Possible mechanisms of interaction include cisplatin-mediated increases in the intracellular content of the reduced folate pool, enhanced DNA damage, and interference with repair of cisplatin-DNA adducts. In some preclinical models, concurrent exposure to both drugs produces synergy, whereas other models suggest that preexposure to 5-FU before cisplatin administration is superior to the opposite sequence. Clinical synergy between infusional 5-FU and cisplatin is evident in tumor types that are sensitive to both drugs, such as squamous cell cancers of the head and neck and esophagus, whereas randomized trials in colorectal cancer show no benefit with the addition of cisplatin. The influence of sequence of cisplatin and 5-FU on therapeutic outcome has not been carefully studied in clinical trials.

The salvage enzyme thymidine kinase converts thymidine to thymidine monophosphate, thereby bypassing the TS-mediated inhibition of *de novo* thymidylate production. In tissue culture models, thymidine (10 to 20 μM) is frequently used to replete dTTP pools and thus negate its potential contribution to toxicity. In some models, pharmacologic concentrations of thymidine promote 5-FU RNA incorporation (by feedback inhibition of thymidine kinase and RR).[74] *In vivo*, however, thymidine (and its catabolite thymine) increased the half-life of 5-FU by interfering with the catabolism of 5-FU to dihydrofluorouracil, leading to a marked increase in 5-FU toxicity with no improvement in antitumor activity. Simultaneous exposure to pharmacologic concentrations of uridine may antagonize the RNA-directed cytotoxicity of 5-FU by decreasing its activation to the ribonucleotide level by uridine kinase; furthermore, expanded UTP pools may decrease FUTP incorporation into RNA. Delayed administration of uridine increases the rate of recovery from 5-FU–associated inhibition of both RNA and DNA synthesis in some models.[115] Delayed administration of oral uridine to patients decreases the myelosuppression associated with weekly bolus 5-FU, but the effect on therapeutic activity has yet to be determined.[116]

Interferons (IFNs) enhance the *in vitro* and *in vivo* activity of 5-FU and FUdR in a cell-line–dependent manner.[117] Heterogeneity exists among cancer cell lines as to the specific type of IFN that enhances fluoropyrimidine toxicity. IFN-α may increase the activity of thymidine and uridine phosphorylases, and increased FdUMP formation has been reported in some cell lines. In other models, IFN-α may enhance fluoropyrimidine-mediated DNA damage in the absence of a direct effect on FdUMP pools or the extent of TS inhibition. In a human colon cancer cell line, IFN-γ abrogated the acute increase in TS protein accompanying 5-FU exposure, and in so doing, enhanced the cytotoxic effects of 5-FU.[118] IFN-α may decrease the clearance of 5-FU in some individuals in a dose- and schedule-dependent manner, particularly with consecutive daily administration of IFN-α in conjunction with bolus 5-FU. Initial clinical trials appeared promising, although the toxicity of IFN-α–modulated 5-FU was substantial. The final results from several randomized trials evaluating IFN-α–modulated 5-FU alone or with LV in advanced colorectal cancer reveal no benefit of IFN to 5-FU therapy in terms of overall response rate and survival.[119,120] Moreover, toxicity was significantly increased with the addition of IFN. A large randomized trial testing the contribution of IFN-α to a daily schedule for 5 days of bolus 5-FU/LV has been conducted by the National Surgical Adjuvant Breast and Bowel Project in the adjuvant treatment of colon cancer. The results from this trial have been published, and as in the case of advanced disease, IFN-α therapy is of no added benefit in the adjuvant setting.[121]

Preexposure to inhibitors of *de novo* pyrimidine synthesis, such as N-(phosphonoacetyl)-L-aspartic acid and brequinar, results in depletion of UTP, CTP, dUMP, and dCTP pools. These biochemical effects are associated with enhanced anabolism of 5-FU to FUTP, increased 5-FU-RNA incorporation, and enhanced DNA-directed cytotoxicity. Although promising results were initially reported with a weekly schedule of low-dose N-(phosphonoacetyl)-L-aspartic acid (250 mg/m^2 intravenously) given 1 day before a 24-hour infusion of 5-FU (2600 mg/m^2), a randomized phase II trial conducted by the Southwest Oncology Group failed to demonstrate an improvement in response rate compared with the same schedule of 5-FU alone.[122] Results from other multiinstitutional phase III trials are pending.

Preclinical studies show that 5-FU enhances the cytotoxicity of ionizing radiation, and both preclinical and clinical studies have revealed that radiosensitization appears to be enhanced with prolonged exposure. The underlying mechanisms for this synergistic interaction may include increased DNA damage, inhibition of DNA repair, and accumulation of cells in S phase.[74,123,124] Some work suggests that the G_1/S checkpoint may play a critical role in determining the ability of 5-FU to enhance the cytotoxic effects of radiation therapy. Moreover, this effect may not depend on normal p53 function, but instead, may rely on intact cyclin E-dependent kinase activity. One example highlighting the successful clinical application of this approach is the use of protracted infusional 5-FU during pelvic radiation in the adjuvant treatment of rectal cancer.[125]

STRATEGIES TO PERMIT ORAL ADMINISTRATION OF FLUOROPYRIMIDINES

TEGAFUR, URACIL, 5-FLUOROURACIL

Administration of 5-FU by the oral route has generally been avoided because of erratic bioavailability. Several strategies to allow oral dosing by decreasing the catabolism of 5-FU are being explored. One approach involves the drug tegafur, uracil, 5-fluorouracil (UFT), a combination of Ftorafur (1-[2-tetrahydrofuryl]-5-fluorouracil, tegafur; see Fig. 19.5-3), a 5-FU prodrug, in a 1:4 molar ratio with uracil. Preclinical studies indicated that UFT resulted in significantly higher tumor-to-serum 5-FU ratios than Ftorafur alone. UFT is administered orally in divided doses, and it has been given daily for 5 to 28 days. With oral doses ranging from 50 to 300 mg/m^2, maximum plasma levels of Ftorafur and 5-FU occur between 0.6 and 2.1 hours. Ftorafur levels (2.7 to 20.0 μg/mL) exceed 5-FU levels (0.025 to 0.9 μg/mL, 0.2 to 7.0 μM), and Ftorafur clearance is approximately 70 mL/min. Combined phase II data from 438 patients treated with UFT in Japan reveal the drug has single-agent activity (19% to 32% response rate) in adenocarcinomas arising in the gastrointestinal tract and breast.

Hematologic toxicity is mild. Gastrointestinal toxicity includes anorexia (24%), nausea and vomiting (12.5%), and diarrhea (12%). UFT in combination with LV has been tested here in the United States in both phase I and phase II studies. When UFT was used at a dose of 300 mg/m^2/d with 150 mg/d LV in patients with advanced colorectal cancer, an overall response rate of 42% was observed.[126] This treatment was well tolerated, and there was only a 24% incidence of grade 3 gastrointestinal toxicity, as manifested by diarrhea, vomiting, and abdominal cramps, and asthenia and fatigue. The results of two randomized, phase III studies comparing oral UFT (300 mg/m^2/d) and oral LV (75 or 90 mg/d) for 28 days every 35 days with the Mayo Clinic regimen of 5-day bolus 5-FU (425 mg/m^2/d) and LV (20 mg/m^2/d) given every 35 days in previously untreated patients with metastatic colorectal cancer show that the oral and intravenous regimens have similar response rates, time to disease progression, and overall survival. However, the oral regimen was associated with a significantly lower incidence of severe neutropenia and need for hospitalization.[127] Thus, UFT/LV is an acceptable alternative to intravenous 5-FU/LV for treatment of advanced colorectal cancer. Studies are ongoing to determine its potential role in the adjuvant therapy of early-stage colorectal cancer.

CAPECITABINE (XELODA)

Capecitabine (Xeloda) represents another oral prodrug of 5-FU that was designed with the rationale of generating selective 5-FU activation in tumor tissue.[128] When administered orally, it is absorbed intact through the intestinal mucosa, metabolized by a carboxylesterase enzyme in the liver to 5'-deoxy-5-fluorocytidine, and then converted to 5'-deoxy-5-fluorouridine by cytidine deaminase, an enzyme principally located in the liver. 5'-Deoxy-5-fluorouridine is then converted directly at the tumor site by the thymidine-metabolizing enzyme, thymidine phosphorylase, a protein that has been shown to function as an angiogenic factor.

Preclinical studies have shown that tumor 5-FU concentrations are significantly higher than those measured in plasma. Moreover, this oral prodrug has shown activity against a broad spectrum of human tumor xenografts with relatively mild host toxicity. Currently, this agent is approved for use as a third-line agent in the treatment of anthracycline- and taxane-resistant advanced breast cancer.[129] Studies are ongoing to determine the role of this compound in the therapy of advanced colorectal cancer. Preliminary results of a randomized phase III North American trial comparing capecitabine (2500 mg/mg^2/d for 14 days every 3 weeks) with a Mayo Clinic regimen of a daily dose for 5 days show that overall response rates are significantly higher for capecitabine (23.2%) versus 5-FU/LV (15.5%).[130] Both the duration of response and progression-free survival are similar. Although survival data remains immature at this time, capecitabine appears to have a more favorable toxicity profile than intravenous 5-FU/LV and the most common toxicities observed were hand-foot syndrome (17.7%) and diarrhea (16.3%), with myelosuppression being relatively uncommon.

S1

S1 is an oral formulation composed of the 5-FU prodrug Ftorafur, the DPD inhibitor 5-chloro-2,4-dihydroxypyridine, and oxonic acid.[75] 5-Chloro-2,4-dihydroxypyridine is a competitive, reversible inhibitor of DPD that helps to significantly prolong the half-life of 5-FU and improve oral bioavailability. Oxonic acid is an inhibitor of pyrimidine phosphoribosyltransferase, and it acts to prevent 5-FU phosphorylation and subsequent incorporation of 5-FU metabolites into the RNA of normal tissues in the gastrointestinal tract. Given its mechanism of action, the goal of oxonic acid is to protect against 5-FU–mediated gastrointestinal toxicity. Phase I studies revealed that the dose-limiting toxicity was myelosuppression mainly in the form of neutropenia. In Japan, where this drug was initially developed, phase II trials have been conducted in several malignancies, including gastric, colorectal, breast, and head and neck cancer. Response rates have ranged between 30% and 50%, and toxicity has been generally mild, with myelosuppression predominating. Phase I and II studies are under way in the United States to confirm its clinical activity.

5-ETHYNYLURACIL

The uracil analogue 5-ethynyluracil (Eniluracil, EU, GW776, 776C85) is a potent, mechanism-based inhibitor of DPD.[75] On binding of EU to DPD (apparent K_m approximately 2 μM), an unstable intermediate is formed, following which the drug becomes covalently linked to the enzyme. Administration of EU to both animals and humans results in complete inhibition of total body DPD, as evidenced by inhibition of DPD enzyme activity in peripheral mononuclear cells and by up to 100-fold elevations of plasma uracil levels.[131,132] Treatment with EU completely inhibits DPD enzyme activity in both the tumors and peripheral lymphocytes of patients with colorectal cancer, a finding that confirms the use of peripheral mononuclear cells as an accurate and reliable surrogate marker for tumoral DPD activity. Preclinical studies *in vivo* show that treatment with EU significantly improves 5-FU pharmacokinetics, resulting in a marked elevation of both the plasma half-life and area under the concentration time curve of 5-FU.

This work has been extended to the clinical setting in which phase I studies investigating the combination of 5-FU and EU have been performed. EU significantly increased 5-FU plasma half-life by up to 20-fold and decreased 5-FU clearance by 18-fold, leading to a prolonged half-life of 4 to 6 hours.[133] Moreover, in the presence of EU, the oral bioavailability of 5-FU approaches 100%. This then allows for effective oral administration of 5-FU. The 5-FU/EU combination has subsequently been advanced to the phase II setting in patients with metastatic colorectal cancer. When 5-FU and EU were administered for 28 days on an every 35-day cycle at the respective doses of 1.0 and 10.0 mg/m^2/d, a 29% objective response rate was observed. Treatment was relatively well tolerated, and grade 3 to 4 diarrhea was noted in 16% of patients, stomatitis and mucositis in 4%, and neutropenia in 4%.

EU is a promising biochemical modulator of 5-FU, and clinical studies suggest that it may help to improve the antitumor activity and host toxicity profile of 5-FU chemotherapy. Currently, there are two large randomized, phase III studies comparing 5-FU and EU with either the Mayo Clinic daily for 5 days regimen of 5-FU and LV or with protracted infusional 5-FU. The results from these studies will provide critical insights as to the precise role of the 5-FU and EU combination in the therapeutic armamentarium of patients with metastatic colorectal cancer. Moreover, this combination may find clinical application in the treatment of other solid tumors such as advanced breast cancer.[133a]

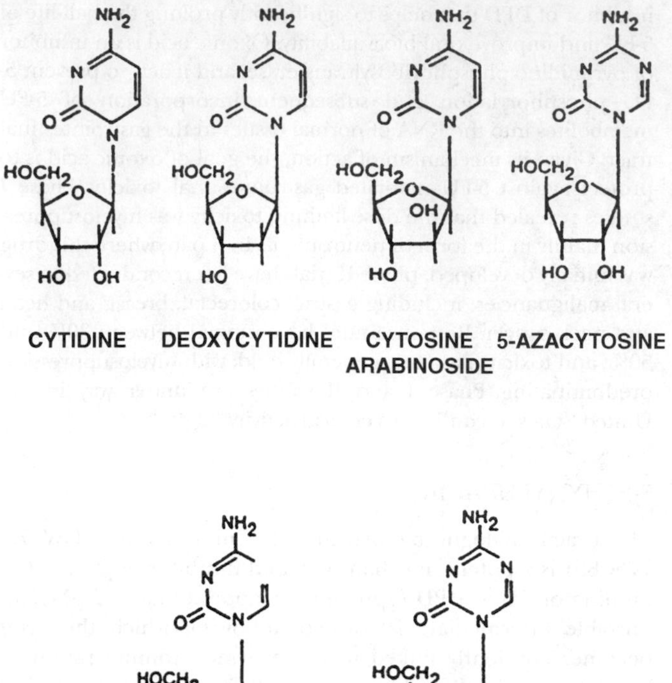

FIGURE 19.5-5. Structures of deoxycytidine analogues of clinical interest.

CYTARABINE

Cytarabine (1-β-D-arabinofuranosylcytosine, Ara-C) is one of several arabinose nucleosides isolated from the sponge *Cryptothethya crypta*,[134] differing from its physiologic counterpart by virtue of a stereotypic inversion of the 2'-hydroxyl group of the sugar moiety (Fig. 19.5-5). Ara-C is regarded as one of the most important drugs in the treatment of acute myelogenous leukemia (AML). A regimen of Ara-C combined with an anthracycline, given as a 5- or 7-day continuous infusion is considered the standard induction treatment for AML. Furthermore, Ara-C is used in the treatment of other hematologic malignancies, such as non-Hodgkin's lymphoma, chronic myelogenous leukemia, and acute lymphocytic leukemia.

Intracellular Metabolism and Mechanism of Action

As with other nucleoside analogues and their physiologic counterparts, Ara-C enters cells via nucleoside-specific transmembrane transport proteins, the most important one being the es (equilibrative inhibitor-sensitive) receptor. Studies with blasts from patients with acute leukemias have shown a strong correlation between expression of es transporters and *in vitro* sensitivity to Ara-C.[135]

Once within the cytoplasm, Ara-C requires activation for its cytotoxic effects. The first metabolic step is the conversion of Ara-C to ara-cyyidine monophosphate (Ara-CMP) by the enzyme deoxycytidine kinase (dCK) (Fig. 19.5-6). This enzyme is the rate-limiting step in intracellular anabolism of Ara-C. This metabolic step is saturable, and the K_m is approximately 20 μM.[136] Ara-CMP is subsequently phosphorylated to ara-cytidine diphosphate (Ara-CDP) and Ara-CTP by the enzymes pyrimidine monophosphate kinase and pyrimidine diphosphate kinase, respectively. Ara-CTP competes with the native substrate deoxycytidine triphosphate (dCTP) for DNA incorporation by DNA-directed DNA polymerase (K_i approximately 1 μM). The incorporated Ara-CTP residue is a potent inhibitor of DNA polymerase α (involved in Okazaki fragment synthesis on the lagging strand of the replication fork), DNA polymerase δ (the leading strand replicase), and DNA polymerase β (involved in the repair of chemically induced DNA damage).[137–139] Inhibition of DNA polymerases, in turn, interferes with DNA chain elongation during both semiconservative DNA replication and DNA repair.[140] The incorporated Ara-CTP residue functions as a relative DNA chain terminator, and interference with chain elongation is influenced by sequence specificity of the DNA template.[138,140] Initiation of new DNA replication intermediates continues, however, with accumulation of nascent DNA fragments.[140] This process may result in abnormal duplication of limited portions of DNA, thus increasing the possibility of recombination, crossover, and gene amplification. Over time, the nascent DNA strand can be extended beyond the arabinosylnucleotide residue, and digestion of DNA reveals the presence of Ara-CMP in the internucleotide (internal) position.[138–140] In some human leukemic cell lines, Ara-C–mediated DNA damage is accompanied by a pattern of internucleosomal DNA fragmentation typical of apoptosis (programmed cell death).[141] There is evidence suggesting that Ara-C metabolism in AML blasts differs from that in normal bone marrow mononuclear cells and CD34+ hematopoietic stem cells.[142] The total levels of phosphorylated Ara-C metabolites, including Ara-CMP, Ara-CDP, Ara-CTP, Ara-CDP-choline, and Ara-UMP, were two- to fourfold higher in leukemic blast cells when compared with normal bone marrow cells, both at standard and high doses of Ara-C. The most striking difference was found with the Ara-CDP-choline metabolite in the setting of Ara-C dose escalation. The level of this metabolite was 4.3-fold higher in leukemic blast cells.[142]

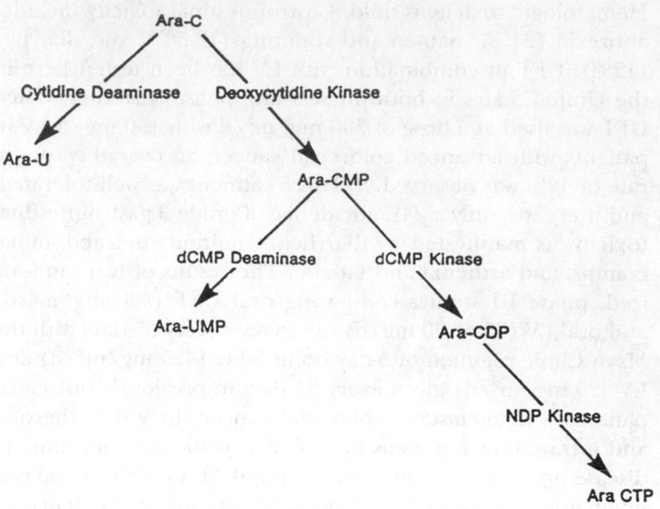

FIGURE 19.5-6. Metabolism of Ara-C. Gemcitabine shares the same metabolic pathway as Ara-C. Ara-CDP, ara-cytidine diphosphate; Ara-CTP, ara-cytidine triphosphate; Ara-U, ara-uridine; Ara-UMP, ara-uridine monophosphate; dCMP, deoxycytidine monophosphate.

In animal studies, Ara-CMP inhibits transfer of galactose, N-acetylglucosamine, and sialic acid to cell surface glycoproteins. Ara-CTP (0.1 to 1.0 mM) inhibits synthesis of CMP-acetyl-neuraminic acid, and Ara-CDP choline can be incorporated into membranes. These effects on phospholipid synthesis and incorporation into membranes may possibly affect membrane structure and function.

Catabolism of Ara-C involves two key enzymes, cytidine deaminase and deoxycytidylate deaminase. They convert Ara-C and Ara-CMP into their respective nontoxic two metabolites, Ara-U and Ara-UMP. Other catabolic enzymes that may affect Ara-C metabolism include dCTP pyrophosphatase, 5'-nucleotidase, and alkaline and acid phosphatases. The balance between intracellular activation and degradation is critical in determining the amount of drug that is ultimately converted to Ara-CTP and, thus, its subsequent cytotoxic and antitumor activity (see Fig. 19.5-6).

Mechanisms of Resistance

Ara-C is most active during the S phase of the cell cycle.[134] The rate of DNA synthesis influences Ara-C cytotoxicity, with maximum effects observed when cells are exposed to Ara-C during periods of rapid DNA synthesis. Longer exposures allow a greater proportion of cells to enter S phase and are associated with enhanced incorporation of Ara-CTP into DNA.[143] Therefore, the duration of Ara-C exposure seems to be a critical determinant of its cytotoxicity.

Several mechanisms of resistance to Ara-C have been described. Impaired transmembrane transport, decreased rate of anabolism, increased rate of catabolism, or all three may result in the development of Ara-C resistance. *In vitro* studies have demonstrated that amplification of the cytidine deaminase gene with resultant overexpression of the corresponding protein product leads to Ara-C resistance.[144] The level of cytidine deaminase enzyme activity has been shown to correlate with clinical response in patients with AML undergoing induction chemotherapy with Ara-C–containing regimens.[145] Blasts from patients who attained complete remission and from those with previously untreated leukemia had significantly higher levels of cytidine deaminase than blasts from patients with refractory disease.

Deletion of the gene encoding deoxycytidine kinase, expansion of CTP and dCTP pools, overexpression of bcl-2, and decreased intracellular half-life of Ara-CTP after drug removal are mechanisms that have been implicated in Ara-C resistance.[143,146,147] The cytotoxicity of Ara-C in leukemic cells isolated from patients correlates well with both the extent of DNA incorporation and the intracellular retention of Ara-CTP after drug exposure.[148]

Cellular sensitivity to Ara-C can also be influenced by the concomitant use of other drugs. For example, all-*trans*-retinoic acid was found to enhance Ara-C cytotoxicity, as well as Ara-C–induced apoptosis in HL-60 human leukemia cells.[149] However, the mechanism by which this sensitization is mediated remains unknown. The sensitivity of human leukemic cell lines to Ara-C has also been tested in the presence of stem cell factor. The addition of stem cell factor to a suspension culture system leads to a significant increase in the toxicity of Ara-C to self-renewing blast progenitors, especially when associated with high concentrations of Ara-C.[150] Although limited in its current clinical application, 6-mercaptopurine (6-MP) has shown a positive interaction with Ara-C. By inhibiting cytidine deaminase enzyme activity in L1210 murine leukemic cells, 6-MP is able to maintain high concentrations of Ara-C in the culture medium. This effect results in enhanced incorporation of Ara-C into cells and subsequent activation to Ara-CTP.[141]

Clinical Pharmacology and Pharmacokinetics

Ara-C has poor oral bioavailability (approximately 20%) due to extensive deamination within the gastrointestinal tract. Consequently, Ara-C is administered via the intravenous route. The drug can also be given subcutaneously. After intravenous bolus administration, Ara-C is rapidly cleared with biphasic elimination: The initial half-life is approximately 12 minutes, whereas the terminal half-life is approximately 2 hours. Within 24 hours, 78% of a bolus dose is excreted in the urine (71% as Ara-U, 7% as Ara-C). During continuous intravenous infusion, steady-state plasma levels of Ara-C increase linearly to 5 to 10 μM, and drug clearance is approximately 1000 $mL/min/m^2$. Thereafter, deamination is saturated, and plasma levels can increase unpredictably.[151] With continuous infusion of doses from 100 to 200 $mg/m^2/d$, steady-state plasma levels range from 0.2 to 1.0 μM, and CSF levels are approximately 50% of the plasma levels.[134,152]

When administered as a high-dose (greater than 2 g/m^2) intravenous infusion over 1 to 3 hours, the plasma elimination is triphasic: α, β, and γ half-lives are 16 minutes, 1.8 hours, and 6 hours, respectively.[152,153] The mean plasma concentration at the end of infusion ranges from approximately 60 to 150 μM, but 12 hours later falls to less than 0.5 μM. Ara-C crosses the blood–brain barrier when used at high doses, with CSF levels between 7% to 14% of plasma levels, reaching peak levels of up to 10 μM. Because cytidine deaminase enzyme activity is nearly completely absent in CSF, the drug displays a longer half-life in the CSF (approximately 2 to 4 hours).[153]

Ara-C can also be given intrathecally as prophylaxis against CNS tumor involvement and to treat leptomeningeal disease of both hematologic and solid malignancies. The usual dose is anywhere from 30 to 60 mg in 5 to 10 mL diluent twice weekly until documentation of three consecutively negative CSF cytology results. Intrathecal administration of 50 mg/m^2 Ara-C yields peak concentrations of 1 mM, and cytotoxic concentrations (0.4 μM or above) are maintained for 24 hours.[134] Of note, the diluent supplied with commercial formulations of Ara-C contains 0.945% benzyl alcohol. Given the potential toxicity of benzyl alcohol, diluents containing this preservative should not be used for intrathecal administration in neonates or with high-dose regimens. In these situations, preservative-free 0.9% sodium chloride injection or other isotonic buffered diluents should be used to reconstitute the drug. Finally, Ara-C can also be used intraperitoneally. This approach is commonly used as second-line treatment for ovarian cancer patients presenting primarily with intraperitoneal disease, and it is usually given in combination with cisplatin.

Toxicity

The toxicity profile of Ara-C is highly dependent on the dose and schedule of administration. Myelosuppression is the dose-limiting toxicity with a standard regimen of 100 to 200 $mg/m^2/d$ for 7 days. Leukopenia and thrombocytopenia are the most severe cytopenias, with the nadir occurring between days 7 and 14 after drug administration. However, the duration of the nadir can be significantly influenced by the concomitant use of other cytotoxic agents and also by previous treatment with chemotherapy.

Gastrointestinal toxicity commonly manifests as a mild to moderate degree of anorexia, nausea, and vomiting. Mucositis, diarrhea, ileus, and abdominal pain can also be observed. Less commonly, epithelial ulceration can occur, ranging from superficial ulceration to intramural hematoma formation and perforation. Transient hepatic dysfunction, manifested as elevation of liver enzymes, may also occur with Ara-C given at conventional doses. Acute pancreatitis has been associated with Ara-C, mostly when given as a continuous infusion. The Ara-C syndrome has been described in pediatric patients receiving Ara-C for hematologic malignancies and is characterized by fever, myalgia, bone pain, maculopapular rash, conjunctivitis, malaise, and occasional chest pain. These symptoms usually begin within 12 hours after Ara-C infusion. This syndrome most likely represents an allergic reaction to Ara-C, as patients usually develop symptoms months after the first dose, and corticosteroids can prevent its onset.[154]

Administration of Ara-C at high doses (2 to 3 g/m^2 intravenously over 1 to 3 hours, every 12 hours; 100 mg/m^2/h for 24 hours) produces severe myelosuppression, sometimes with prolonged nadirs. Severe gastrointestinal toxicity in the form of mucositis, diarrhea, or both, is also frequently observed. Neurologic toxicity is significantly more common with high-dose Ara-C than with standard doses. The clinical manifestations of neurologic toxicity are diverse and include seizures, cerebral and cerebellar dysfunction, peripheral neuropathy, bilateral rectus muscle palsy, aphasia, and Parkinsonian symptoms.[155] Clinical signs of cerebellar dysfunction occur in up to 15% of patients within 8 days and include dysarthria, dysdiadochokinesia, dysmetria, and ataxia.[156] Change in alertness and cognitive ability, memory loss, and frontal lobe release signs reflect cerebral toxicity. Despite discontinuation of therapy, clinical recovery is incomplete in up to 30% of affected patients. The severity of peripheral neuropathy increases with higher cumulative Ara-C doses. Electromyography and nerve conduction test results suggest a demyelinating polyneuropathy with axonal degeneration. Significant neurotoxicity appears uncommon at cumulative doses of 36 g/m^2 or less. Neurotoxicity may also be reduced by prolonged intravenous administration (over 3 hours or more). Patients older than 50 years and patients with elevated serum creatinine levels are particularly susceptible to neurologic toxicity.

Other side effects are less commonly seen. Pulmonary complications may include noncardiogenic pulmonary edema, acute respiratory distress, and pneumonia, resulting from *Streptococcus viridans* infection.[157] Other side effects associated with high-dose Ara-C include conjunctivitis (often responsive to topical corticosteroids), a painful hand-foot syndrome, and, rarely, anaphylactic reactions. A fatal case of toxic epidermal necrolysis has been described. Neutrophilic eccrine hydradenitis, an unusual cutaneous reaction manifested as plaques or nodules, can occur during the second week after high-dose Ara-C.

Intrathecal administration of Ara-C is usually uneventful. However, it may produce fever, seizures, and alterations in mental status within the first 24 hours of administration. Ara-C is teratogenic in animals. Although Ara-C produces chromosomal breaks in both cultured cells and bone marrow, it is not an established carcinogen in humans.

Drug Interactions

In vitro studies and animal tumor model systems have provided evidence for synergistic activity between Ara-C and alkylating agents, platinum compounds, purine analogues, antifolates, and fluoropyrimidines. More recently, synergism has also been observed with Ara-C and other agents, such as bryostatin 1, fludarabine, and paclitaxel. The use of IFN-α combined with Ara-C in low doses is useful in the treatment of patients with early chronic phase chronic myelogenous leukemia, despite the existence of *in vitro* data suggesting a negative interaction for these two drugs.[158] Specific biochemical, cellular, or both, kinetic mechanisms have been described for each of these interactions, and the sequence of drug administration seems to be critical in some cases. Ara-C enhances the cytotoxicity of various DNA-damaging agents, including alkylating agents (cyclophosphamide, carmustine), topoisomerase II inhibitors (amsacrine, etoposide), cisplatin, and ionizing radiation. The mechanism underlying these positive interactions appears to be interference by Ara-C with the process of DNA repair, resulting in enhanced DNA damage.

The metabolism of Ara-U, the main catabolic by-product of Ara-C, is important for the metabolism and toxicity of Ara-C. Ara-U is mainly excreted in the urine. High concentrations of Ara-U can decrease deamination of Ara-C through feedback inhibition of cytidine deaminase, thus resulting in increased intracellular levels of Ara-CTP.[146,178] Ara-U also increases the fraction of murine leukemic cells entering S phase, thereby enhancing Ara-C cytotoxicity.[159] Accumulation of high levels of Ara-U may occur in both plasma and CSF in patients receiving high-dose Ara-C, with a possible increase in Ara-CTP formation in brain tissue.[153,160] These observations may explain the increased risk of neurotoxicity with high-dose Ara-C, especially in those with impaired renal function.

Interference with the DNA incorporation of Ara-C (e.g., by pretreatment with TS inhibitors) may antagonize its cytotoxicity.[161] MTX pretreatment, however, may increase Ara-CTP formation. Antimetabolites that decrease the competing pools of dCTP may enhance Ara-C anabolism, DNA incorporation, and its subsequent cytotoxicity. Such agents include inhibitors of RR (fludarabine, hydroxyurea, and high-dose thymidine), and inhibitors of CTP synthase (the investigational drugs acivicin, cyclopentenol cytosine, and 3-deazauridine).

Interactions between various cytokines and Ara-C may have potential clinical implications. A 24-hour exposure of human myeloid leukemic cells to pIXY 321, a fusion protein combining granulocyte-macrophage colony-stimulating factor and interleukin-3, enhances high-dose Ara-C–mediated induction of apoptosis.[162]

GEMCITABINE

Gemcitabine (2',2'-difluorodeoxycytidine, dFdC, Gemzar) is a difluorinated analogue of deoxycytidine (see Fig. 19.5-5). This compound has shown significant preclinical and clinical activity against several human solid tumors, including cancer of the pancreas, small cell and non–small cell lung cancer, and bladder cancer. In contrast to Ara-C, the spectrum of antitumor activity of gemcitabine is much broader, despite the similarities in structure, metabolism, and mechanism of action.[163] The most commonly used schedule in clinical practice is 1000 mg/m^2

intravenously administered weekly for 3 weeks, followed by a 1-week rest. This schedule seems to provide the most acceptable toxicity profile with the greatest dose intensity. This compound has been moved rapidly from phase I/II studies into phase III studies, mostly in combination with other established anticancer agents.

Intracellular Metabolism and Mechanism of Action

Transport of gemcitabine into cells requires the nucleoside transporter system. Nucleoside transport–deficient cells are highly resistant to the drug. Furthermore, the specific type of nucleoside transporter expressed on the cell surface may be an important determinant of drug sensitivity.[164,165] The intracellular concentration of adenosine triphosphate (ATP) may also be an additional sign of the sensitivity to gemcitabine. In head and neck cancer cell lines, ATP-replete cells accumulated significantly less gemcitabine, when compared with ATP-deplete cells. This finding suggests the existence of an active efflux mechanism for gemcitabine.[166] Gemcitabine is fivefold more lipophilic than Ara-C, a feature that is thought to contribute to the 65% greater rate of accumulation of gemcitabine in cells when compared with Ara-C.

Gemcitabine requires intracellular activation for its cytotoxic effects. The steps involved in its metabolic activation of gemcitabine are similar to those observed with Ara-C, with both drugs being activated by the same enzymatic machinery. Deoxycytidine kinase converts dFdC into dFdCMP.[166,167] The drug is subsequently phosphorylated by nucleoside monophosphate and diphosphate kinases to the respective 5'-diphosphate (dFdCDP) and 5'-triphosphate derivatives (dFdCTP).[166,167] dFdCTP is the major cellular metabolite of dFdC. The intracellular concentration of dFdCTP determines to a large extent its subsequent metabolism. In cells with lower concentrations of this metabolite (less than 100 μmol/L) the main route of elimination is by deamination, whereas in cells with higher concentrations (greater than 100 μmol/L) dephosphorylation and urinary excretion predominate. Furthermore, dFdCTP, by inhibiting dCMP deaminase, establishes a mechanism of self-potentiation, with a marked prolongation of its terminal half-life from 3.6 hours to 19.0 hours. This phenomenon may explain, at least in part, the differences observed between Ara-C and dFdC in their spectrum of clinical activity.

dFdCDP is an inhibitor of RR, and thus decreases the intracellular pools of deoxynucleotide triphosphates (dNTPs). Depletion of dCTP, as a consequence of RR inhibition, leads to decreased feedback inhibition of deoxycytidine kinase and increased phosphorylation of dFdC. dFdCTP directly inhibits deoxycytidylate deaminase; as dCTP is a required activator of this enzyme, dFdCDP-mediated depletion of dCTP also diminishes deoxycytidylate deaminase activity. dFdCTP competes with dCTP for incorporation into DNA by DNA polymerase, and depletion of dCTP favors incorporation of dFdCTP. Inhibition of DNA synthesis may result from both perturbations of deoxynucleotide pools and interference with DNA chain elongation.[168,169] The majority of incorporated residues are found in the internucleotide linkage (internal position). Incorporation of [^{3}H]dFdC into purified RNA has also been reported.[170] At equimolar concentrations of Ara-C and dFdC, dFdCTP formation is greater than Ara-CTP, and dFdCTP is retained for a much longer period after drug removal.[166]

In vitro primer extension studies indicate that dFdCTP competes with dCTP for incorporation into growing DNA strands by purified DNA polymerases α and ε (involved in DNA replication and repair).[168] The exonuclease activity of DNA polymerase ε is unable to remove the incorporated dFdC residue, and a major pause in the polymerization process occurs once the primer is extended by one deoxynucleotide beyond the dFdC residue. Incorporation of dFdC into a synthetic DNA template strand interferes with base insertion by bacterial DNA polymerase (Klenow fragment). Thermal denaturation measurements show that dFdCMP•dGMP base pairs are less stable than dCMP•dGMP base pairs. In intact HL-60 cells, dFdC markedly slowed nascent DNA chain elongation as monitored by pH step alkaline elution.[170] Pulse-chase experiments with [^{3}H]dFdC indicate that a nascent DNA fragment containing [^{3}H]dFdC progressed over time into larger DNA intermediates and ultimately into genomic-length DNA.[170] Thus, dFdC does not function as an absolute chain terminator in intact cells. Cytidine deaminase converts dFdC to the inactive uridine metabolite, dFdU. The drug is cell-cycle specific, and blocks cells in the G_1/S interface. Cytotoxicity is schedule dependent and increases with increasing duration of exposure. In a T-cell lymphoblastoid line, dFdC-DNA incorporation was necessary for induction of apoptosis.

Mechanisms of Resistance

Several mechanisms of resistance to gemcitabine in cell lines have been described. Nucleoside transport–deficient cells are highly resistant to gemcitabine.[164] Furthermore, the efficiency of gemcitabine uptake can vary significantly according to the specific nucleoside transporter expressed on the cell surface.[164]

Several enzymes involved in the intracellular metabolism of gemcitabine have been implicated in the development of resistance to this drug. Initial *in vitro* studies suggested that dCK enzyme activity deficiency was the most important cause of resistance to gemcitabine. Gemcitabine-sensitive human ovarian carcinoma cell lines express tenfold higher dCK enzyme activity than gemcitabine-resistant cells.[171] However, experiments using human epidermoid carcinoma KB cells suggest that the enzyme RR may play an important role as well. RR is an S-phase–specific, rate-limiting enzyme of the DNA synthesis pathway. Cells exhibiting resistance to gemcitabine demonstrated a ninefold overexpression of RR mRNA, a twofold overexpression of RR protein, and a 2.3-fold higher RR enzyme activity when compared with gemcitabine-sensitive cells.[172] The potential role of RR as a determinant of drug resistance has been confirmed in the human erythroleukemia K562 cell line, where high RR enzyme activity was directly correlated with resistance.[173]

The pattern of cross-resistance between various nucleoside analogues may have potential clinical implications. For example, gemcitabine was found to have higher antitumor activity than Ara-C in both Ara-C–sensitive (L1210 and BCLO) and Ara-C–resistant (LA46 and Bara-C) cell lines.[174] In another *in vitro* experiment, human promyelocytic leukemia HL-60 cells were made cladribine resistant, resulting in two resistant sublines (R13 and R23). Neither subline was found to have cross-resistance to gemcitabine.[175] Enzymatic characterization of these sublines revealed that both dCK and 5'-nucleotidase enzymatic activities are likely to be involved. The ratio of dCK to 5'-nucleotidase activity was reduced by approximately 65% in both sublines.

Clinical Pharmacology and Pharmacokinetics

dFdC can be measured in plasma samples by HPLC and an enzyme-linked immunosorbent assay. As dFdC is rapidly deaminated, blood collection tubes must contain tetrahydrouridine for accurate determination of plasma drug levels. After a 30-minute intravenous infusion of dFdC at doses ranging from 50 to 1000 mg/m^2, the plasma concentration versus time curve (area under the concentration time curve) increases in a linear fashion.[176] The compound is rapidly eliminated from plasma, mainly by deamination. The median half-life and clearance of dFdC are 8 minutes and 119 L/h/m^2, respectively.[176] Renal clearance of parent drug is less than 10% of the systemic clearance. dFdU, the main catabolic by-product, is eliminated by biphasic kinetics characterized by a long terminal phase (half-life of 14 hours). The pharmacokinetics and toxicity of dFdC in patients with impaired hepatic and renal function has not yet been determined. The accumulation of dFdCTP in circulating mononuclear cells appears to be saturated when plasma levels exceeded 15 to 20 μM; the median half-life for intracellular retention was 4.7 hours.[176]

A phase I trial of dFdC in cancer patients explored the maximally tolerated duration of dFdC infused at a dose rate of 10 mg/m^2/min, calculated to produce steady-state levels of 20 μM. The maximally tolerated duration was 8 hours (total dose of 4800 mg/m^2), with mean steady-state plasma levels of approximately 26 μM and median clearance of 149 L/h. Cellular pharmacokinetics of dFdCTP in circulating leukemic cells vary considerably among patients. In eight patients with linear dFdCTP elimination, the median half-life was 4.6 hours. In seven patients with biphasic dFdCTP elimination, the median initial and terminal phase half-life values were 2.5 hours and 6.8 hours.

Toxicity

Although gemcitabine is a relatively well-tolerated drug when used as a single agent, its toxicity profile can vary significantly according to the schedule of administration. The most commonly used schedule is a weekly dose of 800 to 1250 mg/m^2, administered intravenously over 30 minutes, for 3 weeks on an every 4-week cycle. With this schedule, myelosuppression is the dose-limiting toxicity, and all three lineages can be affected. A published series of more than 3000 patients treated with gemcitabine for pancreatic carcinoma revealed that nonhematologic side effects are relatively uncommon. They include fever (7.3%), pain (6.8%), asthenia (6.0%), abdominal pain (5.5%), dyspnea (5.0%), vomiting (3.9%), anorexia (3.6%), and deep venous thrombosis (3.2%).[177] A particularly unusual side effect of dFdC is anal pruritus, which may be prevented with the use of corticosteroids.

Although dyspnea is a relatively uncommon side effect of gemcitabine, its development during the treatment with the drug may require discontinuation of the treatment. Continuation of treatment once dyspnea develops may lead to a fatal outcome.[178] Patients usually present with a clinical picture consistent with acute respiratory distress syndrome, with hypoxemia, pulmonary infiltrates, and no evidence of left ventricular failure. The onset of acute respiratory distress syndrome in these patients can take place anywhere between 2 and 40 days after the first dose of the drug. Thus, close monitoring of patients for any change in baseline respiratory status is crucial.

A rare yet potentially fatal complication of dFdC is hemolytic-uremic syndrome (HUS).[179] The incidence of this complication has been estimated to be less than 1%. Early recognition of HUS is important and should prompt the immediate discontinuation of therapy to prevent death from HUS-related complications.

Drug Interactions

Gemcitabine has been combined with various chemotherapeutic agents in the treatment of several solid tumors. Preclinical *in vitro* studies have provided evidence of synergism between gemcitabine and various anticancer agents to support these associations. Cisplatin is one of the agents most commonly used in combination with gemcitabine. *In vitro* studies with different human cancer cell lines have shown synergistic interaction between gemcitabine and cisplatin.[179–181] This synergism is thought to be mainly due to an increase in platinum-DNA adduct formation, which in turn results from dFdC incorporation into DNA.[180] Synergism has also been demonstrated between gemcitabine and etoposide in human ovarian and lung cancer cell lines.[182] Moreover, sequencing of agents in this combination is important as the synergism is maximum when cells are exposed first to etoposide and then to gemcitabine.[182] This may be due to the fact that cells exposed first to etoposide have low levels of dCTP in the cytoplasm, which then allow for enhanced phosphorylation of dFdC and subsequent incorporation of dFdCTP into DNA.[182]

6-THIOPURINES

The development of the purine analogues in cancer chemotherapy began in the early 1950s with the synthesis of the thiopurines. For this seminal work, Hitchings and Elion received the Nobel Prize in Medicine in 1988. The purine analogues, 6-MP and 6-thioguanine (6-TG) continue to be used principally in the management of acute leukemia.[183] 6-MP has an important role in the maintenance therapy of acute lymphoblastic leukemia (ALL), whereas 6-TG is active in remission induction and in the maintenance therapy of AML. These analogues have a single substitution of a thiol group in place of the 6-hydroxyl group of the purine base (Fig. 19.5-7). 6-MP is a structural analogue of hypoxanthine, whereas 6-TG is an analogue of guanine. Azathioprine is a derivative of 6-MP and acts as a prodrug to provide sustained release of 6-MP.

Intracellular Metabolism and Mechanism of Action

6-MP and 6-TG act similarly with regard to their cellular biochemistry. In their respective monophosphate nucleotide form, they inhibit *de novo* purine synthesis and purine interconversion reactions, whereas the nucleotide triphosphate metabolites are incorporated directly into nucleic acids. The relative contribution of each of these actions to the mechanism of cytotoxicity of these agents is unclear.[183] Both 6-MP and 6-TG are converted to their respective monophosphate forms by hypoxanthine-guanine phosphoribosyl transferase (HGPRT) (Fig. 19.5-8). These ribonucleotide monophosphates inhibit the first step of *de novo* purine synthesis catalyzed by glutamine phosphoribosylpyrophosphate aminotransferase and block the conversion of inosinic acid to adenylic acid or to guanylic acid.

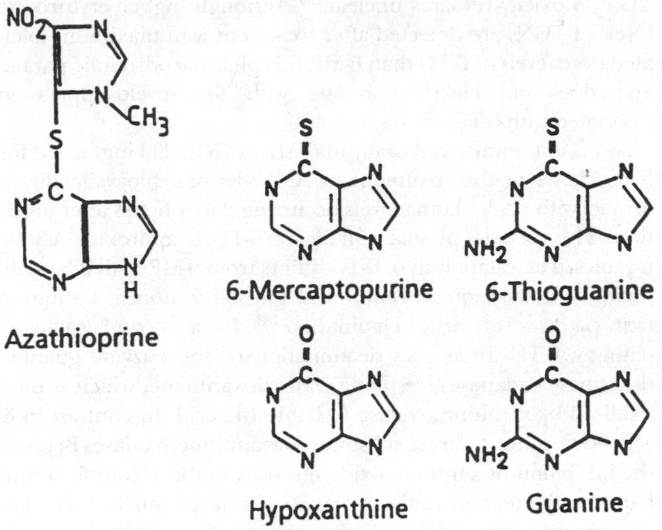

FIGURE 19.5-7. Purine analogues and their physiologic counterparts, hypoxanthine and guanine.

Inhibition of purine nucleotide synthesis leads to the build-up of PRPP, which facilitates the activation of 6-MP and 6-TG to their active nucleotide forms by HGPRT.

Inhibitors of *de novo* purine biosynthesis, such as MTX, interact in a synergistic manner with 6-thiopurines because the MTX-induced block in purine synthesis expands the PRPP pool required for thiopurine activation. Both ribonucleotide and deoxyribonucleotide metabolites of the thiopurines are formed, which can then be incorporated into cellular RNA and DNA. Incorporation of fraudulent nucleotides into DNA interferes with DNA replication and results in the formation of DNA strand breaks.[184] In some model systems, incorporation of thiopurine nucleotides into DNA correlates with cytotoxicity.

In addition to 6-MP effects on DNA biosynthesis, there is now evidence that the glycolytic pathway may also be affected. 6-Phosphofructo-2-kinase, an essential enzyme for carbohydrate metabolism, is inhibited by 6-MP.[185] Finally, this class of compounds may inhibit the process of angiogenesis, as studies have shown *in vivo* antiangiogenic activity of a thiopurine metabolite, methylmercaptopurine riboside, in a human endometrial adenocarcinoma xenograft model.[186]

Mechanisms of Resistance

Biochemical resistance to 6-thiopurines results from a decreased ability to form cytotoxic nucleotide metabolites. In experimental systems, resistant cells express either a complete or partial deficiency of HGPRT.[187] An alteration in the affinity of HGPRT for 6-thiopurines has also been described.[188] Studies have shown that decreased transmembrane transport of 6-TG can also result in drug resistance.[189] In the HHUA, DLD-1, and HCT 166 human cancer cell lines, MMR-defective cells exhibited higher levels of drug resistance and increased mutagenic response at the HGPRT locus to 6-TG when compared with their MMR-proficient counterparts. Thus, the inability to properly repair damaged or mutant DNA may provide a selective growth advantage for MMR-defective cells. Moreover, this finding may provide a mechanism by which 6-TG treatment results in the development of secondary malignancies.[190]

In clinical samples derived from patients with AML, drug resistance has also been associated with either increased concentrations of a membrane-bound alkaline phosphatase or a conjugating enzyme, 6-thiopurine methyltransferase (TPMT).[191] Patients who express high levels of TPMT activity are unable to form sufficiently high levels of active nucleotide metabolites after treatment with 6-MP. As such, they may be more likely to benefit from treatment with 6-TG.[192]

Clinical Pharmacology and Pharmacokinetics

HPLC analysis using the phenylmercury or sulfonated derivatives of the thiopurines is able to detect plasma drug levels as low as 0.1 mM. An HPLC method was developed to measure thiopurine levels in erythrocytes in the 18 to 20 pmol range.[193] Oral doses of 6-MP of 70 to 100 $mg/m^2/d$ are commonly used in the maintenance therapy of ALL. Oral absorption of 6-MP is highly erratic, with only 16% to 50% of the administered dose reaching the systemic circulation. This effect is mainly due to rapid first-pass metabolism in the liver.[194] Food intake and coadministration with the antibiotic cotrimoxazole significantly reduce drug absorption. The variable bioavailability of oral 6-MP may be an important determinant of therapeutic outcome, because low plasma drug concentration over time measurements correlate with an increased risk of relapse in children with ALL.[195] 6-MP bioavailability is increased when combined with high-dose (2 to 5 g/m^2 intravenous) MTX.[196] Studies have shown that MTX

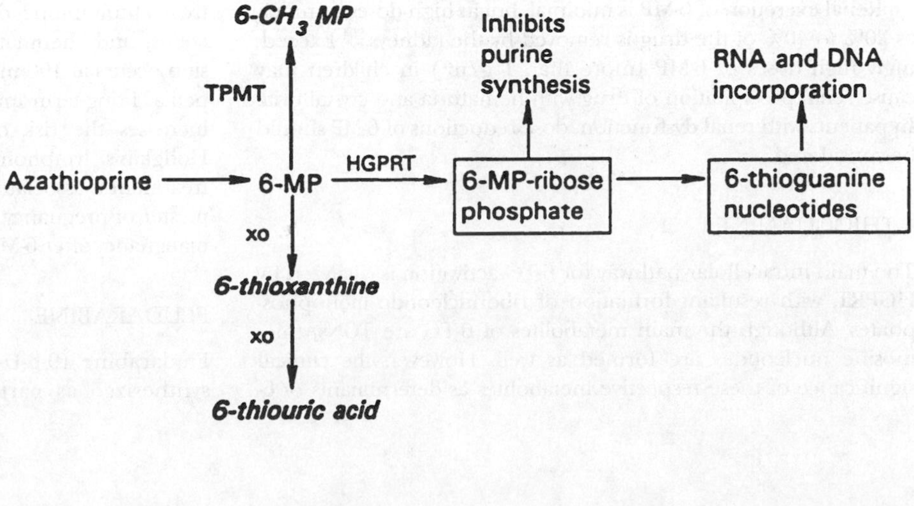

FIGURE 19.5-8. Metabolic pathways for activation and degradation of 6-mercaptopurine (6-MP). HGPRT, hypoxanthine-guanine phosphoribosyl transferase; TPMT, 6-thiopurine methyltransferase.

inhibits xanthine oxidase, an enzyme important in the catabolism of thiopurines.[197]

Oral 6-MP is well distributed into most body compartments, with the exception of the CSF. With high-dose intravenous 6-MP (200 mg/m^2 bolus followed by 800 mg/m^2 over 8 hours), a CSF to plasma ratio of 0.15 is achieved. This schedule is currently being used to prevent CNS relapse in ALL.[198] Approximately 30% of the drug binds weakly to plasma proteins. The plasma half-life is approximately 50 minutes after intravenous injection and 90 minutes after oral administration. When studied in children with ALL, plasma concentrations and erythrocyte thioguanine nucleotide levels are highly variable and independent from dose.[199]

The major route of drug elimination is via metabolism by several enzymatic pathways. 6-MP is oxidized to the inactive metabolite 6-thiouric acid by xanthine oxidase. Enhanced 6-MP toxicity may result from the concomitant administration of both oral and intravenous 6-MP and the xanthine oxidase inhibitor allopurinol.[200] In patients receiving both 6-MP and allopurinol, the 6-MP dose should be reduced by at least 50–75%.

6-MP also undergoes S-methylation by the enzyme TPMT to yield 6-methylmercaptopurine. After further phosphorylation, 6-methylmercaptopurine nucleotides are, themselves, capable of inhibiting *de novo* purine biosynthesis, but to a lesser extent than thioguanine nucleotides (TGNs). TPMT plays a similar role in 6-TG and azathioprine metabolism.[201] It has been shown that TPMT enzyme activity may vary considerably between patients. Moreover, the levels of TPMT enzyme activity correlate inversely with intracellular levels of TGNs and with the duration of 6-MP–induced cytopenia, suggesting that the level of inherited TPMT activity may affect directly 6-MP cytotoxicity and host toxicity.[191] Due to an autosomal codominant genetic polymorphism, a series of TPMT phenotypes, with alleles of differing enzymatic activity, are present in the general population. Point mutations or loss of alleles of TPMT resulting in altered enzyme activity correlate with a defect in thiopurine metabolism, thus defining a true pharmacogenetic syndrome.[202] A polymerase chain reaction–based method is widely used for the genetic detection of these TPMT mutations.[203] Approximately 0.3% of the white population expresses either a homozygous deletion or mutation of both alleles of the TPMT gene. In these patients, grossly elevated TGN concentrations, profound myelotoxicity with pancytopenia, and extensive gastrointestinal symptoms are seen after only a brief course of thiopurine treatment.[201] An estimated 10% of patients may be at increased risk for toxicity due to heterozygous loss of the gene or a mutant allele coding for a less enzymatically active TPMT.[202,203] Drug interactions affecting TPMT activity have also been reported with aspirin, sulfasalazine, 5-aminosalicylic acid, furosemide, and disulfiram.[201]

Renal excretion of 6-MP is minimal, but at high doses, as much as 20% to 40% of the drug is removed by the kidneys.[204] Exceedingly high doses of 6-MP (more than 1 g/m^2) in children may cause renal precipitation of drug with hematuria and crystalluria. In patients with renal dysfunction, dose reductions of 6-MP should be considered.

6-THIOGUANINE

The main intracellular pathway for 6-TG activation is catalyzed by HGPRT, with resultant formation of ribonucleotide monophosphates. Although the main metabolites of 6-TG are TGNs, thioinosine nucleotides are formed as well. However, the clinical significance of these respective metabolites as determinants of 6-TG cytotoxicity remains unclear.[205] Although higher erythrocyte levels of TGNs are detected after treatment with maximum tolerated dose levels of 6-TG than 6-MP, this pharmacodynamic parameter does not clearly correlate with the myelosuppression associated with 6-TG.[206]

6-TG is administered orally in doses of 75 to 200 mg/m^2/d for 5 to 7 days in the treatment of AML. Its oral bioavailability is erratic, with peak plasma levels occurring 2 to 4 hours after ingestion. The median plasma half-life of 6-TG is approximately 90 minutes. The catabolism of 6-TG differs from 6-MP in that S-methylation with subsequent removal of the sulfur atom is an important pathway of drug elimination.[183] In a second catabolic pathway, 6-TG undergoes deamination by the enzyme guanine deaminase (guanase), resulting in 6-thioxanthene, which is then oxidized by xanthine oxidase to 6-thiouric acid. In contrast to 6-MP, 6-TG is not a direct substrate for xanthine oxidase. Because the inhibition of xanthine oxidase results in the accumulation of 6-thioxanthene, an inactive metabolite, adjustments in 6-TG dosage are not required for patients receiving allopurinol.

Toxicity

The major dose-related toxicities of 6-MP are myelosuppression and gastrointestinal toxicity. Leukopenia and thrombocytopenia are maximal 7 days after treatment. Full hematologic recovery usually occurs after 14 days. In TPMT-deficient patients, dose reduction to 5% to 25% of the standard dose (75 mg/m^2/d) is necessary to prevent excessive toxicity.[207] Gastrointestinal toxicities include nausea and vomiting, anorexia, diarrhea, and stomatitis. 6-MP hepatotoxicity occurs in up to 30% of adult patients and is manifested as mainly cholestatic jaundice, although elevations of hepatic transaminases may also be seen. Hepatotoxicity is usually mild and reversible after discontinuation of 6-MP, but frank hepatic necrosis can occur after high doses of the drug. Combinations of 6-MP with other known hepatotoxic agents should be avoided, and liver function test results should be closely monitored. The mechanism of liver toxicity is not known, but may relate to the P-450-dependent metabolism of 6-MP to a hepatotoxic metabolite or accumulation of 6-MP metabolites in the liver.[183] 6-TG also causes dose-limiting bone marrow suppression but is associated with fewer gastrointestinal side effects and less hepatotoxicity than 6-MP.

As a class of drugs, the 6-thiopurine analogues are potent suppressors of cell-mediated immunity. As such, prolonged therapy results in an increased predisposition to bacterial and parasitic infections. Given their immunosuppressive effects, these agents have been used to prevent rejection of transplanted organs and to treat autoimmune diseases, such as Crohn's disease, ulcerative colitis, and rheumatoid arthritis. Therapeutic immunosuppression occurs at 100 mg/d, a dose associated with only mild leukopenia. Long-term immunosuppressive therapy with azathioprine increases the risk of squamous carcinoma of the skin, non-Hodgkin's lymphoma, and Kaposi's sarcoma. Chronic 6-MP treatment is associated with teratogenic effects during the first trimester of pregnancy, and AML has been reported as a secondary malignancy after 6-MP treatment for Crohn's disease.[208]

FLUDARABINE

Fludarabine (9-β-D-arabinosyl-2-fluoroadenine, Fludara) was synthesized as part of a rational process to develop more

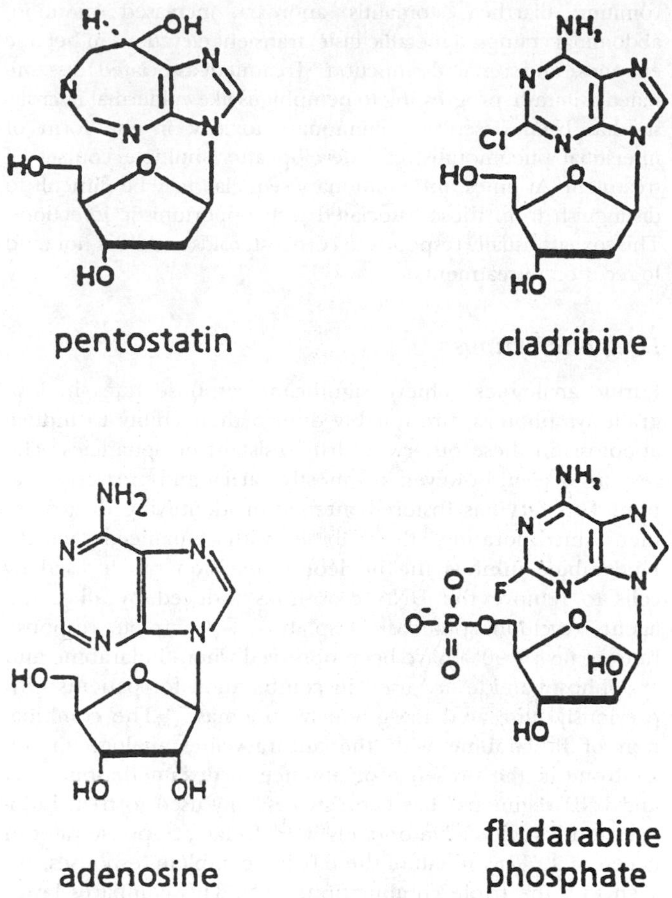

FIGURE 19.5-9. Structures of adenosine analogues.

active analogues of cytarabine (Fig. 19.5-9).[209] The first compound in this series was adenine arabinoside (vidarabine; Ara-A). However, this compound was deaminated to its inactive form to a significant extent, thereby negating its clinical application. The 2'-fluoro derivative of Ara-A was subsequently found to be relatively resistant to deamination, but was difficult to formulate and poorly soluble. Addition of a 5'-monophosphate moiety to the sugar group yielded fludarabine, which is relatively resistant to deamination and displays enhanced solubility.

Mechanism of Action

After intravenous administration, F-Ara-adenosine monophosphate (F-Ara-AMP) is rapidly dephosphorylated to F-Ara-A, which enters cells by nucleoside-specific membrane transport mechanisms. The *es* and *ei* nucleoside transporter systems facilitate the cellular uptake of the hydrophilic nucleoside analogues.[210] F-Ara-A is then rephosphorylated by dCK to F-Ara-AMP, which is subsequently metabolized to the triphosphate form. This nucleotide is the active metabolite of the drug. It competes with deoxyadenosine triphosphate (dATP) for incorporation into DNA, and serves as a highly effective chain terminator. In addition, F-Ara-ATP directly inhibits DNA polymerases involved in DNA synthesis and repair, such as DNA polymerase α and β, and inhibits other enzymes involved in DNA synthesis, such as DNA primase, DNA ligase I and RR. DNA polymerase ε is unable to remove F-Ara-AMP from the 3'-end of DNA even in the presence of excess enzyme and substrate nucleotides, resulting in the formation of dead-end complexes.[211]

Fludarabine is also incorporated into RNA, causing inhibition of RNA function, processing, and mRNA translation.[212] In contrast to other antimetabolites, fludarabine is also active against nondividing lymphocytes. In fact, the primary effect of fludarabine may result from activation of apoptosis, as evidenced by the presence of typical apoptotic fragmentation of DNA into high-molecular-weight fragments, after drug treatment.[213] The induction of apoptosis may explain the activity of this drug in indolent lymphoproliferative diseases with relatively low S-phase fractions.[214]

Mechanisms of Resistance

Fludarabine-resistant cell lines, such as JOK-1 [human hairy cell leukemia (HCL)], K562 (human erythroleukemia), and L1210 (murine leukemia) have been established. In these resistant lines, nucleoside transport of F-Ara-A is intact, and no alterations in intracellular drug accumulation or multidrug-resistant (mdr 1) expression are observed. However, decreased dCK activity with diminished intracellular formation of F-Ara-ATP is the principal mechanism of resistance in each of these cell lines.[215] Subsequent work has shown that deletion of one allele of deoxycytidine kinase is sufficient to result in decreased expression of dCK. Of note, a high degree of cross-resistance develops to multiple nucleoside analogues requiring activation by dCK, including Ara-C, 2-CdA, and gemcitabine.[216] Fludarabine resistance in WSU-CLL xenografts in SCID mice can be decreased by pretreatment with bryostatin, a macrocyclic lactone.[217] Although the underlying mechanisms for this interaction remain to be defined, preliminary studies suggest that bryostatin may induce differentiation of B-CLL cells into HCL-like cells, with expression of CD11c, CD25, and tartrate-resistant acid phosphatase (TRAP), markers typically seen in HCL.

Clinical Pharmacology and Pharmacokinetics

Peak concentrations of F-Ara-A are reached 3 to 4 hours after intravenous or oral administration. Mean plasma levels are proportional to dose. After intravenous administration, the decline in plasma levels has been reported to be bi-exponential, with a distribution half-life of 0.6 to 2.0 hours and a terminal half-life of 6.9 to 19.7 hours. However, other reports describe a three-compartment model with a terminal half-life between 10 and 30 hours.[212,218] The rate-limiting step in elimination is release from tissues and renal function affecting clearance. Dose adjustment in the setting of renal impairment is recommended, and a 30% dose reduction in patients with a serum creatinine above 1.5 mg/dL or creatinine clearance below 70 mL/min should be considered.

The median peak concentration of F-Ara-ATP in lymphocytes of leukemic patients occurs approximately 4 hours after the start of a 30-minute intravenous infusion of 25 mg/m^2. Intracellular F-Ara-ATP elimination exhibits a single phase with a dose-dependent terminal phase. The oral bioavailability of liquid fludarabine is 60% to 80%, leading to approximately two-thirds of the intracellular F-Ara-ATP levels in chronic lymphocytic leukemia (CLL) cells achieved with intravenous administration.[219]

Treatment

Fludarabine is the most active single agent in the treatment of CLL.[220–222] It is also active against indolent non-Hodgkin's lymphoma,[223,224] prolymphocytic leukemia, cutaneous T-cell lymphoma, and Waldenström's macroglobulinemia.[225] This agent has shown promising activity in approximately one-third of patients with mantle cell lymphoma, albeit with relatively brief response.[226] In contrast to its activity in hematologic malignancies, this compound displays minimal activity against common solid tumors.

Toxicity

In initial trials, fludarabine, when administered as a single 260 mg/m^2 dose or 112 mg/m^2 given daily for 5 days, resulted in profound myelosuppression. This effect was not initially predicted from preclinical *in vivo* studies in mice and beagle dogs, given the extensive tissue binding and relatively low renal excretion in humans. In addition, a dose range of 75 to 150 mg/m^2 four times a day for 5 to 7 days resulted in severe prohibitive neurotoxicity characterized by delayed onset cortical blindness, seizures, coma, and death.[227] Subsequent trials demonstrated that fludarabine could be safely administered at much lower doses of 25 to 30 mg/m^2 daily for 5 days every 28 days. At standard doses, neurotoxicity occurs in approximately 15% of patients. This toxicity is rarely severe, generally reversible, and usually presents as headache, somnolence, or peripheral neuropathy.[228]

At currently used doses, myelosuppression and immunosuppression are the major side effects of fludarabine.[229] Dose-limiting and possibly cumulative lymphopenia and thrombocytopenia are well established.[218] Suppression of the immune system affects T-cell more than B-cell function. Fevers, often in the setting of neutropenia, occur in 20% to 30% of patients. Lymphocyte counts, particularly CD4+ cells, decrease rapidly after initiation of therapy, and levels can drop to as low as 150/µL by approximately 6 months.[230] CD4+ cell recovery is slow and may take longer than 1 year to recover to normal levels. Common opportunistic pathogens include herpes zoster, *Candida*, and *Pneumocystis carinii*.[229] The addition of prednisone to fludarabine does not improve the response rate or survival, but significantly increases the risk of opportunistic infections, notably listeriosis and *Pneumocystis carinii*.[230] If concurrent corticosteroids are necessary, such as in patients with autoimmune anemia or thrombocytopenia, long-term prophylaxis against *Pneumocystis carinii* is mandatory. Hemolytic anemia has been observed, and in some instances, has resulted in death on rechallenge with fludarabine.[231] Thrombocytopenia, precipitation of Evan's syndrome, and fulminant fatal myelofibrosis have also been reported. The prolonged immunosuppression experienced with fludarabine has raised the possibility of an increased incidence of secondary malignancies. However, this increased risk is now thought to be due to the underlying immune defects of the malignancy and not to the carcinogenic effects of the nucleoside analogue.[232]

Tumor lysis syndrome occurs in less than 1% of patients, and in some cases, it can be fatal. However, this event does not usually recur on retreatment with fludarabine. Prophylaxis is not uniformly effective. Other uncommon toxicities include rash, nausea, vomiting, diarrhea, stomatitis, anorexia, increased salivation, abdominal cramps, a metallic taste, transient elevations in hepatic enzymes, and renal dysfunction. Treatment-associated disseminated skin rash, progressing to pemphigus-like epidermal necrolysis, has been described. Pulmonary toxicity, in the form of interstitial pneumonitis, can develop after multiple courses of treatment. At times, the pulmonary sequelae may be difficult to distinguish from those associated with opportunistic infections. This toxicity usually responds to corticosteroids and does not tend to recur on retreatment.

Drug Interactions

Purine analogues achieve significant response rates in low-grade lymphomas, presumably due to their ability to induce apoptosis in these otherwise drug-resistant malignancies. The responses seen, however, are mostly partial and of short duration. This fact has fostered interest in identifying drug regimens incorporating fludarabine with enhanced activity. Fludarabine inhibits the nucleotide excision repair used by cells to remove the DNA cross-links induced by alkylating agents (cyclophosphamide, cisplatin).[233] Complete response rates of nearly 90% have been observed when fludarabine and cyclophosphamide are used in combination for patients with previously untreated low-grade lymphomas.[234] The combination of fludarabine with the anthracycline analogue mitoxantrone in the presence or absence of dexamethasone (FN and FND regimens) has been successfully used to treat indolent non-Hodgkin's lymphomas.[235-236] In fact, response rates in excess of 90%, with half of these being complete responses, are seen with the triple combination, FND. This compares favorably with the 60% to 70% response rate observed with single-agent fludarabine.[224]

Fludarabine-induced dCTP depletion increases deoxycytidine kinase activity in K562 human leukemic cells. This enzyme, in addition to playing a key role in generating active fludarabine metabolites, is also capable of phosphorylating Ara-C into its active metabolite, Ara-CTP. The resulting synergistic effect of fludarabine on Ara-C is now established both *in vitro*[237] and *in vivo* in leukemic blast cells derived from patients with AML.[238] This combination has clinical efficacy in childhood AML in combination with idarubicin,[239] in adult CLL,[240] in refractory or relapsed AML,[241,242] and perhaps in patients with myelodysplastic syndromes.

The immunosuppressive effect of fludarabine is being used in a novel, nonmyeloablative bone marrow transplant preparative regimen called *transplant lite*. The goal of this approach is to achieve allogeneic stem cell engraftment and graft-versus-leukemia/lymphoma effect in patients with CLL and low-grade lymphomas. In a pilot study, engraftment was achieved in 11 of 15 patients, with eight showing complete response.[243]

CLADRIBINE

2-Chlorodeoxyadenosine (Cladribine, 2-CdA) is a deoxyadenosine purine nucleoside analogue. A single substitution of a chlorine atom for a hydrogen atom at the 2 position of the purine ring of deoxyadenosine renders this compound resistant to adenosine deaminase (ADA) (see Fig. 19.5-9). It was developed initially as an immunosuppressive agent. 2-CdA exhibits a dose-dependent *in vitro* inhibition of lymphoid neoplasms and human leukemic cell lines,[244] but has no activity against solid tumors. Currently, it is the drug of choice in HCL with activity in low-grade lymphoproliferative disorders as well.

Mechanism of Action

Deoxyadenosine is cleaved within cells by the enzyme ADA, to the deoxyinosine form. A deficiency of this enzyme leads to toxic accumulation of deoxyadenosine in lymphocytes, manifesting as the severe combined immunodeficiency clinical syndrome. 2-CdA enters cells via the nucleoside transporter system.[245] Given its resistance to deamination by ADA, an ADA-deficiency-like state develops, in which 2-CdA accumulates within cells, eventually reaching lymphotoxic levels. On entry into the cell, it first undergoes conversion to cladribine-monophosphate (Cld-AMP), which is then eventually metabolized to the active metabolite, cladribine-triphosphate (Cld-ATP).[246] The rate-limiting step is catalyzed by dCK. In contrast, catabolism of 2-CdA is mediated by a 5'-nucleotidase. The greatest accumulation of Cld-ATP is observed in cells with high levels of dCK and low 5'-nucleotidase activity. Cld-ATP competitively inhibits incorporation of the normal nucleotide dATP into DNA, a process that results in termination of chain elongation.[213] Progressive accumulation of Cld-ATP leads to an imbalance in deoxyribonucleotide pools, thereby inhibiting further DNA synthesis and repair.[247] At concentrations of 0.3 μM, 2-CdA inhibits DNA synthesis by 90% within 30 minutes.[248] The accumulation of unrepaired DNA breaks over time may initiate the apoptosis of quiescent, nondividing lymphocytes. Activation of the caspase-3 proteolytic cascade has been implicated as a potential mechanism for the onset of apoptosis.[249] Finally, 2-CdA is a potent inhibitor of RR, and in so doing, it may further inhibit the synthesis of key nucleotide substrates required for DNA biosynthesis.

Mechanisms of Resistance

Resistance to 2-CdA has been attributed to altered intracellular metabolism of the drug. A reduction in dCK activity, the enzyme responsible for generating cytotoxic nucleotide metabolites, is a major determinant of acquired resistance.[250] Cld-AMP and Cld-ATP are dephosphorylated by the cytoplasmic enzyme, 5'-nucleotidase. WSU-CLL cells, derived from a patient with CLL, exhibit both low levels of dCK expression, and high-levels of 5'-nucleotidase, and accordingly, they are resistant to 2-CdA. Interestingly, restoration of 2-CdA chemosensitivity by pretreatment of WSU-CLL cells *in vitro* with bryostatin has been reported. Bryostatin may induce differentiation of CLL cells into a hairy cell–like phenotype, evidenced by the induced expression of TRAP, CD11c, and CD25 in WSU-CLL cells.[251]

Clinical Pharmacology and Pharmacokinetics

Pharmacokinetic analysis suggests a two-compartment model, with mean α and β half-lives of 35 ± 12 minutes and 6.5 ± 2.5 hours, respectively. The steady-state concentration after a 2- or 24-hour infusion of 0.14 mg/kg was 22.5 ± 11.1 n*M*. After a 2-hour infusion of 0.14 mg/kg, the mean maximum plasma concentrations were in the range of 100 to 400 nmol/L. The disposition of 2-CdA in plasma remains linear over a dose range of 0.2 to 2.5 mg/m^2, with limited interindividual variability.[252] Although there seems to be a close relationship between dose and plasma steady-state concentrations, the relationship between dose and clinical activity remains to be defined.[253] When mean plasma concentrations were fitted to a three-compartment model, the half-lives of the α, β, and γ phases ranged between 3 and 12 minutes, 0.7 to 1.5 hours, and 5.7 to 19.0 hours, respectively.

The dose of 2-CdA used in early clinical trials was 0.09 to 0.10 mg/kg/d administered as a 7-day continuous infusion. As the long terminal half-life suggested the feasibility of intermittent infusions, 2-CdA has also been tested as a 2-hour infusion of 0.09 to 0.10 mg/kg/d for 5 to 7 days or a 1-hour infusion at 6 mg/m^2 for 5 days with a 28-day cycle. A dose-escalation study of bolus daily cladribine established no dose-limiting nonhematologic toxicity up to 21.5 mg/m^2/d, given on a daily 1-hour intravenous bolus infusion for 5 days to patients with advanced hematologic malignancies. At higher dose levels, prolonged cytopenias and severe infections define the upper dose limit of the drug.[254] In a small series of patients with HCL, no significant difference in response rate or toxicity was observed between a 7-day continuous infusion and a daily 2-hour bolus for 5 days. The daily dose for 5 days appears to be better suited as an outpatient regimen. After a 2-hour or a continuous infusion of 0.12 mg/kg in patients with CLL, mean intracellular concentrations of 2-CdA nucleotides are 12.2 and 10.8 μmol/L, respectively. Intracellular concentrations of phosphorylated CdA derivatives thus exceed plasma concentrations of the metabolites by several hundredfold.[255]

In circulating leukemic cells of CLL patients treated with 2-CdA for 10 mg/m^2/d for 3 days, Cld-AMP and Cld-ATP median half-lives of 15 and 10 hours were observed, respectively. While maximum plasma 2-CdA and intracellular Cld-AMP concentrations correlate well, no clear relationship exists between the level of deoxycytidine kinase activity, the levels of the intracellular metabolites (Cld-AMP, Cld-ATP), and response to treatment.[253] These findings indicate that other, as yet, unknown determinants of clinical efficacy may be present.

2-CdA is effectively cleared by the kidneys. Renal clearance is approximately 50%, while 20% to 35% of the drug is excreted unchanged in the urine.[252] 2-CdA is able to cross the blood–brain barrier and penetrates into the CSF. While CSF concentrations in patients, in the absence of meningeal disease, reach only 25% of detected plasma levels, CSF levels exceed plasma levels in patients with meningeal involvement.[252]

The bioavailability of the drug is almost 100% when given at a dose of 0.14 mg/kg via the subcutaneous route. The area under the curve achievable with subcutaneous administration is almost identical to that of the intravenous route.[256] Oral 2-CdA reaches lower, but clinically relevant levels of bioavailability at 37% to 51%. Absorption of the oral form is decreased by gastric pH values below 2, an effect that cannot be prevented or reversed with concomitant proton pump inhibitor use. The bioavailability of oral 2-CdA correlated linearly with dosing in a small study with oral and intravenous cross-over design.[257] Oral dosing showed no cumulative peak concentration or toxicity, and its pharmacokinetics are well-described by a three-compartment model. An oral dose of 0.28 mg/kg achieved similar peak concentrations and area under the concentration time curve as 0.14 mg/kg given either intravenously or subcutaneously.[256] The overall feasibility of intermittent intravenous, subcutaneous, or oral dosing suggests that these different routes of administration may compete with and possibly replace continuous infusional schedules.

Treatment

A single course of CdA achieves durable complete remissions in 65% to 91% of patients with HCL.[258–260] Salvage treatment of patients previously treated with IFN-α or splenectomy is as effective as first-line treatment. Maintenance therapy is not required. Although minimal residual disease is often found on reexamination of bone marrow specimens of HCL patients in clinical complete response, relapse rates are low. Retreatment with cladribine results in complete response in up to 60% of relapsing patients.[261] However, it remains unclear whether cladribine offers any significant long-term survival benefit over another nucleoside analogue, pentostatin. Responses in patients with CLL and non-Hodgkin's lymphoma tend to be brief, and salvage of relapsed or refractory disease is less efficacious than in HCL.[262,263] 2-CdA achieves high response rates in pediatric patients with AML, but not in adult patients. 2-CdA has minimal activity against solid tumors.

Toxicity

At conventional doses, myelotoxicity is dose limiting. Decreased counts in all three cell lines are typically observed. Thrombocytopenia usually recovers within 2 to 4 weeks, and neutropenia in 3 to 5 weeks, after a single course of the drug. Severe, prolonged myelotoxicity is reported, however, after repeated cycles of cladribine used in the treatment of CLL or low-grade lymphomas.[229] Severe autoimmune hemolytic anemia with fatal bone marrow aplasia has been described in CLL patients receiving repeated cycles of the drug, as CdA-induced lymphopenia may exacerbate autoimmune hemolysis. Of note, foci of bone marrow hypoplasia are seen in cladribine-treated patients, although the long-term clinical significance of this effect remains unclear.

Immunosuppression accounts for the late morbidity observed in CdA-treated patients. Lymphocyte counts, particularly CD4+ cells, decrease within 1 to 4 weeks of drug administration and may remain depressed for several years.[264] After discontinuation of cladribine, a median time of up to 40 months may be required for complete recovery of normal CD4+ counts.[229] Fevers occur in 40% to 50% of patients, typically correlating with the duration of granulocytopenia. These episodes may be profound, prolonged, and cumulative.[259] Opportunistic infections are common, although usually seen less frequently than with fludarabine. Herpes zoster is most typical, and a variety of other pathogens are also seen, including *Candida, Pneumocystis, Pseudomonas aeruginosa, Listeria monocytogenes, Cryptococcus neoformans, Aspergillus,* cytomegalovirus, and common bacterial infections. Infectious complications correlate with decreases in CD4+ count, and they are more frequent with repeated courses of therapy.[229] Treatment-related deaths have been reported in more than 30% of patients.[265]

In patients with HCL and CLL, long-term studies have failed to identify an increase in drug-related mortality. Specifically, initial concerns about an increased risk for secondary malignancies have not been confirmed, as the incidence of second cancers is not higher than what would be expected from the underlying hematologic disorder.[232,266]

Severe neurotoxicity was encountered at high doses of 2-CdA in phase I trials, with quadriparesis and paraparesis, proximal neuromyopathy, and rarely, Brown-Séquard and Guillain-Barré syndromes. At currently recommended doses, mild to moderate neurotoxicity occurs in 15% of patients and is, at least, partly reversible with discontinuation of the drug.[228]

Tumor lysis syndrome is rare, tends to occur after the first course, and is generally mild and reversible. However, in rare instances, this process may be fatal, even in patients with prior therapy. Cardiotoxicity is uncommon, but cardiac deaths have been reported, mainly in patients with a prior cardiac history. Pulmonary complications of 2-CdA therapy are uncommon, but in some cases, they have been fatal. Rashes, although uncommon, may be severe and can present as fatal toxic epidermal necrolysis. Mild to severe gastrointestinal toxicities occur in 15% of patients, with nausea, vomiting, and diarrhea, and there have been rare reports of anorexia, severe mucositis, or both. Transient elevations in hepatic enzymes may occur, with exacerbation of hepatitis B, which may be fatal. Renal failure occurs only at high doses.

Drug Interactions

Inhibition of RR by 2-CdA depletes intracellular dCTP pools. This effect leads to compensatory increases in intracellular dCK activity. dCK activity plays a critical role in the formation of the active intracellular Ara-C metabolite, Ara-CTP. Synergistic interaction between 2-CdA and Ara-C was observed in leukemic blast cells isolated from patients with AML, in which 2-CdA pretreatment led to increases of intracellular Ara-CTP pools by up to 40%, with sustained inhibition of DNA synthesis in the circulating leukemia blasts.[267] Studies are ongoing to translate the positive interaction between Ara-C and 2-CdA into the clinical setting.

2'-DEOXYCOFORMYCIN

2'-Deoxycoformycin (Pentostatin), a fermentation product of *Streptomyces antibioticus*, was developed as a potent inhibitor of ADA (see Fig. 19.5-9).[268] ADA is present in high concentrations in lymphoid tissues, and this enzyme plays a vital role in the differentiation of both T and B cells. Genetic absence of ADA leads to severe combined immunodeficiency disorder in children, and this syndrome is characterized by profound T- and B-cell lymphopenia. Inhibition of this enzyme leads to an accumulation of deoxyadenosine as there is no alternate route for its metabolic conversion to deoxyinosine and uric acid. Deoxyadenosine is subsequently phosphorylated by deoxycytidine kinase to deoxyadenosine monophosphate, which is then further metabolized to the triphosphate form. This metabolite accumulates within cells and inhibits RR, a key enzyme in DNA synthesis.[212,268]

Mechanism of Action

Pentostatin enters cells via the nucleoside transport system, and once within the cell, it forms a tight inhibitory complex with ADA.[268] Exposure of both murine L1210 leukemic cells and normal resting human lymphocytes results in progressive accumulation of DNA breaks along with a decrease in RNA synthesis. In response to drug treatment, DNA repair is activated, resulting in depletion of critical intracellular nicotinamide-adenine dinucleotide levels. This then leads to exhaustion of ATP pools, resulting in eventual cell death.

Clinical Pharmacology and Pharmacokinetics

After rapid intravenous infusions (1 to 9 minutes), pentostatin shows dose-independent first-order elimination, with a biphasic decay characteristic of a two-compartment open model. The rapid disposition phase is short, with a mean half-life of 8.72 minutes and a mean terminal half-life of 4.93 hours. The mean volume of distribution is 23.1 ± 6.16 L/m^2, and the mean steady-state volume of distribution is 20.0 ± 5.31 L/m^2. Nearly 100% of an administered dose is excreted in the urine, and there is a significant correlation between plasma levels and creatinine clearance.[269]

Treatment

Initial clinical trials with high doses of pentostatin in patients with ALL and HCL revealed prohibitive myelosuppression and neurotoxicity, the latter manifesting as somnolence, lethargy, confusion, seizures, and coma.[270] Current standard regimens consist of 4 mg/m^2 doses every 1 or 2 weeks.[271] With this schedule, pentostatin exhibits remarkable activity against HCL. In phase II studies, durable response rates over 90% are routinely achieved, and maintenance treatment is not required. On relapse, retreatment with the drug can be effective.[272] In a large, prospective phase III trial, pentostatin achieved significantly higher response rates (79% vs. 38%) and relapse-free-survival than IFN-α_{2a}. However, this effect was not translated into overall survival benefit.[273] Although a small number of pentostatin-pretreated patients show good response to cladribine, pentostatin use in patients who have progressed on cladribine has not been investigated in a systematic manner. Minimal residual disease on immunohistochemical examination of bone marrow specimens is detectable in 20% to 40% of HCL patients, who achieve complete response after pentostatin treatment. Although minimal residual disease may be associated with an increased risk of relapse, it remains unclear whether treatment of asymptomatic patients with minimal residual disease provides clinical benefit.[274]

Pentostatin is also active in CLL, prolymphocytic leukemia, cutaneous T-cell lymphoma, indolent non-Hodgkin's lymphoma, chronic myelogenous leukemia, and Langerhans' cell histiocytosis.[268,275] Overall response rates in these malignancies are less than that achieved with either fludarabine and cladribine or that observed with pentostatin in HCL. No significant activity is seen in multiple myeloma or in solid tumors.

Toxicity

The profound immunosuppression associated with pentostatin may persist for several years after therapy is discontinued.[276] T-cell function is affected more than B-cell or natural killer cell function, perhaps because of higher baseline levels of ADA in T cells. A standard course of pentostatin is associated with more prolonged immunosuppression than that observed with a single-course of cladribine treatment in patients with HCL. The mean time of recovery of CD4+ cells to normal levels is up to 50 months after completion of treatment.[277] Myelosuppression with neutropenia and thrombocytopenia is commonly described. Thrombotic thrombocytopenic purpura and HUS and persistent bone marrow failure with myelodysplastic features have been reported. Neutropenic fever is seen in up to 30% of cases, and opportunistic infections occur with *Candida*, herpes zoster, *Pneumocystis carinii*, and a variety of other pathogens.[229] Although an increased incidence of second cancers is noted in pentostatin-treated patients, the relative risk is similar to that observed with the underlying disease in the absence of nucleoside analogue treatment.[232]

Ocular complications include conjunctivitis, desquamative keratitis, or periorbital edema. Dermatologic toxicity in the form of skin rash, photosensitivity reactions, and a case of fatal erythroderma have been reported. Nausea and vomiting with pentostatin are dose dependent. Other uncommon side effects include stomatitis, constipation, diarrhea, cardiac toxicity, pulmonary toxicity, renal insufficiency, urate nephropathy, and allergic reactions. Transient and reversible increases in hepatic enzymes and fulminant hepatic failure have been described.

REFERENCES

1. Farber S, Diamond LK, Mercer RD, Sylvester RF, Wolff JA. Temporary remissions in acute leukemia in children produced by folic acid antagonist, 4-aminopteroylglutamic acid (aminopterin). *N Engl J Med* 1948;238:787.
2. Chu E, Allegra CJ. Antifolates. In: Chabner BA, Longo DL, eds. *Cancer chemotherapy and biotherapy: principles and practice.* Philadelphia: Lippincott–Raven, 1996:109.
3. Chu E, Drake JC, Boarman D, et al. Mechanism of thymidylate synthase inhibition by methotrexate in human neoplastic cell lines and normal human myeloid progenitor cells. *J Biol Chem* 1990;256:8470.
4. Jolivet J, Chabner BA. Intracellular pharmacokinetics of methotrexate polyglutamates in human breast cancer cells: selective retention and less dissociable binding of 4-N-10-CH_3-pteroylglutamate$_4$ and 4-NH_2-10-CH_3-pteroylglutamate$_5$ to dihydrofolate reductase. *J Clin Invest* 1983;72:773.
5. Winick NJ, Kamen BA, Balis FM, et al. Folate and methotrexate polyglutamate tissue levels in rhesus monkeys following chronic low-dose methotrexate. *Cancer Drug Deliv* 1987;4:25.
6. Allegra CJ, Hoang K, Yeh GC, et al. Evidence for direct inhibition of de novo purine synthesis in human MCF-7 breast cells as a principal mode of metabolic inhibition by methotrexate. *J Biol Chem* 1987;262:13520.
7. Goulian M, Bleile B, Tseng BY. Methotrexate-induced misincorporation of uracil into DNA. *Proc Natl Acad Sci U S A* 1980;77:1956.
8. Smith SG, Lehman NL, Moran RG. Cytotoxicity of antifolate inhibitors of thymidylate synthase and purine synthesis to WiDr colonic carcinoma cells. *Cancer Res* 1993;1993:5697.
9. Fiskerstrand T, Ueland PM, Refsum H. Folate depletion induced by methotrexate affects methionine synthase activity and its susceptibility to inactivation by nitrous oxide. *J Pharmacol Exp Ther* 1997;202:1305.
10. Schalinske KL, Steele RD. Methotrexate alters carbon flow through the hepatic folate-dependent one-carbon pool in rats. *Carcinogenesis* 1996;17:1695.
11. Nesher G, Osborn TG, Moore TL. *In vitro* effects of methotrexate on polyamine levels in lymphocytes from rheumatoid arthritis patients. *Clin Exp Rheumatol* 1996;14:395.
12. Fung KP, Lam WP, Choy YM, Lee CY. Effect of methotrexate on the intracellular phosphoribosyl pyrophosphate level and glucose transport of Ehrlich ascites tumor cells *in vitro*. *Oncology* 1996;53:27.
13. Murray RC, Williams FMR, Flintoff WF. Structural organization of the reduced folate carrier gene in Chinese hamster ovary cells. *J Biol Chem* 1996;271:19174.
14. Zhao R, Seither R, Brigle KE, et al. Impact of overexpression of the reduced folate carrier (RFC1), an anion exchanger, on concentrative transport in murine L1210 leukemia cells. *J Biol Chem* 1997;272:21207.
15. Jansen G, Mauritz RM, Assaraf YG, et al. Regulation of carrier-mediated transport of folates and antifolates in methotrexate-sensitive and –resistant leukemia cells. *Adv Enzyme Regul* 1997;37:59.
16. Dixon KH, Lanpher BC, Chiu J, et al. A novel cDNA restores reduced folate carrier activity and methotrexate sensitivity to transport-deficient cells. *J Biol Chem* 1994;269:17.
17. Antony AC. The biological chemistry of folate receptors. *Blood* 1992;79:2807.
18. Page ST, Owen WC, Price K, Elwood PC. Expression of the human placental folate receptor transcript is regulated in human tissues. Organization and full nucleotide sequence of the gene. *J Mol Biol* 1993;229:1175.
19. Shen F, Ross JF, Wang X, Ratnam M. Identification of a novel folate receptor, a truncated receptor, and receptor type β in hematopoietic cells: cDNA cloning, expression, immunoreactivity, and tissue specificity. *Biochemistry* 1994;33:1209.
20. Wang X, Janses G, Fan J, et al. Variant GPI structure in relation to membrane-associated functions of a murine folate receptor. *Biochemistry* 1996;35:16305.
21. Weitman SD, Lark RH, Coney LR, et al. Distribution of the folate receptor GP38 in normal and malignant cell lines and tissues. *Cancer Res* 1992;52:3396.
22. Ross JF, Chaudhuri PK, Ratnam M. Differential regulation of folate receptor isoforms in

normal and malignant tissues in vivo and in established cell lines. Physiologic and clinical implications. *Cancer* 1994;73:2432.

23. Spinella MJ, Brigle KE, Freemantle SJ, et al. Comparison of methotrexate polyglutamylation in L1210 leukemia cells when influx is mediated by the reduced folate carrier or the folate receptor. Lack of evidence for influx route-specific effects. *Biochem Pharmacol* 1996;52:703.
24. Sierra EE, Brigle KE, Spinella MJ, Goldman ID. pH dependence of methotrexate transport by the reduced folate carrier and the folate receptor in L1210 leukemia cells. Further evidence for a third route mediated at low pH. *Biochem Pharmacol* 1997;53:223.
25. Saxena M, Henderson GB. Identification of efflux systems for large anions and anionic conjugates as the mediators of methotrexate efflux in L1210 cells. *Biochem Pharmacol* 1996;51:974.
26. Pinedo HM, Zaharko DS, Bull JM, et al. The reversal of methotrexate cytotoxicity to mouse bone marrow cells by leucovorin and nucleosides. *Cancer Res* 1976;36:4418.
27. Widemann BC, Balis FM, Murphy RF, et al. Carboxypeptidase-G2, thymidine, and leucovorin rescue in cancer patients with methotrexate-induced renal dysfunction. *J Clin Oncol* 1997;15:2125.
28. Hsueh C-T, Dolnick BJ. Regulation of folate-binding protein gene expression by DNA methylation in methotrexate-resistant KB cells. *Biochem Pharmacol* 1994;47:1019.
29. Moscow JA, Connolly T, Myers TG, et al. Reduced folate carrier gene (RFC1) expression and anti-folate resistance in transfected and non-selected cell lines. *Int J Cancer* 1997;72:184.
30. Flintoff WF, Bertino JR. Defective transport is a common mechanism of acquired methotrexate resistance in acute lymphocytic leukemia and is associated with decreased reduced folate carrier expression. *Blood* 1997;89:1013.
31. Wong SC, McQuade R, Proefke SA, et al. Human K562 transfectants expressing high levels of reduced folate carrier but exhibiting low transport activity. *Biochem Pharmacol* 1997;53:199.
32. Cowan KH, Jolivet J. A methotrexate-resistant human breast cancer cell line with multiple defects, including diminished formation of methotrexate polyglutamates. *J Biol Chem* 1984;259:10793.
33. Pizzorno G, Mini E, Coronnello M, et al. Impaired polyglutamylation of methotrexate as a cause of resistance in CCRF-CEM cells after short-term, high-dose treatment with this drug. *Cancer Res* 1989;48:2149.
34. Rhee MS, Wang Y, Nair MG, et al. Acquisition of resistance to antifolates caused by enhanced gamma-glutamyl hydrolase activity. *Cancer Res* 1993;53:2227.
35. Li W-W, Lin TJ, Tong WP, et al. Intrinsic resistance to methotrexate in human soft tissue sarcoma cell lines. *Cancer Res* 1992;52:3908.
36. Dicker AP, Waltham MC, Volkenandt M, et al. Methotrexate resistance in an *in vivo* mouse tumor due to a non-active-site dihydrofolate reductase mutation. *Proc Natl Acad Sci U S A* 1993;90:11797.
37. Morris JA, McIvor RS. Saturation mutagenesis at dihydrofolate reductase codons 22 and 31: a variety of amino acid substitutions conferring methotrexate resistance. *Biochem Pharmacol* 1994;47:1207.
38. Haber DA, Schimke RT. Unstable amplification of an altered dihydrofolate reductase gene associated with double-minute chromosomes. *Cell* 1981;26:355.
39. Drummond JT, Genschel J, Wolf E, Modrich P. DHFR/MSH3 amplification in methotrexate-resistant cells alters the hMutSα/hMutSβ ratio and reduces the efficiency of base-base mismatch repair. *Proc Natl Acad Sci U S A* 1997;94:10144.
40. Melera PW, Davide JP, Oen H. Antifolate-resistant Chinese hamster cells: molecular basis for the biochemical and structural heterogeneity among DHFRs produced by drug-sensitive and drug-resistant cell lines. *J Biol Chem* 1987;262:1978.
41. Domin BA, Grill SP, Bastow KF, Cheng YC. Effect of methotrexate on dihydrofolate reductase activity in methotrexate resistant human KB cells. *Mol Pharmacol* 1982;21:478.
42. Cowan KH, Goldsmith ME, Ricciardone MD, et al. Regulation of dihydrofolate reductase in human breast cancer cells and in mutant hamster cells transfected with a human dihydrofolate reductase minigene. *Mol Pharmacol* 1986;30:69.
43. Chu E, Takimoto CH, Voeller D, et al. Specific binding of human dihydrofolate reductase protein to dihydrofolate reductase messenger RNA in vitro. *Biochemistry* 1993;32:4756.
44. Ercikan-Abali EA, Banerjee D, Waltham MC, et al. Dihydrofolate reductase protein inhibits its own translation by binding to dihydrofolate reductase mRNA sequences within the coding region. *Biochemistry* 1997;36:12317.
45. Simonian PL, Grillot DAM, Nunez G. Bcl-2 and Bcl-XL can differentially block chemotherapy-induced cell death. *Blood* 1997;90:1208.
46. Curt GA, Jolivet J, Carney DN, et al. Determinants of the sensitivity of human small-cell lung cancer cell lines to methotrexate. *J Clin Invest* 1985;76:1323.
47. Horns RC Jr, Dower WJ, Schimke RT. Gene amplification in a leukemic patient treated with methotrexate. *J Clin Oncol* 1984;2:2.
48. Galpin AJ, Schuetz JD, Mason E, et al. Differences in folylpolyglutamate synthetase and dihydrofolate reductase expression in human B-lineage versus T-lineage leukemic lymphoblasts: mechanisms for lineage differences in methotrexate polyglutamylation and cytotoxicity. *Mol Pharmacol* 1997;52:155.
49. Matherly LH, Taub JW, Wong SC, et al. Increased frequency of expression of elevated dihydrofolate reductase in T-cell versus B-precursor acute lymphoblastic leukemia in children. *Blood* 1997;90:578.
50. Chabner BA, Stoller RG, Hande KR, et al. Methotrexate disposition in humans: case studies in ovarian cancer and following high-dose infusion. *Drug Metab Rev* 1978;8:107.
51. Fossa SD, Heilo A, Bormer O. Unexpectedly high serum methotrexate levels in cystectomized bladder cancer patients with an ileal conduit treated with intermediate doses of the drug. *J Urol* 1990;143:498.
52. Sholar PW, Baram J, Seither R, et al. Inhibition of folate-dependent enzymes by 7-OH-methotrexate. *Biochem Pharmacol* 1988;37:3531.
53. Calvert AH, Bondy PK, Harrap KR. Some observations on the human pharmacology of methotrexate. *Cancer Treat Rep* 1977;61:1647.
54. Browman GP, Goodyear MDE, Levine MN, et al. Modulation of the antitumor effect of methotrexate by low dose leucovorin in squamous cell head and neck cancer: a randomized placebo-controlled clinical trial. *J Clin Oncol* 1990;8:203.
55. DeAngelis LM, Tony WP, Lin S, et al. Carboxypeptidase-G2 rescue after high-dose methotrexate. *J Clin Oncol* 1996;14:2145.
56. Shapiro WR, Young D, Mehta BM. Methotrexate distribution in cerebrospinal fluid after intravenous ventricular and lumbar injections. *N Engl J Med* 1975;293:161.
57. Bleyer WA. The clinical pharmacology of methotrexate. *Cancer* 1978;41:36.
58. Walker RW, Allen JC, Rosen G, et al. Transient cerebral dysfunction secondary to high-dose methotrexate. *Cancer* 1984;53:1849.
59. Marshall JL, DeLap RJ. Clinical pharmacokinetics and pharmacology of trimetrexate. *Clin Pharmacokinet* 1994;26:190.
60. Takimoto CH, Allegra CJ. New antifolates in clinical development. *Oncology* 1995;9:649.
61. Takimoto CH. Antifolates in clinical development. *Semin Oncol* 1997;24(Suppl 18):S18.
62. Punt CJA, Keizer HJ, Douma J, et al. Multicenter randomized trial of 5-fluorouracil (5FU) and leucovorin (LV) with or without trimetrexate (TMTX) as first line treatment in patients with advanced colorectal cancer (ACC). *Proc Am Soc Clin Oncol* 1999;18:262.
63. Jackman AL, Taylor GA, Gibson W, et al. ICI D1694, a quinazoline antifolate thymidylate synthase inhibitor that is a potent inhibitor of L1210 tumor cell growth in vitro and in vivo. *Cancer Res* 1991;51:5579.
64. Jackman AL, Kelland LR, Kimbell R, et al. Mechanisms of acquired resistance to the quinazoline thymidylate synthase inhibitor ZD1694 (Tomudex) in one mouse and three human cell lines. *Br J Cancer* 1995;71:914.
65. Lu K, Yin MB, McGuire JJ, et al. Mechanisms of resistance to N-[5-[N-(3,4-dihydro-2-methyl-4-oxoquinazolin-6-ylmethyl)-N-methylamino]-2-thenoyl]-L-glutamic acid (ZD1694), a folate-based thymidylate synthase inhibitor, in the HCT-8 human ileocecal adenocarcinoma cell line. *Biochem Pharmacol* 1995;50:391.
66. Blackledge G. New developments in cancer treatment with the novel thymidylate synthase inhibitor raltitrexed ('Tomudex'). *Br J Cancer* 1998;77:29.
67. Cunningham D. Mature results from three large controlled studies with raltitrexed ('Tomudex'). *Br J Cancer* 1998;77:15.
68. Cocconi G, Cunningham D, Van Custem E, et al. Open, randomized, multicenter trial of raltitrexed versus fluorouracil plus high-dose leucovorin in patients with advanced colorectal cancer. Tomudex Colorectal Cancer Study Group. *J Clin Oncol* 1998;16:2943.
69. Grant SC, Kris MG. New antineoplastic agents in lung cancer. *Cancer Treat Res* 1995;72:323.
70. Shih C, Chen VJ, Gosset LS, et al. LY231514, a pyrollo[2,3-d]pyrimidine-based antifolate that inhibits multiple folate-requiring enzymes. *Cancer Res* 1997;57:1116.
71. McDonald AC, Vasey PA, Adams L, et al. A phase I and pharmacokinetic study of LY231514, the multitargeted antifolate. *Clin Cancer Res* 1998;4:605.
72. Postmus PE, Green MR. Overview of MTA in the treatment of non-small cell lung cancer. *Semin Oncol* 1999;26:31.
73. Heidelberger C, Chandhari NK, Dannenberg P, et al. Fluorinated pyrimidines: a new class of tumor inhibitory compounds. *Nature* 1957;179:663.
74. Sotos GA, Grogan L, Allegra CJ. Preclinical and clinical aspects of biomodulation of 5-fluorouracil. *Cancer Treat Rev* 1994;20:11.
75. Lamont EB, Schilsky RL. The oral fluoropyrimidines in cancer chemotherapy. *Clin Cancer Res* 1999:5:2289.
76. Santi DV, McHenry CS, Raines RT, Ivanetich KM. Kinetics and thermodynamics of the interaction of 5-fluoro-2'-deoxyuridylate and thymidylate synthase. *Biochemistry* 1987; 26:8606.
77. Piedbois P, Buyse M, Rustum Y, et al. for the Advanced Colorectal Cancer Meta-Analysis Project. Modulation of fluorouracil by leucovorin in patients with advanced colorectal cancer: evidence in terms of response rate. *J Clin Oncol* 1992;10:896.
78. Bleiberg H. Role of chemotherapy for advanced colorectal cancer: new opportunities. *Semin Oncol* 1996:23;42.
79. Kufe DW, Major PP. 5-Fluorouracil incorporation into human breast carcinoma RNA correlates with cytotoxicity. *J Biol Chem* 1981;256:9802.
80. Will CL, Dolnick BJ. 5-Fluorouracil inhibits dihydrofolate reductase precursor mRNA processing and/or nuclear mRNA stability in methotrexate-resistant KB cells. *J Biol Chem* 1989;264:21413.
81. Doong SL, Dolnick BJ. 5-Fluorouracil substitution alters pre-mRNA splicing in vitro. *J Biol Chem* 1988;263:4467.
82. Patton JR. Ribonucleoprotein particle assembly and modification of U2 small nuclear RNA containing 5-fluorouridine. *Biochemistry* 1993;32:8939.
83. Wu XP, Dolnick BJ. 5-Fluorouracil alters dihydrofolate reductase pre-mRNA splicing as determined by quantitative polymerase chain reaction. *Mol Pharmacol* 1993;44:22.
84. Ghoshal K, Jacob ST. An alternative molecular mechanism of action of 5-fluorouracil a potent anticancer drug. *Biochem Pharmacol* 1997;53:1569.
85. Canman CE, Lawrence TS, Shewach DS, et al. Resistance to fluorodeoxyuridine-induced DNA damage and cytotoxicity correlates with an elevation of deoxyuridine triphosphatase activity and failure to accumulate deoxyuridine triphosphate. *Cancer Res* 1993;53:5219.
86. Mauro DJ, De Riel JK, Tallarida RJ, Sirover MA. Mechanisms of excision of 5-fluorouracil by uracil DNA glycosylase in normal human cells. *Mol Pharmacol* 1993;43:854.
87. Canman CE, Tang HY, Normolle DP, et al. Variations in patterns of DNA damage induced in human colorectal tumor cells by 5-fluorodeoxyuridine: implications for mechanisms of resistance and cytotoxicity. *Proc Natl Acad Sci U S A* 1992;89:10474.
88. Lowe SW, Ruley HE, Jacks T, Housman DE. p53-Dependent apoptosis modulates the cytotoxicity of anticancer agents. *Cell* 1993;74:957.
89. Fisher TC, Milner AE, Gregory CD, et al. Bcl-2 modulation of apoptosis induced by anticancer drugs: resistance to thymidylate stress is independent of classical resistance pathways. *Cancer Res* 1993;53:3321.
90. Houghton JA, Harwood FG, Tillman DM. Thymineless death in colon carcinoma cells is mediated via Fas signaling. *Proc Natl Acad Sci U S A* 1997;94:8144.
91. Leichman L, Lenz H-J, Leichman CG, et al. Quantitation of intratumoral thymidylate synthase expression predicts for response to protracted infusion of 5-fluorouracil and

weekly leucovorin in disseminated colorectal cancers: preliminary report from an ongoing trial. *Eur J Cancer* 1995;31:1306.

92. Chu E, Allegra CJ. Mechanisms of clinical resistance to 5-FU chemotherapy. In: Hait WN, ed. *Advances in cancer research.* Norwell, MA: Kluwer Academic, 1996:175.
93. Beck A, Etienne MC, Chéradame S, et al. A role for dihydropyrimidine dehydrogenase and thymidylate synthase in tumour sensitivity to fluorouracil. *Eur J Cancer* 1994;30:1517.
94. Aschele C, Sobrero A, Faderan MA, Bertino JR. Novel mechanisms of resistance to 5-fluorouracil in human colon cancer (HCT-8) sublines following exposure to two different clinically relevant dose schedules. *Cancer Res* 1992;52:1855.
95. Wang F-S, Aschele C, Sobrero A, Chang Y-M, Bertino JB. Decreased folylpolyglutamate synthetase expression: a novel mechanism of fluorouracil resistance. *Cancer Res* 1993;53:3677.
96. Barbour KW, Berger SH, Berger FG. Single amino acid substitution defines a naturally occurring genetic variant of human thymidylate synthase. *Mol Pharmacol* 1990;37:515.
97. Copur S, Aiba K, Drake JC, Allegra CJ, Chu E. Thymidylate synthase gene amplification in human colon cancer cell lines resistant to 5-fluorouracil. *Biochem Pharmacol* 1995:49;1419.
98. Chu E, Drake JC, Koeller DM, et al. Induction of thymidylate synthase associated with multidrug resistance in human breast and colon cancer cell lines. *Mol Pharmacol* 1991;39:136.
99. Chu E, Koeller DM, Johnston PG, Zinn S, Allegra CJ. Regulation of thymidylate synthase in human colon cancer cells treated with 5-fluorouracil and interferon-gamma. *Mol Pharmacol* 1993;43:527.
100. Keyomarsi K, Samet J, Moinar G, Pardee AB. The thymidylate synthase inhibitor, ICI D 1694, overcomes translational detainment of the enzyme. *J Biol Chem* 1993;268:15142.
101. Swain SM, Lippman ME, Chabner BA, et al. Fluorouracil and high-dose leucovorin in previously treated patients with metastatic breast cancer. *J Clin Oncol* 1989;7:890.
102. Chu E, Koeller DM, Casey JL, et al. Autoregulation of human thymidylate synthase messenger RNA translation by thymidylate synthase. *Proc Natl Acad Sci U S A* 1991;88:8977.
103. Chu E, Allegra CJ. The role of thymidylate synthase as an RNA binding protein. *BioEssays* 1996;18:191.
104. Van Groeningen CJ, Pinedo HM, Heddes J, et al. Pharmacokinetics of 5-fluorouracil assessed with a sensitive mass spectrometric method in patients on a dose escalation schedule. *Cancer Res* 1988;48:6956.
105. Harris BE, Carpenter JT, Diasio RB. Severe 5-fluorouracil toxicity secondary to dihydropyrimidine dehydrogenase deficiency as a potentially more common pharmacogenetic syndrome. *Cancer* 1993;68;499.
106. Diasio RB, Lu ZH. Dihydropyrimidine dehydrogenase activity and fluorouracil chemotherapy. *J Clin Oncol* 1994; 12:2239.
107. Ridge SA, McLeod HL, Gonzalez FJ, et al. Dihydropyrimidine dehydrogenase pharmacogenetics in patients with colorectal cancer. *Br J Cancer* 1998;77:497.
108. Ensminger WD, Rosowsky A, Raso VO, et al. A clinical pharmacological evaluation of hepatic arterial infusion of 5-fluoro-2'-deoxyuridine and 5-fluorouracil. *Cancer Res* 1978;38:3784.
109. Kemeny NE. Regional chemotherapy of colorectal cancer. *Eur J Cancer* 1975;31:1271.
110. Wadler S, Benson III AB, Engelking C, et al. Recommended guidelines for the treatment of chemotherapy-induced diarrhea. *J Clin Oncol* 1998;16:3169.
111. Lokich JJ, Ahlgren JD, Gullo JJ, et al. A prospective randomized comparison of continuous infusion fluorouracil with a conventional bolus schedule in metastatic colorectal carcinoma: a Mid-Atlantic Oncology Program Study. *J Clin Oncol* 1989;7:425.
112. Takimoto CH, Lu ZH, Zhang R, et al. Severe neurotoxicity following 5-fluorouracil-based chemotherapy in a patient with dihydropyrimidine dehydrogenase activity. *Clin Cancer Res* 1995;2:477.
113. Marsh JC, Bertino JR, Katz KH, et al. The influence of drug interval on the effect of methotrexate and fluorouracil in the treatment of advanced colorectal cancer. *J Clin Oncol* 1991;9:371.
114. Piedbois P, Buyse M, Blijham G, et al. Meta-analysis of randomized trials testing the biochemical modulation of fluorouracil by methotrexate in metastatic colon cancer for the Advanced Colorectal Cancer Meta-Analysis Project. *J Clin Oncol* 1994;12:960.
115. Nord LK, Stolfi RL, Martin DS. Biochemical modulation of 5-fluorouracil with leucovorin or delayed uridine rescue. *Biochem Pharmacol* 1992;43:2543.
116. Van Groeningen CJ, Peters GJ, Pinedo HM. Reversal of 5-fluorouracil-induced toxicity by oral administration of uridine. *Ann Oncol* 1993;4:317.
117. Wadler S, Schwartz E. Antineoplastic activity of the combination of interferon and cytotoxic agents against experimental and human malignancies: a review. *Cancer Res* 1990;50:3473.
118. Chu E, Zinn S, Boarman D, Allegra CJ. Interaction of interferon and 5-fluorouracil in the H630 human colon carcinoma cell line. *Cancer Res* 1990;50:5834.
119. Hill M, Norman A, Cunningham D, et al. Royal Marsden Phase III trial of fluorouracil with or without interferon alfa-2b in advanced colorectal cancer. *J Clin Oncol* 1995;13:1297.
120. Corfu-A Study Group. Phase III randomized study of two fluorouracil combinations with either interferon alfa-2a or leucovorin for advanced colorectal cancer. *J Clin Oncol* 1995;13:921.
121. Wolmark N, Bryant J, Smith R, et al. Adjuvant 5-fluorouracil and leucovorin with or without interferon alfa-2a in colon carcinoma: National Surgical Adjuvant Breast and Bowel Project Protocol C-05. *J Natl Cancer Inst* 1998;90:1810.
122. Leichman CG, Fleming TR, Muggia FM, et al. Phase II study of fluorouracil and its modulation in advanced colorectal cancer: a Southwest Oncology Group Study. *J Clin Oncol* 1995;131:1303.
123. Lawrence TS, Tepper JE, Blackstock AW. Fluoropyrimidine-radiation interactions in cells and tumors. *Semin Radiat Oncol* 1997;7:260.
124. Rich TA. Irradiation plus 5-fluorouracil: cellular mechanisms of action and treatment schedules. *Semin Radiat Oncol* 1997;7:267.
125. O'Connell MJ, Martenson JA, Wieand HS, et al. Improving adjuvant therapy for rectal cancer by combining protracted infusion fluorouracil with radiation therapy after curative surgery. *N Engl J Med* 1994;331:502.
126. Pazdur R, Lassere Y, Rhodes V, et al. Phase II trial of uracil and tegafur plus oral leucovorin: an effective oral regimen in the treatment of metastatic colorectal carcinoma. *J Clin Oncol* 1994;12:2296.
127. Pazdur R, Douillard JY, Skillings JR, et al. Multicenter phase III study of 5-fluorouracil (5-FU) or UFT in combination with leucovorin (LV) in patients with metastatic colorectal cancer. *Proc Am Soc Clin Oncol* 1999;18:263a.
128. Budman DR, Meropol NJ, Reigner B, et al. Preliminary studies of a novel oral fluoropyrimidine carbamate: capecitabine. *J Clin Oncol* 1998;16:1795.
129. Blum JL, Buzdar AU, Lorusso PM, et al. A multicenter phase II trial of Xeloda (capecitabine) in paclitaxel-refractory metastatic breast cancer (MBC). *Proc Am Soc Clin Oncol* 1997;17;476.
130. Cox JV, Pazdur R, Thibault A, et al. A phase III trial of XELODA (Capecitabine) in previously untreated advanced/metastatic colorectal cancer. *Proc Am Soc Clin Oncol* 1999;18:265a.
131. Baccanari DP, Davis ST, Knick V, Spector T. 5-Ethynyluracil (776C85): a potent modulator of the pharmacokinetics and antitumor efficacy of 5-fluorouracil. *Proc Natl Acad Sci U S A* 1993;90:11064.
132. Ahmed FY, Johnston SJ, Cassidy J, et al. Eniluracil treatment completely inactivates dihydropyrimidine dehydrogenase in colorectal tumors. *J Clin Oncol* 1999;17:2439.
133. Schilsky R, Hohneker J, Ratain MJ, et al. Phase I clinical and pharmacology study of eniluracil plus fluorouracil in patients with advanced cancer. *J Clin Oncol* 1998;16:1450.
133a. Burris HA, Ravdin P, Gutheil J, et al. Eniluracil/5-FU in anthracycline and taxane refractory breast cancer. *Proc Am Soc Clin Oncol* 1999;18:107a.
134. Chabner BA. Cytidine analogues. In: Chabner BA, Longo DL, eds. *Cancer chemotherapy and biotherapy: principles and practice,* 2nd ed. Philadelphia: Lippincott–Raven, 1996:213.
135. Gati WP, Paterson AR, Belch AR, et al. Es nucleoside transporter content of acute leukemia cells: role in cell sensitivity to cytarabine (araC). *Leuk Lymphoma* 1998;32:45.
136. Plunkett W, Liliemark JO, Estey E, Keating MJ. Saturation of ara-CTP accumulation during high-dose ara-C therapy: pharmacologic rationale for intermediate-dose araC. *Semin Oncol* 1987;14(Suppl 1):159.
137. Townsend AJ, Cheng Y-C. Sequence-specific effects of ara-5-aza-CTP and ara-CTP on DNA synthesis by purified human DNA polymerases in vitro: visualization of chain elongation on a defined template. *Mol Pharmacol* 1987;32:330.
138. Ohno Y, Spriggs D, Matsukage A, et al. Effects of 1-β-D-arabino furanosylcytosine incorporation on elongation of specific DNA sequences by DNA polymerase. *Cancer Res* 1988;48:1494.
139. Mikita T, Beardsley GP. Functional consequences of the arabinosylcytosine structural lesion in DNA. *Biochemistry* 1988;27:4698.
140. Ross DD, Cuddy DP, Cohen N, Hensley DR. Mechanistic implications of alterations in HL-60 cell nascent DNA after exposure to 1-β-D-arabinofuranosylcytosine. *Cancer Chemother Pharmacol* 1992;31:61.
141. Nakamura T, Takauji R, Kamiya K, et al. Intracellular pharmacodynamics of ara-C and flow cytometric analysis of cell cycle progression in leukemia chemotherapy. *Leukemia* 1997;11(Suppl 3):548.
142. Braess J, Wegendt C, Feuring-Buske M, et al. Leukaemic blasts differ from normal bone marrow mononuclear cells and CD34+ haematopoietic stem cells in their metabolism of cytosine arabinoside. *Br J Haematol* 1999;105:388.
143. Grem JL, Geoffroy F, Politi P, et al. Determinants of sensitivity to 1-β-D-arabinofuranosylcytosine in human colon carcinoma cell lines. *Mol Pharmacol* 1995;48:305.
144. Momparler RL, Laliberte J, Eliopoulos N, et al. Transfection of murine fibroblast cells with human cytidine deaminase cDNA confers resistance to cytosine arabinoside. *Anticancer Drugs* 1996;7:266.
145. Schroder JK, Kirch C, Seeber S, Schutte J. Structural and functional analysis of the cytidine deaminase gene in patients with acute myeloid leukemia. *Br J Haematol* 1998;103:1096.
146. Richel DJ, Colly LP, Arkesteijn GJA, et al. Substrate-specific deoxycytidine kinase deficiency in 1-β-D-arabinofuranosylcytosine-resistant leukemic cells. *Cancer Res* 1990;50:6515.
147. Kufe DW, Spriggs D, Egan EM, Munroe D. Relationships among ara-CTP pools, formation of (ara-C)DNA, cytotoxicity of cytosine arabinoside in human leukemic cells. *J Clin Invest* 1987;79:380.
148. Plunkett W, Iacoboni S, Estey E, Lilliemark JO, Keating MJ. Pharmacologically directed ara-C therapy for refractory leukemia. *Semin Oncol* 1985;12(Suppl 3):20.
149. Freund A, Rossig C, Lanvers C, et al. All-trans-retinoic acid increases cytosine arabinoside cytotoxicity in HL-60 human leukemia cells in spite of decreased cellular ara-CTP accumulation. *Ann Oncol* 1999;10:335.
150. Viallard JF, Grosset C, Lacombe F, et al. Effect of stem cell factor on leukemic progenitor cell growth and sensitivity to cytosine-arabinoside. *Leuk Res* 1996;20:915.
151. Donehower RC, Karp JE, Burke PJ. Pharmacology and toxicity of high-dose cytarabine by 72-hour continuous infusion. *Cancer Treat Rep* 1986;70:1059.
152. Capizzi RL, White JC, Powell BL, Perrino F. Effect of dose on the pharmacokinetic and pharmacodynamic effects of cytarabine. *Semin Hematol* 1991;28(Suppl 4):54.
153. Damon LE, Plunkett W, Linker CA. Plasma and cerebrospinal fluid pharmacokinetics of 1-β-arabinofuranosylcytosine and 1-β-D-arabino-furanosyluracil following the repeated intravenous administration of high- and intermediate dose 1-β-D-arabinofuranosylcytosine. *Cancer Res* 1991;51:4141.
154. Castleberry RP, Crist WM, Holbrook T, et al. The cytosine arabinoside (Ara-C) syndrome. *Med Pediatr Oncol* 1981;9:257.
155. Baker WJ, Royer GL, Weiss RB. Cytarabine and neurologic toxicity. *J Clin Oncol* 1991;9:679.
156. Herzig RH, Hines JD, Herzig GP, et al. Cerebellar toxicity with high-dose cytosine arabinoside. *J Clin Oncol* 1987;5:927.
157. Kern W, Kurrle E, Schmeiser T. Streptococcal bacteremia in adult patients with leukemia undergoing aggressive chemotherapy: a review of 55 cases. *Infection* 1990;18:138.
158. Hassan HT, Grell S, Borrmann-Danso U, Freund M. Interferon-alpha enhances the cytotoxic and cytostatic activities of chemotherapeutic drugs in human myeloid leukemia cells. *J Interferon Cytokine Res* 1996;16:139.
159. Yang JL, Cheng EH, Capizzi RL, Cheng Y-C, Kute T. Effect of uracil arabinoside on metabolism and cytotoxicity of cytosine arabinoside in L5178Y murine leukemia. *J Clin Invest* 1985;75:141.

160. Capizzi RL, Yang J-L, Cheng E, et al. Alteration of the pharmacokinetics of high-dose ara-C by its metabolite ara-U in patients with acute leukemia. *J Clin Oncol* 1983;12:763.
161. Grem JL, Allegra CJ. Sequence-dependent interaction of 5-fluorouracil and arabinosyl-5-azacytosine or 1-β-D-arabinofuranosylcytosine. *Biochem Pharmacol* 1991;42:409.
162. Bhalla K, Tang C, Ibrado AM, et al. Granulocyte-macrophage colony-stimulating factor/interleukin-3 fusion protein (pIXY 321) enhances high-dose ara-C-induced programmed cell death or apoptosis in human myeloid leukemia cells. *Blood* 1992;80:2883.
163. Plunkett W, Huang P, Searcy CE, Gandhi V. Gemcitabine: preclinical pharmacology and mechanisms of action. *Semin Oncol* 1996;23(Suppl 10):3.
164. Mackey JR, Mani RS, Selner M, et al. Functional nucleoside transporters are required for gemcitabine influx and manifestation of toxicity in cancer cell lines. *Cancer Res* 1998; 58:4349.
165. Hammond JR, Lee S, Ferguson PJ. [^{3}H]gemcitabine uptake by nucleoside transporters in a human head and neck squamous carcinoma cell line. *J Pharmacol Exp Ther* 1999;288:1185.
166. Heinemann V, Hertel LW, Grindey GB, Plunkett W. Comparison of the cellular pharmacokinetics and toxicity of 2',2'-difluorodeoxycytidine and 1-β-D-arabinofuranosylcytosine. *Cancer Res* 1988;48:4024.
167. Heinemann V, Xu Y-Z, Chubb S, et al. Cellular elimination of 2',2'-difluorodeoxycytidine 5'-triphosphate: a mechanism of self-potentiation. *Cancer Res* 1992;52:533.
168. Huang P, Chubb S, Hertel LW, et al. Action of 2',2'-difluorodeoxycytidine on DNA synthesis. *Cancer Res* 1991;51:6110.
169. Ross DD, Cuddy DP. Molecular effects of 2'-2'-difluorodeoxycytidine (gemcitabine) on DNA replication in intact HL-60 cells. *Biochem Pharmacol* 1994;48:1619.
170. Ruiz van Haperen VWT, Veerman G, Vermorken JB, Peters GF. 2',2'-difluorodeoxycytidine (gemcitabine) incorporation into RNA and DNA of tumour cell lines. *Biochem Pharmacol* 1993;46:762.
171. Ruiz van Haperen VW, Veerman G, Eriksson S, et al. Development and molecular characterization of a 2',2'-difluorodeoxycytidine-resistant variant of the human ovarian carcinoma cell line A2780. *Cancer Res* 1994;54:4138.
172. Goan YG, Zhou B, Hu E, et al. Overexpression of ribonucleotide reductase as a mechanism of resistance to 2,2-difluorodeoxycytidine in the human KB cancer cell line. *Cancer Res* 1999;59:4204.
173. Bergman AM, Pinedo HM, Jongsma AP, et al. Decreased resistance to gemcitabine (2',2'-difluorodeoxycitidine) of cytosine arabinoside-resistant myeloblastic murine and rat leukemia cell lines: role of altered activity and substrate specificity of deoxycytidine kinase. *Biochem Pharmacol* 1999;57:397.
174. Schirmer M, Stegmann AP, Geisen F, Konwalinka G. Lack of cross-resistance with gemcitabine and cytarabine in cladribine-resistant HL60 cells with elevated 5' nucleotidase activity. *Exp Hematol* 1998;26:1223.
175. Abbruzzese JL, Grunewald R, Weeks AE, et al. A Phase I clinical, plasma, and cellular pharmacology study of gemcitabine. *J Clin Oncol* 1991;9:491.
176. Storniolo AM, Enas NH, Brown CA, et al. An investigational new drug treatment program for patients with gemcitabine. Results for over 3000 patients with pancreatic carcinoma. *Cancer* 1999;85:1261.
177. Kaye SB. Gemcitabine: current status of phase I and II trials. *J Clin Oncol* 1994;12:1527.
178. Pavlakis N, Bell DR, Millward MJ, Levi JA. Fatal pulmonary toxicity resulting from treatment with gemcitabine. *Cancer* 1997;80:286.
179. Fung MC, Storniolo AM, Nguyen B, et al. A review of hemolytic uremic syndrome in patients treated with gemcitabine therapy. *Cancer* 1999;85:2023.
180. Van Moorsel CJA, Pinedo HM, Veerman G, et al. Mechanisms of synergism between cisplatin and gemcitabine in ovarian and non-small cell lung cancer cell lines. *Br J Cancer* 1999;80:981.
181. Bergman AM, Ruiz van Haperen VW, Veerman G, et al. Synergistic interaction between cisplatin and gemcitabine in vitro. *Clin Cancer Res* 1996;2:521.
182. van Moorsel CJ, Pinedo HM, Veerman G, et al. Combination chemotherapy studies with gemcitabine and etoposide in non-small cell lung and ovarian cancer cell lines. *Biochem Pharmacol* 1999;57:407.
183. Hande KR, Garrow GC. Purine antimetabolites. In: Chabner BA, Longo DL, eds. *Chemotherapy and biotherapy: principles and practice.* Philadelphia: Lippincott–Raven, 1996:235.
184. Christie NT, Drake S, Meyn RE, et al. 6-Thiopurine-induced DNA damage as a determinant of cytotoxicity in cultured Chinese hamster ovary cells. *Cancer Res* 1984;44:3665.
185. Mojena M, Bosca L, Rider MH, et al. Inhibition of 6-phosphofructo-2-kinase activity by mercaptopurines. *Biochem Pharmacol* 1992;43:671.
186. Presta M, Rusnati M, Belleri M, et al. Purine analogue 6-methylmercaptopurine riboside inhibits early and late phases of the angiogenesis process. *Cancer Res* 1999;59:2417.
187. Van Diggelen OP, Donahue TF, Shin SI. Basis for differential cellular sensitivity to 8-azaguanine and 6-thioguanine. *J Cell Physiol* 1979;98:59.
188. Calabresi P, Chabner BA. Chemotherapy of neoplastic diseases. In: Gilman AG, Rall TW, Nies AS, Taylor P, eds. *The pharmacologic basis of therapeutics.* New York: Pergamon Press, 1990:1202.
189. Bemi V, Turchi G, Margotti E, et al. 6-thioguanine resistance in a human colon carcinoma cell line with unaltered levels of hypoxanthine guanine phosphoribosyltransferase activity. *Int J Cancer* 1999;82:556.
190. Glaab WE, Risinger JI, Umar A, et al. Resistance to 6-thioguanine in mismatch-repair deficient human cancer cell lines correlates with an increase in induced mutations at the HPRT locus. *Carcinogenesis* 1998;19:1931.
191. Lennard L, Lillyman JS. Are children with lymphoblastic leukemia given enough 6-mercaptopurine? *Lancet* 1987;2:785.
192. Lennard L, Lilleyman JS. Individualizing therapy with 6-mercaptopurine and 6-thioguanine related to the thiopurine methyltransferase genetic polymorphism. *Ther Drug Monitoring* 1996;18:328.
193. Mawatari H, Kato Y, Nishimura S, et al. Reverse-phase high-performance liquid chromatographic assay method for quantitating 6-mercaptopurine and its methylated and non-methylated metabolites in a single sample. *J Chromatography* 1998;716:392.
194. Zimm S, Collins JM, Riccardi R, et al. Variable bioavailability of oral 6-mercaptopurine: is maintenance chemotherapy in acute lymphoblastic leukemia being optimally delivered? *N Engl J Med* 1983;308:1005.
195. Koren G, Ferrazini G, Sulh H, et al. Systemic exposure to mercaptopurine as a prognostic factor in acute lymphocytic leukemia in children. *N Engl J Med* 1990;323:17.
196. Innocenti F, Danesi R, Di Paolo A, et al. Clinical and experimental pharmacokinetic interaction between 6-mercaptopurine and methotrexate. *Cancer Chemother Pharmacol* 1996;37:409.
197. Lewis AS, Murphy L, McCalla C. Inhibition of mammalian xanthine-oxidase by folate compounds and amethopterin. *J Biol Chem* 1984;259:12.
198. Jacqz-Aigrain E, Nafa S, Medard Y, et al. Pharmacokinetics and distribution of 6-mercaptopurine administered intravenously in children with lymphoblastic leukemia. *Eur J Clin Pharm* 1997;53:71.
199. Balis FM, Holcenberg JS, Poplack DG, et al. Pharmacokinetics and pharmacodynamics of oral methotrexate and mercaptopurine in children with lower risk acute lymphoblastic leukemia: a Joint Children's Cancer Group and Pediatric Oncology Branch Study. *Blood* 1998;92:3569.
200. Keuzenkamp-Jansen CW, DeAbreu RA, Bokkerink JP, et al. Metabolism of intravenously administered high-dose 6-mercaptopurine with and without allopurinol treatment in patients with non-Hodgkin's lymphoma. *J Pediatr Hematol Oncol* 1996;18:145.
201. Lennard L. Clinical implications of thiopurine methyltransferase—optimization of drug dosage and potential drug interactions. *Ther Drug Monit* 1998;20:527.
202. Krynetski EY, Evans WE. Pharmacogenetics as a molecular basis for individualized drug therapy: the thiopurine S-methyltransferase paradigm. *Pharm Res* 1999;16:342.
203. Yates CR, Krynetski EY, Loennechen T, et al. Molecular diagnosis of thiopurine S-methyltransferase deficiency: genetic basis for azathioprine and mercaptopurine intolerance. *Ann Intern Med* 1997;126:608.
204. Coffey JJ, White CA, Lesk AB, et al. Effect of allopurinol on the pharmacokinetics of 6-mercaptopurine (NSC 755) in cancer patients. *Cancer Res* 1972;32:1283.
205. Erb N, Harms DO, Janka-Schaub G. Pharmacokinetics and metabolism of thiopurines in children with acute lymphoblastic leukemia receiving 6-thioguanine versus 6-mercaptopurine. *Cancer Chemother Pharmacol* 1998;42:266.
206. Lancaster DL, Lennard L, Rowland K, et al. Thioguanine versus mercaptopurine for therapy of childhood lymphoblastic leukemia: a comparison of haematological toxicity and drug metabolite concentrations. *Br J Haematol* 1998;102:439.
207. Andersen JB, Szumlanski C, Weinshilboum RM, Schmiegelow K. Pharmacokinetics, dose adjustments, and 6-mercaptopurine/methotrexate drug interactions in two patients with thiopurine methyltransferase deficiency. *Acta Pediatr* 1998;87:108.
208. Heizer WD, Peterson JL. Acute myeloblastic leukemia following prolonged treatment of Crohn's disease with 6-mercaptopurine. *Digest Dis Sci* 1998;43:1791.
209. Montgomery JA, Hewson K. Nucleosides of 2-fluoroadenine. *J Med Chem* 1969;12:498.
210. Belt JA. Heterogeneity of nucleoside transport in mammalian cells. Two types of activity in L1210 and other cultured neoplastic cells. *Mol Pharmacol* 1983;24:479.
211. Kamiya K, Huang P, Plunkett W. Inhibition of the 3'→5' exonuclease of human DNA polymerase epsilon by fludarabine-terminated DNA. *J Biol Chem* 1996;271:19428.
212. Plunkett W, Gandhi V. Cellular metabolism of nucleoside analogs in CLL: implications for drug development. In: Cheson BD, ed. *Chronic lymphocytic leukemia: scientific advances and clinical developments.* New York: Marcel Dekker, 1993:197.
213. Huang P, Robertson LE, Wright S, Plunkett W. High molecular weight DNA fragmentation: a critical event in nucleoside analog-induced apoptosis in leukemia cells. *Clin Cancer Res* 1995;1:1005.
214. Dighiero G. Adverse and beneficial immunological effects of purine nucleoside analogues. *Hematol Cell Ther* 1996;38(Suppl 2):S75.
215. Bai L, Yamaguchi M, Tatsumi M, et al. Mechanisms responsible for resistance of sublines derived from leukemia cell lines to an antitumor agent, 9-β-D-arabinofuranosyl-2-fluoroadenine. *J Cancer Res Clin Oncol* 1998;124:367.
216. Dumontet C, Fabianowska-Majewska K, Mantincic D, et al. Common resistance mechanisms to deoxynucleoside analogs in variants of the human erythroleukaemic line K562. *Br J Haematol* 1999;106:78.
217. Mohammad RM, Limvarapuss C, Hamdy N, et al. Treatment of a de novo fludarabine-resistant CLL xenograft model with bryostatin 1 followed by fludarabine. *Int J Oncol* 1999;14:945.
218. Malspeis L, Grever MR, Staubus AE, Young D. Pharmacokinetics of 2-F-ara-A (9-β-D-arabinofuranosyl-2-fluoroadenine) in cancer patients during the phase I clinical investigation of fludarabine phosphate. *Semin Oncol* 1990;17(Suppl 8):18.
219. Kemena A, Keating MJ, Plunkett W. Plasma and cellular bioavailability of oral fludarabine. *Blood* 1991;78(Suppl 1):52.
220. Hiddemann W, Johnson S, Smith A, et al. Fludarabine versus cyclophosphamide, adriamycin, prednisone (CAP) for the treatment of chronic lymphocytic leukemia—results of a multinational prospective randomized trial. *Blood* 1993;82(Suppl 1):199a.
221. Keating MJ, O'Brien S, Kantarjian H, et al. Long-term follow-up of patients with chronic lymphocytic leukemia treated with fludarabine as a single agent. *Blood* 1993;81:2878.
222. Rai KR, Peterson B, Kolitz J, et al. Fludarabine induces high complete remission rate in previously untreated patients with active chronic lymphocytic leukemia (CLL): a randomized inter-group study. *Blood* 1995;86(Suppl 1):607.
223. Hochster HS, Kim K, Green MD, et al. Activity of fludarabine in previously treated non-Hodgkin's low-grade lymphoma: results of an Eastern Cooperative Oncology Group study. *J Clin Oncol* 1992;10:28.
224. Solal-Celigny P, Brice P, Brousse N, et al. Phase II trial of fludarabine monophosphate as first-line treatment in patients with advanced follicular lymphoma: a multicenter study by the Groupe d'Etude des Lymphomes de l'Adulte. *J Clin Oncol* 1996;14:514.
225. Chun HG, Leyland-Jones B, Cheson BD. Fludarabine phosphate: a synthetic purine antimetabolite with significant activity against lymphoid malignancies. *J Clin Oncol* 1991;9:175.
226. Foran JM, Rohatiner AZ, Coiffier B, et al. Multicenter phase II study of fludarabine phosphate for patients with newly diagnosed lymphoplasmacytoid lymphoma, Waldenström's macroglobulinemia, and mantle-cell lymphoma. *J Clin Oncol* 1999;17:546.

227. Spriggs DR, Stopa E, Mayer RJ, Schoene W, Kufe DW. Fludarabine phosphate (NSC 312878) infusions for the treatment of acute leukemia: phase I and neuropathological study. *Cancer Res* 1986;46:5953.
228. Cheson BD, Vena D, Foss F, Sorensen JM. Neurotoxicity of purine analogs: a review. *J Clin Oncol* 1994;12:2216.
229. Cheson B. Immunologic and immunosuppressive complications of purine analogue therapy. *J Clin Oncol* 1995;13:2431.
230. O'Brien S, Kantarjian H, Beran M, et al. Results of fludarabine and prednisone therapy in 264 patients with chronic lymphocytic leukemia with multivariate analysis derived prognostic model for response to treatment. *Blood* 1993;82:1695.
231. Weiss RB, Freiman J, Kweder SL, et al. Hemolytic anemia after fludarabine therapy for chronic lymphocytic leukemia. *J Clin Oncol* 1998;16:1885.
232. Cheson BD, Vena DA, Barrett J, Freidlin B. Second malignancies as a consequence of nucleoside analog therapy for chronic lymphocytic leukemias. *J Clin Oncol* 1999;17:2454.
233. Li L, Liu X, Glassman AB, et al. Fludarabine triphosphate inhibits nucleotide excision repair of cisplatin-induced DNA adducts in vitro. *Cancer Res* 1997;57:1487.
234. Hochster H, Oken M, Bennett J, et al. Efficacy of cyclophosphamide (CYC) and fludarabine (FAMP) as first-line therapy of low-grade non-Hodgkin's lymphomas (NHL) ECOG 1491. *Blood* 1994;84(Suppl 1):383.
235. McLaughlin P, Hagemeister FB, Romaguera JE, et al. Fludarabine, mitoxantrone, and dexamethasone: an effective new regimen for indolent lymphoma. *J Clin Oncol* 1996;14:1262.
236. Emmanouilides C, Rosen P, Rasti S, et al. Treatment of indolent lymphoma with fludarabine/mitoxantrone combination: a phase II trial. *Hematol Oncol* 1998;16:107.
237. Gandhi V, Huang P, Chapman AJ, et al. Incorporation of fludarabine and 1-β-D-arabinofuranosylcytosine-5'-triphosphates by DNA polymerase alpha: affinity, interaction, and consequences. *Clin Cancer Res* 1997;3:1347.
238. Gandhi V, Estey E, Du M, et al. Minimum dose of fludarabine for the maximal modulation of 1-β-D-arabinofuranosylcytosine phosphate in human leukemia blasts during therapy. *Clin Cancer Res* 1997;3:1539.
239. Dinndorf PA, Avramis VI, Wiersma S, et al. Phase I/II study of idarubicin given with continuous infusion fludarabine followed by continuous infusion cytarabine in children with acute leukemia: a report from the Children's Cancer Group. *J Clin Oncol* 1997;15:2780.
240. Gandhi V, Robertson LE, Keating MJ, Plunkett W. Combination of fludarabine and arabinosylcytosine for treatment of chronic lymphocytic leukemia: clinical efficacy and modulation of arabinosylcytosine pharmacology. *Cancer Chemother Pharmacol* 1994;34:30.
241. Estey E, Plunkett W, Gandhi V, et al. Fludarabine and arabinosylcytosine therapy of refractory and relapsed acute myelogenous leukemia. *Leuk Lymphoma* 1993;9:343.
242. Visani G, Tosi P, Zinzani PL, et al. FLAG (fludarabine, high-dose cytarabine, G-CSF): an effective and tolerable protocol for the treatment of poor risk acute myeloid leukemia. *Leukemia* 1994;8:1842.
243. Khouri IF, Keating M, Korbling M, et al. Transplant-lite: induction of graft-versus-malignancy using fludarabine-based nonablative chemotherapy and allogeneic blood progenitor-cell transplantation as treatment for lymphoid malignancies. *J Clin Oncol* 1998;16:2817.
244. Carson DA, Wasson DB, Beutler E. Antileukemic and immunosuppressive activity of 2-chloro-2'-deoxyadenosine. *Proc Natl Acad Sci U S A* 1984;81:2252.
245. Griffiths M, Beaumont N, Yao SYM, et al. Cloning of a human nucleoside transporter, implicated in the cellular uptake of adenosine and chemotherapeutic drugs. *Nat Med* 1997;3:89.
246. Kawasaki H, Carrera CJ, Piro LD, et al. Relationship of deoxycytidine kinase and cytoplasmic 5'-nucleotidase to the chemotherapeutic efficacy of 2-chlorodeoxyadenosine. *Blood* 1993;81:597.
247. Seto S, Carrera CJ, Kubota M, Wasson DB, Carson DA. Mechanism of deoxyadenosine and 2-chlorodeoxyadenosine toxicity to nondividing human lymphocytes. *J Clin Invest* 1985;75:377.
248. Griffig J, Koob R, Blakley RL. Mechanisms of inhibition of DNA synthesis by 2-chlorodeoxyadenosine in human lymphoblastic cells. *Cancer Res* 1989;49:6923.
249. Leoni LM, Chao Q, Cottam HB, et al. Induction of an apoptotic program in cell-free extracts by 2-chloro-2'-deoxyadenosine 5'-triphosphate and cytochrome C. *Proc Natl Acad Sci U S A* 1998;95:9567.
250. Talbot DC, Orr RM, Serafinowski P, Harrap KR. Characteristics of acquired resistance to 2-chloro-2'-deoxyadenosine in lymphoid cell lines. *Proc Am Assoc Cancer Res* 1993;305.
251. Mohammad RM, Katato K, Almatchy VP, et al. Sequential treatment of human chronic lymphocytic leukemia with bryostatin 1 followed by 2-chlorodeoxyadenosine: preclinical studies. *Clin Cancer Res* 1998;4:445.
252. Liliemark J. The clinical pharmacokinetics of cladribine. *Clin Pharmacokinet* 1997;32:120.
253. Albertioni F, Lindemalm S, Reichelova V, et al. Pharmacokinetics of cladribine in plasma and its 5'-monophosphate and 5'-triphosphate in leukemic cells of patients with chronic lymphocytic leukemia. *Clin Cancer Res* 1998;4:653.
254. Larson RA, Mick R, Spielberger RT, et al. Dose-escalation trial of cladribine using five daily intravenous infusions in patients with advanced hematologic malignancies. *J Clin Oncol* 1996;14:188.
255. Liliemark J, Juliusson G. Cellular pharmacokinetics of 2-chloro-2'-deoxyadenosine nucleotides: comparison of intermittent and continuous intravenous infusion and subcutaneous and oral administration in leukemia patients. *Clin Cancer Res* 1995;1:385.
256. Liliemark J, Albertioni F, Hassan M, et al. On the bioavailability of oral and subcutaneous 2-chloro-2'-deoxyadenosine in humans; alternative routes of administration. *J Clin Oncol* 1992;10:1514.
257. Saven A, Cheung WK, Smith I, et al. Pharmacokinetic study of oral and bolus intravenous 2-chlorodeoxyadenosine in patients with malignancy. *J Clin Oncol* 1996;14:978.
258. Piro LD, Carrera CJ, Carson DA, Beutler E. Lasting remissions in hairy cell leukemia induced by a single infusion of 2-chlorodeoxyadenosine. *N Engl J Med* 1990;322:1117.
259. Estey EH, Kurzrock R, Kantarjian HM, et al. Treatment of hairy cell leukemia with 2-chlorodeoxyadenosine (2-CdA). *Blood* 1992;79:882.
260. Juliusson G, Heldal D, Hippe E, et al. Subcutaneous injections of 2-chlorodeoxyadenosine for symptomatic hairy cell leukemia. *J Clin Oncol* 1995;13:989.
261. Saven A, Burian C, Koziol JA, Piro LD. Long-term follow-up of patients with hairy cell leukemia after cladribine treatment. *Blood* 1998;92:1918.
262. Saven A, Lemon RH, Kosty M, Beutler E, Piro LD. 2-Chlorodeoxyadenosine activity in patients with untreated chronic lymphocytic leukemia. *J Clin Oncol* 1995;13:570.
263. Tallman MS, Hakimian D, Zonzig C, et al. Cladribine in the treatment of relapsed or refractory chronic lymphocytic leukemia. *J Clin Oncol* 1995;13:983.
264. Betticher DC, Fey MF, von Rohr A, et al. High incidence of infections after 2-chlorodeoxyadenosine (2-CDA) therapy in patients with malignant lymphomas and chronic and acute leukaemias. *Ann Oncol* 1994;5:57.
265. Juliusson G, Liliemark J. High complete remission rate from 2-chloro-2'-deoxyadenosine in previously treated patients with B-cell chronic lymphocytic leukemia: response predicted by rapid decrease in blood lymphocyte count. *J Clin Oncol* 1993;11:679.
266. Kurzrock R, Strom SS, Estey E, et al. Second cancer risk in hairy cell leukemia: analysis of 350 patients. *J Clin Oncol* 1997;15:1803.
267. Gandhi V, Estey E, Keating ML, et al. Chlorodeoxyadenosine and arabinosylcytosine in patients with acute myelogenous leukemia: pharmacokinetic, pharmacodynamic, and molecular interactions. *Blood* 1996;87:256.
268. Dillman RO. A new chemotherapeutic agent: deoxycoformycin (pentostatin). *Semin Hematol* 1994;31:16.
269. Malspeis L, Weinrib AB, Staubus AE, et al. Clinical pharmacokinetics of 2'-deoxycoformycin. *Cancer Treat Symp* 1984;2:7.
270. Cassileth PA, Chenwart B, Spiers AS, et al. Pentostatin induces durable remissions in hairy-cell leukemia. *J Clin Oncol* 1991;9:243.
271. Tallman MS, Peterson LC, Hakimian D, et al. Treatment of hairy-cell leukemia: current views. *Semin Hematol* 1999;36:155.
272. Ribeiro P, Bouaffia P, Peaud PY, et al. Long term outcome of patients with hairy cell leukemia treated with pentostatin. *Cancer* 1999;85:65.
273. Flinn IW, Kopecky KJ, Foucar MK, et al. Long-term results in hairy cell leukemia (HCL) treated with pentostatin. *Blood* 1997;90:578a.
274. Tallman MS, Hakimian D, Kopecky KJ, et al. Minimal residual disease in patients with hairy cell leukemia in complete remission treated with 2-chlorodeoxyadenosine or 2-deoxycoformycin and prediction of early relapse. *Clin Cancer Res* 1999;5:1665.
275. Cortes J, Kantarjian H, Talpaz M, et al. Treatment of chronic myelogenous leukemia with nucleoside analogs deoxycoformycin and fludarabine. *Leukemia* 1997;11:788.
276. Kraut EH, Neff JC, Bouroncle BA, Gochnour D, Grever MR. Immunosuppressive effects of pentostatin. *J Clin Oncol* 1990;8:848.
277. Seymour JF, Talpaz M, Kurzrock R. Response duration and recovery of CD4+ following deoxycoformycin in interferon-resistant hairy-cell leukemia: 7-year follow-up. *Leukemia* 1997;11:42.

SECTION **6**

CLINTON F. STEWART
MARK J. RATAIN

Topoisomerase Interactive Agents

Isolation and characterization of the topoisomerase enzymes have provided a basis for development of anticancer drugs that contribute to the treatment of patients with a wide range of malignancies.[1] Simply stated, the topoisomerase enzymes control and modify the topologic states of DNA.[2] The mechanisms of these enzymes involve DNA cleavage and strand passage through the break, followed by religation of the cleaved DNA. The precise manner by which these complicated events occur in a single cell is the source of intense research, and the results of this research promise to provide additional targets for anticancer drug therapy.

The length and intricate structure of DNA in eukaryotic cells requires efficient organization to fit in the nucleus. This organization presents a challenge to the cell to access and segregate portions of DNA required for cellular functions, especially because it is done within an extremely complex and dense intracellular milieu. The DNA topoisomerases are nuclear enzymes that assist

TABLE 19.6-1. Characteristics and Comparison of Mammalian DNA Topoisomerases

Characteristic	*Topoisomerase I*	*Topoisomerase II*[a]
Size	100 kd, monomer	170 kd, dimer
Catalytic intermediate	DNA single-strand break; covalent linkage to 3' DNA terminus	DNA double-strand break; covalent linkage to 5' DNA terminus
Energy dependent	No	ATP-dependent
Co-factor requirements	Divalent metal ions (e.g., Mg^{2+}) stimulate activity but are not essential	Requires divalent metal ions (e.g., Mg^{2+})
Activities	Releases DNA torsional strain; replication; transcription; recombination	Releases DNA torsional strain; transcription; chromosomal condensation; recombination

ATP, adenosine triphosphate.
[a]Two isoforms of topoisomerase II exist, topoisomerase α and β (see text). Properties listed in this table primarily reflect topoisomerase α.

in these cellular functions. These enzymes reduce DNA twisting and supercoiling that occur in selected regions of DNA as a result of essential cellular processes such as transcription, replication, and repair recombination. All known DNA topoisomerases possess two characteristics: to cleave and reseal the phosphodiester backbone of DNA; and to form a covalent enzyme-DNA linkage, which allows the passage of another single- or double-strand DNA through the nicked DNA. Thus, topoisomerases enable the DNA within a cell to be tightly packed and yet still accessible for processes necessary for proper cellular function.

The first DNA topoisomerase was discovered in the early 1970s.[3] Since then, many different DNA topoisomerases have been found in eukaryotic and prokaryotic cells. In mammalian cells, these enzymes have been differentiated into two types—type I and type II—based on their mechanistic and physical properties. The characteristics of each topoisomerase are summarized and compared in Table 19.6-1.[4]

The type I topoisomerase (top I) found in mammals is a monomeric protein encoded by a single-copy gene located on chromosome 20; its activity is adenosine triphosphate (ATP)–independent.[5] This enzyme binds preferentially to double-stranded DNA and cleaves one of the DNA strands of the duplex, simultaneously forming an enzyme-DNA covalent bond between a tyrosine residue and the 3'-phosphate of the cleaved DNA. Through a swivel mechanism, the unbroken strand can pass through this enzyme-mediated nick and release the torsional stress of the DNA double helix.[6] Top I has been shown to be regulated at the transcriptional, translational, and posttranslational levels. Phosphorylation-dephosphorylation and poly(adenosine-diphosphoribo)sylation are important mechanisms of top I regulation *in vitro*, but the therapeutic implications of these findings are not known.

Numerous reports have shown malignant tissue to contain higher levels of top I than its normal counterpart. Specifically, this was observed for colon and ovarian carcinoma, chronic lymphocytic leukemia, and diffuse histiocytic lymphoma.[7,8] This initial observation of increased levels of top I in malignant tissues suggested to investigators that use of top I interactive agents might lead to a selective antitumor effect; however, results from subsequent clinical trials have not supported this hypothesis. In fact, more recent studies *in vitro* suggest that the apparent high level of top I in malignant tissue might be related to differences in malignant compared to normal tissue. Other factors, such as rate of DNA synthesis, repair of drug-induced double-strand breaks, or presence of drug transporters, are also potential determinants of drug activity in the cell.

Two top II isoenzymes have been identified in humans.[9] The α form, which has an apparent molecular weight of 170 kd, is encoded by a single-copy gene located on chromosome 17q21-22. The β form has a molecular weight of 180 kd and has been mapped to chromosome 3p4. Top II α and β have different subnuclear distributions and DNA binding patterns, supporting the hypothesis that each isoform has a specific cellular function, but these precise functions are not known. Whereas top IIβ is relatively constant over cell and growth cycles, top IIα increases in rapidly proliferating cells.[10]

In contrast to type I topoisomerase, the function of type II topoisomerases is ATP-dependent.[11] Once top II binds to duplex DNA, nucleophilic reactions sequentially cleave the two complementary strands of DNA 4 base pairs apart, and the resulting 5'-phosphoryl groups become covalently linked to a pair of tyrosine groups, one in each half of the dimeric top II enzyme. Once the double-strand break has been made, the cleaved ends must be moved apart by at least 2 nm (the diameter of a double-stranded DNA helix) and a second double-strand segment of DNA passed through the break. DNA strand passage is completely dependent on the binding of magnesium and ATP. Once strand passage is complete, the cleaved DNA is religated. As with top I, top II is a phosphoprotein, and casein kinase II and protein kinase C can phosphorylate it *in vitro*, resulting in an enhancement of enzyme activity.

MECHANISM OF ACTION OF TOPOISOMERASE INTERACTIVE AGENTS

Although much is known about the biochemical effects of the topoisomerase interactive agents, very little is known about the actual mechanism by which cell death mediated by these agents occurs. Presumably, the damage done to DNA ultimately leads to necrosis or apoptosis through a series of cellular processes, such as cell cycle perturbations (possibly involving cyclins or cyclin-dependent kinases) or DNA repair deficiency. Figure 19.6-1 is a diagrammatic depiction of the normal activities of the topoisomerases and the effect of topoisomerase interactive agents.

Top I interactive agents, thus far consisting primarily of camptothecin analogues, interact with the enzyme-DNA complex.[12] This interaction prevents the resealing of the top I–mediated DNA single-strand breaks. However, these breaks result in cell death only if DNA synthesis is ongoing. A collision between the advancing replication fork and the drug-stabilized

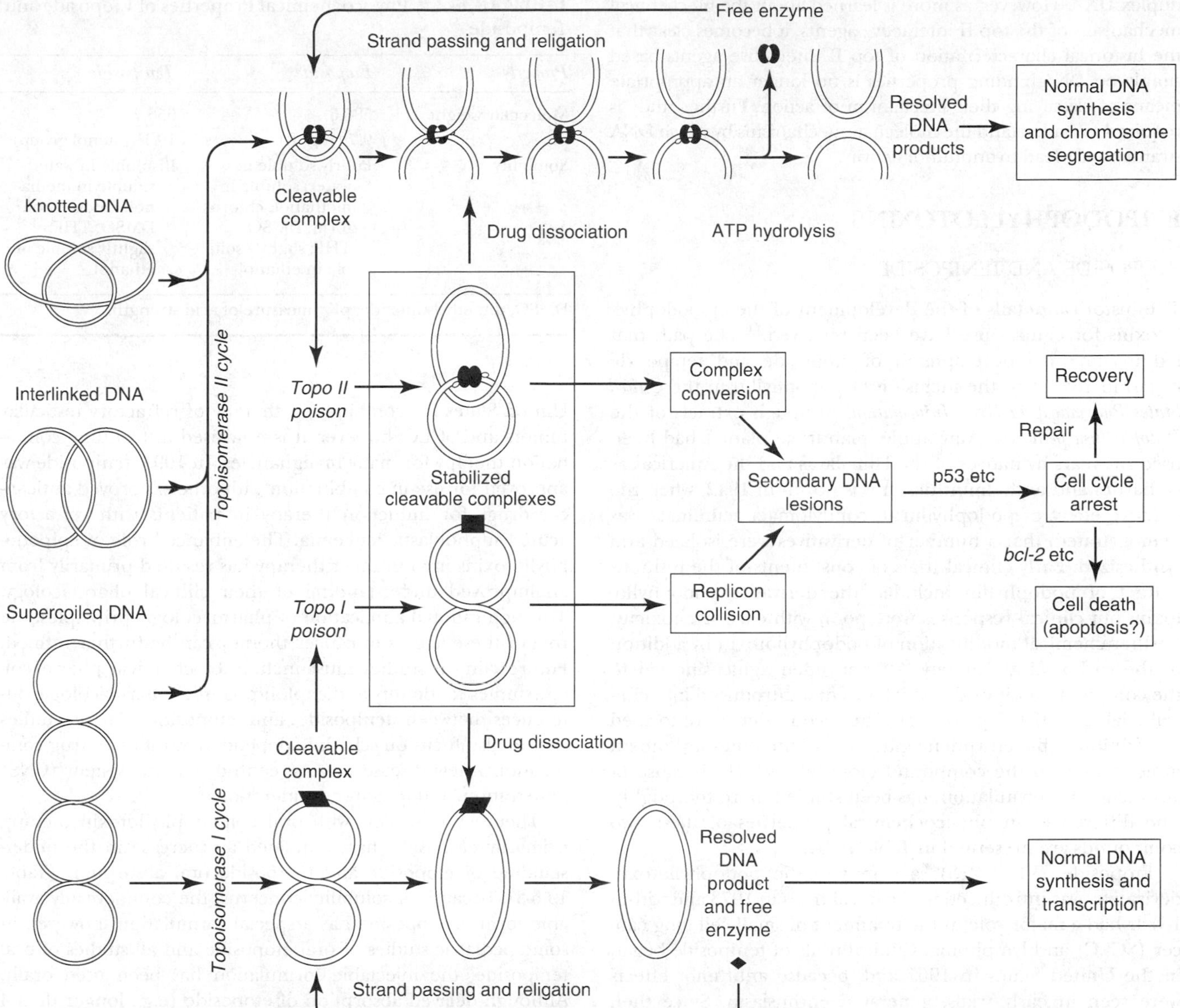

FIGURE 19.6-1. Diagrammatic representation of the normal activities of type I and type II topoisomerases, the effects of specific topoisomerase interactive agents, and the cellular consequences of trapping topoisomerase-DNA complexes. ATP, adenosine triphosphate. (From ref. 152, with permission.)

single-strand break in DNA results in replication fork breakage and double-strand breaks in the DNA. Treatment of mammalian cells with top I inhibitors induces inhibition of DNA synthesis, cell cycle arrest in G_2, and cell death by apoptosis. Drug-induced G_2 arrest has been associated with a failure to activate cdc2 kinase. Because the cytotoxicity associated with top I interactive agents is highly dependent on DNA synthesis, any deregulation of cyclins, cell cycle–regulated kinases, or phosphatases may influence the cytotoxicity of top I interactive agents (see Fig. 19.6-1). Several other types of chemotherapeutic agents, such as doxorubicin or actinomycin D, inhibit both top I and top II by a similar mechanism, but at different sites in the DNA.

Top II is the molecular target for many anticancer drugs, such as the aminoacridines, anthracyclines, and epipodophyllotoxins.[13] These drugs inhibit religation of DNA cleaved by top II and induce protein-linked breaks in the DNA, as documented by DNA alkaline elution assays. When drug is removed, these breaks are reversible. The demonstration that drug-induced, protein-associated strand breaks were mediated through interaction with top II occurred when Chen and Liu[3] were able to show that the protein covalently bound to DNA fragments induced by these drugs was top II. They used the term *cleavable complex* to refer to these lesions because the enzyme-DNA complex could be isolated (cleaved) after protein denaturation. The cleavable complex *in situ* is a covalent topoisomerase-DNA complex.

In addition to the top II interactive agents that stabilize top II–DNA complexes, other inhibitors apparently inhibit the enzyme before covalent binding to DNA occurs. However, these agents have not yet proven useful clinically. Except for the epipodophyllotoxins, all mammalian top II inhibitors are DNA intercalators that insert a planar moiety between two adjacent base pairs in duplex DNA. However, as more is learned about the biochemical mechanisms of the top II interactive agents, it becomes clear that the historical characterization of top II interactive agents based simply on DNA-binding properties is no longer an appropriate means of classifying their mechanism of action. Further study is required to understand the molecular mechanisms by which DNA strand breaks lead to antitumor activity.

EPIPODOPHYLLOTOXINS

ETOPOSIDE AND TENIPOSIDE

The historical details of the development of the epipodophyllotoxins for clinical use have been reviewed.[14] The path that led to the final development of etoposide and teniposide began in 1820 with the inclusion of podophyllin in the *United States Pharmacopeia Drug Information.* Although extracts of the *Podophyllum peltatum* (May apple, mandrake plants) had been used for years by natives of the Himalayas and the Americas as cathartics and anthelminthics, it was not until 1942, when the curative effect of podophyllin in condylomata acuminata was demonstrated, that a number of derivatives were isolated and synthesized. Early clinical trials of constituents of the resinous extract of podophyllin included the derivative podophyllotoxin, but clinical responses were poor, with excessive toxicity. Further chemical modification of podophyllotoxin by addition of the carbohydrate moiety β-D-thenylidene glucoside led to the compound teniposide, which was first introduced into clinical trials in 1970 (Fig. 19.6-2). The second derivative formed by addition of β-D-ethylidene glucoside to the podophyllotoxin molecule led to the compound etoposide, which, because of advantages in formulation, has been studied more thoroughly. The differences in physicochemical properties of these two compounds are presented in Table 19.6-2.

Etoposide (VP-16-213), a semisynthetic podophyllotoxin derivative, was introduced into clinical trials in 1973 and within 1 year had a major role in the treatment of small cell lung cancer (SCLC) and lymphoma. Clinical trials of teniposide began in the United States in 1967 and, because antitumor effects were seen in early trials, generated enthusiasm. Since then more aggressive teniposide dosing regimens have been evaluated, and teniposide has shown activity as a single agent in the treatment of SCLC. In 1983 etoposide was approved in the United States for combination therapy of refractory testicular tumors and SCLC; however, it is now used in frontline combination therapy for many malignancies. In 1993, teniposide was approved for use in combination with other approved anticancer drugs for induction therapy in patients with refractory acute lymphoblastic leukemia. The enhanced role of epipodophyllotoxins in anticancer therapy has resulted primarily from an improved understanding of their clinical pharmacology. Through rational application of pharmacologic principles, the role of these agents in cancer therapy can be further refined. Future clinical studies must include biochemical pharmacology studies to identify and exploit potential pharmacologic differences between teniposide and etoposide. These studies should also focus on schedule dependency, rational drug combinations, new disease targets, central nervous system (CNS) penetration, and toxicity considerations.[15]

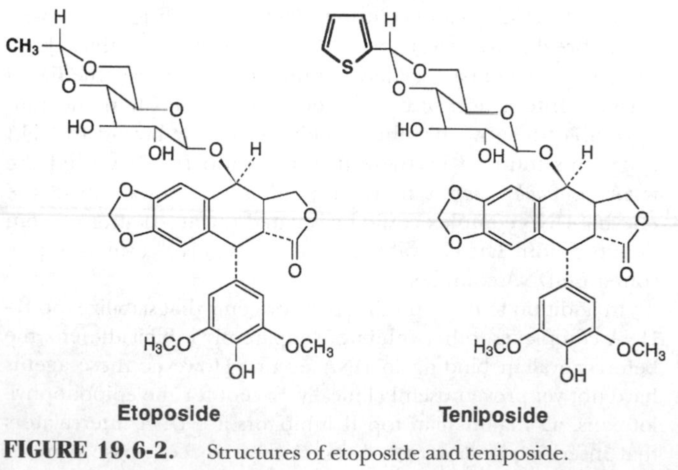

FIGURE 19.6-2. Structures of etoposide and teniposide.

TABLE 19.6-2. Physicochemical Properties of Etoposide and Teniposide

Property	*Etoposide*	*Teniposide*
Molecular weight	588.6	656.7
pK_a	9.7 (ring E)	10.1 (phenol group)
Solubility	Poorly soluble in water; soluble in methanol, chloroform, DMSO, THF; slightly soluble in ethanol	Insoluble in water; soluble in methanol, chloroform, DMSO, THF; slightly soluble in ethanol

DMSO, dimethylsulfoxide; pK_a, measure of acid strength.

Therapeutic success with oral epipodophyllotoxin therapy, primarily etoposide, has stimulated an increase in the understanding of etoposide and teniposide oral absorption (Table 19.6-3). Because of solubility concerns, the commercially available form of etoposide has a special formulation; however, in some pediatric studies of oral etoposide and all studies of oral teniposide, the injectable formulation has been used orally. Although delayed absorption of etoposide (e.g., longer than 4 hours) has been observed in patients receiving concurrent narcotics, the basis for this observation is unknown.[16] Marked intrapatient and interpatient variability characterizes both etoposide and teniposide oral bioavailability.[17] Oral absorption of etoposide and teniposide is nonlinear, with less than a proportional increase in etoposide in the area under the plasma concentration-time curve (AUC) with increased oral dose. The cause for these findings is unknown, but they suggest that more frequent oral administration of low doses are preferable to less frequent administration of high doses to increase dose intensity.

Etoposide and teniposide have comparable distribution properties within the body (Table 19.6-4); however, the extent of plasma protein binding is different between the two drugs. Etoposide is highly bound to plasma proteins, with approximately 6% to 8% of the total drug concentration not bound to plasma proteins;[18,19] whereas less than 1% of the total teniposide concentration is unbound.[20] The etoposide binding ratio measured in patients correlated directly with serum albumin concentration, consistent with *in vitro* studies that show etoposide primarily binds to albumin.[21] Hyperbilirubinemia (e.g., total bilirubin >10 mg/dL) is associated with an increased eto-

TABLE 19.6-3. Comparison of Oral Absorption between Etoposide and Teniposide

Oral Absorption Property	*Etoposide*	*Teniposide*
Formulation	Liquid filled, soft gelatin capsules containing etoposide in a vehicle consisting of citric acid, glycerin, purified water, and polyethylene glycol 400	No oral formulation; intravenous formulation has benzyl alcohol, N,N-dimethylacetamide, polyoxyethylated castor oil, maleic acid, absolute alcohol
Bioavailability	Median 50%; interpatient variability 24–137%; intrapatient variability 16–53%	Approximately 40%; interpatient variability 20–70%; intrapatient variability 3–14%
Time to peak concentrations	0.5–4.0 h	1.0–1.5 h
Dose proportionality	Nonlinear F = 0.76 at 100 mg/m^2 F = 0.48 at 400 mg/m^2	Nonlinear F = 0.36 at 120 mg/m^2 F = 0.24 at 240 mg/m^2

poside percent unbound. *In vitro* studies confirmed that bilirubin displaces etoposide from binding sites on albumin, leading to an increased percent unbound. A model to predict etoposide percent unbound, based on serum albumin and total bilirubin, has been prospectively validated in cancer patients.[22] This model provides clinicians and investigators with a method of estimating a patient's etoposide plasma protein binding using easily accessible patient data.

The activity of etoposide against tumors of the CNS in preclinical and clinical studies is intriguing because etoposide penetrates poorly into the cerebrospinal fluid (CSF) after standard and high intravenous doses or oral doses (e.g., CSF to plasma concentration ratio of approximately 2%).[23] The CSF penetration of teniposide is lower (i.e., CSF to plasma concentration ratio of 0.03% to 0.55%)[24]; however, after intravenous doses of 50 to 100 mg/m^2 significant amounts of teniposide were found in cerebral tumor samples. Teniposide demonstrated a greater penetration into tumor tissue than peritumoral tissue, suggesting further evaluation of teniposide for use in treatment of patients with brain tumors,[25,26] although more recent work suggests that presence of blood in tissue specimens may hinder the accurate assessment of teniposide penetration into brain tumor tissue.[27]

Nonrenal clearance accounts for 70% to 90% of etoposide and teniposide elimination, respectively. The exact extent and clinical relevance of this route of elimination are unknown.

TABLE 19.6-4. Comparison of Clinical Pharmacokinetic Parameters between Etoposide and Teniposide

Pharmacokinetic Parameters	*Etoposide*	*Teniposide*
Vd_{ss} (L/m^2)	6.7–12.6	3–16
Percent unbound	6–8[a] (up to 40 in patients with hypoalbuminemia and hyperbilirubinemia)	0.44–1.25[a] (more than 2 in patients with hypoalbuminemia)
Terminal half-life (hr)	4.1–11.0	5.2–13.9
Cl_s (mL/min/m^2)	17.7–31.8	9.4–15.4
Cl_r (mL/min/m^2)	3.4–7.4	0.97
Cl_{nr} (mL/min/m^2)	10.3–28.4	8.4–14.4

Cl_s, systemic clearance; Cl_r, renal clearance; Cl_{nr}, nonrenal clearance; Vd_{ss}, steady-state volume of distribution.
[a]In patients with normal albumin and hepatic function.

Numerous metabolites of etoposide have been identified, although they comprise only a minor percentage of the administered dose and have little, if any, inherent cytotoxic activity. Similarly, only trace quantities of teniposide metabolites have been found in humans.[28] More recent work with *in vitro* incubation of etoposide or teniposide with human liver microsomes has shown that O-demethylation by cytochrome P-450 enzymes leads to formation of a catechol metabolite.[29] Further studies with a panel of prototypical substrates and inhibitors demonstrated the catechol formation is catalyzed by human CYP3A4.[30] Formation of these reactive metabolites may have important clinical consequences because they covalently bind to DNA and cellular protein and have intrinsic cytotoxic activity.[31,32] Renal clearance of etoposide is greater than teniposide. Approximately 10% or 50% of an administered dose is recovered in the urine as unchanged teniposide or etoposide, respectively.

The disposition of etoposide in patients with renal and hepatic dysfunction has been extensively studied, whereas little is known about the effect of organ dysfunction on teniposide.[33–39] From early reports, etoposide clearance in patients with chronic renal failure was not altered by hemodialysis[40,41]; however, this may be attributed to poor dialyzer efficiency, lack of penetration of etoposide into the dialysis membrane, or high protein binding. Etoposide systemic clearance is significantly correlated with creatinine clearance[42]; however, few of these studies have reported the clinical relevance of altered renal function on etoposide toxicity. In a study of patients with normal albumin and hepatic transaminases, an increase in etoposide AUC was seen in patients with serum creatinine greater than 1.4 mg/dL.[43] Based on increased myelosuppression seen in the patients with elevated creatinine, the authors recommend a 30% decrease in etoposide dose for patients with serum creatinine greater than 1.4 mg/dL. Other approaches to adjusting etoposide dosage for altered renal function include use of measured renal function [e.g., ^{51}Cr-EDTA clearance],[44,45] or adaptive control dosing based on measured plasma concentrations.[46] These approaches provide more accurate methods of determining patient-specific dose reductions for renal dysfunction; furthermore, they allow for dose escalation in patients with unusually rapid renal function. Thus far, all dosage adjustment recommendations for etoposide in patients with renal dysfunction are based on hematopoietic toxicity; whether adjusting etoposide dosage compromises antitumor efficacy is unknown.

Although etoposide is renally excreted (approximately 50%), a significant nonrenal or metabolism component exists

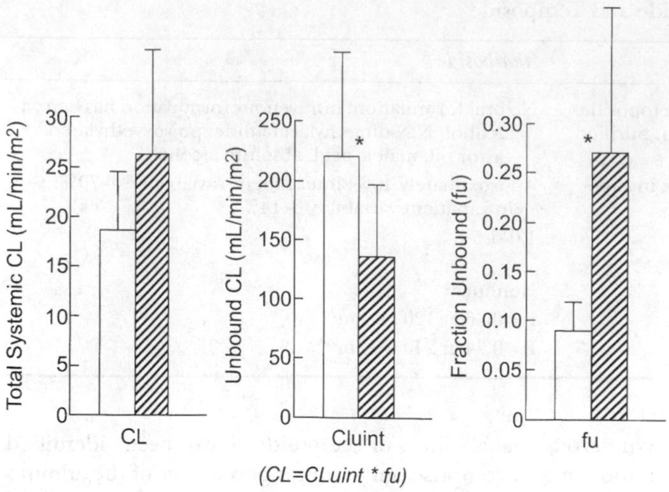

FIGURE 19.6-3. Bar graphs relating changes in etoposide total systemic clearance (CL), unbound clearance, and fraction unbound for patients with total bilirubin levels of more than 1.0 mg/dL (*striped bar*), and patients with total bilirubin levels of less than 1.0 mg/dL (*solid bar*). Statistically significant differences were noted (*asterisks*) for unbound etoposide clearance and fraction unbound (*t* test $P<.05$). (From ref. 37, with permission.)

(primarily etoposide glucuronide formed in the liver and excreted in the urine).[47] However, data from three studies show that total etoposide clearance and half-life are not significantly altered in patients with hepatic dysfunction (i.e., total bilirubin 2 to 32 mg/dL and elevated transaminases) compared with controls. This seeming contradiction of no change in etoposide total systemic clearance in patients with hepatic dysfunction could be explained by concomitant increases in unbound drug (e.g., bilirubin displacement or hypoalbuminemia) countering a reduction of nonrenal clearance (e.g., hepatocellular metabolism of unbound drug). The relationship between reduced unbound clearance and increased fraction unbound, leading to offsetting changes in total drug clearance, is depicted in Figure 19.6-3.

Etoposide dosage adjustment in patients with organ dysfunction should not be made solely on changes in etoposide pharmacokinetics, although they can aid in the understanding of altered drug toxicity and therapeutic efficacy associated with impairment of renal and hepatic function. Quantitation of the relation between pharmacokinetics and clinical outcome (pharmacodynamics) provides the clinician with a model to optimize etoposide dosage for an individual patient. The three primary determinants of etoposide disposition, and presumably pharmacologic effect, include excretion (renal), metabolism (hepatic), and protein binding. In a clinical situation in which excretion or metabolism is altered, the pharmacologic effect of etoposide could also be affected. In the absence of prospectively validated dosing recommendations, any recommendations for dosage alterations can only be considered as guidelines for initial dosing. Clinical effects and patient tolerance should guide subsequent etoposide dosing. Other clinical considerations include the current condition of the patient (e.g., performance status), previous cytotoxic chemotherapy, and the therapeutic goal (palliation vs. cure). Arbitrary reductions in etoposide dosage based solely on estimates of renal and hepatic function without regard to pharmacologic effect may lead to overdosing and toxicity or to underdosing and inadequate antitumor effects. Table 19.6-5 summarizes what effect different clinical conditions may have on etoposide protein binding and suggested dosage adjustments.

The results of *in vitro* cell culture studies and murine tumor models have firmly established a relation between epipodophyllotoxin exposure and cytotoxicity[48]; however, most clinical pharmacodynamic studies focus on the relation between etoposide exposure (e.g., AUC, steady-state drug concentration (Cp_{ss}), time above a particular concentration, or trough concentration) and toxicity (e.g., neutropenia or thrombocytopenia). One clinical pharmacodynamic study of continuous infusion teniposide in children with acute leukemia, lymphoma, or neuroblastoma, showed the median Cp_{ss} was higher in responding patients (24 vs. 8 μ*M*), presumably due to a greater teniposide clearance in the nonresponder group.[49] From this study, a range of teniposide systemic exposure associated with a high probability of response and an acceptable degree of reversible myelotoxicity was defined. In another study, teniposide unbound systemic exposure was significantly correlated with percent decrease in white blood cell count (WBC), whereas total systemic exposure was not as well correlated.[50]

Inclusion of patient-specific variables, such as serum albumin in pharmacodynamic models,[51,52] provides indirect evidence for the importance of protein binding to etoposide pharmacodynamics. Because only unbound drug is active, systemic exposure to unbound drug should be more informative of response in a patient population in which protein binding might be considered to be variable. In a number of clinical trials, a statistically significant mathematical relation between systemic exposure to unbound etoposide and myelosuppression

TABLE 19.6-5. Examples of Clinical Conditions in Which Etoposide Elimination, Metabolism, or Protein Binding Are Affected, and the Anticipated Pharmacologic Effect[a]

Excretion (Renal)	*Metabolism (Hepatic)*	*Fraction of Etoposide Not Bound to Protein*	*Anticipated Pharmacologic Effect*
Normal	Normal	Increased (e.g., hypoalbuminemia)	Unchanged
Decreased	Normal	Normal	Increased
Normal	Decreased	Normal	Increased
Decreased	Normal	Increased (e.g., hypoalbuminemia)	Increased (±)
Normal	Decreased	Increased (e.g., hypoalbuminemia)	Increased (±)
Decreased	Decreased	Increased (e.g., hypoalbuminemia)	Increased (+)

[a]Excretion and metabolism are assumed to remove etoposide from the body, and no active metabolites are formed via metabolism. Pharmacologic effect is against both normal tissue (toxicity) and tumor tissue (efficacy).

has been observed.[53–55] Thus, in patients with anticipated variable etoposide protein binding (e.g., hypoalbuminemia), measured unbound etoposide systemic exposure could be a more informative measure of drug effect than total systemic exposure.

The effect of schedule on etoposide activity has been the source of intense investigation. Although an early study[56] suggested prolonged schedules of etoposide were more effective in patients with SCLC, convincing evidence for schedule dependency came from two studies of single-agent intravenous etoposide in previously untreated SCLC.[57,58] In the first study, 500 mg/m^2 was given either as a 24-hour infusion or in five daily 2-hour infusions. The systemic exposure to total etoposide was identical between the two treatment arms, but the duration of exposure to putatively cytotoxic concentrations (1 μg/mL) was 95 hours in the daily arm compared to 46 hours in the 24-hour infusion arm. Furthermore, the overall response rate in the 5-day arm was 89%, compared with only 10% in the 24-hour arm. Confirmation of this observation was derived from a randomized trial of 500 mg/m^2 given intravenously over either a 5-day or an 8-day schedule.[58] No difference in antitumor activity was noted between the two schedules, although hematologic toxicity was more severe in the 5-day schedule.

Etoposide total systemic clearance is increased in the presence of the anticonvulsants (e.g., phenytoin or phenobarbital) often administered with high-dose chemotherapy. Because etoposide undergoes hepatic metabolism, induction of hepatic enzymes by anticonvulsants may be of clinical relevance. Median etoposide systemic clearance in adults receiving phenytoin was approximately 40% greater than in patients not receiving anticonvulsants as part of their bone marrow conditioning regimen.[59] In children, median etoposide systemic clearance was 77% higher in those receiving phenobarbital or phenytoin than in those not taking anticonvulsants.[60] The increased systemic clearance associated with anticonvulsant coadministration translates into a lower systemic exposure at the same dose. Thus, patients receiving anticonvulsants or other drugs known to induce hepatic enzymes need a higher dose of etoposide to achieve a similar systemic exposure to that attained in the absence of this interaction. In contrast, etoposide systemic clearance is decreased in patients receiving cyclosporine[61] or its analogue valspodar,[62] suggesting inhibition of P-450 metabolism, disruption of P glycoprotein function, or modulation of other mechanisms of etoposide elimination.[63]

Etoposide and cisplatin are widely used to treat solid tumors. Because cisplatin causes both acute and chronic decreases in renal function, numerous studies have investigated the potential for it to alter etoposide excretion. The concurrent infusion of cisplatin with high-dose etoposide (i.e., 350 mg/m^2/d for 5 consecutive days) did not alter the pharmacokinetics of cisplatin or etoposide.[64,65] However, etoposide systemic clearance was significantly lower in the first 48 hours after cisplatin, as compared to 21 days later.[66] Early studies suggested cumulative cisplatin exposure was associated with lower etoposide systemic clearance[67]; however, data from more patients have failed to demonstrate a persistent decrease in clearance with up to 360 mg/m^2 cisplatin. Whether etoposide excretion would be affected by larger cumulative cisplatin doses remains to be determined.

Phenylbutazone and sodium salicylate (at pharmacologic concentrations) were able to displace etoposide from plasma protein binding sites.[68] Other drugs (e.g., ifosfamide, indomethacin, nafcillin) were able to displace etoposide, but only at suprapharmacologic plasma concentrations. Unpublished data suggest that therapeutically relevant concentrations of tolbutamide, sodium salicylate, and sulfamethiazole can displace protein-bound teniposide in fresh human serum. The clinical relevance of this displacement is unknown.

Myelosuppression is the dose-limiting toxicity for etoposide and teniposide, and only at very high doses is mucositis dose-limiting (i.e., >1000 mg/m^2). Granulocyte nadir counts occur between 5 and 15 days after intravenous drug administration, and recovery is usually complete by day 28. After continuous oral administration, the nadir granulocyte count occurs between day 21 and 28, and in most patients, recovery is sufficient by day 35 for retreatment.[69–71] Thrombocytopenia occurs less often, with nadir counts observed within 9 to 16 days after drug administration. Regardless of route of administration, myelosuppression is reversible and usually not cumulative. To avoid the potential of severe myelosuppression, consideration should be given to reducing the etoposide dosage for patients who have received extensive prior myelosuppressive chemotherapy or radiation to marrow-bearing areas of the skeleton. Mild to moderate nausea and vomiting occur in approximately 30% to 40% of patients and may be more frequent with oral than intravenous administration. Other gastrointestinal toxicities, including constipation, diarrhea, stomatitis, and anorexia, have been reported but are infrequent at standard intravenous doses; however, with divided-dose oral etoposide, diarrhea and mucositis were dose-limiting. At etoposide dosages used in bone marrow transplantation regimens, mucositis occurs more frequently, and as the dosage increases, the severity also increases. Two patients receiving high-dose etoposide (cumulative dose at least 6.8 g/m^2) had elevations in bilirubin, alkaline phosphatase, and aminotransferase levels that reversed within 12 weeks.[72]

Hypersensitivity reactions (including vasomotor changes), symptoms related to the gastrointestinal tract, and pulmonary symptoms are observed after therapy with etoposide. Although the rate reported in adults is less than 3%, children with acute lymphocytic leukemia have an incidence as high as 51%[73]; however, children appear to develop more frequent reactions to etoposide than adults.[74] Premedication with histamine (H_1 and H_2) blockers and a slower infusion rate may reduce the risk of further hypersensitivity reactions upon rechallenge with etoposide, although patients developing bronchospasm, urticaria, and severe hypotension or in whom symptom resolution was slow probably should not be rechallenged.

Therapy-associated acute nonlymphocytic leukemia (t-ANLL) has been described after epipodophyllotoxin-containing therapy for both solid tumors and acute lymphocytic leukemia.[75–80] The incidence of t-ANLL varies widely from 1.6% to as high as 25%. These leukemias appear relatively early after diagnosis of the primary tumor (<5 years), present in overt leukemia without preceding myelodysplasia, and are usually French-American-British (FAB) subtypes of M4 and M5. Relationships between the cumulative dose and schedule of etoposide therapy and development of t-ANLL have been described. Cumulative etoposide doses greater than 2 g/m^2 or 3 g/m^2 have been associated with a greater incidence of t-ANLL, although this association has not been found in all studies. A relationship between schedule of administration and development of t-ANLL also has been suggested, with frequent administration of high-dose intravenous epipodophyllotoxin associated with an increased incidence of t-ANLL. Reports suggest that t-ANLL may also occur with oral etoposide therapy.[81,82] If the metabolism of the epipodophyllotoxins has prognostic significance to the development of t-ANLL, as suggested by some investigators,[83] then pharmacogenetic differences may be important.[84]

A somewhat unexpected adverse event associated with teniposide is characterized by somnolence, hypotension, and metabolic acidosis and has been described in three children receiving more than 500 mg/m^2 of intravenous teniposide over 4 hours.[85] Due to poor water solubility, teniposide is formulated with polyoxyethylated castor oil (Cremophor EL) and 42.7% (volume to volume ratio) dehydrated ethanol, and in these patients, clinically significant (i.e., >60 mg/dL) ethanol concentrations were detected at the time of the adverse event. To avoid high ethanol and teniposide concentrations, teniposide doses of more than 500 mg/m^2 should be given over 8 hours. With the exception of this acute, vehicle-related reaction, the pattern of toxicity for teniposide and etoposide are identical.

ETOPOSIDE PHOSPHATE

Because of poor water solubility, etoposide is formulated with modified polysorbate 80 (Tween 80), polyethylene glycol 300, and ethanol. Preparation of an etoposide prodrug by modification of the etoposide molecule to add a phosphate group at the 4 position in the E ring led to a more water-soluble compound.[86] Etoposide phosphate is rapidly and completely converted by endogenous phosphatases to etoposide. Initial studies have evaluated parenteral administration, but etoposide phosphate can also be given orally.[87–89]

In early phase I studies, etoposide generated from etoposide phosphate showed the same pharmacokinetic and toxicity pattern as etoposide, but with a number of advantages over the parent compound.[90–92] Excipients known to be toxic are not found in etoposide phosphate. The drug can be given by intravenous bolus (i.e., 5 minutes vs. 30 to 60 minutes), reducing the cost of drug preparation and increasing patient convenience. Etoposide phosphate is more stable and can be given at high concentrations, making it ideal for high-dose therapy or continuous infusion regimens. Whether these advantages will translate into improved clinical efficacy remains to be answered.

CAMPTOTHECIN ANALOGUES

The antitumor activity of 20(S)-camptothecin, a plant alkaloid isolated from *Camptotheca acuminata*, has been recognized for more than 20 years.[93,94] Although 10-hydroxycamptothecin demonstrated activity in studies conducted primarily in China, its use was associated with severe and unpredictable toxicity. Several camptothecin derivatives have been evaluated in clinical trials, including 9-amino-20(S)-camptothecin (9-AC), 9-nitrocamptothecin (rubitecan), lurtotecan (GI 147211), 9-dimethylaminomethyl-10-hydroxycamptothecin (topotecan), and 7-ethyl-10-(4-[1-piperidino]-1-piperidino)-carbonyloxy-camptothecin (irinotecan) (Fig. 19.6-4). The two camptothecin analogues approved for clinical use (topotecan and irinotecan) contain the camptothecin pentacyclic structure with a lactone (closed ring) moiety in the E ring. This lactone is essential for cytotoxicity because the open ring, or hydroxy acid form, is inactive. Because of logistical difficulties in stabilizing the lactone ring before analysis, many investigators have chosen to acidify the plasma sample, which makes all hydroxy acid convert back to the lactone form. Thus, these investigators measure the sum of lactone and hydroxy acid, or *total* drug. The clinical pharmacokinetics of the camptothecin analogues are summarized in Table 19.6-6. Many different doses, routes, and schedules of administration have been evaluated for the camptothecin analogues, and controversy exists over which is optimal.

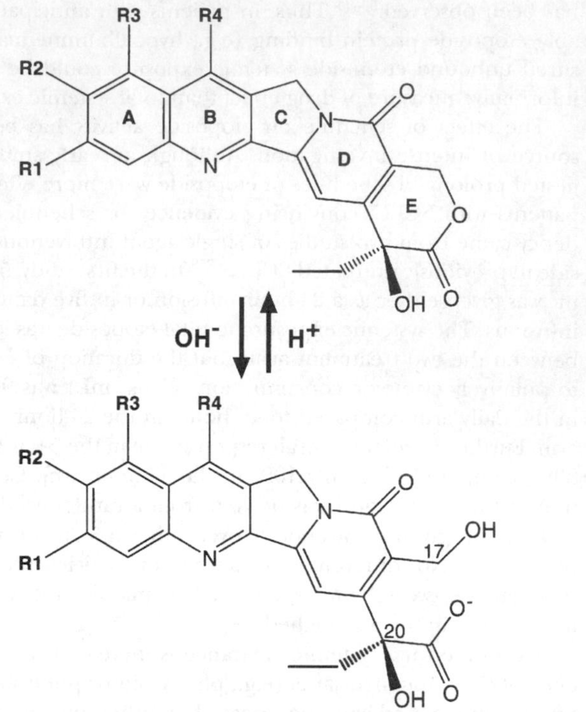

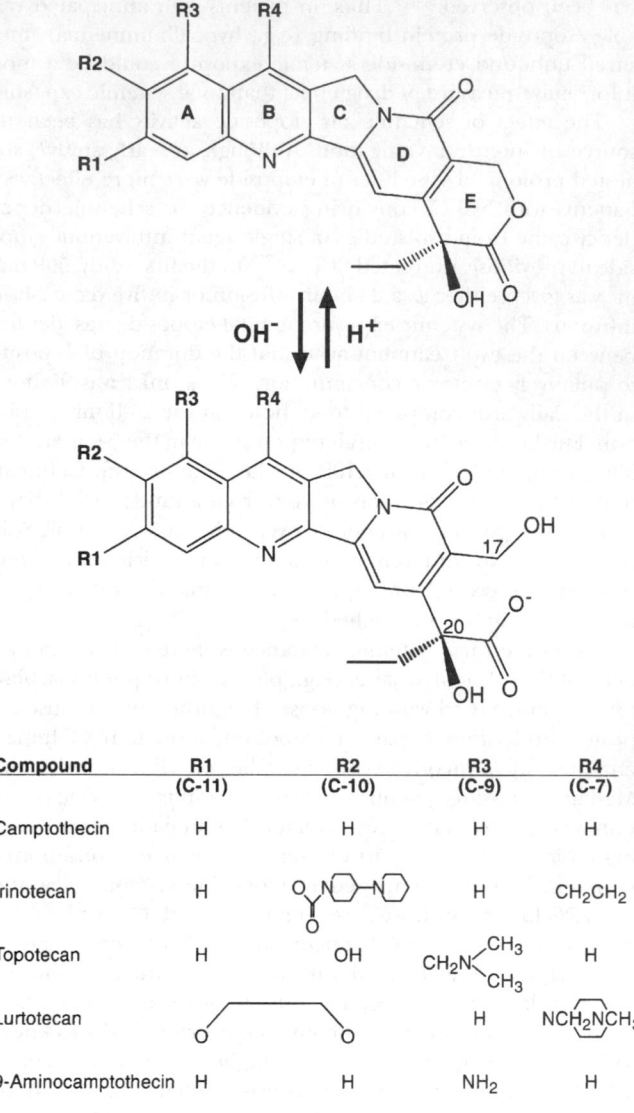

Compound	R1 (C-11)	R2 (C-10)	R3 (C-9)	R4 (C-7)
Camptothecin	H	H	H	H
Irinotecan	H	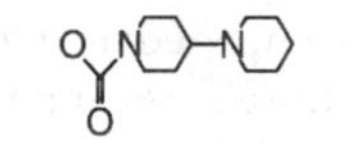	H	CH_2CH_2
Topotecan	H	OH	$CH_2N(CH_3)_2$	H
Lurtotecan			H	NCH_2NCH_3
9-Aminocamptothecin	H	H	NH_2	H
9-Nitrocamptothecin	H	H	NO_2	H

FIGURE 19.6-4. Camptothecin analogues.

Studies of low-dose, protracted topotecan in mice bearing xenografts of human tumors have shown less toxicity and equal or greater antitumor activity over shorter, more intense courses,[95–97] stimulating interest in oral administration of camptothecin analogues. Clinical studies of oral topotecan show a variable time to peak concentration[98,99] and have marked interpatient variability. However, in a study of either 15 or 21 days of oral topotecan in children, intrapatient variability for the oval topotecan AUC and bioavailability (F) was

TABLE 19.6-6. Comparison of Clinical Pharmacokinetic Parameters between Topotecan and Irinotecan

Parameter	*Topotecan*	*Irinotecan*
Bioavailability (F)	0.19–0.91	NA
Vd_{ss} (L/m^2)	—	—
Lactone	15–68	160–266
Total	16–70	85–209
Percent unbound	~40–60	~50[a]
$t_{1/2b}$ (h)	—	—
Lactone	1.5–3.7	1.4–8.3
Total	3–12	1.5–13.8
Cl_s (L/hr/m^2)	—	—
Lactone	19–34	31–67
Total	3–14	9.0–24.9
Major metabolites	N-desmethyl topotecan, topotecan O-glucuronide	SN-38, SN-38 glucuronide, APC, NPC

Cl_s, systemic clearance; NA, not available; Vd_{ss}, steady-state volume of distribution.
[a]Active metabolite, SN-38, is approximately 2% unbound.

smaller than interpatient variability.[100] In most clinical trials, topotecan is administered on an empty stomach, although in one study, co-administration of topotecan gelatin capsules with a high-fat meal led to a small decrease in the rate, but not extent, of absorption.[101] Pharmacokinetic data from a study of the oral absorption of intravenous irinotecan showed that irinotecan was rapidly absorbed, and peak irinotecan concentrations were observed within 1 to 2 hours of adminstration.[102] The relative extent of conversion of irinotecan to SN-38 was high, with mean ratios of 0.8 and 0.7 on days 1 and 5, respectively. This compares with values of 0.02 and 0.07 after intravenous administration[103] and suggests that presystemic formation of SN-38 occurs after oral administration. Preliminary results of a small pediatric study suggest that the absolute bioavailability of intravenous irinotecan administered orally is approximately 10%, which is in agreement with preclinical studies in the mouse.[104]

Topotecan and irinotecan both have a large steady-state volume of distribution (Vd_{ss}), consistent with either extensive plasma protein or tissue binding. Topotecan and irinotecan are approximately 20% and 50% bound to plasma protein, respectively, thus the high Vd_{ss} is most likely due to extensive tissue binding; SN-38 is approximately 98% bound to plasma proteins.[105] The impact of human serum albumin on the conversion of the lactone to carboxylate form is an important aspect of camptothecin drug-protein interactions.[106,107] Variations in the camptothecin molecular structure may alter these interactions, with SN-38 lactone having enhanced stability in the presence of human serum albumin, compared with irinotecan or topotecan. The δ-lactone ring moiety of 9-aminocamptothecin hydrolyzes almost immediately (more than 99.5%) in the presence of human serum albumin, substantially reducing the pharmacologically active lactone form in human blood. In contrast, topotecan does not associate with human serum albumin, resulting in a higher level of lactone stability in human plasma.[108] The clinical significance of variability in serum albumin concentrations on camptothecin toxicity and antitumor activity is presently unknown.

Topotecan CSF penetration in children was determined from the ratio of CSF to plasma AUC during a 24- and 72-hour continuous topotecan infusion.[109] The median CSF penetration of topotecan lactone was 29% (range, 10% to 59%) and 42% (range, 11% to 97%) for the 24- and 72-hour continuous infusions, respectively. The degree of penetration is consistent with that reported for the nonhuman primate model.[110]

The primary route of elimination from the body varies between topotecan and irinotecan. For topotecan, 50% to 65% of a dose is recovered in the urine; thus, renal excretion is a major route of elimination.[111–113] Although topotecan has been measured in human bile, the importance of biliary excretion is unknown. Approximately 30% to 40% of topotecan is eliminated by nonrenal pathways, and the N-desmethyl metabolite of topotecan has been isolated from urine of patients receiving topotecan.[114] This metabolite has antitumor activity equal to that of the parent compound, and its formation is catalyzed by the cytochrome P-450 system. The maximum plasma concentration of total (sum of lactone and hydroxy acid) N-desmethyl topotecan is only 0.5% of total topotecan, and the average urinary recovery is less than 5% of the administered dose. Two other metabolites, topotecan O-glucuronide and N-desmethyl topotecan O-glucuronide have been reported; however, they accounted for only 13.5% of the urinary recovery of the administered dose.[115] Thus, other nonrenal routes (e.g., metabolism) of topotecan elimination are yet to be identified.

In contrast, irinotecan itself has little *in vitro* cytotoxicity[116] and requires conversion, by the carboxylesterase enzyme, to 7-ethyl-10-hydroxycamptothecin (SN-38) for antitumor activity. *In vitro* studies have shown decreased carboxylesterase activity may be a mechanism of cellular resistance to irinotecan.[117] Furthermore, transfection of carboxylesterases into tumor cells increases the activation and cytotoxicity of irinotecan.[118,119] SN-38 is conjugated to glucuronic acid at the C_{10} position by UGT1A1, and this metabolite has no intrinsic antitumor activity.[120] The extent of conversion of SN-38 to its glucuronide has been inversely correlated with the risk of severe diarrhea, because the other major route of SN-38 excretion is biliary excretion by canalicular multispecific organic anion transporter (cMOAT)[121,122] (presumably leading to mucosal injury).[123] In addition to SN-38 and SN-38 glucuronide, 7-ethyl-10-[4-N-(5-aminopentanoic acid)-1-piperidino]carbonyloxycamptothecin (APC) and 7-ethyl-10-(4-amino-1-piperidino)carbonyloxycamptothecin (NPC) are oxidative metabolites of irinotecan formed by CYP3A4.[124,125] Renal excretion is a minor route of elimination for irinotecan and SN-38.

The disposition of topotecan in patients with renal and hepatic dysfunction has been studied in adults receiving intravenous topotecan daily for 5 consecutive days.[126–128] Patients with renal dysfunction were placed into three groups according to their creatinine clearance (20 or below, 21 to 40, or 41 to 60 mL/min), and hepatic dysfunction was defined as a total bilirubin greater than 1.5 mg/dL. A control group of patients with normal renal and hepatic function was also studied. Topotecan disposition and hematologic toxicity were not significantly altered in patients with hepatic dysfunction (as defined by elevated total bilirubin); therefore, no dosage alteration is recommended for these patients. Severe neutropenia was observed in patients with moderate to severe renal dysfunction treated at one-third of the adult maximal tolerated dosage (i.e., 0.5 mg/m^2/d). Based on the results of this study, the investigators recommended an initial topotecan dosage of 0.75 mg/m^2/d when given daily for 5 consecutive days to patients with moderate renal dysfunction (i.e., creatinine clearance <39 mL/min). In another study of patients with renal dysfunction, no correlation was found between total topotecan clearance and a more specific measure of glomerular filtration rate [technetium Tc 99m DPTA clearance]. Furthermore, one patient studied with a technetium clearance of 19 mL/min/m^2 had a normal topotecan total clearance, suggesting topotecan may undergo renal tubular secretion in addition to glomerular filtration. Results of a study in mice showed that probenecid would inhibit renal tubular secretion of topotecan and decrease topotecan renal and systemic clearance, leading to an increase in topotecan lactone systemic exposure.[129] Irinotecan undergoes significant hepatic metabolism, and preliminary pharmacokinetic and toxicity results of a study of irinotecan administration in adults with liver dysfunction suggest that the irinotecan dosage should be reduced by one-third in patients with total bilirubin more than three times the upper limit of normal.[130]

As with the epipodophyllotoxins, results of preclinical studies of the camptothecin analogues show a definite relationship between dose and antitumor effect in mice bearing human tumor xenografts. These studies have evaluated a variety of schedules and routes of administration, and the results suggest that the camptothecin analogues are highly schedule-dependent.[131] Early clinical studies of the relationship between systemic exposure and pharmacologic effect reported a statistically significant and clinically relevant relationship between drug exposure and myelosuppression (i.e., percentage change in absolute neutrophil count and platelets).[132,133] A significant correlation was reported between systemic exposure to 9-aminocamptothecin lactone and the extent of neutropenia observed after a 72-hour continuous infusion.[134] Few studies have looked at the relationship between drug exposure and antitumor efficacy; however, one study of continuous infusion topotecan in children with relapsed acute leukemia found a correlation between topotecan lactone systemic exposure and toxicity and topotecan lactone systemic exposure and oncolytic effect (Fig. 19.6-5).[135]

The presence of the pH-sensitive lactone ring present in the two commercially available camptothecin analogues, topotecan and irinotecan, raises the question of whether lactone or total systemic exposure is a better representation of pharmacologic effect. The advantage of measuring total drug is the elimination of the more cumbersome determination of the lactone concentrations, which require immediate sample processing. Total concentrations (lactone plus hydroxy acid) may be determined without immediate processing, and assays may be performed several weeks or months later, thus, making it feasible to do large population studies. Use of total drug as a surrogate for systemic exposure to the active lactone has potential drawbacks (e.g., presence of active metabolites, intrapatient variability), although the lactone and hydroxy acid exist in a pH-dependent equilibrium that varies little at physiologic pH.

Reversible myelosuppression, with both neutropenia and thrombocytopenia, is the dose-limiting toxicity observed with topotecan. After intravenous dosing of topotecan, the neutrophil nadir occurs between 8 and 10 days, and recovery is usually complete by day 21. On a schedule of extremely high doses given daily for 5 days, hemolytic anemia was observed as a dose-limiting toxicity.[136] Reversible moderate to severe anemia also has been reported with topotecan. The use of growth factors to further escalate the topotecan dose has been used with mixed

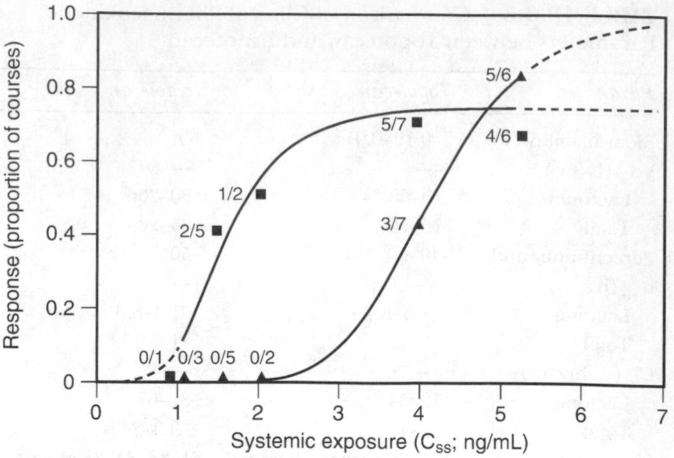

FIGURE 19.6-5. Plot of topotecan lactone systemic exposure (C_{ss}; steady-state concentration) versus proportion of courses of therapy with either an oncolytic response (*upper curve*, ■) or grade 2 to 4 mucositis (*lower curve*, ▲). Twelve courses of topotecan were associated with an oncolytic response, defined as greater than 75% reduction in circulating blast count or a complete or partial response based on bone marrow aspirate. In this figure, the number of courses associated with a response or mucositis is shown in the numerator over the total number of courses at each level of systemic exposure. (From ref. 135, with permission.)

success.[137] With oral topotecan, prolonged oral administration (i.e., twice daily for 21 days every 28 days) resulted in gastrointestinal side effects as the dose-limiting toxicity, whereas, when given in the short term (i.e., once daily for 5 days every 21 days), myelosuppression was the dose-limiting toxicity.[138] For topotecan, the only nonhematologic dose-limiting toxicity reported is mucositis, but only after a 120-hour continuous topotecan infusion.[139,140]

The major dose-limiting toxicities for irinotecan are myelosuppression and diarrhea. Irinotecan-induced diarrhea is generally of two types. The first type has an early onset, beginning during or immediately after the irinotecan infusion. This is often accompanied by facial flushing and abdominal cramping characteristic of diarrhea associated with vasoactive compounds. Standard-dose anticholinergic drugs, such as scopolamine or atropine, can be used to control this diarrhea, which is caused by the cholinergic effects of irinotecan. The second type of diarrhea, a cholera-like syndrome unresponsive to loperamide or codeine, is often dose-limiting. Many therapeutic approaches have been tried to ameliorate or prevent the diarrhea associated with irinotecan, including the use of the cyclooxygenase inhibitor indomethacin and the enkephalinase inhibitor acetorphan, but none has been universally successful.[141,142] Modulation of irinotecan pharmacokinetics by inhibitors of SN-38 biliary excretion or inducers of SN-38 glucuronidation may be another method to reduce the severity of irinotecan-associated diarrhea.[143–145]

Other nonhematologic toxicities seen with the camptothecin analogues are generally reversible and not dose-limiting. Mild nausea and vomiting have occurred in approximately 20% to 30% of patients. Low-grade fever has been observed in approximately 20% of patients, and alopecia occurs at higher doses. Other mild toxicities observed include fatigue, anorexia, and skin rash. Top I interactive agents have not been in clinical use long enough for therapy-associated malignancies to be reported; however, sister chromatid exchanges and gene deletions or rearrangements have been induced *in vitro*.[146]

Topotecan systemic clearance and the formation of the N-desmethyl topotecan metabolite are increased in the presence of enzyme-inducing anticonvulsants (e.g., phenytoin).[147] Although hepatic metabolism is a relatively minor component of topotecan disposition, the steep exposure-response relationship observed with topotecan makes this interaction clinically relevant. Patients concomitantly administered enzyme-inducing anticonvulsants may require an increase in topotecan dose to achieve a similar pharmacologic effect as a patient not receiving anticonvulsants. This interaction with anticonvulsants was also observed in a group of patients receiving 9-aminocamptothecin, a camptothecin analogue that has no known hepatic metabolism. In this study, patients receiving 9-aminocamptothecin and anticonvulsants did not have the expected extent of myelosuppression. On further study of 9-aminocamptothecin pharmacokinetics, it was found that the median steady-state 9-aminocamptothecin plasma concentrations in patients on anticonvulsants (25.3 n*M*) was significantly lower than patients not receiving anticonvulsants (76.5 n*M*).[148] Anticonvulsants also increased irinotecan clearance in a study of patients with glioma, which led to a decrease in the mean irinotecan and SN-38 AUC.[149] Although the numbers of patients studied were small, it appears that phenobarbital may have a different effect from carbamazepine and phenytoin, in that phenobarbital increased SN-38 glucuronide and APC AUC by 1.6- and 2.6-fold, respectively. In another study of adults with malignant glioma receiving irinotecan and anticonvulsants and dexamethasone, the irinotecan clearance was twofold and the systemic exposure to irinotecan, SN-38, and SN-38 glucuronide was statistically lower compared with a historical control group of patients with non-CNS tumors.[150]

ANTHRACYCLINES AND RELATED COMPOUNDS

Anthracyclines, anticancer agents consisting of a pigmented aglycone, an amino sugar, and a lateral chain (Fig. 19.6-6), have been in clinical practice since the 1960s and represent one of the most commonly used classes of anticancer drugs.[151] The first anthracyclines in clinical use, doxorubicin and daunorubicin, were produced by the *Streptomyces* species, and the anthracyclines have thus been classified as antitumor antibiotics; however, classification by mechanism of action is more rational, especially because the second-generation anthracyclines (e.g., idarubicin, epirubicin) are synthetic. The first anthracycline, doxorubicin, still remains the most widely used and is the benchmark against which new analogues are compared.

The anthracyclines induce formation of covalent topoisomerase-DNA complexes and prevent the enzyme from completing the religation portion of the ligation-religation reaction. These agents are also DNA intercalators that insert part of their planar structures between two adjacent base pairs in DNA, causing single-stranded and double-strand breaks. The anthracyclines can undergo chemical reduction through enzymatically catalyzed or iron-catalyzed pathways to yield reactive free radical intermediates. Through hydrogen peroxide and hydroxyl radicals, these free radical intermediates can cause oxidative damage to cellular proteins. Under hypoxic

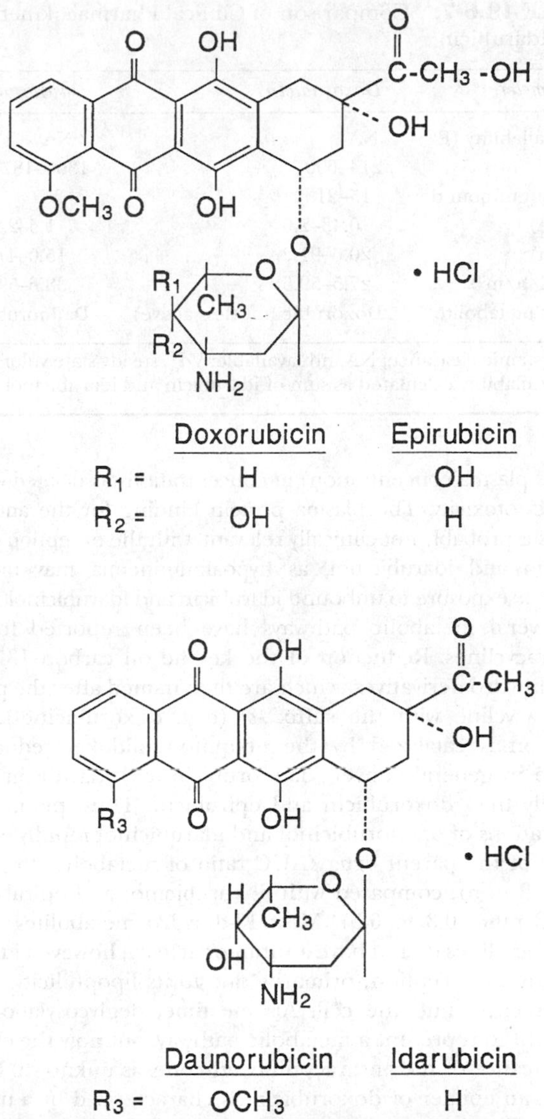

FIGURE 19.6-6. Structures of the four anthracyclines in current clinical use. Epirubicin differs from doxorubicin in the steric position of the 4'-OH group, whereas idarubicin differs from daunorubicin in lacking an A-ring methoxy substitution.

conditions, these free radicals can rearrange to form metabolites capable of covalently binding to DNA. Although the anthracyclines are associated with all of these reactions, it is their interaction with top II that is the most important mechanism of cytotoxicity.[152]

With the exception of idarubicin, none of the anthracyclines are administered orally. Idarubicin, a synthetic analogue of daunorubicin, has increased lipophilicity compared to daunorubicin, which allows it to be readily absorbed from the gastrointestinal tract.[153] Absorption of idarubicin is erratic and incomplete (Table 19.6-7); however, higher concentrations of its active metabolite, idarubicinol, are achieved after oral than intervenous administration because of first-pass hepatic metabolism.

Anthracyclines as a class are unable to cross the blood–brain barrier either because of low lipophilicity, the presence of P glycoprotein in the cells of brain endothelial vessels, or both.[154] However, after intravenous administration of idarubicin, its metabolite, idarubicinol, can be detected in the CSF (1% to 13% simulta-

TABLE 19.6-7. Comparison of Clinical Pharmacokinetic Parameters between Doxorubicin, Daunorubicin, Epirubicin, and Idarubicin

Parameter	*Doxorubicin*	*Daunorubicin*	*Epirubicin*	*Idarubicin*
Bioavailability (F)	NA	NA	NA	28–45[a]
Vd_{ss} (L/m^2)	214–690	1300–1877	583–2964	362–2556
Percent unbound	15–21	~30	NA	3 (6 for idarubicinol)
$t_{1/2b}$ (h)	0.43–2.0	1.5–2.2	0.49–3.1	0.9–6.0
$t_{1/2g}$ (h)	20.6–91.2	15.0–47.7	18.3–44.8	6.2–42.7
Cl_s (L/h/m^2)	27.5–59.6	38.6–59.0	30.5–94.9	39.0–122.0
Major metabolite	Doxorubicinol (less active)	Daunorubicinol (inactive)	Epirubicinol (low cytotoxicity)	Idarubicinol (cytotoxic)

Cl_s, systemic clearance; NA, not available; Vd_{ss}, steady-state volume of distribution.
[a]Bioavailability calculated as sum of idarubicin and idarubicinol.

neous plasma concentration) at concentrations associated with *in vitro* cytotoxicity. The plasma protein binding for the anthracyclines is probably not clinically relevant, with the exception of idarubicin and idarubicinol, as hypoalbuminemia may increase systemic exposure to unbound idarubicin and idarubicinol.

Several metabolic pathways have been reported for the anthracyclines. Reduction of the ketone on carbon 13 yields 13S-dihydro derivatives, which are then named after the parent anthracycline with the suffix *-ol* (e.g., doxorubicinol). This reaction is catalyzed by the ubiquitous aldoketoreductases, which in general convert daunorubicin and idarubicin more rapidly than doxorubicin and epirubicin. Thus, plasma concentrations of daunorubicinol and idarubicinol rapidly exceed those of the parent drug (AUC ratio of metabolite to parent drug, 2 to 5), compared with doxorubicinol and epirubicinol (AUC ratio, 0.3 to 0.5). Most 13-dihydro metabolites of the anthracyclines do not have antitumor activity; however, idarubicinol is an exception, primarily due to its lipophilicity, which allows entry into the cell. At one time, deglycosylation was thought to represent a metabolic pathway, but now the clinical significance of the anthracycline aglycones is unknown. Epirubicin, an epimer of doxorubicin, is characterized by a unique metabolic step present only in humans. The equatorial position of the 4' hydroxyl group allows epirubicin to be conjugated to glucuronic acid. The glucuronide AUC is similar to that of the parent compound, potentially explaining the lower myelotoxic and cardiotoxic properties of epirubicin compared with doxorubicin; however, the exact clinical significance of this metabolic step is unknown.

Elimination of the anthracyclines proceeds primarily through the bile, with urinary excretion accounting for less than 10% of the total dose administered. No evidence for enterohepatic recirculation has been observed. Although epirubicin is excreted in the bile, a larger proportion of an injected dose is recovered in the urine relative to the other anthracyclines, due to formation of soluble glucuronides.[155]

In patients with hyperbilirubinemia or reduced renal function, dose reduction recommendations for daunorubicin and doxorubicin are provided in the package literature. These dose reductions are based on retrospective data and have not been prospectively validated. The results of a study of patients with hyperbilirubinemia receiving doxorubicin raise questions about the validity of adjusting doses in patients with hyperbilirubinemia.[156] The systemic clearance of epirubicin and idarubicin in patients with liver disease is decreased, and although a dosage reduction is recommended based on bilirubin or serum aspartate, as with doxorubicin, it is unclear if a dosage reduction is clinically indicated. Whereas renal impairment reduces the clearance of epirubicin and idarubicin, only idarubicin has been adequately studied to provide dosing guidelines.

As with other anticancer drugs, few clinical studies have related exposure to anthracyclines and antitumor effect. Early studies suggested doxorubicin concentration, peak or 3 hours after end of infusion, was associated with outcome of remission induction or reduction of tumor mass, respectively. These findings have led investigators to speculate that improved tumor response might be linked to high initial plasma doxorubicin concentrations. The contribution of the anthracycline metabolite to the overall effect depends on the anthracycline under study. As discussed previously, idarubicinol has significant cytotoxic activity; patients with a low rate of epirubicin glucuronidation had a lower percent change in neutrophils and better tumor response. The only pharmacodynamic relation between doxorubicin systemic exposure and toxicity (e.g., decrease in WBC) was noted after continuous doxorubicin infusion.[157] A positive correlation was noted between the AUC for epirubicin, or epirubicin and epirubicinol, and logarithm of the WBC survival fraction.[158]

Although a number of drugs have been reported to interact with doxorubicin, most of these have been in experimental systems, so their clinical significance is unknown. Of the drug interactions reported in patients with cancer, only a few are of clinical consequence. Despite numerous studies showing pharmacologic prevention of anthracycline-induced cardiotoxicity, only dexrazoxane has been able to significantly retard development of cardiotoxicity. The reversal of doxorubicin-induced multidrug resistance has been attempted using a variety of pharmacologic modulators, such as trifluoperazine, verapamil, and cyclosporine, and has met with mixed success.

The dose-limiting acute toxicity of the anthracyclines is myelosuppression, primarily affecting the neutrophils; in the treatment of leukemia, however, this may be considered a desirable side effect. The onset of myelosuppression is usually 7 days after administration, with maximum effect seen at approximately day 10 to 14. Recovery is usually complete by day 21 to 28. Gastrointestinal toxicities are common, including nausea and vomiting, diarrhea, and mucositis. Although not dose-limiting, alopecia also occurs in almost all patients. Although not always readily apparent when it occurs, extravasation of the anthracyclines can lead to severe local tissue damage and deep ulcerations that progress over weeks. These lesions are slow to heal and often require skin grafting, although the graft is not always successful. Once an extravasation has been discovered, the optimal method of management is unknown, although most agree that local measures such as ice packs and subcutaneous injections of saline, steroids, or bicarbonate may be useful. Topical dimethylsulfoxide has been suggested to be a safe and effective approach to reducing the tissue damage associated with anthracycline-induced extravasation.[159,160] The best approach to avoiding extravasation is to take all possible precautions when administering an anthracycline, such as ensuring good blood return on the intravenous line, monitoring the intravenous site carefully, and good patient education.

The anthracyclines are associated with both acute and chronic cardiac toxicity. The less common acute cardiac toxicity includes nonspecific electrocardiographic changes that may be observed during or immediately after the infusion. In its extreme form, this acute toxicity can include a pericarditis-myocarditis syndrome with onset of fever, pericarditis, and congestive heart failure.[161] No association between the acute toxicity and later development of chronic toxicity has been shown. Besides symptomatic management, no specific therapy is recommended for this relatively rare syndrome.

Anthracyclines also produce a dose-dependent congestive myopathy that often leads to congestive heart failure. This typically becomes apparent 4 to 8 weeks after the last anthracycline dose, although it may occur during treatment or years later. The clinical significance of this chronic toxicity has been its inability to treat it, leading to a drug-induced mortality ranging in early reports from 33% to 70%, and in more recent reports to less than 30%. If a sufficiently high cumulative dose is administered, all anthracyclines can cause cardiac toxicity; however, idarubicin and epirubicin are associated with a lower incidence than doxorubicin and daunorubicin. The mechanisms of the chronic cardiotoxicity have been reviewed extensively. To summarize, they include enzymatic-mediated formation of oxygen free radicals that initiate lipid peroxidation and a nonenzymatic pathway for free radical formation.[162] Iron is central to both pathways; it is required to begin hydroxyl radical production in the first pathway, and to form an iron-drug complex in the second. The risk of anthracycline-associated congestive heart failure is increased by the presence of preexisting heart disease or hypertension, prior radiation to the heart or mediastinum, age (generally, children younger than 4 years are more susceptible), prior cyclophosphamide therapy (questionable), and cumulative anthracycline dose. For doxorubicin, a cumulative dose of less than 450 mg/m^2, in the absence of other risk factors, is rarely associated with cardiomyopathy, whereas as the cumulative dose increases to 550, 600, and 700 mg/m^2, the incidence increases to 7%, 15%, and 30%, respectively. For daunorubicin, the overall incidence of congestive heart failure is low (approximately 1.2% in a population of 5613 patients), and the incidence was related to the cumulative daunorubicin dose administered.[163] At daunorubicin doses of 550 mg/m^2, the incidence of congestive heart failure was 4%, whereas at a total dose of 1050 mg/m^2, the incidence increased to 14%. A retrospective study of idarubicin cardiotoxicity found few clinically significant symptoms at cumulative doses of 290 mg/m^2, although left ventricular ejection fraction (LVEF) decreased during therapy. A metaanalysis of studies comparing epirubicin and doxorubicin found epirubicin as active as doxorubicin (1:1) and less cardiac toxic (1:1.8).[164]

Patients receiving anthracyclines should be monitored for the onset of cardiomyopathy. The most useful noninvasive test is serial radionuclide angiocardiography, which provides a reproducible measure of LVEF and is sensitive to subclinical cardiac dysfunction. This technique and others have done much to allow earlier detection of subclinical cardiac toxicity and to reduce the mortality associated with it. Management of the cardiomyopathy involves bed rest and afterload reduction. With continued conservative management, patients may experience a gradual improvement; this improvement, however, may take more than 1 year.

Many different approaches have been tried to prevent anthracycline-induced cardiac toxicity, including analogue synthesis, altering dosing schedules, and the use of biochemical antagonists. Although many of the anthracycline analogues are associated with a lower incidence of toxicity, they still are associated with decreased LVEF, albeit asymptomatic. The use of continuous infusion schedules of anthracyclines has reduced the incidence of cardiac toxicity somewhat, providing a pharmacokinetic basis for the hypothesis that high peak concentrations are associated with an increased incidence of cardiotoxicity.[165] However, this approach is not widely used because of concern over compromising antitumor efficacy, unpredictable toxicities, and logistical issues.

Dexrazoxane (ICRF-187) is the first biochemical antagonist shown in a randomized clinical trial to dramatically reduce the incidence of cardiac toxicity in patients with breast cancer, without altering the antitumor activity of the doxorubicin combination regimen. Although its mechanism is not fully elucidated, dexrazoxane either acts as a free radical scavenger or prevents formation of free radicals.

In addition to oral and intravenous administration, doxorubicin and epirubicin have been administered via the intraarterial route for well-defined, nonresectable metastatic and primary tumors of the liver. Consistent with their metabolic profile, the systemic toxicity for doxorubicin was not reduced using this route of administration, whereas relatively low levels of epirubicin were produced because of substantial first-pass effect. Intrapleural doxorubicin has been used to treat malignant pleural effusions, and intravesical administration is an effective therapy for recurrent, superficial transitional cell bladder carcinoma.

MITOXANTRONE AND LOSOXANTRONE

Cumulative cardiotoxicity limits the clinical use of the anthracyclines, and much work has been directed at synthesizing related compounds less prone to undergo reductive metabolism to form free radicals.[166–168] Mitoxantrone, a member of the anthracenedione class of synthetic antitumor compounds, is an example of one effort. It lacks the sugar moiety of the anthracycline drugs, but retains the planar polycyclic aromatic ring structure that permits its intercalation into DNA. More important, mitoxantrone lacks the ability to produce the quinone-type free radicals thought to be responsible for anthracycline-associated cardiac toxicity. Losoxantrone (biantrazole; CI-941) is a member of the anthrapyrazole group of antitumor agents, which are structurally similar to the anthracyclines. The anthrapyrazoles were synthesized to have antitumor activity similar to the anthracyclines, but without cardiotoxicity. The

TABLE 19.6-8. Comparison of Clinical Pharmacokinetic Parameters between the Two Anticancer Drugs Mitoxantrone and Losoxantrone

Pharmacokinetic Parameter	*Mitoxantrone*	*Losoxantrone*
Vd_{ss} (L/m^2)	450–5288	17–409
Percent unbound	~4	5
Terminal half-life (h)	42–189	6–38
Cl_s (mL/min/m^2)	180–2450	132–936
Percent dose in urine	4–10	1–16

Cl_s, systemic clearance; Vd_{ss}, steady-state volume of distribution.

rationale underlying the development of the anthrapyrazoles was to make the electron-deficient quinone chromophore of the anthracyclines more resistant to enzymatic reduction by forming a quasi-iminoquinone. The planar conformation and cationic nature of the anthracyclines, necessary for intercalative binding to DNA, is retained in the anthrapyrazoles. Losoxantrone can also cause cytotoxicity by inhibition of top II.[169] Preclinical studies demonstrated that a number of anthrapyrazoles had a spectrum of activity and potency similar to doxorubicin and were superior to mitoxantrone.

The clinical pharmacokinetics of mitoxantrone and losoxantrone are summarized in Table 19.6-8. Both compounds have very large distribution volumes and are highly protein bound (percentage unbound, <5%).[170,171] Both compounds undergo hepatic metabolism, but the clinical relevance of these metabolites is unknown, as is whether the dosage of either compound should be reduced in patients with hepatic dysfunction. The low urinary recovery for both compounds suggests no dosage adjustment is necessary for patients with mild to moderate renal dysfunction.

The primary dose-limiting toxicity of both compounds is myelosuppression, primarily neutropenia, although thrombocytopenia has been reported.[172,173] Cumulative myelosuppression was not noted. At higher doses, moderate nausea and vomiting have been reported, but only mild nausea and vomiting at lower doses. Although mitoxantrone is associated with less cardiotoxicity than the anthracyclines, it can cause decreases in LVEF. For losoxantrone, data for 183 patients showed mild to severe cardiotoxicity in 25 and congestive heart failure in 2 patients.

DACTINOMYCIN (ACTINOMYCIN D)

Dactinomycin is a member of a class of compounds first isolated from *Streptomyces parvullus*. The only member to be clinically useful, dactinomycin is highly effective in the treatment of Wilms' tumor, Ewing's sarcoma, embryonal rhabdomyosarcoma, and gestational choriocarcinoma. Responses have also been reported in testicular cancer, Kaposi's sarcoma, and lymphoma.[174]

Dactinomycin is composed of a planar tricyclic ring chromophore (phenoxazone) to which two identical cyclic polypeptides are attached.[175] The compound binds to DNA by intercalation, depending on a specific interaction between the polypeptide chains and deoxyguanosine. This interaction blocks the ability of DNA to act as a template for RNA and DNA synthesis in a concentration-dependent manner. Low drug concentrations inhibit RNA synthesis more than higher drug concentrations, which block both RNA and DNA syntheses. Dactinomycin can also cause topoisomerase-mediated single-strand breaks in DNA, although the contribution of these breaks to cytotoxicity is unclear.[176] *In vitro* studies suggest that concomitant actinomycin D and hyperthermia (e.g., 42° or 43°C) resulted in an increased uptake and prolonged retention of actinomycin D.[177]

After an intravenous bolus, dactinomycin has a rapid disappearance phase followed by a long elimination half-life of 36 hours.[178] Dactinomycin is minimally metabolized, is concentrated in nucleated red blood cells, and does not cross the blood–brain barrier. Dactinomycin is primarily eliminated by renal and biliary excretion, although only 30% has been recovered in the urine and stool over the week after a dose. Inadequate data exist to formulate dosage recommendations for use of dactinomycin in patients with renal or hepatic dysfunction.

The dose-limiting toxicity for dactinomycin is myelosuppression, affecting both platelets and neutrophils. Severe nausea and vomiting occur during the first few hours after administration, but these side effects are responsive to antiemetic therapy. Gastrointestinal toxicity manifests primarily as stomatitis, accompanied by pain, and diarrhea may occur. Extravasation of this drug after intravenous use may result in severe soft tissue damage and ulceration. Dactinomycin is a radiation sensitizer, leading to enhanced skin and gastrointestinal toxicity when administered concurrently with radiation.[179] In addition, late radiation damage to lung and liver appears increased, potentially because of the ability of dactinomycin to block repair of radiation-mediated DNA damage. This recall reaction can be observed even when months separate radiation therapy and dactinomycin administration.

REFERENCES

1. Cumming J, Smyth JF. DNA topoisomerase I and II as targets for rational design of new anticancer drugs. *Ann Oncol* 1993;4:533.
2. Wang JC. DNA topoisomerases. *Annu Rev Biochem* 1996;65:635.
3. Chen AY, Liu LF. DNA topoisomerases: essential enzymes and lethal targets. *Annu Rev Pharmacol Toxicol* 1994;34:191.
4. Pommier Y, Leteurtre F, Fesen MR, et al. Cellular determinants of sensitivity and resistance to DNA topoisomerase inhibitors. *Cancer Invest* 1994;12:530.
5. Gupta M, Fujimori A, Pommier Y. Eukaryotic DNA topoisomerases I. *Biochim Biophys Acta* 1995;1262:1.
6. Berger JM. Structure of DNA topoisomerases. *Biochim Biophys Acta* 1998;1400:3.
7. Husain I, Mohler JL, Seigler HF, Besterman JM. Elevation of topoisomerase I messenger RNA, protein, and catalytic activity in human tumors: demonstration of tumor-type specificity and implications for cancer chemotherapy. *Cancer Res* 1994;54:539.
8. Giovanella BC, Stehlin JS, Wall ME, et al. DNA topoisomerase I–targeted chemotherapy of human colon cancer in xenografts. *Science* 1989;246:1046.
9. Takano H, Kohno K, Matsuo K, Matsuda T, Kuwano M. DNA topoisomerase-targeting antitumor agents and drug resistance. *Anticancer Drugs* 1992;3:323.
10. Burden DA, Osheroff N. Mechanism of action of eukaryotic topoisomerase II and drugs targeted to the enzyme. *Biochim Biophys Acta* 1998;1400:139.
11. Wigley DB. Structure and mechanism of DNA topoisomerases. *Annu Rev Biophys Biomol Struct* 1995;24:185.
12. Pommier Y. Diversity of DNA topoisomerases I and inhibitors. *Biochimie* 1998;80:255.
13. Corbett AH, Osheroff N. When good enzymes go bad: conversion of topoisomerase II to a cellular toxin by antineoplastic drugs. *Chem Res Toxicol* 1993;6:585.
14. Stahelin HF, von Wartburg A. The chemical and biological route from podophyllotoxin glucoside to etoposide: ninth Cain memorial award lecture. *Cancer Res* 1991;51:5.
15. Muggia FM. Teniposide: overview of its therapeutic potential in adult cancers. *Cancer Chemother Pharmacol* 1994;34:127.
16. Sonnichsen DS, Ribeiro RC, Luo X, Mathew P, Relling MV. Pharmacokinetics and pharmacodynamics of 21-day continuous oral etoposide in pediatric patients with solid tumors. *Clin Pharmacol Ther* 1995;58:99.
17. Hande K, Messenger M, Wagner J, Krozely M, Kaul S. Inter- and intrapatient variability in etoposide kinetics with oral and intravenous drug administration. *Clin Cancer Res* 1999;5:2742.
18. Liu B, Earl HM, Poole CJ, Dunn J, Kerr DJ. Etoposide protein binding in cancer patients. *Cancer Chemother Pharmacol* 1995;36:506.

19. Stewart CF, Pieper JA, Arbuck SG, Evans WE. Altered protein binding of etoposide in patients with cancer. *Clin Pharmacol Ther* 1989;45:49.
20. Petros WP, Rodman JH, Relling MV, et al. Variability in teniposide plasma protein binding is correlated with serum albumin concentrations. *Pharmacotherapy* 1992;12:273.
21. Fleming RA, Evans WE, Arbuck SG, Stewart CF. Factors affecting *in vitro* protein binding of etoposide in humans. *J Pharm Sci* 1992;81:259.
22. Stewart CF, Fleming RA, Arbuck SG, Evans WE. Prospective evaluation of a model for predicting etoposide plasma protein binding in cancer patients. *Cancer Res* 1990;50:6854.
23. Relling MV, Mahmoud H, Pui CH, et al. Etoposide achieves potentially cytotoxic concentrations in cerebrospinal fluid of children with acute lymphoblastic leukemia. *J Clin Oncol* 1996;14:399.
24. Holthuis JJM, de Vries EGE, Postmus PE. Pharmacokinetics of high-dose teniposide. *Cancer Treatment Rep* 1987;71:599.
25. Zuchetti M, Rossi C, Knerich R, et al. Concentrations of VP16 and VM26 in human brain tumors. *Ann Oncol* 1991;2:63.
26. Stewart DJ, Richard MT, Hugenholtz H, et al. Penetration of teniposide (VM-26) into human intracerebral tumors. *J Neuro-Oncol* 1984;2:315.
27. van Tellingen O, Boogerd W, Nooijen WJ, Beijnen JH. The vascular compartment hampers accurate determination of teniposide penetration into brain tumor tissue. *Cancer Chemother Pharmacol* 1997;40:330.
28. Splinter TAW, Holthuis JJM, Kok TC, Post MH. Absolute bioavailability and pharmacokinetics of oral teniposide. *Semin Oncol* 1992;19:28.
29. Relling MV, Evans R, Dass C, Desiderio DM, Nemec J. Human cytochrome P450 metabolism of teniposide and etoposide. *J Pharmacol Exp Ther* 1992;261:491.
30. Relling MV, Nemec J, Schuetz EG, et al. O-Demethylation of epipodophyllotoxins is catalyzed by human cytochrome P450 3A4. *Mol Pharmacol* 1994;45:352.
31. Mans DRA, Lafleur MVM, Westmijze EJ, et al. Reactions of glutathione with the catechol, the *ortho*-quinone and the semi-quinone free radicals of etoposide. *Biochem Pharmacol* 1992;43:1761.
32. van Maanen JMS, deVries J, Pappie D, et al. Cytochrome P450-mediated O-demethylation: a route in the metabolic activation of etoposide. *Cancer Res* 1987;47:4658.
33. Arbuck SG, Douglass HO, Crom WR, et al. Etoposide pharmacokinetics in patients with normal and abnormal organ function. *J Clin Oncol* 1986;4:1690.
34. D'Incalci M, Rossi C, Zucchetti M, et al. Pharmacokinetics of etoposide in patients with abnormal renal and hepatic function. *Cancer Res* 1986;46:2566.
35. Hande KR, Wolff SN, Greco FA, et al. Etoposide kinetics in patients with obstructive jaundice. *J Clin Oncol* 1990;8:1101.
36. Pfluger KH, Schmidt L, Merkel M, Jungclas H, Havemann K. Drug monitoring of etoposide (VP 16-213): correlation of pharmacokinetic parameters to clinical and biochemical data from patients receiving etoposide. *Cancer Chemother Pharmacol* 1987;20:59.
37. Stewart CF, Arbuck SG, Fleming RA, Evans WE. Changes in the clearance of total and unbound etoposide in patients with liver dysfunction. *J Clin Oncol* 1990;8:1874.
38. English MW, Lowis SP, Peng B, et al. Pharmacokinetically guided dosing of carboplatin and etoposide during peritoneal dialysis and haemodialysis. *Br J Cancer* 1996;73:776.
39. Suzuki S, Koide M, Sakamoto S, Matsuo T. Pharmacokinetics of carboplatin and etoposide in a haemodialysis patient with Merkel-cell carcinoma. *Nephrol Dial Transplant* 1997;12:137.
40. Brindley CJ, Antoniw P, Newlands ES, Bagshawe KD. Pharmacokinetics and toxicity of the epipodophyllotoxin derivative etoposide (VP 16-213) in patients with gestational choriocarcinoma and malignant teratoma. *Cancer Chemother Pharmacol* 1985;15:66.
41. Holthuis JJM, Van de Vyver FL, van Oort WJ, et al. Pharmacokinetic evaluation of increasing dosages of etoposide in a chronic hemodialysis patient. *Cancer Treat Rep* 1985;69:1279.
42. Pfluger KH, Hahn M, Holz JB, et al. Pharmacokinetics of etoposide: correlation of pharmacokinetic parameters and clinical conditions. *Cancer Chemother Pharmacol* 1993;31:350.
43. Joel SP, Shah R, Slevin ML. Etoposide dosage and pharmacodynamics. *Cancer Chemother Pharmacol* 1994;34:S69.
44. Lowis SP, Pearson ADJ, Newell DR, Cole M. Etoposide pharmacokinetics in children: the development and prospective validation of a dosing equation. *Cancer Res* 1993;53:4881.
45. Kintzel PE, Dorr RT. Anticancer drug renal toxicity and elimination: dosing guidelines for altered renal function. *Cancer Treat Rev* 1995;21:33.
46. Ratain MJ, Schilsky RL, Choi KE, et al. Adaptive control of etoposide administration: impact of interpatient pharmacodynamic variability. *Clin Pharmacol Ther* 1989;45:226.
47. Hande KR, Bennett R, Hamilton R, Grote T, Branch R. Metabolism and excretion of etoposide in isolated, perfused rat liver model. *Cancer Res* 1988;48:5692.
48. Wolff SN, Grosh WW, Prater K. *In vitro* pharmacodynamic evaluation of VP-16-213 and implications for chemotherapy. *Cancer Chemother Pharmacol* 1987;19:246.
49. Rodman JH, Abromowitch M, Sinkule JA, et al. Clinical pharmacodynamics of continuous infusion teniposide: systematic exposure as a determinant of response in a phase I trial. *J Clin Oncol* 1987;5:1007.
50. Evans WE, Rodman JH, Relling MV, et al. Differences in teniposide disposition and pharmacodynamics in patients with newly diagnosed and relapsed acute lymphocytic leukemia. *J Pharmacol Exp Ther* 1992;260:71.
51. Ratain MJ, Mick R, Schilsky RL, Vogelzang NJ, Berezin F. Pharmacologically based dosing of etoposide: a means of safely increasing dose intensity. *J Clin Oncol* 1991;9:1480.
52. Karlsson MO, Port RE, Ratain MJ, Sheiner LB. A population model for the leukopenic effect of etoposide. *Clin Pharmacol Ther* 1995;57:325.
53. Stewart CF, Arbuck SG, Fleming RA, Evans WE. Relation of systemic exposure to unbound etoposide and hematologic toxicity. *Clin Pharmacol Ther* 1991;50:385.
54. Aita P, Robieux I, Sorio R, et al. Pharmacokinetics of oral etoposide in patients with hepatocellular carcinoma. *Cancer Chemother Pharmacol* 1999;43:287.
55. Nguyen L, Chatelut E, Chevreau C, et al. Population pharmacokinetics of total and unbound etoposide. *Cancer Chemother Pharmacol* 1998;41:125.
56. Cavalli F, Sonntag RW, Jungi F. VP-16-213 monotherapy for remission induction of small cell lung cancer: a randomised trial using three dosage schedules. *Cancer Treat Rep* 1978;62:473.
57. Slevin ML, Clark PI, Joel SP, et al. A randomized trial to evaluate the effect of schedule on the activity of etoposide in small-cell lung cancer. *J Clin Oncol* 1989;7:1333.
58. Clark PI, Slevin ML, Joel SP, et al. A randomized trial of two etoposide schedules in small-cell lung cancer: the influence of pharmacokinetics on efficacy and toxicity. *J Clin Oncol* 1994;12:1427.
59. Mross K, Bewermeier P, Kruger W, et al. Pharmacokinetics of undiluted or diluted high-dose etoposide with or without busulfan administered to patients with hematologic malignancies. *J Clin Oncol* 1994;12:1468.
60. Rodman JH, Murry DJ, Madden T, Santana VM. Altered etoposide pharmacokinetics and time to engraftment in pediatric patients undergoing autologous bone marrow transplantation. *J Clin Oncol* 1994;12:2390.
61. Lum BL, Kaubisch S, Yahanda AM, et al. Alteration of etoposide pharmacokinetics and pharmacodynamics by cyclosporine in a phase I trial to modulate multidrug resistance. *J Clin Oncol* 1992;10:1635.
62. Advani R, Saba HI, Tallman MS, et al. Treatment of refractory and relapsed acute myelogenous leukemia with combination chemotherapy plus the multidrug resistance modulator PSC 833 (Valspodar). *Blood* 1999;93:787.
63. Lum BL, Fisher GA, Brophy NA, et al. Clinical trials of modulation of multidrug resistance. Pharmacokinetic and pharmacodynamic considerations. *Cancer* 1993;72:3502.
64. Gouyette A, Deniel A, Pico JL, et al. Clinical pharmacology of high-dose etoposide associated with cisplatin. Pharmacokinetic and metabolic studies. *Eur J Cancer Clin Oncol* 1987;23:1627.
65. Holthuis JJM, Postmus PE, van Oort WJ. Pharmacokinetics of high dose etoposide (VP16-213). *Eur J Cancer Clin Oncol* 1986;22:1149.
66. Relling MV, McLeod HL, Bowman LC, Santana VM. Etoposide pharmacokinetics and pharmacodynamics after acute and chronic exposure to cisplatin. *Clin Pharmacol Ther* 1994;56:503.
67. Sinkule JA, Hutson P, Hayes FA, Etcubanas E, Evans WE. Pharmacokinetics of etoposide (VP-16) in children and adolescents with refractory solid tumors. *Cancer Res* 1984;44:3109.
68. Gaver RC, Deeb G. The effect of other drugs on the *in vitro* binding of ^{14}C-etoposide to human serum proteins. *Proc Am Assoc Cancer Res* 1989;30:536(abst).
69. Shaklai S, Bairey O, Blickstein D, et al. Severe myelotoxicity of oral etoposide in heavily pretreated patients with non-Hodgkin's lymphoma or chronic lymphatic leukemia. *Cancer* 1996;77:2313.
70. Ashley DM, Meier L, Kerby T, et al. Response of recurrent medulloblastoma to low-dose oral etoposide. *J Clin Oncol* 1996;14:1922.
71. Johnson DH, Greco FA, Strupp J, Hande KR, Hainsworth JD. Prolonged administration of oral etoposide in patients with relapsed or refractory small-cell lung cancer: a phase II trial. *J Clin Oncol* 1990;8:1613.
72. Johnson DH, Greco FA, Wolff SN. Etoposide-induced hepatic injury: a potential complication of high-dose therapy. *Cancer Treat Rep* 1983;67:1023.
73. Kellie SJ, Crist WM, Pui CH, et al. Hypersensitivity reactions to epipodophyllotoxins in children with acute lymphoblastic leukemia. *Cancer* 1991;67:1070.
74. de Souza P, Friedlander M, Wilde C, Kirsten F, Ryan M. Hypersensitivity reactions to etoposide. A report of three cases and review of the literature. *Am J Clin Oncol* 1994;17:387.
75. van Leeuwen FE, Chorus AMJ, van den Belt-Dusebout AW, et al. Leukemia risk following Hodgkin's disease: relation to cumulative dose of alkylating agents, treatment with teniposide combinations, number of episodes of chemotherapy, and bone marrow damage. *J Clin Oncol* 1994;12:1063.
76. Pui CH, Ribeiro RC, Hancock ML, et al. Acute myeloid leukemia in children treated with epipodophyllotoxins for acute lymphoblastic leukemia. *N Engl J Med* 1991;325:1682.
77. Chak LY, Sikic BI, Tucker MA, Horns RC, Cox RS. Increased incidence of acute nonlymphocytic leukemia following therapy in patients with small cell carcinoma of the lung. *J Clin Oncol* 1984;2:385.
78. Ratain MJ, Kaminer LS, Bitran JD, et al. Acute nonlymphocytic leukemia following etoposide and cisplatin combination chemotherapy for advanced non–small cell carcinoma of the lung. *Blood* 1987;70:1412.
79. Pedersen-Bjergaard J, Daugaard G, Hansen SW, et al. Increased risk of myelodysplasia and leukaemia after etoposide, cisplatin, and bleomycin for germ-cell tumors. *Lancet* 1991;338:359.
80. Froelich-Amon SJ, Osheroff N. Topoisomerase poisons: harnessing the dark side of enzyme mechanisms. *J Biol Chem* 1995;270:21429.
81. Goto H, Shimazaki C, Tatsumi T, et al. Acute myelomonocytic leukemia after treatment with chronic oral etoposide: are MLL and LTG9 genes targets for etoposide? *Int J Hematol* 1994;60:145.
82. Yagita M, Ieki Y, Onishi R, et al. Therapy-related leukemia and myelodysplasia following oral administration of etoposide for recurrent breast cancer. *Int J Oncol* 1998;13:91.
83. Relling MV, Yanishevski Y, Nemec J, et al. Etoposide and antimetabolite pharmacology in patients who develop secondary acute myeloid leukemia. *Leukemia* 1998;12:346.
84. Felix CA, Walker AH, Lange BJ, et al. Association of *CYP3A4* genotype with treatment-related leukemia. *Proc Natl Acad Sci U S A* 1998;95:13176.
85. McLeod HL, Baker DK, Pui CH, Rodman JH. Somnolence, hypotension, and metabolic acidosis following high-dose teniposide treatment in children with leukemia. *Cancer Chemother Pharmacol* 1991;29:150.
86. Schacter LP, Igwemezie LN, Seyedsadr M, et al. Clinical and pharmacokinetic overview of parenteral etoposide phosphate. *Cancer Chemother Pharmacol* 1994;34:S58.
87. de Jong RS, Mulder NH, Uges DR, et al. Randomized comparison of etoposide pharmacokinetics after oral etoposide phosphate and oral etoposide. *Br J Cancer* 1997;75:1660.
88. Sessa C, Zucchetti M, Cerny T, et al. Phase I clinical and pharmacokinetic study of oral etoposide phosphate. *J Clin Oncol* 1995;13:200.
89. Chabot GG, Armand JP, Terret C, et al. Etoposide bioavailability after oral administration of the prodrug etoposide phosphate in cancer patients during a phase I study. *J Clin Oncol* 1996;14:2020.
90. Fields SZ, Igwemezie LN, Kaul S, et al. Phase I study of etoposide phosphate (Etopophos) as a 30-minute infusion on days 1, 3, and 5. *Clin Cancer Res* 1995;1:105.

91. Thompson DS, Greco FA, Miller AA, et al. A phase I study of etoposide phosphate administered as a daily 30-minute infusion for 5 days. *Clin Pharmacol Ther* 1995;57:499.
92. Budman DR, Igwemezie LN, Kaul S, et al. Phase I evaluation of a water-soluble etoposide prodrug, etoposide phosphate, given as a 5-minute infusion on days 1, 3, and 5 in patients with solid tumors. *J Clin Oncol* 1994;12:1902.
93. Potmesil M. Camptothecins: from bench research to hospital wards. *Cancer Res* 1994;54:1431.
94. Wall ME, Wani MC. Camptothecin and taxol: discovery to clinic. Thirteenth Bruce F. Cain Memorial Award Lecture. *Cancer Res* 1995;55:753.
95. McCabe FL, Johnson RL. Comparative activity of oral and parenteral topotecan in murine tumor models: efficacy of oral topotecan. *Cancer Invest* 1994;12:308.
96. Thompson J, Stewart CF, Houghton PJ. Animal models for studying the action of topoisomerase I targeted drugs. *Biochim Biophys Acta* 1998;1400:301.
97. Houghton PJ, Cheshire PJ, Hallman JD, et al. Efficacy of topoisomerase I inhibitors, topotecan and irinotecan, administered at low dose levels in protracted schedules to mice bearing xenografts of human tumors. *Cancer Chemother Pharmacol* 1995;36:393.
98. Schellens JHM, Creemers GJ, Beijnen JH, et al. Bioavailability and pharmacokinetics of oral topotecan: a new topoisomerase I inhibitor. *Br J Cancer* 1996;73:1268.
99. Gerrits CJ, Burris H, Schellens JH, et al. Five days of oral topotecan (Hycamtin), a phase I and pharmacological study in adult patients with solid tumours. *Eur J Cancer* 1998;34:1030.
100. Zamboni WC, Bowman LC, Tan M, et al. Interpatient variability in bioavailability of the intravenous formulation of topotecan given orally to children with recurrent solid tumors. *Cancer Chemother Pharmacol* 1999;43:454.
101. Herben VM, Rosing H, ten Bokkel Huinink WW, et al. Oral topotecan: bioavailability and effect of food co-administration. *Br J Cancer* 1999;80:1380.
102. Drengler RL, Kuhn JG, Schaaf LJ, et al. Phase I and pharmacokinetic trial of oral irinotecan administered daily for 5 days every 3 weeks in patients with solid tumors. *J Clin Oncol* 1999;17:685.
103. Rivory LP, Haaz MC, Canal P, et al. Pharmacokinetic interrelationships of irinotecan (CPT-11) and its three major plasma metabolites in patients enrolled in phase I/II trials. *Clin Cancer Res* 1997;3:1261.
104. Stewart CF, Zamboni WC, Crom WR, Houghton PJ . Disposition of irinotecan and SN-38 following oral and intravenous dosing in mice. *Cancer Chemother Pharmacol* 1997;40:259.
105. Zamboni WC, Crom WR, Houghton PJ, Thompson JC, Stewart CF. Plasma protein binding of SN-38: the active metabolite of irinotecan. *Pharmacotherapy* 1996;16:500(abst).
106. Burke TG, Munshi CB, Mi Z, Jiang Y. The important role of albumin in determining the relative human blood stabilities of the camptothecin anticancer drugs. *J Pharm Sci* 1995;84:518.
107. Burke TG, Mi Z. The structural basis of camptothecin interactions with human serum albumin: impact on drug stability. *J Med Chem* 1994;37:40.
108. Mi Z, Malak H, Burke TG. Reduced albumin binding promotes the stability and activity of topotecan in human blood. *Biochemistry* 1995;34:13722.
109. Baker SD, Heideman RL, Crom WR, et al. Cerebrospinal pharmacokinetics and penetration of continuous infusion topotecan in children with central nervous system tumors. *Cancer Chemother Pharmacol* 1996;37:195.
110. Blaney SM, Cole DE, Balis FM, Godwin K, Poplack DG. Plasma and cerebrospinal fluid pharmacokinetic study of topotecan in nonhuman primates. *Cancer Res* 1993;53:725.
111. Rowinsky EK, Grochow LB, Hendricks CB, et al. Phase I and pharmacologic study of topotecan: a novel topoisomerase I inhibitor. *J Clin Oncol* 1992;10:647.
112. van Warmerdam LJ, Verweij J, Schellens JH, et al. Pharmacokinetics and pharmacodynamics of topotecan administered daily for 5 days every 3 weeks. *Cancer Chemother Pharmacol* 1995;35:237.
113. Stewart CF, Baker SD, Heideman RL, et al. Clinical pharmacodynamics of continuous infusion topotecan in children: systemic exposure predicts hematologic toxicity. *J Clin Oncol* 1994;12:1946.
114. Rosing H, Herben VMM, van Gortel-van Zomeren DM, et al. Isolation and structural confirmation of N-desmethyl topotecan, a metabolite of topotecan. *Cancer Chemother Pharmacol* 1997;39:498.
115. Rosing H, van Zomeren DM, Doyle E, Bult A, Beijnen JH. O-glucuronidation, a newly identified metabolic pathway for topotecan and N-desmethyl topotecan. *Anticancer Drugs* 1998;9:587.
116. Tanizawa A, Fujimori A, Fujimori Y, Pommier Y. Comparison of topoisomerase I inhibition, DNA damage, and cytotoxicity of camptothecin derivatives presently in clinical trials. *J Natl Cancer Inst* 1994;86:836.
117. Ogasawara H, Nishio K, Kanzawa F, et al. Intracellular carboxyl esterase activity is a determinant of cellular sensitivity to the antineoplastic agent KW-2189 in cell lines resistant to cisplatin and CPT-11. *Jpn J Cancer Res* 1995;86:124.
118. Danks MK, Morton CL, Pawlik CA, Potter PM. Overexpression of a rabbit liver carboxylesterase sensitizes human tumor cells to CPT-11. *Cancer Res* 1998;58:20.
119. Danks MK, Morton CL, Krull EJ, et al. Comparison of activation of CPT-11 by rabbit and human carboxylesterases for use in enzyme/prodrug therapy. *Clin Cancer Res* 1999;5:917.
120. Iyer L, King CD, Whitington PF, et al. Genetic predisposition to the metabolism of irinotecan (CPT-11): role of uridine diphosphate glucuronosyltransferase isoform 1A1 in the glucuronidation of its active metabolite (SN-38) in human liver microsomes. *J Clin Invest* 1999;101:847.
121. Chu XY, Kato Y, Niinuma K, et al. Multispecific organic anion transporter is responsible for the biliary excretion of the camptothecin derivative irinotecan and its metabolites in rats. *J Pharmacol Exp Ther* 1997;281:304.
122. Sugiyama Y, Kato Y, Chu X. Multiplicity of biliary excretion mechanisms for the camptothecin derivative irinotecan (CPT-11), its metabolite SN-38, and its glucuronide: role of canalicular multispecific organic anion transporter and P-glycoprotein. *Cancer Chemother Pharmacol* 1998;42[Suppl]:S44.
123. Gupta E, Lestingi TM, Mick R, et al. Metabolic fate of irinotecan in humans: correlation of glucuronidation with diarrhea. *Cancer Res* 1994;54:3723.
124. Rivory LP, Riou JF, Hazz MC, et al. Identification and properties of a major plasma metabolite of irinotecan (CPT-11) isolated from the plasma of patients. *Cancer Res* 1996;56:3689.
125. Dodds HM, Haaz MC, Riou JF, Robert J, Rivory LP. Identification of a new metabolite of CPT-11 (irinotecan): pharmacological properties and activation to SN-38. *J Pharmacol Exp Ther* 1998;286:578.
126. O'Reilly S, Rowinsky EK, Slichenmeyer W, et al. Phase I and pharmacologic study of topotecan in patients with impaired renal function. *J Clin Oncol* 1996;14:3062.
127. O'Reilly S, Rowinsky E, Slichenmyer W, et al. Phase I and pharmacologic studies of topotecan in patients with impaired hepatic function. *J Natl Cancer Inst* 1996;88:817.
128. Slichenmyer WJ, Rowinsky EK, Grochow LB, Kaufmann SH, Donehower RC. Camptothecin analogues: studies from The Johns Hopkins Oncology Center. *Cancer Chemother Pharmacol* 1994;34:S53.
129. Zamboni WC, Houghton PJ, Johnson RK, et al. Probenecid alters topotecan systemic and renal disposition by inhibiting tubular secretion. *J Pharmacol Exp Ther* 1998;284:89.
130. Raymond E, Vernillet L, Boige V, et al. Phase I and pharmacokinetic (PK) study of irinotecan (CPT-11) in cancer patients (pts) with hepatic dysfunction. *Proc Am Soc Clin Oncol* 1999;18:165a(abst).
131. Houghton PJ, Stewart CF, Zamboni WC, et al. Schedule dependent efficacy of camptothecins in models of human cancer. *N Y Acad Sci* 1996;803:188.
132. Haas NB, LaCreta FP, Walczak J, et al. Phase I/pharmacokinetic study of topotecan by 24-hour continuous infusion weekly. *Cancer Res* 1994;54:1220.
133. Wall JG, Burris HA III, Von Hoff DD, et al. A phase I clinical and pharmacokinetic study of topoisomerase I inhibitor topotecan (SK&F 104864) given as an intravenous bolus every 21 days. *Anticancer Drugs* 1992;3:337.
134. Takimoto CH, Dahut W, Harold N, et al. Pharmacodynamics and pharmacokinetics of a 72-hour infusion of 9-aminocamptothecin in adult cancer patients. *J Clin Oncol* 1997;15:1492.
135. Furman WL, Baker SD, Pratt CB, et al. Escalating systemic exposure to topotecan following a 120-hr continuous infusion in children with relapsed acute leukemia. *J Clin Oncol* 1996;14:1504.
136. Rowinsky EK, Kaufmann SH, Baker SD, et al. A phase I and pharmacological study of topotecan infused over 30 minutes for five days in patients with refractory acute leukemia. *Clin Cancer Res* 1999;2:1921.
137. Saltz L, Sirott M, Young C, et al. Phase I clinical and pharmacology study of topotecan given daily for 5 consecutive days to patients with advanced solid tumors, with attempt at dose intensification using recombinant granulocyte colony-stimulating factor [published erratum appears in *J Natl Cancer Inst* 1993;85:1777]. *J Natl Cancer Inst* 1993;85:1499.
138. Gerrits CJ, Schellens JH, Burris H, et al. A comparison of clinical pharmacodynamics of different administration schedules of oral topotecan (Hycamtin) [see comments]. *Clin Cancer Res* 1999;5:69.
139. Kantarjian HM, Beran M, Ellis A, et al. Phase I study of Topotecan, a new topoisomerase I inhibitor, in patients with refractory or relapsed acute leukemia. *Blood* 1993;81:1146.
140. Rowinsky EK, Adjei A, Donehower RC, et al. Phase I and pharmacodynamic study of the topoisomerase I-inhibitor topotecan in patients with refractory acute leukemia. *J Clin Oncol* 1994;12:2193.
141. Sakai H, Diener M, Gartmann V, Takeguchi N. Eicosanoid-mediated Cl– secretion induced by the antitumor drug, irinotecan (CPT-11), in the rat colon. *Arch Pharmacol* 1995;351:309.
142. Conclaves E, Da Costa L, Abigerges D, Armand JP. A new enkephalinase inhibitor as an alternative to loperamide in the prevention of diarrhea induced by CPT-11. *J Clin Oncol* 1995;13:2144.
143. Gupta E, Wang X, Ramirez J, Ratain MJ. Modulation of glucuronidation of SN-38, the active metabolite of irinotecan, by valproic acid and phenobarbital. *Cancer Chemother Pharmacol* 1997;39:440.
144. Ratain MJ, Goh BC, Iyer L, et al. A phase I study of irinotecan with pharmacokinetic modulation by cyclosporine A and phenobarbital. *Proc Am Soc Clin Oncol* 1999;18:202a(abst).
145. Gupta E, Safa AR, Wang X, Ratain MJ. Pharmacokinetic modulation of irinotecan and metabolites by cyclosporin A. *Cancer Res* 1996;56:1309.
146. Hashimoto H, Chatterjee S, Berger NA. Mutagenic activity of topoisomerase I inhibitors. *Clin Cancer Res* 1995;1:369.
147. Zamboni WC, Gajjar AJ, Heideman RL, et al. Phenytoin alters the disposition of topotecan and *N*-desmethyl topotecan in a patient with medulloblastoma. *Clin Cancer Res* 1998;4:783.
148. Grossman SA, Hochberg F, Fisher J, et al. Increased 9-aminocamptothecin (9-AC) dose requirements in patients on anticonvulsants (AC). *Cancer Chemother Pharmacol* 1997;42:118.
149. Reid J, Buckner J, Schaaf L, et al. Pharmacokinetics of irinotecan (CPT-11) in recurrent glioma patients: results of an NCCTG phase II trial. *Proc Am Soc Clin Oncol* 1999;18:141a(abst).
150. Friedman HS, Petros WP, Friedman AH, et al. Irinotecan therapy in adults with recurrent or progressive malignant glioma. *J Clin Oncol* 1999;17:1516.
151. Robert J, Gianni L. Pharmacokinetics and metabolism of anthracyclines. *Cancer Surv* 1993;17:219.
152. Smith PJ, Soues S. Multilevel therapeutic targeting by topoisomerase inhibitors. *Br J Cancer* 1994;23:S47.
153. Robert J. Clinical pharmacokinetics of idarubicin. *Clin Pharmacokinet* 1993;24:275.
154. Cersosimo RJ. Idarubicin: an anthracycline antineoplastic agent. *Am J Hosp Pharm* 1992;11:152.
155. Robert J. Clinical pharmacokinetics of epirubicin. *Clin Pharmacokinet* 1994;26:428.
156. Johnson PJ, Dobbs N, Kalayci C, et al. Clinical efficacy and toxicity of standard dose Adriamycin in hyperbilirubinaemic patients with hepatocellular carcinoma: relation to liver tests and pharmacokinetic parameters. *Br J Cancer* 1992;65:751.
157. Ackland SP, Ratain MJ, Vogelzang NJ. Pharmacokinetics and pharmacodynamics of long-term continuous infusion doxorubicin. *Clin Pharmacol Ther* 1989;45:340.
158. Jakobsen P, Steiness E, Bastholt L, et al. Multiple-dose pharmacokinetics of epirubicin at four different dose levels: studies in patients with metastatic breast cancer. *Cancer Chemother Pharmacol* 1991;28:63.

159. Lawrence HJ, Walsh D, Zapotowski KA, et al. Topical dimethylsulfoxide may prevent tissue damage from anthracycline extravasation. *Cancer Chemother Pharmacol* 1989;23:316.
160. Olver IN, Aisner J, Hament A, et al. A prospective study of topical dimethyl sulfoxide for treating anthracycline extravasation. *J Clin Oncol* 1988;6:1732.
161. Basser RL, Green MD. Strategies for prevention of anthracycline cardiotoxicity. *Cancer Treat Rev* 1993;19:57.
162. Allen A. The cardiotoxicity of chemotherapeutic drugs. *Semin Oncol* 1992;19:529.
163. Von Hoff DD, Layard M. Risk factors for development of daunorubicin cardiotoxicity. *Cancer Treat Rep* 1981;65[Suppl 4]:19.
164. Launchbury AP, Habboubi N. Epirubicin and doxorubicin: a comparison of their characteristics, therapeutic activity and toxicity. *Cancer Treat Rev* 1993;19:197.
165. Workman P. Infusional anthracyclines: is slower better? If so, why? *Ann Oncol* 1992;3:591.
166. Graham MA, Newell DR, Butler J, Hoey B, Patterson LH. The effect of the anthrapyrazole antitumour agent CI941 on rat liver microsome and cytochrome P-450 reductase mediated free radical processes. *Biochem Pharmacol* 1987;36:3345.
167. Fisher GR, Patterson LH. Lack of involvement of reactive oxygen in the cytotoxicity of mitoxantrone, CI941 and ametantrone in MCF-7 cells: comparison with doxorubicin. *Cancer Chemother Pharmacol* 1992;30:451.
168. Herman EH, Zhang J, Hasinoff BB, et al. Comparison of the chronic toxicity of piroxantrone, losoxantrone and doxorubicin in spontaneously hypertensive rats. *Toxicology* 1998;128:35.
169. Leteurtre F, Kohlhagen G, Paull KD, Pommier Y. Topoisomerase II inhibition and cytotoxicity of the anthrapyrazoles DuP 937 and DuP 941 (Losoxantrone) in the National Cancer Institute preclinical antitumor drug discovery screen. *J Natl Cancer Inst* 1994;86:1239.
170. Graham MA, Newell DR, Foster BJ, et al. Clinical pharmacokinetics of the anthrapyrazole CI-941: factors compromising the implementation of a pharmacokinetically guided dose escalation scheme. *Cancer Res* 1992;52:603.
171. Shenkenberg TD, Von Hoff DD. Mitoxantrone: a new anticancer drug with significant clinical activity. *Ann Intern Med* 1986;105:67.
172. Allan SG, Cummings J, Evans S, et al. Phase I study of the anthrapyrazole biantrazole: clinical results and pharmacology. *Cancer Chemother Pharmacol* 1991;28:55.
173. Talbot DC, Smith IE, Mansi JL, et al. Anthrapyrazole CI941: a highly active new agent in the treatment of advanced breast cancer. *J Clin Oncol* 1991;9:2141.
174. Farber S, Selman A. Waksman Conference on Actinomycins: their potential for cancer chemotherapy. Opening remarks. *Cancer Chemother Rep* 1974;58:5.
175. Anton DL, Friedman PA. Actinomycin. *Cancer Growth Prog* 1989;10:131.
176. Ross WE, Bradley MO. DNA double-strand breaks in mammalian cells after exposure to intercalating agents. *Biochim Biophys Acta* 1981;654:129.
177. Matsuoka H, Abe R, Furusawa M, et al. Increased uptake and prolonged retention of actinomycin D by concomitant hyperthermia related to cytotoxic enhancement. *Int J Hyperthermia* 1993;9:403.
178. Tattersall NHM, Sodergren JE, Segupta SK. Pharmacokinetics of actinomycin D in patients with malignant melanoma. *Clin Pharmacol Ther* 1975;17:701.
179. Cohen JJ, Loven D, Schoenfeld T. Dactinomycin potentiation of radiation pneumonitis: a forgotten interaction. *Pediatr Hematol Oncol* 1991;8:187.

SECTION **7**

ERIC K. ROWINSKY
ANTHONY W. TOLCHER

Antimicrotubule Agents

The microtubule is increasingly recognized as a strategic subcellular target against which to direct therapeutic efforts, owing to the widespread use of the vinca alkaloids in both curative and palliative chemotherapeutic regimens and the successful incorporation of the taxanes in cancer chemotherapeutics. This chapter reviews the vinca alkaloids, taxanes, and estramustine and other novel antimicrotubule agents in early development.

MICROTUBULES

Microtubules are integral components of the mitotic spindle, which can be disrupted by the vinca alkaloids, taxanes, and an increasing number of both natural products and synthetic compounds, resulting in metaphase arrest in dividing cells.[1–3] However, they are also involved in nonmitotic functions, such as chemotaxis, membrane and intracellular scaffolding, transport, secretory processes, anchorage of subcellular organelles and receptors, cell adhesion, and locomotion transmission of receptor signaling. Antimicrotubule agents may disrupt a range of these nonmitotic functions.[1–3]

Microtubules are polymers of dimeric subunits of α- and β-tubulin (each tubulin subunit consisting of approximately 450 amino acids with a molecular weight of 50,000 D) that are arranged into 13 protofilaments (Fig. 19.7-1).[1,4] The dimers are aligned side by side around an apparently hollow core with the β subunit of one dimer in contact with the α-tubulin subunit of the next. The microtubule polymer is in a dynamic equilibrium with the intracellular pool of tubulin dimers, which results in the simultaneous incorporation of free dimers into the polymerized structures and release of dimers into the soluble tubulin pool. The direction of the equilibrium—toward polymerization or depolymerization—is influenced by several cofactors, including guanosine triphosphate (GTP), the ionic environment, and microtubule-associated proteins (MAPs), which is a family of proteins that regulate tubulin polymerization and microtubule function (discussed later in the section Microtubule-Associated Proteins and Microtubule Motors). Microtubule growth occurs spontaneously at the plus end, resulting in the hydrolysis of GTP, which weakens the binding affinity of tubulin for adjacent molecules. This, in turn, favors the opposing process: depolymerization. Net shortening occurs at the opposite minus end. In essence, microtubules are under the control of two dynamic processes. The first is dynamic instability, which is the process whereby microtubule ends switch spontaneously and stochastically between slowly growing and rapidly shrinking states.[4] The rate of dynamic instability is accelerated during some processes, such as mitosis, so that chromosomes can readily be "captured" by growing microtubules, thereby leading to the formation of mitotic spindles; dynamic instability is suppressed, perhaps by MAPs, during nonproliferative processes (e.g., differentiation). When both these actions occur simultaneously, the microtubule is said to be *treadmilling*, which plays a role in the polar movement of the chromosomes during anaphase.[5]

There are at least six isotypes of both α- and β-tubulin in humans; they are distinguished by slightly different amino acid sequences and appear to be encoded by different genes.[6–9] The C-terminal amino acid sequence of β-tubulin is the most variable in terms of amino acid composition, and both posttranslational modifications, including phosphorylation and glutamylation (which may account in part for their structural diversity) have been described.[9,10] Equivalent isotypes expressed in specific tissues of different species are highly conserved, indicating that expression of tubulin isotypes may be important in specific microtubule functions.[7–10] Analysis of tubulin isotype expression in various tissues has demonstrated a complex pattern of isotype distribution, suggesting functional specificity.[7–10] In neurons, for example, isotype segregation within cells, and both differential isotype synthesis and posttranslational modification during neurite outgrowth, suggest functional specialization. A third member of the tubulin superfamily, γ-tubulin, which is less abundant

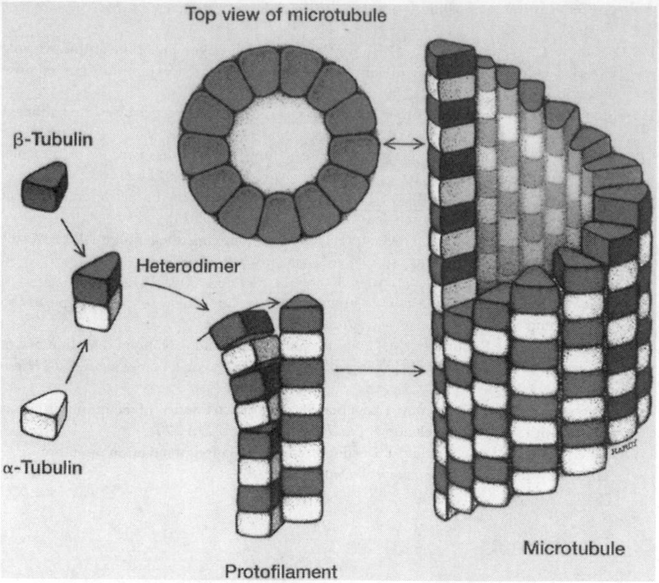

FIGURE 19.7-1. Microtubles are composed mainly of dimeric subunits of α- and β-tubulin that are arranged into protofilaments. The cylindric microtubule is approximately 25 nm in diameter and may reach several micrometeres in length. (From I Ringel, IR Horwitz, Paclitaxel affects microtuble dynamics and apoptosis. *Adv Oncol* 1999;15:1, with permission.)

than the α and β forms, completes the microtubule-organizing center (MTOC) or centrosome.[11] Although tubulin can polymerize into microtubules in acellular preparations, they are polymerized from, and nucleated by, the MTOC, with minus ends located at the MTOC.[12] The MTOC in the cytoplasm of mammalian cells duplicates and separates before cell division, forming the two poles of the mitotic spindle.

MICROTUBULE-ASSOCIATED PROTEINS AND MICROTUBULE MOTORS

The dynamic behavior of microtubules is regulated by a variety of MAPs.[1–3] The number of MAPs identified is increasing rapidly, and these proteins appear to be diverse, differing from species to species and cell type to cell type. Among the best characterized MAPs are those that come from mammalian brain, including the tau proteins, MAP1, MAP1c (an adenosine triphosphatase), MAP2, MAP4, and dynein (a GTPase), which promote tubulin polymerization and microtubule stability. Some MAPs, such as the dyneins and kinesins, function as microtubule motors, transmitting chemical energy to mechanical sliding force and moving various solutes and subcellular organelles along the microtubule.[1–3,13] Motor proteins function in many types of cellular events, such as mitosis, premeiotic events, and organelle transport.

VINCA ALKALOIDS

The vinca alkaloids are naturally occurring or semisynthetic compounds that are found in minute quantities in the periwinkle plant *Catharanthus roseus* g. Don.[14–23] The early medicinal uses of this plant led to the screening of these compounds for their hypoglycemic activity, which was of little importance as compared to their cytotoxic effects. Although many vinca alkaloids have been investigated clinically, only vincristine (VCR), vinblastine (VBL), and vinorelbine (VRL) are approved for use in the United States. The vinca alkaloids are dimeric molecules composed of two multiringed units (Fig. 19.7-2), an indole nucleus (catharanthine) and a dihydroindole nucleus (vindoline). VCR and VBL are structurally identical except for a single substitution on the vindoline nucleus, where VCR and VBL possess formyl and methyl groups, respectively. Despite this small difference, these two agents significantly differ in their antitumor and toxicologic profiles. VCR is used more commonly in pediatric oncology than in adults with cancer, most likely owing to the higher level of sensitivity of pediatric malignancies to VCR and to the better tolerance of higher VCR doses in children. VCR is an essential part of the combination chemotherapeutic regimens used for acute lymphocytic leukemia and lymphoid blast crisis of chronic myeloid leukemia and plays an important role in the treatment of both Hodgkin's and non-Hodgkin's lymphomas. The agent also plays a role in the multimodality therapy of Wilms' tumor, Ewing's sarcoma, neuroblastoma, and rhab-

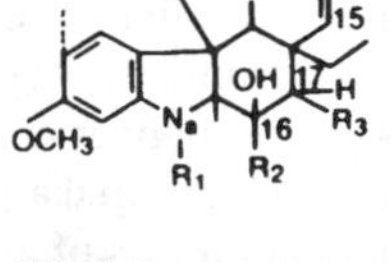

Vindoline nucleus

Catharanthine nucleus

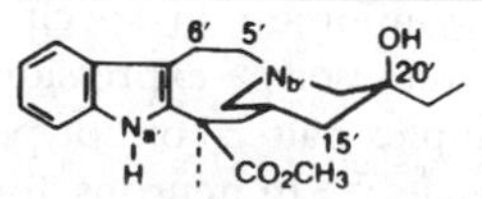

	R_1	R_2	R_3
Vindesine	CH_3	$CONH_2$	OH
Vincristine	CHO	CO_2CH_3	$OCOCH_3$
Vinblastine	CH_3	CO_2CH_3	$OCOCH_3$
Vinorelbine	CH_3	CO_2CH_3	$OCOCH_3$

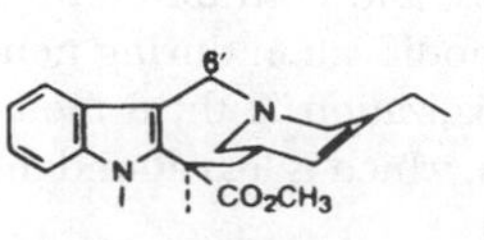

FIGURE 19.7-2. Structural modifications of the vindoline and catharanthine rings in various vinca alkaloids.

domyosarcoma in children, as well as in the treatment of multiple myeloma and small cell lung cancer in adults. VBL has been an integral component of chemotherapeutic regimens for germ cell malignancies and advanced lymphoma and is used in combination with other agents to treat Kaposi's sarcoma and bladder, brain, and breast cancers.[14–17]

Deacetyl VBL (vindesine, or VDS), initially identified as a metabolite of VBL, was introduced in the 1970s.[18] VDS is registered in many countries but available only for investigational purposes in the United States. The agent is most commonly used in combination with other agents, particularly the platinating agents or mitomycin C (or both), in treating non–small cell lung cancer, but it is also active in several hematologic and solid neoplasms.[17,18] The semisynthetic VBL derivative VRL (5'-norhydro-VBL), which is structurally modified on its catharanthine nucleus, is approved in the United States for treating non–small cell lung cancer as either a single agent or in combination with cisplatin and has been registered for advanced breast cancer in many other countries.[19,20] VRL has also demonstrated anticancer activity in advanced ovarian carcinoma and lymphoma; however, a unique role in the therapy of these malignancies has not been defined.

MECHANISM OF ACTION

The principal mechanism of cytotoxicity of the vinca alkaloids is by interacting with tubulin and disrupting microtubule function, particularly of microtubules that compose the mitotic spindle apparatus, leading to metaphase arrest.[21–25] However, they are also capable of many other biochemical and biologic activities that may or may not be related to their effects on microtubules.[26] In support of antimicrotubule actions or, more specifically, antimitotic actions as the principal cytotoxic effect of the vinca alkaloids is that the dissolution of the mitotic spindle apparatus, appearance of mitotic figures, and cytotoxicity strongly correlate with both the duration and concentration of drug treatment.[26] Nevertheless, the vinca alkaloids and other antimicrotubule agents also affect both nonmalignant and malignant cells in the nonmitotic cell cycle, which is not surprising, as microtubules are involved in many nonmitotic functions.

The vinca alkaloids bind to sites on tubulin that are distinct from the binding sites of the taxanes, colchicine, podophyllotoxin, and GTP.[20–25] Binding is rapid and readily reversible. There appear to be two binding sites per mole of tubulin dimer. Vinca alkaloid binding to tubulin induces tubulin to self-associate into nonmicrotubule polymers and ordered aggregates through a self-association pathway, which in turn increases the affinity of one of the binding sites for the drug. The vinca alkaloid self-association of tubulin can lead to the formation of paracrystalline structures *in vitro*, which generally occurs at high drug concentrations. The vinca alkaloids bind to their binding sites in intact microtubules with different affinities, depending on whether the binding sites are located at the microtubule ends or situated along the microtubule surface.[25] There are approximately 16 to 17 high-affinity binding sites per microtubule (K_d, 1 to 2 μmol) located at the ends of each microtubule. Binding of the vinca alkaloids to these sites disrupts microtubule assembly. The main effect of low drug concentrations is to decrease the rates of both growth and shortening at the assembly end of the microtubule, which in effect produces a "kinetic cap" and suppresses function.[21–25] The potent kinetic suppression of tubulin exchange that occurs at low vinca alkaloid concentrations (<1 μmol) is almost certainly due to drug binding at the high-affinity sites at the microtubule ends. This action suppresses dynamic instability and increases the time that microtubules spend in a state of attenuated activity, neither growing nor shortening. The disruptive effects of the vinca alkaloids on microtubule dynamics, particularly at the ends of the mitotic spindle, which leads to metaphase arrest, occur at drug concentrations below those that decrease microtubule mass. There are also one to two low-affinity binding sites per mole of tubulin dimer (K_d, 0.25 to 3.0 mmol) along the microtubule surface.[25] Binding of the vinca alkaloids to these sites appears to be responsible for the splaying of microtubules into spiral aggregates or spiral protofilaments, which leads to microtubule disintegration. This effect occurs at high drug concentrations (>1 to 2 μmol) by a self-propagated mechanism, initially involving drug binding to a limited number of sites, which progressively weakens the lateral interactions between the protofilaments and thereby exposes new sites. Spiral protofilaments may then associate to form paracrystals.

Despite the wide range of sensitivities of different tissues to the actions of the vinca alkaloids *in vivo*, the qualitative effects of these agents on tubulin, as well as both tubulin-binding and inhibitory constants, are similar. The differential sensitivities of various tissues appear to be multifactorial. One of the most likely explanations is that each tissue type has a distinct tubulin isotype composition and that vinca alkaloid sensitivity is, in part, tubulin isotype–dependent. In addition, differences in the tissue content of cofactors, such as MAPs and GTP, which may influence drug interactions with tubulin, and variability in cellular permeation and retention may influence the formation and stability of vinca alkaloid-tubulin complexes.[26–36] Differences in the pharmacokinetics between the vinca alkaloids may also contribute to differential tissue sensitivity.

The vinca alkaloids are rapidly taken up into cells and then accumulate intracellularly, with intracellular-extracellular concentration ratios as high as 5- to 500-fold, depending on the cell type.[37–39] In murine leukemia cells, the intracellular concentrations of VCR are 5- to 20-fold higher than the extracellular concentrations, and this ratio has been reported to range from 150- to 500-fold for other vinca alkaloids in human leukemia cell lines.[40] In isolated human hepatocytes, VRL is more rapidly taken up and metabolized than other vinca alkaloids.[39,40] There are also marked differences in cellular retention between the vinca alkaloids.[31,39,41,42,43] VBL is retained to a much greater degree than either VCR or VDS. Overall, the most important determinant of the rates of drug accumulation and retention is lipophilicity.[39] Drug uptake and retention may also be tissue-specific as well as drug-specific, as illustrated by studies indicating that the accumulation and retention of VRL in neurons are much less than with other vinca alkaloids.[31]

It was originally believed that the vinca alkaloids entered cells by both energy-dependent and temperature-dependent transport processes.[39] However, it appears that temperature-independent, nonsaturable mechanisms, analogous to simple diffusion, account for the majority of drug transport, and temperature-dependent, saturable processes are less important.[39–41] Although the drug concentration and duration of treatment are important determinants of both drug accumulation and cytotoxicity, the duration of drug exposure above a critical threshold concentration appears to be the most important determinant.[41,42]

TABLE 19.7-1. Vinca Alkaloids: Comparative Pharmacokinetic and Toxicologic Characteristics

	Vincristine	*Vinblastine*	*Vindesine*	*Vinorelbine*
Standard adult dose (range, mg/m²/wk)	1–2	6–8	3–4	15–30
Pharmacokinetic behavior	Triphasic	Triphasic	Triphasic	Triphasic
Plasma half-lives				
α (min)	<5	<5	<5	<5
β (min)	50–155	53–99	55–99	49–168
γ (h)	23–85	20–64	20–24	18–49
Clearance (L/kg/h)	0.16	0.74	0.25	0.4–1.29
Primary route	Hepatic metabolism and biliary elimination	Hepatic metabolism and biliary elimination	Hepatic metabolism and biliary elimination	Hepatic metabolism and biliary elimination
Principal toxicity	Neurotoxicity	Neutropenia	Neutropenia	Neutropenia
Other toxicities	Constipation, SIADH	Alopecia, neurotoxicity, mucositis	Alopecia, neurotoxicity	Neurotoxicity, vomiting, constipation, mucositis

SIADH, syndrome of inappropriate secretion of antidiuretic hormone.

MECHANISMS OF RESISTANCE

Two mechanisms of resistance to the vinca alkaloids *in vitro* have been well characterized. The first is pleiotropic or multidrug resistance (MDR), which can be innate or acquired. MDR-mediating proteins include permeability glycoprotein (P-gp), MDR protein, and lung resistance protein, which are overexpressed in resistant cells and function as drug efflux pumps.[43–50] The best characterized mechanism is mediated by the 170-kD P-gp drug efflux pump that is encoded by the *mdr1* gene and results in decreased drug accumulation. The MDR phenotype confers varying degrees of cross-resistance to other structurally bulky natural products, such as the taxanes, anthracyclines, epipodophyllotoxins, and colchicine.[44–50] The amino acid sequence of the specific P-gp associated with resistance to the vinca alkaloids differs slightly from P-gp of cells selected for resistance to other agents.[47,48] These proteins also undergo posttranslational modifications, resulting in further structural diversity, which may explain the greater degree of resistance for the specific agent, in which resistance was selected against, and the variable degrees of resistance to agents aside from that specific agent. The composition of membrane gangliosides in VCR-resistant cells has also been demonstrated to be different from wild-type cells, which may have functional significance.[49] The clinical ramifications of these mechanisms are not entirely known. In one study in childhood acute lymphoblastic leukemia, VCR resistance measured *in vitro* did not correlate with P-gp overexpression.[50] Although many types of agents reverse resistance conferred by P-gp *in vitro* and the role of MDR modulators has been a source of great contemporary interest, the interpretation of clinical studies of resistance modulation has been confounded by the fact that MDR modulators also enhance drug uptake in normal cells, decrease biliary elimination and drug clearance, and lead to enhanced toxicity.[51,52] Overall, strategies aimed at reversing resistance to the vinca alkaloids in the clinic with pharmacologic modulators of MDR have been disappointing.[52]

Structural and functional alterations in α- and β-tubulins, resulting from either genetic mutations or posttranslational modifications, have also been identified in tumor cells with acquired resistance to the vinca alkaloids.[53–55] Tubulin alterations may result in either decreased drug-binding affinity of the altered tubulin or increased resistance to microtubule disassembly. These "hyperstable" microtubules are collaterally sensitive to the taxanes, which inhibit microtubule disassembly (discussed later in Taxanes, Mechanisms of Resistance). Although the precise mechanisms that lead to cell death after treatment with the vinca alkaloids are not entirely clear, these mechanisms appear similar to those that have been elucidated for the taxanes and involve the action of such genes as *p53, bcl-2, and bcl-x* and gene products that trigger programmed cell death or apoptosis after significant microtubule disruption.[56,57]

PHARMACOLOGY

General Overview

The vinca alkaloids are usually administered intravenously as a brief infusion, and their pharmacokinetic behavior in plasma is optimally described by three-compartment models. Table 19.7-1 displays several pertinent pharmacokinetic features of these agents. At conventional adult doses, peak plasma concentrations range from 100 to 500 nmol, but levels of this magnitude are sustained in plasma for only short periods (alpha half-lives, <5 minutes).[15,17–19,40,58–61] The vinca alkaloids share many pharmacokinetic characteristics, including large volumes of distribution, high clearance rates, and long terminal half-lives, which reflect the high magnitude and avidity of drug binding in peripheral tissues. There is also great interindividual and intraindividual variability in their pharmacologic behaviors, which has been attributed to many factors, including differences in protein binding and both hepatic and biliary clearance.[40] Although it has been proposed that prolonged infusion schedules may avoid excessive toxic peak concentrations and increase the duration of drug exposure in plasma above biologically relevant threshold concentrations for any given tumor, there is little (if any) evidence to support the notion that prolonged infusion schedules are more effective than bolus schedules. This approach has primarily been directed at achieving plasma concentrations that likely underestimate drug concentrations in peripheral tissues where binding is high and avid, owing to the ubiquitous nature of tubulin.

In comparative studies of the vinca alkaloids, VCR had the longest terminal half-life and the lowest clearance rate, VBL had the shortest terminal half-life and the highest clearance rate, and VDS had intermediate characteristics.[15,18–20,59,60] Comparable values for VLR overlap with those of VDS and VBL. The longest half-life and lowest clearance rate of VCR may account for its greater propensity to induce neurotoxicity,[58,59] but there are many other nonpharmacologic determinants of tissue sensitivity (discussed earlier in the section Mechanism of Action under Vinca Alkaloids).

Vincristine

After conventional doses of VCR (1.4 mg/m^2) given as brief infusions, peak plasma levels approach 0.4 μmol.[15,17,18,62,63] VCR binds extensively to both plasma proteins (48%) and formed blood elements, particularly platelets, which contain high concentrations of tubulin and led, in the past, to the use of VCR-loaded platelets for treating disorders of platelet consumption, such as idiopathic thrombocytopenia purpura.[17] The platelet count inversely has been demonstrated to influence drug exposure.[17,64] Penetration of VCR across the blood–brain barrier is poor, probably because of its large size and the fact that it is an avid substrate for the multidrug transporter pumps that maintain the integrity of the blood–brain barrier.[15,18,40,64–69] Plasma clearance is slow, and terminal half-lives range from 23 to 85 hours.[15,17,18,40,58,59,62]

VCR is metabolized and excreted primarily by the hepatobiliary system. Seventy-two hours after the administration of radiolabeled VCR, approximately 12% of the radiolabel is excreted in the urine (50% of which consists of metabolites), and approximately 70% is excreted in the feces (40% of which consists of metabolites).[15,18,40,63,65,69,70] The nature of the VCR metabolites identified to date, as well as the results of metabolic studies *in vitro*, indicate that VCR metabolism is mediated by hepatic cytochrome P-450 CYP3A.[15,18,40] There has been conflicting, albeit sparse, evidence indicating that peak VCR plasma concentration or systemic exposure correlates positively with the degree of neurotoxicity.[15]

Vinblastine

The clinical pharmacology of VBL is similar to that of VCR. Binding of VBL to plasma proteins and formed elements of blood is extensive.[40,71,72] Peak plasma drug concentrations are approximately 0.4 μmol after rapid intravenous injections of VBL at standard doses. Distribution is rapid, and terminal half-lives range from 20 to 24 hours.[17,40,58,59,66,72,73] Tissue sequestration appears to be greater for VBL than VCR, with 73% of radioactivity retained in the body 6 days after treatment with radiolabled drug.[72] Like VCR, VBL disposition is principally through the hepatobiliary system.[40] Fecal excretion of the parent compound is low, indicating that the metabolism is significant. *In vitro* studies indicate that the cytochrome P-450 CYP3A isoform is primarily responsible for the drug biotransformation.[40,73] Although the metabolic fate of VBL has not been fully characterized, 4-deacetyl-VBL, or VDS, which appears to be as active as the parent compound, is the principal metabolite of VBL.[72]

Vindesine

VDS is rapidly distributed to tissues, and terminal half-lives range from 20 to 24 hours.[18,40,58,59,69,74–79] The large volume of distribution, low renal clearance, and long terminal half-life of VDS suggest that it undergoes extensive tissue binding and delayed elimination and that drug accumulation may occur with repeated administration at short intervals. Although peak VDS concentrations ranging from 0.1 to 1.0 μmol are achieved with rapid injections, levels typically decline to less than 0.1 μmol in 1 to 2 hours after treatment. Plasma levels achieved with rapid injections are approximately 16-fold higher than those achieved with protracted infusions; however, prolonged periods of exposure above concentrations resulting in cytotoxicity *in vitro* (0.01 to 0.1 μmol) are readily achieved using protracted infusions (1.2 to 2.0 mg/m^2/d for 2 to 5 days).[18,40,62,76–80] Renal clearance is negligible, accounting for 1% to 12% of drug disposition.[18,40,77,79] Similar to the other vinca alkaloids, VDS disposition is primarily by hepatic metabolism and biliary clearance, and the cytochrome P-450 isoform CYP3A plays a major role in drug metabolism.[18,40,67,81,82]

Vinorelbine

The pharmacologic behavior of VRL is essentially similar to that of the other vinca alkaloids, with plasma concentrations declining in either a biexponential or triexponential manner.[17,19,20,40,83–85] After intravenous administration, there is a rapid decay of VRL concentrations followed by a much slower elimination phase (terminal half-life, 18 to 49 hours). Plasma protein binding has been reported to range from 80% to 91%, with binding primarily to α_1-acid glycoprotein, albumin, and lipoproteins,[19,20,40,86] and drug binding to platelets is also extensive. The unbound fraction has been reported to range from 0.09 to 0.20.[19]

VRL is widely distributed, and high concentrations are found in virtually all tissues, except brain.[19,20,40,87,88] The wide distribution of VRL reflects the agent's lipophilicity, which is among the highest of the vinca alkaloids.[22] In fact, drug concentrations in human lung have been demonstrated to be 300-fold greater than plasma levels and 3.4- to 13.8-fold higher than lung concentrations achieved with VDS and VCR, respectively.[87] As with other vinca alkaloids, the liver is the principal excretory organ, and 33% to 80% of the drug is excreted in the feces, whereas urinary excretion represents only 16% to 30% of total drug disposition, the bulk of which is unmetabolized VLR.[18,19,40,89,90] Studies in humans indicate that 4-O-deacetyl-VRL, 3,6-epoxy-VRL, and several hydroxy-VRL isomers are the principal metabolites.[19,20,90] Although most metabolites are inactive, deacetyl-VRL may be as active as VRL. The cytochrome P-450 CYP3A isoenzyme appears to be principally involved in biotransformation.[19,20,40] Human studies of powder- and liquid-filled gelatin capsules have shown that bioavailability of the parent compound is 43% for the powder-filled and 27% for the liquid-filled capsules.[85,91] Plasma concentrations peak within 1 to 2 hours after oral treatment, and interindividual variability is moderate.

DRUG INTERACTIONS

Methotrexate accumulation in tumor cells is enhanced *in vitro* by the presence of VCR or VBL, an effect mediated by a vinca alkaloid–induced blockade of drug efflux; however, the minimal concentrations of VCR required to achieve this effect occur only transiently *in vivo*.[92–94] The vinca alkaloids also inhibit the cellular influx of the epipodophyllotoxins *in vitro*, resulting in less cytotoxicity, but the clinical ramifications of this effect are unknown.[95] L-Asparaginase may reduce the hepatic clearance of the vinca alkaloids, particularly VCR, which may result in increased toxicity. To minimize the possibility of this interaction, VCR should be given 12 to 24 hours before L-asparaginase.

Treatment with the vinca alkaloids has precipitated seizures associated with subtherapeutic plasma phenytoin concentrations.[94,96,97] Reduced plasma phenytoin levels have been noted from 24 hours to 10 days after treatment with both VCR and VBL. Because of the importance of the cytochrome P-450 CYP3A isoenzyme in vinca alkaloid metabolism, administration of the vinca alkaloids with erythromycin and other inhibitors of CYP3A may lead to severe toxicity.[98] Concomitantly administered drugs, such as pentobarbital and H_2-receptor antagonists, may also influence VCR clearance by modulating hepatic cytochrome P-450 metabolic processes.[94,99] Another potential drug interaction may occur in patients who have Kaposi's sarcoma related to acquired immunodeficiency syndrome (AIDS) and are receiving concurrent treatment with 3' azido-3'-deoxythymidine (AZT) and the vinca alkaloids, as the vinca alkaloids may inhibit glucuronidation of AZT to its 5'-O-glucuronide metabolite.[100]

TOXICITY

Despite close similarities in structure, the vinca alkaloids differ significantly in their toxicologic profiles. VCR principally induces neurotoxicity characterized by a peripheral, symmetric mixed sensory-motor, and autonomic polyneuropathy.[15,17–20,101–105] The primary pathologic effects are axonal degeneration and decreased axonal transport due to interference with microtubule function. Initially, only symmetric sensory impairment and paresthesias in a length-dependent manner (distal extremities first) usually are encountered. Neuritic pain and loss of deep tendon reflexes may develop with continued treatment, which may be followed by foot drop, wrist drop, motor dysfunction, ataxia, and paralysis. Back, bone, and limb pains occasionally occur. Nerve conduction velocities are usually normal, although diminished amplitude of sensory and motor nerve action potentials and prolonged distal latencies, suggesting axonal degeneration, may be noted.[15,101,104,105] Cranial nerves may be affected rarely, resulting in hoarseness, diplopia, jaw pain, and facial palsies. The uptake of VCR into the brain is low, and central nervous system effects, such as confusion, mental status changes, depression, hallucinations, agitation, insomnia, seizures, coma, inappropriate secretion of antidiuretic hormone (SIADH), and visual disturbances, are rare.[15,65–67,106] Acute, severe autonomic neurotoxicity is uncommon but may arise as a consequence of high-dose therapy (>2 mg/m^2) or in patients with altered hepatic function. Toxic manifestations include constipation, abdominal cramps, paralytic ileus, urinary retention, orthostatic hypotension, and hypertension.[107–109] Laryngeal paralysis has also been reported.[110]

In adults, neurotoxic effects may begin with cumulative doses as little as 5 to 6 mg, and manifestations may be profound after cumulative doses of 15 to 20 mg. Children may be less susceptible than adults, but the elderly are particularly prone. However, the apparent influence of age may, in fact, be due to previously inadequate dose calculation by body weight in children and adults and by body surface area in infants.[103,104,111,112] In infants, VCR doses are calculated now according to body weight. Patients with antecedent neurologic disorders, such as Charcot-Marie-Tooth disease, hereditary and sensory neuropathy type 1, Guillain-Barré syndrome, and childhood poliomyelitis, are highly predisposed.[113,114] VCR treatment in patients with hepatic dysfunction or obstructive liver disease is associated with an increased risk of developing neuropathy because of impaired drug metabolism and delayed biliary excretion.

The only known treatment for VCR neurotoxicity is discontinuation of the drug or reduction of the dose or frequency of treatment.[116] Although a number of antidotes, including thiamine, vitamin B_{12}, folinic acid, and pyridoxine, have been used, these treatments have not been clearly shown to be effective.[15,17,116] However, results with several other protective agents appear promising.[15,17,115,116] In one randomized, double-blind trial, coadministration of glutamic acid and VCR has been demonstrated to decrease neurotoxicity.[15,117] The adrenocorticotropic hormone (4-9) analogue ORG 2766 has also been shown to protect against VCR-induced neuropathy both in an animal model and in cancer patients in a double-blind, placebo-controlled pilot study.[15] However, the younger age of the ORG 2766–treated group as compared to the placebo group may have accounted for this result. Experimental results indicate that several other agents, such as nerve growth factor, insulin-like growth factor I, and amifostine, might alter the natural course of drug-induced neurotoxicity.[15]

The manifestations of neurotoxicity are similar for the other vinca alkaloids; however, they are typically less common and severe.[15,17–20] Severe neurotoxicity is observed infrequently with both VBL and VDS. VRL has been shown to have a lower affinity for axonal microtubules than either VCR or VBL, which seems to be confirmed by clinical observations.[31,118] Mild to moderate peripheral neuropathy, principally characterized by sensory effects, occurs in 7% to 31% of patients, and constipation and other autonomic effects are noted in 30% of subjects, whereas severe toxicity occurs in 2% to 3%. Muscle weakness, jaw pain, and discomfort at tumor sites may also occur. In a study in patients with non–small cell lung cancer randomly assigned to treatment with either VRL alone, VRL plus cisplatin, or VDS plus cisplatin, the rate of severe neurotoxicity was lower in both the single-agent VRL and VRL plus cisplatin arms than in the VDS plus cisplatin arm.[119] Furthermore, the addition of cisplatin did not significantly increase the incidence of severe toxicity in excess of that observed with VRL alone.

Neutropenia is the principal dose-limiting toxicity of VBL, VDS, and VRL. Thrombocytopenia and anemia are usually less common and less severe. The onset of neutropenia is usually 7 to 11 days after treatment, and recovery is generally by days 14 to 21. Myelosuppression is not typically cumulative.

Gastrointestinal toxicities, aside from those caused by autonomic dysfunction, may be caused by all the vinca alkaloids.[15–20,120] Gastrointestinal autonomic dysfunction, as manifested by bloating, constipation, ileus, and abdominal pain, occur most commonly with VCR or high doses of the other vinca alkaloids. Mucositis occurs more frequently with VBL than with VRL or VDS and is least common with VCR. Nausea, vomiting, and diarrhea may also occur to a lesser extent. Pancreatitis has also been reported with VRL.[121]

All vinca alkaloids are potent vesicants and may cause significant tissue damage if extravasation occurs. If extravasation occurs or is suspected, treatment should be discontinued, and aspiration of any residual drug remaining in the tissues should be attempted.[122,123] The application of local heat and the injection of hyaluronidase, 150 mg subcutaneously, in a circumferential manner around the needle site are thought to minimize both discomfort and latent cellulitis. Phlebitis may also occur along the course of an injected vein, with resultant sclerosis. The risk of phlebitis may increase if veins are not adequately flushed after treatment.

Mild and reversible alopecia occurs in approximately 10% and 20% of patients treated with VLR and VCR, respectively. Acute cardiac ischemia, chest pains without evidence of ischemia, fever without an obvious source, acute pulmonary effects (alone or in combination with mitomycin C), Raynaud's phenomenon, hand-foot syndrome, and both pulmonary and liver toxicity have also been reported with the vinca alkaloids.[124–131] All the vinca alkaloids have been implicated as a cause of SIADH, and patients who are receiving intensive hydration are particularly prone to severe hyponatremia secondary to SIADH.[15,17–20] This entity has been associated with elevated plasma levels of antidiuretic hormone and usual remits in 2 to 3 days. Hyponatremia generally responds to fluid restriction, as with hyponatremia associated with SIADH due to other causes.

ADMINISTRATION

VCR is commonly administered to children weighing more than 10 kg as a bolus intravenous injection at a dose of 1.5 to 2.0 mg/m^2 weekly, whereas 0.05 to 0.65 mg/kg weekly is commonly used in smaller children. For adults, the conventional weekly dose is 1.4 mg/m^2. A restriction of the absolute dose of VCR to 2.0 to 2.5 mg in children and 2.0 mg in adults (often called *capping*) has been adopted based on early reports of substantial gastrointestinal toxicity in small numbers of patients treated at higher doses. However, this practice is largely unfounded, and available evidence suggests that it should be reconsidered, particularly in light of the wide interpatient variability in pharmacokinetic behavior and tolerance.[103] There is significant interpatient variability in the clearance of VCR (as much as 11-fold), and some patients are able to tolerate much higher doses with little or no toxicity. Moreover, the safety and efficacy of treatment regimens that do not employ capping at 2.0 mg have been documented in adults.[132] In any case, doses should not be reduced for mild peripheral neurotoxicity, particularly if the agent is being used in a potentially curative setting. Instead, doses should be modified for manifestations indicative of more serious neurotoxicity, including severe symptomatic sensory changes, motor and cranial nerve deficits, and ileus, until toxicity resolves. In clearly palliative situations, dose reductions, lengthened dosing intervals, or selection of an alternative agent may be justified in the event of moderate neurotoxicity. A routine prophylactic regimen to prevent severe autonomic toxicity, particularly severe constipation, is also recommended.

The most common schedule for VBL in combination chemotherapeutic regimens uses a rapid intravenous injection at a dose of 6 mg/m^2 weekly. Approved dosing recommendations for weekly dosing are 2.5 and 3.7 mg/m^2 for children and adults, respectively, followed by gradual escalation in increments of 1.8 and 1.25 mg/m^2 weekly based on hematologic tolerance. It is recommended that weekly VBL doses of 18.5 mg/m^2 in adults and 12.5 mg/m^2 in children not be exceeded as a single agent; however, these doses are substantially higher than most patients can tolerate because of myelosuppression, even on less-frequent schedules of administration. Because the severity of leukopenia that may occur with identical VBL doses varies widely, VBL should probably not be given more frequently than once each week.

VDS has been administered intravenously on many schedules, including weekly and biweekly bolus and prolonged infusion schedules. The agent has also been given in fractionated doses as either an intermittent or a continuous infusion over 1 to 5 days. VDS is most commonly administered as a single intravenous dose of 2 to 4 mg/m^2 every 7 to 14 days. Intermittent or continuous infusion schedules usually employ VDS doses of 1 to 2 mg/m^2/d for 1 to 2 days or 1.2 mg/m^2/d for 5 days every 3 to 4 weeks.[62]

VRL is usually administered at a dose of 30 mg/m^2 on a weekly or biweekly schedule as a 6- to 10-minute intravenous injection through a side-arm port into a running infusion (alternatively, a slow bolus injection followed by flushing the vein with 5% dextrose or 0.9% sodium chloride solutions) or as a short infusion over 20 minutes.[17–20] It appears that the more rapid infusions are associated with less local venous toxicity. Oral doses of 80 to 100 mg/m^2 given weekly are generally well tolerated, but an acceptable oral formulation has not yet been approved. Other dosing schedules that have been evaluated include chronic oral administration of low doses, intermittent high dose, and prolonged intravenous infusion schedules.

The vinca alkaloids are potent vesicants and should not be administered intramuscularly, subcutaneously, intravesically, or intraperitoneally. Direct intrathecal injection of VCR and other vinca alkaloids, which has occurred as an inadvertent clinical mishap, induces a severe myeloencephalopathy characterized by ascending motor and sensory neuropathies, encephalopathy, and rapid death.[133]

Although it has not been carefully evaluated, the major role of the liver in the disposition of the vinca alkaloids implies that dose modifications should be considered for patients with hepatic dysfunction.[134] However, firm guidelines have not been established. A 50% dose reduction is often recommended for patients with total bilirubin levels between 1.5 and 3.0 mg/dL (50% dose reduction for bilirubin levels between 2.0 and 3.0 mg/dL is recommended for VRL), and at least a 75% dose reduction for plasma total bilirubin levels greater than 3.0 mg/dL. Dose reduction for renal dysfunction is not indicated.

THE TAXANES

The unique chemical structure and mechanism of action of the taxanes, coupled with their antitumor activities against a broad range of cancers, has rendered the taxanes one of the most important new classes of anticancer agents. Interest in the taxanes began in 1963, when a crude extract of the bark of the Pacific yew tree, *Taxus brevifolia*, was shown to have broad activity in preclinical tumor models. In 1971, paclitaxel was identified as the active constituent of the bark extract.[135,136] The initial development of paclitaxel was hampered by the limited supply of its primary source; the difficulties inherent in large-scale isolation, extraction, and preparation of bulk compound for a natural product; and its poor aqueous solubility.[135–137] Interest was maintained during this time by the characterization of its novel mechanism of cytotoxic action and the availability of an adequate drug supply for requisite preclinical and limited clinical evaluations. The early search for taxanes derived from more

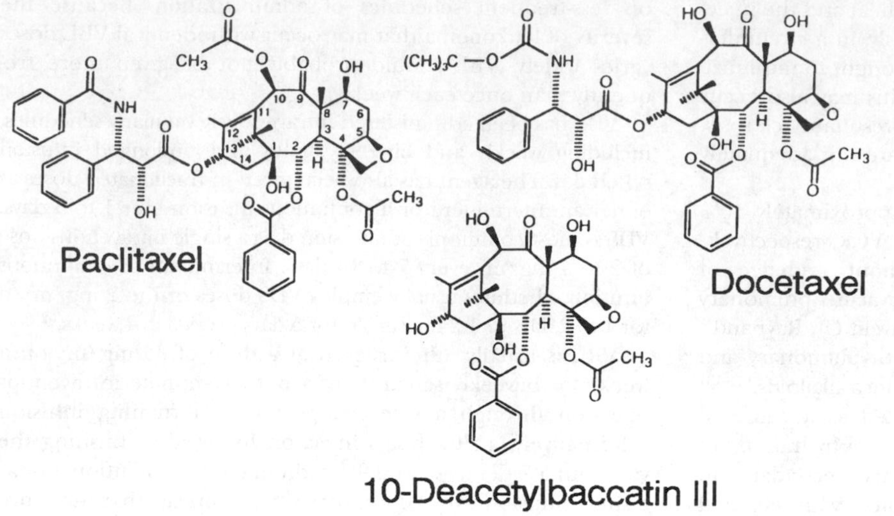

FIGURE 19.7-3. Structures of paclitaxel, docetaxel, and a precursor 10-deacetylbaccatin III.

abundant and renewable resources led to the development of docetaxel, which is synthesized by the addition of a side chain to 10-deacetylbaccatin III, an inactive taxane precursor found in the needles and other components of more abundant yew species.[137,138] The supply of paclitaxel is no longer a limiting issue because the agent is also produced semisynthetically from 10-deacetylbaccatin III and other abundant precursors.

The structures of paclitaxel, docetaxel, and their precursor 10-deacetylbaccatin III are shown in Figure 19.7-3. The taxanes are complex esters consisting of a 15-member taxane ring system linked to an unusual 4-member oxetan ring. The taxane rings of both paclitaxel and docetaxel (but not 10-deacetylbaccatin III) are linked to an ester side chain attached to the C13 position of the ring, which is essential for antimicrotubule and antitumor activity. The structures of paclitaxel and docetaxel differ in substitutions at the C10 taxane ring position and on the ester side chain attached at C13.

The most impressive clinical activity of paclitaxel has been in patients with ovarian and breast cancers.[135–141] Paclitaxel initially received regulatory approval in the United States and many other countries for the treatment of patients with ovarian cancer after failure of first-line or subsequent chemotherapy. It subsequently received regulatory approval for patients with advanced breast cancer after failure of combination chemotherapy or at relapse within 6 months of adjuvant chemotherapy. Its use in combination with a platinum compound as primary induction therapy in suboptimally debulked stage III or IV ovarian cancer and as a component of adjuvant chemotherapy after primary local treatment in high-risk patients with early-stage breast cancer has demonstrated a survival advantage in randomized phase III studies.[139,141] Paclitaxel has also received regulatory approval in the United States for second-line treatment of Kaposi's sarcoma associated with AIDS, in combination with cisplatin as primary treatment of non–small cell lung cancer, and as a component of adjuvant chemotherapy in high-risk lymph node–positive breast cancer.[139–143]

Docetaxel initially received regulatory approval in the United States for patients with metastatic breast cancer that has progressed on or relapsing after anthracycline-based chemotherapy, which was later broadened to a general second-line indication.[137,138] Its role as a component of adjuvant and neoadjuvant chemotherapy after local treatment of early-stage breast cancer and first-line chemotherapy for locally advanced or metastatic breast cancer is being evaluated. Furthermore, docetaxel has received regulatory approval in many countries for treatment of locally advanced or metastatic non–small cell lung carcinoma and in the United States for treatment of non–small cell lung cancer after failure of cisplatin-based therapy. The clinical antitumor spectra for paclitaxel and docetaxel are similar, with activity noted in many other diverse tumor types that are generally refractory to conventional therapies, including lymphoma, and small cell lung, head and neck, esophageal, endometrial, bladder, and germ cell carcinomas.

MECHANISMS OF ACTION

Schiff et al.,[144] Schiff and Horwitz,[145] and Manfredi et al.[146] initially identified the unique mechanism of action for paclitaxel in 1979. The taxanes bind to tubulin polymers (microtubules) at binding sites that are distinct from exchangeable GTP, colchicine, podophyllotoxin, and the vinca alkaloids. Paclitaxel binds preferentially to the N-terminal 31 amino acids of the β-tubulin subunit, although additional sites of interaction on β-tubulin and α-tubulin may also be involved.[147,148] The binding of paclitaxel to polymerized tubulin is reversible, with a binding constant of approximately 1 μmol.[146,149] Docetaxel, which most likely shares the same tubulin-binding site as paclitaxel, appears to have a 1.9-fold higher affinity for the site.[149] Tubulin assembly induced by docetaxel also proceeds with a critical protein concentration that is 2.1-fold lower than that of paclitaxel.[149] However, these differences may not translate into greater therapeutic indices for docetaxel in the clinic, as greater potency may also portend more severe toxicity at identical drug concentrations *in vivo*. Nevertheless, the results of both preclinical and clinical studies suggest that the taxanes may not be completely cross-resistant.[150,151]

The taxanes stabilize the microtubule against depolymerization, thereby disrupting normal microtubule dynamics.[2,25,144–146,152–157] They profoundly alter the tubulin dissociation rate constants at both ends of the microtubule, suppressing both treadmilling and dynamic instability. Association rate constants are not appreciably affected. The ability of the taxanes to induce polymerization is associated with stoichiometric drug binding to microtubules, which occurs at submicromolar concentrations that are readily achieved in the clinic. At substoichiometric concentrations, the taxanes suppress microtubule dynamics without increasing the amount of polymerized tubulin.[152] Taxane-treated microtubules are very stable, resisting depolymerization by cold, calcium ions, dilution, and other mitotic drugs. This stability inhibits the dynamic reorganization of the microtubule network, which is essential for normal function during both mitosis and interphase.

Both stoichiometric and substoichiometric binding of the taxanes inhibit the proliferation of cells, principally by inducing a sustained mitotic block at the metaphase-anaphase boundary; however, the taxanes also affect interphase microtubules in nonproliferating cells.[25,144,152] Distinct morphologic evidence that the taxanes affect microtubules during interphase and mitosis include the formation of microtubule bundles during the nonmitotic cell cycle phases and multiple mitotic spindle asters during mitosis.[154] Many taxane-induced disturbances in cellular processes lead to apoptosis or programmed cell death (discussed later in the section Taxanes, Drug Resistance, and in Chapter 7).[56,57,157–166] On removal of the drug after treatment, even at substoichiometric concentrations that do not increase microtubule mass, cells exit from mitosis but do not continue to proliferate. Instead, the cells undergo apoptosis, and cell death ensues in 2 to 3 days. Although the precise mechanism by which microtubule disturbances lead to apoptosis has not been determined, the taxanes interact with numerous substances, including regulatory molecules and oncogenes that bind to the mitotic apparatus. Paclitaxel has been reported to induce transcription factors and enzymes that govern proliferation, apoptosis, and inflammation and, interestingly, some of these effects, such as the induction of tumor necrosis factor-α.[157,167] The taxanes also inhibit angiogenic activity at concentrations below those that induce cytotoxicity.[165,168,169]

Both paclitaxel and docetaxel have been shown to enhance the effects of ionizing radiation *in vitro* at clinically achievable concentrations (<50 nmol) and *in vivo*, which may related to the inhibition of cell-cycle progression in the G_2 phase, which is the most radiosensitive phase of the cell cycle.[170–172]

MECHANISMS OF RESISTANCE

The best characterized mechanism of resistance to the taxanes is the MDR phenotype, mediated by the 170-kD P-gp efflux pump, encoded by the *mdr*1 gene (discussed previously in the section Vinca Alkaloids, Mechanisms of Resistance).[44–49,173,174] The MDR protein has been shown to be an efficient transporter of the vinca alkaloids but not of the taxanes.[45,175,176] The results of early studies evaluating the role of MDR in the clinic indicate that cross-resistance to the taxanes and anthracycline is incomplete, which has significant clinical ramifications in treating breast cancer.[140] Strategies aimed at reversing drug resistance in the clinic with various types of P-gp substrates and inhibitors are also being evaluated, but the interpretation of the results is confounded by the effects of P-gp modulators on taxane clearance.[177,178]

Several taxane-resistant mutant cell lines that have structurally altered α- and β-tubulin proteins and an impaired ability to polymerize into microtubules also have been identified (discussed previously in the section Vinca Alkaloids, Mechanisms of Resistance).[54,157,179] These mutants lack normal interpolar mitotic spindles and have an inherently slow rate of microtubule assembly, which is normalized in the presence of the drug. Mutants with "hypostable" microtubules exhibit collateral sensitivity to the vinca alkaloids. A number of cell lines resistant to tubulin-binding agents, including the taxanes, have been shown to have alterations in tubulin content, expression of tubulin isotypes, tubulin polymerization dynamics, or tubulin isotype content.[180–185] Mutations of tubulin isotype genes have also been reported in taxane-resistant cell lines, and β-tubulin gene mutations have been reported to be a strong determinant of paclitaxel resistance in a series of patients with non–small lung cancer.[186]

The regulation and integrity of genes that regulate apoptosis, such as *p53, bcl-2, and bcl-x*, may be determinants of sensitivity to the taxanes.[56,57,157,162–164,187,188] MAPs are also likely to be involved in these mechanisms of resistance to drug-induced apoptosis, as illustrated by the fact that MAP4, which is negatively regulated by wild-type *p53*, has been shown to increase the sensitivity to paclitaxel.[189,190] It has been proposed that paclitaxel induces apoptosis through two different mechanisms—a *p53*-independent pathway in cells blocked in prophase and a *p53*-dependent mechanism in cells that accumulate in the G_1 cell-cycle phase—and requires functional *p53*.[157,191] However, there are conflicting experimental data as to the role of *p53* as a determinant of cell sensitivity to paclitaxel and other antitumor agents. Several lines of experimental evidence suggest that the induction of p53 in cells treated with paclitaxel represents a mechanism of drug resistance.[192,193] The taxanes have been also shown to modulate the function of genes involved in apoptotic regulation and in the disruption of microtubule dynamics by paclitaxel and other antimicrotubule drugs, and docetaxel results in the phosphorylation of such regulatory proteins as Bcl-x_L and Bcl-2, thereby annulling the antiapoptotic functions of these regulators.[194,195]

Interestingly, paclitaxel-resistant cell lines, which have mutations in tubulin and fail to exhibit phosphorylation of Bcl-x_L after paclitaxel treatment, have been described.[56] These cells demonstrate Bcl-x_L phosphorylation in the presence of other antimicrotubule agents, suggesting that apoptosis mediated by paclitaxel is related to the drug's ability to interact with microtubules.

PHARMACOLOGY

The taxanes are commonly administered by intravenous infusion at doses ranging from 175 to 225 mg/m^2 over 3 hours (for paclitaxel) or 75 to 100 mg/m^2 over 1 hour (for docetaxel) every 3 weeks. Various other administration schedules have been evaluated (discussed later in the section Administration, Dose, and Schedule). The oral bioavailability of both paclitaxel and docetaxel is poor, owing in part to the constitutive overexpression of P-gp by enterocytes or first-pass metabolism in the liver or intestines (or both). However, biologically relevant plasma concentrations are transiently achieved if the taxanes are administered orally after treatment with oral cyclosporin or other modulators of P-gp and cytochrome P-450 mixed-function oxidases.[196,197] As shown in Table 19.7-2, paclitaxel and docetaxel share the following pharmacologic characteristics: large volumes of distribution, rapid and avid binding to all tissues except for the unperturbed central nervous system, long terminal half-lives and substantial hepatic metabolism, biliary excretion, and fecal elimination.

Paclitaxel

Pharmacologic studies of paclitaxel on both long and short administration schedules have been performed (discussed later

TABLE 19.7-2. Taxanes: Comparative Pharmacokinetic and Toxicologic Characteristics

	Paclitaxel	*Docetaxel*
Standard adult dose range (mg/m²/3 wk)	135 (24-h infusion), 175–225 (3-h infusion)	75–100 (1-h infusion)
Pharmacokinetic behavior	Saturable elimination and distribution	Triphasic
Plasma half-lives (terminal)	10–20 h	10–20 h
Clearance	20–25 L/h[a]	36 L/h
Primary route	Hepatic metabolism and biliary elimination	Hepatic metabolism and biliary elimination
Principal toxicity	Neutropenia	Neutropenia
Other toxicities	Alopecia, neurotoxicity, myalgia, hypersensitivity reactions, asthenia	Alopecia, skin and nail toxicity, asthenia, myalgia, fluid retention, neurotoxicity, hypersensitivity reactions

[a]Dose schedule: 175 mg/m² over 3 hours.

in the section Administration, Dose, Schedule). In early studies that principally evaluated prolonged (6- and 24-hour) schedules, substantial interpatient variability was noted, and nonlinear, dose-dependent behavior was not observed.[136,137,198] In these studies, drug disposition was characterized as a biphasic process, with values for alpha and beta half-lives averaging approximately 20 minutes and 6 hours, respectively. However, more recent studies of paclitaxel administered on shorter schedules, particularly as a 3-hour infusion, indicate that the pharmacokinetic behavior of paclitaxel is nonlinear.[199–203] Nonlinearity occurs with all administration schedules, but it is more apparent with shorter infusions that result in higher plasma paclitaxel concentrations that more effectively saturate both drug elimination and tissue distribution processes. Both saturable distribution and elimination processes may be, in part, responsible for paclitaxel's nonlinear behavior, with tissue distribution becoming effectively saturated at lower drug concentrations (achieved with paclitaxel doses <175 mg/m² over 3 hours) compared to elimination processes that are effectively saturated at higher concentrations (achieved with paclitaxel doses >175 mg/m² over 3 hours). The use of shorter infusion schedules also results in higher plasma concentrations of paclitaxel's polyoxyethylated castor oil vehicle, which may also be responsible for this nonlinearity.[202] This nonlinear profile may have several important clinical implications, particularly regarding dose modifications, because dose escalation may result in a disproportionate increase in drug exposure and hence toxicity, whereas dose reductions may result in a disproportionate decrease in drug exposure, thereby decreasing antitumor activity.

Paclitaxel's volume of distribution is much larger than the volume of total body water, indicating extensive drug binding to plasma proteins or other tissue elements, probably tubulin. Plasma protein binding is high (>95%) and readily reversible.[198] Drug binding to platelets is extensive and saturable, and animal distribution studies with radiolabeled paclitaxel indicate extensive drug uptake and retention by virtually all tissues, except for the normal brain and testes.[204] In humans, peak plasma concentrations achieved with 3- to 96-hour schedules (>0.05 to 10 μmol) and drug concentrations in third-space fluid collections, such as ascites (>0.1 μmol), are capable of inducing significant biologic effects *in vitro*, but drug penetration into the normal central nervous system is negligible.[198,204,205]

The liver is the principal organ involved with paclitaxel clearance, which metabolizes and excretes both paclitaxel and metabolites into the bile.[198,206–209] Ninety-eight percent of radioactivity is recovered from feces collected for 6 days after rats are treated with radiolabeled paclitaxel, and approximately 71% of an administered dose of paclitaxel is excreted in the feces over 5 days as either parent compound or metabolites in humans, with 6α-hydroxypaclitaxel being the largest component and accounting for 26% of the dose. Only 5% is unchanged paclitaxel. Renal clearance of paclitaxel and metabolites is minimal, accounting for 14% of the administered dose.[198] In humans, cytochrome P-450 mixed-function oxidases are responsible for the bulk of drug disposition, specifically the isoenzymes CYP2C8, and CYP3A4, which metabolize paclitaxel to hydroxylated 6α-hydroxypaclitaxel (major) and another hydroxylated metabolite, both of which are inactive.

Pharmacodynamic analyses as part of individual phase I and II trials demonstrated that several pharmacokinetic indices of drug exposure can be related to the various toxicities of paclitaxel, the most important and consistent of which is the relationship between the severity of neutropenia and the duration of drug exposure above biologically relevant plasma concentrations ranging from 0.05 to 0.1 μmol.[198–201,210] However, a prospective analysis of pharmacokinetic determinants of outcome in several hundred patients with advanced non–small cell lung cancer treated with the combination of cisplatin and paclitaxel at either 135 or 250 mg/m² over 24 hours demonstrated that the magnitude of the steady-state plasma paclitaxel concentration correlated poorly with antitumor activity, disease-free survival, and overall survival.[211]

Docetaxel

The pharmacokinetics of docetaxel on a 1-hour schedule are linear at doses of 115 mg/m² or less and optimally fit a three-compartment model.[137,138,212–216] Terminal half-lives ranging from 11.1 to 18.5 hours have been reported. In one population study, plasma concentration data were optimally fit by a three-compartment model, and the following pharmacokinetic parameters were generated: $t_{1/2\gamma}$ of 12.4 hours, clearance of 1 L/h/m², and steady-state volume of distribution of 74 L/m².[212–214] The most important determinants of docetaxel clearance were the body surface area, hepatic function, and plasma α1–acid glycoprotein concentration, whereas age and albumin level had significant (albeit minor) influences on clearance. As with paclitaxel, plasma protein binding is high (>80% to 90%), and binding is primarily to α1–acid glycoprotein, albumin, and lipoproteins.[213] Docetaxel is also distributed to all tissues except the central nervous system.[212,217] In both dogs and mice treated with radiolabeled drug, fecal excretion accounts for 70% to 80% of total radioactivity, whereas urinary excretion accounts for 10% or less.[212,217] The hepatic cytochrome P-450 mixed-function oxidases, particularly isoforms CYP3A4 and CYP3A5, are primarily involved in biotransformation that, in contrast to paclitaxel, principally affects the C13 side chain and not the taxane ring.[212,213,218–220]

The main pharmacokinetic determinants of toxicity, particularly the principal toxicity neutropenia, are drug exposure and the time that plasma concentrations exceed biologically relevant concentrations.[213,214] A population pharmacodynamic analysis of determinants of outcome in phase II trials of docetaxel revealed that the most important determinants of the time to progression in patients with metastatic breast cancer are the pretreatment plasma concentration of α1–acid glycoprotein, number of prior chemotherapeutic regimens, and number of disease sites, whereas both drug exposure and the pretreatment plasma concentration of α1–acid glycoprotein were strong positive determinants of time to progression in patients with advanced lung cancer treated with docetaxel.[214] Conversely, the pretreatment plasma level of α1–acid glycoprotein was negatively—albeit significantly—related to the probability of experiencing both severe neutropenia and febrile neutropenia.

DRUG INTERACTIONS

Both sequence-dependent pharmacokinetic and toxicologic interactions between paclitaxel and several other chemotherapy agents have been noted.[198] The sequence of cisplatin followed by paclitaxel (24-hour schedule) induces more profound neutropenia than the reverse sequence, which is explained by a 33% reduction in the clearance of paclitaxel after cisplatin.[221] The least toxic sequence—paclitaxel before cisplatin—was demonstrated to induce more cytotoxicity *in vitro*; therefore, this drug sequence was selected for further clinical development.[222] However, sequence dependence does not appear to be a clinically relevant phenomenon on shorter schedules. Treatment with paclitaxel on either a 3- or 24-hour schedule followed by carboplatin has been demonstrated to produce equivalent neutropenia and less thrombocytopenia as compared to carboplatin as a single agent, which is not explained by pharmacokinetic interactions.[223,224] Although sequence dependence has not been noted with carboplatin and paclitaxel in clinical studies, this phenomenon has been noted with other paclitaxel-based chemotherapy combinations, the most important of which involve the anthracyclines.[225] Both neutropenia and mucositis are more severe when paclitaxel on a 24-hour schedule is administered before doxorubicin, compared to the reverse sequence, which is most likely due to an approximately 32% reduction in the clearance of doxorubicin and doxorubicinol when it is administered after paclitaxel.[225,226] Although neither sequence-dependent pharmacologic interactions nor toxicologic interactions between doxorubicin and paclitaxel on a shorter (3-hour) schedule have been noted, pharmacologic interactions occur with both sequences, and combined treatment with paclitaxel (3-hour schedule) and doxorubicin as a bolus infusion has been associated with a higher frequency of congestive cardiotoxicity than would have been expected from an equivalent cumulative doxorubicin dose given without paclitaxel (discussed later in the section Toxicity).[227] Similar decrements in the clearance of epirubicin and its metabolites have also been noted in studies of paclitaxel combined with epirubicin, but a similar enhancement of cardiotoxicity has not been observed.[228] The precise etiology for these interactions is unclear; however, competition for the hepatic or biliary P-gp transport of the anthracyclines with paclitaxel or its polyoxyethylated castor oil vehicle (or both) is a logical explanation.[226,229] The vehicle is suspected because similar effects have not been noted with docetaxel, which is not formulated in polyoxyethylated castor oil. Hematologic toxicity has been more profound with the sequence of cyclophosphamide before paclitaxel (24-hour schedule) than the reverse sequence.[230] In human tumor xenografts, both paclitaxel and docetaxel have been demonstrated to induce thymidine phosphorylase activity, which may increase the metabolic activation of the oral fluoropyrimidine prodrug capecitabine.[231]

Drug interactions may also result from the effects of other classes of drugs on the cytochrome P-450–dependent metabolism of the taxanes. Various inducers of cytochrome P-450 mixed-function oxidases, such as the anticonvulsants phenytoin and phenobarbital, accelerate in the metabolism of both paclitaxel and docetaxel in human microsomal studies and in both children and adults who are concurrently receiving treatment with these anticonvulsants, as manifested by rapid drug clearance and tolerance of high drug doses.[209,219,232–234] Conversely, many types of agents that inhibit cytochrome P-450 mixed-function oxidases, such as orphenadrine, erythromycin, cimetidine, testosterone, ketoconazole, fluconazole, midazolam, polyoxyethylated castor oil, and corticosteroids, interfere with the metabolism of paclitaxel and docetaxel in human microsomes *in vitro*; however, the inhibitory concentrations of these agents exceed those achieved in clinical practice, and the clinical relevance of these findings is not known.[207–209,217–220,235] Although there has been concern that the use of corticosteroids and different H_2-receptor antagonists with variable cytochrome P-450 inhibitory activities as components of premedication regimens may differentially affect drug clearance and hence toxicity, neither toxicologic nor pharmacologic differences between the agents were noted in a randomized clinical trial.[236]

TOXICITY

Myelosuppression is the principal toxicity of paclitaxel and docetaxel. However, despite similar structures, these agents differ modestly in their toxicity spectra.

Paclitaxel

Neutropenia is the principal toxicity of paclitaxel. The onset is usually on days 8 to 10, and recovery is generally complete by days 15 to 21. The main clinical determinant for the severity of neutropenia is the extent of prior myelosuppressive therapy. Neutropenia is noncumulative, and the duration of severe neutropenia, even in heavily pretreated patients, is usually brief. The most important pharmacologic determinant of the severity of neutropenia is the duration that plasma concentrations are maintained above biologically relevant levels (0.05 to 0.10 μmol; discussed earlier in the section Pharmacology), which may explain why neutropenia is more severe with longer infusion schedules.[237] This does not necessarily mean that longer schedules will portend optimal antitumor activity in the clinic. Instead, most randomized clinical data do not indicate that there is an optimal schedule for any particular tumor, although treatment with higher doses should be considered if shorter schedules are used.[238] At paclitaxel doses exceeding 175 mg/m^2 on a 24-hour schedule and 225 mg/m^2 on a 3-hour schedule, nadir neutrophil counts are typically less than 500 µL for fewer than 5 days in most courses, even in untreated patients. Even patients who have received extensive prior therapy can usually tolerate paclitaxel doses of 175 to 200 mg/m^2 over 3 or 24 hours. More frequent administration schedules (e.g., weekly treatment) have been associated with less severe neutropenia as compared to single-dose schedules (discussed later in the section Administration, Dose, and Schedule). Severe thrombocytopenia and anemia are unusual, except in heavily pretreated patients.

Although the incidence of major hypersensitivity reactions in early phase I trials approached 30%, the incidence is 1% to 3% with effective prophylaxis.[135,136,237,239,240] Most major reactions, which are characterized by dyspnea with bronchospasm, urticaria, and hypotension, occur within the first 10 minutes after the first (and less frequently after the second) treatment and resolve completely after stopping treatment and occasionally occur after treatment with antihistamines, fluids, and vasopressors. Patients who have major reactions have been rechallenged successfully after receiving high doses of corticosteroids, but this approach has not always been successful.[241,242] Although minor reactions, such as flushing and rashes, have been noted in as many as 40% of patients, minor hypersensitivity reactions do not portend the development of major reactions. The hypersensitivity reactions are most likely caused by a nonimmunologically mediated release of histamine or histamine-like substances, owing to the taxane moiety or, more likely, its polyoxyethylated castor oil vehicle, possibly through complement activation.[243] Although the incidence of major hypersensitivity reactions is reduced with lower administration rates and longer infusion durations, the rates of major reactions are low on both 3- and 24-hour schedules when patients are premedicated with corticosteroids and both H_1- and H_2-receptor antagonists (discussed later in the section Administration, Dose, and Schedule).[237] In an assessment of the relative safety of two different paclitaxel schedules (3 vs. 24 hours), the rates of major reactions were low and similar (2.1% vs. 1.0%) in patients receiving paclitaxel for 3 or 24 hours, respectively, with premedication.[237]

Paclitaxel induces a peripheral neuropathy characterized by sensory symptoms, such as numbness in a symmetric glove-and-stocking distribution.[244–246] Neurologic examination reveals sensory loss and loss of deep tendon reflexes. Neurophysiologic studies support a primary disruption of neuronal microtubules resulting in axonal degeneration and demyelination as the primary pathogenic mechanism; however, manifestations suggestive of microtubule disruption resulting in a neuronopathy may be noted, particularly at higher doses or when combined with other neurotoxic agents, such as cisplatin.[245] Severe neurotoxicity is uncommon when paclitaxel is given alone at doses below 200 mg/m^2 on a 3- or 24-hour schedule every 3 weeks or below 100 mg/m^2 on a continuous weekly schedule, but almost all patients experience mild or moderate effects. Symptoms may begin as soon as 24 to 72 hours after treatment with higher doses (250 mg/m^2 or greater) but usually occur only after multiple courses at 135 to 250 mg/m^2 every 3 weeks. Neurotoxicity is generally more pronounced when paclitaxel is administered on short infusion schedules, indicating that peak plasma concentration is a principal determinant. The combination of paclitaxel on a 3-hour schedule and cisplatin is particularly neurotoxic. Motor and autonomic dysfunction may occur, especially at high doses and in patients with preexisting neuropathies due to diabetes mellitus and alcoholism. Transient myalgia, usually noted 24 to 48 hours after therapy, is also common, and a myopathy has been described in patients receiving high doses with cisplatin. Although several measures, such as the administration of amifostine, glutamate, and pyridoxine, appear to reduce the neurotoxic effects of paclitaxel in experimental models, there is no convincing clinical evidence that any specific measure is effective at ameliorating existing manifestations or preventing the development or worsening or neurotoxicity.[244,246] Optic nerve disturbances, manifested by scintillating scotoma, may also occur.[247,248] Acute encephalopathy, which can progress to coma and death, has been reported after treatment with high doses (600 mg/m^2 or greater).[249]

Paclitaxel causes cardiac rhythm disturbances, but the clinical relevance of these effects is not known.[239,250–252] The most common rhythm disturbance, a transient bradycardia, was noted in 29% of patients in one trial. [239,250,251] Isolated asymptomatic bradycardia without hemodynamic effects does not appear to be an indication for discontinuing paclitaxel. More important bradyarrhythmias, including Mobitz type I (Wenckeback syndrome), Mobitz type II, and third-degree heart block, have been noted, but the incidence in a large National Cancer Institute database was only 0.1%.[251] Most documented episodes have been asymptomatic. These events primarily occurred in patients enrolled in early trials that required continuous cardiac monitoring, indicating that second- and third-degree heart block are likely underreported because such monitoring is not usually performed. These bradyarrhythmias are probably caused by paclitaxel, as related taxanes affect cardiac automaticity and conduction, and similar disturbances have occurred in humans and animals who have ingested various species of yew plants. Myocardial infarction, cardiac ischemia, atrial arrhythmias, and ventricular tachycardia have been noted, but whether there is a causal relationship between paclitaxel and these events is uncertain.

There is no evidence that chronic, long-term treatment with paclitaxel causes progressive cardiac dysfunction. Routine cardiac monitoring during paclitaxel therapy is not necessary but is advisable for patients who may not be able to tolerate bradyarrhythmias, such as those with atrioventricular conduction disturbances or ventricular dysfunction. Although patients with a wide range of cardiac abnormalities and cardiac histories were broadly and empirically restricted from participating in early clinical trials, paclitaxel treatment has been reported to be well tolerated in a small series of gynecologic cancer patients with major cardiac risk factors.[252] On the other hand, repetitive treatment of patients with the combined regimen of paclitaxel on a 3-hour schedule and doxorubicin as a brief infusion is associated with a higher frequency of congestive cardiotoxicity than would be expected to occur with the same cumulative doxorubicin dose given without paclitaxel (discussed previously in the section Drug Interactions).[226,227] In one study of previously untreated women with advanced breast cancer treated with escalating doses of paclitaxel as a 3-hour infusion and doxorubicin, 60 mg/m^2 to a cumulative dose of 480 mg/m^2, which would be predicted to result in a less than 5% incidence of congestive cardiotoxicity in patients treated with doxorubicin alone, the incidence of congestive cardiotoxicity was approximately 25%.[227] However, the incidence of cardiotoxicity was less than 5% when similar patients received identical schedules of paclitaxel and doxorubicin, but the cumulative doxorubicin dose did not exceed 360 mg/m^2. Both experimental and early clinical results suggest that dexrazoxane may reduce the cardiotoxicity of the doxorubicin and paclitaxel combination.[253,254] The incidence of congestive heart failure was also significantly higher in breast cancer patients treated with the combination of trastuzumab and paclitaxel than paclitaxel alone in a phase III trial; therefore, careful monitoring of patients receiving this combination is warranted.[255]

Drug-related gastrointestinal effects, such as vomiting and diarrhea, are uncommon. Higher paclitaxel doses may cause mucositis, especially in patients with leukemia who may be more prone to mucosal barrier breakdown or in patients receiving 96-hour infusions.[256,257] Rare cases of neutropenic enterocolitis and gastrointestinal necrosis have been noted, particularly in patients given high doses of paclitaxel in combination with doxorubicin or cyclophosphamide.[230,239,258,259] Severe hepatotoxicity and pancreatitis have also been noted, but these events are rare.[260,261] Acute bilateral pneumonitis has been reported in fewer than 1% of patients treated on a 3-hour schedule in one series, and both interstitial and parenchymal pulmonary toxicity have been reported, but clinically significant pulmonary effects are uncommon.[262,263]

Paclitaxel also induces reversible alopecia of the scalp, but all body hair is usually lost with cumulative therapy. Although the agent is often not considered a vesicant, extravasation of large volumes can cause moderate soft tissue injury. Inflammation at the injection site and along the course of an injected vein may occur. Alopecia occurs in most patients. Nail disorders have been reported, particularly in patients treated on weekly schedules.[264] Recall reactions in previously irradiated sites have also been noted.

Docetaxel

Neutropenia is the principal toxicity of docetaxel.[137,138,265] At a dose of 100 mg/m^2, neutrophil counts are below 500/μL in most patients. Similar to paclitaxel, the onset of neutropenia occurs on approximately day 8, and complete resolution typically occurs by days 15 to 21. As with paclitaxel, neutropenia is significantly less when low doses are administered frequently (i.e., on a weekly schedule; discussed later in the section Administration, Dose, and Schedule). The most important determinant of neutropenia is the extent of prior treatment. Significant effects on platelets and red blood cells are uncommon.

Although docetaxel is not formulated in polyoxyethylated castor oil, hypersensitivity reactions have been reported in approximately 31% of patients receiving docetaxel without premedications in early phase II studies.[137,138,265] As with paclitaxel, major reactions characterized by dyspnea, bronchospasm, and hypotension typically occur during the first two courses and within minutes after the start of treatment. Signs and symptoms generally resolve within 15 minutes after cessation of treatment, and docetaxel is usually able to be reinstituted without sequelae, occasionally after treatment with an H_1-receptor antagonist. However, most hypersensitivity reactions are minor. Both the incidence and severity of hypersensitivity reactions appear to be reduced by premedication with corticosteroids and H_1- and H_2-receptor antagonists (discussed later in the section Administration, Dose, and Schedule). Like paclitaxel, patients who experience major reactions have been retreated successfully after the resolution of symptoms and after treatment with corticosteroids and H_1-receptor antagonists.

Docetaxel induces a unique fluid retention syndrome characterized by edema, weight gain, and third-space fluid collection.[137,138,265–267] Fluid retention is cumulative and does not appear to be due to hypoalbuminemia or cardiac, renal, or hepatic dysfunction. Instead, several lines of evidence indicate that it is due to increased capillary permeability.[266] Capillary filtration studies in patients who were not receiving corticosteroid premedication have revealed a two-stage process, with progressive congestion of the interstitial space by proteins and water starting between the second and fourth course, followed by insufficient lymphatic drainage.[266] In early studies in which prophylactic medication was not used, fluid retention was not usually significant at cumulative docetaxel doses below 400 mg/m^2; however, the incidence and severity of fluid retention increased sharply at cumulative doses of 400 mg/m^2 or greater and often resulted in the delay or termination of treatment. Prophylactic treatment with corticosteroids with or without H_1- and H_2-receptor antagonists have been demonstrated to reduce the overall incidence of fluid retention and increase the number of courses and cumulative docetaxel dose before the onset of this toxicity (discussed later in the section Administration, Dose, and Schedule).[267] Fluid retention typically resolves slowly after docetaxel is stopped, with complete resolution occurring several months after treatment in patients with severe toxicity. Aggressive and early treatment with progressively more potent diuretics starting with potassium-sparing diuretics has been successfully used to manage fluid retention. The incidence of fluid retention appears to be lower in studies using lower doses (60 to 75 mg/m^2) of docetaxel during each course, but this may be due to the administration of lower overall cumulative doses, and the effects of lower doses on antitumor activity are unknown.

Skin toxicity may occur in as many as 50% to 75% of patients[137,138,265,268]; however, premedication may reduce the overall incidence of this effect. An erythematous pruritic maculopapular rash that affects the forearms, hands, or feet is typical. Other cutaneous effects include desquamation of the hands and feet, palmar-plantar erythrodysesthesia that may respond to pyridoxine or cooling,[269,270] and onychodystrophy characterized by brown discoloration, ridging, onycholysis, soreness, and brittleness and loss of the nail plate.

Both neurosensory and neuromuscular effects are generally less frequent and less severe with docetaxel as compared to paclitaxel. Mild to moderate peripheral neurotoxicity occurs in approximately 40% of previously untreated patients,[137,138,265,271,272] and patients who were previously treated with cisplatin appear to be particularly susceptible, with the incidence approaching 74% in one trial.[273] The neurotoxicity is qualitatively similar to that of paclitaxel. Patients typically complain of paresthesia and numbness, but peripheral motor effects may also occur. Severe toxicity has been unusual after repetitive treatment with docetaxel doses less than 100 mg/m^2, except in patients with antecedent disorders, such as alcohol abuse. Transient arthralgia and myalgia are occasionally noted within days after treatment. Malaise or asthenia have been prominent complaints in patients who have been treated with large cumulative doses, particularly when docetaxel is administered on a continuous weekly schedule.[137,138,265,274] Stomatitis appears to occur more frequently with docetaxel than paclitaxel, particularly with prolonged infusions, which are utilized rarely. Mild to moderate conjunctivitis, which is responsive to topical corticosteroids, may also occur, particularly with weekly administration. Nausea, vomiting, and diarrhea have also been observed, but severe gastrointestinal toxicity is rare.

ADMINISTRATION, DOSE, AND SCHEDULE

Paclitaxel

Many investigations have focused on optimal dosing and scheduling since the regulatory approval of paclitaxel.[238] Early clinical studies were limited to the 24-hour schedule, largely owing to an apparent increased rate of severe hypersensitivity reactions on shorter schedules, but the development of effective premedication regimens has facilitated evaluations of a broad range of dosing schedules. Although paclitaxel, 135 mg/m^2 on a 24-hour schedule, was initially approved for patients with refractory and recurrent ovarian cancer, regulatory approval was subsequently obtained for paclitaxel, 175 mg/m^2 on a 3-hour schedule. In patients with advanced breast and ovarian cancers, the cumulative body of randomized study results indicate that both schedules are equivalent, particularly with regard to event-free survival and overall survival, although response rates have occasionally been superior with the 24-hour infusion.[238,275]

Intriguing results were initially obtained with more protracted schedules, such as a 96-hour infusion schedule in patients with advanced breast cancer.[140,238,276] The development of such schedules was based on the observation that duration of exposure above a biologically relevant threshold is one of the most important determinants of cytotoxicity *in vitro* (discussed earlier in the section Pharmacology), but there has been no clear evidence that protracted infusion schedules are superior to shorter schedules with regard to clinical efficacy or toxicity.[238,276–278] The extensive and rapid distribution of the taxanes to peripheral tissues and the avid and protracted tissue binding of these agents may explain the lack of substantial differences in antitumor activity between short and more protracted administration schedules despite substantial differences *in vitro*. There has also been considerable interest in intermittent schedules, particularly those in which paclitaxel is administered as a 1-hour infusion weekly, which results in substantially less myelosuppression than conventional 3- and 24-hour every 3-week schedules.[279,280] However, the reports that antitumor activity on weekly schedules is superior to that noted with less frequent schedules are largely anecdotal, and randomized trials are in progress. Nevertheless, the weekly schedule may be advantageous for patients who are at high risk of developing severe myelosuppression.

Paclitaxel is generally administered every 3 weeks at a dose of 175 mg/m^2 over 3 hours or 135 to 175 mg/m^2 over 24 hours. Several phase III studies in patients with advanced lung, head and neck, and ovarian cancers have consistently failed to show that paclitaxel doses greater than 135 to 175 mg/m^2 on a 24-hour schedule are superior to conventional doses.[143,238,281] Nearly identical results have been obtained in a phase III study in patients with metastatic breast cancer, in which efficacy was not increased in patients treated with paclitaxel doses greater than 175 mg/m^2 on a 3-hour schedule.[155,277,326] The following doses have been recommended on less conventional schedules: 200 mg/m^2 over 1 hour as either a single dose or 3 divided doses every 3 weeks; 140 mg/m^2 over 96 hours every 3 weeks; and 80 to 100 mg/m^2 weekly. The most common schedules evaluated in patients with AIDS-associated Kaposi's sarcoma are paclitaxel, 135 mg/m^2 over 3 or 24 hours every 3 weeks, and 100 mg/m^2 every 2 weeks.[142] Paclitaxel has also been administered into the pleural and peritoneal cavities.[282,283] Biologically relevant plasma concentrations have been achieved with intraperitoneal administration, and concentrations in the peritoneal cavity are several orders of magnitude greater than plasma concentrations.[282]

The following premedication is recommended to prevent major hypersensitivity reactions: dexamethasone, 20 mg orally or intravenously, 12 and 6 hours before treatment; an H_1-receptor antagonist (such as diphenhydramine, 50 mg intravenously) 30 minutes before treatment; and an H_2-receptor antagonist (such as cimetidine, 300 mg; famotidine, 20 mg; or ranitidine, 150 mg intravenously) 30 minutes before treatment. A single dose of a corticosteroid (dexamethasone, 20 mg intravenously) administered 30 minutes before treatment has been reported to confer very effective prophylaxis of major hypersensitivity reactions.[284,285] Contact of paclitaxel with plasticized polyvinyl chloride equipment or devices must be avoided because of the risk of patient exposures to plasticizers that may be leached from polyvinyl chloride infusion bags or sets. Paclitaxel solutions should be diluted and stored in glass or polypropylene bottles or suitable plastic bags (polypropylene or polyolefin) and administered through polyethylene-lined administration sets that include an in-line filter with a microporous membrane not greater than 0.22 μm.

The extensive involvement of hepatic metabolism and biliary excretion in the disposition of paclitaxel—similar to that of other anticancer drugs, such as the vinca alkaloids—in which dose modifications are required indicates that doses should be modified in patients with hepatic dysfunction. Official recommendations have not been formulated, but prospective evaluations indicate that patients with moderate to severe elevations in serum concentrations of hepatocellular enzymes or bilirubin (or both) are more likely to develop severe toxicity than patients without hepatic dysfunction.[286,287] Therefore, it would be prudent to reduce paclitaxel doses by at least 50% in patients with moderate or severe hepatic excretory dysfunction (hyperbilirubinemia) or significant elevations in hepatic transaminases. Renal clearance contributes minimally to overall clearance (5% to 10%), and patients with severe renal dysfunction do not appear to require dose modification.[288] Based on the pharmacologic behavior, particularly the wide distributive properties of the taxanes, dose modifications are not required solely for peripheral edema and third-space fluid collections.

Docetaxel

In the United States, docetaxel is indicated at a dose range of 60 to 100 mg/m^2 and 75 mg/m^2 over 1 hour in patients with breast and non–small cell lung cancers, respectively, but most early clinical trials in advanced breast, ovarian, and non–small cell lung cancers evaluated doses in the higher end of this range (75 to 100 mg/m^2), with scant data available for patients treated at 60 mg/m^2.[137,138,265] Although some untreated or minimally pretreated patients generally tolerate docetaxel at a dose of 100 mg/m^2 without severe toxicity, emerging data indicate poorer tolerance in more heavily pretreated patients in

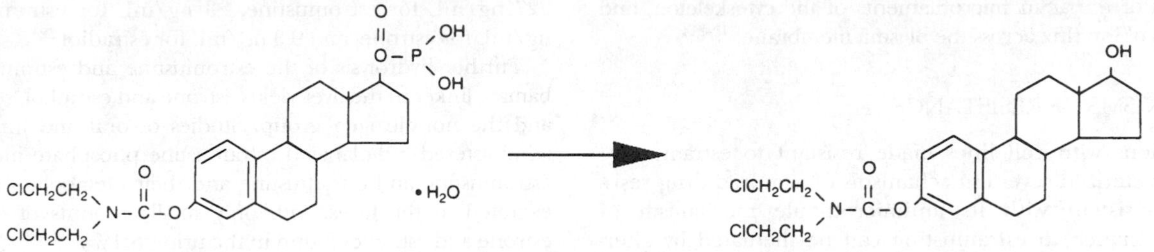

FIGURE 19.7-4. Structure of estramustine phosphate undergoing dephosphorylation to estramustine.

whom 75 mg/m^2 appears to be more reasonable from a toxicologic perspective.[289] Like paclitaxel, docetaxel has also been administered as a 1-hour infusion weekly. Although there are no clear benefits of chronic weekly drug administration in terms of antitumor activity, hematologic toxicity is much less than with conventional dose schedules, with a high incidence of cumulative asthenia and neurotoxicity noted with docetaxel doses exceeding 36 mg/m^2/wk.[274] Despite the use of a polysorbate 80 formulation instead of polyoxyethylated castor oil, which is used to formulate paclitaxel, a relatively high rate of hypersensitivity reactions and profound fluid retention in patients who did not receive premedication has led to the use of several effective premedication regimens, the most popular of which is dexamethasone, 8 mg orally twice daily for 3 or 5 days starting 1 or 2 days, respectively, before docetaxel, with or without both H_1- and H_2-receptor antagonists given 30 minutes before docetaxel.[267]

A retrospective review of docetaxel pharmacokinetics in patients without hyperbilirubinemia demonstrated that docetaxel clearance is reduced by approximately 25% in patients with elevations in serum concentrations of both hepatic transaminases (1.5-fold or greater) and alkaline phosphatase (2.5-fold or greater), regardless of whether the elevations are due to hepatic metastases.[212–214] Therefore, dose reductions by at least 25% are recommended for such individuals. More substantial reductions (50% or greater) may be required in patients who have moderate or severe hepatic excretory dysfunction (hyperbilirubinemia).[287] As with paclitaxel (discussed previously in the section Administration, Dose, and Schedule, Paclitaxel), there is no rationale for dose modification solely for renal deficiency or third-space fluid accumulation (or both). Also similar to the case with paclitaxel, glass bottles or polypropylene or polyolefin plastic products should be used for preparation and storage, and docetaxel should be administered through polyethylene-lined administration sets.

ESTRAMUSTINE PHOSPHATE

Estramustine phosphate (Fig. 19.7-4) is a conjugate of the alkylating agent nornitrogen mustard linked to 17β-estradiol by a carbamate ester. This agent was originally designed so that estramustine would accumulate specifically in estrogen receptor–bearing breast cancer cells via the 17β-estradiol component followed by degradation of the carbamate ester and release of the alkylating nor-nitrogen mustard moiety. Estramustine phosphate, however, did not demonstrate useful anticancer activity in clinical trials in breast cancer and, thereafter, it was determined that alkylation of DNA did not occur.[290] Further investigations later established that preferential accumulation of radiolabeled estramustine phosphate in the ventral prostate of rats occurred unrelated to the estrogen receptor.[291] This selective accumulation was mediated by the presence of a specific protein in prostate tissue, subsequently labeled *estramustine-binding protein* (EMBP).[291,292] Clinical studies of estramustine phosphate were initiated in advanced prostate cancer based on this unique pattern of drug distribution.[293,294] Anticancer activity was subsequently demonstrated in prostate cancer patients with disease refractory to diethylstilbestrol.

MECHANISMS OF ACTION

Several mechanisms of cytotoxic activity have been attributed to estramustine phosphate. The preponderance of data indicates that cell death is principally mediated through a direct effect on microtubules. Estramustine is known to inhibit mitotic microtubule networks and to depolymerize interphase microtubules.[296,297] Consonant with other antimicrotubule agents, estramustine-treated cells arrest in the G_2/M phase of the cell cycle and then undergo apoptosis. Estramustine inhibits microtubule function through direct binding to β-tubulin independent of MAPs while also inhibiting microtubule function through an interaction with MAPs.[298–302] Once bound to tubulin, estramustine inhibits the dynamic growth and shortening of microtubules. Like the taxanes, estramustine can also exert an antiproliferative effect via stabilization of spindle microtubules.[300] The binding of estramustine to β-tubulin, however, occurs at a unique site distinct from those of the taxanes, colchicine, and vinca alkaloids.[303] Finally, the antimicrotubule effects of estramustine are mediated by the intact conjugate and not the individual nor-nitrogen or estradiol components.[304]

The specific binding of estramustine and its metabolite, estromustine, to EMBP permits tissue selectivity for estramustine accumulation and action.[304,305] After exposure to estramustine, cell lines that contain high levels of EMBP exhibit a greater fraction of cells arresting in the G_2/M phase as compared to those with low levels of EMBP expression.[304–306] Proteins similar to EMBP have also been found in other tumors, including gliomas and astrocytomas.[307–309] Because estramustine phosphate induces a G_2/M block, crosses the blood–brain barrier, and accumulates in gliomas and astrocytomas, the potential for estramustine selectively to sensitize central nervous system tumor cells to irradiation is an area of active investigation.[310,311]

Other proposed mechanisms of action attributed to estramustine include interaction and disruption of the nuclear matrix, alterations of the actin microfilaments of the cytoskeleton, and alterations of ion flux across the plasma membrane.[312–314]

MECHANISMS OF RESISTANCE

Investigations with cell lines made resistant to estramustine have characterized several mechanisms of acquired drug resistance. Consistent with its antimicrotubule mechanism of action, resistance to estramustine can be mediated by alterations at the site of estramustine-tubulin interaction, increased microtubule stability through overexpression of specific tubulin isotypes, or alterations in MAPs. A drug efflux mechanism, distinct from classical MDR has been described.

The targets of estramustine—β-tubulins—are composed of multiple isotypes encoded by separate cellular genes. An increase in β_{III}- and β_{IVa}-tubulin isotypes relative to other β-tubulin isotypes occurs in human prostate cancer cells rendered eight- to ninefold resistant to estramustine.[301] Although the precise site of estramustine binding is not known, microtubules containing β_{III}-tubulin isotypes appear to bind estramustine less efficiently as compared to either other β-tubulins or α-tubulin.[301] Furthermore, tubulin isotypes differ from one another principally at MAP binding sites. Because the binding of different β-tubulin subtypes to α-tubulin alters the dynamic properties of microtubule growth and stability, a change in the relative β-tubulin isotypes may counter the inhibitory and destabilizing effects of estramustine on microtubule assembly.[315,316]

Some prostate cancer cell lines with acquired resistance to estramustine overexpress the MAP tau. The capacity to maintain microtubule stability and kinetics involves the interaction of tubulin with MAPs. Exposure to estramustine induces both quantitative and qualitative changes in tau, leading to a sevenfold increase in estramustine resistance in some cell lines.[317] To what extent alterations in tau or other altered MAPs contribute to clinical estramustine resistance is not known.

Although estramustine can bind to the classical MDR efflux pump, P-gp-overexpressing cells are not cross-resistant to estramustine.[318–320] Estramustine may, in fact, act as a competitive inhibitor of P-gp action, reducing the efflux of other cytotoxic agents subject to P-gp-mediated resistance.[318,320] A drug efflux mechanism distinct from P-gp has been described that is distinct from P-gp and can mediate estramustine resistance.[321] Some cell lines with acquired estramustine resistance exhibit a sixfold resistance to estramustine commensurate with the degree of overexpression of the gene encoding this new efflux pump.

PHARMACOLOGY

After oral administration, estramustine phosphate undergoes rapid dephosphorylation within the gastrointestinal tract, as shown in Figure 19.7-4. The bioavailability of oral estramustine phosphate is 37% to 75%.[322,323] The majority of absorbed estramustine is rapidly metabolized to an oxidized isomer, estromustine, which is the principal component detected in the plasma.[324] Maximal estromustine plasma concentrations are reached within 2 to 4 hours after oral consumption, and the mean elimination half-life is 14 hours.[322] Estromustine pharmacokinetics are linear over the usual administered oral doses of estramustine phosphate. Peak plasma concentrations in patients treated chronically with oral estramustine phosphate at 560 mg/d have been 227 ng/mL for estromustine, 23 ng/mL for estramustine, 95 ng/mL for estrone, and 9.3 ng/mL for estradiol.[324]

Further hydrolysis of the estromustine and estramustine carbamate linker in the liver yields estrone and estradiol, respectively, and the nor-nitrogen group. Studies of oral and intravenously administered radiolabeled estramustine phosphate indicate that estromustine and estramustine and their metabolites are largely excreted in the feces, with only small amounts of conjugated estrone and estradiol found in the urine (<1%).[322–325]

In contrast to oral administration, intravenous estramustine phosphate delivers significantly higher plasma concentrations of estramustine phosphate and metabolites while reducing the marked interpatient variability noted for the oral route.[322–325] Intravenous estramustine phosphate is currently investigational in the United States.

DRUG INTERACTIONS

Coadministration of food or dairy products significantly impairs the absorption of estramustine phosphate.[326] Calcium-rich foods appear to lead to the formation of a poorly absorbable calcium complex. Current recommendations include fasting before the oral administration of estramustine phosphate and avoidance of calcium-rich foods and calcium antacids.[326]

Preliminary evidence suggests that oral estramustine phosphate, when coadministered with intravenous docetaxel, significantly delays the clearance of docetaxel, with disproportionate increases in docetaxel concentrations.[327] This has led to a reduction in the recommended dose for docetaxel when combined with estramustine phosphate despite the fact that, for the most part, these two agents have nonoverlapping toxicities. The mechanism by which estramustine impairs docetaxel clearance is not known.

TOXICITY

Nausea and vomiting, which are the principal toxicities encountered with oral estramustine phosphate, may infrequently necessitate discontinuation. At conventional dosing schedules, nausea and vomiting can be prevented by antiemetic therapy. Diarrhea has also been observed in some patients with chronic use. Myelosuppression is not associated with estramustine phosphate when administered as a single agent.

Commonly observed estrogenic side effects of estramustine therapy include gynecomastia, nipple tenderness, and fluid retention. Caution should be exercised in prescribing estramustine phosphate to patients with congestive heart failure because of the risk for fluid retention and edema. Thromboembolic complications represent the most hazardous toxicity of estramustine phosphate therapy and may occur in as many as 10% of patients. These include venous thrombosis, pulmonary emboli, and cerebrovascular and coronary thrombotic events. Transient elevations in hepatic transaminases occur in approximately one-third of patients receiving estramustine phosphate therapy. The rate of hepatic toxicity is similar to that described for diethylstilbestrol in a randomized study of estramustine phosphate versus diethylstilbestrol.[328]

ADMINISTRATION, DOSE, AND SCHEDULE

Estramustine phosphate is approved for the treatment of metastatic prostate cancer, particularly hormone-refractory disease.

The recommended daily dose of estramustine phosphate (available as a 140-mg capsule) is 14 mg/kg of body weight given in three to four divided doses, though most patients are usually treated in the dosing range of 10 to 16 mg/kg. Patients should be instructed to take estramustine phosphate with water at least 1 hour before or 2 hours after meals. Patients are generally treated for 30 to 90 days before assessment of therapeutic benefit. Chronic oral therapy can be maintained for months or even years as long as the favorable response continues. Abbreviated 5-day courses of oral estramustine phosphate have been proposed for use with such chemotherapy agents as docetaxel. This schedule allows for the concurrent administration of estramustine phosphate with intravenous chemotherapeutic agents while reducing some of the toxicity of chronic oral administration.

NOVEL COMPOUNDS TARGETING MICROTUBULES

Many other structurally—and functionally—unique antimicrotubule compounds are the focus of discovery efforts, preclinical development, and clinical evaluations. Although the majority of efforts are being directed toward agents that interfere with tubulin, other potential strategic components of the microtubule, including motor proteins, are the focus of discovery and developmental efforts.[13]

The successes with the taxanes have provided the impetus to discover new chemotypes that work by a similar mechanism but yet have higher therapeutic indices. Several natural products that are structurally dissimilar to the taxanes, share their mechanism of action, and show comparable activities have been identified. For example, rhazinilam, like paclitaxel, originates from tree bark but is the first nontaxane identified that induces cold-stable tubulin polymerization *in vitro* and microtubule bundling in cells.[329] Unlike paclitaxel, rhazinilam is capable of inducing tubulin polymerization at 0°C; however, the resulting polymerized product is unstable. In contrast, discodermolide, which originates from a marine sponge, polymerizes tubulin at 37°C *in vitro* more potently and rapidly than does paclitaxel, yielding polymerization products that are cold-stable, and it polymerizes tubulin almost as rapidly at 0°C.[330] Unlike rhazinilam, discodermolide-induced tubulin polymers are completely stable to treatment with calcium ions and are composed of very short microtubules instead of tubulin spirals. The epothilones A and B, which are derived by microbial fermentation, appear to be more like the taxanes in their polymerization products.[331,332] The microtubules they induce are relatively long, rigid, and resistant to destabilization by cold temperature and calcium ions. These epothilones and their analogues are at least as potent as paclitaxel and cause mitotic arrest and microtubule bundling. Epothilone B analogues are currently undergoing clinical evaluation. The marine soft coral–derived natural products—sarcotidicytins A and B and eleutherobin also promote tubulin polymerization in a manner analogous to that of paclitaxel.[333]

All the aforementioned compounds are likely substrates for P-gp to some extent, expressing varying degrees of cross-resistance against P-gp–expressing cells. However, other marine-derived, microtubule-stabilizing cytotoxins, such as laulimalide and isolaulimalide, appear to be poor substrates for the P-gp drug efflux pump.[334] Because eleutherobin, epothilones A and B, and discodermolide competitively inhibit [^{3}H]paclitaxel binding to microtubules, a common pharmacophore has been sought and identified and may enable the development of hybrid constructs with more desirable biologic characteristics.[335]

Other natural products and semisynthetic antimicrotubule compounds under evaluation interact with tubulin in the vinca alkaloid– or colchicine-binding domains. Among the most potent are the cryptophycins, which are a family of cyanobacterial macrolides that deplete microtubules in intact cells, including cells with the MDR phenotype.[336,337] The cryptophycins compete for the binding of [^{3}H]VBL, but neither for radiolabeled paclitaxel nor for colchicine, and inhibit GTP hydrolysis by isolated tubulin. They also have excellent activity against several types of tumor xenografts, including tumors resistant to the vinca alkaloids. One semisynthetic analogue, cryptophycin-52, is currently undergoing initial clinical evaluation.[336] The dolastatins constitute a series of oligopeptides isolated from the sea hare, *Dolabela auricularia*.[337–340] Two of the most potent dolastatins, dolastatin-10 and -15, noncompetitively inhibit the binding of vinca alkaloids to tubulin, inhibit tubulin polymerization and tubulin-dependent GTP hydrolysis, stabilize the colchicine-binding activity of tubulin, and possess cytotoxic activity in the picomolar to low nanomolar range. Dolastatin-10 and semisynthetic dolastatin analogues are undergoing preclinical development and clinical evaluation.[340] Phomopsin A, halichondrin B, homohalichondrin B, and spongistatin 1, which interact with tubulin in the vinca alkaloid–binding domain and with the natural products combretastatin and steganacin and the synthetic compounds pyridine and pyridazine, and the pentafluorophenylsulfonamides, which interact with tubulin at the colchicine-binding domain, are currently being evaluated in preclinical or early clinical evaluations.[341,342]

REFERENCES

1. Gelfand VI, Bershadsky AD. Microtubule dynamics: mechanism, regulation, and function. *Annu Rev Cell Biol* 1991;7:93.
2. Hyams JF, Lloyd CW. *Microtubules.* New York: Wiley-Liss, 1993.
3. Nogales E, Whittaker M, Milligan RA, Downing KH. High-resolution model of the microtubule. *Cell* 1999;96:78.
4. Mitchison T, Kirchner M. Dynamic instability of microtubule growth. *Nature* 1984;312:237.
5. Margolis RL, Wilson L. Microtubule treadmilling: what goes around comes around. *Bioessays* 1998;20:830.
6. Raff EC. Genetics of microtubule systems. *J Cell Biol* 1984;99:1.
7. Ludena RF. Are tubulin isotypes functionally significant? *Mol Biol Cell* 1983;4:445.
8. Luduena RF. Multiple forms of tubulin: different gene products and covalent modifications. *Int Rev Cytol* 1998;178:207.
9. Raff, EC. The role of multiple tubulin isoforms in cellular microtubule function. In: Hyams JF, Lloyd CD, eds. *Microtubules.* New York: Wiley-Liss, 1993:89.
10. Olmsted JB. Microtubule-associated proteins. *Annu Rev Cell Biol* 1986;2:421.
11. Zheng Y, Jung MK, Oakley BR. Gamma-tubulin is present in *Drosophila melanogaster* and *Homo sapiens* and is associated with the centrosome. *Cell* 1991;65:817.
12. Kellogg DR, Moritz M, Alberts BM. The centrosome and cellular organization. *Annu Rev Biochem* 1994;63:639.
13. Vale RD. Microtubule motors: many new models off the assembly line. *Trends Biochem Sci* 1992;17:300.
14. Johnson IS. Historical background of vinca alkaloid research and areas of future interest. *Cancer Chemother Rep* 1968;52:455.
15. Gidding CE, Kellie SJ, Kamps WA, de Graaf SS. Vincristine revisited. *Crit Rev Oncol Hematol* 1999;29:267.
16. Johnson IS, Armstrong JG, Gorman M, et al. The vinca alkaloids: a new class of oncolytic agents. *Cancer Res* 1963;23:1390.
17. Rowinsky EK, Donehower RC. The clinical pharmacology and use of antimicrotubule agents in cancer chemotherapeutics. *Pharmacol Ther* 1992;52:35.
18. Joel S. The comparative clinical pharmacology of vincristine and vindesine: Does vindesine offer any advantage in clinical use? *Cancer Treat Rev* 1995;21:513.
19. Budman DR. Vinorelbine (Navelbine): a third-generation vinca alkaloid. *Cancer Invest* 1997;15:475.
20. Johnson SA, Harper P, Hortobagyi GN, Pouillart P. Vinorelbine: an overview. *Cancer Treat Rev* 1996;22:127.
21. Himes RH. Interactions of the catharanthus (vinca) alkaloids with tubulin and microtubules. *Pharmacol Ther* 1991;51:256.

22. Jordan MA, Thrower D, Wilson L. Mechanism of inhibition of cell proliferation by the vinca alkaloids. *Cancer Res* 1991;51:2212.
23. Donoso RJ, Jordan MA, Farrell KW, Matsumoto B, Wilson L. Kinetic stabilization of the microtubule dynamic instability in vitro by vinblastine. *Biochemistry* 1993;32:1285.
24. Jordan MA, Thrower D, Wilson L. Effects of vinblastine, podophyllotoxin and nocodazole on mitotic spindles. Implications for the role of microtubule dynamics in mitosis. *J Cell Sci* 1992;102:401.
25. Wilson L, Jordan MA. Pharmacological probes of microtubule function. In: Hyams JF, Lloyd CD, eds. *Microtubules*. New York: Wiley-Liss, 1993:59.
26. Howard SMH, Theologides A, Sheppard JR. Comparative effects of vindesine, vinblastine, and vincristine on mitotic arrest and hormone response of L1210 leukemia cells. *Cancer Res* 1980;40:2695.
27. Beck WT. Alkaloids. In: Fox BW, Fox M, eds. *Antitumor drug resistance*. Berlin: Springer-Verlag, 1984:589.
28. Ferguson PJ, Cass CE. Differential cellular retention of vincristine and vinblastine by cultured human promyelocytic leukemia HL-60/C-1 cells: the basis of differential toxicity. *Cancer Res* 1985;45:5480.
29. Himes RH, Kersey RN, Heller-Bettinger I, Sampson FE. Action of the vinca alkaloids, vincristine and vinblastine, and desacetyl vinblastine amide on microtubules in vitro. *Cancer Res* 1976;36:3798.
30. Jordan MA, Himes RH, Wilson L. Comparison of the effects of vinblastine, vincristine, vindesine, and vinepidine on microtubule dynamics and cell proliferation in vitro. *Cancer Res* 1985;45:2741.
31. Ferguson PJ, Philips JR, Seiner M, Cass CE. Biochemical effects of Navelbine on tubulin and associated proteins. *Cancer Res* 1984;44:3307.
32. Gout PW, Wijck LL, Beer CT. Differences between vinblastine and vincristine in distribution in the blood of rats and binding by platelets and malignant cells. *Eur J Cancer* 1978;14:1167.
33. Gout PW, Noble RL, Bruchovsky N, Beer CT. Vinblastine and vincristine growth-inhibitory effects correlate with their retention by cultured Nb2 node lymphoma cells. *Int J Cancer* 1984;34:245.
34. Lobert S, Vulevic B, Correria JJ. Interaction of vinca alkaloids with tubulin: a comparison of vinblastine, vincristine, and vinorelbine. *Biochemistry* 1996;35:6806.
35. Bowman LC, Houghton JA, Houghton PJ. GTP influences the binding of vincristine in human tumor cytosols. *Biochem Biophys Res Commun* 1986;135:695.
36. Bowman LC, Houghton JA, Houghton PJ. Formation and stability of vincristine-tubulin complex in kidney cytosols. Role of GTP and GTP hydrolysis. *Biochem Pharmacol* 1988;37:1251.
37. Lengfeld AM, Dietrich J, Schultze-Maurer B. Accumulation and release of vinblastine and vincristine in HeLa cells: light microscopic, cinematographic, and biochemical study. *Cancer Res* 1982;42:3798.
38. Bleyer WA, Frisby SA, Oliverio VT. Uptake and binding of vincristine by murine leukemia cells. *Biochem Pharmacol* 1975;24:633.
39. Zhou XJ, Placidi M, Rahmani R. Uptake and metabolism of vinca alkaloids by freshly isolated human hepatocytes in suspension. *Anticancer Res* 1994;14:1017.
40. Rahmani R, Zhou XJ. Pharmacokinetics and metabolism of vinca alkaloids. In: Workman P, Graham, M, eds. *Cancer surveys, vol 17: pharmacokinetics and cancer chemotherapy*. Plainview, NY: Cold Spring Harbor Laboratory Press, 1993:269.
41. Ferguson PJ, Cass CE. Differential cellular retention of vincristine and vinblastine by cultured human promyelocytic leukemia HL-60/C-1 cells: the basis of differential toxicity. *Cancer Res* 1985;45:5480.
42. Jackson DV, Bender RA. Cytotoxic thresholds of vincristine in a murine and human leukemia cell line in vitro. *Cancer Res* 1979;39:4346.
43. Inaba M, Fujikura R, Sakurai Y. Active efflux common to vincristine and daunorubicin in vincristine-resistant P388 leukemia. *Biochem Pharmacol* 1981;30:1863.
44. Safa AR, Glover CJ, Meyers MB, et al. Vinblastine photoaffinity labeling of a high molecular weight surface membrane glycoprotein specific for multidrug-resistant cells. *Biochemistry* 1987;262:13685.
45. Grant CE, Validmarsson G, Hipfner R, et al. Overexpression of multidrug resistance–associated protein (MRP) increases resistance to natural product drugs. *Cancer Res* 1994;54:356.
46. Scheper RJ, Broxterman HJ, Scheffer GL. Overexpression of a Mr 110000 vesicular protein in non-P-glycoprotein-mediated multidrug resistance. *Cancer Res* 1993;53:1475.
47. Greenberger LM, Williams SS, Horwitz SB. Biosynthesis of heterogeneous forms of multidrug resistance associated glycoproteins. *J Biol Chem* 1987;262:13685.
48. Choi K, Chen C, Kriegler M, Roninson IB. An altered pattern of cross-resistance in multidrug-resistant human cells results from spontaneous mutations in the mdr1 (P-glycoprotein) gene. *Cell* 1988;53:519.
49. Peterson RHF, Meyers MB, Spengler BA. Alterations of plasma membrane glycopeptides and gangliosides of Chinese hamster cells accompanying development of resistance to daunorubicin and vincristine. *Cancer Res* 1983;43:222.
50. Pieters R, Hongo T, Loonen AH, et al. Different types of non-P-glycoprotein mediated multiple drug resistance in children with relapsed acute lymphoblastic leukaemia. *Br J Cancer* 1992;65:691.
51. Betrand Y, Capdeville R, Balduck N, et al. Cyclosporin A used to reverse drug resistance increases vincristine neurotoxicity. *Am J Hematol* 1992;40:158.
52. Pinkerton CR. Multidrug resistance reversal in childhood malignancies—potential for a real step forward? *Eur J Cancer* 1996;32A:641.
53. Houghton JA, Houghton PJ, Hazelton BJ, Douglas EC. In situ selection of a human rhabdomyosarcoma resistant to vincristine with altered α-tubulins. *Cancer Res* 1985;45:2706.
54. Cabral FR, Barlow SB. Resistance to the antimitotic agents as genetic probes of microtubule structure and function. *Pharmacol Ther* 1991;52:159.
55. Reichle A, Diddens H, Altmayr F, et al. Beta-tubulin and P-glycoprotein: major determinants of vincristine accumulation in B-CLL cells. *Leukemia Res* 1995:19:823.
56. Poruchynsky MS, Wang EE, Rudin CM, Blagosklonny MV, Fojo T. Bcl-xL is phosphorylated in malignant cells following microtubule disruption. *Cancer Res* 1998;58:3331.
57. Wang LG, Liu XM, Kreis W, Budman DR. The effect of antimicrotubule agents on signal transduction pathways of apoptosis: a review. *Cancer Chemother Pharmacol* 1999;44:355.
58. Nelson RL, Dyke RW, Root MA. Comparative pharmacokinetics of vindesine, vincristine, and vinblastine in patients with cancer. *Cancer Treat Rev* 1980;7[Suppl]:17.
59. Nelson RL. The comparative clinical pharmacology and pharmacokinetics of vindesine, vincristine, and vinblastine in human patients with cancer. *Med Pediatr Oncol* 1982;10:115.
60. Rahmani R, Bruno R, Iliadis A, et al. Clinical pharmacokinetics of the antitumor drug Navelbine (5′-noranhydrovinblastine). *Cancer Res* 1987;47:5796.
61. Jehl F, Quoix E, Leveque D, et al. Pharmacokinetic and preliminary metabolic fate of Navelbine in humans as determined by high performance liquid chromatography. *Cancer Res* 1991;51:2073.
62. Jackson DV Jr. The periwinkle alkaloids. In: Lokich JJ, ed. *Cancer Chemotherapy by Infusion*. Chicago: Precept Press Inc, 1990:155.
63. Bender RA, Castle MC, Margileth DA, Oliverio VT. The pharmacokinetics of [^{3}H]-vincristine in man. *Clin Pharmacol Ther* 1977;22:430.
64. Sethi VS, Jackson DV, White CT, et al. Pharmacokinetics of vincristine sulfate in adult cancer patients. *Cancer Res* 1981;41:3551.
65. Castle MC, Margileth DA, Oliverio VT. Distribution and excretion of [^{3}H]vincristine in the rat and the dog. *Cancer Res* 1976;36:3684.
66. Jackson DV, Sethi VS, Spurr CL, McWhorter JM. Pharmacokinetics of vincristine in the cerebrospinal fluid of humans. *Cancer Res* 1981;41:1466.
67. Rahmani R, Zhou XJ, Placidi M, et al. In vivo and in vitro pharmacokinetics and metabolism of vinca alkaloids in rat. I. Vindesine (4-deacetyl-vinblastine 3-carboxyamide). *Eur J Drug Metab Pharmacokinet* 1990;15:49.
68. Zhou XJ, Martin M, Placidi M, et al. In vivo and in vitro pharmacokinetics and metabolism of vinca alkaloids: II. Vinblastine and vincristine. *Eur J Drug Metab Pharmacokinet* 1990;15:323.
69. Owellen RJ, Root MA, Hains FO. Pharmacokinetic of vindesine and vincristine in humans. *Cancer Res* 1977;37:2603.
70. Jackson DV, Castle MC, Bender RA. Biliary excretion of vincristine. *Clin Pharmacol Ther* 1978;24:101.
71. Owellen RJ, Hartke CA, Hains FO. Pharmacokinetics and metabolism of vinblastine in humans. *Cancer Res* 1977;37:2597.
72. Owellen RJ, Hartke CA. The pharmacokinetics of 4-acetyl tritium vinblastine in two patients. *Cancer Res* 1975;35:975.
73. Zhou-Pan XR, Seree E, Zhou XJ, et al. Involvement of human liver cytochrome P450 3A in vinblastine metabolism: drug interactions. *Cancer Res* 1993;53:5121.
74. Hande K, Gay J, Gober J, Greco FA. Toxicity and pharmacology of bolus vindesine injection and prolonged vindesine infusion. *Cancer Treat Rev* 1980;7:25.
75. Nelson RL, Dyke RW, Root MA. Clinical pharmacokinetics of vindesine. *Cancer Chemother Pharmacol* 1979;2:243.
76. Jackson DV Jr, Sethi VS, Long TR, et al. Pharmacokinetics of vindesine bolus and infusion. *Cancer Chemother Pharmacol* 1994;13:114.
77. Ohnuma T, Norton L, Andrejczuk A, Holland JF. Pharmacokinetics of vindesine given as an intravenous bolus and 24-hour infusion in humans. *Cancer Res* 1985;45:464.
78. Dyke RW, Nelson RL, Brade WP. Vindesine: a short review of preclinical and first clinical data. *Cancer Chemother Pharmacol* 1979;2:229.
79. Rahmani R, Kleisbauer JP, Cano JP, et al. Clinical pharmacokinetics of vindesine infusion. *Cancer Treat Rep* 1985;69:839.
80. Rahmani R, Martin M, Favre R, et al. Clinical pharmacokinetics of vindesine: repeated treatments by intravenous bolus injections. *Eur J Cancer Clin Oncol* 1984;20:1409.
81. Culp HW, Daniels WD, McMahon RE. Disposition and tissue levels of [^{3}H]-vindesine in rats. *Cancer Res* 1977;37:3053.
82. Zhou XJ, Zhou-Pan XR, Gauthier T, et al. Human liver microsomal cytochrome P450 3A isoenzymes mediated vindesine biotransformation: metabolic drug interactions. *Biomed Pharmacol* 1993;4:853.
83. Levêque D, Jehl F. Clinical pharmacokinetics of vinorelbine. *Clin Pharmacokinet* 1996;31:184.
84. Jehl F, Quoix E, Levêque D, et al. Pharmacokinetic and preliminary metabolic fate of Navelbine in humans as determined by high performance liquid chromatography. *Cancer Res* 1991;51:2073.
85. Rowinsky EK, Noe DA, Lucas VS, et al. A phase I, pharmacokinetic and absolute bioavailability study of oral vinorelbine (Navelbine) in solid tumor patients. *J Clin Oncol* 1994;12:1754.
86. Urien S, Bree F, Breillout F, et al. Vinorelbine high-affinity binding to human platelets and lymphocytes: distribution in human blood. *Cancer Chemother Pharmacol* 1988;23:247.
87. Levêque D, Quoiz E, Dumont P, et al. Pulmonary distribution of vinorelbine in patients with non-small lung cancer. *Cancer Chemother Pharmacol* 1993;33:176.
88. Rahmani R, Gueritte F, Martin M, et al. Comparative pharmacokinetics of antitumor vinca alkaloids: intravenous bolus injections of Navelbine and related alkaloids to cancer patients and rats. *Cancer Chemother Pharmacol* 1986;16:223.
89. Levêque D, Merle-Melet M, Bresler L, et al. Biliary elimination and pharmacokinetics of vinorelbine in micropigs. *Cancer Chemother Pharmacol* 1993;32:487.
90. Krikorian A, Rahmani R, Bromet M, et al. Pharmacokinetics and metabolism of Navelbine. *Semin Oncol* 1989;16[Suppl 4]:21.
91. Favre R, Delgado J, Besenval M, et al. Phase I trial of escalating doses of orally administered Navelbine (NVB): II. Clinical results. *Proc Am Soc Clin Oncol* 1989;8:246(abst).
92. Bender RA, Bleyer WA, Frisby SA. Alteration of methotrexate uptake in human leukemia cells by other agents. *Cancer Res* 1975;35:1305.
93. Zager RF, Frisby SA, Oliverio VT. The effects of antibiotics and cancer chemotherapeutic agents on the cellular transport and antitumor activity of methotrexate in L1210 murine leukemia. *Cancer Res* 1973;33:1670.
94. Chan JD. Pharmacokinetic drug interactions of vinca alkaloids. Summary of case reports. *Pharmacotherapy* 1998;18:1304.
95. Yalowich JC. Effect of microtubule inhibition on etoposide accumulation and DNA damage in human K562 cells in vitro. *Cancer Res* 1987;47:1010

96. Bollini R, Riva R, Albani R, et al. Decreased phenytoin levels during antineoplastic therapy: a case report. *Epilepsia* 1983;24:75.
97. Jarosinski PF, Moscow JA, Alexander MS, et al. Altered phenytoin clearance during intensive chemotherapy for acute lymphoblastic leukemia. *J Pediatr* 1988;112:996.
98. Tobe SW, Siu LL, Jamal SA, et al. Vinblastine and erythromycin: an unrecognized serious drug interaction. *Cancer Chemother Pharmacol* 1995;35:188.
99. Crom WR, De Graaf SSN, Synold T, et al. Pharmacokinetics of vincristine in children and adolescents with acute lymphocytic leukemia. *J Pediatr* 1994;125:642.
100. Rajaonarison JF, Lacarelle B, Catalin J, et al. Effect of anticancer drugs on the glucuronidation of 3'azido-3'-deoxythymidine in human liver microsomes. *Drug Metab Dispos* 1993;21:823.
101. Legha SS. Vincristine neurotoxicity. Pathophysiology and management. *Med Toxicol* 1986;1:421.
102. Tuxen MK, Hansen SW. Neurotoxicity secondary to antineoplastic drugs. *Cancer Treat Rev* 1994;20:191.
103. Sulkes A, Collins JM. Reappraisal of some dosage adjustment guidelines. *Cancer Treat Rep* 1987;71:229.
104. Bradley WG, Lassman LP, Pearce GW. The neuromyopathy of vincristine in man: clinical electrophysiological and pathological studies. *J Neurol Sci* 1970;10:107.
105. Casey EB, Jellife AM, Le Quesne PM, Millett YL. Vincristine neuropathy, clinical and electrophysiological observations. *Brain* 1973;96:69.
106. Greig NH, Soncrant TT, Shetty HU, et al. Brain uptake and anticancer activities of vincristine and vinblastine are restricted by their low cerebrovascular permeability and binding to plasma constituents in rat. *Cancer Chemother Pharmacol* 1990;26:263.
107. Hironen HE, Saknu TT, Heinonen E, et al. Vincristine treatment of acute lymphoblastic leukemia induces transient autonomic cardioneuropathy. *Cancer* 1988;64:801.
108. Gottlieb RJ, Cuttner J. Vincristine-induced bladder atony. *Cancer* 1971;28:674.
109. Carmichael SM, Eagleton L, Ayers CR, Mohler D. Orthostatic hypotension during vincristine therapy. *Arch Intern Med* 1970;126:290.
110. Burns BV, Shotton JC. Vocal fold palsy following vinca alkaloid treatment. *J Laryngol Otol* 1998;112:485.
111. Morgan E, Baum E, Breslow N, et al. Chemotherapy-related toxicity in infants treated according to the second national Wilms' tumor study. *J Clin Oncol* 1988;6:51.
112. Woods WG, O'Leary M, Nesbit ME. Life-threatening neuropathy and hepatotoxicity in infants during induction therapy for acute lymphoblastic leukemia. *J Pediatr* 1981;98:642.
113. Griffiths JD, Stark RJ, Ding JC, Cooper IA. Vincristine neurotoxicity in Charcot-Marie Tooth syndrome. *Med J Aust* 1985;143:305.
114. McGuire SA, Gospe SM Jr, Dahl G. Acute vincristine neurotoxicity in the presence of hereditary motor and sensory neuropathy type I. *Med Pediatr Oncol* 1989;17:520.
115. Desai ZR, Van den Berg HW, Bridges JM, et al. Can severe vincristine neurotoxicity be prevented? *Cancer Chemother Pharmacol* 1982;8:211.
116. Boyle FM, Wheeler HR, Shenfield GM. Glutamate ameliorates experimental vincristine neuropathy. *J Pharmacol Exp Ther* 1996;279:410.
117. Jackson DV, Wells HB, Atkins JN, et al. Amelioration of vincristine neurotoxicity by glutamic acid. *Am J Med* 1988;84:1016.
118. Binet S, Fellous A, Lataste H, et al. In situ analysis of the action of Navelbine on various types of microtubules using immunofluorescence. *Semin Oncol* 1989;16[Suppl 4]:5.
119. Le Chevalier T, Brisgand D, Douillard J-Y, et al. Randomized study of vinorelbine and cisplatin versus vindesine and cisplatin versus vindesine and cisplatin versus vinorelbine alone in non-small cell lung cancer: results of a European multicenter trial including 612 patients. *J Clin Oncol* 1994;12:360
120. Sharma RK. Vincristine and gastrointestinal transit. *Gastroenterology* 1988;95:1435.
121. Tester W, Forbes W, Leighton J. Vinorelbine-induced pancreatitis: a case report. *J Natl Cancer Inst* 1997;89:1631.
122. Dorr RT, Alberts DS. Vinca alkaloid skin toxicity: antidote and drug disposition studies in the mouse. *J Natl Cancer Inst* 1985;74:113.
123. Bellone JD. Treatment of vincristine extravasation. *JAMA* 1981;245:343.
124. Hoff PM, Valero V, Ibrahim N, Willey, Hortobagyi GN. Hand-foot syndrome following prolonged infusion of high doses of vinorelbine. *Cancer* 1998;85:965.
125. Karminsky N, Merimsky O, Kovner F, Inbar M. Vinorelbine-related acute cardiopulmonary toxicity. *Cancer Chemother Pharmacol* 1999;43:180.
126. Tassinari D, Sartori S, Gianni L, Pasguini E, Ravaioli A. Is acute dyspnea a rare side effect of vinorelbine? *Ann Oncol* 1997;8:503.
127. Kouroukis C, Hings I. Respiratory failure following vinorelbine tartrate infusion in a patient with non-small cell lung cancer. *Chest* 1997;112:846.
128. Subar M, Muggia FM. Apparent myocardial ischemia associated with vinblastine administration. *Cancer Treat Rep* 1986;70:690.
129. Hantel A, Rowinsky EK, Donehower RC. Nifedipine and oncologic Raynaud's phenomenon. *Ann Intern Med* 1988;108:767.
130. Israel RH, Olson JP. Pulmonary edema associated with intravenous vinblastine. *JAMA* 1978;240:1585.
131. Raderer M, Kornek G, Hejna M, et al. Acute pulmonary toxicity associated with high-dose vinorelbine and mitomycin C. *Ann Oncol* 1996;7:973.
132. Sweet DL, Golumb HM, Ultmann JE, et al. Cyclophosphamide, vincristine, methotrexate with leukovorin rescue, and cytarabine (COMLA) combination sequential chemotherapy for advanced diffuse histiocytic lymphoma. *Ann Intern Med* 1980;92:785.
133. Meggs WJ, Hoffman RS. Fatality resulting from intraventricular vincrisitine administration. *J Toxicol Clin Toxicol* 1998;36:243.
134. Shibata SI, Synold TW, Carroll M, et al. A pilot study of the tolerability and pharmacokinetics of vinorelbine in patients with varying degrees of liver dysfunction. *Proc Am Soc Clin Oncol* 1999;18:190a(abst).
135. Rowinsky EK, Donehower RC. Drug therapy: paclitaxel (Taxol). *N Engl J Med* 1996;332:1004.
136. Rowinsky EK, Cazenave LA, Donehower RC. Taxol: a novel investigational antineoplastic agent. *J Natl Cancer Inst* 1990;82:1247.
137. Eisenhauer EA, Vermorken JB. The taxoids. Comparative clinical pharmacology and therapeutic potential. *Drugs* 1998;55:5.
138. Cortes JE, Pazdur R. Docetaxel. *J Clin Oncol* 1995;13:2643.
139. McGuire WP, Hoskins WJ, Brady MF, et al. Cyclophosphamide and cisplatin compared with paclitaxel and cisplatin in patients with stage III and IV ovarian cancer. *N Engl J Med* 1996;334:1.
140. Seidman AD. The emerging role of paclitaxel in breast cancer therapy. *Clin Cancer Res* 1995;1:247.
141. Henderson IC, Berry D, Demetri G, et al. Improved disease-free survival and overall survival from the addition of sequential paclitaxel, but not from the escalation of doxorubicin dose level in the adjuvant chemotherapy of patients with node-positive primary breast cancer. *Proc Am Soc Clin Oncol* 1998;17;101a(abst).
142. Jie C, Tulpule A, Zheng T, et al. Treatment of epidemic AIDS-related Kaposi's sarcoma. *Curr Opin Oncol* 1997;9:433.
143. Bonomi P, Kim K, Fariclough D, et al. Comparison of survival and quality of life in advanced non-small cell lung cancer patients treated with two dose levels of paclitaxel combined with cisplatin versus etoposide with cisplatin: results from an Eastern Cooperative Oncology Group trial. *J Clin Oncol* 2000;18:623.
144. Schiff PB, Fant J, Horwitz SB. Promotion of microtubule assembly in vitro by taxol. *Nature* 1979;22:665.
145. Schiff PB, Horwitz SB. Taxol stabilizes microtubules in mouse fibroblast cells. *Proc Natl Acad Sci U S A* 1980;77:1561.
146. Manfredi JJ, Parness J, Horwitz SB. Taxol binds to cellular microtubules. *J Cell Biol* 1982;94:688.
147. Rao S, Krauss NE, Heerding JM, et al. 3'-(*p*-Azidobenzamido)taxol photolabels the N-terminal 31 amino acids of β-tubulin. *J Biol Chem* 1994;269:3132.
148. Rao S, Orr GA, Chaudhary AG, et al. Characterization of the Taxol binding site on the microtubule: 2-(m-azidobenzoyl)taxol photolabels a peptide (amino acids 217-231) of beta tubulin. *J Biol Chem* 1995;270:20235.
149. Diaz JF, Andreu JM. Assembly of purified GDP-tubulin into microtubules induced by taxol and taxotere: reversibility, ligand stoichiometry and competition. *Biochemistry* 1993;32:2747.
150. Vanhoerfer U, Cao S, Harstrict A, Seeber S, Rustum YM. Comparative antitumor efficacy of docetaxel and paclitaxel in nude mice bearing human tumor xenografts that overexpress the multidrug resistant protein. *Ann Oncol* 1997;8:1221.
151. Valero V, Jones SE, Von Hoff DD, et al. A phase II study of docetaxel in patients with paclitaxel-resistant metastatic breast cancer. *J Clin Oncol* 1998;16:3362.
152. Jordan MA, Toso RJ, Thrower D, Wilson L. Mechanism of mitotic block and inhibition of cell proliferation by taxol at low concentrations. *Proc Natl Acad Sci U S A* 1993;90:9552.
153. Ringel I, Horwitz SB. Studies with RP56976 (Taxotere): a semisynthetic analogue of taxol. *J Natl Cancer Inst* 1991;83:288.
154. Rowinsky EK, Donehower RC, Jones RJ, Tucker RW. Microtubule changes and cytotoxicity in leukemic cell lines treated with taxol. *Cancer Res* 1988;48:4093.
155. Jordan MA, Wilson L. Use of drugs to study the role of microtubule assembly dynamics in living cells. *Methods Enzymol* 1998;298:252.
156. Jordan A, Hadfield JA, Lawrence NJ, McGowan AT. Tubulin as a target for anticancer drugs which interact with the mitotic spindle. *Med Res Rev* 1998;18:259.
157. Dumontet C, Sikic B. Mechanism of action and resistance to antitubulin agents: microtubule dynamics, drug transport, and cell death. *J Clin Oncol* 1999;17:1061.
158. Bhalla K, Ibrado AM, Tourkina E, et al. Taxol induces internucleosomal DNA fragmentation associated with programmed cell death in human myeloid leukemia cells. *Leukemia* 1993;7:563.
159. Jordan MA Wendell K, Gardiner S, et al. Mitotic block induced in HeLa cells by low concentrations of paclitaxel (Taxol) results in abnormal mitotic exit and apoptotic cell death. *Cancer Res* 1996;56:816.
160. Zhang CC, Yang JM, Bash-Babula J, et al. DNA damage increases sensitivity to vinca alkaloids and decreases sensitivity to taxanes through p53-dependent repression of microtubule-associated protein 4. *Cancer Res* 1999;59:3663.
161. Strobel T, Swanson L, Korsmeyer S, Cannistra SA. BAX enhances paclitaxel-induced apoptosis through a p53-independent pathway. *Proc Natl Acad Sci U S A* 1996;93:14094.
162. Strobel T, Kraeft SK, Chen LB, Cannistra SA. BAX expression is associated with enhanced intracellular accumulation of paclitaxel: a novel role for BAX during chemotherapy-induced cell death. *Cancer Res* 1998;58:4776.
163. Scatena CD, Stewart ZA, Mays D, et al. Mitotic phosphorylation of Bcl-2 during normal cell cycle progression and Taxol-induced cell growth arrest. *J Biol Chem* 1998;273:30777.
164. Torres K, Horwitz SB. Mechanisms of Taxol-induced cell death are concentration dependent. *Cancer Res* 1998;58:3620.
165. Griffon-Etienne G, Boucher Y, Brekken C, et al. Taxane-induced apoptosis decompresses blood vessels and lowers interstitial fluid pressure in solid tumors: clinical implications. *Cancer Res* 1999;59:776.
166. Moos PJ, Fitzpatrick FA. Taxane-mediated gene induction is independent of microtubule stabilization: induction of transcription regulators and enzymes that modulate inflammation and apoptosis. *Proc Natl Acad Sci USA* 1998;95:3896.
167. Burkhart CA, Berman JW, Cwindell CS, et al. Relationship between taxol and other taxanes on induction of tumor necrosis factor-α gene expression and cytotoxicity. *Cancer Res* 1994;54:5779.
168. Belotti D, Vergani V, Drudis T, et al. The microtubule-affecting drug paclitaxel has antiangiogenic activity. *Clin Cancer Res* 1996;2:1843.
169. Klauber N, Paragni S, Flynn E, Hamel E, D'Amato RJ. Inhibitor of angiogenesis and breast cancer in mice by the microtuble inhibitors 2-methoxyestradiol and taxol. *Cancer Res* 1997;57:81.

170. Tishler RB, Geard CR, Hall EJ, Schiff PB. Taxol sensitizes human astrocytoma cells to radiation. *Cancer Res* 1992;52:3595.
171. Niero A, Emiliani E, Monti G, et al. Paclitaxel and radiotherapy: sequence-dependent efficacy—a preclinical model. *Clin Cancer Res* 1999;5:2213.
172. Mason KA, Hunter NR, Milas M, Abbruzzese JL, Milas L. Docetaxel enhances tumor radioresponse in vivo. *Clin Cancer Res* 1997;3:2431.
173. Horwitz SB, Cohen D, Rao S, et al. Taxol: mechanisms of action and resistance. *Monogr Natl Cancer Inst* 1993;15:63.
174. Roy SN, Horwitz SB. A phosphoglycoprotein with taxol resistance in J774.2 cells. *Cancer Res* 1985;45:3856.
175. Cole SPC, Sparks KE, Fraser K, et al. Pharmacological characterization of multidrug resistant MRP-transfected human tumor cells. *Cancer Res* 1994;54:5902.
176. Lorico A, Rappa G, Flavell RA, et al. Double knockout of the *MRP* gene leads to increased drug sensitivity in vitro. *Cancer Res* 1996;56:5351.
177. Rowinsky EK, Smith L, Chaturvedi P, et al. Pharmacokinetic and toxicologic interactions between the multidrug resistance reversal agent VX-710 and paclitaxel in cancer patients. *J Clin Oncol* 1998;16:2964.
178. Patnaik A, Oza AM, Warner E, et al. A phase I dose-finding and pharmacokinetic study of paclitaxel and carboplatin with oral PSC 833 in patients with advanced solid tumors. *J Clin Oncol* 2000 (*in press*).
179. Cabral F, Wible L, Brenner S, Brinkley BR. Taxol-requiring mutants of Chinese hamster ovary cells with impaired mitotic spindle activity. *J Cell Biol* 1983;97:30.
180. Kavallaris M, Kuo DYS, Burkhart CA, et al. Taxol-resistant ovarian tumors are associated with altered expression of specific beta-tubulin isotypes. *J Clin Invest* 1997;100:1282.
181. Haber M, Burkhart CA, Regl DL, et al. Altered expression of Mβ2, the class II β-tubulin isotype, in a murine J774.2 cell line with a high level of taxol resistance. *J Biol Chem* 1995;270:31269.
182. Blade K, Menick DR, Cabral F. Overexpression of class I, II, or IVb beta-tubulin isotypes in CHO cells is insufficient to confer resistance to paclitaxel. *J Cell Sci* 1999;112:2213.
183. Kavallaris M, Burkhart CA, Horwitz SB. Antisense oligonucleotides to class III beta-tubulin sensitize drug resistant cells to Taxol. *Br J Cancer* 1999;80:1020.
184. Dumontet C, Jaffrezou JP, Tsuchiya E, et al. Resistance to microtubule-targeted cytotoxins in a K562 leukemia cell variant associated with altered tubulin expression and polymerization. *Elec J Oncol* 1998;2:44.
185. Giannakakou P, Sackett DL, Kang YK, et al. Paclitaxel-resistant human ovarian cancer cells have mutant beta-tubulins that exhibit impaired paclitaxel-driven polymerization. *J Biol Chem* 1997;272:17118.
186. Monzo M, Rosell R, Sánchez JJ, et al. Paclitaxel resistance in non–small cell lung cancer associated with beta tubulin gene mutations. *J Clin Oncol* 1999;17:1786.
187. Liu Q-Y, Stein CA. Taxol and estramustine-induced modulation of human prostate cancer cell apoptosis via alteration in bcl-x_L and bax expression. *Clin Cancer Res* 1997;3:2039.
188. Tang C, Willingham MC, Reed JC, et al. High levels of p26BCL-2 oncoprotein related Taxol-induced apoptosis in human pre-B leukemia cells. *Leukemia* 1994;8:1960.
189. Murphy M, Hinmann A, Levine AJ. Wild-type p53 negatively regulates the expression of a microtubule-associated protein. *Genes Dev* 1996;10:2971.
190. Zhang CC, Yang JM, White E, et al. The role of MAP4 expression in the sensitivity to paclitaxel and resistance to vinca alkaloids in p53 mutant cells. *Oncogene* 1998;16:1617.
191. Woods CM, Zhu J, McQueney PA, et al. Taxol-induced mitotic block triggers rapid onset of a p53-independent apoptotic pathway. *Mol Med* 1995;1:506.
192. Blagosklonny MV, Schulte TW, Nguyen P, et al. Taxol-induction of p21 WAF1 and p53 requires c-raf-1. *Cancer Res* 1995;55:4623.
193. Tisher RB, Lamppu DM, Park S, et al. Microtubule-active drugs Taxol, vinblastine, and nocodazole increase the level of transcriptionally active p53. *Cancer Res* 1995;55:6021.
194. Srivastava RK, Srivastava AR, Korsmeyer SJ, et al. Involvement of microtubules in the regulation of Bcl2 phosphorylation and apoptosis through cyclic AMP-dependent protein kinase. *Mol Cell Biol* 1998;18:3509.
195. Haldar S, Basu A, Croce CM. Bcl-2 is the guardian of microtubule integrity. *Cancer Res* 1997;57:229.
196. Van Asperen J, van Tellingen O, van der Valk M, et al. Enhanced oral absorption and decreased elimination of paclitaxel in mice cotreated with cyclosporin A. *Clin Cancer Res* 1998;4:2293.
197. Meerum Terwogt JM, Malingre MM, Beokmem JH, et al. Co-administration of oral cyclosporin enables therapy with paclitaxel. *Clin Cancer Res* 1999;5:3379.
198. Rowinsky EK. Pharmacology and metabolism. In: McGuire WG, Rowinsky EK, eds. *Paclitaxel in cancer treatment.* New York: Marcel Dekker, 1995:91.
199. Huizing MT, Keung ACF, Rosing H, et al. Pharmacokinetics of paclitaxel and metabolites in a randomized comparative study in platinum-pretreated ovarian cancer patients. *J Clin Oncol* 1993;11:2127.
200. Gianni L, Kearns C, Gianni A. et al. Nonlinear pharmacokinetics and metabolism of paclitaxel and its pharmacokinetic/pharmacodynamic relationships in humans. *J Clin Oncol* 1995;13:180.
201. Sonnichsen D, Hurwitz C, Pratt C, Relling MV. Saturable pharmacokinetics and paclitaxel pharmacodynamics in children with solid tumors. *J Clin Oncol* 1994;12:532.
202. Van Tellingen O, Huizing MT, Panday VR, et al. Cremophor EL causes (pseudo-) nonlinear pharmacokinetics of paclitaxel in patients. *Br J Cancer* 1999;81:330.
203. Ohtsu T, Sasaki Y, Tamura T, et al. Clinical pharmacokinetics and pharmacodynamics of paclitaxel: a 3-hour infusion versus a 24-hour infusion. *Clin Cancer Res* 1995;1:599.
204. Lesser G, Grossman SA, Eller S, Rowinsky EK. The neural and extra-neural distribution of systemically administered [^{3}H]paclitaxel in rats: a quantitative autoradiographic study. *Cancer Chemother Pharmacol* 1995;34:173.
205. Glantz MJ, Choy H, Kearns CM, et al. Paclitaxel disposition in plasma and central nervous systems of humans and rats with brain tumors. *J Natl Cancer Inst* 1995;87:1077.
206. Monsarrat B, Alvinerie P, Dubois J, et al. Hepatic metabolism and biliary clearance of taxol in rats and humans. *Monograph Natl Cancer Inst* 1993;15:39.
207. Cresteil T, Monsarrat B, Alvinerie P, et al. Taxol metabolism by human liver microsomes: identification of cytochrome P450 isoenzymes involved in its biotransformation. *Cancer Res* 1994;54:386.
208. Walle T, Walle UK, Kumar GN, Bhalla KN. Taxol metabolism and disposition in cancer patients. *Drug Metab Dispos* 1995;23:506.
209. Harris JW, Rahman A, Kim B-R, Guengerich P, Collins JM. Metabolism of taxol by human hepatic microsomes and liver slices: participation of cytochrome P450 3A4 and an unknown P450 enzyme. *Cancer Res* 1994:15:4026.
210. Kerns CM, Gianni L, Egorin M. Paclitaxel pharmacokinetics and pharmacodynamics. *Semin Oncol* 1995;22:16.
211. Rowinsky EK, Bonomi P, Jiroutek M, et al. Paclitaxel steady-state plasma concentration as a determinant of disease outcome and toxicity in lung cancer patients treated with paclitaxel and cisplatin. *Clin Cancer Res* 1999;5:767.
212. Bruno R, Sanderink GJ. Pharmacokinetics and metabolism of Taxotere (docetaxel). In: Workman P, Graham MA, eds. *Cancer surveys, vol 17: pharmacokinetics and cancer chemotherapy.* New York: Cold Spring Harbor Laboratory Press, 1993.
213. Clarke SJ, Rivory LP. Clinical pharmacokinetics of docetaxel. *Clin Pharmacokinet* 1999;36:99.
214. Bruno R, Hille D, Riva A, et al. Population pharmacokinetic/pharmacodynamics of docetaxel in phase II studies in patients with cancer. *J Clin Oncol* 1998;16:186.
215. Baille P, Bruno R, Schellens JHM, et al. Optimal sampling strategies for Bayesian estimation of docetaxel (Taxotere) clearance. *Clin Cancer Res* 1997;3:1535.
216. McLeod HL, Kearns CM, Kuhn JG, Bruno R. Evaluation of the linearity of docetaxel pharmacokinetics. *Cancer Chemother Pharmacol* 1998;42:155.
217. Marland M, Gaillard C, Sanderink G, et al. Kinetics, distribution, metabolism and excretion of radiolabeled Taxotere (^{14}C-RPR 56976) in mice and dogs. *Proc Am Assoc Cancer Res* 1993;34:393(abst).
218. Sparreboom A, Van Tellingen O, Scherrenburg EJ, et al. Isolation, purification and biological activity of major docetaxel metabolites from human feces. *Drug Metab Dispos* 1996;24:655.
219. Royer I, Bonsarrat B, Sonnier M, Wright M, Cresteil T. Metabolism of docetaxel by human cytochromes P450: interactions with paclitaxel and other antineoplastic agents. *Cancer Res* 1996;56:58.
220. Shou M, Martinet M, Korzekwa KR, et al. Role of cytochrome P450 3A4 and 3A5 in the metabolism of taxotere and its derivatives: enzyme specificity, interindividual distribution and metabolic contribution in human liver. *Pharmacogenetics* 1998;8:391.
221. Rowinsky EK, Gilbert M, McGuire WP, et al. Sequences of taxol and cisplatin: a phase I and pharmacologic study. *J Clin Oncol* 1991;9:1692.
222. Rowinsky EK, Citardi M, Noe DA, Donehower RC. Sequence-dependent cytotoxicity between cisplatin and the antimicrotubule agents taxol and vincristine. *J Cancer Res Clin Oncol* 1993;119:737.
223. Kearns CM, Egorin MJ. Considerations regarding the less-than-expected thrombocytopenia encountered with combination paclitaxel/carboplatin chemotherapy. *Semin Oncol* 1997;24[Suppl 2]:S2.
224. Belani CP, Kearns CM, Zuhowski EG, et al. Phase I trial, including pharmacokinetic and pharmacodynamic correlations, of combination paclitaxel and carboplatin in patients with metastatic non-small-cell lung cancer. *J Clin Oncol* 1999;17:676.
225. Holmes FA, Madden T, Newman RA, et al. Sequence-dependent alteration of doxorubicin pharmacokinetics by paclitaxel in a phase I study of paclitaxel and doxorubicin in patients with metastatic breast cancer. *J Clin Oncol* 1996;14:2713.
226. Gianni L, Vigano L, Locatelli A, et al. Human pharmacokinetic characterization and in vitro study of the interactions between doxorubicin and paclitaxel in patients with breast cancer. *J Clin Oncol* 1997;15:1906.
227. Gianni L, Munzone E, Capri G, et al. Paclitaxel by 3-hour infusion in combination with bolus doxorubicin in women with untreated metastatic breast cancer: high antitumor efficacy and cardiac effects in a dose- finding and sequence-finding study. *J Clin Oncol* 1995;13:2688.
228. Gennari A, Salvadori B, Donati S, et al. Cardiotoxicity of epirubicin/paclitaxel-containing regimens: role of cardiac risk factors. *J Clin Oncol* 1999;11:3596.
229. Webster LK, Cosson EJ, Stokes KH, Millward MJ. Effect of the paclitaxel vehicle, Cremophor EL, on the pharmacokinetics of doxorubicin and doxorubicinol in mice. *Br J Cancer* 1996;73:522.
230. Kennedy MJ, Zahurak ML, Donehower RC, et al. Phase I and pharmacologic study of sequences of paclitaxel and cyclophosphamide supported by granulocyte colony-stimulating factor in women with previously treated metastatic breast cancer. *J Clin Oncol* 1995;14:783.
231. Sarvada N, Ishikawa T, Fukase Y, et al. Induction of thymidine phosphorylase activity and enhancement of capecitabine efficacy by taxol/taxotere in human cancer xenografts. *Clin Cancer Res* 1998;4:1013.
232. Fettel MR, Grossman SA, Fisher J, et al. Pre-irradiation paclitaxel in glioblastoma multiforme (GBM): efficacy, pharmacology, and drug interactions. *J Clin Oncol* 1997;15:3121.
233. Prados MD, Schold SC, Spence AM, et al. Phase II study of paclitaxel in patients with recurrent malignant glioma. *J Clin Oncol* 1996;14:2316.
234. Monsarrat B, Chatelut E, Royer I, et al. Modification of paclitaxel metabolism in a cancer patient by induction of cytochrome P450 3A4. *Drug Metab Dispos* 1998;26:229.
235. Desai PB, Duan JZ, Zhu YW, Kouzi S. Human liver microsomal metabolism of paclitaxel and drug interactions. *Eur J Drug Metab Pharmacokinet* 1998;23:417.
236. Slichenmyer W, McGuire W, Donehower R, Chen T-L, Rowinsky EK. Pretreatment H2 receptor antagonists that differ in P450 modulation activity: comparative effects on paclitaxel clearance rates. *Cancer Chemother Pharmacol* 1995;36:227.
237. Eisenhower E, ten Bokkel Huinink W, Swenerton KD, et al. European-Canadian randomized trial of taxol in relapsed ovarian cancer: high vs low dose and long vs. short infusion. *J Clin Oncol* 1994;12:2654.
238. Rowinsky EK. The taxanes: dosing and scheduling considerations. *Oncology* 1997; 11[Suppl 2]:1.
239. Rowinsky EK, Eisenhauer EA, Chaudhry V, Arbuck SA, Donehower RC. Clinical toxicities encountered with taxol. *Semin Oncol* 1993;20[Suppl 3]:1.

240. Weiss R, Donehower RC, Wiernik PH, et al. Hypersensitivity reactions from taxol. *J Clin Oncol* 1990;8:1263.
241. Peereboom D, Donehower RC, Eisenhauer EA, et al. Successful retreatment with taxol after major hypersensitivity reactions. *J Clin Oncol* 1993;11:885.
242. Olson JK, Sood AK, Sorosky JI, Anderson B, Buller RE. Taxol hypersensitivity: rapid retreatment is safe and cost effective. *Gynecol Oncol* 1998;68:25.
243. Szebeni J, Muggia FM, Alving CR. Complement activation by Cremophor EL as a possible contributor to hypersensitivity to paclitaxel: an in vitro study. *J Natl Cancer Inst* 1998;90;300.
244. Rowinsky EK, Chaudhry V, Cornblath DR, Donehower RC. The neurotoxicity of taxol. *Monogr Natl Cancer Inst* 1993;15:107.
245. Chaudhry V, Rowinsky EK, Sartorious SE, Donehower RC, Cornblath DR. Peripheral neuropathy from taxol and cisplatin combination chemotherapy: clinical and electrophysiological studies. *Ann Neurol* 1994;35:490.
246. Gelmon K, Eisenhauer E, Bryce C, et al. Randomized phase II study of high-dose paclitaxel with or without amifostine in patients with metastatic breast cancer. *J Clin Oncol* 1999;17:3038.
247. Capri G, Munzone E, Tarenzi E, Fulgaro F, Gianni L. Optic nerve disturbances: a new form of paclitaxel neurotoxicity. *J Natl Cancer Inst* 1994;86:1099.
248. Hofstra LS, de Vries EG, Willemse PH. Ophthalmic toxicity following paclitaxel infusion. *Ann Oncol* 1997;8:1053.
249. Nieto Y, Cagnoni PJ, Bearman SI, Shpall EJ. Acute encephalopathy: a new toxicity associated with high-dose paclitaxel. *Clin Cancer Res* 1999:5:501.
250. Rowinsky EK, McGuire WP, Guarnieri T, Christian MA, Donehower RC. Cardiac disturbances during the administration of taxol. *J Clin Oncol* 1991;9:1704.
251. Arbuck SG, Strauss H, Rowinsky EK, et al. A reassessment of the cardiac toxicity associated with taxol. *Monogr Natl Cancer Inst* 1993;15:117.
252. Markman M, Kennedy A, Webser K, et al. Paclitaxel administration to gynecologic cancer patients with major cardiac risk factors. *J Clin Oncol* 1998;16:3483.
253. Sparano JA, Speyer J, Gradishar WJ, et al. Phase I trial of escalating doses of paclitaxel plus doxorubicin and dexrazoxane in patients with advanced breast cancer. *J Clin Oncol* 1999;17:880.
254. Della Torre P, Imondi AR, Bernardi C, Podesta A, et al. Cardioprotection by dexrazoxane in rats treated with doxorubicin and paclitaxel. *Cancer Chemother Pharmacol* 1999;44:138.
255. Jeriah S, Keegan P. Cardiotoxicity associated with paclitaxel/trastuzumab combination chemotherapy. *J Clin Oncol* 1999;17:1647.
256. Rowinsky EK, Burke PJ, Karp JE, et al. Phase I and pharmacodynamic study of taxol in refractory adult acute leukemia. *Cancer Res* 1989;49:4640.
257. Wilson WH, Berg S, Bryant G, et al. Paclitaxel in doxorubicin-refractory or mitoxantrone-refractory breast cancer: a phase I/II trial of 96 hour infusion. *J Clin Oncol* 1994;12:1621.
258. Pestalozzi BC, Sotos GA, Choyke PL, et al. Typhlitis resulting from treatment with taxol and doxorubicin in patients with metastatic breast cancer. *Cancer* 1993;71:1797.
259. Seewaldt VL, Cain JM, Goff BA, et al. A retrospective review of paclitaxel-associated gastrointestinal necrosis in patients with epithelial ovarian cancer. *Gynecol Oncol* 1997;67:137.
260. Feenstra J, Vermeer RJ, Stricker BH. Fatal hepatic coma attributed to paclitaxel. *J Natl Cancer Inst* 1997;16;582.
261. Hoff PM, Valero V, Homes FA, Whealin Hudis C, Hortobagyi GN. Paclitaxel-induced pancreatitis: a case report. *J Natl Cancer Inst* 1997;89:91.
262. Ramanathan RK, Belani CP. Transient pulmonary infiltrates: a hypersensitivity reaction to paclitaxel. *Ann Intern Med* 1996;124:278.
263. Ayoub JP, North L, Greer J, Cabanillas F, Younes A. Pulmonary changes in patients with lymphoma who receive paclitaxel. *J Clin Oncol* 1997;15:2476.
264. Luftner D, Flath B, Akrivakis C, et al. Dose-intensified weekly paclitaxel induces multiple nail disorders. *Ann Oncol* 1998;9:1139.
265. Schrijvers D, Wanders J, Dirix L, et al. Coping with toxicities of docetaxel (Taxotere). *Ann Oncol* 1993;4:610.
266. Semb KA, Aamdal S, Oian P. Capillary protein leak syndrome appears to explain fluid retention in cancer patients who receive docetaxel treatment. *J Clin Oncol* 1998;16:3426.
267. Piccart MJ, Klijn J, Paridaens R, et al. Corticosteroids significantly delay the onset of docetaxel-induced fluid retention: final results of a randomized study of the European Organization for Research and Treatment of Cancer, Investigational Drug Branch for Breast Cancer. *J Clin Oncol* 1997;15:149.
268. Zimmerman GC, Keeling JH, Barris HA, et al. Acute cutaneous reactions to docetaxel, a new chemotherapeutic agent. *Arch Dermatol* 1995;131:202.
269. Vukeljia SJ, Baker WJ, Burris HA III, Keeling JH, Von Hoff DD. Pyridoxine therapy for palmar-plantar erythrodysesthesia associated with Taxotere. *J Natl Cancer Inst* 1993;85:1432.
270. Zimmerman GC, Keeling JH, Lowry M, et al. Prevention of docetaxel-induced erythrodysesthesia with local hypothermia. *J Natl Cancer Inst* 1994;86:557.
271. New PZ, Jackson CE, Rinaldi D, Burris H, Barohn RJ. Peripheral neurotoxicity secondary to docetaxel. *Neurology* 1996;46:108.
272. Hilkens PH, Verweij J, Stoter G, et al. Peripheral neurotoxicity induced by docetaxel. *Neurology* 1996;46:104.
273. Frances P, Schneider J, Hann L, et al. Phase II trial of docetaxel in patients with platinum-refractory advanced ovarian cancer. *J Clin Oncol* 1994;12:2201.
274. Hainsworth JD, Burris HA, Greco FA. Weekly administration of docetaxel (Taxotere): summary of clinical data. *Semin Oncol* 1999;26[Suppl 10]:19.
275. Smith RE, Brown AM, Mamounas EP, et al. Randomized trial of 3-hour versus 24-hour infusion of high-dose paclitaxel in patients with metastatic or locally advanced breast cancer: National Surgical Adjuvant Breast and Bowel Project Protocol B-26. *J Clin Oncol* 1999;17:3403.
276. Seidman AD, Hochhauser D, Gollub M, et al. Ninety-six-hour paclitaxel infusion after progression during short taxane exposure: a phase II pharmacokinetic and pharmacodynamic study in metastatic breast cancer. *J Clin Oncol* 1996;14:1877.
277. Markman M, Rose PG, Jones E, et al. Ninety-six-hour infusional paclitaxel as salvage therapy of ovarian cancer patients previously failing treatment with 3-hour or 24-hour paclitaxel infusion. *J Clin Oncol* 1998;16:1849.
278. Holmes FA, Valero V, Buzdar AU, et al. Final results: randomized phase III trial of paclitaxel by 3-hr versus 96-hr infusion in patients with metastatic breast cancer. *Proc Am Soc Clin Oncol* 1999;18:110a(abst).
279. Seidman AD, Hudis CA, Albanel J, et al. Dose-dense therapy with weekly 1-hour paclitaxel infusions in the treatment of metastatic breast cancer. *J Clin Oncol* 1998;16:3353.
280. Greco FA, Thomas M, Hainsworth JD. One-hour paclitaxel infusions: review of the safety and efficacy. *Cancer Sci Am* 1999;5:179.
281. Winer E, Berry D, Duggan D, et al. Failure of higher dose paclitaxel to improve outcome in patients with metastatic breast cancer—results from CALGB 9342. *Proc Am Soc Clin Oncol* 1998;17:101a(abst).
282. Francis P, Rowinsky E, Schneider J, et al. Phase I feasibility and pharmacologic study of intraperitoneal paclitaxel: a Gynecologic Oncology Group study. *J Clin Oncol* 1995;13:2961.
283. Markman M, Brady MF, Spirtos NM, Hanjani P, Rubin SC. Phase II trial of intraperitoneal paclitaxel in carcinoma of the ovary, tube, and peritoneum: a Gynecologic Oncology Group study. *J Clin Oncol* 1998;16:2620.
284. Bookman MA, Kloth DD, Kover PE, Smolinski S, Ozols RF. Short-course intravenous prophylaxis for paclitaxel-related hypersensitivity reactions. *Ann Oncol* 1997;8:611.
285. Rosenberg P, Andersson H, Boman K, et al. A randomized multicenter study of single agent paclitaxel (Taxol) given weekly versus every three weeks to patients with ovarian cancer previously treated with platinum therapy. *Proc Am Soc Clin Oncol* 1999;18:368a(abst).
286. Venock AP, Egorin MJ, Rosner GL, et al. Phase I and pharmacokinetic trial of paclitaxel in patients with hepatic dysfunction. Cancer and leukemia group B 9264. *J Clin Oncol* 1998;16:1811.
287. Baker SD, Ravdin P, Aylesworth, C, et al. A phase I and pharmacokinetic study of docetaxel in cancer patients with liver dysfunction due to malignancies. *Proc Am Soc Clin Oncol* 1998;17:192(abst).
288. Woo MH, Gregornik D, Shearer PD, Meyer WH, Relling MV. Pharmacokinetics of paclitaxel in an anephric patient. *Cancer Chemother Pharmacol* 1999;43:92.
289. Salminen E, Bergman M, Huhtala S, et al. Docetaxel: standard recommended dose of 100 mg/m^2 is effective but not feasible for some metastatic breast cancer patients heavily pretreated with chemotherapy-A phase II single-center study. *J Clin Oncol* 1999;17:1127.
290. Fex H, Hogberg B, Konyves I. Estramustine phosphate—historical overview. *Urology* 1984;23:4.
291. Forsberg JG, Hoisaeter PA. Effects of hormone-cytostatic complexes on the rat ventral prostate in vivo and in vitro. *Vitam Horm* 1975;33:137.
292. Forsgren B, Bjork P, Carlstrom K, et al. Purification and distribution of a major protein in rat prostate that binds estramustine, a nitrogen mustard derivative of estradiol-17 beta. *Proc Natl Acad Sci USA* 1979;76:3149.
293. Lindberg B. Treatment of rapidly progressing prostatic carcinoma with estracyt. *J Urol* 1972;108:303.
294. Nilsson T, Muntzing J. Initial clinical studies with estramustine phosphate. *Urology* 1984;23:49.
295. Hartley-Asp B. Estramustine-induced mitotic arrest in two human prostatic carcinoma cell lines DU 145 and PC-3. *Prostate* 1984;5:93.
296. Kanje M, Deinum J, Wallin M, et al. Effect of estramustine phosphate on the assembly of isolated bovine brain microtubules and fast axonal transport in the frog sciatic nerve. *Cancer Res* 1985;45:2234.
297. Stearns ME, Tew KD. Antimicrotubule effects of estramustine, an antiprostatic tumor drug. *Cancer Res* 1985;45:3891.
298. Stearns ME, Wang M, Tew KD, Binder LI. Estramustine binds a MAP-1-like protein to inhibit microtubule assembly in vitro and disrupt microtubule organization in DU 145 cells. *J Cell Biol* 1988;107:2647.
299. Stearns ME, Tew KD. Estramustine binds MAP-2 to inhibit microtubule assembly in vitro. *J Cell Sci* 1988;89:331.
300. Panda D, Miller HP, Islam K, Wilson L. Stabilization of microtubule dynamics by estramustine by binding to a novel site in tubulin: a possible mechanistic basis for its antitumor action. *Proc Natl Acad Sci USA* 1997;94:10560.
301. Laing N, Dahllof B, Hartley-Asp B, Ranganathan S, Tew KD. Interaction of estramustine with tubulin isotypes. *Biochemistry* 1997;36:871.
302. Friden B, Wallin M. Dependency of microtubule-associated proteins (MAPs) for tubulin stability and assembly: use of estramustine phosphate in the study of microtubules. *Mol Cell Biol* 1991;105:149.
303. Dahllof B, Billstrom A, Cabral F, Hartley-Asp B. Estramustine depolymerizes microtubules by binding to tubulin. *Cancer Res* 1993;53:4573.
304. Walz PH, Bjork P, Gunnarsson PO, Edman K, Hartley-Asp B. Differential uptake of estramustine phosphate metabolites and its correlation with the levels of estramustine binding protein in prostate tumor tissue. *Clin Cancer Res* 1998;4:2079.
305. Eklov S, Mahdy E, Wester K, et al. Estramustine-binding protein (EMBP) content in four different cell lines and its correlation to estramustine induced metaphase arrest. *Anticancer Res* 1996;16:1819.
306. Yoshida D, Cornell-Bell A, Piepmeier JM. Selective antimitotic effects of estramustine correlate with its antimicrotubule properties on glioblastoma and astrocytes. *Neurosurgery* 1994;34:863.
307. Bjork P, Borg A, Ferno M, Nilsson S. Expression and partial characterization of estramustine-binding protein (EMBP) in human breast cancer and malignant melanoma. *Anticancer Res* 1991;11:1173.
308. Johansson M, Bergenheim AT, D'Argy R, et al. Distribution of estramustine in the BT4C rat glioma model. *Cancer Chemother Pharmacol* 1998;41:317.
309. Vallbo C, Bergenheim AT, Bergstrom P, Gunnarsson PO, Henriksson R. Apoptotic tumor cell death induced by estramustine in patients with malignant glioma. *Clin Cancer Res* 1998;4:87.

310. Yoshida D, Piepmeier J, Weinstein M. Estramustine sensitizes human glioblastoma cells to irradiation. *Cancer Res* 1994;54:1415.
311. Bergenheim AT, Zackrisson B, Elfverson J, Roos G, Henriksson R. Radiosensitizing effect of estramustine in malignant glioma in vitro and in vivo. *J Neurooncol* 1995;23:191.
312. Pienta KJ, Lehr JE. Inhibition of prostate cancer growth by estramustine and etoposide: evidence for interaction at the nuclear matrix. *J Urol* 1993;149:1622.
313. Stearns ME, Jenkins DP, Tew KD. Dansylated estramustine, a fluorescent probe for studies of estramustine uptake and identification of intracellular targets. *Proc Natl Acad Sci U S A* 1985;82:8483.
314. Sandstrom PE, Jonsson O, Grankvist K, Henriksson R. Identification of potassium flux pathways and their role in the cytotoxicity of estramustine in human malignant glioma, prostatic carcinoma and pulmonary carcinoma cell lines. *Eur J Cancer* 1994;30A:1822.
315. Ranganathan S, Dexter DW, Benetatos CA, et al. Increase of beta(III)- and beta(IVa)-tubulin isotopes in human prostate carcinoma cells as a result of estramustine resistance. *Cancer Res* 1996;56:2584.
316. Ranganathan S, Dexter DW, Benetatos CA, Hudes GR. Cloning and sequencing of human betaIII-tubulin cDNA: induction of betaIII isotype in human prostate carcinoma cells by acute exposure to antimicrotubule agents. *Biochim Biophys Acta* 1998;1395:237.
317. Sangrajrang S, Denoulet P, Millot G, et al. Estramustine resistance correlates with tau over-expression in human prostatic carcinoma cells. *Int J Cancer* 1998;77:626.
318. Yang CP, Shen HJ, Horwitz SB. Modulation of the function of P-glycoprotein by estramustine. *J Natl Cancer Inst* 1994;86:723.
319. Speicher LA, Sheridan VR, Godwin AK, Tew KD. Resistance to the antimitotic drug estramustine is distinct from the multidrug resistant phenotype. *Br J Cancer* 1991;64:267.
320. Speicher LA, Barone LR, Chapman AE, et al. P-glycoprotein binding and modulation of the multidrug-resistant phenotype by estramustine. *J Natl Cancer Inst* 1994;86:688.
321. Laing NM, Belinsky MG, Kruh GD, et al. Amplification of the ATP-binding cassette 2 transporter gene is functionally linked with enhanced efflux of estramustine in ovarian carcinoma cells. *Cancer Res* 1998;58:1332.
322. Gunnarsson PO, Andersson SB, Johansson SA, Nilsson T, Plym-Forshell G. Pharmacokinetics of estramustine phosphate (Estracyt) in prostatic cancer patients. *Eur J Clin Pharmacol* 1984;26:113.
323. Forshell GP, Muntzing J, Ek A, Lindstedt E, Dencker H. The absorption, metabolism, and excretion of Estracyt (NSC 89199) in patients with prostatic cancer. *Invest Urol* 1976;14:128.
324. Dixon R, Brooks M, Gill G. Estramustine phosphate: plasma concentrations of its metabolites following oral administration to man, rat and dog. *Res Commun Chem Pathol Pharmacol* 1980;27:17.
325. Gunnarsson PO, Forshell GP. Clinical pharmacokinetics of estramustine phosphate. *Urology* 1984;23:22.
326. Gunnarsson PO, Davidsson T, Andersson SB, Backman C, Johansson SA. Impairment of estramustine phosphate absorption by concurrent intake of milk and food. *Eur J Clin Pharmacol* 1990;38:189.
327. Petrylak DP, Macarthur RB, O'Connor J, et al. Phase I trial of docetaxel with estramustine in androgen-independent prostate cancer. *J Clin Oncol* 1999;17:958.
328. Smith PH, Suciu S, Robinson MR, et al. A comparison of the effect of diethylstilbestrol with low dose estramustine phosphate in the treatment of advanced prostatic cancer: final analysis of a phase III trial of the European Organization for Research on Treatment of Cancer. *J Urol* 1986;136:619.
329. Bruno D, Sevenet T, Morgat M, et al. Rhazinilam mimics the cellular effects of Taxol by different mechanisms of action. *Cell Motil Cytoskelton* 1994;28:317.
330. Kowalski RJ, Giannakakou P, Gunasekera SP, et al. The microtubule-stabilizing agent discodermolide competitively inhibits the binding of paclitaxel (Taxol) to tubulin polymers, enhances tubulin nucleation reactions more potently than paclitaxel, and inhibits the growth of paclitaxel-resistant cells. *Mol Pharmacol* 1997;52:613.
331. Kowalski RJ, Giannakakou P, Hamel E. Activities of the microtubule-stabilizing agents epothilones A and B with purified tubulin and in cells resistant to paclitaxel (Taxol). *J Biol Chem* 1997;272:2534.
332. Chou TC, Zhang XG, Harris CR, et al. Desoxyepothilone B is curative against human tumor xenografts that are refractory to paclitaxel. *Proc Natl Acad Sci U S A* 1998;95:15798.
333. Hamel E, Sackett DL, Vourloumis D, Nicolaou KC. The coral-derived natural products eleutherobin and sarcodictyins A and B: effects on the assembly of purified tubulin with and without microtubule-associated proteins and binding at the polymer taxoid site. *Biochemistry* 1999;38:5490.
334. Mooberry SL, Tien G, Hernandez AH, et al. Laulimalide and isolaulimalide, new paclitaxel-like microtubule-stabilizing agents. *Cancer Res* 1999;59:653.
335. Ojima I, Chakravarty S, Inoue T, et al. A common pharmacophore for cytotoxic natural products that stablize microtubules. *Proc Natl Acad Sci U S A* 1999;96:4256.
336. Panda D, DeLuca K, Williams D, Jordan MA, Wilson L. Antiproliferative mechanism of action of cryptophycin-52: kinetic stabilization of microtubule dynamics of high-affinity binding to microtubule ends. *Proc Natl Acad Sci U S A* 1998;95:9313.
337. Bai R, Schwartz, RE, Kepler JA, et al. Characterization of the interaction of cryptophycin 1 with tubulin: binding in the vinca domain, competitive inhibition of dolastatin 10 binding, and an unusual aggregation reaction. *Cancer Res* 1996;56;4398.
338. Aherne GW, Hardcastle A, Valenti M, et al. Antitumour evaluation of dolastatins 10 and 15 and their measurements in plasma by radioimmunoassay. *Cancer Chemother Pharmacol* 1996;38:225.
339. Pitot HC, McElroy AE Jr, Reid JM, et al. Phase I trial of dolastatin-10 (NSC 376128) in patients with advanced solid tumors. *Clin Cancer Res* 1999;5:525.
340. Villalona-Calero MA, Baker SD, Hammond L, et al. Phase I and pharmacokinetic study of the water soluble dolastatin-15 analog LU103793 in patients with advanced solid malignancies. *J Clin Oncol* 1998;16:2770.
341. Hamel E. Natural products which interact with tubulins in the vinca domain: maytansine, rhizoxin, phomopsin A, dolastatin 10-15 and halicondrin B. *Pharmacol Ther* 1992;55:31.
342. Shan B, Medina JC, Santha E, et al. Selective, covalent modification of beta-tubulin residue Cys-239 by T138067, an antitumor agent with in vivo efficacy against multidrug-resistant tumors. *Proc Natl Acad Sci U S A* 1999;96:5686.

SECTION 8

BRUCE D. CHESON

Miscellaneous Chemotherapeutic Agents

HOMOHARRINGTONINE

Homoharringtonine (HHT) and its congener, harringtonine, are cephalotaxine esters isolated from the evergreen tree *Cephalotaxus fortunei* Hook F, which is distributed throughout southern and northeastern China. The two esters differ by only a single methylene group, and they have similar activity against murine leukemia.[1] The greater availability of HHT led to its further testing in the United States.

The primary action of HHT appears to be inhibition of protein synthesis, with degradation of polyribosomes, delayed inhibition of initiation of protein synthesis, and inhibition of chain elongation by interference with peptide bond formation.[2] DNA effects may also be important, with a block in progression of cells from G_1 into S phase and from G_2 phase into M phase.[3] Prolonged drug exposure is necessary for maximal antileukemic effect *in vitro*. Preclinical toxicology identified toxicities of the bone marrow, gastrointestinal tract, kidneys, and heart.[4,5]

Radiolabeled HHT exhibits a triphasic plasma decay, with a terminal half-life of 65.3 hours and an apparent volume of distribution of 2.4 L/kg.[6] In early phase I studies, HHT was administered as a daily 10- to 360-minute infusion for up to 10 days.[7] Dose-limiting cardiovascular toxicity with hypotension began 4 or more hours after drug administration, which is presumed secondary to vasodilatation with a compensatory increase in cardiac output. Hypotension is ameliorated by interrupting the infusion or by fluid administration, or both, and prolonging the duration of administration. The major dose-limiting toxicity with currently used infusion schedules is myelosuppression.

Initial clinical studies with HHT conducted in China identified activity against acute myeloid leukemia and chronic-phase chronic myelogenous leukemia (CML).[8] Clearing of central nervous system blasts occurred after intrathecal administration. Variable activity was observed in the initial series of phase II trials in U.S. pediatric and adult patients with acute leukemia or myelodysplastic syndrome.[8–10] In late chronic-phase CML, a continuous intravenous infusion of HHT, 2.5 $mg/m^2/d$, for 10 to 14 days each month induces complete hematologic remission in 72% of cases, with cytogenetic response in 31%.[11] HHT is being combined with interferon or cytarabine in early chronic-phase CML. O'Brien et al.[12] reported that HHT followed by interferon did not achieve a higher cytogenetic response rate than previously observed with HHT alone.

Nonmyelosuppressive toxicities have been minimal, including diarrhea, hyperglycemia, nausea and vomiting, tachycardia, chest pain, headache, and fatigue.

SURAMIN

Suramin is a polysulfonated napthylurea first used for the treatment of onchocerciasis and trypanosomiasis in the 1920s. Its use against parasites and discoid lupus erythematosus was abandoned because of the availability of more effective drugs. Its inhibition of reverse transcriptase and other RNA polymerases led to trials in patients with autoimmune deficiency syndrome.[13] However, initial clinical enthusiasm was not substantiated by additional study.[14,15]

The precise mechanism of suramin's antitumor action is unknown. The drug binds nonspecifically to a wide variety of plasma proteins and enzymes. It inhibits the binding and mitogenic action of many polypeptide autocrine growth factors, including platelet-derived growth factor, fibroblast growth factor, transforming growth factor-α and -β, epidermal growth factor, insulin-like growth factor-1 and -2, interleukin-2, transferrin, and nerve growth factor.[16] It is capable of dissociating growth factors from their receptors, with higher affinity to heparin binding growth factors. It interferes with glycosaminoglycan catabolism, leading to an accumulation in the liver and blood of heparan sulfate and dermatan sulfate, which are thought to be related to cell proliferation. Suppression of bone resorption may contribute to the decreased pain reported in patients with prostate cancer.

Suramin exhibits antitumor activity against a number of cell lines, notably growth factor–responsive tumors, but low doses induce proliferation in some cell lines. It inhibits the growth of malignant, but not normal, prostate cells. Early clinical trials suggested activity against adrenal, renal, and other cancers.[16] Activity in prostate cancer has led to phase III studies.

CLINICAL PHARMACOLOGY

Suramin has limited absorption from the gastrointestinal tract. The intravenous route is recommended because of better bioavailability.

The original dosing schedule of 1 g weekly for 6 weeks resulted in plasma concentrations that fell over the first few hours after administration but gradually increased over time, with increasing trough levels before each injection.[17] The pharmacokinetics were described by a two-compartment model, with an initial (distribution) half life ($t_{1/2}\alpha$) of 2 days and an elimination half life ($t_{1/2}\beta$) of 48 days (range, 44 to 54 days). Suramin is 99.7% protein bound, primarily to albumin, and may persist in the blood for 3 months after administration, with no evidence of metabolism and 80% renal clearance. The total body clearance is only 0.41 mL/min, with little interpatient variability. Suramin does not cross the blood–brain barrier. It may displace other highly protein-bound drugs.

DOSE AND SCHEDULE

The optimal schedule of administration is still being determined.[18–24] Earlier schedules used adaptive control feedback[25] in which the timing and calculated dose were pharmacologically computed for individual patients to maintain plasma concentrations in the range of 200 to 300 μg/mL. Labor-intense pharmacologic monitoring was used because of concern that the severe neurologic toxicity with suramin was directly correlated with high blood levels. More recently, other pharmacokinetic correlations have been postulated, including time above a threshold concentration, total dose, and others.[26] The relative importance of free drug concentration is unknown. However, several phase I studies have determined that concentrations in the 200 to 300 μg/mL range are better tolerated overall. Phase I studies have demonstrated little pharmacokinetic variability, making complex adaptive control algorithms unnecessary. This observation has led to investigation of a wide variety of schedules, including a 14-day continuous infusion, intermittent short infusions, and intermittent bolus administration.[20,27–29]

Suramin has modest activity in patients with prostate cancer.[19,27,28,30,31] Combinations with other agents have been studied in prostate cancer and other solid tumors, but without clear additive benefit.[32–37] The future of this drug is uncertain.

TOXICITY

The most serious toxic effect of suramin is a polyneuropathy, which may begin within several weeks of therapy and peaks in severity 3 to 6 months after the drug is discontinued. It ranges from mild stocking-glove paresthesia to paralysis requiring mechanical ventilation, and it is an indication to discontinue treatment.[38,39] At 350 mg/m^2/d by continuous infusion, a Guillain-Barré syndrome occurred in 11% of patients; the incidence increased to 40% with levels of more than 350 μg/mL .[38] Suramin may lead to a progressive, reversible myopathy; hyperesthesia of palms and soles; headache; and altered taste. Adrenal insufficiency is very common and may be irreversible. All patients receive concurrent corticosteroids until normal adrenal function can be documented.

Infections are frequent with suramin therapy because the drug induces lymphocytotoxicity and myelosuppression and inhibits phagocytosis and bacterial killing, which is compounded by the addition of hydrocortisone.

Other common toxicities include renal dysfunction, transaminase elevations, and coagulopathy.[40,41] Prophylactic vitamin K has been used to minimize the contribution from other causes. Bleeding is managed by replacement of blood and plasma. Heparin can be given safely using careful monitoring. An increase in serum creatinine or the development of a coagulopathy necessitates interruption of therapy. Other serious toxicities include supraventricular arrhythmias, especially atrial fibrillation, pericardial effusions, and deep venous thromboses.

Rash has been reported, occasionally with desquamation or toxic epidermolysis as well as keratoacanthomas and superficial actinic keratoses. Vortex keratopathy, which resolves after therapy, also has been reported. Metabolic consequences include hyponatremia, hypokalemia, hypocalcemia, hypermagnesemia, hypophosphatemia, hypouricemia, and elevations in amylase and lipase. Rash and renal dysfunction may not recur if the drug is resumed.

BLEOMYCIN

The bleomycins are a group of glycopeptides originally extracted from a strain of *Streptomyces verticillus* from culture broths obtained from the soil of a Japanese coal mine.[42] The most active agent was a mixture of peptides now known as *bleomycin*, with a molecular weight of 1200.

The primary action of bleomycin is to produce single- and double-strand DNA breaks, which result from the production of free radicals by an Fe(II)-bleomycin complex intercalated between opposing strands of DNA. It is ineffective in producing strand breaks of native RNA or synthetic ribonucleotide polymers. Cells are most sensitive to bleomycin during the G_2 and M phases and least sensitive in the G_1 phase.[43] Noncycling cells may be more sensitive than cycling cells. The observation that cells were killed during G_2 suggested an advantage for a continuous infusion, which was not supported by clinical trials.

CELLULAR PHARMACOLOGY

Bleomycin is taken up by cells slowly and inactivated by an aminohydrolase found in normal and malignant cells.[44] Hydrolase levels are higher in animal species resistant to the pulmonary toxicity of bleomycin and is low in lung and skin, the two organs most susceptible to bleomycin toxicity. Levels in tumor cell lines do not appear to correlate with drug resistance.

CLINICAL PHARMACOLOGY

Using a 4- to 5-day continuous intravenous infusion, the steady-state concentration is approached approximately 12 hours after initiation of infusion and ranged from 0.132 to 0.312 mμ/mL. After an intravenous bolus of 15 U/m^2, peak plasma concentrations reach 1 to 10 mμ/mL, with a rapid two-phase disappearance from plasma with a half-life of elimination of approximately 3 hours. Approximately two-thirds of excretion is renal, and the half-life increases rapidly in patients with a creatinine clearance of less than 25 to 35 mL/min. There is increased pulmonary toxicity with renal insufficiency, but no formal guidelines for dose reduction have been determined. Bleomycin is absorbed rapidly after intramuscular administration, resulting in peak plasma concentrations approximately one-third to one-half of those obtained after rapid intravenous administration. One hour after intramuscular injection, maximum serum levels range from 0.13 to 0.35 mμ/ml, with no drug detectable in the serum 24 hours after injection. Absorption after subcutaneous injection has not been clearly defined. Intracavitary administration of bleomycin achieves levels 10- to 22-fold higher than simultaneous plasma levels and is effective in the control of malignant effusions.[45–49] Approximately 45% of the intracavitary dose is absorbed into systemic circulation. Bleomycin also has been applied topically.[50] No pharmacologic advantage to intraperitoneal administration has been reported.

TOXICITY

A test dose of 1 mg of bleomycin is generally administered before a weekly or twice-weekly dose of 5 to 15 U/m^2 because of the risk of hypersensitivity with urticaria, periorbital edema, and bronchospasm. The dose-limiting toxicity of bleomycin is pulmonary fibrosis of uncertain pathogenesis, which occurs in 10% of patients and is more common in patients older than 70 years, with doses of more than 400 U, or in those with a history of chest radiotherapy and in the postoperative period.[51–59] The onset is usually delayed, and the initial physical examination and chest x-ray may be normal. Eventually, rales, rhonchi, and pleural friction rubs are noted, and abnormal pulmonary function, with decreased lung capacity and increased lung stiffness, is seen. Clinical parameters better predict outcome than pulmonary function studies. Chest x-ray may reveal increased interstitial markings, patchy reticulonodular infiltrates, consolidation, or nodules indistinguishable from metastatic lesions, which may cavitate. Biopsy findings are nonspecific. After the drug is discontinued, reversal may take months, and fibrosis may be only partially reversible and may be fatal. A number of investigational approaches are being evaluated to prevent or reduce the severity of this complication.[54,55,60–62]

Myelosuppression and immunosuppression are not prominent. Fevers occur in 20% to 50% of patients, occasionally with hyperpyrexia. Mucocutaneous toxicities are common, with mucositis; alopecia; and hyperpigmentation, erythema, induration, hyperkeratosis, and peeling that may progress to ulceration. The digits, hands, joints, and areas of prior radiation or surgery are most affected. Acute arthritis may occur.

L-ASPARAGINASE

The growth of malignant and normal cells depends on the availability of specific nutrients and cofactors required for protein synthesis. Some nutrients can be synthesized within the cell, whereas others, such as essential amino acids, require exogenous sources. L-asparagine is a nonessential amino acid synthesized by the transamination of L-aspartic acid by a reaction catalyzed by the enzyme L-asparagine synthetase. The ability to synthesize asparagine is notably lacking in malignancies of lymphoid origin. In 1953, Kidd[63] first reported that the growth of transplantable lymphomas of rat and mouse was inhibited by guinea pig serum, and subsequent experiments demonstrated that the responsible factor was L-asparaginase. Subsequent purification from *Escherichia coli* and *Erwinia carotovora* permitted production of large quantities of the enzyme for clinical use. The purified bacterial enzyme has a molecular weight of 133,000 to 141,000 daltons and is composed of four subunits, each with one active site. The enzymes are specific for the L-isomer. Asparaginase catalyzes the conversion of L-asparagine to aspartic acid and ammonia. The enzyme does not enter cells, instead degrading circulating asparagine to aspartic acid, which cannot be converted to asparagine by the cancer cell. In contrast, most normal cells can synthesize asparagine from aspartic acid by induction of asparagine synthetase. This metabolic difference is not absolute, as demonstrated by the toxicity profile of the agent. Resistance occurs through increased expression of the asparagine synthetase gene, which is transcriptionally silent in most tissues and leads to increased enzyme synthesis in response to a decrease in intracellular L-asparagine levels.[64] Resistance may also be mediated by the formation of asparaginase antibodies that alter asparaginase pharmacokinetics.

CLINICAL PHARMACOLOGY

L-asparaginase is administered either intravenously or intramuscularly. The intramuscular route produces peak blood levels 50% lower than the intravenous route, but the former may be less immunogenic and is more commonly used. Three preparations of L-asparaginase are in clinical use. The most widely used is derived from *E coli*, and an *Erwinia* preparation is available for patients who develop hypersensitivity to the *E coli*–

derived agent. The usual doses are 6000 IU/m^2 three times weekly for 3 to 4 weeks, or daily doses of 5000 to 20,000 IU/m^2 for 10 to 20 days. The optimal dose and schedule are unknown. Intermittent schedules with less frequent administration are associated with reduced efficacy and increased anaphylaxis. An *E coli* preparation modified by the covalent attachment of polyethylene glycol (PEG) has a prolonged half-life, thus permitting lower doses and less frequent administration.[65] The approved dose of PEG-asparaginase is 2500 IU/m^2 every 14 days, either intravenously or intramuscularly.

L-asparaginase concentration in plasma is proportional to a total dose up to 200,000 IU/m^2 and falls with a primary half-life of 14 to 22 hours after administration. Blood levels of the *E coli* enzyme are detectable for 1 to 2 weeks after a single dose, and concentrations of L-asparagine fall below 1 mmol within minutes of enzyme injection and remain low for 7 to 10 days after completion of therapy. The half-life is independent of the dose administered, disease status, renal or hepatic function, age, or gender. The pharmacokinetics of asparaginase depend on the preparation.[66–68] With *E coli*–derived enzyme, the $t_{1/2}$ (1.14 to 1.35 days) administered by the intramuscular route is the same irrespective of dose (2500 or 25,000 IU/mL) or with repeated doses. Peak serum levels are reached in 24 to 48 hours and are no longer detectable in serum by 10 to 14 days. Extremely low levels are found in the urine at 24 hours, suggesting clearance of L-asparaginase by mechanisms other than urinary excretion. Cerebrospinal fluid levels disappear rapidly. The serum $t_{1/2}$ for *Erwinia* is 0.65 days, and enzyme was no longer detectable by 7 days. This value is shorter than the *E coli* preparation, although similar schedules are often used. The serum $t_{1/2}$ of PEG-modified L-asparaginase as an initial dose was 5.73 days, which is significantly longer than after subsequent doses.[66]

Patients who experience a hypersensitivity reaction to *E coli* asparaginase have a decreased $t_{1/2}$ subsequently with PEG asparaginase.[66,69] Serum L-asparaginase activity is undetectable in the week after an anaphylactoid reaction. And even a "silent" anaphylactoid reaction to *E coli* may result in neutralizing antibodies and reduced drug efficacy.[70]

TOXICITIES

L-asparaginase has no effect on bone marrow function. Hypersensitivity is the most serious toxicity, and it occurs in fewer than 10% of patients. It is manifested by urticaria, nausea, vomiting, and chills, and less often by a serum sickness–like reaction or by anaphylaxis with hypotension, laryngospasm, and cardiac arrest, which is fatal in fewer than 1% of patients. Reactions generally occur during the second week of treatment or later, and they mandate a change to another preparation. The risk of hypersensitivity is greater when the drug is used as a single agent than with concurrent immunosuppressive agents (steroids, 6-mercaptopurine), at doses higher than 6000 IU/m^2/d administered by the intravenous route and with repeated courses of treatment. Neither skin testing nor antibody levels have been sufficiently predictive. The PEG formulation is the least immunogenic[71,72] and may be more cost-effective.[73] The development of an allergic reaction does not appear to compromise the efficacy of the agent.[74]

Decreased protein synthesis leads to reduced albumin and serum lipoprotein concentrations. A reduction in vitamin K–dependent clotting factors, a fall in fibrinogen levels, and decreased platelet aggregation to collagen may lead to bleeding. Decreases in antithrombin III, proteins C and S, and increased endogenous thrombin generation are associated with venous thrombosis and embolism.[75–81] Other toxic effects include confusion, aphasia, stupor, or coma in 25% to 33% of patients[82,83]; hyperlipidemia[84,85]; and abnormal liver enzymes with fatty metamorphosis. L-asparaginase is contraindicated in patients with a history of pancreatitis because of the risk of acute pancreatitis.[86]

AMIFOSTINE

Amifostine is a phosphorylated aminothiol prodrug analogue of cysteamine. It was developed by the Walter Reed Army Medical Institute (thus the military code name WR-2721) during the cold war as part of a classified research project to identify an agent that would protect military personnel from radiation in the event of nuclear war. Amifostine was found to afford greater protection against radiation than more than 4000 other compounds screened. Nevertheless, the army terminated development of this compound in 1988 because of its poor oral bioavailability and the prohibitive nausea, vomiting, diarrhea, and abdominal cramps noted with the oral formulation.

When administered intravenously, the pharmacokinetics (PK) of amifostine varies somewhat with dose.[87] The clearance from plasma is rapid (distribution and elimination phases in humans of $t_{1/2}\alpha$, less than 1 minute; $t_{1/2}\beta$, 8.8 minutes), with a plasma half-life of 1 minute and almost all drug cleared by the plasma within 10 minutes. Bioavailability from the subcutaneous route is high but variable.[87,88]

Amifostine is dephosphorylated at the tissue level to its active metabolite, the free thiol WR-1065, by membrane-bound alkaline phosphatase. WR-1065 is rapidly taken up by cells and is thought to be the major cytoprotective metabolite. WR-1065 protects normal cells by acting as a free radical scavenger and by hydrogen donation to repair damaged target molecules.[89,90]

Preclinical studies with amifostine suggested that the agent could protect normal tissues from radiation and chemotherapy toxicity without protecting tumors.[91–97] Phosphorylation of the aminothiol contributes substantially to the selective uptake of WR-1065 by normal kidneys, bone marrow, heart, and salivary glands compared with tumor tissues. Several explanations have been postulated for this preferential uptake, such as that concentrations of alkaline phosphatase are higher in normal tissues compared with malignant tissues. The hypovascular, hypoxic nature of tumors results in anaerobic metabolism and a low interstitial pH, which are associated with a low rate of prodrug activation by alkaline phosphatase.

Separate phase I trials of amifostine were conducted in conjunction with radiotherapy or chemotherapy. A true maximum tolerated dose was not identified in either setting, but the recommended dose ranges from 740 mg/m^2 to 910 mg/m^2.[98–101] No clear therapeutic advantage to the higher doses has been determined.[100,102,103] Drug-related toxicity appears to correlate with the duration of the infusion.[104]

CHEMOTHERAPY-RELATED NEPHROTOXICITY

Amifostine has been evaluated for its ability to prevent chemotherapy-related nephrotoxicity, especially that induced by cisplatin.[100–102,105] In the only phase III trial, Kemp et al.[106] randomized 242 women with advanced ovarian cancer to six cycles of chemotherapy, with or without amifostine, 910 mg/m^2, before each cycle. The severity of renal toxicity was reported to be lower in the group receiving amifostine. Fewer patients discontinued therapy on the amifostine arm because of toxicity. The response rates and survival durations were comparable between the two arms. However, the doses of cisplatin used in this study are higher than the dose currently recommended, and this regimen is less commonly used than other less nephrotoxic programs.

NEUROLOGIC TOXICITIES AND OTOTOXICITY

Several small phase II studies and one phase III trial suggest that amifostine may offer modest protection against the neurologic toxicities of cisplatin, but with no effect on ototoxicity.[101,105,106]

NEUTROPENIA AND THROMBOCYTOPENIA

Various phase I, II, and III trials suggest a myeloprotective effect from amifostine. Glover et al.[103] conducted a phase II trial of amifostine in combination with cyclophosphamide with 21 patients used as their own controls; 90% had an improved white blood cell count with the second course of cyclophosphamide compared with the first course. Whether these findings are clinically meaningful is questionable.[103,106,107] In a study conducted by the Cancer and Leukemia Group B,[108] patients with solid tumors were treated with high-dose cyclophosphamide with amifostine alone or with amifostine and granulocyte-macrophage colony-stimulating factor. No additional protection was noted with the combination.

Preliminary phase I data suggest less thrombocytopenia in patients treated with carboplatin and amifostine.[109] However, the aggregate data from subsequent studies provide less support for clinically meaningful benefit.[108,110–113]

ADDITIONAL OBSERVATIONS

Limited data suggest that amifostine may modulate the cardiotoxicity of doxorubicin and the pulmonary toxicity of bleomycin.[54,55,114]

RADIOPROTECTION

Amifostine has been evaluated in combination with radiation therapy or combined modality treatment for patients with head and neck and lung cancers.[111,115–124] The suggestion has been made of a reduction in esophagitis in lung cancer patients and less xerostomia and loss of taste with amifostine, but with no clear impact on mucositis or salivary gland function.[117–119] There is no clear radioprotective effect in patients with rectal cancer.[98,125]

TOXICITIES

The major toxicities associated with amifostine include nausea and vomiting, hypotension, hypocalcemia, and allergic reactions. The onset of nausea and vomiting is generally within 15 to 30 minutes of the start of the infusion, and they resolve spontaneously. Pretreatment with dexamethasone and a 5-hydroxytryptamine receptor antagonist is recommended.

Hypotension is a potentially serious side effect. It is generally systolic, lasting 5 to 15 minutes, without central nervous system, renal, or cardiovascular consequences. Administration issues that influence the frequency and severity of hypotension include patient hydration, infusion duration, position of patient, and antiemetic pretreatment. Patients should not be receiving agents that potentiate the potential for hypotension, and the drug should not be administered to patients who cannot be without antihypertensive medications for at least 24 hours. Dehydrated patients should not receive the drug until the problem has been corrected. Patients should be hydrated before administration of amifostine. Patients should remain supine or reclining during amifostine therapy.

Hypocalcemia is clinically significant in approximately 1% of patients and can be managed with oral calcium carbonate and vitamin D. The drug has been used successfully to treat hypercalcemia.[126]

Allergic reactions occur in fewer than 1% of patients and are successfully treated with diphenhydramine.

DRUG ADMINISTRATION

Amifostine should be administered over 15 minutes, 5 to 30 minutes before cytotoxic chemotherapy. The patient should be well hydrated and in a reclining position, with frequent blood pressure monitoring. The recommended dose with radiation therapy is 200 mg/m^2/d, as a slow intravenous push over 3 minutes, 15 to 30 minutes before each radiation fraction. Bolus schedules have been studied as well.[127]

MYELODYSPLASTIC SYNDROMES

Amifostine stimulates hematopoiesis in animal models, and in *in vitro* studies it stimulates the formation of hematopoietic progenitors from myelodysplastic syndrome bone marrow.[128] In a phase I/II study,[129,130] the drug was administered at doses of 100, 200, or 400 mg/m^2 three times per week, or 740 mg/m^2 weekly for 3 weeks. Hematologic improvement was observed in 83% of patients with the thrice-weekly schedule, including either an increase in neutrophils or a reduction in red blood cell transfusion requirements. More than 40% of patients had a rise in their platelet counts. Acceleration to acute myeloid leukemia was noted in several patients with RAEB-T (refractory anemia with excess of blasts in transformation). In a subsequent multicenter trial,[131] there was single or multilineage improvement in 35%. A poor response rate was reported using a continuous schedule of eight uninterrupted thrice-weekly doses of 300 to 450 mg/m^2.[132] The role of this agent in myelodysplastic syndrome is being elucidated.

RECOMMENDATIONS FOR THE USE OF AMIFOSTINE

Based on a careful review of the data, the American Society of Clinical Oncology made the following recommendations regarding the use of amifostine[133]:

- It may be considered for the reduction of nephrotoxicity in patients receiving cisplatin-based chemotherapy.
- Although it may be considered for the reduction of neutropenia in patients receiving alkylating agents, chemotherapy dose reduction or growth factor use should be considered as an alternative to the use of amifostine.

- Present data are insufficient to recommend the use of amifostine for protection against thrombocytopenia or the routine use of amifostine to prevent cisplatin-associated neurotoxicity or ototoxicity. Similarly, the data were felt to be insufficient to support the use of amifostine for the prevention of paclitaxel-associated neurotoxicity.
- The use of amifostine may be considered to decrease the incidence of acute and late xerostomia in certain patients undergoing fractionated radiation therapy in the head and neck region, although the present data are insufficient to recommend the use of amifostine to prevent radiation therapy–associated mucositis.

REFERENCES

1. Powell RG, Weisleder D, Smith CR Jr, Rohwedder WK. Structures of harringtonine, isoharringtonine, and homoharringtonine. *Tetrahedron Lett* 1970;11:815.
2. Huang MT. Harringtonine, an inhibitor of initiation of protein biosynthesis. *Mol Pharmacol* 1975;11:511.
3. Baaske DM, Heinstein P. Cytotoxicity and cell cycle specificity of homoharringtonine. *Antimocrob Agents Chemother* 1977;12:298.
4. Hacker MP, Stewart JA, Newman RA, et al. Toxicologic studies of homoharringtonine in humans and rats. *Proc AACR* 1983;24:325.
5. O'Dwyer PJ, King SA, Hoth DF, Suffness M, Leyland-Jones B. Homoharringtonine—perspectives on an active new natural product. *J Clin Oncol* 1986;4:1563.
6. Savaraj N, Lu K, Dimery I, et al. Clinical pharmacology of homoharringtonine. *Cancer Treat Rep* 1986;70:1403.
7. Neidhart JA, Young DC, Kraut E, Howinstein B, Metz EN. Phase I trial of homoharringtonine administered by prolonged continuous infusion. *Cancer Res* 1986;46:967.
8. Grem JL, Cheson BD, King SA, Leyland-Jones B, Suffness M. Cephalotaxine esters: antileukemic advance or therapeutic failure? *J Natl Cancer Inst* 1988;80:1095.
9. Feldman E, Arlin Z, Ahmed T, et al. Homoharringtonine is safe and effective for patients with acute myelogenous leukemia. *Leukemia* 1992;6:1185.
10. Feldman E, Deiter KP, Ahmed T, Baskind P, Arlin ZA. Homoharringtonine in patients with myelodysplastic syndrome (MDS) and MDS evolving to acute myeloid leukemia. *Leukemia* 1996;10:40.
11. O'Brien S, Kantarjian H, Keating M, et al. Homoharringtonine therapy induces responses in patients with chronic myelogenous leukemia in late chronic phase. *Blood* 1995;86:3322.
12. O'Brien S, Kantarjian H, Koller C, et al. Sequential homoharringtonine and interferon-alpha in the treatment of early chronic phase chronic myelogenous leukemia. *Blood* 1999;93:4149.
13. De Clercq E. Suramin: a potent inhibitor of the reverse transcriptase of RNA tumor viruses. *Cancer Lett* 1979;8:9.
14. Broder S, Yarchoan R, Collins JM, et al. Effects of suramin on HTLV-III/LAV infection presenting as Kaposi's sarcoma or AIDS-related complex: clinical pharmacology and suppression of virus replication *in vivo*. *Lancet* 1985;2:627.
15. Cheson BD, Levine AM, Mildvan D, et al. Suramin therapy in AIDS and related disorders. Report of the U.S. Suramin Working Group. *JAMA* 1987;258:1347.
16. Stein CA, LaRocca RV, Thomas R, McAtee N, Myers CE. Suramin: an anticancer drug with a unique mechanism of action. *J Clin Oncol* 1989;7:499.
17. Collins JM, Klecker RW Jr, Yarchoan R, et al. Clinical pharmacokinetics of suramin in patients with HTLV-III/LAV infection. *J Clin Pharmacol* 1986;26:22.
18. Vogelzang NJ, Small EJ, Halabi S, et al. A phase III trial of three different doses of suramin (SUR) in metastatic hormone refractory prostate cancer (HRPC): safety profile of CALGB 9480. *Proc ASCO* 1998;17:347a(abst 1339).
19. Sinibaldi VJ, Long GS, Chaudry V, et al. Phase I and pharmacologic evaluation of a monthly, daily times five days (D), schedule (SCH) of suramin (S) in patients with hormone refractory prostate cancer (HRPC). *Proc ASCO* 1998;17:218a(abst 841).
20. Reyno LM, Egorin MJ, Eisenberger MA, et al. Development and validation of a pharmacokinetically based fixed dosing scheme for suramin. *J Clin Oncol* 1995;13:2187.
21. Kobayasi K, Vokes EE, Vogelzang NJ, et al. Phase I study of suramin given by intermittent infusion without adaptive control in patients with advanced cancer. *J Clin Oncol* 1995;13:2623.
22. Kobayashi K, Vokes EE, Vogelzang NJ, Janisch L, Ratain MJ. Suramin (SUR) without adaptive control: three different intermittent infusion (II) schedules (sched) are equally safe. *Proc ASCO* 1999;16:211a(abst 738).
23. Jodrell DI, Reyno LM, Sridhara R, et al. Suramin: development of a population pharmacokinetic model and its use with intermittent short infusions to control plasma drug concentration in patients with prostate cancer. *J Clin Oncol* 1994;12:166.
24. Eisenberger MA, Sinibaldi VJ, Reyno LM, et al. Phase I and clinical evaluation of a pharmacologically guided regimen of suramin in patients with hormone-refractory prostate cancer. *J Clin Oncol* 1995;13:2174.
25. Eisenberger MA, Sinibaldi VJ, Reyno LM, et al. Phase I and clinical evaluation of a pharmacologically guided regimen of suramin in patients with hormone-refractory prostate cancer. *J Clin Oncol* 1995;13:2174.
26. Bitton RJ, Figg WD, Venzon DJ, et al. Pharmacologic variables associated with the development of neurologic toxicity in patients treated with suramin. *J Clin Oncol* 1995;13:2223.
27. Kelly WK, Curley T, Leibretz C, et al. Prospective evaluation of hydrocortisone and suramin in patients with androgen-independent prostate cancer. *J Clin Oncol* 1995;13:2208.
28. Kelly WK, Scher HI, Mazumbdar M, et al. Suramin and hydrocortisone: determining drug efficacy in androgen-independent prostate cancer. *J Clin Oncol* 1995;13:2214.
29. Kobayashi K, Vokes EE, Vogelzang NJ, et al. Phase I study of suramin given by intermittent infusion without adaptive control in patients with advanced cancer. *J Clin Oncol* 1995;13:2196.
30. Garcia-Schurmann JM, Schultze H, Haupt G, et al. Suramin treatment in hormone- and chemotherapy-refractory prostate cancer. *Urology* 1999;53:535.
31. Eisenberger M, Meyer M, Lenehan P, et al. Suramin induced decrease in PSA is associated with prolonged objective progression-free (OPFS) and overall survival in hormone-refractory prostate cancer (HRPC). *Proc ASCO* 1999;18:314a(abst 1208).
32. Dawson NA, Figg WD, Cooper MR, et al. Phase II trial of suramin, leuprolide, and flutamide in previously untreated metastatic prostate cancer. *J Clin Oncol* 1997;15:1470.
33. Dawson N, Figg WD, Brawley OW, et al. Phase II study of suramin plus aminoglutethimide in two cohorts of patients with androgen-independent prostate cancer: simultaneous antiandrogen withdrawal and prior antiandrogen withdrawal. *Clin Cancer Res* 1998;4:37.
34. Falcone A, Antonuzzo A, Danesi R, et al. Suramin in combination with weekly epirubicin for patients with advanced hormone-refractory prostate carcinoma. *Cancer* 1999;86:470.
35. Long GS, Sinibaldi VJ, O'Reilly S, et al. Phase I and pharmacologic study of suramin (S) and topotecan (T) in patients (PTS) with hormone refractory prostate cancer (HRPC). *Proc ASCO* 1998;17:247a(abst 948).
36. Miglietta L, Canobbio L, Granetto C, et al. Suramin/epidoxorubicin association in hormone-refractory prostate cancer: preliminary results of a pilot phase II study. *J Cancer Res Clin Oncol* 1997;123:407.
37. Tu SM, Pagliaro LC, Banks ME, et al. Phase I study of suramin combined with doxorubicin in the treatment of androgen-independent prostate cancer. *Clin Cancer Res* 1998;4:1193.
38. La Rocca RV, Cooper MR, Stein CA, et al. A pilot study of suramin in the treatment of progressive refractory follicular lymphomas. *Ann Oncol* 1992;3:571.
39. Bitton RJ, Figg WD, Venzon DJ, et al. Pharmacologic variables associated with the development of neurologic toxicity in patients treated with suramin. *J Clin Oncol* 1995;13:2223.
40. Horne MK III, Stein CA, LaRocca RV, Myers CE. Circulating glycosaminoglycan anticoagulants associated with suramin treatment. *Blood* 1988;71:273.
41. Horne MK III, Wilson OJ, Cooper M, Gralnick HR, Myers CE. The effect of suramin on laboratory tests of coagulation. *Thromb Haemost* 1992;67:434.
42. Umezawa H, Maeda K, Takeuchi T, Okami Y. New antibiotics, bleomycin A and B. *J Antibiot (Tokyo)* 1966;19:200.
43. Barlogie B, Drewinko B, Schumann J, Freireich EJ. Pulse cytophotometric analysis of cell cycle perturbation with bleomycin *in vitro*. *Cancer Res* 1976;36:1182.
44. Yoshioka O, Amano N, Takahashi K, Matsuda A, Umezawa H. Intracellular fate and activity of bleomycin. In: Carter SK, Crooke ST, eds. *Bleomycin: current status and new developments*. New York: Academic Press, 1978:35.
45. Emad A, Rezaian GR. Treatment of malignant pleural effusions with a combination of bleomycin and tetracycline. A comparison of bleomycin or tetracycline alone versus a combination of bleomycin and tetracycline. *Cancer* 1996;78:2498.
46. Martinez-Moragon E, Aparicio J, Rogado MC, et al. Pleurodesis in malignant pleural effusions: a randomized study of tetracyclines versus bleomycin. *Eur Respir J* 1997;10:2380.
47. Moffett MJ, Ruckdeschel JC. Bleomycin and tetracycline in malignant pleural effusions: a review. *Semin Oncol* 1992;19[Suppl 2]:62.
48. Noppen M, Degreve J, Mignolet M, Vincken W. A prospective randomised study comparing the efficacy of talc slurry and bleomycin in the treatment of malignant pleural effusions. *Acta Clin Belg* 1998;52:258.
49. Zimmer PW, Hill M, Casey K, Harvey E, Low DE. Prospective randomized trial of talc slurry vs bleomycin in pleurodesis for symptomatic malignant pleural effusions. *Chest* 1997; 112:430.
50. Epstein JB, Gorsky M, Wong FL, Millner A. Topical bleomycin for the treatment of dysplastic oral leukoplakia. *Cancer* 1998;83:629.
51. Blum RH, Carter SK, Agre K. A clinical review of bleomycin—a new antineoplastic agent. *Cancer* 1973;31:903.
52. Parvinen LM, Kilkku P, Makinen E, Liukko P, Gronroos M. Factors affecting the pulmonary toxicity of bleomycin. *Acta Radiol Oncol* 1983;22:417.
53. Bloor AJ, Seale JR, Marcus RE. Two cases of fatal pneumonitis complicating the treatment of non-Hodgkin's lymphoma. *Clin Lab Haematol* 1998;20:119.
54. Nici L, Santos-Moore A, Kuhn C, Calabresi P. Modulation of bleomycin-induced pulmonary toxicity in the hamster by the antioxidant amifostine. *Cancer* 1998;83:2008.
55. Nici L, Calabresi P. Amifostine modulation of bleomycin-induced lung injury in rodents. *Semin Oncol* 1999;26[Suppl 7]:28.
56. Sato E, Koyama S, Masubuchi T, et al. Bleomycin stimulates lung epithelial cells to release neutrophil and monocyte chemotactic activities. *Am J Physiol* 1999;276(Pt 1):L941.
57. Saxman SB, Nichols CR, Einhorn LH. Pulmonary toxicity in patients with advanced-stage germ cell tumors receiving bleomycin with and without granulocyte colony stimulating factor. *Chest* 1997;111:657.
58. Simpson AB, Paul J, Graham J, Kaye SB. Fatal bleomycin pulmonary toxicity in the west of Scotland 1991–1995: a review of patients with germ cell tumors. *Br J Cancer* 1998; 78:1061.
59. Takamizawa A, Koyama S, Sato E, et al. Bleomycin stimulates lung fibroblasts to release neutrophil and monocyte chemotactic activity. *J Immunol* 1999;162:6200.
60. Keane MP, Belperio JA, Moore TA, et al. Neutralization of the CXC chemokine, macrophage inflammatory protein-2, attenuates bleomycin-induced pulmonary fibrosis. *J Immunol* 1999;162:5511.
61. Tran PL, Weinbach J, Opolon P, et al. Prevention of bleomycin-induced pulmonary fibrosis after adenovirus-mediated transfer of the bacterial bleomycin resistance gene. *J Clin Invest* 1997;99:608.

62. Wang Q, Wang Y, Hyde DM, et al. Reduction of bleomycin induced lung fibrosis by transforming growth factor beta soluble receptors in hamsters. *Thorax* 1999;54:805.
63. Kidd JG. Regression of transplanted lymphomas induced *in vivo* by means of normal guinea pig serum. I. Course of transplanted cancers of various kinds given guinea pig serum, horse serum, or rabbit serum. *J Exp Med* 1953;98:565.
64. Haskell CM, Canellos GP. L-asparaginase resistance in human leukemia—asparagine synthetase. *Biochem Pharmacol* 1969;18:2578.
65. Ho DH, Brown NS, Yen A, et al. Clinical pharmacology of polyethylene glycol-L-asparaginase. *Drug Metab Dispos* 1986;14:349.
66. Asselin BL, Whitin JC, Coppola DJ, et al. Comparative pharmacokinetic studies of three asparaginase preparations. *J Clin Oncol* 1993;11:1780.
67. Boos J, Werber G, Ahlke E, et al. Monitoring of asparaginase activity and asparagine levels in children on different asparaginase preparations. *Eur J Cancer* 1996;32A:1544.
68. Boos J. Pharmacokinetics and drug monitoring of L-asparaginase treatment. *Int J Clin Pharmacol Ther* 1997;35:96.
69. Kurtzberg J, Asselin B, Poplack D, et al. PEG-L-asparaginase (PEG-ASP) pharmacology in pediatric patients with acute lymphoblastic leukemia (ALL). *Proc ASCO* 1994;13:144(abst 370).
70. Kurtzberg J, Asselin B, Poplack D, et al. Antibodies to asparaginase alter pharmacokinetics and decrease enzyme activity in patients on asparaginase therapy. *Proc AACR* 1993;34:304.
71. Koerholz D, Brueck M, Nuernberger W, et al. Chemical and immunological characteristics of four different L-asparaginase preparations. *Eur J Haematol* 1989;42:417.
72. Ettinger LJ, Kurtzberg J, Voute PA, Jurgens H, Halpern SL. An open-label, multicenter study of polyethylene glycol-L-asparaginase for the treatment of acute lymphoblastic leukemia. *Cancer* 1995;75:1176.
73. Peters BG, Goeckner BJ, Ponzillo JJ, Velasquez WS, Wilson AL. Pegespargase versus asparaginase in adult ALL: a pharmacoeconomic assessment. *Formulary* 1995;30:388.
74. Larson RA, Fretzin MH, Dodge RK, Schiffer CA. Hypersensitivity reactions to L-asparaginase do not impact on the remission duration of adults with acute lymphoblastic leukemia. *Leukemia* 1998;12:660.
75. Homans AC, Ryback ME, Baglini RL, et al. Effect of L-asparaginase administration on coagulation and platelet function in children with leukemia. *J Clin Oncol* 1987;5:811.
76. Vigano'D'Angelo S, Gugliotta L, Mattioli Belmonte M, et al. L-asparaginase treatment reduces the anticoagulant potential of the protein C system without affecting vitamin K–dependent carboxylation. *Thromb Res* 1990;59:985.
77. Mitchell L, Hoogendoorn H, Giles AR, Vegh P, Andrew M. Increased endogenous thrombin generation in children with acute lymphoblastic leukemia: risk of thrombotic complications in L-asparaginase-induced antithrombin III deficiency. *Blood* 1994;83:386.
78. Nowak-Gottl U, Ahlke E, Klosel K, Jurgens H, Boos J. Changes in coagulation and fibrinolysis in childhood acute lymphoblastic leukemia re-induction therapy using three different asparaginase preparations. *Eur J Pediatr* 1997;156:848.
79. Oner AF, Gurgey A, Kirazli S, Okur H, Tunc B. Changes in hemostatic factors in children with acute lymphoblastic leukemia receiving combined chemotherapy including high dose methylprednisolone and L-asparaginase. *Leuk Lymphoma* 1999;33(3–4):361.
80. Alberts SR, Bretscher M, Wiltsie JC, et al. Thrombosis related to the use of L-asparaginase in adults with acute lymphoblastic leukemia: a need to consider coagulation monitoring and clotting factor replacement. *Leuk Lymphoma* 1999;32(5–6):489.
81. Nowak-Gottl U, Wermes C, Junker R, et al. Prospective evaluation of the thrombotic risk in children with acute lymphoblastic leukemia carrying the MTHFR TT 677 genotype, the prothrombin G20210A variant, and further prothrombotic risk factors. *Blood* 1999;93:1595.
82. Feinberg WM, Swenson MR. Cerebrovascular complications of L-asparaginase therapy. *Neurology* 1988;38:127.
83. Kingma A, Tamminga RY, Kamps WA, Le Coultre R, Saan RJ. Cerebrovascular complications of L-asparaginase therapy in children with leukemia: aphasia and other neuropsychological deficits. *Pediatr Hematol Oncol* 1993;10:303.
84. Tozuka M, Yamauchi K, Midaka H, et al. Characterization of hypertriglyceridemia induced by L-asparaginase therapy for acute lymphoblastic leukemia and malignant lymphoma. *Ann Clin Lab Sci* 1997;27:351.
85. Hoogerbrugge N, Jansen H, Hoogerbrugge PM. Transient hyperlipidemia during treatment of ALL with L-asparaginase is related to decreased lipoprotein lipase activity. *Leukemia* 1997;11:1377.
86. Sahu S, Saika S, Pai SK, Advant SH. L-asparaginase (Leunase) induced pancreatitis in childhood acute lymphoblastic leukemia. *Pediatr Hematol Oncol* 1998;15:533.
87. Shaw LM, Bonner HS, Schuchter L, Schiller J, Lieberman R. Pharmacokinetics of amifostine: effects of dose and method of administration. *Semin Oncol* 1999;26[Suppl 7]:34.
88. Shaw LM, Turrisi AT, Glover DJ, et al. Human pharmacokinetics of WR-2721. *Int J Radiat Oncol Biol Phys* 1986;12:1501.
89. DeNeve WJ, Everett CK, Suminski JE, et al. Influence of WR-2721 on DNA cross-linking by nitrogen mustard on normal mouse bone marrow and leukemia cells *in vivo*. *Cancer Res* 1988;48:6002.
90. Treskes M, Nijtmans LG, Fichtinger-Schepman AM, van der Vijgh WJ. Effects of the modulating agent WR2721 and its main metabolites on the formation and stability of cisplatin-DNA adducts *in vitro* in comparison to the effects of thiosulphate and diethyldithiocarbamate. *Biochem Pharmacol* 1992;43:1013.
91. Yuhas JM, Storer JB. Differential chemoprotection of normal and malignant tissues. *J Natl Cancer Inst* 1969;42:331.
92. Yuhas JM. Differential protection of normal and malignant tissues against the cytotoxic effects of mechlorethamine. *Cancer Treat Rep* 1979;63:971.
93. Yuhas JM, Culo F. Selective inhibition of the nephrotoxicity of *cis*-dichlorodiammineplatinum (II) by WR-2721 without altering its antitumor properties. *Cancer Treat Rep* 1980;64:57.
94. Yuhas JM. Active versus passive absorption kinetics as the basis for selective protection of normal tissues by S-2-(3-aminopropylamino)-ethylphosphorothioic acid. *Cancer Res* 1980;40:1519.
95. Yuhas JM, Spellman JM, Culo F. The role of WR-2721 in radiotherapy and/or chemotherapy. *Cancer Clin Trials* 1980;3:211.
96. Yuhas JM, Spellman JM, Jordan SW, et al. Treatment of tumors with the combination of WR-2721 and cisdichlorodiammineplatinum. *Br J Cancer* 1980;42:574.
97. Grdina DJ, Hunter N, Kataoka Y, Murley JS, Milasz L. Chemopreventive doses of amifostine confers no cytoprotection to tumor nodules growing in the lungs of mice treated with cyclophosphamide. *Semin Oncol* 1999;26[Suppl 7]:22.
98. Kligerman MM, Liu T, Liu Y, et al. Interim analysis of a randomized trial of radiation therapy of rectal cancer with/without WR-2721. *Int J Radiat Oncol Biol Phys* 1992; 22:799.
99. Blumberg AL, Nelson DF, Gramkowski M, et al. Clinical trials of WR-2721 with radiation therapy. *Int J Radiat Oncol Biol Phys* 1982;8(3–4):561.
100. Glover D, Glick J, Weiler C, Yuhas J, Kligerman MM. Phase I trials of WR-2721 and cisplatinum. *Int J Radiat Oncol Biol Phys* 1984;10:1781.
101. Glover D, Glick JH, Weiler C, et al. Phase I/II trials of WR-2721 and cis-platinum. *Int J Radiat Oncol Biol Phys* 1986;12:1509.
102. Glover DJ, Glick JH, Weiler C, Fox K, Guerry D. WR-2721 and high dose cisplatin: an active combination in the treatment of metastatic melanoma. *J Clin Oncol* 1987;5:574.
103. Glover D, Glick JH, Weiler C, Hurowitz S, Kligerman MM. WR-2721 protects against the hematologic toxicity of cyclophosphamide: a controlled phase II trial. *J Clin Oncol* 1986;4:584.
104. Turrisi AT, Glover DJ, Hurwitz S, et al. Final report on phase I trial of WR-2721 [S-2-(3-aminopropylamino)ethylphosphorothiotic acid]. *Cancer Treat Rep* 1986;70:1389.
105. Mollman JE, Glover DJ, Hogan WM, Furman RE. Cisplatin neuropathy: risk factors, prognosis, and protection by WR-2721. *Cancer* 1988;61:2192.
106. Kemp G, Rose P, Lurain J, et al. Amifostine pretreatment for protection against cyclophosphamide-induced and cisplatin-induced toxicities: results of a randomized control trial in patients with advanced ovarian cancer. *J Clin Oncol* 1996;14:201.
107. Glick JH, Glover D, Weiler C, et al. Phase I controlled trials of WR-2721 and cyclophosphamide. *Int J Radiat Oncol Biol Phys* 1984;10:1777.
108. Budman DR, Rosner GL, Lichtman SM, et al. Evaluation of amifostine as a chemoprotective agent in combination with cyclophosphamide and melograstim. *Cancer Ther* 1998;1:164.
109. Budd GT, Ganapathi R, Bauer L, et al. Phase I study of WR-2721 and carboplatin. *Eur J Cancer* 1993;29A:1122.
110. Shpall EJ, Stemmer SM, Hami L, et al. Amifostine (WR-2721) shortens the engraftment period of 4-hydroperoxycyclophosphamide-purged bone marrow in breast cancer patients receiving high-dose chemotherapy with autologous bone marrow support. *Blood* 1994;83:3132.
111. Betticher DC, Anderson H, Ranson M, et al. Carboplatin combined with amifostine, a bone marrow protectant, in the treatment of non-small-cell lung cancer: a randomized phase II study. *Br J Cancer* 1995;72:1551.
112. Budd GT, Ganapathi R, Adelstein DJ, et al. Randomized trial of carboplatin plus amifostine versus carboplatin alone in patients with advanced solid tumors. *Cancer* 1997; 80:1134.
113. Budd GT, Ganapathi R, Wood L, et al. Approaches to managing carboplatin-induced thrombocytopenia: focus on the role of amifostine. *Semin Oncol* 1999;26[Suppl 7]:41.
114. De Lana M, Catino A, Lorusso V, et al. Amifostine (AMF) protects against doxorubicin (D) toxicity with preservation of therapeutic activity in advanced breast cancer (ABC) patients. *Proc ASCO* 1998;17:137a(abst 521).
115. Brizel D, Sauer R, Wannenmacher M, et al. Randomized phase III trial of radiation ± amifostine with head and neck cancer. *Proc ASCO* 1998;17:386a(abst 1487).
116. Buntzel J, Kuttner K, Russell L, et al. Selective cytoprotection by amifostine in the treatment of head and neck cancer with simultaneous radiochemotherapy. *Proc ASCO* 1997;16: 393a(abst).
117. McDonald S, Meyerowitz C, Smudzin T, et al. Amifostine preserves the salivary gland function during irradiation of the head and neck. *Eur J Cancer* 1995;31A[Suppl 5]:415(abst).
118. Giglio R, Mickiewicz E, Pradier E, et al. Alternating chemotherapy + radiotherapy (RT) with amifostine (A) protection for head and neck cancer (HN). Early stop of a randomized trial. *Proc ASCO* 1998;16:1369(abst).
119. Buntzel J, Glatzel M, Kuttner K, et al. Selective cytoprotection with amifostine in concurrent radiochemotherapy of head and neck cancer. *Ann Oncol* 1998;9:505.
120. Sauer R, Wannenmacher M, Wasserman T, et al. Randomized phase III trial of radiation ± amifostine in patients with head and neck cancer. *Proc ASCO* 1999;18:392a(abst 1516).
121. Anderson H, Mercer V, Russell L, Oster W, Thatcher N. A phase III randomized study of carboplatin and amifostine vs carboplatin and G-CSF in patients with inoperable non–small cell lung cancer. *Blood* 1996;88[Suppl 1]:350a(abst 1387).
122. Schiller JH, Storer B, Berlin J, et al. Amifostine, cisplatin, and vinblastine in metastatic non–small cell lung cancer. A report of high response rates and prolonged survival. *J Clin Oncol* 1996;14:1913.
123. Tannehill SP, Mehta MP, Larson M, et al. Effect of amifostine on toxicities associated with sequential chemotherapy and radiation therapy for unresectable non-small-cell lung cancer. Results of a phase II trial. *J Clin Oncol* 1997;15:2850.
124. Fishman DA, Calhoun E, Golub R, et al. Cost-utility assessment of amifostine in first-line therapy for ovarian cancer. *Proc ASCO* 1998;17:417a(abst 1608).
125. Liu T, Liu Y, He S, et al. Use of radiation with or without WR-2721 in advanced rectal cancer. *Cancer* 1992;69:2820.
126. Glover DJ, Shaw L, Glick JH, et al. Treatment of hypercalcemia in parathyroid cancer with WR-2721, S-2-(3-aminopropylamino)ethyl-phosphorothioic acid. *Ann Intern Med* 1985;103:55.

127. Wagner W, Radmard A, Schonekaes KG. A new administration schedule for amifostine as a radioprotector in cancer therapy. *Anticancer Res* 1999;19(3B):2281.
128. List AF, Heaton R, Glinsmann-Gibson B, et al Amifostine stimulates formation of multipotent and erythroid bone marrow progenitors. *Leukemia* 1998;12:1596.
129. List AF, Heaton R, Glinsmann-Gibson B, Capizzi R. Amifostine stimulates formation of multipotent progenitors and generates macroscopic colonies in normal and myelodysplastic bone marrow. *Proc ASCO* 1996;15:449(abst 1403).
130. List AF, Brasfield F, Heaton R, et al. Stimulation of hematopoiesis by amifostine in patients with myelodysplastic syndrome. *Blood* 1997;90:3364.
131. List AF, Holmes H, Vempaty H, Greenberg PL, Bennett JM. Phase II study of amifostine in patients with myelodysplastic syndromes (MDS): impact on hematopoiesis. *Proc ASCO* 1999;18:51a(abst 190).
132. Bowen DT, Denzlinger C, Brugger W, et al. Poor response rate to a continuous schedule of amifostine therapy for "low/intermediate risk" myelodysplastic patients. *Br J Haematol* 1998;103:785.
133. Hensley ML, Schucter LM, Lindley C, et al. American Society of Clinical Oncology Clinical Practice guidelines for the use of chemotherapy and radiotherapy protectants. *J Clin Oncol* 1999;17:3333.

CHAPTER 20

Pharmacology of Cancer Biotherapeutics

SECTION 1

JOHN M. KIRKWOOD

Interferons

RATIONALE FOR INVESTIGATION OF INTERFERONS: DIRECT REGULATION OF CELL GROWTH, DIFFERENTIATION, ANTIGEN EXPRESSION; INDIRECT EFFECTS MEDIATED THROUGH MODULATION OF THE HOST IMMUNE RESPONSE

The interferons (IFNs) are a complex family of inducible natural host proteins that have been traced in phylogeny to prevertebrate species. The physical and chemical immunologic and biologic differences among the IFNs have served as a basis for speciation of these molecules, long before the knowledge of intracellular signaling pathways that have been more recently elucidated was known.[1,2] These intercellular pathways activated by the IFNs (signal transducers and activators of transcription)[3,4] are triggered by a large number of signaling polypeptides, but are activated in different patterns by different signaling polypeptides, to induce precise cellular responses in mammalian (as well as insect and slime mold) cells, demonstrating critical roles in different phases of cell biology. Disruption of the STAT genes in the mouse has shown roles in viral/bacterial defense (STAT 1).[5,6] Early lethality has been reported for STAT 2 and 3 lesions, whereas disruption of TH1 has been identified as a consequence of disruption of STAT 4,[7,8] and TH2 function has been assigned to STAT 6.[9–11] The role of IFN-induced gene regulation in many diverse tissues is likely to account for the effects of IFNs on a variety of neoplastic, viral, and angiogenic conditions in which IFN therapeutic activity has been clinically observed since the 1980s.

The IFNs have been empirically tested as therapies for a multitude of hematologic and solid neoplasms, demonstrating therapeutic benefits in more than a dozen cancers, leading to regulatory approval in multiple countries across the world. This chapter reviews the biology and preclinical effects of the IFNs, discussing the multiple mechanisms of potential relevance to cancer and the therapeutic advances that have been made with IFNs as single agents and combined with chemotherapy, radiotherapy, and other biologic agents, including vaccines, particularly as these relate to the solid tumors.

INTERFERONS OF TYPE I: INTERFERON-α, -β, -τ, AND -ω

Human IFN-α comprises a complex array of subspecies, each of approximately 165 to 166 amino acids encoded by a superfamily of closely related genes located with the IFN-α and -β genes on the short arm of human chromosome 9 that are variably modified by posttranslational glycosylation.[12–14] In the human, 14 nonallelic IFN-α genes and four pseudogenes are clustered together with genes for IFN-α. A variable mixture of IFN-α species is induced in leukocytes and other host cells by a range of stimuli classically including virus or nucleic acids. The biologic effects of the many subspecies are overlapping in large part, despite differences in relative antiviral, antiproliferative, antigen-modulating, and immunomodulating effects to be discussed later in this chapter.[15,16]

IFN-α and -β bind with high affinity (dissociation constant of 10^{-10} to 10^{-12} mol/L) to a single receptor of 110 kD specified on chromosome 21,[17,18] ranging in density from 100 to 10,000 receptors per cell. A range of cellular processes induced by IFNs follow the production of a new set of proteins, after binding and internalization. Knowledge of the events that occur after binding of IFN to its receptor has advanced significantly.[1,19–21] A multimeric transcription activator ISGF3 is stimulated to translocate to the nucleus, where it binds *cis* to the IFN response element of DNA and induces genes that make up the array of IFN-stimulated genes.[21–25] The cytoplasmic and nuclear components of the transcription-activating factor ISGF3 associated with IFN-α are activated, such that ISGF3-γ (the component of the complex specifically recognizing the ISRE) and ISGF3-α (which contains three polypeptides activated specifically on phosphorylation) interact and translocate to the nucleus without the requirement of protein synthesis to activate the IFN response element.

INTERFERON-BINDING RECEPTOR OF TYPE II: INTERFERON-γ

IFN-γ binds a receptor that is discrete from that bound by type I IFNs. Evidence for two classes of receptors, one with low (10^{-9} mol/L) and one with high (10^{-11} mol/L) affinity, has been reported.[26] The *in vitro* and *in vivo* immunomodulatory activity of IFN-γ in experimental animals as well as the human has been one of the most potent of all IFNs,[27] leading to expectations that IFN-γ would also be the most therapeutically active of all IFNs against cancer. Trials of IFN-γ in patients with advanced metastatic melanoma and renal cell carcinoma, as well as adjuvant trials in patients with a high risk of relapse, have been conducted, but have not shown therapeutic effects equivalent to the IFN-α_2 molecule. Reasons for this may relate to effect on antigen presumption and the proteosome complex.

The pleiotropism of the IFNs has posed significant challenges in their quantification and the definition of mechanism of action. The specific activity of various IFN preparations may be expressed in terms of differing functions (e.g., antiviral, antiproliferative, differentiating, effector cell activating, antigen augmenting, and enzyme inducing). Antiviral activity has been accepted as the basis of IFN standardization, although it is far from clear that this function is related to the effects of IFN-γ in cancer therapy. Units of antiviral activity determined against reference standards of the Center for Biologics (Washington, DC) are commonly used to quantify IFN-α and -β, but recombinant IFN-γ and newer polyethylene glycol (PEG) bound forms of IFN-α_2 are generally reported in terms of mass. The various species, subspecies, and molecular variants (muteins) of IFNs argue for adoption of functional standardization in terms of alternative mechanisms relevant to antitumor activity for clinical trials.

MECHANISMS RELEVANT TO ANTITUMOR ACTION

The pleiotropic actions of IFNs may be separated into several categories that are useful in analyzing preclinical and clinical data, as summarized in Table 20.1-1. Direct effects of the IFNs include antiproliferative and differentiating effects that may be demonstrated against fresh melanoma tissues or cultured cell lines *in vitro*. Effects have been designated as *composite* that result in alterations in tumor cell surface antigen expression without direct effect on tumor cell growth, invasion, and metastasis. These effects may permit host recognition and response *in vivo*. Each of three major categories of IFN effects that are potentially relevant to melanoma has been studied in some detail and may provide a basis for understanding the outcome of therapeutic trials (as discussed). Indirect effects of the IFNs are those that are mediated by the host immune system, including the cellular elements such as the large granular lymphocyte or natural killer (NK)/lymphokine-activated killer cell, macrophage/dendritic cell, neutrophil, and T and B cells.[28–31]

DIRECT EFFECTS ON TUMOR CELL PROLIFERATION AND ENZYME AND SIGNALING PATHWAYS

The actual mechanism(s) responsible for the antitumor action of IFNs in human cancer remain uncertain. Nonrecombinant IFN-α and -β and recombinant subspecies of IFN-α_2, -β, and -γ have been evaluated *in vitro* for their antiproliferative activity against cultured and fresh solid tumor cells. These demonstrate comparable growth-inhibitory activity, and one may draw the general observations that (1) there exists a direct dose-response tumor-inhibiting relationship for each species; (2) there is considerable heterogeneity among different tumors regarding sensitivity to inhibition; and (3) solid tumors are generally sensitive to IFNs *in vitro* if exposed to high levels (greater than 500 μ/mL) of IFN-α_2.

TABLE 20.1-1. Pleiotropy of Interferons: Direct, Composite, and Indirect Effects

Direct (Tumor Cell)	*Composite (Tumor Cell Antigens)*	*Indirect (Immune)*	*Indirect (Vascular)*
Antiproliferative	Major histocompatibility complex class I and II cell surface antigens	Nonantigen-specific effector activation	Antiangiogenic
Differentiating	Tumor-restricted cell surface antigens	Macrophage–monocyte/dendritic cell	
Antiviral	Adhesion molecules	Large granular lymphocyte	
	Intracellular adhesion molecule-1	FcR expression	
		Major histocompatibility complex class I and II expression	
		Antigen-specific effector modulation	
		T cell	
		B cell	

Molecular pathways of IFN signaling have been defined, allowing analysis of the proximate intracellular pathways of action, which may prove more informative than the measurement of IFN-induced enzymes such as oligoadenylate synthetase, and more distal effects such as induction of major histocompatability complex (MHC) antigen expression. Studies of cultured *in vitro* tumor cells have suggested acquired defects in the STAT signaling pathway and the absence of STAT that may be associated with IFN resistance. By contrast, studies of human tumor tissues *in vivo* have revealed the constitutive activation of STAT pathways and nuclear correlation of STAT, in melanocytic nevi tissues of patients untreated with IFN as well as in solid tumor tissues (squamous carcinoma of the upper aerodigestive tract). The analysis of signal transduction intermediates of the IFNs in tumor cells of patients undergoing therapy with the IFNs is now feasible. The prospective evaluation and correlation of these intermediate end points of IFN action with clinical evidence of response, progression, or both will be of interest in future trials.[32]

Enzyme Induction

A number of enzyme pathways are activated after induction of the IFN response element, including some that have been evaluated in clinical trials. These include 2'5' oligoadenylate synthetase (2'5' oligo-As) and protein kinase (p67).[33] Two molecular forms of 2'5' oligo-As of 33 kD and 110 kD have been identified differing in subcellular localization and activation requirements.[34,35] The role of the different forms of 2'5' oligo-As as in relation to antitumor effects of IFNs has yet to be established. Indoleamine 2,3, dioxygenase is induced by IFNs in a dose- and time-dependent fashion; this enzyme alters tryptophan metabolism[36] and with xanthine oxidase generates superoxides that may relate to both therapeutic and toxic effects of IFN, as well as depression of cytochrome P-450 enzymes levels.[37,38] Neopterin production induced by IFN-γ may provide an additional biochemical tool for the analysis of intermediate effects of IFN-γ *in vivo.*

Antiproliferative Effects of Interferons in Combination with Chemotherapy and Other Biologic Agents In Vitro

The presence of additive or synergistic effects of chemotherapeutic agents has been examined with IFNs *in vitro* using isobologram plots to compare various combinations for synergistic, additive, or subadditive effects against tumor cells.[39] Although synergism and additive effects have been identified with some combinations[40–44] and negative interactions[40] for others, there is no compelling evidence that these *in vitro* effects have been useful in the development of therapeutic regimens for the clinic.

IFN-γ has been shown to potentiate apoptotic cell death and DNA fragmentation induced by tumor necrosis factor (TNF),[45] whereas IFN-α and -γ potentiate the tumor-cytotoxic activity of TNF in clonogenic stem cell assays.[46]

Differentiation In Vitro *and* In Vivo

Differentiative and growth regulatory or apoptotic effects of the IFNs have become focal points of interest in multiple solid and hematopoietic neoplasms. A number of adhesion molecules, growth factors, and receptors have been identified in the process of malignant progression that are subject to IFN regulation. The receptor-ligand pairs may serve as paracrine or autocrine growth-stimulating circuits[47,48] that may be interrupted at various stages. IFN-α and retinoic acid inhibit epidermal growth factor receptor expression, and retinoids as well as IFNs are under study as potential inhibitors of progression.

COMPOSITE (ANTIGENIC) ANTITUMOR MECHANISMS: MODULATION OF MELANOMA-ASSOCIATED CELL SURFACE ANTIGENS

The antitumor effects of IFNs have been attributed to their effects on cell surface antigens of several tumors. The histocompatability complex is among the most consistent and sensitive targets of the IFNs. It is well established that MHC class I antigens are inducibly type I IFNs, whereas MHC class II antigens are the target of type II IFNs (IFN-γ).[49–54] *In vivo* studies have suggested an even broader pleiotropy type of the IFNs than *in vitro,* in which induction of both MHC class I (ABC) and II (DR, DP, DQ) antigens have been reported with IFN-α_2.[55,56]

IFNs modulate the expression of many cell surface molecules, not all of which have been assigned physiologic functions, and a number of which play roles in the progression from neoplastic to invasive neoplastic disease.[51,57–60]

The clinical implications of altered MHC antigen expression relate to their pivotal function in intercellular immunologic recognition and communication at multiple levels. Antigen presentation to T cells by Langerhans'/dendritic cells of the macrophage monocyte lineage and B cells is associated with the expression of MHC class I and II antigens, adhesion molecules, and costimulating molecules (B7.1/7.2, CD80, CD86). Antitumor effects of IFNs may thus occur through MHC class I and II antigens even if the tumor antigens recognized by the immune system are not themselves upregulated.[61,62] Decreased susceptibility to NK cells is associated with induction of class I major histocompatability antigen expression,[63,64] and IFN-γ protects human tumor cells that are otherwise susceptible to NK cell lysis within hours.[65,66]

The induction of MHC class I and II antigens by IFNs may increase the immunogenicity of tumor cells used for vaccination, outweighing effects on susceptibility to NK/lymphokine-activated killer effector cells in experimental models.[67,68] Thus, induction of increased MHC class I and II tumor cell surface antigen expression may account for the enhanced efficacy of host T-cell–mediated immunity or tumor cell elimination by means of a composite mechanism, irrespective of the modulation of effector cell functions. To date, studies have not resolved these issues in human clinical trials.

INDIRECT IMMUNOMODULATORY EFFECTS

Natural Killer, Macrophage, and Dendritic Cells

The macrophage is a key target of IFN-γ, which was earlier described as macrophage activating factor[69–71] (see Table 20.1-1). The large granular lymphocyte known as the *NK cell* is a well-recognized target of the type I and II IFNs.[72,73] Clinical relevance of the effects of IFNs on NK activity has been sought for many years, both *in vitro* and *in vivo* for IFN-α, -β, and -γ. NK activity measurements performed in the context of multiple trials has depended on assay conditions, effector cell manipulation, and the delay from blood-drawing to assay (*rest period*). To date, no convincing evidence of a relationship between NK cell activity *in vivo* and the therapeutic activity of IFNs in patients with solid tumors has been documented.[74–77] Antibody-dependent cellular cytotoxicity of peripheral blood lymphocytes is mediated in part by NK cells and augmented *in vitro* and *in vivo* by IFN-α, as well as interleukin-2 (IL-2).[78] As trials of antitumor antibodies are further developed, the optimization of NK activity and antibody-dependent cellular cytotoxicity with IFNs, IL-2, as well as IL-12, and other newer biologic agents will continue to be important.

The dendritic cell, a central antigen-presenting cell, is influenced by multiple cytokines, including granulocyte-macrophage colony-stimulating factor, IL-4, IL-12, and IFN-α. The immunomodulatory effects of IFN-α may thus be due to altered numbers or functional capacities of dendritic cells,[79] although studies *in vivo* during IFN therapy have yet to be performed to evaluate this potential mechanism.

T Cell

Specific T-cell–mediated immunity has been implicated as the basis of antitumor effects of the IFNs in many solid tumors. Durable complete responses have been reported in multiple clinical trials of IFN-α for chemotherapy-refractory solid tumors, including renal cell carcinoma and melanoma. Shifts in T-cell subsets (CD4 to CD8 ratio increased) have been correlated with clinical antitumor response to IFN-α and -γ.[80–88] IFN-α modulates mixed leukocyte reactions *in vitro*,[89] and the modulation of specific cytotoxic T-cell immune responses to solid tumors by IFN-α_2 remains a leading hypothetical basis for the durable antitumor effects observed clinically with IFN-α_2 in melanoma, renal cell carcinoma, and other solid tumors. This is prospectively being evaluated in the context of current trials for several solid tumors.[29,30,90–95] The prognostic importance of CD4+ T-cell infiltrates in predicting response of melanoma and other solid tumors has been suggested by Hakansson et al.[87] and is now being tested prospectively as a means to select a more IFN-responsive population. The definition of both MHC class I–restricted and MHC class II (DR)–restricted epitopes recognized by CD4+ T cells in melanoma, renal cell carcinoma/H/N cancer, and other solid tumors adds a new dimension to the expanse of CD8+ T-cell–defined MHC class I–restricted epitopes for analysis of IFN-modulated effector functions.[96]

In preclinical systems, Belardelli and Gresser et al.[97–99] have shown that IFN prevents the outgrowth of experimental murine tumors that does not correlate with the tumor cell susceptibility to direct tumor growth inhibition by IFN. This effect depends critically on the presence of an intact immune system in the host and particularly the CD4 T cell. Tumor response suggesting that tumor regression induced by IFN in this system is dependent on immunologic effects of IFN on the tumor and host.

B Cell

IFN-γ increases production of IgG2a and decreases that of IgG3, IgG1, IgG2b, and IgE by human B cells.[100] Several tumor vaccines have been evaluated in conjunction with IFN-α_2 to evaluate the immunomodulatory role (and possible inhibitory effects) of IFN-α_{2b} administered together with or following GM2 vaccine (Eastern Cooperative Oncology Group trial E2696: GMK, Progenics, Tarrytown, NY). The results of these trials have established the feasibility of this combination and the absence of inhibitory interactions between ganglioside GM2 vaccination and high-dose IFN-α_{2b} in regard to serologic IgM and IgG response and pave the way for IFN combinations in other disease settings.

The specific effects of IFN-α, -β, and -γ on specific immune function against autologous solid tumors have not been examined due to the complexity of measuring immune responses to autologous tumor cell surface antigens in clinical trials. Analyses of specific immune responses to tumor-associated antigens will be essential to interpret therapeutic responses to IFN, much as it is critical to the analysis of an array of vaccine trials underway for many solid tumors.

ROLE OF INTERFERON-γ AS A MEDIATOR OF CLINICAL EFFECTS OF OTHER CYTOKINES

IFN-γ induction by IL-2 and IL-12 has been documented *in vivo* in humans.[101,102] Ambient levels of 1 to 7 U/mL have been demonstrated after continuous intravenous infusion of IL-2 and are likely to be a major component of the dose-limiting toxicity of IL-12.[102,103] The IFN-γ induced during therapy with IL-2, IL-12, and other cytokines may play a role in therapeutic as well as toxic effects of a number of biologic agents.

DENDRITIC CELL MODULATION

A cell that has taken center stage and is central to antigen presentation is the dendritic antiangiogenic actions of the IFN-α cell[104]; this cell, regulated by a series of cytokines, including granulocyte-macrophage colony-stimulating factor, IL-4, IL-12, and IFN-α, has the ability to promote T-cell immune responses in naive subjects.

IFN-α is one of the earliest antiangiogenic agents established in clinical trials in experimental and human systems. Angiogenesis associated with tumor progression[105] is a logical mechanism for evaluation, although direct evidence of a role for antiangiogenic effects of IFNs in the clinical therapy of human solid tumors has yet to be documented. The observation that IFN-α is able to cause regression of hemangiomas of childhood remains a clinical foundation for the exploration of antitumor antiangiogenic effects of IFN in malignant neoplasms.[106] A balance between proangiogenic (basic fibroblast growth factor) and antiangiogenic (IFN-α) effects has been proposed on the basis of preclinical studies that may have implications for the optimal administration of IFN-α in bladder cancer, ovarian cancer, and melanoma, among other solid tumors.[107,108]

CLINICAL EVALUATION

TOXICITY AND PHARMACOKINETICS OF THE INTERFERONS

General

The clinical toxicity of the different species of IFNs involves a similar range of target organs, although the relative components of toxicity differ from species to species and in the human from individual to individual[109,110] (Table 20.1-2). Acutely, a flu-like constitutional syndrome with fever, chills, headache, malaise, myalgias, arthralgias, and fatigue occurs in the majority of patients and diminishes over time with continued daily or alternate-daily administration. For this reason, therapy is best tolerated in many patients at bedtime. Low back pain and headache

TABLE 20.1-2. Toxicities of Interferons

Acute/Subacute	*Chronic*
Symptoms	
Fever, chills	Anorexia
Headache	Dysgeusia
Myalgia	Fatigue
Nausea/vomiting	Depression
Diarrhea	
Signs	
Hyperthermia	Weight loss
Tachycardia	Alopecia
Anemia	Hypothyroidism
Neutropenia	
Rash	
Rarer	
Rhabdomyolysis	Nephrotic syndrome
Subacute hepatic necrosis	

with severe rigors have been associated with IFN-α in particular. Metabolic alterations in the blood lipid profile have been noted with hypertriglyceridemia, and elevated low-density lipoprotein is seen due to inhibition of lipoprotein lipase.[111] IFN-α may depress the plasma cholesterol in 15% to 40% of patients, with a parallel decrement in both high- and low-density cholesterol, without alteration of very low-density lipoproteins.[112–114] Long-term toxicity of IFN consists in constitutional flu-like symptoms compounded by anorexia, weight loss, and fatigue. These late toxicities are the result of dysgeusia, low-grade fever, and nutritional compromise and may be difficult to differentiate from the appearance of thyroid dysfunction or other endocrine pathology on the basis of autoimmune processes associated with IFN-α (as for IL-2). Neuropsychiatric toxicity ranges from mild cognitive deficits to frank depression and psychosis (see Neurologic Effects, later in this chapter).

Hematologic Effects

Hematologic toxicities of the IFNs include leukopenia and, less frequently, thrombocytopenia and anemia; infections are a recognized complication of the leukopenia, but bleeding complications have been rare. Diminished colony-forming capacity and hypocellularity have been noted in the bone marrow, which are rapidly reversible on withdrawal of IFN.[115,116]

Hepatic Effects

Hepatotoxicity observed at high doses frequently includes elevated circulating transaminase enzyme levels that are dose related and reversible on withdrawal of the agent, without evidence of cholestasis. Rarely, subacute hepatic necrosis and cholestatic liver failure with death have been observed when IFN has been administered in the face of hepatotoxicity with hyperbilirubinemia or a history of antecedent viral or alcoholic liver disease. Careful observation of hepatic function generally permits the avoidance of such problems, with treatment modification according to signs and symptoms of toxicity.[29,117] Indeed, after the initial report of two cases of fatal hepatotoxicity of high-dose IFN in the pivotal E1684 adjuvant trial for high-risk melanoma,[118] the confirmatory intergroup trial E1690 was completed without any instance of life-threatening hepatotoxicity, and the only two toxic fatalities noted were cardiovascular and cerebrovascular, occurring with low-dose IFN.

Cardiac and Renal Effects

Cardiovascular, renal, and CNS toxicity are less common. Supraventricular tachyarrhythmias noted with the IFNs may be direct effects or the consequence of fever or nutritional and fluid imbalances. Complex conduction disturbances have been observed with IFN-γ, including bradycardia with high-grade heart block.[93] Cardiotoxicity is increased among elderly patients and patients with underlying heart disease or prior exposure to cardiotoxic agents, but the mechanism has not been defined.[119,120] Hypotension occurs through at least two separate mechanisms: acute hypotension, occurring 1 to 2 hours after administration of IFNs, may be related to peripheral vasodilatation and responds to fluid repletion or rarely may require pressors. Hypotension during chronic administration of IFNs is related to subclinical low-grade fever with insidious fluid losses, anorexia, dysgeusia, and diminished fluid intake. Proteinuria is the most common renal manifestation of the IFNs and is generally reversible on withdrawal of IFN.[121–124] Rarely, interstitial nephritis and nephrotic syndrome have been reported with IFN-α and -γ.[119,125]

Neurologic Effects

CNS toxicity associated with global changes in mentation is often subtle. The cognitive dysfunction induced by IFN may be documented in formal testing, but is often more apparent to family and friends of patients.[126] Stupor and coma with diffuse slowing of the electroencephalographic pattern have infrequently been reported and are reversible on discontinuation of IFN.[120,127] Mild peripheral neuropathy has also been noted, with paraesthesia and slowing of nerve conduction velocity. Most recently, reversible retinal microvascular toxicity has been noted during studies of IFN-α administered for macular degeneration, which may indicate the need for ophthalmologic evaluation of patients with visual changes during IFN-α therapy in other settings.[128]

Musculoskeletal Effects

Rhabdomyolysis has rarely been reported in association with IFN-α_2 at high dosages.[129] However, the significance and even the attribution of such occurrences is difficult to resolve at this time, as this complication has been reported as early as the first week into IFN-α_2 therapy in postoperative patients in whom it is difficult to exclude other contributory factors. Although monitoring for elevations in creatine phosphokinase enzymes has been suggested, this has not been adopted in practice because of the rarity of the event and the early occurrence of the event, which would preclude use of laboratory values to monitor treatment and supportive care.

PHARMACOLOGY AND DOSAGE

Recombinant Interferon of the First Generation

The maximum tolerated dose for IFN-α lies between 10 and 20 μ/m² daily and 50 μ/m² on alternating days for periods of weeks to months, regardless of subspecies. The half-life of IFN-α_2 is 6 hours in the blood and has allowed alternate-daily schedules of outpatient administration by intramuscular and subcutaneous routes. The maximum tolerated dose for IFN-α varies according to the industrial preparation used, schedule, and route; acceptable absorption and activity have been reported with IFN-γ administered intravenously or intramuscularly.[130,131] Early pharmacokinetic studies of IFN-α_2 have demonstrated that peak levels at 5 μ/m^2 obtained by the intravenous route do not reach 100 μ/mL, whereas by the intramuscular and subcutaneous routes generally adopted for therapy they remain under 50 μ/mL. By contrast, the administration of doses of 20 μ/m^2 (or 36 μ/dose in early pharmacodynamic studies) achieves serum levels approaching 10,000 μ/mL.[132] This difference in the pharmacodynamics and peak levels has been the focus of considerable interest, as the positive results of trials using the intravenous administration of 20 μ/m^2 have shown the first survival benefits in melanoma, whereas lower dosages administered by alternative routes have yielded antitumor effects in terms of delayed recurrence (during therapy) without significant survival prolongations.

Recombinant Interferons of the Second Generation

A second generation of recombinant IFN-α_2 therapy is currently unfolding, with intense exploration of linear polyethylene glycol–conjugated IFN-α_{2b} (PEG-Intron, Schering Plough Corporation, Kenilworth, NJ) and larger branched chain formulations of IFN-α_{2a} (Pegasys, Roche Laboratories Inc., Nutley, NJ) entering multicenter trials in the United States, Canada, and Europe. The half-life of these species is substantially prolonged, allowing twice weekly and weekly administration, with concentration time products that are significantly higher than can be achieved with the first-generation recombinant IFN-α_2 species as initially formulated, regardless of route. Clinical studies, accompanied by more sophisticated molecular laboratory corollaries, are under way in the context of these trials in leukemia (chronic myelogenous leukemia), solid tumors (melanoma, renal cell carcinoma), and viral diseases (hepatitis).

ANTIBODIES

The development of anti-IFN neutralizing serum antibodies has been correlated with loss of toxicity and antitumor effects in chronic myelogenous leukemia. The role of anti-IFN antibodies appears to vary with the disease state as well as the species of IFN used. In representative series, antibodies have been detected in from 0% to 5% of subjects after 2 to 6 months of therapy[133,134] without demonstrable adverse consequences for therapeutic effects in patients with most solid tumors to date. Strategies to reduce the immunogenicity and increase the likelihood of tolerance to recombinant IFN-α have included the initial use of intravenous, as opposed to subcutaneous or intramuscular, routes and continuous as opposed to interrupted schedules. Despite the delayed release and depot-like behavior of polyethylene glycol–bound IFN-α_2, the immunogenicity of polyethylene glycol–bound IFN formulations appears to be less than that of the parent recombinant IFN-α_2 species.

TABLE 20.1-3. Efficacy of Interferon-α_2 in Human Cancer

Role	*Solid Tumors*	*Hematologic Neoplasm*
Advanced disease	Kaposi's sarcoma	Hairy cell leukemia
	Renal cell carcinoma[a]	Chronic myelopenia leukemia
	Melanoma[b]	Non-Hodgkin's lymphoma
	Carcinoid	T cell
	Ovarian cancer	B cell
Postoperative adjuvant setting	Melanoma stage II and III	
	Bladder carcinoma	

[a]With vinblastine chemotherapy.
[b]With polychemotherapy and interleukin-2 greater than 50% response; alone, 16% response; and 5% complete.

CLINICAL EFFICACY OF INTERFERONS ADMINISTERED SYSTEMATICALLY

Nonrecombinant IFN-α was initially brought to clinical trial against several solid tumors in 1978, when the American Cancer Society began a series of trials of buffy coat leukocyte IFN produced by Cantell with the Finnish Red Cross. These trials were limited by the extremely short supply of the agent (the trials lasted for only 6 weeks) from which no firm conclusions can be drawn. The trials served as an important impetus for the pharmaceutical industry to begin commercial production of IFN-α, as well as IFN-β, -γ, and other biologic agents, using recombinant DNA technology. The large-scale production of IFNs by recombinant DNA technology enabled the first systematic evaluation of appropriate dose, route, and schedule of IFN-α_2, as well as the other major subspecies of IFN-α, -β, and -γ.

Phase II trials have documented the antitumor activity of recombinant IFN-α_2 in many solid tumors as documented elsewhere in this volume. Table 20.1-3 lists the applications of IFN-α that have received approval by the U.S. Food and Drug Administration in the United States.[80,109,134–141] General principles that can be drawn from this experience are that the hematologic neoplasms appear to respond to lower dosages than the solid tumors and to respond on the basis of direct effects that are either antiproliferative, prodifferentiative, or proapoptotic. The mechanism for IFN-α_2 antitumor activity in solid tumors appears to be indirect, as the result of antigenic modulation (MHC), modulation of host immune responses (CD4/CD8 T cell), or both, or antigen presentation (dendritic cell), although vascular effects may also be implicated.

REGIONAL THERAPY WITH INTERFERON-α

Intralesional administration of IFN-α[142] at 6 to 10 Mu twice or three times weekly has been used for refractory solid tumors such as melanoma,[143] but offers little advantage over systemic therapy. Regional *in transit* disease of the extremity is an infrequent manifestation of melanoma that continues to be studied with hyperthermic isolated limb perfusion using combinations of chemotherapy (melphalan) and two cytokines (TNF, together with IFN-γ). IFN-γ was given for the original theoretical purpose of modulating TNF receptor expression for subsequent isolated limb perfusion with TNF. The role of IFN-γ in this combination is debated, but the reported response rates of 90% with the original combination have been confirmed by investigators in the United States[144,145] and the Netherlands.[146,147] TNF given alone at comparable doses has shown only brief and limited antitumor activity,[148] suggesting that melphalan, or melphalan and IFN-γ, may be critical to the therapeutic effects of the triple combination. Fraker and colleagues are undertaking a controlled study of isolated limb perfusion that will allow more definitive conclusions.[144,149]

COMBINATIONS

Phase II Trials of Combinations of Biologic Agents: Types I and II, Interferon-α_2 Plus Interferon-γ

Combinations of IFNs of types I and II (IFN-α_2 or -β, and -γ, respectively) have been of theoretical interest, given the potential synergism of IFNs interacting through the two separate classes of IFN receptor. The modulation of receptors for IFN-α_2 by IFN-γ and elucidation of signal transduction pathways through which IFN-γ and IFN-α act at a molecular level[22] provide a further impetus for exploration of combined IFN therapy. The molecular synergism of IFN-γ and IFN-α through signal transducer and transcriptional activators of IFN summarized by Darnell is currently under investigation with IFN-α_2 and IL-12 (an inducer of IFN-γ).[19,21–25,150–152]

Clinical studies of combinations of IFN-α and -γ have previously followed two strategies: concurrent and sequenced administration. Increased toxicity without apparent therapeutic benefit was seen with concurrent regimens,[153–156] whereas sequenced regimens have improved therapeutic and immunomodulatory activity in renal cell carcinoma.[85,157]

Modulation of Antitumor and Immunologic Effects of Interferons by Biologic Agents, Cytotoxic Drugs, and Nonsteroidal Antiinflammatory Drugs

The pleiotropic effects of IFN-α_2 include the induction of a variety of feedback mechanisms of immunosuppression that may be associated with prostaglandins for which nonsteroidal antiinflammatory drugs might be of benefit. In addition, it has been hoped that these agents might alleviate some of the significant constitutional toxicity and flu-like symptoms of IFN therapy.

Miller et al.[158] have conducted a randomized controlled trial of indomethacin with IFN-α_2, demonstrating neither clinical nor immunologic untoward interactions. Dexamethasone has been assiduously avoided in most trials of IFN-α, -β, and -γ as a consequence of its potent immunosuppressive effects. IFN-α has been used with corticosteroids for multiple myeloma and lymphoma, diseases in which corticosteroids have an established role. Corticosteroids abrogate the benefit of IFN in experimental animals, and it appears prudent to avoid corticosteroids during IFN-α_2 therapy for solid tumors.[158,159]

Combinations of Interferon-α and Retinoids

Broad interest exists in the potential applications of retinoids for therapy and prevention of squamous carcinomas of aerodigestive tract skin, carcinoma of the cervix, and other epithelial neoplasms. There have been unexpected and dramatic clinical responses of acute promyelocytic leukemia with the retinoids, and this disorder is associated with a lesion in the chromosomal region coding for the retinoic acid receptor. The retinoic acid receptors exhibit sequence homology with the corticosteroid hormone receptor superfamily, suggesting that both may function through the regulation of gene transcription, although the mechanism and optimal combination of retinoids and IFN-α have not been established.[160–162]

Combined Modality Therapy

Given the differing presumed mechanisms and nonoverlapping toxicities of cytotoxic chemotherapy and IFN regimens available for hematologic neoplasms and solid tumors as well as the lack of a survival effect of previous combination chemotherapy,[163] the combination of chemotherapy and IFN-α_2 has been an obvious one. The combination has shown mixed results.[164–171] The Eastern Cooperative Oncology Group has tested combinations of tamoxifen, IFN-α, or both versus dacarbazine in a factorial two-by-two study that demonstrates a lack of any advantage of IFN (high-dose) (or hormonal combination therapy with tamoxifen) over standard chemotherapy in melanoma.[172] Combinations of IFN-α and chemotherapy have suggested improved duration of response in myeloma[173] and non-Hodgkin's lymphoma.[174,175]

In melanoma, combination chemotherapy has been found to induce complete responses in a small fraction (less than 5%), and IL-2 has been shown to achieve a durable complete response in 6%.[176] IFN-α_2 with IL-2 and combination chemotherapy has been associated with complete responses in more than 10%, and overall complete and partial responses in more than 50% of patients in multiple single-institution trials, leading to exploration of the role of IFN-α_2 plus IL-2 with cisplatin, vinblastine, and dacarbazine, as opposed to polychemotherapy alone, in the current intergroup E3695 trial for metastatic melanoma.[177,178]

A number of regimens have evaluated the role of IFN-α_2 in combination with complex cisplatin-based polychemotherapy regimens, with or without IL-2. These regimens have generally exacted greater toxicity than the binary regimens, requiring hospitalization for administration of IL-2 when administered by continuous intravenous infusion or high-dose bolus schedules.[179–181]

More complex regimens using multiple cytotoxic agents, IFN-α_2, and IL-2 have been reported from multiple centers in the United States and Europe.[177,178] Regimens known collectively as biochemotherapy have consistently achieved response rates greater than 50% with complete response in 10% or greater, at the cost of significant toxicity and hospitalization for metastatic melanoma. Intergroup study E3695 of the Eastern Cooperative Oncology Group and Southwest Oncology Group is evaluating whether IL-2 as a continuous infusion at high dosage for 4 days and IFN-α_{2b} at a daily dosage of 5 μ/m^2 subcutaneously prolongs the survival of patients with metastatic melanoma over cisplatin, vinblastine, and dacarbazine polychemotherapy.

The application of IFN as systemic adjuvant therapy is currently focused on melanoma, in which the precision of prognostic assessment for regional lymph node disease has advanced substantially. The risk category of patients with nodal metastasis defined using sentinel node mapping has improved substantially.[182]

Melanoma risk may be categorized as very high, high, intermediate, and low, according to 5-year relapse and mortality. The prognosis of clinically localized primary melanoma may be estimated rather precisely by the Breslow depth of primary tumor invasion (in millimeters) at the site of origin, the presence or absence of ulceration, and sentinel lymph node status. The poor prognosis for cure for deep or ulcerated primary disease, or node-positive patients has provided the rationale for postoperative adjuvant therapy of these categories of high-risk patients.[183,184]

ADJUVANT TRIALS OF INTERFERON-α_2 IN MELANOMA

On the basis of the antitumor activity of IFN-α_2 in metastatic melanoma and the gradient of response with patients having the smallest size and number of metastases exhibiting the highest response rates, multiple trials of IFN-α_2 for prevention of melanoma relapse were commenced in the United States and international cooperative groups during the 1980s. The three largest and most mature studies of IFN-α_2 conducted to date adopted similar entry criteria, including patients with deep (T4) primary lesions or pathologically proven involvement of regional lymph nodes. The groups that have undertaken these studies were the Eastern Cooperative Oncology Group, North Central Cancer Treatment Group, and the World Health Organization.

Eastern Cooperative Oncology Group

E1684 accrued 287 patients between 1984 and 1990, was unblinded and reported to the American Society of Clinical Oncology in 1993[185] at 5 years of median follow-up, and published in 1996 at 6.9 years median follow-up. This trial used an aggressive therapy of 1 year's duration, 20 μ/m² intravenously daily for 5 days a week for 1 month, then 10 μ/m² subcutaneously t.i.w. for the balance of the year with IFN-α_{2b} or observed as the reference standard of care. Risk groups were defined by lymph node pathology (reviewed in all cases) and stratified to allow the analysis of therapeutic effect in homogeneous groups of patients whose susceptibility to this therapy was postulated to be potentially related to tumor burden and disease extent.[186,187]

The analysis of treatment effect for high-dose IFN-α_{2b} on relapse for the overall trial revealed a highly significant reduction of relapse rate (P_2 = .004) and a significant survival benefit in the intention-to-treat analysis (P_2 = .046). A Cox multivariate analysis demonstrated significant improvement in the disease-free and overall survival (P = .001 to .01) and estimated the relative improvement in continuous relapse-free survival to be 50%.

The median interval to relapse with IFN-α_{2b} adjuvant therapy was prolonged from 0.9 to 1.6 years, whereas the median survival of treated patients has been prolonged from 2.62 to 3.78 years. A retrospective quality-adjusted analysis of time spent without symptoms or toxicity (Q-TWiST) study has been conducted in the context of this trial.[188,189] After 84 months, the group of patients receiving IFN-α_{2b} gained a mean of 8.9 months quality-adjusted time without relapse (P = .03) and 7 months of overall survival time (P = .02) compared with the observation group.

Economic analyses of the E1684 regimen[190–192] projected incremental cost comparable with other accepted adjuvant therapies of breast and colorectal cancer. This therapy has been approved for resected high-risk melanomas by regulatory authorities across North and South America, Europe, and Australia.

To confirm and extend the preliminary results of the E1684 trial, the two intergroup trials were initiated: E1690, comparing the high-dose regimen of IFN-α_{2b} with a low-dose regimen of 3 μm subcutaneous IFN-α_{2b} three times a week, which accrued 642 patients between 1990 and 1995, with 608 evaluable at 52 months' median follow-up, as the study was recently reported. An improvement in relapse-free survival for the high-dose IFN-α_{2b} was noted that is significant (P_2 = .03 by Cox analysis) only for high-dose IFN-α_{2b}. Neither the high-dose arm nor the low-dose arm showed an improvement in overall survival, as compared with observation, in this trial, which included a substantial fraction (25%) who had deep primary melanoma, most of whom were not surgically and pathologically staged at elective lymph node dissection (as had been mandated in the first trial E1684). Postrelapse salvage surgery was feasible in these patients, followed by extensive use of IFN in patients who had relapsed after initial assignment to observation. The systematic and unbalanced pursuit of IFN salvage therapy in observation patients, more than IFN-assigned patients (P = .004), was associated with prolonged survival that may have confounded efforts to detect differences between survival of those who were assigned originally to high-dose IFN, not observation. The World Health Organization trial 16 of low-dose IFN showed no significant survival or relapse-intense prologation in a study of similar size.[193] Most recently, the intergroup E1694 trial has been concluded, in which the overall survival and relapse-free survival benefit of the high-dose E1684 IFNα_2 1 year regimen, with P = .009 and P = .0015, in the largest study of high-dose IFNα_2 conducted to date (u = 880).

Vaccine: Interferon Contributions as Adjuvant Therapy for Melanoma

The attractiveness of vaccines for melanoma is broad and theoretically compelling, although no randomized controlled trial of vaccine has yet shown benefit in melanoma. Eastern Cooperative Oncology Group trial E2696 has tested the anti-GM2 antibody IgG and IgM response induced by the vaccine alone, in comparison with the vaccine combined with or followed by IFN-α_{2b} at high dosage as in E1684/E1690. This trial has been completed and analyzed, demonstrating no significant inhibition of the immunogenicity of the GMK vaccine in terms of anti-GM2 antibody immunoglobulin G and immunoglobulin M.[194] Thus, it is reasonable to consider the combined use of vaccine, and high-dose IFN-α_{2b} in future adjuvant trials, as any vaccine has been demonstrated to be of benefit in appropriate randomized controlled trials, alone.

REFERENCES

1. Darnell JE Jr. STATs and gene regulation. *Science* 1997;277:1630.
2. Leaman DW, Leung S, Li X, Stark GR. Regulation of stat-dependent pathways by growth factors and cytokines. *FASEB J* 1996;10:1578.
3. Darnell JE Jr, Kerr IM, Stark GR. Jak-stat pathways and transcriptional activation in response to IFNs and other extracellular signaling proteins. *Science* 1994;264:1415.
4. Schindler C, Darnell JE. Transcriptional responses to polypeptide ligands: the JAK-STAT pathway. *Annu Rev Biochem* 1995;64:621.
5. Meraz M, White JM, Sheehan K, et al. Trageted disruption of stat1 gene in mice reveals unexpected physiologic specificity in the JAK-STAT signaling pathway. *Cell* 1996;84:431.
6. Durbin JE, Hackenmiller R, Simon M, Levy DE. Targeted disruption of the mouse Stat1 gene results in compromised innate immunity to viral disease. *Cell* 1996;84:443.
7. Kaplan MH, Sun Y, Hoey T, Gruss JG. Impaired IL-12 responses and enhanced development of Th2 cells in Stat4-deficient mice. *Nature* 1996;382:174.
8. Thierfelder W, van Deursen J, Yamamoto K, et al. Requirement for Stat4 in interleukin-12-mediated responses of natural killer and T cells. *Nature* 1996;382:171.
9. Kaplan MH, Schindler U, Smiley S, Grusby MJ. Stat6 is required for mediating responses to IL-4 and for development of Th2 cells. *Immunity* 1996;4:313.
10. Takeda K, Tanaka T, Shi W, et al. Essential role of STAT 6 in IL-4 signalling. *Nature* 1996;380:627.
11. Wakao H, Gouilleaux F, Groner B. Mammary gland factor (MGF) is a novel member of the cytokine regulated transcription factor gene family and confers the prolactin response. *EMBO J* 1994;13:2182.
12. Zoon KC, Bekisz J, Miller D. Human interferon alpha family: protein structure and function. In: Baron S, Coppenhaver DH, Dianzani F, et al., eds. *Interferon:principles and medical applications*, 1st ed. Galveston, TX: The University of Texas Medical Branch, 1992:95.

13. Dron M, Tovey MG. Interferon α/β, gene structure and regulation. In: Baron S, Coppenhaver DH, Dianzani F, et al., eds. *Interferon: principles and medical applications,* 1st ed. Galveston, TX: The University of Texas Medical Branch, 1992:33.
14. Mariano TM, Donnelly RJ, Soh J, Pestka S. Structure and function of the type I interferon receptor. In: Baron S, Coppenhaver DH, Dianzani F, et al., eds. *Interferon: principles and medical applications,* 1st ed. Galveston, TX: The University of Texas Medical Branch, 1992:129.
15. DeGrado WF, Wasserman ZR, Chowdry V. Sequence and structural homologies among type I and II interferons. *Nature* 1982;300:379.
16. Revel M. The interferon system in man: nature of the interferon molecules and mode of action. In: Becker Y, ed. *Antiviral drugs and interferon.* Amsterdam: Martinus Nijhoff, 1988:358.
17. Epstein LB, Epstein CJ. Localization of the gene AVG for the antiviral expression of immune and classical interferon to the distal part of the long arm of chromosome 21. *J Invest Dermatol* 1976;133(Suppl):56.
18. Weil J, Tucker G, Epstein LB, Epstein CJ. Interferon induction of (2'-5') oligoisoadenylate synthetase in diploid and trisomy 21 human fibroblasts: relation to dosage of the interferon receptor gene *(IRFC). Hum Genet* 1983;65:108.
19. Levy DE. Cytoplasmic events in signal transduction leading to IFN α-induced gene expression. In: Baron S, Coppenhaver DH, Dianzani F, et al., eds. *Interferon: principles and medical applications,* 1st ed. Galveston, TX: The University of Texas Medical Branch, 1992:161.
20. Fuchs E. Clues to b-cell memory. *Nat Med* 1996;2:743.
21. Darnell JE Jr. STATs and gene regulation. *Science* 1997;277:1630.
22. Schindler C, Shuai K, Prezioso VR, Darnell JE Jr. Interferon-dependent tyrosine phosphorylation of a latent cytoplasmic transcription factor. *Science* 1992;257:809.
23. Pine R, Decker T, Kessler DS, Levy DE, Darnell JE. Purification and cloning of interferon-stimulated gene factor 2 (ISGF2): ISGF2 (IRF-1) can bind to the promoters of both beta interferon- and interferon-stimulated genes but is not a primary transcriptional activator of either. *Mol Cell Biol* 1990;10:2448.
24. Fu X-Y, Kessler DS, Veals SA, Levy DE, Darnell JE Jr. ISGF3, the transcriptional activator induced by interferon α, consists of multiple interacting polypeptide chains. *Proc Natl Acad Sci U S A* 1990;87:8555.
25. Levy D, Darnell JE Jr. Interferon-dependent transcriptional activation: signal transduction without second messenger involvement? *New Biol* 1990;2:923.
26. Aiyer RA, Serrano LE, Jones PP. Interferon-gamma binds to high and low affinity receptor components on murine macrophages. *J Immunol* 1986;136:3329.
27. Kirkwood JM, Bryant J, Schiller JH, et al. Immunomodulatory function of interferon gamma in patients with metastatic melanoma: results of a phase I trial in subjects with metastatic melanoma (EST 4987). *J Immunother* 1997;20:146.
28. Herberman RB. *Natural cell-mediated immunity against tumors.* New York: Academic, 1980.
29. Müllbacher A. The long-term maintenance of cytotoxic T cell memory does not require persistence of antigen. *J Exp Med* 1994;179:317.
30. Ernstoff MS, Fusi S, Kirkwood JM. Parameters of interferon action: II. Immunological effects of recombinant leukocyte interferon (IFN alpha-2) in phase I/II trials. *J Biol Resp Mod* 1983;2:540.
31. Ortaldo JR, Woodhouse C, Morgan AC, et al. Analysis of effector cells in human antibody-dependent cellular cytotoxicity with murine monoclonal antibodies. *J Immunol* 1987;138:3566.
32. Kirkwood JM, Farkas DL, Chakraborty A, et al. Systemic interferon-alpha (IFN-alpha) treatment leads to Stat3 inactivation in melanoma precursor lesions. *Mol Med* 1999;5:11.
33. Merritt JA, Borden EC, Ball LA. Measurement of 2',5'-oligoadenylate synthetase in patients receiving interferon-alpha. *Journal of Interferon Research* 1985;5:191.
34. St.Laurent G, Yoshie U, Floyd-Smith G. Interferon action: two (2'5') A (A)n synthetase specified by distinct mRNAs in Erhlich ascites tumor cells treated with interferon. *Cell* 1983;33:95.
35. Ilson DH, Torrence PF, Vilcek J. Two molecular weight forms of human 2'5'-oligoadenylate synthetase have different activation requirements. *Journal of Interferon Research* 1986;6:5.
36. Yoshida R, Imanishi J, Oku T, Kishida T, Hayaishi O. Induction of pulmonary indoleamine 2,3, dioxegenase by interferon. *Proc Natl Acad Sci U S A* 1981;78:129.
37. Yasui H, Takai K, Yoshida R, Hayaishi O. Interferon enhances tryptophan metabolism by inducing pulmonary indoleamine 2,3-dioxygenase: its possible occurrence in cancer patients. *Proc Natl Acad Sci U S A* 1986;83:6622.
38. Ghezzi P, Bianchi M, Montovani A, Spreaficio F, Salmona M. Enhanced xanthine oxidase activity in mice treated with interferon and interferon inducers. *Biochem Biophys Res Commun* 1984;119:144.
39. Berens ME, Saito T, Welander CE, Modest EJ. Antitumor activity of new anthracycline analogues in combination with interferon alfa. *Cancer Chemother Pharmacol* 1987;19:301.
40. Saito T, Berens ME, Welander EC. Characterization of the indirect antitumor effect of gamma-interferon using ascites-associated macrophages in a human tumor clonogenic assay. *Cancer Res* 1987;47:673.
41. Fleischmann WR. Potentiation of the direct anticellular activity of mouse interferons: mutual synergism and interferon concentration dependence. *Cancer Res* 1982;42:869.
42. Czarniecki CW, Fennie CW, Powers DB, Estell DA. Synergistic antiviral and antiproliferative activities of *Escherichia coli*-derived human alpha, beta, and gamma interferons. *J Virol* 1984;49:490.
43. Schiller JH, Willson JKV, Bittner G, et al. Antiproliferative effects of interferons on human melanoma cells in the human tumor colony-forming assay. *Journal of Interferon Research* 1986;6:615.
44. Nachbaur DM, Denz HA, Gastl G, et al. Combination effects of human recombinant interferon (alpha-2-arg, gamma) and cytotoxic agents on colony formation of human melanoma and hypernephroma cell lines. *Cancer Lett* 1989;44:49.
45. Dealtry GB, Naylor MS, Fiers W, Balkwill FR. DNA fragmentation and cytotoxicity caused by tumor necrosis factor is enhanced by interferon-gamma. *Eur J Immunol* 1987;17:689.
46. Bregman MD, Meyskens FL Jr. Human recombinant alpha- and gamma-interferons enhance the cytotoxic properties of tumor necrosis factor on human melanoma. *J Biol Resp Mod* 1988;7:384.
47. Wang Y, Rao U, Mascari R, et al. Molecular analysis of melanoma precursor lesions. *Cell Growth and Differentiation* 1996;7:1733.
48. Elder DE, Rodeck U, Thurin J, et al. Antigenic profile of tumor progression in human melanocytic nevi and melanomas. *Cancer Res* 1989;49:5091.
49. Giacomini P, Aguzzi A, Pestka S, Fisher PB, Ferrone S. Modulation by recombinant DNA leukocyte (a) and fibroblast (b) interferons of the expression and shedding of HLA- and tumor-associated antigens by human melanoma cells. *J Immunol* 1984;133:1649.
50. Giuffré L, Isler P, Mach J-P, Careel S. A novel IFN-gamma regulated human melanoma associated antigen gp33-38 defined by monoclonal antibody Mel4-D12. I. Identification and immunochemical characterization. *J Immunol* 1988;141:2072.
51. Matsui M, Temponi M, Ferrone S. Characterization of a monoclonal antibody-defined human melanoma-associated antigen susceptible to induction by immune interferon. *J Immunol* 1987;139:2088.
52. Audette M, Carrel S, Hayoz D, et al. A novel interferon-gamma regulated human melanoma-associated antigen, gp33-38, defined by monoclonal antibody Me14-D12. II. Molecular cloning of a genomic probe. *Mol Immunol* 1989;26:515.
53. Dolei A, Ameglio F, Capobianchi MR, et al. Human β-type interferon enhances the expression and shedding of Ia-like antigens, comparison to HLA-A, B, C and β_2-microglobulin. *Antivir Res* 1981;1:367.
54. Basham TY, Bourgeade MF, Creasey AA, Merigan TC. Interferon increases HLA synthesis in melanoma cells: interferon-resistant and -sensitive cell lines. *Proc Natl Acad Sci U S A* 1982;79:3265.
55. von Stamm U, Bröcker EB, von Depka Prondzinski M, et al. Effects of systemic interferon-α (IFN-α) on the antigenic phenotype of melanoma metastases. EORTC melanoma group cooperative study No. 18852. *Melanoma Res* 1993;3:173.
56. Kirkwood JM, Sosman J, Ernstoff M, et al. E2690: a study of the mechanism of IFN alfa-2b in high risk melanoma in the ECOG/intergroup trial E1690. *Proc Am Assoc Cancer Res* 1995;36:641.
57. Graf LH Jr, Rosenberg CD, Mancino VA, Ferrone S. Transfer and co-amplification of a gene encoding a 96-kDa immune IFN-inducible human melanoma-associated antigen. Preferential expression by mouse melanoma host cells. *J Immunol* 1988;141:1054.
58. Friess GG, Brown TD, Wrenn RC. Improvement in cardiac ectopy during gamma interferon infusion: a case report. *Cancer Treat Rep* 1986;70:1463.
59. Murray JL, Stuckey SE, Pillow JK, Rosenblum MG, Gutterman JU. Differential in vitro effects of recombinant α-interferon and recombinant gamma-interferon alone or in combination on the expression of melanoma-associated surface antigens. *J Biol Resp Mod* 1988;7:152.
60. Maio M, Gulwani B, Langer JA, et al. Modulation for interferons of HLA antigen, high-molecular-weight melanoma-associated antigen, and intercellular adhesion molecule 1 expression by cultured melanoma cells with different metastatic potential. *Cancer Res* 1989;49:2980.
61. Houghton AN, Thomson TM, Gross D, Oettgen HF, Old LJ. Surface antigens of melanoma and melanocytes. Specificity of induction of Ia antigens by human gamma-interferon. *J Exp Med* 1984;160:255.
62. Anichini A, Castelli C, Sozzi G, Fossati G, Parmiani G. Differential susceptibility to recombinant interferon-gamma-induced HLA-DQ antigen modulation among clones from a human metastatic melanoma. *J Immunol* 1988;140:183.
63. Taniguchi K, Petersson M, Höglund P, et al. Interferon gamma induces lung colonization by intravenously inoculated B16 melanoma cells in parallel with enhanced expression of class I major histocompatibility complex antigens. *Proc Natl Acad Sci U S A* 1987;84:3405.
64. Gorelik E, Gunji Y, Herberman RB. H-2 antigen expression and sensitivity of BL6 melanoma cells to natural killer cell cytotoxicity. *J Immunol* 1988;140:2096.
65. Taramelli D, Fossati G, Mazzocchi A, et al. Classes I and II HLA and melanoma-associated antigen expression and modulation on melanoma cells isolated from primary and metastatic lesions. *Cancer Res* 1986;46:433.
66. De Fries RU, Golub SH. Characteristics and mechanism of IFN-gamma-induced protection of human tumor cells from lysis by lymphokine-activated killer cells. *J Immunol* 1988;140:3686.
67. Zöller M, Strubel A, Hämmerling G, et al. Interferon gamma treatment of B16 melanoma cells: opposing effects for non-adaptive and adaptive immune defense and its reflection by metastatic spread. *Int J Cancer* 1988;41:256.
68. Zoller M. IFN-treatment of B16-F1 versus B16-F10: relative impact of non-adaptive and T-cell-mediated immune defense in metastatic spread. *Clin Exp Metast* 1988;6:411.
69. Kleinschmidt WJ, Schultz RM. Similarities of murine gamma interferon and the lymphokine that renders macrophages cytotoxic. *J Interferon Res* 1982;2:291.
70. Talmadge KW, Gallati H, Sinigaglia F, Walz A, Garotta G. Identity between human interferon-gamma and "macrophage-activating factor" produced by human T lymphocytes. *Eur J Immunol* 1986;16:1471.
71. Spear GT, Paulnock DM, Jordan RL, et al. Enhancement of monocyte class I and II histocompatibility antigen expression in man by *in vivo* β-interferon. *Clin Exp Immunol* 1987;69:107.
72. Sayers TJ, Mason AT, Ortaldo JR. Regulation of human natural killer cell activity by interferon-gamma: lack of a role in interleukin 2-mediated augmentation. *J Immunol* 1986;136:2176.
73. Platsoucas CD. Regulation of natural killer cytotoxicity by *Escherichia coli*-derived human interferon gamma. *Scand J Immunol* 1986;24:93.
74. Maluish AE, Ortaldo JR, Conlon JC, et al. Depression of natural killer cytotoxicity after in vivo administration of recombinant leukocyte interferon. *J Immunol* 1983;131:503.
75. Silver HK, Connors JM, Kong S, Karim KA, Spinelli JJ. Survival, response and immune effects in a prospectively randomized study of dose strategy for alpha-N1 interferon. *Br J Cancer* 1988;58:783.
76. Kirkwood JM, Bryant J, Schiller J, et al. Determination of phenotypic and functional correlates of interferon gamma (IFNγ) therapy of metastatic melanoma in a multi-institutional phase Ib trial (ECOG 4987/4687). *Proc Am Soc Clin Oncol* 1991;10:218.
77. Seitz DE. Trimetrexate: a critical appraisal of the phase II clinical trial experience: evidence of drug discovery—clinical development disjunction. *Cancer Invest* 1994;12:657.

78. Herberman RB, Ortaldo JR, Bonnard GD. Augmentation by interferon of human natural and antibody-dependent cell-mediated cytotoxicity. *Nature* 1979;227:221.
79. Chakrabarti D, Hultgren B, Stewart TA. IFN-α induces autoimmune T cells though the induction of intracellular adhesion molecule- and B7.2. *J Immunol* 1996;157:522.
80. Hersey P, Hasic E, MacDonald M, et al. Effects of recombinant leukocyte interferon (rIFN-aA) on tumour growth and immune responses in patients with metastatic melanoma. *Br J Cancer* 1985;51:815.
81. Mittleman A, Krown SE, Cirrincione C, et al. Analysis of T cell subsets in cancer patients treated with interferon. *Am J Med* 1983;75:966.
82. Kirkwood JM, Ernstoff MS. The role of interferons in the management of melanoma. In: Nathanson L, ed. *Management of advanced melanoma.* New York: Churchill Livingstone, 1986:209.
83. Creagan ET, Ahmann DL, Frytak S, Long HJ, Itri LM. Recombinant leukocyte A interferon (rIFN-aA) in the treatment of disseminated malignant melanoma: Analysis of complete and long-term responding patients. *Cancer* 1986;58:2576.
84. Neefe JR, Phillips EA, Treat J. Augmentation of natural immunity and correlation with tumor response in melanoma patients treated with human lymphoblastoid interferon. *Diagn Immunol* 1986;4:299.
85. Ernstoff MS, Nair S, Bahnson RR, et al. A phase IA trial of sequential administration recombinant DNA-produced interferons: combination recombinant interferon gamma and recombinant interferon alfa in patients with metastatic renal cell carcinoma. *J Clin Oncol* 1990;8:1637.
86. Fuchs HJ, Debs R, Patton JS, Liggitt HD. The pattern of lung injury induced after pulmonary exposure to tumor necrosis factor-α depends on the route of administration. *Diag Microbiol Infect Dis* 1990;13:397.
87. Hakansson A, Gustafsson B, Krysander L, Hakansson L. Tumor-infiltrating lymphocytes in metastatic malignant melanoma and response to interferon alpha treatment. *Br J Cancer* 1996;74:670.
88. Hakansson A, Gustafsson B, Krysander L, et al. On down-regulation of the immune response to metastatic malignant melanoma. *Cancer Immunol Immunother* 1999;48:253.
89. Chen BP, Sondel PM. Recombinant DNA-derived interferons-α and -β modulate the alloactivated proliferative response of bulk and cloned human lymphocytes. *J Biol Resp Mod* 1985;4:287.
90. Laszlo J, Huang AT, Brenckman WD, et al. Phase I study of pharmacological and immunological effects of human lymphoblastoid interferon given to patients with carcinoma. *Cancer Res* 1983;43:4458.
91. Maluish AE, Ortaldo JR, Sherwin SA, Oldham RK, Herberman RB. Changes in immune function in patients receiving natural leukocyte interferon. *J Biol Resp Mod* 1983;2:418.
92. Edwards BS, Merritt JA, Fuhlbrigge RC, Borden EC. Low doses of interferon alpha result in more effective clinical natural killer cell activation. *J Clin Invest* 1985;75:1908.
93. Ernstoff MS, Trautman T, Davis CA, et al. A randomized phase I/II study of continuous versus intermittent intravenous interferon gamma in patients with metastatic melanoma. *J Clin Oncol* 1987;5:1804.
94. Zarour H, Richards T, Whiteside T, et al. E2690: intergroup immunological evaluation of IFNα2b dose-response in patients (Pts) with high-risk melanoma. *Proc Am Soc Clin Oncol* 1999;18.
95. Kirkwood JM, Ibrahim J, Sondak V, et al. Preliminary analysis of the E1690/S9111/C9190 Intergroup postoperative adjuvant trial of high - and low-dose IFNa2b (HDI and LDI) in high-risk primary or lymph node metastatic melanoma. *Proc Am Soc Clin Oncol* 1999;18:537A.
96. Creagan ET, Ahmann DL, Green SJ, et al. Phase II study of recombinant leukocyte A interferon (rIFN-aA) in disseminated malignant melanoma. *Cancer* 1984;54:2844.
97. Belardelli F, Gresser I, Maury C, Maunoury MT. Antitumor effects of interferon in mice injected with interferon-sensitive and interferon-resistant Friend leukemia cells. II. Role of host mechanisms. *Int J Cancer* 1982;30:821.
98. Gresser I, Maury C, Belardelli F. Anti-tumor effects of interferon in mice injected with interferon-sensitive and interferon-resistant Friend leukemia cells. VI. Adjuvant therapy after surgery in the inhibition of liver and spleen metastases. *Int J Cancer* 1987;39:789.
99. Gresser I, Maury C, Carnaud C, et al. Anti-tumor effects of interferon in mice injected with interferon-sensitive and interferon-resistant friend erythroleukemia cells. VIII. Role of the immune system in the inhibition of visceral metastases. *Int J Cancer* 1990;46:468.
100. Snapper CM, Paul WE. Interferon-gamma and B cell stimulatory factor-1 reciprocally regulate Ig isotype production. *Science* 1987;236:944.
101. Konrad MW, DeWitt SK, Bradley ED, et al. Interferon-gamma induced by administration of recombinant interleukin-2 to patients with cancer: kinetics, dose dependence, and correlation with physiological and therapeutic response. *J Immunother* 1992;12:55.
102. Atkins MB. Interleukin-2 in metastatic melanoma: establishing a role. *CA Cancer J* 1998;3:S7.
103. Atkins MB, Lotze M, Wiernick P, et al. High-dose IL-2 therapy alone results in long-term durable complete responses in patients with metastatic melanoma. *Proc Am Soc Clin Oncol* 1997;16:494a.
104. Steinman RM. Dendritic cells and immune-based therapies. *Exp Hematol* 1996;24:859.
105. Hanahan D, Folkman J. Patterns and emerging mechanisms of the angiogenic switch during tumorigenesis. *Cell* 1996;86:353.
106. Folkman J. Successful treatment of an angiogenic disease. *N Engl J Med* 1989;320:1211.
107. Yoneda J, Kuniyasu H, Crispens MA, et al. Expression of angiogenesis-related genes and progression of human ovarian carcinomas in nude mice. *J Natl Cancer Inst* 1997;90:447.
108. Dinney CPN, Bielenberg DR, Perrotte P, et al. Inhibition of basic fibroblast growth factor expression, angiogenesis, and growth of human bladder carcinoma in mice by systemic interferon-a administration. *Cancer Res* 1998;58:808.
109. Legha SS, Papadopoulos NEJ, Plager C, et al. Clinical evaluation of recombinant interferon alfa-2a (Roferon-a) in metastatic melanoma using two different schedules. *J Clin Oncol* 1987;5:1240.
110. Creagan ET, Ahmann DL, Frytak S, et al. Phase II trials of recombinant leukocyte A interferon in disseminated malignant melanoma: results in 96 patients. *Cancer Treat Rep* 1986;70:619.
111. Creagan ET, Buckner JC, Hahn RG, et al. An evaluation of recombinant leukocyte A interferon with aspirin in patients with metastatic renal cell cancer. *Cancer* 1988;61:1787.
112. Massaro ER, Borden EC, Hawkins MJ, Wiebe DA, Shrago E. Effects of recombinant interferon-alpha$_2$ treatment upon lipid concentrations and lipoprotein composition. *J Interferon Res* 1986;6:655.
113. Ehnholm C, Aho K, Huttunen JK, et al. Effect of interferon on plasma lipoproteins and on the activity of postheparin plasma lipases. *Arteriosclerosis: A Journal of Vascular Biology and Thrombosis* 1982;2:68.
114. Dixon RM, Borden EC, Keim NL, et al. Decreases in serum high-density-lipoprotein cholesterol and total cholesterol resulting from naturally produced and recombinant DNA derived leukocyte interferons. *Metabolism* 1982;2:68.
115. Ernstoff MS, Kirkwood JM. Changes in the bone marrow of cancer patients treated with recombinant interferon alpha-2. *Am J Med* 1984;76:593.
116. Ernstoff MS, Gallicchio V, Kirkwood JM. Analysis of granulocyte macrophage progenitor cells in patients treated with recombinant interferon alpha-2. *Am J Med* 1985;79:167.
117. Krown SE, Burk MW, Kirkwood JM, et al. Human leukocyte (alpha) interferon in metastatic malignant melanoma: the American Cancer Society phase II trial. *Cancer Treat Rep* 1984;68:723.
118. Kirkwood JM, Strawderman MH, Ernstoff MS, et al. Interferon alfa-2b adjuvant therapy of high-risk resected cutaneous melanoma: the Eastern Cooperative Oncology Group Trial EST 1684. *J Clin Oncol* 1996;14:7.
119. Kirkwood JM, Ernstoff MS. Interferons in the treatment of human cancer. *J Clin Oncol* 1984;2:336.
120. Mattson K, Niiranen A, Levanainen M, et al. Neurotoxicity of interferon. *Cancer Treat Rep* 1983;67:958.
121. Sumpio BE, Ernstoff MS, Kirkwood JM. Urinary excretion of interferon, albumin, and β_2-microglobulin during interferon treatment. *Cancer Res* 1984;44:3599.
122. Ault BH, Stapleton FB, Gaber L, et al. Acute renal failure during therapy with recombinant human gamma interferon. *N Engl J Med* 1988;319:1397.
123. Taylor AE, Wiltshaw E, Gore ME, Fryatt I, Fisher C. Long-term follow-up of the first randomized study of cisplatin versus carboplatin for advanced epithelial ovarian cancer. *J Clin Oncol* 1994;12:2066.
124. Kurzrock R, Quesada JR, Rosenblum MG, Sherwin SA, Gutterman JU. Phase I study of iv administered recombinant gamma interferon in cancer patients. *Cancer Treat Rep* 1986;70:1357.
125. McDermott DF, Mier JW, Lawrence DP, et al. A phase II pilot trial of concurrent biochemotherapy with cisplatin, vinblastine, dacarbazine (CVD), interleukin-2 (IL-2) and interferon alpha-2b (IFN) in patients with metastatic melanoma. *Proc Am Soc Clin Oncol* 1997;16:490a.
126. Bender CM, Yasko JM, Kirkwood JM, et al. Cognitive function and quality of life in interferon therapy for melanoma. *Clin Nursing Res* 2000;9:350.
127. Rohatiner AZS, Balkwill FR, Griffin DB, et al. A phase I study of human lymphoblastoid interferon administered by continuous intravenous infusion. *Cancer Chemother Pharmacol* 1982;9:97.
128. Guyer DR, Tiedeman J, Yannuzzi LA, et al. Interferon-associated retinopathy. *Arch Opthalmol* 1993;111:350.
129. Reinhold U, Hartl C, Hering R, Hoeft A, Kreysel HW. Fatal rhabdomyolsis and multiple organ failue associated with adjuvant high-dose interferon alfa in malignant melanoma. *Lancet* 1997;349:540.
130. Thompson JA, Cox WW, Lindgren CG, et al. Subcutaneous recombinant gamma interferon in cancer patients: toxicity, pharmacokinetics, and immunomodulatory effects. *Cancer Immunol Immunother* 1987;25:47.
131. Wagstaff J, Smith D, Nelmes P, Loynds P, Crowther D. A phase I study of recombinant interferon gamma administered by s.c. injection three times per week in patients with solid tumours. *Cancer Immunol Immunother* 1987;25:54.
132. Wheeler A, Rubenstein EB. Current management of disseminated intravascular colgulation. *Oncology* 1994;8:69.
133. Breslow A. Thickness, cross-sectional areas and depth of invasion in the prognosis of cutaneous melanoma. *Ann Surg* 1970;172:902.
134. Coates A, Rallings M, Hersey P, Swanson C. Phase II study of recombinant alpha 2-interferon in advanced malignant melanoma. *J Interferon Res* 1986;6:1.
135. Creagan ET, Ahmann DL, Green SJ, et al. Phase II study of low-dose recombinant leukocyte A interferon in disseminated malignant melanoma. *J Clin Oncol* 1984;2:1002.
136. Sertoli MR, Bernengo MG, Ardizzoni A, et al. Phase II trial of recombinant alpha-2b interferon in the treatment of metastatic skin melanoma. *Oncology* 1989;46:96.
137. Elsasser-Beile U, Drees N, Neumann HA, Schopf E. Phase II trial of recombinant leukocyte A interferon in advanced malignant melanoma. *J Cancer Res Clin Oncol* 1987;113:273.
138. Steiner A, Wolf C, Pehamberger H. Comparison of the effects of three different treatment regimens of recombinant interferons (r-IFN alpha, r-IFN gamma, and r-IFN-alpha + cimetidine) in disseminated malignant melanoma. *J Cancer Res Clin Oncol* 1987;113:459.
139. Kirkwood JM, Ernstoff MS, Davis CA, et al. Comparison of intramuscular and intravenous recombinant alpha-2 interferon in melanoma and other cancers. *Ann Intern Med* 1985;103:32.
140. Dorval T, Palangic T, Jouve M, et al. Clinical phase II trial of recombinant DNA interferon (interferon alfa 2b) in patients with metastatic malignant melanoma. *Cancer* 1986;58:215.
141. Robinson WA, Mughal TI, Thomas MR, Johnson M, Spiegel RJ. Treatment of metastatic malignant melanoma with recombinant interferon alpha-2. *Immunobiology* 1986;172:275.
142. Fogler WE, Sun LK, Klinger MR, Ghrayeb J, Daddona PE. Biological characterization of a chimeric mouse-human IgM antibody directed against the 17-1A antigen. *Cancer Immunol Immunother* 1989;30:43.
143. von Wussow P, Block B, Hartmann F, Deicher H. Intralesional interferon-alpha therapy in advanced malignant melanoma. *Cancer* 1988;61:1071.
144. Fraker DL, Alexander HR. The use of tumor necrosis factor in isolated limb perfusions for melanoma and sarcoma. *Cancer Principles and Practice of Oncology* 1993;7:1.
145. Lejeune FJ. Administration of high-dose tumor necrosis factor alpha by isolation perfusion of the limbs: rationale and results. *Journal of Infusional Chemotherapy* 1994.
146. Lienard D, Eggermont AM, Schrafford T, Koops H, Lejeune FJ. High dose of rTNF-alpha, rINF-gamma and melphalan in isolation perfusion produce 90% CR in melanoma in-transit metastasis. *Ann Oncol* 1992;3(Suppl 5):160(abst).

147. Buzaid AC, Bedikian A, Houghton AN. Systemic chemotherapy and biochemotherapy. In: Balch CM, Houghton AN, Sober AJ, et al., eds. *Cutaneous melanoma*, 3rd ed. St. Louis: Quality Medical Publishing, 1998:405.
148. Posner MC, Lienard D, Lejeune FJ, Rosenfelder D, Kirkwood JM. Hypothermic isolated limb perfusion with tumor necrosis factor alone for melanoma. *Cancer J* 1995;1:274.
149. Thom AK, Alexander HR, Andrich MP, et al. Systemic toxicity and cytokine levels in patients undergoing isolated limb perfusion (LIP) with dose TNF, IFN gamma and melphalan. *Proc Am Soc Clin Oncol* 1993;12:389.
150. Carson JJ, Gold LH, Barton AB, Biss RT. Fatality and interferon a for malignant melanoma. *Lancet* 1998;352:1443.
151. Knost JA, Reynolds V, Greco FA, Oldham RK. Adjuvant chemoimmunotherapy stage I/II malignant melanoma. *J Surg Oncol* 1982;19:165.
152. Fisher RI, Terry WD, Hodes RJ, et al. Adjuvant immunotherapy or chemotherapy for malignant melanoma: preliminary report of the National Cancer Institute randomized clinical trial. *Surg Clin North Am* 1981;61:1267.
153. Schiller JH, Storer B, Bittner G, Willson JKV, Borden EC. Phase II trial of a combination of interferon-β_{ser} and interferon-γ in patients with advanced malignant melanoma. *J Interferon Res* 1988;8:581.
154. Creagan ET, Loprinzi CL, Ahmann DL, Schaid DJ. A phase I-II trial of the combination of recombinant leukocyte A interferon and recombinant human interferon-gamma in patients with metastatic malignant melanoma. *Cancer* 1988;62:2472.
155. Osanto S, Jansen R, Naipal AMIH, et al. In vivo effects of combination treatment with recombinant interferon-gamma and -alpha in metastatic melanoma. *Int J Cancer* 1989;43:1001.
156. Kurzrock R, Rosenblum MG, Quesada JR, et al. Phase I study of a combination of recombinant interferon-alpha and recombinant interferon-gamma in cancer patients. *J Clin Oncol* 1986;4:1677.
157. Ernstoff MS, Gooding W, Nair S, et al. Immunological effects of treatment with sequential administration of recombinant interferon gamma and alpha in patients with metastatic renal cell carcinoma during a phase I trial. *Cancer Res* 1992;52:851.
158. Miller RL, Steis RG, Clark JW, et al. Randomized trial of recombinant α2b-interferon with or without indomethacin in patients with metastatic malignant melanoma. *Cancer Res* 1989;49:1871.
159. Eddy B, Ernstoff MS, Logan T, et al. A randomized phase I trial of recombinant interferon gamma (IFNγ, Biogen, Inc. Cambridge, MA) with indomethacin (I), dexamethasone (D) or acetaminopen (A) in patients (PT) with melanoma (M) and renal cell carcimona (RCC). *Proc Am Soc Clin Oncol* 1987;6:243.
160. Gambacorti-Passerini C, Hank JA, Albertini MR, et al. A pilot phase II trial of continuous-infusion interleukin-2 followed by lymphokine-activated killer cell therapy and bolus-infusion interleukin-2 in renal cancer. *J Immunother* 1993;13:43.
161. Izzo J, Khuri FR, Hong WK. Adjuvant biological therapy of head and neck cancer. In: Kirkwood JM, ed. *Strategies in adjuvant therapy*. Malden, MA: Martin Dunitz, 2000:153.
162. Dhingra K, Papadopoulos N, Lippman S, Lotan R, Legha SS. Phase II study of alpha-interferon and 13-cis-retinoic acid in metastatic melanoma. *Invest New Drugs* 1993;11:39.
163. Kirkwood JM, Agarwala S. Systemic cytotoxic and biologic therapy melanoma. *Cancer Principles and Practice of Oncology* 1993;7:1.
164. Kirkwood JM, Ernstoff MS, Guiliano A, et al. Clinical trials of interferon alfa-2B (Intron A, alpha-IFN) in melanoma: review of phase I, II, and III studies. *Proceedings of the XIV International Cancer Congress (Budapest)* August 1986.
165. Kirkwood JM, Ernstoff MS, Guiliano A, et al. Interferon α-2a and dacarbazine in melanoma [letter]. *J Natl Cancer Inst* 1990;82:1062.
166. Thompson D, Adena M, McLeod GRC, et al. Interferon alpha-2a does not improve response or survival when added to dacarbazine in metastatic melanoma: results of a multi-institutional Anstrahan randomized trial. *Proc Am Soc Clin Oncol* 1992;11:343.
167. Bajetta E, Negretti E, Giannotti B, et al. Phase II study of interferon α-2a and dacarbazine in advanced melanoma. *Am J Clin Oncol* 1990;13:405.
168. Gundersen S, Flokkmann A. Interferon plus dacarbazine in advanced malignant melanoma: a phase I-II study. *Eur J Cancer* 1991;27:220.
169. Mulder NH, deVries EGE, Sleijfer DTH, et al. Dacarbazine (DTIC), human recombinant interferon alpha 2a (roferon) and 5-fluorouracil for disseminated malignant melanoma. *Br J Cancer* 1992;65:303.
170. Sertoli MR, Queirolo P, Bajetta E, et al. Dacarbazine with or without recombinant interferon alpha-2a at different dosages in the treatment of stage IV melanoma patients. *Proc Am Soc Clin Oncol* 1992;11:345.
171. Bajetta E, Zampino MG, Di Leo A, et al. A phase III study with dacarbazine (DTIC) ± r-interferon alpha-2a (r-IFN) at different doses in advanced melanoma. *Ann Oncol* 1992;3:612.
172. Falkson CI, Ibrahim J, Kirkwood JM, et al. Phase III trial of dacarbazine versus dacarbazine with interferon α-2b versus dacarbazine with tamoxifen versus dacarbazine with interferon α-2b and tamoxifen in patients with metastatic malignant melanoma: an Eastern Cooperative Oncology Group Study (E3690). *J Clin Oncol* 1998;16:1743.
173. Oken MM, Kyle RA, Greipp PR, et al. Complete remission induction with combined VBMCP chemotherapy and interferon (rIFN alpha 2b) in patients with multiple myeloma. *Leukemia Lymphoma* 1996;20:447.
174. Solal-Celigny P, Lepage E, Brousse N, et al. Doxorubicin-containing regimen with or without interferon alfa-2b for advanced follicular lymphomas: final analysis of survival and toxicity in the Groupe d'Etude des Lymphomes Folliculaires 86 Trial. *J Clin Oncol* 1998;16:2332.
175. Smalley RV, Andersen JW, Hawkins MJ, et al. Interferon alfa combined with cytotoxic chemotherapy for patients with non-Hodgkin's lymphoma. *N Engl J Med* 1992;327:1336.
176. Agarwala SS, Atkins MB, Kirkwood JM. Current approaches to advanced and high-risk melanoma. *Proc Am Soc Clin Oncol* 2000.
177. Richards JM, Mehta N, Ramming K, et al. Sequential chemoimmunotherapy in the treatment of metastatic melanoma. *J Clin Oncol* 1992;8:1338.
178. Pyrhonen S, Hahka-Kemppinen M, Muhonen T. A promising interferon plus four-drug chemotherapy regimen for metastatic melanoma. *J Clin Oncol* 1992;10:1919.
179. Khayat D, Borel C, Tourani JM, et al. Sequential chemoimmunotherapy with cisplatin, interleukin-2, and interferon alfa-2a for metastatic melanoma. *J Clin Oncol* 1993;11:2173.
180. Nordlund JJ, Kirkwood JM, Forget BM. Vitiligo in patients with metastatic melanoma: a good prognostic sign. *J Am Acad Dermatol* 1983;9:689.
181. Harris J, Bines S, Das Gupta T. Therapy of disseminated malignant melanoma with recombinant alfa-2b interferon and piroxicam: clinical results with a report of an unusual response-associated feature (vitiligo) and unusual toxicity (diffuse pulmonary interstitial fibrosis). *Med Pediatr Oncol* 1994;22:103.
182. Figlin RA. Biotherapy with interferon in solid tumors. *Oncol Nurs Forum* 1987;14:23.
183. Karjalainen S, Hakulinen T. Survival and prognostic factors of patients with skin melanomas. *Cancer* 1988;62:2274.
184. Ryan L, Kramar A, Borden E. Prognostic factors in metastatic melanoma. *Cancer* 1993;71:2995.
185. Kirkwood J, Hunt M, Smith T, et al. A randomized controlled trial of high-dose IFN alfa-2b for high-risk melanoma: the ECOG trial EST-1684. *Proc Am Soc Clin Oncol* 1993;12:390.
186. Day CL Jr, Lew RA, Mihm MC Jr, et al. A multivariate analysis of prognostic factors for melanoma patients with lesions ≥3.65 mm in thickness: the importance of revealing alternate Cox models. *Ann Surg* 1982;195:44.
187. Day CL Jr, Sober AJ, Lew RA, et al. Malignant melanoma patients with positive nodes and relatively good prognoses: microstaging retains prognostic significance in clinical stage I melanoma patients with metastases to regional nodes. *Cancer* 1981;47:955.
188. Cole BF, Gelber RD, Kirkwood JM, et al. A quality-of-life-adjusted survival analysis of interferon alfa-2b adjuvant treatment for high-risk resected cutaneous melanoma: an Eastern Cooperative Oncology Group Study (E1684). *J Clin Oncol* 1996;14:2666.
189. Kilbridge KL, Sock D, Kirkwood J, et al. Patient utilities for adjuvant interferon (IFN) treatment for high-risk melanoma. *Proc Am Soc Clin Oncol* 1999.
190. Hillner BE, Kirkwood JM, Atkins MB, Johnson ER, Smith TJ. Economic analysis of adjuvant interferon alfa-2b in high-risk melanoma based on projections from ECOG 1684. *J Clin Oncol* 1997;15:2351.
191. Messori A, Becagli P, Trippoli S, Tendi E. A retrospective cost-effectiveness analysis of interferon as adjuvant therapy in high-risk resected cutaneous melanoma. *Eur J Cancer* 1997;33:1373.
192. Messori A, Becagli P, Trippoli S. Cost-effectiveness of interferon-alpha as maintenance therapy in chronic myelogenous leukemia. *Ann Intern Med* 1997;126:664.
193. Cascinelli N, Bufalino R, Morabito A, MacKie R. Results of adjuvant interferon study in WHO melanoma programme. *Lancet* 1994;343:913.
194. Chapman PB, Morrissey D, Ibrahim J, et al. Eastern Cooperative Oncology Group phase II randomized adjuvant trial of GM2-KLH + QS21 (GMK) vaccine ± high dose interferon-α 2b (HD IFN) in melanoma (MEL). *Proc Am Soc Clin Oncol* 1999;538a.

SECTION 2

JAMES W. MIER
MICHAEL B. ATKINS

Interleukin-2

Interleukin-2 (IL-2) is the first agent available for the treatment of metastatic cancer that functions solely through the activation of the immune system. Originally described as a growth factor for activated T cells, IL-2 was subsequently found to exert multiple effects on cellular immune function and to induce tumor regression in mice. Subsequent clinical trials in patients with renal cell carcinoma and malignant melanoma demonstrated sufficient efficacy to establish IL-2 as a U.S. Food and Drug Administration (FDA)-approved treatment for both of these malignancies.

ISOLATION, CHARACTERIZATION, AND CLONING OF INTERLEUKIN-2

In 1976, Morgan et al.[1] demonstrated the existence of a growth factor present in the conditioned medium of lectin-stimulated human peripheral blood mononuclear cells that could sustain indefinitely the *ex vivo* proliferation of human T cells. This initial report was followed in short order by the isolation, biochemical characterization, and, ultimately, the cloning of what was then termed *T-cell growth factor.*[2,3] Subsequently designated *IL-2*, this factor was shown to be a 15-kD polypeptide made up of 153 amino acids, the first 20 of which form a signal sequence that is proteolytically cleaved during secretion. Natural IL-2 is glycosylated, although the attachment of sugar moieties is not essential for biologic activity. The molecule has cysteine residues at positions 58, 105, and 125, the first two of which form an intramolecular disulfide bridge. The third cysteine is not essential for biologic activity and can be replaced with alternative amino acids to minimize polymerization and increase shelf life. Crystallographic analysis indicates that IL-2 is a spherical molecule comprised of six α helical regions.

INTERLEUKIN-2 RECEPTOR

The various biologic effects of IL-2 are the result of the binding of the lymphokine to specific surface receptors.[4] As with IL-2 itself, the expression of high-affinity IL-2 receptors is induced as a result of signaling through the T-cell antigen receptor. With the exception of a minor population of memory T cells that presumably were activated *in vivo* by a prior antigen exposure, freshly isolated peripheral blood T cells do not constitutively express high-affinity IL-2 receptors.[5]

The high-affinity IL-2 receptor consists of three distinct subunits designated the α, β, and γ chains (Fig. 20.2-1). The α chain[6] is a 251 amino acid polypeptide with a large extracellular domain, a transmembrane span, and a short 13-residue cytoplasmic tail. The extracellular domain of this protein binds IL-2 with low affinity. The cytoplasmic domain of this receptor has no known biologic function and is dispensable for IL-2–induced signaling.

The IL-2 receptor β chain has a 214 amino acid extracellular domain, a transmembrane motif, and a large 286-residue cytoplasmic tail.[7] In contrast to the cytoplasmic domain of the α chain, that of the β chain is essential for IL-2 signaling. The IL-2 receptor β chain has paired cysteines at two sites within the extracellular domain and a perimembrane WSXWS motif characteristic of the members of an enlarging cytokine receptor superfamily that includes the receptors for IL-3, IL-4, IL-6, IL-7, granulocyte-macrophage colony-stimulating factor, prolactin, erythropoietin, and growth hormone.

The γ chain is a novel 64-kD protein that physically associates with the β chain. Like the β chain, the γ chain is a member of the cytokine receptor superfamily.[8] These two together bind IL-2 with intermediate affinity. When cotransfected along with the complementary DNAs of the α and β chains, the complementary DNA encoding the γ chain yields a high-affinity IL-2 receptor that transduces signals and is internalized in response to IL-2 binding. More recent studies have demonstrated that this receptor chain is shared by the receptors for several lymphokines, including IL-4, IL-7, IL-9, and IL-15, as well as IL-2.[9] Mutations in the gene encoding this receptor chain account for most, if not all, cases of X-linked severe combined immunodeficiency.[10] Using antibodies against these receptor chains, resting T cells were found to constitutively express low levels of the IL-2 receptor γ chain, but not the α or β chains. All three chains are upregulated as a result of antigenic stimulation. Resting natural killer cells constitutively express the β chain, and both the α and γ chains are induced in these cells by exposure to IL-2 or IL-12.[11]

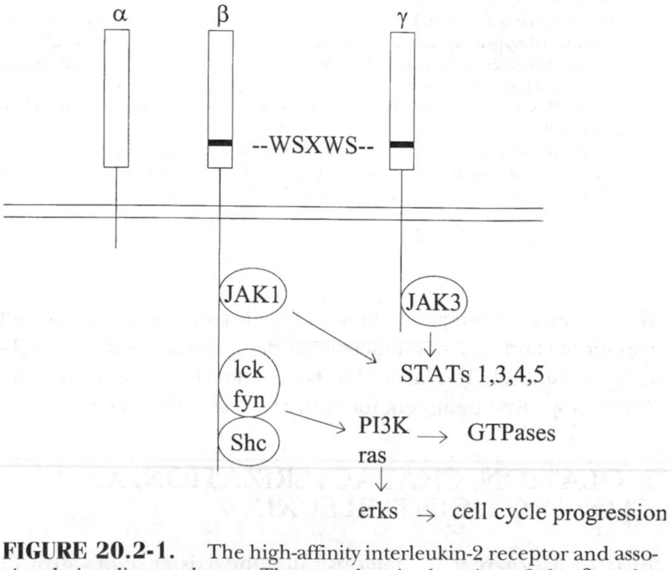

FIGURE 20.2-1. The high-affinity interleukin-2 receptor and associated signaling pathways. The cytoplasmic domains of the β and γ chains contain several tyrosines that, when phosphorylated, provide docking and activation sites for numerous downstream kinases that affect cell proliferation, gene expression, and cell motility. GTPases, guanosine triphosphatases; JAK, Janus kinase; PI3K, phosphoinositide 3 kinase; STAT, signal transduction and activators of transcription.

INTERLEUKIN-2–ACTIVATED SIGNALING PATHWAYS

The binding of IL-2 to its receptor induces the tyrosine phosphorylation of numerous cellular proteins, including the IL-2 receptor β chain itself. Because all three chains of the IL-2 receptor lack intrinsic tyrosine kinase activity, these events must be transduced through kinases that physically associate with the cytoplasmic domains of the receptor subunits (see Fig. 20.2-1). Indeed, the *src* family member $p56^{lck}$ has been shown to associate with the β chain, and its kinase activity is augmented by IL-2.[12] IL-2 also induces the recruitment and subsequent tyrosine phosphorylation of the adapter protein *Shc* to the IL-2R β chain. This particular association is thought to be largely responsible for the activation of $p21^{ras}$ and the downstream mitogen-activated protein kinases *erk-1* and *erk-2* in response to IL-2.[13] The IL-2 receptor γ chain is also essential for IL-2–induced signaling, because T-cell lines expressing the α and β chains and a mutant version of the γ chain lacking the C-terminal 68 residues fail to express the protooncogenes *c-fos*, *c-jun*, and *c-myc* when stimulated with IL-2.[14]

In addition to the association with *src* family tyrosine kinases, both the β and γ receptor chains associate with members of the Janus kinase family of tyrosine kinases.[15] Janus kinase family member JAK3 associates with the C-terminus of the IL-2 receptor γ chain, and both JAK1 and JAK2 associate with the β chain. JAK1 has been shown to bind to a specific serine-rich domain present in the membrane-proximal region of the β chain. Janus kinases activate various members of the signal transduction and activators of transcription (STAT) family of transcription factors. The binding of IL-2 to its receptor results in the activation of STAT1, STAT3, and STAT5 in T cells, and an additional member, STAT4, in natural killer (NK) cells.[16]

IN VITRO EFFECTS OF INTERLEUKIN-2

IL-2 was originally isolated based on its ability to induce the growth of previously activated T cells.[1] In addition to its proliferative effects, IL-2 induces the synthesis of an array of secondary cytokines, such as IL-1, tumor necrosis factor (TNF), IL-6, and lymphotoxin.[17] Several of these secondary cytokines are detectable in the circulation of cancer patients receiving IL-2 immunotherapy (see later, Toxicity of High-Dose Interleukin-2 Administration) and are thought by many investigators to contribute to the side effects of IL-2.[18]

The biologic effect of IL-2 arguably most pertinent to its use as an antitumor agent may be its ability to enhance the cytolytic activity of antigen-specific cytotoxic T lymphocytes and NK cells.[19,20] The biochemical basis for this enhanced cytolytic function is currently unclear, but it is thought to be due in part to the increased expression of genes encoding the lytic components of cytotoxic granules (e.g., perforin, granzymes) as well as adhesion molecules (lymphocyte function-associated antigen 1) that facilitate the binding of activated leukocytes to tumor endothelium and the tumor cells themselves. In addition to increasing the HLA-restricted cytolytic activity of cytotoxic T lymphocytes for cells expressing a particular antigen and that of NK cells for susceptible tumor cell targets, IL-2 markedly diversifies the range of target cells susceptible to killing by these effectors.[21,22] Indeed, human peripheral blood lymphocytes exposed only to high concentrations of IL-2 without prior exposure to tumor cells are able to kill virtually all tumor cell lines and most freshly isolated tumor cells *in vitro*, regardless of the particular HLA class I alleles expressed by the target cell. Some nontransformed cells, in particular cultured endothelial cells, are similarly susceptible to IL-2–primed peripheral blood lymphocytes in isotope release assays.[23] The cells responsible for this HLA-unrestricted killing in response to IL-2 have been termed *lymphokine-activated killer* (LAK) cells.[21,22] LAK cells appear to be a mixture of activated NK cells and CD3+/CD8+ cytotoxic T cells, the relative contributions of which depend on the duration of culture in IL-2 and whether human peripheral blood lymphocytes or murine spleen suspensions are used as a LAK cell source. As described below, these *ex vivo*–activated LAK cells featured prominently in the early clinical trials carried out with IL-2 in cancer patients.

PRECLINICAL STUDIES WITH INTERLEUKIN-2 IN TUMOR-BEARING MICE

The results of the *in vitro* studies demonstrating that IL-2 could enhance the cytolytic activity of NK cells and tumor-specific cytotoxic T cells suggested that systemically administered IL-2 might induce tumor regression in tumor-bearing mice. IL-2 has since undergone extensive evaluation as an antitumor agent in a variety of murine tumor models. IL-2 has been used alone, in combination with other cytokines, and in conjunction with the adoptive transfer of various *ex vivo*–activated lymphoid preparations to eradicate a wide range of local and metastatic tumors. Early studies demonstrated that IL-2 used alone could reduce or eliminate pulmonary metastases from methylcholanthrene-induced sarcoma and melanoma cell lines and that this antitumor effect was strictly dependent on the dose of IL-2 administered.[24] In another early study, IL-2 was able to cure 50% of mice inoculated with FBL-3 leukemia cells.[25] In this study, mice cured of leukemia by IL-2 were resistant to the subsequent inoculation of the same tumor cell line, suggesting that IL-2 treatment had effectively immunized the tumor-bearing mice against this particular tumor. In more recent studies in which mice were immunized with dendritic cells pulsed with tumor lysates, the concurrent systemic administration of IL-2 was shown to enhance the efficacy of the vaccine.[26]

In several studies, the effects of IL-2 could be enhanced by the concurrent administration of LAK cells generated by culturing splenocytes *ex vivo* in IL-2–containing media.[27] Mice bearing hepatic micrometastases from poorly immunogenic MCA-105 or MCA-102 sarcomas or MCA-38 adenocarcinoma cells, for example, were highly responsive to treatment with the combination of IL-2 and LAK cells but were unresponsive to LAK cells alone and only partially responsive to IL-2.

Lymphocytes present within tumor infiltrates are presumably enriched for effector cells capable of killing tumor cells.[28] When isolated and tested *in vitro* for cytolytic activity against autologous tumor cells, these tumor-infiltrating lymphocytes (TILs) are 50- to 100-fold more potent than IL-2–activated splenocytes (LAK cells). This apparent superiority was also evident *in vivo*. The infusion of 2×10^6 TILs with IL-2, for example, completely eradicated the pulmonary metastases of mice previously inoculated with MCA-105 sarcoma cells.[29] As many as 2×10^8 LAK cells were required for a comparable effect.

CLINICAL APPLICATIONS OF INTERLEUKIN-2

The potent immunomodulatory and antitumor effects of IL-2 in the *in vitro* experiments and preclinical animal tumor models described in the previous two sections prompted the rapid movement of IL-2 into the clinical setting. Early clinical trials involving the brief administration of modest doses of purified, cell-derived IL-2 produced only transient fever and lymphopenia, but no sustained ill effects or tumor responses.[30] Because preclinical trials had shown that tumor responses were dose-dependent and maximal when IL-2 was combined with LAK cells, the advent of recombinant IL-2 led quickly to a series of trials using higher doses of IL-2, with and without LAK cells.

CLINICAL INVESTIGATIONS INVOLVING HIGH-DOSE INTERLEUKIN-2

Investigators at the National Cancer Institute (NCI) Surgery Branch developed a regimen that involved the administration of high-dose intravenous bolus IL-2.[31,32] In this regimen, IL-2 [aldesleukin (Proleukin); Cetus/Chiron, Emeryville, CA] was administered at 600,000 to 720,000 IU/kg intravenously every 8 hours on days 1 to 5 and 15 to 19 of a treatment course. A maximum of 28 to 30 doses per course was administered; however, doses were frequently withheld for excessive toxicity. Treatment courses were repeated at 8- to 12-week intervals in responding patients. During initial studies, patients underwent daily leukaphereses on days 8 to 12, during which large numbers of lymphocytes were obtained to be cultured in IL-2 for 3 to 4 days to generate LAK cells; these LAK cells were then reinfused into the patient during the second 5-day period of IL-2 administration.

This high-dose IL-2 regimen, with or without LAK cells, produced overall tumor responses in 15% to 20% of patients with metastatic melanoma or renal cell cancer in clinical trials conducted at either the NCI Surgery Branch or within the Cytokine Working Group (formerly the Extramural IL-2 and LAK Working Group).[32–34] Complete responses were noted in 4% to 6% of patients with each disease and were frequently durable. Rare responses, usually partial and of shorter duration, were also noted in patients with either Hodgkin's or non-Hodgkin's lymphoma,[35] or non–small cell lung, colorectal, or ovarian carcinoma.[36] Randomized and sequential clinical trials comparing IL-2 plus LAK cells with high-dose IL-2 alone did not show sufficient benefit for the addition of LAK cells to justify their continued use.[37–39] The quality and durability of tumor responses to this high-dose IL-2 regimen led to IL-2 receiving FDA approval for the treatment of metastatic renal cell carcinoma in 1992 and metastatic melanoma in 1998.[40,41]

TOXICITY OF HIGH-DOSE INTERLEUKIN-2 ADMINISTRATION

The utility of high-dose IL-2 has been limited by toxicity, many features of which resemble bacterial sepsis. Side effects are dose-dependent and largely predictable and rapidly reversible. Common side effects include fever, chills, lethargy, diarrhea, nausea, anemia, thrombocytopenia, eosinophilia, diffuse erythroderma, hepatic dysfunction, and confusion.[42,43] Myocarditis also occurs in approximately 5% of patients. IL-2 therapy also commonly produces a "capillary leak syndrome," leading to fluid retention, hypotension, early adult respiratory distress syndrome, prerenal azotemia, and, occasionally, myocardial infarction. As a consequence of these side effects, few patients are able to receive all of the proposed therapy. IL-2 also has been shown to produce a neutrophil chemotactic defect that predisposes patients to infection with gram-positive and, occasionally, gram-negative bacteria.[44,45] Early high-dose IL-2 studies were associated with 2% to 4% mortality, largely related to infection or cardiac toxicity.[40–43] The routine use of antibiotic prophylaxis, more extensive cardiac screening, and more judicious IL-2 administration have greatly enhanced the safety of this therapy; since 1990, the mortality rates at experienced treatment centers have been less than 1%[46] (Table 20.2-1). Nonetheless, the considerable toxicity of the high-dose IL-2 regimen has continued to limit its application to highly selected patients with excellent performance status and

TABLE 20.2-1. Safety of High-Dose Intravenous Bolus Recombinant Interleukin-2 Therapy[a]: The National Cancer Institute Experience[b]

Adverse Event[c]	*1985 Incidence (%)*	*1997 Incidence (%)*
Hypotension	81	31
Diarrhea	92	12
Neuropsychiatric toxicity	19	8
Line sepsis	18	4
Pulmonary complications	12	3

[a]720,000 IU/kg every 8 hours.
[b]With patient selection and experience in managing side effects, high-dose recombinant interleukin-2 is safe. No treatment-related deaths in 809 consecutive patients.
[c]Incidence of grade 3–4 adverse events has been greatly reduced.
Data from ref. 46.

adequate organ function treated at medical centers with considerable experience with this approach.

Laboratory studies have suggested that IL-2 toxicity appears to be mediated, at least in part, by the release of secondary cytokines such as TNF-α, IL-1, and IL-6 and the generation of nitric oxide.[47–49] Nonetheless, attempts to block the toxicity of IL-2 by the co-administration of selective inhibitors of the biologic effects of these secondary cytokines have been largely unsuccessful to date.[50–52]

MANAGEMENT OF PATIENTS RECEIVING HIGH-DOSE INTERLEUKIN-2

The management of patients undergoing high-dose IL-2 therapy begins at the time of patient selection. This therapy should be limited to patients without significant cardiac disease (prior myocardial infarction, angina, congestive heart failure, or serious cardiac arrhythmias). Patients older than age 40 years should have a normal cardiac stress test. In addition, patients should have no evidence of central nervous system metastases; adequate pulmonary, renal, and hepatic function (forced expiratory volume in 1 second of more than 2 L, serum creatinine less than 1.6 mg/dL, serum bilirubin less than 1.5 mg/dL); and good performance status (Eastern Cooperative Oncology Group scale, 0 or 1).

Concomitant therapy typically includes acetaminophen and indomethacin to prevent rigors and fever, H_2 blockers to prevent gastritis, and prophylactic antibiotics to prevent catheter-related infections. Patients should also receive antiemetics, antidiarrheals, and skin care on an as-needed basis. Steroids should be avoided because they interfere with immune activation. Patients typically require fluid administration to support their blood pressure. Hypotension unresponsive to fluid administration is treated with intravenous dopamine hydrochloride and, when necessary, intravenous phenylephrine hydrochloride. Sodium bicarbonate administration is often necessary to keep the serum HCO_3 concentration higher than 18 mEq/L. Severe toxicities, such as hypotension requiring multiple pressor agents, confusion, cardiac arrhythmias or myocarditis, metabolic acidosis, or dyspnea, are usually managed by withholding doses of IL-2. Once these problems resolve, treatment usually can be resumed (omitted doses of IL-2 are not replaced).

With careful patient selection and judicious treatment of toxicity, most patients can safely receive an adequate amount of high-dose IL-2; however, because of the unusual nature and potential severity of these side effects, the use of this therapy by inexperienced physicians and nurses should be discouraged.

LOWER-DOSE OR ALTERNATIVE INTERLEUKIN-2 REGIMENS

Because of the significant toxicity associated with high-dose intravenous bolus IL-2 regimens and the expense involved with the necessary hospitalization and intensive monitoring, various investigators have attempted to establish active regimens using lower doses of IL-2. In these regimens, IL-2 was administered either by lower-dose intravenous bolus, continuous intravenous infusion, or subcutaneous injection in an effort to maintain or enhance antitumor effects while decreasing toxicity. Table 20.2-2 lists a variety of the more commonly used lower-dose IL-2 regimens.[53–59]

The maximum tolerated dose for IL-2 when administered by a 5-day (120-hour) continuous infusion was shown to be 18

TABLE 20.2-2. Commonly Used Treatment Regimens of Interleukin-2 (IL-2) Alone

Regimen	*IL-2 Dose*	*IL-2 Schedule*	*Clinical Setting*
High-dose IV bolus IL-2	600,000–720,000 IU/kg	IV q8h days 1–5, 15–19	ICU-like
Continuous infusion IL-2	18 MIU/m²/d	CIV infusion days 1–5, 15–19	ICU-like
Low-dose IV bolus IL-2	72,000 IU/kg	IV q8h days 1–5, 15–19	Ward
Subcutaneous IL-2	250,000 IU/kg/d	SC days 1–5, wk 1	Outpatient
	125,000 IU/kg/d	SC days 1–5, wk 2–6	
Decrescendo IL-2	18 MIU/m²/6 h	CIV infusion × 1 d	Ward
	18 MIU/m²/12 h	CIV infusion × 1 d	
	18 MIU/m²/24 h	CIV infusion × 1 d	
	4.5 MIU/m²/24 h	CIV infusion × 3 d	
Ultra-low-dose IL-2	≤1 MIU/d	CIV infusion × 14–42 d	Outpatient

CIV, continuous intravenous; ICU-like, intensive care unit or specialized unit capable of providing blood pressure support.

MIU/m²/d or only approximately one-fifth the total amount of IL-2 tolerated by intravenous bolus IL-2 regimens.[53] Although continuous infusion IL-2 regimens were shown to produce response rates similar to the high-dose intravenous bolus IL-2 regimen, the toxicity was also generally comparable.[53–55] Other regimens, such as those using lower doses of IL-2 administered either by intravenous bolus or subcutaneous injection, are much better tolerated, enabling treatment to be provided in a routine ward or even an outpatient setting. The side effects are generally limited to the flu-like symptoms and constitutional symptoms already described, allowing treatment to be provided safely, even to patients with more limited cardiac, pulmonary, and renal function. These regimens have produced roughly comparable response rates in patients with renal cell carcinoma; however, the quality and durability of these responses have yet to be shown to be comparable to the responses observed with high-dose intravenous regimens.[56,57] Lower-dose IL-2 regimens have been largely inactive in patients with metastatic melanoma.[60]

BIOLOGY AND PHARMACOKINETICS OF INTERLEUKIN-2

Although only the recombinant IL-2 manufactured by Chiron (Proleukin) is currently FDA approved for clinical use, several different IL-2 preparations have been used in clinical trials. These preparations differ in potency and, in some instances, biologic activity. By convention,[60] the following conversion factors are used: 1 Cetus unit = 6 IU; 1 Hoffman-LaRoche unit = 1 Biologic Response Modifier Program = 2.6 IU. It has become apparent, however, that many other differences may exist between these preparations[61] and, therefore, these simple conversions may not be entirely valid.

Yang et al.[56] examined the pharmacokinetics of IL-2 (Proleukin) administered to patients with advanced renal cell carcinoma on three distinct treatment regimens (Fig. 20.2-2). Patients undergoing treatment with high-dose intravenous IL-2 (720,000 IU/kg) achieved peak serum concentrations of 4680 ± 1188 IU/mL shortly after the first injection. Subsequent clearance was biphasic, with an initial half-life of 12.6 ± 5.4 minutes and a terminal half-life of 1.6 ± 0.4 hours. Patients receiving low-dose intravenous IL-2 (72,000 IU/kg) exhibited peak levels of 486 ± 198 IU/mL after the first injection, with a similar clearance pattern and rates. Those patients receiving IL-2 administered subcutaneously at a dose of 250,000 IU/kg had peak serum levels of 61 ± 34 IU/mL 2 to 3 hours after the injection, with a half-life of 5.3 ± 1.9 hours. Levels in excess of 18 IU/mL were maintained between injections in patients receiving either the high-dose intravenous or the subcutaneous regimen cited, but not the low-dose intravenous regimen. The relationship of these differing pharmacokinetic profiles to the biologic and antitumor effects of IL-2 remains to be determined.

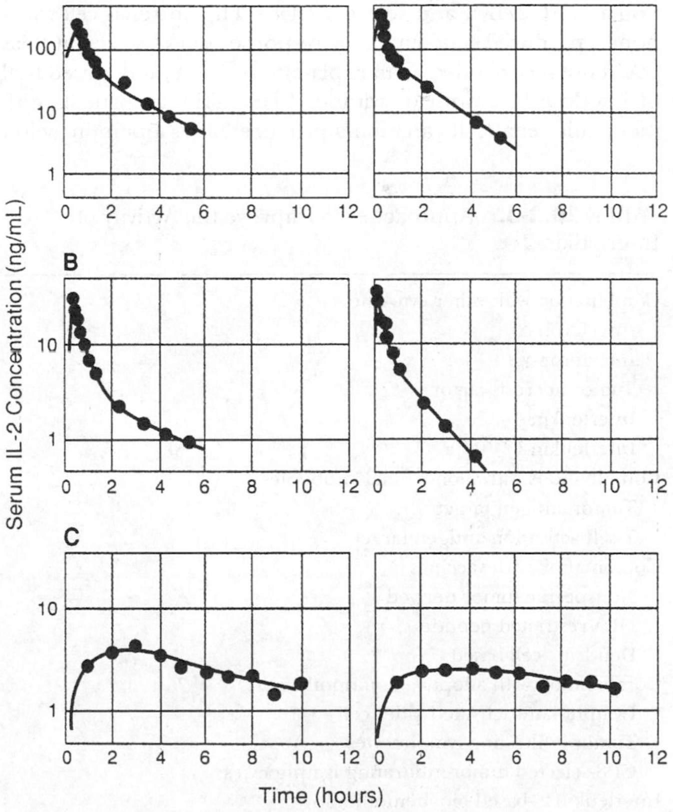

FIGURE 20.2-2. Examples of pharmacokinetic studies on representative patients with metastatic renal cell carcinoma measuring biologically active serum interleukin (IL)-2 levels after the first administration of recombinant IL-2 at **(A)** 720,000 IU/kg by intravenous bolus, **(B)** 72,000 IU/kg by intravenous bolus, or **(C)** 250,000 IU/kg by subcutaneous injection. (From ref. 56, with permission.)

ATTEMPTS TO IMPROVE ACTIVITY OF INTERLEUKIN-2–BASED THERAPY

A number of approaches have been tried in an effort to improve the activity of IL-2–based therapy. These are listed in Table 20.2-3. Although preclinical laboratory and animal studies provided a strong rationale for the clinical investigations involving the combination of IL-2 and interferon-α (IFN-α),[62] and early clinical studies appeared promising,[63] subsequent clinical trials have not shown superiority for this combination relative to high-dose IL-2.[64–66] Nonetheless, combinations of low-dose IL-2 with IFN have been developed that can be administered safely in an outpatient setting, and they appear to possess sufficient antitumor activity to enable them to be considered by many as an alternative to high-dose IL-2.[67–69] In addition, low-dose IL-2 and IFN regimens have been better able to accommodate the addition of other potentially active agents, such as chemotherapy or cellular therapy.

Efforts to combine IL-2 with other potentially active cytokines, such as IFN-γ, TNF, and IL-4, have been largely unsuccessful to date,[70] whereas clinical trials involving combinations of IL-2 and IL-12 are ongoing. Likewise, combinations of IL-2 with a variety of monoclonal antibodies directed either against tumor antigens (GD2 or GD3 gangliosides) or T-cell activation antigens (CD3) have been disappointing.[71] Although IL-2 and TIL combinations were extremely promising in animal tumor models, results of human investigations with this approach have been mixed. Although preliminary studies involving IL-2 and TILs in melanoma or IL-2/IFN and selected CD8+ TILs in renal cell carcinoma produced encouraging response rates, selection bias could not be excluded as an explanation.[72–74] A randomized trial of low-dose IL-2, with or without CD8+ TILs, in patients with metastatic renal cell carcinoma produced a disappointingly low response rate for both treatment arms[75]; a similar study has yet to be performed in patients with metastatic melanoma.

Despite their limited therapeutic utility, TILs have proven to be a valuable tool for identifying melanoma-associated tumor regression antigens.[76] Extensive research at the NCI Surgery Branch and elsewhere has identified HLA-restricted melanocyte lineage–specific antigens that are recognized by the cellular immune system in patients exhibiting a response to IL-2–based therapy.[77] Active immunization trials with immunodominant peptides derived from these tumor regression antigens have produced some encouraging results.[78,79] For example, vaccination with a mutated version of the *gp100* peptide antigen, together with high-dose IL-2, produced tumor responses in more than 40% of patients.[80] Confirmatory trials examining either a variety of schedules of peptide vaccination and IL-2 administration or comparing this combination to high-dose IL-2 alone are currently under way. In addition, trials examining combinations of similarly HLA-restricted antigens or antigen-presenting cells pulsed with these peptides together with IL-2 have been initiated.

Another promising approach has involved the combination of IL-2–based immunotherapy and cytotoxic chemotherapy—so called biochemotherapy. Efforts in renal cell cancer patients have focused on the addition of 5-fluorouracil–based chemotherapy,[79] whereas in melanoma, investigations have primarily examined IL-2 together with cisplatin- and dacarbazine-based cytotoxic chemotherapy.[81,82] Response rates as high as 40% in patients with renal cell carcinoma and 50% to 60% in patients with metastatic melanoma have been reported with these regimens. These encouraging results from multiple phase II trials and metaanalyses[83,84] await confirmation in ongoing large-scale phase III clinical trials. If biochemotherapy proves superior to chemotherapy alone in either disease, it might conceivably provide a rationale for examining IL-2–based biochemotherapy regimens in other 5-fluorouracil– or cisplatin-sensitive malignancies. In addition, these or other approaches mentioned here might show sufficient activity in the metastatic setting to justify their being examined in the high-risk adjuvant setting in which tumor burden and associated immune suppression may be less and, consequently, the potential for clinical impact may be greatly enhanced.

TABLE 20.2-3. Approaches to Improve the Activity of Interleukin-2

Combination with other cytokines
Interferon-α
Interferon-γ
Tumor necrosis factor
Interleukin-4
Interleukin-12
Combinations with monoclonal antibodies
Tumor antigen target
T-cell activation antigen target
Combination with vaccines
Nonspecific tumor derived
HLA-restricted peptide
Dendritic cell based
Combination with adoptive immunotherapy
Lymphokine-activated killer cell
Tumor-infiltrating lymphocytes
CD8-selected tumor-infiltrating lymphocytes
Interleukin-2–based biochemotherapy
5-Fluorouracil based
Cisplatin/dacarbazine based
Expansion to other diseases
Adjuvant therapy

REFERENCES

1. Morgan D, Ruscetti FW, Gallo R. Selective *in vitro* growth of T-lymphocytes from normal bone marrows. *Science* 1976;193:1007.
2. Mier J, Gallo R. Purification and some characteristics of human T cell growth factor (TCGF) from PHA-stimulated lymphocyte conditioned media. *Proc Natl Acad Sci U S A* 1980;77:6134.
3. Taniguchi T, Matsui H, Fujita T, et al. Structure and expression of a cloned cDNA for human interleukin-2. *Nature* 1983;302:305.
4. Taniguchi T, Minami Y. The IL-2/IL-2 receptor system: a current overview. *Cell* 1993;73:5.
5. Gootenberg J, Ruscetti F, Mier J, Gazdar A, Gallo R. Human cutaneous T-cell lymphoma and leukemia cell lines produce and respond to T-cell growth factor. *J Exp Med* 1981;154:1403.
6. Leonard WJ, Depper J, Uchiyama T, et al. A monoclonal antibody that appears to recognize the receptor for T cell growth factor: partial purification of the receptor. *Nature* 1982;300:267.
7. Hatakeyama M, Tsudo M, Minamoto S, et al. Interleukin-2 receptor beta chain gene: generation of three receptor forms by cloned human alpha and beta chain cDNAs. *Science* 1989;244:551.
8. Takeshita T, Asao H, Ohtani K, et al. Cloning of the gamma-chain of the human IL-2 receptor. *Science* 1992;257:379.
9. Lodolce JP, Boone DL, Chai S, et al. IL-15 receptor maintains lymphoid homeostasis by supporting lymphocyte homing and proliferation. *Immunity* 1998;9:669.
10. Noguchi M, Yi H, Rosenblatt HM, et al. Interleukin-2 receptor gamma chain mutation results in X-linked severe combined immunodeficiency in humans. *Cell* 1983;73:147.
11. Nakarai T, Robertson MJ, Streuli M, et al. Interleukin-2 receptor gamma chain expression on resting and activated lymphoid cells. *J Exp Med* 1994;180:241.
12. Hatakeyama M, Kono T, Kobayashi N, et al. Interaction of the IL-2 receptor with the *src*-family kinase $p56^{lck}$: identification of novel intermolecular association. *Science* 1991;252:1523.

13. Friedmann MC, Migone TS, Russell SM, Leonard WJ. Different interleukin-2 receptor beta chain tyrosines couple to at least two signaling pathways and synergistically mediate interleukin-2-induced proliferation. *Proc Natl Acad Sci U S A* 1996;93:2077.
14. Asao H, Takeshita T, Ishii N, et al. Reconstitution of functional interleukin 2 receptor complexes on fibroblastoid cells: involvement of the cytoplasmic domain of the gamma chain in two distinct signaling pathways. *Proc Natl Acad Sci U S A* 1993;90:4127.
15. Russell SM, Johnston JA, Noguchi M, et al. Interaction of IL-2 receptor beta and gamma c chains with JAK1 and JAK3: implications for XSCID and XCID. *Science* 1994;266:1042.
16. Wang KS, Ritz J, Frank DA. IL-2 induces STAT4 activation in primary NK cells and NK cell lines, but not in T cells. *J Immunol* 1999;162:299.
17. Numerof R, Aronson F, Mier J. Interleukin-2 stimulates the production of interleukin-1 alpha and interleukin-1 beta by human peripheral blood mononuclear cells. *J Immunol* 1988;141:4250.
18. Gemlo BT, Palladino MA, Jaffe HS, Espevik TP, Rayner AA. Circulating cytokines in patients with metastatic cancer treated with recombinant interleukin-2 and lymphokine-activated killer cells. *Cancer Res* 1988;48:5864.
19. Strasser JL, Rosenberg SA. *In vitro* growth of cytotoxic human lymphocytes. I. Growth of cells sensitized *in vitro* to alloantigens. *J Immunol* 1978;121:1951.
20. Lotze MT, Grimm EA, Mazumder A, Strausser JL, Rosenberg SA. Lysis of fresh and cultured autologous tumor by human lymphocytes cultured in T-cell growth factor. *Cancer Res* 1981;41:4420.
21. Grimm EA, Mazumder A, Zhang HZ, Rosenberg SA. Lymphokine-activated killing phenomenon: lysis of natural killer resistant fresh solid tumor cells by interleukin-2 activated autologous human peripheral blood lymphocytes. *J Exp Med* 1982;155:1823.
22. Grimm EA, Robb RJ, Roth JA, et al. The lymphokine activated killer cell phenomenon. III. Evidence that IL-2 alone is sufficient for direct activation of PBL into lymphokine-activated killer cells. *J Exp Med* 1983;158:1356.
23. Aronson F, Libby P, Brandon E, Janicka M, Mier J. Interleukin-2 rapidly induces natural killer cell adhesion to human endothelial cells: a potential mechanism for endothelial injury. *J Immunol* 1988;141:158.
24. Rosenberg SA, Mule JJ, Spiess PJ, Reichert CM, Schwarz SL. Regression of established pulmonary metastases and subcutaneous tumors mediated by the systemic administration of high-dose recombinant interleukin-2. *J Exp Med* 1985;161:1169.
25. Thompson JA, Peace DJ, Klarnet JP, et al. Eradication of disseminated murine leukemia by treatment with high dose interleukin-2. *J Immunol* 1986;137:3675.
26. Shimizu K, Fields RC, Giedlin M, Mule JJ. Systemic administration of interleukin-2 enhances the therapeutic efficacy of dendritic cell-based tumor vaccines. *Proc Natl Acad Sci U S A* 1999;96:2268.
27. Lafreniere R, Rosenberg SA. Adoptive immunotherapy of murine hepatic metastases with lymphokine activated killer (LAK) cells and recombinant interleukin-2 (RIL-2) can mediate the regression of both immunogenic and nonimmunogenic sarcomas and an adenocarcinoma. *J Immunol* 1985;135:4273.
28. Belldegrun A, Muul LM, Rosenberg SA. Interleukin-2 expanded tumor infiltrating lymphocytes in human cancer: isolation, characterization and antitumor activity. *Cancer Res* 1988;48:206.
29. Spiess PJ, Yang JC, Rosenberg SA. *In vivo* antitumor activity of tumor-infiltrating lymphocytes expanded in recombinant interleukin-2. *J Natl Cancer Inst* 1987;79:1067.
30. Lotze MT, Frana LW, Sharrow SO, et al. *In vivo* administration of purified human interleukin 2. I. Half-life and immunologic effects of the Jurkat cell line-derived interleukin 2. *J Immunol* 1985;134:157.
31. Rosenberg SA, Lotze MT, Muul LM, et al. Observations on the systemic administration of autologous lymphokine-activated killer cells and recombinant interleukin-2 to patients with metastatic cancer. *N Engl J Med* 1985;313:1485.
32. Rosenberg SA, Yang JC, Topalian SL, et al. Treatment of 283 consecutive patients with metastatic melanoma or renal cell cancer using high-dose bolus interleukin-2. *JAMA* 1994;271:907.
33. Parkinson D, Abrams J, Wiernik P, et al. Interleukin-2 therapy in patients with metastatic malignant melanoma: a phase II study. *J Clin Oncol* 1990;8:1650.
34. Dutcher JP, Creekmore S, Weiss GR, et al. A phase II study of interleukin-2 and lymphokine activated killer (LAK) cells in patients with metastatic malignant melanoma. *J Clin Oncol* 1989;7:477.
35. Benyunes MC, Fefer A. Interleukin-2 in the treatment of hematologic malignancies. In: Atkins MB, Mier JW, eds. *Therapeutic applications of interleukin-2.* New York: Marcel Dekker Inc, 1993:163.
36. Sznol M, Hawkins MJ. Interleukin-2 in malignancies other than melanoma and renal cell carcinoma. In: Atkins MB, Mier JW, eds. *Therapeutic applications of interleukin-2.* New York: Marcel Dekker Inc, 1993:177.
37. Rosenberg SA, Lotze MT, Muul LM, et al. A progress report on the treatment of 157 patients with advanced cancer using lymphokine-activated killer cells and interleukin-2 or high dose interleukin-2 alone. *N Engl J Med* 1987;316:889.
38. McCabe MS, Stablein D, Hawkins MJ, et al. The modified group C experience phase III randomized trials of IL-2 vs. IL-2/LAK in advanced renal cell carcinoma and advanced melanoma. *Proc Am Soc Clin Oncol* 1991;10:213(abst).
39. Rosenberg SA, Lotze MT, Yang JC, et al. Prospective randomized trial of high-dose interleukin-2 alone or in conjunction with lymphokine-activated killer cells for the treatment of patients with advanced cancer. *J Natl Cancer Inst* 1993;8:622.
40. Fyfe G, Fisher RI, Rosenberg SA, et al. Results of treatment of 255 patients with metastatic renal cell carcinoma who received high-dose recombinant interleukin-2 therapy. *J Clin Oncol* 1995;13:688.
41. Atkins MB, Lotze M, Dutcher J, et al. High-dose recombinant interleukin-2 therapy for metastatic melanoma: analysis of 270 patients treated from 1985–1993. *J Clin Oncol* 1999;17:2105.
42. Schwartzentruber DJ. Biologic therapy with interleukin-2. Clinical applications: principles of administration and management of side effects. In: DeVita V, Hellman S, Rosenberg SA, eds. *Biologic therapy of cancer,* 2nd ed. Philadelphia: JB Lippincott, 1995:235.
43. Margolin K. The clinical toxicities of high-dose interleukin-2. In: Atkins MB, Mier JW, eds. *Therapeutic applications of interleukin-2.* New York: Marcel Dekker Inc, 1993:331.
44. Klempner M, Noring R, Mier J, Atkins MB. An acquired neutrophil chemotactic defect in patients receiving immunotherapy with interleukin-2. *N Engl J Med* 1990;322:959.
45. Snydman DR, Sullivan B, Gill M, et al. Nosocomial sepsis associated with interleukin-2. *Ann Intern Med* 1990;112:102.
46. Kammula US, White DE, Rosenberg SA. Trends in the safety of high dose bolus interleukin-2 administration in patients with metastatic cancer. *Cancer* 1998;83:797.
47. Numerof RP, Aronson FR, Mier JW. IL-2 stimulates the production of IL-1 alpha and IL-1 beta by human peripheral blood mononuclear cells. *J Immunol* 1988;141:4250.
48. Mier J, Vachino G, Van der Meer J, et al. Induction of circulating tumor necrosis factor (TNF) as the mechanism for the febrile response to interleukin-2 (IL-2) in cancer patients. *J Clin Immunol* 1988;8:426.
49. Hibbs JB, Westenfelder C, Taintor R, et al. Evidence for cytokine inducible nitric oxide synthesis from L-arginine in patients receiving interleukin-2 therapy. *J Clin Invest* 1992;89:867.
50. Margolin K, Atkins M, Sparano J, et al. Prospective randomized trial of lisophylline for the prevention of toxicities of high-dose interleukin 2 therapy in advanced renal cancer and malignant melanoma. *Clin Cancer Res* 1997;3:565.
51. DuBois J, Trehu EG, Mier JW, et al. Randomized placebo-controlled clinical trial of high-dose interleukin-2 (IL-2) in combination with the soluble TNF receptor IgG chimera (TNFR:Fc). *J Clin Oncol* 1997;15:1052.
52. McDermott D, Trehu E, DuBois J, et al. Phase I clinical trial of the soluble IL-1 receptor either alone or in combination with high-dose IL-2 in patients with advanced malignancies. *Clin Cancer Res* 1998;5:1203.
53. West WH, Tauer KW, Yannelli JR, et al. Constant-infusion recombinant interleukin-2 in adoptive immunotherapy of advanced cancer. *N Engl J Med* 1987;16:898.
54. Dillman RO, Church C, Oldham RK, et al. In patient continuous infusion IL-2 in 788 patients with cancer. The national biotherapy study group experience. *Cancer* 1993;71:2358.
55. Legha SS, Gianan MA, Plager C, et al. Evaluation of interleukin-2 administered by continuous infusion in patients with metastatic melanoma. *Cancer* 1996;77:89.
56. Yang JC, Rosenberg SA. An ongoing prospective randomized comparison of interleukin-2 regimens for the treatment of metastatic renal cell cancer. *Cancer J Sci Am* 1997;3:S79.
57. Sleijfer DT, Janssen RAJ, Buter J, et al. Phase II study of subcutaneous interleukin-2 in unselected patients with advanced renal cell cancer on an outpatient basis. *J Clin Oncol* 1992;10:1119.
58. Keilholz U, Scheibenbogen C, Tilgen W, et al. Interferon-a and interleukin-2 in the treatment of metastatic melanoma: comparison of two phase II trials. *Cancer* 1993;72:607.
59. Caligiuri MA, Murray C, Robertson MJ, et al. Selective modulation of human natural killer cells *in vivo* following prolonged infusion of low-dose recombinant interleukin 2. *J Clin Invest* 1993;91:123.
60. Atkins MB, Shet A, Sosman JA. IL-2 clinical applications: melanoma. In: Rosenberg SA, ed. *Principles and practice of biologic therapy of cancer,* 3rd ed. Philadelphia: Lippincott Williams & Wilkins, 2000.
61. Hank JA, Surfus J, Gan J, et al. Distinct clinical and laboratory activity of two recombinant interleukin-2 preparations. *Clin Cancer Res* 1999;5:281.
62. Cameron RB, McIntosh JK, Rosenberg SA. Synergistic anti-tumor effects of combination immunotherapy with recombinant interleukin-2 and a recombinant hybrid alpha-interferon in the treatment of established murine hepatic metastases. *Cancer Res* 1988;48:5810.
63. Rosenberg SA, Lotze MT, Yang JC, et al. Combination therapy with interleukin-2 and interferon for the treatment of patients with advanced cancer. *J Clin Oncol* 1989;7:1863.
64. Atkins MB, Sparano J, Fisher RI, et al. A randomized phase II trial of high dose IL-2 either alone or in combination with interferon alpha 2B in advanced renal cell carcinoma. *J Clin Oncol* 1993;11:661.
65. Sparano JA, Fisher RI, Sunderland M, et al. Randomized phase III trial of treatment with high dose interleukin-2 either alone or in combination with alfa-2A in patients with advanced melanoma. *J Clin Oncol* 1993;11:1969.
66. Marcinola FM, White DE, Wise AP, Rosenberg SA. Combination therapy with interferon alfa-2A and interleukin-2 for the treatment of metastatic cancer. *J Clin Oncol* 1995;13:1110.
67. Karp SE. Low-dose intravenous bolus interluekin-2 with interferon-alpha therapy for metastatic melanoma and renal cell carcinoma. *J Immunotherapy* 1998;21:56.
68. Atzpodien J, Lopez HE, Kirchner H, et al. Multi-institutional home therapy trial of recombinant human interleukin-2 and interferon alfa-2 in progressive metastatic renal cell carcinoma. *J Clin Oncol* 1995;13:497.
69. Dutcher JP, Fisher RI, Weiss G, et al. Outpatient subcutaneous interleukin-2 plus alpha interferon in metastatic renal cell cancer: three-year follow-up of the Cytokine Working Group study. *Cancer J Sci Am* 1997;3:157.
70. Atkins MB, Trehu EG, Mier JW. Combination cytokine therapy. In: DeVita VT Jr, Hellman S, Rosenberg SA, eds. *Biologic therapy of cancer principles and practice,* 2nd ed. Philadelphia: JB Lippincott, 1995:443.
71. Sosman J, Weiss G, Margolin K, et al. Phase 1B clinical trial of anti-CD3 followed by high dose interleukin-2 in patients with metastatic melanoma and advanced renal cell carcinoma: clinical and immunologic effects. *J Clin Oncol* 1993;11:1496.
72. Rosenberg SA, Schwartz SL, Spiess PJ. Combination immunotherapy for cancer: synergistic antitumor interactions of interleukin-2, alfa interferon, and tumor-infiltrating lymphocytes. *J Natl Cancer Inst* 1988;80:1393.
73. Figlin RA, Pierce WC, Kaboo R, et al. Treatment of metastatic renal cell carcinoma with nephrectomy, interleukin-2 and cytokine-primed or CD8(+) selected tumor infiltrating lymphocytes from primary tumor. *J Urology* 1997;158:740.
74. Atkins MB. Immunotherapy and experimental approaches for metastatic melanoma. *Hematol Oncol Clin North Am* 1998;12:877.
75. Figlin RA, Thompson JA, Bukowski RM, et al. Multicenter, randomized, phase III trail of CD8+ tumor-infiltrating lymphocytes in combination with recombinant interleukin-2 in metastatic renal cell carcinoma. *J Clin Oncol* 1999;17:2521.

76. Kawakami Y, Eliejahu S, Jennings C, et al. Recognition of multiple epitopes in the human melanoma antigen gp100 by tumor infiltrating T-lymphocytes associated with *in vivo* tumor regression. *J Immunol* 1995;154:3461.
77. Zhai Y, Yang JC, Kawakami Y, et al. Antigen-specific tumor vaccines: development and characterization or recombinant adenovirus encoding MART-1 or gp100 for cancer therapy. *J Immunol* 1996;156:700.
78. Parkhurst MR, Salgaller ML, Southwood S, et al. Improved induction of melanoma-reactive CTL with peptides from the melanoma antigen gp100 modified at HLA-A* 0201-binding residues. *J Immunol* 1996;157:2539.
79. Rosenberg SA, Yang JC, Schwartzentruber DJ, et al. Immunologic and therapeutic evaluation of a synthetic peptide vaccine for the treatment of patients with metastatic melanoma. *Nat Med* 1998;4:321.
80. Atzpodien J, Kirchner H, Hanninen EL, et al. Interleukin-2 in combination with interferon-a and 5-fluorouracil for metastatic renal cell cancer. *Eur J Cancer* 1993;29A[Suppl 5]:S6.
81. Atkins MB. The role of cytotoxic chemotherapeutic agents either alone or in combination with biological response modifiers. In: Kirkwood JM, ed. *Molecular diagnosis, prevention and therapy of melanoma.* New York: Marcel Dekker Inc, 1998:219.
82. Legha SS, Buzaid AC. Role of recombinant interleukin-2 in combination with interferon-alfa and chemotherapy in the treatment of advanced melanoma. *Semin Oncol* 1993;2[Suppl 9]:27.
83. Allen IE, Kupelnick B, Kumashiro M, et al. Efficacy of interleukin-2 in the treatment of metastatic melanoma: systematic review and meta-analysis. *Cancer Ther* 1998;1:168.
84. Keilholz U, Conradt C, Legha SS, et al. Results of interleukin-2 based treatment in advanced melanoma: a case record-based analysis of 631 patients. *J Clin Oncol* 1998;16:2921.

SECTION **3**

CHARLES ERLICHMAN
CHARLES L. LOPRINZI

Hormonal Therapies

There are many hormonal agents used in the treatment of patients with cancer. The primary use of these agents is in hormonally responsive cancers such as breast, prostate, or endometrial carcinomas. Other uses for some hormonal therapies include paraneoplastic syndromes, such as carcinoid syndrome, or symptoms caused by cancer, including anorexia. This chapter discusses the major hormonal agents for such therapy, first with a general overview of their use in practice, then with more detailed pharmacologic information regarding them.

SELECTIVE ESTROGEN RECEPTOR MODULATORS

TAMOXIFEN

Tamoxifen is most frequently used in the adjuvant treatment of women with resected breast cancer. There is general consensus, at present, that tamoxifen should be continued for 5 years. Tamoxifen is also used for treating patients with metastatic breast cancer if their disease has characteristics that would suggest hormonal responsiveness.[1,2] In addition, tamoxifen has undergone prospective evaluation as a potential breast cancer chemoprevention drug.[3] The study reported that tamoxifen decreased the incidence of breast cancer by approximately 50%. Nonetheless, this treatment has not been widely used to date in clinical practice for several reasons, including: (1) the vast majority of treated patients do not get benefit; (2) there is not yet any significant effect on patient survival; (3) the economic cost of the drug is high; (4) toxicities occur from this drug; and (5) the findings of this study have not been confirmed by two ongoing European trials (which underwent interim analyses).

The standard dose of tamoxifen is 20 mg. The long terminal half-life of the drug indicates that this can be given once daily. Tamoxifen is among the least toxic antineoplastic agents. Randomized, placebo-controlled trials have demonstrated that it does not cause any more gastrointestinal symptoms than placebo. The most prominent toxicity from tamoxifen is hot flashes, which affect approximately one-half of women. These hot flashes are of varying intensity and varying duration. Tamoxifen-induced hot flashes appear to increase over the first 3 months of therapy and then plateau.[1] They appear to be more prominent in women with a prior history of hot flashes or a prior history of using estrogen replacement. They can be ameliorated by the concurrent use of low doses of megestrol.[4,5]

The estrogenic properties of tamoxifen are responsible for both beneficial and deleterious side effects. The most prominent deleterious one, endometrial cancer, is increased approximately threefold in incidence over the general population. It has not yet been determined if progestins can prevent this toxicity of tamoxifen as they do with estrogen treatment. Beneficial estrogenic effects from tamoxifen include a decrease in total cholesterol,[6,7] a suggestion of decreased cardiovascular disease,[8] and a preservation of bone density in postmenopausal women.[9,10] In premenopausal women, tamoxifen appears to have a negative effect on bone density.[11] Although most patients do not complain of vaginal symptoms, a few complain of vaginal dryness, whereas others have increased vaginal secretions with a resultant vaginal discharge. An uncommon effect from tamoxifen is retinal toxicity. This has usually been associated with high drug doses or prolonged drug use.[12] Tamoxifen may predispose to thromboembolic phenomena, especially if used with concomitant chemotherapy. Depression has also been described, but this association with tamoxifen is not clear. Although liver cancers have been noted in laboratory animals, there is no clear-cut association between tamoxifen and liver cancers in humans.

Pharmacology

The chemical structure of tamoxifen is shown in Figure 20.3-1. It acts by blocking estrogen stimulation of breast cancer cells, inhibiting both translocation and nuclear binding of the estrogen receptor. This alters transcriptional and posttranscriptional events mediated by this receptor.[13,14] *In vivo*, tamoxifen activity is complicated by the potential actions of the metabolite *trans*-4-hydroxy-tamoxifen, which is a potent antiestrogen. Tamoxifen has agonistic, partial agonistic, or antagonistic effects depending on the species, target, or end points that have been assessed. Other effects that have been attributed to tamoxifen include inhibition of the conversion of estrone sul-

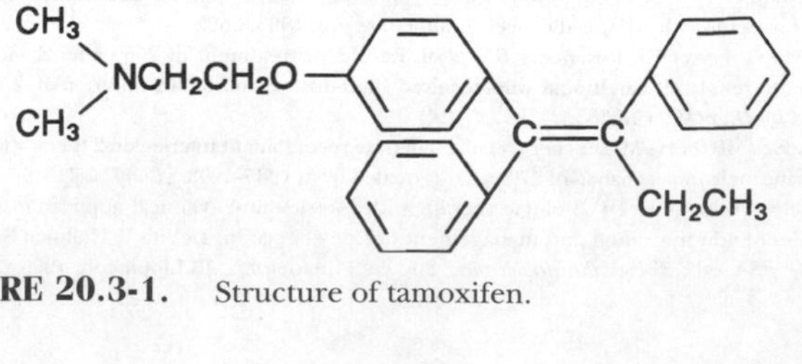

FIGURE 20.3-1. Structure of tamoxifen.

fate to estradiol,[15] inhibition of protein kinase C,[16] and reversal of multidrug resistance.[17,18]

Resistance to tamoxifen develops with resultant recurrence or progression of metastatic breast cancer.[19] Several mechanisms for this resistance have been proposed.[20,21] At each step of the signal transduction pathway with which tamoxifen interferes, there is potential for an alteration in response. Tamoxifen binds to the estrogen receptor, and subsequent translocation of this complex to the nucleus and binding to the estrogen response element occur. This binding prevents transcriptional activation of estrogen-responsive genes. Decreased tamoxifen metabolism to the potent antiestrogen *trans*-4-hydroxy-tamoxifen and increased metabolism to estrogenic compounds such as metabolite E have been proposed as possible mechanisms of resistance.[22–24] In some cases resistance occurs after loss of estrogen receptor-positive cells.[25,26] Although estrogen receptor mutation has been suggested as a mechanism of resistance, two groups have found little evidence for such changes in the estrogen receptor.[27,28] Phosphorylation of the estrogen receptor can mediate the hormone binding, DNA binding, and ultimately transcriptional activation. Alterations in this phosphorylation mediated by changes in protein kinase A and C could lead to resistance. Finally, modifications of the estrogen-response element such as sequence alteration or element duplication may lead to binding of the tamoxifen-estrogen receptor complex with increased transcription of the estrogen-response genes. At present, the primary mechanisms of tamoxifen action remain unknown, and further studies are needed.

The carcinogenic potential of tamoxifen has been recognized in rat studies[29–31] and in humans.[32] Although the mechanism of these carcinogenic effects is not understood, it has been proposed that generation of reactive intermediates that bind covalently to macromolecules underlies the process. Such reactive intermediates have been demonstrated *in vitro*.[33–35] In addition, induction of covalent DNA adducts in rat livers treated with tamoxifen has been reported.[36] Both constitutive and inducible cytochrome P-450 enzymes have been implicated in the formation of metabolites with tamoxifen,[37,38] and the flavine-containing monooxygenase has been implicated in the formation of the N-oxide of tamoxifen. Reactive intermediates from such metabolic steps are being evaluated for their carcinogenic potential *in vitro* and *in vivo*.

The pharmacokinetics of tamoxifen have not been fully elucidated despite clinical use of the drug for more than 20 years. The oral bioavailability is not known. Results from animal studies suggest that the drug is well absorbed.[39] Oral administration of [^{14}C]tamoxifen results in only 30% of radioactive material detectable in feces and approximately 11% in urine.[40] Whereas oral absorption may be good, first-pass metabolism may significantly alter exposure *in vivo*. The metabolic pathway of tamoxifen outlined in Figure 20.3-2 is dependent on the cytochrome P-450 3A subfamily-mediated demethylation and hydroxylation (possibly by an as yet undetermined cytochrome P-450 isoenzyme) followed by glucuronidation and biliary excretion. 4-Hydroxy-tamoxifen, which exists as two stereoisomers, is a potent antiestrogen[41] as the *trans*-isomer, but is much less potent as the *cis*-isomer.[42,43] The predominant species in serum are N-desmethyl-tamoxifen and N-desdimethyl-tamoxifen whereas 4-hydroxy-tamoxifen and 4-hydroxy-N-desmethyl-tamoxifen and metabolite Y, which are more hydrophilic, are found in lower concentrations. Metabolism affects the actions of tamoxifen

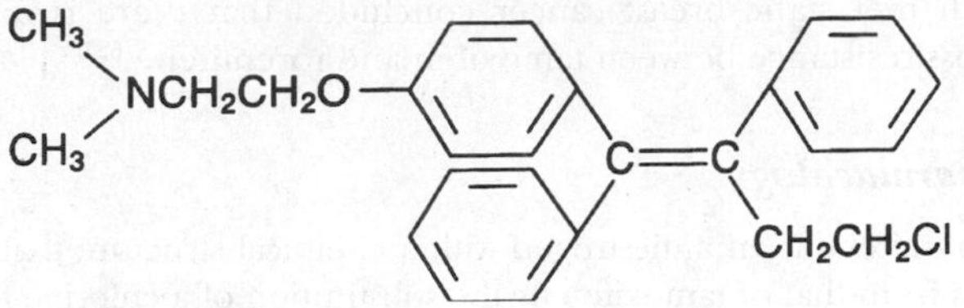

FIGURE 20.3-2. Tamoxifen metabolism.

because the hydroxylated metabolites have higher affinity for the estrogen receptor than the parent compound.[44] Tamoxifen is 98% bound to human serum albumin.[45,46] α_1-acid glycoprotein binding by tamoxifen may have an impact on its clinical activity because the presence of α_1-acid glycoprotein in tissue cultures abolishes the inhibitory effect of tamoxifen and toremifene on P glycoprotein.[17]

Peak plasma levels of tamoxifen (C_{max}) are seen 3 to 7 hours after oral administration. Assuming an oral bioavailability of 30%, the volume of distribution has been calculated to be 20 L/kg, and plasma clearance ranges from 1.2 to 5.1 L/h.[60] The terminal half-life of tamoxifen has been reported to range between 4 and 11 days.[47,48] The elimination half-life of tamoxifen increases with successive doses.[47,49] This finding is consistent with tamoxifen inhibition of its own metabolism. The drug's distribution in tissues is extensive. Levels of the parent drug and metabolites have been reported to be higher in tissue than in plasma in animal studies.[50,51] Reports of tamoxifen concentrations 10- to 60-fold higher than plasma concentrations in liver, lung, brain, pancreas, skin, and bone have appeared.[52,53] Concentrations of tamoxifen in pleural, pericardial, and peritoneal effusions approach those in plasma, with effusion to serum ratios ranging between 0.2 and 1.0. These findings are consistent with the large calculated volume of distribution. Elevated levels of tamoxifen with biliary obstruction have been reported.[54]

Tamoxifen has been reported to interact with coumadin,[55–58] digitoxin, phenytoin,[59] and medroxyprogesterone.[58] Lien et al.[60] have reported that tamoxifen serum concentrations and those of metabolites Y, 4-hydroxy-tamoxifen, 4-hydrox-N-desmethyl-tamoxifen, N-desmethyl-tamoxifen, and N-desdimethyl-tamoxifen are markedly reduced after aminoglutethimide administration. The mean increase in tamoxifen clearance was 249% when administered with aminoglutethimide. Each of these clinical drug interactions is consistent with an effect at the level of cytochrome P-450 3A. Inasmuch as progestational agents, such as megestrol acetate, are cytochrome P-450 3A substrates, these agents may also alter tamoxifen metabolism and ultimately elimination. This indicates that administration of tamoxifen to individuals taking medication dependent on cytochrome P-450 3A metabolism may alter drug levels extensively, and careful consideration of this should be made when prescribing tamoxifen.

TOREMIFENE

Toremifene, an agent similar to tamoxifen, is thought to be a more pure antiestrogen. It has become available in the United States for the treatment of patients with metastatic breast cancer. A randomized comparison of toremifene and tamoxifen in metastatic breast cancer suggested that these two medications were equivalent.[61] Clinical trials in postmenopausal women with metastatic breast cancer concluded that there is major cross-resistance between tamoxifen and toremifene.[62,63]

Pharmacology

Toremifene is an antiestrogen with a chemical structure that differs from that of tamoxifen by the substitution of a chlorine for a hydrogen atom that is retained when toremifene undergoes metabolism.[64] Like tamoxifen, toremifene is metabolized by cytochrome P-450 3A.[65] Toremifene and its 4-hydroxylated metabolite both bind to the estrogen receptor.[66] Although the oral bioavailability has not been defined, toremifene's oral absorption appears to be good. The time to peak plasma concentrations after oral administration ranges from 1.5 to 6.0 hours,[67] with the terminal half-lives for toremifene and one metabolite, 4-hydroxy toremifene, being 5 to 6 days.[68,69] The apparent clearance is 5.1 L/h. The terminal half-life for the major metabolite, N-desmethyl-toremifene, is 21 days.[70] Time to reach plasma steady-state concentrations is 1 to 5 weeks. Plasma protein binding is more than 99%. As with tamoxifen, toremifene tissue distribution in rats has been studied and found to be extensive and in high concentrations. Consistent with this is the high apparent volume of distribution, 958 L. Seventy percent of the drug is excreted in feces as metabolites. Studies in patients with impaired liver function secondary to alcoholic cirrhosis and in patients on anticonvulsants known to induce cytochrome P-450 3A have been undertaken.[70] Those patients with hepatic dysfunction had decreased clearance of toremifene and N-desmethyl-toremifene, whereas those patients on anticonvulsants had an increased clearance. Interestingly, toremifene appears to be less carcinogenic than tamoxifen in preclinical models.[35,71,72]

RALOXIFENE

Raloxifene is an estrogen agonist and antagonist that was initially developed as an anti–breast cancer agent. Initial studies were not promising regarding this approach, but large placebo-controlled randomized studies have reported that this drug does retard osteoporosis in women at risk for such. These studies demonstrated an apparent reduction in breast cancer in treated women, leading to the development of a second-generation breast cancer chemoprevention trial in which it will be compared with tamoxifen in high-risk postmenopausal women. Although this drug is relatively well tolerated, it can produce hot flashes. A potential advantage for raloxifene over tamoxifen is that it does not appear to induce endometrial cancer.

Pharmacology

Raloxifene is partially estrogenic in bone[73] and lowers cholesterol.[74] It is antiestrogenic in mammary tissue[75,76] and uterine tissue.[77] The mechanism whereby raloxifene exerts tissue-selective effects is not clear. Several hypotheses have been proposed. Coactivators and corepressor proteins are involved in the transcription complex when estrogen receptor is bound. There may be differential distribution of these coactivators or corepressors, which are responsible for the changes in estrogenicity seen in tissue. The discovery of a second estrogen, estrogen receptor-β, with 55% homology between it and estrogen receptor-α raises the possibility that there is a differential expression of these two estrogen receptors in different tissue.[78] This presence of two forms of the receptor also raises the possibility that there are different downstream effectors when one or the other estrogen receptor is activated.[79,80]

The pharmacokinetics of raloxifene have been studied principally in postmenopausal women.[81–84] Pharmacokinetic parameters of raloxifene show considerable interindividual variation. Limited information is available on the pharmacokinetics of raloxifene in individuals with hepatic impairment, renal impairment, or both.

Raloxifene is rapidly absorbed from the gastrointestinal tract. Because raloxifene undergoes extensive first-pass glucuronidation, oral bioavailability of unchanged drug is low. While approximately 60% of an oral dose is absorbed, absolute bioavailability as unchanged raloxifene is only 2%. However, systemic availability of raloxifene may be greater than that indicated in bioavailability studies because circulating glucuronide conjugates are converted back to the parent drug in various tissues.

Following oral administration of a single 120- or 150-mg dose of raloxifene hydrochloride, peak plasma concentration of raloxifene and its glucuronide conjugates are achieved at 6 and 1 hours, respectively. Plasma concentrations of raloxifene's glucuronide conjugates exceed those of the parent drug, and the time to achieve maximum concentrations of the drug and glucuronide metabolites depends on the extent and rate of systemic interconversion and enterohepatic circulation. Following oral administration of radiolabeled raloxifene, less than 1% of total circulating radiolabeled material in plasma represents parent drug.

Area under the curve (AUC) for plasma concentration-time of raloxifene following a single dose is the same as the AUC following multiple doses of the drug. Increasing the dose of raloxifene hydrochloride over a range of 30 to 150 mg results in a slightly less than proportional increase in the AUC of raloxifene. Administration of raloxifene with a standardized high-fat meal increases the raloxifene peak plasma concentration by 28% and AUC by 16%, when compared with administration on an empty stomach, but does not result in clinically important changes in systemic exposure.

Results of a single-dose study in patients with cirrhosis of the liver (Child-Pugh class A) and total serum bilirubin concentrations of 0.6 to 2.0 mg/dL indicate that plasma raloxifene concentrations correlate with serum bilirubin concentrations and are 2.5 times higher in such individuals compared with individuals with normal hepatic function. In postmenopausal women receiving raloxifene in clinical trials, plasma concentrations of raloxifene and the glucuronide conjugates in those with renal impairment (i.e., estimated creatinine clearance values as low as 23 mL/min) were similar to values in women with normal renal function.

Distribution of raloxifene into body tissues and fluids has not been fully characterized. Raloxifene and raloxifene 4'-glucuronide have been detected in saliva following oral administration of radiolabeled drug. In studies in rats given radiolabeled raloxifene 6-glucuronide, the liver contained the highest concentration of radioactivity, followed by serum, lung, and kidney. While bone and the uterus contained relatively low concentrations of radiolabeled metabolite, 24% of the radioactivity in bone, 14% in the uterus, and 23% in the liver represented raloxifene. Results of this study indicate that the conversion of metabolite to parent drug occurs readily in a variety of tissues including the liver, lung, spleen, kidney, bone, and uterus. The apparent volume of distribution following oral administration of single doses of raloxifene hydrochloride, 30 to 150 mg, is 2348 L/kg, suggesting extensive tissue distribution. The volume of distribution is not dose dependent over a dosage range of 30 to 150 mg daily.

Raloxifene and its monoglucuronide conjugates are more than 95% bound to plasma proteins. Raloxifene binds to albumin and α_1-acid glycoprotein.

Raloxifene undergoes extensive first-pass metabolism to the glucuronide conjugates raloxifene 4'-glucurone, 6-glucuronide, and 6,4'-diglucuronide. Metabolism of raloxifene does not appear to be mediated by cytochrome P-450 enzymes, since metabolites other than glucuronide conjugates have not been identified.

The plasma elimination half-life of raloxifene at steady state averages 32.5 hours (range, 15.8 to 86.6 hours).

Raloxifene is excreted principally in feces as unabsorbed drug and via biliary elimination as glucuronide conjugates, which subsequently are metabolized by bacteria in the gastrointestinal tract to the parent drug. Following oral administration, less than 0.2% of a raloxifene dose is excreted as parent compound and less than 6% as glucuronide conjugates in urine.

MEDROXYPROGESTERONE AND MEGESTROL

Medroxyprogesterone and megestrol are 17-OH-progesterone derivatives differing in a double bond between C6 and C7 positions in megestrol. Megestrol has been most commonly used as a hormonal agent for patients with advanced breast cancer; usually at a total daily dose of 160 mg/d. It has also been used frequently for the treatment of hormonally responsive metastatic endometrial cancer, at a dosage of 320 mg/d. In addition, dosages of 160 mg/d are occasionally used as a hormonal therapy for prostate cancer.[85] Megestrol has also been extensively evaluated for the treatment of anorexia-cachexia related to cancer or acquired immunodeficiency syndrome.[86–89] Various dosages ranging from 160 to 1600 mg/d have been used. Prospective studies have demonstrated dose-response relationship with doses up to 800 mg/d.[90] Low dosages of megestrol (40 mg/d) have been shown to be an effective means of reducing hot flashes in women with breast cancer and in men who have undergone androgen ablation therapy.[5] Although megestrol historically had been commonly administered four times per day, the long terminal half-life supports that once per day dosing is reasonable.

Megestrol is a relatively well-tolerated medication, with its most prominent side effect being appetite stimulation and resultant weight gain. While this may be a beneficial effect in patients with anorexia-cachexia, it can be an important problem in patients with breast or endometrial cancers. Another side effect of megestrol acetate is the marked suppression of adrenal steroid production by suppression of the pituitary-adrenal axis.[91] While this appears to be an asymptomatic state in the majority of patients, reports suggest that this adrenal suppression can cause clinical problems in some patients.[92] This drug has been abruptly stopped for decades without recognizing untoward sequelae in patients, and it seems reasonable to continue this practice. Nonetheless, if Addisonian signs or symptoms develop after drug discontinuation, corticosteroids should be administered. Furthermore, if patients receiving megestrol have a significant infection, experience trauma, or undergo surgery, then corticosteroid coverage should be administered. There may be a slight increased incidence of thromboembolic phenomena in patients receiving megestrol alone.[90] This risk appears to be higher if megestrol is administered with concomitant cytotoxic therapy.[93] There are conflicting reports regarding megestrol causing edema.[94] If it does, it is generally minimal and easily handled with a mild diuretic. Megestrol may cause impotence in some men.[95] The incidence of this is controversial, although it is generally agreed that this is a reversible situation. Megestrol can cause menstrual irregularities, the most prominent of which is withdrawal menstrual bleeding within a few weeks of drug discontinuation.[5] Although nausea and vomiting have been attributed as a toxicity, there are good data to demonstrate that this drug has antiemetic properties.[86,89,93] In terms of magnitude, megestrol appears to decrease both nausea and vomiting in advanced-stage cancer patients by approximately two-thirds.

Medroxyprogesterone has many of the same properties, clinical uses, and toxicities as megestrol acetate. It is not used commonly in the United States, but has been used more in Europe. Medroxyprogesterone is available in 2.5- and 10.0-mg tablets and in injectable formulations of 100 and 400 mg/L. Dosing for treatment of metastatic breast or prostate cancer is 400 mg/wk or more and for metastatic endometrial cancer, 1000 mg/wk or more. Smaller injectable or daily oral doses have been used for controlling hot flashes.

PHARMACOLOGY

The exact mechanism of antitumor effect of medroxyprogesterone and megestrol is unclear. These drugs have been reported to suppress adrenal steroid synthesis,[96] suppress estrogen receptor levels,[97] alter tumor hormone metabolism,[98] enhance steroid metabolism,[99] and directly kill tumor cells.[100] In addition to this, progestins may influence some growth factors,[101] suppress plasma estrone sulfate formation, and, at high concentrations, inhibit P glycoprotein.

The oral bioavailability of these progestational agents is unknown, although absorption appears to be poor for medroxyprogesterone relative to megestrol.

The terminal half-life for megestrol is approximately 14 hours[102,103] with a t_{max} of 2 to 5 hours after oral ingestion.[104] The AUC for a single megestrol dose of 160 mg is between 2.5- and 8-fold higher than that for single-dose medroxyprogesterone at 1000 mg. Of the radioactive dose of megestrol, 50% to 78% is found in the urine after oral administration, and 8% to 30% in the feces. Three glucuronide metabolites of megestrol have been identified in the urine: megestrol hydroxylated in the 2 position and the 6-methyl position, or both. They account for only 5% to 8% of the radioactive dose administered.

Metabolism and excretion of medroxyprogesterone have been incompletely characterized. In humans, 20% to 50% of a [3H] medroxyprogesterone dose is excreted in the urine and 5% to 10% in the stool following intravenous administration.[105–108] Metabolism of medroxyprogesterone occurs via hydroxylation, reduction, demethylation, and combinations of these different reactions.[109] The major urinary metabolite is a glucuronide. Less than 3% of the dose is excreted as unconjugated medroxyprogesterone in humans. Clearance of medroxyprogesterone has been reported to range between 27 and 70 L/h.[108] The initial volume of distribution is between 4 and 8 L in humans. The mean terminal half-life is 60 hours. The t_{max} for medroxyprogesterone occurs 2 to 5 hours after oral administration. Medroxyprogesterone appears to be concentrated in small intestine, colon, and adipose tissue in human autopsy studies.[110] Drug interactions of medroxyprogesterone have been reported with aminoglutethimide, which decreases plasma medroxyprogesterone levels.[111] Medroxyprogesterone may reduce the concentration of the N-desmethyl-tamoxifen metabolite concentration. Progestational agents also may increase plasma coumadin levels.[112] These reports are consistent with cytochrome P-450 3A being the site of interaction.

AROMATASE INHIBITORS

AMINOGLUTETHIMIDE

Aminoglutethimide was the first clinically used aromatase inhibitor. When it became available, it was used to cause a *medical adrenalectomy.* A 32% response rate in metastatic breast cancer[113] has been reported. Aminoglutethimide is infrequently used for treating metastatic breast cancer because there are other available hormonal treatments with less toxicity. Aminoglutethimide has also occasionally been used to try to reverse excess hormone production by adrenocortical cancers.[114]

For treatment of metastatic breast cancer before other aromatase inhibitors became available, aminoglutethimide commonly was started at a dose of 250 mg/d, increasing doses every couple of days to twice a day, then three times a day, and sometimes four times a day. Replacement hydrocortisone was often started at 100 mg/d for a week and then decreased to 40 mg/d. Aminoglutethimide doses less than 500 mg/d did not require corticosteroid replacement.[115] For suppression of hormone production by adrenocortical cancers, doses may be increased to 2 g/d.

Toxicities most frequently associated with aminoglutethimide are lethargy, orthostatic hypertension, nausea, vomiting, hypothyroidism, reversible agranulocytosis, and rash.[116,117] The rash is generally self-limited and usually disappears despite the continuation of aminoglutethimide. However, a severe rash leading to a Stevens-Johnson syndrome can occur.

Pharmacology

Aminoglutethimide (Fig. 20.3-3) suppresses postmenopausal estrogen synthesis by inhibiting the conversion of circulating androgens into estrogens. Androstenedione is peripherally converted to estrone by cytochrome P-450 aromatase. Estrone can be further converted to estradiol by the enzyme, hydroxysteroid dehydrogenase. Aromatase inhibitors block estrogen production in postmenopausal women or oophorectomized premenopausal women by 90% inhibition of peripheral conversion of androstenedione to estrone, whereas ovarian estrogen synthesis is maintained by gonadotropin release in the premenopausal women with intact ovarian function. Another biochemical effect of aminoglutethimide includes the inhibition of several enzymes in adrenal steroid synthesis, which may lead to mineralocorticoid deficiency.[118,119] Aminoglutethimide effect on adrenal steroid synthesis is complex.[120] Suppression of circulating plasma cortisol may occur,[121] but a compensatory increase in pituitary corticotropin (previously adrenocorticotropic hormone) levels may overcome this suppression. Because aminoglutethimide is a competitive inhibitor of aromatase, increased adrenal steroid synthesis may compete with aminoglutethimide at the level of the aromatase. Concomitant replacement doses of hydrocortisone addresses both potential effects on adrenal steroid synthesis. Aminoglutethimide is administered as a racemic mixture with different biologic effects.[121] The *d* form is the more potent inhibitor of adrenal steroid synthesis and aromatase activity. The pharmacokinetic characteristics of the separate enantiomers have not been characterized. Aminoglutethimide is absorbed well, with 80% to 98% of a radioactive dose recovered in the urine within 72 hours. Only 1% of the drug is excreted unchanged in the feces. Of the administered aminoglutethimide dose, 12% to 20% is excreted unmetabolized in the urine, and 3% to 7% is excreted as the N-acetyl-aminoglutethimide.[122] The C_{max} occurs 0.5 to 4.0 hours after oral administration in fasting patients. The clearance of the drug ranges from 1.5 to 6.0 L/h with a mean of 3 L/h. The volume of distribution is 66 to 70 L. Aminoglutethimide undergoes acetylation[123] and is cleared more rapidly in fast acetylators [half-life ($t_{1/2}$) = 12.6 hours] than in slow acetylators ($t_{1/2}$ = 19.5 hours). After 7 days of treatment, the half-life in slow acetylators decreased from 19.5 to 14.3 hours and in fast acetylators, from 12.6 to 8.6 hours. This was associated with an increased apparent systemic clearance of chronically administered aminoglutethimide and indicates autoinduction of this drug's metabolism.[122,124] Lønning and associates[125] have reported a decrease in volume of distribution on repeated dosing, which may also contribute to the decreased terminal half-life. Aminoglutethimide is approximately 25% bound to plasma proteins. Little is known about aminoglutethimide tissue distribution in humans. The erythrocyte to plasma concentration ratio is 0.83:1. Aminoglutethimide induces mixed function oxidases, enhancing the metabolism of coumadin, dexamethasone, theophylline, and digitoxin. Also, aminoglutethimide has been reported to decrease concentrations of progestational agents and tamoxifen.[60,99] These drug interactions implicate cytochrome P-450 3A in aminoglutethimide metabolism. The increased clearance of progestational agents and tamoxifen in the presence of aminoglutethimide makes the interpretation of studies that combine this aromatase inhibitor with tamoxifen or progestins difficult. Alterations in the blood levels of antiestrogen or progestational agents may have decreased their contribution to any therapeutic benefit.

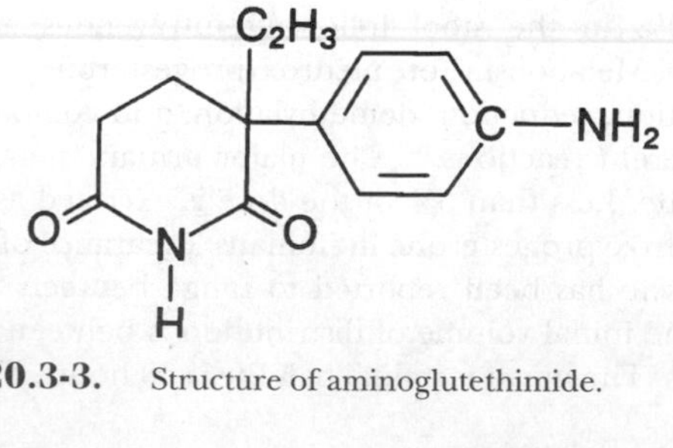

FIGURE 20.3-3. Structure of aminoglutethimide.

A series of second-generation aromatase inhibitors have been synthesized and many are undergoing clinical trials. These include rogletimide, formestane, fadrozole, letrozole, exemestane, vorozole, and anastrozole.[120,126,127]

LETROZOLE AND ANASTROZOLE

Letrozole and anastrozole are available in the United States for women with metastatic breast cancer. These second-generation aromatase inhibitors have basically replaced aminoglutethimide for breast cancer given their better toxicity profile. Headaches were the most common toxicity in a phase I trial.[128] It is not necessary to give replacement doses of corticosteroids as was previously done with aminoglutethimide. Letrozole and anastrozole appear to be similar drugs in clinical practice. Randomized trials have demonstrated that they are better hormonal agents for treating tamoxifen-resistant breast cancer than is megestrol acetate.

Letrozole is a nonsteroidal aromatase inhibitor with a high specificity for inhibition of estrogen production. Letrozole is 180 times more potent than aminoglutethimide as an inhibitor of aromatase *in vitro.* Aldosterone production *in vitro* is inhibited by concentrations 10,000 times higher than those required for inhibition of estrogen synthesis.[129,130] In a normal male volunteer study, letrozole was shown to decrease estradiol and serum estrone levels to 10% of baseline with a single 3-mg dose. In phase I studies,[131,132] letrozole caused a significant decline in plasma estrone and estradiol within 24 hours of a single oral dose of 0.1 mg. Following 2 weeks of treatment, the blood levels of estradiol, estrone, and estrone sulfate were suppressed 95% or more from baseline. This continued over the 12 weeks of therapy. There was no apparent alteration in plasma levels of cortisol and aldosterone with letrozole or following corticotropin stimulation.[131] In postmenopausal women with advanced breast cancer, the drug did not have any effect on follicle-stimulating hormone (FSH), luteinizing hormone (LH), thyrotropin (previously thyroid-stimulating hormone), cortisol, 17-α-hydroxyprogesterone, androstenedione, or aldosterone blood levels.[128,133,134]

Anastrozole is an aromatase inhibitor that is 200-fold more potent than aminoglutethimide.[135] No effect on the adrenal glands has been detected. In human studies, the t_{max} is 2 to 3 hours after oral ingestion.[136] Elimination is primarily via hepatic metabolism, with 85% excreted by that route and only 10% excreted unchanged in urine. The main circulating metabolite is triazole after cleavage of the two rings in anastrozole by N-dealkylation. Linear pharmacokinetics have been observed in the dose range of 1 to 20 mg and do not change with repeat dosing. The terminal half-life is approximately 50 hours and steady-state concentrations are achieved in approximately 10 days with once a day dosing and are three to four times higher than peak concentrations after a single dose. Plasma protein binding is approximately 40%.[137] Anastrozole 1 mg and 10 mg daily inhibits *in vivo* aromatization by 96.7% and 98.1%, respectively, and plasma estrone and estradiol levels were suppressed 86.5% and 83.5% regardless of dose.[138] Thus, 1 mg of anastrozole achieves near maximal aromatase inhibition and plasma estrogen suppression in breast cancer patients.

VOROZOLE

Vorozole is another aromatase inhibitor that is not currently available for clinical use, but is undergoing clinical trial evaluation.

Pharmacology

Vorozole, a racemic mixture of (+) and (−) enantiomers, is approximately 1000 times more effective than aminoglutethimide in the inhibiting human placental aromatase. The aromatase inhibitory activity is primarily due to the (+) enantiomer.[139] This drug does not appear to affect cytochrome P-450–dependent cholesterol synthesis, cholesterol side-chain cleavage, 7-α-hydroxylation of cholesterol, or 21-hydroxylase.[140] In rat ovarian, testicular, and adrenal cell cultures, vorozole affects progesterone, androgen, and glucocorticoid production at concentrations at least 1000 times greater than that required to inhibit aromatase.[139,141] In initial human studies, doses of 5 mg of the racemic mixture of vorozole resulted in 94.4% inhibition of peripheral aromatization, and, in healthy male volunteers, a single dose of the racemic mixture lowered plasma estradiol levels to the detection limits of the assay between 4 and 8 hours after drug administration. Johnston and associates[142] reported a similar inhibition of plasma estradiol, estrone, and estrone sulfate with no significant effect on aldosterone, testosterone, androstenedione, 17-α-hydroxyprogesterone, or thyroid-stimulating hormone. Vorozole is rapidly absorbed, with peak plasma concentrations obtained 1 hour after oral intake. Peak plasma concentrations and AUC of vorozole increase proportionately with the dose. Vorozole displays a biphasic disposition curve with a mean terminal half-life ranging from 4.7 to 7.5 hours. The total body clearance ranges from 6.1 to 11.8 L/h in a single dose study in normal healthy male volunteers.[143]

GONADOTROPIN-RELEASING HORMONE ANALOGUES

Gonadotropin-releasing hormone (GnRH) analogues result in a *medical orchiectomy* in men and are used as a means of providing androgen ablation for metastatic prostate cancer.[144] Because the initial agonist activity of GnRH analogues can cause a *tumor flare* from temporarily increased androgen levels, concomitant use of the antiandrogen, flutamide, has been used to prevent this effect. GnRH analogues can also cause tumor regressions in hormonally responsive breast cancers[145] and have recently received U.S. Food and Drug Administration approval for treatment of metastatic breast cancer in premenopausal women. Emerging data suggest that these drugs may be useful as adjuvant therapy of premenopausal women with resected breast cancer.[146]

The primary toxicities of GnRH analogues are secondary to the ablation of sex steroid concentrations and include hot flashes, sweating, and nausea.[147] These symptoms can be reversed with low doses of progestational analogues.[5]

GnRH analogues available for clinical use include goserelin[148,149] and leuprolide.[150] Both are available in depot intramuscular preparations to be given at monthly intervals. The recommended monthly dose of leuprolide is 7.5 mg and for goserelin is 3.6 mg. There are also longer acting depot preparations that only need to be administered every 3 months.

PHARMACOLOGY

Analogues of the decapeptide GnRH[149–151] have been synthesized by modifications of position 6 in which the L-glycine has been exchanged for a D-amino acid and the C-terminal amino acid has been either replaced by an ethylamide or substituted for a modified amino acid. These changes increase the affinity of the analogue for the GnRH receptor and decrease the susceptibility to enzymatic degradation. There is an amino acid structure of GnRH with the substitutions for leuprolide and goserelin. Initial administration of these compounds results in stimulation of gonadotropin release. However, prolonged administration has led to profound inhibition of the pituitary-gonadal axis.[152] Plasma estradiol and progesterone are consistently suppressed to postmenopausal or castrate levels after 2 to 4 weeks of treatment with goserelin or leuprolide.[153–155] These drugs are administered intramuscularly or subcutaneously in a parenteral sustained-release microcapsule preparation because parenteral administration of the parent drug otherwise is associated with rapid clearance. The GnRH analogues are metabolized in the liver, kidney, hypothalamus, and pituitary gland by neutral peptidase cleavage of the peptide bond between the tyrosine in the 5 position and the amino acid in position 6, and a postproline cleaving enzyme that cleaves the peptide bond between proline in the 9 position and the glycine-NH_2 in the 10 position. Substitutions at the glycine 6 position and modification of the C-terminal make these analogues more resistant to this enzymatic cleavage.

Leuprolide is approximately 80 to 100 times more potent than endogenous GnRH. It induces castrate levels of testosterone in men with prostate cancer within 3 to 4 weeks of drug administration after an initial sharp increase in LH and FSH. The mechanisms of action include pituitary desensitization following reduction in pituitary GnRH receptor-binding sites and possibly a direct antitumor effect in estrogen receptor-positive human breast cancer cells.[150] The depo form results in a dose rate of 210 μg of leuprolide per day. Peak concentrations of the depo form that are achieved at approximately 3 hours after drug administration have been reported to range between 13.1 and 54.5 μg/L. There appears to be a linear increase in the AUC for doses of 3.75, 7.5, and 15.0 mg in the depo form. The parenteral bioavailability of subcutaneously injected leuprolide is 94%. The volume of distribution ranges from 27.4 to 37.1 L. In human studies, leuprolide urinary excretion as a metabolite was the primary route of clearance.

Goserelin is approximately 100 times more potent than the naturally occurring GnRH. Like leuprolide, it causes stimulation of LH and FSH acutely, and with subsequent administration, GnRH receptor numbers decrease and the pituitary becomes desensitized with decreasing LH and FSH levels. Castrate levels of testosterone are achieved within 1 month. In women, goserelin inhibits ovarian androgen production, but serum levels of dihydroepiandrosterone sulfate, and to a lesser extent androstenedione, are preserved. *In vitro*, goserelin has demonstrated antitumor activity in estrogen-dependent MCF-7 human breast cancer cells and LNCaP-2 prostate cancer cells. The drug is released at a continuous mean rate of 120 μg/d in the depo form, with peak concentrations in the range of 2 to 3 μg/L achieved. The mean volume of distribution in six patients has been reported to be 13.7 L,[156] consistent with extracellular fluid volume. Goserelin is principally excreted in the urine, with a mean total body clearance of 8 L/h in patients with normal renal function. The total body clearance is reduced by approximately 75%, with renal dysfunction and the elimination half-life increased two- or threefold. However, dose adjustment for renal insufficiency does not appear to be necessary. The 5 to 10 hexapeptide and the 4 to 10 hexapeptide were detected in urine in animal studies.[157] The terminal half-life of goserelin is approximately 5 hours after subcutaneous injection. Protein binding is low, and no known drug interactions have been documented.

ANTIANDROGENS

FLUTAMIDE

The antiandrogen flutamide is used in men with metastatic prostate cancer either as initial therapy, combined with GnRH analogue administration, or when the metastatic prostate cancer is unresponsive despite androgen ablation therapy. The recommended dosage is 250 mg orally three times a day. In patients whose prostate cancer is growing despite flutamide use, stopping flutamide can clearly cause a flutamide-withdrawal response.

The most common toxicity seen with flutamide is diarrhea with or without abdominal discomfort. Gynecomastia, which can be tender, frequently occurs in men who are not receiving concomitant androgen ablation therapy.[158] Flutamide can rarely cause hepatotoxicity, a condition that is reversible if detected early, but can also be fatal.[159] There is no accepted clinically recommended testing schedule to screen for flutamide-induced hepatotoxicity other than being aware of this phenomenon and testing for liver function if hepatic symptoms develop.

Pharmacology

Flutamide is a pure antiandrogen with no intrinsic steroidal activity.[160] Flutamide's mechanism of action is as an androgen-receptor antagonist. This binding prevents the dihydrotestosterone binding and subsequent translocation of the androgen-receptor complex into the nuclei of cells. Because it is a pure antiandrogen, it acts only at the cellular level with no progestational effects. Administration by flutamide alone leads to increased LH and FSH production and a concomitant increase in plasma testosterone and estradiol levels. Plasma protein binding of flutamide ranges between 94% and 96%, and for 2-hydroxy-flutamide, its major metabolite ranges between 92% and 94%. When the drug is administered three times a day, steady-state levels are achieved by day 6. The steady-state C_{max} is 112.7 ng/L and occurs at approximately 1.13 hours after drug administration. The steady-state C_{max} is between three and five times higher than after the first dose. The elimination half-life at steady state is 7.8 hours. 2-Hydroxy-flutamide achieves concentrations 50 times higher than the parent drug at steady state and has a potency equal to or greater than that of flutamide.[160] The mean C_{max} averaged 1719 ng/mL at steady state and was achieved 1.9 hours after drug administration. The elimination half-life for the metabolite is 9.6 hours. The high plasma concentrations of 2-hydroxy-flutamide, as compared with flutamide, suggest that the therapeutic benefits of flutamide are mediated primarily through its active metabolite.[161]

BICALUTAMIDE (CASODEX)

Casodex is another nonsteroidal antiandrogen that has been approved by the U. S. Food and Drug Administration for use in the United States. The recommended dose is one 50-mg tablet per day. One randomized trial reported that Casodex compared favorably with flutamide in patients with advanced prostate cancer.[162] Casodex appears to be relatively well tolerated and is associated with a lower incidence of diarrhea than is flutamide.

Pharmacology

Casodex[163,164] has a binding affinity to the androgen receptor in the rat prostate that is four times greater than that of 2-hydroxyflutamide. *In vivo,* Casodex caused marked inhibition of growth of accessory sex organs in rats with a potency five to ten times greater than flutamide. Unlike flutamide, Casodex did not cause a significant increase in LH or testosterone in rats. Casodex bioavailability in humans has not been defined. The drug has a long plasma half-life of 5 to 7 days such that the drug may be administered on a weekly schedule. Pharmacokinetics of the drug showed a dose-dependent increase in mean peak plasma concentrations, and the AUC increased linearly with dose. The half-life of Casodex in humans was approximately 6 days, and the drug clearance was not saturable at plasma concentrations up to 1000 ng/mL. Daily dosing of the drug led to an approximately ten-fold accumulation after 12 weeks of administration. In contrast to rats, serum concentrations of testosterone and LH increased significantly from baseline at all dose levels tested in humans. Whereas serum FSH concentrations remained essentially unchanged, the median serum estradiol concentrations increased significantly.[165]

NILUTAMIDE

Nilutamide represents the third variation of antiandrogens available for use in patients with prostate cancer. Although it may be less expensive than the other antiandrogens, it has two unique toxicities, night blindness and pulmonary toxicity, which limit its utility.

Pharmacology

Nilutamide[166,167] is a newer nonsteroidal antiandrogen that has a high bioavailability with moderate plasma protein binding. It is extensively metabolized with less than 2% of parent drug administered isolated in urine over 5 days. Oxidation of a methyl group forms two stereoisomeric metabolites whose pharmacokinetics and pharmacodynamics are not characterized. Sixty-two percent of oral drug is eliminated in the urine as metabolites. The terminal half-life varies from 38 to 59 hours. Steady-state levels are achieved in 2 to 4 weeks with 150 mg given twice a day with approximately a twofold accumulation of drug over that time.

FLUOXYMESTERONE

Fluoxymesterone is an androgen that has been used in women with metastatic breast cancer who have hormonally responsive cancers and who have progressed on other hormonal therapies such as tamoxifen, an aromatase inhibitor, and megestrol acetate. The usual dose is 10 mg given twice daily. Although the overall response rate is low for fluoxymesterone used in this clinical situation,[168] there are some patients who have substantial antitumor responses lasting for months or even years.

Toxicities associated with fluoxymesterone are those that would be expected with an androgen: hirsutism, male-pattern baldness, voice lowering (hoarseness), acne, enhanced libido, and erythrocytosis. Fluoxymesterone can also cause elevated liver function test results in some patients and rarely has been associated with hepatic neoplasms.

PHARMACOLOGY

Fluoxymesterone is a chlorinated synthetic analogue of testosterone with potent androgenic and anabolic activity in humans. Limited pharmacologic information is available on this agent. Colburn,[169] using a radioimmunoassay, studied two subjects after a single oral administration of a 50-mg dose. Peak serum concentrations were achieved between 1 and 3 hours after administration, with the average peak concentrations being 335 ng/mL. By 5 hours after drug administration, serum levels had declined to approximately 50% of the peak concentration. Urinary excretion of a 10-mg dose can be detected for 24 hours; and at least 6-hydroxy, 4 ene, 3 β, and 11 hydroxy metabolites of fluoxymesterone have been detected.[170]

DIETHYLSTILBESTROL AND ESTRADIOL (ESTRACE)

Diethylstilbestrol (DES) used to be the primary hormonal therapy for postmenopausal metastatic breast cancer. Randomized comparative trials demonstrated that it had a similar response rate as tamoxifen.[171,172] However, based on these trials, DES use was supplanted by tamoxifen primarily because DES has more toxicity. DES is occasionally used in metastatic breast cancer patients who have hormonally sensitive cancers that have failed to respond to multiple other hormonal therapies. The usual dose in this situation is 15 mg/d (either as a single dose or as divided doses). DES was also used as androgen ablation therapy in men with metastatic prostate cancer.[173] Doses of approximately 3 mg/d result in testosterone levels that are seen in an anorchid state.

In women, DES may cause a number of toxicities. One of the most common is nausea and vomiting. It also can cause breast tenderness and a darkening of the nipple-areolar complex. DES increases the risk of thromboembolic phenomenon, and this may result in life-threatening complications. In men, DES results in increased thromboembolic events and mortality, thus limiting its use. It also causes painful gynecomastia. Although breast irradiation before DES administration appears to prevent this toxicity, it does not appear to help if it is given after the toxicity develops.

DES has not been clinically available in the United States in recent years but similar antitumor effects and toxicities are seen with Estrace, 1 mg orally three times a day.

PHARMACOLOGY

DES disposition studies in humans have been limited.[174] In animal studies, the oral absorption is approximately 20%. The drug undergoes hepatic metabolism and is excreted as dienestrol and hydroxydienestrol in urine.[175] The parent compound has been detected in feces. After administration of a radioactive dose of DES, approximately 40% of the drug was found in urine in the first 24 hours, with 87% of this being in the form of glucuronides. The peak plasma concentrations were achieved approximately 20 hours after ingestion and the terminal half-life for the radioactivity ranged between 2 and 3 days.

Estrace is a micronized form of estradiol. The pharmacology of estradiol has been extensively described in other texts.[176,177]

OCTREOTIDE

Octreotide is a somatostatin analogue that has revolutionized the therapy of carcinoid syndrome and other hormonal excess syndromes associated with some pancreatic islet cell cancers and acromegaly. Response rates are high and, on average, last for several months, sometimes for years. Occasionally, antitumor responses temporarily related to octreotide are seen with these tumors. Octreotide is being investigated as a potential therapy for other cancers such as breast or pancreas, but is not recommended for routine treatment of these tumors. Finally, octreotide appears to help to alleviate 5-fluorouracil–induced severe diarrhea in some patients.[178,179]

Octreotide can be administered intravenously or subcutaneously. Initial doses of 50 μg are given two to three times on the first day. The dose is titrated upward with a usual daily dose of 300 to 450 μg/d for most patients. At times, doses up to 1500 μg/d have been given. A depot preparation is available, allowing doses to be administered at monthly intervals. Octreotide is generally well tolerated overall. It appears to cause more toxicity in acromegalic patients, with such problems as bradycardia, diarrhea, hypoglycemia, hyperglycemia, hypothyroidism, and cholelithiasis.

Pharmacology

Octreotide is an 8 amino acid synthetic analogue of the 14 amino acid peptide somatostatin.[21] Octreotide has a similar high affinity for somatostatin receptors as does its parent, with a concentration that inhibits the receptor by 50% (IC_{50}) in the subnanomolar range. Octreotide inhibits insulin, glucagon, pancreatic polypeptide, gastric inhibitory polypeptide, and gastrin secretion. It has a much longer duration of action than the parent compound because of its greater resistance to enzymatic degradation. Its absorption following subcutaneous administration is rapid, and bioavailability is 100% after subcutaneous injection. Peak concentrations of 4 μg/L after a 100-μg dose occur within 20 to 30 minutes of subcutaneous injection and are 20% to 40% of the corresponding intravenous injection. Both peak concentration and AUC for octreotide increase linearly with dose. The total body clearance in healthy volunteers is 9.6 L/h. Hepatic metabolism of octreotide accounts for 30% to 40% of the drug's disposition, and 11% to 20% is excreted unchanged in the urine. The volume of distribution ranges between 18 and 30 L and the terminal half-life is reported to be between 72 and 98 minutes. Sixty-five percent of the drug is protein bound primarily to the lipoprotein fraction.[180,181] Because of the short half-life, classic octreotide is administered subcutaneously two or three times per day.[182] A slow-release form of octreotide, designed for once per month administration, is now evaluable.[183]

REFERENCES

1. Kiang DT, Kennedy BJ. Tamoxifen (antiestrogen) therapy in advanced breast cancer. *Ann Intern Med* 1977;87:687.
2. Mouridsen H, Palshof T, Patterson J, et al. Tamoxifen in advanced breast cancer. *Cancer Treat Rev* 1978;5:131.
3. Fisher B, Constantino JP, Wickerham DL, et al. Tamoxifen for prevention of breast cancer: report of the National Surgical Adjuvant Breast and Bowel Project P-1 study. *J Natl Cancer Inst* 1998;90:1371.
4. Love RR, Cameron L, Connell B. Symptoms associated with tamoxifen treatment in postmenopausal women. *Arch Intern Med* 1991;151:1842.
5. Loprinzi CL, Michalak JC, Quella SK, et al. Megestrol acetate for the prevention of hot flashes. *N Engl J Med* 1994;33:347.
6. Dewar JA, Horobin JM, Preece PE, et al. Long term effects of tamoxifen on blood lipid values in breast cancer. *BMJ* 1992;305:225.
7. Love RR, Weibe DA, Newcomb PA, et al. Effects of tamoxifen on cardiovascular risk factors in postmenopausal women. *Ann Intern Med* 1991;115:860.
8. McDonald CC, Stewart HJ for the Scottish Breast Cancer Committee. Fatal myocardial infarction in the Scottish adjuvant tamoxifen trial. *BMJ* 1991;303:435.
9. Love RR, Mazess RB, Tormey DC, et al. Bone mineral density in women with breast cancer treated with adjuvant tamoxifen for at least two years. *Breast Cancer Res Treat* 1988;12:297.
10. Ward RL, Morgan G, Dalley D, et al. Tamoxifen reduces bone turnover and prevents lumbar spine and proximal femoral bone loss in early postmenopausal women. *Bone Miner* 1993;22:87.
11. Powles TJ, Hickish TF, Kanis JA, Ashley S. Tamoxifen preserves bone mineral density in postmenopausal women but causes loss of bone density in premenopausal women. *Program/Proc Am Soc Clin Oncol* 1995;14:165(abst).
12. Kaiser-Kupfer MI, Lippman ME. Tamoxifen retinopathy. *Cancer Treat Rep* 1978;62:315.
13. Jaiyesimi IA, Buzdar AU, Decker DA, et al. Use of tamoxifen for breast cancer: twenty-eight years later. *J Clin Oncol* 1995;13:513.
14. Tonetti DA, Jordan VC. Possible mechanisms in the emergence of tamoxifen-resistant breast cancer. *Anticancer Drugs* 1995;6:498.
15. Gelly C, Pasqualini JR. Effect of tamoxifen and tamoxifen derivatives on the conversion of estronesulfate to estradiol in the R-27 cells, a tamoxifen-resistant line derived from MCF=n7 human breast cancer cells. *J Steroid Biochem* 1988;30:321.
16. Horgan K, Cooke E, Hallett MB, et al. Inhibition of protein kinase C mediated signal transduction by tamoxifen. *Biochem Pharmacol* 1986;35:4463.
17. Chatterjee M, Harris AL. Reversal of acquired resistance to adriamycin in CHO cells by tamoxifen and 4-hydroxy tamoxifen-role of drug interaction with alpha-1 acid glycoprotein. *Br J Cancer* 1990;62:712.
18. DeGregorio MW, Ford JM, Benz CC, et al. Toremifene: pharmacologic and pharmacokinetic basis of reversing multidrug resistance. *J Clin Oncol* 1989;7:1359.
19. Wiebe VJ, Osborne CK, Fuqua SA, et al. Tamoxifen resistance in breast cancer. *Crit Rev Oncol Hematol* 1993;14:173.
20. Osborne CK, Fuqua SA. Mechanisms of tamoxifen resistance. *Breast Cancer Res Treat* 1994;32:49.
21. Reid AD, Horobin JM, Newman EL, et al. Tamoxifen metabolism is altered by simultaneous administration of medroxyprogesterone acetate in breast cancer patients. *Breast Cancer Res Treat* 1992;22:153.
22. Osborne CK. Mechanisms for tamoxifen resistance in breast cancer: possible role of tamoxifen metabolism. *J Steroid Biochem Mol Biol* 1993;47:83.
23. Osborne CK, Jarman M, McCague R, et al. The importance of tamoxifen metabolism in tamoxifen-stimulated breast tumor growth. *Cancer Chemother Pharmacol* 1994;34:89.
24. Osborne CK. Tamoxifen metabolism as a mechanism for resistance. *Endocr Relat Cancer* 1995;2:53.
25. Encarnacion CA, Fuqua SA. Estrogen receptor variants in breast cancer. *Cancer Treat Res* 1994;71:97.
26. Encarnacion CA, Ciocca DR, McGuire WL, et al. Measurement of steroid hormone receptors in breast cancer patients on tamoxifen. *Breast Cancer Res Treat* 1993;26:237.
27. Watts CKW, Handel ML, King RJB. Oestrogen receptor gene structure and function in breast cancer. *J Steroid Biochem Mol Biol* 1992;41:529.
28. Karnik PS, Kulkarni S, Liu XP, et al. Estrogen receptor mutations in tamoxifen-resistant breast cancer. *Cancer Res* 1994;54:349.
29. Williams GM. Tamoxifen experimental carcinogenicity studies: implications for human effects. *Proc Soc Exp Biol Med* 1995;208:141.
30. Williams GM, Iatropoulos MJ, Djordjevic MV, et al. The triphenylethylene drug tamoxifen is a strong liver carcinogen in the rat. *Carcinogenesis* 1993;14:315.
31. Fendl KC, Zimniski SJ. Role of tamoxifen in the induction of hormone-independent rat mammary tumors. *Cancer Res* 1992;52:235.
32. Rutqvist LE, Johansson H, Signomklao T, et al. Adjuvant tamoxifen therapy for early stage breast cancer and second primary malignancies. Stockholm Breast Cancer Study Group. *J Natl Cancer Inst* 1995;87:645.
33. Mani C, Kupfer D. Cytochrome p-450-mediated activation and irreversible binding of the antiestrogen tamoxifen to proteins in rat and human liver: possible involvement of flavin-containing monooxygenases in tamoxifen activation. *Cancer Res* 1991;51:6052.
34. Mani C, Pearce R, Parkinson A, et al. Involvement of cytochrome P4503A in catalysis of tamoxifen activation and covalent binding to rat and human liver microsomes. *Carcinogenesis* 1994;15:2715.
35. Styles JA, Davies A, Lim CK, et al. Genotoxicity of tamoxifen, tamoxifen epoxide and toremifene in human lymphoblastoid cells containing human cytochrome P450s. *Carcinogenesis* 1994;15:5.
36. Han XL, Liehr JG. Induction of covalent DNA adducts in rodents by tamoxifen. *Cancer Res* 1992;52:1360.
37. Mani C, Gelboin HV, Park SS, et al. Metabolism of the antimammary cancer antiestrogenic agent tamoxifen. I. Cytochrome P-450-catalyzed N-demethylation and 4-hydroxylation. *Drug Metab Dispos* 1993;21:645.
38. Mani C, Hodgson E, Kupfer D. Metabolism of the antimammary cancer antiestrogenic agent tamoxifen. II. Flavin-containing monooxygenase-mediated N-oxidation. *Drug Metab Dispos* 1993;21:657.
39. Fromson JM, Pearson S, Bramah S. The metabolism of tamoxifen (I.C.I. 46474) part I: in laboratory animals. *Xenobiotica* 1973;3:693.
40. Fromson JM, Pearson S, Bramah S. The metabolism of tamoxifen (I.C.I. 46,474) part II: in female patients. *Xenobiotica* 1973;3:711.

41. Jordan VC, Collins MM, Rowsby L, et al. A monohydroxylated metabolite of tamoxifen with potent antiestrogenic activity. *J Endocrinol* 1977;75:305.
42. Robertson DW, Katzenellenbogen JA, Long DJ, et al. Tamoxifen antiestrogens: a comparison of the activity, pharmacokinetics, and metabolic activation of the cis and trans isomers of tamoxifen. *J Steroid Biochem* 1982;16:1.
43. Katzenellenbogen JA, Carlson KE, Katzenellenbogen BS. Facile geometric isomerization of phenolic non-steroidal estrogens and antiestrogens: limitations to the interpretation of experiments characterizing the activity of individual isomers. *J Steroid Biochem* 1985;22:589.
44. Robertson DW, Katzenellenbogen JA, Long DJ, et al. Tamoxifen antiestrogens: a comparison of the activity, pharmacokinetics, and metabolic activation of the cis and trans isomers of tamoxifen. *J Steroid Biochem* 1982;16:1.
45. Lien EA, Solheim E, Lea OA, et al. Distribution of 4-hydroxy-N-desmethyltamoxifen and other tamoxifen metabolites in human biological fluids during tamoxifen treatment. *Cancer Res* 1989;49:2175.
46. Shah IG, Parsons DL. Human albumin binding of tamoxifen in the presence of a perfluorochemical erythrocyte substitute. *J Pharm Pharmacol* 1991;43:790.
47. Adam HK, Patterson JS, Kemp JV. Studies on the metabolism and pharmacokinetics of tamoxifen in normal volunteers. *Cancer Treat Rep* 1980;64:761.
48. Patterson JS, Settatree RS, Adam HK, et al. Serum concentrations of tamoxifen and major metabolite during long term Nolvadex therapy, correlated with clinical response. In: Mouridsen HT, Palshof T, eds. *Breast cancer; experimental and clinical aspects.* Oxford: Permagon Press, 1980:89.
49. Camaggi CM, Strocchi E, Pannuti F. Tamoxifen pharmacokinetics in advanced breast cancer patients. In: Pannuti F, ed. *Anti-oestrogens in oncology, past: present and prospects.* Amsterdam: Excerpta Medica, 1985:90.
50. Lien EA, Solheim E, Ueland PM. Distribution of tamoxifen and its metabolites in rat and human tissues during steady-state treatment. *Cancer Res* 1991;51:4837.
51. Lien EA, Wester K, Lønning PE, Solheim E, Ueland PM. Distribution of tamoxifen and metabolites into brain tissue and brain metastases in breast cancer patients. *Br J Cancer* 1991;3:641.
52. Daniel CP, Gaskell SJ, Bishop H, et al. Determination of tamoxifen and biologically active metabolites in human breast tumours and plasma. *Eur J Cancer Clin Oncol* 1981;17:1183.
53. Robinson SP, Langan-Fahey SM, Johnson DA, et al. Metabolites, pharmacodynamics, and pharmacokinetics of tamoxifen in rats and mice compared to the breast cancer patient. *Drug Metab Dispos* 1991;19:36.
54. DeGregorio MW, Wiebe VJ, Venook AP, et al. Elevated plasma tamoxifen levels in a patient with liver obstruction [Letter]. *Cancer Chemother Pharmacol* 1989;23:194.
55. Lodwick R, McConkey B, Brown AM, et al. Life threatening interactions between tamoxifen and warfarin. *BMJ* 1987;295:1141.
56. Ritchie LD, Grant SMT. Tamoxifen-warfarin interaction: the Aberdeen hospitals drug file. *BMJ* 1989;298:1253.
57. Tenni P, Lalich DL, Byrne MJ. Life threatening interaction between tamoxifen and warfarin. *BMJ* 1989;298:93.
58. Camaggi CM, Strocchi E, Canova N, et al. Medroxyprogesterone acetate (map) and tamoxifen (tmx) plasma levels after simultaneous treatment with 'low' tmx and 'high' map doses. *Cancer Chemother Pharmacol* 1985;14:229.
59. Rabinowicz AL, Hinton DR, Dyck P, et al. High-dose tamoxifen in treatment of brain tumors—interaction with antiepileptic drugs. *Epilepsia* 1995;36:513.
60. Lien EA, Anker G, Lønning PE, et al. Decreased serum concentrations of tamoxifen and its metabolites induced by aminoglutethimide. *Cancer Res* 1990;50:5851.
61. Hayes DF, Vanzyl JA, Hacking A, et al. Randomized comparison of tamoxifen and two separate doses of toremifene in postmenopausal patients with metastatic breast cancer. *J Clin Oncol* 1995;13:2556.
62. Stenbygaard LE, Herrstedt J, Thomsen JF, et al. Toremifene and tamoxifen in advanced breast cancer—a double-blind cross-over trial. *Breast Cancer Res Treat* 1993;25:67.
63. Vogel CL, Shemano I, Schoenfelder J, et al. Multicenter phase II efficacy trial of toremifene in tamoxifen-refractory patients with advanced breast cancer. *J Clin Oncol* 1993;11:345.
64. Kangas L. Review of the pharmacological properties of toremifene. *J Steroid Biochem* 1990;36:191.
65. Berthou F, Dreano Y, Belloc C, et al. Involvement of cytochrome P450 3A enzyme family in the major metabolic pathways of toremifene in human liver microsomes. *Biochem Pharmacol* 1994;47:1883.
66. Simberg NH, Murai JT, Siiteri PK. In vitro and in vivo binding of toremifene and its metabolites in rat uterus. *J Steroid Biochem* 1990;36:197.
67. Kohler PC, Hamm JT, Wiebe VJ, et al. Phase I study of the tolerance and pharmacokinetics of toremifene in patients with cancer. *Breast Cancer Res Treat* 1990;16(Suppl):19.
68. Wiebe VJ, Benz CC, Shemano I, et al. Pharmacokinetics of toremifene and its metabolites in patients with advanced breast cancer. *Cancer Chemother Pharmacol* 1990;25:247.
69. Tominaga T, Abe O, Izuo M, et al. A phase I study of toremifene. *Breast Cancer Res Treat* 1990;16(Suppl):27.
70. Anttila M, Laakso S, Nylanden P, et al. Pharmacokinetics of the novel antiestrogenic agent toremifene in subjects with altered liver and kidney function. *Clin Pharmacol Ther* 1995;57:628.
71. Montandon F, Williams GM. Comparison of DNA reactivity of the polyphenylethylene hormonal agents diethylstilbestrol, tamoxifen and toremifene in rat and hamster liver. *Arch Toxicol* 1994;68:272.
72. Hard GC, Iatropoulos MJ, Jordan K, et al. Major difference in the hepatocarcinogenicity and DNA adduct forming ability between toremifene and tamoxifen in female Crl: CD(BR) rats. *Cancer Res* 1993;53:4534.
73. Delmas PD, Bjarnason NH, Mitlak BH, et al. Effects of raloxifene on bone mineral density, serum cholesterol concentrations, and uterine endometrium in postmenopausal women. *N Engl J Med* 1997;337:1641.
74. Draper MW, Flowers DE, Huster WJ, et al. A controlled trial of raloxifene (LY139481) HCl: impact on bone turnover and serum lipid profile in healthy postmenopausal women. *J Bone Miner Res* 1996;11:835.
75. Gottardis MM, Jordan VC. Antitumor actions of keoxifene and tamoxifen in the N-nitrosomethylurea-induced rat mammary carcinoma model. *Cancer Res* 1987;47:4020.
76. Anzano MA, Peer CW, Smith JM, et al. Chemoprevention of mammary carcinogenesis in the rat: combined use of raloxifene and 9-cis-retinoic acid. *J Natl Cancer Inst* 1996;88:123.
77. Black LJ, Jones CD, Falcone JF. Antagonism of estrogen action with a new benzothiophene derived antiestrogen. *Life Sci* 1983;32:1031.
78. Kuiper GG, Carlsson B, Grandien K, et al. Comparison of the ligand binding specificity and transcript tissue distribution of estrogen receptors alpha and beta. *Endocrinology* 1997;138:863.
79. Paech K, Webb P, Kuiper GG, et al. Differential ligand activation of estrogen receptors ER-alpha and ER-beta at AP1 sites. *Science* 1997;277:1508.
80. Webb P, Lopez GN, Uht RM, et al. Tamoxifen activation of the estrogen receptor/AP-1 pathway: potential origin for the cell-specific estrogen-like effects of antiestrogens. *Mol Endocrinol* 1995;9:443.
81. Forgue ST, Rudy AC, Knadler MP, et al. Rasloxifene pharmacokinetics in healthy postmenopausal women. *Pharmaceut Res* 1996;13:S429.
82. Ni L, Allerheiligen SRB, Basson R, et al. Pharmacokinetics of raloxifene in men and postmenopausal women volunteers. *Pharmaceut Res* 1996;13:S430.
83. Allerheilgen S, Geiser J, Knadler M, et al. Rasloxifene (RAL) pharmacokinetics and the associated endocrine effects in premenopausal women treated during the follicular, ovulatory and luteal phases of the menstrual cycle. *Pharmaceut Res* 1996;13:S430.
84. Hochner-Celnikier D. Pharmacokinetics of raloxifene and its clinical application. *Eur J Obstet Gynecol Reprod Biol* 1999;85:23.
85. Bonomi P, Pessis D, Bunting N, et al. Megestrol acetate used as primary hormonal therapy in stage D prostatic cancer. *Semin Oncol* 1985;12:36.
86. Loprinzi CL, Ellison NM, Schaid DJ, et al. Controlled trial of megestrol acetate for the treatment of cancer anorexia and cachexia. *J Natl Cancer Inst* 1990;82:1127.
87. Bruera E, Macmillan K, Kuehn N, et al. A controlled trial of megestrol acetate on appetite, caloric intake, nutritional status, and other symptoms in patients with advanced cancer. *Cancer* 1990;66:1279.
88. Feliu J, Gonzalez-Baron M, Berrocal A, et al. Usefulness of megestrol acetate in cancer cachexia and anorexia. *Am J Clin Oncol* 1992;15:436.
89. Tchekmedyian NS, Hickman M, Siau J, et al. Megestrol acetate in cancer anorexia and weight loss. *Cancer* 1992;69:1268.
90. Loprinzi CL, Michalak JC, Schaid DJ, et al. Phase III evaluation of four doses of megestrol acetate as therapy for patients with cancer anorexia and/or cachexia. *J Clin Oncol* 1993;11:762.
91. Loprinzi CL, Jensen MD, Jiang NS, et al. Effect of megestrol acetate on the human pituitary-adrenal axis. *Mayo Clin Proc* 1992;67:1160.
92. Leinung MC, Liporace R, Miller CH. Induction of adrenal suppression by megestrol acetate in patients with AIDS. *Ann Intern Med* 1995;122:843.
93. Rowland KM Jr, Loprinzi CL, Shaw EG, et al. Randomized double-blind placebo controlled trial of cisplatin and etoposide plus megestrol acetate/placebo in extensive stage small cell lung cancer: a North Central Cancer Treatment Group Study. *J Clin Oncol* 1995;14:135.
94. Loprinzi CL, Johnson P, Jensen M. Megestrol acetate for anorexia and cachexia. *Oncology* 1992;49(Suppl 2):46.
95. Von Roenn JH, Armstrong D, Kotler DP, et al. Megestrol acetate in patients with AIDS-related cachexia. *Ann Intern Med* 1994;121:393.
96. Alexieva-Figusch J, Blankenstein MA, Hop WC, et al. Treatment of metastatic breast cancer patients with different dosages of megestrol acetate; dose relations, metabolic and endocrine effects. *Eur J Cancer Clin Oncol* 1984;20:33.
97. Tseng L, Gurpide E. Effect of progestins on estradiol receptor levels in human endometrium. *J Clin Endocrinol Metab* 1975;41:402.
98. Gurpide E, Tseng L, Gusberg SB. Estrogen metabolism in normal and neoplastic endometrium. *Am J Obstet Gynecol* 1977;129:809.
99. Gordon GG, Altman K, Southren AL, et al. Human hepatic testosterone A-ring reductase activity: effect of medroxyprogesterone acetate. *J Clin Endocrinol Metab* 1971;32:457.
100. Allegra JC, Kiefer SM. Mechanism of action of progestational agents. *Semin Oncol* 1985;12:3.
101. Ewing TM, Murphy LJ, Ng ML, et al. Regulation of epidermal growth factor receptor by progestins and glucocorticoids in human breast cancer cell lines. *Int J Cancer* 1989;44:744.
102. Martin F, Adlercreutz H. Aspects of megestrol acetate and medroxyprogesterone acetate metabolism. In: Garattini S, Berendes HW, eds. *Pharmacology of steroid contraceptive drugs.* New York: Raven Press, 1977:99.
103. Adlercreutz H, Eriksen PB, Christensen MS. Plasma concentration of megestrol acetate and medroxyprogesterone acetate after single oral administration to healthy subjects. *J Pharm Biomed Anal* 1983;1:153.
104. Gaver RC, Pittman KA, Reilly CM, et al. Bioequivalence evaluation of new megestrol acetate formulation in humans. *Semin Oncol* 1985;12:17.
105. Fotherby K, Kamyab S, Littleton P, et al. Metabolism of synthetic progestational compounds in humans. *J Reprod Fertil* 1968;5(Suppl):51.
106. Fukushima DK, Levin J, Liang JS, et al. Isolation and partial synthesis of a new metabolite of medroxyprogesterone acetate. *Steroids* 1979;34:57.
107. Slaunwhite WR, Sandberg AA. Disposition of radioactive 17α-hydroxyprogesterone, 6α-methyl-prednisolone in human subjects. *J Clin Endocrinol Metab* 1961;21:753.
108. Utaaker E, Lundgren S, Kvinnsland S, et al. Pharmacokinetics and metabolism of medroxyprogesterone acetate in patients with advanced breast cancer. *J Steroid Biochem* 1988;31:437.
109. Sturm G, Haberlein H, Bauer T, et al. Mass spectrometric and high-performance liquid chromatographic studies of medroxyprogesterone acetate metabolites in human plasma. *J Chromatogr* 1991;562:351.

110. Pannuti F, Camaggi CM, Strocchi E, et al. Medroxyprogesterone acetate pharmacokinetics. In: Pelligrini A, et al., eds. *Role of medroxyprogesterone in endocrine related tumors.* New York: Raven Press, 1984:43.
111. Lundgren S, Lønning PE, Aakvaag A, et al. Influence of aminoglutethimide on the metabolism of medroxyprogesterone acetate and megestrol acetate in post-menopausal patients with advanced breast cancer. *Cancer Chemother Pharmacol* 1990;27:101.
112. Lundgren S, Kvinnsland S, Utaaker E, et al. Effect of oral high-dose progestins on the disposition of antipyrine, digitoxin, and warfarin in patients with advanced breast cancer. *Cancer Chemother Pharmacol* 1986;18:270.
113. Santen RJ. Suppression of estrogens with aminoglutethimide and hydrocortisone (medical adrenalectomy) as treatment of advanced breast carcinoma: a review. *Breast Cancer Res Treat* 1981;1:183.
114. Schteingart DE, Cash R, Coon JW. Aminoglutethimide and metastatic adrenal cancer. *JAMA* 1966;198:1007.
115. Hoffken K, Kempf H, Miller AA, et al. *Cancer Treat Rep* 1986;70:1153.
116. Santen RJ, Worgul TJ, Samojlik E, et al. A randomized trial comparing surgical adrenalectomy with aminoglutethimide plus hydrocortisone in women with advanced breast cancer. *N Engl J Med* 1981;305:545.
117. Lawrence B, Santen RJ, Lipton A, et al. Pancytopenia induced by aminoglutethimide in the treatment of breast cancer. *Cancer Treat Rep* 1978;62:1581.
118. Lønning PE, Kvinnsland S. Mechanisms of action of aminoglutethimide as endocrine therapy of breast cancer. *Drugs* 1988;35:685.
119. Santen RJ, Worgul TJ, Lipton A, et al. Aminoglutethimide as treatment of postmenopausal women with advanced breast carcinoma. *Ann Intern Med* 1982;96:94.
120. Goss PE, Gwyn KM. Current perspectives on aromatase inhibitors in breast cancer. *J Clin Oncol* 1994;12:2460.
121. Graves PE, Salhanick HA. Stereoselective inhibition of aromatase by enantiomers of aminoglutethimide. *Endocrinology* 1979;105:52.
122. Adam AM, Rogers HJ, Amiel SA, et al. The effect of acetylator phenotype on the disposition of aminoglutethimide. *Br J Clin Pharmacol* 1984;18:495.
123. Coombes RC, Foster AB, Harland SJ, et al. Polymorphically acetylated aminoglutethimide in humans. *Br J Cancer* 1982;46:340.
124. Murray FT, Santner S, Samojlik E, et al. Serum aminoglutethimide levels studies of serum half-life, clearance, and patient compliance. *J Clin Pharmacol* 1979;19:704.
125. Lønning PE, Schanche JS, Kvinnsland S, et al. Single-dose and steady-state pharmacokinetics of aminoglutethimide. *Clin Pharmacokinet* 1985;10:353.
126. Coombes RC, Jarman M, Dowsett M, et al. New endocrine agents for the treatment of breast cancer. *Recent Results Cancer Res* 1993;127:267.
127. Dowsett M, Smithers D, Moore J, et al. Endocrine changes with the aromatase inhibitor fadrozole hydrochloride in breast cancer. *Eur J Cancer* 1994;30A:1453.
128. Iveson TJ, Smith IE, Ahern J, et al. Phase I study of the oral nonsteroidal aromatase inhibitor CGS 20267, in post menopausal patients with advanced breast cancer. *Cancer Res* 1993;53:266.
129. Bhatnagar AS, Hausler A, Schieweck K, et al. Highly selective inhibition of estrogen biosynthesis by cgs 20267, a new nonsteroidal aromatase inhibitor. *J Steroid Biochem Mol Biol* 1990;37:1021.
130. Bhatnagar AS, Hausler A, Schieweck K. Inhibition of aromatase in vitro and in vivo by aromatase inhibitors. *J Enzym Inhib* 1990;4:179.
131. Demers LM. Effects of Fadrozole (CGS 16949A) and Letrozole (CGS 20267) on the inhibition of aromatase activity in breast cancer patients. *Breast Cancer Res Treat* 1994;30:95.
132. Lipton A, Demers LM, Harvey HA, et al. Letrozole (CGS 20267). A phase I study of a new potent oral aromatase inhibitor of breast cancer. *Cancer* 1995;75:2132.
133. Bhatnagar AS, Hausler A, Trunet P, et al. *Inhibitors of estrogen biosynthesis: CGS 16949 and CGS 20267, preclinical and clinical endocrine effects, in aromatase inhibition: past, present, and future, symposium.* 15th International Cancer Congress, Hamburg, Germany, 1990:13.
134. Trunet P, Muller PH, Bhatnagar A, et al. Phase I study in healthy male volunteers with the non-steroidal aromatase inhibitor GCS 20267. *Eur J Cancer* 1990;26:173.
135. Dukes M, Edwards PN, Large M, et al. The preclinical pharmacology of "Arimidex" (anastrozole; ZD1033)—a potent, selective aromatase inhibitor. *J Steroid Biochem Molec Biol* 1996;58:439.
136. Yates RA, Dowsett M, Fisher GV, et al. Arimidex (ZD1033): a selective, potent inhibitor of aromatase in postmenopausal female volunteers. *Br J Cancer* 1996;73:543.
137. Lønning PE, Geisler J, Dowsett M. Pharmacological and clinical profile of anastrozole. *Breast Cancer Res Treat* 1998;49(Suppl 1):S53.
138. Geisler J, King N, Dowsett M, et al. Influence of anastrozole (Arimidex), a selective, non-steroidal aromatase inhibitor, on in vivo aromatization and plasma oestrogen levels in postmenopausal women with breast cancer. *Br J Cancer* 1996;74:1286.
139. Wouters W, De Coster R, Beerens D, et al. Potency and selectivity of the aromatase inhibitor R 716713. A study in human ovarian, adipose, stromal, testicular and adrenal cells. *J Steroid Biochem* 1990;36:57.
140. Vanden Bossche H, Willemsens G, Roels I, et al. R 76713 and enantiomers: selective, non-steroidal inhibitors of the cytochrome P450-dependent oestrogen synthesis. *Biochem Pharmacol* 1990;40:1707.
141. Wouters W, Van Ginckel R, Krekels M, et al. Pharmacology of vorozole. *J Steroid Biochem Mol Biol* 1993;44:617.
142. Johnston SR, Smith IE, Doody D, et al. Clinical and endocrine effects of the oral aromatase inhibitor vorozole in postmenopausal patients with advanced breast cancer. *Cancer Res* 1994;54:5875.
143. Wouters W, Snoeck E, De Coster R. Vorozole, a specific non-steroidal aromatase inhibitor [Review]. *Breast Cancer Res Treat* 1994;30:89.
144. Ahmann FR, Citrin DL, deHaan HA, et al. Zoladex: a sustained-release, monthly luteinizing hormone-releasing hormone analogue for the treatment of advanced prostate cancer. *J Clin Oncol* 1987;5:912.
145. Corbin A. From contraception to cancer: a review of the therapeutic applications of LHRH analogues as antitumor agents. *Yale J Biol Med* 1982;55:27.
146. Davidson N, O'Neill A, Vukov A, et al. Effect of chemohormonal therapy in premenopausal, node (+), receptor (+) breast cancer: an Eastern Cooperative Oncology Group phase III intergroup trial (E5188, INT-0101). *Proc Am Soc Clin Oncol* 1999;18:67a.
147. Harvey HA, Lipton A, Max DT, et al. Medical castration produced by the GnRh analogue Leuprolide to treat metastatic breast cancer. *J Clin Oncol* 1985;3:1068.
148. Vogelzang NJ, Chodak GW, Soloway MS, et al. Goserelin versus orchiectomy in the treatment of advanced prostate cancer: final results of a randomized trial. Zoladex Prostate Study Group. *Urology* 1995;46:220.
149. Brogden RN, Faulds D. Goserelin—a review of its pharmacodynamic and pharmacokinetic properties and therapeutic efficacy in prostate cancer. *Drugs Aging* 1995;6:324.
150. Plosker GL, Brogden RN. Leuprorelin: a review of its pharmacology and therapeutic use in prostatic cancer, endometriosis and other sex hormone-related disorders. *Drugs* 1994;48:930.
151. Brogden RN, Buckley MM, Ward A. Buserelin: a review of its pharmacodynamic and pharmacokinetic properties, and clinical profile. *Drugs* 1990;39:399.
152. Nillius SJ. The therapeutic uses of gonadotropin-releasing hormone and its analogues. In: Beardwell C, Robertson GL, eds. *Clinical endocrinology 1: the pituitary.* London: Butterworth, 1981:211.
153. Harvey H, Lipton A, Max DT. LH-RH agonist treatment breast cancer: a phase II study in the USA. In: Klijn JGM, et al. eds. *Hormonal manipulation of cancer.* New York: Raven Press, 1987:321.
154. Klign JGM, DeJong FH, Blankenstein MA, et al. Anti-tumor and endocrine effects of chronic LHRH agonist treatment (buserelin) with or without tamoxifen in premenopausal metastatic breast cancer. *Breast Cancer Res Treat* 1984;4:209.
155. Nicholson RI, Walker KJ. Use of LH-RH agonists in the treatment of breast cancer. *Proc R Soc Edinburgh* 1989;95B:271.
156. Clayton RN, Bailey LC, Cottam J, et al. A radioimmunoassay for GnRH agonist analogue in serum patients with prostate cancer treated with D-Ser (tBu) AZA Gly[10] GnRH. *Clin Endocrinol* 1985;22:453.
157. Chrisp P, Goa KL. Goserelin: a review of its pharmacodynamic and pharmacokinetic properties, and clinical use in sex hormone-related conditions. *Drugs* 1991;41:254.
158. Brogden RN, Clissold SP. Flutamide: a preliminary review of its pharmacodynamic and pharmacokinetic properties, and therapeutic efficacy in advanced prostatic cancer. *Drugs* 1989;38:185.
159. Wysowski DK, Freiman JP, Tourtelot JB, et al. Fatal and nonfatal hepatotoxicity associated with flutamide. *Ann Intern Med* 1993;118:860.
160. Brogden RN, Chrisp P. Flutamide: a review of its pharmacodynamic and pharmacokinetic properties, and therapeutic use in advanced prostatic cancer. *Drugs Aging* 1991;1:104.
161. Radwanski E, Perentesis G, Symchowicz S, et al. Single and multiple dose pharmacokinetic evaluation of flutamide in normal geriatric volunteers. *J Clin Pharmacol* 1989;29:554.
162. Schellhammer P, Sharifi R, Block N, et al. A controlled trial of bicalutamide versus flutamide, each in combination with luteinizing hormone-releasing hormone analogue therapy, in patients with advanced prostate cancer. *Urology* 1995;45:745.
163. Furr BJ. Casodex: preclinical studies. *Eur Urol* 1990;18(Suppl 3):2.
164. Furr BJ. "Casodex" (ICI 176,334)—a new, pure, peripherally-selective anti-androgen: preclinical studies. *Horm Res* 1989;32(Suppl 1):69.
165. Kennealey GT, Furr BJA. Use of the nonsteroidal anti-androgen casodex in advanced prostatic carcinoma. *Urol Clin North Am* 1991;18:99.
166. Mahler C, Verhelst J, Denis L. Clinical pharmacokinetics of the antiandrogens and their efficacy in prostate cancer. *Clin Pharmacokinet* 1998;34:405.
167. Dole EJ, Holdsworth MT. Nilutamide: an antiandrogen for the treatment of prostate cancer. *Ann Pharmacother* 1997;31:65.
168. Kennedy BJ. Hormonal therapies in breast cancer. *Semin Oncol* 1974;1:119.
169. Colburn WA. Radioimmunoassay for fluoxymesterone (Halotestin). *Steroids* 1975;25:43.
170. Kammerer RC, Merdink JL, Jagels M, et al. Testing for fluoxymesterone (Halotestin) administration to man: identification of urinary metabolites by gas chromatography-mass spectrometry. *J Steroid Biochem* 1990;36:659.
171. Ingle JN, Ahmann DL, Green SJ, et al. Randomized clinical trial of diethylstilbestrol versus tamoxifen in post menopausal women with advanced breast cancer. *N Engl J Med* 1981;304:16.
172. Stewart HJ, Forrest APM, Gunn JM, et al. The tamoxifen trial: a double-blind comparison with stilboestrol in postmenopausal women with advanced breast cancer. In: Mouridsen HT, Palshof T, eds. *Breast cancer: experimental and clinical aspects.* Oxford: Pergamon Press, 1980:83.
173. Byar DP. Proceedings: the Veterans Administration Cooperative Urological Research Group's studies of cancer of the prostate. *Cancer* 1973;32:126.
174. Marselos M, Tomatis L. Diethylstilboestrol. I. Pharmacology, toxicology and carcinogenicity in humans. *Eur J Cancer* 1992;28A:1182.
175. Metzler M. Metabolic activation of carcinogenic diethylstilbestrol in rodents and humans. *J Toxicol Environ Health* 1976;(Suppl 1):21.
176. Williams CL, Stancel GM. *Estrogens and progestins.* New York: McGraw-Hill, 1996.
177. Hardman, Linbud, Molinoff, et al., eds. *Good and Gilman's The pharmacologic basis of therapeutics.* 9th ed. New York: McGraw-Hill, 1996.
178. Cascinu S, Fedeli A, Luzi Fedeli S, et al. Control of chemotherapy induced diarrhea with octreotide in patients receiving 5-fluorouracil. *Eur J Cancer* 1992;28:482.
179. Cascinu S, Fedeli A, Fedeli SL, et al. Octreotide versus loperamide in the treatment of fluorouracil-induced diarrhea: a randomized trial. *J Clin Oncol* 1993;11:148.
180. Chanson P, Timsit J, Harris AG. Clinical pharmacokinetics of octreotide. Therapeutic applications in patients with pituitary tumours. *Clin Pharmacokinet* 1993;25:375.
181. Harris AG. Somatostatin and somatostatin analogues: pharmacokinetics and pharmacodynamic effects. *Gut* 1994;35:S1.
182. Marbach P, Briner U, Lemaire M, et al. From somatostatin to Sandostatin: pharmacodynamics and pharmacokinetics. *Digestion* 1993;54(Suppl 1):9.
183. Rubin J, Ajani J, Schirmer W, et al. Octreotide acetate long-acting formulation versus open-label subcutaneous octreotide acetate in malignant carcinoid syndrome. *J Clin Oncol* 1999;17:600.

SECTION 4

RAYMOND P. WARRELL, JR.

Differentiation Agents

Chemotherapy treatment of certain tumors (notably germ cell cancers and neuroblastoma) is occasionally associated with persistence of residual tumors that on biopsy reveal only differentiated cells. These clinical observations, combined with *in vitro* data that morphologic differentiation can be induced in many cancer cell lines, have led to a resurgence of interest in the concept of induced cytodifferentiation as a means of cancer treatment. The identification of drugs that can induce an irreversible commitment to terminal differentiation (and consequently programmed cell death) has yielded some noteworthy successes.

RETINOIDS

Retinoids, which are natural or synthetic derivatives of vitamin A (retinol), induce cellular differentiation, suppress carcinogenesis, or inhibit proliferation of a number of cell lines, including epithelial cancers, melanoma, neuroblastoma, leukemia, germ cell, bone, and breast cancers.[1] These findings have generated widespread interest in these agents for cancer treatment and prevention. Several retinoids (all-*trans* retinoic acid [RA] and 9-*cis* RA) are normally found in plasma at nanomolar concentrations. Most retinoids bind to nuclear proteins that are RA receptors (RARs).[2,3] Cofactors, called *retinoid X receptors* (RXRs),[4] dimerize with RARs (Fig. 20.4-1), as well as receptors for thyroid hormone, vitamin D, and peroxisome proliferation activators. These receptor dimers bind specific DNA segments within target genes known as *retinoid response elements.* Activation of the receptor requires binding of its ligand, which then regulates transcription in part via recruitment of histone acetyltransferases.[5] Importantly, nonactivated receptors have important roles in silencing basal transcription of target genes via interaction with nuclear corepressor proteins that recruit histone deacetylases.[6]

ALL-*TRANS* RETINOIC ACID

The most striking success of the clinical application of differentiation therapy has been in acute promyelocytic leukemia (APL)[7] (see Chapter 46.2) where all-*trans* RA induces complete remission in a high proportion of patients with APL. Resistance to all-*trans* RA in a previously untreated patient is exceptionally rare, and failure is almost exclusively because of early death.[7,8] In APL, reciprocal translocations between the long arms of chromosomes 15 and 17 result in a fusion between genes that encode a RAR (RAR-α) and a transcription factor known as PML.[9,10] The resulting fusion protein, PML-RAR-α, blocks myeloid differentiation at the promyelocyte stage, which is relieved by pharmacologic (but not physiologic) concentrations of all-*trans* RA.

The initial response to all-*trans* RA in APL is associated with induced differentiation of leukemic cells.[11] This process is obvious, both in the bone marrow and in the peripheral blood, with the appearance of cells that are intermediate in maturation between promyelocytes and neutrophils. Prominent features of these intermediate cells are indented nuclei, loss of azurophilic granularity, and nuclear and cytoplasmic vacuolation.[7] Cell surface immunophenotyping of the neoplastic cells shows progression from a pattern of immature antigen expression at presentation toward the appearance of mature granulocytic markers during remission.[11]

The plasma half-life of all-*trans* RA is approximately 40 minutes,[12] and continuous dosing induces a progressive decrease in the plasma drug concentration.[13] Remissions induced by all-*trans* RA in patients with APL who do not receive additional anticancer therapy are brief and average 3 to 5 months in duration.[14] The mechanisms of clinically acquired retinoid resistance may be multifactorial,[15] but point mutations in the ligand-binding domain of the PML-RAR-α have been described in a few patients.[16] Combined sequential treatment programs that use all-*trans* RA (with or without chemotherapy) for induction, followed by anthracycline-based chemotherapy for consolidation, have yielded a two- to threefold increase in the proportion of patients cured of this disease.[17–19] Further administration of all-*trans* RA as maintenance therapy during the first year of remission makes a further, albeit modest,[8,17] contribution to relapse-free survival. Regrettably, the high single-agent activity of all-*trans* RA observed in APL has not been replicated in other neoplastic diseases.

13-*CIS* RETINOIC ACID

Of all retinoids, 13-*cis* RA has undergone the most extensive clinical examination; however, the single-agent activity of this drug in established cancer is quite limited. In the hematologic cancers, modest single-agent activity has been observed in patients with cutaneous T-cell lymphoma (mycosis fungoides)[20,21]; however, responses are usually partial and limited in duration. Studies of 13-*cis* RA in patients with myelodysplastic syndromes[22,23]; chronic myelocytic leukemia[24]; germ cell cancer and neuroblastoma[25,26]; and carcinomas of the head and neck, lung, and bladder [27–29] have had negative results. Modest activity has been observed in patients with epidermoid skin cancers, alone and in combination with interferon-α.[30–32]

The drug has also been explored as a means of cancer prevention, either as primary (to prevent an initial cancer) or secondary (to reduce the risk of recurrence) therapy. Treatment with 13-*cis* RA (1 to 2 mg/kg/d for 3 months) in heavy tobacco users reverses oral leukoplakia,[33] a known precursor to squamous carcinoma of the oral cavity. Because this dose causes considerable mucocutaneous toxicity, follow-up studies have used a high-dose induction course followed by a lower dose (0.5 mg/kg/d) maintenance program.[34] However, the duration of the clinical response is frequently brief, and most patients relapse when the drug is withdrawn. In an important preliminary study, adjuvant treatment with 13-*cis* RA (1 mg/kg/d) in patients who had undergone primary surgical excision, radiation treatment, or both for head and neck cancer significantly reduced the incidence of second primary tumors of the aerodigestive tract.[35] However, a large randomized multicenter study has not confirmed these findings.

OTHER RETINOIDS

The natural ligand of the RXRs is 9-*cis* RA, an isomer of all-*trans* RA[36] (see Fig. 20.4-1). Because 9-*cis* RA also binds to RARs, this

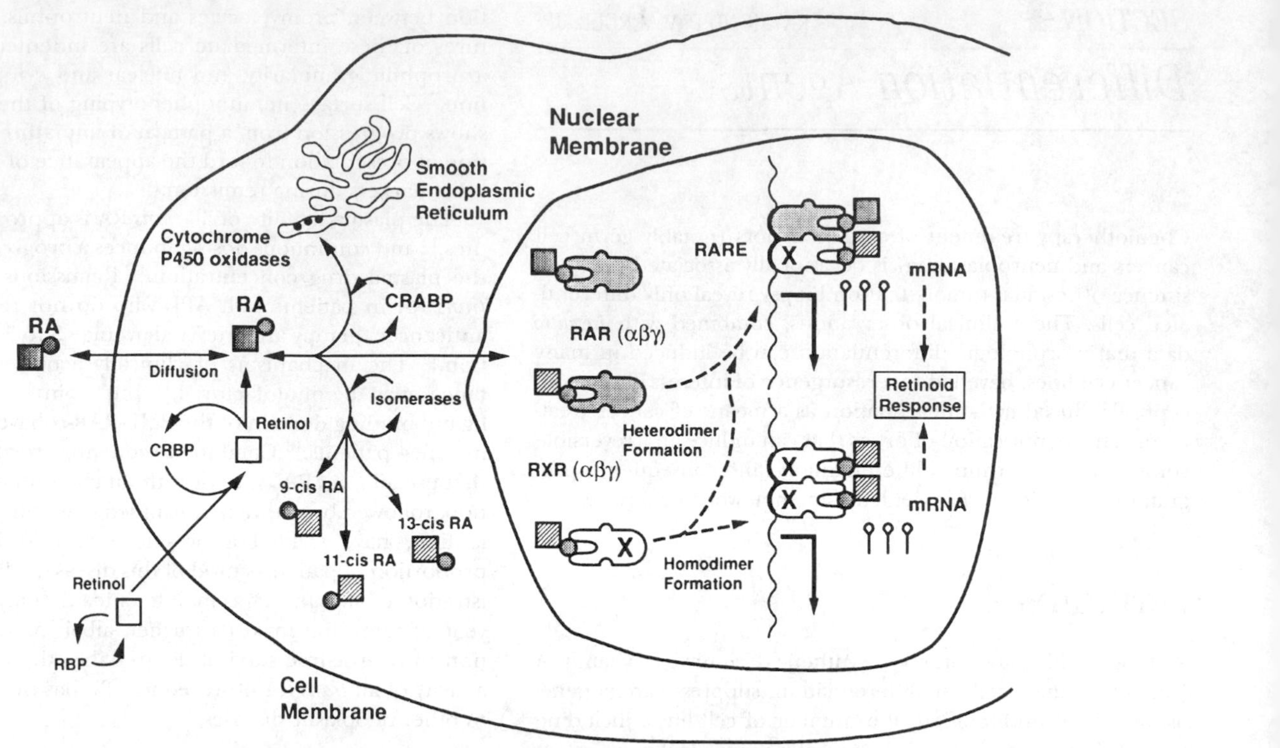

FIGURE 20.4-1. Metabolism of all-*trans* retinoic acid (RA). RA enters the cell by simple diffusion or by conversion from retinol (vitamin A) that has been absorbed from the gastrointestinal tract, bound in circulating form to retinol-binding proteins (RBP), and rebound intracellularly to cellular retinol-binding proteins (CRBP). RA can be immediately metabolized on binding to cellular retinoic acid–binding proteins (CRABP) and oxidized by cytochrome P-450 enzymes located in smooth endoplasmic reticulum. Alternatively, RA (or its isomers) enter the cell nucleus and bind to retinoic acid receptors (RARs) or retinoid X receptors (RXRs). On dimerization of these receptors (i.e., formation of a RAR-RXR heterodimer or RXR-RXR homodimer), RA-activated receptors bind with high affinity to specific DNA segments [the retinoic acid response element (RARE)] and effect messenger RNA (mRNA) transcription. Ultimately, the retinoid response is mediated by primary target genes, by interference with other transcription factors, or by control of certain posttranscriptional actions. (From ref. 1, with permission.)

property as a receptor pan-agonist suggested potentially broad biologic effects. Early clinical trials of 9-*cis* RA showed activity comparable with all-*trans* RA in APL, but the drug has not reversed clinically acquired retinoid resistance in this disease.[37] Toxicity of the two compounds has also been similar (see Adverse Effects of Retinoids, later in this chapter).[38,39] The drug was recently approved for topical use in patients with Kaposi's sarcoma related to acquired immunodeficiency syndrome. A number of relatively selective retinoid receptor agonists have also been synthesized[39] and are under active development. In contrast, fenretinide (N-[4-hydroxyphenyl], Retinamide) is a synthetic retinoid whose receptor has not yet been identified, but that has exhibited some chemopreventive activity against carcinomas of the breast, prostate, oral cavity, and bladder.[40] A large Italian study showed that fenretinide did not reduce the incidence of contralateral breast cancer, although an unexpected reduction of ovarian carcinoma was observed.[41] Fenretinide lowers serum retinol levels, which can cause temporary night blindness.[42]

ADVERSE EFFECTS OF RETINOIDS

Retinoids share many common side effects (Table 20.4-1). Most reactions are relatively mild; however, serious and occasionally fatal reactions have occurred. Headache that occurs several hours after drug ingestion is the most common side effect of all-*trans* and 9-*cis* RA.[7,38,43,44] This effect is less prominent with 13-*cis* RA in which mucositis is the most common reaction. Although narcotics are occasionally required, mild analgesics generally control the headaches, and tolerance to this effect develops within the first week of dosing. Pseudotumor cerebri has been documented in several patients (especially children)[44] who have required treatment with lumbar punctures and high-dose corticosteroids.

Dry skin, itching, flaking, nasal stuffiness, xerostomia, and cheilitis are relatively common with both all-*trans* and 13-*cis* RA. These reactions have been managed with topical lubricants and moisturizing agents, but some patients may require a decrease in drug dose. Genital ulcerations have been observed with all-*trans* RA. Bone pain occurs in 10% to 20% of APL patients receiving all-*trans* RA.[7] Like headache, this effect tends to occur early, remits with continued therapy, but can be quite severe, requiring parenteral narcotics for relief. Although bone pain is less common with 13-*cis* RA, protracted treatment with that agent has caused formation of bone spurs on vertebral bodies and the calcaneus.[45] Hypercalcemia has been reported with many RA isomers.[46]

Hypertriglyceridemia has been observed with all-*trans* RA, 9-*cis* and 13-*cis* RA, and also with RXR-selective agonists[7,38]; hypercholesterolemia is less striking. Cardiovascular consequences specifically related to hyperlipidemia have not yet been described, although acute pancreatitis has been reported.[38]

TABLE 20.4-1. Adverse Clinical Effects of the Retinoids

Skin/mucous membranes	
	Skin dryness, itching, peeling
	Penile/scrotal excoriations
	Angular cheilitis, lip cracking
	Skin/lymph node (especially tonsillar) infiltration with leukocytes
Neurologic	
	Headache
	Intracranial hypertension (*pseudotumor cerebri*)
	Night blindness[a]
Metabolic	
	Hypertriglyceridemia
	Hypercholesterolemia
	Hypercalcemia
Hematologic[b]	
	Leukocytosis
	Thrombosis
Gastrointestinal	
	Hepatic toxicity (increased serum glutamic-oxaloacetic transaminase, alkaline phosphatase, bilirubin)
Cardiovascular[b]	
	Congestive heart failure
	Fluid overload
	Lower extremity edema
	Episodic hypotension
	Weight gain
	Pericardial effusion
Pulmonary[b]	
	Respiratory distress
	Pleural effusion
	Radiographic infiltrates
Musculoskeletal	
	Bone pain
	Hyperostosis
	Myalgia

[a]Effect of fenretinide only.
[b]Occurs in patients with acute myelocytic leukemias only.

These complications may assume increasing importance as retinoids are used in more patients for extended periods. Hepatic toxicity, usually manifested by a transient increase in serum transaminase, alkaline phosphatase, or bilirubin, is a well-known side effect of all retinoids. Generally, this reaction occurs during the first several weeks of therapy and reverses after the drug is stopped. As with vitamin A itself,[47] retinoids are exceptionally potent teratogens, but this reaction is more important during treatment of nonmalignant conditions. The risk of fetal malformation (usually craniofacial abnormalities) appears to be highest in the first trimester and quite low in the third trimester.[48,49]

Leukocytosis (peripheral blood leukocytes greater than or equal to 10,000 cells/mm^3) occurs in approximately one-half of APL patients treated with all-*trans* RA[50] who do not receive concurrent cytotoxic chemotherapy. This finding is usually the first clinical sign of a biologic response. Cytotoxic therapy specifically directed toward lowering the leukocyte count is not required; however, patients who present with leukocyte counts greater than or equal to 5000 cells/mm^3 should be treated with full-dose chemotherapy (including an anthracycline) rather than low-dose chemotherapy (e.g., hydroxyurea or cytosine arabinoside), as the latter can trigger the onset of a lethal coagulopathy.[50]

More than one-half of patients with APL treated with all-*trans* RA experience the *RA syndrome*, a disorder characterized by fluid retention, weight gain, respiratory distress, radiographic pulmonary infiltrates, hectic fever, and pleural or pericardial effusions.[51] Leukocytosis is frequently but not invariably associated with this syndrome, and chemotherapy does not reduce the risk of this problem.[8,17,50–52] Early recognition of the syndrome before the onset of dyspnea (especially fever or weight gain) is critical. These signs should prompt immediate treatment with corticosteroids (dexamethasone, 10 mg intravenously every 12 hours for 3 or more days), which halts progression of the syndrome in most patients. RA need not be discontinued, but recurrence of the syndrome is common, requiring an additional course of corticosteroids.

ARSENIC TRIOXIDE

After a resurgence of interest owing to studies in China,[53,54] intravenous arsenic trioxide has been shown to induce complete remissions in a high proportion of patients with APL.[55] In APL, the drug is given intravenously as a 1- to 2-hour infusion at a dose of 0.15 mg/kg once per day until visible evidence of leukemic cells has been eliminated from the bone marrow. The duration of treatment in relapsed patients has ranged from 12 to 60 days, with a median of approximately 32 days.[55,56] Recovery of the peripheral leukocyte and platelet counts usually follows cessation of drug therapy. One or more additional treatment courses, each of a fixed duration of 25 cumulative days, is usually started approximately 3 weeks after discontinuing the initial series of infusions. These later infusions have been administered on a weekdays-only schedule without any apparent decrease in efficacy to date.

Arsenic trioxide has proved surprisingly potent in APL; indeed, the proportion of patients who achieve a molecular remission (as manifest by a negative reverse transcriptase–polymerase chain reaction result for the PML-RAR-α rearrangement) considerably exceeds that of patients on all-*trans* RA.[56] In APL, the drug is associated with induction of partial nonterminal differentiation, degradation of the PML-RAR-α fusion protein, and caspase activation.[55] The drug is currently being studied in other conditions and in different dosing schedules.[57,58]

When administered in the low-dose daily schedule described previously, the drug has generally been well tolerated. Fatigue is common. Lightheadedness during the infusion can be ameliorated by increasing its duration. A characteristic maculopapular skin eruption over the neck and torso occasionally occurs that resolves on discontinuation of the drug. Arsenic can cause peripheral neuropathy when administered for prolonged periods or higher doses, and severe neuropathic reactions, including quadriparesis,[59] have been reported from overdosage. Prolongation of the QT interval may occur, which may require treatment with parenteral potassium and magnesium supplements, especially in patients after amphotericin B therapy. APL patients treated with arsenic trioxide may also develop leukocytosis and the RA syndrome.[60] Management of these problems is identical to that described previously.

HISTONE DEACETYLASE INHIBITORS

The enzymatic addition of acetyl groups to histones, nuclear proteins closely associated with DNA, is known to have a per-

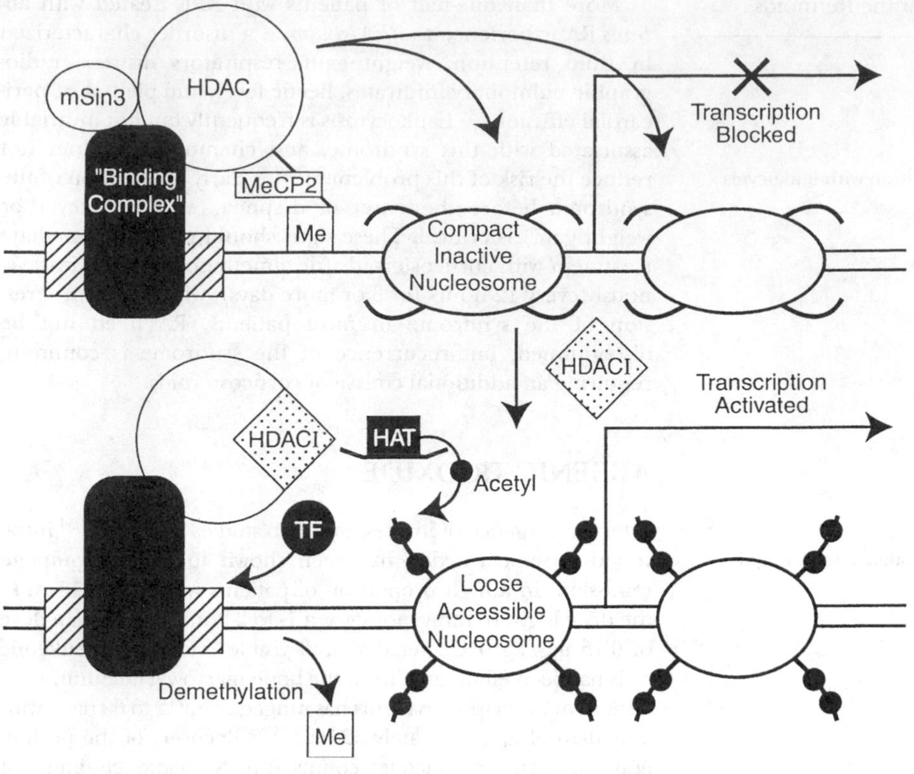

FIGURE 20.4-2. Mechanism of transcriptional repression by DNA methylation and histone deacetylation. In a transcriptionally inactive state, DNA is tightly coiled around core histones in the nucleosome. To activate transcription, the compact inactive nucleosome must undergo conformational relaxation, which may facilitate the binding of transcription factors (TF). Chromatin relaxation is associated with histone acetylation by histone acetyltransferases (HAT). A variety of normal DNA-binding proteins or oncogene products can complex with other proteins, and these complexes recruit histone deacetylases (HDACs), which cleave acetyl groups from histones, thereby preventing chromatin relaxation and blocking gene transcription. Treatment with a HDAC may prevent such cleavage, thereby yielding a loose accessible nucleosome whose DNA is then accessible for gene activation and transcription. Last, gene methylation (Me) in the promoter region has long been known to suppress gene activation in cancer. These two processes (i.e., gene methylation and histone deacetylation) have now been linked by the discovery of a protein (MeCP2) that forms a bridge between HDAC and methylated DNA. Inhibition of both processes may be required in cases wherein inhibition of only one process is insufficient to activate the target gene.

missive effect for messenger RNA transcription.[61] Histone hyperacetylation may induce site-specific conformational relaxation of tightly coiled DNA that facilitates binding of transcription factors.[62] Conversely, histone deacetylation has been linked to gene repression, and a number of oncogenes (as well as normal genes) silence transcription by recruiting histone deacetylases.[63,64] Furthermore, a link between gene methylation, a recognized mechanism of transcriptional repression, and histone deacetylation has now been established[65] (Fig. 20.4-2). Thus, DNA demethylation and inhibition of histone deacetylation offer potential targets for anticancer therapy. Azacytidine is the best-studied agent that induces demethylation, and the drug has shown modest single-agent activity in patients with various myelodysplastic syndromes.[66] Trichostatin A is the prototypic inhibitor of histone deacetylase,[67] but the agent has not been used clinically. In addition to the drugs noted in the following sections, other inhibitors include the trapoxins,[67] depudecins,[68] and depsipeptides.[69]

BUTYRATES AND OTHER FATTY ACIDS

Butyric acid induces differentiation in various cell lines,[70] but high concentrations (0.3 mM) have been required to reliably induce these effects. Butyrates have been widely studied as a treatment for thalassemia[71] and certain hyperammonemic states in children.[72] Several clinical studies have suggested that sodium phenylbutyrate has little single-agent activity in patients with advanced cancer or myelodysplasia.[73,74]

Histone deacetylase was shown to mediate transcriptional repression in APL,[75–77] as well as other cancers.[78–83] One report has shown that sodium phenylbutyrate reversibly induced histone hyperacetylation in leukemic cells and induced a complete remission in a child with retinoid-resistant APL when used in combination with all-*trans* RA.[84] Studies have suggested that these drugs act synergistically to induce cytodifferentiation,[85,86] and this combination is currently undergoing additional clinical testing. The major side effects of sodium phenylbutyrate are fluid overload and central nervous system depression, including transient somnolence and confusion.

Phenylbutyrate exhibits pleiotropic effects, and the agent is a prodrug for phenylacetate,[87] which promotes *in vitro* differentiation of certain cell lines.[88] High doses of phenylacetate itself (250 to 550 mg/kg/d) have been used clinically[89] with low single-agent activity in malignant gliomas[90] and prostate cancer.[91] Tributyrin is a major constituent of dietary butterfat, which yields three molecules of butyrate after hydrolysis. The relatively high butyrate concentrations that are achievable in the colon have suggested a potential chemopreventive utility for colon cancer.[92]

HYBRID POLAR COMPOUNDS

Certain hybrid polar compounds have broad *in vitro* activity as differentiating agents. The prototype compound of this class, hexamethylene bisacetamide,[93] has required relatively high concentrations (1 to 5 mM). Renal insufficiency, central nervous system toxicity, and thrombocytopenia were dose-limiting in early studies,[94] but some responses were observed in patients with myelodysplastic syndromes using 10-day infusion schedules.[95] Newer synthetic derivatives have more potent activity than hexamethylene bisacetamide, and several are potent inhibitors of histone deacetylase.[96]

VITAMIN D

1,25-Dihydroxyvitamin D_3, the active form of the hormone, facilitates differentiation in a variety of cell types.[97] Vitamin D receptors have been identified in a variety of cell types.[98,99] Circumstantial evidence has suggested that vitamin D can decrease the incidence of some tumor types.[100,101] Vitamin D decreases growth of leukemia,[102,103] breast,[104] colon,[105] and prostate[106] cancer cell lines. In HL60 cells, vitamin D induces differentiation into monocytes and macrophages,[107] unlike retinoids and dimethyl sulfoxide, which induce granulocytoid differentiation.

Few clinical trials of vitamin D have been conducted. Several responses were observed in a study of patients with myelodysplastic syndromes treated at a dose of 2 mg/d, but intolerable hypercalcemia proved limiting.[102] New analogues of vitamin D_3 have become available that retain differentiating activity while causing minimal effects on calcium metabolism.[108,109]

CYTOKINES AND OTHER PROTEINS

Colony-stimulating factors induce a variety of responses in their target cells, including a commitment to terminal differentiation.[110] Both granulocyte colony-stimulating factor (filgrastim) and granulocyte-macrophage colony-stimulating factor (sargramostim) have been studied clinically. Neither agent has proved dramatically effective in either myelodysplastic syndromes or acute myeloid leukemias; however, mature populations of granulocytes and monocytes can be regularly increased in many patients, sometimes with clinical benefit (e.g., reduced infectious complications).[111]

REFERENCES

1. Warrell RP Jr. Retinoids in cancer. In: Kimball ES, ed. *Immunopharmaceutical.* Boca Raton, FL: CRC Press, 1995:101.
2. Petkovich M, Brand NJ, Krust A, et al. A human retinoic acid receptor which belongs to the family of nuclear receptors. *Nature* 1987;330:444.
3. Giguere V, Ong ES, Segui P, et al. Identification of a receptor for the morphogen retinoic acid. *Nature* 1987;330:624.
4. Mangelsdorf DJ, Ong ES, Dyck JA, et al. Nuclear receptor that identifies a novel retinoic acid response pathway. *Nature* 1990;345:224.
5. Wolffe AP, Pruss D. Targeting chromatin disruption: transcription regulators that acetylate histones. *Cell* 1996;84:817.
6. Ptashne M, Gann A. Transcriptional activation by recruitment. *Nature* 1997;386:569.
7. Chen JD, Evans RM. A transcriptional co-repressor that interacts with nuclear hormone receptors. *Nature* 1995;377:454.
8. Warrell RP Jr, de Thé H, Wang Z-Y, et al. Acute promyelocytic leukemia. *N Engl J Med* 1993;329:177.
9. Tallman MS, Andersen JW, Schiffer CA, et al. All-*trans* retinoic acid in acute promyelocytic leukemia. *N Engl J Med* 1997;337:1021.
10. de Thé H, Chomienne C, Lanotte M, et al. The t(15;17) translocation of acute promyelocytic leukaemia fuses the retinoic acid receptor α gene to a novel transcribed locus. *Nature* 1990;347:558.
11. Warrell RP Jr, Frankel SR, Miller WH Jr, et al. Differentiation therapy of acute promyelocytic leukemia with tretinoin (all-*trans* retinoic acid). *N Engl J Med* 1991;324:1385.
12. Muindi J, Frankel S, Huselton C, et al. Clinical pharmacology of oral all-*trans* retinoic acid in patients with acute promyelocytic leukemia. *Cancer Res* 1992;52:2138.
13. Muindi J, Frankel SR, Miller WH Jr, et al. Continuous treatment with all-*trans* retinoic acid results in a progressive decrease in plasma concentrations: implications for relapse and retinoid "resistance" in acute promyelocytic leukemia. *Blood* 1992;79:299.
14. Warrell RP Jr, Maslak P, Eardley A, et al. All-*trans* retinoic acid for treatment of acute promyelocytic leukemia: an update of the New York experience. *Leukemia* 1994;8:929.
15. Warrell RP Jr. Acquired retinoid resistance in acute promyelocytic leukemia: new mechanisms, strategies, and implications. *Blood* 1993;82:1949.
16. Ding W, Li Y-P, Nobile LM, et al. Leukemic cellular retinoic acid resistance and missense mutations in the PML-RARα fusion gene after relapse of acute promyelocytic leukemia from treatment with all-*trans* retinoic and intensive chemotherapy. *Blood* 1998;92:1172.
17. Fenaux P, Chastang C, Sanz M, et al. Effect of ATRA in newly diagnosed acute promyelocytic leukemia (APL): validation of short term effect in a large multicenter trial (APL 93 trial) and assessment of long term benefit (APL 91 trial). *Blood* 1996;88(Suppl 1):209a.
18. Mandelli F, Diverio D, Avvisati G, et al. Molecular remission in PML/RAR alpha-positive acute promyelocytic leukemia by combined all-*trans* retinoic acid and idarubicin (AIDA) therapy. *Blood* 1997;90:1014.
19. Soignet S, Fleischauer A, Polyak T, et al. All-*trans* retinoic acid significantly increases 5-year survival in acute promyelocytic leukemia: an updated analysis of the New York study. *Cancer Chemother Pharmacol* 1997;40(Suppl):S25.
20. Warrell RP Jr, Coonley CJ, Kempin SJ, et al. Isotretinoin in cutaneous T-cell lymphoma. *Lancet* 1983;1:629.
21. Molin L, Thomsen K, Volden G, et al. Oral retinoids in mycosis fungoides and Sezary syndrome: a comparison of isotretinoin and etretinate. A study from the Scandinavian Mycosis Fungoides group. *Acta Derm Venereol* 1987;67:232.
22. Picozzi VJ, Swanson GF, Morgan R, et al. 13-*Cis* retinoic acid treatment for myelodysplastic syndromes. *J Clin Oncol* 1986;4:589.
23. Koeffler HP, Heitjan D, Mertelsmann R, et al. Randomized study of 13-*cis* retinoic acid *v* placebo in the myelodysplastic disorders. *Blood* 1988;71:703.
24. Arlin ZA, Mertelsmann R, Berman E, et al. 13-*Cis* retinoic acid does not decrease the true response rate and the duration of true remission (induced by cytotoxic chemotherapy) in patients with chronic myelogenous leukemia. *J Clin Oncol* 1987;3:473.
25. Gold EJ, Bosl GJ, Itri LM. Phase II trial of 13-*cis* retinoic acid in patients with advanced nonseminomatous germ cell tumors. *Cancer Treat Rep* 1984;68:1287.
26. Finklestein JZ, Krailo MD, Lenarsky C, et al. 13-*cis* retinoic acid (NSC 122578) in the treatment of children with metastatic neuroblastoma unresponsive to conventional chemotherapy: report from the Children's Cancer Study Group. *Med Pediatr Oncol* 1992;20:307.
27. Lippman SM, Kessler JF, Al-Sarraf M, et al. Treatment of advanced squamous cell carcinoma of the head and neck with isotretinoin: a phase II randomized trial. *Invest New Drugs* 1988;6:13.
28. Grunberg S, Itri L. Phase II study of isotretinoin in the treatment of advanced non-small cell lung cancer. *Cancer Treat Rep* 1987;71:1097.
29. DiSilverio F, Concolino G, Tenaglia R, et al. Retinoids in recurrences of superficial bladder tumors. *Proceedings of the 5th International Conference on the Adjuvant Therapy of Cancer*, Tucson, AZ, March 11–14, 1987:75.
30. Lippman SM, Meyskens FM Jr. Treatment of advanced squamous cell carcinoma of the skin with isotretinoin. *Ann Intern Med* 1987;107:499.
31. Lippman SM, Parkinson DR, Itri LM, et al. 13-*Cis*-retinoic acid and interferon α-2a: effective combination therapy for advanced squamous cell carcinoma of the skin. *J Natl Cancer Inst* 1992;84:235.
32. Lippman SM, Kavanagh JJ, Paredes-Espinosa M, et al. 13-*Cis* retinoic acid plus interferon-alpha 2a: highly active systemic therapy for squamous cell carcinoma of the cervix. *J Natl Cancer Inst* 1992;84:241.
33. Hong WK, Endicott J, Itri LM, et al. 13-*Cis*-retinoic acid in the treatment of oral leukoplakia. *N Engl J Med* 1986;315:1501.
34. Lippman SM, Batsakis JG, Toth BB, et al. Comparison of low-dose isotretinoin with beta carotene to prevent oral carcinogenesis. *N Engl J Med* 1993;328:15.
35. Hong WK, Lippman SM, Itri LM, et al. Prevention of second primary tumors with isotretinoin in squamous cell carcinoma of the head and neck. *N Engl J Med* 1990;323:795.
36. Heyman R, Mangelsdorf D, Dyck J, et al. 9-*Cis* retinoic acid is a high affinity ligand for the retinoid X receptor. *Cell* 1992;68:397.
37. Miller WH Jr, Jakubowski A, Benedetti F, et al. 9-*Cis* retinoic acid induces complete remission in acute promyelocytic leukemia but does not reverse clinically acquired resistance to all-*trans* retinoic acid. *Blood* 1995;85:3021.
38. Miller VA, Rigas JR, Benedetti FM, et al. Initial clinical trial of the retinoid receptor pan-agonist, 9-*cis* retinoic acid. *Clin Cancer Res* 1996;2:471.
39. Boehm MF, Zhang L, Zhi L, et al. Design and synthesis of potent retinoid X receptor selective ligands that induce apoptosis in leukemia cells. *J Med Chem* 1995;38:3146.
40. Moon RC, Mehta RG. Chemoprevention of experimental carcinogenesis. *Prev Med* 1989;18:576.
41. De Palo G, Camerini T, Marubini E, et al. Chemoprevention trial of contralateral breast cancer with fenretinide: rational, design, methodology, organization, data management, statistics, and accrual. *Tumori* 1997;83:884.
42. Formelli F, Clerici M, Campa T, et al. Five-year administration of fenretinide: pharmacokinetics and effects on plasma retinol concentrations. *J Clin Oncol* 1993;11:2036.
43. Lee JS, Newman RA, Lippman SM, et al. Phase I evaluation of all-*trans* retinoic acid in adults with solid tumors. *J Clin Oncol* 1993;11:959.
44. Smith MA, Adamson PC, Balis FM, et al. Phase I and pharmacokinetic evaluation of all-*trans* retinoic acid in pediatric patients with cancer. *J Clin Oncol* 1992;10:1666.
45. DiGiovanna J, Helfgott R, Gerber L, et al. Extraspinal tendon and ligament calcification associated with long-term therapy with etretinate. *N Engl J Med* 1986;315:1177.
46. Niesvizky R, Siegel DS, Busquets X, et al. Hypercalcaemia and increased serum interleukin-6 levels induced by all-*trans* retinoic acid in patients with multiple myeloma. *Br J Haematol* 1995;89:217.
47. Rothman KJ, Moore LL, Siinger MR, et al. Teratogenicity of high vitamin A intake. *N Engl J Med* 1995;333:1369.
48. Dai WS, LaBraico JM, Stern RS. Epidemiology of isotretinoin exposure during pregnancy. *J Am Acad Dermatol* 1992;26:599.
49. Stentoft J, Nielsen JL, Hvidman LE. All-*trans* retinoic acid in acute promyelocytic leukemia in late pregnancy. *Leukemia* 1994;8:1585.
50. Vadhat L, Eardley A, Maslak P, et al. Early mortality and the "retinoic acid syndrome" in acute promyelocytic leukemia: impact of leukocytosis, low-dose chemotherapy, PML/RAR-α isoform, and CD13 expression in patients treated with all-*trans* retinoic acid. *Blood* 1994;84:3843.

51. Frankel SR, Eardley A, Lauwers G, et al. The "retinoic acid syndrome" in acute promyelocytic leukemia. *Ann Intern Med* 1992;117:292.
52. Tallman MS, Andersen JW, Schiffer CA, et al. Clinical description of 44 patients with acute promyelocytic leukemia who developed the retinoic acid syndrome. *Blood* 2000;95:90.
53. Zhang P, Wang SY, Hu XH. Arsenic trioxide treated 72 cases of acute promyelocytic leukemia. *Chin J Hematol* 1996;17:58.
54. Shen Z-X, Chen G-Q, Ni J-H, et al. Use of arsenic trioxide (As_2O_3)in the treatment of acute promyelocytic leukemia (APL): II. clinical efficacy and pharmacokinetics in patients at relapse. *Blood* 1997;89:3354.
55. Soignet SL, Maslak P, Wang Z-G, et al. Complete remission after induction of nonterminal differentiation and apoptosis in acute promyelocytic leukemia by arsenic trioxide. *N Engl J Med* 1998;339:1341.
56. Soignet S, Kantarjian H, Frankel S, et al. Arsenic trioxide in acute promyelocytic leukemia: results of initial U.S. pilot and multicenter trials. *Blood* 1998;92(Suppl):483a.
57. Soignet S, Calleja E, Cheung N-K, et al. A phase 1 study of arsenic trioxide in patients with solid tumors. *Proc Am Soc Clin Oncol* 1999;18:228a.
58. Soignet S, Wang Z-G, Nagy J, et al. Dose-ranging study of arsenic trioxide in advanced hematologic cancers: clinical pharmacokinetic and biological effects. *Blood* 1998;92(Suppl):598a.
59. Westervelt P, Pollock J, Haug J, et al. Response and toxicity associated with dose escalation of arsenic trioxide in the treatment of resistant acute promyelocytic leukemia. *Blood* 1997;90(Suppl 1):249b.
60. Warrell RP Jr, Chanel S, Ho R, Soignet S. Leukocytosis and "retinoic acid syndrome" in patients with acute promyelocytic leukemia treated with arsenic trioxide. *Proc Am Soc Clin Oncol* 1999;18:21a.
61. Grunstein M. Histone acetylation in chromatin structure and transcription. *Nature* 1997;389:349.
62. Lee DY, Hayes JJ, Pruss D, et al. A positive role for histone acetylation in transcription factor access to DNA. *Cell* 1993;72:73.
63. Alland L, Muhle R, Hou H Jr, et al. Role for N-CoR and histone deacetylase in Sin3-mediated transcriptional repression. *Nature* 1997;387:49.
64. Heinzel T, Lavinsky RM, Mullen TM, et al. A complex containing N-CoR, mSin3 and histone deacetylase mediates transcriptional repression. *Nature* 1997;387:43.
65. Nan X, Ng H-H, Johnson CA, et al. Transcriptional repression by the methyl-CpG-binding protein MeCP2 involves a histone deacetylase complex. *Nature* 1998;393:386.
66. Zagonel V, Lo Re G, Marotta G, et al. 5-aza-2'-deoxycytidine (decitabine) induces trilineage response in unfavourable myelodysplastic syndromes. *Leukemia* 1993;7(Suppl 1):30.
67. Yoshida M, Horinouchi S, Beppu T. Trichostatin A and traopoxin: novel chemical probes for the role of histone deacetylation in chromatin structure and function. *Bio Essays* 1995;17:423.
68. Kwon HJ, Owa T, Hassig CA, et al. Depudecin induces morphological reversion of transformed fibroblasts via the inhibition of histone deacetylase. *Proc Natl Acad Sci U S A* 1998;95:3356.
69. Nakajima H, Kim YB, Terano H, et al. FR901228, a potent antitumor antibiotic, is a novel histone deacetylase inhibitor. *Exp Cell Res* 1998;241:126.
70. Samid D, Yeh A, Prasanna P. Induction of erythroid differentiation and fetal hemoglobin production in human leukemic cells treated with phenylacetate. *Blood* 1992;80:1576.
71. Dover GJ, Brusilow S, Samid D. Increased fetal hemoglobin in patients receiving sodium 4-phenylbutyrate. *N Engl J Med* 1992;327:569.
72. Maestri NE, Brusilow SW, Clissold DB, et al. Long-term treatment of girls with ornithine transcarbamylase deficiency. *N Engl J Med* 1996;335:855.
73. Gore SD, Miller CB, Weng L-J, et al. Improved hematopoiesis in patients with myelodysplastic syndromes (MDS) and acute myeloid leukemia (AML) following administration of the putative differentiating agent sodium phenylbutyrate (SPB). *Blood* 1996;88(Suppl):582a.
74. Carducci M, Bowling M, Eisenberger M, et al. Oral sodium phenylbutyrate (PB) for refractory solid tumors: phase 1 and bioavailability assessment. *Proc Am Soc Clin Oncol* 1998;17:215a.
75. Lin RJ, Nagy L, Inoue S, et al. Role of the histone deacetylase complex in acute promyelocytic leukaemia. *Nature* 1998;391:811.
76. Grignani F, De Matteis S, Nervi C, et al. Fusion proteins of the retinoic acid receptor-α recruit histone deacetylase in promyelocytic leukaemia. *Nature* 1998;391:815.
77. He L-Z, Guidez F, Tribioli C, et al. Distinct interactions of PML-RARα with co-repressors determine differential responses to RA in APL. *Nature Genet* 1998;18:126.
78. Borrow J, Stanton VP Jr, Andresen JM, et al. The translocation t(8;16)(p11;p13) of acute myeloid leukaemia fuses a putative acetytransferase to the CREB-binding protein. *Nature Genet* 1996;14:33.
79. Sobulo OM, Borrow J, Tomek R, et al. MLL is fused to CBP, a histone acetyltransferase, in therapy-related acute myeloid leukemia with a t(11;16)(q23;p13.3). *Proc Natl Acad Sci U S A* 1997;94:8732.
80. Dhordain P, Albagli O, Lin RJ, et al. Corepressor SMRT binds the BTB/POZ repressing domain of the LAZ3/BCL6 oncoprotein. *Proc Natl Acad Sci U S A* 1997;94:10762.
81. Ayer DE, Lawrence QA, Eisenman RN. Mad-max transcriptional repression is mediated by ternary complex formation with mammalian homologs of yeast repressor Sin3. *Cell* 1995;80:767.
82. Schreiber-Agus N, Chin L, Chen K, et al. An amino-terminal domain of Mxil mediates anti-Myc oncogenic activity and interacts with a homolog of the yeast transcriptional repressor Sin3. *Cell* 1995;80:777.
83. Laherty CD, Yang WM, Sun JM, et al. Histone deacetylases associated with the mSin3 corepressor mediate Mad transcriptional repression. *Cell* 1997;83:349.
84. Warrell RP Jr, He L-Z, Richon V, et al. Therapeutic targeting of transcription in acute promyelocytic leukemia using an inhibitor of histone deacetylase. *J Natl Cancer Inst* 1998;90:1621.
85. Weng LJ, Yu K, Fu S, et al. Synergy between retinoic acid (RA) and the putative differentiating agent sodium phenylbutyrate (SPB) promotes maximal cytostasis and differentiation of myeloid cells at clinically achievable doses of SPB. *Blood* 1996;90(Suppl):329a.
86. Sidell N, Chang B, Yamashiro JM, et al. Transcriptional upregulation of retinoic acid receptor β (RARβ) expression by phenylacetate in human neuroblastoma cells. *Exp Cell Res* 1998;239:169.
87. Samid D, Shack S, Sherman LT. Phenylacetate: a novel nontoxic inducer of tumor cell differentiation. *Cancer Res* 1992;52:1988.
88. Shack S, Liu L, Miller A, et al. Differentiation therapy using the aromatic fatty acids phenylacetate and phenylbutyrate as an alternative treatment for multiple drug resistant tumors. *Proc Am Assoc Cancer Res* 1995;36:319.
89. Thibault A, Cooper MR, Figg WD, et al. A phase I and pharmacokinetic study of intravenous phenylacetate in patients with cancer. *Cancer Res* 1994;54:1690.
90. Samid D, Ram Z, Hudgins WR, et al. Selective activity of phenylacetate against malignant gliomas: resemblance to fetal brain damage in phenylketonuria. *Cancer Res* 1994;54:891.
91. Olsson IL, Breitman TR. Induction of differentiation of the human histiocytic lymphoma cell line U-937 by retinoic acid and cyclic adenosine 3':5'-monophosphate-inducing agents. *Cancer Res* 1982;42:3924.
92. Freeman JJ. Effects of differing concentrations of sodium butyrate on 1,2-dimethylhydrazine-induced rat intestine neoplasia. *Gastroenterology* 1986;91:596.
93. Marks PA, Richon VM, Kiyokawa H, et al. Inducing differentiation of transformed cells with hybrid polar compounds: a cell-cycle-dependent process. *Proc Natl Acad Sci U S A* 1994;91:10251.
94. Young CW, Fanucchi MP, Walsh TD, et al. Phase I trial and clinical pharmacological evaluation of hexamethylene bisacetamide administration by ten-day continuous intravenous infusion at twenty-eight-day intervals. *Cancer Res* 1988;48:7304.
95. Andreeff M, Stone R, Michael J, et al. Hexamethylene bisacetamide in myelodysplastic syndrome (MDS) and acute myelogenous leukemia (AML): a phase II clinical trial with a differentiation inducing agent. *Blood* 1992;80:2604.
96. Richon VM, Emiliani S, Verdin E, et al. A class of hybrid polar inducers of transformed cell differentiation are potent inhibitors of histone deacetylases. *Proc Natl Acad Sci U S A* 1998;95:3003.
97. Reichel H, Koeffler HP, Norman AW. The role of vitamin D endocrine system in health and disease. *N Engl J Med* 1989;320:980.
98. Kizaki M, Norman AW, Bishop JE, et al. 1,25-dihydroxyvitamin D_3 receptor RNA: expression in hematopoietic cells. *Blood* 1991;77:1238.
99. Evans SRT, Nolla J, Hanfelt J, et al. Vitamin D receptor expression as a predictive marker of biological behavior in human colorectal cancer. *Clin Cancer Res* 1998;4:1591.
100. Garland C, Shekelle RB, Barrett-Connor E, et al. Dietary vitamin D and calcium and risk of colorectal cancer: a 19 year prospective study in men. *Lancet* 1985;1:307.
101. Corder EH, Guess HA, Hulka BS, et al. Vitamin D and prostate cancer: a prediagnostic study with stored sera. *Cancer Epidemiol Biomarkers Prev* 1993;2:467.
102. Koeffler HP, Hirji K, Itri L, et al. 1,25-dihydroxyvitamin D_3: in vivo and in vitro effects on human preleukemic and leukemic cells. *Cancer Treat Rep* 1985;69:1399.
103. Elstner E, Lee YY, Hashiya M, et al. 1α,25-dihydroxy-20-epi-vitamin D_3: an extraordinarily potent inhibitor of leukemic cell growth in vitro. *Blood* 1994;84:1960.
104. Elstner E, Linker-Israeli M, Said J, et al. 20-epi-vitamin D_3 analogues: a novel class of potent inhibitors of proliferation and inducers of differentiation of human breast cancer cell lines. *Cancer Res* 1995;55:2822.
105. Wali RK, Bissonnette M, Khare S, et al. 1α,25-dihydroxy-16-ene-23-yne-26,27-hexafluorocholecalciferol, a noncalcemic analogue of 1α,25-dihydroxyvitamin D_3, inhibits azoxymethane-induced colonic tumorigenesis. *Cancer Res* 1995;55:3050.
106. Miller GJ, Stapleton GE, Hedlund TE, et al. Vitamin D receptor expression 24-hydroxylase activity, and inhibition of growth by 1α,25-dihydroxyvitamin D_3 in seven human prostatic carcinoma cell lines. *Clin Cancer Res* 1995;1:997.
107. Manglesdorf DJ, Koeffler HP, Donaldson CA, et al. 1,25-dihydroxyvitamin-D_3-induced differentiation in a human promyelocytic leukemia cell (HL-60): receptor-mediated maturation to macrophage-like cells. *J Cell Biol* 1984;98:391.
108. Wilkerson CL, Darjatmoko SR, Lindstrom MJ, et al. Toxicity and dose-response studies of 1,25-$(OH)_2$-16ene-23-yne vitamin D_3 in transgenic mice. *Clin Cancer Res* 1998;4:2253.
109. Asou H, Koike M, Elstner E, et al. 19-nor vitamin-D analogs: a new class of potent inhibitors of proliferation and inducers of differentiation of human myeloid leukemia cell lines. *Blood* 1998;92:2441.
110. Metcalf D. The molecular control of cell division, differentiation commitment and maturation in haemopoietic cells. *Nature* 1989;339:27.
111. Estey E, Thall PF, Kantarjian H, et al. Treatment of newly diagnosed acute myelogenous leukemia with granulocyte-macrophage colony-stimulating factor (GM-CSF) before and during continuous infusion high-dose ara-C + daunorubicin: comparison to patients treated without GM-CSF. *Blood* 1992;79:2246.

SECTION **5**

LOUIS M. WEINER
GREGORY P. ADAMS
MARGARET VON MEHREN

Therapeutic Monoclonal Antibodies: General Principles

Antibody-based therapeutics are coming of age. Antibodies have provided an important means to exploit the capacity of the immune system to specifically recognize and direct antitumor responses. Antibody therapy studies were among the earliest attempts to explicitly target cancers based on the structural and biologic properties that distinguish neoplastic cells from their normal counterparts. Although the early clinical studies yielded inconsistent and often disappointing clinical results, more recent work has identified a number of important and useful applications for antibody-based cancer therapy. Unconjugated antibodies directed against the lymphocyte antigen CD20 have significant clinical activity in patients with low-grade lymphomas.[1] The U.S. Food and Drug Administration (FDA) has approved one of these antibodies, rituximab, for clinical use. Radioimmunoconjugates directed against CD20 demonstrate significant clinical activity in patients with chemotherapy-pretreated lymphomas as well.[2,3] A chemoimmunoconjugate containing an anti-CD33 antibody and calicheamicin has impressive activity in acute myelogenous leukemia (AML).[4] Finally, the anti-HER2/*neu* antibody trastuzumab has single-agent activity in metastatic breast cancer and potentiates the antitumor effects of Taxol chemotherapy.[5,6] This antibody also received FDA approval for clinical use. These results provide ample evidence that a number of strategies using unconjugated antibodies or antibody conjugates carrying toxic payloads, such as radiation or chemotherapy agents, have clinical benefits. At this time, the mechanisms underlying the clinical benefits of rituximab and trastuzumab are not understood, but both antibodies mediate antibody-dependent cellular cytotoxicity (ADCC) *in vitro* and may do so in the clinical setting as well.[7]

Antibodies are produced by B cells. These proteins arise in response to exposure to a variety of structures, termed *antigens,* as a result of a series of recombinations of V, D, and J germline genes. Somatic hypermutation occurs with each subsequent exposure to the antigen and introduces further variation that can increase binding affinity or alter target antigen specificity. The resulting proteins exhibit selective targeting of a variety of potential antigens and can direct the clearance or immune recognition of such antigens. Various isotypes of antibodies have specialized functions [e.g., immunoglobulin A (IgA) molecules play important roles in mucosal immunity, and IgE molecules are involved in anaphylaxis]. IgG molecules are most commonly used as the working backbones of current therapeutic monoclonal antibodies (MABs).

Before 1975, the ability of antibodies to specifically target immunogens for therapeutic applications was inconsistently exploited because the available antibody preparations were derived from polyclonal antisera obtained from immunized animals. The advent of hybridoma technology by Kohler and Milstein[8] made it possible to produce large quantities of antibodies with high purity and monospecificity for a single binding region (epitope) on an antigen.

IMMUNOGLOBULIN STRUCTURE: STRUCTURAL AND FUNCTIONAL DOMAINS

IgG antibodies are comprised of two identical light chains and two identical heavy chains. The variable region contains hypervariable regions, or complementarity determining regions (CDRs), in which the antigen-contact residues reside. Antibodies achieve diversity due to variations in the amino acid sequences of the CDRs resulting from the VDJ recombinations and somatic hypermutations previously described. The Fc domain is composed of the CH2 and CH3 regions of the antibody's heavy chains. This portion of the antibody mediates its effector functions, transport across cellular barriers, and biologic half-life. The different isotypes of immunoglobulins are defined by the structure and function of their Fc domains. The types of immune effector cells that interact with IgG and the results of the interactions are dictated by cellular Fc receptor expression patterns. Developments in the field of molecular biology have led to the production of a wide variety of novel antibody-based targeting structures (Fig. 20.5-1). These include chimeric human-murine antibodies with human constant regions and murine variable regions,[9] humanized antibodies in which murine CDR sequences have been grafted into human IgG molecules and entirely human antibodies derived from human hybridomas and more recently from transgenic mice expressing human immunoglobulin genes.[10] Additionally, a large number of recombinant immunoglobulin-based structures have been produced from the variable or constant domains of antibodies. These range in size from CDR-based peptides[11] to bispecific antibodies (BsAb) with dual antigen specificities. Some of the more promising structures include monovalent single-chain Fv (scFv), derived from murine hybridomas[12–14] or phage-display libraries,[15,16] and multivalent dimeric Fv [$(scFv)_2$],[17] diabodies,[18,19] triabodies,[20] and minibodies.[21] This technology also has resulted in the creation of a number of antibody-based fusion proteins designed to target cytokines [e.g., interleukin (IL)-2] to the tumor.[22]

FACTORS REGULATING ANTIBODY-BASED TUMOR TARGETING

Although great progress has been made since initial treatment trials of MAB therapy, a number of obstacles to treatment efficacy have been identified in preclinical studies and in clinical trials. It is not surprising that obstacles have been identified for a concept that attempts to introduce an unprecedented degree of targeting specificity while using large proteins whose sizes greatly exceed those of conventional pharmaceuticals. It should be emphasized that the identification of obstacles is not a reason for discouragement, but rather is a necessary prelude to the cycles of molecular and strategy refinements that are inherent in the development of any new therapeutic modality.

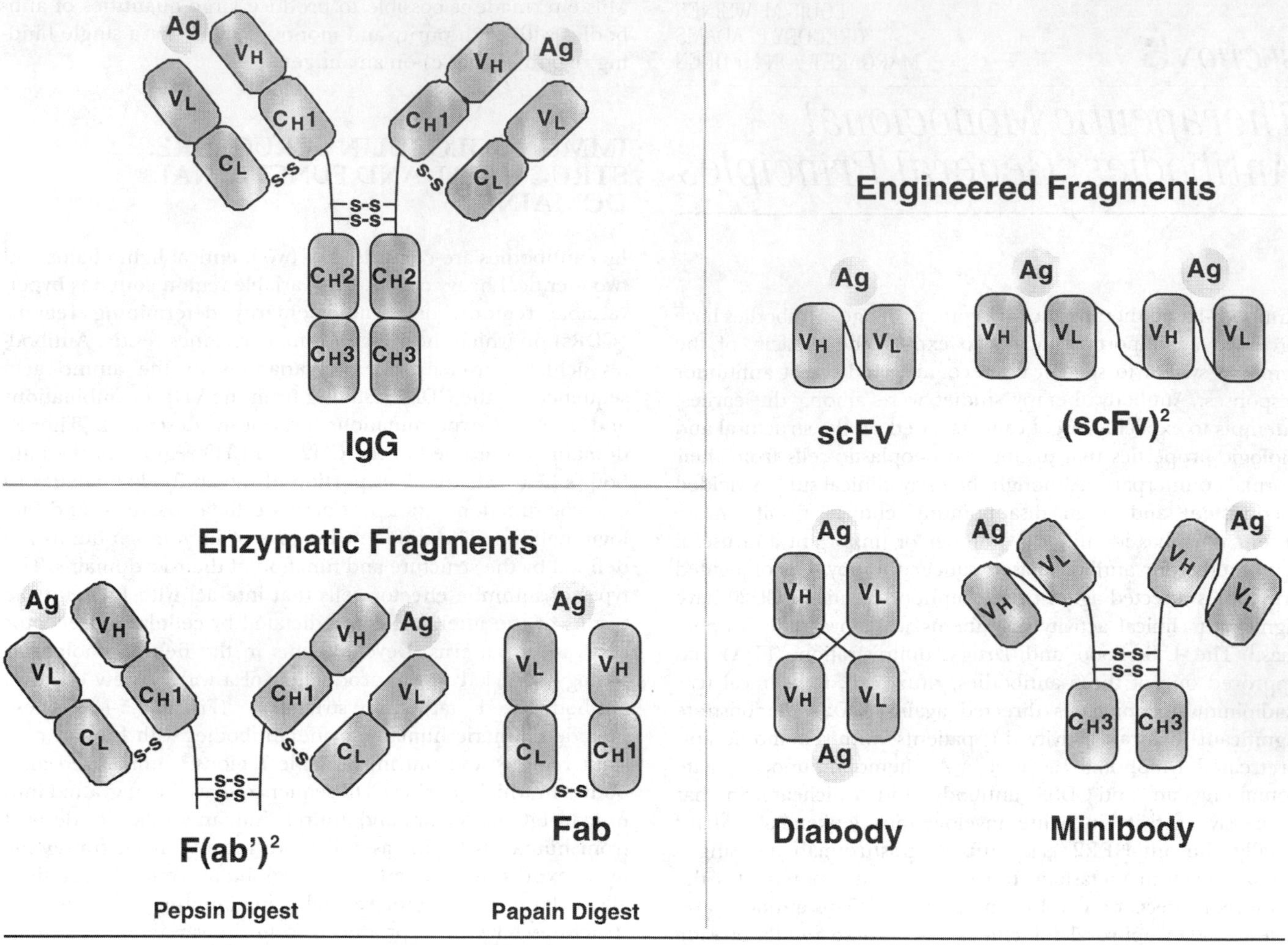

FIGURE 20.5-1. Antibody-based targeting proteins. Ag, target antigen; C, constant; Fab, fragment (of IgG involved in) antigen binding; $F(ab')_2$, fragment (of IgG) after digestion with the enzyme pepsin; H, heavy chain; IgG, immunoglobulin G; L, light chain; scFv, single-chain Fv; $(scFv)_2$, dimeric scFv; V, variable.

IMPAIRED DISTRIBUTION AND DELIVERY OF ANTIBODY TO TUMOR SITE

IgG molecules are large proteins of approximately 150 kD in mass; most chemotherapy agents have a molecular weight of less than 1 kD. Accordingly, MABs would be expected to have significantly slower kinetics of distribution and severely limited tissue penetration properties as compared to small molecules. Indeed, nonuniform uptake of systemically administered antibody is generally observed in biopsied specimens of solid tumors. Although inhomogenous tumor antigen expression can be a factor, physiologic barriers to MAB penetration bear the greatest responsibility for the limited distribution of MABs within a tumor mass. Heterogeneous tumor blood supply limits uniform antibody delivery to tumors, and elevated interstitial pressures in the centers of tumors oppose inward diffusion.[23] Furthermore, the relatively large transport distances in the tumor interstitium combine with the above factors to increase the time required for these large macromolecules to reach target cells. For example, the diffusion of an intact IgG molecule into a solid tumor is limited to 100 μm in 1 hour, 1 mm in approximately 2 days, and 1 cm in approximately 7 to 8 months.[24] These physiologic barriers pose substantial obstacles to antibody penetration in the majority of solid tumors and bulky lymphomas. Thus, it can be anticipated that the therapy of patients with large tumors using MABs will be compromised. These concepts also hold true for potentially cytotoxic leukocytes to accumulate at tumor sites; as a result, physiologic barriers can represent a major limitation to the effective clinical exploitation of ADCC.

The poor tumor penetration of MABs has been addressed by using the smaller antibody-based constructs and fragments (discussed earlier in Immunoglobulin Structure: Structural and Functional Domains). As shown in Figure 20.5-1, commonly used antibody-based structures include $F(ab')_2$ [fragment (of IgG) after digestion with the enzyme pepsin], Fab [fragment (of IgG involved in) antigen binding], and scFv molecules. These derivative structures usually exhibit binding affinity for target antigen that is of the same order of magnitude as the intact parental immunoglobulin. These molecules exhibit systemic clearance that accelerates with decreasing size. In general, the smaller molecules have the advantages of improved tumor penetration, rapid systemic clearance, and improved specificity of tumor targeting during the terminal phases of elimination. These advantages are counterbalanced by decreased quantitative tumor targeting.[25,26] The ideal size of tumor-targeting antibodies will most probably depend on the intended therapeutic application. When prolonged inhibition of a tumor-associated function is intended, larger molecules with slow clearance might be preferred, whereas the administration of a highly potent immunotoxin might be facilitated if the molecule is small and rapidly clears from normal organs.

TUMOR ANTIGENS

The properties of the tumor antigen can be a major factor in regulating the success or failure of antibody-based therapies. Heterogeneity of antigen expression by tumor cells can restrict the percentage of cells that can be reliably targeted by antibodies. This is manifested not only as the presence or absence of antigen on a cell, but also by the degree of its expression on a given cell. The density of antigen expression may be a critical determinant of therapeutic effect for a variety of antibody-based applications. The ultimate fate of a cell surface antigen (e.g., whether it is shed from the membrane or internalized) can also impact on the degree of targeting and therapeutic efficacy of an antibody. For example, large concentrations of shed antigen in the tumor microenvironment may saturate the antibody's binding sites and prevent binding to the cell surface. In contrast, a rapidly internalized antigen may deplete the quantity of cell surface MABs capable of initiating ADCC or cytotoxic signal transduction events. Finally, additional obstacles relate to the tumor specificity of the targeted antigens. Antibody targets may be *tumor-associated* or *tumor-specific*. Tumor-associated targets have most frequently been identified and typically are oncofetal antigens or overexpressed growth factor receptors with extracellular membrane domains. Tumor-associated antigens usually are relatively overexpressed on tumor cells but are found to a lesser extent on normal cellular counterparts and by other normal cells. Potential consequences of targeting this class of antigens with toxic immunoconjugates can include decreased targeting specificity and unacceptable normal tissue cytotoxicity. Tumor-specific antigens that exhibit high levels of expression limited to malignant tissue are both highly desirable and rare. Typically, these antigens arise as a result of unique genetic recombinations that are the cause or consequence of oncogenic transformation. Examples of tumor-specific antigens include clonal immunoglobulin idiotypes expressed on the surface of B-cell lymphomas[27] and tumor-specific mutations, such as the epidermal growth factor receptor (EGFR)-VIII deletion mutant of the EGFR that is present in a small proportion of tumors, including glioblastoma and non–small cell lung carcinoma.[28,29] The advent of new techniques for identifying genetic abnormalities in malignancies will no doubt uncover numerous tumor-specific mutations, some of which will provide accessible protein targets for antibody therapy.

IMMUNOLOGIC RESPONSES TO MONOCLONAL ANTIBODIES

The initial clinical trials of MABs used murine proteins produced by hybridoma technology. Treatment with murine MABs and their derivatives often induces human antimouse antibody (HAMA) responses within 2 to 3 weeks after the initial infusion. These responses, which are directed to any portion of the antibody, can impair targeting and accelerate MAB clearance. The induction of HAMA has precluded the continued successful application of MAB therapy in several instances.[30] Considerable effort has been expended to overcome HAMA by creating human or nearly human antibodies (discussed earlier in Immunoglobulin Structure: Structural and Functional Domains) or by suppressing the human immune response to the mouse MAB. As a result, the majority of the MABs currently entering the clinic bear human or humanized structures.

Although the field of antibody therapy is progressing beyond murine MABs and their associated drawbacks, analysis of the HAMA responses in clinical trials has led to the development of a novel therapeutic strategy. Although most of the HAMAs generated during these immune responses recognize conserved sequences, a small percentage of the antibodies are specific for the idiotypic or hypervariable sequences that comprise the active binding site of the antibody. Some of these antiidiotypic antibodies mimic the original antigen completely enough to be capable of inducing an immune response that is capable of reacting with the original tumor antigen.[31] Stimulation of this "idiotypic network," originally postulated by Jerne,[31] offers some specificity advantages when compared with immunization strategies that directly make use of the tumor antigens.

UNCONJUGATED ANTIBODIES

ANTIBODY-DEPENDENT CELLULAR CYTOTOXICITY

In the process of ADCC, the antibody Fab domains engage tumor antigen and the Fc domain binds to cellular Fc receptors to bridge effector and target cells. This bridging induces effector cell activation and natural killer (NK) cell–mediated cytotoxicity or phagocytosis by neutrophils, monocytes, or macrophages.[10]

In addition to rituximab and trastuzumab, many other antibodies have been clinically tested to exploit their ADCC properties, but without consistent clinical benefit in the setting of advanced disease.[32] ADCC continues to be a potent *in vitro* phenomenon that should provide a powerful antitumor mechanism, if it can be replicated or mimicked in the *in vivo* setting. Advances in the understanding of human Fc receptor and T-cell receptor structures and functions have made it possible to refine antibody-directed cellular activation strategies, particularly given the improved flexibility afforded by antibody engineering techniques. Human Fcγ and Fcα receptors can trigger cellular cytotoxicity,[33–35] as can elements of the T-cell receptor/CD3 complex,[36,37] CD28 on T cells,[38] and CD44 on NK cells.[39] It is now possible to create a wide variety of recombinantly produced antibody binding site–based targeting proteins, including IgG, $F(ab')_2$, Fab, and scFv formats, with an equally formidable choice of approaches to create multimeric, monospecific, or bispecific binding proteins. The affinity properties of the binding sites can be manipulated through chain-shuffling or site-directed mutagenesis.[40] The HAMA response can be circumvented by the production of chimeric antibodies or by the use of human antibodies prepared by fusion techniques or from human phage display libraries.[41]

BISPECIFIC ANTIBODIES

In the years since the pioneering work of Segal and colleagues,[42] numerous BsAb targeting tumor antigens and effector cell trigger molecules have been developed and shown to redirect cellular cytotoxicity. For example, BsAb can target tumor antigens and human effector cell trigger molecules on T cells via CD3/TcR[39,40,42] and CD28.[41] BsAb directed against FcγRI[36] trigger tumor cytotoxicity by neutrophils, monocytes, and macrophages. BsAb targeting FcγRIII[37,43] promote tumor lysis by macrophages and NK cells, and BsAb targeting CD44[42] promote tumor cytotoxicity by NK cells. Typically, BsAb promote *in vitro* cytotoxicity at low concentrations and have been shown to cause either growth delays or tumor regressions in appropriate animal models.[44–46] These properties have led to the testing of several BsAb in human clinical trials.

Several early reports of CD3-directed BsAb suggested possible applications in glioblastoma[46] and ovarian cancer.[47] However, subsequent trials of a number of intact CD3-directed BsAb have yielded few objective responses, and treatment has been limited by toxicities reminiscent of the first-dose effect seen with OKT3 antibody therapy. The first-dose effect is characterized by the release of massive amounts of cytokines, such as tumor necrosis factor-α (TNF-α). Treatment with an $F(ab')_2$ anti-CD3 BsAb, which is bereft of Fc domains and Fc domain–dependent cellular cross-linking properties, also has led to toxicities at low BsAb doses. This finding indicates that the engagement of some T-cell activating molecules on circulating T cells can produce unacceptable dose-limiting toxicity.[48] A series of clinical trials used the BsAb 2B1, a murine IgG that is dually specific for extracellular domain epitopes on the human tumor antigen HER2/*neu* and the human Fc receptor FcγRIII. Whereas therapy with 2B1 yielded a handful of objective responses, BsAb-induced cross-linking of Fc receptors on circulating leukocytes led to massive cytokine release and associated toxicities. 2B1-promoted antigen presentation led to the induction of anti-HER2/*neu* antibodies, but only in patients treated with 2B1 doses exceeding the ultimate maximum tolerated dose.[49,50]

The clinical experience with the MDX-210 BsAb provides a useful additional perspective to the results previously described. MDX-210 targets the same epitope on HER2/*neu* as does 2B1, and it targets human FcγRI on neutrophils and mononuclear phagocytes. In contrast to 2B1, MDX-210 is a chemically conjugated $F(ab')_2$. Because it lacks an Fc domain, MDX-210 cannot activate leukocyte Fcγ receptors in the absence of tumor antigen engagement. Like 2B1, MDX-210 is a potent mediator of *in vitro* cytotoxicity and phagocytosis. Because much higher doses of this BsAb can be given safely in comparison with 2B1, monomeric FcγRI engagement may have different consequences than do FcγR aggregation or CD3 engagement.[51] Like 2B1, MDX-210 therapy leads to antigen presentation and the induction of anti-HER2/*neu* antibodies. Again, as with 2B1, clinical responses have been seen with BsAb targeting FcγRI, and the results obtained with MDX-210 indicate that the Fc domain of a BsAb is not required for Fc receptor–dependent antigen presentation.

PROMOTION OF TUMOR INFLAMMATION

A number of strategies can be considered to promote selective tumor inflammation. Experiences with systemic cytokines have shown that the selectivity of effects at tumor sites is usually low, as evidenced by work with high-dose IL-2.[52] With IL-2 and other cytokines, such as TNF-α, toxicities caused by systemic leukocyte activation have limited the doses that can safely be administered. Several groups have attempted to address this fact by producing immunocytokines, which are composed of engineered antibodies fused to cytokines. Antibody/IL-2 fusion proteins have exhibited promising preclinical results.[25,53] However, a potential limitation to this strategy is that these large (e.g., greater than 150-kD) proteins will have relatively prolonged half-lives. As a result, functionally intact IL-2 will circulate predominantly in the vasculature, leading to systemic leukocyte activation that at least partially offsets any targeting advantages conferred by the antibody binding property. Less progress has been reported regarding the creation of antibody-targeted vasoactive or chemotactic conjugates or fusion proteins. Conjugates containing antibody binding sites and F-M-L-P[54] and RANTES[55] have been reported but have not undergone extensive preclinical testing or clinical trials.

Several antibodies that have been used clinically are capable of fixing serum complement, and this mechanism of action has been postulated to be relevant to the *in vivo* mechanisms of action of antibodies directed against gangliosides and against CD20 as well, as discussed in the section on Antiganglioside Antibodies.

GROWTH FACTOR RECEPTOR SIGNALING PERTURBATION

Antibodies directed against selected growth factor receptors, such as the EGFR, directly inhibit the growth of receptor-bearing tumors *in vitro* and *in vivo*, and they synergize with a number of antineoplastic agents. EGFR is overexpressed on many cancers. The receptor and its ligands, EGF and TGF-α, act in an autocrine loop to stimulate the growth of breast cancer cells. *In vitro*, some anti-EGFR antibodies have been shown to inhibit the binding of the receptor ligands.[56,57] Antibodies that block the binding of EGFR ligands limit receptor activation by tyrosine kinases and inhibit growth of normal fibroblasts,[58] as well as tumor cells in culture.[59] Also, combining anti-EGFR antibodies with cisplatin leads to a significant decrease in the IC_{50} (concentration that inhibits 50%) of cisplatin,[60] and cures of established tumors are seen when anti-EGFR antibodies are combined with cisplatin[61] or doxorubicin.[62] *In vitro* and *in vivo* studies also have suggested anti-EGFR antibodies may lead to terminal differentiation of squamous cell carcinoma cells, with accumulation of cells in G_0 to G_1 phases of the cell cycle and expression of cell surface markers, such as involucrin and cytokeratin-10.[63]

The anti-EGFR antibody MAB225 blocks *in vitro* phosphorylation of the EGFR and induces receptor internalization, as occurs with binding of the natural ligand.[64] However, receptor processing is slower with antibody engagement than with natural ligand engagement.[65] Smaller bivalent $F(ab')_2$ and univalent Fab forms of this antibody also inhibit growth and decrease receptor phosphorylation, although the bivalent form is superior to the monovalent form.[66] Because the smaller fragments lead to tumor regressions, the efficacy of antibody therapy is not dependent on ADCC, as these smaller fragments lack the Fc portion of the antibody required for ADCC. Rather, the efficacy of this antibody is due to its ability to inhibit binding of the natural ligand, limit receptor phosphorylation, and thus downstream signals, and induce receptor internalization.

The chimeric form of MAB225, C225, has been evaluated *in vitro* and *in vivo* in hormone-sensitive and hormone-refractory prostate cancer.[67] EGF is a strong chemoattractant for prostate cancer cells. Blocking the EGFR receptor with C225 *in vitro* results in decreased migration of prostate cancer cells in a dose-dependent manner due to decreased phosphorylation of the EGFR.[68] This antibody also has been shown to lead to cell-cycle arrest and decreased proliferation of prostate cancer cells.[69,70] The binding of C225 to the EGFR results in multiple events leading to a decrease in proliferation and, possibly, decreased metastatic potential in prostate cancer. Preclinical animal models also have suggested a potential therapeutic role for anti-EGF antibodies in combination with radiation therapy for the treatment of gliomas.[71] Other studies have demonstrated increased efficacy with topotecan,[72] antisense oligonucleotides targeting CRIPTO[73] and protein kinase A,[74] and Trastuzomab.[75] C225 also has been shown to have antiangiogenic properties.[76]

C225 has been tested in phase I studies in recurrent head and neck cancer in combination with cisplatin. Four of seven patients exhibited clinical responses.[77] The safety of C225 in combination with radiation therapy has been documented in head and neck carcinoma in preliminary reports.[78]

ICR62, a rat monoclonal IgG, has been shown *in vitro* to block binding of the ligands of EGFR, inhibit growth of tumor cell lines that overexpress EGFR, and to cause differentiation of malignant cells to a normal phenotype. This antibody was evaluated in a phase I trial of patients with squamous head and neck and lung cancer. Evidence was found of localization of antibody to tumor sites at doses of 40 to 100 mg, accompanied by the development of anti-rat antibodies.[79] Another anti-EGFR antibody, RG 83853, has been used to treat patients with non–small cell lung cancer and head and neck cancer in a phase I setting. In this study, patients received up to 600 mg/m^2 by continuous infusion over 5 days without significant toxicity.[80] Saturation of at least 50% of the EGFR was noted at doses of 200 mg/m^2 or more. EGFR-expressing tumor cells demonstrate increased sensitivity to chemotherapy[81] and to radiation therapy[82] in the presence of EGF. In two of five patients with pre- and posttherapy biopsies of tumor, evidence was found for increased tyrosine kinase activity of EGFR, providing a rationale for combined modality therapy.

Similar strategies have been developed for MAB directed against another member of the EGFR family, the HER2/*neu* (c-erbB-2) receptor, as discussed later in the section Breast Cancer. It has been shown that intracellular antibodies can interfere with the expression of proteins that are critical for the maintenance of the neoplastic phenotype. For example, Curiel and coworkers[83] have packaged the gene for an anti–c-erbB-2 antibody in viral vectors and infected c-erbB-2–expressing tumor cells *in vitro* and *in vivo.* The infected cells express the encoded antibody, which is engineered to contain signals for its retention in the endoplasmic reticulum of the target cells. This approach efficiently inhibits c-erbB-2 expression and exhibits potent antitumor activity in preclinical models.[83]

ANTIIDIOTYPE ANTIBODIES

MAB can be used as the basis for creating tumor vaccines by inducing the idiotypic network. The antigen-combining site of each antibody, the idiotype, is a unique, clonally derived structure that stimulates the production of a series of host antibodies, some of which bind to the idiotype. Accordingly, an idiotype-containing antibody (i.e., Ab1) that binds to a tumor antigen induces the production of antiidiotype antibodies (i.e., Ab2).[36] Ab1 can be used to immunize mice and create Ab2-secreting hybridomas. The resulting Ab2, a portion of which contains a surrogate tumor epitope recognized by the Ab1, can be used to immunize patients, leading to the production of anti-antiidiotype antibodies (i.e., Ab3) that in part bind to the tumor epitope against which the Ab1 was directed. Based on this idiotypic network put forth by Lindenmann and Jerne,[31] various investigators have created antiidiotypic antibodies to serve as vaccines.[84–86] Antiidiotype antibody strategies that mimic a number of tumor antigens have been generated and are under investigation as cancer vaccines. This approach offers the practical advantages of an abundant supply of highly purified immunogen that stimulates an immune response against carefully defined tumor antigen epitopes. This approach may be preferable to immunization with tumor antigens, because the immune response to the whole antigen may include reactivity with epitopes on the antigen that are shared by other structures that are not selectively expressed by tumors.

Results are available for several clinical trials of antiidiotype antibodies. Herlyn and colleagues[87] treated 30 patients with advanced colorectal carcinoma with serial injections of polyclonal goat antibody induced by immunizations with murine 17-1A MAB. Six patients experienced brief clinical responses, and all 30 developed antibodies directed against the immunizing goat antibody.[87] Mittelman and colleagues[88] treated 15 patients with metastatic melanoma using a murine antiidiotype MAB directed against an antibody recognizing a high-molecular-weight human melanoma–associated antigen. Seven of these patients developed Ab3, and three patients exhibited partial responses (PRs) to therapy.[88] Similar findings have been observed using antibodies directed against the carcinoembryonic antigen (CEA) system.[89] It is noteworthy that these strategies induce not only the desired immunologic responses, but also possess clinical activity in some patients with advanced solid tumors. If these results hold up with further testing, this general strategy will merit testing in the adjuvant, high-risk setting.

An antiidiotypic antibody, created using an antibody directed against the gp72 antigen, has been used to treat patients with advanced colorectal cancer,[90] as well as rectal cancer patients in an adjuvant setting.[91] The antibody 105AD7 was produced by fusion of plasma cells from patients treated with an anti-gp72 antibody 791T/36 with EL41, a mouse-human heterohybrid. The 105AD7 hybridoma was found to produce a human IgG1 that bound to the binding site of the 791T/36 antibody. In 13 patients with metastatic colorectal cancer treated with the vaccine, survival was 12 months as compared to 4 months for patients in a contemporary control cohort; the significance of this increase in survival is unknown because this was not a prospectively randomized study. *In vitro* immunologic correlates demonstrated evidence of cellular responses as indicated by lymphocyte proliferation to gp72-expressing tumor cells and IL-2 production. In the adjuvant setting, six patients were vaccinated preoperatively. In a follow-up study, the immunologic responses and progression-free survival rate in patients were superior in patients who received a 100-μg versus a 200-μg dose of vaccine.[92]

Foon[89,93] has evaluated an anti-idiotypic vaccine strategy for CEA expressing tumors. The antiidiotypic antibody 3H1 was derived from a murine antibody that targets a highly restricted epitope of CEA, which is not found on normal adult tissues or hematopoietic cells. Patients with advanced colorectal cancer treated with 3H1 injections developed both humoral and cellular responses against CEA.[89] This response was not abrogated by concurrent chemotherapy.[93] An ongoing phase II randomized study is evaluating 3H1 plus granulocyte-macrophage colony-stimulating factor (GM-CSF), or alum-precipitated 3H1 antibody with GM-CSF, in patients with stage II or stage III colorectal cancer. This trial is the first to evaluate an antibody as a vaccine in the adjuvant setting. Patients were found to have a cellular, but not a humoral, response to the immunization.

The impact of antiidiotypic vaccines remains to be clarified. Most of the vaccines use nonhuman antibodies for the vaccine, which may help stimulate an immune response against the antibody. However, as has been seen with intravenously administered antibodies, multiple administrations of the antiidiotype vaccine may be limited by the immune response against the constant regions of the antibody (e.g., HAMA response). Also, although *in vitro* data supporting the induction immune responses have been demonstrated, no clear evidence exists for the induction of clinically meaningful responses. Clinical trials with various antibodies have demonstrated antiidiotypic cascades after therapy.[53] There are also examples of antibodies with specificity for the tumor antigen that are being used as vaccines.[94–96] The infused antibody may allow for *in vivo* immunization, and the induction of these antiidiotypic antibodies may serve to amplify the antigenic stimulus to the immune system. For example, ovarian and breast cancer patients receiving high-dose chemotherapy followed by stem cell transplantation have been immunized with Theratope STn-KLH, an antibody directed against a MUC-1 epitope. Eleven of 26 patients developed STn-specific T-cell responses.[97] It remains to be determined if such responses are components of therapeutic responses.

IMMUNOCONJUGATES

The use of antibodies as "magic bullets" has captured the scientific and public imagination for some time. In contrast to the immunologically oriented strategies already described, antibodies used in immunoconjugates are designed to provide targeting specificity to cytotoxic processes. The toxic payloads used in clinically tested immunoconjugates have included catalytic toxins, chemotherapy agents, and radionuclides.

RADIOIMMUNOCONJUGATES

To a large extent, both immunotoxins and drug immunoconjugates kill by single-cell mechanisms. Thus, less opportunity exists for the destruction of "innocent bystander" antigen-negative tumor cells at the tumor site. Radioimmunoconjugates address this potential deficiency by virtue of the long track lengths of many of the commonly used radionuclides, so that toxic effects can extend over several cell diameters from the radiation source. Most radioimmunoconjugates do not require internalization to be effective, and the cytotoxic effects do not require the presence of an intact, functional immune system. Radioimmunotherapy (RIT) has been the most extensively studied immunoconjugate treatment strategy and has been the source of several exciting clinical results, particularly in the treatment of chemotherapy-refractory lymphomas. In the past, most RIT studies used iodine 131, but improvements in chelation technology have enabled the study of yttrium 90 conjugates. ^{90}Y is preferred because of its long track length, high-energy β-emissions, lack of volatility, and the relative ease and safety of its conjugation to antibodies and subsequent patient administration.

Early studies of RIT have shown that partial, short-lived clinical responses can be achieved in some patients with advanced, solid tumors. Hematologic neoplasms are more responsive than are solid tumors. Bone marrow suppression is the common dose-limiting toxicity of RIT. The HAMA response can limit the use of multiple rounds of RIT in some patients. Lymphomas and leukemias remain the most sensitive tumor targets for RIT, presumably because of their intrinsic sensitivity to radiation and the relatively good access of radioimmunoconjugates to the malignant cells that comprise these neoplasms. Patients with hematologic neoplasms are less likely to mount HAMA responses and frequently can be re-treated with MAB.

IMMUNOTOXINS

One approach to immunoconjugates involves coupling MAB (or fragments) to highly lethal cellular toxins. A number of plant and bacterial catalytic toxins have been used, but most clinical trials to date have been conducted using immunotoxins containing either the plant toxin ricin or the bacterially derived *Pseudomonas* exotoxin. These toxins require transport and intracellular processing to exert their effects and, generally, act by inhibiting protein synthesis via interruption of ribosomal elongation factor-2. Toxins of this type are extremely efficient and potent and usually contain two chains. One chain facilitates cell binding and intracellular transport, whereas the other chain is responsible for the catalytic activity of the toxin. Substituting an antibody binding domain for the cell binding chain of the toxin creates immunotoxins. The antibody specificity directs the cellular targeting of the catalytic chain of the toxin. Immunotoxins have been prepared by chemical conjugation of antibodies or their fragments to the catalytic toxin chains, or by the creation of recombinant fusion proteins linking either Fab or sFv antibody fragments to native or modified catalytic toxin chains. Nanomolar concentrations of immunotoxins are capable of eradicating tumor cells *in vitro*, and low doses are extremely effective in preclinical animal models.

Clinical trials have been performed using immunotoxins in patients with breast cancer, ovarian cancer, colorectal cancer, melanoma, and lymphoproliferative disorders. In a landmark study, Vitetta and colleagues[98] treated 14 patients with B-cell lymphoma using an anti-CD22 MAB conjugated to ricin A chain and observed clinical responses in five patients. In a separate study, patients with B-cell lymphomas were treated using a continuous infusion of an immunotoxin composed of an anti-CD19 MAB conjugated to whole ricin with a blocked B chain, so that the toxin's entrance into cells was conferred solely by the antibody binding specificity. In 34 patients with B-cell neoplasms, two complete and three PRs were noted.[99]

The results of trials in patients with solid tumors have been less impressive. Toxicities have limited the doses of immunotoxins that have been used, and such dose limits must be overcome before the full therapeutic benefit of this highly potent therapy approach can be obtained. These toxicities include vascular leak syndrome, fevers, rigors, malaise, occasional hepatotoxicity, rhabdomyolysis, and rare but potentially devastating central nervous system effects. These effects are thought to arise from unintended uptake of the toxins by normal cells and can be caused by low levels of targeted antigen expression by such cells, or by poorly understood nonspecific uptake. Further improvements in toxin selection and design, coupled with more knowledgeable selections of tumor antigen targets and the development of recombinant antibody-based proteins, are likely to address many of the impediments to effective therapy that have been observed to date.[100] It may prove more difficult to overcome the potent human antitoxin immune response that these plant or bacterial proteins elicit. However, overcoming this response is necessary to permit multiple cycles of therapy.

CHEMOIMMUNOCONJUGATES

One of the major potential advantages of immunotoxins is that such toxins work catalytically, so that the antitumor effects can be amplified *in situ.* Paradoxically, the potent toxicity of these molecules may make it difficult to identify an appropriate therapeutic window that permits efficacy within the tolerable host range. An alternate strategy is to use antibody-based targeting to deliver conventional chemotherapy agents to tumor sites. These molecules have well-understood pharmacology and can be administered safely in native form, so that it should be feasible to administer high, tumor-cytotoxic doses of antibody-conjugated agent within acceptable host toxicity ranges. For example, promising preclinical results were obtained using the immunoconjugate BR96-doxorubicin, with exceptional activity *in vitro* and in a variety of preclinical rodent models.[101] This agent has been examined in a series of phase I clinical trials, and the dose-limiting toxicity was gastritis, possibly related to the Fc domain of the intact IgG BR96 molecule.[102] More recently, highly potent calicheamicin-antibody conjugates have been tested in leukemia and other cancers and are undergoing clinical evaluation.[103,104]

THERAPEUTIC APPLICATIONS

HEMATOLOGIC MALIGNANCIES

Initial studies using antibodies directed against B-cell determinants showed that the passive administration of these antibodies led to clearance of circulating tumor cells and rare objective clinical responses.[105] In a series of landmark studies, Levy and colleagues[106] prepared customized antibodies reactive with a given lymphoma patient's idiotype that was uniquely expressed on the surface of the malignant B-cell clone. Each patient's idiotype served as a tumor-specific signature that could be targeted by a customized MAB. The procedures for preparing such antibodies for each patient were laborious, but approximately 50% of treated patients experienced significant clinical responses, with some patients achieving durable complete remissions.[106] The addition of chemotherapy agents, interferon (IFN), or other cytokines did not appreciably improve treatment outcomes. Effective therapy had to overcome circulating lymphoma idiotype proteins that diverted antibodies from their cellular targets, and resistance to therapy resulted in part from the emergence of idiotype-negative variants. The mechanisms underlying responses to these antibodies have not been completely elucidated, but may include mechanisms such as ADCC and perturbation of signal transduction through idiotype engagement.[107] Because of the immunosuppression of lymphoma patients, relatively few patients developed HAMAs that interfered with repeated therapeutic antibody administration. This exciting approach was very cumbersome, because it required the generation of patient-customized reagents. These results could not be replicated by using antibodies that recognize shared idiotypes expressed by a large proportion of lymphoma patients.[108] Despite this set of impediments, these important observations have informed much of the subsequent work in this field.

Other antibodies directed against B-cell surface determinants have been developed and clinically tested. For example, Lym-1 recognizes an HLA-DR10 determinant and promotes ADCC. Clinical trials with this antibody have shown interesting response profiles in low-, intermediate-, and high-grade lymphoma, respectively.[109]

CAMPATH-1

The CAMPATH-1 antibody has specificity for CD52, a glycopeptide that is highly expressed on T and B lymphocytes. It has been tested as a therapeutic agent for chronic lymphocytic and promyelocytic leukemias, as well as other non-Hodgkin's lymphomas, and as a means to deplete T cells from allogeneic transplantation grafts. One-half of the patients with fludarabine-resistant chronic lymphocytic leukemia or B-prolymphocytic leukemia exhibited clinical responses to CAMPATH-1.[110]

A phase II multicenter study of CAMPATH-1H in previously treated patients with low-grade non-Hodgkin's lymphomas has been reported.[111] Fifty patients with relapsed or refractory disease were treated with 30 mg of CAMPATH-1H three times weekly for up to 12 weeks. Infection, anemia, and thrombocytopenia were common, and myocardial infarction occurred in a patient with a prior history of angina and congestive heart failure. A 16% PR rate and a 4% complete response (CR) rate were reported, for an overall response rate of 20%. Responses were short in duration, with a median time to progression of 4 months. Patients with mycosis fungoides responded more frequently and had a longer time to progression (10 months) than did patients with low-grade non-Hodgkin's lymphoma (4 months). Treatment was associated with reactivation of herpes simplex, oral candidiasis, *Pneumocystis carinii* pneumonia, cytomegalovirus pneumonitis, pulmonary aspergillosis, disseminated tuberculosis, and seven cases of pneumonia and septicemia.

CAMPATH-1 has been used to deplete T cells from allogeneic transplantation grafts in patients with hematologic malignancies.[112,113] The initial study suggested that the addition of CAMPATH-1 can significantly decrease graft rejection and graft-versus-host disease compared with conventional therapy. However, the frequency of graft rejection and graft failure may be higher. A retrospective review of patients with acute lymphocytic leukemia or AML who underwent allogeneic transplantation with CAMPATH-1–purged marrow suggested no impact on the graft-versus-leukemia effect, because no increase in leukemia relapse was found.[114] Additionally, the development of Epstein-Barr virus–related lymphoproliferative disorders was decreased in allogeneic transplantation patients who had T-cell depletion with CAMPATH-1 therapy compared with other methods of T-cell depletion (e.g., E-rosettes or other MABs).[115] CAMPATH-1 eliminates B cells within the graft, thus eliminating a potential reservoir of Epstein-Barr virus or targets for subsequent infection.

Anti-CD20 Antibodies

The testing and evaluation of the chimeric anti-CD20 antibody, IDEC-C2B8, also known as *rituximab*, has led to significant excitement within the field.[116,117] Rituximab was the first antibody therapy approved by the FDA for use in treating human malignancy. Other anti-CD20 antibodies had demonstrated responses of low-grade non-Hodgkin's lymphomas; however, therapy was limited because of the induction of HAMAs. By reducing immunogenicity through the substitution of human for murine constant domain sequences, rituximab allows for the safe administration of multiple doses of therapy. The phase I study that set out to determine the maximum tolerated dose used four weekly infusions.[119] Thrombocytopenia and B-cell lymphocytopenia were observed. The lymphocytopenia persisted for 3 to 6 months. Six of 18 patients (33%) demonstrated PRs. Phase II studies using the maximum tolerated dose, 375 mg/m^2, confirmed the efficacy of this therapy, demonstrating 46% and 48% response rates in two separate studies.[118,119] Although the numbers of circulating B cells were reduced by therapy, no changes were documented in serum immunoglobulin levels. Bacterial and viral infections were seen in patients with relapsed indolent lymphomas, but in contrast to the CAMPATH-1 experience, treatment with rituximab did not result in significant morbidity due to infections. However, patients with small lymphocytic B-cell lymphoma had lower response rates, likely related to the lesser expression of CD20 on these tumor cells. A different multiinstitutional phase II study using a 375-mg/m^2 dose for eight weekly treatments in low-grade or follicular non-Hodgkin's lymphoma with relapsed or primary refractory disease also demonstrated minimal toxicity, with an overall response rate of 57%.[120]

In another phase II trial, 54 patients with relapsing or refractory diffuse large B-cell lymphoma, mantle cell lymphoma, or other intermediate- or high-grade B-cell non-Hodgkin's lymphomas were treated.[121] The study randomized patients to either eight weekly treatments of 375 mg/m^2 intravenous rituximab, or to 375 mg/m^2 rituximab intravenously in week 1 followed by seven weekly intravenous infusions of 500 mg/m^2. Five CRs and 12 PRs were observed, for an overall response rate of 31%; no evidence of superiority of either treatment regimen was demonstrated. Patients with refractory disease and those with histologies other than diffuse large B-cell lymphoma appeared to have lower response rates.

Peak levels of circulating antibody inversely correlate with pretreatment B-cell counts and the bulk of tumor.[121,122] Greater numbers of peripheral lymphocytes or larger tumor bulk serve as an antigen sink and therefore remove antibody from the circulation. For patients with bulky disease, future consideration of a higher antibody dose or a greater number of cycles may be warranted, because patients with lower serum antibody concentrations have had statistically significant lower response rates. In some patients with circulating blood tumor cells, however, rituximab therapy has induced an infusion-related syndrome characterized by fever, rigors, thrombocytopenia, tumor lysis, bronchospasm, and hypoxemia requiring discontinuation of the antibody infusion. Symptoms typically resolve with supportive care, and patients may continue further therapy without sequelae.[122] Another case report has documented rapid tumor lysis in a patient with B-cell chronic lymphocytic leukemia with a pretreatment lymphocytosis of more than 100×10^9 cells per liter.[123]

Rituximab therapy rarely selects for the emergence of an antigen-negative population of tumor cells. This phenomenon has been documented in a patient with a follicular mixed small and large cell lymphoma treated with rituximab after progression through multiple chemotherapy regimens.[124]

Rituximab has been tested in conjunction with chemotherapy.[125] Preclinical data have shown this antibody can sensitize chemotherapy-resistant cell lines to the cytotoxic effects of chemotherapy.[126] Forty patients with low-grade or follicular B-cell non-Hodgkin's lymphoma received six cycles of the cyclophosphamide, doxorubicin, vincristine, and prednisone (CHOP) regimen every 21 days, with six infusions of rituximab at a dose of 375 mg/m^2 given before, during, and after the completion of chemotherapy. Thirty-eight patients received therapy, with three patients not completing treatment because of intercurrent infections (n = 2) and patient choice (n = 1). The overall response rate was 95% (38 of 40) with a 55% CR and a 40% PR, with fewer CRs noted in patients with bulky disease. Median response duration and time to progression had not been reached after more than 29 months of follow-up. Seven of eight patients initially positive for the bcl-2 translocation became negative for the translocation by polymerase chain reaction assay after therapy; this finding has not been seen previously with CHOP chemotherapy alone.[127]

Unconjugated antibodies directed against CD20 and other B-lymphocyte antigens have exhibited exciting and clinically important antitumor activity in patients with low-grade lymphomas (Table 20.5-1).[128]

Radiolabeled Antibodies

Press and colleagues[2,129] used high, marrow-ablative RIT doses in patients with biodistributions that predicted favorable tumor dosimetry within tolerable host toxicity ranges in the setting of autologous bone marrow transplantation. In a group of 42 patients with chemotherapy-refractory lymphomas, 24 had favorable biodistributions and 19 received high-dose RIT. A remarkable 84% of these patients experienced complete remissions, and

TABLE 20.5-1. Antibody Therapy of B-Cell Lymphomas: Selected Results

Treatment	*References*
Unconjugated	
Antiidiotype	Miller[106]; Vuist[107]; Swisher[108]
CAMPATH-1	Bowen[110]; Lundin[111]
Anti-CD26	Shih[128]
Rituximab	Maloney[1,116,117]; McLaughlin[118]; Berinstein[119]; Piro[120]; Coiffier[121]; Jensen[123]; Davis[124]; Czuczman[125]; Demiden[126]
Interleukin-2 receptor	Waldmann[143]; Junghans[144]
Radiolabeled conjugates	
Iodine 131 B1	Kaminski[3,131]; Press[2,129]; Liu[132]
Yttrium 90 C2B8	Knox[133]
Iodine 131 Lym-1	DeNardo[134,135]
Immunotoxins	
Anti-CD19 dgA	Vitetta[98]
Blocked ricin A chain	Grossbard[99]

an additional 11% had partial remissions. More recent updates suggest that many of the complete remissions are durable, with a 62% progression-free survival rate at 2 years. Preliminary studies in patients with AML suggest that RIT may be useful as a conditioning regimen before bone marrow transplantation.[130]

These exciting results illustrate the potential of RIT in appropriately selected patients, and they certainly contradict any pessimism regarding the role of antibody-based targeted therapeutics in the management of cancer. Further advancements in antibody design, chelation chemistry, choice of radioligand, and selection of appropriate candidates and clinical setting for therapy can be safely predicted to expanded indications for antibody-based RIT in the treatments of patients with hematologic neoplasms.

^{131}I-B1 (anti-CD20) treatment has caused 50% and 79% CR rates for patients with chemotherapy-refractory B-cell lymphoma treated with low-dose nonmyeloablative[3,131] and high-dose ablative[2,132] RIT followed by autologous transplantation, respectively. The median CR duration of a single nonmyeloablative dose was 16.5 months. Patients were pretreated with unlabeled anti-CD20 to enhance the targeting of ^{131}I-B1 to tumor by prolonging blood and whole body radioisotope clearance through the saturation of nonspecific binding sites, nonmalignant B cells, and other potential antigenic sinks.[3] CD20 antigen does not internalize after antibody binding, allowing for extended retention of intact ^{131}I-B1 at the targeted cell. Minimal myelosuppression was observed in all patients treated at nonmyeloablative doses.[3,134] Toxicity in the high-dose trials[2,132] was modest compared to total body irradiation. The myeloablative doses delivered less than 27.25 Gy to dose-limiting normal organs. Further dose escalation was limited by cardiopulmonary toxicity. Sixty percent of patients have developed elevated thyroid-stimulating hormone levels, and 2 of 29 patients have developed second malignancies (bladder and colon cancer) several years after therapy. Acute leukemias or myelodysplastic syndromes have been documented at a median of 42 months after therapy.[132] Responses have been attributed to the tumoricidal effects of the MAB itself and to the selective delivery of irradiation by the radiolabeled MAB. The murine anti-CD20 antibody C2B8, which was chimerized to create rituximab, has been conjugated to ^{90}Y, and the resulting radioimmunoconjugate has shown impressive antitumor activity in patients with chemotherapy-refractory B-cell lymphomas.[133]

Therapy with ^{131}I Lym-1 in phase I/II clinical trials has shown significant antitumor activity as well. Low-dose fractionated treatment of 30 patients (25 with non-Hodgkin's lymphoma, five with chronic lymphocytic leukemia) resulted in three CRs and 14 PRs.[134] At the nonmyeloablative maximally tolerated dose of 100 mCi/m^2, 11 of 21 patients exhibited clinical responses.[135]

CD33 is expressed on most myeloid leukemic blasts and leukemic progenitor cells. This tumor-associated antigen is also present on committed normal myelomonocytic and erythroid progenitor cells and is expressed at low levels on early hematopoietic stem cells. M195, a murine anti-CD33 MAB, has been used to deliver therapeutic doses of ^{131}I in combination with busulfan or cyclophosphamide to eliminate residual leukemia before bone marrow transplantation.[136] More recently, a humanized form of M195, HuM195, has been radiolabeled and used as a single agent in the treatment of AML and chronic myeloid leukemia. In these studies, 8 of 12 patients treated with ^{90}Y-conjugated MAB and 13 of 18 patients treated with bismuth 213–conjugated MAB exhibited minor responses.[137,138]

Other Approaches

CD15 and CD33 have been used as targets in AMLs.[139,140] PM-81, or MDX-11, is an IgM with specificity for CD15.[133] It was evaluated before induction therapy in patients with AML. The number of peripheral blasts decreased transiently. Two patients at the highest dose level, 1.5 mg/m^2, had grade 4 toxicities of hypotension or rhabdomyolysis. Unconjugated HuM195 recognizes CD33.[142] Patients with persistent disease after chemotherapy were treated with daily infusions 4 days a week for 2 weeks. One of ten patients had a CR. More recently, this antibody has been conjugated to a recombinant form of gelonin, a single-chain plant catalytic toxin that inactivates the 60S ribosomal subunit.[141] *In vitro* experiments using HuM195-rGel with CD33-expressing AML cell lines, as well as primary cultures of human AML blasts, demonstrated effective cell killing. There was also enhanced killing of AML blasts after exposure to HuM195-rGel for 24 hours followed by freeze thawing of cells compared with freeze thawing alone. This approach may have applicability in purging autologous bone morrow products for transplantation, particularly because CD33 is not expressed on stem cells.[142]

Anti-Tac is a MAB that recognizes the IL-2 receptor. Infection with human T-cell leukemia virus type I can result in the development of adult T-cell leukemia. The majority of leukemic blasts in adult T-cell leukemia have been found to express large numbers of IL-2 receptor. Waldmann and colleagues[143] reported on the use of anti-Tac for treatment of patients with adult T-cell leukemia. Of 19 treated patients, four PRs, two CRs, and seven mixed responses were reported. Responding patients also demonstrated a lowering of elevated calcium levels. The Tac receptor can be shed in the serum and decrease the available unbound anti-Tac antibody available for binding at the tumor site.[143] However, the antibody can be exchanged from soluble Tac to tumor-bound Tac.[144] This antibody may have therapeutic potential in other hematologic disorders, such as T- and B-cell leukemia, myelogenous leukemia derived from monocytes and granulocytes, hairy cell leukemia, Hodgkin's disease, and histiocytic and mixed cell diffuse lymphoma, all of which overexpress IL-2 receptors.

SOLID TUMORS

Breast Cancer

HER-2/*neu* (c-erbB-2), a member of the EGFR family, has been targeted for antibody therapy because it is overexpressed on 25% of adenocarcinomas. Recombinant human MAB (rhuMAB) HER-2[145], also known as *trastuzumab*, is a humanized antibody derived from 4D5, a murine MAB that recognizes HER-2/*neu*. In a phase II trial in women with metastatic breast cancer, Basegla and associates[5] reported an objective response rate of 11.6%, with responses seen in the liver, mediastinum, lymph nodes, and chest wall metastases. Patients typically received ten or more treatments with the antibody, and none developed an antibody response against trastuzumab.[5] Cobleigh and coworkers[146] treated 222 women with metastatic breast cancer, finding an objective response rate of 16%. The median response duration

TABLE 20.5-2. Selected 17-1A Clinical Trials

Phase	*Dose and Schedule*	*Disease*	*Number of Patients*	*Responses*	*References*
I	25–200 mg IV	Met GI	4	1 MR	Sears[150]
I	15–1000 mg IV	Met GI	20	3 CR	Sears[153]
I	400 mg IV + FAM chemotherapy	Pancreas	16	2 PR	Paul[151]
I	400 mg IV	Pancreas	25	4	Sindelar[152]
II	500 mg IV t.i.w. × 8 wk	Pancreas	28	1 PR	Weiner[154]
II	400 mg IV day 3 + GM-CSF days 1–10	Colorectal	20	2 CR	Ragnhammar[155]
II	150 mg IV days 2–4 + IFN-γ days 1–4 IV	Colorectal	19	None	Weiner[180]
II	150 mg IV days 2–4 + IFN-γ days 1–4 IV	Pancreas	30	1 CR	Tempero[156]
III	500 mg IV × 1, then 100 mg IV q4wk × 4	Dukes' C colorectal	189	Improved DFS and OS	Riethmuller[163]

CR, complete response; DFS, disease-free survival; FAM, 5-fluorouracil, Adriamycin, and mitomycin; GI, gastrointestinal; GM-CSF, granulocyte-macrophage colony-stimulating factor; IFN-γ, interferon-γ; MR, minor response; NR, not reported; OS, overall survival; PR, partial response.

was 9.1 months with a median overall survival rate of 13 months, which is superior to results reported for second-line chemotherapy in metastatic breast cancer.[146]

Preclinical data with trastuzumab suggested enhanced clinical activity in combination with cisplatin chemotherapy. A phase II study in patients with chemotherapy-refractory breast cancer that overexpressed HER2/*neu* has been completed.[147] Nine of 37 assessable patients achieved a PR, and nine additional patients exhibited a minor response or stable disease. The median response duration was 3.3 months. Toxicities were largely attributable to cisplatin. No evidence was found for cisplatin-related alteration of antibody pharmacokinetics.

A large, randomized, phase III trial comparing cytotoxic chemotherapy alone or with trastuzumab (anti-HER-2/*neu*) has been completed.[148] Patients receiving initial therapy for metastatic breast cancer were treated with doxorubicin or epirubicin and cyclophosphamide, or with paclitaxel if they had received an anthracycline in the adjuvant setting. Patients were randomized to receive chemotherapy alone or in combination with weekly antibody therapy. The addition of trastuzumab improved response rates for combination therapy from 42.1% to 64.9% for the anthracycline-based regimens and from 25.0% to 57.3% for the taxane regimen. Myocardial dysfunction seen with anthracycline therapy was observed with increased frequency in patients receiving antibody alone[149] or with doxorubicin or epirubicin, and therefore trastuzumab is not recommended in combination with anthracyclines.

Colorectal Cancer

Ep-CAM is a glycoprotein normally found on the basolateral surface of the nonsquamous epithelium of the lung, gastrointestinal tract, pancreas, ovary, kidney, sweat glands, biliary tract, and thymus. Most recently it has been detected in prostatic intraepithelial neoplasia and prostatic adenocarcinoma. 17-1A, a murine antibody that targets an extracellular epitope of this antigen, has undergone extensive clinical trials in metastatic colorectal cancer and pancreatic cancer as a single agent,[150–154] or in combination with GM-CSF[155] or IFN-γ.[156]

The therapeutic administration of 17-1A also has been shown to induce potentially effective antiidiotypic antibodies[157–159] with increased titers when GM-CSF was coadministered with the 17-1A.[160] T-cell responses against antiidiotypic epitopes have been demonstrated by *in vitro* proliferation assays, IFN-γ production, and *in vivo* delayed-type hypersensitivity responses.[161] In a small study of ten patients, those with T-cell proliferation against antiidiotypic antibodies demonstrated clinical responses, contrasting with patients without a T-cell response who had no clinical response.[159]

Initial phase I studies with 17-1A demonstrated occasional responses in metastatic cancers of the gastrointestinal tract after only one intravenous dose of antibody. Therapy was well tolerated, with mild side effects of nausea, vomiting, or diarrhea. Phase II studies in colon and pancreatic cancers were less encouraging (Table 20.5-2). The overall lack of efficacy seen in these studies may have resulted from the large tumor burden or the associated immunosuppression seen in these patients with metastatic disease.

Riethmuller and colleagues[162] have evaluated 17-1A in the adjuvant setting in patients with colorectal cancer. Patients with lymph node–positive cancers were randomized to observation or to therapy with 17-1A for 5 months. After 5 years, the death rate in the 17-1A group was 36% versus 51% in the observation group.[162] The decreased death rate persisted at 7 years—43% versus 63%.[163] This result translated to a 30% reduction in death ($P = .04$) and a 27% reduction in recurrence ($P = .03$). This study has been criticized for the higher than expected death rate in the observation group and the lack of adjuvant chemotherapy. Currently, a clinical trial is comparing 17-1A to observation in patients with lymph node–negative cancers. Another ongoing study is evaluating lymph node–positive colorectal cancer patients, randomizing patients to standard adjuvant chemotherapy alone or in conjunction with 17-1A. These trials will define the role of this antibody therapy in the adjuvant setting. If the encouraging outcomes of the original randomized study are confirmed, it will signify a paradigm shift. In this new paradigm, high objective response rates in patients with metastatic disease will not be required to provide an activity signal that warrants testing in the adjuvant setting when the agent involved acts to stimulate immune responses.

Ovarian Cancer

The majority of patients with ovarian cancer relapse even after receiving adjuvant chemotherapy and even when they present with limited disease. RIT using HMFG1, which recognizes a polymorphic epithelial mucin, has been evaluated in patients with stage Ic to IV ovarian cancer after standard chemotherapy.[164] The radiolabeled antibody was given once as an intraperitoneal injection. Compared with a retrospective matched control group, the estimated survival at 10 years was superior for the patients treated with RIT. Further prospective studies are needed to confirm this initial observation.

Antiganglioside Antibodies

Significant promise has been associated with MAB directed against ganglioside antigens in patients with melanoma and neuroblastoma.[165–167] In these trials, the induction of complement-mediated cytotoxicity has been suggested as a possible mechanism of response. Gangliosides have a limited distribution within the body and normally can be found only on peripheral nerves at low densities. In contrast, gangliosides (GD2) are overexpressed on melanomas, neuroblastomas, osteosarcoma, and small cell lung cancers. Antibodies targeting gangliosides have unique toxicities resulting from peripheral nerve tissue targeting, and treatment is associated with severe pain, often requiring narcotic analgesia. Long-term neurologic deficits have been observed, although rarely. Murray et al.[167] treated 18 patients who demonstrated GD2 tumor expression by prior radionuclide imaging using the murine MAB 14.G2a. Toxicities included pain, fever, hyponatremia, paresthesias, and postural hypotension. Treatment with the anti-GD2 ganglioside antibodies 3F8 and Ch14.18 has been associated with lesser toxicities, although pain during infusion has been described. All studies have demonstrated responses in patients with neuroblastoma. Cheung and colleagues[168] have evaluated 3F8 in metastatic neuroblastoma, observing PRs as well as long-term, unmaintained remissions and survivals of 79 to 130 months. More recently, this group reported on the use of 3F8 in patients with metastatic disease treated in conjunction with chemotherapy at the time of relapse.[169] Two-thirds of patients with occult disease had evidence of response after 3F8 treatment. One-third of the patients are progression-free 40 to 130 months after completion of therapy. Treatment with 3F8 antibody, alone or radiolabeled, has not resulted in the selection of GD2-negative tumor clones. Ongoing studies with 3F8 are evaluating its effectiveness as a consolidation therapy after bone marrow transplantation.

The human chimeric antibody Ch14.18 has been tested in neuroblastoma and osteosarcoma.[168,169] The first study[168] reported on nine patients with previously treated stage IV neuroblastoma. Pain in the abdomen and joints controlled by intravenous morphine defined the maximally tolerated dose of 50 mg/m^2. Two patients with bone and paravertebral disease had complete remissions lasting 2 months and more than 14 months, respectively. Two other patients with bone and adrenal metastases had PRs, and one other patient had a minor response of an adrenal metastasis. These results were essentially replicated in a second phase I trial,[169] in which five of seven patients with metastases to bone marrow had evidence of minor to CRs in the bone marrow as assessed by repeated bone marrow biopsies. This agent also has been used as consolidation therapy after bone marrow transplantation following high-dose chemotherapy and ^{131}I-metaiodobenzylguanidine with encouraging preliminary results.[170]

GD3 ganglioside has been targeted by the R24 antibody, which promotes ADCC and complement deposition. Therapy with R24 has induced occasional tumor regressions in patients with metastatic melanoma.[171] Soiffer and associates[172] reported on a trial in metastatic melanoma combining IL-2 at both high and low doses with R24. Treatment was limited by IL-2–related toxicities, particularly catheter-related infections. Treatment led to the expansion and activation of NK cells and T lymphocytes. In spite of this *in vitro* immune activation, only one PR was observed.

IFN-α given in an adjuvant setting may decrease the risk of melanoma recurrence in patients free of disease after the resection of lymph node–positive primary disease. The combination of IFN-α, R24, and IL-2 was studied in patients with metastatic melanoma.[173] Patients were treated with R24 by continuous intravenous infusion, followed by approximately 3 weeks of therapy with IL-2 and IFN-α. The cytokine therapy was designed to enhance the proliferation and cytotoxicity of T lymphocytes infiltrating melanoma lesions after R24 MAB therapy. However, pre- and posttreatment biopsies of these lesions showed no evidence of augmentation in the composition or biologic features of the effector cell population after the combination therapy in comparison with cytokine or MAB therapy alone. No objective tumor responses were observed. M-CSF also has been administered in combination with R24.[174] In this study, M-CSF was given as a 14-day continuous intravenous infusion, adding R24 on days 6 to 10. Three of 19 treated patients had a minor tumor response in metastases to the breast, liver, and lymph nodes. In yet another study evaluating combination therapies with R24, treatment combining R24 and GM-CSF demonstrated increased ADCC *in vitro* after therapy.[175] Two PRs were seen in 20 patients treated. Similar results have been obtained with ch14.18.[176,177]

FUTURE DIRECTIONS

The initial clinical studies using antibodies and their derivatives have identified a number of applications that promise to make significant impacts in the management of patients with cancer. Patience was required to acquire the results, understand the reasons for disappointment or success, and refine the treatment strategies to obtain results that provide legitimate causes for encouragement. These promising results represent the most advanced clinical antibody therapy programs, but a wealth of innovative strategies using recombinantly prepared antibody molecules with novel effector functions are in earlier stages of clinical evaluation. Some of these approaches, such as modulating growth factor receptor functions or inducing immune responses using BsAb, show considerable promise and are expected to add to the list of novel agents available for the treatment of malignancies in which previously conventional therapeutic strategies have proven inadequate.

In the past, antibody development has focused on identification of targets on the cancer cell itself. There are now an increasing number of targets in the extracellular matrix and local tumor environment. The most developed approach targets the vascular endothelial growth factor, a mediator of tumor neovascularization. An antibody-targeting tenascin, a class of extracellular matrix proteins, has been tested in a RIT trial in patients with primary or metastatic brain tumors.[178]

Antibodies against osteoclast integrins can prevent osteoclastic bone resorption.[179] Such approaches offer additional causes for optimism about antibody-based therapeutics.

REFERENCES

1. Maloney DG, Liles TM, Czerwinski DK, et al. Phase I clinical trial using escalating single-dose infusion of chimeric anti-CD20 monoclonal antibody (IDEC-C2B8) in patients with recurrent B-cell lymphoma. *Blood* 1994;84:2457.
2. Press OW, Eary JF, Appelbaum FR, et al. Radiolabeled-antibody therapy of B-cell lymphoma with autologous bone marrow support. *N Engl J Med* 1993;329:1219.
3. Kaminski MS, Zasady KR, Francis IR, et al. Radioimmunotherapy of B-cell lymphoma with ^{131}I-anti-B1 (anti-CD20) antibody. *N Engl J Med* 1993;329:459.
4. Sievers EL, Bernstein JD, Spielberger RT, et al. Dose escalation phase I study of recombinant engineered human anti-CD33 antibody-calicheamicin drug conjugate (CMA-676) in patients with relapsed or refractory acute myeloid leukemia (AML) *Proc ASCO* 1997;16:A8.
5. Baselga J, Tripathy D, Mendelsohn J, et al. Phase II study of weekly intravenous recombinant humanized anti-p185^{HER2} monoclonal antibody in patients with HER2/*neu*-overexpressing metastatic breast cancer. *J Clin Oncol* 1996;14:737.
6. Slamon DJ, Leyland-Jones B, Shak S, et al. Addition of Herceptin (humanized anti-HER2 antibody) to first line chemotherapy for HER2 overexpressing metastatic breast cancer (HER2+/MBC) markedly increased anticancer activity: a randomized, multinational controlled phase III trial. *Proc ASCO* 1998;17:A377.
7. Sliwkowski MX, Lofgren JA, Lewis GD, et al. Nonclinical studies addressing the mechanism of action of Trastuzomab (Herceptin). *Semin Oncol* 1999;26[Suppl 12]:60.
8. Kohler G, Milstein C. Continuous cultures of fused cells secreting antibody of predefined specificity. *Nature* 1975;256:495.
9. LoBuglio AF, Wheeler RH, Trang J, et al. Mouse/human chimeric monoclonal antibody in man: kinetics and immune response. *Proc Natl Acad Sci U S A* 1989;86:4220.
10. Kudo T, Saeki H, Tachibana T. A simple and improved method to generate human hybridomas. *J Immunologic Methods* 1991;145:119.
11. Hussain R, Courtenay-Luck NS, Siligardi G. Structure-function correlation and biostability of antibody CDR-derived peptides as tumour imaging agents. *Biomed Pept Proteins Nucleic Acids* 1996;2:67.
12. Huston JS, Levinson D, Mudgett-Hunter M, et al. Protein engineering of antibody binding sites: recovery of specific activity in an anti-digoxin single-chain Fv analogue produced in *Escherichia coli*. *Proc Natl Acad Sci U S A* 1988;85:5879.
13. Begent RH, Verhaar MJ, Chester KA, et al. Clinical evidence of efficient tumor targeting based on single-chain Fv antibody selected from a combinatorial library. *Nat Med* 1996;2:979.
14. Mack M, Riethmuller G, Kufer P. A small bispecific antibody construct expressed as a functional single-chain molecule with high tumor cell cytotoxicity. *Proc Natl Acad Sci U S A* 1995;92:7021.
15. Schier R, Marks JD, Wolf EJ, et al. *In vitro* and *in vivo* characterization of a human anti-c-erbB-2 single-chain Fv isolated from a filamentous phage antibody library. *Immunotechnology* 1995;1:73.
16. Clackson T, Hoogenboom HR, Griffiths AD, Winter G. Making antibody fragments using phage display libraries. *Nature* 1991;352:624.
17. Pluckthun A, Pack P. New protein engineering approaches to multivalent and bispecific antibody fragments. *Immunotechnology* 1997;3:83.
18. Hollinger P, Prospero T, Winter G. "Diabodies": small bivalent and bispecific antibody fragments. *Proc Natl Acad Sci U S A* 1993;90:444.
19. Adams GP, Schier R, McCall AM, et al. Prolonged *in vivo* tumor retention of a human diabody targeting the extracellular domain of human HER2/neu. *Br J Cancer* 1998;77:1405.
20. Iliades P, Kortt AA, Hudson PJ. Triabodies: single chain Fv fragments without a linker form trivalent trimers. *FEBS Lett* 1997;409:437.
21. Hu S, Shively L, Raubitschek A, et al. Minibody: a novel engineered anti-carcinoembryonic antigen antibody fragment (single-chain Fv-CH3) which exhibits rapid, high-level targeting of xenografts. *Cancer Res* 1996;56:3055.
22. Gillies SD, Reilly EB, Lo KM, Reisfeld RA. Antibody-targeted interleukin 2 stimulates T-cell killing of autologous tumor cells. *Proc Natl Acad Sci U S A* 1992;89:1428.
23. Jain RK. Transport of molecules in the tumor interstitium: a review. *Cancer Res* 1987;47:3039.
24. Jain RK. Transport of molecules across tumor vasculature. *Cancer Metastasis Rev* 1987;6:559.
25. Colcher DR, Bird R, Roselli M, et al. *In vivo* tumor targeting of a recombinant single-chain antigen-binding protein. *J Natl Cancer Inst* 1990;82:1191.
26. Adams GP, McCartney JE, Tai MS, et al. Highly specific *in vivo* tumor targeting by monovalent and divalent forms of 741F8 anti-c-erbB-2 single-chain Fv. *Cancer Res* 1993;53:4026.
27. Miller RA, Maloney DG, et al. Treatment of B-cell lymphoma with monoclonal anti-idiotype antibody. *Med Intelligence* 1982;306:517.
28. Humphrey PA, Wong AJ, Vogelstein B, et al. Anti-synthetic peptide antibody reacting at the fusion junction of deletion-mutant epidermal growth factor receptors in human glioblastoma. *Proc Natl Acad Sci U S A* 1990;87:4207.
29. Garcia de Palazzo IE, Adams GP, Sundareshan P, et al. Expression of mutated epidermal growth factor receptor by non–small cell lung carcinomas. *Cancer Res* 1993;53:3217.
30. Khazaeli MB, Conry RM, LoBuglio AF. Human immune response to monoclonal antibodies. *J Immunother* 1994;15:42.
31. Jerne NK. Towards a network theory of the immune system. *Ann Immunol* 1974;125:373.
32. Yang XD, Jia XC, Corvalan JR, et al. Eradication of established tumors by a fully human monoclonal antibody to the epidermal growth factor receptor without concomitant chemotherapy. *Cancer Res* 1999;59:1236.
33. Shen L, Guyre PM, Anderson CL, Fanger MW. Heteroantibody-mediated cytotoxicity: antibody to the high affinity Fc receptor for IgG mediates cytotoxicity by human monocytes that is enhanced by interferon-γ and is not blocked by human IgG. *J Immunol* 1986;137:3378.
34. Garcia de Palazzo I, Gercel-Taylor C, Kitson J, Weiner LM. Potentiation of tumor lysis by a bispecific antibody that binds to CA19-9 antigen and the Fcγ receptor expressed by human large granular lymphocytes. *Cancer Res* 1990;50:7123.
35. Valerius T, Stockmeyer B, van Spriel AB, et al. FcalphaRI (CD89) as a novel trigger molecule for bispecific antibody therapy. *Blood* 1997;90:4485.
36. Lanzavecchia A, Scheidegger D. The use of hybrid hybridomas to target human cytotoxic T lymphocytes. *Eur J Immunol* 1987;17:105.
37. Link BK, Weiner GJ. Production and characterization of a bispecific IgG capable of inducing T-cell-mediated lysis of malignant B cells. *Blood* 1993;81:3343.
38. Renner C, Jung W, Sahin U, van Lier R, Pfreundschuh M. The role of lymphocyte subsets and adhesion molecules in T cell–dependent cytotoxicity mediated by CD3 and CD28 bispecific monoclonal antibodies. *Eur J Immunol* 1995;25:2027.
39. Sconocchia G, Titus JA, Segal DM. CD44 is a cytotoxic triggering molecule in human peripheral blood NK cells. *J Immunol* 1994;153:5473.
40. Schier R, McCall A, Adams GP, et al. Isolation of picomolar affinity anti-c-erbB-2 single-chain Fv by molecular evolution of the complementarity determining regions in the center of the antibody binding site. *J Mol Biol* 1996;263:551.
41. Schier R, Marks JD, Wolf EJ, et al. *In vitro* and *in vivo* characterization of a human anti-c-erbB-2 single-chain Fv isolated from a filamentous phage antibody library. *Immunotechnology* 1995;1:73.
42. Segal DM, Wunderlich JR. Targeting of cytotoxic cells with heterocrosslinked antibodies. *Cancer Invest* 1988;6:83.
43. Hombach A, Jung W, Pohl C, et al. A CD16/CD30 bispecific antibody induces lysis of Hodgkin cells by unstimulated natural killer *in vitro* and *in vivo*. *Int J Cancer* 1993;55:830.
44. Weiner LM, Holmes M, Adams GP, et al. A human tumor xenograft model of therapy with a bispecific monoclonal antibody c-erbB-2 and CD-16. *Cancer Res* 1993;53:94.
45. Weiner GJ, Kostelny SA, Hillstrom JR, et al. The role of T cell activation in anti-CD3 x antitumor bispecific antibody therapy. *J Immunol* 1994;152:2385.
46. Nitta T, Sato K, Yagita H, Okumura K, Ishii S. Preliminary trial of specific targeting therapy against malignant glioma. *Lancet* 1990;335:368.
47. Canevari S, Stoter G, Arienti F, et al. Regression of advanced ovarian carcinoma by intraperitoneal treatment with autologous T lymphocytes retargeted by a bispecific monoclonal antibody. *J Natl Cancer Inst* 1995;87:1463.
48. Tibben JG, Boerman OC, Claessens RAMJ, et al. Cytokine release in an ovarian carcinoma patient following intravenous administration of bispecific antibody OC/TR $F(ab')_2$. *J Natl Cancer Inst* 1993;85:1003.
49. Weiner LM, Clark JI, Davey M, et al. Phase I trial of 2B1, a bispecific monoclonal antibody targeting c-erbB-2 and FcγRIII. *Cancer Res* 1995;55:4586.
50. Clark JI, Alpaugh RK, von Mehren M, et al. Induction of multiple anti-c-erbB2 specificities accompanies a classical idiotypic cascade following 2B1 bispecific monoclonal antibody treatment. *Cancer Immunol Immunother* 1997;44:265.
51. Valone FH, Kaufman PA, Guyre PM, et al. Phase Ia/Ib trial of bispecific antibody MDX-210 in patients with advanced breast or ovarian cancer that overexpresses the proto-oncogene HER-2/*neu*. *J Clin Oncol* 1995;13:2281.
52. Fyfe G, Fisher RI, Rosenberg SA, et al. Results of treatment of 255 patients with metastatic renal cell carcinoma who received high-dose recombinant interleukin-2 therapy. *J Clin Oncol* 1995;13:688.
53. Sabzevari H, Gillies SD, Mueller BM, Pancook JD, Reisfeld RA. A recombinant antibody-interleukin 2 fusion protein suppresses growth of hepatic neuroblastoma metastases in severe combined immunodeficiency mice. *Proc Natl Acad Sci U S A* 1994;91:9626.
54. Obrist R, Schmidli J, Obrecht JP. Chemotactic monoclonal antibody conjugates: a comparison of four different f-Met-peptide-conjugates. *Biochem Biophys Res Commun* 1988;155:1139.
55. Chalitta-Eid P, Abboud CA, Morrison SL, et al. A RANTES-antibody fusion protein retains antigen specificity and chemokine function. *J Immunol* 1998;161:3729.
56. Modjtahedi H, Komurasaki T, Toyoda H, Dean C. Anti-EGFR monoclonal antibodies which act as EGF, TGF alpha, HB-EGF, and BTC antagonists block the binding of epiregulin to EGFR-expressing tumours. *Int J Cancer* 1998;75:310.
57. Teramoto T, Onda M, Tokunaga A, Asano G. Inhibitory effect of an anti-epidermal growth factor receptor antibody on human gastric cancer. *Cancer* 1996;77:1639.
58. Sato JD, Kawamoto T, Le AD, et al. Biologic effect *in vitro* of monoclonal antibodies to human EGF receptors. *Mol Biol Med* 1983;1:511.
59. Artega CL, Corondo E, Osbore CK. Blockade of the epidermal growth factor receptor inhibits transforming growth factor a—induced but not estrogen-induced growth of hormone-dependent human breast cancer. *Mol Endocrinol* 1988;2:1064.
60. Hoffman T, Hafner D, Ballo H, Haas I, Bier H. Antitumor activity of anti-epidermal growth factor receptor monoclonal antibodies and cisplatin in ten human head and neck squamous cell carcinoma lines. *Anticancer Res* 1997;17:4419.
61. Fan Z, Baselga J, Masui H, Mendelsohn J. Antitumor effect of anti–epidermal growth factor receptor monoclonal antibodies plus cis-diamminedichloroplatinum on well established A431 cell xenografts. *Cancer Res* 1993;53:4637.
62. Baselga J, Norton L, Masui H, et al. Antitumor effects of doxorubicin in combination with anti–epidermal growth factor receptor monoclonal antibodies. *J Natl Cancer Inst* 1993;85:1327.
63. Modjtahedi H, Eccles S, Sandle J, et al. Differentiation or immune destruction: two pathways for therapy of squamous cell carcinomas with antibodies to the epidermal growth factor receptor. *Cancer Res* 1994;54:1695.
64. Sunada H, Magun G, Mendelsohn J, et al. Monoclonal antibody against the EGF receptor is internalized without stimulating receptor phosphorylation. *Proc Natl Acad Sci U S A* 1986;83:3825.

65. Sunada H, Yu P, Peacock JS, et al. Modulation of tyrosine serine and threonine phosphorylation and intracellular processing of the epidermal growth factor receptor by anti-receptor monoclonal antibody. *J Cellular Physiol* 1990;142:284.
66. Fan Z, Masui M, Altas I, Mendelsohn J. Blockade of the epidermal growth factor receptor function by bivalent and monovalent fragments of 225 anti–epidermal growth factor receptor monoclonal antibodies. *Cancer Res* 1993;53:4322.
67. Prewett M, Rockwell RF, Giorgio NA, et al. The biologic effects of C225, a chimeric monoclonal antibody to the EGFR, on human prostate carcinoma. *J Immunother Emphasis Tumor Immunol* 1996;19:419.
68. Zolfaghari A, Djakiew D. Inhibition of chemomigration of a human prostatic carcinoma cell (TSU-pr1) line by inhibition of epidermal growth factor receptor function. *Prostate* 1996;28:232.
69. Peng D, Fan Z, Lu Y, et al. Anti–epidermal growth factor receptor monoclonal antibody 225 up-regulates p27KIP1 and induces G1 arrest in prostatic cancer cell line DU145. *Cancer Res* 1996;56:3666.
70. Wu X, Rubin M, Fan Z, et al. Involvement of p27KIP1 in G1 arrest mediated by an anti–epidermal growth factor receptor monoclonal antibody. *Oncogene* 1996;12:1397.
71. Raben D, Buchsbaum DJ, Gillepsie Y, Saleh M, Waksal H. Treatment of human intracranial gliomas with chimeric monoclonal antibody against the epidermal growth factor receptor increases survival of nude mice when treated concurrently with irradiation. *Proc AACR* 1999;40:A1224.
72. Ciardiello F, Bianco R, Damiano V, et al. Antitumor activity of sequential treatment with topotecan and anti–epidermal growth factor receptor monoclonal antibody C225. *Clin Cancer Res* 1999;5:909.
73. Normanno N, Tortora G, De Luca A, et al. Synergistic growth inhibition and induction of apoptosis by a novel mixed backbone antisense oligonucleotide targeting CRIPTO in combination with C225 anti-EGFR monoclonal antibody and 8-Cl-cAMP in human GEO colon cancer cells. *Oncol Rep* 1999;6:1105.
74. Tortora G, Caputo R, Pomatico G, et al. Cooperative inhibitory effect of novel mixed backbone oligonucleotide targeting protein kinase A in combination with docetaxel and anti–epidermal growth factor-receptor antibody on human breast cancer cell growth. *Clin Cancer Res* 1999;5:875.
75. Ye D, Mendelsohn J, Fan Z. Augmentation of a humanized anti-HER2 mAb 4D5 induced growth inhibition by a human-mouse chimeric anti-EGF receptor mAb C225. *Oncogene* 1999;18:731.
76. Perrotte P, Matsumoto T, Inoue K, et al. Anti–epidermal growth factor receptor antibody C225 inhibits angiogenesis in human transitional cell carcinoma growing orthotopically in nude mice. *Clin Cancer Res* 1999;5:257.
77. Mendelsohn J, Shin DM, Donato N, et al. A phase I study of chimerized anti–epidermal growth factor receptor (EGFr) monoclonal antibody, C225, in combination with cisplatin (CDDP) in patient (PTS) with recurrent head and neck squamous cell carcinoma (SCC). *Proc Am Assoc Clin Oncol* 1999;18:A1502.
78. Ezekiel MP, Robert F, Merideth RF, et al. Phase I study of anti–epidermal growth factor receptor antibody C225 in combination with irradiation in patients with advanced squamous cell carcinoma of the head and neck. *Proc ASCO* 1998;17:A1522.
79. Modjtahedi H, Hickish T, Nicolson M, et al. Phase I trial and tumour localisation of the anti-EGFR monoclonal antibody ICR62 in head and neck or lung cancer. *Br J Cancer* 1996;73:228.
80. Perez-Soler R, Donato NJ, Shin DM, et al. Tumor epidermal growth factor receptor studies in patients with non–small cell lung cancer or head and neck cancer treated with monoclonal antibody RG83852. *J Clin Oncol* 1994;12:730.
81. Christen RD, Hom DK, Porter DC, et al. Epidermal growth factor regulates the *in vitro* sensitivity of human ovarian carcinoma cells to cisplatin. *J Clin Invest* 1990;86:1632.
82. Kwok TT, Sutherland RM. Differences in EGF related radio-sensitization of human squamous carcinoma cells with high and low numbers of EGF receptors. *Br J Cancer* 1991;64:251.
83. Deshane J, Cabrera G, Grim JE, et al. Targeted eradication of ovarian cancer mediated by intracellular expression of anti-erbB-2 single-chain antibody. *Gynecol Oncol* 1995;59:8.
84. Austin EB, Robins RA, DurRant LG, Price MR, Baldwin RW. Human monoclonal anti-idiotypic antibody to the tumour-associated antibody 791T/36. *Immunology* 1989;67:525.
85. Herlyn D, Wettendorff M, Schmoll E, et al. Anti-idiotype immunization of cancer patients: modulation of the immune response. *Proc Natl Acad Sci U S A* 1987;84:8055.
86. Munn RK, Hutchins L, Garrison J, et al. Immune responses in patients with breast cancer treated with an anti-idiotype antibody that mimics the human milk fat globule (HMFG) antigen. *Proc Am Soc Clin Oncol* 1998;17:A1648.
87. Herlyn D, Wettendorf M, Schmoll E, et al. Anti-idiotype immunization of cancer patients: modulation of the immune response. *Proc Natl Acad Sci U S A* 1987;84:8055.
88. Mittelman A, Chen ZJ, Kageshita T, et al. Active specific immunotherapy in patients with melanoma: a clinical trial with mouse antiidiotypic monoclonal antibodies elicited with syngeneic anti-high-molecular-weight-melanoma-associated antigen monoclonal antibodies. *J Clin Invest* 1990;86:2136.
89. Foon KA, Chalaraborty M, John WJ, et al. Immune response to the carcinoembryonic antigen in patients treated with an anti-idiotype antibody vaccine. *J Clin Invest* 1995;96:334.
90. Denton GW, Durrant LG, Hardcastle JD, et al. Clinical outcome of colorectal cancer patients treated with human monoclonal anti-idiotypic antibody. *Int J Cancer* 1994;57:10.
91. Durrant LG, Buckley TJ, Denton GW, et al. Enhanced cell-mediated tumor killing in patients immunized with human monoclonal anti-idiotypic antibody 105AD7. *Cancer Res* 1994;54:4837.
92. Durrant LG, Buckley DJ, Spendlove I, Robins RA. Low doses of 105AD7 cancer vaccine preferentially stimulate anti-tumor T-cell immunity. *Hybridoma* 1997;16:23.
93. Foon KA, John WJ, Chakraborty M, et al. Clinical and immune responses in surgically resected colorectal cancer (CRC) patients treated with an anti-idiotype (ID) monoclonal antibody that mimics carcinoembryonic antigen (CEA) with or without 5-fluorouracil (5-FU). *Proc Am Soc Clin Oncol* 1998;17:A1678.
94. Madiyalakan R, Yang R, Schultes BC, Baum RP, Noujaim AA. OVAREX MAb-B43, 13:IFN-gamma could improve the ovarian tumor cell sensitivity to CA125-specific allogenic cytotoxic T cells. *Hybridoma* 1997;16:41.
95. Livingston P. Ganglioside vaccines with emphasis on GM2. *Semin Oncol* 1998;25:636.
96. MacLean GD, Reddish MA, Koganty RR, Longenecker BM. Antibodies against mucin-associated sialyl-Tn epitopes correlate with survival of metastatic adenocarcinoma patients undergoing active specific immunotherapy with synthetic STn vaccine. *J Immunother* 1996;19:59.
97. Sandmaier BM, Oparin DV, Holmberg LA, et al. Evidence of a cellular immune response against sialyl-Tn in breast and ovarian cancer patients after high-dose chemotherapy, stem cell rescue, and immunization with Theratope STn-KLH cancer vaccine. *J Immunother* 1999;22:54.
98. Vitetta ES, Stone M, Amlot P, et al. Phase I immunotoxin trial in patients with B-cell lymphoma. *Cancer Res* 1991;51:4052.
99. Grossbard ML, Lambert JM, Goldmacher VS, et al. Anti-B4-blocked ricin: a phase I trial of 7-day continuous infusion in patients with B-cell neoplasms. *J Clin Oncol* 1993;11:726.
100. Fitzgerald D, Pastan I. Targeted toxin therapy for the treatment of cancer. *J Natl Cancer Inst* 1989;81:1455.
101. Trail PA, Willner D, Lasch SJ, et al. Cure of xenografted human carcinomas by BR96-doxorubicin immunoconjugates. *Science* 1993;261:212.
102. Tolcher AW, Sugarman S, Gelmon KA, et al. Randomized phase II study of BR96-doxorubicin conjugate in patients with metastatic breast cancer. *J Clin Oncol* 1999;17:478.
103. Hinman LM, Hamann PR, Wallace R, et al. Preparation and characterization of monoclonal antibody conjugates of the calicheamicins: a novel and potent family of antitumor antibiotics. *Cancer Res* 1993;53:3336.
104. Sievers EL, Bernstein ID, Spielberger RT, et al. Dose escalation phase I study of recombinant engineered human anti-CD33 antibody-calicheamicin drug conjugate (CMA-676) in patients with relapsed or refractory acute myeloid leukemia (AML) *Proc ASCO* 1997;16:A8.
105. Nadler LM, Stashenko P, Hardy R, et al. Serotherapy of a patient with a monoclonal antibody directed against a human lymphoma-associated antigen. *Cancer Res* 1980;40:3147.
106. Miller RA, Maloney DG, Levy R, et al. Treatment of B-cell lymphoma with monoclonal anti-idiotype antibody. *Med Intelligence* 1982;306:517.
107. Vuist WM, Levy R, Maloney DG. Lymphoma regression induced by monoclonal anti-idiotypic antibodies correlates with their ability to induce Ig signal transduction and is not prevented by tumor expression of high levels of bcl-2 protein. *Blood* 1994;83:899.
108. Swisher EM, Shawler DL, Collins HA, et al. Expression of shared idiotypes in chronic lymphocytic leukemia and small lymphocytic lymphoma. *Blood* 1991;77:1977.
109. DeNardo GL, DeNardo SJ, Goldstein DS, et al. Maximum-tolerated dose, toxicity, and efficacy of (131)I-Lym-1 antibody for fractionated radioimmunotherapy of non-Hodgkin's lymphoma. *J Clin Oncol* 1998;16:3246.
110. Bowen AL, Zomas A, Emmett E, et al. Subcutaneous CAMPATH-1H in fludarabine-resistant/relapsed chronic lymphocytic and B-prolymphocytic leukaemia. *Br J Haematol* 1997;96:617.
111. Lundin J, Osterborg A, Brittinger G, et al. CAMPATH-1H monoclonal antibody in therapy for previously treated low-grade non-Hodgkin's lymphomas: a phase II multicenter study. *J Clin Oncol* 1988;16:3257.
112. Hale G, Zhang MJ, Bunjes D, et al. Improving the outcome of bone marrow transplantation by using CD52 monoclonal antibodies to prevent graft-versus-host disease and graft rejection. *Blood* 1998;92:4581.
113. Naparstek E, Delukina M, Or R, et al. Engraftment of marrow allografts treated with Campath-1 monoclonal antibodies. *Exp Hematol* 1999;27:1210.
114. Novitzky N, Thomas V, Hale G, Waldmann H. *Ex-vivo* depletion of T-cells from bone marrow grafts with Campath-1 in acute leukemia: graft-versus-host disease and graft-versus-leukemia effect. *Transplantation* 1999;67:620.
115. Hale G, Waldmann H. Risks of developing Epstein-Barr virus–related lymphoproliferative disorders after T-cell-depleted marrow transplants. *Blood* 1998;91:3079.
116. Maloney DG, Grillo-López AJ, Bodkin DJ, et al. IDEC-C2B8: results of a phase I multiple-dose trial in patients with relapsed non-Hodgkin's lymphoma. *J Clin Oncol* 1997;15:3266.
117. Maloney DG, Grillo-López AJ, White CA, et al. IDEC-C2B8 (rituximab) anti-CD20 monoclonal antibody therapy in patients with relapsed low-grade non-Hodgkin's lymphoma. *Blood* 1997;90:2188.
118. McLaughlin P, Grillo-López AJ, Link B, et al. Rituximab chimeric anti-CD20 monoclonal antibody therapy for relapsed indolent lymphoma: half of patients respond to a four-dose treatment program. *J Clin Oncol* 1998;16:2825.
119. Berinstein NL, Grillo-López AJ, White CA, et al. Association of serum rituximab (IDEC-C2B8) concentration and anti-tumor response in the treatment of recurrent low-grade or follicular non-Hodgkin's lymphoma. *Ann Oncol* 1998;9:995.
120. Piro LD, White CA, Grillo-López AJ, et al. Extended rituximab (anti-CD20 monoclonal antibody) therapy for relapsed or refractory low-grade or follicular non-Hodgkin's lymphoma. *Ann Oncol* 1999;10:619.
121. Coiffier B, Haioun C, Ketterer N, et al. Rituximab (anti-CD20 monoclonal antibody) for the treatment of patients with relapsing or refractory aggressive lymphoma: a multicenter phase II study. *Blood* 1998;92:1927.
122. Byrd JC, Wasenko JK, Maneatis TA, et al. Rituximab therapy in hematologic malignancy patients with increased circulating blood tumor cells: association with increased infusion-related side effects and rapid tumor lysis. *Blood* 1998;92[Suppl 1]:106a.
123. Jensen M, Winkler U, Manze O, Diehl V, Engert A. Rapid tumor lysis in a patient with B-cell chronic lymphocytic leukemia and lymphocytosis treated with an anti-CD20 monoclonal antibody (IDEC-C2B8, rituximab). *Ann Hematol* 1998;77:89.
124. Davis TA, Czerwinski DK, Levy R. Therapy of B-cell lymphoma with anti-CD20 antibodies can result in the loss of CD20 antigen expression. *Clin Cancer Res* 1999;5:611.
125. Czuczman MS, Grillo-López AJ, White CA, et al. Treatment of patients with low-grade B-cell lymphoma with the combination of chimeric anti-CD20 monoclonal antibody and CHOP chemotherapy. *J Clin Oncol* 1999;17:268.

126. Demidem A, Lam T, Alas S, et al. Chimeric anti-CD20 (IDEC-C2B8) monoclonal antibody sensitizes a B cell lymphoma cell line to cell killing by cytotoxic drugs. *Cancer Biother Radiopharm* 1997;12:177.
127. Gribben J, Freedman A, Woo S, et al. All advanced stage non-Hodgkin's lymphomas with a polymerase chain reaction amplifiable breakpoint of bcl-2 have residual cells containing the bcl-2 rearrangement at evaluation and after treatment. *Blood* 1991;78:3275.
128. Shih LB, Lu HH, Xuan H, Goldenberg DM. Internalization and intracellular processing of an anti-B-cell lymphoma monoclonal antibody, LL2. *Int J Cancer* 1994;56:538.
129. Press OW, Eary JF, Appelbaum FR, et al. Phase II trial of ^{131}I-B1 (anti-CD20) antibody therapy with autologous stem cell transplantation for relapsed B cell lymphomas. *Lancet* 1995;346:336.
130. Nikula TK, McDevitt MR, Finn RD, et al. Alpha-emitting bismuth cyclohexylbenzyl DTPA constructs of recombinant humanized anti-CD33 antibodies: pharmacokinetics, bioactivity, toxicity and chemistry. *J Nucl Med* 1999;40:166.
131. Kaminski MS, Zasadny KR, Francis IR, et al. Iodine-131-anti-B1 radioimmunotherapy for B-cell lymphoma. *J Clin Oncol* 1996;14:1974.
132. Liu SY, Eary JF, Petersdorf SH, et al. Follow-up of relapsed B-cell lymphoma patients treated with iodine-131 labeled anti-CD20 antibody and autologous stem cell rescue. *J Clin Oncol* 1998;16:3270.
133. Knox SJ, Goris ML, Trisler K, et al. Yttrium-90-labeled anti-CD20 monoclonal antibody therapy of recurrent B-cell lymphoma. *Clin Cancer Res* 1996;2:457.
134. DeNardo GL, DeNardo SJ, Lamborn KR, et al. Low-dose fractionated radioimmunotherapy for B-cell malignancies using ^{131}I-Lym-1 antibody. *Cancer Biother Radiopharm* 1998;13:239.
135. DeNardo GL, DeNardo SJ, Goldstein DS, et al. Maximum-tolerated dose, toxicity, and efficacy of (131)I-Lym-1 antibody for fractionated radioimmunotherapy of non-Hodgkin's lymphoma. *J Clin Oncol* 1998;16:3246.
136. Jurcic JG, Caron PC, Nikula TK, et al. Radiolabeled anti-CD33 monoclonal antibody M195 for myeloid leukemia. *Cancer Res* 1995;55[Suppl]:5908s.
137. Jurcic JG, Divgi CR, McDevitt MR, et al. Potential for myeloablation with yttrium-90-labeled HuM195 (anti-CD33): a phase I trial in advanced myeloid leukemias. *Blood* 1998;92:613A.
138. Jurcic JG, McDevitt MR, Sgouros G, et al. Phase I trial of targeted alpha-particle therapy for myeloid leukemias with bismuth-213-HuM195 (anti-CD33). *Proc ASCO* 1999;18:7A.
139. Ball ED, Selvaggi K, Hurd D, et al. Phase I clinical trial of serotherapy in patients with acute myeloid leukemia with an immunoglobulin M monoclonal antibody to CD15. *Clin Cancer Res* 1995;1:965.
140. Caron PC, Dumont L, Scheinberg DA. Supersaturating infusional humanized anti-CD33 monoclonal antibody HuM195 in myelogenous leukemia. *Clin Cancer Res* 1998;4:1421.
141. Stirpe F, Olsnes SE, Phil A. Gelonin, a new inhibitor of protein synthesis, nontoxic to intact cells. *J Biol Chem* 1980;255:6947.
142. Pagilaro LC, Liu B, Munker R, et al. Humanized M195 monoclonal antibody conjugated to recombinant gelonin: an anti-CD33 immunotoxin with antileukemic activity. *Clin Cancer Res* 1998;4:1971.
143. Waldmann TA, White JD, Goldman CK, et al. The interleukin-2 receptor: a target for monoclonal antibody treatment of human T-cell lymphotrophic virus I–induced adult T-cell leukemia. *Blood* 1993;82:1701.
144. Junghans RP, Carrasquillo JA, Waldmann TA. Impact of antigenemia on the bioactivity of infused anti-Tac antibody: implication for dose selection in antibody immunotherapies. *Proc Natl Acad Sci U S A* 1998;95:1752.
145. Carter P, Presta L, Gorman CM, et al. Humanization of an anti-p185HER2 antibody for human cancer therapy. *Proc Natl Acad Sci U S A* 1992;89:4285.
146. Cobleigh MA, Vogel CL, Tripathi D, et al. Efficacy and safety of Herceptin (humanized anti-HER2 antibody) as a single agent in 222 women with HER2 overexpression who relapsed following chemotherapy for metastatic breast cancer. *Proc ASCO* 1998;17:A376
147. Pegram MD, Lipton A, Hayes DF, et al. Phase II study of receptor-enhanced chemosensitivity using recombinant humanized anti-p185$^{HER2/neu}$ monoclonal antibody plus cisplatin in patients with HER2/*neu*-overexpressing metastatic breast cancer refractory to chemotherapy treatment. *J Clin Oncol* 1998;16:2659.
148. Slamon D, Shak S, Paton V, et al. Addition of Herceptin (humanized anti-HER2 antibody) to first line chemotherapy for HER2 overexpressing metastatic breast cancer (HER2+/MBC) markedly increases anticancer activity: a randomized multinational controlled phase III trial. *Proc Am Soc Clin Oncol* 1998;17:A377.
149. Ewer MS, Gibbs HR, Swafford J, Benjamin RS. Cardiotoxicity in patients receiving Trastuzomab (Herceptin): primary toxicity, synergistic or sequential stress, or surveillance artifact? *Semin Oncol* 1999;26[Suppl 12]:96.
150. Sears HF, Herlyn D, Steplewski Z, Koprowski H. Effects of monoclonal antibody immunotherapy on patients with gastrointestinal adenocarcinoma. *J Biol Response Mod* 1984;3:138.
151. Paul AR, Engstrom PF, Weiner LM, et al. Treatment of advanced measurable or evaluable pancreatic carcinoma with 17-1A murine monoclonal antibody alone or in combination with 5-fluorouracil, Adriamycin, and mitomycin (FAM). *Hybridoma* 1986;5[Suppl 1]:S171.
152. Sindelar WF, Maher MM, Herlyn D, et al. Trial of therapy with monoclonal antibody 17-1A in pancreatic carcinoma: preliminary results. *Hybridoma* 1986;5[Suppl 1]:125.
153. Sears HF, Herlyn D, Steplewski Z, Koprowski H. Phase II clinical trial of a murine monoclonal antibody cytotoxic for gastrointestinal adenocarcinoma. *Cancer Res* 1985;45:5910.
154. Weiner LM, Harvey E, Padavic-Shaller K, et al. Phase II multicenter evaluation of prolonged murine monoclonal antibody 17-1A therapy in pancreatic carcinoma. *J Immunother* 1993;13:110.
155. Ragnhammar P, Fragerberg J, Frodin JE, et al. Effect of the monoclonal antibody 17-1A and granulocyte monocyte colony stimulating factor in patients with colorectal carcinoma. Long lasting complete remissions can be induced. *Int J Cancer* 1993;53:751.
156. Tempero MA, Sivinski C, Steplewski Z, et al. Phase II trial of interferon gamma and monoclonal antibody 17-1A in pancreatic cancer: biologic and clinical effects. *J Clin Oncol* 1990;8:2019.
157. Frodin JE, Faxas ME, Hagstrom B, et al. Induction of anti-idiotypic (ab2) and anti-anti-idiotypic (ab3) antibodies in patients treated with the mouse monoclonal antibody 17-1A (ab1). Relation to the clinical outcome—an important antitumoral effector function? *Hybridoma* 1991;10:421.
158. Hanzawa Y, Tsujisaki M, Tokuchi S, et al. Detection of xenogeneic anti-idiotypic antibodies specific to murine monoclonal antibody 17-1A in patients with gastrointestinal cancer. *Tumour Biol* 1992;13:226.
159. Fagerberg J, Frodin JE, Wigzell H, Mellstedt H. Induction of an immune network cascade in cancer patients treated with monoclonal antibodies (ab1). I. May induction of ab-1 reactive T cells and anti-anti-idiotypic antibodies (ab3) lead to tumor regression after mAb therapy? *Cancer Immunol Immunother* 1993;37:264.
160. Ragnhammar P, Fagerberg J, Frodin JE, et al. Granulocyte monocyte colony stimulating factor augments the induction of antibodies, especially anti-idiotypic antibodies to therapeutic monoclonal antibodies. *Cancer Immunol Immunother* 1995;40:367.
161. Fagerberg J, Frodin JE, Ragnhammar P, et al. Induction of an immune network cascade in cancer patients treated with monoclonal antibodies (ab1). II. Is induction of anti-idiotype reactive T cells (T3) of importance for tumor response to mAb therapy? *Cancer Immunol Immunother* 1994;38:149.
162. Reithmuller G, Schneider-Gadicke E, Schlimok G, et al. Randomized trial of monoclonal antibody for adjuvant therapy of resected Dukes' C colorectal carcinoma. *Lancet* 1994;343:1177.
163. Reithmuller G, Holz E, Schlimok G, et al. Monoclonal antibody therapy for resected Dukes' C colorectal cancer: seven-year outcome of a multicenter randomized trial. *J Clin Oncol* 1998;16:1788.
164. Nicholson S, Gooden CS, Hird V, et al. Radioimmunotherapy after chemotherapy compared to chemotherapy alone in the treatment of advanced ovarian cancer: a matched analysis. *Oncol Rep* 1998;5:223.
165. Handgretinger R, Anderson K, Lang P, et al. A phase I study of human/mouse chimeric anti-ganglioside GD2 antibody ch 14.18 in patients with neuroblastoma. *Eur J Cancer* 1995;31A:261.
166. Yu AL, Uttenreuther-Fischer MM, Huang CS, et al. Phase I trial of human-mouse chimeric anti-disialoganglioside monoclonal antibody ch14.18 in patients with refractory neuroblastoma and osteosarcoma. *J Clin Oncol* 1998;16:2169.
167. Murray JL, Cunningham JE, Brewer H, et al. Phase I trial of murine monoclonal antibody 14.G2a administered by prolonged intravenous infusion in patients with neuroectodermal tumors. *J Clin Oncol* 1994;12:184.
168. Cheung NK, Kushner BH, Yeh SDJ, Larson SM. 3F8 monoclonal antibody treatment of patients with stage 4 neuroblastoma: a phase II study. *Int J Oncol* 1998;12:1299.
169. Cheung NK, Kushner BH, Cheung IY, et al. Anti-G(D2) antibody treatment of minimal residual stage 4 neuroblastoma diagnosed at more than 1 year of age. *J Clin Oncol* 1998; 16:3053.
170. Klingebiel T, Bader P, Bares R, et al. Treatment of neuroblastoma stage 4 with ^{131}I-meta-iodobenzylguanidine high-dose chemotherapy and immunotherapy. A pilot study. *Eur J Cancer* 1998;34:1398.
171. Vadhan-Raj S, Cordon-Cardo C, Carswell E, et al. Phase I trial of a mouse monoclonal antibody against GD3 ganglioside in patients with melanoma: induction of inflammatory responses at tumor sites. *J Clin Oncol* 1988;6:1636.
172. Soiffer RJ, Chapman PB, Murray C, et al. Administration of R24 monoclonal antibody and low-dose interleukin 2 for malignant melanoma. *Clin Cancer Res* 1997;3:17.
173. Alpaugh RK, von Mehren M, Palazzo I, et al. Phase IB trial for malignant melanoma using R24 monoclonal antibody, interleukin-2/α-interferon. *Med Oncol* 1998;15:191.
174. Minasian LM, Yao TJ, Steffens TA, et al. A phase I study of anti-GD3 ganglioside monoclonal antibody R24 and recombinant human macrophage-colony stimulating factor in patients with metastatic melanoma. *Cancer* 1995;75:2251.
175. Chachoua A, Oratz R, Liebes L, et al. Phase Ib trial of granulocyte-macrophage colony-stimulating factor combined with murine monoclonal antibody R24 in patients with metastatic melanoma. *J Immunother* 1994;16:132.
176. Albertini MR, Hank JA, Schiller JH, et al. Phase IB trial of chimeric antidisialoganglioside antibody plus interleukin 2 for melanoma patients. *Clin Cancer Res* 1997;3:1277.
177. Murray JL, Kleinerman ES, Jia SF, et al. Phase Ia/Ib trial of anti-GD2 chimeric monoclonal antibody 14.18 (ch 14.18) and recombinant human granulocyte-macrophage colony-stimulating factor (rhGM-CSF) in metastatic melanoma. *J Immunother* 1996;19:206.
178. Bigner DD, Brown MT, Friedman AH, et al. Iodine-131-labeled antitenascin monoclonal antibody 81C6 treatment of patients with recurrent malignant gliomas: phase I trial results. *J Clin Oncol* 1998;16:2202
179. Helfrich MH, Nesbitt SA, Lakkakorpi PT, et al. Beta 1 integrins and osteoclast function: involvement in collagen recognition and bone resorption. *Bone* 1996;19:317.
180. Weiner LM, Moldofsky P, Gatenby R, et al. Antibody delivery and effector cell activation in a phase II trial of recombinant interferon-gamma and the murine monoclonal antibody CO17-1A in advanced colorectal carcinoma. *Cancer Res* 1988;48:2568.

SECTION **6** JUDAH FOLKMAN

Antiangiogenesis Agents

The second half of the twentieth century witnessed an explosion of knowledge about the cause and development of cancer at the biochemical, genetic, and molecular levels. Numerous studies have revealed the elegant wiring plan of the normal cell and have uncovered the subtle but complex events that transform normal cells into the neoplastic state. Virtually all of these studies have focused on the cancer cell. Therapy also has been directed almost exclusively against the cancer cell. When taken together, these results give hope that eventually molecular solutions to the cancer problem will be found. An example of such a molecular therapy would be some manipulation that would revert cancer cells to normal cells or would selectively cause cancer cells to undergo apoptosis without damage to normal cells. However, no one knows how far off such therapy is, or if it is even possible. I do not believe that we can ever paint a complete picture of cancer by the reductionist approach alone.

Therefore, it has seemed prudent to explore the cancer problem at a different level. Linus Pauling taught his students that an intractable problem may yield to a change in the level of exploration.[1] Furthermore, Alvin Feinstein emphasizes that, in medical practice, a disconnect often exists between understanding the cause of a disease and having effective therapy for it.[2] Compare, for example, appendicitis to sickle cell anemia. In the former, epidemiology, genetics, and direct cause are poorly understood, but the cure rate is very high. In the latter, a precise molecular cause is known, but therapy is unsatisfactory.

To examine the cancer problem at a different level, consider a cancer cell that has progressed through numerous checkpoints and through a long series of mutations so that many of its oncogenes are overexpressed and its suppressor genes are mutated or deleted. Assuming that this cancer cell is immortal *in vitro* and tumorigenic *in vivo*, we can ask, Are these neoplastic properties necessary and sufficient for a cancer cell to expand into a population that is detectable, symptomatic, or lethal? Experimental evidence now argues that these neoplastic properties may only be *necessary*, but *not sufficient* for a cancer cell to be lethal. This evidence shows that the microvascular endothelial cell acts as a critical control point in tumor growth and dictates to a microscopic *in situ* population of tumor cells whether they can continue to expand the primary tumor, metastasize, or kill their host.[3–5] In the final analysis, the capacity of a tumor to switch to the angiogenic phenotype and to recruit its own private blood supply determines whether a tumor remains undetectable or becomes symptomatic and potentially lethal. Nonangiogenic tumor cells may not be inherently dangerous; they usually remain *in situ*.

Because it is now understood that the microvascular endothelial cell is a critical determinant of tumor growth *in vivo*, this cell has become a second target for cancer therapy. It is the target for which novel angiogenesis inhibitors have been developed as therapeutic anticancer agents. At this writing, at least 20 angiogenesis inhibitors are currently in clinical trials in the United States, and seven of them are in phase III (see Clinical Trials of Angiogenesis Inhibitors, later in this chapter) (Fig. 20.6-1).

GUIDELINES TO THE BIOLOGIC BASIS OF ANTIANGIOGENIC THERAPY

Because a wide variety of different angiogenesis inhibitors are currently being evaluated in clinical trials for patients with advanced cancer in the United States, the United Kingdom, and Europe, it is important for clinicians to understand certain fundamental principles of the angiogenic process that form the scientific basis of this translation from laboratory to clinical application.

Phase I

Drug	Sponsor	Mechanism
COL-3	Collagenex, NCI	Synthetic MMP inhibitor; tetracycline derivative
BMS-275291	Bristol-Myers Squibb	Synthetic MMP inhibitor
SU6668	Sugen	Blocks VEGF, FGF & EGF receptor signaling
Endostatin	EntreMed	Inhibits endothelial proliferation
EMD 121974	Merck KCgaA	Blocks an endothelial integrin
Angiostatin	EntreMed	Inhibits endothelial proliferation
2-methoxy-estradiol	EntreMed	Inhibits microtubule function

Phase II

Squalamine	Magainin	Inhibits Na/H exchanger
TNP-470	TAP Pharm.	Fumagillin analogue; inhibits endothelial proliferation
Combretastatin	Oxigene	Apoptosis in proliferating endothelium
Interleukin-12	Genetics Inst.	Induces IFN-gamma and IP-10
CAI	NCI	Inhibits calcium influx
Anti-VEGF Ab	Genentech	Monoclonal antibody to VEGF

Phase III

Marimastat	British Biotech	Synthetic MMP inhibitor
AG3340	Agouron	Synthetic MMP inhibitor
Neovastat	Aeterna	Natural MMP inhibitor
Interferon-alfa	Commercially available	Inhibition of bFGF production
IM862	Cytran	Endothelial inhibitor
Thalidomide	Celgene	Unknown
SU5416	Sugen	Blocks VEGF receptor signaling

FIGURE 20.6-1. Angiogenesis inhibitors in clinical trial in the United States as of April 2000. bFGF, basic fibroblast growth factor; EGF, epidermal growth factor; FGF, fibroblast growth factor; IFN, interferon; IP-10, interferon-γ–inducible protein-10; MMP, matrix metalloproteinase; NCI, National Cancer Institute; VEGF, vascular endothelial growth factor. (Data from the National Cancer Institute.)

TUMORS AND THEIR METASTASES ARE ANGIOGENESIS-DEPENDENT

I first proposed the hypothesis that tumor growth is angiogenesis-dependent in 1971.[6,7] In its simplest terms, this hypothesis predicted that, beyond the size of a microscopic *in situ* cancer in humans or after "tumor take" in experimental animals, every further increase in tumor population must be *preceded* by the growth of new microvessels that converge on the tumor. Since 1971, many experiments that support this hypothesis have been reported. The first evidence was mostly indirect, because it was based on *in vitro* studies of tumor spheroids, measurements of the prevascular stage of tumors *in vivo,* and mechanical separation of tumors from their vascular bed.[8–26] Direct experimental evidence did not appear until the late 1980s, when it first became possible to inhibit angiogenesis by biochemical and molecular methods. These experiments were based on: (1) administration of molecules that inhibited angiogenesis specifically or selectively, (2) blockade of tumor-derived angiogenic factors, (3) transfection of dominant-negative receptors for an angiogenic factor into endothelial cells in the tumor bed, (4) transfection of angiogenesis inhibitor proteins into tumor cells, and (5) antiangiogenic therapy of spontaneous tumors in transgenic mice.[27–41]

Three decades after publication of the hypothesis that tumors are angiogenesis-dependent, elegant proofs continue to be published. Two such studies appeared in 1999. One of these is a gene knockout experiment.[42] Mice deficient in one allele of Id1 and two alleles of Id3 are unable to mount an angiogenic response to 100 million inoculated tumor cells. The tumors take, but remain dormant and nonangiogenic and do not metastasize. Placental angiogenesis is unaffected. In a second experiment, human cancer cells are transfected with thrombospondin-1 and/or thrombospondin-2, both of which inhibit angiogenesis. The transfected cells are then inoculated into immunodeficient mice.[43] Tumor growth is inhibited in direct proportion to the level of thrombospondin secreted. Tumor cell apoptosis is inversely proportional to tumor angiogenesis (i.e., apoptosis increases as angiogenesis decreases). Tumor cell proliferation, however, is independent of angiogenesis and apoptosis (Fig. 20.6-2).

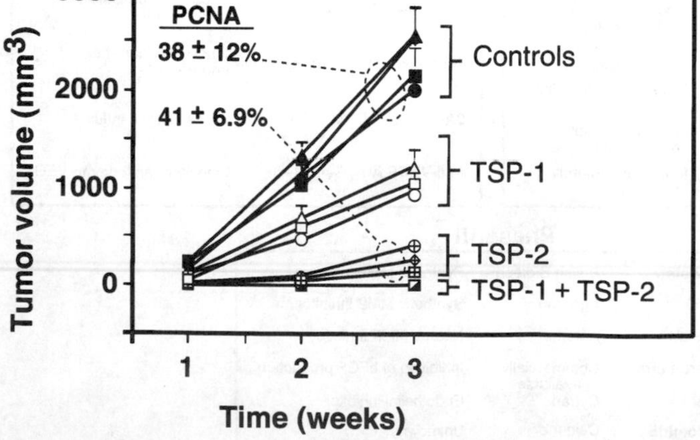

FIGURE 20.6-2. Transfection of squamous cell carcinoma cells by thrombospondin-1 (TSP-1), thrombospondin 2 (TSP-2), or both. PCNA, proliferating cell nuclear antigen. (From ref. 43, with permission.)

MICROVASCULAR ENDOTHELIAL CELLS CONTROL A TUMOR'S SUPPLY OF OXYGEN, NUTRIENTS, AND GROWTH FACTORS

Oxygen and Nutrients

Virtually every cell in the body lives adjacent to a capillary endothelial cell, or at least a distance no greater than the oxygen diffusion limit of 100 to 200 μm.[20] This arrangement permits *perfused* vessels to deliver oxygen and nutrients and to remove catabolites over short distances. This proximity of tissue cells to microvessels is accomplished by at least three common configurations and some rare configurations (Fig. 20.6-3). One category includes cells such as pancreatic islet cells, fat cells, and certain skeletal muscle cells, which are surrounded by two or more microvessels. A second category includes hepatic cells and cells of other solid organs. Each hepatic cell abuts a microvessel on one side and another hepatocyte on the other side. Epithelial cells exposed to the environment make up a third category (e.g., keratinocytes in the skin; mucosal cells in the gastrointestinal tract and bladder; and cells that line a wide variety of ducts, such as those in the breast or prostate). These cells exist in an avascular compartment (e.g., epidermis) separated from underlying microvessels (e.g., in the dermis) by a basement membrane. The basal cells lying on the basement membrane are closest to the microvessels beneath it and receive oxygen and nutrients across a short distance defined by the limits of oxygen diffusion (100 to 200 μm). However, the cells in the upper layers lie beyond the oxygen diffusion limit and are undergoing apoptosis. In contrast, tumor cells form multiple layers that encircle a microvessel until these cell layers (three to six or more), reach the absolute limits of oxygen diffusion. In the outermost cell layer, tumor cells are completely anoxic and are dying. This has been quantified by infrared spectroscopy in transparent skin chambers in experimental animals.[20] A gradient of tumor cell proliferation also is present in these multiple layers. The highest rate of proliferation is found in tumor cells closest to the microvessel.[19] Tumor cells may continue to proliferate and die in this *in situ* configuration, but they cannot expand the tumor mass beyond 0.2 to 2.0 mm until they have induced endothelial cell migration, proliferation, and sprout formation.[44,45] Therefore, a general rule is that any expansion of tumor mass beyond a microscopic size is dependent on two cell compartments growing in tandem: tumor cells and microvascular endothelial cells.

Growth Factors and Antiapoptotic Factors

Endothelial cells not only guard the entry of oxygen and nutrients as well as the exit of catabolites, these cells also elaborate mitogens and survival factors for tumor cells. This *paracrine* activity of microvascular endothelial cells includes the mobilization of basic fibroblast growth factor (bFGF), platelet-derived growth factor, insulin-like growth factor-1 and -2, and cytokines such as interleukin-6 and granulocyte-macrophage colony-stimulating factor. At least 20 paracrine factors are known to be produced by vascular endothelial cells.[46–52]

Antiangiogenic therapy can cause either arrest or regression of growing blood vessels,[39,53] which would shut down the supply of endothelial-derived paracrine factors and contribute to tumor cell apoptosis. In an *in vitro* experiment, the withdrawal of insulin-like growth factor-1 from *myc*-dependent lymphoma cells caused them to undergo apoptosis.[54] Because one microvascular

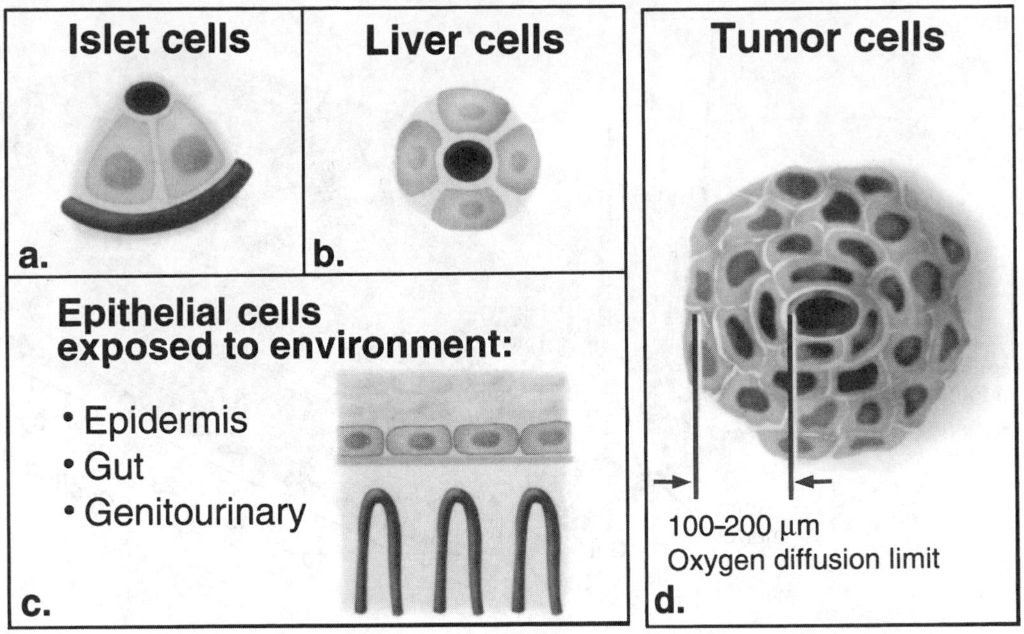

FIGURE 20.6-3. Common patterns of normal tissue cells (**A,B,C**) illustrating how they are apposed to capillaries in comparison to tumor cells (**D**). (See Color Fig. 20.6-3 in the CD-ROM and on the Web at www.LWWoncology.com.)

endothelial cell can support up to 5 to >100 tumor cells, antiangiogenic therapy directed solely against endothelial cells is amplified in contrast to conventional chemotherapy, which attacks tumor cells directly.[55,56]

ANTIANGIOGENIC THERAPY OPERATES OVER A WIDE THERAPEUTIC WINDOW

In animal studies and in human clinical trials, antiangiogenic therapy generally has fewer side effects than conventional cytotoxic chemotherapy. Endostatin, for example, showed no detectable side effects in tumor-bearing animals. At this writing, no significant side effects have been reported during the first 6 months of a phase I clinical trial of endostatin in five cancer centers.

Turnover Times of Endothelium in a Tumor Bed versus Endothelium in Other Regions of the Vasculature

One reason for this predicted lack of toxicity in antiangiogenic therapy is that, under normal conditions, vascular endothelial cells, which form a monolayer of approximately 1000 m^2, are not dividing. Their turnover time is more than 1000 days.[57,58] In contrast, bone marrow cells and mucosal cells in the gastrointestinal tract are among the most rapidly proliferating cells in the body. Bone marrow cells undergo approximately 6 billion cell divisions per hour, and the entire bone marrow is turned over in 5 days. During ovulation and in wound healing, microvascular endothelial cells may grow almost as rapidly as bone marrow cells, but for short periods (days). During tumor angiogenesis, microvascular endothelial cells undergo sustained rapid proliferation that persists for as long as the tumor is present. In Figure 20.6-4, proliferation rates of cells in various human tissues are plotted as turnover times on the horizontal axis. Relative size of tissue mass is plotted on the vertical axis. The tissues turning over most rapidly, in descending order, are gut mucosa, bone marrow, and skin. Cancer of the esophagus (depicted in blue) contains a subset of tumor cells that are rapidly cycling, as well as tumor cells with slower cycling times and some tumor cells that are not cycling. Conventional cytotoxic chemotherapy targets proliferating cells in a tumor but is limited by coincidental injury to normal tissues according to their individual proliferation rates. Rapidly cycling tissues succumb first, then more slowly cycling tissues, as cytotoxic therapy continues.

A second limitation of conventional cytotoxic therapy is that only a small fraction of tumor cells are in cycle when chemotherapy is administered (e.g., in human prostate cancer, fewer than 2% of cells are in cycle).[59] After these cells are killed, they may be replaced by cycling cells. Thus, repeated therapy is required, followed by intervals off of the drug to recover bone marrow and gut. In contrast, antiangiogenic therapy, which either selectively or specifically targets the microvascular endothelial cells in a tumor bed, restricts growth of all tumor cells, regardless of their cycling state.

Differences in Specificity of Angiogenesis Inhibitors

Because a drug is an angiogenesis inhibitor *per se* does not guarantee its freedom from side effects. Certain synthetic small molecules designed to inhibit an angiogenic target (such as a receptor for an angiogenic factor), may induce side effects that are related to the structure of the molecule and not to its antiangiogenic function.

The more specifically that an angiogenesis inhibitor targets growing endothelial cells to the exclusion of resting endothelium or other cell types, such as smooth muscle or fibroblasts, the less is the risk of side effects. Although the pharmaceutical industry generally prefers to develop small synthetic molecules instead of proteins as therapeutic anticancer agents, certain proteins are advantageous because they inhibit angiogenesis specifically. Endostatin is an example. This 20-kD internal fragment of the carboxy-terminus of collagen XVIII is one of the most highly specific and least toxic of the known angiogenesis inhibitors.[37,39,60] Doses of endostatin that produce tumor dormancy or tumor regression have no effect on pregnant mice. Normal babies are born and their growth is not delayed by treating them with endostatin (R. Rohan and R. D'Amato, personal

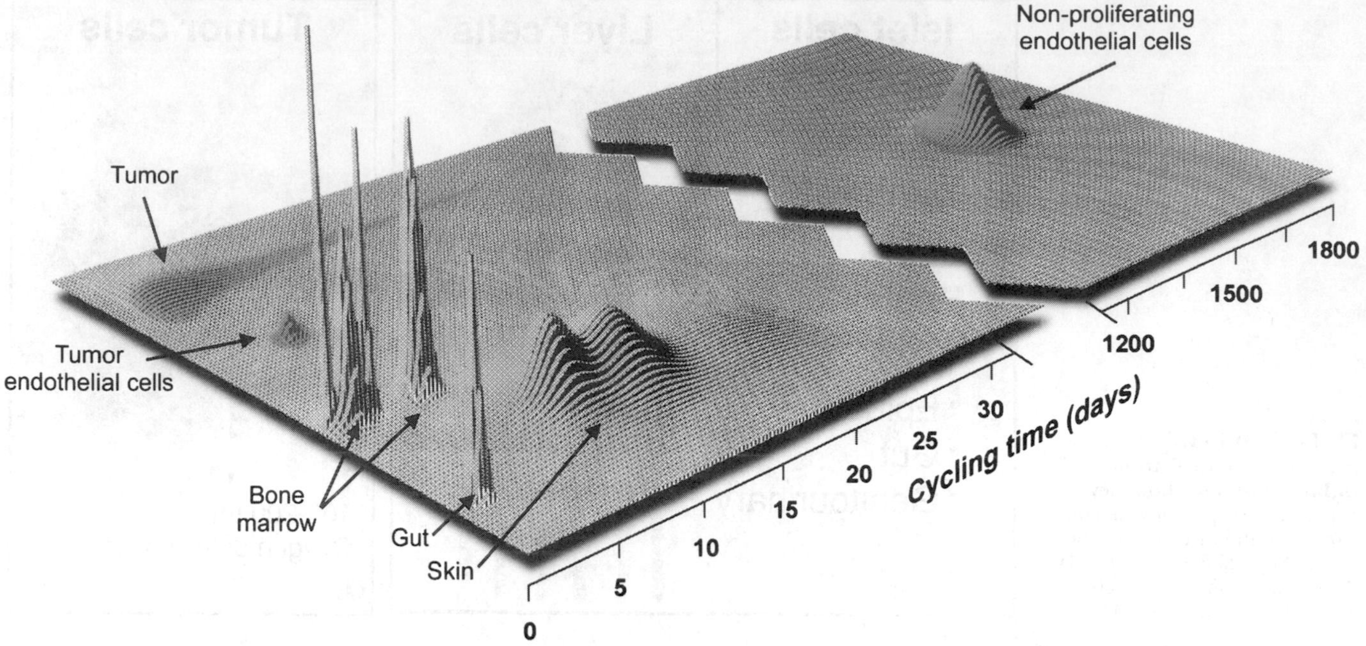

FIGURE 20.6-4. Turnover times of various tissues plotted against tissue mass. (See Color Fig. 20.6-4 in the CD-ROM and on the Web at www.LWWoncology.com.) (From ref. 58, with permission.)

communication, 1998). Furthermore, wound healing is not delayed by endostatin (J. Marler, personal communication, unpublished data, 1999). Therefore, endostatin is not only a specific angiogenesis inhibitor, but it also appears to be a selective inhibitor of tumor neovascularization. Not all angiogenesis inhibitors are free of effects on healing wounds. For example, the fumagillin analogue TNP-470 slows tumor growth by approximately 65% to 75% in a wide variety of tumor-bearing mice,[28] but it also delays wound healing by at least 15% to 17%.[61] In addition, it causes 5% weight loss.

Differences in Types of Angiogenesis Generated by the Host

Why should tumor and wound vessels respond differently to a specific angiogenesis inhibitor such as endostatin? A possible explanation is that these two types of neovascular beds may be controlled in part by different ratios of certain endothelial regulatory proteins, such as the angiopoietins. Angiopoietin-1 is a 70-kD ligand that binds to a specific tyrosine kinase expressed only on endothelial cells, called *Tie2* (also called *Tek*).[62–66] (A ligand for Tie1 has not been elucidated.) Like vascular endothelial growth factor (VEGF), angiopoietin-1 is an endothelial cell–specific growth factor. Angiopoietin-1 is not a direct endothelial mitogen *in vitro,* but it induces endothelial cells to recruit pericytes and smooth muscle cells to appose themselves to the wall of a microvessel. This process can convert a capillary vessel to a venule. Pericyte and smooth muscle recruitment are mediated by endothelial production of platelet-derived growth factor-BB (and probably other factors) when Tie2 is activated by angiopoietin-1.[67] In mice that overexpress angiopoietin-1 in the skin, increased vascularization is noted.[65] The vessels are significantly larger than normal and the skin is reddened. The vessels are not leaky and no skin edema is present, in contrast to dermal vessels of mice overexpressing VEGF. In transgenic mice expressing both angiopoietin-1 and VEGF in the skin, dermal angiogenesis is increased in an additive manner, but the vessels do not leak.[68] This model closely approximates angiogenesis in healing wounds (i.e., relatively nonleaky vessels coated by pericytes and some perivascular smooth muscle cells). In contrast, tumor vessels are leaky and thin-walled with a paucity of pericytes. Angiopoietin-2 blocks the Tie-2 receptor on endothelial cells,[66] which initiates a chain of events so that pericytes and smooth muscle cells are repelled. Angiopoietin-2 is produced by vascular endothelium in a tumor bed, but a putative "angiopoietin-inducing factor" from tumor cells is unknown. Nevertheless, tumor vessels remain as thin "endothelial-lined tubes," even though some of these microvessels reach the diameter of venules. Angiopoietin-2 and VEGF acting together increase angiogenesis. However, if VEGF is antagonized or withdrawn at this point, endothelial cells may undergo apoptosis and new microvessels can regress.[68] In summary, endostatin may regress tumor neovascularization that is under the control of angiopoietin-2, but it may have little or no effect on wound neovascularization regulated by angiopoietin-1.

Differences in Angiogenic Response at Different Sites in the Host

In animals, it has been shown that the same tumor type may elicit different intensities of angiogenesis when implanted at different sites in the body. For example, subcutaneous tumors implanted on the dorsum between the scapulae may grow at four times the rate of tumor implanted more caudally between the iliac crests.[69] Human colon cancers implanted subcutaneously (in immunodeficient mice) do not become neovascularized and remain dormant at a microscopic size. In contrast, when these tumors are transplanted to the surface of the

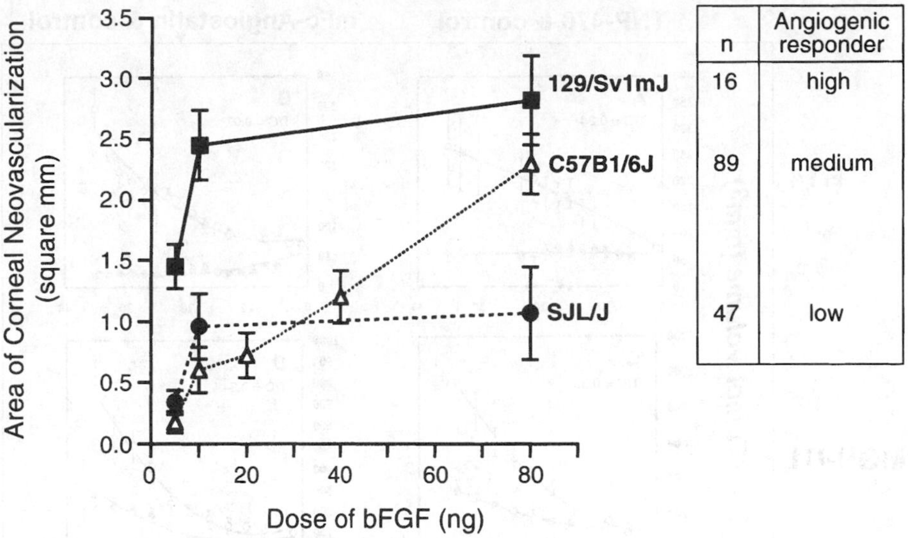

FIGURE 20.6-5. Genetic heterogeneity of angiogenesis in different genetic strains of mice. bFGF, basic fibroblast growth factor. (From ref. 71, with permission.)

colon, they become neovascularized and grow to a large size.[70] This tumor uses bFGF as its major angiogenic mediator but is unable to induce angiogenesis in the subcutaneous position because of high levels of interferon-β in the keratinocytes, which is not found in the colon wall. Interferon-β, like its commercially available relative interferon-α, down-regulates bFGF messenger RNA and protein production by colon cancer cells,[70] thus acting as a natural suppressor of any angiogenesis mediated by bFGF. In this experiment, the colon cancer cells lacked a receptor for bFGF. If these findings apply to patients, metastases in different sites (e.g., lung vs. bone), may respond differently to a given dose of angiogenesis inhibitor. Conversely, different doses of inhibitor may be required for inhibition of metastases at different organ sites.

Genetic Differences in Host Angiogenic Response

D'Amato and Rohan in our department of surgery at Children's Hospital, Boston, demonstrated that certain strains of mice (e.g., 129/SvImJ) produce an intense angiogenic response to the same dose of an angiogenic protein (bFGF) that induces a low angiogenic response in mice of a different genetic background (SJL/J).[71] At least a tenfold difference is seen between the high and low responders, with other strains of mice responding in the middle range (Fig. 20.6-5).

TOTAL ANGIOGENIC OUTPUT OF A TUMOR MAY DETERMINE ITS RESPONSE TO ANTIANGIOGENIC THERAPY

When taken together, the experimental findings cited above indicate that the total angiogenic output of a tumor may be a sum of (1) the balance of positive and negative angiogenic regulators that the tumor cells generate, (2) the genetic heterogeneity of angiogenic responsiveness in the host, and (3) the angiogenic heterogeneity at the tumor site. If these results are extrapolated to cancer patients, metastases in one site (e.g., lungs) may respond to a given angiogenesis inhibitor before metastases at another site (e.g., bone) in the same patient. Furthermore, two patients with the same tumor type may respond differently to a given dose of an angiogenesis inhibitor. Therefore, in principle, optimal therapeutic efficacy would be achieved by administering antiangiogenic therapy at a dose that would match the total angiogenic output of the tumor. In practice, however, it is not currently feasible to determine the total angiogenic output of a tumor. Therefore, those angiogenesis inhibitors that have little or no side effects could possibly be increased to whatever dose level causes a tumor response (i.e., stable disease or tumor regression).

ANTIANGIOGENIC THERAPY MAY BYPASS ACQUIRED DRUG RESISTANCE

The genetic instability and high mutation rate of tumor cells is responsible, in part, for the frequent emergence of acquired drug resistance with conventional cytotoxic anticancer therapy. However, vascular endothelial cells, like bone marrow cells, are genetically stable and have a low mutation rate. Therefore, Kerbel[72] proposed a hypothesis in 1991 that antiangiogenic therapy would be a strategy to bypass drug resistance. Subsequently, my laboratory validated this concept in tumor-bearing mice treated with endostatin.[39]

ANTIANGIOGENIC THERAPY IS INDEPENDENT OF TUMOR CELL CYCLE

Conventional cytotoxic chemotherapy is generally cell cycle–dependent. Indolent tumors with a low percentage of cycling tumor cells are more refractory to cytotoxic chemotherapy than are rapidly growing tumors. This property is thought to explain the high efficacy of chemotherapy in fast-growing mouse tumors compared to the relatively low efficacy in adult human tumors, with success against pediatric tumors viewed as somewhere in between. It has been widely assumed that antiangiogenic therapy would be similar to chemotherapy. Experimental studies, however, reveal just the opposite. Slowly growing tumors in mice require lower doses of antiangiogenic therapy to bring them to dormancy than do faster growing tumors, which require higher doses (Fig. 20.6-6).[73]

Furthermore, during tumor inhibition by antiangiogenic therapy, tumor cell proliferation usually remains unchanged from the

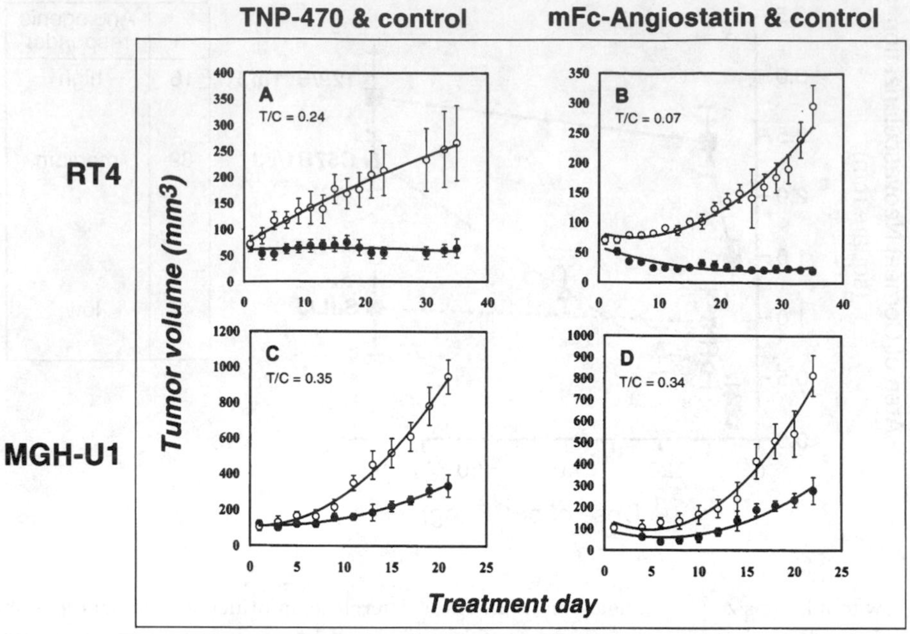

FIGURE 20.6-6. The effect of antiangiogenic therapy on slowly growing (RT4) **(A,B)** versus rapidly growing (MGH-U1) **(C,D)** human bladder cancer in mice.

pretreated state.[14,44] When mice bearing drug-sensitive tumors were treated with cyclophosphamide on a "conventional" schedule, tumor cell proliferation was significantly decreased[74] (see Cytotoxic Chemotherapy May Be Angiogenesis Dependent, later in this chapter). However, when the same tumor was made highly resistant to cyclophosphamide, the tumor cell proliferation rate did not decrease, despite the fact that tumors regressed under an "antiangiogenic" schedule of the same drug.

MICROVESSEL DENSITY IS A USEFUL PROGNOSTIC INDICATOR BUT MAY NOT BE A USEFUL INDICATOR OF EFFICACY OF ANTIANGIOGENIC THERAPY

The first quantitative method for histologic grading of tumor angiogenesis was reported by Steven Brem and colleagues[75] from my laboratory in 1972. They correlated neovascularization in human brain tumors with tumor grade. It was not until thirteen years later that a second report describing histologic quantification of tumor angiogenesis was published.[76] This report was followed 3 years later by the first report of the use of tumor vascularity as a prognostic marker (cutaneous melanoma).[77] In 1991, Noel Weidner and I used specific antiendothelial antibodies to highlight tumor vasculature and showed that microvessel density was a prognostic marker for human breast cancer.[78] Since then, the majority of reports (52 different studies) have confirmed that microvessel density is a powerful and often an independent prognostic indicator for many different types of human cancer. However, other reports fail to show that microvessel density is a prognostic indicator (seven studies), especially for certain types of tumors. Many of the negative reports may be methodological. Others may result from poorly understood biologic differences, such as the possible coexistence of angiogenesis inhibitors and stimulators in certain tumors. Gasparini and Harris[79] analyzed the variables in quantitation of tumor angiogenesis in histologic sections, and they have summarized the reports up to 1999. These reports are also summarized in tabular form.[4] The basis of the prognostic value of quantifying the areas of highest microvessel density ("hot spots") in a tumor may be that these areas represent the most angiogenic clones of tumor cells. Such clones have the highest probability of being angiogenic metastases.

However, because microvessel density of a tumor is a prognostic marker for the risk of metastasis or death of a patient does not necessarily make it a useful indicator of efficacy of antiangiogenic therapy. Microvessel density is largely determined by intercapillary distance, which itself is governed by the thickness of the cuff of tumor cells surrounding a microvessel (50 to 200 μm). In experimental animals, microvessel density may remain constant as a tumor is regressing under antiangiogenic therapy. Despite ongoing capillary dropout in a shrinking tumor mass, residual tumor cells can assemble around the remaining microvessels, thus leaving the microvessel density relatively unchanged. Furthermore, microvessel density may not distinguish between certain benign and malignant tumors. For example, normal human pituitary has a higher microvessel density than a pituitary adenoma, which has a higher microvessel density than a pituitary carcinoma.[80] One explanation of this apparent paradox is that, in most normal tissues, the perivascular cuff is usually one or two cells thick. In some normal tissues, therefore, intercapillary distance is small, leading to a high microvessel density. In contrast, in many tumors the perivascular cuff thickness increases as tumor cells adapt to lower oxygen tension and survive at an increasing distance from the nearest open capillary. The cuff thickness of a murine breast carcinoma (MCa-IV) reaches 100 μm or more, which approaches the limit of oxygen diffusion.[81] For other tumors, such as breast carcinoma, microvessel density is significantly higher in the cancer than in normal breast.[78,82] In certain animal tumors, angiogenic output appears to exceed the growth capacity of the tumor cells so that treatment with an angiogenesis inhibitor initially induces a significant decrease in microvessel density as tumor growth is inhibited or arrested. Because all of these variables are not fully understood, it may not be prudent at this time to use microvessel density as a surrogate marker for efficacy of antiangiogenic therapy.

STABLE DISEASE OR TUMOR DORMANCY CAN BE SUSTAINED BY BLOCKED ANGIOGENESIS

Increasing evidence shows that experimental tumors can be maintained at a stable size or at a microscopic dormant size by uninterrupted antiangiogenic therapy or by blocked angiogenesis.[35–37,39,42,43] For the purpose of this chapter, *stable disease* may be defined as tumor that has stopped expanding but is grossly visible or radiologically detectable. A definition of *tumor dormancy* is nonexpanding tumor that can be detected only microscopically. In either event, recruitment of new vessels is sufficiently restricted that tumor cells surviving on residual vessels exist in a steady state of proliferation and apoptosis that prohibits further expansion of tumor mass, regardless of whether it is a primary tumor or a metastasis. It is too early to say whether prolonged stable disease or durable tumor dormancy can be achieved by antiangiogenic therapy in cancer patients. Nevertheless, it may be prudent to include these states as possible end points in clinical protocols for antiangiogenic therapy. A close approximation to tumor dormancy in experimental animals may be the regression of a recurrent giant cell tumor of the mandible by interferon-α administered at a low dose of 3 million units per day for 1 year.[83] Interferon-α is an angiogenesis inhibitor by virtue of its ability to block overproduction of bFGF.[53,70]

LEUKEMIA IS ANGIOGENESIS DEPENDENT

The conventional wisdom has been that, because leukemia is regarded as a liquid tumor, it does not require angiogenesis. However, in children with newly diagnosed untreated acute lymphoblastic leukemia, bone marrow biopsies revealed a six- to sevenfold increase in microvessel density in the leukemic marrows in contrast to control bone marrows from children undergoing staging evaluations at the time of diagnosis of solid tumor.[84] Microvessels in leukemic bone were surrounded by a perivascular cuff of tumor cells not unlike solid tumors. This configuration was best observed by confocal microscopy. bFGF was approximately sevenfold higher in the leukemic children than in controls. Interestingly, acute myeloid leukemia in adults is also associated with intense bone marrow neovascularization.[85–88] Cellular levels of the angiogenic factor VEGF are abnormally elevated and provide an independent predictor of outcome.[89] The myeloproliferative diseases polycythemia vera, chronic myelocytic leukemia, and myelofibrosis also have significantly increased neovascularity.[90] The close configuration of bone marrow cells and microvessels may permit a two-way paracrine pathway between vascular endothelial cells, which can release granulocyte colony-stimulating factor[52] (a mitogen for bone marrow cells), and bone marrow cells, which release bFGF (a mitogen for vascular endothelial cells).[91]

These results show that leukemia (and other proliferative diseases of the bone marrow) are angiogenic. They do not, however, prove that leukemia is angiogenesis dependent. The first experimental evidence in support of this concept is by Browder and colleagues,[74] who demonstrated that L1210 leukemia can be eradicated by an antiangiogenic schedule of chemotherapy, but not by the conventional schedule of maximum tolerated dosing. Unpublished preliminary data by Browder suggests that endostatin, a specific angiogenesis inhibitor, can significantly prolong survival of mice bearing murine leukemias.

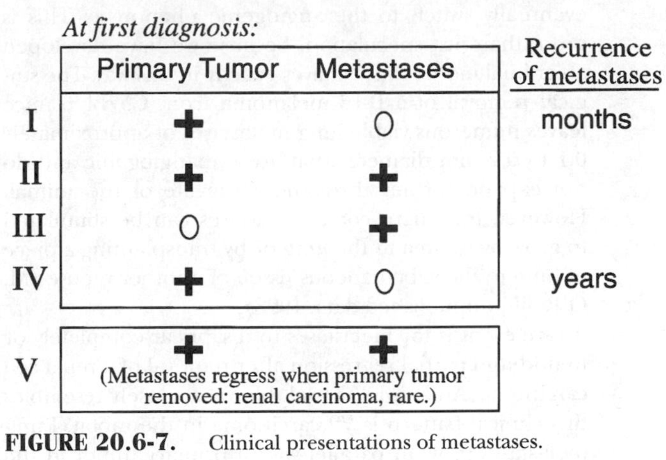

FIGURE 20.6-7. Clinical presentations of metastases.

These observations provide a conceptual basis for the potential future use of angiogenesis inhibitors in leukemia, perhaps first in patients for whom all conventional therapy has been unsuccessful, and later as an adjunct to conventional therapy.

CLINICAL PATTERNS OF METASTASIS PRESENTATION MAY BE ANGIOGENESIS DEPENDENT

Cancer metastases may present at least four common clinical patterns and one rare pattern (Fig. 20.6-7). These clinical observations have previously been unrelated to each other, but we can now propose that they may all be explained on the basis of angiogenic principles.[92]

1. The patient whose metastases appear a few months after surgical removal of a primary tumor may have undergone a decrease in a circulating angiogenesis inhibitor that was generated by the primary tumor. A murine Lewis lung carcinoma that generates angiostatin is a model of this type of clinical presentation.[35]
2. When metastases are already present at the first diagnosis of a primary tumor (i.e., parallel tumor growth), the primary tumor may have lost or down-regulated its ability to generate a circulating angiogenesis inhibitor and therefore is incapable of suppressing distant metastases. The experimental analogue would be a subline of Lewis lung carcinoma that has lost the ability to generate angiostatin.[35]
3. When metastases present in the absence of a primary tumor (i.e., a pattern known as the *occult primary*),[93] this finding may be similar to mice in which tumor cells are injected intravenously and are allowed to take as lung metastases before a primary tumor is implanted subcutaneously.[94] In this experiment, growth of the subcutaneous tumor appears to be inhibited by the extensive metastatic growth. However, it has not yet been ascertained whether the inhibition was mediated by a circulating inhibitor. In a patient presenting with this metastatic pattern, the total mass of metastases would need to expand faster than the primary tumor to produce sufficient quantities of circulating angiogenesis inhibitor that could suppress the primary tumor.
4. The patient whose metastases do not appear until years after removal of the primary tumor may harbor dormant metastases that are not angiogenic for many years but

eventually switch to the angiogenic phenotype. This is more than just speculation, because we have developed an animal model that behaves exactly in this way. The surgical removal of a B-16 melanoma from C57Bl/6 mice leaves numerous viable lung metastases of approximately 0.1 to 0.2 mm diameter that are nonangiogenic and do not expand further throughout the life of the animal. However, the microscopic metastases can be stimulated to grow by trauma to the lung or by transplanting a piece of lung to the subcutaneous tissue of another mouse (M. O'Reilly, unpublished data, 1998).

5. A rare event is for metastases to disappear completely or to undergo partial regression after removal of a renal cell carcinoma. An animal model that most closely resembles this clinical pattern is V2 carcinoma in the rabbit. Lung metastases grow in parallel with a primary tumor in the thigh. However, lung metastases regress after the primary is completely resected (H. Verheul, R. D'Amato, and D. Panigrahy, unpublished data, 1998). This finding does not appear to be an immune reaction, because fresh tumor can be successfully grown in the same rabbit. One explanation may be that the metastases were dependent on high production of a circulating angiogenic factor(s), such as the high tissue levels of bFGF that have been found to correlate with high mortality in renal cancer.[95]

By describing these patterns of metastatic presentation in patients, I have tried to provide a possible unifying mechanism to explain them. The experimental evidence for the animal models is discussed in more detail by Holmgren et al.[14] It must be emphasized that the similarity of such animal models to human patterns of metastatic presentation does not prove that the human patterns are based on the same angiogenic principles as the animal models. However, this arrangement of the human metastatic patterns will hopefully stimulate other investigators to find additional clinical or experimental evidence to support or refute the general hypothesis. Thus, the heuristic value of Figure 20.6-7 is its potential inclusion in the design of clinical trials of angiogenesis inhibitors. These observations also provide an alternative to the widely held assumption that tumor cells in a dormant microscopic tumor are not cycling and remain in G_0. In fact, dormant animal tumors with blocked angiogenesis maintain a high apoptosis rate balanced by a high proliferation rate in the tumor cells.[14]

CYTOTOXIC CHEMOTHERAPY MAY BE ANGIOGENESIS-DEPENDENT

Conventional cytotoxic chemotherapeutic drugs target tumor cells, but the effect of these drugs on microvascular endothelial cells has received little attention until the 1990s. Baguley et al.[96] demonstrated in 1991 that vinblastine caused more than 90% necrosis of drug-resistant solid tumors within hours but had no direct effect on the tumor cells as demonstrated when the cells were grown as ascites. In 1992, Steiner showed that vincristine, vinblastine, doxorubicin, mitoxantrone, and etoposide had short-term antiangiogenic activity in the chick embryo.[97] Also, *in vitro* antiendothelial effects have been reported for cyclophosphamide,[98] 5-fluorouracil,[99] and mitomycin C.[99,100] Short-term *in vivo* antiangiogenic effects have been reported for paclitaxel,[101–103] 6-methylmercaptopurine,[104] tegafur,[105] 9-amino-20(S)-camptothecin,[106] topotecan,[106] and combretastatin A-4.[107,108]

The question was raised by Browder as to why those cytotoxic chemotherapeutic agents with antiangiogenic activity still induced acquired drug resistance. Specific angiogenesis inhibitors do not usually induce drug resistance.[39,72] Vascular endothelial cells, like bone marrow cells, do not develop drug resistance, in part because of their low mutation rate. Browder hypothesized that the usual dose-schedule regimen for chemotherapeutic agents is not conducive to sustained blockade of angiogenesis. Conventional chemotherapy is traditionally administered at maximum tolerated doses followed by an extended treatment-free interval to permit recovery of hematopoietic progenitors and gastrointestinal tract mucosa. Browder proposed, however, that *during this off-therapy interval, microvascular endothelial cells in the tumor bed could also resume growth and nourish tumor recurrence.* Virtually all animal experiments show that antiangiogenic therapy is most successful when it is given over short intervals (e.g., daily or every other day) without off-therapy gaps. Browder demonstrated that 5-fluorouracil and 6-mercaptopurine are nearly devoid of antiangiogenic activity when given as bolus injections, but they reveal potent antiangiogenic efficacy when the same dose is given as a continuous infusion.[74]

He further showed that a standard cytotoxic agent, cyclophosphamide, can be administered to animals bearing Lewis lung carcinoma at a dose and schedule that is optimized for more sustained apoptosis of *endothelial* cells but not of tumor cells. This was named the *antiangiogenic schedule.* The *conventional schedule* is a maximum tolerated dose administered every other day for three doses followed by 21 days off-therapy to rescue bone marrow. The antiangiogenic schedule consists of a lower dose administered every 6 days. A drug-sensitive Lewis lung carcinoma became drug resistant on the conventional schedule and killed all mice, but it was eradicated on the antiangiogenic schedule. No detectable tumor was detected after 657 days, when the animals reached the end of their natural lifespan. When the tumor was made drug resistant before therapy, the antiangiogenic schedule suppressed tumor growth three time more effectively than the conventional schedule. When an angiogenesis inhibitor, TNP-470, was added at a dose 86% lower than its effective dose alone, the drug-resistant tumor was eradicated in 84% of mice.[74] This finding is provocative because TNP-470 alone, even at its full dose, slows Lewis lung carcinoma by only 65% and cannot cause regression. Thus, a cytotoxic chemotherapeutic agent administered in an antiangiogenic dose schedule can more effectively control tumor growth in mice, whether or not its tumor cells are drug resistant, an improvement that has come from using new logic for an old drug. In summary, the new logic is that the antiangiogenic properties of certain conventional cytotoxic agents are not revealed unless the drugs are administered frequently, without a prolonged off-therapy period. Frequent administration requires lower doses. Klement et al.[109] in Robert Kerbel's laboratory have demonstrated this new logic with a different experimental system. For a commentary on antiangiogenic chemotherapy, see Hanahan et al.[110] They showed that continuous low-dose therapy with vinblastine and an antibody to VEGF receptor-2 induced sustained regression of neuroblastoma without overt toxicity. No evidence of acquired drug resistance was found throughout the 6 months' course of treatment.

When taken together, these results in mice may help to explain why some patients who are receiving long-term maintenance or even palliative chemotherapy continue to have stable disease beyond the time that the tumor cells would have been expected to develop drug resistance. However, because conventional schedules of combination chemotherapy have led to profound increases in the survival of children with cancer and have improved the survival of adults with certain types of cancer, we do not believe that these clinical protocols should be changed for the sake of increasing the antiangiogenic efficacy of any given drug.[74] Formal clinical trials with patients whose tumor has become refractory to conventional chemotherapy or radiotherapy will be necessary to find an optimum antiangiogenic dose and schedule and to demonstrate whether it is an improvement over conventional chemotherapy dose schedules.

CLINICAL TRIALS OF ANGIOGENESIS INHIBITORS

At this writing, 20 angiogenesis inhibitors produced by the biotechnology and pharmaceutical industry are in clinical trial for patients with advanced metastatic cancer, and seven are in phase III trials (see Fig. 20.6-1).

Three general strategies have been used to develop these inhibitors. A target molecule in the angiogenic pathway is identified and then is counteracted by a synthetic inhibitor or by an antibody (e.g., an antibody to the angiogenic factor VEGF or its receptor). A second approach is to identify antiangiogenic activity in a drug previously used for a different effect. Examples are thalidomide and interferon-α. Slamon showed that Herceptin has antiangiogenic activity in addition to its direct antitumor effect on breast cancer cells: It interferes with the activity of at least three angiogenic proteins produced by breast cancer cells (D. Slamon, Plenary Address before the American Association of Cancer Research, San Francisco, April 2000). A third approach is to discover specific endogenous angiogenesis inhibitors that are already in the circulation or in matrix. In fact, several of these are internal fragments of larger proteins that have different functions. Some examples are thrombospondin-1, a 140-kD protein under the control of p53[111]; angiostatin, a 38-kD fragment of plasminogen[35]; endostatin, a 20-kD fragment of collagen XVIII[37]; pigment epithelium-derived factor, a 50-kD serine protease inhibitor[112]; antiangiogenic antithrombin III, a 53-kD cleaved or latent conformation of the 58-kD antithrombin III[40]; restin, a 22-kD internal fragment of collagen XV[113]; canstatin, a 24-kD fragment of the α_2-chain of type IV collagen[114]; and maspin, a 42-kD gene product of normal breast epithelium, also under the control of p53 and silenced during breast cancer progression.[115,116] A longer list would include SPARC (*s*ecreted *p*rotein *a*cidic and *r*ich in *c*ysteine),[117] VEGI (*v*ascular *e*ndothelial cell *g*rowth *i*nhibitor),[118] IP-10 (interferon-γ-inducible protein-10),[119] interleukin-18,[120] and 16-kD prolactin.[121]

The angiogenesis inhibitors operate by quite different mechanisms, which reveal that multiple pathways in the angiogenic process are vulnerable to attack.[4] As of this writing, it is too soon to say which of the angiogenesis inhibitors currently in clinical trial will receive U.S. Food and Drug Administration approval. However, because angiogenesis inhibitors can be added to chemotherapy, radiotherapy, immunotherapy, or gene therapy, as well as to each other, there is likely to be a future need for a group of angiogenesis inhibitors from which physicians can choose. The eventual possibility also exists that antiangiogenic therapy may be used as long-term maintenance therapy, like tamoxifen, to reduce the risk of recurrences.

REFERENCES

1. Hager T. *Force of nature: the life of Linus Pauling.* New York: Simon & Schuster, 1995.
2. Feinstein A. The intellectual crisis in clinical science: medaled models and muddled mettle. *Perspect Biol Med* 1987;30:215.
3. Folkman J. Angiogenesis in breast cancer. In: Bland KI, Copeland EM III. *The breast, comprehensive management of benign and malignant diseases,* 2nd ed. Philadelphia: WB Saunders, 1998:586.
4. Folkman J. Tumor angiogenesis. In: Holland JF, Frei E III, Bast RC, et al., eds. *Cancer medicine,* 5th ed. Hamilton, Ontario: BC Decker, 2000.
5. Hanahan D, Weinberg RA. The hallmarks of cancer. *Cell* 2000;100:57.
6. Folkman J. Tumor angiogenesis: therapeutic implications. *N Engl J Med* 1971;285:1182.
7. Folkman J. Anti-angiogenesis: new concept for therapy of solid tumors. *Ann Surg* 1972;175:408.
8. Algire GH, Chalkely HW, Legallais FY, Park H. Vascular reactions of normal and malignant tumors *in vivo.* I. Vascular reactions of mice to wounds and to normal and neoplastic transplants. *J Natl Cancer Inst* 1945;6:73.
9. Folkman J. What is the evidence that tumors are angiogenesis dependent? *J Natl Cancer Inst* 1990;82:4.
10. Folkman J, Hochberg M. Self-regulation of growth in three dimensions. *J Exp Med* 1973;138:745.
11. Adam JA, Maggelakis AA. Diffusion of regulated growth characteristics of a spherical prevascular carcinoma. *Bull Math Biol* 1990;52:549.
12. Sutherland RM. Cell and environment interactions in tumor microregions: the multicell spheroid model. *Science* 1988;240:177.
13. Sutherland RM, McCredie JA, Inch WR. Growth of multicell spheroids in tissue culture as a model of nodular carcinomas. *J Natl Cancer Inst* 1971;46:113.
14. Holmgren L, O'Reilly MS, Folkman J. Dormancy of micrometastases: balanced proliferation and apoptosis in the presence of angiogenesis suppression. *Nat Med* 1995;1:149.
15. Gimbrone MA Jr, Cotran R, Leapman S, Folkman J. Tumor growth and neovascularization: an experimental model using rabbit cornea. *J Natl Cancer Inst* 1974;52:413.
16. Gimbrone MA Jr, Leapman S, Cotran RS, Folkman J. Tumor dormancy *in vivo* by prevention of neovascularization. *J Exp Med* 1972;136:261.
17. Brem S, Brem H, Folkman J, Finkelstein D, Patz A. Prolonged tumor dormancy by prevention of neovascularization in the vitreous. *Cancer Res* 1976;36:2807.
18. Folkman J. Tumor angiogenesis factor. *Cancer Res* 1974;34:2109.
19. Tannock IF. Population kinetics of carcinoma cells, capillary endothelial cells, and fibroblasts in a transplanted mouse mammary tumor. *Cancer Res* 1970;30:2470.
20. Helmlinger G, Yuan F, Dellian M, Jain RK. Interstitial pH and pO_2 gradients in solid tumors *in vivo*: high-resolution measurements reveal a lack of correlation. *Nat Med* 1997;3(2):177.
21. Knighton D, Ausprunk D, Tapper D, Folkman J. Avascular and vascular phases of tumour growth in the chick embryo. *Br J Cancer* 1977;35:347.
22. Lien W, Ackerman NB. The blood supply of experimental liver metastases. II. A microcirculatory study of normal and tumor vessels of the liver with the use of perfused silicone rubber. *Surgery* 1970;68:334.
23. Folkman J, Watson K, Ingber D, Hanahan D. Induction of angiogenesis during the transition from hyperplasia to neoplasia. *Nature* 1989;339:58.
24. Thompson WD, Shiach KJ, Fraser RA, Mintosh LC, Simpson JG. Tumors acquire their vasculature by vessel incorporation, not vessel ingrowth. *J Pathol* 1987;151:323.
25. Skinner SA, Tutton PJ, O'Brien PE. Microvascular architecture of experimental colon tumors in the rat. *Cancer Res* 1990;50:2411.
26. Holash J, Maisonpierre PC, Compton D, et al. Vessel cooption, regression, and growth in tumors mediated by angiopoietins and VEGF. *Science* 1999;284:1994.
27. Ingber DM, Fujita T, Kishimoto S, et al. Synthetic analogues of fumagillin that inhibit angiogenesis and suppress tumour growth. *Nature* 1990;348:555.
28. Folkman J. Tumor angiogenesis. In: Wells SA Jr, Sharp PA, eds. *Accomplishments in cancer research.* Philadelphia: Lippincott Williams & Wilkins, 1998:32.
29. Hori A, Sasada R, Matsutani E, et al. Suppression of solid tumor growth by immuno-neutralizing monoclonal antibody against human basic fibroblast growth factor. *Cancer Res* 1991;51:6180.
30. Kim KJ, Li B, Winer J, et al. Inhibition of vascular endothelial growth factor–induced angiogenesis suppresses tumour growth *in vivo. Nature* 1993;362:841.
31. Plate KH, Breier G, Millauer B, Ullrich A, Risau W. Up-regulation of vascular endothelial growth factor and its cognate receptors in a rat glioma model of tumor angiogenesis. *Cancer Res* 1993;53:5822.
32. Millauer B, Shawver LK, Plate KH, Risau W, Ullrich A. Glioblastoma growth inhibited *in vivo* by a dominant-negative Flk-1 mutant. *Nature* 1994;367:576.
33. Dameron KM, Volpert OV, Tainsky MA, Bouck N. Control of angiogenesis in fibroblasts by p53 regulation of thrombospondin-1. *Science* 1994;265:1582.
34. Brooks PC, Montgomery AMP, Rosenfeld M, et al. Integrin alpha v beta 3 antagonists promote tumor regression by inducing apoptosis of angiogenic blood vessels. *Cell* 1994;79:1157.
35. O'Reilly MS, Holmgren L, Shing Y, et al. Angiostatin: a novel angiogenesis inhibitor that mediates the suppression of metastases by a Lewis lung carcinoma. *Cell* 1994;79:315.

36. O'Reilly MS, Holmgren L, Chen C, Folkman J. Angiostatin induces and sustains dormancy of human primary tumors in mice. *Nat Med* 1996;2:689.
37. O'Reilly MS, Boehm T, Shing Y, et al. Endostatin: an endogenous inhibitor of angiogenesis and tumor growth. *Cell* 1997;88:277.
38. O'Reilly MS, Brem H, Folkman J. Treatment of murine hemangioendotheliomas with the angiogenesis inhibitor AGM-1470. *J Pediatr Surg* 1994;30:325.
39. Boehm T, Folkman J, Browder T, O'Reilly MS. Antiangiogenic therapy of experimental cancer does not induce acquired drug resistance. *Nature* 1997;390:404.
40. O'Reilly MS, Pirie-Shepherd S, Lane WS, Folkman J. Antiangiogenic activity of the cleaved conformation of the serpin antithrombin. *Science* 1999;285:1926.
41. Cao Y, O'Reilly MS, Marshall B, et al. Expression of angiostatin cDNA in a murine fibrosarcoma suppresses primary tumor growth and produces long-term dormancy of metastases. *J Clin Invest* 1998;101:1055.
42. Lyden D, Young AZ, Zagzag D, et al. Id1 and Id3 are required for neurogenesis, angiogenesis and vascularization of tumour xenografts. *Nature* 1999;401:670.
43. Streit M, Riccardi L, Velasco P, et al. Thrombospondin-2: a potent endogenous inhibitor of tumor growth and angiogenesis. *Proc Natl Acad Sci U S A* 1999;96:14888.
44. Li CY, Shan S, Huang Q, et al. Initial stages of tumor cell–induced angiogenesis: evaluation via skin window chambers in rodent models. *J Natl Cancer Inst* 2000;92:143.
45. Folkman J. Incipient angiogenesis. *J Natl Cancer Inst* 2000;92:94.
46. Nicosia RF, Tchao R, Leighton J. Interactions between newly formed endothelial channels and carcinoma cells in plasma clot culture. *Clin Exp Metastasis* 1986;4:91.
47. Hamada J, Cavanaugh PG, Lotan O, Nicolson GL. Separable growth and migration factors for large-cell lymphoma cells secreted by microvascular endothelial cells derived from target organs for metastasis. *Br J Cancer* 1992;66:349.
48. Rak JW, St. Croix BD, Kerbel RS. Consequences of angiogenesis for tumor progression, metastasis and cancer therapy. *Anticancer Drugs* 1995;6:3.
49. Schweigerer L, Neufeld G, Friedman J, et al. Capillary endothelial cells express basic fibroblast growth factor, a mitogen that promotes their own growth. *Nature* 1987;25:257.
50. Motro B, Itin A, Sachs L, Keshet E. Pattern of interleukin 6 gene expression *in vivo* suggests a role for this cytokine in angiogenesis. *Proc Natl Acad Sci U S A* 1990;87:3092.
51. Podor TJ, Jirik FR, Loskutoff DJ, Carson DA, Lotz M. Human endothelial cells produce IL-6. Lack of responses to exogenous IL-6. *Ann N Y Acad Sci* 1989;557:374.
52. Zsebo KM, Yuschenkoff VN, Schiffer S, et al. Vascular endothelial cells and granulopoiesis: interleukin-1 stimulates release of G-CSF and GM-CSF. *Blood* 1988;71:99.
53. Folkman J, Mulliken JB, Ezekowitz RAB. Antiangiogenic therapy of haemangiomas with interferon A. In: Stuart-Harris R, Penny R, eds. *The Clinical applications of the interferons.* London: Chapman & Hall Medical, 1997:255.
54. Evans GI. Old cells never die, they just apoptose. *Trends Cell Biol* 1994;4:191.
55. Folkman J. Tumor angiogenesis and tissue factor. *Nat Med* 1996;2:167.
56. Modzelewski RA, Davies P, Watkins SC, et al. Isolation and identification of fresh tumor-derived endothelial cells from a murine RIF-1 fibrosarcoma. *Cancer Res* 1994;54:336.
57. Denekamp J. Vascular attack as a therapeutic strategy for cancer. *Cancer Metastasis Rev* 1990;3:267.
58. Folkman J, Hahnfeldt P, Hlatky L. The logic of anti-angiogenic gene therapy. In: Friedman T, ed. *The development of human gene therapy.* Cold Spring Harbor, NY: Cold Spring Harbor Laboratory Press, 1998:527.
59. Berges JR, Vukanovic J, Epstein JI, et al. Implication of cell kinetic changes during the progression of human prostatic cancer. *Clin Cancer Res* 1995;1:473.
60. Ding YH, Javaherian K, Lo KM, et al. Zinc-dependent dimers observed in crystals of human endostatin. *Proc Natl Acad Sci U S A* 1998;95:10443.
61. Brem H, Folkman J. Analysis of experimental antiangiogenic therapy. *J Pediatr Surg* 1993;28:445.
62. Davis S, Aldrich TH, Jones PF, et al. Isolation of angiopoietin-1, a ligand for the TIE2 receptor, by secretion-trap expression cloning. *Cell* 1996;87:1161.
63. Sato TN, Tozawa Y, Deutsch U, et al. Distinct roles of the receptor tyrosine kinases Tie-1 and Tie-2 in blood vessel formation. *Nature* 1995;376:70.
64. Koblizek TI, Weiss C, Yancopoulos GD, Deutsch U, Risau W. Angiopoietin-1 induces sprouting angiogenesis *in vitro. Curr Biol* 1998;8:529.
65. Suri C, McClain J, Thurston G, et al. Increased vascularization in mice overexpressing Angiopoietin-1. *Science* 1998;282:468.
66. Maisonpierre PC, Suri C, Jones PF, et al. Angiopoietin-2, a natural antagonist for Tie2 that disrupts *in vivo* angiogenesis. *Science* 1997;277:55.
67. Folkman J, D'Amore P. Blood vessel formation: what is its molecular basis? *Cell* 1996;87:1153.
68. Thurston G, Suri C, Smith K, et al. Leakage-resistant blood vessels in mice transgenically overexpressing angiopoietin-1. *Science* 1999;286:2511.
69. Auerbach R, Auerbach W. Regional differences in the growth of normal and neoplastic cells. *Science* 1982;215:127.
70. Singh RK, Gutman M, Bucana CD, et al. Interferons alpha and beta down-regulate the expression of basic fibroblast growth factor in human carcinomas. *Proc Natl Acad Sci U S A* 1995;92:4562.
71. Rohan RM, Fernandez A, Udagawa T, Yuan J, D'Amato RJ. Genetic heterogeneity of angiogenesis in mice. *FASEB J* 2000;14:871.
72. Kerbel RS. Inhibition of tumor angiogenesis as a strategy to circumvent resistance to anticancer therapeutic agents. *Bioessays* 1991;1:31.
73. Beecken WDC, Fernandez A, Joussen AM, et al. Effect of antiangiogenic therapy on slow growing, poorly vascularized tumors in mice. *J Natl Cancer Inst* 2000 (*in press*).
74. Browder T, Butterfield CE, Kraling BM, et al. Antiangiogenic scheduling of chemotherapy improves efficacy against experimental drug-resistant cancer. *Cancer Res* 2000;60:1878.
75. Brem S, Cotran R, Folkman J. Tumor angiogenesis: a quantitative method for histologic grading. *J Natl Cancer Inst* 1972;48:347.
76. Mlynek M, van Beunigen D, Leder LD, Streffer C. Measurement of the grade of vascularization in histological tumour tissue sections. *Br J Cancer* 1985;52:945.
77. Srivastava A, Laidler P, Davies RP, Horfan K. The prognostic significance of tumor vascularity in intermediate-thickness (0.76–4.0 mm thick) skin melanoma. A quantitative histologic study. *Am J Pathol* 1988;133:419.
78. Weidner N, Semple JP, Welch WR, Folkman J. Tumor angiogenesis correlates with metastasis in invasive breast carcinoma. *N Engl J Med* 1991;324:1.
79. Gasparini G, Harris AL. Prognostic significance of tumor vascularity. In: Teicher BA, ed. *Antiangiogenic agents in cancer therapy.* Totowa, NJ: Humana Press, 1999:317.
80. Turner HE, Nagy Z, Gatter KC, et al. Angiogenesis in pituitary adenomas and the normal pituitary gland. *J Clin Endocrinol Metab* 2000;85:1159.
81. Hashizume H, Baluk P, Morikawa S, et al. Openings between defective endothelial cells explain tumor vessel leakiness. *Am J Pathol* 2000;156:1363.
82. Weidner N. Current pathologic methods for measuring intratumoral microvessel density within breast carcinoma and other solid tumors. *Breast Cancer Res Treat* 1995;36:169.
83. Kaban LB, Mulliken JB, Ezekowitz RA, et al. Antiangiogenic therapy of a recurrent giant cell tumor of the mandible with interferon alfa-2a. *Pediatrics* 1999;103:1145.
84. Perez-Atayde AR, Sallan SE, Tedrow U, et al. Spectrum of tumor angiogenesis in the bone marrow of children with acute lymphoblastic leukemia. *Am J Pathol* 1997;150:815.
85. Vacca A, Ribatti D, Roncali L, et al. Bone marrow angiogenesis and progression in multiple myeloma. *Br J Haematol* 1994;87:503.
86. Vacca A, Ribatti D, Roncali L, Dammacco F. Angiogenesis in B cell lymphoproliferative diseases: biological and clinical studies. *Leuk Lymphoma* 1995;20:27.
87. Munshi N, Wilson CS, Penn J, et al. Angiogenesis in newly diagnosed multiple myeloma: poor prognosis with increased microvessel density (MVD) in bone marrow biopsies. *Blood* 1998;92[Suppl 1]:98A(abst).
88. Vacca A, Ribatti D, Presta M, et al. Bone marrow neovascularization, plasma cell angiogenic potential and matrix metalloproteinae-2 secretion parallel progression of human multiple myeloma. *Blood* 1999;93:3064.
89. Aguayo A, Estey E, Kantarjian H, et al. Cellular vascular endothelial growth factor is a predictor of outcome in patients with acute myeloid leukemia. *Blood* 1999;94:3717.
90. Lundberg LG, Lerner R, Sundelin P, et al. Bone marrow in polycythemia vera, chronic myelocytic leukemia and myelofibrosis has an increased vascularity. *Am J Pathol* 2000; 157:15.
91. Brunner G, Metz CN, Nguyen H, et al. An endogenous glycosylphosphatidylinositol-specific phospholipase D releases basic fibroblast growth factor–heparan sulfate proteoglycan complexes from human bone marrow cultures. *Blood* 1994;83:2115.
92. Folkman J. Angiogenesis in cancer, vascular, rheumatoid and other disease. *Nat Med* 1995;1:27.
93. Hess KR, Abbruzzese MC, Lenzi R, Raber MN, Abbruzzese JL. Classification and regression tree analysis of 1000 consecutive patients with unknown primary carcinoma. *Clin Cancer Res* 1999;5:3403.
94. Yuhas JM, Pazmino NH. Inhibition of subcutaneously growing line 1 carcinoma due to metastatic spread. *Cancer Res* 1974;34:2005.
95. Nanus DM, Schmitz-Drager BJ, Motzer RJ, et al. Expression of basic fibroblast growth factor in primary human renal tumors: correlation with poor survival. *J Natl Cancer Inst* 1993;85:1597.
96. Baguley BC, Holdaway KM, Thomsen LL, Zhuang L, Zwi LJ. Inhibition of growth of colon 38 adenocarcinoma by vinblastine and colchicine: evidence for a vascular mechanism. *Eur J Cancer* 1991;27:482.
97. Steiner R. Angiostatic activity of anticancer agents in the chick embryo chorioallantoic membrane (CHE-CAM) assay. In: Steiner R, Weisz PB, Langer R, eds. *Angiogenesis. Key principles—science—technology—medicine.* Basel, Switzerland: Birkhauser Verlag, 1992:449.
98. Kachel DL, Martin WJ II. Cyclophosphamide-induced lung toxicity: mechanism of endothelial cell injury. *J Pharmacol Exp Ther* 1994;268:42.
99. Nuyts RMMA, Pels E, Greve EL. The effects of 5-fluorouracil and mitomycin C on the corneal endothelium. *Curr Eye Res* 1992;11:565.
100. Hoorn C, Wagner JG, Petry TW, Roth RA. Toxicity of mitomycin C toward cultured pulmonary artery endothelium. *Toxicol Appl Pharmacol* 1995;130:87.
101. Belotti D, Vergani V, Drudis T, et al. The microtubule-affecting drug paclitaxel has antiangiogenic activity. *Clin Cancer Res* 1996;2:1843.
102. Klauber N, Parangi S, Hamel E, Flynn E, D'Amato RJ. Inhibition of angiogenesis *in vivo* by the microtubule inhibitors 2-methoxyestradiol and Taxol. *Cancer Res* 1997;57:81.
103. Lau DH, Xue L, Young LJ, Burke PA, Cheung AT. Paclitaxel (Taxol): an inhibitor of angiogenesis in a highly vascularized transgenic breast cancer. *Cancer Biother Radiopharm* 1999;14:31.
104. Presta M, Rusnati M, Belleri M, et al. Purine analogue 6-methylmercaptopurine riboside inhibits early and late stages of the angiogenesis process. *Cancer Res* 1999;59:2417.
105. Yonekura K, Basaki Y, Chikahisa L, et al. UFT and its metabolites inhibit the angiogenesis induced by murine renal cell carcinoma, as determined by a dorsal air sac assay in mice. *Clin Cancer Res* 1999;5:2185.
106. O'Leary JJ, Shapiro RL, Ren CJ, et al. Antiangiogenic effects of camptothecin analogues 9-amino-20(S)-camptothecin, topotecan, and CPT-11 studied in the mouse cornea model. *Clin Cancer Res* 1999;5:181.
107. Iyer S, Chaplin DJ, Rosenthal DS, et al. Induction of apoptosis in proliferating human endothelial cells by the tumor-specific antiangiogenesis agent combretastatin A-4. *Cancer Res* 1998;58:4510.
108. Chaplin DJ, Pettit GR, Hill SA. Anti-vascular approaches to solid tumour therapy: evaluation of combretastatin A4 phosphate. *Anticancer Res* 1998;58:4510.
109. Klement G, Baruchel S, Rak J, et al. Continuous low-dose therapy with vinblastine and VEGF receptor-2 antibody induces sustained tumor regression without overt toxicity. *J Clin Invest* 2000;105:R15.
110. Hanahan D, Bergers G, Bergsland E. Less is more, regularly: metronomic dosing of cytotoxic drugs can target tumor angiogenesis in mice. *J Clin Invest* 2000;105:1045.

111. Rastinejad F, Polverini P, Bouck NP. Regulation of the activity of a new inhibitor of angiogenesis by a cancer suppressor gene. *Cell* 1989;56:345.
112. Dawson DW, Volpert OV, Gillis P, et al. Pigment epithelium-derived factor: a potent inhibitor of angiogenesis. *Science* 1999;285:245.
113. Ramchandran R, Dhanabal M, Volk R, et al. Antiangiogenic activity of restin, NC10 domain of human collagen XV: comparison to endostatin. *Biochem Biophys Res Commun* 1999;255:735.
114. Kamphaus GD, Colorado PC, Panka DJ, et al. Canstatin, a novel matrix-derived inhibitor of angiogenesis and tumor growth. *J Biol Chem* 2000;275:1209.
115. Zhang M, Volpert O, Shi YH, Bouck N. Maspin is an angiogenesis inhibitor. *Nat Med* 2000;6:196.
116. Hendrix MJ. De-mystifying the mechanism(s) of maspin. *Nat Med* 2000;6:374.
117. Jendraschak E, Sage EH. Regulation of angiogenesis by SPARC and angiostatin: implications for tumor cell biology. *Semin Cancer Biol* 1996;7:139.
118. Zhai Y, Yu J, Iruela-Arispe L, et al. Inhibition of angiogenesis and breast cancer xenograft tumor growth by VEGI, a novel cytokine of the TNF superfamily. *Int J Cancer* 1999;82:131.
119. Angiolillo AL, Sgadari C, Tosato G. A role for the interferon-inducible protein 10 in inhibition of angiogenesis by interleukin-12. *Ann N Y Acad Sci* 1996;795:158.
120. Cao R, Farnebo J, Kurimoto M, Cao Y. Interleukin-18 acts as an angiogenesis and tumor suppressor. *FASEB J* 1999;13:2195.
121. Clapp C, Weiner RI. A specific, high affinity, saturable binding site for the 16-kilodalton fragment of prolactin on capillary endothelial cells. *Endocrinology* 1992;130:1380.

CHAPTER 21

Clinical Trials in Cancer

SECTION 1

RICHARD SIMON

Design and Analysis of Clinical Trials

Clinical trials are experiments to determine the value of treatments. There are two key components to the experimental approach. First, results rather than plausible reasoning are required to support conclusions. Second, experiments should be prospectively planned and conducted under controlled conditions in order to provide definitive answers to well-defined questions. Comparing the survival rates (based on tumor registry data) of prostate cancer patients treated with surgery to those of patients receiving radiotherapy is an example of an observational study, not a clinical trial. In an observational study, the investigators are passive observers. Treatment assignments, staging workup, and follow-up procedures are out of the control of the investigators and are conducted with no considerations about the validity of the subsequent attempt at comparison. The statistical associations resulting from such studies are, consequently, a weak basis for causal inferences about relationships between the treatments administered and the outcomes observed. Treatments usually are selected on the basis of subjective assessment of the prognosis of the patient, specialties of the physician, and various diagnostic evaluations. Unknown patient selection factors generally are more important determinants of patient outcome than are differences between treatments.

Observational studies are generally the only feasible approach for epidemiologic assessment of disease etiology. Acute observations in poorly structured therapeutic settings can also lead to the development of valuable ideas that can be tested in the laboratory and in clinical trials. However, observational studies rarely are satisfactory substitutes for clinical trials.[1–3] As pointed out by MacMahon and Pugh[4]:

> Only a minority of statistical associations are causal. . . . Once a statistical association has been demonstrated, how can it be determined whether or not it is causal. . . . The most satisfactory procedure is a direct experiment. . . . The evaluation of the causal nature of a relationship, in the absence of direct experiment, is neither easy nor objective. . . . The field of cancer therapy is replete with examples of new modalities that were taken up with enthusiasm and proved worthless only after they had resulted in many years of futile cost and suffering.

Clinical trials require careful planning. The first result of the planning process is a written protocol. Typical subject headings for the protocol are shown in Table 21.1-1. The protocol should define treatment and evaluation policies for a well-defined set of patients. It also should define the specific questions to be answered by the study and should directly justify that the number of patients and the nature of the controls are adequate to answer these questions. Some clinical trials are really only guidelines for clinical management supplemented by lofty objectives with no scientific meaning and no realistic chance of providing a reliable answer to a well-defined medical question. Such studies do not warrant the expenditure of limited clinical research dollars and represent a disservice to the patients who may be willing to undergo some inconvenience in order to contribute to the welfare of future patients. In this section, we attempt to provide information that will help to avoid such clinical trials.

PHASE I CLINICAL TRIALS

The objective of a phase I trial is to determine a dose that is appropriate for use in phase II trials. Patients with advanced disease that

TABLE 21.1-1. Subject Headings for a Protocol

Introduction and scientific background
Objectives
Selection of patients
Design of study (including schematic diagram)
Treatment plan
Drug information
Toxicities to be monitored and dosage modifications
Required clinical and laboratory data and study calendar
Criteria for evaluating the effect of treatment and end point definition
Statistical considerations
Informed consent and regulatory considerations
Data forms
References
Study chairperson, collaborating participants, addresses, and telephone numbers

is resistant to standard therapy are included in such trials, but it is important that the patients have normal organ function.

There are several different types of phase I trials. The most common is the phase I trial of a new cytotoxic drug. Such studies usually are performed by starting with a low dose not expected to produce serious toxicity in any patients. A starting dose of one-tenth the lethal dose (expressed as milligrams per square meter of body surface area) in the most sensitive species usually is used.[5] The dose is increased for subsequent patients according to a series of preplanned steps. Dose escalation for subsequent patients occurs only after sufficient time has passed to observe acute toxic effects for patients treated at lower doses. Cohorts of three to six patients are treated at each dose level. Usually, if no dose-limiting toxicity (DLT) is seen at a given dose level, the dose is escalated for the next cohort. If the incidence of DLT is 33%, then three more patients are treated at the same level. If no further cases of DLT are seen in the additional patients, then the dose level is escalated for the next cohort. Otherwise, dose escalation stops. If the incidence of DLT is greater than 33% at a given level, then dose escalation also stops. The phase II recommended dose often is taken as the highest dose for which the incidence of DLT is less than 33%. Usually, six or more patients are treated at the recommended dose.

The dose levels themselves commonly are based on a modified Fibonacci series.[6] The second level is twice the starting dose; the third level is 67% greater than the second; the fourth level is 50% greater than the third; the fifth is 40% greater than the fourth; and each subsequent step is 33% greater than that preceding it. Escalating doses for subsequent courses in the same patient is generally not done, except at low doses before any DLT has been encountered.

There is no compelling scientific basis for the approach just outlined, except that experience has shown it to be safe. Traditional phase I trials have three limitations: (1) They sometimes expose too many patients to subtherapeutic doses of the new drug; (2) the trials may take a long time to complete; and (3) they provide very limited information about interpatient variability and cumulative toxicity. New trial designs have been developed to address these problems. One class of designs, *accelerated titration designs,* permit within-patient dose escalation and use only one patient per dose level until grade 2 or greater toxicity is seen.[7] Doses are titrated within patients to achieve grade 2 toxicity. The analysis consists of fitting a statistical model to the full set of data that includes all grades of toxicity for all courses of a patient's treatment. The model includes parameters that represent the steepness of the dose-toxicity curve, the degree of interpatient variability in the location of the dose-toxicity curve, and the degree (if any) of cumulative toxicity. All these parameters are estimated from the data.

In developing the accelerated titration designs, Simon et al.[7] fit a stochastic model to data from 20 phase I trials of nine different drugs. New data then were simulated using the model with the parameters estimated from the actual trials, and the performance of alternative phase I designs on this simulated data was evaluated. Four designs were evaluated. Design 1 was a conventional design using cohorts of three to six patients with 40% dose-step increments and no intrapatient dose escalation. Designs 2 through 4 included only one patient per cohort until one patient experienced dose-limiting toxicity or two patients experienced grade 2 toxicity (during their first course of treatment for designs 2 and 3 or during any course of treatment for design 4). Designs 3 and 4 use 100% dose steps during this initial accelerated phase. After the initial accelerated phase, designs 2 through 4 resort to standard cohorts of three to six patients with 40% dose-step increments. Designs 2 through 4 use intrapatient dose escalation if the worst toxicity is grade 0 to 1 in the previous course for that patient.

Only three of the actual trials showed any evidence of cumulative toxicity. The average number of patients required was reduced from 39.9 for design 1 to 24.4, 20.7, and 21.2 for designs 2, 3, and 4, respectively. The average number of patients who had grade 0 to 1 toxicity as their worst toxicity grade over three cycles of treatment was 23.3 for design 1 but only 7.9, 3.9, and 4.8 for designs 2, 3, and 4, respectively. The average number of patients with a worst toxicity grade of 3 increased from 5.5 for design 1 to 6.2, 6.8, and 6.2 for designs 2, 3, and 4, respectively. The average number of patients with a worst toxicity grade of 4 increased from 1.9 for design 1 to 3.0, 4.3, and 3.2 for designs 2, 3, and 4, respectively. Accelerated titration designs appear to be effective in reducing the number of patients who are undertreated, speeding the completion of phase I trials, and providing increased information. These advantages are achieved with some increase in the number of patients experiencing grade 3 and 4 toxicities.

Some phase I trials are very complex in that they involve the simultaneous escalation of two or more drugs. The design of such trials has been discussed by Korn and Simon.[8]

So-called phase IB trials attempt to determine the relationship between dose of a biologic agent and both toxicity and immunologic effect. Such trials often suffer from two flaws. One is that it is assumed that cohorts of three to six patients are sufficient for relating dose to immunologic effects, without consideration of interpatient variability and measurement error of the immunologic assays. The second problem is that there is often little information about what immunologic end points actually are relevant for antitumor effects. Such studies have little potential for producing meaningful information about the dose of a biologic that should be used for subsequent trials.

Some phase I trials attempt to answer comparative questions. For example, should paclitaxel be administered before or after doxorubicin in a two-drug combination? Because of the small sample sizes of phase I trials, the maximum tolerated doses (MTDs) generally are determined imprecisely. This, combined with the nonrandomized nature of such trials, means that reliable comparative conclusions can be expected only if the differences are large.

PHASE II CLINICAL TRIALS

PATIENT SELECTION

Whereas phase I trials need not be performed separately by tumor type, this is not the case for phase II trials, because the biologic response of interest is that of the tumor itself. When a drug enters phase II trials, it should be tested in the patient group that is most likely to show a favorable effect but for whom no effective therapy is available. This is best accomplished by patients with maximum performance status and a minimum amount of prior chemotherapy. Full-dose chemotherapy is often impossible in patients debilitated by prior treatment, and lack of chemotherapeutic activity in previously treated patients may not indicate lack of clinical usefulness in earlier disease. This issue was well illustrated by etoposide in small cell lung carcinoma.[9,10] For the less chemosensitive cancers, chemotherapy offers little or no palliative benefit, and initial phase II trials should be conducted in patients with no prior chemotherapy. In more sensitive tumors, such as breast, small cell lung, or ovarian carcinoma or non-Hodgkin's lymphoma, it is desirable to evaluate new drugs in patients with no more than one prior treatment for advanced disease. For very chemosensitive tumors, the window-of-opportunity design sometimes is used, in which patients not previously treated are given one or two courses of a phase II drug and then are switched to a standard combination. In general, agents should be shown to be active in a favorable population of patients before they are given to a less favorable group. Adherence to this principle saves patients with advanced disease from exposure to inactive agents for which the likelihood of toxicity is much greater than the likelihood of benefit.

TRIALS OF SINGLE AGENTS

There is much confusion about the appropriate objectives of phase II trials. It often is useful to distinguish between phase II trials of single agents and phase II trials of combinations. Both are called *phase II trials* because eligibility is limited to patients with a specific diagnosis and there is no internal control group. For most single-agent phase II trials, however, the objective is simply to determine whether the drug has activity against the tumor type in question. For this objective, response rate is an appropriate end point for evaluating the question posed by the trial. It is important to recognize, however, that tumor response is not a direct measure of patient benefit and, hence, it cannot be assumed that response rate is an appropriate end point for drawing conclusions about treatment efficacy. A treatment that causes partial responses is not necessarily beneficial to the patient, and analyses that demonstrate that responders live longer than nonresponders are invalid for concluding that a treatment extended survival.[11,12] First, responders, by definition, have lived long enough to achieve that status. Second, responders may have more favorable prognostic factors. Finally, treatment may shorten survival of nonresponders while not influencing survival of responders. To demonstrate that treatment extends survival, it must be demonstrated that the treated group as a whole lives longer than an appropriate control group. Phase II trials do not have an internal control group and, hence, drawing conclusions about survival from such trials is very problematic.

A variety of statistical accrual plans and sample size methods that have been developed for phase II trials have been reviewed by Simon.[13] One of the most popular approaches is the optimal two-stage design.[14] A number (n_1) of evaluable patients is entered into study in the first stage of the trial. If fewer than a specified r_1 responses are obtained among these n_1 patients, then accrual terminates and the drug is rejected as being of little interest. Otherwise, accrual continues to a total of n evaluable patients. At the end of the second stage, the drug is rejected if the observed response rate is less than or equal to r/n, where r and n are determined by the design employed.

Tables 21.1-2 and 21.1-3 illustrate some of these optimized designs. To select a design, researchers must specify a target activity level of interest, p_1, and also a lower activity level, p_0. The first row of each triplet of optimal designs provides designs with probability $\leq .10$ of accepting drugs worse than p_0 and probability $\leq .10$ of rejecting drugs better than p_1. Subject to these two constraints, the optimal designs minimize the average sample size. The average sample size is calculated at the lower activity level p_0 in order to optimize protection of patients from exposure to inactive drugs. The tables show for each design the optimal values of r_1, n_1, r, and n, the average sample size, and the probability of stopping after the first stage for a drug with activity level p_0.

These tables also show the "minimax" designs, which provide the smallest maximum sample size n that satisfies the two constraints just described. Although minimax designs have somewhat larger average sample sizes than do optimal designs, in some instances they are preferable because the small increase in average sample size is more than compensated for by a large reduction in maximum sample size.

The designs shown in Tables 21.1-2 and 21.1-3 are two-stage designs with the potential for early stopping for lack of activity. Other two-stage designs have been described that provide for early termination for inactivity or for early evidence for activity.[15] Also, optimized three-stage designs have been described.[16]

When sufficient numbers of patients and several treatments are available to test, there are advantages to randomized phase II trials.[17] Although phase II trials are not comparative, in selecting the most promising treatment or schedule to pursue, it is advantageous to evaluate the candidates on comparable patients. Table 21.1-4 shows the number of patients per treatment arm required to ensure that the best treatment will have the highest observed response rate. This calculation assumes that the true response probability for the best treatment is 10 percentage points better than for the others. Simon et al.[17] provide similar tables for 15% differences. This selection approach is useful when one treatment will be carried forward and the treatments are similar with regard to cost and toxicity.

TRIALS OF COMBINATION REGIMENS

Many so-called phase II trials of combination regimens are conducted. The objectives of such trials are often unclear. One reasonable objective is sometimes merely to ensure that the combination is feasible and tolerable when used in a multiinstitution setting before embarking on a phase III trial. Achieving

TABLE 21.1-2. Simon Two-Stage Phase II Designs for $p_1 - p_0 = .20^a$

		Optimal Design				*Minimax Design*			
		Reject Drug if Response Rate				Reject Drug if Response Rate			
p_0	p_1	$\leq r_1/n_1$	$\leq r/n$	EN (p_0)	PET (p_0)	$\leq r_1/n_1$	$\leq r/n$	EN (p_0)	PELLT (p_0)
.05	.25	0/9	2/24	14.5	.63	0/13	2/20	16.4	.51
		0/9	2/17	12.0	.63	0/12	2/16	13.8	.54
		0/9	3/30	16.8	.63	0/15	3/25	20.4	.46
.10	.30	1/12	5/35	19.8	.65	1/16	4/25	20.4	.51
		1/10	5/29	15.0	.74	1/15	5/25	19.5	.55
		2/18	6/36	22.5	.71	2/22	6/23	26.2	.62
.20	.40	3/17	10/37	26.0	.55	3/19	10/36	28.2	.46
		3/13	12/43	20.6	.75	4/18	10/33	22.3	.50
		4/19	15/54	30.4	.67	5/24	13/45	31.2	.66
.30	.50	7/22	17/46	29.9	.67	7/28	15/39	35.0	.36
		5/15	18/46	23.6	.72	6/19	16/39	25.7	.48
		8/24	24/63	34.7	.73	7/24	21/53	36.6	.56
.40	.60	7/18	22/46	30.2	.56	11/28	20/41	33.8	.55
		7/16	23/46	24.5	.72	17/34	20/39	34.4	.91
		11/25	32/66	36.0	.73	12/29	27/54	38.1	.64
.50	.70	11/21	26/45	29.0	.67	11/23	23/39	31.0	.50
		8/15	26/43	23.5	.70	12/23	23/37	27.7	.66
		13/24	36/61	34.0	.73	14/27	32/53	36.1	.65
.60	.80	6/11	26/38	25.4	.47	18/27	24/35	28.5	.82
		7/11	30/43	20.5	.70	8/13	25/35	20.8	.65
		12/19	37/53	29.5	.69	15/26	32/45	35.9	.48
.70	.90	6/9	22/28	17.8	.54	11/16	20/25	20.1	.55
		4/6	22/27	14.8	.58	19/23	21/26	23.2	.95
		11/15	29/36	21.2	.70	13/18	26/32	22.7	.67

[a]For each value of (p_0, p_1), designs are given for three sets of error probabilities (α, β). The first, second, and third rows correspond to error probability limits (.10, .10), (.05, .20), and (.05, .10), respectively. α is the probability of accepting a drug with response probability p_0. β is the probability of rejecting a drug with response probability p_1. For each design, EN (p_0) and PET (p_0) denote the expected sample size and the probability of early termination when the true response probability is p_0.

this objective does not require many patients. An alternative objective is to determine whether the new regimen is promising enough to warrant a phase III trial. Achieving this objective requires considerable planning. Consequently, many phase II trials of this type are not adequately planned and analyzed to serve any real scientific objective.

Investigators often do not distinguish between phase II trials of combinations of active agents and phase II trials of new single agents. Consequently, protocols often are written to distinguish between inactivity of the combination (e.g., $p_0 = .05$ or .10) and some modest level of activity (e.g., $p_1 = .20$ or .25). Since the drugs being combined are generally already known to be active, this makes little sense. If response rate is the primary end point, then the level of no interest (p_0) should generally represent the level of activity of the most active single-agent component or the level of activity of previously studied combination regimens (as presumably the new regimen would be considered promising only if it is promising relative to other existing regimens).

With the lower limit of activity, p_0, defined as described earlier, Tables 21.1-2 and 21.2-3 can be used for the design of phase II trials of combination regimens. One problem with this approach, however, is the uncertainty in specifying a meaningful value of p_0 to be used for trial design and analysis. Because the conclusions of phase II trials of combinations are essentially comparative, it is important that the comparison be based on a prognostically similar group of patients given standard treatment. Hence, the planning of such a trial should include the prospective identification of such a group of patients. Although such historical control comparisons are not considered reliable enough to eliminate the need for phase III trials, if done carefully they will provide better decisions about which new regimens are worthy of phase III evaluation. For comparative trials of response rates using historical controls, appropriate tables for sample size planning are given by Makuch and Simon[18] and are summarized in Table 21.1-5. This table is for achieving 80% power with a one-sided 5% significance level. If the historical control group of 50 patients showed a response rate of 30%, and the target level of improvement is a 50% response rate, then 69 patients should be treated with the experimental regimen. If there were 100 appropriate historical control patients, then only 48 new patients are required. If there were only 30 historical control patients, then 137 new patients are needed for the experimental treatment. If the uncertainty in the level of response achievable with standard treatment is substantial because of the limited number of appropriate historical controls, then it is not efficient to con-

TABLE 21.1-3. Simon Two-Stage Phase II Designs for $p_1 - p_0 = .15^a$

		Optimal Design				*Minimax Design*			
		Reject Drug if Response Rate				Reject Drug if Response Rate			
p_0	p_1	$\leq r_1/n_1$	$\leq r/n$	EN (p_0)	PET (p_0)	$\leq r_1/n_1$	$\leq r/n$	EN (p_0)	PET (p_0)
.05	.20	0/12	3/37	23.5	.54	0/18	3/32	26.4	.40
		0/10	3/29	17.6	.60	0/13	3/27	19.8	.51
		1/21	4/41	26.7	.72	1/29	4/38	32.9	.57
.10	.25	2/21	7/50	31.2	.65	2/27	6/40	33.7	.48
		2/18	7/43	24.7	.73	2/22	7/40	28.8	.62
		2/21	10/66	36.8	.65	3/31	9/55	40.0	.62
.20	.35	5/27	16/63	43.6	.54	6/33	15/58	45.5	.50
		5/22	19/72	35.4	.73	6/31	15/53	40.4	.57
		8/37	22/83	51.4	.69	8/42	21/77	58.4	.53
.30	.45	9/30	29/82	51.4	.59	16/50	25/69	56.0	.68
		9/27	30/81	41.7	.73	16/46	25/65	49.6	.81
		13/40	40/110	60.8	.70	27/77	33/88	78.5	.86
.40	.55	16/38	40/88	54.5	.67	18/45	34/73	57.2	.56
		11/26	40/84	44.9	.67	28/59	34/70	60.1	.90
		19/45	49/104	64.0	.68	24/62	45/94	78.9	.47
.50	.65	18/35	47/84	53.0	.63	19/40	41/72	58.0	.44
		15/28	48/83	43.7	.71	39/66	40/68	66.1	.95
		22/42	60/105	62.3	.68	28/57	54/93	75.0	.50
.60	.75	21/34	47/71	47.1	.65	25/43	43/64	54.4	.46
		17/27	46/67	39.4	.69	18/30	43/62	43.8	.57
		21/34	64/95	55.6	.65	48/72	57/84	73.2	.90
.70	.85	14/20	45/59	36.2	.58	15/22	40/52	36.8	.51
		14/19	46/59	30.3	.72	16/23	39/49	34.4	.56
		18/25	61/79	43.4	.66	33/44	53/68	48.5	.81
.80	.95	5/7	27/31	20.8	.42	5/7	27/31	20.8	.42
		7/9	26/29	17.7	.56	7/9	26/29	17.7	.56
		16/19	37/42	24.4	.76	31/35	35/40	35.3	.94

[a]For each value of (p_0, p_1), designs are given for three sets of error probabilities (α, β). The first, second, and third rows correspond to error probability limits (.10, .10), (.05, .20), and (.05, .10), respectively. α is the probability of accepting a drug with response probability p_0. β is the probability of rejecting a drug with response probability p_1. For each design, EN (p_0) and PET (p_0) denote the expected sample size and the probability of early termination when the true response probability is p_0.

duct a phase II trial of the new regimen. It would be more efficient to conduct a randomized phase II or phase III trial of the new regimen and the standard treatment.

Thall et al.[19,20] have developed Bayesian methods for planning and conducting trials in which the precision in the response probability p_0 is quantified by a "prior probability distribution." These Bayesian designs provide for continual analysis of results after evaluation of response for each patient. This is difficult logistically for multiinstitution trials but provides a valid statistical basis for the intensive monitoring of cancer center or pharmaceutical industry trials in which patients may be limited or time may be critical. One begins with a prior probability distribution of response for p_1 that is flat over the range 0 to 1. After each patient is evaluated on the experimental regimen, the "posterior probability distribution" for p_1 is updated. This permits calculation of the posterior probability distribution for $p_1 - p_0$.

Let δ denote the difference in response probabilities that is of interest. If, at some point during the trial, the posterior probability that $p_1 - p_0 \geq \delta$ becomes small—say less than 0.05—one might terminate the trial and conclude that the new regimen is not promising. If, at some point during the trial, the posterior probability that $p_1 - p_0 \geq 0$ becomes large—say greater than 0.95—one might terminate the trial and conclude that the new regimen appears better than the historical control. In this case, one could continue entry of patients if it were desirable to study the regimen further in a phase II setting.

The trial is designed with a maximum number of patients, n_{max}, that limits sample size even if neither early termination condition occurs. Table 21.1-6 shows an example of the operating characteristics of a design of this type. In this example, the historical data indicate that the expected response probability for the control regimen is .20 and that the width of the 90% confidence interval around .20 for the true value is approximately 0.20. The table also represents targeting a 20–percentage point improvement in response probability (δ = 0.20). The maximum sample size is set at 65, and it is assumed that the trial is arbitrarily not terminated before ten patients are evaluated. As can be seen from the table, the median number of patients required is 12 under the null hypothesis that the response probability for the experimental regimen is .20 and is only 13 under the alter-

TABLE 21.1-4. Number of Patients per Treatment Group for Selecting Better Treatment When True Response Probabilities Differ by 10 Percentage Points [a]

Baseline Response Probability	*85% Probability of Correct Selection*	*90% Probability of Correct Selection*
.05	20	29
.10	28	42
.15	35	53
.20	41	62
.30	49	75
.40	54	82
.50	54	82
.60	49	75
.70	41	62
.80	28	53

[a]Assumes that investigator is indifferent to treatment selected when true response probabilities differ by less than 10 percentage points.

native hypothesis. The table also indicates that 75% of the time the trial will terminate by the evaluation of 20 to 22 patients. Bayesian continuing-monitoring phase II designs have also been developed for simultaneously monitoring multiple end points, including efficacy and toxicity. Designs of this type used in actual clinical trials have been illustrated in the work of Thall et al.[19]

Some investigators and statisticians do not like to use approaches based on explicit comparison to historical controls. Phase II trials of combinations are inherently comparative, however. Going through the exercise of explicitly quantifying the basis of comparison, which these methods require, clarifies beforehand whether the uncertainty in outcome for the control group is so great that a phase II trial is not useful. Phase II trials of combinations are problematic. Only by using methods that provide more careful statistical planning of such trials can we streamline the drug development process.

Many reports in the literature of phase II trials of combination regimens conclude that the treatment is effective. As noted, response rates generally are not a measure of patient benefit. Such reports generally fail to make any meaningful attempt at determining outcome on standard treatment for a prognostically comparable set of patients. Often these trials are not conducted as a prelude to a phase III evaluation, and hence their value to clinical therapeutics is difficult to identify.

For some diseases, it has been noted that combination regimens that produce high response rates in phase II trials do not result in improved survival in phase III trials as compared to standard treatment. This has led to interest in using survival directly as an end point for phase II trials to evaluate the promise of a regimen. In some types of cancer, response rate is difficult to measure, and many patients do not have measurable disease (e.g., brain, ovarian, gastric, and prostate cancer). Dixon and Simon[21] have developed tables for planning historically controlled phase II comparative studies with a survival or time-to-progression end point.

DESIGN OF PHASE III CLINICAL TRIALS

Good clinical therapeutic research requires asking important questions and getting reliable answers. This chapter attempts to provide guidance on the components necessary for getting reliable answers. As noted earlier in Trials of Combination Regimens, many phase II trials of combination regimens do not provide reliable answers. Some phase III trials, however, do not ask important questions. The most important clinical trials are often the most difficult to conduct.[22] They may involve withhold-

TABLE 21.1-5. Number of Patients Needed in an Experimental Group for 80% Power to Detect (One-Sided $\alpha = 0.05$) a Specified Difference in Success Rates

Proportion of Success for Historical Controls	*No. of Historical Controls (patients)*						
	20	30	40	50	75	100	200
0.10	[a]	223[b]	108	80	58	50	42
	116	53[c]	40	35	29	27	24
	39	27[d]	23	21	18	18	16
	22	17[e]	15	14	13	13	12
0.20	[a]	[a]	285	167	101	83	65
	385	98	67	55	44	40	35
	67	40	33	30	26	24	22
	31	23	21	19	18	17	16
0.30	[a]	[a]	554	259	137	108	80
	882	137	87	69	54	48	42
	86	49	39	35	30	29	26
	31	27	24	22	20	19	18
0.40	[a]	[a]	699	303	153	120	88
	913	147	92	74	58	52	44
	85	50	41	36	32	30	27
	36	27	24	22	21	20	19
0.50	[a]	[a]	538	267	145	115	86
	455	122	83	68	55	50	43
	67	44	37	34	30	28	26
	30	24	22	20	18	18	17
0.60	[a]	[a]	295	185	117	97	76
	179	83	63	55	46	42	38
	45	33	29	27	25	24	22
	22	19	17	17	15	15	15

[a]Required sample size >1000.
[b]Number of patients needed for the new treatment to detect a difference in success rate of 15 percentage points.
[c]Number of patients needed to detect a difference in success rate of 20 percentage points.
[d]Number of patients needed to detect a difference in success rate of 25 percentage points.
[e]Number of patients needed to detect a difference in success rate of 30 percentage points.

TABLE 21.1-6. Thall-Simon Bayesian Phase II Design

	Sample Size Percentiles			*Probability Reject Regimen*	*Probability Accept Regimen*
p_1	25%	50%	75%		
.20	10	12	20	.92	.07
.40	10	13	22	.15	.83

ing a treatment established by tradition, potentially transferring patient management responsibility across specialties, standardizing procedures among physicians who believe that their way is best, and sharing recognition with a large group of collaborators.

Phase III trials attempt to provide guidance to practicing physicians to help them make treatment decisions with their patients. Consequently, the trials should provide reliable information concerning end points of relevance to the patients. The major end points for evaluating the effectiveness of a treatment should be direct measures of patient welfare. Survival and symptom control are two such end points. The latter is not routinely used because of the difficulty of measuring it reliably and because it may be influenced by concomitant treatments. As stated, tumor shrinkage usually is not an appropriate end point for phase III trials because it may have little or no relation to patient benefit. Torri et al.[23] performed a metaanalysis of the relationship between difference in response rates and difference in median survivals for randomized clinical trials of advanced ovarian carcinoma. They found that large improvements in response rates corresponded to very small improvements in median survival. Hence, use of response rate as an end point results in giving patients increasingly intensive and toxic therapy with little or no net benefit to them.

It is usually important that the results of phase III trials be applicable to patients seen in the community outside of clinical research settings. This is accomplished by conducting the trials in multiinstitution settings that include community physician participation. The eligibility criteria established for the trial also has a bearing on the generalizability of the conclusions; trials conducted with narrow eligibility criteria tend to be less generalizable. Narrow eligibility criteria also complicate trials logistically. Narrow eligibility criteria tend to require extensive and expensive patient workups and thereby do not facilitate broad participation, especially in an era of closely monitored medical costs. For these and other reasons, there is a trend toward broadened eligibility criteria for phase III clinical trials. In the United Kingdom, many trials are designed using the *uncertainty principle*, an approach that leaves much of the decision making about eligibility to the treating physician. There may be guidelines for eligibility, but the ultimate decision will be made by the treating physician; if he or she is uncertain about which treatment is more appropriate for the patient, then the patient is eligible.

RANDOMIZATION

To determine whether a new treatment cures any patients with a disease that is uniformly and rapidly fatal, history is a satisfactory control. Once we leave this setting of complete determinism, however, the definition of an adequate nonrandomized control group becomes problematic. In studies using nonrandomized controls, often diagnostic and staging procedures, supportive care, secondary treatments, and methods of evaluation and follow-up are different for the controls and for the new patients. There is generally differential bias in the selection of patients to be treated resulting from judgments by the physicians, self-selection by the patients, and differences in referral patterns. There may be bias in treatment ineligibility rates. Current patients sometimes are excluded from analysis for not meeting eligibility criteria, not receiving "adequate" treatment, refusing treatment, or committing a major protocol violation. The control group, on the other hand, generally contains all the patients. There may be differences in the distribution of known and unknown prognostic factors between the controls and the current treatment group. Often there is inadequate information to determine whether such differences are present, and current known prognostic factors may not have been measured for the controls. It generally is difficult or impossible to determine whether the controls would have been eligible for the current study and in what way they represent a selection of all eligible patients.

Formation of the control group by random treatment assignment as an integral part of the planned study can avoid most of the systematic biases just mentioned.[24–29] Randomization does not ensure that the study will include a representative sample of all patients with the disease, but it does help to ensure an unbiased evaluation of the relative merits of the two treatments for the types of patients entered.

It is sometimes said that randomization is unnecessary because matched historical or concurrent controls can be selected. However, matching can be done only with regard to known prognostic factors, and these generally are not sufficient for the construction of prognostically homogeneous groups of patients.[30] Matching with regard to known factors gives no assurance that the distributions of unknown factors are similar between the groups. It also is sometimes said that randomization is not effective in ensuring that the treatment groups are similar with regard to unknown prognostic factors unless the number of patients is large. This is true but reflects a misunderstanding of the purpose of randomization. Randomization does not ensure that the groups are medically equivalent, but it distributes the unknown biasing factors according to a known random distribution so that their effects can be rigorously allowed for in significance tests and confidence intervals. This is true regardless of the study size. A significance level represents the probability that differences in outcome can be the result of random fluctuations. Without a randomized treatment allocation, a "statistically significant difference" may be the result of a nonrandom difference in the distribution of unknown prognostic factors.

Many investigators today see a useful role for both nonrandomized and randomized clinical trials. The nonrandomized format is used for determining which regimens are sufficiently promising for randomized phase III evaluation and for use in clinical settings where outcome is uniformly poor. For major questions of public health importance, unless the treatment effects are huge, the need for reliable answers dictates the use of randomized phase III trials.

Randomization of a patient should be performed after the patient has been found eligible and has consented to participate in the trial and to accept either of the randomized options. A truly random and nondecipherable randomization procedure should be used and implemented by calling a central randomization office staffed by individuals who are independent of participating physicians.

STRATIFICATION

When important prognostic factors are known for patients in a randomized trial, it is often advisable to stratify the randomization to ensure equal distribution of these factors. This is usually accomplished by preparing a separate randomization list (or set of cards in sealed envelopes) for each stratum of patients. Each list must be balanced so that after each block of four to ten patients within the stratum, the treatment groups contain equal numbers of patients. Within the blocks, the sequence of treatment assignments is random. The stratification factors must be known for each patient at the time of randomization.

It generally is best to limit stratification to those factors definitely known to have important independent effects on outcome. If two factors are closely correlated, only one need be included. Peto[31,32] believes that stratification is an unnecessary complication because adjustment for imbalances of known factors can be made in the analysis. This is true for large trials. Stratification helps to ensure balance for interim analyses when the sample sizes may be limited and provides the medical audience with confidence in the results, which often is not available when depending on complex adjustment methods to deal with prognostic imbalances. Stratification also is a convenient way of specifying *a priori* what are considered the important prognostic factors. Subsequent "subset analyses" can then be limited to the patient subsets determined by the stratification factors.

Many clinical trials use adaptive stratification methods. These methods permit effective balancing by many prognostic factors, although they typically require a computer program for their use. Simon[33] and Kalish and Begg[34] have reviewed the various stratification methods that are available. Kalish and Begg[35] have also studied analytic aspects of adaptive stratification methods.

SAMPLE SIZE

The protocol for a phase III trial should specify the number of patients to be accrued and the duration of follow-up after the close of accrual when the final analysis will be performed. Methods of sample size planning are based on the assumption that at the conclusion of the follow-up period, a statistical significance test will be performed comparing the experimental treatment to the control treatment with regard to a single primary end point. A statistical significance level of .05 has the following meaning: If there is no true difference in treatment effectiveness, the probability of obtaining a difference in outcomes as extreme as that observed in the data is .05. The significance level does not represent the probability that the null hypothesis is true; it represents a probability of an observed difference, assuming that the null hypothesis is true. Conventional statistical theory ascribes no probabilities to hypotheses, only to data.

A one-sided significance level represents the probability, by chance alone, of obtaining a difference as large as and in the same direction as that actually observed. A two-sided significance level represents the probability of obtaining by chance a difference in either direction as large in absolute magnitude as that actually observed. The two-sided significance level is usually twice the one-sided significance level. Controversy exists over the appropriateness of one-sided or two-sided significance levels. Although this is a somewhat trivial issue, a two-sided significance level of .05 has become widely accepted as a standard level of evidence.

With few patients in the trial, the difference in observed outcomes must be extreme in order to obtain statistical significance. Consequently, the probability of obtaining a statistically significant result may be low even when a substantial true difference in effectiveness exists. The probability of obtaining a statistically significant result when the treatments differ in effectiveness is called the *power* of the trial. As the sample size and extent of follow-up increases, the power increases. The power depends critically, however, on the size of the true difference in effectiveness of the two treatments. Generally, one sizes the trial so that the power is either .80 or .90 when the true difference in effectiveness is the smallest size that is considered medically important to detect.

TABLE 21.1-7. Number of Events Needed for Comparing Survival Curves

Percentage Reduction in Hazard of Death	*Ratio of Median Survival for Exponential Distributions*	*No. of Total Deaths to Observe*[a]
20	1.25	846
30	1.43	330
33	1.50	257
40	1.67	162
50	2.0	88

[a]Total number of deaths in both groups to have power .90 for detecting ratio of median survival. Type I error $\alpha = .05$ (two-sided).

A number of statisticians have developed useful methods for planning sample size to compare survival curves or disease-free survival curves in phase III trials. Table 21.1-7 demonstrates results that are valid whenever the *hazard ratio,* the ratio of forces of mortality for the two treatment groups, is constant over time.[36,37] The table shows the total number of deaths that must occur in a given cohort to reflect 90% power for detecting a specified reduction in the hazard for the experimental treatment relative to the control treatment. For exponential distributions, the percentage reduction in hazard of death can be expressed as a ratio of median survivals, which is displayed in the second column of Table 21.1-7. For comparing disease-free survival curves, *deaths* should be replaced by *events,* wherein death, disease recurrence, or development of second cancer usually are considered events. The translation of the number of deaths or events required among the number of patients depends on the actual shape of the survival distributions, the rate of accrual, and the duration of follow-up after close of accrual. Generally, however, it is best to specify the time of the final analysis as the time when the specified number of deaths or events are obtained, not in terms of absolute calendar time.

In some cases, it may be convenient to think in terms of specifying the smallest medically important improvement—for instance, an increase in the proportion of patients who survive beyond some landmark time, such as 5 years. Tables 21.1-8 and 21.1-9 provide required numbers of patients for clinical trials planned on this basis. This approach is less flexible for studies in which survival or disease-free survival is the end point, as it presumes that all patients will be followed for the landmark time as a minimum. These tables can, however, be used generally for detecting differences in a binary end point, denoted *success rate* in the tables. Table 21.1-8 is for one-sided significance tests, and Table 21.1-9 is for two-sided tests. For comparing treatments, differences of more than 15 percentage points usually are unrealistic.

Sample size planning with good statistical power for detecting realistically expected treatment improvements is important. Numerous published "negative" results are actually uninterpretable because the sample sizes are too small.[38] For trials comparing a standard treatment to a more conservative or less invasive

TABLE 21.1-8. Number of Patients in Each of Two Treatment Groups (One-Sided Test)

Smaller Success Rate	*Larger Minus Smaller Success Rate*									
	0.05	0.10	0.15	0.20	0.25	0.30	0.35	0.40	0.45	0.50
0.05	512[a]	172	94	62	45	35	28	23	19	16
	381[b]	129	72	48	35	27	22	18	15	13
0.10	786	236	121	76	54	40	31	25	21	17
	579	176	91	58	41	31	24	20	16	14
0.15	1026	292	144	88	60	44	34	27	22	18
	752	216	108	66	46	34	26	21	17	14
0.20	1231	339	163	98	66	48	36	29	23	19
	900	250	121	73	50	37	28	22	18	15
0.25	1402	377	178	105	70	50	38	29	23	19
	1024	278	132	79	53	38	29	23	18	15
0.30	1539	407	189	111	73	52	38	30	23	19
	1122	300	141	83	55	39	30	23	18	15
0.35	1642	429	197	114	74	52	38	29	23	18
	1196	315	146	85	56	40	30	23	18	14
0.40	1711	441	201	115	74	52	38	29	22	17
	1246	324	149	86	56	39	29	22	17	14
0.45	1745	446	201	114	73	50	36	27	21	16
	1271	327	149	85	55	38	28	21	16	13
0.50	1745	441	197	111	70	48	34	25	19	15
	1271	324	146	83	53	37	26	20	15	12

[a]Upper figure: significance level = .05, power = .90.
[b]Lower figure: significance level = .05, power = .80.

therapy, small reductions in effectiveness will be medically important because survival time or cure probability is being traded for convenience or cosmesis. High statistical power for detecting small differences requires large trials. False acceptance of the null hypothesis of equivalence may result in erroneous adoption of a new, more conservative, and less effective therapy. The burden of proof for therapeutic equivalence trials should generally be on showing that results are similar, not on demonstrating that they are different. These trials should be planned using the specialized methods described later in the section Therapeutic Equivalence Trials. If standard frequency methods are used to analyze such trials, rather than the Bayesian methods described in the section Therapeutic Equivalence Trials, confidence intervals rather than statistical significance tests should be used. The confidence interval for the true difference of effectiveness gives a much clearer picture of which differences are consistent with the data. Makuch and Simon[39] and Durrleman and Simon[40] discuss this approach for planning and monitoring therapeutic equivalence trials.

FACTORIAL DESIGNS

In a two-by-two factorial design, there are actually four treatment groups. The first factor represents two alternative interventions, such as amputation and resection. The second factor represents two other alternatives superimposed on the first factor, such as adjuvant chemotherapy and no chemotherapy. In another example, the first factor might be chemotherapy regimen A or B, and the second factor might be the duration of treatment, 6 or 12 months. Although there are actually four treatment groups, the average effect of each treatment factor can be evaluated using all of the patients and pooling with regard to the other factor (or by accounting for the influence of the other factor in the analysis by stratification, but not by separate analyses for each level of the other factor).[41,42] The usefulness of this analysis of average effects is proportional to whether the comparison between the two levels of one factor depends in any important way on the level of the other factor. If the effects of the two factors do interact, then the analysis of main effects may not be meaningful. Usually, the sample size for a two-by-two factorial trial is computed assuming that there is no interaction between the effects of the factors. This sample size will not provide enough patients to test adequately the assumption of no interaction between the factors. Consequently, the factorial design offers the possibility of answering two questions for the cost of one, but there is a risk of ambiguity in the interpretation of results.[43–45] For situations in which interactions are unlikely or in which it is unlikely that both factors will have substantial effects, the factorial design can provide a substantial improvement in the efficiency of clinical trials.

The use of a factorial design for a clinical trial is often controversial. Proponents sometimes indicate that factorial designs are ideal for studying interactions. Others have questioned how factorial trials can provide meaningful information about interactions when the trials are sized only to detect main effects. Brittain and Wittes[45] noted that the power for detecting an effect of treatment A is substantially impaired by a negative interaction with treatment B, as compared to an experiment wherein all the patients are randomly allocated to either treatment A or placebo, with no use of treatment B. Consequently, factorial designs

TABLE 21.1-9. Number of Patients in Each of Two Treatment Groups (Two-Sided Test)

Smaller Success Rate	*Larger Minus Smaller Success Rate*									
	0.05	0.10	0.15	0.20	0.25	0.30	0.35	0.40	0.45	0.50
0.05	620[a]	206	113	74	54	42	33	27	23	19
	473[b]	159	88	58	43	33	27	22	18	16
0.10	956	285	146	92	64	48	38	30	25	21
	724	218	112	71	50	38	30	24	20	17
0.15	1250	354	174	106	73	53	41	33	26	22
	944	269	133	82	57	42	32	26	21	18
0.20	1502	411	197	118	79	57	44	34	27	22
	1132	313	151	91	62	45	34	27	22	18
0.25	1712	459	216	127	84	60	45	35	28	23
	1289	348	165	98	65	47	36	28	22	18
0.30	1880	495	230	134	88	62	46	36	28	22
	1414	375	175	103	68	48	36	28	22	18
0.35	2006	522	239	138	89	63	46	35	27	22
	1509	395	182	106	69	49	36	28	22	18
0.40	2090	537	244	139	89	62	45	34	26	21
	1571	407	186	107	69	48	36	27	21	17
0.45	2132	543	244	138	88	60	44	33	25	19
	1603	411	186	106	68	47	34	26	20	16
0.50	2132	537	239	134	84	57	41	30	23	17
	1603	407	182	103	65	45	32	24	18	14

[a]Upper figure: significance level = .05, power = .90.
[b]Lower figure: significance level = .05, power = .80.

often are used only when one can assume with confidence that there will be no interactions between the effects of the factors and can determine sample size on the basis of that assumption.

Simon and Freedman[46] developed a Bayesian method for the design and analysis of factorial clinical trials. Their approach avoids the need to dichotomize one's assumptions that interactions either do or do not exist and provides a flexible approach to the design and analysis of such clinical trials. The Bayesian method encourages the quantification of prior belief about the size of interactions that may exist. Rather than forcing the investigator to adopt one of two extreme positions regarding interactions, it provides for the specification of intermediate positions. The Bayesian approach also avoids a preliminary test of interaction having poor power.

The Bayesian model suggests that in planning a factorial trial where interactions are unlikely but cannot be excluded, the sample size should be increased by at least 30% as compared to a simple two-arm clinical trial for detecting the same size of treatment effect. This is less extreme than doubling the sample size but is a recommendation that differs greatly from current usage. The 30% figure allows for a 5% prior probability of a medically important, qualitative interaction between the treatment effects.

Factorial designs can also be useful in phase II trials when an internal control is needed. For example, consider the investigation of antiangiogenic agents A and B for patients in partial remission after induction chemotherapy. With a factorial design, there would be four treatment groups. One group would receive neither agent, one would receive A, one group would receive B, and one group would receive both A and B. Patients are randomized to the four groups. For analyzing the effect of A, the time to progressive disease for the two arms that received A are compared to the time to progressive distribution for the two arms that did not receive A. Analyzing the effect of B is performed analogously. The single-arm phase II trial is problematic when the end point is disease stabilization or time to progression. It is easy to come up with a definition of disease stabilization, but just defining it does not make it valid for measurement of treatment effect. Data are needed that demonstrate that such stabilization does not occur in the absence of treatment in a comparable group of patients. This is difficult to do reliably because of the usual difficulties of identifying comparable historical controls and because of special difficulties involved with documenting stabilization or measuring time to disease progression in a consistent manner, comparable to the way it was done with historical controls. Consequently, the use of disease stabilization or time to progression as an end point in single-arm phase II trials is particularly problematic. A better approach is use of the factorial design, because the factorial design is internally controlled for evaluating the effects of the factors and, hence, the use of time to progression is not problematic.

THERAPEUTIC EQUIVALENCE TRIALS

The objective of a therapeutic equivalence trial is generally to demonstrate that a new treatment is equivalent to a standard therapy with regard to a specified clinical end point. This is contrasted to bioequivalence trials in which the objective is to demonstrate equivalence of serum concentrations of the active moiety. In some cases, investigators would like to demonstrate that the new treatment is effective as compared to no treatment but, because use of a no-treatment arm is not feasible, they attempt to demonstrate therapeutic equivalence to a standard treatment.

Therapeutic equivalence trials are problematic because it is impossible to demonstrate equivalence. If the outcomes for the two treatments are similar, one can only conclude that results are consistent with differences within specified limits.

In conventional trials, rejection of the null hypothesis leads to change in the treatment of future patients. The implications of failure to reject the null hypothesis are more difficult to interpret. Failure to reject the null hypothesis often is interpreted as a demonstration of therapeutic equivalence and grounds for adoption of the new regimen but may merely reflect inadequate sample size or ineffectiveness of the standard treatment for the patients in the clinical trial.

Large sample sizes often are needed for meaningful therapeutic equivalence trials. For example, consider a cancer trial evaluating tumor resection as an alternative to amputation of the organ containing the tumor in a setting in which amputation is the standard therapy known to be curative in a large number of cases. Tumor resection may have clear advantages with regard to quality of life, but few patients would be interested in these advantages unless they were assured that any reduction in the chance of cure would be very small. Hence, the appropriate trial should focus on distinguishing the null hypothesis in which the difference in efficacy is expressed as $\Delta = 0$ from that in which the difference in efficacy is expressed as $\Delta = \delta$, where δ is very small. Consequently, this trial would have to be very large.

In a therapeutic equivalence trial, there is no internal validation of the assumption that the control treatment *C* is actually effective for the patient population at hand. It is not enough for the experimental treatment *E* to be therapeutically equivalent to *C*; we want equivalence coupled with the effectiveness of *E* and *C* relative to no treatment or to whatever was standard before the adoption of *C*.

None of the conventional approaches to the design and analysis of therapeutic equivalence trials is satisfactory. These approaches depend on the specification of a minimal difference (δ) in efficacy that one is willing to tolerate but do not address how δ should be determined. Simon[47] has recently developed a general Bayesian approach to the utilization of information from previous trials in the design and analysis of therapeutic equivalence trials. The effectiveness of the control treatment *C* relative to no treatment or to the previous standard before *C* was adopted is represented by a parameter β. We will denote the previous standard by P. The effectiveness of *C* relative to P will not be known with certainty and may vary among trials. The information about β is summarized by a prior distribution, which is normal with mean μ_β and standard deviation σ_β. The parameter γ represents the effectiveness of the new experimental treatment *E* relative to P. Usually, it is assumed that there is no prior information about γ.

The result of the therapeutic equivalence trial is summarized by a value *y*, which estimates the effectiveness of *E* relative to *C*.

Two major objectives of active controlled trials can be distinguished. The first is to determine whether the experimental treatment is effective relative to P. This requires explicit use of prior information about outcomes of trials comparing P to the active control. Meaningful interpretation of active control trials is impossible without consideration of such information. Establishing whether or not the experimental treatment is effective relative to P is a first requirement. The second objective is to determine whether any medically important portion of the treatment effect for the active control is lost with the experimental treatment. In some cases, this objective is unrealistic because the size of the treatment effect (relative to P) for the active control is imprecisely determined.

If there is no prior information about the effectiveness of *E* relative to P(γ), then after the equivalence trial is completed γ has a posterior normal distribution with mean $\mu_\beta + y$. This is the expected effectiveness of *C* relative to *P* plus the estimate of the effectiveness of *E* relative to *C* based on the therapeutic equivalence trial. The variance of the posterior distribution of γ is $\sigma_\beta^2 + \sigma^2$, where σ_β^2 is the variance of the prior distribution of β and σ is the standard error of *y*. The size of the trial may be planned in this case using the result

$$\frac{1.645\sqrt{1+r+z}}{\sqrt{r}} = -0.84$$

where *z* is μ_β/σ_β, which is the *z* value for comparison of the active control *C* to P in the previous trial (or metaanalysis of previous trials), with a positive value of *z* corresponding to superiority of *C*. The parameter *r* represents the ratio of the required sample size of the therapeutic equivalence trial to the effective sample size of the previous trials demonstrating the superiority of *C* to P. When the *z* value is 3 (corresponding to a two-sided significance level of .0027 for the effectiveness of *C* relative to P), the ratio *r* equals 1.25, indicating that the therapeutic equivalence trial needs to be 25% larger than the previous trial. If, however, the *z* value is only 2 (corresponding to a two-sided significance level of approximately .05), then the ratio *r* equals 10, indicating that the therapeutic equivalence trial needs to be ten times as large as the previous trial that established the effectiveness of *C*. Consequently, unless the evidence for the effectiveness of *C* is highly statistically significant, the therapeutic equivalence trial is not feasible or appropriate.

An important implication of the new approach is that reliable therapeutic equivalence trials are not practical unless evidence of the effectiveness of the control treatment is substantial and consistent. Conventional methods for planning therapeutic equivalence trials often miss this point, because they take the maximum likelihood estimate of the effectiveness of the control treatment as if it were a value known with certainty. This ignores the fact that the degree of effectiveness of the control treatment is known only imprecisely unless the effect is overwhelmingly significant. For example, if the effect is of borderline significance, then the confidence interval for the size of the effect almost includes zero. Consequently, many planned therapeutic equivalence trials, even large multicenter trials, cannot demonstrate clinically relevant objectives. Superiority trials, rather than therapeutic equivalence trials with marginally effective control treatments, are strongly preferred whenever possible.

ANALYSIS OF PHASE III CLINICAL TRIALS

INTENTION-TO-TREAT ANALYSIS

One of the important principles in the analysis of phase III trials is called the *intention-to-treat* principle. This indicates that all randomized patients should be included in the primary analysis of the trial. For cancer trials, this has often been interpreted to mean all "eligible" randomized patients. Because eligibility requirements sometimes are vague and unverifiable by an external auditor, excluding "ineligible" patients can itself result in bias. However, excluding patients from analysis because of treatment deviations, early death, or patient withdrawal can severely distort the results.[32,48,49] Often, excluded patients have poorer outcomes than do those who are not excluded. Investigators frequently rationalize that the poor outcome experienced by a patient was due to lack of compliance to treatment, but the direction of causality may be the reverse. For example, in the Coronary Drug Project, the 5-year mortality for poor adherents to the placebo regimen was 28.3%, significantly greater than the 15.1% experienced by good adherents to the placebo regimen.[50] In randomized trials, there may be poorer compliance in one treatment group than the other, or the reasons for poor compliance may differ. Excluding patients, or analyzing them separately (which is equivalent to excluding them), for reasons other than eligibility is generally considered unacceptable. The intention-to-treat analysis with all eligible randomized patients should be the primary analysis. If the conclusions of a study depend on exclusions, then these conclusions are suspect. The treatment plan should be viewed as a policy to be evaluated. The treatment intended cannot be delivered uniformly to all patients, but all eligible patients should generally be evaluable in phase III trials.

INTERIM ANALYSES

If statistical significance tests are performed repeatedly, the probability that the difference in outcomes will be found to be statistically significant (at the .05 level) at some point may be considerably greater than 5%. This probability is called the *type I error* of the analysis plan. Fleming et al.[51] have shown that the type I error can be as great as 26% if a statistical significance test is performed every 3 months of a 3-year trial that compares two identical treatments. Many trials are published without stating the target sample size, without indicating whether a target sample size was stated in the protocol, and without describing whether the published analysis represented a planned final analysis or was one of multiple analyses performed during the course of the trial. In such cases, one must suspect that the investigators were not aware of good statistical practices and the dangers of informal multiple analyses. Consequently, the statistical significance reported in such trials must be discounted as uninterpretable.

Interim analyses can be very misleading, and the significance levels of interim analyses cannot be taken at face value. Nevertheless, the random trends often seen in interim analyses can destroy accrual to a clinical trial and interfere with a physician's attempt to state honestly to the patient that there is no reliable evidence indicating that one treatment option or the other is preferable. For these reasons, it has become standard in multicenter clinical trials to have a data-monitoring committee review interim results, rather than having the monitoring done by participating physicians. This approach helps to protect patients by having interim results carefully evaluated by an experienced group of individuals and helps to protect the study from damage that ensues from misinterpretation of interim results. Generally, interim outcome information is available to only the data-monitoring committee. The study leaders are not part of the data-monitoring committee, because they may have a perceived conflict of interest in continuing the trial. The data-monitoring committee determines when results are mature and should be released. These procedures are used only for phase III trials.

A number of useful statistical designs have been developed for monitoring interim results. The simplest is that of Haybittle.[32,52] Interim differences are discounted unless the difference is statistically significant at the two-sided $P<.0025$ level. If the interim differences are not significant at that level, the trial continues until its originally intended size. The final analysis is performed without regard to the interim analyses, and the type I error is almost unaffected by the monitoring.

Others have developed group-sequential methods for interim monitoring based on a prespecified number of planned interim analyses.[53–55] The critical P value for determining whether an interim difference should be judged statistically significant depends on the number of analyses that will be performed during the trial. For a five-stage trial—four interim analyses and one final analysis—the critical P values are shown in Table 21.1-10.

Extreme treatment differences at an interim analysis are unusual in cancer clinical trials. It is more common to find that interim results do not support the hypothesis that the experimental treatment is substantially better than the control. The method of stochastic curtailment[56] was developed for evaluating such a circumstance. At any interim analysis, the probability of rejecting the null hypothesis at the end of the trial is computed. This probability is calculated as being conditional on the data already obtained and on the assumption that the alternative hypothesis of superiority of the experimental treatment used initially in planning the sample size for the trial is true. If this conditional power is less than approximately 0.20, then the trial may be terminated with acceptance of the null hypothesis. The 0.20 cutoff can be raised substantially to at least 0.40 if this type of interim analysis is performed only a few times during the course of the trial. With stochastic curtailment, interim analyses need not be equally spaced, and the number of interim analyses need not be specified in advance.

Several investigators have developed other designs for early termination of the clinical trial if results are not promising for the experimental treatment.[57–60] For example, Table 21.1-11 shows some of the two-stage designs developed by Thall et al.[59] for clinical trials with dichotomous end points. The first two columns show the hypothesized success rates for the control and experimental treatments. The remaining columns show the first-stage sample size per treatment and the maximum sample size per treatment. In all instances, the clinical trial is terminated after the first stage, and the experimental treatment is rejected as superior, if the one-sided significance level for comparing success rates is no less than approximately .38. If the one-sided significance level is less than .38, then a second stage of patient

TABLE 21.1-10. Nominal Two-Sided Significance Levels for Interim Monitoring Methods That Maintain an Overall Type I Error Level of .05

Analysis Number	*Pocock*[53]	*Peto et al.*[32] *and Haybittle*[52]	*O'Brien and Fleming*[54]	*Fleming et al.*[55]
1	.016	.0027	.00001	.0051
2	.016	.0027	.0013	.0061
3	.016	.0027	.008	.0073
4	.016	.0027	.023	.0089
Final	.016	.049	.041	.0402

TABLE 21.1-11. Two-Stage Early Termination Designs

		Power .80		*Power .90*	
Success Rate Control	*Success Rate Experimental Treatment*	Stage 1 Sample Size per Treatment	Maximum Sample Size per Treatment	Stage 1 Sample Size per Treatment	Maximum Sample Size per Treatment
0.2	0.35	48	116	73	157
0.2	0.40	28	68	43	92
0.3	0.45	56	137	85	185
0.3	0.50	33	78	48	106
0.4	0.55	61	146	92	197
0.4	0.60	33	82	51	110
0.5	0.65	59	143	89	193
0.5	0.70	33	78	49	106
0.6	0.75	53	128	81	173
0.6	0.80	28	68	42	72

accrual is conducted to give the maximum sample size per group shown. When the treatments are equivalent, the chance of early termination is generally 60% to 65% with this design.

Schaid et al.[57] and Wieand et al.[61] developed designs for early termination when results are not promising in survival studies. Schaid's design provides for multiple experimental treatment arms, as do the designs of Thall et al.[62,63] Such designs have been reviewed by Simon.[43] Jennison and Turnbull[64] have presented methods for calculating confidence intervals for treatment differences at interim analyses. Such confidence intervals can be useful in deciding when to terminate the trial.

Stochastic curtailment is based on computing the conditional probability of rejection of the null hypothesis calculated under the alternative hypothesis of the trial.[56] The probability is conditioned on the data available at that point but, because the probability is computed under the originally specified alternative hypothesis that the new regimen E is superior, stochastic curtailment is conservative. Bayesian biostatisticians have argued that the conditional probability should be computed under a distribution of the treatment difference that itself reflects the data available at that point. That distribution is called the *posterior distribution.* The Bayesian predictive probability is the probability of rejecting the null hypothesis if the trial is continued to its target number of events, conditional on the data available at that point and computed and averaged with regard to a range of hypotheses about the true difference δ as determined by the posterior distribution of δ given the data at that point. Computing the posterior distribution of δ, however, requires specification of a prior distribution for δ before the trial begins. The need to specify a prior distribution in a satisfactory manner has limited the applicability of Bayesian methods in clinical trials.

Phase III trials are supposed to be definitive and objective; if we could believe the subjective opinions of experts, we would not need to conduct phase III clinical trials. Recently, it has been recognized that a single prior distribution is not necessary for using Bayesian monitoring. It has been found useful to think in terms of one prior distribution of δ for "enthusiasts" for the experimental regimen E and a different prior distribution for "skeptics."[65] The investigators conducting the trial often are enthusiasts, whereas other investigators or practicing physicians may be more skeptical. If a trial is to terminate early with a claim that E is more effective than C, then the data from the trial should be strong enough to convince skeptics. On the other hand, if the trial is to terminate early with a claim that E is not more effective than C, then the data from the trial should be strong enough to convince enthusiasts. Although this is a somewhat oversimplified view (some enthusiasts or skeptics will never be convinced), it serves as a useful basis for interim monitoring. For computing the Bayesian predictive probability of rejection of the null hypothesis at the end of the trial if it is continued, it would be useful to use an enthusiast's prior distribution to ensure that the data are sufficiently compelling.

Stopping trials when the experimental regimen E is not appearing more effective than C but is not statistically significantly worse than C is sometimes controversial. Statisticians tend to want data as definitively as possible. One must also be cautious that with survival or disease-free survival end points, early parts of the survival curve may not reflect latter parts. Another argument for continuing such trials even if it is clear that E will not be found to be significantly better than C is that additional data will provide narrower confidence intervals for the true difference δ. The alternative point of view is that it is not appropriate to continue to expose patients to a more toxic and debilitating treatment E if the essential outcome of the trial is well assured. Data-monitoring committees are charged with helping to make these difficult judgments.[66]

SIGNIFICANCE LEVELS, HYPOTHESIS TESTS, AND CONFIDENCE INTERVALS

Medical decision making is complicated, and clinicians frequently misinterpret statistical significance tests in search of clear-cut answers from ambiguous data. A statistical significance level for comparing outcomes represents the probability of obtaining a difference as large as that actually observed if the treatments were actually of equal efficacy and differences occur merely by chance. If differences in either direction as large in absolute value as the one actually obtained are included, the significance level is called *two-sided.* If the probability is calculated only for differences in the same direction as that actually obtained, the significance level is called *one-sided.* Generally, the two-sided significance level is twice the one-sided level.

After significance tests had been used for many years, Neyman and Pearson[67] formalized a mathematical theory of hypothesis testing. In this theory, a study must prespecify a null

TABLE 21.1-12. Life-Table Method for Estimating a Survival Distribution

Years After Randomization $x - l$ *to* x	*No. Alive at Beginning of Interval* l_x	*No. Lost to Follow-up or Withdrawn Alive During Interval* w_x	*No. Died During Interval* d_x	*Effective No. Exposed to Risk of Dying During Interval (Col 2 −* ½ *Col 3)*	*Proportion Dying (Col 4/Col 5)* q_x	*Proportion Surviving (Col 1 − Col 6)* p_x	*Cumulative Proportion Surviving from Randomization through End of Interval* ($p_1 \times p_2 \times \ldots \times p_x$) S_x
0–1	252	38	94	233	0.40	0.60	0.60
1–2	120	34	10	103	0.10	0.90	0.54
2–3	76	30	4	61	0.07	0.93	0.50
3–4	42	18	4	33	0.12	0.88	0.44
4–5	20	12	0	14	0.00	1.00	0.44
5–6	8	8	0	4	0.00	1.00	0.44

Col, column.

hypothesis, an alternative hypothesis, and a decision rule for accepting one hypothesis and rejecting the other based on the data obtained. The theory has appealed to clinicians because it simplifies complex medical decision making by providing yes or no answers; either the difference is statistically significant or it is not. The distinction between one- and two-sided decision rules becomes crucial because a one-sided $P = .05$ is simply nonsignificant if a type I error of .05 based on a two-sided decision rule is prespecified.

The concept of prespecification of hypotheses is important for medical experimentation. However, the accept-reject nomenclature of the Neyman-Pearson theory provides an oversimplified and sometimes misleading interpretation of the data. Significance levels can serve as useful aids to interpretation of results, but quibbling about whether a one-sided $P = .04$ is significant makes little sense. Significance levels are influenced by sample sizes, and failure to reject the null hypothesis does not mean that the treatments are equivalent. There is no simple index of truth for interpreting results. Some attempt to use the notion of statistical significance in this way, but thorough presentation, skeptical evaluation, and cautious interpretation of results always are required.

Confidence intervals are generally much more informative than are significance levels. A confidence interval for the size of the treatment difference provides a range of effects consistent with the data. The significance level tells nothing about the size of the treatment effect because it depends on the sample size. However, it is the size of the treatment effect, as communicated by a confidence interval, that should be used in weighing the costs and benefits of clinical decision making. Many so-called negative results are actually noninformative, and confidence intervals help to determine when this is the case. Simon[68] has presented a nontechnical discussion of how to calculate confidence intervals for treatment differences with the types of end points commonly used in cancer clinical trials.

CALCULATION OF SURVIVAL CURVES

Most cancer clinical trials display results by showing survival curves or disease-free survival curves. Survival curves display the probability of surviving beyond any specified time, with time shown on the horizontal axis. In disease-free survival curves, it is the time until recurrence or death that is shown. Other time-to-event distributions can be similarly represented using the same methods. The usual statistical methods are not appropriate for analyzing survival because they ignore the fact that surviving patients have a limited follow-up period after which their survivals are "censored."

The most satisfactory way of representing such data is to estimate the survival function *S(t)*. This function represents the probability of surviving more than *t* time units. Time *t* is measured from diagnosis, start of treatment, or some other meaningful time point. For randomized studies, it is best to measure time from the date of randomization. There are basically two satisfactory methods for estimating *S(t)*. The first is the life-table or actuarial method. It frequently is attributed to Berkson and Gage[69] or Cutler and Ederer[70] and is appropriate when the number of patients is large. The other method is the product limit method of Kaplan and Meier.[71] This method is appropriate for any number of patients, but it involves more effort than the life-table method when the number of patients is large.

The first step in the application of either method is the calculation of survival time for all patients. Survival is the duration from the chosen baseline (e.g., date of randomization) until death or date last known to be alive for patients who are not known to have died. To use the life-table method, intervals for the grouping of survival times are determined. The life table, shown in Table 21.1-12, is then filled out. This sample life table is prepared with yearly intervals in the first column. The number of patients alive at the beginning of the interval is entered in column 2. The number who died in the interval is entered in column 4. Patients dying exactly at a time that represents a boundary between two intervals (e.g., 365 days) are considered to have died in the preceding interval (e.g., 0 to 1 year). Column 3 contains the number of patients who are lost to follow-up during the interval or who are alive with maximum follow-up duration included in the interval. These latter patients are referred to as *withdrawn alive* in the conventional life-table terminology. The life-table method assumes that patients lost to follow-up or withdrawn alive during the interval are at risk of death for half of the interval. Hence, column 5, the number alive at the start of the interval minus half the number lost or withdrawn during the interval, represents an approximate number of patients at risk of death during the interval. Col-

TABLE 21.1-13. Kaplan-Meier Method for Estimating a Survival Distribution

Months After Randomization	*No. Alive at Beginning of Interval* l_x	*No. Lost to Follow-up or Withdrawn Alive During Interval* w_x	*No. Died During Interval* d_x	*Effective No. Exposed to Risk of Dying Just Before End of Interval (Col 2 – Col 3)*	*Proportion Dying (Col 4/Col 5)* q_x	*Proportion Surviving (Col 1 – Col 6)* p_x	*Cumulative Proportion Surviving from Randomization through End of Interval* ($p_1 \times p_2 \times \ldots \times p_x$) S_x
0–3	10	0	2	10	0.2	0.8	0.8
3–5	8	1	1	7	0.14	0.86	0.68
5–6	6	0	1	6	0.17	0.83	0.57
6–10	5	2	2	3	0.67	0.33	0.19

Col, column.

umn 6 gives the ratio of the number of patients who died during the interval to the number at risk during the interval. Column 7 gives the estimated probability of surviving the interval for patients alive at the start of the interval.

Column 8 should be studied carefully, because it provides the life-table estimate of the survival distribution and indicates the logic behind the method. The probability of surviving more than 3 years after randomization, for example, equals the entry in the third row of column 8 (0.50). The logic is as follows: To survive 3 full years, the patients must survive through the first year; and given that they have survived the first year, they must survive the second year; and given that they have survived the second year, they must survive the third year. Consequently, the probability of surviving for at least 3 years is estimated by the product $P_1 \times P_2 \times P_3$ of factors in column 7. By using this product, the life-table method takes maximal advantage of the mortality experience of patients with limited follow-up. The entry S_x in column 8, row x, represents the life-table estimate of the probability of surviving more than x years from randomization. Computational shortcuts to observe are those for column 8—$S_x = P_x \times S_{x-1}$—and for column 2—$l_{x+1} = l_x - w_x - d_x$.

The product limit method of Kaplan and Meier[71] is similar in concept to the life-table method. With the Kaplan-Meier approach, however, the intervals are defined by the actual survival times of patients who have died. Suppose, for example, that the survivals are 3, 3, 3+, 5, 6, 8+, 8+, 10, 10, and 12+ months, where a plus sign follows survivals for patients still alive. Then the intervals are 0 to 3, 3 to 5, 5 to 6, and 6 to 10 months, as shown in Table 21.1-13. With the Kaplan-Meier method, deaths occur only at the ends of intervals. The entry in column 5 equals $l_x - w_x$ rather than $l_x - 2w_x$ for the life-table method. This is because deaths occur only at the ends of intervals here, and the number of patients at risk of death just before the interval end is $l_x - w_x$. In the entry w_x in column 3 for the Kaplan-Meier method, patients who are lost to follow-up or withdrawn alive at the end of an interval are considered not lost or withdrawn until the following interval. These differences between the Kaplan-Meier and life-table methods render the former more appropriate for studies with fewer patients.

Once the values S_x have been calculated for the Kaplan-Meier method, they may be graphed with time on the horizontal axis. The graph is a step function that starts at time zero and ordinate 1.0. It drops to value S_x at time x, where x is the time at the right end of an interval. The survival curve corresponding to Table 21.1-14 is shown in Figure 21.1-1. The tic marks are placed on the curve at 3, 8, and 12 months to represent the follow-up times of living patients. The step function can be extended horizontally out to 12 months to represent follow-up of the last patient, but the right-hand end of the curve usually is very imprecisely estimated, and concluding that a plateau exists at the level shown on the curve is often erroneous.

For any time t, the Kaplan-Meier curve is an estimator of the true unknown value of $S(t)$. The estimator is approximately normally distributed in large samples. If m patients remain alive at time x, the standard error of the estimate can be conservatively estimated[32] as

$$S_x\sqrt{(1-S_x)/m}$$

The Kaplan-Meier estimate of a survival distribution is based on the assumption that censoring is noninformative, which means that the censoring time is independent of the prognosis of the patient. Most censoring in a randomized clinical trial results from the fact that some patients are alive and still being followed at the time of analysis. This is noninformative censoring. However, if patients are lost to follow-up, if they fail to return to clinic when they are too sick to travel, then the censoring is informative and all the usual methods of survival analysis are invalidated. Consequently, it is essential to obtain follow-up information actively on *all* patients before analysis. If some patients have not been contacted for many months and their status is unknown, that information should be obtained

TABLE 21.1-14. Probability of Obtaining at Least One Statistically Significant ($P < .05$) Difference by Chance Alone in Multiple Comparisons of Two Equivalent Treatments

Comparisons	*Probability of at Least One "Significant" Difference (%)*
1	5
2	9.7
3	14.3
4	18.5
5	22.6
10	40
20	64.1

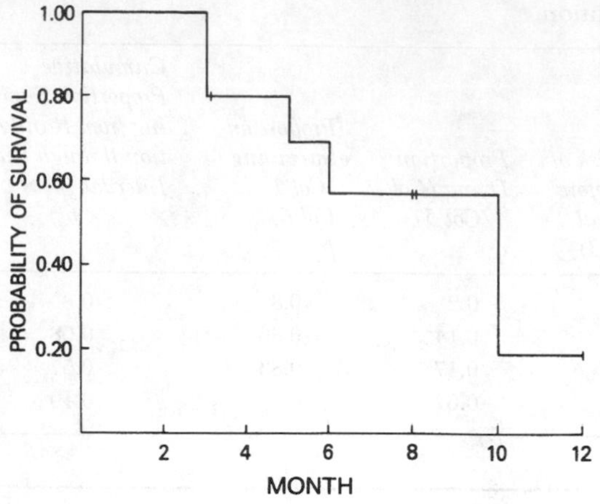

FIGURE 21.1-1. Example of estimated survival distribution.

before any analysis is performed. Examining the distribution of time since the last contact for patients not known to have died is a good way to examine the adequacy of follow-up.

The issue of informative censoring also arises in considering end points other than death. For example, one may be attempting to estimate the distribution of time until tumor recurrence in the central nervous system (CNS) in a pediatric leukemia trial. How should one handle patients whose disease recurs in the marrow without evidence of CNS recurrence? One may be tempted to censor the time to CNS recurrence of such patients at their time of marrow recurrence, but that implicitly assumes that the censoring is noninformative. Because CNS and marrow recurrence may be biologically linked, the assumption of noninformative censoring may not be valid. Other issues of informative censoring can be similarly problematic. Clearly, one should never censor patients because of lack of compliance with therapy, as this can severely bias results.

More extensive, but fairly nontechnical, discussions of statistical methods for the analysis of clinical trial data are given by Anderson et al.[72] and by Harrington and Anderson.[73]

MULTIPLE COMPARISONS

Table 21.1-14 shows the probability of obtaining one statistically significant ($P < .05$) difference by chance alone as a function of the number of independent comparisons of two equivalent treatments. With only five comparisons, the chance of at least one false-positive conclusion is 22.6%. When the number of end points, interim analyses, and patient subsets are considered in the analysis of clinical trials, these results are disturbing.[74] The comparisons performed in clinical trials are not entirely independent, but this does not have much effect on ameliorating the problem. Fleming and Watelet[75] performed a computer simulation to determine the chance of obtaining a statistically significant treatment difference when two equivalent treatments in six subsets determined by three dichotomous variables are compared. The chance of a statistically significant difference between treatments in at least one subset was 20% at the final analysis and 39% in the final or one of the three interim analyses. Subset analysis, comparison of treatments with regard to multiple end points, and multiple interim analyses are common sources of erroneous conclusions. The primary end point should be defined in the protocol. Subset analyses and analyses with regard to secondary end points should be specified in advance, and statistical significance should be declared only for significance levels much more extreme than the conventional .05. The simplest approach to multiple comparisons is to declare statistical significance only if the P value is less than $.05/n$, where n denotes the number of comparisons to be made. For example if $n = 10$, then .005 should be the threshold for declaring significance for a secondary analysis. The number of comparisons planned in the protocol is represented by n. Comparisons not preplanned should not be considered significant in any case and represent hypothesis generation to be tested in subsequent trials.

Interaction tests are statistical procedures that test for lack of homogeneity of treatment effect across subsets of patients. A statistically significant interaction should be documented before claiming that treatment effects vary among subsets. Such tests are described by Simon[76,77] and by Gail and Simon.[78]

Generally, it is not valid to adjust the analysis by characteristics measured after the start of treatment (e.g., compliance, dose delivered, toxicity). New approaches to subset analysis and multiple end point analysis using Bayesian methods have been described by Simon et al.[79,80]

REPORTING RESULTS OF CLINICAL TRIALS

Effective reporting of results is an integral part of good research. Unfortunately, numerous reviews have indicated that the quality of reporting of clinical trial results is poor.[49,81–83] Pocock et al.[84] concluded that "overall, the reporting of clinical trials appears to be biased toward an exaggeration of treatment differences." Barr and Tannock[48] have given a clear illustration of how this is easily done. Simon and Wittes[85] developed a set of methodologic guidelines for reports of clinical trials, and these guidelines have been adopted by major cancer journals. These nine guidelines are summarized below:

1. Authors should discuss briefly the quality control methods used to ensure that the data (including response assessments) are complete and accurate.
2. All patients registered on study should be accounted for.
3. The study should not have an inevaluability rate of greater than 15% for major end points.
4. In randomized trials, the report should include a comparison of survival and other major end points for all eligible patients as randomized, with no exclusions other than those not meeting eligibility criteria.
5. The sample size should be sufficient to establish or conclusively rule out the existence of effects of clinically important magnitude. For "negative" conclusions in therapeutic comparisons, the adequacy of sample size should be demonstrated by presenting confidence limits for the true treatment differences.
6. The report should indicate the initial target sample size. It should specify how many interim analyses were performed and how the decisions to stop accrual and report results were made.
7. Claims of therapeutic efficacy should not be made based on nonrandomized phase II trials, unless the disease is so rare or the prognosis so poor that properly controlled randomized trials are not possible. In the latter case, nonrandomized trials should use explicit his-

torical controls for which comparability of patients can be thoroughly evaluated. Comparison of survival between responders and nonresponders is not a valid way of establishing therapeutic efficacy.[11,12,86]

8. The patients studied should be adequately described. Applicability of conclusions to the general population of patients should be carefully discussed. Claims of subset-specific treatment differences should be carefully documented statistically as more than the random result of multiple significance testing.[74]
9. The methods of statistical analysis should be described in detail sufficient that a knowledgeable reader could reproduce the analyses if the data were available.

EPIDEMIOLOGY OF CLINICAL TRIALS

Several authors have pointed out that many of the positive results reported from small trials are expected to be false-positive results.[76,87,88] In 100 trials, suppose that there are 10 in which the experimental treatment is sufficiently better than the control such that there is an 80% chance of the difference being detected in a small or moderate-sized clinical trial. Of these 10 trials, obtaining a statistically significant difference in 8 cases (0.80×10) is expected. Of the remaining 90 trials, it is assumed that the treatments are approximately equivalent to the control. We would expect to obtain a statistically significant difference in 5% (4.5) of these cases. Hence, of the 12.5 (8 + 4.5) trials that yield statistically significant results, the finding is false-positive in 4.5 or 36% of the cases (4.5/12.5). The 36% false-positive result is striking. It depends on the assumption that only 10% of the trials represent important advances, but this assumption does not seem overly pessimistic.

An additional factor to consider is that of publication bias,[89] which denotes the preference of journals to publish positive rather than negative results. A negative result may not be published at all, particularly from a small trial. If it is published, it is likely to appear in a less widely read journal than it would if the result were positive.

These observations emphasize that results in the medical literature often cannot be accepted at face value. It is essential to recognize that "positive" results need confirmation, particularly positive results of small studies, before they can be believed and applied to the general population.

METAANALYSIS

A metaanalysis is a quantitative summary of research in a particular area. It is distinguished from the traditional literature review by its emphasis on quantifying results of individual studies and combining results across studies. Key components of this approach are to include only randomized clinical trials, to include all relevant randomized clinical trials that have been initiated, regardless of whether they have been published, to exclude no randomized patients from the analysis, and to assess therapeutic effectiveness based on the average results pooled across trials.[90]

Attention is restricted to randomized trials, because the bias from nonrandomized comparisons may be larger than the small to moderate therapeutic effects likely to be present. Including all relevant randomized trials that have been initiated in a geographic area (e.g., the world, or the Americas and Europe) represents an attempt to avoid publication bias. Avoiding exclusion of any randomized patients also functions to avoid bias. Assessing therapeutic effectiveness based on average pooled results is an attempt to make the evaluation on the totality of evidence rather than on extreme isolated reports. In calculating average treatment effects, a measure of difference in outcome between treatments is calculated separately for each trial. For example, an estimate of the logarithm of the hazard ratio can be computed for each trial. A weighted average of these study-specific differences then is computed, and the statistical significance of this average is evaluated. This approach to metaanalysis requires access to individual patient data for all randomized patients in each trial. It also requires collaboration of the leaders of all the relevant trials and is very labor-intensive. Nevertheless, it represents the gold standard for metaanalysis methodology.

A major issue of concern in metaanalyses is whether the individual trials are sufficiently similar to make calculation of average effects medically meaningful. If the therapeutic interventions or control treatments differ too greatly or if the patient populations are too different, then the results may not be medically meaningful as a basis for making treatment decisions for individual patients. Often in cancer therapeutics, the studies will not be identical in their treatment regimens or their patient populations, but they will not be so different as to make the results meaningless. In this case, the metaanalysis may be useful for answering important questions about a class of treatments that the individual trials cannot address reliably. For example, trials evaluating adjuvant treatment of primary breast cancer often are designed to detect differences in disease-free survival, and a metaanalysis is often required to evaluate survival. Similarly, subset analysis can usually be meaningfully evaluated only in the context of a metaanalysis, because individual trials are not sized for this objective.

Metaanalysis is *not* an alternative to properly designed and sized randomized clinical trials. Some have suggested that one need not be concerned about computing sample size in the traditional ways, as small randomized trials can be pooled for metaanalysis. Because most investigators would prefer to "do their own thing," this would lead to a proliferation of diverse trials of inconsequential individual size that were too heterogeneous to permit a meaningful metaanalysis. Given that sufficient large, randomized clinical trials of very similar treatment regimens have been conducted, metaanalysis can provide supplemental information about a given class of treatments that is not available from the individual trials.

REFERENCES

1. Bull JP. The historical development of clinical therapeutic trials. *J Chronic Dis* 1959;10:218.
2. Byar DP. Why data bases should not replace randomized clinical trials. *Biometrics* 1980; 36:337.
3. Dambrosia JM, Ellenberg JH. Statistical considerations for a medical data base. *Biometrics* 1980;26:323.
4. MacMahon B, Pugh TF. *Epidemiology: principles and methods.* Boston: Little, Brown and Company, 1970.
5. Leventhal BG, Wittes RE. *Research methods in clinical oncology.* New York: Raven Press, 1988.
6. Schneiderman MA. Mouse to man: statistical problems in bringing a drug to clinical trial. In: *Proceedings of the fifth Berkeley symposium on mathematical statistical probability.* Berkeley: University of California, 1967:855.
7. Simon R, Freidlin B, Rubinstein L, et al. Accelerated titration designs for phase I clinical trials in oncology. *J Natl Cancer Inst* 1997;89:1138.
8. Korn EL, Simon R. Using the tolerable-dose diagram in the design of phase I combination chemotherapy trials. *J Clin Oncol* 1993;11:794.
9. Ettinger DS. Evaluation of new drugs in untreated patients with small-cell lung cancer: its time has come. *J Clin Oncol* 1990;8:374.

10. Wittes RE, Marsoni S, Simon R, et al. The phase II trial. *Cancer Treat Rep* 1985;69:1235.
11. Anderson JR, Cain KC, Gelber RD. Analysis of survival by tumor response. *J Clin Oncol* 1983;1:710.
12. Simon R, Makuch RW. A nonparametric graphical representation of the relationship between survival and the occurrence of an event: application to responder versus non-responder bias. *Stat Med* 1984;3:1.
13. Simon R. How large should a phase II trial of a new drug be? *Cancer Treat Rep* 1987;71:1079.
14. Simon R. Optimal two-stage designs for phase II clinical trials. *Control Clin Trials* 1989;10:1.
15. Fleming TR. One sample multiple testing procedure for phase II clinical trials. *Biometrics* 1982;38:143.
16. Ensign L, Gehan EA, Kamen D, Thall PF. An optimal three-stage design for phase II clinical trials. *Stat Med* 1994;13:1727.
17. Simon R, Wittes RE, Ellenberg SS. Randomized phase II clinical trials. *Cancer Treat Rep* 1985;69:1375.
18. Makuch RW, Simon R. Sample size considerations for nonrandomized comparative studies. *J Chronic Dis* 1980;33:171.
19. Thall PF, Simon R, Estey E. Bayesian sequential monitoring designs for single-arm clinical trials with multiple outcomes. *Stat Med* 1995;14:357.
20. Thall P, Simon R, Estey E. New statistical strategy for monitoring safety and efficacy in single-arm clinical trials. *J Clin Oncol* 1996;14:296.
21. Dixon DO, Simon R. Sample size considerations for studies comparing survival curves using historical controls. *J Clin Epidemiol* 1988;41:1209.
22. Simon R. Randomized clinical trials in oncology: principles and obstacles. *Cancer* 1994;74:2614.
23. Torri V, Simon R, Russek-Cohen E, Midthune D, Friedman M. Relationship of response and survival in advanced ovarian cancer patients treated with chemotherapy. *J Natl Cancer Inst* 1992;84:407.
24. Pocock SJ. Randomized clinical trials. *Br Med J* 1977;1:1161.
25. Byar DP, Simon RM, Friedewald WT, et al. Randomized clinical trials: perspectives on some recent ideas. *N Engl J Med* 1976;295:74.
26. Chalmers TC, Block JB, Lee S. Controlled studies in clinical cancer research. *N Engl J Med* 1972;287:75.
27. Lasagna L. The controlled clinical trial: theory and practice. *J Chronic Dis* 1955;1:353.
28. Hill AB. The clinical trial. *Br Med J* 1951;7:278.
29. Saks H, Chalmers TC, Smith H. Randomized versus historical controls for clinical trials. *Am J Med* 1982;72:233.
30. Simon R. The importance of prognostic factors in cancer clinical trials. *Cancer Treat Rep* 1984;68:185.
31. Peto R, Pike MC, Armitage P, et al. Design and analysis of randomized clinical trials requiring prolonged observation of each patient: I. Introduction and design. *Br J Cancer* 1976;34:585.
32. Peto R, Pike MC, Armitage P, et al. Design and analysis of randomized clinical trials requiring prolonged observation of each patient: II. Analysis and examples. *Br J Cancer* 1977;35:1.
33. Simon R. Restricted randomization designs in clinical trials. *Biometrics* 1979;35:503.
34. Kalish LA, Begg CB. Treatment allocation methods in clinical trials: a review. *Stat Med* 1985;4:129.
35. Kalish LA, Begg CB. The impact of treatment allocation procedures on nominal significance levels and bias. *Control Clin Trials* 1987;8:121.
36. George SL, Desu MM. Planning the size and duration of a clinical trial studying the time to some critical event. *J Chronic Dis* 1974;27:15.
37. Rubenstein LV, Gail MH, Santner TJ. Planning the duration of a comparative clinical trial with loss to follow-up and a period of continued observation. *J Chronic Dis* 1981;34:469.
38. Frieman JA, Chalmers TC, Smith HJ. The importance of beta, the type II error, and sample size in the design and interpretation of the randomized control trial: survey of 71 "negative" trials. *N Engl J Med* 1978;299:690.
39. Makuch R, Simon R. Sample size requirements for evaluating a conservative therapy. *Cancer Treat Rep* 1978;62:1037.
40. Durrleman S, Simon R. Planning and monitoring of equivalence studies. *Biometrics* 1990;46:329.
41. Peto R. Clinical trial methodology. *Biomedicine* 1978;28:24.
42. Byar DP, Piantadosi S. Factorial designs for randomized clinical trials. *Cancer Treat Rep* 1985;69:1055.
43. Simon R. Designs for efficient clinical trials. *Oncology* 1989;3:34.
44. Simon R. A critical assessment of approaches to improving the efficacy of cancer clinical trials. In: Baum M, Kay R, Scheurlen H, eds. *Recent results in cancer research,* vol 3. Heidelberg: Springer-Verlag, 1988:18.
45. Brittain E, Wittes J. Factorial designs in clinical trials: the effects of non-compliance and subaddictivity. *Stat Med* 1989;8:161.
46. Simon R, Freedman LS. Bayesian design and analysis of 2 by 2 factorial clinical trials. *Biometrics* 1997;53:456.
47. Simon R. Bayesian design and analysis of active control clinical trials. *Biometrics* 1999;55:484.
48. Barr J, Tannock I. Analyzing the same data two ways: a demonstration model to illustrate the reporting and misreporting of clinical trials. *J Clin Oncol* 1989;7:969.
49. Tannock I, Murphy K. Reflections on medical oncology: an appeal for better clinical trials and improved time of their results. *J Clin Oncol* 1983;1:66.
50. Group CDR. Influence of adherence to treatment and response of cholesterol on mortality in the coronary drug project. *N Engl J Med* 1980;302:1038.
51. Fleming TR, Green SJ, Harrington DP. Considerations of monitoring and evaluating treatment effects in clinical trials. *Control Clin Trials* 1984;5:55.
52. Haybittle JL. Repeated assessment of results in clinical trials of cancer treatment. *J Radiol* 1971;44:793.
53. Pocock SJ. Interim analyses for randomized clinical trials. *Biometrics* 1982;38:153.
54. O'Brien PC, Fleming TR. A multiple testing procedure for clinical trials. *Biometrics* 1979;35:549.
55. Fleming TR, Harrington DP, O'Brien PC. Designs for group sequential tests. *Control Clin Trials* 1984;5:348.
56. Lan KKG, Simon R, Halperin M. Stochastically curtailed tests in long-term clinical trials. *Commun Stat Sequen Anal* 1982;1:207.
57. Schaid DJ, Wieand S, Therneau TM. Optimal two-stage screening designs for survival comparisons. *Biometrics* 1990;77:507.
58. Storer BE. A sequential phase II/III trial for binary outcomes. *Stat Med* 1990;9:229.
59. Thall PF, Simon R, Ellenberg SS, Shrager R. Optimal two-stage designs for clinical trials with binary response. *Stat Med* 1988;7:571.
60. Wieand S, Therneau T. A two-stage design for randomized trials with binary outcomes. *Control Clin Trials* 1987;8:20.
61. Wieand S, Schroeder G, O'Fallon JR. Stopping when the experimental regimen does not appear to help. *Stat Med* 1994;13:1453.
62. Thall PF, Simon R, Ellenberg SS. Two-stage selection and testing designs for comparative clinical trials. *Biometrics* 1988;75:303.
63. Thall PF, Simon R, Ellenberg SS. A two-stage design for choosing among several experimental treatments and a control in clinical trials. *Biometrics* 1989;45:537.
64. Jennison C, Turnbull BW. Repeated confidence intervals for group sequential clinical trials. *Control Clin Trials* 1984;5:33.
65. Spiegelhalter D, Freedman L, Parmar M. Bayesian approaches to randomized trials. *J R Stat Soc [A]* 1994;157:357.
66. Smith M, Ungerleider R, Korn E, Rubinstein L, Simon R. The role of independent data monitoring committees in randomized clinical trials sponsored by the National Cancer Institute. *J Clin Oncol* 1997;15:2736.
67. Neyman J, Pearson ES. On the use and interpretation of certain test criteria. *Biometrika* 1928;201:175.
68. Simon R. Confidence intervals for reporting results from clinical trials. *Ann Intern Med* 1986;105:429.
69. Berkson J, Gage RP. Calculation of survival rates for cancer. *Proc Mayo Clin* 1950;25:270.
70. Cutler SJ, Ederer F. Maximum utilization of the life table method in analyzing survival. *J Chronic Dis* 1958;8:699.
71. Kaplan EI, Meier P. Nonparametric estimation from incomplete observations. *J Am Stat Assoc* 1958;53:457.
72. Anderson JR, Crowley JJ, Propert KJ. Interpretation of survival date in clinical trials (with discussion by R Simon). *Oncology* 1991;5:104.
73. Harrington DP, Anderson JW. Common methods of analyzing response data in clinical trials (with discussion by R Simon). *Oncology* 1990;4:95.
74. Tannock IF. False-positive results in clinical trials: multiple significance tests and the problem of unreported comparisons. *J Natl Cancer Inst* 1996;88:206.
75. Fleming TR, Watelet L. Approaches to monitoring clinical trials. *J Natl Cancer Inst* 1989;81:188.
76. Simon R. Randomized clinical trials and research strategy. *Cancer Treat Rep* 1982;66:1083.
77. Simon R. Statistical tools for subset analysis in clinical trials. In: Baum M, Kay R, Scheurlen H, eds. *Recent results in cancer research,* vol 3. Heidelberg: Springer-Verlag, 1988:55.
78. Gail M, Simon R. Testing for qualitative interactions between treatment effects and patient subsets. *Biometrics* 1985;41:361.
79. Dixon DO, Simon R. Bayesian subset analysis. *Biometrics* 1991;47:871.
80. Simon R. Discovering the truth about Tamoxifen: problems of multiplicity in the evaluation of biomedical data. *J Natl Cancer Inst* 1995;87:627.
81. Zelen M. Guideline for publishing papers on cancer clinical trials: responsibilities of editors and authors. *J Clin Oncol* 1983;1:164.
82. Begg CB, Pocock SJ, Freedman L, Zelen M. State of the art in comparative cancer clinical trials. *Cancer* 1987;60:2811.
83. Begg CB. Quality of clinical trials. *Ann Oncol* 1990;1:319.
84. Pocock SJ, Hughes MD, Lee RJ. Statistical problems in the reporting of clinical trials: a survey of three medical journals. *N Engl J Med* 1987;317:426.
85. Simon R, Wittes RE. Methodologic guidelines for reports of clinical trials. *Cancer Treat Rep* 1985;69:1.
86. Weiss GB, Hokanson JA. Comparing survival of responders and non-responders after treatment: a potential source of confusion in interpreting cancer clinical trials. *Control Clin Trials* 1983;4:43.
87. Staquet MJ, Rosencweig M, Hoff DDV. The delta and epsilon errors in the assessment of cancer clinical trials. *Cancer Treat Rep* 1984;63:1917.
88. Zelen M. Strategy and alternative randomized designs in cancer clinical trials. *Cancer Treat Rep* 1982;66:1095.
89. Begg CB, Berlin JA. Publication bias and dissemination of clinical research. *J Natl Cancer Inst* 1989;81:107-115.
90. Collins R, Gray R, Godwin J, Peto R. Avoidance of large biases and large random errors in the assessment of moderate treatment effects: the need for systematic overviews. *Stat Med* 1987;6:245.

SECTION **2**

DOUGLAS HAGEMAN
DIANNE M. REEVES

Research Data Management

Historically, discussions of data management have focused on an inherently manual process. Questions pertaining to data collection form layout, transport of information, and the role of computers were paramount. Now the questions relate to information technology's assumed role in research data management. Data can be collected in real time from study sites worldwide. Data quality can be verified at time of input or collection. The human interface between clinical care data (the hospital-clinic systems) and clinical research data (the subset of clinical data dictated by protocol) can be significantly assisted by the electronic interchange of data between computers. Still, the fundamentals of data management remain fairly constant and can be applied throughout the steps in the clinical trial life cycle. The clinical trial life cycle begins with protocol development and continues through patient recruitment, screening and registration, protocol implementation, and analysis and publication.

PROTOCOL DEVELOPMENT

Data management begins with the protocol document and the events prescribed in that document. The protocol defines study objectives, patient selection and eligibility, and the temporal sequence of events. Data to be collected must be prospectively identified. Common elements in treatment protocols include a précis or summary of the protocol, schema, protocol objectives, study design, definition of patient population, the protocol intervention, drug information, toxicities and dosage modifications, methods of evaluation against study end points, data collection, and statistical considerations (see protocol outline in Table 21.2-1).[1,2] Each component has an impact on research data management and defines requirements to be carried out during the study. In fact, data management begins with the process of authoring, reviewing, and approving the protocol document itself. This process often depends on coordination with associate investigators, internal review committees, institutional review boards, and external sponsors. It is often time-consuming and driven by multiple levels of review. Document templates, electronic document routing, electronic signature, and the use of structured text in the protocol-authoring step of the life cycle could mean that protocols can be conducted more quickly with higher-quality information at every level. The National Cancer Institute (NCI) is pursuing development of information systems that may help to evolve this lengthy process into a faster one.[3]

PHASE OF PROTOCOL

The protocol phase determines the type of data collected to evaluate study end points. Phase I is not disease-specific. Major end points are maximum tolerated dose of the treatment. The data collection will be focused on measurement and categorization of toxicities. The study size will be small, composed of groups (usually fewer than six participants) at each dose level until maximum tolerated dose is reached.

Phase II is tumor- and diagnosis-specific. The major end points are response of the tumor to the intervention. Phase II studies do not require a control group. The data collection will be to evaluate biologic effect and tumor response.

Phase III is disease- and diagnosis-specific, and its major end points are efficacy, survival, and symptom control. Phase III studies yield results that can be generalized to the population. This imposes the need for a dramatically larger sample size and, possibly, randomization of study subjects to create a control group. The implications for data management are huge: To achieve protocol accrual in a reasonable time, phase III studies are usually conducted in multiple centers.[1,4] A coordinating center is responsible for the management and monitoring of study accrual and conduct of the randomization process. Phase IV studies are designed for postmarketing surveillance of approved drugs.

STUDY OBJECTIVES

This section includes scientific background and defines study. The end points will drive study conduct as well as determine the data required.

STUDY DESIGN

The study design specifies study population, sample size, enrollment, treatment administration and schema, data collection, and analysis. Each component will require specific data management events or tasks.

The study population is determined by the use of inclusion and exclusion criteria: what patient diagnoses or characteristics are required to participate in the study (inclusion) and which will eliminate someone from participating (exclusion). Data management tasks include the evaluation and recording of these criteria for each prospective patient.

TREATMENT ADMINISTRATION AND SCHEMA

Treatment administration and schema outline the study intervention and the temporal sequence in which events must occur. The impact on data management is the resultant schedule sequence for data collection. Schedule delays and intervention modification will be described in sufficient detail to render these directives operational.

PROCEDURAL ISSUES

The protocol should identify procedural issues for the study conduct, such as documentation of eligibility, enrollment and registration procedures, study schedule, and detailed data collection and handling methods. The tools (forms, procedures, computer applications) for data collection will be included, as well as documentation about computerized systems used to handle trial data.[5] All processes, data requirements, sequence of events, data collection instruments, database, and electronic system usage in a study should be identified prospectively as intended, to support only the stated study objectives.[6]

TABLE 21.2-1. Protocol Outline, National Cancer Institute Division of Clinical Sciences, Bethesda, MD

PATIENT RECRUITMENT, SCREENING, AND REGISTRATION

Once the protocol is approved and ready for patient accrual, the life cycle moves to the step of patient recruitment. The goal here is to apply the study population parameters—inclusion and exclusion criteria—to potential patients. Matching eligibility criteria with a particular patient requires that criteria be expressed in a standard way. As appropriate within the study design, rendering the entrance criteria as nonspecific as possible will facilitate study accrual.[6] An additional challenge is the display of protocol information based on very specific patient characteristics. Without this capability, information may not narrow study choices sufficiently for patients and their physicians to make informed preliminary decisions. For example, one test using the NCI's Physician Data Query protocol search at http://cancernet.nci.nih.gov/trialsrch.shtml to enter a search for breast cancer trials returned 140 trials, but when the search was limited to only phase III trials for stage II breast cancer, the return dropped significantly. To the extent that the patient population specified in the protocol can be expressed via minimal criteria, the study-patient matching can be facilitated.

TABLE 21.2-2. Data Management for Support of the Protocol Life Cycle

Life Cycle Step	*Data Management Tasks*
Protocol development	Protocol authoring; document routing, mark-up, and approval; definition of protocol data requirements; study categorization (phase, disease, identification of study population)
Patient recruitment	Patient-study matching; information dissemination for patients and for physicians; contact management
Patient screening and registration	Documentation of first patient encounter; collection of demographic information; collection of patient history; eligibility assessment; protocol enrollment-registration
Protocol implementation	Protocol-specific data collection forms; reuse of existing patient information (from patient record, laboratory, ancillary hospital services); automatic grading of laboratory toxicities; data elements defined in data dictionary and applied uniformly; data dictionary in support of standards across patients and studies
Analysis and publication	Predefined report formats; user-defined reports; *ad hoc* query; data plotting; data export to external statistical applications

Prospective registration (before study intervention) ensures that the patient selection process does not bias the results. Given the methodologic issues and the administrative challenges associated with tracking study accrual, an independent registration office or coordinating center is recommended. A common model is for a coordinating center to record patient registration to a study. After registration, notification to the pharmacy allows study agents to be released to the patient. Additionally, randomization assignments can be made by the coordinating center at time of registration, independently of the study team.

PROTOCOL IMPLEMENTATION

The protocol life cycle approach allows the researcher to reap the benefit of advance planning at the point of protocol implementation (Table 21.2-2). Study design and questions drive the collection of research data and the creation of study-specific data management tools,[1] while U.S. Food and Drug Administration (FDA) recommendations and international guidelines define good clinical practices (GCPs) that must be operational in clinical research.[7]

Clinical research data constitute a subset of the patient's medical information, so the requirement in the design of data management tools and processes is to be selective. The desire to capture interesting but unused data will dilute the ability to answer the study's scientific questions and will overwhelm study personnel with unnecessary workloads.

A data management approach that supports the protocol life cycle will reuse elements identified in the concept and protocol documents, maintaining focus on the study design. It also supports minimal redundancy of data entry, using data harmonization to add standardized meaning to terminology. Researchers understand the strength of this approach in their long-term ability to share information with other investigators and to apply the same analytic procedures across protocols, and in their ability to enroll patients and conduct clinical trials across organizational and geographic constraints.

The heart of data management is the effort of personnel using a set of tools and work processes. Processes must support the sophistication of the tools (electronic or paper-based) used and facilitate the collection and entry of clinical research data.

DATA COLLECTION

Case report forms (CRFs) represent the industry's standard approach that has been adopted by most research institutions for the collection of clinical research data. The CRF is a layout, or template, of the data elements that are to be captured by personnel working with clinical research data. Items may be categorized and grouped in a logical work flow and order.[8] Items collected or abstracted from source documents should be contiguous on the forms,[9] encouraging the capture of complete data sets and lessening the risk of missing elements. Consistency across protocols will be reflected in a similar display of generic items on forms, use of the same coding conventions across studies, and standardized definition of terms across protocols and across forms for a single study. Figure 21.2-1 is an example of a CRF used for collecting a patient's prior therapy information. Notice that acceptable choices for certain categories (prior therapy type and response) are identified at the top of the form, in addition to other specific instructions supplied at the bottom of the form.

In recent years, many institutions have moved to the use of electronic CRFs to enter, view, and monitor clinical research data. The automated approach offers such advantages as the ability to aggregate data for reports, the ability to search for patient-specific data as needed, and the ability to share information rapidly. The use of paper CRFs as retrievable, auditable signs of data abstraction is a powerful reminder of the benefits of a paper approach.

Electronic CRFs that are customized for a protocol yet retain some measure of generic content to support cross-study aggregate views of the data are appealing to investigators and clinical trial teams. A presentation of data collection needs that is driven by the study, and not a cloned set of data points used for all trials, supports principles of data integrity. The electronic replacement of paper CRFs and data discrepancy forms with computers requires the same attention to coding conventions, work flow, and consistency as do approaches with paper tools. Additionally, the electronic approach permits front-end validation processes, such as range checking, simple edit checks, and cross-validation between variables measured on repeated occasions.[8,10]

The decision to move from paper to electronic CRFs and automated data management processes requires an organizational commitment to reengineer work processes. Hammer and Champy[11] noted that most organizations view technology through the "lens of existing processes." They should not ask how they can use technology to do what they are doing now but rather how they can improve what they are doing now and achieve entirely new goals.[12] Electronic CRFs may enable organizations to streamline their work flow, introduce new data quality practices, or prepare auditors before monitoring visits. In 1996, 95% of all clinical trials still used paper.[12] Moving to the electronic arena requires personnel to overcome fears about change, to reengineer processes, and to create radically new goals.[13] It is possible to redefine data management to make the paper CRF obsolete and create electronic access for personnel to enter clinical data directly from the source document into the computer. Auditors could review an activity log and electronic CRFs as well as view aggregate data before a site visit. Data abstracted in a paper-based system could be replaced by direct data entry without abstraction onto CRFs.[12] These technologic advancements must be accompanied by process reengineering, so that personnel are comfortable with these changes and the benefits they offer. They may enable geographically distant sites, patients, and researchers to collaborate on clinical trial accrual, using Internet-based technologies and multisite-consistent work practices.[14]

Data Collection Instruments

A collection of data values from the conduct of clinical research is a logically coherent, meaningful collection of related data. It is designed and populated for a specific purpose. Data are entered and stored so that they may be retrieved and used in meaningful ways. Clinical research data are composed of discrete pieces of raw material gathered through investigation. If the data are ambiguous, incomplete, or erroneous, processing cannot turn the data into valid information. There are strategies an institution can adapt to validate data at the point of abstraction and entry.

Data Standards

Data must be accurate, precise, current, and complete. CRFs (electronic or paper) must be constructed to encourage correct entries, supplying user instructions and cues. Instructions should be unambiguous and written in terminology useful for personnel completing the forms. Form identifiers and landmarks must be consistent and clearly define required items. When choice lists are used to code or list items, they must be readily available for review. The sequence of items on a form must be logical and mimic source documents or work processes used to capture these items.[8,10] Elements captured together must be contiguous on the CRFs, to enter a complete set of data points.

Duplication must be avoided. To increase efficiency and eliminate the need to cross-check items across forms, data should be collected without redundancy. Data should be entered once and reused, not reentered. To indicate the presence of mandatory items, elements can be set in bold-face type or displayed in some consistent manner.

PROTOCOL QUESTIONS AND END POINTS

Data must be targeted to answer protocol questions. Forms must focus on the data needed to answer questions central

Pt's Initials: A.B. **Protocol ID:** 99C#### **Site ID:** ABCD **Date:** 03/10/2000

PATIENT LABEL HERE

PRIOR THERAPY

Prior Therapy Type:		Response:	
A	Antiretroviral	CR	Complete Response
C	Chemotherapy	CRU	Complete Response Unconfirmed
G	Gene Therapy	MR	Minimal Response
H	Hormonal Therapy	NA	Not Assessed
I	Immunotherapy	NE	Not Evaluable
A	Alternative Therapy	PD	Progressive Disease
O	Other	PR	Partial Response
R	Radiation	SD	Stable Disease
S	Surgery	TE	Too Early
B	Bone Marrow Transplant		

_____ (check here) IF NO PRIOR THERAPY

Type	Start	Stop	Agent	Alternative Therapy	Schedule	Dose	Site	Response
*1.	MM/DD/YYYY	MM/DD/YYYY						*2.
C	04/15/1996	10/15/1996	Cyclophosphamide					PR

Additional Form Instructions

*1.	Type: Include only the "Type" codes listed at the top of this form
*2.	Response: Use only "Response" codes listed at the top of this form
3.	Make all entries in ink
4.	record dates in mm/dd/yyyy format

Signature/Date:

FIGURE 21.2-1. Sample case report form: prior therapy.

to the study conduct. Study end points must be defined with specificity and then decomposed to yield the components needing collection on a defined schedule. Element definitions and coding conventions must be recorded consistently across the protocol, to ensure that outcomes can be replicated and results generalized and to attest to the proper conduct of the protocol. Data harmonization and standardization should be reflected in data validation approaches that focus on the interpretation of results across single or multiple protocols. The use of a data dictionary or inventory of well-defined data elements could help to impose standards critical for study outcomes.

Whether in paper or electronic form, data collection instruments combined with quality control offer an integrated approach to the capture and entry of clinical research data.

QUALITY CONTROL

GCPs are codes, regulations, and guidelines that supply structure and requirements to the clinical research process. Scientific questions and data that must be collected add the direction and level of detail required for personnel to conduct clinical research. International standards have emerged from the International Conference on Harmonisation, a union of the United States, the European Union, and Japan. This group has formulated global standards for the conduct of clinical research[7] that have been adopted by many industry and academic groups worldwide.

The International Conference on Harmonisation defines a GCP as "A standard for the design, performance, monitoring, auditing, recording, analyses, and reporting of clinical trials to provide assurance that the data and reported results are credible and accurate."[15] Study performance, monitoring, and auditing are components of quality control activities pivotal to the conduct of clinical research. Long impugned as undesirable or even noncontributing measures of research integrity, quality control topics have found new disciples in an environment sensitized to the disasters that can occur when they are missing.

Quality control activities merit a plan for each level of personnel to handle clinical research data according to guidelines. Clinical data systems and processes have the potential to improve the quality and costs of research by influencing medical decisions at the point they are being made.[16] Quality control processes must be integrated into daily work assignments, not approached as an additional requirement. This approach views quality control within an organizational philosophy, a continuum of events resulting in process improvement and the professional development of personnel.

MONITORING AND AUDITS

Monitoring and audit activities fit the traditional profile of quality assurance activities. Whether it is the submission of current data or the retrospective audit of source documents and forms, these activities reflect an ongoing process and the expectation of never reaching perfect compliance. Monitoring activities reflect the scientific and administrative rigor an organization imposes on itself to measure the quality of its research programs.

Monitoring is a primary means of quality control for clinical research studies. It is an activity performed by the study monitor of a clinical research organization with the formal responsibility of monitoring the conduct of research trials. Monitoring visits can focus on a variety of protocol-centered elements. Data can be inspected for their completeness and comparison to expected values. Values that fall outside the range of acceptance as well as missing values will generate data clarification forms for the submitting organization. The creation of clarifications or data discrepancy reports and the resolution of clarifications with resultant resubmission of corrected and validated data back to the monitoring agency creates a continual loop for process improvement at the organizational level. Monitoring activities can focus on protocol administrative and regulatory aspects, the availability and completeness of standard operating procedures, institutional and regulatory approvals and reviews, and adverse-event reporting or can even compare electronic data entry screens to reports submitted by the institution.[17]

An audit is one means of quality assurance, to assess the quality of the research process, and must be conducted by personnel independent of a clinical trial.[17] While the terms *audit* and *monitoring* often are used interchangeably, most literature conveys the relationship to be many audits or auditing activities within the realm of a monitoring plan.

ANALYSIS AND PUBLICATION

Data management tasks associated with analysis and publication in the life cycle are centered on data retrieval. An investigator or clinical research team will have predetermined and preformatted views or reports that they use to examine data, producing validated views of the data as important data management tasks. More flexible queries or simple graphic plots may be required. Report creation on an *ad hoc*, as-needed basis is a common requirement. However, producing reports and views of the research data does not in any way replace the efforts of appropriate biostatistical support and analysis. One of the primary data management tasks for this step may be simply exporting clean, validated data in a format requested by the biostatistician.

INFORMATION TECHNOLOGY

The information technology architecture required to support clinical trials will depend on the research portfolio and the number of studies and centers involved. Supporting a single study can be accomplished using commercially available office automation software, such as desktop database applications or spreadsheets. There are also applications specifically for management of clinical trials well suited for a single trial or a small study portfolio. More common is the clinical trial portfolio of multiple studies coordinated through a cooperative group or a cancer center. In this case, the burden of managing multiple studies and patients at multiple centers increases the challenges, both administratively and from the clinical data collection and management perspectives. Data management tools available over a Web browser can assist the coordination of multicenter trials.

Information technology is the key to producing better information faster and to finding the answers to research questions more rapidly. If we step away from the view of data management as one step in a process and toward the protocol life cycle model, information technology can be more broadly applied and important to the success of the studies.

BASIC CONCEPTS

To the extent possible, software applications for clinical research should support work processes, not dictate the process. They should provide study-specific display and collection of information. To support ease of use as well as enforce security, research data management systems should render information and functions based on the role of the user. For example, a registered system user would see only the functions appropriate for a role (e.g., data collection, accrual monitoring, audit, report generation). This role should allow access to only those protocols and patients for which there is an appropriate need to know. Rules-based validation must be technologically supported. As studies are conducted in large or multiple institutions, remote data entry can speed data collection and assimilation. This is increasingly being accomplished via Internet-based technologies.

INTERNET TECHNOLOGIES

Web-based data collection and management for single and multicenter trials is being increasingly used.[14,18] This approach supports the collection and display of complex medical information unconstrained by geographic location. Additionally, it permits display of complex medical information textually or graphically, managed from a central database.[19] Since it can operate from any site that has an Internet connection and a Web browser, it may be the best answer for large randomized multicenter trial data collection and administration. It can be platform-independent and stores system logic and data centrally.[20] Given the match of flexible and almost universally available Internet technology with the requirement for collecting data from multiple sites, use of Web technology will continue to increase exponentially in the next few years. Lowe[14] describes this as a paradigm shift in medicine toward Internet-based solutions for information management. "Perhaps the two most important applications to emerge in the next decade will be Internet-based clinical trials (in which patients and researchers, though geographically distributed, will be linked via secure Internet-based data collection, review and reporting systems) and the Internet-based multimedia electronic medical record."[14]

DATA CLASSIFICATION

As information is collected from multiple studies, sites, investigators, and the like, the issues of data standards and data classification become more important. If data are to be collected or aggregated across multiple patients at different centers or multiple studies over time, concepts and terms must be expressed with as little ambiguity as possible. While there is still no consensus on national or international standards for medical vocabularies, there are some dominant candidates to consider, depending on the medical concept being described.[21] One example is the NCI Cancer Therapy Evaluation Program's adverse event reporting requirement, which uses Common Toxicity Criteria (CTC) and the Medical Dictionary for Regulatory Activities (MedDRA). Classification of diagnoses, procedures, morphology, and medications are areas in which fairly mature internationally or commercially maintained vocabularies exist.

Realizing that there is much change occurring in classification of medical terminology, there is no guarantee that a standard used today will be the universally accepted standard tomorrow. However, implementation of a current classification standard is highly recommended over using a home-grown standard or no standard at all. Using an existing standard brings a high likelihood that it will be accounted for should a master thesaurus, such as the Unified Medical Language System, become the standard. Whichever particular scheme is used for data classification on one or a group of studies, adherence to the chosen classifications, enforced by a system data dictionary, will ensure consistent use.

U.S. FOOD AND DRUG ADMINISTRATION RECOMMENDATIONS

The FDA has adopted guidelines for clinical trial computer systems that report data to that agency.[5] While only guidelines, they are a benchmark against which data management systems can be measured. Areas to underscore include a recommendation that standard operating procedures be established for system setup, system maintenance, data collection, data backup and recovery, and data security. Systems should use electronic signatures to verify that persons entering, viewing, or updating data are authorized to do so. This also ensures attribution so that data entered under electronic signature can be tracked back to the person entering or updating the data.

Audit trails allow recreation of the data history.[5] By viewing the audit trail, a user can determine what was recorded at any point in time and who changed the data.

DATA VALIDATION

Systems should provide validation logic to be applied to data at time of entry or in batch edit, a process that records data that fail built-in validation rules. Validation can be simple range checking or algorithms that alert users when certain conditions are present. One example of this is the application of the NCI Common Toxicity Criteria; the software prompts the user to file an adverse event report based on a laboratory value falling sufficiently out of range. Data corrections or other actions taken at time of entry are enforced in real time, but this may or may not be desirable. If the person entering data does not have the expertise or documentation to answer computer-driven queries, a preferred process would be to record queries centrally and ensure that they be addressed later (i.e., batch edit). Several types of validation can be easily applied in a computer-based system. These include detection of missing data, data artifacts (outside the usual range), data that contradict other data, and data trends (conflicting data from one encounter to the next).[2]

Validation checks for the presence of data in these fields should be displayed to personnel using clear instructions. When using electronic CRFs, data that fail validation attempts should generate a message in natural language that will identify delinquent items.

Simple edit checks can verify that text fields are not filled with numbers or dates, that future dates are detected, and that values fall within specified acceptable ranges. Because it is difficult to apply edit check logic to free text, responses translated into coding lists can help in the application of edit check rules.

Cross-checks can be used in the context of relationships between data points. The value in one field may constrain the entry of a value in another field, so that the content of these fields can be compared. There can also be cross-validation between variables expected to correlate. For example, if the response to "Prior Chemotherapy?" is yes, the CRF may require that details of a chemotherapy treatment regimen be entered on the CRF. Other cross-validation would occur between variables measured on repeated occasions (e.g., lesion measurements on repeated cycle visits) and other context-specific checks.

Double data entry is another form of validation used to minimize data entry. However, double entry procedures may not be sufficient or even necessary for the production of high-quality clinical research data. Day et al.[10] used exploratory data analysis techniques on simulated clinical data measurements and found that while the double entry approach does detect some errors, many others occur during the transcription process that are not detectable by double entry processes. The use of systems with computerized CRFs to enter data directly from source documents also lessens the benefit of a double entry approach. While the double data entry practice may offer some benefit, other methods to validate data integrity and validity should be mandatory.

DIRECT DATA CAPTURE

Electronic transfer of data from hospital laboratory or other systems into the research data management system is known as *direct data capture.* When direct data capture is used, it can result in higher-quality data through reduction of the errors produced when data are rekeyed. Where this model is used, the data management system must be able to indicate whether and where data have been changed after import.[5]

SECURITY

Data management systems should control security at the physical and logical levels. *Physical security* applies to controlling and safeguarding the physical computer resources and data storage, enforced via off-site storage of backup data and fire walls that prevent unauthorized access to data and computing resources. *Logical access* refers to those persons who have access to data through the assignment of system-based roles.[5] Spriet and Dupen-Spriet[2] described required security as (1) operational (proper maintenance, virus protection, and proper use); (2) physical (protection against physical harm by fire, water damage, and the like and safeguarding backup data); and (3) malice (protection against theft, piracy, or sabotage).[2]

SUMMARY

Each step of the clinical trial life cycle creates distinct data management tasks and processes specified during protocol development. Supporting these tasks can be accomplished with manual (paper-based) processes, completely automated with computer systems, or through some combination of both. The model chosen at the organizational level will depend on principles of good clinical practice and quality control need. The acceptance and use of Internet systems is increasing the acceptance of computer systems as data management facilitators. The product of clinical research is data, and proper data management can help to turn the data into information.

REFERENCES

1. Simon RM. Clinical trials in cancer. In DeVita VT, Hellman S, Rosenberg S, eds. *Cancer: principles and practices of oncology,* 5th ed. Philadelphia: Lippincott-Raven Publishers, 1997:513.
2. Spriet A, Dupen-Spriet T. *Good practice of clinical drug trials.* Farmington, CT: Karger, 1997.
3. Silva JS. Fighting cancer in the information age. An architecture for national scale clinical trials. *MD Comput* 1999;16(3):43.
4. Friedman LM, Furberg CD, DeMets DL. *Fundamentals of clinical trials.* New York: Springer-Verlag, 1998.
5. Food and Drug Administration. *Guidance for industry, computerized systems used in clinical trials.* April 1999.
6. Knatterud GL, Rockhold FW, George SL, et al. Guidelines for quality assurance on multicenter clinical trials: a position paper. *Control Clin Trials* 1998;19:477.
7. International Conference on Harmonisation. Good clinical practice: consolidated guideline. *Fed Reg* 1997;62(90):1.24.
8. Rotmensz N, ed. *Data management and clinical trials. EORTC Study Group on Data Management.* Amsterdam: Elsevier Science, 1989.
9. FitzHenry F, Snyder J. Improving organizational processes for gains during implementation. *Comput Nurs* 1996;14(3):171.
10. Day S, Fayers P, Harvey D. Double data entry: what value, what price? *Control Clin Trials* 1998;19:15.
11. Hammer M, Champy J. *Reengineering the corporation.* New York: HarperCollins, 1993.
12. Vogel R. Remote data capture. *Appl Clin Trials* 1997;6(5):36.
13. Bartruff B. Issues in clinical trials management: I. Clean data: the mark of excellence. *Res Nurs* 1999;5(2):12.
14. Lowe HJ. Transforming the cancer center in the 21st century. *MD Comput* 1999;16(3):40.
15. Hawkins K. Defining good clinical practice. *Res Nurs* 1999;5:(5):1.
16. Classen D. Clinical decision support systems to improve clinical practice and quality of care. *JAMA* 1998;280:1360.
17. Bohaychuk W, Ball G. *Conducting GCP-compliant clinical research.* New York: John Wiley and Sons, 1999.
18. Santoro E, Nicolis E, Franzosi MG, Tognoni G. Internet for clinical trials: past, present, and future. *Control Clin Trials* 1999;19:194.
19. Vissers MC, Hasman A, Stapert JW. Presenting treatment protocols with Web technology. *Med Inf* 1998;9(1):521.
20. Sippel H, Ohmann C. A Web-based data collection system for clinical studies using Java. *Med Inf* 1998;23(3):223.
21. Degoulet P, Fieschi M. *Introduction to clinical informatics.* New York: Springer-Verlag, 1997.

PART 3

PRACTICE OF ONCOLOGY

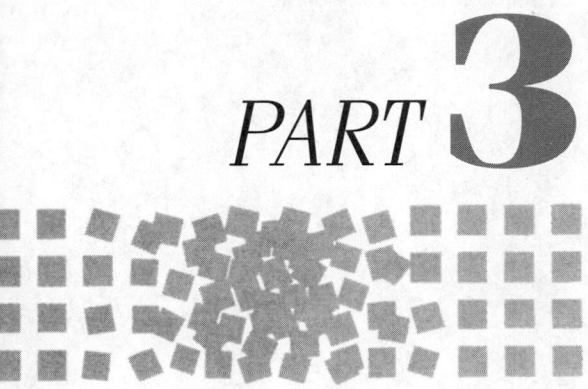

Howard K. Koh
Christine Kannler
Alan C. Geller

CHAPTER **22**

Cancer Prevention: Preventing Tobacco-Related Cancers

Tobacco addiction ranks as the greatest public health catastrophe of our time. The practice of inhaling cigarette smoke, which gained widespread acceptance only during the twentieth century, has generated devastating cancer outcomes for our society. Specifically, lung cancer, previously rare, has risen to become the leading cancer killer in American men and women.[1,2] Worldwide estimates suggest that the annual deaths attributable to smoking, currently 2.5 million, will rise to 12 million by the year 2050.[3–5] Future medical historians undoubtedly will recall the 1900s as the Tobacco and Cancer Century.[2]

A healthier twenty-first century requires a societal commitment to reducing and eradicating tobacco addiction. This chapter reviews the impact of tobacco on cancer and individual and societal strategies for tobacco control.

TOBACCO AND NICOTINE ADDICTION

Tobacco and tobacco smoke contain at least 4000 chemicals, of which 55 are known carcinogens identified by the International Agency for Research on Cancer.[6] The most notable carcinogen classes include polycyclic aromatic hydrocarbons (PAHs), N-nitrosamines, and miscellaneous organic compounds. Of the PAHs, benzo(a)pyrene (BaP) is the most extensively studied lung carcinogen. Of the N-nitrosamines, 4-(methylnitrosamino)-1-(3-pyridyl)-1-butanone (NNK) is best known. Metabolic activation of these agents can incite DNA adduct formation, gene mutations, and a sequence of events that can lead to cancer. The balance between detoxification and metabolic activation determines, in part, the susceptibility of smokers to cancer.[6]

Though nicotine in tobacco is itself not carcinogenic, addiction to nicotine exposes the user to carcinogens, which increases the likelihood of cancer. Nicotine addiction fulfills the physiologic, behavioral, and social characteristics of a dependence syndrome.[7] The American Psychiatric Association's *Diagnostic and Statistical Manual of Mental Disorders* (*DSM*, third edition) requires a minimum of three of seven diagnostic symptoms for drug dependency: (1) tolerance, (2) withdrawal, (3) greater use than intended, (4) persistent desire to quit, (5) great amounts of time spent smoking, (6) activities given up or reduced due to smoking, and (7) continued smoking despite knowledge of having persistent physical or psychological problems with the substance.[7] The 1988 Surgeon General's report focused on the concept of nicotine addiction and its clinical ability to produce brief, pleasurable psychoactive effects; its continued use despite known adverse health outcomes; development of tolerance during early usage; and occurrence of withdrawal symptoms on cessation of use.[8] Withdrawal symptoms include nervousness, restlessness, anxiety, impaired cognition, headache, drowsiness, gastrointestinal disturbances, nicotine cravings, increased appetite and weight gain, and anxiety.[7–9]

Opinions expressed are those of the authors and do not represent the opinions of the Massachusetts Department of Public Health.

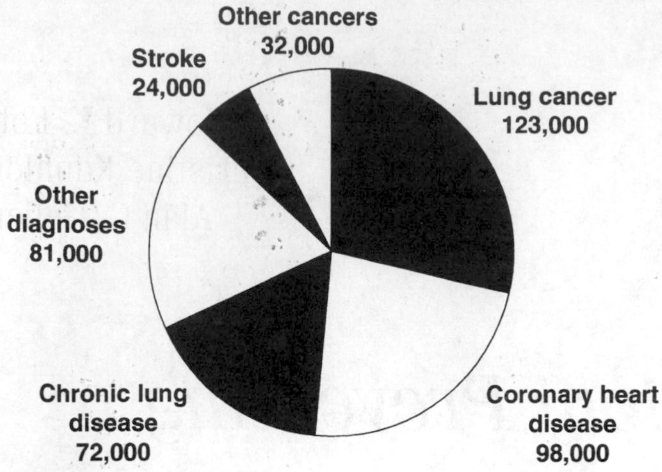

FIGURE 22-1. 430,000 U.S. deaths are attributable each year to cigarette smoking.

HEALTH EFFECTS

As early as 1928, Lombard and Doering[10] reported higher smoking rates among patients with cancer than among controls. Later, the pioneering epidemiologic work of Doll and Hill,[11] Wynder and Graham,[12] and Hammond and Horn[13] led to further investigations, which culminated in the 1964 U.S. Surgeon General's report on smoking and health.[14] This report concluded that cigarette smoking was the major cause of lung cancer in men and was causally related to laryngeal cancer and oral cancer in men.[14]

In total, more than 60,000 studies and two dozen additional reports of the Surgeon General have confirmed the devastating impact of tobacco use on human health. Tobacco use, causing approximately 30% of all deaths and more than 400,000 deaths annually, is the leading cause of preventable death in this country (Fig. 22-1).[1,15,16] Tobacco use kills more Americans each year than do alcohol, cocaine, crack, heroin, homicide, suicide, car accidents, firearms, and the acquired immunodeficiency syndrome (AIDS) combined.[17]

Smoking causes more than 85% to 90% of lung cancers, with a clear dose-response relationship between risk and daily cigarette consumption.[18] People who smoke more than a pack of cigarettes per day have a risk that is as much as 20 times that of nonsmokers.[18] In smokers exposed to other carcinogens in the workplace (e.g., pipefitters exposed to asbestos; uranium workers exposed to radon), the risk for lung cancer is raised in a synergistic fashion.[19–22]

Lung cancer is the leading cause of cancer mortality in both men and women. U.S. estimates for 2000 include approximately 157,000 lung cancer deaths. Lung cancer incidence rates vary widely by race and ethnicity, from a high of 73.9 per 100,000 in African Americans to a low of 27.6 among Hispanics.[1] Gender differences exist as well. Male lung cancer incidence rates peaked in 1984 (86.5 per 100,000) and have decreased since then. Similarly, male lung cancer mortality rates peaked in 1990 at 75.2 per 100,000.[1] In contrast, female lung cancer incidence and mortality continue to rise. Of note, in the late 1980s, lung cancer surpassed breast cancer as the leading cause of cancer death among U.S. women.[1] The histologic profile of lung cancer has shifted, with declining rates of squamous cell carcinoma but increasing rates of adenocarcinoma.[23]

In addition, smoking is accepted as the major cause of cancers of the larynx, pharynx, oral cavity, and esophagus, and is a contributory factor in cancers of the pancreas, bladder, kidney, stomach, colon, and uterine cervix and in acute leukemia.[24,25] A synergistic, multiplicative effect appears to exist between smoking and drinking.[26] For example, the risk for developing cancer of the larynx is as much as 75% higher in people who use tobacco and alcohol as compared with people using either substance alone.[24,26]

The use of pipes, cigars, and spit tobacco in its various forms (plug tobacco, loose-leaf tobacco, twist tobacco, and moist snuff) also causes cancers of the oral cavity.[18,24–28] Tobacco use is responsible for more than 90% of tumors of the oral cavity among men and 60% among women.[27] Spit tobacco is a significant cause of leukoplakia,[27–30] an abnormal thickening and keratinization of the oral mucosa that is recognized as a precursor of malignancy. Even after cessation of tobacco exposure, the "field cancerization effect" elevates the risk of cancer of the entire epithelium of the upper aerodigestive tract for years.[31]

Other adverse health outcomes from tobacco addiction include increased risks of cardiovascular disease.[32–34] The Nurses' Health Study found a 2.5-fold increased risk of fatal coronary heart disease and nonfatal myocardial infarction and up to three times the risk of cerebrovascular disease in smokers as compared to nonsmokers. Smoking also contributes to peripheral vascular disease, aortic aneurysm, impotence, Buerger's disease (thromboangiitis obliterans), and skin aging.[32–34]

Americans spend an estimated $50 billion annually on direct medical care for smoking-related illnesses.[35] Lost productivity and forfeited earnings due to smoking-related disability account for another $47 billion per year.[36]

SMOKING RATES AND TRENDS

With the vigorous promotion of the blended cigarette in the twentieth century, the annual adult per capita consumption of cigarettes has skyrocketed from 54 cigarettes in 1900 to 4345 cigarettes in 1963, the peak of American consumption per individual smoker.[35] Although consumption has declined, approximately 500 billion cigarettes were sold in the United States in 1995.[6] Historically, smoking rates in men have far exceeded those in women, but the gender difference has narrowed as male rates declined and female rates rose.[1,35] Rates for most races and ethnic groups have decreased since 1978, although the rate of decrease recently has ebbed (Fig. 22-2).[37] The tobacco industry's attempts to recruit women range from the American Tobacco Company's advertising campaign, "To keep a slender figure, reach for a Lucky Strike instead of a sweet" (1920s) to Philip Morris's Virginia Slims slogan, "You've come a long way, baby."[38]

ADULTS

Approximately 1 billion smokers are found worldwide.[39] According to the 1995 National Health Interview Study, in the United States, nearly 47 million adults (24.7%) currently smoke, either daily (20.1%) or on some days (4.6%).[37] Currently, men (27.0%) are more likely to smoke than are women (22.6%). Among racial and ethnic groups, American Indians and Alaskan natives had the highest prevalence (36.2%), whereas Asian Americans

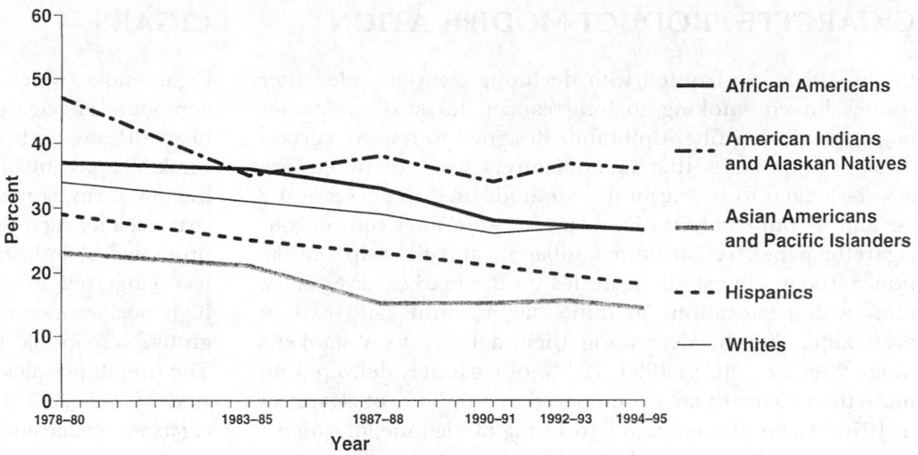

FIGURE 22-2. Current cigarette smoking among adults, National Health Interview Surveys, United States 1978–1995 aggregate data.

and Pacific Islanders had the lowest (16.6%).[37] Educational level is the most important predictor of smoking prevalence.[9] High school dropouts had the highest prevalence (41.9% and 33.7% for men and women, respectively), whereas college graduates had the lowest (14.3% and 13.7%, respectively).[37]

Since the landmark 1964 Surgeon General's report, overall U.S. smoking prevalence has declined by half, from 50.2% (1965) to 25% (1998), although adult smoking rates reached a plateau in the 1990s.[1] Declines in smoking prevalence were greater among African American, Hispanic, and white men who were high school graduates than among those with less education.[1] In fact, in the United States during 1965 through 1994, smoking prevalence in adults younger than 65 years declined in every demographic category except those with less than 12 years of education.[7]

CHILDREN, ADOLESCENTS, AND COLLEGE STUDENTS

Tobacco use qualifies as a pediatric disease.[40] Its current prevalence among adolescents (cigarettes, cigars, or smokeless tobacco) is an astonishing 42.7%.[1,41] The 1997 Youth Risk Behavior Survey showed smoking rates for girls and boys as 69.3% and 70.9% for lifetime cigarette use and 34.7% and 37.7% for current cigarette use.[41] Nearly 90% of adult smokers begin smoking by the age of 18 years. Even by grade 9, 67% of children have experimented with cigarettes.[41] It is estimated that of nearly 3000 young people who start smoking each day, 1 in 3 will die prematurely.[42,43] At least 3 million American teenagers smoke regularly.[9]

Numerous surveys document increased smoking among children and adolescents in recent years.[41] The national 1997 Youth Risk Behavior Survey indicated that cigarette smoking prevalence among U.S. high school students increased from 27.5% in 1991 to 36.4% in 1997.[41] This rise occurred in all racial and ethnic groups [e.g., whites (30.9% to 39.7%), African Americans (12.6% to 22.7%), and Hispanics (25.3% to 34.0%)]. In 1997, the prevalence of current cigar use was 22.0%. Monitoring the Future Project data (an analysis of high school seniors from 1976 to 1995) show that the smoking rate among high school seniors (defined as smoking in the past 30 days) rose from 28.3% in 1991 to 34% in 1996, and rates for grades 8 and 10 show similar or larger increases.[43]

Notably, the age of smoking initiation has declined over the past four decades, for both whites (by 2.4 years) and African Americans (by 1 to 3 years). The decline is particularly striking for girls (5.4 years and 4.6 years for whites and African Americans, respectively).[9] Also, half of the nation's 6 million smokeless tobacco users were younger than 21 years, and several national surveys show an increase in prevalence, especially among boys.[9]

Predictors of future tobacco use include a number of behavioral risk factors.[42–48] These factors include the child's own certainty about smoking or not smoking in the future, low self-image, poor academic career, receptivity to tobacco advertising, peer pressure, and the use of promotional items.[42–49] Individual personality traits such as risk taking and deviant behaviors and perceptions of maturity, attractiveness, and independence also play a role in a child's susceptibility to tobacco use. In white youngsters, peer pressure (estimated by the number of friends who smoke) and a low grade point average were important risk factors. Among African Americans, a greater risk-taking attitude was an important predictor of tobacco use.[48] Acculturation or integration into American society is associated with increased smoking by Latin and Asian women.[48]

Tobacco use in children is linked to alcohol and illegal drug use.[44,45] Among boys especially, aggressive or disruptive classroom behavior as early as first grade has been found to predict later tobacco and other heavy drug use, as well as antisocial behavior and criminality.[44] The National Household Study on Drug Abuse from 1985 showed children who smoke are 3 times more likely to drink alcohol, 8 times more likely to smoke marijuana, and 22 times more likely to use cocaine.[48] Children's tobacco and alcohol use also were associated with less effective parenting behaviors in the children's families and with parental use of tobacco and alcohol.[45]

Newer data point to increasing smoking rates among college students.[50] In serial surveys of nearly 15,000 randomly selected college students, Wechsler et al.[50] found that the prevalence of current cigarette smoking rose by 27.8% (from 22.3% to 28.5% during the period 1993 through 1997). Defying earlier trends, 11% of college smokers had their first cigarette and 28% began to smoke regularly at or after age 19 years. Half of current college smokers tried to quit in the previous year; 18% had made five or more attempts to quit.[50]

CIGARETTE PRODUCT MODIFICATION

In the 1950s, confronted with declining cigarette sales after studies linked smoking to lung cancer, tobacco companies began producing filter-tip brands designed to remove certain smoke components that manufacturers had not heretofore acknowledged to be harmful.[51] Methods used to decrease the tar and nicotine content in cigarettes were filter tips, porous cigarette paper, reconstituted tobacco, and filter-tip ventilation.[52] Today, almost all cigarettes on the market have filters, most with perforations to dilute tar, nicotine, and carbon monoxide, thereby decreasing their delivery to a smoker's lungs.[53] As a result, in 1995, 72.7% of cigarettes delivered no more than 15 mg of tar, as compared to only 3.6% of cigarettes in 1970.[1] Cigarettes contain 6 to 11 mg of nicotine, of which a smoker typically absorbs 1 to 3 mg, irrespective of nicotine yield ratings. To satisfy the level of nicotine needed, smokers modified their smoking behavior by inhaling more deeply and blocking filter vents with their fingers or lips to increase nicotine yield. These behaviors now are suspected to be linked to rising rates of adenocarcinoma of the lung, which currently is the most common type of lung cancer in the United States.[23] Nevertheless, the tobacco industry has continued to suggest health benefits to consumers through the creation and promotion of "light," "ultralight," "mild," "medium," "slim," and "superslim" cigarettes.[25]

SPIT TOBACCO

Spit tobacco (smokeless tobacco), available as snuff or chewing tobacco, has gained great popularity over the last few decades.[54–58] Snuff dipping, the practice of sucking on a pinch of powdered, flavored tobacco in the cavity between gum and cheek, has increased. Consumption of snuff products nearly tripled between 1972 and 1991.[56] The 1997 Youth Risk Behavior Survey documented a 9.3% prevalence of current spit tobacco use among high school students, with 21% of boys ages 11 to 19 defined as experimenters.[57] The consumption of chewing tobacco, which involves a "chaw" held in the inner cheek area, has also increased.[56,58]

Use of both snuff and chewing tobacco requires continual expectoration—hence the term *spit tobacco*.[55] Manufacturers prefer the term *smokeless tobacco,* to imply a safe alternative to smoking. However, the nicotine in snuff is 2 times the dose in cigarettes, whereas the nicotine in chewing tobacco is 15 times that found in cigarettes.[58] Users tend to be white male adolescents aged 18 to 24 years, persons of low socioeconomic status, current cigarette smokers, residents of the southern United States, baseball players, and American Indians.[57]

Spit tobacco can accelerate a litany of destructive oral changes, from local nonmalignant effects (gingival recession, loss of periodontal attachments, periodontal bone and soft tissue destruction, halitosis, tooth staining, tooth abrasion) to leukoplakia and frank oral cancer. Leukoplakia typically occurs on the cheek mucosa, alveolar ridge, and gingiva, where the snuff is placed. In contrast, tobacco chewers tend to have bilateral lesions of leukoplakia, which is associated with a 3% to 6% progression to squamous cell carcinoma.[58]

CIGARS

Cigar smoke, which contains the same carcinogenic and toxic compounds as cigarettes, also increases risk of cancer, coronary heart disease, and pulmonary pathologic processes.[8,59–61] Cigar smoking is potentially addicting and is associated with cancers of the oral cavity, larynx, esophagus, and lung.[8,59,61] Reversing a 20-year decline, cigar sales increased by 50% from 1993 to 1997,[61] prompted by industry marketing and the belief that cigars are less dangerous than cigarettes. Young to middle-aged men of high socioeconomic status, teenagers, and women are the groups responsible for the increased consumption of cigars.[60] The overall prevalence of current cigar use among high school students was 22% in 1997. Teenagers most at risk of smoking cigars were male and those students who smoke cigarettes.[60]

ENVIRONMENTAL TOBACCO SMOKE

The 1986 U.S. Surgeon General's report defined *environmental tobacco smoke* (ETS), also called *secondhand smoke,* as the combination of sidestream smoke (released from a burning cigarette between puffs) and the fraction of mainstream smoke exhaled by the smoker.[62] The more hazardous sidestream smoke has double the amount of nicotine than mainstream smoke and a higher concentration of carcinogens.[62] Most people spend 90% of their time in the two microenvironments of home and work, where ETS exposure usually occurs.[63] Those at greatest risk for harm from ETS are those who live with smokers in homes where smoking is allowed. Levels of serum cotinine, a nicotine metabolite, are increased in nonsmokers who live with smokers and are correlated to the number of cigarettes smoked.[64]

An increasing number of studies have documented the health risks of the nonsmoker exposed to ETS.[62–68] Case-control studies first noted that nonsmoking wives of smoking husbands had increased risk of lung cancer.[64] In 1992, the U.S. Environmental Protection Agency (EPA), in the most thoroughly documented analysis ever undertaken of the effects of exposure to ETS, concluded that secondhand smoke can cause lung cancer in nonsmoking adults and can impair the respiratory systems of children. The EPA classified ETS as a group A carcinogen, a designation reserved for agents such as asbestos. Of 30 studies analyzed in the EPA report, 24 found an increased risk of lung cancer for nonsmoking wives of husbands who smoked, and each of the 17 studies that examined risk based on exposure level reported increased lung cancer among those most exposed.[67]

The EPA report and other ETS studies now attribute approximately 3000 deaths to lung cancer, up to 62,000 deaths to ischemic heart disease, and up to 2700 deaths to sudden infant death syndrome.[67] The 1997 California Environmental Protection Agency Report also notes that ETS is responsible for new cases of low-birth-weight infants (up to 18,600 cases per year), new cases of childhood asthma (up to 26,000 new cases per year), exacerbation of childhood asthma (up to 1 million new cases per year), and bronchitis or pneumonia in children aged 18 months and younger (up to 300,000 cases per year). Workers at great risk for harm from ETS include flight attendants, casino workers, and restaurant and bar workers, among others.[68]

TOBACCO INDUSTRY ADVERTISING STRATEGIES

Tobacco companies have dedicated considerable resources to corner new markets, because an estimated 3500 Americans quit smoking and an additional 1200 customers die of smoking-related illness each day. During the last two decades, the tobacco industry has nearly quadrupled its marketing expenditures (Fig. 22-3).[69,70] The 1994 U.S. Surgeon General's report, "Preventing Tobacco Use Among Young People," summarized the research on the impact of tobacco advertising and promotional activities on youth[71]:

- Young people constitute a highly strategic market for the tobacco industry.
- Young people are continuously exposed to cigarette messages through print media and promotional activities.
- Cigarette advertising uses images, not information, to portray the attractiveness of smoking.
- Cigarette advertisements capitalize on the disparity between an ideal and actual self-image, implying that smoking may close the gap.
- Cigarette advertising appears to affect young people's perceptions of the pervasiveness, image, and function of smoking. Such misperceptions increase young people's risk of smoking.

Most adolescents now experiment with tobacco almost as a rite of passage and have high recollection of tobacco industry promotional messages. Nearly 70% of children aged 13 reported at least moderate receptivity to marketing materials, indicating susceptibility.[72] Adolescents and youth are susceptible to image advertising and promotional themes as they seek to find their own identities.[49] One study found 6-year-old children were as likely to identify Joe Camel as they were Mickey Mouse.[73]

In addition, adolescents smoke the most heavily advertised brands.[49] Pierce et al.[49] provided the first longitudinal evidence that tobacco promotional activities are causally related to the onset of smoking. A total of 1752 adolescents who had never smoked and who were not susceptible to smoking when first interviewed in 1993 were reinterviewed in 1996. Nearly 50% progressed toward smoking, by becoming susceptible, by experimenting, or by consuming at least 100 cigarettes. The authors attributed 34% of all adolescent tobacco experimentation in California from 1993 through 1996 to industry promotional activities.[49]

Tobacco marketing strategies include magazine and newspaper advertising, outdoor advertising, sponsorship of sporting events and public entertainment, and distribution of free samples of cigarettes in public places. Promotions and specialty items include mailings and giveaways of multiple packs (buy one, get one free) and coupon reductions for attractive specialty items (such as T-shirts, caps, calendars, and sporting goods).[9,42,74] Surveys have found that half of all adolescent smokers and one-fourth of adolescent nonsmokers owned at least one tobacco promotional item.[42] Tobacco companies also pay retailers for shelf space and engage them to promote point-of-sale advertising, a technique that places the tobacco products in convenient visible (usually self-service) racks and in point-of-purchase displays.[9,42]

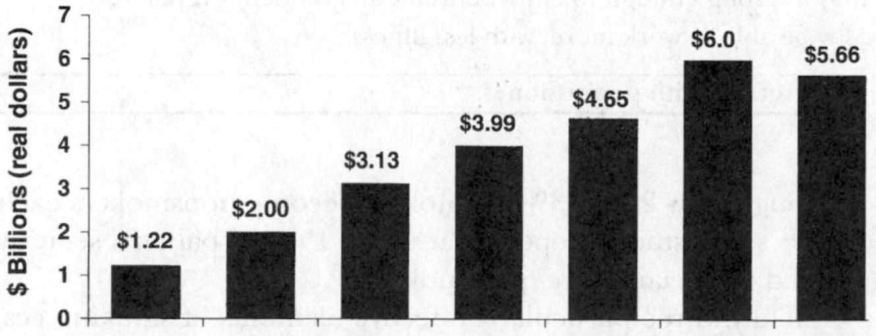

FIGURE 22-3. Cigarette advertising and promotion expenditures in the United States have more than quadrupled in 22 years.

One of the first studies to examine systematically the relationship between cigarette brand–specific advertising and youth readership found that youth brands were more likely than adult brands to be advertised in magazines having a higher percentage of young readers (ages 12 to 17 years). The authors recommended that cigarette advertising in all youth magazines be eliminated.[75]

The tobacco industry also uses its considerable financial and legal resources to influence local and national policy.[35,76–78] Industry magnates frame the increasing public debate about smoking regulations around rights and liberty rather than health, portray adversaries as extremists, and invest millions of dollars in campaign contributions to the leading political parties.[35,76–79] They successfully solicit allies (including advertisers, civil libertarians, and restaurant owners) to help lobby or advance arguments that oppose regulation.[77]

The tobacco industry has generally escaped strong government legislation. Federal legislation, including the Controlled Substances Act (1970), Consumer Product Safety Act (1972), and Toxic Substances Control Act (1976) all exclude tobacco from regulation.[78] The landmark 1965 Federal Cigarette Labeling and Advertising Act, the first federal statute enacting labeling requirements for cigarette packages, contained a federal preemption clause preventing individual states from making laws to regulate tobacco advertising.[78]

STRATEGIES FOR TOBACCO CONTROL

For decades, the concept of tobacco control focused solely on cessation strategies for individual smokers. More recently, the emphasis has broadened to encompass prevention strategies that stress denormalization of tobacco use for the entire community. Hence, key dimensions now include individual approaches that expand the role of the clinician in smoking cessation services, which include pharmacologic cessation therapies; community and state interventions; policy strategies; tobacco taxes that fund comprehensive statewide tobacco control programs; mass media and counter-advertising; and tobacco litigation and the tobacco settlement.[78]

INDIVIDUAL APPROACHES

Each year, approximately 20 million (of the 50 million smokers in the United States) try to quit smoking.[79–81] In addition, 77% of smokers would like to quit, and 65% have made at least one serious attempt at quitting. Yet, studies indicate that one-third relapse after 24 hours and another third relapse after 48 hours.[79–81] Of all smokers that attempt to quit each year, fewer than 10% are successful. Cigarette smokers who have successfully quit made, on average, seven serious attempts before achieving abstinence.[79–81]

Even young smokers want to quit.[42,82,83] The 1989 and 1993 Teenage Attitudes and Practice Surveys did show that nearly 75% of 12- to 18-year-olds had seriously thought about quitting smoking; more recent surveys found that 73% of young smokers had tried to quit smoking.[42,82,83]

Smoking cessation restores a chance of living a full, healthy life.[84] Quitting smoking reduces the risk of lung cancer by 50% at 5 years, and by 10 years, lung cancer risk drops almost to the rate for nonsmokers.[35] After a year, mortality from heart disease decreases by half, and by 5 years it equals the rate for nonsmokers.

CLINICIANS' ROLE

Physicians and health professionals should view smoking cessation as a cornerstone of their practice.[85] Providing a brief physician intervention to all smokers could more than double annual quit rates.[86] Seventy percent of smokers see their doctors at least once annually, thereby granting physicians ample opportunity for smoking cessation counseling.[87] If only one-half of all U.S. physicians gave brief advice to their patients regarding smoking cessation, leading to success in 10%, clinician intervention would account for 2 million new nonsmokers in the United States each year.[88,89]

The Agency for Health Care Policy and Research (AHCPR) smoking cessation guidelines incorporate the National Cancer Institute's (NCI's) four *A*s: ask, advise, assist, and arrange.[85] The physician should *ask* each patient about his or her smoking status; *advise* the patient to stop and educate him or her regarding the long-term health consequences of smoking; *assist* by helping the patient to set a stop date, prescribing pharmacologic interventions, and supplying self-help pamphlets; and *arrange* follow-up.[90] This NCI manual provides good reasons for quitting smoking, targeted to different groups (Table 22-1).[90] Other groups recommend the four *R*s: The physician discusses with the patient the *relevance* of a stop-smoking program to health, the smoking *risks*, and the *rewards* of quitting, and continues *repetition* of the stop-smoking message.[91]

Clinicians should determine and document the tobacco use status of every patient treated in a health care setting.[85] To remind physicians, Fiore[92] has recommended that smoking status be included as part of a routine patient vital sign assessment. Other researchers recommend flagging smokers' charts to ensure necessary smoking interventions (Fig. 22-4).[36] Ahluwalia et al.[93] have found that placing a smoking stamp on patients' charts significantly increases (from 45.6% to 78.4%) the likelihood that a physician will ask patients whether they smoke.

The AHCPR guidelines also stipulate that effective cessation treatments should be offered to every patient who smokes.[85] Brief cessation treatments *are* effective. At least a minimal intervention should be provided for every patient who uses tobacco.

As described in the AHCPR guidelines, a dose-response relationship exists between the intensity and duration of treatment and its effectiveness.[85] In general, more intense intervention leads to more effective long-term abstinence from tobacco. The success of an intervention also is maximized by proper training and education of physicians and medical students, by increasing the number of modalities used and the number of professionals involved, and by the creation of office-based systems.[36,92–96]

TABLE 22-1. Good Reasons to Stop Smoking

FOR TEENAGERS
Bad breath
Stained teeth
Cost
Lack of independence, controlled by cigarettes
Sore throats
Cough
Dyspnea (might affect participation in sports)
Frequent respiratory infections
FOR PREGNANT WOMEN
Increased rate of spontaneous abortion and fetal death
Increased risk of low birth weight
FOR PARENTS
Increased coughing and respiratory infections among children of smokers
Poor role model for child
FOR NEW SMOKERS
Easier to stop now
FOR LONG-TERM SMOKERS
Decreased risk of heart disease and cancer if you stop
FOR MEMBERS OF A FAMILY WITH HISTORY OF HEART DISEASE, CANCER, ETC.
Risk of death increased even more by smoking
FOR ASYMPTOMATIC ADULTS
Twice the risk of heart disease
Six times the risk of emphysema
Ten times the risk of lung cancer
Shortened life span by 5–8 years
Cost of cigarettes
Cost of sick time
Bad breath
Socially unacceptable
Wrinkles
FOR SYMPTOMATIC ADULTS (*Correlate current symptoms with:*)
Upper respiratory infections, cough
Sore throats
Dyspnea
Ulcers
Angina
Claudication
Osteoporosis
Esophagitis
Gum disease
FOR ANY SMOKER
Money saved by stopping
Improved health (feel better)
Improved ability to exercise
May live long enough to enjoy retirement, grandchildren, etc.
May be able to work more, with less illness

From ref. 90, with permission.

Although only 2% to 3% of smokers become nonsmokers each year,[81] some studies report that up to 15% of patients seen by trained physicians have quit smoking.[96]

Finally, three particularly effective elements of smoking cessation treatment are (1) nicotine replacement therapy (NRT), (2) social support (clinician-provided encouragement and assistance), and (3) skills training and problem-solving techniques

Vital Signs

Temperature: ____
Blood Pressure: ____
Pulse: ____
Respiratory Rate: ____
Smoking Status: Current Former Never

FIGURE 22-4. Smoking status included in the vital signs (a proposal by Fiore[92]).

for achieving and maintaining abstinence.[36] Individualizing the message to the patient increases the likelihood for success.[25] Studies have shown that 3 minutes or less of advice increased quit rates from 7.9% to 10.2%.[96] For example, quit rates of 50% to 63% 6 months after a myocardial infarction can increase to 65% to 75% for those patients who received other interventions in addition to physician contact. Blum[25] recommends that physicians ask nonthreatening questions, such as "What brand do you buy?" and "How much do you spend on cigarettes?" The term *inhalation count* can remind a pack-a-day patient that he or she will breathe in as many as 1 million doses of cyanide, ammonia, carcinogens, and carbon monoxide in less than 15 years. To the construction worker, the physician could link smoking cessation to the likelihood of fewer lost paydays, greater physical strength, and greater ability to work. A high school student, unresponsive to discussions of future emphysema and lung cancer, might be more receptive to the cosmetic unattractiveness of yellow teeth, bad breath, loss of athletic ability, or the financial drain of cigarettes (with costs for a pack-a-day smoker in excess of $1460 a year, calculated at $4 per pack).[25]

Also, the physician needs to tailor the message to the patient's readiness to change, according to the Prochaska and DiClemente[97] model: precontemplation, contemplation, action, and maintenance. During *precontemplation,* the patient has not considered quitting. During the *contemplation* phase, the patient is thinking about quitting. In the *action* phase, the patient is preparing and attempting to quit, and, during *maintenance,* the patient is avoiding relapse. Patients do not necessarily pass through each stage in orderly fashion; they may skip a stage or regress.[97]

NICOTINE REPLACEMENT THERAPY

Approximately 300 cessation methods are reported in the literature, ranging from group therapy, hypnosis, and self-help manuals to acupuncture.[25] The introduction of nicotine-based medications in the form of chewing gum or a transdermal patch, combined with counseling, now provides cessation rates roughly double that of a control group (a factor of 1.4 to 2.6) as compared to placebo treatments. However, 70% to 80% of smokers who use these therapies still start to smoke again.[98,99]

By providing a substitute source of nicotine, NRT lessens the withdrawal symptoms associated with quitting and improves the cessation process. As dozens of published studies have demonstrated its efficacy, safety, and utility, the Smoking Cessation Clinical Practice Guideline of AHCPR recommends NRT as a first-line treatment for tobacco dependence "except in the presence of special circumstances."[85] Most commonly, NRT is used in the form of nicotine (polacrilex) gum [first approved by the U.S. Food and Drug Administration (FDA) in 1984] or the transdermal nicotine patch (FDA-approved in 1991). In 1996, both of these medications became available as over-the-counter products,[79,80] greatly increasing access. In a metaanalysis, Fiore et al.[99] studied 42 randomized controlled trials of nicotine gum, as well as trials with fewer subjects using a transdermal patch and nasal spray inhaled nicotine. From their studies of nearly 18,000 persons, the authors concluded that NRT was effective, either as a sole therapy or as an adjunct to other therapeutic approaches.[99,100] Dosing of nicotine gum should initially be titrated by the level of nicotine dependence and then adjusted if withdrawal symptoms are not relieved. The Fagerstrom Test for Nicotine Dependence (which features such questions as "How soon after you wake up do you smoke your first cigarette?") helps guide dosing decisions.[81]

Other agents also show promising results. Recent attention has focused on bupropion, an antidepressant, in combination with the nicotine patch. A recent double-blind, placebo-controlled smoking cessation trial found 12-month abstinence rates of 15.6% for placebo, 16.4% for the nicotine patch alone, 30.3% for sustained-release bupropion (Zyban) alone, and 35.5% for bupropion in conjunction with the nicotine patch. Treatment consisted of 9 weeks of bupropion (150 mg/d) for the first 3 days and then 150 mg twice daily.[98]

COMMUNITY LEVEL AND STATE INTERVENTIONS

The Community Intervention Trial for Smoking Cessation (COMMIT) and the American Stop Smoking Intervention Study for Cancer Prevention (ASSIST), two NCI-funded efforts to change social norms regarding tobacco use in the community, marked a societal shift toward viewing tobacco control as a public health prevention issue.[101–104] The 4-year COMMIT study involved 11 matched pairs of communities, randomly assigning one community to active intervention while the other served as the control site. The hypothesis was that a community-level, multichannel intervention (involving media, public education, work-site intervention, and other means) would increase quit rates among smokers, particularly heavy smokers. In 1995, the trial concluded with equal smoking prevalence rates in both groups of communities. Although no increase in the quit rates of heavy smokers was documented, a testament to the powerful nature of nicotine addiction, a statistically significant decrease was realized in the smoking rates of the light to moderate smokers in intervention communities.[101,102]

From 1991 through 1999, the NCI (with logistic support from the American Cancer Society) conducted ASSIST, a nonrandomized study. The project funded health departments in 17 states to implement tobacco control programs that included cessation classes, mass media campaigns, and public policy such as clean indoor air campaigns, efforts to prohibit youth access to tobacco products, and tax increases. Though the goal of reducing adult smoking prevalence to 15% by the year 2000 was not reached, the ASSIST initiative helped public health officials to gain valuable knowledge in statewide tobacco control planning and to move toward statewide denormalization of tobacco use.[103,104]

RESTRICTING YOUTH ACCESS

Preventing youth access to tobacco products should affect youth smoking rates.[105–107] All states prohibit the sale and distribution of tobacco products to minors under the age of 18. In several dozen states, additional laws prevent youth access by designating enforcement authorities, enforcing license suspension or revocation for sales to minors, banning vending machines in areas accessible to minors, or restricting advertising. However, one study found that even when 82% of merchants complied with laws banning sales to minors, teenagers reported only a small decrease in their ability to purchase tobacco and no decline in its use.[107] More data are needed to verify the effectiveness of reducing sales to minors in actually limiting adolescents' access.

RESTRICTING SMOKING IN PUBLIC PLACES

Restricting smoking in workplaces has the potential to decrease greatly human exposure to ETS. Data show that in 1994, of 122 million full-time workers in the United States, nearly 100 million worked indoors.[108] The 1994 National Health Interview Survey showed that smoking prevalence of indoor workers was 26%, and 59% of workers (59 million) worked in buildings where smoking was not permitted.[108] A review of 19 studies of the impact of smoke-free workplaces found that almost all reported declines in daily smoking rates and smoking prevalence. Approximately 13% of the national decline in cigarette consumption in the United States between 1988 and 1994 was attributed to smoke-free workplaces.[108]

An ongoing challenge is to guarantee that smoke-free policies have strength at the local level and are not subject to preemption (i.e., legislation that prevents any local jurisdiction from enacting restrictions that are more stringent than the state law). The Centers for Disease Control and Prevention (CDC), by including tobacco control laws and policies as part of their surveillance efforts, note that from 1993 through 1996, the number of tobacco control laws with a preemption provision increased significantly to cover 30 states currently.[109]

TOBACCO TAXES THAT FUND DEDICATED, COMPREHENSIVE STATEWIDE TOBACCO CONTROL PROGRAMS

Many public health experts regard tobacco taxes to be the single most effective measure for decreasing tobacco consumption.[78] Economic research documents price elasticity (i.e., a 10% increase in cigarette price generally reduces overall consumption by 4%).[110] Studies show that youth, lower-income smokers, young adults, and minority smokers are more likely than others to be encouraged by a price increase to quit smoking.[111] Government has traditionally taxed tobacco to fund government services, but public health professionals support increased taxes on tobacco products to deter consumption. The Canadian tobacco tax experience in the 1980s and early 1990s demonstrated the potential health impact. The combined average federal and provincial tax reached close to $3.00, pushing the average price per pack to more than $4.00. As a result, per capita cigarette consumption (adjusted for estimates of tobacco smuggling) dropped by 38% (1982 to 1992).[110,112]

In contrast, among the world's industrialized countries, the United States has one of the lowest cigarette tax rates, with an average combined federal and state tax on cigarettes in 1993 of 53¢ per pack, as compared to countries such as Denmark and Norway, where taxes exceed $3.00 per pack. U.S. federal cigarette taxes, currently 24¢ per pack, will rise to 39¢ by 2002. Other forms of tobacco such as snuff, chewing tobacco, and pipe tobacco also are taxed.[113]

To some degree, the state's dependence on tobacco production determines the level of state tax, which currently ranges from 2.5¢ in Virginia to $1.00 per pack in Alaska and Hawaii (nationwide average, 38.9¢ per pack). The cigarette tax–to–price ratio, which assesses the relative contribution of the total (state and federal) taxes to the full price of cigarettes, has declined from 49.8% in 1960 to 29.6% in 1997.[113]

In general, the public is willing to increase tobacco taxes if those extra revenues are earmarked for specific purposes such as health programs.[114] To date, four states—Arizona, California, Massachusetts, and Oregon—have passed tobacco tax initiatives and used the revenue to develop statewide comprehensive tobacco control programs.[115,116] The CDC recently studied state experiences and disseminated best practices for comprehensive tobacco control programs.[117]

CALIFORNIA

California voters approved a 1988 ballot initiative that increased the state cigarette tax by 25¢, allocating 20% of the revenue to establish a comprehensive statewide tobacco education and prevention program.[118,119] The initiative also funded mass media antitobacco campaigns, assistance to local health agencies for providing technical support and monitoring adherence to antismoking laws, community-based interventions, smoking cessation services (including a statewide quit-smoking telephone hot line), and enhancement of school-based prevention programs.[118,119] As a result, an analysis of per capita cigarette consumption indicated that the start of the California Tobacco Control Program in 1989 was associated with a 50% more rapid rate of decline in cigarette consumption than was seen in the rest of the country. Both the tax increase and the funded tobacco control program contributed to this decline. However, the post-1993 rate of decline, while still significantly more rapid in California than in the rest of the United States (where the decline in consumption halted), slowed to less than one-third of the rate seen in 1989 through 1993. Pierce et al.[120] attributed the slowing to reduced program funding, increased tobacco industry expenditures for advertising and promotion, industry pricing, and political activities.

MASSACHUSETTS

Massachusetts voters approved a special 25¢ tax that helped to fund the Massachusetts Tobacco Control Program (MTCP).[114] The MTCP had three major goals: to prevent onset of tobacco use by children, to assist smokers in quitting, and to guard against the harm of ETS. Like California's program, the MTCP consisted of funding for local cessation efforts and local coalitions, a statewide quit-smoking telephone hot line, funding of local boards of health, a statewide public awareness and counter-advertising campaign, and comprehensive school-based programs.[121] Adult per capita tobacco consumption in Massachusetts declined by 20% from the program's inception in 1992 through 1996, reflecting a threefold increase over the reduction observed at the national level.[122] The number of cities and towns that have adopted ordinances restricting youth access to cigarette vending machines has doubled. Recently, data showed the prevalence of current smoking among adults in Massachusetts was 19.1% in 1999, down from 23% in 1993, one of the lowest rates in all the 50 states.[123]

OTHER STATES

Similar results accompanied a successful 1996 ballot measure in Oregon that increased the excise tax by 30¢ per pack of cigarettes. After passage, per capita consumption has declined 11.3% in Oregon, or the equivalent of 200 cigarettes per capita.[124] Arizona's ballot initiative in 1994 raised cigarette prices by 40¢.[116] Funds from a settled Medicaid lawsuit launched the Florida Pilot Program on Tobacco Control, which is credited with sparking significant declines in tobacco use among middle school and public high school students, declines attributed primarily to a youth-oriented, counter-advertising media campaign, community partnerships in all 67 Florida counties, and enhanced enforcement of youth access laws.[125] From 1998 to 1999, the prevalence of cigarette use among middle school students declined from 18.5% to 15.0% ($P < .01$); among high school students, use declined from 27.4% to 25.2% ($P = .02$).[125]

MASS MEDIA AND COUNTER-ADVERTISING

All the statewide tobacco control programs just cited have incorporated counter-advertising efforts through mass media. Minnesota (1986) and Michigan (1994) also have initiated limited tax-funded media campaigns.[116] Such efforts counter the tobacco industry's efforts to normalize a lethal product through advertising and promotional cigarette sales. A counter-advertising public health approach aims to reduce tobacco use by deglamorizing and denormalizing use of the product. To be effective, such mass media antismoking campaigns should provide consistent messages from multiple sources, repeatedly and over a long period, and should work in concert with other interventions and policies, with the goal of changing societal norms.[74]

The effects of these counter-advertising media campaigns, especially those in California and Massachusetts, have been striking. Of the California Tobacco Control Program's decline in cigarette consumption, approximately 20% was estimated to be attributable to the media campaign.[74,126,127] One study of California adults who successfully quit smoking (1990 and 1991) found that in 41%, the media counter-advertising campaign had influenced their decision to stop.[128]

The effectiveness of counter-advertising first emerged in 1967 when the Federal Communications Commission invoked the Fairness Doctrine to require broadcasters to air one antismoking message for every three cigarette commercials aired.[74] When such antismoking advertising prompted a decline in per capita cigarette consumption of at least 5%, the tobacco industry then agreed (in 1970) to Congressional legislation to ban all tobacco advertising on television and radio, thereby eliminating the need for free antismoking ads.[74]

Later, research in Vermont and Minnesota showed that community- and school-based interventions highlighted by prominent mass media campaigns could reduce smoking in young persons by up to 40%.[74,129,130] However, such mass media campaigns before 1988 usually occurred on a sporadic basis. Also, institutionalizing counter-advertising campaigns has posed a public health challenge, as funding for such campaigns can be subjected to legislative diversion.[74] Typically, public service announcements on television did not air during prime time and therefore reached smaller audiences.[74]

Goldman and Glantz[131] have concluded that messages challenging social norms are more successful than are those aimed at changing individual behavior to improve health. Focus groups analysis by these researchers found that the most effective themes stressed the tobacco industry's manipulation of young persons, the negative impact of secondhand smoke, and the burden of cigarette addiction. Such advertisements can be controversial yet memorable and, ultimately, effective.[74,131]

TOBACCO LITIGATION AND TOBACCO SETTLEMENT

Public health lawyers have advocated bringing suits against tobacco companies as a cancer prevention strategy.[132] The last half century of tobacco litigation can be divided into three waves. Wave 1 (1954 through 1973) featured a number of individual lawsuits against an industry that maintained that tobacco products had never been proven to cause disease. The industry claimed that smokers chose to smoke, hence assuming risk for themselves. In essence, the 1965 Federal Cigarette Labeling and Advertising Act, which requires warning labels on all cigarette packaging and labeling, ironically served as a shield from liability. Wave 2 (1983 through 1992) featured *Cipollone v. Liggett Group Inc.*, a suit brought by a smoker and continued by her husband after her death. Although the original jury verdict of $400,000 favored the plaintiff, it was reversed on appeal and the case finally was dropped after years of litigation.

Wave 3 (1994 to the present) capitalizes on the release of internal industry documents and subsequent industry concessions that tobacco is addictive and causes cancer and that tobacco companies had consciously marketed their products to children. From this ensued an increasing number of individual lawsuits and class action suits. Among the class action suits is *Broin v. Philip Morris*, which was brought on behalf of flight attendants injured by ETS and was settled for $349 million. The money realized from this suit will establish a foundation for the study of diseases associated with tobacco.[133–135] *Engle v. R.J. Reynolds* is a suit brought on behalf of addicted and sick smokers in Florida. In the first phase of this massive class action suit, the industry was found liable for punitive damages, with the award potentially in the hundreds of billions of dollars.[136] In addition, in 1999, the Justice Department filed a $20 billion lawsuit against the nation's tobacco companies to recover federal costs of treating smoking-related illness.

The most notable litigation to date has been lawsuits brought by states' attorneys general against the tobacco industry to recoup Medicaid costs for the treatment of ill smokers.[137,138] In a remarkable turn of events, the major tobacco manufacturers first settled individually with Mississippi, Texas, Minnesota, and Florida at a cost of $40 billion over 25 years. Then the industry signed a Master Settlement Agreement with 46 state attorneys general in November 1998, agreeing to pay $206 billion over 25 years in exchange for no future state litigation. Other conditions included some advertising restrictions (e.g., bans on billboard advertisements) and the establishment of a national foundation to reduce teen smoking.

As the twentieth century ends, states are embroiled in historic discussions of how best to spend the settlement money. The Master Settlement Agreement expressly states that parties "have agreed to settle their respective lawsuits and potential claims pursuant to terms which will achieve for the Settling States and their citizens significant funding for the advancement of public health, the implementation of important tobacco-related public health measures, including the enforcement of mandates and restrictions related to such measures, as well as funding for a national foundation dedicated to significantly reducing the use of tobacco products by youth...."[138] However, to date, in most states, the debate has been dominated by proposals to fund civic projects such as debt reduction, school construction, teacher retirement funds, prison construction, and sidewalk repair.[137] As the suits were launched and settled for reasons of tobacco and health, the most fitting outcome would be to dedicate such funds to tobacco control and health programs.

PROPOSED U.S. FOOD AND DRUG ADMINISTRATION REGULATION

Under Commissioner David Kessler, the FDA first investigated whether to regulate nicotine as a drug. The Federal Food, Drug and Cosmetic Act defines a drug as "an article (except for food) intended to affect the structure and function of the body."[135] Universal scientific consensus indicates that nicotine is an addictive drug. Evidence of the intent of the industry had been supported by the release of internal documents showing that tobacco manufacturers knew that nicotine caused significant pharmacologic effects and designed their products to provide pharmacologically active doses.[80,135] In 1996, the FDA proposed strategies to restrict access to tobacco products and advertising to youth. The first step, effected in part in 1997, involved stricter enforcement of laws affecting minors. The remaining proposed steps included banning free samples, restricting advertising within 1000 feet of schools and playgrounds, and limiting to black and white text print advertising in youth publications. The U.S. Supreme Court recently rejected these proposals, saying the FDA had never received authority from congress to regulate tobacco products.[139]

CONCLUSION

The dawn of the twenty-first century offers us a new opportunity to create a smoke-free society. All health care professionals, and indeed all citizens, can work to achieve this goal and prevent cancer. At the individual level, we must maximize access to cessation services for all smokers and promote further research into improving nicotine replacement therapies and other pharmacologic approaches. Health care professionals can raise awareness and promote cessation with every clinical opportunity. Reducing and even eliminating nicotine from cigarettes is also technically feasible and may hold the future to eradicating the potential for addiction.

On a broader societal level, communities can commit to changing permanently to a nonsmoking social norm. Such efforts include restricting tobacco advertising and promotion to children, prohibiting tobacco access by youth and teenagers, enhancing public education, raising tobacco excise taxes, and controlling tobacco exports. Dedication of tobacco settlement funds to statewide tobacco control programs nationwide can reduce cigarette consumption and promote prevention, as has been done in California and Massachusetts. Key to such comprehensive programs are broad-scale counter-advertising programs that deglamorize tobacco use.

On the legal front, multiple individual and class action suits ultimately may change the tobacco industry's ability to conduct business as usual. In light of the U.S. Supreme Court's decision as to the authority of the FDA to regulate tobacco, we now await study of this issue by the U.S. Congress.

It is hoped that all these combined efforts will cause the decline and prevention of tobacco-related cancers in the new millennium. Medical historians then can mark the end of the so-called Tobacco and Cancer Century and celebrate the beginning of a new smoke-free chapter in public health.

REFERENCES

1. Wingo PA, Ries LA, Giovino GA, et al. The annual report to the nation on the status of cancer 1973–1996 with a special section on lung cancer and tobacco smoking. *J Natl Cancer Inst* 1999;91:675.
2. Koh HK. The end of the "Tobacco and Cancer" century. *J Natl Cancer Inst* 1999;91:60.
3. Peto R, Lopez AD, Boreham J, et al. Mortality from tobacco in developed countries: indirect estimation from national vital statistics. *Lancet* 1996;39:1268.
4. Peto R. Smoking and death: the past 40 years and the next 40. *BMJ* 1994;309:937.
5. Peto R, Lopez AD, Boreham J, et al. Mortality from smoking worldwide. *Br Med Bull* 1996;52:12.
6. Hecht SS. Tobacco smoke carcinogens and lung cancer. *J Natl Cancer Inst* 1999;91:1194.
7. Bergen AW, Caporaso N. Cigarette smoking. *J Natl Cancer Inst* 1999;91:1365.
8. Report of the surgeon general: the health consequences of smoking: nicotine addiction. Pub. No. CDC 88-8406. Washington, DC: Department of Health and Human Services, 1988.
9. Novotny TE, Shane P, Daynard RA, Connolly GN. Tobacco use as a sociologic carcinogen: the case for a public health approach. *Cancer Prev* 1992:1.
10. Lombard HL, Doering CR. Cancer studies in Massachusetts: habits, characteristics, and environment of individuals with and without cancer. *N Engl J Med* 1928;198:481.
11. Doll R, Hill AB. Lung cancer and other causes of death in relation to smoking: second report on mortality of British doctors. *Br Med J* 1956;2:1071.
12. Wynder EL, Graham EA. Tobacco smoking as a possible etiologic factor in bronchogenic carcinoma. *JAMA* 1950;143:329.
13. Hammond EL, Horn D. Smoking and death rates: report on forty-four months of follow-up of 187,783 men. *JAMA* 1958;166:1294.
14. US Department of Health, Education, and Welfare. Smoking and health: report of the Advisory Committee to the Surgeon General. Atlanta: Centers for Disease Control (Public Health Service), 1964.
15. Average annual number of deaths, 1990–1994. *MMWR* 1997;46:448.
16. Cigarette brand use among adult smokers—United States, 1986. *MMWR* 1990;39:665.
17. Epps RP, Manley MW, Glynn TJ. Tobacco use among adolescents. *Pediatr Clin North Am* 1995;42:389.
18. US Department of Health and Human Services. The health consequences of smoking: cancer. A report of the surgeon general, 1982. DHHS Pub. No. (PHS)82-50179. Rockville, MD: US Department of Health and Human Services, Public Health Service, Office of Smoking and Health, 1982.
19. Steenland K. Age specific interactions between smoking and radon among United States uranium miners. *Occup Environ Med* 1994;51:192.
20. Berry G, Newhouse ML, Antonis P. Combined effect of asbestos and smoking on mortality from lung cancer and mesothelioma in factory workers. *Br J Med* 1985;42:12.
21. Selikoff IJ, Seidman H, Hammond EC. Mortality effects of cigarette smoking among amosite asbestos factory workers. *J Natl Cancer Inst* 1980;65:507.
22. US Department of Health and Human Services. The health consequences of smoking: cancer and chronic lung disease in the workplace. A report of the surgeon general.

DHHS Pub. No. (PHS)85-50207. Washington, DC: US Department of Health and Human Services, Public Health Service, Centers for Disease Control, Office of Smoking and Health, 1985.

23. Thun M, Lally C, Flannery J, et al. Cigarette smoking and changes in the histopathology of lung cancer. *J Natl Cancer Inst* 1997;89:1580.
24. US Department of Health, Education, and Welfare. Smoking and health: a report of the surgeon general. DHEW(PHS) 79-50066. Washington, DC: Public Health Service, Office of the Assistant Secretary for Health, Office on Smoking and Health, 1979.
25. Blum A. Cancer prevention: preventing tobacco-related cancers. In: DeVita C, Hellman S, Rosenberg S, eds. *Cancer principles and practice of oncology,* 5th ed. Philadelphia: Lippincott–Raven Publishers, 1997.
26. Flanders WD, Rothman KJ. Interaction of alcohol and tobacco in laryngeal cancer. *Am J Epidemiol* 1982;115:371.
27. US Department of Health and Human Services. The health consequences of smokeless tobacco: a report of the Advisory Committee to the Surgeon General. NIH Publication No. 86-2874. Washington, DC: US Department of Health and Human Services, Public Health Service, 1986.
28. US Department of Health and Human Services. Reducing the health consequences of smoking: 25 years of progress. A report of the surgeon general. DHHS(CDC)89-8411,1989. Washington, DC: US Department of Health and Human Services, Public Health Service, Centers for Disease Control, Office of Smoking and Health, 1989.
29. Banoczy J, Sugar L. Progressive and regressive changes in Hungarian oral leukoplakias in the course of longitudinal studies. *Community Dent Oral Epidemiol* 1975;3:194.
30. Roed-Petersen B, Banoczy J, Pindborg JJ. Smoking habits and histological characteristics of oral leukoplakia in Denmark and Hungary. *Br J Cancer* 1973;28:575.
31. Hays GL, Lippman SM, Flaitz CM, et al. Cocarcinogenesis and field cancerization: oral lesions offer first signs. *J Am Dent Assoc* 1995;126:47.
32. Bartecchi CE, MacKenzie TD, Schrier RW. The human costs of tobacco use, part 1. *N Engl J Med* 1994;330:907.
33. MacKenzie TD, Bartecchi CE, Schrier RW. The human costs of tobacco, part 2. *N Engl J Med* 1994;330:975.
34. Davis B, Koh HK. Faces going up in smoke. *Arch Dermatol* 1992;128:1106.
35. Bartecchi CE, MacKenzie TD, Schrier RW. The global tobacco epidemic. *Sci Am* May 1995.
36. US Department of Health and Human Services, Public Health Service, Agency for Health Care Policy and Research. Smoking cessation: a systems approach. A guide for health care administrators, insurers, managed care organizations, and purchasers. AHCPR Pub. No. 97-0698. Washington, DC: US Department of Health and Human Services, Public Health Service, April 1997.
37. Centers for Disease Control and Prevention. Cigarette smoking among adults—United States, 1995. *MMWR* 1997;46:1217.
38. Ernster VL. Mixed messages for women: a social history of cigarette smoking and advertising. *NY State J Med* 1985;85:335.
39. World Health Organization. The tobacco epidemic: a global public health emergency. Tobacco alert. Geneva: World Health Organization, April 1998. http://www.who.int/archives/tobalert/apr96/fulltext.htm
40. Kessler DA, Natanblut SL, Wilkenfield JP, et al. Nicotine addiction: a pediatric disease. *J Pediatr* 1997;130:518.
41. Tobacco use among high school students—United States, 1997. *MMWR* 1998;47:229.
42. *Growing up tobacco free: preventing nicotine addiction in children and youths.* Washington, DC: Institute of Medicine, National Academy Press, 1994.
43. An LC, O'Malley PM, Schulenberg JE, et al. Changes at the high end of risk in cigarette smoking among US high school seniors, 1976–1995. *Am J Public Health* 1999;89:699.
44. Kellam SG, Anthony JC. Targeting early antecedents to prevent tobacco smoking: findings from an epidemiologically based randomized field trial. *Am J Public Health* 1998;88:1490.
45. Jackson C, Henriksen L, Dickinson D, et al. The early use of alcohol and tobacco: its relation to children's competence and parents' behavior. *Am J Public Health* 1997;87:59.
46. Coogan PF, Adams M, Geller AC, et al. Factors associated with smoking among children and adolescents in Connecticut. *Am J Prev Med* 1998;15:17.
47. Jackson C, Henriksen L, Dickinson D, et al. A longitudinal study predicting patterns of cigarette smoking in late childhood. *Health Educ Behav* 1998;25:436.
48. Bachman JG, Wallace JM, O'Malley PM, et al. Racial/ethnic differences in smoking, drinking, and illicit drug use among American high school seniors, 1976–1989. *Am J Public Health* 1991;81:372.
49. Pierce JP, Choi WS, Gilpin EA, et al. Tobacco industry promotion of cigarettes and adolescent smoking. *JAMA* 1998;279:511.
50. Wechsler H, Rigotti NA, Gledhill-Hoyt J, et al. Increased levels of cigarette use among college students. *JAMA* 1998;280:1673.
51. Miller GH. The 'less hazardous' cigarette: a deadly delusion. *NY State J Med* 1985;85:313.
52. Hoffmann D, Djordjevic MV, Hoffman I. The changing cigarette. *Prev Med* 1997;26:427.
53. Filter ventilation levels in selected U.S. cigarettes, 1997. *MMWR* 1997;46:1043.
54. State-specific prevalence among adults of current cigarette smoking and smokeless tobacco use and per capita tax-paid sales of cigarettes–United States, 1997. *MMWR* 1998;47:922.
55. Blum A. Smokeless tobacco. *JAMA* 1980;244:192.
56. Spangler J, Salisbury P. Smokeless tobacco: epidemiology, health effects and cessation strategies. *Am Fam Physician* 1995;52:1421.
57. Tomar S, Giovino G. Incidence and predictors of smokeless tobacco use among U.S. youth. *Am J Public Health* 1998;88:20.
58. Smokeless (spit) tobacco: a review of the state of the science. Proceedings of a symposium during the seventy-fourth general session of the International Association for Dental Research, San Francisco, CA, March 13, 1996. *Adv Dent Res* 1997;11:305.
59. Iribarren C, Tekaiva I, Sidney S, et al. Effect of cigar smoking on the risk of cardiovascular disease, chronic obstructive pulmonary disease and cancer in men. *N Engl J Med* 1999;340:1773.
60. Cigar smoking among teenagers—United States, Massachusetts, and New York, 1996. *MMWR* 1997;46:433.
61. Satcher D. Cigars and public health. *N Engl J Med* 1999;340:1829.
62. US Department of Health and Human Services. The health consequences of involuntary smoking: a report of the surgeon general. Pub. No. (CDC)87-8398. Washington, DC: Public Health Service, Centers for Disease Control, Office on Smoking and Health, Department of Health and Human Services, 1986.
63. Davis RM. Exposure to environmental tobacco smoke: identifying and protecting those at risk. *JAMA* 1998;280:1947.
64. Brownson RC, Eriksen MP, Davis RM, et al. Environmental tobacco smoke: health effects and policies to reduce exposure. *Annu Rev Public Health* 1997;18:163.
65. National Research Council, National Academy of Sciences. *Environmental tobacco smoke: measuring exposures and assessing health effects.* Washington, DC: National Academy Press, 1986.
66. California Environmental Protection Agency. Health effects of exposure to environmental tobacco smoke. *Tob Control* 1997;6:346.
67. US Environmental Protection Agency. Respiratory health effects of passive smoking: lung cancer and other disorders. Environmental Protection Agency Pub. EPA/600/6-90/006F. Washington, DC: Environmental Protection Agency, Office of Air and Radiation, 1992.
68. California Environmental Protection Agency. Health effects of exposure to environmental tobacco smoke. Sacramento: California Environmental Protection Agency, Office of Environmental Health Hazard Assessment, 1997.
69. Federal Trade Commission. Report to Congress for 1991: pursuant to the Federal Cigarette Labeling and Advertising Act. Washington DC: Federal Trade Commission, 1994.
70. Federal Trade Commission. Pursuant to the Comprehensive Smokeless Tobacco Health Education Act of 1986. Washington, DC: Federal Trade Commission, 1993.
71. Centers for Disease Control and Prevention. Preventing tobacco use among young people: a report of the surgeon general, 1994. S/N 017-001-004901-0. Washington, DC: US Government Printing Office, 1994:175.
72. Feighery E, Borzekowski DL, Schooler C, et al. Seeing, wanting, owning: the relationship between receptivity to tobacco marketing and smoking susceptibility in young people. *Tob Control* 1998;7:123.
73. Difranza JR, Richards JW, Paulman PM, et al. RJR Nabisco's cartoon camel promotes camel cigarettes to children. *JAMA* 1991;266:3149.
74. Siegel M. Mass media antismoking campaigns: a powerful tool for health promotion. *Ann Intern Med* 1998;129:128.
75. King C, Siegel M, Celebucki C, et al. Adolescent exposure to cigarette advertising in relation to youth readership. *JAMA* 1998;279:516.
76. Bloch M, Daynard R, Roemer R. A year of living dangerously: the tobacco control community meets the global settlement. *Public Health Rep* 1998;113:488.
77. Arno PS, Brandt AM, Gostin LO, et al. Tobacco industry strategies to oppose federal regulation. *JAMA* 1996;275:1258.
78. Emmons KM, Kawachi I, Barclay G. Tobacco control: a brief review of its history and prospects for the future. *Hematol Oncol Clin North Am* 1997;11:177.
79. Cincirpini PM, McClure JB. Smoking cessation: recent developments in behavioral and pharmacologic interventions. *Oncology* 1998;12:249.
80. Cinciripini PM, Hecht SS, Henningfield JE, et al. Tobacco addiction: implications for treatment and cancer prevention. *J Natl Cancer Inst* 1997;89:1852.
81. Henningfield J. Nicotine medication for smoking cessation. *N Engl J Med* 1995;333:1196.
82. Zhu SH, Sun J, Billings S, et al. Predictors of smoking cessation in US adolescents. *Am J Prev Med* 1999;16:202.
83. Selected cigarette smoking initiation and quitting behaviors among high school students—United States, 1997. *MMWR* 1998;47:386.
84. Skaar K, Tsoh J, Cinciripini P, et al. Current approaches in smoking cessation. *Curr Opin Oncol* 1996;8:434.
85. Agency for Health Care Policy and Research, Smoking Cessation Clinical Practice Guideline Panel and Staff. Smoking cessation clinical practice guideline. *JAMA* 1996;275:1270.
86. Fiore MC, Bailey WC, Cohen SC, et al. Smoking cessation: clinical practice guideline no. 18. AHCPR Pub. No. 96-0692. Rockville, MD: Agency for Health Care Policy and Research, April 1996.
87. Sherin K. Smoking cessation: the physician's role. *Postgrad Med* 1982;11:71.
88. Fiore MC, Novotny TE, Pierce JP, et al. Methods used to quit smoking in the United States. *JAMA* 1990;263:2760.
89. Glynn TJ. Methods of smoking cessation—finally, some answers. *JAMA* 1990;263:2795.
90. Glynn TJ, Manley MW. *How to help your patients stop smoking: a National Cancer Institute manual for physicians.* Washington, DC: US Department of Health and Human Services, Public Health Service, National Institutes of Health, 1993.
91. US Department of Health and Human Services. The health benefits of smoking cessation: a report of the surgeon general. DHHS CDC 90-8416. Atlanta: US Department of Health and Human Services, Public Health Service, Centers for Disease Control and Prevention, Centers for Chronic Disease Prevention and Health Promotion, Office of Smoking and Health,1990.
92. Fiore MC. The new vital sign. Assessing and documenting smoking status. *JAMA* 1991;266:3183.
93. Ahluwalia JS, Gibson CA, Kenney RE, et al. Smoking status as a vital sign. *J Gen Intern Med* 1999;14:402.
94. Ferry LH, Grissino LM, Runfola PS. Tobacco dependence curricula in US undergraduate medical education. *JAMA* 1999;282:825.
95. Fiore MC, Epps RP, Manley MW. A missed opportunity: teaching medical students to help their patients successfully quit smoking. *JAMA* 1994:271:624.
96. Ockene JK, Zapka JG. Physician-based smoking intervention: a rededication to a five-step strategy to smoking research. *Addict Behav* 1997;22:835.

97. Prochaska JO, DiClemente CC, Norcross JC. In search of how people change. Applications to addictive behaviors. *Am Psychol* 1992;47:1102.
98. Jorenby DE, Leischow SJ, Nides MA, et al. A controlled trial of sustained-release bupropion, a nicotine patch, or both for smoking cessation. *N Engl J Med* 1999;340:685.
99. Fiore MC, Bailey WC, Cohen SJ, et al. Smoking cessation, Clinical Practice guideline no. 18. Rockville, MD: AHCPR Publ. No. 96-0692.
100. Shiffman S, Mason KM, Henningfield JE. Tobacco dependence treatments: review and prospects. *Annu Rev Public Health* 1998;19:335.
101. Community Intervention Trial for Smoking Cessation (COMMIT): I. Cohort results from a four-year community intervention. *Am J Public Health* 1995;85:183.
102. Fisher E Jr. The results of the COMMIT trial [Editorial]. *Am J Public Health* 1995;85:159.
103. Eyre H. Building on the foundation of ASSIST. *Tob Control* 1997;6:341.
104. Manley M, Pierce JP, Gilpin EA, et al. Impact of the American Stop Smoking Intervention Study on cigarette consumption. *Tob Control* 1997;6[Suppl 2]:S12.
105. Fishman JA, Allison H, Knowles SB, et al. State laws on tobacco control—United States, 1998. *MMWR* 1999;48(SS-3):22.
106. Forster JL, Wolfson M. Youth access to tobacco: policies and politics. *Annu Rev Public Health* 1998;19:203.
107. Rigotti N, DiFranza J, Chang Y, et al. The effect of enforcing tobacco-sales laws on adolescents: access to tobacco and smoking behavior. *N Engl J Med* 1997;337:1044.
108. Chapman S, Borland R, Scollo M, et al. The impact of smoke-free workplaces on declining cigarette consumption in Australia and the U.S. *Am J Public Health* 1999;89:1018.
109. Preemptive state tobacco-control laws—United States, 1982–1998. *MMWR* 1999;47:1112.
110. Grossman M, Chaloupka FJ. Cigarette taxes. The straw to break the camel's back. *Public Health Rep* 1997;112:290.
111. Farrelly M, Bray J. Response to increases in cigarette prices by race/ethnicity, income and age groups, United States 1976–1993. *MMWR* 1998;47:605.
112. Kaiserman MJ, Rogers B. Tobacco consumption declining faster in Canada than in the US. *Am J Public Health* 1991;81:902.
113. Pierce-Lavin C, Geller AC, Hyde J, et al. Creating statewide tobacco control programs after passage of a tobacco tax. *Cancer* 1998;83[Suppl]:2666.
114. Koh HK. An analysis of the successful 1992 Massachusetts tobacco tax initiative. *Tob Control* 1996;5:220.
115. Pierce-Lavin C, Geller AC. Creating statewide tobacco control programs after passage of a tobacco tax: executive summary. *Cancer* 1998;83[Suppl]:2659.
116. Nicholl J. Tobacco tax initiatives to prevent tobacco use. A study of eight statewide campaigns. *Cancer* 1998;83[Suppl]:2666.
117. Best practices for comprehensive tobacco control programs. Atlanta: Centers for Disease Prevention and Control, Office of Smoking and Health, August 1999.
118. Bal DG, Kizer KW, Felten PG, et al. Reducing tobacco consumption in California. Development of a statewide anti-tobacco use campaign. *JAMA* 1990;264:1570.
119. Flewelling RL, Kenney E, Elder JP, et al. First-year impact of the 1989 California cigarette tax increase on cigarette consumption. *Am J Public Health* 1992;82:867.
120. Pierce JP, Gilpin EA, Emery SL, et al. Has the California Control Program reduced smoking? *JAMA* 1998;280:893.
121. Connolly G, Robbins H. Designing an effective statewide tobacco control program—Massachusetts. *Cancer* 1998;83[Suppl]:2722.
122. Cigarette smoking before and after an excise tax increase and an antismoking campaign—Massachusetts, 1990–1996. *MMWR* 1996;45:966.
123. Beiner L. Personal communication, 1999.
124. Decline in cigarette consumption following implementation of a comprehensive tobacco prevention and education program—Oregon, 1996–1998. *MMWR* 1999;48:140.
125. Tobacco use among middle and high school students—Florida, 1998 and 1999. *MMWR* 1999;48:248.
126. Hu T, Keeler TE, Sung H, et al. The impact of California anti-smoking legislation on cigarette sales, consumption, and prices. *Tob Control* 1995;4[Suppl 1]:S34.
127. Hu T, Sung HY, Keeler TE. Reducing cigarette consumption in California: tobacco taxes versus an anti-smoking media campaign. *Am J Public Health* 1995;85:1218.
128. Popham WJ, Potter LD, Bal DG, et al. Do anti-smoking media campaigns help smokers quit? *Public Health Rep* 1993;108:510.
129. Secker-Walker RH, Worden JK, Holland RR, et al. A mass media program to prevent smoking among adolescents: costs and cost effectiveness. *Tob Control* 1997;6:207.
130. Flynn BS, Worden JK, Secker-Walker RH, et al. Mass media and school interventions for cigarette smoking prevention: effects 2 years after completion. *Am J Public Health* 1994;84:1148.
131. Goldman LK, Glantz SA. Evaluation of antismoking advertising campaigns. *JAMA* 1998;279:772.
132. Kelder GE, Daynard RA. Tobacco litigation as a public health and cancer control strategy. *J Am Med Womens Assoc* 1996;51:57.
133. Glantz SA, Barnes DE, Bero L, et al. Looking through a keyhole at the tobacco industry. The Brown and Williamson documents. *JAMA* 1995;274:219.
134. Hurt R, Robertson CR. Prying open the door to the tobacco industry's secrets about nicotine: the Minnesota tobacco trial. *JAMA* 1998;280:1173.
135. Kessler DA, Barnett PS, Witt A, et al. The legal and scientific basis for FDA's assertion of jurisdiction over cigarettes and smokeless tobacco. *JAMA* 1997;277:405.
136. Broder J. Cigarette maker concedes smoking can cause cancer. *New York Times* 1998 Nov 14:1.
137. Meier B. Tobacco windfall begins tug-of-war among lawmakers. *New York Times* 1999 Jan 10:1.
138. Multistate Master Settlement Agreement, November 23, 1998. National Association of Attorneys General website: http://www.naag.org/cigna.rtf
139. Greenhouse L. High court holds FDA can't impose rules on tobacco. *New York Times* 2000 March 22:1.

CHAPTER 23

Cancer Prevention: Diet and Chemopreventive Agents

SECTION 1

WALTER C. WILLETT

Fat

In recent years, reduction in dietary fat has been at the center of cancer prevention efforts. In the landmark 1982 National Academy of Sciences review of diet, nutrition, and cancer,[1] reduction in fat intake to 30% of calories was the primary recommendation; this objective has been echoed in subsequent dietary recommendations as well.[2]

Interest in dietary fat as a cause of cancer began in the first half of the twentieth century when studies by Tannenbaum and colleagues[3,4] indicated that diets high in fat could promote tumor growth in animal models. In this early work, energy (caloric) restriction also profoundly reduced the incidence of tumors. A vast literature on dietary fat and cancer in animals has subsequently accumulated (reviewed elsewhere).[1,5–8] Dietary fat has a clear effect on tumor incidence in many models, although not in all[9,10]; however, a central issue has been whether this is independent of the effect of energy intake. An independent effect of fat has been seen in some animal models,[5,7,11] but this has been either weak[12] or nonexistent[13] in some studies designed specifically to address this issue.

In the 1970s, the possible relation of dietary fat intake to cancer incidence gained greater attention as the large international differences in rates of many cancers were noted to be strongly correlated with apparent per capita fat consumption.[14,15] Particularly strong associations were seen with cancers of the breast, colon, prostate, and endometrium, which include the most important cancers in affluent countries not caused by smoking.[16] These correlations were observed to be limited to animal, not vegetable, fat.[17] Complementing these correlational observations, studies of populations migrating from low- to high-incidence areas indicated that the migrating groups adopted the cancer rates of the new environment. This provided powerful evidence that the large international differences in cancer incidence were not due to genetic factors and therefore that the high rates of specific cancers in affluent countries were potentially avoidable. Although such evidence did not directly implicate dietary factors, the animal studies noted previously made the area of diet a strong suspect.

A principal limitation of both the international correlational and migrant studies is the potential for confounding; many other differences besides dietary fat exist between the low-fat (less affluent) and high-fat (more affluent) countries. Indeed, the correlations with gross national product are similar to those for fat intake.[15] Among the many factors that differ between low- and high-fat countries, reproductive behaviors, physical activity level, and body fatness are particularly notable and are strongly associated with specific cancers.[18,19] The quality of dietary data used in the international correlations has also been problematic; this information is not based on actual intakes, but rather on estimated production figures.

Despite their limitations, the suggestive findings of at least some animal models as well as the international correlations and migrant studies have clearly indicated the need for more detailed studies in humans. In particular, studies that can control for the confounding influences of lifestyle factors other than fat intake are important. Two general approaches, discussed elsewhere in detail,[20] are available: case-control or cohort epidemiologic studies and randomized trials. Both case-control and cohort studies are dependent on a reasonably valid assessment of dietary intake. Although for some nutrients, biochemical measurements can be used to assess intake, for total fat consumption a useful biochemical indicator does not exist. Since 1980, considerable effort has been given to the development of standardized questionnaires for measuring intake of fat and other dietary factors and numerous studies have been conducted to assess the validity of these methods.[20–23] These investigations have clearly demonstrated that an informative range of fat exists within the populations of the United States and other countries and that standardized food frequency questionnaires can reasonably measure differences among subjects. Although the range of fat intake that can be studied is restricted to the range of diets in the study population, this typically includes both the levels that have often been recommended (less than 30% of energy) as well as more traditional U.S. levels (more than 40% of energy).[24] Moreover, by combining the data from multiple large prospective studies, the range of fat has been extended from less than 20% of energy to more than 45% of energy), which is similar to the current range observed internationally.[25]

In principle, the most definitive approach to evaluate the relation between fat intake and cancer is to conduct a large randomized trial. However, many practical problems exist in conducting such a trial, the most important being the need to maintain a difference in fat intake between the intervention and control groups for many years; the experience of the Multiple Risk Factor Intervention Trial heart disease prevention study and the pilot studies for the Women's Health Initiative[26,27] indicates this may be difficult. Moreover, the necessary duration for such a trial is not known; much evidence suggests that factors acting from childhood through postmenopausal years can influence breast cancer risk. Because trials of cancer prevention require tens of thousands of subjects to be randomized and the costs of instruction in dietary change is high, such studies are extremely expensive; for example, the Women's Health Initiative will cost well over half a billion dollars.[26]

Since 1985 information on fat intake and cancer has grown rapidly and will continue to accrue exponentially as the populations of ongoing cohort studies age and as recently started cohort studies begin to report their findings. In the following sections, current data on the relation of fat intake to cancers of the breast, colon, and prostate are briefly reviewed as these are the cancers for which the current evidence is most abundant.

FAT AND BREAST CANCER

Breast cancer is the most frequent malignancy among women in Western countries, and incidence rates have been increasing for decades.[28,29] Rates in most parts of Asia, South America, and Africa have been only approximately one-fifth as high as that of the United States,[30,31] but in almost all these areas rates of breast cancer are also increasing. Populations that migrate from low- to high-incidence countries develop breast cancer rates that approximate those of the new host country.[32,33] However, among Japanese immigrants to the United States, not until the second or third generation do rates approach those of the general U.S. population.[34] This slower rate of change for Japanese immigrants may indicate delayed acculturation, although a similar delay in increase is not observed for colon cancer.

A major rationale for the dietary fat hypothesis has been the international correlation between fat consumption and national breast cancer mortality.[15] However, in a study of 65 Chinese counties,[35] in which both dietary assessment and mortality were measured using standardized methods, and per capita fat intake varied from 6% to 25% of energy, only a weak positive association was seen between fat intake and breast cancer mortality. Notably, four counties consumed approximately 25% of energy from fat, yet experienced rates of breast cancer far below those of U.S. women with similar fat intake,[24] thus providing strong evidence that factors other than fat intake account for the large international differences.

Breast cancer incidence rates increased substantially in the United States during the twentieth century, as have the estimates of per capita fat consumption based on food disappearance data.

However, surveys based on reports of individual actual intake, rather than food disappearance, indicate that consumption of energy from fat, either as absolute intake or as a percentage of energy, has actually declined in the last several decades,[36,37] a time during which breast cancer incidence has increased.[38]

CASE-CONTROL STUDIES

A number of case-control studies have been performed to investigate the dietary fat effect on breast cancer. The largest study so far is that of Graham et al.,[39] who used a food frequency questionnaire to compare the fat intake of 2024 women with breast cancer with that reported by 1463 women controls entering the hospital with benign conditions. Both animal fat and total fat intake were essentially identical in the two groups. The results from 12 smaller case-control studies have been summarized in a metaanalysis by Howe et al.,[40] which included 4312 cases and 5978 controls. The pooled relative risk was 1.35 ($P < .0001$) for a 100-g increase in daily total fat intake, although the risk was somewhat stronger for postmenopausal women (relative risk = 1.48; $P < .001$). This magnitude of association, however, could potentially be compatible with biases due to recall of diet or the selection of controls.[41]

COHORT STUDIES

A substantial body of data from cohort studies is now available to assess the relation between dietary fat intake and breast cancer in developed countries. Because of the prospective design, most of the methodologic biases of case-control studies are avoided. In a pooled analysis of the seven prospective studies with more than 200 cases of breast cancer, which included 337,000 women who developed 4980 incident cases of breast cancer,[25] no overall association was seen for fat intake over the range of less than 20% to greater than 45% of energy (Fig. 23.1-1). A similar lack of association was seen among postmenopausal women only and for specific types of fat. Only among the small number of women consuming less than 15% of energy from fat was a significant association seen; breast cancer risk was elevated twofold in this group. An update of the Nurses' Health Study included 14 years of follow-up, during which 2956 women developed breast cancer.[42] Because repeated assessments of diet were obtained at 2- to

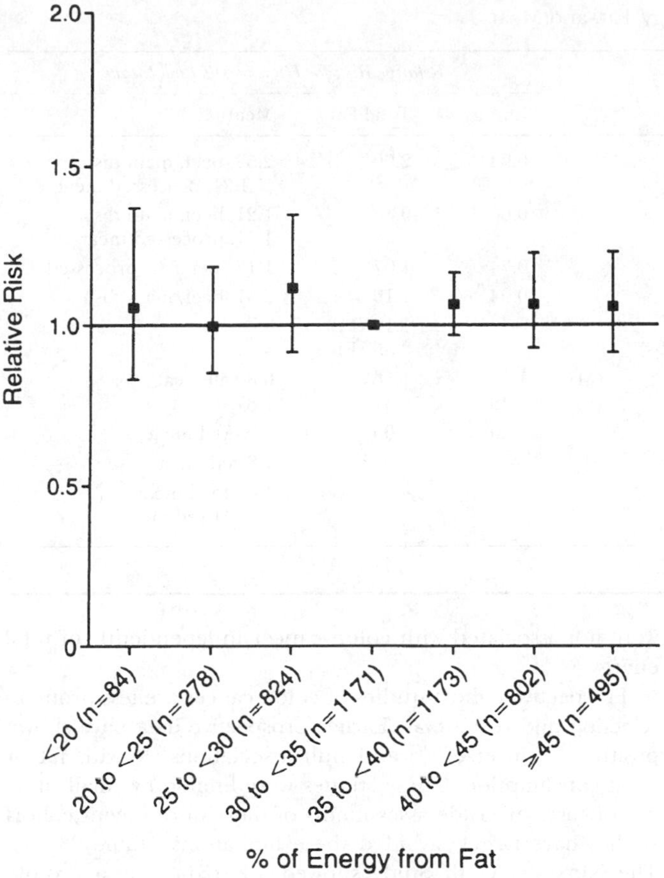

FIGURE 23.1-1. Pooled relative risks and 95% confidence intervals for various levels of energy from fat. A level of 30% to less than 35% of total energy from fat was designated as the reference category. (From ref. 25, with permission.)

4-year intervals, this provided a particularly detailed evaluation of the fat intake over an extended period in relation to breast cancer risk. For total fat intake, the overall association was weakly inverse and statistically significant. There was no suggestion of any reduction in risk at intakes below 25% of energy. These cohort findings therefore do not support the hypothesis that dietary fat is an important cause of breast cancer.

Estrogen level in blood has now been established as a factor for breast cancer.[43] Thus, the effects of fat and other dietary factors on estrogen levels are of potential interest. Vegetarian women, who consume higher amounts of fiber and lower amounts of fat, have lower blood levels and reduced urinary excretion of estrogens, apparently due to increased fecal excretion.[44] A metaanalysis has suggested that reduction in dietary fat may reduce plasma estrogen levels,[45] but the studies included were plagued by the lack of concurrent controls, short duration, and confounding by negative energy balance.[46] In a large randomized trial among postmenopausal women with a previous diagnosis of breast cancer, reduction in dietary fat did not affect estradiol levels when appropriately analyzed.[47,48]

DIFFERENT TYPES OF FAT

In animal mammary tumor models, the tumor-promoting effect of fat intake has been observed primarily for polyunsaturated fats when fed in the presence of high-fat diets containing approximately 45% of energy.[6,49,50] In a metaanalysis of animal studies, monosaturated fat had no significant effect on mammary carcinogenesis, and the effect of saturated fat was weak.[6]

In several prospective cohort studies, an inverse association between monounsaturated fat and breast cancer has been present.[24,51] This is an intriguing observation because of the relatively low rates of breast cancer in Southern European countries with high intakes of monounsaturated fats due to the use of olive oil as the primary fat. In case-control studies in Spain, Greece, and Italy, women who used more olive oil had reduced risks of breast cancer.[52–54] Also, olive oil has been protective relative to other sources of fats in several animal studies.[5,6] Further examination is needed of the hypothesis that monounsaturated fats, and perhaps olive oil in particular, may protect against breast cancer.

FAT AND AGE AT PUBERTY

An earlier age at menarche is an established risk factor for breast cancer. Although the relative risks associated with early menarche are generally modest, usually less than approximately 1.5 for the earliest compared with the latest age groups within a population, this is likely to be due to the limited range of age at menarche within a population. For example, in the United States, the average age is between 12 and 13 years,[55] but in rural China the typical age is approximately 17 to 18 years.[56] Further, the average age at menarche has been declining worldwide for the last 200 years,[55] thus suggesting that increasing breast cancer rates that occur with increasing industrialization are in part due to a decreasing average age at menarche.

For this reason, nutritional factors that influence age at menarche are of particular interest. Nutritional factors have been examined as potential predictors of age at menarche in several prospective cohort studies. Body mass index, height, and weight have consistently been strong determinants of age at menstruation.[57–59] In the United States,[57] as well as in the Canadian cohorts,[59] no association was found between the fat composition of the diet and occurrence of menarche, but a suggestion of earlier onset with higher fat intake was seen in the German study.[58] Collectively, these studies provide strong evidence that rapid growth rates before puberty play an important role in determining future risk of breast cancer, but that overall energy balance rather than fat intake is most important.

FAT AND BREAST CANCER SURVIVAL

High intake of dietary fat has been hypothesized to affect survival adversely in patients with breast cancer, in part because of observations that, adjusted for stage, survival is lower in the United States than in Japan.[60] However, obesity has often been associated with adverse survival from breast cancer, which provides an alternative hypothesis as Japanese women tend to be substantially leaner than U.S. women, and other dietary and lifestyle factors have differed substantially between the United States and Japan.

At present, studies of dietary fat intake and survival from breast cancer are few and have substantial limitations. Most were not specifically designed for this purpose, but instead are based on the follow-up of the control series of case-control or cohort studies of breast cancer incidence. Thus, they usually

TABLE 23.1-1. Large Prospective Studies of Colon Cancer: Energy, Fat, and Meat

				Relative Risk for High versus Low Intake		
	Population	*Cases*		Energy	Total Fat	Meat
Willett et al., 1990[99]	88,751 U.S. women	150		0.94	2.00	2.52, beef, main dish; 1.21, processed meat
Bostick et al., 1994[101]	35,215 U.S. women	212		0.60	0.88	1.21, beef, main dish 1.51, processed meat
Goldbohm et al., 1994[100]	120,852 Dutch men and women	215		0.74	1.07	1.17 (per s.d.) processed
Giovannucci et al., 1994[102]	47,949 U.S. men	205		0.94	1.19	3.57, beef, main dish
Thun et al., 1992[103]	764,343 U.S. men and women	1150 (deaths)		—	1.14 (M) 0.85 (F)	— —
Gaard et al., 1996[134]	50,535 Norwegian men and women	143	(M) (F)	1.13 1.49	1.16 0.47	0.80 all meat 1.87
Kato et al., 1997[135]	14,727 New York women	100		1.20	1.05	1.23 red meat
Hsing et al., 1998[136]	17,633 Minnesota men	120		—	—	1.8 red meat
Singh and Fraser, 1998[137]	32,051 Adventist men and women	157		—	—	1.85 total meat; 1.41 red meat

F, female; M, male.

refer to premorbid diet assessed either before or at about the time of diagnosis rather than to diet after diagnosis and, moreover, most studies have been small in terms of the failure end points. Mixed results have been seen in the published work; positive associations have been seen in several studies,[61–66] but not in others.[67–70] In a report from the Nurses' Health Study,[71] fat intake after diagnosis was not significantly associated with survival, but a modest effect could not be excluded. Unexpectedly, higher protein intake was associated with improved survival. A randomized trial has been started to evaluate the effect of a diet low in fat (15% of energy from fat is the dietary goal) on survival of breast cancer patients.[72]

FAT AND COLON CANCER

In comparisons among countries, rates of colon cancer are strongly correlated with national per capita disappearance of animal fat and meat, with correlation coefficients ranging between 0.8 and 0.9.[15,17] Rates of colon cancer rose sharply in Japan after World War II, paralleling a 2.5-fold increase in fat.[31] Based on these epidemiologic investigations and animal studies, a hypothesis has developed that dietary fat increases excretion of bile acids, which can be converted to carcinogens or promoters.[73] However, more recent evidence from many studies that obesity and low levels of physical activity increase risk of colon cancer risk means that at least part of the high rates in affluent countries previously attributed to fat intake are probably due to sedentary lifestyle.

With some exceptions,[74–77] case-control studies have generally shown an association between risk of colon cancer and intake of fat[78–85] or red meat.[86–91] However, in many of these studies, a positive association between total energy intake and risk of colon cancer has also been observed,[78–82,84,85] raising the question of whether it is general overconsumption of food or the fat composition of the diet that is etiologically important. A metaanalysis by Howe of 13 case-control studies found a significant association between total energy and colon cancer, but saturated, monounsaturated, and polyunsaturated fat were not associated with colon cancer independently of total energy.[92]

Prospective cohort studies of colon cancer are less prone to selection and recall bias. Earlier prospective data have shown positive,[93,94] inverse,[95,96] and null associations[97,98] with fat or meat consumption. These studies were limited by small number of cases or crude assessments of diet. More recent cohort studies have largely avoided these limitations (Table 23.1-1). The Nurses' Health Study showed approximately a twofold higher risk of colon cancer among women in the highest compared with those in the lowest quintile of animal fat intake.[99] In a multivariate analysis of these data, which included red meat and animal fat intakes in the same model, red meat intake remained significantly predictive of risk of colon cancer, whereas the association with animal fat was eliminated. A cohort study from the Netherlands showed a significant direct association between intake of processed meats and risk of colon cancer, but no relationship was observed for fresh meats or overall fat intake.[100] A cohort study in Iowa women also found a direct association with processed meats, although this was not statistically significant.[101] Among a large cohort study of men, a direct association between red meat consumption and risk of colon cancer was seen, but no association was observed with other sources of fat.[102] In this study, no overall relationship existed between total or saturated fat and colon cancer despite a substantial range in fat intake. A similar association was noted for colorectal adenomas in the same cohort of men.[73] In the large American Cancer Society Cohort,[103] little relation was seen between either meat or fat intake and mortality caused by colon cancer, but the dietary questionnaire was brief and of uncertain validity. As noted in Table 23.1-1, other cohort studies have also failed to support an association with fat intake, even though positive associations with red meat were usually observed.

The apparently stronger association with red meat compared with fat intake in most recent cohort studies needs further confirmation, but could result if the fatty acids or nonfat components of meat (e.g., the heme iron or carcinogens created by cooking) were the primary etiologic factors. This issue

TABLE 23.1-2. Prospective Studies of Dietary Fat and Prostate Cancer Risk

			Relative Risk for High versus Low Intake	
Study	*Population*	*Cases*	Total Fat	Saturated Fat
Severson et al., 1989[116]	8000	174	0.9	1.0
Mills et al., 1989[117]	14,000	180	—	1.4 (animal fat)
Giovannucci et al., 1993[118]	52,000	126 (aggressive cases)	1.8	1.6
Le Marchand et al., 1994[119]	20,316	198	—	1.6 (animal fat)

does have major practical implications as current dietary recommendations[104] support the daily consumption of red meat as long as it is lean. Virtually no data exist on the relation of dietary fat to survival from colon cancer.

FAT AND PROSTATE CANCER

Consumption of animal fat, but not vegetable fat, is strongly correlated with prostate cancer mortality internationally.[15] Associations with fat intake have been seen in many case-control studies,[105–114] but sometimes only in subgroups. In a large case-control study among various ethnic groups within the United States,[115] consistent associations with prostate cancer risk were seen for saturated fat, but not with other types of fat.

The association between fat intake and prostate cancer risk has been assessed in only a few cohort studies (Table 23.1-2). In a cohort of 8000 Japanese men living in Hawaii, no association was seen between intake of total or unsaturated fat.[116] However, diet was assessed with a single 24-hour recall in this study so the lack of association may not be informative. In a study of 14,000 Seventh-Day Adventist men living in California, a positive association between the percentage of calories from animal fat and prostate cancer risk was seen, but this was not statistically significant.[117] More recently, three large prospective studies have been published. In the Health Professionals Follow-up Study of 51,000 men, a positive association was seen with intake of red meat and total and animal fat, which was largely limited to aggressive prostate cancers.[118] No association was seen with vegetable fats. In another cohort from Hawaii, increased risks of prostate cancer were seen with consumption of beef and animal fat.[119] In contrast, no relation was seen between intakes of either total or saturated fat and incidence of prostate cancer in a large Dutch cohort.[120]

Although further data are desirable, the evidence from international correlations, case-control, and cohort studies provides some support for an association between consumption of fat-containing animal products and prostate cancer incidence. This evidence does not generally support a relation with intake of vegetable fat, which suggests that either the type of fat or other components of animal products are responsible. Some evidence also suggests that animal fat consumption may be most strongly associated with aggressive prostate cancer, which suggests an influence on the transition from the widespread indolent form to the more lethal form of this malignancy. No data are available on fat intake in relation to the probability of survival after the diagnosis of prostate cancer.

OTHER CANCERS

Rates of other cancers that are common in affluent countries, including those of the endometrium and ovary, are, of course, also correlated with fat intake internationally. Although these have been studied in a small number of case-control investigations, consistent associations with fat intake have not been seen.[121–130] In a prospective study among Iowa women,[131] no evidence of a relation between fat intake and risk of endometrial cancer was observed. Positive associations have been hypothesized between fat intake and risks of skin cancer[132] and lung cancer, but relevant data in humans are limited.

SUMMARY

Based largely on the results of animal studies, international correlations, and a few case-control studies, great enthusiasm developed in the 1980s that modest reductions in fat intake would have a major effect on breast cancer incidence. However, as the findings from large prospective studies have become available, support for this relationship has weakened considerably. For colon cancer, the associations seen with animal fat internationally have been supported in numerous case-control and cohort studies. However, more recent evidence has suggested that this might be explained by factors in red meat other than simply its fat content. Further, the importance of physical activity and leanness as protective factors against colon cancer indicates that international correlations probably overstate the contribution of diet to differences in colon cancer incidence. At present, the available evidence most strongly suggests an association between animal fat consumption and risk of prostate cancer, particularly the aggressive form of this disease. As with colon cancer, the possibility remains that other factors in animal products contribute to risk.

Despite the large body of data on dietary fat and cancer that has accumulated since 1985, any conclusions should be regarded as tentative because we are dealing with disease processes that are poorly understood, but that are likely to take many decades to develop. As almost all of the reported literature from prospective studies is based on less than 15 years of follow-up, further evaluation of the effects of diet earlier in life and at longer intervals of observation will be needed to understand fully these complex relationships. Nevertheless, persons interested in reducing their risk of cancer could be advised, as a prudent measure, to minimize their intake of foods high in animal fat, particularly red meat. Such a dietary pattern is also likely to be beneficial from the standpoint of cardiovascular disease. On the other hand, unsaturated fats (with the exception of *trans* fatty acids) reduce blood low-density lipoprotein cholesterol levels and risk of cardiovascular disease[133] and little evidence suggests that they adversely affect cancer risk. Thus, efforts to reduce unsaturated fat intake do not appear to be warranted at this time and may have adverse effects on cardiovascular disease. As excess adiposity adversely affects risks of several cancers and cardiovascular disease, balancing calories from any source with adequate physical activity is extremely important.

REFERENCES

1. Committee on Diet Nutrition and Cancer, Assembly of Life Sciences, National Research Council. *Diet, nutrition, and cancer.* Washington, DC: National Academy Press, 1982.
2. U.S. Department of Agriculture, U.S. Department of Health and Human Services. *Nutrition and your health: dietary guidelines for Americans.* Washington, DC: U.S. Government Printing Office, 1995.
3. Tannenbaum A. The genesis and growth of tumors. III. Effects of a high fat diet. *Cancer Res* 1942;2:468.
4. Tannenbaum A, Silverstone H. Nutrition in relation to cancer. *Adv Cancer Res* 1953;1:451.
5. Welsch CW. Relationship between dietary fat and experimental mammary tumorigenesis: a review and critique. *Cancer Res* 1992;52(Suppl 7):2040S.
6. Fay MP, Freedman LS. Meta-analyses of dietary fats and mammary neoplasms in rodent experiments. *Breast Cancer Res Treat* 1997;46:215.
7. Birt DF. Dietary fat and experimental carcinogenesis: a summary of recent in vivo studies. *Adv Exp Med Biol* 1986;206:69.
8. Albanes D. Total calories, body weight, and tumor incidence in mice. *Cancer Res* 1987;47:92.
9. Sonnenschein E, Glickman L, Goldschmidt M, et al. Body conformation, diet, risk of breast cancer in pet dogs: a case-control study. *Am J Epidemiol* 1991;133:694.
10. Appleton BS, Landers RE. Oil gavage effects on tumor incidence in the National Toxicology Program's 2-year carcinogenesis bioassay. *Adv Exp Med Biol* 1986;206:99.
11. Freedman LS, Clifford C, Messina M. Analysis of dietary fat, calories, body weight, and the development of mammary tumors in rats and mice: a review. *Cancer Res* 1990;50:5710.
12. Ip C. Quantitative assessment of fat and calorie as risk factors in mammary carcinogenesis in an experimental model. In: Mettlin CJ, Aoki K, eds. *Recent progress in research on nutrition and cancer.* Proceedings of a workshop sponsored by the International Union Against Cancer, Nagoya, Japan, November 1–3, 1989. New York: Wiley-Liss, 1990:107.
13. Boissonneault GA, Elson CE, Pariza MW. Net energy effects of dietary fat on chemically induced mammary carcinogenesis in F344 rats. *J Natl Cancer Inst* 1986;76:335.
14. Carroll MD, Abraham S, Dresser CM. *Dietary intake source data: United States, 1976–1980.* Series 11. National Center for Health Statistics, 1983.
15. Armstrong B, Doll R. Environmental factors and cancer incidence and mortality in different countries, with special reference to dietary practices. *Int J Cancer* 1975;15:617.
16. Prentice RL, Sheppard L. Dietary fat and cancer. Consistency of the epidemiologic data, and disease prevention that may follow from a practical reduction in fat consumption. *Cancer Causes and Control* 1990;1:81.
17. Rose DP, Boyar AP, Wynder EL. International comparisons of mortality rates for cancer of the breast, ovary, prostate, and colon, and per capita food consumption. *Cancer* 1986;58:2263.
18. Giovannucci E, Ascherio A, Rimm EB, et al. Physical activity, obesity, and risk for colon cancer and adenoma in men. *Ann Intern Med* 1995;122:327.
19. Harris JR, Lippman ME, Veronsei U, et al. Breast cancer. *N Engl J Med* 1992;327:319.
20. Willett WC. *Nutritional epidemiology.* New York: Oxford University Press, 1990.
21. Rimm EB, Giovannucci EL, Stampfer MJ, et al. Reproducibility and validity of an expanded self-administered semiquantitative food frequency questionnaire among male health professionals. *Am J Epidemiol* 1992;135:1114.
22. Pietinen P, Hartman AM, Haapa E, et al. Reproducibility and validity of dietary assessment instruments. I. A self-administered food use questionnaire with a portion size picture booklet. *Am J Epidemiol* 1988,128:655.
23. Block G. A review of validations of dietary assessment methods. *Am J Epidemiol* 1982;115:492.
24. Willett WC, Hunter DJ, Stampfer MJ, et al. Dietary fat and fiber in relation to risk of breast cancer: an 8-year follow-up. *JAMA* 1992;268:2037.
25. Hunter DJ, Spiegelman D, Adami HO, et al. Cohort studies of fat intake and the risk of breast cancer: a pooled analysis. *N Engl J Med* 1996;334:356.
26. Michels KB, Willett WC. The Women's Health Initiative: daughter of politics or science? *Principles and Practices of Oncology* 1992;6:1.
27. Multiple Risk Factor Intervention Trial Research Group. Multiple Risk Factor Intervention Trial: risk factor changes and mortality results. *JAMA* 1982;248:1465.
28. Sondik EJ. Breast cancer trends—incidence, mortality, and survival. *Cancer* 1994;74 (Suppl S):995.
29. Garfinkel L, Boring CC, Heater CW. Changing trends—an overview of breast cancer incidence and mortality. *Cancer* 1994;74(Suppl s):222.
30. Anonymous. Cancer incidence on five continents. In: *International Agency for Research on Cancer.* Lyon, France: IARC Scientific, 1987;5:882.
31. Aoki K, Hayakawa N, Kurihara M, et al. Death rates for malignant neoplasms for selected sites by sex and five-year age group in 33 countries, 1953–57 to 1983–87. International Union Against Cancer. Nagoya, Japan: University of Nagoya Coop Press, 1992.
32. Staszewski J, Haenszel W. Cancer mortality among the Polish-born in the United States. *J Natl Cancer Inst* 1965;35:291.
33. Adelstein AM, Staszewski J, Muir CS. Cancer mortality in 1970–1972 among Polish-born migrants to England and Wales. *Br J Cancer* 1979;40:464.
34. Buell P. Changing incidence of breast cancer in Japanese-American women. *J Natl Cancer Inst* 1973;51:1479.
35. Marshall JR, Qu Y, Chen J, et al. Additional ecological evidence: lipids and breast cancer mortality among women aged 55 and over in China. *Eur J Cancer* 1992;28A:1720.
36. Stephen AM, Wald NJ. Trends in individual consumption of dietary fat in the United States, 1920–1984. *Am J Clin Nutr* 1990;52:457.
37. McDowell MA, Briefel RR, Alaimo K, et al. *Energy and macronutrient intakes of persons ages 2 months and over in the United States*: third national health and nutrition examination survey, phase I 1988–1991. National Center for Health Statistics, Centers for Disease Control, Public Health Service, U.S. Department of Health and Human Services, Hyattsville, MD, 1994.
38. American Cancer Society. *Cancer facts and figures.* Atlanta, GA: American Cancer Society, 1994.
39. Graham S, Marshall J, Mettlin C, et al. Diet in the epidemiology of breast cancer. *Am J Epidemiol* 1982;116:68.
40. Howe GR, Hirohata T, Hislop TG, et al. Dietary factors and risk of breast cancer: combined analysis of 12 case-control studies. *J Natl Cancer Inst* 1990;82:561.
41. Giovannucci E, Stampfer MJ, Colditz GA, et al. A comparison of prospective and retrospective assessments of diet in the study of breast cancer. *Am J Epidemiol* 1993;137:502.
42. Holmes MD, Hunter DJ, Colditz GA, et al. Association of dietary intake of fat and fatty acids with risk of breast cancer. *JAMA* 1999;281:914.
43. Hankinson SE, Willett WC, Manson JE, et al. Plasma sex steriod hormone levels and risk of breast cancer in postmenopausal women. *J Natl Cancer Inst* 1998;90:1292.
44. Goldin BR, Aldercreutz H, Gorbach SL, et al. Estrogen excretion patterns and plasma levels in vegetarian and omnivorous women. *N Engl J Med* 1982;307:1542.
45. Wu AH, Pike MC, Stram DO. Meta-analysis: dietary fat intake, serum estrogen levels, and the risk of breast cancer. *J Natl Cancer Inst* 1999;91:529.
46. Holmes MD, Schisterman EF, Spiegelman D, et al. Re: Meta-analysis: dietary fat intake, serum estrogen levels, and the risk of breast cancer [Letter]. *J Natl Cancer Inst* 1999;91:1511.
47. Rose DP, Connolly JM, Chlebowski RT, et al. The effects of a low fat dietary intervention and tamoxifen adjuvant therapy on the serum estrogen and sex hormone-binding globulin concentrations of postmenopausal breast cancer patients. *Breast Cancer Res Treat* 1993;27:253.
48. Willett WC. Dietary fat and breast cancer. *Nutritional epidemiology.* 2nd ed. New York: Oxford Press, 1998.
49. Hopkins GJ, Carroll KK. Relationship between amount and type of dietary fat in promotion of mammary carcinogenesis induced by 7,12-dimethylbenz (a) anthracene. *J Natl Cancer Inst* 1979;62:1009.
50. Hopkins GJ, Kennedy TG, Carroll KK. Polyunsaturated fatty acids as promoters of mammary carcinogenesis induced Sprague-Dawley rats by 7,12 dimethylbenz[a]anthracene. *J Natl Cancer Inst* 1981;66:517.
51. Wolk A, Bergstrom R, Hunter D, et al. A prospective study of association of monounsaturated and other types of fat with risk of breast cancer. *Arch Intern Med* 1998;158:41.
52. Martin-Moreno JM, Willett WC, Gorgojo L, et al. Dietary fat, olive oil intake and breast cancer risk. *Int J Cancer* 1994;58:774.
53. Trichopoulou A, Katsouyanni K, Stuver S, et al. Consumption of olive oil and specific food groups in relation to breast cancer risk in Greece. *J Natl Cancer Inst* 1995;87:110.
54. La Vecchia C, Negri E, Franceschi S, et al. Olive oil, other dietary fats, and the risk of breast cancer (Italy). *Cancer Causes Control* 1995;6:545.
55. Wyshak G, Frisch RE. Evidence for a secular trend in age of menarche. *N Engl J Med* 1982;306:1033.
56. Chen J, Campbell TC, Junyao L, et al. Diet, life-style, and mortality in China: a study of the characteristics of 65 Chinese counties. Oxford, England: Oxford University Press, 1990.
57. Maclure M, Travis LB, Willett WC, et al. A prospective cohort study of nutrient intake and age at menarche. *Am J Clin Nutr* 1991;54:649.
58. Merzenich H, Boeing H, Wahrendorf J. Dietary fat and sports activity as determinants for age at menarche. *Am J Epidemiol* 1993;138:217.
59. Moisan J, Meyer F, Gingras S. Diet and age at menarche. *Cancer Causes Control* 1990;1:149.
60. Chlebowski RT, Rose D, Buzzard IM, et al. Adjuvant dietary fat intake reduction in postmenopausal breast cancer patient management. The Women's Intervention Nutrition Study (WINS). *Breast Cancer Res Treat* 1992;20:73.
61. Nomura AMY, Marchand LL, Kolonel LN, et al. The effect of dietary fat on breast cancer survival among Caucasian and Japanese women in Hawaii. *Breast Cancer Res Treat* 1991;18:S135.
62. Gregorio DI, Emrich LJ, Graham S, et al. Dietary fat consumption and survival among women with breast cancer. *J Natl Cancer Inst* 1985;75:37.
63. Verreault R, Brisson J, Deschenes L, et al. Dietary fat in relation to prognostic indicators in breast cancer. *J Natl Cancer Inst* 1988;80:819.
64. Holm LE, Nordevang E, Hjalmar ML, et al. Treatment failure and dietary habits in women with breast cancer. *J Natl Cancer Inst* 1993;85:32.
65. Jain M, Miller AB, To T. Premorbid diet and the prognosis of women with breast cancer. *J Natl Cancer Inst* 1994;86:1390.
66. Zhang S, Folsom AR, Sellers TA, et al. Better breast cancer survival for postmenopausal women who are less overweight and eat less fat. *Cancer* 1995;76:275.

67. Newman SC, Miller AB, Howe GR. A study of the effect of weight and dietary fat on breast cancer survival time. *Am J Epidemiol* 1986;123:767.
68. Rohan TE, Hiller JE, McMichael AJ. Dietary factors and survival from breast cancer. *Nutr Cancer* 1993;20:167.
69. Ewertz M, Gillanders S, Meyer L, et al. Survival of breast cancer patients in relation to factors which affect the risk of developing breast cancer. *Int J Cancer* 1991;49:526.
70. Kyogoku S, Hirohata T, Nomura Y, et al. Diet and prognosis of breast cancer. *Nutr Cancer* 1992;17:271.
71. Holmes MD, Stampfer MJ, Colditz GA, et al. Dietary factors and the survival of women with breast carcinoma. *Cancer* 1999;86:826.
72. Chlebowski RT, Blackburn GL, Buzzard IM, et al. Adherence to a dietary fat intake reduction program in postmenopausal women receiving therapy for early breast cancer—the Women's Intervention Nutrition Study. *J Clin Oncol* 1993;11:2072.
73. Giovannucci E, Stampfer MJ, Colditz GA, et al. Relationship of diet to risk of colorectal adenoma in men. *J Natl Cancer Inst* 1992;84:91.
74. Macquart-Moulin G, Riboli E, Cornee J, et al. Case-control study on colorectal cancer and diet in Marseilles. *Int J Cancer* 1986;38:183.
75. Berta JL, Coste T, Rautureau J, et al. Diet and rectocolonic cancers. Results of a case-control study. *Gastroenterol Clin Biol* 1985;9:348.
76. Tuyus AJ, Haelterrnan M, Kaaks R. Colorectal cancer and the intake of nutrients: oligosaccharides are a risk factor, fats are not. A case-control study in Belgium. *Nutr Cancer* 1987;10:181.
77. Meyer F, White E. Alcohol and nutrients in relation to colon cancer in middle-aged adults. *Am J Epidemiol* 1993;138:225.
78. Jain M, Cook GM, Davis FG, et al. A case-control study of diet and colo-rectal cancer. *Int J Cancer* 1980;26:757.
79. Potter JD, McMichael AJ. Diet and cancer of the colon and rectum: a case-control study. *J Natl Cancer Inst* 1986;76:557.
80. Lyon JL, Mahoney AW, West DW, et al. Energy intake: its relationship to colon cancer risk. *J Natl Cancer Inst* 1987;78:853.
81. Graham S, Marshall J, Haughey B, et al. Dietary epidemiology of cancer of the colon in western New York. *Am J Epidemiol* 1988;128:490.
82. Bristol JB, Emmett PM, Heaton KW, et al. Sugar, fat, and the risk of colorectal cancer. *BMJ (Clin Res Ed)* 1985;291:1467.
83. Kune GA, Kune S, Watson LF. The nutritional causes of colorectal cancer: an introduction to the Melbourne Study. *Nutr Cancer* 1987;9:5.
84. West DW, Slattery ML, Robison LM, et al. Dietary intake and colon cancer: sex- and anatomic site-specific associations. *Am J Epidemiol* 1989;130:883.
85. Peters RK, Pike MC, Garabrandt D, et al. Diet and colon cancer in Los Angeles County, California. *Cancer Causes Control* 1992;3:457.
86. Manousos O, Day NE, Trichopoulos D, et al. Diet and colorectal cancer: a case-control study in Greece. *Int J Cancer* 1983;32:1.
87. La Vecchia C, Negri E, Decarli A, et al. A case-control study of diet and colo-rectal cancer in northern Italy. *Int J Cancer* 1988;41:492.
88. Miller AB, Howe GR, Jain M, et al. Food items and food groups as risk factors in a case-control study of diet and colo-rectal cancer. *Int J Cancer* 1983;32:155.
89. Young TB, Wolf DA. Case-control study of proximal and distal colon cancer and diet in Wisconsin. *Int J Cancer* 1988;42:167.
90. Benito E, Obrador A, Stiggelbout A, et al. A population-based case-control study of colorectal cancer in Majorca. I. Dietary factors. *Int J Cancer* 1990,45:69.
91. Lee HP, Gourley L, Duffy SW, et al. Colorectal cancer and diet in an Asian population—a case-control study among Singapore Chinese. *Int J Cancer* 1989;43:1007.
92. Howe GR. Meeting Presentation. *Advances in the biology and therapy of colorectal cancer.* M.D. Anderson's Thirty-seventh Annual Clinical Conference. M.D. Anderson Cancer Center, Houston, TX, 1993.
93. Gerhardsson M, Floderus B, Norell SE. Physical activity and colon cancer risk. *Int J Epidemiol* 1988;17:743.
94. Bjelke E. Epidemiology of colorectal cancer, with emphasis on diet. In: Davis W, Harrup KR, Stathopoulos G, eds. *Human cancer. Its characterization and treatment.* Amsterdam, Congress Series No. 484: Exerpta Medica, 1980:158.
95. Stemmermann GN, Nomura AM, Heilbrun LK. Dietary fat and the risk of colorectal cancer. *Cancer Res* 1984;44:4633.
96. Hirayama T. A large-scale study on cancer risks by diet—with special reference to the risk reducing effects of green-yellow vegetable consumption. In: Hayashi Y, Magao M, Sugimura T, et al., eds. *Diet, nutrition, and cancer.* Tokyo: Japan Scientific Societies Press, 1986:41.
97. Garland C, Shekelle RB, Barrett-Conner E, et al. Dietary vitamin D and calcium and risk of colorectal cancer: a 19-year prospective study in men. *Lancet* 1985;1:307.
98. Phillips RL, Snowdon DA. Association of meat and coffee use with cancers of the large bowel, breast, and prostate among Seventh-Day Adventists: preliminary results. *Cancer Res* 1983;43(Suppl):2403S.
99. Willett WC, Stampfer MJ, Colditz GA, et al. Relation of meat, fat, and fiber intake to the risk of colon cancer in a prospective study among women. *N Engl J Med* 1990;323:1664.
100. Goldbohm RA, van den Brandt PA, vans Veer P, et al. A prospective cohort study on the relation between meat consumption and the risk of colon cancer. *Cancer Res* 1994;54:718.
101. Bostick RM, Potter JD, Kushi LH, et al. Sugar, meat, and fat intake, and non-dietary risk factors for colon cancer incidence in Iowa women (United States). *Cancer Causes Control* 1994;5:38.
102. Giovannucci E, Rimm EB, Stampfer MJ, et al. Intake of fat, meat, and fiber in relation to risk of colon cancer in men. *Cancer Res* 1994;54:2390.
103. Thun MJ, Calle EE, Namboodiri MM, et al. Risk factors for fatal colon cancer in a large prospective study. *J Natl Cancer Inst* 1992;84:1491.
104. U.S. Department of Agriculture. The food guide pyramid. *Home and Garden Bulletin* 252. Washington, DC: Government Printing Office, 1992:30.
105. Talamini R, La Vecchia C, Decarli A, et al. Nutrition, social factors, and prostatic cancer in a Northern Italian population. *Br J Cancer* 1986;53:817.
106. Rotkin ID. Studies in the epidemiology of prostatic cancer: expanded sampling. *Cancer Treat Rep* 1977;61:173.
107. Mishina T, Watanabe H, Araki H, et al. Epidemiological study of prostate cancer by matched-pair analysis. *Prostate* 1985;6:423.
108. Talamini R, Franceschi S, La Vecchia C, et al. Diet and prostatic cancer: a case-control study in Northern Italy. *Nutr Cancer* 1992;18:277.
109. Schuman LM, Mandel JS, Radke A, et al. Some selected features of the epidemiology of prostatic cancer: Minneapolis-St. Paul, Minnesota case-control study, 1976–1979. In: Magnus K, ed. *Trends in cancer incidence: causes and practical implications.* Washington, DC: Hemisphere Publishing, 1982:345.
110. Graham S, Haughey B, Marshall J, et al. Diet in the epidemiology of carcinoma of the prostate gland. *J Natl Cancer Inst* 1983;70:687.
111. Ross RK, Shimizu H, Paganini-Hill A, et al. Case-control studies of prostate cancer in Blacks and Whites in Southern California. *J Natl Cancer Inst* 1987;78:869.
112. West DW, Slattery ML, Robison LM, et al. Adult dietary intake and prostate cancer risk in Utah: a case-control study with special emphasis on aggressive tumors. *Cancer Causes Control* 1991;2:85.
113. Kolonel LN, Yoshizawa CN, Hankin JH. Diet and prostatic cancer: a case-control study in Hawaii. *Am J Epidemiol* 1988;127:999.
114. Heshmat MY, Kaul L, Kovi J, et al. Nutrition and prostate cancer: a case-control study. *Prostate* 1985;6:7.
115. Whittemore AS, Kolonel LN, Wu AH, et al. Prostate cancer in relation to diet, physical activity, and body size in blacks, whites, and Asians in the United States and Canada. *Natl Cancer Inst* 1995;87:652.
116. Severson RK, Nomura AMY, Grove JS, et al. A prospective study—demographics, diet, and prostate cancer among men of Japanese ancestry in Hawaii. *Cancer Res* 1989;49:1857.
117. Mills PK, Beeson WL, Phillips RL, et al. Cohort study of diet, lifestyle, and prostate cancer in Adventist men. *Cancer* 1989;64:598.
118. Giovannucci E, Rimm EB, Colditz GA, et al. A prospective study of dietary fat and risk of prostate cancer. *J Natl Cancer Inst* 1993;85:1571.
119. Le Marchand L, Kolonel LN, Wilkens LR, et al. Animal fat consumption and prostate cancer: a prospective study in Hawaii. *Epidemiology* 1994;5:276.
120. Schuurman AG. *Association of energy and fat intake with prostate carcinoma risk.* American Cancer Society, 1999:1019.
121. Cramer DW, Welch WR, Hutchison GB, et al. Dietary animal fat in relation to ovarian cancer risk. *Obstet Gynecol* 1984;63:833.
122. La Vecchia C, Decarli A, Negri E, et al. Dietary factors and the risk of epithelial ovarian cancer. *J Natl Cancer Inst* 1987;79:663.
123. Shu XO, Gao YT, Yuan JM, et al. Dietary factors and epithelial ovarian cancer. *Br J Cancer* 1989;59:92.
124. Byers T, Marshall J, Graham S, et al. A case-control study of dietary and nondietary factors in ovarian cancer. *J Natl Cancer Inst* 1983;71:681.
125. Slattery ML, Schuman KL, West DW, et al. Nutrient intake and ovarian cancer. *Am J Epidemiol* 1989;130:497.
126. Risch HA, Jain M, Marrett LD, Howe GR. Dietary fat intake and risk of epithelial ovarian cancer. *J Natl Cancer Inst* 1994;86:1409.
127. Levi F, Franceschi S, Negri E, et al. Dietary factors and the risk of endometrial cancer. *Cancer* 1993;71:3575.
128. Barbone F, Austin H, Partridge EE. Diet and endometrial cancer: a case-control study. *Am J Epidemiol* 1993;137:393.
129. Potischman N, Swanson CA, Brinton LA, et al. Dietary associations in a case-control study of endometrial cancer. *Cancer Causes Control* 1993;4:239.
130. Shu XO, Zheng W, Potischamn N, et al. A population based case-control of dietary factors and endometrial cancer in Shanghai, People's Republic of China. *Am J Epidemiol* 1993;137:155.
131. Zheng W, Kushi LH, Potter JD, et al. Dietary intake of energy and animals foods and endometrial cancer incidence. *Am J Epidemiol* 1995;142:388.
132. Black HS, Herd JA, Goldberg LH, et al. Effect of a low-fat diet on the incidence of actinic keratosis. *N Engl J Med* 1994;330:1272.
133. Willett WC. Diet and coronary heart disease. In: Willett WC, ed. *Nutritional epidemiology.* 2nd ed. New York: Oxford University Press, 1998.
134. Gaard M, Tretli S, Løken EB. Dietary factors and risk of colon cancer: a prospective study of 50,535 young Norwegian men and women. *Eur J Cancer Prev* 1996;5:445.
135. Kato I, Akhmedkhanov A, Koenig K, et al. Prospective study of diet and female colorectal cancer: the New York University Women's Health Study. *Nutr Cancer* 1997;28:276.
136. Hsing AW, McLaughlin JK, Chow W-H, et al. Risk factors for colorectal cancer in a prospective study among U.S. white men. *Int J Cancer* 1998;77:549.
137. Singh PN, Fraser GE. Dietary risk factors for colon cancer in a low-risk population. *Am J Epidemiol* 1998;148:761.

SECTION 2

PETER GREENWALD

Dietary Fibers

The hypothesis linking high intakes of dietary fiber with reduced risk of colorectal cancer in humans was advanced in the early 1970s by Burkitt, who observed that certain chronic diseases common to westernized societies, including colon cancer, diverticular disease, gallstones, and ischemic heart disease, were rare among African populations whose diets consisted predominantly of high-fiber foods.[1] Since that time, a compelling body of epidemiologic evidence, experimental data, and clinical research has found that diets high in fiber, grains, cereals, and fresh vegetables and fruits are associated with reduced risk of several cancers, including cancers of the colon, rectum, and breast, and possibly with lowered risk for additional cancers of the alimentary canal (mouth, esophagus, pharynx, stomach) and other hormone-sensitive cancers (ovarian, endometrial, and prostate cancers).[2–9]

Despite a substantial body of research suggesting that diets high in fiber-rich foods protect against certain cancers, results from epidemiologic and animal studies investigating the effect of dietary fiber on cancer risk are not entirely consistent.[6,9–12] The type or source of fiber consumed, temporal nature of consumption (current versus past intake), overall eating patterns, familial predisposition to certain cancers, cancer site, and other nutrients found in high-fiber foods (e.g., folate; antioxidants such as vitamins C and E and selenium; and phytochemicals such as carotenoids, phytoestrogens, organosulfides, and isothiocyanates) may all influence cancer risk.[5,8,10,13] Also at issue are the complexities of fiber and the lack of standardized analytical methods for extracting and quantifying the fiber content of food; the differential effects of the various types of fiber on gut physiology; the effect of storage, processing, and food preparation on the physical and chemical nature of fiber; the lack of comprehensive food composition data on types of dietary fiber and total fiber; and problems with dietary assessment methods, such as recall bias.[14,15] Inconsistencies in animal studies may be related to the species and strain of animal used; the type (i.e., an initiator versus promoter) and amount of carcinogen administered; the type and amount of fiber; the overall composition of the animal's diet; the timing of administration of fiber, in relation to the carcinogenic process; and the length of the study.[16]

SOURCES AND TYPES OF DIETARY FIBER

Dietary fiber is a heterogeneous mixture of complex, plant-based carbohydrates that are resistant to digestion by human intestinal enzymes. High-fiber foods include whole grains, vegetables, fruits, beans, nuts, and seeds (Table 23.2-1). The skins of many vegetables and fruits and the bran layers of grains also are good sources of fiber. Components of dietary fiber in plant foods vary with plant species, stages of maturity, and parts of the plant. Further, although one or two types of fiber may predominate in a particular food, most plants contain a variety of fiber types or components. Grains, roots, green leafy vegetables, legumes, and some fruits such as apples contain high levels of cellulose and hemicelluloses. Another component of fiber, lignin, is found in the walls of plant cells and increases as the plant matures. Most fruits contain pectin, but citrus fruits and apples contain the highest amounts of this fiber component.

The two primary types of fiber are categorized as soluble and insoluble, according to their degree of solubility in water.[5,17] Fibers also are described in terms of their fermentability characteristics (Table 23.2-2). Soluble fibers attract water, form a gel during digestion, and generally are fermentable. Insoluble fibers, in contrast, are insoluble in water and usually are nonfermentable. Different types of dietary fibers in commonly consumed plant foods are grouped further according to their chemical structure, as nonstarch polysaccharides and lignin, a polymer of aromatic alcohols. Nonstarch polysaccharide plant fibers include cellulose, hemicelluloses, pectins, gums, mucilages, and other miscellaneous polysaccharides. Soluble, fermentable gel-forming fibers include pectins, gums, starches, some hemicelluloses, and other polysaccharides and are present at the highest levels in fruits, oats, beans, and vegetables. Whole grains and whole-grain foods are primary sources of insoluble, nonfermentable *structural* fibers such as cellulose, most hemicelluloses, and lignins.[5]

The type and characteristics of the fiber contained in different foods influence normal gut activity and appear to have a differential effect on cancer risk, as discussed in the following sections.[5,11,17,18]

DIETARY FIBER AND COLORECTAL CANCER

SUMMARY OF EPIDEMIOLOGIC AND EXPERIMENTAL EVIDENCE

International colon cancer incidence rates vary by a factor of 20 or more, and a large proportion of that difference is believed to be a result of various dietary factors, including certain types of fiber.[8,10] Overall, results of international comparisons and correlation and case-control studies support the hypothesis that high-fiber intakes reduce risk for colorectal cancer. In these studies, total dietary fiber intake and consumption of cereal fiber and whole grains show a consistent reduction in risk for colorectal cancer.[3,7] A metaanalysis of data from 13 case-control studies reported a 50% reduction in risk for colorectal cancer when the highest versus lowest quintiles of fiber intake were compared.[19] Results of prospective cohort studies are mixed, with most showing either only weak protective associations[20,21] or no statistically significant relationship[22,23] between fiber intake and risk of cancers of the colon or rectum. Differences in the findings of these and other epidemiologic studies likely result in part not only from the heterogeneous nature of fiber, the way in which fiber is measured, and the problems associated with collection of dietary intake data, but also with the relatively homogeneous fiber intakes across the study cohorts.[8]

Data from both epidemiologic and basic research studies suggest that the various types of fiber confer a differential effect on colorectal cancer risk. One international study of 20 populations in 12 countries reported a strong inverse relationship between starch consumption and risk for colorectal cancer.[24] Another study found that soluble but not insoluble fiber,

TABLE 23.2-1. Dietary Fiber Content of Commonly Consumed Vegetables, Fruits, and Whole-Grain Products

Foods	*Serving Size*	*Fiber (g)*	*Foods*	*Serving Size*	*Fiber (g)*
VEGETABLES			**FRUITS**		
Beans, with pork and tomato sauce	1/4 cup	4.8	Peaches, dried	5 halves	5.3
Spinach, cooked	1/2 cup	4.0	Raisins, seedless	2/3 cup	5.3
Black-eyed peas, canned	1/2 cup	3.7	Pears, raw	1 fruit	4.3
Butterbeans	1/2 cup	3.7	Strawberries, raw	1 cup	3.9
Sweet potato, canned	1 cup	3.6	Figs, uncooked, dry	2 fruits	3.4
Great Northern beans, canned	1/4 cup	3.5	Blackberries, raw	1/2 cup	3.3
Brussels sprouts, fresh or frozen, cooked	1/2 cup	3.4	Apples, raw with skin	1 medium	3.0
Lima beans, boiled	1/4 cup	3.3	Prunes, dried, stewed, unsweetened	5 prunes	3.0
Peas, green, frozen, boiled	1/2 cup	3.0	Oranges, raw, Valencia	1 medium	2.9
Peas, green, canned	1/2 cup	2.9	Raspberries, raw, red	1/2 cup	2.9
Squash, winter, all varieties, frozen, cooked	1/2 cup	2.9	Papayas, raw	1 medium	2.8
Squash, acorn, baked, cubed	1/2 cup	2.9	Kiwi fruit, raw	1 fruit	2.6
Carrot, raw	1 carrot	2.3	Nectarines, raw	1 fruit	2.2
Potato, baked, flesh	1 medium	2.3	Mango, raw	1 fruit	2.2
Peas, green, boiled	1/2 cup	2.2	Dates, dried	5 dates	2.1
Turnip greens, fresh or frozen, cooked	1/2 cup	2.2	Pineapple, canned, chunks, juice packed	1 cup	1.9
Broccoli, fresh or frozen, cooked	1/2 cup, chopped	2.0	Applesauce, canned, unsweetened	1/2 cup	1.8
Baby lima beans, mature	1/4 cup	1.9	Bananas, raw	1 medium	1.8
Beans, white, cooked	1/4 cup	1.9	Cherries, raw, sweet	1/2 cup	1.8
Lentils, mature seeds, cooked	1/4 cup	1.9	Blueberries, raw	1/2 cup	1.6
Black beans, boiled	1/4 cup	1.8	Peaches, raw	1 medium	1.4
Cabbage, green or red, cooked	1/2 cup	1.8	Cantaloupe, raw	1 cup pieces	1.3
Pinto beans, cooked	1/4 cup	1.7	Grapefruits, raw, white	1/2 medium fruit	0.7
Kidney beans, red, cooked	1/4 cup	1.6	Watermelon, raw	1 cup	0.6
Navy beans, boiled	1/4 cup	1.6	Plums, canned, juice packed	3 fruits	0.4
Tomato, raw	1 medium	1.6	Grapefruit sections, canned, juice packed	1/2 cup	0.3
Turnips, fresh, cooked	1/2 cup	1.6			
Corn, sweet, canned, cream style	1/2 cup	1.5	**GRAIN PRODUCTS**		
Great Northern beans, boiled	1/4 cup	1.5	Whole-wheat flour	1 cup	15.2
Cauliflower, fresh or frozen, cooked	1/2 cup	1.4	Rye flour, medium or light	1 cup	14.9
Garbanzo beans, chickpeas, boiled	1/4 cup	1.4	High-fiber bran cereal	1/2 cup (1 oz)	14.0
Spinach, raw	1 cup	1.4	Cornmeal, whole-grain	1 cup	13.4
Onion, fresh, chopped	1/2 cup	1.3	Wheat bran	1/2 cup	12.7
Squash, summer, cooked	1/2 cup	1.3	Bran cereal	1/3 cup (1 oz)	10.0
Asparagus, canned	1/2 cup	1.2	Cornmeal, degermed	1 cup	7.2
Beans, green, cut, fresh, boiled	1/2 cup	1.1	Wheat germ	1/4 cup	4.4
Beans, snap, cooked in a small amount of water	1/2 cup	1.1	Wheat, shredded, cereal	2 biscuits	4.4
Corn, sweet, canned or frozen, cooked	1/2 cup	1.1	Oats, rolled, cooked	2/3 cup	4.2
Beets, cooked slices, canned	1/2 cup	0.9	Bran muffin, with raisins	1 medium (2 oz)	3.9
Tomatoes, whole, peeled, canned	1/2 cup	0.8	Rice, brown, long-grain, cooked	1 cup	3.3
Mushrooms, canned, drained	1/2 cup	0.7	Whole-wheat bread	2 slices	3.2
			Rye bread, Jewish, with seeds	2 slices	2.6
			Macaroni, enriched, cooked	1 cup	2.2
			Noodles, egg and spinach, cooked	1 cup	2.2
			Rice, brown	2/3 cup	2.2
			Spaghetti, enriched, cooked	1 cup	2.2
			Cracked-wheat bread	2 slices	2.1
			Corn tortilla, enriched	1 tortilla	1.0
			Rice, white	2/3 cup	0.5

(From Pennington JAT. In: *Bowes & Church's food values of portions commonly used*, 16th ed. Philadelphia: Lippincott, 1994, with permission.)

TABLE 23.2-2. Benefits and Examples of Good Sources of Both Soluble and Insoluble Fiber

	Soluble Fiber	*Insoluble Fiber*
Natural fiber components	Gums, mucilages, pectins, some hemicelluloses	Cellulose, lignins, some hemicelluloses
Benefits	May help in reducing blood cholesterol and controlling blood glucose levels	May help prevent colon cancer; helps prevent constipation
Good sources	Oat bran, beans (navy, kidney, pinto, or lima), barley, vegetables, and fruits	Whole-wheat bread, beans (navy, kidney, pinto, or lima), cereals, and the skins of vegetables and fruits

(From ref. 17, with permission.)

and fiber from fruits but not vegetables, had a protective effect on the development of distal colon adenoma in men.[25] Results of a case-control study of nearly 2000 patients with confirmed colorectal cancer and more than 4100 controls with no history of cancer indicated that total fiber intake, and particularly intake of cellulose, soluble noncellulose polysaccharides, and fiber of vegetable and fruit origin, was associated with a reduction in the risk of cancers of the colon and rectum.[26] Reviews of animal studies investigating the effect of different types of dietary fiber on colon tumorigenesis generally report that the greatest protective effect, as measured by lowered incidence (number of animals with tumors) and multiplicity (number of tumors per animal with tumors) of small intestine and colon tumors, is conferred by insoluble fibers, in particular wheat bran, whereas soluble fibers may increase risk.[5,8,16,27]

The growing interest in the potential effect of wheat bran fiber on colorectal cancer risk has been the focus of several reviews.[16,28,29] Wheat bran, which contains more than 70% of the fiber of the whole grain, is rich in lignin and polysaccharides.[29] Numerous animal studies show wheat bran fiber to be as or more effective than other fiber sources, such as corn and oat, in inhibiting or preventing colon tumor growth.[16,27,29,30] In some studies, however, dietary wheat bran fiber either had no effect on the development of colon tumors in rats or increased colon tumorigenesis.[16,27] Several epidemiologic studies and clinical interventions also have investigated the effect of different dietary fibers, including wheat bran, on factors associated with increased risk for colorectal cancer, including colonic or rectal cell proliferation, bile acid excretion, fecal mutagens, and activity of several intestinal bacterial enzymes linked with the production of carcinogenic substances.[16] Results of these studies indicate that wheat bran has a favorable, and sometimes more favorable, effect when compared with other sources of fiber, on these factors. The cancer-protective effects of wheat bran may be the result, at least in part, of various compounds, including the fermentation product butyrate[16] and certain constituents of wheat bran, including phytic acid,[31,32] phenolic acids,[29] and phytoestrogens,[33,34] all of which have shown a cancer-protective effect in either, or both, epidemiologic and animal studies.

POTENTIAL INFLUENCES OF DIETARY FIBER ON GENETICALLY LINKED COLORECTAL CANCERS

Approximately 10% to 15% of all cases of colorectal cancers are believed to result from genetic predisposition to these cancers.[35,36] Two inherited genetic forms of colorectal cancer, familial adenomatous polyposis and hereditary nonpolyposis colon cancer, are associated with up to an 80% lifetime risk of developing the disease.

The potential of a high-fiber diet, or fiber supplementation, to modulate cancer risk in at-risk or high-risk individuals who have a genetic predisposition to colorectal cancer has been studied and further investigations are under way. One clinical trial found that supplementing the diet with at least 11 g of wheat bran fiber per day significantly reduced the recurrence of rectal adenomas in patients with familial adenomatous polyposis.[37] Results of the Australian Polyp Prevention Project indicated that consuming high levels of dietary fiber supplementation (25 g wheat bran fiber per day) or a low-fat diet (25% of total calories) for 2 to 4 years reduced risk (but not to a level of statistical significance) of developing new, large adenomas (diameter greater than or equal to 10 mm) in healthy individuals who had had at least one colonic polyp removed before the start of the study.[38] Participants following a combined low-fat, high-fiber diet had no large adenomas at both 2 and 4 years, a finding that was statistically significant ($P<.03$). The European Concerted Action Polyp Prevention studies are examining the role of a variety of preventive strategies, including daily dietary supplementation with resistant starch, in high-risk persons with a family history of either familial adenomatous polyposis or hereditary nonpolyposis colon cancer.[35,36]

PROPOSED MECHANISMS OF ACTION

Several mechanisms by which dietary fiber may protect against colon cancer have been proposed.[5,18,29,39] These mechanisms include both direct and indirect actions on the alimentary and gastrointestinal canals that are related to properties of fiber, such as solubility and fermentability; actions may occur at the physical, chemical, cellular, and/or molecular levels.

One direct mechanism by which fiber may reduce the risk of colorectal cancer is through the absorption of water by insoluble dietary fiber; this action increases fecal bulk, diluting the concentration of carcinogens in the feces, and decreases transit time, reducing the effective interaction of carcinogens with colonic mucosal cells.[5,11,17,18] The direct binding of carcinogens to insoluble dietary fibers, such as wheat bran, cellulose, and lignin, similarly reduces the potential interaction between carcinogens and cells within the bowel.[5,40] Indirect mechanisms by which dietary fiber may lower colorectal cancer risk include stimulation of microbial growth, which increases fecal bulk and the production of short chain fatty acids (SCFAs); alteration of bile acid production; influence on the production of factors that affect cell proliferation, such as diacylglycerol, p21, and protein kinase C; and reduction of luminal pH, largely as a result in increases in SCFAs, especially butyrate.[5,16,39–43]

Products of fiber fermentation, particularly butyrate, appear to have a beneficial, antineoplastic effect in the bowel.[44] Several studies suggest that, compared with other SCFAs, butyrate most consistently protects against the development of colon tumors in the rat by acting through a variety of mechanisms, including blocking the proliferative action of carcinogens and other cancer-promoting agents such as bile acids, inducing cell differentiation, lowering concentrations of secondary bile acids, reducing the mutagenicity of fecal water, and enhancing programmed cell death (apoptosis) in human colorectal cancer cell lines.[5,16,18,36,39,44,45] Acting at the molecular level, butyrate stimulates histone acetylation by inhibiting the enzyme histone deacetylase, which, in turn, makes certain sections of the DNA molecule more accessible to factors (e.g., proteins known as *transcription factors*) that control gene expression.[46] The effects of butyrate on histones appear to be through induction of the *p21* gene and subsequent production of the p21 protein, which slows the growth of cancer cells.[46,47] Butyrate also decreases the expression of the transcription factors c-fos and c-jun, acting, in turn, to reduce proliferative activity.[5,36,39]

Experimental data show that dietary wheat bran fiber reduces the formation of early markers of colon cancer associated with carcinogen-induced disease, such as the number of aberrant crypts or foci, and alters the colonic environment in several other ways, such as increasing fecal bulk, decreasing transit time, adsorbing to carcinogens, and stimulating the production of butyric acid.[27,29,45] In epidemiologic and clinical intervention studies, wheat bran fiber supplementation favorably modified several putative makers of colorectal cancer, including fecal mutagenicity,[48] concentrations of total and secondary fecal bile acids,[49,50] the activity of bacterial enzymes associated with the production of carcinogenic substances,[49] and rectal proliferation in high-risk individuals.[28,51]

DIETARY FIBER AND COLORECTAL CANCER AT SPECIFIC SITES

The incidence of cancers at different colon subsites varies by geographic region, with higher proportions of proximal tumors found in less developed countries that have low rates of colorectal cancer and higher proportions of distal and right-sided tumors reported in developed, affluent countries where colorectal cancer rates are high.[8,41] Such observations suggest the possibility of differences in risk factors for colonic tumors at different anatomic subsites. Although data are limited, some studies report that certain dietary constituents may contribute to this variable, site-specific risk.

A possible role for dietary fiber in differential risk for cancers in the proximal versus distal colon is suggested primarily from animal studies.[45,52] Soluble fibers, such as guar gum, oat bran, and pectin, are fermented by anaerobic bacteria in the proximal colon, producing large amounts of SCFAs, which are absorbed almost entirely in the proximal colon. In contrast, insoluble and poorly soluble fibers, such as wheat bran, cellulose, and lignin, are fermented along the length of the gut, providing a more continuous supply of SCFAs throughout the intestine, which, in turn, assists in maintaining normal colonocyte proliferation and differentiation. Such fiber-related maintenance of normal cell function and activity likely contributes to the inhibition of tumors in the distal colon in rats fed wheat bran compared with other fiber sources, such as oat bran.[52]

Results of dietary epidemiologic studies have not consistently found similar associations. One case-control study found no difference in risk of cancers of the right colon, transverse and descending colon, sigmoid colon, rectosigmoid junction, or rectum according to total fiber intake.[26] Another case-control study reported the strongest inverse associations between consumption of dietary fiber, whole grains, and vegetables and risk of proximal tumors in both men and women; and between soluble fiber, insoluble fiber, and pectin intake and risk of proximal tumors in women.[53] In contrast, a prospective study of 16,448 men from the Health Professionals Follow-up Study reported a reduced risk of distal colon adenoma as intake of fiber from fruit increased ($P < .03$ for trend) and an inverse association between soluble, but not insoluble, fiber intake and distal colon adenoma (P for trend, .007).[25] This study did not examine or compare associations according to other intestinal subsites.

DIETARY FIBER AND CALCIUM: POTENTIAL INTERACTIONS

An association between dietary calcium or calcium supplementation and reduced colorectal cancer risk has been suggested from the results of epidemiologic, clinical, and experimental research studies.[18,54–57] Mechanisms by which calcium may inhibit colorectal carcinogenesis are similar to those of dietary fiber and include the ability of calcium to bind potentially carcinogenic compounds, such as secondary bile acids; slow proliferation of colonic epithelial cells; and enhance cell differentiation.[54,55,57–59] These effects of calcium have been reported in both animal and human studies and in *in vitro* experiments.[54,58] Animal experiments further suggest that calcium and fiber may act synergistically in their effect on the colonic environment.[56]

The roles of calcium and fiber on markers for colorectal cancer risk are being studied in several clinical trials. The multicenter European Cancer Prevention Calcium Fibre Polyp Prevention Study is testing the efficacy of oral calcium (2 g/d) or oral dietary fiber supplements (as 3.8 g ispaghula husk, a mucilaginous substance) on adenoma recurrence, colonic cell proliferation, and stool bile acid and sterol concentration.[60,61] Participants include patients from nine European countries who are between 35 and 75 years old at study entry and have at least two adenomas greater than 5 mm in diameter. Preliminary results of another clinical trial showed that high doses of wheat bran fiber (13.5 g/d) or calcium (1500 mg/d), or high doses of fiber plus high doses of calcium, increased both fecal bile acid concentrations and excretion rates.[50] The strongest statistical effect, reflecting an approximate 50% reduction in fecal concentrations of total bile acids and deoxycholic acid, was seen in the high-fiber group. The effect of the combined high-fiber and high-calcium diet on mean fecal bile acid parameters was less than that for either factor alone; the reason for this lack of additivity between the two supplements is not clear but may be caused by cross-interference with each agent's putative effects on bile acids. A subsequent analysis of the same study reported that neither level of wheat bran fiber or calcium supplementation significantly reduced [^{3}H]thymidine labeling index percentages in rectal mucosal crypts.[62] These preliminary findings suggest that a primary mechanism by which wheat bran fiber and calcium may protect against colon cancer is through reducing fecal bile acid concentrations.

ONGOING NATIONAL CANCER INSTITUTE CLINICAL TRIALS

The National Cancer Institute (NCI) is evaluating the role of dietary fiber in the prevention of colorectal cancer in humans through several clinical trials. The Polyp Prevention Trial, for example, allows for the simultaneous investigation of the effect of three dietary components on recurrence of polyps in the large bowel.[63–65] Polyp Prevention Trial study participants include men and women at least 35 years old who have had one or more adenomas removed within 3 months of randomization. The primary objective of the Polyp Prevention Trial is to determine whether a diet that is low in fat (20% of calories from fat), high in fiber (18 g fiber/1000 calories), and high in vegetable and fruit intake (five to eight daily servings) will decrease the recurrence of large bowel polyps. The trial also is evaluating the relationship between dietary modification and biochemical markers in the blood and validating promising intermediate endpoint markers of large bowel carcinogenesis with respect to polyp recurrence.

Another NCI-supported study, the Women's Health Initiative Clinical Trial and Observational Study, is investigating several strategies for the prevention and control of cancer, cardiovascular disease, and osteoporotic fractures in postmenopausal women 50 to 79 years old.[66] The Clinical Trial, which anticipates an enrollment of 64,500 participants, is a randomized, controlled evaluation of three interventions: (1) a goal of a low-fat (20% of calories) eating pattern that includes at least five servings of vegetables and fruits and six or more servings of grain products per day, hypothesized to prevent breast cancer and colorectal cancer and, secondarily, coronary heart disease; (2) hormone replacement therapy; and (3) calcium (1000 mg/d) *and* vitamin D_3 (400 IU/d) supplementation (or placebo), hypothesized to prevent hip fractures and, secondarily, other fractures and colorectal cancer. A prospective surveillance (the Observational Study) will enroll an additional 100,000 women to identify new etiologic factors and biologic predictors of disease and community-based interventions. The Women's Health Initiative was initiated in 1992 and is scheduled to end in 2007.

The double-blind, placebo-controlled Arizona Phase III cancer prevention trial, also funded by NCI, is examining how supplementing the diet with large versus small doses of wheat bran fiber (13.5 vs. 2.0 g/d) alters the molecular genetics of polyp tissue in patients with previously resected adenomatous colon polyps.[67,68] Genetic changes will be compared with dietary factors and bile acid profiles. Approximately 945 participants have fulfilled all aspects of the study protocol in this 3-year dietary intervention, which is nearing completion.

DIETARY FIBER AND BREAST CANCER

SUMMARY OF EPIDEMIOLOGIC AND EXPERIMENTAL RESEARCH

Evidence from both epidemiologic and experimental studies suggests a protective role for fiber in the prevention of breast cancer, although the exact role of fiber on breast cancer development is not yet clear.[2,12,69] One review, a metaanalysis of the original data from 12 case-control studies of populations with widely varying breast cancer risks and dietary habits, reported a significant reduction in breast cancer risk among women in the highest versus lowest quintiles of fiber intake, both before and after adjusting for fat intake.[70] A more recent review found that four of four ecological studies and nine of ten case-control studies showed an inverse correlation between either cereal consumption or fiber intake and breast cancer risk; in the five case-control studies reporting a statistically significant decrease in breast cancer risk among women consuming a high-fiber diet, the odds ratios ranged from 0.46 to 0.60. All four prospective cohort studies included in this review reported either no change in breast cancer risk or a nonsignificant decrease in risk in association with cereal or fiber intake.[9] Another study of international breast cancer mortality data and dietary intake data found that both current and past cereal intake were inversely correlated ($P < .0001$) with breast cancer mortality.[12] Further evidence suggests that diets rich in fruits and vegetables, particularly green vegetables, protect against the development of breast cancer.[8]

The combination of a high-fiber, low-fat diet also has been associated with reduced risk for breast cancer, with evidence from both epidemiologic and animal studies suggesting that the proposed protective effect of fiber may occur independently of dietary fat content.[8,71,72] It also has been postulated that a high-fiber diet may modulate the risk of breast cancer associated with a high-fat diet.[73] Experiments in rats support the hypotheses that dietary fiber, including wheat bran and psyllium,[74,75] protects against breast cancer and that dietary fiber may block the promotion of mammary tumors by fat.[72]

PROPOSED MECHANISMS

Research indicates that reproductive hormones, especially estrogens, are involved in the development of breast cancer.[8,76] The mechanisms by which fiber alters hormone production, metabolism, and bioavailability focus on the ability of fiber to bind estrogen in the small intestine, thereby both increasing the excretion and reducing the enterohepatic circulation of hormones,[9,77,78] and on the biologic activity of phytoestrogens, compounds present in fiber-rich foods that possess weak estrogenic and antiestrogenic activity.[33,77,79]

High-fiber intake and diets rich in fiber and low in fat or high in vegetables, fruits, and soy-based foods are associated with low plasma levels of all major biologically active sex hormones, including free estradiol and testosterone; high levels of sex-hormone binding globulin; and low urinary and high fecal estrogen and androgen excretion.[9,80,81] In one intervention study, the diets of 62 premenopausal women were supplemented with 15 g of wheat, corn, or oat bran per day, essentially doubling daily intake of fiber.[82] Luteal phase serum levels of both estrone and estradiol were significantly reduced following addition of fiber to the diet. A subsequent study found that supplementing the diet of premenopausal women with 10 or 20 g of wheat bran fiber per day for 1 to 2 months significantly reduced serum estrone during both the luteal and follicular phases of the menstrual cycle; serum sex-hormone binding globulin concentrations were unaffected.[83]

Dietary phytoestrogens (i.e., isoflavonoids and plant lignans) are found in a variety of high-fiber foods such as fruits, berries, seeds, soy products, and flaxseed and in grain and vegetable fibers.[33] Two common isoflavonoids are genistein and daidzein; two mammalian lignans, enterolactone and enterodiol, are formed from plant lignans by the action of intestinal bacteria. Urinary concentrations of these lignans have been found to correlate directly with consumption of foods containing phytoestrogens.[79,84,85] A review of 26 animal studies in which the animals' diets were supplemented with soy or soybean isoflavonoids found a cancer-protective effect in 65% of the studies, as reflected by reductions in tumor incidence, latency, or number.[34] Results of both *in vitro* and *in vivo* animal studies suggest that phytoestrogens mimic the activity of and compete with endogenous estrogens by binding to estrogen receptors.[33] Although the affinity of phytoestrogens to estrogen receptors is tens to thousands of times lower than that of endogenous estrogens, the ability of these plant-based compounds to bind to estrogen receptors permits a dual, dose-dependent effect on mammary tumor initiation and growth. At lower doses, *in vitro* experiments show that phytoestrogens can increase the mitogenic activity of breast cancer cells.[86] In contrast, higher doses of phytoestrogens inhibit mammary tumor development,[77] suppress the growth of established tumors,[77] and inhibit the proliferation of human breast cancer cells that require estrogen to replicate.[33,34] Phytoestrogens also induce the production of sex-hormone binding globulin in the liver and inhibit the enzyme aromatase, which catalyzes the conversion of androstenedione to estrogen and testosterone to estradiol; through these two actions, phytoestrogens indirectly reduce the concentration and availability of circulating sex hormones and possibly contribute to reduced risk for breast cancer.[77]

DIETARY FIBER AND OTHER CANCERS

Limited epidemiologic evidence suggests that high-fiber intake, consumption of fiber-rich foods, or both may lower risk of cancers of the mouth, esophagus, pharynx, larynx, stomach,[6,8,87] ovary, endometrium, and prostate.[6,7,88,89] The evidence for a cancer-protective role of fiber at these sites is not as strong as for colorectal or breast cancer, however.[8] Dietary fiber may protect against these alimentary canal cancers through many of the same mechanisms suggested for the modulation of colorectal cancer risk and influence risk of these hormone-dependent cancers by affecting the bioavailability of both estrogens and androgens.[5]

PUBLIC HEALTH IMPLICATIONS

In addition to its proposed protective effects against colorectal cancer, breast cancer, and possibly other cancers, dietary fiber as total fiber, whole grains, cereal fiber, soluble fiber, undigested fiber, fiber-rich foods, psyllium, or dietary flavonoids has been associated with reduced risk of other conditions important to public health, including cardiovascular diseases[90,91] and type II diabetes.[90] Because of the significant health benefits afforded by fiber-rich foods, individuals and the public at large are encouraged to consume a diet that includes a wide variety of vegetables, fruits, and whole grains, with a goal of meeting the NCI's recommended 20 to 30 g of fiber per day.[92] Results of the 1992 National Health Interview Survey, cosponsored by the Census Bureau, the National Center for Health Statistics, and the NCI, indicate that adult Americans consume an average of 10.4 g of fiber per day. The U.S. Department of Agriculture's (USDA) Nationwide Food Consumption Survey found a higher overall consumption rate for fiber among American adults, with a mean intake of 14 g/d.[93] Although these values are well below the recommended intake levels, it is encouraging that fiber intake increased among all Americans and in all subgroups in the National Health Interview Survey between 1987 and 1992[94] and among all surveyed in the USDA's Continuing Survey of Food Intake by Individuals between 1989 through 1991 and 1994.[95]

Several national programs have been instituted to increase both fiber intake and consumption of fiber-rich fruits and vegetables. For example, the 5 A Day for Better Health Program, sponsored by the NCI in partnership with the Produce for Better Health Foundation, includes retail, community, and research components as well as a national media campaign that encourages Americans to eat five or more servings of vegetables and fruits each day as part of a low-fat, high-fiber diet.[96–98] The USDA's Food Guide Pyramid suggests that fiber-containing breads and grains, followed by vegetables and fruits, should form the foundation of an individual's diet. Recommended are 6 to 11 servings of breads and grains per day, 2 to 4 servings of fruits per day, and 3 to 5 servings of vegetables per day.[99] The 1989 through 1991 USDA Continuing Survey of Food Intakes in Individuals found that, overall, Americans met the minimum basic recommended intakes for breads and grains (mean, 5.7 servings per day) and vegetables (mean, 3.3 servings per day), but failed to meet the recommended intake for fruits (mean, 1.3 servings per day).[100] The subsequent 1994 USDA survey reported significant ($P < .0005$) increases in intakes of vegetables, fruits, and grains when compared with data from the 1989 through 1991 survey.[95] A comprehensive review of seven nationally representative surveys of food and nutrient consumption among Americans similarly reported significant ($P < .0001$) increases in per capita intakes of vegetables (19%), fruits (22%), and grain products (47%) during the 24-year period from 1970 to 1994.[95]

To help consumers increase fiber intake, the Food and Drug Administration required fiber content to be included on the nutrition facts panel on food labels. In addition, foods containing 10% of the daily value for fiber (i.e., 2.5 g of fiber per serving) may be labeled a "good source" of fiber, and products containing 20% or more of the daily value for fiber (at least 5 g of fiber per serving) can claim to be "high in," "rich in," or "an excellent source" of fiber.[90] The Food and Drug Administration also allows manufacturers to make certain health claims related to fiber intake and lowered risk of cancer and other health conditions for foods meeting specific eligibility criteria.[91]

Results of successful nutritional intervention programs incorporating components of the 5 A Day for Better Health Program and other similar guidance, in conjunction with data from national dietary intake surveys, suggest that Americans are receiving and implementing messages designed to promote healthier eating patterns that include increased consumption of fiber, vegetables, fruits, and whole grains. Research, including ongoing clinical trials, will continue to augment current knowledge and refine recommendations. While such research is being conducted, the complement of data indicates that a varied diet that is low in fat and high in plant-based foods likely protects against several cancers, most notably colorectal cancer, as well as other major diseases, including cardiovascular diseases and diabetes.

REFERENCES

1. Burkitt DP. Epidemiology of cancer of the colon and rectum. *Cancer* 1971;28:3.
2. Steinmetz KA, Potter JD. Vegetables, fruit, and cancer prevention: a review. *J Am Diet Assoc* 1996;96:1027.
3. Hill MJ. Cereals, cereal fibre and colorectal cancer risk: a review of the epidemiological literature. *Eur J Cancer Prev* 1998;7:S5.
4. Caygill CPJ, Hill MJ. Fish, n-3 fatty acids and human colorectal and breast cancer mortality. *Eur J Cancer Prev* 1995;4:329.
5. Moore MA, Park CB, Tsuda H. Soluble and insoluble fiber influences on cancer development. *Crit Rev Oncol Hematol* 1998;27:229.

6. La Vecchia C, Chatenoud L. Fibres, whole-grain foods and breast and other cancers. *Eur J Cancer Prev* 1998;7:S25.
7. Jacobs DR Jr, Marquart L, Slavin J, et al. Whole-grain intake and cancer: an expanded review and meta-analysis. *Nutr Cancer* 1998;30:85.
8. World Cancer Research Fund. Food, nutrition and the prevention of cancer: a global perspective. Washington, DC: American Institute for Cancer Research, 1997.
9. Gerber M. Fibre and breast cancer. *Eur J Cancer Prev* 1998;7:S63.
10. Potter JD. Nutrition and colorectal cancer. *Cancer Causes Control* 1996;7:127.
11. Kritchevsky D. Dietary fibre and cancer. *Eur J Cancer Prev* 1997;6:435.
12. Caygill CPJ, Charlett A, Hill MJ. Relationship between the intake of high-fibre foods and energy and the risk of cancer of the large bowel and breast. *Eur J Cancer Prev* 1998;7:S11.
13. Block G, Patterson BH, Subar AF. Fruit, vegetables, and cancer prevention: a review of the epidemiological evidence. *Nutr Cancer* 1992;18:1.
14. Kaaks R. The epidemiology of diet and colorectal cancer: review and perspectives for future research using biologic markers. *Annali Dell Istituto Superiore* 1996;32:111.
15. Willett WC. Nutritional epidemiology. In: Rothman KJ, Greenland S, eds. *Modern epidemiology*. Philadelphia: Lippincott–Raven, 1998:623.
16. Reddy BS. Role of dietary fiber in colon cancer: an overview. *Am J Med* 1999;106:16S.
17. Greenwald P, Clifford C. Fiber and cancer: prevention research. In: Kritchevsky D, Benfield C, eds. *Dietary fiber in health and disease*. St.Paul: Eagen Press, 1995:159.
18. Chaplin MF. Bile acids, fibre and colon cancer: the story unfolds. *J R Soc Health* 1998;118:53.
19. Howe GR, Enrique B, Castelleto R, et al. Dietary intake of fiber and decreased risk of cancers of the colon and rectum: evidence from the combined analysis of 13 case-control studies. *J Natl Cancer Inst* 1992;84:1887.
20. Giovannucci E, Rimm EB, Stampfer MJ, et al. Intake of fat, meat, and fiber in relation to risk of colon cancer in men. *Cancer Res* 1994;54:2390.
21. Sellers TA, Bazyk AE, Bostick RM, et al. Diet and risk of colon cancer in a large prospective study of older women: an analysis stratified on family history (Iowa, United States). *Cancer Causes Control* 1998;9:357.
22. Fuchs CS, Giovannucci EL, Colditz GA, et al. Dietary fiber and the risk of colorectal cancer and adenoma in women. *N Engl J Med* 1999;340:169.
23. Kato I, Akhmedkhanov A, Koenig K, et al. Prospective study of diet and female colorectal cancer: the New York University Women's Health Study. *Nutr Cancer* 1997;28:276.
24. Cassidy A, Bingham SA, Cummings JH. Starch intake and colorectal cancer risk: an international comparison. *Br J Cancer* 1994;69:937.
25. Platz EA, Giovannucci E, Rimm EB, et al. Dietary fiber and distal colorectal adenoma in men. *Cancer Epidemiol Biomark Prev* 1997;6:661.
26. Negri E, Tzonou A, Beral V, et al. Hormonal therapy for menopause and ovarian cancer in a collaborative re-analysis of European studies. *Int J Cancer* 1999;80:848.
27. Kritchevsky D. Protective role of wheat bran fiber: preclinical data. *Am J Med* 1999;106:28S.
28. Macrae F. Wheat bran fiber and development of adenomatous polyps: evidence from randomized, controlled clinical trials. *Am J Med* 1999;106:38S.
29. Ferguson LR, Harris PJ. Protection against cancer by wheat bran: role of dietary fibre and phytochemicals. *Eur J Cancer Prev* 1999;8:17.
30. Chapkin RS, Clark AE, Davidson LA, et al. Dietary fiber differentially alters cellular fatty acid-binding protein expression in exfoliated colonocytes during tumor development. *Nutr Cancer* 1998;32:107.
31. Jenab M, Thompson LU. The influence of phytic acid in wheat bran on early biomarkers of colon carcinogenesis. *Carcinogenesis* 1998;19:1087.
32. Owen RW, Spiegelhalder B, Bartsch H. Phytate, reactive oxygen species and colorectal cancer. *Eur J Cancer Prev* 1998;7:S41.
33. Barrett J. Phytoestrogens. *Environ Health Perspect* 1996;104:478.
34. Wiseman H. Role of dietary phyto-oestrogens in the protection against cancer and heart disease. *Biochem Soc Trans* 1996;24:795.
35. Burn J, Chapman PD, Mathers J, et al. The protocol for a European double-blind trial of aspirin and resistant starch in familial adenomatous polyposis: the CAPP study. *Eur J Cancer* 1995;31A:1385.
36. Burn J, Chapman PD, Bishop DT, et al. Diet and cancer prevention: the Concerted Action Polyp Prevention (CAPP) studies. *Proc Nutr Soc* 1998;57:183.
37. DeCosse JJ, Miller HH, Lesser ML. Effect of wheat fiber and vitamins C and E on rectal polyps in patients with familial adenomatous polyposis. *J Natl Cancer Inst* 1989;81:1290.
38. MacLennan R, Macrae F, Bain C, et al. Randomized trial of intake of fat, fiber, and beta carotene to prevent colorectal adenomas. *J Natl Cancer Inst* 1995;87:1760.
39. Kritchevsky D. Cereal fibres and colorectal cancer: a search for mechanisms. *Eur J Cancer Prev* 1998;7:S33.
40. Nagengast FM, Grubben MJAL, Van Munster IP. Role of bile acids in colorectal carcinogenesis. *Eur J Cancer* 1995;31A:1067.
41. Kanazawa K, Konishi F, Mitsuoka T, et al. Factors influencing the development of sigmoid colon cancer. *Cancer* 1996;77:1701.
42. Pickering JS, Lupton JR, Chapkin RS. Dietary fat, fiber, and carcinogen alter fecal diacylglycerol composition and mass. *Cancer Res* 1995;55:2293.
43. Assert R, Kotter R, Bisping G, et al. Anti-proliferative activity of protein kinase C in apical compartments of human colonic crypts: evidence for a less activated protein kinase C in small adenomas. *Int J Cancer* 1999;80:47.
44. Scheppach W, Bartram HP, Richter F. Role of short-chain fatty acids in the prevention of colorectal cancer. *Eur J Cancer* 1995;31A:1077.
45. Lupton JR, Turner ND. Potential protective mechanisms of wheat bran fiber. *Am J Med* 1999;106:24S.
46. Hassig CA, Tong JK, Schreiber SL. Fiber-derived butyrate and the prevention of colon cancer. *Chem Biol* 1997;4:783.
47. Archer MC, Bruce WR, Chan CC, et al. Aberrant crypt foci and microadenoma as markers for colon cancer. *Environ Health Perspect* 1992;98:195.
48. Reddy BS, Engle A, Katsifis S, et al. Biochemical epidemiology of colon cancer: effects of types of dietary fiber on fecal mutagens, acid, and neutral sterols in healthy subjects. *Cancer Res* 1989;49:4629.
49. Reddy BS, Engle A, Simi B, et al. Effect of dietary fiber on colonic bacterial enzymes and bile acids in relation to colon cancer. *Gastroenterology* 1992;102:1475.
50. Alberts DS, Ritenbaugh C, Story JA, et al. Randomized, double-blind, placebo-controlled study of effect of wheat bran fiber and calcium on fecal bile acids in patients with resected adenomatous colon polyps. *J Natl Cancer Inst* 1996;88:81.
51. Alberts DS, Einspahr J, Rees-McGee S, et al. Effects of dietary wheat bran fiber on rectal epithelial cell proliferation in patients with resection for colorectal cancer. *J Natl Cancer Inst* 1990;82:1280.
52. Zoran DL, Turner ND, Taddeo SS, et al. Wheat bran diet reduces tumor incidence in a rat model of colon cancer independent of effects on distal luminal butyrate concentrations. *J Nutr* 1997;127:2217.
53. Slattery ML, Potter JD, Coates A, et al. Plant foods and colon cancer: an assessment of specific foods and their related nutrients (United States). *Cancer Causes Control* 1997;8:575.
54. Szilagyi A. Altered colonic environment, a possible predisposition to colorectal cancer and colonic inflammatory bowel disease: rationale of dietary manipulation with emphasis on disaccharides. *Can J Gastroenterol* 1998;12:133.
55. Bostick RM. Human studies of calcium supplementation and colorectal epithelial cell proliferation. *Cancer Epidemiol Biomark Prev* 1997;6:971.
56. Kleibeuker JH, Cats A, van der Meer R, et al. Calcium supplementation as prophylaxis against colon cancer? *Dig Dis* 1994;12:85.
57. Govers MJAP, Termont DSML, Lapré JA, et al. Calcium in milk products precipitates intestinal fatty acids and secondary bile acids and thus inhibits colonic cytotoxicity in humans. *Cancer Res* 1996;56:3270.
58. Lipkin M, Newmark H. Calcium and the prevention of colon cancer. *J Cell Biochem Suppl* 1995;22:65.
59. Newmark HL, Lipkin M. Calcium, vitamin D, and colon cancer. *Cancer Res* 1992;52(Suppl 7):2067s.
60. Faivre J, Couillault C, Kronborg O, et al. Chemoprevention of metachronous adenomas of the large bowel: design and interim results of a randomized trial of calcium and fibre. *Eur J Cancer Prev* 1997;6:132.
61. Faivre J, Giacosa A. Primary prevention of colorectal cancer through fibre supplementation. *Eur J Cancer Prev* 1998;7:S29.
62. Alberts DS, Einspahr J, Ritenbaugh C, et al. The effect of wheat bran fiber and calcium supplementation on rectal mucosal proliferation rates in patients with resected adenomatous colorectal polyps. *Cancer Epidemiol Biomark Prev* 1997;6:161.
63. Schatzkin A, Lanza E, Ballard-Barbash R. The case for a dietary intervention study of large bowel polyps. *Cancer Prev* 1990;1:84.
64. Schatzkin A, Lanza E, Freedman LS, et al. The Polyp Prevention Trial I: rationale, design, recruitment, and baseline participant characteristics. *Cancer Epidemiol Biomark Prev* 1996;5:375.
65. Lanza E, Schatzkin A, Ballard-Barbash R, et al. The Polyp Prevention Trial II: dietary intervention program and participant baseline dietary characteristics. *Cancer Epidemiol Biomark Prev* 1996;5:385.
66. The Women's Health Initiative Study Group. Design of the Women's Health Initiative clinical trial and observational study. *Controlled Clin Trials* 1998;19:61.
67. Earnest DL, Sampliner RE, Roe DJ, et al. Progress report: the Arizona Phase III study of the effect of wheat bran fiber on recurrence of adenomatous colon polyps. *Am J Med* 1999;106:43S.
68. Martinez ME, Reid ME, Guillen-Rodriguez J, et al. Design and baseline characteristics of study participants in the Wheat Bran Fiber trial. *Cancer Epidemiol Biomark Prev* 1998;7:813.
69. Wiseman H, Lim P, O'Reilly J. Inhibition of liposomal lipid peroxidation by isoflavonoid type phyto-oestrogens from soybeans of different countries of origin. *Biochem Soc Trans* 1996;24:392S.
70. Howe GR, Hirohata T, Hislop TG, et al. Dietary factors and risk of breast cancer: combined analysis of 12 case-control studies. *J Natl Cancer Inst* 1990;82:561.
71. Hannah JS. Beyond calories: other benefits of macronutrient substitutes—effects on chronic disease. *Ann N Y Acad Sci* 1997;819:221.
72. Cohen LA, Kendall ME, Zang E, et al. Modulation of *N*-nitrosomethylurea-induced mammary tumor promotion by dietary fiber and fat. *J Natl Cancer Inst* 1991;83:496.
73. Rose DP. Dietary fiber and breast cancer. *Nutr Cancer* 1990;13:1.
74. Cohen LA, Zhao Z, Zang EA, et al. Wheat bran and psyllium diets: effects on *N*-methylnitrosourea-induced mammary tumorigenesis in F344 rats. *J Natl Cancer Inst* 1996;88:899.
75. Zile MH, Welsch CW, Welsch MA. Effect of wheat bran fiber on the development of mammary tumors in female intact and ovariectomized rats treated with 7,12-dimethylbenz(a)anthracene and in mice with spontaneously developing mammary tumors. *Int J Cancer* 1998;75:439.
76. Jones LA, Gonzalez R, Pillow PC, et al. Dietary fiber, Hispanics, and breast cancer risk? *Ann N Y Acad Sci* 1997;837:524.
77. Rose DP. Dietary fiber, phytoestrogens, and breast cancer. *Nutrition* 1992;8:47.
78. Lewis SJ, Heaton KW, Oakey RE, et al. Lower serum oestrogen concentrations associated with faster intestinal transit. *Br J Cancer* 1997;76:395.
79. Adlercreutz H. Phytoestrogens: epidemiology and a possible role in cancer protection. *Environ Health Perspect* 1995;103:103.
80. Ross JK, Pusateri DJ, Shultz TD. Dietary and hormonal evaluation of men at different risks for prostate cancer: fiber intake, excretion, and composition, with *in vitro* evidence for an association between steroid hormones and specific fiber components. *Am J Clin Nutr* 1990;51:365.
81. Dorgan JF, Judd JT, Longcope C, et al. Effects of dietary fat and fiber on plasma and urine androgens and estrogens in men: a controlled feeding study. *Am J Clin Nutr* 1996;64:850.
82. Rose DP, Goldman M, Connolly JM, et al. High-fiber diet reduces serum estrogen concentrations in premenopausal women. *Am J Clin Nutr* 1991;54:520.

83. Rose DP, Lubin M, Connolly JM. Effects of diet supplementation with wheat bran on serum estrogen levels in the follicular and luteal phases of the menstrual cycle. *Nutrition* 1997;13:535.
84. Hutchins AM, Lampe JW, Martini MC, et al. Vegetables, fruits, and legumes: effect on urinary isoflavonoid phytoestrogen and lignan excretion. *J Am Diet Assoc* 1995;95:769.
85. Hutchins AM, Slavin JL, Lampe JW. Urinary isoflavonoid phytoestrogen and lignan excretion after consumption of fermented and unfermented soy products. *J Am Diet Assoc* 1995;95:545.
86. Martin PM, Horwitz KB, Ryan DS, et al. Phytoestrogen interaction with estrogen receptors in human breast cancer cells. *Endocrinology* 1978;103:1860.
87. Jacobs DR Jr, Meyer KA, Kushi LH, et al. Whole-grain intake may reduce the risk of ischemic heart disease death in postmenopausal women: the Iowa Women's Health Study. *Am J Clin Nutr* 1998;68:248.
88. Goodman MT, Hankin JH, Wilkens LR, et al. Diet, body size, physical activity, and the risk of endometrial cancer. *Cancer Res* 1997;57:5077.
89. Goodman MT, Wilkens LR, Hankin JH, et al. Association of soy and fiber consumption with the risk of endometrial cancer. *Am J Epidemiol* 1997;146:294.
90. Papazian R. Bulking up fiber's healthful reputation: more benefits of "roughage" are discovered. *FDA Consum* 1998;31.
91. Kurtzweil P. Staking a claim to good health: FDA and science stand behind health claims on foods. *FDA Consum* 1998;32:16.
92. Butrum RR, Clifford CK, Lanza E. NCI dietary guidelines: rationale. *Am J Clin Nutr* 1988;48:888.
93. Krebs-Smith SM, Cleveland LE, Ballard-Barbash R, et al. Characterizing food intake patterns of American adults. *Am J Clin Nutr* 1997;65:1264.
94. Norris J, Harnack L, Carmichael S, et al. U.S. trends in nutrient intake: the 1987 and 1992 National Health Interview Surveys. *Am J Public Health* 1997;87:740.
95. Krebs-Smith SM. Progress in improving diet to reduce cancer risk. *Cancer* 1998;83:1425.
96. Subar AF, Heimendinger J, Patterson BH, et al. Fruit and vegetable intake in the United States: the Baseline Survey of the Five A Day for Better Health program. *Am J Health Promot* 1995;9:352.
97. Havas S, Heimendinger J, Reynolds K, et al. 5 A Day for Better Health: a new research initiative. *J Am Diet Assoc* 1994;94:32.
98. Heimendinger J, Van Duyn MA, Chapelsky D, et al. The national 5 A Day for Better Health Program: a large-scale nutrition intervention. *J Public Health Manag Pract* 1996;2:27.
99. Slavin JL. Implementation of dietary modifications. *Am J Med* 1999;106:46S.
100. Cleveland LE, Cook DA, Krebs-Smith SM, et al. Method for assessing food intakes in terms of servings based on food guidance. *Am J Clin Nutr* 1997;65:1254.

SECTION **3**

SUSAN TAYLOR MAYNE
SCOTT M. LIPPMAN

Retinoids, Carotenoids, and Micronutrients

Cancer chemoprevention can be defined as pharmacologic intervention with specific nutrients or other chemicals to suppress or reverse carcinogenesis and to prevent the development of invasive cancer.[1] Two basic concepts support this cancer control strategy: multistep and field carcinogenesis. Carcinogenesis is a chronic, multistep process characterized by the accumulation of specific genetic and phenotypic alterations that can evolve over a 10- to 20-year period from the first initiating event. The premise of human chemoprevention is that one can intervene (and suppress) at many steps in the carcinogenic process and over many years. Field carcinogenesis is a concept that was first described in the early 1950s in the head and neck site as *field cancerization* and subsequently found to apply to many epithelial sites. The concept is that patients at high risk for an epithelial cancer have a wide surface area of carcinogenic tissue change that can be detected at the gross (oral premalignant lesions, polyps), microscopic (metaplasia, dysplasia), and molecular (gene loss or amplification) levels. More recent molecular studies detecting profound genetic alterations in histologically normal tissue from high-risk individuals have provided strong support for the field carcinogenesis concept. The implication is that multifocal, genetically distinct premalignant lesions can progress over a broad tissue region. The clinical importance is best illustrated in head and neck squamous cancer, for which both synchronous and metachronous second primary tumors are common. The latter develop at an annual rate of 5% to 7% in prospective studies[2] and account for the principal cause of cancer death in early-stage disease and in long-term survivors of head and neck cancer, regardless of stage of diagnosis of the first cancer. The essence of chemoprevention, then, is intervention within the multistep carcinogenic process and throughout a wide field.

To date, retinoids (the natural derivatives and synthetic analogues of vitamin A) and one member of the carotenoid class, β-carotene, are among the best-studied agents in human chemoprevention (Fig. 23.3-1). This review focuses on these compounds, with a brief discussion of other micronutrients that have often been evaluated for chemopreventive efficacy along with the retinoids and carotenoids, namely vitamins E and C and the trace mineral selenium.

HISTORICAL PERSPECTIVE

Vitamin A was first recognized as an essential nutrient in 1913 and has been the subject of considerable research in the ensuing years. In 1925, Wolbach and Howe described the histopathologic changes in epithelia associated with vitamin A deficiency.[3] This led to the identification of retinol and some of its naturally occurring retinoid derivatives (see Fig. 23.3-1) and a large body of research aimed at understanding the role of vitamin A and retinoids in cellular differentiation and in neoplastic transformation. Epidemiologic studies of vitamin A and cancer began to emerge in the 1970s, when it was shown that computed indices of total vitamin A intake were associated significantly with lower cancer risk, particularly for lung cancer.[4]

Vitamin A is a nonspecific term embracing two families of dietary factors: preformed vitamin A (chiefly retinyl esters, but also retinol and retinal) and the other family consisting of the various provitamin A carotenoids (β-carotene and those other carotenoids that can be metabolic precursors of retinol). Preformed vitamin A is found predominantly in foods of animal origin, whereas provitamin A carotenoids are found predominantly in fruits and vegetables.

Epidemiologic studies conducted in the 1980s and 1990s evaluated the independent associations of preformed retinol and provitamin A carotenoids with cancer in humans. Dietary intake of provitamin A carotenoids, such as β-carotene, but not of retinol, was associated with a lower risk of cancer.[4,5] Interpretation of observational epidemiologic studies is difficult as carotenoids are consumed in the form of fruits and vegetables, which contain numerous other substances, many of which may have cancer preventive properties.[6] In contrast, the primary dietary sources of retinol are animal products, consumption of

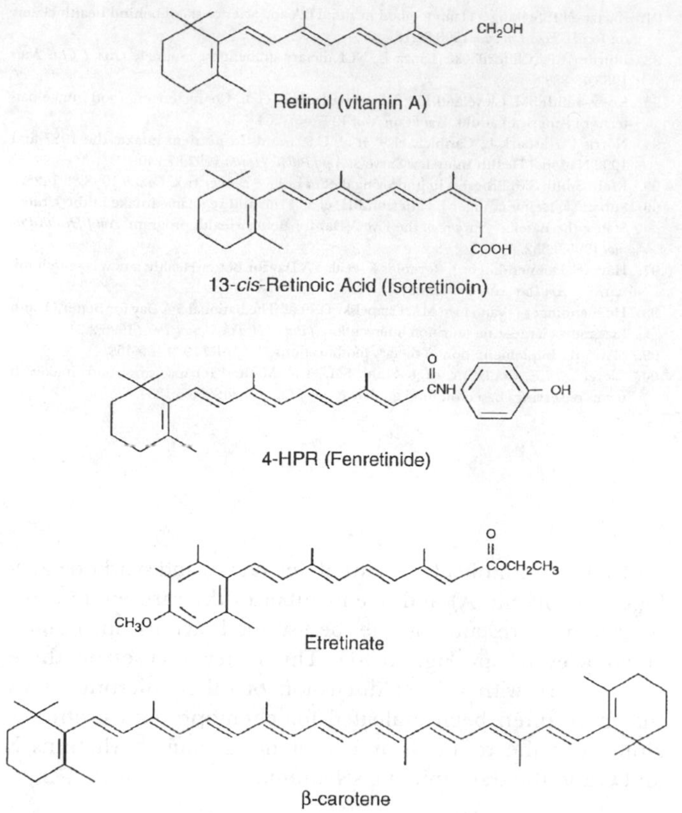

FIGURE 23.3-1. Structures of selected retinoids and the carotenoid, β-carotene. Retinol, 13-*cis* retinoic acid, and β-carotene are naturally occurring; 4HPR and etretinate are synthetic retinoids.

which tends to be associated positively with cancer risk. Also, blood levels of carotenoids increase with increasing dietary intake, whereas blood levels of retinol are regulated homeostatically. Thus, in evaluating the chemopreventive efficacy of carotenoids and retinoids, one must consider evidence from epidemiologic studies, clinical trials, animal models, and mechanistic considerations. This chapter reviews briefly the biology and pharmacology of retinoids and carotenoids and then focuses on randomized cancer prevention clinical trials involving carotenoids, retinoids, and other selected micronutrients.

RETINOID BIOLOGY AND PHARMACOLOGY

Retinoids are required for the maintenance of normal cell growth, differentiation, and loss within epithelial tissues. Various retinoids have been shown to suppress or reverse epithelial carcinogenesis and prevent the development of invasive cancer in many animal systems, including skin, lung, oral cavity, esophagus, bladder, mammary gland, cervix, stomach, prostate, pancreas, and liver. Retinoids act primarily in the postcarcinogen (postinitiation) phases of promotion and progression, which are most relevant to human cancer chemoprevention. Significant single-agent activity has been observed with natural [e.g., all-*trans*-retinoic acid (ATRA), 13-*cis* retinoic acid (13cRA), 9-*cis* retinoic acid (9cRA), retinyl palmitate] and synthetic [e.g., N-(4-hydroxyphenyl) retinamide or fenretinide (4HPR)] retinoids. Additive to synergistic increases in chemopreventive activity have been achieved by combining retinoids with other agents,[7–11] such as the combination of 4HPR or 9cRA with tamoxifen in mammary carcinogenesis systems.

The term *retinoid* was redefined in 1985 by Sporn and Roberts[12] to include a substance that binds and activates one or more specific receptors, the latter producing a biologic response. Much has been learned about the specific receptors and mechanisms of action for the retinoids. The retinoid molecular mechanism of action is similar to that of steroid/thyroid hormones in that retinoid nuclear receptors are members of the steroid receptor superfamily.[13,14] These elusive nuclear receptors were discovered simultaneously by two groups of investigators and reported in 1987. The subsequent studies indicate that retinoid receptors are unique from other members of the steroid receptor family in that there are two receptor classes, RARs and RXRs. Each receptor contains α, β, and γ subtypes, and several of these subclasses have multiple isoforms. These receptors are DNA-binding transcription factors that can activate or suppress the expression of many genes, the products of which mediate retinoid effects on cell growth, differentiation, and apoptosis. Different retinoids bind to the different receptor classes and subclasses with different affinities. This receptor complexity and great diversity in ligand binding, activation, and receptor function has important preventive and therapeutic implications.

As with other members of the steroid family, retinoid receptors are active only as dimers. Two retinoid receptor dimer types have been identified: RAR-RXR heterodimers, and RXR-RXR homodimers (RAR-RAR homodimers have not been identified). Part of the retinoid receptor binds to the ligand, and part binds to specific DNA sequences (RARE or RXRE) and either induces or suppresses gene transcription. The best characterized pathway involves RAR-RXR heterodimers. RXRs have been shown to form heterodimers with other members of the steroid receptor family, including the vitamin D receptor and thyroid hormone receptor. RXRs and their ligands, therefore, can modulate the activities of other steroid hormones.[15] The different ligand-binding patterns can be illustrated with the three major natural retinoic acid derivatives, 13cRA, ATRA, and 9cRA, which are found endogenously in human plasma, albeit at low physiologic levels. RARs bind ATRA and 9cRA, and RXRs bind only 9cRA. 13cRA does not bind directly to nuclear receptors, but is rapidly isomerized to ATRA. Ligand binding stabilizes the receptor dimers and activates gene transcription.[13,14]

The retinoid receptor distribution pattern in normal and neoplastic human tissue is under intense study. The tissue distribution of these receptor classes, subclasses, and isoforms varies greatly in normal and pathologic conditions and in different sites within the human body. In normal tissue, RAR-α is expressed in most tissues, RAR-β expression is more limited (e.g., not expressed in the skin), and RAR-γ is expressed predominantly in the skin. In cancer, these normal tissue patterns can change (e.g., RAR-β is lost in aerodigestive tract carcinogenic progression).

More than 1000 retinoids have been synthesized.[7,12,16–18] Current intensive efforts to develop more active and less toxic retinoids for cancer prevention and therapy are directed to the study of which retinoid receptors mediate retinoid effects on cell growth, differentiation, and apoptosis in different systems and the synthesis of new receptor-selective ligands to obtain the desired retinoid pharmacologic effect.[17,18] An exciting development for chemoprevention is the finding that certain retinoids can interfere with the activity of certain transcription factors such as AP-1 and, therefore, inhibit neoplastic cell proliferation.[17] Mechanistic studies of retinoid pharmacology provide a basis for rational retinoid development programs for chemoprevention.[18]

CAROTENOID BIOLOGY AND ACTIONS

As described by Krinsky,[19] carotenoids have both biologic functions and actions. Carotenoids function as accessory pigments in photosynthesis, via singlet excited carotenoid; offer protection against photosensitization, via triplet excited carotenoid; and some serve as provitamin A compounds, via central and eccentric cleavage. Mechanisms for these functions are reasonably well characterized. Carotenoids also have been reported to have a number of biologic actions, including antioxidant activity, immunoenhancement, inhibition of mutagenesis and transformation, and regression of premalignant lesions. In contrast to the carotenoid functions, mechanisms of carotenoid action are far from clear. Some of the actions of carotenoids, such as regression of premalignant lesions, are shared by the retinoids, with the potential for a similar mechanism of action. The identification of retinoid cleavage products from carotenoids[20] certainly suggests that retinoids and carotenoids may share not only structural similarities and *vitamin A* activity, but perhaps other mechanisms of action that are not fully appreciated at present. However, carotenoids and retinoids also have distinct differences in action, the most notable of which includes antioxidant activity.

Many carotenoids including β-carotene have the ability to quench singlet oxygen, a highly reactive form of oxygen. The quenching involves a physical reaction in which the energy of the excited oxygen is transferred to the carotenoid, forming an excited state molecule.[19] Quenching of singlet oxygen is the basis for β-carotene's well-known therapeutic efficacy in erythropoietic protoporphyria, a photosensitivity disorder.[21] The ability of β-carotene and other carotenoids to quench excited oxygen, however, is limited, because the carotenoid itself can be oxidized during the process (auto-oxidation). Burton and Ingold[22] and others have shown that β-carotene auto-oxidation *in vitro* is dose dependent and dependent on oxygen concentrations.

In addition to singlet oxygen, carotenoids are also thought to quench oxygen free radicals. A relatively large body of literature has linked oxygen free radicals with carcinogenesis,[23] thus there is considerable interest in antioxidant compounds and antioxidant activity as a mechanism for cancer prevention. Despite the focus on antioxidants and cancer and clear evidence of chemopreventive efficacy of β-carotene in some animal carcinogenesis models,[24] it is not clear that antioxidant activity is responsible for the chemoprotective effects observed in the animal studies. For example, β-carotene–induced immunologic enhancement could have a significant role in tumor inhibition by increasing natural killer cells and activating immunoregulatory lymphocytes important in host defense.[25] Various carotenoids have been reported to affect gap junctional communication, related to their ability to up-regulate the expression of the connexin43 gene.[26] This activity was not related to the antioxidant activities of the various carotenoids. Supplementary β-carotene also has been reported to increase the expression of transforming growth factor-β_1 in cervical biopsy specimens.[27] These and other potential mechanisms reviewed elsewhere[24] suggest that it is biologically plausible that carotenoids may have chemopreventive activity, although we know far less about mechanisms of action for the carotenoids than the retinoids.

Given the interest in antioxidant activity as a potential mechanism for chemopreventive effects, it is not surprising that other dietary antioxidants have been studied for chemopreventive efficacy, particularly vitamins E and C and selenium. These agents are often evaluated in combination. However, as is the case with β-carotene, these micronutrients may have biologic actions independent of antioxidant activity.

CLINICAL TRIALS

A number of randomized cancer prevention trials involving carotenoids and retinoids and a few of other micronutrients are ongoing or have been completed. Completed trials involving retinoids are summarized in Table 23.3-1 and those involving carotenoids in Table 23.3-2. Retinoid trials have tested efficacy of several retinoids, including retinol, retinyl palmitate, ATRA, 13cRA, etretinate, and 4HPR. Cancer prevention trials with carotenoids, however, are limited to β-carotene at present. The focus on β-carotene, one of more than 600 carotenoids thus far identified, is based on practical considerations: β-Carotene has been the only carotenoid that is commercially available in large quantities for which human data supporting safety existed. Several other carotenoids (e.g., lycopene) have been suggested to have chemopreventive efficacy in animal models, but are only beginning to be evaluated in human chemoprevention studies (see New Retinoids and Carotenoids, later in this chapter).

HEAD AND NECK TRIALS: PREMALIGNANCY

Oral premalignant lesions include leukoplakias and erythroplakias. Small hyperplastic leukoplakia lesions have a 30% to 40% spontaneous regression rate, and less than a 5% risk of malignant transformation. Erythroleukoplakia and dysplastic leukoplakia lesions, however, are associated with a low rate of spontaneous regression and a 30% to 40% long-term risk of oral cancer.[2,28,29] High-risk, diffuse, and multifocal disease, accounting for 10% to 15% of all oral premalignant lesions, often is not controlled adequately by local therapy. Oral premalignant lesions are markers of field carcinogenesis, since patients with oral premalignancy develop squamous cancers at the site of the lesions as well as in distant sites within the upper aerodigestive tract. Thus, regression of oral premalignant lesions can be used to screen agents that may have utility in the prevention of upper aerodigestive tract cancers. The frequency of micronuclei (an indicator of genotoxic damage) in exfoliated cells from buccal mucosa is another premalignant end point that has been used in head and neck chemoprevention trials.[28]

Studies in the 1980s in populations at high risk of oral cancer (tobacco chewers, betel quid chewers) demonstrated that supplemental β-carotene and retinol significantly reduced the frequency of oral micronuclei.[30–32] As for premalignant lesions, nine trials have investigated the effects of supplemental β-carotene, alone or

TABLE 23.3-1. Randomized Trials of Retinoids in Human Cancer Chemoprevention[a]

Reference	*Population*	*Intervention*	*No.*	*End Point*	*Result*	*P Value*
Hong et al. (1986)[42]	U.S., oral leukoplakia	13cRA (2 mg/kg/d)	24	Regression	67% (response)	= .0002
		Placebo	20		10%	
Stich et al. (1988)[46]	India, oral leukoplakia	Vitamin A (200,000 IU/d)	21	Regression	57% (CR)	<.05
		Placebo	33		3%	
Han et al. (1990)[47]	China, oral leukoplakia	4HCR (40 mg/d)	31	Regression	87% (CR)	<.01
		Placebo	30		17%	
Lippman et al. (1993)[43]	U.S., oral leukoplakia	13cRA (0.5 mg/kg/d)	24	Progression after 13cRA induction	8%	<.001
		β-Carotene (30 mg/d)	29		55%	
Chiesa et al. (1993)[44b]	Italy, oral leukoplakia	4HPR (200 mg/d)	74	Recurrence and new lesion	6% (failure)	<.05
		No treatment control	79		30%	
Zaridze et al. (1993)[40]	Uzbekistan, oral leukoplakia	β-Carotene (40 mg/d) + retinol (100,000 IU/wk) + vitamin E (80 mg/wk)	384	Leukoplakia prevalence	OR = 0.62 (0.39–0.98)	<.05
	Esophagitis	Placebo	291	Progression/stable vs. regression	OR = 0.65 (0.29–1.48)	= NS
Hong et al. (1990, 1994)[48,49]	U.S., prior HNSCC	13cRA (50–100 mg/m²/d)	49	Second primary tumor	4% (32 mo); 14% (55 mo)[c]	= .005 (32 mo)
		Placebo	51		24% (32 mo); 31% (55 mo)	= .042 (55 mo)
Bolla et al. (1994)[51]	France, prior HNSCC	Etretinate (50/25 mg/d)	156	Second primary tumor	18% (41 mo)[c]	= NS
		Placebo	160		18%	
van Zandwijk et al. (1999)[71b]	Europe, prior HNSCC, NSCLC	Vitamin A, 300,000/150,000 IU/d	2592 total	Second primary tumor	NS	= NS
		N-acetylcysteine, 600 mg/d 2 × 2 factorial				
McLarty et al. (1995)[53]	U.S., male asbestos workers	Retinol (25,000 IU qod) + β-carotene (50 mg/d)	755 total	Sputum atypia	OR = 1.24 (0.78–1.96)	= NS
		Placebo				
Arnold et al. (1992)[57]	Canada, bronchial metaplasia	Etretinate (25 mg/d)	75	Improvement	32%	= NS
		Placebo	75		30%	
Lee et al. (1994)[58]	U.S., bronchial metaplasia	13cRA (1 mg/kg/d)	41	Improvement	54%	= NS
		Placebo	45		59%	
Kurie et al. (1999)[59b]	U.S., bronchial metaplasia	4HPR (200 mg/d)	33	Improvement	42%	= NS
		Placebo	35		51%	
Omenn et al. (1996)[62]	U.S., smokers and asbestos workers	β-Carotene (30 mg/d) + retinol (25,000 IU/d)	18,314 total	Lung cancer	RR = 1.28 (1.04–1.57)	<.05
		Placebo				
Pastorino et al. (1993)[70]	Italy, prior NSCLC	Retinyl palmitate (300,000 IU/d)	150	Second primary tumor	Longer time to second primary tumor	= .045
		No treatment control	157			
Veronesi et al. (1999)[76]	Italy, prior breast cancer	4HPR (200 mg/d)	1432	Contralateral breast cancer	RR = 0.92 (0.66–1.29)	= NS
		No treatment	1435			
Moriarty et al. (1982)[82]	Ireland, actinic keratosis	Etretinate (75 mg/d)	44	Regression	84%	<.05
		Placebo	42		5%	

TABLE 23.3-1. (*Continued*)

Reference	*Population*	*Intervention*	*No.*	*End Point*	*Result*	*P Value*
Watson (1986)[83]	Australia, actinic keratosis	Etretinate (75 mg/d)	15 total	Regression	93%	<.05
		Placebo (crossover)			13%	
Kligman and Thorne (1991)[81]	U.S., actinic keratosis	Topical ATRA (.05%)	266	Regression	42%	= NS
		Vehicle control	261		34%	
Kligman and Thorne (1991)[81]	U.S., actinic keratosis	Topical ATRA (0.10%)	226	Regression	55%	<.001
		Vehicle control	229		41%	
Tangrea et al. (1992)[87]	U.S., prior BCC	13cRA (10 mg/d)	490	Second BCC	0.94 tumor/patient/y	= NS
		Placebo	491		0.96	
Moon et al. (1997)[89]	U.S., prior actinic keratosis	Retinol (25,000 IU/d)	2298 total	Second SCC	RR 0.74 (0.56–0.99) = 1	= .04 (SCC)
		Placebo		Second BCC	RR 1.06 (0.86–1.32) = 1	= .36 (BCC)
Levine et al. (1997)[88]	U.S., prior BCC/SCC	13cRA (5–10 mg/d)	525 total	Second skin cancer	n = 40 SCC; n = 103 BCC	= NS (both arms)
		Retinol (25,000 IU/d)			n = 41 SCC; n = 106 BCC	
		Placebo			n = 41 SCC; n = 110 BCC	
Bouwes Bavinck et al. (1995)[86]	Netherlands, renal transplant patients	Acitretin (30 mg/d)	19	Skin cancer	2 patients	=.01
		Placebo	19		9 patients	
Lamm et al. (1994)[95]	U.S., prior bladder transitional cell carcinoma	Megadose vitamins (40,000 IU retinol/d)	35	Recurrence	41%	=.0014
		Recommended dietary allowance vitamins	30		91%	
Alfthan et al. (1983)[93]	Finland, prior bladder cancer	Etretinate (25–50 mg/d)	15	Preventive rate (complete and partial) of recurrence	73%	<.01
		Placebo	15		27%	
Pedersen et al. (1984)[92]	Denmark, prior bladder cancer	Etretinate (50 mg/d)	33	Proportion free of recurrence at 8 mo	27%	= NS
		Placebo	40		37%	
Studer et al. (1984)[94]	Switzerland, prior bladder cancer	Etretinate (25–50 mg/d)	38	Recurrence	29% (recur)/35%/29%[d]	<.02[e]
		Placebo	40		40%/55%/56%	
Meyskens et al. (1994)[97]	U.S., CIN 2,3	Topical ATRA (0.372%)	150	Complete response	43% (CIN 2); 25% (CIN 3)	= .041 (CIN 2)
		Placebo	151		27% (CIN 2); 31% (CIN 3)	= NS (CIN 3)
Munoz et al. (1985, 1987)[102,105]	Huixian, China, high risk	Retinol (50,000 IU/wk) + riboflavin (200 mg/wk) + zinc (50 mg/wk)	610 total	Precancerous esophageal lesions	48.9%	= NS (dysplasia)
		Placebo			45.3%	<.05 (esophageal micronuclei)

ATRA, all-*trans*-retinoic acid; BCC, basal cell carcinoma; CIN, cervical intraepithelial neoplasia; CR, complete response; HNSCC, head and neck squamous cell carcinoma; NSCLC, non–small cell lung cancer; OR, odds ratio; RR, relative risk; SCC, squamous cell carcinoma; 4HCR, N-4-(hydroxycarbophenyl) retinamide; 4HPR, N-(4-hydroxyphenyl) retinamide; 13cRA, 13-*cis* retinoic acid.

[a]Trials including β-carotene are also listed in Table 23.3-2 for completeness.

[b]Ongoing and/or reported in abstract only.

[c]Median study follow-up in months.

[d]Tumor recurrence 3 months/12 months/24 months.

[e]*P* value given for 12-month rates of multifocal (greater than three tumors) recurrence.

TABLE 23.3-2. Randomized Trials of β-Carotene in Human Cancer Chemoprevention[a]

Reference	*Population*	*Intervention*	*No.*	*End Point*	*Result*	*P Value*
Stich et al. (1984)[30]	Philippines, betel quid users	β-Carotene (180 mg/wk)	25	Oral micronuclei	Decreased 66%	<.001
		Placebo	18		Decreased 1%	
Stich et al. (1985)[31]	Inuits, smokeless tobacco users	β-Carotene (180 mg/wk)	23	Oral micronuclei	Decreased 60%	<.001
		Placebo	31		Decreased 0.5%	
Stich et al. (1988)[32]	India, betel nut chewers	β-Carotene (180 mg/wk)	31	Oral micronuclei	Decreased 71%/ decreased 75%[b]	<.001
		β-Carotene and retinol (100,000 IU/ wk)	51		Decreased 71%/ decreased 71%	<.001
		Placebo	30		Increased 8%/ decreased 7%	
Stich et al. (1988)[32]	India, betel nut chewers	β-Carotene (180 mg/wk)	27	Oral leukoplakia (complete remission)	14.8%	= NS
		β-Carotene and retinol (100,000 IU/ wk)	51		27.5%	<.05
		Placebo	33		3%	
Sankaranarayanan et al. (1997)[39]	India, tobacco chewers	β-Carotene (360 mg/wk)	55	Oral leukoplakia (complete regression)	β-Carotene 33%	<.0001
		Retinyl acetate (300,000 IU/wk)	50		Vitamin A 52%	
		Placebo	55		Placebo 10%	
Zaridze et al. (1993)[40]	Uzbekistan, oral leukoplakia, esophagitis	β-Carotene (40 mg/ d) + retinol (100,000 IU/wk) + vitamin E (80 mg/wk)	384	Leukoplakia prevalence	OR = 0.62 (0.39–0.98)	<.05
		Placebo	291	Progression/stable vs. regression	OR = 0.66 (0.37–1.16)	= NS
McLarty et al. (1995)[53]	U.S., male asbestos workers	Retinol (25,000 IU q.o.d.) + β-carotene (50 mg/d)	755 total	Sputum atypia	OR = 1.24 (0.78–1.96)	= NS
		Placebo				
Van Poppel et al. (1992)[54]	Netherlands, male smokers	β-Carotene (20 mg/ d)	114 total	Sputum micronuclei	Decreased 27%	<.05
		Placebo			(9–41%)	
Alpha-Tocopherol, Beta Carotene Cancer Prevention Study Group (1994)[60]	Finland, male smokers	β-Carotene (20 mg/ d) ± vitamin E (50 mg/d)	29,133 total	Lung cancer	β-Carotene RR = 1.18 (1.03–1.36)	<.05
		Placebo				
Omenn et al. (1996)[62]	U.S., smokers and asbestos workers	β-Carotene (30 mg/ d) + retinol (25,000 IU/d)	18,314 total	Lung cancer	RR = 1.28 (1.04–1.57)	<.05
		Placebo				
Hennekens et al. (1996)[63]	U.S., male physicians	β-Carotene (50 mg/ q.o.d.)	22,071 total	Total cancer	RR = 0.98 (0.91–1.06)	= NS
		Placebo				
Lee et al. (1999)[64]	U.S., female health professionals	β-Carotene (50 mg/ q.o.d.)	19,939	All cancers	RR = 1.03 (0.89–1.18)	= NS
		Placebo	19,937			

TABLE 23.3-2. ***(Continued)***

Reference	*Population*	*Intervention*	*No.*	*End Point*	*Result*	*P Value*
Greenberg et al. (1990)[90]	U.S., prior skin cancer	β-Carotene (50 mg/d)	1805 total	Second skin cancer	RR = 1.05 (0.91–1.22)	= NS
		Placebo				
DeVet et al. (1991)[98]	Netherlands, CIN	β-Carotene (10 mg/d)	278 total	Regression	OR = 0.68[c] (0.28–1.60)	= NS
		Placebo				
Romney et al. (1997)[99]	U.S., CIN	β-Carotene (30 mg/d)	39	Persistent CIN	OR = 1.53 (0.38–6.18)	= NS
		Placebo	30			
Mackerras et al. (1999)[100]	Australia, CIN 1 or minor squamous atypia of the cervix	β-Carotene (30 mg/d) ± vitamin C (500 mg/d)	141 total (60 on β-carotene)	Regression rate	RR = 1.58 (0.86–2.93)	= NS
		Placebo		Progression rate	RR = 1.75 (0.57–5.36)	= NS
Blot et al. (1993)[103]	Linxian County, China, general population	β-Carotene (15 mg/d) + vitamin E (30 mg/d) + selenium (50 μg/d)	29,584 total	Stomach cancer death	RR = 0.79 (0.64–0.99)	<.05
		Placebo		Esophageal cancer death	RR = 0.96 (0.78–1.18)	= NS
Li et al. (1993)[104]	Linxian County, China, esophageal dysplasia	Multivite/multimineral + β-carotene (15 mg/d)	3318 total	Stomach cancer death	RR = 1.18 (0.76–1.85)	= NS
		Placebo		Esophageal cancer death	RR = 0.84 (0.54–1.29)	= NS
Greenberg et al. (1994)[107]	U.S., resected adenoma	β-Carotene (25 mg/d) ± vitamin C (1 g/d) + vitamin E (400 mg/d)	751 total	Recurrent adenoma	β-Carotene RR = 1.01 (0.85–1.20)	= NS
		Placebo				
Kikendall et al. (1991)[109]	U.S., resected adenoma	β-Carotene (15 mg/d)	132[d]	Recurrent polyps	29%	= NS
		Placebo	125		24%	
MacLennan et al. (1995)[108]	Australia, resected adenoma	β-Carotene (20 mg/d) ± fat reduction ± fiber (25 g/d)	390 total	Recurrent adenoma	RR = 1.4 (0.8–2.3)	= NS
		Placebo		Adenoma >10 mm	RR = 1.5 (0.3–4.2)	
				Adenoma with moderate or severe dysplasia	RR = 0.8 (0.3–2.2)	

CIN, cervical intraepithelial neoplasia; OR, odds ratio; RR, relative risk.
[a]Trials including retinoids are also listed in Table 23.3-1 for completeness.
[b]Change in leukoplakia and normal mucosa, respectively.
[c]Based on broad definition of regression (major and minor).
[d]Number completing 36 months.

in combination with other agents, on regression of oral leukoplakia. Six nonrandomized studies[33–38] reported response rates ranging from 44% to 97%. The response rates from these uncontrolled studies, however, must be interpreted cautiously for three reasons: (1) leukoplakias can regress spontaneously; (2) varying response criteria were used; and (3) there was no apparent dose-response relationship. Three placebo-controlled trials of β-carotene and oral leukoplakia are available. Stich et al.[32] reported that the combination of β-carotene plus retinol produced complete remissions in 27.5%, β-carotene alone in 14.8%, and placebo in 3.0% of subjects (partial remissions were not reported) with a 6-month intervention. Sankaranarayanan et al.[39] got better response rates with an even longer duration of intervention (12 months), consisting of 33% complete regression with β-carotene and 52% with retinyl palmitate versus 10% in the placebo arm. In a trial in Uzbekistan,[40] 6 months of treatment with the combination of retinol, β-carotene, and vitamin E led to a significant reduction in the prevalence odds ratio of oral leukoplakia [odds ratio = 0.62; 95% confidence interval (CI) = 0.39 to 0.98]. The risk of progression or no change versus regression also was reduced by 40% by this intervention, although not statistically significant (odds ratio = 0.60; 95% CI = 0.23 to 1.63). Vitamin E was evaluated by itself in a single-arm trial in oral leukoplakia in which both clinical and histologic responses were observed.[41]

Retinoids have been studied extensively in the reversal of oral premalignant lesions.[2,28,29] One of the first such trials, reported in 1986,[42] was a 3-month placebo-controlled study of 13cRA (2 mg/kg/d). The complete plus partial response rate in the 44 evaluable patients was 67% in the retinoid arm and 10% in the placebo arm (P = .0002). The histopathologic improvement rate (e.g., reversal of dysplasia) was also higher in the retinoid arm (54% vs. 10%, P = .01). There were two major problems, however, with this high-dose, short-term approach. First, high-dose 13cRA toxicity was substantial and not acceptable in this clinical setting. Second, over one-half of the responders had recurrences or developed new lesions within 3 months of stopping the intervention.

Based on the results of this placebo-controlled trial, a randomized maintenance trial was designed.[43] In this trial, patients initially received a 3-month induction course of high-dose 13cRA (1.5 mg/kg/d), followed by a 9-month maintenance course with low-dose 13cRA (0.5 mg/kg/d) or β-carotene (30 mg/d) in patients with responding or stable lesions during the high-dose induction phase. The induction-phase response rate was 55% (95% CI = 42% to 67%). During the maintenance phase, 2 (8%) of the patients in the retinoid group progressed versus 16 (55%) in the β-carotene group (P<.001). Toxic effects of low-dose 13cRA maintenance therapy were mild, although greater than for β-carotene, with no patients discontinuing therapy because of toxicity.

4HPR, a promising new retinoid, is also being evaluated in oral premalignancy. A randomized study was begun in 1988 at the Milan Cancer Institute to evaluate the efficacy of 52 weeks of systemic 4HPR maintenance therapy (vs. no intervention) after complete laser resection of oral premalignant lesions. The most recent report on this ongoing study included data from 153 randomized patients.[44,45] A 3-day drug holiday at the end of each month was prescribed to avoid the adverse effects (night blindness) of lowering serum retinol by 4HPR treatment. The rate of treatment failure (recurrence plus new lesion rate) among those patients who completed the 12-month intervention was 6% in the 4HPR group and 30% in the control group.

Two other randomized studies involving retinol[39,46] and another involving the retinoid N-4-(hydroxycarbophenyl) retinamide (4HCR)[47] have been reported; all observed significant retinoid chemopreventive activity.

HEAD AND NECK TRIALS: MALIGNANCY

There have been only two phase III adjuvant chemoprevention trials of retinoids in head and neck cancer. The first, reported by Hong et al., tested high-dose 13cRA in 103 head and neck cancer patients.[48] Following definitive local therapy of stage I to IV (M0) disease with surgery, radiotherapy, or both, patients were assigned randomly to 12 months of 13cRA (50 to 100 mg/m^2/d) or placebo. At a median follow-up of 32 months, there were no significant differences in primary disease recurrence (local, regional, or distant) or survival. The rate of second primary tumors, however, was significantly lower in the retinoid arm than in the placebo group, developing in two (4%) of the 13cRA-treated patients compared with 12 (24%) of the placebo-treated patients (P = .005). More than 70% of second primary tumors occurred in the carcinogen-exposed aerodigestive tract fields of the head and neck, lungs, and esophagus. Side effects were substantial and included skin dryness and peeling, cheilitis, conjunctivitis, and hypertriglyceridemia. Approximately 30% of the retinoid-treated patients required dose reduction and 18% did not complete the 12-month intervention because of toxicity.

This trial has been reanalyzed with a longer median follow-up of 55 months.[49] With the additional follow-up, each group had one more second primary tumor in the aerodigestive tract, resulting in a cumulative total of three of the retinoid group and 13 of the placebo group (P = .008).

Based on this high-dose adjuvant trial[48,49] and the low-dose 13cRA trial in oral premalignancy,[43] a multicenter large-scale phase III National Cancer Institute trial was designed and is ongoing to evaluate low-dose 13cRA as adjuvant chemoprevention in stage I and II head and neck cancer.[50]

The other randomized trial studied the synthetic retinoid etretinate in 316 patients following definitive therapy of stage I to III (T1,2, N0,1) squamous cell carcinoma of the oral cavity and oropharynx.[51] In this French trial, the etretinate dose was 50 mg/d for 1 month, then 25 mg/d for 2 years. The etretinate was well tolerated. At a median follow-up of 41 months, the rate of second primary tumor development in the two arms was not significantly different. The lack of a retinoid effect on second primary tumors in this trial is in contrast to the result of the earlier high-dose 13cRA trial and could be attributable to differences in the patient populations and differing dose levels. A more likely reason for the difference, however, involves the pharmacokinetics and mechanisms of action of the two retinoids studied. 13cRA leads to transcriptional activation via rapid isomerization to ATRA. In contrast, etretinate is known not to be transcriptionally active and is not known to isomerize to ATRA or any other transcriptionally active retinoid.

The most recently reported trial (Euroscan) included head and neck and lung cancer–associated second primary tumors and is discussed in detail in a following section called Lung Trials: Malignancy.

Two trials involving β-carotene and head and neck cancer prevention have completed intervention, but results have not yet been released, one in the United States[52] and one in Italy (Dr. S. Toma, unpublished data). Both are designed to determine whether supplemental β-carotene reduces the incidence of second malignant cancers of the oral cavity, pharynx, larynx, esophagus, and lung in patients who have been "cured" of an early-stage head or neck cancer. A total of 264 patients were randomized in the U.S. trial and 211 in the Italian trial. Results are expected shortly.

LUNG TRIALS: PREMALIGNANCY

The Tyler (Texas) Chemoprevention Trial randomized 755 asbestos workers to receive β-carotene (50 mg/d) and retinol (25,000 IU every other day) versus placebo, to see if the nutrient combination could reduce the prevalence of atypical cells in sputum. After a mean intervention period of 58 months, there was no difference in the two groups in the prevalence of sputum atypia.[53] In another randomized, placebo-controlled trial, 14 weeks of supplemental β-carotene (20 mg/d) significantly reduced micronuclei counts in sputum from heavy smokers.[54] β-Carotene was not found, however, to reduce oxidative damage as measured by urinary excretion of 8-oxo-7, 8-dihydro-2'-deoxyguanosine,[55] suggesting that antioxidant activity was not responsible for the reduction in micronuclei.

In a French trial, chronic smokers with squamous metaplasia of the bronchial epithelium detected in initial bronchoscopy specimens were treated with etretinate (25 mg/d) for 6 months.[56] In this uncontrolled trial, a decline in the extent of squamous metaplasia was observed in most treated patients. The positive result of this French study led to three randomized trials: one of etretinate in Canada and one of 13cRA and one of 4HPR in the United States. The Canadian study evaluated the ability of 25 mg of etretinate per day for 6 months to reverse sputum atypia in chronic smokers.[57] Toxicity was mild and the number of subjects requiring dose reductions or dropping out was small and similar in both arms. No difference in the degree of atypia occurred between the etretinate and placebo groups. In the U.S. 13cRA study, chronic smokers underwent bronchoscopy with endobronchial biopsies taken from six specific anatomic sites within the proximal lung field,[58] as reported in the earlier single-arm French study.[56] Ninety-three of the 152 chronic smokers who underwent bronchoscopic biopsies had squamous metaplasia or dysplasia. Eligible smokers with metaplasia or dysplasia were randomized to 6 months of 13cRA or placebo. The extent of metaplasia decreased similarly (in approximately 50% of subjects) in both study arms. Only smoking cessation (confirmed biochemically), which occurred in 16 patients (ten in the 13cRA group and six in the placebo group), was associated significantly with a reduction in the metaplasia index during the 6-month intervention. 4HPR was involved in the most recent study (reported in abstract only[59]). This study was similar to the earlier isotretinoin study with respect to overall design (excepting the drug) and the negative primary result.[58] Although the retinoid arm results were consistent with the French findings in showing a decline in metaplasia with treatment, the use of a placebo control group in the randomized trials suggested no specific retinoid effect. These findings underscore the critical importance of placebo-controlled designs to establish drug activity in chemoprevention trials using intermediate end points.

LUNG TRIALS: MALIGNANCY

Two large trials using incident lung cancer as a primary end point have now been completed. The first involved 29,133 men aged 50 to 69 years old from Finland,[60] who were heavy cigarette smokers at entry (average one pack per day for 36 years). The study design was a two-by-two factorial with participants randomized to receive either supplemental β-carotene (20 mg/d), α-tocopherol (50 mg/d), the combination, or placebo for 5 to 8 years. Unexpectedly, participants receiving β-carotene (alone or in combination with α-tocopherol) had a statistically significant 18% increase in lung cancer incidence (relative risk [RR] = 1.18; 95% CI = 1.03 to 1.36) and 8% increase in total mortality (relative risk [RR] = 1.08; 95% CI = 1.01 to 1.16) relative to participants receiving placebo. Supplemental β-carotene did not appear to affect the incidence of other major cancers occurring in this population. Although not the primary outcome of this trial, an interesting observation was made with regard to vitamin E and prostate cancer: Men randomized to receive α-tocopherol had a 32% decrease in prostate cancer incidence and a 41% decrease in prostate cancer mortality.[61] This promising finding will be followed up in future trials (see Conclusions, later in this chapter).

The finding of an increased incidence of lung cancer in β-carotene–supplemented smokers was apparently replicated in another major trial. The Carotene and Retinol Efficacy Trial was a multicenter lung cancer prevention trial of supplemental β-carotene (30 mg/d) plus retinol (25,000 IU/d) versus placebo in asbestos workers and smokers.[62] The Carotene and Retinol Efficacy Trial was terminated nearly 2 years early in January 1996, because interim analyses of the data indicated that should the trial have continued for its planned duration, it is highly unlikely that the intervention would have been found to be beneficial. Furthermore, the interim results indicated that the supplemented group was developing more lung cancer, not less, consistent with the results of the Finnish trial. Overall, lung cancer incidence was increased by 28% in the supplemented subjects (RR = 1.28; 95% CI = 1.04 to 1.57) and total mortality was also increased (RR = 1.17; 95% CI = 1.03 to 1.33). The increase in lung cancer following supplementation with β-carotene and retinol was observed for current but not former smokers. Major findings of one additional trial, the Physicians' Health Study of supplemental β-carotene versus placebo in 22,071 male U.S. physicians, are also now available.[63] There was no significant effect, positive or negative, of 12 years of supplementation of β-carotene (50 mg every other day) on total cancer, lung cancer, or cardiovascular disease. The relative risk for lung cancer in current smokers randomized to β-carotene was 0.90 (95% CI = 0.58 to 1.40). Among nonsmokers, the relative risk was 0.78 (95% CI = 0.34 to 1.79). The apparent lack of an effect of long-term supplementation of β-carotene on lung cancer incidence, even in baseline smokers who took the supplements for up to 12 years, is noteworthy and is discussed further here. A similar lack of effect of supplemental β-carotene on overall cancer incidence was seen in the Women's Health Study, although the duration of intervention was short (median, 2.1 years).[64]

In contrast, more encouraging results for lung cancer prevention come from an esophageal and gastric cancer prevention trial in China (see Esophagus and Stomach Trials, later in this chapter). The relative risk of death from lung cancer was 0.55 (95% CI = 0.26 to 1.14) among those receiving the combination of β-carotene, α-tocopherol, and selenium.[65] However, this result is not statistically significant, based on only 31 total lung cancer deaths.

A clear mechanism to explain the apparent enhancement of lung carcinogenesis by supplemental β-carotene, alone or in combination with retinol, in smokers has yet to emerge. As detailed elsewhere,[66] it should be noted that the two trials that observed this enhancing effect had higher median plasma β-carotene concentrations in their intervention groups than did the trials that did not observe an enhancing effect. Thus, it is possible that high tissue concentrations of β-carotene in the presence of strongly oxidative tobacco smoke cause an interaction that affects carcinogenesis. Wang et al. have used the ferret to model β-carotene/tobacco interactions in lung and noted a relative lack of both retinoic acid and RAR-β expression in the lung of smoke-exposed ferrets given high-dose β-carotene.[67] The authors suggested that oxidative metabolites of β-carotene might cause diminished retinoid signaling and thus increase tumorigenesis. Other groups are also studying β-carotene oxidation products, for example Salgo et al.[68] reported that under some conditions β-carotene oxidation products, but not β-carotene, enhanced binding of cytochrome P-450–catalyzed metabolites of benzo[a]pyrene to DNA. While mechanistic studies continue,[69] it is prudent to recommend that heavy smokers, particularly those from well-nourished populations, should avoid high-dose supplements of β-carotene for lung cancer chemoprevention.

Retinoids have not been tested as single agents in primary prevention trials of lung cancer; however, one trial of retinyl palmitate in adjuvant chemoprevention of lung cancer is available.[70] Following surgery, patients with stage I non–small cell lung cancer (n = 307) were assigned randomly to treatment with retinyl palmitate (300,000 IU) for 1 year of observation. At a median follow-up of 46 months, survival trends favored retinyl palmitate over no therapy in estimated 5-year disease-free survival (64% vs. 51%, $P = .054$) and overall survival (62% vs. 54%, $P = .44$). Eighteen patients in the retinyl palmitate arm developed a second primary tumor compared with 29 patients developing 33 second primaries in the control group. Reduction of tobacco-associated second primary tumors was more pronounced. At a median follow-up of 46 months, tobacco-associated second primary tumors developed in 13 patients in the retinyl palmitate arm compared with 25 control patients. The time to development of tobacco-related second primary tumors also favored the retinyl palmitate arm ($P = .045$). Retinyl palmitate toxicity was frequent, occurring in the majority of treated patients; however, more than 80% of patients maintained regular drug intake during the first 12 months, indicating that the intervention was tolerable.

Based on the encouraging second primary tumor results and retinoid activity in related carcinogenic systems, two large-scale phase III retinoid trials were implemented in the setting of second primary tumor prevention. One of these trials, called Euroscan, has been completed in Europe. Euroscan[71] was an open-label multicenter trial employing a two-by-two factorial design to test 2 years of retinyl palmitate and N-acetylcysteine in preventing second primary tumors in 2592 patients. Patients had completed definitive therapy of early-stage head and neck cancer (larynx Tis, T1 to 3, N0 to 1; oral cavity T1 to 2, N0 to 1) and non–small cell lung cancer (T1 to 2, N0 to 1, and T3, N0). Retinyl palmitate, N-acetylcysteine, or both produced no improvement in event-free survival, survival, or incidence of second primary tumors. The other related trial is still ongoing in the United States. This is a multicenter trial (intergroup NCI I91-0001) of low-dose isotretinoin to prevent second primary tumors after definitive therapy of stage I non–small cell lung cancer.[72] Currently, new phase III chemoprevention trials in the non–small cell and small cell lung cancer settings are being designed.[73] In addition, new retinoid formulations and delivery systems (e.g., aerosolized) and potential secondary lung benefits are under active study.[74,75]

BREAST TRIALS

The retinamide 4HPR is a potent apoptosis-inducing retinoid with retinoid receptor-dependent and receptor-independent activities. Moon and colleagues first showed that 4HPR was among the most active cancer chemopreventive agents for the breast, having a high therapeutic index and synergistic interaction with tamoxifen in mammary carcinogenesis model studies.[7] This laboratory work led to a large-scale randomized trial of 4HPR (vs. no treatment) for 5 years to prevent contralateral breast cancer in women aged 30 to 70 years with a history of resected early breast cancer and no prior adjuvant therapy.[76] The intervention produced no significant overall effect. Subset analyses suggested that reduced contralateral and ipsilateral breast cancer rates occurred in premenopausal women and that an opposite trend occurred in postmenopausal women.[76] Promising new retinoids for breast cancer prevention include other potent apoptosis-inducing retinoids and RAR-subtype-selective, RXR-selective, and anti-AP-1 retinoids.[77]

As for β-carotene, observational data have suggested that higher intake of β-carotene from foods is an important prognostic factor in breast cancer.[78,79] Given this, randomized trials aimed at increasing vegetable intake to prevent breast cancer recurrence are under way.[80] These interventions clearly influence circulating carotenoid concentrations and illustrate a food-based approach to investigate potential chemopreventive efficacy.

SKIN TRIALS

Data suggest that topical ATRA has significant dose-related activity in reversing premalignant skin lesions (e.g., actinic keratoses, which undergo a malignant transformation rate of 5%).[81] Systemic retinoid therapy has produced significant activity in the two reported randomized trials.[82,83] Several small, single-arm studies have found that 13cRA and etretinate can reduce skin cancer incidence significantly in high-risk patients with xeroderma pigmentosum (XP) and in renal transplant recipients, respectively.[84,85]

The XP trial, published in 1988, was a landmark trial for the field of chemoprevention in general in that it was the first human trial to establish a significant reduction in tumor development.[84] Although including only five XP patients, the extremely high rate of skin cancer development and rigorous documentation of skin tumor rates before, during, and after the 2-year high-dose (2 mg/kg/d) 13cRA intervention provided statistically valid results. The overall average reduction in skin cancer incidence during therapy was 63% ($P = .019$). Two major problems were evident from this trial: Severe, acute mucocutaneous toxicity occurred with this high 13cRA dose, and the preventive effect of the retinoid was lost after stopping retinoid therapy, as indicated by a mean 8.5-fold increase in the annual rate of skin tumor development ($P = .007$). The retinoid chemopreventive effect in this study was greatest in the XP patients with the highest frequency of *de novo* skin tumor development, and, in subsequent studies, was found to be dose related.

Based on positive single-arm retinoid data,[85] a randomized, placebo-controlled trial of the retinoid acitretin (30 mg/d for 6 months) was conducted in 38 renal transplant recipients.[86] The retinoid group had significant reductions in (1) premalignant lesions ($P = .008$); (2) the number of patients with skin cancer ($P = .01$); and (3) the cumulative number of skin cancers ($P = .009$). Nine of the 19 placebo patients developed a total of 18 skin cancers and 2 of the 19 retinoid patients developed skin cancer, one cancer each. After completing the intervention, the rate of skin cancer development in the retinoid arm increased and became similar to that of the placebo arm. Toxicity in the retinoid group was frequent but mild in degree, and the retinoid had no adverse effect on renal function.

Three large-scale randomized phase III trials of retinoids and skin cancer have been reported. A trial of very low-dose 13cRA (10 mg/d)[87] and one of retinol (25,000 IU/d) or 13cRA (5 to 10 mg/d) versus placebo in patients with prior skin cancers[88] were negative. The third trial, involving retinol in patients with prior actinic keratoses, did see a significant reduction of squamous but not basal skin cancers in the retinoid arm.[89] The contrasting results of the phase III retinoid trials in skin cancer chemoprevention suggest the importance of retinoid dose, biologic timing of intervention, and target histopathology.

Greenberg and colleagues[90] conducted a large randomized clinical trial of supplemental β-carotene (50 mg/d for 5 years) in 1805 persons with a previous nonmelanoma skin cancer. There was no difference between the two groups in the rate of occurrence of the first new nonmelanoma skin cancer (RR = 1.05; 95% CI = 0.91 to 1.22).

Selenium is another nutrient that has been evaluated for efficacy in the prevention of second skin cancers.[91] Clark et al. randomized a total of 1312 patients with a history of nonmelanoma skin cancer to 200 μg selenium per day or placebo. Selenium did not affect the incidence of second skin cancers (RR = 1.10 for basal cell carcinoma and RR = 1.14 for squamous cell carcinoma). However, there was a significant reduction in total cancer mortality (RR = 0.50; 95% CI = 0.31 to 0.80), mainly due to reductions in incident lung, colorectal, and prostate cancers. Other selenium trials are now getting under way (see Conclusions, later in this chapter), given these promising results.

BLADDER TRIALS

Data from *in vivo* animal, *in vitro*, and epidemiologic studies suggested efficacy of retinoids for bladder cancer prevention. Three randomized clinical trials have tested the retinoid etretinate in patients following resection of their superficial (noninvasive) bladder tumors, which recur in 40% to 90% of cases. All three studies were limited substantially because of mucocutaneous toxicity.[92–94] However, in two of the three trials, prolonged (greater than 1 year) low-dose etretinate (25 mg/d) apparently was effective. These positive results require a cautious reading, because of small patient numbers and short-term follow-up.

Another chemoprevention trial randomized 65 patients with biopsy-confirmed transitional cell carcinoma of the bladder to a multivitamin (recommended dietary allowance levels) alone or supplemented with 40,000 IU of retinol, 100 mg of pyridoxine, 2000 mg of ascorbic acid, 400 IU of α-tocopherol, and 90 mg of zinc.[95] The 5-year estimate of tumor recurrence was 91% in the recommended dietary allowance arm versus 41% in the megadose arm ($P = .0014$). These results are promising in that the intervention was essentially nontoxic, with only one patient (3%) requiring dose reduction for mild stomach upset. Further research is needed to identify which vitamin(s) were responsible for chemopreventive efficacy.

Studies in the bladder of newer synthetic retinoids with better therapeutic ratios are also anticipated. One such leading candidate is 4HPR,[7,10] which tests as one of the strongest anticarcinogenic retinoids in the rodent bladder, is less toxic than either etretinate or isotretinoin in humans, and has produced promising results in a phase IIA trial.[96]

CERVICAL TRIALS

Many randomized and nonrandomized chemoprevention studies have been conducted in cervical dysplasia. Randomized trials include two studies of folic acid, four of interferons, three of β-carotene, and one of ATRA. Only one of these trials, using topical ATRA,[97] found a significant treatment effect. Three hundred one patients with moderate (cervical intraepithelial neoplasia 2) and severe (cervical intraepithelial neoplasia 3) dysplasia were randomly assigned to topical ATRA versus placebo. This trial administered a 0.372% β-ATRA solution by collagen sponge in a cervical cap delivery system for 4 days initially, then for 2 days at months 3 and 6. Patients were evaluated by serial colposcopy, Pap cytology, and cervical biopsy. The ATRA dose, schedule, and delivery system were determined by prior single-arm phase I and II studies. The major finding was a higher complete response rate in the ATRA group (43%) than in the placebo group (27%; $P = .041$) among the 141 patients with moderate dysplasia. No significant differences in dysplasia regression rates between the two study arms were detected in patients with severe dysplasia. Acute toxicity was infrequent, mild, and reversible consisting primarily of local (vaginal and vulvar) irritation occurring in less than 5% of treated subjects. Major problems with compliance (e.g., 52 patients lost to follow-up), however, have limited somewhat the interpretation of this trial.

Three randomized trials involving β-carotene have been published. The first was a trial from the Netherlands that randomized women with a histologic diagnosis of cervical dysplasia to either 10 mg of β-carotene per day for 3 months or placebo. After 3 months of intervention, there was no detectable effect of supplemental β-carotene on the regression and progression of cervical dysplasia.[98] Romney et al.[99] randomized women with cervical dysplasia to 30 mg of β-carotene per day (n = 39) or placebo (n = 30). After 9 months of intervention, there was no beneficial effect of β-carotene supplementation. An Australian trial used a factorial design to investigate the effects of supplemental β-carotene (30 mg/d) or vitamin C (500 mg/d) in 141 women with minor cervical abnormalities.[100] There was no significant effect of either agent in this trial. In contrast are results from a nonrandomized phase II intervention trial of cervical dysplasia[101] that reported a striking 70% response rate following 6 months of supplementation with 30 mg of β-carotene per day. The results of the randomized trials suggest that this impressive response rate may reflect spontaneous regression rather than an effect of the β-carotene.

ESOPHAGUS AND STOMACH TRIALS

Certain regions of China (Huixian and Linxian) have strikingly high incidence rates of esophageal and gastric cancers; moreover, intake and blood levels of various micronutrients are consistently low in these populations. These observations have led to three esophageal and esophageal and gastric cancer prevention trials in China.[102–104] The first was in high-risk Chinese subjects from Huixian and tested the combination of retinol, riboflavin, and zinc for 13.5 months. After the intervention, there was no overall difference between the two arms in the occurrence of premalignant lesions or the prevalence or severity of dysplasia.[102] However, esophageal (but not oral) micronuclei frequency decreased in the intervention arm.[105]

Two more recent trials were done in Linxian county. The first trial was conducted in residents from the general population.[103] Nearly 30,000 men and women aged 40 to 69 took part in the study, which tested the efficacy of four different nutrient combinations at inhibiting the development of esophageal and gastric cancers. The nutrient combinations included retinol plus zinc, riboflavin plus niacin, ascorbic acid plus molybdenum, and the combination of β-carotene, selenium, and α-tocopherol. After a 5-year intervention period, those who were given the combination of β-carotene, vitamin E, and selenium had a 13% reduction in total cancer deaths (RR = 0.87; 95% CI = 0.75 to 1.00), a 4% reduction in esophageal cancer deaths (RR = 0.96; 95% CI = 0.78 to 1.18), and a 21% reduction in gastric cancer deaths (RR = 0.79; 95% CI = 0.64 to 0.99). None of the other nutrient combinations reduced gastric or esophageal cancer deaths significantly in this trial. The finding that vitamin supplements reduced cancer deaths in this population provides compelling data supporting the concept of cancer prevention via nutrients; however, the applicability of these results for populations with adequate nutritional status and for other tumor sites may be limited. Also, it is unclear which nutrient(s) (β-carotene, vitamin E, or selenium) was responsible for the observed protection. It is perhaps of interest that selenium was not deficient in this population.

The other Linxian trial was done to determine whether a multivitamin and multimineral preparation plus β-carotene (15 mg) reduced esophageal and gastric cardia cancers in 3318 residents with esophageal dysplasia.[104] Cumulative esophageal and gastric cardia death rates after the 6-year intervention period were 8% lower (RR = 0.92; 95% CI = 0.67 to 1.28), esophageal cancer mortality was 16% lower (RR = 0.84; 95% CI = 0.54 to 1.29), and total cancer mortality was 4% lower (RR = 0.96; 95% CI = 0.71 to 1.29) in the supplemented group. Surprisingly, stomach cancer mortality was 18% higher (RR = 1.18; 95% CI = 0.76 to 1.85) in the supplemented group. None of the results were statistically significant.

Repeat endoscopic surveys were carried out 2 and 6 years after randomization in a subsample of participants in the dysplasia trial.[106] At baseline (1983, 2 years before randomization), all of the subjects had a cytologic diagnosis of dysplasia (98% squamous). In the 1987 survey (n = 768), 61.3% of the participants who were endoscoped and on the active arm were found to have normal cytology, compared with 57.6% of those on the placebo arm. In the 1991 survey (n = 396), 17.8% of the participants who were endoscoped and on the active arm were found to have normal cytology, compared with 20.6% on the placebo arm. The striking degree of apparent regression observed in the placebo arm, particularly in the 1987 survey, again underscores the importance of placebo controls in trials of intermediate end points.

In addition to the Chinese trials, a trial from Uzbekistan used a factorial design to study the combination of β-carotene, retinol, and α-tocopherol, with and without riboflavin, in subjects with chronic esophagitis.[40] The risk of progression or no change versus regression was nonsignificantly decreased by 34% in those receiving retinol, β-carotene, and α-tocopherol (OR = 0.66; 95% CI = 0.37 to 1.16) versus those who did not receive these agents.

COLORECTAL TRIALS

Three randomized trials aimed at the prevention of recurrent colorectal adenomas with supplemental β-carotene have been completed. The largest trial studied 751 patients who had had an adenoma diagnosed and removed within the previous 3 months.[107] Participants were randomized using a two-by-two factorial design, with the active treatments being β-carotene (25 mg/d), and the combination of 1 g of vitamin C plus 400 mg of vitamin E. There was no evidence that either β-carotene or vitamins C and E reduced the incidence of adenomas in this 4-year trial. The relative risk for β-carotene was 1.01 (95% CI = 0.85 to 1.20); for vitamins C and E it was 1.08 (95% CI = 0.91 to 1.29). The Australian Polyp Prevention Project evaluated the efficacy of reducing dietary fat to 25% of total calories, and supplementing the diet with 25 g of wheat bran, 20 mg of β-carotene, or both daily, in a factorial design.[108] β-Carotene did not reduce the incidence of adenomas; at 24 months 50 patients on the β-carotene arm had adenomas versus 36 patients on the placebo arm. However, patients taking β-carotene had a statistically significantly lower proportion of positive nuclei in the upper rectal crypt compartments than those taking placebo, suggesting that β-carotene modified preneoplastic mucosal proliferation rather than adenoma growth. Another trial (n = 291) using a lower dose of 15 mg of β-carotene per day also failed to see a reduction in adenomas with supplementation.[109]

TRANSLATIONAL AND INTERMEDIATE END POINT STUDIES IN RETINOID CHEMOPREVENTION

Clinical-laboratory translational research is critical for developing new and better chemopreventive agents and for moving them more quickly into standard care; the oral premalignancy model appears to be an excellent model for translational studies.[28,110–112] Advanced oral lesions can be visualized, biopsied, and monitored prospectively; they are linked to carcinogenesis throughout the aerodigestive tract; and activity of retinoids and β-carotene has been demonstrated in randomized trials. Work in the retinoid oral premalignancy system offers a paradigm for clinical and laboratory collaboration in other tumor sites and with other agents. One aspect relates to an understanding of the predictive value of biomarker modulation in terms of clinical outcome and correlation of various markers within the same system.

Basic research in the retinoid oral premalignancy model will increase our knowledge of the biology of epithelial carcinogenesis and agent mechanisms, and, it is hoped, will lead to valid intermediate end point biomarkers. As reviewed in detail elsewhere, intermediate end point biomarkers are short-term markers of chemopreventive agent activity. Criteria include (1) differential expression in high- and low-risk tissue, (2) pattern and degree of expression correlating with histopathologic stage (e.g., hyperplasia, degree of dysplasia, cancer), (3) low rate of spontaneous change, (4) ability to be modulated, and (5) technical and logistic feasibility.[1,111] The most substantial work in the retinoid oral premalignancy model involves RAR-β and p53.

The discovery and early descriptions of nuclear receptors came from molecular *in vitro* studies in several systems. These receptors are also being studied intensively in clinical specimens from many cancer types and sites. The best-studied site in chemoprevention is the head and neck. Xu and colleagues employed a nonradioactive RNA *in situ* hybridization method to study the expression of all six human retinoid receptors in squamous cell carcinoma and surrounding premalignant and normal tissue contained in surgical resection specimens.[113] All six receptors were strongly expressed in 100% of oral tissue from normal, nonsmoking volunteers. In premalignant and malignant specimens, however, there was a selective, histopathologic

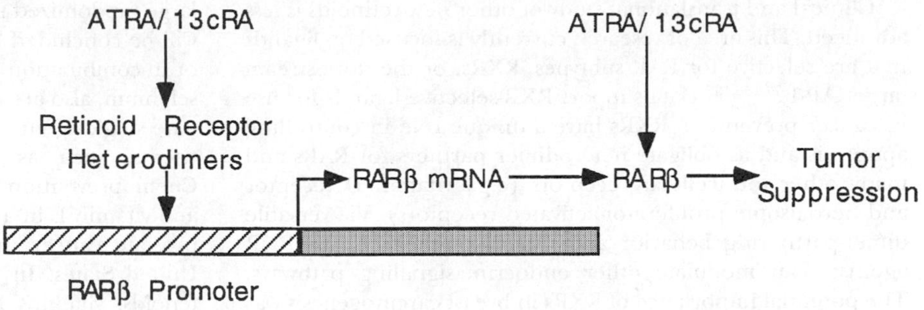

FIGURE 23.3-2 Molecular model of retinoid chemoprevention. ATRA, all-*trans*-retinoic acid; 13cRA, 13-*cis*retinoic acid; RAR-β, retinoic acid receptor beta.

stage-dependent loss of RAR-β mRNA expression, with expression detected in 72% of histologically normal and hyperplastic tissue adjacent to squamous cell carcinomas, 56% of dysplastic tissue, and 35% of squamous cell carcinomas ($P<.05$).

This finding, suggesting an apparent tumor suppressor function in carcinogenic progression, led to a translational study of RAR-β that had three major findings.[114] First, in contrast to 100% expression in normal controls, RAR-β mRNA was detected in only 40% (21 of 52) of oral premalignant lesions ($P = .003$). The expression of the other five receptors, detected in 70% (RXR-β) to 100% (RXR-α) of oral premalignant lesions did not differ significantly from normal controls. RAR-β loss in oral premalignant lesions was not associated significantly with tobacco use. Second, there was a striking retinoid up-regulation of RAR-β expression after 3 months of high-dose 13cRA, from 40% to 90%. Third, RAR-β up-regulation was associated with clinical response: Receptor up-regulation was observed in 82% of responding lesions (including all four complete responses) and 47% of nonresponding lesions ($P = .039$). The early and progressive loss of RAR-β in premalignant tissues and significant 13cRA up-regulation (in association with lesion response) meets several major criteria for a potential intermediate end point. Similar findings have been reported in the lung in two randomized studies in smokers.[115,116] Future long-term validation trials will determine if early RAR-β up-regulation is associated with late lesion response and a reduction in cancer incidence.

These translational RAR-β findings in the retinoid and oral premalignant system are consistent with *in vitro* data. The RAR-β promoter has a DR5 response element and is the most tightly retinoid-regulated receptor. Mutations, deletions, or structural changes in the RAR-β gene or its promoter, however, have not been identified. More recent data suggest that loss of RAR-β expression in oral premalignant lesion is related to a defect in intracellular vitamin A metabolism (and reduced levels of retinoic acid in premalignant cells), which can be corrected by pharmacologic doses of retinoic acid.[117] These translational findings are consistent with preclinical data in vitamin A–deficient animals.

The available *in vitro* and *in vivo* data suggest a molecular model of retinoid chemoprevention in the head and neck (Fig. 23.3-2). *In vitro* transfection studies in lung cancer and other experimental systems suggest that RAR-β, which is located on chromosome 3p, may have tumor suppressor activity,[118,119] contributing to suppression of the premalignant phenotype. RAR-β loss may enhance the progression of carcinogenesis by rendering the epithelium resistant to physiologic retinoic acid levels. Pharmacologic doses of retinoic acid, administered systemically, can enter premalignant cells and, via residual retinoic acid receptors (e.g., RAR-γ), induce the synthesis of RAR-β via heterodimer binding to the RAR-β promoter and subsequent activation of RAR-β gene transcription. Although 13cRA does not bind directly to RARs, it is isomerized to ATRA. 13cRA can activate RAR-β RARE transcription *in vitro* at levels comparable with ATRA. This model of RAR-β up-regulation and tumor suppressor activity may represent the basis of retinoid chemoprevention in the head and neck.

p53 chromosome instability and loss of heterozygosity are also under intensive study in aerodigestive tract carcinogenesis.[120–122] As indicated previously, translational research in the retinoid oral premalignancy model is a paradigm for chemoprevention research in general. Future goals include increasing our knowledge of the biology of carcinogenesis and agent mechanisms of action, establishing effective screens for response and resistance to agents, and establishing valid intermediate end point biomarkers. Valid intermediate markers will be necessary for reducing the size and duration, and therefore, the tremendous costs, of future chemoprevention trials. Perhaps of greater importance, valid intermediate markers will help focus limited research resources on only the most promising candidate agents.

NEW RETINOIDS AND CAROTENOIDS

The retinamide 4HPR is a promising new retinoid now in clinical trials for human chemoprevention.[1,2,7–10,44,45,76,96,123–134] It has a unique mechanism of action and a favorable toxicity profile and has already generated significant chemopreventive activity in several animal carcinogenesis systems including mammary, bladder, lung, and prostate models. Several clinical chemoprevention trials targeting cervix, skin, bladder, and lung are currently in progress.

4HPR has potent apoptosis-inducing activity in several neoplastic systems (including leukemia, neuroblastoma, melanoma, small cell lung cancer, and cervical and head and neck squamous cell carcinoma) including those resistant to ATRA and 9cRA.[123–128] The finding that 4HPR is a potent inducer of apoptosis has exciting clinical implications.[135] Eliminating premalignant, genetically damaged cells by apoptosis may be more effective in cancer prevention than suppressing proliferation. Clinical effects of current chemopreventive agents, most of which primarily suppress proliferation, cease on stopping the drug. Apoptosis-inducing agents such as 4HPR, on the other hand, could allow shorter term effective chemoprevention with less toxicity. An understanding of the mechanism(s) by which 4HPR induces apoptosis is not yet available, but would facilitate the design of future preventive approaches, using rational combinations of 4HPR with other agents.

Clinical and translational study of other new retinoids is less advanced. This area of research currently is focused on ligands that are selective for RAR subtypes, RXRs, or the downstream target AP-1.[77,136,137] Data support RXR-selective ligands for use in cancer prevention. RXRs have a unique role in controlling apoptosis and as obligate heterodimer partners for RARs and many other intracellular receptors (e.g., vitamin D receptor and peroxisome proliferator-activated receptors). Via versatile dimer-partnering behavior and other complex effects, RXR agonists can modulate other endocrine-signaling pathways. The potential importance of RXRs in breast carcinogenesis was first illustrated by mammary carcinogenesis studies suggesting that the RAR-RXR panagonist 9cRA is more active than RAR agonists. Findings of subsequent prevention studies of selective RXR agonists in a rat mammary carcinoma model were as follows: less toxic and more active than 9cRA; inhibited estrogen- and tamoxifen-stimulated uterine proliferation; activity in tamoxifen-resistant disease and similar to that of tamoxifen; and supra-additive effects when combined with tamoxifen. This study of RXR agonists has led to intensive study of their combination with selective estrogen receptor modulators.[77]

Several carotenoids also appear to have promising chemopreventive activity. For example, epidemiologic as well as preclinical (*in vitro* and *in vivo*) studies suggest that α-carotene may have chemopreventive efficacy. Lycopene, a carotenoid found primarily in tomato and tomato products, is of great interest as a potential agent for the prevention of prostate[138] and other cancers.[139] In one article, 57 of 72 studies reviewed reported inverse associations between tomato intake or blood lycopene levels and the risk of cancer; 35 of these inverse associations were statistically significant.[139] Small intervention trials of lycopene in men with prostate cancer have been initiated.[140] Other carotenoids including crocetin, canthaxanthin, fucoxanthin, and α-carotene have been found to inhibit tumorigenesis in animal models.[19] While there is considerable interest in these and other carotenoids for cancer prevention, large-scale human trials should be undertaken with great caution, given the lack of a clear understanding of the apparent mechanism of β-carotene in promoting lung carcinogenesis.

CONCLUSIONS

A number of chemoprevention trials involving retinoids and the carotenoid β-carotene are ongoing or have been completed. Although many of the trials have reported chemopreventive efficacy for various retinoids and for β-carotene, particularly in oral premalignancy, other trials have been negative or have even suggested promotional effects. This suggests that the patient population, tumor site, histopathology, choice of agent(s), dose, duration, and timing of intervention may be critical in determining efficacy. Although our understanding of mechanisms of action for retinoids has increased dramatically in the last decade, the same is not true for the carotenoids, and additional research is needed in this area. Nonrandomized phase I and II trials provide useful information regarding toxicity, feasibility, and suggestions of drug activity; however, randomized phase IIB and III trials[1] are clearly necessary for rigorous evaluation of efficacy. This is particularly true for trials using intermediate end points, as uncontrolled trials are difficult to interpret and may produce spurious findings. Several large randomized trials of retinoids in the prevention of cancer will be concluded by 2003. Others involving β-carotene, alone or in combination with other agents such as vitamins E, C, and selenium, also are ongoing. Trials will soon be initiated to evaluate single-agent efficacy of some of the less-studied micronutrients, such as the planned Selenium and Vitamin E Chemoprevention Trial (select), which will examine selenium and vitamin E in a factorial design aimed at the prevention of prostate cancer in 32,400 healthy male participants in the United States. In the meantime, the use of retinoids, carotenoids, vitamins E, C, and selenium for cancer prevention remains investigational.

REFERENCES

1. Lippman SM, Benner SE, Hong WK. Cancer chemoprevention. *J Clin Oncol* 1994;12:851.
2. Lippman SM, Spitz MR, Huber M, Hong WK. Strategies for chemoprevention study of premalignant lesions and second primary tumors in the head and neck. *Curr Opin Oncol* 1995;7:234.
3. Wolbach SB, Howe PR. Tissue changes following deprivation of fat soluble A vitamin. *J Exp Med* 1925;42:753.
4. Ziegler RG, Mayne ST, Swanson CA. Diet and lung cancer. *Cancer Causes and Control* 1996;7:157.
5. Mayne ST, Graham S, Zheng T. Dietary retinol: prevention or promotion of carcinogenesis in humans? *Cancer Causes and Control* 1991;2:443.
6. Dragsted LO, Strube M, Larsen JC. Cancer protective factors in fruits and vegetables: biochemical and biologic background. *Pharmacol Toxicol* 1993;72(Suppl):s116.
7. Moon RC, Mehta RG, Rao KV. Retinoids and cancer in experimental animals. In: Sporn MB, Roberts AB, Goodman DS, eds. *The retinoids.* 2nd ed. New York: Raven Press, 1994:573.
8. Pollard M, Luckert PH, Sporn MB. Prevention of primary prostate cancer in Lobund-Wistar rats by N-(4-hydroxyphenyl) retinamide. *Cancer Res* 1991;51:3610.
9. Slawin K, Kadmon D, Park SH, et al. Dietary fenretinide, a synthetic retinoid, decreases the tumor incidence and the tumor mass of ras+myc-induced carcinomas in the mouse prostate reconstitution model system. *Cancer Res* 1993;19:4461.
10. Kelloff GJ, Crowell JA, Boone CW, et al. N-(4-hydroxyphenyl)retinamide (4HPR): clinical development plan. *J Cell Biochem* 1994;(Suppl 20):176.
11. Anzano MA, Byers SW, Smith JM, et al. Prevention of breast cancer in the rat with 9-cis-retinoic acid as a single agent and in combination with tamoxifen. *Cancer Res* 1994;54:4614.
12. Sporn MB, Roberts AB. What is a retinoid? *CIBA Foundation Symposium* 1985;113:1.
13. Mangelsdorf DJ, Umesono K, Evans RM. The retinoid receptors. In: Sporn MB, Roberts AB, Goodman DS, eds. *The retinoids.* 2nd ed. New York: Raven Press, 1994:319.
14. Chambon P. The retinoid signaling pathway: molecular and genetic analyses. *Semin Cell Biol* 1994;5:115.
15. Demirpence E, Balaguer P, Trousse F, et al. Antiestrogenic effects of all-trans-retinoic acid and 1,25-dihydroxyvitamin D_3 in breast cancer cells occur at the estrogen response element level but through different molecular mechanisms. *Cancer Res* 1994;54:1458.
16. Lippman SM, Kessler JF, Meyskens FL Jr. Retinoids as preventive and therapeutic anticancer agents. *Cancer Treat Rep* 1987;71:391,493.
17. Fanjul A, Dawson MI, Hobbs PD, et al. A new class of retinoids with selective inhibition of AP-1 inhibits proliferation. *Nature* 1994;372:107.
18. Lippman SM, Heyman RA, Kurie JM, Benner SE, Hong WK. Retinoids and chemoprevention: clinical and basic studies. *J Cell Biochem* 1995;22:1.
19. Krinsky NI. Actions of carotenoids in biologic systems. In: Olsen RE, Bier DM, McCormick DB, eds. *Annual review of nutrition.* Palo Alto: Annual Reviews, 1993;13:561.
20. Wang X-D, Krinsky NI, Benotti PN, Russell RM. Biosynthesis of 9-cis-retinoic acid from 9-cis-beta-carotene in human intestinal mucosa in vitro. *Arch Biochem Biophys* 1994;313:150.
21. Mathews-Roth MM. Carotenoids in erythropoietic protoporphyria and other photosensitivity diseases. *Ann N Y Acad Sci* 1993;691:127.
22. Burton GW, Ingold KU. Beta-carotene: an unusual type of lipid antioxidant. *Science* 1984;224:569.
23. Floyd RA. Role of free radicals in carcinogenesis and brain ischemia. *FASEB J* 1990;4:2587.
24. International Agency for Research on Cancer (IARC). *IARC handbooks of cancer prevention.* Carotenoids. Vol. 2. North Carolina: Oxford University Press, 1998.
25. Watson RR, Rybski J. Immunomodulation by retinoids and carotenoids. In: Chandra RK, ed. *Nutrition and immunology.* New York: Alan R. Liss, 1988:87.
26. Zhang LX, Cooney RV, Bertram JS. Carotenoids up-regulate connexin43 gene expression independent of their provitamin A or antioxidant properties. *Cancer Res* 1992;52:5707.
27. Comerci JT, Runowicz CD, Fields AL, et al. Induction of transforming growth factor beta-1 in cervical intraepithelial neoplasia in vivo after treatment with beta-carotene. *Clin Cancer Res* 1997;3:157.
28. Lippman SM, Hong WK. Retinoid chemoprevention of upper aerodigestive tract carcinogenesis. In: DeVita VT, Hellman S, Rosenberg SA, eds. *Important advances in oncology.* Philadelphia: Lippincott, 1992:93.
29. Vokes EE, Weichselbaum RR, Lippman SM, Hong WK. Head and neck cancer. *N Engl J Med* 1993;328:184.
30. Stich HF, Rosin MP, Vallejera MO. Reduction with vitamin A and beta-carotene administration of proportion of micronucleated buccal mucosal cells in Asian betel nut and tobacco chewers. *Lancet* 1984;1:1204.

31. Stich HF, Hornby AP, Dunn BP. A pilot beta-carotene intervention trial with Inuits using smokeless tobacco. *Int J Cancer* 1985;36:321.
32. Stich HF, Rosin MP, Hornby P, et al. Remission of oral leukoplakias and micronuclei in tobacco/betel quid chewers treated with beta-carotene and with beta-carotene plus vitamin A. *Int J Cancer* 1988;42:195.
33. Garewal HS, Meyskens FL, Killen D, et al. Response of oral leukoplakia to beta-carotene. *J Clin Oncol* 1990;8:1715.
34. Toma S, Benso S, Albanese E, et al. Treatment of oral leukoplakia with beta-carotene. *Oncology* 1992;49:77.
35. Garewal H, Katz RV, Meyskens F, et al. Beta-carotene produces sustained remissions in patients with oral leukoplakia—results of a multicenter prospective trial. *Arch Otolaryngol Head Neck Surg* 1999;125:1305.
36. Malaker K, Anderson BA, Beecroft WA, Hodson DI. Management of oral mucosal dysplasia with beta-carotene and retinoic acid: a pilot cross-over study. *Cancer Detect Prev* 1991;15:335.
37. Kaugars GE, Silverman S Jr, Lovas JGL, et al. A clinical trial of antioxidant supplements in the treatment of oral leukoplakia. *Oral Surg Oral Med Oral Pathol* 1994;78:462.
38. Barth TJ, Zoller J, Kubler A, Born IA, Osswald H. Redifferentiation of oral dysplastic mucosa by the application of the antioxidants beta-carotene, alpha-tocopherol and vitamin C. *Int J Vit Nutr Res* 1997;67:368.
39. Sankaranarayanan R, Mathew B, Varghese C, et al. Chemoprevention of oral leukoplakia with vitamin A and beta carotene: an assessment. *Oral Oncol* 1997;33:231.
40. Zaridze D, Evstifeeva T, Boyle P. Chemoprevention of oral leukoplakia and chronic esophagitis in an area of high incidence of oral and esophageal cancer. *Ann Epidemiol* 1993;3:225.
41. Benner SE, Winn RJ, Lippman SM, et al. Regression of oral leukoplakia with alpha-tocopherol: a community clinical oncology program chemoprevention study. *J Natl Cancer Inst* 1993;85:44.
42. Hong W, Endicott J, Itri LM, et al. 13-cis retinoic acid in the treatment of oral leukoplakia. *N Engl J Med* 1986;315:1501.
43. Lippman SM, Batsakis JG, Toth BB, et al. Comparison of low-dose isotretinoin with beta carotene to prevent oral carcinogenesis. *N Engl J Med* 1993;328:15.
44. Chiesa F, Tradati N, Marazza M, et al. 4HPR in chemoprevention of oral leukoplakia. *J Cell Biochem Suppl* 1993;17F:255.
45. Costa A, Formelli F, Chiesa F, et al. Prospects of chemoprevention of human cancers with the synthetic retinoid fenretinide. *Cancer Res* 1994;54:2032.
46. Stich HF, Hornby AP, Mathew B, et al. Response of oral leukoplakias to the administration of vitamin A. *Cancer Lett* 1988;40:93.
47. Han J, Lu Y, Sun Z, et al. Evaluation of N-4-(hydroxycarbophenyl) retinamide as a cancer prevention agent and as a cancer chemotherapeutic agent. *In Vivo* 1990;4:153.
48. Hong WK, Lippman SM, Itri LM, et al. Prevention of second primary tumors with 13cRA in squamous-cell carcinoma of the head and neck. *N Engl J Med* 1990;323:795.
49. Benner SE, Pajak TF, Lippman SM, Earley C, Hong WK. Prevention of second primary tumors with isotretinoin in patients with squamous cell carcinoma of the head and neck: long term follow-up. *J Natl Cancer Inst* 1994;86:140.
50. Khuri FR, Lee JJ, Winn RJ, et al. Interim analysis of randomized chemoprevention trial of HNSCC. *Proc Am Soc Clin Oncol* 1999;18:389a(abst).
51. Bolla M, Lefur R, Ton Van J, et al. Prevention of second primary tumours with etretinate in squamous cell carcinoma of the oral cavity and oropharynx. Results of a multicentric double-blind randomised study. *Eur J Cancer* 1994;30A:767.
52. Mayne ST, Zheng T, Janerich DT, et al. A population-based trial of beta-carotene chemoprevention of head and neck cancer. In: Newell GR, Hong WK, ed. *The biology and prevention of aerodigestive tract cancers.* New York: Plenum Press, 1992:119.
53. McLarty JW, Holiday DB, Girard WM, et al. Beta-carotene, vitamin A and lung cancer chemoprevention: results of an intermediate endpoint study. *Am J Clin Nutr* 1995;62(Suppl):1431S.
54. Van Poppel G, Kok FJ, Hermus RJ. Beta-carotene supplementation in smokers reduces the frequency of micronuclei in sputum. *Br J Cancer* 1992;66:1164.
55. Van Poppel G, Poulsen H, Loft S, Verhagen H. No influence of beta carotene on oxidative DNA damage in male smokers. *J Natl Cancer Inst* 1995;87:310.
56. Misset JL, Mathe G, Santelli G, et al. Regression of bronchial epidermoid metaplasia in heavy smokers with etretinate treatment. *Cancer Detect Prev* 1986;9:167.
57. Arnold AM, Browman GP, Levine MN, et al. The effect of the synthetic retinoid etretinate on sputum cytology: results from a randomized trial. *Br J Cancer* 1992;65:737.
58. Lee JS, Lippman SM, Benner SE, et al. Randomized placebo-controlled trial of isotretinoin in chemoprevention of bronchial squamous metaplasia. *J Clin Oncol* 1994;12:937.
59. Kurie JM, Lee JS, Khuri FR, et al. 4-Hydroxyphenylretinamide (4-HPR) in the reversal of bronchial metaplasia and dysplasia in smokers. *Proc Am Soc Clin Oncol* 1999;18:473a(abst).
60. The Alpha-Tocopherol, Beta Carotene Cancer Prevention Study Group. The effect of vitamin E and beta carotene on the incidence of lung cancer and other cancers in male smokers. *N Engl J Med* 1994;330:1029.
61. Heinonen OP, Albanes D, Virtamo J, et al. Prostate cancer and supplementation with alpha-tocopherol and beta-carotene: incidence and mortality in a controlled trial. *J Natl Cancer Inst* 1998;90:440.
62. Omenn GS, Goodman GE, Thornquist MD, et al. Effects of a combination of beta carotene and vitamin A on lung cancer and cardiovascular disease. *N Engl J Med* 1996;334:1150.
63. Hennekens CH, Buring JE, Manson JE, et al. Lack of effect of long-term supplementation with beta carotene on the incidence of malignant neoplasms and cardiovascular disease. *N Engl J Med* 1996;334:1145.
64. Lee IM, Cook NR, Manson JE, Buring JE, Hennekens CH. Beta-carotene supplementation and incidence of cancer and cardiovascular disease: the Women's Health Study. *J Natl Cancer Inst* 1999;91:2102.
65. Blot WJ, Li J-Y, Taylor PR, Li B. Lung cancer and vitamin supplementation [Letter]. *N Engl J Med* 1994;331:614.
66. Mayne ST. Beta-carotene, carotenoids, and cancer prevention. *Principles and Practice of Oncology Updates* 1998;12:1.
67. Wang XD, Liu C, Bronson RT, et al. Retinoid signaling and activator protein-1 expression in ferrets given beta-carotene supplements and exposed to tobacco smoke. *J Natl Cancer Inst* 1999;91:60.
68. Salgo MG, Cueto R, Winston GW, Pryor WA. Beta carotene and its oxidation products have different effects on microsome mediated binding of benzo[a]pyrene to DNA. *Free Radical Biol Med* 1998;26:162.
69. Paolini M, Cantelli-Forti G, Peroccot P, et al. Co-carcinogenic effect of b-carotene [Letter]. *Nature* 1999;398:760.
70. Pastorino U, Infante M, Maioli M, et al. Adjuvant treatment of stage I lung cancer with high-dose vitamin A. *J Clin Oncol* 1993;11:1216.
71. van Zandwijk N, Pastorino U, De Vries N, et al. Randomized trial of chemoprevention with vitamin A and N-acetylcysteine in patients with cancer of the upper and lower airways: the Euroscan study. *Proc Am Soc Clin Oncol* 1999;18:464a(abst).
72. Lippman SM, Lee JJ, Karp DD, et al. Phase III Intergroup trial of 13-cis-retinoic acid to prevent second primary tumors in stage I non-small cell lung cancer (NSCLC): Interim Report of NCI #I19-0001. *Proc Am Soc Clin Oncol* 1998;17:456a(abst):1753.
73. Lippman SM. Not yet standard: retinoids versus second primary tumors. *J Clin Oncol* 1993;11:1204.
74. Parthasarathy R, Gilbert B, Mehta K. Aerosol delivery of liposomal all-trans-retinoic acid to the lungs. *Cancer Chemother Pharmacol* 1999;43:277.
75. Massaro GD, Massaro D. Retinoic acid treatment abrogates elastase-induced pulmonary emphysema in rats. *Nat Med* 1997;3:675.
76. Veronesi U, De Palo G, Marubini E, et al. Randomized trial of fenretinide to prevent second breast malignancy in women with early breast cancer. *J Natl Cancer Inst* 1999;91:1847.
77. Lippman M, Brown PH. Tamoxifen prevention of breast cancer: an instance of the fingerpost. *J Natl Cancer Inst* 1999;91:1809.
78. Ingram D. Diet and subsequent survival in women with breast cancer. *Br J Cancer* 1994;69:592.
79. Jain M, Miller AB, To T. Premorbid diet and the prognosis of women with breast cancer. *J Natl Cancer Inst* 1994;86:1390.
80. Pierce JP, Faerber S, Wright FA, et al. Feasibility of a randomized trial of a high-vegetable diet to prevent breast cancer recurrence. *Nutr Cancer* 1997;28:282.
81. Kligman AM, Thorne EG. Topical therapy of actinic keratosis with tretinoin. In: Marks R, ed. *Retinoids in cutaneous malignancy.* Cambridge, MA: Blackwell Scientific, 1991:66.
82. Moriarty M, Dunn J, Darragh A, et al. Etretinate in treatment of actinic keratosis: a double blind crossover study. *Lancet* 1982;1:364.
83. Watson AB. Preventative effect of etretinate therapy on multiple actinic keratoses. *Cancer Detect Prev* 1986;9:161.
84. Kraemer KH, DiGiovanna JJ, Moshell AN, et al. Prevention of skin cancer in xeroderma pigmentosum with the use of oral isotretinoin. *N Engl J Med* 1988;318:1633.
85. Kelly JW, Sabto J, Gurr FW, Bruce F. Retinoids to prevent skin cancer in organ transplant recipients. *Lancet* 1991;338:1407.
86. Bouwes Bavinck JN, Tieben LM, Van Der Woude FJ, et al. Prevention of skin cancer and reduction of keratotic skin lesions during acitretin therapy in renal transplant recipients: a double-blind, placebo-controlled study. *J Clin Oncol* 1995;13:1933.
87. Tangrea JA, Edwards BK, Taylor PR, et al. Long-term therapy with low-dose isotretinoin for prevention of basal cell carcinoma: a multicenter clinical trial. *J Natl Cancer Inst* 1992;84:328.
88. Levine N, Moon TE, Cartmel B, et al. Trial of retinol and isotretinoin in skin cancer prevention: a randomized, double-blind, controlled trial. Southwest Skin Cancer Prevention Study Group. *Cancer Epidemiol Biomarkers Prev* 1997;6:957.
89. Moon TE, Levine N, Cartmel B, et al. Effect of retinol in preventing squamous cell skin cancer in moderate-risk subjects: a randomized, double-blind, controlled trial. *Cancer Epidemiol Biomarkers Prev* 1997;6:949.
90. Greenberg ER, Baron JA, Stukel TA, et al. and the Skin Cancer Prevention Study Group. A clinical trial of beta carotene to prevent basal cell and squamous cell cancers of the skin. *N Engl J Med* 1990;323:789.
91. Clark LC, Combs GF, Tumbull BW, et al. Effects of selenium supplementation for cancer prevention in patients with carcinoma of the skin. *JAMA* 1996;24:1957.
92. Pedersen H, Wolf H, Jensen SK, et al. Administration of a retinoid as prophylaxis of recurrent non-invasive bladder tumors. *Scand J Urol Nephrol* 1984;18:121.
93. Alfthan O, Tarkkanen J, Grohn P, et al. Tigason (etretinate) in prevention of recurrence of superficial bladder tumors. *Eur Urol* 1983;9:6.
94. Studer UE, Biedermann C, Chollet D, et al. Prevention of recurrent superficial bladder tumors by oral etretinate: preliminary results of a randomized, double blind multicenter trial in Switzerland. *J Urol* 1984;131:47.
95. Lamm DL, Riggs DR, Shriver JS, et al. Megadose vitamins in bladder cancer: a double-blind clinical trial. *J Urol* 1994;151:21.
96. Decensi A, Bruno S, Costantini M, et al. Phase IIa study of fenretinide in superficial bladder cancer, using DNA flow cytometry as an intermediate end point. *J Natl Cancer Inst* 1994;86:138.
97. Meyskens FL, Surwit E, Moon TE, et al. Enhancement of regression of cervical intraepithelial neoplasia II (moderate dysplasia) with topically applied all-trans-retinoic acid: a randomized trial. *J Natl Cancer Inst* 1994;86:539.
98. DeVet HCW, Knipschild PG, Willebrand D, Schouten HJA, Sturmans F. The effect of beta-carotene on the regression and progression of cervical dysplasia: a clinical experiment. *J Clin Epidemiol* 1991;44:273.
99. Romney SL, Ho GYF, Palan PR, et al. Effects of beta-carotene and other factors on outcome of cervical dysplasia and human papillomavirus infection. *Gynecol Oncol* 1997; 65:483.
100. Mackerras D, Irwig L, Simpson JM, et al. Randomized double-blind trial of beta-carotene and vitamin C in women with minor cervical abnormalities. *Br J Cancer* 1999;79:1448.

101. Meyskens FL Jr, Manetta A. Prevention of cervical intraepithelial neoplasia and cervical cancer. *Am J Clin Nutr* 1995;62:1417S.
102. Munoz N, Wahrendorf J, Bang LJ, et al. No effect of riboflavin, retinol and zinc on prevalence of precancerous lesions of oesophagus: randomized double-blind intervention study in high-risk population of China. *Lancet* 1985;2:111.
103. Blot WJ, Li J-Y, Taylor PR, et al. Nutrition intervention trials in Linxian, China: supplementation with specific vitamin/mineral combinations, cancer incidence, and disease-specific mortality in the general population. *J Natl Cancer Inst* 1993;85:1483.
104. Li J-Y, Taylor PR, Li B, et al. Nutrition intervention trials in Linxian, China: multiple vitamin/mineral supplementation, cancer incidence, and disease-specific mortality among adults with esophageal dysplasia. *J Natl Cancer Inst* 1993;85:1492.
105. Munoz N, Hayashi M, Bang LJ, et al. Effect of riboflavin, retinol and zinc on micronuclei of buccal mucosa and of esophagus: a randomized double-blind intervention study in China. *J Natl Cancer Inst* 1987;79:687.
106. Dawsey SM, Wang G-Q, Taylor PR, et al. Effects of vitamin/mineral supplementation on the prevalence of histological dysplasia and early cancer of the esophagus and stomach: results from the dysplasia trial in Linxian, China. *Cancer Epidemiol Biomarkers Prev* 1994;3:167.
107. Greenberg ER, Baron JA, Tosteson TD, et al. and the Polyp Prevention Study Group. A clinical trial of antioxidant vitamins to prevent colorectal adenoma. *N Engl J Med* 1994;331:141.
108. MacLennan R, Macrae F, Bain C, et al. Randomized trial of intake of fat, fiber and beta carotene to prevent colorectal adenomas. *J Natl Cancer Inst* 1995;87:1760.
109. Kikendall JW, Mobarhan S, Nelson R, Burgess M, Bowen PE. Oral beta carotene does not reduce the recurrence of colorectal adenomas. *Am J Gastroenterol* 1991;36:1356(abst).
110. Hong WK, Lippman SM, Hittelman WN, Lotan R. Retinoid chemoprevention of aerodigestive cancer: from basic research to the clinic. *Clin Cancer Res* 1995;1:677.
111. Lippman SM, Lee JS, Lotan R, et al. Biomarkers as intermediate end points in chemoprevention trials. *J Natl Cancer Inst* 1990;82:555.
112. Hong WK, Lippman SM, Wolf GT. Recent advances in head and neck cancer-larynx preservation and cancer chemoprevention. *Cancer Res* 1993;53:5113.
113. Xu X-C, Ro JY, Lee JS, et al. Differential expression of nuclear retinoic acid receptors in normal, premalignant, and malignant head and neck tissues. *Cancer Res* 1994;54:3580.
114. Lotan R, Xu X-C, Lippman SM, et al. Suppression of retinoic acid receptor-b in premalignant oral lesions and its upregulation by isotretinoin. *N Engl J Med* 1995;332:1405.
115. Xu X-C, Lee JS, Lee JJ, et al. Nuclear retinoid receptor beta in bronchial epithelium of smokers before and during chemoprevention. *J Natl Cancer Inst* 1999;91:1317.
116. Ayoub J, Jean-Francois R, Cormier Y, et al. Placebo-controlled trial of 13-cis-retinoic acid activity on retinoic acid receptor-beta expression in a population at high risk: implications for chemoprevention of lung cancer. *J Clin Oncol* 1999;17:3546.
117. Xu X-C, Zile MH, Lippman SM, et al. Anti-retinoic acid (RA) antibody binding to human premalignant oral lesions, which occurs less frequently than binding to normal tissue, increases after 13-cis-RA treatment in vivo and is related to RA receptor beta expression. *Cancer Res* 1995;55:5507.
118. Houle B, Rochette-Egly C, Bradley WE. Tumor-suppressive effect of the retinoic acid receptor beta in human epidermoid lung cancer cells. *Proc Natl Acad Sci U S A* 1993;90:985.
119. Frangioni JV, Moghal N, Stuart-Tilley A, et al. The DNA binding domain of retinoic acid receptor b is required for ligand-dependent suppression of proliferation: application of general purpose mammalian co-expression vectors. *J Cell Sci* 1994;107:827.
120. Lippman SM, Shin DM, Lee JJ, et al. p53 and retinoid chemoprevention of oral carcinogenesis. *Cancer Res* 1995;55:16.
121. Mao L, Lee JS, Fan YH, et al. Frequent microsatellite alterations at chromosome 9p21 and 3p14 in oral premalignant lesions and its value in cancer risk assessment. *Nat Med* 1996;2:682.
122. Mao L, Lee JS, Kurie JM, et al. Clonal genetic alterations in the lungs of current and former smokers. *J Natl Cancer Inst* 1997;89:857.
123. Delia D, Aiello A, Lombardi L, et al. N-(4-hydroxyphenyl)retinamide induces apoptosis of malignant hemopoietic cell lines including those unresponsive to retinoic acid. *Cancer Res* 1993;53:6036.
124. Delia D, Aiello A, Formelli F, et al. Regulation of apoptosis induced by the retinoid N-(4-hydroxyphenyl)retinamide and effect of deregulated Bcl-2. *Blood* 1995;85:359.
125. Oridate N, Lotan D, Xu X-C, Hong WK, Lotan R. Differential induction of apoptosis by all-trans-retinoic acid and N-(4-hydroxyphenyl) retinamide in human head and neck squamous cell carcinoma cell lines. *Clin Cancer Res* 1996;2:855.
126. Ponzoni M, Bocca P, Chiesa V, et al. Differential effects of N-(4-hydroxyphenyl)retinamide and retinoic acid on neuroblastoma cells: apoptosis versus differentiation. *Cancer Res* 1995;55:853.
127. Mariotti A, Marcora E, Bunone G, et al. N-(4-hydroxyphenyl)retinamide: a potent inducer of apoptosis in human neuroblastoma cells. *J Natl Cancer Inst* 1994;86:1245.
128. Kalemkerian GP, Slusher R, Ramalingam S, Gadgeel S, Mabry M. Growth inhibition and induction of apoptosis by fenretinide in small-cell lung cancer cell lines. *J Natl Cancer Inst* 1995;87:1674.
129. Newton DL, Henderson WR, Sporn MB. Structure-activity relationships of retinoids in hamster tracheal organ culture. *Cancer Res* 1980;40:3413.
130. Veronesi U, De Palo G, Costa A, et al. Chemoprevention of breast cancer with retinoids. *J Natl Cancer Inst* 1992;12:93.
131. Rotsmensz N, De Palo G, Formelli F, et al. Long-term tolerability of fenretinide (4-HPR) in breast cancer patients. *Eur J Cancer* 1991;27:1127.
132. De Palo G, Costa A, Veronesi U. Five-year administration of fenretinide: pharmacokinetics and effects on plasma retinol concentrations. *J Clin Oncol* 1993;11:2036.
133. Dowlatshahi K, Mehta RG, Thomas CF, et al. Therapeutic effect of N-(4-hydroxyphenyl)retinamide on N-methyl-N-nitrosourea-induced rat mammary cancer. *Cancer Lett* 1989;47:187.
134. Formelli F, Carsana R, Costa A, et al. Plasma retinol level reduction by the synthetic retinoid fenretinide: a one year follow-up study of breast cancer patients. *Cancer Res* 1989;49:6149.
135. Lotan R. Retinoids and apoptosis: implications for cancer chemoprevention and therapy. *J Natl Cancer Inst* 1995;87:1655.
136. Lippman SM, Lee JJ, Sabichi AL. Cancer chemoprevention: progress and promise. *J Natl Cancer Inst* 1998;90:1514.
137. Hong WK, Sporn MB. Recent advances in chemoprevention of cancer. *Science* 1997;278:1073.
138. Giovannucci E, Ascherio A, Rimm EB, et al. Intake of carotenoids and retinol in relation to risk of prostate cancer. *J Natl Cancer Inst* 1995;87:1767.
139. Giovannucci E. Tomatoes, tomato-based products, lycopene, and cancer: review of the epidemiologic literature. *J Natl Cancer Inst* 1999;91:317.
140. Kucuk O, Sakr W, Sarkar F, et al. Lycopene supplementation in men with localized prostate cancer (PCa) modulates grade and volume of prostatic intraepithelial neoplasia (PIN) and tumor, level of serum PSA and biomarkers of cell growth, differentiation and apoptosis. *Proc Am Assoc Cancer Res* 1999;40:2706(abst).

SECTION **4**

PETER GREENWALD

Naturally Occurring Dietary Anticarcinogens

Experimental research has identified hundreds of food-derived compounds as having inhibitory effects on carcinogens.[1] In humans, these cancer-protective compounds are typically consumed as components within a complex diet, rather than as high-dose supplements. Because the variety and complexity of the diet of free-living humans limits direct experimental intervention of food intake, observational studies of eating patterns are often used to infer the role of particular dietary components. Epidemiologic studies emphasizing overall dietary intake or consumption of specific foods, rather than investigation of a particular nutrient or dietary supplement, do, however, provide consistent evidence that populations consuming higher levels of fruits and vegetables are at decreased risk of various cancers relative to populations with lesser intakes.[2] A growing body of research indicates that certain nonnutritive phytochemicals, including those found in the everyday diet, have marked cancer-preventive properties. This chapter examines some of the current evidence for the link between dietary anticarcinogens and cancer risk, with particular emphasis on selected nonnutritive phytochemicals.

CAROTENOIDS

Commonly consumed green, yellow-red, and yellow-orange vegetables and fruits contain more than 40 carotenoids, including β-carotene, lutein, lycopene, and the xanthins.[3] Various carotenoids may serve as cancer-preventive agents,[4] and a comprehensive review of experimental and epidemiologic studies examining their properties has been published.[5] Among the most promising of these carotenoids is lycopene, commonly found in tomatoes and tomato-based products; the biochemical and metabolic characteristics of lycopene have been summarized.[6] Epidemiologic studies have found an inverse relationship between intake of tomatoes or plasma lycopene level and risk of cancer at various sites, particularly the prostate, lung, and stomach.[7] *In vitro* studies have found a synergistic inhibitory effect of lycopene and α-tocopherol on growth of two human prostate carcinoma cell lines.[8] Mechanisms of action of carotenoids that may explain their potential cancer-preventive effects include antioxidant activity; modulation of carcinogen metabolism; and effects on cell transformation, differentiation, and communication.[5] More definitive conclusions regarding the role of lycopene in cancer prevention await controlled clinical trials.

Lutein displays anticarcinogenic properties that include enhancement of immune function, inhibition of the auto-oxidation of cellular lipids, and protection against oxidant-induced cell damage. In mice, dietary lutein inhibited mammary tumor growth,[9] and, among humans, high plasma lutein is associated with increased expression of estrogen receptors in breast cells and better survival rates and response to hormone therapy.[10]

PHYTOESTROGENS

Sources for two major categories of phytoestrogens, isoflavonoids and lignans, include legumes, whole grains, fruits, and berries.[11] Phytoestrogens exhibit both weak estrogenic and antiestrogenic effects.[11,12] Evidence for the role of phytoestrogens as cancer-preventive agents, from experimental and epidemiologic studies, has been the subject of a number of reviews.[12–15]

ISOFLAVONOIDS

Isoflavonoids, common in soy-based foods, inhibit angiogenesis, cell-cycle progression, and aromatase enzyme; stimulate sex hormone–binding globulin synthesis; and have antioxidant properties.[14] The primary isoflavonoid associated with cancer prevention is genistein.[16] Although the specific molecular mechanisms have yet to be elucidated, genistein displays multiple biochemical properties that inhibit the proliferation of cancer cells in various tissue cultures.[17,18] Genistein also possesses nonestrogenic properties, including inhibition of ribosomal S6 kinase activity and induction of differentiation of malignant cells.[19] Epidemiologic studies of populations that regularly consume soy-based foods reveal markedly lower incidence rates for breast, colon, and prostate cancer, when compared with populations with lesser intake of soy products.[12,17,19]

LIGNANS

In addition to their estrogen-like properties, lignans possess a wide range of other biologic activities, including antioxidant, antiproliferative, antiangiogenic, antiaromatase, antiestrogenic, antimitotic, and antiviral properties. High-fiber diets in Western countries provide a substantial proportion of lignan precursors, and the lower incidence of cancer in countries consuming high vegetarian or semi-vegetarian diets may be partially attributable to such fiber-associated substances. Flaxseed flour is a particularly good source of certain lignans, and dietary flaxseed is being investigated as a potential anticancer agent in humans.[20]

The relationship between phytoestrogens and breast cancer has been of particular interest, given the ability of phytoestrogens to mimic the properties of natural estrogens and the hormonal factors determining disease risk, respectively. Numerous animal and human studies indicate that increased consumption of phytoestrogens, particularly soy-based products, is associated with decreased breast cancer risk.[13] The traditional Western diet, having as a component low soy consumption, may adversely affect risk of certain hormone-dependent cancers. For example, the risk of breast cancer is less among Asian women born in Asia, where soy consumption is higher, relative to Asian women born in the United States, where soy consumption is lower.[21] In experimental studies, soy positively affects various physiologic parameters (e.g., menstrual cycle length, hormone levels of follicle-stimulating hormone and luteinizing hormone), and inhibits the proliferation of human breast cancer cells.[12] One potential mechanism for the protective effect of phytoestrogens involves inhibition of *ras* gene expression.[13]

Like breast cancer, prostate cancer risk also may be influenced by dietary consumption of phytoestrogens. Men living in Asian countries where consumption of soy-based foods is higher display a lesser risk of disease relative to men in Western countries where soy consumption is lower.[13] More research into the molecular and biochemical characteristics of the various phytoestrogens, and valid data on their consumption in the typical diet, are required.

ORGANOSULFUR AND ORGANOSELENIUM COMPOUNDS

Both experimental and epidemiologic studies support the cancer-preventive ability of certain organosulfur compounds.[22,23] Garlic, a member of the genus *Allium*, is rich in organosulfides, and diallyl sulfide (DAS) is the most frequently investigated sulfur compound found in garlic. In animals and humans, DAS and related compounds inhibit chemical carcinogenesis through an array of mechanisms, in various tissues, and against a variety of specific carcinogens. For example, studies have demonstrated protective effects of DAS against human colon tumor cells[24] and murine skin carcinogenesis.[25] Studies of the related compound diallyl disulfide (DADS) have noted that it suppresses human colon, skin, and lung tumor cell proliferation; the effect possibly being attributable to the ability of DADS to induce G_2/M arrest and depress $p34^{cdc2}$ kinase activity.[24] Epidemiologic studies have found an inverse association between garlic consumption and risk of gastric cancer, possibly a result of the antibacterial properties of garlic that inhibit conversion of nitrate to nitrite in the stomach, thereby limiting formation of carcinogenic nitrosamines.[23] Organosulfide preventive agents also are present in *Brassica* vegetables (e.g., broccoli, cabbage, cauliflower, and Brussels sprouts). Sulphoraphane, for example, inhibits carcinogen-induced mammary tumorigenesis in rats,[26] and induced phase 2 enzymes in murine hepatoma cells.[27] Selenium inhibits various types of tumors in rodents,[28] and, in humans, low plasma levels of selenium are associated with increased risk of polyps[29] and possibly prostate cancer.[30,31] A sampling of additional studies of organosulfur and organoselenium compounds is found in Table 23.4-1.

TABLE 23.4-1. Studies of the Anticarcinogenic Effect of Organosulfur and Organoselenium Products

Substance	*Target*	*Effect*	*Reference*
Diallyl sulfide	Colon tumor cells[a]	Depression of p34^{cdc2} kinase activity	24
	Skin carcinogenesis[b]	Protective effect	25
Diallyl sulfide, diallyl disulfide	Colon tumor cells[a]	Inhibition of NAT activity	78
	Hepatic tissue[c]	Reduction of hepatic DNA breaks	79
Sodium selenite	Colonic mucosa[a]	Antiproliferative effect	29
1,4-phenylenebis(methylene)selenocyanate	NNK-induced lung tumorigenesis[d]	Preventive effect	80
Selenite/selenate	Aberrant crypt formation[c]	Protective effect	28
S-allylcysteine	GST activity in liver, small intestine, and colon[c]	Increase in GST activity	81

GST, glutathione S-transferase; NAT, N-acetyltransferase; NNK, (4-methylnitrosamino)-1-(3-pyridyl)-1-butanone.
[a]Human.
[b]Mouse.
[c]Rat.
[d]Rodent.

PHENOLIC COMPOUNDS

Almost all fresh fruits, vegetables, and grains contain measurable amounts of natural plant phenolics, some of which display cancer-inhibitory properties.[32,33] The metabolic, bioavailability, antioxidant, and chemical properties of phenolic compounds have been reviewed,[34] as have potential mechanisms accounting for their anticarcinogenic activity.[33] For example, resveratrol, a triphenolic common in grapes, displays strong antioxidant and antiinflammatory properties and has received considerable attention as a potential cancer-preventive agent in humans.[35] Although the exact mechanism(s) for its antitumorigenic effects are not fully known, its growth inhibitory and antiproliferative properties may be attributable to induction of apoptotic cell death.[36] Resveratrol exhibits a chemical structure similar to diethylstilbestrol, and thus may also be classified as a phytoestrogen. Resveratrol has shown variable amounts of estrogen receptor agonism in different test systems.[37] Resveratrol inhibited the development of preneoplastic lesions in carcinogen-treated mouse mammary glands in culture, and inhibited tumorigenesis in a mouse skin cancer model.[35]

SIMPLE PHENOL AND PHENOLIC ACIDS

The simple phenols include the monophenols, found in fruits (e.g., raspberry, blackberry); the diphenols; and vanillin. Ellagic acid, a phenolic acid found in nuts and berries, possesses a number of anticarcinogenic properties, and different parts of the ellagic acid molecule may be responsible for assorted putative anticarcinogenic effects.[38] In animal studies, ellagic acid inhibited DNA-carcinogen adduct formation[39]; lung tumorigenesis induced by nicotine-derived nitrosamine in mice[40]; and development of an esophageal-specific carcinogen.[41] Other phenolics also have shown antioxidant, antimutagenic, and anticarcinogenic effects (Table 23.4-2).

FLAVONOIDS

Flavonoids represent the most important single group of phenolics in food[33]; more than 4000 different types have been identified.[42] Potential mechanisms for the anticancer effects of flavonoids include interaction with the cytochrome P-450 mixed function oxidase system and inhibition of tyrosine protein kinase activity and phosphoinositide phosphorylation.[43–45] Like phytoestrogens, flavonoids display structural properties that allow them to bind to estrogen receptors, potentially decreasing the risk of certain estrogen-dependent cancers.[46]

Experimental and epidemiologic studies of quercetin, the most common and biologically active dietary flavonol, have been reviewed.[42] Quercetin has multiple biochemical effects in mammalian cells and has shown antiproliferative activity against ovarian, breast, and stomach cancer cell lines *in vitro*[44] and against human ovarian cancer primary cultures *ex vivo*.[43] In a phase I clinical trial, quercetin inhibited tyrosine kinase activity and showed evidence of antitumor activity.[44] Other flavonoids, particularly tangeretin and nobiletin, appear to inhibit proliferation of the human breast cancer cell lines MDA-MB-435 and MCF-7.[43]

Long-term studies of the preventive ability of silymarin, a flavonoid isolated from artichoke or milk thistle, indicate its ability to protect against tumor promotion in mouse skin models of carcinogenesis.[47] Protective effects of common citrus flavonoids (e.g., naringen, hesperitin, hesperidin) include actions against B16F10 melanoma cells in mice, *in vitro* inhibition of MDA-MB-435 human breast cell cancer proliferation, and a preventive effect against oral carcinogenesis in rats.[48] Additional studies involving the anticarcinogenic properties of the flavonoids are summarized in Table 23.4-2.

GREEN TEA POLYPHENOLS

Experimental studies supporting the antimutagenic and anticarcinogenic activities of tea polyphenols, and epidemiologic data indicating an association between tea consumption and cancer risk, have been reviewed.[49] Studies on the catechin (-)-epigallocatechin-3-gallate, the primary green tea polyphenol (GTP), indicate that its growth inhibitory effects are selective, operating on cancerous but not on normal cells.[50] Although various GTPs individually exhibit inhibitory effects,[51] certain catechins act synergistically to reduce cancer risk, indicating that green tea is a more effective protective agent than any of its individual components.[52] Studies of the anticarcinogenic properties of green tea and its constituents are summarized in Table 23.4-2.

Characteristics of GTPs that may account for their anticarcinogenic properties include scavenging of carcinogenic electro-

TABLE 23.4-2. Studies of the Anticarcinogenic Effect of Phenolic Compounds

Substance	*Target*	*Effect*	*Reference*
PHENOLS			
Resveratrol	Promyelocytic leukemia (HL60) cells[a]	Decreased viability and DNA synthesis	36
Caffeic acid	COX-2[a]/prostaglandin synthesis[b]	Suppression	82
Ellagic acid, tannic acid, caffeic acid, ferulic acid	Skin tumors[c]	Inhibition	32
Apigenin, tangeretin	Liver epithelial cells[b]	Antagonism of tumor-induced inhibition of intercellular communication	83
FLAVONOIDS			
Flavopiridol	Prostate carcinoma cells[a]	Antitumor activity in *in vivo* and *in vitro* models	84
Hesperidin	Skin[c]	Inhibition of polycyclic aromatic hydrocarbon-induced tumor initiation	85
Quercetin	MCF-7 breast cancer cells[a]	Decrease in cell protein content; inhibition of protein, DNA, and RNA synthesis	45
Rutin	Nuclear DNA[b]	Reduction of aflatoxin B_1 and N-nitrosodimethylamine–induced single-strand breaks	86
TEA POLYPHENOLS			
Green tea/green tea polyphenols	Lung tumor formation[c]	Inhibition	87
EGCG	Lung cancer cells[a]	Increased apoptosis, growth inhibition	52
	Prostate cancer cell lines[a]	Apoptosis	88
Black tea	Lung tumor formation[c]	Inhibition	87

EGCG, epigallocatechin gallate.
[a]Human.
[b]Rat.
[c]Mouse.

philes, inhibitory action against nitrosation, modulation of carcinogen-metabolizing enzymes, trapping of ultimate carcinogens, inhibition of growth-related signal transduction pathways, modulation of enzymes associated with cell proliferation, and stimulation of phase II detoxifying enzymes.[53,54] Epidemiologic studies support the potential preventive effect of green tea against cancer at a number of sites, including the lung, esophagus, stomach, and skin.[54] Although GTPs have been the focus of most studies, black tea is consumed more commonly in the West; its potential cancer-protective properties, however, have yet to be fully explored. Animal studies indicate that certain black tea polyphenols, the theaflavins, are associated with significant inhibition of lung adenomas, both *in vivo*[55] and *in vitro*.[56] Additional research involving black tea polyphenols may be warranted.[57]

CURCUMINOIDS

Curcumin, the major yellow pigment in turmeric and curry, is a common spice, coloring agent, and herbal drug, particularly in Asia. Curcumin has multiple effects on the carcinogenic process, including antioxidant activity, reduction in polyamine synthesis,[58] and inhibition of tumor initiation and promotion.[59] The molecular mechanism explaining the action of curcumin is complex and varied, but it is known to inhibit cyclooxygenase- and lipoxygenase-dependent metabolism of arachidonic acid to prostaglandins and hydroxyeicosatetraenoic acids and to moderately enhance interleukin-4 production.[58] Additional work has shown that curcumin inhibits colon carcinogenesis during the postinitiation phase[60] and has a cytostatic effect at G_2/M against MCF-7 human breast tumor cells.[61]

MONOTERPENES

Monoterpenes are found in the essential oils of citrus fruits and other edible plants.[62] The most common monocyclic monoterpene, *d*-limonene, and its metabolite perillyl alcohol have shown effectiveness as cancer-protective agents against rodent cancers of the mammary, skin, liver, lung, forestomach, pancreas, and prostate.[22,62] In human breast cancer cell lines, limonene-related monoterpenes exhibited a dose-dependent inhibition on cell proliferation.[63] Multiple mechanisms may account for the actions of the monoterpenes, depending on tumor type.[62] The blocking effects of *d*-limonene and other monoterpenes during the initiation phase of mammary carcinogenesis may result from induction of phase II carcinogen-metabolizing enzymes and subsequent carcinogen detoxification; in the postinitiation phase, tumor-suppressive activity may be a result of induction of apoptosis and inhibition of the posttranslational isoprenylation of proteins that regulate cell growth.[64] Other cancer-preventive mechanisms include actions on the mevalonate[62] and *ras* signal transduction pathways.[65]

ISOTHIOCYANATES AND INDOLES

Epidemiologic studies have consistently found strong, inverse relationships between high consumption of cruciferous vegetables and cancer incidence.[66] Cruciferous vegetables contain three groups of glucosinolate-derived compounds likely to be cancer-protective: indole-3-carbinol (I3C) and related indole compounds; phenylethyl isothiocyanate (PEITC) and related isothiocyanates, such as benzyl isothiocyanate (BITC); and dithiolthione and other thiol-containing compounds.[67] The mechanisms by which cruciferous vegetables exert their anticarcinogenic effects have been reviewed.[68] The isothiocyanates and indoles have shown promising results against cancer at a number of sites, in both animals and humans. For example, indoles reduce mammary tumor formation in laboratory animals[67]; PEITC inhibits nitrosamine-induced esophageal cancer in rats[69] and may be protective against lung cancer among smokers[70]; and dithiolthiones reduce mammary and pulmonary tumorigenesis in rodents.[71] Mechanisms for the cancer-preventive actions of the isothiocyanates and indoles include induction of phase II detoxifying enzymes.[71,72]

PROTEASE INHIBITORS

In vivo, in vitro, and epidemiologic studies examining the suppression of neoplastic growth by soy-based protease inhibitors (PIs) have been summarized.[15,73] Actions of protease inhibitors include alteration of the expression of certain oncogenes and proteolytic activities that are elevated in carcinogen-exposed tissues; interference with oxyradical formation by neutrophils; and modulation of adenosine diphosphate ribosyltransferase,[74] possibly through the induction of synthesis and distribution of endogenous PIs by dietary PIs.[73] The soybean-derived Bowman-Birk inhibitor (BBI), a major protease inhibitor, may be at least partially responsible for the differences noted in cancer incidence between Asian and Western populations.[75] BBI and its concentrated form (BBIC) have exhibited suppressive effects in a number of carcinogenic models, including animals with a known genetic susceptibility to cancer.[75]

IMPLICATIONS FOR CANCER PREVENTION

Primary prevention represents the most desirable and cost-effective means of decreasing cancer incidence. Toward this end, the human diet contains anticarcinogens capable of reducing cancer risk, but substantial basic science research will be required to elucidate the mechanisms by which any particular phytochemical exerts its anticancer effect. In the absence of specific knowledge of anticarcinogenic dietary components and their mechanisms, consumption of a wide variety of fruits and vegetables is highly encouraged,[1] because several agents having weak effects *in vitro* may, in combination, prove more effective than any single agent.[76] Such a "polypharmaceutical" approach to cancer prevention is most likely to minimize cancer risk.[77]

Because phytochemicals are consumed, not in the form of high-dose supplements, but rather as constituents within a complex matrix of nutrients, the difficulty in identifying any particular component as being "a" primary preventive agent can be profound, particularly given the attendant problems of valid dietary assessment, confounding, and interaction with other factors. This is not to say, however, that such research cannot, or should not, be conducted. The further elucidation of naturally occurring dietary anticarcinogens represents a key element in efforts to decrease cancer incidence through primary preventive means. Additional epidemiologic and experimental research involving dietary anticarcinogens holds great potential for future cancer prevention efforts.

REFERENCES

1. Committee on Comparative Toxicity of Naturally Occurring Carcinogens, Estabrook RW, Birt D, et al. Conclusion, recommendations, and future directions. In: *Carcinogens and anticarcinogens in the human diet: a comparison of naturally occurring and synthetic substances.* Washington, DC: National Academy Press, 1996;335.
2. Potter JD. Cancer prevention: epidemiology and experiment. *Cancer Lett* 1997;114:7.
3. Khachik F, Nir Z, Ausich RL, et al. Distribution of carotenoids in fruits and vegetables as a criterion for the selection of appropriate chemopreventive agents. In: Ohigashi H, Osawa T, Terao J, et al., eds. *Food factors for cancer prevention.* New York: Springer-Verlag New York, 1997;204.
4. Krinsky NI. Overview of lycopene, carotenoids, and disease prevention. *Proc Soc Exp Biol Med* 1998;218:95.
5. IARC Working Group on the Evaluation of Cancer-Preventive Agents. *IARC handbooks of cancer prevention—carotenoids.* Lyon, France: International Agency for Research on Cancer, 1998.
6. Clinton SK. Lycopene: chemistry, biology, and implications for human health and disease. *Nutr Rev* 1998;56:35.
7. Giovannucci E. Tomatoes, tomato-based products, lycopene, and cancer: review of the epidemiologic literature. *J Natl Cancer Inst* 1999;91:317.
8. Pastori M, Pfander H, Boscoboinik D, Azzi A. Lycopene in association with α-tocopherol inhibits at physiological concentrations proliferation of prostate carcinoma cells. *Biochem Biophys Res Commun* 1998;250:582.
9. Park JS, Chew BP, Wong TS. Dietary lutein from marigold extract inhibits mammary tumor development in BALB/c mice. *J Nutr* 1998;128:1650.
10. Rock CL, Saxe GA, Ruffin MT IV, et al. Carotenoids, vitamin A, and estrogen receptor status in breast cancer. *Nutr Cancer* 1996;25:281.
11. Clarke R, Hilakivi-Clarke L, Cho E, et al. Estrogens, phytoestrogens, and breast cancer. In: American Institute for Cancer Research, ed. *Dietary phytochemicals in cancer prevention and treatment.* New York: Plenum Publishing, 1996:63.
12. Wiseman H. Role of dietary phyto-oestrogens in the protection against cancer and heart disease. *Biochem Soc Trans* 1996;24:795.
13. Bingham SA, Atkinson C, Liggins J, et al. Phyto-oestrogens: where are we now? *Br J Nutr* 1998;79:393.
14. Murkies AL, Wilcox G, Davis SR. Clinical review 92: phytoestrogens. *J Clin Endocrinol Metab* 1998;83:297.
15. Fournier DB, Erdman JW Jr, Gordon GB. Soy, its components, and cancer prevention: a review of the *in vitro*, animal, and human data. *Cancer Epidemiol Biomarkers Prev* 1998; 7:1055.
16. Fritz WA, Coward L, Wang J, Lamartiniere CA. Dietary genistein: perinatal mammary cancer prevention, bioavailability and toxicity testing in the rat. *Carcinogenesis* 1998;19:2151.
17. Onozawa M, Fukuda K, Ohtani M, et al. Effects of soybean isoflavones on cell growth and apoptosis of the human prostatic cancer cell line LNCaP. *Jpn J Clin Oncol* 1998;28:360.
18. Davis JN, Singh B, Bhuiyan M, Sarkar FH. Genistein-induced upregulation of $p21^{WAF1}$, downregulation of Cyclin B, and induction of apoptosis in prostate cancer cells. *Nutr Cancer* 1998;32:123.
19. Shao ZM, Wu J, Shen ZZ, Barsky SH. Genistein exerts multiple suppressive effects on human breast carcinoma cells. *Cancer Res* 1998;58:4851.
20. Harris RK, Greaves J, Alexander D, et al. Development of stability-indicating analytical methods for flaxseed lignans and their precursors. In: Ho CT, Osawa T, Huang MT, Rosen RT, eds. *Food phytochemicals for cancer prevention II—teas, spices, and herbs.* Washington, DC: American Chemical Society, 1994:295.
21. Wu AH, Ziegler RG, Horn-Ross PL, et al. Tofu and risk of breast cancer in Asian-Americans. *Cancer Epidemiol Biomarkers Prev* 1996;5:901.
22. Wargovich MJ. Experimental evidence for cancer preventive elements in foods. *Cancer Lett* 1997;114:11.
23. Block E. Recent results in the organosulfur and organoselenium chemistry of genus *Allium* and *Brassica* plants. Relevance for cancer prevention. In: American Institute for Cancer Research, ed. *Dietary phytochemicals in cancer prevention and treatment.* New York: Plenum Publishing, 1996:155.
24. Knowles LM, Milner JA. Depressed $p34^{cdc2}$ kinase activity and G_2/M phase arrest induced by diallyl disulfide in HCT-15 cells. *Nutr Cancer* 1998;30:169.
25. Singh A, Shukla Y. Antitumour activity of diallyl sulfide on polycyclic aromatic hydrocarbon-induced mouse skin carcinogenesis. *Cancer Lett* 1998;131:209.
26. Fahey JW, Zhang Y, Talalay P. Broccoli sprouts: an exceptionally rich source of inducers of enzymes that protect against chemical carcinogens. *Proc Natl Acad Sci U S A* 1997;94:10367.
27. Zhang Y, Talalay P. Mechanism of differential potencies of isothiocyanates as inducers of anticarcinogenic phase 2 enzymes. *Cancer Res* 1998;58:4632.
28. Davis CD, Feng Y, Hein DW, Finley JW. The chemical form of selenium influences 3,2'-dimethyl-4-aminobiphenyl-DNA adduct formation in rat colon. *J Nutr* 1999;129:63.
29. Bartram HP, Draenert R, Dusel G, et al. Effects of sodium selenite on deoxycholic acid-induced hyperproliferation of human colonic mucosa in short-term culture. *Cancer Epidemiol Biomarkers Prev* 1998;7:1085.
30. Clark LC, Combs GF Jr, Turnbull BW, et al. Effects of selenium supplementation for cancer prevention in patients with carcinoma of the skin. *JAMA* 1996;276:1957.
31. Yoshizawa K, Willett WC, Morris SJ, et al. Study of prediagnostic selenium level in toenails and the risk of advanced prostate cancer. *J Natl Cancer Inst* 1998;90:1219.
32. Kaul A, Khanduja KL. Polyphenols inhibit promotional phase of tumorigenesis: relevance of superoxide radicals. *Nutr Cancer* 1998;32:81.
33. Newmark HL. Plant phenolics as potential cancer prevention agents. In: American Institute for Cancer Research, ed. *Dietary phytochemicals in cancer prevention and treatment.* New York: Plenum Publishing, 1996:25.
34. Bravo L. Polyphenols: chemistry, dietary sources, metabolism, and nutritional significance. *Nutr Rev* 1998;56:317.

35. Jang M, Cai L, Udeani GO, et al. Cancer chemopreventive activity of resveratrol, a natural product derived from grapes. *Science* 1997;275:218.
36. Surh YJ, Hurh YJ, Kang JY, et al. Resveratrol, an antioxidant present in red wine, induces apoptosis in human promyelocytic leukemia (HL-60) cells. *Cancer Lett* 1999;140:1.
37. Gehm BD, McAndrews JM, Chien PY, Jameson JL. Resveratrol, a polyphenolic compound found in grapes and wine, is an agonist for the estrogen receptor. *Proc Natl Acad Sci U S A* 1997;94:14138.
38. Barch DH, Rundhaugen LM, Stoner GD, Pillay NS, Rosche WA. Structure-function relationships of the dietary anticarcinogen ellagic acid. *Carcinogenesis* 1996;17:265.
39. Constantinou A, Stoner GD, Mehta R, et al. The dietary anticancer agent ellagic acid is a potent inhibitor of DNA topoisomerases *in vitro*. *Nutr Cancer* 1995;23(2):121.
40. Castonguay A, Boukharta M, Jalbert G. Comparative study of ellagic acid and its analogues as chemopreventive agents against lung tumorigenesis. In: Huang MT, Osawa T, Ho CT, Rosen RT, eds. *Food phytochemicals for cancer prevention I—fruits and vegetables.* Washington, DC: American Chemical Society, 1994:294.
41. Stoner GD, Morse MA. Isothiocyanates and plant polyphenols as inhibitors of lung and esophageal cancer. *Cancer Lett* 1997;114:113.
42. Wang HK, Xia Y, Yang ZY, et al. Recent advances in the discovery and development of flavonoids and their analogues as antitumor and anti-HIV agents. In: Manthey JA, Buslig BS, eds. *Flavonoids in the living system.* New York: Plenum Publishing, 1998:191.
43. Guthrie N, Carroll KK. Inhibition of mammary cancer by citrus flavonoids. In: Manthey JA, Buslig BS, eds. *Flavonoids in the living system.* New York: Plenum Publishing, 1998:227.
44. Ferry DR, Smith A, Malkhandi J, et al. Phase I clinical trial of the flavonoid quercetin: pharmacokinetics and evidence for *in vivo* tyrosine kinase inhibition. *Clin Cancer Res* 1996;2:659.
45. Rodgers EH, Grant MH. The effect of flavonoids, quercetin, myricetin and epicatechin on the growth and enzyme activities of MCF7 human breast cancer cells. *Chem Biol Interact* 1998;116:213.
46. Le Bail JC, Varnat F, Nicolas JC, Habrioux G. Estrogenic and antiproliferative activities on MCF-7 human breast cancer cells by flavonoids. *Cancer Lett* 1998;130:209.
47. Lahiri-Chatterjee M, Katiyar SK, Mohan RR, Agarwal R. A flavonoid antioxidant, Silymarin, affords exceptionally high protection against tumor promotion in the SENCAR mouse skin tumorigenesis model. *Cancer Res* 1999;59:622.
48. Montanari A, Chen J, Widmer W. Citrus flavonoids: a review of past biologic activity against disease. In: Manthey JA, Buslig BS, eds. *Flavonoids in the living system.* New York: Plenum Publishing, 1998:103.
49. Kuroda Y, Hara Y. Antimutagenic and anticarcinogenic activity of tea polyphenols. *Mutation Res* 1999;436:69.
50. Chen ZP, Schell JB, Ho CT, Chen KY. Green tea epigallocatechin gallate shows a pronounced growth inhibitory effect on cancerous cells but not on their normal counterparts. *Cancer Lett* 1998;129:173.
51. Valcic S, Timmermann BN, Alberts DS, et al. Inhibitory effect of six green tea catechins and caffeine on the growth of four selected human tumor cell lines. *Anticancer Drugs* 1996;7:461.
52. Suganuma M, Okabe S, Kai Y, et al. Synergistic effects of (-)-epigallocatechin gallate with (-)-epicatechin, sulindac, or tamoxifen on cancer-preventive activity in the human lung cancer cell line PC-9. *Cancer Res* 1999;59:44.
53. Yu R, Jiao JJ, Duh JL, et al. Activation of mitogen-activated protein kinases by green tea polyphenols: potential signaling pathways in the regulation of antioxidant-responsive element-mediated phase II enzyme gene expression. *Carcinogenesis* 1997;18:451.
54. Yang CS, Chen L, Lee MJ, Landau JM. Effects of tea on carcinogenesis in animal models and humans. In: American Institute for Cancer Research, ed. *Dietary phytochemicals in cancer prevention and treatment.* New York: Plenum Publishing, 1996:51.
55. Yang GY, Liu Z, Seril DN, et al. Black tea constituents, theaflavins, inhibit 4-(methylnitrosamino)-1-(3-pyridyl)-1-butanone (NNK)-induced lung tumorigenesis in A/J mice. *Carcinogenesis* 1997;18:2361.
56. Sazuka M, Imazawa H, Shoji Y, et al. Inhibition of collagenases from mouse lung carcinoma cells by green tea catechins and black tea theaflavins. *Biosci Biotech Biochem* 1997;61:1504.
57. Blot WJ, McLaughlin JK, Chow WH. Cancer rates among drinkers of black tea. *Crit Rev Food Sci Nutr* 1997;37:739.
58. Man-Ying M, Fong D. Anti-inflammatory and cancer-preventive immunomodulation through diet—effects of curcumin and T lymphocytes. In: Ho CT, Osawa T, Huang MT, Rosen RT, eds. *Food phytochemicals for cancer prevention II—teas, spices, and herbs.* Washington, DC: American Chemical Society, 1994:222.
59. Lin JK, Huang TS, Shih CA, Liu JY. Molecular mechanism of action of curcumin. Inhibition of 12-*O*-tetradecanoylphorbol-13-acetate-induced responses associated with tumor promotion. In: Ho CT, Osawa T, Huan MT, Rosen RT, eds. *Food phytochemicals for cancer prevention II—teas, spices, and herbs.* Washington, DC: American Chemical Society, 1994:196.
60. Kawamori T, Lubet R, Steele VE, et al. Chemopreventive effect of curcumin, a naturally occurring anti-inflammatory agent, during the promotion/progression stages of colon cancer. *Cancer Res* 1999;59:597.
61. Simon A, Allais DP, Duroux JL, et al. Inhibitory effect of curcuminoids on MCF-7 cell proliferation and structure-activity relationships. *Cancer Lett* 1998;129:111.
62. Crowell PL. Antitumorigenic effects of limonene and perillyl alcohol against pancreatic and breast cancer. In: American Institute for Cancer Research, ed. *Dietary phytochemicals in cancer prevention and treatment.* New York: Plenum Publishing, 1996:131.
63. Bardon S, Picard K, Martel P. Monoterpenes inhibit cell growth, cell cycle progression, and cyclin D1 gene expression in human breast cancer cell lines. *Nutr Cancer* 1998;32:1.
64. Crowell PL. Prevention and therapy of cancer by dietary monoterpenes. *J Nutr* 1999;129:775S.
65. Hohl RJ. Monoterpenes as regulators of malignant cell proliferation. In: American Institute for Cancer Research, ed. *Dietary phytochemicals in cancer prevention and treatment.* New York: Plenum Publishing, 1996:137.
66. Steinmetz KA, Potter JD. Vegetables, fruit, and cancer prevention: a review. *J Am Diet Assoc* 1996;96:1027.
67. Michnovicz JJ, Bradlow HL. Dietary cytochrome P-450 modifiers in the control of estrogen metabolism. In: Huang MT, Osawa T, Ho CT, Rosen RT, eds. *Food phytochemicals for cancer prevention I—fruits and vegetables.* Washington, DC: American Chemical Society, 1994:282.
68. Verhoeven DTH, Verhagen H, Goldbohm RA, et al. A review of mechanisms underlying anticarcinogenicity by brassica vegetables. *Chem Biol Interact* 1997;103:79.
69. Stoner GD, Adams C, Kresty LA, et al. Inhibition of *N'*-nitrosonornicotine-induced esophageal tumorigenesis by 3-phenylpropyl isothiocyanate. *Carcinogenesis* 1998;19:2139.
70. Hecht SS. Chemoprevention of cancer by isothiocyanates, modifiers of carcinogen metabolism. *J Nutr* 1999;129:768S.
71. Kohlmeier L, Simonsen N, Mottus K. Dietary modifiers of carcinogenesis. *Environ Health Perspect* 1995;103(suppl 8):177.
72. Huang C, Ma W, Li J, et al. Essential role of p53 in phenethyl isothiocyanate-induced apoptosis. *Cancer Res* 1998;58:4102.
73. Clawson GA. Protease inhibitors and carcinogenesis: a review. *Cancer Invest* 1996;14:597.
74. Kennedy AR. Prevention of carcinogenesis by protease inhibitors. *Cancer Res* 1994;54:1999S.
75. Kennedy AR. The Bowman-Birk inhibitor from soybeans as an anticarcinogenic agent. *Am J Clin Nutr* 1998;68(suppl):1406S.
76. Chesson A, Collins A. Assessment of the role of diet in cancer prevention. *Cancer Lett* 1997;114:237.
77. Potter JD. Cancer prevention: epidemiology and experiment. *Cancer Lett* 1997;114:7.
78. Chen GW, Chung JG, Hsieh CL, Lin JG. Effects of the garlic components diallyl sulfide and diallyl disulfide on arylamine *N*-acetyltransferase activity in human colon tumour cells. *Food Chem Toxicol* 1998;36:761.
79. Martinez ME, Reid ME, Guillen-Rodriguez J, et al. Design and baseline characteristics of study participants in the Wheat Bran Fiber Trial. *Cancer Epidemiol Biomarkers Prev* 1998;7:813.
80. Rosa JGV, Prokopczyk B, Desai DH, et al. Elevated 8-hydroxy-2'-deoxyguanosine levels in lung DNA of A/J mice and F344 rats treated with 4-(methylnitrosamino)-1-(3-pyridyl)-1-butanone and inhibition by dietary 1,4-phenylenebis(methylene)selenocyanate. *Carcinogenesis* 1998;19:1783.
81. Hatono S, Jimenez A, Wargovich MJ. Chemopreventive effect of *S*-allylcysteine and its relationship to the detoxification enzyme glutathione *S*-transferase. *Carcinogenesis* 1996;17:1041.
82. Michaluart P, Masferrer JL, Carothers AM, et al. Inhibitory effects of caffeic acid phenethyl ester on the activity and expression of cyclooxygenase-2 in human oral epithelial cells and in a rat model of inflammation. *Cancer Res* 1999;59:2347.
83. Chaumontet C, Droumaguet C, Bex V, et al. Flavonoids (apigenin, tangeretin) counteract tumor promoter-induced inhibition of intercellular communication of rat liver epithelial cells. *Cancer Lett* 1997;114:207.
84. Drees M, Dengler WA, Roth T, et al. Flavopiridol (L86-8275): selective antitumor activity *in vitro* and activity *in vivo* for prostate carcinoma cells. *Clin Cancer Res* 1997;3:273.
85. Berkarda B, Koyuncu H, Soybir G, Baykut F. Inhibitory effect of hesperidin on tumour initiation and promotion in mouse skin. *Res Exp Med* 1998;198:93.
86. Webster RP, Gawde MD, Bhattacharya RK. Protective effect of rutin, a flavonol glycoside, on the carcinogen-induced DNA damage and repair enzymes in rats. *Cancer Lett* 1996;109:185.
87. Yang CS, Yang GY, Landau JM, et al. Tea and tea polyphenols inhibit cell hyperproliferation, lung tumorigenesis, and tumor progression. *Exp Lung Res* 1998;24:629.
88. Paschka AG, Butler R, Young CYF. Induction of apoptosis in prostate cancer cell lines by the green tea component, (-)-epigallocatechin-3-gallate. *Cancer Lett* 1998;130:1.

SECTION 5

PETER GREENWALD

Dietary Carcinogens

With the exception of tobacco, no environmental exposure to potential carcinogens is comparable to sources in the diet.[1] Although the public often attributes the source of carcinogens in the food supply to food additives, synthetic pesticides, and various environmental contaminants, these chemicals are estimated to represent less than 1% of the carcinogens found in foods. In fact, most known dietary carcinogens either occur naturally in plants or are produced during food preparation.[2,3] Dietary carcinogens in both groups are discussed, with a review of common food sources, mechanisms of action, human exposure, and degree of human risk. A brief overview of issues regarding synthetic carcinogens in the diet is also provided.

In many cases, current knowledge is incomplete and does not allow reliable estimates of risk. First, no concentration data exist for many potentially carcinogenic constituents of foods. In addition, determining human exposure levels is difficult and sometimes inconclusive.[4] Dietary assessment tools are subjective and often biased,[5] the food levels of some substances can vary from year to year,[6] and exposure to mixtures of substances at low doses might be more important than exposure to single agents.[4] High-dose animal testing has been used to approximate human risk, and the Carcinogenic Potency Database currently includes results for approximately 1298 chemicals tested in long-term animal experiments (http://potency.berkeley.edu/app14.html). However, this information cannot predict human risk with a high degree of confidence.[7,8] Extrapolation from the near-toxic doses used in animal tests to human risk at low-dose exposure is difficult, and some critics believe its use has sometimes led to overemphasis of potentially minimal risks.[1] One challenge relates to differences in the carcinogenic mechanisms involved. For example, mitogens likely act by increasing cell proliferation, but only at near-toxic levels, whereas mutagens can damage DNA at low doses. As a result, animal tests involving mutagens may have more significance for human risk.[7,8]

To increase the reliability of exposure estimates, biomarkers are being developed to mark internal dose, putative early response, and susceptibility. For example, DNA-carcinogen adducts have been used as measurable end points in laboratory studies and, to a more limited extent, in humans, to assess dietary carcinogen exposure, carcinogen metabolism, mutagenesis, and tumorigenesis.[9,10] In addition, genetic and acquired susceptibility traits have been shown to affect carcinogen metabolism, DNA damage, and repair.[11] In fact, more than a dozen polymorphic gene/phenotypes related to the metabolism of dietary carcinogens are possible actors in the complex process of carcinogenesis at many sites.[12–14] Although related technology is just emerging and more study is needed,[4,15] approaches such as these have already affected understanding of the substances discussed in the following sections.

TABLE 23.5-1. Food Sources of Naturally Occurring Dietary Carcinogens

NATURAL PESTICIDES	
Caffeic acid	Apples, pears, plums, cherries, carrots, celery, lettuce, potatoes, endive, grapes, eggplant, thyme, basil, anise, sage, dill, caraway, rosemary, tarragon, coffee beans
Allyl isothiocyanate	Cabbage, cauliflower, Brussels sprouts, mustard, horseradish
Saffrole	Nutmeg, mace, pepper, cinnamon, natural root beer
Estragole	Basil, fennel, tarragon
Carvacrol	Marjoram
Furocoumarins	Lime, citrus oils, carrots, celery, parsley, parsnips
Hydrazines	Mushrooms
Pyrrolizidine	Herbal teas (comfrey)
MYCOTOXINS	
Aflatoxins	Corn, peanuts, seed nuts, peanut butter
Ochratoxin A	Grains, green coffee beans
T-2 toxin	Barley, maize, safflower seeds, cereals
Zearalenone	Feed grains, soybean, maize, wheat
Fumonisins	Corn
Deoxynivalenol	Wheat, maize
Nivalenol	Wheat, maize, barley

(Data from refs. 2, 3, 16, 22, 73–75.)

NATURALLY OCCURRING DIETARY CARCINOGENS

Most naturally occurring dietary carcinogens are either "natural pesticides," produced by plants for protection against fungi, insects, and animal predators, or mycotoxins, secondary metabolites produced by molds in foods. Table 23.5-1 lists some of the most common substances in both categories.

NATURAL PESTICIDES

Animal studies have provided evidence for the carcinogenicity of a large number of individual plant constituents fed at high doses. However, no firm conclusions can be drawn about the overall effects of most of these substances on human health. Plant foods contain thousands of phytochemicals representing various chemical classes and exhibiting diverse molecular structures, and only a small fraction of potential carcinogens produced by plant foods have been tested systematically.[3] In addition, the difficulties previously described in assessing human risk are well illustrated by naturally occurring pesticides. Caffeic acid, which has been shown to cause forestomach squamous cell carcinomas in rats as well as renal tubular cell hyperplasia and adenomas in mice, is a good example. The relevance of the animal findings to humans is uncertain, because data are not available on carcinogenicity in humans, very high doses were used in the animal studies, humans do not have a forestomach, and the renal lesions were related to toxic lesions.[16] In addition, *in vitro*, caffeic acid may act either as a pro- or antioxidant, and it has been observed to be both protective and enhancing when administered orally in combination with known carcinogens.[16] Another confounding factor is the fact that many foods containing caffeic acid also contain compounds believed to be protective, which might affect its ultimate human impact.

Despite such challenges, with additional information on factors such as exposure levels, concentration levels, mechanisms of action, and human clinical experience, researchers can draw conclusions on human risk from natural pesticides. For example, studies of coumarin—a substance with many food sources (particularly cinnamon) that has been found to be carcinogenic in rats and mice—have concluded that it poses no health risk to humans. Known exposure levels and differences in coumarin metabolism between susceptible rodent species and humans contributed to this finding.[17] Other studies are elucidating some of the important factors in assessing human risk, particularly regarding mechanisms of action in animals. For instance, researchers rationalized the restriction of allyl isothiocyanate–related bladder tumors to male rats compared with female rats and both sexes of mice on the basis of a species difference in metabolism and a sex difference in exposure to allyl isothiocyanate metabolites.[18] Other studies have found that the hepatocarcinogenicity of hydrazine is linked to the hypomethylation of total target organ DNA that occurs with chronic exposure and that the hypomethylation is dose-related to the development of liver cancer.[19] Methylation is believed to be a factor in aberrant gene expression and the development of tumors.

From a public health perspective, dietary exposure to natural pesticides can generally be controlled by selecting genetic strains of plants that produce lower concentrations and by reducing plant stress during the growing season. Particular natural pesticides that are carcinogenic in animals might be bred out of crops if research indicates they could be hazardous to humans.[8] Increasing the level of natural pesticides by breeding as an alternative to synthetic pesticides must be considered cautiously in view of their potential health effects. Consumers also could be informed of the relative risks associated with food products such as herbal teas, for which both protective and toxic effects have been documented.[20]

MYCOTOXINS

Mycotoxins are structurally diverse toxic fungal metabolites that are common contaminants of ingredients in animal feed and human food; to date, more than 300 mycotoxins have been identified.[21] The mycotoxins listed in Table 23.5-1 are among those shown to have carcinogenic potential in animals. However, only aflatoxin B_1 (AFB_1) and naturally occurring mixtures of aflatoxins are known to be genotoxic and carcinogenic to humans. Fumonisins and ochratoxin A have been shown to be possibly carcinogenic to humans.[22]

Aflatoxins

AFB_1 is a potent carcinogen in many species of animals, including rodents, nonhuman primates, and fish. Epidemiologic studies show a strong direct association between AFB_1 intake in Africa and China and risk for primary liver and lung cancer in humans.[23,24] Synergistic interactions of AFB_1 with both viral B hepatitis and alcohol consumption in humans also have been demonstrated.[23] High levels of AFB_1, produced by the *Aspergillus* species, are found in regions of Africa, southeast Asia, and southern China, where the foods they contaminate are dietary staples for humans and animals. In fact, human exposure to AFB_1 in southern China (either directly or through eating the products of animals that ate contaminated feed) can be as high as 75 to 250 μg/d, compared with 25 to 75 ng/d in the United States, where aflatoxin contamination levels are lower.[25]

The aflatoxins have been extensively characterized with respect to chemistry, biology, and toxicology. Like most other mycotoxins with the exception of fumonisins, aflatoxins are genotoxic agents, and substantial research has been conducted on the genetic damage created by AFB_1 in liver and lung tumors. A key biomarker, the predominant AFB_1-DNA adduct (AFB_1-N^7-Gua), has been identified and correlated with the incidence of hepatic tumor in trout and rats.[21] Formation of the AFB_1-DNA adduct requires metabolic activation of AFB_1 to its carcinogenic form, the 8,9-epoxide.[26] A review of data from animal and human studies that measured urinary excretion of aflatoxin-DNA adducts by molecular dosimetry suggested that these adducts are useful markers of exposure.[15] For instance, a prospective study of more than 18,000 men in Shanghai, China, demonstrated a significant increase in risk [relative risk (RR) = 3.4] for liver cancer in individuals in whom urinary aflatoxin-DNA adducts were detected.[23]

Striking species differences exist in the oncogenic mutations involving AFB_1. For example, a considerable amount of evidence shows that dietary AFB_1 exposure can produce codon 249 (AGG to AGT) *p53* tumor suppressor gene mutations during human liver carcinogenesis.[27] In rat liver tumors, however, codon 12 of K-*ras* appears to be the "hot spot" for AFB_1-induced mutations.[28] In mice exposed to AFB_1, preneoplastic lesions contained mutations in codon 61 of the Ha-*ras* gene, and *in vitro* studies show that metabolically activated AFB_1 in humans is capable of mutating this proconcogene to its oncogenic form, although no such mutations have been reported *in vivo*.[26] Thus, although these mutations are clearly associated with exposure, their significance in terms of mechanistic involvement in tumorigenesis needs further elucidation.[29]

Elimination of exposure to aflatoxins is not possible given the ubiquitous nature of the molds that produce them. Primary prevention methods have included developing aflatoxin-resistant plants, building better storage facilities for grains, and establishing regulatory and testing programs around the world.[23]

Fumonisins and Ochratoxin A

Of the six fumonisins identified, fumonisin B_1 has been shown to be carcinogenic in rats and mice at high doses, primarily targeting the liver and kidneys. It also has been linked in ecologic studies to esophageal cancer in humans in high corn-consuming regions of China and Africa where high levels of contamination are documented, but no convincing evidence of causality has been presented to date.[30]

Fumonisins, which are produced by *Fusarium moniliforme*, do not appear to be genotoxic, but they may induce cancer through disturbing the signal transduction pathways.[21] As with other dietary carcinogens, difficulties exist with available technologies for assessing exposure, and the search for biomarkers is a rapidly growing area of research. Fumonisins in urine and altered sphingolipid metabolism (sphinganine-sphingosine ratio) in urine and blood are two potential markers currently under investigation.[30,31] The co-occurrence of fumonisins and aflatoxins in corn-based foods has been demonstrated and a synergistic effect postulated.[30]

Ochratoxins are produced by *Aspergillus ochraceus* and related species. Ochratoxin A (OA) has induced renal adenomas and kidney cancers in mice and rats. Carcinogenic effects in humans are suspected based on findings of high levels of OA in the blood of patients with Balkan endemic nephropathy, who also have a high incidence of varied carcinomas.[21] The search for DNA adducts as biomarkers of OA also is ongoing.[21] The relative lack of information on fumonisins, ochratoxins, and other mycotoxins compared with aflatoxins does not mean that their public health risk is necessarily less. Rather, it indicates that more investigation of these mycotoxins is needed.

PRODUCTS OF FOOD PREPARATION AND PROCESSING

Food preparation and preservation are major sources of dietary carcinogens, including heterocyclic aromatic amines (HAA), formed during frying, broiling, and grilling high-protein foods and more prevalent in well-done meats; polycyclic aromatic hydrocarbons (PAH), formed during broiling and smoking food; and N-nitrosocompounds (NOC), formed in smoked, salted, and pickled foods cured with nitrate or nitrite.[32,33] NOCs are also formed endogenously at sites such as the stom-

TABLE 23.5-2. Dietary Carcinogens Produced during Food Preparation: Sources and Cooking Methods

Urethene	All fermented and yeast-leavened foods: wines, yogurt, soy sauce, sake, ale, beer, bread
Heterocyclic aromatic amines	
2-amino-3-methylimidazo [4,5-*f*]quinoline	Broiled beef and salmon; fried ground beef and fish
2-amino-3,8-dimethylimidazo [4,5-*f*]quinoxaline	Barbecued chicken, fish, pork; broiled beef, chicken, mutton, pork; fried bacon, ground beef, fish
2-amino-3,4,8-trimethylimidazo [4,5-*f*]quinoxaline	Barbecued chicken, pork; broiled chicken, mutton; fried bacon, fish; smoked mackerel
2-amino-1-methyl-6-phenylimidazo[4,5-*b*]pyridine	Barbecued pork, fish; broiled beef, chicken, mutton, fish; fried bacon, fish, ground beef, ground pork
2-amino-9H-pyrido[2,3-*b*]indole	Barbecued fish; broiled beef, chicken, mutton
Polycyclic aromatic hydrocarbons	
Pyrene	Charcoal-broiled/grilled steak, beef patties, chicken, frankfurters, pork; bacon; liquid smoke; smoked fish
Benz(a)anthracene	Charcoal-broiled/grilled steak, beef patties, chicken, frankfurters, pork; liquid smoke; smoked fish
Chrysene	Charcoal-broiled/grilled steak, beef patties, chicken, frankfurters, pork; bacon; smoked fish
Benz(a)pyrene	Charcoal-broiled/grilled steak, beef patties, chicken, frankfurters, pork; liquid smoke; smoked fish
N-Nitrosocompounds	
N-Nitrosomethylamine	Cured meats; fried bacon; millet flour, grain products; dairy, cheese products; pickled/fermented vegetables; beer, whiskey
N-Nitrosoethylamine	Cured meats, salami; millet flour, grain products
N-Nitrosobutylamine	Cured meats; smoked chicken; dried fish
N-Nitrosopyrrolidine	Cured meats; fried bacon; broiled squid; pickled vegetables; mixed spices; dried chilies
N-Nitrosopiperidine	Cured meats; fried bacon; peppered salami; pepper; mixed spices; pickled vegetables

(Data from refs. 2, 3, 16, 22, 58, 73–75.)

ach from nitrites and amines in the diet.[34] Table 23.5-2 lists common carcinogens produced during food preparation and related food sources and cooking methods. Although human risk from these compounds is not always well understood, it may be prudent to minimize exposure by modifying meat cooking methods and eating fewer foods containing NOCs.

HETEROCYCLIC AROMATIC AMINES

HAAs are potent mutagens and animal carcinogens, causing cancers of the liver, colon, mammary gland, skin, Zymbal gland, large intestine, prostate, lymphoid tissues, oral cavity, lung, and clitoral gland in rodent models.[35,36] Approximately 20 HAAs have been isolated[33]; the major subclass found in the human diet comprises the aminoimidazoazaarenes (AIA). Four of these are possibly carcinogenic to humans, including 2-amino-3-methylimidazo[4,5-*f*]quinoline (IQ); 2-amino-3,4-dimethylimidazo[4,5-*f*]quinoline (MeIQ); 2-amino-3,8-dimethylimidazo[4,5-*f*]quinoxaline (8-MeIQx); and 2-amino-1-methyl-6-phenylimidazo[4,5-*b*]pyridine (PhIP).[33,37] However, the etiologic role of HAAs in human cancer is unclear, in part because of a lack of information on the effect of typical cooking methods and degree of doneness on concentrations of HAAs as well as on variation in exposure.[38–40]

Animal studies have demonstrated formation of HAA-DNA adducts in numerous tissues, and a review reports that all of the AIAs studied adduct to the guanine base, with the major adduct being formed at the C8 atom of guanine. Two AIAs, IQ and MeIQx, also form minor adducts at the N^2 position of guanine.[35] Studies of animal tumors have begun to relate AIA-DNA adduct-induced mutagenic events with the mutations found in critical genes associated with oncogenesis, and AIA-DNA adduct levels in target tissues are strongly related to tumor incidence.[35] Dietary fat also has been implicated as a promotional factor in HAA-related carcinogenesis in animal studies, but the data remain difficult to interpret.[41,42]

Although HAA-DNA adducts can be useful biomarkers, their detection in humans has proved difficult. Some adducts have been documented, however.[35] For example, one report indicates that MeIQx forms DNA adducts in the human colon at a low dose and that the human colon may be more sensitive to MeIQx than the colon of mice or rats.[43] In addition, using accelerator mass spectrometry, it has been possible to detect AIA-DNA adducts in tissues after dosing animals with amounts equivalent to human dietary exposures. Such studies confirm that AIAs are potentially genotoxic and carcinogenic at specific target sites at doses derived from the human diet.[35]

Metabolic activation is necessary to the formation of HAA-DNA adducts in animals and humans and is critical to the mutagenicity and carcinogenicity of HAAs.[4,35] The metabolic activation of HAAs varies among species, but activation in humans appears to occur via N-oxidation to form N-hydroxy metabolites followed by O-acetylation to form N-acetoxy arylamines that bind to DNA. These steps are catalyzed by cytochrome P-450A2 and N-acetyltransferase-2 (NAT-2), respectively.[39,44]

There is wide interindividual variation in the capacity of human tissues to activate HAAs, and polymorphisms of related enzymes in humans have been investigated for potential relationship to cancer risk. In some studies, but not in others, individuals who were both rapid N-oxidizers and rapid acetylators had a greater risk of colon cancer than those who were both slow N-oxidizers and slow acetylators.[4,45–47] In one study, rapid acetylators had an increased risk only with a high intake of meat.[41] Some data suggest that variations in susceptibility to pancreatic and prostate cancer also are associated with genetic differences of carcinogen-metabolizing enzymes, although these areas require further investigation.[48,49] In breast cancer, differential susceptibility in rapid versus slow acetylators has been found in some studies, but not in others.[50–53]

Urinary excretion of cooking-associated HAAs and their metabolites is being investigated as a possible biomarker of human exposure, and studies have shown measurable excretion of MeIQx and its metabolites after consumption of proteins cooked at high temperatures.[15,54] Although researchers found a dose-response relationship between the bacon intake of African American, white, and Asian American men and MeIQx excretion,[55] no such relationship was seen in the same group of men for consumption of any type of cooked meat and PhIP.[54]

POLYCYCLIC AROMATIC HYDROCARBONS

PAHs, several of which have been found to be carcinogenic in animal studies, have a widespread distribution throughout the environment, both as a by-product of cooking meats over an open flame and as a contaminant in animal and human foods.[56,57] However, available exposure and carcinogenicity data are insufficient to allow a reliable estimate of dietary PAH risk for humans at this time.

It is clear that fat dripping onto the coals and the subsequent deposition of PAHs that rise with smoke onto the meat contribute significantly to PAH exposure.[15] Benzo(a)pyrene, the most carcinogenic PAH, has been reported at levels of up to 50 μg/kg in charbroiled steaks and ground beef, five times greater than levels in some less fatty pork cuts and chicken.[58]

In addition, several studies have demonstrated a consistent association between recent consumption of charbroiled foods and increased PAH-DNA adduct concentrations in peripheral white blood cells and excretion of 1-hydroxypyrene in urine.[15,59,60] One review suggests a correlation between PAH-DNA adducts and *ras* oncogene mutations.[61] Some evidence points to an antioxidant response element playing a significant role in PAH carcinogenesis.[62] It also has been suggested that the *hGSTP1* gene, which has been shown to be polymorphic in humans, may be an important factor in differential susceptibility to PAH-related cancers, although study conclusions differ. The chemical composition of the PAH mixtures to which humans are exposed can include cigarette smoke and industrial emissions as well as dietary sources, and differences in mixtures may affect the involvement of the *hGSTP1* gene.[63]

N-NITROSOCOMPOUNDS

NOCs administered orally in animals, including nonhuman primates, consistently elicit carcinogenic responses.[64] These compounds also may be a significant risk factor for human cancers of the stomach, esophagus, colon and rectum, nasopharynx, urinary bladder, and liver.[22,65,66] One review found that, although the epidemiologic evidence overall remains inconclusive, an association between NOCs and human cancer cannot be ruled out. The author postulated that inadequate available data may be obscuring a small to moderate carcinogenic effect of NOCs.[34]

The formation of endogenous NOCs may be inhibited by naturally occurring compounds in foods, such as ascorbic acid, tocopherols, retinoids, phenolic compounds, sulfhydryl compounds, tea, orange peel, and certain fruits and vegetables.[67] This may in part explain the generally protective effect of vegetables and fruits consistently observed in epidemiologic studies.[68,69]

SYNTHETIC CARCINOGENS IN THE DIET

Animals and humans also are exposed to a variety of synthetic chemicals in their foods from food additives. Direct (intentional) synthetic additives include antioxidants, colorants, flavor ingredients, artificial sweeteners, solvents, and humectants. Regulation of synthetic or natural chemicals intentionally added to food has led to extensive data on exposure. Indirect (unintentional) synthetic additives include pesticides, solvents, and packaging-derived chemicals. These chemicals, which number more than 2000, enter the food supply during production, processing, packaging, and storage from a variety of sources. Very little data exist on exposure to these chemicals. Pesticides are of major concern to the public and regulatory agencies compared with other indirect food additives. Most, if not all, pesticides have possible human toxicity, including carcinogenic potential. In general, levels encountered are below allowable tolerances, although actual estimates of risk are problematic.[16] Packaging materials, including vinyl chloride, and several phthalate esters used as plasticizers have gained attention from researchers as another possible unintentional addition to packaged foods with potential risks to human health.

Synthetic chemical contamination of water has been another concern, principally focused on trihalomethanes, which are disinfection by-products, in public water supplies and pesticides in well water.[70–72]

The National Research Council classifies synthetic chemicals as genotoxic, which directly affect DNA, form DNA adducts, and increase cancer risk, and nongenotoxic, which do not directly affect DNA, but which may affect carcinogenesis through other posited mechanisms.[16] Some synthetic chemicals can exhibit both genotoxic and nongenotoxic activity.

The metabolic pathways involved in the biotransformation of both synthetic and naturally occurring chemicals are similar, and evidence to date suggests that the processes of carcinogenesis also are similar, if not identical. Not surprisingly, the difficulties that complicate risk prediction for naturally occurring dietary carcinogens also apply to the synthetic carcinogens.[16]

FUTURE RESEARCH NEEDS

It is clear from human epidemiologic data that diet contributes to an appreciable portion of cancer; however, continuing research is needed for better identification of the risk to humans from specific carcinogens in the diet. Although we have begun to understand some of the key factors affecting risk estimation for some of the phytochemicals in plant foods, both naturally occurring and synthetic chemicals are numerous and diverse. The National Research Council suggests that new concepts and methods must be developed and extensive research conducted before results obtained in various model systems can be extrapolated with greater reliability to humans.[16]

REFERENCES

1. Lindsay DG. Dietary contribution to genotoxic risk and its control. *Food Chem Toxicol* 1996;34:423.
2. Scheuplein RJ. Perspectives on toxicological risk—an example: foodborne carcinogenic risk. *Crit Rev Food Sci Nutr* 1992;32:105.
3. Ames BN, Gold LS. Dietary carcinogens, environmental pollution, and cancer: some misconceptions. *Med Oncol Tumor Pharmacother* 1990;7:69.
4. Vineis P. Biomarkers, low-dose carcinogenesis and dietary exposures. *Eur J Cancer Prev* 1997;6:147.
5. Egan KM, Giovannucci E. Dietary mutagens and the risk of breast cancer. *J Natl Cancer Inst* 1998;90:1687.

6. Omer RE, Bakker MI, van't Veer P, et al. Aflatoxin and liver cancer in Sudan. *Nutr Cancer* 1998;32:174.
7. Abbott PJ. Carcinogenic chemicals in food: evaluating the health risk. *Food Chem Toxicol* 1992;30:327.
8. Ames BN, Gold LS. Animal cancer tests and cancer prevention. *J Natl Cancer Inst Monogr* 1992;12:125.
9. Eder E. Intraindividual variations of DNA adduct levels in humans. *Mutat Res* 1999;424:249.
10. Otteneder M, Lutz WK. Correlation of DNA adduct levels with tumor incidence: carcinogenic potency of DNA adducts. *Mutat Res* 1999;424:237.
11. Hirvonen A. Polymorphisms of xenobiotic-metabolizing enzymes and susceptibility to cancer. *Environ Health Perspect* 1999;107:37.
12. Sinha R, Caporaso N. Diet, genetic susceptibility and human cancer etiology. *J Nutr* 1999;129:556S.
13. Lai C, Shields PG. The role of interindividual variation in human carcinogenesis. *J Nutr* 1999;129:552S.
14. Lunn RM, Langlois RG, Hsieh LL, et al. XRCC1 polymorphisms: effects on aflatoxin B_1-DNA adducts and glycophorin A variant frequency. *Cancer Res* 1999;59:2557.
15. Strickland PT, Groopman JD. Biomarkers for assessing environmental exposure to carcinogens in the diet. *Am J Clin Nutr* 1995;61:710S.
16. Committee on Comparative Toxicity of Naturally Occurring Carcinogens, Board on Environmental Studies and Toxicology, Commission on Life Sciences, National Research Council. *Carcinogens and anticarcinogens in the human diet.* Washington, DC: National Academy Press, 1996.
17. Lake BG. Coumarin metabolism, toxicity and carcinogenicity: relevance for human risk assessment. *Food Chem Toxicol* 1999;37:423.
18. Bollard M, Stribbling S, Mitchell S, Caldwell J. The disposition of allyl isothiocyanate in the rat and mouse. *Food Chem Toxicol* 1997;35:933.
19. FitzGerald BE, Shank RC. Methylation status of DNA cytosine during the course of induction of liver cancer in hamsters by hydrazine sulfate. *Carcinogenesis* 1996;17:2703.
20. Manteiga R, Park DL, Ali SS. Risks associated with consumption of herbal teas. *Rev Environ Contam Toxicol* 1997;150:1.
21. Wang JS, Groopman JD. DNA damage by mycotoxins. *Mutat Res* 1999;424:167.
22. International Agency for Research on Cancer Working Group. *IARC monographs on the evaluation of carcinogenic risks to humans,* vol. 56. Lyon, France: International Agency for Research on Cancer, 1993.
23. Groopman JD, Scholl P, Wang JS. Epidemiology of human aflatoxin exposures and their relationship to liver cancer. *Prog Clin Biol Res* 1996;395:211.
24. Wang LY, Hatch M, Chen CJ, et al. Aflatoxin exposure and risk of hepatocellular carcinoma in Taiwan. *Int J Cancer* 1996;67:620.
25. Gonzalez FJ. Genetic polymorphism and cancer susceptibility: fourteenth Sapporo Cancer Seminar. *Cancer Res* 1995;55:710.
26. Riley J, Mandel HG, Sinha S, et al. *In vitro* activation of the human Harvey-*ras* proto-oncogene by aflatoxin B_1. *Carcinogenesis* 1997;18:905.
27. Hussain SP, Harris CC. Molecular epidemiology of human cancer. *Toxicol Lett* 1998;102/103:219.
28. Donnelly PJ, Devereux TR, Foley JF, et al. Activation of K-*ras* in aflatoxin B_1-induced lung tumors from AC3F1 (A/JxC3H/HeJ) mice. *Carcinogenesis* 1996;17:1735.
29. Stanley LA, Mandel HG, Riley J, et al. Mutations associated with *in vivo* aflatoxin B_1-induced carcinogenesis need not be present in the *in vitro* transformations by this toxin. *Cancer Lett* 1999;137:173.
30. Turner PC, Nikiema P, Wild CP. Fumonisin contamination of food: progress in development of biomarkers to better assess human health risks. *Mutat Res* 1999;443:81.
31. Wang E, Riley RT, Meredith FI, Merrill AH Jr. Fumonisin B_1 consumption by rats causes reversible, dose-dependent increases in urinary sphinganine and sphingosine. *J Nutr* 1999; 129:214.
32. Zheng W, Gustafson DR, Sinha R, et al. Well-done meat intake and the risk of breast cancer. *J Natl Cancer Inst* 1998;90:1724.
33. Skog KI, Johansson MAE, Jagerstad MI. Carcinogenic heterocyclic amines in model systems and cooked foods: a review on formation, occurrence and intake. *Food Chem Toxicol* 1998;36:879.
34. Eichholzer M, Gutzwiller F. Dietary nitrates, nitrites, and *n*-nitroso compounds and cancer risk: a review of the epidemiologic evidence. *Nutr Rev* 1998;56:95.
35. Schut HAJ, Snyderwine EG. DNA adducts of heterocyclic amine food mutagens: implications for mutagenesis and carcinogenesis. *Carcinogenesis* 1999;20:353.
36. Shirai T, Sano M, Tamano S, et al. The prostate: a target for carcinogenicity of 2-amino-1-methyl-6-phenylimidazo[4,5-*b*]pyridine (PhIP) derived from cooked foods. *Cancer Res* 1997;57:195.
37. De Stefani E, Ronco A, Mendilaharsu M, et al. Meat intake, heterocyclic amines, and risk of breast cancer: a case-control study in Uruguay. *Cancer Epidemiol Biomarkers Prev* 1997; 6:573.
38. Augustsson K, Skog K, Jägerstad M, et al. Dietary heterocyclic amines and cancer of the colon, rectum, bladder, and kidney: a population-based study. *Lancet* 1999;353:703.
39. Adamson RH, Thorgeirsson UP, Sugimura T. Extrapolation of heterocyclic amine carcinogenesis data from rodents and nonhuman primates to humans. *Arch Toxicol Suppl* 1996;18:303.
40. Byrne C, Sinha R, Platz EA, et al. Predictors of dietary heterocyclic amine intake in three prospective cohorts. *Cancer Epidemiol Biomarkers Prev* 1998;7:523.
41. Roberts-Thomson SJ, Snyderwine EG. Effect of dietary fat on codon 12 and 13 Ha-*ras* gene mutations in 2-amino-1-methyl-6-phenylimidazo-[4,5-*b*]pyridine-induced rat mammary gland tumors. *Mol Carcinog* 1997;20:348.
42. Pence BC, Landers M, Dunn DM, et al. Feeding of a well-cooked beef diet containing a high heterocyclic amine content enhances colon and stomach carcinogenesis in 1,2-dimethylhydrazine-treated rats. *Nutr Cancer* 1998;30:220.
43. Mauthe RJ, Dingley KH, Leveson SH, et al. Comparison of DNA-adduct and tissue-available dose levels of MeIQx in human and rodent colon following administration of a very low dose. *Int J Cancer* 1999;80:539.
44. Lang NP, Butler MA, Massengill J, et al. Rapid metabolic phenotypes for acetyltransferase and cytochrome P4501A2 and putative exposure to food-borne heterocyclic amines increase the risk for colorectal cancer or polyps. *Cancer Epidemiol Biomarkers Prev* 1994;3:675.
45. Kampman E, Slattery ML, Bigler J, et al. Meat consumption, genetic susceptibility, and colon cancer risk: a United States multicenter case-control study. *Cancer Epidemiol Biomarkers Prev* 1999;8:15.
46. Hubbard AL, Moyes C, Wyllie AH, et al. *N*-acetyl transferase 1: two polymorphisms in coding sequence identified in colorectal cancer patients. *Br J Cancer* 1998;77:913.
47. Rafter J, Glinghammar B. Interactions between the environment and genes in the colon. *Eur J Cancer Prev* 1998;7:S69.
48. Bartsch H, Malaveille C, Lowenfels AB, et al. Genetic polymorphism of *N*-acetyltransferases, glutathione *S*-transferase M1 and NAD(P)H:quinone oxidoreductase in relation to malignant and benign pancreatic disease risk. *Eur J Cancer Prev* 1998;7:215.
49. Fukutome K, Watanabe M, Shiraishi T, et al. *N*-acetyltransferase 1 genetic polymorphism influences the risk of prostate cancer development. *Cancer Lett* 1999;136:83.
50. Stone EM, Williams JA, Grover PL, et al. Interindividual variation in the metabolic activation of heterocyclic amines and their N-hydroxy derivatives in primary cultures of human mammary epithelial cells. *Carcinogenesis* 1998;19:873.
51. Gertig DM, Hankinson SE, Hough H, et al. *N*-acetyl transferase 2 genotypes, meat intake and breast cancer risk. *Int J Cancer* 1999;80:13.
52. Huang CS, Chern HD, Shen CY, et al. Association between *N*-acetyltransferase 2 (*NAT2*) genetic polymorphism and development of breast cancer in post-menopausal Chinese women in Taiwan, an area of great increase in breast cancer incidence. *Int J Cancer* 1999;82:175.
53. Dubuisson JG, Gaubatz JW. Bioactivation of the proximal food mutagen 2-hydroxyamino-1-methyl-6-phenylimidazo[4,5-*b*]pyridine (N-OH-PhIP) to DNA-binding species by human mammary gland enzymes. *Nutrition* 1998;14:683.
54. Kidd LCR, Stillwell WG, Yu MC, et al. Urinary excretion of 2-amino-1-methyl-6-phenylimidazo[4,5-*b*]pyridine (PhIP) in white, African-American, and Asian-American men in Los Angeles County. *Cancer Epidemiol Biomarkers Prev* 1999;8:439.
55. Ji H, Yu MC, Stillwell WG, et al. Urinary excretion of 2-amino-3,8-dimethylimidazo[4,5-*f*]quinoxaline in white, black, and Asian men in Los Angeles County. *Cancer Epidemiol Biomarkers Prev* 1994;3:407.
56. Dipple A, Peltonen K, Cheng SC, et al. Chemical and mutagenic specificities of polycyclic aromatic hydrocarbon carcinogens. *Adv Exp Med Biol* 1994;354:101.
57. Schoket B. DNA damage in humans exposed to environmental and dietary polycyclic aromatic hydrocarbons. *Mutat Res* 1999;424:143.
58. Lijinsky W. The formation and occurrence of polynuclear aromatic hydrocarbons associated with food. *Mutat Res* 1991;259:251.
59. Dingley KH, Curtis KD, Nowell S, et al. DNA and protein adduct formation in the colon and blood of humans after exposure to a dietary-relevant dose of 2-amino-1-methyl-6-phenylimidazo[4,5-*b*]pyridine. *Cancer Epidemiol Biomarkers Prev* 1999;8:507.
60. Rothman N, Correa-Villaseñor A, Ford DP, et al. Contribution of occupation and diet to white blood cell polycyclic aromatic hydrocarbon-DNA adducts in wildland firefighters. *Cancer Epidemiol Biomarkers Prev* 1993;2:341.
61. Ross JA, Nesnow S. Polycyclic aromatic hydrocarbons: correlations between DNA adducts and *ras* oncogene mutations. *Mutat Res* 1999;424:155.
62. Burczynski ME, Lin HK, Penning TM. Isoform-specific induction of a human aldo-keto reductase by polycyclic aromatic hydrocarbons (PAHs), electrophiles, and oxidative stress: implications for the alternative pathway of PAH activation catalyzed by human dihydrodiol dehydrogenase. *Cancer Res* 1999;59:607.
63. Hu X, Xia H, Srivastava SK, et al. Catalytic efficiencies of allelic variants of human glutathione *S*-transferase P1-1 toward carcinogenic *anti*-diol epoxides of benzo[*c*]phenanthrene and benzo[*g*]chrysene. *Cancer Res* 1998;58:5340.
64. Thorgeirsson UP, Dalgard DW, Reeves J, Adamson RH. Tumor incidence in a chemical carcinogenesis study of nonhuman primates. *Regul Toxicol Pharmacol* 1994;19:130.
65. Knekt P, Jarvinen R, Hakulinen T. Risk of colorectal and other gastro-intestinal cancers after exposure to nitrate, nitrite and *N*-nitroso compounds: a follow-up study. *Int J Cancer* 1999;80:852.
66. De Stefani E, Boffetta P, Mendilaharsu M, et al. Dietary nitrosamines, heterocyclic amines, and risk of gastric cancer: a case-control study in Uruguay. *Nutr Cancer* 1998;30:158.
67. Xu GP, Song PJ, Reed PI. Effects of fruit juices, processed vegetable juice, orange peel and green tea on endogenous formation of *N*-nitrosoproline in subjects from a high-risk area for gastric cancer in Moping County, China. *Eur J Cancer Prev* 1993;2:327.
68. Steinmetz KA, Potter JD. Vegetables, fruit, and cancer prevention: a review. *J Am Diet Assoc* 1996;96:1027.
69. World Cancer Research Fund. *Food, nutrition and the prevention of cancer: a global perspective.* Washington, DC: American Institute for Cancer Research, 1997.
70. Paulu C, Aschengrau A, Ozonoff D. Tetrochloroethylene-contaminated drinking water in Massachusetts and the risk of colon-rectum, lung, and other cancers. *Environ Health Perspect* 1999;107:265.
71. Boorman GA, Dellarco V, Dunnick JK, et al. Drinking water disinfection byproducts: review and approach to toxicity evaluation. *Environ Health Perspect* 1999;107:207.
72. Cantor KP. Drinking water and cancer. *Cancer Causes Control* 1997;8:292.
73. Wagstaff DJ. Dietary exposure to furocoumarins. *Regul Toxicol Pharmacol* 1991;14:261.
74. Tricker AR, Preussmann R. Carcinogenic *N*-nitrosamines in the diet: occurrence, formation, mechanisms and carcinogenic potential. *Mutat Res* 1991;259:277.
75. Stavric B. An update on research with coffee/caffeine (1989–1990). *Food Chem Toxicol* 1992;30:533.

MICHAEL J. THUN
CHARLES H. HENNEKENS

SECTION **6**

Aspirin and Other Nonsteroidal Antiinflammatory Drugs and the Risk of Cancer Development

Since the late 1970s, researchers have been interested in whether regular ingestion of aspirin or other nonsteroidal antiinflammatory drugs (NSAIDs) can decrease the risk of cancer, especially colorectal cancer.[1] This hypothesis was stimulated by basic research[2–5] and uncontrolled clinical observations[6] beginning in the mid-1970s. Further support derives from numerous observational epidemiologic studies[7–34] and mechanistic insights in the 1990s, and from several randomized clinical trials showing that the aspirin-like prodrug sulindac[35–38] and the novel selective cyclooxygenase-2 (COX-2) inhibitor celecoxib[39] suppress adenomatous polyps among patients with familial adenomatous polyposis (FAP). More recent data indicate that NSAIDs increase apoptosis,[40–43] inhibit angiogenesis,[44,45] and reduce metastasis in various experimental models of carcinogenesis.[46,47]

No randomized trials have been completed to test whether aspirin or other NSAIDs inhibit colorectal cancer. The Physician's Health Study, a randomized trial of aspirin designed to evaluate the primary prevention of cardiovascular end points,[48] found no reduction in colorectal cancer among male physicians randomized to 325 mg aspirin or placebo every other day for 5 years and followed for 12 years.[49] However, the short duration and low dose of randomized treatment limit the interpretability of this finding. At least five ongoing randomized clinical trials are testing whether nonselective NSAIDs, such as aspirin and sulindac, or novel selective inhibitors of inducible COX reduce the recurrence of adenomatous polyps among patients with previous sporadic polyps. Trials of intermediate end points in high-risk populations have the advantage of decreasing the necessary sample size and duration of treatment but have the disadvantage of not directly measuring the effect of NSAIDs on cancer.

This chapter reviews the experimental, clinical, epidemiologic, and randomized trial evidence relevant to NSAIDs and cancer, particularly colorectal cancer. We also consider the limited evidence available on lowest effective dose, treatment criteria, and the balance of potential benefits to risk of prolonged NSAID treatment. Although extensive evidence now indicates that NSAIDs inhibit neoplasia in several experimental settings and in the clinical context of FAP, we believe that aspirin and other NSAIDs are presently promising but unproven candidates for the chemoprevention of colorectal and perhaps other cancers in high-risk populations.

PHARMACOLOGY AND TOXICITY OF NONSTEROIDAL ANTIINFLAMMATORY DRUGS

NSAIDs are a chemically diverse group of drugs effective in the relief of pain, inflammation, and fever.[50] The analgesic, antiinflammatory, and antipyretic properties of salicylate in willow bark and other plant extracts were recognized in ancient Egypt and Greece.[51] NSAIDs also have dose-related toxicity to the gastrointestinal (GI) tract and kidney. The chemist Felix Hoffman was reportedly motivated to synthesize aspirin (acetylsalicylic acid) from sodium salicylate in the late nineteenth century because of the GI toxicity experienced by his father during treatment with salicylate for arthritis.[52] NSAIDs can also affect hemostasis, reproduction, childbirth, and asthma.[50] Efforts to minimize stomach irritation and to prolong the half-life of these drugs have motivated the development of many new NSAIDs in addition to aspirin.[53] Nonselective NSAIDs, such as ibuprofen, indomethacin, naproxen, piroxicam, and sulindac, now compete with novel, selective COX inhibitors that are reputed to lack major GI toxicity.[54]

The common pharmacologic action of NSAIDs is to inhibit COX, the initial and rate-limiting enzymatic step in the metabolism of arachidonic acid into a complex group of signaling proteins termed *prostaglandins*.[55–57] Arachidonic acid derives from meat or linoleic acid in the diet. It is normally tightly bound to cell membranes until being hydrolyzed by phospholipases as free arachidonic acid (arachidonate). Arachidonate can then be metabolized through COX pathways into prostaglandins and thromboxane; through lipoxygenase into leukotrienes and other lipid mediators; or by nonenzymatic pathways. Metabolites of arachidonic acid are called *eicosanoids*.

Prostaglandins and their derivatives modulate many functions within cells (autocrine) or across neighboring tissues (paracrine).[58] They differ from systemic hormones in that they are produced and destroyed almost instantaneously. Most tissues produce only a few prostaglandins in abundance. The function of the same prostaglandin may differ in different organs. Thromboxane-A_2 (TXA_2) produced by platelets enhances platelet aggregation, clot formation, and hemostasis; prostacyclin (prostaglandin I_2) from vascular endothelial cells enhances vasodilatation and prevents the aggregation of platelets. Prostaglandin E_2 (PGE_2) is a potent vasodilator in most vascular beds and also relaxes tracheobronchial and uterine muscle and protects gastric epithelium from acid. Prostaglandin G and prostaglandin D contract smooth muscle and modulate renal blood flow and sodium and water retention by the kidney.[58]

The diverse homeostatic and reactive functions of prostaglandins have prompted pharmacologists to seek drug and treatment regimens that improve NSAID specificity. One such strategy is to use low-dose aspirin (40 to 100 mg daily) to inhibit COX activity and TXA_2 production by platelets as they pass through the enterohepatic circulation.[59] Aspirin is the only NSAID that covalently acetylates and permanently inhibits COX. Platelets lack a nucleus and cannot synthesize new enzyme during their 7- to 10-day lifespan. At antiplatelet doses, virtually all of the absorbed aspirin is metabolized by the liver and does not reach the systemic circulation.

A second strategy is to develop new NSAIDs that selectively target a single isoform of the COX enzyme.[53] Until 1991, only one isoform of COX was recognized. Then a second isoform was identified[57] that increased in many tissues during inflammation, wound healing, and neoplasia.[60–64] These isoforms were named *COX-1* and *COX-2*, reflecting the sequence with which their structure was characterized by x-ray crystallography. The original enzyme, COX-1,[65] is expressed constitutively in most tissues of the body. It plays a central role in gastric cytoprotection and platelet aggregation and contributes to vascular dilatation, renal sodium and water balance, and other homeostatic functions.[66] The second isoform, COX-2,[67] has substantial sequence homology with COX-1[68] but is encoded by a different gene. COX-2 is not expressed under basal conditions in many tissues, but is up-regulated by inflammatory cytokines, growth factors, tumor promoters, and other physiologic stimuli.[54,69]

The paradigm that COX-2 is merely a "bad" enzyme that causes inflammatory and neoplastic processes, whereas COX-1 is a "good" enzyme essential for homeostasis now appears to be oversimplified.[54] COX-2 is expressed constitutively in the brain and kidney. It is known to be essential in ovulation and fertilization and implantation of the embryo, and it has as yet poorly understood homeostatic functions in the kidney, brain, cartilage, and bone.[66] The main distinction between the COX isoforms is that COX-1 is expressed constitutively in most tissues, whereas COX-2 is more often induced on demand.[66]

Most conventional NSAIDs inhibit both COX-1 and COX-2 with variable potency.[61,62] Aspirin is a relatively selective COX-1 inhibitor, except at antiinflammatory doses of 1 g/d or more. Novel selective COX-2 inhibitors have been introduced that cause GI symptoms but are thought not to cause serious GI ulceration.[70,71] Prototypes of these, such as celecoxib (SC-58635) and rofecoxib, are considerably more expensive than conventional NSAIDs. These drugs are proving informative in mechanistic studies to identify the enzymatic target(s) by which NSAIDs inhibit carcinogenesis in experimental models.

HISTORICAL EVOLUTION OF THE HYPOTHESIS THAT NONSTEROIDAL ANTIINFLAMMATORY DRUGS INHIBIT CANCER

EICOSANOIDS IN HUMAN TUMORS

The hypothesis that certain cancers might overproduce specific prostaglandins and thereby promote their own growth arose in the mid-1970s when Bennett and colleagues[3,4] observed higher concentrations of PGE_2 in some human colorectal carcinomas than in surrounding normal mucosa. Subsequent studies confirmed that certain human colon cancer cell lines[72] and tumor tissues[2,56,73] overproduce PGE_2. The idea that tumor prostaglandins might accelerate the growth and invasion of the cancer was further supported by the observation of Narisawa et al.[74] that PGE_2 in venous blood draining human colorectal carcinomas is higher in vivo when the cancers are large and locally invasive.

NONSTEROIDAL ANTIINFLAMMATORY DRUGS AND CHEMICALLY INDUCED CANCER IN RODENTS

Extensive experimental evidence confirms that many NSAIDs suppress tumor development in animal models and cell culture. More than 40 experiments in rodents show that aspirin, other nonaspirin NSAIDs, and selective COX-2 inhibitors suppress intestinal tumorigenesis in rats and mice exposed to chemical carcinogens.[39,47] Colorectal cancers produced in these rodent experiments[75–107] resemble human cancer, except for a lower tendency to metastasize.[108] Tumor inhibition is greatest when NSAID treatment is begun before exposure to the carcinogen and continued without interruption throughout the experiment.

UNCONTROLLED CLINICAL STUDIES OF SULINDAC IN PATIENTS WITH FAMILIAL ADENOMATOUS POLYPOSIS

The early rodent experiments prompted Waddell and Loughry[6] to test whether the prodrug sulindac inhibits adenomatous polyps in the rare hereditary condition of FAP. Adenomatous polyps are the precursor to most human colorectal cancers. Patients with FAP inherit a germline mutation inactivating one allele of the adenomatous polyposis coli (APC) gene. Loss of the remaining functional APC allele results in hundreds to thousands of adenomatous polyps by the second or third decade of life. Patients who do not undergo prophylactic colectomy almost invariably develop colorectal cancer by the age of 40 to 50 years.[109,110] FAP patients who have undergone total colectomy still have increased risk of adenomatous polyps; cancer of the rectal stump and small intestine; and nonmalignant, primitive desmoid tumors.

In FAP, sulindac reduces the number and size of new polyps and even causes existing polyps to regress. This finding has been reported in thirteen case studies[1] and in three small randomized crossover trials.[35,37,38] Sulindac also suppresses the formation of desmoid tumors in these reports. However, sulindac does not prevent all polyp growth in FAP patients, just as conventional NSAIDs do not inhibit all chemically induced colorectal cancer in the rodent model. Some polyps may grow during treatment[111] or be transformed into carcinoma.[112,113] Most adenomatous polyps typically increase in number and size after sulindac is discontinued.

EPIDEMIOLOGIC STUDIES OF NONSTEROIDAL ANTIINFLAMMATORY DRUGS IN THE GENERAL POPULATION

At least 25 observational epidemiologic studies have compared people who regularly use aspirin or other NSAIDs to those who do not with respect to colorectal cancer[7–34] (Tables 23.6-1 and 23.6-2) or colorectal adenomatous polyps.[16,18,23,31–34,114] All but one of the published studies finds 30% to 50% lower incidence or mortality rates from colorectal cancer (Fig. 23.6-1) or lower incidence of adenomatous polyps (Fig. 23.6-2). The consistency of these observational studies is striking, despite different researchers using varied study designs in different parts of the world. Interestingly, the single observational study that did not find reduced risk of colorectal cancer or adenomatous polyps among aspirin users also did not find reduced risk of myocardial infarction among the elderly subjects (median age of 70 years at enrollment) who reported taking one aspirin daily.[10,11]

Several observational studies report a dose-response gradient of decreasing risk of colorectal cancer or adenomatous polyps among individuals who report more prolonged[18,26,30,115] or frequent[12,20,23,30,114] NSAID use. Factors that influence self-selection for or against NSAID use could, in principle, confound this observation. Perhaps a more important limitation of the analyses by dose and duration is that none of the studies have simultaneously taken into account both aspirin and nonaspirin NSAIDs, prescription and nonprescription medications, and changes in the frequency or dose of NSAID use over time. Two large prospective studies[18,115] and one case-control study[30] found the largest reductions in colorectal cancer in persons who have used aspirin for at least 10 or even 20 years. Another large prospective

TABLE 23.6-1. Cohort Studies on the Use of Nonsteroidal Antiinflammatory Drugs and the Risk for Colorectal Cancer in General Populations

Reference	*Population*	*Study Size*	*End Point*	*Drug*	*Frequency*	*Results*[a]	*Comments*
Isomaki et al. (1978)[7]	Rheumatoid arthritis, Finland, 34,618 women and 11,483 men, 1967–1973	Women 33 cases 20 cases Men 11 cases 7 cases	Colon cancer Rectal cancer (incidence) Colon cancer Rectal cancer (incidence)	Therapy for arthritis	Heavy use	0.84 (NS) 0.58 (*P*<.05) 1.1 (NS) 0.64 (NS)	
Gridley et al. (1993)[8]	Rheumatoid arthritis, Sweden, 7933 women and 3750 men, 1965–1984	44 cases 28 cases	Colon cancer Rectal cancer (incidence)	Therapy for arthritis	Heavy use	0.63 (0.5–0.9) 0.72 (0.5–1.1)	Risk for stomach cancer also reduced
Paganini-Hill et al. (1989, 1991)[9,10]; Paganini-Hill (1995)[11]	U.S. retirement community, 13,987 elderly men and women, 1981–1987	181 cases	Colon cancer (incidence)	Aspirin	Daily	1.5 (1.1–2.2)	Median age, 73 y; no data on aspirin after baseline
Thun et al. (1991, 1992, 1994)[12–14]	American Cancer Society, 662,424 U.S. adults, 1982–1988	950 deaths 138 deaths	Colon cancer (mortality) Rectal cancer (mortality)	Aspirin Aspirin	≥16 times/mo	0.58 (0.45–0.74) 0.66 (0.37–1.20)	Multivariate estimates Multivariate estimates; no data on aspirin after baseline; decreased risk mostly confined to users of ≥10 y
Schreinemachers and Everson (1994)[15]	12,688 U.S. adults, 1971–1987	169 cases	Colorectal cancer (incidence)	Aspirin	Last 30 d	0.74 (0.4–1.1)	RR reduced under age 65
Giovannucci et al. (1994)[16]	Harvard Health Professionals, 47,900 U.S. men, 1986–1991	251 cases	Colorectal cancer (incidence)	Aspirin	≥2 tablets/wk	0.68 (0.52–0.92)	All cancers and metastatic or fatal cancers
Giovannucci et al. (1995)[18]	U.S. Nurses Health Study, 89,446 women, 1984–92	297 cases	Colorectal cancer (incidence)	Aspirin	≥2 tablets/wk ≥20 y	0.56 (0.36–0.90)	Risk decreased with duration but not with dose >2–4 mo

NS, not significant; RR, relative risk.
[a]In parentheses, 95% confidence level.

study based on prescription drug records in the United Kingdom between 1994 and 1997 found reduced risk of colorectal cancer in patients prescribed at least 300 mg aspirin daily compared to nonusers, but not among current users of less than 300 mg aspirin daily.[20] The U.K. study lacked information on long-term use of aspirin or other NSAIDs. It is important to define the lowest effective dose and optimal duration, because the GI toxicity of NSAIDs increase with dose, and risk accumulates with duration. The use of antiplatelet doses of aspirin (100 mg or less) to prevent cardiovascular events did not begin until the late 1980s and

TABLE 23.6-2. Case-Control Studies on the Use of Nonsteroidal Antiinflammatory Drugs (NSAIDs) and the Risk for Colorectal Cancer in the General Population

Reference	*Population*	*Study Size*	*End Point*	*Drug*	*Frequency*	*Results (RR)*[a]	*Comments*
Kune et al. (1988)[21]	Population-based, Melbourne, Australia, 1980–1981	715 cases 727 controls	Colorectal cancer (incidence)	Aspirin	Not stated	0.60 (0.44–0.82) 0.77 (0.60–1.01)	Adjusted for diet
				NSAIDs	Not stated		Not adjusted for aspirin use
Rosenberg et al. (1991)[22]	Hospital-based, four cities in eastern United States, 1977–88	1326 cases 4891 controls	Colorectal cancer (incidence)	Mostly aspirin	≥4 d/wk ≥3 mo	0.5 (0.4–0.8)	Trend with duration NS; risk increased after cessation
Suh et al. (1993)[23]	Hospital-based, Roswell Park Cancer Institute (Buffalo, New York), 1982–1991	830 cases 1138 clinic controls 524 hospital controls	Colorectal cancer (incidence)	Aspirin	≥1 per day in 4 y before study	0.24 (0.12–0.50)	Men
						0.54 (0.26–1.10)	Women
Peleg et al. (1994)[24]	Hospital-based, Atlanta, 1988–1990	97 cases 388 controls	Colorectal cancer (incidence)	Aspirin and nonaspirin	Used aspirin >624 d in 4 y before study	0.08 (0.01–0.59)	Urban poor
					Used NSAIDs >313 d in 4 y before study	0.25 (0.09–0.73)	
Muscat et al. (1994)[26]	Hospital-based, American Health Foundation, 1989–1992	511 cases 500 controls	Colorectal cancer (incidence)	NSAIDs	≥3 times/wk for ≥1 y	0.64 (0.42–0.97)	Men
						0.32 (0.18–0.57)	Women
Muller et al. (1994)[25]	Hospital-based, U.S. veterans, 1988–1992	12,304 cases 49,216 controls	Colon cancer (incidence)	NSAIDs	Not stated	0.52–0.91	Range of RR estimates comparing patients with six conditions treated with aspirin to those treated with anticoagulants
Reeves et al. (1996)[27]	Population-based, women in Wisconsin, 1991–1992	184 cases 293 controls	Colorectal cancer (incidence)	Aspirin and nonaspirin	≥1 tablet at least twice week for ≥1 y	0.65 (0.40–1.00)	Nonaspirin NSAIDs more strongly associated than aspirin
Bansal and Sonnenberg (1996)[28]	Hospital-based, U.S. veterans, 1981–1993	371 cases (with IBD) 11,075 controls	Colorectal cancer (incidence) (mortality)	NSAIDs	Not stated	0.84 (0.65–1.08)	Controls have IBD but not colon cancer
		52,243 controls				0.68 (0.65–0.72)	Controls have colon cancer but not IBD
Collet et al. (1999)[30]	Saskatchewan Prescription Drug Plan	3844 cases 15,373 controls	Colon cancer (incidence)	NSAIDs, prescription	≥30% maximum dose	0.57 (0.36–0.89)	
		1971 cases 7882 controls	Rectal cancer (incidence)			0.26 (0.11–0.61)	

IBD, inflammatory bowel disease; NS, not significant; RR, relative risk.
[a]In parentheses, 95% confidence level.

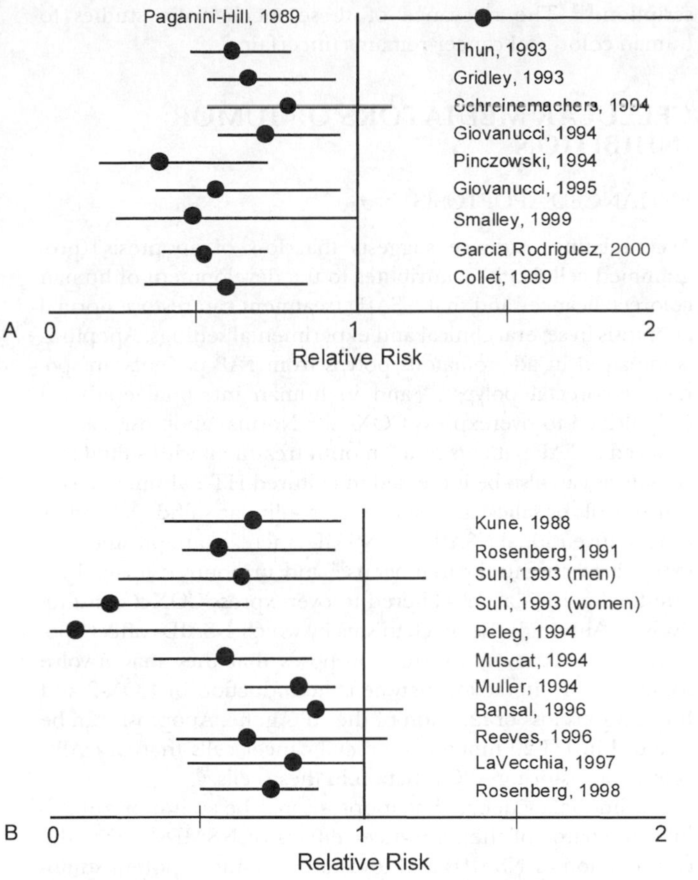

FIGURE 23.6-1. Epidemiologic studies of nonsteroidal antiinflammatory drugs and colorectal cancer. **A:** Prospective cohort trials. **B:** Retrospective case-control trials.

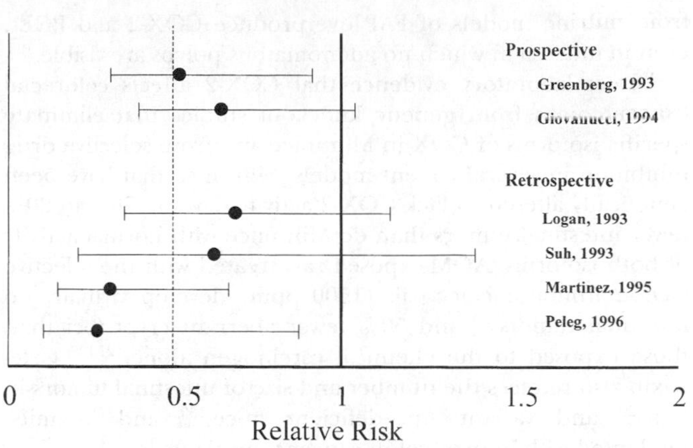

FIGURE 23.6-2. Epidemiologic studies of nonsteroidal antiinflammatory drugs and adenomatous polyps.

cannot yet be evaluated with respect to colorectal cancer. However, even antiplatelet doses of aspirin (80 to 100 mg/d) causes some increase in GI[116] and intracerebral bleeding,[117] especially with prolonged treatment of large numbers of healthy people. If NSAIDs are proven to be effective in preventing colorectal cancer in the future, it is likely that long-term prophylaxis could produce a net benefit only in persons with substantially increased risk of colorectal cancer, or because of a combination of other factors that may affect individual risk and benefit.[118]

COMPLETED AND ONGOING RANDOMIZED TRIALS

Several randomized clinical trials show that sulindac[35–38] and the novel selective COX-2 inhibitor celecoxib[39] reduce the number and size of adenomatous polyps in FAP patients and causes existing polyps to regress. Only one randomized clinical trial of aspirin in the primary prevention of cardiovascular end points has been sufficiently large to measure incidence or death rates from colorectal cancer, although the aspirin arm of this trial was terminated after 5 years. The Physicians' Health Study showed no reduction in either invasive or *in situ* colorectal cancer incidence, nor a reduction in colorectal cancer mortality among 22,071 male physicians randomized to 325 mg aspirin or placebo every other day for 5 years and followed for 12 years.[48] The short duration of randomized treatment and relatively low dose of aspirin limit the interpretability of these results.

Several randomized clinical trials are now testing whether aspirin or other NSAIDs inhibit adenomatous polyps among patients with previous sporadic polyps or FAP. Trials of intermediate end points in high-risk populations have the advantage of decreasing the necessary sample size and duration of treatment, but have the disadvantage of not directly measuring the effect of NSAIDs on cancer.

STUDIES OF MECHANISM

Debate is ongoing over the mechanisms by which NSAIDs inhibit carcinogenesis in various experimental and clinical models. This debate is further complicated in that NSAIDs may affect several stages in the adenoma-carcinoma sequence, perhaps by different mechanisms. Most evidence suggests that COX, particularly the inducible COX-2 isoform, is probably the major enzymatic target by which NSAIDs inhibit cancer in various models. Effects mediated through COX could explain why numerous NSAIDs with diverse chemical structures all inhibit COX activity and nearly all suppress colorectal carcinogenesis. There is also debate about which cellular targets and functions may be most relevant to NSAID tumor inhibition in humans.

Studies Implicating Cyclooxygenase-2

Circumstantial evidence that the inducible isoform of COX contributes to colorectal neoplasia is that COX-2 is up-regulated as normal intestinal mucosa progresses to invasive colorectal cancer in humans.[47] COX-2 protein and messenger RNA are undetectable in normal colonic mucosa, yet are present in approximately 40% of human adenomatous polyps[119] and more than 80% of colorectal cancers.[119–121] COX-1, in contrast, is expressed at constant basal levels in all of these tissues. COX-2 is expressed constitutively by at least one human colon cancer cell line (HT-116) and can be induced in four other human tumor cell lines by exogenous agonists.[122] COX-2 concentration in human colorectal carcinomas has been reported to increase with larger tumor size and deeper invasion, although not with evidence of metastases.[123] In rodent models, COX-2 expression is up-regulated after exposure of rats to azoxymethane (AOM).[124] COX-2 is also expressed at an early stage in APC^{min} and $APC^{\Delta}716$ mice.[125] Intestinal cells from murine models of FAP overproduce COX-2 and PGE_2, even in mucosa in which no adenomatous polyps are visible.[126]

Direct laboratory evidence that COX-2 affects colorectal cancer comes from genetic knockout studies that eliminate specific isoforms of COX in Min mice and from selective drug inhibition in several rodent models. Min mice that have been genetically altered to lack COX-2 activity develop 70% to 80% fewer intestinal tumors than do Min mice with normal activity of both isoforms. AOM-exposed rats treated with the selective COX-2 inhibitor celecoxib (1500 ppm) develop virtually no intestinal tumors[102] and 50% fewer aberrant crypt foci than those exposed to the chemical carcinogen alone.[127,128] Celecoxib also reduces the number and size of intestinal tumors in Min[129] and variant Apc–deficient mice,[130] and in mice implanted with human colon cancer transplants.[131]

Studies Implicating Cyclooxygenase-1

More limited experimental and epidemiologic evidence suggests that COX-1 activity may also contribute to the development of colorectal and other cancers.[132] Homozygous inactivation of either COX-1 or COX-2 produces an equivalent 70% to 80% reduction in intestinal tumors compared to Min mice with both COX isoforms intact.[132] No experimental studies have tested selective COX-1 inhibitors in various rodent models of carcinogenesis. However, participants in several epidemiologic studies who report taking 365 mg of aspirin daily experience fewer adenomatous polyps or colorectal cancers than those who do not take NSAIDs.[18,20] Aspirin is predominantly a COX-1 inhibitor at this dosage. Epidemiologic studies cannot yet assess whether prolonged use of aspirin at doses of 100 mg or less is also associated with reduced incidence of colorectal cancer or adenomatous polyps. Clinical studies report that people given low-dose aspirin (80 mg) for up to 3 months,[133,134] or 325 mg daily for 60 days,[135] have lower concentrations of PGE_2 and $PGF_{2\alpha}$ in rectal mucosa than were present in biopsy specimens taken before aspirin administration. These studies are limited in interpretability, however, in that rectal epithelial specimens are likely to have been contaminated by platelets, possibly accounting for the observed changes in eicosanoid levels.

Evidence for Noncyclooxygenase Mechanisms

Some research suggests that NSAIDs may inhibit neoplasia through pathways other than COX or that a mix of prostaglandin-independent and -dependent mechanisms may exist.[1] Sulindac sulfone, the sulfone metabolite of sulindac, is believed to have little inhibitory activity against COX,[136,137] yet high oral concentrations (1000 and 2000 ppm in food) inhibit intestinal tumors[106,107] and aberrant crypt formation[138] in AOM-exposed rats, and inhibit chemically induced mammary cancer in mice.[139] In one of these studies,[107] no suppression was found in PGE_2 or the activity of COX, lipoxygenase, and phospholipase A_2. In other studies, supraphysiologic concentrations of sulindac sulfone in cell culture inhibit the growth of human HT-29 tumor cells,[140] as well as other human cell lines that do not express COX or produce prostaglandins.[41,141] NSAIDs also have been postulated to inhibit colorectal cancer by influencing nitric oxide metabolism[142] or binding with the peroxisome proliferator–activated receptor δ (PPAR δ).[143] The latter is postulated to be a common target by which NSAIDs can mimic the effects of the APC gene and down-regulate transcription.[143] The relevance of these mechanistic studies to human colorectal cancer remains uncertain.

CELLULAR MEDIATORS OF TUMOR INHIBITION

ENHANCED APOPTOSIS

Accumulating evidence suggests that loss of apoptosis (programmed cell death) contributes to the development of human colorectal cancer and that NSAID treatment can restore normal apoptosis in several clinical and experimental settings. Apoptosis is impaired in adenomatous polyps from FAP patients, in sporadic colorectal polyps,[144] and in human intestinal epithelial cells altered to overexpress COX-2.[145] Normal apoptosis can be restored in FAP patients by a 3-month treatment with sulindac.[40] Apoptosis can also be increased in cultured HT-29 human colon cancer cells by salicylate,[41] sulindac or sulindac sulfide,[146] and by other conventional NSAIDs.[146] NSAIDs increase apoptosis in rats exposed to chemical carcinogens[42] and in nontransformed rat intestinal epithelial cells altered to overexpress COX-2 constitutively.[145] Although the mechanisms by which NSAIDs affect apoptosis are unknown, Taketo[47] proposes that they may involve some critical interaction between the induction of COX-2 and homozygous loss of function of the APC gene. Apoptosis can be induced in HT-29 human colorectal cancer cells that lack APC activity by restoring APC function in these cells.[43]

Additional evidence that apoptosis may be an important cellular mediator of the anticancer effects of NSAIDs is that the combination of NSAIDs and lovastatin is a more potent stimulus for apoptosis, experimentally, than either agent alone.[147] Lovastatin is a cholesterol-reducing hepatic 3-hydroxy-3-methylglutaryl coenzyme A (HMG-CoA) reductase inhibitor. The combination of lovastatin and sulindac amplifies several-fold the stimulatory effect of sulindac alone on apoptosis in three human colon cancer cell lines (HCT-116, SW 480, and LoVo) and in AOM-exposed rodents.[147] Agarwal et al.[147] suggest that combining NSAIDs with an HMG-CoA reductase inhibitor may increase the effectiveness of chemoprevention or allow the use of lower, less toxic doses of NSAID.

Furthermore, experimental evidence suggests that NSAIDs cause cell-cycle arrest and accumulation of cells in the G_0/G_1 phase, potentially contributing to enhancement of apoptosis.[41,146] Indomethacin has long been known to induce reversible cell-cycle arrest in the G_1 phase in cultured, transformed rat hepatoma and nontransformed human fibroblast cells.[148,149] NSAIDs such as sulindac and sulindac sulfide also reduce the level and activity of several cyclin-dependent kinases that regulate cell-cycle progression and induction of apoptotic cell death in human HT-29 colon cancer cells.[146] These effects on cell-cycle progression require concentrations of salicylate between 1 and 5 mmol/L[41]; thus, the extent to which these effects are relevant to human colon cancer remains unclear.

INHIBITION OF ANGIOGENESIS

Another cellular function by which NSAIDs may inhibit cancer involves the suppression of angiogenesis and neovascularization.[44,45] A selective COX-2 inhibitor (NS-398) suppresses production of angiogenic factors such as vascular endothelial growth factor, basic fibroblast growth factor, transforming growth factor-β, platelet-derived growth factor, and endothelin-1 by human cul-

TABLE 23.6-3. Cohort Studies of Use of Nonsteroidal Antiinflammatory Drugs and Risks for Esophageal and Gastric Cancers[a]

Reference	*Population*	*Study Size*	*End Point*	*Drug*	*Frequency*	*Results (RR)*[b]	*Comments*
Isomaki et al. (1978)[7]	Rheumatoid arthritis, Finland, 34,618 women and 11,483 men, 1967–1973	5 cases	Esophageal cancer	Therapy for arthritis	Heavy use	0.67 (NS)	
		51 cases	Gastric cancer (incidence)			1.1 (NS)	
Gridley et al. (1993)[8]	Rheumatoid arthritis, Sweden, 8787 women and 3750 men, 1965–1984	11 cases	Esophageal cancer	Therapy for arthritis	Heavy use	1.3 (0.7–2.4)	
		39 cases	Gastric cancer (incidence)			0.63 (0.5–0.9)	
Thun et al. (1993)[13]	American Cancer Society, 635,031 U.S. adults, 1982–1988	176 deaths	Esophageal cancer (fatal)	Aspirin	≥16 times/mo	0.78 (0.42–1.40)	Multivariate estimates
		308 deaths	Gastric cancer (fatal)	Aspirin		0.49 (0.22-1.12)	No data on aspirin after baseline; decreased risk mostly confined to users of ≥10 y
Schreinemachers and Everson (1994)[15]	12,688 U.S. adults, 1971–1987	20 cases	Gastric cancer (incidence)	Aspirin	Last 30 d	0.93 (0.49–1.70)	
Funkhouser and Sharp (1995)[160]	12,688 U.S. adults, 1971–1987	15 cases	Esophageal cancer	Aspirin	Last 30 d	0.10 (0.01–0.76)	Multivariate estimate, also for alcohol use and smoking

NS, not significant; RR, relative risk.
[a]Modified from International Agency for Research on Cancer.
[b]In parentheses, 95% confidence level.

tured colon cancer cells that express COX-2. COX-2 expression greatly increases the production of angiogenic factors by these cells. In the same experiment, aspirin at concentrations thought to inhibit COX-1 selectively suppressed endothelial tube formation by human umbilical endothelial cells exposed to these growth factors. The inhibitory effect of NSAIDs on angiogenesis may involve several mechanisms, such as a COX-2 pathway that affects the production of angiogenic factors by tumor cells and a COX-1 pathway involving the endothelial cell response.

EFFECTS ON METASTASIS

Relatively little research has examined the effect of NSAIDs on cancer metastases, although this area of experimental research has been active. Also limited has been research on the potential of aspirin or other NSAIDs as adjuvant therapy in treating cancers. A small randomized clinical trial found no improvement in the survival of 66 patients with Duke's class B2 or C invasive colorectal cancer with aspirin treatment of 600 mg twice daily.[150]

NONSTEROIDAL ANTIINFLAMMATORY DRUGS AND CANCERS OTHER THAN COLORECTAL CANCER

A few studies have examined the relationship between the use of aspirin and other NSAIDs and the digestive tract cancers other than that of the large intestine. Table 23.6-3 lists the studies pertaining to cancers of the esophagus and stomach. In the American Cancer Society study, aspirin use was inversely associated with fatal cancers of the esophagus and stomach as well as colon and rectum, but not generally with fatal cancers outside the GI tract.[13] The limited evidence that NSAIDs may inhibit cancers throughout the digestive tract is interesting in light of the common embryologic derivation of GI tissues[47] and observations that COX-2 is also prominently expressed in cancers of the esophagus[151,152] and stomach.[153,154]

The results of nonrandomized studies relating breast cancer to NSAID use have been less consistent, with two case-control studies reporting some reduction in risk, but other large prospective studies finding no association (Fig. 23.6-3). Extensive evidence indicates that eicosanoids affect several aspects of carcinogenesis in mouse models of mammary carcinoma[155] and that both COX-1 and COX-2 are moderately up-regulated in some human breast tumors.[156] However, the current evidence that NSAIDs may be useful in the prevention or treatment of breast cancer in humans is limited.

DOSE AND DURATION ISSUES IN CHEMOPREVENTION

Because the GI toxicity of NSAIDs is dose-dependent, at least two strategies have emerged for minimizing the toxicity of NSAID treatment while maintaining therapeutic effectiveness. One has been the development of "designer" drugs, such as

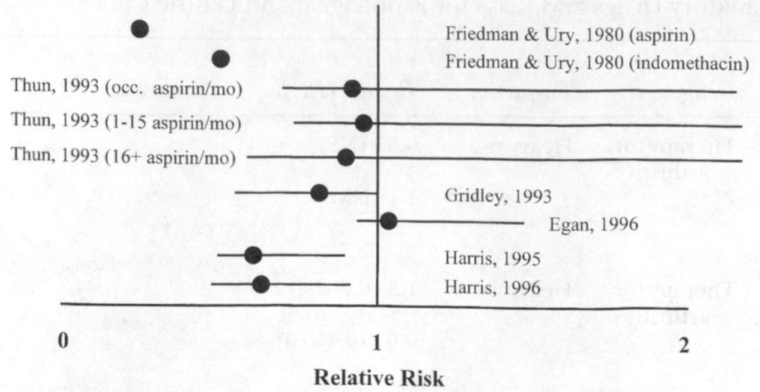

FIGURE 23.6-3. Epidemiologic studies of nonsteroidal antiinflammatory drugs and breast cancer. occ., occasional.

the novel selective COX-2 inhibitors that are thought to be less ulcerogenic than conventional NSAIDs. A second approach, used effectively in preventing cardiovascular disease with aspirin, has been to identify a sufficiently low dose of NSAID that is effective therapeutically yet has minimal GI toxicity. Antiplatelet doses not exceeding 100 mg aspirin daily have the largest absolute benefit in populations at high risk of cardiovascular events, because the large, immediate reduction in cardiovascular risk far outweighs the small increase in GI bleeding that occurs even with low-dose aspirin.

With respect to the chemoprevention of colon cancer, researchers have not yet identified the lowest effective dose or optimal NSAID treatment regimen. Resolving these uncertainties becomes critically important when large numbers of people might consider taking a chemopreventive drug for several decades. In this context, the balance of cumulative benefit to risk is highly susceptible to the lowest effective dose of the drug, the toxicity at this dosage, the probability of serious adverse effects in a particular individual,[154] and the probability of the event being prevented. None of these clinical questions has yet been adequately answered with respect to NSAIDs and colorectal or other cancers.

REFERENCES

1. International Agency for Research on Cancer. Non-steroidal anti-inflammatory drugs. *IARC Handbooks of Cancer Prevention*, vol 1. Lyon, France: IARC Press, 1997.
2. Jaffe BM. Prostaglandins and cancer: an update. *Prostaglandins* 1974;6:453.
3. Bennett A, del Tacca M. Proceedings: prostaglandins in human colonic carcinoma. *Gut* 1975;16:409.
4. Bennett A, Tacca MD, Stamford IF, Zebro T. Prostaglandins from tumors of human large bowel. *Br J Cancer* 1977;35:881.
5. Bennett A, Civier A, Hensby CN, et al. Measurement of arachidonate and its metabolites extracted from human normal and malignant gastrointestinal tissues. *Gut* 1987;28:315.
6. Waddell WR, Loughry RW. Sulindac for polyposis of the colon. *J Surg Oncol* 1983;24:83.
7. Isomaki HA, Hakulinen T, Joutsenlahti U. Excess risk of lymphomas, leukemia and myeloma in patients with rheumatoid arthritis. *J Chronic Dis* 1978;31:691.
8. Gridley G, McLaughlin JK, Ekbom A. Incidence of cancer among patients with rheumatoid arthritis. *J Natl Cancer Inst* 1993;85:307.
9. Paganini-Hill A, Chao A, Ross RK, Henderson BE. Aspirin use and chronic diseases: a cohort study of the elderly. *BMJ* 1989;299:1247.
10. Paganini-Hill A, Hsu G, Ross RK, Henderson BE. Aspirin use and incidence of large-bowel cancer in a California retirement community [Letter]. *J Natl Cancer Inst* 1991;83:1182.
11. Paganini-Hill A. Aspirin and colorectal cancer. The Leisure World cohort revisited. *Prev Med* 1995;24:113.
12. Thun MJ, Namboodiri MM, Heath CW Jr. Aspirin use and reduced risk of fatal colon cancer. *N Engl J Med* 1991;325:1593.
13. Thun MJ, Namboodiri MM, Calle EE, Flanders WD, Heath CW Jr. Aspirin use and risk of fatal cancer. *Cancer Res* 1993;53:1322.
14. Thun MJ. Aspirin, NSAIDs, and digestive tract cancers. *Cancer Metastasis Rev* 1994;13:269.
15. Schreinemachers DM, Everson RB. Aspirin use and lung, colon, and breast cancer incidence in a prospective study. *Epidemiology* 1994;5:138.
16. Giovannucci E, Rimm EB, Stampfer MJ, et al. Aspirin use and the risk for colorectal cancer and adenoma in male health professionals. *Ann Intern Med* 1994;121:241.
17. Giovannucci E, Willett WC. Dietary factors and risk of colon cancer. *Ann Intern Med* 1994;26:443.
18. Giovannucci E, Egan KM, Hunter DJ, et al. Aspirin and the risk of colorectal cancer in women. *N Engl J Med* 1995;333:609.
19. Giovannucci E, Rimm EB, Ascherio A, et al. Alcohol, low-methionine and low-folate diets, and risk of colon cancer in men. *J Natl Cancer Inst* 1995;87:265.
20. Garcia Rodriguez LA, Huerta-Alvarez C. Reduced risk of colorectal cancer among long-term users of aspirin and non-aspirin nonsteroidal anti-inflammatory drugs: a pooled analysis of epidemiologic studies and a new population based study. *JAMA* 1999 (*in press*).
21. Kune GA, Kune S, Watson LF. Colorectal cancer risk, chronic illnesses, operations, and medications: case control results from the Melbourne Colorectal Cancer Study. *Cancer Res* 1988;48:4399.
22. Rosenberg L, Palmer JR, Zauber AG, et al. A hypothesis: nonsteroidal anti-inflammatory drugs reduce the incidence of large-bowel cancer. *J Natl Cancer Inst* 1991;83:355.
23. Suh O, Mettlin C, Petrelli NJ. Aspirin use, cancer, and polyps of the large bowel. *Cancer* 1993;72:1171.
24. Peleg II, Maibach HT, Brown SH, Wilcox CM. Aspirin and nonsteroidal anti-inflammatory drug use and the risk of subsequent colorectal cancer. *Arch Intern Med* 1994;154:394.
25. Muller AD, Sonneberg A, Wasserman IH. Diseases preceding colon cancer: a case-control study among veterans. *Dig Dis Sci* 1994;39:2480.
26. Muscat JE, Stellman SD, Wynder EL. Nonsteroidal antiinflammatory drugs and colorectal cancer. *Cancer* 1994;74:1847.
27. Reeves MJ, Newcomb PA, Trentham-Diez A, Storer BE, Remington PL. Nonsteroidal anti-inflammatory drug use and protection against colorectal cancer in women. *Cancer Epidemiol Biomarkers Prev* 1996;5:955.
28. Bansal P, Sonnenberg A. Risk factors of colorectal cancer in inflammatory bowel disease. *Am J Gastroenterol* 1996;91:44.
29. Coogan PF, Rosenberg L, Louik C, et al. NSAIDs and risk of colorectal cancer according to presence or absence of family history of the disease. *Cancer Causes Control* 2000;11:249.
30. Collet JP, Sharpe C, Belzile E, et al. Colorectal cancer prevention by non-steroidal anti-inflammatory drugs: effects of dosage and timing. *Br J Cancer* 1999;81:62.
31. Greenberg ER, Baron JA, Freeman DH Jr, Mandel JS, Haile R. Reduced risk of large-bowel adenomas among aspirin users. *J Natl Cancer Inst* 1993;85:912.
32. Logan RFA, Little J, Hawtin PG, Hardcastle JD. Effect of aspirin and non-steroidal anti-inflammatory drugs on colorectal adenomas: case-control study of subjects participating in the Nottingham faecal occult blood screening programme. *BMJ* 1993;307:285.
33. Martinez ME, McPherson RS, Levin B, Annegers JF. Aspirin and other nonsteroidal anti-inflammatory drugs and risk of colorectal adenomatous polyps among endoscoped individuals. *Cancer Epidemiol Biomarkers Prev* 1995;4:703.
34. Garcia Rodriguez LA, Huerta-Alvarez C. Reduced incidence of colorectal adenoma among long-term users of nonsteroidal anti-inflammatory drugs: a pooled analysis of published studies and a new population based study. *Epidemiology* 2000;11:376.
35. Labayle D, Fischer D, Vielh P, et al. Sulindac causes regression of rectal polyps in familial adenomatous polyposis. *Gastroenterology* 1991;101:635.
36. Rigau J, Pique JM, Rubio E, Tarrech JM, Bordas JM. Effects of long-term sulindac therapy on colonic polyposis. *Ann Intern Med* 1991;115:952.
37. Giardiello FM, Hamilton SR, Krush AJ, et al. Treatment of colonic and rectal adenomas with sulindac in familial adenomatous polyposis. *N Engl J Med* 1993;328:1313.
38. Nugent KP, Farmer KC, Spigelman AD, Williams CB, Phillips RK. Randomized controlled trial of the effect of sulindac on duodenal and rectal polyposis and cell proliferation in patients with familial adenomatous polyposis. *Br J Surg* 1993;80:1618.
39. *New drug approvals—Celebrex.* U.S. Food and Drug Administration Center for Drug Evaluation and Research. World Wide Web URL: http://www.fda.gov/cder/foi/label/1999/21156lbl.pdf, 1999.
40. Pasricha PJ, Bedi A, O'Connor K, et al. The effects of sulindac on colorectal proliferation and apoptosis in familial adenomatous polyposis. *Gastroenterology* 1995;109:994.
41. Elder DJ, Hague A, Hicks DJ, Paraskeva C. Differential growth inhibition by the aspirin metabolite salicylate in human colorectal tumor cell lines: enhanced apoptosis in carcinoma and *in vitro*-transformed adenoma relative to adenoma cell lines. *Cancer Res* 1996;56:2273.
42. Samaha HS, Kelloff GJ, Steele V, Rao CV, Reddy BS. Modulation of apoptosis by sulindac, curcumin, phenylethyl-3-methylcaffeate, and 6-phenylhexyl isothiocyanate: apoptotic index as a biomarker in colon cancer chemoprevention and promotion. *Cancer Res* 1997;57:1301.
43. Morin PJ, Vogelstein B, Kinzler KW. Apoptosis and APC in colorectal tumorigenesis. *Proc Natl Acad Sci U S A* 1996;93:7950.
44. Tsujii M, Kawano S, Tsuji S, Hori M, DuBois R. Cyclooxygenase regulates angiogenesis induced by colon cancer cells. *Cell* 1998;93:705.
45. Jones MK, Wang H, Peskar BM, et al. Inhibition of angiogenesis by nonsteroidal anti-inflammatory drugs: insights into mechanisms and implications for cancer growth and ulcer healing. *Nat Med* 1999;5:1418.
46. Taketo M. Cyclooxygenase-2 inhibitors in tumorigenesis (part I). *J Natl Cancer Inst* 1998;90:1529.
47. Taketo M. Cyclooxygenase-2 inhibitors in tumorigenesis (part II). *J Natl Cancer Inst* 1998;90:1609.
48. Steering Committee of the Physicians' Health Study Research Group. Final report on the aspirin component of the ongoing Physicians' Health Study. *N Engl J Med* 1989;321:129.

49. Sturmer T, Glynn RJ, Lee IM, Buring JE, Hennekens CH. Aspirin use and colorectal cancer: post-trial follow-up data from the Physicians' Health Study. *Ann Intern Med* 1998;128:713.
50. Insel PA. Analgesic-antipyretics and antiinflammatory agents; drugs employed in the treatment of rheumatoid arthritis and gout. In: Goodman L, Gilman A, eds. *Pharmacological basis of therapeutics.* London: Macmillian Co, 1995:638.
51. Vane JR, Flower RJ, Botting RM. History of aspirin and its mechanism of action. *Stroke* 1990;21[suppl 4]:12.
52. Jack DB. One hundred years of aspirin. *Lancet* 1997;350:437.
53. Vane J. Pharmacology: towards a better aspirin. *Nature* 1994;367:215.
54. Hawkey CJ. Cox-2 inhibitors. *Lancet* 1999;353:307.
55. Vane JR. Inhibition of prostaglandin synthesis as a mechanism of action for aspirin-like drugs. *Nat New Biol* 1971;231:232.
56. Marnett LJ. Aspirin and the potential role of prostaglandins in colon cancer. *Cancer Res* 1992;52:5575.
57. Smith WL, Garavito RM, DeWitt DL. Prostaglandin endoperoxide H synthases (cyclooxygenases)-1 and -2. *J Biol Chem* 1996;271:33157.
58. Campbell WB. Lipid-derived autacoids: eicosanoids and platelet-activating factor. In: Goodman L, Gilman A, eds. *Pharmacological basis of therapeutics.* London: Macmillan Co, 1995:600.
59. Patrono C. Aspirin as an antiplatelet drug. *N Engl J Med* 1994;330:1287.
60. Xie W, Robertson DL, Simmons DL. Mitogen-inducible prostaglandin G/H synthase: a new target for nonsteroidal antiinflammatory drugs. *Drug Dev Res* 1992;25:249.
61. Meade EA, Smith WL, DeWitt DL. Differential inhibition of prostaglandin endoperoxide synthase (cyclooxygenase) isozymes by aspirin and other non-steroidal anti-inflammatory drugs. *J Biol Chem* 1993;268:6610.
62. Mitchell JA, Akarasereenont P, Thiemermann C, Flower RJ, Vane JR. Selectivity of nonsteroidal antiinflammatory drugs as inhibitors of constitutive and inducible cyclooxygenase. *Proc Natl Acad Sci U S A* 1993;90:11693.
63. Masferrer JL, Isakson PC, Seibert K. Cyclooxygenase-2 inhibitors: a new class of anti-inflammatory agents that spare the gastrointestinal tract. *Gastroenterology Clin North Am* 1996;25:363.
64. Chan CC, Boyce S, Brideau C, et al. Pharmacology of a selective cyclooxgenase-2 inhibitor, L-745,337: a novel nonsteroidal anti-inflammatory agent with an ulcerogenic sparing effect in rat and nonhuman primate stomach. *J Pharmacol Exp Ther* 1995;274:1531.
65. Picot D, Loll PJ, Garavito RM. The x-ray crystal structure of the membrane protein prostaglandin H2 synthase-1. *Nature* 1994;367:243.
66. Lipsky PE, Abramson SB, Crofford SB, et al. The classification of cyclooxygenase inhibitors. *J Rheumatol* 1998;25:2298.
67. Luong C, Miller A, Barnett J, et al. The structure of human cylooxygenase-2; conservation and flexibility of the NSAID binding site. *Nat Struct Biol* 1996;3:927.
68. Kujubu DA, Fletcher BS, Varnum BC, Lim RW, Herschman HR. TIS10, a phorbol ester tumor promoter–inducible mRNA from Swiss 3T3 cells, encodes a novel prostaglandin synthase/cyclooxygenase homologue. *J Biol Chem* 1991;266:12866.
69. Smalley WE, DuBois RN. Colorectal cancer and nonsteroidal anti-inflammatory drugs. *Adv Pharmacol* 1997;39:1.
70. Lanza FL, Rack MF, Callison DA, et al. A pilot endoscopic study of the gastroduodenal effect of SC-58635, a novel COX-2-selective inhibitor. *Gastroenterology* 1997;112[suppl 4]:A194.
71. Kalgutkar AS, Crews BC, Rowlinson SW, et al. Aspirin-like molecules that covalently inactivate cyclooxygenase-2. *Science* 1998;280:1268.
72. Hubbard WC, Alley MC, McLemore TL, et al. Profiles of prostaglandin biosynthesis in sixteen established cell lines derived from human lung, colon, prostate and ovarian tumors. *Cancer Res* 1988;48:4770.
73. Rigas B, Goldman IS, Levine L. Altered eicosanoid levels in human colon cancer. *J Lab Clin Med* 1993;122:518.
74. Narisawa T, Kusaka H, Yamazaki Y, et al. Relationship between blood plasma prostaglandin E_2 and liver and lung metastases in colorectal cancer. *Dis Colon Rectum* 1990;33:840.
75. Pollard M, Luckert PH. Indomethacin treatment of rats with dimethylhydrazine-induced intestinal tumors. *Cancer Treat Rep* 1980;64:1323.
76. Pollard M, Luckert PH. Effect of indomethacin on intestinal tumors induced in rats by the acetate derivative of dimethylnitrosoamine. *Science* 1981;214:558.
77. Pollard M, Luckert PH. Treatment of chemically-induced intestinal cancers with indomethacin. *Proc Soc Exp Biol Med* 1981;167:161.
78. Pollard M, Luckert PH. Prolonged antitumor effect of indomethacin on autochthonous intestinal tumors in rats. *J Natl Cancer Inst* 1983;70:1103.
79. Pollard M, Luckert PH, Schmidt MA. The suppressive effect of piroxicam on autochthonous intestinal tumors in the rat. *Cancer Lett* 1983;21:57.
80. Pollard M, Luckert PH. Effect of piroxicam on primary intestinal tumors induced in rats by N-methylnitrosourea. *Cancer Lett* 1984;25:117.
81. Pollard M. Antitumor effect of indomethacin in rats with autochthonous intestinal tumors. In: Levin B, Riddell R, eds. *Frontiers in gastrointestinal cancer.* New York: Elsevier, 1984:91.
82. Pollard M, Luckert PH. Prevention and treatment of primary intestinal tumors in rats by piroxicam. *Cancer Res* 1989;49:6471.
83. Kudo T, Narisawa T, Abo S. Antitumor activity of indomethacin on methylazoxymethanol-induced large bowel tumors in rats. *Gann* 1980;71:260.
84. Narisawa T, Sato M, Tani M, Takahashi T, Goto A. Inhibition of development of methylnitrosourea-induced rat colon tumors by indomethacin treatment. *Cancer Res* 1981;41:1954.
85. Narisawa T, Sato M, Sano M, Takahashi T. Inhibition of development of methylnitrosourea-induced rat colonic tumors by peroral administration of indomethacin. *Gann* 1982;73:377.
86. Narisawa T, Satoh M, Sano M, Takahashi T. Inhibition of initiation and promotion by N-methylnitrosourea-induced colon carcinogenesis in rats by non-steroid anti-inflammatory agent indomethacin. *Carcinogenesis* 1983;4:1225.
87. Narisawa T, Hermanek P, Habs M, Schmahl D. Reduction of carcinogenicity of N-nitrosomethylurea by indomethacin and failure of resuming effect of prostaglandin E_2 (PGE_2) against indomethacin. *J Cancer Res Clin Oncol* 1984;108:239.
88. Metzger U, Meier J, Uhlschmid G, Weihe H. Influence of various prostaglandin synthesis inhibitors on DMH-induced rat colon cancer. *Dis Colon Rectum* 1984;27:366.
89. Nigro ND, Bull AW, Boyd ME. Inhibition of intestinal carcinogenesis in rats: effect of difluoromethylornithine with piroxicam or fish oil. *J Natl Cancer Inst* 1986;77:1309.
90. Reddy BS, Maruyama H, Kelloff G. Dose related inhibition of colon carcinogenesis by dietary piroxicam, a nonsteroidal antiinflammatory drug, during different stages of rat colon tumor development. *Cancer Res* 1987;47:5340.
91. Reddy BS, Nayini J, Tokumo K, al et. Chemoprevention of colon carcinogenesis by concurrent administration of piroxicam, a nonsteroidal anti-inflammatory drug with D,L,-difluoromethylornithine decarboxylase inhibitor, in diet. *Cancer Res* 1990;50:2562.
92. Reddy BS, Tokumo K, Kulkarni N, Aligia C, Kelloff G. Inhibition of colon carcinogenesis by prostaglandin synthesis inhibitors and related compounds. *Carcinogenesis* 1992;13:1019.
93. Reddy BS, Rao CV, Rivenson A, Kelloff G. Inhibitory effect of aspirin on azoxymethane-induced colon carcinogenesis in F344 rats. *Carcinogenesis* 1993;14:1493.
94. Craven P, DeRubertis FR. Effects of aspirin on 1,2-dimethylhydrazine-induced colonic carcinogenesis. *Carcinogenesis* 1992;13:541.
95. Moorghen M, Ince P, Finney KJ, et al. A protective effect of sulindac against chemically induced primary colonic tumors in mice. *J Pathol* 1988;156:341.
96. Moorghen M, Ince P, Finney KJ, et al. The effect of sulindac on colonic tumor formation in dimethylhydrazine-treated mice. *Acta Histochem Suppl* 1990;39:195.
97. Skinner SA, Penney AG, O'Brien PE. Sulindac inhibits the rate of growth and appearance of colon tumors in the rat. *Arch Surg* 1991;126:1094.
98. Rao CV, Tokumo K, Rigotty J, et al. Chemoprevention of colon carcinogenesis by dietary administration of piroxicam α-difluoromethylornithine, 16-fluoro-5-androsten-17-one, and ellagic acid individually and in combination. *Cancer Res* 1991;51:4528.
99. Rao CZ, Rivenson A, Simi B, et al. Chemoprevention of colon carcinogenesis by sulindac, a nonsteroidal anti-inflammatory agent. *Cancer Res* 1995;55:1464.
100. Davis AE, Patterson F. Aspirin reduces the incidence of colonic carcinoma in the dimethylhadrazine rat animal model. *Aust N Z J Med* 1994;24:301.
101. Hursting S, Velasco M, Woods C, Wang K, Wargovich M. Chemoprevention of azoxymethane-induced aberrant crypt foci and colon tumors in p53-deficient mice by sulindac. *Am Soc Prev Oncol* 1998 (abst).
102. Kawamori T, Rao CV, Seibert K, Reddy BS. Chemopreventive activity of celecoxib, a specific cyclooxygenase-2 inhibitor, against colon carcinogenesis. *Cancer Res* 1998;58:409.
103. Li H, Kramer PM, Steele VE, et al. Effect of duration of treatment with piroxicam on azoxymethane-induced colon cancer, aberrant crypt foci, apoptosis and cell proliferation in rats. *Proc Am Assoc Cancer Res* 1998;39:23(abst).
104. Li H, Schut HAJ, Conran P, et al. Prevention by aspirin and its combination with α-difluoromethylornithine of azoxymethane-induced tumors, aberrant crypt foci and prostaglandin E_2 levels in rat colon. *Carcinogenesis* 1999;20:425.
105. Barnes CJ, Lee M. Determination of an optimal dosing regimen for aspirin chemoprevention of 1,2-dimethylhydrazine-induced colon tumours in rats. *Br J Cancer* 1999; 79:1646.
106. Reddy BS, Kawamori T, Lubet RA, et al. Chemopreventive efficacy of sulindac sulfone against colon cancer depends on time of administration during carcinogenic process. *Cancer Res* 1999;59:3387.
107. Piazza GA, Alberts DS, Hixson LJ, et al. Sulindac sulfone inhibits azoxymethane-induced colon carcinogenesis in rats without reducing prostaglandin levels. *Cancer Res* 1997;57:2909.
108. Weisburger JH, Reddy BS, Joftes DL. *Colorectal cancer.* UICC Technical Report 19. Geneva, Switzerland: Union Internationale Contre le Cancer, 1975.
109. Smalley W, Ray WA, Daugherty J, Griffin MR. Use of nonsteroidal anti-inflammatory drugs and incidence of colorectal cancer. *Arch Intern Med* 1999;159:161.
110. Thun MJ. NSAIDs use and decreased risk of gastrointestinal cancers. *Gastroenterol Clin North Am* 1996;25:333.
111. Tonelli F, Valanzano R. Sulindac in familial adenomatous polyposis [Letter]. *Lancet* 1993;342:1120.
112. Lynch HT, Thorson AG, Smyrk T. Rectal cancer after prolonged sulindac chemoprevention. *Cancer* 1995;75:936.
113. Thorson AG, Lynch HT, Smyrk TC. Rectal cancer in FAP patient after sulindac. *Lancet* 1994;343:180.
114. Peleg II, Lubin MF, Cotsonis GA, Clark WS, Wilcox CM. Long-term use of nonsteroidal antiinflammatory drugs and other chemopreventors and risk of subsequent colorectal neoplasia. *Dig Dis Sci* 1996;41:1319.
115. Thun MJ, Heath CW. Aspirin use and reduced risk of gastrointestinal tract cancers in the American Cancer Society prospective studies. *Prev Med* 1995;24:116.
116. Gutthann SP, Garcia Rodriguez LA, Raiford DS. Individual nonsteroidal antiinflammatory drugs and other risk factors for upper gastrointestinal bleeding and perforation. *Epidemiology* 1997;8:18.
117. He J, Whelton PK, Vu B, Klag MJ. Aspirin and risk of hemorrhagic stroke—a meta-analysis of randomized controlled trials. *JAMA* 1998;280:1930.
118. Thun MJ. Beyond willow bark—aspirin in the prevention of chronic disease. *Epidemiology* 2000;11:376.
119. Eberhart CE, Coffey RJ, Radhika A, et al. Up-regulation of cyclooxygenase 2 gene expression in human colorectal adenomas and adenocarcinomas. *Gastroenterology* 1994;107:1183.
120. Kargman SL, O'Neill GP, Vickers PJ, et al. Expression of prostaglandin G/H synthase-1 and -2 protein in human colon cancer. *Cancer Res* 1995;55:2256.
121. Sano H, Kawahito Y, Wilder RL, et al. Expression of cyclooxygenase-1 and -2 in human colorectal cancer. *Cancer Res* 1995;55:3785.
122. Kutchera W, Jones DA, Matsunami N, et al. Prostaglandin H synthase 2 is expressed abnormally in human colon cancer: evidence for a transcriptional effect. *Proc Natl Acad Sci U S A* 1996;93:4816.

123. Fujita T, Matsui M, Takaku K, et al. Size- and invasion-dependent increase in cyclooxygenase 2 levels in human colorectal carcinomas. *Cancer Res* 1998;58:4823.
124. DuBois RN, Radhika A, Reddy BS, Entingh AJ. Increased cyclooxygenase-2 levels in carcinogen-induced rat colonic tumors. *Gastroenterology* 1996;110:1259.
125. Williams CS, Luongo C, Radhika A, et al. Elevated cyclooxygenase-2 levels in Min mouse adenomas. *Gastroenterology* 1996;111:1134.
126. Boolbol SK, Dannenberg AJ, Chadburn A, et al. Cyclooxygenase-2 overexpression and tumor formation are blocked by sulindac in a murine model of familial adenomatous polyposis. *Cancer Res* 1996;56:2556.
127. Reddy BS, Rao CV, Seibert K. Evaluation of cyclooxygenase-2 inhibitor for potential chemopreventative properties in colon carcinogenesis. *Cancer Res* 1996;56:4566.
128. Takahashi M, Fukutake M, Yokota S, et al. Suppression of azoxymethane-induced aberrant crypt foci in rat colon by nimesulide, a selective inhibitor of cyclooxygenase 2. *J Cancer Res Clin Oncol* 1996;122:219.
129. Jacobasch G, Schmehl K, Schmidt U. Influence of meloxicam on loss of apoptotic activity during carcinogenesis. *Proc Am Assoc Cancer Res* 1998;39:197.
130. Oshima M, Dinichuk JE, Kargman SL, et al. Suppression of intestinal polyposis in ApcD716 knockout mice by inhibition of cyclooxygenase (COX-2). *Cell* 1996;87:803.
131. Sheng H, Shao J, Kirkland SC, et al. Inhibition of human colon cancer cell growth by selective inhibition of cyclooxygenase-2. *J Clin Invest* 1997;99:2254.
132. Langenbach R, Loftin C, Lee C, Tiano H. Cyclooxygenase knockout mice: models for elucidating isoform-specific functions. *Biochem Pharm* 1999;58:1237.
133. Ruffin MT, Krishnan K, Rock CL, et al. Suppression of human colorectal mucosal prostaglandins: determining the lowest effective aspirin dose. *J Natl Cancer Inst* 1997;89:1152.
134. Barnes CJ, Hamby-Mason RL, Hardman WE, et al. Effect of aspirin on prostaglandin E_2 formation and transforming growth factor a expression in human rectal mucosa from individuals with a history of adenomatous polyps of the colon. *Cancer Epidemiol Biomarkers Prev* 1999;8:311.
135. Frommel TO, Dyavanapalli M, Oldham T, et al. Effect of aspirin on prostaglandin E_2 and leukotriene B_4 production in human colonic mucosa from cancer patients. *Clin Cancer Res* 1997;3:209.
136. Shen TY, Winter CA. Chemical and biological studies of indomethacin, sulindac and their analogs. *Adv Drug Res* 1977;12:90.
137. Duggan DE, Hare LE, Ditzler CA, Lei BW, Kwan KC. The disposition of sulindac in man. *Clin Pharmacol Exp Ther* 1977;21:326.
138. Charalambous D, O'Brien PE. Inhibition of colon cancer precursors in the rat by sulindac sulphone is not dependent on inhibition of prostaglandin synthesis. *J Gastoenterol Hepatol* 1996;11:307.
139. Thompson HJ, Briggs S, Paranka NS, et al. Sulfone metabolite of sulindac inhibits mammary carcinogenesis. *J Natl Cancer Inst* 1995;87:1259.
140. Piazza GA, Rahm AL, Krutzsch M, et al. Antineoplastic drugs sulindac sulfide and sulfone inhibit cell growth by inducing apoptosis. *Cancer Res* 1995;55:3110.
141. Hanif R, Pittas A, Feng Y, et al. Effects of nonsteroidal anti-inflammatory drugs on proliferation and on induction of apoptosis in colon cancer cells by a prostaglandin-independent pathway. *Biochem Pharmacol* 1996;52:237.
142. Bak AW, McKnight W, Li P, et al. Cyclooxygenase-independent chemoprevention with an aspirin derivative in a rat model of colonic adenocarcinoma. *Life Sci* 1998;62:367.
143. He TC, Chan TA, Vogelstein B, Kinzler K. PPAR is an APC-regulated target of nonsteroidal anti-inflammatory drugs. *Cell* 1999;99:335.
144. Bedi A, Pasricha PJ, Akhtar AJ, et al. Inhibition of apoptosis during development of colorectal cancer. *Cancer Res* 1995;55:1811.
145. Tsujii M, DuBois RN. Alterations in cellular adhesion and apoptosis in epithelial cells overexpressing prostaglandin endoperoxide synthase 2. *Cell* 1995;83:493.
146. Shiff SJ, Qiao L, Tsai LL, Rigas B. Sulindac sulfide, an aspirin-like compound, inhibits proliferation, causes cell cycle quiescence, and induces apoptosis in HT-29 colon adenocarcinoma cells. *J Clin Invest* 1995;96:491.
147. Agarwal B, Rao CV, Bhendwal S, et al. Lovastatin augments sulindac-induced apoptosis in colon cancer cells and potentiates chemopreventive effect of sulindac. *Proc Am Assoc Cancer Res* 1999;40:380(abst).
148. Bayer BM, Beaven MA. Evidence that indomethacin reversibly inhibits cell growth in the G_1 phase of the cell cycle. *Biochem Pharmacol* 1978;28:441.
149. Bayer BM, Kruth HS, Vaughn M, Beaven MA. Arrest of cultured cells in the G_1 phase of the cell cycle by indomethacin. *J Pharmacol Exp Ther* 1979;210:106.
150. Lipton A, Scialla S, Harvey H, al et. Adjuvant antiplatelet therapy with aspirin in colorectal cancer. *J Med* 1982;23:419.
151. Wilson KT, Fu S, Ramanujam KS, Meltzer SJ. Increased expression of inducible nitric oxide synthase and cyclooxygenase-2 in Barrett's esophagus and associated adenocarcinomas. *Cancer Res* 1998;58:2929.
152. Zimmermann KC, Sarbia M, Weber AA, et al. Cyclooxygenase-2 expression in human esophageal carcinoma. *Cancer Res* 1999;59:198.
153. Ristimaki A, Honkanen N, Jankala H, Sipponen P, Harkonen M. Expression of cyclooxygenase-2 in human gastric carcinoma. *Cancer Res* 1997;57:1276.
154. Shimakura S, Boland CR. Eicosanoid production by the human gastric cancer cell line AGS and its relation to cell growth. *Cancer Res* 1992;52:1744.
155. Kawamori T, Nakatsugi S, Ohta T, Sugimura T, Wakabayashi K. Chemopreventive properties of a selective cyclooxygenase-2 inhibitor, nimesulide on PhIP-induced mammary carcinogenesis in rats. *Proc Am Assoc Cancer Res* 1999;40:2373(abst).
156. Hwang D, Scollard D, Byrne J, Levine E. Expression of cyclooxygenase-1 and cyclooxygenase-2 in human breast cancer. *J Natl Cancer Inst* 1998;90:455.
157. Pinczowski D, Ekbom A, Baron J, Yuen J, Adami H-O. Risk factors for colorectal cancer in patients with ulerative colitis: a case-control study. *Gastroenterology* 1994;107:117.
158. La Vecchia C, Negri E, Franceschi S, et al. Aspirin and colorectal cancer. *Br J Cancer* 1997;76:675.
159. Rosenberg L, Louik C, Shapiro S. Nonsteroidal antiinflammatory drug use and reduced risk of large bowel carcinoma. *Cancer* 1998;82:2326.
160. Funkhouser EM, Sharp GB. Aspirin and reduced risk of esophageal carcinoma. *Cancer* 1995;76:1116.
161. Friedman GD, Ury HK. Initial screening for carcinogenicity of commonly used drugs. *J Natl Cancer Inst* 1980;65:723.
162. Egan KM, Stampfer MJ, Giovannucci E, Rosner BA, Colditz, GA. Prospective study of regular aspirin use and the risk of breast cancer. *J Natl Cancer Inst* 1996;88:988.
163. Harris RE, Namboodiri KK, Farrar WB. Nonsteroidal antiinflammatory drugs and breast cancer. *Epidemiology* 1996;7:203.

SECTION 7

GRAHAM A. COLDITZ

Physical Activity and Body Weight

The 1994 report of the U.S. Surgeon General concludes that lack of physical activity is causally related to increased risk of coronary heart disease, diabetes, and colon cancer.[1,2] Other cancers are listed as having a suggestive relation, including breast cancer, whereas there is lack of evidence for a relation between activity and either rectal or prostate cancers. The evidence for colon and breast cancers is therefore summarized in detail.

COLON CANCER

Numerous studies have illustrated a relation between physical activity and colon cancer. Higher levels of physical activity are related to lower rates of colon cancer,[1,3] the fourth most common cancer diagnosed in the United States.

The rates of colon cancer vary considerably among countries. During the 1960s and 1970s, there was a gradual increase in colon cancer in most industrialized countries, and in European countries with low rates there was an increase in the rates observed in high-risk countries, such as the United States and England. Low incidence is reported from India and China, whereas high rates are observed in the United States, Australia, and Western Europe.[4] Numerous lifestyle factors have been proposed to explain this large international variation.[5]

PHYSICAL ACTIVITY

Epidemiologic studies have measured activity in two ways: by occupation and by leisure-time activities. These measures may represent somewhat different patterns of energy expenditure. Activity demanded by employment in a certain occupation may be relatively constant from week to week and year to year, whereas leisure-time activity is far more labile, changing from week to week, season to season, and year to year. In the epidemiologic study of a disease like colon cancer, long-term patterns of activity may be the relevant factor in determining disease risk. Therefore, occupational activity may be a better marker of cancer-determining activity level than is self-reported leisure-time activity. Both the methods used to measure activity and the validity or accuracy of the methods vary considerably. Similar methodologic issues arose in the study of heart disease[6]: When poor measures of activity were used, studies tended to underestimate the true impact of activity on health. In other words, studies using poor measures of physical activity fail to measure true activity levels and then fail to provide data showing a strong association with activity, even though physical activity is, in truth, protective against heart disease.[1]

Likewise for colon cancer, when less accurate measures of physical activity are used, the estimated benefit from this activity is smaller than its probable true benefit. Thus, the protection by physical activity is underestimated. Nonetheless, as summarized in the following section, the most precise studies using validated measures of physical activity have shown, overall, that higher levels of physical activity are related to lower levels of colon cancer.

Validity of Activity Measures

The validity of activity measures has been assessed and is quite variable.[7,8] Among the better measures, one observes a correlation between the self-reported measure of activity and an independent gold standard (such as 28 days of activity diary) in the range of 0.5 to 0.7. Thus, the epidemiologic associations observed with these measures of activity and disease outcome are considerably attenuated, perhaps by as much as one-half. For example, Giovannucci et al.[9] reported a relative risk that was 0.88 [95% confidence interval (CI), 0.81 to 0.95] per 10 metabolic equivalent of task (MET) increase in physical activity. After correcting for measurement error, the relative risk was strengthened to 0.65 (0.48 to 0.88).

A systematic review of published literature through March 1997 identified studies that reported a measure of physical activity and outcomes of colon cancer or colorectal cancer. A review of these studies presents summary data for each, including the relative risk for each level of activity.[2]

CASE-CONTROL STUDIES. Overall, the published case-control studies suggest a consistent inverse relation between both occupational and leisure-time activity and colon cancer risk among men and women. These results have been replicated across a wide range of countries, including China, Japan, New Zealand, Spain, Sweden, Turkey, and the United States.

COHORT STUDIES. Cohort studies generally enroll healthy individuals to assess elements of lifestyle, behavior, environment, and occupation that are thought to influence later development of disease. The initial follow-up of college athletes by Polednak[10] did not show any protection against colon cancer, although data were not available on lifestyle characteristics (including family history, diet, smoking, etc.). The other 17 studies through 1997 show a reduction in risk similar to that observed in the case-control studies. Higher activity in adult life is generally related to reduced risk of colon cancer, although the cohort results are less consistent than are those from the case-control studies. Inconsistency may, in part, be attributed to studies that focused on college activity and cancer risk many years later,[10,11] or that included both colon and rectal cancer in a single outcome category.[11,12] (An inverse association between activity and rectal cancer is generally not seen when rectal cancer is analyzed as a separate outcome variable.) When occupation was used to categorize activity in a study of Swedish men, those with higher activity had a lower risk of colon cancer [relative risk (RR) = 0.8].[13] In that study, the strongest contrast was based on a joint classification of occupation and recreational activity. Men in the highest activity group for both occupation and recreation had a relative risk that was 0.3 (0.1 to 0.8) representing a 70% reduction in risk compared with men who were inactive at work and engaged in little recreational activity.

Leisure-time activity is addressed separately in the Harvard Alumni Study, a cohort of graduates from Harvard College followed since 1960 to study activity and chronic diseases; Lee and colleagues observed a strong inverse association among men who were active both in the 1960s and in 1977 when surveys were administered.[14] Men expending more than 2500 kcal per week in leisure activity had a 50% reduction in risk of colon cancer compared with those expending less than 1000 kcal per week.

Overall, the cohort studies conducted in Denmark, Norway, Sweden, Switzerland, and the United States support a dose-response relation across increasing activity levels: Higher activity levels are related to lower levels of colon cancer risk. Those in the highest activity category have approximately a 40% to 50% reduction in risk of colon cancer compared to the least active category.[2]

Although historically data have suggested that the association between physical activity and reduced risk of colon cancer is stronger in men than in women, this finding may, in part, reflect the small number of women in the high-activity category. Data from Norway show a stronger relation between total physical activity and colon cancer among women than among men,[15] and data from the Nurses' Health Study show similar magnitude of reduction in risk in women as observed among men in a parallel study using comparable methods for activity assessment.[16]

SITE-SPECIFIC RISK. Studies that examined activity in relation to site of cancer in the colon suggest that the relation between higher activity and lower risk of cancer may be stronger for the left than for the right colon. One large case-control study shows no difference in the strength of association between vigorous activity and proximal or distal colon cancer.[17] The association is stronger for the colon than it is for the rectum, for which activity is at best only very weakly associated.

Interpretation

Despite the variable and often poor measures of activity used, a consistent reduction in risk is observed across different study design and different populations and across occupational and leisure-time activity. A consistent dose-response relation emerges, indicating that those at higher levels of activity are at reduced risk of colon cancer. Across the studies, the evidence suggests that the relation is stronger for the left colon and weaker or absent for rectal cancer. Few studies have addressed the relation between specific activities and cancer risk (e.g., Is swimming less protective than jogging?) or the importance of the age at which a person is active in determining the likelihood of cancer (e.g., Is activity more protective in youth, middle age, or years immediately before the diagnosis of cancer?). Three studies that address physical activity during early adulthood show no relation.[10,11,18] Although these studies failed to control for several colon cancer risk factors, the results are consistent with an effect of activity later in the pathway to cancer. Evidence from Lee and colleagues[14] also supports a role later in the pathway to cancer. Men who had increased their level of activity during follow-up of the cohort had a suggestion of lower risk of colon cancer during subsequent follow-up. More data are needed, however, to refine the understanding of the time course between change in physical activity and change in risk of cancer. In general, the studies based on classification of activity by occupation show a stronger dose response than those based on leisure-time activity and support a protective effect across the wide range of activities encompassed by the high-activity occupations.

How do we know that physical activity is actually protecting subjects from developing colon cancer? Is it possible that active men and women are also healthier in other ways (e.g., eating less red meat and more folate) and that these factors are the real reason for the observed protection from physical activity? Several studies have reported analyses that address the independent relation between activity and colon cancer risk—that is, they control for other lifestyle factors [body mass index (BMI), alcohol, and diet] that may be related to higher levels of physical activity and could therefore bias or distort the protection attributed to physical activity. Activity is independent of dietary fat and fiber intake in these studies and is also independent of BMI, a measure of adiposity. Although not all studies examined for the independence of activity from other lifestyle factors, the magnitude of the inverse relation is not materially altered when investigators have controlled for diet, BMI, and other factors. The one exception is the analysis by Whittemore et al.,[19] who saw a shift in the magnitude of association after control for diet in the case-control data from the People's Republic of China, but no substantial change in effect after control for diet in the United States. In a detailed analysis of the Health Professionals Follow-Up Study, a cohort of some 50,000 men followed to study relations between diet and chronic diseases, Giovannucci et al. showed that individuals with higher physical activity were more likely to use multivitamins, had lower intake of saturated fat, higher intake of fiber, lower prevalence of cigarette smoking, and lower BMI (men were leaner).[9] After controlling for these risk factors, as well as use of aspirin and family history, the protection was reduced from 56% to 47% [the relative risk changed from 0.4 (0.3 to 0.7) to 0.5 (0.3 to 0.9)]. In other words, the protection remained at almost 50% despite controlling for all the other factors known to relate to colon cancer risk. The inverse trend in risk with increasing activity remained statistically significant. Thus, we conclude that activity is not merely a marker of healthier lifestyle, but exerts an independent protective effect.

Mechanisms

Several biologic mechanisms have been proposed for the protective effect of physical activity, reflecting changes in physiologic measures after physical activity. Among these is the bowel transit time that decreases with physical activity. It is then proposed that the reduced transit time alters the environment within the colon and thereby reduces exposure to carcinogens.[20,21]

A second mechanism may be that abdominal obesity and low physical activity are independently related to insulin resistance. Across a gradient of physical activity, insulin sensitivity improves with exercise.[22] Furthermore, insulin is a strong growth factor for colon mucosal cells in laboratory studies and an animal model of colon cancer.[23] Thus, it is possible that activity exerts its protective effect through reduced insulin levels.[24,25]

Another possible mechanism is the effect of prostaglandins on colon cell proliferation. Physical activity produces an increase in prostaglandin $F_{2\alpha}$, which increases intestinal motility, and a decrease in prostaglandin E_2, which in cell culture can act to stimulate colon cell proliferation. Further support for this possible mechanism comes from laboratory studies on rats and evidence in humans that aspirin and nonsteroidal anti-inflammatory drugs, also inhibitors of prostaglandin synthesis, reduce risk of colon cancer.[26,27]

With this large body of epidemiologic data and supporting laboratory studies, it appears that low levels of physical activity are causally related to increased risk of colon cancer. Causal considerations include a consistent decrease in risk with higher levels of physical activity, either measured as occupational activity or leisure-time activity, a dose-response relation with hours of activity per week or level of occupational physical activity, specificity for the relation with colon and not rectum, and a temporal relation such that activity measures precede the onset of colon cancer by years, although relations are stronger for more recent activity rather than distant past activity.

BREAST CANCER

Regular physical activity has been hypothesized to prevent breast cancer, largely by reducing circulating levels of sex hormones. The mechanisms by which physical activity reduces exposure to hormones vary by period of life. Young girls participating in strenuous athletic training such as running and ballet dancing have delayed menarche,[28–30] which is known to reduce the risk of breast cancer, and even moderate-intensity physical activity may also delay menstruation.[31] A later menarche is associated with a later onset of regular ovulatory cycles and lower serum estrogen concentrations during adolescence.[32] Once menstruation has been established, anovulatory and irregular menstrual cycles may be more frequent among moderately and strenuously active women than among inactive women,[28,33,34] although there is disagreement regarding the degree to which the intensity of physical activity influences menstrual abnormalities.[35] Among older women, levels of past and current physical activity influence fat stores,[29,30,36–39] which after menopause are the locus of conversion of androstenedione to estrogen.[40,41]

Despite the evidence that higher levels of physical activity are associated with lower levels of circulating ovarian hormones, epidemiologic studies relating physical activity to risk of breast cancer are inconsistent.[42] Methodologic differences in physical activity assessment are likely to have contributed to these inconsistencies. Studies have differed in the ages at which physical activity was assessed; methods for measuring intensity, frequency, and duration of physical activity; definition and categorization of physical activity levels; and age of breast cancer diagnosis. Furthermore, the ranges of physical activity that are typically studied are very limited in comparison with the levels of hard labor typically practiced by women in traditional agrarian societies.

To date, the strongest reduction in breast cancer risk associated with increased physical activity has been reported in a population-based case-control study of women younger than age 40 years in Southern California.[43] The RR was 0.42 (95% CI, 0.27 to 0.64) when comparing women with a lifetime average of 3.8 hours or more of physical activity per week to those with an average of 0 hours per week. This has been the only study explicitly devoted to the relationship between physical activity and breast cancer, and it used a detailed physical activity assessment instrument to quantify the average number of hours per week of recreational physical activity over the reproductive life span, beginning at menarche. Activities such as housework, gardening, and easy walking not for the explicit purpose of physical exercise were not counted in the measure of physical activity. Bernstein et al.[43] concluded from their various analyses that lifelong physical activity is the critical exposure of interest with regard to breast cancer risk.

In contrast to the detailed measurement instrument previously described, a relatively simple measure of physical activity was used in a prospective cohort study of Norwegian women aged 20 to 54 years at baseline.[44] Over a period of 3 to 5 years, women were administered two surveys about their patterns of physical activity during leisure hours. The RR was 0.63 (95% CI, 0.42 to 0.95) for consistently active women compared to consistently sedentary women, which is the second-strongest inverse association reported in the literature. This study is also the only prospective cohort study of the five reported to date[12,44–47] to find a substantial inverse association between physical activity and breast cancer risk.

Most studies fall between these two studies[43,44] with regard to the detail of physical activity measurement and categorization. For instance, in two population-based case-control studies[48,49] conducted among younger women, physical activity both early in life and in the period immediately before the interview was assessed. However, neither of these studies found an inverse association between physical activity (in either period) and breast cancer risk, despite defining physical activity categories in various ways.

Because of the potential public health significance of an association between a modifiable lifestyle risk factor such as physical activity and breast cancer, future studies will need to address important methodologic issues surrounding physical activity measurement.

Although the relation between physical activity and risk of breast cancer remains unsettled, indirect evidence relating higher physical activity to risk of postmenopausal breast cancer is strong because of the important role of activity in controlling weight gain, an important cause of postmenopausal breast cancer. This, in addition to many other benefits of staying lean and fit, provide sufficient justification for including regular physical activity in daily life.

OBESITY

A strong and consistent relation has been reported between obesity and mortality from all cancers among men and women.[50] Due to the relationship of obesity with postmenopausal breast cancer and endometrial cancer, the relation is stronger among women than among men.[51]

Attained weight and weight change in adults provide sensitive measures of the balance between long-term energy intake and expenditure. Although the relation between these variables and breast cancer risk has been complex and confusing, findings provide a coherent picture and indicate a major contribution of weight gain to risk of postmenopausal breast cancer risk. Two reproducible findings have been particularly enigmatic: (1) In affluent Western populations with high rates of breast cancer, measures of body fatness have been *inversely* related to risk of premenopausal breast cancer, and (2) body fatness has been only weakly related to postmenopausal breast cancer risk despite strong associations between body fat and endogenous estrogen levels.

The inverse relation between body weight (typically determined as BMI, calculated as weight in kg divided by height in meters,^{2} to account for variation in height) and incidence of premenopausal breast cancer has been consistently seen in recent prospective studies,[52] and in a metaanalysis of both case-control and cohort studies.[53] Little relation between BMI and breast cancer mortality has been observed in premenopausal women, probably because delayed detection and diagnosis in heavier women counterbalances the lower incidence among heavier women. Heavier premenopausal women, even at the upper limits of what are considered to be healthy weights, have more irregular menstrual cycles and increased rates of anovulatory infertility,[54] suggesting that their lower risk may be due to fewer ovulatory cycles and less exposure to ovarian hormones. Increased rates of menstrual irregularity and anovulatory infertility also are seen among very lean women, but such women are uncommon in Western populations. In case-control studies, a consistent relation between menstrual cycle regularity and breast cancer risk has not emerged, which could cast doubt on this explanation, but this may be due to the indirect relation between menstrual regularity and ovulation and to difficulties in remote recall. In a prospective study among younger women, compared with regular cycles of approximately 28 days, both short and longer or irregular cycles were associated with reduced risk of breast cancer,[55] lending support to irregular anovulation as the explanation for the lower risk in heavier women.

In both case-control and prospective studies conducted in affluent Western countries, the association between BMI and risk of breast cancer among postmenopausal breast cancer has been only weakly positive or nonexistent.[56,57] The lack of a stronger association has been surprising because obese postmenopausal women have plasma levels of endogenous estrogens nearly twice as high as lean women, due to conversion of androstenedione to estrogens in adipose tissue and also lower levels of sex-hormone binding globulin.[58] However, the lack of a stronger positive association now appears to be due to two factors.

First, like the protective effect of early pregnancy, the reduction in breast cancer risk associated with being overweight in early adult life appears to persist throughout later life.[52,59] Thus, an elevated BMI in a postmenopausal woman represents two opposing risks: a protective effect due to the correlation between early weight and postmenopausal weight and an adverse effect due to elevated estrogens after menopause. For this reason, weight *gain* from early adult life to after menopause should be more strongly related to postmenopausal breast cancer risk than would attained weight. Indeed, the relation between weight gain and risk of postmenopausal breast cancer has been consistently supported by both case-control[60] and prospective studies.[52,59,61]

A second reason for failing to appreciate a greater adverse effect of excessive weight or weight gain on risk of postmenopausal breast cancer is that the use of postmenopausal hormones obscures the variation in endogenous estrogens due to adiposity and elevates breast cancer risk regardless of body weight.[52] To appreciate fully the impact of weight or weight gain, an analysis should be limited to women who never used postmenopausal hormones. Thus, among women who never used postmenopausal hormones in the Nurses' Health Study, those who gained 25 kg or more after age 18 years had double the risk of breast cancer compared with women who maintained their weight within 2 kg.[52] In this population, the combination of either using postmenopausal hormones or gaining weight after age 18 years accounted for one-third of postmenopausal breast cancer cases.

The relation between body weight and breast cancer risk among lower risk, mainly non-Western, countries has been observed to be somewhat different in higher risk countries.[62] In general, the inverse relation between weight and premenopausal breast cancer risk has not been observed, and the association between weight and postmenopausal risk has been stronger. This difference is likely to be due to the lower prevalence of obesity among premenopausal women in these low-risk countries; few women are likely to be sufficiently overweight so as to cause anovulation and a reduction in premenopausal breast cancer risk. As a result, BMI after menopause would only reflect the adverse effects of high endogenous estrogens, unopposed by a residual protective effect due to correlation with overweight in early adult life.

RELATIONSHIP BETWEEN OBESITY AND CARCINOMA

As in animal studies, energy balance appears to play an important but complex role in the causation of human breast cancer. During early adult life, obesity is associated with a lower incidence of breast cancer before menopause, but no reduction in breast cancer mortality. However, weight gain after age 18 years is associated with a graded and substantial increase in postmenopausal breast cancer that is seen most clearly in the absence of hormone replacement therapy.

The relationship between obesity and risk of endometrial cancer follows from the excess exposure to estrogen that is associated with adiposity. This direct relation has been long observed.

The relationship between obesity and colon cancer has been observed among both women and men and persists even after control for physical activity and dietary patterns.[9,16] It is postulated that excess weight gain may act through increased insulin resistance and hyperinsulinemia to promote colon carcinogenesis.[24,25]

Evidence for a relationship between obesity and prostate cancer is less consistent. At this time, the inconclusive evidence precludes a definite assertion of any important relation.

CONCLUSIONS

Lack of physical activity and adult weight gain are harbingers of our Western culture and both act to increase risk of major malignancies. Through numerous mechanisms, these two lifestyle factors contribute substantially to the risk of colon and breast cancer. The evidence is strong for obesity and endometrial cancer, and less consistent for other major malignancies.

REFERENCES

1. U.S. Department of Health and Human Services, Centers for Disease Control and Prevention, National Center for Chronic Disease Prevention and Health Promotion, The President's Council on Physical Fitness and Sports. *Physical activity and health: a report of the surgeon general.* Washington, DC: Office of the Surgeon General, 1996.
2. Colditz G, Cannuscio C, Frazier A. Physical activity and reduced risk of colon cancer: implications for prevention. *Cancer Causes Control* 1997;8:649.
3. Macfarlane G, Lowenfels A. Physical activity and colon cancer. *Eur J Cancer Prev* 1994;3: 393.
4. Muir C, Waterhouse J, Mack T, et al., eds. *Cancer incidence in five continents* (IARC scientific publications, no. 88). Lyon, France: International Agency for Research on Cancer, 1987.
5. Potter JD, Slattery ML, Bostick RM, Gapstur SM. Colon cancer: a review of the epidemiology. *Epidemiol Rev* 1993;15:499.
6. Berlin J, Colditz G. A meta-analysis of physical activity in the prevention of coronary heart disease. *Am J Epidemiol* 1990;132:612.
7. Wolf A, Hunter D, Colditz GA, et al. Reproducibility and validity of a self-administered physical activity questionnaire. *Int J Epidemiol* 1994;23:991.
8. Chasan-Taber S, Rimm EB, Stampfer MJ, et al. Reproducibility and validity of a self-administered physical activity questionnaire for male health professionals. *Epidemiology* 1996;7:81.
9. Giovannucci E, Ascherio A, Rimm EB, et al. Physical activity, obesity, and risk for colon cancer and adenoma in men. *Ann Intern Med* 1995;122:327.
10. Polednak AP. College athletics, body size, and cancer mortality. *Cancer* 1976;38:382.
11. Paffenbarger RSJ, Hyde RT, Wing AL. Physical activity and incidence of cancer in diverse populations: a preliminary report. *Am J Clin Nutr* 1987;45(suppl):312.
12. Albanes D, Blair A, Taylor PR. Physical activity and risk of cancer in the NHANES I population. *Am J Public Health* 1989;79:744.
13. Gerhardsson M, Floderus B, Norell SE. Physical activity and colon cancer risk. *Int J Epidemiol* 1988;17:743.
14. Lee IM, Paffenbarger RS Jr, Hsieh CC. Physical activity and risk of developing colorectal cancer among college alumni. *J Natl Cancer Inst* 1991;83:1324.
15. Thune I, Lund E. Physical activity and risk of colorectal cancer in men and women. *Br J Cancer* 1996;73:1134.
16. Martinez ME, Giovannucci E, Spiegelman D, et al. Leisure-time physical activity, body size, and colon cancer in women. Nurses' Health Study Research Group. *J Natl Cancer Inst* 1997;89:948.
17. Slattery M, Potter J, Caan B, et al. Energy balance and colon cancer—beyond physical activity. *Cancer Res* 1997;57:75.
18. Marcus P, Newcomb P, Storer B. Early adulthood physical activity and colon cancer risk among Wisconsin women. *Cancer Epidemiol Biomark Prev* 1994;3:641.
19. Whittemore AS, Wu-Williams AH, Lee M, et al. Diet, physical activity and colorectal cancer among Chinese in North America and China. *J Natl Cancer Inst* 1990;82:915.
20. Reddy BS, Wynder EL. Metabolic epidemiology of colon cancer. Fecal bile acids and neutral sterols in colon cancer patients and patients with adenomatous polyps. *Cancer* 1977;39:2533.
21. Zaridze DG. Environmental etiology of large-bowel cancer. *J Natl Cancer Inst* 1983;70:389.
22. Kriska A, Bennett P. An epidemiologic perspective on the relationship between physical activity and NIDDM: from activity assessment to intervention. *Diabetes Metab Rev* 1992;8:355.
23. Tran T, Medline A, Bruce W. Insulin promotion of colon tumors in rats. *Cancer Epidemiol Biomark Prev* 1996;5:1013.
24. Giovannucci E. Insulin and colon cancer. *Cancer Causes Control* 1995;6:164.
25. McKeown-Eyssen G. Epidemiology of colorectal cancer revisited: are serum triglycerides and/or plasma glucose associated with risk? *Cancer Epidemiol Biomark Prev* 1994;3:687.
26. Giovannucci E, Rimm EB, Stampfer MJ, et al. Aspirin use and the risk for colorectal cancer and adenoma in male health professionals. *Ann Intern Med* 1994;121:241.
27. Giovannucci E, Egan KM, Hunter DJ, et al. Aspirin and the risk of colorectal cancer in women. *N Engl J Med* 1995;333:609.
28. Malina R, Spirduso E, Tate C, Baylor A. Age at menarche and selected menstrual characteristics in athletes at different competitive levels and in different sports. *Med Sci Sports Exer* 1978;10:218.
29. Frisch RE, Wyshak G, Vincent L. Delayed menarche and amenorrhea in ballet dancers. *N Engl J Med* 1980;303:17.
30. Frisch RE, Gotz-Welbergen AV, McArthur JW, et al. Delayed menarche and amenorrhea of college athletes in relation to age of onset of training. *J Am Med Assoc* 1981;246:1559.
31. Merzenich H, Boeing H, Wahrendorf J. Dietary fat and sports activity as determinants for age at menarche. *Am J Epidemiol* 1993;138:217.
32. Apter D, Vihko R. Early menarche, a risk factor for breast cancer, indicates early onset of ovulatory cycles. *J Clin Endocrinol Metab* 1983;57:82.
33. Bernstein L, Ross R, Lobo R, et al. The effects of moderate physical activity on menstrual cycle patterns in adolescence: implications for breast cancer prevention. *Br J Cancer* 1987;55:681.
34. Harlow S, Matanoski G. The association between weight, physical activity and stress and variation in the length of the menstrual cycle. *Am J Epidemiol* 1991;133:38.
35. Cumming D, Wheeler G, Harber V. Physical activity, nutrition, and reproduction. *Ann N Y Acad Sci* 1994;709:55.
36. Broocks A, Pirke KM, Schweiger U, et al. Cyclic ovarian function in recreational athletes. *J Appl Physiol* 1990;68:2083.
37. Feicht CB, Johnson TS, Martin BJ, et al. Secondary amenorrhoea in athletes [Letter]. *Lancet* 1978;2:1145.
38. Bullen BA, Skrinar GS, Beitins IZ, et al. Induction of menstrual disorders by strenuous exercise in untrained women. *N Engl J Med* 1985;312:1349.
39. Russell JB, Mitchell D, Musey PI, Collins DC. The relationship of exercise to anovulatory cycles in female athletes: hormonal and physical characteristics. *Obstet Gynecol* 1984;63:452.
40. Siiteri PK. Adipose tissue as a source of hormones. *Am J Clin Nutr* 1987;45(suppl):277.
41. Cauley JA, Gutai JP, Kuller LH, et al. The epidemiology of serum sex hormones in postmenopausal women. *Am J Epidemiol* 1989;129:1120.
42. Brinton L, Bernstein L, Colditz G. Summary of workshop on physical activity and breast cancer, November 13–14, 1997. *Cancer* 1998;83(suppl):595.

43. Bernstein L, Henderson BE, Hanisch R, et al. Physical exercise and reduced risk of breast cancer in young women. *J Natl Cancer Inst* 1994;86:1403.
44. Thune I, Brenn T, Lund E, Gaard M. Physical activity and the risk of breast cancer. *N Engl J Med* 1997;336:1269.
45. Rockhill B, Willett WC, Hunter DJ, et al. Physical activity and breast cancer risk in a cohort of young women. *J Natl Cancer Inst* 1998;90:1155.
46. Dorgan JF, Brown C, Barrett M, et al. Physical activity and risk of breast cancer in the Framingham Heart Study. *Am J Epidemiol* 1994;139:662.
47. Paffenbarger RS Jr, Lee IM, Wing AL. The influence of physical activity on the incidence of site-specific cancers in college alumni. In: Jacobs MM, ed. *Exercise, calories, fat and cancer.* New York: Plenum Publishing, 1992:7.
48. Chen CL, White E, Malone KE, Daling JR. Leisure-time physical activity in relation to breast cancer among young women (Washington, United States). *Cancer Causes Control* 1997;8:77.
49. Gammon MD, Schoenberg JB, Britton JA. Recreational physical activity and breast cancer risk among women under age 45 years. *Am J Epidemiol* 1998;147:273.
50. Lew EA, Garfinkel L. Variations in mortality by weight among 750,000 men and women. *J Chronic Dis* 1979;32:563.
51. Calle E, Thun M, Petrelli J, et al. Body-mass index and mortality in a prospective cohort of U.S. adults. *N Engl J Med* 1999;341:1097.
52. Huang Z, Hankinson SE, Colditz GA, et al. Dual effects of weight and weight gain on breast cancer risk. *JAMA* 1997;278:1407.
53. Ursin G, Longnecker MP, Halies RW, Greenland S. A meta-analysis of body mass index and risk of premenopausal breast cancer epidemiology. *Epidemiology* 1995;6:137.
54. Rich-Edwards JW, Goldman MB, Willett WC, et al. Adolescent body mass index and ovulatory infertility. *Am J Obstet Gynecol* 1994;171:171.
55. Garland M, Hunter DJ, Colditz GA, et al. Menstrual cycle characteristics and history of ovulatory infertility in relation to breast cancer risk in a large cohort of women. *Am J Epidemiol* 1998;147:636.
56. Howe GR, Hirohata T, Hislop TG, et al. Dietary factors and risk of breast cancer: combined analysis of 12 case-control studies. *J Natl Cancer Inst* 1990;82:561.
57. Hunter DJ, Willett WC. Diet, body size, and breast cancer. *Epidemiol Rev* 1993;15:110.
58. Hankinson SE, Willett WC, Manson JE, et al. Alcohol, height, and adiposity in relation to estrogen and prolactin levels in postmenopausal women. *J Natl Cancer Inst* 1995;87:1297.
59. Barnes-Josiah D, Potter JD, Sellers TA, Himes JH. Early body size and subsequent weight gain as predictors of breast cancer incidence (Iowa, United States). *Cancer Causes Control* 1995;6:112.
60. Ziegler RG, Hoover RN, Nomura AMY, et al. Relative weight, weight change, height, and breast cancer risk in Asian-American women. *J Natl Cancer Inst* 1996;88:650.
61. Le Marchand L, Kolonel LN, Earle ME, Mi MP. Body size at different periods of life and breast cancer risk. *Am J Epidemiol* 1988;128:137.
62. Pathak DR, Whittemore AS. Combined effects of body size, parity, and menstrual events on breast cancer incidence in seven countries. *Am J Epidemiol* 1992;135:153.

Richard M. Sherry

CHAPTER 24

Cancer Prevention: Role of Surgery in Cancer Prevention

Prophylactic is a word derived from Greek (*pro-* "before" and *phylassin-* "to guard") meaning "advanced guard." The current status of prophylactic surgery to prevent malignant disease is limited and often controversial. Clinicians have long recognized that certain conditions, such as inflammatory bowel disease and cryptorchidism, confer on patients an increased risk of developing fatal organ-specific malignancies. Advances in molecular biology coupled with an increased appreciation that cancer is a genetic disorder have made accurate risk evaluation with genetic screening a reality for certain malignancies. As our understanding of cancer susceptibility has advanced, so too has our appreciation of the complexity of the associated social and clinical issues. Progress in the laboratory has often outpaced our ability to use these new insights in the clinic. These factors have created a new impetus to develop practical strategies to prevent cancer.

That surgery can and should be used to prevent cancer is obvious (Table 24-1). The fact that colonoscopic polypectomy can help prevent colorectal cancer is now accepted and largely taken for granted.[1] However, the efficacy of many other interventions is not as convincing. Although the role of prophylactic surgery is largely undefined, it is certain to evolve. The focus of this chapter is the current use of surgery to prevent cancer.

MULTIPLE ENDOCRINE NEOPLASIA 2 AND FAMILIAL MEDULLARY THYROID CARCINOMA

Multiple endocrine neoplasia (MEN) is characterized by the development of multiple tumors in endocrine organs in a patient and close relatives. The syndrome is divided into three types: MEN 1, MEN 2a, and MEN 2b. MEN 2 is defined by the combination of tissues affected and the presence of developmental abnormalities and has been the focus of extensive genetic analysis. MEN 2a is associated with medullary carcinoma of the thyroid and with hyperparathyroidism. Individuals with MEN 2b have medullary carcinoma of the thyroid, pheochromocytoma, and developmental abnormalities involving hyperplasia of intestinal autonomic nerve plexuses and growth of nerve axons in the lips, oral mucosa, and conjunctiva, which give rise to the characteristic facies. A syndrome related to MEN 2 is familial medullary thyroid carcinoma, in which patients have only medullary carcinoma of the thyroid. MEN 2a, MEN 2b, and familial medullary thyroid carcinoma have an autosomal dominant pattern of inheritance and account for approximately 25% of all cases of medullary carcinoma of the thyroid.[2]

In 1993, it was established that mutations in the RET protooncogene were responsible for the hereditary predisposition to medullary thyroid cancer.[3,4] This genetic breakthrough has allowed accurate identification of kindreds at high risk for developing medullary carcinoma of the thyroid and has permitted families to consider the risks and benefits of prophylactic thyroidectomy.

In 1994, Wells et al.[5] reported the first experience with prophylactic thyroidectomy based on identification of RET protooncogene mutations. Thirteen patients were confirmed to carry a mutation in the RET protooncogene in association with MEN 2a and underwent immediate thyroidectomy. In each patient, the resected thyroid gland demonstrated C-cell hyperplasia. No metastases were found in regional nodes, and all patients had normal postoperative stimulated plasma calcitonin

TABLE 24-1. Prophylactic Surgery for the Prevention of Cancer

Clinical Condition	*Associated Malignancy*	*Recommendations for Prophylactic Surgery*
MEN 2a, MEN 2b; familial medullary thyroid cancer	Medullary thyroid cancer	Total thyroidectomy at approximately 6 years of age for patients with RET protooncogene mutations.
Barrett's esophagus	Adenocarcinoma of the esophagus	Esophagectomy should be considered for healthy patients with high-grade dysplasia.
BRCA1, BRCA2 mutations	Breast cancer	Bilateral total mastectomy is a reasonable option in selected patients.
	Ovarian cancer	Bilateral oophorectomy is a reasonable option in selected patients after childbearing.
Ulcerative colitis	Colon cancer	Colectomy should be considered if associated with dysplasia, at 10 years for patients with pancolitis, and for most patients at 20 years.
Familial adenomatous polyposis	Colon cancer	Colectomy in teenage years or earlier if polyps are detected on endoscopy.
HNPCC	Colon cancer	Surveillance colonoscopy/polypectomy reduces the risk of cancer. The role of prophylactic colectomy is controversial.
Cryptorchidism	Testicular cancer	Orchiectomy for *nonpalpable* undescended testicles. Orchiopexy is recommended for most patients.

HNPCC, hereditary nonpolyposis colorectal cancer; MEN, multiple endocrine neoplasia.

levels. Subsequent reports have confirmed the validity of this approach, and prophylactic thyroidectomy is now recommended for these patients at approximately 6 years of age.

Kebebew et al.[6] reported a review of ten published series of patients that had prophylactic thyroidectomy for RET protooncogene germline mutations. Two hundred and nine patients were included in this review, and only 3.4% of these patients had normal thyroid histology. A central node dissection was performed on 139 of these patients, and 12 individuals (8.6%) were found to have cervical node metastases. These 12 patients ranged in age from 14 to 70 years. Overall, the morbidity from total thyroidectomy was low. These investigators have recommended that a central node dissection be included when prophylactic total thyroidectomy is performed for patients with RET protooncogene mutations.

A second technical issue is whether to include the routine use of total parathyroidectomy and parathyroid autotransplantation in asymptomatic children with MEN 2a. Decker et al.[7] reported on the strategy of leaving parathyroid tissue preserved *in situ*. These authors recommended this approach because only 10% to 20% of these individuals develop parathyroid disease, and when parathyroid disease does develop in this population, it is usually focal.[7]

Prophylactic thyroidectomy has become the treatment of choice for patients with RET protooncogene mutations and, if done at an early age, the cure rate should be 100%. The identification and management of these patients is perhaps the best example of prophylactic surgery in patients known to be at risk for an inherited malignancy. Genetic testing allows the accurate identification of patients at high risk of developing an invasive cancer, and the organ at risk is removed surgically with low morbidity.

BARRETT'S ESOPHAGUS AND ESOPHAGEAL CANCER

Barrett's esophagus is a premalignant condition in which the stratified squamous epithelium in the distal esophagus is replaced to a variable extent by metaplastic columnar epithelium. It is significant from an oncologic perspective because of the close association between Barrett's esophagus and the development of adenocarcinoma of the esophagus. Barrett's esophagus develops as a sequela of chronic inflammation caused by reflux of gastric contents, including acid, pepsin, and bile acids. Esophageal motility studies and pH monitoring suggest that these patients exhibit weak lower esophageal sphincter tone and slow clearance of gastric acid.[8–12] Although Barrett's esophagus can be recognized or suspected by its appearance on endoscopy, a definitive diagnosis of Barrett's esophagus must be based on biopsy and histologic analysis. The histologic features of Barrett's esophagus should include a demonstration of goblet cells interspersed among mucin-type columnar cells. This represents the so-called specialized columnar epithelium and is pathognomonic of the process.[13]

It is difficult to determine the incidence of Barrett's esophagus. The majority of individuals with Barrett's esophagus in the general population are probably asymptomatic and therefore do not seek medical attention.[14]

Historically, Barrett's esophagus has been taken to mean specialized columnar epithelium that was determined to be more than 3 cm in length, and consequently, much of the published information regarding the incidence and natural history was generated by analyzing patients with long segments of the disease. It is now recognized that intestinal metaplasia of less than 3 cm in length should be classified as Barrett's. It has been reported that up to 33% of all patients undergoing upper endoscopy may have histologic evidence of Barrett's esophagus.[15–18] Approximately 10% of patients with frequent reflux symptoms will have a long segment of Barrett's esophagus identified.[19]

Numerous reports have confirmed that patients with Barrett's esophagus are at increased risk to develop adenocarcinoma of the esophagus.[20–23] In a review of 18 published series, Tytgat[22] estimated the median incidence of esophageal adenocarcinoma in patients with the disease to be approximately 1 cancer per 100 patient-years of follow-up. The overall risk was approximately 40 times higher than that of the general population.[22] The annual rate of cancer development in these patients is estimated to be approximately 0.8%.[23] Information on the risk of developing adenocarcinoma in short segments (less than 3 cm) of Barrett's esophagus is more limited, but the available data suggest it is associated with significant potential for malignant degeneration.[20,21]

The detection of esophageal epithelial dysplasia is an important clinical factor used to stratify patients with Barrett's esophagus. Dent et al.[24] reviewed eight published series and reported the outcome of 50 patients with high-grade dysplasia in Barrett's esophagus. These individuals were followed for up to 5 years, and adenocarcinoma developed in 16 patients (32%). Eleven patients had a resection for dysplasia where no malignancy was found in the specimen.[24] Hameeteman et al.[25] published a prospective study of 50 patients with Barrett's esophagus. All patients were without carcinoma at entrance to the study and were followed for a mean of 5.2 years. Six patients had low-grade dysplasia, and one patient had high-grade dysplasia at the start of the study. By the end of the observation period, five patients had developed adenocarcinoma, ten scored as low-grade dysplasia, and three were scored as high-grade dysplasia.[25] Thus, it is suggested that low-grade dysplasia may be helpful in identifying individuals who are likely to progress to high-grade dysplasia or adenocarcinoma. It is clear, however, that not all high-grade dysplasia progresses to cancer, and regression of a short segment of Barrett's esophagus that contained high-grade dysplasia has been reported.[26,27]

The optimal management of Barrett's esophagus has not been established. No prospective randomized trials have compared alternative treatment strategies. Comparing published series can be problematic because of biopsy sampling errors, differences in pathologic interpretation, and variations and improvements in endoscopic and surgical techniques. Although complete agreement has not been reached regarding the best approach for these patients, most experts depend on the degree of dysplasia associated with Barrett's esophagus to guide treatment recommendations.

BARRETT'S ESOPHAGUS WITHOUT DYSPLASIA

No role for esophagectomy has been established in patients with Barrett's esophagus and no evidence of dysplasia. The clinical issues surrounding these patients involve questions about the efficacy of screening and the effects of medical or surgical therapy to prevent progression to dysplasia. The exact risk of a patient with Barrett's esophagus without dysplasia for developing cancer is unknown, but it has been estimated to be 0.2% to 2.1% per year, which is an incidence 30 to 125 times that of the general population.[28] Consequently, most patients who are surgical candidates are enrolled into surveillance programs. Currently, most patients are treated medically with weight reduction, head of bed elevation, and H_2-receptor antagonists or protein pump inhibitors. The goal of therapy is symptomatic relief of gastroesophageal reflux. Although symptoms of reflux often improve with therapy, no evidence suggests that medical therapy consistently induces regression of the metaplastic columnar epithelium.[22,29,30] In addition, there is little evidence to suggest that antireflux surgery has an important impact on this process. DeMeester[31] reported a review of 11 published series that followed patients with Barrett's esophagus after an antireflux procedure. A total of 340 patients were followed for a mean of 4.4 years. Seventy-four percent of these patients showed no change in their Barrett's mucosa, 17% showed progression, 12% showed partial regression, and only 4% achieved a complete regression of Barrett's esophagus.

The current recommendation for patients with Barrett's esophagus without dysplasia is to have endoscopic surveillance and biopsy performed every 1 to 2 years. This recommendation assumes that the patient is a satisfactory surgical candidate.[23,24]

BARRETT'S ESOPHAGUS WITH LOW-GRADE DYSPLASIA

There is no role for esophagectomy in patients with low-grade dysplasia associated with Barrett's esophagus. Clearly, the risks of developing severe dysplasia or adenocarcinoma of the esophagus are significant. Medical therapy and antireflux procedures do not appear to influence the natural history of the condition. The current recommendation for healthy patients with low-grade dysplasia associated with Barrett's esophagus is to undergo histologic surveillance every 6 to 12 months. Innovative techniques, such as mucosal ablation, photodynamic therapy, and chemoprevention, are under active investigation.

BARRETT'S ESOPHAGUS WITH HIGH-GRADE DYSPLASIA

The treatment of patients with high-grade dysplasia associated with Barrett's esophagus is controversial. Most experts recommend that healthy patients undergo esophagectomy by an experienced surgeon. The pathologic diagnosis should be independently confirmed.[23,24,31,32] Because a wide spectrum of mortality has been reported after esophagectomy (1.4% to 21.0%) and because not all patients with high-grade dysplasia develop adenocarcinoma, some experts have made a case for aggressive surveillance for these patients. Levine et al.[33,34] described and reported on an aggressive biopsy protocol with up to 12 biopsy specimens per centimeter of Barrett's mucosa in patients with high-grade dysplasia. Seventy patients with high-grade dysplasia were followed, and 12 were found to have early-stage adenocarcinomas of the esophagus within an average of 2 months after the diagnosis. In the remaining 58 patients, 15 (23%) progressed to early-stage cancer after an average of 1.1 years of follow-up. None of the remaining 43 patients (74%) developed cancer when followed an average of 2.5 years. These results have not been confirmed at other institutions. It should be noted that more than 25% of these patients developed esophageal adenocarcinoma. In addition, the described surveillance protocol may be impractical for most physicians to follow. Physicians managing healthy patients with severe dysplasia associated with Barrett's esophagus should seriously consider prophylactic esophagectomy.

The recommendation for surgery or surveillance should take into account the mortality and morbidity of esophagectomy weighed against the risk and expected prognosis associated with invasive cancer. Most surgical series report an operative mortality of less than 10% when esophagectomy is performed for malignant disease. The mortality for prophylactic esophagectomy may be less than the mortality associated with surgery for malignant disease, because many patients with malignant disease are debilitated. In addition, prophylactic esophagectomy does not require an extensive nodal dissection. Either a transhiatal or multiincisional approach with cervical anastomosis appears to be appropriate. The reported 5-year survival rate for patients undergoing esophagectomy for known invasive cancer is estimated to be 18% to 32%.[35] The survival of patients with invasive adenocarcinoma detected during a rigorous surveillance program may be higher.

BREAST CANCER

It has been estimated that 5% to 10% of women with breast cancer have hereditary breast cancer.[36–39] BRCA1 was identified on the long arm of chromosome 17 (17q21) in 1990, and more than 500 different mutations in this gene have been identified.[37–39] BRCA1 is transmitted as an autosomal dominant gene with high penetrance, so that 50% of the children of carriers inherit the trait. It has been estimated that women with a BRCA1 gene mutation have between a 56% to 85% lifetime risk of developing breast cancer.[39,40] Frequently, these patients develop invasive cancer before the age of 50.[41]

A second breast cancer susceptibility gene, BRCA2, was identified and localized to the long arm of chromosome 13 (13q12-13).[42–44] Women with BRCA2 germline mutations are estimated to have a lifetime risk of breast cancer that is similar to that of BRCA1 carriers.

The optimal management strategy for patients with BRCA1 and BRCA2 mutations has not been established. The clinical options for managing a patient known to have a BRCA1 or BRCA2 mutation are obvious and include increased surveillance or prophylactic bilateral total mastectomy. No prospective trials have compared these options. Furthermore, serious questions remain regarding the efficacy of both surveillance and prophylactic mastectomy in this patient population. Chemoprevention using tamoxifen has been shown to reduce the incidence of breast cancer in women at high risk for breast cancer, but the results in women with an inherited susceptibility to breast cancer are not known. Clearly, counseling regarding any option must take into account the uncertainties associated with the estimation of cancer risk; the lack of definitive research regarding risk; and the social, medical, and psychological status of the patient. Ideally these factors should be reviewed during counseling that occurs before genetic screening.

The most obvious management strategy, and one that appears currently to be most popular among clinicians, is for patients with BRCA1 or BRCA2 mutations to depend on increased surveillance. This strategy is based on the assumption that an invasive cancer will be detected at an early stage, which is associated with a good prognosis. The current recommendations for surveillance in these women include monthly self-examination beginning by age 18, annual or semiannual clinician breast examination, and annual mammography beginning at age 25 to 35 years.[45]

These recommendations reflect a commonsense approach to attempt to reduce the risk of breast cancer–related mortality. However, the evidence to support such a strategy is limited. The one randomized trial that assessed the efficacy of breast self-examination showed no difference in the stage of detected cancers and no reduction in mortality from breast cancer in the trained cohort.[46] The sensitivity of clinician breast cancer examination varies widely based on tumor size, breast density, and experience of the clinician.[47,48] Palpation of a breast mass of less than 10 mm is problematic, even for the most experienced clinician.

Mammography has been firmly established to reduce breast cancer mortality by up to 30% to 40% when used for women 50 to 70 years of age.[49] For women 40 to 49 years of age, the benefit of mammography has been inconsistent.[50–52] Screening mammography has not been effective in younger women, because the density of their breast tissue limits the quality of x-rays. The sensitivity and specificity of mammography for detecting nonpalpable breast cancers in young women with BRCA1 or BRCA2 mutations is unknown.

Prophylactic mastectomy is a second option for reducing breast cancer risk. This procedure had fallen out of favor because of multiple case reports of breast cancer after prophylactic mastectomy, combined with a lack of credible evidence to support the efficacy of the intervention. Breast tissue can be detected in the chest wall, axilla, and abdomen, which are distant to the typical surgical field during subcutaneous or total mastectomy. Residual breast tissue remains after mastectomy, with larger amounts of breast tissue presumed to be present after subcutaneous mastectomy compared to total mastectomy.[53–55]

TABLE 24-2. Efficacy of Bilateral Prophylactic Mastectomy (BPM) in Women with a Family History of Breast Cancer—The Mayo Clinic Experience, 1960–1993

	Patients Undergoing BPM	*Female Siblings Controls*	*Reduction in Risk*
Patients at high risk for breast cancer (family history suggested inherited breast cancer)			
Number of patients	214	403	—
Observed cases of breast cancer	3 (1.4%)	156 (38%): 115 before sib's BPM; 38 after sib's BPM; 3 diagnosis date unknown	90%
Observed deaths from breast cancer	2	10.5–19.4[a]	81–94%
	Patients Undergoing BPM	*Gail Model Prediction*[b]	*Reduction in Risk*
Patients at moderate risk for breast cancer (all other patients electing BPM)			
Number of patients	425	—	—
Observed cases of breast cancer	4 (0.9%)	37.4 expected cases	89.5%
Observed deaths from breast cancer	0	10.4 expected deaths	70–100%

[a]Adjusted for ascertainment bias.
[b]The Gail model was used to predict the incidence and risk of death from breast cancer.

Hartmann et al.[56] published a retrospective study based on the Mayo Clinic experience with prophylactic mastectomy (Table 24-2). This report represents the first indication that prophylactic mastectomy may reduce the incidence of breast cancer in women at high risk for developing invasive cancer. The study included 639 women that had undergone prophylactic mastectomy between 1960 and 1993. Patients were assigned into either a high- or moderate-risk group based on family history. The high-risk cohort had a family history that suggested an autosomal dominant predisposition to breast cancer. All other women were considered to be at moderate risk for developing breast cancer. A control study group of sisters was used for the analysis of the high-risk probands. The Gail model was used to predict the expected number of breast cancers and breast cancer–related deaths for women in the moderate-risk group. The authors found that four breast cancers developed in the 425 moderate-risk patients, although the Gail model predicted 37.4 cases of cancer. In the high-risk group, 3 of 214 women developed breast cancer after prophylactic mastectomy. Among their 403 sisters who had not undergone a prophylactic mastectomy, 115 cases of breast cancer were diagnosed before their sibling's decision for prophylactic surgery, 38 cases were diagnosed after their sibling's decision for prophylactic surgery, and the time of diagnosis was unknown in three. The authors concluded that bilateral prophylactic mastectomy was associated with at least a 90% reduction in the incidence of breast cancer for these women. Women in both the high-risk and moderate-risk cohorts appeared to have a significant reduction in the risk of dying from breast cancer after prophylactic surgery. Interestingly, all seven women who developed breast cancer after prophylactic surgery had undergone bilateral subcutaneous mastectomy. No patient who had bilateral total mastectomy developed breast cancer (7 of 575 vs. 0 of 64; $P = .38$). Most experts recommend bilateral total mastectomy as the procedure of choice for patients who choose prophylactic mastectomy.

Additional support for preventative surgery can be found in a report by Robson et al.[57] These investigators followed women of Ashkenazi Jewish descent who underwent lumpectomy and radiation therapy for invasive breast cancer. Outcomes were compared for women with or without BRCA1 or BRCA2 mutations. Women with BRCA1 or BRCA2 mutations were more likely to develop ipsilateral local cancer recurrence, although this finding was not statistically significant. Women with mutations were also significantly more likely to have cancer before the age of 50, were more likely to develop contralateral breast cancer, and were more likely to have metastatic nodal involvement. Distant disease-free survival and breast cancer–specific survival rates were shorter at 10 years for women with BRCA1 or BRCA2 mutations.

Two reports of the estimated benefit of prophylactic mastectomy for women with BRCA1 or BRCA2 mutations have been based on decision analysis using a Markov model to determine survival. Grann et al.[58] estimated the probability of developing breast cancer based on a literature review of women with BRCA1 or BRCA2 gene mutations and based on the mortality rates associated with breast cancer from Surveillance, Epidemiology, and End Results data. They assumed a 90% reduction of risk with the procedure and concluded that a 30-year-old woman would improve her survival by 2.8 to 3.4 years.[58] Schrag et al.,[59] using a similar model, estimated an 85% reduction in breast cancer incidence with prophylactic mastectomy and concluded that a 30-year-old woman with a BRCA1 or BRCA2 mutation would gain 2.9 to 5.3 years of life expectancy from the surgery.

The psychological effects of prophylactic surgery in patients have not been thoroughly evaluated. Reconstructive surgical techniques that include autologous tissue transfer have dramatically improved the cosmetic results of breast surgery. Although the surgical morbidity associated with bilateral mastectomy is low, it is inevitably increased when breast reconstruction is added. There is a clear need to define the efficacy of surveillance strategies, as well as the efficacy of chemoprevention and prophylactic surgery in this challenging population. Until more accurate clinical information is available, women must be counseled based on the limited information available.

LOBULAR CARCINOMA *IN SITU*

Lobular carcinoma *in situ* (LCIS) is a histopathologic entity characterized by cellular proliferation originating in the lobules and terminal ducts of the breast. Women found to have LCIS on breast biopsy are known to be at increased risk of developing invasive ductal and lobular carcinoma of the breast. The critical clinical features of LCIS are that it is a noninvasive process, frequently found to be multifocal and bilateral, and it generally lacks clinical and mammographic signs. The precise incidence of LCIS is unknown, but it is estimated to be identified in approximately 0.5% to 1.5% of all benign breast biopsies and in approximately 2% of breast specimens obtained for mammographic abnormalities.[60–62]

Women with LCIS are clearly at increased risk for developing subsequent invasive carcinoma. Six series of women with LCIS who were followed for an average of at least 15 years have been published. These series reported that between 12.5% and 34.5% of women with LCIS developed invasive breast cancers.[60–65] A metaanalysis of 389 cases of LCIS followed for a mean of 10.9 years noted that invasive breast cancers developed in 16.4% of these women, and the breast cancer mortality rate was 2.8%.[66]

Treatment options for patients with LCIS remain controversial. Close observation with or without tamoxifen is currently the most popular choice. Evidence from the National Surgical Adjuvant Breast Project tamoxifen prevention trial noted that women with LCIS treated with tamoxifen demonstrated a decrease in the incidence of invasive cancer from 12.99 per 1000 to 5.69 per 1000.[67] Bilateral prophylactic mastectomy is an appropriate choice for healthy women who are unwilling to accept the risks associated with LCIS or with tamoxifen chemoprevention.

OVARIAN CANCER

Women identified as carrying the BRCA1 or BRCA2 mutation are at high risk for developing ovarian cancer as well as breast cancer. The lifetime risk of developing ovarian cancer for a woman with a BRCA1 mutation is approximately 30% to 60%, although some estimates are as high as 85%.[39,41,67,68] Patients with BRCA2 mutations have an estimated lifetime ovarian cancer risk of approximately 10% to 20%.[42,69]

The optimal management strategy for a woman with an inherited susceptibility to ovarian cancer is unclear. To date, no convincing evidence demonstrates that surveillance for ovarian cancer is effective. This may reflect the low ovarian cancer incidence of approximately 1 in 70 women in the general population.[70] Screening for ovarian carcinoma has been hampered by the low sensitivity and specificity of the available techniques, which include pelvic examination, serum CA-125 determinations, and transvaginal ultrasound. In addition, a laparoscopy or a laparotomy is required to make the diagnosis. Currently, routine screening in the general population has not been shown to impact on the morbidity and mortality associated with ovarian cancer, and it is not recommended. The utility of increased surveillance for patients with BRCA1 and BRCA2 mutations has not been thoroughly investigated. It is known, however, that approximately 70% of patients diagnosed with ovarian cancer have stage III or IV disease and that these patients generally have poor 5-year median survival rates.

Faced with a lack of effective screening for ovarian cancer and the poor prognosis of advanced disease, prophylactic oophorectomy has been suggested as a reasonable alternative for women considered to be at high risk for invasive cancer. The National Institutes of Health Consensus Panel on Ovarian Cancer[70] and the American College of Obstetricians and Gynecologists[71] have concluded that prophylactic bilateral oophorectomy should be recommended to women older than 35 or after childbearing is completed if there is an inherited predisposition for ovarian cancer. The Cancer Genetics Consortium reviewed the same information and concluded that the evidence is insufficient to recommend for or against prophylactic oophorectomy as a measure to reduce ovarian cancer risks.[45]

It is clear that prophylactic bilateral oophorectomy does not completely eliminate the risk of developing abdominal carcinomatosis that histologically resembles ovarian cancer. Tobarman et al.[72] reported that, among the 16 potentially inherited ovarian cancer families studied at the National Cancer Institute, prophylactic oophorectomy had been performed on 28 women. Three of these women developed ovarian-like carcinomatosis 1 to 11 years after oophorectomy.[72] This finding may reflect the fact that the peritoneum has the same embryologic origin as the ovarian epithelium and that the entire peritoneum may be at risk for malignant degeneration. Alternatively, occult ovarian cancer may have been present at the time of surgery. Struewing et al.[73] reported an analysis of 12 families with inherited breast/ovarian cancers and noted a reduction in ovarian cancer in oophorectomized women compared with women who had not undergone surgery. Compared with adjusted Connecticut Tumor Registry data, a 24-fold excess of ovarian cancer was found among nonoophorectomized women, and a 13-fold excess of "ovarian-like" cancer was found among the women who had undergone oophorectomy.[73] These results were not statistically significant.

Patients with BRCA1 and BRCA2 mutations are obviously at risk for both breast and ovarian cancer. Clinical decisions regarding prophylactic surgery are difficult when breast and ovary are considered independently, and the decisions become more challenging when they are considered together. Rebbeck et al.[74] analyzed 43 women with BRCA1 mutations who underwent bilateral prophylactic oophorectomy and had not had bilateral prophylactic mastectomy. Control subjects included women with BRCA1 mutations who had not had oophorectomy and had no prior history of breast or ovarian cancer. These authors reported a statistically significant reduction in breast cancer risk after oophorectomy when compared to the control cohort. The reduction in breast cancer risk appeared to increase over time. The use of hormone replacement therapy did not negate the reduction in breast cancer risk after oophorectomy in these patients.[74]

Evidence indicates that the use of oral contraceptives is associated with a decreased risk of ovarian cancer. The use of oral contraceptives has not been analyzed in patients with BRCA1 and BRCA2 mutations, and what effect, if any, these medications would have on the incidence of breast cancer in these patients is unknown.

COLORECTAL CANCER

Approximately 75% of all colorectal cancers occur in patients with no known risk factors for colon cancer. Individuals with ulcerative colitis, familial adenomatous polyposis (FAP), and hereditary nonpolyposis colorectal cancer (HNPCC) are at increased risk for developing the disease, but these patients probably account for fewer than 10% of all colorectal cancer cases. Despite the low incidence of these conditions in the general population, understanding and managing these patients has provided insights into the etiology of cancer and the potential role of surgery in the prevention of cancer.

ULCERATIVE COLITIS

Ulcerative colitis is a nonspecific inflammatory bowel disease of unknown etiology that involves the rectum, usually all or part of the colon, and, frequently, the distal terminal ileum as a result of colonic reflux. The clinical course of ulcerative colitis is variable, ranging from intermittent to chronic, and the severity of attacks also vary widely from mild to fulminant. The incidence of ulcerative colitis is relatively low at approximately 8 to 15 cases per 100,000 people.[75–78] From an oncologic perspective, ulcerative colitis is important because of its association with colorectal cancer. Although only a small fraction of colon cancer occurs in the setting of ulcerative colitis, colorectal cancer is the major cause of the increased morbidity and mortality of patients with this inflammatory disease.[78–80]

It is difficult to precisely determine the risk of colorectal cancer in patients with ulcerative colitis. Most but not all[81,82] studies have noted a significant increase in the risk of colorectal cancer in this population. The duration of disease and the extent of colonic involvement at the time of diagnosis are the two most important clinical factors that determine the degree of increased cancer risk. In patients with pancolitis, the cancer risk is approximately 0.5% to 1.0% per year after 10 years of disease.[83] A disease duration of 20 years in patients with pancolitis is associated with an estimated cumulative incidence of malignancy of between 5% and 35%.[78,84,85] The cumulative risk of malignancy increases over time and is reported to be as high as 75% after 40 years of disease.[86]

Patients with pancolitis are known to be at higher risk of developing cancer compared with patients with left-sided colitis. Ulcerative colitis, when limited to the left colon, is associated with an estimated cumulative incidence of cancer of between 1% and 5% at 20 years.[78,85,87] Patients with only proctitis appear to be at only average risk for colorectal cancer compared with the general population.[85] The impact of other related clinical factors, including the age of onset of the disease and family history of colon cancer, is not known.[88]

The optimal management strategy for patients with longstanding ulcerative colitis remains controversial and varies from prophylactic colectomy after 10 to 20 years of disease to vigilant surveillance with colonoscopic examination and multiple random biopsies to exclude dysplasia. In the latter strategy, colectomy is recommended based on the presence and degree of dysplasia. The differences in management strategies is not surprising given the heterogeneous nature of inflammatory bowel disease and the patient population and the absence of randomized clinical trials to support one strategy over another.

There is widespread agreement that colonic dysplasia is a strong but imperfect marker for identifying patients likely to develop colorectal cancer. Colonic surveillance is performed with the assumption that a dysplastic lesion can be detected before invasive cancer has developed. Invasive cancer can be found in approximately 10% of patients with ulcerative colitis at initial screening. Patients with no dysplasia identified on biopsy have a 3% cumulative risk of developing cancer when followed over time. Patients found to have indefinite or low-grade dysplasia are thought to progress to invasive cancer or severe dysplasia between 16% and 54% at the time. Forty percent to 45% of patients with ulcerative colitis identified to have high-grade dysplasia or dysplasia associated with a mucosal mass develop colorectal cancer. Many of these patients already have evidence of nodal metastasis.[89–91] It is also important to recognize that although the risk of developing colorectal cancer if there is no histologic evidence of dysplasia appears to be low, up to 25% of patients with ulcerative colitis–associated invasive cancer demonstrate no dysplasia in the resected specimens.[90,92,93]

No well-controlled trials have been conducted that confirm the efficacy of colonic surveillance to reduce the mortality of ulcerative colitis–associated colorectal cancer. Lennard-Jones[94] reported a review of four published series that included 423 patients who were screened regularly by colonoscopy over a period of 12 to 15 years. Eleven patients were operated on for precancerous lesions, and only three Duke's class A lesions and one Duke's class B lesion were found. No cancer deaths were reported during the surveillance period. The author suggested that surveillance colonoscopy should be performed only in individuals with long-standing ulcerative colitis involving the entire colon.[94]

Despite the limitations and lack of data to support surveillance for colonic dysplasia, physicians appear reluctant to recommend prophylactic colectomy for patients with long-standing ulcerative colitis. The fact that surgery eliminates the symptoms of ulcerative colitis, including bleeding, diarrhea, anemia, steroid dependence, and cyclosporin therapy, as well as eliminating the risk of colorectal cancer may be underappreciated. Several surgical alternatives are available for patients undergoing colectomy, and the operation should be tailored to the individual and the clinical situation. In the setting of acute colitis, for example, most surgeons recommend a subtotal colectomy and ileostomy. In the elective surgical setting, many options are available, including protocolectomy and ileostomy, colectomy and ileorectal anastomosis (assuming the rectum is free of inflammation), protocolectomy and Kock continent ileostomy, or ileal pouch–anal anastomosis. Each procedure is associated with reported complications; however, surgery for ulcerative colitis is extremely safe for most patients, and the reported operative mortality is less than 1%, even in the emergency setting.[95] Although comparing the outcomes of each procedure is difficult and controlled studies do not exist, most patients report a high quality of life regardless of the procedure performed.

It is evident that some consideration of colectomy should be taken 10 years after the diagnosis of ulcerative colitis in patients with pancolitis. After a 20-year disease interval, a stronger case for prophylactic colectomy can be made for patients, even in the absence of dysplasia. Colonic surveillance for dysplasia is an option favored by many clinicians, and it is most appropriate for patients with disease limited to the left colon or rectum and for patients with a short duration of disease. Any surveillance strategy that recommends colectomy based on histologic evidence of dysplasia will miss some patients with invasive cancer. The precise number of patients in this situation is unknown. If surveillance is the adopted strategy, then it is recommended that, in the absence of dysplasia, colonoscopy and multiple biopsies should be performed every 2 years until 20 years of disease. At 20 years of disease, surveillance colonoscopy should be performed annually.[91]

HEREDITARY COLORECTAL CANCER

It is estimated that up to 20% of patients with colorectal cancer may have some form of inherited susceptibility.[96] Hereditary colon cancer currently includes FAP and HNPCC. Although many of the clinical issues surrounding these syndromes are similar, each syndrome is considered separately because of differences in the genetics, in the phenotypic presentations, and in the accepted management strategy.

FAMILIAL ADENOMATOUS POLYPOSIS

FAP is a rare autosomal dominant inherited disease in which patients develop hundreds to thousands of adenomatous polyps. The clinical diagnosis is based on the histologic confirmation of at least 100 adenomas. These polyps are similar on histologic examination to sporadic adenomatous polyps and usually appear during the second or third decade of life.[97] The genetic cause of FAP is a mutation of the adenomatous polyposis coli (APC) gene located on chromosome 5 (5q21).[98] The genetic alterations found in patients with FAP are similar to those identified in sporadic colon cancer, except an APC mutation is present as a germline mutation.[99] Genetic tests for APC mutations are commercially available.

The obvious phenotypic appearance of FAP coupled with the fact that more than 90% of patients with FAP develop colon cancer by age 40 has helped to establish standard treatment for this disease.[100] Elective prophylactic colectomy is the current mainstay of therapy and has been performed for FAP since the 1930s. No trials have compared surgery with surveillance. The current recommendations for treatment of this genetic disorder include annual sigmoidoscopy beginning by age 10 years and prophylactic colectomy in the teen years or when colonic polyps are detected at endoscopy.[101] Patients that elect to have colectomy and ileorectal anastomosis face the risk of subsequently developing rectal cancer. Estimates of the risk of rectal cancer after subtotal colectomy vary widely and have been reported to be as high as 55% at 30 years. Patients with ileorectal anastomosis require lifelong endoscopic surveillance.

The choice of operations for patients with FAP includes proctocolectomy with ileostomy, proctocolectomy with ileal distal rectal anastomosis, and proctocolectomy with ileal-anal anastomosis. Each of these operations has strengths and weaknesses. Overall, these procedures are performed with low morbidity. The choice of operations should be tailored to patient preference and the experience of the operating surgeon.

FAP is associated with extracolonic manifestations of disease, which can include desmoid tumors and osteomas. Polyps may occur at other intestinal locations, and carcinomas of the upper intestine have been reported as the most common fatal malignancy in patients after prophylactic colectomy.[102] It is recommended that these patients undergo upper endoscopy every 6 months to 3 years starting by age 20.[101] Many agents, including sulindac, vitamin C, and indomethacin, have been investigated as chemopreventive agents. Although some agents have shown promise, none has been proven to be effective in reducing the number of polyps or the risk of cancer in FAP patients.[103]

HEREDITARY NONPOLYPOSIS COLORECTAL CANCER

HNPCC describes a clinical syndrome of colorectal cancer that occurs with early onset and in multiple family members. In contrast to FAP, HNPCC has no antecedent phenotype, and malignancy develops in the absence of adenomatosis of the colon and rectum. The expression of disease may be limited to the colorectum (Lynch syndrome I) or coexist with extracolonic tumors, typically endometrial cancer (Lynch syndrome II). Other associated malignancies include stomach, small intestine, hepatobiliary, pancreas, breast, ovary, brain, and skin cancers.[103–106]

In 1991, the International Collaborative Group on HNPCC established the minimum clinical criteria required to help identify families with HNPCC. The so-called Amsterdam criteria are: (1) colorectal cancer in three or more relatives, one of whom is the first-degree relative of the other two; (2) at least two generations of affected individuals with colorectal cancer; and (3) one or more of the cancers has been diagnosed before the age of 50. FAP must be excluded.[107] One genetic cause of the syndrome was identified in 1993. Peltomaki et al.[108] identified a locus on chromosome 2 that was linked to HNPCC in several families. The genetic basis of HNPCC has been identified as a germline mutation in one of a set of genes responsible for DNA mismatch repair.[109–113] Additional loci have since been identified. More than 90% of the identified mutations are in two genes, MSH2 (MutS homologue 2) and MLH1 (MutL homologue 1), located on chromosome 2p and 3p, respectively.[114] These genes are dominantly inherited, with a penetrance of approximately 90%. Consequently, gene carriers have a 90% likelihood of developing colorectal cancer.[115] Patients suspected of carrying an APC mutation can be tested for at least two mismatch repair gene mutations in commercial laboratories.

HNPCC gene carriers develop colorectal cancer at an average age of 45 years. These tumors occur more commonly in the right colon and tend to be more poorly differentiated.[116,117] Synchronous and metachronous cancers are frequent, and should a segmental colectomy be performed for a primary cancer, there is a 45% risk for a new primary cancer within 10 years.[115] Lynch and Smyrk[118] have reported that colonic polyps can be identified in up to 17% of first-degree relatives during colonoscopic screening. Adenomas are more likely to grow and progress to invasive cancer in this patient population than in the general population.[119,120]

The optimal management strategy for HNPCC gene carriers has yet to be established. Substantial evidence from uncontrolled studies suggests that surveillance colonoscopy and polypectomy are effective in reducing the risk of invasive cancer in these patients. Jarvinen et al.[120] reported a 62% decrease in the diagnosis of colorectal cancer in HNPCC patients in a screening program at a medium follow-up of 117 months compared with patients not followed by colonoscopy at 10 years. Bulow et al.[121] reported a decreased incidence of cancer and improved survival rate of patients with HNPCC who had surveillance and experiments compared with probands. Therefore, it has been recommended that surveillance colonoscopy be performed on gene carriers starting at age 20 and be repeated every 1 to 2 years. Patients older than 35 years of age should have annual colonoscopy.[115,122]

Currently, no consensus among experts has been reached regarding the role of prophylactic subtotal colectomy for patients with HNPCC.[115,123] Given the high penetrance of the disorder and the high rate of synchronous and metachronous disease among mutation carriers, a strong case can be made for prophylactic surgery in patients with this disease. A subtotal colectomy is currently the procedure of choice, and it can be performed with minimal morbidity and mortality. Patients who elect to undergo a subtotal colectomy require colonoscopic surveillance of the remaining rectum. Patients undergoing prophylactic surgery may still face the risk of extracolonic cancers. Patients electing not to consider prophylactic surgery must commit to lifelong surveillance, and should a colon cancer be detected, a subtotal colectomy is then indicated. No prospective clinical trials in patients with HNPCC have been conducted, and given our current understanding of the increased risk of colorectal and extracolonic malignancy in these patients, the suggested benefit of surveillance colonoscopy, and the low morbidity of prophylactic subtotal colectomy, either vigilant surveillance or prophylactic surgery are reasonable management strategies.

TESTICULAR CANCER AND CRYPTORCHIDISM

Cryptorchidism, or undescended testis, is characterized by absence of at least one testis in the scrotum and is the most common genitourinary disorder of childhood. Approximately 3% of children born at full term and up to 30% of children born prematurely will have an undescended testis.[124] A well-known but poorly understood association has been made between cryptorchidism and testicular cancer. In 1929, Cooper[125] noted that the longer a testis remained cryptorchid and the higher the testis lay from the scrotum, the more likely it was to be histologically abnormal. The reported risk for malignancy in cryptorchidism is 48.9 per 100,000, which is more than 20 times the risk of testicular cancer in the general population.[126] It has been estimated that approximately 10% of testicular tumors arise from an undescended testis.[127]

Either orchiopexy in association with observation or observation alone is recommended for patients with cryptorchidism. There are multiple reasons for correcting an undescended testis in a child, including the desire to correct a visible defect, to prevent psychological problems associated with the defect, to enhance the possibility of future fertility, and to place the testis in a site where it can be easily examined. Correction of an undescended testicle may be achieved using hormonal therapy or surgery. Most experts agree that this should be accomplished as early as 12 months of age.[128]

It is not clear that correction of an undescended testicle alters the risk of developing testicular cancer. Reports in the literature conflict regarding the protective effects of correcting cryptorchidism, and virtually no information is available on patients who had an undescended testicle corrected at younger than 2 years of age.[129–131] Most reports are population-based case-controlled studies. It is known that patients with unilateral cryptorchidism have been found to have an increased risk of testicular cancer in both the undescended and the normally descended testis.[132,133]

Management of an undescended testis in a postpubertal patient population has been extensively addressed by Farrer et al.[133] These authors completed a statistical analysis that compared the estimated risk of death from a germ cell testis tumor in patients with cryptorchidism to the risk of death from an orchiectomy. They concluded that the risk of death from orchiectomy is greater than the risk of death from testicular cancer in patients older than 32 years of age. The authors recommended that orchiectomy be considered only for patients younger than 32 years with postpubertal unilateral cryptorchidism.[133] Other experts recommend orchiopexy or observation in older patients, depending on patient preference and assuming the testicle is palpable.[134] General agreement exists that a nonpalpable undescended testicle should be removed.

REFERENCES

1. Winawer SJ, Zauber AG, Ho MN, et al. Prevention of colorectal cancer by colonoscopic polypectomy. *N Engl J Med* 1993:329:1977.
2. Marsh DJ, Leagroyd DL, Robinson BG. Medullary thyroid carcinoma: recent advances and management update. *Thyroid* 1995;5:407.
3. Mulligan LM, Kwok JBJ, Healey CS, et al. Germ-line mutations of the RET proto-oncogene in multiple endocrine neoplasia type 2A. *Nature* 1993;363:458.
4. Donis-Keller H, Dou S, Chi D, et al. Mutations in the RET proto-oncogene are associated with MEN 2A and FMTC. *Hum Mol Genet* 1993;2:851.
5. Wells SA Jr, Chi DD, Toshima K, et al. Predictive DNA testing and prophylactic thyroidectomy in patients at risk for multiple endocrine endoplasia type 2A. *Ann Surg* 1994;220:237.
6. Kebebew E, Tresler PA, Siperstein AE, et al. Normal thyroid pathology in patients undergoing thyroidectomy for finding a RET gene germ line mutation: a report of three cases and review of the literature. *Thyroid* 1999;9:127.
7. Decker RA, Geiger JD, Cox CE, et al. Prophylactic surgery for multiple endocrine neoplasia type IIA after genetic diagnosis: is parathyroid transplantation indicated? *World J Surg* 1996;20:814.
8. Iascone C, DeMeester TR, Little AG, Skinner DB. Barrett's esophagus: functional assessments, proposed pathogenesis and surgical therapy. *Arch Surg* 1983;118:543.
9. Gillen P, Keeling P, Byrne PJ, Hemmess JPJ. Barrett's esophagus: profile. *Br J Surg* 1987;74:774.
10. Vaaezi MF, Richter JC. Role of acid and duodenal-gastroesophageal reflux in gastroesophageal reflux disease. *Gastroenterology* 1996;111:1192.
11. Fiorucli S, Santucci L, Farroni F, Peli MA, Movelli A. Effect of omeprazole on gastroesophageal reflux in Barrett's esophagus. *Am J Gastroenterol* 1989;84:1263.
12. Dent J, Holloway RH, Toouli J, Dodds WJ. Mechanism of lower esophageal sphincter incompetence in patients with symptomatic gastroesophageal reflux. *Gut* 1988;29:1020.
13. Antonioli DA, Wang HH. Morphology of Barrett's esophagus and Barrett's associated dysplasia and adenocarcinoma. *Gastroenterol Clin North Am* 1997;26:495.
14. Cameron AJ, Zinsmeister AR, Ballard DJ, et al. Prevalence of columnar-lined esophagus, comparison of population-based clinical and autopsy findings. *Gastroenterology* 1990;99:918.
15. Cameron AJ, Kamath PS, Carpenter HE. Barrett's esophagus: the prevalence of short and long segments in reflux patients. *Gastroenterology* 1996;108:A65.
16. Johnston MH, Hammond AS, Lasker W, et al. The prevalence and clinical characteristics of short segments of specialized intestinal metaplasia in the distal esophagus on routine endoscopy. *Am J Gastroenterol* 1996;91:1507.
17. Nandurkar S, Ng T, Adams S, et al. Short segment Barrett's esophagus: prevalence, diagnosis and association. *Gastroenterology* 1996;110:A27.
18. Heies SK, Seif F, Webber S, et al. Short segment Barrett's esophagus: clinical and histologic findings. *Gastroenterology* 1996;99:110:A132.
19. Cameron AJ. Management of Barrett's esophagus. *Mayo Clin Proc* 1998;73:457.
20. Clark GWB, Ireland AP, Peters JH, et al. Short segment Barrett's esophagus: a prevalent complication of gastroesophageal reflux disease with malignant potential. *J Gastrointest Surg* 1997;1:113.
21. Sharma P, Movales TG, Samplings RE. Short segment Barrett's esophagus—the need for standardization of the definition of endoscopic criteria. *Am J Gastroenterol* 1998;93:1033.
22. Tytgat GN. Does endoscopic surveillance in esophageal columnar metaplasia have any real value? *Endoscopy* 1995;27:19.
23. Spechler SJ. Barrett's esophagus. *Semin Oncol* 1994;21:431.
24. Dent J, Bremner CG, Collon MJ, et al. Working party report to the world congress of gastroenterology: Barrett's esophagus. *J Gastroenterol Hepatol* 1991;6:1.
25. Hameeteman W, Tatgat GN, Houthoff HJ, et al. Barrett's esophagus: development of dysplasia and adenocarcinoma. *Gastroenterology* 1989;96:1249.
26. Levine DS, Haggitt RC, Irvine S, et al. Natural history of high grade dysplasia in Barrett's esophagus. *Gastroenterology* 1996;110:A550.
27. Levine DS, Haggin RC, Radinovitch PS, et al. Complete regression of high grade dysplasia, DNA content abnormalities, and Barrett's esophagus. *Gastroenterology* 1995;108:A496.
28. Provenzale D, Kemp A, Arora S, et al. A guide for surveillance of patients with Barrett's esophagus. *Am J Gastroenterol* 1994;89:670.
29. Gore S, Healey CJ, Sutton R, et al. Regression of columnar-lined esophagus with continuous omeprazole therapy. *Aliment Pharmacol Ther* 1993;7:623.
30. Galmiche JP, Dumas R, Boyer J, et al. Long-term omeprazole effects on Barrett's mucosa. *Gastroenterology* 1993;104:A85.
31. DeMeester SR, DeMeester TR. The diagnosis and management of Barrett's esophagus. *Adv Surg* 1999;33:29.
32. DeMeester TR. The surgical treatment of dysplasia and adenocarcinoma. *Gastroenterol Clin North Am* 1997;26:669.
33. Levine DS, Hagg HRC, Blount PL, et al. An endoscopic biopsy protocol can differentiate high grade dysplasia from early adenocarcinoma in Barrett's esophagus. *Gastroenterology* 1993;105:40.
34. Levine DS. Management of dysplasia in the columnar-lined esophagus. *Gastroenterol Clin North Am* 1997;26:613.
35. Naunheim KS. Barrett's esophagus. In: Cameron JL, ed. *Current surgical therapy.* St. Louis: Mosby, 1998:62.
36. Newman B, Austin MA, Lee M, King MC. Inheritance of breast cancer: evidence for autosomal dominant transmission in high risk families. *Proc Natl Acad Sci U S A* 1988;85:3044.
37. Hall JM, Lee MK, Newana B, et al. Linkage of early asset breast cancer to chromosome 17q21. *Science* 1990;250:1684.
38. Miki Y, Swensen J, Shattuck E, et al. A strong candidate for the breast and ovarian cancer susceptibility gene BRCA1. *Science* 1994;226:66.
39. Ford D, Easton DF, Stratton M, et al. Genetic heterogenicity and penetrance analysis of the BRCA1 and BRCA2 genes in breast cancer families. *Am J Hum Genet* 1998;62:676.
40. Strauewing JP, Hartge P, Waholder S, et al. The risk of cancer associated with specific mutation of BRCA1 and BRCA2 among Ashkenazi Jews. *N Engl J Med* 1997;336:1401.
41. Easton DF, Ford D, Bishop DT, et al. Breast and ovarian cancer incidence in BRCA1 mutation carriers. *Am J Hum Genet* 1995;56:265.
42. Wooster R, Bignell G, Lancaster J, et al. Identification of the breast cancer susceptibility gene BRCA2. *Nature* 1995;378:789.
43. Phelum CM, Lancaster JM, Tonin P, et al. Mutational analysis of BRCS2 gene in 49 site specific breast cancer families. *Nat Genet* 1996;13:120.
44. Tavtigian SV, Simard J, Rommens J, et al. The BRCA2 gene and mutation in chromosome 12q-linked kindreds. *Nat Genet* 1996;12:333.
45. Burke W, Daly M, Garber J, et al. Recommendations for follow-up care of individuals with an inherited predisposition to cancer. II. BRCA1 and BRCA2. Cancer Genetics Studies Consortium. *JAMA* 1997;277:997.
46. Thomas DB, Gao DE, Self SQ, et al. Randomized trial of breast self examination in Shanghai: methodology and preliminary results. *J Natl Cancer Inst* 1997;89:355.
47. Miller AB, Baines CJ, Turnball C. The role of the nurse examiner in the National breast screening study. *Can J Public Health* 1991;82:162.
48. Campbell HS, Fletcher SW, Liu S, et al. Improving physicians and nurses clinical breast examination. *Am J Prev Med* 1991;7:1.
49. Kerlikowske E, Grady D, Rubin SM, et al. Efficacy of screening mammography: a meta-analysis. *JAMA* 1995;273:149.
50. Elwood JM, Cox B, Richardson AK. The effectiveness of breast cancer screening by mammography in younger women. *Online J Curr Clin Trials* 1993;32:93.
51. Eckhardt S, Badellino F, Murphy GP. Breast cancer screening in pre menopausal women in developed countries. *Int J Cancer* 1994;56:1.
52. Smart CR, Hendrick RE, Rutledge JH, Smith RA. Benefit of mammography in women ages 40 to 49 years current evidence from randomized trials. *Cancer* 1995;75:1619.
53. Eldar S, Meguid MM, Beatty JD. Cancer of the breast after prophylactic subcutaneous mastectomy. *Am J Surg* 1984;148:6932.
54. Goodnight JE, Quagliana JM, Monton DL. Failure of subcutaneous mastectomy to prevent the development of breast cancer. *J Surg Oncol* 1984;26:198.
55. Ziegler LD, Kroll SS. Primary breast cancer after prophylactic mastectomy. *Am J Clin Oncol* 1991;14:451.
56. Hartmann LC, Schaid DJ, Woods JE, et al. Efficacy of bilateral prophylactic mastectomy in women with a family history of breast cancer. *N Engl J Med* 1999;340:77.
57. Robson M, Levin D, Federici M, et al. Breast conservation therapy for invasive breast cancer in Ashkenazi women with BRCA gene founder mutations. *J Natl Cancer Inst* 1999;91:2112.
58. Grann VR, Pamageas KS, Whang W, et al. Decision analysis of prophylactic mastectomy and oophorectomy in BRCA1 or BRCA2 position patients. *J Clin Oncol* 1998;16:979.
59. Schrage D, Kuntz KM, Gardaz JE, Weeks JC. Decision analysis—effects of prophylactic mastectomy and oophorectomy a life expectancy among women with BRCA1 or BRCA2 mutations. *N Engl J Med* 1997;336:1465.
60. Anderson JA. Lobular carcinoma *in situ* of the breast: an approach to rational treatment. *Cancer* 1977;39:2597.
61. Page SL, Kidd TE Jr, Puport UD, et al. Lobular neoplasia of the breast: higher risk for subsequent invasive cancer predicted by more extensive disease. *Hum Pathol* 1991;22:1232.

62. Fryberg ER, Bland KI. *In situ* breast carcinoma. *Adv Surg* 1993;26:29.
63. Wheeler JE, Enterline HT, Roreman JM, et al. Lobular carcinoma *in situ* of the breast: long term follow up. *Cancer* 1974;34:554.
64. Rosen PP, Kosloff C, Lieberman PH, et al. Lobular carcinoma *in situ* of the breast. Detailed analysis of 99 patients with average follow up of 24 years. *Am J Surg Pathol* 1978;3:225.
65. Bodian CA, Perizin KH, Luttes R. Lobular neoplasia long-term risk of breast cancer and related to other forms. *Cancer* 1996;78:1024.
66. Bradley SJ, Weaver DW, Bouwman DE. Alternatives on the surgical management of *in situ* breast cancer. A meta analysis of outcome. *Am Surg* 1990;56:428.
67. Fisher B, Costantino JP, Wickerham DE, et al. Tamoxifen for the prevention of breast cancer: report of the National Surgical Adjuvant Breast and Bowel Project P-1 study. *J Natl Cancer Inst* 1998;90:1271.
68. Ford D, Easton DF, Bishop DT, et al. Risks of cancer in BRCA1 mutation carriers. Breast cancer linkage consortium. *Lancet* 1994;363:692.
69. Ford D, Easton DF. The genetics of breast and ovarian cancer. *Br J Cancer* 1995;72:805.
70. NIH Consensus Development Panel on Ovarian Cancer. Ovarian cancer: screening, treatment, and follow up. *JAMA* 1995;273:491.
71. American College of Obstetricians and Gynecologists committee on quality assessment. ACOQ criteria set for prophylactic bilateral oophorectomy to prevent epithelial carcinoma. *Int J Gynecol Obstet* 1996;52:101.
72. Tobarman JK, Greene MH, Tucker MA, et al. Intraabdominal carcinomatosis after prophylactic oophorectomy in ovarian cancer prone families. *Lancet* 1982;2:795.
73. Struewing JP, Watson P, Easton DF, et al. Prophylactic oophorectomy in inherited breast/ovarian cancer families. *J Natl Cancer Inst Monogr* 1995;17:33.
74. Rebbeck TR, Levin AM, Eisen A, et al. Breast cancer risk after bilateral prophylactic oophorectomy in BRCA1 mutation carriers. *J Natl Cancer Inst* 1999;91:1475.
75. Stonnington CM, Phillips SF, Melton LJ III, Zinsmeister AR. Chronic ulcerative colitis: incidence and prevalence in a community. *Gut* 1997;28:402.
76. Langhel B, Munlcholm P, Neilsen GH, et al. Incidence and prevalence of ulcerative colitis in Copenhagen County from 1962 to 1987. *Scand J Gastroenterol* 1991;26:1247.
77. Kitalosa T, Ulsunomiya T, Yakota A. Epidemiological study of ulcerative colitis in Japan: incidence and familial occurrence. *J Gastroenterol* 1995;30[Suppl 8]:5.
78. Devroede GJ, Taylor UF, Saucer WG, et al. Cancer risk and life expectancy of children with ulcerative colitis. *N Engl J Med* 1971;285:17.
79. Ekbom A, Helmick CG, Zack M, Adam HO. Extra colonic malignancies in inflammatory bowel disease. *Cancer* 1991;67:2015.
80. Eekbom A, Helmick CG, Zack M, et al. Survival and causes of death in patients with inflammatory bowel disease. A population based study. *Gastroenterology* 1992;103:954.
81. Bonnevie O, Binder V, Anthonisen P, Riis P. The prognoses of ulcerative colitis. *Scand J Gastroenterol* 1974;9:81.
82. Langholtz E, Munkholm P, Davidsen M, Binder V. Colorectal cancer and mortality in patients with ulcerative colitis. *Gastroenterology* 1992;103:1444.
83. Kornbluth A, Sachar DB. Ulcerative colitis practice guidelines in adults. *Am J Gastroenterol* 1997;92:204.
84. Lennard-Jones JE, Melville DM, Moison BC, et al. Precancer and cancer in extensive colitis: findings among 401 patients over 22 years. *Gut* 1990;31:800.
85. Ekbom A, Helmick C, Zack M, et al. Ulcerative colitis and colorectal cancer: a population-based study. *N Engl J Med* 1990;323:1228.
86. Devroede G. Risk of cancer in inflammatory bowel disease. In: Winawer SJ, Schottenfeld D, Sherlock P, eds. *Colorectal cancer: prevention, epidemiology, and screening.* New York: Raven Press, 1980;325.
87. Gyde S, Prior P, Dew MJ, et al. Mortality in ulcerative colitis. *Gastroenterol* 1982;83(Pt 1):36.
88. SSAT, AGA, ASCD, ASGE, AHPBA Consensus Panel. Ulcerative colitis and colon carcinoma: epidemiology surveillance, diagnosis and treatment. *J Gastroenterol Surg* 1998;2:305.
89. Bernstein CN, Shanahan F, Weinstein WM. Are we telling patients the truth about surveillance colonoscopy in ulcerative colitis? *Lancet* 1994;343:71.
90. Connell UR, Lennard-Jones JE, William CB, et al. Factory affecting the outcome of endoscopic surveillance for cancer in ulcerative colitis. *Gastroenterology* 1994;107:934.
91. Bernstein CN. How do we assess the values of surveillance techniques in ulcerative colitis? *J Gastroenterol Intest Surg* 1998;2:318.
92. Ranshoff DF, Riddell RH, Levin B. Ulcerative colitis and colonic cancer problems in assessing the diagnostic usefulness of mucosal dysplasia. *Dis Colon Rectum* 1985;28:383.
93. Taylor BA, Pembertory JH, Carpenter HA, et al. Dysplasia in chronic ulcerative colitis. implications for surveillance. *Dis Colon Rectum* 1992;35:950.
94. Lennard-Jones JE. Is colonoscopic cancer surveillance in ulcerative colitis essential for every patient? *Eur J Cancer* 1995;31A(7–8):1178.
95. Mcleod RS. Chronic colitis. In: Cameron JL, ed. *Current surgical therapy.* St. Louis. Mosby, 1998:179.
96. Peterson SM, Brensinger JD, Johnson KA, Giardiello FM. Genetic testing and counseling for hereditary form of colorectal cancer. *Cancer* 1999;86[Suppl]:2540.
97. Kinzler KW, Vogelstein B. Colorectal tumors. In: *The genetic bases of human cancers.* New York: McGraw-Hill, 1998:565.
98. Kinzler KW, Nilbert MC, Su LK, et al. Identification of FAP locus genes from chromosome 5q21. *Science* 1991;253:661.
99. Powell SM. Clinical application of molecular genetics in colorectal cancer. *Semin Colon Rectal Surg* 1995;6:2.
100. Lindor NM, Greene MH. The cancer handbook of family cancer syndromes. Mayo familial cancer program. *J Natl Cancer Inst* 1998;90:1039.
101. Tardiman JP, Conrad PG, Sleisenger MH. Gastric testing in hereditary colorectal cancer: indication and procedures. *Am J Gastroenterol* 1999;94:2344.
102. Spigelman AD, Williams CB, Talbot IC, et al. Upper gastrointestinal cancer in patients with familial adenomatous polyposes. *Lancet* 1989;2:783.
103. Hawk E, Lubet R, Limburg P. Chemoprevention in hereditary colorectal cancer syndromes. *Cancer* 1999;86[Suppl]:2551.
104. Lynch HT, Lynch PM, Pestar J, Fusaro RM. The cancer family syndrome: rare cutaneous phenotypic linkage of Toss's syndrome. *Arch Intern Med* 1981;141:607.
105. Vasen HFA, Offerhaus GJA, den Hartog Jager FCA, et al. The tumor spectrum in hereditary nonpolyposis colorectal cancer: a study of 24 kindreds in the Netherlands. *Int J Cancer* 1990;46:31.
106. Lynch HT, Smyrk TC, Watson P, et al. Genetics, natural history, tumor spectrum, and pathology of hereditary nonpolyposis colorectal cancer: an updated review. *Gastroenterology* 1993;104:1535.
107. Watson P, Lynch HT. Extracolonic cancer in hereditary nonpolyposis colorectal cancer. *Cancer* 1993;71:677.
108. Vasen HF, Mecklin JP, Khan PM, Lynch HT. The international collaborative group on hereditary nonpolyposis colorectal cancer: an international cooperative study of 165 families. *Dis Colon Rectum* 1993;36:1.
109. Peltomaki P, Aaltonen LA, Sistenen P, et al. Genetic mapping of a locus predisposing to human colorectal cancer. *Science* 1993;290:610.
110. Fishel R, Lescoe MK, Rao MR, et al. The human mutator gene homolog MSH2 and its association with hereditary nonpolyposis colon cancer. *Cell* 1993;75:1027.
111. Leach FS, Nicolaides NC, Papadopoulos N, et al. Mutation of a mut S homolog in hereditary nonpolyposis colorectal cancers. *Cell* 1993;75:215.
112. Bronner CE, Baker SM, Mossison PT, et al. Mutation in the DNA mismatched repair gene homologous hMLH1 is associated with hereditary nonpolyposis colon cancer. *Nature* 1994;368:258.
113. Nicolaides NC, Papadopoulos N, Liu B, et al. Mutation of two PMS homologous in hereditary nonpolyposis colon cancer. *Nature* 1994;371:75.
114. Miyaki M, Konishi M, Tanaka K, et al. Germline mutations of MSH6 on the cancer of hereditary nonpolyposis colorectal cancer. *Nat Genet* 1997;17:271.
115. Peltomaki P, Vasen HF. Mutations predisposing to hereditary nonpolyposis colorectal cancer. Data and results of a collaborative study. The international collaborative group or hereditary nonpolyposis colorectal cancer. *Gastroenterology* 1997;113:140.
116. Lynch HT. Is there a role for prophylactic subtotal colectomy among hereditary nonpolyposis colorectal cancer germ line mutation carriers? *Dis Colon Rectum* 1996;39:109.
117. Jass JR, Smyrk TC, Stewart SM, et al. Pathology of hereditary nonpolyposis colorectal cancers. *Anticancer Res* 1994;14:1631.
118. Merklin JT, Jarvinen H. Treatment and follow-up strategies in hereditary nonpolyposis colorectal carcinomas. *Dis Colon Rectum* 1993;36:927.
119. Lynch HT, Smyrk T. Hereditary nonpolyposis colorectal cancer (Lynch syndrome): an updated review. *Cancer* 1996;78:1149.
120. Kinzler KW, Vogelstein B. Lessons from hereditary colorectal cancer. *Cell* 1996;87:159.
121. Jarvinen HJ, Mecklin JP, Sistonen P. Screening reduces colorectal cancer in hereditary nonpolyposis colorectal cancer families. *Gastroenterology* 1995;108:1405.
122. Bulow S, Bulow C, Nielson TF, et al. Centralized registration results in improved prognosis in familial adenomatosis polyposis. *Scand J Gastroenterol* 1995;30:989.
123. Burtz W, Peterson G, Lynch HT, et al. Recommendation for follow-up care for individuals with an inherited predisposition to cancer. Hereditary nonpolyposis colon cancer. *JAMA* 1997;277:915.
124. Rodriguez-Bigas MA. Prophylactic colectomy for gene carriers in hereditary nonpolyposis colorectal cancer. Has the time come? *Cancer* 1996;78:199.
125. Scorer CG. The descent of the testis. *Arch Dis Child* 1964;39:605.
126. Cooper ER. The histology of the retained testis in the human subject at different sizes and its comparison with the testis. *J Anat* 1929;64:5.
127. Gill B, Kogan S. Cryptorchidism: current concepts. *Pediatr Clin North Am* 1997;44:1211.
128. Abratt RP, Reddi VB, Sarembock LA. Testicular cancer and cryptorchidism. *Br J Urol* 1992;70:656.
129. Action Committee Report of the Urology Section, American Academy of Pediatrics. Timing of elective surgery on the genitalia of male children with particular reference to the risks, benefits and psychological effects of surgery and anesthesia. *Pediatrics* 1997;97:590.
130. United Kingdom Testicular Cancer Study Group. A etiology of testicular cancer association with congenital abnormalities, age of puberty, infertility and exercise. *BMJ* 1994;308:1393.
131. Pike MC, Chilvers C, Peckham MIIJ. Effects of age at orchiopexy on risk of testicular cancer. *Lancet* 1986;1:1246.
132. Depue RH, Pike MC, Henderson BE. Cryptorchidism and testicular cancer. *J Natl Cancer Inst* 1986;77:830.
133. Chilvers C, Pike MC. Epidemiology of undescended testis. In: Oliver RTD, Blandy JP, Hope-Stone HF, eds. *Urological and genital cancer.* Oxford: Blackwell Science, 1989:306.
134. Farrer JH, Walker AH, Rajfer J. Management of the post-pubertal cryptorchid testis: a statistical review. *J Urol* 1985;134:1071.
135. Rajfer J. Congenital anomalies of the testis and scrotum. In: Walsh PC, Retik AB, Vaughan ED, Wein AJ, eds. *Campbell's urology.* Philadelphia: WB Saunders, 1998;2172.

Barbara K. Rimer
Joellen Schildkraut
Robert A. Hiatt

CHAPTER **25**

Cancer Screening

The goal of cancer screening is a very practical one—to detect cancer at an early stage when it is treatable and curable. However, the reality is quite complex. For a screening test to be useful, the test or procedure should detect cancer earlier than would occur otherwise *and* there should be evidence that earlier diagnosis results in an improved outcome.[1] Advances in genetics and molecular biology herald the era when it may be possible to detect cancer at earlier and earlier stages along the carcinogenesis pathway. Because of this progress, the line between prevention and screening may narrow further. Moreover, screening will be used to detect susceptibility as well as early markers of disease. Yet, in spite of the promises of molecular diagnostics, screening still must be evaluated according to its present reality, which is to detect asymptomatic disease when it is potentially curable.

The purpose of this chapter is to provide an overview of cancer screening—what it is, key terms, measures of effectiveness, and consequences. We also review briefly the status of screening for several prevalent cancers (breast, cervical, skin, prostate, colorectal, and lung). The recommendations are for the general population, but not for people with identified mutations in cancer susceptibility genes. Currently, no randomized clinical trial data are available to guide practice in this area. However, the Cancer Genetics Studies Consortium, sponsored by the National Human Genome Research Institute, issued provisional recommendations for individuals who are known to carry the breast cancer gene mutations *BRCA1* or *BRCA2*.[2] Generally, it is recommended that people with these and other relevant mutations (e.g., *HNPCC*, *p53*) be screened at an earlier age, and more frequently, for the cancers to which they are predisposed.

This chapter cannot provide comprehensive information on any of the cancer sites reviewed, because the literature for each is vast. Rather, the chapter provides a succinct summary of the field and a perspective for clinicians to use in determining the efficacy of particular screening tests. Several texts provide good overviews of the issues related to screening for specific kinds of cancer.[3] The National Cancer Institute's (NCI) Physician Data Query (PDQ) [World Wide Web site http://cancernet.nci.nih.gov/pdq.htm] also is an excellent source for the latest data on the specific screening tests discussed here.

WHAT IS CANCER SCREENING?

Appropriate cancer screening should lead to the early detection of asymptomatic or unrecognized disease by the application of acceptable, inexpensive tests or examinations in a large number of persons.[4,5] The results of a screening test should then be applied expeditiously to separate apparently well persons who probably have disease from those who probably do not. The main objective of cancer screening is to reduce the morbidity and mortality from a particular cancer among the persons screened. The screening procedure itself is not diagnostic, and positive or suspicious findings must be evaluated further to determine diagnosis and appropriate treatment. Characteristics that distinguish screening tests from diagnostic tests are listed in Table 25-1.

Several characteristics make particular cancers suitable for screening. These include (1) substantial morbidity and mortality; (2) a high prevalence in a detectable preclinical state; (3) the possibility of effective and improved treatment because of early detection; and (4) the availability of a good screening test with high sensitivity and specificity, low cost, and little inconvenience and discomfort. Although there are more than 100 different cancers, most of them lack proven screening interventions. Only cancers of the breast, cervix, skin, colon-rectum, prostate, and

TABLE 25-1. Characteristics of Screening Tests Versus Diagnostic Tests

Screening	*Diagnosis*
Applied to asymptomatic groups	Applied to symptomatic individuals
Lower cost per test	Higher cost; all necessary tests applied to identify disease
Lower yield per test	Higher probability of case detection
Lower adverse consequences of error	Failure to identify true positives can delay treatment and worsen prognosis

TABLE 25-2. Definitions of Criteria for Evaluating a Screening Test

	Truth (Diagnostic Classification)	
Screening Test Results	Cancer Present	Cancer Absent
Positive	TP	FP
Negative	FN	TN
Sensitivity = TP/TP + FN × 100		
Specificity = TN/FP + TN × 100		
PV+ = TP/TP + FP × 100		
PV– = TN/TN + FN × 100		
Accuracy = TP + TN/TP + TN + FP + FN × 100		

FN, false-negative (number of subjects with cancer who are incorrectly classified as cancer-free by the test); FP, false-positive (number of cancer-free subjects who are incorrectly classified as having cancer by the test); TN, true-negative (number of cancer-free subjects who are correctly classified by the test); TP, true-positive (number of subjects with cancer who are correctly classified by the test).

testes have widely accepted screening interventions,[6] and there is controversy over some aspects of each. Only breast, cervical, and colorectal screening have met the rigorous criteria of the U.S. Preventive Services Task Force.[7]

The benefits of the investment in cancer screening occur over many years.[8] Cancer screening affords both benefits and disadvantages; therefore, it is important to evaluate the effectiveness of screening programs by specifying criteria to meet the program's objectives. For screening to be a benefit, treatment given during the detectable preclinical phase must result in a better prognosis than therapy given after symptoms develop, thereby possibly requiring less radical treatment. Cervical cancer is a good example of a disease with a preclinical phase that can be detected in a preinvasive stage, in this case, using the Papanicolaou (Pap) smear.[9] Finally, there are economic costs associated with cancer screening, and these should be evaluated before a cancer screening test is recommended on a population basis.

EVALUATION OF A SCREENING TEST

In the evaluation of a screening test, it is essential to answer questions concerning the test's ability to accurately predict the presence or absence of disease. If the test is *abnormal*, what are the chances that disease is present? If the test result is *normal*, what are the chances that the disease is absent? The validity of a screening test is measured by its ability to classify correctly those persons who have preclinical disease as test-positive and those without the preclinical disease as test-negative.

Sensitivity and *specificity* address the validity of the test. Sensitivity is the probability of testing positive if the disease is truly present. As the sensitivity of the test increases, the number of persons with the disease who are classified as test-negative (false-negative) decreases. Specificity is the probability of screening negative if the disease is truly absent. A highly specific test rarely is positive in the absence of disease and therefore results in a lower proportion of persons without disease who are incorrectly classified as test-positive (false-positive). Two measures that directly address the estimation of probability of disease are the *positive predictive value* (PV+) and the *negative predictive value* (PV–). The PV+ is an estimate of the accuracy of the test in predicting the presence of disease, and the PV– is an estimate of the accuracy of the test in predicting the absence of disease. The predictive value is a function of the sensitivity, specificity, and prevalence of disease. The *accuracy* of a test is a measure of the percent of all results that are true results, whether positive or negative, or the total correct test results. Table 25-2 summarizes the relationship between results of a screening test and the actual presence of disease as determined by an appropriate diagnostic test.

Sources of bias are of particular importance in the evaluation of a screening program. People who choose to participate in screening programs (volunteers) are likely to be different from the general population in ways that pertain to survival; thus, *volunteer bias* is a concern.[4] *Lead-time bias* is defined as the interval between diagnosis of disease at screening and when it would have been detected due to the development of symptoms.[4] If lead-time bias is not taken into account, survival may appear to be erroneously increased among screen-detected cases as compared to unscreened cases. Finally, *length bias* is the overrepresentation among screen-detected cases of those with a long preclinical period (thus less rapidly fatal), leading to the incorrect conclusion that screening was beneficial.[4]

MEASURES OF EFFECTIVENESS

Several measures have been used to judge the effectiveness of screening. The most definitive measure of the efficacy of a breast cancer screening program and least subject to bias is breast cancer mortality as determined by the comparison of screened and unscreened groups in a randomized clinical trial.[4,10] There are excellent epidemiology texts[4,11] and reviews[10] that discuss the measures in more detail than can be presented here.

Other outcome measures have been proposed, including case finding and survival. Each has limitations. The problem with case finding is that it is subject to lead-time bias. Survival may appear to have been advanced, but only because cancer is found earlier in the screened group.[11] Because of length bias, screening may appear effective, but in fact, it has not made a difference in mortality; slow-growing cancers may contribute to the apparent success of the screened group. Thus, length bias limits the value of survival data as outcome measures. Survival, in itself, does not establish that the natural history of the disease has been altered or that mortality has been reduced.[12]

Another potential outcome is improved quality of life (QOL).[13] However, none of the international breast cancer screening trials have good QOL data. These data are being collected as part of the NCI's Prostate, Lung, Colorectal, Ovarian Cancer (PLCO) screening trial. This is an important area for further exploration and, in future trials, QOL should be measured. Cost per quality-adjusted life-years saved would be a good measure, but it has been used rarely.[14] QOL may include a reduction in psychologic morbidity for a woman and her family.[15] QOL also may be enhanced by providing better or more acceptable treatment choices. For example, Tabar and colleagues[16] have argued that even if mammography does not reduce breast cancer mortality for women in their 40s, it may be beneficial because it avoids disfiguring and debilitating surgery. And de Koning and colleagues[17] showed that breast cancer screening could reduce health care costs and improve QOL by preventing advanced disease, which also could be true for cervical and colorectal cancer screening. However, Harris[18] has expressed concern that a woman's QOL could be diminished by living longer with breast cancer.

In assessing the effectiveness of screening technologies, the randomized clinical trial (RCT) has been the gold standard. It is the most powerful methodology for demonstrating the value of screening in comparison to an unscreened group.[19] RCTs overcome the biases inherent in other designs. The RCT with the end point of mortality avoids the two most important biases noted earlier, lead-time and length bias,[19] as well as selection bias and overdiagnosis.[20] However, case-control studies also can provide useful information, and at less cost than RCTs, and may be used to supplement RCT data. In addition, increasingly sophisticated statistical modeling techniques may be appropriate to assess the impact of screening, especially in situations where large RCTs cannot be conducted. The U.S. Preventive Services Task Force,[7] the PDQ system,[21] and others have ranked levels of evidence; the RCT is uniformly regarded as the highest level of evidence.

POSITIVE AND NEGATIVE CONSEQUENCES OF SCREENING

Every medical activity has positive and negative consequences, and screening is no exception. The benefits include (1) improved prognosis for those with screen-detected cancers, (2) the possibility of less radical treatment, (3) reassurance for those with negative test results, and (4) resource savings if treatment costs are reduced because of less radical diagnosis. The optimal outcome is a reduction in cancer mortality. The assumption is that screening can detect cancer when it is early and curable, if cancer is present, or indicate that cancer is not present, if that indeed is the case. But because no medical test is perfect, there are several potential negative consequences of screening that also must be considered. These include the economic and psychologic consequences of false-positives[22–26] and false-negatives,[27,28] the potential for overdiagnosis,[29–32] the potential carcinogenic effects of screening, and the labeling phenomenon.

Screening in the community usually means that many people will require additional tests for what will later be recognized as false-positives.[33] This is one of the predictable costs of cancer screening. A consideration of the negative consequences of screening is essential,[34] because screening is offered to presumably healthy people.[8,11] The negative consequences should not override the potential benefits. However, accumulating evidence in the area of breast cancer screening suggests that although there are negative psychologic consequences of abnormal test results, they appear to be relatively short-lived.[35] On the plus side, abnormal results may increase the likelihood that women will be screened in the future.[24,36,37] However, the data regarding negative psychological consequences are still sparse and related primarily to breast cancer. More data are needed in other areas, such as colorectal cancer screening. Overdiagnosis is an important area that has not been well studied. As understanding of cancer biology increases, it will become easier to classify overdiagnosis.

For all kinds of cancer screening, physicians should engage patients in discussions of the risks and benefits of cancer screening. Because most people overestimate the risks for certain types of cancers (e.g., breast),[38] they may inflate both the need for screening and the potential benefits.[39] For some cancers, such as colorectal cancer, people may underestimate their personal susceptibility and may need encouragement to consider screening, with both the positive and negative consequences. In the case of prostate cancer, where the evidence is still equivocal and population-based screening is not recommended, it is especially important that men understand the limitations of screening.[40] Harris[39] encouraged that screening discussions begin with the possible outcomes of screening, making sure the patient's information is accurate. Then, the physician should define and clarify the patient's perceptions and values. Together, the patient and physician then weigh the benefits of screening versus the costs and benefits. This has been called *shared decision making*.[41]

Austoker[42] outlined the topics that should be included when helping patients to make informed decisions about cancer screening. These include the purpose of screening; the likelihood of positive and negative findings and the possibility of false-positive or false-negative results; the uncertainties and risks involved; any significant medical, social, or financial implications of screening; and follow-up plans.

BREAST CANCER SCREENING

In 1999, 176,000 new invasive cases of breast cancer and approximately 43,700 deaths due to the disease were reported in the United States.[43] Widely accepted techniques for breast cancer screening, but with differing levels of evidence, include mammography, clinical breast exam (CBE), and breast self-examination (BSE). As with other screening techniques, the purpose of breast cancer screening is to find breast cancer early, while the disease is curable, to reduce mortality for breast cancer. As Tabar et al.[44] and others have shown, tumor size, lymph node status, and malignancy grade are major prognostic factors in survival. No cancer screening test has been studied more than mammography (with or without CBE). Yet, after more than 35 years of trials, many questions remain regarding at what age and at what interval women should be screened. The breast cancer screening trials provide clear evidence of benefit for screening women older than age 50 until approximately age 70, and increasing evidence of a small but statistically significant benefit of mammography for women aged 40 to 49 years.

Eight randomized trials have been conducted over more than 35 years to assess the impact of mammography. Together, these trials have included more than 500,000 women, with 180,000 women aged 40 to 49.

The eight international randomized clinical trials have varied greatly[27] (Table 25-3). Most trials have included women in

TABLE 25-3. Selected Characteristics of Eight Randomized Controlled Trials of Breast Cancer Screening

Study (Year Begun)	*Age at Entry (y)*	*Screening Modality*	*Periodicity (mo)*	*Randomization*	*Sample Size* Study	*Sample Size* Control	*Screened at First Examination (%)*	*Years of Follow-Up*
HIP (1963)	40–64	2-view MM and CBE	12	Individual	30,239	30,756	67	18.0
Sweden, two-county: Ostergotland and Kopparberg (1977)	40–74	1-view MM	24 (age <50 y) 33 (age ≥50 y)	Cluster: geographic	78,085	56,782	89	14.2 15.2
Malmö (1976)	45–69	2-view MM	18–24	Cluster: birth cohort	21,088	21,195	74	12.7
Stockholm (1981)	40–64	1-view MM	28	Cluster: birth cohort	39,164	19,943	81	11.4
Gothenburg (1982)	40–59	2-view MM	18	Individual (age 40–49 y); cluster (age 50–59 y)	20,724	28,809	84	12.0
Edinburgh (1976)	45–64	2-view MM initially (later usually 1-view MM)	12 (CBE); 24 (MM)	Cluster: by physician practices	23,226	21,904	61	14.0
Canada NBSS1 (1980)	40–49	2-view MM and CBE	12	Individual: volunteers	25,214	25,216	~100[a]	10.5
Canada NBSS2 (1980)	50–59	2-view MM and CBE versus CBE only	12	Individual: volunteers	19,711	19,694	~100[a]	10.5

CBE, clinical breast examination; HIP, Health Insurance Plan of New York; MM, mammography; NBSS1 and -2, first and second Canadian National Breast Cancer Screening Study.
[a]Study design included randomization of volunteers after clinical breast examination; accordingly, virtually 100% had their first screening examination.
(Adapted from ref. 27; and Rimer BK. Breast cancer screening. In: Harris JR, Lippman ME, Morrow M, eds. *Diseases of the breast.* Philadelphia: Lippincott–Raven Publishers, 1996:311.)

their 40s, although two trials began accrual at 45, and one of the Canadian trials [the first National Breast Cancer Screening Study (NBSS1)] was designed to examine mammography and CBE versus usual care for women in their 40s, with a separate study (NBSS2) to assess mammography and CBE versus CBE only for women aged 50 to 59. The studies also varied in (1) whether they used one-view or two-view mammography; (2) the screening interval, which varied from 12 to 24 months; and (3) the level of compliance achieved. The problems in the trials also have varied. For example, cluster randomization resulted in socioeconomic status differences with the study groups in the Edinburgh trial.[45] Other trials experienced higher than desired contamination, most often because of higher than expected levels of screening in the control groups. For most of the studies, women's breast cancer risk factors were not known; only the Health Insurance Plan of New York (HIP) and NBSS assessed and published data on the breast cancer risk factors for women in the study.[46]

RANDOMIZED CLINICAL TRIALS

Although mammography was first reported in 1913, it was not until 1963 that the first RCT—and the only U.S. RCT—commenced at HIP. HIP included women aged 40 to 64 at entry. Nearly 62,000 women were randomized to the study (two-view mammography and CBE) or control group (usual care). Two-view mammography and physical examination were offered every 12 months during the 4-year study period, and follow-up was continued for 18 years.[27]

The Swedish Two-County Trial in Kopparberg and Ostergotland began in 1977–1978 with an enrollment of almost 135,000 women randomized to one-view mammography every 24 months (younger than age 50) or 33 months (older than age 50). Within those geographic areas, all women were invited to enroll by letters of invitation, using the population registry list. Screening continued for four rounds for younger women and three rounds for older women.[47] The Kopparberg arm used single-view mammography without grids; Ostergotland used a grid.[48]

The Malmö Trial was begun in 1976 in one city in Sweden.[27,28,49] It was one of only two trials that began screening at age 45, and it stopped entry at age 69. It used two-view mammography every 18 to 24 months for five rounds; randomization was by cluster based on birth cohort. Approximately 59,000 women were enrolled in this trial.

The Stockholm Study began in 1981 and enrolled approximately 43,000 women aged 40 to 64 who received single-view mammography every 28 months. Like the Malmö trial, randomization was by birth cohort within clusters.[27]

The final Swedish study was conducted in Gothenburg, starting in 1982. The trial began with nearly 50,000 women aged 40 to 59 who received two-view mammography every 18 months. Randomization of women aged 40 to 49 was by individual, whereas clustered randomization was used for women aged 50 to 59. Verified results have not yet been published,[47] but additional data were provided in 1997 for the National Institutes of Health Consensus Conference on Breast Cancer Screening in women aged 40 to 49.

The Edinburgh Trial began in 1978 as a randomized component of the larger, nonrandomized United Kingdom trial of The Early Detection of Breast Cancer. Approximately 25,000 women aged 45 to 64 were randomized to two-view mammography plus CBE on either a 12- or 24-month schedule. The purpose was to assess the impact of mammography and CBE in reducing mortality from breast cancer.[50–52]

The National Breast Cancer Screening Study (NBSS1) was designed to examine the value of two-view mammography and CBE compared to usual care in women aged 40 to 49. Nearly 53,000 women were enrolled, starting in 1980, and received follow-up yearly for 5 years. Unlike the other trials, the women were recruited as volunteers and then randomized. As Miller and colleagues[53] have reported, these women were different from the Canadian population in several ways—for example, they were less likely to smoke, and they had higher levels of education.

The second Canadian study, the NBSS2, also begun in 1980, enrolled nearly 43,000 women aged 50 to 59 and was designed to compare two-view mammography and CBE against CBE only. In other words, the question was whether there is a benefit of mammography over and above CBE in this age group. This is the only trial planned to assess the additive impact of mammography in addition to CBE.[32] Critiques of this trial have appeared by several authors.[54,55] The criticisms are probably overstated, and the results should not be discounted.

NONRANDOMIZED CLINICAL TRIALS

A number of nonrandomized trials have been conducted around the world. Much can be learned from these studies. However, because of a number of design limitations, they should not be used alone in establishing screening guidelines and policies.[56] The largest study of mammography and CBE was the U.S. Breast Cancer Detection Demonstration Project (BCDDP): 280,000 women aged 35 and older were recruited and screened in 28 centers annually with mammograms and CBE during the 1970s.[20,49] The BCDDP was sponsored jointly by the NCI and the American Cancer Society (ACS). Because the BCDDP participants were not a random sample of the population, there were some important differences from women in the general population. Most notably, the BCDDP population was at much higher risk, with a substantially higher incidence of breast cancer. Moreover, because it was not an RCT, the case fatality rate was used to assess the impact of screening. A subset of women were followed as part of a case-control study conducted by Morrison and colleagues[57] to examine case fatality rates within the BCDDP. Breast cancer mortality was approximately 20% less than expected from national data.[57] There was a benefit for younger women, but it was less than for older women.

EVIDENCE FOR MAMMOGRAPHY

More than 3.5 million women-years of observation have been recorded for women of all ages, and more than 2.7 million women-years for women aged 40 to 49 at entry from the breast cancer screening RCTs.[27,58] One of the challenging aspects of tracking these trials is the constantly shifting nature of the data. The trialists provide updates at different points in time, and some reports use nonverified data. Thus, at any given point, review articles may vary substantially in the numbers they report. Figures 25-1 and 25-2 illustrate the mortality outcomes for women of all ages and for those younger than age 50, with 18 years of follow-up for HIP,[46] 14 years for the Edinburgh trial,[45] 10.5 years for the Canadian trials,[59] and 7 to 13 years for the Swedish trials.

In 1993, the International Workshop on Breast Cancer Screening[27] created considerable controversy when it concluded that for women aged 40 to 49, randomized controlled trials consistently demonstrated no benefit from screening in the first 5 to 7 years after entry and a marginal benefit after that. More recently, in reviewing the same trials, Kerlikowske and colleagues[60] confirmed this conclusion and suggested that the same benefit could be achieved by screening women after age 50. However, several years later, with most of the international RCTs now having more than 10 years of follow-up, the trends are clearer: Six of the trials show reductions in mortality for women who were in their 40s at entry. But a large variability remains in the relative risk of dying from breast cancer for women younger than 50. There also is significant controversy over many of the reported numbers.

Although the randomized trials have included too few women older than age 70 to offer guidance about screening for older women, the Forum on Breast Cancer Screening[61] recommended regular mammograms for women aged 70 years who are otherwise healthy. A case-control analysis in the Nijmegen study[62] confirmed the benefit of mammography for women older than 70.

Six different published metaanalyses, including the two mentioned earlier, have examined the effect of the mammography trials on women aged 40 to 49 (Table 25-4). When Elwood and colleagues[19] conducted a metaanalysis and included all the data except for the controversial Canadian study, they found an overall relative risk of 0.99, suggesting no difference between the screened and control groups. With the Canadian data included, there was a slight increase in the relative risk for the experimental group (relative risk, 1.08). The overall relative risks found in the metaanalyses have ranged from 0.85 to 0.99 without the NBSS data and 0.93 to 1.08 with the NBSS data. Eckhardt and colleagues[63] found a nonsignificant 7% reduction in mortality. In a 1995 metaanalysis, Smart and colleagues[64] found a significant 24% mortality reduction for women in their 40s. Hendrick et al.[58] combined recent follow-up data on women aged 40 to 49 at entry. They found a statistically significant 18% mortality reduction. This is similar to the 18% reduction Berry[8] found when an assumption of homogeneity was made. However, the benefit was not statistically significant when he assumed heterogeneity. The benefit occurs approximately 15 years after the start of screening.[21] The benefit for women in their 50s is larger and also significant: an approximately 25% to 30% reduction in mortality. It is reasonable to conclude that there is a small but statistically significant reduction in mortality for women in their 40s. Nevertheless, most of the benefit actually is achieved when they are in their 50s.[65] For women in their 50s and 60s, there is general agreement about the benefits of mammography.

BREAST CANCER SCREENING GUIDELINES

The question, "At what age should women begin getting regular mammograms?" has been one of the most contentious in science and medicine. The issue became even more inflamed

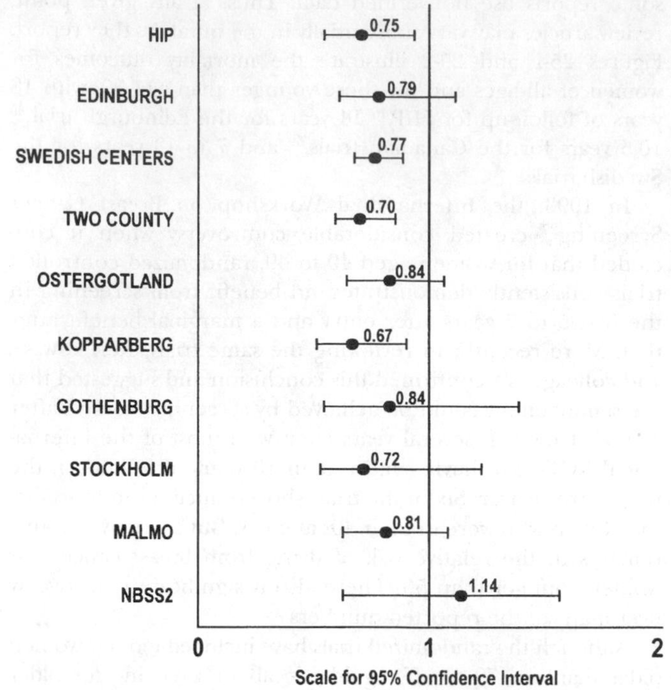

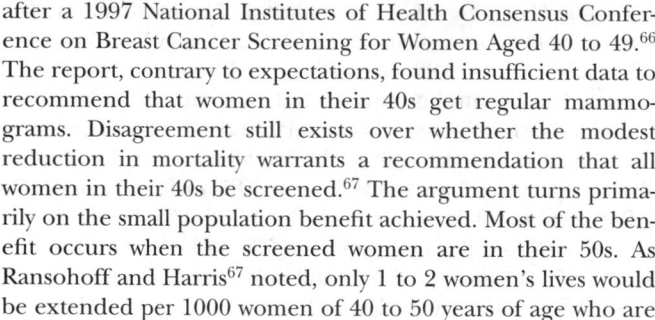

FIGURE 25-1. Mortality impact of the randomized clinical trials (all ages) by relative risk and upper and lower confidence intervals. Adjusted for socioeconomic status differences.[45] HIP, Health Insurance Plan of New York; NBSS2, second Canadian National Breast Cancer Screening Study.

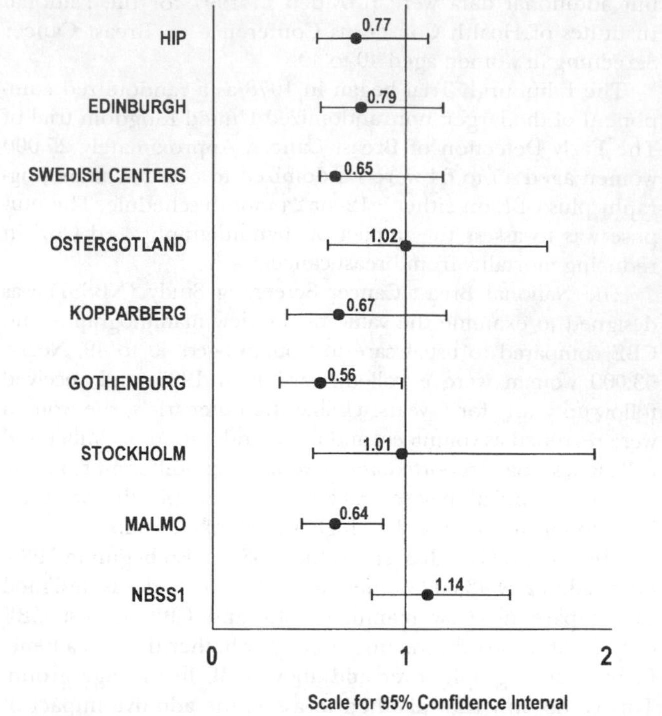

FIGURE 25-2. Mortality impact of the randomized clinical trials (women aged 40 to 49 years at entry) by relative risk and upper and lower confidence intervals. Adjusted for socioeconomic status differences.[45] HIP, Health Insurance Plan of New York; NBSS1, first Canadian National Breast Cancer Screening Study.[58]

after a 1997 National Institutes of Health Consensus Conference on Breast Cancer Screening for Women Aged 40 to 49.[66] The report, contrary to expectations, found insufficient data to recommend that women in their 40s get regular mammograms. Disagreement still exists over whether the modest reduction in mortality warrants a recommendation that all women in their 40s be screened.[67] The argument turns primarily on the small population benefit achieved. Most of the benefit occurs when the screened women are in their 50s. As Ransohoff and Harris[67] noted, only 1 to 2 women's lives would be extended per 1000 women of 40 to 50 years of age who are screened annually for 10 years. However, in agreeing on a reduction in breast cancer mortality of 18%, both the ACS and the NCI changed their screening recommendations, with the ACS now advising annual mammograms for women aged 40 and older. Annual screening for women in their 40s is based on the assumption of a shorter lead time for younger women.[44] The NCI recommends mammograms every 1 to 2 years for average-risk women aged 40 and older.[68] For the first time since 1993, however, the recommendations are compatible; both organizations now endorse regular mammograms for women older than age 40 (Table 25-5).

TABLE 25-4. Metaanalyses of Trials for Women Aged 40 to 49 Years

Description	*Author*	*Relative Risk*	*Confidence Interval (%)*	*Reduction in Mortality Rate (%)*
Without NBSS	Miller et al., 1992[53]	0.85	0.68–1.08	15[a]
With NBSS	Eckhardt et al., 1994[63]	0.93	0.76–1.15	7[a]
Without NBSS	Elwood et al., 1993[19]	0.99	0.74–1.32	No difference
With NBSS	Elwood et al., 1993[19]	1.08	0.85–1.39	No difference
Without NBSS	Smart et al., 1995[64]	0.76	0.62–0.95	24[b]
With NBSS	Hendrick et al., 1997[58]	0.82	0.71–0.95	18[b]
With NBSS	Berry 1998[8]	0.82 (assuming homogeneity)	0.71–0.95	18[b]
Totals		0.82	0.64–1.01	18[b]

NBSS, National Breast Cancer Screening Study (Canada).
[a]Nonsignificant.
[b]Significant.

TABLE 25-5. Screening Guidelines for Breast, Colorectal, Prostate, and Cervical Cancers for Selected Health Care Organizations

	American Cancer Society[43]	*American College of Obstetricians and Gynecologists*	*U.S. Preventive Health Services Task Force*[7]	*National Cancer Institute's Physician Data Query (PDQ) System*[1]	*American College of Radiology*	*American Academy of Family Physicians*
Breast cancer	Mammography and CBE yearly for women age 40 and older. CBE every 3 y ages 20–39; every year age 40 and older. Monthly BSE for all women age 20 and older.	Mammography should be performed every 1–2 y for women ages 40–49, and then annually thereafter.	Mammography every 1–2 y with or without CBE for women ages 50–69.	Mammography every 1–2 y for women age 40 and older. Women at higher risk should talk with their physicians about schedule.	Yearly mammography for asymptomatic women age 40 and older. It is reasonable to institute screening mammography at an earlier age in women with high-risk factors.	Counsel about potential risks and benefits of mammography and CBE for women ages 40–49. Offer mammography and CBE every 1–2 y for women ages 50–69.
Cervical cancer	Pap test and pelvic examination yearly for all women who are, or have been, sexually active or who have reached age 18. After three consecutive normal smears, Pap test less often at the discretion of physician.	Pap test and pelvic examination yearly for all women who are, or have been, sexually active or who have reached age 18. After three consecutive normal smears, Pap test less often at the discretion of physician.	Pap test every 1–3 y for all women who are sexually active and/or who have a cervix. No evidence to support an upper limit, but age 65 can be defended in women with a history of normal and regular Pap tests.	Evidence strongly suggests a decrease in mortality for regular screening with Pap tests in women who are sexually active or who have reached age 18. The upper limit at which such screening ceases to be effective is unknown.	N/A	Offer Pap test at least every 3 y for women who have ever had sex and have a cervix.
Colorectal cancer	One of the following schedules for men and women age 50 and over: FOBT yearly and sigmoidoscopy every 5 y; colonoscopy every 10 y; double-contrast barium enema every 5–10 y (DRE at time of screening except for FOBT). Those with high risk for colorectal cancer should begin screening earlier and/or more frequently.	After the age of 50 years, a DRE should accompany the pelvic examination, and an annual FOBT should be performed; sigmoidoscopy should be performed every 3–5 y.	FOBT and/or sigmoidoscopy yearly at age 50 and older. There is insufficient evidence to determine which screening method is preferable or whether the combination produces greater benefit than either one alone.	FOBT either annually or biennially using rehydrated or nonrehydrated stool specimens in people ages 50–80 decreases mortality for colorectal cancer. Regular screening by sigmoidoscopy in people older than age 50 may decrease mortality from colorectal cancer. There is insufficient evidence to determine the optimal interval for such screening.	N/A	Screen for colorectal cancer annually with FOBT, sigmoidoscopy, colonoscopy, or barium enema in adults age 50 and older.
Prostate cancer	Men age 50 and older with at least a 10-y life expectancy should talk with their health care professional about having a DRE and PSA blood test every year. Those with high risk for prostate cancer should consider beginning these tests at an earlier age.	N/A	Screening is not recommended.	Insufficient evidence to establish that a decrease in mortality occurs with screening by DRE, transrectal ultrasound, or PSA.	Ultrasound examination is best reserved to evaluate those patients who have abnormal DRE or an abnormal PSA level. A combination of DRE examination and PSA level should be used as an initial screening procedure.	Counsel about the known risks and uncertain benefits of screening for prostate cancer for men ages 50–65.

BSE, breast self-examination; CBE, clinical breast examination; DRE, digital rectal examination; FOBT, fecal occult blood test; N/A, not applicable; PSA, prostate-specific antigen.

The evidence suggests that a 5% to 20% additional benefit in mortality reduction can be achieved by adding a high-quality CBE.[19,27] Although the recommendations of different medical organizations vary, it seems prudent to encourage women to have a CBE yearly (see Table 25-3).

CERVICAL CANCER SCREENING

In 1999, an estimated 12,800 new cases of invasive disease and 4800 deaths resulted from cervical cancer.[43] A steady decline in mortality was observed after the initiation of widespread Pap testing in the mid-twentieth century.[69] From 1970 through 1995, mortality continued to decrease by 40%.[69] This decline represents a major success in cancer control in the United States. Mortality associated with invasive cervical cancer is no longer common compared to other cancers. However, cervical cancer is the second most common cancer worldwide,[70] and fatalities from this disease in developed countries should be entirely avoidable with currently available technology. Continued efforts to improve cervical cancer screening practices are, therefore, well justified both nationally and internationally.

Dr. George Papanicolaou introduced the test that bears his name in the 1930s. An RCT has never been conducted to confirm its efficacy because wide-scale adoption and diffusion of the Pap test into medical practice made assignment to a non-screened control group unethical and, therefore, untenable. Nevertheless, one would expect screening to be effective because cervical cancer is accessible and has a relatively long preclinical detectable phase. Numerous observational studies have demonstrated its efficacy beyond a reasonable doubt. Large national screening programs in Nordic countries, Canada, and the United States have been associated with marked drops in mortality from cervical cancer.[69,71,72] Analysis of these studies and others suggested that the probability of invasive cancer could be reduced up to 90% for frequencies up to every 3 years.[73,74] Case-control studies of women with invasive cervical cancer in varied geographic areas, including Italy, Columbia, Scotland, and Denmark, have documented risks three to ten times greater associated with women who have not been screened.[75–78]

Controversy remains about the appropriate screening interval for Pap testing. Guidelines from major expert groups have continued to recommend annual screening, with less frequent intervals after three normal smears (at the discretion of the physician). However, after its review of the evidence, the U.S. Preventive Services Task Force left the interval from 1 to 3 years[7] (see Table 25-5). The literature that bears on this question is limited.

Inadequate data are available to recommend an upper age limit for regular screening. Because mortality increases with advancing age and 40% to 50% of all women who die from cervical cancer are older than 65 years of age,[79] it seems prudent to screen older women. However, national survey data document a marked fall-off in regular screening for older women.[80] There is concern that Pap testing is less sensitive in older women who have a receded squamocolumnar junction of the cervix. However, it is likely that the primary reason for invasive cervical cancer in older women is lack of screening.

For women who have had hysterectomies, the practice of cytologic screening with vaginal smears is still common. However, at least for women who have had a hysterectomy for benign conditions, the likelihood of detecting vaginal dysplasia is extremely low and the false-positive rate is high,[81] thus suggesting that the practice is unnecessary.

SKIN CANCER SCREENING

The incidence of skin cancer has increased worldwide, with U.S. incidence data mirroring this trend.[82,83] In the United States, the incidence rate of melanoma has increased approximately 4% per year since the early 1970s, with a 162% increase in male melanoma cases and 95% in women.[43,84] It is unclear whether this increase is due to actual changes in prevalence or is a function of increased awareness with subsequent diagnosis, improved reporting by tumor registries, or both. In 1999, 54,000 new cases of skin cancer were projected, with 44,200 new cases of melanoma and 7300 deaths.[43] Melanoma now ranks sixth in incidence among cancers in males and seventh in incidence among cancers in females.[43] Approximately 800,000 nonmelanoma skin cancers are diagnosed each year.[43,85] The United States lags behind many other countries in the creative application of interventions to reduce the incidence of and mortality from melanoma and other skin cancers. Australia, which has the highest reported incidence of melanoma anywhere, has mounted successful population-based programs that have had dramatic effects.[86,87]

Although national data are lacking on either population or health professional behavior, at least one study suggests that most physicians do not examine the areas of the skin where melanoma is likely to occur, and most people do not routinely examine their skin for changes. Skin cancer screening consists of a medical history and a whole body examination under strong lighting.[85,88–91] There is a lack of consensus about the routine provision of preventive services in dermatologists' offices.[92] Although no randomized trials proving the impact of skin cancer screening have been performed to date, research results from the efficacy studies that have been conducted suggest that skin cancer screening may lower mortality from skin cancer, especially melanoma, by improving rates of early detection.[93–99] However, more evidence is needed.

Experts have not agreed about screening guidelines for skin cancer. The U.S. Preventive Services Task Force recommends "routine screening for individuals at high risk" (e.g., those having a family or personal history of skin cancer, clinical evidence of precursor lesions, and increased exposure to sunlight). The Task Force neither defines what is meant by routine screening nor reports on the specific recommendations for skin self-examination.[7,85,100,101] The ACS recommends a cancer-related checkup, including a skin examination, every 3 years and "more frequently" for persons at risk.[43,101] The ACS further suggests that "screening for the presence of skin cancer is well within the domain of the well-trained generalist."[101] The NCI also recognizes the benefits of skin cancer screening, but offers no specific guidelines for such screening.[102] Other experts recommend yearly skin cancer screenings,[90,97,99] regular screening for the elderly,[87,103,104] and skin cancer screening for every new patient seen by a dermatologist.[105]

PROSTATE CANCER SCREENING

Prostate cancer is the most commonly diagnosed cancer among men in the United States and is the second leading cause of male cancer deaths. In 1999, 179,000 new cases of prostate cancer were identified, and there were 37,000 deaths. However, consensus is lacking concerning recommendations for prostate cancer screening. There are several reasons for the controversy surrounding screening tests for prostate cancer. First, no definitive evidence suggests that prostate cancer screening results in improved clinical outcomes, especially a reduction in mortality from the disease.[106–109] Second, the incidence of prostate cancer is on the rise largely due to the detection of latent, asymptomatic cases with uncertain clinical relevance, thus putting the value of screening in doubt.[110,111]

SCREENING TESTS FOR PROSTATE CANCER

The three main screening modalities for prostate cancer include digital rectal examination (DRE), serum prostate-specific antigen (PSA), and endorectal (transrectal) ultrasonography (TRUS). The most widely used and oldest technique for detection of prostate cancer is the DRE. Wide ranges in estimates of sensitivity (33% to 69%) and specificity (49% to 97%) of the DRE have been reported. Ultimately, only one in three patients with a positive DRE has prostate cancer.[112–116] With the development and application of intraluminal (rectal) probes with high resolution, studies have shown that small, nonpalpable malignant lesions of the prostate could be detected.[117–119] TRUS has fallen short of expectations, with a large variation in reports of sensitivity and specificity, both ranging from 41% to 79%.[119,120] Despite this, TRUS is considered an excellent ancillary modality to increase accuracy of biopsy over the digital guidance alone.[112] The PSA test is a blood test that allows for earlier detection of many prostate cancers. Interest in the PSA grew in the late 1980s. Impressively, PSA levels were shown to drop to undetectable levels after prostatectomy.[121,122] However, normal PSA values are found in approximately one-third of men with localized cancers, and PSA levels are often elevated in men with noncancerous conditions, such as benign prostatic hyperplasia.[112,122,123] Some investigators have argued that integration of the DRE with determination of PSA levels and the use of TRUS in selected cases would improve prostate cancer detection.[122,124] A new approach for using PSA based on age-dependent thresholds has been suggested and may be promising.[125]

Nonrandomized Studies

Two nonrandomized studies are ongoing to evaluate screening tests for prostate cancer (the ACS National Prostate Cancer Detection Project[126] and a multicenter study headquartered at Washington University[127] involving six university medical centers). Results of these trials will not be available until the first decade of the twenty-first century. Thus, clinicians and patients must make decisions in the absence of RCT data. Table 25-6 summarizes the sensitivity, specificity, and predictive value of these data.

Randomized Clinical Trials

The NCI's PLCO trial is a 16-year randomized control study that began on November 16, 1993.[131] It is accruing 74,000 men 60 to 74 years of age and has a design power of 90% to determine 20% reduction of prostate cancer mortality. This trial will provide important information about the efficacy of screening.

Trends and What They Mean

National data from 1990 to 1996 show that prostate cancer incidence peaked in 1992 at 190.8 per 100,000 and declined at an average rate of 8.5% from 1992 to 1996.[130] A series of related reports in the *Journal of the National Cancer Institute*, based on data from the Surveillance, Epidemiology and End Results Cancer Registry Program, indicates a decline in the incidence of distant stage disease,[107] as well as a decline in incidence-based mortality of distant stage disease and flat incidence-based mortality trends of localized and distant-stage disease.[108] Statistical methods were applied to consider the effect of screening by limiting some analyses to the contribution from cases diagnosed since 1987 when widespread screening using the PSA test had begun. Thus, some evidence shows improved prognosis for the screen-detected cases. However, alternative interpretations, such as the possibility that cause-of-death misclassification could explain these findings, cannot be ruled out.

PROSTATE CANCER SCREENING RECOMMENDATIONS

In light of the limitations of prostate cancer screening, it is important to consider the natural history of this disease and subgroups of men at high risk for developing prostate cancer. These considerations are critical for determining public health policy.[132,133]

Not surprisingly, no consensus has been reached about prostate cancer screening (see Table 25-5). Several groups, including the U.S. Preventive Services Task Force,[7] American College of Physicians,[132] and Canadian Task Force on the Periodic Health Examination,[133] have recommended against routine PSA screening. The NCIPDQ does not recommend PSA screening to the general population.[1] The ACS[43] has modified its guidelines and now recommends that men age 50 and older who have at least a 10-year life expectancy should talk with their health care professionals about having a DRE of the prostate gland and a PSA blood test every year. Men who are at high risk for prostate cancer (African Americans or men who have a history of prostate cancer in close family members) should consider beginning these tests at an earlier age.

COLORECTAL CANCER SCREENING

Increased emphasis on the importance of screening for colorectal cancer during the 1990s has followed studies documenting the efficacy of both fecal occult blood testing (FOBT) and sigmoidoscopy. Cancers of the colon and rectum account for the third largest number of new cancer cases after lung, with 94,700 and 34,700 cases estimated, respectively, in 1999.[43] Substantially fewer people now die from the disease, indicating the promise of screening and treatment (47,900 and 8700 estimated deaths in 1999 for colon and rectum, respectively).[43] A slow decrease has been seen in both incidence and mortality since the late 1970s. Incidence has decreased at a rate of approximately 1.4% per year for the period from 1991 to 1995.

As with cervical and prostate cancers, the long preclinical and detectable phase makes colorectal cancer ideal for screen-

TABLE 25-6. Estimates of Screening Test Performance for Prostate Cancer

Investigation	*Screening Test*	*Sample Size*	*Ages (y)*	*Sensitivity (%)*	*Specificity (%)*	*Positive Predictive Value (%)*	*Detection Rate (%)*
Cancer Detection Study; Jenson et al., 1960[112]	DRE	4367	>50	NA	NA	94	0.8
Cancer Detection Study; Gilbertsen, 1971[113]	DRE	5856	>45	NA	NA	NA	1.3
Chodak and Schoenberg, 1984[114]	DRE	811	41–85	NA	NA	29	1.7
Thompson et al., 1984[115]	DRE	2005	40–70	NA	NA	26	0.8
Mueller et al., 1988[128]	DRE	4843	40–79	NA	NA	39	2.5
Lee et al., 1988[116]	DRE			45	97	34	1.3
	TRUS	784	60–86	91	94	31	2.6
Carter et al., 1989[118]	TRUS	59 (all cancer)	NA	92	NA	54	NA
Cooner et al., 1990[123]	DRE			77	53	43	14.6 (overall)
	TRUS	1807	50–89	NA	NA	32	
	PSA			80	61	48	
	DRE/PSA			90	64	62	
Catalona et al., 1991[122]	DRE			84	51	37	2.2 (overall)
	TRUS	1653	≥50	90	27	30	
	PSA			79	60	33	
Catalona et al., 1994[127]	DRE	6630	≥50	55	45	21	3.2
	PSA			82	48	32	
Mettlin et al., 1991[129]	DRE	2425	55–70	58	96	28	4.6
Babaian et al., 1992[126]	TRUS	2425	55–70	77	89	15	2.4 (overall)
	PSA			67	82	43	

DRE, digital rectal examination; NA, not available; PSA, prostate-specific antigen; TRUS, transrectal ultrasonography.

ing. Like cervical (but unlike prostate) cancer, the specificity of existing screening procedures minimizes the necessity of additional procedures necessary for the follow-up of false-positives. Increased risk for colorectal cancer is found for persons with personal histories of colorectal cancer, adenomatous polyps, or inflammatory bowel disease, as well as those with family histories of adenomas,[134] colorectal cancer, or hereditary colorectal cancer syndromes (i.e., familial adenomatous polyposis and hereditary nonpolyposis colorectal cancer.[135,136]

SCREENING TESTS FOR COLORECTAL CANCER

Four tests are currently in use for colon cancer screening: FOBT, sigmoidoscopy, colonoscopy, and high-contrast barium enema. RCT data are not available for colonoscopy or barium enema. A fifth test, the DRE, is a low-cost, low-harm practice that is well ingrained into routine medical evaluation, but no evidence from controlled studies indicates that it is useful in preventing mortality from rectal cancer.[137] The FOBT, based on the use of guaiac to detect heme in the stool, can detect occult bleeding from early-stage colorectal cancers. Flexible sigmoidoscopy involves the use of a 60-cm fiber-optic endoscope that can view up to the splenic flexure of the colon and at the same time provide access for biopsy and removal of polyps.[138] A comprehensive review of colorectal cancer screening with clinical guidelines has been developed by a multidisciplinary panel under the aegis of the Agency for Health Care Policy and Research.[139]

Fecal Occult Blood Test

Support for the use of FOBT comes from several large randomized controlled trials, including a Minnesota trial of 46,501 participants between the ages of 50 and 80 years of age.[140,141] This study found that annual FOBT with rehydration of the samples decreased the 13-year cumulative mortality from colorectal cancer by 33% and biennial screening by 21%.[140,141] Most (75% to 84%) of this reduction resulted from the test rather than from incidental discovery of cancers by follow-up colonoscopy.[142] Earlier RCTs in England of 152,850 individuals,[143] as well as a large study of 62,000 persons in Denmark,[144] demonstrated that biennial FOBT without rehydration reduced mortality by 15% to 18%. An additional study of 27,000 persons in Sweden, aged 60 to 64 years of age, is ongoing.[145] A fifth trial in the United States evaluated FOBT as a supplement to annual rigid sigmoidoscopy in 21,756 subjects and found a nonsignificant decrease in colorectal cancer mortality.[146] Data from case-control studies are generally consistent with the conclusions of these trials. In a health plan population, a decreased mortality of 31% was associated with having had at least one screening FOBT in the previous 5 years.[147,148] Other case-control studies in Japan and Washington also have demonstrated protective effects on mortality.[149,150]

When used in unscreened populations the FOBT is positive in 1% to 5%; 2% to 10% of these have cancer and 20% to 30% have adenomas.[151,152] Concern remains about the lack of specificity of FOBT and the necessity to follow positive results with colonoscopic examination or barium enema.[153] However, the evidence is mounting that FOBT saves lives from colorectal cancer. Physicians must weigh the benefits of possible early detection of colorectal cancer against the possible complications and expense of follow-up procedures.[138]

Flexible Sigmoidoscopy

The advantage of sigmoidoscopy screening over FOBT is that it frequently includes the actual removal of cancer or a precancerous lesion in a biopsied polyp, thus combining prevention (through removal of polyps), screening, and treatment in one step.[146] Another advantage is that it needs to be performed infrequently, perhaps every 5 to 10 years.[147,148]

At least two large randomized trials of flexible sigmoidoscopy screening are in progress. The NCI's PLCO trial is evaluating the efficacy of examinations every 3 years in 74,000 men and women, 55 to 74 years of age, with an equal number of controls.[154] A trial in the United Kingdom, with 200,000 men and women aged 55 to 64 years, is evaluating the efficacy of one sigmoidoscopy delivered for reducing colorectal cancer mortality.[155]

Meanwhile, supporting evidence for efficacy comes from several case-control studies. In the first, screening sigmoidoscopy, primarily with the rigid sigmoidoscope, reduced mortality from cancer of the rectum and distal colon by 60% (adjusted odds ratio, 0.41; 95% confidence interval, 0.25 to 0.69) in a large Kaiser Permanente California health plan population.[148] Confirmation came from a smaller second study of 66 cases and 196 controls in another health plan population in Wisconsin.[156] A third large case-control study in American veterans, with 4358 cases and 16,199 matched controls, reported a 59% reduction in mortality from any prior colorectal procedure.[157] The first two case-control studies were judged sufficiently convincing that the U.S. Preventive Services Task Force upgraded the evidence and recommends screening with sigmoidoscopy or FOBT annually for persons older than 50.[7]

LUNG CANCER SCREENING

Lung cancer screening is not currently recommended due to lack of evidence that any available screening procedure, even for smokers, can identify tumors early enough to reduce mortality. This remains a major challenge to research and technology because of the tremendous burden caused by this cancer. In 1999, an estimated 171,600 new cases of disease and 158,900 deaths were due to lung cancer, making it by far the most common killer from cancer in both men and women and accounting for 28% of all cancer deaths.[43]

The decision to actively discourage lung cancer screening by x-ray was made based on the results of RCTs performed in the 1970s.[158] None of four randomized trials showed any benefit of reducing mortality from lung cancer.[159–162] The Mayo Lung Project, the primary trial contributing to this evidence, demonstrated that screening with either chest x-rays or chest x-rays plus sputum cytology could lower the stage at presentation and increase survival. Neither approach had any effect on lung cancer mortality.[162] The lack of connection between improved survival and the absence of a mortality benefit can be attributed to lead-time and length biases. This study and its contemporaries have, however, been criticized because of study design and analytic issues, including a lack of statistical power.[163] Recent preliminary results from the Early Lung Cancer Action Project in New York indicated that low-dose spiral computed tomography used in 1000 symptom-free former smokers older than age 60 detected 27 cancer cases versus 7 cases detected by chest radiograph.[164] Although this is not an RCT and, therefore, susceptible to lead-time and length-time bias, these preliminary results suggest that newer noninvasive imaging technologies may hold promise. Efforts to prevent initiation of smoking, especially by young people, and cessation of tobacco use remain the physician's main tools for combating this most common of all cancers.

THE FUTURE OF SCREENING

Many challenges lie ahead for cancer screening. Better detection methods are urgently needed, and molecular detection methods may surpass current techniques. At the same time, more effort is required to encourage adherence to the proven cancer screening modalities. Adherence to screening is less than optimal for all the major recommended screening techniques.[165] With the discovery of mutations in susceptibility genes that predispose for cancer, new challenges in cancer screening arise with the need for appropriate screening recommendations and programs for high-risk subgroups. Not only are those who have inherited a mutation for cancer susceptibility at higher risk for developing some cancers, but often the age at onset among such individuals is younger than the age at onset in the general population. This creates challenges for those who recommend and promote screening regimens. The example of the *BRCA1* susceptibility gene for breast cancer illustrates a perplexing situation in which recommendations for screening with mammography do not address the early age at onset of this disease. Moreover, there are no good population data on which to base guidelines. Further study is needed to establish efficacious screening protocols for those who are genetically predisposed to cancer. Finally, there are new screening modalities on the horizon, such as low-dose helical computed tomography scans for detecting early lung cancers.[164] Among the challenges of the future is how to evaluate new screening technologies in a world where large RCTs may be increasingly difficult to conduct. In screening, as in other areas of medicine and public health, the inclination to recommend screening tests on the basis of an intriguing and promising study must be balanced by a careful assessment of the evidence.

Acknowledgments

Support was provided in part by 1-RO1-CA-63781-03, 1-P50CA-68438-01, and CA720-99.

REFERENCES

1. Kramer BS. *The screening editorial board of the physician data query: NCI state-of-the-art statements on cancer screening.* Bethesda, MD: National Cancer Institute, 1995.
2. Burke W, Daly M, Garber J, et al., for the Cancer Genetics Studies Consortium. Recommendations for follow-up care of individuals with an inherited predisposition to cancer. II. BRCA1 and BRCA2. *JAMA* 1997;277:997.
3. Kramer BS, Gohagan JK, Prorok PC, eds. *Cancer screening: theory and practice.* New York: Marcel Dekker Inc, 1999.
4. Hennekens CH, Buring JE. *Epidemiology in medicine.* Boston: Little, Brown and Company, 1987.

5. Hulka BS. Screening for cancer: lessons learned. *J Occup Med* 1986;28:687.
6. Rimer BK, Demark-Wahnefried W, Egert JR. Acceptance of cancer screening. In: *Handbook of health behavior research: provider determinants.* New York: Plenum Publishing, 1997.
7. U.S. Preventive Services Task Force. *Guide to clinical preventive services.* Alexandria, VA: International Medical Publishing, 1996.
8. Berry DA. Benefits and risks of screening mammography for women in their forties: a statistical appraisal. *J Natl Cancer Inst* 1998;90:1431.
9. Koss LG. The Papanicolaou test for cervical cancer detection: a triumph and a tragedy. *JAMA* 1989;261:737.
10. Hurley SF, Kaldor JM. The benefits and risks of mammographic screening for breast cancer. *Epidemiol Rev* 1992;14:101.
11. Greenberg RS, Daniels SR, Flanders D, Eley JW, Boring JR. *Medical epidemiology.* Norwalk, CT: Appleton & Lange, 1993.
12. Baines CJ. The Canadian National Breast Screening Study: a perspective on criticisms. *Ann Intern Med* 1994;120:326.
13. Hakama M, Elovainio L, Kajantie R, Louhivuori K. Breast cancer screening as public health policy in Finland. *Br J Cancer* 1991;64:962.
14. Ellman R. Clinical cost-benefit of screening programs. In: Stoll B, ed. *Women at high risk to breast cancer.* Boston: Kluwer Academic Publishers, 1991.
15. Swanson GM. May we agree to disagree, or how do we develop guidelines for breast cancer screening in women? [Commentary]. *J Natl Cancer Inst* 1994;86:903.
16. Tabar L, Fagerberg G, Duffy S, Day N. The Swedish two-county trial of mammographic screening for breast cancer: recent results and calculation of benefit. *J Epidemiol Community Health* 1989;43:107.
17. de Koning HJ, van Ineveld BM, de Haes JC, et al. Advanced breast cancer and its prevention by screening. *Br J Cancer* 1992;65:950.
18. Harris R. Breast cancer among women in their forties: toward a reasonable research agenda. *J Natl Cancer Inst* 1994;86:410.
19. Elwood JM, Cox B, Richardson AK. The effectiveness of breast cancer screening by mammography in younger women. *Online J Curr Clin Trials* 1993;Doc. No. 32.
20. Miller A. Mammography: reviewing the evidence. Epidemiology aspect. *Can Fam Physician* 1993;39:85.
21. Physicians Data Query. *Cancer screening.* Bethesda, MD: National Cancer Institute, 1997.
22. Eddy DM, Hasselblad V, McGivney W, Hendee W. The value of mammography screening in women under age 50 years. *JAMA* 1988;259:1512.
23. Kuni CC. Mammography in the 1990s: a plea for objective doctors and informed patients. *Am J Prev Med* 1993;9:185.
24. Lerman C, Trock B, Rimer BK, et al. Psychological and behavioral implications of abnormal mammograms. *Ann Intern Med* 1991;114:657.
25. Paskett E, Rimer BK. Psychosocial effects of abnormal Pap tests and mammograms: a review. *J Women's Health* 1995;4:73.
26. Fletcher SW. False-positive screening mammograms: good news, but more to do. *Ann Intern Med* 1999;131:60.
27. Fletcher SW, Black W, Harris R, Rimer BK, Shapiro S. Report of the International Workshop on Screening for Breast Cancer. *J Natl Cancer Inst* 1993;85:1644.
28. Andersson I, Aspegren K, Janzon L, et al. Mammographic screening and mortality from breast cancer: the Malmö mammographic screening trial. *BMJ* 1988;297:943.
29. Peeters PH, Verbeek AL, Straatman H, et al. Evaluation of overdiagnosis of breast cancer in screening with mammography: results of the Nijmegen programme. *Int J Epidemiol* 1989;18:295.
30. National Cancer Institute. Greenwald P, Kramer BS, Weed DL, eds. *Cancer prevention and control.* New York: Marcel Dekker Inc, 1995.
31. Donovan D, Middleton J, Ellis D. Edinburgh trial of screening for breast cancer [Letter]. *Lancet* 1990;335:1298.
32. Miller AB, Baines CJ, To T, Wall C. Canadian National Breast Screening Study. 2. Breast cancer detection and death rates among women aged 50 to 59 years. *Can Med Assoc J* 1992;147:1477.
33. Sjonell G, Stahle L. Mammography screening does not significantly reduce breast cancer mortality in Swedish daily practice. *Lakartidningen* 1999;96:904, 908.
34. Feig SA. Low-dose mammography: assessment of theoretical risk. In: Feig A, McLelland R. *Breast carcinoma: current diagnosis and treatment.* New York: Masson Publishing, 1983.
35. Rimer BK, Bluman LG. The psychosocial consequences of mammography. *J Natl Cancer Inst Monogr* 1997;22:131.
36. Pisano ED, Earp J, Schell M, Vokaty K, Denham A. Screening behavior of women after a false-positive mammogram. *Radiology* 1998;208:245.
37. Burman ML, Taplin SH, Herta DF, Elmore JG. Effect of false-positive mammograms on interval breast cancer screening in a health maintenance organization. *Ann Intern Med* 1999;131:1.
38. Lipkus IM, Rimer BK, Strigo TS. Relationships among objective and subjective risk for breast cancer and mammography stages of change. *Cancer Epidemiol Biomarkers Prev* 1996;5:1005.
39. Harris R. Decision-making about screening: individual and policy levels. In: Kramer BS, Gohagan JK, Prorok PC, eds. *Cancer screening: theory and practice.* New York: Marcel Dekker Inc, 1999.
40. Volk RJ, Cass AR, Spann SJ. A randomized controlled trial of shared decision making for prostate cancer screening. *Arch Fam Med* 1999;8:333.
41. Deber RB. Shared decision making in the real world. *J Gen Intern Med* 1996;11:377.
42. Austoker J. Gaining informed consent for screening is difficult—but many misconceptions need to be undone. *BMJ* 1999;319:722.
43. American Cancer Society. *Cancer facts & figures: 1999.* Atlanta: American Cancer Society, 1999.
44. Tabar L, Duffy SW, Vitak B, Chen HH, Prevost TC. The natural history of breast carcinoma: what have we learned from screening? *Cancer* 1999;86:449.
45. Alexander FE, Anderson TJ, Brown HK, et al. 14 years of follow-up from the Edinburgh randomised trial of breast-cancer screening. *Lancet* 1999;353:1903.
46. Shapiro S. Periodic screening for breast cancer: the HIP randomized controlled trial. *J Natl Cancer Inst Monogr* 1997;22:27.
47. Tabar L, Fagerberg G, Duffy S, et al. Update of the Swedish two-county program of mammographic screening for breast cancer. *Radiol Clin North Am* 1992;30:187.
48. Tabar L, Duffy SW, Burhenne LW. New Swedish breast cancer detection results for women aged 40–49. *Cancer* 1993;72:1437.
49. Smart C. The role of mammography in the prevention of mortality from breast cancer. *Cancer Prev* 1989;1.
50. Roberts MM, Alexander FE, Anderson TJ, et al. Edinburgh trial of screening for breast cancer: mortality at seven years. *Lancet* 1990;335:241.
51. Alexander F, Roberts M, Lutz W, Hepburn W. Randomisation by cluster and the problem of social class bias. *J Epidemiol Community Health* 1989;43:29.
52. Alexander FE, Anderson TJ, Brown HK, et al. The Edinburgh randomised trial of breast cancer screening: results after 10 years of follow-up. *Br J Cancer* 1994;70:542.
53. Miller AB, Baines CJ, To T, Wall C. Canadian National Breast Screening Study. 1: Breast cancer detection and death rates among women aged 40 to 49 years. *Can Med Assoc J* 1992;147:1459.
54. Burhenne LJ, Burhenne HJ. The Canadian National Breast Screening Study: a Canadian critique. *AJR Am J Roentgenol* 1993;161:761.
55. Kopans DB. The Canadian screening program: a different perspective [Commentary]. *AJR Am J Roentgenol* 1990;155:748.
56. Prorok PC, Kramer BS, Gohagan JK. Screening theory and study design: the basics. In: *Cancer screening: theory and practice.* New York: Marcel Dekker Inc, 1999.
57. Morrison AS, Brisson J, Khalid N. Breast cancer incidence and mortality in the breast cancer detection demonstration project. *J Natl Cancer Inst* 1988;80:1540.
58. Hendrick RE, Smith RA, Rutledge JH III, Smart CR. Benefit of screening mammography in women aged 40–49: a new meta-analysis of randomized controlled trials. *J Natl Cancer Inst Monogr* 1997;22:87.
59. Miller AB, To T, Baines CJ, Wall C. The Canadian National Breast Screening Study: update on breast cancer mortality. *J Natl Cancer Inst Monogr* 1997;22:37.
60. Kerlikowske K, Grady D, Barclay J, et al. Positive predictive value of screening mammography by age and family history of breast cancer. *JAMA* 1993;270:2444.
61. Costanza ME. The extent of breast cancer screening in older women. *Cancer* 1994;74[Suppl 7]:2046.
62. Van Dijck JA, Holland R, Verbeek AL, Hendriks JH, Mravunac M. Efficacy of mammographic screening of the elderly: a case-referent study in the Nijmegen program in the Netherlands. *J Natl Cancer* Inst 1994;86:934.
63. Eckhardt S, Badellino F, Murphy GP. UICC meeting on breast-cancer screening in premenopausal women in developed countries. *Int J Cancer* 1994;56:1.
64. Smart CR, Hendrick RE, Rutledge JH, Smith RA. Benefit of mammography screening in women ages 40 to 49 years: current evidence from randomized controlled trials. *Cancer* 1995;75:1619.
65. Dickersin K. Breast screening in women aged 40–49 years: what next? *Lancet* 1999;353:1896.
66. National Institutes of Health. Proceedings of the National Institutes of Health Consensus Conference on Breast Cancer Screening for Women Ages 40–49, Bethesda, MD, January 21–23, 1997. *J Natl Cancer Inst Monogr* 1997;22:vii, 1.
67. Ransohoff DF, Harris RP. Lessons from the mammography screening controversy: can we improve the debate? *Ann Intern Med* 1997;127:1029.
68. National Cancer Institute. *National Cancer Advisory Board (NCAB) mammography recommendations for women ages 40 to 49.* Bethesda, MD: National Cancer Institute, 1997.
69. Ries LA, Kosary CL, Hankey BF, et al., eds. *SEER cancer statistics review 1973–1995.* Bethesda, MD: National Cancer Institute, 1998.
70. Bosch FX, Manos MM, Munoz N, et al. Prevalence of human papillomavirus in cervical cancer: a worldwide perspective. *J Natl Cancer Inst* 1995;87:796.
71. Laara E, Day NE, Hakama M. Trends in mortality from cervical cancer in the Nordic countries: association with organised screening programmes. *Lancet* 1987;1:1247.
72. Miller AB, Lindsay J, Hill GB. Mortality from cancer of the uterus in Canada and its relationship to screening for cancer of the cervix. *Int J Cancer* 1976;17:602.
73. Eddy DM. Screening for cervical cancer. *Ann Intern Med* 1990;113:214.
74. International Agency for Research on Cancer. Working Group on Evaluation of Cervical Cancer Screening Programmes: Screening for squamous cervical cancer: duration of low risk after negative results of cervical cytology and its implications for screening policies. *BMJ* 1986;293:6599.
75. Aristizabal N, Cuello C, Correa P, Collazos T, Haenszel W. The impact of vaginal cytology on cervical cancer risks in Cali, Colombia. *Int J Cancer* 1984;34:5.
76. Clarke EA, Anderson TW. Does screening by "Pap" smears help prevent cervical cancer? A case-control study. *Lancet* 1979;2:1.
77. La Vecchia C, Franceschi S, Decarli A, et al. "Pap" smear and the risk of cervical neoplasia: quantitative estimates from a case-control study. *Lancet* 1984;2:779.
78. Herrero R, Brinton LA, Reeves WC, et al. Screening for cervical cancer in Latin America: a case-control study. *Int J Epidemiol* 1992;21:1050.
79. Remington P, Lantz P, Phillips JL. Cervical cancer deaths among older women: implications for prevention. *Wis Med J* 1990;89:30, 32.
80. Centers for Disease Control and Prevention. Use of cervical and breast cancer screening among women with and without functional limitations—United States, 1994–1995. *MMWR Morb Mortal Wkly Rep* 1998;47:853.
81. Pearce KF, Haefner HK, Sarwar SF, et al. Cytopathological findings on vaginal Papanicolaou smears after hysterectomy for benign gynecologic disease. *N Engl J Med* 1996;335:1559.
82. Burton RC, Coates MS, Hersey P, et al. An analysis of a melanoma epidemic. *Int J Cancer* 1993;55:765.

83. Miller DL, Weinstock MA. Nonmelanoma skin cancer in the United States: incidence. *J Am Acad Dermatol* 1994;30:774.
84. National Cancer Institute. *SEER cancer statistics review 1973–1995.* Bethesda, MD: National Cancer Institute, 1999.
85. Ferrini RL, Perlman M, Hill L. American College of Preventive Medicine policy statement: screening for skin cancer. *Am J Prev Med* 1998;14:80.
86. Hill D, White V, Marks R, Borland R. Changes in sun-related attitudes and behaviours, and reduced sunburn prevalence in a population at high risk of melanoma. *Eur J Cancer Prev* 1993;2:447.
87. Marks R. Two decades of the public health approach to skin cancer control in Australia: why, how and where are we now? *Australas J Dermatol* 1999;40:1.
88. Emmett EA. Dermatological screening. *J Occup Med* 1986;28:1045.
89. Mihm MC Jr, Fitzpatrick TB. Early detection of malignant melanoma. *Cancer* 1976;37[Suppl]:597.
90. Friedman RJ, Rigel DS, Kopf AW. Early detection of malignant melanoma: the role of physician examination and self-examination of the skin. *CA Cancer J Clin* 1985;35:130.
91. Mackie R. Screening for skin cancer. *Occup Health* (Lond) 1992;44:202, 206.
92. Polster AM, Lasek RJ, Quinn LM, Chren MM. Reports by patients and dermatologists of skin cancer preventive services provided in dermatology offices. *Arch Dermatol* 1998;134:1095.
93. Koh HK, Caruso A, Gage I, et al. Evaluation of melanoma/skin cancer screening in Massachusetts: preliminary results. *Cancer* 1990;65:375.
94. Koh HK, Mackie RM, Reintgen DS. The prevention and early detection of melanoma: screening for melanoma. *Cancer Screening* 1993;18:72.
95. Koh HK, Geller AC, Miller DR, et al. Who is being screened for melanoma/skin cancer? Characteristics of persons screened in Massachusetts. *J Am Acad Dermatol* 1991;24:271.
96. Cummings SR, Tripp MK, Herrmann NB. Approaches to the prevention and control of skin cancer. *Cancer Metastasis Rev* 1997;16:309.
97. Wolfe JT. The role of screening in the management of skin cancer. *Curr Opin Oncol* 1999;11:123.
98. Balanda KP, Lowe JB, Stanton WR, Gillespie AM. Enhancing the early detection of melanoma within current guidelines. *Aust J Public Health* 1994;18:420.
99. Koh HK, Geller AC. Public health interventions for melanoma. Prevention, early detection, and education. *Hematol Oncol Clin North Am* 1998;12:903.
100. Hill L, Ferrini RL. Skin cancer prevention and screening: summary of the American College of Preventive Medicine's practice policy statements. *CA Cancer J Clin* 1998;48:232.
101. McDonald CJ. American Cancer Society perspective on the American College of Preventive Medicine's policy statements on skin cancer prevention and screening. *CA Cancer J Clin* 1998;48:229.
102. National Cancer Institute. *PDQ cancer screening/prevention summary: skin cancer screening.* Bethesda, MD: National Cancer Institute, 1994.
103. Beers MH, Fink A, Beck JC. Screening recommendations for the elderly. *Am J Public Health* 1991;81:1131.
104. Girgis A, Clarke P, Burton RC, Sanson-Fisher RW. Screening for melanoma by primary health care physicians: a cost-effectiveness analysis. *J Med Screen* 1996;3:47.
105. Howell JB. Spotting sinister spots: a challenge to dermatologists to examine every new patient at increased risk for signs of early melanoma. *J Am Acad Dermatol* 1986;15:722.
106. Woolf SH. Public health perspective: the health policy implications of screening for prostate cancer. *J Urol* 1994;152:1685.
107. Hankey BR, Feuer EJ, Clegg LX, et al. Cancer surveillance series: interpreting trends in prostate cancer—Part I. Evidence of the effects of screening in recent prostate cancer incidence, mortality, and survival rates. *J Natl Cancer Inst* 1999;91:1017.
108. Feuer EJ, Merrill RM, Hankey BF. Cancer surveillance series: interpreting trends in prostate cancer—Part II. Cause of death misclassification and the recent rise and fall in prostate cancer mortality. *J Natl Cancer Inst* 1999;91:1025.
109. Etzioni R, Legler JM, Feuer EJ, et al. Cancer surveillance series: interpreting trends in prostate cancer—Part III. Quantifying the link between population prostate-specific antigen testing and recent declines in prostate cancer mortality. *J Natl Cancer Inst* 1999;91:1033.
110. Waterbor JW, Bueschen AJ. Prostate cancer screening (United States). Cancer Causes *Control* 1995;6:267.
111. Walther PJ. Prostate cancer screening: why the controversy? *Surg Oncol Clin North Am* 1995;4:315.
112. Jenson CB, Shahon DB, Wangensteen OH. Evaluation of annual examinations in the detection of cancer. *JAMA* 1960;174:91.
113. Gilbertsen VA. Cancer of the prostate gland. Results of early diagnosis and therapy undertaken for cure of the disease. *JAMA* 1971;215:81.
114. Chodak GW, Schoenberg HW. Early detection of prostate cancer by routine screening. *JAMA* 1984;252:3261.
115. Thompson IM, Ernst JJ, Gangai MP, Spence CR. Adenocarcinoma of the prostate: results of routine urological screening. *J Urol* 1984;132:690.
116. Lee R, Littrup PJ, Torp-Pedersen ST, et al. Prostate cancer: comparison of transrectal US and digital rectal examination for screening. *Radiology* 1988;168:389.
117. Rifkin MD. *Ultrasound of the prostate.* New York: Raven Press, 1988.
118. Carter HB, Hamper UM, Sheth S, et al. Evaluation of transrectal ultrasound in the early detection of prostate cancer. *J Urol* 1989;142:1008.
119. Cupp MR, Oesterling JE. Prostate-specific antigen, digital rectal examination, and transrectal ultrasonography: their roles in diagnosing early prostate cancer. *Mayo Clin Proc* 1993;68:297.
120. Stamey TA, Yang N, Hay AR, et al. Prostate-specific antigen as a serum marker for adenocarcinoma of the prostate. *N Engl J Med* 1987;317:909.
121. Lange PH, Ercole CJ, Lightner DJ, Fraley EE, Vessell R. The value of serum prostate specific antigen determinations before and after radical prostatectomy. *J Urol* 1989;141:873.
122. Catalona WJ, Smith DS, Ratliff TL, et al. Measurement of prostate-specific antigen in serum as a screening test for prostate cancer. *N Engl J Med* 1991;324:1156.
123. Cooner WH, Mosley BR, Rutherford CL Jr, et al. Prostate cancer detection in a clinical urological practice by ultrasonography, digital rectal examination and prostate specific antigen. *J Urol* 1990;143:1146.
124. Mettlin C, Murphy GP, Lee F, et al. Characteristics of prostate cancer detected in the American Cancer Society National Prostate Cancer Detection Project. *J Urol* 1994;152:1737.
125. Oesterling JE, Jacobsen SJ, Chute CG, et al. Serum prostate-specific antigen in a community-based population of healthy men. Establishment of age-specific reference ranges. *JAMA* 1993;270:860.
126. Babaian RJ, Mettlin C, Kane R, et al. The relationship of prostate-specific antigen to digital rectal examination and transrectal ultrasonography. Findings of the American Cancer Society National Prostate Cancer Detection Project. *Cancer* 1992;69:1195.
127. Catalona WJ, Richie JP, Ahmann FR, et al. Comparison of digital rectal examination and serum prostate specific antigen in the early detection of prostate cancer: results of a multicenter clinical trial of 6,630 men. *J Urol* 1994;151:1283.
128. Mueller EJ, Crain TW, Thompson IM, Rodriguez F. An evaluation of serial digital rectal examinations in screening for prostate cancer. *J Urol* 1988;140:1445.
129. Mettlin C, Lee F, Drago J, Murphy GP. The American Cancer Society National Prostate Cancer Detection Project. Findings on the detection of early prostate cancer in 2425 men. *Cancer* 1991;67:2949.
130. Wingo PA, Ries LAG, Giovino GA, et al. Annual report to the nation on the status of cancer, 1973–1996, with a special section on lung cancer and tobacco. *J Natl Cancer Inst* 1999;91:675.
131. Gohagan JK, Prorok PC, Kramer BS, Cornett JE. Prostate cancer screening in the prostate, lung, colorectal and ovarian cancer screening trial of the National Cancer Institute. *J Urol* 1994;152:1905.
132. Clinical Efficacy Assessment Project. Screening for prostate cancer: American College of Physicians. *Ann Intern Med* 1997;126:480.
133. Canadian Task Force on the Periodic Health Examination. Periodic health examination, 1991 update: 3. Secondary prevention of prostate cancer. *CMAJ* 1991;145:413.
134. Ahsan H, Neugut AI, Garbowski GC, et al. Family history of colorectal adenomatous polyps and increased risk for colorectal cancer. *Ann Intern Med* 1998;128:900.
135. Fuchs CS, Giovannucci EL, Colditz GA, et al. A prospective study of family history and the risk of colorectal cancer. *N Engl J Med* 1994;331:1669.
136. Byers T, Levin B, Rothenberger D, et al. American Cancer Society guidelines for screening and surveillance for early detection of colorectal polyps and cancer: update 1997. *CA Cancer J Clin* 1997;47:154.
137. Herrinton LJ, Selby JV, Friedman GD, et al. Case-control study of digital-rectal screening in relation to mortality from cancer of the distal rectum. *Am J Epidemiol* 1995;142:961.
138. Toribara NW, Sleisenger MH. Screening for colorectal cancer. *N Engl J Med* 1995;332:861.
139. Winawer SJ, Fletcher RH, Miller L, et al. Colorectal cancer screening: clinical guidelines and rationale. *Gastroenterology* 1997;112:594.
140. Mandel JS, Bond JH, Church TR, et al. Reducing mortality from colorectal cancer by screening for fecal occult blood. Minnesota Colon Cancer Control Study. *N Engl J Med* 1993;328:1365.
141. Mandel JS, Church TR, Ederer F, et al. Colorectal cancer mortality: effectiveness of biennial screening for fecal occult blood. *J Natl Cancer Inst* 1999;91:434.
142. Ederer F, Church TR, Mandel JS. Fecal occult blood screening in the Minnesota study: role of chance detection of lesions. *J Natl Cancer Inst* 1997;89:1423.
143. Hardcastle JD, Chamberlain JO, Robinson MH, et al. Randomised, controlled trial of faecal occult blood screening for colorectal cancer. *Lancet* 1996;348:1472.
144. Kronborg O, Fenger C, Olsen J, et al. Randomised study of screening for colorectal cancer with faecal-occult-blood test. *Lancet* 1996;348:1467.
145. Kewenter J, Bjork S, Haglind E, et al. Screening and rescreening for colorectal cancer: a controlled trial of fecal occult blood testing in 27,700 subjects. *Cancer* 1988;62:645.
146. Winawer SJ, Flehinger BJ, Schottenfeld D, Miller DG. Screening for colorectal cancer with fecal occult blood testing and sigmoidoscopy. *J Natl Cancer Inst* 1993;85:1311.
147. Selby JV, Friedman GD, Quesenberry CP, Weiss NS. Effect of fecal occult blood testing on mortality from colorectal cancer. *Ann Intern Med* 1993;118:1.
148. Selby JV, Friedman GD, Quesenberry CP Jr, Weiss NS. A case-control study of screening sigmoidoscopy and mortality from colorectal cancer. *N Engl J Med* 1992;326:653.
149. Saito H, Soma Y, Koeda J, et al. Reduction in risk of mortality from colorectal cancer by fecal occult blood screening with immunochemical hemagglutination test. A case-control study. *Int J Cancer* 1995;61:465.
150. Lazovich DA, Weiss NS, Stevens NG, et al. A case-control study to evaluate efficacy of screening faecal occult blood. *J Med Screen* 1995;2:84.
151. Allison JE, Tekawa IS. Hemoccult screening in detecting colorectal neoplasm: sensitivity, specificity, and predictive value: long-term follow-up in a large group practice setting. *Ann Intern Med* 1990;112:328.
152. Eddy DM. Screening for colorectal cancer. *Ann Intern Med* 1990;113:373.
153. Levin B. Colorectal cancer screening: sifting through the evidence. *J Natl Cancer Inst* 1999;91:399.
154. Gohagan JK, Prorok PC, Kramer BS, et al. The Prostate, Lung, Colorectal, and Ovarian Cancer Screening Trial of the National Cancer Institute. *Cancer* 1995;75[Suppl 7]:1869.
155. Atkin WS, Hart A, Edwards R, et al. Uptake, yield of neoplasia and adverse effects of flexible sigmoidoscopy screening. *Gut* 1998;42:560.
156. Newcomb PA, Norfleet RG, Storer BE, Surawicz TS, Marcus PM. Screening sigmoidoscopy and colorectal cancer mortality. *J Natl Cancer Inst* 1992;84:1572.
157. Muller AD, Sonnenberg A. Protection by endoscopy against death from colorectal cancer. A case-control study among veterans. *Arch Intern Med* 1995;155:1741.
158. Eddy DM. Screening for lung cancer. *Ann Intern Med* 1989;111:232.

159. Melamed MR, Flehinger BJ, Zaman MB, et al. Screening for early lung cancer: results of the Memorial Sloan-Kettering Study in New York. *Chest* 1984;86:44.
160. Tockman MS, Levin ML, Frost JK, et al. Screening and detection of lung cancer. In: Aisner J, ed. *Lung cancer.* New York: Churchill Livingstone, 1985:25.
161. Kubik A, Parkin DM, Khlat M, et al. Lack of benefit from semi-annual screening for cancer of the lung: follow-up report of a randomized controlled trial on a population of high-risk males in Czechoslovakia. *Int J Cancer* 1990;45:26.
162. Fontana RS. Screening for lung cancer: recent experience in the United States. In: Hansen HH, ed. *Lung cancer: basic and clinical aspects.* Boston: Martinus Nijhoff Publishers, 1986:91.
163. Smith IE. Screening for lung cancer: time to think positive. *Lancet* 1999;354:86.
164. Henschke CI, McCauley DI, Yankelevitz DF, et al. Early Lung Cancer Action Project: overall design and findings from baseline screening. *Lancet* 1999;354:99.
165. Breen N, Kessler L. Trends in cancer screening—United States, 1987 and 1992. *Oncology* 1996;10:328.

José Costa
Carlos Cordon-Cardo

CHAPTER 26

Cancer Diagnosis: Molecular Pathology

The traditional role of the surgical pathologist has been the morphologic evaluation of human tumors in a search for clues of their histogenesis and anticipated behavior. Over the years, this quest has benefited from the application of specialized techniques, which have become part of the pathologist's armamentarium. The diagnosis of cancer involves the analysis of tissue and cytology samples for features correlated with malignant transformation. Specimens of tissues and cells are obtained through several procedures, including surgical biopsy, endoscopic biopsy, core or aspirational needle biopsy, venipuncture, spinal tap, scraping of tissue surfaces, and collection of exfoliative cells from urine or sputum. The acquired tissue or cell specimens are subjected to a series of analytic modalities for diagnostic purposes.

Light microscopy, assessing morphologic features of the procured specimens, was used as almost the sole approach for many years, and it remains the standard diagnostic method to which all novel methods must be compared. The use of enzyme histochemistry and electron microscopy expanded the primary microanatomic evaluation to include biochemical and subcellular structural features. More recently, cytogenetics, analysis of DNA content, molecular genetic assays, and immunohistochemistry (IHC) have been added as valuable adjuncts to light microscopy in cancer diagnosis. These methods, particularly the latter, have greatly enhanced our ability to precisely define the lines of differentiation of human tumors, which constitutes the basis for the current classification schemes. As important as the "histogenetic" categorization provided by these techniques is, it addresses only indirectly other aspects of human neoplasia that are more relevant to their biologic behavior and response to therapy. These include rate of proliferation, capacity for invasion and metastases, and development of resistance mechanisms to certain treatment agents. This chapter reviews the contributions of novel approaches to the diagnosis and classification of tumors.

ROLE OF MOLECULAR PATHOLOGY IN CLINICAL ONCOLOGY AND TRANSLATIONAL RESEARCH

Molecular pathology studies the origins and pathogenesis of disease at the molecular level. Because cancer is a hereditary disease of the cell, much of the mechanistic studies of the cancer cell are based on the characterization of acquired or somatic mutations and subsequent structural or regulatory alterations of the gene products. In this regard, it differs from medical genetics, in which the main objective is to determine the genetic abnormalities associated with inherited disorders and carried as germline mutations. Molecular pathology of neoplasia aims at identifying and understanding those aberrations involved in the development and progression of neoplastic diseases. Clinically relevant objectives include (1) establishing a definitive diagnosis and classification of tumors based on the recognition of complex profiles ("fingerprints") or unique molecular alterations that occur in specific tumor types; (2) providing early detection of tumor cells using sensitive molecular techniques, thus anticipating therapeutic intervention; (3) rendering prognostic information of clinical relevance through the assessment of molecular predictors of outcome; and (4) assisting in the selection of individualized treatment regimens, saving unnecessary drug toxicity. Protocols based on molecular markers increase the chances for cure by opting for the right management approach, and they improve the quality of life of patients with cancer.

Molecular pathology also serves as a bridge between clinical and basic biomedical sciences. The translational aspects of research in molecular pathology are bidirectional, involving both the active transfer of relevant observations that are the result of the analysis of primary tumors and clinicopathologic correlations to basic laboratory studies, as well as the effective transfer of laboratory findings into clinical analyses and protocols. In promoting such transfers, molecular biology facilitates and maximizes the transfer of biologic discoveries into diagnostic, prognostic, and therapeutic applications.

The use of molecular techniques has led to remarkable progress in the understanding of cell growth, differentiation, maintenance of genomic integrity, and programmed cell death, these being key issues in tumor development and progression. Biologic markers, such as alterations of TP53, which correlate with tumor behavior when detected in specific tumor types, await validation studies. Similarly, prospective clinical analyses using well-characterized cohorts of patients and properly selected pairs of normal and tumor samples are needed to better delineate the role of mutations occurring in these genes, because they may impact on the management of patients affected with cancer. The implementation of objective predictive assays to the diagnostic and prognostic tools will enhance the ability to assess tumor biologic activities and to design effective treatment regimens.

USE OF HUMAN TISSUE SAMPLES FOR MOLECULAR ANALYSES

Discrepancies of reported results aimed at the identification of gene mutations and altered patterns of gene expression in primary tumors could be explained by the use of distinct probes and methods. Critical caveats include assurance for the presence of viable tumor, extent of necrosis, normal cell to tumor cell ratio, and the stage and grade of the lesion being studied. Often, distinct methods are available to detect a given marker, these approaches differing in specificity, sensitivity, speed and cost, and appropriateness for particular clinical situations.

Strategies have been developed whereby, from a single tissue sample, different techniques can be performed in search of the molecular phenotype and genotype.[1,2] One of these strategies is illustrated in Figure 26-1. Briefly, using consecutive tissue sections cut at different thicknesses and deposited either on glass slides or microtubes, one can (1) evaluate morphology (i.e., hematoxylin and eosin staining), (2) perform expression assays [i.e., IHC and *in situ* hybridization (ISH)], (3) identify molecular alterations [i.e., Southern blot, polymerase chain reaction/ single-strand conformation polymorphism (PCR-SSCP), and sequencing], and (4) conduct high-throughput assays (i.e., expression array technologies). Tissue microdissection assays can be implemented to remove normal contaminating cells, enriching the neoplastic cell content of the tumor sample when needed.[3] This method can also be used to study low-grade and high-grade tumor foci in a single tissue sample or to analyze minimal lesions, such as carcinoma *in situ*. Evaluation of gene mutations and altered patterns of expression can be performed using a combination of techniques, including deletion studies by restriction fragment length polymorphism and comparative multiplex PCR, point mutation screening by PCR-SSCP and confirmation by direct sequencing, and assessment of altered expression by IHC and ISH. More recently, the introduction of microchips and other technologies allows the detection of missense mutations in certain genes with great sensitivity.[4]

Manual microdissection of tumor samples, to enrich neoplastic cell aliquots to be used in specific techniques, is achieved by the use of a magnifying lens and sterilized scalpels. It can be also performed using scraping devices mounted on specially designed stereotactic microscopes. More refined, laser-based microdissection instruments have been developed and are commercially available (Fig. 26-2). One of the strategies, the laser-capture method, is based on adhering cells to a material after it is thermally activated by a laser beam.[3] Tissues to be microdissected are viewed through a video microscope, and the position of the slide is adjusted so that the desired cells are under the targeting light. Activation of the laser causes the desired cells to adhere to the special coverslip, which is mounted on a plastic cap and positioned over the targeted cells. The cap is then separated from the tissue section, pulling the desired cells for study. The dissected material can be reviewed for morphology and nonspecific transfers before placing it in a tube containing the appropriate digestion buffer for nucleic acid extraction. Protocols for the dissection of tumor cells from frozen and formalin-fixed paraffin-embedded tissue have been developed that allow the extraction of nucleic acids, mainly DNA. It is possible to select cell populations based on their phenotypic features determined by IHC. Isolation of intact RNA transcripts is difficult, if not impossible, to achieve through this procedure. The distortion produced during the application of the laser beam appears to be responsible for the partial degradation of most RNA species.

The application of the full spectrum of molecular-based methods to the evaluation of tissue and cell specimens, and the implementation of novel therapeutic modalities aimed at specific molecular targets, has led to changes in the established patterns of tissue procurement, processing, and tissue banking. Advanced diagnostic technology should be included in tissue analysis carried out during the diagnostic investigation of any potentially neoplastic lesion. Diagnosticians should "think molecular." Protocols should be implemented and constantly updated to guarantee that samples are handled in a way that will not preclude optimal application of molecular testing. In daily practice, this means that part of the specimen, whenever possible, should be set aside prospectively for advanced diagnostics. The advent of advanced diagnostics is forcing operational changes that ensure fast delivery of specimens to the laboratory, where pathologists can select an aliquot of tissue or cells that will be used to resolve questions pertinent to the management of the lesion or set aside a sample "in reserve" for molecular analysis if necessary.

One of the most common ways to preserve samples is by snap freezing in liquid nitrogen. However, this procedure does not allow for preservation of microanatomic detail. Rapid freezing of tissue in a block with cryopreservative solution maintains morphology and yields frozen sections that can be

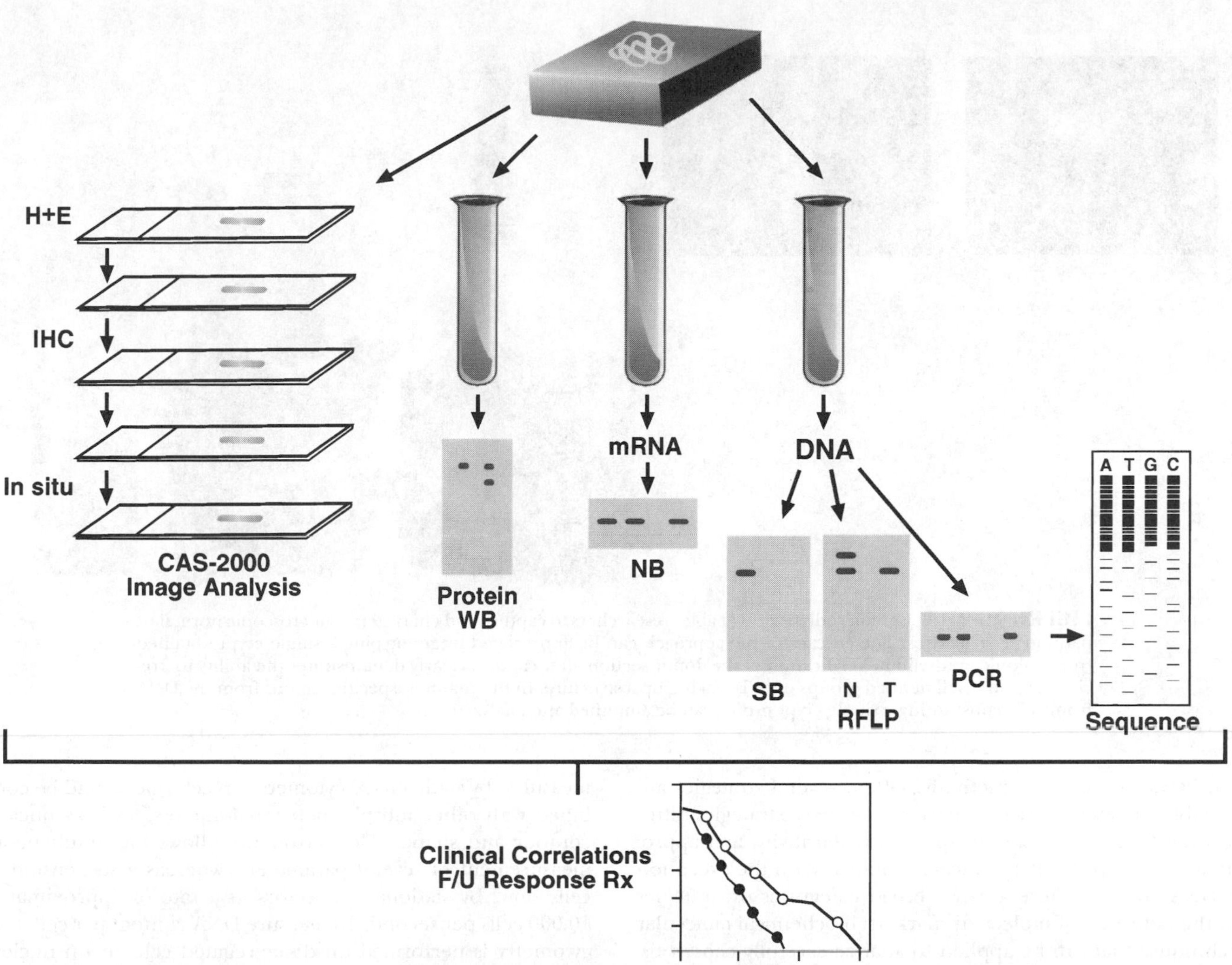

FIGURE 26-1. Use of tissue for research and diagnostic purposes can be prepared to yield a variety of tissue-derived products that can be treated using different technological approaches. The ability to analyze nucleic acids and proteins from small numbers of cells makes it possible to obtain a comprehensive profile of the tissue. These data can then be correlated to the histopathologic appearance and to clinical characteristics of the lesion. Properly annotated samples stored in a tissue bank constitute a precious resource to test the efficacy of newly discovered biomarkers and diagnostic or predictive tests. F/U, follow-up; H&E, hematoxylin and eosin; IHC, immunohistochemical; NB, Northern blot; PCR, polymerase chain reaction; RFLP, restriction fragment length polymorphism; Rx, medication; SB, Southern blot; WB, Western blot.

used for different assays. This method is favored in building frozen tumor banks from which enough genomic DNA or complementary DNA (cDNA) can be generated from a thick section to produce useful reagents for subsequent analyses. In addition, monoclonal antibodies, purified antisera, and riboprobes can easily be used on thin sections, usually 5 μm, by implementing IHC or ISH protocols. In today's practice, one of the ideal moments to procure tissue is at the time of an intraoperative consultation, when tissue is sampled for diagnostic frozen section examination. It is important to realize that the tissue procured for advanced diagnostics remains usable when and if required for routine morphologic analysis. Tissue procurement and tissue banking are different tasks that should be well delineated if this kind of valuable resource is to be implemented with maximum efficiency.

When using archival tissue for research, including both discovery and validation studies, issues of patient confidentiality and informed consent should be carefully considered and resolved through established institutional and national guidelines. Institutional review boards and human investigation committees must be made aware of the ever-growing complexities involved in the use of human tissues for research. These issues grow in complexity because of the rapid development of new technology and bioinformatics. The existence of large databanks containing comprehensive information on disease susceptibility, pharmacogenomics, and other biologic data that can be potentially linked to an individual are of obvious concern to researchers and ethicists.

OVERVIEW OF THE TECHNOLOGICAL APPROACHES TO MOLECULAR DIAGNOSTICS

The value of molecular markers for cancer diagnosis and patient management depends on their accessibility to detec-

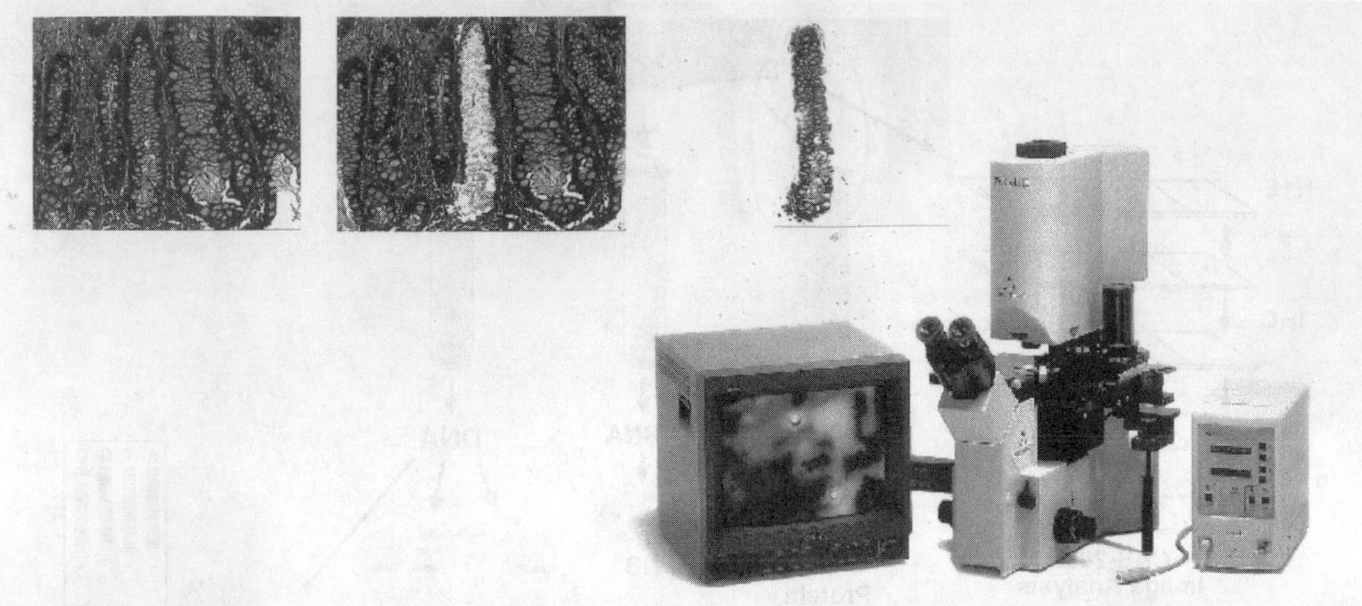

FIGURE 26-2. Laser microdissection enables researchers to capture and characterize microscopic normal or pathologic structures. The efficacy of the approach can be appreciated in genotyping a single crypt obtained from colonic epithelium. Verification of the donor section after capture clearly demonstrates the ability to precisely capture well-defined groups of cells making up a structure. In this manner, specific regions from the DNA from cells constituting a single crypt profile can be amplified and analyzed.

tion by various analytic methods. Often, several strategies are available to detect the same marker, and these strategies differ in several aspects, including specificity, sensitivity, and appropriateness for particular clinical situations. With the exception of DNA content, there are two broad categories of strategies for the detection of molecular markers: biochemical molecular techniques that can be applied to analyze carefully chosen tissue samples or, alternatively, reagents can be applied *in situ* on tissues, cells, or chromosomes to detect and demonstrate the presence and spatial distribution of the marker. At present, the development of new clinical tests depends mainly on low-throughput assays, but it seems likely that the high-throughput, comprehensive analytic techniques described in the following sections will have a major impact in the near future. Some understanding of these techniques is central for the appreciation of their capabilities, advantages, and limitations when analyzing clinical material.

LOW-THROUGHPUT TECHNIQUES

DNA Content and Flow Cytometry

Individual cells harboring many genetic alterations, including genes regulating growth and apoptosis programs, often contain an abnormal amount of nuclear DNA that can be measured by flow cytometry. Deviations in cell DNA content relative to normal cells (DNA index) may indicate duplications or losses of individual chromosomes (aneuploidy) or extra haploid sets of chromosomes (polyploidy). In addition, the profile of DNA content among the cells of a tissue reflects the fraction of cells in S and G_2 phases of the cycle. A high number of cells in these fractions correlate with poorer prognosis in certain cancers.[5,6] The amount of DNA per cell can also be measured by static image cytometry on cell smears and be combined with other morphometric parameters, such as nuclear contour and shape.[7] Flow cytometry allows for simultaneous measurement of several parameters, whereas a suspension of cells flows by stationary detectors at a rate of approximately 10,000 cells per second. To measure DNA content per cell, flow cytometry is performed on disaggregated cells or on nuclear suspensions. The latter can be obtained fresh or from paraffin blocks.[8] In either case, the cells are stained with dyes that bind stoichiometrically to DNA—fluorescent dyes for flow cytometry, and Feulgen dyes for static measurements through a specially equipped light microscope. The data acquired from each individual cell are compiled in a histogram, indicating the distribution of the DNA content among the cells in the tissue. Total DNA measurements permit the evaluation of ploidy and an estimation of the fraction of cells traversing the S phase of the cell cycle. Both parameters have been found to be of prognostic relevance in certain tumors, such as breast cancer, and aneuploidy has been reported as a favorable prognostic feature in neuroblastoma.[9]

DNA Alterations and Detection Assays

Native DNA extracted from either tissues or cells can be directly sequenced or analyzed by Southern blotting, restriction fragment length polymorphism, and comparative genomic hybridization (CGH). These techniques are capable of detecting alterations present in the genome of neoplastic cells that serve as markers, including point mutations, translocations, amplifications, deletions, microsatellite length instability, and altered methylation. Point mutations are the most common dominant oncogene alterations found in human cancer. The amino acid change produced by the mutations causes the gain of function that contributes to the transformed state of the cell. Amplification of an oncogene is usually associated with protein overexpression and is another mechanism for gain of function. Amplification constitutes an easily detectable and measurable change; thus, it is a good diagnostic and potential prognostic marker. In translocations, protooncogenes are subjected to a strong promoter-enhancer or removed from a physiologic regulatory control element. The net effect is an inappropriate increase in product that provides excess function.

Alternatively, a translocation can produce a novel gene by fusion of the two partners participating in the translocation and generate a chimeric product with aberrant function. Missense or nonsense point mutations can cause loss of function of tumor suppressor genes that are important in maintaining control of cell growth and differentiation. In the case of a dominant-negative tumor suppressor gene, the product of the allele inactivated by mutation suffices to contribute to the neoplastic state by binding and abrogating the function of the wild-type product. For the majority of tumor suppressor genes, however, inactivation of the second allele is necessary to completely lose function. The second hit is often effected by the deletion of genomic information, often registered by loss of heterozygosity assays. Loss of function can also be produced by hypermethylation of the promoter or intragenic regions, resulting in silencing or extinction of its expression. The genetic instability inherent to many cancer cells can be manifested by microsatellite instability. Changes in the length of repeats can be caused by lesions in the DNA repair genes (i.e., hMSH1, hMSH2, hPMS1, hPMS2) giving rise to the so-called mutator phenotype.

An additional category of markers is based on the clonal nature of neoplastic proliferations. When there is a question about whether abnormal cells are the consequence of nontumoral tissue response (regenerative atypia) or represent a neoplastic proliferation, clonality assays may provide the answer. If the suspicious cells or tissues can be shown to be clonal, they are likely to represent a neoplastic process, because cells in hyperplastic or reactive lesions are polyclonal. Assays of clonal markers measure the fraction of cells within a tissue or cytology sample that carry the same form of the marker and are thus presumed to be issued from a single cell. Prime examples of diagnostically useful clonal markers are antigen receptor gene rearrangements in lymphoid proliferations.[10] Inactivation of the X chromosomes in females heterozygous for some X-linked genes have been widely used to confirm the clonality of tumors by the examination of isotypes of proteins or the analysis of methylation in X chromosome DNA.[11] If a tumor is known to harbor a specific mutation in a given gene, the altered sequence can, under some conditions, also serve as a marker for clonality. The fundamental requirements are (1) that the sequence be altered early in the genesis of the tumor; (2) that the sequence should not be further altered or lost during tumor progression; and (3) that there be enough diversity in the observed mutations of the specific gene to make it unlikely that two diverse populations of cells, arising from two independent metachronous tumors, would harbor the same mutated sequence.

Southern blotting[12] is the procedure that identifies a specific DNA by using a complementary sequence (probe) that hybridizes to a fragment of the DNA after it has been transferred from an agarose gel to a nitrocellulose filter. This technique was one of the first used for diagnostic testing. It still provides a robust way for detecting changes in DNA nucleotide sequence, particularly when these differences involve rearrangements of sizable stretches of DNA (translocations, large deletions, or amplifications). The major drawback of the Southern blot is its relative lack of sensitivity, because it can detect only 1 cell in 100. Another limitation is the requirement of several micrograms of DNA per test. The term *restriction fragment length polymorphism* defines the use of specific restriction enzymes to cut recognizable DNA fragments, followed by a blotting procedure, and it is mainly used for deletion analysis.

Fluorescence In Situ *Hybridization*

Fluorescence *in situ* hybridization (FISH) overcomes many of the practical problems of conventional cytogenetics by permitting the specific staining of any given region of the genome.[13,14] In addition, the staining can be done using metaphases or interphase nuclei. ISH of DNA probes to metaphase chromosomes deposited on microscope slides or to chromatin within intact interphase cells in smears or tissue sections is usually monitored by fluorescence, and it is therefore referred to as FISH. The DNA probes used for FISH may consist of mixtures of DNA fragments covering whole chromosomes, fragments containing chromosome-specific repeated sequences, or fragments containing unique nonrepetitive sequences. The lower limit of fragment size for unique sequence fragments is approximately 4 kilobases (kb), but in practice, fragments of approximately 25 kb, such as those propagated in bacterial cosmids or in yeast artificial chromosomes, give the most consistent results. The probes hybridized to specific chromosomal sequences are tagged with a marker (digoxigenin or biotin) that can be detected with an antibody specific to the tag and labeled with a fluorochrome. Up to seven probes can be used simultaneously, and changes not detectable in expanded banding preparations can be identified with this approach. The number of simultaneous probes that can be applied is growing, and with the aid of confocal microscopy and image processing, this method can be carried out in paraffin-embedded tissue sections. Used on histologic sections, FISH allows for correlation of genetic findings with the histology, a feature not shared by the analysis of metaphase chromosomes. FISH is well suited for the detection of numerical changes in chromosomes or regions of chromosomes, including microdeletions. In addition, chromosomal translocations can be detected by the simultaneous use of two probes containing DNA sequences known to reside on either side of a translocation breakpoint in one of the two reciprocal translocation products. Apposition of two of the four dots present in diploid cells indicates the presence of a translocation. Identification of such a result is facilitated by labeling the two probes with different tags that are recognized with antibodies conjugated to two different fluorochromes. When used in interphase cells, for the diagnostic or monitoring purposes discussed in the following section, FISH has the advantage over PCR that it is a quantitative technique, because the results can be expressed as the percentage of a class of cells containing the diagnostic abnormality.[15]

The limitation of FISH—providing information only on the regions covered by the probe(s) used—is partially overcome by CGH.[16,17] In this procedure, tumor DNA ultimately recognized by a red fluorochrome and normal DNA recognized by a green fluorescent dye are mixed at equimolar concentrations and then allowed to compete for hybridizing to a normal metaphase spread. If a region of the genome is equally represented in the tumor and in the normal DNA, the chromosomal region appears painted in an orange-yellow signal. If a gene is missing in the tumor, it is painted green. In contrast, if a region of the genome is amplified many-fold in the tumor, this region appears in red. CGH allows assessment of the entire genome, albeit at a relatively rough scale, but it is a technically demanding and lengthy procedure. Although it constitutes a powerful research and discovery tool, it is unlikely to receive widespread diagnostic application as a clinical test.

The simultaneous use of probes labeled with different fluorochromes and cameras capable of sensing and computing different spectra have made it possible to paint each chromosome (or chromosomal regions) with a different color attributed to the individual spectra. This technique, known as *spectral karyotypic analysis*,[18] adds considerable ease, specificity, and potential automation to the detection and identification of translocations and other chromosomal anomalies (see Molecular Biology of Cancer: Cytogenetics chapter).

The application of molecular techniques to diagnosis has been greatly facilitated by the introduction of the PCR.[19–21] PCR-based approaches make it possible to use very small samples of tissue, and therefore, well-defined microscopic lesions can be used as the source of nucleic acid to be analyzed. The products of PCR can be investigated by a variety of methods. PCR can be designed to demonstrate (1) genetic alterations, including microsatellite instability (i.e., using single-strand conformation polymorphism or PCR-SSCP, which reveals band shifts in tumor lanes when compared to normal tissue lanes); (2) point mutations (i.e., using PCR products in sequencing assays); and (3) loss of genetic material (i.e., using multiplex PCR). PCR combined with Southern blot analysis is capable of detecting a unique target sequence within the total DNA of approximately 100,000 human genes in a single reaction. These numbers are only limited by the amount of DNA (approximately 2 μg, equivalent to 2×10^6 cells) that can be tested in a single amplification reaction; selection procedures to restrict the target DNA to the genomic fragment of interest allows a significant expansion of the sample to be analyzed. The extreme sensitivity of PCR-based techniques constitutes their main drawback. Because a single template can give rise to a positive result, contamination of the reaction by exogenous amplifiable sequences can be a problem, even in laboratories that exercise the greatest care to guard against such occurrences. In most instances, the source of contamination is the inadvertent transfer of small amounts of product from one reaction to the ingredients of another reaction that uses the same primers. Measures taken to prevent artifactual results caused by contamination include ultraclean and separate rooms for pre-PCR, PCR, and post-PCR manipulation of the samples; use of pipetting devices containing aerosol barriers; and UV irradiation of the reaction mixture before addition of the polymerase and template DNA. Additionally, control reactions from which template DNA is omitted should always be performed and analyzed in parallel with any PCR test to ensure that the reagents, other than the template, are not contaminated. Products can also be precisely sized on gels, analyzed by Southern blot hybridization, or subjected to nucleotide sequence analysis to distinguish bona fide products expected for a specific amplification reaction from artifactual products that may have been amplified during the reactions. The advantages of PCR, however, far outweigh the

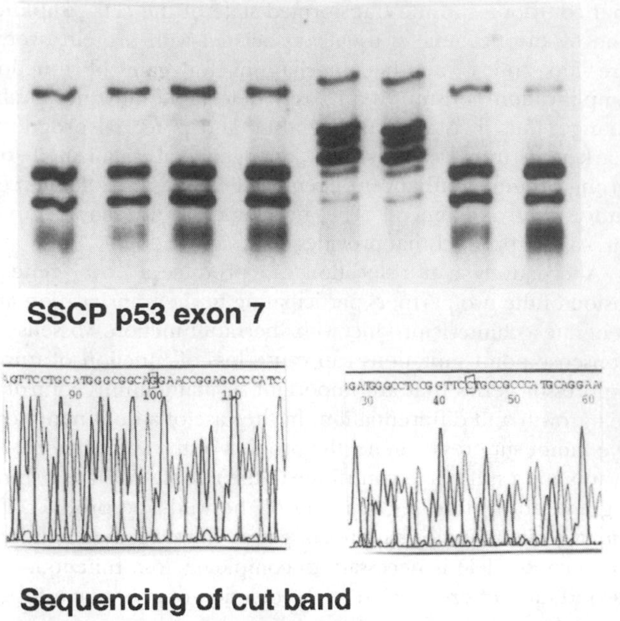

FIGURE 26-3. Cytologic samples that are suspicious but not diagnostic of cancer can be resolved when known genetic alterations are found in a significant proportion of the cell population examined. In the proper clinical context, a mutation in a tumor gene present at the 10% level or higher is a reliable indicator of tumor. DNA obtained from a portion of the cytology sample has been extracted, and exons 5 to 7 of the p53 gene amplified and examined by single-strand confirmation polymorphism (SSCP). A mutation in exon 7 (ATG → AGG transversion) is confirmed by repeating the procedure and sequencing the anomalous migrating band.

disadvantages. The amplification capabilities of the procedure mean that very small numbers of total cells are sufficient for analysis. The small size of the amplification target (as small as 40 to 50 base pairs) makes PCR possible on partially degraded DNA or on the highly fragmented DNA normally obtained when extracting from formalin-fixed paraffin-embedded tissue. PCR is a fast procedure, because standard amplifications that comprise 25 to 30 cycles can be completed in a few hours, facilitating timely turnaround of tests. Furthermore, if maximum sensitivity is not a concern, analysis can be carried out with nonradioactive probes. For all these reasons, PCR has been used in most of the molecular diagnostic tests relevant to cancer. It is the sensitivity of PCR that makes it the method of choice for the staging of cancer, as well as for the monitoring of residual disease after therapy.

A productive application of PCR has been to amplify specific genomic sequences obtained from paraffin sections by microdissection (Fig. 26-3). By using random primers, the entire DNA extracted from a small number of cells can be amplified in an unbiased fashion. Efficient protocols for "whole genomic amplification" make it possible to perform CGH experiments, starting from a microscopic lesion.[22]

RNA-Based Methods

ISH is performed to detect RNA transcripts within cells deposited on microscope slides or on tissue sections.[22–24] The probe can be radiolabeled or linked to a molecular tag, such as biotin. The main diagnostic application is for the tissue typing of neoplasms, revealing the specific transcript for a determined cell product, or demonstrating viral nucleic acids. In the tumors known to be associated with viruses, viral nucleic acids, as well as their encoded proteins, can be used as tumor markers. The most significant viruses in this context are human T-cell leukemia virus type I (associated with adult T-cell leukemia/lymphoma), Epstein-Barr virus (associated with Burkitt's lymphoma and with non-Hodgkin's lymphoma in immunosuppressed patients and those with Hodgkin's disease), and papillomavirus strains associated mainly with cervical cancer. Viral proteins synthesized in the tumor cell contribute to the transformation process, and infection with the virus precedes the development of the tumor. In some instances, such as the case of Epstein-Barr virus infection in nasopharyngeal cancer, the viral integration site serves as a clonal marker for the tumor cells.

A more quantitative estimation of a specific message is obtained by Northern blotting.[25,26] In an analogous way to the Southern procedure, Northern blots identify specific RNA sequences by hybridization against a panel of RNA molecules spread on a gel. The synthesis of cDNA from messenger RNA (mRNA) using reverse transcriptase makes it possible to analyze the messenger molecules after PCR amplification, a procedure known as *reverse transcriptase-PCR* (RT-PCR).[27,28] This technique makes possible the detection of few transcripts coding for a specific message against a large background of mRNAs. In this fashion, a few circulating tumor cells can be detected in peripheral blood. The mRNA coding a cell-specific protein serves as a target that can be used to detect a specific cell type in a background of 10 million cells. This strategy has been used to detect circulating melanoma cells by demonstrating tyrosinase transcripts in peripheral blood, circulating prostatic cells (detecting prostate-specific antigen mRNA), thyroid cells (identifying thyroglobulin mRNA), and breast cancer (finding mRNA for keratin 19).[29–31] The advent of real-time PCR instrumentation has brought quantitative PCR to the laboratory and obviates one of the shortcomings of this kind of amplification technology.[32]

Analysis of Proteins

One of the most favored techniques for unraveling the phenotype, based on detection of specific protein sequences and preserving the microanatomic detail, is IHC. The ever-increasing number of commercially available antisera and monoclonal antibodies is expanding the resolution capabilities of this assay by demonstrating the presence of antigenic determinants in cells and tissue components (Table 26-1). Everything from surface receptors to intercellular matrix components to hormones can now be determined with relative ease and used to pinpoint the cell type, the degree of immunophenotypic differentiation, and even the functional state of the cell. IHC has greatly reduced the number of undifferentiated or unclassified tumors and has been of major assistance in defining metastatic tumors of unknown primary site. The category of unclassified sarcomas has been reduced from approximately 15% of cases to less than 5%. A relatively simple battery of antibodies recognizing intermediate filaments and surface antigens is very effective in sorting out undifferentiated carcinomas from anaplastic lymphomas, melanomas, and sarcomas, thus reducing the number of undifferentiated malignant tumors. Perhaps the best-established use of IHC has been in the diagnosis and classification of lymphomas. The demonstration of surface lymphoid determinants continues to be important in the everyday practice of diagnostic hematopathology. For example, the demonstration of the CD5 surface determinant is helpful in distinguishing mantle cell tumors (positive) from nodular lymphoma (negative).[33] In solid tumors, such as breast carcinomas, IHC is becoming a required complement of predictive clinical value, determining estrogen and progesterone receptor status, and, more recently, with the advent of antibody-based anti-Her-2/Neu therapy, also assessing the expression pattern of this tyrosine-kinase receptor.[34,35]

IHC is a powerful tool to dissect the different cell components present in tumoral tissues. It can show two different phenotypes of tumor cell differentiation most dramatically when two antigens specific for each cell type are shown simultaneously on the same slide, and thus, it has contributed to the elucidation of the composition of tumors showing diverse lines of differentiation. It can also separate reactive cells infiltrating the tumor when distinction of tumor cells from reactive cells is unreliable using routine histologic stains. Such an instance is seen in the so-called T-cell–rich B-cell lymphomas, which consist of neoplastic lymphocytes of B lineage accompanied by a heavy infiltrate of nonneoplastic T cells. The latter sometimes constitute the majority of the cellular elements visible on a slide. At least some of the cases classified as malignant histiocytosis on the basis of finding neoplastic cells admixed with "atypical" histiocytes demonstrating erythrophagocytosis have been shown to be T-cell lymphomas infiltrated by activated histiocytes.[36]

IHC can sometimes contribute to the distinction between benign and malignant tumors. The demonstration of the ectopic chorionic gonadotropin-β subunit in islet cell tumors of the pancreas strongly suggests malignancy.[37] Many tumor markers can be localized in tumoral tissues, contributing to both tumor classification and identification of tumor cells in distant sites. Demonstration of cells containing neuron-specific enolase antigenic determinants in their cytoplasm has increased the sensitivity of detecting bone marrow involvement in neuroblastoma, thus improving the precision of the staging of children with this tumor. Pathologic staging has become more precise when the involvement of lymph nodes is established using IHC to detect breast tumor cells in axial lymph nodes. IHC is a very useful diagnostic adjunct to resolve controversial cases in cell type and to unequivocally identify the presence of small numbers of tumor cells. To maximize the efficiency and usefulness of IHC in clinical practice, it is best to use batteries of antisera chosen to solve specific problems in a critical and systematic fashion. Together with the availability of automated staining devices, this algorithmic approach helps manage the laboratory and facilitates periodic evaluation of test performance and efficiency of operations.

With the explosion of molecular medicine, IHC used mostly to investigate disease in a correlative mode is progressively being applied to attack mechanistic questions. Monoclonal antibodies are capable of recognizing subtle structural changes that are directly related to the function of the molecule and are thus excellent tools for molecular analysis. An example of dissection of molecular function using antibodies is provided

TABLE 26-1. Selected Antigens Analyzed by Immunohistochemistry in the Diagnosis and Characterization of Tumors

Antigen	*Comments on Tissue and Tumor Specificities*
Actin	Isoform specific for smooth muscle and myofibroblasts; sarcomeric isoform specific for striated muscle
α-Fetoprotein	Liver, visceral endoderm; yolk sac tumors, hepatocellular carcinoma
α-Lactalbumin	Breast epithelium, ductal and lobular carcinoma of the breast; hidradenoma papilliferum
CA 19.9	Monosialo Lewis A antigen; pancreaticobiliary carcinoma, transitional cell tumors
CA125	Mucinous epithelial tumors of the ovary, cervix, endometrium, gastrointestinal tract, breast
Cadherin	Carcinoma; expression inversely correlated to differentiation
Carcinoembryonic antigen	Adenocarcinoma; gastrointestinal tract and pancreas, lung, medullary thyroid carcinoma
CD31	Endothelial cells
CD34	Endothelial cells, bone marrow stem cells
Chromogranins	Neuroendocrine tumors
Cytokeratins	Epithelial tumors, less commonly other types
Desmin	Striated and parenchymal smooth muscle
Epithelial membrane antigen	Adenocarcinomas, mesothelioma meningioma
Factor VIII	Megakaryocytes, platelets, mast cells, endothelium; endothelial tumors
Factor XIII	Megakaryocytes, fibroblasts, macrophages, dermal fibrous histiocytomas
Glialfribrillary acidic protein	Glial cells, astrocytomas, oligodendrogliomas, ependymomas, schwannomas
GCDFP-15	Apocrine differentiation in breast and skin; some breast carcinomas
HMB-45	Melanoma, angiomyolipoma, some neural crest tumors
Hormone receptors	Estrogen: carcinoma of the breast, desmoid tumor; progesterone: carcinoma of the breast
Human chorionic gonadotropin-β	Trophoblast; germ cell tumors, ectopic production in lung and other carcinomas
Human placental lactogen	Trophoblast; germ cell tumors, gastric and lung carcinomas
Immunoglobulins	Lymphoid and plasma cell tumors
Integrins	Expressed in tumors according to cell lineage
Ki-67	Proliferation antigen in cycling cells, all tumor types
Laminin	Basement membrane component, epithelial; smooth muscle and endothelial tumors
Leucocyte common antigen	Panlymphocytic; negative in other cell types
LeuM-1	Hodgkin's disease, adenocarcinoma
Leu-7	Neural and neuroendocrine tumors, prostatic carcinoma
MyoD-1	Skeletal muscle tumors, alveolar soft part sarcoma
Myoglobin	Skeletal and myocardial muscle
Myosin	Isoforms specific for smooth and striated muscle
Neurospecific enolase	γ/γ and γ/α predominantly in neural and neuroendocrine tumors; present in many other tumor types
Notch	Present in some stem cells; stains epithelial tumors and lymphomas
p53	Prolonged half-life in many tumor types
P glycoprotein	Normal colon, endothelial, and adrenal cells; associated with multidrug resistance
Placenta-like alkaline phosphatase	Present in gonadal and extragonadal germ cell tumors; marker of *in situ* germ cell neoplasia
Prostate-specific antigen	Present in normal, hyperplastic, and neoplastic prostate; specific for that organ
Prostatic acid phosphatase	Carcinoma of the prostate, transitional cell carcinoma, carcinoids and other tumors
S-100	Peripheral nerve sheath tumors, central gliomas, cartilaginous and adipose tumors; marks myoepithelial cells
Surfactant apoprotein	Primary pulmonary adenocarcinoma
Synaptophysin	Neuroectodermal and neuroendocrine tumors
Thyroglobulin	Thyroid tumors of follicular cell origin
Vimentin	Mesenchymal tumors; high-grade epithelial tumors
Numerous antigens for stages of B- and T-lymphocytic lineage and activation	Hematolymphoid tumors

by monoclonal antibodies directed to the phosphorylated peptides of growth factor receptors. The erbB-2 receptor is phosphorylated on activation. Antibodies that discriminate between the phosphorylated and nonphosphorylated protein provide an accurate assessment of the number of activated molecules present in a cell. Preliminary data suggest that this measurement will provide a better predictor of prognosis than the estimation of total erbB-2 in the tumor cells of patients with breast cancer.[38]

Antibodies directed against the proteins involved in the regulation of the cell cycle are playing an increasing role in the pathologic evaluation of tumors. Antibodies to cyclins D1 and E have been reported to be of interest in the evaluation of breast carcinoma and squamous cell carcinoma of the head and neck.[39,40] IHC also has been used to assess the status of tumor suppressor genes, such as p53 and RB (retinoblastoma). Numerous studies suggest the relevance of determining the patterns of expression of these genes to determine the prognosis in a variety of tumors. We are near to being able to determine the status (overexpression or absence) of many of the key proteins controlling the progression through the cell cycle, and thus we are poised to extensively characterize tumors and guide therapy accordingly.

The expression patterns of gene products involved in accessing apoptotic pathways can also be investigated by IHC. Such an evaluation is likely to be relevant, because drugs and radiation therapy cause apoptotic cell death. Hence, the inability of a cell to access the pathway after DNA damage can cause resistance to certain therapies. Data are beginning to accumulate and indicate that the status of p53 as assessed by IHC in several tumor types, such as breast and bladder carcinomas, correlates with the ability to respond to therapy. Bcl-2, a protooncogene that extends cell survival, is overexpressed in many tumor types, and its detection has been associated with lack of response to therapy and poor outcome.[41]

All the advantages of IHC can be nullified if it is used with lack of technical rigor and in an uncritical fashion. Strict adherence to laboratory practices must also be observed. Results must always be interpreted in the appropriate context, and the use of antibody panels is recommended when first characterizing a diagnostically problematic lesion. Technical advances in antigen retrieval augment the power of tissue immunohistology but also increase the potential for false-positive results. The possibility of antigenic loss that is known to occur in precut preparations is sometimes ignored as a cause of false-negative results.

Another method that allows quantitation and verification of the antigen being identified is Western blotting, also known as *immunoblotting*.[42] This technique combines the resolution of gel electrophoresis with the specificity of immunochemical detection. In this procedure, proteins are first extracted from cells or tissue samples and resolved in an electrophoresis gel. The products are then transferred to a membrane support, usually nitrocellulose membranes or nylon sheets. After blocking nonspecific binding sites, membranes are incubated with appropriately diluted primary antibodies, which are detected by the subsequent application of labeled secondary antibodies. The major limitation of this method, when using clinical samples, is that it requires a significant amount of tissue to obtain a suitable quantity of extracted proteins.

Assessment of Apoptotic Index

Apoptotic cell death can be demonstrated at the microanatomic levels by the application of the terminal transferase to elongate and label the double-stranded DNA cut at the internucleosomal regions. The incorporated labeled nucleotides are detected with an immunoenzymatic approach. This type of assay, also known as in situ *DNA nick end labeling*,[43,44] can quantitate the fraction of cells in apoptosis and may serve to predict behavior or response to therapy.

HIGH-THROUGHPUT TECHNIQUES

The manual sequencing method most widely used is the Sanger dideoxy sequencing technique.[45] This procedure uses base-specific termination during *in vitro* synthesis of DNA and is also known as the *chain termination method*. The basis for terminating the elongation of the DNA chain is the use of a nucleoside triphosphate containing a reduced ribose sugar termed *dideoxyribonucleoside triphosphate* (ddNTP). When such ddNTPs are mixed with the four normal dNTPs at the appropriate concentrations, chain termination occurs. The four normal dNTPs are mixed with the respective ddNTPs in four different test tubes, and reactions are compared for the growing DNA chain. In these reactions, the normal dNTPs are labeled at the α position, usually with phosphorus 32, to incorporate the radioactive signal needed for detection. These products are separated using acrylamide gel electrophoresis. The gels are dried and then imaged using autoradiography, producing a ladder sequence. Besides the technological restraints, this procedure has several drawbacks, including the resolution of the bands and the "compressed" or clustered migrated bands in the top and bottom of the gel. New, automated high-throughput technologies have been developed to increase the sensitivity and speed the analysis of gene sequencing. Incorporating a fluorescent-labeled nucleotide in the newly synthesized DNA strand and coupling a fluorescence emission detector next to gel, fluorescence can be identified while the gel runs. Instead of a photographic image, electropherograms are automatically read and printed. The use of capillary machines and four-color automated fluorescent sequencing produce well-defined peaks in a highly sensitive and reliable fashion. Several genetic analyzers, or automated sequence detection systems, are commercially available that greatly enhance the analytical ability with respect to mutation detection. Moreover, the use of fluorescent-labeled dNTPs allows laboratories to move away from radioactive, gel-based systems. Using fluorescent-labeled microsatellite markers, some of these apparatus also have the capability of detecting genetic losses.[46]

The main technological revolution of more recent years has been the development and implementation of DNA and expression microchip technologies.[47,48] Oligonucleotide microchips are miniaturized devices that enable large genomic studies. These systems allow sequencing analysis of determined genes and expression analysis of mRNA transcripts, including genes or expressed sequence tags. Expression studies can monitor quantitatively and simultaneously the expression of thousands of genes and sequences. Each transcript is typically represented on a microarray by multiple probe pairs, which differentiate among closely related members of gene families. These thousands of oligonucleotide-selected probes hybridize with complementary genetic information provided by the mRNA extracted from the target tissue or cell sample to be analyzed. Expression arrays typically use 20 pairs of specific oligonucleotide probes to interrogate each transcript, minimizing the effects of nonspecific hybridization and background signal. Probe arrays identify mRNA expression changes of greater than twofold between experiments and are able to detect transcript levels, even if only a few copies per cell are present.[49–51] The software linked to such automated systems allows processing and analysis of data, thus enabling control of the whole procedure and providing high quality and reproducible results.[52–54] These programs often interface raw data with online databases, such as GenBank, converting data acquired to expression levels, base calls, or genotype. The inclusion of reference standard genes as intraassay and interassay controls normalizes data, allowing comparison of multiple different experiments on a quantitative level. The gene-chip arrays (Affimetrix) are constructed so as to allow quantitative and robust monitoring of the expression level of thousands of genes simultaneously.

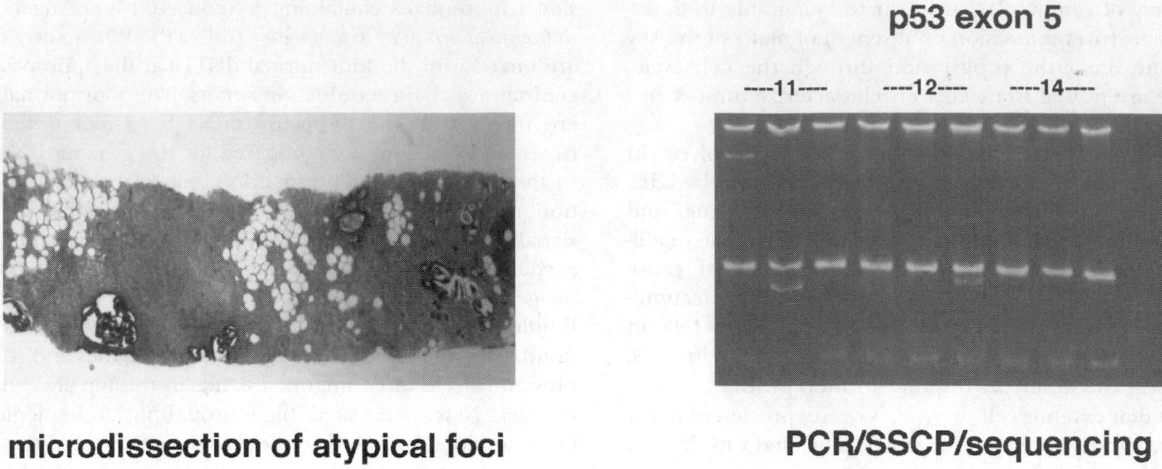

FIGURE 26-4. Microdissection of preneoplastic lesions makes it possible to test whether demonstration of genetic lesions accumulated in the somatic cells enhances the microscopic interpretation of the lesion and allows a more accurate prediction of its potential for progression. Core needle biopsy of a mammographically detected lesion with the phenotypic features of "atypical ductal hyperplasia" shows an abnormal acquired genotype. Microdissection and analysis of stromal cells showing a normal genotype rules out the possibility of an inherited germline mutation. PCR, pathologically confirmed complete remission; SSCP, single-strand conformation polymorphism; WT, wild-type. (Courtesy of Dr. Deborah Dillon, Yale University School of Medicine, New Haven, CT.)

These arrays are made using a combination of semiconductor-based lithography and solid-phase chemical synthesis. Specific DNA probes are synthesized, and then each probe is affixed to a predefined position in the array. An alternative process that brings great flexibility to the construction of cDNA microarrays is the spotting of PCR-prepared arrayable DNA or the spotting of synthetic oligonucleotides on glass slides that are then used for hybridization with labeled RNAs. The synthesis of oligonucleotide probes bypasses the need for handling a large number of clones and PCR products. In addition, probes can be specifically designed to detect alternatively spliced species of mRNA.[55,56] The construction of oligonucleotide arrays lends itself as a target for "artificial CGH." Instead of using normal metaphase chromosomes as a target, an array of DNA, such as provided by yeast artificial chromosomes (YACs) or bacterial artificial chromosomes (BACs), can be used as the target for competition between normal and genomic DNA. The option of using thousands of synthetic oligonucleotides will no doubt be reduced to practice in the near future.

The acquisition and processing of hybridization intensity data obtained by probe arrays is being applied in multiple areas, including the study of differential expression patterns and genotyping or analysis of polymorphisms. The potential for generating a novel molecular nosology of tumors, selecting the most effective therapy for an individual patient, determining molecular staging and grading, and discovering new therapeutic strategies is great and, to many, self-evident. For the data to be analyzed, correlated, and exchanged, however, a unified informatics platform must exist for collecting, storing, retrieving, and interrogating the databases. The development of a specific branch of bioinformatics designed to handle a large volume of data, create appropriate clusters to define entities, and find ways to display the results is common to many of the comprehensive technologies, such as proteomics and even tissue arrays.

Two-dimensional gel electrophoresis of proteins has held the promise of comprehensive analysis of the protein constituents of a tissue or a population of living cells. The development of immobilized pH gradients lowered the barrier to the widespread application of two-dimensional gel analysis to tumors.[57,58] The potential value of proteomics for the accurate classification of tumors was well demonstrated in the mid-1980s by the use of polypeptide phenotyping of acute leukemia in children.[59] Advances in two-dimensional gel analysis and biophysical instrumentation suggest that comprehensive analysis of the proteins expressed in a tissue or population of cells will yield information capable of differentiating different tumor types. As in the case of mRNA profiling, it is hoped that this technique may help select therapies and identify novel targets for therapy. A promising advance is the use of MALDI-TOF (matrix-assisted laser desorption/ionization–time of flight) technology and variations thereof to construct "protein chips" that detect and identify proteins at the femtomole scale directly from their native environments.[60,61] By using modified surfaces to capture molecules on the basis of specific binding kinetics, this type of approach can probe the function of some molecules in an exquisite way, thus significantly contributing to the knowledge of functional genomics. Technological platforms for nucleic acid identification can be modified to greatly enhance the sensitivity of IHC, and molecular counting can be made possible on the basis of rolling circle amplification (RCA) technology.

As a consequence of genomics and proteomics, antibodies will be raised against a very large number of novel antigenic determinants. The task of characterizing the patterns of tissue reactivity and the prevalence of the potential marker in even the most common tumor types appears out of reach of most laboratories. Although still in its early stages of development, tissue microarrays may enable investigators to rapidly characterize novel antisera. Tissue microarrays (Fig. 26-4) make it possible to analyze hundreds, even thousands, of tissue specimens from patients in different stages of disease and to assess the diagnostic, prognostic, and therapeutic importance of emerging cancer gene candidates.[62] *In situ* detection of DNA, RNA, and protein can be performed on consecutive sections of

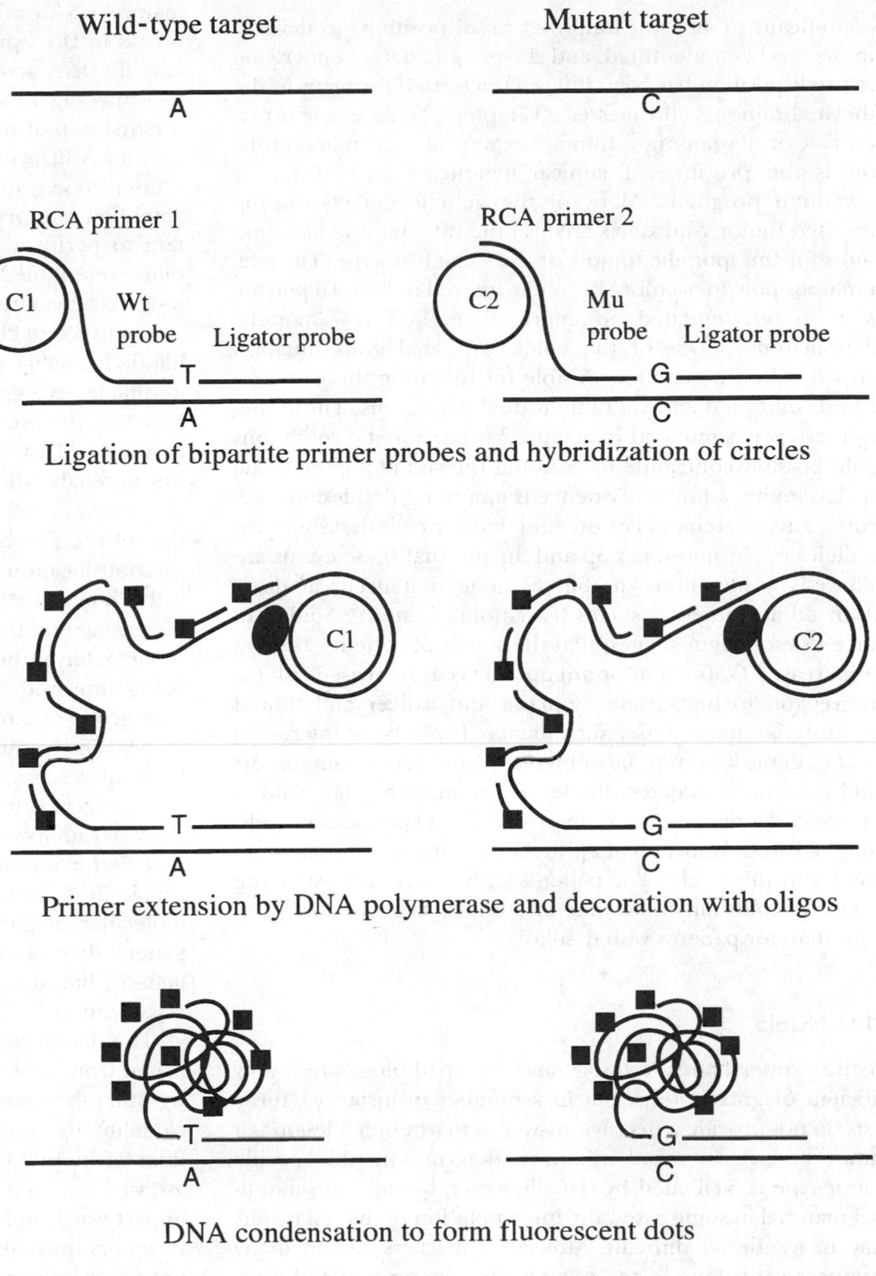

FIGURE 26-5. Schematic representation of the potential application of rolling circle amplification (RCA) for the demonstration of mutations by *in situ* hybridization. It is relatively simple to construct two independent reporter systems for two sequences differing by a single nucleotide. The fact that the RCA reaction is tethered to the target renders the system ideal for the topologic demonstration of mutations. C, circle; Mu, mutant; oligos, oligonucleotides; Wt, wild-type. (Courtesy of Dr. Paul Lizardi, Yale University School of Medicine, New Haven, CT.)

tissue microarrays. In this fashion, hundreds to thousands of samples can be analyzed simultaneously. Although the labor needed to construct a tissue microarray is considerable, and many issues in array design, image acquisition, and data storage are yet to be resolved, it is clear that all barriers will be lowered to facilitate the widespread use of this approach. One of the advantages of tissue arrays is that each human tissue sample is greatly expanded. A regular paraffin block can easily yield twenty 0.2-mm cores, and 300 sections can be obtained from a microarray master block. Thus, 6000 sections can be analyzed from each tumor block. Mutation detection in cytologic specimens and in tissues is now a possibility using a new reporter system, the RCA.[63] RCA is an isothermal amplification driven by a polymerase that replicates circularized oligonucleotide probes. The reaction can be set up to take place with either linear or geometric kinetics and is amenable to use in a variety of formats ranging from surface immobilized DNA to cytologic specimens (Fig. 26-5).

APPLICATIONS OF MOLECULAR MARKERS: DIAGNOSTIC MOLECULAR PATHOLOGY

Molecular markers and the techniques to demonstrate them in cells and tissues can be exploited for a series of paradigmatic clinical purposes that are succinctly discussed in the following paragraphs. As knowledge of the basic pathogenesis of human tumors advances and technology develops, new applications will come to the fore and molecular diagnosis can be truly described as a rapidly evolving and expanding field.

RISK ASSESSMENT

A significant number of inherited predispositions to develop tumors has been identified, and the genetic defect underlying the predisposition has been fully characterized for many of the inherited tumor syndromes (see Chapter 13). Assessing inherited risk of developing a tumor because of a germline mutation is the province of clinical geneticists and of cancer prevention programs. Many of the genetic defects causing inherited tumor syndromes are also the rate-limiting initiating events for the sporadic tumors of the same histotype. The adenomatous polyposis coli (APC) gene altered in familial polyposis is found mutated in more than 90% of sporadic adenomatous polyps of the colon. An analogous situation exists for the Rb gene responsible for initiating the mutation of both inherited and sporadic retinal neoplasms. Thus, finding these genes mutated in acquired preneoplastic conditions could possibly contribute to assessing the risk of a given tissue for developing a tumor. Evidence is emerging that lesions preceding adenocarcinoma of the lung harbor cells that show loss of alleles in chromosomes 3p and 9p and that these events are followed by mutations in the ras gene that occur at more advanced morphologic stages (carcinoma *in situ*).[64] Studies in Barrett's esophagus suggest that the subset of patients showing an increased G_2 fraction or aneuploidy is at increased risk for progression to high-grade dysplasia and cancer and should therefore be under closer surveillance. It will be of interest to see if patients known to be at increased risk for certain tumors can be screened to detect the lesions at an early stage. Studies suggest that detection of microsatellite expansion in cells sloughed from transitional epithelium lining the urinary tract may fulfill this goal.[65] For patients with severe, long-standing ulcerative colitis, microsatellite instability has been more prevalent than for patients with dysplasia.

DIAGNOSIS

In the proper hands, cytology and histopathology are highly efficient diagnostic tests, but in a number of instances, these tests do not provide a decisive answer as to whether a lesion is a tumor or not. In many instances, determining the specific tumor type is facilitated by IHC; however, because of suboptimal material in some cases, the interpretation of the test results may be rendered difficult. Molecular markers can in many instances contribute to the reliable characterization and diagnosis of a sample.

Among the most useful markers are the different translocations that are specific for certain tumor types. Among the cancers on which molecular diagnostics has had the greatest impact is chronic myelogenous leukemia (CML). The marker of this disease has been the Philadelphia chromosome (Ph1) t(9;22) (q34;q11), demonstrable in 95% of cases of CML.[66,67] The translocation is demonstrable by conventional cytogenetics, FISH, Southern blot hybridization, and PCR. The Philadelphia translocation joins the 5' portion of the BCR gene located on chromosome 22 to the 3' portion of the ABL gene on chromosome 9. The chimeric gene is transcribed into a novel 8.5-kb mRNA, which in turn is translated into a 210-kD protein. The precise position of the breakpoints within the DNA varies considerably from case to case. This is due to the fact that the breaks occur within introns, the sequence of which is excised from the initial forms of the BCR-ABL transcript to produce a mature 8.5-kb mRNA. The variability in the positions of the breaks in DNA preclude the use of a single pair of primers to amplify DNA across the breakpoint. To circumvent this problem, investigators have devised the so-called reverse PCR. In the first step of the procedure, BCR-ABL mRNA is transcribed with an ABL primer into single-stranded cDNA using reverse transcriptase. Nucleotide sequences in the cDNA are then amplified with primers for the BCR and ABL exons. It is important to perform control amplifications using primers for an omnipresent mRNA to ensure that the quality of the RNA to be tested is adequate.

Up to 6% of children and 20% of adults with acute lymphoblastic leukemia (ALL) also have a Ph1 chromosome indistinguishable cytogenetically from the one found in CML. However, the precise position of the breakpoints in DNA differ between CML and ALL, and molecular techniques are the only way to reliably distinguish a lymphoid blast crisis of CML from *de novo* ALL. Other practical contributions of the demonstration of the Ph chromosome in ALL is that ALL patients with the translocation seem to have a poorer prognosis than those with Ph-negative ALL. Protocols for the demonstration of an increasing number of translocations linked to the pathogenesis of hematolymphoid neoplasms are available and constantly being improved.[68]

A group of tumors that very often presents a diagnostic challenge is the so-called small round cell tumors of childhood. By light microscopy, it is often very difficult to distinguish rhabdomyosarcoma from lymphoma and from primitive neuroectodermal tumors or Ewing's sarcoma. Translocations that are specific for a number of malignant tumors of the soft tissues (Table 26-2) are beginning to bring the resolutive power of molecular diagnostics to this area. Defining the underlying genetic defects in these tumors not only clarifies their pathogenesis, but also provides the tool for a precise and decisive classification.[69,70]

The demonstration that a mass lesion is composed of cells issued from a single progenitor cell is the single most reliable sign that the mass is a tumor. Hence, methods to demonstrate clonality are important adjuncts to the morphologic evaluations of bioptic tissues. The first tumor in which clonality as assessed by molecular methods had a significant diagnostic impact was lymphoma. Clonal rearrangement of B- and T-cell receptors indicates that a lymphoid mass is a tumor, although not necessarily malignant, and also provides information as to the lymphoid cell lineage of the neoplasm. PCR protocols to demonstrate monoclonal populations are available for both B- and T-cell receptors.[71] This technique makes it possible to determine clonality in small tissue samples, and the demonstration of monoclonality helps to establish the neoplastic nature of lymphoid proliferations of the stomach.

Clonality assays applied to cell smears promise to greatly enhance the diagnostic efficiency of cytology. The differential diagnosis between reactive mesothelial cells and mesothelioma can be resolved by showing clonality of the cells by FISH.

Demonstration of point mutations in the Ki-RAS gene can be an important diagnostic feature of malignant pancreatic tumors. Determining that mutated alleles of the Ki-ras gene are present in cells aspirated from a pancreatic mass strongly suggests a malignant tumor, and the efficiency of diagnosis of pancreatic masses by fine-needle aspiration is significantly increased by the

TABLE 26-2. Selected Molecular Genetic Markers in Cancer Diagnosis Listed by Disease

Disease	*Marker*[a]	*Means of Detection*	*Principal Applications*
Hematologic cancer			
Chronic myelogenous leukemia	t(9;22)(q34;q11) [*BCR/ABL*]	SB, RT-PCR, FISH	Primary diagnosis, residual disease
Chronic lymphocytic leukemia	ARGs	SB, PCR	Primary diagnosis
	Trisomy 12	FISH	Primary diagnosis
Acute lymphoblastic leukemia			
B	AGRs	SB, PCR	Primary diagnosis, residual disease
	t(9;22)(q34;q11) [*BCR/ABL*]	RT-PCR, FISH	Primary diagnosis, residual disease
	t(1;19)(q23;p13) [*E2A/PBX*]	RT-PCR, FISH	Primary diagnosis, residual disease
	t(8;14)(q24;q32), t(2;8)(p11;q24), t(8;22)(q24;q11) [*MYC, IGH, IGK, IGL*]	SB, FISH	Primary diagnosis
	t(4;11)(q21;q23) [*MLL/AF2*]	RT-PCR, FISH	Primary diagnosis, residual disease
T	AGRs	SB, PCR	Primary diagnosis, residual disease
	t(1;14)(p32;q11) del (1p32) [*TAL1;TCRA*]	SB, PCR, FISH	Primary diagnosis, residual disease
Acute myeloblastic leukemia			
M2	t(8;21)(q22;q22) [*AML1/ETO*]	SB, RT-PCR, FISH	Primary diagnosis, residual disease
M3	t(15;17)(q21;q11) [*PML/RARA*]	SB, RT-PCR, FISH	Primary diagnosis, residual disease
M4	inv 16(p13q22) t(16;16)(p13;q22) [*MYH11/CBFb*]	SB, RT-PCR, FISH	Primary diagnosis, residual disease
M4Eo	t(6;9)(p23;q34) [*DEK/CAN*]	SB, FISH	Primary diagnosis
Non-Hodgkin's lymphoma			
All cases	AGRs	SB, PCR	Primary diagnosis, residual disease
Follicular	t(14;18)(q32;q21) [*BCL2/IGH*]	SB, PCR	Primary diagnosis, residual disease
Burkitt's	t(8;14)(q24;q32)	SB	Primary diagnosis, residual disease
	t(2;8)(p11;q24), t(8;22)(q24;q11) [*MYC; IGH, IGK, IGL*]	SB, FISH	Primary diagnosis
	EBV DNA	SB, PCR, ISH	Primary diagnosis
Intermediate	t(11;14)((q13;q32) [*BCL1;IGH*]	SB	Primary diagnosis
Large cell	t(3;14)(q27;q32) [*BCL6/IGH*]	SB	Primary diagnosis
Lymphomas associated with immunosuppression	EBV DNA	SB, PCR, ISH	Primary diagnosis
Adult T-cell leukemia/lymphoma	HTLV1	SB, PCR, ISH	Primary diagnosis
Solid cancers			
Ewing's sarcoma PNET	t(11;22)(q24;q12) [*FL11/EWS*]	SB, RT-PCR	Primary diagnosis, residual disease
Neuroblastoma	*MYCN* amplification	SB, FISH	Prognosis
Breast cancer	*HER2/NEU/ERBB2* amplification	SB, FISH	Prognosis
Prostate cancer	PSA mRNA	RT-PCR	Staging
Bladder cancer	*TP53* mutation	PCR/oligonucleotide hybridization	Staging, monitoring for relapse
	Microsatellite repeat changes	PCR/oligonucleotide hybridization	Primary diagnosis, monitoring for relapse
Squamous cancer of the head and neck	*TP53* mutation	PCR/oligonucleotide hybridization	Staging
Colon cancer	*KRAS* mutation	PCR/oligonucleotide hybridization	Monitoring for relapse
Esophageal cancer	*TP53* mutation	PCR/SSCP PCR/sequence analysis	Prognosis (risk of progression to cancer in Barrett's esophagitis)
Familial cancers			
Breast	*BRCA1, BRCA2* mutation		
Colonic	*APC, MSH2, MLH1, PMS1, PMS2* mutation		
Retinoblastoma, various sarcomas	*RB* mutation	PCR/SSCP	Diagnosis of hereditary predisposition
	WTI mutation	PCR/BRC	
Wilms' tumor	*TP53* mutation	PCR/DGGE	
Li-Fraumeni syndrome	*RET* mutation	PCR/sequence analysis	
MEN 1 and 2	*VHL* mutation		
Kidney cancer	*NF1, NF2* mutation		
Neurofibrosarcoma			

ARGs, antigen receptor gene rearrangements; BRC, bacteriophage resolvase cleavage; DGGE, denaturing gradient gel electrophoresis; EBV, Epstein-Barr virus; FISH, fluorescence *in situ* hybridization; HTLV, human T-cell leukemia; ISH, *in situ* hybridization; MEN, multiple endocrine neoplasia; PNET, peripheral neuroepithelioma; PSA, prostate-specific antigen; SB, Southern blot hybridization; RT-PCR, reverse transcriptase-polymerase chain reaction; SSCP, single-stranded conformational polymorphism.

[a]Genes are indicated by italicized capital letters; genes involved in translocations are shown in brackets.

simultaneous use of Ki-ras assessment and carcinoembryonic antigen levels.

Microsatellite DNA markers are useful clonal markers for the detection of cancer, and microsatellite changes matching those found in the primary tumor can be detected in the urine sediment of 95% of patients diagnosed with bladder cancer. It is of interest that, in the same series of patients, conventional cytology was positive in only 50% of the patients. Thus, microsatellite analysis might possibly be a viable method to screen for bladder cancer.[72]

MOLECULAR GRADING AND STAGING

The purpose of grading is to predict the risk for local and distant spread of a tumor. Improving the capacity to predict whether a tumor has metastasized will have a significant impact on therapy and prognosis. The concept that neoplasia is accumulation of mutations makes it possible to think that, if the molecular pathways of tumor progression are defined, determining the alterations present in a tumor could provide accurate indication of the stage of progression and, thus, complement and refine the prognosis based on conventional grading and staging. It has been suggested that a certain class of mutations of the Ki-ras gene encountered in colorectal cancer could identify the more aggressive neoplasms.[73]

Evaluation of the expression of proteins linked to cell division, such as Ki-67 (MB) and PECAN, have been extensively used to evaluate the percentage of proliferating tumor cells in biopsies or resection specimens. In lymphomas, for example, when the percentage of Ki-67–positive cells is high, the prognosis is significantly worse. For many tumors, a high percentage of cycling cells correlates with bad prognosis. This finding is not surprising and is in keeping with the number of mitotic figures, one of the classic parameters used for tumor grading.

Genotypic characteristics can sometimes predict the behavior of a lesion, as illustrated in the case of fibromatosis. Trisomy of chromosome 8 is found in lesions that recur, whereas lesions with low potential for recurrence have a balanced genetic complement. The status of TP53 (wild-type vs. mutated) has been found to contribute prognostic information in bladder, colon, and breast carcinoma.[74–76] Abrogation of TP53 function can lead to a loss of G_1 arrest in response to DNA damage or can interfere with apoptosis. In the first instance, mitosis without repair could fix mutations contributing to the cumulation of genetic lesions in the same cell. Loss of apoptosis could contribute to an increase in cell number and lack of responsiveness to therapy. The concept that loss of competence for apoptosis could contribute to tumor formation has led to investigation of the pathogenetic role of genes involved in cell survival, such as BCL-2.[77] Overexpression of BCL-2 has been found to correlate with lymph node metastases in ductal carcinoma of the breast.

Neuroblastoma is perhaps the tumor that is most often graded by molecular means in many centers. The status of N-MYC amplification and the level of expression of TRK-A are among the most significant prognostic parameters for tumors of matched stage and morphology. Together with ploidy and loss of chromosome 1p, they complete the molecular staging and grading of neuroblastoma.[78,79]

Gene expression array profiling studies are being reported, disclosing the potential contributions they may be able to make in the molecular classification of neoplastic diseases. They also offer significant novel information regarding differentiation states; global alterations affecting particular cellular programs, such as growth regulation; and host response mechanisms. If current classification schemes still lump together different diseases with distinct clinical phenotypes, differential gene expression will distinguish molecular heterogeneity and produce biologically more accurate, and probably clinically more useful, diagnostic and predictive information.

Few original studies have been reported as proof of principle for the approach using specific entities as "test cases." For example, Golub et al.[80] attempted to produce a molecular classification of acute leukemias based on gene expression monitoring by DNA microarrays and containing 6817 human genes. After producing a teaching set of genes highly correlated with acute myeloblastic leukemia (AML)-ALL class distinction, these investigators then tested the validity of such a class of predictors. The final 50-gene set of predictors derived from cross-validation tests correctly assigned 36 of 38 samples as either AML or ALL, the remaining two cases resulting in "uncertain" phenotypes.[80] The authors concluded that class prediction provides an unbiased general approach to prognostic tests. They also cautioned that sample collection, appropriate histopathologic documentation, and integrity of data sets are critical requirements for reaching robust conclusions. In a more recent study, Alizadeh et al.[81] reported the distinct molecular nature of diffuse, large B-cell lymphomas (DLBCLs), an aggressive malignancy of mature B lymphocytes. This group of investigators had previously produced a specialized microarray, the so-called lymphochip, which holds selected genes preferentially expressed in lymphoid cells and their derived malignancies. Using a modification of this basic tool, they were able to molecularly subclassify DLBCLs into two groups: germinal-center B-like tumors and activated peripheral B-like cell neoplasms. Moreover, this molecular classification not only pointed out what was previously an ill-defined histogenesis, but it also incorporated novel data relating to proliferation and state of differentiation. Patients with germinal-center B-like DLBCL had a significant prolonged overall survival when compared to those with activated B-like DLBCL, revealing the clinical significance of molecular subtyping of neoplastic diseases.[81]

To reach acceptance and clinical applicability, individual tumor markers and "class prediction sets" of biologic determinants must undergo methodical analysis. However, stringent criteria for the development of such studies, which should bring basic laboratory findings to clinical investigations and finally to standard of care, have not been well delineated. Certain groups of clinical investigators have proposed using a strategy similar to the one used by drug discovery programs for evaluating and implementing new therapeutic agents. In this exercise, phases of development and clinical application are well defined (see Chapter 17). Briefly, phase I deals with toxicity, phase II determines dose escalation and definition of therapeutic index, phase III is designed to ascertain efficacy, and phase IV is the final validation before commercialization and routine use. A similar analogy could be implemented that would take into account the process of discovery through validation of any given biologic predictor. Phase I should deal with issues regarding biologic properties of the marker and the methodologies that could better identify the marker in the context of using clinical material. Phase II should include pilot studies aimed at determining the specificity and sensitivity of such an assay; the definition of the cutoff value, if needed; and the potential clinical significance of detecting the marker as an adjunct to the already available clinicopathologic information. Phase III studies should aim at validating the marker by using (if possible) set(s) of well-characterized, prospectively accrued cases in specific clinical protocols designed for such a purpose. Finally, phase IV studies should incorporate multiinstitutional efforts to delineate intra- and interlaboratory variability, define and implement a standardized assay (using the selected cutoff value, if required), and demonstrate the clinical usefulness of the marker. This does not signify a final proposal of the sequential steps that must be fulfilled by a potentially clinical significant tumor marker or set of markers. It is just meant to draw attention to the lack of specific criteria for such an exercise and the need to reach some generally approved system if it is thought that such applications deserve to be translated to the routine clinical practice.

DETECTION OF MINIMAL DISEASE

Detection of minimal disease has benefited greatly from the availability of molecular markers and, perhaps with diagnosis, is one of the most fruitful areas of expansion in molecular diagnostics. It plays a role in three clinical circumstances: (1) evaluation of minimal residual disease, (2) early detection of recurrence, and (3) evaluation of local extension. These applications are based on the high specificity of the molecular markers and the very high sensitivity afforded by the PCR-based techniques.

Detection of circulating cells harboring the bcl-2 translocation is an important prognostic predictor of relapse in patients with t(14:18)-positive B-cell lymphoma treated with high-dose chemotherapy and autologous bone marrow or peripheral blood stem cell support.[82] A correlation exists between the relapse rate and both the degree of contamination of the autograft and the efficacy of purging, suggesting that contamination is in part responsible for treatment failures. Similar strategies are being explored for other malignancies.[83–85] Detection of cytokeratin 19 transcripts by RT-PCR in a sample of bone marrow, peripheral stem cells, or peripheral blood, indicates the presence of epithelial cells for patients with breast carcinoma.[82] Other tumor-specific transcripts, such as tyrosinase for melanoma,[83] prostate-specific antigen for prostate cancer,[84] and thyroglobulin for thyroid cancer,[85] also have been exploited for the detection of circulating cells. In general, these assays achieve the detection of one tumor cell in a background of 10^{10} cells. Circulating soluble Ki-RAS DNA bearing the same mutated sequences as the primary tumor can be detected in plasma and other fluids of patients with pancreatic carcinoma or ovarian cancer.[86] The clinical significance of these findings is not yet established, but when quantitative assays become available, the level of circulating tumor-specific DNA can perhaps be used as a marker to follow therapy and for early detection of recurrence.

A different use of the ability to detect tumor cells with high sensitivity is the analysis of tissues for the presence of a specific mutation that identifies the primary tumor being treated. It is indeed possible to verify the local spread of a tumor by testing the surgical margins, not just by light microscopy but also using the sensitive PCR-based approach. Proof of the worthiness of this strategy is provided by studies in head and neck cancer that show that "molecular margins" are superior in predicting local recurrence when compared to the conventional approach of assessing resection margins by intraoperative frozen section.[87] Should sequencing of short cDNA fragments in minutes become feasible, intraoperative molecular assessment of margins for tumors genotyped at the time the first diagnostic biopsy is obtained may possibly become a real option.

RECURRENCE VERSUS SECOND PRIMARY

With cure rates and survival rates of patients with malignant tumors increasing, it is more important in clinical practice to identify second primary tumors. When a second tumor has its presentation in the same organ system as the first, the question invariably arises about distinguishing between a recurrence and a second primary. Morphologic comparison and an extended immunophenotypical profile of the two lesions can sometimes resolve the question, but the presence of a clonal mutation or a broader constellation of genetic alterations is the most direct way to establish a link between the two lesions or to strongly suggest that the metachronous tumors represent independent events. An adenocarcinomatous lesion in the lung of a patient in long-term remission for a primary adenocarcinoma elsewhere is another situation that benefits from a molecular approach to distinguish between a second primary and a metastasis. Clearly, it is best not to rely on the alterations present on a single gene but to attempt to establish a broad genotypic characterization of the two lesions to maximize the effectiveness of the interpretation of the results. Microsatellite alterations at multiple loci can be useful. Relying on differences or similarities in gene sequence in genes that show a wide spectrum of mutations (e.g., TP53) clearly is more effective than using genes exhibiting a limited repertoire of mutations (e.g., Ki-RAS). Molecular analysis of multiple tumors of the transitional epithelium in the urinary bladder has demonstrated that the multiple lesions arise from a single progenitor cell that seeds the bladder mucosa, explaining the high risk for recurrence encountered in these patients.[88,89]

CONSIDERATIONS FOR THE FUTURE

The practice of conventional histopathology based on light microscopy was changed and complemented in the second half of the twentieth century by three technological advances: ultrastructure, IHC, and molecular diagnostics. The first two represented incremental gains in diagnostic power and efficiency but did not force substantial changes in the practice of morphologic tissue analysis. However, molecular medicine is profoundly changing the approach to tissue analysis. Perhaps more important, molecular medicine is altering the pathway for advancement. The elucidation of the molecular pathogenesis of tumors has led directly to the discovery and application of molecular tumor markers. Diagnosis and prognosis have, in many cases, been enhanced by the use of the marker(s). Finally, the marker (e.g., Her-2/neu) may constitute a therapeutic target. With the advances in biotechnology and bioinformatics, the preceding sequence of events can be predicted to change. Rather than elucidating a molecular pathway, we will have a complete view of the molecular biology of a given tumor type. This comprehensive understanding will lead to the development of specific therapies and to the rational selection of therapeutic modalities for a specific patient. Molecular tests will allow an accurate assessment of the response and modification of therapy when required. The detailed molecular knowledge of the natural history of tumors will yield markers for inherited and acquired risks, and these, in turn, will make improved design and monitoring of prevention a reality.

REFERENCES

1. Slamon DJ, Godolphin W, Jones LA, et al. Studies of the HER-2/neu proto-oncogene in human breast and ovarian cancer. *Science* 1989;244:707.
2. Cordon-Cardo C, Dalbagni D, Saez GT, et al. TP53 mutations in human bladder cancer: genotypic versus phenotypic patterns. *Int J Cancer* 1994;56:347.
3. Emmert-Buck MR, Bonner RF, Smith PD, et al. Laser capture microdissection. *Science* 1996;274:998.
4. Cheng J, Fortina P, Surrey S, Kricka LJ, Wilding P. Microchip-based devices for molecular diagnosis of genetic diseases. *Mol Diagn* 1996;1:183.
5. Wheeless LL, Badalament RA, de Vere White RW, Fradet Y, Tribukait B. Consensus review of the clinical utility of DNA cytometry in bladder cancer. Report of the DNA Cytometry Consensus Conference. *Cytometry* 1993;14:478.
6. Bauer KD, Bagwell CB, Giaretti W, et al. Consensus review of the clinical utility of DNA flow cytometry in colorectal cancer. *Cytometry* 1993;14:486.
7. Stephenson RA, Gay H, Fair WR, Melamed MR. Effect of section thickness on quality of flow cytometric DNA content determinations in paraffin-embedded tissues. *Cytometry* 1986;7:41.
8. Halvorsen OJ, Hostmark J, Haukaas S, Hoisaeter PA, Akslen LA. Prognostic significance of p16 and CDK4 proteins in localized prostate carcinoma. *Cancer* 2000;88:416.
9. Askin FB, Perlman EJ. Neuroblastoma and peripheral neuroectodermal tumors. *Am J Clin Pathol* 1998;109:23.
10. Medeiros LJ, Carr J. Overview of the role of molecular methods in the diagnosis of malignant lymphomas. *Arch Pathol Lab Med* 1999;123:1189.
11. Gale RE. Evaluation of clonality in myeloid stem-cell disorders. *Semin Hematol* 1999;36:361.
12. Southern EM. Detection of specific sequences among DNA fragments separated by gel electrophoresis. *J Mol Biol* 1975;98:503.
13. Ilson DH, Motzer RJ, Rodriguez E, Chaganti RS, Bosl GJ. Genetic analysis in the diagnosis of neoplasms of unknown primary tumor site. *Semin Oncol* 1993;20:229.
14. Glassman AB. Cytogenetics, *in situ* hybridization and molecular approaches in the diagnosis of cancer. *Ann Clin Lab Sci* 1998;28:324.
15. Ried T. Interphase cytogenetics and its role in molecular diagnostics of solid tumors. *Am J Pathol* 1998;152:325.
16. Kallioniemi OP, Kallioniemi A, Piper J, et al. Optimizing comparative genomic hybridization for analysis of DNA sequence copy number changes in solid tumors. *Genes Chromosomes Cancer* 1994;10:231.
17. Isola J, DeVries S, Chu L, Ghazvini S, Waldman F. Analysis of changes in DNA sequence copy number by comparative genomic hybridization in archival paraffin-embedded tumor samples. *Am J Pathol* 1994;145:1301.
18. Schrock E, Veldman T, Padilla-Nash H, et al. Spectral karyotyping refines cytogenetic diagnostics of constitutional chromosomal abnormalities. *Hum Genet* 1997;101:255.
19. Mullis K, Faloona F, Scharf S, et al. Specific enzymatic amplification of DNA *in vitro*: the polymerase chain reaction. *Cold Spring Harb Symp Quant Biol* 1986;51(Pt 1):263.
20. Bustin SA, Dorudi S. Molecular assessment of tumour stage and disease recurrence using PCR-based assays. *Mol Med Today* 1998;4:389.
21. Appelbaum FR. Molecular diagnosis and clinical decisions in adult acute leukemia. *Semin Hematol* 1999;36:401.
22. Kim SH, Godfrey T, Jensen RH. Whole genome amplification and molecular genetic analysis of DNA from paraffin-embedded prostate adenocarcinoma tumor tissue. *J Urol* 1999;162:1512.
23. Capodieci P, Magi-Galluzzi C, Moreira G Jr, Zeheb R, Loda M. Automated *in situ* hybridization: diagnostic and research applications. *Diagn Mol Pathol* 1998;7:69.
24. Fletcher JA. DNA *in situ* hybridization as an adjunct in tumor diagnosis. *Am J Clin Pathol* 1999;112:11.
25. Bartow SA. Diagnostic and prognostic applications of oncogenes in surgical pathology. *Am J Surg Pathol* 1990;14:5.
26. Scarpa A, Tognon M. Molecular approach in human tumor investigation: oncogenes, tumor suppressor genes and DNA tumor polyomaviruses. *Int J Mol Med* 1998;1:1011.
27. van Dongen JJ, Macintyre EA, Gabert JA, et al. Standardized RT-PCR analysis of fusion gene transcripts from chromosome aberrations in acute leukemia for detection of minimal residual disease. Report of the BIOMED-1 Concerted Action: investigation of minimal residual disease in acute leukemia. *Leukemia* 1999;13:1901.
28. Ghossein RA, Carusone L, Bhattacharya S. Review: polymerase chain reaction detection of micrometastases and circulating tumor cells: application to melanoma, prostate, and thyroid carcinomas. *Diagn Mol Pathol* 1999;8:165.
29. Millon R, Jacqmin D, Muller D, et al. Detection of prostate-specific antigen- or prostate-specific membrane antigen-positive circulating cells in prostatic cancer patients: clinical implications. *Eur Urol* 1999;36:278.
30. Ringel MD, Ladenson PW, Levine MA. Molecular diagnosis of residual and recurrent thyroid cancer by amplification of thyroglobulin messenger ribonucleic acid in peripheral blood. *J Clin Endocrinol Metab* 1998;83:4435.
31. Zach O, Kasparu H, Krieger O, et al. Detection of circulating mammary carcinoma cells in the peripheral blood of breast cancer patients via a nested reverse transcriptase polymerase chain reaction assay for mammaglobin mRNA. *J Clin Oncol* 1999;17:2015.
32. Raggi CC, Bagnoni ML, Tonini GP, et al. Real-time quantitative PCR for the measurement of MYCN amplification in human neuroblastoma with the TaqMan detection system. *Clin Chem* 1999;45:1918.
33. Campo E, Raffeld M, Jaffe ES. Mantle-cell lymphoma. *Semin Hematol* 1999;36:115.
34. Osborne CK. Steroid hormone receptors in breast cancer management. *Breast Cancer Res Treat* 1998;51:227.
35. Ross JS, Fletcher JA. HER-2/neu (c-erb-B2) gene and protein in breast cancer. *Am J Clin Pathol* 1999;112:53.
36. Diaz JI, Muro-Cacho CA. Macrophage expression of interleukin-1 in lymphoepithelioid cell ("Lennert's") lymphoma. *Leuk Lymphoma* 1996;21:305.
37. Taylor H, Heaton N, Farrands P, Kirkham N, Fletcher M. Elevated human chorionic gonadotrophin levels in a patient with pancreatic carcinoma presenting with a testicular metastasis. *Postgrad Med J* 1990;66:1073.
38. Bangalore L, Tanner AJ, Laudano AP, Stern DF. Antiserum raised against a synthetic phosphotyrosine-containing peptide selectively recognizes p185neu/erbB-2 and the epidermal growth factor receptor. *Proc Natl Acad Sci U S A* 1992;89:11637.
39. Porter PL, Malone KE, Heagerty PJ, et al. Expression of cell-cycle regulators p27Kip1 and cyclin E, alone and in combination, correlate with survival in young breast cancer patients. *Nat Med* 1997;3:222.
40. Nishimura G, Tsukuda M, Zhou LX, Furukawa S, Baba Y. Cyclin D1 expression as a prognostic factor in advanced hypopharyngeal carcinoma. *J Laryngol Otol* 1998;112:552.
41. Cordon-Cardo C. Molecular alterations in bladder cancer. *Cancer Surv* 1998;32:115.
42. Monni O, Franssila K, Joensuu H, Knuutila S. BCL2 overexpression in diffuse large B-cell lymphoma. *Leuk Lymphoma* 1999;34:45.
43. Sola B, Salaun V, Ballet JJ, Troussard X. Transcriptional and post-transcriptional mechanisms induce cyclin-D1 over-expression in B-chronic lymphoproliferative disorders. *Int J Cancer* 1999;83:230.
44. Gorczyca W, Bedner E, Burfeind P, Darzynkiewicz Z, Melamed MR. Analysis of apoptosis in solid tumors by laser-scanning cytometry. *Mod Pathol* 1998;11:1052.
45. Sanger F, Nicklen S, Coulson A. DNA sequencing with chain-terminating inhibitors. *Proc Natl Acad Sci U S A* 1977;74:5463.
46. Eisenbarth I, Beyer K, Krone W, Assum G. Toward a survey of somatic mutation of the NF1 gene in benign neurofibromas of patients with neurofibromatosis type 1. *Am J Hum Genet* 2000;66:393.
47. Lander ES. Array of hope. *Nat Genet* 1999;21:3.
48. Khan J, Saal LH, Bittner ML, et al. Expression profiling in cancer using cDNA microarrays. *Electrophoresis* 1999;20:223.
49. Pollack JR, Perou CM, Alizadeh AA, et al. Genome-wide analysis of DNA copy-number changes using cDNA microarrays. *Nat Genet* 1999;23:41.
50. Sgroi DC, Teng S, Robinson G, et al. *In vivo* gene expression profile analysis of human breast cancer progression. *Cancer Res* 1999;59:5656.
51. Khan J, Simon R, Bittner M, et al. Gene expression profiling of alveolar rhabdomyosarcoma with cDNA microarrays. *Cancer Res* 1998;58:5009.
52. Loftus SK, Chen Y, Gooden G, et al. Informatic selection of a neural crest–melanocyte cDNA set for microarray analysis. *Proc Natl Acad Sci U S A* 1999;96:9277.
53. Bubendorf L, Kolmer M, Kononen J, et al. Hormone therapy failure in human prostate cancer: analysis by complementary DNA and tissue microarrays. *J Natl Cancer Inst* 1999;91:1758.
54. Bassett DE Jr, Eisen MB, Boguski MS. Gene expression informatics—it's all in your mine. *Nat Genet* 1999;21:51.
55. Sun L, Goodman PA, Wood CM, et al. Expression of aberrantly spliced oncogenic ikaros isoforms in childhood acute lymphoblastic leukemia. *J Clin Oncol* 1999;17:3753.
56. Kraus A, Neff F, Behn M, et al. Expression of alternatively spliced mdm2 transcripts correlates with stabilized wild-type p53 protein in human glioblastoma cells. *Int J Cancer* 1999;80:930.
57. Celis JE, Celis P, Ostergaard M, et al. Proteomics and immunohistochemistry define some of the steps involved in the squamous differentiation of the bladder transitional epithelium: a novel strategy for identifying metaplastic lesions. *Cancer Res* 1999;59:3003.
58. Ryu DD, Nam DH. Recent progress in biomolecular engineering. *Biotechnol Prog* 2000;16:2.
59. Hanash SM, Teichroew D. Mining the human proteome: experience with the human lymphoid protein database. *Electrophoresis* 1998;19:2004.
60. Melis R, White R. Characterization of colonic polyps by two-dimensional gel electrophoresis. *Electrophoresis* 1999;20:1055.
61. Garvin AM, Parker KC, Haff L. MALDI-TOF based mutation detection using tagged *in vitro* synthesized peptides. *Nat Biotechnol* 2000;18:95.
62. Moch H, Schraml P, Bubendorf L, et al. High-throughput tissue microarray analysis to evaluate genes uncovered by cDNA microarray screening in renal cell carcinoma. *Am J Pathol* 1999;154:981.
63. Lizardi PM, Huang X, Zhu Z, et al. Mutation detection and single-molecule counting using isothermal rolling-circle amplification. *Nat Genet* 1998;19:225.
64. Euhus DM, Maitra A, Wistuba II, et al. Use of archival fine-needle aspirates for the allelotyping of tumors. *Cancer* 1999;87:372.
65. Steiner G, Schoenberg MP, Linn JF, Mao L, Sidransky D. Detection of bladder cancer recurrence by microsatellite analysis of urine. *Nat Med* 1997;3:621.
66. Pasternak G, Hochhaus A, Schultheis B, Hehlmann R. Chronic myelogenous leukemia: molecular and cellular aspects. *J Cancer Res Clin Oncol* 1998;124:643.
67. Sinclair PB, Nacheva EP, Leversha M, et al. Large deletions at the t(9;22) breakpoint are common and may identify a poor-prognosis subgroup of patients with chronic myeloid leukemia. *Blood* 2000;95:738.

68. Morgan GJ, Pratt G. Modern molecular diagnostics and the management of haematological malignancies. *Clin Lab Haematol* 1998;20:135.
69. Rowley JD. Cytogenetic and molecular analysis of pediatric neoplasms: diagnostic and clinical implications. *Pediatr Pathol* 1994;14:167.
70. Ladanyi M. The emerging molecular genetics of sarcoma translocations. *Diagn Mol Pathol* 1995;4:162.
71. Sharp JG, Chan WC. Detection and relevance of minimal disease in lymphomas. *Cancer Metastasis Rev* 1999;18:127.
72. Mao L, Schoenberg MP, Scicchitano M, et al. Molecular detection of primary bladder cancer by microsatellite analysis. *Science* 1996;271:659.
73. Ahnen DJ, Feigl P, Quan G, et al. Ki-ras mutation and p53 overexpression predict the clinical behavior of colorectal cancer: a Southwest Oncology Group study. *Cancer Res* 1998;58:1149.
74. Sarkis AS, Dalbagni G, Cordon-Cardo C, et al. Nuclear overexpression of p53 protein in transitional cell bladder carcinoma: a marker for disease progression. *J Natl Cancer Inst* 1993;85:53.
75. Esrig D, Elmajian D, Groshen S, et al. Accumulation of nuclear p53 and tumor progression in bladder cancer. *N Engl J Med* 1994;331:1259.
76. Bergh J, Norberg T, Sjogren S, Lindgren A, Holmberg L. Complete sequencing of the p53 gene provides prognostic information in breast cancer patients, particularly in relation to adjuvant systemic therapy and radiotherapy. *Nat Med* 1995;1:1029.
77. Pui CH, Evans WE. Genetic abnormalities and drug resistance in acute lymphoblastic leukemia. *Adv Exp Med Biol* 1999;457:383.
78. Kramer K, Cheung NK, Gerald WL, et al. Correlation of MYCN amplification, Trk-A and CD44 expression with clinical stage in 250 patients with neuroblastoma. *Eur J Cancer* 1997;33:2098.
79. Gallego S, Parareda A, Munell F, Sanchez de Toledo J, Reventos J. Clinical relevance of molecular markers in neuroblastoma: results from a single institution. *Oncol Rep* 1999;6:891.
80. Golub TR, Slonim DK, Tamayo P, et al. Molecular classification of cancer: class discovery and class prediction by gene expression monitoring. *Science* 1999;286:531.
81. Alizadeh AA, Eisen MB, Davis RE, et al. Distinct types of diffuse large B-cell lymphoma identified by gene expression profiling. *Nature* 2000;403:503.
82. Akasaka T, Akasaka H, Yonetani N, et al. Refinement of the BCL2/immunoglobulin heavy chain fusion gene in t(14;18)(q32;q21) by polymerase chain reaction amplification for long targets. *Genes Chromosomes Cancer* 1998;21:17.
83. Ghossein RA, Coit D, Brennan M, et al. Prognostic significance of peripheral blood and bone marrow tyrosinase messenger RNA in malignant melanoma. *Clin Cancer Res* 1998;4:419.
84. Ghossein RA, Osman I, Bhattacharya S, et al. Detection of prostatic specific membrane antigen messenger RNA using immunobead reverse transcriptase polymerase chain reaction. *Diagn Mol Pathol* 1999;8:59.
85. Ringel MD, Balducci-Silano PL, Anderson JS, et al. Quantitative reverse transcription-polymerase chain reaction of circulating thyroglobulin messenger ribonucleic acid for monitoring patients with thyroid carcinoma. *J Clin Endocrinol Metab* 1999;84:4037.
86. Minamoto T, Mai M, Ronai Z. K-ras mutation: early detection in molecular diagnosis and risk assessment of colorectal, pancreas, and lung cancers. *Cancer Detect Prev* 2000;24:1.
87. Brennan JA, Mao L, Hruban RH, et al. Molecular assessment of histopathological staging in squamous-cell carcinoma of the head and neck. *N Engl J Med* 1995;332:429.
88. Dalbagni G, Presti J, Reuter V, et al. Genetic alterations in bladder cancer. *Lancet* 1993;324:469.
89. Tsai YC, Simoneau AR, Spruck CH 3rd, et al. Mosaicism in human epithelium: macroscopic monoclonal patches cover the urothelium. *J Urol* 1995;153:1697.

CHAPTER **27**

Cancer Diagnosis: Imaging

SECTION **1**

ELLIOT K. FISHMAN
BRUCE A. URBAN

Computed Tomography

Computed tomography (CT) has long been a mainstay of diagnostic imaging in cancer patients. CT offers noninvasive and accurate results for most disease processes and is both widely available and relatively low in cost. The number of CT examinations performed in the United States continues to increase at a rate of approximately 10% per year.[1] CT has remained a vital and important imaging modality because it has continued to evolve, with spiral (helical) CT, multiphase imaging, and multidetector scanning being the notable recent innovations.[2–4] The current diagnostic capabilities and the accuracy of CT continue to improve. With spiral CT, data acquisition can be timed with the administration of contrast material during multiple phases of enhancement, optimizing cancer detection and diagnosis. In addition, new techniques centered on three-dimensional (3D) and virtual CT imaging are being refined to take advantage of some of the capabilities of spiral CT.[5–7] These techniques will prove valuable in planning surgical procedures and radiation therapy. CT is also ideally suited for the guidance of interventional procedures often necessary to confirm malignancy and allow subtyping of tumors.[1] This section reviews some of the key current applications of CT scanning and defines its role in patient treatment and management.

LIVER

Spiral CT currently is the study of choice for the evaluation of the liver and biliary tree. Spiral CT can both detect and characterize hepatic pathology by providing detailed information as to the presence, extent, and vascularity of a lesion. Accurate localization of tumor to specific hepatic segments can be performed when key vascular structures are defined. The enhancement pattern, as well as lesion attenuation values, allow specific classification of a lesion as benign (cyst or hemangioma) or malignant (primary vs. metastases) in most cases. Specific CT characteristics may also suggest whether a lesion is a primary or metastatic lesion, although there is significant overlap in many cases.[8–11] Identification of the characteristics that differentiate benign from malignant lesions is critical because many smaller liver lesions (1 cm or less), even in oncology patients, are benign (Figs. 27.1-1, 27.1-2).[12,13]

There has been much discussion over the last several years, with various conclusions, as to the optimum imaging protocol for the detection of hepatic tumors. Before the introduction of spiral CT, the optimal CT technique for imaging the liver was CT during arterial portography.[14,15] The limitations of that technique include the need for catheterization of the superior mesenteric artery as well as problems with flow-related defects in up to 25% of patients. Newer CT techniques have essentially the same detection rate (or better) but without the related limitations. Kuszyk et al.[16] found that with portal-phase contrast-enhanced spiral CT, 91% of lesions larger than 1 cm can be detected. Hollett et al.[17] found that by using a dual-phase CT technique, almost 10% more lesions were detected than with portal-phase images only. As CT technology is constantly evolving, the prospect of greater accuracy

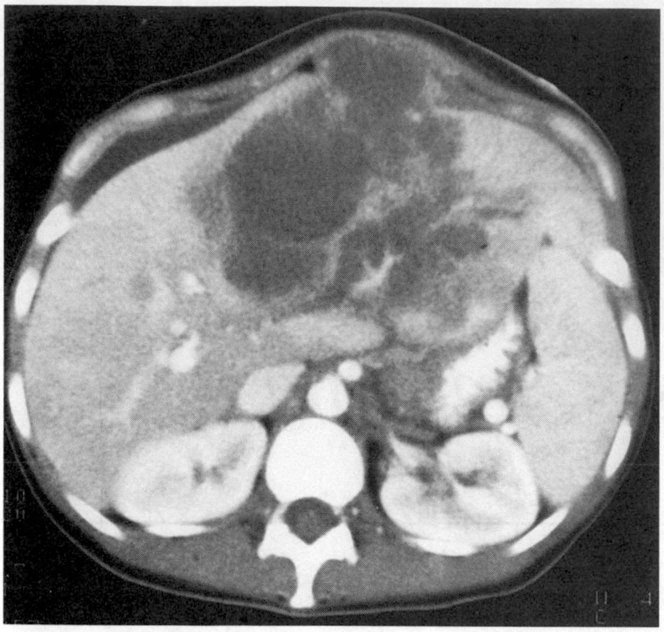

FIGURE 27.1-1. Adenocarcinoma of the liver. Cystic tumor mass grows through the liver capsule. Ascites is also seen.

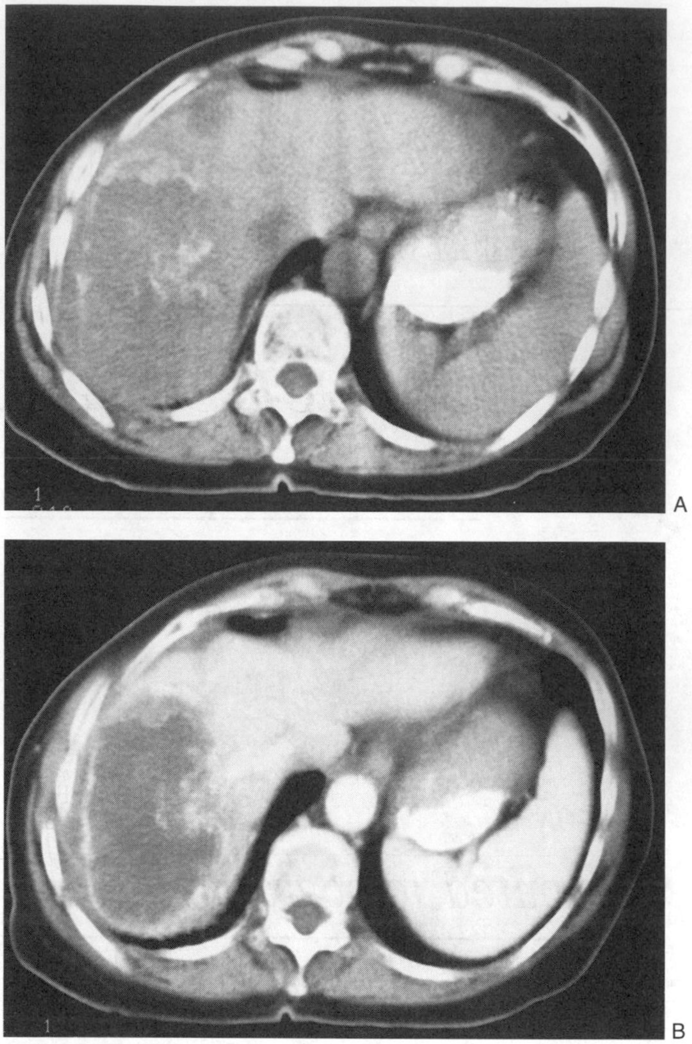

FIGURE 27.1-2. Cholangiocarcinoma of the liver. **A:** A 10-cm intrahepatic mass is partially calcified on non–contrast-enhanced scans. **B:** After infusion of contrast, the vascularity and necrotic nature of the tumor are best defined.

in the ability to detect lesions is fairly optimistic. The most recent work, utilizing multidetector spiral CT scanning, uses very narrow collimation (2.5 mm) for optimal lesion detection, with excellent results.[4]

In addition to the detection of tumor, CT coupled with 3D reconstruction of data represents the next step in CT imaging. The image data are presented in a form that combines the best of angiography and CT scanning.[18] These 3D images can be displayed in real time and can be supplemented by stereoscopic displays to optimize lesion definition and extent. The information generated can help with surgical planning. By combining a vascular map from the arterial phase with a venous map from the portal phase, the radiologist can generate key road maps and vascular anatomy in a noninvasive format. With technical advances such as this, curative resection of some primary and metastatic tumors is now possible. In addition, the number of relatively invasive preoperative studies often needed to document tumor resectability, including conventional angiography and CT portography, have been markedly reduced.[1]

CT is also valuable in monitoring patient treatment. Accurate tumor volumetrics can be accomplished and captured to measure and quantify therapeutic response accurately. Three-dimensional size measurements have been shown to be reproducible and clinically useful for following up response of liver tumors to treatment.[19] Enhancement pattern changes as well as changes in normal liver volumes also are often helpful in assessing treatment success. New techniques to measure liver enhancement after intravenous (IV) injection of contrast material can be used to quantify arterial blood flow to the liver and may be useful in determining which patients are at risk for subsequent development of liver metastases.[20]

PANCREAS

The role of CT in the evaluation of the pancreas typically centers on the detection and staging of pancreatic adenocarcinoma. Although the 5-year survival rate for pancreatic cancer in general remains poor, in selected patients, survival can be increased. Patients with a mass of 2 cm or less limited to the pancreatic head or patients without major vessel encasement or spread to lymph nodes who are treated with a pancreaticoduodenectomy (Whipple procedure) have a 30% or greater 5-year survival.[21] The key roles for CT in this patient population are accurate staging and triage.

The use of spiral CT has increased the accuracy of CT in staging pancreatic cancer by allowing detection of smaller lesions and by its ability to improve definition of vascular encasement.[22–24] With modern spiral CT scanners, tumor detection approaches 96%.[24] The number of indeterminate cases (i.e., the inability to distinguish between glandular enlargement due to inflammation and carcinoma) based on spiral CT findings has also decreased substantially. Pancreatic adenocarcinoma is usually a hypodense lesion relative to the normally enhancing pancreatic gland.[25] In the past, a pancreatic mass was typically detected based on a gross contour change within the pancreatic gland. However, such an obvious contour change usually indicated a relatively large mass. With the optimal IV contrast delivery of spiral CT, smaller lesions can now be detected.

Optimal IV contrast enhancement also provides for better assessment of key arterial and venous structures, such as the portal vein, celiac axis, and superior mesenteric artery, to help to determine their patency and relation to tumor extension (Fig. 27.1-3). The degree of major vascular involvement by pancreatic cancer is useful in predicting which patients will have surgically resectable tumors. Major vessels with less than one-fourth of their circumference involved by tumor are almost always resectable; tumors that surround more than three-fourths of the circumference are almost always unresectable.[23] Hommeyer et al.[26] analyzed the caliber of the peripancreatic veins and found that dilation of these vessels to more than 7 mm also suggests early vascular invasion and unresectability.[26] Conventional angiography is no longer necessary for preoperative planning in most cases, since the sensitivity of CT and that of angiography are nearly identical, and 3D imaging can produce angiography-like images (Fig. 27.1-4). Metastatic disease to the liver and lymph nodes is easier to detect, particularly for lesions that are hypodense and measure at least 1 cm in diameter. The characteristic CT appearance of other pancreatic masses may allow a diagnosis on the basis of appearance alone. CT can also be used to monitor response to adjuvant therapy and to detect any potential sites of tumor recurrence.

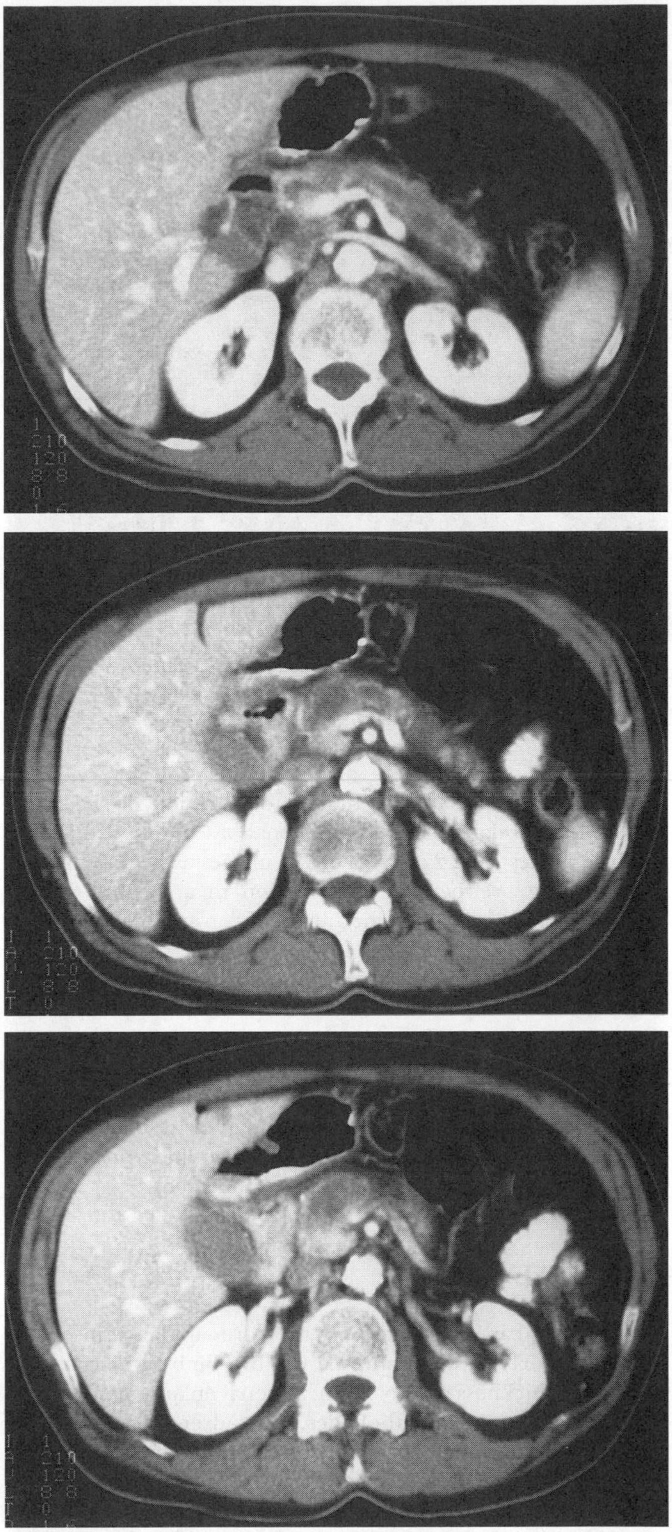

FIGURE 27.1-3. Adenocarcinoma of the pancreas. Sequence of spiral computed tomography scans demonstrate a 2.5-cm low-density mass in the body of the pancreas, with a dilated distal pancreatic duct.

KIDNEY

One of the major roles of CT in the oncology patient is in detecting, classifying, and staging renal tumors (Figs. 27.1-5, 27.1-6, and 27.1-7).[27] Common diagnostic problems in renal imaging are the detection and the characterization of a renal mass. Spiral CT has been shown to be accurate for the evaluation of renal masses and accurately can distinguish between a simple cyst and a solid tumor. In a small percentage of cases, there is an overlap, and an indeterminate diagnosis is made. In these cases, ultrasonography or magnetic resonance imaging (MRI) may be helpful, although usually these techniques are subject to the same limitations as CT.

One of the current controversies in imaging the kidney is the timing of data acquisition in relation to contrast injection.[28–30] Specific acquisitions can be obtained during the arterial phase, nephrogenic phase, or delayed phase of renal enhancement. Most authors now agree that scans during two, if not all three, of these phases are necessary for optimal CT imaging of renal masses.[31] Lesion detection approaches 100% with modern CT scanners.[31] Arterial-phase images (20 to 30 seconds after IV contrast administration) are crucial for evaluating renal artery and tumor vascularity. Nephrogenic phase imaging (90 to 120 seconds after IV contrast administration) is ideal for lesion detection in the central portions of the kidney. Suspected renal vein or inferior vena cava involvement and collecting system opacification require a more delayed scan (3 to 5 minutes after IV contrast administration).

In addition, spiral CT serves as an excellent modality for multiplanar reconstruction and 3D imaging of the kidneys. These techniques are important if such procedures as partial nephrectomy are being considered.[32] The 3D spiral CT study

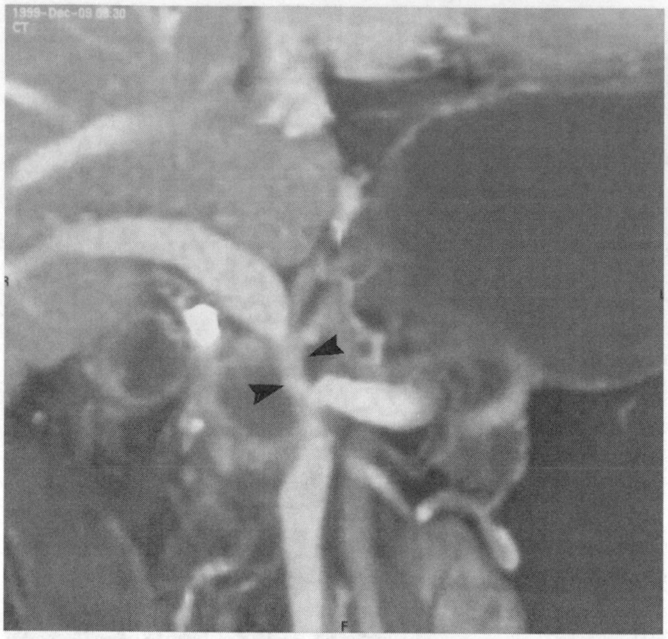

FIGURE 27.1-4. Pancreatic adenocarcinoma. Three-dimensional image reveals narrowing of the confluence of the portal vein and superior mesenteric vein (*arrowheads*) from an unresectable cancer.

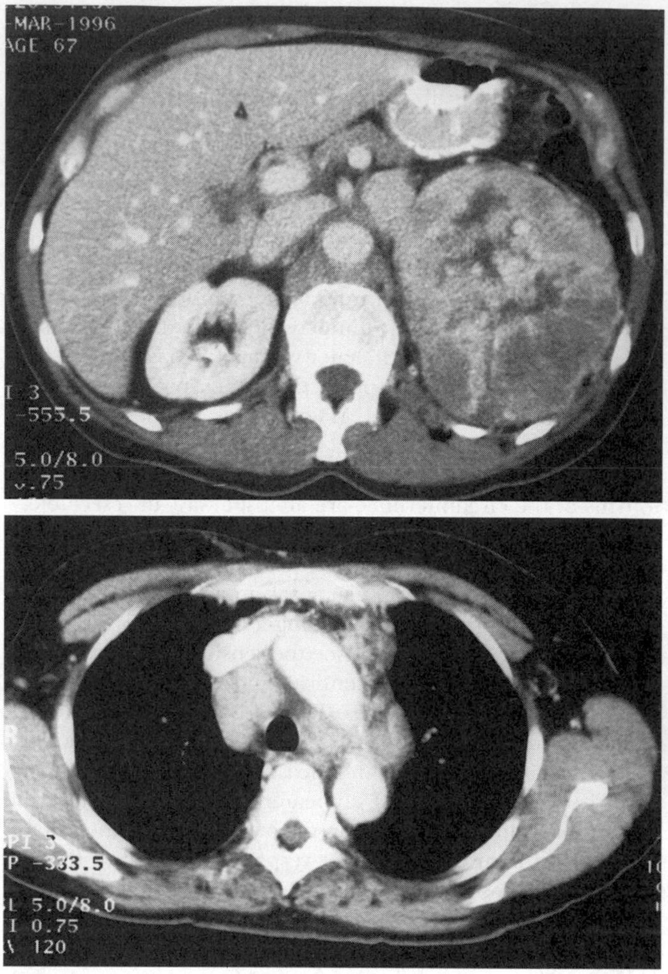

FIGURE 27.1-5. Renal cell carcinoma. Computed tomography demonstrates a vascular tumor of the left kidney, with paraaortic nodes. Metastases to the mediastinal nodes are also seen.

provides a valuable tool to define the location of the renal mass and its relationship to the renal vasculature and perinephric tissues (Fig. 27.1-8). The 3D images assist the surgeon by providing preoperative information in a flexible display that aids in determining whether nephron-sparing surgery is possible.[32]

CT is also useful for evaluation of tumors in the renal pelvis and collecting system, such as transitional cell carcinoma.[33] In these cases, delayed CT scans are necessary to define accurately the true extent of tumor infiltration. Metastases to the kidney from such processes as lymphoma or lung cancer are best detected on these delayed scan examinations, especially since these tumors may not distort the renal outline and are best seen only with differential contrast enhancement.

ADRENAL GLAND

CT scanning can clearly identify the adrenal glands in nearly all patients. The normal adrenal has two limbs, which have a maximum thickness of 3 to 4 mm. Adrenal enlargement can be due to a wide range of pathologies, from adrenal adenoma and hyperplasia to primary and metastatic adrenal tumors.[34–36] The specific clinical criteria used to characterize an adrenal mass include patient history, age, medical history, and the presence of any biochemical or physiologic abnormalities. The specific CT criteria used include mass size, whether it is unilateral or bilateral, the density of the mass, the presence of calcification or fat within the lesion, and the presence of other signs suggestive of malignancy.

Even in the oncology patient, the most common adrenal mass is a benign adrenal adenoma. Adenomas range in size from 1 to 5 cm and are typically of low CT attenuation (–20 to 20 Hounsfield units) values. Several articles have reported successfully differentiating benign from malignant adrenal masses based on CT attenuation of the mass.[37,38] In these studies, all small adrenal masses with CT attenuation below 18 HU on noncontrast evaluation were benign. In practice, then, adrenal masses that are 4 cm or less and are of low CT attenuation can be followed up conservatively with follow-up CT scanning. In the remaining patients with a potentially significant indeterminate adrenal mass, chemical shift MR imaging can be used to characterize the lesion confidently.[39] Percutaneous biopsy may still be necessary in some patients.

Malignant adrenal lesions can be divided into primary and metastatic lesions (Figs. 27.1-9, 27.1-10).[34–36] It may be impossible to distinguish a primary adrenal carcinoma from a metastatic lesion based on its CT appearance alone. Other adrenal tumors that can be confused with a primary adrenal malignancy include pheochromocytoma (which is malignant in up to 10% of cases), neuroblastoma (usually in younger patients), and myelolipoma (usually containing fat and calcification).

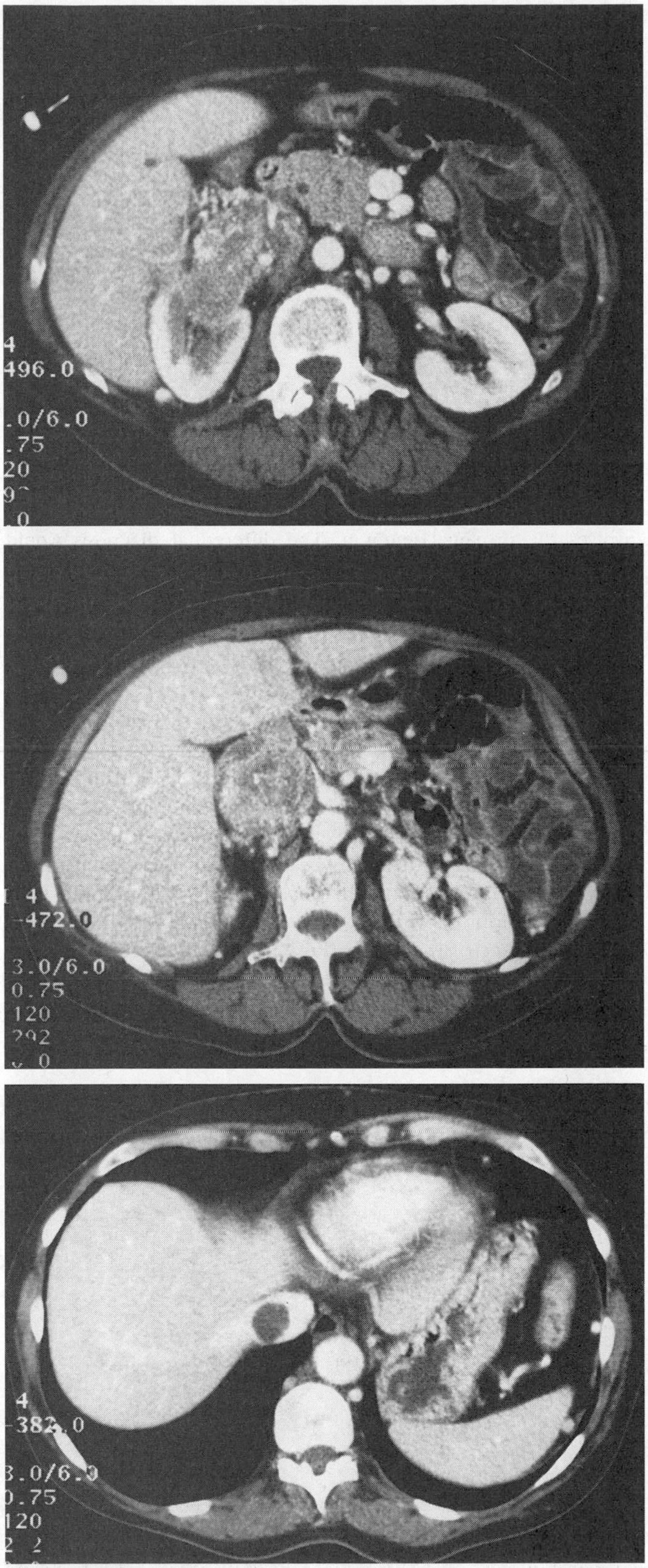

FIGURE 27.1-6. Renal cell carcinoma. Sequence of computed tomography scans demonstrates tumor extension into the renal vein and the inferior vena cava. Tumor extends up to but does not involve the right atrium.

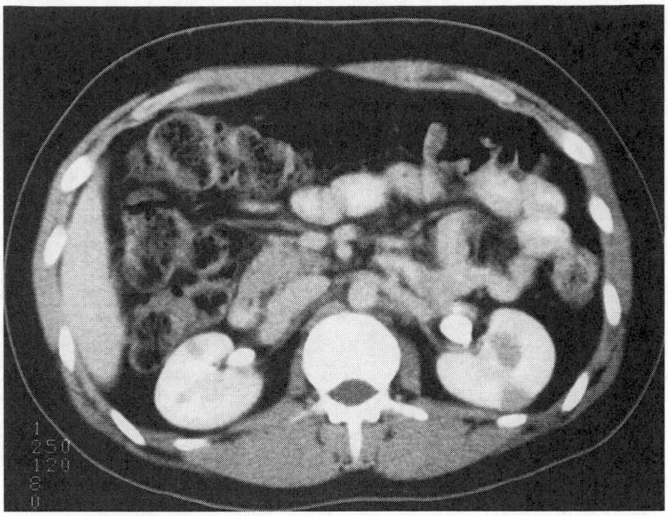

FIGURE 27.1-7. Non-Hodgkin's lymphoma involving the kidneys. Multiple solid bilateral renal masses are due to lymphoma. The kidneys are not enlarged.

SMALL BOWEL AND COLON

CT is typically not the first study to suggest the presence of a small bowel or colon neoplasm. Nevertheless, with the increased use of CT as the initial study for bowel obstruction or an acute abdomen, there has been an increased detection rate of primary gastrointestinal tract tumors.[40,41] In most cases, CT is used in tumor staging to define the extent of the primary

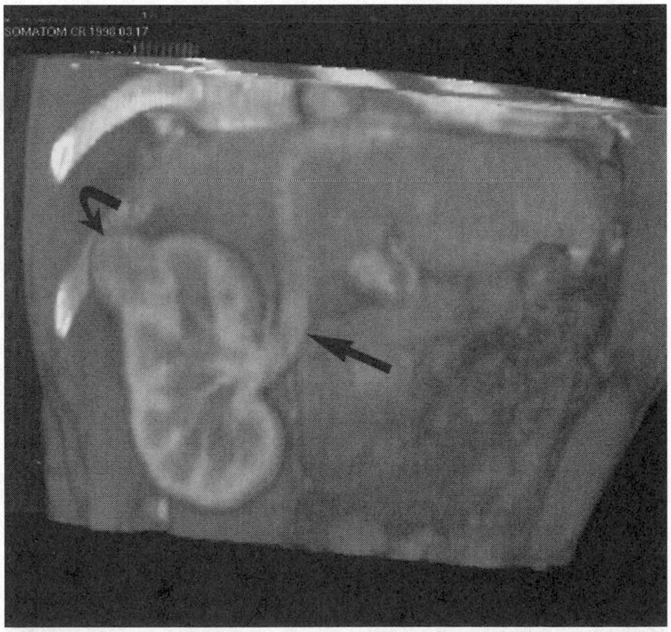

FIGURE 27.1-8. Renal cell carcinoma. Three-dimensional image demonstrates mass in the upper pole of the right kidney (*curved arrow*). The renal vein (*straight arrow*) is patent. Three-dimensional images such as this are valuable for preoperative planning.

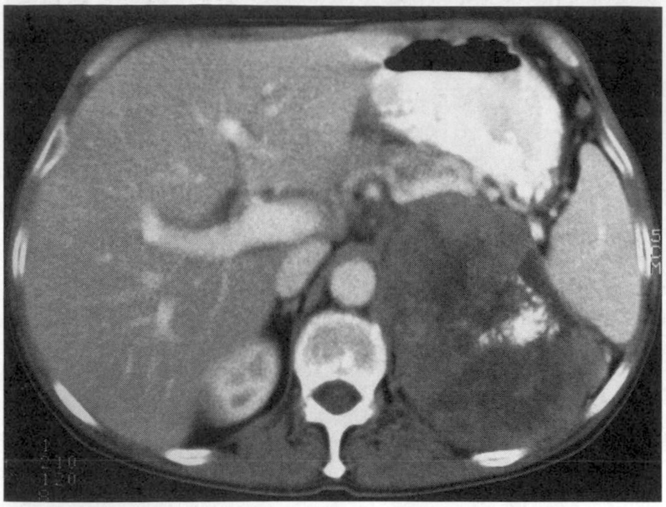

FIGURE 27.1-9. Primary adrenal carcinoma. A 12-cm, left upper quadrant mass with foci of calcification can be seen. The left kidney (not shown) was displaced inferiorly.

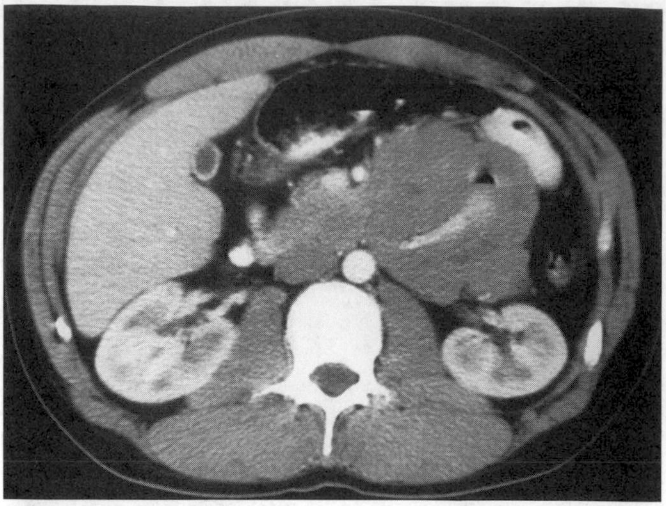

FIGURE 27.1-11. Small bowel lymphoma. Large ulcerating mass involves the proximal jejunum. The differential diagnosis would include a small bowel adenocarcinoma.

mass and to define spread to adjacent structures. Although the CT appearances of small bowel tumors may overlap, several signs are indicative of the etiology of the mass. Small bowel carcinoid tumor, for example, will typically present with an associated calcified mesenteric mass with a desmoplastic reaction.[42] Small bowel adenocarcinoma is variable in appearance and may be an infiltrating lesion, a bulky mass, or an ulcerating lesion. Lymphoma of the small bowel also varies in appearance but is usually bulkier and more extensive than an adenocarcinoma (Fig. 27.1-11).

Adenocarcinoma of the colon is a diagnosis usually made by colonoscopy or barium enema, with CT typically reserved for staging spread of disease (Fig. 27.1-12). In some centers, double-contrast CT of the colon is performed, to stage better the extent of tumor locally and local spread. In other centers, the key role of CT is the detection of extracolonic disease, particularly to the liver or lung.[43]

Recent advances in rapid volumetric CT scanning, combined with 3D imaging and computer graphics, have extended CT imaging into the "virtual" realm. Perhaps no other area has generated as much clinical interest and promise as that of virtual colonoscopy.[44,45] With this technique, CT combined with 3D visualization provides a virtual endoscopic view of the mucosal surface of the colon (Fig. 27.1-13). This rapidly growing application has gained attention as a noninvasive test for screening of colon polyps and cancer. It has also proven effec-

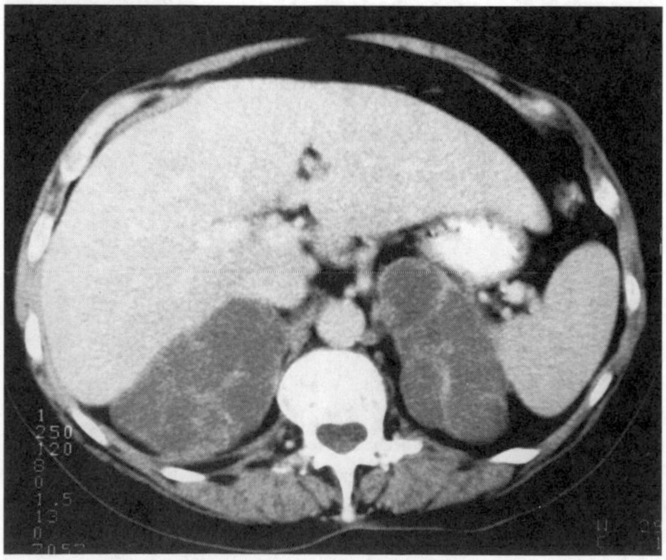

FIGURE 27.1-10. Bilateral adrenal metastases from a non–small cell lung cancer. The masses are unusually cystic.

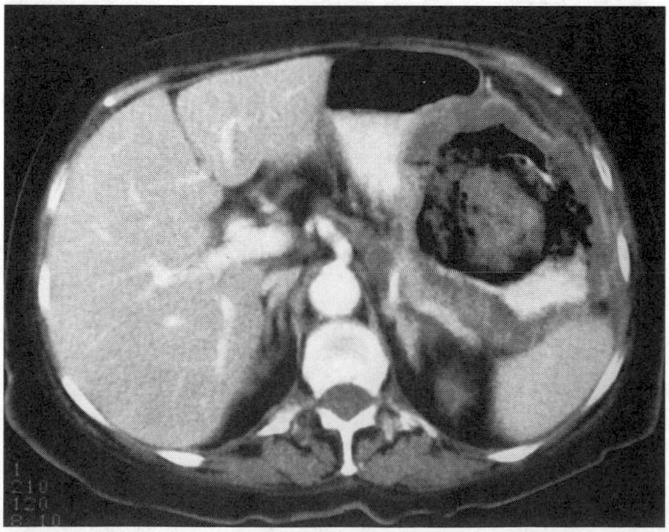

FIGURE 27.1-12. Adenocarcinoma of the transverse colon. Large necrotic left upper quadrant mass invaded the stomach, producing a gastrocolic fistula.

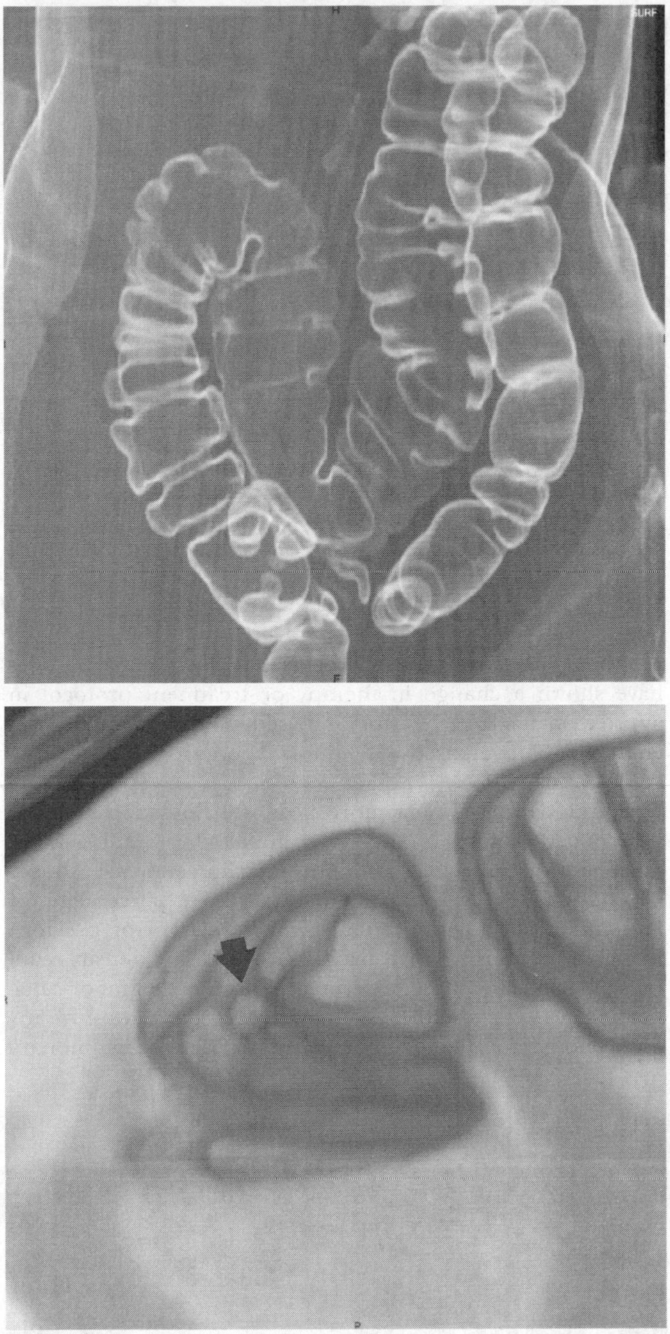

A

B

FIGURE 27.1-13. Virtual colonoscopy. Data from spiral computed tomography can be manipulated with three-dimensional imaging to produce images that simulate the appearance of a barium enema (**A**) or colonoscopy (**B**). The virtual colon view demonstrates a small polyp (*arrow*).

tive in evaluating portions of the colon not accessible or readily seen at conventional colonoscopy.[46] Authors have reported 84% to 100% sensitivity for the detection of polyps larger than 10 mm and 70% to 95% sensitivity for polyps ranging from 6 to 9 mm.[44] Sensitivity remains poor for polyps measuring less than 5 mm but, with such technologic innovations as rapid-speed multidetector CT scanning and improved computer processing, there is great hope for improvement in the detection of tiny polyps.

ESOPHAGUS AND STOMACH

The role of CT in evaluating the upper gastrointestinal tract is somewhat controversial. Published results on the accuracy of CT for staging esophageal and gastric cancer have been variable and depend in large part on the extent of disease and the specific parameter evaluated.[47,48] For example, in the evaluation and staging of esophageal cancer, CT has been shown to be fairly accurate in detecting invasion of the trachea and airway as well as in detecting nodes in the region of the gastrohepatic ligament. Recently, CT has been used increasingly for the follow-up and monitoring of patient status after therapy for esophageal cancer, whether with surgery, chemotherapy, or radiation therapy. Recent progress suggests that CT can be used not only to monitor response but for treatment planning.

Technologic advances have expanded the clinical role of CT in evaluation of the stomach (Figs. 27.1-14, 27.1-15, and 27.1-16). The use of double-contrast spiral CT produces a more detailed evaluation of the stomach than conventional CT. Initial studies suggest that this technique permits earlier detection and more accurate staging of small gastric tumors.[49] The most commonly encountered stomach tumor is adenocarcinoma. Less common malignancies include lymphoma, leiomyosarcoma, and metastases.[50,51] The CT appearance of each of these lesions has findings that are often helpful for diagnosis. Despite these features, there may be some overlap between all these tumors and other malignancies, such as metastatic disease to the stomach, or benign processes, such as *Helicobacter pylori,* which can simulate a malignant process.[52]

LUNGS AND MEDIASTINUM

CT remains the study of choice for a wide range of oncology challenges in the thorax.[53–58] Spiral CT has further enhanced the potential of CT in thoracic studies because of the single breath-hold capability, which essentially eliminates the problem of patient motion and breathing misregistration responsible for suboptimal examination.[59–61] There are four major indications for CT scanning in the oncology patient with thoracic pathology: (1) staging a known tumor, such as lung cancer, lymphoma, or thymoma; (2) detecting possible lung metastases from an extrathoracic primary tumor, such as a renal cell carcinoma; (3) evaluating a known or suspected mediastinal mass (i.e., widened mediastinum on a routine chest radiograph); and (4) evaluating by high-resolution CT the lung parenchyma in suspected complications of therapy, including radiation injury, drug reactions, and such secondary infections as in the immunosuppressed bone marrow transplantation patient.

For staging most chest tumors, IV contrast material is required (Figs. 27.1-17, 27.1-18, and 27.1-19). Contrast delineates the normal vascular structures and defines the presence and extent of tumor and lymphadenopathy. Spiral CT can accurately depict the hilar lymph nodes and their major anatomic relationships.[62] In lung cancer staging, we can determine the extent of disease, including vascular encasement or chest wall involvement. CT scans can also be used as a guide for fiberoptic bronchoscopy to optimize tissue sampling. CT combined

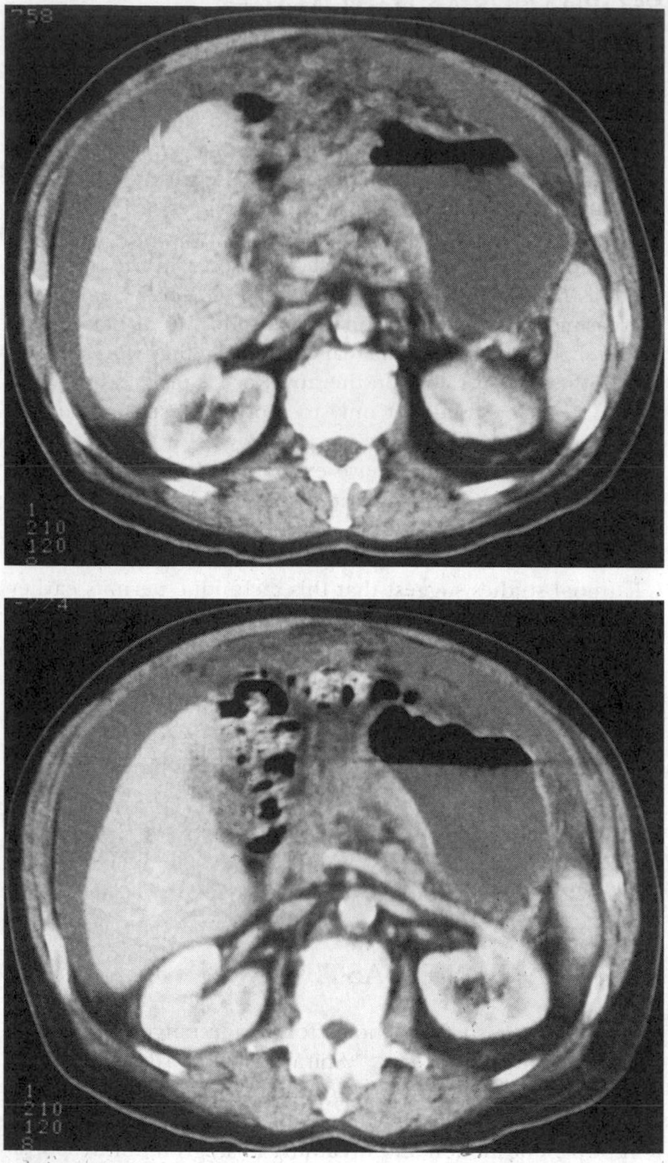

FIGURE 27.1-14. Adenocarcinoma of the stomach. The patient presented with gastric outlet obstruction. Tumor encases the gastric antrum, with carcinomatosis seen.

with 3D visualization can provide a virtual endoscopic view of the trachea and can be useful for evaluating areas beyond high-grade tumor stenoses (Fig. 27.1-20).[63]

CT evaluation of primary mediastinal masses is useful in defining the extent of disease and can suggest a specific diagnosis in many cases. Specific CT findings, including location of the mass (anterior, middle, or posterior mediastinum), the presence of fat or calcification, enhancement characteristics, and mass size and other sites of disease are often helpful in diagnosis.[64,65] Clinical history (e.g., myasthenia gravis), patient age, and medical history are also critical for achieving the correct diagnosis. CT can stage most of these processes and is a useful guide for planning appropriate therapy, such as surgery, radiation therapy, or chemotherapy. CT also plays a major role in monitoring response to therapy.

Another major advantage of CT is the ability to display an entire cross section of anatomy. This is especially important

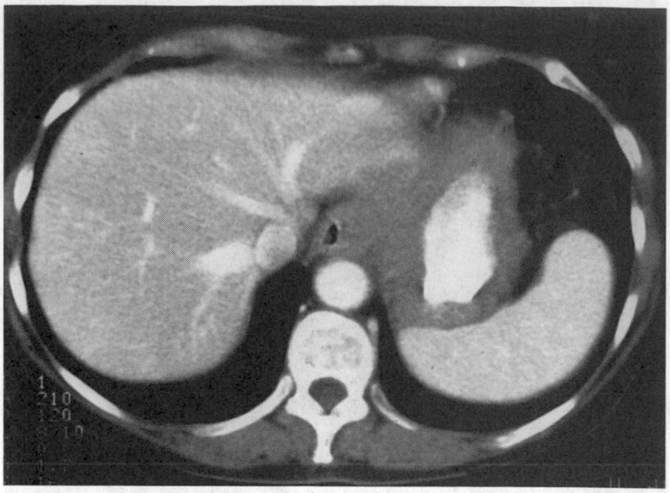

FIGURE 27.1-15. Gastric lymphoma. Computed tomography demonstrates diffuse involvement of the gastric fundus extending into the gastroesophageal junction.

when staging such disease processes as lymphoma. Studies have shown a change in therapy or treatment protocol in approximately 10% of patients based on information from chest CT, as compared with information from chest radiographs only.[66–69]

Spiral CT provides a more accurate detection rate for pulmonary nodules than conventional chest radiography. Small nodule detection is important clinically, as lesions 1 cm or smaller are malignant in a large percentage of patients, especially in patients with a history of previous malignancy.[70] Spiral CT also allows for accurate density readings of lesions to aid in detecting the presence of fat or calcification, which is helpful in determining the nature of any given nodule. Enhancement characteristics of pulmonary

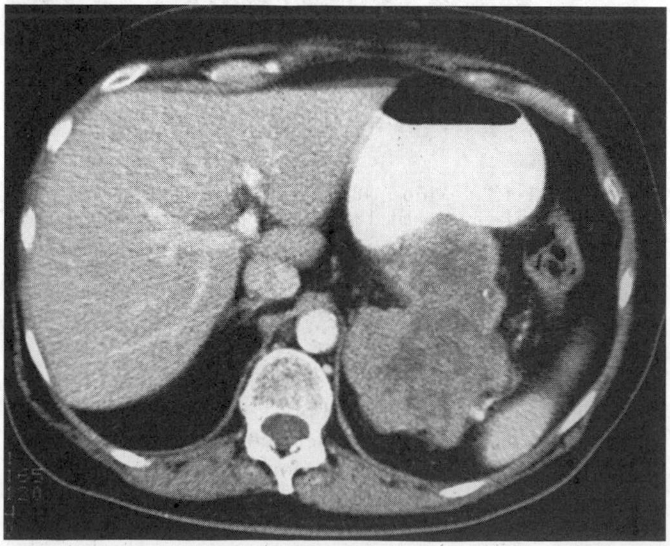

FIGURE 27.1-16. Gastric leiomyosarcoma. Large necrotic mass arises off the gastric fundus. A small focus of calcification is seen in the mass.

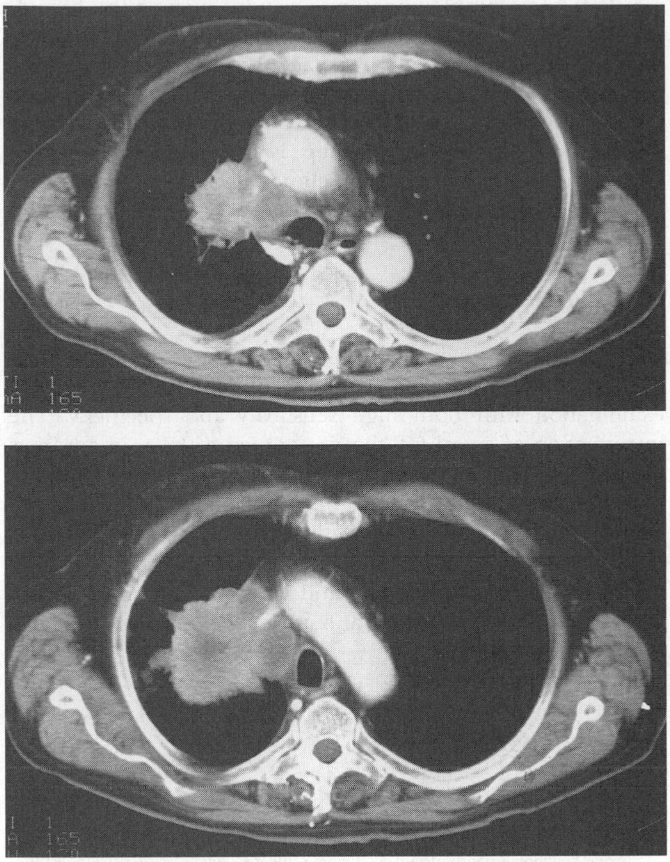

FIGURE 27.1-17. Superior vena cava syndrome due to small cell lung cancer. Spiral computed tomography demonstrates tumor encasement of the superior vena cava. The azygous vein is enlarged.

nodules can also be used to characterize and predict their malignant potential.[71] Recently, much attention has been focused on the use of "low-dose" spiral CT as a screening test for patients at high risk for the development of lung cancer. Spiral CT with dose reduction to 10% to 25% of standard CT has been shown to be very accurate in the detection of pulmonary nodules and can be used to exclude or confirm the presence of a nodule in a patient with an equivocal chest radiograph.[72]

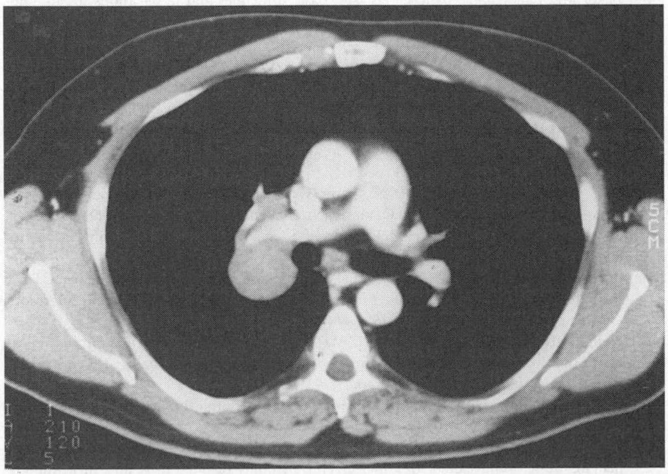

FIGURE 27.1-18. Hodgkin's lymphoma. Computed tomography demonstrates right hilar adenopathy. Vascular enhancement optimizes definition of the nodes.

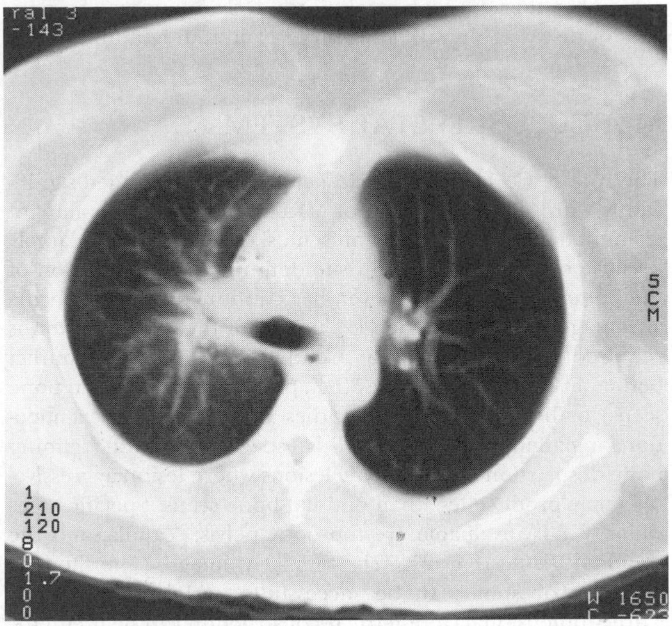

FIGURE 27.1-19. Metastatic breast cancer. Computed tomography demonstrates lymphangitic spread of tumor into the right upper lung.

Finally, the use of what is commonly referred to as *high-resolution CT scanning* is particularly valuable in detecting and defining the presence of parenchymal lung injury, whether from radiation therapy (radiation pneumonitis) or from infections, such as invasive pulmonary aspergillosis after a bone marrow transplant. This CT technique uses very thin sections and a high spatial resolution algorithm. It is important to

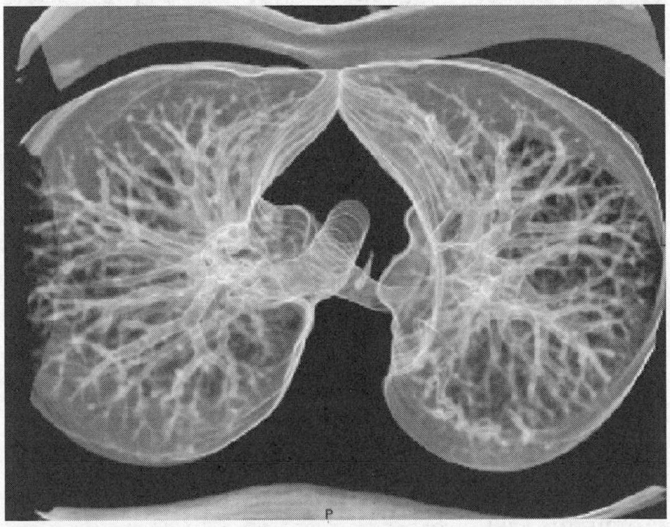

FIGURE 27.1-20. Virtual bronchoscopy. Three-dimensional image from spiral computed tomography data can produce images that can see the inside of the trachea and bronchi.

remember that the high-resolution CT scanning may be positive for disease even with a "normal" plain radiograph.

MUSCULOSKELETAL SYSTEM

The role of CT in the musculoskeletal system changed significantly with the introduction of MRI. It became the dominant examination for staging musculoskeletal tumors, largely because of its superior soft tissue definition and evaluation of the bone marrow. CT, however, has continued to have specific advantages, especially when evaluation of the bony skeleton is required. CT is particularly useful when there is a conflict between radiographic studies (i.e., plain radiographs and bone scans) or between radiology studies and the clinical examination or patient complaints. CT is especially good at defining bone destruction in purely lytic lesions where lesion aggressiveness may produce less than optimal bone scans. Specific areas where CT is invaluable are the bony pelvis, scapula, and the shoulder girdle (Fig. 27.1-21). Similarly, imaging the thoracic and lumbar spine can be successfully performed with CT. Three-dimensional volumetric reconstruction can be useful for preoperative planning and surgical simulation.

CENTRAL NERVOUS SYSTEM

CT became the dominant force in neurooncologic imaging in the early 1980s, before the introduction of clinical MRI. However, with the diffusion of MR technology, MRI is now the dominant force in imaging the central nervous system. CT, however, still has specific applications, particularly when a detailed analysis of the calvarium or spine is required. CT, with high-resolution bone detail algorithms, provides an optimal look at a complex anatomic region, such as the base of the skull, the temporal bone, or the maxillofacial region. Subtle destruction or invasion by adjacent tumor is easily defined on these studies. Similarly, involvement of the spine by primary or metastatic disease may be detected with CT. In these cases, CT may be used when there is a question as a result of bone scan findings or when clinical symptoms and other study results are contradictory.

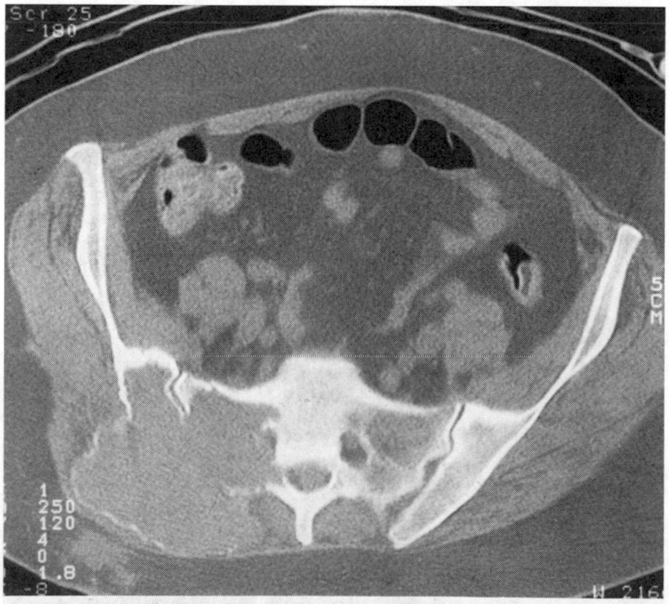

FIGURE 27.1-21. Giant cell tumor. A large lytic lesion involves both the right iliac wing and the sacrum. The study was conducted to emphasize bony detail.

SUMMARY

CT scanning is a mainstay in oncology imaging because of its ability to survey multiple organs and organ systems in a single examination with both high sensitivity and specificity. The introduction of spiral CT that is coupled with rapid advancements in 3D imaging technology ensures that CT will continue to remain a key study in both the detection and staging of diseases. Future progress likely will center on organ-specific contrast agents as well as blood pool agents. Newer technologies, such as real-time 3D imaging and virtual reality displays, will surely expand the role of CT and move it from a diagnostic to a therapeutic modality.

REFERENCES

1. Federle, MP. Opening Plenary Session: 1997. Current status and future trends in abdominal CT. *Radiographics* 1998;18:1555.
2. Kalendar WA, Seissler W, Klotz E, et al. Spiral volumetric CT with single-breath hold technique, continuous transport, and continuous scanner rotation. *Radiology* 1990;176:181.
3. Heiken JP, Brink JA, Vannier MW. Spiral (helical) CT. *Radiology* 1993;189:647.
4. Weg N, Scheer MR, Gabor MP. Liver lesions: improved detection with dual-detector-array CT and routine 2.5-mm thin collimation. *Radiology* 1998; 209:417.
5. Dunco DM. Virtual reality imaging: new techniques in diagnostic imaging. *Appl Radiol* 1996;25:51.
6. Rubin GD, Dake MD, Napel SA, McDonnell CH, Jeffrey RB Jr. Three-dimensional spiral CT angiography of the abdomen: initial clinical experience. *Radiology* 1993;186:147.
7. Johnson PT, Heath DG, Bliss DF, Cabral B, Fishman EK. Computers in radiology. Three-dimensional CT: real-time interactive volume rendering. *AJR Am J Roentgenol* 1996;167:581.
8. Heiken JP, Weyman PJ, Lee JKT, et al. Detection of hepatic masses: prospective evaluation with CT, delayed CT, CT during arterial portography, and MR imaging. *Radiology* 1989;171:47.
9. Soyer P, Bluemke DA, Hruban RH, Sitzmann JV, Fishman EK. Hepatic metastases from colorectal cancer: detection and false-positive findings with helical CT during arterial portography. *Radiology* 1994;193:71.
10. Baker ME, Palley R. Hepatic metastases. Basic principles and implications for radiologists. *Radiology* 1995;197:329.
11. Soyer P, Elias D, Zeiton G, Roche A, Levesque M. Surgical treatment of hepatic metastases: impact of intraoperative sonography. *AJR Am J Roentgenol* 1993;160:511.
12. Jones EC, Chezmar JL, Nelson RC, Bernardino ME. The frequency and significance of small (≤15 mm) hepatic lesions detected by CT. *AJR Am J Roentgenol* 1992;158:535.
13. Schwartz LH, Gandras EJ, Colangelo SM, Ercolani MC, Panicek DM. Prevalence and importance of small hepatic lesions found at CT in patients with cancer. *Radiology* 1999; 210:71.
14. Soyer P, Bluemke DA, Hruban RH, Sitzmann JV, Fishman EK. Primary malignant neoplasms of the liver: detection with helical CT during arterial portography. *Radiology* 1994;192:389.
15. Soyer P, Lacheheb D, Levesque M. False-positive CT portography: correlation with pathologic findings. *AJR Am J Roentgenol* 1993;160:285.
16. Kuszyk BS, Bluemke DA, Urban BA, et al. Portal-phase contrast-enhanced helical CT for the detection of malignant hepatic tumors: sensitivity based on comparison with intraoperative and pathologic findings. *AJR Am J Roentgenol* 1996;166:91.
17. Hollett MD, Jeffrey RB Jr, Nino-Murcia M, Jorgensen MJ, Harris DP. Dual-phrase helical CT of the liver; value of arterial phase scans in the detection of small (≤1.5 cm) malignant hepatic neoplasms. *AJR Am J Roentgenol* 1995;164:879.
18. Fishman EK, Kuszyk BS, Heath DG, Cabral B, Gao L. Surgical planning for liver resection. *Computer* 1996;29(1):64.
19. Van Hoe L, Van Cutsem E, Vergote I, et al. Size quantification of liver metastases in patients undergoing cancer treatment: reproducibility of one-, two-, and three-dimensional measurements determined with spiral CT. *Radiology* 1997;202:671.
20. Platt JF, Francis IR, Ellis JH, Reige KA. Liver metastases: early detection based on abnormal contrast material enhancement at dual-phase helical CT. *Radiology* 1997;205:49.

21. Bluemke DA, Cameron JL, Hruban RH, et al. Potentially resectable adenocarcinoma: spiral CT assessment with surgical and pathologic correlation. *Radiology* 1995;197:381.
22. Nishiharu T, Yamashita Y, Abe Y, et al. Local extension of pancreatic carcinoma: assessment with thin-section helical CT versus with breath-hold fast MR imaging—ROC analysis. *Radiology* 1999;212:445.
23. O'Malley ME, Boland GWL, Wood BJ, et al. Adenocarcinoma of the head of the pancreas: determination of surgical unresectability with thin-section pancreatic-phase helical CT. *AJR Am J Roentgenol* 1999;173:1513.
24. Tabuchi T, Itoh K, Ohshio G, et al. Tumor staging of pancreatic adenocarcinoma using early- and late-phase helical CT. *AJR Am J Roentgenol* 1999;173:375.
25. Freeny PC, Traverso LW, Ryan JA. Diagnosis and staging of pancreatic adenocarcinoma with dynamic computed tomography. *Am J Surg* 1993;165:600.
26. Hommeyer SC, Freeny PC, Crabo LG. Carcinoma of the head of the pancreas: evaluation of the pancreaticoduodenal veins with dynamic CT-potential for improved accuracy in staging. *Radiology* 1995;196:233.
27. Zagoria RJ, Bechtold RE, Dyer RB. Staging of renal adenocarcinoma: role of various imaging procedures. *AJR Am J Roentgenol* 1995;164:363.
28. Silverman SG, Lee BY, Seltzer SE, et al. Small renal masses: correlation of spiral CT features and patient findings. *AJR Am J Roentgenol* 1994;163:597.
29. Cohan RH, Sherman LS, Korobkin M, Bass JC, Francis IR. Renal masses: assessment of corticomedullary-phase and nephrographic phase CT scans. *Radiology* 1995;196:445.
30. Urban BA. The small renal mass: what is the role of multiphasic helical CT? *Radiology* 1997;202:22.
31. Kopka L, Fischer U, Zoeller G, et al. Dual-phase helical CT of the kidney: value of the corticomedullary and ephrographic phase for evaluation of renal lesions and preoperative staging of renal cell carcinoma. *AJR Am J Roentgenol* 1997;169:1573.
32. Smith PA, Marshall FF, Corl FM, Fishman EK. Planning nephron-sparing renal surgery using 3D helical CT angiography. *J Comput Assist Tomogr* 1999;23(5):649.
33. Buckley J, Urban BA, Soyer P, Scherrer A, Fishman EK. Transitional cell carcinoma of the renal pelvis: a retrospective look with pathologic correlation. *Radiology* 1996;201:194.
34. Oliver TW Jr, Bernardino ME, Miller JI, Mansour K, Greene D, Davis WA. Isolated adrenal masses in non small-cell bronchogenic carcinoma. *Radiology* 1984;153:217.
35. Dunnick NR, Heaston D, Halvorsen R, Moore AV, Korobkin M. CT appearance of adrenal cortical carcinoma. *J Comput Assist Tomogr* 1982;6:978.
36. Fishman EK, Deutch BM, Hartman DS, et al. Primary adrenocortical carcinoma: CT evaluation with clinical correlation. *AJR Am J Roentgenol* 1987;148:531.
37. Korobkin M, Brodeur FJ, Francis IR, et al. CT time-attenuation washout curves of adrenal adenomas and nonadenomas. *AJR Am J Roentgenol* 1998;170:747.
38. Korobkin M, Brodeur FJ, Yutzy GG, et al. Differentiation of adrenal adenomas from nonadenomas using CT attenuation values. *AJR Am J Roentgenol* 1996;166:531.
39. Korobkin M, Lombardi TJ, Aisen AM, et al. Characterization of adrenal masses with chemical shift and gadolinium-enhanced MR Imaging. *Radiology* 1995;197:411.
40. Megibow AJ, Balthazar EJ, Cho KC, et al. Bowel obstruction: evaluation with CT. *Radiology* 1991;180:313.
41. Gulliver DJ, Baker KA. CT of the small bowel. *Appl Radiol* 1994;11:39.
42. Pantongrag-Brown L, Buetow PC, Carr NJ, Lichtenstein JE, Buck JL. Calcification and fibrosis in mesenteric carcinoid tumor: CT findings and pathologic correlation. *AJR Am J Roentgenol* 1995;164:387.
43. Balthazar EJ, Megibow AJ, Hulnick D, Naidich DP. Carcinoma of the colon: detection and preoperative staging by CT. *AJR Am J Roentgenol* 1988;150:301.
44. Fenlon HM, Ferrucci JT. First international symposium on virtual colonoscopy. *AJR Am J Roentgenol* 1999;173:565.
45. McFarland EG, Brink JA. Helical CT colonography (virtual colonoscopy): the challenge that exists between advancing technology and generalizability. *AJR Am J Roentgenol* 1999;173:549.
46. Macari M, Berman P, Dicker M, Milano A, Megibow AJ. Usefulness of CT colonography in patients with incomplete colonoscopy. *AJR Am J Roentgenol* 1999;173:561.
47. Noh HM, Fishman EK, Forastiere AA, Bliss DF, Calhoun PS. CT of the esophagus: spectrum of disease with emphasis on esophageal carcinoma. *Radiographics* 1995;15:1113.
48. Balthazar EJ, Siegel SE, Megibow AJ, Scholes J, Gordon R. CT in patients with scirrhous carcinoma of the GI tract: imaging findings and value for tumor detection and staging. *AJR Am J Roentgenol* 1995;165:839.
49. Tsuda K, Hori S, Muasrakami T, et al. Intramural invasion of gastric cancer: evaluation by CT with water-filling method. *J Comput Assist Tomogr* 1995;19(6):941.
50. Kleinhaus U, Militianu D. Computed tomography in the preoperative evaluation of gastric carcinoma. *Gastrointest Radiol* 1988;13:97.
51. Dorfman RE, Alpern MB, Gross BH, Sandler MA. Upper abdominal lymph nodes: criteria for normal size determined by CT. *Radiology* 1991;180:319.
52. Urban BA, Fishman EK, Hruban RH. *Helicobacter pylori* gastritis mimicking gastric carcinoma at CT evaluation. *Radiology* 1991;179:689.
53. Hirakata K, Nakata H, Nakagawa T. CT of pulmonary metastases with pathological correlation. *Semin Ultrasound CT MR* 1995;16(5):379.
54. Fishman EK, Kuhlman JE, Jones RJ. CT of lymphoma: spectrum of disease. *Radiographics* 1991;11:647.
55. Cabanillas F, Fuller LM. The radiologic assessment of the lymphoma patient from the standpoint of the clinician. *Radiol Clin North Am* 1990;28:683.
56. Fishman EK, Kuhlman JE, Schuchter LM, Miler JA III, Magid D. CT of malignant melanoma in the chest, abdomen, and musculoskeletal system. *Radiographics* 1990;10:603.
57. Kawashima A, Fishman EK, Kuhlman JE, Nixon MS. CT of posterior mediastinal masses. *Radiographics* 1991;11:1045.
58. Sones PJ Jr, Torres WE, Colvin RS, et al. Effectiveness of CT in evaluating intrathoracic masses. *AJR Am J Roentgenol* 1982139:469.
59. Zeiberg AS, Silverman PM, Sessions RB, et al. Helical (spiral) CT of the upper airway with three-dimensional imaging: technique and clinical assessment. *AJR Am J Roentgenol* 1996;166:293.
60. Remy-Jardin M, Remy J, Giraud F, Marquette CH. Pulmonary nodules: detection with thick-section spiral CT versus conventional CT. *Radiology* 1993;187:513.
61. Buckley JA, Scott WW Jr, Siegelman SS, et al. Pulmonary nodules: effect of increased data sampling on detection with spiral CT and confidence in diagnosis. *Radiology* 1995;196:395.
62. Remy-Jardin M, Duyck P, Remy J, et al. Hilar lymph nodes: identification with spiral CT and histologic correlation. *Radiology* 1995;196:387.
63. Fleiter T, Merkle EM, Aschoff AJ, et al. Comparison of real-time virtual and fiberoptic bronchoscopy in patients with bronchial carcinoma: opportunities and limitations. *AJR Am J Roentgenol* 1997;169:1591.
64. David R, Lamki N, Fan S, et al. The many faces of neuroblastoma. *Radiographics* 1989;9:859.
65. Rosado-de-Christenson ML, Templeton PA, Moran CA. Mediastinal germ cell tumors: radiologic and pathologic correlation. *Radiographics* 1992;12:1013.
66. Castelino RA. Imaging techniques for staging abdominal Hodgkin's disease. *Cancer Treat Rep* 1982;66:697.
67. Castelino RA, Blank N, Hoppe RT, Cho C. Hodgkin disease: contributions of chest CT in the initial staging evaluation. *Radiology* 1986;160:603.
68. Khoury MB, Godwin JD, Halvorsen R, Hanun Y, Putman CE. Role of chest CT in non-Hodgkin lymphoma. *Radiology* 1986;158:659.
69. Aronberg DJ, Glazer HS, Sagel SS. MRI and CT of the mediastinum: comparisons, controversies, and pitfalls. *Radiol Clin North Am* 1985;23:439.
70. Munden RF, Pugatch RD, Liptay MJ, Sugarbaker DJ, Le LU. Small pulmonary lesions detected at CT: clinical importance. *Radiology* 1997;202:105.
71. Zhang M, Kono M. Solitary pulmonary nodules: evaluation of blood flow patterns with dynamic CT. *Radiology* 1997;205:471.
72. Diederich S, Lenzen H, Windmann R, et al. Pulmonary nodules: experimental and clinical studies at low-dose CT. *Radiology* 1999;213:289.

SECTION **2**

ARTHUR E. LI
DAVID A. BLUEMKE

Magnetic Resonance Imaging

BASIC PRINCIPLES

Magnetic resonance imaging (MRI) is based on the effect of large magnetic fields on the spinning motion of certain nuclei within biologic tissues. Due to the laws of electromagnetics, spinning nuclei with odd mass numbers have a net charge and align themselves in the presence of an external magnetic field. In the human body, the hydrogen nucleus (mass number of 1) is most often used in clinical MRI due to its abundance in water and lipid tissues. When a patient is placed in the bore of a magnet, the hydrogen nuclei partially align themselves with the direction of the external magnet, which generates the net magnetization vector (NMV) of the patient. In addition, these hydrogen molecules are spinning (a process called *precession*) at a specific frequency that varies with the strength of the external magnetic field. This frequency is called the *Larmor frequency*. Based on the principle of resonance, a radiofrequency pulse emitted by a transmitter at the Larmor frequency can displace the alignment of the hydrogen nuclei NMV through a flip angle that depends on the amplitude and duration of the radiofrequency pulse. Once the pulse is turned off, the hydrogen nuclei relax back into their previous alignment with the external magnetic field. It is during this process of relaxation that the spinning hydrogen nuclei produce a radiofrequency electromagnetic signal, which can be detected by a receiver coil placed on or around the patient. The information from this signal can be processed by a computer to generate an image via a mathematical algorithm known as a *Fourier transform.*

The magnetization of the NMV exists in the planes of three-dimensional space. When the NMV is aligned with the external magnetic field, the magnetization is said to be in the longitudinal plane. After a radiofrequency pulse, the NMV is usually flipped into the transverse plane. When the pulse is turned off, the relaxation of the NMV back into the longitudinal plane is called *T1 relaxation.* The decay of transverse plane magnetization is called *T2 relaxation.* Different tissues in the body relax at different rates. Fat has very short T1 and T2 relaxation times, whereas water has considerably longer T1 and T2 relaxation times. Neoplastic tissue also generally relaxes at rates different from the tissues surrounding it. The varying relaxation times of tissues generate different strengths of signal at specific points in measurement times. Hence, it is the difference in relaxation between tissues and the varying strength of the signals they generate that determine the contrast between tissues on MR images. Tissues that appear bright on MR images are said to have high signal intensity, whereas dark-appearing tissues demonstrate low signal intensity. In addition to relaxivity times, the strength of tissue signal also depends on the number of hydrogen nuclei present in the tissue (i.e., "proton density"). The ability of MRI to demonstrate superior contrast between different tissue types (Table 27.2-1) constitutes a major advantage over other cross-sectional imaging modalities, such as computed tomography (CT).

It is possible to "weight" an image by varying the repetition time (TR) between radiofrequency pulses and varying the time to sample the signal, called the *echo time* (TE) (Fig. 27.2-1). One can choose the weighting of an image to emphasize the T1 relaxivity properties of tissues, the T2 relaxivity, or the proton density. Tissues with short T1 relaxivity times, such as fat, appear brighter on T1-weighted images. Tissues exhibiting long T2 relaxivity, such as water, appear brighter on T2-weighted images

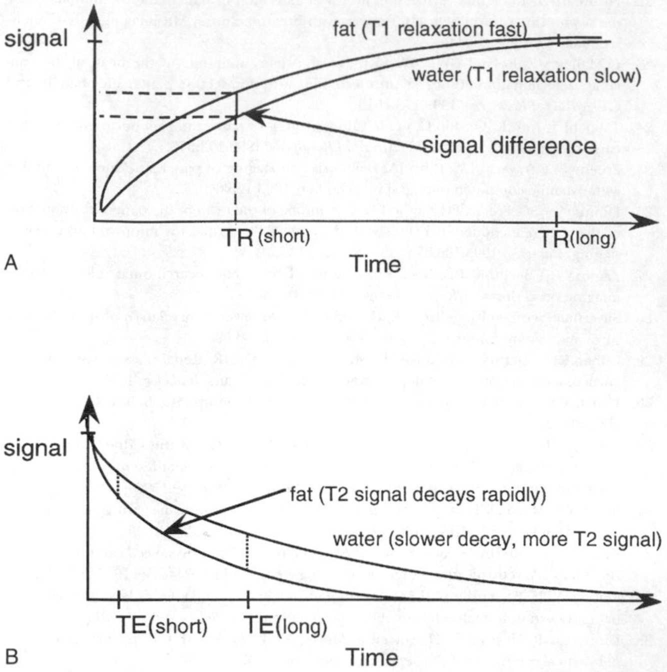

FIGURE 27.2-1. The basis of T1 and T2 weighting. **A:** Because fat has a shorter T1 relaxivity than does water, a short repetition time (TR) can maximize the T1 signal difference between fat and water, prior to full recovery of longitudinal magnetization. Hence, a short TR [and a short echo time (TE), which minimizes T2 effects] results in T1 weighting of a magnetic resonance image. **B:** The T2 signal decay of fat is faster than that of water; hence, a long TE can maximize signal differences from T2 signal between fat and water. As a result, a long TE (in combination with a long TR, which minimizes T1 effects) results in T2 weighting of an image.

(Table 27.2-2). In general, T1 weighting is useful for demonstrating anatomic detail, whereas T2 weighting may be preferred when imaging pathology, such as neoplastic tissue.

The use of contrast agents can also improve the detection of tumors and other pathology by MRI. The most commonly used agent is gadolinium, a paramagnetic rare earth metal that slows the tumbling of adjacent hydrogen molecules. This results in a large reduction in the T1 and T2 relaxivities of the tissues that take up the contrast. Hence, tissues into which gadolinium diffuses appear bright on T1-weighted images. MRI of tumors exploits this property of gadolinium because tumors are often hypervascular and demonstrate increased contrast agent uptake relative to the surrounding normal tissues. Further, tumor vessels are disorganized and "leaky," so that there is increased extracellular fluid in the tumor. Hence, many tumors "enhance" after contrast administration. The distinct enhancement pattern of some tumors on sequential images taken at multiple time points after contrast administration (known as *dynamic MRI*) can also separate tumor from surrounding tissues. The risks and side effects of gadolinium are minimal as compared with those of iodinated contrast agents used for CT.

An ever-increasing number of different radio frequency pulse sequences are available for use in MRI. The gold standard for most imaging is the spin-echo pulse sequence, in

TABLE 27.2-1. Relative Signal Intensities of Tissues

Tissue	*T1-Weighted*	*T2-Weighted*
Adrenal	Intermediate	Moderately bright
Cervix (stroma)	Dark	Dark
Brain		
Cerebrospinal fluid	Dark	Very bright
Gray matter	Intermediate to dark	Intermediate to bright
White matter	Bright	Intermediate to dark
Cortical bone	Very dark	Very dark
Muscle	Dark	Dark
Lung	Very dark	Very dark
Liver	Intermediate to bright	Intermediate to dark
Pancreas	Intermediate to bright	Intermediate to dark
Prostate		
Central	Intermediate	Dark
Peripheral	Intermediate	Bright
Spleen	Intermediate	Bright

Adapted from Schwartz LH, Castellino RA. Magnetic resonance imaging. In: DeVita VT, Hellman S, Rosenberg SA, eds. *Cancer: principles and practice of oncology,* 5th ed. New York: Lippincott–Raven, 1997.

TABLE 27.2-2. Characteristics of Image Weighting

TR	*TE*	*Image Type*	*Fat*	*Water*
Short	Short	T1-weighted	Bright	Dark
Short	Long	Proton density	Intermediate	Intermediate
Long	Short	Proton density	Intermediate	Intermediate
Long	Long	T2-weighted	Intermediate-dark	Bright

TE, echo time; TR, repetition time.
Note: Short TR: 400–800 msec; long TR: >1500 msec; short TE: <30 msec; long TE: >90 msec.

which an initial 90-degree radiofrequency pulse is followed by a 180-degree pulse. Subsequent to the initial 90-degree radiofrequency pulse, the nuclei begin to fall out of phase from each other, which decays the signal produced. The 180-degree pulse rephases the nuclei to generate an "echo," which is the signal detected by the receiver coil. The time between the initial 90-degree pulse and the generation of the echo signal is called the *echo time,* and the time between each succeeding 90-degree pulse is called the *repetition time.* As discussed, the TR and TE can be varied to produce T1-, T2-, or proton density–weighted images. Another important pulse sequence is the gradient echo, in which an initial variable flip-angle pulse is rephased by a magnetic gradient to produce an echo signal. Gradient echo sequences reduce scan times and are particularly useful for demonstrating flow on MR angiograms. The most recent advances have been made in developing very fast pulse sequences that can acquire several image slices in a single breath hold. Faster imaging reduces artifacts from breathing and other movements, and new ultrafast sequences are continually expanding the applications and widening the range of anatomy that can be accurately imaged by MRI.

The basic MR imager consists of the gantry, operating console, and computer with software that coordinates the acquisition and processing of images. During imaging, the patient is placed inside the gantry, surrounded by the primary magnetic coils that generate the main external magnetic field and by the secondary magnetic coils that generate various magnetic field gradients. These magnetic gradients are what allow signal to be localized to precise locations within the patient. The use of gradients also allows MR images to be obtained in multiple planes, including coronal, axial, sagittal, and oblique. Most commercially available "high-field" MRI magnets use field strengths of 1.0 or 1.5 tesla. "Low-field" and "open" MRIs use magnetic strengths from 0.2 to 0.5 tesla. Different radiofrequency receiver coils are available, depending on the anatomy to be imaged, and commonly include shoulder, body, or head coils placed on the patient. Exposure to the magnetic fields of an MR imager is generally considered much safer than exposure to the ionizing radiation of some other imaging modalities. However, MRI is contraindicated in patients with pacemakers and may pose problems for patients with aneurysm clips made prior to 1980 and with several other ferromagnetic implants.

BRAIN

MRI is the imaging technique of choice for evaluating brain tumors. MRI has significant advantages over CT, such as multiplanar capabilities, which allow better assessment of the origin of tumors and their involvement of adjacent structures. In addition, MRI offers both better imaging detail of posterior fossa tumors and superior tissue contrast. MRI can also show the secondary effects of some brain tumors, such as hydrocephalus, hemorrhage, and edema. MRI is also useful in identifying the best location for surgical biopsy. Two disadvantages of MRI are difficulties in detecting calcifications that occur in some tumors, such as oligodendrogliomas, and decreased ability to delineate tumor invasion into bone. In such cases, a CT scan, which can detect these phenomena, can be complementary to MRI.

The characteristic MRI appearance of the majority of brain tumors is a hyperintense signal on T2-weighted images. In addition, gadolinium contrast is used in every MRI workup of brain tumors. Most normal brain tissue does not take up contrast, owing to the integrity of the blood–brain barrier. However, with malignancy, there is breakdown of the blood–brain barrier and neovascularity and, hence, most tumors enhance. Some tumors would not be seen without contrast administration. Gadolinium contrast administration can also help to distinguish tumor margins from surrounding edema on T1-weighted images. The intensity of contrast enhancement correlates in a rough sense with the tumor grade, probably because generally higher-grade lesions have increased neovascularity. Therefore, higher-grade lesions may enhance more intensely than well-differentiated brain tumors. In addition, the amount of vasogenic edema and hemorrhage adjacent to tumor may roughly correlate with the degree of malignancy. Hence, a low-grade fibrillary astrocytoma may demonstrate little contrast enhancement and no edema or hemorrhage, whereas a high-grade glioblastoma may show intense heterogeneous contrast enhancement, with prominent edema and hemorrhage. However, this rule is not always reliable. An exception is low-grade pilocytic astrocytoma, which shows a paradoxical marked contrast enhancement (Fig. 27.2-2). Hence, MRI can help to assess the aggressiveness of brain tumors, but tumor diagnosis and grading must depend on the histopathologic analysis of surgical material.

Other brain tumors may demonstrate some distinguishing characteristics on MRI. Meningiomas are isointense to normal brain on all pulse sequences but enhance intensely with contrast administration. Meningiomas can also demonstrate a focal thickened collar of enhancement adjacent to the tumor's dural attachment, known as the *dural tail sign.*[1] Ependymomas and choroid plexus papillomas may be associated with hydrocephalus seen on MRI. Metastatic lesions often appear at the gray-white interface, enhance intensely, and can demonstrate edema. MRI is the most sensitive modality for imaging brain metastasis,[2] and single lesions on CT can sometimes be

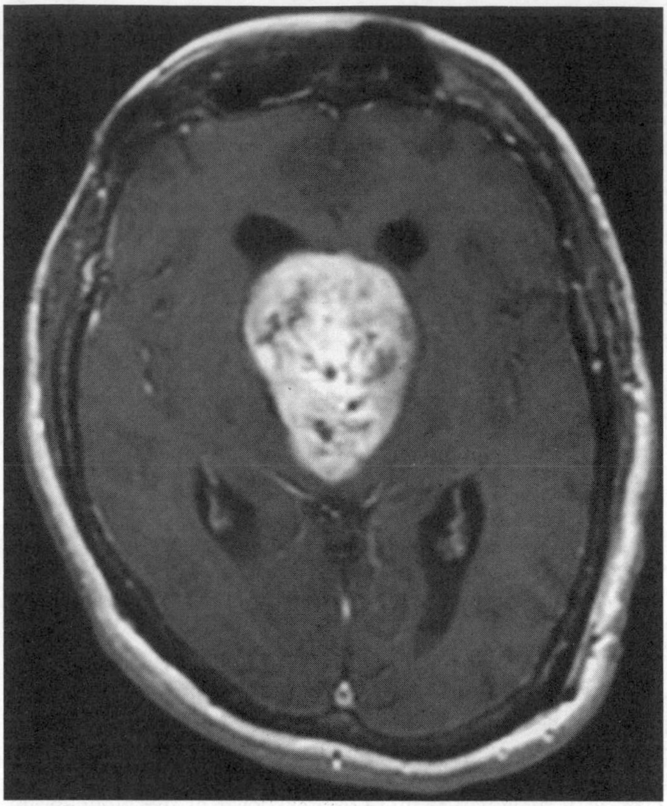

FIGURE 27.2-2. Pilocytic astrocytoma. A large enhancing mass is present, arising from the region of the hypothalamus. Gadolinium contrast has been administered, resulting in heterogeneous enhancement of the mass. The extent of the tumor is well depicted on magnetic resonance imaging, as is the adjacent mass effect on the brain, with mild dilatation of the lateral ventricles.

revealed as multiple intracranial lesions when imaged with contrast-enhanced MRI.

MRI is also useful in assessing patients after surgery, irradiation, or chemotherapy. However, changes secondary to both surgery and irradiation can cause findings that may mimic residual or recurrent tumor.[3] One solution is to reimage the postoperative patient within 4 days after surgery to establish a baseline prior to the development of postoperative processes simulating tumor.[4] In addition, positron emission tomography scanning may be able to differentiate recurrent tumor from the changes of radiation injury.[5]

SPINE

MRI is the primary imaging technique used to evaluate neoplastic disease of the spine. MRI is preferred over CT and plain-film myelography and does not require the infusion of intrathecal contrast. Intramedullary tumors appear with decreased signal intensity relative to cord on T1-weighted images. Cord expansion by tumor can also be seen. Contrast enhancement aids in the detection and characterization of tumors and is also helpful in detecting "drop metastases" that have spread from intracranial and extracranial tumors to the spine via the subarachnoid space. Common extramedullary-intradural tumors (e.g., schwannomas and meningiomas) and extradural tumors (e.g., osseous hemangioma, myeloma) can also be detected on images. MRI accurately assesses for the presence of spinal cord compression by neoplasm (Fig. 27.2-3), with a reported sensitivity of 92% and specificity of 90%.[6]

HEAD AND NECK

MRI is now a primary imaging modality for evaluating many tumors of the head and neck, including tumors of the sinuses, oropharynx, nasopharynx, salivary glands, and larynx. The abilities of MRI to image in multiple planes and to detect subtle differences in soft tissue boundaries render MRI superior to CT in staging and localizing many tumors for guidance in therapeutic decision making. The main advantage of MRI of the sinuses is that malignant tissue can be distinguished from adjacent inflammatory disease and secretions in the sinuses.[7] This is because on T2-weighted images, most sinus tumors have little intercellular and intracellular free water and appear hypointense, whereas inflammatory tissues are high in free

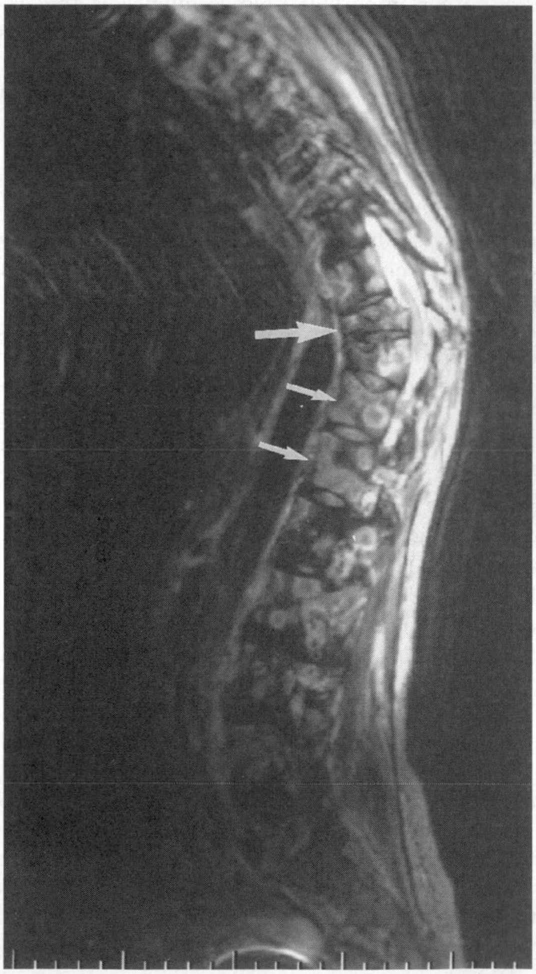

FIGURE 27.2-3. Breast cancer metastatic to spine. The T2-weighted sagittal view of the spine shows areas of increased signal intensity diffusely throughout the spine, owing to metastatic disease (e.g., *small arrows*). In the lower thoracic spine, a pathologic compression fracture has occurred (*large arrow*), resulting in mild compression of the spinal cord at this level.

water and appear hyperintense. Squamous cell carcinomas of the sinuses can erode into bone, a critical finding that affects treatment choices. MRI can demonstrate bony erosion by the absence of signal void normally present within cortical bone. However, in evaluating certain critical areas, such as the orbit, pterygopalatine fossa, and central skull base, a CT should be ordered to improve detection of small focal bony erosions.[8] In the oropharynx, MRI can image without artifacts from dental amalgam and without beam-hardening artifacts from the mandible, both of which limit CT examination of this area. In the nasopharynx, MRI is superior to CT at identifying tumor infiltration beyond the pharyngobasilar fascia, detecting enlarged retropharyngeal lymph nodes, and demonstrating possible intracranial involvement.[9] MRI has replaced CT for imaging major salivary glands.[10] MRI is often used to determine the location of salivary gland tumors relative to the facial nerve so as to optimize treatment approaches that will preserve facial nerve function. The larynx and hypopharynx are regions that are readily accessed by clinical examination, which makes possible the diagnosis of malignancy through endoscopy and biopsy. However, coronal MRI images can complement clinical examination by delineating the depth of extension and submucosal involvement of laryngeal and hypopharyngeal tumors.[11]

BREAST

Contrast-enhanced MRI is the most sensitive imaging modality for detecting breast pathology and can improve the detection of breast cancer in selected patient populations. The majority of invasive carcinomas are hypervascular and demonstrate intense enhancement with contrast administration. When morphologic criteria are combined with characteristic tumor enhancement patterns, MRI in many studies demonstrates greater than 90% sensitivity for detecting invasive breast carcinomas.[12,13] Despite the improved sensitivities of MRI over mammography for detecting breast cancer, MRI should not be used for cancer detection in unselected patient populations, owing to false-positive rates and the higher cost of the examination. Instead, MRI is primarily indicated for detecting malignancy in high-risk patients when mammography is compromised owing to radiographically dense breasts, silicone-augmented breasts, or scarring due to remote surgery or trauma. MRI can detect many tumors that mammography may miss in these patients. When combined MRI and conventional imaging are used in these patients, sensitivities greater than 98% can be routinely achieved for detecting invasive breast carcinomas.[14] MRI may also be useful in the search for a primary tumor when a patient presents with positive axillary nodes but no evidence of breast cancer on conventional imaging or physical examination (Fig. 27.2-4).[15]

There are also a number of emerging indications for the use of MRI in the preoperative staging and posttreatment monitoring of breast cancer, based on preliminary investigations. In considering breast conservation therapy, it is important to determine preoperatively whether a detected breast malignancy is unifocal, multifocal, or multicentric, as multicentric disease is a contraindication for breast conservation therapy. MRI appears to be markedly more sensitive than mammography in detecting multifocality or multicentricity within breast carcinomas.[16–18] The preoperative staging of breast cancer by MRI in one study was shown to alter the subsequent treatment in 18% of cases.[18] MRI also has shown promise in assessing the results of induction chemotherapy in reducing tumor burden prior to breast conservation surgery.[19] A recent review has suggested using MRI prior to lumpectomy to help to decrease the number of reexcisions due to positive pathologic margins.[20] In addition, the use of high-resolution RODEO (rotating delivery of off resonance) MRI has recently been demonstrated to improve the evaluation of ductal carcinoma *in situ.*[21] After conservative breast surgery, MRI has been shown to be superior to mammography in diagnosing recurrent malignant foci. In one study, 4 of 11 local recurrences were detected only by MRI.[22] However, MRI should be performed not less than 6 months after surgery and 12 months after irradiation to reduce false-positive rates.[23]

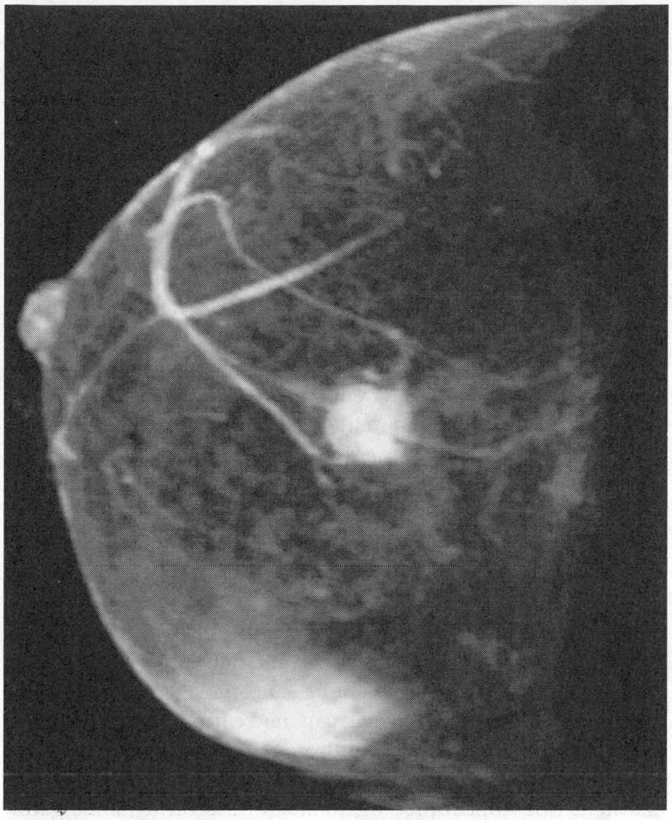

FIGURE 27.2-4. Breast cancer. On a sagittal image of the breast, an intensely enhancing focus of invasive ductal carcinoma is present. This patient had enlarged lymph nodes in the axilla, which were subjected to biopsy and were found to be positive for breast cancer. However, mammogram results were negative. In this circumstance, magnetic resonance imaging is useful for detecting the primary lesion. Although magnetic resonance imaging should not be used for screening for breast cancer, it is useful in younger patients with dense breast tissue and, in certain cases, in determining the extent of the lesion before planned lumpectomy versus mastectomy.

LIVER

With the development of fast breath-hold scanning techniques that reduce motion artifact, the role of MRI in detecting and characterizing focal hepatic lesions has advanced greatly. MRI may be superior to CT and sonography in detecting hepatocellular carcinoma (HCC), as T2-weighted images may demonstrate characteristic morphologic features of HCC, such as mosaic or nodules-in nodule patterns of signal intensity.[24] In addition, HCC demonstrates a pattern of dynamic signal enhancement distinct from the surrounding liver after bolus injection of contrast agents, owing to a prominent arterial blood supply for HCC. MRI can also detect early HCC arising within regenerating nodules associated with cirrhosis, even when the α-fetoprotein level is normal and biopsy is negative for tumor.[25]

Metastatic lesions can appear mildly hypointense on T1-weighted images and hyperintense on T2-weighted images (Fig. 27.2-5) and can contain areas of central necrosis of different intensity from the surrounding tumor. New contrast agents containing superparamagnetic iron oxide particles have recently been approved for clinical use and have improved the accuracy of hepatic metastasis detection.[26] These particles are taken up selectively by Kupffer cells within the liver, causing dropout in the signal of normal liver. Metastatic lesions, which do not contain Kupffer cells and do not take up the particles, appear as high-intensity signal against the low signal of the surrounding liver.

Cavernous hemangiomas are the most common benign tumors of the liver. They are often incidentally discovered on various abdominal imaging studies and must be distinguished from malignant lesions. MRI can make this distinction with greater than 90% sensitivity and specificity, owing to the inherently higher T2 values of hemangiomas (Fig. 27.2-6) and to the characteristic appearance of hemangiomas on dynamic gadolinium-enhanced images.[27]

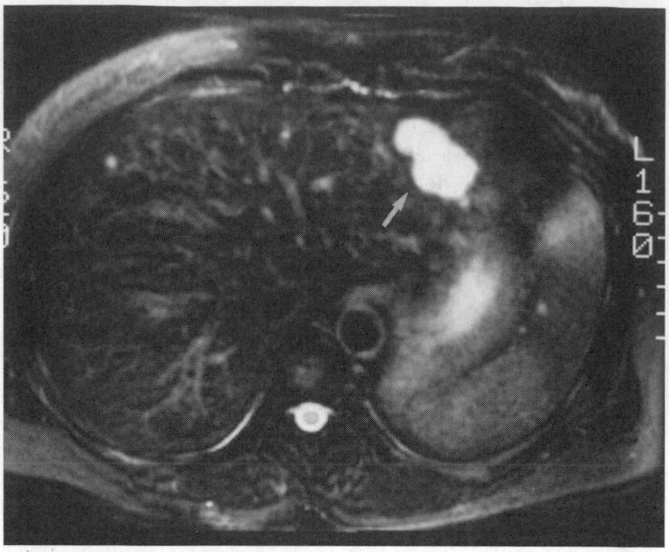

FIGURE 27.2-6. Hemangioma of the liver. In the left lobe of the liver, there is an intensely bright lobulated lesion on this T2-weighted image (*arrow*). Hemangiomas are extremely common, present in approximately 5% of patients. Frequently, these present diagnostic dilemmas on computed tomography scans of the liver. On magnetic resonance imaging, the appearance is characteristic and diagnostic, so biopsy of these lesions can be avoided.

ADRENAL GLANDS

With the use of chemical shift imaging, MRI has become the most effective noninvasive method for distinguishing between commonly found benign adrenal adenomas and malignant masses. MRI can accurately make this distinction, owing to the fact that, unlike malignant adrenal tumors, most adrenal adenomas contain a large amount of cytoplasmic lipid. On application of chemical shift imaging techniques to MRI of the adrenals, tissues that contain both lipid and water demonstrate low signal intensity relative to other tissues containing mostly water. This is because fat and water protons have different precessional frequencies, owing to the size differences in the electron clouds surrounding them. When the appropriate TE is chosen, fat and water are maximally out of phase, and their radiofrequency waves cancel each other, resulting in signal loss. Most adenomas, which contain both fat and water, demonstrate signal loss on chemical shift imaging (Fig. 27.2-7), whereas both primary adrenal malignancies and metastatic lesions, which do not contain fat, have signal intensities similar to other organs, such as liver and spleen. Exploiting this difference, chemical shift MRI has been reported to have a sensitivity for identifying benign adrenal lesions of 80% and a specificity of 100%.[28]

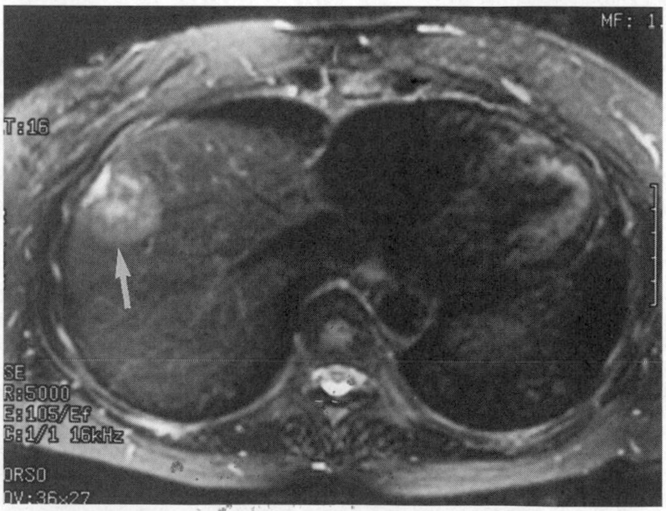

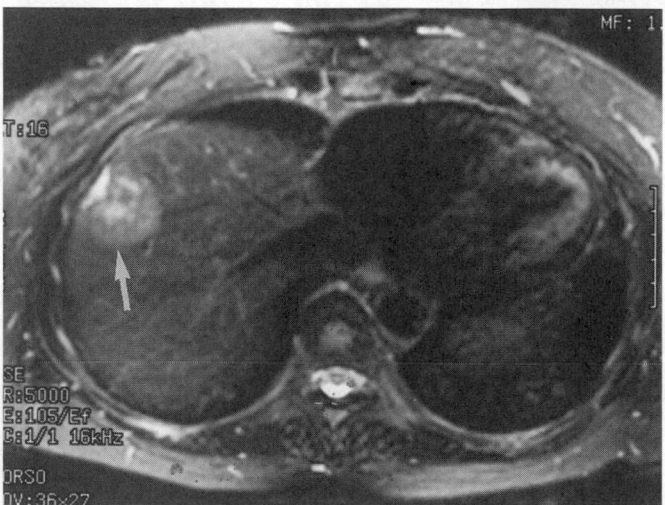

FIGURE 27.2-5. Metastatic colon cancer to the liver. In the right lobe of the liver, there is a rounded lesion (*arrow*) with an internal area of high signal intensity characteristic of metastatic disease in the liver for presurgical evaluation as well as to evaluate indeterminate lesions on computed tomography scan. In addition, patients with parenchymal liver disease, such as cirrhosis, benefit by magnetic resonance imaging scans of the liver, owing to increased detection rate of hepatocellular cancer, compared to other noninvasive imaging modalities.

MRI is particularly useful for characterizing incidental adrenal masses found in patients with known malignancies. In these patients, the finding of a metastatic lesion to the adrenals may profoundly influence treatment of the primary tumor. To date, no lesion metastatic to the adrenals has demonstrated signal loss with chemical shift imaging comparable to that demonstrated by benign lesions. This allows accurate differentiation of metastases from adenomas. In the case of fat detected on chemical shift MRI, an adrenal biopsy is unnecessary. In addition to this application, MRI is the imaging modality of choice in localizing pheochromocytoma and extraadrenal paraganglioma and for evaluating vascular invasion by adrenal carcinoma.

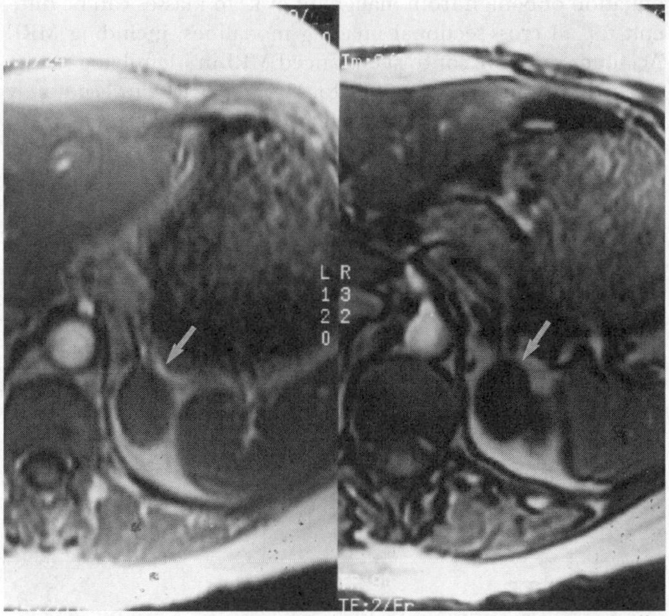

FIGURE 27.2-7. Adrenal adenoma. A 3-cm left adrenal mass is present (*arrows*). On the left-hand images, the mass shows similar signal intensity as compared to the spleen. On the right-hand image, chemical shift imaging was used. In areas that contained fat and water at the cellular level, there is decreased signal using this technique. On the right-hand image, the adrenal lesion is now seen to have lower signal intensity as compared to the spleen. This method is chemically specific for intracellular lipid and is diagnostic of adrenal adenoma. The specificity of this technique approaches 100%.

KIDNEY

In staging renal cell carcinoma (RCC), CT and MRI are comparably accurate, their accuracy ranging from 67% to 96%.[29] Hence, given its lower cost, CT is generally the preferred modality for staging RCC. However, because of its high tissue contrast and multiplanar imaging capabilities, MRI offers improvement over CT for delineation of RCC extension into the renal veins, inferior vena cava, and right atrium (Fig. 27.2-8).[30] MRI can also distinguish tumor thrombus from bland thrombus in the inferior vena cava[31] and offers improved detection of venous wall invasion. Hence, MRI is the preferred modality for RCC staging when iodine contrast is contraindicated, CT results are inconclusive, or it is necessary to determine the extent of venous invasion by tumor to guide surgical approaches for thrombectomy.

UTERUS

T2-weighted images depict three distinct zones of signal intensity within the uterus. A central hyperintense stripe corresponds to the endometrium. This is surrounded by a hypointense zone representing the junctional zone, which is the inner myometrial layer. The remaining segment of the myometrium is of intermediate signal intensity. Endometrial carcinoma can be identified as tissue with signal intensity intermediate between normal endometrium and myometrium. By use of MRI, tumor can be seen confined to the endometrium

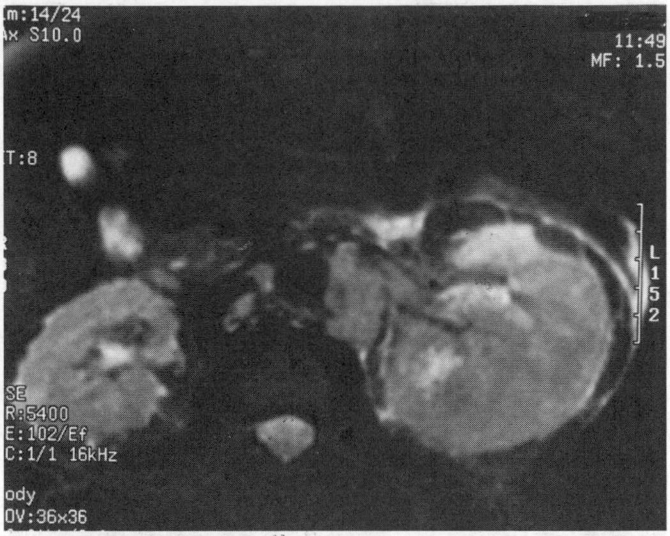

FIGURE 27.2-8. Renal cell cancer. A large mass obscuring the normal anatomy of the left kidney is present. In addition, there is adenopathy surrounding the aorta. However, there is no evidence of linear or tubular involvement of the left renal vein, and the inferior vena cava is not involved by the tumor. Magnetic resonance imaging is very sensitive for detecting renal vein involvement by renal cell cancer. Staging examinations can depict the extent of tumor in the inferior vena cava if present, to determine surgical management of the patient.

(Fig. 27.2-9), extending into the junctional zone, or invading into the deep myometrium.

The primary indication for MRI in patients with proven uterine carcinoma is preoperative staging. Importantly, the presence of greater than 50% myometrial invasion predicts poorer prognosis and requires more extensive surgery, including paraaortic lymphadenectomy. MRI can make this determination with an accuracy of 75% to 95%.[32,33] In addition to determining the depth of myometrial invasion, MRI accurately depicts the extension of endometrial carcinoma to endocervical glands and to cervical stroma. However, MRI staging accuracy is limited when the zonal architecture of the uterus is distorted by uterine anomalies or leiomyomas or when the junctional zone is absent, which can occur in postmenopausal women.[34] Because the MRI appearance of noninvasive endometrial carcinoma is nonspecific, MRI cannot be used as a screening technique.[35]

CERVIX

On T2-weighted images, the normal cervix demonstrates an inner hyperintense signal zone representing the endocervical canal. Adjacent to this is a hypointense zone that corresponds to the cervical stroma. The outer zone, which is continuous with the myometrium, is isointense to myometrium. Parametrial tissues (composed of vessels, ligaments, and fat) surround the cervix and are hyperintense. Most cervical carcinomas have at least intermediate or high signal intensity on T2-weighted images, which provides good contrast between tumor and the hypointense cervical stroma.

MRI is considered the most reliable imaging modality for staging cervical cancer and planning its treatment. In a com-

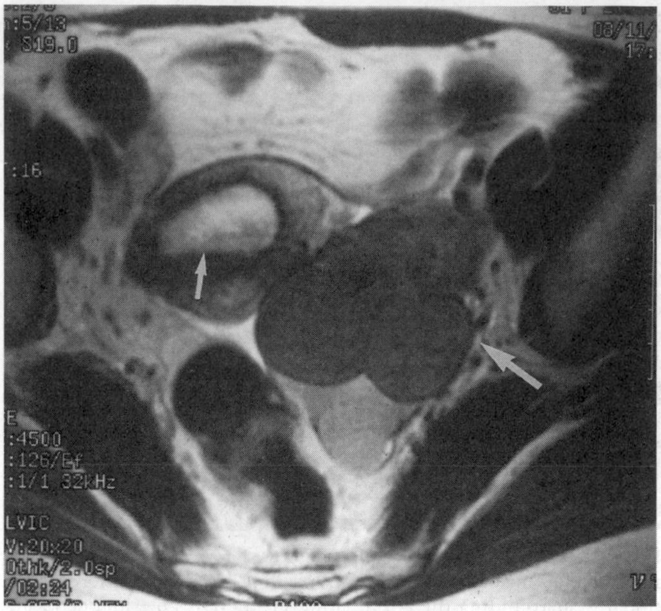

FIGURE 27.2-9. Endometrial cancer. Within the uterus, the central signal due to high signal glandular tissue is markedly thickened (*small arrow*). The darker ring around the inner portion of the uterus, termed the *junctional zone*, is intact, indicating that the cancer has not spread into the superficial layer of the myometrium. Additionally, there is a large mass in the left adnexa due to endometriosis involving the left ovary (*large arrow*). MRI has been found to be useful for staging endometrial cancer. For ovarian tumors, lesions containing fat, such as dermoids, can be specifically identified and determined to be benign in certain cases.

parative study, the overall staging accuracy of MRI (83%) was higher than CT (63%) or clinical staging (70%).[36] Although preinvasive microscopic disease (stage IA) is not well identified on T2-weighted images, MRI can accurately depict the depth of stromal invasion (stage IB), the presence of parametrial extension (stage IIB), invasion of the vagina or pelvic wall (stages IIA and III), and bladder or rectal invasion (stage IV).[37] Of particular importance is determining whether tumor has extended to the parametrium, as patients who present with parametrial invasion are not usually surgical candidates. The presence of a completely intact ring of hypointense cervical stroma excludes parametrial involvement.[38] However, there are false-positive outcomes associated with disruption of the stromal ring. MRI is also useful for distinguishing recurrent tumor from fibrosis if imaged 12 months or more after treatment. The use of MRI has been shown to decrease the number of procedures and invasive studies ordered (e.g., excretory urography, barium enema, lymphography), with a resultant cost benefit.[39]

OVARY

In the evaluation of ovarian masses, MRI is useful in delineating the internal architecture of ovarian tumors. MRI can depict complex tumor structures, such as irregular mural thickening, septations, and solid components, as well as associated findings, such as ascites, visceral lesions, adenopathy, and peritoneal implants.[40] Such findings can be associated with malignancy. However, these findings can be nonspecific; hence, the differentiation of benign from malignant ovarian masses can be difficult for all cross-sectional imaging modalities, including MRI. Accuracy rates for contrast-enhanced MRI in identifying malignancy have ranged from 78% to 95%.[41,42] MRI can accurately identify some benign ovarian masses, such as dermoid cysts, endometriomas, and fibromas. MRI identifies dermoid cysts with an accuracy of 99% by demonstrating the presence of intraluminal fat.[43] In addition, MRI can determine whether a mass is truly ovarian in origin and can accurately differentiate subserosal leiomyomas from ovarian masses. In the preoperative staging of ovarian malignancy, MRI and CT demonstrate generally equivalent accuracy; hence, CT is the primary imaging modality for preoperative staging, given its lower cost and ready availability. Regarding postoperative monitoring, MRI can often detect macroscopic recurrent tumors larger than 2 cm (considered nonresectable), thus eliminating the need for second-look surgery in such patients.[44] However, MRI is less successful in detecting smaller implants or microscopic disease.

PROSTATE

The most common indication for MRI of the prostate is for staging prostate cancer after a biopsy diagnosis has been made (Fig. 27.2-10). The use of an endorectal surface coil alone or with anterior phased-array coils allows MRI identification of the tumor, the prostate capsule, the neurovascular bundles, and the seminal vesicles. Capsular penetration is demonstrated on MRI with the finding of gross tumor extension into the periprostatic fat or with capsular thickening, irregularity, or bulging.[45] Tumor invasion of the neurovascular bundles can manifest as asymmetric enlargement of the bundle. Signs of seminal vesicle invasion on T2-weighted images include a low-

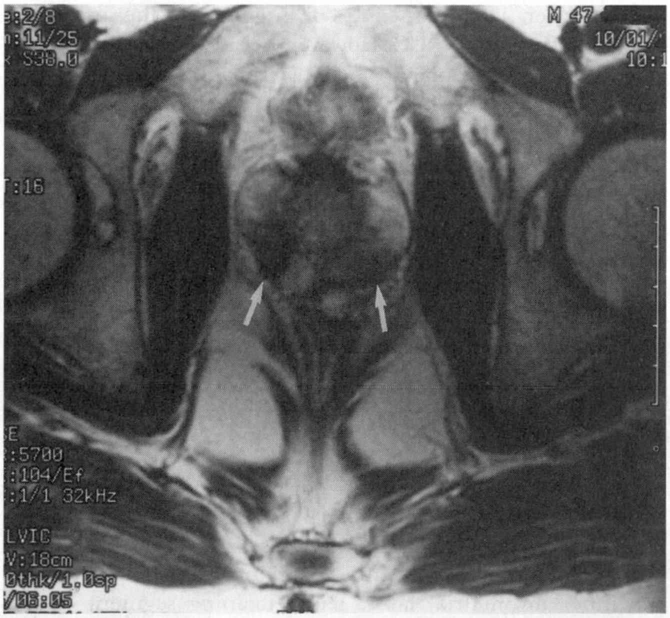

FIGURE 27.2-10. Prostate cancer. T2-weighted magnetic resonance image of the pelvis showed low signal intensity in the peripheral zone of the prostate, owing to multifocal cancer (*arrows*). The tumor is contained within the capsule of the prostate.

signal-intensity mass within the seminal vesicle or wall thickening. MRI can also screen for the presence of enlarged pelvic lymph nodes and bone metastases but cannot detect the presence of tumor in normal-sized nodes. Because MRI offers superior anatomic detail, owing to improved soft tissue contrast, it is considered by some to be superior to CT and ultrasonography in staging prostate cancer.[46] However, there have been wide ranges of sensitivities and specificities reported for MRI staging of prostate cancer, with accuracy ranging from 51% to 92%.[47,48] These variations are in part dependent on the experience of the radiologist performing the readings.[49] Some have proposed that MRI data are best used in combination with other clinical parameters, such as patient's age, prostate-specific antigen, digital rectal examination, and the biopsy Gleason score. In particular, D'Amico et al.[50] have reported that MRI improves staging accuracy for patients at intermediate clinical risk for invasive disease, as indicated by prostate-specific antigen levels of 10 to 20 ng/mL and Gleason scores of 5 to 7. Similar to CT and ultrasonography, MRI is not recommended for initial cancer detection and screening because of its low sensitivity for demonstrating central zone cancers and its difficulty in distinguishing malignant from benign lesions.

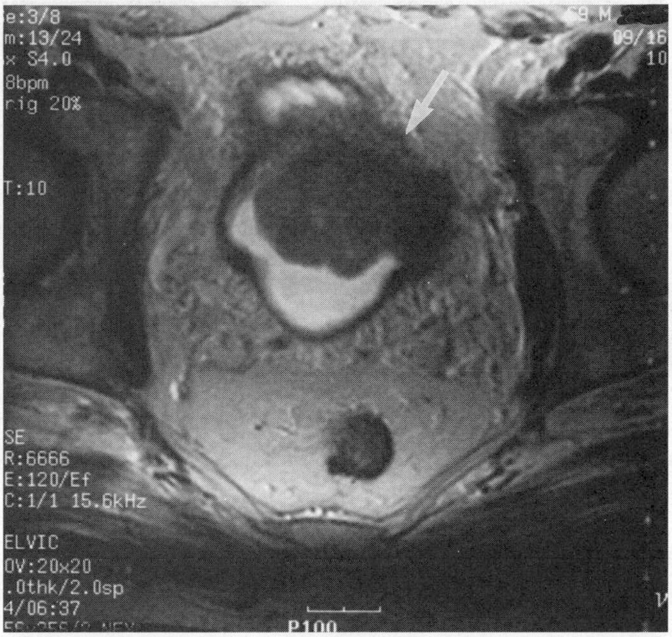

FIGURE 27.2-11. Bladder cancer. T2-weighted image of the base of the bladder shows a large mass (*arrow*) primarily within the bladder. There is a high degree of contrast between the fluid in the bladder, which is bright, and the darker surrounding cancer. The margins of the bladder are obscured at the 12-o'clock to 3-o'clock position, indicating extension of cancer into the perivesical fat.

BLADDER

The use of dynamic imaging after the administration of gadolinium has improved the evaluation of bladder carcinoma with MRI. The tumor usually enhances prior to enhancement of the remainder of normal bladder wall after contrast administration. MRI is the most accurate imaging modality for staging bladder carcinoma and has superior ability to detect perivesical spread and to assess the penetration of tumor through the deep muscle layers of the bladder (Fig. 27.2-11).[51] Precise staging is critical to the selection of the therapy most appropriate for bladder cancer. Recent studies have demonstrated MRI staging accuracy of 84% to 93%.[52,53] A challenge for MRI has been the differentiation between postbiopsy or irradiation changes and tumor. However, the use of dynamic, fast gradient-echo sequences has recently improved the ability of MRI to make this distinction.[54]

MUSCULOSKELETAL SYSTEM

Plain film, MRI, and nuclear medicine play complementary roles in the evaluation of bone tumors. When a bone tumor is suspected, plain film is the initial study to show the lesion and its origin, location, morphology, and aggressivity. After plain film, if the lesion may be something other than an inactive asymptomatic benign tumor, MRI can confirm the initial plain-film findings and add additional diagnostic information. In known malignant lesions, MRI is the best study to determine accurate tumor localization and staging,[55] which is critical to optimizing the success of limb salvage techniques and other surgery. MRI can accurately determine the intraosseous extent of lesions, as bone marrow demonstrates high contrast with tumor. MRI can delineate tumor from adjacent fascia and muscle. "Skip" lesions, which can occur with osteosarcomas, can be detected with sagittal and coronal views that image long bones in their entirety. The detection of neurovascular bundle involvement and the determination of lesion distance from the joint are also MRI capabilities useful in surgical planning. MRI can show the response of tumor to adjuvant chemotherapy prior to resection and can detect residual or recurrent tumor after resection. T1-weighted images are very accurate for detecting metastatic lesions within the marrow compartment (Fig. 27.2-12). Hence, MRI is indicated in symptomatic patients with suspected bony metastases or positive bone scans but with negative or inconclusive plain films. MRI is also extremely sensitive in detecting marrow replacement by myeloma, leukemia, or lymphoma on T1-weighted images and can differentiate these lesions from osteoporosis.[56] MRI is, however, similar to CT in that it is generally nonspecific in determining tumor cell type. A common pitfall of MRI is that it is possible for some bony lesions to appear benign when, in actuality, the lesion represents a high-grade malignancy. This is particularly true in patients older than 40, in whom even benign-appearing lesions commonly represent metastases or myeloma.[57] In younger patients, however, lesion morphology correlates in a very rough sense with its malignancy potential, though MRI still at times over- or underestimates tumor malignancy.

Owing to excellent soft tissue contrast, MRI displays outstanding anatomic detail of soft tissue lesions and is, therefore, the imaging modality of choice for evaluating soft tissue tumors.[55] Plain films, however, should still be additionally obtained. MRI is diagnostic of several common benign tumors, including lipomas (Fig. 27.2-13), ganglion cysts, some hemangiomas, and simple neurofibromas.[58] There is some debate about whether MRI can consistently distinguish lipoma from liposarcoma.[59,60] In general, a thin-rimmed homogeneous high signal on T2-weighted images may represent a simple cyst. Het-

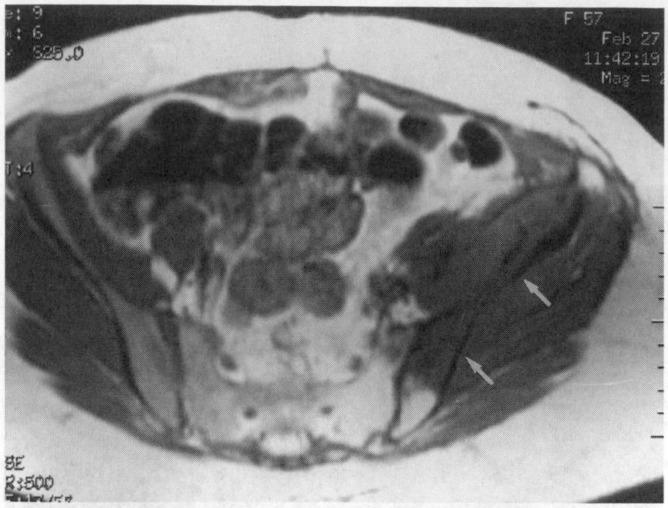

FIGURE 27.2-12. Bone metastasis. This patient had a primary leiomyosarcoma in the abdomen and presented with pelvic pain. T1-weighted magnetic resonance images show a large lesion (*arrows*) involving the left iliac bone as well as extension to the adjacent iliacus and gluteal muscles. The extent of bone involvement is precisely delineated on the magnetic resonance images. T1-weighted images are extremely sensitive for bone metastasis in adult patients and are frequently used in conjunction with nuclear medicine bone scan to determine precisely the extent and location of metastatic bone lesions. Magnetic resonance imaging is particularly useful in the pelvis, where overlapping structures can render diagnosis on plain radiographs difficult.

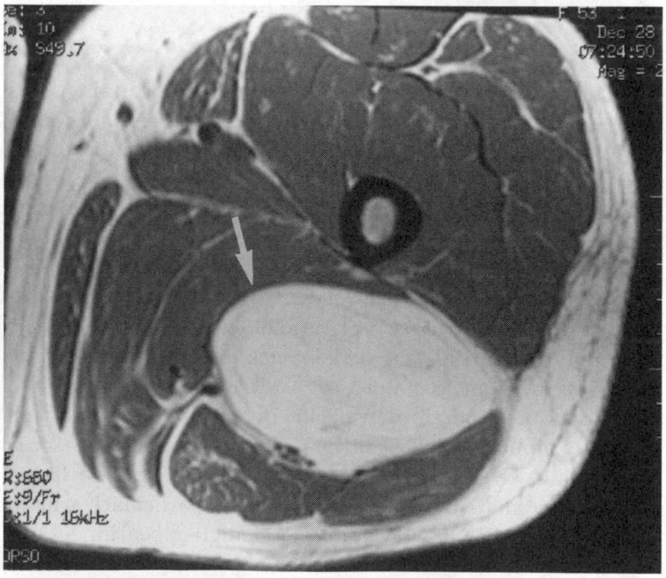

FIGURE 27.2-13. Lipoma of the posterior thigh. This patient felt an enlarging mass in the thigh, which was palpable on clinical examination. Magnetic resonance imaging examination showed a high-signal-intensity mass (*arrow*) on this T1-weighted image. The appearance on magnetic resonance imaging is chemically specific for lipoma due to the presence of macroscopic fat. In the case of a characteristic soft tissue mass, such as lipoma, a biopsy is not necessary for diagnosis, given the magnetic resonance imaging findings.

erogeneous high internal signal on T2-weighted images may indicate a solid lesion with high water or mucin content, a complex thick-walled lesion, calcification, necrosis, or hemorrhage, all of which can be associated with malignancy. MRI can be indeterminate in many of these cases, and MRI is helpful in determining the need for biopsy in suspicious-appearing lesions. In cases of known sarcoma, MRI is the best imaging modality to stage the mass accurately, determining its location relative to fascial planes and muscular structures, invasion into neurovascular or osseous tissues, and the distance of lesions from joints.[55] It is possible for some high-grade sarcomas, however, to display a nonaggressive, benign appearance.

REFERENCES

1. Goldsher D, Litt AW, Pino RS, et al. Dural "tail" associated with meningiomas on Gd-DTPA-enhanced MR images: characteristics, differential diagnostic value and possible implications of treatment. *Radiology* 1990;176:547.
2. Yokoi K, Kaniya N, Matsuguma H, et al. Detection of brain metastasis in potentially operable non-small cell lung cancer: a comparison of CT and MRI. *Chest* 1999;115:714.
3. Sherman JL. Evaluation of the postoperative brain. In: Bradley WG, Muroff LR, eds. *MRI of brain tumors and tumor mimics.* Tampa: Gilham Press, 1994:14.
4. Forsting M, Albert F, Kunze S, et al. Extirpation of glioblastoma: MR and CT follow up of residual tumor and regrowth patterns. *Am J Neuroradiol* 1993;14:77.
5. Shwartz RB, Carvalho PA, Alexander E, et al. Radiation necrosis versus recurrent glioma: dual isotope SPECT. *Am J Neuroradiol* 1991;12:1187.
6. Carmody R, Yang P, Seeley GW, et al. Spinal cord compression due to metastatic disease: diagnosis with MR imaging versus myelography. *Radiology* 1989;173:225.
7. Som PM, Shapiro MD, Biller HF, et al. Sinonasal tumors and inflammatory tissues: differentiation with MR imaging. *Radiology* 1988;167:803.
8. Chow JM, Leonetti JP, Matee MF. Epithelial tumors of the paranasal sinus and nasal cavity. *Radiol Clin North Am* 1993;31(1):61.
9. Tenesi L, Lufkin RB, Vimela F, et al. MR imaging of the nasopharynx and floor of the middle crania fossa: II. Malignant tumors. *Radiology* 1987;164:817.
10. Casselman JW, Mancuso AA. Major salivary gland masses: comparison of MR imaging and CT. *Radiology* 1987;165:183.
11. Castelijns JA, Geritsen GJ, Kaiser MC, et al. MRI of normal or cancerous laryngeal cartilages: histopathological correlation. *Laryngoscope* 1987;97:1085.
12. Harms SE, Flamig DP, Hesley KL, et al. MR imaging of the breast with rotating delivery of excitation off resonance: clinical experience with pathologic correlation. *Radiology* 1993;187:493.
13. Kacl GM, Liu P, Debatin JF, et al. Detection of breast cancer with conventional mammography and contrast enhanced MRI. *Eur Radiol* 1998;8:194.
14. Heywang-Kobrunner SH, Viehweg P, Heinry A, et al. Contrast-enhanced MRI of the breast: accuracy, values, controversies, solutions. *Eur J Radiol* 1997;24:94.
15. Schorn C, Fischer U, Luftner-Nagel S, et al. MRI of the breast in patients with metastatic disease of unknown primary. *Eur Radiol* 1999;9:470.
16. Harms SE, Flamig DP, Evans WP, et al. MR imaging of the breast: current status and future potential. *AJR Am J Roentgenol* 1994:163:1039.
17. Esserman L, Hylton N, Yassa L, et al. Utility of MRI in the management of breast cancer: evidence for improved preoperative staging. *J Clin Oncol* 1999;17:110.
18. Tan JE, Orel SG, Schnall MD, et al. Role of MRI and MRI-guided surgery in the evaluation of patients with early stage breast cancer for breast conservation treatment. *Am J Clin Oncol* 1999;22:414.
19. Tsuboi N, Ogawa Y, Inomata T, et al. Changes in the findings of dynamic MRI by preoperative CAF chemo for patients with breast cancer of stage II and III: pathologic correlation. *Oncol Rep* 1999;6:727.
20. Harms SE. Breast magnetic imaging. *Semin Ultrasound CT MR* 1998;19(1):104.
21. Soderstrom CE, Harms SE, Farrell RS, et al. Three-dimensional RODEO breast MRI of lesions containing ductal carcinoma in situ. *Radiology* 1996;20:427.
22. Heywang-Kobrunner SH, Shlegel A, Beck R, et al. Contrast-enhanced MRI of the breast after limited surgery and radiation therapy. *J Comput Assist Tomogr* 1993;17(6):891.
23. Viehweg P, Hernig A, Lampe D, et al. Retrospective analysis for evaluation of the value of CE-MRI in patients treated with breast conservative treatment. *Magma* 1998;7:141.
24. Choi BI, Lee GK, Kim ST, et al. Mosaic pattern of encapsulated hepatocellular carcinoma: correlation of MRI and pathology. *Gastrointest Radiol* 1990;15:238.
25. Mitchell DG, Plazzo J, Hann HYL, et al. Hepatocellular tumors with high signal on T_1-weighted MR images: chemical shift MRI and histologic correlation. *J Comput Assist Tomogr* 1991;15;762.
26. Ros PR, Freeny PC, Harms SE, et al. Hepatic MR imaging with ferrumoxides: a multicenter clinical trial of the safety and efficacy in the detection of local hepatic lesions. *Radiology* 1995;196:481.
27. MacFarland EG, Mayo-Smith WW, Saini S, et al. Hepatic hemangiomas and malignant tumors: improved differentiation with heavily T_2-weighted conventional spin echo MR imaging. *Radiology* 1994;193:43.
28. Schwartz LH, Panicek PM, Koutcher J, et al. Adrenal masses in patients with malignancy: a prospective comparison of echo-planar fast spin echo and chemical shift MR imaging. *Radiology* 1995;197:421.
29. Zagoria RJ, Bechtold RE. The role of imaging in staging renal adenocarcinoma. *Semin Ultrasound CT MR* 1997;18(2):91.
30. Kallman DA, King BF, Hattery RR, et al. Renal vein and inferior vena cava tumor thrombus in renal cell carcinoma: CT, US, MRI and vena cavography. *J Comput Assist Tomogr* 1992;16:240.
31. Zagoria RJ, Wolfman NT, Karstaedt N, et al. CT features of renal cell carcinoma with emphasis on relation to tumor size. *Invest Radiol* 1990;25:261.

32. Hricak H, Rubenstein LV, Gherman GM, et al. MRI evaluation of endometrial carcinoma: results of an NCI cooperative study. *Radiology* 1991;179:829.
33. Sironi S, Taccagni GL, Gorancini P, et al. Myometrial invasion by endometrial carcinoma: assessment by MRI. *AJR Am J Roentgenol* 1992;158:565.
34. Scoutt LM, McCarthy S, Long F, et al. Pitfalls in staging of endometrial cancer in MR imaging. *Radiology* 1992;185:183.
35. Hricak H, Stern JL, Fisher MR, et al. Endometrial carcinoma staging by MR imaging. *Radiology* 1987;162:297.
36. Subak LL, Hricak H, Powell CB, et al. Cervical carcinoma: computed tomography and MR imaging for preoperative staging. *Obstet Gynecol* 1995;86:43.
37. Togashi K, Morikawa K, Kataoka ML, Konishi J. Cervical cancer. *J Magn Reson Imaging* 1998;8:391.
38. Kim SH, Choi BI, Han JK, et al. Preoperative staging of uterine cervical carcinoma: comparison of CT and MRI in 99 patients. *J Comput Assist Tomogr* 1993;17:633.
39. Hricak H, Powell CB, Yu KK, et al. Invasive cervical carcinoma: role of MR imaging in pretreatment work-up: cost minimization and diagnostic efficacy analysis. *Radiology* 1996;198:403.
40. Outwater EK, Dunton CJ. Imaging of the ovary and adnexa: clinical issues and applications of MR imaging. *Radiology* 1995;194:1.
41. Stevens SK, Hricak H, Stern JL. Ovarian lesions: detection and characterization with gadolinium-enhanced MR imaging at 1.5 T. *Radiology* 1991;181:481.
42. Yamashita Y, Torashima M, Hatanaka K, et al. Adnexal masses: accuracy of characterization with transvaginal US and precontrast and postcontrast MR imaging. *Radiology* 1995;194:557.
43. Scoutt LM, McCarthy SM, Lange R, et al. MR evaluation of clinically suspected adnexal masses. *J Comput Assist Tomogr* 1994;18:609.
44. Prayer L, Kainz C, Kramer J, et al. CT and MR accuracy in the detection of tumor recurrence in patients treated for ovarian cancer. *J Comput Assist Tomogr* 1993;17:626
45. Yu KK, Hricak H, Alagappan R, et al. Detection of extracapsular extension of prostate carcinoma with endorectal and phased-array coil MR imaging: multivariate feature analysis. *Radiology* 1997;202:697.
46. Bates TS, Gillett DA, Cavanagh PM. A comparison of endorectal MRI and TRUS in the local staging of prostate cancer with histopathological correlation. *Br J Urol* 1997;79:927
47. Rifkin MD, Zerhouni EA, Gatsonis CA, et al. Comparison of magnetic resonance imaging and ultrasonography in staging early prostate cancer. *N Engl J Med* 1990;323:621.
48. Bezzi M, Kressel HY, Allen KS, et al. Prostate carcinoma: staging with MR imaging at 1.5 T. *Radiology* 1989;169:339.
49. Seltzer SE, Getty DJ, Tampany CMC, et al. Staging prostate cancer with MR imaging: a combined radiologist-computer system. *Radiology* 1997;202:219.
50. D'Amico A, Whittington R, Schnall M, et al. The impact of the inclusion of endorectal coil magnetic resonance imaging in a multivariate analysis to predict clinically unsuspected extraprostatic cancer. *Cancer* 1995;75:2368.
51. Tanimoto A, Yuasa Y, Imai Y, et al. Bladder tumor staging: comparison of conventional and gadolinium-enhanced dynamic MR imaging and CT. *Radiology* 1992;85:741.
52. Barentsz JO, Jager GJ, Mugler JP II, et al. Staging urinary bladder cancer: value of T_1-weighted 3D MP-Rage and 2D SE sequences. *AJR Am J Roentgenol* 1995;164:109.
53. Barentsz JO, Jager GJ, Van Vierzen PBJ, et al. Staging urinary bladder after transurethral biopsy: value of fast dynamic CE-MRI. *Radiology* 1996;201:185.
54. Barentsz JO, Jager GJ, Van Vierzen PBJ, et al. Staging urinary bladder cancer: value of fast dynamic contrast-enhanced MR imaging. *Radiology* 1996;201:185.
55. Ma LD. Magnetic resonance imaging of musculoskeletal tumors: skeletal and soft tissue masses. *Curr Probl Diagn Radiol* 1999;34.
56. Bobman SA, Riederer SJ, Lee JN, et al. Synthesized MR images: comparison with acquired images. *Radiology* 1985;155:731.
57. Ma LD, Frassica FJ, Scott WW, et al. Differentiation of benign and malignant musculoskeletal tumors: potential pitfalls with MR imaging. *Radiographics* 1995;15:349.
58. Van Slyke MA, Moser RP, Madewell JE. MR imaging of periarticular soft tissue lesions in musculoskeletal soft tissue imaging. *Magn Reson Imaging Clin N Am* 1995;3:651.
59. Haggar AM, Froelich JW. MR imaging strategies in primary and metastatic malignancy. *Radiol Clin North Am* 1998;26:689.
60. Bolen JW Jr, Delange EE, Frierson HF Jr. Infiltrating angiolipoma of skeletal muscle: MR findings. *J Comput Assist Tomogr* 1988;12:681.

SECTION **3**

MARTIN G. POMPER

Functional and Metabolic Imaging

Unique to functional imaging is the provision of unperturbed physiologic information. While pathologists increasingly apply the highly sensitive and accurate techniques of molecular biology to histologic examination, those techniques, when applied to functional imaging, promise even more relevant and timely data. Together with advances in molecular biology, advances in the generation of new imaging agents and in imaging science compel us to rethink cancer diagnosis and treatment. Soon, cancer patients will no longer be categorized according to the primary organ involved; rather, their disease will be diagnosed and treated according to their predominant underlying genetic abnormality. In this fashion and in the spirit of molecular medicine (i.e., the idea that human disease proceeds from biochemical imbalance), the diagnosis and staging of cancer will be tailored to each patient. Tumor characterization will consequently become more accurate and treatment more effective.

The uses of functional imaging in current cancer practice include (1) detection of malignancy, particularly if the primary site is unknown; (2) differential diagnosis of lesions found on anatomic imaging studies; (3) tumor grading; (4) disease staging; (5) assessing for recurrence; and (6) therapeutic monitoring.[1] Table 27.3-1 lists metabolic processes amenable to measurement in humans by functional imaging. Only [^{18}F]fluorodeoxyglucose–positron emission tomography (FDG-PET) and proton magnetic resonance spectroscopy (MRS) are used in routine clinical practice for oncology. Optical imaging techniques are also being developed but have been applied to humans on a limited basis to date.

TECHNIQUES FOR FUNCTIONAL AND METABOLIC IMAGING

POSITRON EMISSION TOMOGRAPHY

Technical Considerations and Imaging Protocol

PET is the most sensitive functional imaging technique used in clinical practice, with the ability to quantify processes that occur at subnanomolar concentrations. Although its resolution is an order of magnitude inferior to that of magnetic resonance imaging (MRI), that obtained with current PET scanners approaches 4 mm. As with many other functional techniques, the initial application of PET was to the study of brain physiology and pathology.[2] PET relies on the detection of coincident photons that result from the annihilation of a positron and an electron.[3] Because the annihilation event occurs up to several millimeters away from the site of decay and the coincident photons do not separate at an angle of precisely 180 degrees, physical and geometric constraints limit the resolution of imaging with PET.[4] Nevertheless, neither clinical nor even high-resolution small-animal imaging systems have reached the resolution limit imposed by those constraints.[5] Radionuclides most commonly used include ^{11}C, ^{13}N, ^{15}O, and ^{18}F, all of which are isotopes of atoms that are found in molecules of biologic importance (^{11}C, ^{13}N, and ^{15}O) or that can be substituted without significant disruption of molecular structure (^{18}F). Because the physical half-lives of radionuclides for PET range from 2 minutes (^{15}O) to 110 minutes (^{18}F), a pre-

TABLE 27.3-1. Physiologic Processes Accessible in Humans by Functional and Metabolic Imaging

Physiologic Processes	*Methods*
Glucose metabolism	FDG-PET[a]
Blood flow or volume	[^{15}O]H_2O-PET, perfusion MRI
Tissue oxygenation	Nitroimidazole-PET, fMRI
Tissue pH	^{31}P-MRS
Protein synthesis	Amino acid–PET
Cell proliferation (mitotic rate)	Thymidine-PET
Receptor concentration or occupancy	PET
Enzyme kinetics	PET
Endogenous metabolite concentration	MRS(I)[a]
Water diffusion	DWI
Tissue anisotropy	DTI
Drug pharmacokinetics/dynamics	PET, MRS
Vascular permeability	Dynamic MR

DTI, diffusion tensor imaging; DWI, diffusion-weighted MR imaging; FDG, [^{18}F]fluorodeoxyglucose; fMRI, functional magnetic resonance imaging; MR, magnetic resonance; MRS(I), magnetic resonance spectroscopy–spectroscopic imaging; PET, positron emission tomography.
[a]Technique used routinely in clinical practice for oncology.

mium is placed on synthetic efficiency. Images are generally reconstructed using algorithms, such as filtered back-projection. PET imaging is performed increasingly frequently on dual-head coincidence (DHC) gamma cameras.[6] Although FDG-DHC imaging is less expensive than is dedicated FDG-PET, the resolution of the former system is lower (13.5 mm vs. 4 mm), suggesting that FDG-DHC not be recommended for detection of lesions less than 1.5 cm in size.

FDG is the mainstay of PET oncologic imaging. As with all radiopharmaceuticals, distribution of FDG throughout the body obeys the tracer principle: It is administered in such small amounts (<10 μg) that while portraying the pathway of interest, it leaves that pathway completely intact. There is no pharmacologic or toxic effect. Neoplastic cells undergo accelerated glycolysis, even under aerobic conditions, a phenomenon known as the *Warburg effect*.[7] That metabolic difference between normal and cancer cells is exploited in FDG-PET imaging. Increased levels of glucose transporters and hexokinase and decreased levels of glucose-6-phosphatase contribute to the relatively increased glucose metabolism of cancer cells.[8] Unlike glucose, because FDG lacks a hydroxyl group at the 2 position, it cannot undergo further metabolism (phosphorylation) and remains trapped within the cell.

Because glucose competes with FDG for glucose transporters and hexokinase, elevated blood glucose levels tend to decrease FDG uptake.[9] Patients are fasted for 4 hours before intravenous administration of FDG (370 MBq, 10 mCi) and for 12 hours to reduce interfering myocardial uptake when searching for mediastinal adenopathy. The study is not performed if blood glucose levels exceed 200 mg/dL. Careful measurement and titration of blood glucose levels with insulin are unnecessary and may actually confound the study, owing to propagation of errors in blood glucose measurement.[10] Patients are scanned approximately 1 hour after FDG administration.

Deep organs may experience a 50-fold attenuation in photon detection relative to those at the surface.[11] Transmission scans using a ^{68}Ge source are accordingly performed to account for such geometric distortions. Transmission scans are time-consuming, particularly for whole body imaging that requires 10 gantry positions (for a 15-cm axial field-of-view scanner), each in turn requiring an 8- to 10-minute transmission scan. Transmission scans are not generally obtained for whole body imaging, and their use is controversial. Nevertheless, attenuation correction is necessary for coregistration of PET images with other modalities and for application of semiquantitative measurements, such as the standard uptake value (SUV).[12] True quantification of FDG-PET data, including kinetic modeling and arterial blood sampling or other surrogate methods for determining the input function, is noted frequently in the recent literature.[13–15] For those reasons, attenuation correction will likely be applied increasingly to clinical imaging. Furthermore, acquiring postinjection transmission scans or using iterative reconstruction methods, such as ordered-subset expectation maximum,[16] on both the emission and transmission scans may save time.

An important issue in clinical PET imaging centers around the necessity of reporting quantitative information (i.e., regional glucose metabolic rate). Currently, PET images are interpreted in a fashion similar to that of other nuclear medicine studies (i.e., areas of increased radiopharmaceutical uptake are reported as abnormal, accounting for the known physiologic distribution of tracer). Along with its high sensitivity, the quantitative capabilities of PET are constantly showcased, but the latter are seldom used clinically, particularly in oncology. As suggested, truly quantitative data are difficult to acquire because tracer uptake reflects more than merely what can be seen and measured by the PET scanner. The images produced also depend on blood flow to the organ of interest, metabolism of the tracer, dispersion of the activity bolus, and the compartmental residence of the tracer (i.e., blood pool vs. target receptor vs. nonspecific binding). To uncover the true concentration of tracer in the region of interest (ROI) requires arterial blood from the patient, which is nontrivial to obtain. Quantitative PET techniques were originally developed for the brain, a homogeneous structure as compared to a tumor. Tissue heterogeneity renders quantification more challenging in tumors. Zasadny and Wahl[12] developed the SUV as somewhat of a compromise between the extremes of true quantification and visual inspection. The SUV is the activity in the lesion (expressed in milliCuries per milliliter) divided by the weight of the patient (in kilograms) and the dose of FDG (in milliCuries). Because of initial concerns over its inappropriate use, the SUV has been refined to account for lean body mass, since FDG distribution differs between fat and muscle.[17] Also, using the maximum intensity pixel, rather than the average value distributed throughout an ROI, and carefully accounting for the time after injection at which the ROI was analyzed, have improved use of the SUV as an objective, semiquantitive measurement. As long as a baseline study is obtained, quantitative PET data may not be necessary for therapeutic monitoring.[18]

Clinical Applications

FDG-PET is superior to anatomic imaging for a variety of tumors and indications (Table 27.3-2).[19–22] Notable is that PET

TABLE 27.3-2. Comparison of [^{18}F]Fluorodeoxyglucose–Positron Emission Tomography and Anatomic Techniques

	Positron Emission Tomography		*Anatomic*		
Tumor	Sensitivity (%)	Specificity (%)	Sensitivity (%)	Specificity (%)	*Study*
Brain (recurrence)	80 (73–86)	39 (22–56)	—	—	19
Lung (solitary nodule)	94 (90–100)	87 (83–90)	NPV[a] = 88 (82–100)	—	20
NSCLC (staging)	90 (76–100)	97 (86–100)	64 (47–81)	83 (56–96)	20
Colorectal (staging)	94 (90–100)	88 (67–100)	78 (69–86)	85 (58–100)	21
Breast (detection)	78 (61–92)	92 (86–97)	—	—	20
Breast (staging)	92 (57–100)	82 (66-100)	—	—	22
Head and neck (staging)	71 (50–90)	99 (94–99)	63 (40–82)	79 (25–100)	20
Head and neck (recurrence)	92 (80–100)	81 (64–100)	52 (25–73)	89 (75–100)	20
Melanoma (staging)	94 (85–100)	93 (83–100)	66 (55–85)	69 (45–84)	21
Pancreas (detection)	88 (85–92)	82 (77–85)	NPV[a] = 74 (71–76)	—	20, 22

NSCLC, non–small cell lung cancer.
[a]Negative predictive value, rather than sensitivity, is given.
Notes: Anatomic techniques are magnetic resonance imaging or computed tomography (or both). Data represent averages and ranges of studies that appear in the literature after 1995 and include studies that constitute more than ten patients.

can identify metastatic deposits in lymph nodes that are still small (<1 cm) and considered benign by computed tomography (CT). In contrast, PET may recognize large masses, such as posttherapy fibrotic tissue, as benign if minimal FDG uptake is demonstrated. The most serious limitation to tumor detection with PET is that increased FDG uptake can also be demonstrated in inflammatory tissue.[23] In areas endemic to fungal infections of the lung, the specificity of PET for detecting malignancy is decreased.[24]

PET has proved capable of differentiating high- and low-grade brain tumors, of assessing prognosis in patients with brain tumors, and may be useful in guiding stereotactic brain biopsy.[25] PET may be used in therapeutic monitoring after chemotherapy or radiotherapy, with a classic indication being assessment for recurrent tumor versus radiation necrosis.[19] Conventional imaging cannot differentiate recurrent tumor from radiation necrosis. Although the specificity for PET in this regard may seem unacceptably low (see Table 27.3-2), an earlier report indicated a sensitivity of 94%.[26] Combining PET with MR techniques, such as perfusion-weighted imaging and magnetic resonance spectroscopy–spectroscopic imaging [MRS(I)], will likely improve the specificity of detecting recurrent brain tumors.

PET is the most accurate noninvasive technique for detecting and staging lung cancer (Fig. 27.3-1; see Table 27.3-2).[20] Accordingly, it was initially for lung cancer that PET was reimbursed.[22] Low background activity in the thorax renders the chest ideal for study, and visual analysis tends to be equivalent to calculating SUVs.[27] By improving staging, unnecessary thoracotomies, estimated at 30%, may be avoided.[28] The management of their disease is changed after whole body PET in 41% of patients with lung cancer.[27]

PET has changed surgical management in 28% of patients with colorectal cancer by identifying resectable or unresectable metastasis not identified on clinical examination or CT.[22] PET is of higher sensitivity (see Table 27.3-2) than is CT arterial portography (80% to 90%) in detecting intrahepatic metastases.[29]

PET has not proved as useful for breast cancer as for lung cancer, primarily owing to lower glucose utilization in the breast and background activity from concurrent mastopathy.[20] Although PET demonstrates the highest accuracy for axillary staging of breast cancer for any noninvasive test (see Table 27.3-2), node dissection is still required for planning adjuvant therapy.[20]

Anatomic complexity in the head and neck region, particularly after surgery, renders PET evaluation of this area a boon to therapeutic monitoring. Tumors as small as 4 mm have been detected in the head and neck with PET.[30] Detection and localization of head and neck tumors may be improved by applying SUVs and anatomic coregistration (Fig. 27.3-2), in part because significant amounts of FDG are distributed to the salivary glands and adenoids.[31] Care must be taken when applying PET after radiation therapy because of false-positive results due to inflammation and false-negative results due to metabolic “stunning” that might occur. Postirradiation PET is, therefore, recommended 40 days to 4 months or longer after therapy.[31,32]

PET has been successfully applied to detecting subclinical involvement of lymph nodes in melanoma (see Table 27.3-2).[20]

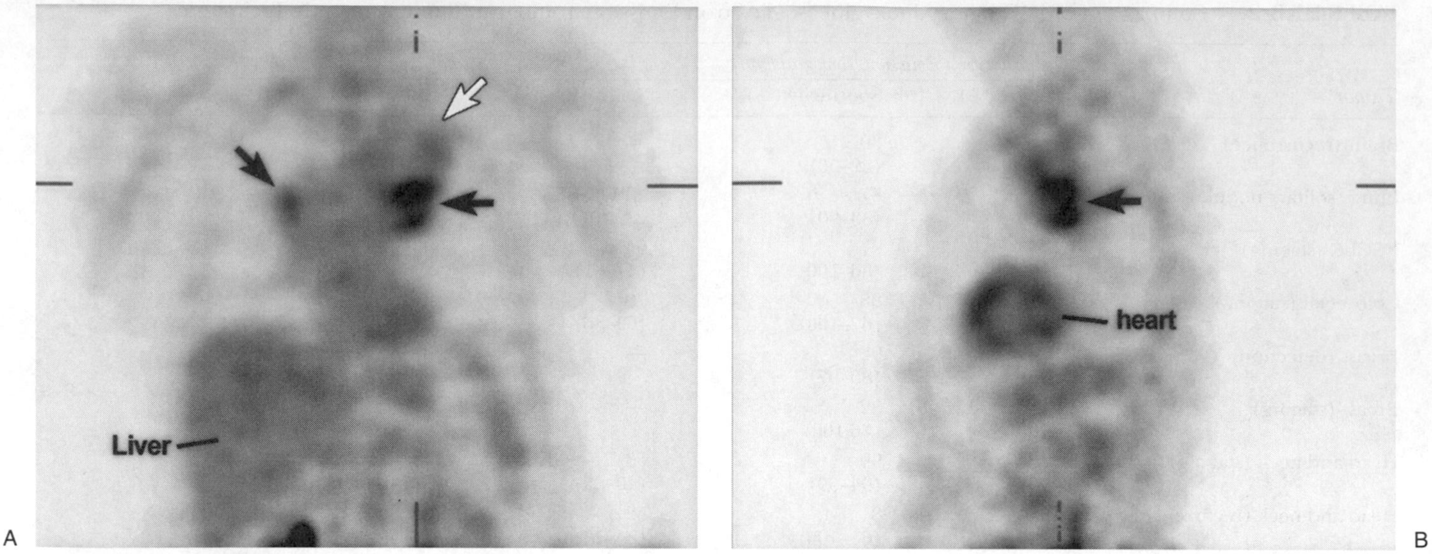

FIGURE 27.3-1. Coronal (**A**) and sagittal (**B**) whole body [18F]fluorodeoxyglucose–positron emission tomography images in a patient with lung cancer and left upper lobe atelectasis (*white arrow* in **A**). The patient was originally thought to have had left hilar and left apical lung masses on CT and was to undergo radiation therapy to the left upper lobe and mediastinum; however, subsequent [18F]fluorodeoxyglucose–positron emission tomography confirmed absence of tumor in the left apex and detected a metastasis in the right mediastinum (*diagonal arrow* in **A**). Horizontal arrows in **A** and **B** depict the left hilar masses. After positron emission tomography, the patient was treated with a different radiation port that spared the left apex but included the left and right mediastinum. (Courtesy of Richard L. Wahl, M.D., Ann Arbor, MI.)

It has proved somewhat less fruitful when applied to pancreatic cancer, likely owing to the presence of concurrent inflammation and high blood glucose levels; however, correction for serum glucose did not significantly improve the accuracy of PET in several studies.[22] PET was more accurate than CT for pancreatic cancer, and surgical management was altered in 43% of cases when PET and CT were used together.[33] PET has also proved useful, even superior to gallium imaging, in staging lymphoma and detecting residual disease after therapy.[20] PET may be useful to evaluate adjuvant therapy in osteosarcoma[34] and in assessing prognosis in malignant pleural mesothelioma.[35] It has proved less useful for genitourinary cancers, primarily because of high background activity in the bladder.[20] Nevertheless, recent applications of PET to cervical and prostate cancers, primarily for detecting local disease recurrence (cervix) and for staging (prostate), show promise.[36,37]

Tracers Other Than FDG

As stated, FDG has limitations. Its tissue uptake may be dictated by factors other than viable tumor cell fraction, such as degree of hypoxia,[38] inflammation,[23] and recent therapy.[32] High FDG levels in cerebral cortex can cloak tumors and metastases. Processes germane to cancer other than glucose uptake (e.g., blood flow, proliferation rate, protein synthesis rate, or tissue oxygenation) may be sought, as they may have prognostic and therapeutic implications as well. For those reasons, new tracers have been developed and include radiolabeled amino acid analogs,[20,39–41] thymidine analogs,[42,43] markers of tissue oxygenation (imidazoles and thiosemicarbazones),[44–46] substrates for multidrug resistance efflux pumps,[47] and such metabolites as choline[48] and acetate.[49] Radiolabeled analogs of chemotherapeutic agents, such as [18F]fluorouracil, have been synthesized to assess for their pharmacokinetics and metabolism. The concentration of [18F]fluorouracil in metastatic colorectal cancer correlated with patient survival.[50] Sex steroid receptor–based imaging agents enable measurement of estrogen receptor status *in vivo* and may be useful in therapeutic monitoring of certain subtypes of breast and prostate cancers.[43]

Among the amino acid analogs, [11C]methionine (MET) and [11C]tyrosine (TYR) have received the most attention. MET may be superior to FDG for brain tumor imaging, particularly for low-grade tumors, owing to minimal brain background activity.[51] Recent studies compared MET and FDG in a variety of tumors.[52–54] MET demonstrates a high negative predictive value (94%) for mediastinal node staging of lung cancer.[55] Because it undergoes less metabolism than MET, TYR may be used to measure protein synthesis rate and has been applied to head and neck cancers and soft tissue sarcomas.[31,56] For metastases due to head and neck cancer, TYR demonstrated higher specificity than FDG.

Developed in search of a noninvasive marker of tumor proliferation, carbon 11–labeled thymidine analogs, particularly those labeled at the 5-methyl moiety, undergo extensive, rapid metabolism, thereby prohibiting routine use.[43] More stable 18F-labeled analogs have been synthesized and have shown promise in an initial study (Fig. 27.3-3).[57]

Future Developments in Oncologic Positron Emission Tomography

Chemists have synthesized a vast array of selective, high-affinity radiopharmaceuticals in positron-emitting form; however, com-

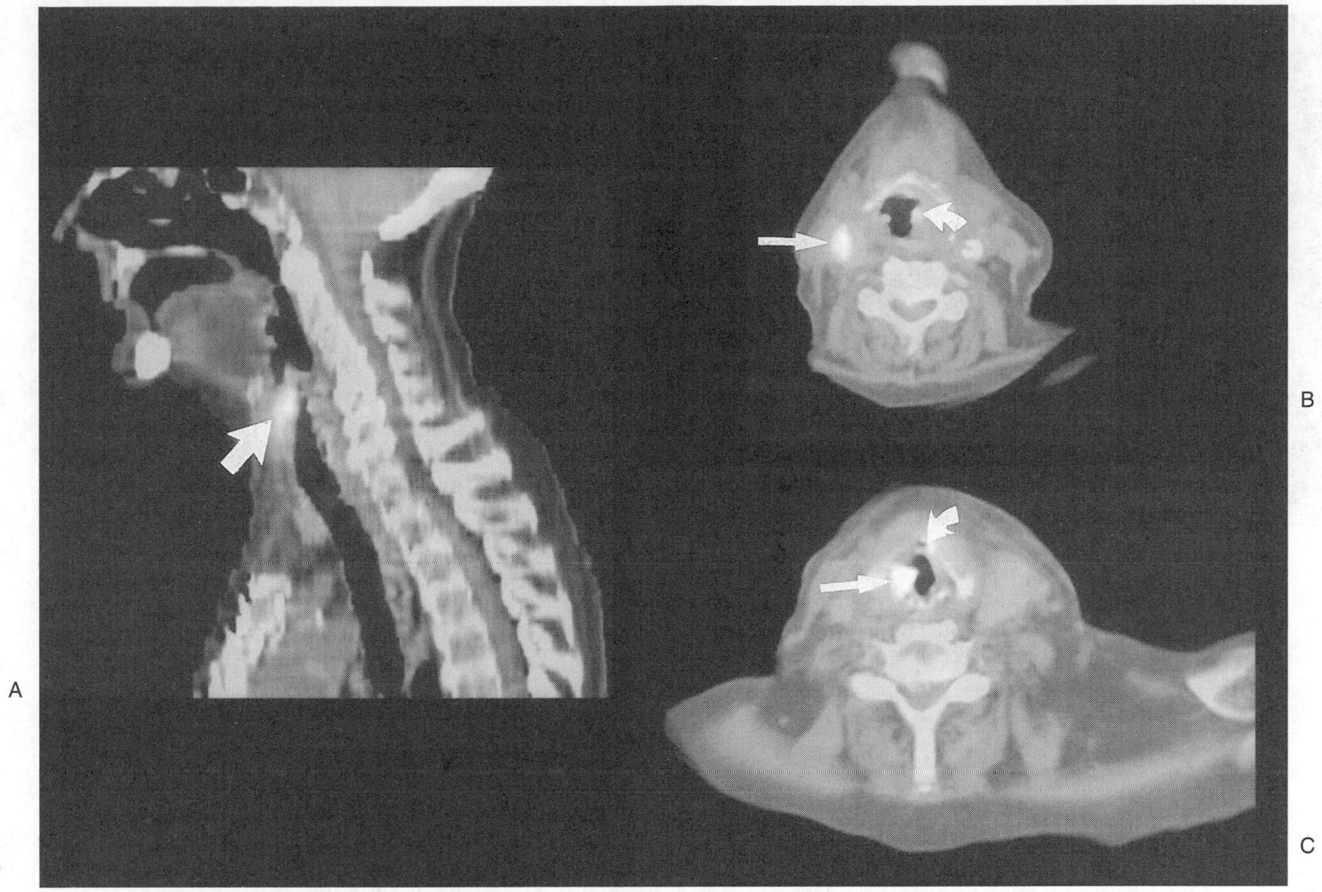

FIGURE 27.3-2. Positron emission tomography–computed tomography (PET-CT) images of a patient with head and neck cancer. CT: 160 mAs; 130 kV; pitch = 1.6; 5-mm slice thickness. PET: 7 mCi [^{18}F]fluorodeoxyglucose (FDG); 2 × 15 min; 3.4-mm slice thickness. False color (*yellow*) depicts the increased FDG uptake on PET. **A:** Sagittal image depicts increased FDG uptake in the anterior larynx (*arrow*). **B:** Axial image depicts increased FDG uptake in the right neck (*arrow*) due to adenopathy. Tumor is also present to a small extent in the left laryngeal mucosa (*curved arrow*). **C:** Axial image at the level of the true vocal cords shows tumor in the right larynx (*arrow*) and, to a lesser extent, in the midline involving thyroid cartilage (*curved arrow*). (See Color Fig. 27.3-2 in the CD-ROM and on the Web at www.LWWoncology.com.) (Courtesy of David Townsend, Ph.D., Pittsburgh, PA.)

binatorial chemistry and phage display libraries will generate even more promising lead molecules for oncologic imaging. More generalized use of old probes, such as [^{18}F]fluoroethylspiperone, may enable gene transcription imaging in tumors with a variety of genetic perturbations.[5] Based on a principle similar to imaging with FDG (i.e., metabolic trapping), radiolabeled herpes simplex virus (HSV) thymidine kinase substrates for imaging gene transfer and expression are nearing clinical trials.[58] Generator-produced PET radionuclides, such as ^{62}Cu, which can render PET available to imaging facilities without a cyclotron on site, have been incorporated into appropriate ligands and used for tumor imaging.[59] Improvements in whole body PET are being sought by performing three-dimensional acquisition, routine attenuation correction, and application of statistical, iterative methods to reconstruct imaging data. If PET is to reach its true potential in oncologic imaging (i.e., measuring genomic events), quantitative techniques developed over the last 15 years for brain imaging must be adapted to tumor imaging. Concurrent recent advances in other imaging modalities and in understanding the microenvironment of tumors (Fig. 27.3-4) are serving to demystify the heterogeneity problem and will facilitate quantitative PET for oncology in the future.

MAGNETIC RESONANCE IMAGING

MR-based techniques are less well established for functional imaging than are those based on PET.[60] They include diffusion-weighted imaging (DWI), perfusion or cerebral blood volume imaging, MRS(I), and functional MR imaging (fMRI). In many ways, those techniques complement PET and attempt to measure similar physiologic phenomena (see Table 27.3-1). Apart from the obvious advantages related to logistics (e.g., no need for synthesis of short-lived radiotracers or for an on-site cyclotron), the MR techniques benefit from not needing anatomic coregistration. The resolution of clinical MR is submillimeter, at least one order of magnitude superior to clinical PET. Quantification of the MR-based techniques is in its infancy, but

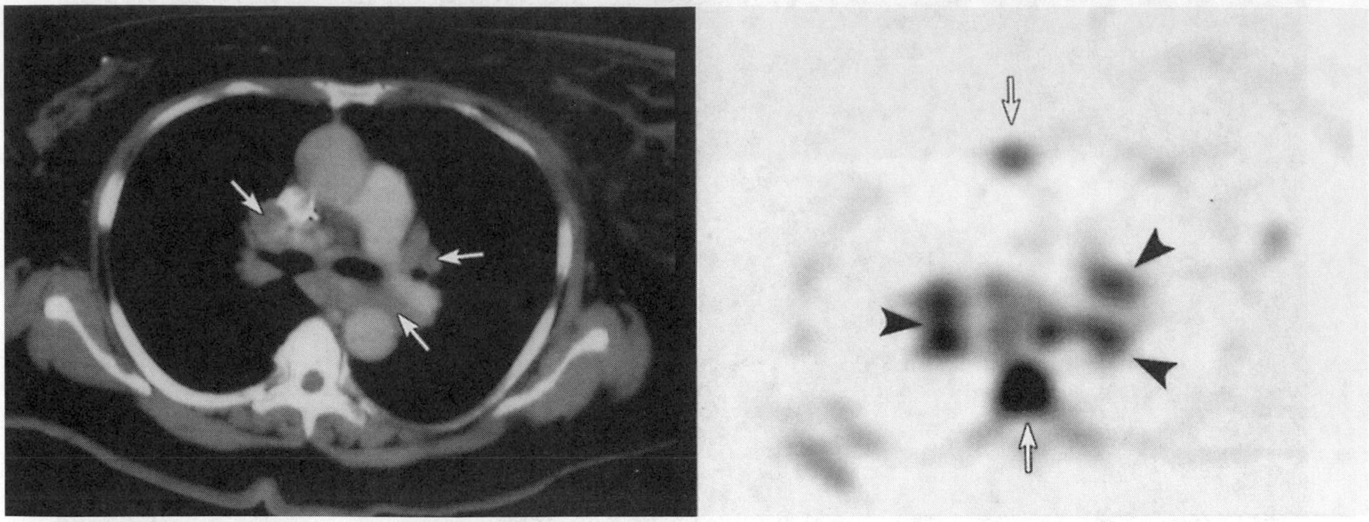

A B

FIGURE 27.3-3. Computed tomography (**A**) and 3'-deoxy-3'-[^{18}F]fluorothymidine–positron emission tomography (FLT-PET) (**B**) images in a patient with breast cancer metastatic to the mediastinal lymph nodes (*arrows* in **A**, *arrowheads* in **B**). The FLT-PET image was obtained 30 to 60 minutes after injection. FLT is retained in normal sternal and vertebral marrow (*top, bottom arrows*, respectively, in **B**) and ribs as well as within mediastinal tumor. (Courtesy of Anthony F. Shields, M.D., Detroit, MI.)

progress is being made, particularly in the assessment of blood flow[61] and metabolite concentrations.[62] As was the case for PET, the brain has been the primary organ of initial inquiry for MR-based techniques, and most of that work, except for MRS(I), has been dedicated to hemodynamics and stroke rather than cancer.

SPECIFIC MAGNETIC RESONANCE–BASED TECHNIQUES

MRS(I) is applied in medicine to determine the concentrations of a relatively few metabolites that are altered in disease.[63–66] In MRS(I), the high-resolution morphologic imaging capabilities of MRI are sacrificed to provide metabolic data that, in many cases, precede structural abnormality. Molecules containing a limited number of nuclei may be imaged, including ^{31}P, ^{23}Na, ^{19}F, and ^{1}H. Among those, ^{31}P-MRS and especially ^{1}H-MRS(I), or MRS(I) have found the most applications in oncology.

Early work focused on ^{31}P-MRS; however, owing to large volumes (voxels) required for analysis, reducing sensitivity, MRS(I) has been developed and used to a greater extent more recently. ^{31}P-MRS still finds applications in oncology because ^{31}P is incorporated into adenosine triphosphate, phosphocreatine, and pyridine dinucleotides (i.e., molecules that reflect tumor energetics). Intracellular tumor pH can be derived from ^{31}P-MRS spectra. Tumors have elevated phosphomonoesters and phosphodiesters. ^{31}P-MRS may find its greatest application in therapeutic monitoring of soft tissue sarcomas, where metabolite changes, which occur soon after the initiation of treatment, correlate with clinical response.[67] ^{31}P-MRS has also been used to detect non-Hodgkin's lymphoma,[68] to study liver metabolism in cancer patients,[69] and to follow up after therapy in patients with breast cancer.[70]

MRS(I) is the most commonly used MR spectroscopic technique because of the high natural abundance of protons. Key metabolites include choline and lactate, which tend to be elevated in tumors. Choline is a membrane constituent, its increase hypothesized to be due to increased cell membrane synthesis in rapidly proliferating tissue. Lactate is generally present only in pathologic tissue, such as necrotic tumors and abscesses, and reflects abnormal carbohydrate metabolism. Preoperative diagnosis and grading are the goals of brain tumor MRS(I); however, MRS(I) currently is best at merely differentiating normal from malignant tissue. Preul et al.[71] obtained remarkable success in grading gliomas by using pattern-recognition analysis rather than simply peak ratios.[71] Nevertheless, that technique is rather sophisticated mathematically and not widely available. MRS(I) is becoming useful in therapeutic monitoring, challenging PET for diagnosis of recurrent tumor versus radiation necrosis in patients with gliomas.[72,73] One recent study showed no false-positive results when using MRS(I) to assess for radiation injury (Fig. 27.3-5).[74] MRS(I) has more recently been applied to head and neck,[75] breast,[76,77] and prostate[78–80] cancers (Fig. 27.3-6). Each of those tumor types displays increased choline that, in the case of head and neck tumors,[75] reflects tissue oxygenation status. Cystic ovarian tumors demonstrated higher levels of lactate and amino acids than their benign counterparts.[81] The high-resolution, multivoxel capabilities of MRS(I) are important in prostate tumor assessment, because the lesions tend to be small and their precise intraglandular location has important therapeutic implications. Difficulty in suppression of lipid peaks outside of the ROI and in shimming continue to challenge extracranial MRS(I).

Clinical studies using ^{19}F-MRS have centered around studying the tumor pharmacokinetics of 5-fluorouracil analogs and

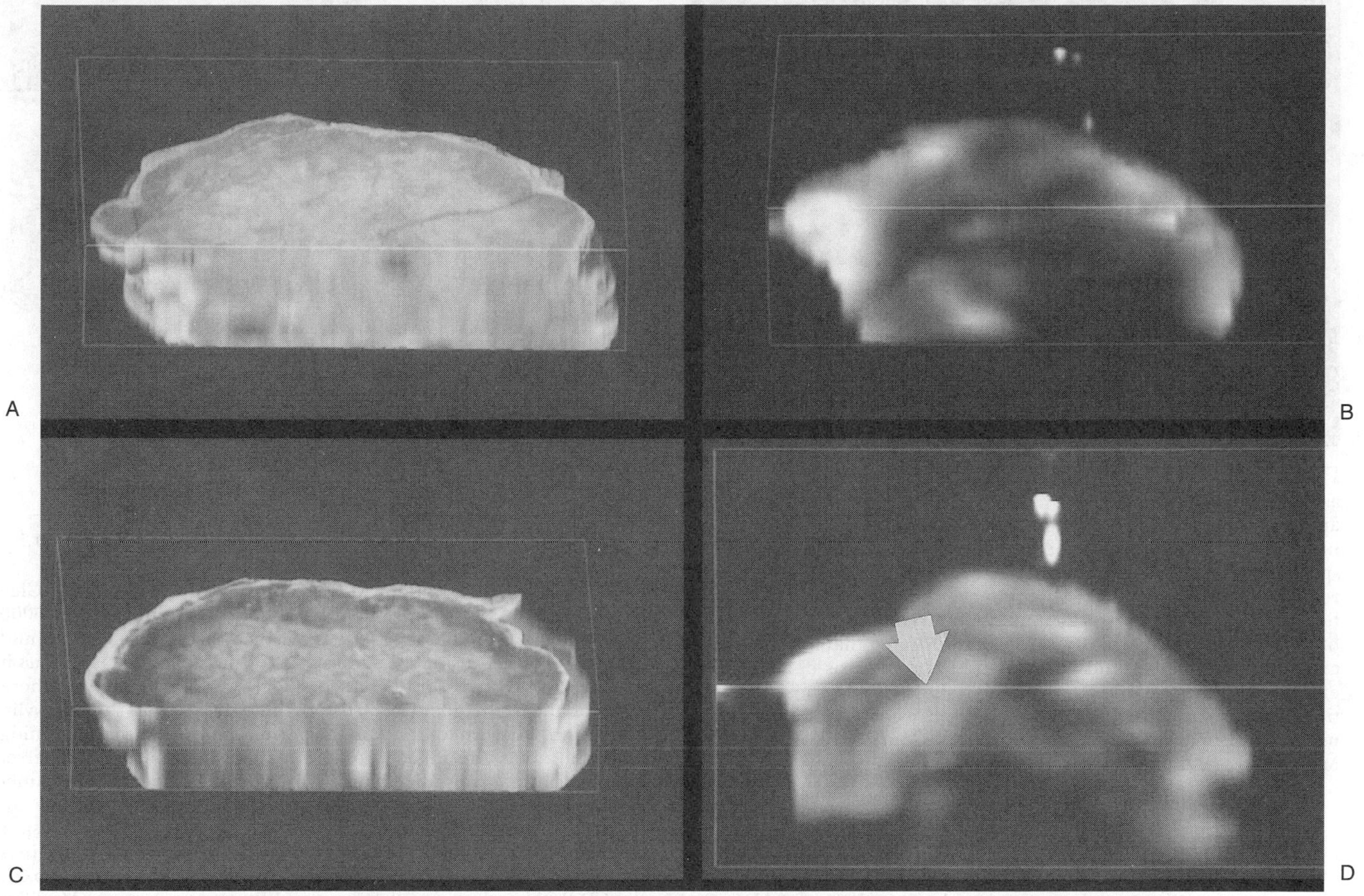

FIGURE 27.3-4. Multimodality, functional radiologic-pathologic correlation of the mammary tumor model MDA-MB-435 in the mammary fat pad of a severe combined immunodeficiency mouse. **A:** Hematoxylin-eosin stain shows a pink hue centrally indicative of dead and dying cells. **B:** Vascular volume map [snapshot–fast low-angle shot (FLASH) magnetic resonance image] with gadolinium-albumin contrast (40 mL/g) shows decreased volume centrally in the area of necrosis. **C:** Vascular endothelial growth factor (VEGF) map generated from polyclonal antibodies to VEGF depicts increased VEGF protein in areas of necrosis. VEGF is a potent modulator of vascular permeability. **D:** Vascular permeability map (snapshot-FLASH magnetic resonance image; 1.27 mL/g/min shows increased vascular permeability (*arrow*) where vascular volume is lowest (i.e., centrally). Such multimodality correlation enables better understanding of the tumor microenvironment. (See Color Figs. 27.3-4*A* and *C* in the CD-ROM and on the Web at www.LWWoncology.com.) (Courtesy of Dmitri Artemov, Ph.D., Meiyappan Solaiyappan, B.E., and Zaver M. Bhujwalla, Ph.D., Baltimore, MD.)

effects of other chemotherapeutic agents on 5-fluorouracil tumor uptake.[82] Those studies are performed with a view to individualizing chemotherapeutic regimens for specific patients. Several groups have used ^{23}Na imaging to characterize brain tumors,[83,84] with new pulse sequences and high-field systems contributing to furthering the sensitivity and resolution for this nucleus.[85]

DWI is among the triad of functional MRI techniques, a triad that also includes perfusion imaging and fMRI.[86,87] Water diffusion is a random event; however, certain structures, such as intracellular organelles and white matter tracts within the brain, may impede diffusion. Applying appropriate pulse sequences and magnetic field gradients, those differences in diffusion may be detected. Resembling free water, necrotic or cystic portions of brain tumors display high apparent diffusion constants (ADCs), while the solid (enhancing) portions have lower ADCs, demonstrating the ability of DWI to distinguish various portions of a single heterogeneous lesion.[88,89] Coupled with the high resolution of MR systems, that finding suggests that DWI may direct biopsies, an important function, as sampling errors now lead to approximately 25% of brain tumors being undergraded.[90] Huang et al.[91] used DWI in conjunction with MRS and perfusion imaging to assess the effects of intracarotid chemotherapy on brain tumors in patients with gliomas or primary central nervous system lymphoma, showing a normalization of ADC values after treatment. In the periphery, hemangiomas (high ADC) can be differentiated from hepatocellular carcinomas (low ADC) of the liver using a turbo-fast low-angle shot sequence with DWI.[92] That technique enabled differentiation of malignant (low-ADC) from benign (high-ADC) ovarian cysts.[93] Other fast MR techniques,

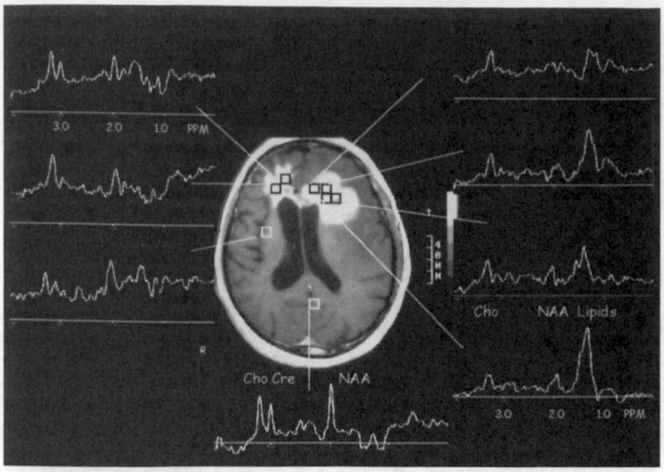

FIGURE 27.3-5. Patient with partial resection of a grade III astrocytoma in 1996 followed by radiotherapy (60 Gy) and chemotherapy. In February 1999, imaging showed a large butterfly-like enhancing mass on magnetic resonance imaging. Magnetic resonance spectroscopy–spectroscopic imaging [MRS(I)] [single slice point-resolved spectroscopy (PRESS) sequence; repetition time = 1500; echo time = 136; slice thickness = 20 mm, nominal resolution of 2 mL (field of view = 160 × 160; matrix 16 × 16)] demonstrated that the enhancing areas contained large lipid peaks; there were no areas of abnormally elevated choline within or outside the lesion. The diagnosis of radiation necrosis was made, and 1 year later, the lesion remained stable by magnetic resonance imaging and MRS(I). (Courtesy of Alberto Bizzi, M.D., Bologna, Italy.)

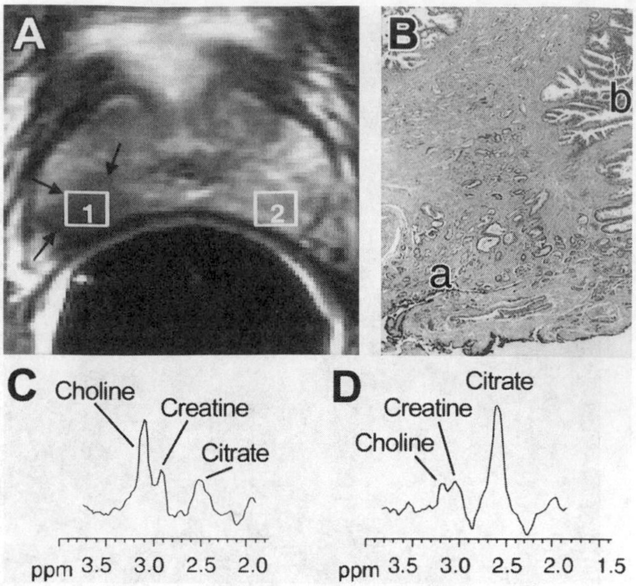

FIGURE 27.3-6. Patient with stage pT3a prostate cancer (Gleason score, 5). **A:** Fast spin-echo T2-weighted (repetition time = 5000; echo time = 102) axial magnetic resonance image through the mid-prostate obtained using an endorectal coil. A tumor focus (*arrows* in **A**) is seen as an area of decreased signal intensity in the peripheral zone of the right gland. **B:** Histopathologic section (hematoxylin-eosin stain) confirmed tumor in the peripheral zone of the right midgland that abuts the inked prostatic margin (a) and is interspersed between normal prostatic glands (b). **C:** 0.24-cm^3 spectrum obtained from area 1 in the image in **A** demonstrates elevated choline and reduced citrate, consistent with cancer. **D:** Magnetic resonance spectrum within the normal left peripheral zone, area 2 in the image in **A**, that shows dominant citrate, as expected. (See Color Fig. 27.3-6*A* in the CD-ROM and on the Web at www.LWWoncology.com.) (Modified from ref. 80, with permission.)

such as echo-planar imaging, are beginning to be applied to extracranial regions, further allowing the calculation of ADC values in abdominal organs.[94]

Once only a function of PET, perfusion imaging is now possible, in some cases quantitatively, with MRI.[95] Perfusion imaging enables calculation of blood volume, which is likely related to tumor angiogenesis, or new blood vessel formation (Fig. 27.3-7). Angiogenesis is a strong indicator of tumor grade.[96] Biopsy of tumor subregions with increased perfusion may prove superior to biopsy of regions of enhancement, the current practice. Areas of perfusion and enhancement often do not coincide, the latter being due to breakdown of the blood–brain barrier in the case of brain tumors. Extracranial studies using perfusion imaging are rare, although several studies of cervical cancer have appeared recently.[97–99] In the latter study, the cervical microcirculatory parameters determined with perfusion imaging did not always correlate with histology; however, they did correlate with patient outcome. Several groups have performed dynamic contrast-enhanced imaging of the breast[100] or prostate[101] in attempting to take advantage of the temporal signature of contrast uptake in tumors relative to neighboring tissue. Dynamic CT with Patlak analysis enabled measurement of perfusion in prostate tumors during therapy.[102]

fMRI detects signals based on the difference in blood oxygen tension that occurs between active and inactive brain regions (i.e., the blood oxygen level dependence effect).[103] Several centers are beginning to use fMRI for preoperative planning of brain tumors because eloquent, or essential, brain regions, such as motor cortex or language areas, may be mapped preoperatively and avoided during surgery for tumors and other lesions.[104,105] Similarly, the nonrandom orientation (anisotropy) of white matter tracts in the brain may be exploited by diffusion tensor imaging,[106] a variant of DWI, for preoperative planning. In diffusion tensor imaging, deep structures, such as the corticospinal tract, well beyond the domain of intraoperative cortical mapping, may be delineated and, consequently, avoided during tumor surgery.[107,108]

FUTURE DEVELOPMENTS IN ONCOLOGIC MAGNETIC RESONANCE IMAGING

In a preliminary study, Enochs et al.[109] used a contrast agent based on long-circulating superparamagnetic iron oxide particles to delineate brain tumors that may differentiate between tumor and postoperative scar tissue. "Smart" MR contrast agents, which may be activated only within the vicinity of an enzyme of interest, are being developed and may prove useful if issues related to pharmacokinetics and metabolism can be resolved.[110] Further application of echo-planar imaging and other rapid MR techniques may enable multiple MR studies [e.g., MRS(I) and perfusion imaging] to be performed within a single 1-hour clinical time slot, permitting collection of correlative data.

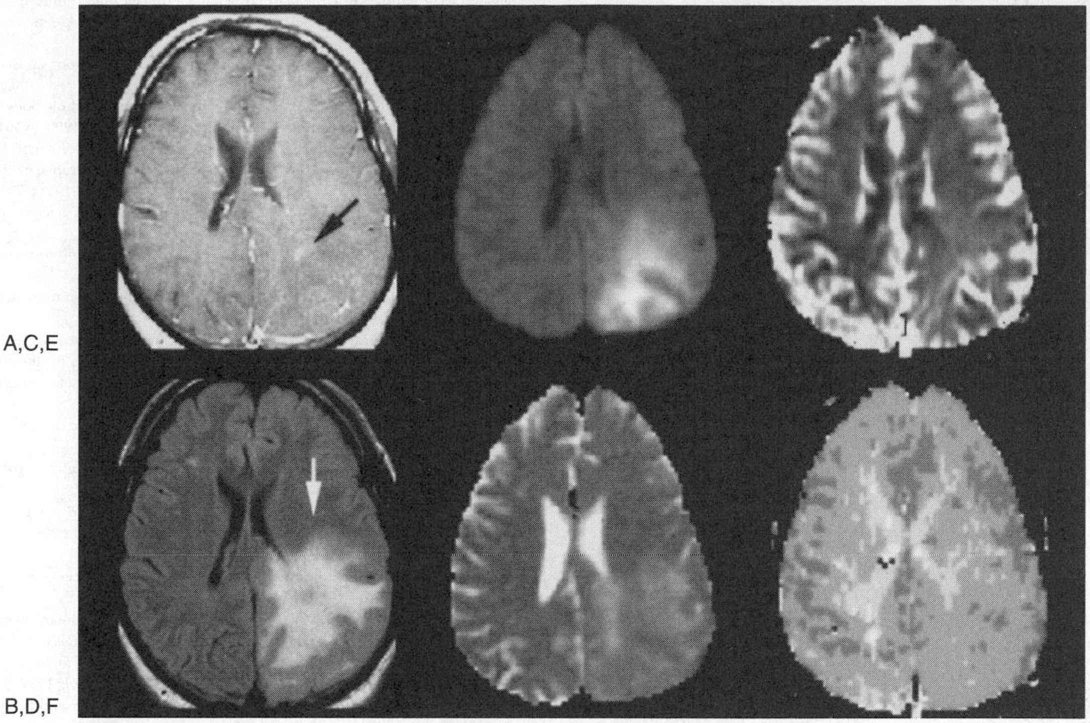

FIGURE 27.3-7. Patient with a left parietal glioma. Postgadolinium T1-weighted image (**A**) [repetition time (TR) = 415; echo time (TE) = 18] demonstrates minimal enhancement (*arrow*) in the left posterior parietal lobe, where a large region of high signal intensity is identified (**B**, *arrow*) on the fluid-attenuated inversion recovery (FLAIR) image [TR = 8800; TE = 130; inversion time(TI) = 2200]. The diffusion-weighted image (**C**) (TR = 9999; TE = 99; B = 1000), calculated apparent diffusion constants map (**D**), and cerebral blood volume perfusion image (**E**) all demonstrate increased signal in the region of the mass favoring the diagnosis of tumor. The time–to–peak perfusion image (**F**) shows delayed perfusion of the mass relative to the neighboring gray matter.

NEW FUNCTIONAL AND METABOLIC IMAGING MODALITIES

Optical imaging techniques are entering the clinical arena. Optical coherence tomography is already being applied to microsurgery[111,112] and cervical cancer[113] (Fig. 27.3-8). Rather than *functional* imaging, however, those techniques are more akin to ultrasonography, except that light is used to obtain the image. Optical coherence tomography may almost be considered a *cellular* imaging technique, owing to its exquisite resolution, approaching cellular dimensions (1 to 15 μm) and one to two orders of magnitude superior to conventional ultrasonography. It is expected to prove invaluable for directed biopsy, decreasing sampling errors.

Either endogenous or exogenous fluorophores may be used to detect fluorescence of malignant tissues. Inaguma and Hashimoto[114] recently applied the former to characterizing oral carcinomas, demonstrating that tumors vary in the amount of a porphyrin-like substance responsible for fluorescence.[114] Andersson-Engels et al.[115] used a porphyrin to delineate basal cell carcinomas. Schantz et al.[116] exploited the endogenous fluorescence of head and neck cancers and demonstrated a correlation between fluorescence maxima and tumor grade and likelihood of recurrence. Tromberg et al.[117] accomplished quantitative functional imaging of breast tumors using near-infrared light in conjunction with photon migration spectroscopy. Low-resolution (0.5- to 1-cm) images of tissue hemoglobin concentration, oxygen saturation, blood volume, and water and fat contents are capable with that technique.

Subtle differences in redox status, oxygenation, and intracellular pH separate normal and malignant tissues.[118] Redox status and oxygenation can be measured by electron paramagnetic resonance.[119] The detection of nitroxides, redox-sensitive probes, has been accomplished using electron paramagnetic resonance–enabled imaging of tumor heterogeneity in a rodent model, with clinical studies on the horizon.[118]

SUMMARY

The use and cost-effectiveness of PET are finally being recognized in the clinic.[120] The proliferation of satellite suppliers of FDG to sites that use DHC gamma cameras and reimbursement for an increasing number of indications may account for the anticipated 30% increase in PET[121] use over the next 5 years. MR techniques are largely replacing PET for indications other than receptor- or enzyme-based imaging (i.e., blood flow) and can provide important complementary information to PET. Recent initiatives of the National Cancer Institute pro-

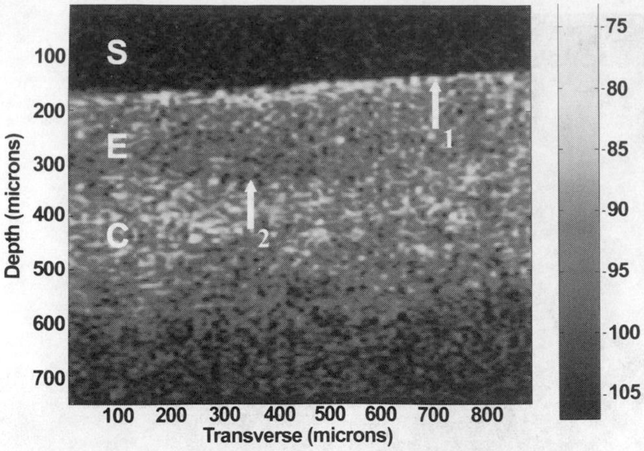

FIGURE 27.3-8. Optical coherence tomography (OCT) images were obtained from fresh tissue samples, within 5 minutes of excision by a loop electrosurgical excision procedure. Image acquisition time was 2.5 seconds. The instrument used delivers and collects 850-nm broadband light via an optical fiber probe that is placed in contact with the sample. Shown is a clinically normal site in the tissue sample. From the top down, the image shows a dark band corresponding to the quartz shield (S) of the optic fiber probe. Next, the surface of the sample is observed (1), followed by a layer of low-scattering epithelial tissue (E) 150 μm deep in this image. Immediately below, approximately 325 μm deep in the image, is the interface with a layer of highly scattering connective (C) tissue (2). This layer occupies the rest of the image, and the signal fades approximately 400 to 500 μm into the tissue. This technique may also be used to demonstrate the optical properties of tissue *in situ.* (See Color Fig. 27.3-8 in the CD-ROM and on the Web at www.LWWoncology.com.) (Courtesy of Rebecca Richards-Kortum, Ph.D., Austin, TX.)

mote the development of research projects and centers dedicated to functional and molecular imaging of cancer. Through synergism of technologic advances, interdisciplinary research, and public support, functional imaging will soon ensure the ultimate goal of the noninvasive characterization of cancer.

REFERENCES

1. Wagner HN. The future. *Semin Nucl Med* 1996;26:194.
2. Di Chiro G, DeLaPaz RL, Brooks RA, et al. Glucose utilization of cerebral gliomas measured by F-18 fluorodeoxyglucose and positron emission tomography. *Neurology* 1982;32:1323.
3. Chandra R. *Introductory physics of nuclear medicine.* Philadelphia: Lea & Febiger, 1992:185.
4. Budinger TF, Brennan KM, Moses WW, et al. Advances in positron tomography for oncology. *Nucl Med Biol* 1996;1996:659.
5. Gambhir SS, Herschman HR, Cherry SR, et al. Imaging transgene expression with radionuclide imaging technologies. *Neoplasia* 2000;2:118.
6. Patton JA, Turkington TG. Coincidence imaging with a dual-head scintillation camera. *J Nucl Med* 1999;40:432.
7. Dang CV, Semenza GL. Oncogenic alterations of metabolism. *Trends Biochem Sci* 1999;24:68.
8. Smith TAD. FDG uptake, tumour characteristics, and response to therapy: a review. *Nucl Med Commun* 1998;19:97.
9. Lindholm P, Minn H, Leskinen-Kallio S, et al. Influence of the blood glucose concentration on FDG uptake in cancer: a PET study. *J Nucl Med* 1993;34:1.
10. Weber WA, Ziegler SI, Thodtmann R, et al. Reproducibility of metabolic measurements in malignant tumors using FDG PET. *J Nucl Med* 1999;40:1771.
11. Wahl RL. To AC or not to AC: that is the question. *J Nucl Med* 1999;40:2025.
12. Zasadny KR, Wahl RL. Standardized uptake values of normal tissues at PET with 2-[fluorine-18]-fluoro-2-deoxy-D-glucose: variations with body weight and a method for correction. *Radiology* 1993;189:847.
13. Hays MT, Segall GM. A mathematical model for the distribution of fluorodeoxyglucose in humans. *J Nucl Med* 1999;40:1358.
14. Sugawara Y, Zasadny KR, Grossman HB, et al. Germ cell tumor: differentiation of viable tumor, mature teratoma and necrotic tissue with FDG PET and kinetic modeling. *Radiology* 1999;211:249.
15. Wahl LM, Asselin MC, Nahmias C. Regions of interest in the venous sinuses as input functions for quantitative PET. *J Nucl Med* 1999;40:1666.
16. Lonneux M, Borbath I, Bol A, et al. Attenuation correction in whole-body FDG oncological studies: the role of statistical reconstruction. *Eur J Nucl Med* 1999;26:591.
17. Keyes JW. SUV: standard uptake or silly useless value? *J Nucl Med* 1995;36:1836.
18. Hoh CK, Schiepers C, Seltzer MA, et al. PET in oncology: will it replace other modalities? *Semin Nucl Med* 1997;27:94.
19. Hustinx R, Alavi A. SPECT and PET imaging of brain tumors. *Neuroimaging Clin N Am* 1999;9:751.
20. Weber WA, Avril N, Schwaiger M. Relevance of positron emission tomography (PET) in oncology. *Strahlenther Onkol* 1999;175:356.
21. Delbeke D. Oncological applications of FDG PET imaging: brain tumors, colorectal cancer lymphoma and melanoma. *J Nucl Med* 1999;40:591.
22. Delbeke D. Oncological applications of FDG PET imaging. *J Nucl Med* 1999;40:1706.
23. Kubota R, Yamada S, Kubota K, et al. Intratumoral distribution of fluorine-18-fluorodeoxyglucose in vivo: high accumulation in macrophages and granulation tissues studied by microautoradiography. *J Nucl Med* 1992;33:1972.
24. Lowe VJ, Naunheim KS. Positron emission tomography in lung cancer. *Ann Thorac Surg* 1998;65:1821.
25. Patronas NJ, Di Chior G, Kufta C, et al. Prediction of survival in glioma patients by means of positron emission tomography. *J Neurosurg* 1985;62:816.
26. Kim EE, Chung SK, Haynie TP, et al. Differentiation of residual or recurrent tumors from post-treatment changes with F-18 FDG PET. *Radiographics* 1992;12:269.
27. Coleman RE. PET in lung cancer. *J Nucl Med* 1999;40:814.
28. Hubner KF. Can ^{11}C-methionine play a role in lung cancer staging? *J Nucl Med* 2000;41:291.
29. Soyer P, Levesque M, Elias D, et al. Detection of liver metastases from colorectal cancer: comparison of intraoperative US and CT during arterial portography. *Radiology* 1992;183:541.
30. Braams JW, Pruim J, Kole AC, et al. Detection of unknown primary head and neck tumors by positron emission tomography. *Int J Oral Maxillofac Surg* 1997;26:112.
31. Chisin R. Nuclear medicine in head and neck oncology: reality and perspectives. *J Nucl Med* 1999;40:90.
32. Kitagawa Y, Sadato N, Azuma H, et al. FDG PET to evaluate combined intra-arterial chemotherapy and radiotherapy of head and neck neoplasms. *J Nucl Med* 1999;40:1132.
33. Delbeke D, Rose DM, Chapman WC, et al. Optimal interpretation of FDG PET in the diagnosis, staging and management of pancreatic carcinoma. *J Nucl Med* 1999;40:1784.
34. Schulte M, Brecht-Krauss D, Werner M, et al. Evaluation of neoadjuvant therapy response of osteogenic sarcoma using FDG PET. *J Nucl Med* 1999;40:1637.
35. Benard F, Sterman D, Smith RJ, et al. Prognostic value of FDG PET imaging in malignant pleural mesothelioma. *J Nucl Med* 1999;40:1241.
36. Sugawara Y, Eisbruch A, Kosuda S, et al. Evaluation of FDG PET in patients with cervical cancer. *J Nucl Med* 1999;40:1125.
37. Heicappell R, Muller-Mattheis V, Reinhardt M, et al. Staging of pelvic lymph nodes in neoplasms of the bladder and prostate by positron emission tomography with 2-[(18)F]-2-deoxy-D-glucose. *Eur Urol* 1999;36:582.
38. Minn H, Clavo AC, Wahl RL. Influence of hypoxia on tracer accumulation in squamous-cell carcinoma: in vitro evaluation for PET imaging. *Nucl Med Biol* 1996;23:941.
39. Cook GJ, Maisey MN, Fogelman I. Normal variants, artefacts and interpretative pitfalls in PET imaging with 18-fluoro-2-deoxyglucose and carbon-11 methionine. *Eur J Nucl Med* 1999;26:1363.
40. Wester HJ, Herz M, Weber W, et al. Synthesis and radiopharmacology of O-(2-[18F]fluoroethyl)-L-tyrosine for tumor imaging. *J Nucl Med* 1999;40:205.
41. Shoup TM, Olson J, Hoffman J, et al. Synthesis and evaluation of [18F]1-amino-3-fluorocyclobutane-1-carboxylic acid to image brain tumors. *J Nucl Med* 1999;40:331.
42. Shields AF, Mankoff DA, Link JM, et al. Carbon-11-thymidine and FDG to measure therapy response. *J Nucl Med* 1998;39:1757.
43. Mankoff DA, Dehdashti F, Shields AF. Characterizing tumors using metabolic imaging: PET imaging of cellular proliferation and steroid receptors. *Neoplasia* 2000;2:71.
44. Rasey JS, Hofstrand PD, Chin LK, et al. Characterization of [18F]fluoroetanidazole, a new radiopharmaceutical for detecting tumor hypoxia. *J Nucl Med* 1999;40:1072.
45. Hustinx R, Eck SL, Alavi A. Potential applications of PET imaging in developing novel cancer therapies. *J Nucl Med* 1999;40:995.
46. Evans SM, Kachur AV, Shiue C-Y, et al. Noninvasive detection of tumor hypoxia using the 2-nitroimidazole [^{18}F]EF1. *J Nucl Med* 2000;41:327.
47. Hendrikse NH, Franssen EJF, van der Graaf WTA, et al. Visualization of multidrug resistance in vivo. *Eur J Nucl Med* 1999;26:283.
48. Roivainen A, Forsback S, Gronroos T, et al. Blood metabolism of [methyl-11C]choline: implications for in vivo imaging with positron emission tomography. *Eur J Nucl Med* 2000;27:25.
49. Shreve PD, Gross MD. Imaging of the pancreas and related diseases with PET carbon-11-acetate. *J Nucl Med* 1997;38:1305.
50. Moehler M, Diitrakopoulou-Strauss A, Gutzler F, et al. 18F-labeled fluorouracil positron emission tomography and the prognosis of colorectal carcinoma patients with metastases to the liver treated with 5-fluorouracil. *Cancer* 1998;83:245.
51. Kaschten B, Stevenaert A, Sadzot B, et al. Preoperative evaluation of 54 gliomas by PET with fluorine-18-fluorodeoxyglucose and/or carbon-11-methionine. *J Nucl Med* 1998;39:778.
52. Sasaki M, Kuwabara Y, Yoshida T, et al. A comparative study of thallium-201 SPET, carbon-11 methionine PET and fluorine-18 fluorodeoxyglucose PET for the differentiation of astrocytic tumours. *Eur J Nucl Med* 1998;25:1261.
53. Kubota K, Tada M, Yamada S, et al. Comparison of the distribution of fluorine-18 fluoromisonidazole, deoxyglucose and methionine in tumour tissue. *Eur J Nucl Med* 1999;26:750.

54. Sasaki M, Kuwabara Y, Ichiya Y, et al. Differential diagnosis of thymic tumors using a combination of 11C-methionine PET and FDG PET. *J Nucl Med* 1999;40:1595.
55. Yasukawa T, Yoshikawa K, Aoyagi H, et al. Usefulness of PET with 11C-methionine for the detection of hilar and mediastinal lymph node metastasis in lung cancer. *J Nucl Med* 2000;41:283.
56. Plaat B, Kole A, Mastik M, et al. Protein synthesis rate measured with L-[1-^{11}C]tyrosine positron emission tomography correlates with mitotic activity and MIB-1 antibody-detected proliferation in human soft tissue sarcomas. *Eur J Nucl Med* 1999;26:328.
57. Shields AF, Grierson JR, Dohmen BM, et al. Imaging proliferation in vivo with [F-18]FLT and positron emission tomography. *Nat Med* 1998;4:1334.
58. Tjuvajev JG, Chen SH, Joshi A, et al. Imaging adenoviral-mediated herpes virus thymidine kinase gene transfer and expression in vivo. *Cancer Res* 1999;59:5186.
59. Welch MJ, McCarthy TJ. The potential role of generator-produced radiopharmaceuticals in clinical PET. *J Nucl Med* 2000;41:314.
60. Pomper MG, Port JD. New techniques in MR imaging of brain tumors. *MRI Clin North Am* 2000 (*in press*).
61. Hoge RD, Atkinson J, Gill B, et al. Investigation of BOLD signal dependence on cerebral blood flow and oxygen consumption: the deoxyhemoglobin dilution model. *Magn Reson Med* 1999;42:849.
62. Soher BJ, Hurd RE, Sailasuta N, et al. Quantitation of automated single-voxel proton MRS using cerebral water as an internal reference. *Magn Reson Med* 1996;36:335.
63. Negendank W. Studies of human tumors by MRS: a review. *NMR Biomed* 1992;5:303.
64. Robinson SP, Barton SJ, McSheehy PMJ, et al. Nuclear magnetic resonance spectroscopy of cancer. *Br J Radiol* 1997;70:S60.
65. Castillo M, Kwock L, Scatliff J, et al. Proton MR spectroscopy in neoplastic and non-neoplastic brain disorders. *MRI Clin North Am* 1998;6:1.
66. Rand SD, Prost R, Li S-J. Proton MR spectroscopy of the brain. *Neuroimaging Clin N Am* 1999;9:379.
67. Sijens PE. Phosphorus MR spectroscopy in the treatment of human extremity sarcomas. *NMR Biomed* 1998;11:341.
68. Negendank WG, Padavic-Shaller KA, Li C-W, et al. Metabolic characterization of human non-Hodgkin's lymphomas *in vivo* with the use of proton-decoupled phosphorus magnetic resonance spectroscopy. *Cancer Res* 1995;55:3286.
69. Dagnelie PC, Sijens PE, Kraus DJ, et al. Abnormal liver metabolism in cancer patients detected by (31)P MR spectroscopy. *NMR Biomed* 1999;12:535.
70. Leach MO, Verrill M, Glaholm J, et al. Measurements of human breast cancer using magnetic resonance spectroscopy: a review of clinical measurements and a report of localized 31P measurements of response to treatment. *NMR Biomed* 1998;11:314.
71. Preul MC, Caramanos Z, Collins DL, et al. Accurate, noninvasive diagnosis of human brain tumors by using proton magnetic resonance spectroscopy. *Nat Med* 1996;2:323.
72. Nelson SJ, Nat DR. Imaging of brain tumors after therapy. *Neuroimaging Clin N Am* 1999;9:801.
73. Nelson SJ, Vigneron DB, Dillon WP. Serial evaluation of patients with brain tumors using volume MRI and 3D ^{1}H MRSI. *NMR Biomed* 1999;12:123.
74. Milanesi I, Erbetta A, Silvani A, et al. H-MRSI is reliable in directing therapy of suspected relapsing neoplasms. Proceedings of the Thirty-Seventh Annual Meeting of the American Society of Neuroradiology, San Diego, 1999; 302(abst):231.
75. Star-Lack JM, Adalsteinsson E, Adam MF, et al. In vivo ^{1}H MR spectroscopy of human head and neck lymph node metastasis and comparison with oxygen tension measurements. *AJNR Am J Neuroradiol* 2000;21:183.
76. Gribbestad IS, Singstad TE, Nilsen G, et al. In vivo ^{1}H MRS of normal breast and breast tumors using a dedicated double breast coil. *J Magn Reson Imaging* 1998;8:1191.
77. Roebuck JR, Cecil KM, Schnall MD, et al. Human breast lesions: characterization with proton MR spectroscopy. *Radiology* 1998;209:269.
78. Kaji Y, Kurhanewicz J, Hricak H, et al. Localizing prostate cancer in the presence of post-biopsy changes on MR images: role of proton MR spectroscopic imaging. *Radiology* 1998;206:785.
79. Scheidler J, Hricak H, Vigneron DB, et al. Prostate cancer: localization with three-dimensional proton MR spectroscopic imaging–clinicopathologic study. *Radiology* 1999;213:473.
80. Kurhanewicz J, Vigneron DB, Nelson SJ. Three-dimensional magnetic resonance spectroscopic imaging of brain and prostate cancer. *Neoplasia* 2000;2:166.
81. Massuger LF, van Vierzen PB, Engelke U, et al. ^{1}H-magnetic resonance spectroscopy: a new technique to discriminate benign from malignant ovarian tumors. *Cancer* 1998;82:1726.
82. Ikehira H, Girard F, Obata T, et al. A preliminary study for clinical pharmacokinetics of oral fluorine anticancer medicines using the commercial MRI system^{19}F-MRS. *Br J Radiol* 1999;72:584.
83. Hashimoto T, Ikehira H, Fukuda H, et al. In vivo sodium-23 in brain tumors: evaluation of preliminary clinical experience. *Am J Physiol Imaging* 1991;6:74.
84. Schuierer G, Ladebeck R, Barfuss H, et al. Sodium-23 MR-imaging of supratentorial lesions at 4.0 T. *Magn Reson Med* 1991;22:1.
85. Hancu I, Boada FE, Shen GX. Three-dimensional triple-quantum-filtered (23)Na imaging of in vivo human brain. *Magn Reson Med* 1999;42:1146.
86. Gray L, MacFall J. Overview of diffusion imaging. *MRI Clin North Am* 1998;6:125.
87. Mori S, Barker PB. Diffusion magnetic resonance imaging: its principles and applications. *Anat Rec* 1999;257:102.
88. Aprile I, Iaiza F, Lavaroni A, et al. Analysis of cystic intracranial lesions performed with fluid-attenuated inversion recovery MR imaging. *AJNR Am J Neuroradiol* 1999;20:1259.
89. Brunburg JA, Chenevert TL, McKeever PE, et al. In vivo MR determination of water diffusion coefficients and diffusion anisotropy: correlation with structural alteration in gliomas of the cerebral hemispheres. *AJNR Am J Neuroradiol* 1995;16:371.
90. Sorensen AG, Tievsky AL, Ostergaard L, et al. Contrast agents in functional MR imaging. *J Magn Reson Imaging* 1997;7:47.
91. Huang W, Roche P, Madajewicz S, et al. Evaluation of brain tumor response to intracarotid chemotherapy using ^{1}H MRS, diffusion and perfusion MRI. Proceedings of the Seventh Scientific Meeting of the International Society for Magnetic Resonance in Medicine, Philadelphia, 1999(abst 903).
92. Moteki T, Ishizaka H, Horikoshi H, et al. Differentiation between hemangiomas and hepatocellular carcinomas with the apparent diffusion coefficient calculated from turbo-FLASH MR images. *J Magn Reson Imaging* 1995;5:187.
93. Moteki T, Ishizaka H. Evaluation of cystic ovarian lesions using apparent diffusion coefficient calculated from reordered turboflash MR images. *Magn Reson Imaging* 1999;17:955.
94. Yamada I, Aung W, Himeno Y, et al. Diffusion coefficients in abdominal organs and hepatic lesions: evaluation with intravoxel incoherent motion echo-planar MR imaging. *Radiology* 1999;210:617.
95. Lev MH, Rosen BR. Clinical applications of intracranial perfusion imaging. *Neuroimaging Clin N Am* 1999;9:309.
96. Aronen HJ, Gazit IE, Louis DN, et al. Cerebral blood volume maps of gliomas: comparison with tumor grade and histologic findings. *Radiology* 1994;191:41.
97. Mayr NA, Yuh WT, Magnotta VA, et al. Tumor perfusion studies using fast magnetic resonance imaging technique in advanced cervical cancer: a new noninvasive predictive assay. *Int J Radiat Oncol Biol Phys* 1996;36:623.
98. Van Vierzen PB, Massuger LF, Ruys SH, et al. Fast dynamic contrast enhanced MR imaging of cervical carcinoma. *Clin Radiol* 1998;53:183.
99. Mayr NA, Hawighorst H, Yuh WTC, et al. MR microcirculation assessment in cervical cancer: correlations with histomorphological tumor markers and clinical outcome. *J Magn Reson Imaging* 1999;10:267.
100. Parker GJM, Suckling J, Tanner SF, et al. MRIW: parametric analysis software for contrast-enhanced dynamic MR imaging in cancer. *Radiographics* 1998;18:497.
101. Turnbull LW, Buckley DL, Turnbull LS, et al. Differentiation of prostatic carcinoma and benign prostatic hyperplasia: correlation between dynamic Gd-DTPA-enhanced MR imaging and histopathology. *J Magn Reson Imaging* 1999;9:311.
102. Harvey C, Dooher A, Morgan J, et al. Imaging of tumour therapy responses by dynamic CT. *Eur J Radiol* 1999;30:221.
103. Thulborn KR, Waterton JC, Mathews PM, et al. Oxygen dependence of the transverse relaxation time of water protons in whole blood at high field. *Biochim Biophys Acta* 1982;714:265.
104. Achten E, Jackson GD, Cameron JA, et al. Presurgical evaluation of the motor hand area with functional MR imaging in patients with tumors and dysplastic lesions. *Radiology* 1999;210:529.
105. Lurito JT, Lowe MJ, Sartorius C, et al. Comparison of fMRI and intraoperative direct cortical stimulation in localization of receptive language areas. *J Comput Assist Tomogr* 2000;24:99.
106. Ulug AM, van Zijl PCM. Orientation-independent diffusion imaging without tensor diagonalization: anisotropy definitions based on physical attributes of the diffusion ellipsoid. *J Magn Reson Imaging* 1999;9:804.
107. Nakada T, Nakayama N, Fujii Y, et al. Clinical application of three-dimensional anisotropy contrast magnetic resonance axonography [Technical note]. *J Neurosurg* 1999;90:791.
108. Inoue T, Shimizu H, Yoshimoto T. Imaging the pyramidal tract in patients with brain tumors. *Clin Neurol Neurosurg* 1999;101:4.
109. Enochs WS, Harsh G, Hochberg F, et al. Improved delineation of human brain tumors on MR images using a long-circulating superparamagnetic iron oxide agent. *J Magn Reson Imaging* 1999;9:228.
110. Louie AY, Huber MM, Ahrens ET, et al. In vivo visualization of gene expression using magnetic resonance imaging. *Nat Biotechnol* 2000;18:321.
111. Boppart SA, Bouma BE, Pitris C, et al. Intraoperative assessment of microsurgery with three-dimensional optical coherence tomography. *Radiology* 1998;208:81.
112. Fujimoto J, Pitris C, Boppart SA, et al. Optical coherence tomography: an emerging technology for biomedical imaging and optical biopsy. *Neoplasia* 2000;2:9.
113. Follen M, Richards-Kortum R. Emerging technologies and cervical cancer. *J Natl Cancer Inst* 2000;92:363.
114. Inaguma M, Hashimoto K. Porphyrin-like fluorescence in oral cancer: in vivo fluorescence spectral characterization of lesions by use of a near-ultraviolet excited autofluorescence diagnosis system and separation of fluorescent extracts by capillary electrophoresis. *Cancer* 1999;86:2201.
115. Andersson-Engels S, Canti G, Eker CU, et al. Preliminary evaluation of two fluorescence imaging methods for the detection and the delineation of basal cell carcinomas of the skin. *Lasers Surg Med* 2000;26:76.
116. Schantz SP, Kolli V, Savage HE, et al. In vivo native cellular fluorescence and histological characteristics of head and neck cancer. *Clin Cancer Res* 1998;4:1177.
117. Tromberg BJ, Shah N, Lanning R, et al. Non-invasive *in vivo* characterization of breast tumors using photon migration spectroscopy. *Neoplasia* 2000;2:26.
118. Kuppusamy P, Afeworki M, Shankar RA, et al. *In vivo* electron paramagnetic resonance imaging of tumor heterogeneity and oxygenation in a murine model. *Cancer Res* 1998;58:1562.
119. Swartz HM, Clarkson RB. The measurement of oxygen in vivo using EPR techniques. *Phys Med Biol* 1998;43:1957.
120. Scott WJ, Shepherd J, Gambhir SS. Cost-effectiveness of FDG-PET for staging non-small cell lung cancer: a decision analysis. *Ann Thoracic Surg* 1998;66:1876.
121. Kritz FL. PET scanning moves into community hospitals. *J Nucl Med* 1999;40:11N.

SECTION **4**

JEAN-FRANCOIS H. GESCHWIND

Interventional Radiology

The field of interventional radiology has continued its rapid expansion into the world of clinical medicine and oncology. In doing so, its focus has shifted from an essentially diagnostic to a primarily therapeutic subspecialty. The interventional radiologist is now involved in direct patient care and, in many instances, has become the patient's primary care physician. This growth of interventional radiology is especially extraordinary in the field of clinical oncology, where many procedures, such as placement of tunneled central venous catheters for infusion of chemotherapy or nutritional support, inferior vena cava (IVC) filters to prevent pulmonary embolism, and catheterization of the biliary or urinary tract to decompress obstructed systems, are now performed by interventional radiologists. In addition, new procedures developed by interventional radiologists, such as transarterial chemoembolization of liver tumors, percutaneous ethanol infusion, radiofrequency ablation, or embolization techniques, have become suitable therapeutic alternatives to other traditional forms of therapy, including systemic chemotherapy, irradiation, or surgery and, in some instances, have become the mainstay of therapy. A wide range of cancer patients benefit from the services of interventional radiology. This chapter first reviews some of the well-established procedures still performed to help diagnose cancer and then addresses the many contributions of interventional radiology in the treatment of cancer patients.

DIAGNOSTIC PROCEDURES

Percutaneous and intraluminal biopsies of suspicious lesions are relatively easy and reliable methods of obtaining tissue for histologic or cytopathologic diagnosis. The lungs, breast, liver, pancreas, adrenal glands, kidney, and retroperitoneum (especially lymph nodes) are the most commonly targeted organs. Ultrasonography, magnetic resonance imaging, and computed tomography (CT) provide excellent image guidance and have made it possible to safely sample focal lesions as small as 5 mm.[1] The majority of percutaneous biopsies can be performed on an outpatient basis. By alleviating the need for diagnostic surgery, biopsy is cost-effective and can have a great impact on patient management.[1] Numerous types and sizes of biopsy needles are commercially available. They vary from the small aspiration needle (19- to 23-gauge), which provides a cellular slurry for cytologic examination when confirmatory diagnosis of malignancy is sought, to the large-core biopsy cutting needle and biopsy gun (18-gauge or less), which provide an actual piece of tissue for cytologic and histopathologic analysis.[2–4] The choice of a specific needle should be made according to the type of tissue to be sampled. Other considerations include the type and vascularity of the target organ, the coagulation status of the patient, and the anticipated course of the needle. Percutaneous biopsy is most commonly performed to provide a definitive diagnosis of malignancy. It can also be used for tumor staging and assessment of tumor response to therapy.

PERCUTANEOUS BIOPSY IN THE THORAX

Despite persistent controversy about its usefulness, transthoracic needle biopsy is still commonly performed to diagnose both benign and malignant disease of the thorax.[5–7] Aspiration or cutting needles can be used to evaluate suspicious lesions adequately in the lung parenchyma, pleura, or mediastinum. Although cutting or core needles generally provide better quality samples than those provided by aspiration needles, they are usually not required to sample parenchymal abnormalities or lung nodules and, in most instances, provide no substantial advantage over needle aspiration.[2,8–11] Only when the diagnosis of malignancy cannot reliably be established by fine-needle aspiration is the use of core needles indicated.[5,7] It is helpful to have the pathologist in attendance during the procedure to determine whether the collected sample can yield a definitive diagnosis.[12] If the initial biopsy sample is negative, the positioning of the needle tip should be checked to ensure that it is within the lesion. Once the needle tip is appropriately redirected, further samples should be collected. Both established and more recent series have shown the sensitivity of transthoracic needle aspiration for the detection of pulmonary parenchymal, hilar, or pleural malignancy to vary between 74% and 97%, its diagnostic accuracy to range from 76% to 99%, and its specificity to approach 100%.[1,2,5–11] Core biopsy marginally increases the diagnostic yield over that obtained with fine-needle aspiration. On the other hand, despite the increased risk of the procedure owing to the larger size of the needle, it is extremely useful when a diagnosis of lymphoma is suspected or to establish a definitive diagnosis of malignancy within the mediastinum.[13–16]

Fluoroscopy, CT scanning, and ultrasonography are the preferred imaging modalities for guidance of needle biopsy in the thorax. All available radiographic studies of the lesion to undergo biopsy should be reviewed before the procedure. For lung nodules, fluoroscopy is the imaging guidance of choice because it provides immediate identification and, thus, rapid sampling of the lesion. If the lesion cannot be identified by fluoroscopy, CT scanning guidance should be used. CT images provide exquisite anatomic details, and vital structures, such as major blood vessels, can thus be avoided.[2] These attributes render CT scanning the imaging guidance of choice for lesions involving the mediastinum, hila, or pleura. Finally, the use of ultrasonography should be reserved for superficial chest wall masses.

Although no absolute contraindications to percutaneous pulmonary biopsy exist, there are several relative contraindications, such as an uncooperative patient, pulmonary hypertension, coagulopathy, and severe bullous emphysematous disease. Severe complications from transthoracic pulmonary biopsy are extremely rare, and the overall mortality ranges from 0.01% to 0.05%.[17–19] On the other hand, the incidence of pneumothorax (by far the most common complication) varies between 14% and nearly 60%, but only 4% to 13% of these cases require treatment by placement of a chest tube.[17–21] Note that the incidence or size of a pneumothorax is not related to either the size of the biopsy needle or the number of passes made during the biopsy.[11] Other complications include hemoptysis (5% of cases) and pleural pain, especially if a pneumothorax is present.[17–21]

BIOPSY OF OTHER ORGAN SYSTEMS

With the advent of high-quality cross-sectional imaging, percutaneous biopsy of suspicious abdominal masses has become a relatively easy, safe, and reliable method of obtaining definitive tissue diagnosis. CT guidance remains by far the most common imaging guidance modality, because it provides superb anatomic details and excellent evaluation of internal structures, thus allowing the operator to plan and choose the safest approach to a biopsy.[22] It is clearly the modality of choice for biopsy of the pancreas, adrenals, lymph nodes, retroperitoneal masses, and liver lesions not seen well by ultrasonography. On the other hand, ultrasonography is the guidance modality of choice for biopsy of the thyroid and breast and is frequently used for biopsy of the liver (especially if the lesions are relatively large and superficial), the pancreas, kidneys, and pelvic organs.[23,24] Ultrasonography offers the advantage of real-time, multiplanar imaging as well as Doppler analysis, which makes it very practical and improves safety by allowing the operator to identify and thus avoid major vessels.[23,24] The role of magnetic resonance imaging in biopsy guidance remains limited by the high cost of nuclear medicine examinations and the need for specialized biopsy needles owing to the magnetic field. Although both fine-needle aspiration and larger cutting needles can theoretically be used for biopsy of abdominal lesions, a fine needle is often preferred because the risk of injury to adjacent vital structures is minimized. Indeed, such structures as the liver, stomach, small bowel, and colon can safely be traversed by a fine needle. Cutting needles should be used if a definitive diagnosis cannot be established with fine-needle aspiration and only if a clear, safe pathway to the target lesion can be established.

Percutaneous biopsy of abdominal or pelvic masses generally yields high diagnostic accuracy rates. In the liver, it ranges from 60% to 84% with fine aspiration needles to 90% to 100% with core or cutting needles.[25–28] In the pancreas, diagnostic accuracy has greatly improved over the last 10 years and now ranges between 85% using fine-needle aspiration and 92% using core needles.[29,30] The diagnostic accuracy for biopsy of the kidney[31] and adrenals is greater than 90%.[32–34] The use of large cutting needles for biopsy of the adrenal glands is not recommended because major vital structures, which surround the adrenal glands, could be transgressed during the procedure, thus causing major complications. For abdominal biopsies, the diagnostic accuracy is directly related to the number of needle passes made during the biopsy.

The complication rate for percutaneous biopsy in the abdomen is low (1% to 3%).[29,32,35–37] It is lowest in the liver (0.1%) and highest in the adrenals (8.4%).[29,32,35–37] Major complications, though extremely rare, include hepatic or renal hemorrhage, pancreatitis, and pneumothorax. They can usually be treated effectively by transcatheter or tract embolization (hemorrhage)[38] or insertion of a drainage catheter (pancreatitis or pneumothorax).[37]

More invasive techniques, such as transjugular liver biopsy[39] and percutaneous transhepatic biopsy of the biliary tree[40] can also be performed to obtain tissue diagnosis in the liver. In cancer patients, transjugular liver biopsy is used mainly to obtain core-like samples of liver tissue to establish the diagnosis of graft-versus-host disease. It is performed via a right internal jugular approach and requires selective hepatic vein catheterization. Once seeded within the hepatic vein, either a biopsy gun or forceps is directed inferiorly and advanced through a vascular sheath directly into the liver parenchyma to collect tissue samples. This technique is especially useful in coagulopathic patients with diffuse liver disease.

Traditional image-guided percutaneous biopsy or endoscopic brush biopsy of the biliary tract have diagnostic yields ranging only from 40% to 70%.[41,42] Benign and malignant biliary strictures have similar cholangiographic appearances, and distinguishing between the two entities can be extremely difficult. Percutaneous transhepatic biliary drainage allows direct access to the biliary tract once satisfactory decompression of the biliary tree has been achieved. Biopsy forceps catheters can then be used through the existing tract to obtain tissue samples of suspicious areas within the biliary tree. Sensitivity and specificity with this technique hover near 85% and 95%, respectively, and are highest when a scope, introduced percutaneously through the established tract, provides direct visualization of the biliary tree.

VISCERAL ANGIOGRAPHY

The role of angiography in the diagnostic evaluation of hepatobiliary or pancreatic neoplastic disease has greatly diminished in the last decades. The advent of sophisticated noninvasive fast imaging modalities, such as CT, ultrasonography, and nuclear medicine, has fulfilled most of the clinician's diagnostic needs. However, angiography continues to be important not only as a visceral diagnostic test but as it provides the basis for many therapeutic interventional procedures. Visceral angiography requires selective catheterization of the celiac axis and superior mesenteric artery after which digital subtraction imaging is performed. Filming should be carried out long enough to visualize the portal venous phase. Visceral angiography is used for detailed evaluation of the splanchnic arterial anatomy, particularly the numerous potential anatomic variations in the arterial supply to the liver (Fig. 27.4-1); documenting patency of the portovenous system; and determination of vascular encasement. When intraarterial chemotherapy administered via a surgically placed pump is being considered for treatment of liver metastases, thorough evaluation of the hepatic arterial anatomy is especially important to ensure appropriate delivery of the chemotherapy to all segments of the liver involved by the tumor.[43] In cases of pancreatic cancer or cholangiocarcinoma, if surgical resection is contemplated, assessment of vascular encasement is critical, since surgery offers the only hope for cure.[44–48] Encasement of the celiac axis, the superior mesenteric artery, portal vein, or superior mesenteric vein (Fig. 27.4-2) usually indicate that the tumor is not amenable to surgical resection for cure, although in some cases and, depending on the surgeon's experience, such findings may not preclude surgical exploration.[44–48]

PORTAL VENOUS SAMPLING

Islet cell tumors of the pancreas can be elusive, and their detection by noninvasive imaging or by conventional angiography often fails. Percutaneous transhepatic portal venous sampling

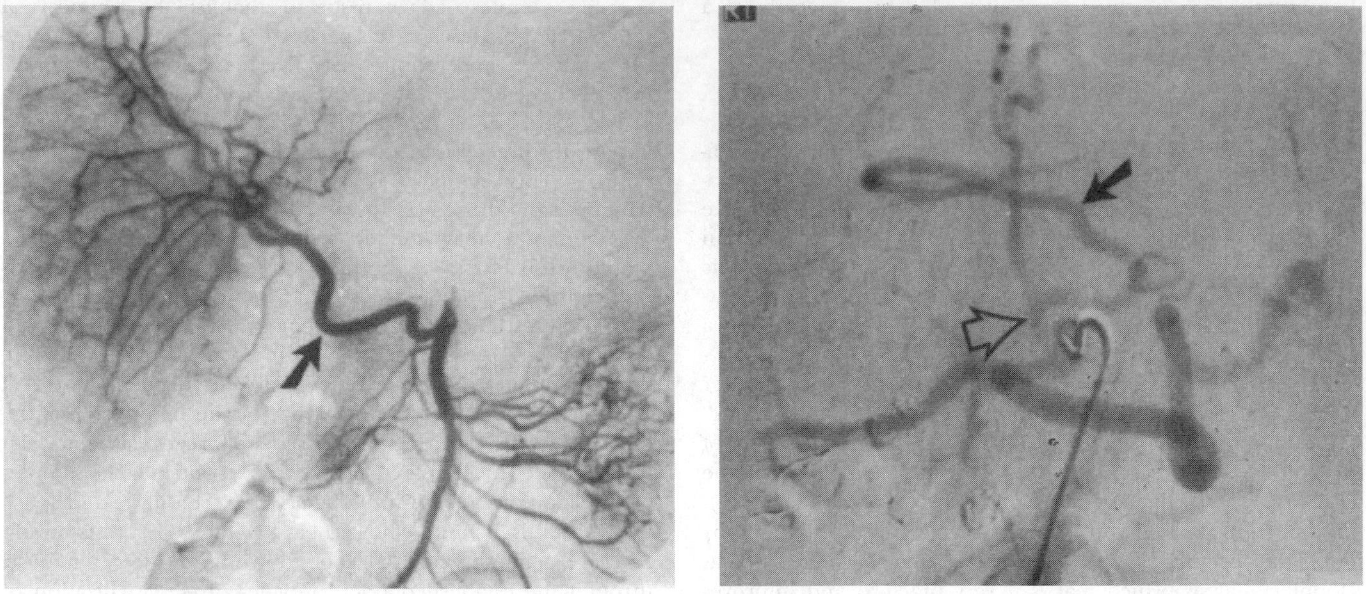

A B

FIGURE 27.4-1. Diagnostic visceral arteriogram: variant arterial anatomy. **A:** Replaced right hepatic artery (*arrow*) off the superior mesenteric artery. **B:** Replaced left hepatic artery (*black arrow*) off the left gastric artery (*open arrow*).

is used to localize islet cell tumors by measuring hormonal levels in the superior mesenteric, splenic, and portal veins. This method has a sensitivity exceeding 95% for localization of islet cell tumors.[49–54] Detection and localization of islet cell tumors is important because patients can be cured once the tumor is resected. Precise anatomic mapping of the hormonal collections is, therefore, essential to accurately locate the tumor, thereby avoiding blind surgical resection and enabling the surgeon to resect the affected segment (head, body, or tail) of the pancreas.[49–54] When the sampling procedure is completed, the transhepatic tract should be embolized with Gelfoam pledgets to prevent excessive bleeding.[49,54]

THERAPEUTIC INTERVENTIONS

The second part of this chapter focuses on the most important contributions of interventional radiology in the treatment and management of hepatic, pancreatic, and biliary malignancies; other gastrointestinal tract cancers; genitourinary tumors; superior vena cava (SVC) syndrome; as well as pulmonary thromboembolic disease.

LIVER CANCER

The management of primary and secondary malignancies of the liver constitutes one of the most difficult challenges for oncologists. First, primary hepatic malignancies frequently escape detection because most patients remain asymptomatic for long periods. Then, if clinical symptoms are present, they may be masked by the patient's underlying liver disease and may, therefore, be difficult to attribute to a malignancy. In addition, clinical outcome is typically poor, with median survival of less than 1 year for all patients and between 3 and 6 months for unresectable presentations.[55–59] Hepatocellular carcinoma (hepatoma) is one of the most common fatal cancers in the world (1.2 million deaths per year) and accounts for approximately 90% of all liver cancers. It is most commonly encountered in Asia and sub-Saharan Africa, where it constitutes 20% to 40% of all malignancies. The high incidence of hepatoma in these regions can be attributed to hepatitis B, which is endemic in these regions of the world. In Europe and North America, the incidence of hepatoma is markedly lower (10,000 to 14,000 cases per year in the United States) and largely related to alcoholic cirrhosis, but it is climbing rapidly and expected to increase further given the recent rise in hepatitis C and its association with hepatoma.[55–60]

Metastatic malignant tumors of the liver are by far the most common type of hepatic malignancies in the United States (at least 20 times that of hepatoma) and occur most often secondary to colorectal carcinoma (155,000 cases and 60,000 deaths per year in the United States),[61] followed by ocular melanoma, neuroendocrine tumors of the pancreas, including carcinoid tumors, as well as both functional and nonfunctional islet cell tumors, and some sarcomas.[62–64] In many of these conditions, the liver is the only site of metastatic involvement, thus justifying a role for locoregional therapy.

Although rare, carcinoid tumor represents the most common of all endocrine tumors of the gastrointestinal tract, and the incidence of metastatic carcinoid tumor is 0.32 to 0.7 per 100,000 with the majority arising from the small bowel.[62,63] The tumor is usually slow growing and, therefore, associated with longer survival than hepatoma or colorectal metastatic disease, but patients can be plagued by severe symptoms due to excessive secretion of serotonin and bradykinin as part of the carcinoid syndrome (4% to 9% of cases). In cases of carcinoid syndrome, the liver is almost always involved, and locoregional palliative therapy with chemoembolization constitutes the only therapeutic option.[62,63]

Ocular melanoma is a very aggressive and highly lethal disease. It usually progresses very rapidly and commonly metastasizes to the liver. Once the liver is involved, fatal hepatic disease

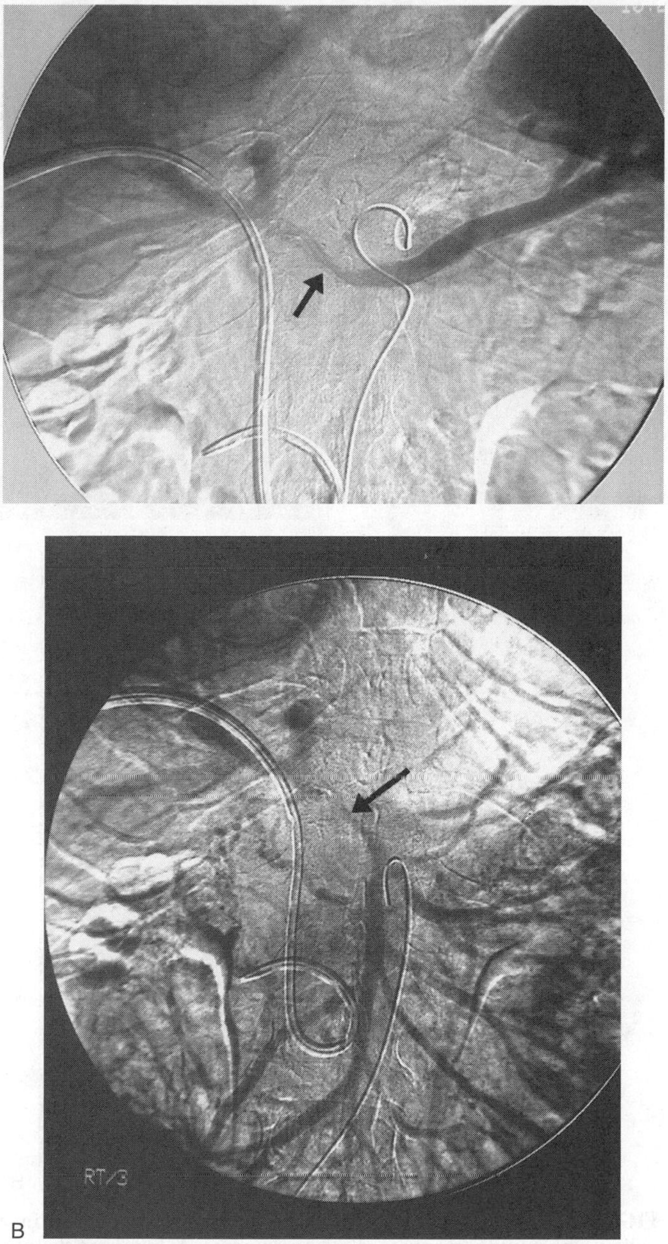

A

B

FIGURE 27.4-2. Diagnostic visceral arteriogram in a patient with pancreatic adenocarcinoma: venous encasement. **A:** Venous phase from splenic arterial injection demonstrates narrowing of the main portal vein consistent with encasement (*arrow*). **B:** Venous phase from superior mesenteric arterial injection demonstrates encasement of main portal vein (*arrow*).

ensues. Median survival ranges from 2 to 6 months.[55,64] As for the other tumors involving the liver, locoregional therapy offers the best option.

For both primary and metastatic liver cancers, such surgical options as resection or transplantation offer the only hope for cure and, at the very least, have a definite impact on survival in operative candidates, with survival rates ranging from 55% to 80% at 1 year and 25% to 50% at 5 years.[61,65–68] Yet, only a minority of patients are surgical candidates (15% to 20% of all patients with either primary or secondary liver cancers).[55,66–68] Criteria used to determine unresectability include the size, location, and volume of the lesion to be resected; multilobar involvement; as well as the presence of limited hepatic reserve due to advanced cirrhosis or chronic hepatitis and significant concurrent disease (especially cardiac or pulmonary disease).[55] In addition, surgical resection continues to be plagued by fairly high morbidity and mortality rates, especially when surgery is performed in patients with underlying liver failure (15% to 30% perioperative mortality), as well as high recurrence rates (75% of patients).[66–68] Liver transplantation remains limited by the scarcity of liver donors (although the development of living-related liver transplantation could remedy this problem) and by a surprisingly high recurrence rate.[67,68] Other therapeutic options, such as systemic chemotherapy and external-beam radiotherapy, have been disappointing. The response rate from single-agent or multidrug chemotherapy is poor, as it does not exceed 15% to 20% and a clear survival benefit has not been demonstrated.[55,67] External-beam irradiation is limited by the extensive damage it causes to the radiosensitive hepatocytes.[55,67]

The limitations of the traditional weapons against cancer (surgery, chemotherapy, and radiotherapy), combined with the fact that the immense majority of patients afflicted by primary or metastatic liver cancer have liver-only disease, have led to the hunt for and development of various locoregional therapies. In addition, patients afflicted by hepatoma usually die of hepatic failure and cachexia as a result of local growth and resultant liver tissue destruction but not of extrahepatic metastatic disease.[66–68] Thus, control of the tumor at the regional level is essential.

The goal of locoregional therapy is to destroy the tumor while preserving as much of the normal liver tissue as possible. This can be accomplished either by direct percutaneous ablative methods, such as percutaneous ethanol injection and radiofrequency ablation, or by intraarterial delivery of embolic material with or without chemotherapeutic agents, such as transcatheter arterial chemoembolization, which is by far the most widely performed procedure in the treatment of unresectable liver cancers.

Transcatheter Arterial Chemoembolization

Transcatheter arterial chemoembolization has truly become the mainstay of therapy for unresectable hepatoma and carcinoid tumors and has shown great promise against colorectal metastases.[55] The concept of chemoembolization evolved from practical experience obtained with two partially effective therapies, intraarterial chemotherapy and embolotherapy. Although many different chemoembolization regimens can be used, the principles and theoretic advantages of chemoembolization are identical and are based on combined infusion of a concentrated dose of chemotherapeutic drugs mixed with iodized oil and an embolic agent directly into the hepatic artery. It is well established that the normal liver draws most of its blood supply from the portal vein (approximately 75%), whereas primary or metastatic liver tumors draw most of their oxygen supply from the hepatic artery (>90%).[69,70] Targeting the hepatic artery for regional delivery with a mixture of chemotherapeutic agents and embolic material is, therefore, not only safe and possible but also extremely attractive to destroy the tumor. The theoretic beneficial effects of chemoembolization include delivery of a high concentration of chemotherapy to the tumor bed, marked increase in contact time between the drugs and the tumor cells, and high first-pass extraction.[55,71,72] These factors combine to increase the drug concentration and the retention rate within the tumor even further (100- to 400-fold increases in drug concentration have been reported), thereby minimizing the systemic toxicity of the chemotherapeutic drugs.[55,71–74] Although many different chemoembolization protocols are being used throughout the world without any compelling evidence of the superiority of one over the other, a generally accepted rule is that the chemoembolization infusion should include a mixture of iodized oil (Ethiodol) and chemotherapeutic agents. Doxorubicin is most commonly used alone in Europe, whereas the combination of cisplatin, doxorubicin, and mitomycin C is favored in the United States. Ethiodol plays a key role in the process since it not only acts as a carrier for the chemotherapeutic agents by creating an emulsion with the agents but it also prolongs contact time between the tumor cells and the agents by clogging the presinusoid arterioportal shunts, thus allowing the agents to slowly diffuse into the tumor.[55,73] Particulate embolization materials (Gelfoam or Ivalon) should also be injected toward the end of the procedure to reduce arterial inflow and, thus, prevent washout of the chemotherapeutic agents.

Since chemoembolization is currently only used as a palliative therapy, its impact on patients' quality of life should be given high priority. The benefits of the procedure should be weighed against the potential complications that could worsen patients' quality of life. Thus, proper patient selection should be conducted to exclude patients who could be adversely affected by the procedure, such as those with clinically apparent jaundice, hepatic encephalopathy, extensive extrahepatic metastases, poor liver function (combination of >50% liver replacement by tumor, aspartate transaminase >100, markedly elevated lactate dehydrogenase, and hyperbilirubinemia), or biliary obstruction.[55]

Patients scheduled to undergo chemoembolization are required to fast overnight. The day of the procedure, vigorous hydration with normal saline, prophylactic antibiotics, antiemetics, and sedatives are administered. A visceral arteriogram is then performed to define the arterial anatomy and to assess portal venous patency. With the advent of hydrophilic guidewires and catheters as well as coaxial systems with smaller diameter catheters, it is now possible to perform superselective catheterization of third- or fourth-order branches. Once the catheter has been advanced beyond the gastroduodenal artery to avoid nontarget embolization and is located within striking distance of the tumor, the chemoembolization material can be injected (Fig. 27.4-3). The infusion should be stopped before thrombosis of the hepatic artery occurs. Patients are then admitted for pain management, continued antibiotic coverage, and hydration. The vast majority of patients requires only a 24- to 48-hour hospital stay. Although most patients experience some degree of pain, nausea, vomiting, and fever as part of the embolization syndrome, which typically lasts 3 to 10 days, chemoembolization is generally relatively well tolerated. True complications, such as liver failure, liver infarction, abscess formation, cholecystitis, nontarget embolization to the gastrointestinal tract, and biliary necrosis, are rare (3% to 4% of cases).[55]

Initial enthusiasm for chemoembolization was generated by early reports[75–82] from Kanematsu,[75] Okamura,[79] and others,[76–78,80–82] who demonstrated that extensive tumor necrosis (60% to 90%) and high radiographic response rates (up to

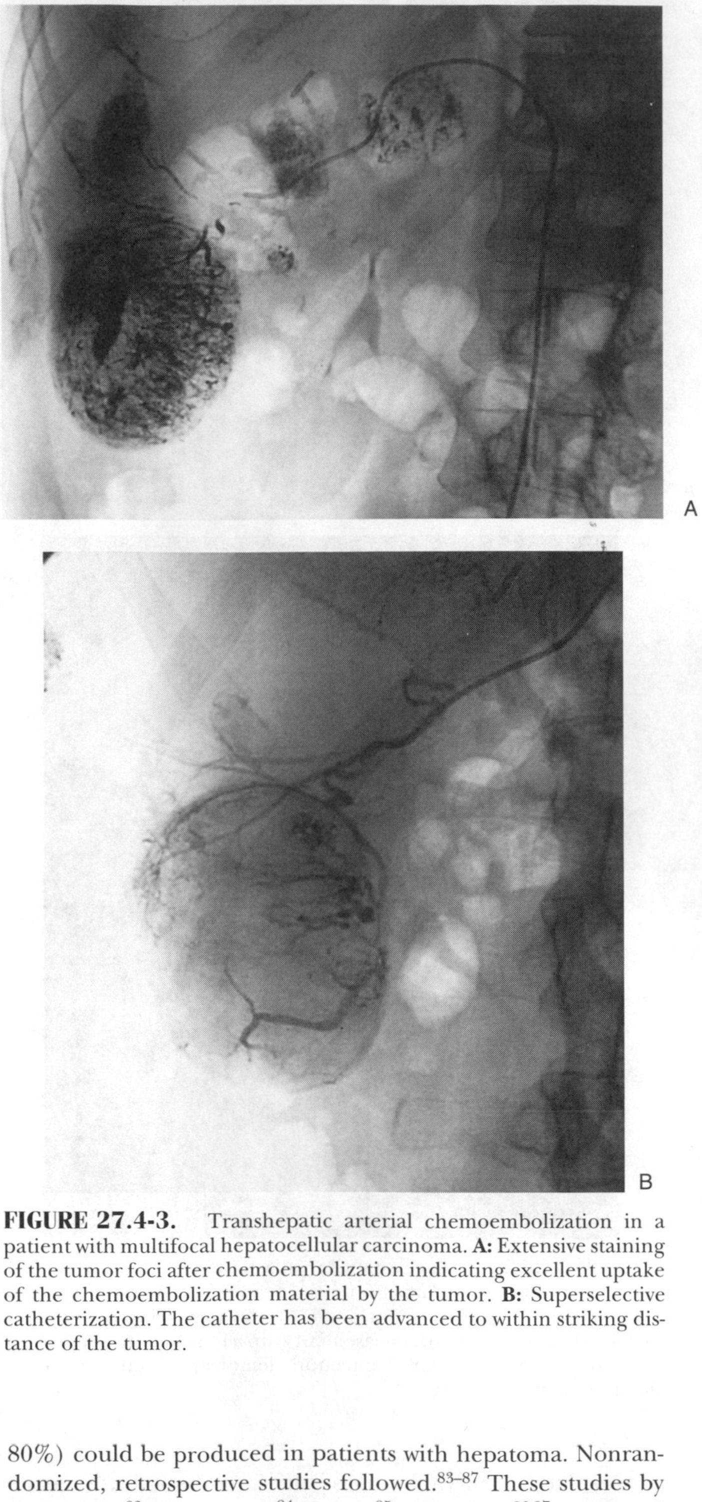

FIGURE 27.4-3. Transhepatic arterial chemoembolization in a patient with multifocal hepatocellular carcinoma. **A:** Extensive staining of the tumor foci after chemoembolization indicating excellent uptake of the chemoembolization material by the tumor. **B:** Superselective catheterization. The catheter has been advanced to within striking distance of the tumor.

80%) could be produced in patients with hepatoma. Nonrandomized, retrospective studies followed.[83–87] These studies by Nakamura,[83] Shimamura,[84] Nakao,[85] and others[86,87] compared chemoembolization to other therapies, such as hepatic artery embolization alone (without added chemotherapeutic agents or iodized oil), using historic controls. They showed that a clear advantage in survival could be established with chemoembolization. Indeed, cumulative probability of survival after chemoembolization ranged from 54% to 88% at 1 year, 33% to 64% at 2 years, and 18% to 51% at 3 years, whereas embolization alone yielded cumulative survival of 44% at 1 year, 29% at 2 years, and 15% at 3 years. These results also compared very favorably with a 1-year survival rate of 13% achieved with systemic chemotherapy. This improvement in survival was accompanied by a decrease in the level of serum α-fetoprotein (AFP) in most cases. These impressive results helped to establish chemoembolization as the treatment of choice for unresectable hepatoma.

Recent prospective randomized trials conducted by Pelletier et al.,[88] Madden et al.,[89] the Groupe d'Etude et de Traitement du Carcinome Hepatocellulaire,[90] and Bruix et al.[91] (the only four randomized trials to date) failed to show a significant survival advantage of chemoembolization over supportive care, although a trend to prolonged survival was detected (63% vs. 44% at 1 year). Each of these studies had significant flaws in their methodology and design, severely limiting their validity. However, they managed to question the utility of chemoembolization in prolonging survival. In a landmark article published in 1991, Vetter[92] reported a case-control study comparing chemoembolization to supportive care, which clearly demonstrated the superiority of chemoembolization over supportive care. Survival at 1 and 2 years was 59% and 30%, respectively, in the treatment arm, whereas it was 0% at 1 year in the supportive care group. Another study by Bartolozzi et al.[93] confirmed the survival benefits of chemoembolization in a group of 53 patients with 93%, 70%, and 43% overall survival rate at 1, 2, and 3 years, respectively. Ngan et al.[60] measured survival as a function of tumor size and found that patients with tumor less than 9 cm had a better survival than those with tumor greater than 9 cm. Overall survival at 1 and 4 years was 67% and 31%, respectively. Solomon et al.[58] focused on the effectiveness of chemoembolization in an exclusively Western population and found cumulative survival of 60% at 1 year, 41% at 2 years, and 16% at 3 years similar to that obtained by studies in Asian populations.

Despite the impact of these studies, the search is still on for one or more specific niches that would help to establish chemoembolization as an uncontested treatment option for hepatoma. For example, the issue of high recurrence after liver transplantation or surgical resection is perplexing, and adequate therapy against such recurrence is lacking. Recent studies[94–97] exploring the role of chemoembolization as a neoadjuvant treatment modality have shown markedly improved disease-free survival when chemoembolization was performed before surgery. Patients treated with chemoembolization before surgical resection had survival rates of 87%, 70%, and 39%, at 1, 3, and 5 years, respectively, whereas patients treated with surgical resection alone had survival rates of 79%, 38%, and 19%. Disease-free survival was also better in the chemoembolization than in the surgery-only group (40% and 28% vs. 20% and 11% at 3 and 5 years, respectively). When chemoembolization was used before liver transplantation, the 1- and 2-year disease-free survival rates were 91% and 84%, respectively.[98] Survival was also significantly improved when chemoembolization was used to treat intrahepatic tumor recurrence that had occurred postoperatively (Figs. 27.4-4, 27.4-5).[99] The 1-, 3-, and 5-year survivals were 75%, 46%, and 30%, respectively, as opposed to 20%, 4%, and 0% when no chemoembolization was administered.[99]

Patients with hepatoma experience a wide spectrum of diseases directly related to the extent of tumor involvement and preexisting nonneoplastic liver disease. There is no doubt that outcome and survival are primarily directly related to these factors, regardless of whether treatment is administered and regardless of the form of therapy selected.[100] However, the available data published to date have clearly helped to define a role for chemoembolization as an effective adjuvant therapy either preoperatively or postoperatively and establish its efficacy as a palliative therapy against unresectable hepatocellular carcinoma.

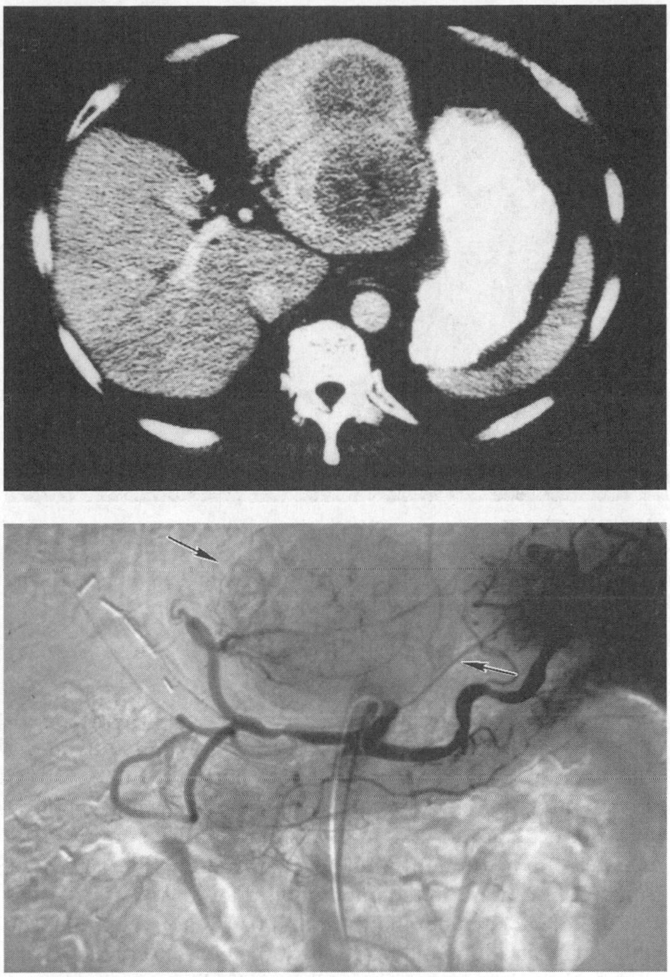
A

B

FIGURE 27.4-4. Transhepatic arterial chemoembolization in a patient with recurrence of hepatocellular carcinoma in the left lobe of the liver 1 year after wedge resection of a solitary hepatocellular carcinoma in the right lobe of the liver. **A:** Two low-density nodules are clearly identified within the left lobe of the liver, consistent with recurrent hepatoma. **B:** Arterial phase from a celiac arteriogram demonstrates hypervascular tumor foci within the left lobe of the liver (*arrows*) consistent with the computed tomography findings.

No controversies exist about the use of chemoembolization in the treatment of metastatic neuroendocrine tumors, such as carcinoid and islet cell tumors, with survival ranges from 27 to 48 months from the time of therapy.[101–105] These tumors are usually hypervascular, thus making them ideal candidates for treatment with chemoembolization; and, unlike patients with hepatoma, patients affected by neuroendocrine tumors are frequently symptomatic. The goal of therapy is clear and consists of alleviating symptoms (pain, anorexia, early satiety) related both to hormonal release and the tumor bulk itself resulting from intrahepatic involvement. Multiple studies by Therasse,[62] Winkelbauer,[101] Mavligit,[102] Stokes,[103] and Perry[104] have clearly demonstrated the effectiveness of chemoembolization against

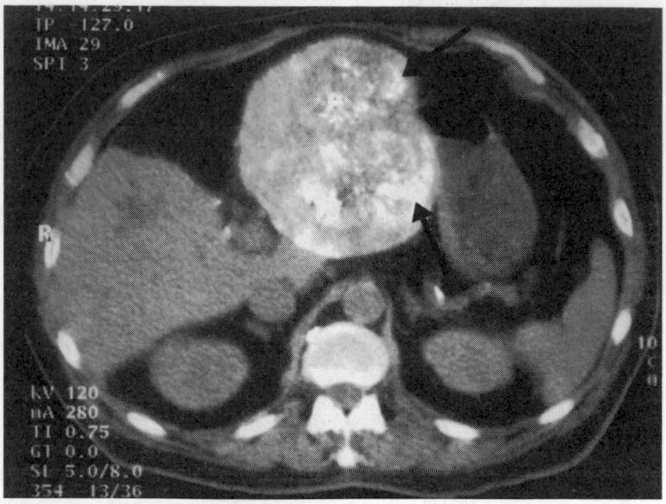

FIGURE 27.4-5. Computed tomography scan of the abdomen without contrast 1 day after chemoembolization in the patient from Figure 27.4-4. Excellent distribution of the chemoembolization material throughout the two tumor nodules (*arrows*).

such tumors. Therasse and Stokes reported a 100% symptomatic response, which lasted for an average of 28 months, and a 90% decrease in hormonal levels after treatment with chemoembolization. Although earlier reports with embolization alone demonstrated high response rates, symptom-free intervals of 5 to 10 months achieved with embolization do not compare favorably with chemoembolization.

The role of chemoembolization in the treatment of colorectal liver metastases is still under investigation at several centers in the United States, and published studies remain sparse. Colorectal carcinoma is especially lethal once it has metastasized to the liver. Indeed, median survival is only 6 months after the diagnosis of hepatic metastasis is made.[61] Systemic chemotherapy with 5-fluorouracil or combination regimens have produced mediocre response rates rarely exceeding the 20% range and have caused significant systemic toxicity.[61] Hepatic artery infusion of chemotherapy with either 5-fluorouracil or 5-fluorodeoxyuridine has been shown to improve response rates to 45%.[61] However, despite encouraging response rates, seven separate randomized phase III studies failed to show survival benefit. Chemoembolization has, therefore, become a sort of last-resort therapy for patients who have liver-dominant disease and have failed to respond to systemic chemotherapy. Enrolling patients with such a deadly disease into clinical trials to demonstrate the worth of chemoembolization is, thus, understandably difficult. Tellez et al.[106] conducted a phase II clinical trial in which 30 patients with colorectal metastases to the liver were treated with chemoembolization. Median survival was 9 months after the initiation of chemoembolization and 29 months after the initial diagnosis of liver metastasis was made. In the largest study to date involving 52 patients, Daniels et al.[107] reported a 78% response rate using biologic criteria (decrease in carcinoembryonic antigen) accompanied by median survival of 11 months from the time of treatment. Despite evidence of promising response rates with chemoembolization, the survival benefit of the procedure is still in question. Only well-designed randomized clinical trials comparing chemoembolization to systemic chemotherapy can answer this question. Such a multicenter trial is now under way in the United States.

Percutaneous Ethanol Injection

Since 1983, when it was first described,[108] percutaneous ethanol injection has been used primarily against unresectable hepatoma[109–121] and occasionally against colorectal metastases.[111,122,123] Ethanol diffuses into the tumor cells, where it causes cellular dehydration and induces coagulative necrosis.[108–110] Ethanol is more effective against hepatoma lesions because they are usually softer than colorectal lesions, thus allowing greater diffusion of the ethanol throughout the tumor.[109,110] Although no specific limitations to the size or number of lesions exists, percutaneous ethanol injection is most effective against tumors measuring less than 3 cm in diameter[109–121] in patients with three or fewer lesions.[113,114,116] The presence of multifocal or diffuse hepatoma, extrahepatic metastases, or severe coagulopathy constitutes absolute contraindications to treatment with percutaneous ethanol.[109–121]

The procedure is usually performed under ultrasonography or CT guidance. A 20- to 22-gauge needle is inserted directly into the tumor, and tumor volume (estimated from the formula on the volume of a sphere) is then calculated to determine the exact amount of ethanol required (Fig. 27.4-6). Once adequate needle placement is confirmed, sterile 95% absolute ethanol is slowly infused. The total volume of ethanol to be injected is determined by the size of the tumor.[124] Volumes of 30 to 40 ml are usually required for tumors greater than 3 cm.[111,125,126] As ethanol diffuses throughout the tumor, the tumor becomes hyperechoic on ultrasonography owing to the presence of microbubbles within the ethanol. Nontarget injection into blood vessels or biliary ducts must be avoided. The procedure can be performed over multiple sessions if necessary, depending on the size of the tumor and the number of lesions to treat. Typically, 4 to 12 sessions are required to treat solitary lesions measuring less than 5 cm. Because the proce-

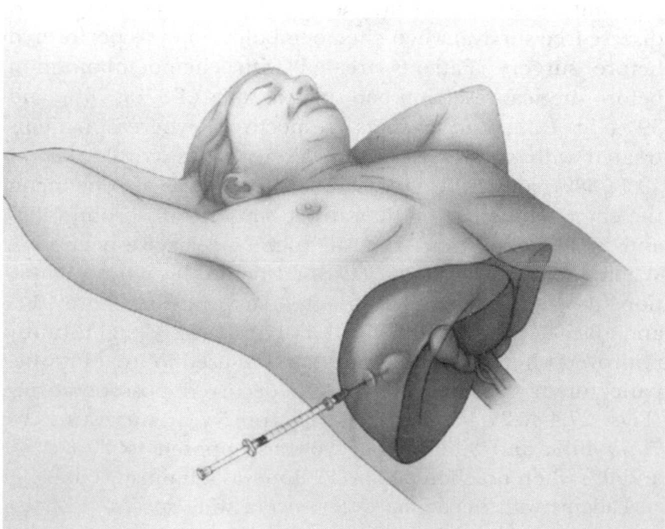

FIGURE 27.4-6. Percutaneous ethanol injection into liver tumor. (Courtesy of Matrix Pharmaceutical, Inc., Fremont, CA.)

dure is minimally invasive and highly specific to the tumor, the normal liver is usually preserved. These features render percutaneous ethanol injection especially attractive in the setting of advanced liver disease. Postprocedure imaging and tumor markers should be obtained at 1 month and then every 4 to 6 months to assess tumor response and potential recurrence. Side effects from the procedure, such as localized pain at the injection site, fever, and alcohol intoxication, are highly variable and can usually be managed conservatively.[109,112,121] Pleural effusion and intraperitoneal hemorrhage are the most commonly reported serious complications but are still very uncommon. In fact, the incidence of severe complications remains less than 2%.[109,111,121]

Large series mostly from Japan and Italy (where percutaneous ethanol injection is most commonly used) have demonstrated that percutaneous ethanol injection can be very effective against hepatoma.[109–126] These studies have also helped to establish clear prognostic factors, such as the number of lesions, tumor size, and the degree of underlying liver disease that have a direct impact on long-term survival rates. In the largest series to date (746 patients) published by Livraghi et al.,[109] survival at 1, 3, and 5 years was 99%, 86%, and 48%, respectively, in patients with a solitary lesion measuring less than 5 cm and minimal underlying liver disease. On the other hand, survival in patients with larger tumors and more severe underlying liver disease fell sharply to 64% at 1 year, 12% at 2 years, and 0 thereafter. Ishii et al.[127] reported similar results in 177 patients with 348 lesions measuring less than 4 cm. Survival rates were 97%, 71%, and 30% at 1, 3, and 5 years, respectively. Another factor that influences survival is the AFP level. Lencioni et al.[128] found long-term survival to be inversely proportional to the initial AFP levels. Percutaneous ethanol injection is, therefore, most potent and effective when used against solitary and small lesions (<3 cm) rather than multiple and large lesions. In addition, patients with the least underlying liver disease fare best in terms of long-term survival.[109–128]

When comparison between percutaneous ethanol injection and supportive care or surgery was made, survival rates achieved with percutaneous ethanol injection were found to be markedly better than those obtained with supportive care and nearly equal to those obtained at surgery. These studies, although retrospective and thus not randomized, attempted to closely match patients between groups based on tumor size, number of lesions, and underlying liver condition. For example, Livraghi et al.[129] found no significant difference in 3-year survival between ethanol injection (79%) and surgical resection (71%) in 391 patients who all had a solitary lesion measuring less than 5 cm. Similar results were reported by Castells et al.[120] who compared clinical outcomes between surgery and ethanol injection in 63 patients with solitary lesions measuring up to 4 cm. Patients treated with ethanol injection had overall survival rates at 1 and 4 years (83% and 34%) nearly equal to those treated with surgical resection (81% and 44%). The high rate of recurrence, which typically varies between 64% and 98% within a 5-year period and is actually similar to recurrence rate after surgery, constitutes a nagging problem.[109,130–132] However, when recurrence does occur, these tumors can be treated repeatedly with ethanol injection (unlike surgery) without damaging liver functions.

The effects of percutaneous ethanol injection and chemoembolization on liver tumors can be synergistically enhanced when the two techniques are combined. Several recent reports have demonstrated the efficacy and potential benefits of such tandem therapy. In a study by Lencioni et al.,[133] 86 patients with mild cirrhosis and a large hepatoma (3 to 8 cm in diameter) were treated with a single cycle of chemoembolization followed by percutaneous ethanol injection. Survival rates were 92% at 1 year, 70% at 3 years, and 47% at 5 years. Tanaka et al.[134] reported 100% and 75% survivals at 3 and 5 years, respectively, in patients with a 3- to 5-cm solitary hepatoma lesion and minimal cirrhosis. Finally, Allgaier et al.[68] compared percutaneous ethanol alone to combined administration of ethanol and chemoembolization and found that patients treated with both therapies had significantly better outcome than those treated with ethanol alone.

Percutaneous ethanol injection has been much less successful against colorectal metastases, and its role in managing these lesions remains, therefore, limited. Recent studies showed that ethanol achieved only 50% necrosis, presumably because of the hard nature of colorectal metastases, which limits the diffusion of ethanol throughout the tumor.[122,123] The impact of ethanol therapy on survival was also somewhat disappointing, as 3-year survival only reached 39%.[122,123]

Percutaneous Radiofrequency Ablation

Radiofrequency ablation, used percutaneously or intraoperatively, offers an alternative method of local tissue destruction by coagulative necrosis. This technique causes frictional heat within the tissue. When the temperature reaches 41°C, a cytotoxic effect is produced, but when the temperature reaches 90°C, immediate coagulative necrosis takes place.[135] The monopolar design of the radiofrequency probe, which could deliver heat only to a small area and, thus, severely restricted the area of tissue destruction, constituted an early limitation of this technique.[136,137] Since then, the design of the probe has been changed to a multipolar one, and extensive research in animals has also been performed to maximize the destructive effects of the probe and increase the volume of tissue necrosis. However, problems inherent to the properties of radiofrequency ablation persist, such as the influence of nearby vessels on heat generation (large vessels can act as a heat sink and prevent the generation of enough heat to destroy the tumor) as well as the creation of excessive heat, which can cause tumor charring.

The procedure is usually performed under ultrasonography or CT guidance (Fig. 27.4-7*A*), and the technical steps are similar to those used for percutaneous ethanol injection. The radiofrequency needle, which generally varies between a 15- and 18-gauge needle, is inserted into the tumor (see Fig. 27.4-7*B, C*). Once within the lesion, multiple electrodes are deployed, and the generator is activated to reach a temperature of 90° to 110°C. Treatment may last up to 15 minutes. The probe can then be moved to a different region of the tumor before further activation of the radiofrequency probe. Complications are rare and, despite a few reported cases of peritoneal hemorrhage, pleural effusion, and fever, the procedure is generally well tolerated.[138–140] Follow-up imaging is similar to that of percutaneous ethanol injection (1 month after procedure and 3 to 4 months thereafter).

Since radiofrequency ablation is a relatively new technique—its use in patients was first described by Rossi[136] in 1993—its impact on long-term survival has not yet been assessed. However,

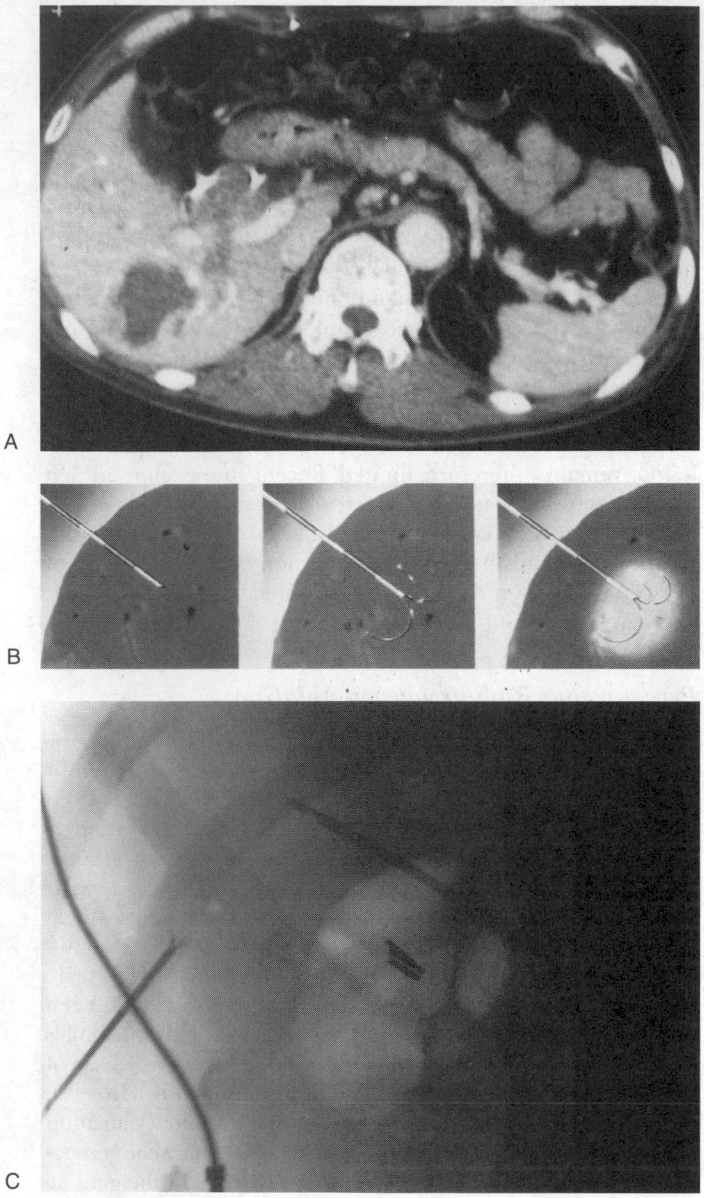

FIGURE 27.4-7. Radiofrequency ablation in a patient with a solitary hepatocellular carcinoma. **A:** Computed tomography scan of the abdomen demonstrates a low-density lesion located in the posterior segment of the right lobe. **B:** Illustration of the radiofrequency probe being advanced into the tumor. **C:** Radiograph of the patient in (**A**), with the probe deployed within the tumor.

several recent studies have shown promising results. Solbiati et al.[139] treated 16 patients with liver metastases of various sizes. Near complete necrosis (80%) was achieved in 84% of lesions, 2-year survival reached 66%, and lesions measuring less than 3 cm responded best to treatment. Livraghi et al.[138] compared percutaneous ethanol injection to radiofrequency ablation in 86 patients with 122 small (≤3 cm) hepatomas. Radiofrequency ablation achieved a greater rate of necrosis (90%) and required fewer treatment sessions (1.2 sessions) than percutaneous ethanol injection (80% necrosis and 4.8 sessions). In addition, these preliminary studies suggest a lower recurrence rate than with percutaneous ethanol injection. In a recent article, Curley et al.[141] used intraoperative radiofrequency ablation to treat primary and metastatic liver lesions and reported the lowest recurrence rate (1.8%) for any sizable clinical series using radiofrequency ablative technique. Such results have yet to be duplicated. Although the data remain scarce and its impact on survival is undetermined, radiofrequency ablation may have a role to play against small primary or metastatic lesions.

Other Techniques

A number of other methods are currently under investigation. These techniques are performed percutaneously and consist of delivering thermal energy via various sources into tumor tissue. They include percutaneous hot saline injection, interstitial laser photocoagulation, percutaneous microwave coagulation, and high-intensity focused ultrasonography. None has shown great promise over the other currently available therapeutic options used to treat liver cancer.

Another method, consisting of direct injection of cisplatin gel into the tumor, offers a radically new approach to the treatment of liver cancer. The injectable gel is actually composed of cisplatin, epinephrine, and a protein carrier matrix, which confers unique diffusion properties to the mixture. The gel is injected percutaneously into the tumor under ultrasonographic or CT guidance and can be used for tumors measuring up to 7 cm in diameter (Fig. 27.4-8). This treatment is currently undergoing a multicenter phase II clinical trial to assess its efficacy against hepatoma in the United States, Europe, and Asia. Early results are promising both in terms of tumor necrosis and impact on survival.[142]

CANCERS OF THE BILIARY TRACT AND PANCREAS

Cancers of the biliary tract, which include gallbladder and bile duct carcinoma or cholangiocarcinoma, are the second most

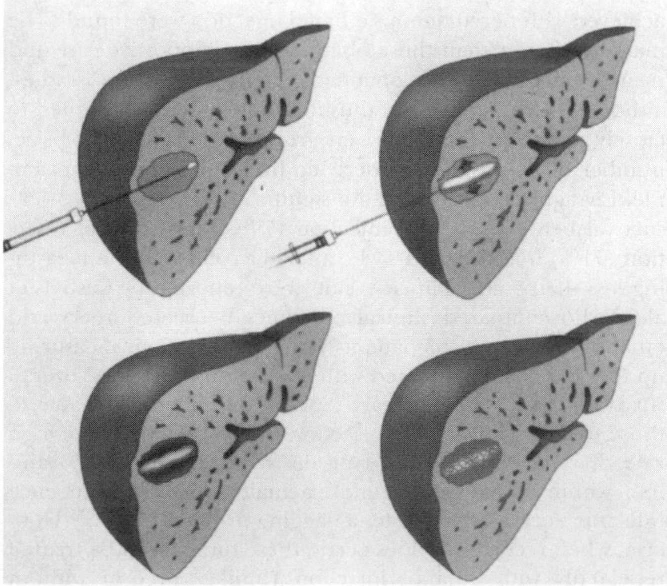

FIGURE 27.4-8. Percutaneous administration of cisplatinum gel (Intra Dose) into a liver tumor. (Courtesy of Matrix Pharmaceutical, Inc., Fremont, CA.)

common primary hepatobiliary cancers after hepatocellular carcinoma.[143] Cholangiocarcinoma is more common in men, whereas gallbladder carcinoma is seen more frequently in women.[144] These differences can be explained by the higher incidence of sclerosing cholangitis in men and gallstones in women, which are well-known risk factors for cholangiocarcinoma and gallbladder carcinoma, respectively.[144] Although gallbladder carcinoma is encountered twice as frequently as cholangiocarcinoma (7500 vs. 2000 to 3000 new cases per year), most patients requiring interventional radiology procedures experience cholangiocarcinoma.[143]

Cholangiocarcinoma is a slow-growing tumor with a peak incidence in the sixth and seventh decades. The tumor is notorious for invading the liver parenchyma as well as hepatic arteries and portal venous system, which renders surgical resection especially difficult.[145] As a result of its infiltrating growth pattern within the biliary ductal system,[146–148] patients with cholangiocarcinoma usually present with symptoms (jaundice, pruritus, and color-altered stools and urine) caused by obstruction of the biliary tree.[149,150] When the tumor involves the common hepatic duct, the common bile duct, or the ampulla, symptoms will occur early in the course of the disease. On the other hand, when the tumor involves the perihilar region, which is the most common area of tumor involvement (approximately two-thirds of the cases), the occurrence of symptoms may be delayed significantly. Other symptoms, such as pain, fatigue, general malaise, and weight loss, are typically seen in advanced disease. Surgical resection is the only therapeutic option associated with improved survival in patients with cholangiocarcinoma. Systemic chemotherapy and external-beam radiotherapy have not significantly improved survival or quality of life.[151] Therefore, palliative therapy plays a critical role in the management of patients who are not surgical candidates.

Carcinoma of the exocrine pancreas carries a dismal prognosis, with median survival from time of diagnosis approaching 6 months.[152] There are no curative treatments, and even surgery, which can be performed only in 10% to 20% of patients with pancreatic carcinoma, does not appear to increase survival.[152] Thus, as for cholangiocarcinoma, the need for effective palliation is critical.

The diagnosis of cholangiocarcinoma or pancreatic carcinoma is usually established by cross-sectional imaging (ultrasonography and CT scanning). Diagnostic visceral angiography and cholangiography are reserved for determining tumor resectability. Depending on the location of the tumor, cholangiography can be performed from a percutaneous transhepatic or an endoscopic approach. The cholangiographic appearance of cholangiocarcinoma is again directly related to the infiltrating-scirrhous nature of its growth pattern.[146–148,153] Thus, cholangiocarcinoma generally presents as a focal stricture, often without a mass,[153] which may mimic sclerosing cholangitis if tumor involvement is diffuse (Fig. 27.4-9).[146] The cholangiographic appearance of pancreatic carcinoma is similar to that of cholangiocarcinoma with a short and irregular stricture, resembling a rat tail, causing massive biliary ductal dilatation (Fig. 27.4-10).[154] Access into the biliary tree also provides an avenue for collection of biopsy samples, which can be extremely useful to differentiate benign from malignant disease. This diagnostic technique is especially useful to distinguish biliary ductal strictures caused by pancreatic carcinoma from those due to pancreatitis.[42] However, in the case of bile

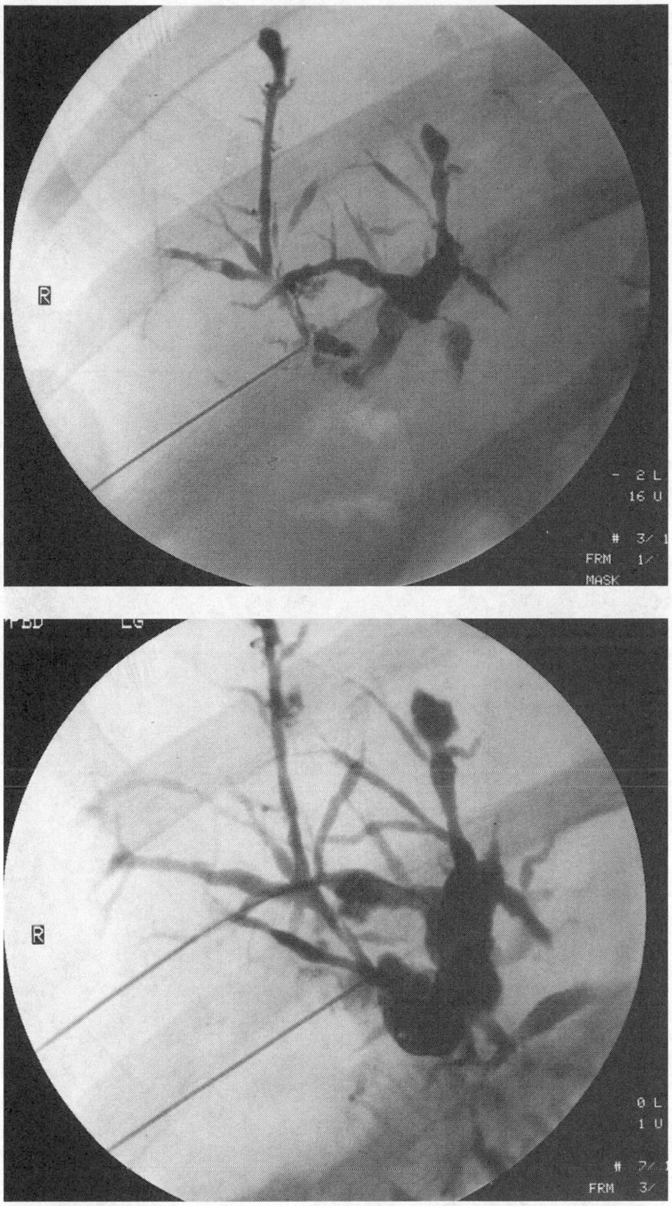

A

B

FIGURE 27.4-9. Percutaneous transhepatic cholangiogram in a patient with diffuse cholangiocarcinoma resembling the appearance of sclerosing cholangitis. **A:** Initial cholangiogram. **B:** Magnified view of the biliary system as the guidewire is being advanced into the biliary tree to secure access.

duct tumors, establishing a definitive diagnosis of cholangiocarcinoma can be difficult owing to the intense desmoplastic reaction that the tumor generates.[155,156] The use of brush biopsies and cytologic examination has increased the diagnostic yield to approximately 40% to 70%.[42,155,156]

The goal of palliative therapy is to relieve the symptoms associated with biliary tract obstruction. This can be accomplished via endoscopic placement of plastic stents or via percutaneous transhepatic placement of internal-external biliary drains or metallic stents. Given the less invasive nature of endoscopic techniques, endoscopic stent placement is preferred as the first line of therapy, especially when the tumor involves the extrahepatic biliary tree, and is successful in 80% to 90% of the

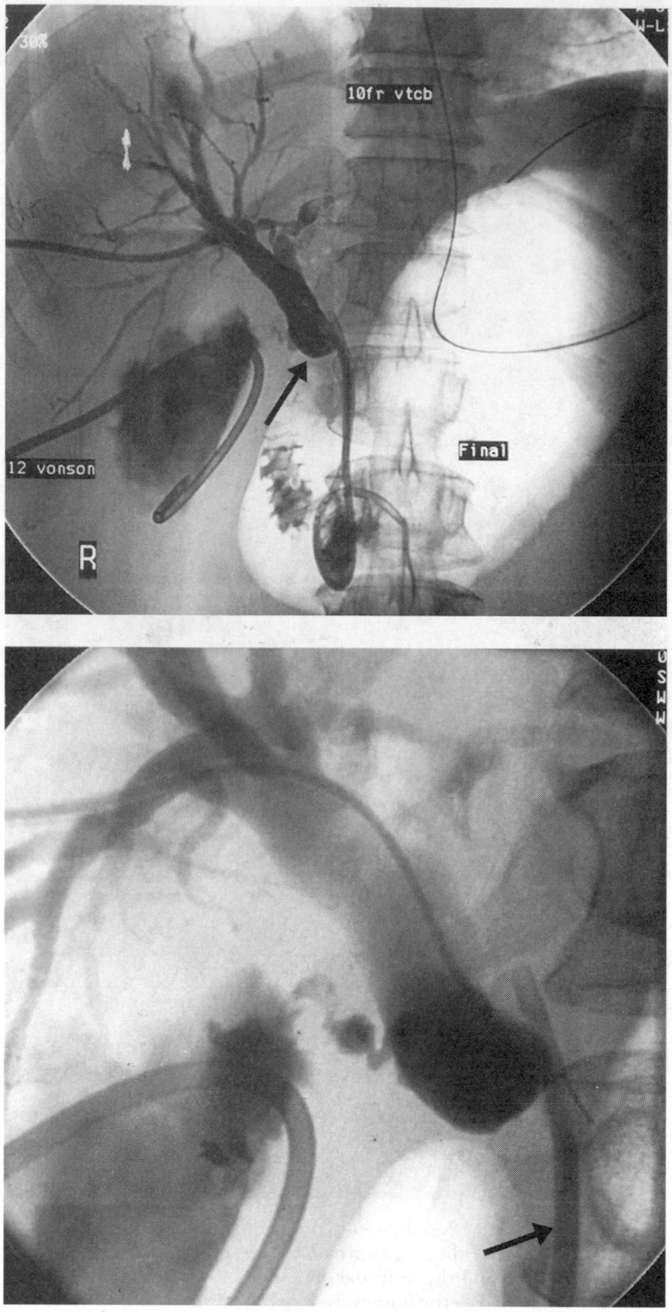

A

B

FIGURE 27.4-10. Percutaneous transhepatic cholangiogram in a patient with pancreatic adenocarcinoma. **A:** Complete obstruction of the common hepatic duct (*arrow*). An internal-external biliary stent has been successfully placed across the obstruction. **B:** Magnification view of the common hepatic duct as the guidewire is being manipulated across the stricture. Note the occluded endoscopically placed plastic stent (*arrow*).

cases.[151,157,158] However, it is usual for these endoscopic stents to become occluded fairly quickly after placement, thus requiring frequent stent replacement (approximately every 3 months).

Percutaneous transhepatic biliary drainage is the procedure of choice in cases of unsuccessful endoscopic stent placement, prior biliary-enteric surgical reconstruction, or high level of biliary obstruction (i.e., above the confluence of the ductal systems). In some centers, such as the Johns Hopkins Hospital, percutaneous biliary drainage is also routinely performed preoperatively to facilitate surgical reconstruction of the biliary tract.[159–163] Indeed, these biliary drainage catheters aid in the creation of biliary-enteric anastomoses by providing anatomic landmarks of the intra- and extrahepatic biliary ducts during surgery, which can be particularly helpful in patients with extensive tumor involvement. Several studies have shown that preoperative percutaneous biliary drainage reduces operative time as well as operative morbidity and mortality.[159–163] One of the critical benefits offered by percutaneous biliary drainage remains the possibility of rapid intervention to decompress the biliary tree (Fig. 27.4-11). The procedure can even be life-saving in cases of acute cholangitis or biliary sepsis. Reestablishment of bile flow usually causes rapid recovery of hepatic function, with decrease in liver enzymes, which in turn leads to relief in patient's symptomatology and improvement in overall health of the patient.[164] Percutaneous biliary drainage can also relieve obstruction in patients with occluded endoscopically placed plastic stents. These stents either can be removed percutaneously (snare technique) (Fig. 27.4-12) or can be pushed into the small bowel (Fig. 27.4-13*A*). Once access into the biliary tree is secured, either internal-external biliary stents or permanent self-expanding metallic internal stents (see Fig. 27.4-13*B*) can be placed to maintain biliary-enteric flow.[151]

Internal-external biliary stents are preferred if surgical resection or debulking of the tumor is contemplated, because they provide immediate access to the surgical site for evaluation of possible complications during the perioperative period and prevent stricture formation at the biliary-enteric anastomosis, which can occur during the late postoperative period. Internal-external biliary stents offer several other advantages, such as allowing for the careful monitoring at the surgical site for possible tumor recurrence in those patients who underwent curative surgery and the exchange of stents when they become occluded. In fact, patients with internal-external stents generally have to undergo routine biliary tube changes every 2 to 3 months to maintain biliary-enteric flow and prevent biliary sepsis. On the other hand, placement of permanent metallic stents is recommended for patients with a limited life expectancy and for whom no surgical options exist.[165] Debilitated or nursing-home patients who cannot care for their internal-external biliary tubes should also be treated with permanent stents if at all possible. These patients usually experience marked improvement in their quality of life owing to the absence of external tubes and their associated risk of skin infection, pericatheter bile leakage, and catheter obstruction or dislodgment. Metallic stents can be deployed atraumatically, since they go through small delivery systems. Once released from the guiding catheter, they self-expand to reach a diameter approximately three times that of plastic stents. Thus, with their larger diameter and inherent radial expansile force, metallic self-expanding stents are favored over endoscopic plastic stents because they tend to stay open longer than endoscopic stents (see Fig. 27.4-13*B*). Several series by Boguth et al.,[166] Schima et al.,[165] and others have reported patency rates for metallic stents of approximately 6 months.[165–169] In addition, metallic stents are very flexible, rendering them especially well suited for tortuous courses. This is particularly useful when the tumor involves the confluence of hepatic ducts (Klatskin tumor). In such cases, massive dilatation of both the right and left intrahepatic bile ducts occurs, and

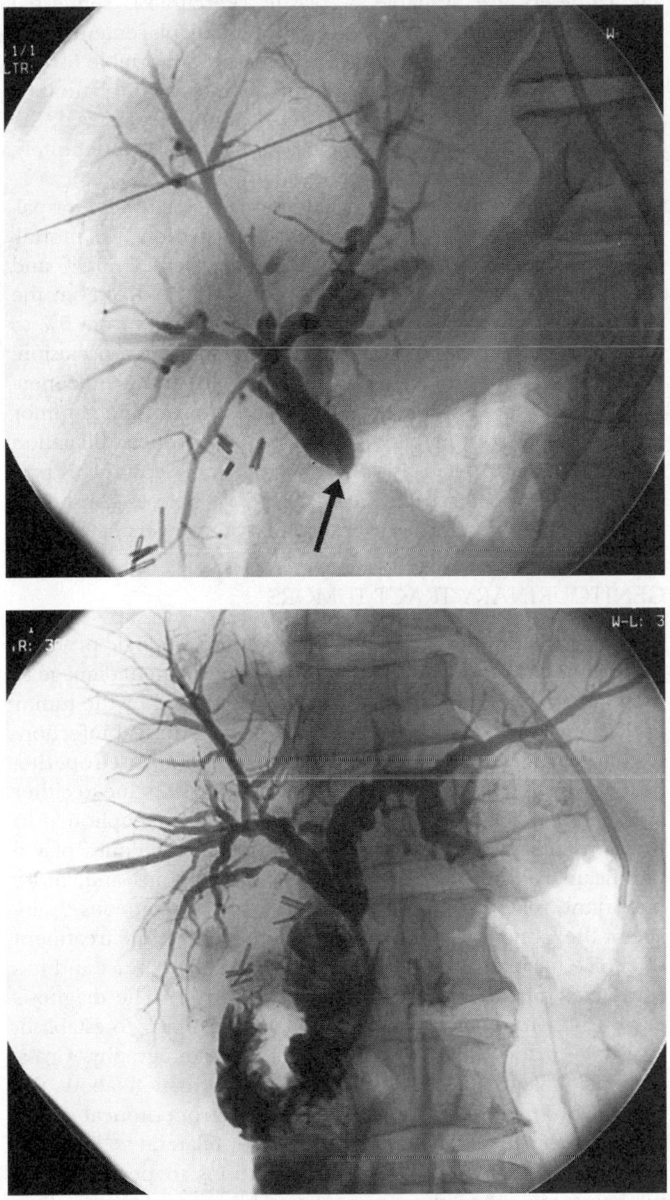

A

B

FIGURE 27.4-11. Percutaneous transhepatic biliary drainage performed emergently secondary to biliary sepsis. **A:** Initial cholangiogram demonstrates complete obstruction of the biliary tree due to cholangiocarcinoma located at the confluence of the hepatic ducts (Klatskin tumor) (*arrow*). **B:** Successful biliary drainage across the obstruction. The patient improved clinically.

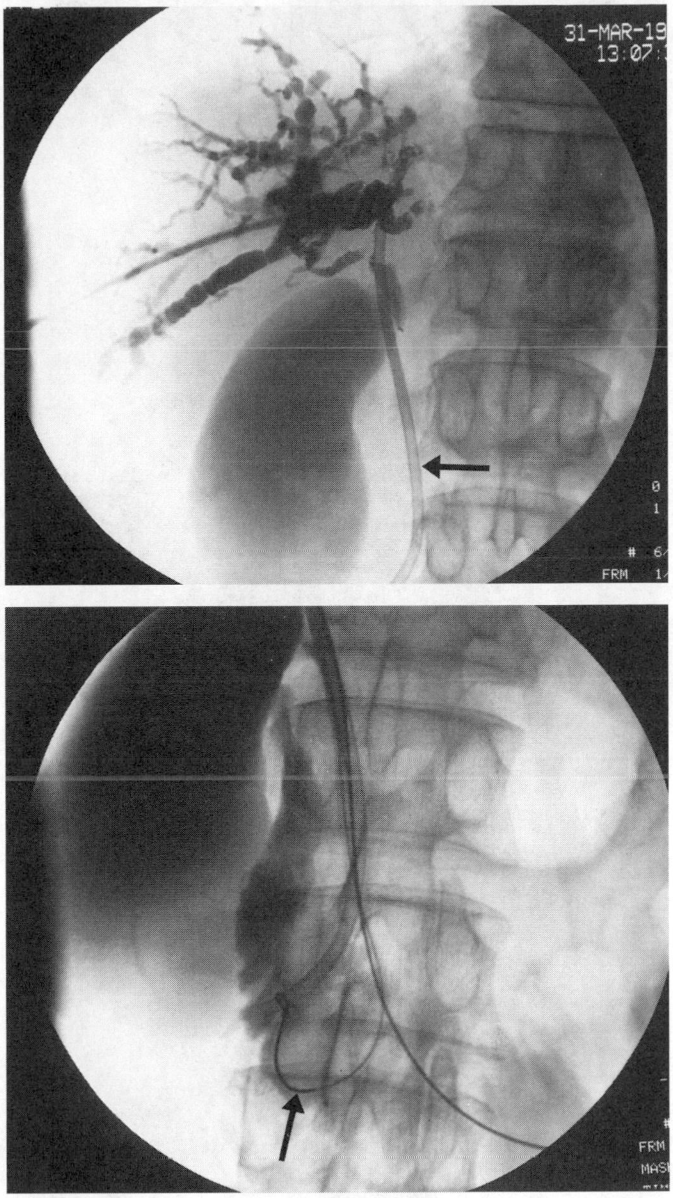

A

B

FIGURE 27.4-12. Percutaneous transhepatic cholangiogram in a patient with pancreatic adenocarcinoma. **A:** Initial cholangiogram demonstrates complete obstruction of the biliary tree. The endostent placed endoscopically is occluded (*arrow*). **B:** Using a snare (*arrow*), the endostent is removed percutaneously (*arrow*).

bilateral access into the biliary tree is necessary to properly relieve the obstruction. Effective palliation with internal stents can then be provided only by self-expanding, flexible stents deployed from above the level of obstruction and extending into the common hepatic duct.[165–169]

Patients scheduled to undergo percutaneous biliary drainage should receive prophylactic broad-spectrum antibiotic coverage, and any coagulopathy should be corrected. Percutaneous transhepatic cholangiography is first performed via a 22-gauge needle inserted from a right midaxillary line. Contrast opacification of the biliary tree provides invaluable information about the nature, location, and extent of the obstructing tumor. After having successfully delineated the anatomy of the biliary tree, a duct within the right posterior ductal system is selected based on its position and course relative to the location of the tumor and accessed using a slightly larger needle (21-gauge). A guidewire is then advanced through the needle into the biliary tree to secure access into the biliary system. Steerable guidewires are then used to cross the obstruction and, thus, gain access into the duodenum. To maintain adequate biliary-enteric flow, a multi-side-hole catheter is placed across the obstruction, with side holes above and below the obstruction. The tube is typically left to external drainage for 12 to 24 hours before it is capped and functions as an internal drainage catheter. Two major types of biliary drain-

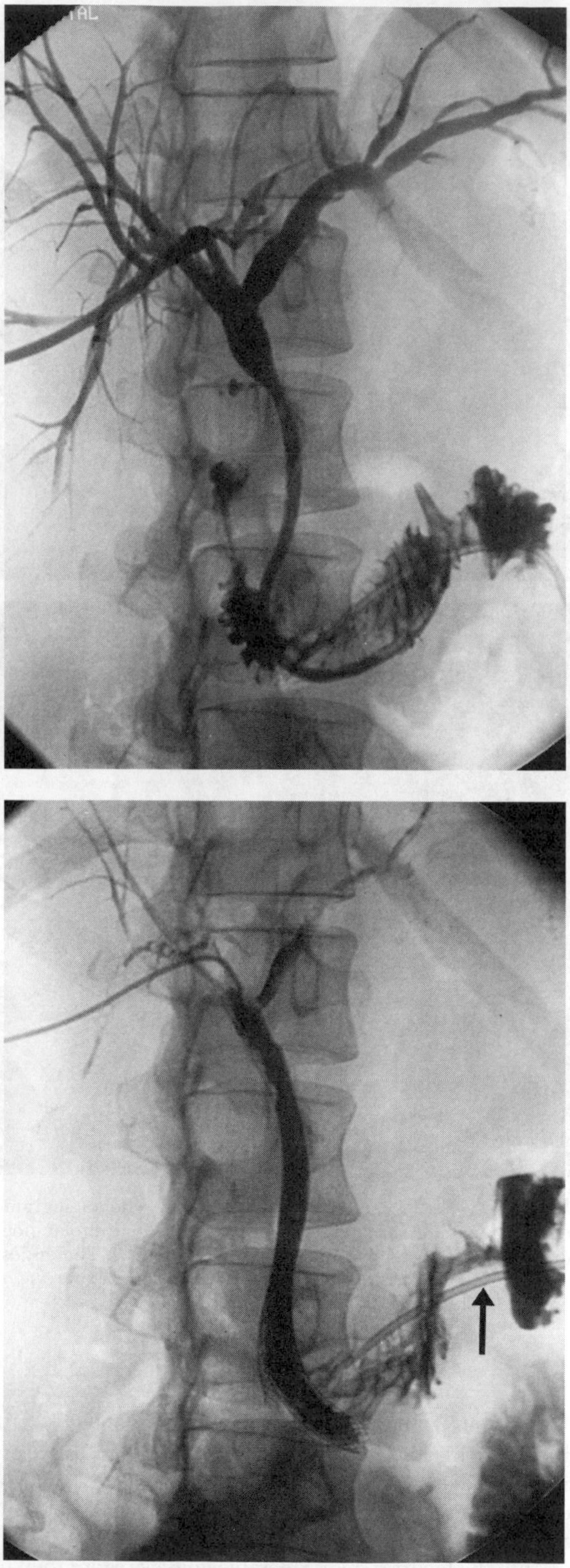

A

B

FIGURE 27.4-13. Placement of a permanent metallic self-expanding biliary stent (Wallstent) in a patient with pancreatic adenocarcinoma. The tumor was found to be unresectable, and the decision was made, therefore, to place a metallic stent. **A:** Successful percutaneous biliary drainage demonstrating the classic appearance of pancreatic adenocarcinoma. **B:** Successful permanent stent placement. Note that the endoscopic stent was pushed into the small bowel (*arrow*).

age catheters are available, a plastic (Percuflex), somewhat stiffer catheter, which is necessary for initial placement, or a softer, silastic catheter, which is much more comfortable for the patient and is generally favored if long-term intubation is required. If access into the duodenum cannot be achieved, the biliary tube must be connected to a drainage bag indefinitely, and oral bile salt replacement must be initiated.

Percutaneous transhepatic biliary drainage performed for palliation is markedly safer than surgical decompression. The mortality rate associated with biliary drainage varies between 0.5% and 3%, as opposed to 20% to 30% for surgery.[170–173] However, the complication rate is not insignificant, since it ranges from 5% to 25%. The most common complications include tube occlusion, tube dislodgment, cholangitis-sepsis, hemobilia, and pseudoaneurysm. Biliary tubes become occluded because of continued tumor growth, blood clots, or bile. As a result, biliary ductal dilatation ensues, leading to bile stasis and cholangitis or sepsis. This process, which has been reported to occur in 23% of cases, constitutes the major indication for performing biliary tube exchange.

GENITOURINARY TRACT TUMORS

Obstruction of the urinary tract is a common urologic problem that requires prompt intervention to avoid permanent damage to the kidney.[174–178] Renal obstruction may be caused by the tumor itself (transitional cell carcinoma), blood clots, fungal infection, fibrotic changes that can occur after radiotherapy, retroperitoneal fibrosis (Fig. 27.4-14), or extrinsic compression due to either enlarged lymph nodes or a tumor mass, such as lymphoma. In these instances, percutaneous interventional techniques play a significant role to alleviate some of the symptoms and, more important, relieve the obstruction. In fact, percutaneous drainage of the kidney or percutaneous nephrostomy is the treatment of choice for malignant obstruction of the urinary tract and has completely replaced surgical nephrostomy.[174–178] The diagnosis of obstruction, which can be somewhat challenging to establish, is usually made with CT scanning or ultrasonography. Cross-sectional imaging studies also provide information about the level of obstruction, the anatomy of the retroperitoneal space, and whether the obstruction is unilateral or bilateral.[174–178]

There are no absolute contraindications to percutaneous nephrostomy other than noncorrectable coagulopathy. Prophylactic antibiotic therapy should be administered before the procedure and continued for at least 24 hours after the procedure. However, in cases of known pyonephrosis or urinary sepsis, antibiotic therapy should be continued for 5 to 7 days. Whether performed under CT, ultrasonography, or fluoroscopy guidance, the goal of the procedure remains the same and consists of gaining access into the renal collecting system via a posterior calyx. Entering the kidney via the posterior calyx is critical to avoid major bleeding complications, since the posterior calyx is less well vascularized than the other calyces. Once the needle is placed within the posterior calyx, an antegrade nephrostogram is performed to define the nature of the obstructing lesion and determine the precise level and extent of the obstruction or stricture. A small-caliber guidewire is then inserted through the needle to secure access into the renal collecting system. Eventually, after successive dilatation of the tract, a pigtail-type nephrostomy catheter is placed and locked into position within the renal pelvis. Initially, a small catheter (8 to 10 Fr.) is typically placed, but it can be safely up-sized to a

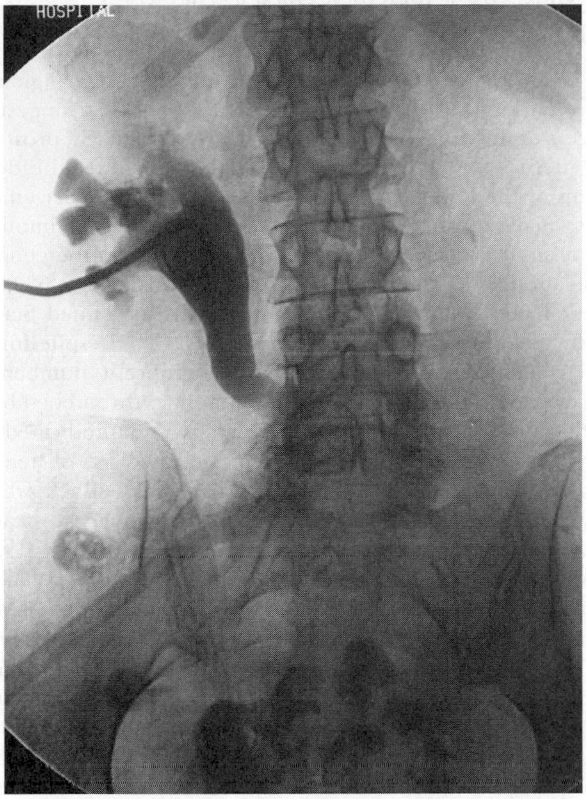

FIGURE 27.4-14. Successful percutaneous nephrostomy in a patient with retroperitoneal fibrosis. The antegrade nephrostogram demonstrates complete obstruction at the level of the proximal ureter.

larger caliber catheter (up to 16 Fr.) if necessary. The nephrostomy catheter usually requires minimal care and drains the urine directly into an external drainage bag, which should be emptied three to six times per day, depending on urine output. Since nephrostomy catheters provide adequate urinary decompression, they can be used indefinitely in chronically obstructed patients without damaging the kidney or altering renal function (see Fig. 27.4-14). However, conversion to a nephroureteral stent, which extends from the renal pelvis through the ureter into the bladder, is desirable and should be attempted whenever possible. The main advantage of nephroureteral stents is that they can function as an internal-external system similar to that described in the biliary system and, therefore, do not require an external bag. These stents can be used only if the obstruction is successfully crossed and require a functioning bladder or reconstructed bladder, such as an ileal loop.[179] The main portion of the stent is located within the patient, and the small portion of catheter residing outside the patient is usually capped off. Multiple side holes exist throughout the entire length of the catheter, allowing urine to bypass the obstruction and collect in the bladder. If fever or flank pain develops, it usually indicates stent occlusion. In such cases, the stent can first be externalized (by attaching a drainage bag) to relieve the symptoms prior to exchanging it for a new one. Common indications for the placement of nephroureteral stents include (1) ureteral strictures, which may develop after pelvic or retroperitoneal surgery or radiotherapy or at the anastomosis after creation of a neobladder and ureteral reimplantation; (2) ureteral fistulae; (3) healing of ureteral injuries postoperatively or after radiotherapy; and (4) reestablishment of urine flow from kidney to bladder in patients with urinary tract obstruction scheduled for definitive surgical repair.[179,180]

Internal-external nephroureteral stents can also be converted to internal double-J nephroureteral stents. These internal stents can be placed from a percutaneous approach via the kidney or from a cystoscopic approach. They offer the advantage of being entirely within the patient, thus relieving the patient of any catheter care and reducing the risk of local or systemic infection. On the other hand, when occluded, they are much more difficult to exchange than internal-external stents. Placement of double-J stents is mostly indicated when long-term drainage of the urinary system is required, such as patients with unresectable malignant urinary tract obstruction, or ureteral injury from surgery or radiotherapy. Internal stents should also be used when patients cannot tolerate or care for them.

Percutaneous nephrostomy is performed successfully in 85% to 98% of the cases and is generally well tolerated, with an incidence of major complications ranging from 4% to 6%. The mortality rate is low (0.2%) as opposed to that of surgical nephrostomy (6%). The most common complications are due to massive hemorrhage requiring surgical treatment or transcatheter embolotherapy (1%), pneumothorax (1%), and peritonitis.[171–178] Minor complications occur in 10% to 28% of the cases and include microscopic or gross hematuria, which usually clears within 24 to 48 hours, unsuspected retroperitoneal or perirenal hematoma, extravasation of urine (<2%), and infection (1.4% to 21%). Infection can be caused by inadequate drainage due to occlusion of the catheter secondary to encrustations or a preexisting urinary tract infection. Flushing the catheter routinely with normal saline solution is useful in preventing catheter occlusion. Finally, if the catheter becomes dislodged, the track should stay open for 72 hours, thus allowing successful reaccess into the renal collecting system.

SUPERIOR VENA CAVA SYNDROME

Venous thrombosis or occlusion is not an uncommon occurrence in cancer patients. It may be due to direct tumor involvement, extrinsic compression by tumor, or lymphadenopathy, fibrosis secondary to radiotherapy, or long-term indwelling central venous catheters, which are often needed for systemic chemotherapy or nutritional support.[181–185] The central veins, such as the subclavian, inominate, SVC, and IVC, are most commonly affected. The severity of symptoms is directly related to the degree of venous obstruction. In the SVC syndrome, most often caused by lung carcinoma with extension into the mediastinum, symptoms are often dramatic. Patients typically present with swelling of the face and neck as well as dilated collateral venous channels readily visible coursing throughout the upper thorax.[181–185] If the degree of obstruction is severe, additional symptoms may be encountered, such as respiratory distress, edema of the conjunctiva, and neurologic disturbances.[181–185] Radiotherapy is the treatment of choice for SVC syndrome, and most patients respond well to therapy.[186] However, when radiotherapy is unsuccessful (failure to clear symptoms, recurrence of symptoms, or presence of benign postirradiation fibrotic changes), percutaneous venous interventions, such as percutaneous transluminal angioplasty or stenting, become the treatment of last resort.[186,187] A diagnostic study, such as central venogram or magnetic resonance venography should first be performed to delineate the extent of the thrombosed or stenosed segment of SVC (Fig. 27.4-15*A*). If concurrent thrombosis of the SVC is present, catheter-directed thrombolytic therapy can be used to reduce the clot burden and allow for better evaluation of the unmasked underlying stenosis. Once the stenosis is successfully crossed, angioplasty of the stenosis is usually first performed (see Fig. 27.4-15*B*). Although some success has been reported with angioplasty alone,[188,189] the recurrence or failure rate after percutaneous transluminal angioplasty is quite high because of the elastic recoil that takes place secondary to the compressing tumor or fibrosis. Therefore, stenting has become the most reliable method of establishing venous continuity. Two types of stent, a self-expandable and a balloon expandable, exist for this purpose. Because of its expansile radial force, the self-expandable stent is more commonly used (Fig. 27.4-16). Improvement in patients' symptomatology may be dramatic and usually occurs within 24 hours of therapy, with complete resolution taking place within 3 days.[184,186,187,190–192] Complications include stent migration or thrombosis and vessel injury or perforation during placement.

Although the technical success rate approaches 100%, long-term results are difficult to evaluate since many of these patients have advanced malignant disease and a limited life expectancy. Percutaneous venous stenting should, therefore, be regarded as a palliative therapy and a successful outcome viewed as a patent SVC at the time of death.

PULMONARY THROMBOEMBOLIC DISEASE AND INFERIOR VENA CAVA FILTERS

The association between venous thrombosis and malignancy has been known for more than a century and is strongest in cancers of the lung, breast, pancreas, colon, stomach, prostate, and uterus.[193–196] When venous thrombosis involves the deep system of the lower extremities, the risk of pulmonary embolism is markedly increased. In fact, the incidence of pulmonary embolism in cancer patients is three times that in the general population.[193–197] There are approximately 570,000 to 630,000 cases of pulmonary embolism annually in the United States, nearly one-third of which are fatal events.[198,199] Despite initial management with anticoagulation, a significant number of cancer patients develop recurrent pulmonary thromboemboli. Furthermore, anticoagulation therapy is contraindicated in many cancer patients because of the associated risk of hemorrhage. It is for these reasons that the use of IVC filters, which prevent thrombi from reaching the lungs, is strongly advocated in cancer patients.[197–203]

Multiple IVC filter designs are commercially available, including the Greenfield stainless steel and titanium filters, the Vena-Tech, the Simon Nitinol, and the Bird's Nest. These filters can be deployed from a femoral or internal jugular approach. A venogram is first performed to measure the diameter of the IVC, to determine the location of the renal veins, and to detect the presence of potential thrombus within the IVC. Filters should be placed immediately below the lowermost renal vein, but they can also be placed above the renal veins if thrombus extends to the level of the renal veins. If the diameter of the IVC exceeds 30 mm, the Bird's Nest filter is the only filter that can be placed; otherwise any of the other filters can be used. Each filter

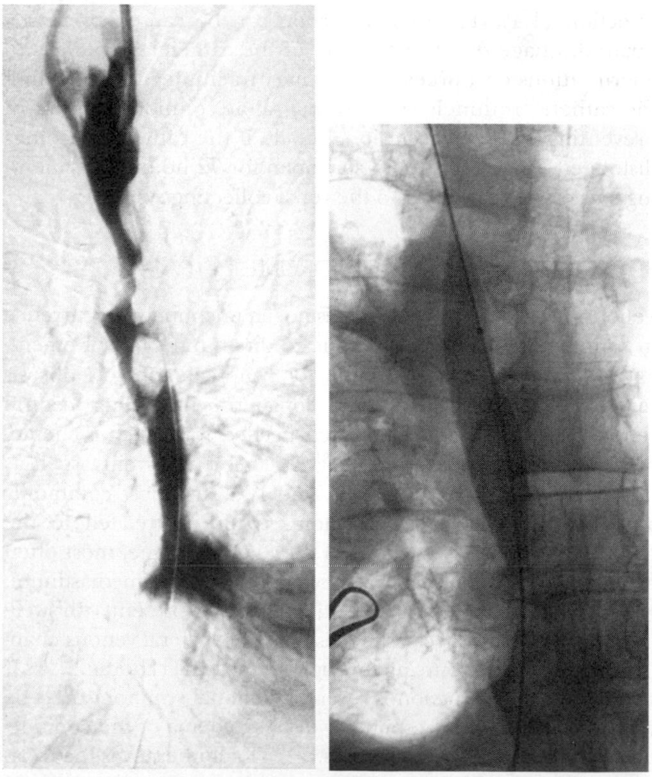

A,B

FIGURE 27.4-15. Superior vena cava syndrome. **A:** Multiple filling defects are visualized within the superior vena cava consistent with metastatic implants from lung carcinoma. The patient was symptomatic, with extensive venous collateral channels identified throughout the torso. **B:** Initial angioplasty is performed to open a channel.

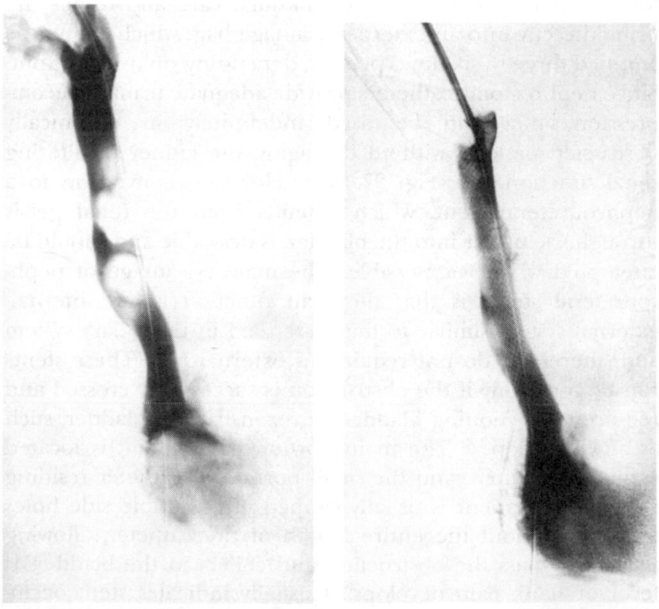

A,B

FIGURE 27.4-16. Superior vena cava syndrome treated with a self-expanding stent (Wallstent). **A:** Venogram performed before stent placement. **B:** After stent placement, venogram demonstrates torrential flow across the obstruction into the right atrium. Symptoms resolved within hours.

has advantages and disadvantages, and selection of a specific filter often depends on the filter availability and experience of the radiologist. Note that the Simon Nitinol filter is the most versatile of the filters since, because of its small delivery system, it can be deployed from virtually any peripheral access site.[204,205]

IVC patency rates vary between 91% and 97% after filter placement. Recurrence of pulmonary embolism occurs in approximately 2% to 4% of the cases. Other complications include filter migration (0% to 30%) and perforation of the IVC (0% to 40%).

REFERENCES

1. Westcott JL, Rao N, Colley DP. Transthoracic needle biopsy of small pulmonary nodules. *Radiology* 1997;202:97.
2. Haaga JR. Interventional CT-guided procedures. In: Haaga JR, Lanzieri CF, Santoris DJ, et al., eds. *Computed tomography and magnetic resonance imaging of the whole body,* 3rd ed. St. Louis: Mosby, 1994.
3. Gazelle GS, Haaga JR, Rowland DY. Effect of needle gauge, level of anticoagulation, and target organ on bleeding associated with aspiration biopsy. Work in progress. *Radiology* 1992;183:509.
4. Andriole JG, Haaga JR, Adams RB, et al. Biopsy needle characteristics assessed in the laboratory. *Radiology* 1983;148(3):659.
5. Conces DJ, Schwenk GR, Doering PR, et al. Thoracic needle biopsy: improved results utilizing a team approach. *Chest* 1987;91:813.
6. Khouri NF, Stitik FP, Erozan YS, et al. Transthoracic needle aspiration biopsy of benign and malignant lung lesions. *AJR Am J Roentgenol* 1985;144:281.
7. Odell MJ, Reid KR. Does percutaneous fine-needle aspiration biopsy aid in the diagnosis and surgical management of lung masses? *Can J Surg* 1999;42(4):297.
8. Staroselsky AN, Schwarz Y, Man A, et al. Additional information from percutaneous cutting needle biopsy following fine-needle aspiration in the diagnosis of chest lesions. *Chest* 1998;113(6):1522.
9. Larscheid RC, Thorpe PE, Scott WJ. Percutaneous transthoracic needle aspiration biopsy: a comprehensive review of its current role in the diagnosis and treatment of lung tumors. *Chest* 1998;114(3):704.
10. Greif J, Marmur S, Schwarz Y, et al. Percutaneous core cutting needle biopsy compared with fine-needle aspiration in the diagnosis of peripheral lung malignant lesions: results in 156 patients. *Cancer* 1998;84(3):144.
11. Swischuk JL, Castaneda F, Patel JC, et al. Percutaneous transthoracic needle biopsy of the lung: review of 612 lesions. *J Vas Interv Radiol* 1998;9(2):347.
12. Austin JH, Cohen MB. Value of having a cytopathologist present during percutaneous fine-needle aspiration biopsy of lung: report of 55 cancer patients and meta-analysis of the literature. *AJR Am J Roentgenol* 1993;160:175.
13. Zinzani PL, Corneli G, Cancellieri A, et al. Core needle biopsy is effective in the initial diagnosis of mediastinal lymphoma. *Haematologica* 1999;84(7):600.
14. Grant TH, Stull MA, Kandallu K, et al. Percutaneous needle biopsy of mediastinal masses using a computed tomography-guided extrapleural approach. *J Thorac Imaging* 1998;13(1):14.
15. Lenglinger FX, Zisch RJ. Technique to avoid iatrogenic pneumothorax during biopsy of mediastinal lesions. *Radiology* 1994;193:878.
16. Bressler EL, Kirkham JA. Mediastinal masses: alternative approaches to CT-guided needle biopsy. *Radiology* 1994;191:391.
17. Weisbrod GL. Transthoracic needle biopsy. *World J Surg* 1993;17:705.
18. Klein JS, Schultz S, Heffner JE. Interventional radiology of the chest: image-guided percutaneous drainage of pleural effusion, lung abscess, and pneumothorax. *AJR Am J Roentgenol* 1995;164:581.
19. Casola G, van Sonnenberg E, Keightley A, et al. Pneumothorax: radiologic treatment with small catheters. *Radiology* 1988;166:89-91.
20. Conces DJ, Tarver RD, Gray WC, et al. Treatment of pneumothoraces utilizing small caliber chest tubes. *Chest* 1988;94:55.
21. Perlmutt LM, Braun SD, Newman GE, et al. Transthoracic needle aspiration: use of a small chest tube to treat pneumothorax. *AJR Am J Roentgenol* 1987;148:849.
22. Welch TJ, Sheedy PF, Johnson CD, et al. CT-guided biopsy: prospective analysis of 1,000 procedures. *Radiology* 1989;171:493.
23. Reading CC, Charboneau JW, James EM, et al. Sonographically guided percutaneous biopsy of small (3 cm or less) masses. *AJR Am J Roentgenol* 1988;151:189.
24. Dodd GD III, Esola CC, Memel DS, et al. Sonography: the undiscovered jewel of interventional radiology. *Radiographics* 1996;16:1271.
25. Burbank F, Kaye K, Belville J, Ekuan J, Blumenfeld M. Image-guided automated core biopsies of the breast, chest, abdomen, and pelvis. *Radiology* 1994;191:165.
26. Martino CR, Haaga JR. Percutaneous biopsy of the liver. *Semin Interv Radiol* 1985;2:245.
27. Pagani JJ. Biopsy of focal hepatic lesions. *Radiology* 1983;147:673.
28. Mueller P, van Sonnenberg E. Interventional radiology in the chest and abdomen. *N Engl J Med* 1990;322:1364.
29. Brandt KR, Charboneau JW, Stephens DH, et al. CT- and US-guided biopsy of the pancreas. *Radiology* 1993;187:99.
30. Ihse I, Axelson J, Dawiskiba S, et al. Pancreatic biopsy: why? When? How? *World J Surg* 1999;23(9):896.
31. Wood BJ, Khan MA, McGovern F, et al. Imaging guided biopsy of renal masses: indications, accuracy and impact on clinical management. *J Urol* 1999;161(5):1470.
32. Welch TJ, Sheedy PF, Stephens DH, et al. Percutaneous adrenal biopsy: review of a 10-year experience. *Radiology* 1994;193:341.
33. Silverman SG, Mueller PR, Pinkney LP. Predictive value of image-guided adrenal biopsy; analysis of results of 101 biopsies. *Radiology* 1993;187:715.
34. Saboorian MH, Katz RL, Charnsangavej C. Fine needle aspiration cytology of primary and metastatic lesions of the adrenal gland. *Acta Cytol* 1995;39:843.
35. Charboneau JW, Reading CC, Welch TJ. CT and sonographically guided needle biopsy; current techniques and new innovations. *AJR Am J Roentgenol* 1990;154:1.
36. Moulton JS, Moore PT. Coaxial percutaneous biopsy technique with automated biopsy device: value in improving accuracy and negative predictive value. *Radiology* 1993;186:515.
37. Smith EH. Complications of percutaneous abdominal fine-needle biopsy. *Radiology* 1991;178:253.
38. Smith TP, McDermott VG, Ayoub DM, et al. Percutaneous transhepatic liver biopsy with tract embolization. *Radiology* 1996;198:769.
39. Corr P, Beningfield SJ, Davey N. Transjugular liver biopsy: a review of 200 biopsies. *Clin Radiol* 1992;45:238.
40. Cope C, Marinelli DL, Weinstein JK. Transcatheter biopsy of lesions obstructing the bile ducts. *Radiology* 1988;169:555.
41. Hall-Craggs MA, Lees WR. Fine-needle aspiration biopsy: pancreatic and biliary tumors. *AJR Am J Roentgenol* 1986;147:399.
42. Savader SJ, Prescott CA, Lund GB, Osterman FA. Intraductal biliary biopsy: comparison of three techniques. *J Vasc Intervent Radiol* 1996;7:743.
43. Daly JM, Kemeny N, Botet JF. Long-term hepatic arterial infusion chemotherapy. *Arch Surg* 1984;152:936.
44. Ring EJ. Vascular disease of the liver. In: Herlinger H, Lunderquist A, Wallace S, eds. *Clinical radiology of the liver.* New York: Marcel Dekker Inc, 1993:953.
45. Okuda K, Obata H, Jinnovichi S, et al. Angiographic assessment of gross anatomy of HCC: comparison of celiac angiograms and liver pathology in 100 cases. *Radiology* 1977;123:21.
46. Cho KJ, Andrews JC, Williams DM, et al. Hepatic arterial chemotherapy: role of angiography. *Radiology* 1989;173:783.
47. Dooley WC, Cameron JL, Lillemoe KD, Venbrux AC, et al. Is preoperative angiography useful in patients with periampullary tumors? *Ann Surg* 1990;211(6):649.
48. Freeny PC. Radiologic diagnosis and staging of pancreatic ductal adenocarcinoma. *Radiol Clin North Am* 1989;27(1):121.
49. Miller DL. Endocrine angiography and venous sampling. *Radiol Clin North Am* 1993;31(5):1051.
50. Rossi P, Allison DJ, Bezzi M, et al. Endocrine tumors of the pancreas. *Radiol Clin North Am* 1989;27(1):129.
51. Cho KJ, Venik AI, Thompson NW, et al. Localization of the source of hyperinsulinism: percutaneous transhepatic portal and pancreatic vein catheterization with hormone assay. *AJR Am J Roentgenol* 1982;139:237.
52. Krudy AG, Doppman JL, Jensen RT, et al. Localization of islet cell tumors by dynamic CT: comparison with plain CT, arteriography, sonography, and venous sampling. *AJR Am J Roentgenol* 1984;143:585.
53. Norton AJ, Doppman JL, Collen MJ, et al. Prospective study of gastrinoma localization and resection in patients with Zollinger-Ellison syndrome. *Ann Surg* 1986;204:468.
54. Roche A, Raisonnier A, Gillon-Savouret MC. Pancreatic venous sampling and arteriography in localizing insulinomas and gastrinomas: procedure and results in 55 cases. *Radiology* 1982;145:621.
55. Soulen MC. Chemoembolization of hepatic malignancies. *Oncology* 1994;8:77.
56. Di Bisceglie AM, Rustgi VK, Koffnagle JH, et al. Hepatocellular carcinoma. *Ann Intern Med* 1988;108:390.
57. Kassianides C, Kew MC. The clinical manifestations and natural history of hepatocellular carcinoma. *Gastroenterol Clin North Am* 1987;16:553.
58. Solomon B, Soulen M, Baum R, et al. Chemoembolization of hepatocellular carcinoma with cisplatin, doxorubicin, mitomycin-C, Ethiodol, and polyvinyl alcohol: prospective evaluation of response and survival in a US population. *J Vasc Intervent Radiol* 1999;10:793.
59. Okuda K, Obata H, Nakajima Y, et al. Prognosis of primary hepatocellular carcinoma. *Hepatology* 1984;4:S3.
60. Ngan H, Lai C, Fan S, et al. Transcatheter arterial chemoembolization in inoperable hepatocellular carcinoma: four-year follow-up. *J Vasc Intervent Radiol* 1996;7:419.
61. Choti MA, Bulkley GB. Management of hepatic metastases. *Liver Transpl Surg* 1999;5(1):65.
62. Therasse E, Breittmayer F, Roche A, et al. Transcatheter chemoembolization of progressive carcinoid liver metastasis. *Radiology* 1993;189:541.
63. Kvols LK, Buck M. Chemotherapy of metastatic carcinoid and islet cell tumors. *Am J Med* 1987;82:77.
64. Mavligit GM, Charnsangavej C, Carrasco CH, et al. Regression of ocular melanoma metastatic to the liver after hepatic arterial chemoembolization with cisplatin and polyvinyl sponge. *JAMA* 1988;260:974.
65. Vogelzang RL, Nemek AA Jr, Lyster M, et al. Hepatic artery chemoembolization for treatment of hepatic malignancy: results with microfibrillar collagen and triple drug therapy. *J Vasc Intervent Radiol* 1993;4:61.
66. Carr BI, Flickinger JC, Lotze MT. Hepatobiliary cancers. In: DeVita VT, Hellman S, Rosenberg SA, eds. *Cancer: Principles & Practice of Oncology.* Philadelphia: Lippincott-Raven Publishers, 1997.
67. Bruix J. Treatment of hepatocellular carcinoma. *Hepatology* 1997;25:259.
68. Allgaier HP, Diebert P, Olschewski M, et al. Survival benefits of patients with inoperable hepatocellular carcinoma treated by a combination of transarterial chemoembolization

and percutaneous ethanol injection–a single-center analysis including 132 patients. *Int J Cancer (Pred Oncol)* 1998;79:601.
69. Breedis C, Young G. The blood supply of neoplasms in the liver. *Am J Pathol* 1954;969.
70. Schenk WG, et al. Direct measurement of hepatic blood flow in surgical patients. *Ann Surg* 1962;156:463.
71. Pentecost MJ. Transcatheter treatment of hepatic metastases. *AJR Am J Roentgenol* 1993;160:1171.
72. Soulen MC. Principles of regional cancer therapy. *Semin Interv Radiol* 1998;15(4):361.
73. Konno T. Targeting cancer chemotherapeutic agents by use of Lipiodol contrast medium. *Cancer* 1990;66:1897.
74. Egawa H, Maki A, Mori K. Effects of intraarterial chemotherapy with a new lipophilic anticancer agent, estradiol-chlorambucil (KM2210), dissolved in Lipiodol on experimental liver tumor in rats. *J Surg Oncol* 1990;44:109.
75. Kanematsu T, Furuta T, Takenaka K, et al. A 5-year experience of lipiodolization: selective regional chemotherapy for 200 patients with hepatocellular carcinoma. *Hepatology* 1989;10:98.
76. Sasaki Y, Imaoka S, Kasugai H, et al. A new approach to chemoembolization therapy for hepatoma using ethiodized oil, cisplatin, and gelatin sponge. *Cancer* 1987;609:1194.
77. Shibata J, Fujiyama S, Sato T, et al. Hepatic arterial injection chemotherapy with cisplatin suspended in an oily lymphographic agent for hepatocellular carcinoma. *Cancer* 1989;64:1586.
78. Kanematsu T, Inokuchi K, Sugimachi K, et al. Selective effects of lipiodolized antitumor agents. *J Surg Oncol* 1984;25:218.
79. Okamura J, Korikawa S, Fujiyama T, et al. An appraisal of transcatheter arterial embolization combined with transcatheter arterial infusion of chemotherapeutic agent for hepatic malignancies. *World J Surg* 1982;6:352.
80. Patt YZ, Chuang VP, Wallace S, et al. Hepatic arterial chemotherapy and occlusion for palliation of primary hepatocellular and unknown primary neoplasms in the liver. *Cancer* 1983;51:1359.
81. Takayasu K, Shima Y, Muramatsu Y, et al. Hepatocellular carcinoma: treatment with intraarterial iodized oil with and without chemotherapeutic agents. *Radiology* 1987;162:345.
82. Onishi K, Tsuchiya S, Nakayama T, et al. Arterial chemoembolization of hepatocellular carcinoma with mitomycin C microcapsules. *Radiology* 1984;152:51.
83. Nakamura H, Hashimoto T, Oi H, et al. Transcatheter oily chemoembolization of hepatocellular carcinoma. *Radiology* 1989;170:783.
84. Shimamura Y, Gunven P, Takenaka Y, et al. Combined peripheral and central chemoembolization of liver tumors. *Cancer* 1988;61:238.
85. Nakao N, Kamino K, Miura K, et al. Recurrent hepatocellular carcinoma after partial hepatectomy: value of treatment with transcatheter arterial chemoembolization. *AJR Am J Roentgenol* 1991;156:1177.
86. Van Beers B, Roche A, Cauqil P, et al. Transcatheter arterial chemotherapy using doxorubicin, iodized oil and Gelfoam embolization in hepatocellular carcinoma. *Acta Radiol* 1989;30:415.
87. Venook AP, Stagg RJ, Lewis BJ, et al. Chemoembolization for hepatocellular carcinoma. *J Clin Oncol* 1990;8:1108.
88. Pelletier G, Roche A, Ink O, et al. A randomized trial of hepatic arterial chemoembolization in patients with unresectable hepatocellular carcinoma. *J Hepatol* 1990;11:181.
89. Madden MV, Krige JEJ, Bailey S, et al. Randomized trial of targeted chemotherapy with lipiodol and 5-epiodoxorubicin compared with symptomatic treatment for hepatoma. *Gut* 1993;34:1598.
90. Groupe d'Etude et de Traitement Du Carcinome Hepatocellulaire. A comparison of Lipiodol chemoembolization and conservative treatment for unresectable hepatocellular carcinoma. *N Engl J Med* 1995;1256.
91. Bruix J, Llovet JM, Castells A, et al. Transarterial embolization versus symptomatic treatment in patients with advanced hepatocellular carcinoma: results of a randomized, controlled trial in a single institution. *Hepatology* 1998;27(6):1578.
92. Vetter D, Wenger J-J, Doffoel M, et al. Transcatheter oily chemoembolization in the management of advanced hepatocellular carcinoma. *Hepatology* 1991;13:427.
93. Bartolozzi C, Lencioni R, Caramella D, et al. Treatment of large HCC: transcatheter arterial chemoembolization combined with percutaneous Ethanol injection versus repeated transcatheter arterial chemoembolization. *Radiology* 1995;197:812.
94. Lu D, Peng Y, Jiang C, et al. Preoperative transcatheter arterial chemoembolization and prognosis of patients with hepatocellular carcinomas: retrospective analysis of 120 cases. *World J Surg* 1999;23:293.
95. DiCarlo V, Ferrari G, Castoldi R, et al. Pre-operative chemoembolization of hepatocellular carcinoma in cirrhotic patients. *Hepatogastroenterology* 1998;45(24):1950.
96. Paye F, Jago P, Vilgrain V, et al. Preoperative chemoembolization of hepatocellular carcinoma. *Arch Surg* 1998;133;767.
97. Oldhafer K, Chavan A, Fruhauf N, et al. Arterial chemoembolization before liver transplantation in patients with hepatocellular carcinoma: marked tumor necrosis, but no survival benefit? *J Hepatol* 1998:953.
98. Harnois DM, Steers J, Andrews JC, et al. Preoperative hepatic artery chemoembolization followed by orthotopic liver transplantation for hepatocellular carcinoma. *Liver Transpl Surg* 1999;5(3):192.
99. Farges O, Regimbeau J, Belghiti J. Aggressive management of recurrence following surgical resection of hepatocellular carcinoma. *Hepatogastroenterology* 1998;45;1275.
100. Okuda K, Ohtsuki T, Obata H, et al. Natural history of hepatocellular carcinoma and prognosis in relation to treatment. *Cancer* 1985;56:918.
101. Winkelbauer FW, Niederle B, Pietschmann F, et al. Hepatic artery embolotherapy of hepatic metastases from carcinoid tumors: value of using a mixture of cyanoacrylate and ethiodized oil. *AJR Am J Roentgenol* 1995;165:323.
102. Mavligit GM, Pollock RE, Evans HL, et al. Durable hepatic tumor regression after arterial chemoembolization-infusion inpatients with islet cell carcinoma of the pancreas metastatic to the liver. *Cancer* 1993;72:375.
103. Stokes KR, Stuart K, Clouse ME. Hepatic arterial chemoembolization for metastatic endocrine tumors. *J Vasc Intervent Radiol* 1993;4:341
104. Perry LJ, Stuart K, Stokes KR, et al. Hepatic arterial chemoembolization for metastatic neuroendocrine tumors. *Surgery* 1994;116:1111.
105. Drougas JG, Anthony LB, Blair TK, et al. Hepatic artery chemoembolization for management of patients with advanced metastatic carcinoid tumors. *Am J Surg* 1998;175(5):408.
106. Tellez C, Benson A, Lyster M, et al. Phase II trial of chemoembolization for the treatment of metastatic colorectal carcinoma to the liver and review of the literature. *Cancer* 1998;82:1250.
107. Daniels S, Pentecost M, Teitelbaum G, et al. Hepatic artery chemoembolization for carcinoma of colon using angiostat collagen and cisplatin, mitomycin and doxorubicin: response, survival and serum drug levels. *Proc Am Soc Clin Oncol* 1992;11;171.
108. Sugiura N, Takara K, Olito M, et al. Percutaneous intratumoral injection of ethanol under ultrasound imaging for treatment of small HCC. *Acta Hepatol Jpn* 1983;24:920.
109. Livraghi T, Giorgio A, Marin G, et al. Hepatocellular carcinoma and cirrhosis in 746 patients: long-term results of percutaneous ethanol injection. *Radiology* 1995;197:101.
110. Livraghi T, Solbiati L. Percutaneous ethanol injection in liver cancer: method and results. *Semin Interv Radiol* 1993;10:69.
111. Redvanly RD, Chezmar JL, Strauss RM, et al. Malignant hepatic tumors: safety of high-dose percutaneous ethanol ablation therapy. *Radiology* 1993;188:283.
112. Lencioni R, Bartolozzi C, Caramella D, et al. Treatment of small hepatocellular carcinoma with percutaneous ethanol injection: analysis of prognostic factors in 105 Western patients. *Cancer* 1995;76:1737.
113. Kotoh K, Sakai H, Morotomi I, et al. The use of percutaneous ethanol injection therapy for recurrence of hepatocellular carcinoma. *Hepatogastroenterology* 1995;42:197.
114. Solmi L, Muratori R, Bertoni F, et al. Echo-guided percutaneous ethanol injection in small hepatocellular carcinoma: personal experience. *Hepatogastroenterology* 1993;40:505.
115. Giorgio A, Tarantino L, Francica G, et al. One-shot percutaneous ethanol injection of liver tumors under general anesthesia: preliminary data on efficacy and complications. *Cardiovasc Intervent Radiol* 1996;19:27.
116. Isobe H, Sakai H, Imari Y, et al. Intratumor ethanol injection therapy for solitary minute hepatocellular carcinoma: a study of 37 patients. *J Clin Gastroenterol* 1994;18:122.
117. Matsuoka Y, Morikawa M, Amamoto Y, et al. Therapeutic ethanol injection of hepatocellular carcinomas undetectable by angiography and Lipiodol computed tomography. *Cardiovasc Intervent Radiol* 1992;15:221.
118. Shiina S, Tagawa K, Unuma T, et al. Percutaneous ethanol injection therapy for hepatocellular carcinoma: a histopathologic study. *Cancer* 1991;68:1524.
119. Vilana R, Bruix J, Bru C, et al. Tumor size determines the efficacy of percutaneous ethanol injection for the treatment of small hepatocellular carcinoma. *Hepatology* 1992;16:353.
120. Castells A, Bruix J, Bru C, et al. Treatment of small hepatocellular carcinoma in cirrhotic patients: a cohort study comparing surgical resection and percutaneous ethanol injection. *Hepatology* 1993;18:1121.
121. Shiina S, Tagawa K, Niwa Y, et al. Percutaneous ethanol injection therapy for hepatocellular carcinoma: results in 146 patients. *AJR Am J Roentgenol* 1993;160:1023.
122. Livraghi T, Vettori C, Lazzaroni S. Liver metastases: results of percutaneous ethanol injection in 14 patients. *Radiology* 1991;179:709.
123. Giovannini M, Seitz JF. Ultrasound-guided percutaneous alcohol injection of small liver metastases: results in 40 patients. *Cancer* 1994;73:294.
124. Livraghi T. Percutaneous ethanol injection in the treatment of hepatocellular carcinoma in cirrhosis. *Hepatogastroenterology* 1998;45:1248.
125. Livraghi T, Benedini V, Lazzaroni S, et al. Long-term results of single session percutaneous ethanol injection in patients with large hepatocellular carcinoma. *Cancer* 1997;83:48.
126. Lee MJ, Mueller PR, Dawson SL, et al. Percutaneous ethanol injection for the treatment of hepatic tumors: indications, mechanism of action, technique, and efficacy. *AJR Am J Roentgenol* 1995;164:215.
127. Ishii H, Okada S, Nose H, et al. Local recurrence of hepatocellular carcinoma after percutaneous ethanol injection. *Cancer* 1996;77:1792.
128. Lencioni R, Caramella D, Bartolozzi C. Hepatocellular carcinoma: use of color Doppler US to evaluate response to treatment with percutaneous ethanol injection. *Radiology* 1995;194:113.
129. Livraghi T, Bolondi, L, Buscarini L, et al. No treatment, resection and ethanol injection in hepatocellular carcinoma: a retrospective analysis of survival in 391 patients with cirrhosis. Italian Cooperative HCC Study Group. *J Hepatol* 1995;22:522.
130. Kotoh K, Sakai H, Sakamoto S, et al. The effect of percutaneous ethanol injection therapy on small solitary hepatocellular carcinoma is comparable to that of hepatectomy. *Am J Gastroenterol* 1994;89:194.
131. Shiina S, Niwa Y, Omata M. Percutaneous ethanol injection therapy for liver neoplasms. *Semin Interv Radiol* 1993;10:57.
132. Tanikawa K, Majima Y. Percutaneous ethanol injection therapy for recurrent hepatocellular carcinoma. *Hepatogastroenterology* 1993:40:324.
133. Lencioni R, Paolicchi A, Moretti M, et al. Combined transcatheter arterial chemoembolization and percutaneous ethanol injection for the treatment of large hepatocellular carcinoma: local therapeutic effect and long-term survival rate. *Eur Radiol* 1998;8(3):439.
134. Tanaka K, Nakamura S, Numata K, et al. The long-term efficacy of combined transcatheter arterial embolization and percutaneous ethanol injection in the treatment of patients with large hepatocellular carcinoma and cirrhosis. *Cancer* 1998;82(1):78.
135. Dickson A, Calderwood S. Thermosensitivity of neoplastic tissues in vivo. In: Storm K, ed. *Hyperthermia in cancer therapy*. Boston: GK Hall, 1983;63.
136. Rossi S, Fornari F, Buscarini L. Percutaneous US-guided radiofrequency electrocautery for the treatment of small hepatocellular carcinoma. *J Intervent Radiol* 1993;8:97.

137. Rossi S, Buscarini E, Garbagnati F, et al. Percutaneous treatment of small hepatic tumors by an expandable RF needle electrode. *AJR Am J Roentgenol* 1998;170:1015.
138. Livraghi T, Goldberg S, Monti F, et al. Saline-enhanced radiofrequency tissue ablation in the treatment of liver metastases. *Radiology* 1997;202:205.
139. Solbiati L, Ierace T, Goldberg S, et al. Percutaneous US-guided radiofrequency tissue ablation of liver metastases: long-term follow-up. *Radiology* 1997;292:195.
140. McGahan J, Schneider P, Brock J, et al. Treatment of liver tumors by percutaneous radiofrequency electrocautery. *Semin Interv Radiol* 1993;10:143.
141. Curley SA, Izzo F, Delrio P, et al. Radiofrequency ablation of unresectable primary and metastatic hepatic malignancies: results in 123 patients. *Ann Surg* 1999;230(1):1.
142. Gores G, Thuluvath P, Geschwind JF, et al. Intradose injectable Gel in treatment of hepatocellular carcinoma. Oral communication: Chemotherapy Foundation Symposium, New York City, November 3, 1999.
143. Landis SH, Murray T, Bolden S, et al. Cancer statistics. *CA Cancer J Clin* 1998;48:192.
144. Henson DE, Albores-Saavedra J, Corle D. Carcinoma of the gallbladder: histologic types, stage of disease, grade, and survival rates. *Cancer* 1992;70:1493.
145. Nunnerley HB, Karani JB. Intraductal radiation in interventional radiology of the biliary tract. *Radiol Clin North Am* 1990;28:1237.
146. Dachman AH. Primary biliary neoplasia In: Friedman AC, Dachman AH, eds. Radiology of the liver, biliary tract and pancreas. St. Louis: Mosby–Year Book, 1994:611.
147. Meyer DG, Weinstein BJ. Klatskin tumors of the bile ducts: sonographic appearance. *Radiology* 1983;148:803.
148. Subramanyam BR, Raghavendra BN, Balthazar EJ, et al. Ultrasonic features of cholangiocarcinoma. *J Ultrasound Med* 1984;3:405.
149. Pitt HA, Dooley WC, Yeo CJ, et al. Malignancies of the biliary tree. *Curr Probl Surg* 1995;32:1.
150. Farley DR, Weaver AL, Nagorney DM. "Natural history" of unresected cholangiocarcinoma: patient outcome after noncurative intervention. *Mayo Clin Proc* 1995;70:425.
151. De Groen PC, Gores GJ, LaRusso NF, et al. Biliary tract cancers. *N Engl J Med* 1999;341:1368.
152. Bell R. Neoplasms of the exocrine pancreas. In: Greenfield LJ, Mulholland M, Oldham KT, et al., eds. *Surgery: scientific principles and practice.* Philadelphia: Lippincott-Raven Publishers, 1997:901
153. Schnur MJ, Hoffman JC, Koenigsberg M. Ultrasonic demonstration of intraductal biliary neoplasms. *J Clin Ultrasound* 1982;10:246.
154. Gudjonnson B. Cancer of the pancreas: 50 years of surgery. *Cancer* 1987;60:2284.
155. Desa LA, Akosa AB, Lazzara S, et al. Cytodiagnosis in the management of extrahepatic biliary stricture. *Gut* 1991;32:1188.
156. Mansfield JC, Griffin SM, Wadehra V, et al. A prospective evaluation of cytology from biliary strictures. *Gut* 1997;40:671.
157. Thuluvath PJ, Rai R, Venbrux AC, et al. Cholangiocarcinoma: a review. *Gastroenterologist* 1997;5(4):306.
158. Stanley J, Gobien RP, Cunnigham J, et al. Biliary decompression: an institutional comparison of percutaneous and endoscopic methods. *Radiology* 1986;158:195.
159. Cameron JL. Proximal cholangiocarcinoma: palliation by transhepatic stenting and hepaticojejunostomy. In: Cameron JL, ed. *Atlas of surgery,* Vol. 1. Philadelphia: BC Decker, Inc, 1990:84.
160. Cameron JL. Resection of a proximal cholangiocarcinoma with hepatic lobectomy and reconstruction utilizing a silastic transhepatic biliary stent and hepaticojejunostomy. In: Cameron JL, ed. *Atlas of surgery,* Vol. 1. Philadelphia: BC Decker, Inc, 1990:72.
161. Nordback IH, Pitt HA, Coleman J, et al. Unresectable hilar cholangiocarcinoma: percutaneous versus operative palliation. *Surgery* 1994;115:597.
162. Grundy SJR, Strodel WE, Knol JA, et al. Efficacy of preoperative biliary tract decompression in patients with obstructive jaundice. *Arch Surg* 1984;119:703.
163. Hatfield ARW, Tobias R, Terblanche J, et al. Pre-operative external biliary drainage in obstructive jaundice. *Lancet* 1982;2:896.
164. Prat F, Chapat O, Ducot B, et al. Predictive factors for survival of patients with inoperable malignant distal biliary strictures: a practical management guideline. *Gut* 1998;42:76.
165. Schima W, Prokesch R, Osterreicher C, et al. Biliary Wallstent endoprosthesis in malignant hilar obstruction: long-term results with regard to the type of obstruction. *Clin Radiol* 1997;52:213.
166. Boguth L, Tatalovic S, Antonucci F, et al. Malignant biliary obstruction: clinical and histopathologic correlation after treatment with self-expanding metal prostheses. *Radiology* 1994;192:669.
167. Rossi P, Bezzi M, Rossi M, et al. Metallic stents in malignant biliary obstruction: results of a multicenter European study of 240 patients. *J Vasc Interv Radiol* 1994;5:279.
168. Lammer J, Klein GE, Kleinert R, et al. Obstructive jaundice: use of expandable metal stents endoprostheses for biliary drainage. *Radiology* 1990;177:789.
169. Kaskarelis IS, Papadaki MG, Papageorgiou GN, et al. Long term followup in patients with malignant biliary obstruction after percutaneous placement of uncovered Wallstent endoprostheses. *Acta Radiol* 1999;40(5):528.
170. Mueller PR, van Sonnenberg E, Gerruci JT Jr. Percutaneous biliary drainage: technical and catheter related problems in 200 procedures. *AJR Am J Roentgenol* 1982;138:17.
171. Ishikawa Y, Oishi I, Miyai M, et al. Experience in 100 cases. *J Clin Gastroenterol* 1980;2:305.
172. Hamlin JA, Friedman M, Stein MG, et al. Percutaneous biliary drainage only: complications of 118 consecutive catherizations. *Radiology* 1986;158:199.
173. Gunther RW, Schild H, Thelen M. Percutaenous transhepatic biliary drainage experience with 311 procedures. *Cardiovasc Interv Radiol* 1988;11:65.
174. Hussain S, Ahmed I. Nephrostomy revisited: cost effective approach. *J Vasc Interv Radiol* 1994;5:394.
175. Reznek RH, Talner LB. Percutaneous nephrostomy. *Radiol Clin North Am* 1984;22:393.
176. Lee WJ, Patel U, Patel S, et al. Emergency percutaneous nephrostomy: results and complications. *J Vasc Interv Radiol* 1994;5:135.
177. Castaneda-Zuniga WR, Brady TM, Thomas R, et al. *Percutaneous uroradiologic techniques. Interventional radiology,* 3rd ed. Baltimore: Williams & Wilkins, 1997.
178. Banner MP, Ramchandani P, Pollack HM. Interventional procedures in the upper urinary tract. *Cardiovasc Interv Radiol* 1991;14(5):267.
179. Kenny B, Lynch N, Hurley GD. Antegrade stenting of malignant ureteral strictures. *Eur Radiol* 1995;5:623.
180. Chang R, Marshall FF, Mitchell SE. Percutaneous management of benign ureteral strictures and fistulas. *J Urol* 1987;137:1126.
181. Lokich JJ, Goodman R. Superior vena cava syndrome: clinical management. *JAMA* 1975;231:58.
182. Davenport D, Ferree C, Blake D, et al. Radiation therapy in the treatment of superior vena caval obstruction. *Cancer* 1978;42:2600.
183. Perez CA, Presant CA, van Amburg AL III. Management of superior vena syndrome. *Semin Oncol* 1978;5:123.
184. Elson JD, Becker GJ, Wholey MH, et al. Vena caval and central venous stenoses: management with palmaz balloons expandable intraluminal stents. *J Vasc Interv Radiol* 1991;2:215.
185. Schraufnagel DE, Hill R, Leech JA, et al. Superior vena caval obstruction: is it a medical emergency? *Am J Med* 1981;70:1169.
186. Irving JD, Dondelinger RF, Reidy JF, et al. Gianturco self-expanding stents: clinical experience in the vena cava and large veins. *Cardiovasc Interv Radiol* 1992;15:328.
187. Rosch J, Bedell JE, Putnam J, et al. Gianturco expandable wire stents in the treatment of superior vena cava syndrome recurring after maximum tolerance radiation. *Cancer* 1987;60:1243.
188. Sherry CS, Diamond NG, Meyers TB, et al. Successful treatment of superior vena cava syndrome by venous angioplasty. *AJR Am J Roentgenol* 1986;147:834.
189. Capek P, Cope C. Percutaneous treatment of superior vena cava syndrome. *AJR Am J Roentgenol* 1989;152:183.
190. Dake MD, Semba CP, Enstrom RJ, et al. Percutaneous treatment of venous occlusive disease with stents. *J Vasc Interv Radiol* 1993;4:42.
191. Trerotola SO, Lund GB, Samphilipo MA, et al. Palmaz stents in the treatment of central venous stenosis; safety and efficacy of redilation. *Radiology* 1994;190:379.
192. Kishi K, Sonomura T, Mitsuzane K, et al. Self-expandable metallic stent therapy for superior vena cava syndrome: clinical observations. *Radiology* 1993;189:531.
193. Moore FD Jr, Osteen RT, Karp DD, et al. Anticoagulants, venous thromboembolism and the cancer patient. *Arch Surg* 1981;116:405.
194. Sack GH, Levin J, Bell WR. Trousseau's syndrome and other manifestation of chronic disseminated coagulopathy in patients with neoplasms: clinical pathophysiologic and therapeutic features. *Medicine* 1977;56:1.
195. Strandness DE, Langlois Y, Cramer M, et al. Long term sequealae of acute deep venous thromboses. *JAMA* 1983:250:1289.
196. Hirsch J, Genton E, Hull R. *Venous thromboembolism.* New York: Grune & Stratton, 1981:63.
197. Savader SJ. Inferior vena cava filters. In: Savader SJ and Trerotola SO, eds. *Venous interventional radiology with clinical perspectives.* New York: Thieme Publishers, 1996; 367.
198. Alpert JS, Smith R, Carlson J, et al. Mortality in patients treated for pulmonary embolism. *JAMA* 1976;236:1477.
199. Dorfman GS, Cronan JJ, Denny DF, et al. Occult pulmonary embolism: a common occurrence in deep venous thrombosis. *AJR Am J Roentgenol* 1987;148:263.
200. Greenfield L. Current indications for and results of Greenfield filter placement. *J Vasc Surg* 1984;1:502.
201. Jones T, Barnes R, Greenfield L. Greenfield vena cava filter: rationale and current indications. *Ann Thorac Surg* 1986;42:S48.
202. Alexander J, Gewerk L, Lu C, et al. New criteria for placement of a prophylactic vena cava filter. *Surg Gynecol Obstet* 1986;163:405.
203. Becker DM, Philbrick JT, Selby JB. Inferior vena cava filters: indications, safety, effectiveness. *Arch Intern Med* 1992;152:1985.
204. Grassi CJ. Inferior vena caval filters: analysis of five currently available devices. *AJR Am J Roentgenol* 1991;156:813.
205. Ferris EJ, McGowan TC, Carver DR, et al. Percutaneous inferior vena cava filters: follow-up of seven designs in 320 patients. *Radiology* 1993;188:851.

SECTION 5

ULRIKE M. HAMPER

Ultrasound

Advances in radiologic techniques have allowed the radiologist to make significant contributions in the diagnosis and management of cancer patients. The applications of ultrasonography (US) in oncology have rapidly increased in recent years, due to development of new technologies and therapeutic regimens as well as easy availability and noninvasiveness of US.[1,2] This chapter gives an overview of the current role of US in the evaluation of the oncologic patient, with particular emphasis on the sonographic diagnosis, staging, and follow-up of superficial or deep masses and discusses US guidance and techniques for abdominal, thoracic, and superficial interventional procedures.

ULTRASONOGRAPHY APPLICATIONS

An evaluation of the diagnostic role of US includes three particular aspects: (1) detection of a mass or lesion, (2) definition of the nature of the lesion, and (3) estimation of the extent of the lesion. Although a large number of organs can be studied by US with good sensitivities, the staging accuracies of US are limited and depend on the site of the organ. Superficial organs (thyroid, parathyroid, breast, testicles) are better evaluated than deep-seated organs. Nevertheless, tumors in the liver, biliary, tree, gallbladder, pancreas and kidney, prostate, and bladder can be detected by US with quite good sensitivities. The results are less favorable in the retroperitoneum and adrenal glands. In deep-seated tumors, US does not provide detailed evaluation of tumor spread, with exception of hepatic hilar node involvement or vascular invasion of the hepatic veins in hepatocellular carcinoma and the renal veins in renal cell carcinoma.[1] US may also play an important role in the follow-up of the oncologic patient in a search for or monitoring of liver metastases as well as for the assessment of response in patients with primary or secondary malignancies treated by intraarterial infusion of cytotoxic drugs. The areas wherein US plays an important role include urologic oncology, gynecologic oncology, medical oncology, and as a guidance modality for interventional diagnostic or therapeutic procedures.

UROLOGIC ONCOLOGY

Ultrasound plays a major role in the oncologic workup of tumors of the kidney, bladder, prostate, and seminal vesicles as well as testes.[3,4]

KIDNEY

When a renal mass is discovered on an intravenous urogram, further evaluation with US is usually performed. A benign renal cyst has a characteristic US appearance, defined as an echo-free fluid-filled lesion with a thin wall and posterior acoustic enhancement (Fig. 27.5-1*A*). Any doubt about the benign nature of a renal mass or the presence of a complex lesion demands further evaluation with computed tomography (CT) to exclude a renal cell carcinoma (see Fig. 27.5-1*B*). Renal lymphoma is usually metastatic or from direct extension from lymphoma in adjacent retroperitoneal lymph nodes. Transitional cell carcinoma arises in the renal pelvis or ureter and presents sonographically as a filling defect in the renal collecting system (Fig. 27.5-2). Doppler and color Doppler US (CDUS) are useful to assess renal vein or inferior vena cava invasion (or both) by tumor (Fig. 27.5-3).[5]

BLADDER

Transabdominal US permits gross evaluation of the bladder to assess for focal masses. US may have difficulty differentiating a hypertrophied median lobe of the prostate from a bladder mass. Cytoscopy is usually performed in cases of hematuria. Transurethral US may be used for staging of bladder cancers.[5]

PROSTATE AND SEMINAL VESICLES

Analysis of transrectal ultrasonography as a screening tool for prostate cancer has been disappointing, due to the low specificity of a hypoechoic lesion for cancer. Likewise, sonographic criteria to predict extracapsular extension of disease or spread into the seminal vesicles have not been reliable, with sensitivities of 65% and 33%, respectively, in some series. Transrectal ultrasonography, however, is an excellent tool to detect mimics of cancer on digital rectal examination, such as cysts, calcification, or abscess, as well as a guidance modality for prostate biopsies and staging biopsies into the seminal vesicles.[6,7]

TESTES

US can detect scrotal masses with an accuracy approaching 100%. The majority of intratesticular masses are malignant, whereas the majority of extratesticular lesions are benign or inflammatory in nature. Testicular tumors account for 1% to 2% of all malignant neoplasms in men and are the most common cancer in 25- to 35-year-olds. The majority of patients present with painless or mildly painful testicular enlargement. Between 90% and 95% of testicular neoplasms are of germ cell origin and include seminomas, embryonal cell cancer, teratomas, choriocarcinomas, or mixed germ cell tumors (Fig. 27.5-4). Leukemia and lymphoma are the most common metastatic tumors to the testis. Malignant lymphoma is the most common secondary neoplasm and most common testicular tumor in men older than 60 years (Fig. 27.5-5). Most are non-Hodgkin's lymphomas, and 50% of patients have extension into the spermatic cord. Leukemia is the most common metastatic testicular neoplasm. Leukemic infiltrates are common in children during bone marrow remission. The testis acts as a sanctuary during chemotherapy because of a blood–gonad barrier inhibiting concentration of chemotherapeutic agents. Other metastases to the testicle are prostate, melanoma, lung, kidney, colon, and pancreas. US is also used for the surveillance of contralateral testicles in patients with testicular tumors and to detect masses in patients with retroperitoneal masses of unknown origin.[8,9]

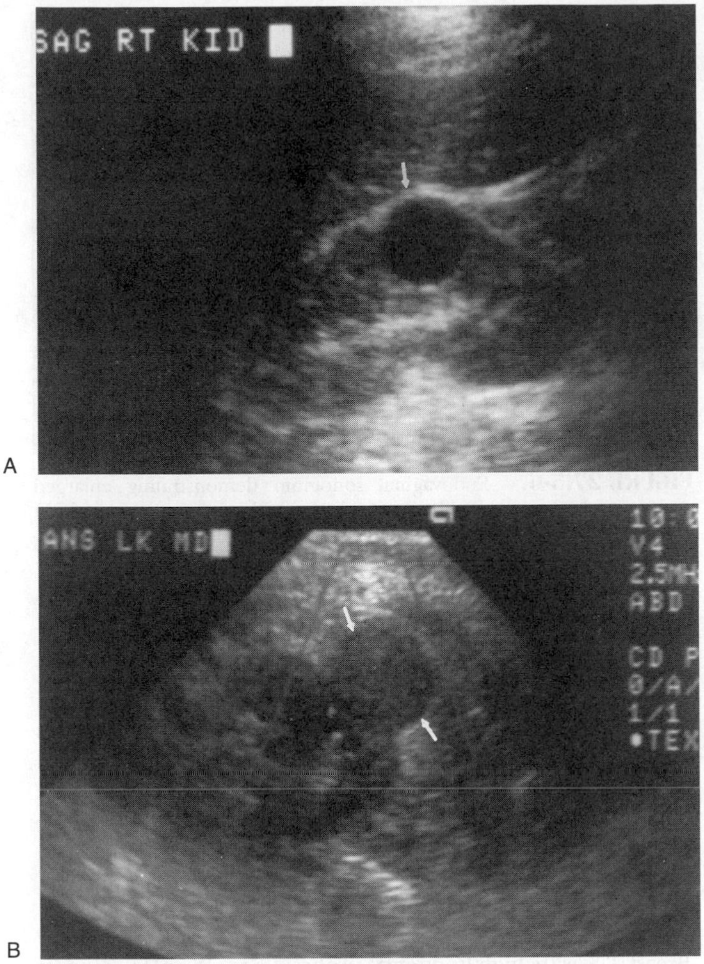

FIGURE 27.5-1. **A:** Sagittal sonogram of a right renal cyst (*arrow*). Note the echo-free appearance and smooth wall. **B:** Solid mass arising from the lower pole of the left kidney (*arrows*), compatible with renal cell carcinoma.

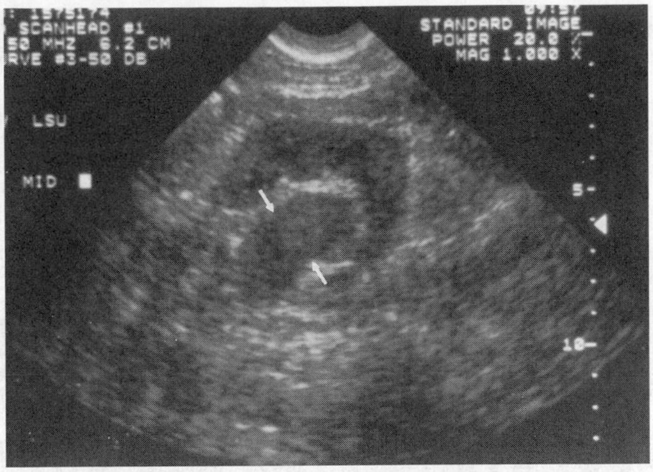

FIGURE 27.5-2. Echogenic mass (*arrows*) filling the left renal collecting system, compatible with transitional cell carcinoma.

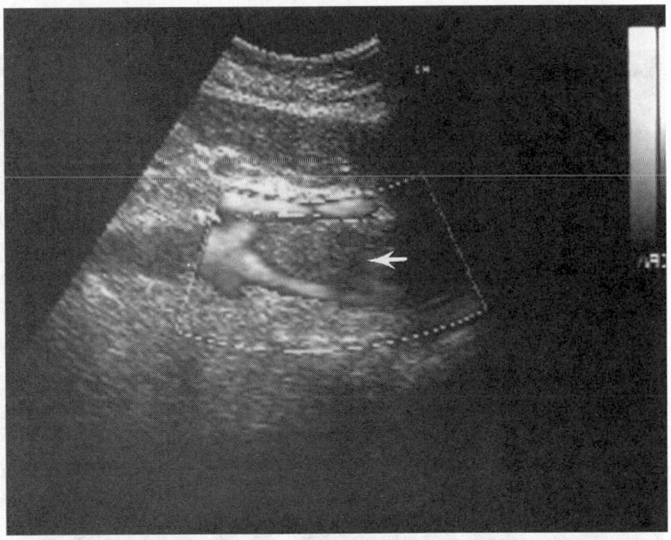

FIGURE 27.5-3. Tumor thrombus (*arrow*) extending into the inferior vena cava in a patient with metastatic leiomyosarcoma to the kidney.

GYNECOLOGIC ONCOLOGY

OVARY

Ovarian cancer is the least frequent but the most lethal of the three common gynecologic malignancies. US has played an increasingly important role in the evaluation of the oncologic patient with an ovarian mass. Scoring systems to differentiate between benign and malignant masses have been reported to provide encouraging results in terms of sensitivity and negative predictive values (95% to 100%); however, significant limitations exist in terms of specificity (73% to 83%) and positive predictive values (32% to 46%).[10] The likelihood of malignancy in an ovarian mass increases with size and complexity of the lesion. Simple cysts are almost always benign. The role of US for screening of early ovarian carcinoma needs yet to be defined. Doppler and CDUS endovaginal techniques to assess blood flow parameters are encouraging; however, the role of endovaginal CDUS for the evaluation of ovarian cancer is controversial, with limited sensitivity and specificity of this technique due to overlaps of flow velocity indices in benign and malignant ovarian masses.[10,11] US is useful to assess local or distant spread and detect ascites. In clinical practice, US is most often used to confirm the presence of an adnexal mass, often with characteristics of malignancy.

ENDOMETRIUM

Endometrial cancer is the most common gynecologic malignancy in the United States. Most patients present with postmenopausal bleeding. On endovaginal US, the endometrium is thickened, inhomogeneous in echotexture, and with irregular hypoechoic areas throughout. Endovaginal US is helpful in staging the degree of myometrial invasion: The presence of an intact subendometrial halo suggests superficial carcinoma without myometrial penetration (Fig. 27.5-6). With advanced invasive cancers, the myometrium becomes heterogeneous, with echogenic areas, and the uterus may have a lobulated appearance.[12] Hysterosonography (instillation of sterile saline into the uterine cavity) allows better detection and character-

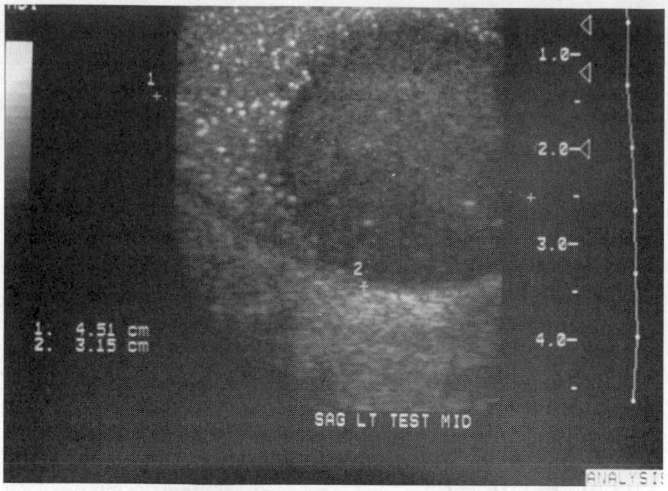

FIGURE 27.5-4. Well-defined hypoechoic mass in the left testicle (*arrows*), compatible with seminoma. Note small, bright, echogenic foci of microlithiasis in the remainder of the testicle.

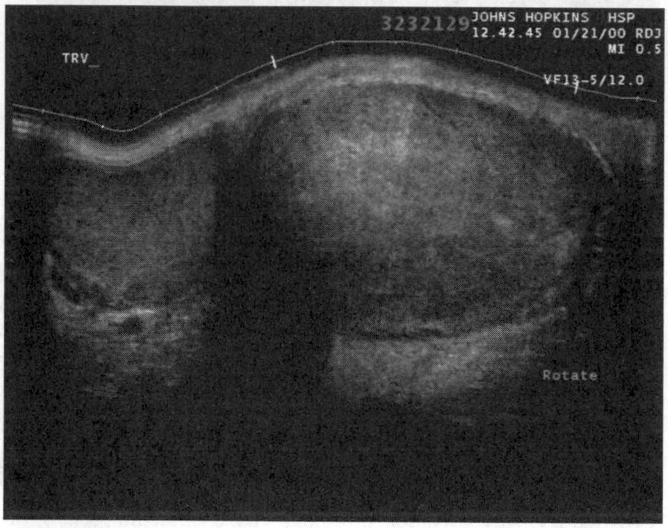

FIGURE 27.5-5. Transverse sonogram of both testicles demonstrating heterogeneous enlargement of the left testicle due to infiltration by B-cell lymphoma.

ization of underlying pathology in a patient with a thickened endometrium.

CERVIX

Cervical cancer is the least frequent of the three common gynecologic malignancies, and most cases can be detected by clinical screening in early stages. US has been shown to be no better than the physical examination to assess the primary tumor, and it has a limited role for staging. Transrectal US has been utilized to identify irregular thickening of the parametria. Endovaginal US may demonstrate secondary signs of a cervical obstructing mass, such as hydro- or hematometra.

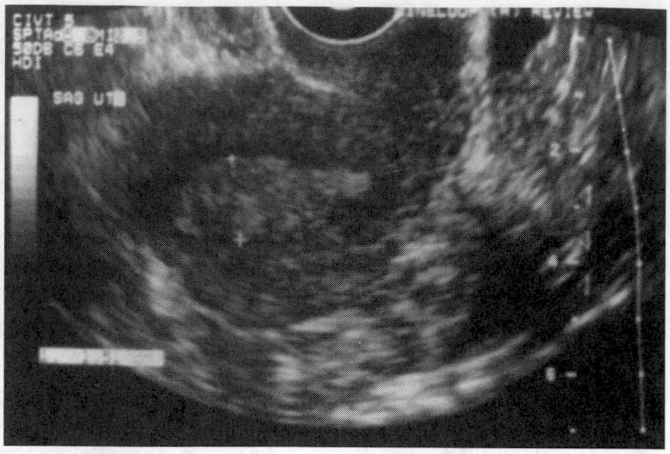

FIGURE 27.5-6. Endovaginal sonogram demonstrating enlarged endometrial echocomplex (between calipers) with posterior irregularity in a patient with endometrial carcinoma with posterior myometrial invasion.

GESTATIONAL TROPHOBLASTIC DISEASE

US has long been the first imaging study to diagnose molar pregnancy, demonstrating hypoechoic grape-like intrauterine structures during the first or second trimester. Recent studies have also demonstrated the use of endovaginal Doppler and color Doppler flow studies in assessing myometrial invasion in patients with persistent human chorionic gonadotropin elevation after dilatation and curettage.

BREAST

Breast US with high-frequency probes (7 to 13 mHz) is most often used to differentiate a cystic from a solid mass detected on palpation or mammography. Recent reports have demonstrated the utility of US to differentiate benign from malignant masses, therefore limiting the need to perform a biopsy on lesions with benign features, such as sharp margins, circumscribed borders, homogeneous internal echotexture and a horizontal orientation of the lesion. Doppler and CDUS studies to differentiate benign from malignant masses are under way.[13] US is an exquisite guidance modality for preoperative needle localization or core biopsy of sonographically visualized and nonpalpable breast masses.

MEDICAL ONCOLOGY

LIVER

Liver and biliary cancers account for only 1.5% of all gastrointestinal malignancies in the United States. Liver cancers are more common in China and Africa, because of higher endemic hepatitis B carrier rates. In the United States, 60% of hepatocellular carcinoma are associated with underlying liver cirrhosis. Hepatic US in conjunction with serum α-fetoprotein has been used to screen patients in Asia and Europe. Sonography in high-risk patients can detect lesions as small as 1 cm in diameter. The sonographic appearance varies with the histologic composition and size. Tumor invasion of the hepatic and portal veins may be demonstrated by CDUS. Most often, biopsy is necessary to make the definitive diagnosis and differentiate these from other benign and malignant liver masses. Hepatic lymphoma is an infiltrative neoplasm, sonographically presenting as focal, multifocal, or diffuse infiltration, often as hypoechoic masses or ill-defined areas of mixed echogenicity (Fig. 27.5-7). Metastases to the liver may be hypoechoic, hyperechoic, or show a diffuse infiltrative pattern. Most common primary tumors are gastrointestinal, renal, pancreas, breast, lung, and thyroid cancer.[14]

GALLBLADDER–BILIARY TREE

Gallbladder carcinoma usually presents with advanced disease. Sonographically, a focal wall mass protruding into the lumen or a diffuse infiltrative mass in the bed may be seen (Fig. 27.5-8). Cholangiocarcinoma may be intrahepatic, nodular, and mass-forming, or it may be infiltrative along the intra- and extrahepatic bile ducts. On US, it is seen as a heterogeneous hypoechoic mass, with or without ductal dilatation.[15]

PANCREAS

Pancreatic cancers include exocrine, endocrine, and cystic neoplasms and most commonly an adenocarcinoma of the exocrine duct. The tumor invades adjacent structures and vessels and commonly metastasizes to the liver. Patients most frequently present with obstructive jaundice. On US, a pancreatic mass, frequently hypoechoic, and a dilated common bile duct and pancreatic duct are identified. Sonography is less sensitive in imaging carcinoma of the body and tail of the pancreas because of overlying bowel gas. Pancreatic endocrine tumors, usually islet cell tumors, may present as small, hypoechoic masses in the gland. Mucinous cystic neoplasms may contain central calcifications.[16] Pancreatic cancers are usually best imaged with CT and biopsies preferably by US, sometimes, however, with CT guidance (Fig. 27.5-9).

ENDOCRINE

Thyroid nodules are not infrequently detected during US performed to evaluate the carotid arteries or in patients with abnormal thyroid function tests or palpable abnormalities. Solitary or suspicious, complex masses are usually biopsied under US guidance. Local lymph node involvement in thyroid malignancies can be exquisitely demonstrated with high-resolution US. Postthyroidectomy local recurrence or lymph node spread can be imaged and proven by US guided biopsy.[17]

Adrenal malignancies are most commonly adrenocortical carcinoma and pheochromocytoma. CT is usually the mainstay for the evaluation of adrenal masses because of its high sensitivity and simultaneous ability to accurately stage extension into adjacent structures. US may be the study on which an adrenal mass is detected incidentally. Small masses are homogeneous, and tumors become progressively heterogeneous with enlargement, due to necrosis and hemorrhage. Right adrenal masses can cause anterior displacement of the inferior vena cava. Metastases from lung primaries are common to the adrenal

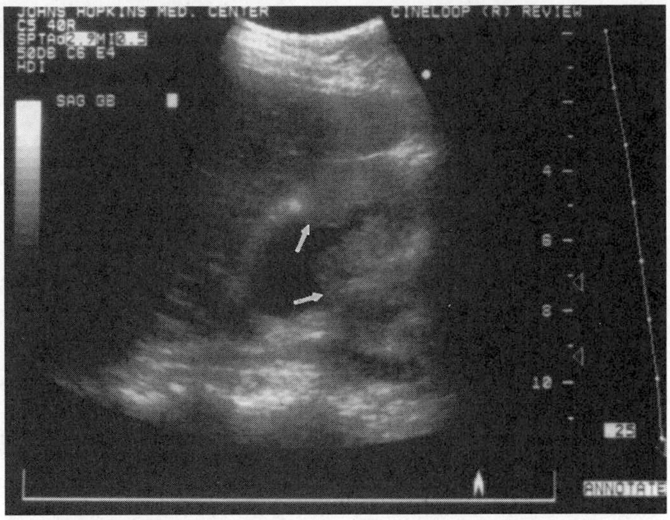

FIGURE 27.5-8. Sagittal sonogram of the gallbladder in patient with gallbladder carcinoma demonstrating thickening of the fundal wall, with mass protruding into the lumen (*arrows*).

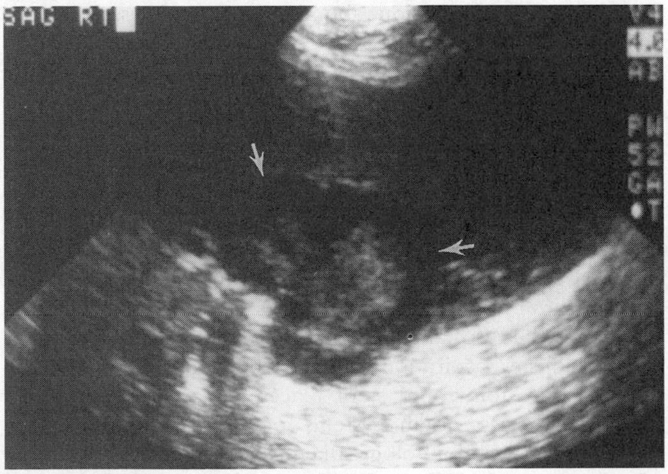

FIGURE 27.5-7. Sagittal sonogram of the right hepatic lobe containing a heterogeneous mass (*arrows*) in this patient 9 years after heart transplantation. Biopsy demonstrated hepatic lymphoma.

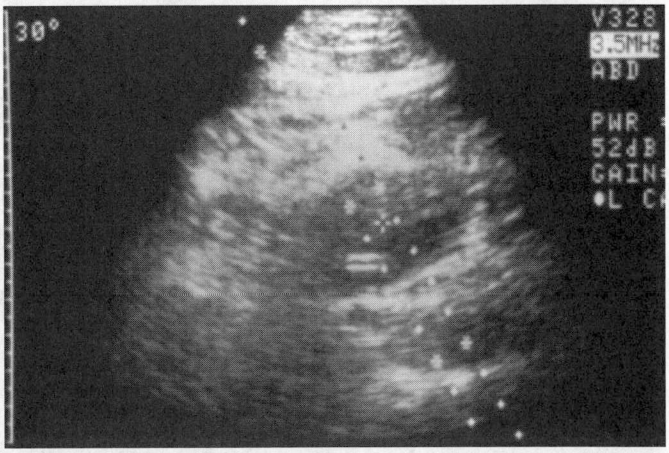

FIGURE 27.5-9. Focal mass in the pancreatic head (*cross-hair*) proven to be metastatic rhabdomyosarcoma. Linear echogenic lines represent indwelling biliary stent.

gland. However, in larger series, one-third to two-thirds of patients with adrenal masses and lung cancer had incidental nonfunctioning adenomas. Fine-needle aspiration biopsy is normally performed in these patients to establish the diagnosis of metastases.[18]

BONE MARROW TRANSPLANT

Sonography is frequently used to evaluate complications of high-dose therapy in bone marrow transplant patients, such as hepatic venoocclusive disease or hemorrhagic cystitis.

Hepatic Venoocclusive Disease

Hepatic venoocclusive disease is caused by high-dose chemotherapy prior to bone marrow transplant salvage. Toxicity to the liver results in hepatic edema, venous compression, and stagnation, with ultimately occlusion of the small hepatic veins. Imaging with CDUS may demonstrate a heterogeneous and enlarged liver, ascites, a thick-walled gallbladder, elevated hepatic artery resistive index (>0.8), decreased hepatic vein flow, and pulsatile or reversal of portal vein flow.[19]

Hemorrhagic Cystitis

Hemorrhagic cystitis is caused by the toxic effect of high-dose steroids to the urothelium, resulting in severe cystitis, hemorrhage, and bladder necrosis. On US, the bladder wall is thickened, and blood clots can be seen as intravesical masses (Fig. 27.5-10). US is also useful to assess the effectiveness of therapy.[20]

ACQUIRED IMMUNODEFICIENCY SYNDROME MALIGNANCIES

The most common neoplasms related to acquired immunodeficiency syndrome (AIDS) are Kaposi's sarcoma and non-Hodgkin's lymphoma. Other malignancies include cervical carcinoma, bronchogenic carcinoma, and Hodgkin's lymphoma with an unusual or aggressive presentation. AIDS patients are also at higher risk to develop testicular neoplasms, such as germ cell tumors or AIDS-related lymphoma (ARL).[21]

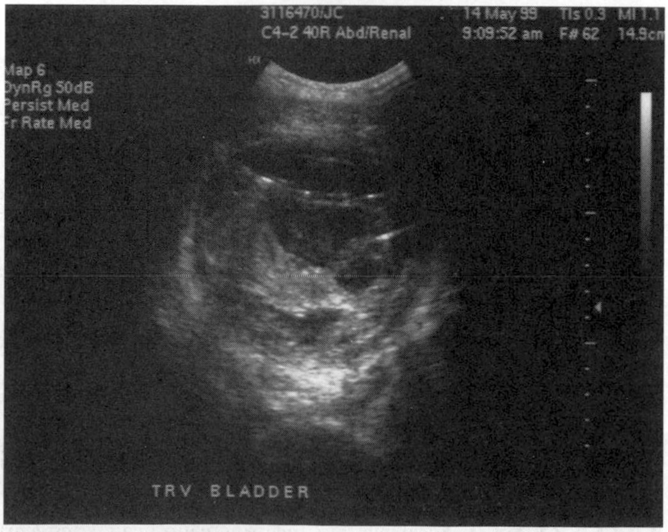

FIGURE 27.5-10. Vesical ultrasonography in a patient with hemorrhagic cystitis. Note bladder wall thickening and heterogeneous mass in the bladder compatible with a large blood clot.

Kaposi's Sarcoma

In AIDS, Kaposi's sarcoma is an aggressive multifocal neoplasm arising from lymphatic endothelial cells. It can involve skin, lymph nodes, gastrointestinal tract, liver, spleen, lung, and pleura. On US, focal liver or splenic masses or infiltrative lesions can be seen. Infiltrative lesions may also be present in the kidney, adrenal, bladder, or prostate.[21]

Acquired Immunodeficiency Syndrome–Related Lymphoma

Isolated or bulky adenopathy is rare and favors chronic infections, such as *Mycobacterium avium–intracellulare* and tuberculosis. Extranodal disease usually involves the gastrointestinal tract, liver, spleen, kidney, and adrenal gland. Chest wall disease involving the spine and sternum as well as pleural effusions are common. On US, hepatic and splenic involvement present as solitary or multiple hypoechoic nodules, which may appear cystic. Renal involvement may demonstrate bilateral parenchymal or perirenal masses. The differential diagnosis for such lesions includes renal cell carcinoma, tuberculosis, candidiasis, aspergillosis, or pyogenic abscesses.[21]

VENOUS COMPLICATIONS

US has become the standard primary imaging technique for the initial evaluation of patients with the clinical suspicion of deep venous thrombosis (DVT) of the extremity veins. Predisposing factors for DVT in the oncologic patient include paraneoplastic syndrome; immobilization; compression or direct invasion by the primary tumor or metastatic masses (pelvis, chest, Pancoast tumor); radiotherapy; and indwelling catheters or stents. The hallmark finding of acute DVT on gray scale, Doppler, and CDUS include distention and noncompressibility of vessels and direct visualization of tumor thrombus. In long-standing venous occlusion, abundant collateral vessels may be seen on US.[22]

ULTRASONOGRAPHICALLY GUIDED INTERVENTIONAL PROCEDURES

Accurate characterization and staging of malignancies has become increasingly important for cancer patients to avail themselves of the increasing advances in treatment options. Precise localization of disease process by fluoroscopy US, CT, and magnetic resonance imaging have made possible percutaneous biopsies, aspirations of fluid collections, abscess drainages, nephrostomy, and stent placement as well as vascular access in many organ systems of the oncology patient. Advances in cytopathology diagnostic techniques and the development of smaller and safer needles coupled with cross-sectional image guidance, particularly US, facilitate accurate and safe needle placement in formerly inaccessible sites. Most biopsies in the oncology patient are performed to confirm

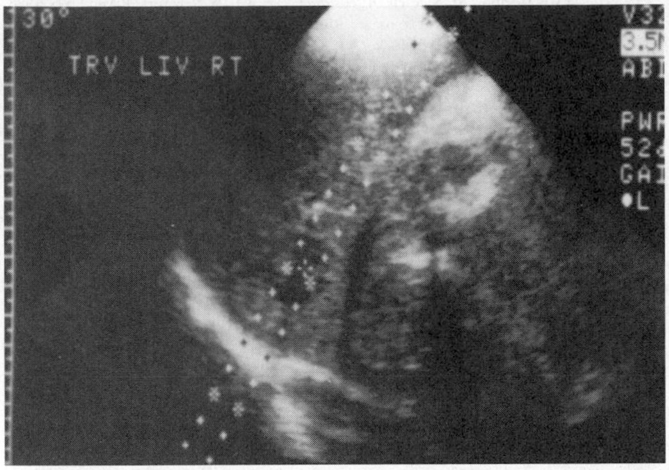

FIGURE 27.5-11. Ultrasonographically guided percutaneous biopsy of a small mass in the liver proved to be metastatic pancreatic carcinoma. Note biopsy trajectory (*dotted lines*).

malignancy in a radiographically suspicious lesion or to obtain a tissue diagnosis in an indeterminate lesion. Growing experience with US as a guidance modality has greatly expanded the role and scope of US-guided interventional masses in deep abdominal and superficial masses, thoracic and mediastinal applications.[23–27] Specific biopsy applications include liver (Fig. 27.5-11) and pancreas; renal, adrenal, retroperitoneal, splenic, neck, and musculoskeletal masses; as well as selected thoracic lesions when pleura-based or mediastinal (Fig. 27.5-12); breast lesions; endocavitary biopsy (endorectal, endovaginal); and recently intraoperative or percutaneous ablations (ethanol, cryosurgery, radiofrequency, laser, and microwave) for hepatic, renal, and prostate lesions.[23–30]

US is an ideal guidance modality for interventional procedures for various reasons. It allows real-time display throughout the procedure with unlimited scan plans, thus allowing creative patient positioning. Speed of the procedure; CDUS for vessel visualization; direct pressure over the lesion with the transducer in case of bleed; portability; lower cost; and nonionizing irradiation are other advantages of US. Future applications include percutaneous US-guided delivery of chemotherapy agents, drug delivery, and gene therapy as well as organ-specific delivery of substances in conjunction with contrast agents and directed local bubble destruction.

SUMMARY

US plays an important role in the diagnostic evaluation and management of cancer patients. With further advances in US technology and an ever-increasing variety of therapeutic options, its use in the oncology patient will expand in the future.

REFERENCES

1. Dalla Palma L, Pozzi Mucelli RS, Ricci C, Zuiani C. Ultrasonography in oncology. *Acta Oncol* 1989;28:157.
2. Berman CG, Brodsky NJ, Clarke RA, eds. *Oncologic imaging.* New York: McGraw-Hill, 1998:349.

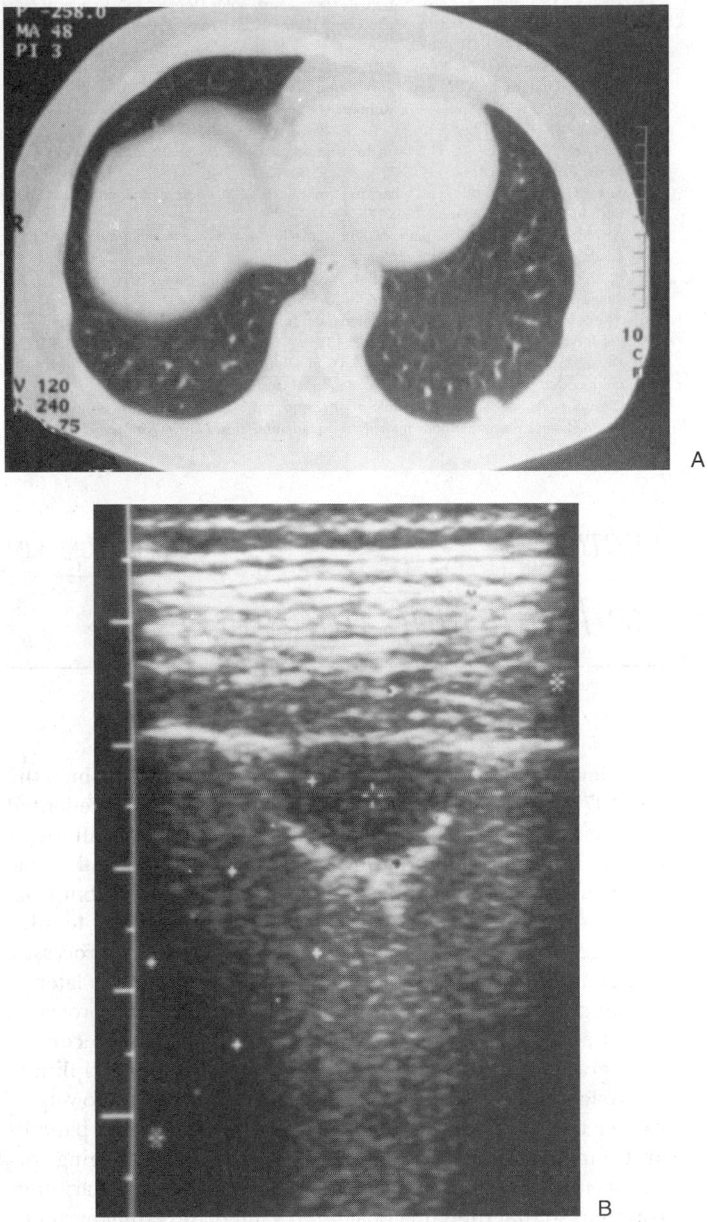

FIGURE 27.5-12. **A:** Computed tomography scan of the chest demonstrating small, left-sided posterior pleural-based lung nodule. **B:** Same nodule imaged by ultrasonography as a hypoechoic mass (*between dotted lines*). Ultrasonographically guided biopsy revealed metastatic squamous cell carcinoma to the lung.

3. Braeckman J, Keuppens F, Chaban M, Denis L. Ultrasound in urological oncology. *Eur J Surg Oncol* 1987;13:475.
4. Abulafia O, Sherer DM, Lee PS. Postoperative color Doppler flow ultrasonographic assessment of ureteral patency in gynecologic oncology patients. *J Ultrasound Med* 1997;16:125.
5. Thurston W, Wilson SR. The urinary tract. In: Rumack CM, ed. *Diagnostic ultrasound,* vol 1. St Louis: Mosby–Year Book, 1998:379.
6. Hamper UM, Sheth S, Walsh PC. Carcinoma of the prostate: value of transrectal sonography to detect extension into the neurovascular bundle. *AJR Am J Roentgenol* 1990;155:1015.
7. Hamper UM. Elevated prostate specific antigen and/or abnormal prostate physical exam. In: Bluth EI, Benson C, Arger P, Siegel M, Ralls P, eds. *The practice of ultrasonography.* New York: Thieme Verlag, 1999:153.
8. Bloom C. Scrotal ultrasonography: a pictorial essay. *Can Assoc Radiol J* 1998;49:12.
9. Hostman WG. Scrotal imaging. *Urol Clin North Am* 1997;24(3):653.
10. Fleischer AC, Rodgers WH, Kepple DM. Color doppler sonography of ovarian masses. A multiparameter analysis. *J Ultrasound Med* 1993;12:41.

11. Hamper UM, Sheth S, Abbas FM, et al. Transvaginal color Doppler sonography of ovarian masses: differences in blood flow impedance in benign and malignant lesions. *AJR AM J Roentgenol* 1993:160:1225.
12. Sheth S, Hamper UM, Kurman RJ. Thickened endometrium in the postmenopausal woman: sonographic-pathologic correlation. *Radiology* 1993;187:135.
13. Mendelson EB. The breast. In: Rumack CM, ed. *Diagnostic ultrasound,* vol 1. St. Louis: Mosby–Year Book, 1998:751.
14. Withers CE, Wilson SR. The liver. In: Rumack CM, ed. *Diagnostic ultrasound,* vol 1. St. Louis: Mosby–Year Book, 1998:87.
15. Laing C. The gallbladder and biliary tree. In: Rumack CM, ed. *Diagnostic ultrasound,* vol 1. St. Louis: Mosby–Year Book, 1998:175.
16. Atri M, Finnegan PW. The pancreas. In: Rumack CM, ed. *Diagnostic ultrasound,* vol 1. St. Louis: Mosby–Year Book, 1998:225.
17. Solbiati L, Charboneau JW, James EM, Hay ID. The thyroid gland. In: Rumack CM, ed. *Diagnostic ultrasound,* vol 1. St. Louis: Mosby–Year Book, 1998:703.
18. Thurston W, Wilson SR. The adrenal glands. In: Rumack CM, ed. *Diagnostic ultrasound,* vol 1. St. Louis: Mosby–Year Book, 1998:431.
19. Deeg KH, Clockel U, Richter R, Bede J. Diagnosis of veno-occlusive disease of the liver by color-coded Doppler sonography. *Pediatr Radiol* 1993;23:134.
20. Cartoni C, Arcese W, Arisati G. Role of ultrasonography in the diagnosis and follow-up of hemorrhagic cystitis after bone marrow transplantation. *Bone Marrow Transplant* 1993;12:463.
21. Federle MP, Megibow AJ, Naidich DP, eds. *Radiology of AIDS.* New York: Raven Press, 1988.
22. Bradley OL. The peripheral veins. In: Rumack CM, ed. *Diagnostic ultrasound,* vol 1. St. Louis: Mosby–Year Book, 1998:943.
23. Christallini EG, Ascani S, Farabi R, et al. Fine needle aspiration biopsy in the diagnosis of intrathoracic masses. *Acta Cytol* 1992;36:416.
24. Athlin L, Blin PJ, Angstrom T. Fine-needle aspiration biopsy of pancreatic masses. *Acta Chir Scand* 1990;156:91.
25. Bognel C, Rougier P, Ledere J. Fine needle aspiration of the liver and pancreas with ultrasound guidance. *Acta Cytol* 1988;32:22.
26. Jaeger HJ, MacFie J, Mitchell CJ, et al. Diagnosis of abdominal masses with percutaneous biopsy guided by ultrasound. *Br Med J* 1990;301:1188.
27. Sheth S, Hamper UM, Stanley DB, Wheeler JH, Smith PA. Sonographic guidance for thoracic biopsies: a valuable alternative to CT. *Radiology* 1999;210:721.
28. Hopper KD. Percutaneous radiographically guided biopsy: a history. *Radiology* 1995;195(3):918.
29. Memel DS, Dodd FD III, Escala CC. Efficacy of sonography as a guidance technique for biopsy of abdominal, pelvic and retroperitoneal lymph nodes. *AJR AM J Roentgenol* 1996;167:957.
30. Lee MJ, Mueller PR, Dawson SK. Percutaneous ethanol injection for the treatment of hepatic tumors: indications, mechanism of action, technique and efficacy. *AJR AM J Roentgenol* 1995;164(1):215.

SECTION 6

E. EDMUND KIM

Radionuclide Imaging

The development of molecular biology and genetics since the late 1970s has provided medical science with an unprecedented chance to understand the molecular basis of disease. Although disease is usually defined as gross structural or histopathologic abnormality, it can now be defined on the basis of abnormal deviation from normal regional biochemistry. Molecular derangements occur at the very beginning of disease processes, and anatomically detectable abnormalities occur much later.

Cancer is viewed as a failure of multiple chemical processes or genetic disease. The care of cancer patients has become a cooperative multidisciplinary endeavor. A multidisciplinary approach to the diagnosis, staging, treatment, and follow-up of cancer takes a great deal of effort, but the rewards to patients and oncologists are tremendous. It is critical for imaging specialists to embrace and participate in the multidisciplinary environment so that they are considered valued and equal partners.

Advanced imaging techniques have made it possible to diagnose localized abnormalities, often before they have produced irreversible damage. Cancers too small to be detected by physical examination can be pinpointed by imaging and treated before metastasis has occurred. Most imaging methods reveal the anatomic extent of an organ or of an abnormality within an organ. Many masses cannot be characterized clearly with imaging studies. This may be a problem when attempting to distinguish residual viable tumor from fibrosis.

Many radionuclide studies have been performed for the detection of primary and metastatic tumors. Most are organ- or receptor-specific but not tumor-specific. A few studies are highly tissue-specific, such as thyroid scans using iodine 131 sodium iodide and adrenal scans using ^{131}I metaiodobenzylguanidine (MIBG) or 6-β-iodomethyl-19-norcholesterol. Radiolabeled antibodies and peptides are potentially tumor-specific. With nonspecific limited agents, abnormalities on scans represent alteration or displacement of normal tissue, and additional scans with other agents are often necessary to evaluate potential involvement of other organs. Extensive effort has been directed toward the development of specific general agents that ideally would be taken up specifically by tumor and that could be used for a broad spectrum of tumor types.

INDIRECT RADIONUCLIDE TUMOR IMAGING

NUCLEAR BONE SCANS

The bisphosphonate bone scan is the most frequently performed radionuclide study, and it is used for the early detection of metastatic bone disease. The positive bone scan (Fig. 27.6-1) reflects levels of blood flow and osteoblastic formation.[1] Magnetic resonance imaging (MRI) has a greater sensitivity and specificity than bone scans in detecting metastatic foci,[2] but bone scans remain the choice for initial screening of bony metastasis because of its ability to easily assess the whole body and because of its availability. In the follow-up of bony metastases, the *flare phenomenon,* in which the patient's clinical condition is improving but the bone scan is worsening, has been described in up to 20% of patients after a therapeutic intervention.[3] Bone single photon emission computed tomography (SPECT) has been helpful and complementary in differentiating degenerative joint disease or facet syndrome from metastasis. Extraskeletal uptake of technetium 99m methylene diphosphonate (MDP) has been reported in many malignant tumors with calcification or increased vascularity. Severe bone pain can be a particularly debilitating effect of metastatic disease. Strontium 89 chloride, samarium 153 ethylene diamine tetramethane phosphoric acid (EDTMP), and rhenium 186 hydroxy ethylene diphosphoric acid (HEDP) and Sn-117m DTPA (diethylenetriamine pentaacetic acid) have been effective in reducing pain in breast and prostate cancer patients.[4]

NUCLEAR LIVER SCANS

Cavernous hemangioma is the most common benign tumor of the liver and consists of dilated endothelium-lined blood-filled spaces. Increasing focal activity over 1 to 2 hours after injection of ^{99m}Tc red blood cells is a typical diagnostic finding. SPECT is cost effective in demonstrating hemangiomas greater than 1 cm when CT or MRI findings are questionable.[5]

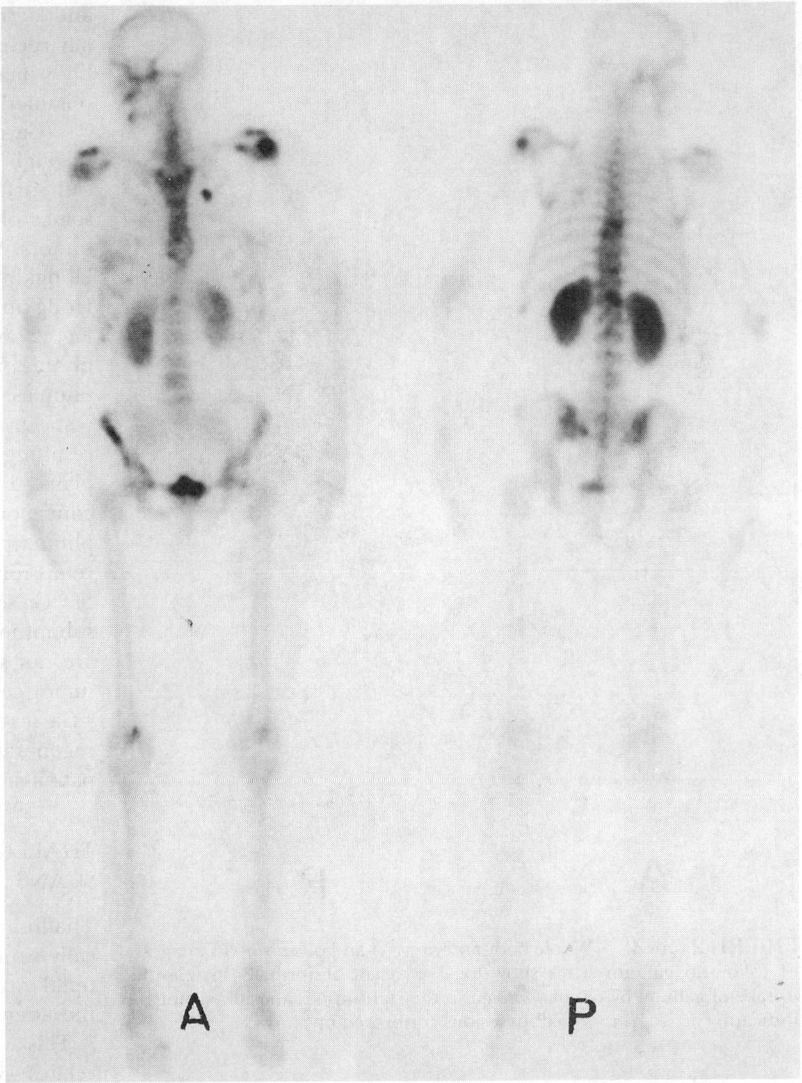

FIGURE 27.6-1. Whole body anterior (A) and posterior (P) images of follow-up bone scans using technetium 99m methylene diphosphonate show focal areas of abnormally increased activities in the left humeral head, T7, T8, T12, left sacrum, and left anterior second rib end, indicating active metastatic lesions. Note also the diffusely increased renal activities suggesting nephrotoxicity in a patient with breast cancer.

Hepatic adenoma and focal nodular hyperplasia show a contrast enhancement on CT or MRI. The adenoma presents as a cold defect on ^{99m}Tc sulfur colloid liver-spleen scans but shows an uptake of ^{99m}Tc iminodiacetic acid hepatobiliary agent because no Kupffer cell is present. On the other hand, focal nodular hyperplasia demonstrates uptake of ^{99m}Tc sulfur colloid because of the presence of Kupffer cells.[6]

HEPATIC PERFUSION SCANS

Intraarterial chemotherapy has been used to treat many tumors in an effort to obtain better results than with systemic chemotherapy. Hepatic tumors derive 99% of their blood supply from the hepatic artery. ^{99m}Tc macroaggregated albumin, usually 10 to 90 mm, is trapped in the first capillary bed and has been useful to detect misplaced or displaced hepatic arterial catheters that require repositioning.[7]

NUCLEAR CARDIOVASCULAR IMAGING

In patients undergoing chemotherapy with doxorubicin (Adriamycin), one risk is developing cardiotoxicity. Radionuclide ventriculography using ^{99m}Tc red blood cells provides the left ventricular ejection fraction, and a 10% to 15% decrease of left ventricular ejection fraction or a decrease to less than 45% is considered significant.[8] Chemotherapy or catheterization increases the risk for thrombus formation in cancer patients. Radionuclide venograms using ^{99m}Tc macroaggregated albumin for lower extremities and ^{99m}Tc sulfur colloid or DTPA for upper extremities have been useful in screening hemodynamically significant venous obstruction.[9] ^{99m}Tc P-829 peptide accumulated in the platelet receptor is now being used to detect acute venous thrombosis.

LYMPHOSCINTIGRAPHY

Approximately 20% of melanoma patients do have clinically undetectable micrometastases in the lymph nodes, and the presence of metastases in the sentinel (first draining) node indicates the need for a regional lymph node dissection. A dose of 0.5 mCi ^{99m}Tc sulfur colloid in 0.25 mL is injected intradermally around the melanoma site, and the lymphatic flow is imaged dynamically for 30 minutes. Subsequent static images demonstrate the draining regional node basin and the location

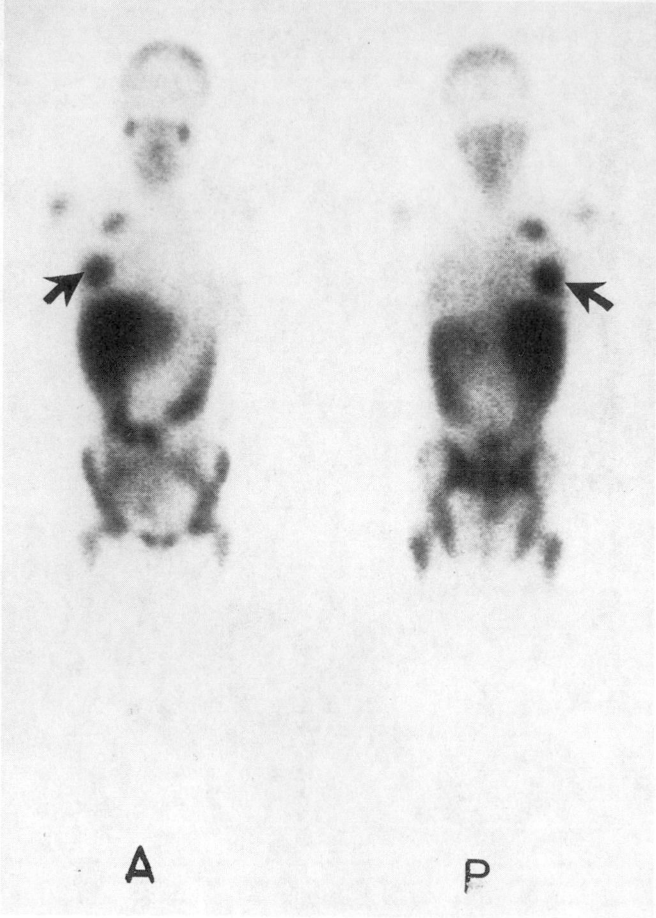

FIGURE 27.6-2. Whole body anterior (A) and posterior (P) images of follow-up gallium scans show focal areas of abnormally increased uptake of gallium 67 citrate (*arrows*) in the right upper and lower lungs, indicating active lymphomatous lesions confirmed by biopsy.

of the sentinel node.[10] The status of regional lymph node remains the most powerful predictor of survival in women with invasive breast cancer. Approximately 14% to 37% of small (less than 1 cm) invasive cancers may have axillary nodal metastases. Lymphatic drainage from breast cancer can be mapped to regional lymph nodes pre- or intraoperatively. The technique involves peritumoral injection of 0.5 mCi ^{99m}Tc sulfur colloid and gamma camera imaging or gamma detection probe. In one study,[11] the sentinel lymph node was identified in 92% of patients, and 32% of them were found to have metastatic diseases.

DIRECT RADIONUCLIDE TUMOR IMAGING

GALLIUM 67 CITRATE SCANS

Gallium 67 citrate has been known to be taken up in varying degrees by many other tumors, and ^{67}Ga scans have been useful as a marker of tumor viability and for evaluating the effectiveness of radiotherapy or chemotherapy. ^{67}Ga citrate binds to serum transferrin, ferritin, and lactoferrin. Approximately 15% to 25% is excreted by kidneys within 24 to 48 hours, and 30% to 40% is cleared slowly through the intestinal tract. ^{67}Ga citrate localizes normally within the reticuloendothelial system and lacrimal and salivary glands. A dose of 5 to 10 mCi is usually recommended for tumor imaging. High-resolution whole body images (Fig. 27.6-2) and SPECT of chest or abdomen are obtained at 48 to 72 hours.

^{67}Ga citrate probably enters the tumor extracellular space through the capillary endothelium and is bound to the tumor cell surface by transferrin receptors. It localizes in the lysosomes of tumor cells and is taken up by viable and growing tumors. ^{67}Ga scans detect nodal and visceral involvement of Hodgkin's disease, and high- and intermediate-grade non-Hodgkin's lymphomas, with approximately 90% sensitivity (see Fig. 27.6-2).[12] The sensitivities for histocytic Burkitt's lymphoma, and poorly and well-differentiated lymphocytic lymphomas, have been reported as 89%, 85%, 70%, and 59%, respectively.[13] SPECT greatly improves contrast resolution, resulting in a 10% to 15% increase of diagnostic accuracy over planar imaging. Persistent ^{67}Ga uptake halfway through the course of chemotherapy in patients with diffuse large cell lymphoma predicts a poor outcome, either by failure to achieve remission or by subsequent relapse.[13] The diagnostic sensitivity of ^{67}Ga scans for lung cancer is 85% to 90%, but ^{67}Ga scans are suboptimal for preoperative staging. However, enlarged nodes are not specific for tumors, and normal-size nodes can carry tumor cells. Most hepatomas and melanomas are Ga-avid, and ^{67}Ga scans can be useful for differentiating hepatomas from regenerative pseudotumor nodules seen on CT in cirrhotic patients.

THALLIUM 201 AND TECHNETIUM 99M SESTAMIBI SCANS

Thallium 201 chloride behaves in a manner that is biologically similar to potassium. Tumor blood flow influences the uptake of ^{201}Tl by tumors, probably related to the action of the adenosine triphosphatase system in the cell membrane. ^{201}Tl is accumulated by viable tumor tissue, and its uptake correlates with the grade of histopathologic differentiation. Planar and SPECT imaging of the lesion is usually obtained at 10 to 30 minutes after the injection of 3 mCi ^{201}Tl chloride. ^{201}Tl scans have been used to determine viability when CT or MRI cannot differentiate residual or recurrent brain or lung tumors from posttreatment changes or infectious lesions (Fig. 27.6-3). ^{201}Tl indices, count-density ratios of tumor to nontumor area, were significantly higher in high-grade tumors than in those patients with low-grade tumors.[14] ^{201}Tl is usually taken up only by tumors, whereas ^{67}GA is taken up in both tumor and inflammatory lesions. ^{201}Tl appears valuable in detecting low-grade non-Hodgkin's lymphoma and also Kaposi's sarcoma. Some studies have found the ^{201}Tl scan to be more sensitive than the ^{131}I scan in the detection of thyroid cancer, although ^{201}Tl is not specific for thyroid cancer and does not give predictive information on the therapeutic potential of ^{131}I sodium iodide.[15]

^{99m}Tc sestamibi uptake is not tumor-specific, but it has been used to detect benign as well as malignant tumors, including parathyroid adenoma and breast cancer. ^{99m}Tc sestamibi is bound by the mitochondrial proteins but is passively transferred across the cell membrane. The sestamibi scan is usually performed at 15 to 30 minutes and 2 to 3 hours after injection of 20 to 29 mCi. ^{99m}Tc sestamibi uptake is inversely proportional to the level of P glycoprotein, which is a product of the

A 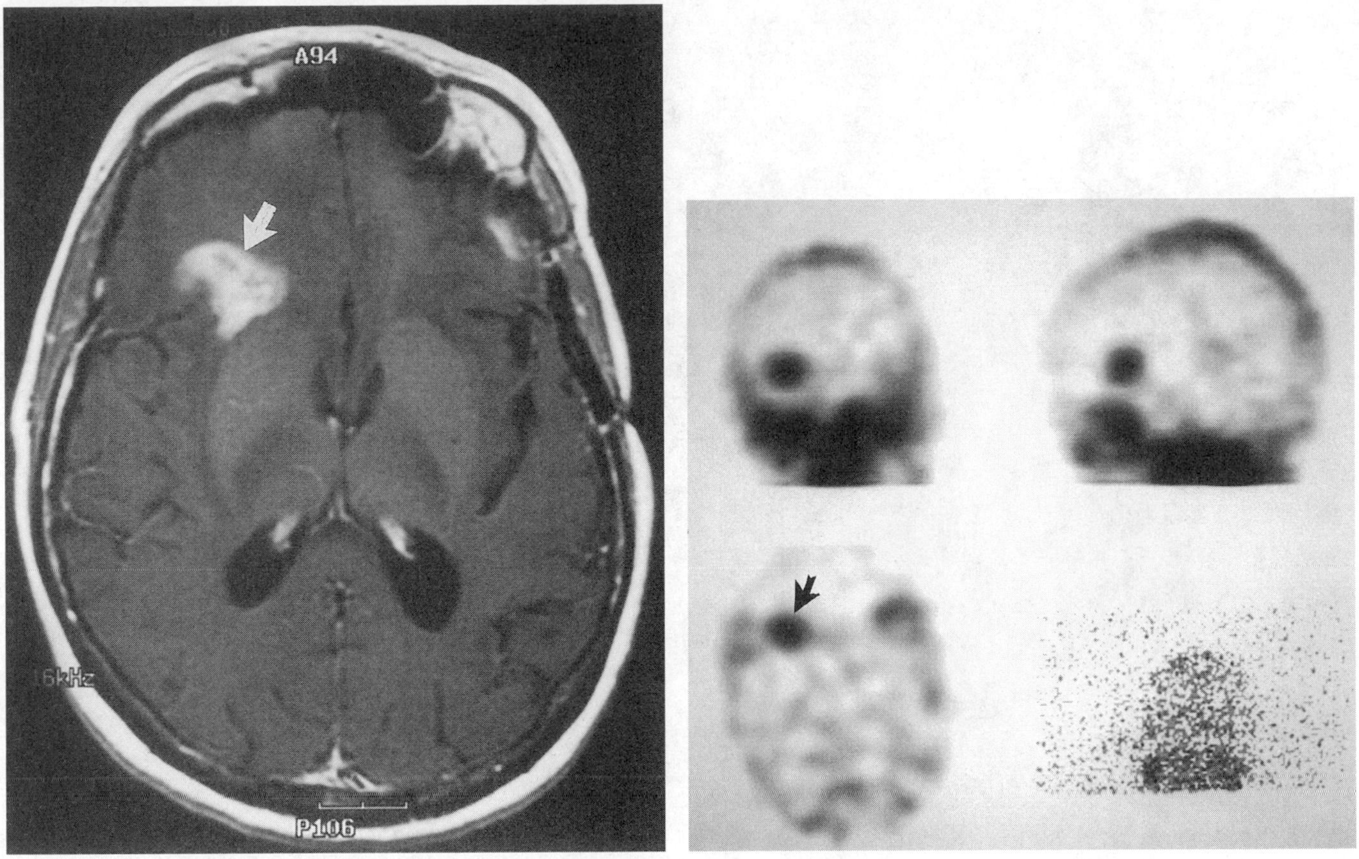 B

FIGURE 27.6-3. **A:** Axial T1-weighted magnetic resonance images of the head show a contrast-enhanced lesion (*arrow*) in the right frontal lobe in a patient who had a treatment for anaplastic astrocytoma. **B:** Selected coronal (*upper left*), sagittal (*upper right*), and axial (*lower left*) single photon emission computed tomography images using thallium 201 chloride show a focal area of markedly increased activity (*arrow*) in the right frontal lobe, indicating active malignant tumor. Biopsy confirmed a recurrent anaplastic astrocytoma.

multidrug resistance gene. Some studies have shown the potential of functional imaging using ^{99m}Tc sestamibi to monitor cancer therapy with the multidrug resistance modulator.[16]

NUCLEAR THYROID AND ADRENAL IMAGING

During the 1990s, it has become apparent that the most cost-effective diagnostic workup of a thyroid nodule is fine-needle aspiration. However, histologic and cellular details of endocrine tumors do not always establish the diagnosis of carcinoma. Both papillary and follicular cancers retain, to varying degrees, the ability to concentrate radioiodine. Medullary and anaplastic carcinomas do not concentrate radioiodine. All types of thyroid cancer do not concentrate radioiodine as avidly as normal thyroid tissue. To enhance radioiodine uptake by thyroid cancer, high levels of circulating thyroid-stimulating hormone are desired (more than 30 μIU/mL).

^{123}I is ideal for imaging because of short physical half-life (13 hours) and optimal photon energy (159 keV). However, it is relatively expensive, and the thyroid imaging is usually performed at 4 to 6 hours after the oral administration of 0.2 mCi ^{123}I sodium iodide. ^{99m}Tc sodium pertechnetate is cheap and ideal for early (30 minutes) imaging with good physical properties (6-hour half-life; 140 keV optimal photon energy), although it is only trapped and not organified. Indications of radionuclide thyroid imaging are functional evaluation of palpable nodules, detection of the primary tumor in patients with known regional or distant thyroidal metastases, detection of thyroid cancer metastases, and assessment of thyroid treatments. Nonfunctioning cold nodules are common, and 6% to 20% of them are usually malignant.[17]

Pheochromocytoma is a tumor of adrenal medulla or sympathetic nervous tissues. Approximately 10% occur in children, 10% are familial, 10% are malignant, 10% are multifocal, and 10% are extraadrenal. CT or MRI is useful in detecting intraadrenal or other abdominal masses. MIBG is an analogue of guanethidine and localizes in cytoplasmic storage vesicles in presynaptic adrenergic nerves through the active amine transport mechanism. ^{123}I- or ^{131}I-labeled MIBG has been useful in surveying the entire body for the localization of pheochromocytoma or paraganglioma.[18]

ANTIBODY AND PEPTIDE IMAGING

Antibodies are glycoproteins produced by plasma cells after exposure to a foreign antigen. Many tumors have antigens expressed on their cell surfaces, thus allowing antibody targeting. Major roles of immunoscintigraphy using indium 111 anti-TAG-12 (OncoScint, Cytogen Co., Princeton, NJ) or ^{99m}Tc anti–carcinoembryonic antigen (CEA) (CEA-scan, Immunomedics Co., Morris Plains, NJ) (Fig. 27.6-4) in colon cancer are: (1) detection of

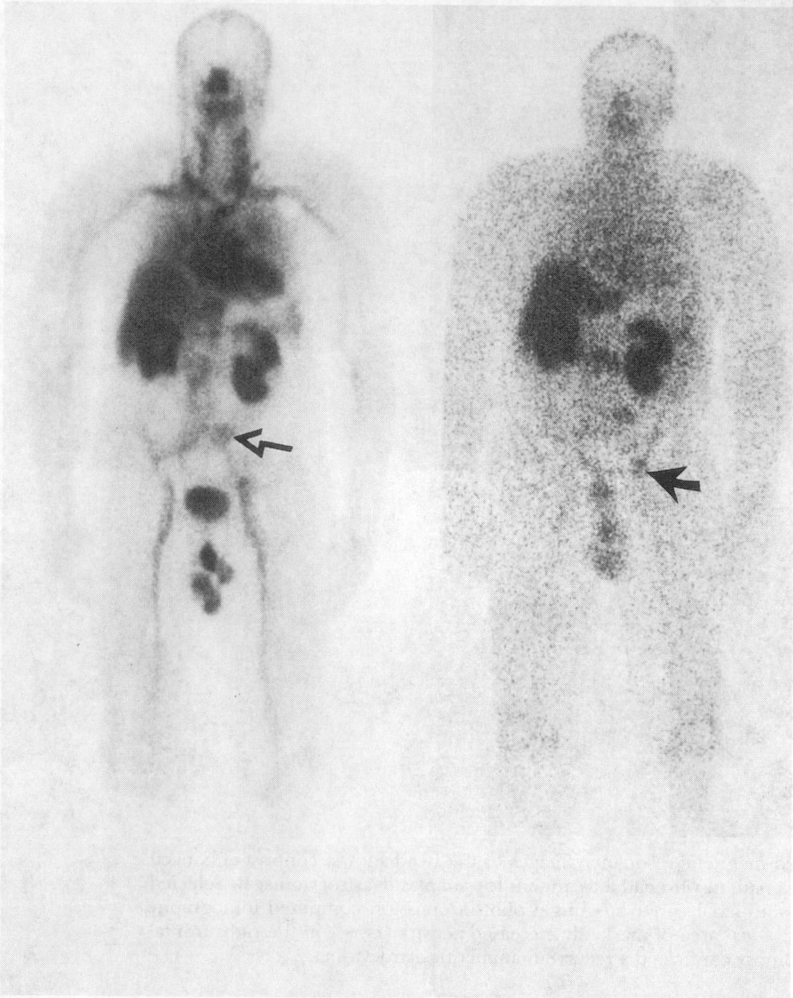

FIGURE 27.6-4. Anterior whole body images at 2 (*left*) and 20 (*right*) hours after the injection of technetium 99m anti–carcinoembryonic antigen (CEA) show focal areas of abnormally increased activity in the left inguinal (*closed arrow*) and iliac (*open arrow*) lymphatic chains in a patient with colon carcinoma and rising serum CEA levels. Note the cystic lesions in the left kidney.

recurrent disease in patients with elevated serum CEA level, and either negative workup or equivocal findings on CT or MRI; (2) differential diagnosis of residual or recurrent disease from posttreatment changes; and (3) exclusion of extraabdominal disease before planned resection of a presumably isolated recurrence. ^{111}In antiprostate membrane antigen (ProstaScint, Cytogen Co.) scans are indicated for patients with proven prostate cancer thought to be localized clinically after standard diagnostic evaluation who are at risk for pelvic node metastasis. It is also indicated in prostate cancer patients with a rising prostate-specific antigen level and negative or equivocal standard metastatic evaluation. Antibody scans generally revealed 70 to 80 T diagnostic sensitivities and should be interpreted in conjunction with CT or MRI studies.[19] Natural somatostatin is a tetradecapeptide produced by hypothalamus and pancreas. Five subtypes of human somatotropin-release inhibiting factor receptors, termed *somatostatin type receptors* (SSTRs), are expressed on many tumors, and SSTR2 is the predominant subtype. Tumors that have been found to express SSTRs include small cell lung cancer, endocrine pancreatic tumor, carcinoid, pituitary adenoma, paraganglioma, lymphoma, and meningioma. Octreotide is a synthetic somatotropin-release inhibiting factor analogue that has been used for treating gastroenteropancreatic tumors. ^{111}In pentetreotide (Octreoscan, Mallinckrodt Co., Hazelwood, MO) has been helpful for detecting neuroendocrine tumors and evaluating their therapeutic response.[20] ^{99m}Tc P-829 peptide has been approved to image somatostatin receptors in lung cancers.[21]

REFERENCES

1. Garrett IR. Bone destruction in cancer. *Semin Oncol* 1993;20:4.
2. Kosuda S, Kaji T, Yokoyama H, et al. Does bone SPECT actually have lower sensitivity for detecting vertebral metastasis than MRI? *J Nucl Med* 1996;37:975.
3. Coleman RE, Mashiter G, Whitaker KB. Bone scan flare predicts successful systemic therapy for bone metastases. *J Nucl Med* 1988;29:1354.
4. Holmes RA. Radiopharmaceuticals in clinical trials. *Semin Oncol* 1993;20:22.
5. Ferrucci JT. Liver tumor imaging: current concepts. *AJR Am J Roentgenol* 1990;160:473.
6. Welch TJ, Sheedy PF, Johnson CM, et al. Focal nodular hyperplasia and hepatic adenoma: comparison of angiography, CT, ultrasound, and scintigraphy. *Radiology* 1985;156:593.
7. Bledin AG, Kim EE, Chuang VP, Wallace S, Haynie TP. Changes of arterial blood flow patterns during infusion chemotherapy, as monitored by intra-arterially injected technetium 99m macroaggregated albumin. *Br J Radiol* 1984;57:197.
8. Schwartz RG, McKenzie B, Alexander J, et al. Congestive heart failure and left ventricular dysfunction complicating doxorubicin therapy. *Am J Med* 1987;82:1109.
9. Knight LC. Scintigraphic methods for detecting vascular thrombus. *J Nucl Med* 1993;34:554.
10. Kapteijin BAE, Nieweg OE, Valdes Olms RA, et al. Reproducibility of lymphoscintigraphy for lymphatic mapping in cutaneous melanoma. *J Nucl Med* 1996;37: 972.
11. Albertini JJ, Lyman GH, Cox C, et al. Lymphatic mapping and sentinel node biopsy in the patients with breast cancer. *JAMA* 1996;276:1818.
12. Front D, Israel O. The role of Ga-67 scintigraphy in evaluating the results of therapy of lymphoma patients. *Semin Nucl Med* 1995;25:60.

13. King SC, Reiman RJ, Prosnitz LR. Prognostic importance of restaging gallium scans following induction chemotherapy for advanced Hodgkin's disease. *J Clin Oncol* 1994;12:306.
14. Takekawa H, Itoh K, Abe S, et al. Tl-201 uptake, histologic differentiation and Na-K ATPase in lung adenocarcinoma. *J Nucl Med* 1996;37:955.
15. Lorberboym M, Murthy S, Cechanick JI, et al. Thallium-201 and iodine-131 scintigraphy in differentiated thyroid carcinoma. *J Nucl Med* 1996;37:1487.
16. Rao VV, Chiu ML, Kronauge JF, Pwinica-Worms D. Expression of recombinant human multidrug resistance P-glycoprotein in insect cells confers decreased accumulation of Tc-99m sestamibi. *J Nucl Med* 1994;35:510.
17. Dworkin HJ, Meier DA, Kaplan M. Advances in the management of patients with thyroid disease. *Semin Nucl Med* 1995;25:205.
18. Freitas JE. Adrenal cortical and medullary imaging. *Semin Nucl Med* 1995;25:235.
19. Zucker LS, DeNardo GL. Trials and tribulations: oncologic antibody imaging comes to the fore. *Semin Nucl Med* 1997;27:10.
20. Olsen JO, Pozderac RV, Inkle G, et al. Somatostatin receptor imaging of neuroendocrine tumors with In-111 pentetreotide. *Semin Nucl Med* 1995;25:251.
21. Vallabhajosula S, Moyer BR, Lister-James J, et al. Preclinical evaluation of Tc-99m labeled somatostatin receptor-binding peptides. *J Nucl Med* 1996;37:1016.

Robert C. Kurtz
Robert J. Ginsberg

CHAPTER 28

Cancer Diagnosis: Endoscopy

UPPER GASTROINTESTINAL ENDOSCOPY

Endoscopy is a rapidly advancing field. Video-recording or electronic instruments use microchip technology to capture high-resolution digitized endoscopic images, leading to more accurate diagnoses and greater ease in documentation and analysis. Many internal organs can be examined by endoscopy with video documentation, endoscopic biopsy, cytology, and endoscopic sonography to determine diagnosis, operability, and staging.

Although diagnostic endoscopy remains the major component of any endoscopy program, therapeutic endoscopy is rapidly catching up. Endoscopic removal of polyps, tumor ablation with laser therapy, luminal stents, control of hemorrhage, relief of biliary obstruction, and enteral nutritional support through endoscopically placed tubes are but some of the therapeutic uses of endoscopy available at large medical centers.

Upper gastrointestinal (GI) endoscopy is the procedure of choice for the diagnosis of symptomatic esophagogastric neoplasia. Benign upper GI conditions that can mimic or complicate cancer are accurately diagnosed. Endoscopy is often the initial diagnostic procedure rather than a follow-up to radiologic examination.[1] Upper GI endoscopes are thin and highly maneuverable, making upper endoscopy comfortable and rapid.[2] Upper GI endoscopy requires only mild sedation and is safe for the patient. Although upper GI endoscopy is more invasive and more expensive than barium upper GI radiography, it is also more accurate and may avoid multiple procedures, with their associated added costs. There is no exposure to radiation, and complications are rare.[3] The ability to perform guided mucosal biopsy and cytology provides tissue diagnosis to complement high-resolution observation and photography.

DIAGNOSTIC UPPER GASTROINTESTINAL ENDOSCOPY

The diagnostic accuracy of endoscopy and biopsy for primary and metastatic upper GI cancer is in the range of 95%.[1] Infiltrating cancers may be less successfully subjected to biopsy, although a tissue diagnosis is still achieved in most cases with large biopsy forceps and needle aspiration cytology.[4] Endoscopy is recommended in all patients with gastric ulcers found on upper GI series, because some benign-appearing gastric ulcers are malignant.[1] If suspicion remains, repeat endoscopy is indicated in 6 to 8 weeks. This is not the case in duodenal ulcer disease, which is only rarely due to cancer, and endoscopy solely to diagnose *Helicobacter pylori* infection is not recommended.

Patients with an identifiable high risk for upper GI cancer, such as those with Barrett's esophagus, prior gastric adenomas, or previous partial gastrectomy, may be considered for periodic screening endoscopy, although the benefits of such screening remain controversial.[5] When high-grade dysplasia is identified on endoscopic biopsy of either the stomach or Barrett's esophagus, surgical management should be considered because there is a high likelihood of developing invasive cancer.[6]

In northern China, where chronic esophagitis and epidermoid carcinoma of the esophagus are endemic,[7] population screening programs for esophageal cancer have been carried out on a large scale with promising results. Screening has been based on esophageal cytology and confirmation with endoscopy.[8] Using these methods, early-stage esophageal cancers with good probability for surgical cure have been detected in asymptomatic persons. Similar screening programs, carried out in heavy smokers and drinkers in the United States, have not proven effective.[9] Endoscopy has identified early asymptomatic esophageal cancer in up to 5% of patients with cancers of the head and neck who are also at risk for esophageal cancer. Endoscopic staining of the esophagus with Lugol's iodine solution before endoscopy may help in detecting small areas of squamous cell malignancy.[10]

In Japan, where gastric cancer is a leading cause of death, mass population screening with radiography and endoscopy has led to a major improvement in the detection of early disease and subsequent survival.[11] Distal gastric cancer in America and Europe has been decreasing in incidence, but there is an increase in cancers affecting the proximal stomach and an increasing incidence of early gastric cancer detection.[12,13] Mass screening is not practical or economically feasible in low-incidence Western countries; the increased detection of early gastric cancer has been attributed to greater physician sensitivity to suggestive symptoms and more aggressive application of radiologic and endoscopic methods.[14]

Whether patients with partial gastrectomy for benign disease are at long-term risk for gastric cancer and merit endoscopic screening is also an open question but, in patients who have dysplasia on endoscopic biopsy, endoscopic surveillance is indicated.[15]

Periodic endoscopic surveillance of the stomach and duodenum in patients with familial adenomatous polyposis (FAP) and Gardner's syndrome is recommended, including the use of a side-viewing duodenoscope for better visualization of the periampullary area. Adenomas of the duodenum are common in patients with FAP. In such cases, the adenomas tend to be very flat and may be numerous.[16] Carcinoma in the duodenum, most often periampullary, has become a major cause of death in patients with FAP who have had a colectomy.

New endoscopic technology is continually being developed. Fluorescence spectroscopy is one such advance currently in clinical trials. Laser-generated light of a specific wavelength is used to stimulate tissue during endoscopy. Differential fluorescence can be detected from benign, dysplastic, and malignant GI tissues. This technology may become a complement to histopathology, especially in sampling large areas of the GI tract before endoscopic biopsy.[17]

As a rule, endoscopy is most effective in evaluating intraluminal GI disease, focal and diffuse, benign and malignant. The procedure can be informative but is less effective in assessing abnormal motility, extrinsic compression by contiguous structures, and degree of luminal obstruction. Barium radiologic and computed tomography (CT) scans provide not only better evaluation of extrinsic lesions that are causing compression and contour defects in the GI tract but better assessment of the degree of obstruction.

THERAPEUTIC UPPER GASTROINTESTINAL ENDOSCOPY

Therapeutic applications of endoscopy include the placement of guidewires, stents, and balloons for the following purposes[18–20]:

1. Dilation of benign and malignant strictures
2. Removal of foreign bodies
3. Removal of polyps by electrocautery
4. Endoscopic strip biopsy of small cancers
5. Vaporization and coagulation of cancerous tissues with neodymium:yttrium aluminum garnet (Nd:YAG) laser or with photodynamic therapy
6. Control of bleeding with electrocautery, heat, or laser probes
7. Injection of epinephrine and sclerosant solutions via needle-tipped catheters for tumor necrosis or treatment of bleeding

In patients with advanced, unresectable cancer of the esophagus or gastric cardia that is unresponsive to primary treatment, endoscopic therapy has assumed a major role in the palliation of concomitant dysphagia. The mainstays of endoscopic palliation have been the placement of endoprostheses, using either plastic stents or self-expanding metallic stents, and laser ablation with Nd:YAG laser energy. There are advantages and disadvantages to both methods. In approximately 70% of patients, laser therapy is more likely to allow a normal diet, but it must be repeated at frequent intervals. Although outpatient treatment is possible, laser sessions become increasingly time-consuming and uncomfortable for the patient as the cancer progresses. Esophageal stents ideally provide a longer-lasting palliation, and they are the treatment of choice for tumors that are primarily infiltrating, submucosal, or extrinsic. They can be used anywhere in the esophagus except near the proximal sphincter. Endoluminal stents are also useful for sealing fistulas into the tracheobronchial tree. In most centers where an Nd:YAG laser is available, laser therapy is performed first, particularly if there is bulky intraluminal tumor. However, some groups preferentially palliate esophageal and esophagogastric malignant stenoses with stents. This is especially true with the advent of self-expanding metal stents, which are easier to insert, cause less trauma, carry a lower perforation rate, but are more expensive initially than polyvinyl stents. Complications, mostly perforations, occur in approximately 5% of those treated with laser and 5% to 18% of those treated with stents.[18,19]

Photodynamic therapy (PDT) uses both photochemical sensitizers that preferentially concentrate in neoplastic tissue and low-powered laser light activation. This technique is, in theory, more selective and safer than the Nd:YAG laser treatment. However, one multicenter study[21] of advanced esophageal cancer showed no difference when the cancers were treated with either PDT or Nd:YAG laser. Perhaps the most effective use of PDT will be in the management of early cancers or premalignant conditions such as Barrett's esophagus.[21,22]

COMPLICATIONS

Upper GI endoscopy is a very safe procedure with few contraindications and only rare complications. The probability of GI perforation is less than 0.1%.[3] This procedure can be performed safely even in patients on anticoagulants or with nadir blood counts, although therapeutic options in these patients may be limited. In weakened or comatose patients, there is an increased risk of aspiration pneumonia.

ENDOSCOPIC ULTRASONOGRAPHY

PRINCIPLES

Endoscopic ultrasonography (EUS) is an important new extension of diagnostic GI endoscopy. Using this modality, it is possi-

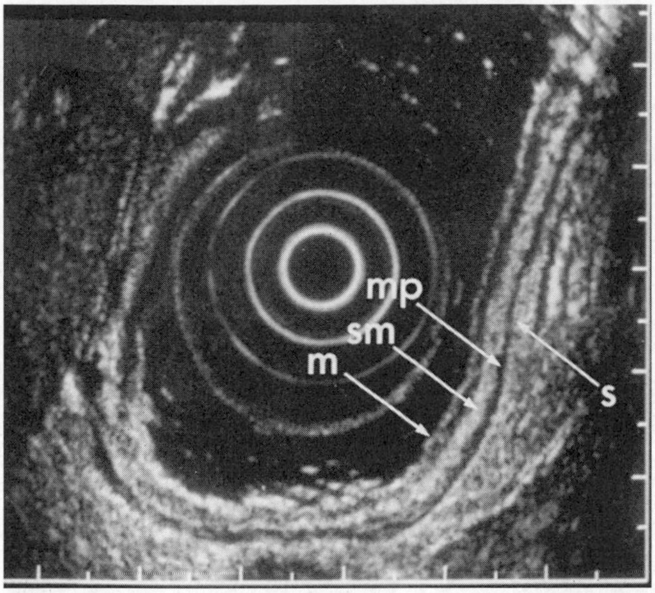

FIGURE 28-1. Endosonographic image of the normal gastric wall. The concentric circles in the center represent the transducer and water-filled balloon in the lumen of the stomach. From the lumen, the first two wall layers correlate with the superficial and deep mucosa (m), the third wall layer represents the submucosa (sm), the fourth layer is the muscularis propria (mp), and the fifth layer is the serosa (s).

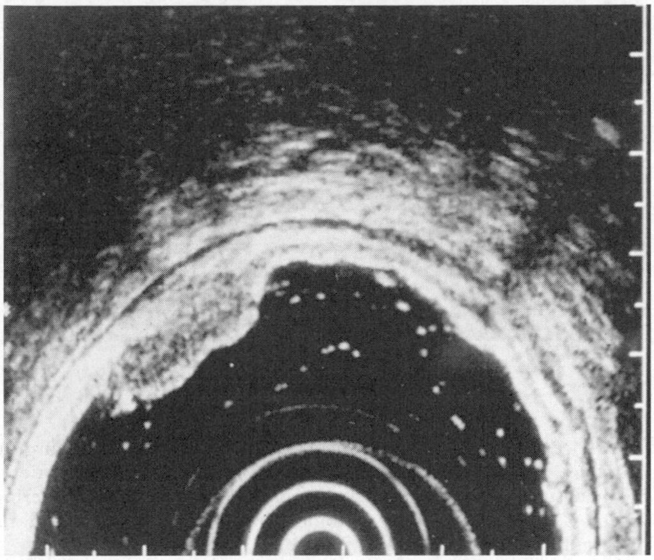

FIGURE 28-2. Endosonographic image shows a polypoid hypoechoic disruption involving only the first three wall layers of the stomach at the angularis. A T1 cancer invading to the submucosa, but not involving the muscularis propria, was confirmed by surgical pathologic examination.

ble for the endoscopist to assess not only mucosal lesions but intramural disease processes deep to the mucosa and extrinsic abnormalities in proximity to the wall of the GI tract.[23–25]

EUS uses high-frequency ultrasound (more than 7 MHz) for high resolution, producing detailed views of the GI wall and surrounding structures that are unmatched by other imaging methods. The higher the ultrasound frequency, the shorter the penetration depth of ultrasound and the more limited the field of view. However, with EUS a limited field is acceptable, because the transducer can be placed immediately adjacent to the area of interest.

Using EUS, the wall of the GI tract can be imaged as a five-layer structure of alternating bright (hyperechoic) and dark (hypoechoic) bands (Fig. 28-1). The echogenic layers consist in part of interface echoes produced as the sound waves travel between tissues of differing densities.[26] For clinical purposes, the first two layers correspond to the superficial and deep mucosa, the third layer to the submucosa, the fourth to the muscularis propria, and the fifth to the serosa or adventitia.

Most clinical studies have been carried out using mechanical sector scan instruments manufactured by the Olympus Corporation, Melville, NY, principally the GF-UM3 instrument. These instruments are combination endoscopes and ultrasound probes that use an acoustic mirror rotating around a transducer with switchable 7.5- and 12-MHz frequencies and produce a 360-degree image.[23–25] In the tubular GI tract, this greatly facilitates orientation of the image. Optics are forward oblique, but the 4-cm rigid tip and the 13-mm diameter make the instrument somewhat difficult to use and limit passage through tightly stenotic areas.

Instruments using linear- or phased-array technology have the advantages of forward-viewing optics and an absence of moving parts but provide a slice-like image, which can make orientation more difficult. Pentax Precision Instruments, Orangeberg, NY, manufactures a linear-array 5- and 7.5-MHz ultrasound endoscope (FG-32UA). Doppler ultrasound technology, to aid in evaluation of vascularity and blood flow, is easily obtained on ultrasound instruments. Blind endosonography probes, rigid and flexible, mechanical and electronic, have been used in the rectum and in the esophagus. Ultrathin miniprobes that can be passed through an endoscope biopsy channel have also been developed. They have a restricted field of view and often produce less-than-satisfactory images.

INDICATIONS AND RESULTS

EUS has been applied most extensively to the staging of esophageal, gastric, and rectal cancer. Data show that EUS is the most accurate imaging modality for staging depth of tumor invasion (T), with preoperative accuracy in the 80% to 90% range when compared with surgical pathology.[27–31] For staging esophageal and gastric cancer, T1 cancers invade the mucosa to submucosa and are imaged as a disruption of the first three endosonographic wall layers (Fig. 28-2). T2 cancers invade the muscularis propria to the subserosa and show a hypoechoic invasion of the fourth layer. T3 cancers invade through the serosa and can be seen to penetrate the fifth layer. T4 cancers directly invade adjacent organs or structures.

At the Memorial Sloan-Kettering Cancer Center (MSKCC), a prospective study used EUS in 50 patients for preoperative staging of esophageal cancer (Fig. 28-3) and in 50 patients for preoperative staging of gastric cancer (Fig. 28-4).[28,29] Results were compared for accuracy with surgical pathology and with CT using rapid scanners, oral contrast, and dynamic technique. EUS was significantly more accurate than dynamic CT in staging tumor extent in esophageal and gastric cancer. Most studies comparing EUS with CT for staging esophageal, gastric, and rectal cancer have found EUS superior for evaluation of tumor extent.[27–31]

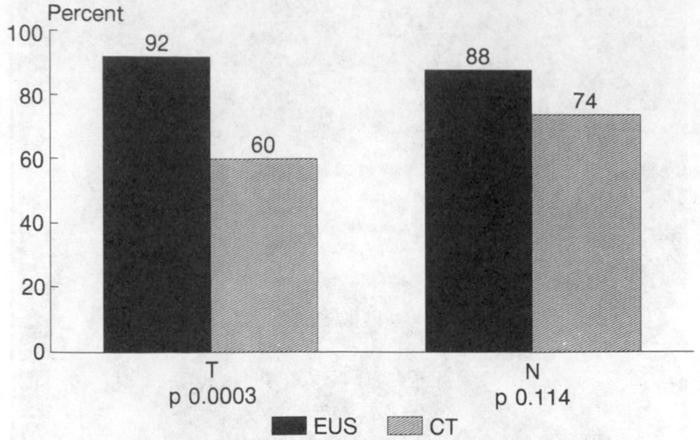

FIGURE 28-3. Esophageal cancer staging concordance with surgical pathology. Results of preoperative staging in 50 consecutive patients who had surgery for esophageal cancer at Memorial Sloan-Kettering Cancer Center. CT, computed tomography; EUS, endoscopic ultrasonography; N, node; T, tumor.

The greatest strength of EUS is in identifying the location of tissues and not the specific histology. Biopsy and histopathologic evaluation are still required to identify the nature of any abnormality. EUS cannot reliably distinguish an inflammatory from a neoplastic process (e.g., determining whether a gastric ulcer is benign or malignant). EUS has proved less accurate in staging lymph nodes than in staging depth of tumor invasion because the node must not only be located but be characterized as benign or malignant. Lymph nodes in the 2- to 3-mm range can be detected with EUS. Some investigators use the echo character of nodes for staging.[27–29] Nodes that are rounded, sharply defined, and hypoechoic are more likely to be malignant (Fig. 28-5). Using such criteria, staging regional lymph node metastases has been more accurate than other imaging modalities, such as CT scan, and is accurate in the range of 70% to 80%.[27–31] EUS is a sensitive method of detecting recurrent upper GI cancer in the area of the surgical anastomosis.[32] There have been false-positive results due to inflammation, and specificity should be improved.

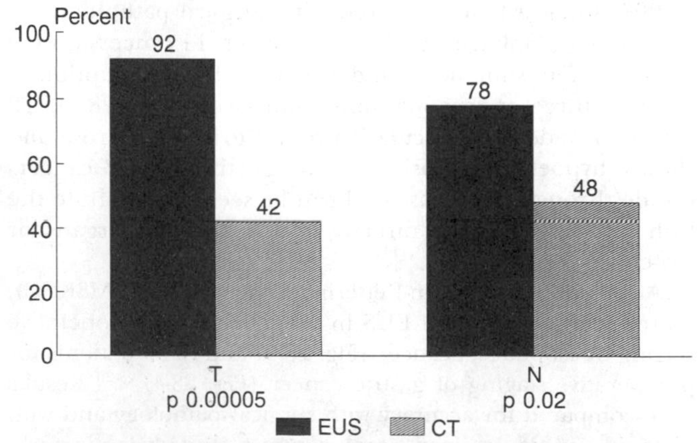

FIGURE 28-4. Gastric cancer staging concordance with surgical pathology. Results of preoperative staging in 50 consecutive patients who had surgery for gastric cancer at Memorial Sloan-Kettering Cancer Center. CT, computed tomography; EUS, endoscopic ultrasonography; N, node; T, tumor.

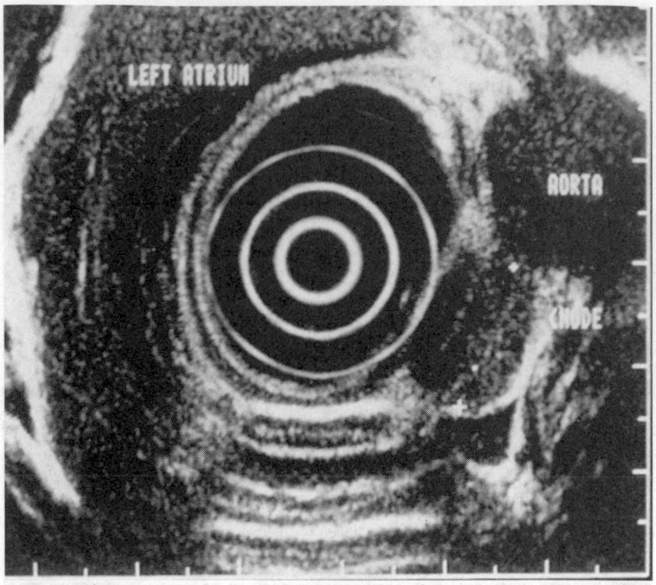

FIGURE 28-5. A round, hypoechoic, sharply defined lymph node measuring 1.4 cm is imaged through the distal esophagus. The posterior node lies between the aorta and azygos vein. The relation of the esophagus to the left atrium is evident posteriorly. The node in a patient with cancer of the esophagogastric junction was malignant at the time of surgical resection.

Characteristic images are recognized for cysts, leiomyomas, and lipomas, but again, it is not always possible to distinguish benign from malignant lesions.[33] On the other hand, large gastric folds due to benign gastropathy can usually be distinguished from malignant infiltration by carcinoma or lymphoma, which tend to destroy the normal tissue architecture.[34] Gastric varices may be readily identified.

Imaging the pancreas through the wall of the stomach and duodenum provides a highly detailed image, allowing the detection of small tumors measuring even less than 1 cm.[35] Although changes due to pancreatitis can be evaluated, once again, it has not been possible reliably to distinguish neoplastic from inflammatory pancreatic masses.[36,37] EUS may play a role in the screening of family members of pancreatic cancer kindreds.[38] Staging of pancreatic, biliary, and ampullary cancer preoperatively[37,39] and the localization of neuroendocrine tumors have been carried out successfully with EUS.[40]

Linear-array endosonographic instruments facilitate the ability to perform fine-needle aspiration of small submucosal lesions or lesions outside of but adjacent to the GI tract. In 50 consecutive patients in whom the combination of EUS and fine-needle aspiration was performed, the highest yield was 93% (14 of 15) in malignant lesions extrinsic to the GI tract.[41] Endosonography is often challenging to perform, and image interpretation can be difficult. However, EUS has become progressively easier and more available as more experience has accumulated and instruments have improved.

SIGMOIDOSCOPY

PRINCIPLES

Rigid and flexible sigmoidoscopies are important for evaluating the distal colon and rectum. Rigid sigmoidoscopes are usually 25 cm long, and flexible instruments are either 35 cm or 60 cm long. Although rigid sigmoidoscopes are less expensive to purchase and maintain and are somewhat easier to use than their flexible counterparts, the flexible instruments offer greater depth of insertion, patient comfort, and acceptance.

INDICATIONS AND RESULTS

Colorectal cancer screening represents one of the most important indications for sigmoidoscopy, because the procedure is highly sensitive and specific.[42] Because of its length, sigmoidoscopy misses proximal colon cancers and polyps. Sigmoidoscopic screening of large population groups remains controversial because most clinical trials have been uncontrolled and because the proposed goal of mortality reduction has not been met. In a case-control trial of rigid sigmoidoscopy, the investigators used data from 261 patients who died of distal colon and rectal cancer. Only 8.8% of these patients underwent sigmoidoscopy, as compared with 24.2% in a control population without cancer. The control patients who had undergone sigmoidoscopy within the preceding 10 years had a 60% to 70% reduction in colorectal cancer mortality.[43] The use of sigmoidoscopy as part of a periodic comprehensive health evaluation to prevent the lethal complications of advanced cancer is case finding and should not be confused with population screening.[44] The American Cancer Society recommends the use of sigmoidoscopic evaluation coupled with annual fecal occult blood testing for average risk, asymptomatic patients every 3 to 5 years, beginning at 50 years of age.[45]

Sigmoidoscopy is a complement to air-contrast barium enema studies performed to evaluate colonic symptoms, such as rectal bleeding. In a comparative study, the combination of sigmoidoscopy and barium enema was almost as effective in identifying colon cancer as was colonoscopy. The identification of small and medium polyps was better with colonoscopy.[46] Sigmoidoscopy is also useful to assess therapy in inflammatory bowel disease patients. It may be therapeutic for sigmoid volvulus, and it is used to follow up patients with FAP after colectomy and ileorectal reconstruction or to evaluate young family members for phenotypic expression.

Sigmoidoscopy is a safe procedure. Flexible sigmoidoscopy can be easily taught to primary care physicians and nurse practitioners.[47] Perforation of the colon during rigid or flexible sigmoidoscopy is possible but extremely unusual. In a series of 5000 flexible sigmoidoscopies, no perforations occurred.[48]

COLONOSCOPY

DIAGNOSTIC COLONOSCOPY

Colonoscopy has become the established method of evaluating and treating diseases of the large intestine. Modern colonoscopes are easier and safer to use, and complete evaluation by direct observation of the rectum and colon to the cecum is the rule. Abnormalities seen may be photographed, subjected to biopsy and, in the case of most polypoid lesions, entirely removed.[49] With aggressive bowel preparation, the patients can often be ready for colonoscopy within 24 hours.

An important indication for colonoscopy is evaluation of abnormal findings on barium enema. When a potential neoplastic lesion is identified on barium enema examination, colonoscopy then is needed to determine the precise nature of the lesion, either by removing it or by biopsy. Colonoscopy also confirms that there are no synchronous lesions elsewhere in the colon. Synchronous adenomas occur in approximately 50% of patients with colon cancer, and separate synchronous colon cancers occur in from 1.5% to 5.0% of patients.[49]

One of the most difficult areas of barium enema interpretation is the differentiation of strictures due to diverticular disease from colon cancer. Barium enema may underestimate the degree and intensity of diverticular inflammation. Colonoscopy, with associated biopsy and cytology, is the most important tool to use in making this distinction. In 44 patients with diverticular disease, Hunt[50] found six (13.6%) with unexpected cancer; he was unable adequately to examine the colon in a similar number of patients.

Hematochezia and melena thought not to be from an upper GI source should be evaluated by colonoscopy. Cancer of the large bowel, particularly in the rectum and left colon, often cause rectal bleeding, whereas cancers involving the right colon are more likely to produce melanotic stools or occult bleeding, with the gradual onset of iron-deficiency anemia. Brand et al.[51] studied by colonoscopy more than 300 patients with recent rectal bleeding and found that the bleeding was due to cancer in approximately 8% of their patients, though in more than 20% it was due to benign colon polyps. Angiodysplasia was also an important cause of large-bowel hemorrhage in their patient population. Tedesco et al.[52] performed colonoscopy in 258 patients with rectal bleeding, negative proctosig moidoscopy, and barium enemas that were either negative or showed only diverticula. In 29 patients (11.2%), cancer was found during colonoscopy.

Asymptomatic patients with a positive fecal occult blood test should also undergo colonoscopy. Data from the New York occult blood screening trial[53] show that, of patients initially tested for occult blood, approximately 50% have a colonic neoplastic lesion. Approximately 12% of these lesions are cancers, and the rest are adenomatous polyps. These rates increase as the age of the study population increases.

Patients who have had a colon cancer or adenomatous polyp resected are at risk for metachronous lesions. Various estimates have placed the risk for metachronous cancer between 5% and 10%, whereas the risk of developing a metachronous adenoma can be as high as 60%, as defined in a study of 383 patients by Fowler and Hedberg.[54] The National Polyp Study (NPS), a multicenter randomized trial, demonstrated a polyp recurrence rate of 29% to 35%, depending on the number of colonoscopies performed and the interval between them. It is clear that these patients should be kept under surveillance by follow-up colonoscopy.[55] Published NPS data have demonstrated that at a follow-up interval of 3 years, as many important colonic lesions were detected as were found at a 1-year interval. Therefore, it is recommended that post-polypectomy surveillance colonoscopy be performed once every 3 years.[56]

Colonoscopic polypectomy, although long thought to help prevent colon cancer, now has been proven to do so. Winawer et al.[57] analyzed the NPS cohort of 1418 patients who had a complete colonoscopy during which at least one polyp was removed. The colon cancer incidence in the study population was compared with the incidence in three reference groups, and reductions in cancer incidence of 76%, 88%, and 90%, respectively, were observed ($P<.001$).

Surveillance for colon cancer in patients with long-standing chronic ulcerative colitis represents a special problem. Although there is disagreement as to the magnitude of the cancer risk in ulcerative colitis, most investigators agree that cancer is unusual during the first 8 to 10 years of the disease and that thereafter the estimated cumulative incidence is approximately 5% at 20 years and 12% at 25 years.[58] Annual surveillance colonoscopy should begin after 10 years. The aim of colonoscopy is to identify those patients who are especially likely to develop colon cancer by finding high-grade dysplastic changes in the colonic mucosa on endoscopic biopsy. Dysplasia is clear-cut neoplastic change in the colonic mucosa, and high-grade dysplasia is generally what triggers intervention. Several studies of colonoscopic surveillance were summarized by Waye.[59] Fifteen percent of patients studied were found to have dysplasia, and 20% of these were found to have colon cancer. However, 10% of colitis patients with cancer had no evidence of dysplasia.

Studies have confirmed that colorectal cancer occurs in first-degree relatives (i.e., parents, children, siblings) of patients with colorectal cancer, with three to four times the frequency expected by chance. There is also an increased risk for adenomatous polyps in first-degree relatives of patients with bowel cancer and an increased risk for colorectal cancer in first-degree relatives with adenomatous polyps.[60,61] Many physicians now recommend colonoscopy, in conjunction with annual fecal occult blood testing, as the primary diagnostic tool for first-degree relatives in colon cancer families.

Screening colonoscopy has been studied in average-risk, asymptomatic patients with negative fecal occult blood studies. In one such study, adenomatous polyps were detected at a rate that was twice that expected from flexible sigmoidoscopy alone.[62] Of 210 patients, 53 (25%) had adenomas, and two had cancers. The larger adenomas and both cancers were found in patients older than 60 years. A follow-up report by the same investigators confirmed the substantial prevalence of colonic neoplasia in asymptomatic people, particularly elderly men, with negative fecal occult blood tests.[63]

THERAPEUTIC COLONOSCOPY: POLYPECTOMY

After a polyp is identified, colonoscopic polypectomy should be performed. If possible, the polyp is totally removed and submitted for histologic assessment. Complete colonoscopy should be performed at polypectomy to identify and remove any synchronous polyps. Biopsy of polyps is not recommended, because the results may be misleading. Small polyps (≤7 mm in diameter) are often removed by "hot biopsy" technique: Electric current is passed through a special biopsy forceps to cauterize the base of the polyp; then the tissue in the forceps is sent to pathology. Larger polyps are removed by snare-cautery technique. A wire loop is passed around the polyp base, and an electric current transects and cauterizes the polyp base. The entire polyp is then retrieved and submitted to pathology for analysis. Most colonic polyps can be managed in this fashion. Large sessile polyps (>2 cm in diameter) may need to be removed with a piecemeal approach. Submucosal saline injection has made this process safer. Occasionally, a large sessile polyp may not be removed safely during colonoscopy, and surgical resection is necessary. Marking the polypectomy site with an injection of sterile india ink has been recommended as an accurate and permanent method for future endoscopic or surgical identification.[64]

COMPLICATIONS

The major complications of colonoscopy are bowel perforation and hemorrhage. In 4713 diagnostic colonoscopies reported by the American Society for Gastrointestinal Endoscopy, perforation occurred in 0.17%.[65] These perforations are usually the result of the mechanical force of the colonoscope shaft on the sigmoid colon, especially a sigmoid colon affected by diverticular disease or adhesions. In 1901 polypectomy patients reported by the American Society for Gastrointestinal Endoscopy, the perforation rate was 0.11%. Perforation almost always occurred at the polypectomy site and was usually related to the removal of a sessile polyp. Hemorrhage occurred more commonly after polypectomy than after diagnostic colonoscopy (2.16% vs. 0.01%). Patients should avoid aspirin for up to 2 weeks after polypectomy. Postpolypectomy abdominal pain, leukocytosis, and fever do not always represent bowel perforation and may be due to a transmural electrocautery burn. Conservative management in this setting is appropriate.[66]

LAPAROSCOPY

PRINCIPLES

Laparoscopy or peritoneoscopy involves the creation of a pneumoperitoneum and the insertion of a thin telescope through a puncture in the anterior abdominal wall. Additional punctures are commonly used for insertion of probes, biopsy needles, and other instruments. For diagnosis and for guided biopsy, laparoscopy can be performed using local anesthesia and mild sedation, similar to that used for other GI endoscopic procedures. This type of laparoscopy should be differentiated from the therapeutic procedure involved in laparoscopic cholecystectomy and other laparoscopic abdominal surgery, which requires general anesthesia.[67] During laparoscopy, the anterior peritoneal space is visualized, with a view of the parietal peritoneum on the anterior abdominal wall and the diaphragm.[68] Most of the liver surface and gallbladder can be examined, along with much of the greater omentum and serosal surfaces of the stomach, small bowel, and colon. The pelvic organs can be visualized. Less completely seen are posterior structures, such as the porta hepatis, pancreas, and spleen. The retroperitoneal lymph nodes and renal system are usually not evaluable.

INDICATIONS AND RESULTS

The ability to see large areas of parietal and visceral peritoneum and to evaluate the cause of ascites have been major indications for laparoscopy. CT scans have a low yield in imaging small peritoneal metastases. Paracentesis and blind peritoneal biopsy are frequently nondiagnostic. Deposits of even a few millimeters in size on the peritoneum are readily identified and undergo biopsy at laparoscopy to distinguish among metastatic cancer, mesothelioma, or infections (such as tuberculosis).[69]

Because so much of the liver surface can be examined in fine detail, primary and metastatic liver cancers are diagnosed with an accuracy in the range of 90%.[4,5] The ability to see and submit for biopsy small lesions on the liver and peritoneum makes laparoscopy particularly useful in staging the extent of malignant disease. Benign focal conditions, such as fibrosis, cirrhosis, and hemangiomas, may be distinguished from malignant disease with high accuracy. Larger biopsy specimens are usually taken at laparoscopy rather than by scan-guided aspiration biopsy. Enough material can be obtained to permit special histopathologic studies. Direct-vision biopsy allows avoidance of vascular areas, and bleeding after biopsy can usually be controlled.[70]

Laparoscopy has been used for preoperative cancer staging, even if CT scans are normal. Experience with laparoscopic staging has been reported in patients with cancer of the pancreas, esophagus, stomach, gallbladder, and rectum.[71–74] Laparoscopy can increase the diagnostic yield of liver biopsy in Hodgkin's disease and non-Hodgkin's lymphoma.[75–78] Normal CT scans, ultrasound scans, or magnetic resonance images do not exclude the possibility that laparoscopic examination may detect liver or peritoneal malignancy.[79]

COMPLICATIONS

Laparoscopy is contraindicated in acute or unstable cardiopulmonary states, although there is a continuum of relative risk in more chronic situations. An uncooperative patient should not have laparoscopy under local anesthesia, nor should patients for whom skin infections interfere with sterile insertion of the laparoscope. The procedure is contraindicated in patients with intestinal obstruction and dilated bowel loops. A small amount of ascites does not present a problem, but tense ascites must first be decreased by diuresis or paracentesis. Coagulation disorders that cannot be corrected are contraindications, but mild abnormalities may be acceptable. A history of generalized peritonitis is an absolute contraindication because of the likelihood of multiple dense adhesions, increasing the risk and decreasing the effectiveness of the procedure. Prior abdominal surgery associated with adhesions represents a relative contraindication.[3]

The overall complication rate from laparoscopy is in the range of 1%, with serious complications that delay discharge or necessitate surgery occurring in approximately 0.2% and with mortality of 0.05%. Subcutaneous emphysema and pneumoomentum are not serious and require no treatment. Mediastinal emphysema, pneumothorax, and air embolism are rare. Abdominal wall bleeding and laceration of blood vessels, organs, or bowel occurs uncommonly but may require surgical management. Biopsy, especially of the liver, accounts for most complications. Tumor implantation at the laparoscopy or biopsy needle insertion site is well described.[67]

ENDOSCOPIC RETROGRADE CHOLANGIOPANCREATOGRAPHY

DIAGNOSTIC ENDOSCOPIC RETROGRADE CHOLANGIOPANCREATOGRAPHY

The technique of endoscopic retrograde cholangiopancreatography (ERCP) was first reported in 1968 and has been an important diagnostic tool for more than 25 years.[80] The skilled endoscopist working with a cooperative patient can often perform a diagnostic ERCP in less than 20 minutes. Success rates for cannulating the common bile duct and pancreatic duct are well in excess of 90%.

A side-viewing electronic duodenoscope is used to afford excellent visualization of the ampulla of Vater. Cannulization of the biliary and pancreatic ducts is then accomplished, and a contrast agent, such as diatrizoate (Renograffin-60), is injected into the desired duct under fluoroscopic control, and radiologic films of the duct anatomy are subsequently obtained. Duct cytology can be obtained, and biopsy of the ampulla, duodenum, and stomach may also be performed.

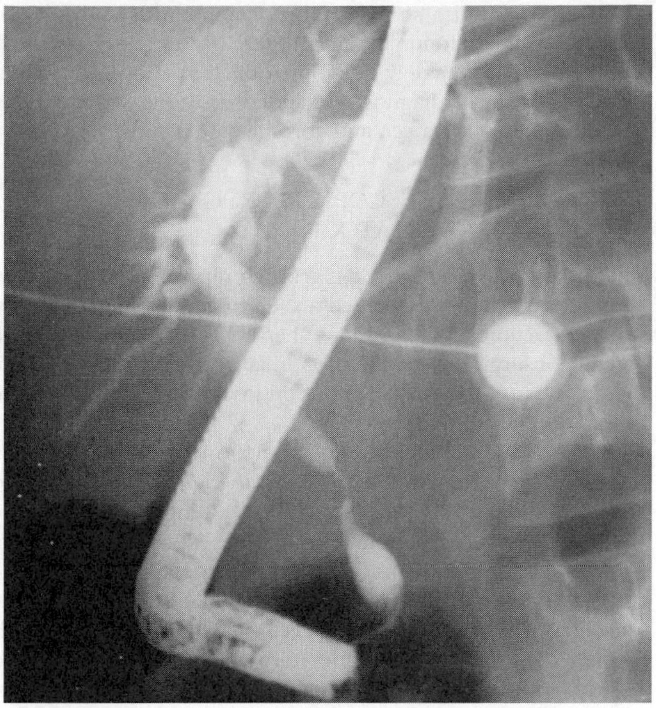

FIGURE 28-6. An endoscopic, retrograde cholangiogram demonstrating a short distal common bile duct stricture caused by a primary bile duct cancer.

Evaluation of the jaundiced patient was one of the more important indications for ERCP. Imaging procedures, such as transabdominal sonography, high-quality CT scans, and magnetic resonance cholangiopancreatography, are replacing diagnostic ERCP (Fig. 28-6).[81] Today, therapeutic ERCP is most commonly performed for endoscopic sphincterotomy, removing bile duct gallstones, or placement of an endobiliary stent across the obstructed bile duct segment.

ERCP may be useful when the patient's symptoms suggest pancreatic cancer and the sonogram or CT scan is not diagnostic. ERCP may be difficult to interpret in the setting of chronic pancreatitis, and cancers can be missed. ERCP is a sensitive and specific diagnostic test for pancreatic cancer. At MSKCC, ERCP had a sensitivity of 92% and a specificity of 97% in the evaluation of 116 patients. In a report by Freeney[82] of 530 patients with pancreatic cancer, normal pancreatograms were seen in only 15 (2.8%). Typical findings include complete occlusion or stenosis of the main pancreatic duct, narrowing or cutoff of the intrapancreatic portion of the common bile duct, and the double-duct sign of stenosis or obstruction of both the main pancreatic duct and the common bile duct. There may also be endoscopic abnormalities, such as a duodenal mass or ulcer that, when subjected to biopsy, document pancreatic cancer.

ERCP is not necessary when the diagnosis appears clear-cut. Frick et al.[83] reported on ERCP used to evaluate 26 patients with indeterminate CT scans and found that ERCP aided the preoperative diagnosis in 25. One pancreatic cancer was missed by

ERCP. In an English study[84] of 140 patients with undiagnosed severe chronic abdominal pain, the ERCP was abnormal in 25 (18%). In approximately one-fourth of the patients, diagnoses were made. These diagnoses included gallstones, peptic ulcer disease, pancreatic cancer, and chronic pancreatitis.

THERAPEUTIC ENDOSCOPIC RETROGRADE CHOLANGIOPANCREATOGRAPHY

The therapeutic use of ERCP is growing rapidly. The major therapeutic procedures performed are endoscopic sphincterotomy, stone extraction, and placement of endobiliary stents for the palliative nonsurgical treatment of biliary obstruction. Approximately 75% of ERCPs done in our endoscopy unit at MSKCC are therapeutic.

Endoscopic sphincterotomy is performed by inserting into the distal common bile duct through the ampulla a specialized cannula containing an electrosurgical cutting wire. When the electrical current is passed through the exposed wire, a controlled incision is made in the sphincter, opening the distal bile duct to allow the endoscopic removal of bile duct stones or the placement of endobiliary stents. Biopsy of ampullary tumors is facilitated by endoscopic sphincterotomy, and the associated obstructive jaundice may be temporarily relieved by this procedure. Bourgeois et al.[85] obtained the correct histologic diagnosis in all 55 patients with periampullary cancer after endoscopic sphincterotomy but in only one-half before sphincterotomy.

Nonsurgical biliary drainage has become an important tool in the palliative management of patients with malignant biliary obstruction. Endoscopic biliary drainage (EBD) (Fig. 28-7) and percutaneous transhepatic drainage (PTD) complement each other and are selected on the basis of the level of the biliary obstruction.[86] In a prospective randomized study comparing EBD with PTD in 75 high-risk patients with malignant biliary obstruction, EBD was significantly more successful in relieving jaundice (81% vs. 61%) and had a significantly lower 30-day mortality rate (15% vs. 33%). The complication rate of EBD was 19%, whereas the morbidity of PTD was 67%.[87]

The location or level of the malignant biliary stricture is very important in determining success and complication rates with nonsurgical biliary drainage. Seventy patients with malignant hilar strictures were stratified by Deviere et al.[88] into three groups. Twenty patients had common hepatic duct lesions (type I), and 50 patients had bifurcation or intrahepatic strictures (types II and III). The type I patients were likely to experience complete drainage, whereas in only approximately 50% of the type II and III patients was drainage adequate. These patients had a higher 30-day mortality, a higher rate of early cholangitis, a higher death rate from sepsis, and a shorter postprocedure survival. Success in adequately draining common bile duct and common hepatic duct strictures should be approximately 90% with large-bore endoprostheses placed during ERCP. The success rate for establishing drainage by ERCP in bifurcation or intrahepatic strictures is much lower. Using an aggressive approach with multiple attempts and combining EBD with PTD increased the success rate of insertion of two or more stents to only approximately 50% of patients with hilar strictures.[88]

EBD has been prospectively compared to surgical biliary bypass. Fifty-two patients with distal common bile duct obstruction were randomly assigned to either EBD or surgical biliary bypass.[89] Survival data for both groups were similar, as was the

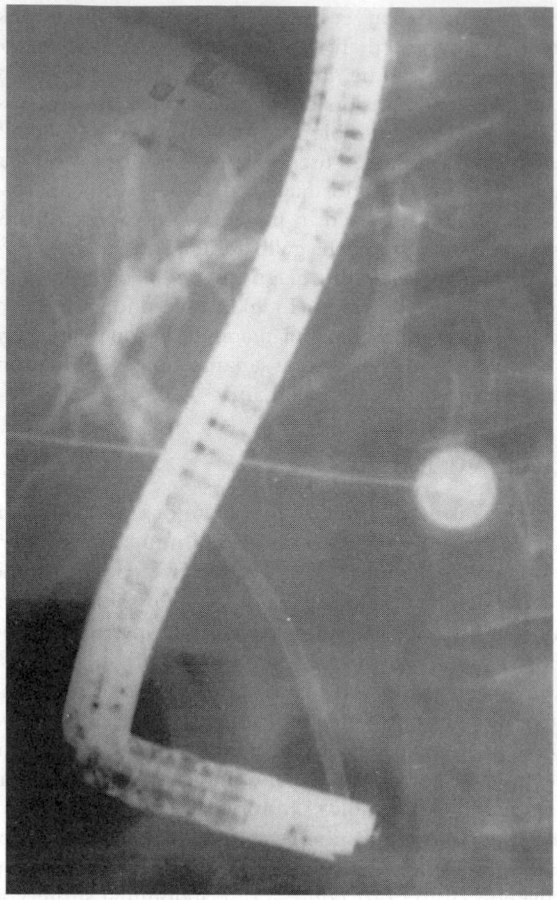

FIGURE 28-7. An endoscopically placed biliary stent is seen in the common bile duct across the malignant stricture shown in Figure 28-6.

90% success rate in relieving jaundice. Patients treated with EBD had a significantly shorter initial hospital stay (5 vs. 13 days; $P < .002$). Readmissions to the hospital were more frequent in the EBD group, but the total hospital stay in days per patient until death was shorter in the EBD group (8 vs. 13 days; $P < .01$). In patients with pancreatic cancer and jaundice who are not candidates for surgical resection, because of either advanced disease or other medical problems, EBD should be the biliary drainage procedure of choice. Metal endoscopic stents are replacing polyethylene stents, especially in those patients who can reasonably be expected to live more than 6 months. The use of metal endobiliary stents should reduce the number of stent replacements. Although EBD affords good palliation for advanced cancer cholestasis, studies have shown that there is no role for preoperative biliary drainage.[90]

COMPLICATIONS

The most common complications of ERCP are cholangitis and sepsis. The rate of cholangitis and sepsis varies, depending on the reason for the ERCP and the underlying pathology. For example, therapeutic ERCP done for biliary obstruction may have a sepsis rate as high as 14%.

The level of the biliary obstruction affects the rate of sepsis. In an MSKCC series[91] looking at PTD after failed EBD, the rate

TABLE 28-1. Comparison of Rigid and Flexible Fiber-Optic Bronchoscopy Technique

Parameter	*Rigid Fiber-Optic Bronchoscopy*	*Flexible Fiber-Optic Bronchoscopy*
Biopsy	Generous specimen	Minute specimen
Visualization of bronchi	Excellent	Excellent
Visualization of segmental bronchi	With angled lenses only	Excellent
Biopsy of peripheral lesions	No	Yes
Anesthesia required	General	Local
Suctioning secretions	Excellent	Good
Complications	Perforation and bleeding reported	Very unusual
Durability of instrument	Durable	Delicate
Training to perform examination	Extensive	Minimal
Management of airway obstruction	Yes	No

of sepsis for patients with intrahepatic and bifurcation strictures was significantly greater than for those with common hepatic or common bile duct lesions (75% vs. 17%; $P = .04$). Another MSKCC study[92] compared the microbiologic data for septic episodes after EBD with septic episodes after PTD. Although enteric gram-negative organisms predominated in both groups, there were significantly more gram-positive organisms noted in the PTD group ($P<.0005$).

Acute pancreatitis is another common complication of ERCP, and it is related to the injection of contrast material into the pancreatic duct. Its frequency varies but generally occurs in fewer than 7% of patients. It is usually self-limited and rarely presents as a serious clinical problem. Clinical trials with such agents as octreotide have not shown a reduction in ERCP-associated pancreatitis.[93]

SMALL INTESTINAL ENDOSCOPY: ENTEROSCOPY

Evaluation of the small intestine beyond the fourth portion of the duodenum is commonly accomplished by barium studies or angiography. Two endoscopic techniques for studying the small bowel have been developed. Dedicated push enteroscopes (Olympus Corp., SIF-10) often can be passed rapidly to approximately 100 cm distal to the ligament of Treitz. Biopsy, polypectomy, diathermy, and Nd:YAG laser treatment can be performed through this instrument. In a study of 56 patients, the median depth of insertion into the small intestine was 45 cm (range, 15 to 90 cm), and procedure times varied from 10 to 45 minutes.[94] Push enteroscopy has been very useful in the evaluation and treatment of GI bleeding due to occult proximal small intestinal sources and in the evaluation of abnormalities seen on barium small intestinal radiographs.

The sonde-type enteroscope is slender and approximately 2.7 m long. It has an inflatable balloon at its tip that helps in passage through the small intestine. Among the several disadvantages of this instrument are its lack of a biopsy channel, the absence of tip deflection, a limited field of view, the need for fluoroscopy, and the 8 hours required for its use.

In using enteroscopy in the evaluation of obscure GI bleeding, one study of push enteroscopy identified the source of bleeding in 15 of 39 patients (38%).[95] The most common cause found was an arteriovenous malformation. The diagnostic yield in a study of 35 patients with obscure GI bleeding using a sonde-type enteroscope was 26%.[96] A study of 258 patients identified nine malignant and four benign tumors to be the cause of the obscure bleeding (5%).[97]

PERCUTANEOUS ENDOSCOPIC GASTROSTOMY

Since its original description by Ponsky and Gauderer[98] in 1981, percutaneous endoscopic gastrostomy (PEG) has become a routine procedure, done in an outpatient setting without general anesthesia, in patients either unable to take oral feedings or in whom parenteral nutritional support is not feasible. PEG and percutaneous endoscopic jejunostomy (PEJ) are rapid and safe endoscopic methods for establishing enteral feeding routes and can eliminate the need for long-term nasal feeding tubes. In a study of 42 patients with dysphagia and cancers of the head and neck, successful use of PEG and PEJ was accomplished in 39.[99] No immediate complications occurred. After a mean follow-up of 4.5 months, only one patient developed pneumonia presumed to be due to aspiration. Complication rates for surgical gastrostomies have been reported to be as high as 75%.[100]

When patients have had previous gastric resections, PEJ may be used. In 115 patients, Shike et al.[101,102] had a success rate with PEJ of more than 90%. PEJ was used in gastric outlet and small bowel obstruction, gastroparesis, and anorexia. Only two patients experienced severe complications of bleeding and abscess formation. Significant caloric intake ranging between 900 and 2400 calories per day could be administered.

BRONCHOSCOPY

Bronchoscopy (Table 28-1) is the single most useful modality for accurately diagnosing lung cancer. With the advent of fiber-optic equipment introduced more than 25 years ago,[103,104] this procedure has been used for diagnosis with increasing frequency.

INDICATIONS

The most common oncologic indication for bronchoscopy is to diagnose and assist in staging lung cancer by direct observation and by obtaining material for cytologic and histologic evaluation.[105] In investigating other upper aerodigestive tumors,

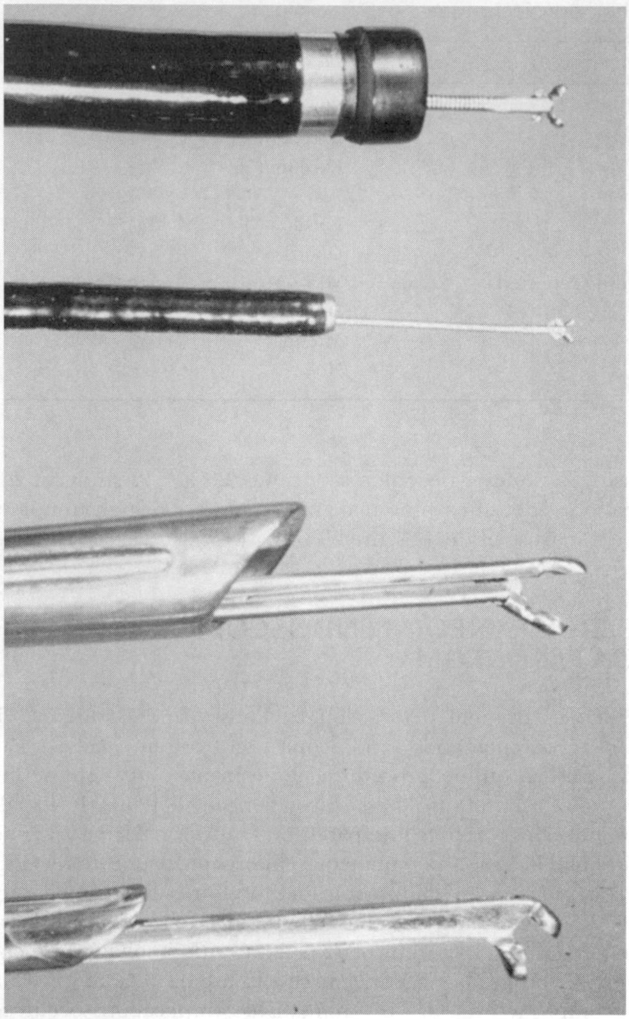

FIGURE 28-8. Comparison of flexible and rigid equipment and of biopsy potential. This photograph illustrates a flexible esophagoscope, flexible bronchoscope, rigid esophagoscope, rigid bronchoscope, and the biopsy forceps that can be used with each endoscope.

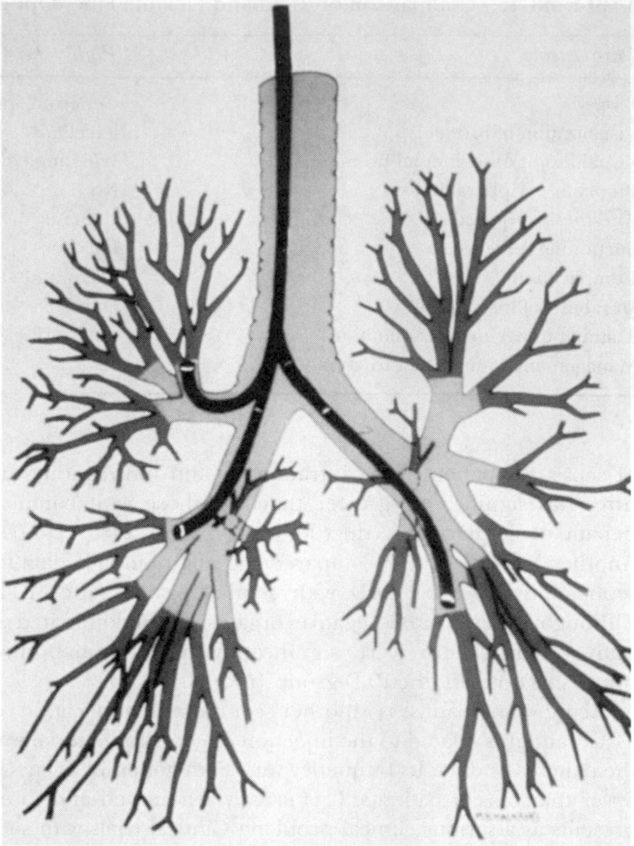

FIGURE 28-9. The range of the flexible bronchoscope within the tracheobronchial tree. The second order of branchings of the tracheobronchial tree can be inspected and subjected to biopsy.

bronchoscopy rules out extension of laryngeal and esophageal carcinomas to the upper airway. Flexible bronchoscopy has been especially important in localizing occult sites of malignancy when sputum cytology results are positive.

Therapeutically, bronchoscopy has been extensively used to remove retained secretions in the postoperative period, to relieve obstructed airways due to malignancy (in conjunction with laser destruction), and to arrest bleeding. This technique is used to deliver anticancer therapy (cauterization, cryotherapy, photocoagulation, and brachytherapy) in the definitive or palliative treatment of endobronchial malignancies.[106,107] Bronchoscopy is also used to insert intraluminal stents when required to maintain airway patency.

TECHNIQUE

Rigid Bronchoscopy

The open-tube rigid bronchoscope, although used less frequently for diagnosis, remains a valuable therapeutic tool. It is especially important in controlling airway hemorrhage and is favored by most endoscopists for mechanical removal and laser coagulation of tumors (Fig. 28-8). It also has the advantages of a large lumen, allowing suctioning of blood or fumes developing during laser coagulation and obtaining larger biopsies. Although the rigid bronchoscope can be introduced under local anesthesia, the preferred approach is general anesthesia.

Flexible Bronchoscopy

Flexible bronchoscopy has become the mainstay of endoscopic airway examination. The flexible equipment is small enough to be introduced transnasally or transorally under local anesthesia with or without sedation. Because of its small diameter (6 mm or smaller), the average flexible bronchoscope can enter all segmental orifices of the tracheobronchial tree. Newer instruments (with an external diameter as small as 2.0 mm) can now extend the visible range to the periphery of the lung and have been used for biopsy of peripheral nodules or infiltrates (Fig. 28-9).[108] These newer instruments no longer use fiberoptics for visualization: Electronic signals are now transmitted from the tip of the bronchoscope to a television monitor.

Most instruments have a 2-mm operating channel for suctioning and to pass brushes and biopsy forceps to obtain pathologic material for examination. Flexible fibers can be passed through the operating channel for Nd:YAG laser treatment and argon beam excitation of hematoporphyrins (PDT) to induce photocoagulation of malignant tissue. The versatility and ease of use of the flexible bronchoscope has allowed this procedure to be performed in an outpatient setting with minimal inconvenience to the patient.

DIAGNOSTIC BRONCHOSCOPY

Malignant lesions of the tracheobronchial tree and pulmonary parenchyma are most often diagnosed using flexible bronchoscopy. Tumors that involve the proximal airways as distal as subsegmental bronchi can usually be seen at the time of flexible bronchoscopy, and specimens can be obtained for histopathology or exfoliative cytology. Those lesions beyond the range of the flexible equipment can be subjected to biopsy under fluoroscopic control, passing biopsy forceps or brushes into the lesion that has been localized using an image intensifier. Diffuse pulmonary infiltrates requiring diagnosis can be easily sampled using similar radiologic techniques, passing biopsy forceps into the pulmonary parenchyma to obtain representative samples (transbronchial biopsy). Wang et al.[109] have popularized the technique of transbronchial needle aspiration for diagnosing malignancy in mediastinal lymph nodes as well as in submucosal lesions inaccessible to direct biopsy or brushing. More recently, localization of mediastinal lymph nodes has been attempted using bronchoscopic ultrasonography. This has proven to be somewhat difficult because the air-containing airway cannot transmit the ultrasound waves, and obstruction of the airway is required to fill the lumen with a fluid-filled balloon to perform the examination. However, subcarinal lymph nodes can be easily accessed by performing endoesophageal ultrasonography with guided endobiopsy.[110]

The success of these techniques is operator-dependent. It is rare for lesions that can be visualized not to yield a diagnosis. Intrapulmonary lesions located more peripherally may be more difficult to diagnose, especially if they are small (<3 cm in diameter) and are probably best diagnosed by percutaneous transthoracic needle aspiration biopsy using radiologic techniques. However, bronchoalveolar lavage with saline and postbronchoscopy sputum samples can provide cytology for examination.

Identification of occult *in situ* malignancies can be enhanced with the use of tumor fluorescence aided by laser light excitation. Injected hematoporphyrin derivatives fluoresce at a specific wavelength (640 nm) emitted by the argon laser beam and, most recently, autofluorescence of tumors using specific wavelengths can identify areas of dysplasia and frank neoplasia (lung imaging fluorescent endoscopy bronchoscopy).[111] This technique is extremely important in identifying occult cancers detected by sputum cytology. This autofluorescence technique is being investigated also as a method of early diagnosis of lung cancer in high-risk individuals (especially patients with previous aerodigestive tumors; Fig. 28-10).[112]

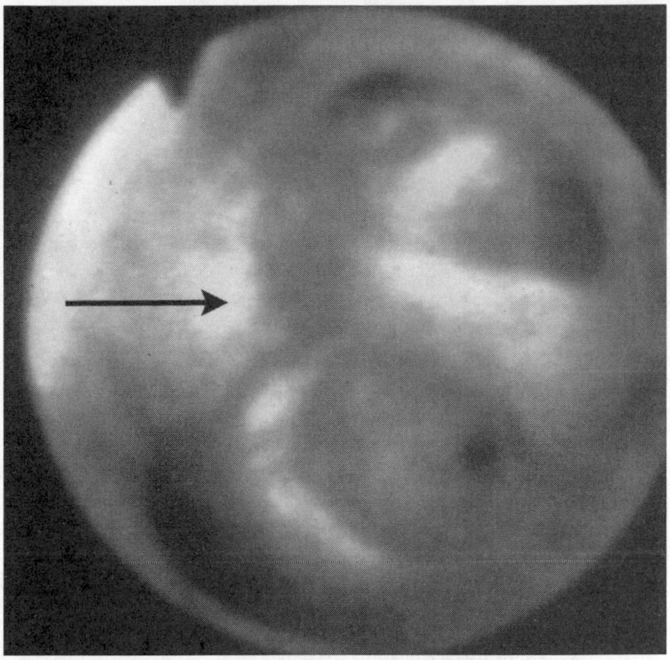

FIGURE 28-10. A lung imaging fluorescent endoscopy bronchoscopic image demonstrating a darkened area of the carina between the anterior and apical segments of the upper right lobe (*arrow*). This proved to be *in situ* carcinoma on biopsy.

THERAPEUTIC BRONCHOSCOPY

The most common oncologic indication for therapeutic bronchoscopy is bronchopulmonary toilet after major pulmonary resections for malignancy. This has become an invaluable bedside tool in the postoperative management of thoracic surgical patients since the introduction of flexible instruments. Bronchoscopy has also been used with success in relieving endobronchial obstruction and in dealing with significant airway hemorrhage.

Endobronchial tumors can be mechanically débrided using the tip of the rigid bronchoscope or a large biopsy forceps.[113] Techniques of tumor coagulation and destruction have been introduced that avoid unnecessary or excessive bleeding. These techniques include cryosurgery, electrocautery and, most recently, carbon dioxide, Nd:YAG, or argon laser destruction.[114] These modalities require significant training in the use of lasers and are best applied when visible endobronchial tumors are present. Extrinsic compression by enlarged mediastinal lymph nodes does not respond to this type of treatment. When extrinsic compression is a major problem, endobronchial stents similar to those used for obstructing esophageal lesions can be inserted. A variety of Silastic and self-expanding metallic stents have been devised. The Silastic stents have the disadvantage of frequent migration. Self-expanding metallic stents, once inserted, cannot be removed but rarely migrate. These stents can be coated with Silastic to avoid growth of tumor through the interstices of the stent (Figs. 28-11 and 28-12). With the expandable metallic stents, instances of tracheoesophageal fistulization have occurred. In properly selected patients, however, these expandable stents are replacing the plastic stents in the management of malignant disease. When either external-beam radiation or internal brachytherapy is added to endobronchial tumor destruction or in conjunction with stents, longer periods of palliation can be achieved, avoiding tumor regrowth and overgrowth.[115] With these techniques, approximately 80% of patients can be relieved of their obstructing symptoms for a median of 3 months.

PDT has also been used to destroy endobronchial tumors. This technique is used as definitive therapy for *in situ* carcinoma and is effective in totally destroying such tumors in approximately 50% of cases.[4] It is now being used with increasing frequency to destroy inoperable tumors obstructing the air-

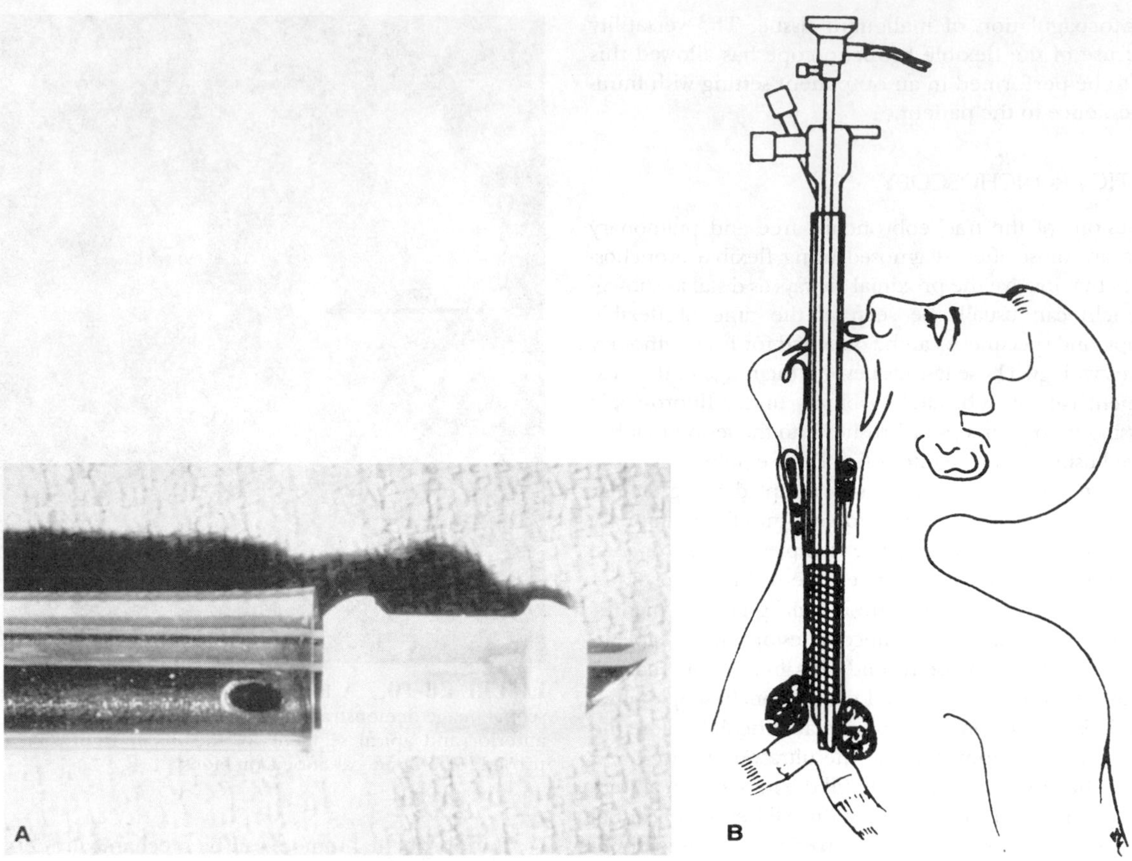

FIGURE 28-11. **A:** An endobronchial stent loaded on the end of a rigid bronchoscope uses a chest tube as an inserter. **B:** Use of an endobronchial stent in extrinsic compression.

A 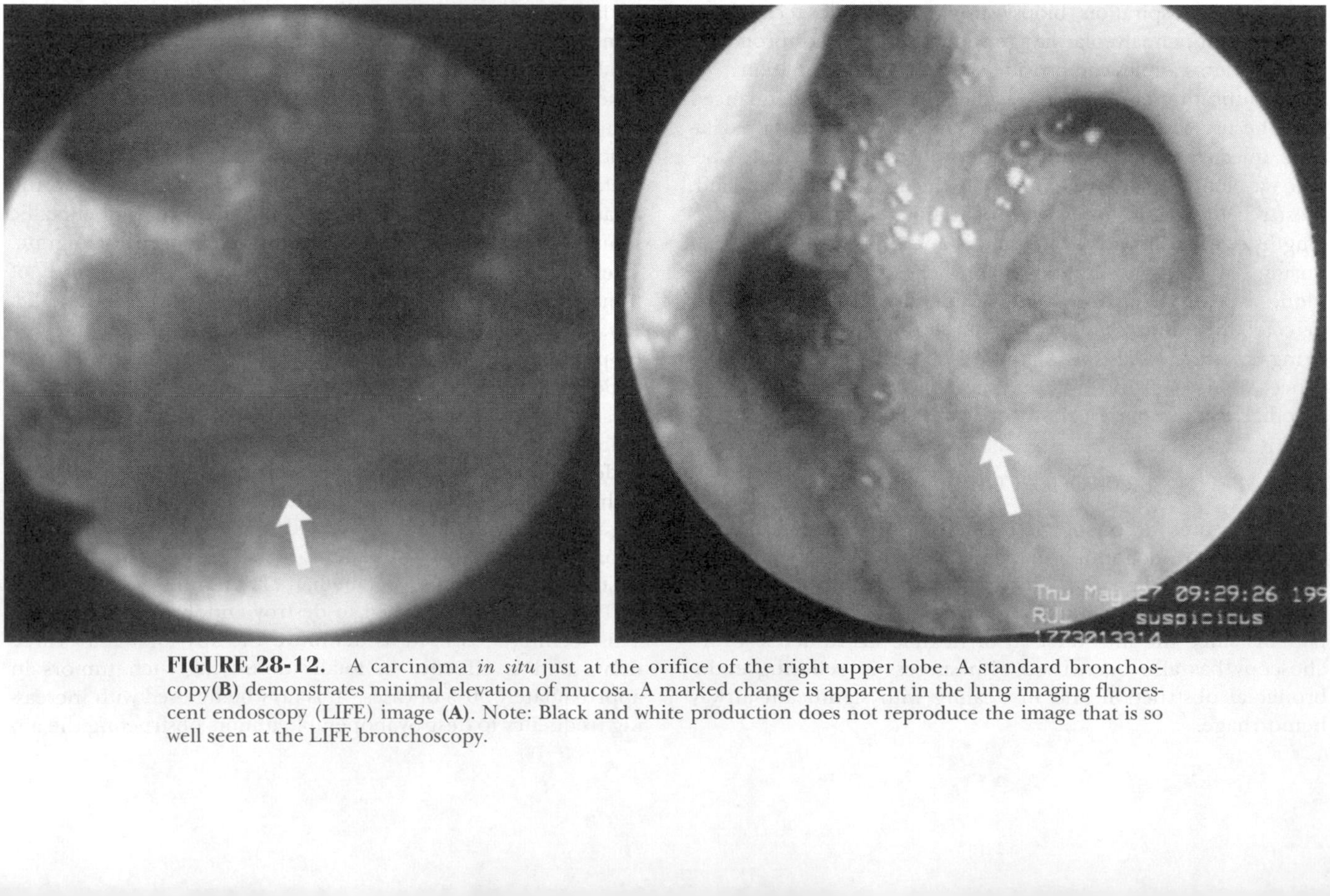 B

FIGURE 28-12. A carcinoma *in situ* just at the orifice of the right upper lobe. A standard bronchoscopy(**B**) demonstrates minimal elevation of mucosa. A marked change is apparent in the lung imaging fluorescent endoscopy (LIFE) image (**A**). Note: Black and white production does not reproduce the image that is so well seen at the LIFE bronchoscopy.

way.[116] Most tumors respond to this therapy, and up to 90% of patients obtain some palliation. With the U.S. Food and Drug Administration release of hematoporphyrins for therapy in North America, significant activity has occurred in investigating this approach for palliation of obstructing tumors and treatment of *in situ* and inoperable stage I proximal tumors. A newer hematoporphyrin, porfimer (Photofrin II), is currently the drug of choice. It is administered 24 to 48 hours before laser illumination of the tumor. This causes an intense and immediate destruction of the tumor, which requires mechanical débridement. In most instances, a second bronchoscopy 24 or 48 hours later completes the débridement. When compared to Nd:YAG laser destruction, it fares very well. Currently, all of these endobronchial-relieving methods are effective, and a combination of two of these (e.g., PDT plus radiotherapy, mechanical or Nd:YAG destruction plus radiotherapy) seems to produce the longest periods of palliation. Metastatic endobronchial tumors are also amenable to these therapies.[117]

COMPLICATIONS

The complications of diagnostic rigid and flexible bronchoscopy are minimal, with fewer than 1.0% of patients experiencing any significant postprocedure problems. Rigid bronchoscopy has the disadvantage of trauma to the teeth, lips, and mouth as well as the larynx. This is completely avoided by using flexible bronchoscopy. Biopsy of lesions can lead to hemorrhage, although bleeding rarely is excessive.[118] As with any other surgical procedure, care must be taken, before bronchoscopy is performed, to evaluate and correct any coagulation abnormalities. Transbronchial biopsy of lung parenchyma can lead to bleeding and pneumothorax; the latter complication occurs rarely if routine precautions are taken to avoid biopsy at the extreme periphery of the lung. In a series from the Cleveland Clinic,[118] only 58 episodes of bleeding occurred in almost 7000 flexible bronchoscopies. Transbronchial biopsy showed a higher incidence of bleeding, though no deaths ensued. In two other large bronchoscopy series, the death rates were 0.1% and 0.3%, respectively.[119,120] In a series of 4000 patients, major complications (pneumothorax, pulmonary hemorrhage, or respiratory failure) occurred in 0.53% of flexible bronchoscopies. After transbronchial biopsy, however, 6.8% of patients experienced either hemorrhage (2.8%) or pneumothorax (4%), and there were no deaths.[121]

MEDIASTINOSCOPY

INDICATIONS

Mediastinoscopy is used most frequently to obtain lymph node samples from the superior mediastinum to assist in the clinical staging of lung cancer. It can be extremely valuable in identifying metastatic malignancy in these lymph nodes, thereby providing histologic evidence of N2 and N3 (stage IIIa and IIIb) disease in patients with lung cancer.[122] Less frequently, this technique is used to diagnose other lesions presenting with mediastinal adenopathy. Lymphomas, primary lung cancers with mediastinal involvement, and a host of benign lesions can be diagnosed using this approach. The procedure can also identify direct mediastinal invasion by a lung tumor and, by extending the mediastinal dissection, can be used for biopsy of lesions in the anterior mediastinum. Either pleural space can be entered through the mediastinum to detect abnormalities, especially in the paramediastinal regions.[123]

TECHNIQUE

The mediastinoscopy technique (Fig. 28-13) is simple and safe in the hands of well-trained thoracic surgeons. A short suprasternal transverse incision is made, dissecting down to the pretracheal fascia, which is opened. Finger dissection in the pretracheal plane precedes the insertion of the mediastinoscope. Direct visualization of all areas of the superior mediastinum then allows appropriate biopsies of tissue in the various mediastinal nodal stations.

Mediastinoscopy is performed under general anesthesia but is usually performed on an outpatient basis. It can also be used just before thoracotomy for final clinical staging in patients suspected of possibly harboring inoperable disease by virtue of mediastinal spread.

RESULTS

With the ability to biopsy mediastinal lymph nodes directly, the accuracy of mediastinoscopy approaches 90% when assessing the mediastinal involvement of lymph nodes in lung cancer.[124] Virtually no false-positive examination results should occur. Because of the inaccessibility of certain areas of the mediastinum, a 10% false-negative rate can be expected. However, those inaccessible mediastinal lymph nodes are usually resectable at the time of surgery. When mediastinoscopy fails to reveal metastatic disease in patients with otherwise operable lung cancer, the resectability rate of such patients approaches 95%. Mediastinoscopy remains the most accurate method of assessing mediastinal involvement by lung cancer and is usually used when CT scanning suggests enlarged mediastinal lymph nodes (>1 cm) to confirm the presence of metastatic disease to the mediastinum.

Since the introduction of positron emission tomography (PET) scanning, many centers have used this technique of staging the superior mediastinum instead of the invasive technique of mediastinoscopy. There are differences of opinion as to whether PET scanning can be depended on to be accurate. Certainly, "positive" PET scans denoting mediastinal spread of tumor should be confirmed by histologic proof. "Negative" PET scans do not rule out microscopic metastatic disease to the superior mediastinum.[125,126]

In expert hands, mediastinoscopy is safe. One retrospective review from Washington University demonstrates the safety of the technique. In more than 2000 mediastinoscopies, there was one treatment-related death in a patient with very extensive mediastinal disease and very few significant complications: Only three patients required a thoracotomy for bleeding and, in all of those patients, the primary tumor was surgically treated at the time of thoracotomy.[127]

ANTERIOR MEDIASTINOTOMY (CHAMBERLAIN PROCEDURE)

Tumors situated in the anterior mediastinum (e.g., lymphomas, germ cell tumors, thymomas) are often diagnosed by percutaneous transthoracic needle aspiration biopsy. The most direct approach to the anterior mediastinum, when incisional

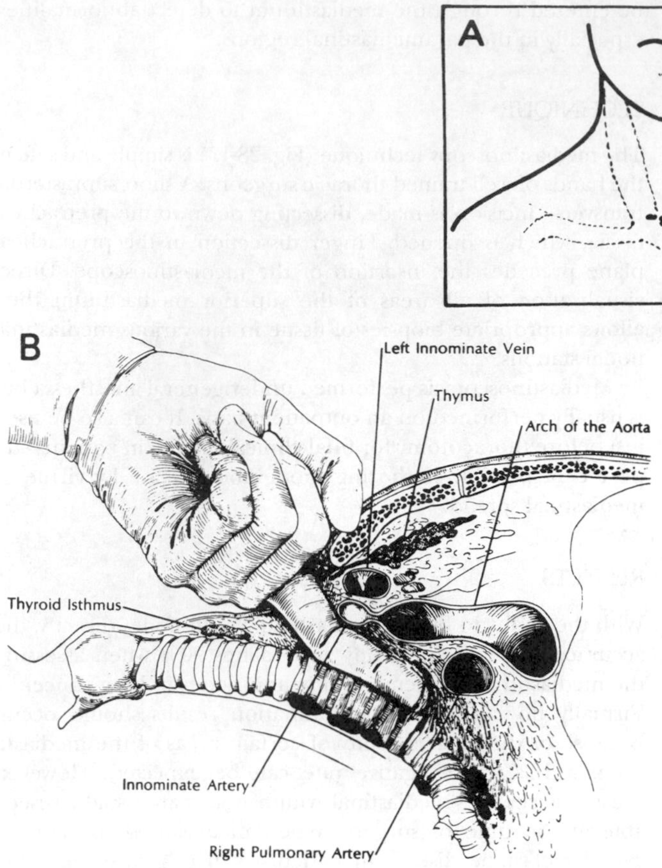

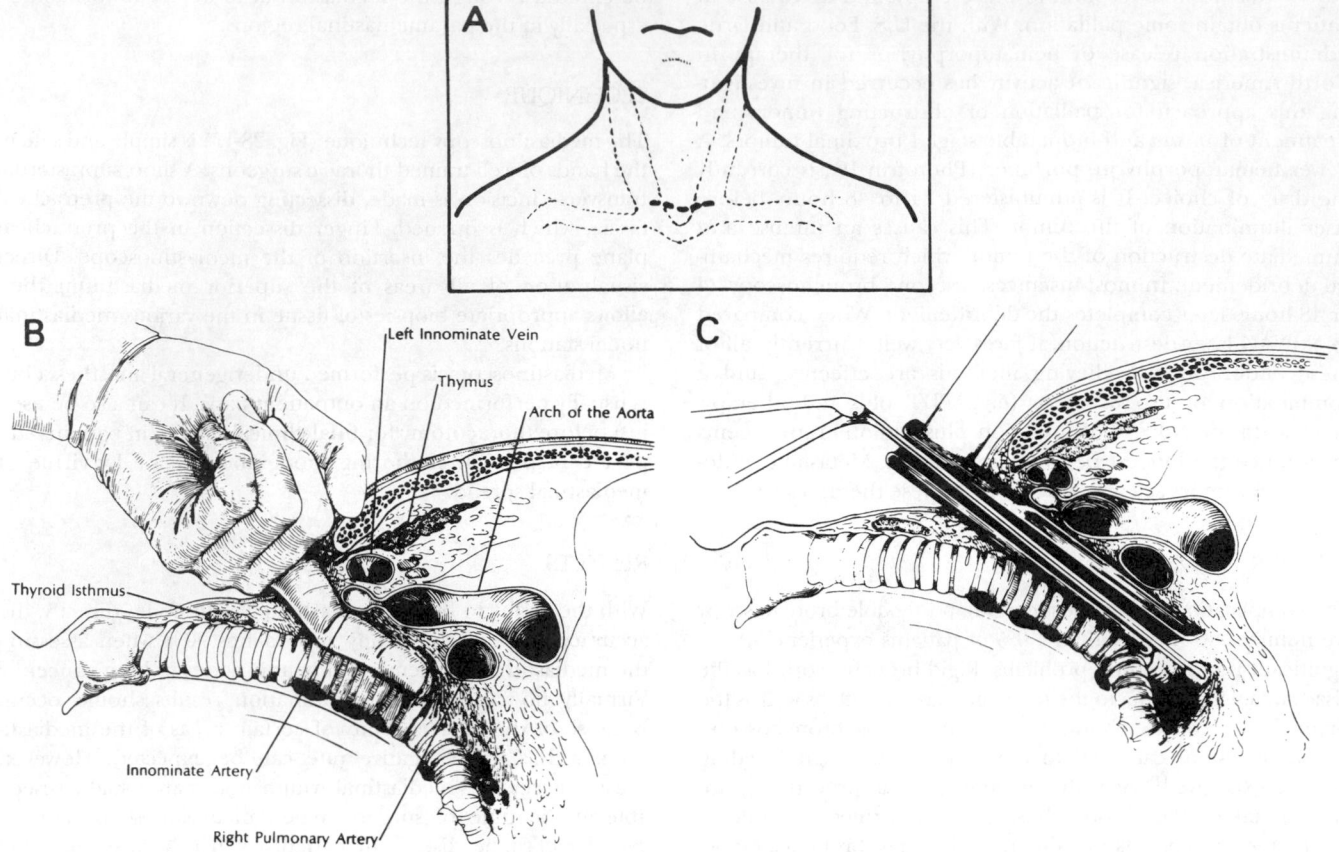

FIGURE 28-13. Technique of mediastinoscopy. **A:** Make a 3- to 4-cm incision just above the manubrium. **B:** Use the finger to dissect bluntly the loose fibrofatty tissue in front of the trachea down to the level of the pulmonary artery. **C:** Introduce the endoscope and take biopsies of suspicious tissues. Needle aspiration of structures before biopsy helps to reduce hemorrhagic complications. (Modified from PA Kerschner. Transcervical approach to the superior mediastinum. *Hosp Pract* 1970;5:61.)

biopsies are required, is a modification of the technique of anterior mediastinotomy described by MacNeill and Chamberlain.[128] A small transverse incision is made in the second intercostal space or over the second or third costal cartilage. The anterior mediastinum is entered, usually without transgressing the pleura, and a biopsy can be obtained. Frequently, left upper lobe tumors do not metastasize to superior mediastinal lymph nodes but to the lymph nodes in the paraaortic area, most accessible by anterior mediastinotomy.

THORACOSCOPY

Thoracoscopy (pleuroscopy) is used most frequently to investigate and treat pleural effusions when simple thoracentesis fails. Until recently, open-tube instruments (e.g., mediastinoscopes) were used for inspection and biopsy. However, the use of thoracoscopy has been extended significantly with the introduction of miniaturized video-recording equipment and improved instrument technology (Fig. 28-14). Learning from the experience developed with laparoscopic surgery, video-assisted thoracoscopic surgery has become a burgeoning enterprise.[115,129] Thoracoscopy has now been used not only for diagnosing pleural disease but for assessing mediastinal spread of lung and esophageal cancer and diagnosing lung disease.[130] The diagnosis of indeterminate pulmonary nodules, previously requiring a thoracotomy, can now be accomplished with relatively minimal invasion using video-assisted techniques. This has become especially important in identifying those nodules so frequently seen on CT scan, only a few millimeters in diameter, inaccessible by any other technique short of thoracotomy. Advanced thoracoscopic techniques can allow partial and total lung resection as well as dissection and removal of mediastinal structures (esophagus, thymus gland, mediastinal lymph nodes, etc.). The ultimate indications for video-assisted thoracoscopic surgery in the treatment of oncologic disease await further investigation and long-term follow-up of efficacy.[131]

TECHNIQUE

Simple thoracoscopy (pleuroscopy) can be performed using a small incision and inserting an open-tube scope (e.g., mediastinoscope) for removal of fluid and simple biopsy of abnormal lesions on the pleural surface. Video-assisted thoracoscopy usually requires the development of a pneumothorax using one-lung anesthesia, three to four small intercostal incisions, and the insertion of multiple trocars to allow the introduction of a videoscope plus a variety of instruments for surgical dissection.

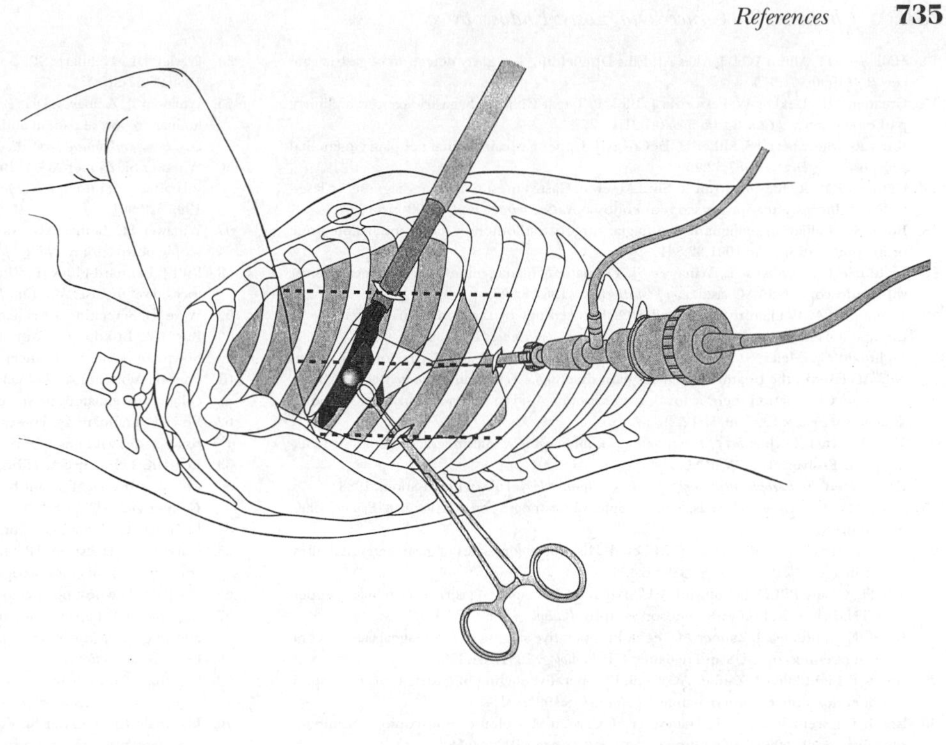

FIGURE 28-14. The video-assisted technique for removing a solitary pulmonary nodule.

With this technique, the total visceral and parietal pleural surfaces can be examined and subjected to biopsy, the mediastinum can be entered and dissected as well as subjected to biopsy, and portions of the lung can be removed, taking advantage of mechanical stapling and cutting devices designed for the purpose.

With very small lesions, difficult to identify at the time of thoracoscopy, transthoracic needles placed radiologically before thoracoscopy can localize the area for resection, similar to the localization techniques used in performing breast biopsies.

RESULTS

Thoracoscopy is an excellent tool to diagnose pleural disease definitively and yields almost a 100% success rate. Peripherally placed lesions of the lung can usually be localized and can be resected for diagnosis, avoiding a major thoracotomy and its attendant morbidity. For this reason, hospital stays are shortened, and the use of expensive medical resources is diminished. The long-term results of thoracoscopic resectional surgery for oncologic disease have yet to be determined. When using this technique for cancer treatment, surgeons must be wary of inadequate resections that may result. In reported series, most surgeons limit video-assisted thoracoscopic resections to early-stage (T1 to T2, N0) tumors. In experienced hands, this approach is safe, and adequate oncologic resections can occur. However, as yet, there is no evidence that this approach provides any benefit to the patient with regard to pain, length of stay, or efficacy. Despite its introduction almost 10 years ago, video-assisted thoracoscopic resections for malignancy are practiced by a very small proportion of thoracic surgeons.[132–134]

COMPLICATIONS

Video-assisted thoracoscopy usually requires general anesthesia, although in diagnosing pleural disease, local anesthetic techniques can be used. The risks of general anesthesia and one-lung ventilation yield some minor morbidity but rarely, if ever, any mortality. Used judiciously, video-assisted thoracoscopy for diagnosis and staging is an extremely safe technique and may be performed on an outpatient basis. Of great concern is its oncologic application. There have been reports of inadequate resections with high local recurrence rates and tumor implantation in thoracoscopic port sites. However, with appropriate techniques, these problems are avoidable. As yet, there is no real evidence of major cost savings or significant long-term benefit using this approach in treating thoracic malignancies. However, the diagnostic abilities of video-assisted thoracoscopic surgery have allowed firm diagnosis to be established with minimal morbidity.

REFERENCES

1. Oguro Y, Takagi K. Recent advances in endoscopic diagnosis of esophagogastric cancer. In: *Endoscopic approaches to cancer diagnosis and treatment.* London: Taylor & Francis, 1990:19.
2. Winawer SJ, Posner G, Lightdale CJ, et al. Endoscopic diagnosis of advanced gastric cancer: factors influencing yield. *Gastroenterology* 1975;69:1183.
3. Silvis SE, Nebel O, Rogers G, Sugawa C, Mandelstam P. Endoscopic complications: results of the 1974 ASGE survey. *JAMA* 1976;235:928.
4. Iishi H, Yamamoto R, Tatsuta M, Okuda S. Evaluation of fine needle aspiration biopsy under direct vision gastrofiberoscopy in diagnosis of diffusely infiltrative carcinoma of the stomach. *Cancer* 1986;57:1365.
5. Lightdale CJ, Winawer SJ. Screening diagnosis and staging of esophageal cancer. *Semin Oncol* 1984;11:101.
6. Kruse P, Boesby S, Bernstein IT, Anderson IB. Barrett's esophagus and esophageal carcinoma: endoscopic and histologic surveillance. *Scand J Gastroenterol* 1993;28:193.
7. Li FP, Shiang EL. Screening for esophageal cancer in 62,000 Chinese. *Lancet* 1979;2:804.
8. Yang CS. Research on esophageal cancer in China: a review. *Cancer Res* 1980;40:2633.
9. Jacob P, Kahrilas PJ, Desai T, et al. Natural history and significance of esophageal squamous cell dysplasia. *Cancer* 1990;65:2731.
10. Shiozaki H, Tahara H, Kobayashi K, et al. Endoscopic screening of early esophageal cancer with the Lugol dye method in patients with head and neck cancers. *Cancer* 1990;66:2068.
11. Kaibara N, Kawaguchi H, Nishidoi H, et al. Significance of mass survey for gastric cancer from the standpoint of surgery. *Am J Surg* 1981;142:543.
12. Blot WJ, Devesa SS, Kneller RW, Fraumeni JF Jr. Rising incidence of adenocarcinoma of the esophagus and gastric cardia. *JAMA* 1991;265:1287.
13. Green PHR, O'Toole KM, Slonim D, Wang T. Increasing incidence and excellent survival of patients with early gastric cancer: experience in a United States medical center. *Am J Med* 1988;85:658.

14. Hallissey MT, Allum WH, Jewkes AJ, Ellis DJ, Fielding JW. Early detection of gastric cancer. *BMJ* 1990;301:513.
15. Craanen ME, Dekker W, Ferwerda J, Blok P, Tytgat GNJ. Early gastric cancer: a clinicopathologic study. *J Clin Gastroenterol* 1991;13:274.
16. Kurtz RC, Sternberg SS, Miller H, DeCosse JJ. Upper gastrointestinal neoplasia in familial polyposis. *Dig Dis Sci* 1987;32:459.
17. Cothren RM, Richard-Kotrum R, Sival M, et al. Gastrointestinal tissue diagnosis by laser-induced fluorescence spectroscopy at endoscopy. *Gastrointest Endosc* 1990;36:105.
18. Bown SG. Palliation malignant dysphagia: surgery, radiotherapy, laser, intubation alone or in combination. *Gut* 1991;32:841.
19. Lightdale CJ, Zimbalist E, Winawer SJ. Outpatient management of esophageal cancer with endoscopic Nd:YAG laser. *Am J Gastroenterol* 1987;82:46.
20. Hamilton FA, Benjamin SB, Castell DO. Proceedings of the consensus conference in therapeutic endoscopy in bleeding ulcers. *Gastrointest Endosc* 1990;36:S1.
21. Lightdale CJ, Meier S, Marcon N, et al. A multicenter phase II trial of PDT versus Nd:YAG laser in the treatment of malignant dysphagia. *Gastrointest Endosc* 1993;39:283.
22. Lightdale CJ. Ablation therapy for Barrett's esophagus: is it time to choose our weapons? *Gastrointest Endosc* 1999:49(1):122.
23. Tio TL, Tytgat GNJ. *Atlas of transintestinal ultrasonography*. Aalsmeer, Netherlands: Drukkenj Mur Kostverloren BV, 1986.
24. Kawai K, ed. *Endoscopic ultrasonography in gastroenterology*. Tokyo: Igaku-Shoin, 1988.
25. Sivak MV Jr, Boyce GA, eds. Endoscopic ultrasonography. *Gastrointest Endosc* 1990; 36[Suppl]:S1.
26. Kimmey MB, Martin RW, Haggitt RC, et al. Histologic correlates of gastrointestinal ultrasound images. *Gastroenterology* 1989;96:433.
27. Tio TL, Coene PPLO, Schouwink MH, Tytgat GNJ. Esophagogastric carcinoma: preoperative TNM classification with endosonography. *Radiology* 1989;173:411.
28. Botet JF, Lightdale CJ, Zauber AG, et al. Preoperative staging of esophageal cancer: comparison of endoscopic US and dynamic CT. *Radiology* 1991;181:419.
29. Botet JF, Lightdale CJ, Zauber AG, et al. Preoperative staging of gastric cancer: comparison of endoscopic US and dynamic CT. *Radiology* 1991;181:426.
30. Rosch T, Lorenz R, Suchy R, Dancygier H, Classen M. Colonic endoscopic ultrasonography: first results of a new technique. *Gastrointest Endosc* 1990;36:382.
31. Tio TL, Tytgat GNJ. Comparison of blind transrectal ultrasonography with endoscopic transrectal ultrasonography in assessing rectal and perirectal disease. *Scand J Gastroenterol* 1986;21[Suppl 123]:104.
32. Lightdale CJ, Botet JF, Kelsen DP, Turnbull AD, Brennan MF. Diagnosis of recurrent upper gastrointestinal cancer at the surgical anastomosis by endoscopic ultrasound. *Gastrointest Endosc* 1989;35:407.
33. Yasuda K, Nakajima M, Yoshida S, Kiyota K, Kawai K. The diagnosis of submucosal tumors of the stomach by endoscopic ultrasonography. *Gastrointest Endosc* 1989;35:10.
34. Tio TL, den Hartog Jager FCA, Tytgat GNJ. Endoscopic ultrasonography of non-Hodgkin lymphoma of the stomach. *Gastroenterology* 1986;91:401.
35. Yasuda K, Mukai H, Fujimoto S, Nakajima M, Kawai K. The diagnosis of pancreatic cancer by endoscopic ultrasonography. *Gastrointest Endosc* 1988;34:1.
36. Lees WR. Endoscopic ultrasonography of chronic pancreatitis and pancreatic pseudocysts. *Scand J Gastroenterol* 1986;21[Suppl 123]:123.
37. Rosch T, Lorenz R, Braig C, et al. Endoscopic ultrasound in pancreatic tumor diagnosis. *Gastrointest Endosc* 1991;37:347.
38. Morales TG, Sampliner RE. Barrett's esophagus: update on screening, surveillance and treatment. *Arch Intern Med* 1999;159(13):141.
39. Tio TL, Cheng J, Wijers OB, Sars PRA, Tytgat GNJ. Endosonographic TNM staging of extrahepatic bile duct cancer: comparison with pathological staging. *Gastroenterology* 1991;100:1351.
40. Lightdale CJ, Botet JF, Woodruff JM, Brennan MF. Localization of endocrine tumors of the pancreas with endoscopic ultrasonography. *Cancer* 1991;68:1815.
41. Wiersema MJ, Wiersema LM, Khurso Q, Cramer HM, Tao L-C. Combined endosonography and fine-needle aspiration cytology in evaluation of gastrointestinal lesions. *Gastrointest Endosc* 1994;40:199.
42. Schottenfeld D, Winawer SJ. Large intestine. In: Schottenfeld D, Fraumeni JF, eds. *Cancer epidemiology and prevention*. Philadelphia: WB Saunders, 1982:703.
43. Selby JV, Friedman GD, Quesenberry CP, Weiss NS. A case control study of screening sigmoidoscopy and mortality from colorectal cancer. *N Engl J Med* 1992;326:653.
44. Winawer SJ, Kern JF. Sigmoidoscopy: case finding versus screening. *Gastroenterology* 1988;95:527.
45. American Cancer Society. Guidelines for the cancer-related checkup: recommendations and rationale. *CA Cancer J Clin* 1980;34:130.
46. Winawer SJ, Lediner SD, Kurtz RC. Comparison of flexible sigmoidoscopy with other diagnostic techniques in the diagnosis of colorectal neoplasia. *Dig Dis Sci* 1979;24:277.
47. Baskin WN, Greenlaw RL, Fraker JT, et al. Flexible sigmoidoscopy training for primary care physicians. *Gastrointest Endosc* 1984;30:141.
48. Traul DG, Davis CB, Pollock JC, et al. Flexible fiberoptic sigmoidoscopy. The Monroe Clinic experience: a prospective study of 5,000 examinations. *Dis Colon Rectum* 1983;26:161.
49. Marks G, Moses ML. The clinical application of flexible fiberoptic colonoscopy. *Surg Clin North Am* 1973;53:735.
50. Hunt RH. The role of colonoscopy in complicated diverticular disease. *Acta Chir Belg* 1979;78:349.
51. Brand EJ, Sullivan BH Jr, Sivak MV Jr, et al. Colonoscopy in the diagnosis of unexplained rectal bleeding. *Ann Surg* 1980;192:111.
52. Tedesco FJ, Waye JD, Raskin JB, et al. Colonoscopic evaluation of rectal bleeding. *Ann Intern Med* 1978;89:907.
53. Winawer SJ, Schottenfeld D, Flehinger BJ. Colorectal cancer screening. *J Natl Cancer Inst* 1991;83:243.
54. Fowler DL, Hedberg SE. Follow-up colonoscopy after polypectomy. *Gastrointest Endosc* 1980;26:67(abst).
55. Winawer SJ, Zauber A, Diaz B, et al. The national polyp study: overview of program and preliminary report of patient and polyp characteristics. In: Steele G, Burt R, Winawer SJ, Karr J, eds. *Basic and clinical perspectives of colorectal polyps and cancer.* New York: Alan R Liss, 1988.
56. Winawer SJ, Zauber AG, O'Brien MJ, et al. Randomized comparison of surveillance intervals after colonoscopic removal of newly diagnosed adenomatous polyps. *N Engl J Med* 1993;328:901.
57. Winawer SJ, Zauber AG, Nah Ho M, et al. Prevention of colorectal cancer by colonoscopic polypectomy. *N Engl J Med* 1993;329:1977.
58. Butt J, Lennard-Jones JE, Ritchie J. A practical approach to the cancer risk in inflammatory bowel disease. *Med Clin North Am* 1980;64:1203.
59. Waye JD. Screening for cancer in ulcerative colitis. *Front Gastrointest Res* 1986;10:243.
60. Burt RW, Bishop DT, Cannon LA, et al. Dominant inheritance of adenomatous colonic polyps and colorectal cancer. *N Engl J Med* 1985;312:1540.
61. Cannon-Albright LA, Skolnick MH, Bishop T, et al. Common inheritance of susceptibility to colonic adenomatous polyps and associated colorectal cancers. *N Engl J Med* 1988;319:533.
62. Rex DK, Lehman GA, Hawes RH, et al. Screening colonoscopy in asymptomatic average-risk persons with negative fecal occult blood test. *Gastroenterology* 1991;100:64.
63. Rex DK, Lehman GA, Ulbright TM, et al. Colonic neoplasia in asymptomatic persons with negative fecal occult blood tests: influence of age, gender and family history. *Am J Gastroenterol* 1993;88:825.
64. Lightdale CJ. India ink colonic tattoo: blots on the record. *Gastrointest Endosc* 1991;37:99.
65. Gilbert GA, Hallsrom AP, Shaneyfelt SL, et al. The national ASGE colonoscopy survey: complications of colonoscopy. *Gastrointest Endosc* 1984;30:156(abst).
66. Waye JD. The post-polypectomy coagulation syndrome. *Gastrointest Endosc* 1981;27:184.
67. Lightdale CJ. Laparoscopy in gastroenterologic practice. In: Sherlock P, Jerzy-Glass G, eds. *Progress in gastroenterology*. New York: Grune & Stratton, 1983:461.
68. Beck K. *Color atlas of laparoscopy*. Philadelphia: WB Saunders, 1984.
69. Lightdale CJ. Indications, contraindications and complications of laparoscopy. In: Sivak M, ed. *Gastroenterological endoscopy*. Philadelphia: WB Saunders, 1987:1030.
70. Lightdale CJ, Winawer SJ, Kurtz RC, Knapper WH. Laparoscopic diagnosis of suspected liver neoplasms: value of prior liver scans. *Dig Dis Sci* 1979;24:588.
71. Riemann JF. Peritoneoscopy in the diagnosis of liver metastases. In: Weiss L, Gilbert H, eds. *Liver metastasis*. Boston: GK Hall, 1982:244.
72. Boyce HW Jr. Laparoscopy. In: Schiff L, Schiff ER, eds. *Diseases of the liver*, 6th ed. Philadelphia: JB Lippincott, 1987:443.
73. Warshaw AL, Tepper JE, et al. Laparoscopy in staging and planning of therapy for pancreatic cancer. *Am J Surg* 1986;151:76.
74. Dagnini G, Martin G, et al. Laparoscopy in the diagnosis of primary carcinoma of the gallbladder. *Gastrointest Endosc* 1984;30:289.
75. DeVita VT, Bagley CM, Goodell B, et al. Peritoneoscopy in the staging of Hodgkin's disease. *Cancer Res* 1971;31:1746.
76. Coleman M, Lightdale CJ, Vinciguerra VP, et al. Peritoneoscopy in Hodgkin's disease. Confirmation of results by laparotomy. *JAMA* 1976;236:2634.
77. Chabner BA, Johnson RE, Young RC, et al. Sequential nonsurgical and surgical staging of non-Hodgkin's lymphoma. *Ann Intern Med* 1976;85:149.
78. Brady PG, Pebbles M, Goldschmid S. Role of laparoscopy in the evaluation of patients with suspected hepatic or peritoneal malignancy. *Gastrointest Endosc* 1991;37:27.
79. Vilardell F, Seres I, Marti-Vicente A. Complications of peritoneoscopy: a survey of 1,455 examinations. *Gastrointest Endosc* 1968;14:178.
80. McCune WS, Short PE, Moscovitz H. Endoscopic cannulation of the ampulla of Vater. *Ann Surg* 1968;167:752.
81. Georgopoulos SK, Schwartz LH, Jarnagin WR, et al. A comparison of magnetic resonance cholangiopancreatography (MRCP) and endoscopic retrograde cholangiopancreatography (ERCP) in malignant pancreaticobiliary obstruction. *Arch Surg* 1999; 134:1002.
82. Freeney PC. Radiology of the pancreas: two decades of progress in imaging and intervention. *AJR Am J Roentgenol* 1988;150:975.
83. Frick MP, Feinberg SB, Goodale RL. The value of endoscopic retrograde cholangiopancreatography in patients with suspected carcinoma of the pancreas and indeterminate computed tomographic results. *Surg Gynecol Obstet* 1982;155:177.
84. Ruddell WSJ, Linott DJ, Axon, ATR. The diagnostic yield of ERCP in the investigation of unexplained abdominal pain. *Br J Surg* 1983;70:74.
85. Bourgeois N, Dunham F, Verhest A, et al. Endoscopic biopsies of the ampulla of Vater at the time of endoscopic sphincterotomy: difficulties in interpretation. *Gastrointest Endosc* 1984;30:163.
86. Dowsett JF, Vaira D, Hatfield ARW, et al. Endoscopic biliary therapy using the combined percutaneous and endoscopic technique. *Gastroenterology* 1989;96:1180.
87. Speer A, Russell RCG, Hatfield A, et al. Randomized trial of endoscopic versus percutaneous stent insertion for malignant obstructive jaundice. *Lancet* 1987;2:57.
88. Deviere J, Baize M, de Toeuf J, et al. Long-term follow-up of patients with hilar malignant strictures treated by endoscopic biliary drainage. *Gastrointest Endosc* 1988;34:95.
89. Sheperd HA, Royle G, Ross APR, et al. Endoscopic biliary endoprosthesis in the palliation of malignant obstruction of the distal common bile duct: a randomized trial. *Br J Surg* 1988;75:1166.
90. Kurtz RC. Preoperative biliary decompression. In: Jacobson IM, ed. *ERCP: diagnostic and therapeutic applications*. New York: Elsevier Science, 1989.
91. Kurtz RC, Botet JB, Gerdes H, et al. Percutaneous biliary drainage following failed endoscopic drainage in malignant biliary obstruction. *Gastroenterology* 1988;34:A189(abst).
92. Levine JG, Kurtz RC, Botet J. Microbiological analysis of sepsis complicating nonsurgical biliary drainage in malignant obstruction. *Gastrointest Endosc* 1990;36:364.
93. Sternlieb JM, Aronchich CA, Retig JN, et al. A multicenter, randomized, controlled trial

to evaluate the effect of prophylactic octreotide on ERCP-induced pancreatitis. *Am J Gastroenterol* 1992;87:1561.
94. Davis FR, Benson MJ, Gertner DE, et al. Diagnostic and therapeutic push type enteroscopy in clinical use. *Gut* 1995;37:346.
95. Foutch PG, Sawyer R, Sanowski RA. Push-enteroscopy for diagnosis of patients with gastrointestinal bleeding of obscure origin. *Gastrointest Endosc* 1990;36:337.
96. Gostout CJ, Schroeder KW, Burton DD. Small bowel enteroscopy: an early experience in gastrointestinal bleeding of unknown origin. *Gastrointest Endosc* 1991;37:5.
97. Lewis BS, Kornbluth A, Waye JD. Small bowel tumors: yield of enteroscopy. *Gut* 1991;32:763.
98. Ponsky JL, Gauderer MWL. Percutaneous endoscopic gastrostomy: a non-operative technique for feeding gastrostomy. *Gastrointest Endosc* 1981;27:9.
99. Shike M, Berner YN, Gerdes H, et al. Percutaneous endoscopic gastrostomy and jejunostomy for long-term feeding in patients with cancer of the head and neck. *Otolaryngol Head Neck Surg* 1989;101:549.
100. Wasiljew BK, Ujiki GT, Beal JM. Feeding gastrostomy: complications and mortality. *Am J Surg* 1982;143:194.
101. Shike M, Schroy P, Ritchie MA, et al. Percutaneous endoscopic jejunostomy in cancer patients with previous gastric resection. *Gastrointest Endosc* 1987;33:372.
102. Shike M, Latkany L, Gerdes H. Direct percutaneous endoscopic jejunostomies (DPEJ): a technique for placement of percutaneous endoscopic tubes directly into the jejunum. *Gastrointest Endosc* 1995;41:312.
103. Ikeda S, Eni Yanai T, Ishikawa S. Flexible bronchofiberscope. *Keio J Med* 1968;17:1.
104. Zavala DC, Richardson RH, Mukerjee PK, et al. Use of the bronchofiberscope for bronchial brush biopsy: diagnostic results and comparisons with other brushing techniques. *Chest* 1973;63:889.
105. Shure D. Fiberoptic bronchoscopy: diagnostic application. *Clin Chest Med* 1987;8:1.
106. Cortese DA. Bronchoscopic photodynamic therapy of early lung cancer. *Chest* 1986;90:629.
107. Seagren SL, Harrell JH, Horn RA. High-dose rate intraluminal irradiation in recurrent endobronchial carcinoma. *Chest* 1985;88:810.
108. Tanaka M, Kawanami O, Satoh M. Endoscopic observation of peripheral airway lesions. *Chest* 1988;93:228.
109. Wong KP, Marsh BR, Summer WR, et al. Transbronchial needle aspiration for diagnosis of lung cancer. *Chest* 1980;80:48.
110. Silvestri GA, Hoffman BJ, Bhutani MS, et al. Endoscopic ultrasound with fine-needle aspiration in the diagnosis and staging of lung cancer. *Ann Thorac Surg* 1996;61:1441.
111. Ginsberg RJ. Evaluation of the mediastinum by invasive techniques. *Surg Clin North Am* 1987;67:1025.
112. Lam S, Kennedy T, Unger M. et al. Localization of bronchial intraepithelial neoplastic lesions by fluorescence bronchoscopy. *Chest* 1998;113:696.
113. Luke WP, Pearson FG, Todd TRJ, et al. Prospective evaluation of mediastinoscopy for assessment of carcinoma of the lung. *J Thorac Cardiovasc Surg* 1986;91:553.
114. Nathanson LK. Basic instrumentation and operative technique for laparoscopic surgery. In: Cuschieri A, ed. *Laparoscopic biliary surgery*. London: Blackwell Science, 1990:33.
115. Nathanson LK, Shimi SM, Wood RAB, Cuschieri A. Video thoracoscopic ligation of bulla and pleurectomy for spontaneous pneumothorax. *Ann Thorac Surg* 1991;52:316.
116. McCaughan JS, Williams TE Jr, Bethel BH. Photodynamic therapy of endobronchial tumors. *Lasers Surg Med* 1986;6:336.
117. McCaughan JS Jr. Survival after photodynamic therapy to non-pulmonary metastatic endobronchial tumors. *Lasers Surg Med* 1999;24(3):194.
118. Cordasco EM, Mehta AC, Ahmad M. Bronchoscopically induced bleeding: a summary of 9 years Cleveland clinical experience and review of a literature. *Chest* 1991;100:1141.
119. Credle WF, Smiddy JF, Elliott RC. Complications of fiberoptic bronchoscopy. *Am Rev Respir Dis* 1974;109:67.
120. Surratt DM, Smiddy JF, Bruber B. Deaths and complications associated with fiberoptic bronchoscopy. *Chest* 1976;69:747.
121. Pue CA, Pacht ER. Complications of fiber-optic bronchoscopy at a university hospital. *Chest* 1995;107:430.
122. Ginsberg RJ. Evaluation of the mediastinum by invasive techniques. *Surg Clin North Am* 1987;67:1025.
123. Ginsberg RJ, Rice TW, Goldberg M, et al. Extended cervical mediastinoscopy: a single staging procedure for bronchial carcinoma of the left upper lobe. *J Thorac Cardiovasc Surg* 1987;94:673.
124. Luke WP, Pearson FG, Todd TRJ, et al. Prospective evaluation of mediastinoscopy for assessment of carcinoma of the lung. *J Thorac Cardiovasc Surg* 1986;91:553.
125. Vansteenkiste JF, Stroobants SG, Dupont PJ, et al. Prognostic importance of the standardized uptake value on 18-F fluoro-2-deoxy-glucose-positron emission tomography scan in NSCLC: an analysis of 125 cases. *J Clin Oncol* 1999;17:3201.
126. Weigel TL, Meltzer CC, Friedman DM, et al. The role of positron emission tomography in evaluating the mediastinum. American Association of Thoracic Surgery. New Orleans, April 18–21, 1999.
127. Hammoud ZT, Anderson RC, Meyers DF, et al. The current role of mediastinoscopy in the evaluation of thoracic disease. *J Thorac Cardiovasc Surg* 1999;118:894.
128. McNeill TM, Chamberlain JM. Diagnostic anterior mediastinotomy. *Ann Thorac Surg* 1966;2:532.
129. Nathanson LK. Basic instrumentation and operative technique for laparoscopic surgery. In: Cuschieri A, ed. *Laparoscopic biliary surgery*. London: Blackwell Science, 1990:33.
130. Hazelrigg SR, Nunchuck SK, LoCicero J, the Video-Assisted Thoracic Surgery Study Group. Video-assisted thoracic surgery study group data. *Ann Thorac Surg* 1993;56:1039.
131. Kirby TJ, Mack MJ, Landreneau RJ, Rice TW. Initial experience with video-assisted thoracoscopic lobectomy. *Ann Thorac Surg* 1993;56:1248.
132. Landreneau RJ, Mack MJ, Dowling RD, et al. The role of thoracoscopy in lung cancer management. *Chest* 1998;113[Suppl 1]:6S.
133. McKenna RJ Jr, Wolf RK, Brenner M, et al. Is lobectomy by video-assisted thoracic surgery an adequate cancer operation? *Ann Thorac Surg* 1998;66:1903.
134. Kaseda S, Aoki T, Hangai N. Video-assisted thoracic surgery (VATS) lobectomy: the Japanese experience. *Semin Thorac Cadiovasc Surg* 1998;10:300.

CHAPTER 29

Specialized Techniques in Cancer Management

SECTION 1

ALAN T. LEFOR

Laparoscopy

Laparoscopy has become an important tool in the diagnosis and treatment of many diseases worldwide since the late 1980s. However, the procedure has been available for nearly 100 years, used mostly by gynecologists, hepatologists, and a few pioneer general surgeons. The first report is from a gynecologic procedure performed by Ott in Russia in 1901.[1] Insufflation was introduced in 1901 by Kelling, in a dog model. The Veress needle was developed in 1938. Older instruments consisted of a metal tube fitted with lenses, which allowed one person at a time to see the hazy images provided. One of the major reasons for the new popularity of laparoscopy is the availability of high-quality images on video monitors, making it easy for a team of surgeons to work together, each with the same view. In addition, the development of long-handled tools that function through ports has rapidly and widely expanded the scope of laparoscopic surgery.[2]

One of the earliest applications of laparoscopy to patients with cancer was by Bagley and coworkers[3] in 1973 who reported 96 cases of peritoneoscopy in the evaluation of lymphoma. Also in 1973, Casirola and colleagues[4] published a series of 38 patients with lymphoma who were evaluated laparoscopically at the University of Pavia. They concluded that laparoscopy should be used routinely in the evaluation of patients with Hodgkin's lymphoma to accurately assess stage. Because of limitations imposed by the available equipment, they were limited to observational staging of the liver surface. Laparoscopy and bone marrow biopsy were advocated as necessary before laparotomy in patients with Hodgkin's disease by several studies as early as 1975.[5,6] The value of laparoscopy in the evaluation of patients with non-Hodgkin's lymphoma (NHL) was further described by Chabner and colleagues[7] from the National Institutes of Health, when they advocated peritoneoscopy as a routine component of a staging procedure. These investigators advocated multiple liver biopsies through the peritoneoscope for patients with negative evaluations for widespread disease, including a history, physical examination, imaging studies, bone marrow biopsies, and a percutaneous liver biopsy. Laparotomy with splenectomy and multiple lymph node biopsies was then recommended for patients with negative peritoneoscopy and liver biopsies.[8]

In 1978, Cuschieri and colleagues[9] reported on the laparoscopic evaluation of 23 patients with pancreatic carcinoma. These pioneers were able to investigate the lesser sac with their primitive instruments and thought that laparoscopy might be used to obviate the need for laparotomy in patients with advanced disease.

Although laparoscopy is applied widely to a large number of surgical conditions and has become the standard surgical approach for cholecystectomy since its introduction to the United States in 1988, its application to patients with cancer remains less well defined. In fact, there are no specific indications for the use of laparoscopy in patients with malignancies.

Two principles guide the use of laparoscopy in the care of the cancer patient. First, as with any procedure, laparoscopy should not be performed simply because it can be done. Second, when laparoscopy is used in the care of the cancer patient for diagnosis, staging, treatment, or palliation, the laparoscopic conduct of the operation should compromise neither the nature of the procedure nor the amount or source of the tissue obtained.

Surgeons have been involved in the diagnosis, staging, treatment, and palliation of malignancies for centuries. Laparoscopy is assuming a role in each of these areas. Laparoscopy has a role in establishing the *diagnosis* of cancer in some situations, allowing biopsy of intraperitoneal and retroperitoneal masses and lymph nodes, biopsy of visceral lesions, and the examination of abdominal contents with ultrasound probes. Laparoscopy is useful in the *staging* of established malignancies, such as pancreatic cancer, Hodgkin's lymphoma, and esophageal cancer. Laparoscopy also has a role in the surgical *treatment* of a variety of malignancies, including gastric carcinoma, pancreatic cancer, renal tumors, adrenal tumors, colon cancer, and gynecologic tumors. Laparoscopy may be the appropriate approach for the definitive therapy of these lesions or may be a way to provide a palliative procedure, such as a cholecystojejunostomy, in a patient with unresectable carcinoma of the pancreas. Lastly, laparoscopy can play an important role in the *palliative care* of the cancer patient as a way of performing procedures such as feeding tube placement or intestinal stoma creation with decreased hospitalization and recovery time.

Although many procedures have been performed successfully using laparoscopic technology, the results obtained should be analyzed objectively and critically. There are advantages and disadvantages to both the open and laparoscopic conduct of many procedures. Most important, the technique selected should benefit the patient maximally. This must be viewed from many angles, including patient comfort, tissue obtained, cost-effectiveness, surgical morbidity, and surgical mortality. At the present time, for most laparoscopic procedures applied to the care of the patient with cancer, insufficient data are available to make quantitative judgments about most of these issues. Therefore, only by critically analyzing the existing data can a practitioner begin to make decisions about what techniques to use for a specific patient.

LAPAROSCOPIC PHYSIOLOGY

CELLULAR EFFECTS

One of the most notable sequelae of laparoscopic surgery is the generally significant decrease in the amount of pain when compared with open procedures. This may easily be attributed to the use of smaller incisions and the lack of retractors holding these incisions open for hours. However, patients who undergo laparoscopic splenectomy and then require an incision for removal of the intact specimen (see later, Laparoscopic Staging of Hodgkin's Lymphoma) also note decreased pain in their incisions. West and colleagues[11] investigated the effect of different insufflation gases on murine peritoneal macrophage intracellular pH and correlated these alterations with alterations in lipopolysaccharide stimulated inflammatory cytokine release. Peritoneal macrophages were incubated for 2 hours in air, helium, or carbon dioxide (CO_2), and the effect on tumor necrosis factor (TNF), interleukin (IL)-1, and cytosolic pH were determined. Macrophages incubated in CO_2 produced significantly less TNF and IL-1 compared with incubation in air or helium. In addition, exposure to CO_2, but not air or helium, produced a marked cytosolic acidification. These authors conclude that cellular acidification induced by peritoneal CO_2 insufflation contributes to the diminished local inflammatory response seen in laparoscopic surgery.

EFFECTS ON HEPATIC BLOOD FLOW

Changes in hepatic blood flow can be significant because the liver plays a central role in the removal of a wide variety of substances from the circulation. Changes in hepatic blood flow could significantly alter the biokinetics of anesthetic and other agents. In an effort to investigate the effect of CO_2 pneumoperitoneum, Tuñón and colleagues[10] evaluated the pharmacokinetics of indocyanine green, an anionic dye frequently used to estimate hepatic blood flow in experimental systems. They found a significantly decreased clearance of indocyanine green in the insufflation and laparoscopic surgery groups compared with the open surgery group, corresponding to a significantly decreased hepatic blood flow in these two groups. They concluded that dose adjustments of many agents may be necessary for patients undergoing laparoscopic procedures, especially those with limited hepatic reserve.

CARDIOPULMONARY EFFECTS

The use of laparoscopy in patients with sepsis may be a significant physiologic challenge. In an effort to assess this experimentally, Greif and Forse[12] studied cardiopulmonary physiologic parameters in a pig model of adult respiratory distress syndrome (ARDS). After inducing ARDS, animals were divided into two groups: One underwent laparoscopy and the other conventional laparotomy. The laparoscopic group demonstrated a significantly decreased pulmonary compliance compared with the laparotomy group, had a higher pCO_2, and was more acidotic. Animals with ARDS demonstrate further compromise in pulmonary physiologic parameters when undergoing laparoscopy, but overall, cardiorespiratory function was preserved.

In a subsequent study, Greif and Forse[13] used a porcine sepsis model to evaluate interventions to ameliorate the effect of laparoscopy on cardiovascular hemodynamics. Specifically, they found that the adverse effects may be mediated by increased pulmonary vascular resistance, diminished venous return, or both. They found that insufflation with air instead of CO_2 to manipulate arterial pH did not improve cardiovascular hemodynamics. Aggressive fluid administration, and administration of prostacyclin or indomethacin, had positive effects on the hemodynamic effects of pneumoperitoneum.

LAPAROSCOPY AND THE SYSTEMIC IMMUNE RESPONSE

The effect of laparoscopy on the activation of the systemic immune response has been studied by a number of investigators. Cytokine levels provide us with one method of evaluating the systemic immune response. The cytokines IL-1, IL-6, C-reactive protein, and TNF are known mediators of the acute-phase response.[14] Peak C-reactive protein levels have been shown to be significantly higher after open cholecystectomy compared with laparoscopic cholecystectomy.[14] Furthermore, these investigators found a significantly prolonged elevation in C-reactive protein levels in patients undergoing open cholecystectomy compared with those undergoing laparoscopic cholecystectomy.

Serum IL-6 levels are early and sensitive markers of tissue damage because they increase proportionally to degree of injury. IL-6 levels also have been shown to correlate with the development of significant complications and mortality. Serum IL-6 levels have been shown to be reduced in patients undergoing laparoscopic cholecystectomy compared with those undergoing open cholecystectomy.[15] There remains a distinct lack of consensus about the meaning of the decreased IL-6 response, and further study is indicated.

The immunosuppression induced by open surgery has been studied in the past and has been well described.[16,17] More recent studies have looked at the effect of laparoscopic surgery on the cellular components of the immune system. Previous studies have shown significant decreases in the CD4 and CD8 cell counts in patients undergoing open cholecystectomy.[17] Vallina and Velasco[16] studied peripheral lymphocyte populations in 11 patients undergoing laparoscopic cholecystectomy and found a transient decrease in the CD4 to CD8 ratio, with no difference in absolute CD4 and CD8 cell counts and a return to preoperative ratio within 1 week of surgery. These studies suggest that laparoscopic surgery may impact less on the cellular components of the immune system than open surgery, but further study is necessary to determine the significance of this information.

PORT-SITE METASTASES

Soon after the laparoscopic treatment of malignancies began throughout the world, a number of reports appeared describing "port-site metastases,"—that is, tumor recurrence at the sites of trocar placement[18–25] in the postoperative period. A large number of such anecdotal reports were published, which subjectively seemed far more common than wound recurrences after open colon resection. The true extent of the problem was difficult to determine. In a large series of open colon resections, Hughes et al.[26] reported 11 (0.7%) wound recurrences of tumor in 1603 patients. Several investigators began to look for port-site recurrences in a prospective manner. Ramos et al.[27] reported 3 recurrences in a series of 208 laparoscopic colon cancer resections. Of these three patients, two had widespread disease. Between 1993 and 1996, 35 cases of port-site recurrence after laparoscopic colectomy for colorectal carcinoma were reported.[28] These observations led to a number of consequences. First, these reports prompted careful scientific evaluation of the procedure and its application to malignancies. Registries were developed to monitor the occurrence of port-site recurrences. Second, a number of investigators began to examine possible mechanisms for this phenomenon in the laboratory.

A retrospective study of 372 patients who underwent laparoscopic colon resection for malignancy was conducted by Nelson and colleagues.[29] This study had relatively short follow-up, with a mean follow-up of just 23 months. The incidence of port-site metastases was 1.1%, which is similar to published data for open surgical resection of colon cancer. This study also demonstrated a 3-year survival rate that was similar, stage for stage, with open colon resection data. In a large prospective study of 533 patients with a variety of intraabdominal malignancies who underwent laparoscopic investigation, port-site recurrences were identified in just four patients (0.8%).[30] The investigators in this study looked at the extent of disease as well, identifying port-site recurrences in 3 of 71 patients with advanced disease compared with just 1 of 462 without advanced disease ($P < .003$), further supporting the concept that this phenomenon may be an indicator of advanced disease.

A number of investigators have attempted to explain this phenomenon using clinical studies and laboratory models of port-site recurrences, specifically looking at the effects of the insufflation gases. In a clinical study of 15 patients with malignancies by Ikramuddin et al.,[31] the insufflation gas effluent was directed through saline. Malignant cells were found in specimens from only two patients, both of whom had carcinomatosis. These authors concluded that tumor cell aerosolization is unlikely to contribute to port-site metastases. In a study of effluent CO_2, another group reported very low levels of tumor cells in the gas, but they did find large numbers of tumor cells on trocars and instruments that were used.[32] They suggest that port-site metastases might be reduced with avoidance of mechanical contamination. In another clinical study, labeled red blood cells were injected in the gallbladder bed in two groups of patients, one with standard CO_2 pneumoperitoneum and one with gasless laparoscopy.[33] Radioactivity was observed in the area of trocar insertion in all patients who underwent standard laparoscopy but was rare in patients who underwent gasless laparoscopy. In a rat model of laparoscopy, peritoneal tumor growth was greater after laparotomy than after CO_2 laparoscopy.[34] The investigators in this study also found that insufflation of CO_2 promotes tumor growth at the peritoneal surface and is associated with more abdominal wall metastases than gasless laparoscopy. Others also have shown that CO_2 pneumoperitoneum significantly increases tumor implantation at trocar sites in a hamster model.[35] In a rat study, the influence of the trocar itself was studied, and investigators found an increase in port-site metastases from the act of withdrawing the port and seeding the wound site.[36] Several studies have looked at the role of the gas used for insufflation with contradictory results. In one study, the gas used was not a contributing factor, comparing CO_2, helium, and air.[37] In another study, helium was associated with reduced tumor growth.[38] Both of these studies suggest the use of gasless laparoscopy for patients with malignancies.

Other investigators have looked at the influence of tissue trauma on the formation of port-site metastases. In a rat experiment, tissue trauma was induced at the port sites, and a significantly greater amount of tumor grew there after insufflation than at port sites without induced trauma.[39] These authors also identified leakage of insufflating gas as a contributing factor. Other investigators also have looked at the influence of tissue injury and found that peritoneal injury enhances peritoneal implantation of tumor cells.[40] A number of investigators have used laboratory models to compare laparotomy and laparoscopy. In the absence of tumor manipulation, no difference was seen in intraperitoneal tumor growth and spread between laparotomy and laparoscopy in a rat model.[41] The possibility of immune mediation has been investigated by one group.[42–44]

These authors found that tumors were established and grew more readily and larger after laparotomy than after insufflation. In one of their studies, altered levels of TNF were found, suggesting an association.[45] The relative immunosuppression of laparotomy may play a role.

A number of explanations have been put forth to explain the phenomenon of port-site metastases. These are outlined briefly in Table 29.1-1. The potential causes of this problem suggest that technical modifications of the procedure may minimize the likelihood of this problem occurring. Early data clearly suggest that the incidence of port-site recurrences after laparoscopic tumor resection is similar to the wound recurrence rate after open resections for colon cancer. Further clinical and experimental studies are in progress to determine the true extent of this problem. Laparoscopic resection of malignancies performed outside of clinical trials should be undertaken "with circumspection" until the true incidence of this problem is known as a result of prospective randomized trials.[28]

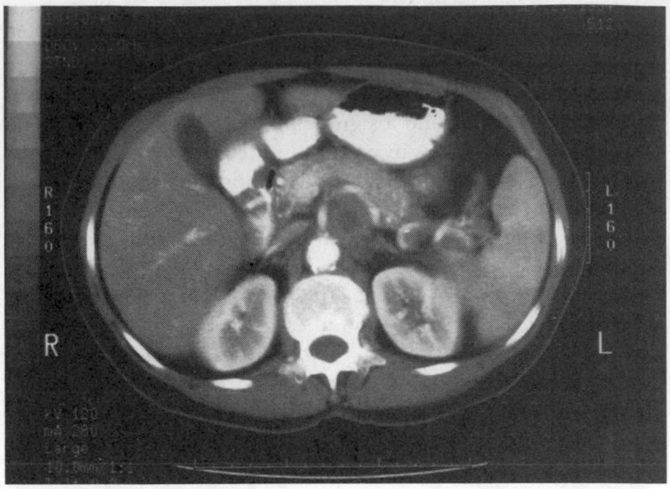

FIGURE 29.1-1. A 70-year-old woman presented with fevers and nonspecific abdominal pain. Workup revealed a negative physical examination, with an enlarged celiac lymph node seen on computed tomography scan. (From ref. 2, with permission.)

LAPAROSCOPY IN THE DIAGNOSIS OF MALIGNANCY

GENERAL CONSIDERATIONS

Patients often present with constitutional symptoms and undergo evaluation by imaging studies in the hopes of identifying an underlying cause. Figure 29.1-1 shows a computed tomography (CT) scan image from a 70-year-old woman who presented with fever and malaise and no evidence of peripheral adenopathy on physical examination. Celiac lymph nodes were sampled laparoscopically (Fig. 29.1-2), establishing the diagnosis of NHL. In this case, the patient underwent a diagnostic procedure and was discharged home the same day with minimal postoperative pain. The use of diagnostic laparoscopy in the evaluation of abdominal malignancies has been reported. In a series by Easter et al.,[46] of 25 patients with suspected malignancies, 17 (68%) had a positive study for cancer; these investigators concluded that patient management had been altered by the laparoscopic finding in 25 patients (100%).

BIOPSY OF MASSES

Masses identified on preoperative imaging studies are often amenable to laparoscopic biopsy. Some studies have evaluated the tactile sensation afforded by laparoscopic instruments and have found it to be almost comparable with open palpation.[47] Techniques available for the biopsy of masses under laparoscopic control include[48]

- Percutaneous insertion of a core biopsy needle with direct puncture of the mass; this is easily performed under the direct vision afforded by the laparoscope.
- Wedge biopsy using the electrocautery; this method should be used cautiously to avoid thermal destruction of the specimen.
- Cup forceps biopsy; careful use of these forceps allows removal of adequate tissue for histopathologic examination while avoiding destruction of the specimen. This technique is extremely useful for the biopsy of small lesions such as those present on peritoneal surfaces (Fig. 29.1-3).

TABLE 29.1-1. Possible Causes of Tumor Cell Dissemination in Laparoscopic Surgery for Cancer

Possible Cause	*Intervention to Potentially Minimize This Cause*
Dispersion of cells by carbon dioxide gas	Avoid sudden loss of pneumoperitoneum
Tumor spillage from manipulation and instrumentation	Avoid excessive manipulation of the tumor
Tumor spillage at extraction site	Protected tumor extraction (plastic bag)
Immunosuppressive effect of pneumoperitoneum	Irrigation of abdomen with tumoricidal solutions[165]

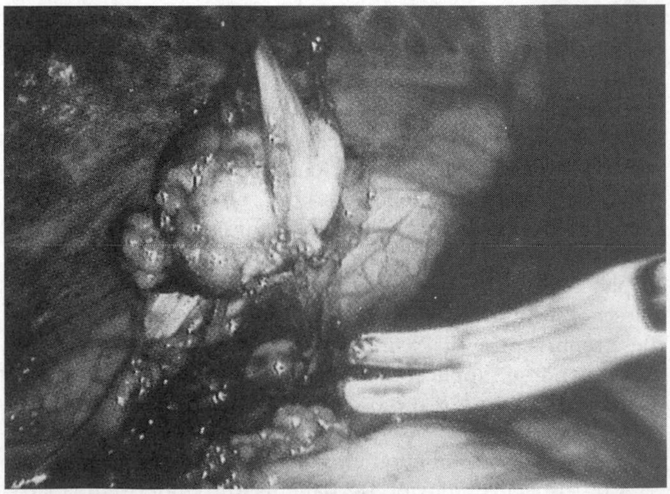

FIGURE 29.1-2. The celiac node was identified laparoscopically and excised. Histopathologic evaluation revealed non-Hodgkin's lymphoma. (From ref. 109, with permission.)

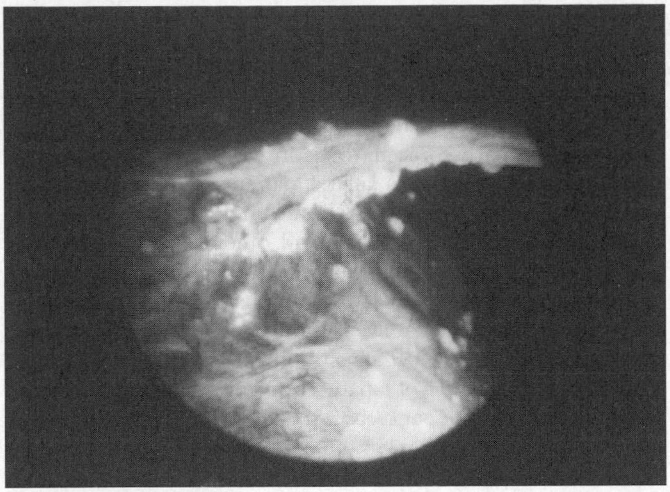

FIGURE 29.1-3. Laparoscopic evaluation of the abdomen can sometimes reveal unexpected widespread metastatic disease, as shown here.

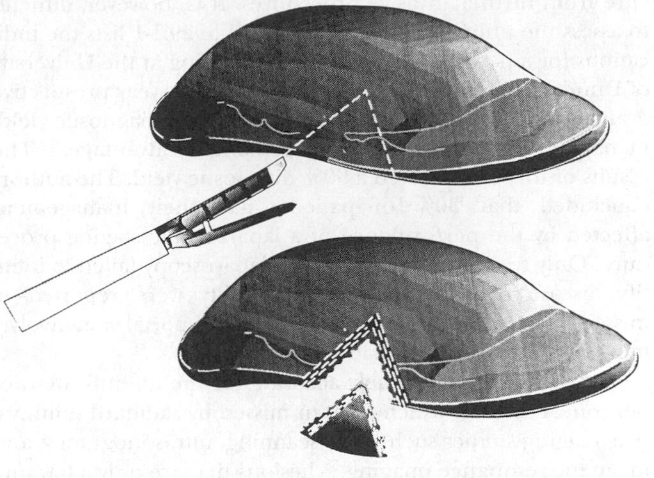

FIGURE 29.1-4. The linear stapler can be used to obtain a wedge biopsy of the liver by firing twice at approximately 90-degree angles. The resulting specimen is of adequate size and lacks burn artifact caused by the use of electrocautery to obtain the specimen. (From ref. 50, with permission.)

Liver Biopsy and Evaluation of Liver Tumors

Laparoscopic investigation of hepatic lesions can include inspection, palpation (with a probe), intraoperative ultrasound (discussed later in Laparoscopic Intracorporeal Ultrasound), and directed biopsy.[49] Lesions that are located on the thin edge of the liver may be easily biopsied using two applications of the linear stapler to avoid destruction of the tissue as shown in Figure 29.1-4.[50] This method is also useful in obtaining blind liver biopsies requiring larger specimens than those available with a core biopsy needle.

Lymph Node Biopsy

With careful dissection, laparoscopic access to most lymph node areas can be obtained. Specifically, mesenteric, portal, iliac, pelvic, peri-aortic, and celiac lymph nodes can be biopsied.[51] In cases in which specific lymph nodes are identified preoperatively with imaging studies, it may be helpful to mark the area of dissection with clips and use intraoperative radiographs as a guide as well as to assure that the desired area has been evaluated.

LAPAROSCOPIC INTRACORPOREAL ULTRASOUND

One of the most important developments in the laparoscopic evaluation of malignancies is the laparoscopic intracorporeal ultrasound (LICU) probe.[52] Intraoperative ultrasound was first described in 1958 and, with advancements in the technology, has had significant impact on the intraoperative management of a number of complex problems.[53] The laparoscopic application of these devices is limited by the size and location of the access ports used. The direct contact of the probe to the liver affords superior resolution compared with that obtained with transabdominal ultrasound imaging. When searching for lymphadenopathy, it is critical to adapt the technique to the specific area being studied, assuring good acoustic contact between the probe and the tissue. Saline solution may be instilled to aid in this process.[52] Doppler techniques are useful to identify blood vessels that will aid the identification of lymph nodes.

The ability to examine the biliary tree with LICU has been described.[54] This report establishes the accuracy of this technique compared with cholangiography in determining common duct size and presence of choledocholithiasis. The use of LICU in 176 patients was reported.[55] In this series, 145 patients underwent laparoscopic cholecystectomy, and 31 patients underwent staging laparoscopy with examination of the liver. From these preliminary studies, it appears that LICU has potential in the intraoperative evaluation of patients with malignancies. It is also clear that the value of this procedure is limited by operator skill.

The use of LICU is clearly complementary to laparoscopy alone, particularly in the evaluation of hepatic lesions. In a study of 50 patients with potentially resectable liver tumors, laparoscopy alone demonstrated factors that rendered the patient unresectable in 23 patients (46%).[56] Of the remaining patients, LICU identified nine patients as unresectable. Patients in this study who underwent combined laparoscopic/LICU staging ultimately had a 93% resectability rate, compared with a 58% resectability rate among a historical group who did not have laparoscopic staging. In another study of 420 patients with a wide range of upper gastrointestinal malignancies, laparoscopy/LICU staging precluded laparotomy in 20% of patients deemed resectable by preoperative imaging studies, with an overall sensitivity of 70%.[57] The results of these studies and others demonstrate that effective use of laparoscopy for tumor diagnosis requires the use of LICU as a complementary technique to evaluate the true extent of disease.

LAPAROSCOPY IN THE STAGING OF MALIGNANCY

GENERAL CONSIDERATIONS

Perhaps the most important benefit of laparoscopic staging is the exclusion of patients with disease that is not resectable for cure from further invasive procedures. It is, however, difficult to assess the utility of this approach. Table 29.1-1 lists the indications for laparoscopic diagnosis and staging at the University of Dundee. This approach was analyzed by a 2-year prospective evaluation, and the parameters assessed were diagnostic yield, management benefit, and management disadvantage.[49] The results of this trial showed a 90% diagnostic yield. The authors concluded that 30% of patients had their management affected by the performance of a laparoscopic staging procedure. Only two cases (4%) in which laparoscopy failed to identify disease that signaled unresectability were reported—a missed hepatic lesion in segment eight, and portal vein involvement by a tumor of the head of the pancreas.

Laparoscopy is extremely accurate for the identification of peritoneal disease, which is often missed by standard noninvasive imaging studies such as CT scanning, ultrasonography, and magnetic resonance imaging.[58] Lesions that are only a few millimeters in size can be biopsied with extreme accuracy. Liver and peritoneal disease are often found in patients with negative CT scans, supporting the use of laparoscopy to identify these lesions.[58] A representative laparoscopic view of such lesions is shown in Figure 29.1-3.

A series of 162 patients with a variety of malignancies, including 98 patients with hepatic lesions and 64 patients with nonhepatic intraabdominal malignancy, underwent laparoscopic staging.[59] All of these patients were believed to be resectable for cure based on a number of preoperative imaging studies. Biopsies were performed in 37% of cases. In 36% of cases, laparoscopy yielded information that prevented unnecessary laparotomy because of the identification of lesions that were unresectable. Conversely, 12% of patients who had laparoscopic findings suggesting resectability were found at laparotomy to be unresectable. Sites missed included positive lymph nodes, hepatic vein involvement, and missed peritoneal metastases. This study supports the use of laparoscopy to prevent unnecessary laparotomy in those patients who will not benefit from resection.

Laparoscopy is facilitated in patients with tense ascites by repeated paracentesis begun 24 hours before surgery.[60] In a series of 47 patients with ascites, laparoscopy revealed carcinomatosis in 22; ovarian cancer in 11; three patients each with mesothelioma, hepatoma, and hepatic myelofibrosis; two patients with pancreatic cancer; and one patient each with squamous cancer, chronic lymphatic leukemia, breast cancer, and lymphoma.[60] The accuracy of laparoscopy in the evaluation of malignant disease presenting as ascites has been reported in one series as 100%.[60]

PANCREATIC CANCER

Laparoscopy has been used in the staging of patients with carcinoma of the pancreas for some time. In fact, the first report of laparoscopy in the United States was the evaluation of a patient with carcinoma of the pancreas.[61] The goal of laparoscopy in the staging of patients with carcinoma of the pancreas is to avoid laparotomy in those patients deemed resectable by preoperative imaging studies. An early report describes the experience of 23 patients with pancreatic cancer.[9] This study was carried out before the widespread use of abdominal CT scan and the advent of quality optics for laparoscopy. This report emphasized the utility of biopsy under direct vision.

In a report of 40 patients with carcinoma of the pancreas, Warshaw and coworkers[62] found 26 patients without evidence of metastatic disease and 14 patients with metastatic disease that precluded a curative resection. Laparoscopy was performed as the final study before laparotomy, but only if the imaging studies were negative for metastatic disease. The negative findings at laparoscopy were confirmed in 23 of 26 patients at laparotomy. The positive laparoscopic findings in 14 of 40 patients altered the therapeutic course of all 14 patients. Findings in these patients were single, small (1 to 2 mm) nodules in the liver (n = 6), peritoneal surfaces (n = 7), and omentum (n = 1), all of which were verified histologically. The three instances of false-negative findings were due to incomplete examination of the liver (n = 2) and a central liver lesion (n = 1). The overall accuracy was 93% and, with negative findings, 88%.

Another application of laparoscopy in the staging of patients with carcinoma of the pancreas is the ability to obtain specimens for cytologic examination. In 40 patients with lesions that were resectable according to the results of preoperative imaging studies, peritoneal washings were obtained (27 at laparoscopy and 13 at laparotomy).[63] Malignant cells were found in 12 (30%) of the specimens. Liver metastases were seen in six patients, all of whom had negative cytology. Interestingly, positive cytology was found in six of eight patients who had previously undergone needle biopsy and in 6 of 32 patients who had not, suggesting that intraperitoneal spread may be enhanced by needle biopsy. Laparoscopy is described as an excellent method to obtain cytologic washings, which may be of importance in the evaluation of patients with carcinoma of the pancreas.

The ability of laparoscopy to detect metastatic disease not otherwise identified has been reported by others.[64] The use of laparoscopy and laparoscopic ultrasonography has been described in the evaluation of 40 consecutive patients felt to have a resectable pancreatic lesion.[65] Resectability was confirmed in 12 patients with negative laparoscopic examinations, for a sensitivity of 100%. Occult metastatic disease was identified in 14 patients, including liver lesions (n = 10), disease on peritoneal surfaces (n = 8), and hilar lymphadenopathy (n = 2). Laparoscopy failed to demonstrate metastatic disease in three patients. As for predicting resectability, laparoscopy alone did not identify the 12 patients with locoregional tumor unresectability, with an overall specificity of only 50%. However, the combined use of laparoscopy and laparoscopic ultrasonography resulted in a sensitivity of 92%, a specificity of 88%, and an accuracy of 89%.

The careful exploration of the abdominal cavity was emphasized in a study by Conlon and coworkers.[61] These investigators performed laparoscopy on 115 patients with radiologically resectable lesions. Unresectability was determined by the presence of any of the following: metastatic lesions, extrapancreatic tumor extension, celiac and portal node involvement, and vascular encasement of the celiac or superior mesenteric vessels. Resection was performed in 76% of patients with a negative laparoscopic evaluation, compared with a historical series of radiologic evaluation only with a resectability rate of 35%.

The importance of laparoscopy combined with LICU was emphasized in a report by John et al.[66] that demonstrated that this combined approach was significantly better than CT in predicting resectability (97% vs. 79%, $P<.005$). LICU was considered indispensable for the detection of occult metastases. Furthermore, these investigators found that LICU is a reliable predictor of tumor unresectability. Others also have affirmed the importance of combined laparoscopy and LICU to evaluate extent of disease.[67]

More recently, several investigators have suggested that laparoscopy be used in a highly selective manner in patients with carcinoma of the pancreas rather than as a standard staging modality.[68,69] Of 398 patients who underwent laparotomy for pancreatic or periampullary carcinoma at one center, 172 patients underwent resection, 150 had a palliative bypass, and 76 underwent exploratory laparotomy only.[69] Local signs of unresectability, identifiable only at laparotomy, were found in 47, leaving 29 patients (7%) who did not require palliation and whose signs of unresectability could have been determined by laparoscopy. The authors of this study concluded that laparoscopy (with or without LICU) should be used selectively in patients considered probably unresectable who do not require a palliative surgical procedure. The laparoscopic conduct of palliative bypass procedures may make laparoscopy somewhat more applicable than these data imply, however. In a retrospective study of 148 patients with pancreatic cancer, survival of patients with clinically resectable pancreatic cancer that was deemed unresectable at laparotomy was evaluated to determine the utility of staging laparotomy.[68] The importance of staging laparoscopy is enhanced if one believes that endoscopic stenting is the best palliation. The authors of this study concluded that extensive laparoscopic evaluation is not necessary, because they contend that operative palliation is superior to endoscopic palliation. Staging laparoscopy is useful only to identify those patients with liver or peritoneal metastases who have an expected survival of approximately 6 months and for whom endoscopic palliation is sufficient.

The use of laparoscopy or combined laparoscopy and laparoscopic ultrasonography appears to be helpful in the identification of lesions that suggest unresectability in patients with negative imaging studies.[70] Although some suggest that laparoscopy be used in a fairly routine manner, data suggest that laparoscopy be used more selectively.

ESOPHAGEAL AND GASTRIC TUMORS

Early laparoscopic studies of the staging of esophageal cancer were usually characterized by little manipulation of the abdominal contents to identify disease and were commonly limited to observation of the parietal peritoneal surfaces. A prospective trial was undertaken to compare the accuracy in diagnosing intraabdominal metastatic disease by scintigraphy, ultrasound scanning, and laparoscopy.[71] Of the 50 patients studied, 23 had esophageal carcinoma, 14 had gastric carcinoma, and 13 had suspected intraabdominal metastatic spread from other lesions. The accuracy of identification of metastatic disease was determined by laparoscopic biopsy, laparotomy, and autopsy. The overall accuracy was 72% for scintigraphy, 75% for ultrasound, and 96% for laparoscopy. Thirteen patients without hepatic metastatic disease had nodal or peritoneal disease diagnosed only by laparoscopy. This study demonstrates the value of laparoscopy and its ability to obviate the need for laparotomy in patients with lesions not resectable for cure.

In another study, 369 patients with carcinoma of the esophagus and cardia of the stomach underwent laparoscopy, revealing single or multiple intraabdominal metastases in 52 patients (14%).[72] This study suggested that intraabdominal metastases become more common as the location of the primary tumor becomes more distal, being greatest in lesions of the cardia. More recent data suggest that abdominal lymph node metastases may be present despite the location of the primary tumor.[73]

The sensitivity, specificity, and accuracy of laparoscopy, ultrasound, and abdominal CT scan were compared in 90 patients with biopsy-proven carcinoma of the esophagus or gastric cardia.[74] Laparoscopy was found to be significantly more sensitive and more accurate ($P<.05$) than either ultrasound or abdominal CT scanning in diagnosing hepatic disease. Peritoneal disease was not identified by ultrasound or CT scan, but laparoscopy identified it in eight (89%) of nine cases. Lymph node metastases were identified most accurately by laparoscopy, although the difference between laparoscopy and CT scanning did not achieve statistical significance. The authors of this study concluded that laparoscopy offers an accurate, reliable, and safe method of preoperative assessment in patients with carcinoma of the esophagus.

Thoracoscopic lymph node staging has been shown to provide accurate pre-resection staging of thoracic node status.[75,76] More recently, laparoscopic lymph node assessment in patients with carcinoma of the esophagus has been combined with thoracoscopic lymph node staging. The use of thoracoscopy in staging accuracy has been validated in a trial comparing thoracoscopy to noninvasive staging techniques that found greater accuracy with thoracoscopic staging.[77] Laparoscopic evaluation of intraabdominal disease was correct in 17 of 18 patients (94%) in a prospective trial.[73] A positive lymph node was not identified in a single patient. Three patients were downstaged as a result of laparoscopic evaluation of intraabdominal lymph nodes. Six of 18 patients (33%) had unsuspected celiac lymph node involvement. Lymph nodes near the diaphragm may be difficult to evaluate without extensive dissection. Furthermore, the laparoscopic staging procedure can be combined with placement of an enteral feeding tube at the same time.

The value of combined laparoscopy and laparoscopic ultrasound has been demonstrated in a number of other studies. In 56 patients with carcinoma of the esophagus (n = 38) and cardia (n = 18), the preoperative stage of disease was altered by laparoscopy in nine (17%) of the overall group of patients.[78] Of the patients with tumors of the gastric cardia (n = 18), laparoscopy altered the stage in seven (41%), but of patients with esophageal tumors (n = 38), stage was altered in just two (6%). The authors of this study concluded that the approach was better suited to tumors of the gastric cardia than of the esophagus. In this study, no attempt was made to perform thoracoscopic staging for lesions of the esophagus, however, and lymphatic drainage patterns may have precluded their ability to identify intraabdominal metastatic disease in patients with more proximal lesions of the esophagus.

In a study of 71 patients with potentially resectable gastric cancer, laparoscopy identified distant disease in 16 patients (23%).[79] The combination of preoperative CT and laparoscopic evaluation resulted in a 93% resectability rate. These authors advocate staging laparoscopy for all patients with potentially resectable gastric cancer. Future studies may use the combination of laparoscopy and laparoscopic ultrasound to improve the results further.

HEPATIC TUMORS

The accurate evaluation of the liver is a critical component of tumor staging for many malignancies of interest to the surgeon, because the presence of metastatic disease in the liver often obviates the need for major resections. Radiologic imaging alone is imperfect, and several studies have demonstrated the scope of the problem. In one series, 63 of 150 of patients (42%) with colorectal carcinoma were found to have unresectable hepatic disease at laparotomy after an imaging evaluation demonstrated resectable lesions.[80] In another series, of 132 patients referred to the National Cancer Institute for liver tumor resection, 107 had negative staging evaluations and were brought to laparotomy. Extrahepatic disease was identified in 28 of these 107 patients (26%).[81] These studies demonstrate one of the major potential benefits of laparoscopic staging—the ability to exclude from laparotomy those patients with unresectable lesions in a way that minimizes postoperative pain and hospitalization.

Of interest, one of the early applications of laparoscopy was for the staging of hepatic lesions, which had been reported as early as 1966 and in 1973 was reported in the evaluation of patients with Hodgkin's lymphoma.[3] Before the advent of modern video systems and laparoscopic instrumentation, it was estimated that 80% of the liver surface could be visualized laparoscopically and, of note, performed in the endoscopy clinic.[58] The sensitivity of laparoscopy in the detection of hepatic metastatic disease was estimated at 70% to 90%.

In a study of 29 patients with hepatic malignancies (12 with hepatoma and 17 with metastatic disease), laparoscopy was undertaken before laparotomy to evaluate the resectability of the lesions.[82] Laparoscopy alone demonstrated unresectability in 14 (48%) of 29 patients evaluated. Unsuspected cirrhosis was identified in four, and unresectable or extrahepatic lesions were found in ten. Not surprisingly, these investigators found that patients who underwent laparoscopy had shorter hospital stays than historical controls who underwent laparotomy that identified unresectable disease, and they concluded that laparoscopy should precede laparotomy for planned resection of hepatic malignancies.

The gold standard for evaluation of the liver is intraoperative palpation combined with intraoperative ultrasonography (LICU). In an experimental study to evaluate the effectiveness of laparoscopy and laparoscopic ultrasonography, liver lesions were induced in 18 pigs.[47] Laparoscopic ultrasound identified the lesions in 17 of 18 animals, for a 94% sensitivity. Two false-negatives were obtained, for a specificity of 78%. In a study of 30 patients undergoing planned hepatic resection and 32 patients undergoing resection of a gastrointestinal primary malignancy, intraoperative ultrasonography was compared with CT angioportography.[83] Of the 30 patients planned to undergo hepatic resection, the procedure was changed or guided by the ultrasonographic result in 20 cases (67%). Of the 32 patients undergoing resection of their primary tumor, five patients (16%) had the stage of their disease altered by the results of intraoperative ultrasonography.

Having demonstrated the value of laparoscopy and intraoperative ultrasonography, combining the two procedures is a natural extension of the technology. In a study of 50 patients undergoing laparoscopic evaluation of hepatic tumors, laparoscopic ultrasonography was performed in 43 patients.[56] Laparoscopy alone demonstrated that lesions shown resectable by preoperative imaging studies were unresectable in 23 patients (46%). Hepatic lesions not visible by laparoscopic examination alone were identified by laparoscopic ultrasonography in 14 patients. Furthermore, the use of laparoscopic ultrasonography provided staging information in addition to that gained by laparoscopy in 18 patients (42%).

In a study combining laparoscopy with laparoscopic ultrasound, 50 patients were evaluated.[84] Of these, 28 patients were deemed resectable on the basis of the laparoscopic studies. At laparotomy, 26 were ultimately resectable, for a false-negative rate of 4%. Of the 22 patients deemed unresectable after laparoscopy, 11 were identified by laparoscopy alone, but 11 more were deemed unresectable after laparoscopic ultrasound. Nodal involvement and vascular invasion were identified by ultrasound, emphasizing the importance of the combined approach for accurate staging.

A study of 420 patients with upper gastrointestinal malignancies evaluated the utility of combined laparoscopy and laparoscopic ultrasound in staging of these tumors.[57] Patients underwent routine imaging studies and were thought to have resectable disease, then underwent laparoscopy and laparoscopic ultrasound. The use of combined laparoscopic staging avoided laparotomy in 20% of patients, with a sensitivity of 70%. Although it was of little use in esophageal tumors—avoiding laparotomy in just 5% of patients and a 42% sensitivity—it appeared beneficial in patients with proximal bile duct tumors, liver tumors, and pancreatic tumors. This study supports the use of combined laparoscopy and laparoscopic ultrasound in the staging of patients with a variety of upper gastrointestinal malignancies.

Up to 90% of metastatic lesions can be seen on the liver surface using laparoscopy.[85] Furthermore, although CT can reliably detect lesions that are at least 10 mm in size, laparoscopy can detect lesions as small as 1 mm. Laparoscopy also facilitates the identification of lesions in areas often missed by CT scan, such as peritoneal, omental, and mesenteric surfaces. Accurate sampling of hepatic lesions with biopsy instruments is greatly facilitated by the direct vision afforded by laparoscopy, and hemostasis can be assured. Finally, the technical problems caused by loops of bowel are avoided when laparoscopy is used compared with external ultrasonography or CT scanning.[85] Thus, laparoscopy is extremely important in the staging of hepatic malignancies of all types.

PROSTATE CANCER

The definitive final staging procedure in the evaluation of prostate cancer is now considered to be pelvic lymphadenectomy. In the past, open bilateral pelvic lymphadenectomy was routinely performed, even with its associated significant morbidity, which included a lengthy recovery time. More recently, laparoscopic pelvic lymph node dissection (LPLND) has become standard practice for many urologists, affording their patients the benefits of decreased hospitalization and recovery times. The technique for this procedure has been described, including the extraperitoneal laparoscopic approach.[86–88]

Laparoscopic detection of positive pelvic lymph nodes may alter the management of patients with prostate cancer. Patients with positive pelvic lymph nodes have been advised to undergo a wide range of therapies, ranging from endocrine treatment to a combination of radical prostatectomy and radiation therapy.[89] An early series of 11 patients found metastatic disease in five, with a resultant change of therapy.[86] This series included one complication, a bladder laceration that was repaired laparoscopically.

The effect of laparoscopic conduct of this procedure on operative morbidity and convalescence has been reported.[90] In a study by Kerbl et al.,[90] the initial 30 patients undergoing LPLND were compared with 16 patients undergoing open node dissections. These authors found that the laparoscopic procedure took longer (mean, 199 minutes) than the open procedure (mean, 102 minutes), but that the blood loss was lower in the laparoscopic group. Furthermore, the laparoscopic group had significantly less postoperative analgesic use, shorter hospital stay, faster return to normal activities, and shorter interval to full recovery compared with the open surgical group. The incidence of complications was higher in the laparoscopic group, but all of these occurred in the first 12 patients of the series. In another series, 54 patients underwent staging laparoscopic pelvic lymphadenectomy for a variety of genitourinary malignancies, with a major complication rate of 17% and a minor complication rate of 18%.[91] Major complications included bleeding requiring transfusion, respiratory failure necessitating intubation, ureteral injury, and small bowel obstruction due to herniation at a trocar site. The ability of CT scan to identify these postoperative complications also has been investigated.[92] Complications were identified in 12 of 85 patients undergoing laparoscopic lymph node dissection, of which eight patients were studied with abdominopelvic CT scans. The CT scan appearance of small bowel herniation, extensive hematomas, urinary ascites, and lymphocele compressing the bladder is described in this review. The CT scan identified the complication in seven of eight patients and is thus an important tool in evaluating the complications of this procedure.

The indications for LPLND have evolved over time, particularly with the advent of widespread prostate-specific antigen (PSA) testing. Before PSA testing, lymph node dissection was indicated in all prostate cancer patients considered candidates for curative therapy.[87] Many urologists limit the conduct of LPLND to patients at high risk for metastatic disease based on clinical stage, a PSA level of greater than 10 mg/dL, and tumor grade (Gleason score ≥7).

TESTICULAR TUMORS

Patients with early-stage nonseminomatous testicular cancer have a 20% to 30% incidence of retroperitoneal spread of disease to paraaortic nodes at the time of diagnosis.[87] Laparoscopic retroperitoneal lymph node dissection has been described to evaluate these patients.[87] At this time, few cases of this procedure have been reported in the literature. No studies to date have carefully compared this technique with its open counterpart. Therefore, this procedure is appropriate only in patients who have a low likelihood of nodal disease based on clinical risk factors.[87]

LYMPHOMA

Lymphomas are a diverse group of malignant disorders of the lymphatic system that arise in nodal tissues. Typically, they are categorized by histology into Hodgkin's lymphoma and NHL. The present role of surgery in the management of lymphoma is to establish a tissue diagnosis or to serve as a diagnostic adjunct when noninvasive diagnostic studies do not accurately define the extent of disease. Definitive treatment based on staged disease then follows.

The histologic type and regional extent of the disease are the primary factors used to determine the prognosis and the treatment selection. Histologic type is usually determined by a regional lymph node biopsy. Evaluating or staging the true extent of the disease has proven more elusive by noninvasive modalities. This is especially true in the determination of an intraabdominal component to the spread of lymphoma. The spleen, for example, is involved in approximately one-third of all cases of Hodgkin's lymphoma.[93] Most involved spleens, however, are of normal size or contain malignant foci whose size is beyond the resolution of present imaging technology.[93] Likewise, lymph node size is a poor determinant of involvement by lymphoma. Many involved lymph nodes are of normal size, whereas normal lymph nodes may be enlarged secondary to a reactive response. Because of this lack of sensitivity and specificity of noninvasive modalities, surgical staging still has a key role in the staging of selected patients with lymphoma. This places the lymphoma staging procedure in the unique position of being one of the few major abdominal surgical procedures that is undertaken strictly for diagnostic purposes.

Indications and techniques for the performance of the staging laparotomy, in attempts to influence the associated morbidity and mortality, have undergone considerable evolution. Although previously performed on 85% of all patients with Hodgkin's disease,[94] staging laparotomy is performed in, at most, only 30% of patients.[95] With refinement of noninvasive imaging techniques, and changes in the medical management of the disease, the value of surgical staging of lymphoma has been reevaluated. Consequently, the subset of patients for whom surgical staging appears to be of value has become much smaller. This reduction has resulted in significant decreases in the proportion of splenectomies performed for staging lymphoma. In a study of the frequency of splenectomy for Hodgkin's lymphoma, Marble et al.[96] reported a rate of 44% during the period from 1979 to 1985, compared with only 26% during the period from 1986 to 1991. The role of splenectomy, however, is still in evolution. Some evidence suggests that combined chemoradiation therapy for Hodgkin's lymphoma may be associated with a significantly increased risk of developing a second malignant disease.[93] If this risk proves to hold true, it follows that surgical staging may again provide significant benefits for patients with Hodgkin's lymphoma by reducing their need for combination therapy. Conversely, some centers are treating every patient with Hodgkin's disease using chemotherapy as a first-line modality, obviating the need for surgical staging.

The role of the surgeon in patients with Hodgkin's lymphoma includes lymph node biopsy to establish a diagnosis and staging laparotomy in a very select group of patients, usually limited to those patients with stage IIB disease after imaging evaluation. Patients with obvious stage III or IV disease should rarely be subjected to staging laparotomy because they will be treated with chemotherapy, and patients with stage I disease are usually treated with radiation alone, obviating the need for staging laparotomy. In some centers, chemotherapy is used to treat all patients with Hodgkin's lymphoma, almost entirely eliminating the need for any surgical staging procedure.

Surgical staging of Hodgkin's lymphoma has been reported to change the pathologic stage of the disease in 30% to 40% of patients, resulting in significant alterations in both prognosis and treatment selection.[97,98] Staging laparotomy is associated with 18% morbidity and up to 0.7% mortality.[93,99] Late complications occur in 5% to 15% of patients.[99,100] These include partial small bowel obstruction in 9.8% of patients, requiring lysis of adhesions in 6.8% of these, and overwhelming post-splenectomy sepsis (OPSS) in 6.8% of patients.[100] Horowitz et al.[101] reported a 52% overall morbidity and a 9% mortality rate after splenectomy for hematologic diseases. Splenic size was the only preoperative factor found to be predictive of postoperative complications.

The conventional technique for the surgical staging for lymphoma has been well described.[102,103] With the smaller incisions used in minimal-access surgery, several potential advantages can be offered to patients undergoing laparoscopic staging of abdominal lymphoma. These include less postoperative pain, earlier ambulation, better breathing, and shorter recovery time. These can be translated into fewer postoperative complications and possibly earlier administration of definitive therapy. However, the procedure remains a technically demanding operation with which no single surgeon will probably gain vast experience. With further advances in laparoscopic technology and refinements in techniques, laparoscopic staging of abdominal lymphoma will become an important tool in the surgical armamentarium.

The laparoscopic approach to this procedure follows the same principles as those delineated for the open procedure.[104] There are no true contraindications to laparoscopic staging. Relative contraindications to laparoscopic staging include abdominal wall sepsis, gastrointestinal distention, intraabdominal sepsis, and extensive adhesions.[105] Laparoscopic staging of abdominal lymphoma has been successfully performed by several groups.[104,106–109] A comparison of laparoscopic and open staging of Hodgkin's disease has demonstrated equivalent oncologic results, and functionally superior results with laparoscopic staging.[104] These investigators found a slightly longer operative time (202 vs. 144 minutes), but significantly shortened postoperative ileus and postoperative hospitalization times. These data strongly support the use of laparoscopy for accurate staging of Hodgkin's disease when indicated.

Techniques for the laparoscopic exploration of other abdominal malignancies, with lymph node retrieval, laparoscopic splenectomy,[110] and laparoscopic wedge biopsy of the liver,[50] were developed. When combined, these procedures complete a laparoscopic staging procedure. The ports, or trocars, are positioned as in Figure 29.1-5. All five ports are 12 mm in diameter. Using identical large ports enables the surgeon the versatility to switch instruments between the different anatomic sites required in this procedure. A sixth port may be, but is not always, necessary for access to the iliac nodes.

Although several groups have advocated preoperative splenic artery embolization, especially for larger spleens,[111–113] most patients with Hodgkin's lymphoma have normal-size spleens, and embolization is usually not indicated. The excised but intact spleen is placed into a stout plastic bag and left in the left upper quadrant for the remainder of the procedure, as shown in Figure 29.1-6. Laparoscopic splenectomy has been widely described and is considered to be the gold standard for splenectomy at this time.[114–118] The identification and removal of accessory spleens has been shown to be effectively carried out using laparoscopic approaches.[119,120] Not only has it been shown that hospital charges for laparoscopic splenectomy are less than charges for open splenectomy, it also has been shown that, over time, charges for laparoscopic splenectomy can be

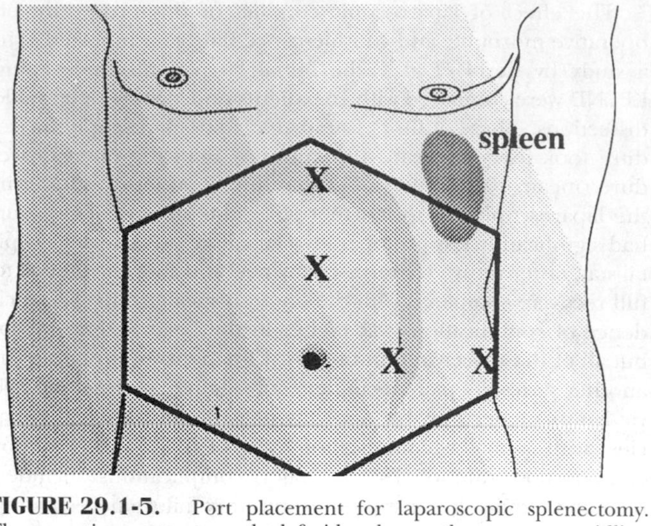

FIGURE 29.1-5. Port placement for laparoscopic splenectomy. The operating ports are on the left side, whereas the two upper midline ports are used for retraction. (From ref. 108, with permission.)

decreased by shorter operating times and judicious use of disposable instruments.[121]

The laparoscopic dissection of lymph nodes can be very challenging because nonpathologic nodes are small and difficult to identify. LPLND is widely used in genitourinary surgery for the staging of prostate cancer and has become well accepted.[87] The magnification afforded by the use of laparoscopic instrumentation has proven to be very helpful. All abnormal nodes on preoperative lymphangiogram should be removed and clips applied as markers. Oophoropexy is then performed in young females by suturing the ovaries to the back of the uterus. The spleen is then removed intact, within the plastic bag, through a small midline incision incorporating the umbilical port site.

The accurate histologic diagnosis of lymphoma requires assessment of the nodal architecture, which requires an intact node capsule. Therefore, whenever possible, one should excise

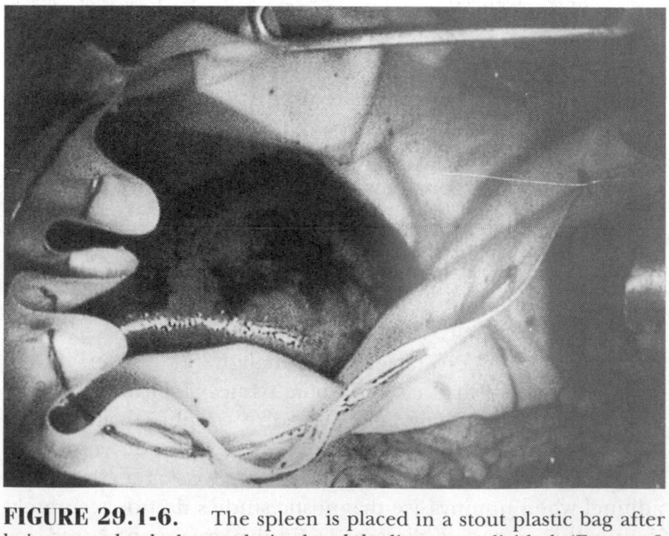

FIGURE 29.1-6. The spleen is placed in a stout plastic bag after being completely devascularized and the ligaments divided. (From ref. 109, with permission.)

an entire intact lymph node. The use of formalin precludes the assessment by flow cytometry, which has become crucial for complete and accurate classification of lymphoma and on which therapeutic decisions may ultimately be based. Therefore, each lymph node should be sent for examination in saline in a fresh state. As mentioned above, the spleen should be sent to the pathologists intact and, usually, in a fresh state. The liver tissue may be placed in formalin for transport to the pathology department. The planning and conduct of the staging procedure involves close cooperation between surgeon, radiologist, medical oncologist, and pathologist.

The morbidity and mortality associated with staging laparotomy is well established.[93,99,100,101,122] A review of staging laparotomy by Multani and Grossbard[123] demonstrated a mortality of 0.3% to 1.0%, major morbidity of 3% to 18%, and minor morbidity of 6% to 19%. Delays to definitive treatment occurred in 5% to 10% of patients.[123] Jockovitch et al.[100] reported surgical complications in 26% of 133 consecutive patients. Complications included atelectasis in 13%, small bowel obstruction in 10% (requiring reoperation in 7%), subphrenic abscesses in 2%, and wound dehiscence in 1%.[100]

OPSS, which can follow any procedure that removes the spleen, remains a serious potential complication. The incidence of OPSS can be decreased by the preoperative administration of the polyvalent pneumococcal vaccine.[100] In addition, vaccinations for *Haemophilus influenzae* and *Neisseria meningitidis* are often administered.[124] These precautions should provide some protection against the three organisms most commonly responsible for OPSS. The optimal timing of such vaccinations remains difficult to define but should probably be administered as long as possible before operation.[124] Patient education is also vitally important. They should be alerted that a low-grade fever might be a harbinger of a serious infection. Although some recommend prophylactic oral penicillin in children, this practice is somewhat controversial. In general, although some question the value of splenectomy because of the risk of OPSS, patients whose therapy depends on accurate staging should undergo splenectomy.[125]

Causes for conversion to an open procedure during splenectomy include densely adherent adjacent structures, technical errors, and cardiopulmonary instability.[126] The most troubling technical errors are those associated with excessive bleeding that makes delineating anatomic structures very difficult. Conversion rates from 0% to 19% have been reported in series of laparoscopic splenectomy alone.[126] Patients about to undergo laparoscopic staging must be apprised of these data as part of the process of informed consent.

Whereas the use of laparoscopic splenectomy in the treatment of idiopathic thrombocytopenia purpura (ITP) has become the standard, some still question the use of laparoscopic approaches in the staging of Hodgkin's disease.[127] More recent data, such as that reported by Baccarini and coworkers,[104] suggest that the laparoscopic operation is equivalent to the open procedure. They demonstrated equivalent lymph node harvest, and on reasonable postoperative follow-up, they found fewer subdiaphragmatic relapses in the laparoscopy group. Although these data are not prospectively randomized, the results are very compelling in support of laparoscopic staging.

The use of laparoscopy in the management of a variety of abdominal lymphoproliferative diseases has been reported by Silecchia et al.[128] These investigators performed laparoscopic investigation on 64 patients with a number of diseases, including retroperitoneal adenopathy, Hodgkin's disease, and non-Hodgkin's disease. Laparoscopic ultrasound was used extensively. They concluded that the interval between diagnosis and treatment was significantly shortened by using a laparoscopic approach. Although this series does not necessarily provide the final word, it again demonstrates the utility of laparoscopy in the evaluation of these patients and suggests the need for further study.

NHL is a diverse group of diseases with a wide range of biologic behaviors. They may be very aggressive and rapidly fatal or behave as one of the most indolent and well-tolerated malignancies afflicting humans.[129] Because the clinical course is variable, the pattern of spread is also unpredictable. NHL is classified into low, intermediate, and high-grade pathologic groups according to the National Cancer Institute's working formulation. Each of these groups is further subdivided based on cell type (e.g., small cell, large cell). The therapy for these patients is still evolving, and surgical staging is generally reserved for the very small minority of patients with localized disease who receive radiation therapy alone. The role of the surgeon in the care of patients with NHL is usually limited to the biopsy of a single peripheral lymph node to establish a tissue diagnosis. In patients with NHL, the precise definition of disease location, unlike Hodgkin's lymphoma, has less impact on therapeutic decision making.[130] In general, NHLs are systemic diseases at the time of diagnosis and require the use of systemic therapy (e.g., chemotherapy) rather than regional therapy (e.g., radiation) for treatment.

Laparoscopy may play a beneficial role in the diagnosis of NHL in a select subgroup of patients. For example, a 70-year-old woman presented to her primary care physician with general malaise, weight loss, and occasional fevers. In the absence of positive findings on physical examination, she was evaluated with an abdominal CT scan (see Fig. 29.1-1), which demonstrated peri-aortic lymphadenopathy.[131] The diagnosis of NHL was made in this patient by laparoscopic lymph node excision as shown in Figure 29.1-2, performed on an outpatient basis, and systemic chemotherapy was begun.

Staging laparoscopy in patients with NHL is restricted to those few patients with clinically limited disease (stage I and II) who are to be treated with radiation therapy alone with curative intent.[93] In these very unusual cases, a staging procedure similar to that performed for patients with Hodgkin's lymphoma may be undertaken laparoscopically. Splenectomy may be omitted from the surgical staging of abdominal NHL because splenic involvement usually does not affect the therapy used,[130] and its removal increases toxicity to patients given combination chemotherapy.[96,132] Laparoscopy may have a role in the evaluation of treatment efficacy because persistent disease is often overdiagnosed by routine imaging studies.[130]

The gastrointestinal tract is involved in 20% of advanced NHL and represents 1% to 4% of all alimentary tract malignancies.[133] When large or small bowel is involved, the typical presenting signs and symptoms are consistent with a bowel obstruction secondary to external compression or intussusception. The most frequent site of involvement is at the ileocecal valve. Complete, curative resection is generally indicated for localized lesions. If the lymphoma is of a diffuse submucosal pattern where systemic therapy is required, resection should be limited to the correction of the mechanical obstruction.

Should the lesion be discovered during a laparoscopic exploration or a laparoscopic staging procedure, laparoscopic resection of the lesion may be feasible if the surgeon has the technical ability and experience.

Laparoscopic localization and laparoscopic-assisted resection of the tumor is another alternative. The entire bowel, however, should be evaluated because skip lesions may exist.[93,94] Gastric lymphoma, on the other hand, may be diagnosed after esophagogastroduodenoscopy, which is usually performed for upper gastrointestinal bleeding or anemia. If the lesion is localized, then laparoscopic resection may be technically feasible. Most patients with NHL are upstaged by staging laparotomy. This upstaging, however, results in no significant impact on the modality of treatment.[130] Therefore, staging laparotomy for NHL has fallen out of favor except for the small, select group of patients whose treatment would be intensified should the liver be involved. The liver can be involved in 20% of patients with NHL.[105] The role of the surgeon for patients with NHL is generally limited to the minimum procedure needed to establish the diagnosis.

GYNECOLOGIC MALIGNANCIES

Although gynecologists have used laparoscopic instrumentation for many years, the use of laparoscopy for the management of gynecologic malignancies is more recent. Several reports of laparoscopic staging for apparent early-stage ovarian cancer have been published.[134] However, the follow-up remains short at this time, and the utility of this technique in ovarian cancer remains unproven. A prospective trial sponsored by the Gynecologic Oncology Group is under way to evaluate the utility of laparoscopy in these patients. The utility of the second-look laparotomy in the assessment of patients who have been treated for ovarian cancer is well established. Several reports of second-look laparoscopy with apparently good results have been published.[134] Further evaluation of this application is currently in progress. Laparoscopy also has been used in the staging of advanced ovarian disease. Patients with cervical cancer have undergone laparoscopic-assisted radical vaginal hysterectomy with LPLND. The utility of this procedure remains to be proven with prospective trials. Patients with early endometrial cancer have been staged by combining laparoscopy with vaginal hysterectomy in a procedure that has been named laparoscopic-assisted surgical staging.[134] Laparoscopy provides the ability to assess the peritoneal cavity, obtain peritoneal washings, and guarantee the removal of the adnexae. Lymph node sampling can also be performed laparoscopically when necessary in these patients. Although laparoscopy has been used in the management of ovarian, cervical, and endometrial malignancies, its potential is unconfirmed at this time. Reports of complications and long-term results are not yet available.[134] The results of ongoing clinical trials must be evaluated before this technique is widely applied in the management of gynecologic malignancies.

LAPAROSCOPY IN THE TREATMENT OF MALIGNANCY

GENERAL CONSIDERATIONS

Laparoscopic approaches have been used to treat a wide variety of malignancies. Many of these techniques were applied with a curative intent, whereas some were conducted as palliative procedures. At the time of this writing, the use of laparoscopic techniques to treat patients with malignancy remains controversial. In an attempt to afford patients with cancer the same benefits afforded patients with cholelithiasis, many investigators have conducted laparoscopic surgery for cancer with curative intent, particularly for carcinoma of the colon. However, this development may have been somewhat premature. The two major concerns about an operation performed laparoscopically for the treatment of cancer are (1) to be sure that the laparoscopic operation meets the same "oncologic" goals of the open procedure (e.g., margins of resection, lymph node harvest, recurrence rate, evaluation of other intraabdominal organs) and (2) to demonstrate an advantage to the patient for having undergone the procedure laparoscopically (e.g., decreased hospital stay, decreased cost, more rapid return to work). To date, few data convincingly demonstrate the validity of these two principles in the laparoscopic treatment of cancer.

GASTRIC CANCER

The application of laparoscopic techniques to gastric resection has been made possible by the rapid advances in stapling technology. The first laparoscopic gastric resection using a Billroth II reconstruction performed intraabdominally was reported in 1992.[135] Since that time, the same group has continued to apply laparoscopic surgical techniques to gastric surgery.[136] In a series of 16 patients, all were operated on for benign disease, although two patients had foci of cancer found at the time of histologic examination. These two patients later underwent open lymphadenectomy. Laparoscopic gastric resection remains a technically demanding procedure, with precise identification of anatomic structures essential to its successful completion.

The use of laparoscopic techniques in the treatment of gastric cancer requires careful selection of patients. Early gastric cancer involving the submucosa requires gastrectomy with removal of the greater omentum and level 1 lymph nodes. Techniques for this procedure have been fully described.[137] More advanced tumors, which require further node dissections, are not amenable to laparoscopic resection. Patients with stage IV disease who require palliative gastric resections are good candidates for laparoscopic resection. Gastric lymphoma and gastric polyps requiring resection are also suitable for laparoscopic resection.[137] The inability to perform extensive lymphadenectomy may limit the applicability of laparoscopic gastric resection to malignancies, but it is clear that advances in technology may make this more feasible.

COLON CANCER

Carcinoma of the colon is a very common disease in the United States, making it an attractive candidate for laparoscopic treatment. Surgical resection of carcinoma of the colon is a well-established procedure. Thus, any surgical approach that can potentially treat this disease with decreased postoperative pain and hospitalization may result in considerable advantages, generating great interest in the laparoscopic resection of colon cancer. It is clear that laparoscopic colon resection is an "advanced" procedure requiring more training, experience, and time than that for procedures such as appendectomy or cholecystectomy.[138] The use of animal models has facilitated the testing of some of these techniques and may be an important educational tool.[139] Intracorporeal anastomotic techniques may be used but remain a greater technical challenge than extracorporeal anastomoses.

Indications for laparoscopic colon resection at this time include segmental resections for diverticular disease, polyps, rectal prolapse, and intestinal volvulus.[140] The role of laparoscopic resections in the management of colonic malignancies remain undefined at this time and should be carried out only in the setting of a prospective trial.[28,140–143] It is reasonable to laparoscopically resect colonic malignancies with synchronous hepatic or pulmonary metastases as a palliative procedure. When performed appropriately, laparoscopic colon resection for cancer should include the following components, just as in open surgical resections: (1) resection of tumor in the bowel wall and adjacent soft tissues, (2) resection of an adequate margin of normal bowel, and (3) an adequate lymph node resection with associated vascular pedicle.[144]

The preoperative factors affecting suitability for laparoscopic colonic surgery are similar to those important in other laparoscopic procedures. The lack of ability to use palpation in the abdominal cavity prompts some to perform a more thorough preoperative evaluation with colonoscopy and CT scan.[144] In general, the surgeon and assistant stand on the side opposite the bowel to be resected. Some prefer the dorsolithotomy position,[144] and others prefer the patient in the supine position.[138] The use of the dorsolithotomy position has two potential advantages. First, intraoperative colonoscopy, facilitated by the use of low stirrups, may be necessary for localizing the lesion in the operating room. Second, one technique demonstrates the utility of the colonoscope in dissecting the hepatic and splenic flexures.[145] The zero-degree laparoscope is used for these procedures.

In general, for a right hemicolectomy, two left-sided and one right-sided port are used in addition to the umbilical camera port (Fig. 29.1-7). The abdomen is explored thoroughly, with special attention paid to the liver, just as is performed with

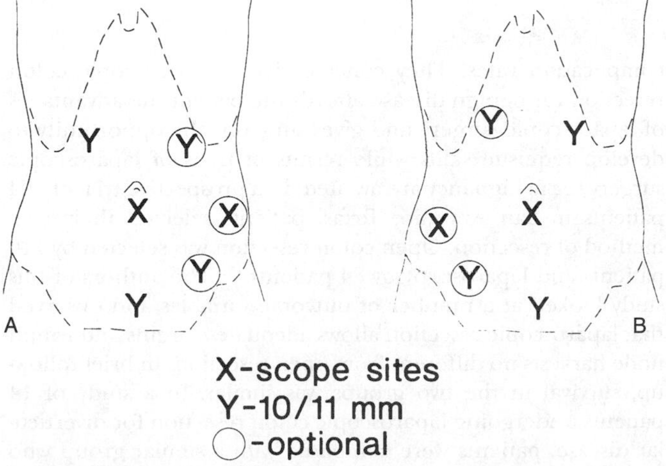

FIGURE 29.1-7. Port placement for laparoscopic colon resection is different for right **(A)** and left **(B)** colon procedures as shown here. (From ref. 148, with permission.)

open surgical approaches. Ports are best placed as they are needed, which allows for flexibility, rather than using a static pattern placing all ports synchronously.[139,141] The bowel is then mobilized and the vascular pedicle to the sigmoid colon divided using a stapler. The bowel is then exteriorized and an extracorporeal anastomosis fashioned.[146]

Technical limitations can hinder the performance of laparoscopic colon resections. In an attempt to define them, Pandya and colleagues[147] examined indications for intraoperative conversion of a laparoscopic colon resection to an open procedure. Two hundred patients who underwent laparoscopic colon resection were reviewed, with 47 (23.5%) converted to an open operation. Indications for conversion included technical problems in 15 patients (hypercarbia, unclear anatomy, and stapler misfire), laparoscopic complications in nine patients (bleeding, cystotomy, and enterotomy), and problems that "exceeded the limits of laparoscopic dissection" in 23 patients (phlegmon, adhesions, obesity, and tumor invasion of adjacent organs). The investigators noted a decreasing conversion rate with experience. After the "learning curve," indications for conversion have included excessive tumor bulk, adhesions, and a massive diverticular phlegmon.

The safety and efficacy of laparoscopic colectomy has been studied retrospectively. A summary of a large number of studies is shown in Table 29.1-2. In a series of 51 laparoscopic colon resections, 24 patients underwent operation for cancer.[148] A majority of these procedures were performed using intracorporeal anastomoses, but 14% were converted to laparoscopic-assisted cases, and 8% were converted to open procedures. This series included right, transverse, left, low, anterior, and abdominoperineal colon resections. Operative time averaged 2.6 hours and hospitalization averaged 4.6 days. Complications were reported in 8% of patients.

In another series, 66 patients underwent attempted laparoscopic colon resections, with a conversion rate to open colectomy in 41%.[149] Major morbidity was reported in 24% of patients, with no mortality. Length of hospitalization, hospital cost, and lymph node harvest was compared with patients who underwent open colon resection. Mean postoperative hospital stay was significantly less in patients with laparoscopic sigmoid and right colectomies than for those patients converted to open operation or for those procedures performed using conventional open techniques. Total hospital cost for patients undergoing conventional open right hemicolectomy was less than that for the converted group but not for those having a laparoscopic resection. Lymph node harvest was comparable in all three groups. The authors of this study concluded that these data demonstrate that laparoscopic colectomy can be performed with acceptable morbidity and mortality, but that there is no definite cost savings.

Laparoscopic colon resection was performed in 80 patients and compared with a control group of 53 patients undergoing conventional open colectomy by the same group of surgeons.[150] Analysis included complications, rate of conversion, length of procedure, duration of postoperative ileus, hospital stay, hospital cost, and adequacy of the specimen obtained. Operations were converted to open procedures in 23% of patients, which decreased to 15% in the second half of the series. The length of procedure was greater in those undergoing laparoscopic resection (mean, 221 minutes) than in those undergoing open colectomy (mean, 183 minutes). Operating

TABLE 29.1-2. Clinical Trials of Laparoscopic Colon Resection

Reference	*Year*	*Patients*	*Indications*	*Outcomes*
Hoffman et al.[158]	1996	238	39 with cancer	2-y follow-up with no adverse patterns of recurrence
Wexner et al.[156]	1996	140	IBD, cancer, diverticular disease, other	11% conversion rate; operative time, 4 hr; hospital stay, 6.8 d
Phillips et al.[148]	1992	51	Cancer, diverticular disease, IBD, polyps	8% conversion rate to open laparoscopy; operative time, 2.3 hr; hospital stay, 4.6 d; 2% mortality
Liberman et al.[153]	1996	14	Diverticular disease	Decrease in costs and postoperative stay
Gellman et al.[162]	1996	102	Cancer, diverticular disease	5.9 d for laparoscopy group; lymph node retrieval same as historical controls
Begos et al.[155]	1996	50	Cancer, diverticular disease	34% conversion rate; single surgeon; hospital stay, 8.3 d
Huscher et al.[159]	1996	200	Cancer, diverticular disease, other	10.5% conversion; multicenter study; mean operative time, 208 min; mean number of nodes, 12.1
Muckleroy et al.[151]	1999	38	Benign disease only	Compared to patients undergoing open colon surgery, decreased length of stay, slightly longer operative time
Lacy et al.[154]	1995	52	Colon cancer	Randomized to laparoscopic (n = 25) and open (n = 26) groups; 16% conversion and longer operative time in laparoscopic cases
Ramos et al.[27]	1994	252	Cancer	All cases from a registry; 1.44% incidence of port-site recurrences (3 of 208)
Kwok et al.[163]	1996	83	Cancer	15.2 mo follow-up
Poulin et al.[160]	1999	135	Cancer	Review of a prospective database; 24 mo median follow-up; no trocar site recurrences; survival curves similar to historical controls
Dean et al.[138]	1994	122	Cancer, diverticular disease	48% conversion rate; longer operative time and shorter length of stay in laparoscopic group compared to those in open group
Franklin et al.[152]	1995	84	Cancer	Total of 194 patients—84 with laparoscopic colon resection and 110 open resection in same nonrandomized group; node harvest similar; margins of resection similar; survival similar at 36 mo
Milsom et al.[166]	1998	42	Cancer	Follow-up of 18 mo; 13% recurrence
Fielding et al.[142]	1997	149	Cancer	7% conversion; 33 mo follow-up; 7% recurrence
Lacy et al.[228]	1998	31	Cancer	Range of follow-up, 11.5 to 21.4 mo; 13% conversion, 16% recurrence

IBD, inflammatory bowel disease.

room and total hospital charges were also greater in those patients undergoing laparoscopic resection compared with those having open colectomy. Patients having a laparoscopic colectomy had an average postoperative stay of 5.2 days, compared with 7.8 days for those having open colectomies. The pathology specimens were similar in all groups. This study further validates that laparoscopic colectomy can be performed safely with shorter hospitalization, but at higher overall cost. Perhaps with greater experience, operating times will decrease, as was suggested by this study.

A number of trials have compared laparoscopic colon resection to traditional open resection. Thirty-eight laparoscopic colon resections were compared with 39 open resections.[151] The authors of this study found slightly longer operative time (161 minutes vs. 131 minutes) in the laparoscopic group, with lower estimated blood loss (122 mL vs. 192 mL) and significantly shorter length of stay (3.3 days vs. 7.4 days), with similar complication rates. They concluded that laparoscopic colon resection for benign disease affords the patient the advantages of laparoscopic surgery and gives surgeons the opportunity to develop requisite skills while results of trials of laparoscopic surgery for malignancy are awaited. In a prospective trial of 194 patients in San Antonio, Texas, patients selected their own method of resection. Open colon resection was selected by 110 patients and laparoscopy by 84 patients.[152] The authors of this study looked at a number of outcome variables and observed that laparoscopic resection allows adequate margins and lymph node harvests no different from open resection. In brief follow-up, survival in the two groups was similar. In a study of 14 patients undergoing laparoscopic colon resection for diverticular disease, patients were compared with a similar group who had undergone open resection.[153] Estimated blood loss, days to oral liquids, and length of stay were significantly less in the laparoscopic group. Mean total hospital charges and costs were also less, suggesting the benefits of laparoscopic colon resection. In a randomized prospective trial, 51 patients underwent colon resection by laparoscopic means or by traditional open techniques.[154] Similar lymph node harvests were reported in the two groups, as were resection margins and adequacy of specimens. Patients were discharged earlier from the hospital in the laparoscopic group as well. Although follow-up was not long, this study suggests that the laparoscopic approach is preferable for patients requiring colon resection. Similar results have been observed by a number of authors.[155–157]

Some of the trials reported to date demonstrate excellent results but lack lengthy follow-up. Hoffman et al.[158] reported 238 patients who underwent laparoscopic colon resections, with 39 patients who underwent resection available for just 24 months of follow-up. They concluded that survival rates were similar to those observed for patients who underwent open colon resection. A single-arm, retrospective multicenter study reported a 10.5% conversion rate, an average of 12.1 lymph nodes resected, and a mean follow-up of 16 months.[159] The authors of this study admitted the need for longer follow-up. In a study of 100 patients, median operative time for laparoscopic resection was 180 minutes, and the conversion rate was 31%,[163] although the conversion rate decreased relatively along the learning curve. Median follow-up was just 15 months in this study, which demonstrated four distant recurrences and one pelvic recurrence. These authors asserted the importance of longer follow-up and a randomized trial to truly establish the benefit of this procedure. In an excellent study of 172 patients who underwent laparoscopic resection for adenocarcinoma of the colon, 25 patients underwent conversion to open resection and 12 patients were lost to follow-up, leaving 135 patients in the study.[160] Median follow-up was 24 months, with observed 2-year survival rates of 100% for stage I, 88% for stage II, 81% for stage III, and 29% for stage IV. Survival rates at 4 years were 100% for stage I, 80% for stage II, 54% for stage III, and 0% for stage IV. No port-site recurrences were observed. Although the authors of this study correctly concluded that early survival curves for patients undergoing laparoscopic resection do not differ from historical controls, they also assert that "further validation is needed."

That laparoscopic colon resection is feasible goes unquestioned. Some studies have pointed out that it remains a technically demanding procedure, considerably more difficult than laparoscopic cholecystectomy, and has a lengthy learning curve. However, the use of laparoscopic resection of the colon for the treatment of malignancies is currently under study. The American Society of Colon and Rectal Surgeons does not endorse the application of laparoscopic technology to cure carcinoma at this time.[140] The studies just described have shown that laparoscopic colon resection is safe, feasible, and obtains pathologic specimens similar to those obtained from open surgery. Although it is tempting to obtain the same benefits of decreased hospitalization and recovery for patients undergoing colon resection as has been shown in patients undergoing cholecystectomy through the use of laparoscopy, there is no evidence at this time to definitively conclude that this is the case. We must also consider the issue of the possibility of compromised cancer control and complications in this discussion.[142] Cancer control issues include extent of lymph node resection, port-site recurrences, and adequacy of intraperitoneal staging in the absence of tactile sensation. The series reviewed above suggest that a lymph node resection similar to that in open surgery is possible. Others have made similar observations regarding lymph node harvests.[158,160–163] The issue of port-site metastases is discussed above in the section Port-Site Metastases, but rates from 0% to 3.2% have been reported, compared with fewer than 1% in open colon resection.[164] The problem with many of the anecdotal reports in the literature is that the overall denominator is not known, and only through a prospective trial can these issues be adequately studied. The 1-year port-site recurrence rate has been reported at less than 1% in the first 252 patients in the registry of the American Society of Colon and Rectal Surgeons.[27] In this series, all of the recurrences were in patients with node-positive disease. Sugarbaker[165] has advocated the use of intraperitoneal chemotherapy based on his work with disseminated gastrointestinal malignancies.

Although laparoscopic surgery has the potential to save hospitalization time and recovery time, such savings must not be made at the expense of overall survival. The prospective trial currently under way at many centers throughout the United States and funded by the National Institutes of Health should address the issues of cancer control, costs, and quality of life.[142] The surgical community is awaiting the results of this trial. This carefully designed prospective trial will answer the significant questions regarding laparoscopic resection of colon cancer. The approach of waiting for the results of this study has been endorsed by a number of authors.[141,142,166,167]

GALLBLADDER CANCER

Although it is rare, the presence of a gallbladder malignancy is a possibility that must always be in the mind of the laparoscopic surgeon while performing a routine laparoscopic cholecystectomy. This disease, most common in older women, is the fifth most common malignancy of the gastrointestinal tract and is associated with a dismal prognosis.[168] It is estimated that carcinoma is present in 1% of all cholecystectomy specimens.[168] Laparoscopic cholecystectomy is the procedure of choice for patients with symptomatic cholelithiasis, but the presence of gallbladder carcinoma remains a contraindication to the laparoscopic conduct of this procedure.[169,170] Preoperative diagnosis of this disease is difficult, because the sensitivity for ultrasonography in early cases is only approximately 20%. In view of the difficulty with which preoperative diagnosis can be made, it is not surprising that the diagnosis is often made only after histologic examination of the surgical specimen.

The optimal treatment for this rare disease remains elusive. In a large retrospective study of 724 patients from a number of European centers, only 4% of patients presented with Tis lesions, but these were the only patients with any hope of long-term survival.[171] Prognosis in stage T1 and T2 was markedly worse, although no data support the use of extended surgical resections in these patients. Furthermore, others have shown that, at the present time, the use of adjuvant chemotherapy or radiation therapy does not significantly affect survival.[172]

The treatment of patients suspected of having carcinoma of the gallbladder preoperatively should include a definitive procedure performed through conventional open surgical techniques as the initial procedure. Clinical data from ten patients with laparoscopically discovered gallbladder carcinoma have been reported.[173] All ten patients were believed to have resectable disease based on preoperative studies and intraoperative findings. The interval to exploration at the referral center was 14 to 74 days, with a median of 30 days. Gross intraperitoneal dissemination was found in four patients. The investigators concluded that patients in whom gallbladder carcinoma is suspected on visual examination of the gallbladder during attempted laparoscopic cholecystectomy should be converted immediately to an open procedure or the procedure terminated and the patient referred for definitive therapy. During the conduct of a laparoscopic cholecystectomy, any evidence for the presence of a carcinoma is cause for conversion to an open procedure.[174] Routine examination of the specimen with frozen section if suspicious areas are present should also be carried out, with conversion to an open procedure if positive for malignancy.[170]

In summary, any patient with a lesion that is preoperatively suspect for malignancy should undergo cholecystectomy by conventional open cholecystectomy.[175] If the diagnosis is suspected during a laparoscopic cholecystectomy based on the appearance of the gallbladder, frozen section should be obtained and the procedure converted to an open cholecystectomy if the histology demonstrates malignancy. If the diagnosis is made only after laparoscopic cholecystectomy is completed, then port sites should be excised at a second procedure.[176] Further surgical or adjuvant therapy may also be indicated.

HEPATIC TUMORS

Whereas the use of laparoscopy in the staging of hepatic lesions, either primary or metastatic, has become fairly widespread, laparoscopic treatment of hepatic malignancies is rarely performed. This is because of the technical difficulty of this procedure as well as the scarcity of patients with lesions amenable to laparoscopic resection. The laparoscopic treatment of hepatic lesions has been reported. A benign liver cyst was fenestrated under laparoscopic guidance and provided effective therapy for a benign condition while avoiding the potential morbidity of a laparotomy.[177] A large series of 43 patients with benign solid and cystic lesions treated laparoscopically has been reported by Katkhouda et al.[178] These authors concluded that laparoscopic surgery is indicated for patients with giant solitary hepatic cysts and select patients with small, benign solid tumors located in anterior liver segments.

A number of techniques can be performed laparoscopically, including wedge excisions using a stapling device[50] or even laparoscopic hepatic segmentectomy. The anterolateral areas of the segments in the Couinaud classification are amenable to laparoscopic resection because of their accessibility.[178]

Although a number of techniques are available for liver resection, the ultrasonic dissector is preferred by some. A randomized prospective trial has shown that a laparoscopic version of this device is effective in laparoscopic cholecystectomy.[179] It is natural that this device may be used for hepatic resection. An animal trial has been reported, demonstrating hepatic resection on pigs using the ultrasonic dissector.[180] The ultrasonic dissector was effective in dissecting the intraparenchymal structures, including vascular structures. A single case of a left lateral segmentectomy in a human performed laparoscopically has been reported.[181] With improved instrumentation becoming available, perhaps more hepatic resections will be performed laparoscopically.

Another application of laparoscopic technology to the treatment of liver lesions is cryotherapy. Cryosurgery has been shown to be effective in the treatment of some hepatic malignancies.[182] Ultrasound monitoring of this procedure is essential. With the advent of laparoscopic ultrasound probes and cryotherapy probes, it is possible to perform cryotherapy of hepatic lesions. However, anatomic limitations may prevent the use of this technology because of limited exposure of certain lesions.

More recently, radio frequency ablation of tumors has been performed for metastatic and primary lesions of the liver.[183,184] This technique is often performed percutaneously, but situations exist in which a lesion is accessible only by using laparoscopic techniques to position the treatment probe accurately. Of 30 patients who underwent radio frequency ablation for primary and metastatic lesions of the liver in one series, 12 were treated laparoscopically, 12 at laparotomy, and six percutaneously.[184]

As laparoscopic technology improves and new modalities are applied to the treatment of hepatic lesions, more applications of minimally invasive surgery may be found for these patients. The role of laparoscopy in the management of malignant lesions of the liver remains undefined.

PANCREATIC CANCER

Resection with the intent for cure is possible in only approximately 10% to 20% of patients who present with carcinoma of the pancreas, and 5-year survival rates of all patients presenting with the disease are only approximately 3%.[185] However, several more recent series have reported 5-year survival rates as high as 20% to 25% for patients who undergo resection for cure. Patients with pathologically negative lymph nodes have an even higher survival rate.[186] Many of the patients who are not resectable for cure often require surgical palliation. Laparoscopic surgery has the potential to provide this palliation while minimizing postoperative pain and length of hospital stay, both especially important considerations in patients with limited life expectancy.

The laparoscopic resection of pancreatic tumors is technically feasible but unlikely to become widely practiced. Gagner and Pomp[187] reported having performed a pylorus-preserving pancreaticoduodenectomy in a patient with chronic pancreatitis and pancreas divisum. Reconstruction was performed with a gastrojejunostomy, hepaticojejunostomy, and pancreaticojejunostomy. The patient's postoperative course was complicated by delayed gastric emptying, and he was discharged on the 30th postoperative day.

Laparoscopic distal pancreatectomy, with or without splenic salvage, has been well described.[188] It is often combined with splenectomy, as described by Cuschieri and colleagues,[189] who reported a series of five patients who underwent laparoscopic distal pancreatectomy and splenectomy using a five-port technique. This procedure is indicated for benign tumors in which the splenic vein cannot be separated from the pancreatic lesion, or in palliative resections of the distal pancreas for lesions such as cystadenoma, neuroendocrine tumors, cysts, and adenocarcinoma of the tail of the pancreas. It is unlikely that minimally invasive surgery will play a large role in the curative resection of malignancies of the head of the pancreas in the near future.

RENAL CELL CARCINOMA

The use of laparoscopic surgical approaches for patients with renal cell carcinoma has been described,[190–192] with investigators demonstrating that nephrectomy can be safely performed using existing laparoscopic instrumentation. In this early series, the procedure took a mean of 5.6 hours to complete, and patients had an average hospital stay of 4.6 days.[190] The kidney is morcellated with an electric morcellator placed through a 10-mm port and extracted using a sturdy bag.

In some cases, preservation of renal parenchyma may be indicated. The laparoscopic enucleation of a renal cell carcinoma also has been described.[193] These investigators concluded that this procedure is relatively easy to perform compared with nephrectomy and, when indicated, may be preferable to perform by a laparoscopic approach.

SPLEEN

Although the spleen rarely harbors primary or secondary tumors in humans, the surgical oncologist is often called on to perform a splenectomy for hematologic diseases. The spleen is well within the reach of the laparoscopic surgeon, and by applying laparoscopic techniques, the patient is afforded the benefits of laparoscopic surgery, including shortened hospitalization and decreased postoperative pain. A number of series in the literature report laparoscopic removal of the spleen.[106,107,110–112,114,121,194–196] These procedures have been performed for a number of indications including staging of Hodgkin's lymphoma, ITP, thrombotic thrombocytopenia purpura, acquired immunodeficiency syndrome–related thrombocytopenia, hereditary spherocytosis, autoimmune hemolytic anemia, leukemia, and splenic abscess. There may be particular subsets of patients for whom laparoscopic splenectomy is particularly beneficial. A case report of successful laparoscopic splenectomy on a patient who is human immunodeficiency virus–positive, a devout Jehovah's witness refusing transfusion, and with a preoperative hematocrit of 8.8% highlights the attractiveness of this technique.[197] In general, laparoscopic splenectomy represents the gold standard for removal of the spleen.[115]

Splenectomy was commonly performed for the staging of lymphomas in the past, and in one series demonstrated a significant increase in the period 1963–1982 compared with 1946–1962.[96] However, more recent trends show that splenectomies are now being performed more often for cytopenic and anemic diseases and less often for Hodgkin's disease.[198] The consequences of splenectomy are poorly understood at an immunologic level, but it is clear that the spleen plays a major role in a wide range of immune responses.[199] Patients should receive a pneumococcal vaccine preoperatively to help avoid the infectious complications of the asplenic state.[125,199] The patient can be positioned in several ways for this procedure, with some groups preferring a right decubitus position.[200]

In one large series, 43 patients were brought to the operating room for laparoscopic splenectomy, and 35 (81%) were successfully completed.[114] The remaining 19% underwent conversion to open splenectomy, usually for bleeding. Laparoscopic splenectomy has become the standard method for splenectomy in some centers. Conversion rates in other series have been reported as 2 (9%) of 22 cases,[195] 2 (12%) of 17,[111] and 3 (19%) of 13.[194] The details of the technique have been adequately described by Flowers et al.[114]

It is important to make a thorough search for accessory splenic tissue, identified in 10% of the patients in one series.[114] Accessory spleens are identified in up to 18% of patients undergoing splenectomy.[201] The magnification afforded by the laparoscope may aid in this task. In a series of 100 patients undergoing open splenectomy for ITP, 13 patients had a poor response to splenectomy, five of which required accessory splenectomy.[202] In one large series of laparoscopic splenectomies for ITP, a positive response was observed in 18 (82%) of 22 patients with ITP.[114] It is difficult to predict who will respond to splenectomy, with no predictive factors being identified, even in large series of patients with ITP.[202]

In a prospective study of operative outcomes, laparoscopic splenectomy using the lateral approach was performed on 147 patients and open splenectomy performed on 63 matched patients at three teaching centers.[194] Laparoscopic splenectomy resulted in longer operative times (145 minutes vs. 77 minutes), reduced blood loss (162 mL vs. 380 mL), shorter postoperative stay (2.4 days vs. 9.2 days), and fewer complications compared with the open procedure. The authors of this study also reported that the mean weighted cost of laparoscopic splenectomy was lower than the open procedure ($3311 vs. $3861). The conversion rate in this series was 2.7%.

Although laparoscopic splenectomy is a technically demanding procedure, it offers the patient the potential for decreased postoperative pain and hospitalization with more rapid return to normal activities of living. Further prospective data are needed to confirm these observations. Surgical alternatives to splenectomy, such as partial splenectomy, have been offered as a way to reduce the incidence of postoperative infections.[203] These techniques may also be approachable with laparoscopic techniques in the future.

ADRENAL TUMORS

Laparoscopic techniques have been used for the resection of adrenal lesions.[204–209] Although the anterior transabdominal approach is considered by some to be a source of postoperative morbidity, the laparoscopic approach may offer some advantages. Adrenal tumors are fairly common, having been found in 2% of patients in autopsy series.[210] Small, asymptomatic tumors are reported in as many as 0.6% of abdominal ultrasound and CT examinations. Those discovered that are less than 4 cm in diameter and in the absence of endocrine syndromes can be observed after a careful evaluation.[210] However, a fair proportion of these lesions may require extirpation, a procedure that has been performed laparoscopically with the apparent advantages of decreased pain and more rapid return to full activity.

Furthermore, a number of laparoscopic approaches have been described. The anterior laparoscopic approach requires mobilization of the colon and, occasionally, other intraabdominal organs. A retroperitoneal laparoscopic approach also has been described, which may be more attractive. One study has compared the two approaches and found no difference in operative time, analgesia requirements, hospital time, recovery time, or complication rate.[205] The retroperitoneal laparoscopic approach may ameliorate some of the negative effects of pneumoperitoneum on the cardiovascular hemodynamics of the patient. However, most surgeons prefer the anterior approach at this time.

In one series of four patients, three patients had unilateral tumors and one had a bilateral pheochromocytoma.[205] Single right adrenalectomy was performed in 2.0 to 2.5 hours, whereas bilateral adrenalectomy lasted 5.5 hours. The hospital stay was 3 to 4 days postoperatively.

Over a 14-month period, Takeda and coworkers[204] removed seven left adrenal glands and three right adrenal glands from ten patients in operations ranging from 165 to 572 minutes (mean, 295 minutes). Conversion to open adrenalectomy was reported in one case (10%). They concluded that laparoscopic adrenalectomy is applicable to cases of primary hyperaldosteronism, but application to other lesions requires further study.

Twenty-five consecutive laparoscopic adrenalectomies performed on 22 patients in a 1-year period were reported by Gagner et al.[206] These surgeries were performed through a lateral decubitus flank approach and four 11-mm trocars and included 12 right and 13 left adrenal glands. The mean operative time for single adrenalectomy was 2.3 hours and for bilateral adrenalectomy was 5.3 hours. Diseases in this series included nonfunctional adenoma, pheochromocytoma, Cushing's disease, Cushing's adenoma, primary aldosteronism, angiomyolipoma, and medullary cyst. Lesions ranged in size from 1 to 15 cm, with a mean of 4.1 cm. Conversion to open laparotomy was required in one patient for lack of exposure, resulting in completion of the procedure in 96% of patients. The median postoperative stay was 4 days. Gagner et al.[206] concluded that laparoscopic adrenalectomy results in less postoperative pain and more rapid return to normal activity compared with open adrenalectomy.

A study compared laparoscopic adrenalectomy with a historical group of posterior adrenalectomies.[207] The two groups were comparable for patient demographics. The median time for posterior adrenalectomy was 120 minutes versus a median of 160 minutes for laparoscopic adrenalectomy. Patients who underwent laparoscopic adrenalectomy had a mean hospital stay of 3 days, a shorter time to return to work, and a lower blood loss than those patients who underwent posterior adrenalectomy with a mean hospital stay of 5 days. The authors of this study concluded that laparoscopic adrenalectomy is the procedure of choice.

One study reported the results of a case-controlled study of 40 laparoscopic and 40 open adrenalectomies.[208] Statistically significant differences were found (laparoscopic vs. open) in operative blood loss (40 mL vs. 172 mL), operating time (147 minutes vs. 79 minutes), hospital stay (12 days vs. 18 days), and late morbidity (0% vs. 48%). The authors of this study found no statistically significant differences in time to oral intake, total cost, and early morbidity. The late morbidity in the open group consisted of wound complications that were absent in the laparoscopic group. The authors concluded that the laparoscopic approach is the method of choice for adrenal masses less than 6 cm in diameter.

A series from the National Cancer Institute reported the learning curve for laparoscopic adrenalectomy. In the first five patients, median operating time was 255 minutes, which dropped to 207 minutes in the second group of five patients and to 143 minutes in the third group of five patients.[209]

The use of minimally invasive surgery for adrenal malignancies remains controversial. *The SAGES Manual* states that laparoscopy is not to be used in the treatment of patients with malignant lesions. Other contraindications to laparoscopic adrenalectomy include masses larger than 10 cm, untreated coagulopathies, and surgeon inexperience.[211] Further study of this technique is clearly needed.

GYNECOLOGIC MALIGNANCIES

The use of laparoscopy in the treatment of gynecologic malignancies has begun relatively recently, particularly in the treatment of endometrial and cervical cancer with the laparoscopic-assisted surgical staging and laparoscopic-assisted radical vaginal hysterectomy trials (described earlier in Gynecologic Malignancies under Laparoscopy in the Staging of Malignancy). At this time, the utility of laparoscopy in the treatment of gynecologic malignancies is unclear, and the results of ongoing prospective trials are awaited.[134]

LAPAROSCOPY IN THE PALLIATION OF MALIGNANCY

PANCREATIC CANCER

The use of laparoscopy in the staging of patients with carcinoma of the pancreas is discussed earlier in Pancreatic Cancer under Laparoscopy in the Staging of Malignancy. In addition, laparoscopic techniques may be useful for palliative surgical procedures. Unfortunately, palliative therapy is all that is indicated for many patients with this disease. It is possible to palliate the three symptoms of this disease—biliary obstruction, gastrointestinal obstruction, and pain—using laparoscopic techniques. As many as 57% of patients who present with this disease undergo palliative surgery.[212] A particularly attractive concept is to stage patients using laparoscopic techniques, and then perform palliative bypass surgery at the same time using a laparoscopic approach in patients found to have unresectable disease.[213,214] Nonoperative palliation of obstructive jaundice using an endoscopically placed stent has been shown effective when compared with surgical palliation, and it also is associated with lower complication rates than surgical palliation.[186]

Palliation for obstructive jaundice may be performed nonoperatively using an endoprosthesis, or it may be carried out using a number of bypass procedures that can be performed laparoscopically. The simplest technique is cholecystojejunostomy, which has been described using both sutured and stapled techniques.[215] Choledochoduodenal or choledochojejunal anastomoses may also be fashioned laparoscopically.[215] The biliary bypass is then combined with a gastroenterostomy, which is performed at the surgeon's discretion. Similarly, the celiac plexus may be injected under laparoscopic guidance to provide pain relief.[216] Such a combined approach was used by Mouiel[215] in 12 patients with excellent results.

FEEDING TUBE PLACEMENT

Enteral feedings are preferable to parenteral feedings in patients who can tolerate them, yet not all patients with cancer are able to take in enough calories by mouth, thereby necessitating placement of a feeding tube. Open surgical gastrostomy is most often performed in the United States by the method of Stamm.[217] This was the only method available until 1980, with the development of the percutaneous endoscopic gastrostomy (PEG).[218] However, placement of a PEG requires upper endoscopy, which is not possible in all patients. Furthermore, the use of a PEG tube, necessitating pulling the tube through the tumor-bearing area, has been reported to result in implantation of the tumor at the PEG site in three cases.[219] In select patients, including patients with head and neck tumors, Zenker's diverticula, and large hiatal hernias, open surgical gastrostomy remains the preferred method of enteral access.

The technique for laparoscopic gastrostomy has been described.[220] Importantly, although formal laparotomy is not needed, the stomach is directly visualized using this technique. A retrospective review established the usefulness of this technique.[218] In this study, 32 patients who underwent laparoscopic gastrostomy and 37 patients who underwent open gastrostomy were reviewed. The underlying illnesses and contraindications to PEG placement were similar in both groups. Operative time was significantly greater in the open gastrostomy group (62 ± 19 minutes) compared with the laparoscopic gastrostomy group (38 ± 7 minutes). Complication rates were 11% in the open group and 6% in the laparoscopic group. The investigators concluded that laparoscopic gastrostomy is a safe and effective alternative procedure in patients unable to undergo placement of a PEG. Laparoscopic placement of jejunostomy tubes also has been described.[221]

LAPAROSCOPIC STOMA CREATION

Decompression of the intestinal tract may be an important procedure in the cancer patient, especially in those with carcinomatosis and resulting intestinal obstruction. The importance of colonic decompression in patients with obstructing carcinomas of the colon has been described.[222] The initial presentation of carcinoma of the colon is obstruction in 15% to 21% of patients, most commonly in the left colon. The 5-year survival rate in these patients is significantly less than that in patients without obstruction. This common situation underscores the importance of palliative procedures that may decrease postoperative pain, incidence of ileus, and recovery time.

Laparoscopic creation of a loop colostomy has been described.[223] In this technique, after the sigmoid colon is mobilized, a drain is passed through its mesentery and is then used to extract the colon through a special 3.5-cm trocar placed in the left lower quadrant. This procedure was modified and described with an associated decrease in postoperative pain and ileus with a rapid recovery.[224]

The use of small laparotomy incisions may be used for the creation of intestinal stomas; however, the presence of metastatic disease or peritoneal implants may make such procedures difficult to perform. The use of a laparoscopic approach makes possible the inspection of the abdominal cavity for other lesions and results in discharge from the hospital within 24 to 48 hours of surgery. In one study, 17 (89%) of 19 patients were successfully diverted using laparoscopic techniques.[225] The remaining two patients had extensive adhesive disease that could not be managed laparoscopically and required conversion to open laparotomy. Other procedures, such as laparoscopic gastrostomy, may also be carried out as needed.

THE FUTURE OF LAPAROSCOPY IN THE CARE OF THE PATIENT WITH CANCER

Exciting technology for laparoscopic surgery now under development will soon be in operating rooms. Cuschieri[226] has pointed out that we need to "see better, feel better, increase the precision of maneuverability and handling, reduce contamination, facilitate specimen extraction and bring order to the present ergonomic chaos in our operating rooms." New developments in the technology of imaging are being applied to laparoscopic surgery. Although head-mounted displays have been tested, they are probably less than optimal for the laparoscopic surgeon because of the isolation created by these devices. Current three-dimensional imaging systems are not without their limitations, but new systems may provide a true improvement in tissue visualization. Continued improvements in instrumentation will certainly be an important part of the evolution of laparoscopic surgery. New methods of tissue extraction include a sleeve system and an extracorporeal pneumoperitoneal access bubble.[226] Both of these systems have potential advantages, especially for the removal of large tumor specimens.

Training of surgeons in these newly emerging techniques remains a complicated problem. Because hospitals decide what procedures may be performed by surgeons, criteria for training and furnishing credentials must be developed.[227] The Society of American Gastrointestinal Endoscopic Surgeons (SAGES) has suggested criteria for training and awarding credentials. It remains to be shown whether some advanced laparoscopic procedures result in a true cost savings when the increased cost of instrumentation and operating room time are factored into the total expenses incurred.

The surgeon has traditionally been involved in the diagnosis, staging, treatment, and palliation of patients with malignancies. Laparoscopy is rapidly becoming an important tool in each of these areas of cancer patient care. The ultimate application of laparoscopic techniques depends on the imagination of surgical investigators and on careful analyses of risks and benefits. Over time, it may be discovered that certain uses for this technology are not ultimately advantageous to the patient compared with traditional open surgical techniques. Only by the conduct of carefully controlled studies, however, will the facts be elucidated, allowing this methodology to be used when it will benefit the patient and avoided when it will not.

REFERENCES

1. Gunning JE. The history of laparoscopy. *J Reprod Med* 1974;12:223.
2. Lefor AT. Laparoscopic surgery for cancer. *PPO Updates* 1995;9:1.
3. Bagley CM, Thomas LB, Johnson RE, Chretien PB, DeVita VT. Diagnosis of liver involvement by lymphoma: results in 96 consecutive peritoneoscopies. *Cancer* 1973;31:840.
4. Casirola G, Ippoliti G, Marini G. Laparoscopy in Hodgkin's disease. *Acta Haematol* 1973;49:1.
5. Spinelli P, Beretta G, Bajetta E, et al. Laparoscopy and laparotomy combined with bone marrow biopsy in staging Hodgkin's disease. *BMJ* 1975;4:554.
6. Castellani R, Bonadonna G, Spinelli P, et al. Sequential pathologic staging of untreated non-Hodgkin's lymphomas by laparoscopy and laparotomy combined with marrow biopsy. *Cancer* 1977;40:2322.
7. Chabner BA, Johnson RE, Young RC, et al. Sequential non-surgical and surgical staging of non-Hodgkin's lymphoma. *Cancer* 1978;42:922.
8. Anderson T, Bender RA, Rosenoff SH, et al. Peritoneoscopy: a technique to evaluate therapeutic efficacy in non-Hodgkin's lymphoma patients. *Cancer Treat Rep* 1977:61:1017.
9. Cuschieri A, Hall AW, Clark J. Value of laparoscopy in the diagnosis and management of pancreatic carcinoma. *Gut* 1978;19:672.
10. Tuñón MJ, Gonzalez P, Jorquera F, et al. Liver blood flow during laparoscopic surgery in pigs. *Surg Endosc* 1999;13:668.

11. West MA, Hackam DJ, Baker J, et al. Mechanism of decreased *in vitro* murine macrophage cytokine release after exposure to carbon dioxide. *Ann Surg* 1997;226:179.
12. Greif WM, Forse A. Cardiopulmonary effects of the laparoscopic pneumoperitoneum in a porcine model of ARDS. *Am J Surg* 1999;177:216.
13. Greif WM, Forse RA. Interventions to improve cardiopulmonary hemodynamics during laparoscopy in a porcine sepsis model. *J Am Coll Surg* 1999;189:450.
14. Cho JM, LaPorta AJ, Clark JR, et al. Response of serum cytokines in patients undergoing laparoscopic cholecystectomy. *Surg Endosc* 1994;8:1380.
15. Vittimberga FJ, Foley DP, Meyers WC, Callery MP. Laparoscopic surgery and the systemic immune response. *Ann Surg* 1998;227:326.
16. Vallina VL, Velasco JM. The influence of laparoscopy on lymphocyte subpopulations in the surgical patient. *Surg Endosc* 1996;10:481.
17. Hansborough JF, Bender EM, Zapata-Sirvent R, Anderson J. Altered helper and suppressor lymphocyte populations in surgical patients: a measure of postoperative immunosuppression. *Am J Surg* 1984;148:303.
18. Fusco MA, Paluzzi MW. Abdominal wall recurrence after laparoscopic-assisted colectomy for adenocarcinoma of the colon. *Dis Colon Rectum* 1993;36:858.
19. Cava A, Roman J, Quintela AG, Martin F, Aramburo P. Subcutaneous metastasis following laparoscopy in gastric adenocarcinoma. *Eur J Surg Oncol* 1990;16:63.
20. Weiss SM, Wengert PA, Harkavy SE. Incisional recurrence of gallbladder cancer after laparoscopic cholecystectomy. *Gastrointest Endosc* 1994;40:244.
21. Nduka CC, Monson JRT, Menzies-Gow N, Darz A. Abdominal wall metastases following laparoscopy. *Br J Surg* 1994;81:648.
22. Stockdale AD, Pocock TJ. Abdominal wall metastasis following laparoscopy. *Eur J Surg Oncol* 1985;11:373.
23. Clair DG, Lautz DB, Brooks DC. Rapid development of umbilical metastases after laparoscopic cholecystectomy for unsuspected gallbladder carcinoma. *Surgery* 1993;113:355.
24. O'Rourke N, Price PM, Kelly S, Sikora K. Tumor inoculation during laparoscopy. *Lancet* 1993;342:368.
25. Pezet D, Fondrinier E, Rotman N, et al. Parietal seeding of carcinoma of the gallbladder after laparoscopic cholecystectomy. *Br J Surg* 1992;79:230.
26. Hughes ESR, McDermott FT, Polglase AL, Johnson WR. Tumor recurrence in the abdominal wall scar tissue after large-bowel cancer surgery. *Dis Colon Rectum* 1983;26:571.
27. Ramos JM, Gupta S, Anthone GJ, et al. Laparoscopy and colon cancer: is the port site at risk? *Arch Surg* 1994;129:897.
28. Johnstone PAS, Rohde DC, Swartz SE, et al. Port site recurrences after laparoscopic and thoracoscopic procedures in malignancy. *J Clin Oncol* 1996;14:1950.
29. Fleshman JW, Nelson H, Peters WR, et al. Early results of laparoscopic surgery for colorectal cancer. Retrospective study of 372 patients after laparoscopic colectomy. *Dis Colon Rectum* 1996;39:S53.
30. Pearlstone DB, Mansfield PE, Curley SA, et al. Laparoscopy in 533 patients with abdominal malignancy. *Surgery* 1999;125:67.
31. Ikramuddin S, Lucas J, Ellison EC, et al. Detection of aerosolized cells during carbon dioxide laparoscopy. *J Gastrointest Surg* 1998;2:580.
32. Reymond MA, Wittekind C, Jung A, et al. The incidence of port site metastases might be reduced. *Surg Endosc* 1997;11:902.
33. Cavina E, Goletti O, Molea N, et al. Trocar site tumor recurrences: may pneumoperitoneum be responsible? *Surg Endosc* 1998;12:1294.
34. Bouvy ND, Marquet RL, Jeekel H, Bonjer HJ. Impact of gasless laparoscopy and laparotomy on peritoneal tumor growth and abdominal wall metastases. *Ann Surg* 1996;224:694.
35. Wu JS, Brasfield EB, Guo LW, et al. Implantation of colon cancer at trocar sites is increased by low pressure pneumoperitoneum. *Surgery* 1997;122:1.
36. Hubens G, Pauwels M, Hubens A, et al. The influence of pneumoperitoneum on the peritoneal implantation of free intraperitoneal colon cancer cells. *Surg Endosc* 1996;10:809.
37. Dorrance HR, Oien K, O'Dwyer PJ. Effects of laparoscopy on intraperitoneal tumor growth and distant metastases in an animal model. *Surgery* 1999;126:35.
38. Neuhaus SJ, Ellis T, Roge AM, et al. Tumor implantation following laparoscopy using different insufflation gases. *Surg Endosc* 1998;12:1300.
39. Tseng LN, Berends FJ, Wittich P, et al. Port site metastases: impact of local tissue trauma and gas leakage. *Surg Endosc* 1998;12:1377.
40. Aoki Y, Shimura H, Li H, et al. A model of port site metastases of gallbladder cancer: the influence of peritoneal injury and its repair on abdominal wall metastases. *Surgery* 1999;125:553.
41. Mutter D, Hajri A, Tassetti V, et al. Increased tumor growth and spread after laparoscopy vs laparotomy. *Surg Endosc* 1999;13:365.
42. Bessler M, Whelan RL, Halverson A, Treat MR, Nowygrod R. Is immune function better preserved after laparoscopic versus open colon resection? *Surg Endosc* 1994;8:881.
43. Allendorf JDF, Bessler M, Kayton ML, et al. Tumor growth after laparotomy or laparoscopy. *Surg Endosc* 1995;9:49.
44. Allendorf JDF, Bessler M, Kayton ML, et al. Increased tumor establishment and growth after laparotomy vs laparoscopy in a murine model. *Arch Surg* 1995;130:649.
45. Bessler M, Allendorf JDF, Chao JD, et al. Permissive tumor growth after laparotomy versus laparoscopy is associated with altered TNF levels. *Surg Forum* 1994;45:486.
46. Easter DW, Cuschieri A, Nathanson LK, Lavalle-Jones M. The utility of diagnostic laparoscopy for abdominal disorders. *Arch Surg* 1992;127:379.
47. Foley EF, Kolecki RV, Schirmer BD. The accuracy of laparoscopic ultrasound in the detection of colorectal cancer liver metastases. *Am J Surg* 1998;176:262.
48. Greene FL, Bianco JE. Laparoscopy's growing role in abdominal tumor diagnosis. *Contemp Oncol* 1994;(Jan):14.
49. Cuschieri A. Diagnosis and staging of tumors by laparoscopy. *Semin Laparosc Surg* 1994;1:3.
50. Lefor AT, Flowers JL. Laparoscopic wedge biopsy of the liver. *J Am Coll Surg* 1994;178:307.
51. Greene FL. Laparoscopy in malignant disease. *Surg Clin North Am* 1992;72:1125.
52. Jakimowicz J. Laparoscopic intraoperative ultrasonography, equipment, and technique. *Semin Laparosc Surg* 1994;1:52.
53. Machi J, Sigel B. Intraoperative ultrasonography. *Radiol Clin North Am* 1992;30:1085.
54. Stiegmann GV, McIntyre RC, Pearlman NW. Laparoscopic intracorporeal ultrasound. *Surg Endosc* 1994;8:167.
55. Jakimowicz JJ. Review: intraoperative ultrasonography during minimal access surgery. *J R Coll Surg Edinb* 1993;38:231.
56. John TG, Greig JD, Crosbie JL, Miles WF, Garden OJ. Superior staging of liver tumors with laparoscopy and laparoscopic ultrasound. *Ann Surg* 1994;220:711.
57. van Dijkum EJ, de Wit LT, van Delden OM, et al. Staging laparoscopy and laparoscopic ultrasonography in more than 400 patients with upper gastrointestinal carcinoma. *J Am Coll Surg* 1999;189:459.
58. Lightdale CJ. Laparoscopy for cancer staging. *Endoscopy* 1992;24:682.
59. Hemming AW, Nagy AG, Scudamore CH, Edelman K. Laparoscopic staging of intraabdominal malignancy. *Surg Endosc* 1995;9:325.
60. Salky BA. Laparoscopic staging of intra-abdominal malignancy. In: Paterson-Brown S, Garden J, eds. *Principles and practice of surgical laparoscopy.* Philadelphia: WB Saunders, 1994.
61. Conlon KC, Dougherty E, Klimstra DG, et al. The value of minimal access surgery in the staging of patients with potentially resectable peripancreatic malignancy. *Ann Surg* 1996;223:134.
62. Warshaw AL, Tepper JE, Shipley WU. Laparoscopy in the staging and planning of therapy for pancreatic cancer. *Am J Surg* 1986;151:76.
63. Warshaw AL. Implications of peritoneal cytology for staging of early pancreatic cancer. *Am J Surg* 1991;161:26.
64. Nishizaki T, Matsumata T, Adachi E, Sugimachi K. Laparoscopy preferable to imaging procedures in detecting metastases of a pancreas carcinoma to the liver. *Surg Endosc* 1994;8:1340.
65. John TG, Greig JD, Carter DC, Garden OJ. Carcinoma of the pancreatic head and periampullary region: tumor staging with laparoscopy and laparoscopic ultrasound. *Ann Surg* 1995;221:156.
66. John TG, Wright A, Allan PL, et al. Laparoscopy with laparoscopic ultrasound in the TNM staging of pancreatic carcinoma. *World J Surg* 1999;23:870.
67. Durup Scheel-Hincke J, Mortensen MB, Qvist N, Hovendal CP. TNM staging and assessment of resectability of pancreatic cancer by laparoscopic ultrasonography. *Surg Endosc* 1999;13:967.
68. Luque de Leon E, Tsiotos GG, Balsiger B, et al. Staging laparoscopy for pancreatic cancer should be used to select the best means of palliation and not only to maximize the resectability rate. *J Gastrointest Surg* 1999;3:111.
69. Rumstadt B, Schwab M, Schuster K, Hagmuller E, Trede M. The role of laparoscopy in the preoperative staging of pancreatic carcinoma. *J Gastrointest Surg* 1997;1:245.
70. Greene FL. Laparoscopic resection. In: DeVita VT, Hellman S, Rosenberg SA, eds. *Cancer: principles and practice of oncology,* 5th ed. Philadelphia: JB Lippincott, 1995.
71. Shandall A, Johnson C. Laparoscopy or scanning in oesophageal and gastric carcinoma. *Br J Surg* 1986;72:449.
72. Dagnini G, Caldironi MW, Marin G, et al. Laparoscopy in abdominal staging of esophageal carcinoma. *Gastrointest Endosc* 1986;32:400.
73. Krasna MJ, Flowers JL, Attar S, McLaughlin JL. Combined thoracoscopic/laparoscopic staging of esophageal cancer. *J Thorac Cardiovasc Surg* 1996;111:800.
74. Watt I, Stewart I, Anderson D, Bell G, Anderson JR. Laparoscopy, ultrasound and computed tomography in cancer of the oesophagus and gastric cardia: a prospective comparison for detecting intra-abdominal metastases. *Br J Surg* 1989;76:1036.
75. Fiocco M, Krasna MJ. Thoracoscopic lymph node dissection in the staging of esophageal carcinoma. *J Laparoendosc Surg* 1992;2:111.
76. Krasna MJ, McLaughlin JS. Thoracoscopic lymph node staging for esophageal cancer. *Ann Thorac Surg* 1993;56:671.
77. Belani CP, White CS, Slawson R, et al. Value of minimally invasive thoracoscopy versus noninvasive staging techniques in esophageal cancer. *Proc Am Soc Clin Oncol* 1994;13:195.
78. Bemelman WA, van Delden OM, van Lanschot JJB, et al. Laparoscopy and laparoscopic ultrasonography in staging of carcinoma of the esophagus and gastric cardia. *J Am Coll Surg* 1995;181:421.
79. Lowy AM, Mansfield PF, Leach SD, Ajani J. Laparoscopic staging for gastric cancer. *Surgery* 1996;119:611.
80. Steele GD, Bleday R, Mayer RJ, et al. A prospective evaluation of hepatic resection for colorectal carcinoma metastases to the liver: gastrointestinal tumor study group protocol 6584. *J Clin Oncol* 1991;9:1105.
81. Lefor AT, Hughes K, Shiloni E, et al. Intra-abdominal extrahepatic disease in patients with colorectal hepatic metastases. *Dis Colon Rectum* 1988;31:100.
82. Babineau TJ, Lewis WD, Jenkins RL, Bleday R, Steele GD. Role of staging laparoscopy in the treatment of hepatic malignancy. *Am J Surg* 1994;167:151.
83. Solomon MJ, Stephen MS, Gallinger S, White GH. Does intraoperative hepatic ultrasonography change surgical decision making during liver resection? *Am J Surg* 1994;168:307.
84. Callery MP, Starsberg SM, Doherty GM, et al. Staging laparoscopy with laparoscopic ultrasonography: optimizing respectability in hepatobiliary and pancreatic malignancy. *J Am Coll Surg* 1997;185:33.
85. Azurin DJ, Go LS, Kirkland ML. Laparoscopic evaluation of the liver. *Surg Rounds* 1995;(Oct):406.
86. Flowers JL, Feldman J, Jacobs SC. Laparoscopic pelvic lymphadenectomy. *Surg Laparosc Endosc* 1991;1:62.
87. Haas CA, Resnick MI. Laparoscopic pelvic and retroperitoneal lymph node dissection. *Semin Laparosc Surg* 1996;3:61.
88. Albala D, Galal HA, Gomella L. Laparoscopic pelvic lymph node dissection for prostate cancer. *Atlas Urol Clin* 1995;3:51.

89. Montie J. Counseling the patient with regional metastasis of prostate cancer. *Cancer* 1993;71[Suppl]:1019.
90. Kerbl K, Clayman RV, Petros JA, Chandhoke PS, Gill IS. Staging pelvic lymphadenectomy for prostate cancer: a comparison of laparoscopic and open techniques. *J Urol* 1993;150:396.
91. Burney TL, Campbell EC, Naslund MJ, Jacobs SC. Complications of staging laparoscopic pelvic lymphadenectomy. *Surg Laparosc Endosc* 1993;3:184.
92. Chow CC, Daly BD, Burney TL, et al. Complications after laparoscopic pelvic lymphadenectomy: CT diagnosis. *AJR Am J Roentgenol* 1994;163:353.
93. Williams SF, Golomb HM. Perspective on staging approaches in the malignant lymphomas. *Surg Gynecol Obstet* 1986;163:193.
94. Bloomfield CD, DeCosse JJ. Staging laparotomy. *Arch Surg* 1978;113:1135.
95. Urba WJ, Longo DL. Hodgkin's disease. *N Engl J Med* 1992;326:678.
96. Marble KR, Deckers PJ, Kern KA. Changing role of splenectomy for hematologic disease. *J Surg Oncol* 1993;52:169.
97. Martin JK, Clark SC, Beart RW, et al. Staging laparotomy in Hodgkin's disease: Mayo Clinic experience. *Arch Surg* 1982;117:586.
98. Schneeberger AL, Girvan DP. Staging laparotomy for Hodgkin's disease in children. *J Pediatr Surg* 1988;23:714.
99. Muskat PC, Johnson RA, Bowers GJ. Staging laparotomy in Hodgkin's lymphoma: 1979–1988. *Am J Surg* 1991;162:603.
100. Jockovich M, Mendenhall NP, Sombeck MD, et al. Long term complications of laparotomy in Hodgkin's disease. *Ann Surg* 1994;219:615.
101. Horowitz J, Smith JL, Weber TK, et al. Postoperative complications after splenectomy for hematologic malignancies. *Ann Surg* 1996;223:290.
102. Huang PP, Urist MM. Evaluation of abdominal Hodgkin's disease. *Surg Oncol Clin North Am* 1993;2:207.
103. Grieco MB, Cady B. Staging laparotomy in Hodgkin's disease. *Surg Clin North Am* 1980;60:369.
104. Baccarini U, Carroll BJ, Hiatt JR, et al. Comparison of laparoscopic and open staging in Hodgkin disease. *Arch Surg* 1998;133:517.
105. Greene FL, Cooler AW. Laparoscopic evaluation of lymphomas. *Semin Laparosc Surg* 1994;1:13.
106. Carroll BJ, Phillips EH, Semer CJ, et al. Laparoscopic splenectomy. *Surg Endosc* 1992:6:183.
107. Tulman S, Holcomb GW, Karamanoukian HL, Reynhout J. Pediatric laparoscopic splenectomy. *J Pediatr Surg* 1993;28:689.
108. Lefor AT, Flowers JL, Heyman M. Laparoscopic staging of Hodgkin's disease. *Surg Oncol* 1993;2:217.
109. Lefor AT. Laparoscopic staging of abdominal lymphomas. In: Greene F, ed. *Minimal access surgical oncology.* Oxford: Radcliffe, 1995.
110. Lefor AT, Flowers JL, Bailey RW, Melvin WS. Laparoscopic splenectomy in the management of immune thrombocytopenia purpura. *Surgery* 1993;114:613.
111. Poulin E, Thibault G, Mamazza J, et al. Laparoscopic splenectomy: clinical experience and the role of preoperative splenic artery embolization. *Surg Laparosc Endosc* 1993;3:445.
112. Poulin EC, Thibault C, Mamazza J. Laparoscopic splenectomy. *Surg Endosc* 1995;9:172.
113. Fujitani RM, Johs SM, Cobb SR, et al. Preoperative splenic artery occlusion as an adjunct for high risk splenectomy. *Am Surg* 1988;54:602.
114. Flowers JL, Lefor AT, Steers JA, et al. Laparoscopic splenectomy in patients with hematologic diseases. *Ann Surg* 1996;224:19.
115. Friedman RL, Fallas MJ, Carrol BJ, Phillips EH. Laparoscopic splenectomy for ITP: the gold standard. *Surg Endosc* 1996;10:991.
116. Diaz J, Eisenstat M, Chung R. A case controlled study of laparoscopic splenectomy. *Am J Surg* 1997;173:348.
117. Saldinger PF, Matthews JB, Mowchenson PM, et al. Stapled laparoscopic splenectomy. *J Am Coll Surg* 1996;182:459.
118. Brunt LM, Langer JC, Quasebarth MA, Whitman ED. Comparative analysis of laparoscopic versus open splenectomy. *Am J Surg* 1996;172:596.
119. Steers JA, Lefor AT, Flowers JL. Laparoscopic accessory splenectomy for recurrent thrombocytopenia. *Surg Rounds* 1994;17:477.
120. Katkhouda N, Hurwitz MB, Rivera RT, et al. Laparoscopic splenectomy: outcome and efficacy in 103 consecutive patients. *Ann Surg* 1998;228:568.
121. Schlinkert RT, Mann D, Weaver A. Laparoscopic splenectomy: reduction of hospital charges. *J Gastrointest Surg* 1998;2:278.
122. Rosenberg SA. Annotation: splenectomy in the management of Hodgkin's disease. *Br J Haematol* 1971;23:271.
123. Multani PS, Grossbard M. Staging laparotomy in the management of Hodgkin's disease: is it still necessary? *Oncologist* 1996;1:41.
124. Shaw JHF, Print CG. Postsplenectomy sepsis. *Br J Surg* 1989;76:1074.
125. Dawson AA, Jones PF, King DJ. Splenectomy in the management of haematologic disease. *Br J Surg* 1987;74:353.
126. Brody FJ, Chekan EG, Pappas TN, Eubanks WS. Conversion factors for laparoscopic splenectomy for immune thrombocytopenic purpura. *Surg Endosc* 1999;13:789.
127. Grossbard ML. Is laparoscopic splenectomy appropriate for the management of hematologic and oncologic disorders? *Surg Endosc* 1996;10:387.
128. Silecchia G, Fantini A, Raparelli L, et al. Management of abdominal lymphoproliferative diseases in the era of laparoscopy. *Am J Surg* 1999;177:325.
129. Rosenberg SA. Non-Hodgkin's lymphoma—selection of treatment on the basis of histologic type. *N Engl J Med* 1979;301:924.
130. Longo DL, DeVita VT, Jaffe ES, et al. Lymphocytic lymphomas. In: DeVita VT, Hellman S, Rosenberg SA, eds. *Cancer: principles and practice of oncology,* 4th ed. Philadelphia: JB Lippincott, 1993:1859.
131. Johna S, Lefor AT. Laparoscopic evaluation of lymphoma. *Semin Surg Oncol* 1998:15:176.
132. Moormeier JA, Williams SF, Golomb HM. The staging of Hodgkin's disease. *Hematol Oncol Clin North Am* 1989;3:237.
133. Palmer ML. Surgical considerations in lymphoma. *Contemp Surg* 1992;41:13.
134. Chi DS. Laparoscopy in gynecologic malignancies. *Oncology* 1999:13:773.
135. Goh PMY, Tekant Y, Kum CK. Totally intraabdominal laparoscopic Billroth II gastrectomy. *Surg Endosc* 1992;6:160.
136. Goh P. Laparoscopic Billroth II gastrectomy. *Semin Laparosc Surg* 1994;1:171.
137. Cuschieri A. Gastric resections. In: Scott-Conner C, ed. *The SAGES manual.* New York: Springer-Verlag New York, 1999:353.
138. Dean PA, Beart RW, Nelson H, Elftmann TD, Schlinkert RT. Laparoscopic assisted segmental colectomy: early Mayo Clinic experience. *Mayo Clin Proc* 1994;69:834.
139. Böhm B, Milsom JW, Kitago K, et al. Use of laparoscopic techniques in oncologic right colectomy in a canine model. *Ann Surg Oncol* 1995;2:6.
140. Elftmann TD, Nelson H, Ota DM, Pemberton JH, Beart RW. Laparoscopic assisted segmental colectomy: surgical techniques. *Mayo Clin Proc* 1994;69:825.
141. Cohen SM, Wexner SD. Laparoscopic right hemicolectomy. *Surg Rounds* 1994;(Nov):627.
142. Fielding GA, Lumley J, Nathanson L, et al. Laparoscopic colectomy. *Surg Endosc* 1997;11:745.
143. Ota DM. Laparoscopic colectomy for cancer: a favorable opinion. *Ann Surg Oncol* 1995;2:3.
144. Jager RM, Ballantyne GH, Fleshman JW, Franklin ME. The technical nuances in laparoscopic colorectal surgery. *Contemp Surg* 1994;45:355.
145. Reissman P, Teoh TA, Piccirillo M, Nogueras JJ, Wexner SD. Colonoscopic assisted laparoscopic colectomy. *Surg Endosc* 1994;8:1352.
146. Weiss EG, Wexner SD. Laparoscopic segmental colectomies, anterior resection and abdominoperineal resection. In: Scott-Conner C, ed. *The SAGES manual.* New York: Springer-Verlag New York, 1999.
147. Pandya S, Murray JJ, Coller JA, Rusin LC. Laparoscopic colectomy: indications for conversion to laparotomy. *Arch Surg* 1999;134:471.
148. Phillips EH, Franklin M, Carroll BJ, et al. Laparoscopic colectomy. *Ann Surg* 1992;216:703.
149. Falk PM, Beart RW, Wexner SD, et al. Laparoscopic colectomy: a critical appraisal. *Dis Colon Rectum* 1993;36:28.
150. Hoffman GC, Baker JW, Fitchett CW, Vansant JH. Laparoscopic assisted colectomy: initial experience. *Ann Surg* 1994;219:732.
151. Muckleroy SK, Ratzer ER, Fenoglio ME. Laparoscopic colon surgery for benign disease: a comparison to open surgery. *JSLS* 1999;3:33.
152. Franklin ME, Rosenthal D, Norem RF. Prospective evaluation of laparoscopic colon resection versus open colon resection for adenocarcinoma. *Surg Endosc* 1995;9:811.
153. Liberman MA, Phillips EH, Carroll BJ, et al. Laparoscopic colectomy vs traditional colectomy for diverticulitis. *Surg Endosc* 1996;10:15.
154. Lacy AM, Garcia-Valdecasas JC, Pique JM, et al. Short-term analysis of a randomized study comparing laparoscopic vs open colectomy for colon cancer. *Surg Endosc* 1995;9:1101.
155. Begos DG, Arsenault J, Ballantyne GH. Laparoscopic colon and rectal surgery at a VA hospital. *Surg Endosc* 1996;10:1050.
156. Wexner SD, Reissman P, Pfeiffer J, Bernstein M, Geron N. Laparoscopic colorectal surgery. *Surg Endosc* 1996;10:133.
157. Pfeifer J, Wexner SD, Reissman P, et al. Laparoscopic vs open colon surgery: costs and outcome. *Surg Endosc* 1996;10:1322.
158. Hoffman GC, Baker JW, Doxey JB, et al. Minimally invasive surgery for colorectal cancer: initial follow-up. *Ann Surg* 1996;223:790.
159. Huscher C, Silecchia G, Croce E, et al. Laparoscopic colorectal resection: a multicenter Italian study. *Surg Endosc* 1996;10:875.
160. Poulin EC, Mamazza J, Schlachta CM, et al. Laparoscopic resection does not adversely affect early survival curves in patients undergoing surgery for colorectal adenocarcinoma. *Ann Surg* 1999;229:487.
161. Greene FL. Laparoscopic management of colorectal cancer. *CA Cancer J Clin* 1999,49:221.
162. Gellman L, Salky B, Edye M. Laparoscopic assisted colectomy. *Surg Endosc* 1996;10:1041.
163. Kwok SP, Carey PD, Li AKC. Prospective evaluation of laparoscopic assisted large bowel excision for cancer. *Ann Surg* 1996;223:170.
164. Berman IR. Laparoscopic colectomy for cancer: some cause for pause. *Ann Surg Oncol* 1995;2:1.
165. Sugarbaker PH. Wound recurrence after laparoscopic colectomy for cancer: new rationale for intraoperative intraperitoneal chemotherapy. *Surg Endosc* 1996;10:295.
166. Milsom JW, Bohm B, Hammerhofer KA, et al. A prospective randomized trial comparing laparoscopic versus conventional techniques in colorectal cancer surgery: a preliminary report. *J Am Coll Surg* 1998;187:46.
167. Ota DM. Laparoscopic colon resection for cancer. *Surg Endosc* 1996;10:1318.
168. Abi-Rached B, Neugut AJ. Diagnostic and management issues in gallbladder carcinoma. *Oncology* 1995;9:19.
169. Targarona EM, Pons MJ, Viella P, Trias M. Unsuspected carcinoma of the gallbladder: a laparoscopic dilemma. *Surg Endosc* 1994;8:211.
170. Copher JC, Rogers JJ, Dalton ML. Trocar site metastasis following laparoscopic cholecystectomy for unsuspected carcinoma of the gallbladder. *Surg Endosc* 1995;9:348.
171. Cubertafond P, Gainant A, Cucchiaro G. Surgical treatment of 724 carcinomas of the gallbladder. *Ann Surg* 1994;219:275.
172. Sariego J, Aharonian A, Byrd M, Matsumoto T, Kerstein M. Adenocarcinoma of the gallbladder. *Contemp Surg* 1994;44:91.
173. Fong Y, Brennan MF, Turnbull A, Coit DG, Blumgart LH. Gallbladder cancer discovered during laparoscopic surgery. *Arch Surg* 1993;128:1054.
174. Yamaguchi K, Chijiiwa K, Ichimiya H, et al. Gallbladder carcinoma in the era of laparoscopic cholecystectomy. *Arch Surg* 1996;131:981.
175. Lomis KD, Vitola JV, Delbeke D, et al. Recurrent gallbladder carcinoma at laparoscopy port sites diagnosed by positron emission tomography. *Am Surg* 1997;63:341.

176. Ferzli GS, Daou R. Laparoscopic cholecystectomy and gallbladder cancer. *Surg Endosc* 1994;8:1357.
177. Tate JJ, Lau WY, Li AK. Transhepatic fenestration of liver cyst: a further application of laparoscopic surgery. *Aust N Z J Surg* 1994;64:264.
178. Katkhouda N, Hurwitz M, Gugenheim J, et al. Laparoscopic management of benign solid and cystic lesions of the liver. *Ann Surg* 1999;229:460.
179. Payne HH. Ultrasonic dissector. *Surg Endosc* 1994;8:416.
180. Baer HU, Metzger A, Barras JP, et al. Laparoscopic liver resection in the large white pig: a comparison between waterjet dissector and ultrasound dissector. *Endosc Surg Allied Technol* 1994;2:189.
181. Azagra JS. Laparoscopic left lateral segmentectomy. Proceedings of the 1st International Congress, European Association of Surgical Sciences, Ischia, Italy, 1994.
182. Ravikumar TS, Kane R, Cady B, et al. A 5-year study of cryosurgery in the treatment of liver tumors. *Arch Surg* 1991;126:1520.
183. Curley SA, Izzo F, Delrio P, et al. Radiofrequency ablation of unresectable primary and metastatic hepatic malignancies: results in 123 patients. *Ann Surg* 1999;230:1.
184. Rose DM, Allegra DP, Bostick PJ, et al. Radiofrequency ablation: a novel primary and adjunctive ablative technique for hepatic malignancies. *Am Surg* 1999;65:1009.
185. Neuberger TJ, Wade TP, Swope TJ, Virgo KS, Johnson FE. Palliative operations for pancreatic cancer in the hospitals of the U.S. Department of Veterans Affairs from 1987 to 1991. *Am J Surg* 1993;166:632.
186. Lillemoe KD. Current management of pancreatic carcinoma. *Ann Surg* 1995;221:133.
187. Gagner M, Pomp A. Laparoscopic pylorus-preserving pancreaticoduodenectomy. *Surg Endosc* 1994;8:408.
188. Salky BA. Distal pancreatectomy In: Scott-Conner C, ed. *The SAGES manual.* New York: Springer-Verlag New York, 1999:307.
189. Cuschieri A, Jakimowicz JJ, van Spreeuwel J. Laparoscopic distal 70% pancreatectomy and splenectomy for chronic pancreatitis. *Ann Surg* 1996;3:280.
190. Clayman RV, Kavoussi LR, McDougall EM. Laparoscopic nephrectomy: a review of 16 cases. *Surg Laparosc Endosc* 1992;2:29.
191. Clayman RV, Kavoussi LR, Soper NJ, et al. Laparoscopic nephrectomy: initial case report. *J Urol* 1991;146:278.
192. Clayman RV, Long SL, Kavoussi LR, et al. Laparoscopic nephrectomy. *N Engl J Med* 1991;324:1370.
193. Luciani RC, Greiner M, Clement JC, Houot A, Didierlaurent JF. Laparoscopic enucleation of a renal cell carcinoma. *Surg Endosc* 1994;8:1329.
194. Phillips EH, Carroll BJ, Fallas MJ. Laparoscopic splenectomy. *Surg Endosc* 1994;8:931.
195. Cadiere GB, Verroken R, Himpens J, et al. Operative strategy in laparoscopic splenectomy. *J Am Coll Surg* 1994;179:668.
196. Park A, Marcaccio M, Sternbach M, Witzke D, Fitzgerald P. Laparoscopic vs open splenectomy. *Arch Surg* 1999;134:1263.
197. Ferzli GS, Hurwitz JB, Fiorillo MA, et al. Laparoscopic splenectomy in a Jehovah's witness with profound anemia. *Surg Endosc* 1997;11:850.
198. Llende M, Santiago-Delpin EA, Lavergne J. Immunobiological consequences of splenectomy. *J Surg Res* 1986;40:85.
199. Weintraub LR. Splenectomy: who, when and why? *Hosp Pract (Off Ed)* 1994;29:27.
200. Hashizume M, Sugimachi K, Kitano S, et al. Laparoscopic splenectomy. *Am J Surg* 1994;167:611.
201. Akwari OE, Itani KMF, Coleman RE, Rosse WF. Splenectomy for primary and recurrent immune thrombocytopenia purpura. *Ann Surg* 1987;206:529.
202. Coon WW. Splenectomy for idiopathic thrombocytopenic purpura. *Surg Gynecol Obstet* 1987;164:225.
203. Hoekstra HJ, Tamminga RYJ, Timens W. Partial splenectomy in children: an alternative for splenectomy in the pathologic staging of Hodgkin's disease. *Ann Surg Oncol* 1994;1:480.
204. Takeda M, Go H, Imai T, Nishiyama T, Morishita H. Laparoscopic adrenalectomy for primary aldosteronism: report of initial ten cases. *Surgery* 1994;115:621.
205. Fernandez-Cruz L, Benarroch G, Torres E, et al. Laparoscopic approach to adrenal tumors. *J Laparoendosc Surg* 1993;3:541.
206. Gagner M, Lacroix A, Prinz RA, et al. Early experience with laparoscopic approach for adrenalectomy. *Surgery* 1993;114:1120.
207. Ting ACW, Lo CY, Lo CM. Posterior or laparoscopic approach for adrenalectomy. *Am J Surg* 1998;175:488.
208. Imai T, Kikumori T, Ohiwa M, et al. A case-controlled study of laparoscopic compared with open lateral adrenalectomy. *Am J Surg* 1999;178:50.
209. Walther MM. Laparoscopic surgery for adrenal disease. *PPO Updates* 1997;11:1.
210. Schmidt N. Strategic management of adrenal tumors. *Oncology* 1994;8:73.
211. Arca MJ, Gagner M. Laparoscopic adrenalectomy. In: Scott-Connor C, ed. *The SAGES manual.* New York: Springer-Verlag New York, 1999:353.
212. Milsom JW, Hammerhofer KA. Role of laparoscopic techniques in colorectal cancer surgery. *Oncology* 1995;9:393.
213. Shima SM, Banting SB, Cuschieri A. Laparoscopy in the management of pancreatic cancer. *Br J Surg* 1992;79:317.
214. Hawasli A. Laparoscopic cholecysto-jejunostomy for obstructing pancreatic cancer. *J Laparoendosc Surg* 1992;1:351.
215. Mouiel J. Palliative laparoscopic surgery for abdominal malignancies. *Semin Laparosc Surg* 1994;1:26.
216. Lillemoe KD, Cameron JL, Kaufman HS, et al. Chemical splanchnicectomy in patients with unresectable pancreatic cancer. *Ann Surg* 1993;217:447.
217. Grant JP. Comparison of percutaneous endoscopic gastrostomy with Stamm gastrostomy. *Ann Surg* 1988;207:598.
218. Murayama K, Schneider PD, Thompson JS. Laparoscopic gastrostomy: a safe method for obtaining enteral access. *J Surg Res* 1995;58:1.
219. Lee DS, Mohit-Tabatabai MA, Rush BF, Levine C. Stomal seeding of head and neck cancer by percutaneous endoscopic gastrostomy tube placement. *Ann Surg Oncol* 1995;2:170.
220. Edelman DS, Unger SW. Laparoscopic gastrostomy. *Surg Gynecol Obstet* 1992;174:401.
221. Ota DM, Evans DB, Mansfield PF. Placement of a feeding jejunostomy. In: Ballantyne GH, Leahy PF, Modlin IM, eds. *Laparoscopic surgery.* Philadelphia: WB Saunders, 1993:467.
222. Leitman IM, Sullivan JD, Brams D, DeCosse JJ. Multivariate analysis of morbidity and mortality from the initial surgical management of obstructing carcinoma of the colon. *Surg Gynecol Obstet* 1992;174:513.
223. Lange V, Meyer G, Shardey HM, Schildberg MD. Laparoscopic creation of a loop colostomy. *J Laparoendosc Surg* 1991;1:307.
224. Lyerly HK, Mault JR. Laparoscopic ileostomy and colostomy. *Ann Surg* 1994;219:317.
225. Ota DM. Laparoscopic management of colon cancer. *Semin Laparosc Surg* 1994;1:18.
226. Cuschieri A. Whither minimal access surgery: tribulations and expectations. *Am J Surg* 1995;169:9.
227. Soper NJ, Brunt LM, Kerbl K. Laparoscopic general surgery. *N Engl J Med* 1994;330:409.
228. Lacy AM, Delgado S, Garcia-Valdecasas JC, et al. Port site metastases and recurrence after laparoscopic colectomy: a randomized trial. *Surg Endosc* 1998;12:1039.

SECTION 2

STEVEN K. LIBUTTI
MCDONALD K. HORNE III

Vascular Access and Specialized Techniques of Drug Delivery

The complex management of the cancer patient frequently relies on the ability to deliver a variety of intravenous or intraarterial agents over a prolonged period. Chemotherapy, anesthesia, analgesics, and total parenteral nutrition may be required alone or in combination. Certain drug delivery systems may be more appropriate than others, depending on the particular situation. Since their introduction in the early 1970s, significant changes and improvements have been made in indwelling catheters and infusion devices.[1,2] All physicians who are involved in caring for cancer patients should have a basic understanding of the uses and limitations of these devices. An understanding of the issues involved in catheter selection, techniques of insertion, routine maintenance, and treatment for catheter-related complications, allows the physician and the patient to optimize the use of these devices.

CATHETER TYPES

A variety of catheter types are available, each with its own intrinsic advantages and disadvantages. The choice of which one to use is based on a variety of factors, including type of agent to be infused, length of time the catheter is to be used, number of concurrent therapies requiring intravascular routes, need for blood draws, desirability of continuous infusion, and patient (or physician) preference. Given the number of available systems, it is convenient to divide catheters into two broad categories. The first group are those catheters having an external component, represented by devices such as the Hickman, Groshong, or Broviac (Bard Access Systems, Salt Lake City, UT). The second group are devices that can be completely internalized or implanted, such as Portacaths and infusion pumps. (Sims Deltec, Inc., St. Paul, MN).

EXTERNAL DEVICES

The simplest and most straightforward central venous access catheter is a single-lumen 16-gauge catheter positioned in either the subclavian, internal jugular, or femoral vein. When inserted using sterile technique, these catheters can generally remain in place for 7 to 10 days, and they allow for the acute infusion of a variety of agents. The catheter is not tunneled, and therefore it is at risk for both infection and migration. Although a simple central line can be very useful, these catheters are not appropriate for long-term or outpatient intravenous therapy.

The Hickman- or Broviac-type catheters are made of barium impregnated silicone rubber (Silastic, Dow Corning Corporation, Midland, MI) and are available as single- or double-lumen devices in both pediatric and adult sizes. These catheters can be tunneled under the skin and have a Dacron cuff, which is implanted in the subcutaneous tissue just above the exit site. This cuff is intended to promote fibrous ingrowth and scarring, which serves to lessen the likelihood of catheter migration and infection. Although some early suggestion was made that silver ion impregnation of the cuff might further reduce the incidence of catheter-related bacteremia,[3,4] prospective randomized studies have not supported any benefit of silver ion impregnation.[5,6] It appears that the mechanical barrier provided by the fibrous reaction to the cuff is sufficient. The Groshong-type catheter is similar to the Hickman and Broviac designs in all respects except for the tip. The Groshong tip is modified with a slit valve to prevent the passive reflux of blood into the lumen (Fig. 29.2-1). The valve only opens when positive or negative pressure is applied to it, such as during infusion or withdrawal of fluid, thereby reducing the frequency with which the catheter must be flushed. These catheters can normally be flushed with saline alone. However, Mayo et al. have

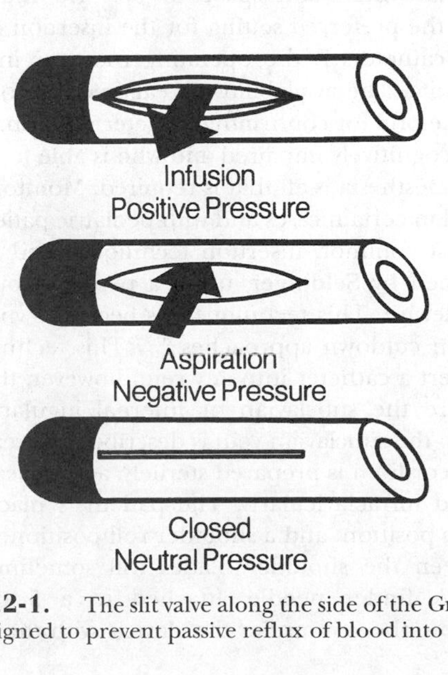

FIGURE 29.2-1. The slit valve along the side of the Groshong catheter tip is designed to prevent passive reflux of blood into the lumen.

shown that the addition of a weekly heparinized saline flush decreased the presence of intraluminal adherent clots and improved the catheter function.[7] This study also demonstrated that the slit valve is frequently incompetent.

Considerable interest has been focused on peripherally inserted central catheters (PICC lines).[8–12] These lines can be inserted in a peripheral vein in the arm using a Seldinger technique or a "through the needle" technique and threaded into the subclavian vein. Advantages include ease of insertion and the low risk of serious complication. Skilled nurses trained in the insertion technique can perform the procedure at the bedside with results similar to those obtained by interventional radiologists.[11] For initial insertions, this approach has proven very cost-effective. If maintained properly, these lines can last for as long as 1 year and can be used for chemotherapy[12] or total parenteral nutrition.[13]

IMPLANTED DEVICES

Since their introduction, implantable ports have become popular with patients and clinicians alike.[14] These devices are constructed from a variety of materials, including titanium and plastic, and can be made compatible with magnetic resonance imaging (MRI) and computed tomography (CT). The general design includes a compressed silicone diaphragm, which can withstand repeated punctures with a Huber needle. A comparison of a typical external catheter device with an implantable port is shown in Figure 29.2-2. The device shown is a single-lumen port; however, dual-lumen models are also available. These ports are typically inserted in the operating room. The technique used for the insertion of the catheter itself is identical to that used for external catheters and is described in detail in the section Insertion Technique. The port housing is placed in a subcutaneous pocket on the chest wall. Care needs to be taken to make sure that the diaphragm of the port can be palpated through the overlying tissue to allow for access to the device. The port housing is anchored to the underlying fascia by several interrupted sutures. Unlike external catheters, removal of a port generally requires a repeat trip to the operating room to perform a cutdown over the port and a removal of the device from the subcutaneous pocket. If the device is removed because of infection, the pocket should be left open to close by secondary intention to prevent the formation of an abscess.

Comparisons have been made between external catheters and implanted ports with respect to infection rates, patency, and long-term complications such as vessel thrombosis.[15–21] Most studies have demonstrated comparable rates of infection between external and implanted devices, with the implanted devices having a longer durability of usage.[19] Overall, the majority of studies have not demonstrated one system to be overwhelmingly superior to the other. The main determinants of catheter survival, regardless of whether the device is external or implanted, are still careful placement and careful maintenance.

Improvements in port design have allowed for the construction of very low profile, small devices that can be implanted in the subcutaneous tissue of the arm with the catheter threaded in a similar fashion as a PICC line. These devices, referred to by their trade name as *Pasports* (Sims Deltec, Inc., St. Paul, MN), can be inserted in the operating room or imaging suite using local anesthesia. Comparisons between these devices, standard Portacaths, and external catheters have shown that both the

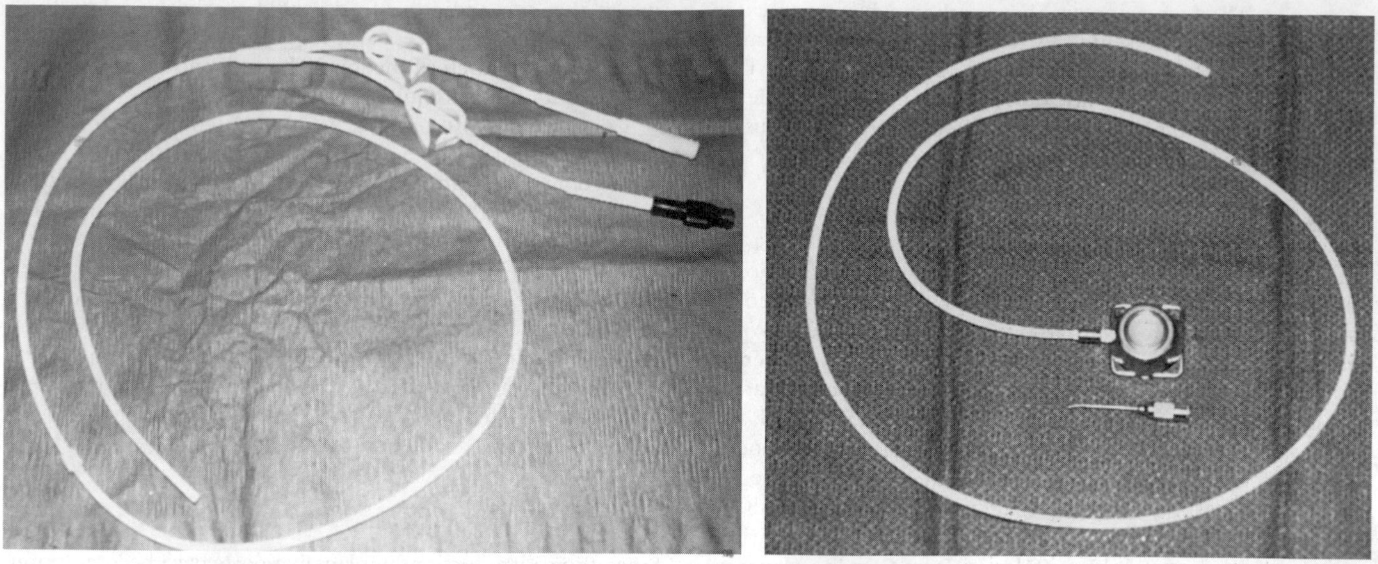

FIGURE 29.2-2. **A:** Dual-lumen 10 Fr. Hickman catheter showing the Dacron cuff. **B:** Implantable venous access device. A noncoring Huber needle is also shown. The housing of the port can be made of titanium (pictured) or plastic.

Portacath and Pasport have a reduced incidence of infectious complications when compared to external catheters.[22]

Implantable Infusion Pumps

Although the implantable ports have been an advance in convenience and comfort for patients, they still must be connected to an external infusion system. This is true whether the port is placed for intravenous or intraarterial access. The reliance on the external pump has been partially supplanted by completely implanted subcutaneous infusion pumps.

The implantable devices are larger, but they resemble infusion ports in many respects (Fig. 29.2-3). The earliest devices were used to deliver long-term heparin therapy for patients with thrombotic complications.[23] Using such a system, patients were able to receive long-term continuous intravenous therapy for periods of up to 1 year.[24]

The first implantable pump to be introduced was manufactured by Infusaid and was known by the same name (it is now produced by Arrow International (Reading, PA).[14] This system weighed slightly less than 200 g when it was empty and was positioned in the subcutaneous tissues of the abdominal wall. The pump delivers a constant rate, determined by internal flow resistors, and is powered by the pressure generated from the expansion of a liquid fluorocarbon to the gaseous phase at body temperature. As the drug reservoir is filled percutaneously through a septum, the surrounding fluorocarbon chamber is recharged as gas is compressed and condensed into the liquid phase. The newest models have a side-access septum that bypasses the infusion system and allows for direct delivery of a flush or bolus of medication.

Although its main use has been in the delivery of intraarterial chemotherapy via the gastroduodenal artery for the regional treatment of liver metastases,[25–28] the Infusaid pump has been used to deliver insulin intravenously,[29] as well as morphine for intractable pain.[30] The current models are smaller than their predecessors, resulting in improved patient comfort (see Fig. 29.2-3). Other implantable systems using battery-powered peristaltic or solenoid pump mechanisms are also available. A telemetry system transmits or receives signals from the totally implanted device, which can turn the pump on or off, adjust the delivery rate, and determine battery voltage.[31] Although these implantable pumps can save patients the inconvenience of carrying an external device and free them from the need to be attached to an intravenous line, they can be expensive. As the number of uses for these devices increases, however, the costs will undoubtedly decline.

INSERTION TECHNIQUE

The single most important aspect of catheter insertion is to strictly adhere to sterile technique. To do this, it is important to have adequate light and space to perform the procedure. Therefore, the preferred setting for the insertion of long-term indwelling catheters is the operating room or interventional radiology suite. The availability of real-time fluoroscopy is also extremely helpful for confirming catheter position. In a patient who is not cognitively impaired and who is able to follow direction, local anesthesia is all that is required. Monitored sedation can be used in certain cases and with pediatric patients.

The most common insertion technique used today is the one described by Seldinger, using a percutaneous approach over a guidewire. This technique has been shown to be superior to open cutdown approaches.[20,32] This technique can be used to insert a catheter into any vein; however, the preferred locations are the subclavian or internal jugular veins. The approach to the subclavian vein is described in greater detail.

The precordium is prepared sterilely, and a local anesthetic is infiltrated infraclavicularly. The patient is placed in Trendelenburg's position, and a shoulder roll positioned longitudinally between the shoulder blades will sometimes facilitate insertion. A finder needle attached to a 5-cc syringe is advanced into the vein under the clavicle with the bevel of the

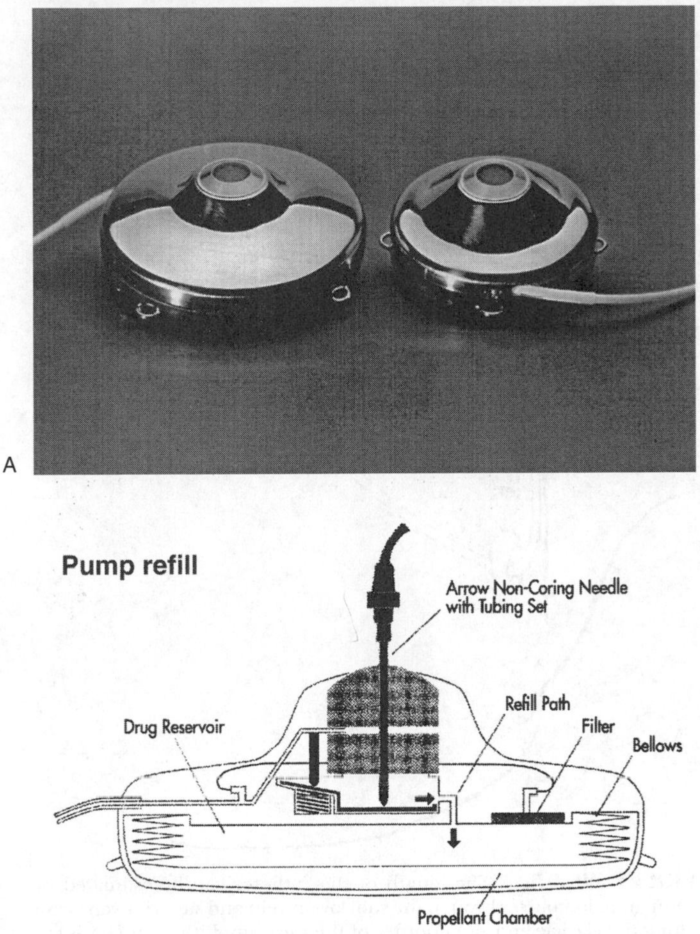

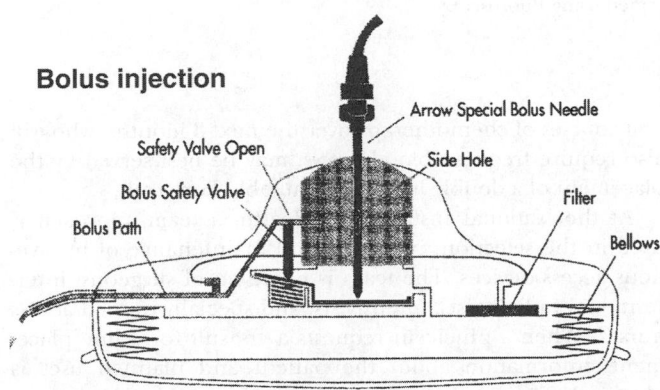

FIGURE 29.2-3. **A:** The implantable infusion pump (Arrow International, Reading, PA), which comes in various sizes. The smaller pump is used for the infusion of narcotic analgesics either intravenously or via an intraspinal route. **B:** A schematic representation of how the pump system works. Body heat causes the propellant to shift from a liquid to a gaseous phase, which compresses the bellows and allows for the drug to be dispensed. When the drug reservoir is refilled, the propellant is compressed and shifts back into a liquid phase.

needle facing up. Gentle aspiration is applied until blood freely flows into the syringe. If there is any question as to whether the needle is in an artery or a vein, a central venous pressure line can be connected to confirm a venous insertion.

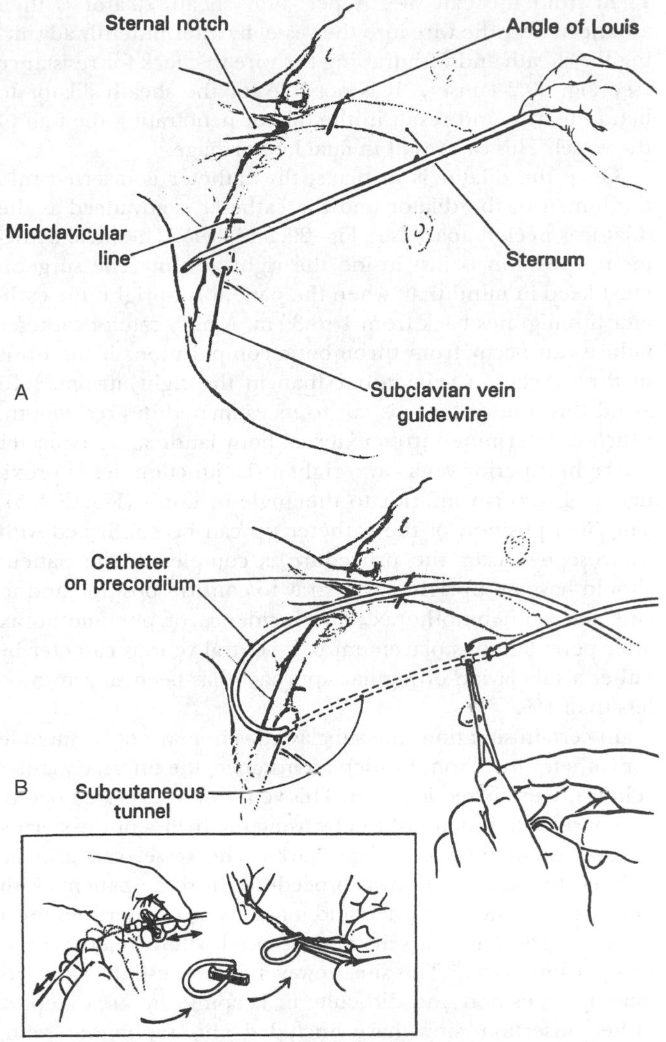

FIGURE 29.2-4. Insertion of a long-term indwelling central venous catheter via a subclavian approach using a percutaneous technique. **A:** After insertion of the guidewire, the catheter is tunneled from the chosen exit site to the venous cannulation site. **B:** The Dacron cuff is placed subcutaneously 1 cm above the exit site. **Inset:** As the sheath/dilator is advanced over the guidewire, care is taken to ensure that the dilator is advancing along the course of the wire by intermittently moving the wire back and advancing the dilator. After trimming the catheter to the proper length, it is advanced through the peel-away sheath.

Once the needle is in the vein, it is rotated 90 degrees and the syringe is disconnected, taking care not to allow air into the vein through the needle. A flexible guidewire is then advanced into the needle. If advancement of the guidewire meets with any resistance, it is not intraluminal and the wire should be removed. The needle should then be repositioned and aspiration of venous blood reconfirmed.

Once the wire has been successfully inserted, its position can be confirmed with fluoroscopy. At this point, a site on the precordium is selected for the catheter exit site (Fig. 29.2-4). After infiltrating the tissues with local anesthetic, a small incision is made at the exit site as well as adjacent to where the wire enters the skin. The catheter is then tunneled under the skin subcutaneously until the Dacron cuff is situated approximately

1 cm from the exit site. A peel-away sheath dilator is then advanced over the wire into the vessel by intermittently advancing the sheath and withdrawing the wire to check for resistance (see Fig. 29.2-4 inset). It is possible for the sheath dilator to bend the wire and result in the dilator penetrating the wall of the vessel. This can result in fatal hemorrhage.

Once the dilator is in place, the catheter is inserted into the lumen of the dilator and the catheter is advanced as the dilator is peeled apart (see Fig. 29.2-4 inset). The ideal catheter tip position is just inside the right atrium. The surgeon must keep in mind that, when the patient is upright, the catheter tip migrates back from 1 to 3 cm. A high rate of catheter failure can occur from thrombotic complications if the tip is in the subclavian vein rather than in the right atrium.[33] To avoid this, the catheter is cut to its estimated desired length, which is determined from external bony landmarks. Typically, the right superior vena cava/right atrial junction lies approximately 4 to 6 cm inferior to the angle of Louis (Fig. 29.2-5). The final position of the catheter tip can be confirmed with fluoroscopy. After the procedure is completed, the patient should have an upright chest x-ray to confirm position and to rule out a pneumothorax. The incidence of pneumothorax after percutaneous placement of a central venous catheter by either a subclavian or jugular approach has been shown to be less than 1%.[34]

In certain situations the subclavian vein may not be suitable for catheter insertion. In such an instance, the internal jugular vein is the preferred location. This vein can be accessed percutaneously in a similar fashion by using the bellies of the sternocleidomastoid muscle as landmarks. The vessel can also be isolated through a cutdown procedure. In some patients with occlusions of the subclavian and jugular veins, other sites must be used. The femoral vein may be used with a relatively low complication rate.[35] This site, however, is less desirable given its anatomic position and difficulty in keeping the area aseptic. Other insertion sites have included the saphenous vein, gonadal vein, intercostal vein, or azygous vein, or direct placement into the inferior vena cava.[35–39]

After the successful placement of a long-term indwelling central venous catheter, certain routine postoperative maintenance procedures should be performed to increase the durability of the catheter. Careful attention should be paid to the maintenance of catheter patency and to the catheter exit site to ensure it is kept clean. Although there is some discrepancy among catheter manufacturers, external catheters are typically flushed daily or every other day with a heparin solution or saline when they are not in use.

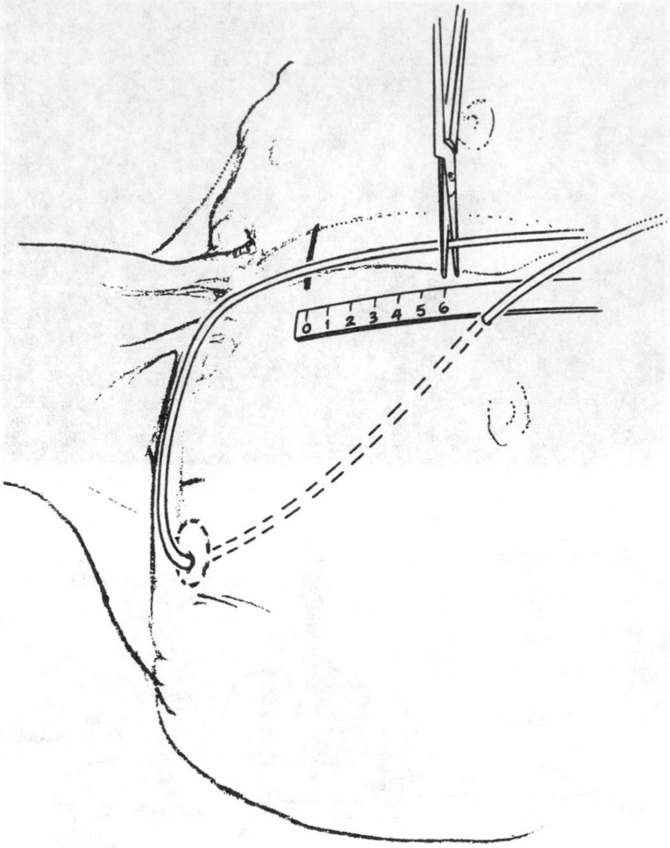

FIGURE 29.2-5. The length of the catheter can be estimated by simulating its course through the subclavian vein and superior vena cava along the clavicle and right border of the sternum. If the catheter is cut 6 cm inferior to the angle of Louis, it approximates a final position at the superior vena caval and atrial junction. Tip position should be confirmed using fluoroscopy.

SELECTING THE APPROPRIATE CATHETER

The selection of the right catheter for a particular patient must be based on an assessment of a number of factors. Consideration must be given to the intended use of the catheter and how long the catheter will be needed. For example, a patient who needs 2 weeks of intravenous antibiotics as an outpatient will probably be best served by having a single-lumen external catheter placed, which can be more easily removed when the course of therapy is completed. Some evidence suggests that single-lumen catheters pose less of an infection risk than dual-lumen devices.[40] In contrast, a patient expected to receive several courses of chemotherapy over the next 3 months, who will also require frequent blood draws, may be best served by the placement of a double-lumen implantable Portacath.

At the National Institutes of Health, a team approach is used in the selection, insertion, and maintenance of intravenous access devices. The team is made up of surgeons, interventional radiologists, intensivists, and specially trained access nurses. When a physician requests a consult for a line placement, information about the patient and planned uses is obtained. The most important issues, in addition to type of agent to be infused and duration of planned use, are history of previous indwelling catheters, patency of central veins (duplex Doppler examinations are obtained if necessary), the patient's ability to maintain the catheter, age of the patient, size of the patient, and need for blood draws. All of these issues are factored into the selection of the appropriate device. The Vascular Access Device (VAD) Service then assists in patient teaching both before and after the device is inserted. Once the device is in place, the VAD Service then tracks information regarding outcome. Programs such as this have been shown to enable the patient and the physician to derive the longest possible benefit from the vascular access device and to minimize complications.[41]

CATHETER-RELATED COMPLICATIONS

CATHETER MALFUNCTION

Catheters leak or break because of defective construction or because they are pinched between the clavicle and first rib when the patient is upright.[42,43] More commonly, infusion through a VAD may be difficult because of a kink in the catheter, a forgotten suture holding it in place, or precipitates of salts or medications obstructing the lumen. The latter can sometimes be removed with instillation of 0.1 N HCl or 70% ethanol.[44,45]

The most common type of VAD malfunction, however, is the inability to withdraw blood from the catheter without difficulty infusing through it. Withdrawal occlusion not only prevents use of the VAD for blood sampling, but also is a sign that fluid injected through the catheter may not be entering freely flowing blood in the superior vena cava. Continuously bathing a small vein with a nonphysiologic solution may lead to chemical phlebitis.[46,47] Withdrawal occlusion is caused by an obstruction at the catheter tip that acts as a one-way valve. It occurs when aspiration pulls the wall of a vein against the catheter orifice. This is especially likely if the catheter tip is in a vein smaller than the superior vena cava. Even if the VAD has been properly placed initially, the catheter tip can migrate into the contralateral innominate or a jugular vein as a result of postural changes.[46,47] More commonly, it can be pulled back into the ipsilateral innominate vein by traction applied by the chest wall, or partially retracted so that the tip is held perpendicular to the superior vena cava wall.[48]

Malpositioning of a catheter can often be identified by a chest x-ray. The problem can be relieved, at least temporarily, by having the patient stand, raise his or her arms, or use Valsalva's maneuver to move the catheter tip. Interventional radiologists can sometimes return a migrant catheter to the superior vena cava with a snare.[42] In the long run, however, poor catheter position is typically associated with recurrent malfunction and ultimately requires replacement of the VAD.

Catheter tips that rub against the vein may stimulate local thrombosis, which can also cause withdrawal occlusion and sometimes anchor the tip to the venous wall. Even in good position, however, catheters virtually always accumulate a coat of fibrin.[49,50] If this "sheath" extends to the catheter orifice, it can act as a one-way valve to obstruct withdrawal.[50] In extreme cases, these fibrin sheaths can extend from the tip of the catheter to the point where it enters the vein. This not only creates withdrawal occlusion but provides a channel for infusates to backtrack and possibly extravasate.[51] Withdrawal occlusion that is not relieved by changing the patient's position, therefore, suggests the possibility that the obstruction is actually due to a fibrin sheath.

An effort can be made to dissolve the obstructing fibrin by instilling a thrombolytic agent through the obstructed catheter into the suspected sheath, where it is left to dwell for 1 to 2 hours before re-attempting withdrawal. Although the traditional thrombolytic agent for this indication has been urokinase, this drug is now unavailable and has been replaced by instillations of recombinant tissue plasminogen activator (rtPA) in a concentration of 1 mg/mL.[52,53] Usually 2 to 3 mL are infused and left for 2 hours before withdrawal is attempted.

If this treatment is not successful, the cause of the withdrawal occlusion should be investigated further. If a chest x-ray has not already been taken, one should be performed to confirm that the catheter tip is properly positioned in the superior vena cava. Then x-ray contrast material should be injected through the obstructed lumen to look for a fibrin sheath, which is detected as a tubular structure filled with contrast encasing the catheter.[51,54] If the presence of a fibrin sheath is confirmed, repeat instillations of rtPA can be tried. In the past, regimens of continuously infused urokinase were often successful in relieving obstructions refractory to routine instillations of the drug.[54] Experience using rtPA in a similar manner, however, is quite limited.

Open-ended catheters have traditionally been flushed with low-dose heparin on a regular schedule to reduce the risk of thrombotic obstruction of the catheter. However, the value of this technique has not been proven, except perhaps with dosing schedules that are not practical on a long-term outpatient basis.[55,56] A reason not to use heparin flushes is the risk, albeit a low one, of heparin-induced thrombocytopenia and thrombosis.[57–59] In addition, coagulation tests cannot be reliably performed with blood drawn through heparinized VADs, even with a large discard volume.[60]

VENOUS THROMBOSIS

Thrombi usually originate at the point where a catheter enters the vein or at any point where it chronically rubs against the venous wall. Symptomatic thrombosis of the catheterized vein develops in 5% to 10% of patients with VADs.[61,62] Most VAD-related venous thrombosis, however, is asymptomatic, occurring in approximately 30% to 70% of patients.[61,62] Thrombi develop soon after the catheter is placed and usually remain clinically silent because abundant collateral veins relieve the pressure as the primary vein becomes obstructed.[62] It is important to be aware of asymptomatic thrombosis as a potential nidus of infection as well as a source of pulmonary emboli.[50,63] Furthermore, because thrombosis may leave the vein permanently obstructed, it may create a problem for an unsuspecting surgeon who attempts to re-catheterize the vein at a later time.[61]

The management of symptomatic VAD-related thrombosis must be individualized. The catheter rarely must be removed immediately and does not necessarily have to be removed until the need for it has passed.[64] Prompt relief of symptoms is often achieved by simply elevating the affected arm overnight. Most patients also receive systemic anticoagulation in the form of heparin, followed by warfarin for several months, with the rationale that this prevents the thrombus from extending.[64–66] However, the risk of extension is unknown. Anticoagulation also is recommended to prevent pulmonary emboli, which are reported to occur in 10% to 15% of patients with upper extremity deep venous thrombosis and can be fatal.[63,67,68] Small emboli, however, frequently occur when the catheters are removed, but the minimal morbidity from these does not justify routine evaluation or therapeutic intervention before explantation.[69] The more threatening emboli appear to be much less commonly associated with the modern silicone and polyurethane catheters.[67] The risk of chronic venous insufficiency due to thrombosis in the axillary-subclavian vein may also be a consideration. On the other hand, the most important issues are often the need for long-term venous access and the risks of antithrombotic treatment.

With the introduction of low-molecular-weight heparin, hospitalization is no longer necessary for initial anticoagulation.[70]

Subcutaneous low-molecular-weight heparin and oral warfarin can be started together and the heparin continued for at least 5 days and until the patient's international normalized ratio has been between 2 and 3 for 2 days. The necessary duration of warfarin therapy is unknown. It can be argued that warfarin should be continued as long as the VAD is in place but that 4 to 6 weeks of warfarin is sufficient if the VAD is removed after the thrombus is discovered.[64,65] However, no clinical trials have tested this recommendation, and extenuating circumstances often dictate the anticoagulant regime for an individual patient.

Thrombolytic therapy of VAD-related thrombosis may be reasonable when salvaging the vein is a high priority because anticoagulation alone will probably not leave the vein patent enough to be used for subsequent VADs (Fig. 29.2-6). A regimen using relatively low doses of rtPA has been published.[71,72] Long-term patency, however, generally requires that the catheter be removed while anticoagulation is continued for several weeks or months.[71]

Of course, effective prophylaxis would eliminate the problem of VAD-related thrombosis. This reportedly can be achieved with very low-dose warfarin (1 mg/day) or with low-molecular-weight heparin.[73–75] However, the benefit of these regimens was demonstrated in patients with an unusually high incidence of symptomatic thrombosis, and therefore it is not clear how easily these results can be generalized. The value of prophylactic warfarin was not apparent in a population of less hypercoagulable patients.[76]

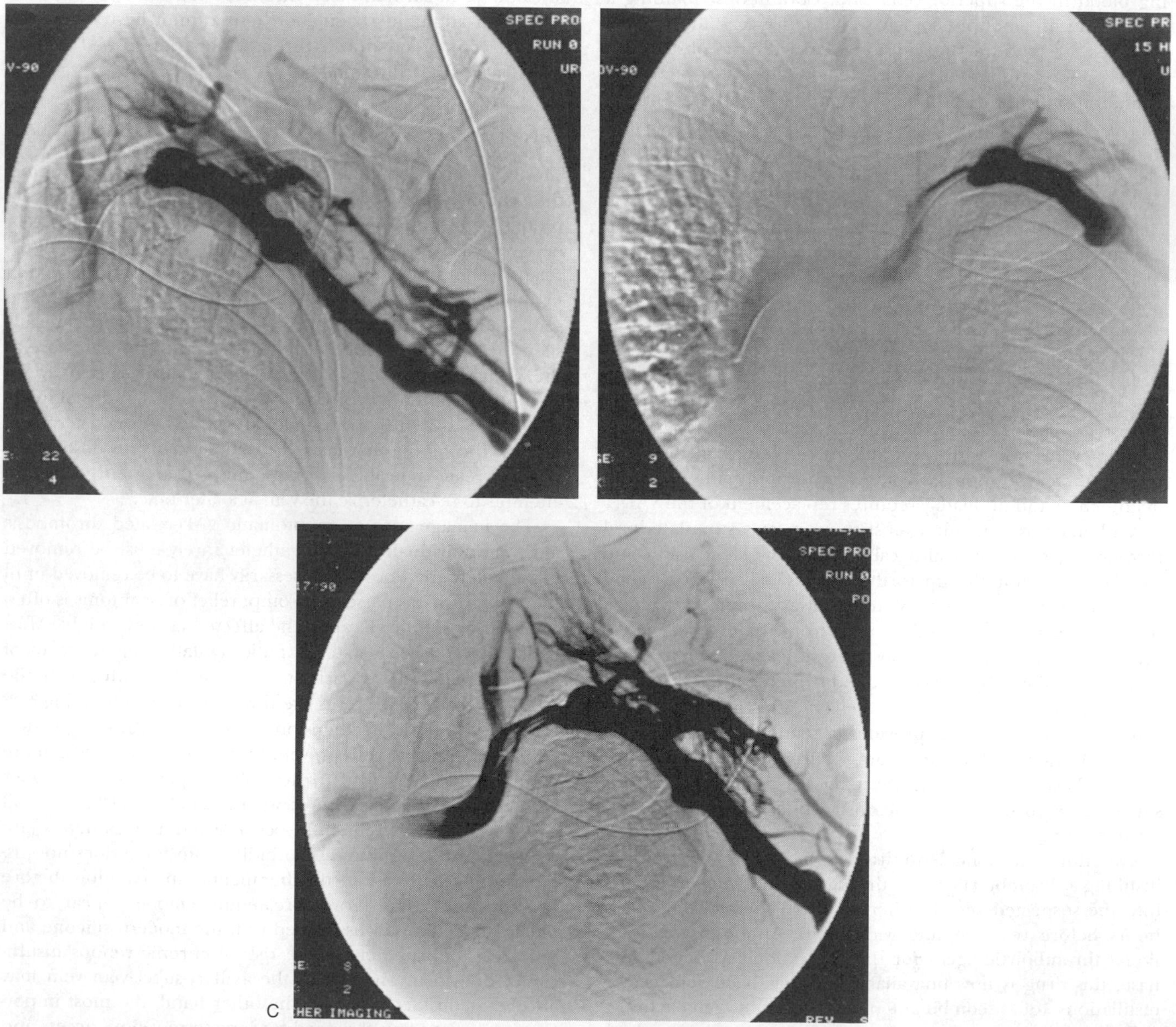

FIGURE 29.2-6. **A:** Catheter-related subclavian vein thrombosis documented by venogram, which shows complete obstruction and collateral venous flow. The patient was treated with urokinase infusion through an ipsilateral forearm vein and, after 16 hours **(B)** and 39 hours **(C)** of urokinase infusion, showed progressive resolution of the thrombosis.

INFECTIONS

Infection is the most common complication of VADs and the most common reason that they are removed prematurely.[77–79] Short-term (i.e., less than 1 month), nontunneled central venous catheters carry the greatest risk of infection, although bonding the catheter material with antimicrobial agents reduces this risk significantly.[80] Among long-term, tunneled VADs the infection rate varies considerably, and in some series, infections are much more common (e.g., approximately 40%) with externalized catheters than for subcutaneous ports (approximately 5% to 10%), with the risk of infection decreasing over time from catheterization.[20,79]

The organisms infecting VADs are most commonly derived from the patient's skin flora or from the hands of health care workers.[81] They migrate along the internal (introduced by accessing the hub) and external (from the skin wound) surfaces of the catheter, secreting a biofilm that protects them from the host's immune system as well as from antibiotics.[82–84] Before the skin is well healed, percutaneous infections are most common, in the form of cellulitis at the insertion site ("exit-site" infections) or deeper in the subcutaneous track of the catheter ("tunnel" infections).[81,85]

Exit-site infections occur at the skin wound, which is the catheter insertion site, or in the case of subcutaneous ports, the needle access site. They present with tenderness and erythema and purulent discharge and are most commonly caused by *Staphylococcus epidermidis.* The site should be cultured and treated with topical antibiotic ointment. The VAD can usually be left in place unless the infection is due to *Pseudomonas* species or atypical mycobacteria.[86,87] If fever or other systemic signs develop, however, blood cultures should be obtained and antibiotics started. If the cultures are negative, an oral cephalosporin may be adequate.[85]

Very serious infections can also develop in the subcutaneous tunnel of the catheter or in the pouch where a port resides. These are usually quite tender and swollen and may be fluctuant. Bacteremia associated with a deep-seated infection requires at least 4 weeks of antibiotics. If fever or bacteremia persists after 3 days of antibiotics, however, catheter removal is usually necessary, particularly when the organism is *Staphylococcus aureus.*[81,88]

Diagnosing catheter-related bacteremia requires obtaining quantitative blood cultures both through the catheter itself and from a peripheral vein. If the number of colonies growing in the catheter-derived culture is more than tenfold greater than the number in the peripheral blood culture, the VAD is implicated as the source of the bacteremia.[81,85] If the catheter is no longer necessary for the patient's care, it should be immediately removed and antibiotics given for 72 hours. However, if retaining the VAD is a priority, it may be left in place and the antibiotics administered through it. If the catheter has several lumens, the antibiotics should be rotated among them. Blood cultures from the catheter should be repeated after 2 to 3 days. If they are sterile, antibiotics should be continued for an additional 7 to 14 days, and the cultures should be repeated 24 to 48 hours after the antibiotics have been discontinued.[85] The most common organism, coagulase-negative staphylococci, can usually be eradicated with vancomycin.

If, however, the patient continues to have positive cultures or does not show prompt symptomatic improvement after antibiotics are started, serious consideration must be given to removing the VAD. An alternative is a trial of local thrombolytic therapy. Skin flora migrating through the catheter to the blood stream tend to adhere to the fibrin sleeve that inevitably coats the catheter surface.[50] Some species add their own secreted proteins to this sleeve.[84] In this matrix, the organisms are relatively protected from phagocytes and antibodies, as well as from antibiotics. Instillations of rtPA into the catheter have been shown to improve the outcome in cases refractory to antibiotics alone.[89,90] rtPA would be expected to provide the same benefit and should be given in the same manner as for treating withdrawal occlusion associated with a fibrin sheath.[53] Another consideration in assessing antibiotic-resistant bacteremia is whether the patient has an infected venous thrombus. A venogram is necessary to evaluate this possibility. If thrombosis is found, the catheter must be removed and antibiotics continued for 4 to 6 weeks. In some cases, the infected clot may require surgical resection.[91]

REFERENCES

1. Broviac JW, Cole JJ, Scribner BH. A silicone rubber atrial catheter for prolonged parenteral alimentation. *Surg Gynecol Obstet* 1973;136:602.
2. Hickman RO, Buckner CD, Clift RA, et al. A modified right atrial catheter for access to the venous system in marrow transplant recipients. *Surg Gynecol Obstet* 1979;148:871.
3. Maki DG, Cobb L, Garman JK, et al. An attachable silver-impregnated cuff for prevention of infection with central venous catheters: a prospective randomized multicenter trial. *Am J Med* 1988;85:307.
4. Flowers RH, Schwenzer KJ, Kopel RF, et al. Efficacy of an attachable subcutaneous cuff for the prevention of intravascular catheter-related infection. A randomized, controlled trial [see comments]. *JAMA* 1989;261:878.
5. Bonawitz SC, Hammell EJ, Kirkpatrick JR. Prevention of central venous catheter sepsis: a prospective randomized trial. *Am Surg* 1991;57:618.
6. Groeger JS, Lucas AB, Coit D, et al. A prospective, randomized evaluation of the effect of silver impregnated subcutaneous cuffs for preventing tunneled chronic venous access catheter infections in cancer patients [see comments]. *Ann Surg* 1993;218:206.
7. Mayo DJ, Horne MK, Summers BL, Pearson DC, Helsabeck CB. The effects of heparin flush on patency of the Groshong catheter: a pilot study. *Oncol Nurs Forum* 1996;23:1401.
8. Masoorli S, Angeles T. PICC lines: the latest home care challenge. *RN* 1990;53:44.
9. Andersen KM, Holland JS. Maintaining the patency of peripherally inserted central catheters with 10 units/cc heparin. *J Intraven Nurs* 1992;15:84.
10. James L, Bledsoe L, Hadaway LC. A retrospective look at tip location and complications of peripherally inserted central catheter lines. *J Intraven Nurs* 1993;16:104.
11. Cardella JF, Cardella K, Bacci N, Fox PS, Post JH. Cumulative experience with 1,273 peripherally inserted central catheters at a single institution. *J Vasc Interv Radiol* 1996;7:5.
12. Banton J. Using midlines and PICC lines for chemotherapy regimens. *Oncol Nurs Forum* 1999;26:514.
13. Alhimyary A, Fernandez C, Picard M, et al. Safety and efficacy of total parenteral nutrition delivered via a peripherally inserted central venous catheter. *Nutr Clin Pract* 1996;11:199.
14. Niederhuber JE, Ensminger W, Gyves JW, et al. Totally implanted venous and arterial access system to replace external catheters in cancer treatment. *Surgery* 1982;92:706.
15. May GS, Davis C. Percutaneous catheters and totally implantable access systems: a review of reported infection rates. *J Intraven Nurs* 1988;11:97.
16. Wurzel CL, Halom K, Feldman JG, Rubin LG. Infection rates of Broviac-Hickman catheters and implantable venous devices. *Am J Dis Child* 1988;142:536.
17. Ross MN, Haase GM, Poole MA, Burrington JD, Odom LF. Comparison of totally implanted reservoirs with external catheters as venous access devices in pediatric oncologic patients. *Surg Gynecol Obstet* 1988;167:141.
18. Shaw JH, Douglas R, Wilson T. Clinical performance of Hickman and Portacath atrial catheters. *Aust N Z J Surg* 1988;58:657.
19. Mirro J Jr, Rao BN, Stokes DC, et al. A prospective study of Hickman/Broviac catheters and implantable ports in pediatric oncology patients. *J Clin Oncol* 1989;7:214.
20. Mirro J Jr, Rao BN, Kumar M, et al. A comparison of placement techniques and complications of externalized catheters and implantable port use in children with cancer. *J Pediatr Surg* 1990;25:120.
21. Alexander HR. Clinical performance of long-term venous access devices. In: *Vascular access in the cancer patient*, vol. 1. Philadelphia: JB Lippincott Co, 1994:18.
22. Sharpe PC, Morris TC. Complications associated with central venous catheters in a haematology unit. *Ulster Med J* 1994;63:144.
23. Rohde TD, Blackshear PJ, Varco RL, Buchwald H. Protracted parenteral drug infusion in ambulatory subjects using an implantable infusion pump. *Trans Am Soc Artif Intern Organs* 1977;23:13.
24. Rohde TD, Blackshear PJ, Varco RL, Buchwald H. One year of heparin anticoagulation. An ambulatory subject using a totally implantable infusion pump. *Minn Med* 1977;60:719.

25. Boyle FM, Smith RC, Levi JA. Continuous hepatic artery infusion of 5-fluorouracil for metastatic colorectal cancer localised to the liver. *Aust N Z J Med* 1993;23:32.
26. Hohn DC, Rayner AA, Economou JS, et al. Toxicities and complications of implanted pump hepatic arterial and intravenous floxuridine infusion. *Cancer* 1986;57:465.
27. Patt YZ, Hoque A, Lozano R, et al. Phase II trial of hepatic arterial infusion of fluorouracil and recombinant human interferon alfa-2b for liver metastases of colorectal cancer refractory to systemic fluorouracil and leucovorin. *J Clin Oncol* 1997;15:1432.
28. Berlin J, Merrick HW, Smith TJ, Lerner H. Phase II evaluation of treatment of complete resection of hepatic metastases from colorectal cancer and adjuvant hepatic arterial infusion of floxuridine: an Eastern Cooperative Oncology Group study (PB083). *Am J Clin Oncol* 1999;22:291.
29. Buchwald H, Rohde TD, Dorman FD, et al. A totally implantable drug infusion device: laboratory and clinical experience using a model with single flow rate and new design for modulated insulin infusion. *Diabetes Care* 1980;3:351.
30. Hassenbusch SJ, Pillay PK, Magdinec M, et al. Constant infusion of morphine for intractable cancer pain using an implanted pump [see comments]. *J Neurosurg* 1990;73:405.
31. Fischell RE. A programmable implantable medication system (PIMS) as a means for intracorporeal drug delivery. In: Tyle P, ed. *Drug delivery devices.* New York: Marcel Dekker Inc, 1988:261.
32. Jansen RF, Wiggers T, van Geel BN, van Putten WL. Assessment of insertion techniques and complication rates of dual lumen central venous catheters in patients with hematological malignancies. *World J Surg* 1990;14:100; discussion 105.
33. Petersen J, Delaney JH, Brakstad MT, Rowbotham RK, Bagley CM Jr. Silicone venous access devices positioned with their tips high in the superior vena cava are more likely to malfunction. *Am J Surg* 1999;178:38.
34. Miller JA, Singireddy S, Maldjian P, Baker SR. A reevaluation of the radiographically detectable complications of percutaneous venous access lines inserted by four subcutaneous approaches. *Am Surg* 1999;65:125.
35. Williard W, Coit D, Lucas A, Groeger JS. Long-term vascular access via the inferior vena cava. *J Surg Oncol* 1991;46:162.
36. Torosian MH, Meranze S, McLean G, Mullen JL. Central venous access with occlusive superior central venous thrombosis. *Ann Surg* 1986;203:30.
37. Lammermeier D, Steiger E, Cosgrove D, Zelch M. Use of an intercostal vein for central venous access in home parenteral nutrition: a case report. *JPEN J Parenter Enteral Nutr* 1986;10:659.
38. Pokorny WJ, McGill CW, Harberg FJ. Use of azygous vein for central catheter insertion. *Surgery* 1985;97:362.
39. Knox MF, Holton JC, Morris WD, Flippin TA. Translumbar inferior vena cava Groshong catheter placement in a patient with superior vena cava occlusion. *J Ark Med Soc* 1989;85:325.
40. Hayward SR, Ledgerwood AM, Lucas CE. The fate of 100 prolonged venous access devices. *Am Surg* 1990;56:515.
41. Groeger JS, Lucas AB, Coit D. Venous access in the cancer patient. In: *Principles and practice of oncology* updates. Philadelphia: Lippincott, 1991;5:1.
42. Boardman P, Hughes J. Pictorial review: radiological evaluation and management of malfunctioning central venous catheters. *Clin Radiol* 1998;53:10.
43. Aitken D, Minton J. The "pinch-off" sign: a warning of impending problems with permanent subclavian catheters. *Am J Surg* 1984;148:633.
44. Duffy L, Kerzner B, Gebus V, Dice J. Treatment of central venous catheter occlusions with hydrochloric acid. *J Pediatr* 1989;114:1002.
45. Pennington CR, Pithie AD. Ethanol lock in the management of catheter occlusion. *JPEN J Parenter Enteral Nutr* 1987;11:507.
46. Currarino G. Migration of jugular or subclavian venous catheters into inferior tributaries of the brachiocephalic veins or into the azygos vein, with possible complications. *Pediatr Radiol* 1996;26:439.
47. Kowalski CM, Kaufman JA, Rivitz SM, Geller SC, Waltman AC. Migration of central venous catheters: implications for initial catheter tip positioning. *J Vasc Interv Radiol* 1997;8:443.
48. Nazarian GK, Bjarnason H, Dietz CA Jr, Bernadas CA, Hunter DW. Changes in tunneled catheter tip position when a patient is upright. *J Vasc Interv Radiol* 1997;8:437.
49. Peters WR, Bush WH Jr, McIntyre RD, Hill LD. The development of fibrin sheath on indwelling venous catheters. *Surg Gynecol Obstet* 1973;137:43.
50. Raad II, Luna M, Khalil SA, et al. The relationship between the thrombotic and infectious complications of central venous catheters. *JAMA* 1994;271:1014.
51. Mayo DJ, Pearson DC. Chemotherapy extravasation: a consequence of fibrin sheath formation around venous access devices. *Oncol Nurs Forum* 1995;22:675.
52. Lawson M, Bottino JC, Hurtubise MR, McCredie KB. The use of urokinase to restore the patency of occluded central venous catheters. *Am J Intraven Ther Clin Nutr* 1982;9:29.
53. Haire WD, Atkinson JB, Stephens LC, Kotulak GD. Urokinase versus recombinant tissue plasminogen activator in thrombosed central venous catheters: a double blinded, randomized trial. *Thromb Haemost* 1994;72:543.
54. Horne MK III, Mayo DJ. Low-dose urokinase infusions to treat fibrinous obstruction of venous access devices in cancer patients. *J Clin Oncol* 1997;15:2709.
55. Smith S, Dawson S, Hennessey R, Andrew M. Maintenance of the patency of indwelling central venous catheters: is heparin necessary? *Am J Pediatr Hematol Oncol* 1991;13:141.
56. Randolph AG, Cook DJ, Gonzales CA, Andrew M. Benefit of heparin in central venous and pulmonary artery catheters: a meta-analysis of randomized controlled trials. *Chest* 1998;113:165.
57. Garrelts JC. White clot syndrome and thrombocytopenia: reasons to abandon heparin i.v. lock flush solution. *Clin Pharm* 1992;11:797.
58. Kadidal VV, Mayo DJ, Horne MK. Heparin-induced thrombocytopenia (HIT) due to heparin flushes: a report of three cases. *J Intern Med* 1999;246:325.
59. Mayo DJ, Cullinane AM, Merryman PK, Horne MK. Serologic evidence of heparin sensitization in cancer patients receiving heparin flushes of venous access devices. *Support Care Cancer* 1999;7:425.
60. Mayo DJ, Dimond EP, Kramer W, Horne MK III. Discard volumes necessary for clinically useful coagulation studies from heparinized Hickman catheters. *Oncol Nurs Forum* 1996;23:671.
61. Horne MK, May DJ, Alexander HR, et al. Venographic surveillance of tunneled venous access devices in adult oncology patients. *Ann Surg Oncol* 1995;2:174.
62. De Cicco M, Matovic M, Balestreri L, et al. Central venous thrombosis: an early and frequent complication in cancer patients bearing long-term silastic catheter. A prospective study. *Thromb Res* 1997;86:101.
63. Horattas MC, Wright DJ, Fenton AH, et al. Changing concepts of deep venous thrombosis of the upper extremity—report of a series and review of the literature. *Surgery* 1988;104:561.
64. Gould JR, Carloss HW, Skinner WL. Groshong catheter–associated subclavian venous thrombosis [see comments]. *Am J Med* 1993;95:419.
65. Becker DM, Philbrick JT, Walker FB. Axillary and subclavian venous thrombosis. Prognosis and treatment. *Arch Intern Med* 1991;151:1934.
66. Hicken GJ, Ameli FM. Management of subclavian-axillary vein thrombosis: a review. *Can J Surg* 1998;41:13.
67. Monreal M, Raventos A, Lerma R, et al. Pulmonary embolism in patients with upper extremity DVT associated to venous central lines—a prospective study. *Thromb Haemost* 1994;72:548.
68. Derish MT, Smith DW, Frankel LR. Venous catheter thrombus formation and pulmonary embolism in children [see comments]. *Pediatr Pulmonol* 1995;20:349.
69. Brismar B, Hardstedt C, Jacobson S. Diagnosis of thrombosis by catheter phlebography after prolonged central venous catheterization. *Ann Surg* 1981;194:779.
70. Savage KJ, Wells PS, Schulz V, et al. Outpatient use of low molecular weight heparin (Dalteparin) for the treatment of deep vein thrombosis of the upper extremity. *Thromb Haemost* 1999;82:1008.
71. Chang R, Horne MK III, Mayo DJ, Doppman JL. Pulse-spray treatment of subclavian and jugular venous thrombi with recombinant tissue plasminogen activator. *J Vasc Interv Radiol* 1996;7:845.
72. Horne MK, Mayo DJ, Cannon RO, et al. Intra-clot recombinant tissue plasminogen activator in the treatment of deep venous thrombosis of the lower and upper extremities. *Am J Med* 2000;108:251.
73. Bern MM, Lokich JJ, Wallach SR, et al. Very low doses of warfarin can prevent thrombosis in central venous catheters. A randomized prospective trial. *Ann Intern Med* 1990;112:423.
74. Monreal M, Alastrue A, Rull M, et al. Upper extremity deep venous thrombosis in cancer patients with venous access devices—prophylaxis with a low molecular weight heparin (Fragmin). *Thromb Haemost* 1996;75:251.
75. Boraks P, Seale J, Price J, et al. Prevention of central venous catheter associated thrombosis using minidose warfarin in patients with haematological malignancies. *Br J Haematol* 1998;101:483.
76. Ratcliffe M, Broadfoot C, Davidson M, Kelly KF, Greaves M. Thrombosis, markers of thrombotic risk, indwelling central venous catheters and efficiency of antithrombotic prophylaxis using low-dose warfarin. *Br J Haematol* 1998;101:79.
77. Wiener ES, McGuire P, Stolar CJ, et al. The CCSG prospective study of venous access devices: an analysis of insertions and causes for removal. *J Pediatr Surg* 1992;27:155; discussion 163.
78. Mueller BU, Skelton J, Callender DP, et al. A prospective randomized trial comparing the infectious and noninfectious complications of an externalized catheter versus a subcutaneously implanted device in cancer patients. *J Clin Oncol* 1992;10:1943.
79. Groeger JS, Lucas AB, Thaler HT, et al. Infectious morbidity associated with long-term use of venous access devices in patients with cancer [see comments]. *Ann Intern Med* 1993;119:1168.
80. Darouiche RO, Raad II, Heard SO, et al. A comparison of two antimicrobial-impregnated central venous catheters. Catheter Study Group [see comments]. *N Engl J Med* 1999;340:1.
81. Raad II, Bodey GP. Infectious complications of indwelling vascular catheters. *Clin Infect Dis* 1992;15:197.
82. Raad II, Costerton W, Sabharwal U, et al. Ultrastructural analysis of indwelling vascular catheters: a quantitative relationship between luminal colonization and duration of placement. *J Infect Dis* 1993;168:400.
83. Vaudaux P, Pittet D, Haeberli A, et al. Host factors selectively increase staphylococcal adherence on inserted catheters: a role for fibronectin and fibrinogen or fibrin. *J Infect Dis* 1989;160:865.
84. Costerton JW, Stewart PS, Greenberg EP. Bacterial biofilms: a common cause of persistent infections. *Science* 1999;284:1318.
85. Jones GR. A practical guide to evaluation and treatment of infections in patients with central venous catheters. *J Intraven Nurs* 1998;21:S134.
86. Benezra D, Kiehn TE, Gold JW, et al. Prospective study of infections in indwelling central venous catheters using quantitative blood cultures. *Am J Med* 1988;85:495.
87. Raad II, Vartivarian S, Khan A, Bodey GP. Catheter-related infections caused by the *Mycobacterium fortuitum* complex: 15 cases and review. *Rev Infect Dis* 1991;13:1120.
88. Jones GR, Konsler GK, Dunaway RP, Lacey SR, Azizkhan RG. Prospective analysis of urokinase in the treatment of catheter sepsis in pediatric hematology-oncology patients. *J Pediatr Surg* 1993;28:350; discussion 355.
89. Jones GR, Konsler GK, Dunaway RP. Urokinase in the treatment of bacteremia and candidemia in patients with right atrial catheters. *Am J Infect Control* 1996;24:160.
90. Verghese A, Widrich WC, Arbeit RD. Central venous septic thrombophlebitis—the role of medical therapy. *Medicine* (Baltimore) 1985;64:394.
91. Dugdale DC, Ramsey PG. *Staphylococcus aureus* bacteremia in patients with Hickman catheters [see comments]. *Am J Med* 1990;89:137.

SECTION 3

H. RICHARD ALEXANDER

Isolation Perfusion

Vascular isolation and perfusion of a cancer-bearing organ or region (i.e., extremity) using a recirculating extracorporeal perfusion circuit has been in clinical use for almost 50 years. It was originally applied to the limb by Creech et al. in the 1950s for patients with high-grade unresectable extremity sarcoma or in-transit melanoma.[1] In the early 1960s additional experience with isolated perfusion of the limb or liver was reported by a small number of centers.[2–4] More recently, the technique has been actively under clinical evaluation for patients with these conditions and has also been used in isolation perfusion of the lung and kidney.[5,6]

Isolation perfusion was initially applied under normothermic conditions using chemotherapeutics alone and subsequently mild to moderate hyperthermia (38.5°C to 42°C) became a routine component of treatment.[7] Over the past 6 years there has been considerable interest in the use of tumor necrosis factor (TNF) used in combination with melphalan and hyperthermia in isolation perfusion.[8–11] This chapter reviews the principles and technique of isolation perfusion and the current status of this treatment modality in clinical practice. The role of the various components of therapy that are routinely used on efficacy and toxicity are reviewed.

PRINCIPLES OF ISOLATION PERFUSION

Isolation perfusion is a specialized surgical technique administered under a general anesthetic and usually for an interval of 60 to 90 minutes. Initially, the vascular supply of a cancer-bearing organ or region such as liver or extremity is identified and isolated and all collateral blood flow to the area is controlled to avoid any leak of perfusate into the systemic circulation or leak of systemic blood into the perfusion circuit. Once the vessels are cannulated they are connected to inflow and outflow lines of an extracorporeal bypass circuit, which consists of an oxygenator, reservoir, heat exchanger, and roller pump. The heat exchanger, which warms the perfusate, is connected to a closed water-recirculating circuit (Fig. 29.3-1). It has become routine practice during isolation perfusion to confirm that complete vascular isolation has been achieved using a continuous intraoperative leak monitoring technique with either radiolabeled ^{131}I human serum albumin or technetium 99–labeled red blood cells.[12–15] Once the perfusion is complete, the vascular bed of the treated region is flushed with several liters of saline and colloid solution to remove any residual intravascular therapeutic agents. Finally, the native vascular blood flow is reestablished to the site and therapy is completed. Because of the need to place indwelling vascular catheters during treatment, the patient must be systemically anticoagulated usually using heparin during perfusion. However, the anticoagulation effects can be effectively reversed with protamine sulfate and thawed fresh frozen plasma.

There are several advantages of isolation perfusion as a treatment technique. In practice, complete separation of the regional and systemic circulation can be achieved in most circumstances. This is particularly true for isolation perfusion of the liver[16] and in patients undergoing isolated limb perfusion (ILP) for in-transit melanoma for high-grade unresectable sarcoma of the extremity.[12] Small, less than 1%, leaks of perfusate into the systemic circulation can be detected using a leak-monitoring system. Klaase and coworkers[12] reported the frequency of perfusate leak in 383 patients who underwent 438 ILPs using a standardized technique. The cumulative overall leak rate was 0.9%. A leak rate of greater than 5% was encountered in 6.2% of ILPs and a leak rate of greater than 10% was observed in only 1.4%. During ILP, leak of perfusate can usually be controlled with various maneuvers such as adjustments in flow rate or tightening of the extremity tourniquet.[17] Because treatment is confined to an organ or region of the body, systemic exposure and toxicity secondary to the therapeutic agents can be eliminated or significantly limited.[18] In addition, dose escalation of the therapeutic agents is limited largely by the tissue tolerance of the perfused organ or the extremity.[19] Finally, isolation perfusion allows one to deliver clinically significant levels of hyperthermia, which has direct cytotoxic[3,20] and synergistic antitumor effects with various chemotherapeutic and biologic agents.[21–24]

ISOLATED LIMB PERFUSION

ILP of the lower extremity is most commonly performed via cannulation of the external iliac vessels and in the arm via the axillary vessels. However, in the lower extremity ILP can be performed via the femoral or popliteal vessels and in the arm via the brachial vessels under certain clinical situations. For the approach to the iliac vessels, a lower abdominal *transplant* incision and a retroperitoneal approach is made. The external iliac artery and vein are carefully dissected from their origin down to the inguinal ligament and small arterial branches and venous tributaries and ligated and divided. This is particularly important in the region of the inguinal ligament to prevent leak of perfusate into the systemic circulation. The hypogastric vein is ligated *in situ* and the hypogastric artery is temporarily occluded with a vascular occluding clamp. If possible, some of the branches of the hypogastric artery in the pelvis should be identified and ligated to prevent collateral flow across the pelvis. These vessels include the vesicular, pudendal, and obturator arteries. A Steinmann pin is anchored into the anterior superior iliac spine and the external iliac vessels are cannulated with the catheter tips positioned just below the inguinal ligament. An Esmarch tourniquet is snugly wrapped at the root of the extremity and the cannulae are connected to the extracorporeal bypass circuit (Fig. 29.3-2).

ISOLATED HEPATIC PERFUSION

Isolated hepatic perfusion (IHP) is a more complex treatment to administer and has not gained as widespread or consistent a clinical evaluation because of the major nature of the operative procedure, the associated morbidity associated with the treatment, and the fact that initial clinical studies did not clearly document efficacy of the therapy. The unique vascular anatomy of the liver, however, does make it an ideally suitable organ for isolated perfusion. The procedure starts with a right subcostal incision and once it has been determined that there are no contraindications

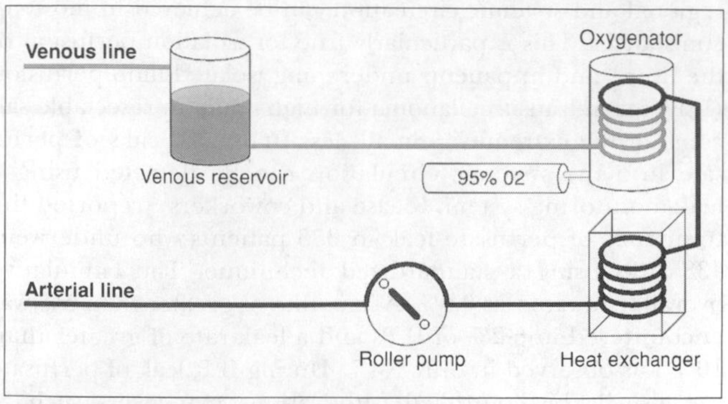

FIGURE 29.3-1. General components of isolated organ perfusion circuit showing the venous reservoir, oxygenator heat exchanger, and roller pump. Blood flow from the perfused site is collected in a venous reservoir by passage drainage. The roller pump on the arterial side of the circuit can be adjusted to increase or decrease flow rates as appropriate. The oxygenator and heat exchanger are in-line components of this circuit, and the latter can effectively heat the perfusate so that tissue hyperthermia can be routinely achieved.

to proceeding with IHP, the incision is extended and the liver is extensively mobilized. This includes division of the diaphragmatic attachments of the left and right hepatic lobes and complete dissection of the retrohepatic vena cava from the level of the renal veins to the diaphragm to prevent any leak of perfusate from the retrohepatic inferior vena cava (Fig. 29.3-3). A cholecystectomy is performed and the portahepatis structures are completely dissected and isolated. This includes complete dissection and division of the surrounding connective tissue and lymphatics, which can serve as a leak of perfusate into the systemic circulation during therapy. Cannulation for inflow to the liver is typically via the gastroduodenal artery alone or the gastroduodenal artery and portal vein.[8] Splanchnic venous flow is shunted to the right atrium using a second veno-veno bypass circuit similar to that used in hepatic transplantation procedures with an inflow cannula positioned in the axillary vein. The venous effluent of the liver is collected from a cannula positioned in an isolated segment of retrohepatic inferior vena cava and, therefore, during treatment the inferior vena cava flow must also be shunted (see Fig. 29.3-3). Originally reports of IHP described the use of a passive double-lumen internal shunt system that may not have provided adequate venous return from the inferior vena cava and the portal vein to the heart.[25] The external veno-veno bypass circuit results in flow rates of approximately 2 L/min and stable cardiac parameters during treatment.[16]

PERFUSION PARAMETERS

The extracorporeal perfusion circuit typically contains 1 L of perfusate, which consists of 700 mL of a balanced salt solution, 1 U of type-matched packed red blood cells, and 1500 U of heparin. The resultant hematocrit of approximately 25% provides adequate tissue oxygen retention and perfusates containing higher hematocrits and provide no additional benefit in preventing regional toxicity.[26] Generally, flow rates in the range of 400 to 800 mL/min are achievable and adjusted depending on line pressure, changes in reservoir volume, or the presence of a systemic perfusate leak based on intraoperative monitoring.

Continuous intraoperative leak monitoring to assess for the presence of leak of the perfusate into the systemic circulation is being used more routinely and is an important component of isolation perfusion therapy when one considers that the perfusate often contains doses of therapeutic agents that are at least tenfold greater than maximally tolerated systemic doses. Careful monitoring of leak can reduce the severity of systemic complications and may improve response rates.[15,18] Standard leak-monitoring techniques using ^{131}I radiolabeled albumin or technetium 99–labeled red blood cells have been described for continuous intraoperative monitoring.[12–14] A gamma detection

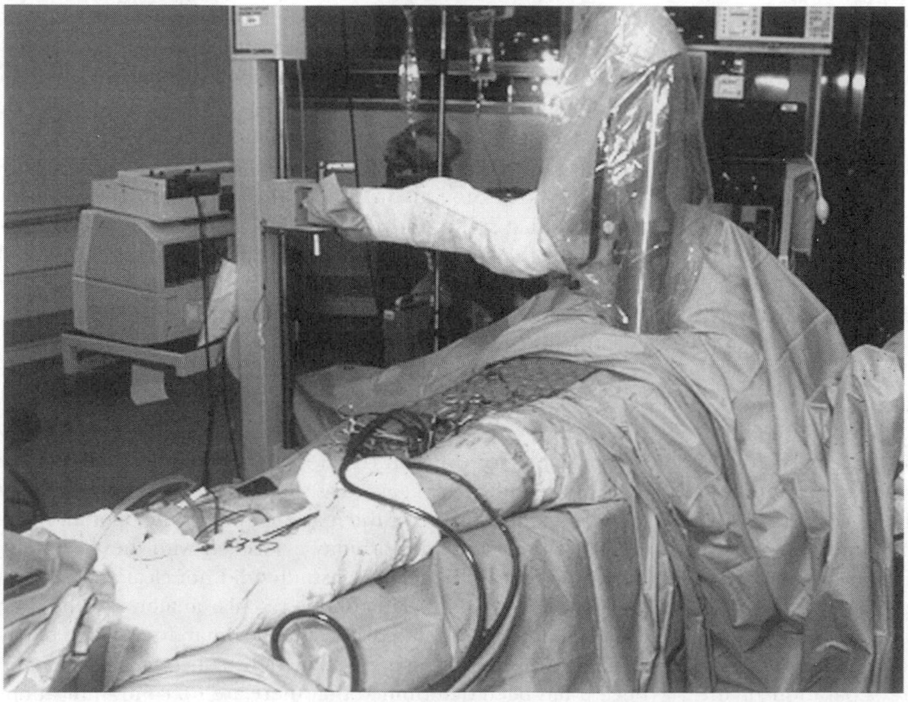

FIGURE 29.3-2. Intraoperative photograph showing an isolated limb perfusion circuit in a patient with in-transit extremity melanoma. Note the leg is wrapped in warming blankets to facilitate tissue warming, and the leak-monitoring gamma detection camera is positioned over the patient's precordium and connected to a strip chart recorder. The extracorporeal bypass circuit (not shown) is positioned by the patient's side during therapy.

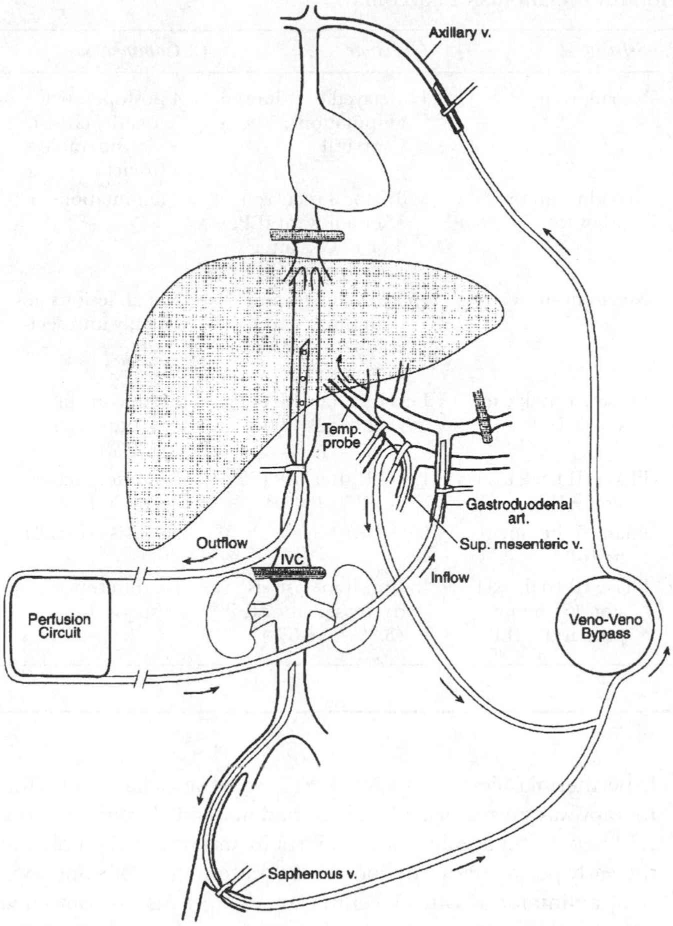

FIGURE 29.3-3. Schematic illustration of the isolated limb perfusion circuit. The arterial inflow is via the gastroduodenal artery, and venous outflow is collected from a cannula positioned in an isolated segment of retrohepatic vena cava. The inflow and outflow cannulae are connected to a perfusion circuit as shown in Figure 29.3-1. On the patient's left is the veno-veno bypass circuit that shunts portal splanchnic and inferior venal caval blood flow back to the systemic circulation during therapy. IVC, inferior vena cava.

camera is positioned either over the precordium of the heart for patients undergoing ILP or over the pump housing of the veno-venous bypass circuit for patients undergoing IHP, both of which serve as a stable reservoir of blood to measure radioactivity (see Fig. 29.3-2). The detection system provides continuous assessment of leak rates and can discriminate leaks less than 1%.[12] Once the gamma detection camera has been positioned, a small dose of radionuclide is given systemically and a baseline level of radioactive counts is measured on a strip chart recorder. Then a tenfold higher dose is administered into the perfusion circuit. Therefore, if a 10% leak of perfusate into the systemic circulation occurs, there will be a doubling of the amount of radioactivity compared with baseline. Leak rates using this system have been shown to correlate with measured leak rates with TNF or melphalan from the perfusate into the systemic circulation.[12,18]

Despite careful preoperative preparation, during ILP the surgeon may encounter several situations that require adjustment in perfusion parameters to minimize a leak of perfusate out of or blood into the perfusion circuit. Flow rates that indirectly affect arterial line pressure, reservoir volume, and leak of perfusate are continuously monitored. If there is leak of systemic blood into the perfusion circuit this is reflected by an increase in the reservoir volume in the circuit and can be remedied by increasing flow rates to increase line pressure, tightening the extremity tourniquet, or increasing venous pressure in the circuit by placing a partial occluding clamp on the venous outflow line. If there is a perfusate leak into the systemic circulation this is manifested by an increase in radioactive counts detected by the gamma camera and the strip chart recorder. In addition, one may see a decrease in reservoir volume in the perfusion circuit, although this is a relatively late manifestation of a perfusate leak. Under these circumstances, one may decrease flow rates to lower the line pressure or tighten the tourniquet to stop systemic leak. Rarely, a two-way leak occurs that is evidenced by changes in reservoir volume (generally a gain) as well as an increase in radioactivity on the strip chart recorder. This can be a particularly difficult and tricky condition to adequately control, and typical steps would include decreasing flow rates to stop any systemic leak of perfusate, tightening the tourniquet, and then placing the partial occluding clamp on the venous outflow line of the perfusion circuit.

RESULTS OF ISOLATION PERFUSION

There are many perfusion and treatment-related factors that may affect efficacy and toxicity of isolation perfusion. The majority of clinical experience with isolation perfusion has been with ILP using chemotherapeutics for in-transit melanoma or sarcoma of the extremity (Table 29.3-1). The early clinical trials of ILP using hyperthermia or chemotherapy for sarcoma were difficult to interpret because of the variability in treatment conditions and patient selection.[27–29] Two early studies of adjuvant ILP using melphalan for patients with melanoma undergoing initial excision of all disease did show a significant reduction in local recurrences with ILP compared with excision alone but suffered from including high- and low-risk patients.[30–32] A large multicenter trial of prophylactic ILP following excision of primary melanoma greater than 1.5 mm in depth showed a decrease in local recurrence with ILP from 6.6% to 3.3% compared with excision alone with no benefit for survival.[33] Based on these results prophylactic ILP has been largely abandoned. There are other components of isolation perfusion that may have substantial effects on outcome including hyperthermia and biologic agents, most notably TNF.

HYPERTHERMIA

Hyperthermia has been used in isolation perfusion alone or in combination with chemotherapeutics and TNF. In experimental models it has direct cytotoxicity against tumor lines[3,20] and has established synergy with various chemotherapeutics and TNF.[21–23,34–37] This later feature is presumed to be the main contribution of hyperthermia in isolation perfusion. Under hyperthermic conditions tumor neovasculature responds differently than native blood vessels. At temperatures up to 46°C normal microvessels dilate and blood flow increases up to sixfold as a compensatory mechanism to diffuse local heat accumulation.[38] In contrast, tumor-associated microvessels have a diminished capacity to vasodilate and at comparable tempera-

TABLE 29.3-1. Results of Selected Trials of Isolated Limb Perfusion for Melanoma or Sarcoma

Author	Year	Diagnosis	Number	Treatment	Setting	Outcome	Comments
Di Filippo[62]	1988	Sarcoma	22	Hyperthermia × 2–4 h	Neoadjuvant	11 delayed excisions; 6 amputations; 50% 5-y survival	4 postoperative deaths (18%); considerable toxicity
Klaase[28]	1989	Sarcoma	29	Doxorubicin/hyperthermia	Neoadjuvant or adjuvant	>50% local recurrence after adjuvant ILP; 4 of 17 CRs after neoadjuvant ILP	3 amputations
Rossi[29]	1994	Sarcoma	23	Doxorubicin/hyperthermia	Neoadjuvant	>50% "radiographic/pathologic necrosis"; 91% limb-sparing surgery	Not all lesions initially unresectable
Ghussen[30,31]	1988	Melanoma	107	Melphalan + hyperthermia	Phase III trial; excision ± ILP	Less LR after ILP (11% vs. 48%; $P = .001$)	LR in control group high (39%)
Hafström[32]	1991	Melanoma	69	Melphalan + hyperthermia	Phase III trial; excision ± ILP	Less LR after ILP (70% vs. 83%; $P = .04$)	No difference in survival
Klaase[61]	1994	Melanoma	120	Melphalan + hyperthermia	Phase II therapeutic ILP	55% CRs	30% 10-y survival
Koops[33]	1998	Melanoma	832	Melphalan + hyperthermia	Phase III trial; excision (>1.5 mm primary) ± ILP	In-transit metastasis decreased after ILP (3.3% vs. 6.6%)	No difference in survival

CR, complete response; ILP, isolated limb perfusion; LR, local recurrence.

tures there is stasis and diminution of blood flow,[38] indicating a differential sensitivity between tumor-associated and normal microvasculature.

Following the original report of normothermic ILP using chemotherapeutics in 1957 by Creech et al.,[1] most investigators subsequently incorporated some degree of hyperthermia as closed circuit water-recirculating heat exchangers became available to replace the use of inefficient warm moist towels and infrared lamps to warm perfusate fluid.[2] Stehlin et al. reported results of ILP in 50 patients in 1969[2] and a follow-up report in 1975 of 165 patients[39] with extremity sarcoma or melanoma in whom significant hyperthermia was delivered to the perfused limb. In the initial series the perfusate was warmed to 46°C and average tissue temperatures of 42°C resulted in severe regional toxicity including pain, edema, blistering, and weakness observed in 70% of patients. When tissue temperatures were reduced to 40°C or less, regional complications were minimal.[39] In 1967 Cavaliere and coworkers[3] reported results of hyperthermia alone ILP with tissue temperatures ranging from 42°C to 44°C. The combination of this degree of hyperthermia, perfusion lasting more than 8 hours, and the lack of a proximal tourniquet resulted in severe regional toxicity and an unacceptable 28% mortality. Stehlin reported that compared with historic controls treated identically at one institution, the addition of hyperthermia during ILP with melphalan in patients with extremity melanoma resulted in an increase in response rates from 35% to 80%.[39] Klaase and coworkers[40] reported an analysis of factors associated with toxicity following ILP for melanoma in 425 patients. Tissue temperature greater than 40°C was the most significant factor associated with increased regional toxicity. In addition, female gender and a decrease in perfusate pH were also associated with worse regional toxicity.

Skibba et al. have reported data on eight patients with unresectable cancer confined to liver and treated with a 4-hour IHP using hyperthermia alone to 42.5°C.[41,42] Toxicity associated with this therapy was substantial; all patients had marked elevation in post-IHP hepatic transaminases and bilirubin and two of eight died in the early postoperative period. There was evidence of some transient antitumor activity by central tumor necrosis on computed tomography scans obtained, in what appears to be, to improve the efficacy chemotherapeutics given via isolation perfusion of the limb or liver. It has marginal, if any, independent antitumor effects, and temperatures higher than 40°C to 41°C are associated with unacceptable toxicity.

TUMOR NECROSIS FACTOR

In 1975 Carswell et al. demonstrated that a circulating factor present in the sera of endotoxin-treated mice caused dramatic hemorrhagic necrosis of tumors when administered to tumor-bearing mice.[43] This factor was termed *TNF*, and after it became available in recombinant form in the mid-1980s it was evaluated in multiple clinical trials via various methods of administration.[44] However, it was found that humans are very sensitive to the toxic effects of TNF, and, at the maximum tolerated doses administered, it had little antitumor activity. Although interest in TNF as a systemically administered antitumor agent waned, enthusiasm for its administration via isolation perfusion grew remarkably in the early 1990s when Liénard et al. reported initial results in 29 patients treated with a combination of TNF, melphalan, and hyperthermia for in-transit melanoma or high-grade sarcoma of the extremity.[45] The overall response rate in that initial trial was 100%, with 89% of patients having a complete response to treatment.

TNF is ideally suited for administration via isolation perfusion and is thought to exert its antitumor activity via effects on the tumor-associated neovasculature. TNF has significant known procoagulant activity[46,47] and increases vascular perme-

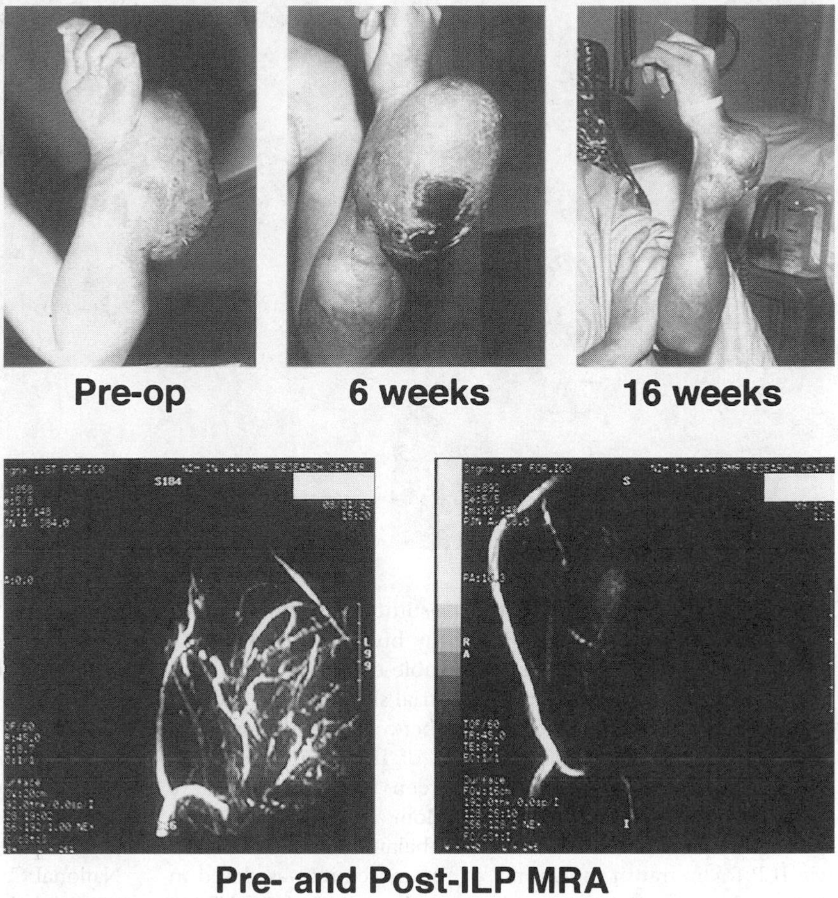

FIGURE 29.3-4. Preperfusion and postperfusion magnetic resonance angiograms showing neovascularity in a large multiply recurrent Ewing's sarcoma arising on the dorsum of a forearm. The patient had small volume pulmonary metastases and was treated with palliative 90-minute hyperthermic isolated limb perfusion using tumor necrosis factor and melphalan. He had a significant regression (*top panel*) that lasted for 2 years until death from systemic disease progression. Three days posttherapy complete obliteration of the tumor neovasculature was observed with no effect of perfusion on the native blood vessels in the extremity (*bottom panel*). ILP, isolated limb perfusion; MRA, magnetic resonance angiography.

ability.[48] In addition, several authors have published data showing selective obliteration of tumor neovasculature following ILP with TNF hyperthermia and melphalan for patients with high-grade unresectable extremity sarcoma (Fig. 29.3-4).[49,50] However, there are few clinical data available using TNF alone via isolation perfusion. Three patients with high-grade extremity sarcoma were treated at our institution with hyperthermic ILP and TNF.[51] One patient had angiographically documented obliteration of tumor-associated neovasculature following ILP; however, he experienced clinical and radiographic tumor progression within 6 weeks, suggesting that the vascular obliteration observed after TNF may not be sufficient for subsequent tumor regression. Posner et al. reported results of ILP with TNF alone in six patients with in-transit melanoma.[52] One had a complete response of 7 months' durations and two others had brief, less than 1 month, partial responses. TNF administered alone via IHP has little antitumor activity. Fraker reported a 20% transient response rate following IHP with escalating doses of TNF.[53] Interestingly, the responses were seen only at the lowest doses of TNF and once perfusate pH was corrected with sodium bicarbonate during treatment, no further responses were seen despite dose escalation of TNF to 2 mg.

When TNF is used in ILP with melphalan it is associated with a rapid time course of response in tumors compared with ILP with melphalan alone, and large tumors form eschar reminiscent of the findings in murine models (Fig. 29.3-5). Because TNF causes increased endothelial permeability[48] and has selective procoagulant effects on tumor-associated vasculature, it has been postulated that during ILP TNF may augment delivery of chemotherapeutics to the tumor by increasing vascular permeability. However, a study reported by Alexander and coworkers[54] evaluated vascular permeability in tumor and unaffected liver tissue obtained from patients undergoing IHP with melphalan alone or TNF and melphalan. After IHP there was a significant increase in permeability in tumor vasculature compared with liver. However, the increase in permeability was similar in those treated with or without TNF, suggesting that the augmentation in permeability occurred via TNF-independent mechanisms.

CURRENT STATUS OF ISOLATED LIMB PERFUSION

The role of TNF in isolation perfusion is still under clinical evaluation and has no conclusively demonstrated benefit in properly designed and conducted prospective random assignment trials. In the initial report from Liénard and Lejeune, results from 29 patients treated with ILP using a combination of TNF, melphalan, and hyperthermia for in-transit melanoma or high-grade sarcoma of the extremity were presented.[45] The overall response rate in that initial trial was 100%, with 89% of patients having a complete response to treatment. In subsequent reports from various institutions, including a follow-up report from Liénard and Lejeune of a larger series of patients, the complete response rates were lower and ranged between 70% and 79% (Table 29.3-2).[18,55,56] A prospective random assignment trial was

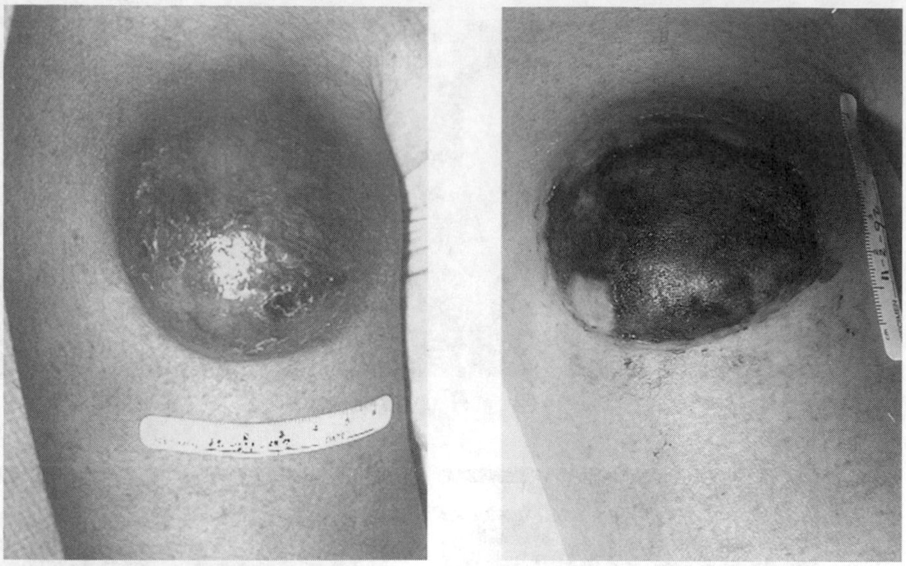

A B

FIGURE 29.3-5. Photographs of a patient treated with isolated limb perfusion using tumor necrosis factor and melphalan for in-transit extremity melanoma. **A:** In-transit site of disease before and **(B)** 5 days after isolated limb perfusion. Note the rapid eschar formation over tumor with sparing of overlying and adjacent normal skin, which is characteristic of the effect of tumor necrosis factor.

initiated at the National Cancer Institute and subsequently expanded to a multiinstitutional study but was closed prematurely in 1997 due to the lack of available clinical-grade TNF in the United States. The results of that trial showed no difference in overall or complete response rates between the groups.[57] It is also noteworthy that in several trials of ILP using melphalan alone, complete response rates between 56% and 82% have been reported.[58–61] A prospective random assignment trial comparing melphalan and TNF with melphalan alone administered via ILP for in-transit melanoma of the extremity was closed in Europe because of low accrual, suggesting a bias that TNF for most patients with this histology does not substantially contribute to efficacy compared with melphalan alone.

ILP has been used for patients with unresectable high-grade extremity sarcoma for palliation, for potential cure in cases of multifocal disease, and as a neoadjuvant therapy to convert an unresectable lesion to a resectable one. Most data reported on ILP using chemotherapeutics alone indicate limited antitumor activity against this histology.[28,62] After the initial reports by Liénard and Lejeune using the combination of TNF, melphalan, and hyperthermia as a neoadjuvant treatment for high-grade unresectable sarcoma, a multiinstitutional trial using this regimen for patients with condition was conducted in Europe and the results reported in two papers by Eggermont and coworkers.[50,63] In more than 219 patients, the overall clinical and pathologic response rate was more than 80% and the limb salvage rate was 84%. Based on these results TNF is now licensed for administration via ILP for high-grade sarcoma in Europe, but no trials are currently being conducted in the United States.

CURRENT STATUS OF ISOLATED HEPATIC PERFUSION

Following the initial experience with TNF and melphalan in ILP several centers have reported results with this regimen used in IHP for patients with unresectable primary or metastatic cancers confined to liver (see Table 29.3-2).[16,64–66] De Vries and coworkers reported results in eight patients treated with melphalan and TNF and one patient treated with TNF alone for 1 hour at 41°C.[66] IHP was associated with a 33% mortality in the series but five of six evaluable patients treated with melphalan and TNF had radiographic evidence of antitumor efficacy. Hafström and coworkers reported results in 11 patients using melphalan and TNF and also reported a high morbidity and mortality of 45% and 18%, respectively.[64] Three patients experienced a radiographic partial response to therapy. A German group reported results in six patients treated with a 60-minute IHP using melphalan and TNF at 40°C to 41°C and had no mortality in this series.[65] Three of six patients had radiographic evidence of significant tumor regression. The largest series reported using TNF and melphalan via IHP comes from the National Cancer Institute; 34 patients underwent IHP with doses of melphalan and TNF that were derived from previously conducted phase I studies and were higher than those used at higher institutions.[16] The treatment lasted for 1 hour and hyperthermia between 39.5°C and 40°C was used in all circumstances. The treatment-related mortality was 4% and the investigators observed an overall radiographic response rate of 75%. The group has presented follow-up data on 44 patients with metastatic unresectable colorectal cancer to the liver.[67] The cohort of patients who had advanced and largely refractory disease had a median number of hepatic lesions of eight, the median diameter of the greatest lesion was 8.5 cm, and one-fourth of patients had more than 50% hepatic replacement by tumor. Furthermore, approximately 45% of patients had failed prior systemic 5-fluorouracil–based chemotherapy. In the 32 patients treated with IHP using TNF and melphalan there was a 74% radiographic partial response rate. The time to liver progression was 8.5 months, and median survival was 16.5 months. In a second cohort of patients, IHP with melphalan alone was administered followed by hepatic artery infusional therapy using floxuridine and leucovorin. The radiographic partial response rate was 90%, with 9 of 11 responses ongoing in the liver at a median follow-up of 11 months.

Although the morbidity and treatment mortality in some of these series are high, the data, for the most part, represent initial institutional experience with a highly technical procedure using agents that have known regional and systemic toxicity. With continued refinement and experience the morbidity and mortality associated with the therapy should decrease. Additional refinements in the technique of IHP, and when combined with potentially effective therapies tailored for specific histologies, the treatment may become a more widely used

TABLE 29.3-2. Selected Series of Isolation Perfusion Using Tumor Necrosis Factor and Melphalan

Author	*Trial Type*	*Agents*	*Assessable*	*Complete Response (%)*	*Partial Response (%)*	*Overall (%)*
		Regimen A				
Liénard[45]	Phase II ILP	Melphalan, 10–13 mg/L	29	90	10	100
	Melanoma/sarcoma	TNF, 3–4 mg				
		IFN, 0.2 mg				
Liénard[68]	Phase III ILP	*Regimen A versus regimen B*				
	Melanoma	Melphalan, 10–13 mg/L	31	78	22	100
		TNF, 3–4 mg	33	69	22	91
Fraker[69]	Phase III ILP	*Regimen A versus*				
	Melanoma	Melphalan, 10–13 mg/L	20	80	10	90
			23	61	39	100
Eggermont[63]	Phase II ILP	*Regimen B*				
	Sarcoma		186	29	53	82
Vaglini[56]	Phase II ILP	Melphalan, 10–13 mg/L	10	70	—	70
	Melanoma	TNF, 0.5–4.0 mg				
		IFN, 0.2 mg				
Alexander[44]	Phase II isolated hepatic perfusion	Melphalan, 1.5 mg/kg	50	2	73	75
	Multiple histologies	TNF, 1.0 mg				
Hill[70]	Phase I ILP	Melphalan, 10–13 mg/L	7	100	—	100
	Melanoma	TNF, 0.125–0.5 mg				
		IFN, 0.2 mg				
Posner[52]	Phase I/II ILP	TNF alone, 1–4 mg	6	16	34	50[a]
	Melanoma					

ILP, isolated limb perfusion; IFN, interferon; TNF, tumor necrosis factor.
[a]All responses short-lived (one 7-month complete response, two 1-month partial responses).

option for patients with unresectable hepatic malignancies from a variety of histologies (see Chapter 52.3).

STATUS OF ISOLATION PERFUSION OF OTHER SITES

There are few data regarding the application of isolation perfusion to other organs. Pass and coworkers from the National Cancer Institute reported results of a phase I isolation lung perfusion with escalating dose TNF for patients with unresectable pulmonary metastases.[6] Twenty patients were treated with unilateral isolated lung perfusion, with TNF doses ranging from 0.3 to 6.0 mg. An oxygenated circuit was used analogous to that in other isolation perfusion settings, and tissue hyperthermia between 38°C and 39.5°C was used. There were no deaths on study, and short-term regression of metastatic nodules was noted in three patients. Walther and coworkers, also from the National Cancer Institute, published a case report of an isolated kidney perfusion with TNF in an individual with localized multifocal renal cell carcinoma for whom renal parenchymal-sparing surgery would normally have been advocated.[5] The patient tolerated the procedure well, but there were no data presented with respect to any antitumor efficacy.

CONCLUSIONS

Isolated perfusion of various organs or the extremity using chemotherapeutics with or without TNF has been shown to have substantial antitumor activity against a variety of histologies. Following the initial studies using TNF there was considerable enthusiasm for its routine use in organ perfusion for the treatment of in-transit melanoma and high-grade extremity sarcoma. Although the data support its importance in treatment of high-grade extremity sarcoma, the benefit of TNF in combination with melphalan against in-transit melanoma has not been conclusively demonstrated. Because of the potential associated toxicity with TNF, its routine use outside of a clinical research trial cannot be advocated. IHP is a promising regional modality for unresectable malignancies confined to the liver, but continued investigation in a clinical research setting is clearly necessary to determine the optimal clinical setting in which to offer this form of therapy. Hyperthermia appears to be an important component of treatment and appears to act primarily by enhancing the tumoricidal effects of melphalan. TNF has no substantial antitumor activity when administered via isolated organ perfusion alone but may enhance the antitumor effects of melphalan against the extremity tumors such as sarcoma.

REFERENCES

1. Creech O, Krementz ET, Ryan RF, Winblad JN. Chemotherapy of cancer: regional perfusion utilizing an extracorporeal circuit. *Ann Surg* 1958;148:616.
2. Stehlin JS. Hyperthermic perfusion with chemotherapy for cancers of the extremities. *Surg Gynecol Obstet* 1969;129:305.
3. Cavaliere R, Ciogatto EC, Giovanelli BC, et al. Selective heat sensitivity of cancer cells. *Cancer* 1967;20:1351.
4. Ausman RK. Development of a technic for isolated perfusion of the liver. *NY State J Med* 1961;61:3393.
5. Walther MM, Jennings SB, Choyke PL, et al. Isolated perfusion of the kidney with tumor necrosis factor for localized renal-cell carcinoma. *World J Urol* 1996;14:S2.

6. Pass HI, Mew DJY, Kranda KC, et al. Isolated lung perfusion with tumor necrosis factor for pulmonary metastases. *Ann Thorac Surg* 1996;61:1609.
7. Alexander HR, Fraker DL, Bartlett DL. Isolated limb perfusion for malignant melanoma. *Semin Surg Oncol* 1996;12:416.
8. Alexander HR, Bartlett DL, Libutti SK. Isolated hepatic perfusion: a potentially effective treatment for patients with metastatic or primary cancers confined to the liver. *Cancer J Sci Am* 1998;4:2.
9. Fraker DL, Alexander HR, Thom AK. Use of tumor necrosis factor in isolated hepatic perfusion. *Circ Shock* 1994;44:45.
10. Liénard D, Eggermont AM, Kroon BBR, Koops HW, Lejeune FJ. Isolated limb perfusion in primary and recurrent melanoma: indications and results. *Semin Surg Oncol* 1998;14:202.
11. Eggermont AM, Schraffordt KH, Klausner JM, et al. Isolation limb perfusion with tumor necrosis factor alpha and chemotherapy for advanced extremity soft tissue sarcomas. *Semin Oncol* 1997;24:547.
12. Klaase JM, Kroon BBR, van Geel AN, Eggermont AMM, Franklin HR. Systemic leakage during isolated limb perfusion for melanoma. *Br J Surg* 1993;80:1124.
13. Alexander C, Omlor G, Berberich R, Gross G, Feifel G. Rapid measurement of blood leakage during regional chemotherapy. *Eur J Nucl Med* 1993;4:606.
14. Hoekstra HJ, Naujocks T, Schraffordt-Koops H, et al. Continuous leaking monitoring during hyperthermic isolated regional perfusion of the lower limb: techniques and results. *Reg Cancer Treat* 1992;4:301.
15. Barker WC, Andrich MP, Alexander HR, Fraker DL. Continuous intraoperative external monitoring of perfusate leak using I-131 human serum albumin during isolated perfusion of the liver and limbs. *Eur J Nucl Med* 1995;22:1242.
16. Alexander HR Jr, Bartlett DL, Libutti SK, et al. Isolated hepatic perfusion with tumor necrosis factor and melphalan for unresectable cancers confined to the liver. *J Clin Oncol* 1998;16:1479.
17. Sorkin P, Abu-Abid S, Lev D, et al. Systemic leakage and side effects of tumor necrosis factor alpha administered via isolated limb perfusion can be manipulated by flow rate adjustment. *Arch Surg* 1995;130:1079.
18. Thom AK, Alexander HR, Andrich MP, et al. Cytokine levels and systemic toxicity in patients undergoing isolated limb perfusion (ILP) with high-dose TNF, interferon-gamma and melphalan. *J Clin Oncol* 1995;13:264.
19. Wieberdink J, Benckhuysen C, Braat RP, van Slooten EA, Olthuis GAA. Dosimetry in isolation perfusion of the limbs by assessment of perfused tissue volume and grading of toxic tissue reactions. *Eur J Cancer Clin Oncol* 1982;18:905.
20. Hahn GM. Metabolic aspects of the role of hyperthermia in mammalian cell inactivation and their possible relevance to cancer treatment. *Cancer Res* 1974;34:3117.
21. Barlogie B, Corry PM, Drewinko B. In vitro thermochemotherapy of human colon cancer cells with cis-dichlorodiammineplatinum(II) and mitomycin C. *Cancer Res* 1980;40:1165.
22. Hahn GM, Strande DP. Cytotoxic effects of hyperthermia and adriamycin on Chinese hamster cells. *J Natl Cancer Inst* 1976;57:1063.
23. Ohno S, Strebetl FR, Stephens C, et al. Increased therapeutic efficacy induced by tumor necrosis factor a combined with platinum complexes and whole-body hyperthermia in rats. *Cancer Res* 1992;52:4096.
24. Sakaguchi Y, Makino M, Kaneko T, et al. Therapeutic efficacy of long duration-low temperature whole body hyperthermia when combined with tumor necrosis factor and carboplatin in rats. *Cancer Res* 1994;54:2223.
25. Aigner K, Walther H, Tonn J, et al. First experimental and clinical results of isolated liver perfusion with cytotoxics in metastases from colorectal primary. *Rec Res Cancer Res* 1983;86:99.
26. Klaase JM, Kroon BBR, van Slooten GW, van Dongen JA. Comparison between the use of whole blood versus a diluted perfusate in regional isolated perfusion by continuous monitoring of transcutaneous oxygen tension: a pilot study. *J Invest Surg* 1994;7:249.
27. Budd GT, Schreiber MJ, Steiger E, Bukowski RM, Weick JK. Phase I trial of intraperitoneal chemotherapy with 5-fluorouracil and citrovorum factor. *Invest New Drugs* 1986;4:155.
28. Klaase JM, Kroon BBR, Benckhuijsen C, et al. Results of regional isolation perfusion with cytostatics in patients with soft tissue tumors of the extremities. *Cancer* 1989;64:616.
29. Rossi CR, Vecchiato A, Foletto M, et al. Phase II study on neoadjuvant hyperthermic-antiblastic perfusion with doxorubicin in patients with intermediate or high grade limb sarcomas. *Cancer* 1994;73:2140.
30. Ghussen F, Nagel K, Groth W, et al. A prospective randomized study of regional extremity perfusion in patients with malignant melanoma. *Ann Surg* 1984;200:764.
31. Ghussen F, Kruger I, Groth W, Stutzer H. The role of regional hyperthermic cytostatic perfusion in the treatment of extremity melanoma. *Cancer* 1988;61:654.
32. Hafström L, Rudenstam C-M, Blomquist E, et al. Regional hyperthermic perfusion with melphalan after surgery for recurrent malignant melanoma of the extremities. *J Clin Oncol* 1991;9:2091.
33. Koops HS, Vaglini M, Suciu S, et al. Prophylactic isolated limb perfusion for localized, high-risk limb melanoma: results of a multicenter randomized phase III trial. *J Clin Oncol* 1998;16:2906.
34. Miller RC, Richards M, Baird C, Martin S, Hall EJ. Interaction of hyperthermia and chemotherapy agents; cell lethality and oncogenic potential. *Int J Hyperthermia* 1994;10:89.
35. Hachiya T, Okada K, Sakurai A, Satomi N, Haranaka K. Antitumor activity of recombinant human tumor necrosis factor in combination with hyperthermia against heterotransplanted human prostatic carcinoma and its lymph node metastasis in nude mice. *Mol Biother* 1992;4:34.
36. Joiner MC, Steel GG, Stephens TC. Response of two mouse tumours to hyperthermia with CCNU or melphalan. *Br J Cancer* 1982;45:17.
37. Klostergaard J, Leroux E, Siddik ZH, Khodadadian M, Tomasovic SP. Enhanced sensitivity of human colon tumor cell lines in vitro in response to thermochemoimmunotherapy. *Cancer Res* 1992;52:5271.
38. Dudar TE, Jain RK. Differential response of normal and tumor microcirculation to hyperthermia. *Cancer Res* 1984;44:605.
39. Stehlin JS, Giovanella BC, de Ipolyi PD, Muenz LR, Anderson RF. Results of hyperthermic perfusion for melanoma of the extremities. *Surg Gynecol Obstet* 1975;140:339.
40. Klaase JM, Kroon BBR, van Geel BN, et al. Patient- and treatment-related factors associated with acute regional toxicity after isolated perfusion for melanoma of the extremities. *Am J Surg* 1994;167:618.
41. Skibba JL, Quebbeman EJ. Tumoricidal effects and patient survival after hyperthermic liver perfusion. *Arch Surg* 1986;121:1266.
42. Skibba JL, Quebbeman EJ, Komorowski RA, Thorsen KM. Clinical results of hyperthermic liver perfusion for cancer in the liver. *Contr Oncol* 1988;29:222.
43. Carswell EA, Old LJ, Kassel RL, et al. An endotoxin-induced serum factor that causes necrosis of tumors. *Proc Natl Acad Sci U S A* 1975;72:3666.
44. Alexander HR, Feldman AL. Tumor necrosis factor: basic principles and clinical application in systemic and regional cancer treatment. In: *Biologic therapy of cancer.* Philadelphia: Lippincott, 2000.
45. Liénard D, Ewalenko P, Delmotti JJ, Renard N, Lejeune FJ. High-dose recombinant tumor necrosis factor alpha in combination with interferon gamma and melphalan in isolation perfusion of the limbs for melanoma and sarcoma. *J Clin Oncol* 1992;10:52.
46. Nawroth PP, Stern DM. Modulation of endothelial cell hemostatis properties by tumor necrosis factor. *J Exp Med* 1986;163:740.
47. Nawroth P, Handley D, Matsueda G, et al. Tumor necrosis factor/cachectin-induced intravascular fibrin formation in meth A fibrosarcomas. *J Exp Med* 1988;168:637.
48. Brett J, Gerlach H, Nawroth P, et al. Tumor necrosis factor/cachectin increases permeability of endothelial cell monolayers by a mechanism involving regulatory G proteins. *J Exp Med* 1989;169:1977.
49. Olieman AFT, van Ginkel RJ, Hoekstra HJ, et al. Angiographic response of locally advanced soft-tissue sarcoma following hyperthermic isolated limb perfusion with tumor necrosis factor. *Ann Surg Oncol* 1997;4:64.
50. Eggermont AMM, Koops HS, Liénard D, et al. Isolated limb perfusion with high dose tumor necrosis factor-α in combination with interferon-gamma and melphalan for irresectable extremity soft tissue sarcomas: a multicenter trial. *J Clin Oncol* 1996;14:2653.
51. Fraker D, Alexander HR, Ross M, et al. A phase II trial of isolated limb perfusion with high dose tumor necrosis factor and melphalan for unresectable extremity sarcomas. *Soc Surg Oncol* 1999;53:22(abst).
52. Posner MC, Liénard D, Lejeune FJ, Rosenfelder D, Kirkwood J. Hyperthermic isolated limb perfusion with tumor necrosis factor alone for melanoma. *Cancer J Sci Am* 1995;1:274.
53. Fraker DL. Isolated hepatic infusion perfusion (IHP) with TNF. *Cambridge Symposia* 1996;1:1(abst).
54. Alexander HR, Brown CK, Bartlett DL, et al. Augmented capillary leak during isolated hepatic perfusion (IHP) occurs via tumor necrosis factor independent mechanisms. *Clin Cancer Res* 1998;4:2362.
55. Liénard D, Lejeune F, Ewalenko I. In transit metastases of malignant melanoma treated by high dose rTNFα in combination with interferon-gamma and melphalan in isolation perfusion. *World J Surg* 1992;16:234.
56. Vaglini M, Santinami M, Manzi R, et al. Treatment of in-transit metastases from cutaneous melanoma by isolation perfusion with tumour necrosis factor-alpha (TNF-α), melphalan and interferon-gamma (IFN-γ). Dose-finding experience at the National Cancer Institute of Milan. *Melanoma Res* 1994;4:35.
57. Fraker DL. Limb perfusion with TNF: current status of United States trials. *Cambridge Symposia* 1996;1:13(abst).
58. Minor DR, Allen RE, Alberts D, et al. A clinical and pharmacokinetic study of isolated limb perfusion with heat and melphalan for melanoma. *Cancer* 1985;55:2638.
59. Lejeune FJ, Deloof T, Ewalenko P, et al. Objective regression of unexcised melanoma intransit metastases after hyperthermic isolation perfusion of the limbs with melphalan. *Rec Res Cancer Res* 1983;86:268.
60. Skene AI, Bulman AS, Williams TR, et al. Hyperthermic isolated perfusion with melphalan in the treatment of advanced malignant melanoma of the lower limb. *Br J Surg* 1990;77:765.
61. Klaase JM, Kroon BBR, van Geel AN, et al. Prognostic factors for tumor response and limb recurrence-free interval in patients with advanced melanoma of the limbs treated with regional isolated perfusion using melphalan. *Surgery* 1994;115:39.
62. di Filippo F, Calabro AM, Cavallari A, et al. The role of hyperthermic perfusion as a first step in the treatment of soft tissue sarcoma of the extremities. *World J Surg* 1988;12:332.
63. Eggermont AMM, Koops HS, Klausner JM, et al. Isolated limb perfusion with tumor necrosis factor and melphalan for limb salvage in 186 patients with locally advanced soft tissue extremity sarcomas. *Ann Surg* 1996;224:756.
64. Hafström L, Naredi P. Isolated hepatic perfusion with extracorporeal oxygenation using hyperthermia TNFα and melphalan: Swedish experience. *Rec Res Cancer Res* 1998;147:120.
65. Oldhafer KJ, Lang H, Frerker M, et al. First experience and technical aspects of isolated liver perfusion for extensive liver metastasis. *Surgery* 1998;123:622.
66. de Vries MR, Borel Rinkes IH, van de Velder CJH, et al. Isolated hepatic perfusion with tumor necrosis factor α and melphalan: experimental studies in pigs and phase I data from humans. *Rec Res Cancer Res* 1998;147:107.
67. Bartlett DL, Libutti SK, Alexander HR. Results of isolated hepatic perfusion (IHP) in patients with regionally advanced unresectable colorectal cancer. *Soc Surg Oncol* 1999:14(abst).
68. Liénard D, Aggermont A, Koops HS, Kroon B, Lejeune FJ. The use of TNF in isolated limb perfusion for treatment of locally advanced melanoma: an update. *Cambridge Symposium* 1996;1:12(abst).
69. Fraker DL, Alexander HR, Bartlett DL, Rosenberg SA. A prospective randomized trial of therapeutic isolated limb perfusion (ILP) comparing melphalan (M) versus melphalan, tumor necrosis factor (TNF) and interferon-gamma (IFN): an initial report. *Soc Surg Oncol* 1996;49:6(abst).
70. Hill S, Thomas JM. Low-dose tumour necrosis factor-alpha (TNF-α) and melphalan in hyperthermic isolated limb perfusion. Results from a pilot study performed in the United Kingdom. *Mel Res* 1994;4:31.

C. CLIFTON LING
CHEN CHUI
THOMAS LOSASSO
CHANDRA BURMAN
MARGIE HUNT
GIGAS MAGERAS
HOWARD IRA AMOLS
MICHAEL J. ZELEFSKY
ZVI Y. FUKS
STEVEN A. LEIBEL

SECTION **4**

Intensity-Modulated Radiation Therapy

In radiotherapy, the sum of experimental and clinical data indicates that the probabilities of local tumor control and normal tissue complications are dose dependent, and that the corresponding dose-response curves are sigmoidal in shape. For some disease sites the curves for local control are at lower dose levels relative to those for associated normal tissue toxicity, underpinning the success of radiotherapy in those cancers. For other sites, where these curves are closer to each other, or when the tumor control curve is less steep (the effect of population averaging due to heterogeneous radiosensitivity among individual tumors), the high doses required for tumor cure may cause unacceptable complications. In the last two decades, the development of three-dimensional conformal radiotherapy (3D-CRT), which substantially reduces the volume of critical organs irradiated to high doses, has partly addressed this issue.[1] In 3D-CRT, patient immobilization, image-guided treatment planning, and computer-controlled treatment delivery have combined to conform the radiation dose to the tumor, while maximally excluding the adjacent normal organs. This approach has permitted the increase of tumor dose without concomitant increase in normal tissue complications. At Memorial Sloan-Kettering Cancer Center (MSKCC), a clinical trial in cancer of the prostate has accrued more than 1100 patients, and the prescription dose has been escalated to 81 Gy with 3D-CRT, and to 86.4 Gy using intensity-modulated radiotherapy (IMRT), with promising results.[2,3]

3D-CRT involves the delineation of target and nontarget structures from patient-specific 3D image data sets [primarily computed tomography (CT), sometimes supplemented with magnetic resonance imaging, positron emission tomography, and so forth], the design of treatment portals using *beam's eye view* (BEV), the calculation and display of dose distributions, the analysis and evaluation of structure-specific dose-volume data [dose-volume histogram (DVH)], radiation delivery with computer-controlled multileaf collimators (MLC), and treatment verification with electronic portal images. However, the dose-distribution conformality achieved with 3D-CRT can be further improved by the use of computer-optimized intensity modulation. In addition, the treatment design phase of 3D-CRT involves several iterative steps and can be time-consuming, particularly when the anatomic geometry is complex. Thus, with the advance in computer technology, there has been much investigation on computer-aided treatment plan optimization.

IMRT is an advanced form of 3D-CRT with two key enhancements: (1) computerized iterative treatment plan optimization, and (2) the use of intensity-modulated radiation beams.[4] Although the overall process of IMRT and 3D-CRT is quite similar, these two ingredients have implications in some aspects of treatment planning and implementation. In this chapter, we describe the process of IMRT as compared with 3D-CRT, identify how they differ, emphasize those features and benefits unique to IMRT, and point to current and future development. At present, there are two primary methods of IMRT delivery: (1) intensity-modulated radiation fields at fixed gantry angles delivered with MLCs,[5] and (2) tomotherapy using beams from 360 degrees and modulated by a slit MLC.[6] Most of our discussion focuses on the former approach.

PROCESS OF INTENSITY-MODULATED RADIOTHERAPY

The process of IMRT, as implemented at MSKCC, is schematically illustrated in Figure 29.4-1. The following is a discussion on each of the steps in the process, and in addition, other information that is pertinent to the development and application of IMRT.

PATIENT SETUP, IMMOBILIZATION, AND IMAGE ACQUISITION

The minimization of patient setup uncertainty is more important in 3D-CRT relative to conventional radiotherapy due to the improved conformality of the dose distribution, and this is even more critical in IMRT, as discussed here. Thus, immobilization devices and precise positioning procedures should be used throughout the process of image acquisition, simulation, and treatment.

The use of simulators may be decreasing in 3D-CRT and IMRT, relative to its use in conventional radiotherapy. If a simulator is used, an initial (pre-CT) simulation may be carried out in conjunction with patient immobilization to establish fiduciary skin marks, define the tentative treatment isocenter, and obtain anteroposterior and lateral radiographic films. A second simulation may be performed, after the treatment plan has been accepted, to position the patient at the established isocenter and acquire reference radiographs of each field for comparison with the corresponding BEV digitally reconstructed radiographs and subsequently, the verification portal films.

A complete 3D CT image set is usually obtained with the patient in the treatment position on a flat couch. The number of CT slices and the interslice spacing are according to protocols, depending on the size, shape, and location of the target and the treatment technique. However, to produce high-resolution digitally reconstructed radiographs, the slices are contiguous with interslice spacing of 3 to 5 mm. For certain sites, magnetic resonance imaging and positron emission tomography are complementary to CT and helpful in defining the extent of disease, especially when used with image-correlation software.

The advent of CT simulation may make the process more efficient, by combining the simulation and CT imaging sessions into one. The CT simulator combines the capabilities of spiral (or helical) scanners for volumetric data acquisition and high-speed workstations for rapid image reconstruction and

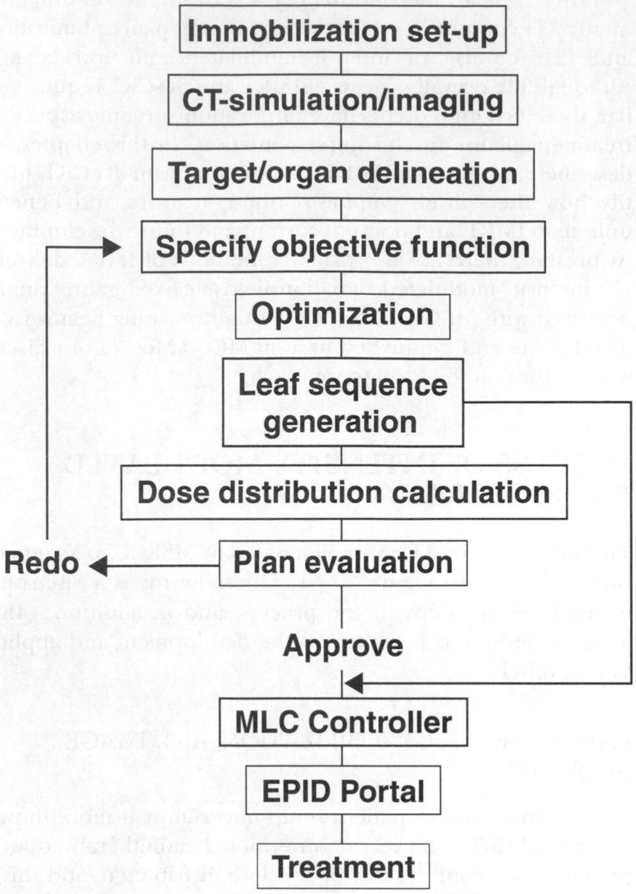

FIGURE 29.4-1. A schematic illustrating step by step the intensity-modulated radiation therapy process. CT, computed tomography; EPID, electronic portal imaging device; MLC, multileaf collimators.

display. This permits the so-called virtual simulation, carried out on a computer workstation using the 3D CT data set (the virtual patient).[7] In this process, a complete 3D CT data set is first obtained with the patient in the treatment position using 3- to 5-mm slice thickness. Then, corresponding to the specific treatment set-up parameters, patient anatomy is reconstructed from the CT data and displayed in BEV, and simulation fluoroscopic and radiographic images are digitally generated for viewing, decision-making, and documentation.

Aside from the improved efficiency, CT simulation eliminates or minimizes systematic uncertainties in the registration of simulation films to CT data sets, and in set-up errors when transferring the patient from one mechanical coordinate system to another. The disadvantage is the degraded image quality of reconstructed radiographs as compared with a conventional simulation film.

DELINEATION OF TREATMENT VOLUME AND SELECTION OF TREATMENT BEAMS

Treatment volumes are derived from the CT images according to the ICRU Report 50 nomenclature,[8] with clinical target volume (CTV) being the visualized tumor plus the regions at risk, and planning target volume (PTV) to include setup and other uncertainties. The manual delineation of these and their adjacent critical organs are time consuming and would benefit from new and improved tools. However, human intervention will likely remain a necessary and important component for defining the CTV and PTV. Other contours needed for treatment planning and dose-distribution calculation such as the outer skin, bone, lungs, and air cavities can be outlined automatically with existing edge detection algorithms.

In 3D-CRT, to facilitate the selection of beam angles and field shapes, various display methods have been developed to represent the PTV and the adjacent critical organs in 3D perspectives. These objects are often displayed as wireframes or solid structures, using colors to differentiate between them and intensity to indicate depth. The treatment geometry is best visualized in the BEV, in which the anatomy is viewed from the perspective of the radiation source.[9,10] Once the beam orientations are chosen, their shapes (apertures) can be determined, again facilitated by the BEV display.

3D image display is probably less critical in IMRT than in 3D-CRT. We believe that as long as there are a sufficient number of radiation fields (five to seven or more), the number of beams and their orientations are less important. This is because the many degrees of freedom in intensity modulation can effectively compensate the less optimal beam direction. Also, field size and shape can be completely defined by the assignment of intensity pattern in the optimization process (see Computer-Aided Plan Optimization in Intensity-Modulated Radiotherapy, later in this chapter). This is true at least for the treatment of cancers of the prostate and of head and neck at MSKCC and likely applies to other disease sites as well. Whether significant improvements in IMRT can be achieved via the use of noncoplanar beams is yet to be demonstrated, although this may likely prove advantageous for brain tumors and possibly other sites.

COMPUTER-AIDED PLAN OPTIMIZATION IN INTENSITY-MODULATED RADIOTHERAPY

The most distinguishing feature in IMRT planning is the use of intensity modulation to improve the dose distribution. An iterative process is invariably used, alternately adjusting the intensity pattern of the beams and assessing the resulting dose distribution until an acceptable plan is devised. The iterative process could be computer automated or could involve significant manual intervention. In general, computer automation is needed in the so-called inverse planning, while user experience and involvement are more important in the forward planning of IMRT. As widespread enthusiasm is primarily for the inverse method, we shall only briefly describe the forward process.

In forward planning, the starting point is a number of open beams and their field shapes. Based on the resultant dose distribution, the user adjusts the intensities in parts of some of the beams and recalculates the dose distribution. This is repeated until an optimal dose distribution is obtained. This approach is sensitive to the experience of the planner and may be restrictive in terms of the number of intensity levels and the complexity of the intensity-modulation pattern.[11]

The inverse method of treatment planning was first proposed by Brahme in 1988.[4] In this approach, the user specifies the number and orientations of the beams, and the desired objectives for the PTV and the critical organs. The computer algorithm divides each beam into individual rays and iteratively

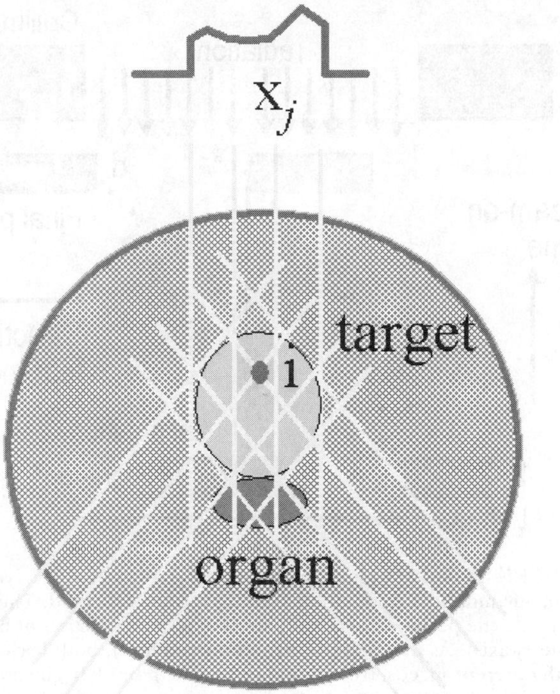

FIGURE 29.4-2. In this illustration of the inverse planning method, the user begins by specifying three beams and their directions. The planning algorithm optimizes the intensities of the different rays (x_j) of each of the beams so that the dose to each point i within the target and the critical organ conform to the user's criteria. The resulting beams are intensity modulated (as shown by the profile of the vertical beam).

alters the ray weights until the composite 3D dose distribution conforms to the specified objectives. The beams derived by this method are intensity modulated (i.e., the pattern of radiation varies within each beam). It is easy to see why the field shapes need not be prespecified; the optimization process determines the edges as well as the intensity patterns within.

Central to the success of computer optimization is the specification of some quantitative measure of the *goodness* of a treatment plan. In inverse planning, the criteria are stated mathematically as objective functions that the optimization algorithm attempts to minimize. At present, most algorithms (including ours) are dose or dose-volume based (i.e., constraints are defined as doses to the target and normal tissues, or to volumes of interest).[12,13] The use of biologically weighted objective functions is in principle more relevant, but is currently limited by the lack of validated biophysical models on tumor control and organ toxicity. The inverse planning method developed by Spirou and Chui at MSKCC is briefly summarized in the section Clinical Experience with the Use of Optimization Criteria, later in this chapter.[13]

The starting point is the specification of the number of beams and their directions, and then the algorithm optimizes the intensities in the different parts of each of the beams. Suppose a patient is treated with three beams as shown in Figure 29.4-2, the computer program first calculates the doses to a matrix of points within the target and the normal organs from each individual rays of the three beams. If the point in question is in the target with a prescribed dose p_i, the goodness of the current set of ray weights is given by the square of the difference between p_i and the current dose. This square of the difference is then summed over all the target points to determine the objective function that describes the goodness of the present set of beam weights. The weights of the individual rays and of each beam are then changed one at the time, with the change accepted if the objective function is reduced. The iterative process continues until the optimal plan is obtained, that is when the objective function is at its minimum.

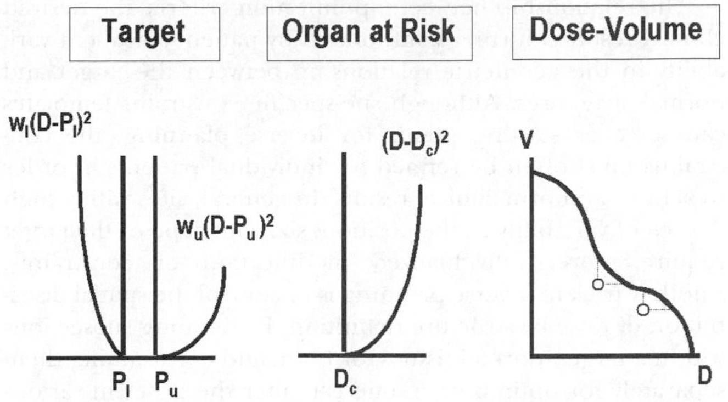

FIGURE 29.4-3. Examples of possible objective functions, illustrated graphically. For the treatment target, doses within the allowable inhomogeneity are permitted, with different penalties (w) assessed for underdose as opposed to overdose. For the normal organ, penalty can be applied if dose exceeds a certain critical value (Dc) or based on dose-volume considerations. D, dose; V, volume.

Constraints for critical organs can be incorporated as added term in the objective function. Dose-volume considerations are typically stated as "no more than q% of the particular organ may receive a dose greater than d_{dv}." To impose such a constraint, at each iteration, the cumulative volume of the organ receiving doses greater than d_{dv} is compared with q. If it exceeds q, a penalty in the form of constraint is added to the objective function, but only for those points that cause the constraint to be violated (i.e., the points beyond the volume q).

Several objective functions are illustrated graphically in Figure 29.4-3. For the treatment target, the graph illustrates the concept of the *allowable inhomogeneity* (i.e., if the dose is between a lower limit P_l and an upper limit P_u, penalty is not assessed). Also, a larger weight can be assigned to penalize underdose as opposed to overdose. For the normal organ, penalty can be applied if dose exceeds a certain critical value (D_c) or based on dose-volume considerations, as discussed previously.

CLINICAL EXPERIENCE WITH THE USE OF OPTIMIZATION CRITERIA

The iterative adjustment of beam modulation by the optimization algorithm is supposed to minimize the user-specified objective function so that the resultant plan would satisfy the specified criteria. However, in our initial experience the resultant plan was often unsatisfactory. There are several reasons for this. First, the initial sets of optimization criteria may not have been realistic. Second, the relationship between the objective function parameters and the resulting dose distribution is complex. Thus, through a trial-and-error process we have developed preliminary criteria templates that are disease-site specific. We have also learned that the optimization criteria must be more stringent than the desired clinical result because no penalty is applied unless the constraint is violated.

The relationship between optimization criteria and desired clinical result is further confounded by patient-to-patient variability in the geometric relationship between the target and normal structures. Although site-specific constraint templates can serve as starting points for inverse planning, the constraints must often be refined for individual patients in order to achieve uniform clinical results. In general, sites with a high degree of variability in the position, size, or shape of the target require more individualized modification of constraints. Another trick in inverse planning is to control the spatial distribution of dose by structure definition. By defining subsections within a target, normal tissues, or both, and constraining them separately for optimization, one can alter the doses in various regions (e.g., to move a high-dose region away from a nearby critical structure). At the present stage of IMRT development, the specification of structures and criteria for optimization are still being studied for the different disease sites, and exactly how patient specificity of such criteria will affect the optimization process needs to be better understood.

TREATMENT PLAN EVALUATION

The process of treatment plan evaluation is continuing to evolve, particularly for IMRT with inverse planning. The tools by which plans are evaluated are largely the same for 3D-CRT and IMRT: two-dimensional (2D) dose distributions superimposed on CT images, 3D volumetric rendering of dose distribution and the PTV (and critical organs), structure-specific DVH, and biologic indices as a rough guide. Additionally, for IMRT plans, inspection of the intensity profiles either from an *observer view* (like a relief map) or by the projection of isointensity lines on a BEV is often useful in evaluating an individual beam's contribution to the dose distribution. Even though the evaluation tools for 3D and IMRT plans are quite similar, the approach and action are quite different.

In the forward process of 3D-CRT or IMRT, the planner and the physician evaluate the initial treatment design(s) with a view to improve on it by altering some of the beam parameters (e.g., directions, weights, shapes, wedges, and so forth). The identification of deficiencies and the devising of remedies rely on the experience and intuition of the planner. The effort-intensive nature of this approach limits the practical number of iterations of evaluation and alteration. On the other hand, the application of class solutions to some disease sites minimizes the alterations needed and facilitates convergence to an acceptable solution within a few cycles.

In the inverse process of IMRT, to exploit the benefits of the increased degrees of freedom with modulated individual ray weights, a significant number of iterations (typically five to ten) are both needed and carried out. As the goal of the iterative adjustment of beam modulation by the optimization algorithm is to minimize the user-specified objective function, the resultant plan should satisfy the clinical criteria of acceptance. Thus, ideally the evaluation process should be primarily checking and approval. However, as discussed previously, this is usually not the case, at least in the developmental phase of IMRT.

Corrective action for an unacceptable IMRT plan would involve alteration of the parameters of the objective functions (instead of the beam parameters in a 3D-CRT plan). As alluded to previously, our observation is that such adjustments are not always consistent with our intuition or past experience in conventional or 3D-CRT treatment planning. One major difference is the lack of control in making coordinate-specific adjustment (i.e., it is difficult to alter the dose level to specific regions in the 3D space by changing the objective function parameters). At present, a trial and error (and time-consuming) approach is used to alter the input parameters and improve the IMRT. However, with improvement in software features and with experience in IMRT planning, we believe that this situation will improve.

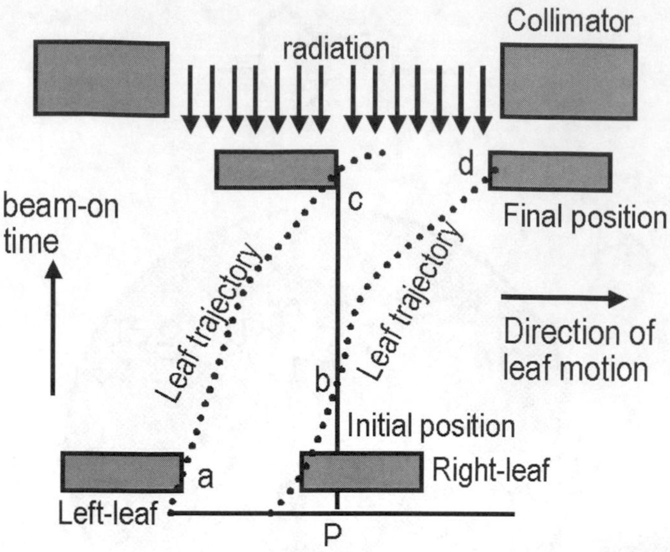

FIGURE 29.4-4. This graph depicts radiation delivery by the dynamic multileaf collimation (sliding window) method. The dotted lines are the positions of a leaf pair (x-axis) as a function of beam-on time (y-axis). As the beam is turned on (point a), both leaves move, with different speeds, from left to right. The point P begins to receive radiation when the right leaf edge moves pass over it (point b). It receives radiation until the left leaf blocks the beam (point c). By controlling the movement of the leaves and therefore the beam-on-time duration between b and c, one can deliver any desired intensity to point P, or any other point under this leaf pair.

DELIVERY OF INTENSITY-MODULATED FIELD WITH DYNAMIC MULTILEAF COLLIMATOR

The intensity-modulated field can be delivered with an MLC.[14–16] The 2D intensity distribution is divided into one-dimensional intensity profiles, with each profile delivered by one pair of leaves. In the dynamic MLC (DMLC or sliding-window) method, the leaves are in continuous motion during radiation delivery. In Figure 29.4-4, the trajectory (the dotted lines) of the left and right leaves of one leaf pair is plotted as a function of beam-on time during radiation delivery, from their initial (instance a) to their final positions (instance d). As the beam is turned on (instance a), both leaves move, with different speeds, from left to right. The point P begins to receive radiation at instance b when the right leaf edge moves past it. It continues to receive radiation until instance c, when the left leaf begins to block the beam from P. By controlling the movement of the leaves and therefore the *exposure* duration (in this case, between b and c), one can deliver any desired intensity to point P, or any other point under this leaf pair. Extending this concept to multiple pairs of leaves, any desired intensity modulation can be produced with designed sequences of leaves positions.

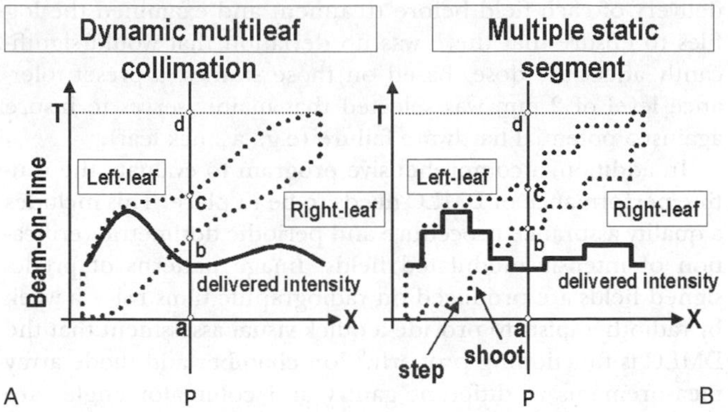

FIGURE 29.4-5. **A:** Illustrating the intensity profile delivered by the leaves' paths shown in Figure 29.4-4 (replotted here as dotted lines). In practice, a leaf-sequencing algorithm is used to translate the desired intensity profiles into computer data file of the leaf positions as a function of monitor units. **B:** Another method using the multileaf collimators to deliver intensity-modulated beams is by multiple static segment (the so-called step-and-shoot method). In the step phase, multileaf collimator travels to discrete positions, then beam-on in the shoot phase (i.e., alternate multileaf collimator movement and radiation delivery). The result is discrete intensity levels, the number of which depends on the step number.

The leaves' paths illustrated in Figure 29.4-4 (replotted in Figure 29.4-5*A* as dotted lines) are planned to produce the intensity profile indicated by the solid line in Figure 29.4-5*A*. In practice, a separate computer program (different from the inverse planning algorithm), sometimes called the *leaf sequencer*, is used to translate the intensity profiles of the intensity-modulated beam into the so-called DMLC file, that contains the data of the leaf position sequence as a function of monitor units (MU).[16] In practice, not all desired intensity profiles are (exactly) achievable because of the constraints on leaf motion imposed by the design of the MLC and the clinical dose rate of the machine. The MLC manufactured by Varian Medical Systems, for example, is constrained by the maximum leaf speed (v_{max} of 2.5 cm/s) and a maximum DMLC field of 14.5 cm (unless movement of the carriage is allowed). Beam delivery systems from other manufacturers may have similar or different limitations and constraints. Some leaf motion patterns may require a large number of MUs to deliver the desired dose (typically two to three times that for static beam conformal therapy), which increases the importance of scatter and leakage dose. Transmissions through the leaves and the rounded leaf ends (see Dose Distribution Calculation, later in this chapter) typically contribute 10% to 15% of the total dose and are compensated for in the leaf sequence translation.

The MLC can also be used to deliver intensity-modulated beams in the multiple static segment (MSS, or the so-called step-and-shoot) mode. In this mode, the MLC travels in a stepwise manner to discrete positions, with the beam turned off during the stepwise movement. As illustrated in Figure 29.4-5*B*, the leaf paths can be approximated by alternate horizontal *step* and vertical *shoot* segments, representing stepwise and alternate MLC movement and radiation delivery. As a result, the delivered intensity profile comprises discrete levels, with its number depending on the number of steps. In either mode, the total beam-on time for this leaf pair is T, and the MU needed for an intensity-modulated field is the largest T among all leaf pairs. It should be noted that there are other methods of MSS leaf sequencing to produce intensity-modulated beams.[17,18]

OTHER METHODS OF DELIVERY OF INTENSITY-MODULATED FIELD

A large number of IMRT treatments have been delivered using the MIMiC collimator from NOMOS.[6] In this schema, a slit beam is used, typically 2-by-20 cm, and intensity modulation is achieved via 20 pairs of leaves. Each of the 40 leaves defines a pencil beam of 1 by 1 cm^2 that is either on or off at any given gantry position. As the gantry rotates through its 360-degree arc, all 40 leaves open and close (in a binary manner, either fully open or fully closed) according to the leaf motion pattern determined during treatment planning. Thus, each gantry arc treats a 2-cm long longitudinal strip of tissue. Treatment fields longer than 2 cm can be delivered by longitudinally translating the patient (with the treatment couch) between multiple arcs. Of extreme importance is the accuracy and stability of patient positioning as the treatment progresses from one axial slice to the next.

Yu proposed the intensity-modulated arc therapy method of IMRT delivery.[19] In this method, the 2D intensity-modulated beams at many equally spaced gantry angles are approximated by a superposition of multiple-shaped radiation fields with uniform intensity. The increments of intensity level are delivered by individual arcs, with the leaf positions changing with gantry angle to produce the shaped fields. As has been pointed out, there are a large number of possible permutations of decomposition patterns for the 2D beams, and therefore the design of the most efficient MLC position sequence in the arc therapy is a challenging problem.

DOSE DISTRIBUTION CALCULATION

To fully account for the intricacies of IMRT dose delivery, the calculation model must accurately predict the incident energy fluence and use a dose kernel that describes the transport of photons and electrons and energy spread in an inhomogeneous medium. One accurate method of dose calculation involves the convolution of pencil beams. In our current dose model, inhomogeneity is accounted for by the traditional equivalent path length method, and pencil beam convolution is used only as a correction factor to account for the variation of intensity as opposed to a flat, uniform field.[20] However, in a highly heterogeneous media such as the lung, the accuracy of this calculation method needs improvement, for which development is in progress. The Monte Carlo method can provide the most accurate dose calculation, but because of the lengthy computation time, its routine use awaits faster computer speed. Nevertheless, the Monte Carlo method is relied on to derive accurate pencil beam kernel and the source function (which predicts the incident intensity pattern), with detailed accounting of the finite source size, extrafocal radiation (from the flattening filters, primary and secondary collimators), beam spectrum, and so forth. For both the DMLC and the MSS methods of IMRT treatment delivery, because small aperture sizes are frequently used, accurate prediction of output factor is important.[21]

Beam-on time calculation for IMRT treatment at MSKCC is an adaptation from our empirical-based method in which the dose D at a point (x,y,z) is given as $D(x,y,z) = MU \times F$, where MU is the monitor unit of radiation beam, and F is a product of several factors, including the field size or output factor, the tissue maximum ratio, the off-center ratio, the inverse-square factor, and so forth. For IMRT, we modify the equation using a factor that accounts for the intensity modulation.

In delivering the intensity-modulated field with an MLC, only a portion of the entire field is exposed at a given time. As a result, the total MU required is usually longer than that normally required. There is no simple relationship between the maximum beam intensity and MU. In practice, the total beam-on time MU is calculated by a computer program, taking into account effects such as leaf transmission, rounded leaf ends, tongue and groove, distributed source, maximum leaf speed, and dose rate. In general, the more complex the intensity modulation, the larger the MU.

For conventional treatment, the independent MU check is typically calculated by hand. For IMRT, however, the intensity distribution is sufficiently complex that hand calculation is not feasible. At MSKCC, the independent check was initially provided by ionization chamber measurement, and subsequently by another computer program. Measurement is a direct assessment of the delivered dose, particularly valuable for new treatment techniques, but extremely time consuming as a routine check. Our computer MU check software was programmed by an independent team. The program first constructs the delivered intensity distribution from the leaf-sequencing files and the beam-on time. Doses to points or to planes at depth in a phantom are then calculated and compared with those of the original plan.

COMMISSIONING AND QUALITY ASSURANCE PROGRAM

Both mechanical and dosimetric measurements are required in the commissioning of IMRT delivery using DMLC.[22–24] Because the dose delivered using DMLC is directly related to the gap widths between pairs of opposing leaves, precise leaf position is much more important in this approach than in treatments using static MLC. Mechanical calibration of the leaf positions can be accomplished using the recommended procedure and software supplied by the manufacturer. We have determined that a precision of 0.2 mm in leaf position is necessary, and that the Varian Mark II MLC satisfies this requirement. Dosimetric characterization of the MLC, using film, ion chambers, or both, includes measurements of radiation transmission through the leaves and their rounded ends, and the determination of head scatter. The dosimetric contribution of these factors, which can amount to as much as 15% of the dose, are accounted for in the leaf sequencer algorithm of the treatment planning system.

Another important consideration of DMLC is the monitoring of the performance of the MLC during treatment. While the beam is on, the Varian MLC control computer checks all leaf positions every 55 msec, compares them to the planned leaf positions in the DMLC file, and records them in a DMLC log file. If any leaf deviates from its planned position beyond a preset tolerance, the control computer invokes a *beam holdoff,* and radiation delivery is withheld until all the leaves are within tolerance again. Deviations that invoke beam holdoff should occur infrequently as the leaf sequencer algorithm, in generating the DMLC file, has duly considered the maximum MLC leaf speed and the nominal dose rate. Tests using clinical fields indicate that deviations of greater than 1 mm occur less than 1% of the time. For the initial group of patients, we tested the delivery of each field before treatment and examined the log files to ensure that there was no deviation that would significantly affect the dose. Based on those studies, a preset tolerance level of 2 mm was selected that mainly serves to insure against a potential hardware failure (e.g., a stuck leaf).

In addition, a comprehensive program to evaluate the routine performance of DMLC needs to be in place. This includes a quality assurance procedure and periodic dosimetric verification of intensity-modulated fields. Image patterns of predesigned fields are produced on radiographic films twice a week by radiotherapists to provide a quick visual assessment that the DMLC is functioning properly.[9] Ion chamber and diode array measurements at different gantry and collimator angles are performed monthly by a physicist to ensure constancy of the DMLC output and to track long-term stability. Ion chamber measurements in solid phantom for patient fields provide a straightforward check on the MU calculations. Film dosimetry, with sufficient spatial resolution for the intensity-modulated patterns, efficiently compares the delivered and the planned dose distributions. It is also used intensively during the testing of new software and new treatment sites for IMRT, as well as for periodic spot checks. The general procedure is to irradiate the film in a homogeneous plastic phantom and to digitize the exposed film with a laser scanner.

TREATMENT DELIVERY WITH DYNAMIC MULTILEAF COLLIMATOR

For treatment implementation, the DMLC files of the intensity-modulated fields are transferred either via a floppy disk or electronically to the MLC control computer of the treatment machine. Also transmitted for each intensity-modulated beam is its fluence aperture, defined as the area with greater than 1% of the maximum intensity, or approximately the MLC aperture with the leading leaves and the trailing leaves at their respective final and initial positions. This fluence aperture is used for acquiring portal image (see Consideration of Treatment Uncertainties, later in this chapter) and for recording and verification purposes by that system.

Before the first treatment, portal localization electronic portal imaging device (EPID) images are taken of each intensity-modulated field with its fluence aperture. The portal localization films are then compared with the corresponding digitally reconstructed radiographs overlaid with the maximal DMLC apertures. This verifies that the radiation is directed properly, relative to the bony anatomy of the patient. During the treatment course, weekly portals are obtained for each field using the EPID. Using the EPID in combination with the MLC allows machine setup and image acquisition to occur without the therapist reentering the room between fields, thereby improving efficiency.

Before the dose delivery in patient treatment, the record and verify computer checks the initial leaf settings and the other machine parameters: the gantry angle, collimator angle, jaw positions, and MU setting. During radiation delivery, the MLC control computer monitors the leaf positions every 55 msec, compares them with the planned positions, and records the result in a DMLC log-file. On completion of the first DMLC field, the record and verify system records the MU delivered and the final positions of the MLC. Without reentering the room, the radiotherapists rotate the gantry to the next orientation, program the accelerator and the MLC for the next intensity-modulated field, and then deliver the radiation. The process is repeated for each of the fields.

CLINICAL EXPERIENCE

CANCER OF THE PROSTATE

Since 1986 we have treated more than 1000 patients with cancers of the prostate using 3D-CRT. An analysis of 743 of these patients showed a significant effect of increased dose (from 64.8 Gy to 81.0 Gy) on response.[3] With the capability of IMRT, we have further escalated the dose and have treated approximately 40 patients to 86.4 Gy. At the same time, a five-field IMRT treatment with a prescription dose of 81.0 Gy has become the standard of care for prostate of the cancer at MSKCC. This summary describes this experience and our preliminary clinical results.

Patients are immobilized in the prone position, simulated, and imaged on a CT simulator. With the CT data transferred electronically to the MSKCC planning system,[30] the PTV, bladder, rectum, bowel, femors, and pelvis are contoured. IMRT planning is performed with the inverse method using a five-field technique (0, 75, 135, 225, and 285 degrees) as detailed previously.[23] The present criteria for optimization are dose uniformity (within 12%) to the PTV, less than 34% of the rectal wall at 75 Gy, and less than 58% of the bladder wall at 81 Gy. The overlap region between the PTV and the rectal wall is separately constrained during optimization to exert greater control over the spatial dose distribution in that region. On approval of the optimized plan, BEV digitally reconstructed radiographs and the fluence apertures are generated, and the DMLC files transmitted to the MLC controller for treatment delivery using DMLC.[16]

We reported the preliminary results of 171 IMRT patients, in comparison with those of 61 3D-CRT patients treated to the same 81 Gy.[25] Comparison of the dose distributions of the five-field IMRT plan and the 3D-CRT plan (six-field primary to 72.0 Gy, plus a 9-Gy boost with the rectum blocked) indicated that IMRT improved the conformality of the 81-Gy isodose line relative to the PTV and decreased the dose to the surrounding normal tissues. A systematic analysis (using the Wilcoxon assigned rank test) of the two types of plans on 20 randomly selected patients demonstrated that significantly higher percentage of the CTV received 81 Gy with IMRT relative to 3D-CRT (98 ± 2% vs. 95 ± 2%, $P<.01$).[25] Concomitantly, the percentages of the rectal wall and bladder wall volumes carried to 75 Gy were significantly decreased with IMRT ($P<.01$). These data support the notion that IMRT significantly improves the conformality of the radiation treatment in prostate cancer.

Figure 29.4-6 is an example of the dose distribution, in a color wash representation, achieved for an IMRT prostate treatment to 81 Gy with five intensity-modulated beams. The dose distributions in the transverse and midsagittal planes are shown, with the PTV (green) and rectum (yellow) outlined. The dose distribution conforms to the PTV and restricts the rectum volume irradiated to high doses. The cumulative DVHs for this plan (Fig. 29.4-7) reinforce this point. Approximately 95% of the PTV receives the prescription dose and the level of dose inhomogeneity is reasonable. DVHs for the rectal and bladder walls are also compliant to acceptable criteria derived from previous 3D-CRT clinical experience. Figure 29.4-8 illustrates the intensity profile of the posterior beam, in the isocentric plane, from the 81-Gy IMRT plan illustrated in Figure 29.4-6.

In terms of clinical outcome, the combined rates of acute grade 1 and 2 rectal toxicity for IMRT were significantly less (45%) than that of 3D-CRT (61%) using the Radiation Therapy Oncology Group morbidity grading scale ($P=.05$).[28] Similarly, there was a highly significant decrease in late grade 2 rectal bleeding to 0.5% with IMRT as compared with 13% for conventional 3D-CRT ($P<.001$). There was one grade 3 rectal toxicity (bleeding requiring laser cauterization) in each treatment group. Based on this experience, we have escalated the dose to 86.4 Gy and have successfully treated 40 patients using IMRT. We now await follow-up data on late reactions before additional patient accrual at this dose level.

Compared with our previous method of 3D-CRT planning for the 81-Gy treatment, IMRT planning is less labor intensive.

A

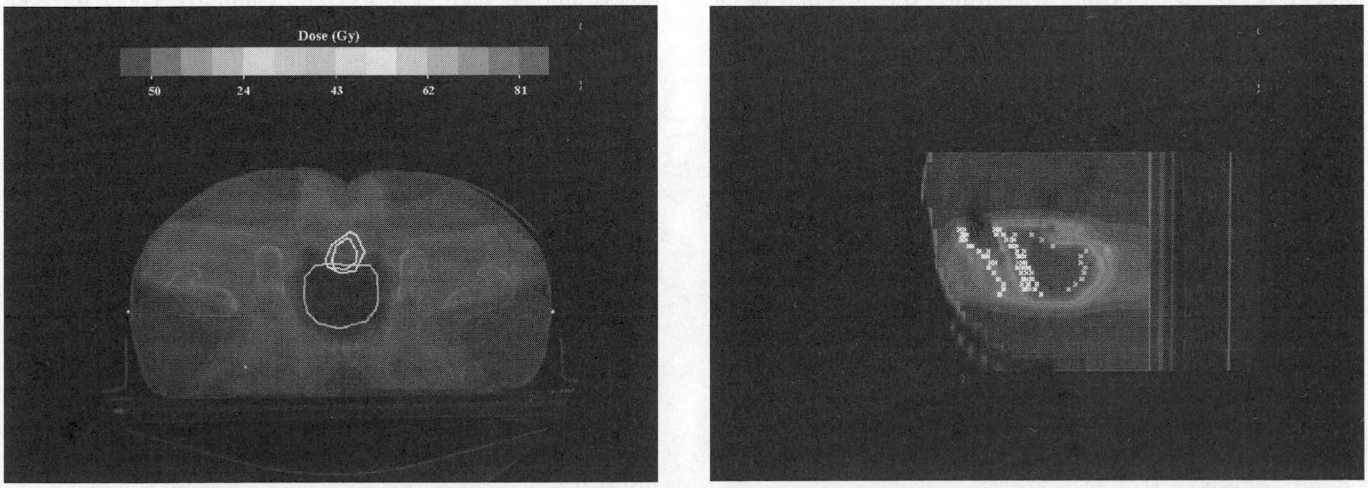

B

FIGURE 29.4-6. An example of the dose distribution, in a color wash representation, for intensity-modulated radiation therapy prostate treatment to 81 Gy with 5 intensity-modulated beams. The dose distributions in the **(A)** transverse and **(B)** midsagittal planes are shown, with the planning target volume (PTV) (green) and rectum (yellow) outlined. (See Color Figs. 29.4-6*A* and *B* in the CD-ROM and on the Web at www.LWWoncology.com.)

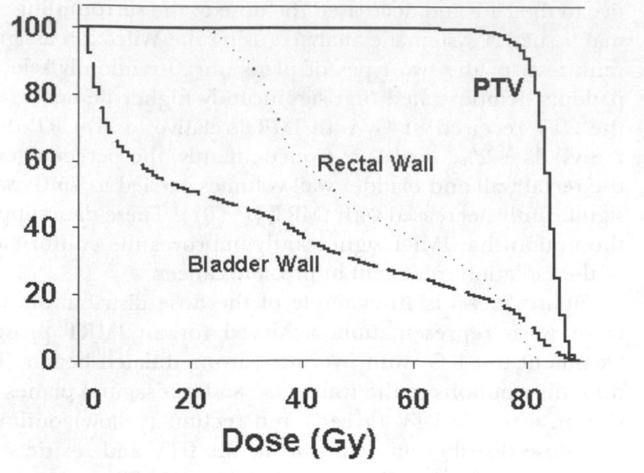

FIGURE 29.4-7. The cumulative dose volume histograms for the 81-Gy intensity-modulated radiation therapy plan illustrated in Figure 29.4-6. The dose-volume histograms for the planning target volume, rectal wall, and bladder wall are shown.

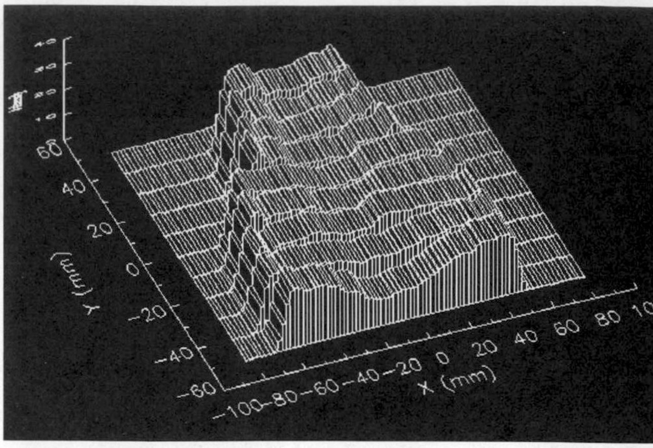

FIGURE 29.4-8. The intensity profile of the posterior beam, in the isocentric plane, from the 81-Gy intensity-modulated radiation therapy plan illustrated in Figure 29.4-6. (See Color Fig. 29.4-8 in the CD-ROM and on the Web at www.LWWoncology.com.)

The 81-Gy 3D-CRT plan was performed in two phases, a standard six-field plan to 72 Gy and a second one for the 9-Gy boost. In contrast, a single IMRT plan for both the 81-Gy or 86.4-Gy treatment course was judged acceptable for both tumor coverage and normal tissue sparing. Thus, the treatment planning effort has been reduced by a factor of two.

In terms of implementation, on average the length of treatment sessions was comparable for the five-field IMRT and the six-field 3D-CRT plans, even though the MUs of IMRT were approximately 2.5-fold higher. The average session for 138 patients treated (April 1995 to March 1996) with 3D-CRT to 75.6 Gy was 17.7 ± 0.1 minutes, compared with 16.5 ± 0.1 minutes for 140 IMRT patients treated (April 1997 to March 1998) to 81 Gy on the same machine, inclusive of the time for setup and weekly portal imaging.

HEAD AND NECK CANCER

Radiotherapy of head and neck cancers is often complex due to target doses of 70 Gy or higher and the close proximity of the spinal cord, brain stem, parotid glands, and optic pathway structures with tolerance doses of 45 to 55 Gy or less. Traditional treatments, consisting of parallel opposed photon fields (with blocks added to shield the spinal cord at 45 Gy) and electron fields to augment the dose to the cervical lymph nodes, are often inadequate in target coverage and in normal tissue sparing. We have previously used a multifield 3D-CRT approach, but since May 1998 have adopted IMRT and DMLC to deliver a uniform target dose with steep dose gradients at target-normal structure interfaces and reduced doses over normal tissues. Approximately one-half of 20 patients have received treatment for primary nasopharynx cancer, with 70 Gy to the gross disease and 54 Gy to the presumed microscopic disease.

Subsequent to CT simulation and image (3-mm increments) acquisition of the immobilized patient, the PTV (the gross disease and adjacent lymph nodes) and the normal structures (spinal cord, brain stem, optic nerves, chiasm, mandible, larynx, and parotid glands) are delineated. The beam arrangement, consisting of seven equally spaced beams directed from the posterior and lateral directions, attempts to create a concave dose distribution that encompasses the nasopharynx, skull base, and regional lymph nodes but encircles and spares the spinal cord and brain stem. When implemented with 3D-CRT, the technique is limited by excessive dose nonuniformity within the PTV (up to 140%) and by both planning and treatment complexities. These limitations are easily overcome with IMRT.

The dose-based criteria for optimization are for the nasopharynx and nodal target volumes to receive the prescription dose with a maximum of 120%, and dose constraints on the normal structures as follows: spinal cord, 40 Gy; brain stem, 50 Gy; optic structures, 50 Gy; and larynx, 45 Gy. The penalties for the spinal cord and brain stem are generally four to five times greater than the penalties for the PTV and other normal tissues. The derived IMRT plan, as assessed by dose distribution and DVH for the PTV and normal structures, demonstrates significant improvements over the traditional approach of parallel opposed primary plus 3D-CRT boost. The dose distributions are highly conformal and constrain the maximum spinal cord and brain stem doses to less than 40 and 50 Gy, respectively, well below maximum acceptable doses. Although there is no specific attempt to decrease the dose to the parotid glands for fear of underdosing nearby lymph nodes, the distribution of dose within the parotid gland is substantially different from that obtained with traditional opposed fields. With traditional parallel opposed beams, nearly the entire parotid gland volume would receive a dose of 70 Gy or more. With IMRT, approximately one-half the gland receives less than 50 Gy. Dose to the mandible is also substantially improved. Although the maximum mandible dose is still approximately 75 Gy, only 10% of the mandible receives more than 60 Gy. Figure 29.4-9 is a 3D display of the 95% isodose surface (blue) for a typical IMRT treatment of nasopharynx. Superimposed are the outer skin surface (purple) and wireframe representation of the PTV (yellow), parotids (green), and the spinal cord (red). The left lateral and cranial views are presented.

BREAST CANCER

Radiation therapy after lumpectomy remains a primary method of treatment for primary breast cancer. Excellent local control is achieved in early-stage disease along with generally good cos-

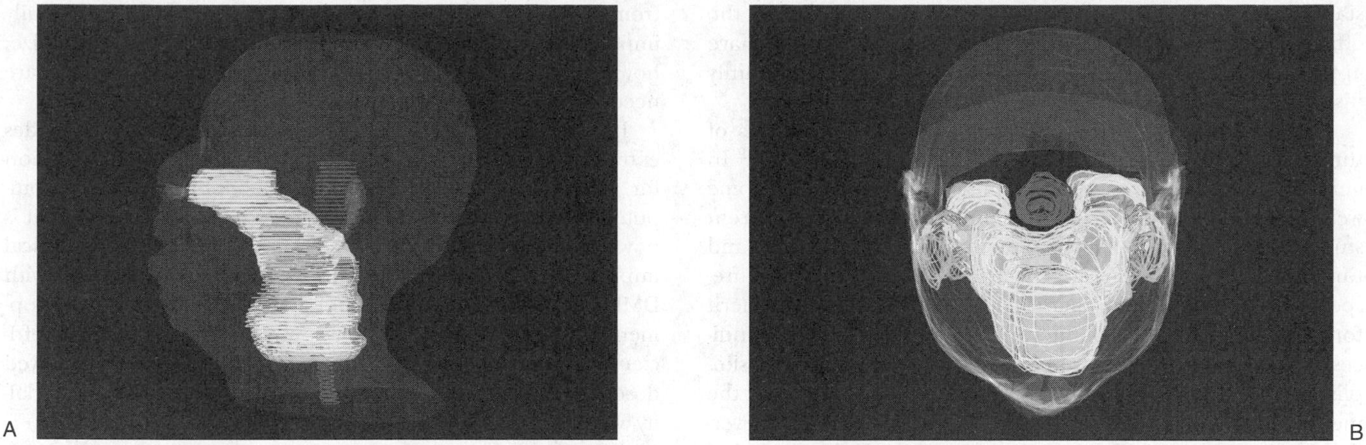

FIGURE 29.4-9. Three-dimensional display of the 95% isodose surface (blue) for an intensity-modulated radiation therapy treatment of nasopharynx. Superimposed are the outer skin surface (purple) and wireframe representation of the planning target volume (yellow), parotids (green), and spinal cord (red). The left lateral **(A)** and cranial **(B)** views are presented. (See Color Figs. 29.4-9*A* and *B* in the CD-ROM and on the Web at www.LWWoncology.com..)

metic results and low toxicity. Nonetheless, improvements are needed, particularly for large-breasted patients with left-sided disease for whom cosmesis and potential cardiac toxicity remain significant issues. Since April 1999, we have treated selected patients with disease in the left breast and with large chest wall diameters with intensity modulation using a standard tangential beam arrangement. All patients undergo CT simulation during which the direction and size of the tangential beams are determined. The PTV is defined to be all tissue encompassed within 0.5 cm of the tangent field borders. The ipsilateral lung and coronary artery regions are defined by the physician using the CT.

The IMRT plan must deliver a uniform dose distribution in the PTV to within 10% of the prescription. Typically, this is achieved by setting an even tighter dose uniformity constraint for the target (of 5%) during optimization. The dose to the coronary artery region is minimized to the extent possible without sacrificing target coverage. Generally, a maximum dose constraint of 95% is used for this structure during optimization. Dose to the apex of the breast is controlled by separately contouring and constraining this region.

The advantages of tangential fields include treatment and setup simplicity and the ability to totally exclude critical structures such as the opposite breast from the treatment fields. Despite the limits imposed by this simple beam geometry, target dose uniformity and normal tissue doses have improved with IMRT. In a study comparing intensity modulation with conventional wedged tangents, an average improvement in target dose homogeneity of 5% was observed with IMRT. The mean dose to the coronary artery region and opposite breast decreased by more than 30% and 35%, respectively. The average volume of ipsilateral lung receiving doses in excess of the prescription decreased by 35%.

CONSIDERATION OF TREATMENT UNCERTAINTIES

To account for treatment uncertainties, arising from patient set-up variation and organ motion, a margin is added to the target in radiotherapy planning.[26] As the dose distributions become more conformal in 3D-CRT and even more so in IMRT, the outcome of the treatment may become more sensitive to these uncertainties. Thus, it is important to quantify them, develop corrective methods to minimize them, and account for the residual component in treatment planning.

Ideally, patient-specific treatment uncertainty data should be used, but practically it would be difficult. Thus, approaches have been developed to quantify treatment uncertainties of a patient population. Set-up errors have been measured for several disease sites using serial portal images and interfraction organ motion by repeated CT scans.[27–29] Based on such data, analysis can be performed to assess the potential effect of treatment uncertainties on treatment outcome using statistical sampling technique.

The previously mentioned population average uncertainty data can also be useful for the calculation of the dose distribution in treatment planning. Specifically, the frequency distribution of treatment uncertainties can be incorporated into the pencil beam kernel, which is equivalent to a convolution of the idealized dose distribution with the frequency distribution of treatment uncertainties. This yields an average dose distribution representing the effects of random, or daily, errors occurring over a treatment course.

DEVELOPMENT AND RESEARCH ISSUES

IMRT is in a developmental phase and there has been limited experience in the use of inverse planning in the radiotherapy community. Although we have had some experience of its use in the treatment of the prostate, each application to a new disease site (head and neck and breast) represented a new challenge, requiring adaptation or new custom features. For example, in the treatment of the breast, an extension of each intensity-modulated field to include a skin flash is needed. Given that our optimization algorithm is developed at MSKCC, we are able to modify the software to meet the unanticipated clinical requirement. We surmise that users of the emerging inverse planning systems may encounter similar experiences and will seek incremental improvement of their algorithms. The situation will likely be system specific and may vary widely among them due to the large number of variables in such systems and in the inverse process. In addition, better understanding in the use of optimization criteria is needed for the efficacious use of the inverse planning technique, and we have approached this by trial and error. Such criteria are certainly disease site specific and probably algorithm specific as well.

There are investigations on the use of biologic models of tumor tissue response as criteria for plan optimization.[30,31] In general, biology-based score functions typically consist of some weighted combination of biologic indices. Two under current study are the normal tissue complication probabilities[32] and tumor control probabilities.[33] These indices condense structure-specific dose-distribution data to yield relative figures of merit for the respective objects of interest. However, both of these indices are at present based on rather rudimentary models with simplistic assumptions. Importantly, clinical data for validating the models and deriving the model parameters are lacking. Nevertheless, the advent of 3D treatment planning and the accrual of patients treated with this modality are beginning to provide clinical outcome data for which dose volume information are available. For example, analysis has been performed on clinical complication data of the lung, liver, and optic pathways.[34–36] Such studies promise to improve the present biologic models, provide better estimates for the model parameters, or both. It is hoped that the iterative process of generating clinical data and refinement and validation of the models will incrementally improve the predictive power of the biologic indices and facilitate the quantitative evaluation of 3D treatment plans.

Certain technical aspects of inverse planning will continue to be investigated. For example, the advantages and disadvantages of gradient-based optimization as compared with simulated annealing.[37–39] The latter method, though much slower computationally, is more likely to yield the global minimum (or the most optimal solution), but this theoretical advantage has not been demonstrated to be clinically important. Another often discussed issue pertains to the optimal number of intensity-modulated beams and their orientations. Again, our view is that given a sufficient number of equally spaced beams (five to seven or more) and the intensity-modulation capability, near optimal plans can be generated.[40]

There is significant interest in developing methods to verify the delivery of intensity-modulated beams. These efforts are benefiting from the gradual maturation of the EPID technology, particularly using amorphous silicon detectors. The ability to verify directly the intensity pattern of the delivered intensity-modulated beams will greatly enhance the confidence in the use of IMRT and lead to wider acceptance of this modality. At present, the electromechanical monitoring of leaf positions during radiation delivery provides similar assurance, albeit indirectly and without providing measured data.

The ability of IMRT to deliver nonuniform dose patterns by design brings to fore the question of how to *dose paint* and *dose sculpt*, leading to the suggestion that *biologic* images may be of assistance.[41] In contrast to the conventional radiologic images that primarily provide anatomic information, biologic images reveal metabolic, functional, physiologic, genotypic, and phenotypic data. Important for radiotherapy, the new and noninvasive imaging methods may yield 3D radiobiologic information. Studies are urgently needed to identify genotypes and phenotypes that affect radiosensitivity and to devise methods to image them noninvasively. Incremental to the concept of gross target volume, CTV, and PTV, we suggest the concept of *biologic target volume* and hypothesize that biologic target volume can be derived from biologic images and that their use may incrementally improve target delineation and dose delivery.[41] We emphasize, however, that much basic research and clinical studies are needed before this potential can be realized.

In conclusion, IMRT is a powerful technique that provides extra degrees of freedom in customizing the dose distribution for photon radiotherapy. With the development of the computer-controlled treatment machines equipped with DMLC, it is now possible to deliver these treatments reliably. The clinical implementation of inverse planning and treatment delivery with DMLC is extremely complex and involves a substantial developmental effort. However, once accomplished, the process is efficient and capable of providing the dual benefits of improved dose distribution and cost savings. It is likely that this new modality will become widely accepted and applied in the future.

REFERENCES

1. Leibel SA, Zelefsky MJ, Kutcher GJ, et al. The biological basis and clinical application of three-dimensional conformal external beam radiation therapy in carcinoma of the prostate. *Semin Oncol* 1994;21:580.
2. Zelefsky MJ, Leibel SA, Kutcher GJ, Fuks Z. Three-dimensional conformal radiotherapy and dose escalation: where do we stand? *Semin Radiat Oncol* 1998;8:107.
3. Zelefsky MJ, Leibel SA, Gaudin PB, et al. Dose escalation with three-dimensional conformal radiation therapy affects the outcome in prostate cancer. *Int J Radiat Oncol Biol Phys* 1998;41:491.
4. Brahme A. Optimization of stationary and moving beam radiation therapy techniques. *Radiother Oncol* 1988;12:129.
5. Ling CC, Burman CM, Chui CS, et al. Conformal radiation treatment of prostate cancer using inversely-planned intensity-modulated photon beams produced with dynamic multileaf collimation. *Int J Radiat Oncol Biol Phys* 1996;35:721
6. Carol M, Grant WH, Pavord D, et al. Initial clinical experience with the Peacock intensity modulation of a 3-D conformal radiation therapy system. *Stereotactic & Functional Neurosurgery* 1996;6:30.
7. Sherouse GW, Bourland JD, Reynolds K, et al. Virtual simulation in the clinical setting: some practical considerations. *Int J Radiat Oncol Biol Phys* 1990;19:1059.
8. ICRU Report 50. *Prescribing, recording, and reporting photon beam therapy.* Bethesda, MD: International Commission on Radiation Units and Measurements, 1993:3.
9. Goitein M, Abrams M, Rowell D, et al. Multidimensional treatment planning. II: beam's eye view, back projection and projection through CT sections. *Int J Radiat Oncol Biol Phys* 1983;9:789.
10. McShan DL, Fraass BA, Lichter AS. Full integration of the beam's eye view concept into computerized treatment planning. *Int J Radiat Oncol Biol Phys* 1990;18:1485.
11. Fraass BA, Kessler ML, McShan DL, et al. Optimization and clinical use of multisegment IMRT for high dose conformal therapy. *Semin Radiat Oncol* 1999;9:60.
12. Bortfeld T, Burkelbach J, Boesecke R, Schlegel W. Methods of image reconstruction from projections applied to conformation radiotherapy. *Phys Med Biol* 1990;35:423.
13. Spirou SV, Chui CS. A gradient inverse planning algorithm with dose-volume constraints. *Med Phys* 1998;25:321.
14. LoSasso T, Chui CS, Kutcher GJ, et al. The use of a multileaf collimator for conformal radiotherapy of carcinoma of the prostate and nasopharynx. *Int J Radiat Oncol Biol Phys* 1993;25:161.
15. Convery D, Rosenbloom M. The generation of intensity modulated fields for conformal radiotherapy by dynamic multileaf collimation. *Phys Med Biol* 1992;37:1359.
16. Spirou S, Chui CS. Generation of arbitrary intensity profiles by dynamic jaws or multileaf collimators. *Med Phys* 1994;21:1031.
17. Galvin JM, Chen XG, Smith RM. Combining multileaf fields to modulated fluence distributions. *Int J Radiat Oncol Biol Phys* 1993;27:697.
18. Bortfeld T, Kahler DL, Waldron TJ, Boyer AL. X-ray field compensation with multileaf collimators. *Int J Radiat Oncol Biol Phys* 1994;28:723.
19. Yu CX. Intensity-modulated arc therapy with dynamic multileaf collimation: an alternative to tomotherapy. *Phys Med Biol* 1995;40:1435.
20. Chui CS, LoSasso T, Spirou S. Dose calculations for photon beams with intensity modulation generated by dynamic jaw or multi-leaf collimations. *Med Phys* 1994;21:1237.
21. Wang X, Spirou S, LoSasso T, Chui CS, Mohan R. Dosimetric verification of an intensity modulated treatment. *Med Phys* 1996;23:317.
22. LoSasso T, Chui CS, Ling CC. Physical and dosimetric aspects of a multileaf collimation system used in the dynamic mode for implementing intensity modulated radiotherapy. *Med Phys* 1998;25:1919.
23. Burman C, Chui CS, Kutcher G, et al. Planning, delivery, and quality assurance of intensity-modulated radiotherapy using dynamic multileaf collimator: a strategy for large scale implementation for the treatment of carcinoma of the prostate. *Int J Radiat Oncol Biol Phys* 1997;39:863.
24. Chui CS, Spirou S, LoSasso T. Testing of dynamic multifleaf collimation. *Med Phys* 1996;23:635.
25. Zelefsky MJ, Fuks Z, Happersett L, et al. Clinical experience with intensity modulated radiation therapy (IMRT) in prostate cancer. *Radiother Oncol* 2000;55:241.

26. Kutcher GJ, Mageras GS, Leibel SA. Control, correction, and modeling of setup errors and organ motion. *Semin Radiat Oncol* 1995;5:134.
27. Zelefsky MJ, Crean D, Mageras GS, et al. Quantification and predictors of prostate position variability in fifty patients evaluated with multiple CT scans during conformal radiotherapy. *Radiother Oncol* 1999;50:225.
28. Hanley J, Lumley MA, Mageras GS, et al. Measurement of patient positioning errors in three-dimensional conformal radiotherapy of the prostate. *Int J Radiat Oncol Biol Phys* 1997;37:435.
29. van Herk M, Bruce A, Kroes APG, et al. Quantification of organ motion during conformal radiotherapy of the prostate by three dimensional (3D) image registration. *Int J Radiat Oncol Biol Phys* 1995;33:1311.
30. Wang X, Mohan R, Jackson A, et al. Optimization of intensity-modulated 3D conformal treatment plans based on biological indices. *Radiother Oncol* 1995;37:140.
31. Niemierko A, Urie M, Goitein M. Optimization of 3D radiation therapy with both physical and biological end points and constraints. *Int J Radiat Oncol Biol Phys* 1992;23:99.
32. Lyman JT. Complication probability as assessed from dose volume histograms. *Radiat Res* 1985;8:104.
33. Niemierko A, Goitein M. Implementation of a model for estimating tumor controlprobability for an inhomogeneously irradiated tumor. *Radiother Oncol* 1993;29:140.
34. Jackson A, Ten Haken RK, Robertson JM, et al. Analysis of clinical complication data for radiation hepatitis using a parallel architecture model. *Int J Radiat Oncol Biol Phys* 1995;31:883.
35. Jackson A, Zelefsky M, Cowan D, et al. Rectal bleeding after conformal radiotherapy of prostate cancer and dose volume histograms. *Int J Radiat Oncol Biol Phys* 1998;42:217.
36. Martel MK, Sandler HM, et al. Dose-volume complication analysis for visual pathway structures on patients with advanced paranasal sinus tumors. *Int J Radiat Oncol Biol Phys* 1997;38:273.
37. Mageras GS, Mohan R. Application of fast simulated annealing to optimization of conformal radiation treatments. *Med Phys* 1993;20:639.
38. Webb S. optimization of conformal radiotherapy dose distributions by simulated annealing. *Phys Med Biol* 1989;34:1349.
39. Webb S. Optimization of simulated annealing of three-dimensional conformal treatment planning for radiation fields defined by multileaf collimator. *Phys Med Biol* 1991;36:1201.
40. Stein J, Mohan R, Wang X-H, et al. Number and orientations of beams in intensity-modulated radiation treatments. *Med Phys* 1997;24:149.
41. Ling CC, Humm J, Larson S, et al. Towards multidimensional radiotherapy (MD-CRT): biological imaging and biological conformality. *Int J Radiat Oncol Biol Phys* 2000;47:551.

CHAPTER 30

Cancer of the Head and Neck

SECTION 1

DAVID SIDRANSKY

Molecular Biology of Head and Neck Tumors

Cancer is a complex genetic disease derived from the accumulation of various genetic changes. These genetic alterations include activation of protooncogenes and inactivation of tumor suppressor genes. Moreover, inactivation of tumor suppressor gene function requires inactivation of both parental alleles, usually by point mutation and a chromosomal deletion. The correlation of these specific genetic changes with the various lesions depicted in the histopathologic progression of colorectal cancer has led to the development of a molecular progression model for this disease.[1] This molecular model now serves as a paradigm for the molecular progression of many other solid neoplasms.

A number of specific genetic events have been identified in the progression of head and neck squamous cell carcinoma (HNSCC). Primary tumor DNA can now be isolated and assessed directly for the presence of chromosomal deletions and amplification, as well as direct characterization of candidate oncogenes. Identification of the critical genetic changes that drive the neoplastic process has provided a preliminary progression model for head and neck cancer. This model now delineates appropriate genetic targets for novel diagnostic, prognostic, and therapeutic strategies.

GENETIC SUSCEPTIBILITY

It has been estimated that up to 10% of all cancers have a strong hereditary component. Generally, familiar clustering of cancer has suggested the possibility of genetic predisposing factors. A clustering of oral cancer has been seen in certain ethnic groups, and an increased risk of cancer has been noted among relatives of patients with one head and neck cancer.[2,3] Several studies have suggested a threefold higher risk of developing an oropharyngeal cancer in populations that have a first-degree relative with HNSCC.[4] There also has been some suggestion of a remarkable increase in the relative risk of cancer in relatives of individuals with multiple primary tumors. Except for the finding of head and neck cancer in some rare cancer syndromes, the basis of this genetic susceptibility has yet to be determined.[5]

An emerging area of study centers on the prevalence of specific polymorphisms in enzymes that are involved in the detoxification of several tobacco smoke–derived carcinogens. One larger study of 162 patients with head and neck cancer and 315 healthy controls suggested that certain glutathione S-transferase (GST) genotypes represented independent risk factors for head and neck cancer.[6] Some studies also have shown a two- to threefold risk for the GST M1 and GST T1 null genotypes, whereas others have shown no increase in HNSCC risk.[7–12] In all these studies, it is difficult to exclude other important risk factors, such as smoking, yet there appears to be a consistent susceptibility based on certain metabolic genotypes. Others also have found that the repair capacity of peripheral lymphocytes or their ability to repair carcinogen-induced chromatical breaks may also define a certain risk for head and neck cancer.[13–15] A more precise contribution of these polymorphisms and other risk factors to the development of head and neck cancer will need to be elucidated in larger studies.

CYTOGENETIC ALTERATIONS

Statistical analysis based on the age-specific incidence of head and neck cancer suggests that HNSCC tumors arise after the accumulation of six to ten independent genetic events.[16] Cytogenetic approaches have given us some insights into potential areas of deletion and amplification involved in the progression of head and neck cancer. Previously, karyotypic studies concentrated on established cell lines with complex chromosomal abnormalities. Unfortunately, different cell culture conditions added substantial variation to these observed chromosomal alterations.[17] Moreover, cultured cells from the primary tumor may represent only a small clone derived from *in vitro* selection pressure that is not representative of the entire cell population. Short-term cultures of primary tumors have proven more reliable for the assessment of complex chromosome abnormalities and rearrangements. These studies have already demonstrated consistent chromosomal abnormalities and the presence of important alterations.[18] Loss of chromosomes 3p, 5q, 8p, 9p, 18q, and 21q has been commonly identified. Preliminary data also suggest that loss of 18q may indicate the presence of a tumor with a poor prognosis.[18] Additionally, multiple chromosomal breakpoints including those on 1p22, 3p21, 8p11, and distal 14q have correlated with decreased radiosensitivity.[19] Fluorescence *in situ* hybridization potentially represents a more sensitive approach for recognizing both chromosomal deletions and amplifications.[20] For example, genomic amplification at the 11q13 region can be detected in preneoplastic lesions and should allow its placement directly into a molecular progression model.

More recently, comparative genomic hybridization has emerged as a comprehensive method for genome-wide evaluation to detect deletions or amplification. In this approach, tumor-normal DNA is mixed and hybridized to metaphase spreads from normal cells. Labeling of tumor-normal DNA by different fluorescent colors allows direct visualization of increased or decreased chromosomal material in neoplastic tissue by fluorescence detection. This approach is complementary to other methods for assessment of both tissue culture and primary tumor material. In addition to the chromosomal areas previously noted, comparative genomic hybridization has demonstrated amplification of 3q, 5p, 11q13, and 19q.[21]

PROTOONCOGENES

Protooncogenes were initially identified as activated cellular genes specifically altered in some human neoplasms.[22] Despite the cloning of dozens of putative protooncogenes involved in the development of human neoplasms, few were found to be altered directly in the progression of primary tumors and cell lines. In addition to activation of oncogenes such as ras by point mutation, amplification is also a mechanism for activation of a protooncogene locus. Definitive studies suggested that the 11q13 amplification was associated with amplification of a critical protooncogene termed *cyclin D1* (PRAD1; CCND1). Although other genes were also coamplified in the same region, only cyclin D1 was consistently amplified in approximately 30% of HNSCC and most other neoplasms.[23,24] Moreover, amplification of this region correlated with increased expression of the cyclin D1 gene and may indicate a likelihood of progression in primary HNSCC.[25]

As previously noted, amplification of 3q has been noted in many squamous cell carcinomas, including head and neck cancer. A p53 homologue (p40/p51/p63) has been cloned and localized to the distal arm of 3q.[26] Although homologous to p53, this genetic locus was found to be amplified in a high frequency of squamous cell cancers (ais), and this amplification correlated with increased expression at the RNA and protein level.[27] Although there has been no evidence of activating point mutations in squamous cell cancers, functional evidence suggests that AIS may in fact be a true oncogene in squamous cell cancers.[27] Interestingly, dominant negative mutations are responsible for a specific hereditary syndrome called *ectrodactyly–ectodermal dysplasia–clefting syndrome.*[28] Knockout mice display a lack of epithelial development consistent with the role of this gene in epithelial renewal.[29] Further studies should establish the role of ais in the genetic progression of head and neck cancers.

The role of cyclin D1 in the progression of human cancer is now well established.[30] Other tumor suppressor genes, including Rb and p16, are negative regulators of the cyclin D1 pathway and often are inactivated in human neoplasms. In head and neck cancer, p16 appears to be a major target of inactivation. Thus, abnormal cycling through this critical G_1/S checkpoint may be a consistent genetic alteration in a majority of primary HNSCC. Although p16 and Rb inactivation are almost always exclusive, cyclin D1 amplification is independent of p16 inactivation in head and neck cancers.[31]

Like other epithelial neoplasms, the role of other protooncogenes has been much less definitive. Few mutations in ras have been identified in primary head and neck tumors. Although epidermal growth factor receptor (EGFR) has been an interesting candidate, increased levels of the receptor at the RNA or protein level rarely correlate with primary DNA amplification.[32] New evidence suggests that activation of signaling through Stat-3 leads to EGFR-mediated cell growth and that antisense suppression of EGFR protein leads to apoptosis (programmed cell death).[33,34] The protein eukaryotic initiation factor (eIF4E) binds to messenger RNA during initial protein synthesis, and its overexpression can result in the up-regulation of proteins essential for cell growth and division. Overexpression of eIF4E has been found in HNSCC, and there has been some evidence of gene amplification and protein overexpression in these tumors.[35,36] Overexpression of the protein in cells can lead to oncogenic transformation and may facilitate the synthesis of angiogenic factors such as vascular epidermal growth factor by enhancing their translation. In at least one study, there was a correlation between increasing eIF4E and vascular epidermal growth factor levels, suggesting its possible role in angiogenesis.[37]

Additionally, several other genes or gene products have been found to be overexpressed in head and neck tumors. High levels of cyclooxygenase (COX)-2, have been seen in squamous cell carcinomas by a competitive reverse transcription assay.[38] GST P1 messenger RNA levels are found to be high in most moderately and poorly differentiated tumors,[39] but only a fraction of these had specific gene amplification. Newer cytogenetic techniques may lead to the identification of important protooncogenes more commonly involved in the progression of HNSCC.

SUPPRESSIVE GROWTH REGULATION

In addition to growth factors with "positive" regulation and augmentation of tumor growth, other growth factor pathways may suppress cell growth. Transforming growth factor-β (TGF-β) is among these growth factors that have been implicated almost universally with suppression of tumor growth. Alterations of the type II TGF-β receptor, one target of TGF-β, were noted in primary colorectal cancers potentially involved in abrogation of this negative regulatory pathway.[40] Initially, some head and neck cancer cell lines were also found to harbor TGF-β receptor mutations, and mutations in the conserved serine/threonine kinase domain were found in 6 of 28 primary tumors.[41,42] The interaction of TGF-β with this critical receptor normally leads to an increase of negative regulators of the cell cycle (e.g., p15, INK4B) and G_1/S arrest; thus, normal negative regulation may be abrogated by mutations in the type II TGF-β receptor.

Through a different mechanism, retinoic acid receptors (RARs) have been implicated in the negative growth regulation of HNSCC. This negative regulation has been the cornerstone of successful chemopreventive approaches to diminish the incidence of second primary tumors by administration of *cis*-retinoic acid to patients with a primary HNSCC tumor.[43] Well-designed studies have demonstrated a significant reduction in the occurrence of second primary tumors in patients who receive retinoic acid. Although the regulation of retinoids is complex, one critical end point may be down-regulation of RAR-β. Studies in patients with premalignant disease (leukoplakia) have suggested that RAR-β levels are closely associated with response to retinoic acid.[44] In particular, those patients with tumors demonstrating low RAR-β levels did not respond to retinoic acid. Further functional studies into the role of retinoic acid and RAR-β may yield important information regarding the role of this pathway in the progression of HNSCC and successful treatment of premalignant lesions.

TUMOR SUPPRESSOR GENES

Molecular analysis has now revolutionized the ability to look at primary neoplasms. Methods that required large amounts of DNA (e.g., Southern blot analysis) have now been supplemented by polymerase chain reaction (PCR)–based approaches that allow access to limited DNA samples. Minute primary specimens from paraffin can be evaluated by rapid and accurate techniques. DNA extracted from these samples can be amplified by PCR to reveal the presence of allelic losses. In practice, maternal and paternal alleles can be distinguished by testing highly polymorphic markers that occur naturally among DNA sequences.[45]

It is now generally believed that these allelic losses (or chromosomal deletions) are markers for inactivation of critical tumor suppressor genes contained within the regions of loss.[46] Testing of highly polymorphic microsatellite markers (small 2- to 4-base pair repeats) from a specific chromosomal region allows rapid assessment of allelic loss by comparing the alleles in tumor DNA to normal DNA. Perhaps the best example of this association is derived from loss of chromosome 17p. These losses led to characterization of p53 as a candidate gene within the deleted area and subsequent identification of point mutations within the remaining allele. Inactivation of p53 now represents the best described and most common genetic change in all of human cancer.[47] Approximately 50% of all primary HNSCCs harbor p53 mutations in the conserved regions (exons 5 to 9).[48,49]

A comprehensive allotype of head and neck cancer has now been completed and refined.[50,51] The most commonly deleted region in head and neck cancer is located at chromosome 9p21-22.[50] Loss of chromosome 9p21 occurs in the majority of invasive tumors and is also present at a high frequency in the earliest definable lesions, including dysplasia and carcinoma *in situ*.[52] Furthermore, homozygous deletions in this region are frequent in HNSCC and represent one of the most common genetic changes identified in all human neoplasms. p16 (*CDKN2*) is contained within this critically deleted region and is a potent inhibitor of cyclin D1/*CDK4* complexes. Thus, p16 has emerged as an excellent candidate tumor suppressor gene within the deleted area.[53] Indeed, germline point mutations of p16 predispose to familial melanoma,[54] and loss of p16 may be necessary for immortalization of keratinocytes.[55]

Although initial enthusiasm for p16 as a target gene in head and neck cancer was diminished when sequence analysis revealed rare point mutation (approximately 10% to 15% of HNSCC tumors),[56,57] alternative mechanisms of inactivation were identified suggesting that abrogation of p16 function may be a common occurrence in head and neck cancer. Homozygous deletion (deletion of both gene copies) and methylation of the 5' CpG region of p16 have been identified, each detected in approximately one-fourth of primary head and neck cancers.[58,59] This methylation is associated with complete block of p16 transcription and appears to be a common mechanism for p16 inactivation. The notion that p16 inactivation is directly involved in the progression of primary tumors has been strengthened. Lack of p16 protein was detected by immunostaining in most primary invasive lesions, and tumors with absent p16 protein contained a homozygous deletion, methylation, or point mutation of p16.[60] Loss of p16 protein has been observed in most advanced premalignant lesions.[61]

It is also possible that a second critical tumor suppressor gene resides at 9p21. We and others have identified an alternative RNA transcript for p16 termed p16 beta.[62] This unique transcript originates from an upstream initiating site in a novel exon 1 and codes for a protein through an alternative rating frame (ARF). Interestingly, introduction of p16 or p16 beta into head and neck cancer cell lines results in potent growth suppression.[63] Although the human transcript is somewhat shorter than the murine protein, functional studies have suggested that ARF binds to MDM2, leading to a decrease in p53 degradation and a subsequent increase in p53 levels.[64,65] Moreover, a knockout ARF mouse develops certain tumors at an increased frequency.[66] In human tumors, homozygous deletion of the p16 locus concomitantly leads to knockout of p16 beta, and thus approximately 30% of HNSCCs have no ARF protein. Evidence in squamous cell carcinoma of the lung suggests that p53 mutations and p16 inactivation are not exclusive, suggesting that, at least at the genetic level, they do not function in the same pathway.[67] Ultimately, further studies will have to be done in primary tumors and human models to establish the precise role of p16 beta inactivation in squamous cell carcinoma.

A second commonly deleted locus occurs on chromosome 3p. Several studies have suggested that this region of loss is complex in head and neck cancer and may in fact be composed of three distinct suppressor regions juxtaposed to one another.[68,69] As for 9p21, analysis of 3p21 losses in HNSCC has revealed frequent loss in early lesions. The 3p21 region is also frequently lost in lung cancer and has been the target of an intensive search for the critical tumor suppressor gene. The *FHIT* gene was found in a critical area of homozygous deletion and was evaluated as possible tumor suppressor gene in many

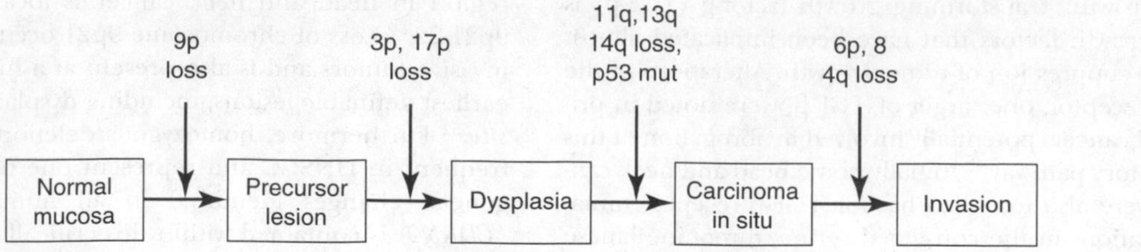

FIGURE 30.1-1. Preliminary progression model for head and neck squamous cell carcinoma. Genetic alterations have been ordered by testing a variety of preinvasive and invasive lesions and determining the frequency of these events at each stage in progression. Inactivation of p16 (chromosome 9p21) and amplification of cyclin D1 (chromosome 11q13q) have not been directly tested in preinvasive lesions. It is the accumulation and not necessarily the order of these genetic changes that determines progression

cancers. Although altered transcripts have been detected in primary tumors and cell lines, specific inactivating mutations of the second allele have not been forthcoming.[70,71] Thus, although many candidate genes have been isolated, none has been demonstrated to be the critical inactivated tumor suppressor gene at 3p involved in the progression of these cancers.

Loss of chromosome 17p is a frequent occurrence in most human cancers, and head and neck cancer is no exception (occurring in 60% of invasive lesions).[48] Although p53 inactivation correlates closely with loss of 17p in invasive lesions, p53 mutations are quite rare in early lesions that contain 17p loss. Some evidence from cell lines also suggests that a distal breakpoint to p53 occurs in head and neck cancer. Together, these data suggest that a second tumor suppressor gene on 17p may be involved early in the progression of this neoplasm. p53 mutations, as in most tumors, generally rise in frequency between the preinvasive to the invasive state. This is consistent with a critical function for p53 in response to DNA damage.[72] p53 mutant tumors are also less likely to respond to local radiation therapy.[73] This model is certain to become more complex, but offers an important insight into the role of p53 in the progression of head and neck cancer and many other tumors.

Loss of chromosomal arm 10q is not uncommon in HNSCC and lung cancer. The *PTEN* gene was cloned and found to be homozygously deleted and inactivated in a variety of different cancers. Homozygous deletion and rare point mutation inactivation have been seen in HNSCC.[74,75] Although only 10% of these cancers have inactivated gene, it seems to be more common in advanced tumors and may harbor a poor prognosis.[74,76]

Loss of 13q also occurs in approximately 60% of primary tumors and the minimal area of loss includes the tumor suppressor gene Rb. However, immunohistochemical analysis of Rb (which detects most Rb alterations) revealed inactivation of Rb in only small percentages of tumors with loss of 13q.[77] Again, as in many other chromosomal regions, there appears to be another tumor suppressor gene near Rb, putatively inactivated in the progression of head and neck cancer.

More recent work has suggested that there may be one or more regions of specific loss on the short arm of chromosome 8 and on 7q31.[78–81] Loss of 18q has been seen, and one of these minimally deleted regions harbors two tumor suppressor genes.[82,83] Homozygous deletions of both *DCC* and *DPC4* have been noted in cell lines but have been rarely seen in primary tumors.[84] Many other areas of chromosomal loss have been seen in head and neck cancer consistent with the occurrence of multiple genetic events in the progression of these neoplasms. Except for those previously noted, critical tumor suppressor genes have not been identified from these loci and remain to be isolated and characterized. Further fine mapping of these deletions, amplifications, and translocations with characterization of critical genes within these areas may provide important information about the biology and clinical behavior of these neoplasms.

We have tested the ten most common allelic loss events in a large number of primary preinvasive lesions and invasive HNSCC to develop a molecular progression model.[85] As seen in Figure 30.1-1, the progression of head and neck cancer involves inactivation of many putative suppressor gene loci. Chromosomes 9p and 3p appear to be lost early, closely followed by loss of 17p. p53 mutations are seen in the progression of the preinvasive to invasive lesions, and many other genetic events occur later in progression. Other specific genetic events, such as amplification of cyclin D1 and inactivation of p16, have been tested predominantly in invasive lesions, and their precise order in the model cannot yet be determined. As noted in the molecular model for colorectal cancer, it is the accumulation and not necessarily the precise order of these genetic events that determine histopathologic progression. This is best exemplified by some early lesions that demonstrated a “late” event as the sole genetic alteration.

To test this model directly, we were able to analyze lesions that demonstrated histologic progression from one area to another. In each of the cases, we confirmed that 9p and 3p loss were early events, with other genetic changes occurring in the more advanced histopathologic lesion. Moreover, lesions biopsied in the same area over time in a few critical patients also demonstrated the same general order of these events. Molecular progression models such as this one allow direct characterization of early genetic events that might be important in diagnostic strategies. Critical events that occur in the progression from the preinvasive state to the invasive state (e.g., p53 mutations) may be useful as prognostic indicators in primary lesions. Losses occurring later in progression, such as 11q, 13q, 14q, and 18q, and loss of p27 protein (another cyclin-dependent kinase inhibitor) have been found to correlate with a decrease in survival.[83–90] Early losses at 3p14 and 9p21 may persist in premalignant lesions exposed to chemoprevention agents and may predict those likely to relapse despite apparent histologic remissions.[91,92] All of these genetic events may one day serve as appropriate targets for novel therapeutic approaches. This model also has given some interesting insights into the well-known phenomenon of field cancerization.

FIELD CANCERIZATION

Patients with head and neck cancer often present with second metachronous and synchronous tumors of the aerodigestive tract. Moreover, patients with primary lesions often have skip areas that are characterized by preinvasive lesions throughout the field. Slaughter[93] originally coined the term *field cancerization* and attributed this to a field defect that allowed independent transformation of epithelial cells at a number of sites. Previous studies in bladder cancer demonstrated that multiple tumors arising in a single patient were derived from the uncontrolled spread of a single transformed cell.[94] These tumors then grew independently with variable subsequent genetic alterations. For head and neck cancer, our working progression model allowed direct assessment of the genetic changes in surrounding areas of histopathologic abnormality. In every case, surrounding lesions appeared to share the same genetic events (e.g., critical breakpoints at chromosomes 9p21 and 3p21) present in the primary tumor, suggesting that a single transformed cell gave rise to the independent and apparently geographically distinct skip areas seen in these patients. Thus, Slaughter's original observations can be explained as follows: A cell is transformed by a critical genetic event and begins to migrate through the mucosa. Additional genetic events in one critical lesion eventually give rise to the clinical tumor that is seen on presentation. However, direct molecular assessment of surrounding regions confirms the presence of clonal cell populations that are not yet fully transformed. Given time, these lesions then arise as other preinvasive or invasive lesions in the same patient.

Although investigators have reported a conformation of this field cancerization effect in head and neck cancer by detection of discordant p53 mutations in multiple tumors,[95] our working model suggests that this conclusion may be premature. Other genetic events, including loss of 9p and 3p, precede inactivation of p53. Thus, one of these early events probably leads to initial cell transformation and replacement of surrounding mucosa, whereas subsequent genetic events including p53 appear to arise independently. Thus, these investigators identified the diversity of subsequent genetic events rather than established the distinct clonal origin of these clinically independent lesions. By examining the pattern of X chromosome inactivation and loss of chromosome 9p21 in multiple tumors from female patients, we demonstrated a common clonal origin in most of these cases.[96] In support of this result, cytogenetic evidence in at least one patient identified the presence of a specific chromosomal marker in both primary neoplasms.[97] More recently, apparent second primary tumors of the lung and even rare esophageal tumors were found to be clonally related to the initial primary HNSCC.[98,99]

If minimally abnormal or benign-appearing premalignant lesions show clonal genetic changes adjacent to a primary HNSCC, it is conceivable that normal-appearing mucosal areas could harbor an occult neoplasm. Clinically detectable cervical lymph node metastases without identification of the primary tumor were assessed by molecular analysis of multiple surveillance biopsies. We investigated whether the site of origin of the primary tumor could be localized by detection of specific losses on some of the key chromosomes described in the molecular progression model.[100] In 10 of 18 patients, at least one pathologically benign biopsy demonstrated a pattern of genetic alterations identical to that present in cervical lymph node metastases. Three of these patients went on to develop primary tumors in the identical or adjacent mucosal region between 1 to 13 years later.[100] These data further support the notion that histopathologically benign mucosa may harbor patches of clonal preneoplastic cells that are genetically related to the metastatic HNSCC and that such mucosal sites are the sites of origin of unknown primary HNSCC.

MOLECULAR EPIDEMIOLOGY

The pattern of specific mutations within a given gene sequence may provide important information concerning the etiology (e.g., effect of a carcinogen) of that particular cancer.[101] The p53 gene can be inactivated by a large variety of distinct mutations and is frequently inactivated in many human cancers, providing an excellent candidate for this type of survey. Analysis of the pattern of the p53 gene mutation in 129 HNSCC patients has demonstrated that the incidence of p53 mutations is much higher among patients exposed to tobacco and alcohol than among those patients who abstained from both.[49] Moreover, we found that the alcohol appeared to augment the effect of smoking, consistent with models in which alcohol is not a carcinogen per se, but might lead to an increase in the absorbance of carcinogens contained within cigarette smoke. Furthermore, we found that CpG mutations are rare among mutations patients who smoke cigarettes, whereas they constituted most of the mutations found in nonsmokers and nondrinkers. C to T mutations at these CpG sites are important because, through methylation and deamination, they are thought to represent potential sites of "endogenous" mutations. These data thus support a growing body of epidemiologic evidence that abstinence from cigarette smoke may help decrease the overall incidence of head and neck cancer.

HUMAN PAPILLOMAVIRUS

Human papillomavirus (HPV) has long been thought to play a role in some head and neck cancers. One study of more than 250 patients used PCR followed by definitive techniques such as sequencing and *in situ* hybridization to search for the presence of HPV in head and neck tumors.[102] HPV was detected in approximately 25% of the lesions and virtually all were "high-risk" oncogenic types (HPV 16). Remarkably, most HPV-positive tumors were in the oropharynx. For these HPV-positive oropharyngeal cancers, they were less likely to occur among heavy smokers and drinkers, less likely to harbor a p53 mutation, and had an improved disease-specific survival. Another group suggested that HPV-positive tumors may also inactivate Rb and harbor a better prognosis.[103] These new data are consistent with previous studies with a smaller number of patients[104] or those that used less definitive determine techniques. It appears that HPV-positive oropharyngeal tumors compose a distinct clinical and pathologic disease entity causally associated with HPV.

DIAGNOSTICS

Clonal genetic alterations can be identified in clinical samples including bodily fluids. These clonal genetic alterations are generally considered to represent specific markers for the presence of neoplastic cells. In many clinical samples, however, the number of neoplastic cells are greatly outnumbered by normal

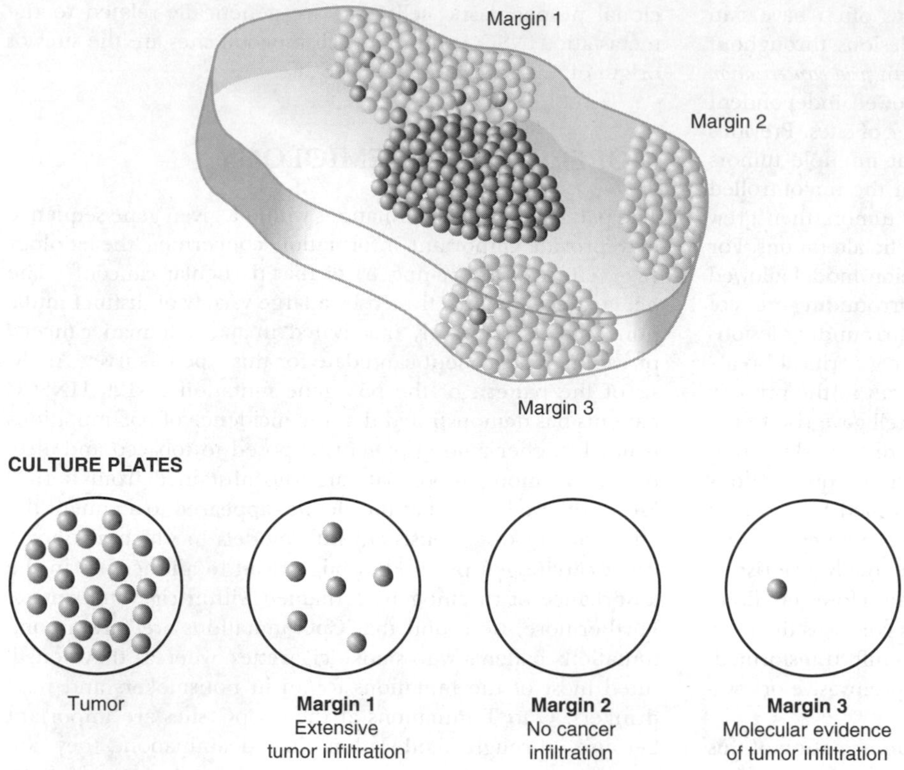

FIGURE 30.1-2. Schematic representation of molecular staging. DNA is extracted from primary clinical (e.g., margin) material and then tested for the presence of infiltrating tumor cells that harbor the identical p53 mutations detected in the primary tumor. This polymerase chain reaction–based approach is much more sensitive than morphologic analysis by standard light microscopy. Patients positive by molecular analysis are at high risk for local regional recurrence

cells within the same specimen. Therefore, we and others have developed very sensitive and specific techniques to detect these rare clonal genetic alterations among many "normal" or wild-type DNA molecules. Clonal ras gene mutations have been detected in the stool of patients with colorectal cancer and p53 mutations in the urine of patients with bladder cancer.[105,106] Moreover, both ras and p53 oncogene mutations were used as targets to detect neoplastic cells in the sputum of patients with lung cancer. In one case, the same clonal cell population containing the identical mutation eventually identified in the primary tumor was detected 1 year before clinical diagnosis in a patient with lung cancer.[107] Analysis of p53 mutations also has confirmed the ability to detect neoplastic clones in the saliva of patients with head and neck cancer.[108]

Telomerase is a ribonuclear protein that maintains telomere length, and reactivation of its activity is associated with escape from cellular senescence. Using a modified PCR-based assay for telomerase activity, 80% to 100% of primary head and neck cancers were found to display telomerase activity.[109,110] Some authors have suggested that most dysplastic lesions and preneoplastic lesions also display telomerase activation.[110] Interestingly, 14 out of 44 (32%) of oral rinses from HNSCC patients were found to harbor telomerase activity, but a small percentage of normal controls also exhibited this telomerase activity.[109] Using a panel of 21 microsatellite markers, clonal genetic changes (loss of heterozygosity or microsatellite instability) were detected in 80% of the saliva samples from the patients with head and neck cancer.[111] Moreover, exfoliative cell samples were subjected to microsatellite analysis and found to contain the identical changes observed in the primary tumors.[112] It is still unknown if these changes can be identified in early lesions or if they can detect recurrence, as has been seen in bladder cancer through urinalysis. Clearly, the continued identification of molecular markers will lead to improved diagnostic techniques for squamous cell carcinoma.

A more pressing problem in HNSCC is the high incidence of local-regional recurrence despite aggressive surgical therapy. We used a similar molecular approach as previously described to probe surgical margins and lymph nodes from patients with primary head and neck cancer after surgical resection.[113] A segment of the p53 gene is amplified by PCR from DNA extracted from the clinical sample. The PCR products are then cloned into phage, transferred to nylon membranes, and probed with a specific oligomer (small DNA strand) able to recognize the same mutation initially identified in the primary tumor. Thus, a unique DNA probe was synthesized and used to test the resected surgical margins and lymph nodes from affected patients. Perhaps not surprisingly, many of the apparently normal margins and lymph nodes by light microscopy were found to contain infiltrating tumor cells by this sensitive molecular analysis (Fig. 30.1-2).

In an initial pilot trial that contained 30 patients, the results were quite interesting. Although all patients were thought to be completely negative by light microscopy, final pathology revealed at least one positive margin in five patients.[113] These five patients had markedly positive margins by molecular analysis and were further excluded from this study. There were 25 remaining patients who were still completely negative by light microscopy. Of these, 13 were positive by molecular analysis and five have recurred within 2 years (average, 9 to 12 months). Of the 12 patients who were completely negative by molecular assessment, none has recurred at 2-year follow-up. As expected, there is a significant improvement in survival for those patients initially negative by molecular analysis (Fig. 30.1-3). Other markers have been used to assess possible recurrence in tumor-free margins. eI4FE (previ-

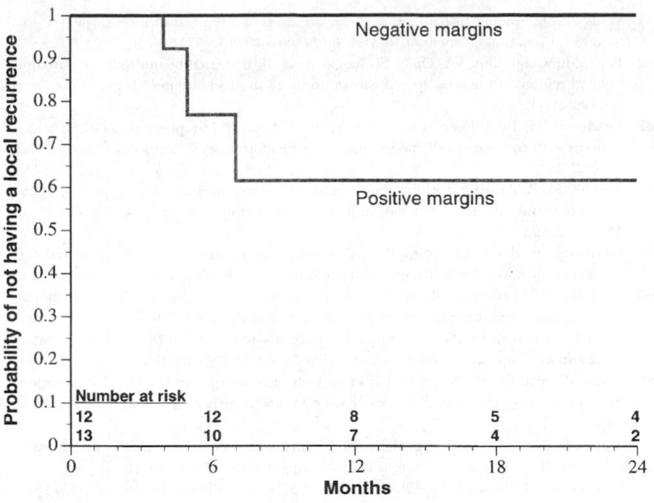

FIGURE 30.1-3. Probability of having no local recurrence, according to the results of the molecular assay. Kaplan-Meier curves are shown for the probability of having no local recurrence in the 25 study patients with surgical margins that were negative by light microscopy but were re-evaluated with molecular probes. The probability of having no local recurrence in patients with positive margins by the molecular assessment was significantly lower than that in patients with negative margins (P = .02 by the log-rank test)

ously described) is associated with increasing overexpression in the progression of head and neck cancer and also has been detected in apparently tumor-free margins.

Although the previous results must be confirmed by a larger prospective trial, the results are already intriguing. Perhaps patients with negative molecular assessment may be spared adjuvant radiation therapy. Moreover, patients with positive margins will benefit from more aggressive chemotherapeutic approaches and perhaps novel approaches, including gene therapy. Because staging is so critical for many types of cancer, this approach may be important for other tumors in addition to head and neck cancer.

The identification of new genes and other molecular markers will help in the early detection of head and neck cancer and may already provide useful prognostic information regarding clinical tumor behavior. As we further understand critical pathways in the genesis of these tumors, chemotherapeutic, pharmacologic, and genetic approaches may all be useful in either reestablishing or abrogating newly established pathways that lead to tumor growth. These discoveries will eventually lead to improved surgical techniques, chemoprevention strategies, and novel therapeutic approaches.

REFERENCES

1. Fearon ER, Vogelstein B. A genetic model of colorectal tumorigenesis. *Cell* 1990;61:759.
2. Ankathil R, Mathew A, Joseph F. Is oral cancer susceptibility inherited? *Eur J Oral Oncol* 1996;32B:63.
3. Gorsky M, Littner M, Sukman Y. The prevalence of oral cancer in relation to the ethnic origin of the Jewish population. *Oral Surg Oral Med Oral Pathol* 1994;78(3):408.
4. Foulkes WD, Brunet JS, Kowalski LP. Family history is a risk factor for squamous cell carcinoma of the head and neck in Brazil: a case control study. *Int J Cancer* 1995;63:769.
5. Jeffries S, Eeles R, Goldgar D, et al. The role of genetic factors in predisposition to squamous cell cancer of the head and neck. *Br J Cancer* 1999;79(5/6):865.
6. Cheng L, Sturgis EM, Eicher SA, et al. Glutathione *S*-transferase polymorphisms and risk of squamous-cell carcinoma of the head and neck. *Int J Cancer* 1999;84:220.
7. Morita S, Yano M, Tsujinaka T, et al. Genetic polymorphisms of drug-metabolizing enzymes and susceptibility to head-and-neck squamous-cell carcinoma. *Int J Cancer* 1999;80:685.
8. Jourenkova-Mironova N, Voho A, Bouchardy C, et al. Glutathione *S*-transferase GSTM3 and GSTP1 genotypes and larynx cancer risk. *Cancer Epidemiol Biomarkers Prev* 1999;8:185.
9. Nazar-Stewart V, Vaughan TL, Burt RD, et al. Glutathione *S*-transferase M1 and susceptibility to nasopharyngeal carcinoma. *Cancer Epidemiol Biomarkers Prev* 1999;8:547.
10. Lazarus P, Sheikh SN, Ren Q, et al. p53, but not p16 mutations in oral squamous cell carcinomas are associated with specific CYP1A1 and GSTM1 polymorphic genotypes and patient use. *Carcinogenesis* 1998;19:509.
11. Jourenkova N, Reinikainen M, Bouchardy C, et al. Larynx cancer risk in relation to glutathione *S*-transferase M1 and T1 genotypes and tobacco smoking. *Cancer Epidemiol Biomarkers Prev* 1998;7:19.
12. Park JY, Muscat JE, Ren Q, et al. CYP1A1 and GSTM1 polymorphisms and oral cancer risk. *Cancer Epidemiol Biomarkers Prev* 1997;6:791.
13. Cloos J, Nieuwenhuis EJ, Boomsma DI, et al. Inherited susceptibility to bleomycin-induced chromatid breaks in cultured peripheral blood lymphocytes. *J Natl Cancer Inst* 1999;91:1125.
14. Cheng L, Eicher SA, Guo Z, et al. Reduced DNA repair capacity in head and neck cancer patients. *Cancer Epidemiol Biomarkers Prev* 1998;7:465.
15. Wang LE, Sturgis EM, Eicher SA, et al. Mutagen sensitivity to benzo(a)pyrene diol epoxide and the risk of squamous cell carcinoma of the head and neck. *Clin Cancer Res* 1998;4:1773.
16. Renan MJ. How many mutations are required for tumorigenesis? Implications from human cancer data. *Mol Carcinog* 1993;7:139.
17. Jin Y, Mertens F, Mandahl N, et al. Chromosome abnormalities in eight-three head and neck squamous cell carcinomas: influence of culture conditions on karyotypic pattern. *Cancer Res* 1993;53:2140.
18. Van Dyke DL, Worsham MJ, Benninger MS, et al. Recurrent cytogenetic abnormalities in squamous cell carcinomas of the head and neck region. *Genes Chromosomes Cancer* 1994;9:192.
19. Cowan JM, Beckett MA, Weichselbaum RR. Chromosome changes characterizing *in vitro* response to radiation in human squamous cell carcinoma lines. *Cancer Res* 1993;53:5542.
20. Visakorpi T, Hyytinen E, Koivisto P, et al. *In vivo* amplification of the androgen receptor gene and progression of human prostate cancer. *Nat Genet* 1995;9:401.
21. Brzoska PM, Levin NA, Fu KK, et al. Frequent novel DNA copy number increase in squamous cell head and neck tumors. *Cancer Res* 1995;55:3055.
22. Bishop JM. Molecular themes in oncogenes. *Cell* 1991;64:235.
23. Berenson JR, Yan J, Micke RA. Frequent amplification of the bcl-1 locus in head and neck squamous cell carcinomas. *Oncogene* 1989;4:1111.
24. Callender T, El-Nagger AK, Lee MS, et al. PRAD-1 (CCND1)/cyclin D1 oncogene amplification in primary head and neck squamous cell carcinoma. *Cancer* (Phila) 1994;74:152.
25. Jares P, Fernández PL, Campo E, et al. PRAD-1/cyclin D1 gene amplification correlates with messenger RNA overexpression and tumor progression in human laryngeal carcinomas. *Cancer Res* 1994;54:4813.
26. Trink B, Okami K, Wu L, et al. A new p53 homologue. *Nat Med* 1998;4:747.
27. Hibi K, Trink B, Patturajan M, et al. AIS is an oncogene amplified in squamous cell carcinoma. *PNAS* (*in press*).
28. Celli J, Dujif P, Hamel B, et al. Heterozygous germline mutations in the p53 homologue p63 are the cause of EEC syndrome. *Cell* 1999;99:143.
29. Yang A, Schweitzer R, Sun D, et al. p63 is essential for regenerative proliferation in limb, craniofacial and epithelial development. *Nature* 1999;398:714.
30. Hunter T, Pines J. Cyclins and cancer. II. Cyclin D and CDK inhibitors come of age. *Cell* 1994;79:573.
31. Okami K, Reed AL, Cairns P, et al. Cyclin D1 amplification is independent of p16 inactivation in head and neck squamous cell carcinoma. *Oncogene* 1999;18:3541.
32. Grandis JR, Tweardy DJ. Elevated levels of transforming growth factor alpha and epidermal growth factor receptor messenger RNA are early markers of carcinogenesis in head and neck cancer. *Cancer Res* 1993;53:3579.
33. He Y, Zeng Q, Drenning SD, et al. Inhibition of human squamous cell carcinoma growth *in vivo* by epidermal growth factor receptor antisense RNA transcribed from the U6 promoter. *J Natl Cancer Inst* 1998;90:1080.
34. Grandis JR, Drenning SD, Chakraborty A, et al. Requirement of Stat3 but not Stat1 activation for epidermal growth factor receptor-mediated cell growth *in vitro*. *J Clin Invest* 1998;102:1385.
35. Sorrells DL, Ghali GE, Meschonat C, et al. Competitive PCR to detect eIF4E gene amplification in head and neck cancer. *Head Neck* 1999;21:60.
36. Sorrells DL, Meschonat C, Black D, Li BD. Pattern of amplification and overexpression of the eukaryotic initiation factor 4E gene in solid tumor. *J Surg Res* 1999;85:37.
37. Nathan CA, Franklin S, Abreo FW, et al. Expression of eIF4E during head and neck tumorigenesis: possible role in angiogenesis. *Laryngoscope* 1999;109:1253.
38. Chan G, Boyle JO, Yang EK, et al. Cyclooxygenase-2 expression is up-regulated in squamous cell carcinoma of the head and neck. *Cancer Res* 1999;59:991.
39. Wang X, Pavelic ZP, Li Y, et al. Overexpression and amplification of glutathione *S*-transferase pi gene in head and neck squamous cell carcinomas. *Clin Cancer Res* 1997;3;111.
40. Markowitz S, Wang J, Myeroff L, et al. Inactivation of the type II TGF-beta receptor in colon cancer cells with microsatellite instability. *Science* 1995;268:1336.
41. Garrigueantar L, Munozantonia T, Antonia SJ, et al. Missense mutations of the transforming growth factor beta type II receptor in human head and neck squamous carcinoma cells. *Cancer Res* 1995;55:3982.
42. Wang D, Song H, Evans JA, et al. Mutation and downregulation of the transforming growth factor beta type II receptor gene in primary squamous cell carcinomas of the head and neck. *Carcinogenesis* 1997;18:2285.
43. Lippman SM, Spitz MR, Huber MH, Hong WK. Strategies for chemoprevention study of premalignancy and second primary tumors in the head and neck. *Curr Opin Oncol* 1995;7:234.

44. Lotan R, Xu XC, Lippman SM, et al. Suppression of retinoic acid receptor-beta in premalignant oral lesions and its up-regulation by isotretinoin. *N Engl J Med* 1995;332:1405.
45. Weber JL, May PE. Abundant class of human DNA polymorphisms which can be typed using the polymerase chain reaction. *Am J Hum Genet* 1989;44:388.
46. Knudson AG Jr. Mutation and cancer: statistical study of retinoblastoma. *Proc Natl Acad Sci U S A* 1971;68:820.
47. Hollstein M, Sidransky D, Vogelstein B, Harris C. p53 mutations in human cancer. *Science* 1991;253:49.
48. Boyle JO, Koch W, Hruban RH, et al. The incidence of p53 mutations increases with progression of head and neck cancer. *Cancer Res* 1993;53:4477.
49. Brennan JA, Boyle JO, Koch WM, et al. Association between cigarette smoking and mutation of the p53 gene in head and neck squamous carcinoma. *N Engl J Med* 1995;332:712.
50. Nawroz H, van der Riet P, Hruban RH, et al. Allelotype of head and neck squamous cell carcinoma. *Cancer Res* 1994;54:1152.
51. Ahsee KW, Cooke TG, Pickford IR, et al. An allelotype of squamous carcinoma of the head and neck using microsatellite markers. *Cancer Res* 1994;54:1617.
52. van der Riet P, Nawroz H, Hruban RH, et al. Frequent loss of chromosome 9p21-22 early in head and neck cancer progression. *Cancer Res* 1994;54:1156.
53. Kamb A, Gruis NA, Weaver-Feldhaus J, et al. A cell cycle regulator potentially involved in genesis of many tumor types. *Science* 1994;264:436.
54. Hussussian CJ, Struewing JP, Goldstein AM, et al. Germline p16 mutations in familial melanoma. *Nat Genet* 1994;8:15.
55. Munro J, Stott FJ, Vousden KH, et al. Role of the alternative INK4A proteins in human keratinocyte senescence: evidence for the specific inactivation of p16INK4A upon immortalization. *Cancer Res* 1999;59:2516.
56. Zhang SY, Kleinszanto AJP, Sauter ER, et al. Higher frequency of alterations in the p16/CDKN2 gene in squamous cell carcinoma cell lines than in primary tumors of the head and neck. *Cancer Res* 1994;54:5050.
57. Cairns P, Mao L, Merlo A, et al. Low rate of p16 (MTS1) mutations in primary tumors with 9p loss. *Science* 1994;265:415.
58. Merlo A, Herman JG, Mao L, et al. 5′ CpG island methylation is associated with transcriptional silencing of the tumour suppressor p16/CDKN2/MTS1 in human cancers. *Nat Med* 1995;7:686.
59. Cairns P, Polascik TJ, Eby Y, et al. Frequency of homozygous deletion at p16/CDKN2 in primary human tumors. *Nat Genet* 1995;11:210.
60. Reed A, Califano J, Cairns P, et al. High frequency of p16CDKN2/MTS-1/INK4A inactivation in head and neck squamous cell carcinoma. *Cancer Res* 1996;56:3630.
61. Papadimitrakopoulou V, Izzo J, Lippman SM, et al. Frequent inactivation of p16INK4a in oral premalignant lesions. *Oncogene* 1997;14:1799.
62. Mao L, Merlo A, Bedi G, et al. A novel p16^{INK4A} transcript. *Cancer Res* 1995;55:2995.
63. Liggett WH Jr, Sewell DA, Rocco J, et al. p16 and p16β are potent growth suppressors of head and neck squamous carcinoma cells *in vitro*. *Cancer Res* 1996;56:4119.
64. Zhang Y, Xiong Y, Yarbrough WG. ARF promotes MDM2 degradation and stabilizes p53: ARF-INK4a locus deletion impairs both the Rb and p53 tumor suppression pathways. *Cell* 1998;92:725.
65. Pomerantz J, Schreiber-Agus N, Liegeois NJ, et al. The INK4a tumor suppressor gene product, p19^{ARF}, interacts with MDM2 and neutralizes MDM2's inhibition of p53. *Cell* 1998;92:713.
66. Kamijo T, Zindy F, Roussel MF, et al. Tumor suppression at the mouse INK4a locus mediated by the alternative reading frame product p19^{ARF}. *Cell* 1997;91:649.
67. Sanchez-Cespedes M, Reed AL, Buta M, et al. Inactivation of the INK4A/ARF locus frequently coexists with TP53 mutations in non–small cell lung cancer. *Oncogene* 1999;18:5843.
68. Maestro R, Gasparotto D, Vuksavljevic T, et al. Three discrete regions of deletion in head and neck cancers. *Cancer Res* 1993;53:5775.
69. Wu CL, Sloan P, Read AP, et al. Deletion mapping on the short arm of chromosome 3 in squamous cell carcinoma of the oral cavity. *Cancer Res* 1994;54:6484.
70. Chen YJ, Chen PH, Lee MD, Chang JG. Aberrant FHIT transcripts in cancerous and corresponding non-cancerous lesions of the digestive tract. *Int J Cancer* 1997;72:955-.
71. Mao L, Fan YH, Lotan R, Hong WK. Frequent abnormalities of FHIT, a candidate tumor suppressor gene, in head and neck cancer cell lines. *Cancer Res* 1996;56:5128.
72. Hartwell LH, Kastan MB. Cell cycle control and cancer. *Science* 1994;266:1821.
73. Koch WM, Brennan JA, Zahurak M, et al. p53 mutation and locoregional treatment failure in head and neck squamous cell carcinoma. *J Natl Cancer Inst* 1996;88:1580.
74. Okami K, Wu L, Riggins G, et al. Analysis of PTEN/MMAC1 alterations in aerodigestive tract tumors. *Cancer Res* 1998;58:509.
75. Shao X, Tandon R, Samara G, et al. Mutational analysis of the PTEN gene in head and neck squamous cell carcinoma. *Int J Cancer* 1998;77:684.
76. Gasparotto D, Vukosavljevic T, Piccinin S, et al. Loss of heterozygosity at 10q in tumors of the upper respiratory tract is associated with poor prognosis. *Int J Cancer* 1999;84:432.
77. Yoo GH, Xu HJ, Brennan JA, et al. Infrequent inactivation of the retinoblastoma gene despite frequent loss of chromosome 13q in head and neck squamous cell carcinoma. *Cancer Res* 1994;54:4603.
78. Wu CL, Roz L, Sloan P, et al. Deletion mapping defines three discrete areas of allelic imbalance on chromosome arm 8p in oral and oropharyngeal squamous cell carcinomas. *Genes Chromosomes Cancer* 1997;20:347.
79. Sunwoo JB, Sun PC, Gupta VK, et al. Localization of a putative tumor suppressor gene in the sub-telomeric region of chromosome 8p. *Oncogene* 1999;18:2651.
80. Ishwad CS, Shuster M, Bockmuhl U, et al. Frequent allelic loss and homozygous deletion in chromosome band 8p23 in oral cancer. *Int J Cancer* 1999;80:25.
81. Wang XL, Uzawa K, Miyakawa A, et al. Localization of a tumour-suppressor gene associated with human oral cancer on 7q31.1. *Int J Cancer* 1998;75:671.
82. Papadimitrakopoulou VA, Oh Y, El-Naggar A, et al. Presence of multiple incontiguous deleted regions at the long arm of chromosome 18 in head and neck cancer. *Clin Cancer Res* 1998;4:539.
83. Pearlstein RP, Benninger MS, Carey TE, et al. Loss of 18q predicts poor survival of patients with squamous cell carcinoma of the head and neck. *Genes Chromosomes Cancer* 1998;21:333.
84. Kim SK, Fan Y, Papadimitrakopoulou V, et al. DPC4, a candidate tumor suppressor gene, is altered infrequently in head and neck squamous cell carcinoma. *Cancer Res* 1996;56:2519.
85. Califano J, van der Riet P, Westra W, et al. A genetic progression model for head and neck cancer: implications for field cancerization. *Cancer Res* 1996;56:2488.
86. Ogawara K, Miyakawa A, Shiba M, et al. Allelic loss of chromosome 13q14.3 in human oral cancer: correlation with lymph node metastasis. *Int J Cancer* 1998;79:312.
87. Lee DJ, Koch WM, Yoo G, et al. Impact of chromosome 14q loss on survival in primary head and neck squamous cell carcinoma. *Clin Cancer Res* 1997;3:501.
88. Lazar AD, Winter MR, Nogueira CP, et al. Loss of heterozygosity at 11q23 in squamous cell carcinoma of the head and neck is associated with recurrent disease. *Clin Cancer Res* 1998;4:2787.
89. Mineta H, Miura K, Suzuki I, et al. Low p27 expression correlates with poor prognosis for patients with oral tongue squamous cell carcioma. *Cancer* 1999;85:1011.
90. Venkatesan TK, Kuropkat C, Caldarelli DD, et al. Prognostic significance of p27 expression in carcinoma of the oral cavity and oropharynx. *Laryngoscope* 1999;109:1329.
91. Mao L, Lee JS, Fan YH, et al. Frequent microsatellite alterations at chromosomes 9p21 and 3p14 in oral premalignant lesions and their value in cancer risk assessment. *Nat Med* 1996;2:682.
92. Mao L, El-Naggar AK, Papadimitrakopoulou V, et al. Phenotype and genotype of advanced premalignant head and neck lesions after chemopreventive therapy. *J Natl Cancer Inst* 1998;90:1545.
93. Slaughter DL, Southwick HW, Smejkal W. "Field cancerization" in oral stratified squamous epithelium: clinical implications of multicentric origin. *Cancer* (Phila) 1953;6:963.
94. Sidransky D, Preisinger AC, Frost P, et al. Clonal origin of metachronous tumors of the bladder. *N Engl J Med* 1992;326:737.
95. Chung KY, Mukhopadhyay T, Kim J, et al. Discordant p53 gene mutations in primary head and neck cancers and corresponding second primary cancers of the upper aerodigestive tract. *Cancer Res* 1993;53:1676.
96. Bedi GC, Westra WH, Gabrielson E, et al. Multiple head and neck tumors: evidence for a common clonal origin. *Cancer Res* 1996;56:2484.
97. Worsham MJ, Wolman SR, Carey TE, et al. Common clonal origin of synchronous primary head and neck squamous cell carcinomas. *Hum Pathol* 1995;26:251.
98. Leong PP, Rezai B, Koch WM, et al. Distinguishing second primary tumors from lung metastases in patients with head and neck squamous cell carcinoma. *J Natl Cancer Inst* 1998;90:972.
99. Califano J, Leong PL, Koch WM, et al. Second esophageal tumors in patients with head and neck squamous cell carcinoma: an assessment of clonal relationships. *Clin Cancer Res* 1999;5:1862.
100. Califano J, Westra WH, Meininger G, et al. Unknown primary head and neck squamous cell carcinoma: molecular identification of the site of origin. *J Natl Cancer Inst* 1999; 91:599.
101. Harris CC, Hollstein M. Clinical implication of the p53 tumor-suppressor gene. *N Engl J Med* 1993;329:1318.
102. Gillison ML, Koch WM, Spafford M, et al. Causal association between human papillomavirus and a subset of head and neck cancers. *JNCI* (*in press*).
103. Andl T, Kahn T, Pfuhl A, et al. Etiological involvement of oncogenic human papillomavirus in tonsillar squamous cell carcinomas lacking retinoblastoma cell cycle control. *Cancer Res* 1998;58:5.
104. Haraf DJ, Nodzenski E, Brachman D, et al. Human papilloma virus and p53 in head and neck cancer: clinical correlates and survival. *Clin Cancer Res* 1996;2:755.
105. Sidransky D, Tokino T, Frost P, et al. Identification of ras oncogene mutations in the stool of patients with curable colorectal tumors. *Science* 1992;256:102.
106. Sidransky D, Von Eschenbach A, Tsai YC, et al. Identification of p53 gene mutations in bladder cancers and urine samples. *Science* 1991;252:706.
107. Mao L, Hruban RH, Boyle JO, et al. Detection of oncogene mutations in sputum precedes diagnosis of lung cancer. *Cancer Res* 1994;54:1634.
108. Boyle JB, Mao L, Brennan JA, et al. Gene mutations in saliva as molecular markers for head and neck squamous cell carcinomas. *Am J Surg* 1994;168:429.
109. Califano JA, Ahrendt S, Meininger G, et al. Detection of telomerase activity in oral rinses from head and neck squamous cell cancer patients. *Cancer Res* 1996;56:5720.
110. Mao L, El-Naggar AK, Fan YH, et al. Telomerase activity in head and neck squamous cell carcinoma and adjacent tissues. *Cancer Res* 1996;56:5600.
111. Spafford MF, Koch WM, Reed AL, et al. Detection of head and neck squamous cell carcinoma in saliva by microsatellite analysis. 2000 (*submitted*).
112. Rosin MP, Epstein JB, Berean K, et al. The use of exfoliative cell samples to map clonal genetic alterations in the oral epithelium of high-risk patients. *Cancer Res* 1997;57:5258.
113. Brennan JA, Mao L, Hruban RH, et al. Molecular assessment of histopathologic staging. *N Engl J Med* 1995;332:429.

SECTION 2

STIMSON P. SCHANTZ
LOUIS B. HARRISON
ARLENE A. FORASTIERE

Tumors of the Nasal Cavity and Paranasal Sinuses, Nasopharynx, Oral Cavity, and Oropharynx

The analysis of cancers within the upper aerodigestive tract reveals a heterogeneity of neoplastic processes. Each bears its own unique set of epidemiologic, anatomic, pathologic, and treatment considerations. This chapter reviews such considerations based on four anatomically defined regions: the nasal cavity and paranasal sinuses; nasopharynx; oral cavity; and oropharynx.

However, there exist general principles regarding these cancers that may be considered here. Such principles involve anatomy (i.e., primarily the anatomy of regional lymph nodes within the head and neck), pathology, staging, and screening, as well as general principles of treatment involving either single modality or multimodality therapy, which are relevant to all sites.

ANATOMY

An understanding of the regional lymph node anatomy is critical to the care of head and neck cancer patients. There are several major lymphatic chains in the neck containing nearly 200 lymph nodes that run parallel to the jugular veins, spinal accessory nerve, and facial artery and into the submandibular triangle (Fig. 30.2-1). To facilitate communication regarding cervical lymph node anatomy, the regions of the neck have been characterized by levels (Fig. 30.2-2).[1–3]

Level I includes nodes within the submental triangle and the submandibular triangle. The submental triangle extends from the midline anteriorly to the anterior belly of the digastric muscle posteriorly. Its third border is formed by the hyoid bone inferiorly. The submandibular triangle is bounded by the mandible superiorly. The anterior and the posterior belly of the digastric muscle complete the triangle.

Level II includes the jugular nodes extending from the subdigastric area down to the carotid bifurcation and the nodes surrounding the spinal accessory nerve from the jugular foramen to the posterior border of the sternocleidomastoid muscle. It includes the lymph nodes in the upper posterior cervical triangle above the entrance of the spinal accessory nerve into this triangle.

Level III represents the nodal area principally along the jugular vein between the carotid and its bifurcation, the posterior border of the sternocleidomastoid muscle, and the omohyoid muscle.

Level IV constitutes nodal areas below the omohyoid muscle above the level of the clavicle and between the carotid vessels anteriorly and the omohyoid muscle posteriorly.

Level V represents nodes in the posterior cervical triangle. Its borders are formed by the posterior edge of the sternocleidomastoid muscle, the level of the entrance of the spinal accessory nerve, the trapezius muscle, and the posterior belly of the omohyoid muscle.

Specific sites within the aerodigestive tract have a predetermined drainage pattern. A knowledge of this pattern aids in diagnosis. It also affects therapy. Drainage patterns are addressed in each of the anatomic subsites detailed in this chapter.

PATHOLOGY

The predominant lesion within these anatomically defined regions is squamous cell carcinoma. Squamous cell carcinoma can be categorized into three classic differentiations. Well-differentiated disease shows greater than 75% keratinization; moderately differentiated disease contributes to the bulk of squamous cell carcinoma and is characterized by 25% to 75% keratinization; and poorly differentiated disease demonstrates less than 25% keratinization. Other variants of squamous cell carcinoma include verrucous carcinoma, sarcomatoid squamous cell carcinoma, and lymphoepithelioma. Additional pathologic criteria of squamous cell carcinoma that is believed to be clinically relevant were developed by Jacobsson and others.[4–7] This includes the number of mitoses, presence of vascular invasion, size of nuclei, degree of inflammatory infiltrate, and pushing or infiltrating borders (Table 30.2-1).

PREMALIGNANCY

A series of pathologic changes from premalignant disease to frank malignancy can occur in the oral cavity. Among the premalignant diseases are leukoplakia, erythroplakia, hyperplasia, and dysplasia. Each of these types has a propensity for malignant transformation.[8] Histopathologic assessment of leukoplakia reveals hyperparakeratosis, which is variably associated with an underlying epithelial hyperplasia. Leukoplakia without underlying dysplastic changes is rarely associated with progression to malignancy (i.e., less than 5% probability of malignant changes).[9,10] Erythroplakia is a condition within the oral cavity and pharynx characterized by red superficial patches adjacent to normal mucosa. Distinct from leukoplakic lesions as identified previously, erythroplakia is commonly associated with underlying epithelial dysplasia. Likewise, it can be associated with carcinoma *in situ* to frank malignancy in nearly 40% of lesions.[9,11]

Dysplasia as compared with the previously mentioned two clinical descriptives is a true histopathologic term that is characterized by several morphologic changes, including the presence of mitoses, pleomorphism, and prominent nucleoli. When dysplasia involves the entire thickness of the mucosa, it is commonly referred to as *carcinoma in situ*. Dysplasia has been associated with a subsequent risk of progression to frank malignancy ranging from 15% to 30% of cases.[12,13]

STAGING AND SCREENING

STAGING

The role and current status of staging for head and neck cancer is undergoing continuous analysis.[14–18] Although standard staging has been defined, there is a growing debate as to what

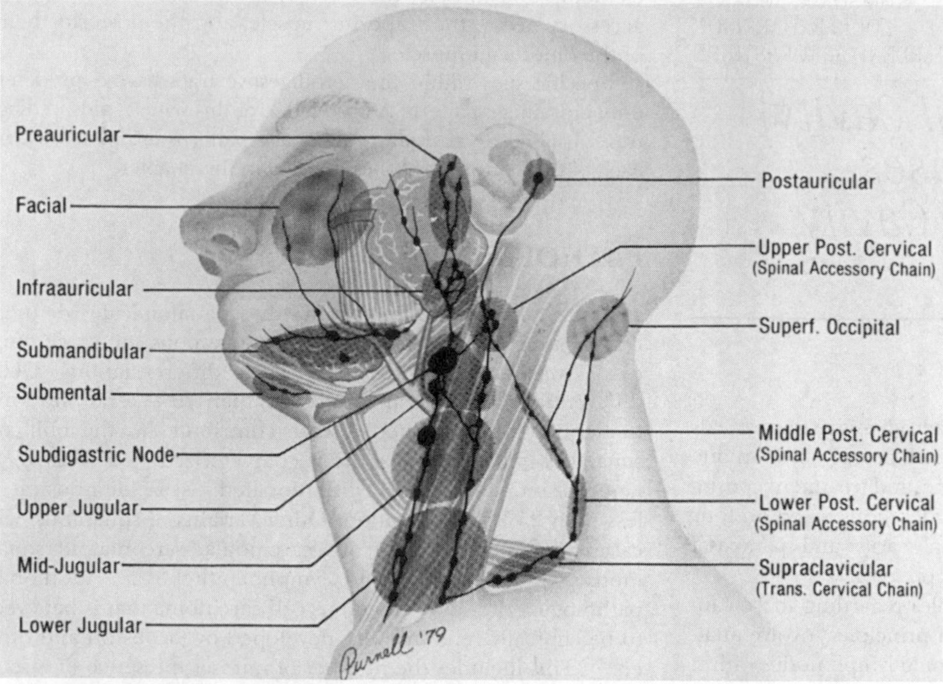

FIGURE 30.2-1. Superficial and deep cervical lymph nodes of the head and neck. (From Shah JP. *A color atlas of head and neck surgery*. Orlando: Grune & Stratton, 1987, with permission.)

the primary function of staging should be. The American Joint Committee on Cancer Staging (AJCC), however, has described the principal goal of staging as a means of defining the natural history of disease. Additional goals include the ability to judge therapeutic results between various centers as well as a means of defining patient prognosis. Revisions to standard staging have continually been offered,[15,16] but today it is based on the TNM classification. T stage represents extent of primary disease. N represents the extent of regional lymph node metastasis and M is a measure of distant metastasis. The AJCC staging system, used for classifying TNM status, is periodically revised.[14]

The current clinical staging system, although based principally on physical examination, has also incorporated specific radiographic observations of disease status. Thus, invasion *through* cortical bone by an oral cavity tumor up-stages a T2 or T3 lesion to T4 (i.e., from stage II or III to stage IV).

Radiographic assessment of cervical lymph node metastases has not been integrated into clinical staging. The benefits of these diagnostic techniques beyond that provided by standard

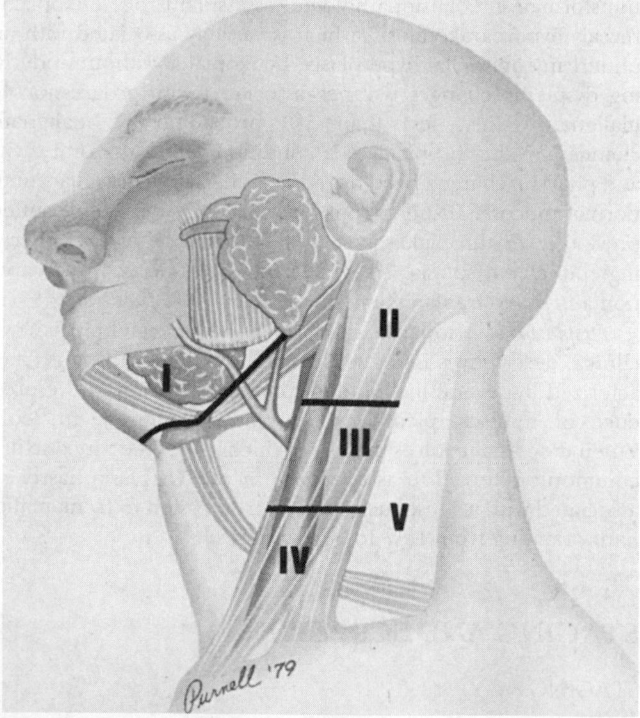

FIGURE 30.2-2. Level classification of regional cervical lymph nodes (see text for description). (From Shah JP. *A color atlas of head and neck surgery*. Orlando: Grune & Stratton, 1987, with permission.)

TABLE 30.2-1. Jacobsson Classification System[a]

Classification	*Score*
TUMOR CELL CHARACTERISTICS	
Degree of keratinization	1–4
Nuclear pleomorphism	1–4
Number of mitoses	1–4
TUMOR-HOST RELATIONS	
Mode of invasion	1–4
Leukocyte infiltration	1–4
TOTAL MALIGNANCY SCORE[b]	
The sum of scores of features	1–5

[a]All features are registered in the most anaplastic areas of invasive sites of the tumors.
[b]A high malignancy score indicates a poorly differentiated tumor. (Modified from ref. 6.)

TABLE 30.2-2. Advantages of Computed Tomographic Scanning and Magnetic Resonance Imaging in the Evaluation of Head and Neck Cancers

CT SCANNING

Fast acquisition time/less motion artifact (especially true for patients with bulky tumors that cause them to continually swallow)

Increased sensitivity to bony destruction?

For patients who cannot tolerate MRI because of claustrophobia, or patients who are not MRI candidates (pacemakers, aneurysm clips)

Cost

Currently CT is better than MRI for evaluating metastatic adenopathy

MRI

No iodinated contrast (contrast allergy renal failure)

No irradiation

Multiplanar capability

No dental amalgam artifact

Superior soft tissue contrast

May be better than CT for primary tumor staging

CT, computed tomography; MRI, magnetic resonance imaging. (From ref. 22, with permission.)

physical examination are under investigation.[17–22] Most would consider the combination of radiographic and clinical assessment to be more accurate than either one alone. Furthermore, growing emphasis is being placed on the advantages of one imaging technique versus another [i.e., the relative merit of magnetic resonance imaging (MRI) vs. computed tomography (CT)].[17] Table 30.2-2 summarizes the relative value of these two techniques in head and neck imaging.

The criteria for T staging within the upper aerodigestive tract differs depending on the primary site. N staging and M staging, however, are uniform and therefore are considered in Table 30.2-3. Table 30.2-4 represents the most current stage classification as defined by the AJCC.[14]

Additional data continue to accrue regarding the effect of comorbidities in prognostication. Data suggest that these host-related factors provide information beyond standard AJCC criteria alone. Host factors include the presence of significant heart disease, liver disease, and severe cerebrovascular disease. Survival rates are significantly reduced if comorbidities exist and are improved with their absence.[23–25] In a study by Singh et al., for instance, involving 70 patients with squamous cell carcinoma of the upper aerodigestive tract, patients with Kaplan-Feinstein comorbidity index grades 2 and 3 had a significantly decreased disease-free survival as compared with those with comorbidity index of grade of 0 to 1.[23] Stage distribution between the two groups was similar.

SCREENING FOR PRIMARY CANCERS

It is intuitive that detection of disease at its earliest stages would improve cancer mortality. Given the degree to which the oral cavity and upper aerodigestive tract can be easily examined, it would also seem that screening for head and neck cancers would be a readily accomplishable goal. Diminished mortality would be readily achievable. The significance of screening as a potentially significant modality is emphasized by a review by Smart, who reported that 94% of head and neck cancer

TABLE 30.2-3. Staging within the Upper Aerodigestive Tract

REGIONAL LYMPH NODES (N)	
NX	Regional lymph nodes cannot be assessed
N0	No regional lymph node metastasis
N1	Metastasis in a single ipsilateral lymph node, 3 cm or less in greatest dimension
N2	Metastasis in a single ipsilateral lymph node, more than 3 cm but not more than 6 cm in greatest dimension; or in multiple ipsilateral lymph nodes, or in bilateral or contralateral lymph nodes, none more than 6 cm in greatest dimension
N2a	Metastasis in a single ipsilateral lymph node more than 3 cm but not more than 6 cm in greatest dimension
N2b	Metastasis in multiple ipsilateral lymph nodes, none more than 6 cm in greatest dimension
N2c	Metastasis in bilateral or contralateral lymph nodes, none more than 6 cm in greatest dimension
N3	Metastasis in a lymph node more than 6 cm in greatest dimension
DISTANT METASTASIS (M)	
MX	Presence of distant metastasis cannot be assessed
M0	No distant metastasis
M1	Distant metastasis

patients had seen a physician at least 1 year before diagnosis.[24] Each patient reported an average of 11 physician visits within a 3-year period before diagnosis. Smart's review emphasizes that with appropriate training and practice of systematic screening habits by examining physicians, head and neck cancer may be diagnosed considerably earlier. In that regard, a study by Prout et al. assessed the value of educational programs for health care providers in the Boston area and provided information that would reinforce that notion.[25] These latter authors noted that health care providers schooled in the oral cancer educational program were significantly more likely to perform systematic oral screening in subsequent years. These studies emphasize the important role of the physician in the early detection of head and neck cancer and that such individuals, if properly motivated, are more likely to perform such screening than those less aware of the significance of oral cancer.

Despite the intuitive benefit that would come with more effective screening, confounding factors may limit success. First, head and neck cancer is a relatively sporadic disease. Mass screening

TABLE 30.2-4. Stage Grouping Based on American Joint Committee on Cancer Staging Criteria

	Classification		
Stage	T	N	M
0	Tis	N0	M0
I	T1	N0	M0
II	T2	N0	M0
III	T3	N0	M0
	T1	N1	M0
	T2	N1	M0
	T3	N1	M0
IV	T4	N0	M0

procedures would detect cancer in only limited instances. Second, individuals at risk tend to be less health conscious. Compliance with health care advice such as avoidance of substance abuse, good nutritional habits, and regular physical evaluation is not readily achieved in this population. Third, head and neck cancer patients can often be characterized by diminished social support systems. Access to medical care is hindered, making routine follow-up by a health care provider difficult. Finally, although it is often stated that a readily identifiable premalignant condition exists (i.e., leukoplakia or erythroplakia), few head and neck cancer cases can be shown to progress through this premalignant clinical stage. Although head and neck cancers tend to occur late in life, these same cancers can occur at any time within a 20-year interval. Knowing which patient and when that patient will develop disease remains a conundrum. Furthermore, whether or not the identification of disease changes its natural history is not clear. We cannot state with certainty the interval required for a tumor to achieve its initially diagnosed stage. We do not know whether the biologic potential of a head and neck cancer follows the same time course within every individual. Ultimate tumor aggressiveness may be determined early in its natural history. The window of opportunity to detect the most lethal cancers may be small. No studies have yet demonstrated that systematic screening diminishes head and neck cancer mortality. Indeed, the Task Force for the Guide to Preventive Services has concluded that routine screening for oral cancer cannot be recommended.[26]

It is not surprising, therefore, that various mass screening programs for head and neck cancer have demonstrated mostly negative results. Jullien et al. and others have made it apparent that the identification of head and neck cancer is only one part of the process.[27–30] In the assessment of nearly 1000 patients as reported by Jullien et al., only 67% of the 12 patients noted to have potentially malignant disease were compliant with follow-up recommendations.[27] The experience in Cuba, likewise, showed similar discouraging results.[28] Annual oral examination had been considered mandatory for all individuals over 15 years of age in Cuba since 1984. The proportion of early-stage disease was noted to increase during this period of more intensive screening. However, overall oral cancer mortality was not altered. As in the study by Jullien et al., a major problem was patient compliance in follow-up examinations once the disease has been diagnosed. The investigators of these large population-based studies conclude that systematic mass screening for head and neck cancer is not a cost-effective process and has little effect on overall cancer mortality.

Perhaps more significant than the screening process itself and in light of the development of more effective behavioral modification approaches, Cowan et al. have demonstrated that screening strategies are valuable in identifying the health care beliefs of the provider.[30] Primary care dentists participating in this study were noted to routinely assess the oral cavity for evidence of disease.[30] However, a minority of dentists routinely recorded information about tobacco and alcohol abuse. The implication of Cowan's study was that screening was already adopted. What should be developed in the primary care setting is a clearer understanding of the benefits of health promotion involving substance abuse modification.

There are, however, novel strategies under development that may enhance screening effectiveness.[31–39] We have previously noted in this brief review that epidemiologic investigations continue to refine risk estimates. Current computer technology may allow for translating previous risk factor assessments into clinical strategies that enhance screening efforts. An example involves the use of neural networks. The Oral Cancer Screening Group in England has demonstrated its potential utility.[31] The performance of the network to identify individuals at increased risk was compared with the results of oral screening by health care specialists. Over 2000 adults were entered into the study and were asked to fill out a questionnaire that identified ten input variables. The overall sensitivity and specificity of the screeners as compared with the neural network were comparable. The use of neural networks could be performed, however, at a fraction of the cost.

Other screening techniques under investigation include the use of genetic markers of increased risk, molecular cytology, serum tumor markers, as well as newer technologies involving optical engineering and the computer sciences.[31–38]

SCREENING FOR SECOND PRIMARY CANCERS

Head and neck cancer patients are characterized by their high risk of developing second primary malignancies. The majority of these cancers occur within tobacco-exposed tissue, including the esophagus, lung, and remaining upper aerodigestive tract. This risk has been well characterized and is known to occur at a rate of 4% per year.[39] Given the high rate of second malignancies within these individuals, numerous screening strategies have been described. Available screening modalities include laryngoscopy, esophagoscopy, contrast studies of the esophagus, chest radiography, sputum cytology, and bronchoscopy. Newer modalities are under investigation including the use of molecular assessments of cells within saliva and sputum.[40] Despite this effort, no agreement exists as to the optimal screening means, including the timing and duration of follow-up. Perhaps the greatest controversy revolves around the role of panendoscopy at the time the patient presents for treatment of the index cancer. Proponents of this procedure, which includes laryngoscopy, esophagoscopy, and bronchoscopy, cite the high rate of identified second cancers, reported in one prospective study to occur in 10% of patients.[41] Disease found in this setting is presumed to be of an earlier stage and more responsive to treatment. Opponents of routine panendoscopy cite the relatively low yield and questionable value in actually altering disease course and survival.[42–44] A prospective study by Benninger et al. provided compelling evidence to support the use of screening procedures based principally on symptomatology (i.e., so-called symptom-directed selective endoscopy).[43] A careful history and physical examination of all newly diagnosed head and neck cancer patients represents the most effective screening method. Although routine panendoscopy cannot be advocated, in certain individuals its use may be more beneficial. This, in our experience, includes patients whose index cancer resides within the pharynx and who admit to a long history of tobacco and alcohol abuse. Special attention should be given to the assessment of the esophagus in these individuals as well as the remaining upper aerodigestive tract.

TREATMENT

PRETREATMENT CONSIDERATIONS

The comprehensive care of the head and neck cancer patient begins with pretreatment considerations including the assessment of general medical conditions, nutritional status, dental health, and the appropriate choice of medical therapies designed to minimize treatment-related complications. It is beyond the scope of this chapter to detail the numerous associated medical illnesses that are typically identified in the head and neck cancer patient. Given the prolonged history of tobacco and alcohol abuse that can be typically identified, diseases involving the pulmonary, cardiovascular, and digestive systems are common. There remain, however, important considerations that should be stressed. This includes the significance of pretreatment dental care, nutritional support, the effect of therapy on the elderly patient, and the choice of preoperative medications (i.e., antibiotics for the patient about to undergo major surgical procedures).

The standard of care today for the head and neck cancer patient is the reduction of oral diseases before initiation of treatment.[45–47] Periodontal diseases, infections, and caries are common in this patient population. This can lead to loss of integrity of the gingival-crevicular tissues. Left unchecked, significant morbidity can result to structural elements of the oral cavity in the face of aggressive therapy. Following initial evaluation by the oncologic team, dentulous patients should be referred to dental colleagues for appropriate oral hygiene. Pretreatment radiographic dental surveys should identify caries and periapical lesions. Other factors that should be considered include defective restorations, ill-fitting prostheses, and impacted molars. It is generally considered prudent to perform necessary dental rehabilitation, including extractions, approximately 2 weeks before the initiation of any radiotherapy. This allows for the appropriate healing of extraction sites and mucosal coverage of exposed bone. In order to minimize delays in the initiation of radiation, dental care can be performed at the time of surgical resection in a patient who is to undergo multimodality therapy.

The assessment of nutritional status and the choice of pretreatment nutritional regimens is more controversial. Several authors report the common finding of malnutrition in the head and neck cancer patient.[48–50] Severe malnutrition has been identified in over 25% of the patients.[48] Furthermore, the presence of severe malnutrition was associated with increased operative morbidity.[50] This has led to efforts to appropriately quantitate nutritional status through the use of documentation of pretreatment weight loss, the measurement of triceps skin fold thickness, and the inclusion of various laboratory measures such as plasma protein levels and the creatinine and height index. To date there has been no conclusive randomized trial of pretherapy nutritional restoration in order to minimize treatment morbidity. However, Goodwin and Byers have stressed that in the severely malnourished patient, attention should be given to a 2-week pretreatment course of nutritional support.[48] Such attempts can most often be achieved through enteral means with the placement of either a nasogastric tube or a percutaneously placed gastrostomy tube.

The care of the elderly patient represents a commonly occurring dilemma.[51–54] The tendency to deny a patient optimal treatment because of the patient's advanced years should be avoided. In a study by McGuirt and Davis, operative mortality was 4% in 217 patients greater than 65 years of age and not significantly different than those less than 65 years.[52] In a subset of patients over the age of 75 and with stage III or IV disease, however, the mortality increased to 6%. A prospective case-control study by Kowalski et al. on elderly patients undergoing head and neck surgery failed to identify any increased frequency of postoperative complications or mortality as compared with younger patients.[51] The choice of treatment should not be predicated on the age of the patient. Rather, it is the patient's general medical condition that remains the most critical consideration, regardless of age. In a more recent article by Clayman, 43 patients who were 80 years of age or older were noted to have no increased postoperative complications than a stage- and site-matched population aged 65 years or less.[54] Of note, the older population was more likely to have a lesser surgical procedure, more likely to have positive pathologic margins, and less likely to receive postoperative radiation therapy (RT). Disease-free survival was also decreased in the older population. The perception of an increased risk of treatment-induced complications may compromise appropriate therapy.

Increasing attention recently has been given to the significance of continued tobacco use in the head and neck cancer population. The data would support the notion that continued tobacco use following diagnosis of the index cancer leads to an adverse patient outcome. This relates to not only the more obvious problem of progressive cardiopulmonary disease, but considerations related to head and neck cancer progression as well. Day et al. and others have provided more information regarding the risk of second primary malignancies in patients who continue to smoke following treatment of their index cancer.[55,56] The risk of second primary malignancies was significantly higher in the smoking population as compared with those who achieved smoking cessation. This difference was apparent only after 5 years following initial treatment.[55] In another study by Browman et al., continued tobacco use was associated with a decreased likelihood to respond to primary therapy.[57] This latter study represents an initial report and is limited by its small population size. It does, however, raise an important consideration in the overall care of these patients, namely, the systematic approach toward achieving smoking cessation. In that regard, several studies have identified characteristics of patients who are likely to continue smoking habits.[59,61–63] Interestingly, Ostroff et al. have reported that it is the patients with the best outlook who seem to be the most recalcitrant.[60] Patients with early-stage disease continued to use tobacco at higher rates than patients with higher stage disease. Strategies are being explored in order to effectively support the patient through this critical period.[58] The hallmark of any approach should include surgeon-delivered advice as well as the judicious use of nicotine replacement.

Finally, head and neck surgical oncologists should critically assess the need for supportive therapies in the patient who is to undergo operative procedures. This has principally related to the choice of perioperative antibiotics. The use of prophylactic antibiotics can only be supported for those individuals undergoing clean-contaminated surgery (i.e., when it is anticipated that the aerodigestive tract is to be entered) or in those circumstances in which there is frank contamination. Postoperative infectious complications may occur in up to 30% of the patients. Several studies have addressed risk factors for infectious complications and found duration of the operative procedure, blood loss, and complexity of the reconstructive procedure to be high-risk variables.[61–63] Common microbials isolated from infected wounds include both aerobes and anaerobes with *Bacteroides fragilis*, *Escherichia coli*, β-hemolytic streptococcus, *Staphylococcus*, and *Pseudomonas* being frequently identified. Perioperative antibiotics should be started before the operative procedure and should continued for 72 hours postoperatively depending on the likelihood of infection. Antibiotic regimens should allow for broad coverage. Regimens include combination sulbactam and ampicillin, metronidazole combined with a cephalosporin, or clindamycin alone. Comparative studies regarding the appropriate antibiotic regimen may be confounded by the definition of infection and rigor in wound assessment. Regardless of the antibiotic regimen one may choose, however, postoperative infection rates should average less than 15%.[64]

GENERAL PRINCIPLES OF SURGERY

In the execution of effective surgical management, the single most significant principle is the adequate preoperative assessment of disease extent. Precise and methodic physical examination of the patient is paramount. Such examination allows for the assessment of adequate extent of surgical excision, which remains for most cancers the fundamental tenet for achieving cure.

An extension of adequate preoperative assessment is optimal intraoperative exposure of disease. The surgeon should consider appropriate means to achieve operative exposure. The choice of incision and the ability to mobilize surrounding anatomic structures to achieve exposure is considered later in the text for each anatomic subsite. Additionally, exposure is facilitated by careful hemostasis. Besides allowing for better operative exposure, minimizing blood loss prevents potential sequelae associated with blood transfusion. Weber et al. reported expected blood loss for various surgical procedures involving cancers of the upper aerodigestive tract.[65] Electrocautery dissection had been used by Weber and colleagues, which may explain the relatively infrequent need for blood transfusion. Electrocautery dissection has been adopted by many experienced surgeons as the preferred extirpative technique.

Additional methods of surgical excision have included the use of the Moh's technique and laser ablation.[66–68] These techniques, however, cannot be considered standard surgical procedure at this time.

Surgical Management of the Cervical Lymph Nodes

General principles of surgery exist involving regional lymph nodes as well. The standard in the surgical control of cervical metastases by which various procedures are judged is the radical neck dissection. The radical neck dissection involves complete removal of the lymphatic pathways within the neck. To ensure complete extirpation, anatomic structures including the sternocleidomastoid muscle, spinal accessory nerve, and jugular vein are routinely sacrificed.

Developments in the management of cervical lymph node disease involve more conservative surgical procedures.[3,69–71] These procedures differ from the classic radical neck dissection principally in the sparing of specific anatomic structures (i.e., principally the spinal accessory nerve and the sternocleidomastoid muscle). Table 30.2-5 provides a classification of currently used selective neck dissection and details removed lymph node regions.

TABLE 30.2-5. Classification of Neck Dissections

Classification	*Level of Lymph Node Removed*
I. Standard radical neck dissection	I, II, III, IV, V
II. Modified radical neck dissection	I, II, III, IV, V
III. Selective neck dissection	
A. Supraomohyoid	I, II, III
B. Lateral type	II, III, IV
C. Posterolateral type	II, III, IV, V
D. Anterior compartment type	VI
IV. Extended neck dissection	

(From Robbins KT. Classification of neck dissection: current concepts and future considerations of neck dissection. *Otolaryngol Clin North Am* 1998;31:639, with permission.)

Surgical Management of Disease in the Neck: N0 Neck

Multiple studies have determined that cancers of the upper aerodigestive tract are associated with an approximately 20% to 30% incidence of occult cervical lymph node metastases, despite clinically negative examination.[72–74] The overall incidence of occult primary disease is influenced by multiple factors including size and location of the primary cancer within the upper aerodigestive tract, depth of invasion, and tumor differentiation.[75] These observations have led to the generally accepted need for elective lymph node neck dissection as part of standard surgical management. Support for this approach has been provided by Spiro et al.[76] Those patients who did not undergo elective dissection were more likely to present with more advanced neck disease when disease recurred as compared with those individuals who underwent prophylactic dissection.[76] It should be emphasized, however, that randomized clinical trials that conclusively support the role of elective cervical lymph node dissection have been limited. Indeed, a study by Vandenbrouck and colleagues failed to find a survival benefit in oral cavity cancer patients randomized to receive elective dissection.[77] This study was limited by the small number of patients entered.

A debate exists as to the type of elective neck dissection that should be performed. The standard radical neck dissection that encompasses lymph node basins I through V as well as the spinal accessory nerve, internal jugular vein, and sternocleidomastoid muscle is not indicated in the treatment of occult disease, principally because of its associated shoulder dysfunction. The debate still exists as to whether to perform modified radical neck dissection versus a more limited selective procedure. Leemans et al., citing a metaanalysis, report a lower incidence of neck recurrence in those patients treated by a modified neck dissection.[78] Others argue that a supraomohyoid neck dissection for cancers of the oral cavity is adequate given the limited likelihood of level V metastases and the limited likelihood of disease recurrence in level V region. In a randomized study conducted by the Brazilian Head and Neck Cancer Study Group, overall survival was the same in patients who underwent a supraomohyoid neck dissection as compared with patients who underwent a standard modified radical neck dissection.[79] This is despite the observation that 50% more lymph nodes were identified in the surgical specimen from the population undergoing modified radical neck dissection. The standard supraomohyoid neck dissection does not, however, encompass level IV nodes. *Skip metastases* may occur in level IV nodes and disease recurrence in this level has been identified. These latter two observations suggest that a selective lymph node dissection in oral cancer patients who are clinically N0 should include levels I to IV.

The value of elective neck dissection is further justified by its low risk ratio. When performed by an experienced head and neck surgeon, the procedure does not require excessively prolonged operative time and can be performed with minimal morbidity. The caveat should be the performance of careful dissection along the spinal accessory nerve. Indeed, advances in the performance of elective neck dissection have been reported by Kraus et al.[80] The authors investigated the probability of metastases in the lymph nodes superior to the spinal accessory nerve in patients who were clinically N0. In 44 patients analyzed, only one individual had disease in this region.

Surgical Management of Disease in the Neck: N+ Neck

The presence of cervical metastases dictates in most instances the use of combination surgery and RT. Surgery alone has been reserved for those situations in which only a single lymph node is involved with disease and in which there is no extension of disease beyond the lymph node capsule. For patients with evidence of disease within cervical lymph nodes the most commonly accepted surgical management involves radical neck dissection. A trend, however, is evolving toward a more oncologically conservative approach designed to preserve shoulder function. Traynor et al. reported on the use of selective neck dissection in the management of the node-positive neck.[81] Twenty-nine patients were retrospectively reviewed in whom 16 had N2 disease or higher. Only one patient developed recurrence. Again, however, experience has been limited by the lack of controlled clinical trials designed to answer the question as to the optimal surgical procedure. Pellitari et al. reviewed their experience with selective neck dissection in 34 patients with multiple pathologically positive lymph nodes who underwent a selective neck dissection.[82] Regional recurrence rates approximated 12%, indicating the adequacy of the surgical resection when used judiciously with postoperative radiation.[83]

A major debate in the management of disease in the neck revolves around the handling of the carotid artery. This includes (1) indications for removal of the carotid as a part of an oncologic procedure and (2) indications and means of carotid artery reconstruction including preoperative assessment determination of cerebral blood flow reserve. There are those who advocate a less aggressive approach to the carotid, indicating that in the majority of circumstances, actual invasion of the carotid wall is rare and with careful dissection disease can be dissected away from the vessel without compromising cancer control. Furthermore, in those situations in which cancer invasion of the carotid artery actually exists, long-term disease control is limited, patients typically die from regional, distant, or both regional and distant metastatic disease. Finally, and most significantly, a conservative approach to the carotid artery minimizes significant incidence of cerebral vascular morbidity. Carew and Spiro reported experience with carotid artery resection at Memorial Sloan-Kettering Cancer Center.[84] In their review of extended neck dissections, the authors noted that in only 3 instances in over 2500 cervical lymph node dissections performed in a 10-year period was carotid artery resection required. Regional disease control in this population of individuals with predominantly N3 cervical lymph node disease was 71% and comparable with those reports in which carotid artery resection is more liberally used. None of the three patients who underwent carotid resection was alive at 2 years. The approach at Memorial Sloan-Kettering Cancer Center also includes the use of brachytherapy implants on the carotid artery in those circumstances in which the surgical peel potentially left macroscopic or microscopic disease. Others use an intermediate approach for disease encasing the carotid. Adams et al., for instance, reserve resection for instances in which there is 70% encasement of the vessel.[85] In those situations in which the patient was noted to tolerate preoperative balloon occlusion, survival was 30% at 2 years. Snyderman et al. have performed a metaanalysis of the reported experience with carotid artery resection in patients with metastatic head and neck cancer.[86] The overall (disease-free) survival for the group of patients reported was 22% and was similar between those who underwent carotid resection versus those who did not. Interestingly, survival has not changed in this group of patients over the last 20 years. The authors emphasize the high complication rate, with major cerebral vascular accidents occurring in 26% of the patients undergoing carotid artery resection. The rate of cerebrovascular accidents was 17% and no difference was seen between the two groups.

There are an increasing number of reports, however, that demonstrate that carotid artery resection in selected circumstances can be performed safely when preceded by appropriate presurgical assessment of collateral blood flow from the opposite cerebral hemisphere through the circle of Willis. This approach is justified by a classic pathologic report by Huvos et al., who showed that metastatic squamous cell carcinoma can be microscopically identified invading the carotid adventitia in up to 30% of cases in which disease is adjacent to the vessel.[87] Vascular surgeons have used pressure flow studies that assess the patency of collateral blood flow, mostly contributed through the circle of Willis, to determine the safety of carotid occlusion. Hays et al. reported that back flow pressure of 50 mm Hg was safe for temporary occlusion and/or ligation.[88] The current protocol of Adams et al. is to perform angiography to demonstrate nonstenotic patent carotid arteries, spontaneous crossover, and an intact circle of Willis. Patients also undergo an angiogram with controlled balloon inflation for 30 minutes. If tolerated, a xenon CT scan to assess the likelihood of successful outcome follows.[85]

GENERAL PRINCIPLES OF RADIATION THERAPY

For early-stage disease, both radiation and surgery are frequently curative and can produce similar rates of cure. Selection of treatment must be individualized to each patient and must consider issues such as cosmetic and functional outcome, quality of life, speed with which treatment can be completed, sequelae of each modality, patient reliability, risk of subsequent cancers, and capacity of salvage therapy should there be a recurrence.

For advanced-stage disease, surgery and radiotherapy are often combined (for resectable cases). When this is done, radiation is usually delivered postoperatively. Peters et al. reported a prospective randomized trial evaluating various dose levels for postoperative radiation in locoregionally advanced head and neck cancer.[89] They found that a dose of 57.6 Gy in daily fractions of 1.8 Gy were superior to doses of 54 Gy. For patients with extracapsular spread in the lymph nodes in the neck, doses of 63 Gy were superior to 57.6 Gy. Doses above 63 Gy did not appear warranted. Typical indications for postoperative radiation include T3 to T4 primary, close or involved margins for any primary, the presence of nodal metastases, especially extracapsular extension, and factors such as perineural invasion, soft tissue extension, and so forth. Ang updated this experience, assessing the effect of a variety of risk factors and total treatment time (surgery plus radiation) on outcome.[90] High-risk features included extracapsular extension, oral cavity primary, positive mucosal margins, nerve invasion, more than one node involved, more than one nodal station involved, node size greater than 3 cm, and greater than a 6-week interval between surgery and radiation. Patients with none of these features did not receive RT. Those with one adverse feature in addition to extracapsular extension were considered intermediate risk, and those with more than one feature plus extracapsular extension were considered high risk. Locoregional control for low-risk patients (no RT) and intermediate-risk patients (57.6 Gy) was greater than 90%, compared with 68% for high-risk (63 Gy) patients ($P = .004$). Actuarial 4-year survival by risk was 83%, 66%, and 43%, respectively. Those who began radiation more than 6 weeks after surgery and whose total therapy time extended beyond 12 to 13 weeks also had worse outcomes.

There are other groups of patients with advanced disease that are treated differently, and these subjects are covered in this chapter. Those with small primary lesions and neck metastases can be treated with definitive RT to the primary and neck, plus a neck dissection. This is especially true for pharyngeal wall, oropharynx, and larynx cancers. Patients who have resectable larynx cancer but who would require total laryngectomy are often treated with organ-preserving therapy combining chemotherapy and radiotherapy. Either that approach or radiation alone (neck dissection) is often used for base of tongue and tonsil lesions, for the purpose of preserving organ function.

A variety of fractionation programs have been used by different groups.[91] The Radiation Therapy Oncology Group (RTOG) reported a prospective trial looking at four different schedules: conventional fractionation (70 Gy/35 fractions/7 weeks) versus hyperfractionation (81.6 Gy/68 fractions/7 weeks) versus accelerated fractionation with split (67.2 Gy/42 fractions/6 weeks including 2 weeks rest after 38.4 Gy) versus accelerated fractionation with concomitant boost (72 Gy/42 fractions/6 weeks), which used a twice a day concomitant boost during the last 12 treatment days.[92] The latter schedule provided better 2-year locoregional control than standard fractionation, and will be the standard treatment in future RTOG trials for locally advanced squamous cell carcinoma of the head and neck.

For unresectable disease, combined chemotherapy and radiotherapy has become the standard of care. Many of these trials are reviewed in this chapter. Interestingly, a combined modality experience using cisplatin and RT has been reported, using a concomitant boost schedule not dissimilar to the RTOG experience. Harrison et al. have reported long-term results of a program using 70 Gy/6 weeks using a concomitant boost during weeks 5 and 6, as well as cisplatin, 100 mg/m^2 on days 1 and 22.[93–95] Three-year local control for unresectable paranormal sinus cancers, T4 nasopharynx cancers, unresectable oropharynx cancers, and unresectable larynx and hypopharynx cancers were 78%, 78%, 64%, and 100%, although there were only six patients in the latter category. Unresectable oral cavity cancers fared poorly.

Merlano et al. reported a prospective, randomized trial comparing radiation alone with an alternating chemotherapy and radiation approach. This trial is reviewed later in this chapter, in Combination Chemotherapy and Radiotherapy, but revealed an improved outcome in the chemotherapy and radiation group.[96]

Side effects of RT are usually separated into acute and late effects. Acute effects generally are related to inflammatory reactions in the tissues within the radiation field (i.e., epidermitis and mucositis). Irradiation of the taste buds can cause loss or diminution of taste, irradiation of the salivary glands causes xerostomia, irradiation of the lacrimal glands can cause dryness in the eye, and epilation can result from irradiating hair-bearing skin. Whether these effects are temporary or permanent are usually dose related and site related. Because RT to the salivary glands and oral cavity can have a significant effect on dentition, all patients receiving this treatment should be seen by a dentist before RT. Any required dental work should be done before the initiation of radiation, and patients should be placed on dental prophylaxis with fluoride applications. It has been clearly shown that fluoride application significantly reduces dental sequela after RT.[97] It has also been clearly shown that dental extractions in an irradiated mandible can lead to osteonecrosis.[98]

Advances in radiotherapy techniques have had a significant effect on head and neck patients. For external-beam treatments, three-dimensional conformal radiation and stereotactic radiotherapy are particularly exciting new areas (Fig. 30.2-3). This allows the physician to plan RT based on three-dimensional reconstruction of the target area, and three-dimensional planning of the radiation beams. As a result, it is frequently possible to lower the dose to surrounding normal tissue while potentially escalating the dose to the tumor.[99] Efforts to use this technique in nasopharyngeal cancer have been particularly interesting and are discussed in that section (see Nasopharynx, later in this chapter). The development of multileaf collimators and on-line portal imaging techniques should make the delivery of three-dimensional RT more efficient. Intensity-modulated radiation is also being developed.

Finally, there are biologic and treatment-related factors that have been emerging as clinically relevant. Anemia has been shown to have a significantly adverse effect on local control[100] and is discussed in greater detail throughout Chapters 30.1 through 30.5. Attempts to overcome tumor hypoxia with hypoxic cell sensitizers concomitant with RT (mitomycin C) have also shown success, all suggestions that tumor oxygenation has significant importance in the success of radiotherapy.[101,102] Also, with respect to reducing the side effects of radiotherapy, Brizel et al. have reported a clinical trial that shows that the daily administration of amifostine with radiotherapy reduced the incidence of acute and chronic xerostomia. This is an area under active investigation.[103]

PRINCIPLES OF CHEMOTHERAPY: RECURRENT AND METASTATIC DISEASE

The median survival for patients with recurrent squamous cell carcinoma of the head and neck is 6 months and the 1-year survival rate is 20%. These statistics have not been affected by the use of chemotherapy. Consequently, patients with recurrent squamous cell carcinoma of the head and neck are candidates for phase I and II trials of experimental therapeutics.

SINGLE-AGENT CHEMOTHERAPY

The activity of older single agents commonly incorporated into combination regimens and newer drugs are listed in Table 30.2-6.[104–139] The older drugs include methotrexate, bleomy-

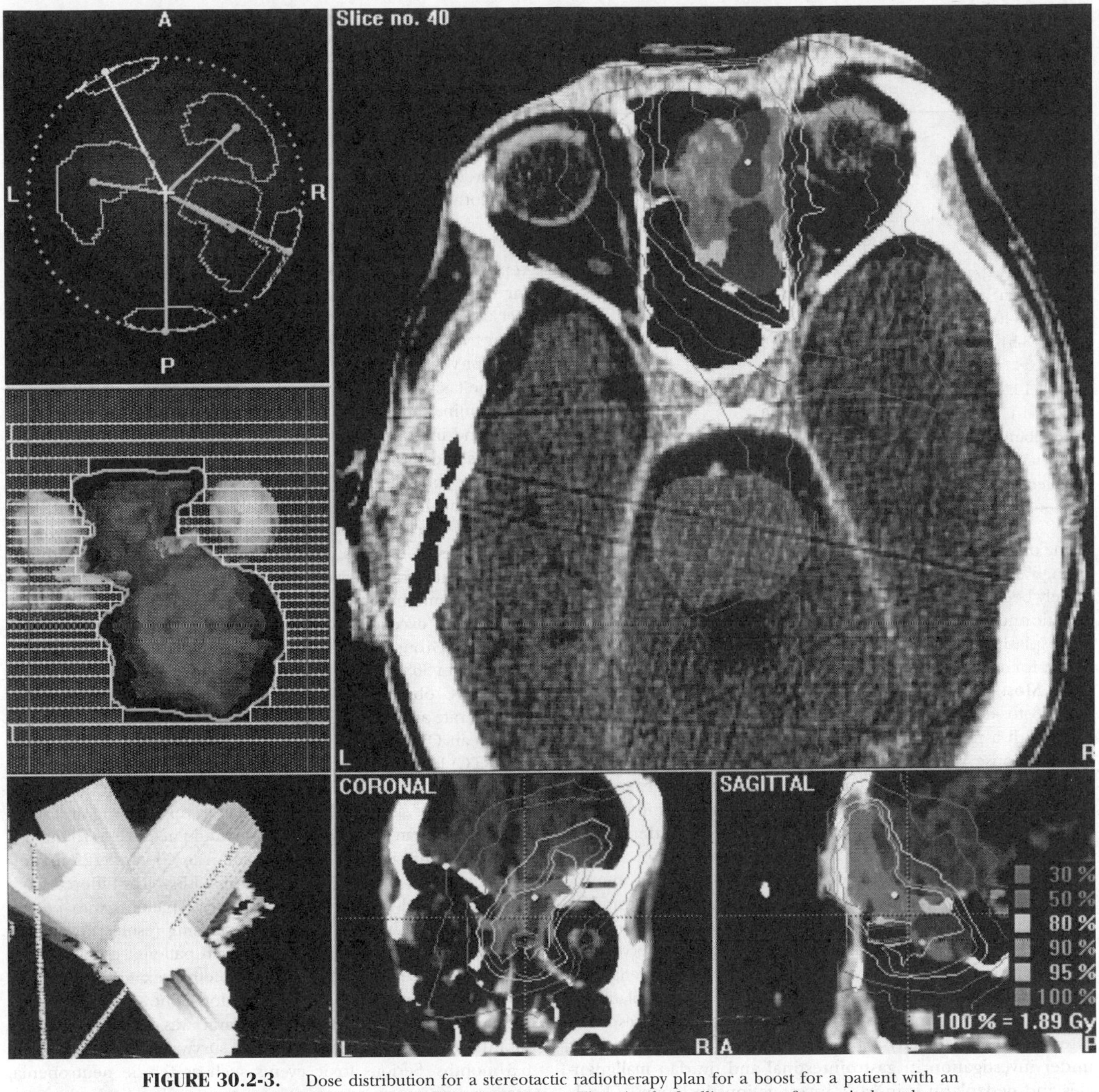

FIGURE 30.2-3. Dose distribution for a stereotactic radiotherapy plan for a boost for a patient with an unresectable squamous cell carcinoma of the frontal sinus. The microleaf collimator conforms nicely to the target. The optic chiasm is well protected, as is the contralateral orbit.

cin, cisplatin, carboplatin, ifosfamide, and 5-fluorouracil (5-FU). The details of these phase II studies may be found in older reviews,[111–113] whereas the activity of newer agents such as the taxanes, vinorelbine, gemcitabine, and topotecan are covered in more recent reviews.[140,141]

Methotrexate is the standard palliative therapy for recurrent squamous cell carcinoma of the head and neck. The standard dose for initiation is 40 mg/m^2/week to be escalated weekly by 10 mg/m^2 increments to 60 mg/m^2/week or until dose-limiting toxicity or an objective response is reached. Therapy with this drug is relatively nontoxic, inexpensive, and convenient. Higher doses of methotrexate in single-arm studies were shown to produce higher response rates.[104–107] Five randomized trials have shown no significant difference in survival rates between higher doses of methotrexate with leucovorin (as much as 5000 mg) and standard-dose methotrexate.[108–110]

The methotrexate analogues trimetrexate,[142] edatrexate,[143] and piritrexim[144–146] have all been tested in small numbers of patients and seem to be active, but have no particular advantage over methotrexate. In a randomized comparison of methotrexate and edatrexate, activity was similar but edatrexate was more toxic.[143]

Bleomycin has been studied extensively as a single agent and in combination in recurrent and metastatic squamous cell carci-

TABLE 30.2-6. Activity of Single Agents in Recurrent and Metastatic Head and Neck Squamous Cell Carcinoma

Chemotherapy	*No. of Patients*	*Response Rate*	*References*
Methotrexate	988	31	104–110
Bleomycin	347	21	111–113
Cisplatin	288	28	111–116
Carboplatin	169	22	111–113, 117
5-Fluorouracil	118	15	111–113
Ifosfamide	120	23	118–124
Paclitaxel (mg/m^2)			
250 (24-h)	73	40	125–127
175 (24-h)	41	20	128
175 (3-h)	60	15	128,129
Docetaxel (mg/m^2)			
100 (1-h)	89	33	130–132
60 (1-h)	23	30	133
Vinorelbine	102	18	134–136
Gemcitabine	54	13	137
Topotecan	43	14	138,139

noma of the head and neck. Response rates as a single agent vary from 6% to 45%, with a pooled average of 21%.[111,112] It has largely been replaced by continuous infusion 5-FU, which is synergistic and more active in combination with cisplatin.

Cisplatin is perhaps the most important chemotherapeutic agent for treating squamous cell carcinoma of the head and neck. Most of the studies have used a dose of 80 to 100 mg/m^2 every 3 to 4 weeks. Response rates have ranged from 14% to 41%, with a pooled average of 28%.[111–113] Whether there is a dose-response relationship is not yet proven. Single-agent cisplatin in doses of up to 200 mg/m^2 produced higher response rates in pilot trials,[114,115] but a randomized trial comparing 60 mg/m^2 doses with 120 mg/m^2 doses found no difference in response or survival.[116]

Carboplatin has significantly less renal, otologic, neurologic, and gastrointestinal toxicity than does cisplatin, but response rates are lower, in the range of 14% to 30%, with an average of 22%.[111,112,117] Carboplatin should be reserved for treatment of patients with peripheral neuropathy or renal dysfunction that prohibits use of cisplatin. Of the other platinum analogues, iproplatin trials have yielded much lower response rates and major toxicity in phase II trials.[147,148] Oxaliplatin is under investigation in gastrointestinal and ovarian malignancies and nedaplatin is in early investigations in Japan.[149] Each drug has its own toxicity profile; the relative advantage over cisplatin and carboplatin will need to be determined in appropriately designed trials in head and neck cancer patients. 5-FU was studied initially using intravenous daily bolus dosing for 5 days or weekly in recurrent squamous cell carcinoma of the head and neck as second- or third-line chemotherapy. Response rates ranged from 0% to 33%, with an average of only 15%.[111,112] The dose-limiting toxicity of this method of administration was myelosuppression. Subsequent studies of 5-FU as a prolonged infusion for 96 to 120 hours at a dose of 1000 mg/m^2/d showed mucositis to be dose-limiting, and antitumor activity was increased. 5-FU was synergistic with cisplatin, leading to the establishment of the now standard combination regimen of cisplatin plus infusional 5-FU.[113]

Ifosfamide, a synthetic analogue of cyclophosphamide, was limited in early clinical trials by the occurrence of hemorrhagic cystitis. With the use of MESNA, a thiol compound that inactivates the urotoxic metabolites, standard doses (less than 10 g) and high doses (17.5 g) have been tested in patients with head and neck cancer. Response rates reported from phase II trials vary widely but average 23%.[118–124] An example are the two most recent reports of single-agent phase II trials conducted in chemotherapy-naive patients. Huber and associates from the M. D. Anderson Cancer Center reported a 26% response rate in 31 patients,[121] whereas the Hoosier Oncology Group reported only a 10% response rate in 21 patients[124] using similar regimens. As with most chemotherapy trials for head and neck cancer, response rates appear to correlate with extent of prior treatment, the antitumor activity is modest, and an advantage for very high doses has not been demonstrated.

The taxanes, paclitaxel and docetaxel, bind to the P subunit of tubulin, induce the formation of stable microtubule bundles, and inhibit microtubule depolymerization. *In vitro,* docetaxel is the more potent analogue. Docetaxel appears to be schedule independent, whereas paclitaxel appears to be more effective with prolonged exposure.[150,151]

Initial paclitaxel trials tested 24-hour infusion paclitaxel repeated every 3 weeks. Three phase II trials evaluating 250 mg/m^2 dose with granulocyte colony-stimulating factor (G-CSF) support in chemotherapy-naive patients with recurrent or metastatic disease and excellent performance status [Eastern Cooperative Oncology Group (ECOG) 0 to 1] reported complete and partial response in 36% to 43% of patients.[125–127] The trial conducted by the ECOG observed a 9-month median survival time and 33% survival rate at 1 year, suggesting a highly active new agent.[125] The European Organization for Research and Treatment of Cancer (EORTC) Head and Neck Cancer Cooperative Group conducted a three-arm randomized phase II trial of single-agent methotrexate, 40 mg/m^2/week with dose escalation up to 60 mg/m^2; paclitaxel, 175 mg/m^2 by 3-hour infusion; and paclitaxel, 175 mg/m^2 by 24-hour infusion.[128] Dose escalation to 200 and 225 mg/m^2 was allowed for the two paclitaxel arms. Eligibility differed from other paclitaxel trials by the inclusion of patients with performance status 2. In contrast to the promising results reported by others, of the 123 evaluable randomized patients, complete and partial response rates were 9.5% for methotrexate, 12.5% for 3-hour infusion paclitaxel, and 19.5% for 24-hour infusion paclitaxel. Median progression-free survival was 2.0, 2.0, and 2.7 months, respectively, and the median survival ranged from 5.4 to 6.3 months. Serious toxic events such as febrile neutropenia, hypersensitivity reaction, or treatment-related death were observed in 34% of 24-hour infusion paclitaxel compared with less than 10% of patients in the other two treatment groups. The authors concluded that the 24-hour infusion schedule was too toxic for further study, and the antitumor activity of 3-hour infusion paclitaxel was no better than standard weekly methotrexate. One other trial tested paclitaxel, 175 mg/m^2 by 3-hour infusion, in 20 patients and reported a 20% response rate.[129]

The optimal infusion schedule for paclitaxel has not been established. It is known that at doses of 135 mg/m^2, adequate plasma concentrations of paclitaxel can be achieved to induce polymerization of microtubules. Studies are in progress evaluating other infusion schedules: 1-hour weekly infusions in doses of 60 to 100 mg/m^2, 3-hour infusions of doses ranging from 175 to 225 mg/m^2 every 3 weeks, and 96-hour infusions of 110 to 150 mg/m^2

every 3 weeks. Toxicities associated with paclitaxel that vary with the infusion schedule include myelosuppression (primarily leukopenia), sensory neuropathy, cardiac conduction disturbances causing bradycardia or arrhythmias, and anaphylaxis that requires premedication with corticosteroids. At present, only the 3-hour infusion schedule every 3 weeks can be recommended.

Phase II trials of docetaxel have been conducted in the United States and Europe. Response rates of 21%,[130] 31%,[131] and 42%[132] were reported in three small trials evaluating 100 mg/m^2 every 3 weeks. A 30% response rate was reported from a fourth study of 60 mg/m^2 every 3 weeks.[133] In addition to myelosuppression, the toxicity profile for docetaxel includes peripheral neuropathy, fluid retention, asthenia, and skin toxicity. Trials using 100 mg/m^2 have been limited to patients with excellent performance status. Lower doses (60 to 75 mg/m^2) are better tolerated and recommended. As with paclitaxel, a weekly dosing schedule of 30 to 40 mg/m^2 is under investigation.

Three other relatively recent drugs with activity in lung cancer and other solid tumors are the semisynthetic vinca alkaloid vinorelbine,[134–136] the pyrimidine antimetabolite gemcitabine,[137] and the topoisomerase I inhibitor topotecan.[138,139] These drugs appear to have only marginal activity in head and neck cancer with response rates under 20%.

Drugs with an uncertain level of activity because they were studied in broad phase I and II trials before uniform response criteria were established include doxorubicin, cyclophosphamide, and hydroxyurea. Response rates of less than 10% have been reported from phase II trials of the plant alkaloids vinblastine and etoposide.[152,153]

COMBINATION CHEMOTHERAPY

Over the last two decades numerous phase II trials of cisplatin-based regimens have been published and detailed in reviews.[111–113,140,141] Most contain small numbers of patients and often the results suggest greater efficacy than would be expected with single-agent cisplatin or methotrexate. In the early 1980s, researchers at Wayne State reported a response rate of 70% and a complete response rate of 27% using cisplatin, 100 mg/m^2 day 1, and 5-FU, 1000 $mg/m^2/d$ for 96 hours repeated every 3 weeks.[154] The compiled results of 12 trials including 365 patients with recurrent or metastatic squamous cell carcinoma show an average response rate of 50% and complete response rate of 16%.[155]

Three large multicenter trials reported by Jacobs et al.,[156] Forastiere et al.,[157] and Clavel et al.[158] compared cisplatin and infusional 5-FU to the single agents cisplatin, 5-FU, or methotrexate. The results of the three trials were remarkably similar. The response rate to cisplatin plus 5-FU was 32% in two of the trials and 31% in the third; all studies demonstrated a significantly higher response rate for cisplatin plus 5-FU compared with the single agents. However, there were no differences in median survival rates (5 to 6 months) or 1-year survival (20%) for any of the treatment arms. These response and survival results serve as the benchmark for comparison of regimens incorporating new agents.

Attempts to improve on the cisplatin plus 5-FU regimen include the addition of leucovorin, continuous infusion bleomycin,[159–161] bleomycin and methotrexate,[162] interleukin-2,[163] and interferon.[164] These three- and four-drug combinations result in enhanced toxicity without indications of survival benefit. More recently, two- and three-drug combinations incorporating paclitaxel or docetaxel have been reported in phase II trials.

Tables 30.2-7 and 30.2-8 list the results of uncontrolled trials of combination chemotherapy regimens that include paclitaxel or docetaxel. Many consist of preliminary findings presented in abstract form at oncology meetings. Some studies include only patients with recurrent or metastatic disease undergoing palliative treatment, whereas others include varying proportions of patients with locally advanced, untreated disease who received two to four cycles before proceeding to radiotherapy, surgery, or both. Nearly all studies were limited to patients with good performance status who had not received prior chemotherapy for treatment of recurrent disease. All paclitaxel studies used the 3-hour infusion schedule and docetaxel was infused over 1 hour.

Trials testing paclitaxel in combination with either cisplatin or carboplatin in recurrent and metastatic disease patients (see Table 30.2-7) demonstrate response in 32% to 39% of patients and complete response rates of less than 10%.[165–168] In contrast, a phase I and II trial of escalating doses of paclitaxel and cisplatin, 75 mg/m^2, reported by Hitt and associates in locally advanced, untreated patients resulted in a 78% overall response rate and 46% clinical complete response rate.[169] Similarly, Dunphy and associates evaluated paclitaxel in doses of 150 to 265 mg/m^2 combined with carboplatin at area under the concentration-time curve (AUC) 7.5 in 33 locally advanced, untreated patients and observed a 54% overall response and 27% complete response rate.[170] The results were quite similar, adding paclitaxel to cisplatin and 5-FU: 38% in recurrent disease patients[171] and 81% in locally advanced, untreated patients evaluated for primary site response before definitive local therapy.[172]

Two successive trials adding ifosfamide to paclitaxel and either cisplatin or carboplatin (TIP or TIC regimens) have been reported by Shin and associates from the M. D. Anderson Cancer Center for the treatment of recurrent disease.[173,174] Both studies combined 175 mg/m^2 of paclitaxel and 1000 mg/m^2 of ifosfamide daily for 3 days with cisplatin, 60 mg/m^2, or carboplatin, AUC 6, repeated at 3- to 4-week intervals. The overall response rate of 55% to 58% and complete response rates of 17% to 18% were encouraging.

Despite the low single-agent activity observed for gemcitabine in head and neck cancer, a 41% response rate was reported by Fountzilas et al. when it was combined with paclitaxel using a day 1 and 8 schedule every 3 weeks.[175]

While the amount of life-threatening toxicity varies with each particular regimen, the data do not suggest that taxane-based regimens are less toxic than older regimens. Myelosuppression and neuropathy are common, particularly with 3-hour infusion paclitaxel combined with cisplatin while the substitution of carboplatin has the potential to augment myelotoxicity. All of the combination regimens should be reserved for patients with good performance status, while patients with poor performance status should be considered for either single-agent chemotherapy or supportive care. The results of these phase I and II series suggest response rates that are similar to what is reported for cisplatin plus 5-FU and certainly no better, for either untreated patients or for patients with recurrent disease. The only exception is the response data from the TIP and TIC regimens[173,174] for patients with recurrent disease that needs to be evaluated further in a larger multiinstitutional trial setting. A randomized trial directly comparing cisplatin plus 5-FU as the standard regimen to pacli-

TABLE 30.2-7. Phase I and II Trials of Paclitaxel Combination Regimens

Author (Reference)	Paclitaxel (3-h)mg/m²	Combination Drug(s) mg/m²	Schedule	No. Evaluable Patients (Previously Untreated)	Response Rate (% Complete Response)
		Cisplatin			
Adamo (165)	175	75	q3wk	23 (3)	39% (0)
Licitra (166)	90	60	q2wk	23 (0)	32% (0)
Hitt (169)	175–300	75	q3wk	27 (27)	78% (46)
		Carboplatin (AUC)			
Fountzilas (167)	200	5	q4wk	49 (0)	33% (8)
Junor (168)	175	5–7	q3–4wk	27 (18)	33% (4)
Dunphy (170)	150–265	7.5	q3wk	33 (33)	54% (27)
		Cisplatin/5-fluorouracil			
Benasso (171)	100–180	Cisplatin, 20–25, days 1–3; 5-fluorouracil, 200–250, days 1–3	q3wk	23 (0)	38%
Hitt (172)	175	Cisplatin 100; 5-fluorouracil, 500, days 1–5	q3wk	42 (42)	81% (67)[a]
		Cisplatin/ifosfamide			
Shin (173)	175	Cisplatin, 60, day 1; ifosfamide, 1000, days 1–3	q3–4wk	52 (2)	58% (17)
		Carboplatin/ifosfamide			
Shin (174)	175	Carboplatin AUC 6, day 1; ifosfamide, 1000, days 1–3	q3–4wk	38 (2)	55% (18)
		Gemcitabine			
Fountzilas (175)	200 days 1 and 8	1100, days 1 and 8	q3wk	44 (0)	41% (11)

[a]Response at primary in previously untreated patients after three cycles.

taxel plus cisplatin completed accrual in January 2000 in the ECOG. This trial will provide important comparative data on response, duration of response, survival, toxicity, and cost.

Phase II trials of docetaxel in combination with other cytotoxic drugs are shown in Table 30.2-8. Similar to the studies in Table 30.2-7 for paclitaxel, many include patients with locally advanced untreated disease for which the overall response rates and complete response are proportionately higher. Only one trial was designed to test docetaxel and cisplatin specifically in patients with recurrent and metastatic disease.[176] A total of 33 patients were enrolled from Johns Hopkins, Vanderbilt, and M. D. Anderson, of whom 5 were previously untreated, presenting with far advanced locoregional disease or metastatic disease. The overall response rate was 52% including a 9% complete response. Toxicity was typical of docetaxel and cisplatin combination regimens with grade 3 to 4 neutropenia observed in 79% of patients, asthenia in 21%, and grade 3 peripheral neuropathy in 9%. Four

TABLE 30.2-8. Phase II Trials of Docetaxel Combination Regimens

Author (Reference)	Docetaxel (mg/m²)	Combination Drug(s) (mg/m²)	Schedule	Evaluable Patients (Previously Untreated)	Response Rate (% Complete Response)
		Cisplatin			
Forastiere (176)	75	75	q3wk	33 (5)	52% (9)
Mel (177)	75	75	q3wk	37 (37)	55% (30)
Manzione (178)	75	100	q3wk	26 (25)	46% (15)
Bauer (179)	80	70	q3–4wk	23 (21)	73% (22)
Schoffski (180)	100	75	q3wk	41 (22)	54% (15)
		5-Fluorouracil			
Fillippi (181)	75	1000 × 5	q3wk	44 (0)	34% (9)
		Vinorelbine			
Airoldi (182)	80	20	q17d	27 (0)	44% (11)
		Cisplatin + 5-fluorouracil			
Janinis (183)	80	Cisplatin, 40, days 1 and 2; 5-fluorouracil, 1000, days 1–3 + granulocyte colony-stimulating factor	q4wk	21 (16)	75% (25)
Schrijvers (184)	75	Cisplatin, 75–100; 5-fluorouracil, 750, days 1–5	q3wk	28 (28)	80% (not reported)

TABLE 30.2-9. Phase III Trials of Combination Regimens versus Single-Agent Cisplatin or Methotrexate in Recurrent and Metastatic Squamous Cell Carcinoma of the Head and Neck

Author (Reference)	*Chemotherapy Regimen*	*Response Rate (%)*	*Median Survival (mo)*
Davis (185)	P	13	NS
	PMB	11	NS
Jacobs (186)	P	18	6.9
	PM	33	6.2
Drelichman (187)	M	33	6.0
	PVcB	41	4.3
Morton (188)	No therapy	—	2.1
	P	24	4.2[a]
	B	14	2.8
	PB	13	4.0
Vogl (189)	M	35	5.6
	PBM	48	5.6
Williams (190)	M	16	7
	PVbB	24	7
Campbell (191)	M	19	2.7
	P	40	8.7[a]
	PM	31	5.3
	PF	33	6.7
Eisenberger (192)	M	25	6
	CM	25	6
Liverpool Study (193)	P	14	6[a]
	PF	12	6[a]
	M	6	2
	PM	11	6[a]
Jacobs (156)	PF	32[a]	5.5
	P	17	5.0
	F	13	6.1
Forastiere (157)	PF	32[a]	6.6
	CF	21	5.0
	M	10	5.6
Clavel (158)	PMBVc	34[a]	7.0
	PF	31	7.0
	P	15	7.0

B, bleomycin; C, carboplatin; F, 5-fluorouracil; M, methotrexate; P, cisplatin; Vb, vinblastine; Vc, vincristine.
[a]Significant difference.

other small phase II trials with previously untreated patients constituting one-half to all patients enrolled reported overall response in 46% to 73% of patients and complete response in 15% to 30%.[177–180]

In separate trials, docetaxel has been combined with 5-day infusional 5-FU[181] and with vinorelbine[182] with response outcomes similar to that achievable with cisplatin plus 5-FU.

Two studies have evaluated the three-drug combination of docetaxel, cisplatin, and 5-FU with or without G-CSF support primarily in patients with locally advanced inoperable disease before treatment with radiotherapy.[183,184] Each study enrolled under 30 patients and reported overall response of 75% and 80% after several cycles of chemotherapy. Whether or not this level of response is superior to cisplatin plus 5-FU in a comparable population of advanced head and neck cancer patients is unknown. The addition of docetaxel clearly leads to a substantial increase in life-threatening toxicities of neutropenia and infection. A large multicenter randomized trial is under way to address this question.

RANDOMIZED TRIALS OF SINGLE AND COMBINATION CHEMOTHERAPY REGIMENS

Randomized trials comparing combination regimens with either single-agent methotrexate or cisplatin are shown in Table 30.2-9.[156–158,185–192] Survival benefit was reported in three trials.[188,191,193] Morton et al. reported median survivals of 4.2 and 4.0 months for patients treated with cisplatin or cisplatin plus bleomycin, respectively, compared with a 2-month median survival for a no-treatment control group.[188] Campbell et al. reported a significant improvement in survival of patients treated with cisplatin (8.7 months) compared with those treated with methotrexate (2.7 months).[191] The Liverpool Head and Neck Oncology Group randomized 200 patients to

TABLE 30.2-10. Phase III Trials Comparing Combination Regimens in Recurrent and Metastatic Squamous Cell Carcinoma of the Head and Neck

Author (Reference)	*Regimen*	*No. of Patients*	*Response (%)*	*Response Duration (mo)*	*Median Survival (mo)*
Kish (194)	PF (bolus)	20	20	—	5.0
	PF (infusion)	18	74	—	6.7
Clavel (195)	MBVc	75	29[a]	4.3	7.3
	MBVcP	85	51[a]	6.8	8.5
Browman (196)	MF (sequential)	14	43	—	—
	MF (simultaneous)	18	67	—	—
Amrein (161)	PF	28	46	—	6.0
	PFMB	27	63	—	6.0
Paccagnella (197)	PMB	19	31	1.5	—
	EMB	47	47	2.3	—
Forastiere (198)	TP (high dose)	105	35	4.1[b]	7.6
	TP (low dose)	104	36	4.0	6.8
Schrijvers (199)	PF	122	47	—	6.3
	PF + IFN	122	38	—	6.0

B, bleomycin; E, epirubicin; F, 5-fluorouracil; IFN, interferon-α_{2b}; M, methotrexate; P, cisplatin; T, paclitaxel; Vc, vincristine.
[a]Statistically significant difference.
[b]Event-free survival.

receive cisplatin alone, methotrexate alone, cisplatin and infusional 5-FU, or cisplatin and methotrexate.[193] Although there were no differences in response rate, survival was significantly better in the three cisplatin-containing arms. In contrast, the three large multicenter trials reported by Jacobs et al.,[156] Forastiere et al.,[157] and Clavel et al.[158] comparing cisplatin plus 5-FU with single agents all showed a significantly increased response rate for combination chemotherapy but no benefit in median or 1-year survival rate. No other trials comparing combination regimens with single agents have been reported since 1994.

Randomized trials comparing combination regimens are shown in Table 30.2-10.[161,194–199] Kish et al. compared cisplatin plus infusional 5-FU versus cisplatin plus bolus 5-FU.[194] The response rate was significantly higher for infusional 5-FU, but median survivals were 6.7 and 5.0 months, respectively. Response rates were also significantly higher for the methotrexate plus bleomycin plus vincristine plus cisplatin regimen compared with methotrexate, bleomycin, and vincristine reported by Clavel et al.,[195] but survival was similar.

To gain perspective on the many trials that have been reported for palliation of patients with recurrent and metastatic squamous cell carcinoma of the head and neck, Browman and Cronin[113] performed a metaanalysis of randomized trials published between 1980 and 1992. Based on this pooled analysis of response and survival data, they concluded that single-agent cisplatin was more efficacious than single-agent methotrexate; the combination of cisplatin and 5-FU was more efficacious than treatment with single agents; and cisplatin and 5-FU was more efficacious than other combinations.

Since then, two additional randomized trials have been reported. The ECOG addressed the questions of dose response and antitumor activity of the combination of paclitaxel and cisplatin in patients with recurrent and metastatic squamous cell carcinoma.[198] A total of 210 patients were randomized to receive either high-dose paclitaxel (200 mg/m^2 over 24 hours) plus cisplatin, 75 mg/m^2, plus G-CSF or low-dose paclitaxel (135 mg/m^2 over 24 hours) plus cisplatin, 75 mg/m^2. No differences were observed in overall response rate, event-free survival, and median and 1-year survival rates. The response rate was 35% for patients in the high-dose paclitaxel arm and 36% for the low-dose paclitaxel group. The median survival of all patients was 7.3 months and 29% of patients were alive at 1 year, suggesting a possible small advantage over the cisplatin plus 5-FU regimen. Myelosuppression was the most frequently encountered toxicity, grade 3 to 4 neutropenia occurring in 70% of patients on the high-dose arm receiving G-CSF support and in 78% of patients on the low-dose arm. These results showed no advantage for the high-dose paclitaxel plus cisplatin regimen, and the toxicities associated with the 24-hour infusion schedule proved excessive for this patient population because of the prevalence of comorbid disease.

The other randomized trial was conducted by Head and Neck Interferon Cooperative Study Group and addressed the question of whether or not the activity of cisplatin and 5-FU could be modulated by interferon-α_{2b} as shown in preclinical experiments.[199] A total of 244 patients with recurrent or metastatic disease were randomized to receive the standard cisplatin (100 mg/m^2) and 5-FU (1000 $mg/m^2/d \times 4$) regimen with or without interferon, 3 million U subcutaneously, days 1 to 5 of each chemotherapy cycle, repeated every 3 weeks. There was no significant difference in response or survival rates between treatment groups.

In summary, cisplatin-based combination chemotherapy is more effective than single agents. Response to cisplatin plus infusional 5-FU occurs in approximately one-third of patients, with complete response in 5% to 15%. An advantage for choosing combination chemotherapy seems to be limited to patients with excellent performance status, no prior chemotherapy for treatment of recurrent disease, and minimal tumor burden. Durable complete responses and prolonged survival are possible in this small subset of patients. Randomized trials directly comparing docetaxel and paclitaxel combination regimens with cisplatin plus 5-FU are in progress. However, it is unlikely that the addition of the taxanes to other conventional cytotoxics will produce substantial gains in survival, reduce toxicity, or otherwise improve patient quality of life. This underscores the need for new therapies to treat this population.

BIOLOGIC TARGETED THERAPIES

An understanding of the molecular and cellular pathways involved in normal and unregulated cell growth is leading to the development of biologically targeted therapies. These novel agents in early clinical trials affect signal transduction, cell-cycle traversal, programmed cell death, transcription regulation, matrix invasion, and angiogenesis. Three targeted therapies in head and neck cancer clinical trials with promising preliminary results are the epidermal growth factor receptor (EGFr) antagonists, cyclin-dependent kinase (cdk) inhibitors, and replication competent adenoviruses.

The EGFr is a transmembrane glycoprotein that is a member of the tyrosine kinase growth factor receptor family encoded by c-erb-B. Activation of the protooncogene results in overexpression of the receptor, which has been demonstrated to occur in over 90% of squamous cell head and neck cancers. Transforming growth factor-α, EGF, and other growth factors bind to the extracellular domain of the EGFr-stimulating tumor growth through autocrine and paracrine pathways.[200,201] Agents that block ligand binding could inhibit cell proliferation. Several monoclonal antibodies against the EGFr are in clinical development.[202–204] The chimeric IgG antibody C225 developed by Mendelsohn has binding affinity that is equal to the natural ligand effectively blocking EGF/transforming growth factor-α binding when administered using a weekly intravenous dosing schedule. Enhanced cytotoxicity is observed in combination with a number of chemotherapeutic agents including cisplatin and paclitaxel, and in combination with radiotherapy.[205] The major toxicity is a follicular rash. Phase I and II trials of C225 with cisplatin are in progress in patients with recurrent disease and in combination with radiotherapy for patients with locally advanced disease.[204,206] The preliminary response rates suggest enhanced antitumor activity, which has prompted the initiation of multicenter double-blind placebo-controlled trials in patients with advanced disease.

Another novel compound in clinical trials that affects signal transduction is the cdk inhibitor flavopiridol.[207,208] Cdks phosphorylate key substances that regulate transition from one cell-cycle phase to the next. *In vitro*, inhibitors of cdks 1, 2, and 4 block cell-cycle progression at G_1/S and G_2/M boundaries. In preclinical testing, flavopiridol induces cell-cycle arrest and p53-independent apoptosis. Flavopiridol is a particularly suitable candidate drug for study in tumors in which cyclin D is overexpressed or in which p16, the endogenous inhibitor of cdk4, is deleted.[209] The most commonly deleted chromosomal region in head and neck cancer is 9p21-22, the locus of p16, and p16 is commonly absent. A phase I trial has been completed by investigators at the National Cancer Institutes, and a phase II trial in head and neck cancer is under way.[210]

A third area of promising clinical research for head and neck cancers involves replication competent viruses. Mutant adenoviruses have been developed that selectively replicate in and cause lysis of cells deficient in p53-suppressor activity.[211] This takes advantage of the high rate (approximately 45%) of p53 mutations in squamous head and neck cancers. Phase I and II clinical studies of intralesional injection of the E1B-deleted adenovirus ONYX-015 have shown tumor cell necrosis and improvement in tumor-related symptoms.[212] There appears to be enhanced antitumor efficacy in studies of systemic chemotherapy combined with ONYX-015 and perhaps more durable responses at the injected tumor sites.[213,214] The status of other novel investigational bioresponse modifiers and gene therapies directly administered to local or regional tumor is discussed in reviews.[215]

PRINCIPLES OF CHEMOTHERAPY: PREVIOUSLY UNTREATED DISEASE

INDUCTION CHEMOTHERAPY

Initial trials of cisplatin-based combination chemotherapy given to newly diagnosed patients before receiving local therapies showed dramatic tumor reduction in 70% to 80% of patients. This observation suggested that sequencing therapies so that chemotherapy was administered before the tumor vasculature was disrupted might improve locoregional control and affect survival. Now, more that two decades since the first randomized trial evaluated induction cisplatin and bleomycin before surgery,[216] we can conclude from many such trials that the induction strategy confers no survival advantage. A role in preservation of the larynx for patients with locally advanced cancers of the larynx or hypopharynx who would otherwise undergo total laryngectomy has emerged and is discussed in Chapter 30.3. Down-staging of the primary and regional node disease with three cycles of cisplatin plus 5-FU chemotherapy has successfully allowed for larynx preservation and a reduction in the rate of development of distant metastases.[217,218]

NONRANDOMIZED TRIALS OF INDUCTION CHEMOTHERAPY

In the early 1980s, Wayne State University investigators reported high response rates with the regimen cisplatin and infusional 5-FU[219,220] administered before local treatment. They achieved a response rate of 88% (complete response 19%)[219] with two courses and 93% (complete response 54%) with three courses of the same regimen.[220] Over the past two decades, thousands of patients have received this regimen (cisplatin, 100 to 120 mg/m^2 day 1, and 5-FU, 1000 mg/m^2/d infused over 96 to 120 hours) in clinical research trials and in community practice. Response occurs in 85% of patients, on average, with complete response in approximately 40%. Two-thirds of clinical complete responses are pathologically confirmed in biopsy or resection specimens. Response varies by site, with the larynx and nasopharynx being most responsive and the oral cavity less responsive. Cisplatin and infusional 5-FU remains the most active regimen in previously untreated patients.[221,222]

Modifications of this regimen to increase the complete response rate have been tested.[223–230] This includes trials of cisplatin, 5-FU, and leucovorin,[223–225] demonstrating overall and compete response rates ranging from 59% to 95% and 24% to 65%, respectively. The initial reports by Vokes et al.,[223] using oral leucovorin, and Dreyfuss et al.,[224] using continuous infusion leucovorin appeared promising; however, long-term follow-up did not demonstrate any striking improvement in survival over cisplatin plus 5-FU. Severe myelosuppression, diarrhea, and mucositis occurred frequently, necessitating dose reductions in most patients.

TABLE 30.2-11. Recent Randomized Trials of Induction Chemotherapy followed by Locoregional Treatment versus Locoregional Treatment Alone

Author (Reference)	*Year*	*No. of Patients*	*Chemotherapy*	*Overall Survival*
Martin (234)	1990	75	FP	No difference
Jortay (235)	1990	187	VBM	No difference
Richard (236)	1991	222	VB(IA)	Advantage: chemotherapy[a]
Mazeron (237)	1991	131	FPBM	No difference
Jaulerry (238)	1992	100	PBVdMi	No difference
Jaulerry (238)	1992	108	FPVd	No difference
Tejedor (239)	1992	42	CpFt	No difference
Depondt (240)	1993	324	FCp	No difference
Di Blasio (241)	1994	69	FP	Advantage: standard treatment
Hasegawa (242)	1994	50	FP	No difference
Paccagnella (243)	1994	237	FP	Advantage: chemotherapy[b]
Dalley (244)	1995	280	FP	No difference
Domenge (245)	1996	166	FP	No difference
Volling (246)	1996	96	FCp	No difference

B, bleomycin; Cp, carboplatin; F, 5-fluorouracil; Ft, ftorafur; IA, intraarterial; M, methotrexate; Mi, mitomycin C; P, cisplatin; V, vincristine; Vd, vindesine.
[a]Floor of mouth cancer patients only.
[b]Unresectable patients only.
(From ref. 233, with permission.)

Cisplatin-based combination regimens that include paclitaxel or docetaxel are being tested in patients with locally advanced, unresectable disease before receiving radiotherapy. The preliminary results of those small phase II studies are listed in Tables 30.2-7 and 30.2-8.[169,170,172,177–179,184] Colevas and associates from the Dana Farber Cancer Institute have published the results of an intensive induction regimen containing docetaxel for patients with stage III or IV squamous cell carcinoma receiving nonsurgical management.[226,227] In a phase I and II trial, the maximum tolerated dose of docetaxel in combination with cisplatin (25 mg/m^2 days 1 to 5), 5-FU (700 mg/m^2 days 2 to 5) and leucovorin was 60 mg/m^2.[226] This regimen required postchemotherapy home infusion of fluids, antibiotics, and G-CSF. In 23 patients, a response rate of 100%, including 61% complete response, was documented after three cycles of chemotherapy. Frequently occurring severe toxicities in addition to myelosuppression included nausea, mucositis, diarrhea, peripheral neuropathy, and sodium-wasting nephropathy. This regimen is of interest because of the remarkably high response rate, but the toxicity is prohibitive for general use. A regimen with more manageable toxicity is being evaluated in a multicenter trial.[228] The preliminary results of docetaxel, 75 mg/m^2, plus cisplatin, 75 mg/m^2 (group A) or cisplatin, 100 mg/m^2 (group B) on day 1, plus 5-FU, 1000 mg/m^2/d, days 1 to 4, were reported by Posner. The response rate for 13 patients in group A was 84%, 23% complete and 61% partial; while all 17 patients in group B responded (47% complete and 53% partial responses). Based on this experience, a phase III trial of taxotere, cisplatinum, and 5-FU versus cisplatin plus 5-FU is being initiated.

RANDOMIZED TRIALS OF INDUCTION CHEMOTHERAPY

Many randomized trials have been conducted to determine if the addition of chemotherapy improves survival, and these are detailed in several reviews.[221,231–233] A listing of 14 randomized trials published since 1990 are shown in Table 30.2-11.[234–246] These trials compared induction chemotherapy followed by definitive local therapy, as dictated by initial resectability status, versus immediate surgery, radiotherapy, or both. Improved survival through a decrease in local and regional failure and distant metastatic rates was the primary goal. Studies designed in the latter half of the 1980s up to 2000 (not included in Table 30.2-7) have focused on organ preservation specifically for primaries in the larynx and hypopharynx.[217,218] The results of these randomized trials are consistent and fail to demonstrate a survival advantage with the addition of induction chemotherapy.

Although many trials have been criticized for methodologic flaws, five used full doses of cisplatin and 5-FU for three to five courses and had adequate power to reach statistical conclusions.[234,241,243–245] Only one of these trials found a significant improvement in survival for chemotherapy-treated patients and that was limited to a subset with unresectable disease.[245] Several studies, however, have found a significant reduction in distant metastases,[216,242,243] but in the absence of improvement in locoregional control this has failed to affect survival. It is noteworthy that both distant metastases and locoregional failure were reduced in the inoperable subset of patients achieving a survival advantage reported by Paccagnella et al.[243]

The following conclusions can be drawn from two decades of experience with induction chemotherapy:

- Induction chemotherapy results in major response rates in 60% to 90% and complete response in 20% to 50% of patients with locally advanced squamous cell carcinoma of the head and neck.
- Pathologic complete response is documented in approximately two-thirds of complete responders determined by clinical assessment, and these patients appear to have a survival advantage.

- Response to induction chemotherapy is predictive of response to subsequent radiotherapy.
- There is no increase in morbidity from surgery or radiotherapy in patients who have received induction chemotherapy.
- Although cancers from all head and neck sites are lumped together in almost all the studies, there is evidence that biologic behavior differs with primary site.
- No significant difference in overall survival has been demonstrated with the use of induction chemotherapy compared with surgery or radiation alone.
- Organ preservation and improved quality of life can result from induction chemotherapy (see Chapter 30.3).

POSTOPERATIVE ADJUVANT TREATMENT

ADJUVANT CHEMOTHERAPY

Chemotherapy administered after a patient has been rendered disease free with surgery, radiation, or both has been evaluated in three large multicenter randomized trials.[247–249] The rationale for this approach was threefold. First, definitive surgery is not delayed. Second, tumor margins may become blurred after response to induction chemotherapy, leaving the extent of required surgery uncertain. Third, up to 20% of patients receiving induction chemotherapy refused surgery once response was achieved and their symptoms abated.

The sequence of surgery followed by adjuvant chemotherapy and then radiation was a strategy developed to avoid these potential disadvantages of induction chemotherapy. The Head and Neck Intergroup tested this strategy using three cycles of cisplatin and infusional 5-FU as adjuvant chemotherapy.[247] From 1985 to 1990, 499 patients with stage III and IV resected squamous cell carcinoma of the oral cavity, oropharynx, hypopharynx, and larynx were stratified into high- and low-risk groups; high-risk was defined as close surgical margins less than 5 mm, cancer *in situ* at margins, or extracapsular nodal extension. Randomization was to immediate radiation or adjuvant chemotherapy followed by radiation. Although the overall comparison of the two treatments showed no significant differences in survival, disease-free survival, or time to locoregional failure, an analysis of treatment effect on high-risk patients suggested benefit. Improved survival and decreased locoregional failure that approached statistical significance was observed for the high-risk subset of patients who received adjuvant chemotherapy compared with those receiving radiation alone. No benefit for adjuvant chemotherapy could be detected for the low-risk patients. Had this trial been limited to high-risk patients, a significant positive outcome may have resulted.

The RTOG[250] retrospectively analyzed survival and locoregional failure rates in three patient cohorts enrolled in RTOG clinical trials: those considered low risk, those at intermediate risk because of two or more involved regional lymph nodes or extracapsular extension of tumor, and those at highest risk because of a positive surgical margin with or without other risk factors. At 3 years, the locoregional recurrence rate was 14% for the low-risk group, 27% for those at intermediate risk, and 49% for the highest risk group. Median survival rates were 5.6 years, 2.6 years, and 1.5 years, respectively, for the three groups.

Two other large randomized trials have been performed by head and neck cancer study groups in Japan and France.[248,249] Japanese investigators evaluated a combination of tegafur and uracil known as *UFT*, 300 mg/d, for 1 year.[248] Three groups of patients were randomized to observation or adjuvant UFT: 424 patients with stage II to IV cancers treated surgically, 111 patients with stage II disease treated with definitive radiotherapy, and 25 patients with nasopharyngeal cancer treated with radiotherapy. Three-year survival results of surgically treated patients showed no significant difference in survival or relapse-free survival, but adjuvant UFT patients had a significantly lower rate of distant metastases (7.9% vs. 14.6%, P = .034). No benefit could be shown in the patients treated with primary radiotherapy.

Reported only in preliminary abstract form, French investigators randomized 287 patients with extracapsular nodal extension to receive postoperative radiation alone or adjuvant cisplatin, bleomycin, and methotrexate after completion of RT.[249] Chemotherapy-treated patients had significantly worse overall survival and an increased rate of distant metastases, but better local regional control.

Several randomized trials that use both induction and adjuvant chemotherapy have been conducted in an attempt to further intensify therapy.[216,251,252] The Head and Neck Contracts Program, a three-arm trial, compared surgery and postoperative radiation to neoadjuvant cisplatin and bleomycin and to treatment with induction chemotherapy plus adjuvant cisplatin for 6 months after surgery and radiation.[216] No differences in overall survival were observed, but a significant decrease in distant metastases was reported for the adjuvant group.

Ervin et al. treated 114 patients with neoadjuvant cisplatin, bleomycin, methotrexate, and leucovorin.[251] After definitive local treatment, patients were randomized to observation or three cycles of adjuvant chemotherapy. The 3-year disease-free survival rates were 55% and 88%, respectively; partial responders to induction chemotherapy showed the greatest benefit. The Southwest Oncology Group conducted a feasibility trial of postoperative radiotherapy and three cycles of concurrent cisplatin followed by three cycles of adjuvant cisplatin plus 5-FU. Compliance was poor, with only 37% of 72 patients completing all six chemotherapy cycles.[252]

In summary, there is no role for adjuvant chemotherapy in low-risk patients (negative margins of resection, neck disease staged N0 or N1 without extracapsular extension). Patients with positive or close margins of resection, two or more involved regional nodes, or extracapsular extension of disease are at increased risk for both locoregional recurrence and distant metastases. It now seems clear from several studies that at least the rate of development of distant metastases can be reduced with systemic chemotherapy, but an effect on overall survival has not been shown perhaps because of the lack of large enough randomized trials enrolling only high-risk patients.

ADJUVANT CHEMORADIOTHERAPY

Improvement in locoregional control through the use of concomitant chemotherapy and radiotherapy may be most feasible in the patient with locally advanced but *resectable* disease. Locoregional recurrence is the most frequent site of failure after surgery and postoperative radiation. Extracapsular extension of tumor in cervical node metastases is well established as an adverse prognostic factor for recurrence.[253–255]

The rationale and potential role of chemotherapy to enhance radiation effects is well known and the clinical experience in head and neck cancer is extensive.[256–259] Before 1999, this experience was almost exclusively limited to patients with bulky unresectable disease. The RTOG conducted a small feasibility study treating 51 patients with resected stage IV disease, positive margins, or both, with postoperative RT and concurrent cisplatin, 100 mg/m^2 every 3 weeks for three cycles.[260] Locoregional control was significantly better compared with matched historic controls. This pilot trial and the positive results of a randomized trial by Bachaud et al.[261] led to a Head and Neck Intergroup Phase III trial now in progress. Resected patients with positive margins, metastases to multiple regional nodes, and the presence of extracapsular spread of disease are randomized to receive postoperative RT with or without concurrent cisplatin (100 mg/m^2 days 1, 22, and 43).

Four randomized trials of postoperative chemoradiation have been published.[261–264] Bachaud et al. randomized 88 patients with extracapsular spread of disease in regional neck node metastases to receive postoperative RT alone or postoperative RT plus cisplatin, 50 mg intravenously weekly.[261] After a minimum follow-up of 5 years, the median survival (22 months vs. 40 months) and 5-year survival (13% vs. 36%) were significantly better for the chemoradiotherapy group. Radiation-treated patients had a higher locoregional failure rate compared with the chemoradiotherapy group, while no differences were observed in the incidence of distant metastases. Randomized trials reported by Weissberg et al.[262] and Haffty et al.[263] evaluated mitomycin C and postoperative RT versus RT alone. Both investigators reported improvement in locoregional control but not survival. A third small trial conducted by Weissler et al. found no benefit for cisplatin and 5-FU plus RT compared with RT alone.[264] These last three trials were not targeted to high-risk patients but included all resected patients with stage III and IV disease.

All postoperative chemoradiotherapy studies reported increased acute toxicity, primarily mucositis, and weight loss with combined therapy. Careful monitoring of patients receiving combined chemoradiotherapy along with psychosocial and nutritional support is essential for these therapies to be successful and to have a high level of patient compliance. Completion of the current Head and Neck Intergroup Trial is crucial to confirm the improved survival reported by Bachaud and to change standard of care.

CONCURRENT CHEMORADIOTHERAPY

The purpose of administering chemotherapy and radiotherapy together is to take advantage of the radiosensitizing capability of many of the active drugs for this disease and effect a substantial enough increase in locoregional control to significantly improve survival. The postulated mechanisms for enhanced cell kill with concurrent chemoradiation strategies have been described for decades and include interference with repair processes after sublethal or potentially lethal damage or with tumor cell synchronization.[257,258] In addition, administering both modalities together may prevent or decrease the emergence of radioresistant or drug-resistant clonagens.

RESULTS FROM METAANALYSES

Since 1992, four metaanalyses evaluating the effect of chemotherapy on survival from randomized trials of induction, adjuvant, and concurrent chemotherapy compared with definitive local therapy alone have been published.[265–268] These analyses covered the period of publication up to 1993; three were literature based,[265–267] while the largest and most comprehensive used updated individual patient data from 63 trials including 10,741 patients.[268] The results of all four analyses were consistent in finding a small survival benefit favoring chemotherapy: 2.8%,[265] 4.0%,[267] 4.0%,[268] and 6.5%.[266] The reduction in risk of death was statistically significant in three of the metaanalyses.[266–268] The survival benefit observed in all of the studies was associated primarily with the patient group receiving concurrent chemoradiation. In the Meta-Analysis of Chemotherapy in Head and Neck Cancer (MACH-NC) analysis based on individual patient data, the absolute survival benefit at 5 years from chemoradiation was 8%.[268] It should be emphasized that the most impressive gains in locoregional control, disease-free survival, and overall survival have been reported since 1995 in large, multicenter randomized trials employing cisplatin-based chemotherapy and concurrent radiotherapy, either standard or altered fractionation.

SINGLE-AGENT CHEMOTHERAPY AND RADIOTHERAPY

Many randomized trials have been published combining the single agents hydroxyurea, methotrexate, bleomycin, 5-FU, mitomycin-C, and cisplatin with radiotherapy compared with radiotherapy alone. These older trials were limited to patients with extensive, locally advanced disease not considered resectable. The results of selected trials with adequate power to demonstrate outcome differences are shown in Table 30.2-12.[269–280] Gupta and associates at the Christie Hospital and Holt Radium Institute in Manchester randomized over 300 patients to concurrent methotrexate or radiotherapy alone.[270] There was a highly significant improvement in local control ($P = .0019$) and survival ($P = .0089$) for patients with oropharyngeal cancers in the methotrexate arm, while survival benefit did not reach statistical significance ($P = .075$) in the overall analysis.

The results of four trials with bleomycin and radiotherapy are conflicting.[271–274] Only the trial reported by Shanta and Krishnamurthi in patients with T3 to T4, N0 to N2 squamous cell carcinoma of the buccal mucosa showed a significant beneficial effect of bleomycin on local control, disease-free survival, and overall survival.[271] Local control and progression-free survival were improved in the Northern California Oncology Group trial reported by Fu et al.,[273] while large trials from the EORTC[274] and the Norwegian Radium Hospital[272] did not observe benefit for any outcome parameter.

Many studies have used 5-FU with concurrent RT. In the study by Lo and associates, local control and 5-year survival were superior in the combined treatment group, but only in patients with oral cavity cancers was the difference significant.[275] Browman and associates of the National Cancer Institute Canada evaluated infusional 5-FU and radiotherapy.[276] The complete response rate was significantly better with combined treatment, but only a trend for improved progression-free and overall survival was observed. Investigators in Barcelona randomized 859 patients with T3 to T4, N0 to N3 cancers to three treatment groups: radiotherapy, 60 Gy in 30 fractions; radiotherapy, 70.4 Gy in 64 fractions; or radiotherapy, 60 Gy in 30 fractions, plus concurrent 5-FU, 250 mg/m^2 every 2 days.[277] The complete response rate and survival were significantly better for the 5-FU–treated group compared with the control group receiving 60-Gy radiotherapy alone, but there was no difference when compared with patients receiving 70.4-Gy radio-

TABLE 30.2-12. Selected Randomized Trials of Concurrent Single-Agent Chemotherapy and Radiotherapy versus Radiotherapy Alone

			Significant Benefit			
Author (Reference)	*No. of Patients*	*Chemotherapy*	Complete Response	Local Control	Progression-Free Survival	Survival
Stefani (269)	150	HU				No
Gupta (270)	313	MTX		Yes		Yes[a]
Shanta (271)	136	Bleo		Yes	Yes	Yes[b]
Vermund (272)	222	Bleo		No		No
Fu (273)	104	Bleo	No[c]	Yes	Yes	No
Eschwege (274)	199	Bleo	No			No
Lo (275)	136	5-FU		Yes[d]		Yes[d]
Browman (276)	175	5-FU	Yes		No[c]	No[c]
Sanchiz (277)	859	5-FU	Yes		Yes	Yes
Weissberg (278)	120	MMC			Yes	No
Haselow (279)	371	Cisplatin	No			No
Al-Sarraf (280)	147	Cisplatin			Yes	Yes[e]

Bleo, bleomycin; 5-FU, 5-fluorouracil; HU, hydroxyurea; MMC, mitomycin C; MTX, methotrexate.
[a]Significant benefit for oropharyngeal primaries only.
[b]Study limited to oral cavity.
[c]Improved but not statistically significant.
[d]Significant benefit for oral cavity primaries only.
[e]Study limited to nasopharyngeal carcinoma.

therapy. Mitomycin C has been shown in trials conducted at Yale to improve progression-free survival but not overall survival.[278]

Cisplatin has been combined with RT because mucositis is not a primary toxicity and experimental data support its effectiveness as a radiosensitizer.[259] As a single agent, cisplatin has been administered using two schedules in head and neck cancer: weekly low doses (20 mg/m^2) or intermittent high doses (100 mg/m^2 every 3 weeks) concomitant with RT. The results of an intergroup randomized trial comparing low-dose weekly cisplatin (20 mg/m^2) during radiation with conventional radiation were reported by Haselow et al.[279] The overall response rate was significantly higher for the cisplatin-treated patients (73% vs. 59%, $P = .007$), but there was no difference in complete response rate (34% vs. 30%) or survival. The lack of benefit may be attributable to the low total dose of cisplatin received (120 to 140 mg/m^2) over the 6 to 8 weeks of radiotherapy. The higher dose of cisplatin (100 mg/m^2 every 3 weeks) during radiotherapy resulted in significant survival benefit for patients with nasopharyngeal carcinoma.[280]

Al-Sarraf et al. reported the findings of an intergroup trial for patients with stage III and IV cancer of the nasopharynx.[280] Patients were randomized to receive standard radiotherapy or cisplatin (100 mg/m^2 days 1, 22, and 43) during radiation followed by three cycles of adjuvant cisplatin and 5-FU. The trial was terminated early after an interim analysis showed a significant improvement in 2-year survival (80% vs. 55%) with combined treatment. Local and distant failure rates were also significantly reduced with combined treatment. These results cannot be generalized to other sites in the head and neck and the contribution of each component (concurrent chemoradiotherapy and adjuvant chemotherapy) to the improvement in survival cannot be determined.

The newer agents paclitaxel, docetaxel, and gemcitabine have radiation-enhancing properties.[281–283] Phase I and II trials are in progress to assess dose-limiting toxicities using various schedules of these drugs as single agents or combined with cisplatin or other drugs concurrent with radiation. The safe dose of gemcitabine for head and neck irradiation has not been determined. Initial dosing in a study at the University of Michigan of 150 to 300 mg/m^2/week was associated with severe late toxicity.[284] Paclitaxel has been studied in low dose as a prolonged infusion,[285] as a weekly low dose by 3-hour infusion, and in combination with cisplatin[286] or carboplatin.[287,288] The optimal schedule for radiosensitization has not been determined.

COMBINATION CHEMOTHERAPY AND RADIOTHERAPY

Administering multiple cytotoxic drugs during radiation substantially increases toxicity and often necessitates frequent interruptions in radiotherapy. Thus, investigators have developed regimens that use split-course RT providing planned breaks in therapy, or regimens that alternate chemotherapy and radiation in order to minimize normal tissue toxicity. The mode of combining the two therapies is an important issue. For head and neck cancer, it has been demonstrated that protracted RT as single modality treatment results in decreased local control rates.[289,290] This is thought to be due to accelerated repopulation of tumor cells surviving the initial treatment. The failure of induction chemotherapy to show any survival benefit in randomized trials may have a similar cause. If RT is considered a non–cross-resistant tumor-killing agent, then alternating it with chemotherapy or simultaneous administration without breaks might circumvent the problem of heterogeneous tumor cell repopulation and primary drug resistance.

Many concomitant chemotherapy and radiation pilot trials have been reported. Some with the longest follow-up that use cisplatin-based combination chemotherapy report promising survival and response data but also severe mucosal toxicity.[291–293] The advantage of multiagent chemotherapy is that in addition to improved local regional control, distant metastases may also be

TABLE 30.2-13. Randomized Trials of Concurrent versus Sequential Chemotherapy and Radiation

Author (Reference)	*Treatment*	*No. of Patients*	*Survival*	*Other Outcomes*
Taylor (294,295)	Concurrent PF/RT	108	NS	Significant improvement in L-R control for T3–4 N0. T1–2 N2 subset with concurrent PF/RT
	Sequential PF → RT	107		
Adelstein (296)	Concurrent PF/RT	24	NS	Significant improvement in disease-free survival with concurrent PF/RT
	Sequential PF → RT	24		
Merlano (297)	Alternating VBM/RT	61	Significant increase	Significant increase in complete response and progression-free survival with alternating VBM/RT
	Sequential VBM → RT	55		
SECOG (298)	Concurrent VBM ± F/RT	136	NS	Disease-free survival improved for larynx with concurrent VBM ± F/RT
	Sequential VBM ± F → RT	131		

B, bleomycin; F, 5-fluorouracil; M, methotrexate; NS, not significant; P, cisplatin; RT, radiation therapy; V, vinblastine.

decreased. Taylor and associates used a regimen of concurrent radiation and cisplatin and 5-FU chemotherapy administered every other week.[291] After a median follow-up of 8 years, 31% of 68 patients had recurrences or progressed. The 5-year progression-free survival was 60% and overall survival 43%. Lavertu and associates reported their 8-year experience from the University Hospitals of Cleveland, Case Western Reserve University, using two courses of cisplatin and 5-FU concurrent with 66- to 72-Gy radiotherapy in 105 patients with stage II, III, and IV cancer.[292] At a median follow-up of 39 months, 66 patients (63%) were disease free. The 4-year disease-specific survival was estimated to be 74% and overall survival 60%. The overall survival with the primary site preserved was 54%. Investigators from the University of Chicago have reported their long-term results with concomitant hydroxyurea and fluorouracil for stage II and III head and neck cancer.[293] At a median follow-up of 52 months, 5-year survival, progression-free survival, and local regional control were 65%, 82%, and 86%, respectively. Only eight patients developed local or regional failure, and three were successfully salvaged with surgery. These results suggest a possible survival advantage over surgery or radiotherapy and the potential for preservation of organ function.

Randomized trials of concurrent or alternating chemotherapy and radiotherapy compared with the induction approach of sequential chemotherapy and radiotherapy are shown in Table 30.2-13.[294–298] Only one of the four trials reported a significant improvement in overall survival for the regimen of vinblastine, bleomycin, and methotrexate alternating with radiotherapy compared with sequential treatment.[297] However, the other three trials showed benefit in complete response rate, locoregional control, or progression-free survival with the concurrent strategy.[294–296,298]

More significant are the results of the randomized trials of concurrent platinum-based chemotherapy and radiotherapy compared with radiotherapy alone in patients with locally advanced disease shown in Table 30.2-14.[299–307] A significant improvement in overall survival has now been reported for three studies in patients with unresectable disease[304–306] and for one trial limited to patients with stage III and IV cancers of the oropharynx.[303] These positive results are reported for standard

TABLE 30.2-14. Randomized Trials of Concurrent Multiagent Chemotherapy and Radiotherapy versus Radiotherapy in Stage III and IV Disease

Author (Reference)	*No. of Patients*	*Study Population*	*Chemotherapy*	*Radiotherapy*	*Local Regional Control (P)*	*Survival (P)*
Keane, 1993 (299)	212	Larynx and hypopharynx	MMC, 5-FU	50 Gy, split	40% vs. 40%	40% vs. 40%
Zakotnik, 1998 (300)	64	Unresectable	MMC, Bleo	66–70 Gy	75% vs. 29% (.007)[d]	38% vs. 10% (.019)[c]
Adelstein, 1999 (301,302)	100	Resectable	Cisplatin, 5-FU	60 Gy, split	77% vs. 45% (<.001)	42% vs. 34% (<.01)[a] (5-y)
Calais, 1999 (303)	226	Oropharynx	Carbo, 5-FU	70 Gy	66% vs. 42% (.03)	51% vs. 31% (.02) (3-y)
Merlano, 1996 (304)	157	Unresectable	Cisplatin, 5-FU (alternating)	60–70 Gy	64% vs. 32% (.038)	24% vs. 10% (.01) (5-y)
Adelstein, 2000 (305)	295	Unresectable	Cisplatin	70 Gy		37% vs. 20% (.016) (3-y)[b]
			Cisplatin, 5-FU	60–70 Gy, split		29% vs. 20% (.13) (3-y)[b]
Wendt, 1998 (306)	270	Unresectable	Cisplatin, 5-FU, L	70 Gy, b.i.d., split	36% vs. 17% (<.004)	48% vs. 24% (<.0003) (3-y)
Brizel, 1998 (307)	116	Resectable and unresectable	Cisplatin, 5-FU	70–75, Gy b.i.d.	70% vs. 44% (.01)	55% vs. 37% (.07) (3-y)

Bleo, bleomycin; Carbo, carboplatin; 5-FU, 5-fluorouracil; L, leucovorin; MMC, mitomycin C.
[a]Survival with primary site preservation.
[b]Preliminary analysis of survival only.
[c]Benefit for patients with oropharyngeal primaries.
[d]Complete response rate.

fractionation radiotherapy as well as altered fractionation radiotherapy. In all studies, toxicity was increased in patients receiving combined treatment, emphasizing the need for aggressive supportive care, ideally at a treatment center familiar with the expected severity of toxicity and potential complications.

Only one study showed no benefit for any outcome parameter.[299] Investigators from the Princess Margaret Hospital compared continuous course radiotherapy with split-course radiotherapy, 50 Gy, and mitomycin and 5-FU in patients with advanced cancers of the larynx and hypopharynx. The lack of a difference may have been due to the 4-week planned break after 25 Gy in the chemotherapy arm, allowing tumor repopulation to occur.[299]

The data from more recently matured trials shown in Table 30.2-14 support the use of concurrent chemotherapy and radiotherapy as the standard of care for the treatment of resectable cancers of the oropharynx when nonsurgical treatment is planned. It must be noted that no randomized trials have been performed or are planned comparing chemoradiotherapy to surgery with reconstruction. The large French cooperative group trial reported by Calais et al.[303] using three courses of carboplatin (70 mg/m^2 days 1 to 4) and 5-FU (600 mg/m^2/d continuous infusion for 4 days) during 70 Gy showed significant survival benefit of 51% versus 31% (P = .02) at 3 years for patients with stage III and IV oropharyngeal cancer. In addition, it is noteworthy that most of patients included in the other positive trials had oropharyngeal primaries. Adelstein et al. using cisplatin and 5-FU on days 1 and 22 of radiotherapy, 66 to 72 Gy, in patients with resectable cancers reported a complete response rate at the primary site in 90% with chemoradiotherapy compared with 66% (P = .03) after radiotherapy alone.[301,302] Recurrence-free interval, local control, and survival with primary site preservation were all significantly better with chemoradiotherapy although overall survival, including salvage surgery for primary site failure, was equivalent in the two treatment groups. What has not been adequately addressed in any trials in patients with resectable disease is speech and swallowing *function.* Preservation of the organ does not equate with preservation of function. Intensive chemoradiotherapy regimens may result in late toxic effects of soft tissue fibrosis that leave patients unable to swallow and thus dependent on gastrostomy tubes. The outcomes of function and quality of life need to be addressed in future trials in addition to survival and local control.[308]

In contrast to the favorable results of chemoradiotherapy achieved with oropharyngeal cancers, oral cavity primaries continue to be managed by a surgical approach. Resection produces less relative organ dysfunction, and these cancers appear somewhat less responsive to cytotoxic therapy. Site-specific trials have not been performed.

The positive results in unresectable patients in five trials[300,304–307] support the use of chemoradiotherapy as the standard of care provided that patients have adequate performance status and psychosocial supports to undergo this more toxic and complex treatment.[308] The large German trial reported by Wendt and associates[306] combining cisplatin, 5-FU, leucovorin, and twice a day radiotherapy compared with the same radiotherapy alone showed significant improvements in locoregional control (36% vs. 17%, P<.004) and survival at 3 years (48% vs. 24%, P<.0003).

The preliminary results of a three-arm intergroup trial, E1392, show significant survival benefit for cisplatin, 100 mg/m^2 on days 1, 22, and 34, during radiotherapy compared with radiotherapy alone in patients with advanced unresectable disease.[305] This trial compared the cisplatin and radiotherapy regimen previously tested in the RTOG[309] and the regimen of cisplatin and 5-FU and split-course radiotherapy tested by Adelstein in the ECOG[310] with standard radiotherapy alone. A total of 295 patients were randomized, and the two investigational therapies were separately compared with the control arm. At a median follow-up of 25 months, there is a significant difference in 2- and 3-year projected survivals for patients in the cisplatin and radiotherapy arm compared with radiotherapy alone, but not for the cisplatin and 5-FU split-course radiotherapy arm. Median survivals were 12.6 months, 19.1 months, and 14 months, respectively, for RT, RT plus cisplatin, and RT plus cisplatin and 5-FU.[304]

In a smaller trial of mitomycin C combined with bleomycin and 66- to 70-Gy radiotherapy compared with the same radiotherapy was reported by Zakotnik and associates.[300] A total of 64 patients with inoperable carcinoma, the majority from oropharyngeal sites, were randomized. The study was closed early because of a significant benefit in complete response (75% vs. 29%, P = .007), disease-free survival at median follow-up of 42 months (48% vs. 10%, P = .001), and overall survival (38% vs. 10%, P = .019) observed for patients with unresectable oropharyngeal cancer in the combined treatment group.

What is apparent in all of these trials is the substantial and significant improvement in local regional control that is of a magnitude (20 to 30 percentage points on average) sufficiently large to affect survival.[308] This is in contrast to the modest increase in local regional control observed in the RTOG radiotherapy trial comparing altered fractionation with concomitant boost or hyperfractionation with standard radiotherapy in over 1200 patients.[311] Local regional control increased from 45% with standard fractionation to 54% with altered fractionation and concomitant boost, but survival was not affected.

Of the various regimens tested in these positive trials, cisplatin, 100 mg/m^2, administered with vigorous hydration and diuretics on days 1, 22, and 43 of standard fractionation radiotherapy (70 Gy) would be a reasonable recommendation for treating unresectable patients. Grade 3 or worse toxicities, particularly mucocutaneous toxicity, can be expected in approximately 75% of patients and thus aggressive support is required with analgesics, oral care, and gastrostomy tube for nutritional support. Patients with poor performance status, complicating comorbid disease, or who lack the psychosocial resources to undergo these complex therapies should be managed with radiotherapy alone.

PRINCIPLES OF CHEMOPREVENTION

Patients at increased risk for developing upper aerodigestive tract cancer may be identified by a history of previous head and neck cancer or exposure to risk factors such as alcohol and tobacco. Because alcohol and tobacco are avoidable risks, there has been considerable interest in developing effective prevention strategies for these patients. One approach currently being tested is chemoprevention, which is the administration of natural or synthetic agents to reverse or suppress carcinogenesis before the development of an invasive cancer. Chemoprevention trials in the upper aerodigestive tract, guided by epidemiologic studies, have often evaluated dietary constituents, such as β-carotene and retinol. The retinoids, natural and synthetic analogues of vitamin A, have been studied extensively as chemopreventive agents. Retinoids can modulate the growth and differentiation of normal, premalignant, and malignant epithelial cells in culture and can suppress carcinogenesis *in vivo* in various human epithelial tissues.[312–314]

Aerodigestive tract epithelial carcinogenesis is an extremely complex, multistep process. The process begins with genetic alterations and proceeds to altered expression of regulatory gene products and dysregulated tissue growth or proliferation and dysregulated differentiation. Gross histologic and clinical markers of this process are observable but not until late in the process. Molecular techniques have revealed specific genetic alterations in the process of epithelial carcinogenesis in which losses of genes on chromosomes 3p, 9p, 11q, 13q, and 17p are common.[315,316] This step-wise process is an accumulation of genetic events that may be reversed or suppressed at any of various points. Advances in the biology of carcinogenesis are leading to the development of reliable intermediate biomarkers that can be quantitatively measured to assess modulation by chemopreventive agents.[317]

CHEMOPREVENTION OF ORAL PREMALIGNANCY

The first chemointervention studies in oral premalignancy began in the mid-1950s and used high doses of topical and systemic natural vitamin A derivatives.[318–320] These early studies reported clinical and histologic activity and response, relapse, and toxicity patterns that are still relevant currently for the reversal of oral leukoplakia. Agents that have been studied in oral premalignancy chemoprevention trials include selenium, α-tocopherol, β-carotene, and six retinoids.[317,321–328] To date, five randomized trials in oral leukoplakia have been reported.[322–326]

Hong et al. reported the first randomized study in 1986 in which 44 patients were entered into a 3-month placebo-controlled trial of 13-*cis* retinoic acid (isotretinoin), 2 mg/m²/d.[322] Differences observed in clinical response rate (67% vs. 10%, $P = .0002$) and histopathologic reversal of dysplasia (54% vs. 10%, $P = .01$) were highly significant between treated and placebo patients, respectively. Toxicity, however, was unacceptable in those patients receiving 2 mg/kg. Cheilitis, facial erythema, and skin dryness and peeling occurred in 88% and conjunctivitis in 76% of patients. Although reversal of the leukoplakic lesions was demonstrated, a relapse rate of higher than 50% occurred within 3 months of stopping the drug.

Hong and coworkers designed a second study to prolong remission with less toxic maintenance therapy. After a 3-month induction phase with high-dose 13-*cis* retinoic acid (1.5 mg/kg/d), responding or stable patients were randomized to a 9-month maintenance program with low-dose 13-*cis* retinoic acid (0.5 mg/kg/d) or β-carotene (30 mg/d).[323] Low-dose 13-*cis* retinoic acid was significantly more effective than β-carotene in maintaining clinicopathologic remission. Only 8% of patients in the 13-*cis* retinoic acid group had progression of their leukoplakia during maintenance, compared with 55% in the β-carotene group ($P < .001$). In addition, the low-dose 13-*cis* retinoic acid regimen was well tolerated, causing only mild and reversible toxicities. The long-term results of this study at a median follow-up of 66 months showed that 17 of 70 patients (24%) developed cancer with an annual rate of 5.8%.[329] The rate of development of cancer in the two treatment groups was not different, 23% for 13-*cis* retinoic acid and 27% for β-carotene.

Four other randomized trials also demonstrated positive results. Stich et al. observed significant activity with natural vitamin A in Asian patients with leukoplakia chewing betel nuts and enrolled in a 6-month placebo-controlled trial: 57.1% complete remission with vitamin A versus 30% for controls ($P < .01$).[324] Benefit was also seen in a second trial from this group comparing β-carotene plus retinol with placebo.[330] Han et al. also noted positive results with a synthetic Retinamide taken for 4 months in a placebo-controlled trial for oral leukoplakia.[325] The most recently completed trial is a randomized maintenance study of the retinoid fenretinide after laser resection of oral premalignant lesions.[326] After 12 months of fenretinide, the relapse rate in 39 treated patients was 8% compared with 29% in 41 control patients. These results are similar to that observed with low-dose 13-*cis* retinoic acid maintenance therapy.

Current research efforts are focusing on the biochemoprevention therapies such as the combination of high-dose 13-*cis* retinoic acid, α-tocopherol, and interferon-α for the treatment of patients with advanced premalignant lesions defined as moderate to severe dysplasia.[331–333] A striking difference in response was noted in favor of laryngeal lesions as compared with oral lesions, suggesting that this may be a promising approach for laryngeal dysplasia.

Chemoprevention of Second Primary Tumors

Regardless of their initial treatment, head and neck cancer patients remain at significantly increased risk for second primary tumor (SPT) development. SPTs occur after treatment for all stages of head and neck cancer, but their effect is most striking in patients treated for early disease.[317,334] SPTs, either synchronous or metachronous, develop conservatively at a constant yearly rate of 2% to 5% in previously treated patients. The long-term risk of developing additional aerodigestive tract malignancies is 10% to 40%.

Investigators at the M. D. Anderson Cancer Center evaluated the role of *cis*-retinoic acid in preventing SPTs.[335,336] Following surgery, radiotherapy, or both, 103 patients with stage I through IV (M0) squamous cell carcinoma of the head and neck were randomized in a double-blind fashion to receive 13-*cis* retinoic acid (100 mg/m²/d) or placebo for 12 months. After a median follow-up of 32 months, there was a significant difference in the development of SPTs (24% vs. 4%, $P = .005$), respectively, for placebo and treated patients.[335] At a median follow-up of 55 months, the retinoid-treated patients continued to have fewer SPTs, within the upper aerodigestive tract (7% vs. 33%, $P = .008$), although the difference in incidence for all SPTs had diminished (14% vs. 31%, $P = .004$).[336] Although these results are impressive, no survival advantage was seen. This may be due to the small sample size and the nature of the study population: One-half of patients had advanced disease.

Bolla and colleagues evaluated etretinate in a placebo-controlled trial to prevent SPTs in patients with squamous cell carcinoma of the oral cavity or oropharynx following local therapy.[337] After a median follow-up of 41 months, the rates of primary disease recurrence and SPTs were the same for both treatment groups.

Two National Cancer Institute–sponsored multicenter placebo-controlled randomized trials evaluating 13-*cis* retinoic acid for the prevention of SPTs were initiated in the early 1990s. Both trials are for patients with stage I or stage II squamous cell carcinoma of the oral cavity, pharynx, or larynx who have been rendered disease free with surgery or radiation. The trial, conducted jointly by M. D. Anderson Cancer Center and the RTOG, randomizes patients between placebo and low-dose 13-*cis* retinoic acid, 30 mg/d (approximately 0.5 mg/kg/d) for 3 years. The trial has completed accrual and is under analysis. The second intergroup trial (ECOG, NCCTG) evaluates very low-dose 13-*cis* retinoic acid, 0.15 mg/kg/d, versus placebo for 2 years. Until these trials are analyzed, there is no role for retinoids in daily practice.

POSTTREATMENT REHABILITATION

Increasing emphasis on the posttreatment rehabilitation of the head and neck cancer patient has taken place over the last decade. No doubt as we see the limitations of current therapeutic strategies to improve on mortality for advanced disease, quality-of-life issues will become increasingly important. Specific approaches to the rehabilitation of the head and neck cancer patient have now been defined.[338–346] The majority of these approaches are based on quantitative assessment of various speech and swallowing parameters (Table 30.2-15).

Optimal rehabilitation approaches for the head and neck patient begin before the initiation of treatment. We have discussed the role of dental examination and hygiene. Another pretreatment assessment should be performed by a speech and swallowing therapist, especially in those circumstances in which resection of critical organs is anticipated, such as the tongue, palate, and pharyngeal wall. Posttreatment rehabilitation should generally be considered within 3 days after treatment depending on the healing and integrity of surgical wounds. Each site within the upper aerodigestive tract must be considered separately.

Appropriate rehabilitation of the oral cavity begins with choice of reconstruction. Resections contribute to intraoral sensory loss, which impairs the initial phases of deglutition. The optimal reconstruction in most circumstances involves primary closure, thereby minimizing large insensate contact surfaces. Teichgraeber et al., however, raised the important consideration of tongue mobility.[343] The degree of swallowing dysfunction correlates with the extent of tongue resection. In certain circumstances, approximation of the residual tongue to lateral soft tissue may serve to further restrict tongue movement. In this setting the use of a split-thickness skin graft to cover the surgical defect may prevent this restricted function. Teichgraeber et al. noted that patients reconstructed with a split-thickness graft had improved articulation and improved swallowing.[343] Resections involving the base of tongue and pharyngeal wall may contribute to velopharyngeal dysfunction (i.e., the inability to build adequate intraoral pressure), which contributes to dysfunction of the pharyngeal phase of swallowing. Reduced capacity for generating normal food bolus propulsion results. Rehabilitation in such circumstances may require several means. The placement of an intraoral prosthesis obturates the defect. The obturator also serves to lower the palate to allow for appropriate contact with the remaining tongue base. Logemann notes that patients with 50% or more of the tongue base resected are likely to benefit from prosthetic rehabilitation.[338] Other rehabilitation approaches to be initiated by the speech and swallowing therapist include the use of exercise programs to improve tongue-base motion. Barium swallow studies should be performed before and following rehabilitation efforts to document both the degree of dysfunction and the extent of improvement.

TABLE 30.2-15. Assessment of Swallowing Capacity after Oral Cavity and Oropharyngeal Surgery

Function	*Measure*
Food intake	—
Oral competence	Water-holding test
Mastication	Food consistency capacity
Tongue mobility	Protrusion
	To upper teeth
	To buccal mucosa
Swallowing	Time interval
	Degree of aspiration
	Pocketing in sulci
Occlusion	Degree of malocclusion
Quality of bolus	Extent of comminution
Speech intelligibility	Diadochokinesis
Trismus	Oral commissure diameter
Laryngeal elevation	Barium swallow

NASAL CAVITY AND PARANASAL SINUSES

EPIDEMIOLOGY

Cancers of the nasal cavity and paranasal sinuses are relatively infrequent cancers with an incidence of 0.75 per 100,000 individuals in the United States.[347] Lesions of the maxillary antrum are twice as frequent as those of the nasal cavity. Cancers of the ethmoid and sphenoid sinuses are the least frequently observed. Disease occurs more frequently in male than in female subjects (2:1 ratio) and primarily involves individuals in the sixth decade of life. It is noted that cancer of the paranasal sinuses is more frequently observed in other regions of the world including Japan and South Africa.[348]

Etiologic factors involved in disease development are multifold. Exposure to nickel has been attributed to cancer development in the nasal cavity.[348,349] Occupations associated with a high incidence of nasal cavity cancers also include those within the furniture, textile, as well as boot and shoe industries.[350–352] Other workers considered at risk include those involved with production of chromium, mustard gas, isopropyl alcohol, and radium.[347] When considering cancers of the paranasal sinuses, the most frequently cited agent has been Thorotrast.[353] Some have attributed maxillary sinus carcinoma to chronic sinusitis.

ANATOMY

The nasal cavity comprises the nasal vestibule, nasal antrum, and turbinates. The paired nasal cavities are separated by septal cartilage. The nasal vestibule is the triangular region of the nasal cavity bounded by the palatine processes of the maxilla inferiorly, the nasal septum medially, and laterally by the fibrofatty tissue called the *nasal ala.* The nasal vestibule represents that portion of the nasal cavity composed of skin (i.e., bearing hair follicles and sweat glands). Its posterior border is demarcated by transition from skin to mucosa.

The nasal antrum represents the remaining portion of the nasal cavity and contains the inferior, middle, and superior turbinates. The superior and middle turbinates are composed of highly vascular tissue overlying fragile bony projections that inset onto the ethmoid air cell bony framework. The inferior turbinate is composed of a separate bone.

The paranasal sinuses include the maxillary, ethmoid, sphenoid, and frontal sinus. More detailed anatomy of this region is provided.[354]

Primary lymphatic drainage of the maxillary sinuses is into the submandibular nodal basin. The ethmoid sinuses drain into the submandibular as well as retropharyngeal nodes. The nasal cavity drains into these regions as well as along the course of the facial blood vessels into the submandibular triangle and to periparotid nodes.

PATHOLOGY

The majority of tumors of the nasal cavity and paranasal sinus are squamous cell carcinomas. Distinct from other sites within the upper aerodigestive tract, however, squamous cell carcinoma is less predominant. A vast variety of histopathologically distinct cancers occur in this region. Tumors found in the superior portion of the nasal cavity include adenocarcinoma and esthesioneuroblastoma. In the paranasal sinuses, additional neoplasms include tumors of minor salivary gland origin including adenocarcinoma, adenoid cystic carcinoma, and mucoepidermoid carcinoma. Rare tumors of this region are lymphoma, mucosal melanoma, teratocarcinomas, angiosarcomas, and various odontogenic and bone tumors.

NATURAL HISTORY

The most common cancers (i.e., squamous cell carcinomas) are usually well differentiated and slow-growing, and the tendency to metastasize is infrequent. Common presenting symptoms include a nonhealing ulcer, occasional bleeding, and unilateral nasal obstruction.

Given the anatomic limitations in making early diagnosis, disease is usually far advanced at time of initial presentation. Other symptoms may reflect growth into the oral cavity causing dental pain, loose teeth, or ill-fitting dentures, or into the orbit leading to ocular symptoms such as diplopia, proptosis, and epiphora. Severe pain and trismus may occur with extension into the pterygoid fossa. Tumors in the superior nasal antrum and paranasal sinuses may invade the cribriform plate and extend into the anterior cranial fossa, causing anosmia or headache.

The regional lymph nodes most frequently involved with metastatic disease are nodes within the periparotid region or within the submandibular triangle. The propensity for spread to regional lymph nodes is dependent on the subsite in which primary disease may occur.[355–357] Approximately 20% of patients with cancers of the nasal vestibule develop clinically evident lymph node disease. Nearly 15% of these patients have bilateral disease. Regional lymph node spread is less frequently seen from tumors of the ethmoid and maxillary sinus, approaching 10% to 15% of patients. The probability of lymph node spread increases with extension of tumors outside the normal confines of the nasal and paranasal cavities, especially with extension into the oral cavity.

TABLE 30.2-16. Staging for Cancer of the Maxillary Sinus

TX	Primary tumor cannot be assessed
T0	No existence of primary tumor
Tis	Carcinoma *in situ*
T1	Tumor limited to antral mucosa with no erosion or destruction of bone
T2	Tumor with erosion of the infrastructure including the hard palate, middle nasal meatus, or both
T3	Tumor invades any of the following: skin of cheek, posterior wall of maxillary sinus, floor or medial wall of orbit, anterior ethmoid sinus
T4	Tumor invades orbital contents, any of the following, or both: cribriform plate, posterior ethmoid or sphenoid sinuses, nasopharynx, soft palate, pterygomaxillary or temporal fossae, or base of skull

Prognoses from nasal cavity lesions are directly proportional to size of the lesion and overall approximate 60% at 5 years.[357,358] The principal determinant of survival is the presence of local recurrence, which is the most frequent site of disease failure. Prognosis for paranasal sinus cancers likewise depends on extent of primary disease at presentation and approximates 30% for advanced T4 lesions.[355,359,360]

STAGING AND SCREENING

Given the infrequency in which primary cancers occur in this region, AJCC classification has been adopted only within the maxillary sinus. For the maxillary sinus, the definition of the TNM system is presented in Table 30.2-16. The regional lymph node (N) and distant metastases (M) staging are identical to other sites within the upper aerodigestive tract and are as stated previously (see Staging, earlier in this chapter).

Careful examination of patients presenting with symptoms referable to the midface may minimize delay in diagnosis of these cancers. Likewise, considerable progress has occurred in the use of diagnostic radiology in the preoperative assessment of tumors of this region. Kraus et al. described how the judicious use of CT, MRI, or both may help to delineate the extent of disease.[361] These authors and others show that CT scan may be optimal for the definition of tumor infiltration of bony architecture (Fig. 30.2-4). MRI, on the other hand, aids in the assessment of tumor invasion of soft tissue structures including orbit, dura brain, and cavernous sinus (Fig. 30.2-5).[361,362] Gadolinium-enhanced MRI is an additional tool to aid the therapist in the pretreatment of patients with paranasal sinus cancers by helping to distinguish inflammatory disease from neoplastic extension.

TREATMENT

Treatment of Tumors of the Nasal Cavity

For tumors of the nasal cavity, the appropriate surgical procedure depends on location of the primary disease. Tumors of the nasal septum can be approached through a lateral rhinotomy or by a midface degloving technique.[363] Cancers of the superior or lateral nasal cavity can be resected by a medial maxillectomy and an *en bloc* ethmoidectomy.[364]

Early tumors of the nasal cavity do not require elective treatment of regional lymph nodes as regional spread of disease is relatively infrequent.

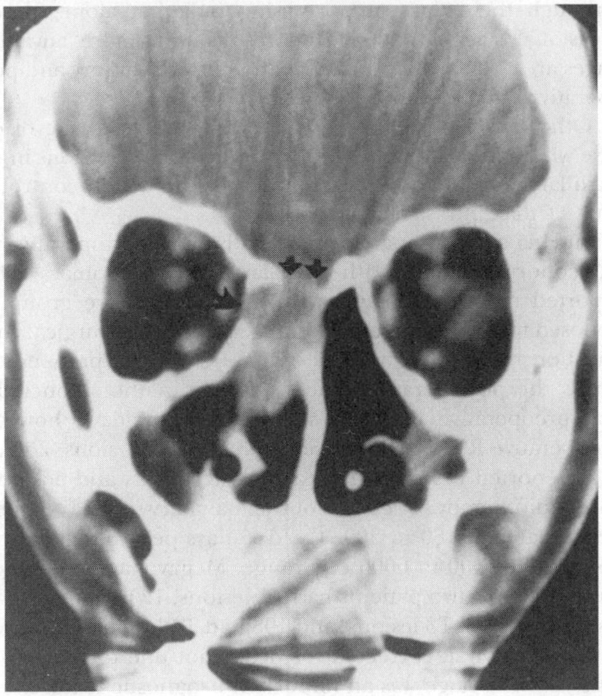

FIGURE 30.2-4. Coronal computed tomographic scan demonstrating bony involvement of the lamina papyracea (*curved arrow*) and intracranial extension (*double arrow*). (From ref. 361, with permission.)

RT and surgical resection yield roughly equivalent results for early lesions. Wong and Cummings have pointed out that most patients presented with lesions that are less than or equal to 5 cm, and less than 10% present with lymph node metastases.[365] When RT is used, treatment can be given by either external-beam techniques, interstitial implants, or a combination of both.

The difficulty with advanced tumors is in obtaining adequate surgical margins. Given the high propensity for local recurrence, combined modality therapy consisting of surgery and radiation should be used in most circumstances.

Treatment of Paranasal Sinus Cancers

For cancers of the maxillary sinus, maxillectomy is the procedure of choice and generally is combined with postoperative radiation. For most lesions, maxillectomy entails a standard Weber-Fergusson incision through skin of the anterior face. The bone cuts used depend on the decision to preserve or resect the orbital floor and orbital contents. It should be recognized that multiple procedures are encompassed by the term *maxillectomy* dependent on the extent or resection of the bony framework (i.e., inferior, medial, anterior, and lateral walls). Spiro et al. have suggested classification schemes indicating limited, subtotal, and total maxillectomy.[366]

Debate in the management of paranasal sinus cancers centers on extent of surgical resection as well as what constitutes resectability. Furthermore, the management of the eye in patients with paranasal sinus cancer remains controversial. For T1 or T2 lesions of the maxilla, the eye can be preserved. Surgeons would advocate resection of orbital contents in patients whose tumors transgress the orbital floor and infiltrate orbital contents. In certain circumstances, however, invasion of orbital floor by maxillary sinus cancers cannot be determined preoperatively.[367]

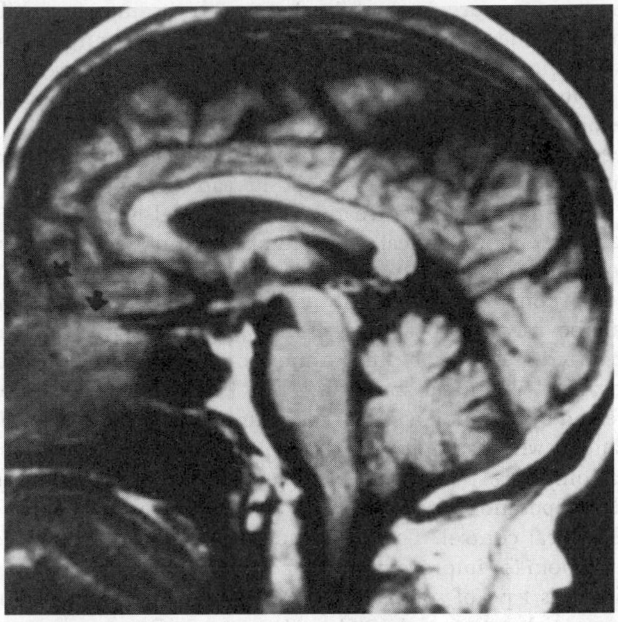

FIGURE 30.2-5. T1-weighted sagittal magnetic resonance image showing dural invasion (*arrows*) within the same patient as in Figure 30.2-4. (From ref. 361, with permission.)

Should disease involve orbital floor and yet not extend into the orbit, resection of the bony floor may be entertained with preservation of globe. However, ocular motion may be impaired and diplopia can result from such a procedure secondary to loss of structural support of orbital contents. This complication has led to numerous procedures for reconstructing the resected orbital floor including median galeal pericranial flaps.[368] The value of one surgical approach versus another is limited by the relative infrequency of these tumors. Tiwari et al. have provided additional insight as to the management of orbital contents in patients whose tumors involves periorbita.[367] The authors, in a careful analysis of anatomic contents of the orbit, note that the periorbita is not the final barrier to tumor invasion, rather, a thin fascia around the periocular fat. This fascial plane is rarely involved in their series, even in the presence of periorbital involvement. The authors note radiographic assessment cannot discriminate involvement of this fascial plane. The authors go on to note that ocular function with preservation of this fascial plane, even when combined with postoperative radiation, is good. Diplopia is not a complicating factor.

With advances in surgical technique and cumulative experience, factors that classically are considered to preclude surgical excision are continually evolving.[369–371] Lund et al., for instance, presented results of craniofacial resection in over 200 patients with a wide variety of tumors of the paranasal sinuses.[371] Actuarial survival in this population was 44%. Lund et al. describe acceptable survival results with acceptable morbidity in patients who underwent skull base resection. Disease involving dura, although associated with an adverse outcome, in selected instances can be controlled surgically. Similar results were noted by McCaffrey et al.[370] Results, however, are significantly influenced by histology. Survival of patients with olfactory neuroblastoma is far superior to those with adenocarcinoma. Involvement of brain parenchyma and extensive involvement of the infratemporal fossa from tumors of the maxillary sinus has not been considered amenable to surgical resection for cure. Each of the decisions regarding resectability should be tempered by the skill of the primary surgeon and availability of neurosurgical and reconstructive expertise.

A major decision in the treatment of paranasal sinus involves reconstruction of the surgical defects. Multiple methods of reconstruction have been advocated including temporal muscle slings, skin grafts, and even composite flaps containing bone.

In general, elective treatment of regional lymph nodes in patients without clinical evidence of lymph node metastases is not indicated.

RT alone is not commonly used for these lesions although it can be used when surgery is not feasible. Roa et al. have reported results of three-dimensional conformal RT for advanced paranasal sinus cancer.[372] For unresectable lesions treated by radiation alone, local control was 32% at 3 years. For patients who had a grossly incomplete resection, local control was only 20%. The group of patients who had a grossly complete operation, leaving only microscopic residual, enjoyed 79% local control. These data suggest that there is considerable room for improvement. In fact, newer programs that combine this type of sophisticated RT with chemotherapy, either sequential or concomitant, have been promising.

Results of Treatment

NASAL CAVITY. Spiro et al. have reviewed the results of therapy for 27 patients with squamous cell carcinoma of the nasal cavity.[373] Surgery alone was the treatment in 21 instances. Five-year determinate cure for nasal cavity lesions were 43%. Local failure remains the most frequent site of failure in the treated surgery, occurring at rates ranging from 10% to more than 40%, emphasizing the need for effective multimodality therapy.[357,358,373,374]

Levendag and Pomp have reported a series of 63 consecutive patients with squamous cell carcinoma of the nasal vestibule who were managed with RT, principally with interstitial implantation.[375] A mean dose of 62 Gy for T1 and 64 Gy for T2 lesions was used. Patients were grouped according to the classification system proposed by Wang.[376,377] Local control was obtained in 97% of T1N0 patients, and 79% of T2N0 patients. Similar results have been observed by others.[365,374] Factors associated with an adverse outcome to primary RT include the presence of nodal metastases and local tumor extension into surrounding anatomic structures such as skin, lip, cartilage, or bone.

PARANASAL SINUS. Results of surgical resection of paranasal sinus cancer have demonstrated local control rates ranging from 10% to 90%, depending on disease stage.[372,373] Surgical series likewise demonstrated that limits of surgical resection could be extended into the anterior as well as the middle cranial fossa with 5-year survival rates approaching 50%.[370,371,378–381]

Parsons et al. have reported on the success of radiation therapy against malignant tumors of the nasal cavity, ethmoid sinus, or sphenoid sinus.[382] The 10- and 15-year actuarial local control for all patients except the adenoid cystic histologies was 52% and 42%, respectively. A 10-year actuarial local control rate for stage I (seven patients) was 100%. The 10-year actuarial local control rate for stage II was 53%, and for stage III it was 30%. Results were dependent on histology, with only a 17% local control in patients with adenoid cystic carcinoma. Although these data support using radiation alone for the occasional stage I patient, the results with more advanced stages are clearly suboptimal. Treatment with surgery and postoperative radiation would be preferred.[382–386]

Other adverse prognostic factors may relate to site of disease within the paranasal sinuses. Suprastructure lesions in the maxillary antrum, for instance, appear more readily controlled with RT than infrastructure lesions.[384]

Yu-Hua et al. compared preoperative and postoperative RT in a cohort of patients with maxillary sinus carcinoma.[385] They reported 64% 5-year survival in the preoperative group, as opposed to 26% in the postoperative group. The surgical complication rate was higher (29% vs. 14%) in the preoperative versus the postoperative groups, but the authors concluded that preoperative radiation was better. Nowadays, however, preoperative RT is seldom used in resectable lesions. Zaharia et al. reported 149 patients treated with surgery and postoperative radiotherapy for cancer of the maxillary sinus.[386] Patients were treated at 180 to 200 cGy/d, 5 days per week, to a total dose in the 5500 to 6000 cGy range. Megavoltage equipment was used. Only two patients had T1 lesions, 12 patients had T2 lesions, 117 had T3 lesions, and 198 had T4 lesions. The 5-year actuarial survival, corrected for death not due to cancer, was 42%. Clinical stage was an important prognostic feature, with survival being 75%, 36%, and 11% for stage II, III, and IV, respectively.

It is clear that the reported local control rates for paranasal sinus tumors are suboptimal. Future results may be improved through the use of CT-based treatment planning. Figure 30.2-6 demonstrates a typical radiation technique for paranasal sinus tumors. A more detailed discussion of treatment planning is available elsewhere.[387]

Chemotherapy for Cancer of the Paranasal Sinuses

Information on the role of chemotherapy in treating paranasal sinus cancer is limited because these patients are usually reported as a subset of a larger series of head and neck cancer patients. For carcinomas of squamous cell histology, there are no data to suggest that the response rate to standard intravenous chemotherapy such as cisplatin and 5-FU is any different from that achievable at other primary sites.

One form of chemotherapy that is specific to paranasal sinus cancer is intraarterial drug delivery. Intraarterial chemotherapy has been studied for almost three decades. The rationale is based on the steep dose-response curve exhibited by most cytotoxic drugs.[388] Regional or intraarterial drug delivery has the potential to increase tumor drug exposure while reducing systemic toxicity. The rationale for using this method of drug delivery for maxillary sinus cancers in particular is to increase local control and to preserve the orbit.

Most of the literature is from trials performed in the 1970s and 1980s using intraarterial bleomycin or 5-FU.[389–395] As an example, Japanese investigators reported cannulating the superficial temporal artery in 68 patients with paranasal sinus cancer and treating with intraarterial 5-FU and RT.[389] In 57 patients, 38 showed disappearance of tumor, and among these, 22 required no further treatment. In 19 cases of residual tumor after therapy, partial resection of the maxilla and intracavitary irradiation were effective in eradicating the tumor. The 2-year survival was 57% compared with 41% in the historic controls treated with surgery and postop-

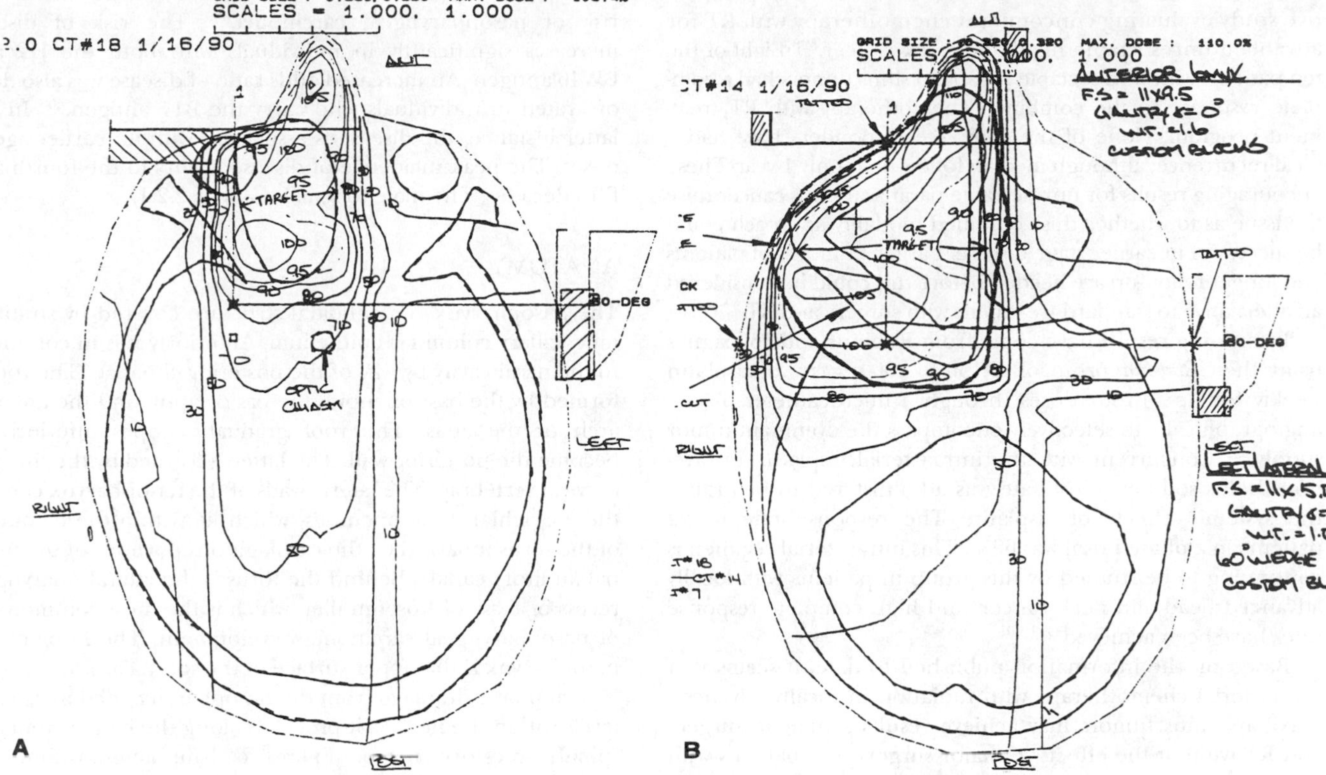

FIGURE 30.2-6. A patient with squamous cell carcinoma of the right maxillary antrum, with disease extension toward the medial portion of the right eye. He underwent a complete resection with close margin near the globe. He was treated with postoperative radiation therapy. The plan is shown here. **A:** A representative cut through the level of the orbit. The plan calls for an anteroposterior field and a left lateral field. The anterior field is weighted over the lateral field 1.6 to 1. The target volume is seen, and the isodose curve shows that the isodose line covers the target volume well. The anterior field has a block for the lateral aspect of the orbit, thereby protecting the lacrimal gland. The medial aspect of the eye is in the target volume well. The left lateral field has blocking for the spinal cord, optic chiasm, and left eye. The dose to the left orbit is less than 10%. A total of 6300 cGy was given, prescribed to the 90% line. This keeps the dose to the optic chiasm well within tolerance. **B:** The same patient, with a cut through a level below the orbits but through the maxillary antrum. The target volume and isodose curves are seen.

erative RT. Similar results were reported by others with intraarterial 5-FU, bleomycin, or methotrexate and RT.[390–393] Many patients avoided radical surgery, which resulted in better cosmesis. In question, however, as cisplatin-based combination chemotherapy regimens evolved, was whether the intraarterial route afforded any advantage over intravenous administration.

More recent trials used intraarterial cisplatin alone or combined with other agents in sequence or simultaneously with radiotherapy. In one trial, intraarterial cisplatin, bleomycin, and intravenous 5-FU infusion were used as an induction regimen.[394] Of a total of 28 evaluable patients, 6 complete and 13 partial responses were observed. After chemotherapy, 13 patients had RT alone and 11 had surgery followed by RT. Overall, 21 patients were rendered free of disease. Of 18 patients who were initially judged to need orbital exenteration, only 7 required it. The median disease-free survival was 42 months. Mortimer et al. employed external carotid artery catheterization to treat 25 patients with intraarterial cisplatin, 100 mg/m^2 every 7 to 14 days for three cycles. The complete response rate was 32% and partial response rate was 50%, which is comparable with that reported for combination chemotherapy administered intravenously.[395]

Wayne State reported its 10-year experience with intravenous cisplatin-based chemotherapy in 24 patients.[396] The response rate was 82% (complete response, 44%; partial response, 38%) for previously untreated patients and 88% (complete response, 38%; partial response, 50%) for patients with recurrent disease. The median survival of untreated patients who achieved complete response was 21 months; for those achieving partial response it was 13 months, and for those achieving no response it was 3 months. For patients treated for recurrent disease who achieved a complete response, the median survival was 16 months; for those who achieved a partial response it was 13.5 months; and for those who achieved no response it was 5 months.

Lee and colleagues from the University of Chicago Hospitals published the results of treatment of 19 consecutive patients with stage III and IV paranasal sinus cancer with multimodality protocols over a 12-year period.[397] Patients received cisplatin-based induction chemotherapy, followed by resection and then concomitant radiotherapy and hydroxyurea and 5-FU. The disease-free survival rate at 5 and 10 years was 66.6% and local control was 76%. Regional and distant control rates were 93% and 95.5%, respectively. These results compared favorably with a 40% survival rate for historic controls treated with surgery and radiotherapy.

Harrison and associates reported the results of a prospective study evaluating concomitant chemotherapy with RT for advanced unresectable head and neck cancer.[398] Eight of the ten patients with unresectable paranasal sinus tumors had a complete response to the combined chemotherapy with RT treatment program. None of the complete responders have had a local recurrence, although median follow-up is only 1 year. These encouraging results for unresectable paranasal sinus cancer raise the issue as to whether this combined modality approach could be successful in earlier stage disease. Larger numbers of patients and longer follow-up are needed before this could be considered an alternative to standard treatment with surgery and RT.

Interesting results have come from Robbins and colleagues using their *Rad-Plat* protocol of 150 to 200 mg/m^2 of cisplatin weekly for up to four doses through a microcatheter placed angiographically to selectively encompass the dominant tumor supply.[399] Concurrent with the intraarterial cisplatin, intravenous bolus sodium thiosulfate was administered to neutralize the systemic effects of cisplatin. The response rate in 22 patients in a phase I trial was 62%. This intraarterial regimen is continuing to be studied by this group in patients with locally advanced head and neck cancer, and high complete response rates have been achieved.[399–401]

Based on the information published to date, it seems that intraarterial chemotherapy with radiation in locally advanced maxillary sinus tumors may achieve results similar to surgery and RT without the effects of major surgery. For patients with paranasal sinus cancer who need orbital exenteration or major craniofacial resection, the option of intraarterial chemotherapy as induction therapy to preserve the eye should be considered as an alternative treatment.

NASOPHARYNX

EPIDEMIOLOGY

The epidemiology of nasopharyngeal carcinoma suggests multiple determinants including diet, viral agents, and genetic susceptibility.[402,403] Endemic areas include Southern China, North Africa, and regions within the far northern hemisphere. The population diets of these regions are what contributes a link to disease development.[404] Populations in endemic areas are characterized by intake of salt-cured fish and meat. The cooking of such food releases volatile nitrosamines that are distributed over nasopharyngeal mucosa when carried by steam.

In addition to diet, considerable epidemiologic evidence incriminates Epstein-Barr virus (EBV) in nasopharyngeal carcinoma development. Old and colleagues first demonstrated the presence of anti-EBV antibodies within the sera of nasopharyngeal carcinoma patients.[405] Knowledge about EBV serology has rapidly progressed, reinforcing the potential causal relationship. More recent advances in molecular biology have provided more direct evidence of the carcinogenic properties of this herpesvirus, including the identification of EBV-related peptides capable of inducing malignant transformation of lymphoblastoid cell lines *in vitro*.[406,407]

Potential genetic determinants of nasopharyngeal carcinoma have been suggested by the increased incidence of disease in individuals with specific major histocompatibility complex profiles.[408] Loci associated with increased relative risk include the H2 locus antigen. Likewise, Simons et al. noted the so-called Singapore antigen, BW46, was associated with a high risk of nasopharyngeal carcinoma.[409] The risk of disease increases significantly in individuals with both the H2 and BW46 antigen. An increased odds ratio of disease was also demonstrated in individuals who carry the B17 antigen.[408] In the latter instance, the disease is associated with an earlier age of onset. The peak incidence of disease occurs in the fourth and fifth decades. The male to female ratio is 2.2:1.

ANATOMY

The nasopharynx is a cuboidal structure covered by stratified mucociliary columnar epithelium. Anteriorly it is in continuity to the nasal cavity by way of the posterior choanae. The roof is formed by the basisphenoid, the basiocciput, and the anterior arch of the atlas. The roof gradually slopes inferiorly to become the posterior wall. The latter is formed by the first two cervical vertebrae. The lateral walls of the nasopharynx contain the eustachian tube openings, which lie within the elevations of the torus tubarii (i.e., the cartilaginous portions of the internal auditory canal). Behind the torus is the lateral pharyngeal recess or fossa of Rosenmüller, which is the most common site of nasopharyngeal carcinoma development. The floor of the nasopharynx is the upper surface of the soft palate.

Lymphatic drainage from the nasopharynx encompasses all levels within the neck as it proceeds along the jugular vein and spinal accessory nerve. Extensive lymphatics within the nasopharynx also drain into the retropharyngeal nodes medial to the carotid artery. It is of note that involvement of these nodes rarely can be detected clinically. Radiologic assessment, either CT or MRI, is the most sensitive diagnostic technique for detecting retropharyngeal node enlargement.

PATHOLOGY

The World Health Organization (WHO) has divided nasopharyngeal carcinoma into three types: type 1, keratinizing squamous cell carcinoma; type 2, nonkeratinizing carcinoma; and type 3, the undifferentiated carcinoma.[410] The latter is the most frequently identified neoplasm. It characteristically is associated with a lymphoid infiltrate that accounts for its more familiar description, lymphoepithelioma. The proportion of type 1 nasopharyngeal carcinoma among the North American population is higher than found in other localities.

Additional cancer types noted include lymphoma, juvenile angiofibroma, plasmacytoma, and adenocarcinomas. The latter is of minor salivary gland origin.

NATURAL HISTORY

Nasopharyngeal cancer grows either by infiltration or by expansion with the former growth pattern predominating. Frequently, mucosal abnormalities may reflect only a small portion of tumor extent. On occasion, no abnormalities of the mucosa are identifiable. In such instances, tumors may exist submucosally and extend into sites outside the confines of the nasopharynx proper.

The most common presenting complaint of nasopharyngeal carcinoma is a mass in the neck occurring in nearly 90% of patients. Additional frequently encountered symptoms include alterations in hearing associated with serous otitis media, tinnitus, nasal obstruction, and pain. Patients may present with symptoms that reflect growth of the disease into the many significant surrounding anatomic structures. Tumors can access the parapharyngeal space through the sinus of Morgagni, an opening in the lateral nasopharyngeal wall through which the eustachian tube courses. Infiltration laterally into paranasopharyngeal space may lead to pterygoid muscle involvement and trismus. Frequently, cranial nerve involvement is manifested with more extensive growth into the skull base. Growth into the cavernous sinus under such circumstances can lead to impairment of cranial nerves II to VI. Additionally, cancer may break through the pharyngobasilar fascia and spread along vascular sheaths (i.e., fascial planes surrounding the jugular vein and carotid artery). Disease extending along these planes may also extend within skull base and lead to cranial nerve involvement.

Any description of the natural history of nasopharyngeal carcinoma must take into account its metastatic potential. Furthermore, the metastatic potential of these tumors is governed by the WHO histopathologic classification. WHO type 1 has a greater propensity for uncontrolled local tumor growth and a lower potential for metastatic spread than the WHO type 2 or 3 cancers. Clinically advanced nodal metastases from WHO type 1 approximates 60%.[411,412] For WHO type 2 and 3 disease, clinical evidence of metastatic disease ranges from 80% to 90%. Distinct from cancers of the oral cavity and oropharynx, metastatic disease frequently presents itself in the posterior triangle. Bilateral neck nodes are present in 53% of patients.[413] Another common location for metastatic disease is in the lymph nodes in the retropharyngeal space, the so-called nodes of Rouviere. Thus, multiple nodal chains can be involved with disease including chains along the special accessory nerve, jugular vein, and the retropharyngeal pathway.

Prognosis for the various WHO classifications of nasopharyngeal carcinoma vary from approximately 15% 5-year survival for type 1 lesions to 60% for type 3 lesions dependent on disease stage.[414,415] The 5-year survival for stage I approximates 67% and decreases to 15% for stage IV.

STAGING AND SCREENING

The regional lymph node (N) and distant metastases (M) staging are identical to other sites within the upper aerodigestive tract (see Staging and Screening, earlier in this chapter; Table 30.2-17).

TREATMENT

RT is the standard treatment of almost all nasopharyngeal carcinomas. Surgery is usually not feasible and cannot provide adequate margins of resection. There is also considerable morbidity to nasopharyngeal surgery, even in the most selected patients.

Modern imaging techniques, including CT and MRI, have dramatically changed RT for this disease. Yu et al. and others have shown that CT scans up-stage more than 50% of T2 and T3 patients.[416,417] In addition, these investigators found that CT identified parapharyngeal extension in more than 60% to 80% of cases. Cellai et al. attempted to study the effect that CT staging and treatment planning had on therapeutic results.[420] They found that patients who were treated with CT treatment plans had improved local control and 5-year survival. This result will not come as a surprise to most radiation oncologists. Because

TABLE 30.2-17. Staging for Nasopharyngeal Cancer

TX	Primary tumor cannot be assessed
T0	No evidence of primary tumor
Tis	Carcinoma *in situ*
T1	Tumor limited to one subsite of nasopharynx
T2	Tumor invades more than one subsite of the nasopharynx
T3	Tumor invades nasal cavity, oropharynx, or both
T4	Tumor invades skull, cranial nerves, or both

CT and MRI scanning have identified disease extensions that were not previously known, the RT plans can now be modified accordingly. An example is shown in Figure 30.2-7. The patient in the figure has parapharyngeal extension. A standard, bilateral opposed field arrangement for the nasopharynx and upper neck would significantly compromise the treatment to the parapharyngeal space. In particular, when the spinal cord block was added, the parapharyngeal extension would be under the block and thereby underdosed. It is not surprising that this would lead to treatment failure. Indeed, Sham and Choy have studied the importance of parapharyngeal extension in the management of nasopharyngeal cancer.[417] This group demonstrated that the degree of parapharyngeal space extension was an important prognostic factor that influenced local tumor control. Using CT scans, they identified four categories of parapharyngeal extension. Type 1 extension involves disease extending up to a line that extends from the medial pterygoid plate to the lateral carotid artery. Type 2 extension goes beyond type 1, up to a line from the medial pterygoid to the styloid process. Type 3 extension goes beyond type 2, up to a line from the lateral pterygoid to the posterior aspect of the ascending ramus of the mandible. Sham and Choy reported that the degree of extension was important, but also that the degree of extension within the T4 group was statistically significant (type 0 and 1 vs. 2 and 3) and approached statistical significance for the T3 group.[417]

In addition to the benefits of target-volume delineation that these new imaging techniques have provided, the advent of three-dimensional RT treatment planning has been vital. Kutcher et al., as well as the experience at Memorial Sloan-Kettering Cancer Center, revealed that multifield conformal plans were able to achieve excellent coverage of tumor, while reducing the normal tissue doses compared with standard treatment techniques.[421] An example of a treatment plan is shown in Figure 30.2-8. It should be pointed out that this is complicated RT. Anywhere from seven to ten fields might be necessary to provide the best dose distribution to the primary site. This needs to be matched to upper neck fields, which then needs to be matched to lower neck fields. The spinal cord must be protected at each junction. Electron beams are required for the posterior neck and these are matched to the photon fields. The result is that up to 15 fields might be required in a single patient. There is some suggestion that RT in a concomitant boost during the last 2 to 2.5 weeks of radiation may provide better local control.[422,430] This allows for the total dose to be increased with a shortened overall treatment time, yielding an enhanced biologic effect. Total doses in the 70-Gy range are usually given to the primary site. The addition of chemotherapy for selected patients with advanced primary and neck disease is discussed later in this section.

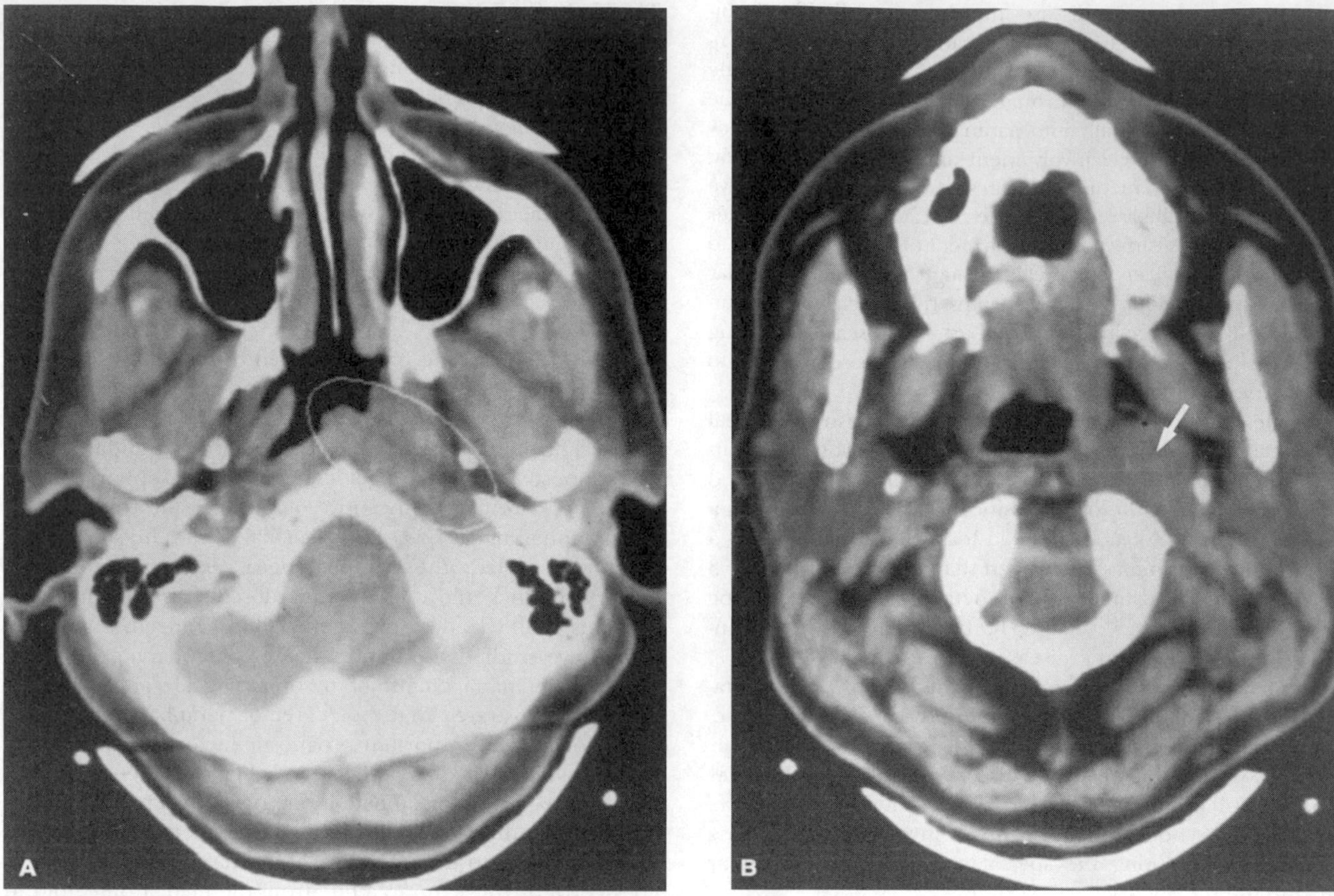

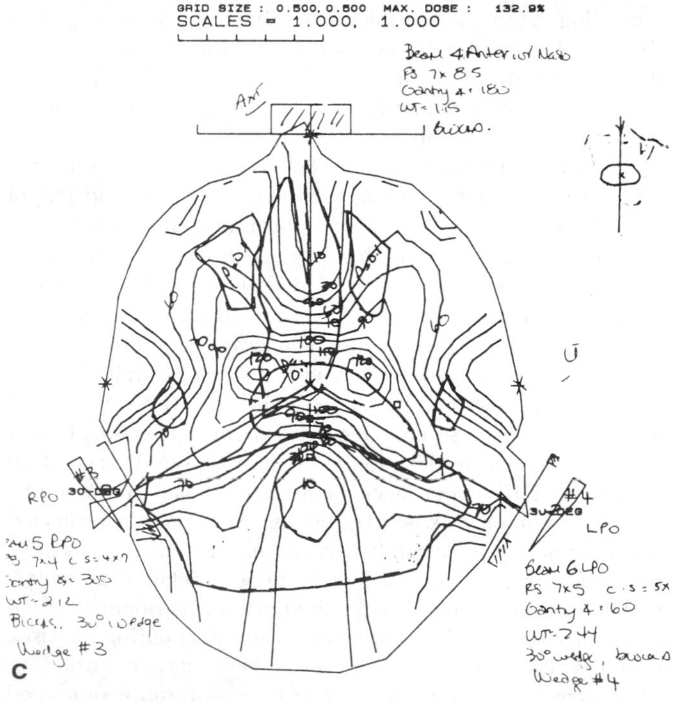

FIGURE 30.2-7. A patient with squamous cell carcinoma of the nasopharynx that was staged as T2N0. **A:** A computed tomographic (CT) scan shows disease extension posteriorly in the parapharyngeal space. If bilateral opposed portals were used for the nasopharynx, the posterior extent of the disease would be undertreated when the spinal cord block is placed. This demonstrates the need for CT scan in all nasopharynx patients. **B:** Another CT scan shows retropharyngeal adenopathy (*arrow*). Again, this disease would be undertreated significantly by conventional, opposed lateral portals with a spinal cord block. **C:** This patient was treated before there was three-dimensional treatment planning. A three-field arrangement was used, which included two posterior oblique portals that protected the spinal cord but treated the posterior extent of disease. A small portion of the posterior aspect of the disease is underdosed by 20%, even with this plan. This area was boosted with an ^{125}I implant. The patient had no evidence of disease at 5 years.

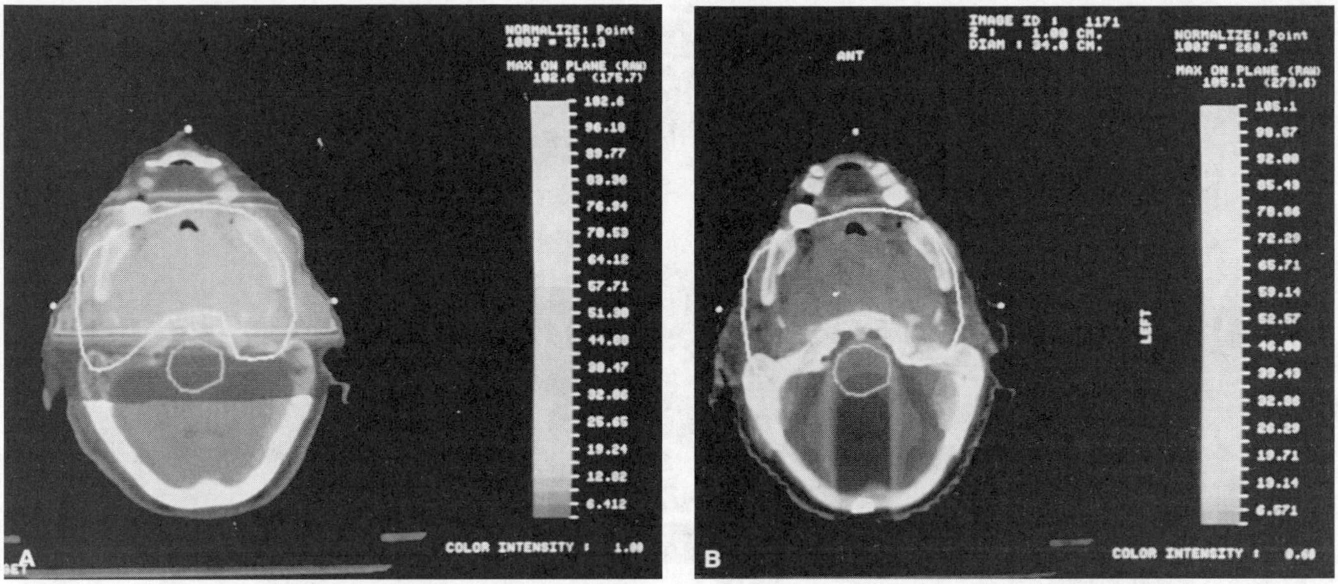

FIGURE 30.2-8. A patient with a T4N0 squamous cell carcinoma of the nasopharynx. The patient has a bulky disease, extending into both retropharyngeal areas. **A:** Computed tomographic scan shows target volume outlines. If bilateral opposed lateral portals were used to treat the nasopharynx, and a spinal cord block was placed at 4500 cGy, the posterior aspect of the target volume is underdosed. The retropharyngeal disease cannot be treated with this technique. **B:** Using a three-dimensional treatment plan, it is possible to encompass the entire retropharyngeal area adequately and still protect the brainstem and the spinal cord. This patient has a complete response to radiation therapy and is doing well 10 months after completion of treatment.

All patients with cancer of the nasopharynx require treatment to both sides of the neck. The overwhelming majority present with either unilateral or bilateral metastases. Those with clinically negative necks still require elective neck irradiation.[418] The pattern of nodal spread is quite orderly with the upper jugulodigastric nodes being involved in the great majority, and the low neck involved far less frequently.[419] It is interesting to note the ability of RT to control neck disease without the need for neck dissection. Neck control is high, even in patients with bulky cervical lymphadenopathy. All patients with nasopharyngeal disease require radiation treatment to regional cervical lymph nodes. Patients with N0 necks are usually treated to 5000 cGy to the entire neck in 180- to 200-cGy daily fractions. Patients with involved necks receive at least 6000 cGy to the region of the involved neck, with boost to higher doses to the gross disease itself. For N1 disease, an additional 500 to 1000 cGy is given. For bulkier necks, doses in the 1000 to 1500 cGy range are added. These additional boost dosages are usually done with electron beams. There has been increasing interest and development of more sophisticated treatment techniques. The role of multileaf and micromultileaf collimators in conformal therapy has allowed for increasing customization and automation of treatment. In particular, micromultileaf systems (leafs less than 5 mm) may be particularly valuable.[423] Three-dimensional intensity-modulated radiotherapy may also be helpful in attempts to maximize tumor dose while decreasing normal tissue dose.[424]

Treatment of Recurrent Disease

For patients with local recurrence, a second course of RT can usually be delivered to the nasopharynx. This can be quite rewarding in selected patients. Wang has shown the importance of high-dose reirradiation in obtaining good results.[425] Five-year survival was 45% in patients who received greater than or equal to 6000 cGy, as compared with zero 5-year survivors in those who receive less than 5000 cGy. Also, the interval of time between the original treatment and the recurrence was of prognostic significance. For patients who had recurrences more than 2 years after their original treatment, 5-year survival could be obtained in 66%. However, only 13% of patients who failed within 2 years of the original treatment were 5-year survivors. Wang emphasizes the importance of combining external beam and brachytherapy in the management of recurrent disease.[425]

Brachytherapy alone has been used for selected patients with local recurrence. Harrison et al. have reported the use of permanent ^{125}I implants for discreet local recurrences in the nasopharynx.[426,427] Either the transoral or the transpalatal approaches can be used. Figure 30.2-9 shows a transpalatal approach. The transnasal approach can also be used.[428] If patients are selected with localized, discreet lesions that are limited to the mucosa, permanent implants can be quite successful. It also has the advantage of limiting the normal tissue that is reirradiated.

In most situations, because the recurrent lesion is not discreet and localized, a combination of external-beam and intracavitary irradiation is important. The field size should be kept as small as possible, preferably smaller than 8 cm in maximum diameter.[429] It would be typical to deliver 4500 to 5000 cGy with external-beam RT, and then boost the nasopharynx with an intracavitary implant with an additional 1000 to 1500 cGy. The techniques for these different brachytherapy approaches have been reviewed by Harrison et al.[430] and Erickson and Wilson.[431] It is important to tailor the implant to the specific location within the nasopharynx that one wants to irradiate. This can help maximize the dose to the target area and minimize the dose to the surrounding normal tissue. The use of charged particle irradiation as well as stereotactic radiosurgery[432] and com-

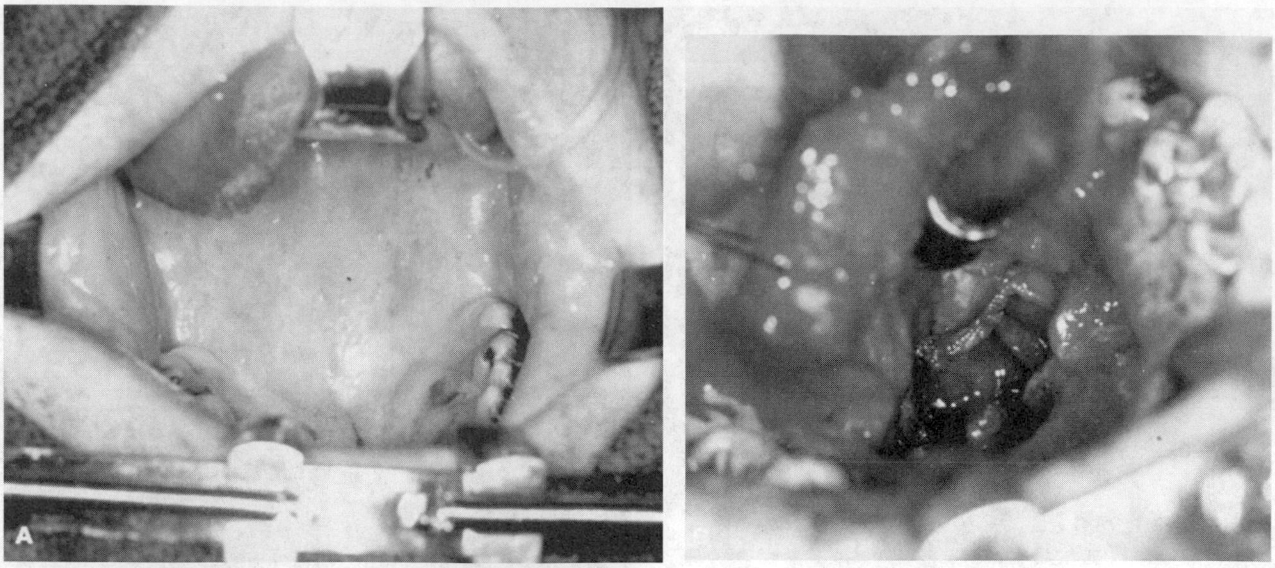

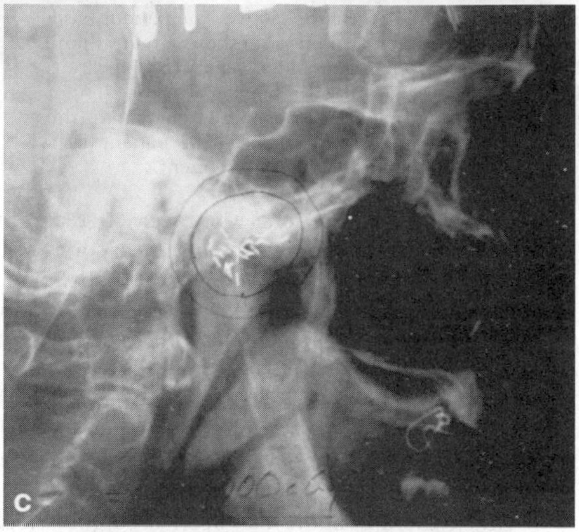

FIGURE 30.2-9. A patient with a discrete mucosal recurrence of a nasopharyngeal cancer. The recurrence was superficial and at the roof of the nasopharynx. It was not accessible through the opened mouth or through the nose. He was treated with an ^{125}I implant via the transplalatal approach. **A:** This view looks into the mouth from above the patient's head, under general endotracheal anesthesia. A mouth retractor holds the mouth open. The tongue is at the top of the figure retracted by the tongue blade. The soft palate is exposed for the incision. **B:** The soft palate has been incised and reflected to expose the interior of the nasopharynx. The torus tubarius is seen, and the glistening mucosa of the nasopharynx is directly visualized. Using this access, ^{125}I seeds are directly implanted into the roof of the nasopharynx. **C:** Localization films of the implant show the position of the seeds in the roof of the nasopharynx.

bining chemotherapy with radiotherapy has been reported. The relative roles of these techniques for patients with recurrent nasopharyngeal carcinoma remain to be determined. The chemotherapy approaches are discussed later in this section.

The role for surgery in nasopharyngeal carcinoma is limited principally to treatment of residual or recurrent disease. Small locally recurrent disease within the nasopharynx has been shown to be amenable to surgical resection with 5-year survival rates of 50% in small patient series.[433–436] Morton et al. have reviewed the various techniques involved in the surgical management of recurrent disease. Various approaches include transpalatal, palatectomy, maxillary swing, infratemporal, and the transcervicomandibulopalatal approach.[435] Complications of such surgery include injury to cranial nerves, cerebral spinal fluid leaks, and hemorrhage secondary to vessel injury.

Management of regional recurrence entails the same considerations as regional recurrence from squamous cell carcinomas elsewhere within the upper aerodigestive tract. If the disease is resectable, an attempt at surgical ablation is indicated. In most instances this requires a radical neck dissection. Brachytherapy can supplement the neck surgery if there is concern about residual disease.

Chemotherapy for Nasopharyngeal Cancer: Metastatic or Recurrent Disease

The natural history of nasopharyngeal carcinoma, WHO types 2 and 3, differs from that of other sites in the head and neck. Local control rates are high, while distant failure is more common and is often the cause of death. The distant metastatic rate at presentation is reported to be 5% to 11%. However, a thorough extent of disease evaluation that includes CT scans of chest and abdomen, a bone scan and bone marrow aspiration, and biopsy reveal distant metastases in up to 40% of patients.[437] Those presenting with bulky or fixed nodes, disease low in the neck, or bilateral involvement are at the greatest risk.[438–441] Bone is the most common site of metastases followed by lung, liver, and extraregional nodes. Autopsy series report distant metastases in up to 87% of patients with nasopharyngeal carcinoma, which is substantially more than found for any other primary site in the head and neck.[442]

TABLE 30.2-18. Combination Chemotherapy in Recurrent and Metastatic Nasopharyngeal Cancer Patients

Author (Reference)	*No. of Patients*	*Chemotherapy*	*% Complete Response + Partial Response (Complete Response)*
Choo (448)	70	30 P-based	70 (22)
		40 Single agents	25 (7.5)
Marchini (449)	26	PF	73 (23)
Cvitkovic (447)	46	FMEP	46 (9)
Boussen (444)	49	PBF	79 (19)
Azli (446)	44	BEP	45 (20)
Gebbia (450)	40	P-based	64 (21)
Fandi (445)	26	F-BEP	69 (35)
Yeo (451)	27	Pac Carbo	59 (11)
Fountzilas (452)	14	Pac Carbo	57 (14)
Yeo (453)	42	Carbo F	38 (17)

B, bleomycin; Carbo, carboplatin; E, epirubicin; F, 5-fluorouracil; M, mitomycin; P, cisplatin; Pac, paclitaxel.

Reports of chemotherapy for treating recurrent and metastatic disease have usually been included with outcome data for other sites. The single agents, cisplatin, doxorubicin, epirubicin, bleomycin, and methotrexate have been shown to be active for this disease, whereas the evidence for the activity of 5-FU, cyclophosphamide, and the vinca alkaloids is less certain.[443]

The most effective combinations are cisplatin based. Using these regimens to treat patients with metastatic disease consistently results in a small proportion of long-term disease-free survivors.[444–447] The results of phase II trials generally show higher complete and partial response rates than are attainable for squamous cell carcinoma from other sites. Selected trials are shown in Table 30.2-18.[444–453]

Choo and Tannock treated 40 patients with single agents or non–cisplatin-containing combinations and reported response in 25%, three complete and seven partial responses.[448] In contrast, the response to cisplatin-based combination chemotherapy in 30 patients was 70%, 7 complete and 14 partial responses.

A multicenter collaborative group led by investigators from the Institut Gustave Roussy-La Grange, France, has performed a sequence of studies evaluating cisplatin-based combination chemotherapy.[444–447] The best results were achieved with a regimen of cisplatin, bleomycin, and 5-FU that resulted in a 20% complete response rate and 79% overall response rate in 49 patients with metastatic or recurrent undifferentiated nasopharyngeal carcinoma.[444] A total of 165 patients with metastatic undifferentiated nasopharyngeal carcinoma were treated on four consecutive protocols between 1985 and 1996. Twenty patients (12%) were long-term disease-free survivors (42+ to 208+ months), demonstrating the chemosensitivity of this disease in patients with visceral or bone metastases.[445]

Investigators from the Prince of Wales Hospital, Hong Kong, evaluated carboplatin, 300 mg/m^2 day 1, and 5-FU, 1000 mg/m^2/d, days 1 to 3 every 3 weeks, in 42 patients with metastatic disease.[453] Complete responses were observed in lung, liver, and distant nodal sites of metastases. The overall response rate of 38% was lower than reported for cisplatin-based combinations; however, both agents were administered in lower total doses than customarily used in the United States. This same group subsequently evaluated paclitaxel, 135 mg/m^2 (3-hour infusion), and carboplatin, AUC 6 dosing every 3 weeks.[451] One-third of the 27 patients enrolled had received prior chemotherapy and yet a 59% response rate was observed with acceptable toxicity. Similar results were reported by Fountzilas and associates using a more intensive regimen of paclitaxel, 200 mg/m^2 (3-hour infusion), carboplatin, AUC 7 dosing, and G-CSF support repeated every 4 weeks.[452]

Combined Modality Therapy for Locally Advanced Disease

Although local control and survival rates are excellent for T1 to T2, N0 to N1 undifferentiated nasopharyngeal carcinoma treated with RT alone, the 5-year survival rate of patients with more advanced disease is unsatisfactory, ranging from 10% to 40%. Because of the high rate of distant metastases, integrating chemotherapy into the primary management is logical. A number of nonrandomized trials evaluating induction, adjuvant, or concomitant chemotherapy and radiotherapy have been performed. Selected trials are shown in Table 30.2-19. These studies and others from older literature may be found in several excellent reviews.[465,466]

Induction Chemotherapy

Reports of two to three cycles of cisplatin-based induction chemotherapy followed by radiotherapy in patients with locally advanced nasopharyngeal carcinoma suggested survival improvement compared with historic controls.[454–459] Overall response rates of 82% to 98% and complete responses in up to 66% of patients were observed. Geara et al. reported the results of a single institution study of 61 patients treated with the standard cisplatin and 120-hour infusion of 5-FU for three courses followed by definitive radiotherapy.[459] The 5-year cumulative incidence of distant metastases was 19% for the chemotherapy patients compared with 34% for the matched historic controls receiving radiotherapy alone. This effect on distant metastases was most notable for patients with N2 to N3 disease. Five-year disease-free and overall survival were also improved (64% vs. 42% and 69% vs. 48%, respectively). However, locoregional control rates were not different.

TABLE 30.2-19. Selected Nonrandomized Trials of Combined Modality Approaches for Advanced Nasopharyngeal Carcinoma

Author (Reference)	*Treatment Strategy*	*No. of Patients*	*Response (% CR)*	*Survival*
			Induction chemotherapy	
Bachouchi (454)	Induction BEP	41	98% (66)	78% (1-y)
Fountizilas (455)	Induction P-based	39	82% (33)	63% (3-y)
Azli (456)	Induction PBF	30	83% (10)	35% (4-y DFS)
Dimery (457)	Induction PF	47	93% (12)	72% (4-y)
Teo (458)	Induction PF	209		55% (5-y)
Geara (459)	Induction PF	61		69% (5-y)
			Response after concurrent therapy	
Al-Sarraf (460)	Concurrent P + RT	27	89% complete	55% (5-y)
			Local control	
Lin (461)	Concurrent P + RT (hyperfractionation)	63	89% 3 y	74% (3-y)
Rahima (462)	Adjuvant CMF or CMB	25		77% vs. 50% HC (3-y DFS)
Droz (463)	Adjuvant P-based	38		71% vs. 47% HC (3-y DFS)
Tsuji (464)	Adjuvant CMU	22		50% vs. 35% HC (5-y DFS)

B, bleomycin; C, cyclophosphamide; DFS, disease-free survival; E, epirubicin; F, 5-fluorouracil; M, methotrexate; P, cisplatin; RT, radiation therapy; U, UFT (Tegafur).

A retrospective comparison was reported by Teo and associates from Hong Kong that also suggested that benefit from chemotherapy was limited to those with advanced disease.[458] Between 1984 and 1989, 209 patients with bulky or low cervical or supraclavicular nodes (less than or equal to 4 cm) were treated with two courses of cisplatin, 100 mg/m^2, and 3 days of infusional 5-FU followed by radiotherapy. In contrast to the findings of Geara et al., a multivariate analysis, after 5.5 years of follow-up, showed significantly fewer local failures in the chemotherapy group for node-positive T3 and stage IV patients when compared with historic controls, but no difference in survival, relapse-free survival, or distant metastases. There was no apparent benefit for stage II or T1 and T2 disease. These divergent results with induction cisplatin and 5-FU may be due to the difference in the number of treatment courses and intensity of the regimens or simply the nature of retrospective comparisons. These findings emphasized the need for randomized trials.

Three prospective randomized trials of induction chemotherapy have been reported and the results are shown in Table 30.2-20.[467–470] The International Nasopharyngeal Cancer Study Group compared three cycles of bleomycin, epirubicin, and cisplatin (BEC) chemotherapy followed by radiotherapy with radiotherapy alone in 339 patients with N2 and N3 staged nasopharyngeal carcinoma (WHO types 2 and 3). This BEC regimen consisted of bleomycin, 15 mg/m^2 intravenous bolus day 1 followed by a 4-day continuous infusion of 12 mg/m^2/d; epirubicin, 70 mg/m^2 day 1; and cisplatin, 100 mg/m^2 day 1 repeated every 3 weeks for three courses. Conventional fractionation radiotherapy was used to a total dose of 65 to 70 Gy to the primary. The overall response rate to chemotherapy was 91%, with 47% complete response. The updated 6-year results showed significant improvement in disease-free survival for chemotherapy patients (41% vs. 30%, $P<.02$) for the control group.[468] BEC induction chemotherapy was associated with substantial toxicity including 8% treatment-related deaths. Fewer distant and local recurrences occurred in the chemotherapy arm, but the magnitude of the effect coupled with severe toxicity was insufficient to produce a statistically significant improvement in overall survival.

The second completed trial was reported by Chan and associates from the Prince of Wales Hospital. From 1988 to 1991, 82 patients with WHO type 3 carcinoma, Ho's N3, or any nodal disease greater than or equal to 4 cm were randomized to receive RT alone or two cycles of cisplatin, 100 mg/m^2 day 1, and 3 days of infusional 5-FU, 1000 mg/m^2/d, followed by RT.[469] Conventional fractionation radiotherapy was given, 66 Gy to the primary with or without brachytherapy. The response rate to chemotherapy was 81% (19% complete response) and 100% after radiation compared with 95% after radiotherapy alone. An updated analysis after a median follow-up of 60 months showed no difference in survival, disease-free survival, or pattern of failure.[466] Only 55% of patients completed the adjuvant chemotherapy phase of treatment. The less intensive nature of this regimen may account for the lower complete response rate and the absence of any difference in survival outcomes.

The third randomized comparison of induction chemotherapy was reported by the Asia-Oceanian Clinical Oncology Association, which included centers from Hong Kong, Thailand, Malaysia, and Indonesia.[470] This study enrolled 334 patients (286 evaluable) with stage III and IV disease or any nodal involvement greater than or equal to 3 cm. All patients had WHO types 2 or 3 histology. The investigational treatment consisted of cisplatin, 60 mg/m^2, and epirubicin, 110 mg/m^2 day 1, repeated every 3 weeks. Response was assessed after two courses with patients demonstrating at least a partial response proceeding to a third cycle before radiotherapy. The total dose of radiotherapy was 70 Gy to the primary tumor; however, the treatment technique was not standardized but left to each participating center. The response rate to chemotherapy was 84%, with 18% complete. There was a trend for improved relapse-free survival for the chemotherapy-treated patients (59% vs. 47%, $P = .06$) at 3 years, but no difference in overall survival, and local or distant failure rates. In a subset analysis of patients with nodal disease greater than or equal to 6 cm, significantly improved survival and relapse-free survival was apparent for the chemotherapy group. This trial has been criticized for the

TABLE 30.2-20. Randomized Trials of Chemotherapy and Radiotherapy for Locally Advanced Nasopharyngeal Carcinoma

Trial (Reference)	*No. of Evaluable Patients*	*Strategy Treatment Arms*	*Percentage Local + Regional Relapse*	*Percentage Distant Metastases*	*Disease-Free Survival*	*Survival*
International Nasopharyngeal Cancer Study Group (467,468)	339	**Induction**			**6-y (*P* <.02)**	**Median**
		RT	23[b]	32[b]	30%	52 mo
		BEP × 3 → RT	15	18	41%	39 mo
Prince of Wales Hospital (469)	77	**Induction and adjuvant**			**5-y**	**5-y**
		RT	15[a]	23[a]	52%	59%
		PF × 2 → RT → PF × 4	16	30	50%	57%
Asia-Oceanian Clinical Oncology Association (470)	286	**Induction**			**3-y**	**3-y**
		RT	29	48	47%	72%
		PE × 2–3 → RT	31	46	59%	81%
Head & Neck Intergroup (280)	147	**Concomitant and adjuvant**			**3-y (*P* <.001)**	**3-y (*P* <.002)**
		RT	33	35	24%	47%
		RT + P → PF × 3	10	13	69%	78%
Prince of Wales Hospital (471)	321	**Concomitant**			**2-y (*P* = .01)**	
		RT			62%	
		RT + P			78%	
Italian National Research Council (472)	229	**Adjuvant**			**4-y**	**4-y**
		Observation	27	17	56%	67%
		VAC × 6	24	20	58%	59%

A, Adriamycin; B, bleomycin; C, cyclophosphamide; E, epirubicin; F, 5-fluorouracil; P, cisplatin; RT, radiation therapy; V, vincristine.
[a]Determined at median follow-up of 28.5 months.
[b]Site of first failure.

lack of standardized radiotherapy technique, nonuniform use of CT for staging and response assessment, and the high number of inevaluable patients.

In summary, the only induction chemotherapy trial with a positive result was the International Nasopharyngeal Cancer Study Group (INSCG) trial of three cycles of BEC followed by radiotherapy in which disease-free survival but not overall survival was improved. Although a high response rate was achieved with BEC, it cannot be recommended because of the associated toxicity and failure to sufficiently improve overall survival. Induction chemotherapy, therefore, remains investigational.

Concurrent Chemotherapy and Radiotherapy

The RTOG conducted a phase II trial of concurrent radiotherapy and cisplatin, 100 mg/m^2 days 1, 22, and 43, in patients with unresectable squamous cell carcinoma from multiple sites. A subset of 27 patients with nasopharyngeal carcinoma had an 89% complete response rate after completing concurrent treatment and a 5-year survival rate of 55%, which was superior to historic controls.[460]

This concept was then tested by the Head and Neck Intergroup. Concomitant chemoradiotherapy and adjuvant chemotherapy (cisplatin, 100 mg/m^2 every 3 weeks for three doses during radiotherapy followed by three cycles of adjuvant cisplatin, 80 mg/m^2, and 5-FU, 1000 mg/m^2/d × 4) were compared with radiotherapy alone.[280] Conventional radiotherapy, total dose 70 Gy, was administered in both arms. This trial was closed in November 1995 when an interim analysis of 138 randomized patients showed a highly significant difference in progression-free survival (52 vs. 13 months) and 2-year survival (80% vs. 55%) favoring the chemotherapy-treated patients. Sixty-three percent of patients received all three doses of cisplatin during radiotherapy and 55% completed adjuvant chemotherapy. When all 185 patients enrolled were included in the analysis, the survival results remained significant: 3-year overall survival was 76% versus 46% (*P* <.001), and progression-free survival was 66% versus 26% (*P* <.001). The population of patients in this study differed from other trials in that approximately one-half had WHO type 1 squamous cell carcinoma, a reflection of the U.S. population. WHO type 1 nasopharyngeal carcinoma is associated with lower sensitivity to chemotherapy and radiotherapy as compared with types 2 and 3 found in endemic areas. Because of the small sample size, a subgroup analysis of these two populations was not feasible. For similar reasons, it is impossible to dissect the contribution of adjuvant chemotherapy to these positive results.

A second randomized trial of concurrent cisplatin and radiotherapy was completed by Chan and colleagues at the Prince of Wales Hospital in Hong Kong.[471] A total of 321 patients with advanced nodal disease were enrolled between 1994 and 1999 and randomized to receive conventional fractionation radiotherapy, 62.5 Gy, plus parapharyngeal boost when indicated, or the same radiotherapy plus concurrent cisplatin, 40 mg/m^2/week for up to eight doses. The preliminary results indicate a significant difference in 2-year disease-free survival (62% vs. 78%, *P* = .01). Further follow-up will be needed to ascertain the effect on overall survival.

Adjuvant Chemotherapy

Adjuvant chemotherapy after radiotherapy is another strategy that is logical to pursue to improve survival given the propensity of this disease for distant spread. Several small institutional phase II adjuvant chemotherapy trials from the 1980s are listed in Table 30.2-19.[462–464] Survival comparisons with historic controls indicated significant improvement in disease-free survival, supporting the need for a prospective randomized trial.

One multicenter randomized trial was reported by Rossi et al. for the Italian National Research Council.[472] A total of 229 patients were treated with radiotherapy or radiotherapy and six cycles of adjuvant vincristine, doxorubicin (Adriamycin), and cyclophosphamide. Seventy-four percent completed the adjuvant chemotherapy. No differences in relapse-free survival, overall survival, or pattern of failure were observed. The results of this single trial of adjuvant chemotherapy are inconclusive regarding the potential benefit of this strategy to reduce the incidence of distant metastases. The vincristine, Adriamycin, and cyclophosphamide regimen would be considered ineffective for this disease. Adjuvant chemotherapy for nasopharyngeal carcinoma requires further formal study using more efficacious regimens.

In summary, three randomized trials evaluating cisplatin-based induction chemotherapy have been performed. Only the INSCG trial used an active regimen optimally (three cycles of BEC)[467,468] and observed significant improvement in disease-free survival. None of the induction trials, however, could demonstrate a survival advantage. The role of adjuvant chemotherapy is unclear as only one randomized trial was designed to specifically address this question, but an ineffective chemotherapy regimen was tested.[472] In contrast, the U.S. Head and Neck Intergroup trial of concurrent cisplatin and radiotherapy was highly positive,[280] and the early, preliminary results of the Prince of Wales Hospital, Hong Kong, trial using concurrent cisplatin on a weekly schedule are supportive. These results now indicate that radiotherapy alone is insufficient treatment for patients with T3 to T4 or node-positive nasopharyngeal cancer. Chemoradiotherapy followed by adjuvant chemotherapy as used in this intergroup trial should be considered the standard of care for this disease.

Results of Treatment

External-beam RT alone has shown to provide excellent local control for T1 and T2 lesions of the nasopharynx.[473–477] Wang reported better results when intracavitary RT is added to external-beam treatment alone.[473] However, results with external-beam plus intracavitary RT are equivalent to the results of external-beam RT alone in other large centers. Well-delivered external-beam RT should provide local control in at least 90% of patients with T1 lesions, and between 85% and 90% of patients with T2 lesions. Doses in the 6500 and 7000 cGy range are used.

For T3 and T4 disease, local control rates have been significantly lower than the earlier stages, ranging from 62% to 73% for T3 lesions and 44% to 71% for T4 lesions.[474–476] There is a suggestion of a dose response curve for RT. Vikram et al.[478] reported a 90% local control rate for T4 patients receiving more than 6700 cGy, although few patients have been followed beyond 4 years. With the use of three-dimensional treatment planning and delivery, dose escalation to 7500 cGy and beyond may be feasible. Investigators at Memorial Sloan-Kettering Cancer Center have had ongoing experience with both three-dimensional conformal radiation alone and in conjunction with concomitant chemotherapy and concomitant boost radiotherapy.[479] Comparison of the outcomes for patients treated with once-daily RT versus concomitant boost RT, both with concurrent chemotherapy, showed a significant advantage to the concomitant boost technique. The implication of these data is that dose escalation alone is not adequate. However, the combination of three-dimensional treatment planning, concomitant boost fractionation, and concurrent chemotherapy are important in improving the outcome.

Results from M. D. Anderson Cancer Center show control of neck disease in all 35 N0 patients, 27 of 30 (90%) for N1, 24 of 26 (92%) for N2a, and 28 of 33 (85%) for N2b. However, patients with N3a metastases in the neck did worse, with only 10 of 16 (63%) being controlled. Today, most patients with N3 neck disease receive chemotherapy along with irradiation. Neck dissection is reserved for salvage for residual disease that persists after radiation or chemoradiation.

ORAL CAVITY

EPIDEMIOLOGY

Oral cavity cancer represents a multiplicity of diseases. Epidemiology as it relates to each of these disease processes likewise differs. However, given that squamous cell carcinoma represents the preponderance of cancers that occur in this region, greater attention is focused on its etiologic determinants.

It is estimated that 30,000 new cases of oral cavity cancer occur annually.[480,481] The relationship between tobacco exposure and disease development has been clearly demonstrated.[482,483] A clear dose-response relationship has been identified with a greater risk being directly proportional to intensity and duration of exposure. Alcohol has been identified as a coagent, most probably through a topical effect.[484] The mucosal areas that are exposed to prolonged contact with alcohol are at greatest risk of cancer development. Readers are referred to reviews on mechanisms of tobacco-induced carcinogenesis for in-depth understanding.[485] Likewise, reviews regarding the role of alcohol in cancer development are available.[482,486]

Cigarette smoking cannot be considered the sole etiologic agent for oral cavity cancer. This fact is made evident by the observation that over 50 million individuals in the United States consume cigarettes. The percentage of the total population that uses tobacco in its various forms is even greater. As mentioned, however, only 30,000 individuals develop oral cavity cancer annually. Other factors must therefore be considered. Arguably it is genetic susceptibility that may be the most significant. Genetic factors associated with increased risk include mutagen sensitivity, which is potentially reflective of an underlying DNA repair deficiency.[487] Syndromes that are characterized by mutagen sensitivity including xeroderma pigmentosum, Fanconi's anemia, and ataxia-telangiectasia have all been associated with oral cavity cancers.[488] Other relevant genetic markers may include inducibility of the cytochrome P-450 enzyme system.[489]

Additional risk factors for oral cavity cancer include diet.[490,491] Patients with vitamin A deficiency have been considered at high risk of malignant transformation of oral mucosa. High dietary consumption of fruits and vegetables have been

TABLE 30.2-21. Staging for Oral Cavity Cancer

TX	Primary tumor cannot be assessed
T0	No existence of primary tumor
Tis	Carcinoma *in situ*
T1	Tumor 2 cm or less in greatest dimension
T2	Tumor more than 2 cm but not more than 4 cm in greatest dimension
T3	Tumor more than 4 cm in greatest dimension
T4(lip)	Tumor invades adjacent structures (e.g., through cortical bone, tongue, skin of neck)
T4(oral cavity)	Tumor invades adjacent structures (e.g., through cortical bone, into deep, extrinsic, muscle of tongue, maxillary sinus, skin)

found to provide a protective effect. Chronic irritants have been considered an etiologic factor, including mouthwash, poor dental hygiene, and syphilis.[492,493] Reports have incriminated marijuana smoking as a contributing factor to oral cavity cancer.[494]

Studies have focused on the viral etiology of cancers within the upper aerodigestive tract. Herpes simplex virus type 1 has long been considered an etiologic agent. The inability to identify herpes simplex virus type 1–related proteins within oral cavity cancers has, however, raised questions as to the significance of this virus.[495] Investigations have identified human papilloma virus within head and neck cancers, specifically types 2, 11, and 16.[496–499] Papilloma transcriptional factors, when inserted within human DNA, can alter normal gene replicative control mechanisms.

ANATOMY

The anatomy of the oral cavity is covered for each specific site.

STAGING

T staging for oral cavity cancer applies to all subsites within the oral cavity unless otherwise stated. For the oral cavity the definition of T staging is presented in Table 30.2-21. The regional lymph node (N) and distant metastases (M) staging are identical to other sites within the upper aerodigestive tract (see Staging and Screening, earlier in this chapter).

PATHOLOGY

The most common cancer within the oral cavity is squamous cell carcinoma. Additionally, cancers can arise from minor salivary glands; these latter cancers include adenoid cystic carcinoma, mucoepidermoid carcinoma, and adenocarcinoma. Rare soft tissue neoplasms include mucosal melanoma, plasmacytoma, and soft tissue sarcomas. Also found within the oral cavity are cancers arising from bone including osteosarcomas.

There also exist neoplastic lesions that are not truly malignant disorders of bone growth such as ameloblastoma. These lesions, however, have a propensity for local expansion and destruction. The principles of sound oncologic surgery and radiation thus apply to these processes.

NATURAL HISTORY

Earliest changes associated with squamous cell carcinoma are associated with erythema and slight mucosal surface irregularities. Many times a punctate lesion also is identified. As disease progresses, several growth patterns emerge that can be typically characterized as exophytic or infiltrative. The latter is more characteristically associated with destruction of surrounding anatomic structures. The exophytic lesions have a less aggressive growth pattern. It should be realized that both patterns are capable of producing metastasis and disease progression. Therapy should be planned accordingly.

Characteristics of the disease are reflected in certain histopathologic criteria. When considering tumor differentiation it has been reported that poorly differentiated disease has a greater propensity for metastasis than well-differentiated disease. This has, however, not been universally accepted. Jacobsson's criteria, as outlined in Table 30.2-1, likewise reflects the natural history of the disease. More specific information regarding natural history is covered in each anatomic subsite.

LIP

EPIDEMIOLOGY

Carcinoma of the lip is second only to skin cancer as a site of neoplasia within the head and neck region. It is noted to occur in approximately 3600 cases per year (i.e., 1.8 persons per 100,000 population annually).[480] The majority of these lesions occur on the lower lip and 95% occur in male subjects. A principal etiologic factor, similar to other upper aerodigestive cancer, has been the use of tobacco, including both pipes and cigars.[500] Sun exposure has also been incriminated and may represent the most significant factor. The latter fact is of potential relevance given the increased incidence of other skin cancers as well as lip cancer. Patients genetically susceptible to skin cancers following sun exposure (i.e., patients with xeroderma pigmentosum) are likewise susceptible to lip cancer.[488] Such an observation emphasizes ultraviolet radiation as an etiologic agent. Disease has likewise been noted in renal and homograft recipients, implicating immune suppression as a determinant.[501]

ANATOMY

The lip is composed of the orbicularis oris muscle and is delineated by the junction of the vermilion border with the skin. Blood supply and sensory nerve supply are by means of the labial artery (a branch of the facial artery) and by cranial nerve V, respectively. The primary lymph node drainage is to levels I and II.

PATHOLOGY

The principal cancer involving the lip is squamous cell carcinoma. Another common lesion is basal cell carcinoma. Rarely, minor salivary gland cancers can occur.

NATURAL HISTORY

Patients most frequently present with either an exophytic or ulcerative lesion of the lower lip. Occasionally, these lesions are associated with bleeding and pain. The latter symptom, however, is a late feature of the disease. These lesions are typically slow-growing lesions. With progression there may be associated numbness of the skin of the chin secondary to involvement of the mental nerve, a branch of the third division of cranial nerve V. Furthermore, progression of disease along the mental nerve may extend into the mental foramen of the mandible. Such involvement leads to enlargement of the foramen with bone destruction and widening of the inferior alveolar canal. A Panorex examination of the mandible is recommended as part of each diagnostic evaluation.

Lymphatic spread occurs relatively infrequently in lip cancer; approximately 5% to 10% of patients develop evidence of nodal involvement.[502–504] Lymph node spread is typically to submandibular nodes or submental nodes. Lesions in the midline may spread bilaterally. The incidence of metastases has been related to histologic grading, with high-grade lesions being at greatest risk. The upper lip tends to metastasize earlier than the lower lip. Upper lesions metastasize to periparotid nodes (i.e., preauricular nodes, in addition to submandibular nodes).

The prognosis from lip cancer is principally dependent on the size of the primary tumor.[505–507] T1 lip cancers have a 5-year survival of 90%. T2 survival is 84%. With evidence of lymph node metastases, survival decreases to 50%. Perineural invasion represents a bad prognostic sign.[508] Likewise, prognosis appears worse in younger adults.[509] Tumors have a greater tendency to metastatic spread in these latter patients.

TREATMENT

Early Disease

Surgery or radiotherapy are the mainstays of therapy. Dysplasias and carcinoma *in situ* can be handled by lip shave (i.e., vermilionectomy with advancement of a mucosal flap). Those lesions that involve less than 30% of the lip can be resected with a V excision and primary closure of resulting defects. For larger lesions transposition flaps are required for reconstruction.

Undoubtedly the challenge in the surgical management of lip cancer resides in the best means of reconstruction. Oral competence remains the primary goal. Those lesions that require resection of 30% to 50% of the lip, can be best handled with a transposition flap drawn from the uninvolved opposing lip. This reconstruction technique is termed Abbe-Estlander.[510–512] When the near total lip is involved (i.e., 50% to 75%), the Karapandzic advancement flap can be used.[513] This has the benefit of providing a competent oral sphincter with an associated neurovascular integrity.

The problem with the Karapandzic reconstruction is the reconstructed lip is tight and significantly foreshortened. Other methods have been devised.[514–516] These vary from simple nasolabial flaps based inferiorly or superiorly to more formal fan-type flaps such as the Gillies flap and Webster cheek advancement flap.[516]

Most T1 to T3 squamous cell carcinomas of the lip can be managed by either RT or surgery. The choice of radiation or surgery may depend on the size and location of disease. If the lesion is quite small and can be easily excised without functional sequelae, surgery would be the chosen treatment. Lesions involving commissures can be irradiated, without the functional sequelae of surgery. However, involvement of the commissure under such circumstances is rare. Brachytherapy alone can be used for early T1 and small T2 lesions. Temporary implantation with ^{192}Ir or localized electron-beam irradiation can be used. Implant doses of 60 Gy over 6 days, or external-beam doses of 50 Gy in seven fractions to 60 Gy can be used. Figure 30.2-10 shows a clinical example of the brachytherapy procedure.

Given the infrequency in which early cancers spread to regional lymph nodes, elective treatment of the neck is not necessarily required.

Advanced Disease

Stage III and IV lip disease are optimally managed with combined surgery and postoperative RT. Selected T3 lesions can be managed with either radiotherapy alone or surgery alone. Reconstructive options are as described in the previous section. Doses in the 6000- to 6300-cGy range, delivered at 180 to 200 cGy per fraction over 6 to 7 weeks, is preferred. If the patient has lymph node metastases in the neck, a neck dissection would be done along with the resection of the primary site. The postoperative RT would then be delivered to both the neck and the primary site. Even if the patient were N0, one should still use elective RT or elective node dissection as part of the management, given the increased risk of microscopic lymph node metastases in these patients.

For patients with T1 to T3 disease who have had an operation, sometimes the radiation oncologist is faced with a positive margin of resection. This can either be managed with brachytherapy alone, or localized superficial external-beam irradiation, with similar doses and techniques as when RT alone is used.

Results of Treatment

The RT results are similar to the reported results of surgical management.[517] Heller and Shah reported approximately 90% local control for T1, T2, and T3 lesions treated with surgery alone.[505] A significant problem in surgical management is local recurrence, which may approach 40% for T3 and T4 lesions.[503] Fitzpatrick has reported the Princess Margaret Hospital experience, which also documents that the results of RT and surgery are basically equivalent.[518]

Jorgensen et al. have reported a series of 869 lip cancers.[519] In 766 patients, treatment was performed entirely with brachytherapy. The remaining cases had external-beam radiation, mainly with orthovoltage beams. The majority of patients had either T1 or T2 lesions, with only 75 having T3 lesions. Local control was in the 90% range. External-beam radiation can also be used. Petrovich et al. reported on 250 patients, most receiving 5100 cGy in 3 weeks with daily fractions of 300 cGy.[520] There were a total of 896 patients in the study, most of whom were treated with orthovoltage beams. Local control was obtained in 94% of T1 and T2 lesions and in 90% of T3 lesions. For T4 disease, 47% of the patients obtained local control with radiation alone, pointing to the need for combined modality treatment for this subset. Sykes et al. reported 26 patients with T1 to T2 squamous cell cancers of the lip treated with electron-beam radiation.[521] With median follow-up of 31 months (range, 1.5 to 60.0 months), there was 100% local control.

ALVEOLAR RIDGE AND RETROMOLAR TRIGONE

EPIDEMIOLOGY

Cancers of the alveolar ridge and retromolar trigone account for approximately 10% of all oral cancers.[522] Male subjects are

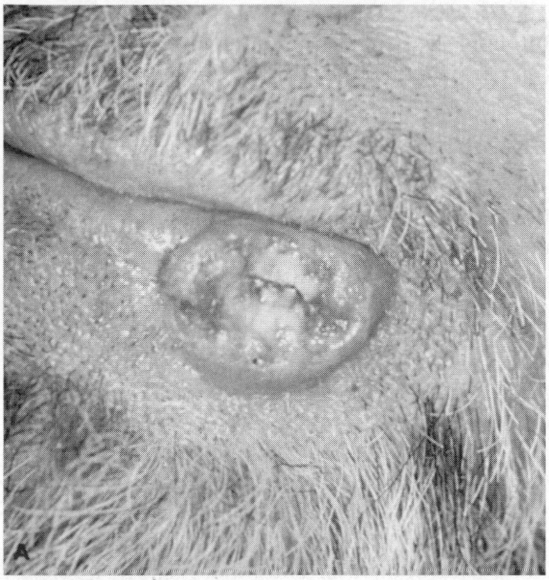

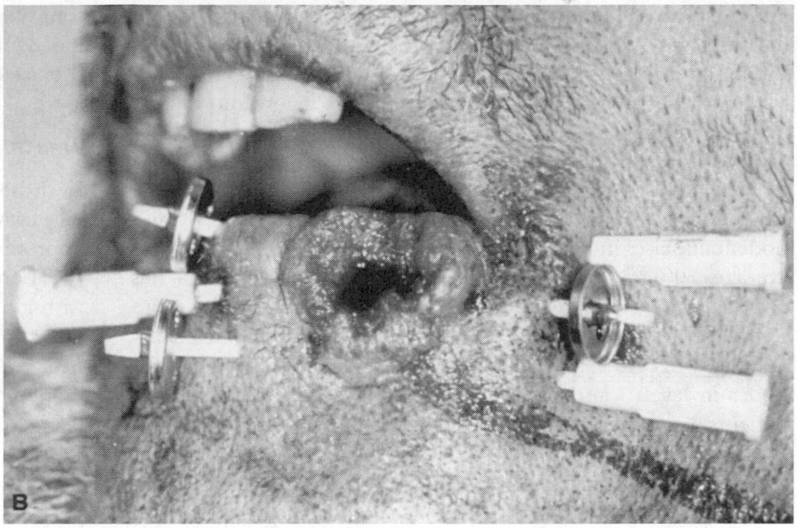

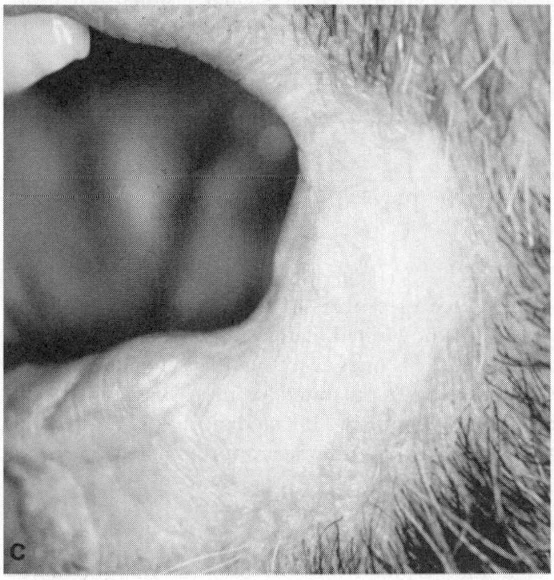

FIGURE 30.2-10. **A:** A patient with a T1N0 squamous cancer of the lower lip. The lesion measured 2 cm in greatest diameter and involved the commissure. **B:** An implant was used as treatment. Under local anesthesia with 2% lidocaine, 14-gauge angiocatheters were placed through the lesion. After localization and planning films were done, ^{192}Ir was loaded into these catheters. A total of 6000 cGy in 67 days was delivered. **C:** The patient had no evidence of disease at 3 years. (From ref. 517, with permission.)

more frequently affected at a ratio of 4:1. An increased frequency in rural women in the southeastern United States has been stated to occur.

ANATOMY

The alveolar ridge consists of an upper and lower portion. The lower alveolar ridge has as its structural basis the alveolar process of the mandible, extending from the ascending ramus to ascending ramus not inclusive of the retromolar trigone. Its borders extend from the gingival-labial sulcus to the free mucosa of the floor of the mouth. The alveolar process of the maxillary bone constitutes the upper alveolar ridge. The retromolar trigone is a triangular area that is composed principally of mucosa overlying the ascending ramus of the mandible. It is bounded superiorly by the hard palate, inferiorly by the alveolar ridge, medially by the anterior tonsillar pillar, and laterally by the gingival buccal sulcus.

Lymphatic drainage of the alveolar ridge and retromolar trigone is principally to levels I and II.

PATHOLOGY

Squamous cell carcinoma represents the near total majority of lesions in this area. Minor salivary gland lesions (i.e., mucoepidermoid carcinomas and adenoid cystic carcinomas) can occur.

NATURAL HISTORY

Squamous cell carcinoma of the alveolar ridge grows in patterns similar to other squamous cell carcinomas of the oral cavity (i.e., either as exophytic lesions or as infiltrative disease). The latter is commonly associated with bony destruction, which occurs in up to 58% of cases. The presenting symptom is primarily pain, which is exacerbated by chewing. Other symptoms include intermittent bleeding as well as loose teeth. In those patients who are edentulous, the principal complaint relates to ill-fitting dentures. The lower alveolus is affected most often in the molar and premolar region. Delay in diagnosis is characteristic because of confusion with inflammatory conditions such as gingivitis or periodontitis.

These lesions have a higher probability of regional lymph node metastases than other cancers within the oral cavity, with the exception of tongue cancer. Overall, the probability of lymph node metastases increases directly with the size of the primary and averages 30%.[523–527] It may increase up to 70% for T4 cancers. It is of note, however, that lymph node metastases tend to occur more frequently from mandibular alveolar ridge cancers than maxillary alveolar ridge disease. Metastatic disease is primarily to lymph nodes in levels I and II. Byers et al. noted that less than 5% of patients develop disease in the posterior cervical triangle.[527]

The prognosis from alveolar ridge carcinoma is reflected by the extent of primary and regional lymph node metastatic disease.[524–527] T1 cancer of the alveolar ridge can be expected to have an 85% survival. T2 lesions and T3 lesions are associated with 80% and 60% survival, respectively. Prognosis with T4 lesions is poor, approximating 20%.

TREATMENT

Early Disease

Surgical management of carcinomas of the alveolar ridge reflects the management principles of cancers of other sites within the oral cavity. The fundamental feature remains the achievement of tumor-free surgical margins with the preservation of critical anatomic structures.

Early T1 or T2 lesions of the alveolar ridge can be managed successfully by surgery alone. With minimal cortical involvement or with involvement by cancer confined to the mucoperiosteum, resection may include a marginal (coronal) mandibulectomy that preserves structural integrity of the mandible. The ability to preserve segments of the mandible is in part dependent on dental status. Not infrequently, edentulous patients present with thin *pipestem* mandibles that preclude all but a segmental resection.

The tendency for bone invasion by alveolar ridge carcinomas through thin mucoperiosteum or through tooth sockets makes primary radiation less feasible. In general, lesions of the gingiva are best managed by surgery. Studies by McGregor and MacDonald have reinforced the notion that a conservative approach to the management of the mandible can only be justified by a thorough understanding of patterns of spread of squamous cell carcinoma into bone.[528]

The need for neck dissection for alveolar ridge carcinomas is enhanced secondary to its tendency to regional nodal spread. The considerations for elective neck dissection as well as the type of neck dissection have been discussed previously in this chapter (see Surgical Management of the Cervical Lymph Nodes, earlier in this chapter). The infrequency of tumor spread to levels IV and V has led to acceptance of selective neck dissection of levels I through III in instances of a clinically N0 neck.

Advanced Disease

Advanced staged tumors generally require multimodality therapy including surgery and radiation. Segmental mandibulectomy is required. Advances in the management of such disease has related to improved reconstructive techniques, principally the use of osteomyocutaneous free-tissue transfer.[529]

Treatment Results

In those studies that report primary surgery results, the actuarial survival for stage I and II was 77% at 5 years, compared with approximately 60% for stage III, and 24% for stage IV.[527,530]

There are relatively few patients reported in the literature with gingival carcinoma who have been managed with primary RT.[530,531] Fuchihata et al. reported a group of patients treated with external-beam irradiation and chemotherapy (bleomycin or peplomycin).[532] Major responders were treated definitively using this approach, whereas others underwent surgery. Responders with T1 and T2 lesions who were not operated on had local control at 3 years of 95%, while those who had surgery had local control of 86%. For T3 and T4 lesions, the nonsurgical group had local control of 45%, while the surgery group had local control of 75%. Thus, there may be a role for nonsurgical management in selected early lesions, but more advanced lesions definitely benefit from surgery followed by postoperative radiation. Early retromolar trigone tumors can be treated successfully by primary radiation, especially when they are superficial. Figure 30.2-11 shows a clinical example.

FLOOR OF MOUTH

EPIDEMIOLOGY

The annual incidence of cancers of the floor of mouth is 0.6 cases per 100,000 in the United States.[480] It occurs in male subjects approximately three times as frequently as female subjects. Reports, however, have demonstrated an increasing incidence of the disease among women.[533] The median age of individuals developing squamous cell carcinoma is approximately 60 years.

ANATOMY

The floor of mouth is delineated by the free margin of the mucosa as it extends from the junction of the mobile tongue to the alveolar process. This margin extends from one anterior tonsillar pillar to the other. Within the floor of mouth anteriorly are the openings of bilaterally located submandibular salivary glands, Wharton's ducts. These ductal openings are significant because anterior lesions of the floor of mouth can frequently obstruct associated salivary flow, leading to tenderness and enlargement of the respective submandibular gland. Also within the floor of mouth are minor salivary glands and the sublingual glands. Distinct from mucosa of the tongue, mucosa of the floor of the mouth is nonkeratinizing stratified squamous epithelium under nonpathologic situations. Musculature making up the floor of mouth include the genioglossus, geniohyoid, and mylohyoid muscles. Blood supply and nerve supply are principally from the paired lingual arteries and lingual nerves, respectively.

PATHOLOGY

Cancers of the floor of mouth account for approximately 10% to 15% of all oral cavity cancers. Squamous cell carcinoma con-

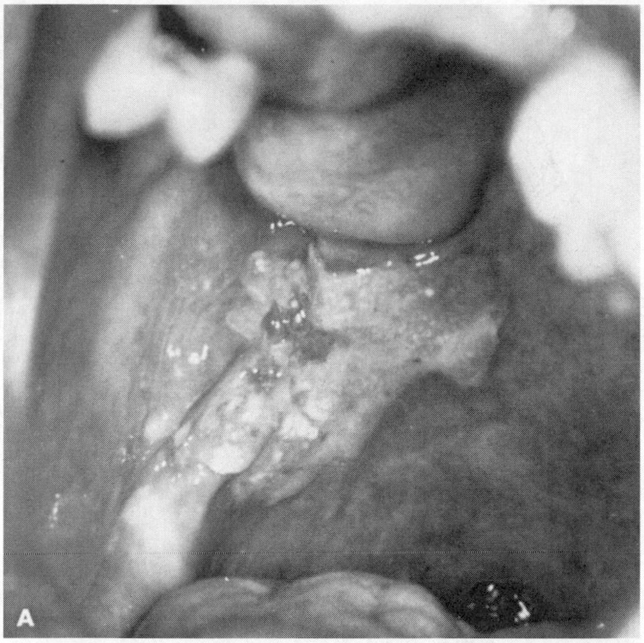
A

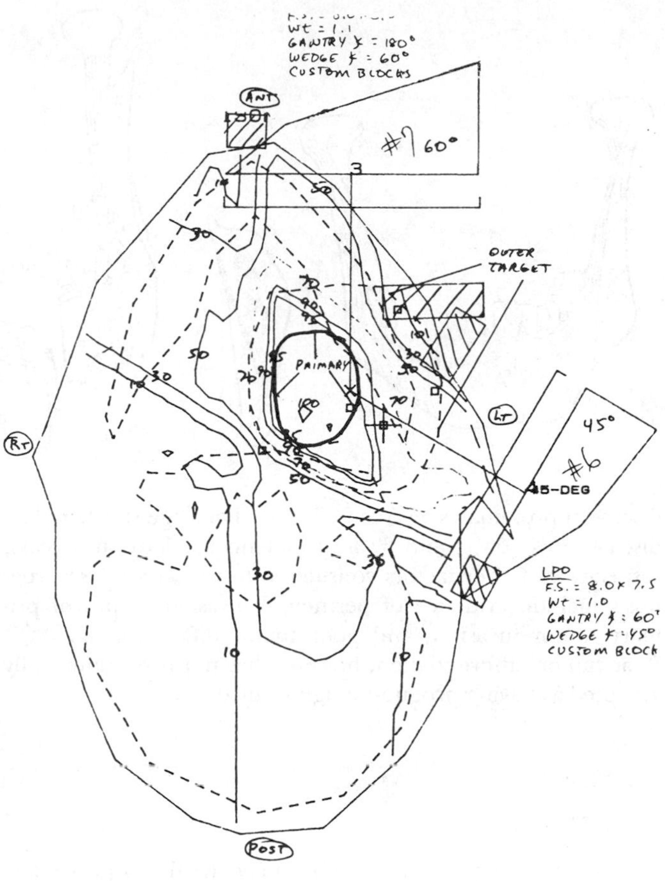

B

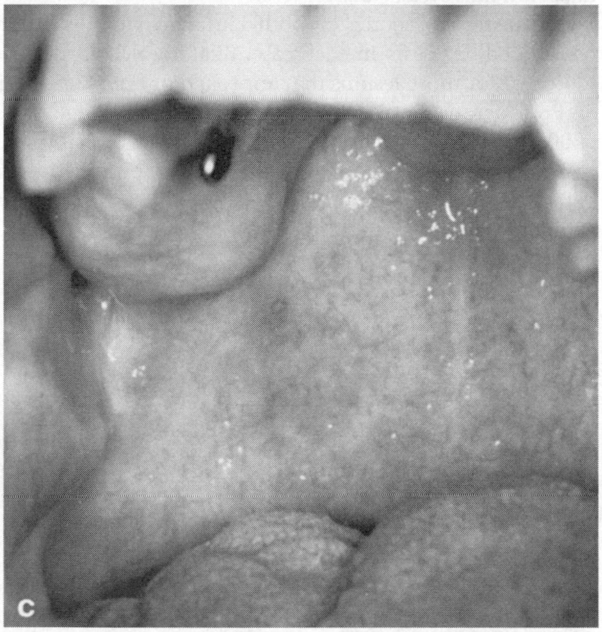
C

FIGURE 30.2-11. **A:** A patient with a T2N0 squamous cancer of the right retromolar trigone. The patient was treated with definitive external-beam radiation therapy to the primary and ipsilateral neck. **B:** The treatment plan involved a wedged photon pair. The boost field is shown. The contralateral parotid area received less than 10% of the dose, thereby avoiding xerostomia. The primary site received 7020 cGy, at 180 cGy per fraction. The right low neck received 5000 cGy over 5 weeks with an ipsilateral low neck field (not shown). **C:** The patient had no evidence of disease at 6.5 years.

stitutes the majority of lesions within the floor of mouth, with the majority of these lesions being moderate to well differentiated. There are several variants of squamous cell carcinoma of the floor of mouth. This includes verrucous and sarcomatoid squamous cell carcinoma. Cancers derived from salivary gland tissue also are encountered including mucoepidermoid carcinomas, adenocarcinomas, and adenoid cystic carcinomas.

NATURAL HISTORY

Squamous cell carcinomas of the floor of mouth typically present as infiltrative lesions that are characteristically painful. These lesions may extend anteriorly to invade bone, deeply to infiltrate muscles of the floor of mouth, or posteriorly to invade tongue. On occasion, an enlarged lymph node in the neck is the presenting symptom.

Floor of the mouth cancers can grow to massive size without metastasizing to cervical lymph nodes. However, approximately 12% of T1 lesions are associated with occult metastatic disease, depending on the thickness of lesion.[74] Metastatic rates to cervical lymph nodes occur in 30%, 47%, and 53% of T2, T3, and T4 cancer, respectively.[74] Lymph nodes in the submandibular and submental triangles represent the first echelon of metastatic sites. Distant metastases is infrequently observed in patients who present with previously untreated disease.

Prognosis is influenced principally by disease stage and presence or absence of histopathologically confirmed regional lymph node metastases. The overall 5-year survival for stage I

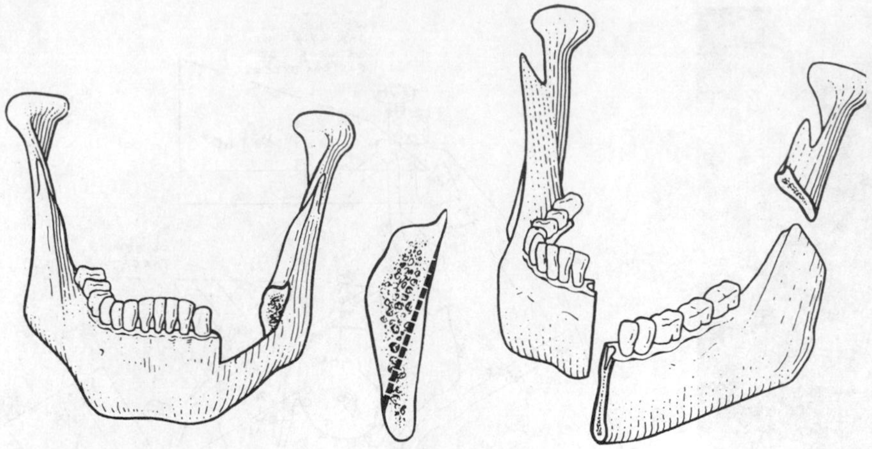

A,B

FIGURE 30.2-12. Types of mandibular resection for squamous cell carcinomas of the floor of mouth. **A:** Marginal resection that preserves mandibular continuity. **B:** Segmental mandibulectomy in which the entire segment of mandible is removed and mandibular continuity is lost. (From Shah JP, Shemen LJ, Strong EW. Surgical therapy of oral cavity tumors. In: Thawley SE, Panje WR, eds. *Comprehensive management of head and neck tumors.* Philadelphia: WB Saunders, 1987:558, with permission.)

disease approximates 85% to 90%.[534,535] For stage II, III, and IV disease, 80%, 66%, and 32% of patients are alive at 5 years, respectively. Other factors considered to reflect a worse prognosis include evidence of perineural invasion, depth of primary tumor invasion, and poor tumor differentiation.[536–539] Poor tumor differentiation, however, has not been universally accepted as having prognostic significance.

TREATMENT

Early Disease

Treatment of floor of the mouth cancers has been principally surgical resection, but may either be surgery or radiation alone. As is true for cancers of the alveolar ridge, superficial involvement of the mandible can be handled by marginal mandibulectomy (Fig. 30.2-12).

When radiation is used for early disease, it has been shown that results are improved when at least a portion of the treatment is delivered by an interstitial implant.[539,540] Interstitial implant alone can also be used.[541] Prostheses can be designed to protect the mandible for brachytherapy (Fig. 30.2-13). Lesions that abut or are tethered to the periosteum of the mandible or lesions that extend onto the gingiva are not good candidates for primary radiotherapy. Implants against the mandible can lead to osteonecrosis.

The treatment of the neck for early cancer of the floor of mouth is controversial. Most advocate elective neck treatment for clinically N0 disease. The value of this approach as compared with observation with neck dissection and RT being performed for clinically developing disease remains unproven. Some have advocated performing neck disscction depending on the thickness of the primary lesion (i.e., greater than 4-mm thickness).

Advanced Disease

For advanced lesions, combined therapy of surgery and radiation is the treatment of choice. Surgical resection generally entails partial glossectomy and segmental mandibulectomy. Identification of the inferior alveolar nerve and frozen section histopathologic assessment should be performed during the operation. This is to ensure that disease has not extended beyond surgical margins by perineural spread. Resection for most advanced lesions requires removal of the entire thickness of the floor of mouth.

New reconstructive techniques have greatly facilitated rehabilitation following surgical excision of advanced tumors. Techniques include myocutaneous flaps as well as osteomyocutaneous free flaps with microvessel anastomoses.[542]

Elective, therapeutic, or both kinds of neck dissections are considered necessary in each case. Bilateral neck dissections are indicated for those lesions that approach or cross the midline.

Postoperative radiation entails doses in the range of 6000 to 6300 cGy at the primary site. In instances of positive surgical margins, our policy is to treat the area of positive margins to 6300 cGy. Certain patients with positive margins may be treated with adjuvant brachytherapy instead of external-beam RT.[543]

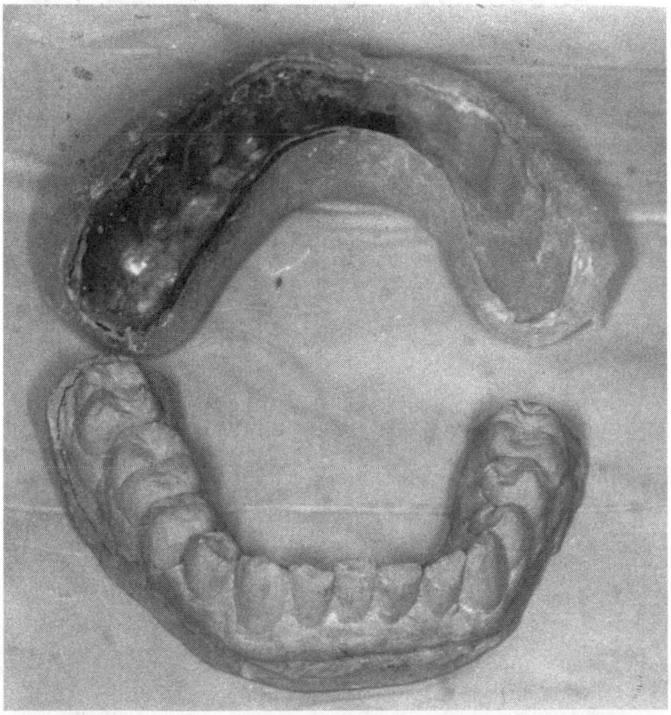

FIGURE 30.2-13. Prosthesis with lead lining that fits onto the lower teeth and serves as mandibular protection for brachytherapy. (Compliments of Dr. Joshua Verona, Dental Service, Beth Israel Medical Center.)

Results of Treatment

Local recurrences after surgical resection of T1 and T2 floor of the mouth cancers are noted in no less than 10% of the patient population.[534,535] As tumors increase in size, the pattern for failure becomes predominately a regional problem. Nearly 40% of failures are solely within regional cervical lymph nodes.[535]

Mazeron et al. have reported a large radiotherapy series.[541] The majority of patients were treated to 65 Gy with ^{192}Ir brachytherapy alone. Local control was 94% for T1 N0, and 74% for T2 N0 lesions and was dependent on size of the lesion as well as the presence or absence of gingival extension. For T2 lesions between 2 and 3 cm, local control was 58%. For lesions with gingival extension, local control was 50%. There is an interest in using high dose-rate brachytherapy for floor of the mouth lesions.[544,545] Inoue et al. reported 2- and 5-year local control of 94% and 94% for a cohort of mainly T1 to T2 lesions treated with high dose-rate brachytherapy alone or combined with 30- to 40-Gy external-beam RT.[545]

Wang et al. have reported excellent results with the use of intraoral cone electron boost and no brachytherapy.[547] The daily dose of radiation via the cone is frequently greater than the conventional 180- to 200-cGy range. Local control was obtained in all 13 patients with T1 lesions, and in 19 of 20 (95%) with T2 lesions.

Fu et al. have published an extensive RT experience with floor of the mouth cancer.[548] When implant was either the only treatment or a part of the treatment, local failure occurred in only 2% (1 of 39 patients) with T1 lesions, 7% (4 of 54 patients) with T2 lesions, and 14% (5 of 35 patients) with T3 lesions. The use of primary radiation may be associated with improved functional outcome as compared with surgery, but this requires more investigation.[546,549,550]

There is a cohort of patients who undergo surgery and are referred for postoperative radiotherapy because the pathology reveals positive or close margins. In this setting, certain patients may be treated with brachytherapy alone, thereby limiting the high-dose region to the area at risk. This is not always technically or oncologically feasible. When it is, it can provide the patient with local control in excess of 80%[543] and can avoid the sequelae of wide field external-beam irradiation to the oral cavity.

TONGUE

EPIDEMIOLOGY

Tongue cancer is estimated to occur in 6200 individuals per year in the United States.[480] Excluding lip, it exceeds all other sites in the oral cavity. The median age for individuals with tongue cancer is approximately 60 years. The male to female ratio is similar to other disease sites, approximately 3:1. It is of interest that an increase in tongue cancer has been reported among young adult men.[551,552] Some have suggested marijuana use as a contributing factor in this latter population.[494]

ANATOMY

The oral tongue represents the mobile portion of the tongue musculature that extends from the line demarcated by the circumvallate papilla posteriorly to the junction of the floor of mouth anteriorly. It is made up of the genioglossus, hyoglossus, styloglossus, and palatoglossus muscles. All of these muscles are innervated by the hypoglossal nerves. Taste and sensation within the tongue are provided by the lingual nerve, a branch of the third division of the cranial nerve V. Blood is supplied principally from the external carotid artery through the paired lingual arteries. Lymphatic drainage is principally to level II, III, and I in decreasing order.

PATHOLOGY

The primary cancer of the tongue is squamous cell carcinoma. Other cancers are frequent and include minor salivary gland cancers such as adenoid cystic carcinoma and adenocarcinoma. Myeloblastoma represents a rare tumor of the tongue.

NATURAL HISTORY

These cancers can grow in both an exophytic and an infiltrative fashion. The primary presenting symptom is pain, although many of these lesions can be painless. Difficulty in speech and deglution is occasionally elicited. It tends to be more rapid in its onset than other cancers within the oral cavity. There may be a history of long-standing leukoplakia before the development of symptoms, especially in younger female subjects.

As compared with other cancers within the oral cavity, tongue cancers have a greater propensity for lymph node metastases. This occurs in ranges from 15% to 75% depending on the extent of primary disease.[553,554] Lymph nodes most frequently involved lie within level II (i.e., jugulodigastric nodes). Nodes within level I, III, and IV are involved in decreasing order. It is of note, however, that all nodes can be involved. The incidence of bilateral nodal metastases occurs in up to 25% of cases. Contralateral nodal metastases are present in 3% of cancers.

Prognosis is principally reflected in extent of nodal metastases, ranging from 75% in early-stage node-negative disease to 30% in those with advanced lesions. Other factors portending more aggressive disease include perineural and vascular invasion and infiltrative versus pushing borders.[555,556] Depth of invasion has likewise been considered significant. Whether or not tongue cancer in young adults represents a worse disease has not been demonstrated.[557]

TREATMENT

Early Disease

It is generally considered that disease-control rates for early disease when using either surgery or RT are equivalent depending on treatment bias. Early stage I and II lesions can usually be removed intraorally. Excision usually entails an hemiglossectomy. Special attention to surgical margins should be exercised as disease may spread along muscle bundles beyond that expected by clinical assessment.

Most T1 lesions can be managed with brachytherapy alone. This generally consists of an ^{192}Ir implant, although high dose-rate implants are also being used.[558–560]

Whether low dose-rate or high dose-rate is used, the catheters themselves are placed in the operating room under general anesthesia. The ^{192}Ir is loaded 1 to 2 days postoperatively. Localization films are taken, and computerized dosimetry is performed. The usual dose rate is in the 40 to 60 cGy/h range, and the usual total dose is 6000 to 7000 cGy. The patient wears a tongue prosthesis during the dwell time of the implant to protect the hard and soft palate as much as possible. For high dose rate, 60 Gy fractions given twice a day over 6 days has yielded good results.[558,559]

As the lesion increases in size when using radiation as primary therapy, it is preferred to combine external-beam irradiation with implant. First, the external beam can be used as elective neck irradiation simultaneous with irradiation to the tongue. The implant then serves as the boost to the tongue. Second, the external beam allows a wider margin of tongue to be treated than does the implant. In these situations, it is typical to treat the primary site and the neck to doses in the 5000-cGy range, followed by a 2000- to 3000-cGy implant boost to the tongue.

For N0 patient, this treatment program manages both the primary site and the neck. For those patients with palpable neck nodes, a neck dissection can be performed at the same as anesthesia for the implant, thereby completing the treatment to the primary site and the neck. This can usually be done approximately 3 weeks after the completion of the external-beam irradiation.

RT is certainly suitable for most T1 lesions. For T2 and T3 lesions, it is most suitable for those tumors that are exophytic or have minimal infiltration. Tumors that are deeply infiltrative are preferably managed with a primary surgical approach, usually with postoperative RT.

Advanced Disease

The surgical management of more extensive lesions requires either a mandibulotomy or a lingual-releasing procedure to gain access to disease. The latter procedure entails removal of neck contents before primary cancer resection. The tongue is delivered into the neck by releasing musculature attachments posteriorly and mucosal attachments within the oral cavity. Large lesions with mandibular involvement require composite resection. The term *composite resection* refers to the removal of tissue involving multiple anatomically defined structures, one of which includes the mandible (Fig. 30.2-14). Typically, it refers to resection of a portion of tongue, floor of the mouth, and segment of mandible.

For patients who require postoperative RT to the primary site alone, this can frequently be done with brachytherapy. This is especially true for the smaller lesions. The decision of how to deliver this irradiation is integrated with the management of the neck. We prefer to use neck dissection as part of the management of all deeply infiltrative or advanced tongue lesions. For the N0 patients, this generally means a staging procedure or a functional neck dissection. For patients who have involved lymph nodes, this means either a radical neck dissection or one of its modifications. Yamazaki et al. have shown a clear relationship between tumor thickness and neck failure in a cohort of patients treated with brachytherapy alone: The incidence of neck metastases was 50%, 40%, and 30% for tumors greater than 11 mm, 6 to 10 mm, and less than or equal to 5 mm, respectively. T stage also correlated with tumor thickness.[560]

Results of Therapy

Decroix and Ghossein from the Curie Institute in Paris have reported on over 600 patients treated with primary RT for T1, T2, or T3 squamous cell carcinoma of the oral tongue.[562] Although the majority of patients had implants alone, a large cohort had combined external-beam irradiation plus implant.

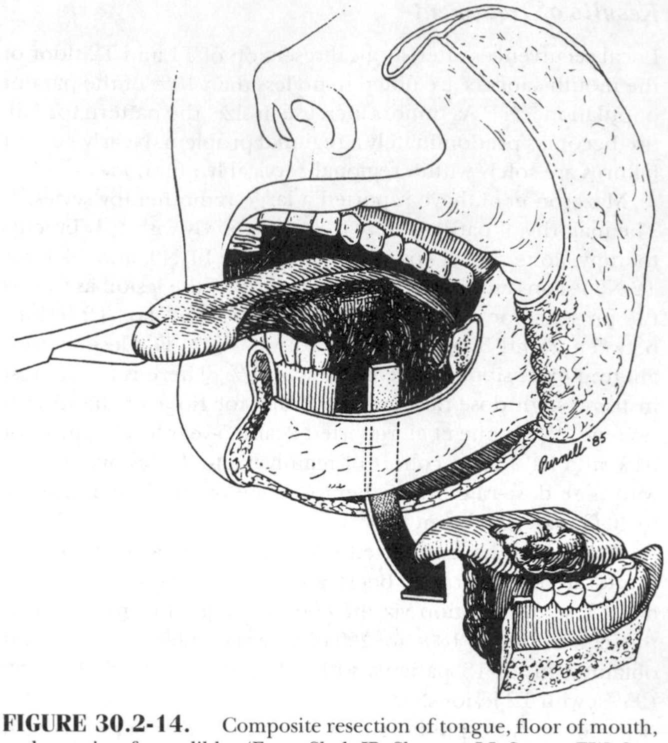

FIGURE 30.2-14. Composite resection of tongue, floor of mouth, and margin of mandible. (From Shah JP, Shemen LJ, Strong EW. Surgical therapy of oral cavity tumors. In: Thawley SE, Panje WR, eds. *Comprehensive management of head and neck tumors.* Philadelphia: WB Saunders, 1987:558, with permission.)

Almost all patients at this center received RT as their primary treatment. Primary control was obtained at 86% for T1, 80% for T2, and 68% for T3. These data compare quite favorably with the results obtained with partial glossectomy.

Pernot et al. have reported a series of 448 patients with brachytherapy alone with or without neck dissection (181 patients) or combined external beam plus brachytherapy (267 patients) for oral tongue cancer.[563] The 5-year local control was 93% for T1, 65% for T2, and 49% for T3 lesions. For T2 lesions managed by brachytherapy alone, local control was 90% versus 50% for those managed by external beam plus implant. These data emphasize the importance of using brachytherapy as a major part of the radiation program, but patient selection factors clearly play a role as well. The 5-year overall survival for T1, T2, and T3 lesions (all N stages) was 69%, 41%, and 25%, respectively. Severe complications were uncommon. While 15% experienced grade 1 soft tissue injury, and 3% had grade 1 bone necrosis, only 1% and 2% had grade 3 soft tissue and bone complications, respectively. Spiro et al. have reviewed the Memorial Sloan-Kettering Cancer Center experience using partial glossectomy as primary management.[564–566] As was true for the Curie Institute series, the Memorial Hospital series is also relatively unselected, with primary surgery being offered to the great majority of patients at that institution. Local control was obtained in 85% for T1, 77% for T2, and 50% for T3. These data serve to highlight the similarity in local control rates for surgery or irradiation for most early tongue lesions.

Although the traditional brachytherapy approach has involved low dose-rate implants,[562] there has been an emergence of interest in high dose-rate brachytherapy for oral tongue.[558,559] Either high dose-rate alone or in combination with moderate doses of external-beam irradiation have been used. Inoue et al. compared low dose-rate versus high dose-rate implants in a small randomized trial of T1 to T2 oral tongue lesions, finding no major differences.[558] A program of 60 Gy in 10 fractions given twice a day over 6 days with high dose-rate yielded 100% local control at 2 years. All tumors had a thickness of 1 mm or less. Leung et al. reported similar local control using the same fractionation program.[559] Mucositis related to these implants can last up to 20 weeks.

There are relatively few recent studies that report the results of therapy for surgery alone for advanced disease.[564,566,567] RT is generally used in the postoperative setting.[570,571] Failure is most often within regional lymph nodes and leads to a 5-year determinate survival of 35% for stage III and IV disease.[565,568]

Ange et al. have reviewed their experience using implants after excisional biopsy for patients with positive or close margins.[569] Local control was obtained in nearly 100% of the cases. When the primary site and the neck require postoperative RT, external-beam techniques must be used. Doses in the 60- to 63-Gy range over 6 to 7 weeks are typically used.

Surgical salvage of radiation failures in the oral tongue can be difficult. Yuen et al. reported 47 patients who underwent attempted salvage for either local recurrence, locoregional recurrence, or regional recurrence.[561] Overall, 62% failed their salvage procedure. The 5-year actuarial survival was 39% for local recurrence alone, 27% for locoregional recurrence, and 68% for regional recurrence alone.

HARD PALATE

EPIDEMIOLOGY

Hard palate cancers account for approximately 5% of all oral cavity cancers.[572] The incidence of the disease in the United States approximates 0.4 per 100,000 population. The male to female ratio is 8:1.

PATHOLOGY

Squamous cell carcinoma accounts for approximately 50% of hard palate tumors. The majority of these lesions are well differentiated. Other cancers occurring in this area include the minor salivary gland lesions such as adenoid cystic and adenocarcinomas, which may be as frequent as squamous cell carcinoma.

NATURAL HISTORY

Cancers of the hard palate grow in a multiplicity of patterns including deeply infiltrating, destructive lesions versus diffuse superficial lesions associated with microscopic invasion.

When considering metastatic squamous cell carcinoma of the hard palate, lymph node metastases is less frequently encountered than cancers of other sites within the oral cavity, ranging clinically from 6% to 29%.[553] Likewise, distant metastasis is infrequent. Prognosis in patients with squamous cell carcinoma is 75%, 46%, 36%, and 11% for stage I through stage IV disease, respectively.[573]

TREATMENT

Early Disease

Surgical management of early disease involves infrastructure maxillectomy (i.e., resection of the palatine process of the maxillary bone). Exposure for such resections is generally obtained through a Weber-Fergusson–type incision.

As stated earlier, carcinoma *in situ* and microinvasive disease can involve a significant portion of the hard palate with extension of disease onto the soft palate and retromolar trigone. Under such circumstances, primary radiation may be used.

Elective treatment of the neck is not generally required unless disease extends beyond the anatomic confines of the hard palate. Selective neck dissection under such circumstances is adequate. Such dissection includes removal of lymph nodes in levels I, II, and III.

Advanced Disease

Surgical resection of advanced disease may involve a near total palatectomy. Generally, however, lesser operations are required. Advances in the surgical therapy of hard palate cancers involve the immediate use of prosthetic obturators that allow for early restoration of adequate speech and swallowing. The need for postoperative radiation is based on the closeness or involvement of tumor margins by tumor, perineural involvement, the presence of regional lymph node metastases, or all three conditions.

Results of Treatment

Generally, incorporating the treatment philosophy described previously, Evans and Shah report an overall survival of 75% for stage I, 46% for stage II, and 36% and 11% for stage III and IV, respectively. The majority of patients who die of disease do so in the face of advanced local recurrence.[573–575]

BUCCAL MUCOSA

EPIDEMIOLOGY

Cancer of the buccal mucosa accounts for approximately 8% of oral cavity cancers in the United States.[572] The disease may be seen much more frequently in other parts of the world such as India depending on tobacco consumption patterns. Indeed, in the southeastern United States, the incidence of buccal mucosal cancer is much higher in women; an observation attributed to the common use of snuff. The median age of individuals with buccal mucosal cancer may be slightly higher than noted in patients with cancers of other sites within the oral cavity.

ANATOMY

The buccal mucosa is composed of a mucous membrane that extends from the lips anteriorly to the retromolar trigone posteriorly. Inferiorly it extends from the lateral alveolar sulcus of the mandible to the lateral sulcus of the maxillary alveolar ridge. Its blood supply and nerve supply are from the facial artery and the third division of cranial nerve V. Lymphatics from the buccal mucosa drain primarily into level II and level I in decreasing order.

PATHOLOGY

As in other sites within the oral cavity, squamous cell carcinoma is the predominant neoplasm. The verrucous variant of squamous cell carcinoma is frequently observed. Only rarely are other cancers, such as minor salivary gland tumors, observed.

NATURAL HISTORY

Cancers of the buccal mucosa are more frequently exophytic than other cancers within the oral cavity. They are also relatively silent in their presentation and thus present rarely as T1 lesions. Pain is the initial presenting complaint and is subsequently followed by bleeding and difficulty chewing. With extension of the disease outside the confines of the buccal mucosa into the pterygoid musculature, patients may present with trismus. Disease not infrequently invades the mandible, maxillary alveolar ridge, or both.

Lymph node metastases are most frequently observed within levels I and II and are observed clinically in 10% of presenting patients.[575]

Five-year survival ranges from 77% to 18% depending on the stage of disease.[577] Urist et al. have shown that tumor thickness is a significant prognostic factor.[576] Patients with tumors less than 6 mm in thickness have significantly better survival rates than those with tumors greater than 6 mm in thickness, regardless of tumor stage.

TREATMENT

Early Disease

Small lesions (T1 and early T2) can be managed with equal effectiveness by either surgery or RT. If the tumor can be excised easily through the open mouth, with minimal functional sequelae, then small lesions are probably best managed in that fashion. Larger T1 lesions and lesions that approach the commissure are best managed with RT. T2 lesions can be managed with RT if they are exophytic or relatively superficial. Deeper lesions are probably best managed by surgery.

In patients with small lesions and a clinically negative neck, the neck can be observed. Neck failure occurs in less than 10% of patients. However, for more advanced lesions, the neck is treated electively with the same therapeutic modality that is used for the primary lesion.

RT can be used with a variety of different techniques. Interstitial brachytherapy, ipsilateral electrons, intraoral cone, or external-beam photon irradiation can all be employed. The exact technique depends on the clinical situation and the expertise of the radiation oncologist.

Advanced Disease

More advanced disease requires surgery as the principal therapeutic modality, usually with postoperative radiation. The initial factor in such treatment relates to adequate operative exposure. This is generally facilitated by dividing the lip in the midline and resecting the cheek posterolaterally in order to gain optimal exposure.

Postoperative radiotherapy is used for patients with close or positive margins, high-grade lesions, positive nodes, bone invasion, and thick (greater than 10 mm) lesions.[577] Adequate locoregional treatment at initial diagnosis is essential, as locoregional failure is a major cause of death for patients with buccal mucosa cancer and few patients can be salvaged.

Care must be taken in assessing the need for resection of surrounding anatomic structures such as skin of face, upper alveolar ridge, and mandible. Invasion of tumor into buccal fat pad and into dermis of cheek skin occurs not infrequently. Such invasion generally requires full-thickness resections including oral mucosa and cheek skin. Such defects can be repaired with myocutaneous flaps. Free-tissue transfer is a relatively recent option for reconstruction.

Ipsilateral neck dissection is advocated in all instances of T3 or T4 primary disease, regardless of the nodal status.

Results of Treatment

Nair et al. have reported on 234 patients with buccal mucosa cancer treated with RT.[578] Disease-free survival at 3 years was 85% for stage I, 63% for stage II, 41% for stage III, and 15% for stage IV disease. All 13 patients with T1 N0 disease were controlled with radiotherapy. Fifty percent of patients with T4 disease failed locally. The presence of nodal metastases clearly affected the local regional failure rate.

Lapeyre et al. reported an experience using definitive brachytherapy for epidermoid cancer of the buccal mucosa.[579] A variety of techniques were employed from 1973 to 1991. The loop technique provided the best results, with only 1 of 22 patients with T1 to T3 lesions having local recurrence. Bloom and Spiro reported the results for 90 patients with buccal mucosa cancer treated by surgery.[580] The 5-year survival rate by stage was 77%, 65%, 27%, and 18% for stages I, II, III, and IV, respectively. Local failure was noted in 47% of patients. Regional failure was observed in 37%.

Dixit et al. performed a comparative study on 176 patients with buccal mucosa cancer, comparing surgery alone with surgery plus postoperative radiation.[577] Postoperative radiation was found to improve local control for patients with positive nodes, close or positive margins, high-grade lesions, bone invasion, and thick tumors greater than 10 mm. Mishra et al. reported a randomized trial comparing surgery alone versus surgery plus postoperative radiotherapy.[581] There was improved disease-free survival (68% vs. 38%, $P<.005$) in those who received radiation. This trial only included patients with stage III and IV disease.

REHABILITATION OF THE ORAL CANCER PATIENT

Over the last decade there has developed an increased effort to address the rehabilitation of the oral cancer patient, the major considerations reflected in speech and swallowing disorders.[582–586] There is no question as to the effect of surgical resection of anatomic components of the oral cavity including the mandible, tongue, and other soft tissue components. The need to preserve function through appropriate reconstructive measures is becoming increasingly apparent. Likewise, rehabilitation efforts have been enhanced by improved quantitative assessments of functional outcomes, as well as through improving rehabilitation techniques. No medical center or treating physicians can truly be considered as providing state-of-the-art therapy unless they are prepared to systematically address these issues.

OROPHARYNX

EPIDEMIOLOGY

The pharynx is divided into three regions: the nasopharynx, oropharynx, and hypopharynx. Our discussion is limited to the oropharynx and its encompassing sites (i.e., the base of tongue,

TABLE 30.2-22. Staging of Tumors of the Oropharynx

T1	Tumor 2 cm or less in greatest dimension
T2	Tumor more than 2 cm but not more than 4 cm in greatest dimension
T3	Tumor more than 4 cm in greatest dimension
T4	Tumor invades adjacent structures (e.g., through cortical bone, soft tissues of neck, deep, extrinsic, muscle of tongue)

tonsil and tonsillar fossa, soft palate, and posterior pharyngeal wall). Cancer of the oropharynx is expected to occur in approximately 4000 patients annually in the United States.[481] Most commonly, the disease involves patients in the fifth through seventh decades of life. Men are afflicted three to five times as frequently as women. The etiology of the disease, to the greatest extent, cannot be distinguished from cancers of the oral cavity. Tobacco and alcohol abuse constitute the most significant risk factors.

STAGING

As was true for staging of oral cavity cancers, staging of tumors of the oropharynx relies on both physical examination as well as a variety of imaging procedures, including CT scan. Staging of the primary tumor is presented in Table 30.2-22. The regional lymph nodes (N) and distant metastases (M) staging are identical to other sites within the upper aerodigestive tract and are as stated in the beginning of this chapter (see Staging and Screening, earlier in this chapter).

BASE OF TONGUE

ANATOMY

The base of tongue is bounded anteriorly by a line demarcated by the circumvallate papillae. Posteriorly, it ends with the epiglottis. Laterally, it extends to the glossopalatini sulcus and includes the pharyngoepiglottic and glossoepiglottic folds. Tongue musculature is composed of the genioglossus, styloglossus, palatoglossus, and hyoglossus muscles. The blood supply and nerve supply are identical to that of the oral tongue and consist of the lingual artery and the hypoglossal nerve, respectively.

Lymphatics are extensive within the base of tongue. Drainage is into numerous node levels including levels II, III, IV, and V in decreasing order. Indeed, disease may involve retropharyngeal lymph nodes in certain instances such as with progression to lateral pharyngeal wall.

PATHOLOGY

Base of tongue cancers are less frequent than cancers of other anatomically defined areas of the tongue. Squamous cell carcinoma represents nearly 95% of those cancers that occur in this subsite. Other cancers in this area include those of minor salivary glands origin (i.e., adenoid cystic and mucoepidermoid carcinoma) and lymphomas.

NATURAL HISTORY

Cancers of the base of tongue are frequently advanced at the time of presentation. This is partly a reflection of the relatively

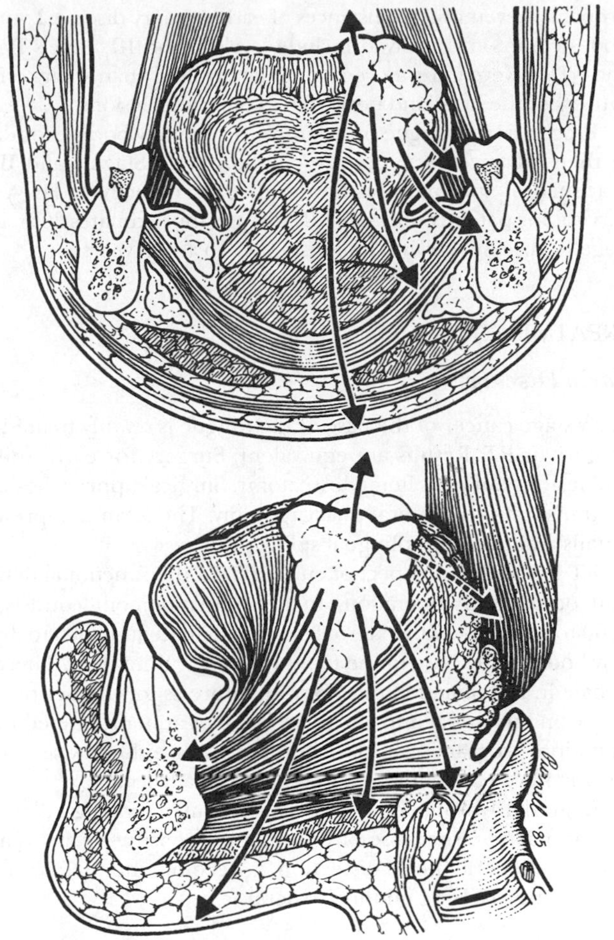

FIGURE 30.2-15. Routes of spread of squamous cell carcinoma of the base of tongue. **A:** Coronal view. **B:** Lateral view. (From Shah JP, Shemen LJ, Strong EW. Surgical therapy of oral cavity tumors. In: Thawley SE, Panje WR, eds. *Comprehensive management of head and neck tumors.* Philadelphia: WB Saunders, 1987:553, with permission.)

silent location of such disease as well as its aggressive tendencies. Patients usually present with symptoms of pain and dysphagia. Not infrequently, as is true for nasopharyngeal carcinomas, individuals present with a mass in the neck. A history of weight loss is common. Likewise, referred otalgia secondary to cranial nerve involvement is common. With progressive laryngeal involvement, a muffled quality of the voice may become apparent.

As is true for other squamous cell carcinomas of the head and neck, cancers of the base of tongue can grow either in an infiltrative or exophytic pattern. Careful physical examination delineates such growth. An important component of that evaluation should include digital and bimanual palpation. This delineates the extent of base of tongue involvement as well as determines whether or not disease has infiltrated into the preepiglottic space. Figure 30.2-15 shows routes of spread for squamous cell cancers for the base of tongue.

Base of tongue tumors have a high propensity for metastatic spread to lymph nodes. Nearly 70% of patients with T1 lesions have clinically palpable disease in the neck. The risk of nodal metastases increases with T stage, approaching 85% for T4 cancers.[553] Likewise, tumors of the base of tongue have a high propensity for bilateral cervical lymph node spread, occurring in approximately 30% of patients.[553] Therapy should account for this propensity even in circumstances of early primary disease. Lymph nodes commonly involved include levels II and III. Levels IV, V, and VI, however, are more frequently involved than many other cancers of the head and neck such as oral cavity lesions.

Prognosis for tongue base tumors is generally poor secondary to their advanced stage at presentation.[587–589] Stage I and II 5-year survival approximates 60% and 40%, respectively. Five-year survival for patients with stage III disease approximates 30%. For stage IV disease, survival diminished to 15% at 5 years.

TREATMENT

Early Disease

Early-stage cancer of the base of the tongue is readily treated by surgery or RT. Results are equivalent. Surgery for early unilateral lesions entails a hemiglossectomy. Surgical approaches can be transoral or by lateral pharyngotomy. The former approach entails a midline labiolingual split.

RT has a high prospect of cure without the functional deficit that occurs with operation. In general, treatment consists of 5000 to 5400 cGy with external-beam radiation and 2000 to 3000 cGy boost to the base of the tongue via an ^{192}Ir implant. There is debate in the radiation oncology literature as to whether or not to use an interstitial implant as the boost treatment. Altered fractionation programs can also be used, with either twice a day treatment or concomitant boost having its advocates.

Regional lymphadenectomy is recommended regardless of the primary size because of the high propensity for metastatic spread. Bilateral neck dissection is recommended for those lesions approaching midline structures.

Advanced Disease

For larger lesions involving the tongue base, primarily T4 lesions, total resection of tongue base, and total laryngectomy may be required. The addition of total laryngectomy may be dictated for several reasons. Tumor may infiltrate through the relatively thin hyoepiglottic ligament and extend well into the preepiglottic space. Laryngectomy is required as part of an *en bloc* procedure necessary to ensure complete extirpation of disease. Additionally, the removal of tongue and soft tissues of the neck (i.e., the preepiglottic space) impairs normal deglutition. With such surgery, chronic aspiration represents a major long-term complication. Total laryngectomy may represent the only means to isolate critical air exchange passages from oral secretions. The need for laryngectomy is increased in patients with diminished cardiopulmonary reserve. Restoring bulk of the base of tongue with myocutaneous flaps or free tissue transfer may minimize aspiration problems.[590] Nowadays, patients who would require a total laryngectomy can be managed with an organ-sparing program of chemotherapy and RT, reserving surgery for salvage.[591]

Extended supraglottic laryngectomy may be performed for smaller lesions involving the vallecula. Disease in such circumstances should not extend along the pharyngoepiglottic fold to involve lateral pharyngeal wall. In the circumstances in which such a procedure is performed, pretreatment assessment must in all circumstances confirm adequate cardiopulmonary reserve.

The need for mandibulectomy as part of the surgical procedure for tongue base tumors is controversial. The traditional surgical management involves the composite (jaw, tongue, neck) resection. Such an *en bloc* procedure ensues more adequate tumor removal, including tumor within surrounding lymphatics. Furthermore, closure of surgical defect is facilitated by such resection (i.e., soft tissues are able to collapse with removal of mandible).

Advances, both surgical and in our understanding of patterns of tumor spread, militate against the need for mandibulectomy. Soft tissue defects can be repaired with free-tissue transfer, thus facilitating wound closure. Studies of lymphatic spread of oropharyngeal tumors have shown that cancer not approximating periosteum rarely infiltrates mandible.[592] Resection of bone is thus not required for oncologic reasons.

Results of Treatment

Surgical results of early base of tongue cancers have been encouraging, with local control rates approximating 85%.[587,592,594] The major determinate of control rate is reflective in tumor growth patterns. Exophytic tumors are controlled in 84% of instances as opposed to 58% with ulcerative-infiltrative disease.[593] With advanced disease, initial surgery is associated with a high probability of positive margins (25%), thus emphasizing the need for combined modality therapy.[615]

Data from Harrison et al.,[595–598] Goffinet et al.,[599] and Puthawala et al.[600] show that the local control rate for T1 to T2 base of tongue tumors is in the 90% range when treated with external-beam RT plus implant. Harrison et al.[595,596] have reported long-term results on 68 patients treated between 1981 and 1995 with combined external-beam RT (54 Gy) plus ^{192}Ir implant (20 to 30 Gy), combined with neck dissection for patients presenting with positive nodes (Fig. 30.2-16 shows a clinical example; Table 30.2-23). Actuarial 5- and 10-year local control is 89% and 89%, distant metastasis-free survival is 91% and 76%, disease-free survival is 80% and 67%, and overall survival is 86% and 52%. All T stages (T1, 17 patients; T2, 32 patients; T3, 17 patients; T4, 2 patients) were combined together, as there were no differences when analyzed by T stage. When survival salvage is included, local control rises to 92%. Lee has reported that all 58 patients who underwent external-beam RT plus neck dissection (all of whom presented with palpable nodes) were regionally controlled at 10 years, and the majority had negative surgical experiences.[610] Harrison et al. reported detailed quality-of-life assessment on these patients, reporting that the majority of patients could maintain their incomes, employment status, and socioeconomic quality of life despite having advanced tongue cancer.[598] Understandability of speech and eating in public were excellent, but xerostomia was a major problem. Horowitz et al. also reported excellent performance status scores for eating in public, understandability of speech, and normalcy of diet for their patients treated with external-beam RT plus brachytherapy.[611] Finally, a comparison of the performance status outcomes of eating in public, understandability of speech, and normalcy of diet showed significant advantages in each category to primary radiotherapy over primary surgery.[598]

External-beam RT alone has its advocates.[607,608] However, the only study that sought to compare external-beam RT alone, external-beam RT plus implant, versus surgery plus postoperative radiation was done by Housset et al.[602] They found that the local control rate for both external-beam RT plus implant or surgery plus postoperative radiation was in the 80% range for

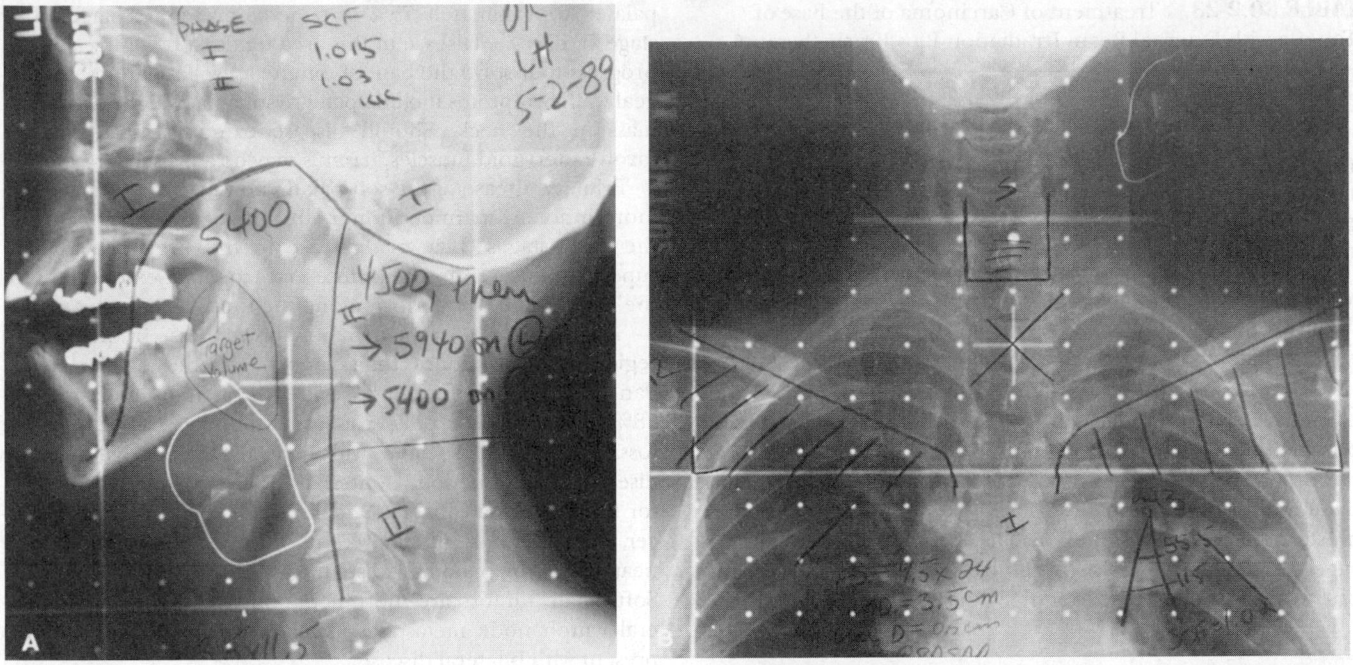

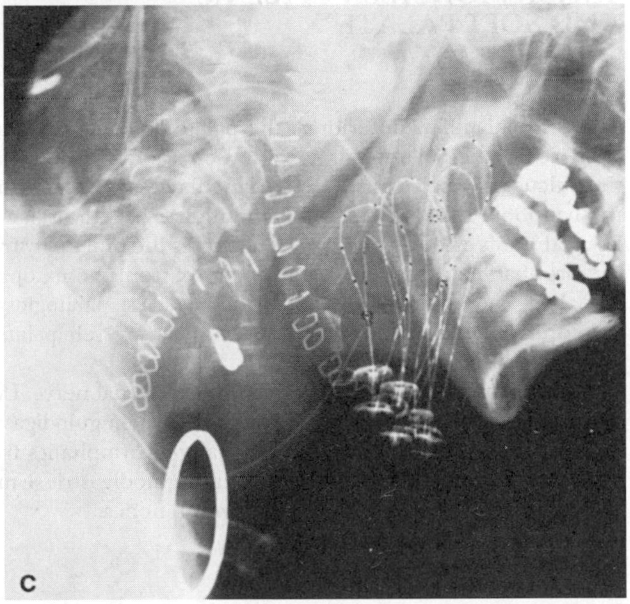

FIGURE 30.2-16. A patient with a T2N2 squamous cancer of the left side of the base of the tongue. The treatment plan consisted of initial external-beam radiation therapy to the primary site and the entire neck bilaterally. This was followed by a left radical neck dissection and an implant, both done with the same anesthesia. **A:** The simulation film shows the primary site outlined and the neck node with wire around it. A bite block is in place. A total of 4500 cGy was given to the primary site and both upper necks, after which a spinal cord block was placed. The primary and upper neck were then treated with 5400 cGy. Fraction size was 180 cGy/d. After that, the bed of the lymph node in the left neck was boosted on the right and to 5940 on the left. **B:** The low neck was treated with a single anterior field to 5000 cGy/5 weeks. A midline block protects the spinal cord at the field junction. **C:** Approximately 3 weeks after the external radiation was completed, the patient was taken to the operating room and a left radical neck dissection and an ^{192}Ir implant were done. The figure shows the catheters looped through the base of tongue by the submental approach. Also visible are the skin staples from the neck surgery. The implant delivered an additional 2800 cGy. The neck specimen was histologically negative. The patient had no evidence of disease at 6 years. He had a soft tissue ulcer in the tongue that healed with conservative management.

T1 and T2 lesions, as opposed to 50% for external-beam RT alone. Survival for external-beam RT alone was 17%, as opposed to more than 50% for the other two approaches.

Various hyperfractionated and accelerated fractionated regimens have been updated.[607–608] Mendenhall reported 5-year local control of 98% for T1, 91% for T2, 81% for T3, and 38% for T4, and advocated that radiotherapy was a better alternative than primary surgery.[607] Moore et al. reported quality-of-life data on the same group of patients, suggesting excellent outcomes with respect to eating in public, understandability of speech, and good outcomes for normalcy of diet.[609] Neck dissection did not have a major effect on the performance status measurements. Morrison has also reported good outcomes using an accelerated fractionation, concomitant boost technique for oropharynx carcinomas of all subsites.[608] However, all patients developed severe mucositis, and there was a growing risk of bone complications and swallowing problems and gastrostomy tube dependence with longer follow-up. Mak et al. reported that this concomitant boost program of 72 Gy in 6 weeks produced local control at 5 years of 76% (T1 = 100%, T2 = 96%, T3 = 67%), with disease-specific survival of 65% and overall survival of 59%.[605]

Implants have also been used for patients who have received prior RT to the oropharynx, who developed either recurrent base of tongue cancers or a second primary cancer in the base of tongue.[601] Housset et al. reported on 55 patients who had received prior irradiation and in whom they performed ^{192}Ir implants.[606] The local control rate was in the 50% to 60% range. Vikram et al. reported on ten patients who had previously treated base of tongue lesions.[603] All ten received

TABLE 30.2-23. Treatment of Carcinoma of the Base of Tongue with External-Beam Irradiation Plus Brachytherapy[a]

T Stage	*Crude Local*[b] Control	*Surgical* Salvage	*Overall Crude* Control
T1	10/11	1/1	11/11
T2	13/14	1/1	14/14
T3	8/10	—	8/10
T4	1/1	—	1/1

[a]Crude local control, including salvage by T stage.
[b]Number of patients controlled/total number of patients.

implants in an attempted salvage maneuver. Local control was obtained in 60% of the patients, with size being the most important prognostic feature. No local failures occurred in patients who had lesions less than or equal to 4 cm, whereas most of the patients with lesions larger than 4 cm were not salvaged. Overall survival in the entire group was poor, mainly due to uncontrolled recurrent neck disease.

TONSIL, TONSILLAR PILLAR, AND SOFT PALATE

ANATOMY

The tonsillar pillars anteriorly (the palatoglossal muscle) and posteriorly (the palatopharyngeal muscle) and the glossopalatini sulcus inferiorly constitute a triangular region that houses the lymphoid tonsillar tissue. Extending from the tonsillar pillars is the soft palate. The latter demarcates the oral cavity from the oropharynx as well as the oropharynx from the nasopharynx. It is composed of the following muscles: palatoglossus, palatopharyngeus, levator veli palatine, tensor veli palatine, and the musculus uvulae.

Nerve supply to this region is via the trigeminal nerve. Lymphatics from the tonsillar region drain into the jugulodigastric basin as well as the submandibular triangle. Lymphatics from the soft palate drain into the upper jugulodigastric lymph nodes as well as the retropharyngeal lymph nodes.

PATHOLOGY

As in other sites within the upper aerodigestive tract, the near total lesions involving this region are squamous cell carcinoma. Occasionally, lymphoepitheliomas have been identified within the tonsillar fossa. Other cancers include lymphomas and those derived from minor salivary glands.

NATURAL HISTORY

Cancers of these three sites may present and spread in a variety of means. Cancers of the tonsillar pillar tend to be more superficial than those of the tonsillar fossa. Tonsillar pillar cancers progress over a broad region including lateral soft palate, retromolar trigone and buccal mucosa, tonsillar fossa, as well as the glossopalatini sulcus.

Tonsillar fossa cancers more often present in advanced-stage disease than either cancers of the tonsillar pillar or soft palate. Approximately 75% of patients present as stage III or stage IV disease. Disease in this area tends to be bulky and can progress to involve the base of tongue as well as lateral pharyngeal wall. Symptoms include pain, dysphagia, weight loss, and a mass in the neck. Should disease extend posteriorly and involve pterygoid muscles, trismus may be a presenting sign.

Primary disease of the soft palate, however, may behave in a more indolent manner. Tumors in this region may remain in the early stages. Likewise, disease in this area may remain superficial, presenting as diffuse erythroplakia extending into the hard palate or inferiorly along the tonsillar pillar.

Tonsillar pillar cancers metastasize less frequently to regional lymph nodes than cancers of the tonsillar fossa. Patients present with clinical evidence of nodal metastases in 38% of T2 tonsillar pillar cancers, while 68% of T2 tonsillar fossa lesions are associated with clinically evident lymph node disease at presentation. Contralateral metastases are common for tonsillar fossa cancers. Nodal disease in tonsillar fossa cancer, likewise, most often presents in an advanced stage with nearly 55% of patients presenting with N2 or N3 disease.[553] Soft palate tumors are more commonly associated with bilateral lymph node metastases. Approximately 20% of patients present with bilateral disease.[553]

Prognosis for tonsillar fossa cancers ranges from 93% for stage I disease to 17% for stage IV disease.[612–615] For soft palate lesions, 5-year survival ranges from 21% to 85% depending on disease stage.[616–618]

TREATMENT

Early Disease

Except in circumstances of early disease, the distinction between cancers arising in the tonsillar fossa versus tonsillar pillar cannot be made. Early cancers of this region can be treated by single modality therapy, either surgery or RT.

Surgical resection of early disease can occasionally be done transorally. Such an approach, however, should be performed only in circumstances in which free surgical margins can be ensured. Better exposure to early cancers of this region may also be obtained through a combined lip-splitting incision coupled with an anterior midline or lateral mandibulotomy. Careful dissection thus proceeds by first identifying anterior lateral margins. If tumors extend to the periosteum of the mandible but remain superficial, partial mandibulectomy may be performed. Partial mandibulectomy includes a coronal resection, which leaves the body and the ascending ramus of the mandible in continuity.

Early squamous cell carcinomas of the tonsillar region can, likewise, be treated with RT. Radiation can be delivered with either external beam, interstitial implant, or a combination of both. In general, radiation is preferred because it offers excellent cure rates and more comprehensive treatment of primary site, retropharyngeal nodes, and neck, all with a potentially better functional outcome.

Given the high propensity for even early cancers of this region to metastasize to cervical lymph nodes, cervical lymphadenectomy should be included as part of the surgical resection. The various types of neck dissections that could be used have been discussed (see Surgical Management of the Cervical Lymph Nodes, earlier in this chapter). Our choice for early lesions in which cervical

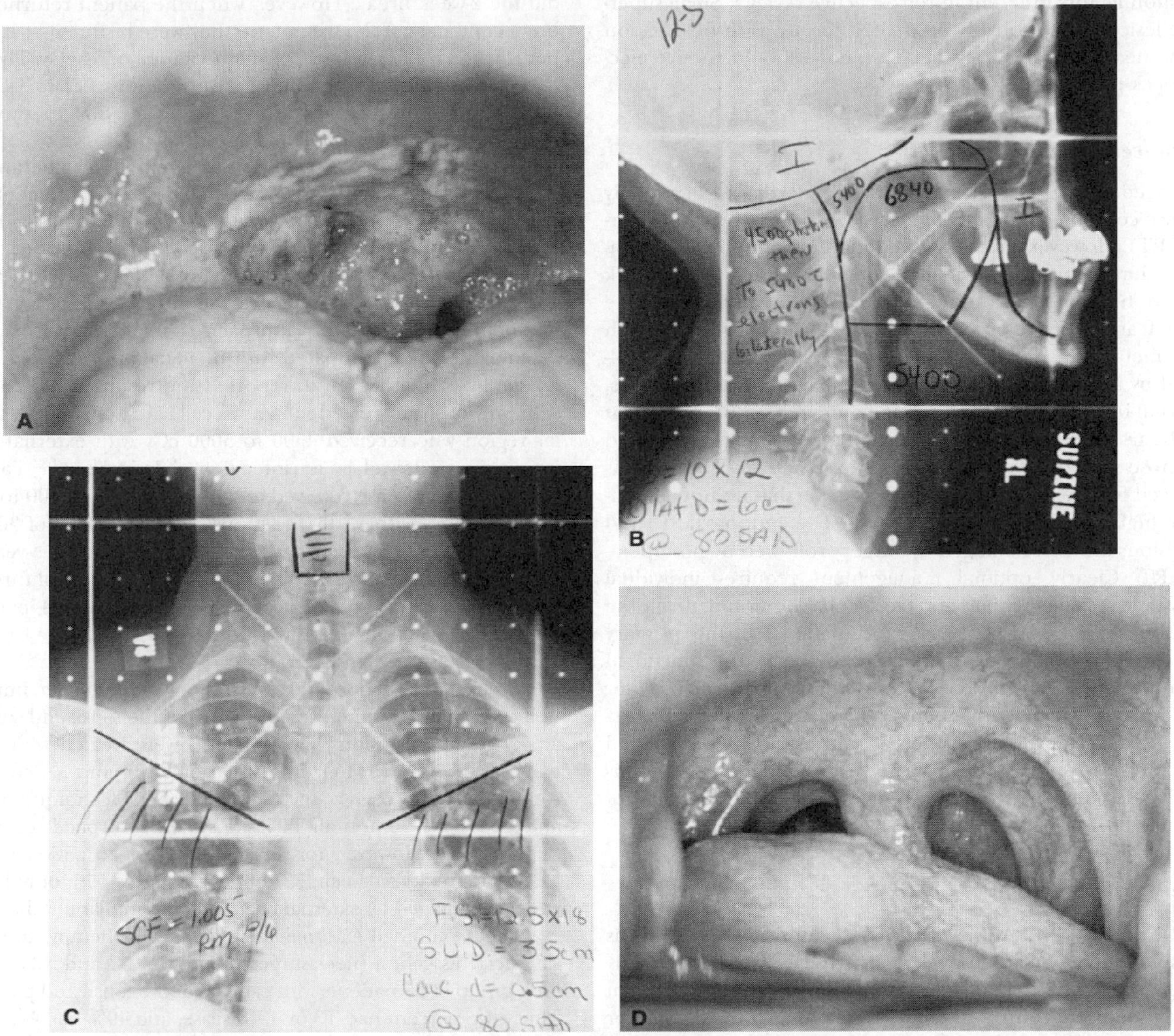

FIGURE 30.2-17. **A:** A patient with a T2N0 squamous cancer of the soft palate. He was treated with external-beam radiation therapy to the primary site and to both necks. Opposed lateral portals were used with a low anterior neck field. **B** and **C:** The simulated fields are shown. The primary site and both upper necks were then treated with 5400 cGy, including the retropharyngeal nodes. The primary site was treated to a total of 6840 cGy. The patient is asked not to swallow during treatment, so the palate remains in position. Adequate margin is placed around the palate in its plane of motion to avoid geographic miss. Fraction size is 180 cG/d. The lower neck is treated with an anterior portal to 5000 cGy/5 weeks, thereby delivering elective nodal irradiation to that site. The posterior necks are boosted with electrons to 5400 cGy to protect the spinal cord. The spinal cord is protected at the junction of the lateral fields with the low anterior neck field by a midline block in the low neck field. This block also protects the larynx. For this purpose, the field is purposely junctioned above the thyroid notch but below the hyoid bone. **D:** The patient had no evidence of disease at 2.5 years.

lymph nodes are not clinically involved with disease would include a modified supraomohyoid neck dissection. Debate exists as to whether or not such dissection should be performed in continuity with extirpation of the primary disease. Where possible, in continuity dissection should be advocated.

When applying RT as the primary treatment modality, it is usually possible to treat the ipsilateral neck alone and avoid contralateral neck irradiation. With such treatment, radiation dosage to the contralateral salivary gland is minimized, thereby reducing the incidence of xerostomia. Due to the rich lymphatic network in the oropharyngeal region, it is standard practice to radiate the neck in all patients. This includes the retropharyngeal nodes. In fact, one advantage of using radiation is the inclusion of these nodes in the treatment, which is not included in primary surgical management.

Early-stage soft palate tumors are readily treated with RT. Treatment can be delivered with external beam, brachytherapy, or a combination of both. Figure 30.2-17 shows the external-beam technique in a typical patient. Most patients do not have palpable cervical lymph node metastases on presentation. It is unclear whether or not all patients require prophylactic neck treatment. Both prophylactic neck irradiation and observation alone have been used by various authors[619,620] with a successful outcome. Of course, this is retrospective and subject to the selection factors inherent in retrospective reviews. Small superficial lesions can probably be treated locally, with observation of the neck. Larger T1 and all T2 lesions should receive elective neck treatment.

Advanced Disease

Advanced cancers (i.e., stage III and stage IV disease) generally require combined modality therapy (i.e., surgery and postoperative RT). However, there has been increasing interest in radiation alone for the primary site, combined with neck dissection.[621–623] Clearly, the choice of treatment relates to the exact T and N stage. For early (T1 to T2) primary lesions with neck metastases, definitive radiation to the primary neck, followed by a neck dissection, is commonly used. For T3 lesions, external-beam radiation alone or combined with an implant can be used for the primary site, with a neck dissection added for those with involved nodes. This approach for T3 lesions is reserved for the exophytic lesions, or those that do not demonstrate highly infiltrative characteristics. The endophytic T3 and T4 lesions are best managed by surgery followed by postoperative RT. Clearly, optimal management requires individual assessment of each patient and close collaboration between the surgeon, radiation oncologist, and patient. If the primary lesion can be managed by radiation, however, the functional outcome with regard to speech and swallowing is usually better than surgically managed patients. The extent of surgical resection should be governed by the size of the primary disease and its pattern of spread. Tumor-free surgical margins generally entail a segmental mandibulectomy in most circumstances of advanced disease in the tonsillar region.

Results of Treatment

TONSILLAR PILLARS AND FOSSA. Surgical resection as the sole modality of therapy for early disease is not frequently used in most series. However, studies have demonstrated that when used, local control rates are excellent.[624] Indeed, even for advanced tumors in highly selected instances, effective local control can approach 80%.[624] The degree to which local control can be obtained depends on disease extension outside the tonsillar fossa. When disease extends to lateral pharyngeal wall or base of tongue, local recurrence approaches 33% and 47%, respectively.[624–626]

Wong et al. have reported the results of definitive external-beam irradiation for 150 patients with previously untreated squamous cell carcinoma of the tonsillar fossa.[627] Most patients were treated with conventional fractionation with total doses in the 6400 to 7200 cGy range. Local control was obtained in 15 of 16 (94%) patients with T1 lesions, and 51 of 52 (79%) patients with T2 lesions. Other series have reported local control rates for T2 lesions approximating 60%.[625,628–632] When surgical salvage is added, local control was 100% for T1 and 85% for T2. Wang has used an accelerated hyperfractionation program for oropharyngeal tumors.[628] During an earlier time period, patients received 1.6 cGy per fraction, two fractions per day, to a total of 38.4 cGy. Due to acute toxicity, a 2-week break was then given. Treatment was then resumed at 1.8 cGy per fraction, one fraction per day, to a total of 65 cGy. This was called the BID-QD program. More recently, the treatment regimen was changed. The initial treatment remained the same, as did the 2-week break. However, when the patient returned for the second part of the treatment, they were resumed at 1.6 cGy per fraction, two fractions per day, to a total of 64 cGy. This was called the BID-BID program. For tonsil lesions (T1 to T4), the 36-month actuarial local control after irradiation therapy was 93% versus 64% for the BID-QD program.

There has been increasing interest in brachytherapy for selected tonsillar lesions.[632–634] Levendag et al. used fractionated high dose-rate or pulsed dose-rate brachytherapy as a boost, combined with external-beam irradiation for a cohort of tonsillar and soft palate lesions.[634] There were 5 T1, 22 T2, 10 T3, and 1 T4 lesions. Local failure occurred in 13% of cases. These authors believed that this approach was superior to external-beam alone when compared with their data for external beam RT alone. Puthawala et al. reported the results of 80 patients with previously untreated squamous cell carcinoma of the tonsillar region who received 4500 to 5000 cGy with external-beam irradiation, followed by an interstitial ^{192}Ir implant.[632] Patients with T1 or T2 disease received an implant boost to 2000 to 2500 cGy, and those with T3 to T4 lesions received a boost of 3000 to 4000 cGy. Overall local control was 84%, and absolute 3-year disease-free survival was 72%. When looked at by stage, all three T1 patients obtained local control. For T2, T3, and T4 patients, local control was obtained in 14 of 15 (93%), 32 of 43 (74%), and 11 of 19 (58%), respectively.

Mazeron et al. reported the results of external beam, implant, or a combination of the two, for lesions of the tonsil and soft palate.[623] For tonsil lesions, most patients were treated with 45-Gy external beam plus 31-Gy interstitial brachytherapy. A comparison was made for each of the radiotherapeutic techniques for T1 and T2 lesions. Almost all T1 lesions were controlled regardless of technique. However, for T2 disease, 7 of 26 patients failed locally after external-beam RT alone, compared with only 1 of 43 patients managed by external-beam RT plus implant. Behar et al. evaluated combined external-beam RT, brachytherapy, and adjuvant neck dissection (neck surgery mainly for N2 and N3 disease) for a group of 37 patients with cancers of the tonsil and palate.[622] Thirty-two percent had T3 or T4 disease, and 49% had N2 or N3 neck metastases. Local control was obtained in 95% of cases, and neck control was achieved in 87%. Actuarial 5-year survival was 64%, and approximately 25% of the patients developed a second primary cancer.

Pernot et al. accumulated a large series of 361 patients with cancers of the tonsil and soft palate who were managed either by brachytherapy alone or a combination of external-beam irradiation (50 Gy) plus a brachytherapy boost (20 to 30 Gy).[621] In total, 64% of patients had T1 to T2 lesions, and 64% were N0. Only two patients had T4 disease. A select group of 18 patients with small T1 lesions were managed by brachytherapy alone, and all were locally controlled. All others received combined external-beam RT plus implant. Local control was 89% for T1, 85% for T2, and 67% for T3 lesions. The group with lesions on the soft palate, tonsillar fossa, and posterior pillar had a better outcome than those with lesions on the anterior pillar and glossotonsillar sulcus. For T3 lesions, the local control with external-beam irradiation falls considerably. However, it would appear that the subset of T3 tumors with tongue involvement have the highest local failure rate. Tong et al. reported that 18 of 39 (46%) T3 patients ultimately had failures in the primary site after external-beam irradiation.[625] Interestingly, all 18 patients who failed had lesions that extended into the base of tongue. Mendenhall has reported that the addition of interstitial implant to the base of tongue, after external-beam irradiation, can improve the local control.[635] In their T3 patients with base of tongue extension, only five of nine patients were controlled with external-beam RT alone, as compared with 13 of 17 who had full-dose external-beam RT plus a localized base of tongue implant. Puthawala et al. reported local control in 16 of 19 patients with T3 N0 lesions, and 5 of 6 patients with T3 N1 lesions, all treated with external-beam RT and implant.[632] Wong et al. reported local control in only 58% of patients with T3 treated with external-beam RT alone.[627] Leborgne analyzed 140 patients with tonsil cancer who received definitive radiation.[654] The subgroup of patients with lingual extension who had an implant as part of their treatment had better local control than those who received external-beam RT alone. Thus, it appears that many T3 lesions and those with lingual extension may be best served with the addition of an implant, if radiation is used as the primary modality. It would therefore appear that the results of external-beam radiation alone for T3 tonsillar cancer are suboptimal. The addition of an interstitial implant may improve the results in selected patients. There may also be a role for a combination of surgery and radiation.

For T1 to T2, N0 to N1 patients, it is usually possible to treat the ipsilateral neck alone and avoid contralateral neck irradiation. By doing this, the radiation dosage to the contralateral salivary gland tissue is minimized, and the incidence of xerostomia is significantly reduced. Murthy and Hendrickson reported that none of their 20 patients with N0 or N1 disease failed in the untreated contralateral neck when the primary and ipsilateral neck were controlled.[636] Tong et al. reported that none of their patients with either T1 N0 or T2 N0 lesions failed in either neck despite the fact that approximately 40% of the cases had ipsilateral treatment only.[625] It is considered safe to omit contralateral neck treatment in most of these early lesions, as long as there is no extension into the base of tongue or significant extension onto the soft palate.

The management of patients with more advanced lesions is somewhat controversial.[635–640] There are advocates of RT alone,[635] reserving surgery for salvage only. Others advocate a approach involving surgery and postoperative radiation.[637,638] Perez et al. analyzed 296 patients with epidermoid carcinoma of the tonsillar fossa.[629] In this group, 127 received radiation alone, 133 were planned to have preoperative RT, and 36 received surgery plus postoperative radiation. There was no statistically significant difference in 3-year disease-free survival for T1 to T2, N0 to N2 patients with radiation alone versus radiation combined with surgery. In patients with T4 or N3 disease, there was an advantage to combined treatment over radiation alone, suggesting a benefit for those who had surgery. The authors concluded that radiation alone was the treatment of choice for early-stage lesions, but there might be an advantage in selected advanced stage patients for a combination of surgery and postoperative irradiation. Dasmahapatra et al., likewise, report that the 5-year survival for patients who had combined radiation and surgery was better than those who had radiation alone in the stage III and IV categories.[637] Spiro and Spiro could not demonstrate a benefit in survival when patients with stage III and IV disease were treated with either radiotherapy alone, surgery alone, or combined surgery and irradiation.[639] This may be a reflection of selection bias, with more advanced and less favorable patients being treated with surgery and radiation combined. The RTOG[574] has performed a prospective randomized trial and analyzed various combinations of radiation and surgery for patients with advanced squamous cell cancer of the oropharynx. Patients with oropharynx tumors were randomized to receive preoperative RT (5000 cGy) plus surgery, surgery plus postoperative RT (6000 cGy), or RT alone (6500 to 7000 cGy) with surgery reserved for salvage. This study revealed that the overall survival, as well as the estimated 4-year local regional control rate, was not statistically different in any of the arms. One of the weaknesses of this study is that it did not stratify the results by subsite within the oropharynx. It is therefore impossible to determine what the specific results would be for tonsil patients. Clearly, treatment must be individualized from patient to patient and should attempt to provide the highest rate of cure as well as the best functional and quality-of-life outcome.

SOFT PALATE. There have been emerging data over the past few years advocating the use of brachytherapy for small soft palate lesions.[619,634,641,642] Mazeron et al. reported on 59 T1 and T2 squamous cancer of the soft palate and uvula treated with definitive irradiation.[633] Sixteen patients had external-beam RT alone, 14 had ^{192}Ir implantation alone, and 29 had a combination of external-beam RT plus brachytherapy. Local failure occurred in 25% (4 of 16) after external irradiation alone, 18% (5 of 19) after combined external-beam RT and implant, but in 0% (0 of 14) in the group selected for ^{192}Ir implant alone. This group preferred the plastic tube technique over the guide gutter technique for implantation. It is unclear exactly how the patients were selected for each of the treatment strategies. The authors believed that severe dry mouth was less frequent in those patients who received all or part of the treatment by implantation compared with those who had external-beam irradiation alone. Similarly, Sealy et al. reported excellent control rates in patients with early squamous cell cancer of the soft palate and uvula treated with ^{192}Ir implants.[641]

Pernot et al. have reported on 277 patients treated for carcinoma of the oropharynx by exclusive RT.[620] The group (212 patients) lumped soft palate and tonsil and posterior pillar lesions together in the reporting of results. Nine percent of these patients had soft palate lesions. In this group, 7% (8 of 121) of the T1 and T2 lesions exhibited recurrence; 27% (23 of 85) recurred in the T3 category. The overall local control at 5 years was 83%. This series has been updated (361 patients) and already quoted in the section on tonsil cancer. Local control was 89% for T1, 85% for T2, and 67% for T3 lesions. All 18 patients managed by brachytherapy alone for small T1 lesions had local control.

The results of the study by Levendag et al.[634] have already been described in the Tonsillar Pillars and Fossa section, but included patients with lesions of either the tonsil or the soft palate. Amdur et al. reported an analysis of 75 patients with squamous cell carcinoma of the soft palate, uvula, or both treated with RT alone or in combination with neck dissection.[643] Most patients received 6000 to 7500 cGy. Local control was obtained in all 8 patients with T1 disease, and 14 of 19 patients with T2 disease. Including surgical salvage, 16 of 19 T2 patients obtained ultimate local control (84%). The results were far worse for T3 and T4 disease, with local control being 45% and 25%, respectively, for continuous course external-beam irradiation. This series highlights the poor results achieved with RT for advanced disease, with quite good results for early-stage disease with external-beam RT alone. Clearly, from an oncologic point of view, there is no definitive proof that brachytherapy is required for early-stage soft palate tumors. However, there may be a rationale for using implant as all or part of the treatment in an effort to improve the functional outcome with regard to salivary gland function. Obviously, brachytherapy spares the major salivary glands from receiving significant doses of radiation and decreases the risk of xerostomia. Proper patient selection is required, and the radiation oncologist must have expertise in performing a palatal implant.

Although the local control is excellent for early-stage disease, the overall survival may not necessarily reflect the high local control rate. Intercurrent illness as well as the problem of second primary malignancies represent a significant cause of mortality in this population.[619,643]

Complications from RT are in the 10% range, with severe complications, principally osteonecrosis of the mandible requiring surgical resection, occurring in 5% or less.[619,641,642]

Whether elective neck treatment is required remains an open question. The probability of neck recurrence in patients with early disease is low, regardless of whether or not the neck is treated prophylactically.[619]

Most advanced soft palate tumors should be treated with combined surgery and postoperative radiation. Amdur et al. reported that the results of external-beam RT alone for T3 and T4 disease were suboptimal.[643]

PHARYNGEAL WALL

EPIDEMIOLOGY

Epidemiologic considerations are as discussed for oropharyngeal cancers.

ANATOMY

The pharyngeal wall within the oropharynx extends from the nasopharynx at a line demarcated by the soft palate to the level of the vallecular. It comprises the posterolateral surfaces of the oropharynx. The pharyngeal constrictor muscles constitute the structural framework of the pharyngeal wall. Nerve supply is from the pharyngeal branches of the ninth and tenth cranial nerves. Blood supply is largely from the ascending pharyngeal and superior thyroid arteries, both emanating from the external carotid artery.

The pharyngeal wall is rich in lymphatics. Primary drainage is to retropharyngeal lymph nodes as well as nodes in levels II and III.

PATHOLOGY

The near total majority of lesions on the pharyngeal wall are squamous cell carcinomas. Occasional minor salivary gland lesions have been identified.

NATURAL HISTORY

Tumors of the posterior pharyngeal wall are generally identified in the late stages. This is due to the silent location in which they develop. Symptoms at presentation include pain and bleeding. Weight loss is common. Likewise, patients may present with a mass in the neck as their initial symptom. Disease spread can be superiorly to involve the nasopharynx. Posteriorly, disease may infiltrate the prevertebral fascia. Inferiorly, disease spreads to involve the pyriform sinuses and hypopharyngeal walls.

Pharyngeal wall tumors have a propensity for cervical lymph node metastases. Clinically palpable disease is identified in 25% of patients with T1 lesions, 30% of T2 lesions, 66% of T3 lesions, and over 75% of patients with T4 disease. Given that most pharyngeal wall tumors extend past the midline, bilateral cervical metastases are common.

Prognosis for pharyngeal wall cancers ranges from 75% for stage I disease, 70% for stage II, 42% for stage III, to 27% for stage IV disease.[644–653]

TREATMENT

Early Disease

Early-stage disease of the pharyngeal wall can be treated by either surgery or radiation. Given the functional impairment that may result from surgical reaction, RT is generally preferred. Surgical resection generally entails a (transhyoid) approach to gain access to the lesion.[645] Wide excision of such lesions includes underlying prevertebral fascia. Split-thickness skin graft coverage is required. A significant morbidity following surgical resection is impaired swallowing secondary to resection of pharyngeal wall musculature.

Bilateral modified neck dissections are indicated in patients with early pharyngeal wall cancers.

An important issue in planning the RT for posterior pharyngeal wall tumors is the proximity of the spinal cord to the primary tumor volume. When opposed lateral fields are used, and the spinal cord block is placed, the posterior edge of the field is dangerously close to the posterior aspect of the tumor. It is important to use a sharp beam edge, so as to avoid underdosing the posterior aspect of the tumor, which can fall in the penumbra of the beam. This is best accomplished by avoiding cobalt 60 and using a 4- or 6-MeV photon beam. Cerrobend blocks are used to define the posterior border. It is also important to make this border as posterior as possible. It has been our practice to place this border at the anterior-most aspect of the spinal cord. This is much closer to the spinal cord than in most other head and neck situations. Frequent portal films must be taken to ensure the accuracy of this field, and for maximal spinal cord protection. This situation represents a difficult challenge to the radiation oncologist. One of the potential advantages to brachytherapy is the delivery of high doses to the tumor with relative sparing of the spinal cord. However, in order for this technique to be useful, tumors have to be relatively small and discrete. Often, this is not the situation.

Advanced Disease

Advanced disease of the posterior pharyngeal wall is best handled by multimodality therapy. Surgery generally involves a total laryngopharyngectomy. Reconstruction under such circumstances includes either a pectoralis major myocutaneous flap, gastric pull-up, or free-flap transposition with microvascular anastomoses. Free-flap transposition entails a jejunal interposition and is becoming the procedure of choice. Rehabilitation and swallowing with the latter procedure is hastened. This allows for more expeditious use of postoperative radiotherapy.

The use of radiotherapy postoperatively is generally recommended. The high incidence of retropharyngeal lymph node metastases and the associated increased local regional failure rate mandates aggressive multimodality treatment.[647]

Results of Treatment

Guillamondegui et al. have reported on the surgical management of pharyngeal wall carcinomas.[644] Twenty-eight percent of the entire patient population developed local regional recurrence. Local recurrence predominated. It was of note in that series that salvage therapy consisting of either surgery or radiation was successful in 9 of 22 patients. The success of therapy was governed by the presence of retropharyngeal nodes, with only 25% of such patients disease free at 2 years.

Meoz-Mendes et al. have reported on 164 patients with squamous cell carcinoma of the pharyngeal walls who were treated with definitive RT at the M. D. Anderson Hospital.[648] Their report included patients with both oropharynx and hypopharynx lesions. The primary sites were generally irradiated to a dose of 7000 to 7500 cGy in 7 to 7.5 weeks. Local control was 71% for T1, 73% for T2, 61% for T3, and 37% for T4. The authors recommended RT alone for T1 and T2 lesions. They concluded that resectable T3 and T4 lesions should be treated with combined surgery and radiation.

Marks et al. reported the experience from Washington University on 51 patients with pharyngeal wall cancer treated between 1964 and 1974.[649] Survival was no different for patients treated with low-dose preoperative radiation plus surgery versus those treated with high-dose radiation alone. However, this was not randomized, and the surgical techniques were not standardized. Survival was also poor, with actuarial 3-year survival of 17%. There was a greater complication rate in the patients receiving surgery, with 31% having pharyngocutaneous fistula, 14% having carotid rupture, and an operative mortality of 14%. Marks et al. updated this series with a total of 89 patients treated between 1964 and 1981.[650] Their update led to the suggestion that combined surgery and radiation might yield better results than high-dose radiation alone. Again, definitive conclusions are difficult to make.

Fein et al. analyzed the treatment factors for 99 patients with pharyngeal wall cancer treated with definitive external-beam irradiation at the University of Florida between 1964 and 1990.[651] The main issues relate to the fractionation schedule (once daily vs. twice daily) and the location of the posterior border of the irradiation field (midvertebral body vs. posterior edge of the vertebral body). Local control is clearly improved when the posterior body of the field is maximally posterior, thus allowing better coverage of the posterior wall. This places significant technical demands on the radiation oncologist, who must verify the safety of this border with respect to the spinal cord on the daily treatment setup. Local control with the border at midvertebral body versus posterior was T1, 100% for both; T2, 57% versus 100%; T3, 46% versus 73%; and T4, 29% versus 75%. Local control for continuous course once daily versus twice daily fractionation was T1, 100% for both; T2, 67% versus 92%; T3, 43% versus 80%; and T4, 17% versus 50%. Clearly, the technical and fractionation parameters were less significant for early lesions, but increasingly important for more advanced lesions.

Spiro et al. reported a 12-year experience from the Memorial Sloan-Kettering Cancer Center.[652] A variety of operations were used over this time. There was no standardized treatment, and at least eight different treatment approaches were used during this time period, representing various combinations of surgery, radiotherapy, and chemotherapy. This heterogeneity of treatment approaches highlights the uncertainty as to the optimal management of this disease and the variety of disease presentations. Five-year survival was 32%, and the overall complication rate was 50%. A small group of patients were treated with ^{125}I implant to the primary site, followed by external-beam RT. The implants were done using surgery for access. Local control in this small group of patients was excellent. Son and Kacinski reported 14 patients treated with a combination of implant and external-beam radiation.[653] Twelve patients had locoregional control, and 18% developed reversible soft tissue and mucosal injury as a result of the RT. It would appear that this technique deserves further investigation. It represents a mechanism for delivering definitive RT with high doses to the tumor. However, it is certainly clear that optimal therapy for tumors in this site has yet to be defined.

REFERENCES

1. Schantz SP, Harrison LH, Forastiere A. Tumors of the nasal cavity and paranasal sinuses, nasopharynx, oral cavity, and oropharynx. In: DeVita VT, Hellman S, Rosenberg SA, eds. *Cancer: principles and practices of oncology.* Philadelphia: Lippincott,1997:742.
2. Shah JP, Strong E, Spiro RH, Vikram B. Neck dissections current status and future possibilities. *Clin Bull* 1981;11:25.
3. Suen JY, Goepfert H. Editorial standardization of neck dissection nomenclature. *Head Neck Surg* 1987;10:75.
4. Jacobsson P, Killander D, Moberger G, et al. Histologisk Klassifikation och malignitets gradering vid larynx cancer. *Proc Swedish Soc Med Radiol* March 11, 1972.
5. Eneroth CM, Moberger G. Histological malignancy grading of squamous cell carcinoma of the palate. *Acta Otolaryngol* 1973;75:293.
6. Anneroth G, Batsakis J, Kyba N. Review of the literature and recommended system of malignancy grading in oral squamous cell carcinoms. *Scand J Dent Res* 1987;95:229.
7. Byrne M, Koppang HS, Lilling R, et al. New malignancy grading is a better prognostic indicator than Broder's grading in oral squamous cell carcinomas. *J Oral Path Oral Med* 1989;18:432.
8. Pindborg JJ. Oral precancer. In: Barnes L, ed. *Surgical pathology of the head and neck.* Vol. 1. New York: Marcel Dekker, 1985:279.
9. Pindborg JJ. *Oral cancer and precancer.* Bristol, John Wright and Sons, 1980.
10. Cawson RA. Premalignant lesions in the mouth. *Br Med Bull* 1975;31:164.
11. Shafer WG, Waldron CA. Erythroplakia of the oral cavity. *Cancer* 1975;36:1021.
12. Mincer HH, Coleman SA, Hopkins KP. Observations on the clinical characteristics of oral lesions showing histologic epithelial dysplasia. *Oral Surg* 1972;33:389.
13. Silverman S, Gorsky M, Lozada F. Oral leukoplakia and malignant transformation: a follow-up study of 257 patients. *Cancer* 1984;53:563.
14. American Joint Committee on Cancer. *Cancer staging manual,* 5th ed. Philadelphia, Lippincott, 1997:21.
15. Piccirillo JF. Purposes, problems, and proposals for purposes in cancer staging. *Arch Otolaryngol Head Neck Surg* 1995;121:145.
16. Bailey BJ. Beyond the TNM classification. *Arch Otolaryngol Head Neck Surg* 1991;117:369.
17. Madison MT, Remley KB, Latchaw RE, Mitchell SL. Radiologic diagnosis and staging of squamous cell carcinoma. *Radiol Clin North Am* 1994;32:163.
18. Som PM. Detection of metastasis in cervical lymph nodes: CT and MR criteria and differential diagnosis. *AJR Am J Roentgenol* 1992;158:961.
19. Close LG, Merkel M, Vuittch MF, Reisch J, Schaefer SD. Computed tomographic evaluation of regional lymph node involvement in cancer of the oral cavity and oropharynx. *Head Neck* 1989;11:309.
20. Brekel van den MWM, Castelijns JA, Croll GA, et al. Magnetic resonance versus palpation of cervical lymph node metastasis. *Arch Otolaryngol Head Neck Surg* 1991;117:666.
21. Brekel van den MWM, Stel HV, Castelijns JA, Croll GJ, Snow GB. Lymph node staging in patients with clinically negative neck examinations by ultrasound and ultrasound-guided aspiration cytology. *Am J Surg* 1991;162:362.
22. Madison MT, Remley KB, Latchaw RE, Mitchell SL. Radiologic diagnosis and staging of head and neck squamous cell carcinoma. *Otolaryngol Clin North Am* 1998;31:727.

23. Sing B, Baya M, Zimbler M, et al. Impact of morbidity on outcome of young patients with head and neck squamous cell carcinoma. *Head Neck* 1998;40:1.
24. Smart CR. Screening for cancer of the aerodigestive tract. *Cancer* 1993;72(Suppl):1061.
25. Prout MN, Morris SJ, Witzburg RA, Hurley C, Chatterjee S. A multidisciplinary educational program to promote head and neck cancer screening. *J Cancer Ed* 1992;7:139.
26. *Screening for oral cancer.* Report of the U.S. Preventive Services Task Force. Baltimore: Williams & Wilkins, 1989:91.
27. Jullien JA, Zakrsewska JM, Downer MC, Speight PM. Attendance and compliance at an oral cancer screening programme in general medical practice. *Eur J Cancer Oral Oncol* 1995;31B:202.
28. Frenandez GL, Sankaranarayanan R, Lence Anta JJ, Rodriguez Salva A, Maxwell Parkin D. An evaluation of the oral cancer control program in Cuba. *Epidemiology* 1995;6:428.
29. Ikeda N, Downer MC, Ishii T, et al. Annual screening for oral cancer and precancer by invitation to 60-year-old residents of a city in Japan. *Comm Dental Health* 1995;12:133.
30. Cowan CG, Gregg TA, Kee F. Prevention and detection of oral cancer: the views of primary care dentists in Northern Ireland. *Br Dental J* 1995;179:338.
31. Speight PM, Elliott AE, Jullien JA, Downer MC, Zakzrewska JM. The use of artificial intelligence to identify people at risk of oral cancer and precancer. *Br Dental J* 1995;179:382.
32. McGuire M, Lydiatt W, Trambert R, Shaha A, Schantz S. Head and neck screening day for the community. *Ann NY Acad Sci* 1995;768:286.
33. Sugarman PB, Savage NW. Exfoliative cytology in clinical oral pathology. *Aust Dental J* 1996;41:71.
34. Bongers V, Snow GB, deVries N, et al. Second primary head and neck squamous cell carcinoma predicted by the glutathione S-transferase expression in health tissue in the direct vicinity of the first tumor. *Lab Invest* 1995;73:503.
35. Sugarman PB, Savage NW. Exfoliative cytology in clinical oral pathology. *Aust Dental J* 1996;41:71.
36. Kurokawa H, Tsuru S, Okada M, Nakamura T, Kajiyama M. Evaluation of tumor markers in patients with squamous cell carcinoma in the oral cavity. *Int J Oral Maxillofasc Surg* 1993;22:35.
37. Schantz SP, Alfano RR. Tissue autofluorescence as an intermediate endpoint in cancer chemoprevention trials. *J Cell Biochem* 1993;(Suppl 17F):199.
38. Kolli V, Savage HE, Yao TJ, Schantz SP. Native cellular fluorescence of neoplastic upper aerodigestive mucosa. *Arch Otolaryngol Head Neck Surg* 1995;121:1287.
39. Tepperman BS, Fitzpatrick PJ. Second respiratory and upper digestive tract cancer after oral cancer. *Lancet* 1981;2:547.
40. Mao L, Hruban RH, Boyle JO, Tochman M, Sidransky D. Detection of oncogene mutations in sputum precedes diagnosis of lung cancer. *Cancer Res* 1994;54:1634.
41. Leipzig B, Zellmer JE, Klug D. The role of endoscopy in evaluating patients with head and neck cancer—a multi-institutional prospective study. *Arch Otolaryngol* 1985;111:589.
42. Shaha AR, Hoover EL, Mitrani M, Marti JR, Krespi YP. Synchronicity, multicentricity, and metachronicity of head and neck cancer. *Head Neck Surg* 1988;10:225.
43. Benninger MS, Enrique RR, Nichols RD. Symptom-directed selective endoscopy of head and neck cancer. *Head Neck* 1993;15:532.
44. deVries N, Gluckman JL, eds. *Multiple primary tumors in the head and neck.* Thieme, Stuttgart, 1990.
45. Lockhart PB, Clark J. Pretherapy dental status of patients with malignant conditions of the head and neck. *Oral Surg Oral Med Oral Pathol* 1994;77:236.
46. Keys HM, McCarland JP. Techniques and results of a comprehensive dental care program in head and neck cancer. *Int J Radiat Oncol Biol Phys* 1976;1:859.
47. Peterson DE. Non-surgical management of head and neck cancer patients. *Dental Clin North Am* 1994;38:435.
48. Goodwin WJ, Byers PM. Nutritional management of the head and neck cancer patient. *Med Clin North Am* 1993;77:597.
49. Goodwin WJ, Torres J. The value of the prognostic nutritional index in the management of patients with advanced carcinoma of the head and neck. *Head Neck Surg* 1984;6:932.
50. Hooley R, Levine H, Flores TC, et al. Predicting postoperative head and neck complications using nutritional assessment. *Arch Otolaryngol* 1983;109:83.
51. Kowalski LP, Alcantara PSM, Magrin J, Parise O. A case-control study on complications and survival in elderly patients undergoing head and neck surgery. *Am J Surg* 1984;168:485.
52. McGuirt WF, Davis SP. Demographic portrayal and outcome analysis of head and neck cancer surgery in the elderly. *Arch Otolaryngol Head Neck Surg* 1995;121:150.
53. Robinson DS. Head and neck considerations in the elderly patient. *Surg Clin North Am* 1994;431.
54. Clayman GL. Surgical outcomes in head and neck cancer patients 80 years of age and older. *Head Neck* 1998;20:216.
55. Day GL, Blot WJ, Shore RE, et al. Second primary cancer following oral and pharyngeal cancers: role of tobacco and alcohol. *J Natl Cancer Inst* 1994;86:131.
56. Cloos J, Leemans CR, van der Sterre MLT, et al. Mutagen sensitivity as a biomarker for second primary tumors after head and neck squamous cell carcinoma. *Cancer Epidemiol Biomarkers Prev* (*in press*).
57. Browman GP, Wong G, Hodson I, et al. Influence of cigarette smoking on the efficiency of radiation therapy in head and neck cancer. *N Engl J Med* 1993;328:159.
58. Gritz ER, Carr CR, Rapkin DA, et al. A smoking cessation intervention for head and neck cancer patients: trial design, patient accrual, and characteristics. *Cancer Epidemiol Biomarkers Prev* 1991;1:67.
59. Gritz ER, Carr CR, Rapkin D, et al. Predictors of long-term smoking cessation in head and neck cancer patients. *Cancer Epidemiol Biomarkers Prev* 1993;2:261.
60. Ostroff JS, Jacobsen PB, Moadel AB, et al. Prevalence and predictors of continued tobacco use following diagnosis of head and neck cancer. *Cancer* 1995;75:569.
61. Clayman GL, Raad II, Hankins PD, Weber RS. Bacteriologic profile of surgical infections after antibiotic prophylaxis. *Head Neck* 1993;15:526.
62. Robbins KT, Byers RM, Cole R, et al. Wound prophylaxis with metronidazole in head and neck surgical oncology. *Laryngoscope* 1988;98:803.
63. Becker GD, Welch WD. Quantitative bacteriology of intraoperative wound tissue in contaminated surgery. *Head Neck* 1990;12:293.
64. Johnson JT, Kachman K, Wagner RL, Myers EN. Comparison of ampicillin/sulbactam versus clindamycin. *Head Neck* 1997;19:367.
65. Weber RS, Lichtiger B, Byers RM, et al. Electro-surgical dissection for reducing blood loss in head and neck surgery. *Head Neck Surg* 1989;11:318.
66. Panje WR, Sher N, Karnell M. Transoral carbon dioxide laser ablation of cancers, tumors and other disease. *Arch Otolaryngol Head Neck Cancer Surg* 1981;115:681.
67. Gluckman JL, Waners M, Shumrick K, et al. Photodynamic therapy: a viable alternative to conventional therapy for early lesions of the upper aerodigestive tract. *Arch Otolaryngol Head Neck Surg* 1986;112:949.
68. Mohs FE, Snow SN. Microscopically controlled surgical treatment of squamous cell carcinoma of the lower lip. *Surg Gynecol Obstet* 1985;160:37.
69. Bocca E, Pignataro O. A conservation technique in radical neck dissection. *Ann Otol Rhinol Laryngol* 1967;76:975.
70. Medina JE. A rational classification of neck dissections. *Otolaryngol Head Neck Surg* 1989;100:169.
71. Robbins KT, Medina JE, Wolfe GT, et al. Standardizing neck dissection terminology. Official report of the Academy's Committee for Head and Neck Surgery and Oncology. *Arch Otolaryngol Head Neck Surg* 1991;117:601.
72. Byers RM, Wolf PF, Ballantyne AJ. Rationale for elective modified neck dissection. *Head Neck Surg* 1988;10:160.
73. Giacomarra V, Tirelli G, Papanikolla L, Bussani R. Predictive factors of nodal metastases in oral cavity and oropharynx carcinomas. *Laryngoscope* 1999;109:795.
74. Suen JY. *Management of the N0 neck.* Proceedings of the Fourth International Conference on Head and Neck Cancer. The Society of Head and Neck Surgeons and American Society of Head and Neck Surgery. Toronto. Madison, WI: Omnipres, 1996:557.
75. Byers RM, El-Naggar A, Lee YY, et al. Can we detect or predict the presence of occult nodal metastases in patients with squamous cell carcinoma of the oral tongue? *Head Neck* 1998;70:138.
76. Lydiatt WJ, Spiro RH, Strong EW, et al. Treatment of Stage I and II oral tongue cancer. *Head Neck* 1993;15:308.
77. Vandenbrouck C, Sancho-Garnier H, Chassange D, et al. Elective versus therapeutic radical neck dissection in epidermoid carcinoma of the oral cavity. Results of a randomized clinical trial. *Cancer* 1980;46:386.
78. Leemans CR, Snow GB. Is selective neck dissection really as efficacious as modified radical neck dissection for elective treatment of clinically negative neck in patients with squamous cell carcinoma of the upper extremity and digestive tracts? *Arch Otolaryngol Head Neck Surg* 1998;124:1042.
79. Brazilian Head and Neck Cancer Study Group. Results of a prospective trial on elective modified radical neck dissection versus supraomohyoid neck dissection in the management of oral squamous carcinoma. *Am J Surg* 1998;176:422.
80. Kraus DH, Rosenberg DB, Davidson BJ, et al. Supraspinal accessory lymph node metastases in supraomohyoid neck. *Am J Surg* 1996;172:646.
81. Traynor SJ, Cohen JI, Gray J, et al. Selective management of the node-positive neck. *Am J Surg* 1996;172:654.
82. Pellitari PK, Robbins KT, Neuman T. Expanded application of selective neck dissection with regard to nodal status. *Head Neck* 1997;19:260.
83. Myers EN, Fagan JJ. Treatment of the N+ neck in squamous cell carcinoma of the upper-aerodigestive tract. *Otolaryngol Clin North Am* 1998;31:671.
84. Carew JF, Spiro RH. Extended neck dissection. *Am J Surg* 1997;174:485.
85. Adams GL, Madison M, Remley K, Gapany M. Preoperative permanent balloon occlusion of internal carotid artery in patients with advanced head and neck squamous cell carcinoma. *Laryngoscope* 1999;109:460.
86. Snyderman CH, et al. Outcome of carotid artery resection for neoplastic disease: a meta-analysis. *Am J Otolaryngol* 1993;14:373.
87. Huvos AG, Leaming RH, Moore OS. Clinicopathologic study of the resected carotid artery: analysis of sixty-four cases. *Am J Surg* 1973;126:570.
88. Hays RJ, Levinson SA, Wylie EJ. Intraoperative measurement of carotid back pressure as a guide to operative management for carotid endarterectomy. *Surgery* 1972;72:953.
89. Peters LJ, Goepfert H, Ang KK, et al. Evaluation of the dose for postoperative radiation therapy of head and neck cancer: first report of a prospective randomized trial. *Int J Radiat Oncol Biol Phys* 1993;26:3.
90. Ang KK, Trotti A, Garden AS, et al. Impact of risk factors and total time for combined surgery and radiotherapy on the outcome of patients with advanced head and neck cancer. *Int J Radiat Oncol Biol Phys* 1999;45(Suppl):199.
91. Tupchong L, Scott C, Blitzer P, et al. Randomized study of pre-operative vs post-operative radiation therapy in advanced head and neck carcinoma: long term follow up of RTOG study 73-03. *Int J Radiat Oncol Biol Phys* 1991;20:21.
92. Fu KK, Pajak TF, Trotti A, et al. A Radiation Therapy Oncology Group (RTOG) phase II randomized study to compare hyperfractionation and two variants of accelerated fractionation to standard fractionation radiotherapy for head and neck squamous cell carcinomas: preliminary results of RTOG 90003. *Int J Radiat Oncol Biol Phys* 1999;45(Suppl):145.
93. Harrison L, Pfister D, Fass D, et al. Concomitant chemotherapy-radiation therapy followed by hyperfractionated radiation therapy for advanced unresectable head and neck cancer. *Int J Radiat Oncol Biol Phys* 1991;21:703.
94. Harrison LB, Pfister DG, Kraus D, et al. Management of unresectable malignant tumors at the skull base using concomitant chemotherapy and radiotherapy with accelerated fractionation. *Skull Base Surg* 1994;4:127.
95. Harrison LB, Raben A, Pfister DG, et al. A prospective phase II trial of concomitant chemotherapy and radiotherapy with delayed accelerated fractionation in unresectable tumors of the head and neck. *Head Neck* 1998;20:497.

96. Merlano M, Benasso M, Corvo R, et al. Alternating radiotherapy and chemotherapy with cisplatin and 5-fluorouracil for advanced inoperable head and neck squamous cell carcinoma: the 5-year update of a randomized trial from the National Institute for Cancer Research of Genoa. J Natl Cancer Institute *(in press).*
97. Regezi JA, Courtney RM, Kerr DA. Dental management of patients radiated for oral cancer. *Cancer* 1976;38:994.
98. Moorish RB, Chan E, Silverman S, et al. Osteonecrosis in patients irradiated for head and neck carcinoma. *Cancer* 1981;47:1980.
99. Leibel SA, Kutcher TJ, Harrison LB, et al. Improved dose distributions for 3-D conformal boost treatment in carcinoma of the nasopharynx. *Int J Radiat Oncol Biol Phys* 1991;20:823.
100. Lee WR, Berkey B, Marcial V, et al. Anemia is associated with decreased survival and increased locoregional failure in patients with locally advanced head and neck carcinoma: a secondary analysis of RTOG 85-27. *Int J Radiat Oncol Biol Phys* 1998;24:1069.
101. Haffty BG, Son YH, Sasaki CT, et al. Mitocycin C as an adjunct to postoperative radiation therapy in squamous cell carcinoma of the head and neck: results from two randomized clinical trials. *Int J Radiat Oncol Biol Phys* 1993;27:241.
102. Weissberg JB, Son YH, Papac RJ, et al. Randomized clinical trial of mitomycin C as an adjunct to radiotherapy in head and neck cancer. *Int J Radiat Oncol Biol Phys* 1989;17:3.
103. Brizel DM, Wasserman TH, Strnad V, et al. Final report of a phase III randomized trial of Amifostine as a radioprotectant in head and neck cancer. *Int J Radiat Oncol Biol Phys* 1999;45(Suppl):147.
104. Mitchell MS, Wawro NW, DeConti RC, et al. Effectiveness of high-dose infusion of methotrexate followed by leucovorin in carcinomas of the head and neck. *Cancer Res* 1968;28:108.
105. Kirkwood JM, Millder D, Pitman S, et al. Initial high dose methotrexate-leucovorin in advanced squamous carcinoma of the head and neck. *Proc Am Assoc Cancer Res* 1978;19:398.
106. Levitt M, Mosher MB, DeConti RC, et al. Improved therapeutics index of methotrexate with "leucovorin rescue." *Cancer Res* 1973;33:1729.
107. Vogle WR, Jacobs J, Moffitt S, et al. Methotrexate therapy with or without citrovorum factor in carcinoma of the head and neck, breast and colon. *Cancer Clin Trials* 1979;2:227.
108. Woods RL, Fox RM, Tattersall MHN. Methotrexate treatment of advanced head and neck cancers: a dose-response evaluation. *Cancer Treat Rep* 1981;65:155.
109. DeConti RC, Schoenfeld D. A randomized prospective comparison of intermittent methotrexate, methotrexate with leucovorin, and a methotrexate combination in head and neck cancer. *Cancer* 1981;48:1061.
110. Taylor SG IV, McGuire WP, Hauck WW, et al. A randomized comparison of high-dose infusion methotrexate versus standard-dose weekly therapy in head and neck squamous cancer. *J Clin Oncol* 1984;2:1006.
111. Al-Sarraf M. Chemotherapeutic management of head and neck cancer. *Cancer Metast Rev* 1987;6:191.
112. Pinto HA, Jacobs CJ. Chemotherapy for recurrent and metastatic head and neck cancer. *Hematol Oncol Clin North Am* 1991;5:667.
113. Browman GP, Cronin L. Standard chemotherapy in squamous cell head and neck cancer: what we have learned from randomized trials. *Semin Oncol* 1994;21:311.
114. Havlin KA, Kuhn JG, Myers JW, et al. High-dose cisplatin for locally advanced or metastatic head and neck cancer: a phase II pilot study. *Cancer* 1989;63:423.
115. Forastiere AA, Takasugi BJ, Baker SR, Wolf GT, Kudla-Hatch V. High dose cisplatin in advanced head and neck cancer. *Cancer Chemother Pharmacol* 1987;19:155.
116. Veronesi A, Zagonel V, Rirelli U, et al. High dose versus low dose cisplatin in advanced head and neck squamous carcinoma. A randomized study. *J Clin Oncol* 1985;3:1105.
117. Al-Sarraf M. Management strategies in head and neck cancer: the role of carboplatin. In: Bunns PA Jr, Canetta R, Ozols PF, Rozencweig M, eds. *Current perspectives and future directions.* Philadelphia: Saunders, 1990.
118. Kish JA, Tapazoglou E, Ensley J, et al. Activity of ifosfamide (NSC-109724) in recurrent head and neck cancer patients. *Proc Am Assoc Cancer Res* 1990;31:190.
119. Verweij J, Alexiera-Figresch J, DeBoer MF. Ifosfamide in advanced head and neck cancer. A phase II study of the Rotterdam Cooperative Head and Neck Cancer Study Group. *Eur J Cancer Clin Oncol* 1988;24:795.
120. Martin M, Diaz-Rubio E, Gonzales Larriba JL, et al. Ifosfamide in advanced epidermoid head and neck cancer. *Cancer Chemother Pharmacol* 1993;31:340.
121. Huber MH, Lippman SM, Benner SE, et al. A phase II study of ifosfamide in recurrent squamous cell carcinoma of the head and neck. *Am J Clin Oncol* 1996;19:379.
122. Buesa JM, Fernandez R, Esteban E, et al. Phase II trial of ifosfamide in recurrent and metastatic head and neck cancer. *Ann Oncol* 1991;2:151.
123. Cervellino JC, Araujo CE, Pirisi C, et al. Ifosfamide and MESNA for the treatment of advanced squamous cell head and neck cancer. *Oncology* 1991;48:89.
124. Bandealy M, Hann M, Arquette M, et al. Phase II trial of ifosfamide in the treatment of advanced or recurrent squamous cell carcinoma of the head and neck: a Hoosier Oncology Group trial. *Proc Am Soc Clin Oncol* 1997;16:396a.
125. Forastiere AA, Shank D, Neuberg D, et al. Final report of a phase II evaluation of paclitaxel in patients with advanced squamous cell carcinoma of the head and neck. *Cancer* 1998;82:2270.
126. Smith R, Thornton D, Allen J, et al. A phase II trial of paclitaxel in squamous cell carcinoma of the head and neck. *Semin Oncol* 1995;22:41.
127. Eisenhauer EA, Vermorken JB. Review: new cytotoxic drugs. *South Am J Cancer* 1997;1:17.
128. Vermorken JB, Catimel G, De Mulder P, et al. Randomized phase II trial of weekly methotrexate versus two schedules of triweekly paclitaxel in patients with metastatic or recurrent squamous cell carcinoma of the head and neck. *Proc Am Soc Clin Oncol* 1999;18:395a.
129. Gebbia V, Testa A, Cannata G, Gebbia N. Single agent paclitaxel in advanced squamous cell head and neck carcinoma. *Eur J Cancer* 1996;32:901.
130. Couteau C, Chouaki N, Leyvraz S, et al. A phase II study of docetaxel in patients with metastatic squamous cell carcinoma of the head and neck. *Br J Cancer* 1999;81:457.
131. Catimel G, Verweij J, Mattijssen V, et al. Docetaxel (Taxotere): an active drug for the treatment of patients with advanced squamous cell carcinoma of the head and neck. *Ann Oncol* 1994;5:533.
132. Dreyfuss A, Clark J, Norris C, et al. Docetaxel: an active drug for squamous cell carcinoma of the head and neck. *J Clin Oncol* 1996;4:1672.
133. Ebihara S, Fujii H, Sasaki Y, et al. A late phase II study of docetaxel (Taxotere) in patients with head and neck cancer. *Proc Am Soc Clin Oncol* 1997;16:A1425.
134. Degardin M, Bastit PH, Rolland F, et al. Phase II study of vinorelbine in patients with metastatic and/or recurrent squamous cell carcinoma of the head and neck. *Eur J Cancer* 1997;33(Suppl 8):S187.
135. Canfield VA, Saxman SB, Kolodziej MA, et al. Phase II trial of vinorelbine in advanced or recurrent squamous cell carcinoma of the head and neck. *Proc Am Soc Clin Oncol* 1997;16:387a.
136. Oliveira J, Geoffrois F, Rolland M, et al. Activity of Navelbine on lesions within previously irradiated fields in patients with metastatic and/or local recurrent squamous cell carcinoma of the head and neck: an EORTC-ECSG study. *Proc Am Soc Clin Oncol* 1997;16:A1449.
137. Catimel G, Vermorken JB, Clavel M, et al. A phase II study of gemcitabine (LYI 88011) in patients with advanced squamous cell carcinoma of the head and neck. *Ann Oncol* 1994;5:543.
138. Smith R, Lew D, Rodriguez G, et al. Evaluation of topotecan in patients with recurrent or metastatic squamous cell carcinoma of the head and neck. A phase II Southwest Oncology Group study. *Invest New Drugs* 1996;14:403.
139. Robert F, Soong SJ, Wheeler RH. A phase II study of topotecan in patients with recurrent head and neck cancer. Identification of an active new agent. *Am J Clin Oncol* 1997;20:298.
140. Schrijvers D, Vermorken JB. Update on the taxoids and other new agents in head and neck cancer therapy. *Curr Opin Oncol* 1998;10:233.
141. Khattab J, Urba SG. Chemotherapy in head and neck cancer: overview of newer agents. *Hematol Oncol Clin North Am* 1999;13:753.
142. Robert F. Trimetrexate as a single agent in patients with advanced head and neck cancer. *Semin Oncol* 1988;15:22.
143. Schomagel JH, Verweij J, Demulder PHM, et al. Randomized phase III trial of edatrexate versus methotrexate in patients with metastatic and/or recurrent squamous cell carcinoma of the head and neck: a European organization for research and treatment of cancer head and neck cancer cooperative group study. *J Clin Oncol* 1995;13:1649.
144. Uen WC, Huang AT, Mennel R, et al. A phase II study of piritrexim in patients with advanced squamous head and neck cancer. *Cancer* 1992;69:1008.
145. Degardin M, Demonge C, Copperlaere P, et al. Phase II piritrexim study in recurrent and/or metastatic head and neck cancer. *Proc Am Soc Clin Oncol* 1992;11:244.
146. Vokes EE, Dimery IW, Jacobs CD, et al. A phase II study of piritrexim in combination with methotrexate in recurrent and metastatic head and neck cancer. *Cancer* 1991;67:2253.
147. Abele R, Clavel M, Rossi A, et al. Iproplatin (CHIP, JM-9) in advanced squamous cell carcinoma of the head and neck: a phase II study of the EORTC early clinical trials group. *Proc Am Soc Clin Oncol* 1986;5:147.
148. Al-Sarraf M, Metch B, Kish J, et al. Platinum analogs in recurrent and advanced head and neck cancer: a Southwest Oncology Group and Wayne State University Study. *Cancer Treat Rep* 1987;71:723.
149. Fujii M, Tokumaru Y, Imanishi Y, et al. Combination chemotherapy with nedaplatin and 5-FU for head and neck cancer. *Gan To Kagaku Ryoho* 1998;25:53.
150. Verweij J, Clavel M, Chevalier B. Paclitaxel (Taxol) and docetaxel (Taxotere): not simply two of a kind. *Ann Oncol* 1994;5:495.
151. Gueritte-Voegelein F, Guenard D, Lavelle F, et al. Relationships between the structure of taxol analogues and their antimitotic activity. *J Med Chem* 1991;4:992.
152. Cobleigh MA, Hill JH, Lad TE, et al. Phase II study of etoposide in previously untreated squamous cell carcinoma of the head and neck. *Cancer Treat Rep* 1987;71:321.
153. Shiu WC, Tsao SY. Etoposide (VP 16-213) in the treatment of advanced nasopharyngeal carcinoma. *Eur J Cancer Clin Oncol* 1988;24:797.
154. Kish JA, Weaver A, Jacobs J, et al. Cisplatin and 5-fluorouracil infusion in patients with recurrent and disseminated epidermoid cancer of the head and neck. *Cancer* 1984;53:1819
155. Urba SG, Forastiere AA. Systemic therapy of head and neck cancer: most effective agents, areas of promise. *Oncology* 1989;3:79.
156. Jacobs C, Lyman G, Velez-Garcia E, et al. A phase III randomized study comparing cisplatin and fluorouracil as single agents and in combination for advanced squamous cell carcinoma of the head and neck. *J Clin Oncol* 1992;10:257.
157. Forastiere A, Metch B, Schuller D, et al. Randomized comparison of cisplatin and 5-fluorouracil versus carboplatin + 5-FU versus methotrexate in advanced squamous cell carcinoma of the head and neck. *J Clin Oncol* 1992;10:1245.
158. Clavel M, Vermorken JB, Cognetti F, et al. Randomized comparison of cisplatin, methotrexate, bleomycin and vincristine (CABO) versus cisplatin and 5-fluorouracil (CF) versus cisplatin (C) in recurrent or metastatic squamous cell carcinoma of the head and neck. *Ann Oncol* 1994;5:521.
159. Vokes EE, Choi KE, Schilsky RL, et al. Cisplatin, fluorouracil, and high-dose leucovorin for recurrent metastatic head and neck cancer. *J Clin Oncol* 1988;6:618.
160. Guthrie TH, Brubaker LH, Porubsky ES, et al. Circadian cisplatin (C), bleomycin (B) and 5-fluorouracil (F) in advanced squamous cell carcinoma of the head and neck (SCCH). *Proc Am Soc Clin Oncol* 1990;9:178.
161. Amrein PC, Fabian RL. Treatment of recurrent head and neck cancer with cisplatin and 5 fluorouracil vs. the same plus bleomycin and methotrexate. *Laryngoscope* 1992:102:901.
162. Hamm JT, Joseph G, Blumenreich MS, et al. Phase II trial of high-dose cisplatinum (CDDP), 5-fluorouracil (F-FU), bleomycin, and methotrexate in advanced/recurrent head and neck cancer. *Proc Am Soc Clin Oncol* 1990;9:175.
163. Dimery I, Martin T, Bradley E, et al. Phase I trial of interleukin-2 (rIL-2) plus cisplatin (CDDP) and 5-fluorouracil (5-FU) in recurrent or advanced squamous cell carcinoma of the head and neck. *Proc Am Soc Clin Oncol* 1989;8:170.
164. Shiriniam M, Choksi AJ, Dimery I, et al. Phase I/II study of cisplatin, 5-fluorouracil, and alpha interferon for recurrent carcinoma of the head and neck. *Invest New Drugs* 1994;12:223.

165. Adamo V, Maisano R, Laudani A, et al. Phase II study paclitaxel (PTX) and cisplatin (Cis) in advanced and recurrent head & neck cancer. *Eur J Cancer* 1999;35:S178.
166. Licitra L, Capri G, Fulfaro F, et al. Biweekly paclitaxel and cisplatin in patients with advanced head and neck carcinoma: a phase II trial. *Ann Oncol* 1997;8:1157.
167. Fountzilas G, Skarlos D, Athanassiades A, et al. Paclitaxel by three-hour infusion and carboplatin in advanced carcinoma of nasopharynx and other sites of the head and neck: a phase II study conducted by the Hellenic Cooperative Oncology Group. *Ann Oncol* 1997;8:451.
168. Junor EJ, Paul J, Robertson A, et al. Phase I dose finding study of paclitaxel in combination with carboplatin in advanced and recurrent squamous carcinoma of the head and neck. *Proc Am Soc Clin Oncol* 1999;18:407a.
169. Hitt R, Paz-Ares L, Hidalgo M, et al. Phase I/II study of paclitaxel/cisplatin as first-line therapy for locally advanced head and neck cancer. *Semin Oncol* 1997;26:S19.
170. Dunphy FR, Boyd JH, Kim HJ, et al. A phase I report of paclitaxel dose escalation combined with a fixed dose of carboplatin in the treatment of head and neck carcinoma. *Cancer* 1997;79:2016.
171. Benasso M, Numico G, Rosso R, et al. Chemotherapy for relapsed head and neck cancer: paclitaxel, cisplatin, and 5-fluorouracil in chemotherapy-naive patients. A dose-finding study. *Semin Oncol* 1997:6:S19.
172. Hitt R, Brandariz A, Paz-Ares L, et al. A phase II study of paclitaxel, cisplatin and 5-fluorouracil in locally advanced head and neck cancer. *Proc Am Soc Clin Onol* 1998;17:382a.
173. Shin DM, Glisson BS, Khuri FR, et al. Phase II trial of paclitaxel, ifosfamide, and cisplatin in patients with recurrent head and neck squamous cell carcinoma. *J Clin Oncol* 1998;16:1325.
174. Shin DM, Khuri FR, Glisson BS, et al. Phase II study of paclitaxel, ifosfamide, and carboplatin in patients with recurrent squamous cell carcinoma of the head and neck. *Proc Am Soc Clin Oncol* 1999;18:394a.
175. Fountzilas G, Stathopoulos G, Nicolaides C, et al. Paclitaxel and gemcitabine in advanced non-nasopharyngeal head and neck cancer: a phase II study conducted by the Hellenic Cooperative Oncology Group. *Ann Oncol* 1999;10:475.
176. Forastiere AA, Glisson B, Murphy B, Frenette G, O'Connell B. A phase II study of docetaxel and cisplatin in patients with squamous cell carcinoma of the head and neck. *Ann Oncol* 1998;9(Suppl 4):75.
177. Mel JR, Rodriguez M, Constenia M, et al. Phase II study of docetaxel and cisplatin as induction chemotherapy in locally advanced squamous cell carcinoma of the head and neck. *Proc Am Soc Clin Oncol* 1999;18:401a.
178. Manzione L, Caponigro F, Massa E, et al. A phase II study of docetaxel + cisplatin in locally advanced and metastatic squamous cell carcinoma of the head and neck. *Proc Am Soc Clin Oncol* 1999;18:398a.
179. Bauer M, Kienzer HR, Schweiger J, et al. First-line therapy in head and neck cancer with docetaxel/cisplatin. *Ann Oncol* 1998;9(Suppl 4):75.
180. Schoffski P, Catimel G, Planting AS, et al. Docetaxel and cisplatin: an active regimen in patients with locally advanced, recurrent or metastatic squamous cell carcinoma of the head and neck. Results of a phase II study of the EORTC Early Clinical Studies Group. *Ann Oncol* 1999;10:119.
181. Filippi MH, Cupissol D, Calais G, et al. A phase II study of docetaxel and 5-fluorouracil in metastatic or recurrent squamous cell carcinoma of the head and neck. *Proc Am Soc Clin Oncol* 1999;18:402a.
182. Airoldi M, Marchionatti S, Pedani F, et al. Docetaxel + vinorelbine in recurrent heavily pre-treated head and neck cancer patients. *Proc Am Soc Clin Oncol* 1999;18:402a.
183. Janinis J, Papadakou M, Panagos G, Boukis C, Xidakis E. A phase II study of combined chemotherapy with docetaxel cisplatin and 5-fluorouracil in patients with advanced squamous cell carcinoma of the head and neck and nasopharyngeal carcinoma. *Proc Am Soc Clin Oncol* 1999;18:402a.
184. Schrijvers D, Van Herpen C, Kerger J, et al. Phase I-II study with docetaxel, cisplatin, and 5-fluorouracil in patients with locally advanced inoperable squamous cell carcinoma of the head and neck. *Proc Am Soc Clin Oncol* 1999;18:394a.
185. Davis S, Kessler W. Randomized comparison of cis-diamminedichloro platinum versus cis-diamminedichloro platinum, methotrexate, and bleomycin in recurrent squamous cell carcinoma of the head and neck. *Cancer Chemother Pharmacol* 1979;3:57.
186. Jacobs C, Meyers F, Hendrickson C, et al. A randomized phase III study of cisplatin without methotrexate for recurrent squamous cell carcinoma of the head and neck. *Cancer* 1983;52:1563.
187. Drelichman A, Cummings G, Al-Sarraf N, et al. A randomized trial of the combination of cisplatinum, oncovin and bleomycin (COB) versus methotrexate in patients with advanced squamous cell carcinoma of the head and neck. *Cancer* 1983;52:399.
188. Morton RP, Rugman F, Dorman EB, et al. Cisplatinum and bleomycin for advanced or recurrent squamous cell carcinoma of the head and neck: a randomized factorial phase III controlled trial. *Cancer Chemother Pharmacol* 1985;15:283.
189. Vogl SE, Schoenfeld DA, Kaplan BH, et al. A randomized prospective comparison of methotrexate with a combination of methotrexate, bleomycin, and cisplatin in head and neck cancer. *Cancer* 1985;56:432.
190. Williams SD, Velez-Garcia E, Essessee I, et al. Chemotherapy for head and neck cancer: comparison of cisplatin plus vinblastine plus bleomycin versus methotrexate. *Cancer* 1986;57:18.
191. Campbell JB, Dorman EB, McCormick M, et al. A randomized phase III trial of cisplatinum, methotrexate, cisplatinum + methotrexate, and cisplatinum + 5-fluorouracil in end-stage head and neck cancer. *Acta Otolaryngol (Stockh)* 1987;103:519.
192. Eisenberger M, Krasnow S, Ellenberg S, et al. A comparison of carboplatin plus methotrexate versus methotrexate alone in patients with recurrent and metastatic head and neck cancer. *J Clin Oncol* 1989;7:1341.
193. Liverpool Head and Neck Oncology Group. A phase III randomized trial of cisplatinum, methotrexate, cisplatinum + methotrexate and cisplatinum + 5-FU in end stage squamous carcinoma of the head and neck. *Br J Cancer* 1990;61:311.
194. Kish JA, Ensley JF, Jacobs J, et al. A randomized trial of cisplatin (CACP) + 5-fluorouracil (5-FU) infusion and CACP + 5-FU bolus for recurrent and advanced squamous cell carcinoma of the head and neck. *Cancer* 1985;56:2740.
195. Clavel M, Cognetti F, Dodion P, et al. Combination chemotherapy with methotrexate, bleomycin and vincristine with or without cisplatin in advanced squamous cell carcinoma of the head and neck. *Cancer* 1987;60:1173.
196. Browman GP, Levin MN, Goodyear MD, et al. Methotrexate/fluorouracil scheduling influences normal tissue toxicity but not antitumor effects in patients with squamous cell head and neck cancer: results from a randomized trial. *J Clin Oncol* 1988;6:963.
197. Paccagnella A, Segati R, Pappagallo GL, et al. Phase II study of epirubicin, methotrexate- and bleomycin (EMB) in recurrent cancer of the head and neck: preliminary results of a randomized GSTTC study. *Proc Am Soc Clin Oncol* 1989;8:175.
198. Forastiere AA, Leong T, Rowinsky E, et al. A phase III comparison of high dose paclitaxel + cisplatin + G-CSF versus low dose paclitaxel + cisplatin in advanced head and neck cancer: an ECOG study. *J Clin Oncol (in press).*
199. Schrijvers D, Johnson J, Jiminez U, et al. Phase III trial of modulation of cisplatin/fluorouracil chemotherapy by interferon alfa-2b in patients with recurrent or metastatic head and neck cancer. Head and Neck Interferon Cooperative Study Group. *J Clin Oncol* 1998;16:1054.
200. Mendelsohn J, Fan Z. Epidermal growth factor receptor family and chemosensitization. *J Natl Cancer Inst* 1997;89:341.
201. Grandis JR, Melhem MF, Gooding WE, et al. Levels of TGF-alpha and EGFR protein in head and neck squamous cell carcinoma and patient survival. *J Natl Cancer Inst* 1998;90:824.
202. Sui LL, Hidalgo M, Nemunaitis J, et al. Dose and schedule-duration escalation of the epidermal growth factor receptor tyrosine kinase inhibitor CP-358, 774: a phase I and pharmacokinetic study. *Proc Am Soc Clin Oncol* 1999;18:388a.
203. Hammond L, Ranson M, Ferry D, et al. ZD1839, an oral epidermal growth factor receptor tyrosine kinase inhibitor: first phase I, pharmacokinetic results in patients. *Proc Am Soc Clin Oncol* 1999;18:388a.
204. Mendelsohn J, Shin DM, Donato N, et al. A phase I study of chimerized anti-epidermal growth factor receptor monoclonal antibody in combination with cisplatin in patients with recurrent head and neck squamous cell carcinoma. *Proc Am Soc Clin Oncol* 1999;18:389a.
205. Mendelsohn J. Epidermal growth factor receptor inhibition by a monoclonal antibody as anticancer therapy. *Clin Cancer Res* 1997;3:2703.
206. Ezekiel MP, Bonner JA, Robert F, et al. Phase I trial of chimerized anti-epidermal growth factor receptor antibody in combination with either once-daily or twice-daily irradiation for locally advanced head and neck malignancies. *Proc Am Soc Clin Oncol* 1999;18:388a.
207. Sausville EA, Zaharevitz D, Gussio R, et al. Cyclin-dependent kinases: initial approaches to exploit a novel therapeutic target. *Pharmacol Ther* 1999;82:285.
208. Senderowicz AM. Flavopiridol: their first cyclin-dependent kinase inhibitor in human clinical trials. *Invest New Drugs* 1999:17:313.
209. Patel V, Senderowicz AM, Pinto D, et al. Flavopiridol, a novel cyclin-dependent kinase inhibitor, suppresses the growth of head and neck squamous cell carcinomas by inducing apoptosis. *J Clin Invest* 1998;102:1674.
210. Senderowicz AM, Headlee D, Stinson SF, et al. Phase I trial of continuous infusion flavopiridol, a novel cyclin-dependent kinase inhibitor, in patients with refractory neoplasms. *J Clin Oncol* 1998;19:2986.
211. Heise CC, Williams AM, Xue S, Propst M, Kirn DH. Intravenous administration of ONYS-015, a selectively replicating adenovirus, induces antitumoral efficacy. *Cancer Res* 1999;59:2623.
212. Kirn D, Nemunaitis J, Ganly I, et al. A phase II trial of intratumoral injection with an E1B-deleted adenovirus, Onyx-015, in patients with recurrent, refractory head and neck cancer. *Proc Am Soc Clin Oncol* 1999;17:391a.
213. Heise C, Sampson-Johannes A, Williams A, et al. ONYX-015, an E1B gene-attenuated adenovirus, causes tumor-specific cytolysis and antitumoral efficacy that can be augmented by standard chemotherapeutic agents. *Nat Med* 1997;3:639.
214. Kirn DH, Khuri F, Ganly I, et al. A phase II trial of ONYX-015, a selectively replicating adenovirus to combination with cisplatin and 5-fluorouracil in patients with recurrent head and neck cancer. *Proc Am Soc Clin* 1999;18:389a.
215. Clayman GL, Dreiling LK. Injectable modalities as local and regional strategies for head and neck cancer. *Hematol Oncol Clin North Am* 1999;13:787.
216. Head and Neck Contracts Program. Adjuvant chemotherapy for advanced head and neck squamous carcinoma: final report of the Head and Neck Contracts Program. *Cancer* 1987;60:301.
217. Department of Veterans Affairs Laryngeal Study Group. Induction chemotherapy plus radiation compared with advanced laryngeal cancer. *N Engl J Med* 1991;324:1685.
218. Lefebvre JL, Chevalier D, Lubomski B, et al. Larynx preservation in hypopharynx and lateral epilarynx cancer: preliminary results of EORTC randomized phase III trial 24891. *J Natl Cancer Inst* 1996;88:890.
219. Kish J, Drelichman A, Jacobs J, et al. Clinical trial of cisplatin and 5-FU infusion as initial treatment for advanced squamous cell carcinoma of the head and neck. *Cancer Treat Rep* 1982;66:471.
220. Kish JA, Ensley JF, Weaver A, et al. Improvement of complete response rate to induction adjuvant chemotherapy for advanced squamous cell carcinoma of the head and neck. *Cancer Treat Rep* 1982;66:471.
221. Dimery IW, Hong WK. Overview of combined modality therapies for head and neck cancer. *J Natl Cancer Inst* 1993;85:95.
222. Tavorath R, Pfister DG. Chemotherapy for recurrent disease and combined modality therapies for head and neck cancer. *Curr Opin Oncol* 1995;7:242.
223. Vokes EE, Schilsky RL, Weichselbaum RR, et al. Induction chemotherapy with cisplatin, fluorouracil, and high-dose leucovorin for locally advanced head and neck cancer: a clinical and pharmacologic analysis. *J Clin Oncol* 1990;8:241.
224. Dreyfuss AI, Clark JR, Wright JE, et al. Continuous-infusion high-dose leucovorin with 5-fluorouracil and cisplatin for untreated stage IV carcinoma of the head and neck. *Ann Intern Med* 1990;112:167.

225. Pfister DG, Bajorin D, Motzer R, et al. Cisplatin, fluorouracil and leucovorin: increased toxicity without improved response in squamous cell head and neck cancer. *Arch Otolaryngol Head Neck Surg* 1994;120:89.

226. Colevas AD, Busse PM, Norris CM, et al. Induction chemotherapy with docetaxel, cisplatin, fluorouracil, and leucovorin for squamous cell carcinoma of the head and neck: a phase I/II trial. *J Clin Oncol* 1998;16:1331.

227. Colevas AD, Norris CM, Tishler RB, et al. Phase II trial of docetaxel, cisplatin, fluorouracil, and leucovorin as induction for squamous cell carcinoma of the head and neck. *J Clin Oncol* 1999;17:3503.

228. Posner MR, Glisson B, Al-Sarraf M, et al. A multi-center phase II study of induction chemotherapy with taxotere (T), cisplatinum (P), and 5-fluorouracil (F) (TPF) for curative treatment of locally advanced squamous cell carcinoma of the head and neck. *Proc Am Soc Clin Oncol* 1999;18:394a.

229. Urba SG, Forastiere AA, Wolf GT, et al. Intensive induction chemotherapy and radiation for organ preservation in patients with advanced resectable head and neck carcinoma. *J Clin Oncol* 1994;12:946.

230. Vokes EE, Ratain MJ, Mick R, et al. Cisplatin, fluorouracil, and leucovorin augmented by interferon alfa-2b in head and neck cancer: a clinical and pharmacologic analysis. *J Clin Oncol* 1993;11:360.

231. Aisner J, Hiponia D, Conley B, et al. Combined modalities in the treatment of head and neck cancers. *Semin Oncol* 1995;22:28.

232. Forastiere AA. Randomized trials of induction chemotherapy: a critical review. *Hematol Oncol Clin North Am* 1991;5:725.

233. Adelstein DJ. Induction chemotherapy in head and neck cancer. *Hematol Oncol Clin North Am* 1999;13:689.

234. Martin M, Hazan A, Vergnes L, et al. Randomized study of 5-fluorouracil and cisplatin as neoadjuvant therapy in head and neck cancer: a preliminary report. *Int J Radiat Oncol Biol Phys* 1990;19:973.

235. Jortay A Demard F, Dalesio O, et al. A randomized EORTC study on the effect of preoperative polychemotherapy in pyriform sinus carcinoma treated by pharyngolaryngectomy and irradiation. Results from 5 to 10 years. *Acta Chir Belg* 1999;90:115.

236. Richard JM, Kramer A, Molinari R, et al. Randomized EORTC Head and Neck Cooperative Group Trial of preoperative intra-arterial chemotherapy in oral cavity and oropharynx carcinoma. *Eur J Cancer* 1991;27:821.

237. Mazeron JJ, Martin M, Brun B, et al. Induction chemotherapy in head and neck cancer: result of a phase lll trial. *Head Neck* 1992;14:85.

238. Jaulcrry C, Rodriquez J, Brunin F, et al. Induction chemotherapy in advanced head and neck tumors: results of two randomized trials. *Int J Radiat Oncol Biol Phys* 1992;23:483.

239. Tejedor M, Murias A, Soria P, et al. Induction chemotherapy with carboplatin and Ftorafur in advanced head and neck cancer. *Am J Clin Oncol* 1992;15:417.

240. Depondt J, Gehanno P, Martin M, et al. Neoadjuvant chemotherapy with carboplatin/5-fluorouracil in head and neck cancer. *Oncology* 1993;50(Suppl):23.

241. Di Blasio B, Barbieri W, Bozzetti A, et al. A prospective randomized trial in resectable head and neck carcinoma: loco-regional treatment with and without neoadjuvant chemotherapy. *Proc Am Soc Clin Oncol* 1994;13:279(abst).

242. Hasegawa Y, Matsuura H, Fukushima M, Kano M, Shimozato K. A randomized trial of neoadjuvant chemotherapy with cisplatin and 5-FU in advanced head and neck cancer. *Proc Am Soc Clin Oncol* 1994;13:286(abst).

243. Paccagnella A, Orlando A, Marchlori C, et al. A phase III trial of initial chemotherapy in stage III or IV head and neck cancer. A study by the gruppo di studio sui tumori della testa e del collo. *J Natl Cancer Inst* 1994;86:265.

244. Dalley D, Beller E, Aroney R, et al. The value of chemotherapy prior to definitive local therapy in patients with locally advanced squamous cell carcinoma of the head and neck. *Proc Am Soc Clin Oncol* 1995;14:297.

245. Domenge C, Coche-Dequeant B, Wibault P, et al. Randomized trial of neoadjuvant chemotherapy before radiotherapy in oropharyngeal carcinoma. *Proceedings of the Fourth International Conference on Head and Neck Cancer.* 1996;99.

246. Volling PM, Schroeder M, Eckel H, et al. Results of a prospective randomized trial with induction chemotherapy in cancer of the oral cavity and the pharynx. *Proceedings of the Fourth International Conference on Head and Neck Cancer.* 1996;179.

247. Laramore G, Scott C, Al-Sarraf M, et al. Adjuvant chemotherapy for resectable squamous cell carcinomas of the head and neck: report on Intergroup study 01034. *Int J Radiat Oncol Biol Phys* 1992;23:705.

248. Tsukuda M, Ogasawara H, Kaneko S, et al. A prospective randomized trial of adjuvant chemotherapy with UFT for head and Neck carcinoma. Head and neck UFT study group. *Gan To Kagaku Ryoho* 1994;21:1169.

249. Domenge C, Marandas P, Vignoud J, et al. Post-surgical adjuvant chemotherapy in extracapsular spread invaded lymph node. (N+R+) of epidermoid carcinoma of the head and neck. A randomized multicentric trial. Second International Conference on Head and Neck Cancer Boston, 1988. *Am Soc Head Neck Surg* 1988;74.

250. Cooper JS, Pajak TF, Forastiere A, et al. Precisely defining high-risk operable head and neck tumors based on RTOG #85-03 and #88-24: targets for postoperative radiochemotherapy? *Head Neck* 1998;20:588.

251. Ervin TJ, Clark JR, Weichulbaum RR, et al. An analysis of induction and adjuvant chemotherapy in the multidisciplinary treatment of squamous cell carcinoma of the head and neck. *J Clin Oncol* 1987;5:10.

252. Kish JA, Benedetti JK, Balcerzak SP, et al. Feasibility trial of postoperative radiotherapy and cisplatin followed by three courses of 5-FU and cisplatin in patients with resected head and neck cancer: a Southwest Oncology Group Study. *Cancer J from Scientific American* 1999;307.

253. Johnson JT, Myers EN, Bedetti CD, et al. Cervical lymph node metastases: incidence and implications of extracapsular carcinoma. *Arch Otolaryngol* 1985;111:534.

254. Snow GB, Annyas AA, Van Slooten EA, et al. Prognostic factors of neck node metastasis. *Clin Otolaryngol* 1982;7:185.

255. Peters LJ, Goepfert H, Ang KK, et al. Evaluation of the dose for postoperative radiation therapy of head and neck cancer: first report of a prospective randomized trial. *Int J Radiat Oncol Biol Phys* 1993;26:3.

256. Brizel DM. Radiotherapy and concurrent chemotherapy for the treatment of locally advanced head and neck squamous cell carcinoma. *Semin Radiat Oncol* 1998;8:237.

257. Fu KK, Phillips TL. Biologic rationale of combined radiotherapy and chemotherapy. *Hematol Oncol Clin North Am* 1991;5:737.

258. Vokes EE, Weichulbaum RR. Concomitant chemoradiotherapy: rationale and clinical experience in patients with solid tumors. *J Clin Oncol* 1990;8:911.

259. Forastiere AA. Cisplatin and radiotherapy in the management of locally advanced head and neck cancer. *Int J Radiat Oncol Biol Phys* 1993;27:465.

260. Al-Sarraf M, Pajak TF, Byhardt RW, et al. Postoperative radiotherapy with concurrent cisplatin appears to improve locoregional control of advanced, resectable head and neck cancer: RTOG 88-24. *Int J Radiat Oncol Biol Phys* 1997;37:777.

261. Bachaud JM, Choen-Jonathan E, Alzieu C, et al. Combined postoperative radiotherapy and weekly cisplatin infusion for locally advanced head and neck carcinoma. Final report of a randomized trial. *Int J Radiat Oncol Biol Phys* 1996;36:999.

262. Weissberg J, Son YH, Papac RJ, et al. Randomized clinical trial of mitomycin C as an adjunct to radiotherapy in head and neck cancer. *Int J Radiat Oncol Biol Phys* 1989;17:3.

263. Haffty B, Son Y, Sasaki C, et al. Mitomycin C as an adjunct to postoperative radiation therapy in squamous cell carcinoma of the head and neck: results from two randomized clinical trials. *Int J Radiat Oncol Biol Phys* 1993;27:241.

264. Weissler M, Melin S, Sailer S, et al. Simultaneous chemoradiotherapy in the treatment of advanced head and neck cancer. *Arch Otolaryngol Head Neck Surg* 1992;118:806.

265. Stell PM. Adjuvant chemotherapy for head and neck cancer. *Semin Radiat Oncol* 1992;2:195.

266. Munro AJ. An overview of randomised controlled trials of trials of adjuvant chemotherapy in head and neck cancer. *Br J Cancer* 1995;71:83.

267. El Sayed S, Nelson N. Adjuvant and adjunctive chemotherapy in the management of squamous cell carcinoma of the head and neck region: a meta-analysis of prospective and randomized trials. *J Clin Oncol* 1996;14:838.

268. Pignon JP, Bourhis J, Domenge C, et al. Chemotherapy as an adjunct to definitive locoregional treatment for head and neck squamous cell carcinoma: results of three meta-analysis using updated individual data. *Lancet* 2000;355:949.

269. Stefani S, Chung TS. Hydroxyurea and radiotherapy in head and neck cancer: long term results of a double-blind randomized prospective study. *J Radiat Oncol Biol Phys* 1980;6:1398.

270. Gupta NK, Pointon RCS, Wilkinson PM. A randomized clinical trial to contract radiotherapy with radiotherapy and methotrexate given synchronously in head and neck cancer. *Clin Radiol* 1987;38:575.

271. Shanta V, Krishnamurthi S. Combined bleomycin and radiotherapy in oral cancer. *Clin Radiol* 1980;156:228.

272. Vermund H, Kaalhus O, Winther F, et al. Bleomycin and radiation therapy in squamous cell carcinoma of the upper aerodigestive tract: a phase III clinical trial. *Int J Radiat Oncol Biol Phys* 1985;11:1877.

273. Fu KK, Phillips TL, Silverberg IJ. Combined radiotherapy and chemotherapy with bleomycin and methotrexate for advanced inoperable head and neck cancer: update of a Northern California Oncology Group randomized trial. *J Clin Oncol* 1987;5:1410.

274. Eschwege F, Sancho-Gamier H, Gerard JP, et al. Ten-year results of randomized trial comparing radiotherapy and concomitant bleomycin to radiotherapy alone in epidermoid carcinomas of theoropharynx: experience of the European Organization for Research and Treatment of Cancer. *Natl Cancer Inst Mongr* 1988;6:275.

275. Lo TCM, Wiley AL Jr, Ainfield FJ, et al. Combined radiation therapy and 5-fluorouracil for advanced squamous cell carcinoma of the oral cavity and oropharynx: a randomized study. *AJR Am J Roentgenol* 1976;126:229.

276. Browman G, Hodson I, Levine M, et al. Placebo-controlled randomized trial of infusional fluorouracil during standard radiotherapy in locally advanced head and neck cancer. *J Clin Oncol* 1994;12:2648.

277. Sanchiz F, Milla A, Roner J, et al. Single fraction per day versus two fractions per day versus radiochemotherapy in the treatment of head and neck cancer. *Int J Radiat Oncol Biol Phys* 1990;19:1347.

278. Weissberg JB, Son YH, Papac RJ, et al. Randomized clinical trial of mitomycin C as an adjunct to radiotherapy in head and neck cancer. *Int J Radiat Oncol Biol Phys* 1989;17:3.

279. Haselow RE, Warshaw MC, Oken MM, et al. Radiation alone versus radiation with weekly low dose cis-platinum in unresectable cancer of the head and neck. *Head Neck Cancer* 1990;2:279.

280. Al-Sarraf M, LeBlanc M, Giri PG, et al. Chemoradiotherapy versus radiotherapy in patients with advanced nasopharyngeal cancer: phase III randomized Intergroup study 0099. *J Clin Oncol* 1998;16:1310.

281. Tishler RB, Geard CR, Hall EJ, Schiff PB. Taxol sensitizes human astrocytoma cells to radiation. *Cancer Res* 1992;52(Suppl 12):3495.

282. Choy H, Rodriguez FF, Loester S, Hilsenbeck S, Von Hoff DD. Investigation of taxol as a potential radiation sensitizer. *Cancer* 1993;71(Suppl 11):3774.

283. Liebmann J, Cook JA, Fisher J, Teague D, Mitchell JB. In vitro studies of taxol as a radiation sensitizer in human tumor cells. *J Natl Cancer Inst* 1994;86:441.

284. Eisbruch A, Shewach DS, Bradford CR, et al. Radiation concurrent with low dose gemcitabine for head and neck cancer: interim results of a phase I study. *Proc Am Clin Oncol* 1998;17:405a.

285. Rosenthal DI, Sinard R, Kavanaugh DY, et al. Dose escalating 7-week continuous infusion paclitaxel with concurrent once-daily radiation therapy for locally advanced squamous carcinoma of head and neck: a phase I study. *Am Soc Clin Oncol* 1999;18:397a.

286. Flood W, Lee DJ, Trotti A, et al. Multimodality therapy of patients with locally advanced squamous cell cancer of the head and neck: preliminary results of two pilot trials using paclitaxel and cisplatin. *Semin Radiat Oncol* 1999;2:64.
287. Conley B, Jacobs M, Suntharalingam M, et al. A pilot trial of paclitaxel, carboplatin, and concurrent radiotherapy for unresectable squamous cell carcinoma of the head and neck. *Semin Oncol* 1997;1:S2-78.
288. Wanebo HJ, Chougule P, Ready N, et al. Preoperative paclitaxel, carboplatin, and radiation therapy in advanced head and neck cancer (stage III and IV). *Semin Radiat Oncol* 1999;2:77.
289. Amdur RJ, Parsons JT, Mendenhall WM, Million RR, Cassissi NJ. Split-course versus continuous-course irradiation in the postoperative setting for squamous cell carcinoma of the head and neck. *Int J Radiat Oncol Biol Phys* 1989;17:279.
290. Pajak TF, Laramore GE, Marcial VA, et al. Elapsed treatment days—a critical item for radiotherapy quality control review in head and neck trials: RTOG report. *Int J Radiat Oncol Biol Phys* 1991;20:13.
291. Taylor SG, Murthy AK, Griem KL, et al. Concomitant cisplatin/5-FU infusion and radiotherapy in advanced head and neck cancer: 8-year analysis of results. *Head Neck* 1997;19:684.
292. Lavertu P, Adelstein DJ, Saxton JP, et al. Aggressive concurrent chemoradiotherapy for squamous cell head and neck cancer: an 8-year single-institution experience. *Arch Otolaryngol Head Neck Surg* 1999;125:142.
293. Haraf DJ, Kies M, Rademaker AW, et al. Radiation therapy with concomitant hydroxyurea and fluorouracil in stage II and III head and neck cancer. *J Clin Oncol* 1999;17:638.
294. Taylor SG IV, Murthy AK, Vannetzel JM, et al. Randomized comparison of neoadjuvant cisplatin and fluorouracil infusion followed by radiation versus concomitant treatment in advanced head and neck cancer. *J Clin Oncol* 1994;12:385.
295. Griem KL, Murthy AK, Varnetzel JM, et al. The five year results of a randomized trial of sequential versus concomitant cisplatin and fluorouracil and radiation in advanced head and neck cancer. *Int J Radiat Oncol Biol Phys* 1995;32(Suppl 1):194.
296. Adelstein DJ, Sharan VM, Earle S, et al. Simultaneous versus sequential combined technique therapy for squamous cell head and neck cancer. *Cancer* 1990;65:1685.
297. Merlano M, Corro R, Bargarino G, et al. Combined chemotherapy and radiation therapy in advanced inoperable squamous cell carcinoma of the head and neck. *Cancer* 1991;67:915.
298. Interim report from the SECOG participants: a randomized trial of combined multi drug chemotherapy and radiotherapy in advanced squamous cell carcinoma of the head and neck. *Eur J Surg Oncol* 1986;12:289.
299. Keane TJ, Cummings BJ, O'Sullivan B, et al. A randomized trial of radiation therapy compared with split course radiation therapy combined with mitomycin and 5-fluorouracil as initial treatment for advanced laryngeal and hypopharyngeal squamous carcinoma. *Int J Radiat Oncol Biol Phys* 1993;25:613.
300. Zakotnik B, Smid L, Budihna M, et al. Concomitant radiotherapy with mitomycin C and bleomycin compared with radiotherapy alone in inoperable head and neck cancer: final report. *Int J Radiat Oncol Biol Phys* 1998;41:1121.
301. Adelstein DJ, Saxton JP, Lavertu P, et al. A phase II randomized trial comparing concurrent chemotherapy and radiotherapy with radiotherapy alone in resectable stage II and IV squamous cell head and neck cancer: preliminary results. *Head Neck* 1997;19:567.
302. Adelstein DJ, Lavertu P, Saxton JP, et al. Long term results of a phase III randomized trial comparing concurrent chemoradiotherpy with radiation therapy alone in squamous cell head and neck cancer. *Am Soc Clin Oncol* 1999;18:394a.
303. Calais G, Alfonsi M, Bardet E, et al. Randomized trial of radiation therapy versus concomitant chemotherapy and radiation therapy for advanced-stage oropharynx carcinoma. *J Natl Cancer Inst* 1999;91:2081.
304. Merlano M, Benasso M, Corvo R, et al. Five-year update of a randomized trial of alternating radiotherapy and chemotherapy compared with radiotherapy alone in treatment of unresectable squamous cell carcinoma of the head and neck. *J Natl Cancer Inst* 1996;88(9):583.
305. Adelstein DJ, Adams GL, Li Y, et al. A phase II comparison of standard radiation therapy versus RT plus concurrent cisplatin versus split-course RT plus concurrent DDP and 5-fluorouracil in patients with unresectable squamous cell head and neck cancer. *Proc Am Soc Clin Oncol* 2000;19:411a.
306. Wendt TG, Grabenbauer GG, Rodel CM, et al. Simultaneous radiochemotherapy versus radiotherapy alone in advanced head and neck cancer: a randomized multicenter study. *J Clin Oncol* 1998:16:1318.
307. Brizel DM, Albers ME, Fisther SR, et al. Hyperfractionated irradiation with or without concurrent chemotherapy for locally advanced head and neck cancer. *N Engl J Med* 1998;42:145.
308. Forastiere AA, Trotti A. Radiotherapy and concurrent chemotherapy: a strategy that improves locoregional control and survival in oropharyngeal cancer. *J Natl Cancer* 1999;91:2065.
309. Marcial VA, Pajak TF, Mohiudin M, et al. Concomitant cisplatin chemotherapy and radiotherapy in advanced mucosal squamous cell carcinoma of the head and neck. Long term results of the Radiation Therapy Oncology Group study 81-17. *Cancer* 1990;66:1862.
310. Adelstein DJ, Kalish LA, Adams GL, et al. Concurrent radiation therapy and chemotherapy for locally unresectable squamous cell head and neck cancer. An Eastern Cooperative Oncology Group pilot study. *J Clin Oncol* 1993;11:2136.
311. Fu KK, Pajak TF, Trotti A, et al. A Radiation Therapy Oncology Group (RTOG) phase III randomized study to compare hyperfractionation and two variants of accelerated fractionation to standard fractionation radiotherapy for head and neck squamous cell carcinomas: preliminary results of RTOG 9003. *Int J Radiat Oncol Biol Phys* 1999;45(Suppl):145.
312. Lotan R. Retinoids in cancer chemoprevention. *FASEB J* 1996;10:1031.
313. Hong WK, Lippman SM, Hittleman W, et al. Retinoid chemoprevention of aerodigestive cancer: from basic research to the clinic. *Clin Cancer Res* 1995;1:677.
314. Papadimitrakopolou V, Hong WK. Retinoids in head and neck chemoprevention. *Proc Soc Exp Biol Med* 1997;216:283.
315. Nawroz H, van der Riet P, Hruban RH, Koch W, Sidransky D. Allelotype of head and neck squamous cell carcinoma. *Cancer Res* 1994;54:1152.
316. Sidransky D. Molecular genetics of head and neck cancer. *Curr Opin Oncol* 1995;7:299.
317. Khuri FR, Lippman SM, Spitz MR, et al. Molecular epidemiology and retinoid chemoprevention of head and neck cancer. *J Natl Cancer Inst* 1997;89:199.
318. Wulf K. Zur vitamin A behandlung der leukoplakien. *Arch Klin Exp Derm* 1957;206:495.
319. Silverman S, Eisenberg E, Renstrup G. A study of the effects of high doses of vitamin A on oral leukoplakia (hyperkeratosis), including toxicity, liver function and skeletal metabolism. *J Oral Ther Pharm* 1965;2:9.
320. Hong WK, Lippman SM, Wolf GT. Recent advances in head and neck cancer. Larynx preservation and cancer chemoprevention. *Cancer Res* 1994;53:5113.
321. Lippman SM, Benner SE, Hong WK. Cancer chemoprevention. *J Clin Oncol* 1994;12:851.
322. Hong WK, Endicott J, Itri LM, et al. 13-cis-retinoic acid in the treatment of oral leukoplakia. *N Engl J Med* 1986;315:1501.
323. Lippman SM, Batsakis JG, Toth BB, et al. Comparison of low-dose isotretinoin with beta carotene to prevent oral carcinogenesis. *N Engl J Med* 1993;328:15.
324. Stich HF, Homby AP, Mathew B, et al. Response of oral leukoplakias to the administration of vitamin A. *Cancer Lett* 1988;40:93.
325. Han J, Lu Y, Sun Z, et al. Evaluation of N-4-(hydroxycarbophenyl) retinamide as a cancer prevention agent and as a cancer chemotherapeutic agent. *In Vivo* 1990;4:153.
326. Costa A, Formelli F, Chiesa F, et al. Prospects of chemoprevention of human cancers with the synthetic retinoid fenretinide. *Cancer Res* 1994;54:2032.
327. Benner SE, Winn RJ, Lippman SM, et al. Regression of oral leukoplakia with alpha-Tocopherol: a community Clinical Oncology Program Chemoprevention Study. *J Natl Cancer Inst* 1993;85:44.
328. Lippman SM, Spitz MR, Huber MH, et al. Strategies for chemoprevention study of premalignancy and second primary tumors in the head and neck. *Curr Opin Oncol* 1995;7:234.
329. Papadimitrakopolou V, Hong WK, Lee JS, et al. Low-dose isotretinoin versus beta-carotene to prevent oral carcinogenesis: longterm follow-up. *J Natl Cancer Inst* 1997;89:257.
330. Stich HF, Rosin MP, Hornby P, et al. Remission of oral leukoplakias and micronuclei in tobacco/betel quid chewers treated with beta-carotene and beta-carotene plus vitamin A. *Int J Cancer* 1988;42:195.
331. Peck R, Bollag W. Potentiation of retinoid-induced differentiation of HL-60 and U937 cell lines by cytokines. *Eur J Cancer* 1992;27:53.
332. Kolla V, Lindner DJ, Xiao W, et al. Modulation of interferon (IFN)-inducible gene expression by retinoic acid. Up regulation of STAT1 protein in IFN-unresponsive cells. A phase II trial from the MD Anderson Cancer Center reported pathologic complete responses in 10 of 30 patients at 6 months and partial responses in 7 patients. *J Biol Chem* 1996;271:10508.
333. Papadimitrakopoulou VA, Clayman GL, Shin DM, et al. Biochemoprevention for dysplastic lesions of the upper aerodigestive tract. *Arch Otolaryngol Head Neck Surg* 1999;125:1083.
334. Cooper JS, Pajak TF, Rubin P, et al. Second malignancies in patients who have head and neck cancers: incidence, effect on survival and implications for chemoprevention based on the RTOG experience. *Int J Radiat Oncol Biol Phys* 1989;17:449.
335. Hong WK, Lippman SM, Itri LM, et al. Prevention of second primary tumors with isotretinoin in squamous cell carcinoma of the head and neck. *N Engl J Med* 1990;323:795.
336. Benner SE, Pajak TF, Lippman SM, et al. Prevention of second primary tumors with isotretinoin in squamous cell carcinoma of the head and neck: long term follow-up. *J Natl Cancer Inst* 1994;86:140.
337. Bolla M, Lefur R, Ton Van J, et al. Prevention of second primary tumours with etretinate in squamous cell carcinoma of the oral cavity and oropharynx. Results of a multicentric double-blind randomized study. *Eur J Cancer* 1994;30A:767.
338. Logemann JA. Rehabilitation of the head and neck cancer patient. *Semin Oncol* 1994;21:359.
339. Rehabilitation of head and neck cancer patients: consensus on recommendation from the international conference on rehabilitation of the head and neck cancer patient. *Head Neck* 1991;13:1.
340. Davis JW, Lazarus C, Logemann JA. Effect of a maxillary glossectomy prosthesis on articulation and swallowing. *J Prosthet Dent* 1987;57:715.
341. Pauloski BR, Logemann JA, Rademaker AW, et al. Speech and swallowing function after oral and oropharyngeal resections: one year follow-up. *J Speech Hear Res* 1993;36:267.
342. Haribhakti VV, Kavarana NM, Tibrewak AN. Oral cavity reconstruction: an objective assessment of function. *Head Neck* 1993;15:119.
343. Teichgraeber J, Bowman J, Goepfert H. Functional analysis of treatment of oral cavity cancer. *Arch Otolaryngol Head Neck Surg* 1986;112:959.
344. Lazarus CL, Logemann JA, Kahrillas PJ, Mittal BB. Swallow recovery in an oral cancer patient following surgery, radiotherapy and hyperthermia. *Head Neck* 1994;16:259.
345. Dodds WJ, Stewart ET, Logemann JA. Physiology and radiology of the normal oral and pharyngeal phases of swallowing. *AJR Am J Roentgenol* 1990;154:953.
346. Effects of chin down posture on aspiration in dysphagic patients. *Arch Phys Med Rehabil* 1993;74:736.
347. Rousch GC. Epidemiology of cancer of the nose and paranasal sinuses. Current concepts. *Head Neck Surg* 1979;2:3.
348. Torjussen W, Haug FMS, Olsen A, Andersen I. Concentration and distribution of heavy metals in nasal mucosa of nickel-exposed workers. *Acta Otolaryngol* 1977;86:449.
349. Pedersen EA, Hogetveit AC, Andersen A. Cancer of the respiratory organs among workers at a nickel refinery in Norway. *Int J Cancer* 1973;12:32.
350. Ironside P, Matthews J. Adenocarcinoma of the nose and paranasal sinuses in woodworkers in the state of Victoria, Australia. *Cancer* 1975;36:1115.
351. Acheson ED, Hadfield EH, Macbeth RG. Carcinoma of the nasal cavity and accessory sinuses in woodworkers. *Lancet* 1967;1:311.
352. Acheson ED, Cowdell RH, Jolles B. Nasal cancer in the Northamptonshire boot and shoe industry. *Br Med J [Clin Res]* 1970;1:385.
353. Buda JA, Conley JJ, Rankow R. Carcinoma of the maxillary sinus following thorotrast instillation. *Am J Surg* 1963;106:868.

354. Moss-Salentijn L. Anatomy and embryology. In: Blitzer A, Lawson W, Friedman WH, eds. *Surgery of the paranasal sinuses.* Philadelphia: Saunders, 1985:1.
355. Sisson GA, Bytell DE, Becker SP, Ruge D. Carcinoma of the paranasal sinuses and cranial-facial resection. *J Laryngol Otol* 1976;90:59.
356. Robin PE, Powell DJ. Regional node involvement and distant metastasis in carcinoma of the nasal cavity and paranasal sinuses. *J Laryngol Otol* 1980;94:301.
357. Jackson RT, Fitz-Hugh GS, Constable WC. Malignant neoplasms of the nasal cavities and paranasal sinuses: a retrospective study. *Laryngoscope* 1977;87:726.
358. Bosch A, Vallecillo L, Frias Z. Cancer of the nasal cavity. *Cancer* 1976;37:1458.
359. Sisson GA, Johnson NE, Amiric S. Cancer of the maxillary sinus: clinical classification and management. *Ann Otol Rhinol Laryngol* 1963;72:1050.
360. Birt BD, Braint TDR. The management of malignant tumors of the maxillary sinus. *Otolaryngol Clin North Am* 1976;9:249.
361. Kraus DH, Lanzieri CF, Wanamaker JR, Little JR, Lavertu P. Complementary use of computed tomography and magnetic resonance imaging in assessing skull base lesions. *Laryngoscope* 1992;102:623.
362. Som PM, Dillon WP, Sze G, et al. Benign and malignant sinonasal lesions with intracranial extension: differentiation with MRI imaging. *Radiology* 1989;172:763.
363. Price JC, Holliday MJ, Johns ME, et al. The versatile midface degloving approach. *Laryngoscope* 1988;98:291.
364. Sessions RB, Humphrey DH. Technical modifications of the medial maxillectomy. *Arch Otolaryngol* 1983;109:575.
365. Wong C, Cummings B. The place of radiation therapy in the treatment of squamous cell carcinoma of the nasal vestibule. *Acta Oncol* 1988;27:203.
366. Spiro RH, Strong EW, Shah JP. Maxillectomy and its classifications. *Head Neck* 1997;19:309.
367. Tiwari R, Van der Waal J, Van der Waal I, Snow G. Studies of the anatomy and pathology of the orbit and carcinoma of the maxillary sinus and their impact on preservation of the eye in maxillectomy. *Head Neck* 1998;20:189.
368. Kirchner JC, Sasaki CT. Reconstructive surgery of the sinuses. In Thawley SE, Panje WR, Batsakis JG, Lindberg RD, eds. *Comprehensive management of head and neck tumors.* Philadelphia: Saunders, 1987:433.
369. Jesse RH, Butler JJ, Healey JE, et al. Paranasal sinuses and nasal cavity. In: MacComb WS, Fletcher GH, eds. In: *Cancer of the head and neck.* Baltimore: Williams & Wilkins, 1967:329.
370. McCaffrey TV, Olsen KD, Yohanan JM, et al. Factors affecting survival of patients with tumors of the anterior skull base. *Laryngoscope* 1994;104:940.
371. Lund VJ, Howard DJ, Wei WI, Cheesman AD. Craniofacial resection for tumors of the nasal cavity and paranasal sinuses—a 7 year experience. *Head Neck* 1998;20:97.
372. Roa W, Hazuka M, Sandler H, et al. Results of primary and adjuvant CT-base 3-dimensional radiotherapy for malignant tumors of the paranasal sinuses. *Int J Radiat Oncol Biol Phys* 1994;28:857.
373. Spiro JD, Soo KC, Spiro RA. Squamous carcinoma of the nasal cavity and paranasal sinuses. *Am J Surg* 1991;158:328.
374. Lewis JS, Castro EB. Cancer of the nasal cavity and paranasal sinuses. *J Laryngol Otol* 1972;86:255.
375. Levendag P, Pomp J. Radiation therapy of squamous cell carcinoma of the nasal vestibule. *Int J Radiat Oncol Biol Phys* 1990;19:1363.
376. Wang CC. Treatment of carcinoma of the nasal vestibule by irradiation. *Cancer* 1976;38:100.
377. Wang CC, Cummings B, Elhakim T, et al. External irradiation for squamous cell carcinoma of the nasal vestibule. *Int J Radiat Oncol Biol Phys* 1986;12:1943.
378. Ketcham AS, Chretien PB, Van Buren JM, et al. The ethmoid sinuses: a re-evaluation of surgical resection. *Am J Surg* 1973;126:469.
379. Terz JJ, Young HF, Lawrence W. Combined craniofacial resection for locally advanced carcinoma of the head and neck. *Am J Surg* 1980;140:618.
380. Clayman GL, et al. Outcome and complications of extended cranial-base resection requiring microvascular free-tissue transfer. *Arch Otolaryngol Head Neck Surg* 1995;121:1253.
381. Kraus DH, Shah JP, Arbit C, Galicich JH, Strong EW. Complications of craniofacial resection for tumor involving the anterior skull base. *Head Neck Surg* 1994;10:307.
382. Parsons J, Mendenhall W, Mancuso A, et al. Malignant tumors of nasal cavity and ethmoid and sphenoid sinuses. *Int J Radiat Oncol Biol Phys* 1988;14:11.
383. Frich J. Treatment of advanced squamous carcinoma of the maxillary sinus by irradiation. *Int J Radiat Oncol Biol Phys* 1982;8:1453.
384. Amendola B, Eisert D, Hazra T, et al. Carcinoma of the maxillary antrum: surgery or radiation therapy? *Int J Radiat Oncol Biol Phys* 1981;7:743.
385. Yu-Hua H, Gui-Yi T, Yu-Quin Q, et al. Comparison of pre- and post-operative radiation in the combined treatment of carcinoma of the maxillary sinus. *Int J Radiat Oncol Biol Phys* 1982;8:1045.
386. Zaharia M, Salem L, Travezan R, et al. Post-operative radiation therapy in the management of cancer of the maxillary sinus. *Int J Radiat Oncol Biol Phys* 1989;17:967.
387. Raben A, Pfister D, Omalley B. Non-surgical management of carcinoma of the nasal vestibule, nasal cavity, and paranasal sinuses. In: Harrison LB, Sessions RB, Hong WK, eds. *Head and neck cancer—a multidisciplinary approach.* Philadelphia: Lippincott–Raven, 1999:595.
388. Collins JM. Pharmacologic rationale for regional drug delivery. *J Clin Oncol* 1984;2:498.
389. Sato Y, Morita M, Takahashi H, et al. Combined surgery, radiotherapy, and regional chemotherapy in carcinoma of the paranasal sinuses. *Cancer* 1970;25:571.
390. Goepfert H, Jesse RH, Lindberg RD. Arterial infusion and radiation therapy in the treatment of advanced cancer of the nasal cavity and paranasal sinuses. *Am J Surg* 1973;126:464.
391. Moseley HS, Thomas LR, Everts EC, et al. Advanced squamous cell carcinoma of the maxillary sinus: results of combined regional infusion chemotherapy, radiation therapy and surgery. *Am J Surg* 1981;141:522.
392. Shibuya H, Suzuki S, Horiuchi JI, et al. Reappraisal of trimodal combination therapy for maxillary sinus carcinoma. *Cancer* 1982;50:2790.
393. Nervi C, Arcangeli G, Badaracco G, et al. The relevance of tumor size and cell kinetics as predictors of radiation response in head and neck cancer: a randomized study on the effect of intraarterial chemotherapy followed by radiotherapy. *Cancer* 1978;41:900.
394. Dimery IW, Lee YY, Van Tassel P, et al. Combined intra-arterial (I.A.) and systemic chemotherapy (CT) for paranasal sinus carcinoma (PNSC). *Proc Am Soc Clin Oncol* 1988;7:150(abst).
395. Mortimer JE, Taylor ME, Schulman S, et al. Feasibility and efficacy of weekly intraarterial cisplatin in locally advanced (stage III and IV) head and neck cancers. *J Clin Oncol* 1988;6:969.
396. LoRusso P, Tapazoglou E, Kish JA, et al. Chemotherapy for paranasal sinus carcinoma: a 10 year experience at Wayne State University. *Cancer* 1988;62:1.
397. Lee MM, Vokes EE, Rosen A, et al. Multimodality therapy in advanced paranasal sinus carcinoma: superior long-term results. *Cancer J Sci Am* 19995:219.
398. Harrison L, Pfister D, Fass D, et al. Concomitant chemotherapy-radiation therapy followed by hyper fractionated radiation therapy for advanced unresectable head and neck cancer. *Int J Radiat Oncol Biol Phys* 1991;21:703.
399. Robbins KT, Storniolo AM, Kerber C, et al. Phase I study of highly selective supradose cisplatin infusions for advanced head and neck cancer. *J Clin Oncol* 1994;12:2113.
400. Samant S, Kumar P, Wan J, et al. Concomitant radiation therapy and targeted cisplatin chemotherapy for the treatment of advanced pyriform sinus carcinoma: disease control and preservation of organ function. *Head Neck* 1999;21:595.
401. Robbins KT, Kumar P, Regine WF, et al. Efficacy of targeted supradose cisplatin and concomitant radiation therapy for advanced head and neck cancer: the Memphis experience. *Int J Radiat Oncol Biol Phys* 1997;38:263.
402. Miller D. The etiology of nasopharyngeal cancer and its management. *Otolaryngol Clin North Am* 1980;13:167.
403. Henderson BE, Louie E, Jing JSH, Buell P, Gardner M. Risk factors associated with nasopharyngeal carcinoma. *N Engl J Med* 1976;295:1101.
404. Yu MC, Ho JHC, Lai SH, Henderson BE. Cantonese-style salted fish as a cause of nasopharyngeal carcinoma: report of a case-control study in Hong Kong. *Cancer Res* 1986;46:956.
405. Old LJ, Boyse EA, Oettgen HF, et al. Precipitating antibody in human serum to an antigen present in cultured Burkitt's lymphoma cells. *Proc Natl Acad Sci U S A* 1966;56:1699.
406. Zur Hausen H, Schulte-Holthausen H, Klein G, et al. Epstein-Barr virus DNA in biopsies of Burkitt tumors and anaplastic carcinoma of the nasopharynx. *Nature* 1970;228:1056.
407. Fahraeus R, Fu HL, Ernberg I, et al. Expression of Epstein-Barr virus-encoded proteins in nasopharyngeal carcinoma. *Int J Cancer* 1988;42:329.
408. Chan SH, Day HE, Kunaratnam N, Chia KB, Simons MJ. HLA and nasopharyngeal carcinoma in Chinese—a further study. *Int J Cancer* 1983;32:171.
409. Simons MJ, Wee GB, Goh EH, et al. Immunogenetic aspects of nasopharyngeal carcinoma. IV. Increased risk in Chinese of nasopharyngeal carcinoma associated with a Chinese related HCA profile (A2, Singapore 2). *J Natl Cancer Inst* 1976;57:977.
410. *International Histological Classification of Tumors,* No. 19: histological typing of upper respiratory tract tumors. World Health Organization, 1978:32.
411. Baker SR. Nasopharyngeal carcinoma: clinical course and results of therapy. *Head Neck Surg* 1980;3:8.
412. Mesic JB, Fletcher GH, Goepfert H. Megavoltage irradiation of epithelial tumors of the nasopharynx. *Int J Radiat Oncol Biol Phys* 1981;7:447.
413. Neel HB III. Nasopharyngeal carcinoma. Clinical presentation, diagnosis, treatment, and prognosis. *Otolaryngol Clin North Am* 1985;18:479.
414. Chen KY, Fletcher GH. Malignant tumors of the nasopharynx. *Radiology* 1971;99:165.
415. Hoppe RT, Williams J, Warnke R, et al. Carcinoma of the nasopharynx—significance of histology. *Int J Radiat Oncol Biol Phys* 1987;4:199.
416. Yu Z, Xu G, Huang Y, et al. Value of computed tomography in staging the primary lesion (T-staging) of nasopharyngeal carcinoma (NPC): an analysis of 54 patients with special reference to the parapharyngeal space. *Int J Radiat Oncol Biol Phys* 1985;11:2143.
417. Sham JST, Choy D. Prognostic value of paranasopharyngeal extension of nasopharyngeal carcinoma on local control and short term survival. *Head Neck* 1991;13:298.
418. Lee A, Sham J, Poon Y, Ho JHC. Treatment of stage I nasopharyngeal carcinoma: analysis of pattern of relapse and the results of withholding elective neck irradiation. *Int J Radiat Oncol Biol Phys* 1989;17:1183.
419. Sham J, Choy D, Wei W. Nasopharyngeal carcinoma: orderly neck node spread. *Int J Radiat Oncol Biol Phys* 1990;19:929.
420. Cellai E, Olmi T, Chiavacci A, et al. Computed tomography in nasopharyngeal carcinoma. II. Impact on survival. *Int J Radiat Oncol Biol Phys* 1990;19:929.
421. Kutcher GJ, Zuks G, Brenner H, et al. Three dimensional photon treatment planning for carcinoma of the nasopharynx. *Int J Radiat Oncol Biol Phys* 1991;21:169.
422. Ang KK, Peters LJ, Weber RA, et al. Concomitant boost radiotherapy schedules in the treatment of carcinoma of the oropharynx and nasopharynx. *Int J Radiat Oncol Biol Phys* 1990;19:1339.
423. Cheung KY, Choi PH, Chau RMC, et al. The roles of multileaf and micro multifleaf collimators in conformal and conventional nasopharyngeal carcinoma radiotherapy treatments. *Med Phys* 1999;26:2077.
424. Sultanem K, Shu HK, Xia P, et al. 3-D intensity modulated radiotherapy (IMRT) in the treatment of nasopharyngeal carcinoma: the UCSF experience. *Int J Radiat Oncol Biol Phys* 1999;45(Suppl):151.
425. Wang CC. Re-irradiation of recurrent nasopharyngeal carcinoma—treatment techniques and results. *Int J Radiat Oncol Biol Phys* 1987;13:953.
426. Harrison LB, Weissberg JB. A technique for interstitial nasopharyngeal brachytherapy. *Int J Radiat Oncol Biol Phys* 1987;13:451.
427. Harrison LB, Sessions RB, Fass DE, et al. Nasopharyngeal brachytherapy using access via a transpalatal flap. *Am J Surg (in press).*
428. Vikram B, Hilaris B. Transnasal permanent interstitial implantation of carcinoma of the nasopharynx. *Int J Radiat Oncol Biol Phys* 1984;10:153.
429. McNeese MB, Fletcher GH. Re-treatment of recurrent nasopharyngeal carcinoma. *Radiology* 1981;138:191.

430. Harrison LB, Nori B, Hilaris B, et al. Nasopharynx. In: The Interstitial Collaborative Working Group, ed. *Interstitial brachytherapy.* New York: Raven, 1990:95.
431. Erickson B, Wilson JF. Nasopharyngeal brachytherapy. *Am J Clin Oncol* 1993;16:424.
432. Castro J, Linstadt D, Bahary J, et al. Experience in charged particle irradiation of tumors of the skull base: 1977–1992. *Int J Radiat Oncol Biol Phys* 1994;29:647.
433. Fee WE, Gilmer PA, Goffinet DR. Surgical management of recurrent nasopharyngeal carcinoma after radiation failure at the primary site. *Laryngoscope* 1988;98:1220.
434. Fisch U. The infratemporal fossa approach for nasopharyngeal tumors. *Laryngoscope* 1983;93:36.
435. Morton RP, et al. Transcervico-mandibulo-palatal approach for surgical salvage of recurrent nasopharyngeal cancer. *Head Neck* 1996;18:352.
436. Wei W. Maxillary swing approach. *Head Neck* 1991;13:204.
437. Cvitkovic E, Bachouchi M, Boussen H, et al. Leukemoid reaction, bone marrow invasion, fever of unknown origin, and metastatic pattern in the natural history of advanced undifferentiated carcinoma of nasopharyngeal type: a review of 255 consecutive cases. *J Clin Oncol* 1993;11:2434.
438. Teo P, Yu P, Lee WY, et al. Significant prognosticators after primary radiotherapy in 903 nondisseminated nasopharyngeal carcinomas evaluated by computer tomography. *Int J Radiat Oncol Biol Phys* 1996;36:2:291.
439. Sham JUST, Choy D, Choi PAK. Nasopharyngeal carcinoma: the significance of neck node involvement in relation to the pattern of distant failure. *Br J Radiol* 1990;63:108.
440. Perez CA, Devonian OR, Marcia-Vega V, et al. Carcinoma of the nasopharynx: factors affecting prognosis. *Int J Radiat Oncol Biol Phys* 1991;23:271.
441. Gear FB, Sanguinity G, Tucker SL, et al. Carcinoma of the nasopharynx treated by radiotherapy alone: determinants of distant metastasis and survival. *Radiat Oncol* 1997;43:53.
442. Ahmad A, Stefani S. Distant metastasis of nasopharyngeal carcinoma. A study of 256 male patients. *J Surg Oncol* 1986;33:194.
443. Fandi A, Altun M, Azli N, Armand JP, Cvitkovic E. Nasopharyngeal cancer: epidemiology, staging, and treatment. *Semin Oncol* 1994;21:382.
444. Boussen H, Cvitkovic E, Wendling JL, et al. Chemotherapy of metastatic and/or recurrent undifferentiated nasopharyngeal carcinoma with cisplatin, bleomycin and fluorouracil. *J Clin Oncol* 1991;9:1675.
445. Fandi A, Bachouchi M, Taamma A, et al. Long term disease-free survivors in metastatic (MTS) undifferentiated carcinoma of nasopharyngeal type (UCNT). *Proc Am Soc Clin Oncol* 1998;17.
446. Azli N, Fandi A, Bachouchi, et al. Final report of a phase II study of chemotherapy with bleomycin, epirubicin and cisplatin for locally advanced and metastatic recurrent undifferentiated carcinoma of the nasopharyngeal type. *Cancer J Sci Am* 1995;1:222.
447. Cvitkovic E, Mahjoubi R, Lianes P, et al. 5-Fluorouracil (FU), mitomycin (M). Epirubicin (E). Cisplatin (P) in recurrent and/or metastatic undifferentiated nasopharyngeal carcinoma (UCNT). *Proc Am Soc Clin Oncol* 1992;11:240.
448. Choo R, Tannock I. Chemotherapy for recurrent or metastatic carcinoma of the nasopharynx. A review of the Princess Margaret Hospital experience. *Cancer* 1991;68:2120.
449. Marchini S, Licitra L, Grandi L, et al. Cisplatin and fluorouracil in recurrent and/or disseminated nasopharyngeal carcinoma. *Proc Am Soc Clin Oncol* 1991;10:202(abst 672).
450. Gebbia V, Zerillo G, Restivo G, et al. Chemotherapeutic treatment of recurrent and/or metastatic nasopharyngeal carcinoma: a retrospective analysis of 40 cases. *Br J Cancer* 1993;68:191.
451. Yeo W, Leung TWT, Chan ATC, et al. Phase II study of combination paclitaxel and carboplatin in advanced nasopharyngeal carcinoma. *Eur J Cancer* 1998;34:2027.
452. Fountzilas G, Skarlos D, Athanassiades A, et al. Docetaxel in combination with fluorouracil for advanced solid tumors. *Oncology* 1997;11:50.
453. Yeo W, Leung TWT, Chan AT, et al. A phase II study of combination paclitaxel and carboplatin in advanced nasopharyngeal carcinoma. *Eur J Cancer* 1998;34(13):2027.
454. Bachouchi M, Cvitkovic E, Azli N, et al. High complete response in advanced nasopharyngeal carcinoma with bleomycin, epirubicin and cisplatin before radiotherapy. *J Natl Cancer Inst* 1990;82:616.
455. Fountzilas G, Daniilidis J, Kosmidis P, et al. Platinum-based chemotherapy followed by radiation therapy of locally advanced nasopharyngeal cancer. A retrospective analysis of 39 cases. *Acta Oncol* 1991;30:831.
456. Azli N, Armand JP, Rahal M, et al. Alternating chemo-radiotherapy with cisplatin and 5-fluorouracil plus bleomycin by continuous infusion for locally advanced undifferentiated carcinoma nasopharyngeal type. *Eur J Cancer* 1992;28A:1792.
457. Dimery IW, Peters L, Goepfert H, et al. Effectiveness of combined induction chemotherapy and radiotherapy in advanced nasopharyngeal carcinoma. *J Clin Oncol* 1993;11:1919.
458. Teo PM, Chan AT, Lee WY, Leung TW, Johnson PJ. Enhancement of local control in locally advanced node-positive nasopharyngeal carcinoma by adjunctive chemotherapy. *Int J Radiat Oncol Biol Phys* 1999;43:261.
459. Geara FB, Glisson BS, Sanguinity G, et al. Induction chemotherapy followed by radiotherapy versus radiotherapy alone in patients with advanced nasopharyngeal carcinoma: results of a matched cohort study. *Cancer* 1997;79:1279.
460. Al-Sarraf M, Paak TF, Cooper JS, et al. Chemo-radiotherapy in patients with locally advanced nasopharyngeal carcinoma: a Radiation Therapy Oncology Group study. *J Clin Oncol* 1990;8:1342.
461. Lin J-C, Chen KY, Jan JS, Hsu CY. Partially hyperfractionated accelerated radiotherapy and concurrent chemotherapy for advanced nasopharyngeal carcinoma. *Int J Radiat Oncol Biol Phys* 1996;35:1127.
462. Rahima M, Rakowski E, Barzilay J, Sidi J. Carcinoma of the nasopharynx. An analysis of 91 cases and a comparison of differing treatment approaches. *Cancer* 1986;58:843.
463. Droz JP, Domenge C, Marin JL, et al. Adjuvant chemotherapy of regionally advanced UCNT with monthly vindesine, adriamycin, bleomycin, cyclophosphamide and cisplatinum: increasing disease-free survival. *Proc Am Soc Clin Oncol* 1987;139:545.
464. Tsuji H, Kamada T, Tsuji H, et al. Improved results in the treatment of nasopharyngeal carcinoma using combined radiotherapy and chemotherapy. *Cancer* 1989;63:1668.
465. Altun M, Fandi A, Dupuis O, et al. Undifferentiated nasopharyngeal cancer (UCNT): current diagnostic and therapeutic aspects. *Int J Radiat Oncol Biol Phys* 1995;32:859.
466. Chang ATC, Teo PML, Johnson PJ. Controversies in the management of loco-regionally advanced nasopharyngeal carcinoma. *Curr Opin Oncol* 1998;10:219.
467. International Nasopharyngeal Cancer Study. Preliminary results of a randomized trial comparing neoadjuvant chemotherapy (cisplatin, epirubicin, bleomycin) plus radiotherapy vs radiotherapy alone in stage IV (> N2, M0) undifferentiated nasopharyngeal carcinoma: a positive effect on progression-free survival. *Int J Radiat Oncol Biol Phys* 1996;35:463.
468. El-Guedari B. Final results of the VUMCA 1 randomized trial comparing neoajuvant chemotherapy plus radiotherapy to RT alone in undifferentiated nasopharyngeal carcinoma. *Proc Am Soc Clin Oncol* 1998;17:1482.
469. Chan ATC, Teo PML, Leung TWT, et al. A prospective randomized study of chemotherapy adjunctive to definitive radiotherapy in advanced nasopharyngeal carcinoma. *Int J Radiat Oncol Biol Phys* 1995;33:569.
470. Chua DTT, Sham JUST, Choy D, et al. Preliminary report of the Asian-Oceanian Clinical Oncology Association randomized trial comparing cisplatin and epirubicin followed by radiotherapy versus radiotherapy alone in the treatment of patient with locoregionally advanced nasopharyngeal carcinoma. *Cancer* 1998;83:2270.
471. Chan ATC, Teo PML, Ngan RKC, et al. A phase III randomized trial comparing concurrent chemotherapy-radiotherapy with radiotherapy alone in locoregionally advanced nasopharyngeal carcinoma. *Proc Am Soc Clin Oncol* 2000 *(in press).*
472. Rossi A, Molinari R, Boracchi P, et al. Adjuvant chemotherapy with vincristine, cyclophosphamide, and doxorubicin after radiotherapy in local-regional nasopharyngeal cancer: result of a 4-year multicenter randomized study. *J Clin Oncol* 1988;10:1401.
473. Wang CC. Improved local control of nasopharyngeal carcinoma after intracavitary brachytherapy boost. *Am J Clin Oncol* 1991;14:5.
474. Hoppe R, Goffinet B, Bagshaw M. Carcinoma of the nasopharynx—eighteen years experience with megavoltage radiation therapy. *Cancer* 1976;37:2605.
475. Bedwinek JM, Perez CA, Keys DJ. Analysis of failure after definitive irradiation for epidermoid carcinoma of the nasopharynx. *Cancer* 1980;45:2725.
476. Mesic JB, Fletcher GH, Goepfert H. Megavoltage irradiation of epithelial tumors of the nasopharynx. *Int J Radiat Oncol Biol Phys* 1981;7:447.
477. Million RR, Cassisi NJ. Nasopharynx. In: Million RR, Cassisi NJ, eds. *Management of head and neck cancer—a multidisciplinary approach.* Philadelphia: Lippincott, 1984:445.
478. Vikram B, Strong E, Manolatos S, et al. Improved survival and carcinoma of the nasopharynx. *Head Neck Surg* 1984;7:123.
479. Wolden SL, Pfister DG, Kraus DH, et al. Improved local control and survival with concomitant boost radiation therapy (CBRT) and chemotherapy (CT) for nasopharyngeal carcinoma (NPC). *Am Soc Clin Oncol* 2000;19:415a.
480. Menck HR, Garfinkel L, Dodd GD. Preliminary report of the National Cancer Data Base. *CA Cancer Clin J* 1991;41:7.
481. *Cancers of the oral cavity and pharynx: a statistics review monograph 1973–1987.* U.S. Department of Health and Human Services.
482. Wynder EL, Stellman SD. Impact of long-term filter cigarette usage on lung and larynx cancer risk. A case-control study. *J Natl Cancer Inst* 1979;62:471.
483. Spitz MR, Fueger JJ, Goepfert H, Hong WK, Newell GR. Squamous cell carcinoma of the upper aerodigestive tract: a case comparison analysis. *Cancer* 1988;61:203.
484. Mashberg A, Garfinkel L, Harris S. Alcohol as a primary risk factor in oral squamous carcinoma. *CA Cancer Clin J* 1981;31:146.
485. Hoffmann D, Hecht SS. Nicotine-derived N-nitrosamines and tobacco-related cancer—current status and future directions. *Cancer Res* 1985;45:935.
486. Schottenfeld D. Alcohol as a co-factor in the etiology of cancer. *Cancer* 1979;43:1962.
487. Schantz SP, Hsu TC. Head and neck cancer patients express increased clastogen-induced chromosome fragility. *Head Neck* 1989;11:337.
488. German J, ed. *Chromosome mutation and neoplasia.* New York: Alan R. Liss, 1983.
489. Guengerich FP. Roles of cytochrome p-450 enzymes in chemical carcinogenesis and cancer chemotherapy. *Cancer Res* 1988;48:2946.
490. McLaughlin JK, Gridley G, Block G, et al. Dietary factors in oral and pharyngeal cancer. *J Natl Cancer Inst* 1988;80:1237.
491. Winn DM, Ziegler RG, Pickle LW, et al. Diet in the etiology of oral and pharyngeal cancer among women from the Southern United States. *Cancer Res* 1984;44:1216.
492. Wynder EL, Hultberg S, Jacobsson F, et al. Oral cancer and mouthwash. *J Natl Cancer Inst* 1983;70:255.
493. Spitz MR, Newell GR. Descriptive epidemiology of squamous cell carcinoma of the upper aerodigestive tract. *Cancer Bull* 1987;39:79.
494. Donald PJ. Marijuana smoking—possible cause of head and neck carcinoma in young patients. *Otolaryngol Head Neck Surg* 1986;94:517.
495. Shillitoe EJ, Greenspan D, Greenspan JS, et al. Immunoglobulin class of antibody to herpes simplex virus in patients with oral cancer. *Cancer* 1983;51:65.
496. DeVilliers EM, Weidauer H, Otta H, et al. Papillomavirus DNA in human tongue carcinomas. *Int J Cancer* 1985;36:575.
497. Dekmezian RH, Batsakis JG, Goepfert H. In situ hybridization of papillomavirus DNA in head and neck squamous cell carcinomas. *Arch Otolaryngol Head Neck Surg* 1987;113:819.
498. Watts SL, Brewer EE, Fry TL. Human papillomavirus DNA types in squamous cell carcinomas of the head and neck. *Oral Surg Oral Med Oral Pathol* 1991;7:701.
499. Bradford CR, Zacks SE, Androphy, EJ, et al. Human papillomavirus DNA sequences in cell lines derived from head and neck squamous cell carcinomas. *Otolaryngol Head Neck Surg* 1990;104:303.
500. Baker SR. Risk factors in multiple carcinoma of the lip. *Otolaryngol Head Neck Surg* 1988;88:248.
501. Berger HM, Goldman R, Gonick HC, Waisman J. Epidermoid carcinoma of the lip after renal transplantation: report of two cases. *Arch Intern Med* 1971;128:609.
502. Sack JG, Ford CN. Metastatic squamous cell carcinoma of the lip. *Arch Otolaryngol* 1978;104:282.

503. Baker SR, Krause CJ. Carcinoma of the lip. *Laryngoscope* 1980;90:19.
504. Nuutinen J, Karja J. Local and distant metastases in patients with surgically treated squamous cell carcinoma of the lip. *Clin Otolaryngol* 1980;6:415.
505. Heller KS, Shah JP. Carcinoma of the lip. *Am J Surg* 1979;138:600.
506. Mendenhall WM, Million RR, Bova EJ. Analysis of time-dose factors in clinically positive neck nodes treated with irradiation alone in squamous cell carcinoma of the head and neck. *J Radiat Oncol Biol Phys* 1984;10:639.
507. Frierson HF Jr, Cooper PH. Prognostic factors in squamous cell carcinoma of the lower lip. *Hum Pathol* 1986;17:346.
508. Byers RM, O'Brien J, Waxler J. The therapeutic and prognostic implications of nerve invasion in cancer of the lower lip. *Int J Radiat Oncol Biol Phys* 1978;4:215.
509. Boddie HW, Fisher EP, Byers RM. Squamous carcinoma of the lower lip in patients under 40 years of age. *South Med J* 1977;70:711.
510. Baker SR, Krause CJ. Carcinoma of the lip. *Laryngoscope* 1980;90:19.
511. Abbé R. A new plastic operation for the relief of deformity due to double hairlip. *Med Rec* 1898;53:477.
512. Estlander JA. Eine Methods aus der einen Lippe Sulstanzverluste der Anderen zu Ersetzen. *Arch Klin Chir* 1872;14:622.
513. Karapandzic M. Reconstruction of lip defects by local arterial flaps. *Br J Plast Surg* 1974;27:93.
514. Baker SR, Krause CJ. Pedicle flaps in reconstruction of the lip. *Facial Plast Surg* 1983;1:61.
515. Webster J. Crescenteric peri-alar cheek excision for upper flap advancement with a short history of upper lip repair. *Plast Reconstr Surg* 1935;27:434.
516. Jackson IT, ed. *Local flaps in head and neck reconstruction.* St. Louis: Mosby, 1985:327.
517. Harrison L, Fass D. Radiation therapy for oral cavity cancer. *Dental Clin North Am* 1990;34:205.
518. Fitzpatrick P. Cancer of the lip. *J Otolaryngol* 1984;13:32.
519. Jorgensen K, Elbrond O, Anderson A. Carcinoma of the lip—a series of 869 cases. *Octaradiol Ther Phys Biol* 1973;12:177.
520. Petrovich Z, Parker R, Luxten G, Kuisk H, Jepson J. Carcinoma of the lip in selective sites of head and neck skin: a clinical study of 896 patients. *Radiol Ther Oncol* 1987;8:11.
521. Sykes AJ, Allan E, Irwin C. Squamous cell carcinoma of the lip: the role of electron treatment. *Clin Oncol* 1996;8:384.
522. Cady B, Catlin D. Epidermoid carcinoma of the gum. A 20-year survey. *Cancer* 1969;23:551.
523. Euch JB, Kragh LV. Results of treatment of squamous cell carcinoma arising in mandibular gingiva. *Arch Surg* 1979;79:100.
524. Willen R, Nathanson A. Squamous cell carcinoma of the gingiva. *Acta Otolaryngol* 1973;75:299.
525. Torabinejad M, Rick GM. Squamous cell carcinoma of the gingiva. *J Am Dent Assoc* 1980;100:870.
526. Nathanson A, Jakobson A, Wersall J. Prognosis of squamous cell carcinoma of the gums. *Acta Otolaryngol* 1973;75:301.
527. Byers RM, Newman R, Russell N, et al. Results of treatment for squamous carcinoma of the lower gum. *Cancer* 1981;47:2236.
528. McGregor AD, MacDonald DG. Patterns of spread of squamous cell carcinoma to the ramus of the mandible. *Head Neck* 1993;15:440.
529. Hidalgo DA. Aesthetic improvements in free-flap mandible reconstruction. *Am Soc Plastic Reconst Surg* 1991;88:574.
530. Soo KC, Spiro RH, King W, et al. Squamous carcinoma of the gingiva: an update. *Am J Surg* 1988;156:281.
531. Million R, Cassisi N. Oral cavity. In: Million RR, Cassissi NJ, eds. *Management of head and neck cancer: a multi-disciplinary approach.* Philadelphia: Lippincott, 1984:295.
532. Fuchihata H, Furukawa S, Murakami S, et al. Results of combined external irradiation and chemotherapy of bleomycin or peplomycin for squamous cell carcinomas of the lower gingiva. *Int J Radiat Oncol Biol Phys* 1994;29:705.
533. Chen J, Katz RV, Krutchkoff DJ. Intraoral squamous cell carcinoma: epidemiologic patterns in Connecticut from 1935 to 1985. *Cancer* 1990;66:1288.
534. Shaha JP, Spiro RH, Shah JP, Strong EW. Squamous carcinoma of the floor of the mouth. *Am J Surg* 1984;148:455.
535. Guillamondegui OM, Oliver B, Hayden R. Cancer of the anterior floor of mouth: selective choice of treatment and analysis of failures. *Am J Surg* 1980;140:56.
536. Soo K, Carter RC, O'Brien CJ, et al. Prognostic implications of perineural spread in squamous carcinoma of the head and neck. *Laryngoscope* 1986;96:1145.
537. Spiro RH, Huvos AG, Wong GY, et al. Predictive value of tumor thickness of squamous carcinoma confined to the tongue and floor of the mouth. *Am J Surg* 1986;152:351.
538. Arthur K, Farr HW. Prognostic significance of histologic grade in epidermoid carcinoma of the mouth and pharynx. *Am J Surg* 1972;124:489.
539. Gilbert E, Goffinet D, Bradshaw M. Carcinoma of the oral tongue and floor of mouth: fifteen years experience with linear excellarator therapy. *Cancer* 1975;35:1517.
540. Mendenhall W, Van Ase W, Bover F, Million R. Analysis of time-dose factors in squamous cell carcinoma of the oral tongue and floor of mouth treated with radiation therapy alone. *Int J Radiat Oncol Biol Phys* 1981;7:1005.
541. Mazeron J, Grimard L, Raynal M, et al. Iridium 192 curietherapy for T1 and T2 epidermoid carcinomas of the floor of mouth. *Int J Radiat Oncol Biol Phys* 1990;18:1299.
542. Salibian AH, Rappaport I, Furnas DW, Auchauer BM. Microvascular reconstruction of the mandible. *Am J Surg* 1980;140:499.
543. Lapeyre M, Peiffert D, Hoffstetter S, et al. Postoperative brachytherapy: a prognostic factor for local control in epidermoid carcinomas of the mouth floor. *Eur J Surg Oncol* 1997;23:243.
544. Klein M, Manneking H, Langford A, Koch K, Stahl H. Treatment of squamous cell carcinoma of the floor of the mouth and tongue by interstitial high-dose-rate irradiation using iridium-192. *Int J Oral Maxillofac Surg* 1998;27:45.
545. Inoue T, Inoue T, Yamazaki H, et al. High dose rate versus low dose rate interstitial radiotherapy for carcinoma of the floor of mouth. *Int J Radiat Oncol Biol Phys* 1998;44:53.
546. Guillamondegui OM, Jesse RH. Surgical treatment of advanced carcinoma of the floor of the mouth. *AJR Am J Roentgenol* 1976;126:1256.
547. Wang CC, Doppke K, Biggs P. Intra-oral cone radiation therapy for selected carcinomas of the oral cavity. *Int J Radiat Oncol Biol Phys* 1983;9:1185.
548. Fu K, Lichter A, Galante M. Carcinoma of the floor of mouth: an analysis of treatment results and the sites and causes of failure. *Int J Radiat Oncol Biol Phys* 1976;1:829.
549. Teichgraber J, Bowman J, Goepfert H. New test series for the functional evaluation of oral cavity cancer. *Head Neck Surg* 1985;8:9.
550. Kramer S, Gelber R, Snow J, et al. Combined radiation therapy and surgery in the management of advanced head and neck cancer: the final report of study 73-03 of the radiation therapy oncology group. *Head Neck Surg* 1987;10:19.
551. Shemen LJ, Klotz J, Shottenfeld D, Strong EW. Increase of tongue cancer in young men. *JAMA* 1984;252:1857.
552. Schantz SP, Byers RM, Goepfert H. Tobacco and cancer of the tongue in young adults. *JAMA* 1988;259:1943.
553. Lindberg R. Distribution of cervical lymph node metastases from squamous cell carcinoma of the upper respiratory and digestive tracts. *Cancer* 1972;29:1446.
554. Strong EW. Carcinoma of the tongue. *Otolaryngol Clin North Am* 1979;12:107.
555. Yamamoto E, Mijakawa, Kohama G. Mode of invasion and lymph node metastasis in squamous cell carcinoma of the oral cavity. *Head Neck Surg* 1984;6:938.
556. Poleksic S, Kalwaic HJ. Prognostic value of vascular invasion in squamous cell carcinoma of the head and neck. *Plast Reconstr Surg* 1978;61:234.
557. Schantz SP, Byers RM, Goepfert H, Shallenberger RS, Beddingfield N. The implication of tobacco use in the young adult with head and neck cancer. *Cancer* 1988;62:1374.
558. Inoue T, Inoue T, Teshima T, et al. Phase III trial of high and low dose rate interstitial radiotherapy for early oral tongue cancer. *Int J Radiat Oncol Biol Phys* 1996;36:1201.
559. Leung TW, Wong VY, Wong CM, et al. High dose rate brachytherapy for carcinoma of the oral tongue. *Int J Radiat Oncol Biol Phys* 1997;39:1113.
560. Yamazaki H, Inoue T, Teshima T, et al. Tongue cancer treated with brachytherapy: is thickness of tongue cancer a prognostic factor for regional control? *Anticancer Res* 1998;18:1261.
561. Yuen AP, Wei WI, Lam LK, Ho WK, Kwong D. Results of surgical salvage of locoregional recurrence of carcinoma of the tongue after radiotherapy failure. *Ann Otol Rhinol Laryngol* 1997;106:779.
562. Decroix Y, Ghossein N. Experience of the Curie Institute in treatment of cancer of the mobile tongue-I. Treatment policy and results. *Cancer* 1981;47:496.
563. Pernot M, Malissard L, Hoffstetter S, et al. The study of tumoral, radiobiological, and general health factors that influence results and complications in a series of 448 oral tongue carcinomas treated exclusively by irradiation. *Int J Radiat Oncol Biol Phys* 1994;29:673.
564. Spiro RH, Strong EW. Surgical treatment of carcinoma of the tongue. *Surg Clin North Am* 1974;54:233.
565. Callery CD, Spiro RH, Strong EW. Changing trends in the management of squamous carcinoma of the tongue. *Am J Surg* 1984;148:449.
566. Spiro R, Strong E. Epidermoid carcinoma of the mobile tongue—treatment by partial glossectomy alone. *Am J Surg* 1971;122:707.
567. Frazell EL, Lucas JC. Cancer of the tongue. Report of the management of 1554 patients. *Cancer* 1962;15:218.
568. Vikram B, Strong EW, Shah JP, Spiro R. Failure at the primary site following multi-modality treatment in advanced head and neck cancer. *Head Neck Surg* 1984;1:720.
569. Ange D, Lindberg R, Guillamondegui O. Management of squamous cell carcinoma of the oral tongue and floor of mouth after excisional biopsy. *Radiology* 1975;116:143.
570. Bamberg M, Schulz U, Scherer E. Post-operative split course radiotherapy of squamous cell carcinoma of the oral tongue. *Int J Radiat Oncol Biol Phys* 1979;5:515.
571. Million R. Squamous cell carcinoma of the head and neck: combined therapy: surgery and post-operative radiation. *Int J Radiat Oncol Biol Phys* 1979;5:2161.
572. Kroll SO, Hoffman S. Squamous cell carcinoma of the oral soft tissues—a statistical analysis of 14,253 cases by age, sex, and race of patients. *J Am Dent Assoc* 1976;92:571.
573. Evans JF, Shah JP. Epidermoid carcinoma of the palate. *Am J Surg* 1981;142:451.
574. Eneroth CM, Hjertman L, Moberger G. Squamous cell carcinoma of the palate. *Acta Otolaryngol* 1972;7:418.
575. Chung CK, Rahman SM, Lim ML, et al. Squamous cell carcinoma of the hard palate. *Int J Radiat Oncol Biol Phys* 1979;5:191.
576. Urist MM, O'Brien CJ, Soong SJ, et al. Squamous carcinoma of the buccal mucosa: analysis of prognostic factors. *Am J Surg* 1987;154:411.
577. Dixit S, Vyas RK, Toparani RB, et al. Surgery versus surgery and postoperative radiotherapy in squamous cell carcinoma of the buccal mucosa: a comparative study. *Ann Surg Oncol* 1998;5:502.
578. Nair M, Sankaranarayanan R, Padmanavhan T. Evaluation of the role of radiation therapy in the management of carcinoma of the buccal mucosa. *Cancer* 1988;61:1326.
579. Lapeyre M, Peiffert D, Malissard L, Hoffstetter S, Pernot M. An original technique of brachytherapy in the treatment of epidermoid carcinoma of the buccal mucosa. *Int J Radiat Oncol Biol Phys* 1995;33:447.
580. Bloom NO, Spiro RH. Carcinoma of the cheek mucosa: a retrospective analysis. *Am J Surg* 1980;140:556.
581. Mishra RC, Singh DN, Mishra TK. Postoperative radiotherapy in carcinoma of the buccal mucosa; a prospective randomized trial. *Eur J Surg Oncol* 1996;22:502.
582. Rehabilitation of head and neck cancer patients: concensus from the International Conference on Rehabilitation of the Head and Neck Cancer Patient. *Head Neck* 1991;13:1.
583. Lazarus CL, Logemann JA, Kahrillas PJ, Mittal BB. Swallow recovery in an oral cancer patient following surgery, radiotherapy, and hyperthermia. *Head Neck* 1994;16:259.
584. Pauloski BR, Logemann JA, Rademaker AW, et al. Speech and swallowing function after oral and oropharyngeal resections: one year follow up. *Head Neck* 1994;16:323.
585. Langius A, Bjorvell H, Lind MG. Functional status and coping in patients with oral and pharyngeal cancer before and after surgery. *Head Neck* 1994;16:559.

586. Lazarus C, Logemann JA, Gibbons P. Effects of maneuvers on swallowing function in a dysphagic oral cancer patient. *Head Neck* 1993;15:419.
587. Whicker JH, DeSanto LW, Devine UD. Surgical treatment of squamous cell carcinoma of the base of the tongue. *Laryngoscope* 1972;82:1853.
588. Harrold CC. Surgical treatment of cancer of the base of tongue. *Am J Surg* 1971;122:487.
589. Riley RW, Fee WE, Goffinet D, Cox R, Goode RI. Squamous cell carcinoma of the base of the tongue. *Otolaryngol Head Neck Surg* 1983;91:143.
590. Sessions DG. Surgical resection and reconstruction for cancer of the base of tongue. *Otolaryngol Clin North Am* 1983;16:309.
591. Pfister DG, Harrison LB, Strong EW, et al. Organ-function preservation in advanced oropharynx cancer: results with induction chemotherapy and radiation. *J Clin Oncol* 1995;13:671.
592. Dupont J, Guillamondegui O, Jesse R. Surgical treatment of advanced carcinoma of the base of tongue. *Am J Surg* 1978;136:501.
593. Weber R, Gidley P, Morrison W, et al. Treatment selection for carcinoma of the base of tongue. *Am J Surg* 1990;160:415.
594. Foote RL, Olson KD, Davis DL, et al. Base of tongue carcinoma: patterns of failure and predictors of recurrence after surgery alone. *Head Neck* 1993;15:300.
595. Harrison L, Sessions R, Strong E, et al. Brachytherapy as part of the definitive management of squamous cancer of the base of tongue. *Int J Radiat Oncol Biol Phys* 1989;17:1309.
596. Harrison L, Zelefsky M, Sessions R, et al. The oncologic and functional outcome of base of tongue cancer treated with external beam radiation plus iridium-192 implant. *Radiology* 1992;184:267.
597. Harrison L, Zelefsky M, Pfister D, et al. Detailed quality of life assessment on long term survivors of primary radiation therapy for cancer of the base of tongue. *Int J Radiat Oncol Biol Phys* 1995;32:78.
598. Harrison L, Zelefsky M, Armstrong J, et al. Performance status after treatment for squamous cell cancer of the base of tongue. A comparison of primary radiation therapy versus primary surgery. *Int J Radiat Oncol Biol Phys* 1994;30:953.
599. Goffinet D, Fee W, Wells J, et al. Iridium 192 pharyngoepiglottic fold implant—the key to successful treatment of base of tongue carcinoma by radiation therapy. *Cancer* 1985; 55:941.
600. Puthawala A, Syed A, Eads D, et al. Limited external beam and interstitial iridium-192 irradiation in the treatment of carcinoma of the base of tongue: a ten year experience. *Int J Radiat Oncol Biol Phys* 1988;14:839.
601. Foote R, Parsons J, Mendenhall W, et al. Interstitial implantation essential for successful radiotherapeutic treatment of base of tongue carcinoma? *Int J Radiat Oncol Biol Phys* 1990;18:1293.
602. Housset M, Baillet F, Dessard-Diana B, et al. A retrospective study of three treatment techniques for T1/T2 base of tongue lesions: surgery plus post-operative radiation, external radiation plus interstitial implantation and external radiation alone. *Int J Radiat Oncol Biol Phys* 1987;13:511.
603. Vikram B, Strong E, Shah J, et al. A non-looping afterloading technique for base of tongue implant: results of the first 20 patients. *Int J Radiat Oncol Biol Phys* 1985;11:1853.
604. List M, Ritter-Sterr C, Lansky S. A performance status scale for head and neck cancer patients. *Cancer* 1990;66:564.
605. Mak A, Morrison W, Garden A, et al. Base of tongue carcinoma: treatment results using concomitant boost radiotherapy. *Int J Radiat Oncol Biol Phys* 1995;33:289.
606. Housset M, Baillet F, Delanian S, et al. Split course interstitial brachytherapy with a source shift: the results of a new iridium implant technique vs single course implant for salvage irradiation of base of tongue cancers in 55 patients. *Int J Radiat Oncol Biol Phys* 1991;20:965-971.
607. Mendenhall WM, Stringer SP, Moore GJ, et al. Squamous cell carcinoma of the base of tongue treated with external-beam radiation therapy: a preferred alternative to surgery. *Int J Radiat Oncol Biol Phys* 1999;45(Suppl):197.
608. Morrison WH, Garden AS, Ang KK, et al. Long-term results of the concomitant boost fractionation schedule for treatment of oropharyngeal carcinoma. *Int J Radiat Oncol Biol Phys* 1999;45(Suppl):197.
609. Moore GJ, Parsons J, Mendenhall WM. Quality of life outcomes after primary radiotherapy for squamous cell carcinoma of the base of tongue. *Int J Radiat Oncol Biol Phys* 1996;36:351.
610. Lee WR, Berkey B, Marcial V, et al. Anemia is associated with decreased survival and increased locoregional failure in patients with locally advanced head and neck carcinoma: a secondary analysis of RTOG 85–27. *Int J Radiat Oncol Biol Phys* 1998;42:1069.
611. Horowitz E, Frazier A, Martinez A, et al. Excellent functional outcome in patients with squamous cell carcinoma of the base of tongue treated with external irradiation and interstitial iodine 125 boost. *Cancer* 1996;78:948.
612. Givens CD, Johns ME, Cantrell RW. Carcinoma of the tonsil. *Arch Otol* 1981;107:730.
613. Whicker JH, DeSanto LW, Devine UD. Surgical treatment of squamous cell carcinoma of the tonsil. *Laryngoscope* 1974;84:90.
614. Healy GB, Strong MS, Uchmakli A, et al. Carcinoma of the palatine arch: the rationale of treatment selection. *Am J Surg* 1976;132:498.
615. Barrs DM, DeSanto LW, O'Fallon WM. Squamous cell carcinoma of the tonsil and tongue-base region. *Arch Otolaryngol* 1979;105:479.
616. Eneroth CM, Hjertman L, Moberger G. Squamous cell carcinoma of the palate. *Acta Otolaryngol* 1972;73:418.
617. Fee WE, Schoeppel SL, Rubenstein R, et al. Squamous cell carcinoma of the soft palate. *Arch Otolaryngol* 1979;105:710.
618. Russ JE, Applebaum EL, Sisson GA. Squamous cell carcinoma of the soft palate. *Laryngoscope* 1977;87:1151.
619. Mazeron J, Marinello G, Crook J, et al. Definitive radiation treatment for early stage carcinomas of the soft palate and uvula: the indications for iridium-192 implantation. *Int J Radiat Oncol Biol Phys* 1987;13:1829.
620. Pernot M, Malissard L, Hoffstetter S, et al. Velotonsillar squamous cell carcinoma: 277 cases treated by combined external irradiation and brachytherapy. Results according to localization, extension and dose rate. *Int J Radiat Oncol Biol Phys* 1991;1:142.
621. Pernot M, Malissard L, Hoffstetter S, et al. Influence of tumoral, radiobiological, and general factors on local control and survival of a series of 361 tumors of the velotonsillar area treated by exclusive irradiation (external beam irradiation and brachytherapy or brachytherapy alone). *Int J Radiat Oncol Biol Phys* 1994;30:1051.
622. Behar R, Martin P, Fee W, Goffinet DR. Iridium-192 interstitial implant and external beam radiation therapy in the management of squamous cell carcinoma of the tonsil and soft palate. *Int J Radiat Oncol Biol Phys* 1994;28:221.
623. Mazeron JJ, Belkacemi Y, Simon J, et al. Place of iridium-192 implantation in definitive irradiation of faucial arch squamous cell carcinomas. *Int J Radiat Oncol Biol Phys* 1993;27:251.
624. Remmler D, Medina JE, Byers RM, Meoz R, Pfalzgraf K. Treatment of choice for squamous cell carcinoma of the tonsillar fossa. *Head Neck Surg* 1985;7:206.
625. Tong D, Laramore G, Griffen T, et al. Carcinoma of the tonsil region. *Cancer* 1982;49:2007.
626. Maltz R, Shumrick D, et al. Carcinoma of the tonsil: results of combined therapy. *Laryngoscope* 1974;84:2172.
627. Wong C, Ang K, Fletcher G, et al. Definitive radiotherapy for squamous cell carcinoma of the tonsillar fossa. *Int J Radiat Oncol Biol Phys* 1989;16:657.
628. Wang CC. Local control of oropharyngeal carcinoma after two accelerated hyperfractionation radiation therapy schemes. *Int J Radiat Oncol Biol Phys* 1988;14:1143.
629. Perez C, Carmichael T, Devinenni V, et al. Carcinoma of the tonsilla fossa: a non-randomized comparison of irradiation alone or combined with surgery: long term results. *Head Neck* 1991;13:282.
630. Perez C, Purdy J, Breaux S, et al. Carcinoma of the tonsillar fossa—a non-randomized comparison of pre-operative radiation and surgery or irradiation alone: long term results. *Cancer* 1982;50:2314.
631. Perez C, Lee F, Ackerman L, et al. Carcinoma of the tonsillar fossa: significance of dose irradiation and volume treated in the control of the primary tumor and metastatic nodes. *Int J Radiat Oncol Biol Phys* 1976;1:817.
632. Puthawala A, Syed A, Eads D, et al. Limited external irradiation and interstitial iridium-192 implant in the treatment of squamous cell carcinoma of the tonsillar fossa. *Int J Radiat Oncol Biol Phys* 1985;11:1595.
633. Mazeron J, Lusinchi A, Marinello G, et al. Interstitial radiation therapy for squamous cell carcinoma of the tonsillar region: The Creteil experience. *Int J Radiat Oncol Biol Phys* 1986;12:895.
634. Levendag PG, Schmitz PI, Jansen PP, et al. Fractionated high-dose rate and pulsed–dose-rate brachytherapy: first clinical experience in squamous cell carcinoma of the tonsillar fossa and soft palate. *Int J Radiat Oncol Biol Phys* 1997;38:497.
635. Mendenhall W, Parsons J, Cassisi N, et al. Squamous cell carcinoma of the tonsillar area treated with radical irradiation. *Radiother Oncol* 1987;10:23.
636. Murthy A, Hendrickson F. Contralateral neck treated necessary in early carcinoma of the tonsil? *Int J Radiat Oncol Biol Phys* 1980;6:91.
637. Dasmahapatra K, Mohit-Tabatabai M, Rush B, et al. Cancer of the tonsil—improved survival with combination therapy. *Cancer* 1986;57:451.
638. Zelefsky M, Harrison L, Armstrong J, Fass D. Post-operative radiation therapy for advanced oropharyngeal carcinoma: long term results. *Cancer* 1992;70:2388.
639. Spiro J, Spiro R. Carcinoma of the tonsillar fossa—an update. *Arch Otol Head Neck Surg* 1989;115:1186.
640. Gluckman J, Zitsch R. Current management of carcinoma of the oropharynx. *Oncology* 1990;4:23.
641. Sealy R, LeRoux T, Hering E, et al. The treatment of cancer of the uvula and soft palate and interstitial radioactive wire implants. *Int J Radiat Oncol Biol Phys* 1984;10:1951.
642. Esche B, Haie C, Gerbaulet A, et al. Interstitial and external radiotherapy in carcinoma of the soft palate and uvula. *Int J Radiat Oncol Biol Phys* 1988;15:619.
643. Amdur R, Mendenhall W, Parsons J, et al. Carcinoma of the soft palate treated with irradiation: analysis of results and complications. *Radiother Oncol* 1987;9:185.
644. Guillamondegui OM, Meoz R, Jesse RH. Surgical treatment of squamous cell carcinoma of the pharyngeal walls. *Am J Surg* 1978;136:474.
645. Ballantyne AJ. Principles of surgical management of cancer of the pharyngeal walls. *Cancer* 1967;20:663.
646. Cunningham MP, Catlin D. Cancer of the pharyngeal wall. *Cancer* 1967;20:1859.
647. Hasegawa Y, Matsuura H. Retropharyngeal node dissection in cancer of the oropharynx and hypharynx. *Head Neck* 1994;16:173.
648. Meoz-Mendez R, Fletcher G, Guillamondegui O, et al. Analysis of the results of irradiation in the treatment of squamous cell carcinomas of the pharyngeal walls. *Int J Radiat Oncol Biol Phys* 1978;4:579.
649. Marks J, Freeman R, Lee F, et al. Pharyngeal wall cancer: an analysis of treatment results complications and patterns of failure. *Int J Radiat Oncol Biol Phys* 1978;4:587.
650. Marks J, Smith P, Sessions D. Pharyngeal wall cancer—reappraisal after comparison of treatment methods. *Arch Otol* 1985;111:79.
651. Fein D, Mendenhall W, Parsons J, et al. Pharyngeal wall carcinoma treated with radiotherapy: impact of treatment technique and fractionation. *Int J Radiat Oncol Biol Phys* 1993;26:751.
652. Spiro R, Kelly J, Vega A, et al. Squamous carcinoma of the posterior pharyngeal wall. *Am J Surg* 1990;160:420.
653. Son Y, Kacinski B. Therapeutic concepts of brachytherapy/megavoltage in sequence for pharyngeal, results of integrated dose therapy. *Cancer* 1987;59:1268.
654. Laborgne JH, Leborgne P, Barlocci L, et al. The place of brachytherapy in the treatment of carcinoma of the tonsil with lingual extension. *Int J Radiat Oncol* 1986;12:1787.

ROY B. SESSIONS
LOUIS B. HARRISON
ARLENE A. FORASTIERE

SECTION 3

Tumors of the Larynx and Hypopharynx

LARYNX

Cancers of the larynx are considerably less frequent than malignancies of other sites, such as lung, breast, prostate, and colon; despite this fact, however, a substantial amount continues to be written on the subject. This seemingly disproportionate body of writing probably reflects the perceived importance of these neoplasms relative to their potential impact on people's communicative skills. It would seem that the mere threat to a person's vocal organ is associated with profound psychological and socioeconomic overtones, and curing the cancer at any cost no longer is accepted casually. More than ever before, a premium is placed on returning the patient to a productive and useful lifestyle (i.e., quality of life after cancer treatment). This attitude is demonstrated more keenly in the treatment of larynx cancer than with almost any other malignancy. In the past, treatment of laryngeal cancer focused predominantly on cure by relentless surgical aggressiveness. That era was followed by the emergence of conservation through larynx-sparing operations, the development of sophisticated radiation methods, and most recently, organ-sparing strategies in which chemotherapeutic, radiotherapeutic, and surgical methods are used in a variety of combinations and sequences.[1–3] The overall 5-year cure rate for patients with laryngeal squamous cell carcinoma (SCC) is almost 70%, and although those data have not changed dramatically during the last decade,[4–6] the treatment options and their sequencing have. As a result, a higher percentage of contemporary patients are retaining their larynx.

EPIDEMIOLOGY AND ETIOLOGY

Although considerable geographic differences exist in the incidence of larynx cancer, the distribution of the disease is consistent within each country. For example, regardless of the culture, this disease most commonly affects middle-aged or older men who have smoked tobacco[7,8] and have consumed excessive alcohol.[9] Laryngeal cancer rarely occurs in people who have done neither. In the United States during the year 2000, more than 12,000 new larynx cancers will be diagnosed, and approximately 10,000 of those cases will be in men. Although this disease has always been more common in men, the gender ratio is changing; in 1956, the ratio was 15:1, whereas current studies show an approximately 5:1 ratio of men to women. This trend is probably due to the predictable effects of the changing smoking patterns of the sexes.[9] Racial differences also exist. Compared with whites, African Americans in the United States have a significantly higher incidence of larynx cancer.[10] Overall, the peak incidence of larynx cancer is in the sixth decade. The disease occurs in young people only rarely.[11]

The etiologic factors that have been implicated in laryngeal cancer are voice abuse and chronic laryngitis[7,12]; dietary factors[13–15]; chronic gastric reflux[16]; and exposure to wood dust, nitrogen mustard, asbestos, and ionizing radiation.[17–20] The carcinogenic effect on the larynx that results from smoking tobacco—whether by pipe, cigarette, or cigar—is, however, the factor most widely held responsible for this malignancy.[17] Larynx cancer only occasionally occurs in patients who have never smoked.[20] Possibly, human papillomavirus is an important cofactor in aerodigestive carcinogenesis in general, and it may be especially significant in the larynx.[21–28]

Heavy alcohol intake appears to be associated with larynx cancer, and it appears to enhance the already present risk factors associated with smoking.[9] On the other hand, some studies have failed to demonstrate an interdependent causal effect for alcohol intake and larynx cancer.[28] The issue of alcohol, smoke, and carcinogenesis is complicated by the nutritional deficiencies that usually occur in alcoholics.[15] In the larynx, this complex issue is more specifically defined by the fact that whatever the role of alcohol, it is apparently more significant in supraglottic than in glottic cancers.[29–32] With the maturation of the current generation of those youngsters using smokeless tobacco, some alteration of the relative incidence in the United States of supraglottic and glottic cancers may be noted. Those worldwide data that show large variations of laryngeal cancer statistics consistently reflect the smoking and drinking habits of the individual country.[33] Also, the sites within the larynx affected by cancers vary considerably between countries. This distribution is shown in Table 30.3-1,[12,24,26,34] which represents a compendium of worldwide data that addresses the relative distributions of cancer within the larynx.

Koufman and Burke[35] make a strong case for a multifactorial etiology, and they have proposed a model that involves tobacco, environmental factors, alcohol, reflux, viral activation, dietary deficiency, and altered host immunity.

RELEVANT ANATOMY

The larynx is a uniquely complicated organ that is strategically located so that significant alteration of its anatomy by either surgery or cancer can have a noticeable impact on vocal, respiratory, and swallowing physiology. The organ consists of three subsites: glottis (paired true vocal cords), supraglottis, and subglottis. Thus, clarification of the subsites within the larynx is essential. Because of different embryologic development and different lymphatic patterns that are subsite-specific, to discuss larynx cancers without specific reference to the exact location(s) within that structure invites inaccuracies in staging and miscalcu-

TABLE 30.3-1. Geographic Variations in Larynx Cancer Sites[a]

		Site (%)		
Country	*Patients*	Supraglottic	Glottic	Subglottic
Japan[19]	6360	49	50	0.9
Finland[23]	638	67	32	1
Yugoslavia[27]	722	62	35	3.5
United States[28]	1645	34	65	1
Sweden[29]	578	11	87	2

[a]Relative incidence of larynx cancer by anatomic site and country. Notice the variation between supraglottic and glottic incidence relative to different countries but the relative consistency of subglottic occurrence.

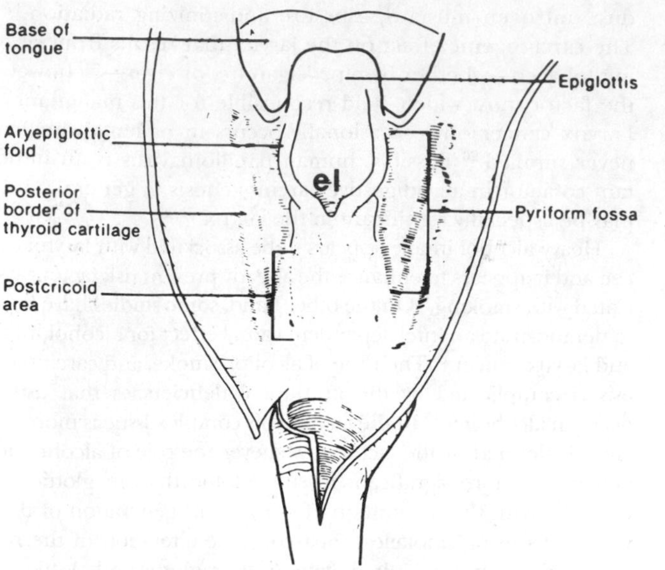

FIGURE 30.3-1. Diagram of internal laryngeal anatomy as viewed posteriorly. Note the endolarynx (el).

lations in treatment planning. Additionally, certain embryologic and anatomic facts are relevant to understanding the natural history of cancers that occur in the larynx. For example, the adjacency of the paraglottic space to the thyroid and cricoid cartilages and to the hypopharynx is critical to the subtle differences between the increasing stages of glottic lesions.

The larynx consists of a complex variety of muscles, an overlying mucous membrane, and a skeletal structure of four cartilages—the cricoid, the epiglottis, the paired arytenoids, and the shield-like thyroid cartilage. Suspended within the endolarynx are the mobile true vocal cords, which are collectively known as the *glottis.* That portion above the glottis, the supraglottis, consists of the false vocal cords, the epiglottis, and the aryepiglottic folds. These folds form the junction (i.e., common partition) between the endolarynx and the hypopharynx. The medial wall of these folds is within the endolarynx, and the lateral wall is actually the medial wall of the adjacent pyriform sinus (Fig. 30.3-1). Those lesions that arise on the rim of the aryepiglottic folds, therefore, have been appropriately referred to as *marginal cancers,* because they bridge the junction between the larynx and the hypopharynx. Those marginal lesions that extend predominantly into the endolarynx behave more like supraglottic cancers, whereas those lesions that spill into the pyriform sinus tend to follow the natural history of the hypopharyngeal malignancies. The subglottis is that portion of the larynx between the underedge of the true vocal cords and the cephalic border of the cricoid cartilage.[36] Although the subglottis is the laryngeal site least likely to harbor a primary cancer, it is critical to the pathogenesis and natural history of glottic (i.e., vocal cord) cancer because it provides an important route of inferior tumor extension.

The true vocal cords are remarkably engineered, although they are somewhat misnamed; rather than cord-like structures, they really are folds of mucosa that cover vocal muscles. These vocal cords (folds) are attached anteriorly to the inner surface of the thyroid cartilage and posteriorly to the arytenoid cartilages. The vocal muscles are complex in their activity, and their dynamic relationship with overlying mucosa is critical to voice production. Any loss of mucosal mobility relative to the underlying muscle, such as that produced by cancer, surgery or, even

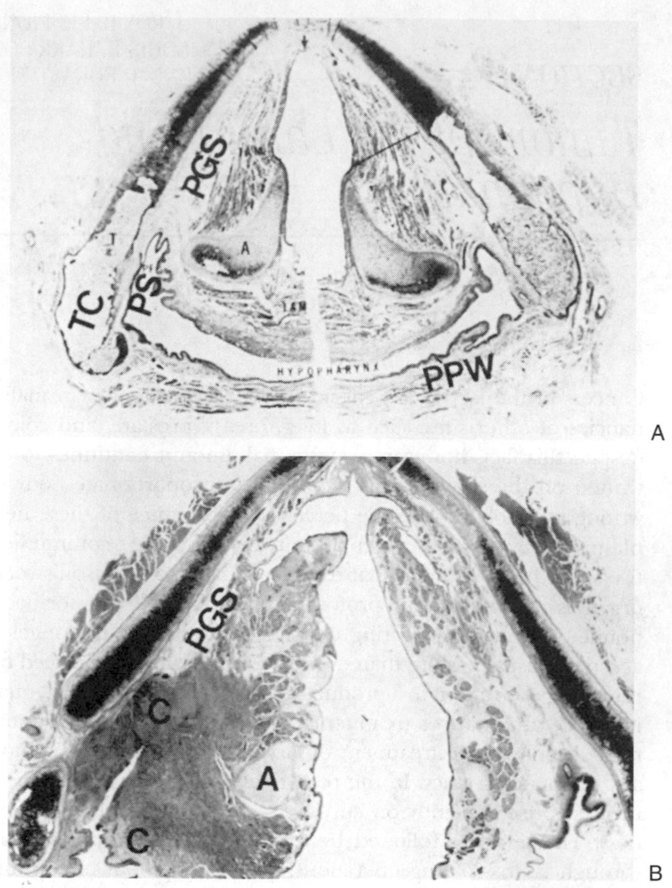

FIGURE 30.3-2. Axial sections of the human laryngopharynx at the level of the glottis. **A:** Notice the relation of the pyriform sinus (PS) to the paraglottic space (PGS) of the endolarynx; the proximity of the lateral wall of the pyriform sinus to the thyroid cartilage (TC); and the relation of the pyriform sinus to the arytenoid (A). Ossification of the area of the thyroid cartilage shown in the axial section renders it vulnerable to skeletal invasion of cancer in this area. The posterior pharyngeal wall (PPW) acts as an extension of the lateral pharyngeal wall and the pyriform sinuses. **B:** Cancer (C) of the pyriform sinus invades the endolarynx (PGS). (Courtesy of Dr. John Kirchner.)

to a lesser extent, by radiation therapy, alters the voice. An appreciation of this fundamental fact is an important component in the selection of treatment of vocal cord cancer.

The lining of the endolarynx consists of respiratory epithelium except on the vibratory edges of the true vocal cords, which typically are lined with pseudostratified squamous epithelium.

The paired arytenoid cartilages each sit on the cephalic rim of the cricoid cartilage and rotate in a relatively horizontal axis around a pivot point. Each arytenoid is attached anteriorly to a true vocal cord, and the clockwise and counterclockwise rotation of these cartilages pulls the respective vocal cord attachment with it, causing abduction and adduction of those structures. Invading cancer can damage any or all of the muscles that are responsible for arytenoid rotation and also the recurrent laryngeal nerve fibers that innervate them. The posterolateral aspect of the larynx is particularly vulnerable to the invasion of cancer because of the adjacency of the medial wall of the pyriform sinus. When cancers of this part of the pyriform sinus extend through the mucosa, they gain direct access to the important laryngeal compartment known as the *paraglottic space,* which leads to all parts of the endolarynx, including the vocal muscles and the preepiglottic space (Fig. 30.3-2). Treatment options for such a tumor are altered significantly because of paraglottic space involvement. Tumors that invade the endolaryngeal muscles or the nerve fibers that innervate them usually create a noticeable effect on vocal cord motion. Of all the findings on laryngeal examination during cancer evaluation, the state of endolaryngeal mobility is one of the most important. This fact has been substantiated by the separate designation that the American Joint Committee on Cancer (AJCC) has assigned to the immobile vocal cord in the staging categorization of this disease.[37]

Another more subtle type of motion alteration pertains to the anatomic relation between the vocal cord musculature and the overlying mucosa. An awareness of this relatively recent knowledge has enhanced the understanding of the pathogenesis and treatment of early glottic cancer.[38] The vibratory mechanism that produces the voice is due to the mobility of the mucous membrane overlying the musculature of the vocal cords. The free edge of the true vocal cord consists of a pseudostratified squamous epithelium, under which is a lamina propria of fibroelastic and gelatinous consistency. This arrangement allows a sliding motion of the mucous membrane, which creates a mucosal wave, the fluidity of which is a direct reflection of the freedom of that layer from the underlying muscle. Any surface cancer that invades through the basement membrane, such as any cancer deeper than carcinoma *in situ* (CIS), affects the mucosal wave by creating a tethering effect. These subtle differences are usually not appreciated by routine laryngeal examination but are obvious with stroboscopic evaluation.[39] An appreciation of these subtleties can translate into the practical matter of determining whether to radiate or microscopically excise certain minimal vocal cord cancers.

Because of the different embryologic origins of the supraglottic from the glottic and subglottic larynx, and also because of the independent lymphatic drainage patterns from each of these subsites, the larynx can be thought of as a compartmentalized structure. These features are important influences in determining the spread of various cancers within that organ.[40]

The lymphatics of the supraglottic larynx are profuse, and the frequency of metastasis associated with cancers of this subsite reflects that fact.[41] Lymphatic spread from the epiglottis is to the false cords, and these channels are directed bilaterally. The drainage from the false cords and the remainder of the supraglottic larynx is lateral and superior, and these channels exit the larynx bilaterally through the thyrohyoid membrane. They then proceed to the adjacent deep cervical nodes. The lymphatics of the infraglottic larynx drain laterally and inferiorly, out of the cricothyroid membrane into the lower deep cervical lymph nodes. The true vocal cords, on the other hand, are unique because they possess little or no lymphatic drainage.[40] From a lymphatic drainage standpoint, the left half of the larynx is essentially independent from the right half, and the supraglottic larynx is independent from the structures below it. These facts are clinically demonstrated: Early-stage supraglottic cancers have little affinity for extension into the lower structures, and those beginning on the true vocal cord do not tend to extend cephalad into the supraglottis.[40,42] Knowledge of this unique pathogenesis has substantial impact on the ability to predict metastasis into various parts of the neck as well as on the planning of the various partial laryngectomies known as *conservation operations.* These techniques combine the removal of laryngeal parts with the preservation of vocal and swallowing functions. Additionally, radiation therapy planning, especially for occult cervical metastasis, is predicated on a thorough knowledge of these and other drainage tendencies of laryngeal cancers.

TABLE 30.3-2. Classification of Laryngeal Malignancies by Histologic Type

Primary malignancies
- Epithelial cancers
  - Squamous cell carcinoma
    - Carcinoma *in situ*
    - Superficially invasive
    - Verrucous carcinoma
    - Pseudosarcoma
    - Anaplastic
    - Transitional cell
    - Lymphoepithelial
  - Adenocarcinoma
    - Mucoepidermoid carcinoma
    - Adenocarcinoma
    - Adenoid cystic carcinoma
  - Neuroendocrine tumors
    - Small cell carcinoma (oat cell)
    - Paraganglioma
    - Carcinoid
  - Oncocytic carcinoma
  - Melanoma
- Nonepithelial cancers
  - Sarcomas
    - Fibrosarcoma
    - Chondrosarcoma
    - Rhabdomyosarcoma
    - Leiomyosarcoma
    - Hemangiosarcoma
    - Giant cell sarcoma
    - Lymphosarcoma

Metastatic malignancies
- Renal cell carcinoma
- Thyroid carcinoma
- Breast
- Lung
- Prostate
- Gastrointestinal tract

PATHOLOGY, PATHOGENESIS, AND NATURAL HISTORY

A variety of laryngeal malignancies, most of which are primary to the larynx and others that are metastatic from other sites, have been reported. A comprehensive classification is shown in Table 30.3-2.

More than 95% of all primary laryngeal malignancies are SCCs, with the remainder being sarcomas, adenocarcinomas, neuroendocrine tumors, and other types.[43] Both spindle cell and verrucous carcinomas probably are variants of SCC.

It should be noted that knowledge and recognition of the neuroendocrine family of malignancies has changed considerably over time, and the exact percentage of these within the overall population of larynx cancers is unknown. In the past, certain tumors were vaguely classified as poorly differentiated malignancies when, in fact, they were neuroendocrine in origin. Modern techniques of immunohistochemical and morphologic analysis will almost certainly lead to the recognition and accrual of more of these tumors in the future, and as a result, they will make up a higher relative percentage of laryngeal malignancies.[44,45]

Laryngeal SCC accounts for approximately one-fourth of all head and neck SCCs.[46] Some variability is seen between series from different institutions and different patient populations; however, more than one-half of laryngeal SCCs present as localized disease without metastasis, one-fourth present as local disease with regional metastasis, and approximately 15% are first seen at an advanced stage with or without distant metastasis. As with other aerodigestive carcinomas, metachronous and synchronous cancers are ongoing considerations in developing appropriate diagnostic and therapeutic strategies. The incidence of metachronous (i.e., second primary aerodigestive SCC) is reported to be between 5% and 35% of all aerodigestive cases,[47–50] with the esophagus being the most common second site overall.[49,50] The larynx, however, seems to demonstrate a more frequent association with lung rather than esophagus carcinoma. This is a logical sequel to the carcinogenic impact of inhaling rather than ingesting offensive chemicals.

Separate consideration must be given to the spectrum of cellular disarray that includes premalignant squamous lesions, CIS, and superficially invasive carcinomas. To discuss the epithelial changes that precede and probably lead to carcinoma of the larynx is of considerable importance because it is with this group of lesions that cancer prevention and conservative management methods are most effective. As our knowledge of this subject has increased, so too has our sophistication in applying the minimal techniques necessary to achieve excellent cure rates in these disorders. The obvious value of a philosophy of preemptive strategies and treatment minimalism is the achievement of an outcome with the least physiologic change. Important also is that, by applying the appropriate minimal treatment, one is able to save radiation in reserve for potential future cancers of the adjacent aerodigestive tissues.[51]

Because the appropriate management strategy for early laryngeal neoplasia depends greatly on a dialogue that is understood by both oncologist and pathologist, the description of the various alterations of the surface epithelium, although not exclusively applicable to the larynx, is important to this discussion. The term *leukoplakia* describes any white lesion on a mucous membrane and does not automatically refer to an associated or underlying malignancy. *Erythroplakia*, on the other hand, is a clinical term that describes any red lesion on a mucous membrane and, in contrast to the white lesions, is often indicative of an underlying malignant tumor. The term *hyperkeratosis* represents an increase in the amount of surface keratin. In the case of the larynx, which normally is lined with a nonkeratinizing epithelium, the use of the term *hyperkeratosis* is redundant; instead, the preferable term is *keratosis*.

Investigators have studied the occurrence of aberrant squamous epithelium in various areas of the larynx, and a predilection seems to exist for carcinogenesis in those respective sites.[52] However, because only those lesions that begin on the true vocal cords are likely to produce early symptoms and signs, the opportunity to treat small cancers on other aerodigestive sites is infrequent. With true vocal cord lesions, however, the early warning symptoms frequently lead to early diagnosis and extraordinary cure rates for glottic malignancies.

The mucosal changes that lead to cancer take years to develop, and that evolution probably follows a consistent pattern. Most laryngeal SCCs result from prolonged exposure to recognized carcinogens that stimulate mucosal hyperplasia and metaplasia. Some of these changes are associated with keratosis, and others are not. In some situations, epithelial atypia or dysplasia may exist, the degree of which probably determines whether a lesion is destined to become malignant.[53–55] In one large study by Sllamniku and colleagues,[56] 3% of patients with vocal cord keratosis unassociated with atypia and 7% with mild atypia developed invasive carcinoma. In those patients with moderate and severe atypia, however, 18% and 24%, respectively, developed carcinoma. Another study by Hjslet and colleagues[57] showed a similar probability of cancer evolution in the group with less atypia and a strikingly higher probability in those patients with severe atypia.

In addition to the morphologic appearance of mucosal alteration, DNA changes seem to show a correlation between cancer potential and cellular aneuploidy. In a study by Munck-Wirland and coworkers,[58] for instance, all of those patients with dysplastic laryngeal lesions that later went on to become carcinoma demonstrated an aneuploid DNA pattern.

Mucosal lesions, whether premalignant or not, have an inconsistent gross appearance; some are white and others are hyperemic. Many investigators believe the risk for cancer development is substantially higher in lesions that are soft and red in appearance.[55] Without histologic study, however, even the most experienced diagnostician cannot consistently predict the presence of cancer or the likelihood of its evolution in any of these lesions. Furthermore, any given point within a lesion does not necessarily represent the balance of that lesion. The facts that CIS is often surrounded by dysplastic epithelium and that many areas of invasive carcinoma are surrounded by zones of both CIS and dysplastic epithelium[59] lend credence to the concept that these morphologic categories of epithelial disturbance are each part of a dynamic spectrum of disorders, each probably related to and possibly representing different stages of the same process. This rationale suggests that dysplasia leads to CIS, which in turn leads to invasive carcinoma.

On the other hand, this concept is challenged vigorously, and contrary thought suggests that the spectrum of abnormal epithelial maturation and individual cellular aberrations can occur in circumstances that may or may not precede invasive carcinoma. *Dysplasia* is a term that is synonymous with atypia, and the degree of dysplasia is graded as mild, moderate, or severe, depending on the extent of involvement of the surface epithelium. In general, the less the degree of dysplasia, the less likely is the transformation to invasive carcinoma. Conversely, the higher the degree of dysplasia, the more likely is such a progression. In the opinion of some investigators, however, severe dysplasia, especially in the larynx, is not a prerequisite for the development of an invasive SCC. In fact, invasive carcinoma can develop in an epithelium with only mild dysplastic changes.

As classically defined, CIS represents full-thickness, mucosal, epithelial, dysplastic change without violation of the basement membrane. For all intents and purposes, severe dysplasia can be synonymous with CIS. Also, CIS is known to arise from the basal epithelial layer in the absence of overlying dysplastic changes. In this setting, therefore, the definition of CIS can be expanded to include those lesions in which the mucosal alterations are so severe as to signal a high probability for the progression to an invasive carcinoma if left untreated. Extension of the dysplastic process to involve the mucoserous glands should still be consid-

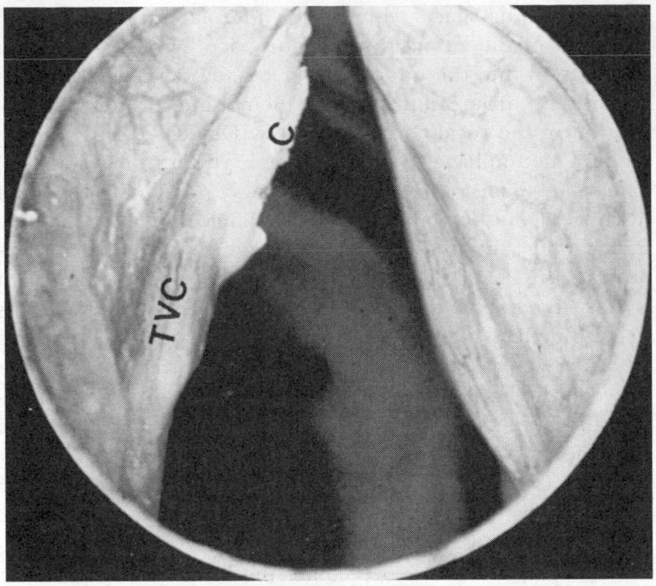

FIGURE 30.3-3. Squamous cell carcinoma (C) of the true vocal cord (TVC). Notice the "surface" appearance of the lesion.

ered CIS and not invasive carcinoma. Such is not the case with transgression across the basement membrane, which is the point at which CIS becomes invasive carcinoma.

It is unknown whether those lesions that have achieved the status of carcinoma continue to grow at the same rate as they did during their premalignant state or whether their growth is accelerated. The growth of a cancer through the basement membrane into the lamina propria constitutes the transition from CIS to microinvasive carcinoma, and accompanying this development is a tethering of vocal cord mucosal motion. The degree of this membrane motion restriction is in direct proportion to the extent of invasion into the underlying lamina propria of the vocal cord.[9] Failure to appreciate these subtle changes can result in the administration of suboptimal treatment. For example, high failure rates that have been reported with mucosal stripping in CIS patients almost certainly represent underestimation of these lesions.[60] Some of those lesions that had been classified in the prestroboscopic era as CIS probably contained areas of invasive carcinoma, and the stripping left behind foci of cancer that resulted in recurrence.

The gross appearance of a given laryngeal lesion is suggestive of its general type. SCCs originate within the mucous membrane and are exophytic or ulcerative, are of surface origin (Fig. 30.3-3), and are frequently adjacent to or surrounded by keratoses. Neuroendocrine cancers and tumors metastatic to the larynx are usually submucosal and, as such, do not resemble lesions of surface origin. Metastatic lesions of various types and neuroendocrine tumors are seen throughout the various subsites within the larynx, although the latter group shows a predilection for the supraglottic area. The distribution of SCC within the various laryngeal subsites varies between different countries, a fact that reflects the different social habits within those cultures. In the United States, for example, the ratio of supraglottic to glottic SCCs is 1:2, whereas the reverse is true in certain European countries (see Table 30.3-1).

The major differences in the natural histories of the various SCCs of the larynx are related largely to the area anatomy and to the lymphatic drainage patterns of the respective subsite(s).

Cellular characteristics vary by site. In the supraglottis, lesions are more likely to be nonkeratinizing and poorly differentiated, and they have more aggressive local behavior in general.[61] Those lesions of the true vocal cords, on the other hand, are more often well differentiated and tend to be less aggressive locally. Although the degree of cellular differentiation is not thought to be the most significant fact in tumor grading, it does seem to correlate with the probability of cervical metastasis,[32,42,62,63] which in turn strongly impacts on survival.[64] Other local characteristics, such as tumor-host interface,[42,61] peritumor inflammatory response,[65] and vascular and perineural invasion,[66] also seem important in determining performance. Finally, the actual tumor thickness and depth of invasion almost certainly have an influence on metastasis and, ultimately, on survival.

A variety of studies have attempted to standardize the predictive value of thickness in SCCs of the upper aerodigestive tract with the probability of cervical metastasis and, therefore, the prognosis.[65,67–70] Although head and neck oncologists have for some time intuitively favored a direct correlation between the two, a number of studies have failed to demonstrate a statistically significant association between tumor thickness and nodal metastasis.[66,71,72] Also, it should be noted that those studies demonstrating a correlation between thickness and metastasis generally focused on sites other than the larynx, and because of the anatomic complexity and embryologic uniqueness of the larynx, one cannot necessarily transpose such data from other head and neck organs.

SPECIFIC SITES

Supraglottis

Lesions of the supraglottic larynx tend to spread locally. If they begin on the epiglottis, they can extend onto the false vocal cords and into the ventricles. Inferior extension beyond the ventricle is initially thwarted, but as growth continues, these cancers can penetrate into the paraglottic space. From there they gain full access to the length of the endolarynx. These cancers often exit the paraglottic space at the top and bottom of the larynx to enter directly into the neck.

Most supraglottic lesions arise on the epiglottis, with fewer being seen on the false vocal cords and aryepiglottic folds. Those lesions that occur on the suprahyoid or upper part of the epiglottis are more often exophytic, whereas those that occur on the lower portion of that structure are likely to be endophytic or ulcerative.[61,73] An endophytic growth pattern is especially significant in this particular area of the epiglottis because of the presence of foramina that lead directly through the cartilage into the preepiglottic space. This space is a compartment continuous with the tongue base. What would appear to be a localized tumor in the endolarynx, therefore, can actually involve considerable unrecognized extralaryngeal extension. Tumors are confined initially to the preepiglottic space by the ligamentous boundaries of that compartment, but once those barriers are overcome, the loosely arranged skeletal muscle fibers of the tongue provide no restriction to further tumor extension.[74] Modern imaging, especially magnetic resonance imaging (MRI), has greatly improved the ability to recognize tumor extension into the preepiglottic space and base of the tongue.

Those lesions that occur on the laryngeal surface of the epiglottis are capable of invading and destroying the cartilage of that structure. Supraglottic cancers, on the other hand, almost never destroy the thyroid cartilage.[75] This feature has an influence on the design of treatment plans. For example, an ossified and invaded thyroid cartilage poses a substantial problem for surgeons attempting to perform partial laryngectomy and also for radiation oncologists attempting to deliver curative therapy.

Aryepiglottic fold cancers are somewhat different in their behavior, more commonly following the tendencies of pyriform sinus lesions by spreading in a more diffuse fashion and metastasizing more frequently than their endolaryngeal counterparts. The particularly ominous natural history of these lesions probably relates as much to the abundant and multidirectional lymphatic drainage of the area as it does to individual cellular peculiarities.[76]

Because of the profuse lymphatic network of the supraglottic larynx, carcinomas of this area metastasize frequently to the cervical lymph nodes, and failure of treatment is usually a result of metastasis rather than local disease.[41,54,77] The incidence of patients with clinically positive lymph nodes at the time of diagnosis is 23% to 50% for all supraglottic sites and stages combined.[76,78–80] A substantial number of those patients with clinically negative necks turn out to have histologic disease as demonstrated when a neck dissection is done, or, if left untreated, they convert to clinically positive necks.[81,82] In supraglottic cancers, the probability of cervical metastasis and the probability of delayed contralateral metastasis increase in direct proportion to the size of the primary (i.e., the T stage).[61,83,84] Lindberg[41] reported impressive overall metastatic rates with various supraglottic carcinomas: Sixty-three percent of T1, 70% of T2, 79% of T3, and 73% of T4 cases metastasized.

In that group of patients with supraglottic lesions that present with a clinically positive cervical node 2 cm in diameter or more, the possibility for contralateral neck metastasis is 40% or higher.[85] The epiglottis is particularly prone to bilateral metastasis, and even in smaller lesions of that site, the incidence of contralateral metastasis is more than 20%.[72] Much of the data on clinically positive necks and on occult metastasis were compiled before the routine use of computed tomography (CT) and MRI of the neck. With the use of these more sophisticated staging methods added to the already 75% to 85% accuracy of physical examination,[86] the overall incidence of metastasis noted at the time of diagnosis will probably become higher than that reported previously.

Glottis

Glottic, or true vocal cord (fold), carcinoma is the most common of all laryngeal cancers encountered in the United States. Although these lesions are usually well differentiated, they can demonstrate an infiltrative growth pattern, even when they appear exophytic and well organized. Most true vocal cord cancers occur on the anterior two-thirds of that structure; a small percentage of them develop on the anterior commissure; and they rarely occur on the posterior commissure.[87]

To a large extent, growth characteristics and the natural history of glottic carcinomas are determined by the unique anatomy of the true vocal cords. First, the sparsity of the lymphatic drainage of the true vocal cords in all areas other than the posterior commissure makes metastasis of early lesions extremely unlikely. Second, the elastic layers (conus elasticus) within the larynx often divert cancers that begin on the free edge of the vocal cord and continue into the underlying vocalis muscle and paraglottic space, which is an inferolateral pathway that leads out of the larynx through the cricothyroid space. With penetration into the underlying tissues, all degrees of motion impairment, from subtle mucous membrane stiffness to frank fixation of the vocal cord, can follow. That increasing impairment of motion has a telling effect on local control and survival data, a fact that is reflected in AJCC staging designations. Much discussion continues about mobility change and its therapeutic implications, and it is in the group of glottic cancers that demonstrate this change that the clinical judgment of the physician is most tested. The final anatomic factor unique to the glottis that influences the growth pattern of certain cancers is the anterior commissure ligament, which forms the bridge between the anterior ends of the true vocal cords. This structure lies immediately against the inner lamina of the thyroid cartilage, and its presence initially retards penetration of cancers into that area, often causing their diversion upward onto the epiglottis or downward onto the cricothyroid membrane. From there, these lesions can escape the larynx into the anterior neck. If the cancer overcomes the ligamentous barrier at the anterior commissure, the cartilage is penetrated.[88] This event is particularly likely in thyroid cartilages that are ossified, and when this does occur, substantial therapeutic implications compromise the effectiveness of radiation therapy and dictate specific surgical approaches.[89,90]

Subglottis

Carcinomas of the subglottic larynx are unusual, making up only approximately 1% to 8% of all laryngeal cancers.[91] These lesions tend to be poorly differentiated and often demonstrate an infiltrative growth pattern unrestricted by tissue barriers. These tumors are, therefore, frequently circumferential and can extend down the trachea. The incidence of cervical metastasis in this group of cancers is reported to be 20% to 30%, but that figure is somewhat obscured by the fact that the primary drainage pattern of these lesions is to the less detectable pretracheal and paratracheal nodes. The actual incidence of metastasis may, therefore, be significantly higher.[85,92,93]

UNUSUAL AND RARE NEOPLASMS

The pathology and pathogenesis of verrucous carcinoma are unique and deserve special consideration. This unusual tumor is poorly understood, and its origin, classification, and response to treatment are controversial.[94,95] Verrucous carcinoma is described as a distinct neoplastic entity of squamous origin that occurs in the oral cavity, larynx, esophagus, and nose and on the genitalia.[47,96–99] Some authorities have suggested the human papillomavirus as its cause.[100] Although there are views to the contrary, most investigators consider verrucous carcinoma to be an entity unto itself.[101] Just because some tumors originally thought to be verrucous carcinoma are discovered to have features of SCC and can metastasize does not, in their opinion, justify combining the two diagnoses (actually, they think that such tumors were always low-grade SCCs rather than verrucous carcinoma).[98] Other investigators, although conceding verrucous carcinoma to be unique, believe it to be only a variant of well-differentiated SCC. Different authors believe that because verrucous carcinomas neither fulfill the histologic and cytologic criteria of malignancy nor possess the capability to metastasize, they should be renamed *verrucous acanthoma.*[102] When

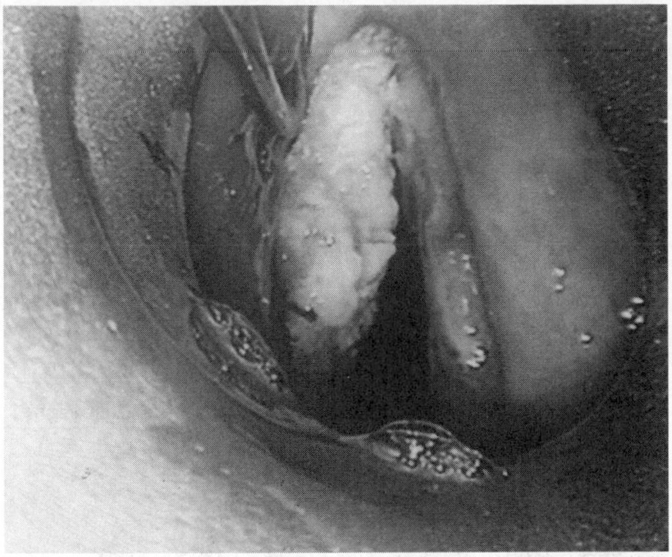

FIGURE 30.3-4. Verrucous carcinoma of the true vocal cord.

this lesion does occur in the larynx, it usually is on the true vocal cord, where it grows slowly and can cause significant local destruction by expanding gradually. Although these lesions often destroy cartilage, they do not tend to metastasize; instead, aggressiveness is directed locally.

Verrucous carcinoma is consistently difficult to diagnose, even when the clinical index of suspicion is high. This observation relates to the fact that these tumors microscopically demonstrate an exuberant and keratinizing hyperplasia that is benign by pure histologic and cytologic criteria.[103] The diagnosis is largely a clinical one and is most effectively achieved by concert between pathologist and surgeon, but usually only after multiple biopsies have been taken.

Verrucous carcinoma is typically a slow-growing but relentless mass, exophytic and warty in appearance, and broad based at its interface with the mucosa (Fig. 30.3-4). Its surface is often necrotic and infected, and the associated inflammation of adjacent tissues can be remarkable. This tendency to cause inflammation can erroneously influence treatment planning. For example, the patient with verrucous carcinoma can demonstrate enlarged adjacent cervical lymph nodes that are worrisome when in fact the adenopathy is only secondary to the inflammatory process. Although this finding has been described in other aerodigestive tumors,[104] the mere presence of lymphadenopathy in the primary drainage area of an impressive primary tumor is worrisome, no matter how benign its histology looks. In such a circumstance, clinical judgment is enhanced greatly by modern imaging and cytopathologic techniques.

This discussion of the nature of verrucous carcinoma has substantial therapeutic implications, especially when the lesion occurs in the larynx. Essentially, SCC is a radiosensitive cancer, a fact that provides treatment options to the oncologist. On the other hand, verrucous carcinoma seems to be somewhat radioresistant, whether found in the mouth or the larynx.[94] Additionally, anecdotal information suggests radiation-induced dedifferentiation into anaplastic cancer in these lesions. This transformation seems to occur in fewer than 10% of verrucous carcinomas[78,96,105–107] and may involve alteration of the DNA that facilitates the integration of the human papillomavirus into host cells.[100] Both the concept of radiation resistance and the transformation into anaplastic cancers are vigorously disputed.[98,108–110]

The neuroendocrine family of tumors represents an evolving database. This is true largely because newer diagnostic techniques have allowed pathologists specifically to label as neuroendocrine a variety of previously undefined cancers. Almost certainly, an immunohistochemical reexamination of laryngeal cancers previously diagnosed as atypical or undifferentiated malignancies would result in the reclassification of many of them as neuroendocrine tumors. The small cell tumors look and act much like their counterpart oat cell lung lesions and, as such, generally are managed by chemotherapy and radiation therapy.[44,111] Surgical procedures do not seem to enhance the likelihood of survival in patients with these tumors.[112–116] The other neuroendocrine tumors that occur in the larynx—carcinoids and paragangliomas—are rare and are best managed surgically.[116–118]

Cartilaginous malignancies,[119] adenocarcinomas,[120] sarcomas,[121] malignant fibrous histiocytomas,[122] plasmacytomas,[123] granular cell tumors,[124] and primary lymphomas[126] have all been reported but are rare. Primary melanomas of the larynx are equally rare. Of all of the laryngeal cancers reported from Memorial Sloan-Kettering Cancer Center between 1949 and 1983, only three were melanomas.[126]

DIAGNOSIS AND EVALUATION

Cancers of the supraglottic larynx usually do not produce early symptoms or signs, and it is common for the first hint of such a cancer to be cervical adenopathy. When symptoms do occur, they are often subtle; pain perceived in the primary site or in the ear (otalgia), a scratchy sensation when swallowing, or merely an alteration of one's tolerance for hot or cold foods may be all that is noticeable. Airway alteration, hoarseness, or a tendency to aspirate liquids are all produced by more advanced lesions.

Cancers of the glottis, on the other hand, are often detected early in the course of the disease because even a slight alteration of the vibratory surface of the true vocal cords produces voice change. Smokers are often hoarse, however, and such alteration of the voice may not alarm them. Anyone with a voice change that persists longer than 2 weeks should have a laryngeal examination. Different than in supraglottic lesions, it is unusual for glottic cancer patients to seek medical attention because of cervical adenopathy. In the latter group, metastasis generally occurs late in the course of the disease, long after the early warning signals.

Subglottic cancers are uncommon, but when they do occur, they do not produce early symptoms; therefore, the disease is often advanced by the time of diagnosis.

Almost all laryngeal cancers are squamous carcinomas and, as such, are surface lesions. Most are obvious with routine laryngeal inspection, but a small percentage are located in obscure areas and, therefore, not readily visible. The modern generation of flexible endoscopes (Fig. 30.3-5) has provided the capability of examining the larynx to a broad range of physicians; thus, the overall process of screening and follow-up after treatment has been enhanced. Importantly, these methods allow the occasional laryngeal examiner to see areas that previously have been visually inaccessible.

It is essential that the larynx be examined in the awake patient who is sitting upright. Direct laryngoscopy under anes-

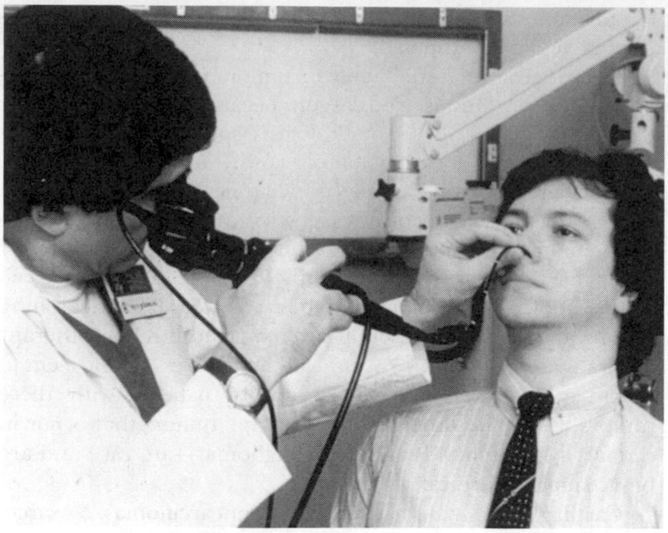

FIGURE 30.3-5. Flexible laryngeal endoscope in use.

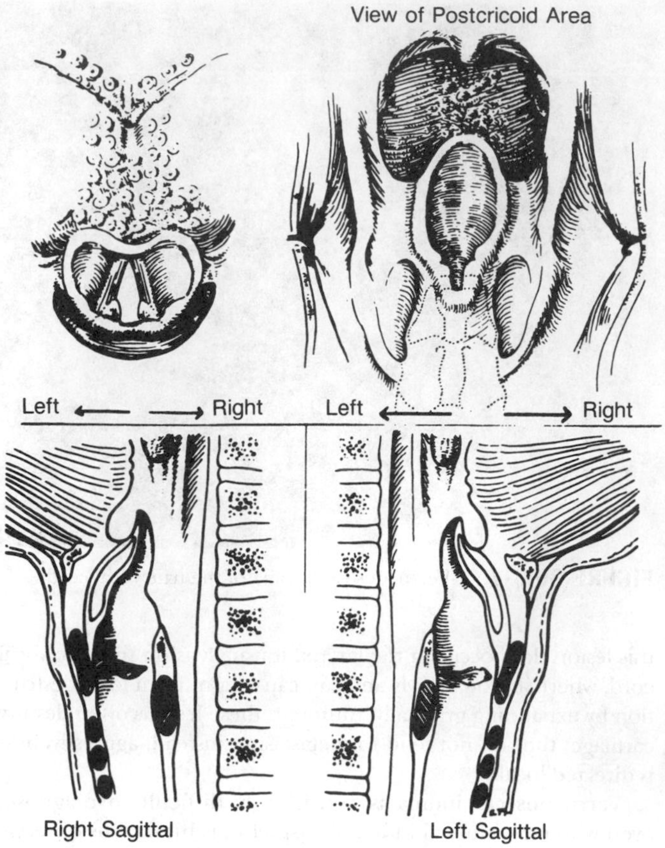

FIGURE 30.3-6. Diagrams of laryngopharynx used for mapping and recording tumors.

thesia should be reserved for biopsy and a more detailed tumor mapping (Fig. 30.3-6). Even when done under local anesthesia, the introduction of a direct laryngoscope distorts the natural position and the relaxed motion of the larynx and, by doing so, tends to disguise subtle motion changes that are important in staging of these tumors. Certain subtleties of contour, such as bulging and tethering, are visually not appreciable during direct laryngoscopy.

The earliest stage of invasive glottic carcinoma through mucosa into the underlying lamina propria is visible as a tethering of the mucous membrane that normally slides over the underlying structures, and the mucosal wave[38] is lost. Although the gross abductive capabilities of the vocal cord may be intact, the early invasive character of a lesion can be appreciated when a stroboscopic examination is used to demonstrate this restrictive feature. As the process of invasion continues into the underlying vocalis muscle, the actual lateral excursion of the vocal cord is limited and eventually lost. The ability of the clinician to view and interpret this scenario is critical to the sophisticated management of vocal cord cancer. Essentially, lesions of the true vocal cord that do not transgress the basement membrane do not cause tethering of the mucosa, and those that enter the underlying lamina propria do cause tethering.[39] Benign lesions and even CIS, therefore, may look extensive topographically, but their lack of depth is revealed by appropriate diagnostic technology. Although contemporary methods of staging tend to emphasize the bulk and topographic size of tumors rather than depth, investigators have begun to focus more on this third dimension. As data are accumulated, more emphasis will be placed on this important matter.

Imaging should not be relied on to detect early larynx cancer, because the routine methods of physical examination are far more suitable. The primary care physician should not, therefore, initially resort to CT or MRI when a laryngeal cancer symptom persists. Instead, someone skilled in the appropriate techniques should examine that patient. Once a lesion is discovered, however, the evaluation of its depth, bulk, and possible cartilage invasion and the status of the regional lymph nodes are often enhanced by CT or MRI. It is not clear which of the two imaging methods is better for larynx cancer evaluation. Both have certain advantages over the other, and both are of limited usefulness in evaluating the radiated larynx. CT of the larynx is most effectively achieved in the axial plane, and because of this, the images are especially efficient in showing lateral tumor extension and the relation of that extension to cervical nodal disease. The axial projection is, therefore, effective in demonstrating the important paraglottic space. CT also effectively demonstrates the vertical extension of tumor, especially in the subglottic and anterior commissure areas. MRI offers the advantages of multiplanal visualization of the larynx and, therefore, is especially valuable in evaluating the preepiglottic space and the adjacent base of the tongue.

Invasion of laryngeal cartilage is important in treatment planning. Determining whether this feature exists has always been difficult because of the inconsistency of the ossification that occurs in the laryngeal framework. Generally, cartilage is vulnerable to tumor invasion in those areas where it is ossified, and it is somewhat resistant where it is not ossified. In fact, healthy, nonossified cartilage provides a considerable natural barrier to cancer invasion. Writings by Castelijns et al.[127] and Towler and Young[125] have suggested that MRI is the method of choice for delineating the important finding of cartilage invasion. Other investigators would dispute this claim. One study correlated MRI findings of cartilage invasion with the effectiveness of radiation treatment, and in so doing, the authors found a surprising number of small glottic lesions with foci of cartilage invasion.[126] Significantly, it was from this group that most of the radiation failures of the series occurred.

Other imaging methods, such as tomography and laryngography, have been surpassed by more elaborate technology and are only of historic interest.

STAGING

The AJCC last updated larynx staging in 1997, and that version is presented in Table 30.3-3. Staging provides a commonality of language that is essential for effective outcomes analysis. The larynx is a complex structure because it involves many anatomic and physiologic factors that impact on performance and, therefore, on staging. Although it is essential that pathologic findings always be compared with preoperative analysis, it should be remembered that the staging referred to and that reported by the AJCC is a clinical one, which is based on performance. The accuracy of clinical staging is periodically updated on the basis of better recognition of performance. For example, Pillsbury and Kirchner[130] studied this question by comparing whole-organ sections of nonradiated larynges and compared the actual pathologic findings with the preoperative staging. They found that 40% of cases had been categorized incorrectly, and most of these inaccuracies reflected understaging. Most commonly, the depth of invasion had been underestimated, and the frequency of cartilage invasion was much higher than previously had been realized. Certainly, as imaging technology improves, so will the ability to stage more accuratcly.[128,129] As clinicians makc usc of adjuvant chemothcrapy treatment protocols for which the assessment of complete versus partial response is required, modern imaging hopefully will enhance the accuracy of that assessment.

Survival in larynx cancer decreases in a linear fashion with increasing stage. The most remarkable change is between stages II and III, the zone that generally represents the occurrence of cervical metastasis.

TREATMENT AND SURVIVAL

Supraglottis

Because the supraglottic larynx is composed of multiple sites, referring to it as one unit is not always accurate when discussing treatment results. Because all of the subsites are intimately related and because the supraglottis is continuous with its neighboring glottic larynx, the hypopharynx, and the oropharynx, it can be difficult to determine the exact site of origin for many larger cancers. For example, when one encounters a lesion that involves the pharyngoepiglottic fold, the aryepiglottic fold(s), and the pyriform sinus(es), it can be difficult to know whether this is a primary hypopharynx cancer extending superiorly or a supraglottic cancer extending inferiorly.

Unlike glottic cancer, in which cervical metastasis is relatively uncommon in early-stage disease, the probability of nodal spread in all supraglottic lesions is substantial.[41,61] A contralateral metastasis is significantly probable in these lesions, and this probability increases in direct proportion to primary tumor size.[83] This finding is especially true for epiglottic lesions, which make up most of the supraglottic carcinomas. It is essential to recognize that the site of treatment failure in supraglottic cancer is usually the neck; therefore, treatment strategies require neck management for virtually all lesions. For the N0 neck, this implies selective neck dissection and/or postoperative radiation, or elective radiation only. For patients with a clinically positive neck(s), this implies neck dissection, therapeutic radiation, or both.

TABLE 30.3-3. Tumor (T), Node (N), Metastasis (M) Staging System for Larynx

Supraglottis	
T1	Tumor limited to one subsite of supraglottis with normal vocal cord mobility
T2	Tumor invades mucosa of more than one adjacent subsite of supraglottis or glottis or region outside the supraglottis (e.g., mucosa of base of tongue, vallecula, medial wall of pyriform sinus) without fixation of the larynx
T3	Tumor limited to larynx with vocal cord fixation and/or invades any of the following: postcricoid area, preepiglottic tissues
T4	Tumor invades through the thyroid cartilage and/or extends into soft tissues of the neck, thyroid, and/or esophagus
Glottis	
T1	Tumor limited to the vocal cord(s) (may involve anterior or posterior commissure) with normal mobility
T1a	Tumor limited to one vocal cord
T1b	Tumor involves both vocal cords
T2	Tumor extends to supraglottis and/or subglottis, and/or with impaired vocal cord mobility
T3	Tumor limited to the larynx with vocal cord fixation
T4	Tumor invades through the thyroid cartilage and/or to other tissues beyond the larynx (e.g., trachea; soft tissues of neck, including thyroid, pharynx)
Subglottis	
Tis	Carcinoma *in situ*
T1	Tumor confined to the subglottic region
T2	Tumor extension to vocal cords, with normal or impaired cord mobility
T3	Tumor confined to larynx, with cord fixation
T4	Massive tumor with cartilage destruction or extension beyond confines of larynx, or both
Stage grouping	
I	T1, N0, M0
II	T2, N0, M0
III	T3, N0, M0
	T1, T2, T3; N1, M0
IV	T4, N0, N1; M0
	Any T, N2, N3; M0
	Any T, any N, M

Note: Differences in T2 glottic cancer allow slight motion alteration, which is different from the subtle mucous membrane motion changes that occur as cancer makes the transition from a surface to an invasive disease. These changes are well appreciated only by stroboscopic visualization[39] and are not represented in the current staging systems. The motion change referred to in the T2 designation reflects gross abduction and adduction alterations that can be seen with the unaided eye.
(Modified from ref. 39.)

Early-stage supraglottic cancers have equivalent cure rates with either conservative (partial laryngectomy) surgery or primary radiation therapy.[131] This is especially true for those lesions on the most cephalic part of the epiglottis (i.e., the suprahyoid epiglottis), but not for those lesions on the lower part of that structure where there are foramina that lead through the cartilage into the preepiglottis space and, ultimately, into the tongue base. For more advanced lesions, a variety of treatment options are available, including radiation therapy alone,[132–134] supraglottic laryngectomy with or without postoperative radiation therapy,[135,136] and chemoradiation therapy programs for patients who would otherwise require a total laryngectomy.[137–140]

The results of primary radiation for supraglottic cancer are well established.[133,134] Mendenhall and colleagues[134] reported 5-year local control of 100% for T1, 83% for T2, 68% for T3, and 56% for T4 lesions. Wang and associates[133] reported 5-year local control of 96% for T1, 86% for T2, 76% for T3, and 43% for T4 lesions. In this particular study, when laryngectomy was added for salvage, local control was 96% for T1, 93% for T2, 88% for T3, and 51% for T4 lesions.

Different criteria create T3 designation of supraglottic laryngeal cancer, and in selected circumstances of this stage in which there is no vocal cord fixation, supraglottic laryngectomy can be applied efficiently; thus, voice sparing is achieved. Three different studies have applied strict standards to the patient selection for supraglottic laryngectomy in T3 lesions, and disease-free survival of approximately 75% at 3 years can be expected.[141–143]

Parsons and coworkers[144] reported on 26 T4 invasive SCCs of the larynx treated with radiation therapy. Only 38% achieved local control at 5 years in this report. Other series also demonstrate the similarity of outcomes of primary radiation therapy and surgery, even for moderately advanced disease.[145,146] Supraglottic lesions that cause vocal cord fixation (T3), those that involve the postcricoid region (T3), those that invade the laryngeal cartilage (T4), or those that extend into extralaryngeal sites (T4) can often be effectively managed with total laryngectomy and postoperative radiation therapy. Today, however, it is the exception rather than the norm to offer a patient a total laryngectomy as an initial treatment option in these advanced-stage cancers. Instead, the organ-sparing strategy of chemoradiation, with laryngectomy reserved for unsuccessful cases, is generally the standard of care. It should be emphasized, however, that each case must be individualized, and certain lesions in certain patients warrant the traditional approach whereby laryngectomy is performed first.

For patients who undergo supraglottic laryngectomy, postoperative radiation therapy is occasionally considered. Excellent local control has been reported with this sequencing in selected T3/T4 lesions[136]; however, the combination of these two treatments is morbid, with increased gastrostomy or tracheostomy dependence, airway problems, and delayed independent swallowing.[135] In general, it is best to choose one or the other (i.e., radiation or surgery) as the definitive local therapy. However, because of the extremely low rate of local recurrence after supraglottic laryngectomy, postoperative radiation to the laryngeal segment is not often used after this operation.

An advantage to radiation as the initial treatment of early-stage supraglottic disease is that bilateral elective neck treatment can be included in the plan with minimal morbidity. If an adequate dose of elective neck radiation is given, neck relapse should be less than 5% in the absence of clinically obvious disease. If surgery is chosen as the treatment for a T1 or T2 supraglottic lesion, the supraglottic laryngectomy should be combined with bilateral selective neck dissections, even when the neck is N0. Postoperative radiation therapy is added to the necks of those patients in whom these staging procedures show metastatic disease. The obvious disadvantage to this approach is that it becomes necessary to use two different treatment modalities compared with the strategy in which radiation therapy is used initially to the primary tumor and necks. The disadvantage to the plan that uses radiation therapy initially is that, when it is unsuccessful, total laryngectomy is needed. Such is the case because supraglottic laryngectomy is contraindicated after full-course radiation therapy to the larynx (complications such as persistent swelling, failure of wound healing, radiation chondritis, and swallowing difficulties are strikingly frequent in this setting).

Pretreatment CT scans can be helpful in predicting outcomes for supraglottic lesions treated with primary radiation therapy. Hermans and colleagues[147] reported that tumor volume derived from CT analysis was the strongest predictor of locoregional failure and that the degree of paraglottic space involvement, subglottic extension, and preepiglottic space involvement all were important prognostic factors demonstrated by this imaging method. Mancuso et al.[148] was able to quantify the correlation between CT findings and local control. For patients with a tumor volume of less than 6 cm^3 who were treated by radiation therapy alone, local control was achieved in 89%. When the tumor volume was 6 cm^3 or greater, the local control was only 52%. A decreased rate of local control and voice preservation was also noted if 25% or more of the preepiglottic space was involved with tumor. A study conducted by Lo and associates[149] also correlated CT tumor volume with radiation failure, but this analysis was unable to demonstrate such a correlation with surgery.

When comparing one type of operation (supraglottic laryngectomy) to the other (total laryngectomy), it is important to note that the former of the two is physiologic and allows retention of vocal and swallowing functions. Furthermore, because of the unique lymphatic drainage patterns of the organ and the presence of certain natural anatomic barriers to tumor spread, this operation is oncologically sound, yielding the same local control rates as achieved by total laryngectomy in comparable lesions.[150,151] Ogura and Biller[151] reported an 85% 3-year control for epiglottis cancers treated with supraglottic laryngectomy, but this result decreased to 71% with extension onto the false cord(s). These figures are comparable to those produced by total laryngectomy for similar lesions.

It is not the mission of this text to provide an elaborate description of the various partial laryngeal surgical techniques used to manage supraglottic cancer; however, the student of this disease should have at least a summary knowledge of the methods known collectively as *conservation laryngeal surgery*. The compartmentalization of the larynx and the directional drainage patterns of the lymph channels within it provide surgeons with the unique opportunity for removing that portion of the larynx above the true vocal cords, and with proper reconstruction, swallowing and vocal functions are retained in the process. Essentially, this procedure is a horizontally directed hemilaryngectomy in which the surgeon removes the upper half of the thyroid cartilage and the contents within it (the false vocal cords, the epiglottis, and the aryepiglottic folds). The edge of the thyroid cartilage is brought up to and attached to the transected base of the tongue. Because the motor nerve supply of the vocal cords comes from below (recurrent laryngeal nerves) and is not in the surgical field, the important vocal cord functions of abduction and adduction are retained, and because of this, voice and the important airway protective functions of glottic closure are preserved.

The supraglottic laryngectomy is, however, physiologically challenging, and patients with chronic pulmonary disease often have difficulty tolerating the aspiration that can follow. Essentially, this elegant technique is oncologically sound in appropriate tumors, but certain patients are not good candidates for its implementation. The correct use of the supraglottic laryngectomy is accomplished only by surgeons properly trained in this methodology and who have the experience to apply the right methods in the right situations. A succinct discussion of the method of selection for all conservation procedures and which patients are suitable for them was developed by Sessions and Parish.[152] Although certain chemoradiotherapy options have been popularized since that discussion was published, the fundamental principles are the same and can be applied to the current philosophy. As those alternative chemoradiation schema are used more frequently, the number of surgeons accomplished in the techniques of conservation laryngeal surgery will diminish. Although the idea of saving more larynges without compromising cure is meritorious, it is worrisome that those subtle skills necessary for achieving excellent functional results with the partial laryngectomies is to some extent being lost by the current generation of head and neck surgeons. A variety of conservation surgery procedures are applied to variations of laryngeal cancer, and although a description of each is beyond the scope of this text, the following classification of these operations should be helpful in placing this important surgical methodology into the proper perspective:

1. Hemilaryngectomy
   a. Horizontal hemilaryngectomy (supraglottic)
   b. Vertical hemilaryngectomy
      i. Lateral hemilaryngectomy
      ii. Frontal hemilaryngectomy
2. Cordectomy
3. Supracricoid laryngectomy[153]
4. Partial laryngopharyngectomy

Just as with the description of specific surgical methods, elaborate details of radiation therapy technique are not appropriate here. In general, patients with early-stage laryngeal disease are treated with once daily continuous course radiation therapy. Opposed lateral fields are used for the primary site and upper neck(s), and a separate anterior field is used for the lower neck(s). In selected total laryngectomies, the stoma is included in this neck treatment plan. The total dose to the primary site is in the 65 to 70 Gy range.[133,134] For more advanced disease, a variety of fractionation schemes have been used, including once daily, twice daily, and concomitant boost techniques.[133,134,154] A Radiation Therapy Oncology Group randomized trial compared four different fractionation schedules for advanced head and neck cancers treated with primary radiotherapy: once daily radiation to a total of 70 Gy in 7 weeks; twice daily radiation using 1.2 Gy per fraction to a total dose of 81.6 Gy; accelerated hyperfractionation technique with a planned break using 1.6 Gy per fraction twice daily up to approximately 38.4 Gy, followed by a 2-week break, and continuing with 1.6 Gy twice daily to 67.2 Gy; and a concomitant boost technique using once daily fractionation in the beginning of the program, followed by twice daily fractionation for the concomitant boost during the final 12 treatment days, up to a total of 72 Gy. The results show better 2-year locoregional control and disease-free survival using the concomitant boost approach. Acute and late toxicity was acceptable, although increased, over standard fractionation.

Glottis

CIS of the true vocal cord is highly curable with equal efficiency by microexcision, laser vaporization,[155] or radiation therapy.[156–158] Pure CIS lesions are unusual, and a frequent association exists, more often than not, between such lesions and invasive carcinoma. Those series that have been reported in which numerous recurrences developed after stripping of vocal cord CIS almost certainly consisted of a heterogeneous group that included lesions containing areas of unrecognized invasive cancer. For this reason, we favor microexcision of the involved membrane over laser vaporization, which destroys the specimen and does not allow for the pathologic analysis needed to identify areas of microinvasion.

True CIS, by definition, remains superficial to the basement membrane, and if mucosal excision techniques are confined to that group of patients, the cure rate should be the same as the best that can be achieved by radiation therapy. The advantages of microexcision over radiation is that it is simpler and that radiation therapy is held in reserve for future use. Considering the incidence of metachronous and synchronous second primary, cancers that occur in the aerodigestive tract, the policy of holding radiation in reserve whenever possible is prudent. The advantages of radiation therapy are that the voice is at least as good and often better than with surgery, and it is a more definitive treatment for invasive cancer that may exist within the lesion. In both microexcision and radiation, when treatment fails, a surgical procedure can still salvage most patients and, in the majority of cases, with a voice-sparing operation.

All things considered, if the diagnosis of pure CIS of the vocal cord(s) is fairly certain, microexcision is probably the treatment of choice. So-called vocal cord stripping often has a crippling effect on the voice and is in violation of the contemporary standard of care. Such is not the case with microexcision, which has minimal impact on vocal quality.

The value of a properly excised piece of tissue to a complete histopathologic analysis cannot be overrated. Importantly, microexcision should include a wide zone around the obvious trouble, followed by a thorough pathologic evaluation of the specimen to look for microinvasive areas. Procedures that excise the underlying vocal cord muscle (i.e., cordectomy) produce a crippling vocal effect and do not offer any oncologic improvement over microexcision or radiation; thus, such a procedure should not be considered as one of the treatment options for vocal cord CIS.

Radiation therapy is used either as the definitive treatment of CIS when microexcision is not possible or is refused, or as a salvage treatment for patients with recurrent CIS following prior surgical procedures.[159,160] Series of CIS patients show that, when radiation therapy is used, it is very effective. Medini and coworkers[158] reported 20 patients with CIS treated with radiotherapy, using a dose of 1.75 Gy per fraction to a median total dose of 68.4 Gy. The 4-year disease-free survival rate was 95%. Improved voice was reported in 16 of 20 patients, with no change noted in the other four. In summary, the standard of care for CIS of the vocal cord consists of a strategy that uses primary surgery for most patients and selective radiation therapy in others.

These authors rely heavily on the preoperative evaluation by videostroboscopy[39] to estimate the depth of the surface cancer. Normal membrane motion (i.e., a normal mucosal wave)[38] suggests confinement of the lesion to that area superficial to the basement membrane (i.e., CIS). On the other hand, if stroboscopy demonstrates tethering of the membrane to the underlying tissue, we consider that a sign of microinvasion (more advanced than CIS). Such a patient receives radiation therapy. If we believe the lesion is entirely superficial to the basement membrane, we do microexcision and examine the specimen carefully for microinvasion. The understaging of CIS in past studies could probably have been avoided by the appropriate use of stroboscopic analysis.

Finally, certain CIS lesions, such as those on the anterior commissure, in the subglottis, or some that extend into the laryngeal ventricle, do not lend themselves to these surgical methods; in these cases, radiation is a better means of initial treatment.

For T1 or T2 invasive glottic cancer, excellent local control is achieved by either radiation therapy or conservation surgery procedures.[156,161–163] It is generally agreed, however, that vocal quality is better after radiation therapy.[164–166] Harrison and colleagues[167] reported an ultimate return to normal voice in nearly all radiated T1 and T2 glottic cancer patients. Even though several patterns of vocal dysfunction existed before, during, and immediately after radiation therapy, normalization of these alterations occurred within 3 months after completion of radiotherapy. Dagli,[164] however, showed that the postradiation voice, although better than the surgically treated counterpart, remains abnormal with respect to various subtle parameters, such as maximum vocal intensity, dynamic vocal intensity range, jitter, and mean fundamental frequency. De Graeff and associates[168] also reported objective improvement of speech after radiotherapy but pointed out that there was short-term, temporary deterioration of physical functioning and fatigue. Tsunoda and coworkers[169] stroboscopically studied the changes of the mucous membrane motion after radiation of early glottic cancers. They demonstrated ultimate return to normal motion in all patients studied. Furthermore, these authors suggested the potential value of stroboscopy for detecting early cancer recurrence, thus corroborating the findings of Sessions et al.[39] in a previously reported study.

Finally, there seem to be predictors of poor vocal quality: Vocal cord stripping (instead of biopsy only) before radiotherapy and continued smoking after radiation therapy predicted worse voice quality as well as substandard stroboscopic performance.[170]

It is important to note that, in those lower-staged (i.e., T1 and T2) glottic lesions that are unsuccessfully treated with radiation, salvage partial laryngectomy (hemilaryngectomy) can be performed successfully in a significant number of patients, thus achieving excellent overall cure rates while retaining voice.[171,172]

Whether achieved by radiation therapy or by surgery, local control rate decreases with increasing tumor bulk. Dickens and coworkers[173] reported the results for early glottic tumors of various sizes and extent. The lesions were categorized by the type of surgical procedure that would have been necessary had surgery been used. This type of analysis provides an excellent basis for comparing the results of surgery and radiation. In patients suitable for hemilaryngectomy, the local control with radiation alone was 94%. This figure increased to 100% when surgical salvage was added. On the contrary, for patients managed by radiation therapy who would have required total laryngectomy, local control rate was only 65%, but it increased to 91% when surgical salvage was added. Extension of these glottic carcinomas onto the anterior and posterior aspects of the larynx lessens the local control rates achieved with radiation therapy.[174] In this study, the surgical procedure required for salvage usually was a total laryngectomy rather than a hemilaryngectomy.

Essentially, the 5-year survival rates for primary surgery (cordectomy or hemilaryngectomy) and primary radiation for T1 lesions are comparable.[161–163,175–178] Local control obtained in this same-stage glottic group using conservation surgical procedures is reported to be 78% by Kirchner and Owen[78] and 87% by Ogura et al.[179] Results obtained for comparable T1 lesions treated by radiation therapy show local control of 91% by Harwood[156] and 93% by Pellitteri.[163]

Sessions and colleagues[180] reported a 5-year survival rate of 74% for T1 and T2 lesions that originated in the anterior commissure of the glottic larynx. This study demonstrated that survival and recurrence rates of anterior commissure lesions correlated with the size and stage of the tumor.[181] Olofsson and associates[182] reported an 80% survival rate at 5 years for early-stage anterior commissure lesions, but this study included those recurrences that had been salvaged by surgery. Those anterior commissure lesions that are thin and of low volume and that do not have substantial subglottic extension probably are treated with equal efficiency by partial laryngectomy or radiation therapy. As lesions become more advanced, the natural barrier of the anterior commissure ligament is overcome and the thyroid cartilage is frequently invaded[183]; therefore, radiation therapy becomes less appealing than surgery as the front-line treatment. Most tumors involving the anterior commissure occur as a result of spread from the true vocal cord. Lesions actually arising in the anterior commissure are unusual, making up 1% to 2% of glottic cancers.[181,183] In summary, the standard for treating T1 glottic cancers is radiation therapy, and partial or total laryngectomy is used as a salvage operation in those patients for whom this first line of treatment is unsuccessful.

The management of T2 lesions, on the other hand, is somewhat more complicated because this group is more heterogeneous. Surgical management usually consists of vertical hemilaryngectomy and is associated with 3-year survival rates of 83%[180] and 82%[179] in two major series. Primary radiation therapy with surgical salvage yields a net 5-year survival rate of 92% in Pellitteri et al.'s series,[163] 72% in Wang's series,[161] and 90% in Fletcher et al.'s series.[162] Because of the heterogeneity of the T2 group, Wang[161] has suggested subdividing these lesions into those with normal mobility (T2A) and those with impaired mobility (T2B). He showed that local control was obtained in 86% of the former and 63% of the latter when primary radiation was used. Similar observations were made by Harwood,[156] whose series yielded 77% and 51% local control rates for T2A and T2B lesions, respectively. Medini and colleagues[158] reported a 5-year disease-free survival rate of 80% for T2A and 64% for T2B lesions. Klintenberg and associates[184] reported local control of 73% for T2 lesions, with subglottic extension being the most important factor. In summary, radiation therapy is usually recommended as the primary treatment modality for T2 lesions with no vocal cord mobility impairment (T2A); however, in those lesions that demonstrate impairment of motion (T2B), hemilaryngectomy is preferred. These criteria are variable, how-

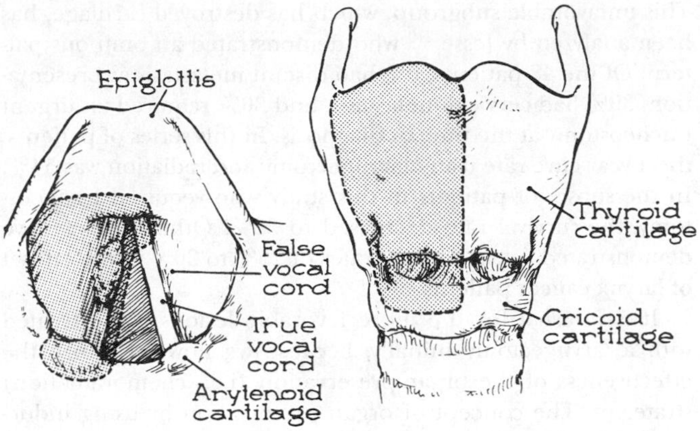

FIGURE 30.3-7. Axial and frontal views of larynx show that portion of the organ removed by a horizontal hemilaryngectomy (*shaded*).

ever, depending on tumor bulk, and in those less bulky T2B lesions, radiation can be used. It should be noted also that, when vocal cord motion is restricted by actual surface tumor bulk rather than by invasion of the underlying muscle, radiation is often effective.

Those conservation surgical procedures that can be applied to the management of glottic cancer are time honored and tested, and when used in the properly selected case of laryngeal cancer, they consistently yield excellent results functionally and oncologically. The most commonly used of these procedures is the vertical hemilaryngectomy, in which the surgeon bisects the larynx and, to a varying degree, removes a portion or all of the true and false vocal cord along with the respective half of the thyroid cartilage. Because most of the lesions for which this operation is performed are located on the anterior two-thirds of the vocal cord, the most posterior resection line usually is in front of the arytenoid cartilage. In those circumstances in which the cancer extends onto the posterior larynx, this cartilage can be resected (Fig. 30.3-7). By using the perichondrium from the external surface of the half of the thyroid cartilage that has been removed, the operated side of the larynx heals in the midline, forming a firm buttress (pseudocord) against which the opposite and normal true vocal cord vibrates.

Just as with surgery, radiation therapy of T2 glottic cancer need not include elective neck treatment. Fein and coworkers[185] reported that, in this group, the incidence of neck failure was 3.7% with elective neck radiation, and 2.6% when no elective treatment was given. The radiation field arrangement is similar to the technique used for T1 disease. The field size must be large enough to encompass the entire extent of disease, and the total dose is usually approximately 70 Gy range.

Various factors seem to be important prognostically for all glottic cancer treated with radiation. Several series[186–188] strongly correlate anemia with poorer outcomes for T1 and T2 glottic cancer treated with radiation, with one series[186] revealing a 6% drop in local control for every 1 g drop in hemoglobin. Similar studies have not been accomplished with surgically treated patients.

Data on other potential prognostic markers include contradictions on whether p53 correlates with radiation failure; some suggest such an ability,[189] whereas others fail to demonstrate a significant relationship.[190,191] Growth factor markers such as Ki-67, an indicator of the proliferation index, may be important and may also be prognostic for surgically treated cases.[192,193]

Radiologic imaging is playing an increasingly important role. CT derived tumor volume correlates with outcome for radiation patients[149,194] and may become increasingly important. Emerging data also suggest that positron emission tomographic scanning may be very useful in assessing patients after radiation therapy and in differentiating radiation-related changes from recurrent tumor.[195–197]

A continued evolution of radiation techniques is largely responsible for the excellent control of early glottic disease in many reported series.[161,163,184,198–201] Individualized treatment planning, isodose contours, and beam compensation are mandatory to optimize local control.[201] Lower-energy photon beams (cobalt 60, ≤ 4-MV linear accelerators) may have an advantage over higher-energy beams,[202] although proper treatment planning may make 6-MV beams acceptable.[185]

Much has been written about the time-dose relationships and the variety of fractionation schemes used.[186,199–201,203–206] The optimal fractionation schedule is not known, although many different programs have been successfully conducted. Most authors agree that dose per fraction of 2 Gy or more is preferable to lower dose per fraction.[201–203] Most institutions use a dose per fraction of 2 Gy or more and a total dose in the 60 to 66 Gy range, with lower total doses in those with higher doses per fraction.[201–203] It seems clear that longer overall treatment times are associated with worse outcomes.[186,200,204–206] Skladowski and colleagues[186] reported that a prolongation of the treatment time from 45 days to 55 days decreased the tumor control probability by 13%. Hayakawa and colleagues[200] reported 5-year local control rates of 95% for those completing treatment in 45 days or less, 81% in 46 to 49 days, and 73% in more than 50 days.

The most commonly used field arrangement is opposed lateral portals measuring between 5.5 × 5.5 cm and 6.0 × 6.0 cm that cover the larynx alone. Patients must be properly immobilized. A larynx contour is taken during simulation, and an appropriate larynx wedge is usually added to keep the dose inhomogeneity to within 5% to 10%.

Involvement of the anterior commissure continues to be a perplexing issue. Certain authors report poorer outcomes,[207,208] whereas others[209] report that proper technique yields satisfactory outcomes not dissimilar to other T1 lesions.

Glottic cancers that cause vocal cord or hemilaryngeal immobilization or fixation (i.e., T3) are substantially more ominous than lesions that do not. At a minimum, such motion impairment reflects vocalis muscle invasion. However, further tumor extension into the paraglottic space is often present, opening the entire larynx and adjacent exit areas to cancer spread. Many of these lesions are associated with thyroid or cricoid cartilage destruction, and the tendency is to underestimate glottic lesions with vocal cord fixation. In Olofsson et al.'s[210] study, a significant number of tumors originally had been understaged as T3 cancers but were actually T4 lesions with extralaryngeal extension. With the unpredictable extent of the disease and the overall high probability of cartilage destruction in mind, surgery, which usually consists of a total laryngectomy, traditionally has been favored over radiation therapy for the primary management of T3 lesions. The overall 5-year survival rate for T3 glottic cancers treated with total laryngectomy is reported to be 55% to 72% in four major series.[78,211] However, it has been shown by Kirchner and Owen[78] that, in carefully selected T3 vocal cord lesions clearly limited to the vocalis muscle and in which no associated cartilage destruction is found, hemilaryngectomy can be performed with oncologic safety. In this series of 22 patients, a 60% cure rate was reported. In another similar study, Som[212] reported a 58% cure rate in 26 patients with selected T3 glottic tumors treated by partial laryngectomy. It should be noted that both of these significant studies were done before the use of CT or MRI. Such technology would almost certainly have made the evaluation of these lesions and the delineation of their dimensions easier and more accurate. Even with this limitation lessened by contemporary technology, the reader should not be led to underestimate the difficulty of correctly selecting the small subset of T3 lesions suitable for hemilaryngectomy. This judgment is appropriately left only to those surgeons with considerable experience in partial laryngeal surgery.

Overall, managing T3 glottic cancer can be challenging. A small number of these lesions can be effectively removed by partial laryngectomy, but because this selection is fraught with hazards, past surgical literature has been slanted toward recommending total laryngectomy. Such is not the case today, however, and those patients with T3 glottic cancer who would require a total laryngectomy are almost always treated with an organ-preservation chemoradiation approach, with laryngectomy being used only for those who are unsuccessful with the former. The survival rate is the same between those that require the three modalities (chemotherapy, radiotherapy, laryngectomy) and those to whom only chemotherapy and radiation are given; however, a substantial percentage of patients retain their larynges in the process.[139,140,213]

A subset of T3 glottic patients can be cured without operation. Van den Bogert et al.[213] reported a local control rate of 53% in a group of patients with operable T3 lesions who had refused surgery. Harwood and colleagues[214] reported a 45% 5-year local control rate for T3 glottic patients, and Wang[215] reported a 36% 5-year actuarial local control rate, which increased to 57% when surgical salvage was added. Mendenhall and associates[216] have reported that T3 glottic cancer treated with radiotherapy alone has a 5-year local control rate of 63%, increasing to 86% with surgical salvage. Pretreatment CT scans helped predict outcome. For tumors whose volume was 3.5 cm^3 or less, local control was 87% compared with 29% for larger-volume lesions. A trend has been noted toward better outcomes with twice daily treatment versus once daily fractionation.[217,218] Finally, no correlation seems to exist between the return of vocal cord mobility and outcome,[217] and it is not uncommon for the vocal cord to remain fixed, even after successful radiation.

T4 tumor designation denotes cartilage destruction or extension of the tumor outside of the confines of the larynx. Grouping together all T4 lesions is misleading, however, because it fails to account for the more favorable tumor of lesser thickness and volume that may have achieved a T4 status only because it originated in a marginal zone and extended to an adjacent area, such as the pyriform sinus or base of the tongue. Just as with T3 supraglottic lesions, there are favorable and unfavorable T4 lesions, and that determination is made appropriately on the basis of tumor volume, depth, and thickness. With this exception in mind, the performance of the group of T4 glottic lesions is expectedly poorer than that of lesser stages. Traditionally, most of the unfavorable lesions are treated with total laryngectomy and some sort of a neck dissection; generally, these patients receive postoperative radiation. This unfavorable subgroup, which has destroyed cartilage, has been analyzed by Jesse,[219] who demonstrated an ominous pattern: Of the 48 patients, 6% had distant metastasis at presentation, 39% had cervical metastasis, and 30% required an urgent tracheostomy at the time of diagnosis. In this series of patients, the 4-year cure rate using laryngectomy and radiation was 54%. In the subset of patients in this study who required tracheostomy, the survival rate decreased to 38%. Other studies have demonstrated 5-year survival rates of 25% to 30% in this subset of larynx cancer patients.[220,221]

It is unusual for the more favorable lesions to be treated with a laryngectomy initially, because we now recognize the effectiveness of the organ-preservation (i.e., chemoradiation) strategies. The concept of organ preservation by using induction chemotherapy to help identify those lesions likely to respond to radiation therapy is a new addition to the treatment armamentarium. Those favorable results of nonrandomized trials[1–3] and the results of the Veterans Administration Cooperative Study Group[222,223] include a number of patients with T4 lesions. Although we must exercise caution in replacing standard and time-honored therapy with new strategies, the concept of organ preservation is today widely accepted as standard therapy in selected advanced larynx and hypopharynx cancers.

Harwood and associates[214] reported local control in 56% of T4, N0 glottic lesions treated with radical radiation therapy. The 5-year survival rate for radiation with surgical salvage was 49%. Within this group, the local control rate for patients classified as T4 from cartilage invasion was 67% at 5 years. This result was significantly better than for those T4 patients who had pyriform sinus involvement. In this latter group, the actuarial local control rate was only 19%. The T4 patients with hypopharyngeal involvement do not seem to be good candidates for radical radiation therapy. This circumstance parallels the dismal performance of the similar group treated surgically and reported by Jesse.[219] It also is similar to a comparably poor performance for those larynx cancer patients with hypopharyngeal extension noted by Pfister et al.[1] in their larynx-preservation study with induction chemotherapy. The same trend of poor chemoradiation performance for those larynx cancer patients with hypopharyngeal extension was noted by Karp and coworkers.[2] Whatever the treatment variation, these patients consistently seem to do poorly.

Subglottis

Although the preponderance of subglottic tumors are SCCs, adenocarcinomas and adenoid cystic carcinomas are seen occasionally.[92] The cure rate for these tumors is poor, despite combination therapy. Total laryngectomy and appropriate neck surgery, including thyroidectomy, are probably the surgical treatment most recommended, and postoperative radiation therapy should probably be administered.[79,93] Mediastinal dissection of the paratracheal nodal groups does not seem to add substantially to survival rates.[92]

Chemotherapy for Preservation of Laryngeal Function—Organ Preservation

Surgical management of locally advanced SCCs of the larynx and hypopharynx has often required total laryngectomy. Organ-preservation trials in the form of uncontrolled feasibility series and prospective randomized controlled trials are now available to guide appropriate use of chemotherapy. In general, two nonsurgical strategies—induction chemotherapy followed by definitive radiation therapy in responding patients, and concurrent radiation therapy and chemotherapy—are the alternatives to laryngectomy.

Concurrent chemoradiation has been used for the treatment of unresectable head and neck cancer for decades. Trials of multiagent cisplatin-based chemoradiation strategies have demonstrated improved locoregional control and survival compared with radiation therapy alone in cancers of the nasopharynx, oropharynx, and in unresectable cancers of all aerodigestive sites.[224–227] For resectable stage III and IV cancers of the larynx and stage II, III, and IV cancers of the hypopharynx, mature data is available on the induction chemotherapy strategies as a means of preserving the larynx. Randomized trials evaluating concurrent chemoradiation are nearing completion in the United States and are in progress in Europe.[228]

The concept of induction chemotherapy as a primary strategy evolved for two main reasons. First, high response rates could be achieved with the standard cisplatin (100 mg/m^2 day 1) and infusional 5-fluorouracil (5-FU) (1000 mg/m^2/d, days 1 to 5) regimen: an 85% overall response rate (complete and partial) and a clinical complete response rate ranging from 30% to 50%.[229–231] A pathologic complete response was confirmed by biopsy or by resection in two-thirds of clinical complete responders. Second, the response to chemotherapy was generally predictive of radiosensitivity.[3,232] These observations led to a number of uncontrolled trials, mostly in patients with advanced laryngeal and hypopharyngeal cancers that were destined for total laryngectomy.[1,2,233–236] These small published series confirmed the feasibility of the concept of induction chemotherapy followed by definitive radiotherapy to preserve speech and swallowing function, and importantly, they suggested that survival was not compromised in the process. Three randomized controlled trials and a metaanalysis provide data from which to draw conclusions and recommend guidelines for patient management.[138,237,238] The general scheme for organ preservation protocols that was conceptualized by Hong and colleagues[3] is outlined in Figure 30.3-8.

Randomized Trials

The first randomized trial[237] using induction chemotherapy for organ preservation was started in 1985 by the Department of Veterans Affairs Laryngeal Study Group in which 332 patients with stage III or IV (M0) cancer of the glottis or supraglottis were analyzed (Table 30.3-4). These were randomly assigned treatments with either surgery (total laryngectomy) and radiation therapy, or induction chemotherapy and radiation therapy. In the experimental arm, partial or complete responders after two cycles of cisplatin and 5-FU received a third cycle of chemotherapy followed by definitive radiation therapy. Laryngectomy was reserved for salvage of persistent or recurrent disease. Patients demonstrating less than a partial response at the primary site after two cycles of chemotherapy underwent immediate laryngectomy.

Various prognostic factors were analyzed for response to chemotherapy, organ preservation, and survival.[239] For surgically treated patients, the one factor in multivariate analysis that was significant for decreased survival was extracapsular extension of nodal disease, whereas no independent predictive

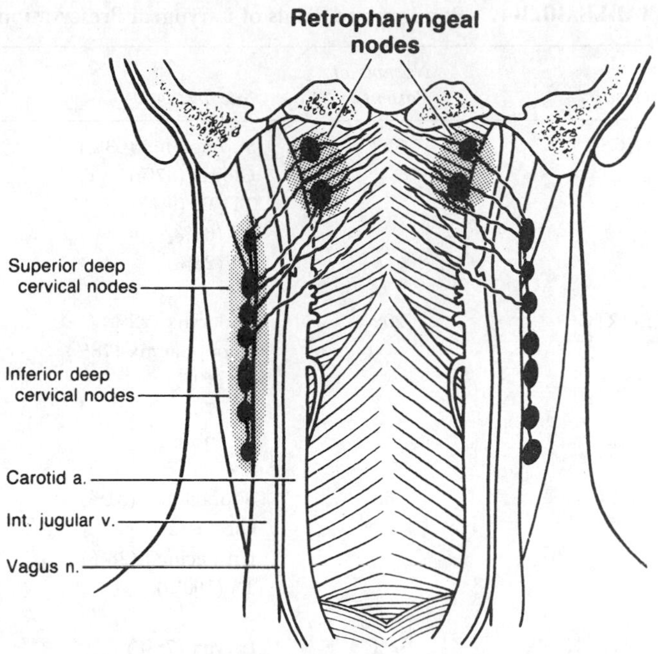

FIGURE 30.3-8. Posterior view of pharynx and great vessels shows retropharyngeal lymph nodes commonly involved in hypopharyngeal cancer. a, artery; Int., internal; n, nerve; v, vein.

factor of survival emerged for chemotherapy-treated patients. Low T class (T1–T3 vs. T4) was the best predictor of response to chemotherapy (relative risk ratio, 5.6; $P = .01$). T class, p53 overexpression, and elevated proliferating cell nuclear antigen index were independent predictors of successful organ preservation with induction chemotherapy and radiotherapy.

The second randomized induction chemotherapy trial of larynx preservation was conducted by the European Organization for Research and Treatment of Cancer (EORTC) in patients with resectable cancers of the pyriform sinus or the aryepiglottic fold (lateral epilarynx)[238] (see Table 30.3-4). A total of 194 patients with stage T2–T4, N0–N2b were randomized to surgery (total laryngectomy plus partial pharyngectomy) and radiation therapy in one study arm or induction chemotherapy (cisplatin + 5-FU) and radiation therapy in responders. A clinical complete response at the primary site after two or three cycles of chemotherapy was required to proceed to radiation, and this was achieved in 54% of patients. Survival equivalence was demonstrated at 3 and 5 years, and a functioning larynx was preserved in 48% at 3 years. A delay in development of distant metastases was noted for the chemotherapy-treated patients, whereas no differences were observed in the rates of local or regional failure between treatment groups.

A third randomized trial of patients with locally advanced larynx cancer was conducted by the Groupe d'Etude des Tumeurs de la Tete et du Cou in France[240] (see Table 30.3-4). This study was limited to patients with T3 tumors and consisted predominately of patients with glottic primaries. This was in contrast to the Veterans Affairs trial in which a majority of the lesions were supraglottic lesions. Laryngectomy was avoided in 41% (15 of 36 patients); however, the trial has been criticized for the small number of patients enrolled, the lack of imaging studies to assess tumor extent before treatment, and the lack of proper response evaluation after chemotherapy and after radiotherapy.

TABLE 30.3-4. Randomized Trials of Laryngeal Preservation

Group	Number of Patients	Site T stage	Treatment	Survival 3 Y	Survival 10 Y	Laryngeal Preservation in Survivors
VACSG[40,139,237]	332	Supraglottic (63%)				
		Glottic (37%)	PF → RT	53%	25%	62% at 5 y
		T1/T2 (9%)	S → RT			
		T3 (65%)				
		T4 (26%)				
				3 y		
EORTC[238]	202	Epilarynx (22%)				
		Hypopharynx (78%)	PF → RT	57%		48% at 3 y
		T2 (19%)	S → RT	43%		
		T3 (75%)				
		T4 (6%)				
				2 y[a]		
GETTEC[240]	68	Supraglottic (31%)				NR
		Glottic (41%)	PF → RT	69%		
		Unspecified (28%)	S → RT	84%		
		T3 (100%)				
				5 y		
MACH-NC[241]	602	Larynx (73%)				58% at 5 y
		Hypopharynx (26%)	PF → RT	39%		
		T1/T2 (12%)	S → RT	45%		
		T3/T4 (77%)				

EORTC, European Organization for Research and Treatment of Cancer; GETTEC, Groupe d'Etude des Tumeurs de la Tete et du Cou; MACH-NC, metaanalysis of chemotherapy in head and neck cancer; NR, not reported; PF, cisplatin + 5-fluorouracil × 2–3 cycles; RT, radiotherapy; S, surgery; VACSG, Veterans Administration Cooperative Study Group.
[a]Statistically significant, $P = .006$.

A metaanalysis by Lefebvre of chemotherapy in head and neck cancer limited to the 602 patients enrolled in these three trials shows a statistically nonsignificant difference in survival after a median follow-up of 5.8 years (45% for surgery patients vs. 39% for the induction chemotherapy group).[241] The larynx was preserved in 58% of surviving patients at 5 years.

From these three randomized studies, one can conclude the following for induction chemotherapy as a strategy to preserve the larynx: Survival is not jeopardized; laryngeal function can be preserved in approximately one-half of surviving patients; and the risk of requiring salvage surgery increases with bulky primary and nodal disease. In effect, these trial results confirm a role for induction chemotherapy using the cisplatin plus 5-FU regimen followed by radiation therapy as an alternative nonsurgical treatment for patients with locally advanced cancers of the larynx (stage III and IV) and hypopharynx (stage II, III, and IV) who would otherwise undergo total laryngectomy. A team approach that includes the surgical, radiation, and medical oncologists; nutritionist; and experts in lifestyle behavior modification is critical to the success of combined modality treatment. So that surgery can be performed promptly in nonresponders and for salvage of recurrent disease, it is essential that the surgeon be involved throughout and after the induction chemotherapy and radiation phases of treatment.

Left unanswered by these trials are the following important questions: (1) What is the precise role of induction chemotherapy?, (2) What is the comparative efficacy of radiation therapy as a single modality for preservation of the larynx?, and (3) What is the potential of concurrent chemotherapy and radiation therapy to improve locoregional control and survival? These questions are being addressed for cancers of the larynx and hypopharynx in randomized trials in the United States and Europe in which cisplatin plus 5-FU induction chemotherapy followed by radiation therapy in responding patients (partial response of the primary tumor) serves as the control arm.[228] The U.S. intergroup trial (R91-11) will complete accrual of 546 patients in the year 2000. This trial will provide data on two treatment alternatives: concurrent radiation therapy plus cisplatin compared to the control group, and radiation therapy alone compared to the control group. Until those trial results mature for larynx cancer specifically, induction chemotherapy sequenced with radiation therapy remains the standard of care. The consistent survival benefit observed in recent multisite and oropharynx randomized trials comparing concurrent chemotherapy and radiotherapy to radiotherapy alone is impressive. This suggests that the concurrent rather than the sequential strategy may emerge as the preferred treatment strategy for larynx and hypopharynx primaries as well.

Chemotherapy in the Treatment of Far Advanced (Unresectable) Locoregional Disease

There is no role for induction chemotherapy in the management of patients with advanced locoregional disease in which clear margins cannot be achieved by resection. Many randomized trials of patients with unresectable disease were carried out in the 1980s, which directly compared induction chemotherapy followed by radiation to radiation therapy alone.[242] Survival benefit was reported in a subset analysis of patients with unresectable disease in only a single randomized trial.[243]

In contrast, prospective randomized trials of patients with unresectable disease clearly demonstrate a substantial increase in locoregional control and significantly improved survival with the use of concurrent chemotherapy and radiation therapy regimens when compared to either standard or altered fractionation schedules of radiation therapy alone.[224–227] Thus, concurrent chemotherapy and radiation therapy can be recommended as the standard of care in this disease setting, provided the patient has sufficient performance status and psychosocial resources to undergo the generally more toxic treatment. At present, the most widely used regimen with proven survival benefit in a multicenter comparative trial is cisplatin 100 mg/m^2 on days 1, 22, and 43, during which radiation is taken to 70 Gy at a rate of 2 Gy/d.[3] Taxane-based regimens are under investigation in phase I and II trials evaluating a variety of doses and infusion schedules combined with varying radiation therapy fractionation schedules.[244–247] However, insufficient data is available on efficacy and toxicity at this time to recommend any taxane-based chemoradiation regimen as a standard of care. For patients with poor performance status, radiation therapy alone or, in some situations, supportive care alone may constitute appropriate management.

In summary, the selection of a treatment strategy for T4 supraglottic and glottic larynx cancers is dependent on a variety of factors, including the following:

1. If there is bulky neck disease and if the primary tumor does not have extensive hypopharyngeal extension, induction chemotherapy followed by radiation therapy to the primary tumor and neck can be used in chemosensitive tumors. This should be followed by a neck dissection(s). In such lesions that are not chemoresponsive, laryngectomy and neck dissection(s) plus postoperative radiation therapy should be used.
2. If substantial hypopharyngeal extension is present, laryngectomy or laryngopharyngectomy plus neck dissection and postoperative radiation therapy is recommended.
3. If no clinical neck disease is present (i.e., T4, N0), induction chemotherapy followed by radiation therapy to the primary tumor and necks in chemoresponsive tumors should be considered. If such a lesion does not respond adequately to induction chemotherapy, then the logical course should be a laryngectomy. The laryngectomy should probably be accompanied by appropriate selective neck dissection for staging[248] and, depending on the result of the histologic analysis of the neck nodes harvested, postoperative radiation therapy.
4. In these large lesions, especially lesions that demonstrate subglottic extension, radiation must be directed to the tracheal stoma, because recurrence here can be seen in a substantial percentage of these patients. Other indications for postoperative radiation are cartilage and extensive soft tissue invasion.

Most of these strategies for treating patients with advanced larynx or hypopharynx cancer and clinically positive necks must be analyzed in light of the dynamic state of the knowledge and experience with the organ-preservation concepts. Hitherto, we have been comfortable with the notion that substantial neck disease usually required surgery of some sort at some stage in the treatment plan. Armstrong and colleagues,[249] however, have published data that parallel the concept of larynx preservation and that suggest that patients with clinically palpable cervical nodal metastases who have a complete response to chemotherapy and who receive high-dose radiation therapy have excellent neck control and may not need neck dissection. To address this issue, they reviewed the neck management of the first 80 patients treated in the larynx preservation trials at Memorial Sloan-Kettering Cancer Center. Of these, 54 patients presented with clinically positive nodes. Of these, 44% had a complete response and 20% had a partial response in the neck to induction chemotherapy. In 63% of the major responders, surgery to the neck was omitted, and radiation alone was used. Neck control was obtained in 91%, with only 1 in 17 complete responders and 1 of 5 partial responders exhibiting neck failure. These data suggest that major responders to induction chemotherapy may possibly avoid neck dissection. These data require supplementation, and data for concomitant chemotherapy and radiotherapy must also be generated before it can be decided if this observation is sustained. Even if these preliminary suggestions are substantiated, however, the definitive question to be asked is whether the morbidity endured with high-dose radiation is justified when moderate-dose neck radiation plus a tailored neck operation is so well tolerated.

Considerations for Neck Surgery

Management of the neck is critical to successful therapy of supraglottic cancer. Levendag and associates[77] studied elective surgical management of the neck in a group of patients with stage I and II supraglottic carcinoma treated with surgery alone at the Memorial Sloan-Kettering Cancer Center. In those patients who underwent elective neck dissection (i.e., the group with clinically negative necks), 32% were found to have histologically positive cervical lymph nodes. One-half of the patients with involved nodes eventually had cancer recurrence in the dissected neck. Additionally, 19% of patients with negative elective neck dissections had cancer recurrence in the contralateral neck. Finally, in a group of 48 patients who did not have elective neck dissection, 29% had cancer recurrence in the neck. Therefore, a total of 35% of the T1, N0 and T2, N0 patients ultimately developed cervical lymph node metastases. Importantly, nearly two-thirds of those who relapsed in the neck eventually died from their cancer. On the other hand, none of the patients without neck relapse died from supraglottic cancer. These investigators compared their experience with a similar patient group from the other studies that showed similar neck failure rates with surgery alone and when radiation therapy was administered to the necks. Less than 5% failure follows electively radiated necks. These reports indicate that even the smallest supraglottic tumors require elective neck management.

A variety of neck operations are currently used in the various treatment plans for laryngeal cancer: the classic radical neck dissection, the modified radical neck dissection, and a group of regional dissections collectively known as *selective neck dissections.* This group of operations has been standardized and endorsed by the American Academy of Otolaryngology–Head and Neck Surgery and the American Head and Neck Society. The monograph outlining the recommended terminology should be studied, and oncologists are strongly urged to incorporate this classification into their lexicon to facilitate interinstitutional data recording and appropriate comparisons.[248]

Considerable diversity of opinion exists in the surgical community as to which of these operations should be applied to which situation. Exact guidelines are not consistently substantiated by the data available. Generalizations are possible, however. The radical neck dissection is almost never used in the clinically negative neck, even in those lesions in which the probability for metastasis is extraordinary. This procedure is usually reserved for necks in which there is gross metastasis, and even then the selective procedures are often used. Most of the time, however, these selective neck dissections are used as staging procedures in which the goal is to harvest and sample the nodal groups at highest risk for metastasis. This philosophy has evolved as a result of our increasing reliance on radiation therapy as the second half of neck treatment whenever disease is discovered in the neck. Only in very limited circumstances is the selective neck dissection thought to be therapeutic; that is to say, in most necks in which any neck disease is present, postoperative radiation is recommended.

The choice of the appropriate selective neck dissection in larynx cancer is based on a knowledge of the consistent patterns of metastasis that are exhibited by the various subsites within the larynx; for example, lesions of the supraglottis are prone to metastasis bilaterally and to levels II and III. Rarely, however, do they spread to level I.[41] Based on this knowledge, the logical staging operation for a supraglottic laryngeal cancer with a clinically negative neck would be designed specifically to clean out those various compartments at highest risk. This is but one example of a tailored approach, and the reader is referred to the classic work by Lindberg,[41] in which he mapped the patterns of metastases of the various aerodigestive SCCs. More recently, Shah and Andersen[250] applied the modern classification to this process of selectivity and have established recommendations for the use of these neck operations.

HYPOPHARYNX

GENERAL

The hypopharynx is the area of the pharynx that lies behind and below the oropharynx, just outside the view provided by tongue blade and flashlight; as such, it is visually inaccessible by routine office examination. Hypopharyngeal cancers are usually aggressive in their behavior, grow in an area of abundant lymphatic drainage, do not produce early symptoms or signs, and usually occur in people who are nutritionally depleted and immunologically compromised. It is not surprising, then, that the survival rates for these cancers are poor and that their treatment is difficult at best.

The hypopharynx extends from the oropharynx above to the esophageal inlet below, is cone shaped, and consists of three regions or subsites: the paired pyriform sinuses, the posterior pharyngeal wall, and the postcricoid area. The larynx is located at the anterior aspect of the hypopharynx, indenting it to create the two lateral sulci that are the pyriform sinuses. Although these sulci lie partially within the framework of the thyroid cartilage, they are actually part of the hypopharynx, and cancers that develop within them behave differently than do those of the larynx. The lateral wall of each pyriform sinus continues around to blend with and become the posterior pharyngeal wall. The apex of the pyriform sinuses extends down to a level just inferior to those endolaryngeal muscles of the adjacent true vocal cord. Above, the medial walls of the pyriform sinuses each form the pharyngeal side of the corresponding aryepiglottic fold, which is the partition between the hypopharynx and endolarynx. Laterally, the pyriform sinuses extend superiorly to the glossoepiglottic fold. The posterior aspect of each pyriform sinus is open and connects with the hypopharyngeal cavity. In effect, each pyriform sinus is a three-walled space that opens into the general hypopharyngeal cavity (see Figs. 30.3-1 and 30.3-2).

The funnel-shaped postcricoid area begins just below the arytenoids and extends to the level of the cricopharyngeus muscle below. It is lined with the mucosa that overlies the posterior lamina of the cricoid cartilage and that continues into the cervical esophagus. Laterally, the postcricoid mucosa blends with that of the pyriform sinuses, and because of this, the same cancer often affects these two areas.

Approximately 70% of hypopharyngeal lesions occur in the pyriform sinuses, and the remaining 20% to 30% occur on the posterior pharyngeal wall and in the postcricoid area.[251] Postcricoid cancers make up a small percentage of the latter group. Cancer of the hypopharynx is uncommon; approximately 2500 new cases are diagnosed in the United States each year. Overall, these lesions occur more often in men by a significant ratio, but there does seem to be a higher incidence of lower hypopharyngeal, or postcricoid, cancers in women. The upper hypopharyngeal lesions are more common in men. Those lower lesions are more often associated with nutritional abnormalities, whereas the lesions in the remainder of the hypopharynx seem to be associated more with heavy smoking and drinking.[252] Those ratios vary somewhat in different countries and change in accordance with the incidence of vitamin deficiencies.[253] For example, a higher incidence of carcinoma of the postcricoid area is seen in patients with Plummer-Vinson syndrome, a condition that includes an iron deficiency anemia. This condition is especially prevalent in northern Europe and is seen in nonsmoking women. Also, other metabolic deficiencies, such as vitamin B_{12} malabsorption, may play a role in the development of these lesions.[254]

PATHOLOGY, PATHOGENESIS, AND NATURAL HISTORY

Almost all hypopharynx malignancies are SCCs that have developed in an environment of deranged mucosa. The generalized effects of the carcinogens encountered over a lifetime can lead to the occurrence of multiple mucosal sites of epithelial disturbances that range from dyskeratosis to frank cancer. The concept of field cancerization is in part responsible for the multiple, synchronous primary malignant lesions that occur in approximately 12% to 20% of hypopharyngeal cancers.[255,256]

Cancers of the hypopharynx are generally aggressive in their behavior and demonstrate a natural history that is characterized by diffuse local spread, early metastasis, and a relatively high rate of distant spread. The anatomy of the area is such that, once a cancer has penetrated the mucosa, little restriction is placed on diffuse tumor extension in the submucosal plane. Because of this fact and also because of the abundant lymphatic network of the region, a localized hypopharyngeal tumor is exceptional rather than expected. An important study by Harrison[256] demonstrated pathologically that, in 40% of hypopharynx lesions, the true extent of the cancer had been underestimated initially.

Tumors of the pharyngeal walls are more often ulcerative than exophytic and are particularly prone to an insidious and deceptive growth pattern characterized by skip metastasis and ill-defined margins; once submucosal, these lesions can resurface at various locations remote from the primary site. They can extend upward in this fashion and can travel all the way to the base of the skull. Cancers of the postcricoid area also tend to spread laterally and can cause vocal cord paralysis by invading the recurrent laryngeal nerve just as it enters the larynx. Postcricoid lesions can extend inferiorly and can develop skip metastases in the cervical esophagus. Gross involvement of the esophagus with postcricoid cancer is uncommon. These lesions usually do not produce early symptoms, and when discovered, they often have caused cricoid cartilage destruction.

It is significant that the lateral walls of the pyriform sinuses lie against that area of the thyroid cartilage that is often ossified, a state that renders the cartilage vulnerable to tumor invasion[257] (see Fig. 30.3-2). In Kirchner and Owen's series[78] of 500 whole-organ larynx sections, more than 50% of the pyriform sinus cancers demonstrated cartilage invasion. This fact is relevant to the strategies of radiation oncologists and surgeons, because cancer involvement in the cartilage probably lessens radiocurability and substantially compromises the potential for conservation laryngeal surgery. Depending on the degree of ossification present, tumor that has invaded the thyroid or cricoid cartilage in one area can permeate the entire framework by extending within the cartilage and can even travel all the way to the opposite lamina of the structure.

Overall, the distribution of metastatic hypopharynx cancer is to all levels of the neck, with the level II (jugulodigastric) nodes being most common; level III the next most common site; and level I, IV, and V the least likely sites of metastasis.[41] Overall, the risk for cervical metastasis from pyriform sinus cancer is 75%; from posterior pharyngeal wall, 60%; and from the postcricoid area, 40%. Because the pyriform sinuses are located laterally, only 10% of these lesions present with bilateral metastasis. Such a pattern of spread occurs more commonly in postcricoid cancers, and it is the norm in posterior pharyngeal lesions.[258] Approximately 60% of posterior pharyngeal wall lesions demonstrate bilateral cervical nodes at the initial examination.[259] Metastasis occurs early in the course of hypopharynx cancers. Approximately 60% of pyriform sinus lesions are associated with clinically positive necks at the time of diagnosis, and many of those that have clinically negative necks turn out to have occult metastasis in the thyroid gland or in the paratracheal node chain.[81,83]

Because a significant number of postcricoid and pyriform sinus apex lesions metastasize to the less obvious paratracheal and thyroid gland lymphatics, the incidence of occult metastasis from those sites is somewhat greater than in the higher pyriform sinus and posterior pharyngeal wall lesions that typically metastasize to the deep jugular nodes.[260,261] Because of this fact, calculating occult metastatic rate is a problem in hypopharyngeal cancers.

The retropharyngeal lymph nodes that are located high in the neck are primary drainage sites for hypopharyngeal cancers and are involved in more than 40% of patients with posterior pharyngeal wall and pyriform sinus lesions.[262] It is, therefore, especially important in the staging and treatment of this particular group of tumors to include these nodes in the field of dissection, radiation, or both. These lymphatics are part of the deep jugular chain, are outside of the constrictor muscles, and are readily visible by imaging (see Fig. 30.3-8). Involvement of the retropharyngeal nodes may produce a symptom complex characterized by pain and stiffness in the neck, with pain radiating to the ipsilateral eye and forehead.

The incidence of distant metastasis from hypopharyngeal cancer is substantial, occurring in 24% of all sites and in all stages. This incidence is initially lower, rising in those subpopulations that live longest.[263,264]

DIAGNOSIS, EVALUATION, AND STAGING

Hypopharyngeal cancer is usually not diagnosed in its early stages. In fact, most series reported include few T1 lesions. This finding is due, in part, to the fact that many patients with these cancers have abused their health by smoking and drinking heavily and therefore they have a high tolerance for throat symptoms; however, it is also true that these lesions are often indolent and produce few symptoms until they are substantial in size. This is especially so for posterior pharyngeal wall cancers. More than 50% of patients with hypopharyngeal cancer have clinically obvious cervical metastasis at the time they are first encountered, and in one-half of these individuals, the neck mass is actually the presenting symptom.[265,266] Pyriform sinus and posterior pharyngeal wall lesions can cause a sensation of irritation and mucus retention that is felt only with swallowing. Otalgia is characteristic of pyriform sinus lesions and is a manifestation of cancer compromising the sensory fibers of the superior laryngeal nerve, the axons of which synapse with sensory nerves of the external auditory canal. The pain generated is typically dull and is perceived by the patient in the posterior and inferior aspects of the canal and on the posterior aspect of the auricle. In the absence of ear findings, persistent pain in these areas must be viewed with suspicion, and a careful examination of the upper aerodigestive tract must be done by someone skilled in the appropriate methods. Voice change associated with pyriform sinus or postcricoid lesions is a late symptom and usually represents impairment of vocal cord function by invasion into the endolarynx or of a recurrent laryngeal nerve. Patients often have lost their ability to swallow comfortably or have a lack of willingness to swallow because of fear of aspiration. Therefore, they often become debilitated during the course of this disease.

Many patients with hypopharyngeal cancer are chronically ill before the development of their lesion, having the pulmonary and hepatic diseases that accompany a lifetime of tobacco and alcohol excesses. Recognition of the compounding nature of these associations with hypopharyngeal cancer is essential in the formulation of an appropriate treatment plan.

Physical examination of the hypopharynx has become much less problematic since the development of the flexible, fiberoptically lighted endoscopes that are easily included in basic outpatient facilities (see Fig. 30.3-5). The crevices and partially hidden areas of the laryngopharynx are effectively visualized using these instruments; however, the conventional hand-held mirror examination is still the state of the art when used by the experienced head and neck diagnostician. For the occasional examiner, however, the benefits of the flexible endoscopes are significant. What is most essential is that the primary care physician not be reassured falsely by a normal tongue blade and light examination. In those patients with persistent symptoms of swallowing alteration or discomfort, otalgia, or voice change, such an examination is inadequate, because only a small part of the hypopharynx and none of the larynx is visualized in such an examination.

Examination of the hypopharynx can reveal pooling of secretions in all lesions of the area, but this finding is especially impressive in postcricoid and pyriform sinus cancers because of impairment of the passage of food and secretions into the esophagus. Often, such pooling is the only sign of a small lesion. In larger tumors, the abundance of secretions sometimes obscures the actual lesion. Occasionally, small and less obvious lesions of the medial wall and apex of the pyriform sinuses cause subglottic edema in the adjacent larynx. Postcricoid carcinomas generally produce esophageal obstructive symptoms sooner than tumors in other areas of the hypopharynx.

In deeply invasive postcricoid or posterior pharyngeal wall cancers, fixation of the larynx and the pharyngeal wall to the prevertebral fascia often is associated with a loss of normal laryngeal crepitation when the examining physician attempts to move the thyroid cartilage from side to side. As with other sites in the head and neck, the importance of lesion thickness and depth is becoming more obvious, especially as the search continues for nonsurgical means of treating these cancers. The thickness, or third dimension, of hypopharyngeal tumors; their lateral extension into the neck; and finally, the status of the adjacent lateral cervical and retropharyngeal nodes are visualized well by CT or MRI.[267]

Barium esophagogram is a relatively effective tool for detecting second primary cancers in the esophagus and also for evaluating postcricoid lesions[268]; however, this study is of limited value because it visualizes only the surface of the area and does not accurately demonstrate the total tumor volume. Because of tissue edema and the resulting image distortion that can be caused by instrumentation, these studies should be obtained before endoscopy and biopsy whenever possible.

Each hypopharyngeal cancer should be examined, staged, and carefully mapped on a permanent record (see Fig. 30.3-6); importantly, this should be accomplished on the awake and upright patient. Direct endoscopy and biopsy should then be done on all patients under general anesthesia, so that adequate tissue can be sampled and the third-dimensional appreciation for the tumor better achieved. Finally, considering the significant incidence of multiple synchronous primary tumors that occur with hypopharyngeal cancer, esophagoscopy and bronchoscope should be done at this time.

STAGING SYSTEM

As with most cancers, a workable staging system is critical to the evaluation of treatment methods and for the comparison of data between institutions (Table 30.3-5). This is especially true now that the use of sophisticated imaging allows for a relative quantification of tumor volume and extension. Although staging based on physical examination alone is fairly accurate, imaging is especially important in those lesions treated by nonsurgical means, because pathologic positivity or negativity of the neck is never proved unless a recurrence develops. Although considerable effort has been expended to develop workable and descriptive terminology, there continue to be limitations to current staging for hypopharyngeal cancers. For example, the system is satisfactory for disease of the pyriform sinuses, but it cannot be applied completely to lesions of the posterior pharyngeal wall, because they usually do not invade the larynx, and fixation is not part of the natural history. Rather, posterior pharyngeal wall tumors would be more appropriately staged by tumor diameter, as is the case with oropharyngeal lesions. According to the current system, a 5 × 4–cm posterior pharyngeal lesion without laryngeal fixation would still be classified as a T1 lesion, but in fact, it would have a prognosis similar to that for a T3 lesion.[37,269] The nodal staging and the stage grouping for the hypopharynx are the same as with other head and neck sites.

TABLE 30.3-5. Hypopharynx Staging

T1	Tumor limited to one subsite of hypopharynx and is 2 cm or less in greatest dimension.
T2	Tumor involves more than one subsite of hypopharynx or an adjacent site, or measures more than 2 cm but not more than 4 cm in greatest diameter without fixation of hemilarynx.
T3	Tumor measures more than 4 cm in greatest dimension or with fixation of hemilarynx.
T4	Tumor invades adjacent structures (e.g., thyroid/cricoid cartilage, carotid artery, soft tissues of neck, prevertebral fascia/muscles, thyroid, and/or esophagus).

(From *American Joint Committee on Cancer Staging,* 5th ed. Philadelphia: Lippincott Williams & Wilkins, 1997, with permission.)

TREATMENT AND SURVIVAL

A variety of prognostic factors have been identified for squamous carcinomas of the hypopharynx. Women and patients younger than 50 years of age seem to have a more favorable outcome. Because these tumors can affect swallowing, significant weight loss can occur, and extreme nutritional deficiency and debilitation may even prevent the delivery of curative therapy. Because many of the symptoms of this disease result from an advanced state, most patients are stage III or IV when diagnosed, and therefore, most are candidates for combined-modality treatment. This treatment involves surgery, radiation therapy and, more recently, chemotherapy programs. Surgeon, radiation oncologist, and medical oncologist must collaborate closely in the multidisciplinary evaluation and treatment of patients with hypopharyngeal cancer.

The fact that most patients with hypopharyngeal cancers currently are managed with combined-treatment modalities probably is not entirely explained by an inherent biologic difference between these tumors and other SCCs in the upper aerodigestive tract; rather, it may also reflect the fact that only a small number of these patients present with T1 or T2 disease. Higher percentages of poorly differentiated carcinomas are seen in the hypopharynx, but cell for cell, it is not entirely clear that these cancers are different from other poorly differentiated SCCs found in other sites. What makes hypopharyngeal cancers particularly ominous is probably related in large part to the anatomy of the area that allows extensive spreading of these tumors. On the other hand, even early-stage lesions do not do as well as other aerodigestive SCCs, and furthermore, in all larynx preservation protocols, the hypopharyngeal lesions fare worse than the larynx lesions. Finally, poor performance relates to debilitation, chronic anemia, to the extensive lymphatic drainage of the area, and to the fact that the diffuse carcinogenic effects that led to the initial problem also create an environment of condemned mucosal multifocality and *de novo* carcinoma formation.

The appropriate therapy for tumors of the hypopharynx is predicated on several factors, such as the patient's performance status, extent of disease, laryngeal involvement, and the presence and extent of metastasis. If, for example, the only surgical option available for removal of a given lesion of the hypopharynx involves a total laryngectomy, then organ preservation strategies using chemotherapy and radiation therapy become more appealing. However, total laryngectomy is not always necessary with resection of hypopharyngeal cancers, and a few selected patients who have tumors of the pharyngeal wall and pyriform sinuses are candidates for partial laryngopharyngectomies. The physiologic stress imposed on older and debilitated patients by these partial operations, however, can be unacceptable. Thin, early-stage cancers of the hypopharynx are probably as curable with radiation therapy as with surgery.

Excision of postcricoid cancers always involves a total laryngectomy. In a select subset of patients, lesions of the posterior pharyngeal wall can be resected even while retaining laryngeal integrity. Even in the smaller of these lesions, however, the larynx can be preserved in only a few cases.[258] Because of the tendency of pharyngeal wall lesions to have ill-defined margins, generous resections are necessary; with such liberal tissue removal, much of the sensory innervation normally used in the act of swallowing is violated. With large T3 and T4 tumors, laryngectomy is mandatory to achieve adequate surgical margins and to avoid the significant chronic aspiration that usually follows pharyngectomy in these cases. With the contemporary techniques of reconstruction in head and neck surgery being as sophisticated as they are, the limitations to this form of surgery do not relate to anatomic realignment; rather, they are physiologic, and an ill-conceived larynx preservation procedure may cure the cancer but condemn the patient to an unacceptable lifestyle. Newer techniques of hypopharyngeal reconstruction are being developed that use reinnervated free flaps. This reconstitution of the sensory apparatus so important to deglutition may to some extent solve the problems currently limiting the ability to resect this area radically.[270]

Limited T1 and T2 lesions on the medial wall of the pyriform sinus may be removed by partial laryngectomy, but either extension to the apex of the sinus or involvement of the adjacent postcricoid area mandates total laryngectomy. These medial wall lesions are particularly prone to penetrate the paraglottic space of the larynx (see Fig. 30.3-2), and when this does occur, partial laryngectomy becomes oncologically unsafe. In a pyriform sinus lesion, any motion change noticed in the vocal cord suggests invasion into the larynx. Some notable surgeons are skeptical of any indication for the use of partial laryngectomy for cancers of the pyriform sinuses. However, whatever the indications, it is fundamental that any attempt to remove a pyriform sinus cancer with less than a total laryngectomy should be done only by those surgeons with considerable experience in making the subtle judgments so often involved in this type of surgery. With the alternatives to surgery that are now available to treat these tumors, and considering our consistent ability to restore voice function after laryngectomy, any oncologic gamble associated with inadvisably trying to save the larynx is unacceptable. Overall, partial laryngopharyngectomy with preservation of voice and swallowing can be justifiably performed in fewer than 5% of all hypopharyngeal cancers.[271]

Radiation therapy is effective for early lesions of the hypopharynx, especially when they are exophytic. Mendenhall and associates[272] report local control in 79% of T1 and 71% of T2 lesions treated with radiation; however, the 5-year survival rate in this group was only 60%. Vandenbrouck and coworkers[273] reported a 5-year survival rate of only 40% in an extensive series of smaller lesions treated with radiation therapy. Itami et al.[274] reported local control of 49% for T1/T2 lesions of the pyriform sinus, which fell to 25% for T3/T4 disease. Doses of 70 Gy or higher are generally used, depending on the fractionation program. Pameijer and colleagues[275] evaluated the role of CT scans in predicting the outcome for patients treated with definitive radiation for T1/T2 disease. Tumor volume was found to be prognostic. For tumors larger than 6.5 mL, local control was 25% compared with 89% for tumors of less than 6.5 mL. These data are similar to those achieved surgically for early disease. For instance, Shah et al.[276] reported 5-year survival rates of 43% and 38%, respectively, for surgically managed TI and T2/T3 (N0) hypopharyngeal disease.

Disease control drops significantly for more advanced lesions. In the series by Mendenhall et al.[272] and Bataini and colleagues,[277] T3 lesions treated with primary radiation therapy had approximately a 40% local control rate but a dismal 5-year survival rate of less than 20%. Results of surgery for advanced disease are not any better. Shah and coworkers[276] reported a 16% 5-year survival rate for patients with T3 disease. When comparing single-modality therapy of hypopharyngeal cancers, results of surgery and radiation therapy are roughly equivalent, with both yielding suboptimal outcomes.

Because of the consistently poor survival data associated with the single-modality methods of treating more advanced hypopharyngeal cancer, combined therapy consisting of radiation administered after pharyngectomy or laryngopharyngectomy is the method currently being practiced in most centers.[272,278,279] The sequencing of the modalities is fairly standard, with the radiation generally administered postoperatively in all but selected circumstances. Essentially, this sequence allows the safe delivery of radiation doses in the 6000- to 7000-cGy range. Various trials from the Radiation Therapy Oncology Group and others have compared preoperative with postoperative therapy, and those data suggest better locoregional control and a trend toward better survival in the group treated with postoperative therapy.[280,281] Select circumstances exist, however, in which radiation therapy is recommended before surgery. For example, in those circumstances in which the primary tumor is small and exophytic and is therefore suitable for definitive radiation therapy, but in which the degree of neck disease precludes management with radiation alone, curative therapy to both the primary tumor and neck followed by neck dissection is an acceptable treatment plan. Mendenhall and associates[272] have reported an 80% 2-year control rate for disease above the clavicle in patients with advanced neck disease and early primary tumors that have been treated in this fashion. Just as with other head and neck sites, the clonal progeny in cervical metastasis is often more prominent than in the primary tumor.

Several groups have reported results of a treatment strategy that consists of primary radiation with surgery being used only for salvage. Keane and colleagues[282] reported 41% disease control using this approach. Most patients (75%) in this series had been staged as T3 or T4. Approximately two-thirds had palpable nodal metastases, and the 5-year survival rate was only 15%.

Traditional treatment programs of surgery and radiation therapy for hypopharyngeal carcinomas have been augmented by organ-preservation induction-chemotherapy strategies. Organ preservation for hypopharyngeal cancer may be feasible, but the percentage of patients who preserve their larynx long term is unsatisfactory. Future trials exploring concomitant chemotherapy and radiotherapy are more likely to yield better locoregional control and to affect survival.

Two randomized trials of organ preservation for patients with cancer of the hypopharynx have been published. The EORTC randomized 202 patients with operable squamous cancers of the pyriform sinus or the aryepiglottic fold (stage T2, T3, or T4 and N0, N1, N2a, or N2b) to receive either induction chemotherapy and radiation or standard treatment with total laryngectomy, partial pharyngectomy, and radiation.[238] In the experimental treatment group, only patients achieving a clinical complete response of the primary tumor proceeded to radiotherapy; all others underwent resection. The preliminary results after a median follow-up of 51 months show no difference in survival for the two treatment groups; 3- and 5-year survival estimates are 57% and 30% for patients randomized to chemotherapy and 43% and 35% for those randomized to surgery. Fifty-four percent of patients had a clinical complete response at the primary site and 52% in the neck after chemotherapy. Three- and 5-year estimates of survival with a functional larynx were 28% and 17%, respectively. If only the deaths from local progression are considered, to account for patients who died with a functional larynx, then these survival estimates with a preserved larynx are 42% and 35%, respectively. The EORTC is now embarking on a trial that will compare sequential to simultaneous chemotherapy and radiotherapy for organ preservation of patients with cancer of the hypopharynx.

Mahe and colleagues[283] evaluated the role of surgery for patients with T3/T4 or N2/N3 cancer of the hypopharynx. Ninety-one patients were randomly assigned treatment with induction chemotherapy followed by surgery and radiation or induction chemotherapy followed by radiation. Median and 5-year survival rates were significantly better with resection: 40 versus 20 months, and 37% versus 19%, respectively. This difference was explained by a significantly higher local failure rate in the nonsurgical group of 61%, compared with 37% in the surgical group. Because of the nature of the study design, no conclusions regarding the impact of induction chemotherapy can be made.

Survival data vary considerably between sites within the hypopharynx. Few postcricoid cancers are treated by radiation, but anecdotal experience suggests that a small subset of patients with smaller thin lesions are treatable with curative therapy. In almost all postcricoid lesions, extensive surgery consisting of laryngopharyngectomy or laryngopharyngoesophagectomy with reconstruction is followed by postoperative radiation and yields a 20% to 25% 5-year survival rate.[284] Posterior pharyngeal wall lesions of earlier stages can be treated with equal effectiveness by radiation or surgery. More advanced lesions are best treated by combined surgery followed by postoperative radiation. Meoz-Mendez and colleagues[285] reported that 91% of T1 and 73% of T2 lesions of the pharyngeal wall can be controlled with primary radiation, requiring a dosage greater than 6500 cGy. For T3 and T4 disease, similar doses controlled 61% and 37%, respectively. Pyriform sinus lesions of early stage are curable by radiation, whereas the much more common advanced lesions are best treated by combined therapy. Data accumulated by Vandenbrouck and coworkers[280] showed a 3-year survival rate of 48%, which dropped to 33% at 5 years for lesions treated with total and partial laryngectomy plus postoperative radiation therapy. In that same series, the 3-year survival rate was 67% in the group treated by partial laryngectomy plus postoperative radiation therapy. This latter statistic probably reflects the increased survival expected in lesser-stage disease.

All treatment plans for hypopharyngeal cancer must consider certain facts: The overwhelming majority of these lesions metastasize to cervical lymph nodes, and in the case of the posterior pharyngeal wall, bilateral metastasis is the rule rather than the exception; 40% of posterior pharyngeal wall lesions and probably an equal number of upper pyriform sinus lesions metastasize to the retropharyngeal nodes; in those patients with clinically negative necks, the incidence of occult metastasis is substantial; and between 20% and 30% of pyriform sinus lesions, and probably an equal number of posterior pharyngeal wall lesions, are associated with distant metastasis. Even in the lesser-stage hypopharyngeal lesions, the high rate of regional metastases requires inclusion of the neck(s) in all management plans.

SPECIFIC TREATMENT METHODS

Patients treated with primary radiation therapy require treatment to the primary site and both necks. The primary site and upper neck fields are treated with bilateral opposed portals, and the low-neck fields are treated with anterior portals. If lymph nodes are involved, a neck dissection usually is added. If no neck dissection is planned, the node-bearing regions must be treated with higher doses.

When patients who have had a total laryngectomy are receiving postoperative radiation, it is important to radiate the tracheal stoma. For postoperative radiation, the total doses recommended to the primary site and involved areas of the neck are between 6000 and 6500 cGy in 6.5 to 7.5 weeks. The tracheal stoma is treated with a total dose of 5000 to 5500 cGy.

Lesions of the hypopharynx often require laryngopharyngectomy or laryngopharyngoesophagectomy, after which the means of reconstruction consist of free jejunal graft with microvascular anastomosis,[286] various myocutaneous flaps or, in the cases that include esophagectomy, gastric transposition.[287] Reconstruction of the hypopharynx has been enhanced greatly by the interposition free jejunal graft, which is less morbid than gastric transposition and is associated with a high rate of success.

Surgical management of the neck is similar to that of other sites in the upper aerodigestive tract. In those patients with substantial and multilevel disease, at least a modified radical neck dissection usually is performed in continuity with the primary resection, unless the primary tumor has been treated with curative radiation. In those patients with minimal neck disease or with clinically negative necks, radiation alone can suffice, or any of a variety of selected neck dissections can be used as a means of removing gross disease from the neck in preparation for radiation.[248]

REFERENCES

1. Pfister D, Strong E, Harrison L. Larynx preservation with combined chemo- and radiotherapy in advanced head and neck cancer. *J Clin Oncol* 1991;9:830.
2. Karp D, Vaughan C, Carter R, et al. Larynx preservation with induction chemotherapy plus radiation as alternative to laryngectomy. *Am J Clin Oncol* 1991;14:273.
3. Hong W, O'Donoghue G, Sheetz S. Sequential response patterns to chemotherapy and radiotherapy in head and neck cancer: potential impact of treatment in advanced laryngeal cancer. *Prog Clin Biol Res* 1985;201:191.

4. Cann C, Fried M, Rothman K. Epidemiology of squamous cell cancer of the head and neck. *Otolaryngol Clin North Am* 1985;18;367.
5. Gloecker Ries L, Miller B, Hankey B. *SEER cancer statistics review, 1973–1991*. Washington, DC: Surveillance Program, Division of Cancer Prevention and Control, National Cancer Institute, 1992.
6. Barclay T, Rao N. The incidence and mortality rates for laryngeal cancer from total cancer registries. *Laryngoscope* 1975;83:254.
7. Krajina Z, Kucar Z, Zonic-Carnelutti V. Epidemiology of laryngeal cancer. *Laryngoscope* 1975;85:11.
8. Iwai H, Koike Y. Primary laryngoplasty. *Laryngoscope* 1975;85:929.
9. Lowry W. Alcoholism in cancer of the head and neck. *Laryngoscope* 1975;85:1275.
10. Clayton L, Byrd W. The African-American cancer crisis. *J Health Care Poor Underserved* 1993;4:830.
11. Austen D. Larynx. In: Schottenfeld P, Aumeni J, eds. *Cancer epidemiology and prevention*. Philadelphia: WB Saunders, 1982:554.
12. Iwamoto H. An epidemiological study of laryngeal cancer in Japan (1960–1969). *Laryngoscope* 1975;85:1162.
13. Hiranandani L. Panel on epidemiology and etiology of laryngeal carcinoma. *Laryngoscope* 1975;85:1197.
14. DeStefani E, Correa P, Oreggia F. Risk factors for laryngeal cancer. *Cancer* 1987;60:3087.
15. Graham S, Mettlin C, Marshall J. Dietary factors in the epidemiology of cancer of the larynx. *Am J Epidemiol* 1981;113:675.
16. Morrison M. Is chronic gastroesophageal reflux a causative factor in glottic carcinoma? *Otolaryngol Head Neck Surg* 1988;99:370.
17. Wynder E, Bross I, Day E. Epidemiological approach to the etiology of cancer of the larynx. *JAMA* 1956;160:1384.
18. Kurozumi S, Harada Y, Sugimoto Y, Saaski H. Airway malignancy in poisonous gas workers. *Laryngol Otol* 1977;91:217.
19. Morgan R, Shettigara P. Occupational asbestos exposure, smoking, and laryngeal carcinoma. *Ann N Y Acad Sci* 1976;271:308.
20. Goolden A. Radiation cancer of the pharynx. *BMJ* 1951;2:1110.
21. Doyle D, Henderson L, LeJeune F. Changes in human papillomavirus typing of recurrent respiratory papillomatosis progressing to malignant neoplasm. *Arch Otolaryngol Head Neck Surg* 1994;120:1273.
22. Fouret P, Dabit D, Sibony M. Expression of p53 protein related to the presence of human papillomavirus infection in precancerous lesions of the larynx. *Am J Pathol* 1995;146:599.
23. Glssman L, Wolnik W, Ikenberg H. Human papilloma virus types 6 and 11 DNA sequences in genital laryngeal papillomas and in some cervical cancers. *Proc Natl Acad Sci U S A* 1983;80:560.
24. Howley P. The human papillomaviruses. *Arch Pathol Lab Med* 1982;106:429.
25. Kashima HD, Tzyy-Choou W, Mounts P. Carcinoma ex-papilloma: histologic and virologic studies in whole-organ sections of the larynx. *Laryngoscope* 1988;98:619.
26. Kashima H, Kutcher M, Keswsis T. Human papillomavirus in squamous cell carcinoma, leukoplakia, lichen planus and clinically normal epithelium of the oral cavity. *Ann Otol Rhinol Laryngol* 1990;99:55.
27. Lynch P. Warts and cancer. *Am J Dermatopathol* 1982;4:55.
28. Spitz M, Fvegers J, Goepfert H, Hong W, Newell G. Squamous cell carcinoma of the upper aerodigestive tract. *Cancer* 1988;61:203.
29. Segi M. Age-adjusted death rates for cancer for selected sites in 46 countries in 1977. Tokyo: Segi Institute for Cancer Epidemiology, 1982:13.
30. Ramadan M, Morton R, Stell P, Phawah P. Epidemiology of laryngeal cancer. *Clin Otolaryngol* 1982;7:417.
31. Pietramtoni L, Fior R. Clinical and surgical problems of cancer of the larynx and hypopharynx. *Acta Otolaryngol* 1958;142:1.
32. Lauerma S. Treatment of laryngeal cancer: a study of 638 cases. *Acta Otolaryngol* 1967;225:140.
33. Wynder E. Toward the prevention of laryngeal cancer. *Laryngoscope* 1975;85:1190.
34. Martensson B. Indications for transconiscopy. In: Alberti P, Bryce D, eds. *Workshops from the Centennial Conference on Laryngeal Cancer.* East Norwalk, CT: Appleton-Century-Crofts, 1976:668.
35. Koufman J, Burke A. Etiology of laryngeal carcinoma. *Otolaryngol Clin North Am* 1997;30:14.
36. Kirchner J. Growth and spread of laryngeal cancer: as related to partial laryngectomy. In: Alberti P, Bryce D, eds. *Workshops from the Centennial Conference on Laryngeal Cancer.* East Norwalk, CT: Appleton-Century-Crofts, 1976:54.
37. American Joint Committee on Cancer. *Manual for staging of cancer,* 3rd ed. Philadelphia: JB Lippincott, 1988.
38. Hirano M. Structure of the vocal fold in normal and disease states. In: Ludlow C, O'Connell H, eds. *Proceedings of the Conference on the Assessment of Vocal Pathology.* Report no. 11. Rockville, MD: American Speech and Hearing Association, 1981:11.
39. Sessions R, Miller S, Martin G, et al. Videostroboscopy in assessment of early glottic carcinomas. *Trans Am Laryngol Assoc* 1989;100:56.
40. Pressman J, Simon M, Moncel C. Anatomical studies related to the dissemination of cancer of the larynx. *Trans Am Acad Ophthalmol Otolaryngol* 1970;64:628.
41. Lindberg R. Distribution of cervical lymph nodes from squamous cell carcinoma of upper respiratory and digestive tracts. *Cancer* 1972;29:1446.
42. Kashima H. The characteristics of laryngeal cancer correlating with cervical lymph node metastasis. In: Alberti P, Bryce D, eds. *Workshops from the Centennial Conference on Laryngeal Cancer.* East Norwalk, CT: Appleton-Century-Crofts, 1976:855.
43. Clinical evaluation of the larynx. In: Thawley S, Panje W, Batsakis J, Lindberg R, eds. *Comprehensive management of head and neck tumors,* vol 1. Philadelphia: WB Saunders, 1987:874.
44. Milroy C, Rode J, Moss E. Laryngeal paragangliomas and neuroendocrine carcinomas. *Histopathology* 1991;18:201.
45. Laccourreye O, Chabardes E, Weinstein G, et al. Synchronous arytenoid and pancreative neuroendocrine carcinomas. *Laryngol Otol* 1991;105:573.
46. Batsakis J. *Tumors of the head and neck: clinical and pathological considerations,* 2nd ed. Baltimore: Williams & Wilkins, 1979:200.
47. Luna M, Tortoledo M. Verrucous carcinoma. In: Gnepp DR, ed. *Pathology of the head and neck.* New York: Churchill Livingstone, 1988:497.
48. Mansel R, Vermeersch H. Panendoscopies for second primaries in head and neck cancer. American Laryngology Society Meeting, Vancouver, British Columbia, May 1981.
49. McGuirt W, Matthews B, Koufman J. Multiple simultaneous tumors in patients with head and neck cancer. *Cancer* 1982;50:1195.
50. Shapsay S, Hong W, Fried M. Simultaneous carcinomas of the esophagus and upper aerodigestive tract. *Otolaryngol Head Neck Surg* 1980;88:373.
51. Healey G, Strong M, Uchmakli A. Carcinoma of the palatine arch: the rationale of therapeutic selection. *Am J Surg* 1978;132:498.
52. Arold-Schneider M, Schall H. Occurrence of non-metaplastic squamous epithelium within the larynx and its relation to the development of cancer. *Laryngol Rhinol Otol* 1990;69:91.
53. Crissman J. Laryngeal keratosis preceding laryngeal carcinoma. *Arch Otolaryngol* 1982;108:445.
54. Crissman J. Laryngeal keratosis and subsequent carcinoma. *Head Neck Surg* 1979;1:386.
55. Hellquist H, Lundgren J, Olofsson J. Hyperplasia, keratosis, dysplasia and carcinoma-*in-situ* of the vocal cords. *Clin Otolaryngol* 1982;7:11.
56. Sllamniku B, Bauer W, Painter C, Sessions D. The transformation of laryngeal keratosis into invasive carcinoma. *Am J Otolaryngol* 1989;10:42.
57. Hjslet P, Nielsen P, Palvio P. Premalignant lesions of the larynx. *Acta Otolaryngol* 1989;107:130.
58. Munck-Wirland E, Krylenstierna R, Lindholm J, Amer G. Image cytometry DNA analysis of dysplastic squamous epithelial lesions of the larynx. *Anticancer Res* 1991;11:597.
59. Baucr W. Concomitant carcinoma *in situ* and invasive carcinoma of the larynx. In: Alberti P, Bryce D, eds. *Workshops from the Centennial Conference on Laryngeal Cancer.* East Norwalk, CT: Appleton-Century-Crofts, 1976:127.
60. Miller A, Fisher H. Clues to the life history of carcinoma *in situ* of the larynx. *Laryngoscope* 1971;81:1475.
61. McGavran M, Bauer W, Ogura J. The incidence of cervical lymph node metastases from epidermoid carcinoma of the larynx and their relationship to certain characteristics of the primary tumor. *Cancer* 1961;14:55.
62. Reid A, Robin P, Powell J, McConkey C, Rockley J. Staging carcinoma: its value. *J Laryngol Otol* 1991;105:456.
63. Hirabayshi H, Koshi K, Uno K. Extracapsular spread of squamous carcinoma in neck nodes: prognostic factors in laryngeal cancer. *Laryngoscope* 1991;101:502.
64. Spiro R, Alfonso A, Farr H, Strong E. Cervical node metastases for epidermoid carcinoma: a critical assessment of current staging. *Am J Surg* 1974;128:566.
65. Mohit-Tabatabai M, Sobel H, Rush B, Mashberg R. Relationship of thickness of floor of mouth stage I and II cancers to regional metastasis. *Am J Surg* 1986;152:351.
66. Close L, Brown P, Vuitch M, Reisch J, Schaefer S. Microscopic invasion and survival in cancer of the oral cavity and oropharynx. *Arch Otolaryngol Head Neck Surg* 1989;115:1304.
67. Spiro R, Huvos A, Wong G, et al. Predictive value of tumor thickness in squamous carcinoma confined to the tongue and floor of the mouth. *Am J Surg* 1986;152:345.
68. Rasgon B, Cruz R, Hilsinger R, Sawicki J. Relation of lymph node metastasis to histopathologic appearance in oral cavity and oropharyngeal carcinoma. *Laryngoscope* 1989;99:1103.
69. Platz H, Fries R, Hudec M, Min Tjoa A, Wagner R. The prognostic relevance of various factors at the time of first admission of the patient. *J Maxillofac Surg* 1983;11:3.
70. Barades S, Leeman D, Chen T, Mohit-Tabatabai M. Significance of tumor thickness in soft palate carcinoma. *Laryngoscope* 1992;103:389.
71. Ravasz L, Hordijk G, Slootweg P, Smit F, Tweel I. Uni- and multivariant analysis of eight indications for post-operative radiotherapy and their significance for local-regional cure in advanced head and neck cancer. *J Laryngol Otol* 1993;107:437.
72. Morton R, Ferguson C, Lambie N, Whitlock R. Rumor thickness in early tongue cancer. *Arch Otolaryngol Head Neck Surg* 1994;120:717.
73. Kirchner J, Cornog J, Holmes R. Transglottic cancer: its growth and spread within the larynx. *Arch Otolaryngol* 1974;99:247.
74. Micheau C, Luboinski B, Sancho H, Cachin Y. Modes of invasion of cancer of the larynx: a statistical, histological, and radioclinical analysis of 120 cases. *Cancer* 1976;38:346.
75. Kirchner J. One hundred laryngeal cancer studies by serial section. *Ann Otol Rhinol Laryngol* 1969;78:689.
76. Ogura J, Sessions D, Spector G. Conservation surgery for epidermoid carcinoma of the supraglottic larynx. *Laryngoscope* 1975;85:1808.
77. Levendag P, Vikram B, Sessions R. The problem of neck relapse in early stage supraglottic cancer—results of different treatment modalities for the clinically negative neck. *Int J Radiat Oncol Biol Phys* 1987;13:1621.
78. Kirchner J, Owen J. Five hundred cancers of the larynx and pyriform sinus. *Laryngoscope* 1977;87:1288.
79. Hansen H. Supraglottic carcinoma of the aryepiglottis fold. *Laryngoscope* 1975;85:1667.
80. Shah J, Tollefsen H. Epidermoid carcinoma of the supraglottic larynx. *Am J Surg* 1974;128:494.
81. Ogura J, Biller H, Wette R. Elective neck dissection for pharyngeal and laryngeal cancers. *Ann Otol Rhinol Laryngol* 1971;80:646.
82. Putney F. Elective versus delayed neck dissection in cancer of the larynx. *Surg Gynecol Obstet* 1961;112:736.
83. Biller H, Davis W, Ogura J. Delayed contralateral cervical metastasis with laryngeal and laryngopharyngeal cancers. *Laryngoscope* 1971;81:1499.
84. Ogura J, Spector G, Sessions D. Conservation surgery for carcinoma of the marginal area. *Laryngoscope* 1975;85:1801.
85. Som M. Conservation surgery for carcinoma of the supraglottis. *J Laryngol Otol* 1970;84:655.
86. Spiro R. Cervical node metastasis from epidermoid carcinoma of the oral cavity and oropharynx. *Am J Surg* 1974;128:562.

87. Lawson W, Biller H, Suen J. Cancer of the larynx. In: Myers G, Suen J, eds. *Cancer of the head and neck,* 2nd ed. New York: Churchill Livingstone, 1989:533.
88. Kirchner J, Fischer J. Anterior commissure cancer. In: Alberti P, Bryce D, eds. *Workshops from the Centennial Conference on Laryngeal Cancer.* East Norwalk, CT: Appleton-Century-Crofts, 1976:679.
89. Jesse R, Lindberg R, Horiot J. Vocal cord cancer with anterior commissure extension: choice of treatment. *Am J Surg* 1971;122:437.
90. Sessions D, Ogura J, Fried M. Laryngeal carcinoma involving anterior commissure and subglottis. In: Alberti P, Bryce D, eds. *Workshops from the Centennial Conference on Laryngeal Cancer.* East Norwalk, CT: Appleton-Century-Crofts, 1976:674.
91. Lawson W, Biller H, Suen J. Cancer of the larynx. In: Myers G, Suen J, eds. *Cancer of the head and neck,* 2nd ed. New York: Churchill Livingstone, 1989:558.
92. Stell P. The subglottic space. In: Alberti P, Bryce D, eds. *Workshops from the Centennial Conference on Laryngeal Cancer.* East Norwalk, CT: Appleton-Century-Crofts, 1976:682.
93. Harrison D. The pathology and management of subglottic cancer. *Ann Otol Rhinol Laryngol* 1971;80:6.
94. Kraus F, Perez-Mesa C. Verrucous carcinoma: clinical and pathological study of 105 cases involving oral cavity, larynx, and genitalia. *Cancer* 1966;19:26.
95. Van Nostrand A, Olofsson J. Verrucous carcinoma of the larynx. *Cancer* 1972;30:691.
96. Biller H, Ogura J, Bauer W. Verrucous cancer of the larynx. *Laryngoscope* 1971;81:1323.
97. Ackerman L. Verrucous carcinoma of the oral cavity. *Surgery* 1948;23:670.
98. Batsakis J, Hybels R, Crissman J, Rice D. The pathology of head and neck tumors: verrucous carcinoma, Part XV. *Head Neck Surg* 1982;5:29.
99. Ferlito, A, Recher G. Ackerman's tumor of the larynx. *Cancer* 1980:46:1517.
100. Vesely J, Sibl O, Kudrmann J, Kremar M. Verrucous carcinoma of the larynx. *Otolaryngology* 1989;38:284.
101. Abramson A, Brandsma J, Steinberg B, Winkler B. Verrucous carcinoma of the larynx. *Arch Otolaryngol* 1985;111:709.
102. Glanz H, Kleinasser O. Verrucous carcinoma of the larynx: a misnomer. *Arch Otorhinolaryngol* 1987;244:108.
103. Myers E, Sobol S, Ogura H. Hemilaryngectomy for verrucous carcinoma of the glottis. *Laryngoscope* 1980;90:693.
104. Sessions R, Hudkins C. Malignant cervical adenopathy. In: Cummings C, ed. *Otolaryngology: head and neck surgery,* 2nd ed. St. Louis: Mosby, 1992:1605.
105. Fonts E, Greenlaw R, Rush B, Rovin S. Verrucous squamous cell carcinoma of the oral cavity. *Cancer* 1969;23:152.
106. Perez C, Kraus F, Evans J. Anaplastic transformation in verrucous carcinoma of the oral cavity after radiation therapy. *Radiology* 1966;86:108.
107. Elliott G, MacDougall J, Elliott J. Problems of verrucous squamous carcinoma. *Ann Surg* 1973;177:21.
108. Rider W. Toronto experience of verrucous carcinoma of the larynx. In: Alberti P, Bryce D, eds. *Workshops from the Centennial Conference on Laryngeal Cancer.* East Norwalk, CT: Appleton-Century-Crofts, 1976:460.
109. Medina J, Dichtel W, Luna M. Verrucous-squamous carcinomas of the oral cavity. *Arch Otolaryngol* 1984;110:437.
110. Burns H, Van Nostrand A, Bryce D. Verrucous carcinoma of the larynx: management by radiotherapy and surgery. *Ann Otol Rhinol Laryngol* 1976;85:538.
111. Myerowitz R, Barnes E, Myers E. Small cell anaplastic (oat cell) carcinoma of the larynx. *Laryngoscope* 1978;88:1697.
112. Gould V, Linnoila R, Memoli V, Warren W. Neuroendocrine components of the bronchopulmonary tract. *Lab Invest* 1983;49:519.
113. Strahlenther O. Primary small cell neuroendocrine carcinoma of the larynx. 1994;170:365.
114. Sole J, Jurgens A, Musulen E, et al. Small cell carcinoma of the larynx. *Bull Cancer Radiother* 1994;81:45.
115. Mullins J, Newman R, Coltman C. Primary oat cell carcinoma of the larynx. *Cancer* 1979;43:711.
116. Goldman N, Hood C, Singleton G. Carcinoid of the larynx. *Arch Otolaryngol* 1969;90:90.
117. Ferlito A, Milroy C, Wenig B, Barnes L, Silver C. Laryngeal paraganglioma versus atypical carcinoid tumor. *Ann Otol Rhinol Laryngol* 1995;104:78.
118. Ferlito A, Barnes L, Wenig B. Identification classification, treatment of laryngeal paraganglioma. *Ann Otol Rhinol Laryngol* 1994;103:525.
119. Devaney K, Ferlito A, Silver C. Cartilaginous tumors of the larynx. *Ann Otol Rhinol Laryngol* 1995;104:251.
120. Obermyer N, Ramadan H. Adenocarcinoma of the larynx. *Head Neck* 1994;16:453.
121. Morland B, Cox G, Randall C, Ramsay A, Radford M. Synovial sarcoma of the larynx. *Med Pediatr Oncol* 1994;23:64.
122. Scott K, Carter C. Malignant fibrous histiocytoma of the larynx. *J Otolaryngol* 1995;2:198.
123. Maniglia A, Xue J. Plasmacytoma of the larynx. *Laryngoscope* 1983;93:741.
124. Booth J, Osborn D. Granular cell myoblastoma of the larynx. *Acta Otolaryngol* 1970;70:279.
125. Anderson H, Maisel R, Cantrell R. Isolated laryngeal lymphoma. *Laryngoscope* 1976;86:1251.
126. Reuter V, Woodruff J. Melanoma of larynx. *Laryngoscope* 1986;96:389.
127. Castelijns J, Gerristen G, Kaiser M, et al. Invasion of laryngeal cartilage by cancer: comparison of CT to MR. *Radiology* 1989;167:199.
128. Towler C, Young S. MRI of the larynx. *Magn Reson* 1989;5:228.
129. Castelijns J, Golding R, Van-Schaik C, Valk J, Snow G. MR findings of cartilage invasion by laryngeal cancer: value of predicting outcome of radiation therapy. *Radiology* 1990;174:669.
130. Pillsbury H, Kirchner J. Clinical versus histologic staging in laryngeal cancer. *Arch Otolaryngol* 1979;105:157.
131. Spriano G, Antognoni P, Piantanida R, et al. Conservative management of T1-T2N0 supraglottic cancer. *Am J Otolaryngol* 1997;18:299.
132. Lera J, Lara P, Perez S, Cabrera J, Santana C. Tumor proliferation, p53 expression, and apoptosis in laryngeal carcinoma: relation to the results of radiotherapy. *Cancer* 1998;83:2493.
133. Wang C, Nakfoor B, Spiro I, Martins P. Role of accelerated fractionated irradiation for supraglottic carcinoma. *Cancer J Sci Am* 1997;3:88.
134. Mendenhall W, Parsons J, Mancuso A, Stringer S, Cassisi N. Radiotherapy for squamous cell carcinoma of the supraglottic larynx: an alternative to surgery. *Head Neck* 1996;18:24.
135. Steinger J, Parnes S, Gardner G. Morbidity of combined therapy for the treatment of supraglottic carcinoma: supraglottic laryngectomy and radiotherapy. *Ann Otol Rhinol Laryngol* 1997;106:151.
136. Adamopoulos G, Yotakis I, Apostolopoulos K, et al. Supraglottic laryngectomy. *J Laryngol Otol* 1997;111:730.
137. Bradford CR, Wolf GT, Fisher SG, McClatchey KD. Prognostic importance of surgical margins in advanced laryngeal squamous carcinoma. *Head Neck* 1996;18:11.
138. Lefebvre J, Wolf G, Luboninski B. Meta-analysis of chemotherapy in head and neck cancer (MACHNC) (2) Larynx preservation using neoadjuvant chemotherapy in laryngeal and hypopharyngeal carcinoma. *Am Soc Clin Oncol* 1998;34:224.
139. Wolf G, Hong W, Fisher S. Neoadjuvant chemotherapy for organ preservation: current status. Fourth International Conference on Head and Neck Cancer. 1996:89.
140. Wolf GT, Forastiere A, Ang K, et al. Workshop report: organ preservation strategies in advanced head and neck cancer—current status and future directions. *Head Neck* 1999;21:689.
141. Lee N, Goepfert H, Awendt C. Supraglottic laryngectomy for intermediate stage cancer: UT M. D. Anderson Cancer Center experience with combined therapy. *Laryngoscope* 1990;100:831.
142. Soo K, Shah J, Gopinath K, et al. Analysis of prognostic variables and results after supraglottic partial laryngectomy. *Am J Surg* 1988;156:301.
143. Bocca E, Pignataro O, Oldini C. Supraglottic laryngectomy: 30 years of experience. *Ann Otol Rhinol Laryngol* 1983;92:14.
144. Parsons J, Mendenhall W, Stringer S, Cassisi N. T4 laryngeal carcinoma: radiotherapy alone with surgery reserved for salvage. *Int J Radiat Oncol Biol Phys* 1998;40:549.
145. Vermund H, Boysen M, Evensen J, et al. Recurrence after different primary treatment for cancer of the supraglottic larynx. *Acta Oncologica* 1998;37:167.
146. Finizia C, Geterud A, Holmberg E, et al. Advanced laryngeal cancer T3-T4 in Sweden: a retrospective study 1986–1990. Survival and locoregional control related to treatment. *Acta Otolaryngol* 1996;116:906.
147. Hermans R, Van den Bogaert W, Rijnders A, Baert A. Value of CT as outcome predictor of supraglottic squamous cell carcinoma treated by definitive radiation therapy. *Int J Radiat Oncol Biol Phys* 1999;44:755.
148. Mancuso A, Mukherji S, Schmalfuss I, et al. Preradiotherapy computed tomography as a predictor of local control in supraglottic carcinoma. *J Clin Oncol* 1999;17:631.
149. Lo S, Venkatesan V, Matthews T, Rogers J. Tumour volume: implications in T2/T3 glottic/supraglottic squamous cell carcinoma. *J Otolaryngol* 1998;27:247.
150. Jankovic I, Merkas Z. Radiotherapy as the primary approach in the treatment of laryngeal cancer. In: Alberti P, Bryce D, eds. *Workshops from the Centennial Conference on Laryngeal Cancer.* East Norwalk, CT: Appleton-Century-Crofts, 1976:881.
151. Ogura J, Biller H. Conservative surgery in cancer of the head and neck. *Otolaryngol Clin North Am* 1969;2:641.
152. Sessions R, Parish R. How are patients chosen for conservation surgery of the larynx? In: Harrison DFN, ed. *Dilemmas in otorhinolaryngology.* London: Churchill Livingstone, 1988:283.
153. Laccourreye H, Laccourreye O, Menard M, et al. Supracricoid laryngectomy with cricohyoidoepiglottopexy: a partial laryngeal procedure for glottic carcinoma. *Ann Otol Rhino Laryngol* 1990;99:421.
154. Fu K, Pajak T, Trotti A, et al. A Radiation Therapy Oncology Group (RTOG) phase III randomized study to compare hyperfractionation and two variants of accelerated fractionation to standard fractionation radiotherapy for head and neck squamous cell carcinomas: preliminary results of RTOG 9003. *Int J Radiat Oncol Biol Phys* 1999;45[Suppl]:145.
155. McGuirt WF, Kaufman JA. Endoscopic laser surgery: an alternative in laryngeal cancer treatment. *Arch Otolaryngol Head Neck Surg* 1987;113:501.
156. Harwood A. Cancer of the larynx: the Toronto experience. *J Otolaryngol* 1982;11:1.
157. Njuyen C, Naghibzadeh B, Black M, Rochon L, Shenouda G. Carcinoma *in situ* of the glottic larynx: excision or irradiation? *Head Neck* 1996;18:225.
158. Medini E, Medini I, Lee CK, Gapany M, Levitt SH. The role of radiotherapy in the management of carcinoma *in situ* of the glottic larynx [Review]. *Am J Clin Oncol* 1998;21:298.
159. Smitt M, Goffinet D. Radiotherapy for cis of glottic larynx. *Int J Radiat Oncol Biol Phys* 1994;28:251.
160. Fein D, Mendenhall W, Parsons J, et al. Carcinoma *in situ* of the glottic larynx: the role of radiation. *Int J Radiat Oncol Biol Phys* 1993;27:370.
161. Wang CC. Treatment of glottic carcinoma by megavoltage radiation therapy and results. *Am J Roentgenol Radium Ther Nucl Med* 1974;120:157.
162. Fletcher G, Lindbert R, Hamberger A, Horiot J. Reasons for irradiation failure in squamous cell carcinoma of the larynx. *Laryngoscope* 1975;85:987.
163. Pellitteri P, Kennedy T, Vrabec D, Beiler D, Hellstrom M. Radiotherapy, the mainstay in the treatment of early glottic carcinoma. *Arch Otolaryngol Head Neck Surg* 1991;117:297.
164. Dagli A, Mahieu H, Festen J. Quantitative analysis of voice quality in early glottic laryngeal carcinomas treated with radiotherapy. *Eur Arch Otorhinolaryngol* 1997;254:78.
165. Morton R. Laryngeal cancer: quality of life and cost effectiveness. *Head Neck* 1997;19:243.
166. Rosier J, Gregoire V, Counoy H, et al. Comparison of external radiotherapy, laser microsurgery and partial laryngectomy for the treatment of T1N0M0 glottic carcinomas: a retrospective evaluation. *Radiother Oncol* 1998;48:175.
167. Harrison L, Solomon B, Miller S, et al. Prospective computer assisted voice analysis for patients with early stage glottic cancer: a preliminary report of the functional result of laryngeal irradiation. *Int J Radiat Oncol Biol Phys* 1990;19:123.
168. de Graeff A, de Leeuw R, Ros W, et al. A prospective study on quality of life of laryngeal cancer patients treated with radiotherapy. *Head Neck* 1997;19:243.
169. Tsunoda K, Soda Y, Tojima H, et al. Stroboscopic observation of the larynx after radiation in patients with T1 glottic carcinoma. *Acta Otolaryngologica* 1997;527[Suppl]:1656.
170. Verdonck-de Leeuw J, Vreeburg G, Bartelink H. Consequences of voice impairment in daily life for patients following radiotherapy for early glottic cancer: voice quality, vocal function, and vocal performance. *Int J Radiat Oncol Biol Phys* 1999;44:1071.

171. Biller H, Barnhill F, Ogura J, Perez C. Hemilaryngectomy following radiation failure for carcinoma of the vocal cords. *Laryngoscope* 1970;80:249.

172. Sorenson H, Hansen H, Thomsen K. Partial laryngectomy following irradiation. *Laryngoscope* 1980;90:1344.

173. Dickens W, Cassisi N, Million R, Bova F. Treatment of early vocal cord carcinoma: a comparison of apples and apples. *Laryngoscope* 1983;93:216.

174. Wang CC. Treatment of squamous cell carcinoma of the larynx by radiation. *Radiol Clin North Am* 1978;16:209.

175. Daly C, Strong E. Carcinoma of the glottic larynx. *Am J Surg* 1975;130:489.

176. Leroux-Robert J. A statistical study of 620 laryngeal carcinomas of the glottic region personally operated upon more than five years ago. *Laryngoscope* 1975;85:1440.

177. Sessions D, Maness G, McSwain B. Laryngofissure in the treatment of carcinoma of the vocal cord. *Laryngoscope* 1964;75:490.

178. Southwick H. Cancer of the larynx: surgical management. In: *Seventh National Cancer Conference proceedings*. Philadelphia: JB Lippincott, 1973:54.

179. Ogura J, Sessions D, Spector G. Analysis of surgical therapy for epidermoid carcinoma of the laryngeal glottis. *Laryngoscope* 1975;85:1522.

180. Sessions D, Ogura J, Fried M. The anterior commissure in glottic carcinoma. *Laryngoscope* 1974;85:1624.

181. Sessions D, Ogura J, Fried M. Laryngeal carcinoma involving the anterior commissure and subglottis. In: Alberti P, Bryce D, eds. *Workshops from the Centennial Conference on Laryngeal Cancer*. East Norwalk, CT: Appleton-Century-Crofts, 1976:674.

182. Olofsson J, Williams G, Rider W, Bryce D. Anterior commissure carcinoma: primary treatment with radiotherapy in 57 patients. *Arch Otolaryngol* 1972;95:230.

183. Olofsson J. Specific features of laryngeal carcinoma involving the anterior commissure and subglottic region. In: Alberti P, Bryce D, eds. *Workshops from the Centennial Conference on Laryngeal Cancer*. East Norwalk, CT: Appleton-Century-Crofts, 1976:626.

184. Klintenberg C, Lundgren J, Adell G, et al. Primary radiotherapy of T1 and T2 glottic carcinoma—analysis of treatment results and prognostic factors in 223 patients. *Acta Oncologica* 1996;35[Suppl]:81.

185. Fein DA, Hanlon AL, Lee WR, Ridge JA, Coia LR. Neck failure in T2N0 squamous cell carcinoma of the true vocal cords: the Fox Chase experience and review of the literature [Review]. *Am J Clin Oncol* 1997;20:1547.

186. Skladowski K, Tarnawski R, Maciejewski B, Wygoda A, Slosarek K. Clinical radiobiology of glottic T1 squamous cell carcinoma. *Int J Radiat Oncol Biol Phys* 1999;43:101.

187. Warde P, O'Sullivan B, Bristow RG, et al. T1/T2 glottic cancer managed by external beam radiotherapy: the influence of pretreatment hemoglobin on local control. *Int J Radiat Oncol Biol Phys* 1998;41:347.

188. Tamawski R, Skladowski K, Maciejewski B. Prognostic value of hemoglobin concentration in radiotherapy for cancer of supraglottic larynx. *Int J Radiat Oncol Biol Phys* 1997;38:1007.

189. Narayana A, Vaughan A, Gunaratne S, et al. Is p53 an independent prognostic factor in patients with laryngeal carcinoma? *Cancer* 1998;82:286.

190. Lera J, Lara P, Perez S, Cabrera J, Santana C. Tumor proliferation, p53 expression, and apoptosis in laryngeal carcinoma: relation to the result of radiotherapy. *Cancer* 1998;83:2493.

191. Pai H, Rochon L, Clark B, Black M, Shenouda G. Overexpression of p53 protein does not predict local regional control or survival in patients with early stage squamous cell carcinoma of the glottic larynx treated with radiotherapy. *Int J Radiat Oncol Biol Phys* 1998;41:37.

192. Kropveld A, Slootweg P, Blankenstein M, Terhaard C, Hordijk G. Ki-67 and p53 in T2 laryngeal cancer. *Laryngoscope* 1998;108:1548.

193. Valente G, Giusti U, Kerim S, et al. High prognostic impact of growth fraction parameters in advanced stage laryngeal squamous cell carcinoma. *Oncol Rep* 1999;6:298.

194. Pameijer FA, Mancuso AA, Mendenhall WK, Parsons JT, Kubilis PS. Can pretreatment computed tomography predict local control in T3 squamous cell carcinoma of the glottic larynx treated with definitive radiotherapy? *Int J Radiat Oncol Biol Phys* 1997;37:1011.

195. Stokkel MP, Terhaard CH, Mertens IJ, Hordijk GJ, van Rijk PP. Fluorine-18-FDG detection of laryngeal cancer postradiotherapy using dual-head coincidence imaging. *J Nucl Med* 1998;39:1385.

196. Kim HJ, Boyd J, Dunphy F, Lowe V. F-18 FDG PET scan after radiotherapy for early-stage larynx cancer. *Clin Nucl Med* 1998;23:750.

197. McGuirt WF, Greven KM, Keyes JW Jr, Williams DW III, Watson N. Laryngeal radionecrosis versus recurrent cancer: a clinical approach. *Ann Otol Rhinol Laryngol* 1998;107:293.

198. Dickens W, Cassisi N, Million R, Bova F. Treatment of early vocal cord carcinoma. *Laryngoscope* 1983;93:216.

199. Medini E, Medini A, Gapany M, Levitt SH. Radiation therapy in early carcinoma of the glottic-larynx T1N0M0. *Int J Radiat Oncol Biol Phys* 1996;36:1211.

200. Hayakawa K, Mitsuhashi N, Akimoto T, et al. The effect of overall treatment time of radiation therapy on local control of T1-stage squamous cell carcinoma of the glottis. *Laryngoscope* 1996;106:1545.

201. Yu E, Shenouda G, Beaudet MP, Black MJ. Impact of radiation therapy fraction size on local control of early glottic carcinoma. *Int J Radiat Oncol Biol Phys* 1997;37:587.

202. Yamamoto M, Joja I, Takemoto M, Kuroda M, Hiraki Y. The results of radiotherapy for T1 glottic cancers: influence of radiation beam energy. *Acta Medica Okayama* 1999;53:91.

203. van der Voet JC, Keus RB, Hart AA, Hilgers FJ, Bartelink H. The impact of treatment time and smoking on local control and complications in T1 glottic cancer. *Int J Radiat Oncol Biol Phys* 1998;42:247.

204. Robertson AG, Robertson C, Perone C, et al. Effect of gap length and position on results of treatment of cancer of the larynx in Scotland by radiotherapy: a linear quadratic analysis. *Radiother Oncol* 1998;48:165.

205. Robertson C, Robertson AG, Hendry JH, et al. Similar decreases in local tumor control are calculated for treatment protraction and for interruptions in the radiotherapy of carcinoma of the larynx in four centers. *Int J Radiat Oncol Biol Phys* 1998;40:319.

206. Saarilahti K, Kajanti M, Lehtonen H, Hamalainen T, Joensuu H. Repopulation during radical radiotherapy for T1 glottic cancer. *Radiother Oncol* 1998;47:155.

207. Marshak G, Brenner B, Shvero J, et al. Prognostic factors for local control of early glottic cancer: the Rabin Medical Center retrospective study on 207 patients. *Int J Radiat Oncol Biol Phys* 1999;43:1009.

208. Le QT, Fu KK, Kroll S, et al. Influence of fraction size, total dose, and overall time on local control of T1-T2 glottic carcinoma. *Int J Radiat Oncol Biol Phys* 1997;39:11526.

209. Jakobsson P, Rneroth G, Kollander D, Moeberger G, Martensson B. A histological classification and grading of malignancy in carcinoma of the larynx. *Acta Radiologica* 1973;12:1.

210. Olofsson J, Lord I, VanNostrand A. Vocal cord fixation in laryngeal carcinoma. *Acta Otolaryngol* 1973;75:486.

211. Mullins J, Newman R, Coltman C. Primary oat cell carcinoma of the larynx. *Cancer* 1979;43:7.

212. Som M. Cordal cancer with extension to vocal process. *Laryngoscope* 1975;85:1298.

213. Van den Bogert W, Ostyn F, Vancer Schuerren E. The primary treatment of advanced vocal cord cancer: laryngectomy or radiotherapy? *Int J Radiat Oncol Biol Phys* 1983;9:329.

214. Harwood A, Hawkins V, Beale F. Management of advanced glottic cancer: a 10-year review of the Toronto experience. *Int J Radiat Oncol Biol Phys* 1979;5:899.

215. Wang C. Radiation therapy of laryngeal tumors. In: Thawley S, Panje W, Batsakis J, Lindberg R, eds. *Comprehensive management of head and neck tumors*. Philadelphia: WB Saunders, 1987:906.

216. Mendenhall W, Parsons J, Mancuso A, et al. Definitive radiotherapy for T3 squamous cell carcinoma of the glottic larynx. *J Clin Oncol* 1997;15:2394.

217. Mendenhall W, Parsons J, Stringer S. Stage T3 squamous cell carcinoma of the glottic larynx: irradiation compared to laryngectomy. *Int J Radiat Oncol Biol Phys* 1991;21[Suppl 1]:142.

218. Terhaard C, Karim A, Hoogenraad S. Local control in T3 laryngeal cancer treated with radical radiotherapy: time-dose relationship—the concept of nominal standard dose and linear quadratic model. *Int J Radiat Oncol Biol Phys* 1991;20:1207.

219. Jesse R. The evaluation of treatment of patients with extensive squamous cancer of the vocal cords. *Laryngoscope* 1975;85:1424.

220. Hawkins N. The treatment of glottic carcinoma: an analysis of 800 cases. *Laryngoscope* 1975;85:1485.

221. Stewart J, Brown J, Palmer M, Cooper A. The management of glottic carcinoma by primary irradiation with surgery in reserve. *Laryngoscope* 1975;85:1477.

222. Jacobs C, Goffinet D, Goffinet L. Chemotherapy as a substitute for surgery in the treatment of advanced resectable head/neck cancer. *Cancer* 1987;60:1178.

223. Wolf G, Hong W, Fisher S, et al. Larynx preservation with induction chemotherapy and radiation in advanced laryngeal cancer: final result of the VA Laryngeal Cancer Study Group cooperative trial. *Proc Am Soc Clin Oncol* 1993;12:277.

224. Adelstein DJ, Adams GL, Li Y, et al. A phase II comparison of standard radiation therapy (RT) versus RT plus concurrent DDP and 5-fluorouracil (5-FU) in patients with unresectable squamous cell head and neck cancer: an intergroup study. *Proc Am Soc Clin Oncol* 2000 (*in press*).

225. Brizel DM, Albers ME, Fisher SR, et al. Hyperfractionated irradiation with or without concurrent chemotherapy for locally advanced head and neck cancer. *N Engl J Med* 1998;338:1798.

226. Merlano M, Vitale V, Rosso R, et al. Treatment of advanced squamous cell carcinoma of the head and neck with alternating chemotherapy and radiotherapy. *N Engl J Med* 1992;327:1115.

227. Wendt TG, Grabenbauer GG, Rodel CM, et al. Simultaneous radiochemotherapy versus radiotherapy alone in advanced head and neck cancer: a randomized multicenter study. *J Clin Oncol* 1998;16:1318.

228. Forastiere AA. Larynx preservation trials: a critical appraisal. *Semin Radiat Oncol* 1998:8:254.

229. Al-Kourainy K, Kish J, Ensley J, et al. Achievement of superior survival for histologically negative versus histologically positive clinically complete responders to cisplatin combination in patients with locally advanced head and neck cancer. *Cancer* 1987;59:233.

230. Kish J, Weaver A, Jacobs J, et al. Cisplatin and 5-fluorouracil infusion in patients with recurrent and disseminated epidermoid cancer of the head and neck. *Cancer* 1984;53:1819.

231. Weaver A, Fleming S, Ensley J, et al. Superior clinical response and survival rates with initial bolus of cisplatin and 120 hour infusion of 5 fluorouracil before definitive therapy for locally advanced head and neck cancer. *Am J Surg* 1984;148:525.

232. Ensley J, Jacobs J, Weaver A, et al. Correlation between response to cisplatinum combination chemotherapy and subsequent radiotherapy in previously untreated patients with advanced squamous cell cancers of the head and neck. *Cancer* 1984;54:811.

233. Demard F, Chauvel P, Santini J, et al. Response to chemotherapy as justification for modification of the therapeutic strategy for pharyngolaryngeal carcinomas. *Head Neck* 1990;12:225.

234. Clayman GL, Weber RS, Guillamondegui O, et al. Laryngeal preservation for advanced laryngeal and hypopharyngeal cancers. *Arch Otolaryngol Head Neck Surg* 1995;121:219.

235. Shirinian MH, Weber RS, Lippman SM, et al. Laryngeal preservation by induction chemotherapy plus radiotherapy in locally advanced head and neck cancer: the MD Anderson Cancer Center experience. *Head Neck* 1994;16:39.

236. De Andres L, Brunet J, Lopez-Pousa A, et al. Function preservation in stage III squamous laryngeal carcinoma: results with an induction chemotherapy protocol. *J Clin Oncol* 1995;13:1493.

237. Wolf GT, Hong WK, Fisher S, et al. Induction chemotherapy plus radiation compared with surgery plus radiation in patients with advanced laryngeal cancer. The Departments of Veterans Affairs Laryngeal Cancer Study Group. *N Engl J Med* 1991;324:1685.

238. Lefebvre JL, Chevalier D, Luboniski B, et al. Larynx preservation in pyriform sinus cancer. Preliminary results of a European Organization for Research and Treatment of Cancer phase III trial. EORTC Head and Neck Cancer Cooperative Group. *J Natl Cancer Inst* 1996;88:890.

239. Bradford CF, Wolf GT, Carey TE, et al. Predictive markers for response to chemotherapy, organ preservation, and survival in patients with advanced laryngeal carcinoma. *Otolaryngol Head Neck Surg* 1999;121:534.

240. Richard J, Sancho-Garnier H, Pessey J, et al. Randomized trial of induction chemotherapy in larynx carcinoma. *Oral Oncol* 1998;34:224.

241. Lefebvre J, Wolf G, Luboninski B. Meta-analysis of chemotherapy in head and neck cancer (MACH-NC): (2) larynx preservation using neoadjuvant chemotherapy in laryngeal and hypopharyngeal carcinoma. *Am Soc Clin Oncol* 1998;17:382a.

242. Adelstein DJ. Induction chemotherapy in head and neck cancer. *Hematol Oncol Clin North Am* 1999;13:689.
243. Paccagnella A, Orlando A, Marchiori C, et al. Phase III trial of initial chemotherapy in stage III or IV head and neck cancers: a study by the Gruppo di Studio sui Tumori della Testa a del Collo. *J Natl Cancer Inst* 1994;86:265.
244. Brockstein B, Haraf D, Stenson K, et al. Phase I study of concomitant chemoradiotherapy with paclitaxel, fluorouracil, and hydroxyurea with granulocyte colony-stimulating factor support for patients with poor-prognosis cancer of the head and neck. *J Clin Oncol* 1998;16:735.
245. Conley B, Jacobs M, Suntharalingam M, et al. A pilot trial of paclitaxel, carboplatin and concurrent radiotherapy for unresectable squamous cell carcinoma of the head and neck. *Semin Oncol* 1997;24:78.
246. Fountzilas G, Athanassiadis A, Samathas E, et al. Paclitaxel and carboplatin in recurrent or metastatic head and neck cancer: a phase II study. *Semin Oncol* 1997;19:28.
247. Hoffman W, Belka C, Schmidberger H, et al. Radiotherapy and concomitant weekly 1-hour infusion of paclitaxel in the treatment of head and neck cancer: result from a phase I trial. *Int J Radiat Oncol Biol Phys* 1997;38:691.
248. Robbins KT, Medina J, Wolfe G. Standardizing neck dissection terminology. *Arch Otolaryngol Head Neck Surg* 1991;117:604.
249. Armstrong J, Pfister D, Strong E, et al. The management of the clinically positive neck as part of a larynx preservation approach. *Int J Radiat Oncol Biol Phys* 1993;26:759.
250. Shah J, Andersen P. The impact of patterns of nodal metastasis on modifications of neck dissection. *Ann Surg Oncol* 1994;1:521.
251. Carpenter R III, DeSanto L. Cancer of the hypopharynx. *Surg Clin North Am* 1977;57:7.
252. Wynder E, Hultberg S, Jacobsson F, Bross I. Environmental factors in cancer of the upper alimentary tract. *Cancer* 1957;10:470.
253. Higginson J, Terracini B, Agthe C. Nutrition and cancer: ingestion of foodborne carcinogens. In: Schottenfeld D, ed. *Cancer epidemiology and prevention.* Springfield, IL: Charles C Thomas Publisher, 1975:177.
254. Larsson L, Sandstrom A, Westling P. Relationship of phenomenon: Vinson disease to cancer of the upper alimentary tract in Sweden. *Cancer Res* 1975;3:3308.
255. Cunningham M, Catlin D. Cancer of the pharyngeal wall. *Cancer* 1967;20:1859.
256. Harrison D. Pathology of hypopharyngeal cancer in relation to surgical management. *J Laryngol Otol* 1970;84:349.
257. Harrison D. Significance and means by which laryngeal cancer invades thyroid cartilage. *Ann Otol Rhinol Laryngol* 1981;93:392.
258. Guillamondegui O, Meoz-Mendez R, Jesse R. Surgical treatment of squamous cell carcinoma of the pharyngeal walls. *Am J Surg* 1978;136:474.
259. McGavarvan M, Bauer W, Spjut H. Carcinoma of the pyriform sinus. *Arch Otolaryngol* 1963;78:826.
260. Ogura J, Jurema H, Watson R. Partial laryngopharyngectomy and neck dissection for pyriform sinus cancer. *Laryngoscope* 1960;70:1399.
261. Byers R, Wolf P, Ballantyne A. Rationale for elective modified neck dissection. *Head Neck Surg* 1988;10:160.
262. Ballantyne A. Methods of repair after surgery for cancer of the pharyngeal wall, post cricoid area, and cervical esophagus. *Am J Surg* 1971;122:482.
263. Marks J, Freeman R, Lee F, Ogura J. Pharyngeal wall cancer: an analysis of treatment results, complications, and patterns of failure. *Int J Radiat Oncol Biol Phys* 1978;4:587.
264. Merino O, Landberg R, Fletcher C. An analysis of distant metastases from squamous cell carcinoma of the upper respiratory and digestive tracts. *Cancer* 1977;40:1415.
265. Keane T. Carcinoma of the hypopharynx. *J Otolaryngol* 1982;11:227.
266. Honvitz S, Caldarelli D, Hendrickson F. Treatment of carcinoma of the hypopharynx. *Head Neck Surg* 1979;2:107.
267. Mancuso A, Harnsberger H, Muraki A, Stevens M. Computed tomography of cervical and retropharyngeal lymph nodes. II. Pathology. *Radiology* 1983;148:709.
268. Grossman T, Kita M, Toohill R. The diagnostic accuracy of pharyngoesophagogram compared to esophagoscopy of patients with head and neck cancer. *Laryngoscope* 1987;97:103
269. Million R, Cassissi N. *Management of head and neck cancer: a multidisciplinary approach.* Philadelphia: JB Lippincott, 1984:85.
270. Urken ML, Weinberg H, Vickery C, et al. The combined sensate radical forearm and iliac crest free flaps for reconstruction of significant glossectomy-mandibulectomy defects. *Laryngoscope* 1992;102:543.
271. Million R, Cassissi N. Radical irradiation for carcinoma of the pyriform sinus. *Laryngoscope* 1981;91:439.
272. Mendenhall W, Parsons J, Devine J. Squamous cell carcinoma of the pyriform sinus treated with surgery and/or radiotherapy. *Head Neck Surg* 1987;10:88.
273. Vandenbrouck C, Eschwege F, DeLaRochfordiere A. Squamous cell carcinoma of the pyriform sinus: retrospective study of 351 cases treated at the Institute Roussy. *Head Neck Surg* 1987;10:4.
274. Itami J, Uno T, Aruga M, Ode S. Local control of piriform sinus cancer treated by radiation therapy alone. *Acta Oncologica* 1997;36:389.
275. Pameijer F, Mancuso A, Mendenhall W, et al. Evaluation of pretreatment computed tomography as a predictor of local control in T1/T2 pyriform sinus carcinoma treated with definitive radiotherapy. *Head Neck* 1998;20:159.
276. Shah J, Shaha A, Spiro R, Strong E. Carcinoma of the hypopharynx. *Am J Surg* 1976; 132:439.
277. Bataini P, Brugere J, Vernier J. Results of radical radiotherapy treatment of carcinoma of the pyriform sinus: experience of the Institute Curie. *Int J Radiat Oncol Biol Phys* 1982;8:1276.
278. Donald P, Haves H, Dhalival R. Combined treatment for pyriform sinus cancer using postoperative irradiation. *Otolaryngol Head Neck Surg* 1980;88:738.
279. Hong W, Dimery I, Kramer A. The role of induction chemotherapy in the treatment of advanced head and neck cancer. In: Salmon S, ed. *Adjuvant therapy of cancer,* 5th ed. Orlando, FL: Grune & Stratton, 1987:79.
280. Vandenbrouck C, Sancho A, LeFur R. Results of a randomized clinical trial of preoperative irradiation versus postoperative in treatment of tumors of the hypopharynx. *Cancer* 1977;39:145.
281. Kramer S, Gelber R, Snow J. Combined radiation therapy in the management of advanced head and neck cancer: final report of study 73-03 of the Radiation Therapy Oncology Group. *Head Neck Surg* 1987;10:19.
282. Keane T, Hawkins N, Beal F. Carcinoma of the hypopharynx: results of primary radical radiation therapy. *Int J Radiat Oncol Biol Phys* 1983;9:659.
283. Mahe M, Peuvrel P, Bergerot P, et al. Final results of a randomized trial comparing chemotherapy plus radiotherapy (ct + rt) versus chemotherapy plus surgery plus radiotherapy (ct + s + re) in locally advanced resectable hypopharyngeal carcinomas. *Proc Am Soc Clin Oncol* 1995;14:295.
284. Harrison D, Thompson A. Pharyngolaryngoesophagectomy with pharyngogastric anastomosis for cancer of the hypopharynx. *Head Neck Surg* 1986;8:418.
285. Meoz-Mendez R, Fletcher G, Guillamondegui O, Peters L. Analysis of the results of irradiation in the treatment of squamous cell carcinoma of the pharyngeal walls. *Int J Radiat Oncol Biol Phys* 1978;4:579.
286. Kato H, Iizuka T, Watanabe H. Reconstruction of the esophagus by microvascular surgery. *Jpn J Clin Oncol* 1984;14:379.
287. Theile D, Robinson D, McCafferty G. Pharyngolaryngectomy reconstruction by revascularized free jejunal graft. *Aust N Z J Surg* 1986;56:849.

SECTION **4**

ROY B. SESSIONS
LOUIS B. HARRISON
ARLENE A. FORASTIERE

Tumors of the Salivary Glands and Paragangliomas

MAJOR SALIVARY GLAND TUMORS

The same neoplasms affect all salivary gland tissue, but with predictable variations for the different anatomic sites. The major salivary glands consist of paired parotids in the preauricular area, paired submandibulars deep and inferior to the mandible, and paired sublinguals in the floor of the mouth. The minor salivary glands, on the other hand, are ubiquitous in the upper aerodigestive tract, occurring throughout the oral and nasal cavities and the paranasal sinuses. The probability of any given salivary neoplasm being malignant is highest in the sublingual glands, next highest in the minor salivary glands, third highest in the submandibular glands, and least in the parotid glands. Overall, salivary cancers make up approximately 3% of all head and neck malignancies that are diagnosed in North America each year; most of these are in the parotid glands. Sublingual and minor salivary gland cancers are unusual.[1]

ANATOMY

The parotid gland is tightly compacted in the area immediately anterior and inferior to the external ear. It is best thought of in three dimensions, with the deep portion extending medially behind the posterior rim of the ascending ramus of the mandi-

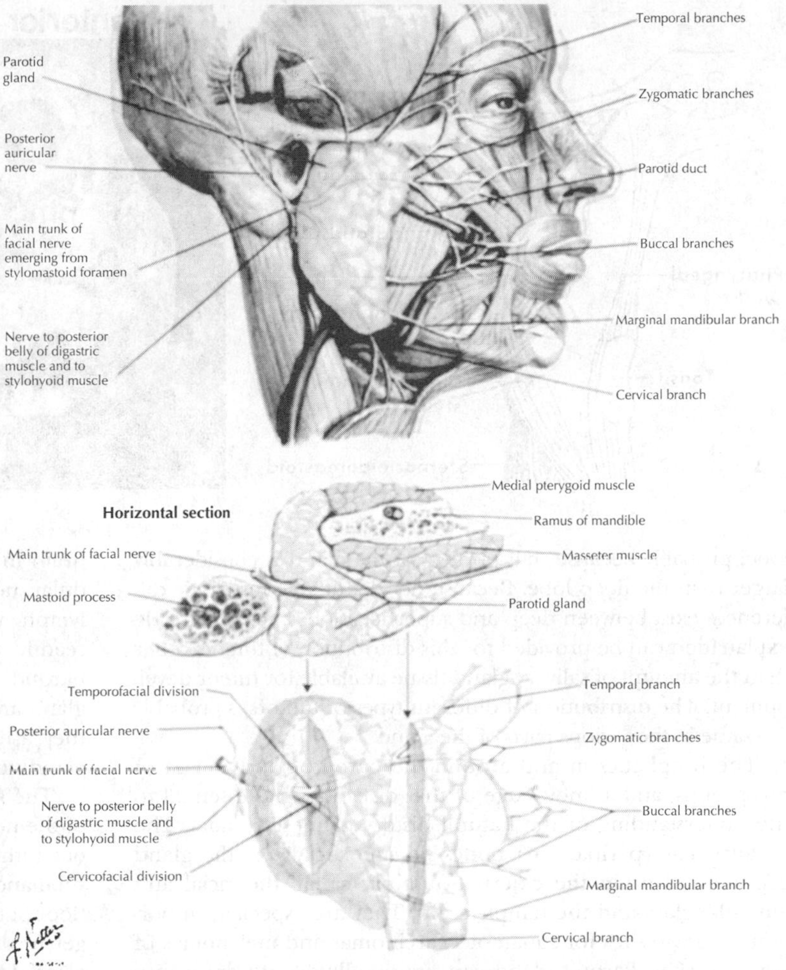

FIGURE 30.4-1. Representation of parotid gland and facial nerve anatomy. Lower part of diagram shows details of the relation of the nerve to the surrounding gland. Various branches of the nerve are directed to various parts of the facial musculature. (CIBA Collection, Frank Netter.)

ble into the parapharyngeal space. The superficial part of the gland lies on the masseter muscle and extends inferiorly to overlie the sternocleidomastoid and digastric muscles (Fig. 30.4-1). The same fascia that engulfs both of these muscles also forms a substantial capsule around both the parotid and submandibular glands, thus forming a barrier that confines tumors to their site of origin. The most inferior extent of the parotid gland extends a variable distance, and in those necks in which this extension is exaggerated, the glandular tail overlies the transverse process of the second cervical vertebrae as well as the deep jugular lymph nodes adjacent to this level. Not infrequently, a prominent transverse process or an enlarged lymph node in this area is misinterpreted as a parotid tail mass. This circumstance is encountered less frequently today, however, because contemporary imaging has helped to define that which is abnormal.

The facial nerve leaves the stylomastoid foramen at the base of the skull and almost immediately penetrates the posterior capsule of the parotid gland. Once within that structure, the nerve divides into five main branches—temporal, zygomatic, buccal, mandibular, and cervical—all of which extend in a consistent direction and depth, and all of which gradually become more superficial as they extend anteriorly. In addition to being more superficial, the more anterior branches of the nerve are more delicate; thus, increased risks are associated with dissection of tumors located more anterior in the gland.

Although no actual lobes are defined by fascial planes, that part of the parotid gland superficial to the facial nerve is arbitrarily referred to as the *superficial lobe.* That portion deep to the nerve is called the *deep lobe.* These facts have considerable bearing on dissections done within the parotid gland (see Fig. 30.4-1). The deep lobe of the parotid gland extends into the parapharyngeal space; thus, tumors of that portion of the gland can come into contact with the carotid sheath and its contents, which form the posterior boundary of that space. These deep lobe tumors can press against the constrictor muscles of the pharynx that normally form the medial wall of the parapharyngeal space (Fig. 30.4-2). A large deep lobe parotid tumor can, therefore, present as a submucosal bulge of the tonsil pillar, a finding that is easily misinterpreted by the inexperienced diagnostician as an oropharyngeal neoplasm (Fig. 30.4-3). The distinction between a deep lobe parotid tumor and an oral lesion becomes clear on either magnetic resonance imaging (MRI) or computed tomography (CT). There is some difficulty, however, in distinguishing these deep lobe neoplasms from tumors that have their origin in the parapharyngeal space. Correct diagnosis depends on the presence or absence of a fat plane between the deep lobe and the tumor. The distinction between the two is important, because the differential diagnosis of tumors that originate in the parapharyngeal space must include lymphomas, neurogenic tumors, and paragangliomas,[2,3] none of which is likely to occur primarily in the parotid gland. Most parotid tumors originate in the superficial

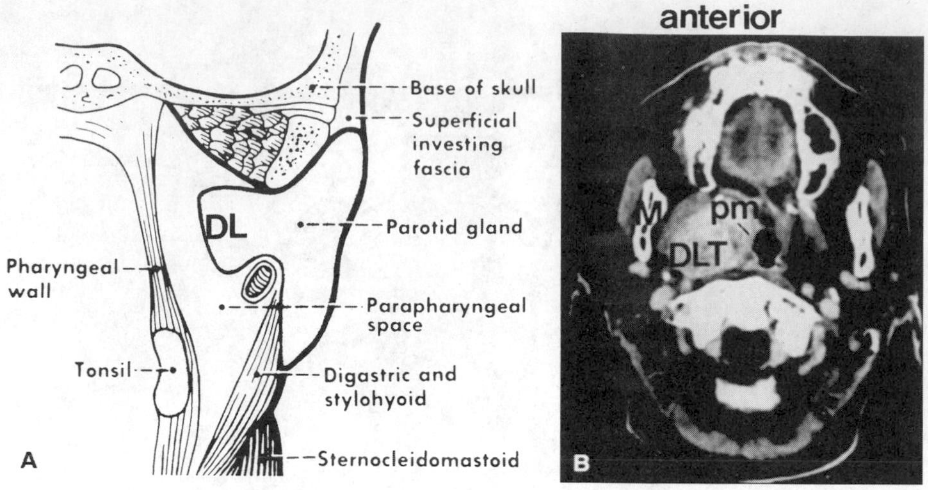

FIGURE 30.4-2. Presentation of deep lobe parotid gland tumors. **A:** Schematic diagram shows frontal view just posterior to mandible where the deep lobe (DL) enters parapharyngeal space. Notice the proximity of the deep lobe to the pharyngeal muscles and the palate. **B:** An axial computed tomographic scan of the skull shows the deep lobe tumor (DLT) occupying parapharyngeal space and pressing against the pharyngeal constrictor muscles (pm). The retromandibular tunnel extends the deep lobe behind the mandible (M).

lobe, probably because that portion of the gland is considerably larger than the deep lobe. Because no identifiable histologic differences exist between deep and superficial lobes, no reasonable explanation can be provided for this distribution of tumors other than the amount of salivary gland tissue available for tumor development. The distribution of different types of tumors is probably the same in the various parts of the gland.

The lymphatics in and around the parotid gland consist of two groups, and a knowledge of that distribution is essential to the understanding of the natural history of these tumors. The preauricular (periparotid) nodes lie superficially to the gland capsule and drain the external auditory canal, the facial and auricular skin, and the temple scalp. They are especially important drainage sites for squamous carcinomas and melanomas of adjacent skin. Parotid gland cancers usually do not drain into these nodes. The second nodal group consists of five to seven intraparotid lymph nodes that do play a role in the pathogenesis of parotid cancer. The efferent channels of the superficial nodes drain into the superficial jugular chain, whereas the intraglandular nodes drain into the upper and middle deep jugular lymph nodes.[1,4] The extraparotid (periparotid) nodes are readily palpable and are distinguished easily from primary parotid tumors; however, nodes within the substance of the gland are not easily palpated and become noticeable only when they are enlarged. Distinguishing them from primary parotid gland tumors by palpation or by imaging can be difficult.

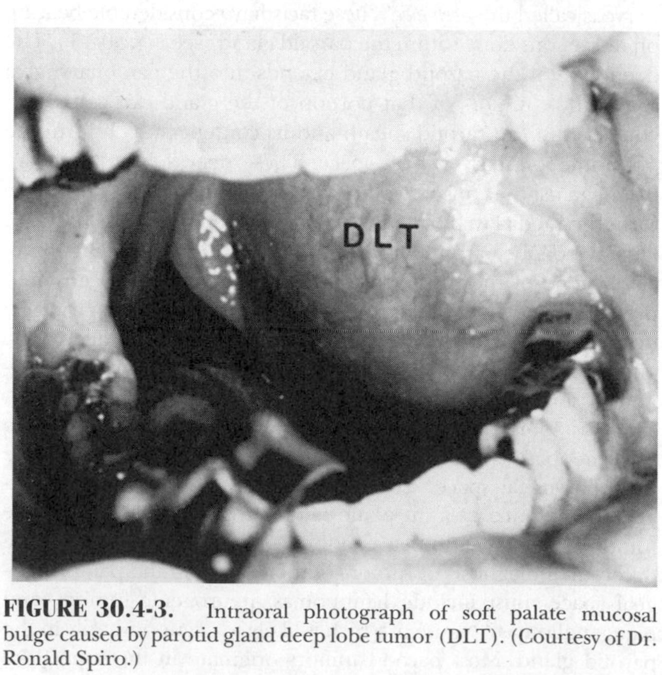

FIGURE 30.4-3. Intraoral photograph of soft palate mucosal bulge caused by parotid gland deep lobe tumor (DLT). (Courtesy of Dr. Ronald Spiro.)

The submandibular gland lies in the submandibular triangle of the neck with its posterior extent adjacent to, but not contiguous with, the tail of the parotid gland. The deep surface of the submandibular gland lies against the muscular diaphragm of the floor of the mouth and is best examined bimanually, with one finger in the mouth and the external hand on the surface of the gland. Lymph nodes do not exist within the submandibular gland, but instead they lie around its surface. A mass outside the submandibular gland may represent a metastatic node from some other site, such as the lateral tongue or the floor of the mouth. Drainage from the submandibular gland goes into the adjacent nodes and upper deep jugular chain. Three important nerves, the marginal mandibular branch of the facial nerve (motor) and the lingual (sensory) and hypoglossal (motor) nerves to the tongue all lie in close proximity to the submandibular gland.

The sublingual glands are located submucosally in the floor of the mouth, just superficially to the muscular diaphragm. They are oval and lie along the inner table of the mandible. The sublingual glands drain into submandibular lymphatics and then into the deep jugular nodes.

ETIOLOGY, PATHOLOGY, AND CLASSIFICATION

The causes of salivary gland cancer have not been determined. Certain factors have been etiologically suggested, including ionizing radiation with all salivary cancers,[5] a familial predisposition in parotid cancer,[6] and chronic wood dust inhalation in certain individuals who develop minor salivary gland adenocarcinomas of the nasal and paranasal sinuses.[7] Proof of cause and effect does not exist, however, in any of these postulated associations, and the etiology of most salivary gland cancers cannot be determined.

Overall, the majority of salivary gland neoplasms are benign, a fact that reflects an overwhelming predominance of

TABLE 30.4-1. Classification of Salivary Gland Neoplasms

BENIGN
Benign mixed tumor (pleomorphic adenoma)
Warthin's tumor (papillary cystadenoma lymphomatosum)
Benign lymphoepithelial lesion
Oncocytoma
Monomorphic adenoma
MALIGNANT
Mucoepidermoid carcinoma
Adenoid cystic carcinoma
Adenocarcinoma
Malignant mixed tumor (or carcinoma expleomorphic adenoma)
Acinic cell carcinoma
Epidermoid carcinoma

parotid tumors, three-fourths of which are nonmalignant. Different classifications of salivary gland neoplasms have been established, but the one that seems to be the most consistently workable is shown in Table 30.4-1.

Benign Tumors

PLEOMORPHIC ADENOMA. Also known as the *benign mixed tumor*, the pleomorphic adenoma is the most common of the neoplasms that originate in the major salivary glands.[8] This tumor is more correctly referred to by its formal name, which describes its multiple histologic components, including myxoid, mucoid, chondroid, and other elements. Although these lesions can occur in all salivary gland tissues, most often they are seen in the parotid gland.

The distinction between this tumor and its malignant counterpart, malignant mixed tumor, is often difficult, but the histologic features that most reliably separate the two include a tendency in the malignant version for perivascular and perineural invasion and significant cellular atypia and mitosis. Malignant lesions can be underinterpreted and their true nature not appreciated until metastasis occurs; even then, the metastases can appear histologically benign.[9–11] At the opposite extreme, a benign but extremely cellular pleomorphic adenoma can be overinterpreted as a malignant mixed tumor. These factors must be critically considered when doing retrospective interinstitutional outcomes research.

The natural history of these tumors is characterized by slow growth and few symptoms. Even when growing to large size, those lesions that remain benign rarely affect clinical facial nerve function. In such tumors, however, the nerve is often stretched around the mass and seems to become more fragile with increasing tumor size. In that circumstance, tumor removal may more likely be associated with postoperative nerve weakness.

There is controversy over the evolution of pleomorphic adenomas into their malignant counterparts. Many authors believe that the latter originates in a preexisting benign setting; hence, the term *carcinoma expleomorphic adenoma*. Other researchers, however, believe that malignant mixed tumor arises *de novo*.[9–12]

PAPILLARY CYSTADENOMA LYMPHOMATOSUM (WARTHIN'S TUMOR). Papillary cystadenoma lymphomatosum (Warthin's tumor) is a slow-growing, often cystic, and usually innocuous tumor that almost always occurs in older men, seems to favor the tail of the parotid gland, and occurs bilaterally in 10% of cases. Because of its benign nature and because it can be easily diagnosed cytologically, surgical removal is not always necessary, especially in older or unhealthy patients.

MONOMORPHIC ADENOMA. The monomorphic adenomas are a group of benign lesions that can have a variety of growth patterns. The most common monomorphic patterns are the basal cell and the oxyphilic adenomas (oncocytomas). Other monomorphic adenomas are the sebaceous lymphadenomas and sebaceous adenomas. The parotid gland is the most common site of these lesions.

BENIGN LYMPHOEPITHELIAL LESION. Benign lymphoepithelial lesion (BLL) was first described in association with systemic conditions such as Sjögren's and Mikulicz's syndromes.[13] An apparent increase in its incidence has been seen in patients with human immunodeficiency virus (HIV). BLL now encompasses a spectrum of cystic changes seen in the parotid glands of HIV-infected persons, the common denominator of which is atypical lymphoid hyperplasia. It is thought that these changes are the direct result of HIV infection of intraparotid lymph nodes.[14]

Several reports of HIV-associated malignancies of the parotid have been published, including non-Hodgkin's lymphoma,[15] Kaposi's sarcoma,[16] and adenoid cystic carcinoma.[17] Some of these have arisen on a background of BLL. Malignancy in association with prior BLL, however, was described before the acquired immunodeficiency syndrome (AIDS) epidemic,[18] and it remains unclear whether HIV infection predisposes this lesion to malignancy.

Treatment of BLL in HIV-infected patients is controversial. Some clinicians cite the association of malignancy as justification for parotidectomy.[19] Others have proposed observation of the lesion with intermittent fine-needle aspirations (FNAs) for decompression of cyst.[20] Still others have recommended low-dose radiation therapy.[21] Optimally, therapy should be individualized, depending on the clinical and diagnostic suspicion of malignancy, the status of the patient's HIV infection (asymptomatic, AIDS-related complex, or AIDS), and risk-benefit analysis for patient and surgeon.

Malignant Tumors

Spiro and Spiro[1] have developed a compendium of the various series of salivary gland cancers reported and, in their survey, have outlined the relative occurrence rates of the various cancers in both the parotid and submandibular glands. The various reports from nine studies total 1778 parotid gland cancers, the distribution of which is abbreviated and summarized in Table 30.4-2. Summarized in Table 30.4-3 are comparable data for the submandibular gland that are taken from eight studies and that, when combined, reflect the relative distribution by type of 383 submandibular gland cancers.

ACINIC CELL CARCINOMA. Acinic cell carcinoma is an uncommon malignancy that probably accounts for fewer than 10% of all salivary gland cancers.[22] Although acinic cell lesions usually are seen in the parotid gland, they occasionally occur in the submandibular gland.[23] They are low grade, only infrequently invade the facial nerve, and are late to metastasize.

TABLE 30.4-2. Relative Prevalence of Histologic Types of Parotid Gland Cancer[a]

Histologic Type	*Prevalence (%)*
Mucoepidermoid	32
Adenocarcinoma	16
Malignant mixed tumor	14
Adenoid carcinoma	11
Acinic carcinoma	11
Undifferentiated + squamous cell	16

[a]Total of 1778 cases from Memorial Sloan-Kettering Cancer Center. (Adapted from ref. 1, with permission.)

When they do metastasize, however, it is usually to the lungs, and under these circumstances, death usually follows. Because of their slow growth, survival data are good when generous surgical excision is performed.[24,25]

MUCOEPIDERMOID CARCINOMA. In major salivary glands, mucoepidermoid carcinoma occurs more frequently than any other malignancy. It is relatively more common in the parotid than in the submandibular gland, where it is third in prevalence after adenoid cystic carcinoma and adenocarcinoma (see Tables 30.4-2 and 30.4-3). Mucoepidermoid carcinoma is unique in that it demonstrates a broad spectrum of aggressiveness, from the low grade that rarely kills to its high-grade counterpart that frequently does. Low-grade mucoepidermoid carcinomas tend to create mostly local problems and can have a long natural history. A locally aggressive surgical approach is usually associated with cure. Although metastasis can occur from these lesions, it is the exception rather than the rule. In fact, such a striking performance gradient is apparent between low- and high-grade mucoepidermoid carcinomas that some investigators believe that the former should be referred to as *mucoepidermoid tumor* rather than *carcinoma.* When low-grade mucoepidermoid cancer metastasizes, however, it can be lethal,[26–28] and to diminish the appreciation of its potential seriousness by this name change seems ill advised. The high-grade and, to a great extent, the intermediate-grade mucoepidermoids are often troublesome because they are locally aggressive and are prone to invasion of nerves and vessels as well as to early metastasis. Spiro[26] have reported that 44% of the previously untreated patients with intermediate- or high-grade mucoepidermoid parotid tumors develop nodal involvement at some stage. Analysis of only the high-grade lesions reveals an incidence of nodal metastasis from all salivary gland sites that is probably even higher.[26,29,30] Because of the propensity for regional nodal metastasis in high-grade mucoepidermoid carcinomas, regional nodal dissection combined with generous local or primary resection plus postoperative radiation therapy is important in the treatment of these lesions.

Grading of mucoepidermoid lesions relates in part to the ratio between epidermoid and glandular elements, the high-grade tumors having a larger proportion of the former.[30] It is common for those higher-grade tumors that demonstrate little glandular component on routine hematoxylin and eosin stains to be misinterpreted as epidermoid or squamous cell carcinomas.

TABLE 30.4-3. Relative Prevalence of Histologic Types of Submandibular Gland Cancer[a]

Histologic Type	*Prevalence (%)*
Adenoid cystic	41
Acinic cell	17
Mucoepidermoid	12
Malignant mixed tumor (carcinoma expleomorphic adenoma)	10
Squamous cell	9
Undifferentiated	9
Adenocarcinoma	2

[a]Total of 383 cases from Memorial Sloan-Kettering Cancer Center. (Adapted from ref. 1, with permission.)

ADENOCARCINOMA. Adenocarcinomas make up approximately 16% of parotid gland and 9% of submandibular gland cancers (see Tables 30.4-2 and 30.4-3). These lesions are encountered more frequently in the minor salivary glands of the nose and paranasal sinuses. A difference in survival seems to correlate with grade, with the high grade having a poorer prognosis and the low grade a much more favorable one.[9,22,31] In the higher-grade tumors, treatment failures result predominantly from distant metastasis. Along with the overall poor performance, this fact is important in helping to judge the degree of aggressiveness with which locoregional disease should be treated.

SQUAMOUS CELL CARCINOMA. Squamous cell carcinomas are uncommon in salivary tissue, making up approximately 7% of parotid gland and 10% of submandibular gland cancers.[22] Individuals with high-grade tumors do poorly and usually present with an advanced stage of cancer.[32,33] Squamous cell carcinomas of the parotid gland frequently are not primary to that gland but instead represent metastasis into parotid nodes from adjacent sites, such as temple, auricular, and facial skin. Skin lesions that come from virtually any site on the face tend to metastasize to the superficial lymph nodes that lie external to the parotid capsule.[34,35]

MALIGNANT MIXED TUMOR. Malignant mixed tumors make up approximately 14% of parotid gland and 12% of submandibular gland cancers (see Tables 30.4-2 and 30.4-3). The diagnosis is often difficult because of the similarities with the tumor's benign counterpart, the pleomorphic adenoma. Many of the malignant mixed tumors seem to originate in previous pleomorphic adenomas (carcinoma ex-pleomorphic adenoma), but just how often they occur *de novo* is not known. Thus, controversy has continued for some time. Those proponents of the malignant transformation theory believe that the evolution of malignancy within a pleomorphic adenoma is the explanation for the circumstance encountered periodically in which a long-standing and stable tumor begins to grow significantly. When this does occur, they believe the assumption of malignant development should be made and management tailored accordingly. Although growth acceleration of a previously dormant salivary mass is not pathognomonic of malignancy, we agree that this behavior pattern dictates such a treatment strategy. The exact probability of any given benign mixed tumor becoming malignant is unknown but probably occurs in approximately 5% of pleomorphic adenoma cases.[36] Survival from malignant mixed tumor must be measured over a lengthy period, because the natural history of this lesion can be characterized by protracted but inexorable growth. Metastasis to regional lymph nodes occurs in more than one-fourth of cases.[22,31,37]

ADENOID CYSTIC CARCINOMA. In most series, adenoid cystic carcinoma accounts for almost one-fourth of the malignant salivary gland tumors treated and constitutes approximately 10% to 15% of all parotid gland malignancies (see Table 30.4-2). This cancer is relatively more common in minor than in major salivary glands. It is unique because of its protracted natural history, even when local recurrence or distant metastasis has developed. For instance, patients are known to live 10 to 20 years despite pulmonary metastasis, the most frequent manifestation of distant spread. When visceral or bone metastasis occurs, however, death usually follows within a relatively short time.[1] The actual cure rate of adenoid cystic carcinoma is poorly defined, because long-term follow-up often is not included in data analyses. Also clouding the issue of cure is the fact that some 10- to 20-year studies have shown disease-related deaths that continue to occur throughout the follow-up period.[30,38] Some investigators believe that most adenoid cystic carcinomas recur if followed long enough. Overall, the rate of pulmonary metastasis from these cancers is approximately 40%.

Adenoid cystic carcinoma has an exceptional capability to invade nerve tissue, and when this occurs, local control and survival are compromised. Such a morphologic finding is the rule rather than the exception in this cancer, and recognition of the tendency is essential in planning treatment, which usually consists of wide surgical excision and radiation therapy. Treatment failure most often occurs in the primary tumor site. Some authors have drawn a correlation between histologic patterns of adenoid cystic carcinoma and clinical behavior.[39] Others, although conceding certain behavior pattern differences in the different histologic variants of adenoid cystic carcinoma, do not believe a correlation exists between these features and long-term outcome.[38]

NATURAL HISTORY, BEHAVIOR STAGING, AND TREATMENT PRINCIPLES

Malignant tumors of major salivary gland origin are a heterogeneous group of diseases; three primary sites and at least eight different histologic patterns have been identified for this relatively uncommon group of cancers. Studies reporting treatment results have, therefore, often grouped primary sites and histologic types. This method is flawed, however, and because the problem often has been compounded by analyzing short-term results in diseases that often have a long natural history, many questions remain unanswered.

Most patients with benign tumors, whether in minor or major salivary glands, present with asymptomatic swelling of the lip or the parotid, submandibular, or sublingual glands (floor of the mouth). Neurologic signs, such as mucosal or tongue numbness, associated with a floor of mouth mass usually indicate a malignancy. In the presence of a lip mass, a numb lower lip can result from tumor involvement of the submental nerve. Facial nerve weakness that is associated with a parotid or submandibular tumor is an ominous finding. Even in huge tumors of the parotid gland that are benign, the facial nerve usually is not affected. Essentially, any compromise in nerve function greatly heightens concern for malignancy. Overall, malignant parotid gland tumors are associated with facial nerve paralysis in 10% to 20% of patients.[40] Although benign tumors occasionally cause facial discomfort, persistent facial pain is strongly suggestive of malignancy in a salivary gland tumor; in fact, approximately 10% to 15% of patients with malignant parotid neoplasms present with pain.[29] Furthermore, those malignancies that are characterized by pain seem to have a worse prognosis.

The majority of parotid tumors, whether benign or malignant, present with an asymptomatic mass in the gland; in fact, this is the case even in the majority of malignant tumors.

The most common benign tumor, the pleomorphic adenoma, can be problematic. Usually a pseudocapsule is found around this lesion, and, importantly, finger-like projections of tumor penetrate into the surrounding glandular parenchyma, whether it is parotid or submandibular. Enucleation of these lesions tends to leave behind foci of tumor that result in frequent local recurrence. It should be remembered that benign mixed tumor, although not classified as malignant, can ultimately cause great hardship for a patient. Multiple recurrences, skull base involvement, facial nerve paralysis, malignant transformation and, ultimately, incurable disease can all result from a casual initial approach to this neoplasm. This tumor should be regarded as locally dangerous, and any operation should provide a wide margin of normal tissue.

Special problems exist with tumors of the parotid deep lobe, because they are frequently surrounded by little or no glandular parenchyma; thus, even the best of operations consists largely of tumor enucleation. In this circumstance, the probability is high for leaving behind histologic disease, and postoperative radiation therapy must be considered.

Malignant tumors of the parotid can be locally aggressive, demonstrating invasiveness that leads to involvement of the facial nerve, skin, bone, and surrounding soft tissue. Prognosis is related to tumor size and stage and is affected by histologic grade. Decreasing survival occurs for many years, especially in patients with adenoid cystic carcinoma and malignant mixed tumor, and in those lesions, distant metastasis may not always represent a terminal event. The treatment of primary disease, therefore, is not necessarily precluded by lung metastasis, especially in adenoid cystic carcinoma.

Overall, the prognosis for parotid gland cancer is better than it is for the submandibular gland lesions: 50% to 81% 5-year survival is reported for the former and 30% to 50% for the latter[29,41]; the 10-year survival rate declines in both sites. The lower survival rate for the submandibular gland group probably relates to the larger proportion of adenoid cystic carcinomas in that group. Spiro and colleagues[42] reported survival results in 474 patients with major salivary gland tumors treated at the Memorial Sloan-Kettering Cancer Center from 1944 to 1986. The 5-, 10-, and 15-year survival rates were 54%, 43%, and 34%, respectively, with determinate survivals of 63%, 47%, and 42%, respectively. Multivariate analysis showed that advanced stage, higher histologic grade, and submandibular location were prognostic for a poorer outcome. In addition, treatment after 1966 was found to be an important prognostic factor and was thought to relate to an increased use of postoperative radiation therapy beginning during this latter period.

Differences in histologic features affect natural history. The prognosis for acinic cell carcinoma is the most favorable for the major salivary cancers; more than 75% 5-year and more than 65%

10-year survivals are reported in various series.[26,37] Low-grade mucoepidermoid carcinomas show 76% to 95% 5-year survival rates, whereas only 30% to 50% of those with high-grade tumors are alive at 5 years.[26,32] The survival rates for intermediate-grade mucoepidermoids are between those of the low and high grades. Adenoid cystic carcinoma, on the other hand, must be analyzed with the realization that 5-year survival rates are always better than 10-year figures, which in turn are better than those at 15 years, and so on. Most series show 50% to 90% 5-year survival rates, 30% to 67% 10-year survival rates, and 25% 15-year survival rates for treated adenoid cystic carcinoma.[38,39,41,43] Patients with adenocarcinomas of major salivary glands show gradual deterioration of survival statistics with the passage of time; 76% to 85% survival at 5 years and 34% to 71% at 10 years.[31] Patients with malignant mixed tumors do not do well; only 31% to 65% survive 5 years and 23% to 30% survive 10 years.[6,41]

Distant metastasis is predictive of a poor prognosis, and it occurs in approximately 20% of parotid malignancies.[44] Distant metastasis is a significant concern in most higher-grade salivary gland malignancies. At least 40% of patients with adenoid cystic carcinoma and 26% to 32% with malignant mixed tumors demonstrate this feature.[38] Even with lower-grade tumors, such as acinic cell carcinoma, a measurable incidence of distant metastasis is found.[9,26] In all of these lesions, the site of distant metastasis is most often the lung(s). Overall, the likelihood of metastasis from the submandibular gland is almost twice that from the parotid gland.[22]

Regional lymphatic metastasis is a subject of considerable importance in relation to malignant salivary gland tumors. In the extensive series reported from Memorial Sloan-Kettering Cancer Center, 14% of patients presented with palpable nodal metastases. Thirty-four percent of the patients with high-grade tumors demonstrated this finding, compared to only 2% of patients with low-grade lesions. Additionally, in the group of patients who had clinically negative necks but underwent elective neck dissections, 49% of the high-grade and 7% of the low-grade tumors turned out to have histologically positive necks.[45,46] These statistically significant figures suggest that the rates of occult and clinically positive node disease are increased with high-grade malignant salivary gland tumors.

With submandibular gland malignancies, as with parotid tumors, prognosis is dependent on a number of factors, the most significant of which seem to be clinical stage and perineural invasion.[47,48]

Spiro and associates believed that the most important prognosticator for survival is tumor stage. Accordingly, in 1975, they proposed a staging system that was later incorporated into the current American Joint Committee on Cancer staging system.[29,49] This system addresses the size of the primary lesion and the presence or absence of fixation or facial nerve dysfunction. It was first applied only to parotid sites but seems to serve all salivary sites. Table 30.4-4 describes the American Joint Committee on Cancer staging system. According to Spiro,[22] cumulative survival exceeds 90% at 10 years for patients with stage I or II disease, whereas only 22% of stage III or IV patients are alive after 10 years.

CLINICAL EVALUATION AND WORKUP

Short of surgical exploration, the physical examination remains the most important tool of the experienced diagnostician. A hard mass with fixation or nerve palsy is likely to be malignant; however, any malignancy can masquerade with a more benign appearance and presentation. Cytologic analysis achieved through FNA is helpful in selected circumstances, especially when the index of suspicion for malignancy is high or when the patient is not a good candidate for surgery. In the latter circumstance, the patient is somewhat reassured by benign cytologic findings and is more secure in choosing a nonsurgical approach. In a patient with disseminated metastatic disease in whom a salivary gland mass also is found, making a diagnosis easily with FNA of the parotid lesion can be of considerable value to the patient. For example, if the FNA reveals lymphoma, the appropriate diagnostic cascade is different than in the nonlymphomatous mass. Finally, if an older patient has FNA findings suggestive of Warthin's tumor, surgery can be avoided. Some concern has been expressed that the false-negative rate with cytologic evaluation of salivary gland cancers is somewhat higher than in other tumor families, and because of the heterogeneity of salivary gland tumors, a negative FNA does not substantially alter the treatment plan in most circumstances. False-positive rates for malignancy, on the other hand, are very low. To know in advance of a malignancy is helpful in both treatment strategizing and in patient education. Malata and colleagues[50] reported 88% sensitivity for FNA-cytologic evaluation for the parotid gland. Overall, the accuracy rate of FNA is extraordinary, and we use it in the vast majority of parotid and submandibular masses.

CT and MRI are helpful in analyzing the important third dimension of larger tumors, especially those that involve the deep lobe of the parotid gland. Imaging technologies are especially important in studying malignant tumors; however, these expensive methods are not necessary for the evaluation of all parotid or submandibular gland tumors. As it pertains to tumors, sialography is of historic interest only and is superfluous.

TREATMENT

The initial treatment for salivary gland neoplasia, whether benign or malignant, whether of minor or major gland origin, is almost always surgical, and whenever possible, removal of parotid, submandibular, and sublingual gland tumors should be excisional rather than incisional. The diagnosis of parotid tumors usually is established by removal of the involved part of the gland, thus avoiding lumpectomy whenever possible. In the case of a lesion of the parotid superficial lobe, for instance, the least extensive or most conservative operation should be superficial parotidectomy. With benign tumors, the diagnostic operation and the definitive operation are, therefore, usually the same. Before surgery, it is helpful for the surgeon to have a sense of whether the tumor is benign or malignant, and this is achieved by physical examination, history, and technological aids such as FNA and imaging.

An important general principle of management that applies particularly to higher-grade adenocarcinomas, malignant mixed tumor, and adenoid cystic carcinoma is that, by combining postoperative radiation therapy with moderate locoregional surgery, mutilation and physiologic compromise are often avoided. The preoccupation with liberal resection of facial nerve, mandible, and other important structures solely because they are in the field no longer dominates surgical philosophy. Instead, the realization that "more" does not necessar-

TABLE 30.4-4. Staging System for Major Salivary Gland Malignancies

PRIMARY TUMOR (T)			
TX	Primary tumor cannot be assessed		
T0	No evidence of primary tumor		
T1	Tumor 2 cm or less in greatest dimension without extraparenchymal extension		
T2	Tumor more than 2 cm but not more than 4 cm in greatest dimension without extraparenchymal extension		
T3	Tumor having extraparenchymal extension without seventh nerve involvement and/or more than 4 cm but not more than 6 cm in greatest dimension		
T4	Tumor invades base of skull, seventh nerve, and/or exceeds 6 cm in greatest dimension		
REGIONAL LYMPH NODES (N)			
NX	Regional lymph nodes cannot be assessed		
N0	No regional lymph node metastasis		
N1	Metastasis in a single ipsilateral lymph node; 3 cm or less in greatest dimension		
N2	Metastasis in a single ipsilateral lymph node, more than 3 cm but not more than 6 cm in greatest dimension; or in multiple ipsilateral lymph nodes, none more than 6 cm in greatest dimension; or in bilateral or contralateral lymph nodes, none more than 6 cm in greatest dimension		
N2a	Metastasis in a single ipsilateral lymph node more than 3 cm but not more than 6 cm in greatest dimension		
N2b	Metastasis in multiple ipsilateral lymph nodes; none more than 6 cm in greatest dimension		
N2c	Metastasis in bilateral or contralateral lymph nodes; none more than 6 cm in greatest dimension		
N3	Metastasis in a lymph node more than 6 cm in greatest dimension		
DISTANT METASTASIS (M)			
MX	Distant metastasis cannot be assessed		
M0	No distant metastases		
M1	Distant metastasis		
STAGE GROUPING			
I	T1	N0	M0
	T2	N0	M0
II	T3	N0	M0
III	T1	N1	M0
	T2	N1	M0
IV	T4	N0	M0
	T3	N1	M0
	T4	N1	M0
	Any T	N2	M0
	Any T	N3	M0
	Any T	Any N	M1

(Adapted from American Joint Committee on Cancer. *Cancer staging manual,* 5th ed. Philadelphia: Lippincott–Raven, 1997, with permission.)

ily improve survival has spawned a form of surgical minimalism. When failure does occur, it is frequently at a distant site and is probably not influenced by the degree of the local treatment. Important anatomic structures are rarely sacrificed unless obviously invaded by tumor. The surgeon's reliance on postoperative radiation therapy to manage histologic disease has dramatically altered the surgical feats required to deal with many malignant salivary gland tumors. It should be pointed out, however, that although local and regional control of these tumors is enhanced by this combined therapy, its impact on the development of distant metastasis and, therefore, on survival is less clear.

Some investigators have proposed the routine use of postoperative radiation therapy for almost all malignant tumors of the parotid,[51] but the absence of randomized data complicates the issue. Armstrong and associates[52] performed a matched-pair analysis comparing surgery alone versus surgery plus postoperative radiotherapy. Patients with stage III/IV disease and those with positive nodes experienced improved locoregional control and survival with postoperative radiation. A trend also was seen toward improved local control for high-grade lesions treated with postoperative radiation (63% vs. 44%). The 5-year determinant survival rate tended to be better for high-grade lesions treated with adjuvant radiotherapy than with surgery alone (57% vs. 28%). No benefits were achieved for lower-grade or lower-stage tumors. Malata and coworkers[50] reported 51 patients with malignant parotid tumors, most of whom (73%) received postoperative radiation. The crude 5- and 10-year survival rates were 68% and 49%, respectively, and 10-year actuarial local control was 79%.

Surgical resection is the mainstay of the management of benign pleomorphic adenoma. Renehan et al.[53] reported the cumulative experience of more than 1400 salivary gland tumors treated at Christie Hospital between 1947 and 1992. For 551 patients with previously untreated parotid pleomorphic adenoma treated by surgery, the recurrence rate (median follow-up of 12.5 years) was 1.6%. The recurrence rate rises to 15% in patients undergoing surgery for recurrence. Dawson and Orr[54] reported long-term outcomes for pleomorphic adenomas treated by "lumpectomy" plus radiotherapy. The 10-year local recurrence rate was 1.5%, with cumulative risk rising to 8% at 20 years. Most late recurrences were malignant, with one of four developing malignant recurrence at 15 years, and three at 18 years. The possibility of radiation-induced malignancy, therefore, must be added to the known possibility of malignant transformation when considering treatment options. Given these considerations, surgery alone seems to be the obvious initial treatment of choice.

Management of parotid pleomorphic adenomas that recur despite surgical removal can be particularly challenging. Generally, recurrences develop slowly, and frequently their appearance is not noted for years after surgery. Furthermore, recurrences often present in the form of multifocal nodules, all of which are inevitably engulfed in scar tissue from the previous surgery, and in this setting, the identification and protection of the facial nerve is substantially more difficult than in the nonoperated circumstance. Leverstein and colleagues[55] reported on 40 patients with recurrent pleomorphic adenoma of the parotid. In three patients, no tumor resection was performed. Two received radiotherapy, and both were controlled. In the remaining 37 cases, *en bloc* resection was done. Pathology remained benign in 36 cases, and 16 received postoperative radiotherapy. None of the patients developed local failure with a median follow-up of 106 months. One patient experienced facial nerve paralysis and two developed malignant transformation. It would seem, therefore, that in high-risk circumstances, such as multifocality, positive surgical margins, and certain deep lobe tumors, selective use of radiation therapy after appropriate surgical excision should be the treatment of choice.

Cervical metastasis is an ominous event in salivary gland malignancy, and the standard management approach is to do a modified radical neck dissection followed by postoperative radiation. In malignant parotid and submandibular tumors in which no clinical adenopathy is present, the first echelon lymph nodes should be sampled because of a surprisingly high rate of occult metastasis. In a multivariate analysis, Armstrong et al.[52] reported that the risk of occult metastasis is 20% in primary malignancies larger than 4 cm, with a 49% risk for high-grade tumors. Frankenthaler and colleagues[56] found a 33% risk of occult metastases for parotid malignancies associated with facial nerve paralysis and 18% risk for high-grade tumors in general. At the present time, however, no compelling data support the benefit of elective neck dissection for the clinically negative neck in malignant high-grade tumors.[57]

Other series consistently have shown improvement in locoregional control when patients with major salivary gland cancers received postoperative radiation therapy.[37,43,58–62] These consistent data are a marked improvement over the substantial local failure rates (39% for parotid gland and 60% for submandibular gland) reported for patients treated by surgery alone.[22]

Specifically, the indications for adding radiation to surgery for management of malignant tumors are positive surgical margins, advanced primary tumor stage (including facial nerve involvement, positive neck nodes, high-grade histology, and deep lobe involvement), and tumor spillage during the operation.

Other data suggest that, for lesions that are locally advanced at the time of initial treatment and for patients with involved margins, intraoperative brachytherapy plus postoperative external-beam radiation therapy might be useful in improving local control.[59] Fu and associates[63] showed that, with positive resection margins, local control improved with the addition of radiation. Overall, only 14% of those with microscopic disease at or close to the surgical margin experienced local recurrence when postoperative radiation therapy was given, as compared with 54% who recurred locally in the surgery-only group. Most patients in this series received total doses between 5000 and 7500 cGy.

Although a detailed technical description of parotidectomy is inappropriate here, several points should be made about this meticulous but safe surgical technique. Were it not for the presence of the facial nerve within the substance of the parotid gland, the procedure would be far less challenging; however, this important motor nerve, along with all of its branches, weave through the parotid parenchyma in such a way that almost all tumor operations involve nerve identification, isolation, and dissection. The approaches vary somewhat, but consistent with all parotid operations is the fundamental surgical tenet of generous and well-planned incision, skin flap elevation, and wide exposure. When well designed, the parotidectomy incision, even though long, leaves little obvious scarring. The incision usually is begun anterior to the auricle, extends behind the edge of the external ear canal to minimize its exposure, then swings along the lower edge of the ear lobe down to the first horizontal crease of the cervical skin and then anteriorly for some distance (Fig. 30.4-4). A skin flap is then lifted anteriorly to an extent that exposes the entire external surface of the parotid gland. The gland is separated from the anterior border of the sternocleidomastoid muscle, and the posterior belly of the diagastric muscle is identified lying deep to the sternocleidomastoid. The diagastric muscle and the cartilaginous ear canal serve as landmarks for identification of the main trunk of the facial nerve as it exits the stylomastoid foramen and extends anteriorly. The various branches of the nerve are dissected and, in the case of the tumors within the superficial lobe of the parotid gland, that lobe and the tumor within it are removed without violating the capsule of the neoplasm. To remove tumors that lie within the deep lobe (i.e., under the nerve), the superficial lobe of the gland is often removed, and various manipulations of the nerve are necessary to remove the tumor under it. For a large, deep lobe neoplasm, other techniques of deep lobe exposure, such as submandibular gland excision, with or without mandibulotomy, may be necessary to accomplish safely and effectively the important goal of *en bloc* tumor removal.

Often, the oncologic principles of wide excision with ample surrounding normal parenchyma are not attainable in deep lobe tumors, and the adequacy of the surgery must be sternly questioned. Generally speaking, one should apply liberal criteria in this circumstance for the use of postoperative radiation therapy. Modern imaging provides the means by which the surgeon can be forewarned about deep lobe involvement, its size, and the probability of needing extended methods, such as mandibulotomy, to extricate the tumor from the parapharyngeal space. Whether partial or total parotidectomy is done, the defect incurred is usually reasonable. With proper attention to detail, dissection of the facial nerve and removal of most tumors can be accomplished with minimal risk of postoperative facial weakness. Closure of the skin incision usually is followed by a pleasing esthetic result.

Radiation therapy techniques vary, depending on the anatomic and pathologic situation. Submandibular lesions are usually treated with parallel opposed portals to cover the entire tumor bed and submandibular/submental area. The cervical lymph nodes are included for node-positive patients, and the occasional, high-risk, node-negative patient. For parotid, treatment-planning CT scans should routinely be done. A variety of techniques have been reported.[59,64] Yaparpalvi and coworkers[65]

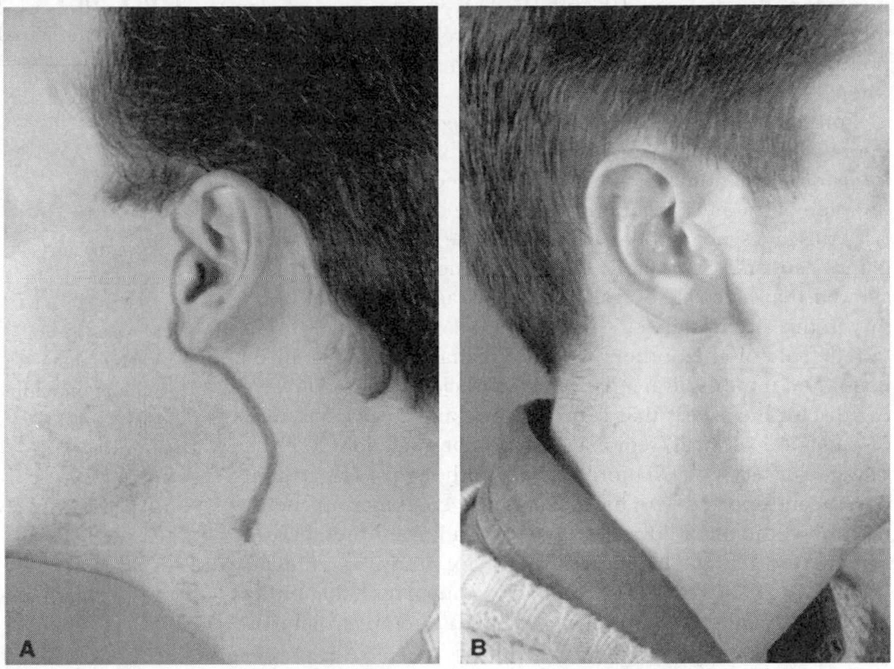

FIGURE 30.4-4. Typical parotidectomy incision. **A:** The drawing of the incision is designed to blend into natural skin folds and minimize visibility. **B:** One-year postoperative result of an actual parotidectomy incision like the one depicted in **A**.

reported a comparison of nine different techniques using dose-volume histogram analysis of exit dose to contralateral parotid, hot spots in mandible and temporal lobe, and other key parameters. They concluded that an ipsilateral wedged pair; a three-field anteroposterior (wedged), posteroanterior (wedged), and lateral portal using 6-MV photons; and a mixed 6-MV photon beam with a 16-MeV electron beam (1:4 weighting) provided the best target coverage with minimal normal tissue dose. Garden et al.[64] reported a preference for ipsilateral mixed beam over the wedged pair technique with respect to complications. Modern conformal techniques should provide excellent coverage of the target area and minimum dose to surrounding normal tissue using either approach.

The exact dose required for postoperative radiation therapy has not been determined. In a study in which patients who received doses of at least 5750 cGy were compared with patients who received smaller doses, Harrison and colleagues[59] compared dose with outcome. The 10-year local control rate for the higher-dose group was 72%, compared with 53% for those in the lower-dose group. However, despite the suggestion of a trend in favor of high doses, the difference was not statistically significant. In another important study, Garden and associates[64] reported no clear dose-response relationship, except in patients with positive margins or tumor involvement of major named nerves, and in those, he noted better local control with doses of more than 60 Gy. Hosokawa and coworkers[66] reported that patients with mucoepidermoid cancer of salivary gland origin experienced no local recurrences with postoperative doses of more than 55 Gy, whereas 3 of 17 patients recurred locally with doses of less than 55 Gy. The difference was statistically significant. McNaney and coworkers[61] reviewed treatment failure and the total dose for patients who received at least 6000 cGy or more. The doses that were associated with treatment failure did not lend themselves to a specific dose-response relation. In general, doses in the 6000 to 6500 cGy range given over 6 to 7 weeks are used for postoperative radiation therapy, except in patients with involved margins or T4 disease, who may require even higher doses. In this subset of patients, the expected high local failure rate that has been reported supports the need for dose intensification with either conformed external-beam techniques or intraoperative brachytherapy/radiotherapy approaches.

Because of the unique natural history of adenoid cystic carcinoma and because of its affinity for neural involvement, this tumor deserves special and separate consideration. Data from three different studies consistently show that postoperative radiation therapy should be added for almost all adenoid cystic carcinomas. When regional nodes are involved, the neck should be included in the treatment planning.[59,67,68] When these nodes are uninvolved, elective neck radiation generally is not recommended.

Management of the neck in general includes the consideration of important variables such as T stage and grade. In a study by Armstrong and associates,[52] 474 patients with major salivary gland cancers were reviewed. High-grade tumors had a 49% risk for occult metastases, as compared with only 7% for intermediate- or low-grade tumors. The risk for epidermoid cancers was 41%, but only 10% for all other histologies combined. Submandibular tumors had a higher risk for occult metastases, occurring in 21% as compared with 9% for parotid tumors. Occult disease was found in 7% of T1 and T2 tumors, 16% of T3 tumors, and 24% of T4 tumors. Most agree that, in patients with clinically positive regional nodes, postoperative radiation therapy should be administered. The question of how to manage the clinically negative neck is less clear, but the thinking is aided by Armstrong's data. In patients who would otherwise need postoperative radiation therapy because of concerns about the primary site, elective neck treatment with radiation can be used. It is appropriate to electively harvest the first echelon nodes in high-risk patients as a means of staging the neck. If histologic nodal examination reveals disease, postoperative radiation therapy to the neck should be added. In Armstrong's study, the periparotid nodes were the ones most commonly involved, and in those that were positive, 25% had positive nodes at levels III and IV. This was because of skip metastases to level III and IV without level II metastases. This point emphasizes the need for treatment of the entire neck when involved nodes are found.

For patients with a clinically positive neck, surgery and postoperative radiation therapy are indicated. Although with squamous cell carcinoma of the head and neck, nodal disease in one side of the neck frequently places the contralateral neck at risk, this does not appear to be the case with major salivary gland cancers. King and Fletcher[69] and Harrison et al.[59] showed that elective contralateral neck radiation is not necessary in this circumstance.

The role of chemotherapy in the management of both the major and minor salivary gland malignancies is limited to treating distant metastasis that is progressing and to circumstances of palliation of local/regional disease not amenable to either salvage surgery or radiation therapy. Although a few patients have been reported who have been given combination chemotherapy in the neoadjuvant setting or as adjuvant therapy after surgery, too few patients are available for study.[70,71] Similarly, no data has been published evaluating concurrent chemotherapy and radiotherapy administered in an attempt to improve outcome by increasing radiation cell kill.

The interpretation of response data from phase II trials of single agents and combination chemotherapy regimens is limited by the heterogeneity of histologic types of salivary gland cancer, by the fact that response probably differs by histologic type, and by the small numbers of patients enrolled in any one study. Mucoepidermoid, adenoid cystic, and adenocarcinoma histologies constitute the bulk of patients referred to medical oncologists and therefore those that are included in clinical trials. Patients with other salivary gland malignancies, such as malignant mixed tumors, epithelial-myoepithelial carcinomas, salivary duct carcinomas, acinic cell carcinomas, and squamous cell carcinomas, are rare and therefore not separated out in the chemotherapy literature.

Mucoepidermoid and squamous cell carcinomas are thought to arise from the salivary excretory duct and generally respond to cisplatin-based chemotherapy regimens used for other sites in the head and neck. Adenoid cystic carcinomas and adenocarcinomas arise from the intercalated ducts of the salivary glands and tend to be lumped together in study reports but often have a different clinical course; adenoid cystic carcinoma may be surprisingly indolent and only manifested by the chronic pain of perineural tumor infiltration. Metastatic adenocarcinoma, on the other hand, generally has a more aggressive course that is reflected in proportionately more obvious responses to chemotherapy.

Table 30.4-5 lists single-agent and combination regimens reported to have activity in salivary gland cancers. Cumulative response rates to single agents range from 10% to 40%, with the higher rates reported from older literature.[72–79] Retrospective reviews of patients treated for adenoid cystic carcinoma before 1980 at both the M. D. Anderson and Princess Margaret hospitals indicated that Adriamycin and 5-fluorouracil were the most effective single agents,[80,81] whereas methotrexate, vincristine, and cyclophosphamide showed little activity. A review published by Suen and Johns[82] in 1982 noted clinical efficacy for cisplatin as well.

In the 1990s, three new agents were tested in multicenter trials with adequate numbers of patients with adenoid cystic carcinoma. The European Organization for Research and Treatment of Cancer (EORTC) conducted a phase II evaluation of epirubicin in 20 patients and reported two responses that lasted 7.5 and 20 months, respectively, and ten patients with disease stabilization.[76] Symptomatic improvement was documented in 29% in this particular study. Phase II trials of mitoxantrone in adenoid cystic carcinoma patients were carried out by the EORTC[77] and the Southwest Oncology Group.[78] EORTC investigators observed four partial responses and 22 with stable disease in a total of 32 patients; the Southwest Oncology Group investigators reported one complete response and 12 patients with stable disease out of the 18 treated.

TABLE 30.4-5. Single Agents and Combination Regimens with Activity in Salivary Gland Malignancies

Single agents	
Cisplatin	80–100 mg/m², or 20 mg/m²/d × 5 q 4wk
5-FU	500 mg/m² q wk, or 225–300 mg/m²/d continuous infusion
Adriamycin	60 mg/m² q 3wk
Epirubicin	30 mg/m² q wk, or 90 mg/m² q 3wk
Mitoxantrone	14 mg/m² q 3wk
Vinorelbine	30 mg/m² q wk
Combination regimens	
CAP (q 4wk): Cyclophosphamide +	400 mg/m² day 1
Adriamycin +	40 mg/m² day 1
Cisplatin	40–60 mg/m² day 1
PAF (q 4wk): Cisplatin +	50 mg/m² day 1 + 8
Adriamycin +	30 mg/m² day 1 + 8
5-FU	500 mg/m² day 1 + 8
PF (q 3–4wk): Cisplatin +	100 mg/m² day 1
5-FU	1000 mg/m²/d continuous infusion days 1–4
PEF (q 3wk): Cisplatin +	60 mg/m² day 1
Epirubicin +	50 mg/m² day 1
5-FU	600 mg/m² day 1
PAB (q 3wk): Cisplatin +	20 mg/m²/d × 5
Adriamycin +	50 mg/m² day 1
Bleomycin	30 mg days 1–5

5-FU, 5-fluorouracil.

Paclitaxel at a dose of 200 mg/m² over 3 hours every 3 weeks was tested in the Eastern Cooperative Oncology Group, using a standard two-stage statistical design, in three patient cohorts: individuals with adenoid cystic carcinoma, adenocarcinoma, or mucoepidermoid carcinoma. The trial was closed for the adenoid cystic carcinoma cohort after no responses were observed in 15 patients, but patients with adenocarcinoma and mucoepidermoid carcinoma continue to be enrolled, with both arms demonstrating responses.[83]

A fourth new drug studied is vinorelbine. Airoldi et al.[79] conducted a phase II trial in 20 patients with salivary gland malignancies (13 adenoid cystic carcinomas, five adenocarcinomas, one malignant mixed tumor, and one undifferentiated carcinoma). Four patients achieved a partial response and nine demonstrate stable disease. In summary, modest activity has been shown for epirubicin, mitoxantrone, and vinorelbine in patients with adenoid cystic carcinoma. Paclitaxel does not appear to be active for adenoid cystic carcinoma, but preliminary findings from the Eastern Cooperative Oncology Group suggest activity for adenocarcinoma and mucoepidermoid carcinoma.

Combinations that include cisplatin, Adriamycin, or 5-fluorouracil (5-FU) have been the cornerstone of palliative treatment for salivary gland malignancies, a fact particularly true in adenoid cystic and adenocarcinomas. Complete and partial response rates in the 30% to 60% range have been reported. In addition, some trials note prolonged disease stabilization and relief of pain among patients with adenoid cystic carcinoma.[76,84,85] Median response duration is in the range of 6 to 9 months, with some responses lasting more than 1 year. It is unknown whether survival is improved with chemotherapy.[86] Two- and three-drug regimens combining cyclophosphamide with Adriamycin and cisplatin (CAP)[17–21]; cisplatin with Adriamycin or epirubicin plus 5-FU (OAF or OEF)[70,87,89,91]; cisplatin plus 5-FU (PF)[3,16,19,21]; or cisplatin, Adriamycin, and bleomycin (PAB)[84] all appear equally effective. Combinations that incorporate mitomycin C or vincristine[71,88,90] or use more than three drugs[92] do not seem to offer any advantage.

In summary, no standard drug therapy has been established for treatment of salivary gland cancer because of the lack of formal trials with adequate numbers of patients. For the treatment of adenoid cystic carcinoma, the information at hand would suggest that combination chemotherapy is superior to single-agent strategies and that two- or three-drug combinations of cisplatin, doxorubicin, and 5 FU would be reasonable initial treatment. The slow growth rate of adenoid cystic carcinoma may be one of the factors that account for the lack of response observed in some studies. Relief of symptoms and stabilization of disease may be more achievable palliative end points for evaluating drug efficacy. Adenocarcinomas of salivary gland origin may be treated with the same regimens. High-grade mucoepidermoid carcinoma appears to be sensitive to the same spectrum of drugs that are commonly used to treat squamous malignancies (cisplatin, bleomycin, methotrexate, and 5-FU).[72,93] Thus, the combination of cisplatin and 5-FU or taxane-based combinations are reasonable regimens to use. No data are available about treatment of the less common malignancies, such as acinic cell carcinoma and malignant mixed tumors. All patients should be considered candidates for trials of investigational new drugs. Studies of adjuvant chemotherapy, particularly for high-grade mucoepidermoid carcinoma, have not been undertaken because of the small number of patients available for study. The optimal way to assess new therapies for salivary gland carcinoma is in a multiinstitutional setting in which patient resources can be pooled and treatments made uniform.

MINOR SALIVARY GLAND TUMORS

Minor salivary gland tumors can occur in any age group, and they have no particular gender predilection. The glands are ubiquitous in the upper aerodigestive tract, so tumors originating in minor glands can occur anywhere in the head and neck; however, the palate is the most common site for both benign and malignant lesions. Rarely, ectopic salivary gland tissue can lead to tumors in such diverse locations as the middle ear or the thyroid area. Table 30.4-6 shows the distribution by site of origin in the Memorial Sloan-Kettering Cancer Center's experience with these tumors. Minor salivary gland lesions occur in the nasal cavities and paranasal sinuses, nasopharynx, larynx, lip, floor of the mouth, trachea, and other sites in the head and neck, but overall, they are most frequently seen in the oral cavity. It is often impossible to differentiate between a primary sublingual tumor and a minor salivary gland tumor in the anterior floor of the mouth.

TABLE 30.4-6. Incidence by Site of Origin of Minor Salivary Gland Tumors[a]

Site	*Benign*	*Malignant*	*Total*
Palate	58	114	172
Tongue	2	62	64
Cheek	9	38	47
Maxillary sinus	1	43	44
Nasal cavity	3	20	23
Gingiva	0	22	22
Floor of mouth	0	21	21
Lip	5	11	16
Larynx	0	15	15
Tonsil	1	9	10
Retromolar trigone	0	9	9
Nasopharynx	0	6	6
Ethmoid sinus	0	5	5
Pharynx	2	3	5
Total	81	378	459

[a]Total of 459 cases from the Memorial Sloan-Kettering Cancer Center. (Adapted from ref. 1, with permission.)

Between 65% and 88% of all of minor salivary gland tumors are malignant.[94] Adenoid cystic carcinoma is the most common histologic type, occurring in as many as 55% of patients with minor salivary gland tumors.[95] Otherwise, the presenting types are the same as for major salivary gland tumors, including mucoepidermoid carcinoma, adenocarcinoma, malignant mixed tumor, and anaplastic carcinoma. Small cell (oat cell) carcinoma of minor salivary gland origin also has been reported.[96] Minor salivary gland tumors tend to present as painless submucosal masses and can be present for many years without change. Malignant tumors can persist without change, but more often they increase in size.

Any submucosal mass in the head or neck should be considered a minor salivary gland tumor until proved otherwise. Malignancies can spread to invade local tissue, including bone and nerve. Tumors of the floor of the mouth or the tongue can extend into the neck and into the mandible. Adenoid cystic carcinoma has a particular tendency to grow along the perineural spaces and to extend great distances from the primary tumor along nerve pathways, and it is important for the surgeon to realize that skip areas of tumor involvement can occur along the nerve. For instance, when this lesion occurs in the lateral aspect of the palate, it can infiltrate the branches of the greater palatine nerve, extend centrally, and can ultimately occupy the gasserian ganglion in the middle cranial fossa. This fact should be taken into account, and treatment planning should include the ganglion. The presence of a negative frozen section taken from the nerve trunk proximal to the originally discovered peripheral nerve lesion does not rule out the possibility that the nerve is involved with tumor more centrally. Adenoid cystic carcinomas can also spread along the haversian canals of bone. Therefore, when involvement of the mandible is questionable in floor of mouth lesions, the surgeon must be prepared to deal with further extension than what is obvious.

Fewer than 20% of patients with minor salivary gland malignancies present with lymph node metastases, and approximately 10% who demonstrate a clinically negative neck subsequently develop nodal metastases. As with major salivary gland tumors, the incidence of nodal metastases is related to grade and tumor size (i.e., stage).

No uniform staging system has been developed for minor salivary gland tumors. Survival seems to correlate with clinical stage. Olsen and coworkers[97] showed that tumor size was significant for mucoepidermoid carcinoma of the oral cavity. In their study, patients with lesions larger than 2 cm did much worse than those with lesions smaller than 2 cm. None in the latter group died from mucoepidermoid carcinoma.

TREATMENT

Surgery is usually the treatment of choice for minor salivary gland tumors, whether benign or malignant. Enucleation is considered inadequate and is associated with a recurrence rate in excess of 93%[106]; therefore, wide excision or regional excision must be performed whenever possible. The surgeon should not hesitate to remove underlying bone, such as palate or sinus wall(s), to achieve such excision. Paranasal sinus malignancies often require partial maxillectomy for complete removal. Speech and swallowing rehabilitation for hard palate defects that have been created by tumor resection is easily accomplished by prosthetic devices. Defects of the soft palate, however, are more problematic.

Limited information exists on the effectiveness of primary radiation treatment. Ellis and colleagues[98] reported their results, in which a total of 20 patients with minor salivary gland malignancies received only radiation therapy for their disease. Seven had early-stage tumors and 13 had advanced tumors. Local control was obtained in six of the seven early-stage lesions (86%), a result that is comparable with those for surgical management. For more advanced lesions, however, radiation alone controlled only 2 of 13 (15%), a result considerably inferior to that following combined therapy. Parsons and associates[99] reported local control in 13 patients treated with radiotherapy alone for adenoid cystic cancer, and five of these patients have follow-up longer than 10 years. A total of 20 of 51 cases treated with radiotherapy alone are locally controlled with follow-up ranging from 2.5 to 21.0 years. Several surgical failures were salvaged with radiotherapy as well. Although this and other limited studies suggest that radiation can be effective for small lesions, surgery usually is considered the treatment of choice whenever possible. Advanced lesions should always be treated initially with surgery, and usually that procedure is followed by postoperative radiation therapy. Exactly which patients should receive postoperative radiation therapy remains unclear. We tend to recommend the guidelines that have been established for major salivary gland tumors: Patients with advanced-stage disease, lymph node metastases, high-grade tumors, or inadequate surgical margins are treated with postoperative radiation. Many patients have a combination of these factors.

Long-term follow-up is now available for patients with minor salivary gland tumors. Parsons and associates[99] reported 20-year local control of 57%. The most important factors affecting local control were tumor stage and combined modality therapy (surgery plus radiotherapy). It is significant that, with longer follow-up, the distant metastasis rate at 12 years was 40%.

Eapen and colleagues[100] reported 70 patients with salivary gland carcinomas. Approximately one-third had minor salivary gland tumors, and the indications cited for postoperative radiation therapy were inconsistent. However, a significant decrease in locoregional recurrence was noted among patients who were given postoperative radiation therapy. The actuarial risk of locoregional recurrence in the nonradiated patients was 62%, as compared with 20% for the radiated group. Ninety percent of the patients received between 5500 and 6590 cGy over 5.0 to 6.5 weeks. In 95% of radiated patients, the regional lymph nodes were treated along with the primary site.

Tran and coworkers[95] reviewed the University of California, Los Angeles, experience with salivary gland tumors of the oral cavity. A total of 62 patients with previously untreated lesions were analyzed, all of whom were treated with primary surgical resection. Twenty-four patients received postoperative radiation therapy owing to advanced local disease, involved margins of resection, or both. Most of the lesions in this series were adenoid cystic carcinomas, and the palate was the most common primary site. Local tumor control in patients with positive margins was 50% for surgery alone, as compared with 71% with combined surgery and postoperative radiation therapy. A trend toward less successful disease control and poorer survival for patients with adenoid cystic carcinoma was noted as compared with the other malignant tumors.

The experience with minor salivary gland tumors of the nasal cavity and paranasal sinuses was also reported by Tran and coworkers.[95] Thirty-five patients seen and treated between 1962 and 1985 were included, most of whom (68%) had adenoid cystic carcinoma. Adenocarcinoma was seen in approximately one-half the ethmoid and nasal cavity lesions. Local control for the combined surgery and radiation group was 62%; for surgery alone, it was 18%, and for radiation alone, it was 9%. This benefit of radiation was present despite the fact that the radiated group had higher-stage disease and fewer patients had adequate surgical margins. Among those with positive margins, local recurrence was seen in 67% with surgery alone and 30% with postoperative radiation therapy.

Just as with the major salivary glands, data on the treatment of adenoid cystic cancer of minor salivary gland origin clearly demonstrate a local control advantage from combined surgery and postoperative radiation therapy over surgery alone. The authors recommend this combined strategy for almost all adenoid cystic carcinomas of minor salivary gland origin. A young patient with a small lesion that is resected completely may be an exception to this rule. Essentially, all treatment decisions must be individualized.

Koss and associates[96] reported 14 patients with small cell carcinoma of minor salivary gland origin. Although no conclusive data were obtained from this or other series, these lesions may be managed optimally with resection, chemotherapy, and local radiation therapy.

The technique of radiation therapy for minor salivary gland tumors is similar to that for squamous cancer at the corresponding primary site. For postoperative radiation, doses in the 6000- to 6500-cGy range are used over 6 to 7 weeks. Wide portals are required, especially for adenoid cystic cancer. The nerve pathways up to and including the base of the skull should be included in the treated portals. When radiation therapy alone is used for early-stage disease, doses of at least 7000 cGy in 7.0 to 7.5 weeks should be used. Brachytherapy can be used for a portion of the treatment, especially for oral cavity lesions. Elective nodal radiation usually is indicated only in selected circumstances, such as the occasional patient with minor salivary gland tumors of the nasopharynx. Whether elective nodal radiation is required here is unclear, but it can certainly be justified on the basis of the rich lymphatic drainage of the nasopharynx.

SPECIFIC STRATEGIES FOR SPECIAL SITUATIONS

Deep lobe parotid tumors, whether benign or malignant, are often inaccessible in standard parotidectomy. In such a circumstance, a variety of mandibulotomy techniques are available to surgeons that provide excellent exposure to the area into which these tumors expand (i.e., the parapharyngeal space). Because deep lobe tumors often are not surrounded by parotid gland parenchyma, removing the lesion without fragmentation can be difficult. Additionally, this potential space is at the skull base, and the carotid sheath forms part of its perimeter.[101] Although these mandibulotomy techniques are seldom required, in selected circumstances the efficient and safe removal of deep lobe tumors is greatly enhanced by their use.

Occasionally, the facial nerve or one of its branches is encased within (but not invaded by) a benign tumor; thus, sparing the nerve requires meticulous and painstaking removal of the neoplasm. Radiation therapy is not usually part of the primary management of benign lesions; however, for a lesion that encases the nerve, for recurrent benign lesions, and when complete gross tumor removal is not possible, radiation therapy is often recommended.[54] Postoperative radiation therapy is probably important for recurrent deep lobe parotid tumors, whether benign or malignant, even though all gross tumor has been removed. Even with gross tumor removal, large pleomorphic adenomas of the deep lobe are associated with a high local recurrence rate. To add radiation after routine and uncomplicated removal of a benign tumor of the superficial lobe of the parotid or from the submandibular gland seems unwarranted.

In cancers that involve the facial nerve or its branches, the involved segment is best resected and grafted with an interposition of nerve harvested from another site. In most cases, however, nerve can be dissected off a tumor surface and, with the use of postoperative radiation therapy, control results are achievable that are similar to those from a more radical approach. However, sacrifice of the facial nerve is rarely required; when it is necessary, the consequence of the surgery and the gravity of the prognosis take on added dimensions. The functional and esthetic results of correctly done nerve grafting, although not perfect, are good in a substantial percentage of cases. Essentially, oncologists are working in an era of surgical minimalism when the tendency is to sacrifice the facial nerve only in extraordinary circumstances. The substantial body of knowledge showing the effectiveness of postoperative radiation therapy has in large part been responsible for this more conservative approach to dealing with the facial nerve in parotid gland surgery. No prospective studies have been done that document the effectiveness of this approach, which has evolved from considerable anecdotal information. It is axiomatic that those patients who require nerve resection and grafting have advanced-staged disease and, therefore, require postoperative radiation therapy. Even though no definitive studies have been done to analyze the impact of external-beam radiation on nerve regeneration, it is generally felt that nerve grafts do equally well despite radiation. The important addition of postoperative radiation therapy for these advanced malignancies should not, therefore, be avoided or even delayed because of concern for neural regeneration.

Although most data for major salivary gland cancers involve the parotid gland, selected reports have focused on submandibular tumors. Sykes and colleagues[51] reported 30 cases of carcinoma of the submandibular gland treated with radiation therapy. Most were treated postoperatively, but 12 patients were radiated after grossly incomplete surgery or after biopsy alone. The 5- and 10-year local control rates were 85% and 73%, respectively. Cancer-specific survival was 79% and 57%, respectively. Late recurrences were seen, especially for those with adenoid cystic histology. Interestingly, 9 of 12 patients radiated for gross disease had local control.

Not infrequently, a particular situation arises in which a patient with a submandibular mass is explored, and for various reasons, only gland resection is done at the initial operation (i.e., none of the adjacent tissue is removed), and pathologic examination later reveals the existence of a malignancy. The literature is not clear in its recommendations, but the value of reoperation usually lies in the removal of gross disease such as that left behind at the primary site or metastatic nodes. To reoperate and radically remove regional nerves such as cranial nerve XII or to remove mandible in the absence of such gross disease does not seem warranted. Neck dissection of some sort is often recommended, and postoperative radiation to the primary bed and neck should be conducted. Considering the potential for locoregional control with this plan, and considering that more radical measures at the locoregional site do nothing to prevent distant metastasis, this moderate approach seems appropriate.[102]

A unique accumulation of data has assessed the value of fast-neutron radiotherapy for malignant salivary gland tumors.[103–107] Douglas et al.'s report[103] of the results of neutron radiotherapy in 148 patients with major salivary gland malignancies is particularly noteworthy. The 5-year actuarial locoregional control rate for patients treated with curative intent for gross tumor was 59%. Tumor size was an important determinant of outcome. Tumors smaller than 4 cm were controlled in 80%, whereas larger tumors were only controlled in 35%. All patients who had complete resection followed by postoperative neutron therapy had local control. In yet another report,[104] Douglas and colleagues assessed fast-neutron radiotherapy for minor salivary tumors. They reported on 84 patients with adenoid cystic cancers treated between 1985 and 1994. Overall 5-year actuarial locoregional control was 59%. For advanced lesions that involved the skull base, cavernous sinus, or nasopharynx, locoregional control was only 15%, whereas it was 63% when these sites were uninvolved. Recurrence-free survival of 53% at 5 years also has been reported for adenoid cystic carcinoma in a European series.[106]

Buchholz and coworkers[108] also reviewed a limited experience of six patients with large, advanced, or recurrent pleomorphic adenoma who, because surgery was deemed excessively morbid, were treated with neutron beam therapy. With median follow-up of 52 months, all tumors are locally controlled.

Although the method is alluring, the unavailability of neutrons precludes most patients from receiving this therapy.

PARAGANGLIOMAS

Throughout modern medical literature, the paragangliomas have been known by a variety of names, including *glomus tumors, chemodectomas, nonchromaffin paragangliomas, glomerocytomas, carotid body* and *tympanic body tumors,* and *receptomas.* These names and others make up a heterogeneous and confusing list that addresses certain individual characteristics of various tumors but does not achieve the necessary consistency of classification.[109–119]

Essentially, these tumors make up a family of neoplasms that develop from the paraganglia tissues, which are themselves chemoreceptor organs that are distributed throughout the body. These organs are of neural crest origin and have similar functions and histologic appearances.[112] Their cells of origin are part of the *diffuse neuroendocrine system* (DNES), a name that has replaced the previous designation of *amine precursor uptake and decarboxylase system.* The newer terminology acknowledges that the primary products of the paraganglia, neuropeptides, and catecholamines may serve as neurotransmitters, neurohormones, hormones, and parahormones.[113]

Paragangliomas can be broadly categorized as either sympathetic or parasympathetic. The former arise from the adrenal medulla (pheochromocytomas), certain extraadrenal sympathetic paraganglia, and visceral autonomic paraganglia.[120] Parasympathetic paraganglia are found throughout the body, and it is this group that gives rise to almost all the paragangliomas of the head and neck.

The chief cell is probably the principal component of the paraganglia, serving as its chemoreceptor. These cells contain acetylcholine, catecholamines, and serotonin. They are of neural crest origin and, hence, are neuroendocrine in nature. The chief cells render the paraganglia receptive to hypoxia and pH changes, and to fluctuations in the blood carbon dioxide concentration.[114]

As members of the DNES, the chief cells of the paraganglia are functionally and ultrastructurally linked with thyroid C cells, ultimobranchial cells, and adrenaline/noradrenaline-producing cells of the adrenal medulla.[121] These chief cells migrate with autonomic ganglion cells and are, therefore, in close association with sympathetic ganglia around the aorta and its main branches.[115] Many head and neck paraganglia, and their respective neoplasms, are distributed in relation to the vessels and cranial nerves of the primitive branchial arches and are therefore referred to as *branchiomeric paraganglia.*[109,116,117] For example, the jugulotympanic paragangliomas are branchiomeric by virtue of their relation to the third gill arch. The intravagal paragangliomas, on the other hand, are not associated with either the gill arches or their arterial derivatives.[109]

Although paragangliomas can be seen in a variety of head and neck locations—orbit, maxilla, larynx, trachea—most are found on the carotid body, the vagus nerve, or in the jugulotympanic area. This follows the consistent sites occupied throughout the body by the paraganglia. They can be classified as follows:

I. Branchiomeric paraganglia
   a. Temporal bone (tympanicum, jugulare)
   b. Carotid body
   c. Other head and neck (orbit, laryngeal, nasal)
   d. Subclavian, aortic, pulmonary

II. Intravagal (upper mediastinal) paraganglia
III. Aorticosympathetic (retroperitoneal) paraganglia
IV. Visceral (pelvic, vagal, mesenteric) paraganglia

The term *glomus* was applied to paragangliomas because it was believed that the chief cells within the paraganglia were derived from specialized pericytes or from blood vessel walls, as is seen in true arteriovenous glomus complexes.[109] Depending on whether they began in the ear or on the jugular bulb, those tumors that develop in the jugulotympanic paraganglia usually are referred to as *glomus tympanicum* or *glomus jugulare tumors,* respectively. The paraganglia from which these neoplasms arise are associated with the tympanic branch of the glossopharyngeal nerve and the auricular branch of the vagus nerve, respectively.[119] The paragangliomas of the intravagal area are often referred to as *glomus intravagal*[122] or *vagal body tumors.*[123] Although the term *glomus* enjoys considerable name recognition, it is deceiving because of the suggestion of pathologic uniqueness. Such is not the case, however, because all the head and neck paragangliomas have similar histologic, ultrastructural, and cytochemical features, irrespective of the site of origin.[109,112,117] In point of fact, location and functional capabilities, rather than appearance, separate them from one another. It is noteworthy that the first description of a temporal bone glomus tumor by Lubbers[124] referred to a carotid body-like tumor that was thought to be metastatic from a contralateral carotid body tumor.

PATHOGENESIS

The word *functional* is used to describe paragangliomas that secrete catecholamines (epinephrine and norepinephrine) and serotonin. Even though the capacity for catecholamine synthesis and secretion has been documented for both jugulotympanic and intravagal paragangliomas, these two tumors actually have the lowest catecholamine content of all paragangliomas.[109,122,123,125,126] Other functional capabilities have been documented in paragangliomas, but the significance of any secretory activity should be evaluated by its clinical impact. The incidence of clinically functional paragangliomas is only 1% to 3%[127]; however, because of the potentially serious consequences of a catecholamine crisis during manipulations of a functional tumor, evaluation of patients with paragangliomas should include screening for symptoms and signs of catecholamine secretion and in selected circumstances, even the measurement of the appropriate blood and urine products.[128] Although all paraganglia are chemically capable of secreting these products, no physiologic function of the jugulotympanic or the intravagal paraganglia has been established. For the carotid body paraganglia, however, a physiologic role is clearly defined. The carotid body and carotid sinus function as complementary chemoreceptor and baroreceptor, respectively, to effect homeostatic regulation of both ventilation and perfusion.

Overall, paragangliomas are uncommon neoplasms that occur as nonfamilial and familial tumors; the former develop more frequently in women and the latter in men. The mode of inheritance is thought to be autosomal dominant with incomplete penetration. The affected gene is probably located in the long arm of chromosome 11, but there have also been abnormalities found in chromosomes 5 and 7.[117,129–134]

Multiple paragangliomas occur synchronously or metachronously, unilaterally or bilaterally, in 25% to 50% of the familial and in approximately 10% of the nonfamilial tumors.[130,132,135–137]

Any combination of two, three, or more sites of origin of synchronous tumors can occur, but the most frequent combination involves concurrent carotid body and jugulotympanic tumors.[131] Synchronous occurrence is seen between paragangliomas and other DNES lesions, such as pheochromocytomas.[130,136] Although this occurrence is unusual, the serious consequences of not being forewarned before surgery mandates screening for this tumor in all paragangliomas. Specifically, in patients with certain catecholamine profiles, the existence of a pheochromocytoma must be ruled out before any surgery is undertaken. Parathyroid adenomas, thyroid carcinomas, and certain other neural crest tumors also can be concurrent with jugulotympanic, intravagal, and carotid body paragangliomas.[117,138,139] Essentially, this group of neoplasms must always be thought of as potentially systemic afflictions, especially in patients with a family history of similar tumors. Carotid body tumors are much more common in people living at high altitudes than in those living at sea level.[140]

CLINICAL BEHAVIOR AND NATURAL HISTORY

Although the clinical behavior of paragangliomas is determined somewhat by cellular characteristics, tumor location is the more influential factor. Malignancy is rare and typically is defined by the existence of metastasis rather than by cellular characteristics. Metastasis is usually to lungs, lymph nodes, liver, bone, or spleen.[139,141,142] Because paraganglia tissue is not usually found in these structures, its presence in them constitutes metastasis. Metastasis apparently is more frequent in intravagal and jugulotympanic paragangliomas than in carotid body tumors,[143] a fact that is probably related to tumor proximity to the jugular vein.[144,145] DNA ploidy studies do not seem to be predictive of behavior.[146] In the final analysis, no criteria other than metastasis can consistently be used to gauge aggressiveness of a primary paraganglioma.[147] Malignancy also varies by site of origin: Up to 13% of carotid body, 7% to 15% of vagal, and a substantially smaller percentage of jugulotympanic paragangliomas are malignant.[148–152] Malignant lesions metastasize to either the regional lymph nodes or to distant sites, the more common of which are lung and bone. Much like the primary paragangliomas, which are late to metastasize, metastatic sites are characterized by a quiescent natural history; some patients with known lung and bone metastases can live as long as 25 years after the lesions are discovered. Spontaneous remission of metastatic paraganglioma has been reported.[153]

The natural history of primary benign paragangliomas usually is characterized by slow and inexorable growth, and the alterations of the structures into or around which they grow determines the clinical symptoms and signs that occur. Furthermore, different lesions have different structure, and this fact probably impacts on the type of expansion that ultimately occurs. For example, carotid body paragangliomas are encapsulated and rubbery, whereas their jugulotympanic counterparts are friable. Regardless of their site of origin, most paragangliomas are extremely vascular and tend to bleed profusely when manipulated. The jugulotympanic tumors extend into the skull, the eustachian tubes, and the normal cracks and furrows of the ear space. If the tumor originates in the hypotympanicum or on the jugular bulb, it often can be seen through the tympanic membrane. A bluish red mass behind the membrane or a polyp in the external ear canal can be but the surface of an extensive paraganglioma, and a casual biopsy or myringotomy can lead to troublesome bleeding. Only by appropriate imaging can the true extent of the tumor be determined.

The jugulotympanic paragangliomas often initially create a sense of fullness in the ear, followed by a conductive hearing loss and pulsatile tinnitus. Destruction of the temporal bone can lead to facial nerve weakness, vertigo, deafness, and intracranial complications such as cerebrospinal fluid leak and meningitis. When a tumor occurs in the jugular bulb area, its otologic manifestations often precede vagal nerve signs.

Paragangliomas of the vagus nerve, on the other hand, almost always create vocal cord paralysis before otologic symptoms and signs occur.[154] That is not to say, however, that vagal nerve paragangliomas always produce vocal cord paralysis; such is not the case. Overall, only approximately 3% of paragangliomas are vagal in origin.[155] These slow-growing tumors occur most often at the base of the skull and in the parapharyngeal space but may arise anywhere along the course of the nerve or its branches. When the tumors are located high on the nerve, they tend to displace the internal carotid artery anteriorly. Such a vagal paraganglioma is demonstrated by the arteriogram shown in Figure 30.4-5*A*. The arteriographic appearance is, therefore, different from that of carotid body paragangliomas, which generally cause splaying of the external and internal carotid arteries (Fig. 30.4-5*B*). Vagal paragangliomas often present as asymptomatic cervical masses,[156] and in the absence of unusually aggressive local behavior, neurogenic signs such as those caused by involvement of the sympathetic trunk and cranial nerves X, XI, and XII usually occur only after extensive growth.

Laryngeal paragangliomas are extremely uncommon.[157] Most originate in the supraglottic portion of that organ and, as such, do not present with early symptoms, such as hoarseness, or with airway compromise. When discovered, they present as a discolored, submucosal mass that is atypical in appearance and is often confused with other tumors, especially neuroendocrine carcinoma. These malignancies have a distinctly different behavioral pattern. Studies have concluded that laryngeal paragangliomas are benign neoplasms.[157] Malignant behavior of these lesions is so unusual as to suggest misdiagnosis. These lesions are effectively managed by surgical excision.

Most commonly, carotid body paragangliomas present as painless masses located deep to the anterior border of the sternocleidomastoid muscle in the upper or midneck. These are generally slow growing and often have been obvious for years before diagnosis. They are usually nonfunctional, but they do have the capability of function.[148] Carotid body paragangliomas actually can grow to impressive dimensions without creating neurologic or vascular findings. Large tumors occasionally produce compressive carotid artery symptoms. These facts are important in determining treatment philosophy, especially in older, asymptomatic patients. They begin in the arterial adventitia, usually at or around the bifurcation of the internal and external carotid arteries. Because these tumors generally develop from the medial aspect of the great vessels, the arteries generally are displaced laterally. This typical appearance of splayed and lateralized vessels distinguishes the carotid body tumors radiographically from vagal nerve paragangliomas (see Fig. 30.4-5). The radiography is important in diagnosis, because it is unique. As these neoplasms become larger, they can occupy the parapharyngeal space, actually presenting as a bulge in the tonsil area, and encroachment into this area can produce dysphagia.

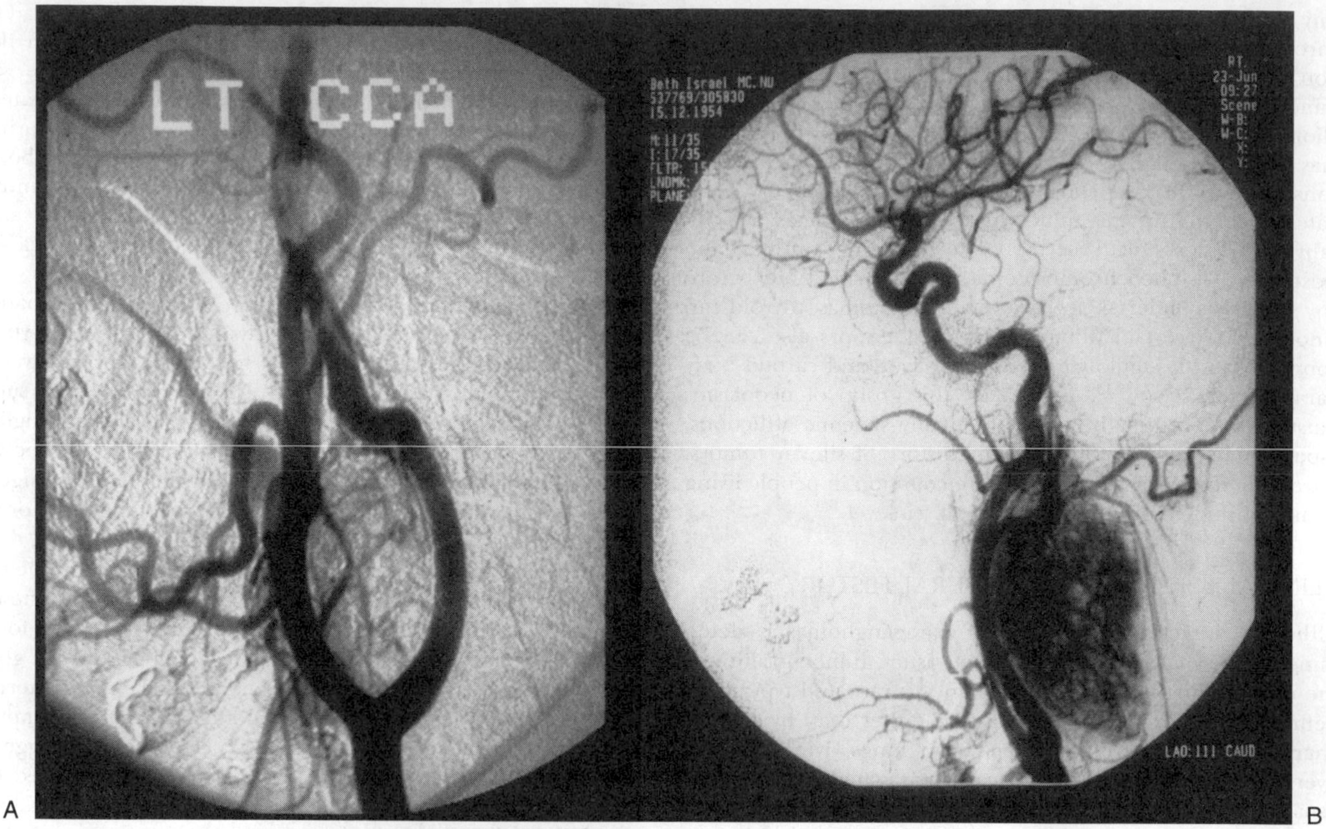

FIGURE 30.4-5. Arteriogram shows vagal paraganglioma and anterior displacement of internal carotid artery (ICA) **(A)** and carotid body paraganglioma **(B)**. Notice the splaying of the ICA and external carotid arteries.

EVALUATION

The diagnostic workup of paragangliomas should consist of CT or MRI and, in selected situations, angiography. Imaging should delineate bone destruction and complete tumor, intracranial and extracranial. CT scanning is more effective for imaging bone, but MRI offers a superior capability in accessing intracranial extension, as well as the relation of tumor to bone. With proper enhancement techniques, one or both of these images plus clinical evaluation can provide sufficient information to plan treatment of most paragangliomas. This point is relevant to overall management strategy; if radiation therapy is the planned treatment, the radiation oncologist must be comfortable enough with the diagnosis to proceed without a biopsy. FNA and cytologic analysis can be helpful, but because of the location medial to the carotid artery and because of the dense vascularity of most of these lesions, this study may not always be practical. Open biopsy becomes necessary when the diagnosis is not achieved by these other means.

Invasive arteriography is valuable in preoperative preparation because it provides a picture of contralateral vascular crossover and because it allows tumor embolization to be done before contemplated surgery. Paragangliomas are usually very vascular, and when surgery is planned, intraluminal embolization of the main arterial supply and the tumor bed is helpful for safe and less morbid removal of large tumors. The continued concern for the purity of the commercial blood supply is such that surgeons should avoid transfusion whenever possible, and preoperative embolization can be extremely helpful in pursuing this goal. This technique has its most impressive impact in the removal of larger carotid body and jugular bulb tumors and is probably unnecessary for most small tumors. The techniques of embolization are beyond the scope of this chapter, and the reader is referred to the literature on the subject; it must be emphasized, however, that use of this technology carries significant risks and should be undertaken only by an experienced interventional radiology team. Finally, embolization of paragangliomas is only an adjunct to surgery and should not be considered primary treatment for these highly vascular tumors, no matter how successful the devascularization. If embolization is not followed promptly by tumor removal, undesirable collateral circulation and vascular shunting can develop, ultimately complicating an already challenging surgical process. In fact, the sooner the surgery follows the embolization, the more effective the hemostasis will be during surgery. If surgery is not to be the treatment of choice, then embolization should probably not be done.

TREATMENT AND RESULTS

Paragangliomas usually are considered benign, and although they can metastasize or be locally aggressive, such is the exception rather than the rule. Traditionally, the mainstay of treatment has been surgical removal,[158,159] but repeated series of cases treated by radiation therapy have demonstrated its effectiveness in achieving local control of these tumors.[160–165] Investigators have reviewed the literature and have compared surgical with radiation therapy results, which show no difference in local control achieved by either modality. Accordingly, treatment decisions should be based on a formula that considers tumor size, patient age and general health, symptoms and signs present before treatment, treatment-related morbidity, and the expertise of those involved in the planned treatment.

Reluctance to use radiation therapy in paragangliomas probably stems from a historic bias against radiating benign tumors. Furthermore, series that have compared the two treatment methods have been somewhat biased because many tumors radiated in various series were not favorable lesions by virtue of their size and recurrent state. As in any study that compares treatment results, an accurate comparison of radiation and surgery should analyze comparable tumors. An important aspect of radiation therapy of paragangliomas relates to the definition of local control. In traditional cancer thinking, sustained complete response after radiation is the criterion by which local control is usually judged. Such cannot be the case, however, with paragangliomas. Instead, these tumors typically partially regress or remain stable after therapy. Because the tumors are composed predominantly of vascular tissue, the proliferative (i.e., neoplastic) elements make up but a minor portion of the overall tumor volume, and although successful radiotherapy kills the proliferative cellular component, the remaining vascular tissue typically does not change significantly. For purposes of assessing local control, therefore, the absence of disease progression with the resolution or even halting of symptoms after radiation is the ultimate goal. In fact, there may even be some short-term postradiation edema or swelling of the involved area, but this generally resolves within several months. When radiation is used as the treatment modality, therefore, it is important that both the treatment team and the patient understand this important aspect of local control, and all concerned should exercise patience in judging the outcome. Some investigators have been skeptical of the persistence palpable tissue after radiation, expressing concern for its capacity to proliferate after 20 to 30 years' dormancy.[166] However, it has never been demonstrated that this has occurred. In the future, genetic mutations of p53, p161NK4A, and others may provide markers for local tumor progression and regression.[167]

Cummings and coworkers[160] have reported 45 patients radiated for glomus tumors. Only three patients (6.6%) have had symptomatic recurrences, two of which were believed to be due to a "geographic miss." The radiation therapy was effective in relieving the presenting symptoms of most patients. For example, 27 of 35 patients (77%) who received 3500 cGy in 3 weeks had complete relief of their tinnitus. The remaining 23% had partial relief or stabilization of symptoms. All patients with pain, vertigo, discharge, bleeding, and abnormalities of the fifth cranial nerve had complete relief of their symptoms with radiation therapy. All patients with abnormalities of cranial nerve IX through XII had partial relief or stabilization of their cranial nerve abnormalities. The authors of this study noted that symptomatic improvement often did not occur until many months after radiation therapy, highlighting the need to follow these patients for a lengthy period. As long as no clinical progression was noted, the authors believed there would be no need to intervene in the postradiation setting.

Kim and associates[161] have analyzed the dose-response relation for radiation of paragangliomas. The literature was reviewed, and the rate of failure was correlated with dose. Overall, the recurrence rate was 25% when the radiation dose was less than 4000 cGy. With doses greater than 4000 cGy, local recurrence was rare. Overall, only 2 of 142 patients (1.4%) who received more than 4000 cGy had local recurrence. The authors recommended doses in the 4000- to 4500-cGy range delivered over 4.0 to 4.5 weeks. Cole and Beiler[163] treated 39 glomus jugulare or vagal tumors with radiotherapy. The last 32 of those patients were treated with megavoltage radiotherapy (cobalt 60) or linear accelerator; the first seven patients had been treated with orthovoltage therapy. In the first seven patients, the results were unpredictable; however, 30 of the 32 later patients show no evidence of recurrence.

Evenson et al.[168] have reported the results of 15 patients with 23 paragangliomas treated with radiotherapy. Eighteen of these tumors were previously untreated, whereas five had been unsuccessfully treated with prior therapy (one with radiation therapy, four with surgery). Most patients received doses in the 15-Gy range over 5 weeks. The local control for previously untreated patients was 100% at 10 years. The cause-specific survival rate was 100% for the 14 patients that were previously untreated. No cranial nerve injuries were seen. The patient who was re-radiated developed a transient lethargy syndrome. Mumber and Greven[169] also reported that all 15 patients treated in their series with definitive radiotherapy had long-term local control. Doses of more than 4500 cGy did not improve the outcome.

Complications are associated with both methods of treatment; most series show the rate to be higher in patients managed by surgery.[170] It should be pointed out, however, that most series have studied cases accumulated over many years, and when many of the earlier surgical cases were done, modern temporal bone and carotid artery bypass techniques had not yet been developed. The contemporary methods of reducing intraoperative bleeding by preoperative embolization usually are not included in these series. The intraoperative precision achieved by using contemporary methods surely render previous complication data invalid. The complications associated with radiation therapy are dose related. Bone and brain necrosis and abscess are the most serious of those reported. Each of these has occurred in approximately 1% of treated patients. These complications should not occur as long as doses in the 4000- to 4500-cGy range are used. Fuller and colleagues[171] reported one fibrosarcoma in their series that was considered a radiation-induced malignancy. Malignant transformation of tissue secondary to radiation has been reported in these tumors, and although unusual, this occurrence is a concern.

The decision to operate or radiate should be based on a formula that considers tumor size and location, patient age and health, symptoms or signs present before treatment, potential morbidity, and the expertise and availability of those involved in treatment. The decision should be made in consultation between the head and neck surgeon and the radiation oncologist and with an appreciation for the fact that this group of tumors is one of the most complex and dangerous head and neck tumors to be treated. To do nothing is an acceptable option in some patients, because these lesions are often tolerated well and for a prolonged period. In general, a reasonable plan in patients with head and neck paragangliomas is to operate and remove those lesions (whether jugulotympanic, intravagal, laryngeal, or carotid body in origin) that are smaller and less likely to be associated with significant operative morbidity. For large tumors that demonstrate extensive bone destruction, intracranial involvement, or both, or in which considerable operative morbidity is expected, radiation therapy is probably the method of choice for achieving local control. In young patients, radiation therapy should be avoided if a reasonable surgical option is available. On the other hand, the risk for radiation-induced cancer is small, and these authors do not hesitate to recommend it to young patients if the surgical procedure required is likely to be associated with unreasonable morbidity. Older patients are especially suited for radiation therapy, because local control usually is sustained throughout the balance of their lifetime.

Removal of jugulotympanic lesions should only be attempted by surgeons trained in otologic and skull base techniques. Those intravagal paragangliomas that are located high in the neck are often very challenging surgical endeavors, being too high to approach by conventional cervical exposure and too low to be handled from an intracranial approach. These are true skull base lesions, often having an epicenter within the jugular foramen. This mostly inaccessible location is best approached by complex but precise and well-described skull base techniques.[159,172] Paragangliomas of the temporal bone can be a challenging group of patients.[173] De Jong and colleagues[174] reported on 38 patients radiated for temporal bone paragangliomas between 1956 and 1991. Fourteen patients were treated primarily, 13 in combination with surgery, and 11 as salvage. Local control was achieved in 79% of the primary radiation group, 100% of the combined therapy group, and 91% in the salvage group. Complications were few and minor.

Because resection of vagal paragangliomas is almost always followed by complete vagal paralysis, the choice of a radiation versus a surgical strategy in these lesions should be based on a particularly flexible paradigm. Rehabilitation after resection of midcervical vagal lesions is more easily accomplished than those at the base of the skull. This is partly because of the fact that, in the latter group, multiple cranial nerve injuries are more common. Older individuals have much more physiologic difficulty after vagal nerve resection than do younger patients, regardless of the part of the nerve involved. One must factor into the decision process the fact that a significant percentage of patients with vagal paragangliomas demonstrate a vagal nerve paralysis at the time of diagnosis, and that fact certainly alters the decision process somewhat.

Surgery of carotid body paragangliomas, although safe overall, is fraught with hazards, and only head and neck surgeons competent in vascular techniques should attempt to remove these lesions, especially in recurrent lesions. Carotid artery bypass or shunt, or even artery resection and reconstruction, are sometimes necessary to achieve complete tumor removal. Additionally, and with regard to the surgical removal of carotid body paragangliomas, the input from both chemoreceptor and baroreceptor mechanisms is mediated via a common neural pathway; therefore, function of the entire system is affected by the resection of tumors involving the intercarotid paraganglia. Whereas the resection of unilateral carotid body lesions is generally well accepted, excision of bilateral tumors or of a unilateral carotid tumor with a contralateral vagal paraganglioma is often problematic from two standpoints: the potential of sustaining bilateral vagal nerve injury and the baroreceptor dysfunction that potentially can result from the bilateral denervation of the carotid sinuses. Labile hypertension and hypotension, headaches, diaphoresis, and emotional anxiety occur in a substantial percentage of patients who undergo bilateral excision.[175] Apparently, the loss of the parasympathetic regulatory system and the subsequent unopposed sympathetic system leads to this cardiovascular syndrome. Surprisingly little emphasis has been placed on this finding in the literature. Considering the gravity of the potential morbidity, we do not recommend bilateral carotid body paraganglioma removal, especially simultaneously. If bilateral surgery is contemplated, the procedures should be staged, both to ensure the functionality of the vagus nerve on the first side, and to minimize the risk of baroreceptor dysfunction. Surgery on one side and radiation therapy to the contralateral lesion is an accepted alternative to bilateral surgery. Finally, one can also consider radiation to both lesions.

Overall, the most accepted treatment for paragangliomas is surgical extirpation; however, radiation therapy is an effective alternative to surgery for achieving local control in certain patients. An asymptomatic paraganglioma in an elderly patient or one in ill health is of questionable concern, and therefore, consideration should be given to observation only.

Malignant paragangliomas are managed most effectively with surgery, radiation therapy, or both. Essentially, chemotherapy has no defined role for treatment at any stage. Patients with disease that cannot be approached with surgery or radiation should be treated when symptoms require palliation, but because these are rarely encountered, only a few anecdotal reports of experience with chemotherapy have been published. These patients should be considered for investigational therapies.

REFERENCES

1. Spiro R, Spiro J. Cancer of the salivary glands. In: Meyers E, Suen J, eds. *Cancer of the head and neck,* 2nd ed. New York: Churchill Livingstone, 1984:645.
2. Som P, Braun I, Shapiro M. Tumors of the parapharyngeal space: MR imaging. *Radiology* 1987;164:823.
3. Work W, Gates G. Tumors of the parotid gland and parapharyngeal space. *Otolaryngol Clin North Am* 1969;2:497.
4. Cassissi N, Dickerson D, Million R. Squamous cell cancer of the skin metastatic to parotid nodes. *Arch Otol* 1978;104:336.
5. Katz A, Preston-Martin S. Salivary gland tumors and previous radiation therapy to the head and neck. *Am J Surg* 1984;147:345.
6. Hollander L, Cunningham M. Management of cancer of the parotid gland. *Surg Clin North Am* 1973;53:113.
7. Klintenber C, Olofsson J, Hellquist H, Sokjer H. Adenocarcinoma of the ethmoid sinuses: a review of 28 cases with special reference to dust exposure. *Cancer* 1984;54:482.
8. Evans R, Cruckshank A. Epithelial tumors of the salivary glands. Philadelphia: WB Saunders, 1970.
9. Batsakis J, Regezi T, Bloch D. The pathology of head and neck tumors, vol 3. *Head Neck Surg* 1979;1:260.
10. Livolsi V, Perzin K. Malignant mixed tumors arising in salivary glands: carcinomas arising in benign mixed tumors. *Cancer* 1971;39:2209.
11. Geraghty R, Scofield H, Brown F, Hennigar C. Malignant mixed tumors of salivary origin. *Cancer* 1969;24:471.
12. Spiro R, Huvos A, Strong E. Malignant mixed tumor of salivary gland origin. *Cancer* 1978;41:924.
13. Godwin J. Benign lymphoepithelial lesion of the parotid gland. *Cancer* 1952;5:1089.
14. Bruner J, Cleary K, Smith F, Batsakis J. Immunocytochemical identification of HIV antigen in parotid lymphoid lesions. *J Laryngol Otol* 1989;103:1063.
15. Finn D. Lymphoma of the head and neck and acquired immunodeficiency syndrome: clinical investigation and immunohistological study. *Laryngoscope* 1995;105:1.
16. Yeh C, Fox P, Fox C, et al. Kaposi's sarcoma of the parotid gland in acquired immunodeficiency syndrome. *Oral Surg Oral Med Oral Pathol* 1989;67:308.
17. McShane D, Vellend H, Dayal V. AIDS, otolaryngology and a case of adenoid cystic carcinoma of the parotid arising in a patient with AIDS-related complex. *J Otolaryngol* 1987;16:10.
18. Gravanis M, Giansanti J. Malignant histopathologic counterpart of the benign lymphoepithelial lesion. *Cancer* 1970;26:1332.
19. Finfer M, Schinella R, Rothstein S, Persky M. Cystic parotid lesions in patients at risk for the acquired immunodeficiency syndrome. *Arch Otolaryngol Head Neck Surg* 1988; 114:1290.
20. Sperling N, Lin P. Parotid disease associated with HIV infection. *Ear Nose Throat J* 1990;69:475.

21. Terry J, Lorec T, Thomas M, Marti J. Major salivary gland lymphoepithelial lesions and the acquired immunodeficiency syndrome. *Am J Surg* 1991;162:324.
22. Spiro R. Salivary neoplasms: overview of 25 years' experience with 2,807 patients. *Head Neck Surg* 1986;8:177.
23. Perzin K, Livoisi V. Acinic cell carcinoma arising in ectopic salivary gland tissue. *Cancer* 1980;45:967.
24. Spiro R, Huvos A, Strong E. Acinic cell carcinoma of salivary origin. *Cancer* 1978;41:924.
25. Chong GC, Beahrs O, Woolner L. Surgical management of acinic cell carcinoma of the parotid gland. *Surg Gynecol Obstet* 1974;136:65.
26. Spiro R, Huvos A, Berk R, Strong E. Mucoepidermoid carcinoma of salivary gland origin. *Am J Surg* 1978;136:461.
27. Eneroth C, Hertman L, Moberger G, Soderberg G. Mucoepidermoid carcinoma of the salivary glands with special reference to the possible existence of a benign variety. *Acta Otolaryngol* 1972;73:68.
28. Thoryaldsson S, Beahrs O, Woolner L, Simons J. Mucoepidermoid tumors of major salivary glands. *Am J Surg* 1970;120:432.
29. Spiro R, Huvos A, Strong E. Cancer of the parotid gland. *Am J Surg* 1975;130:452.
30. Nasomento A, Amarol A, Prado L. Mucoepidermoid carcinoma of salivary glands. *Head Neck Surg* 1986;8:409.
31. Spiro R, Huvos A, Strong E. Adenocarcinoma of salivary gland origin. *Am J Surg* 1982;144:423.
32. Eneroth C. Facial nerve paralysis: a sign of malignancy in parotid tumors. *Arch Otolaryngol* 1972;95:300.
33. Conley T, Hamaker R. Prognosis of malignant tumors of the parotid gland with facial paralysis. *Arch Otolaryngol* 1975;101:39.
34. Conley J, Arena S. Parotid gland as a focus of metastasis. *Arch Surg* 1963;87:757.
35. Nicholas R, Pinnock L, Szymanowski R Metastases to parotid nodes. *Laryngoscope* 1980;90:1324.
36. Duck S, McConnel F. Malignant degeneration of pleomorphic adenoma. *Am J Otolaryngol* 1993;14:175.
37. Borthune A, Kjellevold K, Kaalhus O, Vermurad H. Salivary gland malignant neoplasms: treatment and prognosis. *Int J Radiat Oncol Biol Phys* 1986;12:747.
38. Spiro R, Huvos H, Strong E. Adenoid cystic carcinoma of salivary gland origin. *Am J Surg* 1974;128:512.
39. Matsuba H, Simpson J, Mauney M, Thawley S. Adenoid cystic salivary gland carcinoma: a clinicopathologic correlation. *Head Neck Surg* 1986;8:200.
40. Frankenthaler R, Luna M, Lee S, et al. Prognostic variables in parotid gland cancer. *Arch Otolaryngol Head Neck Surg* 1991;117:1251.
41. Cohen J, Guillamondegui O, Batsakis J, Medina J. Cancer of the minor salivary glands of the larynx. *Am J Surg* 1985;150:513.
42. Spiro R, Armstrong J, Harrison L. Carcinoma of major salivary glands. *Arch Otolaryngol Head Neck Surg* 1989;115:316.
43. Johns M, Coulthard S. Survival and follow-up in malignant tumors of the salivary glands. *Otolaryngol Clin North Am* 1977;10:455.
44. Eisele D, Kleinberg L, O'Malley. Management of malignant salivary gland tumors. In: Harrison L, Sessions R, Hong K, eds. *Head and neck cancer.* Philadelphia: Lippincott Raven Publishers, Chapter 30.
45. Spiro R, Huvos A, Strong E. Malignant mixed tumor of salivary origin. *Cancer* 1977;39:388.
46. Armstrong J, Harrison L, Thaler H, et al. The indications for elective treatment of the neck in cancer of the major salivary glands. *Cancer* 1992;69:615.
47. Van Poorten V, Balm A, Hilgers F, et al. Prognostic factors for long term results of the treatment of patients with malignant submandibular tumors. *Cancer* 1999;85:2255.
48. Camilleri I, Malata C, McLean N, Kelly C. Malignant tumours of the submandibular salivary gland: a 15 year review. *Br J Plastic Surg* 1998;51:181.
49. American Joint Committee for Cancer Staging and End Results. *Manual for staging of cancer.* Chicago: American Joint Committee for Cancer, 1978.
50. Malata C, Camilleri I, McLean N, et al. Malignant tumors of the parotid gland: a 12 year review. *Br J Plastic Surg* 1997;50:600.
51. Sykes A, Slevin N, Birzgalis A, Gupta N. Submandibular gland carcinoma: local control and survival following adjuvant radiotherapy. *Oral Oncol* 1999;35:L187.
52. Armstrong J, Harrison L, Spiro R, et al. The role of postoperative radiation therapy in malignant salivary gland tumors: a matched pain analysis using historic controls. *Int J Radiat Oncol Biol Phys* 1988;15:176.
53. Renehan A, Gleave E, Hancock B, Smith P, McGach M. Long term follow up of over 1000 patients with salivary gland tumors treated in a single center. *Br J Surg* 1996;83:1750.
54. Dawson A, Orr J. Long-term results of local excision and radiotherapy in pleomorphic adenoma of the parotid. *Int J Radiat Oncol Biol Phys* 1985;11:451.
55. Leverstein H, Tiwari R, Snow G, van der Waal J, van der Waal I. The surgical management of recurrent or residual pleomorphic adenomas of the parotid gland. *Eur Arch Otorhinolaryngol* 1997;254:313.
56. Frankenthaler R, Byers R, Luna M, et al. Predicting occult lymph node metastasis in parotid cancer. *Arch Otolaryngol Head Neck Surg* 1993;119:517.
57. Armstrong J, Harrison L, Thaler H, et al. The indications for elective treatment of the neck in cancer of the major salivary glands. *Cancer* 1992;69:615.
58. Fitzpatrick P, Theriault C. Malignant salivary gland tumors. *Int J Radiat Oncol Biol Phys* 1986;12:1743.
59. Harrison L, Armstrong J, Spiro R, Fass D, Strong E. Post-operative radiation therapy for major salivary gland malignancies. *J Surg Oncol* 1990;45:52.
60. North C, Lee D, Piantadosi S, Zahurak M, Johns M. Carcinoma of the major salivary glands treated by surgery or surgery plus post-operative radiotherapy. *Int J Radiat Oncol Biol Phys* 1990;18:1319.
61. McNaney D, McNeese M, Guillamondegui O. Postoperative irradiation in malignant epithelial tumors of the parotid. *Int J Radiat Oncol Biol Phys* 1983;9:1289.
62. Elkon D, Coleman M, Hendrickson F. Radiation therapy in the treatment of malignant salivary gland tumors. *Cancer* 1978;41:502.
63. Fu K, Leibel S, Levine M. Cancer of the major and minor salivary glands. *Cancer* 1977; 40:2882.
64. Garden A, el-Naggar A, Morrison W, et al. Post-operative radiotherapy for malignant tumors of the parotid gland. *Int J Radiat Oncol Biol Phys* 1997;37:79.
65. Yaparpalvi R, Fontanla D, Tyerech S, Boselli L, Beitler J. Parotid gland tumors: a comparison of postoperative radiotherapy techniques using 3 dimensional dose distributions and dose volume histograms. *Int J Radiat Oncol Biol Phys* 1998;40:43.
66. Hosokawa Y, Shirato H, Kagei K, et al. Role of radiotherapy for mucoepidermoid carcinoma of salivary gland. *Oral Oncol* 1999;35:105.
67. Simpson J, Matsuba H, Thawley S. Improved treatment of salivary gland adenocarcinoma: planned confirmation surgery and irradiation. *Laryngoscope* 1986;96:904.
68. Vikram B, Strong E, Shah J, Spiro R. Radiation therapy in adenoid cystic carcinoma. *Int J Radiat Oncol Biol Phys* 1984;10:221.
69. King J, Fletcher G. Malignant tumors of the major salivary glands. *Radiology* 1971;100:381.
70. Venook A, Tseng A, Meyers F. Cisplatin, doxorubicin, and 5-fluorouracil chemotherapy for salivary gland malignancies: a pilot study of the Northern California Oncology Group. *J Clin Oncol* 1987;5:951.
71. Triozzi P, Brantley A, Fisher S. 5-Fluorouracil, cyclophosphamide, and vincristine for adenoid cystic carcinoma of the head and neck. *Cancer* 1987;59:887.
72. Airoldi M, Brando V, Giordano C, et al. Chemotherapy for recurrent salivary gland malignancies: experience of the ENT department of Turin University. *ORL J Otorhinolaryngol Relat Spec* 1994;56:105.
73. Licitra L, Marchini R, Spinazze R, et al. Cisplatin in advanced salivary gland carcinoma. A phase II study of 25 patients. *Cancer* 1991;68:1874.
74. Schramm V, Srodes C, Myers E. Cisplatin therapy for adenoid cystic carcinoma. *Arch Otolaryngol* 1981;107;739.
75. Jones A, Phillips D, Cook J, Helliwell T. A randomized phase II trial of epirubicin and 5 fluorouracil versus cisplatinum in the palliation of advanced and recurrent malignant tumour of the salivary glands. *Br J Cancer* 1993;37:1127.
76. Vermorken J, Verweij J, de Mulder P, et al. Epirubicin in patients with advanced or recurrent adenoid cystic carcinoma of the head and neck: a phase II study of the EORTC Head and Neck Cancer Cooperative Group. *Ann Oncol* 1993;4:785.
77. Venveij J, de Mulder P, de Graeff A, et al. Phase II study on mitoxantrone in adenoid cystic carcinomas of the head and neck. EORTC Head and Neck Cancer Cooperative Group. *Ann Oncol* 1996;7:876.
78. Mattox F, VonHoff D, Balcerzak S. Southwest Oncology Group study of mitoxantrone for treatment of patients with advanced adenoid cystic carcinoma of the head and neck. *Invest New Drugs* 1990;8:105.
79. Airoldi M, Bumma C, Bertetto O, et al. Vinorelbine treatment of recurrent salivary gland carcinomas. *Bull Cancer* 1998;85:892.
80. Tannock I, Sutherland D. Chemotherapy for adenoid cystic carcinoma. *Cancer* 1980;46:452.
81. Rentschler R, Burgess M, Byers R. Chemotherapy of malignant salivary gland neoplasms: a 25 year review of M. D. Anderson Hospital experience. *Cancer* 1977;40:619.
82. Suen J, Johns M. Chemotherapy for salivary gland cancer. *Laryngoscope* 1982;92:235.
83. H Pinto, personal communication.
84. de Haan L, De Mulder P, Vermorken J, et al. Cisplatin-based chemotherapy in advanced adenoid cystic carcinoma of the head and neck. *Head Neck* 1992;14:273.
85. Hill M, Constenla D, A'Hern R, et al. Cisplatin and 5-fluorouracil for symptom control in advanced salivary adenoid cystic carcinoma. *Oral Oncol* 1997;33:275.
86. Belani C, Eisenberger M, Gray W. Preliminary experience with chemotherapy in advanced salivary gland neoplasms. *Med Pediatr Oncol* 1988;16:197.
87. Alberts D, Manning M, Coulthard S. Adriamycin/cisplatinum/cyclophosphamide combination chemotherapy for advanced carcinoma of the parotid gland. *Cancer* 1981;47:645.
88. Creagan E, Woods J, Rubin J. Cisplatin-based chemotherapy for neoplasms arising from salivary glands and contiguous structures in the head and neck. *Cancer* 1988;62:2313.
89. Dreyfuss A, Clark J, Fallon B. Cyclophosphamide, doxorubicin, and cisplatin combination chemotherapy for advanced carcinomas of salivary gland origin. *Cancer* 1987;60:2869.
90. Kaplan M, Johns M, Cantrell R. Chemotherapy for salivary gland cancer. *Otolaryngol Head Neck Surg* 1986;95:165.
91. Airoldi M, Pedani F, Brando V, Gabriele P, Giordano C. Cisplatin, epirubicin and 5-fluorouracil combination chemotherapy for recurrent carcinoma of the salivary gland. *Tumori* 1989;75:252.
92. Dimery I, Legha T, Shirinian M. Fluorouracil, doxorubicin, cyclophosphamide, and cisplatin combination chemotherapy in advanced or recurrent salivary gland carcinoma. *J Clin Oncol* 1990;8:1056.
93. Posner M, Ervin T, Weichselbaum R. Chemotherapy of advanced salivary gland neoplasms. *Cancer* 1982;50:2261.
94. McKenna R. Tumors of the major and minor salivary glands. *CA Cancer J Clin* 1984;34:24.
95. Tran L, Sidrys J, Sadeghi A, et al. Salivary gland tumors of the oral cavity. *Int J Radiat Oncol Biol Phys* 1990;18:413.
96. Koss L, Spiro R, Hajdu S. Small cell (oat cell) carcinoma of minor salivary gland origin. *Cancer* 1972;30:737.
97. Olsen K, Devine D, Weiland L. Mucoepidermoid carcinoma of the oral cavity. *Otolaryngol Head Neck Surg* 1981;89:783.
98. Ellis E, Million R, Mendenhall W, Parsons J, Cassisi N. The use of radiation therapy in the management of minor salivary gland tumors. *Int J Radiat Oncol Biol Phys* 1988;15:613.
99. Parsons J, Mendenhall W, Stringer S, Cassisi N, Million R. Management of minor salivary gland carcinomas. *Int J Radiat Oncol Biol Phys* 1996;35:443.
100. Eapen L, Gerig L, Catton G, Danjoux C, Girard A. Impact of local radiation in the management of salivary gland carcinomas. *Head Neck Surg* 1988;10:239.
101. Biller H, Shugar J, Krespi Y. A new technique for wide-field exposure of the base of the skull. *Arch Otolaryngol* 1981;107:698.
102. Sessions R, Ward P, Johns M, Goeffinet D. Carcinoma of the submaxillary gland, radiation and or surgery? *Head Neck Surg* 1987;10:129.

103. Douglas J, Lee S, Laramore G, et al. Neutron radiotherapy for the treatment of locally advanced major salivary gland tumors. *Head Neck* 1999;21:255.
104. Douglas J, Laramore G, Austin-Seymour M, et al. Neutron radiotherapy for adenoid cystic carcinoma of minor salivary glands. *Int J Radiat Oncol Biol Phys* 1996;36:87.
105. Prott F, Haverkamp U, Willich N, et al. Ten years of fast neutron therapy in Munster. *Bull Cancer Radiother* 1996;835[Suppl]:115s.
106. Krull S, Schwarz R, Engenhart R, et al. European results in neutron therapy of malignant salivary gland tumors. *Bull Cancer Radiother* 1996;835[Suppl]:125.
107. Potter R, Prott F, Micke O, et al. Results of fast neutron therapy of adenoid cystic carcinoma of salivary glands. *Strahlentiver Onkologie* 1999;175[Suppl 2]:65.
108. Buchholz TA, Laramore GE, Griffin TW. Fast neutron radiation for recurrent pleomorphic adenomas of the parotid gland. *Am J Clin Oncol* 1992;15:441.
109. Glenner G, Grimley P. Tumors of the extra-adrenal paraganglion system (including chemoreceptors). In: Hymes V, ed. *Atlas of tumor pathology*, 2nd ser, pt 9. Washington, DC: Armed Forces Institute of Pathology, 1974:1.
110. Mulligan R. Chemodectoma in the dog. *Am J Pathol* 1950;28:680(abst).
111. Rosenwasser H. Glomus jugulare tumors. *Arch Otolaryngol* 1968;88:29.
112. Zak F. An expanded concept of glomus tissue. *N Y State J Med* 1954;54:1153.
113. Pearse A. The diffuse neuroendocrine system: historical review. *Front Horm Res* 1984;12:1.
114. Bleau H, Rougues L, Gerard P. L'angiome du rocher et son aspect radiographique. *Presse Med* 1950;58:1141.
115. Case 14-1975. Case records of the Massachusetts General Hospital. *N Engl J Med* 1975;292:741.
116. Kohn A. Uber den Bau and die Entwicklung der sogenannten Caotisdruse. *Arch Mikr Anat Mika Anat* 1903;62:263.
117. Batsakis J. Paragangliomas of the head and neck. In: Batsakis J, ed. *Tumors of the head and neck: clinical and pathological considerations*, 2nd ed. Baltimore: Williams & Wilkins, 1979:369.
118. Smith P, Schwaber M, Goebel J. Clinical evaluation of glomus tumors of the ear and the base of the skull. In: Thawley S, Panje W, Batsakis J, Lindberg R, eds. *Comprehensive management of head and neck tumors*. Philadelphia: WB Saunders, 1987:207.
119. Guild S. The glomus jugulare, a nonchromaffin paraganglion, in man. *Ann Otol Rhinol Laryngol* 1953;62:1045.
120. Hodge K, Byers R, Peters L. Paragangliomas of the head and neck. *Arch Otolaryngol Head Neck Surg* 1988;114:872.
121. Pearse A. The cytochemistry and ultrastructure of polypeptide hormone-producing cells of the APUD series and the embryologic, physiologic and pathologic implications of the concept. *J Histochem Cytochem* 1969;17:303.
122. Conley J, Clairmont A. Glomus intravagale. *Laryngoscope* 1977;87:2096.
123. Kahn L. Vagal body tumor (nonchromaffin paraganglioma, chemodectoma, and carotid body-like tumor) with cervical node metastases and familial association. *Cancer* 1976;38:2367.
124. Lubbers J. Fezwel van het os petrum met gecombineerede hersenzenuw verlanning. *Ned Tijdschr Gencesk* 1937;81:2566.
125. Cantrell R, Kaplan M, Winn H, Atuk N, Jahrsdoerfer R. Catecholamine-secreting infratemporal fossa paraganglioma. *Ann Otol Rhinol Laryngol* 1984;93:583.
126. Brown J. Glomus jugulare tumors revisited: a ten-year statistical follow-up of 231 cases. *Laryngoscope* 1985;95:284.
127. Schwaber M, Glasscock M, Jackson C, Nissen A, Smith P. Diagnosis and management of catecholamine secreting glomus tumors. *Laryngoscope* 1984;94:1008.
128. Million R, Cassisi N, Wittes R. Cancer of the head and neck. In: DeVita V, Hellman S, Rosenberg S, eds. *Cancer: principles and practice of oncology*, 2nd ed. Philadelphia: JB Lippincott, 1985:407.
129. Brown J. Glomus jugulare tumors: methods and difficulties of diagnosis and surgical treatment. *Laryngoscope* 1967;77:26.
130. Parkin J. Familial multiple glomus tumors and pheochromocytomas. *Ann Otol Rhinol Laryngol* 1981;90:60.
131. Van Baars F, Van den Brock P, Cremers C, Veldman J. Familial non-chromaffinic paragangliomas (glomus tumors): clinical aspects. *Laryngoscope* 1981;91:988.
132. Van Baars F, Cremers C, Van den Brock P, Veldman J. Familiar non-chromaffinic paragangliomas (glomus tumors): clinical and genetic aspects [Abridged]. *Acta Otolaryngol* 1981;91:589.
133. McCaffrey T, Meyer F, Michels V, Piepgras D, Marion M. Familial paragangliomas of the head and neck. *Arch Otolaryngol Head Neck Surg* 1994;120:1211.
134. Zaslav A, Mvssiorek D, Mucia C, Fox J. Cytogenetic analysis of tissues from patients with familial paragangliomas of the head and neck. *Head Neck* 1995;17:102.
135. Spector G, Ciralski R, Maisel R, Ogura J IV. Multiple glomus tumors in the head and neck. *Laryngoscope* 1975;85:1066.
136. Irons G, Weiland L, Brown W. Paragangliomas of the neck. Clinical and pathologic analysis of 116 cases. *Surg Clin North Am* 1977;57:575.
137. Bickerstaff E, Howell J. The neurological importance of tumors of the glomus jugulare. *Brain* 1953;76:576.
138. Revak C, Morris S, Alexander G. Pheochromocytoma and recurrent chemodectomas over a 25-year period. *Radiology* 1971;100:53.
139. El Fiky F, Paparella M. A metastatic glomus jugulare tumor. A temporal bone report. *Am J Otol* 1984;5:197.
140. Arias-Stella J, Valcarel J. Chief cell hyperplasias in human carotid body at high altitudes. Physiologic and pathologic significance. *Hum Pathol* 1976;7:361.
141. Borsanyi S. Glomus jugulare tumors. *Laryngoscope* 1962;72:1336.
142. Taylor M, Alford B, Greenberg S. Metastasis of glomus jugulare tumors. *Arch Otolaryngol* 1965;82:5.
143. Crouzet G, Vasdev A, Lambrinidis M, et al. Spinal metastasis of carotid paragangliomas. *J Neuroradiol* 1989;16:172.
144. Spector G, Sobol S, Thawley S, Maisel R, Ogura J. Panel discussion: glomus jugulare tumors of the temporal bone. *Laryngoscope* 1979;89:1628.
145. Druck N, Spector G, Ciralsky R, Ogura J. Malignant glomus vagale. *Arch Otolaryngol* 1976;102:634.
146. Barnes L, Taylor S. Carotid body paragangliomas: a clinicopathologic and DNA analysis of 13 cases. *Arch Otolaryngol Head Neck Surg* 1990;116:447.
147. Granger J, Houn H. Head and neck paragangliomas: a clinicopathologic study with DNA flow cytometry. *South Med J* 1990;83:1407.
148. Lack E, Cubilla A, Woodruff J. Paragangliomas of the head and neck region. A pathologic study of tumors from 71 patients. *Hum Pathol* 1979;10:191.
149. Kliewer K, Wen D, Cancilla P, Cochran A. Paragangliomas: assessment of prognosis by histologic, immunohistochemical, and ultrastructural techniques. *Hum Pathol* 1989; 20:29.
150. Barnes L. Paraganglioma of the larynx. *ORL J Otorhinolaryngol Relat Spec* 1991;53:220.
151. Someren A, Karcioglu Z. Malignant vagal paraganglioma. *Am J Clin Pathol* 1977;68:400.
152. Heinrich M, Harris A, Bell W. Metastatic intravagal paraganglioma. *Am J Med* 1985;78:1017.
153. Nixon D, York R, McConnel F. Spontaneous remission of metastatic paraganglioma. *Am J Med* 1987;83:805.
154. Leonetti N, Brackman D. Glomus vagale tumor: the significance of early vocal cord paralysis. *Otolaryngol Head Neck Surg* 1989;100:533.
155. Hirsch B, Johnson J, Black F, Meyers E. Paraganglioma of vagal origin. *Otolaryngol Head Neck Surg* 1982;90:708.
156. Nunez D, Lang N, Pollack J. Associated carotid body tumor and pharyngeal pouch. *J Laryngol Otol* 1989;103:531.
157. Ferlito A, Barnes L, Wenig BM. Identification, classification, treatment, and prognosis of laryngeal paraganglioma. Review of the literature and eight new cases. *Ann Otol Rhinol Laryngol* 1994;103:525.
158. Mischkle R, Balkany T. Skull base approach to glomus jugulare tumors. *Laryngoscope* 1987;90:89.
159. Glasscock M, Harris P, Newsome G. Glomus tumors: diagnosis and treatment. *Laryngoscope* 1974;84:2006.
160. Cummings B, Beale F, Garrell P. The treatment of glomus tumors in the temporal bone by megavoltage radiation. *Cancer* 1984;53:2635.
161. Kim J, Elkon D, Lim M. Optimum dose of radiotherapy for chemodectomas of the middle ear. *Int J Radiat Oncol Biol Phys* 1980;6:815.
162. Boyle J, Shimm D, Coulthard S. Radiation therapy for paragangliomas of the temporal bone. *Laryngoscope* 1900;8:896.
163. Cole JM, Beiler D. Long-term results of treatment for glomus jugulare and glomus vagale tumors with radiotherapy. *Laryngoscope* 1994;104:1461.
164. Valdagni P, Amichett M. Radiation therapy of carotid body tumors. *Am J Clin Oncol* 1990;13:45.
165. Peyzant P, Chow J, Easley J. Twenty-five years experience with radiation therapy for temporal bone chemodectomas. *Int J Radiat Oncol Biol Phys* 1989;17:1303.
166. Schwaber M, Gussack G, Kirkpatrick W. The role of radiation therapy in the management of catecholamine secreting glomus tumors. *Otolaryngol Head Neck Surg* 1988;98:150.
167. Guran S, Tali E. p53 and p161NK4A mutations during the progression of glomus tumor. *Pathol Oncol Res* 1999;5:41.
168. Evenson L, Mendenhall W, Parsons J, Cassisi N. Radiotherapy in the management of chemodectomas of the carotid body and glomus vagale. *Head Neck* 1998;20:609.
169. Mumber M, Greven K. Control of advanced chemodectomas of the head and neck with irradiation. *Am J Clin Oncol* 1995;18:389.
170. Wang M, Hussey D, Doornbos J, Vigliotti A, Wen B. Chemodectoma of the temporal bone: a comparison of surgical and radiotherapeutic results. *Int J Radiat Oncol Biol Phys* 1988;14:643.
171. Fuller A, Brown H, Harrison E. Chemodectomas of the glomus jugulare tumors. *Laryngoscope* 1967;77:218.
172. Biller H, Lawson W, Som P, Rosenfeld R. Glomus vagale tumors. *Ann Otol Rhinol Laryngol* 1989;98:21.
173. Jackson C. Basic surgical principles of neurotologic skull base surgery. *Laryngoscope* 1993;103[Suppl 60]:29.
174. de Jong A, Coker N, Jenkins H, Goepfert H, Alford B. Radiation therapy in the management of paragangliomas of the temporal bone. *Am J Otol* 1995;16:283.
175. Netterville J, Reilly M, Reiber M, Armstrong W. Carotid body tumors: a review of 30 patients with 46 tumors. *Laryngoscope* 1995;105:115.

SECTION 5

SUSAN D. MILLER
ROY B. SESSIONS

Rehabilitation after Treatment for Head and Neck Cancer

In the 1980s and 1990s, concern for posttreatment function restoration became a primary part of management of head and neck cancer. Conservation surgery, radiation strategies, reinnervation of free flaps, and larynx-sparing protocols continue to be used under various circumstances in an attempt to maintain or reestablish functional speech, voice, and swallowing in head and neck cancer patients. The ideal multidisciplinary concept requires interactions, therefore, among the surgical, radiation, and medical oncologists, reconstructive surgeons, speech pathologists, maxillofacial prosthodontists, dental oncologists, nutritionists, nurse oncologists, psychologists, audiologists, and social workers during pretreatment assessment and posttreatment intervention. To say the least, the standard for the complete head and neck team is complex.

Pretreatment counseling for persons with oral cavity and pharyngeal cancer is well established; the same should apply to organ preservation patients with laryngeal and hypopharyngeal cancers. Patients benefit from discussions with the speech pathologist regarding swallowing and voice and speech difficulties that can result from radiation therapy and chemotherapy regimens. Regrettably, however, patients entering organ preservation protocols often are inadequately counseled, if at all. Should failure of the treatment protocol occur, surgery is performed immediately, and the patient and family are forced to enter a frightening and stressful period unprepared for either the surgical experience or the rehabilitation that lies ahead. Optimal rehabilitation for all patients requires consideration of future strategies should one particular treatment plan fail.

PRETREATMENT ASSESSMENT

Preoperative consultation with the speech pathologist should be scheduled soon after the physician has made the final diagnosis and a treatment plan is formulated. During this consultation, the speech pathologist reviews what the patient already knows and further explains normal anatomy and physiology as well as the anticipated changes resulting from treatment. Patients with glottic carcinoma who are scheduled to be treated with radiation are counseled regarding vocal changes and swallowing difficulties that might occur during or after the treatment. Patients scheduled to undergo oral, pharyngeal cavity, or conservation laryngeal surgical procedures should be counseled in a special way, with an emphasis on their immediate postsurgical needs that relate to nasogastric, gastrostomy, and tracheostomy tubes. Additionally, short- and long-term rehabilitation strategies for speech, voice, and swallowing are summarily discussed in this initial consultation. The speech pathologist must be sensitive to the fine line between appropriate coverage and information overload; patients labor under a heavy emotional burden at this stage of their treatment and can easily be overwhelmed by someone insensitive to this potential. It is important, however, to accomplish as much of this as possible before the treatment. Depending on the specific treatment used, the patient's ability to communicate may be largely or completely impaired afterward. Even though there are substitute means of communicating during this period, none are as effective as an interactive dialogue between patient and speech pathologist. If loss of oral communication is expected after treatment, patients will need information regarding augmentative or alternative communication methods or devices. Patients scheduled for total laryngectomy learn about alternatives to natural voice: the availability of the electrolarynx and the mastery of esophageal or tracheoesophageal puncture speech (or both). Frequently, patients will consent to trial use of an electrolarynx and will order the recommended device before surgery. We have found that patients who are willing preoperatively to experiment with speech replacement devices feel more empowered and are relieved that they will be able to express their needs immediately after surgery. We frequently incorporate patient volunteers to meet patients and their families, thus allowing them to relate to and question a person who has had a similar treatment experience. Even candidates not scheduled for laryngectomy (i.e., laryngeal preservation protocol patients) should meet with the speech pathologist to discuss potential problems with voice and swallowing during or after the treatment.

DIAGNOSTIC EVALUATION

The correct rehabilitative effort after treatment is enhanced greatly by the initial evaluation of speech and swallowing. In matters pertaining to potential speech rehabilitation, baseline reading samples of standardized articulation sentences, nonnasal and nasal paragraphs, and conversational speech samples are audio-recorded from patients whose tongue, velum, or jaw will be affected by surgery. These recordings serve to establish baseline speech patterns of articulation, fluency, rate, dialect, intonation, and nasality. A spectrogram that portrays frequency, intensity, and format information descriptive of resonant frequencies of the vocal tract provides additional baseline data regarding tongue placement and resonance. Standardized articulation testing typically is not performed for patients undergoing treatment for early- or later-stage laryngeal carcinoma unless modification of the articulators (lips, tongue, cheek, etc.) is planned. The speech pathologist, however, should document any articulation, fluency, rate, or dialectal patterns observed during this conversation with the patient. Additionally, orofacial structures, sensation, and function should be carefully examined. Plans for pretreatment dental care or postoperative radiation are discussed at this time because they also can have an impact on articulation, voice, and deglutition. Finally, because of the fact that patients with hearing deficiencies often have difficulty in monitoring the intelligibility and precision of their articulation, it is important to evaluate hearing before treatment.

If preexisting swallowing problems are present, a modified barium swallow (MBS),[1] fiberoptic endoscopic evaluation of swallowing (FEES),[2] or FEES with sensory testing (FEESST)[3] should be performed. If dysphagia does exist postoperatively, it is important that these studies be performed at the time to aid in the development of a management strategy. The MBS is a videofluoroscopic study of the motor aspects of the oral, pharyngeal, and esophageal stages of the swallow with varying food consistencies. This procedure permits measured amounts of barium bolus to be followed from the lips to the stomach and incorporates the effects of compensatory strategies, such as head position, chin tuck, and the like.[4] Because of its clear documentation of the oral preparatory and oral stages of the swallow, the MBS is ideal for patients with oral-stage dysphagia; in fact, it is the diagnostic test of choice. If pharyngeal or laryngeal swallowing problems exist, however, the FEES or FEESST should be performed. The FEES uses a fiber-optic nasoendoscope to observe the pharyngeal and laryngeal structures directly during the pharyngeal phase of the swallow. A bolus of contrasting color is used to note premature spillage into the hypopharynx or laryngeal vestibule before swallowing and vocal fold closure and the presence of residuum in the hypopharynx and laryngopharynx after a swallow. Although penetration (i.e., aspiration) may be identified during a FEES or MBS examination,[5] the primary purpose of these procedures is to analyze the motor components of swallowing. The FEESST combines the FEES with a technique that determines laryngopharyngeal sensory discrimination thresholds by endoscopically delivering air pulse stimuli to the mucosa that is innervated by the superior laryngeal nerve.[3]

Because vocal and aerodynamic parameters may be affected by the presence of a lesion or a biopsy (or both), baseline acoustic and aerodynamic analysis should be performed on all early glottic cancer patients, regardless of whether destined for radiation, microsurgery, or laser excision. Vocal measures of fundamental frequency, amplitude, frequency perturbation (jitter), amplitude perturbation (shimmer), and noise-to-harmonic ratio are obtained from a sustained vowel *a*. Sophisticated instruments, such as the Computerized Speech Laboratory (Kay Elemetrics Corp., Lincoln Park, NJ), Speech Viewer III (IBM, Austin, TX), Dr. Speech (Tiger Electronics, Seattle, WA), and Speech Master III (Speech-Master, Vero Beach, FL), all obtain and record these measures quickly. Baseline airflow rates, subglottal pressure, and laryngeal resistance are calculated using the Aerophone II (Kay Elemetrics), Glottal Enterprise MS-100 (Syracuse, NY), or Nagashima Phonatory Function Analyzer. Documentation of these measures prior to treatment and at specific intervals during and after treatment is important for objective comparison of vocal changes after surgery or radiation therapy (or both) for glottic carcinoma.

POSTTREATMENT INTERVENTION

SPEECH AND SWALLOWING AFTER ORAL CAVITY SURGERY

Restoration of speech and swallow function after glossectomy appears to be highly dependent on a number of factors: the quantity and mobility of residual tongue after surgery, the particular reconstructive technique used, the integrity of motor and sensory nerve supply to the tissue, the functional recovery after reconstruction, the degree of scarring and fibrosis to the residual tongue musculature after surgery and radiation, the early intervention of speech therapy, and patient psychosocial factors, such as age, medical condition, motivation, and family support.[6–8] Even patients undergoing resection of the anterior portion or less than 50% of the mobile tongue can develop a delayed swallowing reflex and reduced ability to manipulate the bolus in the oral cavity.[5] The return of normal speech intelligibility and deglutition for small, anterior tongue lesions of up to 3 cm has been reported.[9,10] Articulation deficits are mild and often characterized by only a lisp. Speech therapy should focus on oral motor exercises to achieve adequate linguoalveolar and linguopalatal contact for accurate phoneme productions.

Owing to decreased tongue bulk and mobility, patients who have been treated for larger tongue lesions present with poor bolus formation, poor bolus manipulation, delayed elicitation of the swallow reflex, and increased oral transit time.[1] Finally, because of the loss of tongue volume, glossopalatal contact and closure are often severely compromised: Vertical capabilities of the tongue are diminished. Compensatory speech patterns, such as contacting the tongue behind the lower teeth, are used to obtain intelligible linguoalveolar (*t, d, n, l, s, z*) and linguopalatal (*sh, ch*) sound production if the tongue cannot contact the alveolar ridge or palate. If contact remains difficult, a palatal drop prosthesis is often helpful in lowering the contact point of the palate; thus, the vertical deficiency of the tongue is diminished, and linguopalatal contact is achieved.[5,12]

Speech and swallowing difficulties can be profound when more than 50% of the tongue is sacrificed; when the base of tongue, floor of mouth, or lateral pharyngeal walls are altered[13]; or when an extensive oral lesion requires a composite resection that might include total glossectomy, floor-of-mouth resection, radical neck dissection, and mandibulectomy.[14,15] Reconstructive methods for large tongue or floor-of-mouth tumors (or both) in which split-thickness skin grafts, reinnervated free flaps,[10,16] and pectoralis major[17] myocutaneous flaps are used generally provide a speech and swallowing outcome that is superior to those techniques in which the defect is closed primarily.[18,19] In particular, the bilobed, sensate radial forearm flap allows maximum functional speech and swallowing return after extensive oral cavity surgery.[20–22] The design allows for one part of the flap to provide bulk for restoring the floor of the mouth, whereas the other lobe provides volume to the mobile tongue.[23] Excellent speech and swallowing have been reported using the infrahyoid muscle flap for medium-sized defects in the floor of the mouth, tongue, buccal mucosa, and lateral pharyngeal wall.[24] Salibian et al.[25] found that the successful outcome of swallowing and speech correlated with the shape and position of the tongue root and the surface area of the floor of the mouth.

In the realm of nonsurgical treatment of tongue cancer, excellent to good functional speech and swallowing outcomes were reported in 18 of 20 patients with tongue base lesions (11 of 12 patients with stage T1 or T2 cancer; 8 of 9 patients with stage T3 or T4 cancer) treated with external-beam radiation followed by an interstitial implant boost with iodine 125 several weeks later.[26]

As reconstructive techniques and organ preservation protocols proliferate, additional diagnostic studies, such as videosonography,[27] high-speed cineradiography,[28] and perfusion manometry[29] may be needed to measure and compare functional aspects of swallowing recovery accurately after different radiologic and rehabilitative treatments. The short- and long-term effects of radiation therapy, chemotherapy, or surgery on the sensory aspects of swallowing also will become more apparent as FEESST becomes an integral part of cancer management.

VOICE AND SWALLOWING CHANGES AFTER TREATMENT OF LARYNGEAL CANCER

There is general agreement that voice quality in early glottic cancers (T1a and T2b) is better after radiation than before radiation[30–32] and better after radiation than after surgery.[30,31] Studies vary, however, regarding whether the postradiation voice ever becomes normal. Harrison[33] reported an ultimate return to normal voice within 3 months after completion of radiation therapy in nearly all irradiated T1 and T2 glottic cancer patients. Tsunoda[34] found ultimate return of normal mucosal wave motion stroboscopically in his patients with early glottic cancer that had been treated with radiation. Other studies report that voice after radiation therapy cannot be considered normal. Dagli et al.[30] investigated vocal parameters in patients successfully treated with radiation therapy for T1a and T1b glottic carcinoma. They found less than normal values for maximum vocal intensity, dynamic vocal intensity, range, jitter, and mean fundamental frequency. Aref et al.[32] reported abnormal acoustic and aerodynamic measures on T1 glottic cancer patients 3 months to 7 years after completion of radiation therapy. Increased laryngeal resistance that affected communication function was reported in laryngeal cancer patients treated with chemotherapy and radiation.[35] Longitudinal multiinstitutional standardized stroboscopic, acoustic, and aerodynamic investigations of early-stage glottic carcinoma patients are needed to allow more systematic predictions of vocal quality after radiation and surgical treatment. At present, there seem to be several predictors of poor vocal quality: Vocal fold stripping before radiation and continued smoking during and after radiation therapy predicted worse voice quality.[36] Nevertheless, as changes in vocal quality are common among patients after either radiation therapy or laser excision, patients should be seen by the speech pathologist for at least one posttreatment therapy session. Adherence to a vocal hygiene program with certain daily exercises results in a more efficient, resonant voice.

Patients in whom radiation therapy for early glottic carcinoma has failed or selected glottic lesions that are not suitable for radiation are frequently treated with conservation surgery (i.e., hemilaryngectomy). Voice and swallowing problems after hemilaryngectomy vary according to the extent of surgery. For example, if the arytenoid has been resected, the risk for aspiration is greater. If the hemilaryngectomy is isolated to one true vocal fold, one false vocal fold and the ventricle, with preservation of the epiglottis, swallowing may be improved with a chin tuck to assist in airway protection and head turning toward the operated side to direct food from the compromised area.[5] Vocal characteristics of the hemilaryngectomee have been described as rough, low-pitched, and breathy, all of which are probably due to compensatory efforts to achieve adequate glottal adduction.[37] Therapy techniques, such as forced adduction exercises, digital pressure to the side of the thyroid cartilage, decreased speaking rate, and increased phrasing, may decrease vocal strain, improve voice quality, and increase vocal intensity by reducing glottal opening.[5] Surgical augmentation techniques deserve consideration to improve glottal closure.

Those supraglottic cancers that fail radiation are not candidates for supraglottic laryngectomy; however, those nonradiated patients with supraglottic lesions who are able to undergo supraglottic laryngectomy not infrequently experience dysphagia due to the combined effects of supraglottic sensory denervation, incomplete posterior motion of the partially resected tongue base, restricted arytenoid motion, partial closure of the airway, and delays in bolus propulsion from narrowing at the laryngeal entrance.[38] These patients must avoid thin liquids and learn the special techniques and maneuvers of supraglottic[5,39] and supersupraglottic[40,41] swallow to ensure feeding safety. Commercially available thickening agents may be used to thicken the consistency of thin liquids for safer swallowing. Supraglottic laryngectomy patients frequently experience breathiness or hoarseness (or both), which may respond to short-term voice therapy. They may also demonstrate an increase in fundamental frequency, which may result from added tension to the vocal cords, thought to be the result of forced adduction exercises.[5]

It is not widely appreciated that a significant percentage of total laryngectomy patients experience dysphagia. Although they often do not complain of this, various studies have reported that 10% to 58% of laryngectomees have the problem,[42–44] which appears to center around the pharyngoesophageal (PE) segment.[43] Total laryngectomy may produce increased resistance to bolus transfer from stenosis and decrease of negative pressure in the upper esophageal segment. Resections of the hyoid bone and thyroid cartilage further aggravate this problem by allowing the pharyngeal lumen to collapse.[45]

Dysphagia that is secondary to surgery, chemotherapy, radiation therapy, and concomitant chemoradiation can cause swallowing dysfunction by compromising salivary flow; by causing edema, myositis, and fibrosis; by causing a delayed pharyngeal motor response stimulus; by decreasing laryngopharyngeal sensation; by causing pharyngeal incoordination; and by decreasing laryngeal elevation as a result of scaring and fibrosis.[45,49] Patients in whom dysphagia is suspected should undergo objective assessment with MBS, FEES, or FEESST. The MBS and FEES primarily analyze the motor components of swallowing, whereas the FEESST analyzes the sensory component that is frequently present in patients who have undergone conservation laryngeal operations and also in patients treated on preservation protocols. The short- and long-term effects of radiation therapy, chemotherapy or surgery on the sensory aspects of swallowing will almost certainly become more apparent as we learn and extend the range of FEESST-type testing as a routine part of cancer management.

For some laryngectomy patients, concerns regarding loss of speech are more important than survival itself.[47] Alternative voice sources for the laryngectomee include the use of a pneumatic or an electronic speech aid, esophageal speech, or the gold-standard tracheoesophageal puncture (TEP) speech. Patients who have undergone a partial or total glossectomy are unable to use these alternative voice sources, and they should be introduced to computerized speaking systems or talking keyboards.

Artificial Larynges

A 1987 study of voice rehabilitation practices revealed that the use of an artificial speaking device was widely recommended by 90% of 400 head and neck surgeons surveyed, in many cases as a temporary means of communication after total laryngectomy.[48] These battery-operated or pneumatic devices simulate vocal sound, are relatively inexpensive, are easy to operate, and can be used by a patient 1 to 2 days after surgery. These devices continue to serve a useful purpose, and surgeons and speech pathologists should encourage all patients to own an artificial device as a primary or auxiliary speech system. Pneumatic devices consist of a piece that fits over the tracheal stoma, a unit containing a reed that produces sound, and a tube that directs sound into the mouth to be articulated. These particular devices are less popular in the United States than they are in Europe.

On the other hand, a variety of battery-operated, hand-held artificial larynges (electrolarynges) are currently available. Examples are illustrated in Figure 30.5-1. The Cooper-Rand Electronic Speech Aid (Luminaud Inc., Mentor, OH) is an electrolarynx that is used exclusively with an intraoral adapter. This adapter directs sound into the oral cavity through a tube placed in the mouth. The NuVois 1 and NuVois 2 (Mountain Precision Manufacturing, Boise, ID), Servox Inton (Siemens Hearing Instruments, Inc., Prospect Heights, IL), Romet (Romet, Inc., Las Vegas, NV), OptiVox (Bivona Medical Technologies, Gary, IN), TruTone and SolaTone (Griffin Laboratories, Temecula, CA), Denrick (Denrick, Inc., Honolulu, HI), SPKR (UNI Mfg. Co., Ontario, OR; not pictured), and Amplicord model 55 (Amplicord, Inc., Rome, Italy) are neck-type devices that transmit sound through the tissues of the neck into the oral cavity for speech production. These devices are activated with an on-off switch and are equipped with an adapter so that they can be used either as intraoral or when pressed against the neck. The availability of both options is important because patients can use the intraoral adapter immediately after surgery when the neck is edematous. The Amplicord model 95 is pressure-activated as it contacts the neck rather than being activated by a switch. The UltraVoice (UltraVoice, Ltd., Berwyn, PA; Fig. 30.5-2) is an intraoral electrolarynx custom-built into a denture or retainer and activated by a remote control switch.

Esophageal Speech

Esophageal speech involves learning to inject or inhale air into the esophagus through the reservoir created by surgical closure of the PE segment or gullet after laryngectomy. The trapped air is then released through the upper esophageal segment, which is the vibratory source for sound in the laryngectomee.[49–53]

Typically, the speech pathologist encourages the laryngectomee to attempt esophageal sound soon after the patient is able to swallow food comfortably. The details of the techniques taught by speech pathologists are beyond the scope of this text, but certain basic principles should be pointed out. The patient traps air in the mouth and forces it into the esophagus. Some patients learn the inhalation method, in which a lowered pressure in the esophageal segment relative to atmospheric pressure allows air to enter the gullet; thus, the source and the location of vibratory sound are fulfilled.

Even though esophageal speech can be introduced to the patient 1 or 2 weeks after the total laryngectomy, the development of functional capabilities with this method may take from 6 months to 1 year to learn; in fact, some patients never master it. Previous reports regarding the success rate in learning esophageal speech have varied from 26% to 55%[54–57]; however, Fujii[58] found that 74% (51 of 69) of their patients successfully used esophageal speech in daily communication. Age was the most important factor in success and failure. Ninety percent of the patients in this study who were younger than 60 were successful in learning esophageal speech as compared to 10% of those older than 75.[58] Although motivation and age appear to be

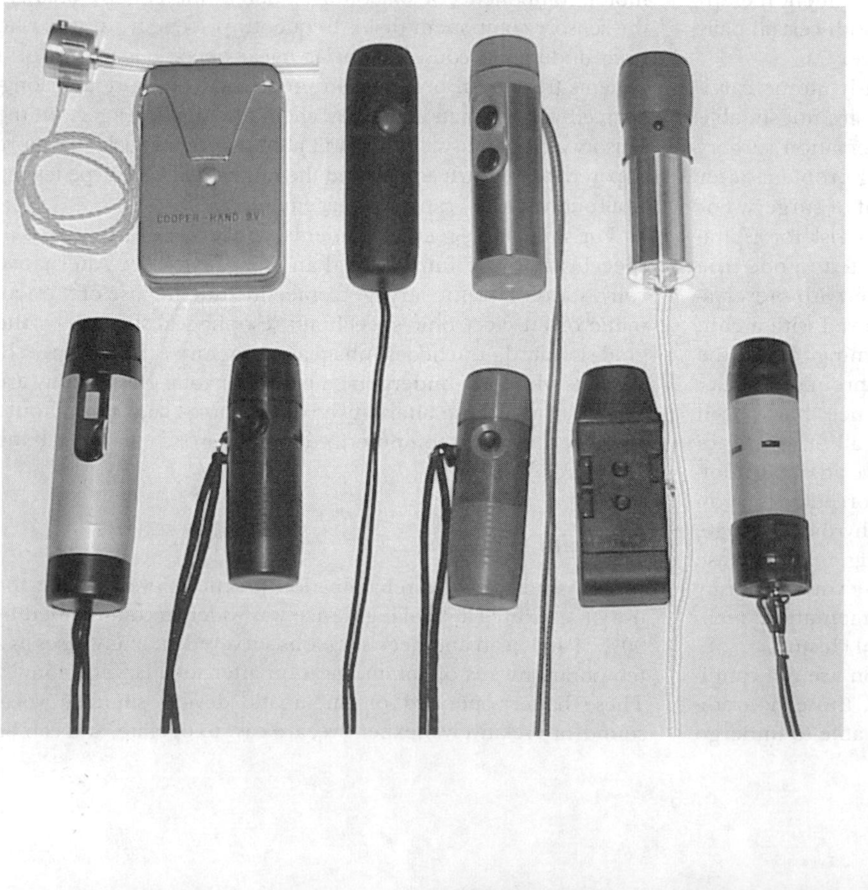

FIGURE 30.5-1. Various speech aids. *Top, left to right,* the Cooper-Rand Electronic Speech Aid (Luminaud Inc., Mentor, OH); the NuVois 2 (Mountain Precision Manufacturing, Boise, ID); the Servox Inton (Siemens Hearing Instruments, Inc., Prospect Heights, IL); the Romet (Romet, Inc., Las Vegas, NV); *bottom, left to right,* the OptiVox (Bivona Medical Technologies, Gary, IN); the TruTone and SolaTone (Griffin Laboratories, Temecula, CA); the Denrick (Denrick, Inc., Honolulu, HI); and the Amplicord model 55 (Amplicord, Inc., Rome, Italy).

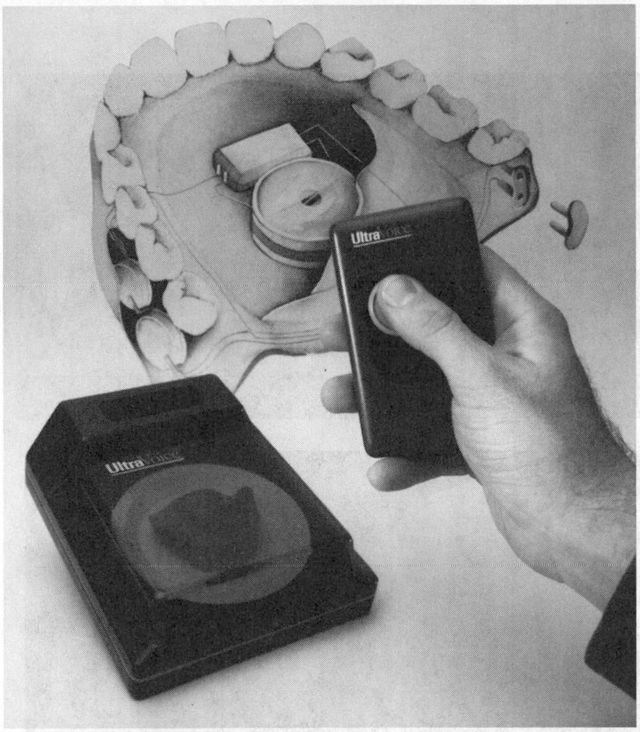

FIGURE 30.5-2. UltraVoice (courtesy of UltraVoice, Ltd., Malvern, PA). (From Miller SD, Levine DK. Rehabilitation of speech, voice and swallowing functions after treatment of head and neck cancer. In: Harrison LB, Sessions RB, Hong WK, eds. *Head and neck cancer.* Philadelphia: Lippincott-Raven Publishers, 1999, with permission.)

important to the achievement of esophageal speech,[56,59] abnormalities of the vibrating esophageal segment—tonic and hypertonic spasms—are the most common reasons cited for esophageal speech failure.[60,61] Botulinum toxin type A injections have been used to combat other muscular spasmodic conditions, including the cricopharyngeus muscle spasm sometimes responsible for failure of TEP patients to achieve satisfactory speech.[62,63] Perhaps some of the speakers who cannot master esophageal speech would benefit from this same treatment.

In patients in whom esophageal speaking has failed, the tonicity or relaxation of that esophageal segment that vibrates (the PE segment) can be accurately evaluated by simultaneous use of videofluoroscopy and esophageal insufflation.[64] This is not routinely performed in the postoperative laryngectomee. An easier and reliable way to assess initial opening pressures of the PE segment is a portable manometry system that can be used 4 weeks after laryngectomy.[65] An initial opening pressure of between 15 and 20 mm Hg has been found to correlate with the production of a good esophageal voice.[65,66]

TRACHEOESOPHAGEAL PUNCTURE

Most head and neck surgeons and most professionals who rehabilitate laryngectomy patients think that in properly selected patients, TEP, introduced by Singer and Blom in 1980,[67] is the standard of care for reconstitution of voice after laryngectomy. Rather than relying on the trapping of air in the esophagus, the creation of a permanent puncture through the tracheoesophageal wall permits the shunting of pulmonary air into and up the esophagus; thus, the basis for noise—vibration of the PE segment walls—is generated. Importantly, unlike esophageal speech, the reservoir of air does not depend on the gulping or trapping of air; instead it is limited only by expiratory capacity and, as such, more closely resembles normal voice. A valved prosthesis is placed into the puncture and, when the tracheal stoma is occluded, directs pulmonary air into the esophagus for speech. The one-way valve design of the prosthesis prevents aspiration from the esophagus into the trachea. An outer housing that contains a soft diaphragm allows normal respiration during silent periods; however, when speech is used, an alteration of the patient's expiratory effort shuts off the diaphragm, thus diverting the air through the tracheoesophageal conduit into the esophagus. This external housing, called a *tracheostoma breathing valve*, was developed in 1982, and is of immeasurable value in rehabilitation of these patients because it eliminates the need for manual occlusion of the stoma during speech.[68] A patient can, therefore, wear normal clothing over the lower neck to cover the apparatus, as there is no need for involvement of the hands. For a historical review of the evolution of voice restoration procedures and prostheses, the reader is referred to Singer[69] and Singer and Blom.[70] Although TEP is the method of choice for voice and speech rehabilitation in the United States, some patients and some cultures are not so enthusiastic about its implementation.

Initially, TEP was performed as a second surgery in patients who had been laryngectomized; however, many surgeons and speech pathologists now prefer that TEP be done at the time of the laryngectomy. The controversy as to the value of the secondary versus primary TEP is ongoing and is unlikely to end. Recently, Chan[71] performed a TEP as an outpatient office procedure using a flexible endoscope with local anesthesia and intravenous sedation. Those surgeons and speech pathologists who advocate secondary or delayed TEP think that waiting for 1 to 3 months after laryngectomy allows better control of factors, such as stoma size, vibration of the PE segment, and migration of the puncture site after radiation. Proponents of the primary puncture argue that patients are psychologically uplifted[72] by the fact that they can speak 3 weeks after surgery. Furthermore, primary TEP proponents cite the value of technical simplicity, effectiveness, low morbidity, and cost-effectiveness of the one-stage procedure. Success rates for both primary and secondary procedures are reported to be between 73% and 95%, respectively.[73–75] Regardless of time of puncture, an average of 7 hours of speech therapy is needed to learn to manage the prosthesis and to obtain optimal communication using the TEP.[73] Researchers have reported a decrease in TEP speech success rates from an initial 84% to 67% at 9 months[74] and 65% at 10 years[75] due to such "patient factors" as delays in seeking medical attention when the valve becomes dislodged and failure to care for the equipment properly. Although the Blom-Singer technique is popular in the United States, specialists in other parts of the world favor different methods to restore phonation.[76] Most interesting was a study by Quer,[77] who performed TEP at the time of the laryngectomy and also provided intensive esophageal speech instruction to 24 patients. Seventy percent of the patients (16 of 23) later chose to use esophageal speech rather than TEP speech even though they agreed that TEP speech was superior to esophageal speech.

Candidacy for Tracheoesophageal Puncture

The success of voice restoration depends on a multidisciplinary team committed to thorough patient assessment, consistent

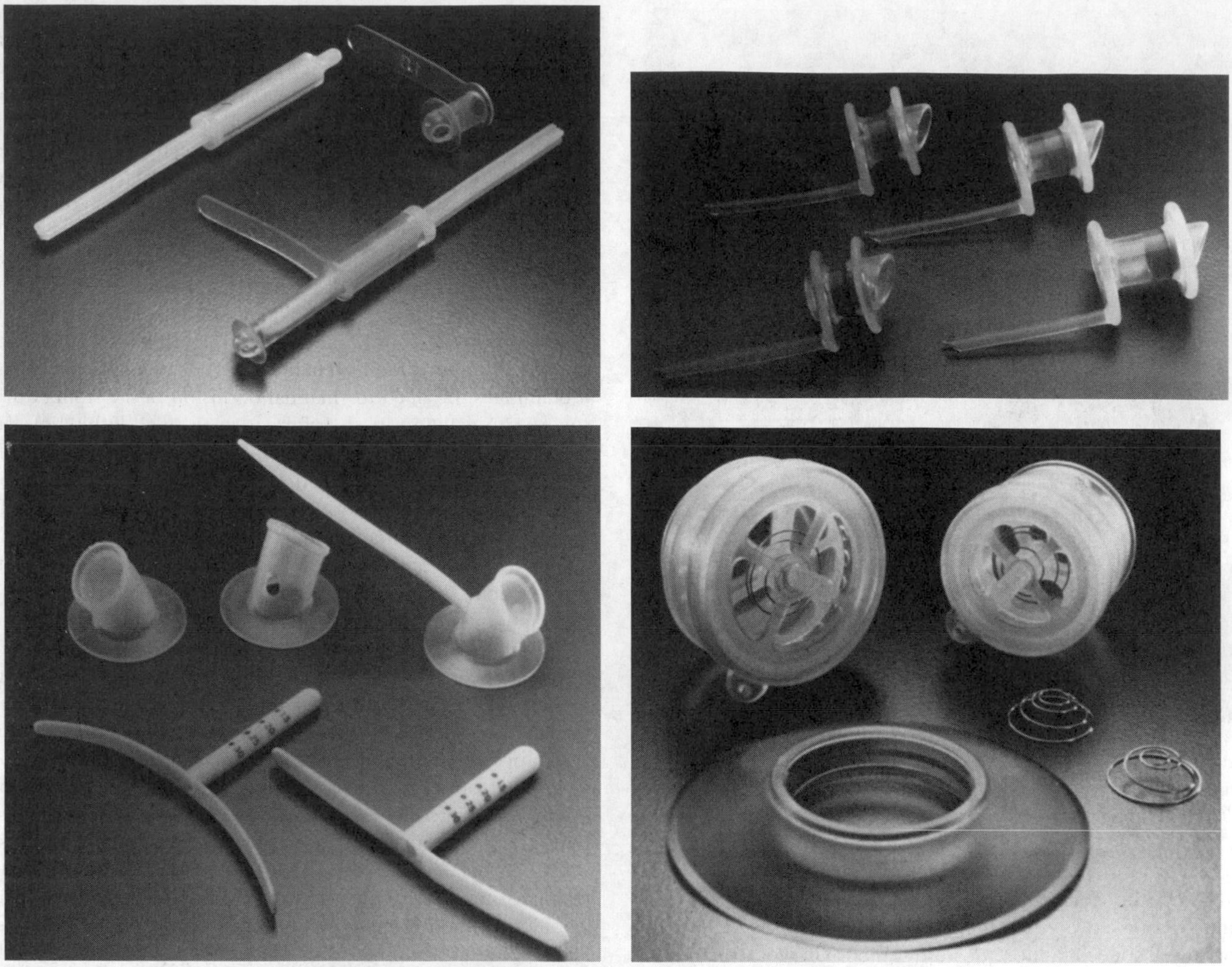

FIGURE 30.5-3. Bivona and Atos voice restoration products. **A:** Bivona ultra-low-resistance prostheses and inserter. **B:** Bivona-Colorado button, template and sizing devices. Bivona-Colorado products are designed in cooperation with Bruce Jafek, M.D. and Bryan Spofford, M.D. **C:** Atos Medical Provox 2 prostheses. **D:** Bivona Tracheostoma Valve II and housing assembly. (Courtesy of Bivona Medical Technologies, Gary, IN.) (From Miller SD, Levine DK. Rehabilitation of speech, voice and swallowing functions after treatment of head and neck cancer. In: Harrison LB, Sessions RB, Hong WK, eds. *Head and neck cancer.* Philadelphia: Lippincott-Raven Publishers, 1999, with permission.)

management, and flexibility in problem solving. Success with TEP depends on good stoma construction, adequate stomal size, and accurate placement and angle of the TEP.[78] The tracheal stoma should be at least 1.5 cm and not retracted behind the manubrium. If stomal stenosis is a problem, a Bivona-Colorado stent can be used by the surgeon to create the puncture. A Bivona-Colorado prosthesis (Fig. 30.5-3), which is built into the tracheostoma vent, is inserted into the puncture.

Patients with emphysema, severe allergies, or pulmonary complications are generally not good TEP candidates, owing to copious amounts of secretions and reduced air volume associated with these conditions. The patient's cognitive status, physical health, and desire for communication should be considered before TEP. The presence or absence of radiation therapy does not seem to have a significant relationship to the success or failure of TEP.[79]

Because of the development of low-resistance, self-retaining prostheses inserted by the speech pathologist or surgeon (or both) and composed of materials designed to last approximately 3 to 6 months, manual dexterity and visual acuity are no longer essential for the use of this technology. These prostheses include Inhealth Indwelling (Inhealth Technologies, Santa Barbara, CA; Fig. 30.5-4); Provox-2[80] (Atos Medical, Sweden, Milwaukee, WI; see Fig. 30.5-4); Voicemaster[81] (Amsterdam, Netherlands), and Nijdam[82] (Sweden; not pictured). The Provox (Atos Medical), and Groningen prostheses (Groningen, Holland; not pictured) are popular indwelling prostheses in Europe.

In following up TEP patients over 13 years, Lavertu[83] found that the absence of PE stricture was the only significant predictor of good to excellent speech. Because the tonicity of the PE segment in a primary puncture patient before the laryngectomy cannot be assessed, surgeons often perform a pharyngeal constrictor myotomy, a unilateral pharyngeal plexus neurectomy, or a unilateral pharyngeal plexus neurectomy with a cricopharyngeal myotomy at the time of surgery. Although all three methods are equally effective in preventing pharyngospasms, Singer et al.[84] advocate use of the pharyngeal plexus neurectomy, as it preserves the vascular supply to the pharyngeal wall and preserves any residual resting tone in the PE segment, resulting in a higher speaking fundamental frequency compared to the other methods.

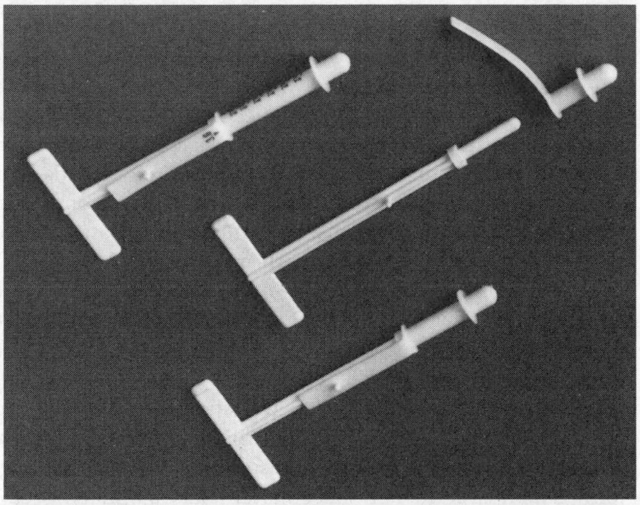
A

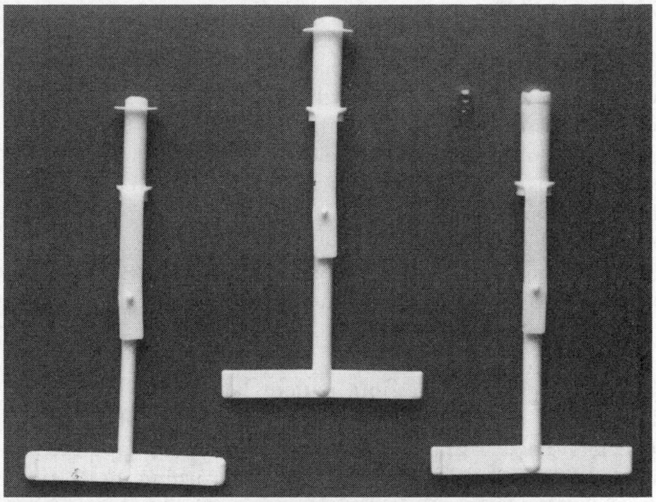
B

C

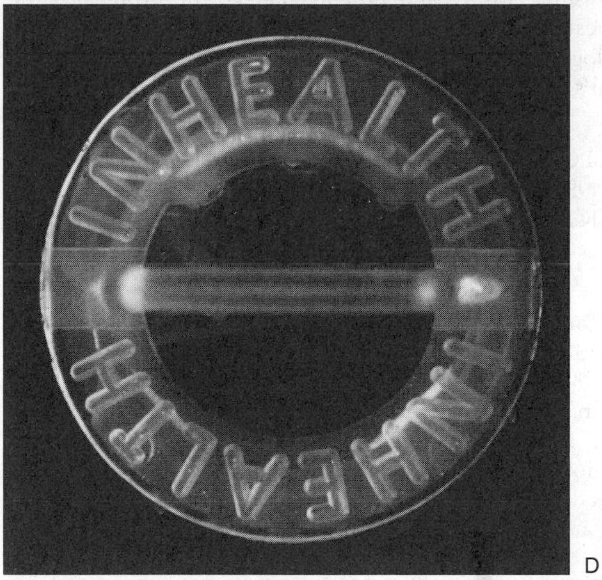

D

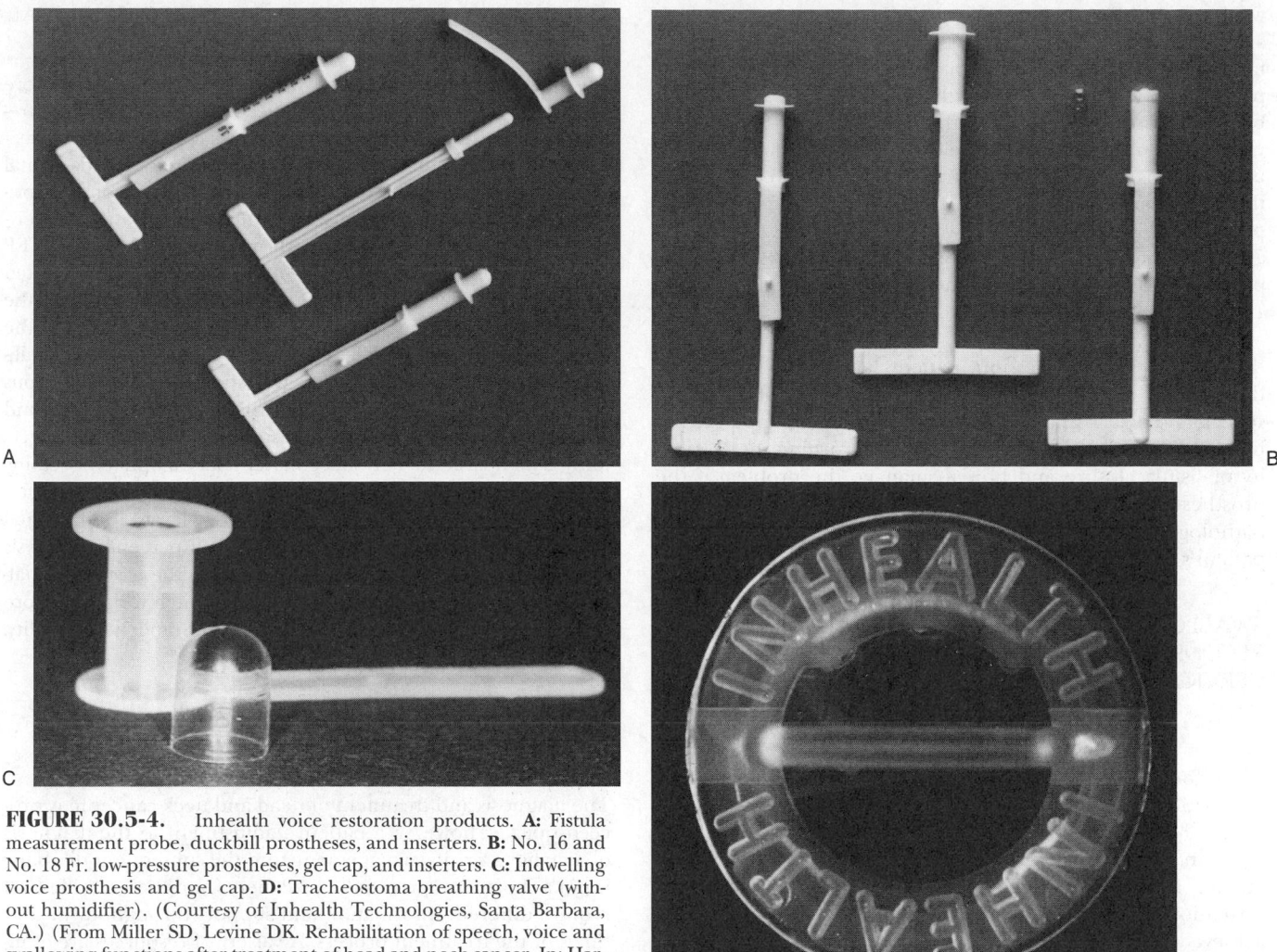

FIGURE 30.5-4. Inhealth voice restoration products. **A:** Fistula measurement probe, duckbill prostheses, and inserters. **B:** No. 16 and No. 18 Fr. low-pressure prostheses, gel cap, and inserters. **C:** Indwelling voice prosthesis and gel cap. **D:** Tracheostoma breathing valve (without humidifier). (Courtesy of Inhealth Technologies, Santa Barbara, CA.) (From Miller SD, Levine DK. Rehabilitation of speech, voice and swallowing functions after treatment of head and neck cancer. In: Harrison LB, Sessions RB, Hong WK, eds. *Head and neck cancer.* Philadelphia: Lippincott-Raven Publishers, 1999, with permission.)

Many speech pathologists perform air insufflation testing before a secondary puncture, although the value of this has been challenged.[85] Lewin[86] reported greater than 90% success in predicting TEP failures when intraesophageal peak pressure levels are obtained in conjunction with the air insufflation test. The air insufflation test is performed by insertion of a transnasal catheter approximately 25 cm into the upper thoracic esophagus. The catheter is attached to a circular tracheostoma housing, which is secured to the patient's skin by an adhesive. As air is insufflated into the catheter, patients are instructed to inhale, occlude the stomal assembly, and sustain a vowel sound for as long as they can. Success is determined by patients' ability to sustain a vowel for 15 to 20 seconds and count from 1 to 15.[67] To ensure optimal results, it is important for the patient to feel relaxed and comfortable with the examiner. Multiple trials and a repeat visit are often necessary to confirm test results.

If insufflation testing fails but speech is achieved in a patient after a pharyngeal plexus nerve block with lidocaine, PE spasm is suspected. This should be confirmed via a videofluoroscopic MBS performed during rest and swallow and during speech with air insufflation. If the PE segment is confirmed to be highly resistant to airflow, botulinum toxin type A injection should be considered as a first-line treatment[87] before consideration of surgical procedures, such as a pharyngeal constrictor myotomy, a unilateral pharyngeal plexus neurectomy, or a unilateral pharyngeal plexus neurectomy with cricopharyngeal myotomy. If speech during the air insufflation test is faint or whispery, the PE segment may be hypotonic. Digital pressure on the outside of the neck may help to produce a stronger sound. The existence of hypotonicity is not a contraindication for TEP, although it may indicate the need for a neck band or digital pressure postoperatively to enhance contact of intraluminal vibratory surfaces.

Post–Tracheoesophageal Puncture Intervention

With primary TEP, a catheter is placed in the newly created fistula that penetrates the posterior wall of the trachea and enters the esophageal lumen. The catheter provides a stent that keeps the fistula open during the weeks in which the tract is regenerating mucosae. Removal of the catheter and fitting of the voice prosthesis in a primary TEP patient generally takes place from 10 to 21 days after surgery.[88] If radiation therapy is planned, the patient should be advised that speech may diminish during the third to fourth week of radiation, owing to mucositis and radiation-induced edema. In the secondary, or delayed, TEP patient, the device is measured and inserted approximately 1 week. The 14-Fr. catheter placed during surgery is removed, and the patency of the tract is assessed by asking the patient to take a breath and say "Ah" on exhalation while the speech pathologist or patient occludes the stoma. If the tract is patent but sound cannot be attained, the patient can be fitted with a prosthesis but should be counseled that speech may not occur until there is further healing of the tissue tract. To determine the proper prosthesis size, the Inhealth fistula measurement probe (see Fig. 30.5-4) or the Bivona fitting kit (see Fig. 30.5-3) are used to measure the length of the fistula tract. Once appropriate length has been determined, the patient is fitted with a 16-Fr. duckbill or lower-resistance prosthesis (see Figs. 30.5-3 and 30.5-4).

During this initial session, patients are taught to occlude their stoma digitally. They are taught how to phrase their speech and how to apply appropriate abdominal support to initiate sound. Patients are also instructed regarding the possibility of fistula closure and how to manage the problem if the prosthesis becomes dislodged. It is essential that the speech pathologist be available for the first few days after fitting of a patient's prosthesis should problems arise.

SWALLOWING AND SPEECH AFTER EXTENSIVE RECONSTRUCTION OF THE PHARYNX OR CERVICAL ESOPHAGUS

Several researchers think that after extensive pharyngeal resection or cervical esophageal resection (or both), the tubed radial forearm free flap maximizes functional rehabilitation of the patient by providing the best swallowing and speech results.[89–91] Free jejunal transfer also has gained wide acceptance in PE reconstruction because the jejunum is well vascularized and is associated with a low incidence of fistula formation and stricture. Voice restoration has been successfully achieved in these jejunal interpositions with the creation of either a primary tracheojejunal shunt at the time of the surgery[92,93] or a secondary procedure.[94] Reconstruction with jejunal interposition and gastric pull-up have demonstrated better swallowing results than those with myocutaneous (pectoralis and latissimus dorsi) flaps, and colon interposition.[29,95] Performance of a TEP in gastric pull-up patients has been successful in certain small heterogeneous patient groups,[96,97] but this is unpredictable, and the overall experience is limited.

Dysphasia in jejunal interposition patients may occur from discoordination of jejunal peristalsis with occasional oral and nasal regurgitation. Regurgitation of food is frequently noted in the gastric pull-up patient, owing to an absent esophagogastric sphincter. These patients are encouraged to eat small meals throughout the day. From a functional and from a morbidity standpoint, the jejunal interposition is generally considered to be a superior method of reconstruction compared to the gastric pull-up.

Patients undergoing total laryngopharyngectomy or laryngopharyngoesophagectomy with jejunal graft reconstruction experience a lack of innervation and muscle in the wall of the jejunum that causes hypotonicity. Therefore, sound may be easier to attain than esophageal speech; however, it is often softer in intensity and limited to fewer syllables per air charge.[198] Voice quality is often described as *wet,* owing to mucus in the jejunum; however, the success rates of primary or secondary tracheojejunal puncture are reported to be 72% to 93%.[99–101]

COMPARISON OF ESOPHAGEAL, TRACHEOESOPHAGEAL PUNCTURE, AND NORMAL SPEECH

Acoustic and temporal studies indicate that TEP speech more closely approximates laryngeal speech in fundamental frequency, intensity, reading rate, percent silent time, and maximum phonation time.[102,103] Significantly higher fundamental frequencies were found during reading in neurectomized primary TEP patients as compared to primary TEP patients receiving myotomy or a neurectomy with myotomy. In addition, TEP speakers using the tracheostoma-breathing valve demonstrated faster speaking rates and fewer pauses. The valve prevents the escape of air sometimes observed with digital occlusion of the tracheostoma.[88] Although TEP speech in general is more intelligible and preferred over esophageal speech, the monotonous tone, voicing errors, and fricative errors are similar in TEP and esophageal speakers.[88] When TEP speech after a total laryngectomy is compared to TEP speech after a laryngopharyngectomy with pectoralis major flap reconstruction, no significant differences were noted for soft and loud intensity levels, fundamental frequency for soft voice, and jitter, although perceptual analysis revealed significant differences.[104] Speech in the tracheojejunal-esophageal puncture patients has even less pitch variation, more noise in the signal, shorter mean phonation time, a wet quality, and a softer intensity voice than TEP speech.[105]

VOLUNTEER AND SUPPORT ORGANIZATIONS

The diagnosis and treatment of head and neck cancer may proceed quickly; however, a patient's adjustment to the diagnosis of a malignancy, its management, and the subsequent disability is not a short-term process.[106–108] Patients and their families will require different information and support throughout various times of the treatment process. A variety of resources are available to laryngectomees and their families.

WRITTEN MATERIALS

Several good books are available for the laryngectomee that may be provided to the patient preoperatively or postoperatively. These guides provide useful information regarding anatomic changes, stoma care, first aid, alternative communication options, practice exercises, and support groups. They include the following titles:

- *Self-Help for the Laryngectomee,* by Edmund Lauder
  Lauder Enterprises, Inc., 11115 Whisper Hollow,
  San Antonio, TX 78230-3609
  800-388-8642
  E-mail: lauder@voicestore.com
  www.voicestore.com
- *A Handbook for the Laryngectomee,* by Robert L. Keith
  PRO-ED, 8700 Shoal Creek Boulevard, Austin, TX 76001
  512-451-8542
- *Looking Forward* by R. Keith, H. Shane, H. Coates, K. Devine.
  Thieme Medical Publishers, Suite 1501,
  381 Park Avenue South, New York, NY 10157-0208
- *Rescue Breathing for Laryngectomees* and *Check the Neck* (videotape)
  IAL, 7822 Ivymount Terrace, Potomac, MD 20854
  301-983-9323

- *The Clinician's Guide of Alaryngeal Speech Therapy,* by Minnie S. Graham
  (available from Lauder Enterprises, Inc.; see first item in this list)
  Butterworth–Heinemann, 225 Wildwood Avenue,
  Woburn, MA 01801-2041
  1-800-388-8642

Booklets about cancer treatment and living with cancer can be obtained free of charge by writing the Office of Cancer Communications, National Cancer Institute, Building 31, Room 1024, Bethesda, MD 20892, or calling 1-800-4-CANCER.

VOLUNTEERS

Patients are encouraged to meet before or after surgery with individuals who have undergone similar procedures. Some otolaryngology or speech pathology departments require that patient volunteers participate in formal volunteer training; other departments choose well-adjusted individuals and attend the patient visit with the volunteer. Many laryngectomee clubs maintain a laryngectomee volunteer-patient visitation program coordinated with medical professionals in local hospitals and clinics.

SUPPORT GROUPS

Patients and their spouses should be encouraged to join the International Association of Laryngectomies (IAL) and the American Cancer Society (ACS). The IAL is a voluntary, nonprofit, organization dedicated to total rehabilitation of laryngectomees. The purpose of the IAL is to facilitate the formation of new laryngectomee clubs, foster improvement of hospital laryngectomee visitor programs, and upgrade standards for teachers of alaryngeal speech. The IAL provides educational support to more than 200 member clubs located throughout the United States, Canada, Europe, South America, Asia, and Australia. The IAL publishes *IAL News*, conducts an annual meeting, and sponsors an annual Voice Rehabilitation Institute. The Voice Rehabilitation Institute is attended by laryngectomees and speech pathologists for alaryngeal speech instructor training. The IAL publishes a directory of certified alaryngeal speech instructors. It can be contacted at International Association of Laryngectomies, 7822 Ivymount Terrace, Potomac, MD 20854; 301-983-9323; www.larynxlink.com.

The various geographic, state divisions, and local units of the ACS assist IAL member clubs and sponsor field work of benefit to laryngectomees. Some ACS offices are able to lend equipment and other types of support. The ACS can be contacted at 1599 Clifton Road NE, Atlanta, GA 30329; 404-320-3333.

The American Speech-Language-Hearing Association (ASHA) is a professional organization that oversees certification of speech pathologists and audiologists. ASHA defines position statements and guidelines for practice standards within the profession. Several policy statements are related to the management of head and neck cancer patients and to instrumental diagnostic procedures for swallowing and evaluation and treatment of tracheoesophageal fistulization and puncture. ASHA can provide patients and their families with speech pathology resources in their area. ASHA can be contacted at 10801 Rockville Pike, Rockville, MD 20852; 1-800-638-6868; or www.asha.org.

REFERENCES

1. Logemann JA. *Manual for the videofluorographic study of swallowing,* 2nd ed. Austin, TX: PRO-ED, 1993.
2. Langmore S, Schatz K, Olson N. Fiberoptic endoscopic evaluation of swallowing safety: a new procedure. *Dysphagia* 1988;2:216.
3. Aviv J, Kim T, Goodhart M, et al. FEESST: a new bedside endoscopic test of the motor and sensory components of swallowing. *Ann Otol Rhinol Laryngol* 1998;107(5):378.
4. Lazarus C, Logemann J, Gibon P. Effects of maneuvers on swallowing function in a dysphagic oral cancer patient. *Head Neck* 1993;15:419.
5. Logemann JA. Speech and swallowing rehabilitation for head and neck tumor patients. In: Myers EN, Suen JY, eds. *Cancer of the head and neck,* 2nd ed. New York: Churchill Livingstone, 1989:1021.
6. Dios PD, Feijoo JF, Ferreiro MC, Alvarez JA. Functional consequences of partial glossectomy. *Am Assoc Oral Maxillofac Surg* 1994;52:12.
7. Urken ML, Biller HF. A new bilobed design for the sensate radial forearm flap to preserve tongue mobility following significant glossectomy. *Arch Otolaryngol Head Neck Surg* 1994;120:26.
8. Urken ML, Moscoso JF, Lawson W, Biller H. A systematic approach to functional reconstruction of the oral cavity following partial and total glossectomy. *Arch Otolaryngol Head Neck Surg* 1994;120:589.
9. Logemann J. Speech and swallowing rehabilitation for head and neck, 2nd ed. 1989:1021.
10. Heller SH, Levy J, Sciubba JJ. Speech patterns following partial glossectomy for small tumors of the tongue. *Head Neck* 1991;13(4):340.
11. Dios PD, Conley JJ. The crippled oral cavity. *Plast Reconstr Surg* 1962:469.
12. Yamamoto Y, Sugihara T, Furuta Y, Fukuda S. Functional reconstruction of the tongue and deglutition muscles following extensive resection of tongue cancer. *Plast Reconstr Surg* 1998;102(4):99.
13. Wheeler R, Logemann JA, Rosen M. Maxillary reshaping prosthesis: effectiveness in improving speech and swallowing of post-surgical oral cancer patients. *J Prosthet Dent* 1980;43:314.
14. Hirano M, Matsuoka H, Kuroiwa Y, et al. Dysphagia following various degrees of surgical resection for oral cancer. *Ann Otol Rhinol Laryngol* 1992;101:138.
15. Teichgraeber J, Bowman J, Geopfert H. Functional analysis of treatment of oral cavity cancer. *Arch Otolaryngol Head Neck Surg* 1986;112:959.
16. Rentschler GJ, Mann MB. The effects of glossectomy on intelligibility of speech and oral perception discrimination. *J Oral Surg* 1980;38:348.
17. Lyos AT, Evans GR, Perez D, Schusterman MA. Tongue reconstruction: outcomes with the rectus abdominis flap. *Plast Reconstr Surg* 1999;103(2):442.
18. Pompei S, Caravelli G, Vigili MG, Ducci M, Marzetti F. Free radial forearm flap and myocutaneous flaps in oncological reconstructive surgery of the oral cavity, comparison of functional results. *Minerva Chir* 1998;53(3):183.
19. Tiwari RM, Greven AJ, Karim ABMF, Snow GB. Total glossectomy: reconstruction and rehabilitation. *J Laryngol Otol* 1989;103:917.
20. Tiwari RM, Karim ABMF, Greven AJ, Snow GB. Total glossectomy with laryngeal preservation. *Arch Otolaryngol Head Neck Surg* 1993;119:945.
21. Urken ML, Vickery C, Weinberg H, Biller HF. The neurofasciocutaneous radial forearm free flap for functional reconstruction of near-total glossectomy defects. *Laryngocope* 1990;100:161.
22. Urken ML, Biller HF. A new bilobed design for the sensate radial forearm flap to preserve tongue mobility following significant glossectomy. *Arch Otolaryngol Head Neck Surg* 1994;120:589.
23. Aviv JE, Keen MS, Rodriquez HP, et al. Bilobed radial forearm free flap for functional reconstruction of near-total glossectomy defects. *Laryngoscope* 1994;104:893.
24. Hell B, Heissler E, Gath H, Menneking H, Langford. The infrahyoid flap. A technique for defect closure in the floor of the mouth, the tongue, the buccal mucosa, and the lateral pharyngeal wall. *Int J Oral Maxillofac Surg* 1997;26(1):35.
25. Salibian AH, Allison GR, Armstrong WB, et al. Functional hemitongue reconstruction with the microvascular ulnar forearm flap. *Plast Reconstr Surg* 1999;104(3):654.
26. Horwitz EM, Frazier AJ, Martinez AA, et al. Excellent functional outcome in patients with squamous cell carcinoma of the base of the tongue treated with external irradiation and interstitial iodine 125 boost. *Cancer* 1996;78(5):948.
27. Neuschaefer-Rube C, Wein BB, Angerstein W, Klajman S, Fischer-Wein G. Sector-related grey scale analysis of video ultrasound recorded tongue movements in swallowing. *HNO* 1997;45(7):556.
28. Krappen S, Remmert S, Gehrking E, Zwaan M. Cinematographic functional diagnosis of swallowing after plastic reconstruction of large tumor defects of the mouth cavity and pharynx. *Laryngorhinootologie* 1997;76(4):229.
29. Sommer K, Burk C, Sommer T, Remmert S. Perfusion manometry in the evaluation of postoperative swallowing function following various reconstructive procedures of the upper aero-digestive tract. *Laryngorhinootologie* 1997;76(3):178.
30. Dagli A, Mahieu H, Festen J. Quantitative analysis of voice quality in early glottic laryngeal carcinomas treated with radiotherapy. *Eur Arch Otorhinolaryngol* 1997:254(2):78.
31. Rydell R, Schalen L, Fex S, Elner A. Voice evaluation before and after laser excision vs. radiotherapy of TIA glottic carcinoma. *Acta Otolaryngol (Stockh)* 1995;115(4):560.
32. Aref A, Dworkin J, Devi S, Denton L, Fontanesi J. Objective evaluation of the quality of voice following radiation therapy for T1 glottic cancer. *Radiother Oncol* 1997; 45(2):149.
33. Harrison L, Sololmon B, Miller S, et al. Prospective computer assisted voice analysis for patients with early stage glottic cancer: a preliminary report of the functional result of laryngeal irradiation. *Int J Radiat Oncol Biol Phys* 1990;19:123.
34. Tsunoda K, Soda Y, Tojima H, et al. Stroboscopic observation of the larynx after radiation in patients with T1 glottic carcinoma. *Acta Otolaryngol Suppl* 1997;527:165.
35. Woodson G, Rosen C, Murry T, et al. Assessing vocal function after chemoradiation for advanced laryngeal carcinoma. *Arch Otolaryngol Head Neck Surg* 1996;122(8):858.

36. Wang M, Hussey D, Doornbos J, et al. Chemodectoma of the temporal bone: a comparison of surgical and radiotherapeutic results. *Int J Radiat Oncol Biol Phys* 1988;14:643.
37. Leeper H, Heeneman H, Reynolds C. Vocal function following vertical hemilaryngectomy: a preliminary investigation. *J Otolaryngol* 1990;19:62.
38. Logemann J, Gibbons P, Rademaker A, et al. Mechanisms of recovery of swallow after supraglottic laryngectomy. *J Speech Hear Res* 1993;37:965.
39. Martin B, Logemann J, Shaker R, et al. Normal laryngeal valving patterns during three breath hold maneuvers: a pilot investigation. *Dysphagia* 1993;8:11.
40. Omae Y, Logemann J, Haqnson D, et al. Effects of two breath-holding maneuvers on oropharyngeal swallow. *Ann Otol Rhinol Laryngol* 19996;105:123.
41. Kahrilas P, Logemann J, Gibbons P. Food intake by maneuver: an extreme compensation for impaired swallowing. *Dysphagia* 1992;7:155.
42. Balfe DM, Koehler RE, Setzen M, Weyman PJ, Raaron RL. Barium examination of the esophagus after total laryngectomy. *Radiology* 1982;143:501.
43. McConnell FM, Mendelsohn MS, Logemann JA. Examination of swallowing after total laryngectomy using manofluorography. *Head Neck Surg* 1986;9:3.
44. Kirchner JA, Scatliff JH, Dey FL, Shedd DP. The pharynx after laryngectomy: changes in its structure and function. *Laryngoscope* 1963;73:18.
45. Broniatowski M, Sonies B, Rubin J, et al. Current evaluation and treatment of patients with swallowing disorders. *Otol Head Neck Surg* 1999;120:464.
46. Lazarus CL, Logemann JA, Kahrilas PJ, Mittal BB. Swallow recovery in an oral cancer patient following surgery, radiotherapy, and hyperthermia. *Head Neck* 1994;16:259.
47. McNeil BJ, Weichselbaum R, Pauker, SG. Speech and survival: tradeoffs between quality and quantity of life in laryngeal cancer. *N Engl J Med* 1981;305:982.
48. Davis R, Vincent M, Shapshay S, Strong M. The anatomy and complication of "T" versus vertical closure of the hypopharynx after laryngectomy. *Laryngoscope* 1982;92:16.
49. Damste PH. Some obstacles to learning esophageal speech. In: Keith RL, Darley FH, eds. *Laryngectomee rehabilitation,* 2nd ed. San Diego: College-Hill Press, 1986:85.
50. Diedrich WM, Youngstrom KA. *Alaryngeal speech.* Springfield, IL: Charles C Thomas Publisher, 1966.
51. Gardner WH. *Laryngectomee speech and rehabilitation.* Springfield, IL: Charles C Thomas Publisher, 1971.
52. Singer MT. The upper esophageal sphincter: role in alaryngeal speech acquisition. *Head Neck Surg* 1988;[Suppl 2]:S118.
53. Gates GA, Ryan W, Cooper JC Jr, et al. Current status of laryngectomee rehabilitation: I. Results of therapy. *Am J Otol* 1982;3:1.
54. Van Weissenbruch R, Albers FW. Vocal rehabilitation after total laryngectomy using Provox voice prosthesis. *Clin Otolaryngol* 1993;18(5):359.
55. Gates GA, Ryan W, Cooper JC Jr, et al. Current status of laryngectomee rehabilitation: I. Results of therapy. *Am J Otol* 1982;3:1.
56. Mjones AB, Olofsson J, Danbolt C, Tibbling L. Oesophageal speech after laryngectomy: a study of possible influencing factors. Clin Otolaryngol 1991;16:442.
57. Salmon SJ. Adjusting to laryngectomy. In: Perkins WH, Northern JL, eds. *Current strategies of rehabilitation of the laryngectomized patient: seminars in speech and language.* New York: Thieme Medical Publishers, 1986.
58. Fujii T, Sato T, Yoshino K, et al. Voice rehabilitation with esophageal speech in the laryngectomized. *Nippon Jibiinkoka Gakkai Kaiho* 1993;96(7):1086.
59. Shanks JC. Evoking esophageal voice. *Semin Speech Lang* 1986;7:1.
60. Cheesman AD, Knight J, McIvor J, Perry A. Tracheo-oesophageal "puncture speech": an assessment technique for failed oesophageal speakers. *J Laryngol Otol* 1986;100:191.
61. Perry A, Cheesman AD, McIvor JL, Charlton R. British experience of surgical voice restoration techniques as a secondary procedure following total laryngectomy. *J Laryngol Otol* 1987;101:155.
62. Blitzer A, Komisar A, Baredes S, Brin MF, Stewart C. Voice failure after tracheoesophageal puncture: management with botulinum toxin. *Otolaryngol Head Neck Surg* 1995;113(6):668.
63. Hoffman HT, Fischer H, VanDenmark D, et al. Botulinum neurotoxin injection after total laryngectomy. *Head Neck* 1997;19(2):92.
64. Sloane PM, Griffin JM, O'Dwyer TP. Esophageal insufflation and videofluoroscopy for evaluation of esophageal speech in laryngectomy patients: clinical implications. *Radiology* 1991;181:433.
65. Morgan DW, Hadley J, Willis G, Cheesman AD. Use of a portable manometer as a screening procedure in voice rehabilitation. *J Laryngol Otol* 1992;106:353.
66. Baugh RF, Lewin JS, Baker SR. Preoperative assessment of tracheo-oesophageal speech. *Laryngoscope* 1987;97:461.
67. Singer MI, Blom ED. An endoscopic technique for restoration of voice after laryngectomy. *Ann Otol Rhinol Laryngol* 1980;89:529.
68. Blom ED, Singer MI, Hamaker R. Tracheostoma valve for postlaryngectomy voice rehabilitation. *Ann Otol Rhinol Laryngol* 1082;91:576.
69. Singer MI. Voice rehabilitation. In: Cummings CW, ed. *Otolaryngology—head and neck surgery,* 2nd ed. St Louis: Mosby, 1993:2190.
70. Singer MI, Blom ED. Medical techniques for voice restoration after total laryngectomy. *CA Cancer J Clin* 1990;40:166.
71. Chan H, Mesko T, Fields K, Barkin J. An improved method of flexible endoscopic creation of tracheoesophageal fistula for voice restoration. *Surg Endosc* 1997;11(10):1034.
72. Yoshida GY, Hamaker RC, Singer MI, Blom ED, Glenwood AC. Primary voice restoration at laryngectomy. *Laryngoscope* 1989;99:1093.
73. Izdebski K, Reed C, Ross J, Hilsinger R. Problems with tracheoesophageal fistula voice restoration in totally laryngectomized patients. *Arch Otolaryngol Head Neck Surg* 1994;120:840.
74. Van Weissenbruch R, Albers FWJ. Vocal rehabilitation after total laryngectomy using the Provox voice prosthesis. *Clin Otolaryngol* 1993;18:359.
75. Lacau St Guily J, Angelard B, El-Bez M, et al. Postlaryngectomy voice restoration. *Arch Otolaryngol Head Neck Surg* 1992;118:252.
76. Mehta AR, Sarkar S, Mehta SA, Bachher GK. The Indian experience with immediate tracheoesophageal puncture for voice restoration. *Eur Arch Otorhinolaryngol* 1995;252(4):209.
77. Quer M, Burgues-Vila J, Garcia-Crespillo P. Primary tracheoesophageal puncture vs esophageal speech. *Arch Otolaryngol Head Neck Surg* 1992;118(3):252.
78. Schultz JR, Harrison J. Defining and predicting tracheoesophageal puncture success. *Arch Otolaryngol Head Neck Surg* 1992;102:704.
79. Artazkoz del Toro JJ, Lopez MR. Surgical voice rehabilitation: influence of postoperative radiotherapy on tracheoesophageal fistulas. Long-term follow-up study. *Acta Otorrhinolaringol Esp* 1997;48(4):299.
80. Hilgers FJ, Ackerstaff AH, Balm AJ, et al. Development and clinical evaluation of a second-generation voice prosthesis (Provox 2), designed for anterograde and retrograde insertion. *Acta Otolaryngol (Stockh)* 1997;117(6):889.
81. Schouwenburg PF, Eelenstein SE, Grolman W. The Voicemaster voice prosthesis for the laryngectomized patient. *Clin Otolaryngol* 1998;23(6):555.
82. Van den Hoogen FJA, Nijdam HF, Veenstr A, Manni JJ. The Nijdam voice prosthesis. A self-retaining valveless voice prosthesis for vocal rehabilitation after total laryngectomy. *Acta Otolaryngol (Stockh)* 1996;116:913.
83. Lavertu P, Guay ME, Meeker SS, et al. Secondary tracheoesophageal puncture: factors predictive of voice quality and prosthesis use. *Head Neck* 1996;18(5):393.
84. Singer MI, Blom ED, Hamaker RC. Pharyngeal plexus neurectomy for alaryngeal speech rehabilitation. *Laryngoscope* 1986;96:50.
85. Callaway E, Truelson JM, Wolf GT, Thomas-Kincaid L, Cannon S. Predictive value of objective esophageal insufflation testing for acquisition of tracheoesophageal speech. *Laryngoscope* 1992;102:704.
86. Lewin JS, Baugh RF, Baker SR. An objective method for prediction of tracheoesophageal speech production. *J Speech Hear Disord* 1990;52:212.
87. Zormeier NM, Melecca RJ, Simpson ML, et al. Botulinum toxin injection to improve tracheoesophageal speech after total laryngectomy. *Otolaryngol Head Neck Surg* 1999;120(3):314.
88. Paulowski BR, Blom ED, Logemann JA, Hamaker RC. Functional outcome after surgery for prevention of pharyngospasms in tracheoesophageal speakers: Part II. Swallow characteristics. *Laryngoscope* 1995;105:1104,
89. Anthony JP, Singer MI, Mathes SJ. Pharyngoesophageal reconstruction using the tubed free radial forearm flap. *Clin Plast Surg* 1994;21(1):137.
90. Kelly KE, Anthony JP, Singer M. Pharyngoesophageal reconstruction using the radial forearm fasciocutaneous free flap: preliminary results. *Otolaryngol Head Neck Surg* 1994;111(1):16.
91. Hussain A, Dolph JL, Padilla JF, Silver S. Tubed, folded radial forearm free flap for pharyngeal reconstruction and voice rehabilitation. *Ann Plast Surg* 1993;30(6):541.
92. Kinishi M, Amatsu M, Tahara S, Makino K. Primary tracheojejunal shunt operation for voice restoration following pharyngolaryngoesophagectomy. *Ann Otol Rhinol Laryngol* 1991;100(6):435.
93. Matsuura K, Yamada A, Hashimoto S, et al. Simultaneous reconstruction of pharyngoesophagus and phonation following laryngopharyngoesophagectomy. *Nippon Jibiinkoka Gakkai Kaiho* 1999;102(2):208.
94. Bleach N, Perry A, Cheesman A. Surgical voice restoration with the Blom-Singer prosthesis following laryngopharyngoesophagectomy and pharyngogastric anastomosis. *Ann Otol Rhinol Laryngol* 1991;100(2):142.
95. Carlson GW, Schusterman MA, Guillamondegui OM. Total reconstruction of the pharynx and cervical esophagus: a 20 year experience. *Ann Plast Surg* 1992;29:408.
96. Medina JE, Nance A, Burns L, Overton R. Voice restoration after total laryngopharyngectomy and cervical esophagectomy using the duckbill prosthesis. *Am J Surg* 1987;154:407.
97. Juarbe C, Sheman L, Wang R, et al. Tracheoesophageal puncture for voice restoration extended laryngopharyngectomy. *Arch Otolaryngol* 1989;115:356.
98. Wilson PS, Bruce-Lockhart FJ, Johnson AP, Physevans PH. Speech reconstruction following total laryngo-pharyngectomy with free jejunal repair. *Clin Otolaryngol* 1994;19:145.
99. Garth RJN, McRae A, Rhysevans PH. Tracheo-esophageal puncture: a review of problems and complications. *J Laryngol Otol* 1991;105:750.
100. Mendolsohn M, Morris M, Gallagher R. A comparative study of speech after total laryngectomy and total laryngopharyngectomy. *Arch Otolaryngol Head Neck Surg* 1981;305:982.
101. Wenig BR, Mullooly V, Levy J, Abramson AL. Voice restoration following laryngectomy: the role of primary versus secondary tracheoesophageal puncture. *Ann Otol Rhinol Laryngol* 1989;98:70.
102. Robbins J, Fisher HB, Blom ED, Singer MI. A comparative acoustic study of normal, esophageal, and tracheoesophageal speech production. *J Speech Hear Disord* 1984; 49:202.
103. Casper J, Colton R. *Understanding voice problems: physiological perspective for diagnosis and treatment.* Baltimore, MD: Williams & Wilkins, 1966.
104. Deschler DB, Doherty ET, Reed CG, Singer MI. Quantitative and qualitative analysis of tracheoesophageal voice following pectoralis major flap reconstruction of the neopharynx. *Otolaryngol Head Neck Surg* 1998;118(6):771.
105. Haughey BH, Fredrickson JM, Sessions DG, et al. A comparative study of speech after total laryngectomy and total laryngopharyngectomy. *Arch Otolaryngol Head Neck Surg* 1993;119:487.
106. Blood GW, Luther AR, Stemple JC. Coping and adjustment in alaryngeal speakers. *Am J Speech Lang Pathol* 1992;1:63.
107. Doyle PC. *Foundations of voice and speech rehabilitation following laryngeal cancer.* San Diego: Singular Publishing Group, 1994.
108. Gunn AE. Cancer rehabilitation: an overview. In: Gunn AE, ed. *Cancer rehabilitation.* New York: Raven Press, 1984:1.

CHAPTER 31

Cancer of the Lung

SECTION 1

YOSHITAKA SEKIDO
KWUN M. FONG
JOHN D. MINNA

Molecular Biology of Lung Cancer

Lung cancer cells have accumulated a number of molecular genetic and epigenetic lesions, which appear necessary to transform normal bronchial epithelium to an overt lung cancer. There is complex interaction between the various molecular changes that ultimately result in the abrogation of key cellular regulatory and growth control pathways. Of the three major classes of human "cancer" genes, the protooncogenes and tumor suppressor genes (TSGs) are involved in lung carcinogenesis, whereas evidence implicating DNA repair genes is not yet conclusive. Many of the protooncogene and TSG changes are present in both major lung cancer subtypes: small cell lung cancer (SCLC) and non–small cell lung cancer (NSCLC), although certain mutations have subtype specificity (Table 31.1-1). Protooncogenes generally encode proteins that are positive effectors of the transformed phenotype and can simplistically be considered positive growth regulators. Their "activation" results in their functional deregulation, leading to a gain in function or "dominant" effect. Conversely, TSG products are negative growth regulators and their "inactivation" results in a loss of function that contributes to malignancy. Interacting with yet other biologic changes, these fundamental molecular events appear to underlie the characteristics of dysregulated growth, clonal expansion, and immortality, which are typical of overt lung cancers. In addition, these, and yet other to be discovered molecular changes, may affect the processes of invasion, metastasis, and resistance against cancer therapy. In translating these laboratory discoveries into the clinic, it is important to identify these various changes, determine the frequency of occurrence, and test whether they have clinically important associations (e.g., with histologic type, stage, survival, response to therapy), as well as to determine if they could be used for early diagnosis, to monitor prevention and treatment efforts, and as targets for the development of new treatments. In addition, these abnormalities will probably also give us important understanding about lung development and differentiation.

GENETIC AND EPIGENETIC ALTERATIONS IN LUNG CANCERS

CHROMOSOMAL ABNORMALITIES

Lung cancer cells display numerical abnormalities (aneuploidy) of chromosomes, which are suggestive of allele loss or gain, as well as structural cytogenetic abnormalities. The latter include nonreciprocal translocations and deletions, whereas the presence of double minutes and homogeneously staining regions indicate gene amplification, such as for the *MYC* gene family.[1] In SCLCs, losses from chromosomes 3p, 5q, 13q, and 17p predominate, but double minutes may be common late in disease. In NSCLCs, deletions of 3p, 9p, and 17p, together with +7, i(5)(p10), and i(8)(q10) are often seen. Molecular cytogenetic analysis with comparative genomic hybridization has identified hitherto unrecognized abnormalities, including deletions at 10q26, 16p11.2, and 22q12.1-13.1 and amplification at 1q24, 3q, 5p, 17q, and Xq26.

It has been proposed that human tumors may be genetically unstable at two levels: at the chromosomal level, including losses and gains (amplification), and at the DNA nucleotide level, including single or several base changes.[2] It will thus be impor-

TABLE 31.1-1. The Most Frequent Acquired Molecular Abnormalities in Lung Cancer

	Small Cell Lung Cancer	*Non–Small Cell Lung Cancer*
Microsatellite instabilities	~35%	~22%
Autocrine loops	GRP/GRP receptor	TGF-α/EGFR; Heregulin/HER2/neu
	SCF/KIT	HGF/MET
RAS point mutation	<1%	15–20%
MYC family overexpression	15–30%	5–10%
p53 inactivation	~90%	~50%
RB inactivation	~90%	15–30%
$p16^{INK4A}$ inactivation	0–10%	30–70%
FHIT inactivation	~75%	~50–75%
Frequent allelic loss	3p, 4p, 4q, 5q, 8p, 10q, 13q, 17p, 22q	3p, 6q, 8p, 9p, 13p, 17p, 19q
Telomerase activity	~100%	80–85%
BCL2 expression	75–95%	10–35%

EGFR, epidermal growth factor receptor; FHIT, fragile histidine triad; GRP, gastrin-releasing peptide; HGF, hepatocyte growth factor; RB, retinoblastoma protein; SCF, stem cell factor; TGF-α, transforming growth factor-α.

tant to determine if aneuploidy and structural cytogenetic abnormalities, apart from targeting key genes, actually represent the phenomenon of chromosomal instability in lung cancers.

MICROSATELLITE INSTABILITY

A genetic change that manifests itself as a mutator phenotype (often called the *replication error repair phenotype*) in human cancers results in widespread microsatellite instability. The result of microsatellite instability is a "laddering" of short-tandem DNA repeat sequences at multiple loci seen on high-resolution polyacrylamide electrophoretic gels. This phenotype is usually due to mutational inactivation of DNA mismatch repair enzymes, resulting in marked instability of these polymorphic DNA repeat sequences. This phenotype was initially reported in hereditary nonpolyposis colon cancers. Lung cancer frequently exhibits microsatellite instability; however, this occurs at only a few loci and results only in "shifts" of individual allelic bands ("microsatellite alterations") compared to normal DNA in the same patient. The abnormal mechanism underlying this phenotype is currently unknown, and apparently mutations in DNA mismatch repair enzymes are very uncommon in lung cancer. The human 8-oxoguanine DNA glycosylase (*hOGG1*) gene, involved in the repair of oxidative DNA damage, is another candidate for involvement in generating multiple lung cancer mutations. However, abnormalities in this gene only rarely occur in lung cancer, and mutations in other DNA repair genes have not yet been reported in lung cancer. Overall, approximately 35% (37 of 106) of SCLCs and 22% (160 of 727) of NSCLCs showed some examples of microsatellite alterations at individual loci.[3] Microsatellite alterations in lung cancer have been reported to be associated with younger age, reduced survival, and advanced tumor stage. Regardless of the underlying mechanism, many groups are testing the possibility of using this microsatellite alteration phenotype for the early diagnosis of lung cancer by detecting these shifted DNA bands in sputum, bronchial washings, or blood.

ABERRANT DNA METHYLATION

DNA methylation involves covalent modification at the fifth carbon position of cytosine residues within CpG nucleotides of DNA, which tend to be clustered around the 5' ends of many housekeeping genes (CpG islands). Hypermethylation in the 5' promoter region of genes is associated with transcriptional silencing and is an alternative mechanism for down-regulating TSG expression rather than gene deletion or mutation.

Hypermethylation of the promoter region of the $p16^{INK4A}$ gene in a subset of NSCLCs results in its down-regulation and may be an early event in lung cancer pathogenesis.[4] Other genes also have been found to undergo aberrant promoter methylation in lung cancer but are not found in the normal lung associated with these tumors, including *DAP* (death associated protein) kinase, *GSTP1* (glutathione S-transferase), and *MGMT* (O^6-methylguanine-DNA-methyltransferase).[5] In addition, DNA containing these methylated sequences could be detected in the corresponding blood samples from the same patients, indicating that the tumor cells had shed DNA into the peripheral blood. Thus, aberrantly methylated DNA sequences, which can be sensitively detected among a background of normal DNA, represent an attractive strategy for early molecular detection. Other sites of hypermethylation, including 3p, 4q34, 10q26, and 17p13, have been implicated in lung cancer pathogenesis, although the precise gene targets are uncertain. In addition to use as an early detection target, it may be possible to reverse methylation pharmacologically. In tissue culture systems, this is routinely done with the demethylating agent 5-aza-2'-deoxycytidine. Clinical trials with such agents have been attempted in other diseases, and agents with less toxicity need to be developed and tested in lung cancer.

Another acquired tumor abnormality is loss of imprinting (loss of methylation) to allow the expression of genes in lung cancer. Methylation plays a role in mediating genomic imprinting, which is a gamete-specific modification causing differential expression of the two alleles of a gene in somatic cells. Loss of genomic imprinting of the insulin-like growth factor-2 (*IGF-2*) gene and the *H19* gene (associated with hypomethylation of its promoter region) also occurs in lung cancer.

PROTOONCOGENES AND GROWTH STIMULATION

The activation of protooncogenes requires mechanisms such as gene amplification or point mutation of a single allele leading to constitutive overexpression. In some cases, however, the mechanisms causing overexpression are still unclear. Protooncogene products include several growth factor receptors, such as epidermal growth factor receptor (EGFR), ERBB2, KIT, and MET. Indeed, many growth factor/receptor systems are expressed by either the lung tumor or adjacent normal cells, thus providing autocrine or paracrine growth stimulatory loops (Fig. 31.1-1). For example, overexpression of the EGFR encoded by the *ERBB1* gene is more common in NSCLC than SCLC and may be related to tumor stage and differentiation. Coexpression of EGFR and their ligands, especially transforming growth factor-α (TGF-α), by

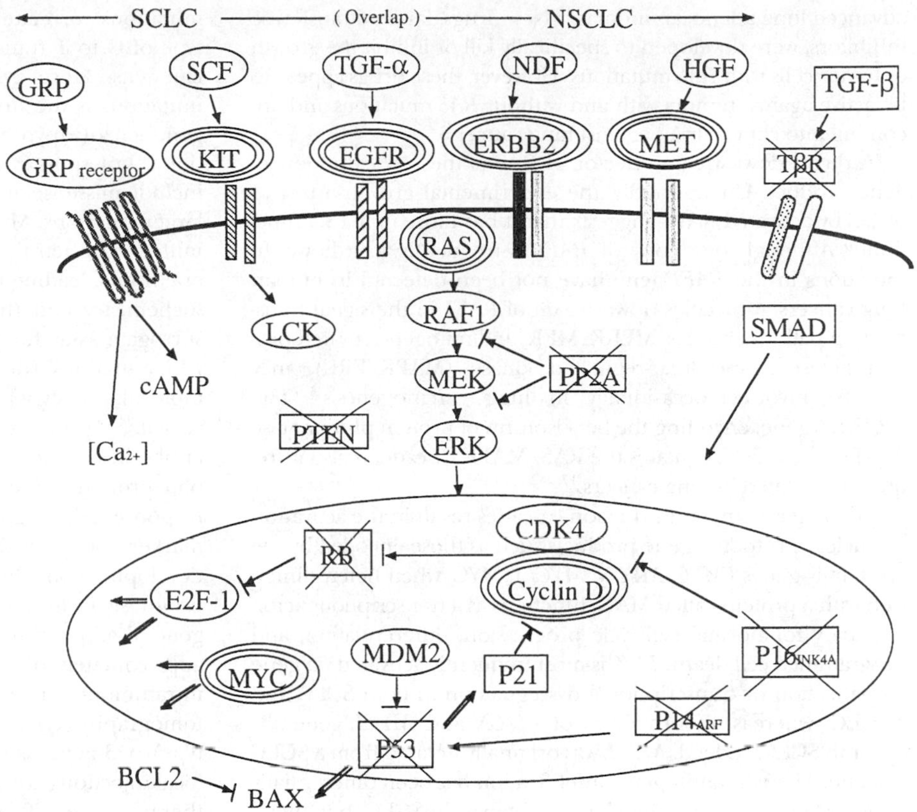

FIGURE 31.1-1. The common growth stimulatory and inhibitory cascades involved in lung cancer cells. A *single circle* denotes growth stimulatory molecules, and *multiple circles* denote activation caused by some tumor-acquired abnormality. A *box* denotes growth inhibitory molecules, whereas their inactivation is indicated by a cross within the box, again acquired (for example) by mutation in the tumor. *Double arrows* indicate transcriptional activation of target genes that regulate cell growth. cAMP, cyclic adenosine monophosphate; CDK4, cyclin-dependent kinase-4; EGFR, epidermal growth factor receptor; ERK, extracellular regulated kinase; GRP, gastrin-releasing peptide; HGF, hepatocyte growth factor; NSCLC, non–small cell lung carcinoma; RB, retinoblastoma protein; SCF, stem cell factor; SCLC, small cell lung carcinoma; TGF-α, transforming growth factor-α.

lung cancer cells indicates the presence of an autocrine (self-stimulatory) growth factor loop. Overexpression of EGFR occurred in 70% of NSCLCs, and overexpression of both EGFR and TGF-α occurred in 38%.[6] Clinically, the presence of this loop had no significant impact on overall survival in early-stage NSCLCs and thus seems to play a role in lung tumor formation rather than tumor progression.[6] ERBB2 (HER2/neu) is highly expressed in more than one-third of NSCLCs, especially adenocarcinomas. Its expression correlates with a shorter survival in lung adenocarcinomas and may also be a marker for intrinsic multidrug resistance in NSCLC cell lines.[7] KIT and its ligand, stem cell factor (SCF), are both preferentially expressed in many SCLCs. Activation of this putative autocrine loop may provide a growth advantage, or it may mediate chemoattraction. The SCF/KIT signal transduction pathway has been shown to be associated with Lck, a src-related tyrosine kinase.[8] MET and its ligand, hepatocyte growth factor (HGF), are involved in fetal lung development. Coexpression of this putative loop is observed in most NSCLCs, and high HGF levels were associated with a poor outcome in resectable NSCLC patients.[9] There are several clinical applications of these growth factor receptor abnormalities that have occurred in other cancers, which also need to be explored as new treatments for lung cancer. These include treatment with humanized monoclonal anti-HER-2/neu receptor antibody Herceptin alone or in combination with chemotherapy, treatment with monoclonal anti-EGF receptor antibody combined with radiotherapy, and new drugs that would inhibit the tyrosine kinase activity of these receptors.

Apart from protooncogene products, other growth stimulatory loops are found in lung cancer. The best known is that governed by gastrin-releasing peptide (GRP) and other bombesin-like peptides, together with their receptors, which participates in lung development and repair as well as promoting SCLC growth via an autocrine loop. This loop represents a future therapeutic target because a clinical trial of an anti-GRP monoclonal antibody showed some antitumor activity in patients with previously treated SCLC.[10]

Because downstream effectors are needed to transduce incoming growth factor/receptor signals to the nucleus, it is not surprising that cytoplasmic signal transduction cascades are also implicated in carcinogenesis. For instance, the receptor tyrosine kinases initially signal the guanosine triphosphate–binding RAS protein. The *RAS* gene family (*KRAS, HRAS,* and *NRAS*) can be activated by point mutations at codons 12, 13, or 61, and one member of this family is mutated in approximately 20% to 30% of NSCLC (particularly adenocarcinomas) but probably never in SCLC.[11] *KRAS* accounts for 90% of the *RAS* mutations in lung adenocarcinomas, with approximately 85% of the *KRAS* mutations affecting codon 12. Characteristically, approximately 70% of *KRAS* mutation are G to T transversions, with the substitution of the normal glycine (GGT) with either cysteine (TGT) or valine (GTT). Similar G to T transversions also affect the *P53* gene in lung cancer and represent the type of DNA damage expected from bulky DNA adducts caused by the polycyclic hydrocarbons and nitrosamines in tobacco smoke. Further evidence for a causative role for tobacco smoke is the correlation of *KRAS* mutations with cigarette consumption. The presence of *KRAS* mutations portends a poor prognosis in both early- and late-stage NSCLCs,[12] although the data conflict.[13] Nonetheless, a metaanalysis of eight studies of 217 (of 881) NSCLC patients positive for *KRAS* mutations suggested a negative prognostic role.[14] A prospective study has shown that neither chemosensitivity or survival correlated with *KRAS* mutation in advanced lung adenocarcinomas.[15] New drugs, farnesyltransferase inhibitors, were developed to specifically kill or inhibit the growth of tumor cells with *RAS* mutations. However, these drugs appear to be active against tumors with and without *RAS* mutations and are coming into clinical trials against lung cancer.

A direct downstream effector of RAS is the *RAF1* protooncogene product. Unexpectedly, the experimental growth arrest of SCLC by activated RAF1 suggests that it has more of a TSG function.[16] Although one copy of *RAF1* is frequently lost; however, mutations in the *RAF1* gene have not been detected in human lung cancers. Molecules downstream of RAF1 in the signal transduction pathway, such as MEKK, MEK, and mitogen-activated protein kinase/extracellular-regulated kinase (MAPK/ERK), may also be involved occasionally in lung carcinogenesis.[3] The *PPP2R1B* gene, encoding the beta isoform of protein phosphatase 2A (PP2A), which regulates the RAS/MAPK cascade, is also infrequently mutated in lung cancers.[17]

Ultimately, signal transduction cascades result in the activation of nuclear protooncogene products such as those encoded by the *myc* family genes (*MYC, MYCN, MYCL*). MYC, when heterodimerized with a protein called MAX, functions as a transcription factor, necessary for normal cell-cycle progression, differentiation, and programmed cell death. *MYC* is most frequently activated via gene amplification or transcriptional dysregulation in both SCLC and NSCLC, whereas abnormalities of *MYCN* and *MYCL* generally occur in SCLC. Indeed, *MYCL* was originally isolated from a SCLC cell line. The *myc* family gene amplification has been differentially observed in the major lung cancer subtypes. In SCLC, one member of the *MYC* family was amplified in 18% of tumors and 31% of cell lines, compared to 8% of NSCLC tumors and 20% of cell lines, respectively.[11] Amplification appears more frequent in patients previously treated with chemotherapy, the "variant" subtype of SCLC, and its presence correlates with adverse survival. In terms of therapy, all-*trans*-retinoic acid (RA) treatment inhibited the *in vitro* growth of a SCLC cell line overexpressing MYC, a process associated with increased neuroendocrine differentiation and increased *MYCL* and decreased *MYC* expression.[18] Lastly, there also have been reports of *MYCL* amplification with rearrangement in which *MYCL* fuses to the *RLF* gene causing a chimeric protein.[19]

Occasional reports have implicated other oncogenes, such as *ERBA, MYB, JUN,* and *FOS* in lung cancer, but data are relatively few.

TUMOR SUPPRESSOR GENES AND GROWTH SUPPRESSION

p53 PATHWAY

p53 (or TP53) maintains genomic integrity in the face of cellular stress from DNA damage (for example caused by γ- and UV irradiation, carcinogens, or chemotherapy). It functions as a transcription factor to activate the expression of genes that control cell-cycle checkpoints (e.g., *p21*$^{WAF1/CIP1}$), apoptosis (*BAX*), DNA repair (*GADD45*), and angiogenesis (thrombospondin). The *p53* gene is the most frequently mutated TSG in human malignancies, and mutations affect approximately 90% of SCLCs and 50% of NSCLCs.[20,21] Most mutations occur in the evolutionarily conserved p53 exons 5 to 8. In NSCLCs, p53 alterations occurred more frequently in squamous cell (51.2%) and large cell (53.7%) carcinomas than adenocarcinomas (38.8%).[21] *p53* mutations correlate with cigarette smoking and most are of the type of G to T transversions expected from tobacco smoke carcinogens. More evidence linking smoking damage with *p53* mutations is the finding that a major cigarette smoke carcinogen, benzo(a)pyrene, selectively forms adducts at the *p53* mutational hot spots.[22] The types of *p53* mutations are varied and include missense, nonsense, and splicing abnormalities as well as larger deletions. Missense mutations (the most common type of mutation) often prolong the half-life of the p53 protein to several hours, leading to increased levels detectable by immunohistochemistry and thus the use of immunohistochemistry as a surrogate assay for *p53* mutation.[23] Whether the occurrence of *p53* mutations (detected by either immunohistochemistry or molecular analysis) in a patient's tumor affect survival is controversial.[24] Approximately 15% of lung cancer patients develop antibodies to the p53 protein, raising the possibility that mutant p53 protein overexpression can lead to a humoral immune response. Although p53 antibodies have been proposed as a marker for early diagnosis[25] and chemoresponsiveness,[26] the development of these antibodies does not appear to improve prognosis in lung cancer.[27] There have been several promising gene therapy clinical trials with objective response rates of approximately 10% to 15% in which lung cancers are treated by intratumoral injection [endobronchially, or by computed tomography (CT)–guided needle injection] with a normal (wild-type) p53 gene using retroviral[28] or adenoviral vectors.[29] These local injections are now being combined with chemo- and radiotherapy to test if gene therapy increases sensitivity to conventional treatments. Also, systemic methods (such as with lipid vesicles) of delivering *p53* gene therapy to disseminated tumors are being developed. In another approach, clinical trials are being conducted to immunize patients against either mutant p53 or RAS proteins occurring in patients' tumors in attempts to generate a tumor-specific cytotoxic T-cell response.

p53 functions in a biochemical pathway; thus it is reasonable to consider that other components of this pathway may be mutated in lung tumors that are wild-type for *p53*. One of the upstream components is the kinase that phosphorylates p53 encoded by the ataxia telangiectasia (*ATM*) gene. However, this gene has not yet been found to be mutated in lung cancer. Other components are the *MDM2* and *p14*^{ARF} genes (see p16^{INK4A}, later in this chapter), which regulate the levels of p53 protein, but so far they have not been implicated in lung cancer. Two proteins homologous to p53—p51 and p73—have been discovered, leading to the hypothesis that they may be mutated in p53 wild-type tumors. However, they are only infrequently, if ever, mutated in lung cancers. Finally, the Li-Fraumeni syndrome of inherited susceptibility to cancer determined by an inherited germline mutation of *p53* may also lead to increased susceptibility to lung cancer in adults in these pedigrees.

THE p16^{INK4A}–CYCLIN D1–CYCLIN-DEPENDENT KINASE-4–RETINOBLASTOMA PROTEIN PATHWAY

p16^{INK4A}

The p16^{INK4A}–cyclin D1–cyclin-dependent kinase-4 (CDK4)–retinoblastoma (RB) protein pathway is a key cell-cycle regulator at the G_1/S phase transition, and one of the components of this pathway is abnormal in the majority of lung cancers. The activation of CDKs by cyclins eventually leads to the phosphorylation (inactivation) of the growth-suppressive RB protein (see Fig. 31.1-1). As p16^{INK4A} is an inhibitor of CDKs, especially CDK4 or CDK6 (which phosphorylate and keep RB in an "inactive" state), its normal role is to positively regulate RB's growth-controlling function by keeping RB unphosphorylated. However, if p16^{INK4A} is inactivated by mutation, RB remains chronically phosphorylated and thus cannot function to regulate growth (see Fig. 31.1-1).

The *p16*^{INK4A} (also called *CDKN2*) gene locus on chromosome 9p21 is frequently abnormal in human malignancies. In lung cancer, *p16*^{INK4A} abnormalities are frequent in NSCLC but rare in SCLC (in which, by contrast, *RB* is mutated in 90% of cases). Thus, these two major histologic lung cancer types have this pathway inactivated by mutation of one or the other gene, and double mutants in the same tumor are very rare. A summary of 20 studies showed that *p16*^{INK4A} point mutations in NSCLCs were observed in only 14% of primary tumors.[3] However, homozygous deletions or aberrant promoter methylation can also down-regulate *p16*^{INK4A}. Indeed, aberrant methylation of *p16*^{INK4A} may be the most frequent as well as an early preneoplastic event in the pathogenesis of squamous cell carcinomas.[4] Taken together, these mechanisms ultimately result in absent p16^{INK4A} expression in approximately 40% of primary NSCLCs,[3] indicating that this may be the most common way to inactivate the p16^{INK4A}-cyclin D1-CDK4-RB pathway in NSCLC. Because of the frequency of the abnormalities, p16^{INK4A} is an attractive clinical trials candidate for replacement gene therapy or induction of re-expression with antimethylation drug therapy.

Complicating matters is the discovery of an alternative reading frame at the *p16*^{INK4A} locus, *p14*^{ARF}, which encodes a protein that binds p53/MDM2 complex, leading to p53 protein stabilization. If *p14*^{ARF} is missing because of mutations in the p16 locus, p53 is less stable and its function diminished. It thus emerges that inactivation of the p53 pathway may also be triggered by abnormalities of the *p16*^{INK4A} gene locus. Another CDK inhibitor gene, *p15*^{INK4B} is situated close to *p16*^{INK4A} and can be co-deleted with *p16*^{INK4A} in NSCLC. However, it appears that the majority of lung cancer abnormalities focus on *p16*^{INK4A} and not on *p15*^{INK4B}.

Cyclin D1 and Cyclin-Dependent Kinase-4

Because cyclin D1/CDK4 complex inhibits RB activity by stimulating its phosphorylation, cyclin D1 or CDK4 overexpression is an alternative way to disrupt this pathway. Immunohistochemically, cyclin D1 is overexpressed in 12% to 47% of primary NSCLCs and, in some cases, cyclin D1 overexpression is associated with a poor prognosis.[30] How this overexpression occurs in lung cancer is unknown.

Retinoblastoma Protein

The RB gene (*RB*), located at chromosomal region 13q14, encodes a growth-suppressive nuclear phosphoprotein. When active (i.e., hypophosphorylated), RB binds and inactivates proteins such as transcription factor E2F-1, which is essential for G_1/S transition of the cell cycle (see Fig. 31.1-1). *RB* mutations (truncation by deletion, nonsense mutation, or splicing abnormalities), together with loss of the wild-type *RB* allele, have been demonstrated in lung cancers, particularly SCLC. The RB protein is absent or structurally abnormal in more than 90% of SCLCs and 15% to 30% of NSCLCs.[31] Absent RB expression may be associated with poor prognosis in NSCLCs, although this is not a consistent finding. The relatively low frequency of *RB* abnormalities in NSCLC is consistent with the frequent disruption of the p16^{INK4A}-cyclin D1-CDK4-RB pathway in these histologic types. Essentially, lung cancers can be characterized as having either *RB* mutation (mostly SCLC) or *p16*^{INK4A} inactivation (mostly NSCLC). Gene therapy with replacement of RB function has been considered, but because of the large size of the *RB* coding region and the necessity for systemic delivery in, for example, typical widely metastatic SCLCs, such therapy has not been actively pursued. Mutations of two other *RB* related genes, *p107* and *RB2/p130,* also have been implicated in lung cancer. In the case of RB2, loss of protein expression and restoration of growth control by genetically re-introducing a normal copy of *RB2* have been demonstrated.[32] Finally, retinoblastoma patients or their relatives who carry a mutant *RB* in the germline have an excess risk of developing small cell lung cancer if they survive into adult life.[33]

PTEN, FHIT, RAR-β, PUTATIVE 3P TUMOR SUPPRESSOR GENES, AND OTHER TUMOR AND GROWTH-SUPPRESSIVE GENE SITES IN LUNG CANCER PATHOGENESIS

Besides the *p53, p16*^{INK4A}*, RB,* and loci, cytogenetic and allelotyping studies show nonrandom, hemiallelic loss at many other chromosome regions in lung cancer. Such tumor-specific somatically acquired loss of heterozygosity is a hallmark feature of traditional TSG inactivation. In other words, the consistent identification of multiple sites of loss of heterozygosity at various chromosomal regions suggests the existence of underlying TSGs in these regions. Usually the remaining allele is silenced by point or small mutations, epigenetic hypermethylation of the promoter region or, less frequently, by a larger deletion. These sites of allele loss have been defined at more than 30 regions dispersed on 21 different chromosomal arms, although the molecular targets of most of these sites is not known.[34] Although several of these chromosomal arms contain known TSGs, including *VHL* (3p25), *APC* (5q21), *WT1* (11p13), *DCC* (18q21), and *NF2* (22q12), these genes are not known to be mutated in lung cancer. The TSG *PTEN,* which encodes a phosphatase, is located at chromosome region 10q23, another common area of allele loss in lung cancer. However, *PTEN* is mutated in only a subset of lung cancers.[35] Frequent loss (60% to 80%) of several 4p and 4q regions were found in thoracic malignancies (particularly SCLC and mesotheliomas); however, the genes involved are not yet known.[36]

Among these chromosomal locations, chromosome 3p allele loss (occurring at more than four different 3p regions) stands out as a very frequent and early event in lung cancer pathogenesis. 3p loss occurs in more than 90% of SCLCs and more than 80% of NSCLCs. In addition, it appears to be the earliest genetic change found in lung cancer development, occurring at great frequency in patches of normal epithelium accompanying lung cancer or in smokers, as well as in sites of hyperplasia, dysplasia, and carcinoma *in situ* of respiratory epithelium (see Molecular Changes in Preneoplasia, later in this chapter). Multiple distinct 3p regions have been identified by allelotyping, including 3p25-26, 3p21.3-22, 3p14, and 3p12. Furthermore, homozygous deletions are found in several lung cancer cell lines (at several 3p21.3 sites, as well as at 3p12 and 3p14.2). Several candidate TSGs have been identified in an approximately 600-kilobase 3p21.3 region homozygously deleted in three SCLCs, and another 800-kilobase deletion region at 3p21 also has been described.[37,38] The *FHIT* (fragile histidine triad) gene is found in the 3p14.2 homozygous deletion region. Forty percent to 80% of lung cancer cells express abnormal *FHIT* messenger RNA transcripts but paradoxically almost always also express wild-type *FHIT* transcripts.[39] Regardless of these molecular complexities, the FHIT protein is absent in many lung cancers, particularly in the squamous cell type (87%) compared to adenocarcinoma (57%) and may also be lost in some preneoplastic lesions. The loss of FHIT protein expression is also strongly associated with smoking.[40,41] Functionally, FHIT may be involved in the regulation of apoptosis and in cell-cycle control.[42] Transfection of wild-type *FHIT* into lung cancers induces apoptosis and blocks tumor formation *in vivo* in mouse models.[43,44] Because of the occurrence of *FHIT* abnormalities early in lung cancer pathogenesis (e.g., in preneoplastic stages), it is possible to consider delivering *FHIT* gene therapy to airways containing multiple preneoplastic lesions by using aerosols.

TGF-β1 is a potent inhibitor of proliferation of most epithelial and hematopoietic cells, and its signal is mediated through TGF-β receptors and subsequently SMAD proteins. In SCLC cells, down-regulation of the type II receptor (TGFβ-RII) located in chromosome region 3p, has been shown to correlate with the resistance to growth inhibition by TGF-β1.[45] However, the TGFβ-RII or SMAD family genes are rarely mutated in lung cancer.

There is considerable evidence of dysfunction of retinoic acid receptor beta (RAR-β), located in chromosome region 3p24, in lung cancers, leading to resistance of lung cancer cells to retinoids and making it an excellent candidate 3p TSG.[46] Although initial studies did not find RAR-β mutations, more recent studies have shown loss of expression of RAR-β protein in approximately 50% of clinically overt lung cancers.[47] It is quite likely that this loss of expression without genomic changes occurs because of methylation of the promoter region. Because of the widespread testing of retinoids as chemoprevention agents, it will be important to characterize the timing of loss of RAR-β function in lung cancer preneoplasia. It is possible that loss of expression of RAR-β may occur at such an early stage that chemoprevention with retinoids cannot succeed.

OTHER BIOLOGIC ABNORMALITIES FOR LUNG CANCER DEVELOPMENT

TELOMERASE ACTIVITY

During normal cell division, telomere shortening leads to cell senescence and thus governs normal cell "mortality." Telomeres are maintained in normal stem cells by the enzyme telomerase. However, with abnormal expression of the enzyme in, for example, tumors, telomerase has been implicated in contributing to human cell immortalization and cancer cell pathogenesis. Telomerase is a ribonucleocomplex, and ectopic expression in tumors of its catalytic subunit, human telomerase reverse transcriptase, appears critical for the cellular immortalization typical of cancer cells. Using the highly sensitive telomere replication amplification protocol assay, approximately 100% of SCLCs and 80% to 85% of NSCLCs were demonstrated to express high levels of telomerase activity. High telomerase activity was associated with increased cell proliferation rates and advanced stage in NSCLCs.[48] Further tests must be performed to conclusively demonstrate that true telomerase-negative NSCLCs exist. If these telomerase-negative tumors truly exist, debulking therapy with surgery and radiotherapy should be considered, even for metastatic disease. It would be predicted that eventually such tumors would "senesce" and stop growing when their telomeres got too short. Telomerase activity and expression of its RNA component are also dysregulated in carcinoma *in situ* lesions associated with lung cancer, indicating that the timing of telomerase activation for lung cancer development can occur in preneoplasia.[49] Because of the nearly ubiquitous expression of telomerase in human tumors, including lung cancer, there is much interest in developing anti-telomerase drugs as new therapeutics.

APOPTOSIS

Unlike normal cells, tumors have acquired the ability to escape from programmed cell death (apoptosis), which usually occurs under adverse conditions such as DNA damage. In addition to p53, other molecules of the complex apoptotic signaling pathways are abnormal in lung cancer cells. For example, the antiapoptotic gene, *BCL2,* can be abnormally overexpressed in SCLCs (75% to 95%) and some NSCLCs (25% to 35% of squamous cell carcinoma and an approximately 10% of adenocarcinoma). Because of the potent role BCL2 plays in suppressing apoptosis and thus also in inhibiting responses to chemotherapy and radiotherapy, there is considerable ongoing effort to develop antisense BCL2 therapeutics, which are entering clinical trials. Also, extracellular matrix proteins may protect SCLC against chemotherapy-induced apoptosis via β_1 integrin–stimulated tyrosine kinase activation.[50] In addition, Fas (CD95) and its ligand (FasL), which play key roles in the initiation of one apoptotic pathway, also have been implicated in lung cancer.[51] In this case, lung cancers express Fas ligand but not the receptor, whereas T cells express the receptor. In this way, lung cancers could cause the clonal deletion of immune T cells that were directed against lung cancer antigens and thus provide a mechanism for escape from immune surveillance.

METASTASIS AND ANGIOGENESIS

Many potential factors influencing metastasis from primary lung cancers have been studied, including cell adhesion molecules. For instance, reduced E-cadherin expression, which can occur by promoter hypermethylation, was associated with tumor dedifferentiation, increased lymph node metastasis, and poor survival in NSCLC patients.[52] Reduced α_3 integrin expression correlated with a poor prognosis of patients with lung adenocarcinoma.[53] Specific CD44 isoforms may be associated with lung cancer metastasis. Meanwhile, matrix metalloproteinases inducing stromal degradation may also be involved in lung cancer invasion: Gelatinase A expression was observed in approximately 50% of SCLCs and 65% of NSCLCs, and stromelysin-3 overexpression was detected in stromal elements of primary NSCLCs. Because of this expression, several ongoing clinical trials of matrix metalloproteinase inhibitors in the treatment of lung cancer are ongoing. Finally, multiple other as yet unidentified genes may also be involved in lung tumor progression and metastases, as evidenced by the development of additional allelic losses (at 2q, 9p, 18q, and 22q) in brain metastases compared to the primary NSCLCs in the same patients.[54]

Tumor angiogenesis is necessary for a tumor mass to grow beyond a few millimeters in size. Currently, angiogenesis is thought to be regulated by the balance of inducers and inhibitors that are released by both tumor cells and host cells. Vascular endothelial growth factor (VEGF) and basic fibroblast growth factor are two major angiogenesis inducers produced by human lung cancers.[55] Angiogenic CXC chemokines, such as interleukin-8, also have been implicated in lung cancer. Mutations in *p53* lead to decreased expression of thrombospondin, a negative regulator of angiogenesis. Overall it is thought that lung cancers produce factors that stimulate angiogenesis and stop producing others that would inhibit this process. Thus, tumor angiogenesis has become a major new therapeutic target for lung cancer. Clinical trials with humanized recombinant anti-VEGF monoclonal antibody combined with chemotherapy in NSCLC are already ongoing. In addition, several new small molecules that inhibit the tyrosine kinase activity of the VEGF receptor(s) are entering clinical trials as new drugs.

CARCINOGENS IN TOBACCO SMOKE AND GENETIC SUSCEPTIBILITY TO LUNG CANCER (GENETIC EPIDEMIOLOGY)

The major cause of lung cancer, of course, comes from smoking, and tobacco smoke contains many substances, including carcinogens, co-carcinogens, and tumor promoters. Among them, 20 carcinogens convincingly cause lung tumors in laboratory animals or humans and are likely to be involved in lung cancer induction.[56] The carcinogenic effects of tobacco smoke in the lung involve the induction of carcinogen-activating and inactivating enzymes, as well as covalent DNA adduct formation, which may cause DNA misreplication and mutation. DNA adducts have been identified in the bronchial tissue of lung cancer patients, and adduct levels correlate with the amount of tobacco smoke exposure. Of great importance is preventing children from starting to smoke. In this regard, it was found that, in former smokers, age at smoking initiation was inversely associated with DNA adduct levels.[57] Thus, after controlling for the amount of smoking, the earlier one started smoking, the worse the long-term damage. In addition, for reasons that are not yet clear, it appears that women are more susceptible to developing lung cancer from cigarette smoking than men.[58] Of the three major classes of carcinogens in tobacco smoke (polycyclic aromatic hydrocarbons, such as benzo[a]pyrene; nitrosamines; and aromatic amines), much interest focuses on the nitrosamines, especially 4-(methylnitrosamino)-1-(3-pyridyl)-1-butanone (NNK), partly because it induces tumors of the lung—primarily adenomas and adenocarcinomas—independent of the route of administration in mice.[56]

The finding that not every heavy smoker develops lung cancer has led to the concept of interindividual variation and the hypothesis that individuals may exhibit genetic polymorphisms in carcinogen-metabolizing pathways that determine individual lung cancer risk. Clearly, such genetic susceptibility operates in close interaction with smoking and other external carcinogenic factors ("gene-environment" interaction, with smoking being the primary environment factor). Among genes for carcinogen-metabolizing enzymes, polymorphisms in the cytochrome P-450 genes *CYP1A1, CYP2D6, CYP2E1* and in mu-class glutathione S-transferase (*GSTM1*) have received the most attention. Although studies have suggested that there may be a modest association of GSTM1 null polymorphism with lung cancer,[59] studying single candidate genes may not be adequate to predict lung cancer risk due to complexity of carcinogen metabolism and gene-gene and gene-environment interactions.[56] In addition to carcinogens, it also appears that persons may inherit different susceptibility to become addicted to nicotine, for example, through polymorphisms in one of the dopamine receptors. Overall, molecular epidemiology, aided by DNA microarray technology together with the Human Genome Project, should in the near future help to identify individuals at highest risk of developing lung cancer. Such information will be of great value in new lung cancer screening trials (for example with spiral CT scans) and in chemoprevention trials.

MOLECULAR CHANGES IN PRENEOPLASIA

Before clinically recognizable lung cancer develops, a series of morphologically distinct changes (hyperplasia, metaplasia, dysplasia, and carcinoma *in situ*) can be observed in the bronchial epithelium of smokers. It is felt that dysplasia and carcinoma *in situ* represent true preneoplastic (precancerous) changes. These sequential changes found with squamous cell cancers arising from central bronchi have long been recognized, whereas other changes in peripheral bronchioles and alveoli (adeno- and large cell cancers), such as adenomatous and alveolar hyperplasia, are more recently described.

It is now clear that preneoplastic cells contain several genetic abnormalities identical to some of the abnormalities found in overt lung cancer cells. Immunohistochemical analysis has confirmed abnormal expression of protooncogenes (cyclin D1) and TSGs (p53) in these lesions.[60] Allelotyping of precisely microdissected, preneoplastic foci of cells shows that 3p allele loss is currently the earliest known change, suggesting that one or more 3p TSGs may act as "gatekeepers" for lung cancer pathogenesis. This loss is followed by 9p allele loss, 8p allele loss, and 17p allele loss (and *p53* mutation) (Fig. 31.1-2).[61] Even the histologically normal bronchial epithelium adjacent to cancers has been shown to have genetic losses. Similarly, atypical alveolar hyperplasia, the potential precursor lesion of adenocarcinomas, also harbors *KRAS* mutations.[62] These observations are also consistent with the multistep model of carcinogenesis and a "field cancerization" process, whereby the whole tissue region is repeatedly exposed to carcinogenic damage (tobacco smoke) and is at risk for developing multiple separate foci of neoplasia. Although all types of lung cancers have associated molecular abnormalities in their normal and preneoplastic lung epithelium, small cell lung cancer patients in particular appear to have multiple genetic alterations occurring in their histologically normal-appearing respiratory epithelium. Molecular changes have been found not only in the lungs of patients with lung cancer but also in the lungs of current and former smokers without lung cancer.[63,64] These molecular alterations are thus important targets for use in the early detection of lung cancer and for use as surrogate biomarkers in following the efficacy of lung cancer chemoprevention. In this regard, it appears that the smoke-damaged lung has thousands of multiple clonal or subclonal patches of approximately 90,000 cells each in the respiratory epithelium containing clones of cells with 3p and other allele loss abnormalities.[65]

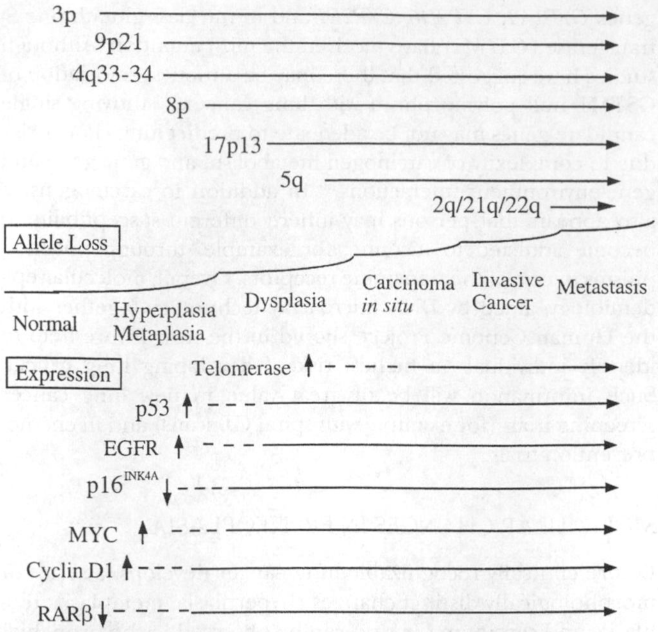

FIGURE 31.1-2. Timing of genetic changes found in preneoplastic lesions in respiratory epithelium, best studied to date in squamous cell lung carcinoma. Note that not every change is necessary, and the sequence may not always be the same. EGFR, epidermal growth factor receptor; RAR-β, retinoic acid receptor beta.

MOLECULAR TOOLS IN THE LUNG CANCER CLINIC

Our understanding of the molecular genetic changes in lung cancer pathogenesis is advancing rapidly. Some abnormalities also occur in other human cancers, whereas others appear more specific for lung cancer. Where their biochemical function is known, the proteins rendered abnormal appear to fall into several growth regulatory pathways. Thus, the "wiring" diagram of the lung cancer cell is becoming clear. There is a substantial effort to translate this current scientific knowledge of these abnormalities from the bench to the bedside. These approaches fall into four general categories:

1. Identification of persons at highest risk of developing lung cancer to enable chemoprevention and intensified smoking cessation efforts. In this regards, with improved methods of molecular identification of true precancerous lesions, our paradigm will become "treatment" of precancerous lesions rather than "chemoprevention." Obviously, because this treatment would occur in individuals without clinically evident cancer, the treatments must have low toxicity and high risk-benefit ratios.
2. Early detection tools to identify primary and recurrent disease (e.g., polymerase chain reaction–based molecular methods for testing body fluids).[5,66] Again, such "early detection" of invasive but clinically occult disease would require careful analysis of risk-benefit ratios. Because only one out of ten cigarette smokers eventually develops lung cancer, the identification of persons with a genetic susceptibility to lung cancer should allow targeting and intensification of smoking cessation, early detection, and chemoprevention efforts. In this regard, the encouraging new information on spiral CT scanning for the early detection of lung cancer[67] should be greatly targeted and enhanced by combining radiologic screening with identification of genetic epidemiology markers and acquired respiratory genetic alterations to identify the individuals at highest risk.
3. Identification of prognostic biomarkers[68] that would also include markers that would predict the response to various therapies such as chemo- and radiotherapy.
4. The designing of new cancer-specific therapies based on knowledge of genetic abnormalities. This includes replacing mutant TSGs; developing drugs targeted against activated protooncogenes; interfering with autocrine or paracrine loops; and inhibiting angiogenesis, metastasis, and apoptotic pathways in cancer cells. Although new therapies may be dramatically effective, it is probably more reasonable to assume that they would complement rather than replace existing therapies.

REFERENCES

1. Testa JR, Liu Z, Feder M, et al. Advances in the analysis of chromosome alterations in human lung carcinomas. *Cancer Genet Cytogenet* 1997;95:20.
2. Lengauer C, Kinzler KW, Vogelstein B. Genetic instabilities in human cancers. *Nature* 1998;396:643.
3. Sekido Y, Fong KM, Minna JD. Progress in understanding the molecular pathogenesis of human lung cancer. *Biochim Biophys Acta* 1998;1378:F21.
4. Belinsky SA, Nikula KJ, Palmisano WA, et al. Aberrant methylation of p16(INK4a) is an early event in lung cancer and a potential biomarker for early diagnosis. *Proc Natl Acad Sci U S A* 1998;95:11891.
5. Esteller M, Sanchez-Cespedes M, Rosell R, et al. Detection of aberrant promoter hypermethylation of tumor suppressor genes in serum DNA from non–small cell lung cancer patients. *Cancer Res* 1999;59:67.
6. Rusch V, Klimstra D, Venkatraman E, et al. Overexpression of the epidermal growth factor receptor and its ligand transforming growth factor alpha is frequent in resectable non–small cell lung cancer but does not predict tumor progression. *Clin Cancer Res* 1997;3:515.
7. Tsai CM, Chang KT, Wu LH, et al. Correlations between intrinsic chemoresistance and *HER-2/neu* gene expression, *p53* gene mutations, and cell proliferation characteristics in non–small cell lung cancer cell lines. *Cancer Res* 1996;56:206.
8. Krystal GW, DeBerry CS, Linnekin D, Litz J. Lck associates with and is activated by Kit in a small cell lung cancer cell line: inhibition of SCF-mediated growth by the Src family kinase inhibitor PP1. *Cancer Res* 1998;58:4660.
9. Siegfried JM, Weissfeld LA, Singh-Kaw P, et al. Association of immunoreactive hepatocyte growth factor with poor survival in resectable non–small cell lung cancer. *Cancer Res* 1997;57:433.
10. Kelley MJ, Linnoila RI, Avis IL, et al. Antitumor activity of a monoclonal antibody directed against gastrin-releasing peptide in patients with small cell lung cancer. *Chest* 1997;112:256.
11. Richardson GE, Johnson BE. The biology of lung cancer. *Semin Oncol* 1993;20:105.
12. Rosell R, Li S, Skacel Z, et al. Prognostic impact of mutated K-*ras* gene in surgically resected non–small cell lung cancer patients. *Oncogene* 1993;8:2407.
13. Graziano SL, Gamble GP, Newman NB, et al. Prognostic significance of K-*ras* codon 12 mutations in patients with resected stage I and II non-small-cell lung cancer. *J Clin Oncol* 1999;17:668.
14. Huncharek M, Muscat J, Geschwind JF. K-ras oncogene mutation as a prognostic marker in non–small cell lung cancer: a combined analysis of 881 cases. *Carcinogenesis* 1999;20:1507.
15. Rodenhuis S, Boerrigter L, Top B, et al. Mutational activation of the K-*ras* oncogene and the effect of chemotherapy in advanced adenocarcinoma of the lung: a prospective study. *J Clin Oncol* 1997;15:285.
16. Ravi RK, Weber E, McMahon M, et al. Activated Raf-1 causes growth arrest in human small cell lung cancer cells. *J Clin Invest* 1998;101:153.
17. Wang SS, Esplin ED, Li JL, et al. Alterations of the *PPP2R1B* gene in human lung and colon cancer. *Science* 1998;282:284.
18. Ou X, Campau S, Slusher R, et al. Mechanism of all-*trans*-retinoic acid–mediated L-*myc* gene regulation in small cell lung cancer. *Oncogene* 1996;13:1893.
19. Makela TP, Hellsten E, Vesa J, et al. The rearranged L-*myc* fusion gene (*RLF*) encodes a Zn-15 related zinc finger protein. *Oncogene* 1995;11:2699.
20. Bennett WP, Hussain SP, Vahakangas KH, et al. Molecular epidemiology of human cancer risk: gene-environment interactions and p53 mutation spectrum in human lung cancer. *J Pathol* 1999;187:8.

21. Tammemagi MC, McLaughlin JR, Bull SB. Meta-analyses of p53 tumor suppressor gene alterations and clinicopathological features in resected lung cancers. *Cancer Epidemiol Biomarkers Prev* 1999;8:625.
22. Denissenko MF, Pao A, Tang M, Pfeifer GP. Preferential formation of benzo[*a*]pyrene adducts at lung cancer mutational hotspots in *P53*. *Science* 1996;274:430.
23. Casey G, Lopez ME, Ramos JC, et al. DNA sequence analysis of exons 2 through 11 and immunohistochemical staining are required to detect all known p53 alterations in human malignancies. *Oncogene* 1996;13:1971.
24. Graziano SL. Non–small cell lung cancer: clinical value of new biological predictors. *Lung Cancer* 1997;17:S37.
25. Lubin R, Zalcman G, Bouchet L, et al. Serum p53 antibodies as early markers of lung cancer. *Nature Med* 1995;1:701.
26. Zalcman G, Schlichtholz B, Tredaniel J, et al. Monitoring of p53 autoantibodies in lung cancer during therapy: relationship to response to treatment. *Clin Cancer Res* 1998;4:1359.
27. Mitsudomi T, Suzuki S, Yatabe Y, et al. Clinical implications of p53 autoantibodies in the sera of patients with non-small-cell lung cancer. *J Natl Cancer Inst* 1998;90:1563.
28. Roth JA, Nguyen D, Lawrence DD, et al. Retrovirus-mediated wild-type *p53* gene transfer to tumors of patients with lung cancer. *Nature Med* 1996;2:985.
29. Swisher SG, Roth JA, Nemunaitis J, et al. Adenovirus-mediated p53 gene transfer in advanced non-small-cell lung cancer. *J Natl Cancer Inst* 1999;91:763.
30. Mishina T, Dosaka-Akita H, Kinoshita I, et al. Cyclin D1 expression in non-small-cell lung cancers: its association with altered p53 expression, cell proliferation and clinical outcome. *Brit J Cancer* 1999;80:1289.
31. Reissmann PT, Koga H, Takahashi R, et al. Inactivation of the retinoblastoma susceptibility gene in non-small-cell lung cancer. *Oncogene* 1993;8:1913.
32. Claudio P, Howard C, Pacilio C, et al. Mutations in the retinoblastoma-related gene RB2/p130 in lung tumors and suppression of tumor growth *in vivo* by retroviral-mediate gene transfer. 2000;60:372.
33. Sanders BM, Jay M, Draper GJ, Roberts EM. Non-ocular cancer in relatives of retinoblastoma patients. *Br J Cancer* 1989;60:358.
34. Kohno T, Yokota J. How many tumor suppressor genes are involved in human lung carcinogenesis? *Carcinogenesis* 1999;20:1403.
35. Forgacs E, Biesterveld EJ, Sekido Y, et al. Mutation analysis of the *PTEN/MMAC1* gene in lung cancer. *Oncogene* 1998;17:1557.
36. Shivapurkar N, Virmani AK, Wistuba II, et al. Deletions of chromosome 4 at multiple sites are frequent in malignant mesothelioma and small cell lung carcinoma. *Clin Cancer Res* 1999;5:17.
37. Sekido Y, Bader S, Latif F, et al. Human semaphorins A(V) and IV reside in the 3p21.3 small cell lung cancer deletion region and demonstrate distinct expression patterns. *Proc Natl Acad Sci U S A* 1996;93:4120.
38. Wei MH, Latif F, Bader S, et al. Construction of a 600-kilobase cosmid clone contig and generation of a transcriptional map surrounding the lung cancer tumor suppressor gene (*TSG*) locus on human chromosome 3p21.3: progress toward the isolation of a lung cancer TSG. *Cancer Res* 1996;56:1487.
39. Fong KM, Biesterveld EJ, Virmani A, et al. *FHIT* and *FRA3B* 3p14.2 allele loss are common in lung cancer and preneoplastic bronchial lesions and are associated with cancer-related *FHIT* cDNA splicing aberrations. *Cancer Res* 1997;57:2256.
40. Sozzi G, Pastorino U, Moiraghi L, et al. Loss of FHIT function in lung cancer and preinvasive bronchial lesions. *Cancer Res* 1998;58:5032.
41. Geradts J, Fong K, Zimmerman P, Minna J. Loss of Fhit expression in non–small cell lung cancer: correlation with other molecular genetic abnormalities and clinico-pathologic features. *Br J Cancer* 2000;82:1191.
42. Sard L, Accornero P, Tornielli S, et al. The tumor-suppressor gene FHIT is involved in the regulation of apoptosis and in cell cycle control. *Proc Natl Acad Sci U S A* 1999;96:8489.
43. Ji L, Fang B, Yen N, et al. Induction of apoptosis and inhibition of tumorigenicity and tumor growth by adenovirus vector-mediated fragile histidine triad (*FHIT*) gene overexpression. *Cancer Res* 1999;59:3333.
44. Siprashvili Z, Sozzi G, Barnes LD, et al. Replacement of Fhit in cancer cells suppresses tumorigenicity. *Proc Natl Acad Sci U S A* 1997;94:13771.
45. Norgaard P, Spang-Thomsen M, Poulsen HS. Expression and autoregulation of transforming growth factor β receptor mRNA in small-cell lung cancer cell lines. *Br J Cancer* 1996;73:1037.
46. Geradts J, Chen JY, Russell EK, et al. Human lung cancer cell lines exhibit resistance to retinoic acid treatment. *Cell Growth Differ* 1993;4:799.
47. Picard E, Seguin C, Monhoven N, et al. Expression of retinoid receptor genes and proteins in non-small-cell lung cancer [see comments]. *J Natl Cancer Inst* 1999;91:1059.
48. Albanell J, Lonardo F, Rusch V, et al. High telomerase activity in primary lung cancers: association with increased cell proliferation rates and advanced pathologic stage. *J Natl Cancer Inst* 1997;89:1609.
49. Yashima K, Litzky LA, Kaiser L, et al. Telomerase expression in respiratory epithelium during the multistage pathogenesis of lung carcinomas. *Cancer Res* 1997;57:2373.
50. Sethi T, Rintoul RC, Moore SM, et al. Extracellular matrix proteins protect small cell lung cancer cells against apoptosis: a mechanism for small cell lung cancer growth and drug resistance *in vivo*. *Nature Med* 1999;5:662.
51. Niehans GA, Brunner T, Frizelle SP, et al. Human lung carcinomas express Fas ligand. *Cancer Res* 1997;57:1007.
52. Sulzer MA, Leers MP, van Noord JA, Bollen EC, Theunissen PH. Reduced E-cadherin expression is associated with increased lymph node metastasis and unfavorable prognosis in non–small cell lung cancer. *Am J Respir Crit Care Med* 1998;157:1319.
53. Adachi M, Taki T, Huang C, et al. Reduced integrin alpha3 expression as a factor of poor prognosis of patients with adenocarcinoma of the lung. *J Clin Oncol* 1998;16:1060.
54. Shiseki M, Kohno T, Adachi J, et al. Comparative allotype of early and advanced stage non–small cell lung carcinomas. *Genes Chromosomes Cancer* 1996;17:71.
55. Mattern J, Koomagi R, Volm M. Association of vascular endothelial growth factor expression with intratumoral microvessel density and tumour cell proliferation in human epidermoid lung carcinoma. *Br J Cancer* 1996;73:931.
56. Hecht SS. Tobacco smoke carcinogens and lung cancer. *J Natl Cancer Inst* 1999;91:1194.
57. Wiencke JK, Thurston SW, Kelsey KT, et al. Early age at smoking initiation and tobacco carcinogen DNA damage in the lung. *J Natl Cancer Inst* 1999;91:614.
58. Zang EA, Wynder EL. Differences in lung cancer risk between men and women: examination of the evidence. *J Natl Cancer Inst* 1996;88:183.
59. Spivack SD, Fasco MJ, Walker VE, Kaminsky LS. The molecular epidemiology of lung cancer. *Crit Rev Toxicol* 1997;27:319.
60. Lonardo F, Rusch V, Langenfeld J, Dmitrovsky E, Klimstra DS. Overexpression of cyclins D1 and E is frequent in bronchial preneoplasia and precedes squamous cell carcinoma development. *Cancer Res* 1999;59:2470.
61. Wistuba II, Behrens C, Virmani AK, et al. Allelic losses at chromosome 8p21-23 are early and frequent events in the pathogenesis of lung cancer. *Cancer Res* 1999;59:1973.
62. Westra WH, Baas IO, Hruban RH, et al. K-*ras* oncogene activation in atypical alveolar hyperplasias of the human lung. *Cancer Res* 1996;56:2224.
63. Wistuba II, Lam S, Behrens C, et al. Molecular damage in the bronchial epithelium of current and former smokers. *J Natl Cancer Inst* 1997;89:1366.
64. Wistuba II, Behrens C, Milchgrub S, et al. Sequential molecular abnormalities are involved in the multistage development of squamous cell lung carcinoma. *Oncogene* 1999;18:643.
65. Park IW, Wistuba II, Maitra A, et al. Multiple clonal abnormalities in the bronchial epithelium of patients with lung cancer. *J Natl Cancer Inst* 1999;91:1863.
66. Ahrendt SA, Chow JT, Xu LH, et al. Molecular detection of tumor cells in bronchoalveolar lavage fluid from patients with early stage lung cancer. *J Natl Cancer Inst* 1999;91:332.
67. Henschke CI, McCauley DI, Yankelevitz DF, et al. Early Lung Cancer Action Project: overall design and findings from baseline screening [see comments]. *Lancet* 1999;354:99.
68. D'Amico TA, Massey M, Herndon JE II, Moore MB, Harpole DH Jr. A biologic risk model for stage I lung cancer: immunohistochemical analysis of 408 patients with the use of ten molecular markers. *J Thorac Cardiovasc Surg* 1999;117:736.

ROBERT J. GINSBERG
EVERETT E. VOKES
KENNETH ROSENZWEIG

SECTION **2**

Non–Small Cell Lung Cancer

EPIDEMIOLOGY

INCIDENCE

Lung cancer is among the most commonly occurring malignancies in the world and is one of the few that continues to show an increasing incidence. In the United States, lung cancer is the leading cause of cancer death in men, and it surpassed breast cancer as the leading cause of cancer death in women in the latter part of the 1980s.[1] In the year 2000, there will be approximately 164,100 new cases and approximately 156,900 deaths from this disease (Fig. 31.2-1).

Excluding this malignancy, most developed countries have shown declines in death rates from cancer in the last 20 years. During the same period in countries such as the United States and Canada, the death rate from lung cancer increased more than threefold but, in the last 5 years, it has finally begun to decline. In developing countries, the death rate from lung cancer continues to accelerate. These changes appear to be affected significantly by the observed difference in smoking habits and cigarette tar levels in developed and developing countries.[2]

The incidence of lung cancer now exceeds 70 per 100,000 men in the United States. As we enter the twenty-first century,

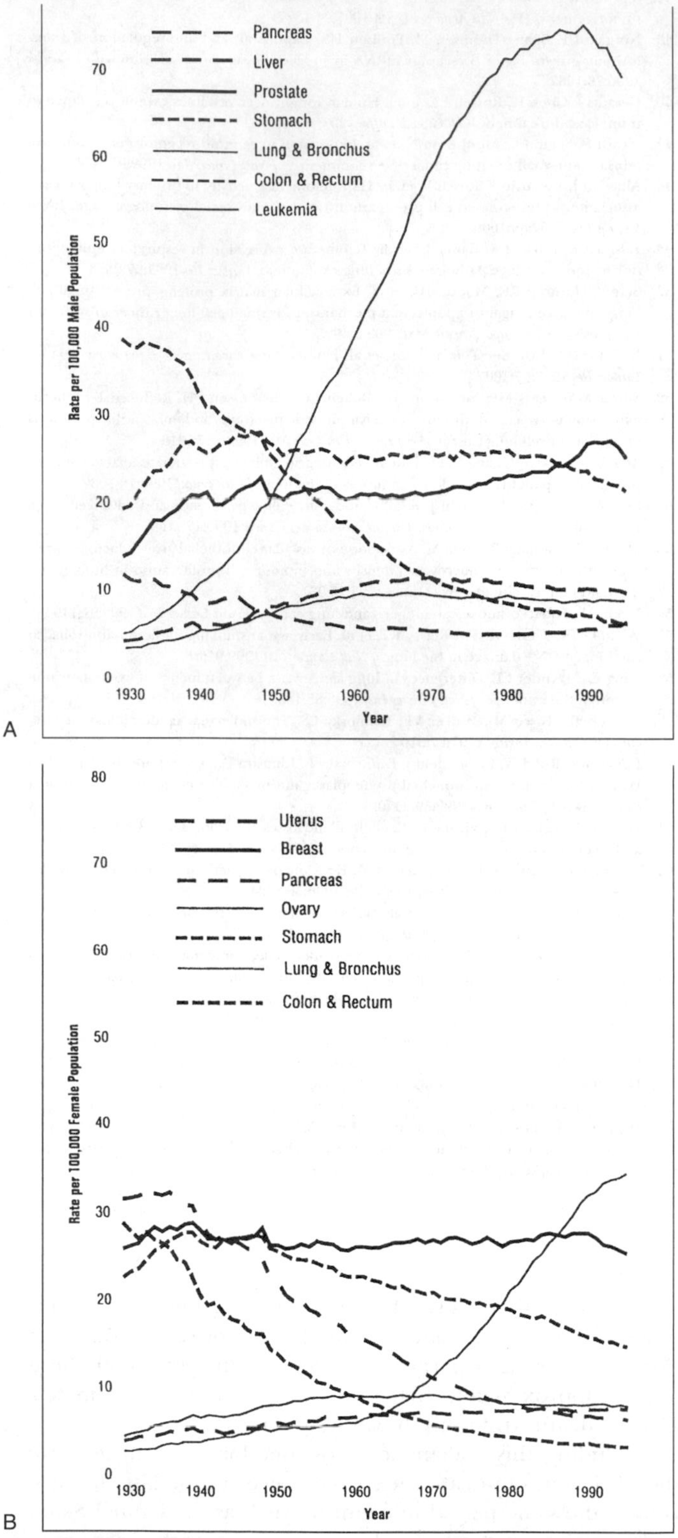

FIGURE 31.2-1. The age-adjusted cancer death rates for selected sites in males (**A**) and females (**B**) in the United States from 1930 to 1996. It appears that lung cancer deaths from smoking are leveling off in males but are continuing to rise in females. Data adjusted to the age distribution of the 1970 U.S. Census Population (U.S. National Center for Health Statistics and U.S. Bureau of the Census).

it is expected that the altered smoking habits of the nation's population during the last two decades and the decreased tar content of cigarettes consumed in the United States will lead to a further decline in lung cancer incidence.

MORTALITY

In the United States, only 14% of patients who develop lung cancer survive 5 years. These mortality rates (>150,000/year) far exceed those of the acquired immunodeficiency syndrome epidemic. However, this survival rate has only slightly increased in the last two decades, and it appears unlikely that marked improvements will occur in the near future. With the anticipated decreased incidence, however, it is hoped that the lung cancer epidemic, at least in developed countries, will abate and that the total number of deaths per year attributed to this cancer will decline even further.

LUNG CANCER CONTROL

With the solid base of scientific information linking cigarette smoking habits to the development of lung cancer, many countries have launched programs to decrease tobacco use and educate the population. Included in these programs are legislative activity (e.g., increased taxes, smoke-free areas, banning tobacco advertisements), educational activities through mass media and schools, and interventional approaches (e.g., smoking-cessation clinics) targeted to groups at the highest risk for developing tobacco-related cancer. The greatest impact on decreased smoking habits appears to be the societal stigma directed at smokers. These activities have reduced the percentage of the U.S. population who smoke from a high of approximately 40% to approximately 30%. However, this decline has now leveled off. The only cohort that has demonstrated an increasing smoking habit in the United States is younger women. It is hoped, however, that with the societal pressures and the educational programs in developed countries, the incidence of smoking will continue to decrease. It is also hoped that a similar trend will occur in developing countries, where smoking activity continues to increase at present.[3]

SMOKING

The epidemiologic data on smoking and lung cancer fulfill the following criteria for causal association: the consistency of results across studies, the strength of the relation and its specificity, the correct temporal sequence between exposure and disease, and the coherence of the association as evidenced by a dose-response relation.[4]

It has been estimated that 80% of lung cancer deaths among men (approximately 65,000 deaths per year) and 75% of lung cancer deaths among women (approximately 27,000 deaths per year) are attributable to smoking.[5] Mattson et al.[6] calculated that a 35-year-old man who smokes 25 or more cigarettes per day has a 13% risk of dying of lung cancer before the age of 75 years, a 10% chance of dying of coronary heart disease, and a 28% chance of dying of smoking-related disease.

There is clear evidence for a dose-response relation between smoking and lung cancer. The risk of lung cancer increases with the number of cigarettes smoked, years of smoking duration, earlier age at onset of smoking, degree of inhalation, tar and nicotine content, the use of unfiltered cigarettes, and passive smoking,[4] and it decreases in proportion to the number of years after smoking cessation.[7] These relationships to lung carcinogenesis are discussed in more detail in Chapter 11 and are incontrovertible.[8–23,24,27]

OCCUPATION

Increases in lung cancer risk accompany exposure to carcinogens, such as asbestos,[28–39] radon,[40–44] bis(chloromethyl)ether, polycyclic aromatic hydrocarbons, chromium, nickel, and inorganic arsenic compounds.[25,26] The association with occupational exposure to these agents appears to be independent of cigarette smoking.

DIET

The role of dietary antioxidant micronutrients in the prevention of lung cancer is reviewed in Chapter 23.3. The presumed mechanism leading to prevention of carcinogenesis by these nutrients is that antioxidant micronutrients, including carotenoids, vitamins C and E, and selenium, have an important role in scavenging free radicals produced endogenously and exogenously by tobacco smoke, solvents, and pollutants. Carotenoids and vitamins C and E trap free radicals and reactive oxygen molecules, whereas selenium is a component of antioxidant enzymes.[45] Analysis of the role of nutrients in the cause of lung cancer is confounded by methodologic problems and by the conflicting results of studies.[45–49] However, to date, chemoprevention studies have failed to have an impact on lung cancer incidence.[50–60]

EVIDENCE FOR A GENETIC PREDISPOSITION

There is limited evidence that genetic factors may contribute to lung cancer risk. Variations in the metabolism of carcinogens have been implicated.[61] The pathways to create these toxic metabolites are genetically determined. The metabolism of the antihypertensive drug debrisoquin is genetically determined by a single gene. The metabolisms of many drugs and chemicals correlate with that of debrisoquin,[61] and this may also apply to carcinogenic components of cigarette smoke (Table 31.2-1), although this has not been proven for any one substance with respect to lung carcinogenesis.[61–65] Several approaches have been adopted to detect a genetic association: studies of familial clustering, studies of naturally occurring antigens, and studies of the metabolism of drugs. Studies of familial clustering have been interpreted as showing no substantial genetic predisposition.[66–68] Braun et al.[66] conducted a twin cohort study and found no genetic factors to be predictive of lung cancer. Highway et al.[69] observed that the allele K-ras occurred in 29% of non–small cell lung cancer (NSCLC) cases, compared with 15% of controls ($P = .03$). Numerous other chromosomal abnormalities (rearrangements and deletions) are present in lung cancer. These abnormalities are thought to result from the effects of carcinogens or the genetic instability observed in malignant transformation.

Although the molecular and genetic events underlying the pathogenesis of lung cancer are an area of active investigation, no genetic abnormality has conclusively defined the risk of lung cancer. In NSCLC, the most frequently identified abnormalities are deregulation of tumor suppressor gene p53, aberrant expression of the epidermal growth factor receptor (EGFR) and one of its ligands, and the presence of K-ras abnormalities in adenocarcinoma (discussed in New Potential Prognostic Markers).[70–74]

APPLICATIONS OF ADVANCES IN LUNG CANCER BIOLOGY TO CLINICAL PRACTICE

Advances in our understanding of the biology of lung cancer have the potential to affect all areas of lung cancer management. The identification of specific mutations related to tobacco exposure has elucidated the possible molecular foundation for the association of cigarette smoking and lung cancer and may allow us better to identify at-risk people for chemoprevention programs. The presence of autocrine growth factor receptors, specific mutations, or chromosomal deletions may provide additional or more accurate means for diagnosing, staging, choosing therapies, and establishing prognosis for patients with lung cancer. The presence of K-ras point mutations has been shown to be associated with a shortened survival in patients with completely resected NSCLC.[72] Clinical trials targeting adjuvant therapies for patients with resected NSCLC with K-ras point mutations are in progress. Monoclonal antibodies or other drugs blocking the action of epidermal growth factor are in clinical trials.[75,76] The activation of cellular receptors for virtually all autocrine growth factors involves the activation of a protein kinase.[77] This observation has given us a new therapeutic target, and the search for agents specifically inhibiting this enzyme is under way. The mutated sequences of p53 provide a unique, tumor-specific antigen at which to direct therapeutic strategies.[78] New treatment approaches using viral vectors to reverse discordant p53 mutations are in progress.

TABLE 31.2-1. Major Mutagens, Carcinogens, and Related Substances in Tobacco Smoke

Substance	*Effect*	*Model*
PARTICULATE PHASE		
Neutral fraction	C	Rodents
Benzo[a]pyrene	C	
Dibenz[a]anthracene	C	
Basic fraction	C	
Nicotine		
Tobacco-specific nitrosamines	C	Rodents
Acidic fraction	CC + TP	
Cathecol		
Unidentified	TP	
Residue	C	
Nickel	C	
Cadmium	C	
^{210}Po	C	
GASEOUS PHASE	C + M	
Hydrazine	C	Mice
Vinyl chloride	M	Ames

C, carcinogenic; M, mutagenic; TP, toxic product.

PATHOLOGY

The World Health Organization (WHO) classification of lung cancer is accepted worldwide (Table 31.2-2). NSCLC includes carcinoma, adenocarcinoma, and large cell (undifferentiated) carcinoma.

HISTOGENESIS

Evidence is increasing that lung cancer is derived from a pluripotent stem cell that is capable of expressing a variety of phenotypes. This epithelial stem cell, in normal histogenesis, differentiates to those cells found in the tracheobronchial tree, including pseudo-

TABLE 31.2-2. World Health Organization Histologic Classification of Epithelial Tumors of the Lung

Preinvasive lesions
- Squamous dysplasia/carcinoma *in situ*
- Atypical adenomatous hyperplasia
- Diffuse idiopathic pulmonary neuroendocrine cell hyperplasia

Invasive malignant lesions
- Squamous cell carcinoma
  - Variants
    - Papillary
    - Clear cell
    - Small cell
    - Basaloid
- Small cell carcinoma
  - Variant
    - Combined small cell carcinoma
- Adenocarcinoma
  - Acinar
  - Papillary
  - Bronchioloalveolar carcinoma
    - Nonmucinous (Clara cell/type II pneumocyte) type
    - Mucinous (goblet cell) type
    - Mixed mucinous and nonmucinous (Clara cell/type II pneumocyte and goblet cell) type, or indeterminate cell type
  - Solid adenocarcinoma with mucin formation
  - Adenocarcinoma with mixed subtypes
  - Variants
    - Well-differentiated fetal adenocarcinoma
    - Mucinous ("colloid") adenocarcinoma
    - Mucinous cystadenocarcinoma
    - Signet ring adenocarcinoma
    - Clear cell adenocarcinoma
- Large cell carcinoma
  - Variants
    - Large cell neuroendocrine carcinoma
    - Combined large cell neuroendocrine carcinoma
    - Basaloid carcinoma
    - Lymphoepithelioma-like carcinoma
    - Clear cell carcinoma
    - Large cell carcinoma with rhabdoid phenotype
- Adenosquamous carcinoma
- Carcinomas with pleomorphic, sarcomatoid, or sarcomatous elements
  - Carcinomas with spindle or giant cells
    - Pleomorphic carcinoma
    - Spindle cell carcinoma
    - Giant cell carcinoma
  - Carcinosarcoma
  - Pulmonary blastoma
- Carcinoid tumours
  - Typical carcinoid
  - Atypical carcinoid
- Carcinomas of salivary gland type
  - Mucoepidermoid carcinoma
  - Adenoid cystic carcinoma
  - Others
- Unclassified

[From WD Travis, TD Colby, B Corrin. *Histologic Typing of Lung and Pleural Tumors—The World Health Organization (WHO) Classification of Lung Cancer 1999* (rev. 10 October 1998). Geneva: World Health Organization, 1999, with permission.]

stratified reserved cells, ciliated goblet columnar cells, neuroendocrine cells, and type I and II pneumocytes seen lining the alveoli. Cells that are capable of division can express hyperplastic, metaplastic, or neoplastic change.[79] Frequently, a lung cancer exhibits two or more histologic patterns. The frequency of this occurrence depends on the assiduity of the pathologist and the number of sections examined. In one study, when at least 10 blocks from each tumor were examined, 45 of the 100 cases demonstrated heterogeneity, and 10% of cases showed elements of both squamous cell carcinoma and adenocarcinoma.[80]

It appears that squamous cell carcinoma and small cell carcinoma have a distinct dose-response relation, with increasing tobacco exposure producing increasing numbers of these histologic subtypes. Worldwide, however, adenocarcinoma appears to be increasing, especially in women, despite the fact that it does not have this significant dose-response relation with smoking. This increasing incidence of adenocarcinoma is especially seen in the United States and is less apparent in Europe and Japan.[81]

Squamous Cell Carcinoma

Although at one time the most frequent of all lung cancers, squamous cell carcinoma in North America has not seen the marked increase observed with adenocarcinoma, the latter tumor accounting for most of the recent increased incidence of lung cancer. Some of these differences may be related to the change from nonfiltered to filtered cigarettes and their relation to site of deposition of the carcinogens. Squamous cell carcinoma arises most frequently in proximal segmental bronchi and is associated with squamous metaplasia. In its earliest form, carcinoma *in situ*, stratified squamous epithelium is replaced by malignant squamous cells without invasion through the basement membrane. Because of the ability of these cells to exfoliate, this tumor can be detected by cytologic examination at its earliest stage. With further growth, the tumor invades the basement membrane and extends into the bronchial lumen, producing obstruction with resultant atelectasis or pneumonia.

Histologically, the squamous cell tumor is composed of sheets of epithelial cells, which may be well or poorly differentiated. Most well-differentiated tumors demonstrate keratin pearls. The more poorly differentiated tumors, if determined to be squamous cell carcinoma, have positive keratin staining (Fig. 31.2-2).

These tumors tend to be slow-growing, and it is estimated that up to 3 or 4 years are required from the development of *in situ* carcinoma to a clinically apparent tumor.

Adenocarcinoma

In North America, adenocarcinoma is the most frequent tumor, accounting for 40% of all cases of lung cancer. Some of this increase is due to the better identification of adenocarcinoma using immunohistochemical staining, with fewer tumors classified as undifferentiated large cell tumors. Most of these tumors are peripheral in origin, arising from alveolar surface epithelium or bronchial mucosal glands; they also can present as peripheral tumors arising in areas of previous infections, so-called scar tumors (Fig. 31.2-3).

Histologically, these tumors form glands and produce mucin. Although they can be subdivided by light microscopy into the classic four types defined by the WHO classification, this has little clinical relevance except for bronchoalveolar carcinoma, which appears to be a distinct clinicopathologic entity

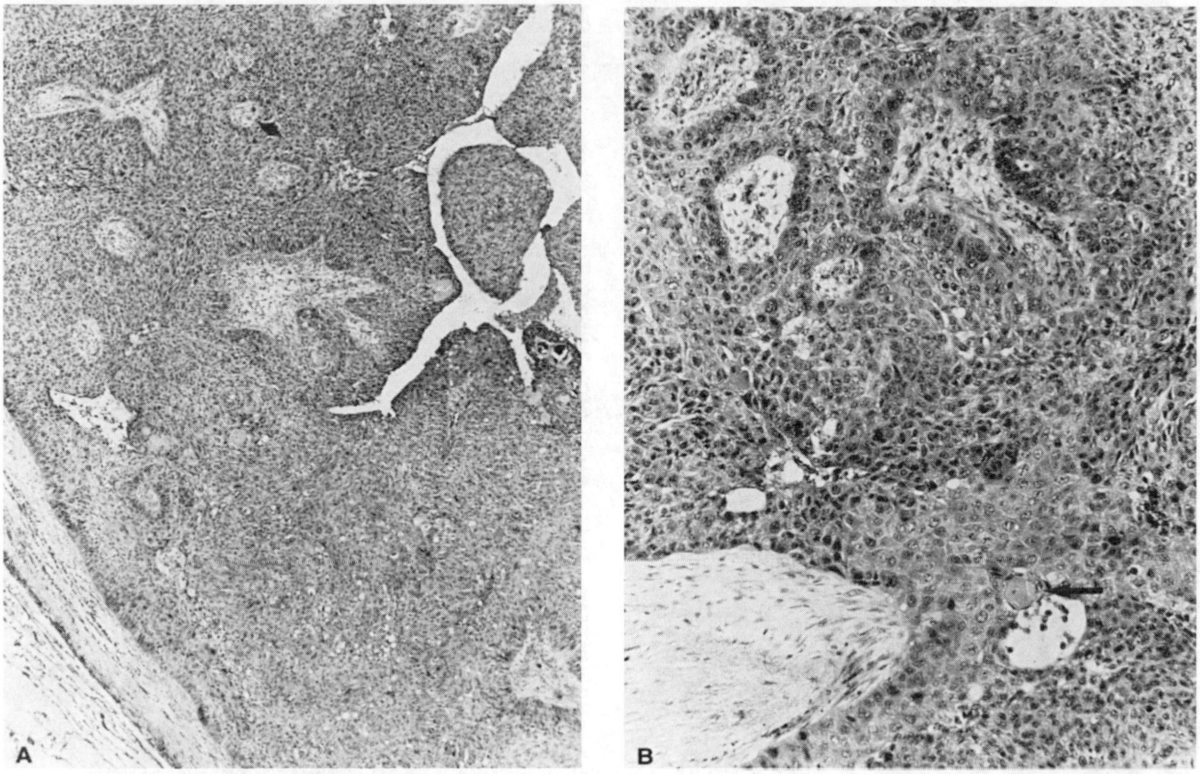

FIGURE 31.2-2. Moderately differentiated squamous cell carcinoma. Sheets of tumor cells with variable amounts of cytoplasm and moderate nuclear atypia are present. Focal keratinization is evident (*arrow*). **A:** Low-power magnification. **B:** High-power magnification.

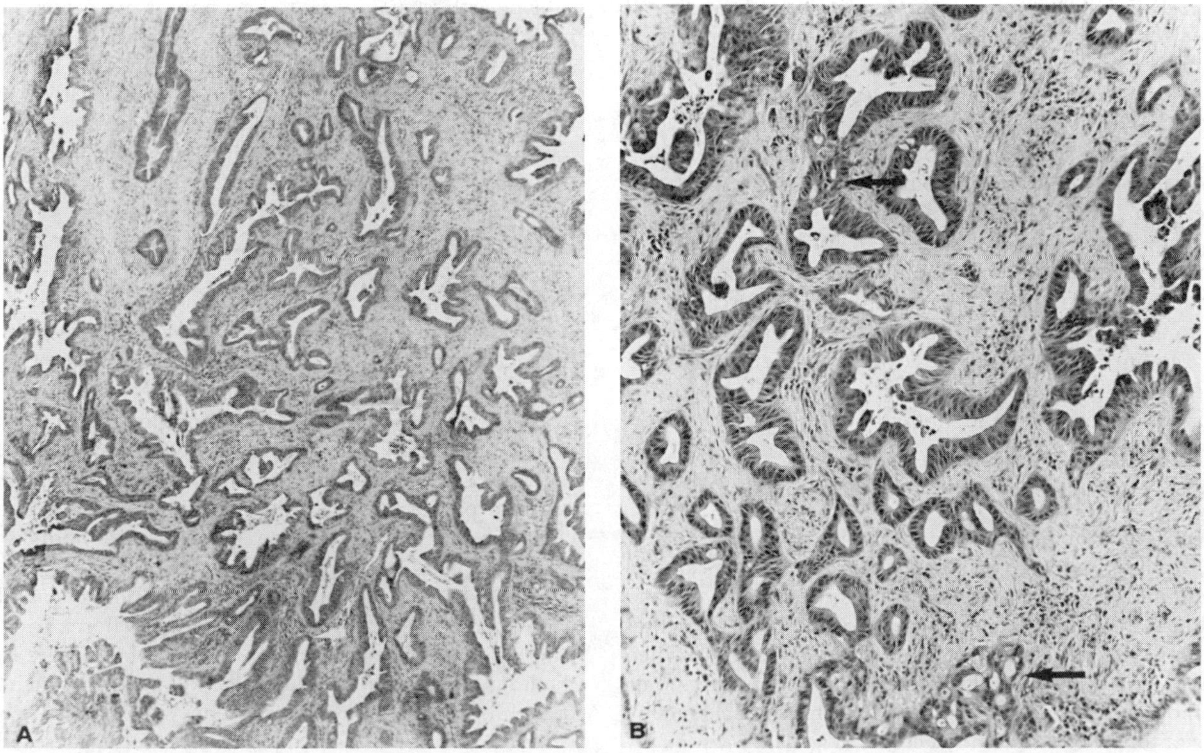

FIGURE 31.2-3. Well-differentiated adenocarcinoma. Well-formed glands with a focal cribriform arrangement (*arrows*) are surrounded by a cellular stroma. **A:** Low-power magnification. **B:** High-power magnification.

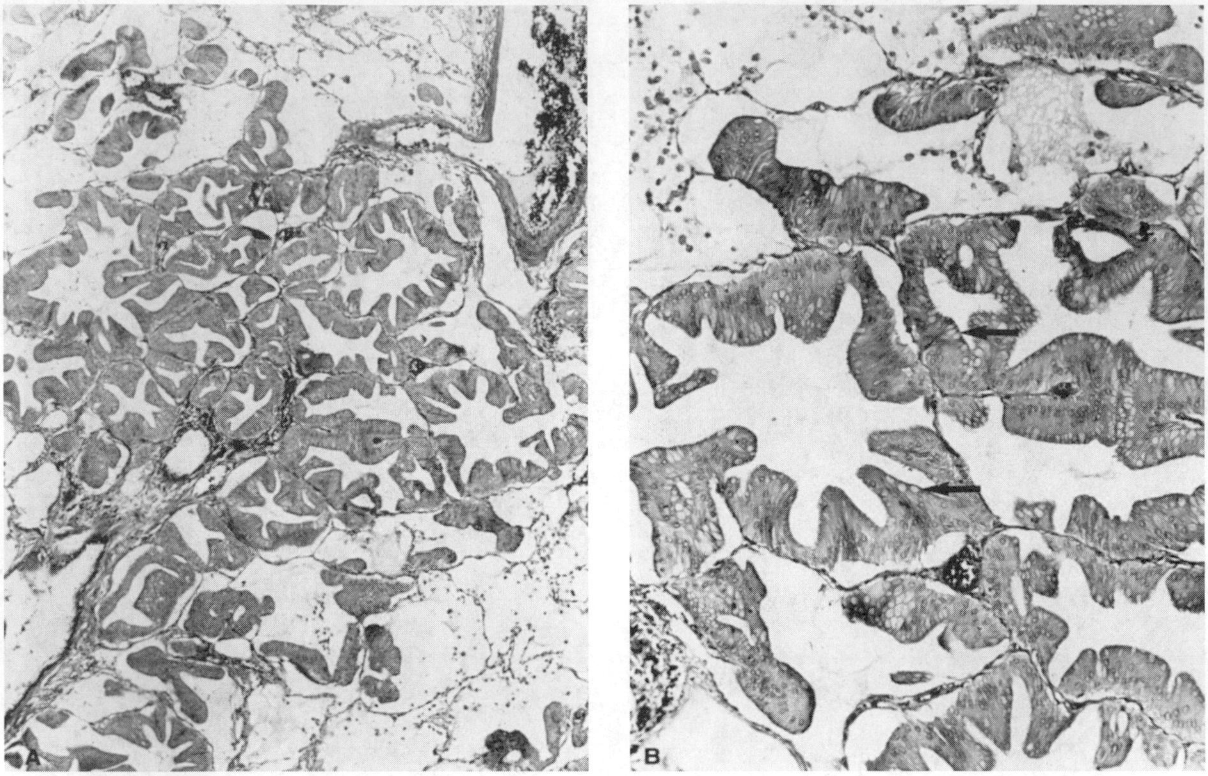

FIGURE 31.2-4. Bronchoalveolar carcinoma. Columnar cells with minimal nuclear atypia are arranged along intact alveolar septa. The lepidic growth pattern is associated with no stromal reaction. Mucin vacuoles are present in the apical cytoplasm (*arrows*). **A:** Low-power magnification. **B:** High-power magnification.

(Fig. 31.2-4).[82] This latter tumor appears to arise from type II pneumocytes, grows along alveolar septa by lepidic growth, and shows little, if any, desmoplastic or glandular change. These tumors are interesting in that they present in three different fashions: a solitary peripheral nodule, multifocal disease, or a rapidly progressive pneumonic form, which appears to spread from lobe to lobe, ultimately encompassing both lungs.

Other than T1N0 tumors, it appears that adenocarcinoma has a somewhat worse prognosis, stage for stage, than does squamous cell carcinoma. Immunohistochemistry and electron microscopy have been used by pathologists with increasing frequency to identify adenocarcinoma.[83] Using these techniques, adenocarcinoma cells stain positive for carcinoembryonic antigen and mucin. Specific monoclonal antibodies recognizing adenocarcinoma have been identified.[84]

Large Cell Carcinoma

Large cell carcinoma is the least common of all NSCLC tumors, accounting for approximately 15% of all lung cancers. With immunohistochemical staining, electron microscopy, and monoclonal antibodies, many tumors previously diagnosed as undifferentiated large cell carcinoma can now be classified more appropriately as poorly differentiated adenocarcinoma or squamous cell carcinoma. For this reason, the incidence of this type of tumor continues to decrease (Fig. 31.2-5).

Although the WHO classification subdivides this group into giant cell and clear cell varieties, these subclassifications have little clinical relevance. Few true giant cell tumors have been identified, although they do represent a poorly differentiated subtype with what appears to be a poorer prognosis. The prognosis of large cell undifferentiated carcinoma appears to be similar to that of adenocarcinoma and, in most clinical trials, these two histologic types are grouped together using immunohistochemical staining. Pathologists are increasingly identifying neuroendocrine features in large cell tumors. These tumors appear to have a worse prognosis, and their relation to small cell lung cancer remains to be defined.

METHODS OF SPREAD

After a variable period as a primary tumor growing within lung parenchyma or within the bronchial wall, the tumor ultimately invades the vascular and lymphatic channels, resulting in spread by these channels to regional draining lymph nodes and distant metastatic sites. Occasionally, airborne or lymphatic metastases (so-called satellite nodules) can be seen in the lung parenchyma near the primary tumor or in ispilateral lobes other than that containing the primary tumor. These satellite nodules auger a worse prognosis and alter the stage of the disease.

In most instances, it appears that lymphatic spread occurs earlier than spread to metastatic sites elsewhere. The regional lymphatic drainage of the lung is outlined in Figure 31.2-6. In the lung tissue, lymphatic drainage follows the bronchoarterial branching pattern, with lymph nodes situated at the origin of these branchings. These lymphatic channels coalesce, draining into lymph nodes situated around segmental and lobar bronchi. Lower lobe lymphatics then drain to the posterior mediastinum and, ultimately, to the subcarinal lymph nodes. In the right upper lobe, lymphatics drain toward the superior medi-

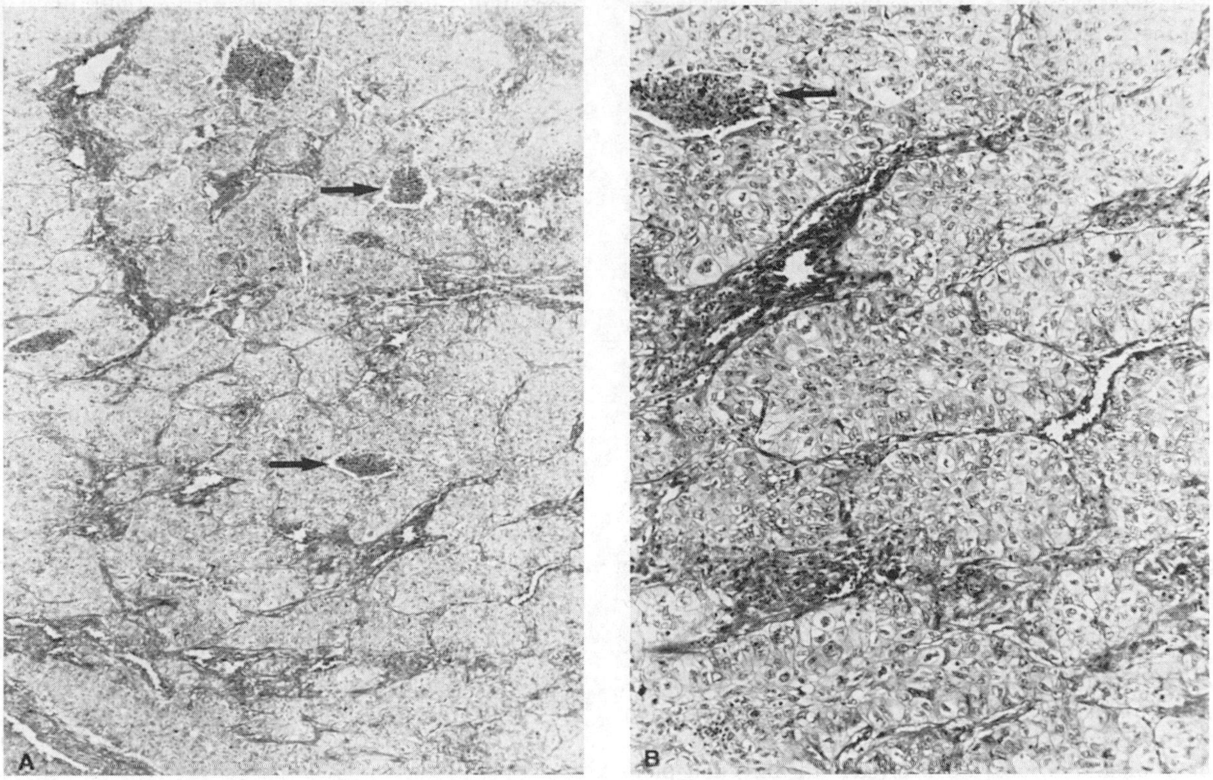

FIGURE 31.2-5. Large cell undifferentiated carcinoma. Sheets of highly atypical cells with focal necrosis (*arrows*) are present. There is no evidence of keratinization of gland formation. **A:** Low-power magnification. **B:** High-power magnification.

astinum; in the left upper lobe, lymphatic channels run anterolateral to the great vessels (aorta and subclavian artery) in the anterior mediastinum as well as along the main bronchus into the superior mediastinum in one-third of cases.

Ultimately, all these lymphatic channels drain to the right lymphatic or left thoracic ducts. Metastatic lymphatic spread of lung cancer follows these lymphatic channels with tumor involving bronchopulmonary (N1), mediastinal (N2-3) and, ultimately, supraclavicular (N3) lymph nodes. Retrograde lymphatic spread to the pleural surface can occur, especially in peripheral tumors.

The primary tumor can also spread locally, ultimately invading contiguous structures, including mediastinal pleura or organs and the chest wall or diaphragm. Once vascular or lymphatic invasion occurs, metastatic spread to distant sites is common. The most frequent sites involved include bone, liver, adrenals, and brain. As demonstrated in autopsy studies, however, lung cancer metastases can be found in every organ sys-

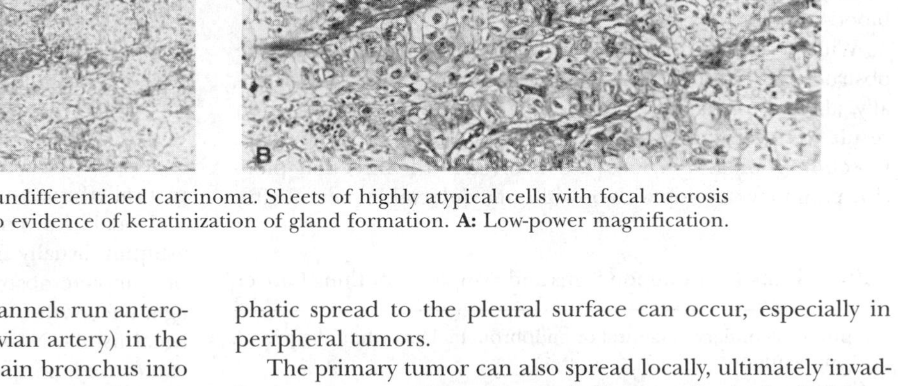

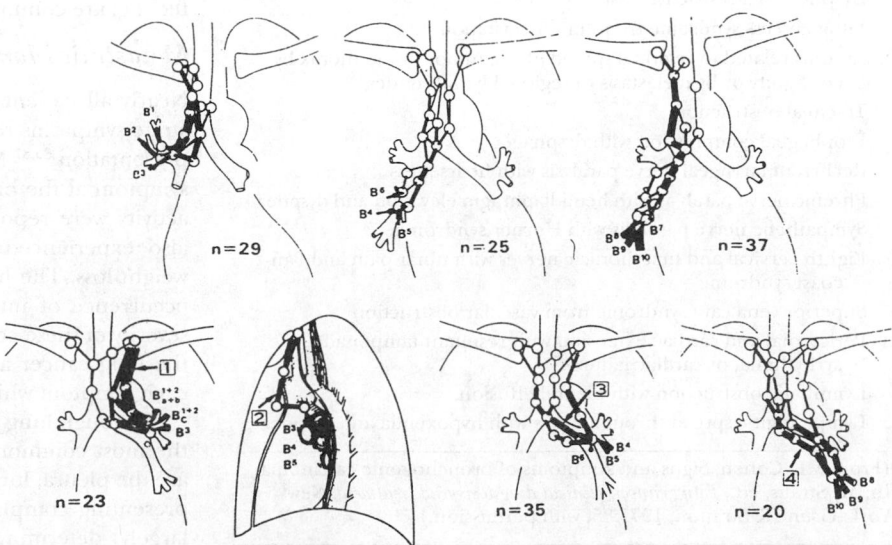

FIGURE 31.2-6. The regional lymphatic drainage of the lung as described by Noel. Most of the lymphatic drainage ultimately reaches the right superior mediastinum and right supraclavicular regions. (From ref. 416, with permission.)

tem.[85] Metastases within the lung are thought to result from a variety of mechanisms, including airborne spread by bronchi, retrograde lymphatic spread, and blood-borne spread.

CLINICAL FEATURES

The signs and symptoms manifested by patients suffering from lung cancer depend on the location of the tumor, its locoregional spread, or the effects of metastatic spread (Table 31.2-3). Lung cancer is associated with paraneoplastic syndromes more frequently than any other tumor. Many patients present with an asymptomatic lesion discovered incidentally on chest radiography.

Locoregional Manifestations

Tumors arising in the larger airways produce symptoms related to the growth of the tumor. Frequently, patients present with a persistent cough. In larger airways, with encroachment of the lumen, a wheeze or stridor may develop. As the tumor grows, areas of necrosis may develop, resulting in bleeding. Massive hemoptysis is a rare event, with most patients experiencing blood-streaked sputum.

With continued tumor growth, airways may become obstructed, resulting in atelectasis, pneumonia and, occasionally, abscess formation. These obstructive complications often result in fevers and the signs and symptoms of pulmonary infection. If pleural surfaces are involved in the infection, pleuritic pain may develop with or without a detectable pleural effusion. With endobronchial obstruction and the failure of ventilation of segments or lobes or even an entire lung, increasing shortness of breath can ensue.

Depending on the location of the primary tumor, adjacent structures, such as the chest wall or mediastinum, may ultimately become involved by direct spread. Radicular chest wall pain then develops. With apical tumors, the classic Pancoast's syndrome (lower brachial plexopathy, Horner's syndrome, and shoulder pain) may become manifest, owing to local invasion of the lower brachial plexus (T1 and C8 nerve roots), chest wall, and stellate ganglion.

Similarly, tumors invading or involving lymph nodes in the mediastinum may encase the phrenic nerve, vagus nerve, or recurrent nerve, resulting in malfunction of the specific end organs (e.g., diaphragm, vocal cord). It is not uncommon for patients to present initially with symptoms of a recurrent nerve palsy, including hoarseness and cricopharyngeal dysphagia, especially with left upper lobe tumors.

Superior vena cava syndrome usually results from mediastinal lymphadenopathy encroaching on this structure rather than primary tumor invasion. Direct invasion of the pericardium or metastases to this structure can occur and lead to a malignant pericardial effusion, with signs and symptoms of pericardial tamponade.

Visceral pleural invasion or retrograde lymphatic spread *can* ultimately result in visceral and parietal pleural seeding. Pleuritic pain or increasing shortness of breath due to a massive pleural effusion can ensue.

Nodal involvement or tumor invasion of the posterior mediastinum, usually from lower lobe tumors, can produce partial or complete obstruction of the esophagus, resulting in dysphagia and, with further invasion, symptoms of a tracheoesophageal fistula. Nodal involvement of the superior mediastinum can cause a nonproductive cough or, when extensive, superior vena cava obstruction.

In addition to these specific symptoms related to the presence of tumor or lymphadenopathy in a locoregional area, nonspecific and vague chest pains, generally referred to the ipsilateral hemithorax, are frequent occurrences in patients suffering from lung cancer. These pains are of visceral origin and are unrelated to invasion of local structures. Other nonspecific symptoms, including weight loss and a general unwell feeling, are common and usually indicate advanced disease.

TABLE 31.2-3. Common Signs and Symptoms of Lung Cancer

Symptoms secondary to central or endobronchial growth of the primary tumor
Cough
Hemoptysis
Wheeze and stridor
Dyspnea from obstruction
Pneumonitis from obstruction (fever, productive cough)
Symptoms secondary to peripheral growth of the primary tumor
Pain from pleural or chest wall involvement
Cough
Dyspnea on a restrictive basis
Lung abscess syndrome from tumor cavitation
Symptoms related to regional spread of the tumor in the thorax by contiguity or by metastasis to regional lymph nodes
Tracheal obstruction
Esophageal compression with dysphagia
Recurrent laryngeal nerve paralysis with hoarseness
Phrenic nerve paralysis with hemidiaphragm elevation and dyspnea
Sympathetic nerve paralysis with Horner syndrome
Eighth cervical and first thoracic nerves with ulnar pain and Pancoast syndrome
Superior vena cava syndrome from vascular obstruction
Pericardial and cardiac extension with resultant tamponade, arrhythmia, or cardiac failure
Lymphatic obstruction with pleural effusion
Lymphangitic spread through lungs with hypoxemia and dyspnea

(From MH Cohen, Signs and symptoms of bronchogenic carcinoma. In: MJ Straus, ed., *Lung cancer: clinical diagnosis and treatment.* New York: Grune & Stratton, 1977:85, with permission.)

Metastatic Manifestations

Nearly all patients with advanced inoperable NSCLC demonstrate symptoms referable to their disease at the time of initial presentation.[86,87] Most patients, in fact, have more than one symptom at the onset of their illness.[87] Fatigue and decreased activity were reported by more than 80%, and most patients also experienced cough, dyspnea, decreased appetite, and weight loss. The high incidence of lung cancer symptoms, the occurrence of multiple symptoms in most patients, and the severity of these complaints demand both prompt treatment of the lung cancer and careful attention to the management of each symptom while definitive therapy is in progress.

Although lung cancer can metastasize to virtually any organ, the most common sites of spread that are clinically apparent are the pleura, lung, bone, brain, pericardium, and liver.[85] The presenting complaints of a patient with metastatic spread are largely determined by the specific metastatic organ site involved. For example, bone metastases present with pain and limitation of function in the affected area.

We cannot explain the high incidence of adrenal metastases in NSCLC, detected in 41% of patients at autopsy.[85] Most adrenal metastases are asymptomatic and are discovered incidentally during a staging evaluation or at autopsy. The computed tomographic (CT) scan is the most frequent method of diagnosis. Fine-needle aspiration provides a safe method to confirm the presence of metastatic disease in the adrenal gland if pathologic documentation is necessary, although other imaging studies, such as magnetic resonance imaging (MRI) and positron emission tomography (PET) can be confirmatory. Adrenal hormone insufficiency due to bilateral adrenal metastases from lung cancer is rare but can occur.[88]

Pericardial complications are due to direct invasion, metastatic spread, or a cancer-associated but nonmalignant pericardial effusion.[89] The presenting complaints of dyspnea, cough, and chest discomfort are identical to those of pulmonary tumors or pleural metastases. Because of its slow evolution, signs of pericardial tamponade are often absent. Electrocardiograms are usually not diagnostic. Enlargement of the cardiac silhouette on chest radiograph is often subtle and apparent only on review of multiple prior studies. The frequent association of a pleural effusion in patients with pericardial involvement further impedes the prompt diagnosis of this condition.[90] The echocardiogram provides a safe and rapid diagnostic test for this condition as well as information on the presence and severity of associated cardiac compromise. Pericardial involvement should be considered in any lung cancer patient with dyspnea, cough, or chest discomfort and should be ruled out if a large pleural effusion is present.

Nonmetastatic Features

The anorexia-cachexia syndrome and generalized weakness and fatigue are the most common and least understood nonmetastatic complications of lung cancer. In addition, a variety of paraneoplastic syndromes associated with epithelial lung cancer have been identified. Many of these conditions are not specific to lung cancer but have been documented to occur frequently in lung cancer patients owing to the large number of patients with this disease (Table 31.2-4).

Hypertrophic pulmonary osteoarthropathy (HPO) occurs frequently in NSCLC patients. Symptoms of bone and joint pain herald the onset of this condition and can be the presenting signs of lung cancer. Clubbing of the digits is observed. The alkaline phosphatase level is commonly elevated, while serum hepatic enzyme levels are normal. Plain radiographs of affected bones demonstrate periosteal inflammation and elevation, and radionuclide bone scans reveal an intense and symmetric generalized increased uptake of the radiolabel, particularly in the distal end of long bones. Symptoms usually respond dramatically to aspirin and other nonsteroidal antiinflammatory agents and disappear after effective definitive treatment of the primary lesion. The digital clubbing is frequently present without other signs of HPO and resolve, as does HPO, with curative therapy.

TABLE 31.2-4. Paraneoplastic Syndromes in Patients with Lung Cancer

ENDOCRINE
Hypercalcemia (ectopic parathyroid hormone)
Cushing's syndrome
Syndrome of inappropriate antidiuretic hormone
Carcinoid syndrome
Gynecomastia
Hypercalcitonemia
Elevated growth hormone
Elevated prolactin, follicle-stimulating hormone, luteinizing hormone
Hypoglycemia
Hyperthyroidism
NEUROLOGIC
Encephalopathy
Subacute cerebellar degeneration
Progressive multifocal leukoencephalopathy
Peripheral neuropathy
Polymyositis
Autonomic neuropathy
Eaton-Lambert syndrome
Optic neuritis
SKELETAL
Clubbing
Pulmonary hypertrophic osteoarthropathy
HEMATOLOGIC
Anemia
Leukemoid reactions
Thrombocytosis
Thrombocytopenia
Eosinophilia
Pure red cell aplasia
Leukoerythroblastosis
Disseminated intravascular coagulation
CUTANEOUS
Hyperkeratosis
Dermatomyositis
Acanthosis nigricans
Hyperpigmentation
Erythema gyratum repens
Hypertrichosis lanuginosa acquista
OTHER
Nephrotic syndrome
Hypouricemia
Secretion of vasoactive intestinal peptide with diarrhea
Hyperamylasemia
Anorexia or cachexia

(Adapted from M Maddaus, RJ Ginsberg, Diagnosis and staging. In: FG Pearson, J Deslauriers, R Ginsberg, eds. *Thoracic surgery.* New York: Churchill Livingstone, 1995:671.)

DIAGNOSIS AND STAGING

In 1985, the American Joint Committee on Cancer, the Union Internationale Contre le Cancer, and the Japanese Cancer Committee agreed to a worldwide tumor, node, metastasis (TNM) staging system.[91] This has been rapidly accepted and is used extensively in the management of lung cancer. A revision of the 1985 version was accepted by the American Joint Committee on Cancer and Union Internationale Contre le Cancer in 1997.

TABLE 31.2-5. Tumor, Node, Metastasis (TNM) Staging System for Lung Cancer; Including Proposed Changes

PRIMARY TUMOR		
TX	Positive malignant cell; no lesion seen	
T1	<3 cm diameter	
T2	>3 cm diameter	
	Distal atelectasis	
T3	Extension to pleura, chest wall diaphragm, or pericardium	
	<2 cm from carina or total atelectasis	
T4	Invasion of mediastinal organs	
	Malignant pleural effusion	
REGIONAL LYMPH NODE INVOLVEMENT		
N0	No nodal involvement	
N1	Ipsilateral bronchopulmonary or hilar	
N2	Ipsilateral or subcarinal mediastinal	
	Ipsilateral supraclavicular nodes	
N3	Contralateral mediastinal hilum or supraclavicular	
METASTATIC INVOLVEMENT		
M0	No metastases	
M1	Metastases present	
Stage	*Descriptors*	*5-Y Survival Rate (%)*
CURRENT SYSTEM		
I	T1–2, N0, M0	60–80
II	T1–2, N1, M0	25–50
IIIA	T3, N0–1, M0	25–40
	T1–3, N2, M0	10–30
IIIB	Any T4 or any N3, M0	<5
IV	Any M1	<5
PROPOSED CHANGES (UICC AND AJCC)		
Ia	T1, N0, M0	>70
Ib	T2, N0, M0	60
IIa	T1, N1, M0	50
IIb	T2, N1, M0	30
	T3, N0–1, M0	40
IIIa	T1 3, N2, M0	10–30
IIIb	Any T4, any N3, M0	<10
		<5
IV	Any M1	<2

AJCC, American Joint Committee on Cancer; UICC, Union Internationale Contre le Cancer.

The primary tumor is subdivided into four categories (T1–4), depending on size, site, and local involvement. Lymph node spread has been subdivided into bronchopulmonary (N1), ipsilateral mediastinal (N2), and contralateral or supraclavicular disease (N3), and metastatic spread is absent (M0) or present (M1; Table 31.2-5; Fig. 31.2-7). Four stages of lung cancer have been identified, with significant differences found in 5-year survival, depending on the stage of disease at diagnosis. The accuracy of these stages in predicting survival has been confirmed by many authors (Fig. 31.2-8). Although the 1979 staging system still lacks uniformity in definition and prognosis in certain subsets of locally advanced disease (T3 vs. T4 and N2 vs. N3),[92] on the whole, it is a functional system that should be used for all patients.

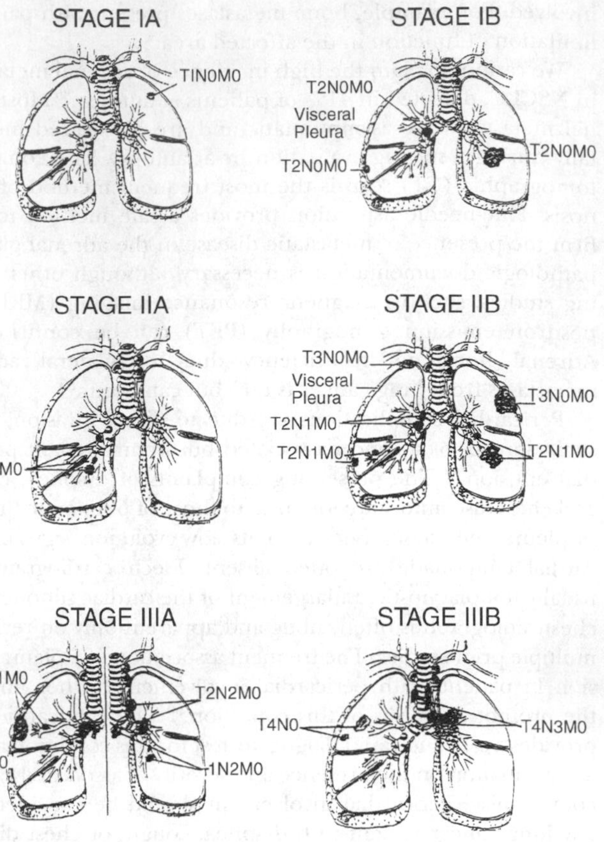

FIGURE 31.2-7. New International Staging System (ISS). Categories of stage IA, IB, IIA, IIB, IIIA, and IIIB disease. (From ref. 91, with permission.)

The TNM staging includes clinical, surgical, and pathologic collection. Even with the use of pretreatment minimally invasive techniques only, a significant percentage of patients are clinically understaged as compared with the ultimate stage identified by surgical and pathologic staging. Despite these inadequacies, it is clinically relevant to stage all lung cancer patients before treatment (clinical) and after therapy (surgical and pathologic).[93,94]

In patients suspected of harboring lung cancer, accurate diagnosis with confirmatory cytology or histology is of supreme importance, as is an estimation of the clinical stage of the disease, since clinical staging will determine treatment. Since many of the modalities used for diagnosis are also important in clinical staging, these are discussed simultaneously (Fig. 31.2-9).

HISTORY AND PHYSICAL EXAMINATION

A detailed history and accurate physical examination remain the most important steps in assessing a patient with lung cancer. Smoking history, past exposure to environmental carcinogens, and family history may suggest a higher probability of lung cancer. New symptoms, including a change in cough, hemoptysis, or history of recurrent respiratory infection, are of concern. Symptoms suggesting locoregional spread include chest pain, symptoms of recurrent nerve palsy, or superior vena cava obstruction. Symptoms suggestive of metastatic disease frequently include focal neurologic symptoms, bone pain, or weight loss. Occasionally, patients suffering from NSCLC

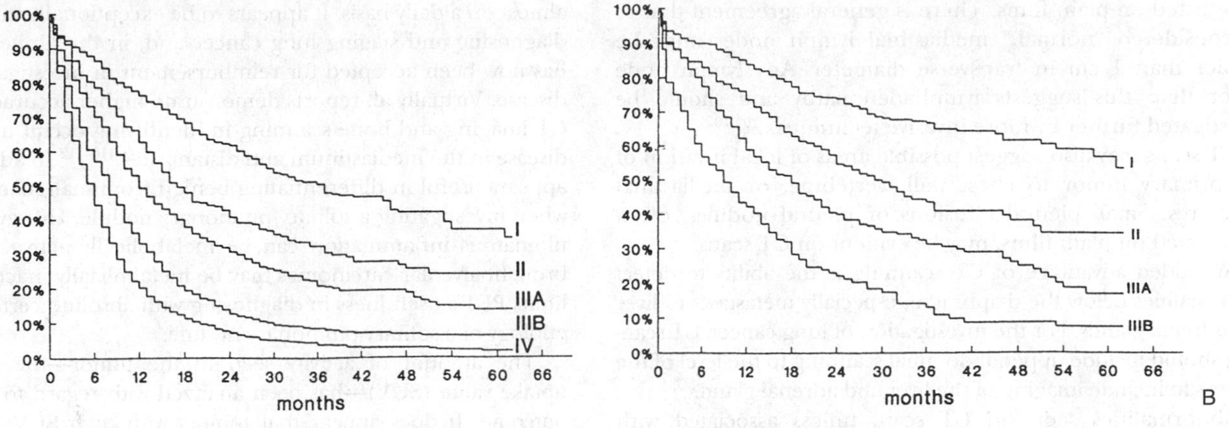

FIGURE 31.2-8. Actuarial survival curves according to different stages (1986 staging). **A:** Survival after clinical staging. **B:** Survival after final pathologic staging. Note that early stages are understaged by clinical staging resulting in a poorer survival than after pathologic staging. However, the higher the stage, the less likely that clinical staging understages the disease. (From ref. 91, with permission.)

present with symptoms and signs of a paraneoplastic syndrome but not as frequently as with small cell tumors.

Physical examination should look for signs of partial or complete obstruction of airways, atelectasis or pneumonia, and pleural effusions. Examination of the head and neck, including the draining regional lymph node areas in the supraclavicular area, may demonstrate lymphadenopathy, indicating regional lymphatic (N3) spread.

SPUTUM CYTOLOGY

Once the disease is suspected, a simple and effective method of obtaining a positive diagnosis of lung cancer is sputum cytology. The yield from sputum cytology depends on many factors, including the ability of the patient to produce sufficient sputum, the size of the tumor, the proximity of the tumor to major airways and, to a lesser extent, the histologic type of the tumor.

With sputum samples, up to 80% of central tumors can be diagnosed. The yield is much smaller for peripheral tumors, dropping to less than 20% for peripheral tumors smaller than 3.0 cm in diameter. A 3-day collection of early morning sputa, preserved in Saccamano's solution, appears to be the optimal method of assessment. Squamous cell tumors, being more proximal, are more frequently diagnosed by cytology than adenocarcinoma or large cell tumors. Another factor affecting the ability of sputum cytology to diagnose malignancy is the experience and training of the cytopathologist. Viral infections and other acute inflammations can produce cellular changes that are difficult to distinguish from malignancy, especially adenocarcinoma. Frequently, severe dysplasia is misinterpreted as a malignancy, and vice versa. Tockman et al.[95–97] have described a monoclonal antibody–staining technique that may more accurately diagnose the presence or absence of malignancy in severely dysplastic cells. This is being tested prospectively in a large North American effort.

IMAGING STUDIES

Chest Radiography

Chest radiography is probably the most valuable tool in the diagnosis of lung cancer. A perfectly normal chest radiograph rules out this diagnosis in most instances, except for the rare occult tumor.[98] Plain chest radiography can reveal peripheral nodules and hilar and mediastinal changes suggestive of lymphadenopathy or pleural effusions, all suggestive of possible malignancy. Areas of subsegmental, segmental, lobar, or lung collapse suggest an endobronchial obstruction. Improvements in plain radiography (e.g., digital radiography) may improve the diagnostic yield of this modality.[99,100]

Computed Tomography

With the introduction of CT scanning in the late 1970s, a giant step was taken in the ability to diagnose and stage lung cancer employing noninvasive imaging techniques. CT imaging can confirm abnormalities seen on plain chest radiographs, can often detect early (<1 cm) lesions that cannot be seen on chest radiographs, and has played an important role in staging of lung cancer, especially spread to areas of the mediastinum

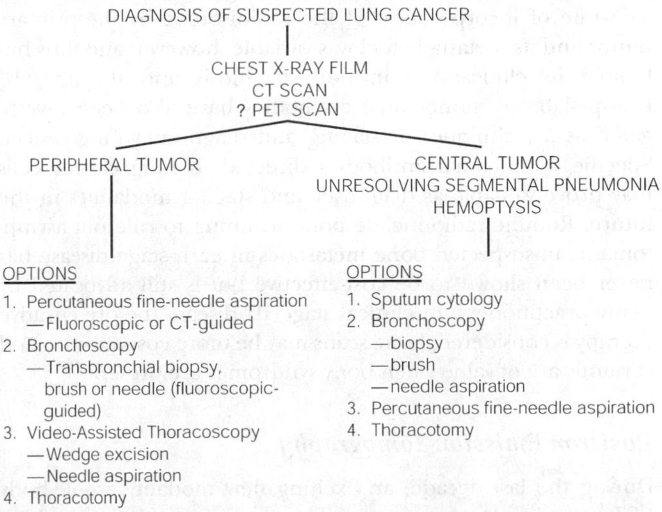

FIGURE 31.2-9. Schema to indicate the diagnostic procedures depending on the presenting lesion. CT, computed tomography. PET, positron emission tomography.

undetected on plain films. There is general agreement that to be considered "normal," mediastinal lymph nodes must be smaller than 1 cm in transverse diameter. Any lymph node larger than this suggests lymphadenopathy and should be investigated further by more invasive techniques.[101,102]

CT scans may also suggest possible areas of local invasion of the primary tumor to chest wall, vertebrae, or mediastinal structures. Small pleural effusions or pleural nodules, often undetected on plain films, may be evident on CT scans.

An added advantage of CT scanning is the ability to detect abnormalities below the diaphragm, especially metastases to liver and adrenal glands. For the investigation of lung cancer, CT scanning should include upper abdominal scanning to the level of the kidneys to include imaging of the liver and adrenal gland.

Abnormalities seen on CT scan, unless associated with unequivocal signs of malignancy, should be confirmed by more invasive cytologic or histologic investigation.[103]

Magnetic Resonance Imaging

MRI investigation of pulmonary lesions has been disappointing and has offered no improvement over CT scanning. Exceptions to this rule include investigation of paravertebral tumors, because imaging of the spinal canal without contrast media is possible. Changes in bone marrow of the vertebrae suggestive of carcinoma can be detected with greater accuracy with MRI. Also, invasion of tissue planes and vascular structures within the mediastinum and at the thoracic inlet can be assessed with greater accuracy using MRI. Routine MRI of all lung cancer is unnecessary and should be reserved for situations in which local tumor invasion of the mediastinum, thoracic inlet, or paravertebral region is questioned on CT scanning.[104–106]

Radionuclide Scanning

Until the advent of PET scanning, the ability of radionuclide scanning to diagnose and stage lung cancer was limited by its lack of specificity. Nuclide scanning with gallium citrate or cobalt-bleomycin previously was used mainly for detecting unsuspected mediastinal spread once the diagnosis had been made. The rate of incorporation of the radioisotope by the primary tumor and its metastatic foci was variable, however, and thus has limited its clinical use in both diagnosis and staging.[107,108] Isotope-labeled monoclonal antibodies have also been investigated as a technique for staging and diagnosing lung cancer. Specific monoclonal antibodies directed to lung cancer cells may prove valuable as diagnostic and staging modalities in the future. Routine radionuclide bone scanning to rule out asymptomatic, unsuspected bone metastases in early-stage disease has never been shown to be cost-effective but is still advocated by many practitioners. In clinical stage III disease, before curative therapy is considered, bone scans may be more cost-effective and certainly are of value when bony syndromes are present.[109]

Positron Emission Tomography

During the last decade, an exciting new modality, whole-body PET scanning, came into use. This scanning technique, which has yet to be completely investigated, is based on the uptake of a radioactive glucose, fluorodeoxyglucose, in metabolically active cells. In North America and Europe, PET centers are opening almost on a daily basis. It appears to be exceptionally valuable in diagnosing and staging lung cancer and, in the United States, has now been accepted for reimbursement in investigating this disease. Virtually all reports demonstrate higher accuracies than CT imaging and bone scanning in identifying occult metastatic disease in the mediastinum and distant sites.[110–112] In addition, it appears useful in differentiating benign from malignant lesions when investigating a solitary pulmonary nodule. However, granulomatous inflammation can be metabolically active, whereas bronchoalveolar carcinomas may be metabolically inactive. This limits PET's usefulness in diagnosing with absolute certainty the etiology of a solitary pulmonary nodule.

The amount of activity seen in the tumor—the standard uptake value (SUV)—has been analyzed with regard to ultimate outcome. It does appear that tumors with high SUV numbers have a poor prognosis, which is independent of other prognostic indices, such as stage of disease. The exact level of SUV activity that is independently prognostic has yet to be defined but appears to be somewhere in excess of 7. In addition, the response to therapy (e.g., induction chemotherapy or radiotherapy) as measured by a declining SUV is being investigated with the use of PET. In the future, chemotherapy response rates may be able to be assessed with repeated PET scans; this is being actively investigated. The response to primary chemoradiotherapy may also be assessed using this technique. The exact place of PET scanning in assessing response to therapy, however, has yet to be defined.[112]

PERCUTANEOUS FINE-NEEDLE ASPIRATION

Fine-needle aspiration biopsy of pulmonary nodules is an excellent method of obtaining cytologic and histologic material for positive identification of malignancy. This is performed using fluoroscopic or CT-guided techniques. The positive yield in experienced hands can be as high as 95%. An indeterminate biopsy, however, cannot be accepted as negative. False-negative examination results are frequent and must be considered indeterminate unless a positive benign diagnosis (e.g., hamartoma, tuberculosis) can be made.[113]

Abnormalities identified by imaging scans in bone, liver, or adrenal gland and suggestive of metastatic disease can be confirmed by fine-needle aspiration biopsy using ultrasonographic or CT-guided techniques, and abnormalities identified on physical examination (e.g., large supraclavicular nodes) are very accessible to fine-needle aspiration. In some centers, confirmation by PET scanning or MRI has been considered accurate enough and has replaced the necessity of biopsy confirmation (e.g., of adrenal tumor).

BRONCHOSCOPY

Although rigid bronchoscopy was used for many years to confirm the diagnosis of lung cancer, the introduction of flexible fiber-optic bronchoscopy more than 20 years ago has revolutionized this approach. The procedure, although invasive, can be performed under local anesthesia with or without sedation and with minimal morbidity and exceptional safety. Using flexible instruments, the proximal tracheobronchial tree can be examined up to the second or third subsegmental division, and cytologic or histologic specimens can be obtained from identified abnormal lesions. The diagnostic yield of fiber-optic bronchoscopy with cytology brushing and biopsy for histology when a visible lesion is identified is higher than 90%. Even with no visible lesion seen, the bronchus draining the area of suspicion can be irrigated and lavaged, yielding cytologic material. With fiber-optic bronchoscopy and image intensification, peripheral lesions can be reached by cytology brushes, needles, or biopsy forceps, and specimens can thus be obtained. This is most effective in lesions larger than 2 cm in diameter.

The increased yield of postbronchoscopy sputum cytology (as compared with routine induction sputum cytology) renders this maneuver valuable as an added diagnostic tool. The bronchoscope is also valuable for staging. The site of the primary tumor in a major airway may affect its stage (T3 vs. T2 vs. T1), and transbronchoscopic needle aspiration through the airway wall, as popularized by Wang, can confirm the presence of malignancy in enlarged mediastinal lymph nodes (N3 vs. N2 vs. N1).[113a,113b] Care must be taken, however, with this latter technique, because false-positive examination results have been reported, and differentiation between resectable N2 and unresectable N2 or N3 disease cannot always be determined by needle aspiration alone; a more invasive approach (e.g., mediastinoscopy, thoracoscopy) may be required.[114]

MEDIASTINOSCOPY AND MEDIASTINOTOMY

Mediastinoscopy was developed by Carlens approximately 45 years ago to facilitate staging of superior mediastinal lymph nodes (N2 or N3) before consideration of therapy in patients with lung cancer. It remains the most accurate lymph node staging technique to assess superior mediastinal lymph nodes, which are frequently involved in this disease. The procedure is simple, safe, and effective in experienced hands. In two large series,[115,116] the mortality rate was 0%, and the major morbidity rate was less than 1%. In patients suspected of having inoperable disease by virtue of mediastinal involvement as detected by CT or PET scanning, confirmation by mediastinoscopy is indicated. Depending on the philosophy of management of patients with minimal mediastinal involvement, mediastinoscopy is used to a greater or lesser extent by individual practitioners. Mediastinoscopy is extremely valuable for accurate staging of the disease before neoadjuvant (induction) chemotherapy.

In the future, PET scanning may replace this invasive procedure as a method of accurately identifying superior mediastinal involvement. However, prospective studies have suggested that in "negative" PET scans related to the superior mediastinum, approximately 10% of individuals will be found to have microscopic mediastinal nodal involvement.[23,117] Whether a negative PET scan result is sufficient to allow primary surgery in patients without the addition of mediastinoscopy is yet to be determined. Granulomatous inflammation within the mediastinal lymph nodes will be identified as increased activity on a PET scan. For this reason, "positive" PET imaging in the superior mediastinum must be confirmed histologically as representing metastatic cancer.

Involvement of anterior mediastinal lymph nodes, which occurs frequently in left upper lobe tumors, can be assessed by the extended mediastinoscopy technique,[118] by an anterior mediastinotomy (as advocated by McNiel and Chamberlain[119]), or by video-assisted thoracoscopy. Because this is the first level of mediastinal lymph nodes involved in disease, many practitioners defer this examination when cervical mediastinoscopy fails to reveal metastatic disease in the superior mediastinum unless these lymph nodes appear involved on imaging studies. Patients without superior mediastinal involvement have a good prognosis after resection, even when anterior mediastinal (first-level) nodes are microscopically involved.[120]

THORACENTESIS

Thoracentesis of a pleural effusion associated with a presumed lung cancer can identify pleural disease (T4). Classically, a bloody pleural effusion is considered malignant; however, unless malignant cells are identified in the cytologic assessment of these pleural effusions, for the sake of the patient, a bloody pleural effusion should be considered traumatic. In these instances, thoracoscopy may be required to prove, without a doubt, the existence of pleural metastases.

THORACOSCOPY

Video-assisted thoracoscopy has been used in the diagnosis and staging of lung cancer. Peripheral nodules can be identified and excised using video-assisted minimally invasive techniques, and mediastinal lymph nodes can be sampled for histologic examination. This technique also can identify suspected pleural disease and has the ability to assess accurately the status of pleural effusions when thoracentesis does not. The exact indications and use of this minimally invasive technique await further prospective studies,[121–123] but it has been used for assessment of mediastinal nodes and T4 status, especially when pleural effusions with nonmalignant cytology are present.

THORACOTOMY

Thoracotomy continues to be used in the diagnosis and staging of lung cancer. With less invasive procedures, however, more than 95% of tumors can be accurately diagnosed and staged prior to thoracotomy. Despite this, there remains a small minority of patients in whom the diagnosis of lung cancer is made only at thoracotomy. At the time of thoracotomy, the diagnosis can be confirmed by fine-needle aspiration, incisional or (preferably) excisional biopsy, and frozen-section analysis. All these techniques can provide tissue that can be rapidly assessed by pathologists.

At the time of thoracotomy, further staging is mandatory by the surgeon by sampling hilar and mediastinal lymph node or performing a complete ipsilateral lymph node dissection. Not infrequently, unsuspected involvement of adjacent structures is recognized only at the time of surgery, identifying a T3 or T4 tumor invading adjacent structures.

EVALUATION OF EXTENT OF DISEASE

Once the diagnosis of lung cancer has been made and before consideration of definitive therapy, a clinical evaluation of extent of disease is required (Fig. 31.2-10). Frequently, the history and physical examination suggest evidence of lymphatic or distant metastatic spread. These symptoms or signs should be confirmed by appropriate radiologic studies directed at the organs suspected to be involved (Fig. 31.2-11).

Regarding patients suspected of having disease localized to the hemithorax, there has been significant debate about the minimum required investigations to prove or disprove meta-

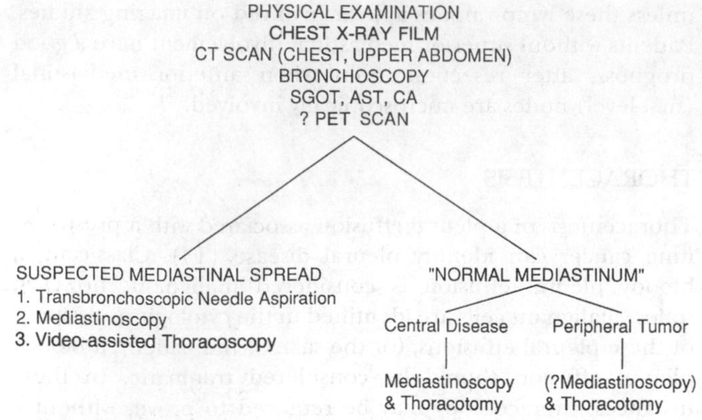

FIGURE 31.2-10. Clinical staging of lung cancer: a schema to indicate extent of disease evaluation. AST, aspartate aminotransferase; CA, serum calcium; CT, computed tomography; PET, positron emission tomography; SGOT, serum glutamic oxaloacetic transaminase.

static spread. After an accurate medical history and physical examination, routine studies should include chest radiographs, hematologic survey, and specific biochemical markers, including serum calcium, alkaline phosphatase, and aspartate aminotransferase. Elevation of these biochemical markers indicates the need for investigation for bony or liver metastases.

In the United States, virtually all patients considered for curative treatment of lung cancer undergo routine CT scanning of the chest and upper abdomen to detect mediastinal lymph node enlargement, unsuspected pulmonary metastases, and unsuspected liver and adrenal metastases. Whether the use of CT scanning is cost-effective in detecting these unsuspected metastases is a moot point. Frequently, abnormalities found with this examination lead to further invasive testing, ultimately revealing a false-positive investigation result. Similarly, the routine use of bone scans despite the absence of clinical or biochemical abnormalities is probably not cost-effective.

PET scanning is being used with increased frequency to assess both regional and metastatic spread of tumor. Because of the inherent high metabolic activity within the brain, this area cannot be accurately assessed by this new imaging technique.

The routine use of mediastinoscopy before surgical intervention for the treatment of lung cancer is also debated. With mediastinoscopy, inoperable superior mediastinal disease can be identified, thereby avoiding some unnecessary thoracotomies. Approximately 10% of patients harbor inoperable unsuspected mediastinal disease if mediastinoscopy is not used as a routine staging operation, despite the use of CT and PET scanning.

In clinical practice, for peripheral nodules smaller than 3 cm in diameter with no other abnormalities detected on chest radiograph, physical examination, or biochemical screening, it

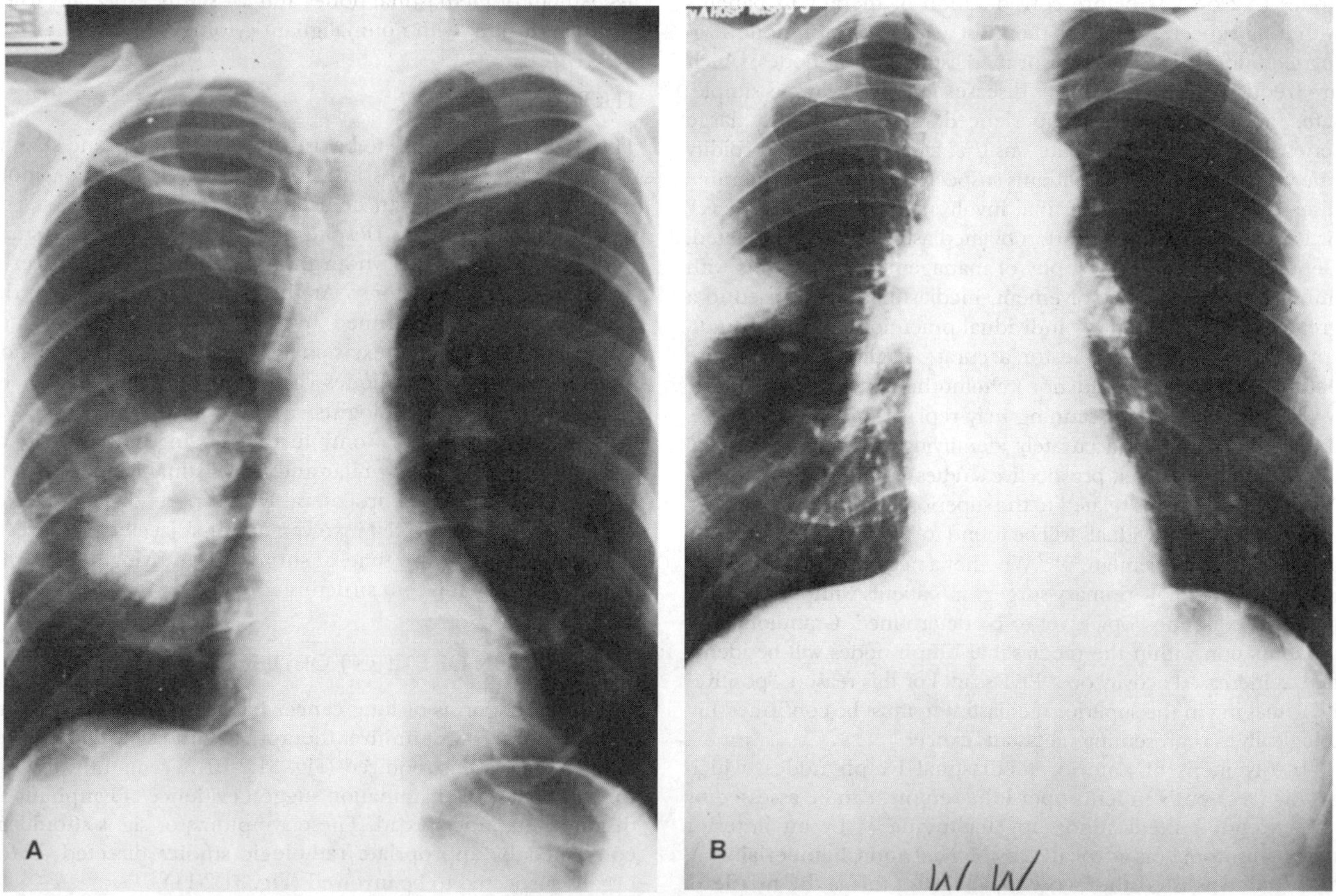

FIGURE 31.2-11. Chest radiographs of patients with different presentations of lung cancer. **A:** A centrally located tumor on cavitation, suggestive of squamous cell carcinoma. **B:** A peripherally located nodule with possible pleural involvement. (*Figure continues*)

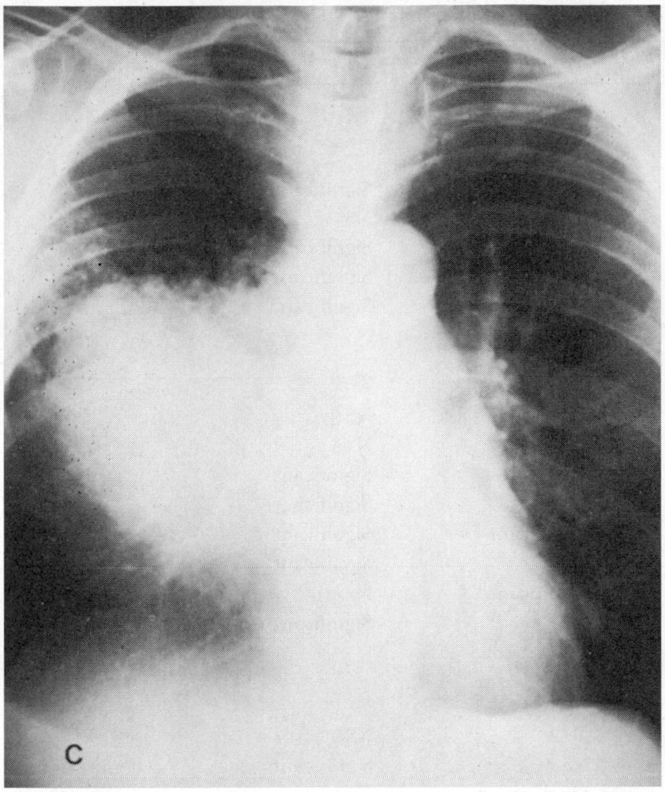

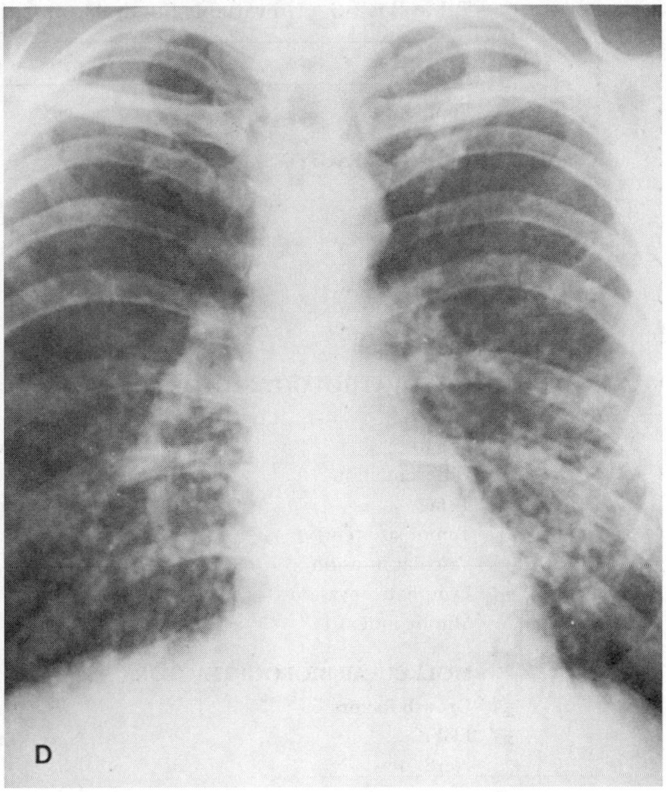

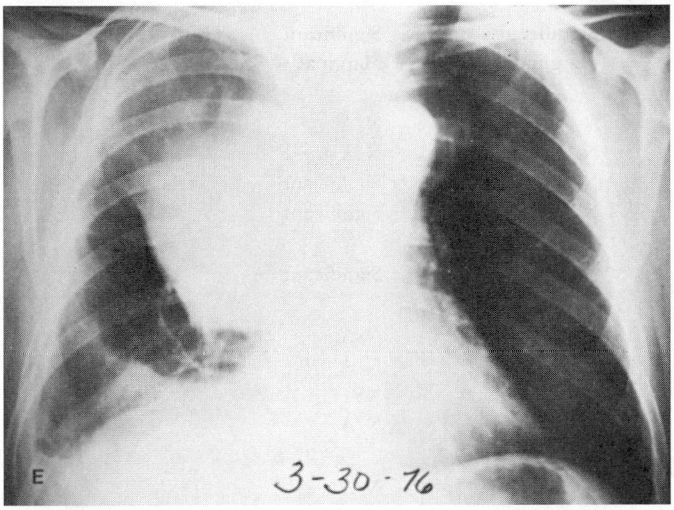

FIGURE 31.2-11. (*Continued*) **C:** A large hilar mass in mediastinal adenopathy, suggesting stage IIIB disease. **D:** Multiple bilateral pulmonary nodules of bronchoalveolar carcinoma. **E:** Small cell lung cancer involving a large, bulky central mass with hilar and mediastinal adenopathy and obstruction of the right upper lobe.

is probably not cost-effective to pursue all these investigations. The role of routine PET scanning in this early stage of disease has yet to be defined.

In patients with more locally advanced disease (clinical stage II or III) and in patients with suggestive adverse prognostic signs (e.g., weight loss), a more complete metastatic survey might be advantageous, although as yet there is no evidence of cost-effectiveness.[124] The routine use of CT scanning or MRI of the brain to detect asymptomatic cerebral metastasis has not been settled but is probably not cost-effective, especially in early-stage (I and II) disease.

PRETREATMENT PROGNOSTIC FACTORS

After establishing the diagnosis and clinical stage of NSCLC, it is desirable to determine the likely clinical course and survival outcome. This is important for both the patient and the treating physician, because this estimate is essential to guide the choice of therapy. Such information is also vital for the design and interpretation of clinical trials when it is necessary to discriminate between the effectiveness of a new therapy and the natural history of disease for a particular group of patients. Several retrospective analyses have evaluated traditional and newer prognostic factors for

Table 31.2-6 Univariable Survival Comparison of Three Large Retrospective Datasets

	Syracuse (1999)	*Dana Farber (1998)*	*Duke (1995, 1999)*
Population	260[a]	250	408
CLINICAL FACTORS			
Gender	NS	Significant	Significant
Age	Significant	NS	NS
Cough	Significant	N/A	Significant
Hemopytsis	N/A	N/A	Significant
Any symptom	N/A	N/A	Significant
Resection type	N/A	Significant	NS
HISTOPATHOLOGY FACTORS			
Histology	NS	NS	NS
Mucin	Significant	Significant	N/A
Differentiation	NS	NS	Significant
T-stage	Significant	NS	Significant
Tumor size (cm)	N/A	Significant	Significant
Vascular invasion	N/A	NS	Significant
Lymphatic invasion	N/A	Significant	N/A
Mitotic index	NS	NS	Significant
MOLECULAR BIOLOGIC FACTORS			
Growth factors			
EGFr	N/A	N/A	NS
Her2/neu	NS	NS	Significant
Kras codon 12	NS	Significant	N/A
Apoptosis factors			
p53	NS	Significant	Significant
Bcl-2	Significant	Marginal	Marginal
Cell-cycle factors			
Ploidy	NS	N/A	N/A
S-Phase	NS	N/A	N/A
Rb	NS	NS	Significant
Kl-67	Significant	N/A	Significant
Angiogenesis/Invasion			
Angiogenesis	NS	N/A	Significant
Differentiation factors			
Neuroendocrine	NS	N/A	N/A
CEA	NS	N/A	N/A
Blood group A	Significant	NS	NS
Lewis^y antigen	NS	N/A	N/A
Adhesion proteins			
E-cadherin	NS	N/A	N/A
CD-44	N/A	N/A	Significant
STn	N/A	N/A	NS

N/A, not available; NS, not significant ($P > .2$); marginal ($P > .05$ and $P \leq .2$), significant, ($P \leq .05$).
[a]Syracuse series incuded 67 stage II patients. Molecular biologic factors were divided by mechanism of action.
Note: Unvariable statistic demonstrated for stage I non–small cell lung cancer.

patients with operable and patients with inoperable NSCLC (Table 31.2-6).[125–130]

EARLY-STAGE (I, II, AND RESECTABLE STAGE III) DISEASE

The major clinical prognostic determinants for patients with early-stage disease are the size of the tumor and the presence or absence of lymph node spread. These features are well captured in the TNM staging classifications.[131] Additional clinical adverse prognostic factors are age older than 60 years and male gender and performance of a wedge resection instead of lobectomy or pneumonectomy.[132] Histologic subtype does not provide consistent additional prognostic information.[133] Expression of mucin has been shown to be a poor prognostic factor.[126,129,134,135] Mucin decreases tumor cell aggregation and may facilitate formation of metastases. Overall, clinical stage remains the most important prognostic tool.[136] However, newer diagnostic techniques are likely to continue to refine our precision in staging patients. For example, the detection of disseminated tumor cells in lymph nodes or the bone marrow using immunohistochemical analysis has been shown to correlate with a poor prognosis,[137,138] as do high SUV numbers in the primary tumors on PET scan.

ADVANCED-STAGE (UNRESECTABLE STAGE III AND IV) DISEASE

Because advanced-stage lung cancer has few 5-year survivors, TNM staging is not as valuable in assessing prognosis within these groups. Several comprehensive evaluations have searched for pretreatment prognostic factors in patients with advanced-stage NSCLC.[139–145] Pretreatment stage, performance status, and weight loss are the most important factors. The definitions of weight loss have varied among the reviews. Many trials evaluated small numbers of women. Those that included larger numbers of women generally found them to survive longer than men.[141,142,144] Serum lactate dehydrogenase, a predictor of survival in small cell lung cancer and many other malignancies, also appears to be an independent survival variable. The use of chemotherapy has also been shown to be of prognostic importance.[144] Histologic subtype is of no prognostic importance.

Whether any specific metastatic disease site confers a survival advantage or disadvantage remains controversial. Bone and liver metastases have been cited most often as predicting shorter survival. The total number of metastatic sites or total tumor burden has been shown to influence prognosis. In particular, patients with a solitary metastasis have a better prognosis, and an aggressive surgical approach should be considered. As yet, there is no clinically meaningful model combining the various independent factors that can be recommended either to select appropriate therapy or predict outcome for individual patients.

NEW POTENTIAL PROGNOSTIC MARKERS

With the increasing availability of sophisticated molecular testing, a variety of novel potential prognostic factors has emerged. These factors have largely been studied in earlier-stage disease, owing to the ready availability of surgical specimens. Activation of oncogenes (RAS, MYC C-ERB B-2, and BCL-2) or loss of the tumor suppressor genes (RB, p53, and p16) have frequently been described.[125–130] Several trials have shown that patients with diploid tumors survive longer than those with aneuploid tumors.[130,146,147] Further study is necessary to define the significance of ploidy and that of specific chromosomal alterations within the lung cancer field.[148,149]

Epidermal Growth Factor Receptors

After the identification of the presence and often increased numbers of EGFRs on lung cancer cells, trials have assessed the impact of EGFR expression on survival. In one trial, patients with operable EGFR-positive tumors survived significantly longer than those with EGFR-negative tumors (median survival, 71 and 28 months, respectively). In a second trial, overexpression of EGFR in primary lung tumors was associated with poor survival.[150,151] The presence of EGFR on lung cancer cells is a common finding and may be an important therapeutic target in the future.

Blood Group Antigen

Investigators have reported that the expression of blood group antigen A in tumors of patients with blood group types A and AB was associated with longer survival after surgical therapy than was seen in patients with blood types A and AB who had no blood group antigen A expressed on their tumor cells.[152] This finding has been confirmed in some studies, while others have not been able to show this.[128,129,153,154] This is also true for expression of Lewis^y antigen.[129,155]

Neuroendocrine Markers

After the observation that tumors with neuroendocrine differentiation, such as small cell lung cancer, are responsive to chemotherapy and the fact that many types of NSCLC contain small cell lung cancer elements, several investigators have looked for evidence of neuroendocrine differentiation in NSCLC. They have done this in the hope of identifying a population of NSCLC patients with enhanced responsiveness to chemotherapy and improved survival. Markers of neuroendocrine differentiation include chromogranin, L-dopa decarboxylase, dense core granules, neuron-specific enolase, and Leu-7.[156] In a group of NSCLC patients treated with a variety of chemotherapeutic agents, neuron-specific enolase, Leu-7, and chromogranin were more commonly expressed in responding patients.[157] In the same study, responding patients with two or more positive markers survived longer. In another study using a monoclonal antibody to define neuroendocrine differentiation, approximately 30% of tumors were positive, and the presence of biopsy specimens containing more than 50% positively staining cells was associated with shortened survival in a multivariable analysis.[158] Although they remain an intriguing and potentially useful area of investigation, neuroendocrine markers cannot be used to select a specific therapy or to determine response or survival in patients with NSCLC.

Genetic Markers

The intensive study of the role of oncogenes in the pathogenesis of human malignancy has led to an investigation of oncogene activation in lung cancer. In one study, *K-ras point mutations* occurred in almost one-third of human lung adenocarcinomas, while it is less common in squamous cell cancers.[159] In a follow-up study, the same authors found that the presence of K-ras point mutations can define a subgroup of operable NSCLC patients at high risk for relapse and overall shortened survival.[72] This has largely been confirmed by other studies.[73,160–166]

Mutation of the *p53* tumor suppressor gene has been frequently investigated. To date, it has no consistent correlation with prognosis.[126,129,132,167,168] Reduced E-cadherin expression has been associated with unfavorable prognosis in one trial.[163] Plakoglobin expression is also thought to play a role in cell adhesion. Its reduced expression has been shown to be associated with a poor prognosis.[169] Expression of *BCL-2* leads to inhibition of apoptosis. It has been described in approximately 20% of patients and is a favorable prognostic factor.[126,129,170,171] *Fas* expression has been suggested to be associated with a good prognosis in resected stage III disease.[172] Angiogenesis is increasingly recognized as an important factor of tumorigenesis. A variety of end points have been evaluated as angiogenic indicators, including microvessel density or immune staining with anti-factor VIII antibodies. Current evidence supports an adverse prognosis correlating with angiogenesis.[173–178]

OCCULT DISEASE

An occult lung cancer is defined as a tumor in a symptom-free patient without radiographic findings. In most instances, this is detected by finding abnormal cells on screening sputum cytologic examination. On occasion, an occult lung cancer may be identified at bronchoscopy that has been performed for other reasons (e.g., screening patients with other aerodigestive tract abnormalities). These occult tumors are usually found at an early stage either as *in situ* disease (Tis) or early T1N0 tumors. A truly occult lung cancer, undetected by radiography and asymptomatic, is almost always found at this early stage of disease. An extremely high proportion (>90%) of such tumors are squamous cell and can be totally cured by surgical removal. In many instances, nonsurgical approaches [e.g., laser ablation, hematoporphyrin ablation, or endobronchial brachytherapy (EBB)] may be employed as curative treatment, especially in noninvasive mucosal tumors.

LUNG CANCER SCREENING

In the hope that the screening of high-risk population groups by sputum cytology and chest radiograph would improve the identification of early-stage lung cancer, the National Cancer Institute Cooperative Early Lung Cancer Group was formed more than 20 years ago and developed protocols for screening high-risk people (e.g., male cigarette smokers older than 45 years). More than 30,000 male volunteers at three centers were recruited and followed up. One-half underwent intensive screening with four monthly sputum examinations and an annual chest radiograph, and the other one-half composed a control group. Each center had different methods of following up the control group, but initial chest radiographs were performed by all study groups.

The results of this trial demonstrated that lung cancers identified by screening methods were more frequently early-stage tumors (40% vs. 15%). Patients who developed lung cancer during the screening period had an overall 5-year survival of 35%, as compared with 13% in the general population. Despite this, there was no impact on overall survival of the two groups when all deaths were considered.[179,180] It was also found that sputum cytology can identify squamous cell carcinomas and that yearly chest radiographs identify with modest accuracy squamous cell carcinoma and adenocarcinomas. Small cell carcinoma is rarely detected at an early stage no matter what the screening technique.

Other mass screening trials using plain chest radiography performed in Europe have also failed to alter the total death rate in screened versus control groups. All trials demonstrated an improved ability to diagnose lung cancer early. Because these screening interventions fail to alter mortality rates, however, mass screening for lung cancer by chest radiography or sputum cytology (or both) cannot be recommended.

Despite the failure of mass chest x-ray screening, most investigators involved in these studies continue to believe that a person at high risk for developing lung cancer would be prudent to undergo annual chest radiography. Sputum cytology may be worthwhile as an initial screen, limiting further sputum cytology follow-up to those patients demonstrating dysplasia.

Chest Radiography

Although there are no specific recommendations from cancer agencies, plain posteroanterior and lateral chest radiographs have been used on a yearly basis in high-risk people in an attempt to provide an earlier diagnosis of lung cancer.[181] Important in this approach is the ability to compare previous radiographs with recent films to detect subtle changes. As yet, routine CT scans of high-risk people have not been performed as a mass screening technique, and the impact of digitized chest radiography has not been assessed.

Computed Tomography Scans

Most recently, two reports of screening using low-dose spiral CT scans have been reported. In a long-term Japanese study, a significant number of very early primary tumors have been identified using this technique, with significantly improved 5-year survival outcome in treated patients. In a more recent U.S. study, the use of low-dose spiral CT scans has confirmed the ability to discover extremely early lung cancers, with a prevalence rate of 30 per 1000 (vs. 3000 to 4000 with plain chest radiographs). These provocative studies have suggested that screening for lung cancer using low-dose, low-cost spiral CT scans is worthwhile in identifying early tumors and, it is hoped, in improving the outcome of patients with lung cancer by virtue of earlier detection. Although the exact cost of this type of mass screening program cannot be estimated in relation to finances or the investigation of other abnormalities identified at the time of CT scan (23% of individuals in the American study had other noncalcified benign nodules requiring investigation), this approach is worthy of further study. Whether the discovery of early treatable cancers ultimately affects the overall long-term mortality in a mass screening population will have to be determined prospectively. However, the 5-year survival of screen-detected stage I lung cancer falls from near 70% to less than 20% if left untreated, suggesting a significant benefit for earlier treatment.[182–185]

Sputum Cytology

The routine use of annual sputum examination for cytologic assessment is not cost-effective in the detection of early lung cancer. Dysplastic changes identified at sputum cytology, however, should be followed up. Severe dysplasia indicates a significant chance of ultimately developing lung cancer.[186] These patients should be followed up extremely closely.[187] As noted, Tockman et al.[95–97] have developed a monoclonal antibody that may improve the yearly detection rate of lung cancer using specific monoclonal antibodies.

Bronchoscopy

Bronchoscopy certainly can identify early mucosal changes suggestive of lung cancer. Tis and T1N0 proximal tumors (usually squamous cell) can be identified with relative ease using flexible bronchoscopy. The improved acuity of video equipment will probably further increase this yield.[188] However, many early lesions can be missed. Hematoporphyrins are preferentially taken up by rapidly dividing cells and, by using hematoporphyrin excitation by specific wavelengths (630 or 410 nm) of light, a characteristic fluorescence occurs in tissue containing the hematoporphyrin sensitizer. This technique can be used to detect these occult neoplasms but has the disadvantages of false-positive results (due to fluorescence of cellular atypia or metaplasia), hematoporphyrin light sensitivity, and limited availability. Only two or three centers have pursued this diagnostic approach.[189,190]

A new approach exploits spectral differences of autofluorescence in dysplastic and malignant cells without using drugs. This technique, called *lung imaging fluorescent endoscopy*, has been shown to identify early cellular changes and is being investigated for the detection and localization of early lung cancer,[191,192] especially proximal squamous cell tumors.

MANAGEMENT

The management of occult lung cancer depends on the stage of disease at diagnosis. Because most of these tumors are early but invasive T1N0 carcinomas, many are treated by surgical excision. Whenever surgery is contraindicated, curative radiotherapy is indicated. With proximal early-stage tumors, the role of brachytherapy alone or to augment the total dose is unknown, but curative treatment can be applied in this fashion.

In patients who have carcinoma *in situ*, hematoporphyrin or neodymium–yttrium aluminum garnet laser destruction of lesions can been used. Hayata et al.[194] found that early lesions should be less than 1 cm^2 in total surface area. Only a complete endobronchial response to such therapy is acceptable. After such a response, local recurrences are rare. Cortese et al.[193] recently reported using photodynamic therapy (PDT) in 21 carefully selected patients with superficial T1N0 lesions, all of which were squamous cell lung cancers. Using PDT, a complete response was identified in 15 of 21 patients at the Mayo Clinic; ultimately, 9 patients were spared an operation, 12 had recurrent disease after treatment, and 6 had complete responses. Recommendations for primary treatment with PDT in minimal occult tumors await further definition.[194,195] Only those patients who have had complete responses should be maintained on this type of treatment protocol, and they should be closely monitored with follow-up bronchoscopies. Whenever possible, surgical treatment is indicated for invasive T1N0 tumors and for all lesions persisting after nonsurgical (e.g., phototherapy, laser destruction, radiotherapy) treatment.

CHEMOPREVENTION

No chemopreventive strategy has been proven effective for NSCLC, either for at-risk people (i.e., smokers or individuals with occupational exposures) or for patients with treated lung cancer who have an increased risk of second primary tumors. No definite link between the dietary intake of carotenoids, vitamins C and E, or selenium and the pathogenesis of lung cancer has yet been established. Chemoprevention trials of carotene, retinol, and the combinations of folic acid plus vitamin B_{12} and carotene plus retinol in lung cancer have failed to demonstrate a chemopreventive effect. In two studies, an adverse risk was associated with carotene use.[47,53]

Recent insights into the biology of lung cancer and cellular differentiation suggest several new lines of research in this area. The most relevant to the chemoprevention of lung cancer appears to be the use of derivatives of retinoic acid, particularly 13-*cis* retinoic acid. This agent has been demonstrated to control leukoplakia (a premalignant epithelial lesion)[196] and to prevent second primary cancers in head and neck cancer patients after treatment of their primary tumors.[197] The association of specific chromosomal deletions, inactivation or loss of tumor suppressor genes, and mutation of specific protooncogenes may allow better definition of people at risk for second lung cancers and development of specific interventions for each genetic event. A nationwide trial in the United States is assessing the value of this association. Early unpublished results appear to be negative.

OVERVIEW OF INVASIVE LUNG CANCER MANAGEMENT: TREATMENT MODALITIES

Surgery and radiotherapy have been used independently to obtain local control of the primary tumor and regional lymphatic drainage. Until recently, chemotherapy had been used in an attempt to prolong symptom-free life in patients with metastatic disease. In the last 20 years, however, combined-modality therapies have become much more prevalent and have spurred intensive investigation. All three modalities are now used as primary therapy and, in combination, have been employed to improve disease-free intervals and ultimate survival.

Historically, surgery has provided the best chance of cure in the management of NSCLC when the tumor can be completely resected. Whenever surgery is not an option because of the inability of the patient to tolerate this approach, primary radiotherapy has been offered for patients with limited locoregional disease. Effective chemotherapy in the management of NSCLC is the last modality to be introduced. Although as a single modality chemotherapy rarely provides a total cure in the management of lung cancer, complete responses do occur with locoregional disease and in patients with metastatic disease. Long-term survival occasionally is possible. This section describes these three treatment modalities and, in general terms, their application. The newer forms of systemic therapy (e.g., biologic therapy) also are discussed.

SURGERY

In NSCLC, when the tumor is limited to the hemithorax and can be totally encompassed by excision, surgery provides the best chance for cure (Fig. 31.2-12). In stage I and stage II disease, when the tumor has not extended beyond the bronchopulmonary lymph nodes, a complete excision is almost always possible. Controversy arises in the management of N2 disease. Ipsilateral (N2) mediastinal lymph node involvement, despite being potentially resectable, remains a contentious issue when indications for surgery are discussed. Whenever a complete excision occurs, the patient is afforded a chance of cure. In clinical staging, it is imperative that the surgeon assess whether the tumor and its involved nodes can be completely removed at operation. N2 disease identified preoperatively (clinical staging), either by imaging studies or mediastinoscopy, affords a much poorer prognosis (<10% 5-year survival rate) than occult N2 disease (30% 5-year survival rate) discovered only at the time of surgery.

Except for a few special circumstances, stage IIIB disease, by virtue of incontrovertible evidence of contralateral lymph node spread (N3) or primary tumor invasion of vital structures (T4), denotes inoperability, with a small likelihood of success after surgical excision. Similarly, lung cancer that has metastasized to distant organs is usually beyond the realm of surgical excision. There has been success, however, in removing the primary tumor as well as a solitary metastatic focus. In selected patients, this affords long-term disease-free control. Surgical approaches are frequently used to palliate symptoms.

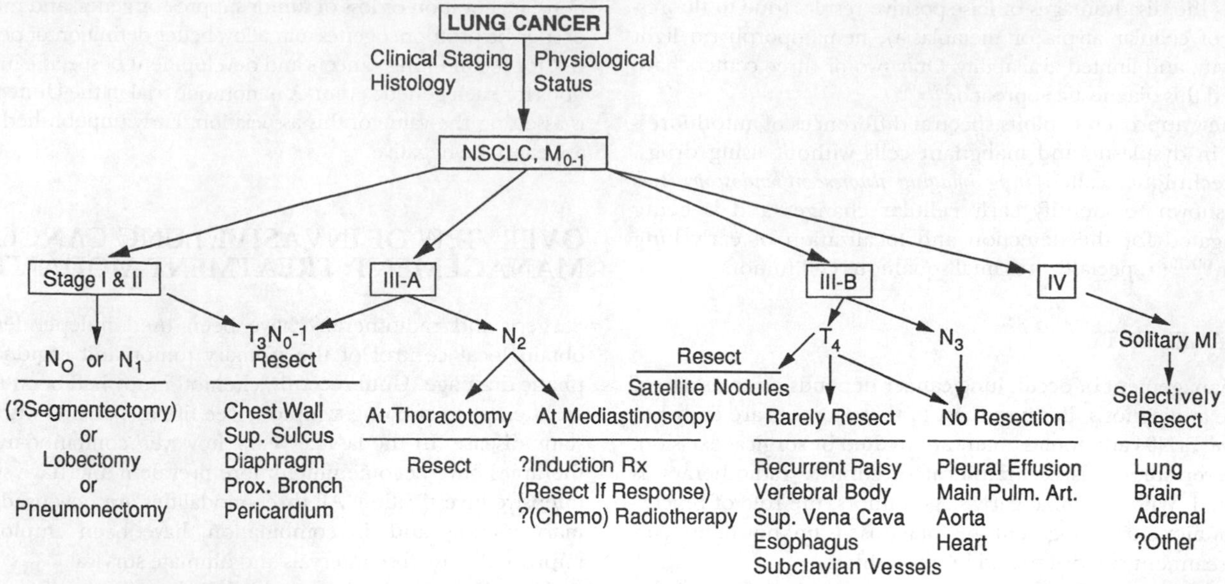

FIGURE 31.2-12. Schema for operability at the various stages of non–small cell lung cancer (NSCLC). See text for details. Chemo, chemotherapy; Prox. Bronch, proximal bronchus; Pulm. Art., pulmonary artery; Rx, therapy; Sup., superior.

Patient Selection

The preoperative assessment of patients considered for surgical treatment of lung cancer includes clinical staging of the disease to assess its resectability, assessment of the cardiopulmonary reserve of the patient to determine whether the intended pulmonary resection is possible, and assessment of the patient with regard to the perioperative risk of the procedure. Traditionally, patients are suitable candidates for pneumonectomy if the predicted forced expiratory volume in 1 second (FEV_1) after pneumonectomy is greater than 1.2 L, the patient does not suffer from hypercapnia, and cor pulmonale is not present.[198–200] Pulmonary function studies best suited to assess these parameters include spirometry, arterial blood gases, diffusion capacity measurements of oxygen uptake with exercise (mVO_2) and, when indicated, ventilation-perfusion scans to estimate the proportions of functioning pulmonary tissue required to be excised.[201] Patients undergoing lobectomy or smaller resection require similar postoperative pulmonary function parameters.[202,203] Prospective analyses, however, have failed to show differences in pulmonary function studies, including FEV_1, after lobectomy or smaller resection.[204,205] The amount of functioning pulmonary tissue removed by lobectomy or smaller resection rarely interferes with ultimate recovery and function and may actually improve pulmonary function,[206] as it does with volume-reduction operations for emphysema.

A more important factor in preoperative assessment is the ability of the patient to tolerate a general anesthetic and the rigors of the early postoperative period. To prevent postoperative cardiopulmonary complications and decrease the chance of other major postoperative problems, care must be taken to determine accurately the patient's cardiopulmonary status before operation. In the hope of ultimately improving the estimate of these risks, mVO_2, cardiac radionuclide studies, and echocardiography have been introduced. The ability of patients to perform the necessary pulmonary toilet (e.g., coughing, deep breathing) after such procedures requires intensive preoperative instruction and a period of rehabilitation when necessary.

Pulmonary complications increase remarkably when the FEV_1–forced vital capacity (FEV_1/FVC) ratio is below 75% of predicted, indicating significant airway obstruction. FEV_1/FVC ratios of less than 50% of predicted lead to significant postoperative morbidity and mortality. Similarly, it appears that an mVO_2 of less than 15 increases morbidity and an mVO_2 of less than 10 leads to significant morbidity and mortality. However, the exact risk for any single patient cannot be estimated. No single test is absolutely predictive. Clinical judgment is extremely important.

Postoperative Care

A major insult to cardiopulmonary reserve reflected by thoracotomy and pulmonary resection demands that patients undergoing such procedures receive assiduous care and monitoring in the postoperative period. This is best served by a 24- to 48-hour period in a monitored setting. With newer forms of pain control (epidural narcotic analgesia, patient-controlled analgesia, intrathoracic analgesia), the potential for less morbidity after pulmonary resection may be realized.

Surgical Procedures

Until 50 years ago, pneumonectomy was considered the surgical excision of choice in managing all lung cancers.[207] Presently, when complete excision can be obtained by lobectomy, thus sparing functioning lung, this is the preferred resection method, with what appears to be an equal opportunity for long-term success.[208] In the last 20 years, there has been a resurgence of interest in smaller resections and lung-conserving operations. Jensik[209] has been the major proponent of segmentectomy for T1–2N0 peripheral tumors. Survival after such a limited resection and the morbidity and mortality of the operation appeared at least equivalent to lobectomy in retrospective analyses.[210] Newer information, however, suggests that locoregional recurrence is increased and survival is decreased when less than a lobectomy is performed.

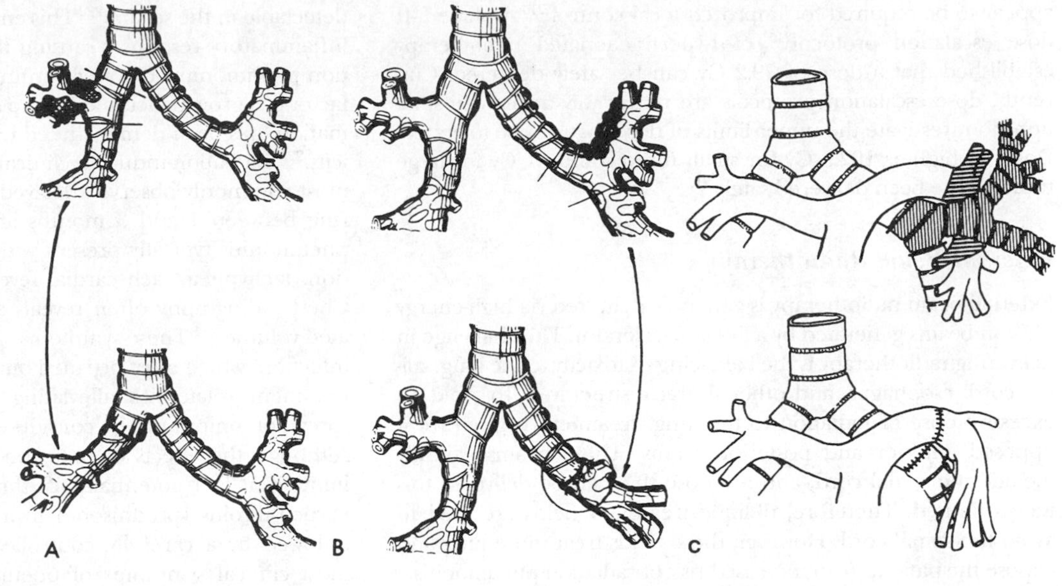

FIGURE 31.2-13. Bronchoplastic and bronchovascular sleeve resections to preserve pulmonary function. **A:** Right upper lobe sleeve resection. **B:** Left upper lobe sleeve resection. **C:** Left upper lobe bronchovascular sleeve resection.

In proximally situated tumors (T3) for which a pneumonectomy may be required for total excision, lung-conserving operations using bronchoplastic procedures to preserve uninvolved lobes (e.g., sleeve lobectomy) have results equivalent to the more extensive pneumonectomy and should be employed when possible. Even when the proximal pulmonary artery is involved, vascular sleeve resections can be used to preserve pulmonary function (Fig. 31.2-13).

With improved surgical and anesthetic technique and perioperative care, the postoperative mortality rate for surgical resections has decreased remarkably during the last 50 years. Today, pneumonectomy can be performed with a mortality rate of less than 6%, lobectomy with less than 3%, and smaller resections with 1% mortality or less. These mortality figures are significantly affected by the age of the patient, stage of the disease, and extent of resection.[211]

The most common complications after resectional surgery are not technical failures of the operation but cardiopulmonary problems, especially supraventricular arrhythmias and respiratory failure. Improved preoperative assessment and postoperative care to identify high-risk patients and to decrease these complications will ultimately lead to lessened operative risks for the patient (Table 31.2-7).[212]

RADIOTHERAPY

Radiotherapy is used for the treatment of NSCLC in various ways. In unresectable disease, it is the primary modality for the cure of tumor. In the postoperative setting, it used as an adjuvant treatment to improve local control. Radiotherapy is also frequently used for the palliation of advanced and metastatic lung cancer.

The vast bulk of radiotherapy for NSCLC is delivered via external-beam radiotherapy, either through a radioactive source, such as cobalt 60, or more commonly via a linear accelerator. Newer techniques, such as three-dimensional conformal radiotherapy (3D-CRT) and intensity-modulated radiotherapy, are essentially improved techniques to deliver external-beam radiotherapy more accurately and with fewer side effects. This allows for a higher dose of radiation to be delivered safely. Brachytherapy is another treatment modality that is used for both curative and palliative intent. Alterations in dose fractionation, such as hyperfractionation, are attempts to take advantage of the biologic behavior of tumors and normal tissue to optimize repair of radiation damage and limit tumor repopulation.

The maximum tolerated dose of radiotherapy to the thorax has yet to be established. Standard therapy for unresected disease in this country and Europe has consisted of 60 to 65 Gy over approximately 6 weeks. When patients receiving 65 Gy without chemotherapy were carefully evaluated for local tumor control, only 15% were free of disease after treatment.[213] Radiation resistance to the dose levels typically used represents a major factor contributing to the high incidence of local failure. Higher doses

TABLE 31.2-7. Postoperative Mortality for Surgical Resections

	Mortality Rate (%)	*Complication Rate (%)*
TYPE OF RESECTION		
Segment or wedge	1.3	10.4
Lobectomy	2.9	15
Pneumonectomy	6.2	15
AGE (Y)		
<50	1.3	3
50–59	1.3	10.7
60–69	4.1	13.0
70–79	7	24.5
>80	8.1	20
PULMONARY FUNCTION		
FEV_1 <1.2	NS	22
FEV_1 1.2–2.0	NS	14
FEV_1 >2	NS	14
DISEASE STAGE		
I	NS	10.6
II	NS	11.2
III	NS	18.6

FEV_1, forced expiratory volume in 1 second; NS, not stated.

appear to be required for improved local control.[214] A phase I–II dose escalation protocol[215] of hyperfractionated radiotherapy established that a dose of 79.2 Gy can be safely delivered. Currently, dose escalation protocols are under way at many institutions to investigate the upper limits of dose that can be tolerated. Doses as high as 102.9 Gy for small tumors and 81 Gy for large tumors have been delivered safely.[216–218]

External-Beam Radiotherapy

External-beam radiotherapy is generally delivered via high-energy photon beams generated by a linear accelerator. The challenge in delivering radiotherapy is the balancing of toxicity to the lung, spinal cord, esophagus, and other thoracic structures. To avoid an excessive dose of radiation to the lung, treatment is given from opposed anterior and posterior beams. These beams typically include the spinal cord, and the dose that can be delivered this way is limited. Therefore, oblique treatment fields are used to avoid the spinal cord. However, these fields treat more lung and expose the patient to an increased risk of radiation pneumonitis.

When a patient is simulated for radiotherapy, the treatment field encompasses the tumor with enough margin to account for tumor motion, patient movement, and set-up error. The tumor can be demarcated by many methods. The most straightforward is observing the tumor under fluoroscopy and on plain films during simulation. This has the advantage of helping to determine tumor motion. However, this method might lead to underestimation of tumor dimensions because of inadequate imaging technique and disease not discernible on plain films. Therefore, CT images should be used to help to localize tumor. With the advent of CT-based simulation, tumors can be outlined in the axial plane of consecutive images. A representation of the tumor in three dimensions can then be placed on a digitally reconstructed radiograph. Recently, new imaging modalities, such as [^{18}F]fluorodeoxyglucose-PET scanning, have been used to help to define tumor volumes.[219] The treatment field should be verified on the treatment machine prior to the initiation of radiotherapy. Treatment fields should also be checked weekly so that adjustments can be made.

Acute side effects occurring during the course of radiotherapy are organ-specific and related to the fractionation scheme, total dose, and use of sequential or concomitant chemotherapy or radiosensitizers. They typically manifest in the second to third week of treatment. A significant concern of combined therapy is the increased toxicity, which may outweigh the benefit from both modalities.

Delayed acute radiation toxicity can occur 1 to 3 months after completing treatment but has been known to occur as late as 6 months after completion of treatment. Organs at risk include normal lung, esophagus, spinal cord, and heart. Radiation factors, including fraction size, overall treatment time, radiation dose, and volume of normal organ treated, contribute to acute delayed toxicity for conventional fractionation with radiotherapy. Similarly, the use of concurrent chemotherapy, as well as novel fractionation regimens, can lower the threshold for delayed tissue reactions.[220]

PULMONARY TOXICITY. Animal models have demonstrated increased vascular permeability after thoracic irradiation.[221] Alveolar surfactant levels also increase after thoracic irradiation and, owing to increased vascular permeability, are detectable in the serum.[222] This endothelial injury may lead to an inflammatory response, causing the clinical syndrome of radiation pneumonitis. Elevated serum levels of transforming growth factor-β, a growth factor known to stimulate connective tissue formation, has been demonstrated in patients developing lung toxicity.[223] Radiation-induced clinical pneumonitis represents the most commonly observed delayed acute reaction, usually occurring between 1 and 3 months after completion. Patients with pneumonitis typically present with shortness of breath on exertion, tachypnea, tachycardia, fever, and nonproductive cough. Chest radiography often reveals an infiltrate within the irradiated volume.[224] These symptoms can mimic an upper respiratory infection, which must be ruled out before embarking on specific treatment related to alleviating pneumonitis. Recurrence or spread of tumor must be considered in the differential diagnosis. Although the effects of radiation pneumonitis are usually self-limiting, it is a potentially life-threatening process. The use of corticosteroids (prednisone) in a starting dose of 1 mg/kg/d, followed by a carefully controlled slow taper, usually resolves most clinical symptoms of pneumonitis. Corticosteroids, however, appear to reduce the ability of alveolar macrophages to release tumor necrosis factor in response to infectious agents, which can lead to recurrent respiratory tract infections in patients treated chronically with these drugs.[225]

Enhancement of radiation damage by chemotherapy in terms of acute and late effects appears to be maximum with concurrent treatment, with a tendency for damage to decline as the interval between drug and radiation is increased.[226,227] Roach et al.[228] analyzed radiotherapy parameters in 24 combined-modality trials completed before 1994, involving more than 1911 patients with both small cell lung cancer and NSCLC, to determine potential risk factors for radiation pneumonitis when radiation is combined with chemotherapy. Multiple fractionation schemes, total doses, and fraction sizes, along with several chemotherapeutic regimens, were used. The overall incidence of pneumonitis was 7.8%. Factors associated with a higher risk included fraction size higher than 2.67 Gy and total dose. Twice-daily radiation, however, appeared to reduce the risk expected if the same total daily dose were given as a single fraction. Based on this analysis, high dose per fraction when combined with chemotherapy should be avoided.

Late radiation injury is related primarily to the dose per fraction and total dose. Most patients who develop clinical pneumonitis eventually become asymptomatic, although nearly all ultimately develop the radiologic evidence of pulmonary fibrosis in the region of the previous pneumonitis. The degree of late pulmonary toxicity and fibrosis is directly proportional to the volume of normal lung irradiated and the total dose delivered, as well as the fraction size. It is not clear whether chemotherapy actually modifies the latency period for the development of late pulmonary reactions or increases the actual incidence. For most patients, pulmonary fibrosis is an expected and unavoidable consequence of high-dose irradiation. For patients presenting with preexisting compromised pulmonary function, however, and for patients who develop severe clinical pneumonitis, a distortion of the pulmonary architecture by fibrosis can have a major impact on the quality of life and functional status.

ESOPHAGEAL TOXICITY. Since the esophagus has a central location, it is exposed to high-dose radiation during the treatment of most NSCLCs and can be a major dose-limiting factor. Radiation may induce acute esophagitis during the course of therapy. Histologic changes occur during the first week of treatment,[229] although clinical symptoms typically begin during the second through fourth weeks of treatment. Esophagitis presents with mild to severe swallowing difficulty requiring diet modification and nonnarcotic or narcotic analgesics, depending on severity. It is caused by an inflammatory response of the esophageal mucosa.[229]

Chemotherapy and radiosensitizers appear to accelerate the onset and severity of symptoms. In a randomized prospective intergroup trial, the rate of grade 3 or worse esophagitis increased from 1.3% to 65% with the addition of concurrent cisplatin and etoposide to 50.4 Gy thoracic radiation.[230] When used concurrently with carboplatin and paclitaxel, the grade 3 or 4 esophageal toxicity has been reported to be approximately 25%.[229] Agents such as 5-fluorouracil, doxorubicin, cisplatin, and mitomycin also enhance radiation-induced esophageal toxicity.[168–170,231–233] Acute esophagitis generally resolves shortly after the completion of radiotherapy, with few patients progressing to chronic esophagitis. The rare patient with chronic esophagitis may require dilatation to relieve stricture formation.

Hyperfractionated treatment has also been shown to increase toxicity. When 60 Gy given via accelerated hyperfractionation was compared to standard fractionation, the grade 3 or worse acute esophageal toxicity increased from 9% to 35% ($P = .0017$).[234]

CUTANEOUS TOXICITY. With the use of megavoltage equipment, treatment rarely causes an acute reaction to the skin, such as erythema or moist desquamation. Moist desquamation can occur in the supraclavicular region after a course of high-dose radiotherapy, owing to the sloping surface of the chest at the level of the thoracic inlet. The addition of chemotherapy or sensitizers may also enhance the effects of radiotherapy on the skin.

NEUROTOXICITY. A transient myelopathic syndrome (Lhermitte's syndrome) can occur during the first 6 months after therapy and is manifested by dysesthesias and paresthesias affecting the upper extremities and shoulder girdles on flexion of the neck.[235] It is related to the total radiation dose, dose per fraction, and length of spinal cord irradiated. Lhermitte's syndrome is self-limiting and does not appear to be related to the development of late radiation myelitis.[236]

The spinal cord can tolerate conventionally fractionated radiotherapy doses in the range of 45 to 50 Gy, and the radiation oncologist should strive to maintain the maximal spinal cord dose at or below this level. In some cases, depending on the volume of spinal cord treated and the dose per fraction, the tolerance has been reported to be as high as 60 Gy; in selected cases in which the tumor is paraspinal, it may be appropriate to treat a small portion of the cord to this dose with the patient's understanding of potential toxicity.[237] Chemotherapy can reduce the tolerance threshold of this organ. There has been a concern that altered fractionation might lead to increased myelitis. Jeremic et al.[238] have reported no cases of radiation myelitis in 158 patients who lived at least 1 year after receiving hyperfractionated radiotherapy in fraction sizes of 1.2 Gy per day to a total dose of 50.4 Gy. Once it develops, radiation-induced transverse myelitis is irreversible.

CARDIAC TOXICITY. Radiation injury to the heart is usually manifested as pericarditis, although other complications, such as myocardial ischemia and chronic pericardial effusions, can occur. The tolerance for the entire heart is approximately 40 Gy; up to one-third of the heart can tolerate approximately 60 Gy.[239]

Three-Dimensional Conformal Radiotherapy

3D-CRT represents an approach to improve the local outcome of radiotherapy in NSCLC.[239a,239b] The major aim of this method is to decrease the risk of underdosing or missing portions of the tumor. In addition, owing to the improved ability to conform the high radiation dose to the target, considerable amounts of normal lung, esophagus, and heart can be effectively excluded from the high-radiation-dose regions. This provides a potential for increasing the tumor dose to levels beyond those feasible with conventional radiotherapy, with a concomitant decrease in the normal tissue complication probability. Single-institution and cooperative group studies of dose escalation are under way[216–218] to evaluate the efficacy of this strategy.

3D-CRT is accomplished using CT to aid in treatment planning. A clinical tumor volume (CTV) is defined in the axial plane of the CT images. A margin is subsequently added to the CTV to generate the planning target volume. This margin compensates for tumor motion during treatment caused by breathing, patient movement, and set-up error. The treatment beams are subsequently constructed using the beam's-eye-view technique.

The use of 3D-CRT also allows investigators to predict more accurately the toxicity of a given course of radiotherapy. The normal tissue complication probability is an estimate of clinical toxicity based on the dose delivered to the volume of normal lung. It has been shown to correlate with incidence of radiation pneumonitis. Other institutions use either the mean lung dose[240] or the dose that a given volume of lung receives as a determinant of lung toxicity. For example, in the Radiation Therapy Oncology Group (RTOG) dose escalation protocol, the volume of lung receiving 20 Gy is used as a guide as to what dose to deliver.[216]

Intensity-Modulated Radiotherapy

Intensity-modulated radiotherapy represents a new approach to radiotherapy wherein the beam within the treatment field is dynamically changed during treatment to give more radiotherapy to areas with tumor and less to areas with normal tissue.[241] Its use is being investigated.

Gated Radiotherapy

Motion of the tumor and of the lung itself during the delivery of each treatment appears to affect the outcome of radiotherapy in inoperable NSCLC. Lung tumors have been shown to move substantially during quiet breathing, causing inaccuracies in treatment delivery.[242,243] Underdosage of the CTV may result if the tumor target moves outside the treatment volume during the administration of radiotherapy. To compensate for this motion, a large margin is usually used, consequently increasing the amount of normal lung tissue in the high-dose volume and limiting the amount of radiation that can be delivered.

To overcome this, techniques have been developed to keep the tumor still during radiotherapy. Two distinct techniques have been used to reduce the effect of respiratory motion. The first involves confining the radiation delivery to a specified phase in the breathing cycle by gating the linear accelerator while the patient breathes freely. Breathing is monitored with devices that trigger radiation delivery during specific phases of the patient's respiratory cycle.[244] The use of gated treatments has been evaluated[244–247] and offers the advantage of allowing patients to breathe freely while the radiation beam is turned on and off. In the second approach, breathing is controlled either voluntarily by the patient[248] or by using an occlusion valve.[249] This technique is less challenging to perform, since it involves no modification to the treatment machine, but it is not suitable for all patients.

Stereotactic Radiotherapy

Stereotactic radiotherapy and stereotactic radiosurgery have been shown to be effective in treating brain metastases. Stereotactic radiotherapy is a technique by which a high dose of radiation is delivered to a small, well-circumscribed lesion with minimal dose to surrounding structures. This technique has been applied to lung tumors with good local control.[250] It will be applicable only in a small subset of patients with very early, small tumors and must be considered investigational at this time.

Neutron Therapy

Fast neutrons have been examined as a potential modality to improve the results of therapy for NSCLC. The biologic properties of neutrons differ from conventional photon energies, possessing advantages of high-linear-energy transfer. This high-linear-energy transfer can lead to a number of biologic effects, including greater relative biologic effectiveness, reduced oxygen enhancement ratio, less sublethal and potentially lethal damage repair, and less cell cycle specificity than photons.[251]

A randomized trial of 200 patients was performed using modern neutrons to a dose of 20.4 neutron Gy as compared to 66 Gy of standard photons.[252] It showed no difference in overall survival between the two groups. Grade 3 or worse radiation pneumonitis occurred in 11% and 24% of the patients in the photon and neutron groups, respectively. Therefore, unless a specific group of patients who might benefit from neutron therapy can be identified, it is unclear whether this modality is useful for patients with NSCLC.

Brachytherapy

INTRAOPERATIVE INTERSTITIAL BRACHYTHERAPY AND RADIOTHERAPY. Intraoperative interstitial brachytherapy has been applied in the curative and palliative treatment of NSCLC. Implantation of radioactive sources offers an advantage over external irradiation because of the limited penetrability from source to prescription point, resulting in rapid dose fall-off and sparing of surrounding normal tissues.

Indications for implantation include unresectable or incompletely resected tumors found at thoracotomy: hilar tumors adherent to major vasculature with no clearance for safe dissection; attachment of tumors to mediastinal structures, such as the trachea, pericardium, or esophagus; extensive tumor involvement of the chest wall, spine, or paravertebral tissue when a complete resection is not possible; and recurrent or metastatic endobronchial lesions.[253]

For curative techniques, the selection of radioactive sources depends on the tumor location and the amount of gross disease left after surgery. In circumstances in which more than 1 cm of tumor is left behind, a permanent volume implant is usually required. The area to be implanted is determined, and its dimensions are measured. A nomogram is applied to determine the number of radioactive sources (^{125}I or ^{103}Pd) needed and the proper spacing of the needles, which in turn are based on the strength of the sources and the average dimension of the tumor volume. Hollow needles are inserted into the tumor, and radioactive sources are permanently implanted. For close and positive margins or in the presence of a minimal plaque of residual gross disease, either a permanent planar or temporary interstitial implant may be used. For situations requiring permanent placement of radioactive sources, ^{125}I seeds encapsulated in Vicryl or ^{103}Pd seeds can either be directly sutured onto the area at risk or sewn into a premeasured Dexon or Vicryl mesh, which in turn is sutured onto the target area. A similar technique employing ^{125}I embedded in a Gelfoam plaque has been described.[254] Both techniques allow implantation of radioactive seeds in areas that are near vital structures that cannot be directly sutured.[255]

Temporary implants use ^{192}Ir or ^{125}I at either a low- or a high-dose-rate method of delivering radiation using afterloading catheters. Temporary implants have been advocated for tumors invading the chest wall, superior sulcus, mediastinum, and paravertebral regions when a complete resection is not certain. In general, the catheters are spaced 1 cm apart, with a 1-cm margin around the defined target, and exit out the chest wall. The patient is then loaded with radioactive sources (^{125}I or ^{192}Ir) approximately 4 or 5 days after surgery to allow for proper wound healing.

INTRALUMINAL BRACHYTHERAPY. Intraluminal brachytherapy or EBB is generally used as a palliative treatment for obstructive recurrent tumors causing such symptoms as dyspnea and hemoptysis. This treatment directly introduces a high-activity ^{192}Ir source directly into the lumen of the tracheal or bronchial airway. Flexible bronchoscopic guidance is used to localize the tumor and to position a catheter beyond the site of disease. Patients are generally treated under a combination of monitored intravenous sedation and the application of local anesthesia to the larynx and trachea. The radioactive ^{192}Ir source is then introduced into the catheter and positioned. Treatment lasts only a couple of minutes, owing to the high activity of the source. High-dose-rate intraluminal brachytherapy has largely replaced both direct interstitial implantation of ^{125}I seeds into endobronchial tumors and low-dose-rate endobronchial irradiation.[256]

Side effects after intraluminal brachytherapy include massive hemoptysis, fistula formation, chronic mucosal sloughing, and airway edema.[257] Langendijk et al.[258] examined risk factors for massive hemoptysis. The highest complication rate occurred in patients receiving EBB for recurrent tumor (43%) or combination external-beam therapy and EBB (25%). They also found that patients receiving a single fraction of 15 Gy prescribed to 1 cm had a 50% rate of massive hemoptysis, whereas patients receiving 7.5 Gy × 2 or 10 Gy in a single fraction had an 11% rate. Hennequin et al.[259] theorized that most massive hemoptysis is from disease progression and not treatment toxicity. They reported a 7% risk of massive hemoptysis and concluded that all but one case had evidence of tumor progression. They also reported an 8.7% rate of radiation bronchitis. The risk factors for toxicity in their series included palliative intent of treatment and the length of bronchus treated.

Intraoperative Radiotherapy

Experience with the use of intraoperative radiotherapy for NSCLC is limited. This modality does not appear to show a significant benefit over external-beam irradiation alone or in combination with chemotherapy. The technique involves the modification of a linear accelerator through the attachment of an intraoperative cone for electron-beam treatment.[260] Both the optimal dose and threshold tolerance of mediastinal structures are unknown; however, one fraction is generally delivered intraoperatively at a dose of 10 to 20 Gy. The published results are conflicting. With no reported phase III trials, this modality must be considered experimental.

CHEMOTHERAPY

General Principles

Chemotherapy for patients with NSCLC has been under investigation for several decades. Conceptually, it has evolved from the administration in the palliative care setting to its integration into combined-modality curative therapy settings in patients with locoregionally advanced disease.

Currently, chemotherapy as a single-treatment modality can be considered standard therapy for most patients with stage IV disease or stage IIIB disease due to pleural effusion or positive scalene lymph nodes.[261–265] In these settings, prolongation of survival time and amelioration of clinical symptoms are the goals of therapy. It has been conclusively demonstrated in randomized clinical trials that chemotherapy prolongs median survival times as compared with "best supportive care" and also increases quality of life (discussed later in Stage IV Disease).

In patients with locoregionally advanced disease (stage IIIA or IIIB), traditional therapy has consisted of surgery and postoperative radiotherapy (PORT) or radiotherapy alone for patients with unresectable disease. In these patients, chemotherapy is now used as a component of multimodality therapy.[266–268] Therapy is given with curative intent, and it is hoped that the integration of chemotherapy will lead not only to an increased overall median survival time but to an increase in the percentage of (cured) patients surviving for long periods (discussed later in "Unresectable" Stage IIIA and IIIB Non–Small Cell Lung Cancer).

Strategies in this setting have included classic adjuvant chemotherapy in patients with fully resected disease and induction (or "neoadjuvant") chemotherapy whereby a specified number of chemotherapy cycles are administered prior to definitive local therapy with surgery, radiotherapy, or both. The simultaneous use of chemotherapy and radiotherapy (concomitant chemoradiotherapy) has also been intensively investigated. In theory, adjuvant and induction chemotherapy are aimed at improving systemic control of occult microscopic metastatic disease. Decreasing the size (downstaging) of the locoregional tumor burden may also be observed with induction chemotherapy. The delay of radiotherapy to allow for administration of induction chemotherapy has been of theoretic concern, since this could lead to the proliferation of clonogenic tumor cells in an unresponsive tumor.[269] Concomitant chemoradiotherapy may also result in systemic antitumor activity.[270] However, this will be realized only if systemically active doses and schedules of the drugs are administered. In clinical practice, the latter has been challenging, since radiation-related toxicities are usually increased in the presence of chemotherapy (i.e., esophagitis and radiation pneumonitis). Therefore, the primary goal of concomitant chemoradiotherapy may be to enhance the antitumor activity of radiation and increase locoregional control (radiation sensitization or enhancement).[270]

It has been conclusively demonstrated that induction chemotherapy followed by radiotherapy prolongs the median survival time in patients with unresectable stage III disease when compared with radiotherapy alone.[213,271–273] Encouraging data also exist to support the administration of combination chemotherapy with concomitant radiotherapy.[274,275] The use of induction chemotherapy in the surgical setting (stage IIIA)[276,277] or with simultaneous radiotherapy[274] remains investigational. Also, the use of adjuvant chemotherapy in patients with resected stage I, stage II, or stage IIIA disease is considered experimental.

Selection of Specific Drugs

Most patients with NSCLC present with metastatic (stage IV) disease at initial diagnosis. There is no known curative therapy for these patients. The treatment goals are, therefore, broadly defined to maximize survival time and maintain acceptable quality of life. Because metastatic NSCLC is a systemic disease, its therapy is logically based on the use of systemic therapy. Additional local therapy is used to palliate specific sites of disease.

Most traditional drugs have at best moderate single-agent activity in NSCLC.[261,263–265,270,278–281] It has been generally accepted that a single agent should have a response rate of approximately 15% for the drug to be considered active.[261–265] This guideline is compromised by the fact that, historically, not all drugs have been studied in rigorously designed and conducted phase II or phase III trials. For example, rigorous testing during the 1990s suggested response rates for cisplatin or carboplatin of only approximately 10%.

Throughout the 1970s and 1980s, only six drugs were thought to have sufficient single-agent activity in NSCLC. Complete responses to single-agent therapy were exceedingly rare. Furthermore, the response duration was short, on average 2 to 3 months. Median survival trials were 6 to 8 months, with no long-term survivors.

Combination chemotherapy was investigated in an attempt to increase response rates.[261–265,270,282] Generally, higher responses were reported, but it remained unclear whether a more pronounced impact on survival was also achieved. One of the earliest combination chemotherapy regimens was the regimen consisting of cyclophosphamide, doxorubicin (Adriamycin), methotrexate, and procarbazine (CAMP). In a single-institution study, a response rate of 26% was noted.[283]

Subsequent clinical trials incorporated cisplatin, which was thought by many investigators to be the most active single agent in NSCLC in the 1980s.[144,282,284] Among the most frequently used combinations were the regimens of cisplatin and etoposide, cisplatin and vinblastine, or (in Europe) cisplatin and vindesine or teniposide.[282,285–287] Three-drug combinations incorporating ifosfamide,[288,289] mitomycin C,[286,290] or leucovorin[291,292] were also investigated (Table 31.2-8).

Most of these regimens have in common the combination of cisplatin with a vinca alkaloid or etoposide. They were based on the incorporation of drugs with known single-agent activity,

TABLE 31.2-8. Combination Chemotherapy Regimens for Non–Small Cell Lung Cancer

Drug Regimen	*Dose*	*Response (%)*
CAP		
Cyclophosphamide	500 mg/m^2 × 1	15–25
Doxorubicin (Adriamycin)	50 mg/m^2 × 1	
Cisplatin (platinum)	50 mg/m^2 × 1	
PV		
Cisplatin (platinum)	120 mg/m^2 × 1	15–30
Vinblastine	6 mg/m^2 × 2	
or Vindesine	3 mg/m^2 × 2	
CE		
Carboplatin	300–375 mg/m^2 × 1	10–30
Etoposide	100–120 mg/m^2 × 3	
EP		
Etoposide	80–100 mg/m^2 × 3	20–30
Cisplatin (platinum)	80–100 mg/m^2 × 1	
MVP		
Mitomycin	8–10 mg/m^2 × 1	30–60
Vinblastine	6 mg/m^2 × 1	
or Vindesine	3 mg/m^2 × 1	
Cisplatin (platinum)	80–120 mg/m^2 × 1	
PFL		
Cisplatin (platinum)	100 mg/m^2 × 1	29
5-Fluorouracil	800 mg/m^2 × 5	
Leucovorin	100 mg PO q4h × 5	
MIP		
Mitomycin	6 mg/m^2 × 1	35–50
Ifosfamide	3 g/m^2 × 1	
Cisplatin (platinum)	50 mg/m^2 × 1	
ICE		
Ifosfamide	4 g/m^2 × 1	25–40
Cisplatin	25 mg/m^2/d × 3	
Etoposide	100 mg/m^2/d × 3	

unlike earlier combinations, such as CAMP. Phase II studies of these regimens frequently resulted in response rates of 30% to 50%, suggesting higher activity than the first-generation combination regimens.[265] Because cisplatin is logistically difficult to administer and can result in severe toxicity, direct comparisons of cisplatin-based regimens with non–cisplatin-containing combinations were performed. Although some studies reported increased response rates with a cisplatin-containing regimen, there was no consistent increase in survival. Only three studies reported superior survival with cisplatin.[293]

Another question of interest was whether there exists a dose-response curve for cisplatin's activity in NSCLC. One early study suggested an increase in response rate when increasing the cisplatin dose from 60 to 120 mg/m^2.[294] A second study, however, did not support this observation.[282] The Southwestern Oncology Group (SWOG) initiated a three-arm comparison of cisplatin administered at 100 mg/m^2 versus 200 mg/m^2 per cycle versus a third arm of high-dose cisplatin and mitomycin based on promising phase II data for high-dose cisplatin.[284] The response rates for the three arms were 12%, 14%, and 27%, respectively, and median survival times were not statistically different at 5 to 7 months.[295] This study discounted the possibility that increasing the cisplatin dose beyond 100 mg/m^2 results in significantly higher activity. Currently, most clinical trials use doses of 75 or 80 mg/m^2 every 3 weeks.

The Eastern Cooperative Oncology Group (ECOG) conducted several comparative studies attempting to identify the most active combination in treating NSCLC. In one such study, a first-generation regimen (CAMP) was compared with three cisplatin-containing regimens, including the combination of mitomycin C, vinblastine, and cisplatin (platinum), or MVP.[296] Although the MVP regimen produced the highest numeric response rate at 31%, the median survival time ranged from 4.5 months (for MVP) to 6.5 months and was not significantly different among the four regimens. In another five-arm study, single-agent carboplatin or iproplatin followed by MVP chemotherapy at the time of first progression was compared with first-line MVP and two other cisplatin-based regimens.[297] Patients treated with initial carboplatin had the longest median survival time; first-line MVP again resulted in the highest response rate but in a lower median survival time (23 weeks, versus 32 weeks for initial carboplatin). Carboplatin and cisplatin are now considered to be of equal activity in NSCLC, with single-agent response rates of approximately 10% and a different spectrum of clinical toxicities.

New Drugs

During the decade of the 1990s, several new drugs with single activity in NSCLC were identified. These include the taxanes, paclitaxel, and docetaxel; the antimetabolite gemcitabine; the topoisomerase I inhibitor irinotecan; and the vinca alkaloid vinorelbine.[261–265] The introduction of these agents into clinical practice generated much enthusiasm, since they are usually tolerated better than cisplatin, have reproducible single-agent activity of 15% to 25% and, in some cases, have novel intracellular targets. Current standard regimens for stage IV disease and most clinical trials in earlier-stage disease involving chemotherapy are focused on combinations including these drugs and are discussed further in the stage-specific segments.

BIOLOGIC THERAPY

Investigators have evaluated both nonspecific and specific means to stimulate the immune system of patients with NSCLC.[298] Despite this effort and the proven ability to modulate immunologic end points, no immunologic agent or approach has been shown to induce regressions or improve survival in epithelial lung cancer patients. As with all other forms of systemic therapy for this illness, immunotherapy remains an investigational approach. Patients should be treated only as part of formal protocols. In addition, because cytotoxic chemotherapy given as initial treatment for metastatic NSCLC can reliably induce regressions and prolong survival, inclusion of chemotherapeutic drugs in the overall treatment plan should be discussed.

Several trials have tested nonspecific agents to enhance immune response. After observations that patients who survive an empyema after lung cancer surgery appear to have prolonged survival,[299] McKneally et al.[300] tested the usefulness of intrapleural bacille Calmette-Guérin (BCG) in stage I NSCLC and found fewer recurrences and deaths in treated patients than in comparable controls. Confirmatory prospective randomized trials have failed to confirm this result and, in fact, demonstrated a decrease in disease-free interval for patients given BCG.[301] Levamisole has also been tested as a nonspecific immunopotentiator in epithelial lung cancer patients, with no evidence of benefit.[302,303]

The combination of BCG and levamisole as adjuvant therapy has been compared to cyclophosphamide, doxorubicin, and cisplatin (CAP) chemotherapy in patients with completely resected stage II and III adenocarcinoma and large cell carcinoma.[304] This trial showed an improvement in both disease-free survival and overall survival among patients randomly assigned to receive CAP chemotherapy. The accumulated data demonstrate that no nonspecific immunostimulating agent tested has been shown to improve symptoms, response, or survival in NSCLC.

Interferons have been tested alone and in combination in patients with epithelial lung cancer. Trials of human leukocyte interferon[305] and recombinant interferon-α[306] or interferon-β[307] have not shown sufficient activity to warrant either use or further study for this indication. The combination of interferon-α and -β given with cisplatin plus etoposide has been compared with the same chemotherapy given alone.[308] No improvement in response or survival and enhanced hematologic toxicity were observed in the combination chemotherapy plus interferon arm of this study. Preclinical data, however, demonstrated additive effects or synergy when interferon was combined with cytotoxic agents, such as fluorouracil or cisplatin, in several tumor types.[309] A therapeutic clinical benefit has not been established.[310–312] At present, there is no evidence that interferon-α, -β, or -γ, given alone or in combination with chemotherapy, can influence the natural history of NSCLC. The use of interferon for this indication remains investigational.

Phase I and phase II trials of interleukins have failed to reveal any significant effect.[313] Current investigations are focused on a possible role for monoclonal antibodies to the EGFR (e.g., IMclone C225) or the Her2/neu antibody herceptin.

SPECIFICS OF LUNG CANCER MANAGEMENT

LOCALIZED "RESECTABLE" (STAGES I, II, AND IIIA) DISEASE

When disease is localized to the lung or includes only regional draining lymphatic channels, treatment of the primary disease and these regional lymphatics employs a surgical or radiotherapeutic approach. However, despite lack of evidence of distant metastatic disease at initial staging, patients fail most frequently after treatment because of distant recurrences that indicate that despite primary control, micrometastatic disease was probably present at the time of initial treatment. For this reason, even with disease that can be completely resected, combined-modality treatments are being investigated with fervor to eliminate these presumed micrometastatic foci at the time of initial therapy.

Primary Surgery

Stage I and II lung cancer denotes disease limited to the hemithorax, with tumor extension no farther than the adjacent resectable structures peripherally (T3) or hilar nodes proximally (N1). In these cases, whenever possible, surgical excision is the treatment of choice.

In most instances, lobectomy is the resection procedure required. When the primary tumor or lymph node involvement extends to the proximal bronchus or proximal pulmonary artery (T3) or cross the major fissure such that a complete resection is only possible by pneumonectomy, this more extensive procedure should be performed. When resectable adjacent structures are involved, an *en bloc* resection of the involved area together with the pulmonary resection is necessary.

The role of mediastinal lymphadenectomy as part of the surgical procedure when hilar or mediastinal nodes are uninvolved is debated. The proponents of complete ipsilateral or bilateral mediastinal lymphadenectomy argue that complete removal of mediastinal lymph nodes improves survival. Certainly, this dissection provides the best possible surgical staging by removing all draining lymph nodes, which can then be analyzed pathologically for metastatic involvement. At minimum, for accurate final surgical and pathologic staging, lymph node sampling of all draining areas should be performed at the time of surgical resection,[314,315] and all lymph nodes involved or suspected to be involved with tumor should be removed. A small randomized trial comparing mediastinal lymphadenectomy to mediastinoscopy plus intraoperative lymph node sampling showed no difference in survival, locoregional recurrence, or accuracy of the two staging procedures as applied to stage I or II lung cancer.[316] A larger phase III trial is under way in North America to address this issue.

In peripheral T1N0 tumors, the role of lesser resection (segmentectomy, wedge excision, or precision cautery dissection) has yet to be fully defined. A randomized trial conducted by the Lung Cancer Study Group (LCSG)[205] showed that after long-term follow-up, the locoregional recurrence rate with limited resection was threefold greater than with lobectomy (15% vs. 5%), and mortality, morbidity, and pulmonary function were equal in both arms. There was a marginally significant long-term survival benefit for lobectomy. For this reason, it is recommended that limited resection be reserved for compromise situations in which the surgeon feels that lobectomy is contraindicated and a complete excision can be performed by a smaller resection (Table 31.2-9). As well, an analysis by the Rush-Presbyterian group also suggests that locoregional recurrence rate after segmentectomy is much higher than that after lobectomy. The value of segmentectomy in preserving lung function in otherwise normal individuals has been questioned. A recent analysis suggests that lobectomy and segmentectomy result in identical pulmonary function 1 year after the surgery.[205,317,318] Except in a few centers, lesser resections (e.g., segmentectomy, wedge excision, precision cautery dissection) have been reserved for situations in which, because of poor cardiopulmonary reserve, it is thought that the patient cannot tolerate a lobectomy. In these situations, this "compromised resection" is certainly indicated, although the risks of locoregional recurrence are higher.

In the LCSG trial, there appeared to be no difference in locoregional recurrence rates whether the tumor measured 1, 2, or 3 cm. However, some surgeons do advocate that for very early tumors (1 cm or less) a lesser resection is justified without the need to perform a lobectomy. However, studies have demonstrated that even in these very early tumors, lymphatic permeation may have occurred within that lobe,[205,317,318] and the patient would have been better served by a formal lobectomy. The exact

TABLE 31.2-9. Results of Limited Pulmonary Resection Performed as an Intentional Procedure, Mainly for T1N0 Tumors

Study	*Patients*	*Estimated 5-Y Survival Rate (%)*	*Operative Mortality Rate (%)*	*Local Recurrence Rate (%)*
Jensik[210]	296	52	1	12
Read et al.[210a]	113	70	4.4	4.4
Wain et al.[210b]	164	<50	5	5
Lung Cancer Study Group[205]	123	70	1	17.5

role of lesser resections in these very small (often CT-detected) tumors (0.5 to 1 cm) has yet to be defined. This will be important in managing CT-screening-identified subcentimeter nodules.

After surgical resection for stage I and II lung cancer, the 5-year survival rate without recurrence exceeds 50% in stage I and 35% in stage II disease. In completely resected T1N0 tumors, 5-year survival rates exceed 70%. Approximately 25% of patients are tumor-free at death, suggesting that surgical resection in T1N0 lung cancer renders 80% of patients tumor-free.

T3N0 Tumors

Tumors that invade the chest wall, the diaphragm, the mediastinal pleura, or the pericardium or are situated within 2 cm of the carina constitute the designation of *T3*. At the Japan National Cancer Center, Naruke et al.[315] reported an overall 5-year survival rate of 26% in 327 patients with this stage of disease. At Memorial Sloan-Kettering Cancer Center (MSKCC), 77 patients with completely resected tumor had a 42% 5-year survival rate, but 48 patients with incomplete resections did not survive beyond 2.5 years. From the literature, it appears that approximately 40% of patients with completely resected T3N0 lesions survive at least 5 years.

CHEST WALL INVASION. Involvement of parietal pleura or chest wall muscle or rib constitutes T3 tumors (Table 31.2-10). The deeper the invasion, the worse is the prognosis. In all instances, it is recommended that the tumor be resected *en bloc* with the involved chest wall, with a minimum of 2 cm of normal chest wall removed in all directions beyond the tumor. When necessary, plastic reconstruction can be used to reconstitute the chest wall. Prognosis is related to the completeness of resection and depth of chest wall invasion, with no patients surviving 5 years after incomplete resection. Whether simple removal of the parietal pleura in tumors only invading this structure is adequate remains a contentious issue. A recent report suggested that with sufficient care and experience, pleurectomy is adequate in selected T3 tumors.[319]

SUPERIOR SULCUS TUMORS. Pancoast described a tumor in the apex of the lung invading the first rib, with associated involvement of the brachial plexus and stellate ganglion, creating Pancoast's syndrome (rib erosion, shoulder pain radiating down the arm, Horner's syndrome). Shaw and Paulson were the first to describe a curative resection in this disease. Since that initial report, most surgeons continue to treat a documented superior sulcus tumor with preoperative radiotherapy of 3000 to 4500 cGy, followed by *en bloc* resection of the involved lung, chest wall and, frequently, the T1 nerve root. Residual disease at the time of resection is treated with PORT or intraoperative brachytherapy,[320] but the results of these R1 or R2 resections are disappointing despite the adjuvant therapy.

The overall survival rate for patients with completely resected tumors is approximately 40% (Table 31.2-11). Adverse prognostic factors include involved mediastinal lymph nodes (stage IIIA) and bony erosion. In a report from MSKCC, lobectomy with *en bloc* chest wall resection proved far superior to smaller resections in treating this disease, and N2 disease severely affected prognosis.[321]

Usual contraindications to surgery for superior sulcus tumors include a T4 tumor (vertebral body invasion, subclavian artery, or vein invasion) or clinically evident N2 disease. On occasion, palliative resection of such lesions may be required for pain relief. More recently, aggressive curative approaches to remove and replace these adjacent structures have been reported, with some long-term survivors.[322]

MEDIASTINAL INVASION. Invasion of the mediastinal pleura, pericardium, or mediastinal fat also constitutes T3 disease. In many instances, *en bloc* resection of the involved mediastinal tissue can accomplish a complete resection. The results of such surgery for this type of invasion are not well-known. At

TABLE 31.2-10. Results after Surgical Treatment for Non–Small Cell Lung Cancer with Chest Wall Invasion (T3)

Study	*Patients*	*Patients with Complete Resection*	*Estimated 5-Y Survival Rate (%)*	*Mortality Rate (%)*
Paone et al.[342a]	32	28	35	3
Patterson et al.[342b]	35	30	38	9
Piehler et al.[342]	93	66	33[a]	15
Van de Wal et al.[342c]	16	NS	12	6
Allen et al.[342d]	52	NS	26	4
Downey et al.[319]	29	175	49[b]	3.8

NS, not stated.
[a]Survival of patients with completely resected tumors (including patients with stage IIIa disease).
[b]Survival of T3N0 patients in whom tumor was completely resected (n = 100).

TABLE 31.2-11. Reported Results after Surgical Treatment for Non–Small Cell Lung Cancer with a Superior Sulcus Lesion (T3)

Study	*Patients*	*Estimated 5-Y Survival Rate (%)*	*Mortality Rate (%)*
Paulson[607]	79	31	3
Anderson et al.[608]	28	34	7
Devine et al.[609]	40	10	8
Rice et al.[610]	36	28	0
Miller[611]	36	31	NS
McKneally[612]	25	51	NS
Ricci et al.[613]	41	34	5
Carrel et al.[614]	37	29	NS
Komaki et al.[615]	25	40	NS
Ginsberg et al.[321]	100	30	NS
Hagan et al.[616]	34	33	0
Darteville et al.[322]	70	34	0
Attar et al.[617]	67	36	NS

NS, not significant.

MSKCC, a review suggested that only approximately 10% of such patients with completely resected disease survive 5 years.[323] From this review of 225 patients with mediastinal invasion, it was apparent that once mediastinal invasion occurs, frequently major structures are involved (T4), or concomitant mediastinal lymph node disease is present (N2 or N3). In such patients, whenever possible, technical resectability should be determined preoperatively. MRI to detect mediastinal invasion value, then CT scanning to detect mediastinal invasion and mediastinoscopy, are indicated before resection of any of these tumors. Of 225 patients analyzed in this series, only 22% had tumors that could be completely resected, 44% had totally unresectable disease and, in 34%, tumors were incompletely resected. In this sole report of the results of mediastinal invasion, brachytherapy was used in incomplete resections, with a surprising 22% survival rate in this small subset of patients. A more recent reanalysis of this group of patients confirmed a 30% to 40% 5-year survival rate in patients with completely resected T3N0 disease.[324]

PROXIMAL AIRWAY INVOLVEMENT. Tumors within 2 cm of the carina can be resected by pneumonectomy but, whenever possible, preservation of distal normal lung is preferred, using sleeve resection of main bronchi (sleeve lobectomy). In the absence of nodal disease, a 50% 5-year survival rate can be expected. Once mediastinal lymph nodes are involved (T3N2), as with other T3 tumors, few if any patients are cured by surgical resection.[325] For tumors in this location, when a complete surgical excision can be obtained with lung-conserving bronchoplastic procedures (vs. pneumonectomy), these should be performed. In retrospective analyses, the cure rate after sleeve lobectomy appears no different than that after pneumonectomy for similar early-stage (N0) disease. The quality of life allowed by such lung-preserving operations suggests that this is the preferable approach whenever possible.

DIAPHRAGMATIC INVASION. Tumors invading the diaphragm frequently spread along the diaphragmatic pleura, and most patients present with a malignant pleural effusion (T4) that usually is unresectable. In the occasional patient, focal diaphragmatic invasion can be completely resected by lobectomy and *en bloc* resection of the diaphragm, replacing this structure with a synthetic mesh or fabric. In a recent analysis of our material at MSKCC, only seven patients were found with diaphragmatic invasion, and in only two was disease localized enough to be resected.[326] There are no reports of results of such surgery in a series large enough to analyze results, but one would anticipate a result similar to that for T3 tumors elsewhere.

Stage IIIA Disease

T3N1 DISEASE. Stage IIIA disease includes T3N1 tumors. As with any other T status, once lymph nodes are involved, the prognosis is much worse, thus categorizing these patients as IIIA rather than IIB. Even with completely resected tumors, of 32 patients with lymphatic metastases in T3 lesions, only 20% survived 5 years, and few if any survive 5 years when mediastinal nodes are involved.[319]

T1–3N2 DISEASE. The existence of N2 disease remains the most controversial area for primary surgical management of lung cancer. Although potentially resectable, once ipsilateral mediastinal or subcarinal lymph nodes (or both) are involved by tumor, the ultimate prognosis is much worse. When disease is diagnosed preoperatively either by noninvasive or invasive staging techniques, fewer than 10% of all patients treated with primary surgery survive 5 years, no matter the adjuvant therapy.

Selectivity is important before considering surgery for patients with preoperatively identified N2 disease. Adverse prognostic factors include multiple levels of N2 disease, multiple lymph nodes at one level involved with tumor, adenocarcinoma, and extranodal spread of disease. More than 75% of patients with N2 disease present with disease extending beyond one lymph node station.

"Minimal" N2 Disease. Single-station lymph node involvement with microscopic foci of disease not clinically apparent on clinical staging constitutes most of the subset of patients with minimal N2 disease. This early-stage disease is usually discovered at the time of thoracotomy or at pretreatment mediastinoscopy. Five-year survival rates after surgical resection are

10% to 20% and are higher when a complete resection is performed (Table 31.2-12). Incomplete (R1, R2) resection results in a noncurative treatment, with few if any patients surviving beyond 3 years. Patients found to have multiple lymph node stations involved at final pathologic staging also fare poorly.

The criteria for resection of minimal N2 disease include no mediastinal involvement seen on CT or PET scan but found to be present at surgery or mediastinoscopy, identifying a single station of lymph nodes involved with only microscopic disease. At the time of surgery, a complete mediastinal lymph node dissection is warranted whenever N2 disease is suspected or known. Proponents of mediastinal lymph node dissection (vs. lymph node sampling) in all patients treated by surgical resection for lung cancer believe that this extended dissection can identify patients with occult N2 disease who might have benefited by complete nodal dissection. One retrospective study[327] suggested a doubling of 5-year survival rates (15.9% vs. 6.7%) when lymph node dissection is carried out in patients with this stage of disease, although this has not been confirmed by other studies.

"Bulky" N2 Disease. Tumors with mediastinal involvement beyond that described as minimal N2 disease constitute the large segment of patients presenting with stage IIIA disease. This more advanced, bulky, or multistation N2 disease usually can be identified preoperatively and is termed *clinical N2 disease.* It is considered by most surgeons to be inoperable by primary surgery, with few 5-year survivors identified after surgical resection.[328–330] Induction therapies before surgery using chemotherapy or chemoradiotherapy have been tested in this group. For most of these patients, primary radiotherapy is still considered the standard treatment for local control.

TABLE 31.2-12. Results after Surgical Treatment for Non–Small Cell Lung Cancer with N2 Disease

Study	*Patients*	*Estimated 5-Y Survival Rate (%)*	*Mortality Rate (%)*
ALL N2			
Kirschner[618]	45	20	0
Sawamura et al.[619]	107	?	25
Mastrorilli et al.[620]	108	?	2
Naruke et al.[315]	426	14	10
Deneffe and Stalpactt[621]	42	9	NS
Levasseur and Regnard[622]	254	18	6
Watanabe et al.[623]	153	17	3
Walker et al.[624]	70	32[a]	10
COMPLETELY RESECTED N2			
Martini and Flehinger[328]	151	30[a]	1
Naruke et al.[315]	242	19	10
Mountain[625]	118	21[b]	NS
Levasseur and Regnard[622]	191	23	6
Watanabe et al.[623]	84	24	3
Miller et al.[626]	14	24[a]	NS
Goldstraw et al.[627]	237	18	5
Riquet et al.[630]	184	20	NS
MEDIASTINOSCOPY + VE N2			
Pearson et al.[628]	79	9	NS
Couglin et al.[629]	28	18	NS

NS, not significant; VE, positive.
[a]Adjusted for noncancer deaths.
[b]Excluded operative deaths.

Combined-Modality Approaches (Including Surgery)

SITES OF FAILURE. Recognition of prognostic and surgical factors that predict for specific anatomic failure patterns can allow selection of patients for local, systemic, or combined therapy. After surgical resection, patients with pathologic stage T1–2N0 tumors who have negative resection margins have survival rates in excess of 50%. For these patients, isolated mediastinal or primary site recurrences are unusual, and there is no rationale for the routine use of PORT. Patients with T1N1 tumors have an isolated local failure rate of 12%. The rate of isolated distant failure for T1N1 patients is 33% and provides a clear need for developing effective prophylactic therapy for systemic and central nervous system spread. For T2N1 disease, the isolated local failure rate is 14%, and the distant failure rate is 36%, again demonstrating the need for effective adjuvant systemic therapy.[331] In view of the fact that isolated N1 metastases are rare in these large surgical series, it is reasonable to consider adjuvant local therapy in patients with documented N1 disease when the mediastinal nodes were neither sampled nor dissected because occult N2 disease may be present.

Survival decreases for patients with N2 disease discovered intraoperatively. When no adjuvant therapy is used for these more advanced patients, thoracic recurrence occurs in approximately 20% of patients even if the resection margins are negative, and distant metastases become even more common, suggesting that both failure patterns need to be addressed if survival is to be improved.[332] Although not proven equally effective, increasingly more conservative resections are being performed for early-stage lung cancers. For sleeve lobectomies, isolated local failure rates are more common than distant failures, ranging from 30% to 52%. Isolated local failure rates are particularly high if the procedure is performed to conserve parenchyma in patients with compromised pulmonary function. This high incidence of isolated local failure provides a basis for the selective use of PORT after sleeve lobectomy. Second primary lung cancers occur frequently in all surviving patients at a rate of approximately 1% each year.[333,334]

ADJUVANT RADIOTHERAPY. *Stage I Disease.* The results for selected patients managed with surgery alone (T1–2N0) are reasonably good, and in general these patients require no further treatment. Randomized trials of PORT including N0 patients have found no benefit with the addition of adjuvant treatment,[335–338] and it is not recommended. In fact, some trials have shown a survival disadvantage in patients receiving PORT, presumably from the toxicity of the radiation. The Medical Research Council recently performed a metaanalysis of nine trials of 2128 patients who underwent complete resection and were randomly assigned to either no treatment or PORT.[339]

Doses of PORT varied from 30 to 60 Gy, and most of the trials used cobalt 60. Patients with stage I disease were included in many of the trials. A significantly increased hazard ratio of mortality in stage I patients receiving PORT was reported.

Stage II and Stage III Disease. The role of adjuvant radiotherapy for stage II (N1) NSCLC is controversial but has been recommended in the past because the incidence of local failure with surgery alone is high. A locoregional intrathoracic failure rate of 31% was observed by the Ludwig Lung Cancer Group for patients with completely resected stage II disease.[340] The Medical Research Council metaanalysis reported a trend toward decreased survival in patients receiving PORT with stage II disease.

The LCSG investigated the efficacy of postoperative mediastinal irradiation in completely resected stage II and III squamous cell carcinoma of the lung. This trial randomly assigned 210 patients to receive 50 Gy in 25 fractions after surgery versus observation alone. The locoregional failure rate (as first site of failure) was reduced from 41% to 3% with radiotherapy for all node-positive patients. Despite this improvement, the increase in locoregional control with radiotherapy did not translate into a survival benefit for stage II patients because more than two-thirds of first failures were distant.[332] The LCSG failed to separate patients with N1 and N2 disease but rather combined and analyzed them as a single group.[332] A trend toward improved survival was observed in N2 patients receiving radiotherapy.

The Medical Research Council of the United Kingdom also completed a randomized adjuvant trial in which 308 patients with stage II and III disease were treated with either 40 Gy or no further therapy, although a trend toward improved survival was seen in the T2N2 subgroup. Again, no overall survival benefit was observed.[341] The metaanalysis performed by the Medical Research Council confirmed these results. The Council reported higher local recurrences in 276 patients in the surgery-only arms of the trials. There were fewer local recurrences in patients receiving PORT. In addition, there was a trend toward improved survival in stage III and N2 patients in this arm, although it did not reach significance.[339] PORT has also been advocated for resected NSCLC invading pleura or chest wall without nodal metastases (T3N0). This issue has never been properly examined in prospective fashion, although the LCSG attempted to address this question in a study that was closed owing to poor patient accrual.[323,342] The survival rate approaches 50% for patients with chest wall tumors undergoing *en bloc* complete resection (R0), and there would appear to be little gained with additional local treatment.[343] Therefore, the role of PORT remains controversial. It has not been shown to produce a benefit in early-stage disease. It has been shown to improve local control in patients with mediastinal nodal disease but has no proven survival benefit. There is likely a subgroup of patients, such as those with micrometastatic disease, who will have an improved survival from PORT; however, this patient population has yet to be identified.

Positive Margins (R1, R2 Resections). The presence of microscopic disease after curative surgery for early-stage disease at the bronchial resection margin, chest wall, or vascular margin may adversely affect the prognosis of patients. Yet, despite data that suggest that adjuvant radiotherapy reduces local recurrence, the retrospective literature regarding the efficacy of radiotherapy to improve local control is conflicting.[344–346]

BRACHYTHERAPY. Intraoperative brachytherapy was used as an adjuvant treatment in 23 patients undergoing video-assisted thoracoscopic limited resections (wedge resections) who were unable to tolerate conventional resections. ^{125}I seeds implanted into a Vicryl mesh were placed thoracoscopically over the tumor bed and resection staple line. A dose of 100 to 120 Gy was delivered. As yet, there have been no local failures in this treatment group.[347]

ADJUVANT CHEMOTHERAPY WITH OR WITHOUT RADIOTHERAPY. Given the large number of patients with resectable disease, few randomized studies of adjuvant chemotherapy in NSCLC have been published. Most of these studies used chemotherapy regimens with limited activity.[348,349]

The LCSG published two large randomized trials using the CAP regimen. The first trial included patients with completely resected stage II or III adenocarcinoma or large cell carcinoma.[304] Patients were randomly assigned to receive either CAP chemotherapy or immunotherapy with intrapleural BCG and levamisole administered for 18 months. In 141 randomly assigned patients, there was a trend for increased time to recurrence and for prolonged overall survival favoring chemotherapy. The survival of the control immunotherapy group was similar to that of earlier patients treated with surgery alone, and the authors attributed the improved survival in the chemotherapy arm to the effects of chemotherapy.

Another study involved patients with incompletely resected disease who were randomly assigned to PORT alone or radiotherapy and six cycles of CAP.[350] Incomplete resection was defined as postoperative residual microscopic or macroscopic disease or disease in the highest resected paratracheal lymph node. One hundred sixty-four patients were analyzed. The chemotherapy group had a significantly longer time to progression ($P = .066$); median survival was only marginally improved with chemotherapy, and there was no 5-year survival benefit.

Studies in patients with less advanced disease have also been published. The LCSG compared four cycles of CAP to no further therapy in 269 patients with stage I disease. No benefit was identified for chemotherapy, but only 53% of assigned patients completed chemotherapy. A study testing a lower-dose, six-cycle CAP regimen in T1–3N0 disease showed a benefit in time to recurrence and survival; however, an imbalance in the randomization process resulted in the assignment of more patients with advanced disease to the observation arm.[351] A metaanalysis of all trials of adjuvant chemotherapy failed to demonstrate a decided advantage (<5%) to this approach.[352]

Since the CAP regimens are no longer considered the most active available regimens in NSCLC, the question of adjuvant chemotherapy in NSCLC remains open. A large intergroup study in the United States is testing the value of four cycles of cisplatin plus etoposide (the first two cycles given with concomitant radiotherapy) versus radiotherapy alone in patients with completely resected N1 or N2 disease. Additional international studies are in progress.

It is possible that recurrence rates in early-stage disease are too low to be effectively influenced by adjuvant chemotherapy. An alternative concept of influencing survival rates in these patients is focused on a reduction in the incidence of second primary malignancies. A large North American intergroup study randomly assigning patients with stage I disease to postoperative placebo versus *cis*-retinoic acid chemopreventive therapy has been completed, but the results have yet to be reported. An interesting Japanese study using 1 to 2 years of oral Tegafur in early-stage lung cancer has demonstrated a survival benefit and reduction of second primary tumors in the treated group.[353]

After complete resection of stage I or II lung cancer or microscopic N2 disease, the current standard must be considered surgery alone without adjuvant treatments. Because of the minimal effect of chemotherapy as assessed in the foregoing recent metaanalysis, larger trials of adjuvant chemotherapy are being carried out in North America and Europe. Patients with completely resected disease should be offered inclusion in these randomized trials whenever possible.

INDUCTION RADIOTHERAPY. After the initial studies were published on the use of preoperative irradiation as a component of treatment of NSCLC, many attempts with this induction approach were initiated in the hope of improving both local control and survival of patients with marginally resectable disease.[354–356] Preliminary acceptance of preoperative irradiation was based on observations of improved resectability as well as on a significant number of complete responses in a surgical specimen after the use of preoperative irradiation. Reports of survival in patients with tumors arising in the superior sulcus after combined preoperative radiotherapy (where no previous survivals occurred) also contributed to the initial enthusiasm of a preoperative radiotherapy-alone approach. Subsequently, a few randomized trials were initiated to answer this question with larger cohorts of patients. The first such major randomized trial was performed by the U.S. Veterans Administration. With a minimum follow-up of 4 years in surviving patients, no increase in survival was noted in the pretreatment group. The overall survival rate was 12.5% in the pretreatment arm, as compared with 21% in the surgery-alone arm, although this was not statistically significant.[356] In 1975, the National Cancer Institute published two separate but integrated multiinstitutional randomized trials addressing the use of preoperative radiotherapy followed by surgery in both operable and inoperable NSCLC without evidence of preoperative radiotherapy advantage.[357]

It is clear from both the nonrandomized and randomized data that preoperative irradiation alone does not improve long-term survival and has no role as a single-induction modality in the management of marginally resectable or unresectable stage IIIA or IIIB disease. The use of radiotherapy as a single preoperative modality is no longer studied consistently, owing to the advent of effective chemotherapeutic agents. Most current trials investigate the use of preoperative concomitant chemoradiotherapy.

Induction Chemotherapy. Phase II studies using a variety of chemotherapeutic regimens have suggested that preoperative chemotherapy could be administered and may be beneficial in locally advanced (N2) disease.[358,359] Martini et al.[360,361] had demonstrated that otherwise resectable patients with ipsilateral mediastinal lymphadenopathy as their sole site of distant spread can have 3-year survival rates of 43% and 5-year survival rates of 24% if both the primary tumor and ipsilateral mediastinal nodes are completely resected and followed by mediastinal irradiation. However, the same studies revealed that patients with ipsilateral mediastinal lymphadenopathy large enough to be clinically apparent on a plain chest radiograph had only an 18% resectability rate and only an 8% 3-year survival rate. A program was developed that used preoperative combination chemotherapy with high-dose cisplatin (120 mg/m^2), vinca alkaloids, and mitomycin (i.e., MVP) in stage IIIA patients with clinically apparent ipsilateral mediastinal spread.[362] In a group of 73 patients, the objective major response rate to MVP chemotherapy was 77%, with a 10% complete response rate. Overall, 60% of patients underwent complete resections, and 12% had pathologic complete responses at surgery. The median survival was 19 months for all patients and 27 months for those with complete resections. The 3-year survival rate for the completely resected patients was 44%, a significant improvement over the prior surgery-only experience, in which the 3-year survival rate for clinically evident N2 disease was only 8% (P = .001).[361] Two treatment-related deaths occurred. Using the same MVP chemotherapy program before surgery, Burkes et al.[363] reported a 69% chemotherapy response rate, a 49% complete resection rate, and a median survival of 19 months for all 35 patients studied. Three randomized trials have compared surgery alone to the combined-modality program of induction chemotherapy before surgery. Despite small numbers of patients in each arm, all reported significant differences in both 2-year survival and distant recurrence rates, favoring the induction chemotherapy arm. These survival advantages have been confirmed in 5-year survival update reports.[276,277,364] Larger trials have yet be reported, but a recent abstract of a very large phase III clinical trial of all resectable stages except T1N0 has failed to confirm this survival advantage in the N2 disease subset.[365] More recent phase II trials of chemotherapy have been reported in T4 disease and earlier stage tumors.[366] Because of these successful outcomes in most phase III trials of induction chemotherapy in stage III disease, this approach is now being investigated in earlier-stage disease. At least three phase III trials in North America and Europe have been instituted, involving patients with clinically evident stage I and II disease, excluding T1N0 tumors.

Induction Chemotherapy with Concomitant Radiotherapy. Cisplatin-based combination chemotherapy has been combined with concomitant radiotherapy in an effort to improve results. In the 1950s, Faber et al.[367] conducted two consecutive trials in clinical N2 NSCLC patients. The first combined 5-fluorouracil, cisplatin, and 40 Gy of chest radiotherapy; the second added etoposide to the regimen. The complete resection rate was 68% in the first trial and 76% in the second program. Median survivals were 21 months and 34 months, respectively. The difference in survival was not significant. Four treatment-related deaths occurred in the two trials. The LCSG combined 5-fluorouracil, cisplatin, and 30 Gy of chest radiotherapy.[368] Overall, 42% of patients underwent a complete surgical resection, and a median survival of 11 months was observed. These results were similar to an earlier trial by the LCSG employing the CAP regimen with 30 Gy of chest irradiation; a 33% resection rate and 11-month median survival were seen in stage III patients.[369] The Cancer and Leukemia Group B (CALGB) tested the combination of 5-fluorouracil, vinblastine, and cisplatin plus 30 Gy of irradiation in 32 stage IIIA patients.[370] The complete resection rate was 62%, and three treatment-related deaths occurred. The SWOG employed 45 Gy with etoposide and cisplatin and documented a 65% complete resection rate.[371]

More recently, a significant effort has been put forth in phase I and II trials to optimize the locoregional therapy in a select group of patients with marginally resectable stage IIIA and IIIB disease. The goals of induction therapy are to convert marginally or unresectable disease, improve locoregional control, and eliminate distant micrometastases.

Sequential Chemotherapy and Radiotherapy. Two phase II trials reported results with induction chemotherapy followed by preoperative radiotherapy and surgery for stage III NSCLC. Skarin et al.[372] treated 41 patients with pathologically determined marginally resectable stage IIIA NSCLC. Included within this group were patients with T3N0 disease and patients with N2 mediastinal metastases. Forty-one patients received two cycles of CAP chemotherapy followed by 30 Gy of irradiation. A complete resection was accomplished in 36 of 41 patients (88%). The median survival was 32 months, and the 3-year survival rate was 30%. Systemic treatment failed in 18 of 36 patients (50%), and local treatment failed in 4 patients. Using a sequential chemotherapy regimen of vinblastine and cisplatin, Sherman et al.[373] treated 21 patients with this neoadjuvant regimen followed by 30 Gy of irradiation to the mediastinum. The observed radiographic response rate, resection rate, and median survival were similar to those reported by Skarin et al.[372]

Concurrent Chemotherapy and Radiotherapy. Several phase II trials have tested the feasibility of combining a variety of induction chemotherapy regimens concurrently with radiotherapy before surgery to maximize induction results through a trimodal strategy. To determine whether surgical resection is a necessary component of a combined-modality approach in the treatment of stage IIIA and select stage IIIB NSCLC, using the SWOG VP-16-platinum regimen, a North American intergroup effort is completing a phase III trial (chemoradiotherapy vs. chemoradiotherapy plus surgery).

It is a challenge to define an optimal regimen from this large group of phase II trials because of the heterogeneity of both the patients entered and the treatments delivered.[374] Different chemotherapeutic regimens were used, with either low-dose cisplatin alone or other agents in a multidrug regimen. Significant variability among the different trials can be seen in the sequencing of the chemotherapy in relation to the radiation, radiation dose, dose per fraction, continuous-course versus split-course strategy, timing of surgery, inclusion by some studies of T3N0 versus clinical N2 disease, inclusion of stage IIIB disease, staging methods, performance criteria, and the toxicity of individual regimens. Although a number of phase II trials report promising results, wide variation also exists in terms of initial response rates (range, 50% to 90%); complete resection rates (range, 28% to 88%); pathologic complete response rates (range, 9% to 21%); median survival rates (range, 13 to 32 months); and 2-year survival rates (range, 20% to 40%).

Recent trials have attempted novel fractionation schemes (especially hyperfractionation) combined with concurrent chemotherapy using a variety of drugs and dosage schemes further to enhance the response rates and optimize resection rates and local control.[375–377] Overall, these trials appear to suggest that a bimodality or trimodality approach combining neoadjuvant chemotherapy with or without radiation and followed by surgery provides a potentially superior method of enhancing resectability and improving locoregional control and survival over radiotherapy alone followed by surgery. Some series also demonstrated a doubling of both local control and survival rates over those reported with primary radiotherapy with or without chemotherapy. The use of altered fractionation also appears to provide greater response rates and local control rates than standard fraction irradiation combined with chemotherapy with acceptable toxicity.

The role of induction therapies followed by surgery in resectable lung cancer remains to be defined. In N2 disease, it does appear to improve long-term survival, although the role of surgery vis-à-vis radiotherapy as the primary control mechanism will be defined only as a result of the aforementioned current phase III trial in North America. Whether induction therapies will have an impact on earlier-stage (non-T1N0) disease has yet to be defined but, once again, it is hoped that current phase III trials will resolve this question.

Primary Radiotherapy

EXTERNAL-BEAM RADIOTHERAPY. *Selection Criteria.* The selection of patients for definitive management with radiotherapy depends on several factors, the most important of which are extent of disease, performance status, and pulmonary function. Accurate staging is required to establish and exclude patients with distant metastasis from undergoing radical treatment. In addition to distant metastases, malignant pleural and pericardial effusions are an absolute contraindication for definitive radiotherapy. In some circumstances, however, a small pleural effusion not seen on chest radiography is discovered on staging CT scanning, rendering the decision to proceed with definitive management less clear. Patients with this finding, in the setting of no other significant clinical, laboratory, or radiographic findings that suggest distant spread, should be considered for curative treatment.[378]

No specific criteria exist to define the extent of tumor bulk as unsuitable for treatment with curative intent using conventional treatment planning. In general, however, intrathoracic tumors 8 cm or larger are considered relatively prohibitive for high-dose treatment (55 to 70 Gy) due to excessive pulmonary toxicity. Patients with such large tumors without evidence of extrathoracic spread should be considered for induction chemotherapy to attempt tumor shrinkage and reduction in the volume of lung that would otherwise be targeted. Large tumors or bulky nodal disease may potentially receive high-dose radiotherapy with 3D-CRT. This approach has the potential to maximize delivery of the prescribed high dose to the target volume and minimize the dose to surrounding normal tissues. Clinical research is addressing this issue in ongoing phase I dose escalation trials.[216–218]

Most patients considered for primary radiotherapy have preexisting compromised lung function from underlying emphysema or chronic obstructive pulmonary disease secondary to a long history of smoking. It remains a difficult challenge for the radiation oncologist to predict accurately which patients will retain the minimum adequate posttreatment functional lung volume to provide basic pulmonary function for normal activity.[379] Physiologic changes in pulmonary function after radiotherapy depend on several factors, including preexisting pulmonary function reserve before radiotherapy, the anatomic region of lung treated, total dose, dose per fraction, prior chemotherapy or the desire to incorporate chemotherapy concurrent with radiotherapy, and the presence of more than a 10% shift of the ventilation or perfusion to the contralateral lung from tumor or nodal disease causing central bronchial or major pulmonary vessel obstruction.[380] Some investigators have found that the decrease in pulmonary function as determined by pulmonary function tests and single-photon emission CT imaging studies correlates with the amount of lung receiving 30 Gy.[381]

For patients with clinical stage I and II NSCLC that otherwise is technically resectable but in whom surgery is prohibitive secondary to severe medical contraindications, as well as for patients who refuse surgery or have clinical but minimal N2 disease, primary radiotherapy alone offers a reasonable alternative approach and potential for locoregional control and cure.[382–398] Although surgery has resulted in the highest reported survival rates in stage I and II disease, no modern randomized studies have compared surgery to radiation in a comparable group of patients. The observed differences in results between surgery and radiation are due in part to selection bias because, in many instances, patients referred for radiation have worse performance status, are less rigorously staged, and have poor pulmonary function combined with comorbid illnesses.[393] In addition, most surgical series report results after pathologic staging. Surgical series reveal that approximately 25% to 50% of clinical stage I patients are upstaged (see Fig. 31.2-8). The rate of occult N1 or N2 disease is as high as 56% if the patient has a positive preoperative bronchoscopy.[399] Therefore, it is important to evaluate cause-specific survival as an end point in these studies, since many patients die of intercurrent disease. In addition, many historical series reporting results with radiation alone used inferior equipment and treatment planning by today's standards and delivered inadequate doses.

More modern series have examined the issues of dose and dose escalation in relation to tumor size, local control, and survival for stage I and II disease. The evidence suggests that radical radiotherapy is an effective treatment primarily for tumors smaller than 3 cm (T1) when treated to doses of 65 Gy or higher. This treatment has a greater probability of complete response rates, local control, and disease-free survival almost comparable to some surgical series.[383] Complete response and local control of larger tumors, however, appear less likely with standard radiation fraction schedules and doses, despite availability of modern equipment and CT-based planning.

The need electively to treat the mediastinum in patients with no evidence of nodal spread has been challenged. The inclusion of large volumes of lung within a radiation port, especially for peripheral T1 and T2 tumors, to prevent regional failure must be balanced against the potential for increased toxicity. The rationale for treating the local tumor volume alone appears justified when the patient's outcome is not subjected to negative impact if the regional lymph nodes are not included. The evidence appears to support the use of smaller target volumes to deliver higher doses without compromise of the regional outcome.[388] The regional failure rate is typically less than 10% in reported series where elective nodal areas were not treated.[388,394,400] In one series,[396] most patients did receive elective nodal irradiation but still had a failure rate approaching 10%, which suggests that a typical elective dose of 40 Gy is not enough to control occult disease. Selection for this approach would be improved by pretreatment invasive mediastinal staging.

The issue of split-course versus continuous-course radiation has also been examined for stage I and II NSCLC with mixed results and has generally been discouraged when treating with curative intent.[385,388] Split-course radiotherapy is a reasonable alternative for elderly patients or patients living at great distances in whom a protracted course of treatment is impractical. It is also potentially more cost-effective.

Results. One of the earliest studies demonstrating the curability of medically inoperable lung cancer with radiation alone was reported by Hilton and Smart in the early 1940s and 1950s. Thirty-eight patients with stage I or II NSCLC were treated with curative intent. Doses of 50 to 55 Gy were prescribed for squamous cell histology, delivered to the primary site only, and doses of 40 to 45 Gy were prescribed for undifferentiated cancers, delivered to the primary site and mediastinum. Despite inadequate doses, frequent treatment breaks to allow recovery for acute reactions, orthovoltage equipment, unsatisfactory staging, and a mix of histologies, the 2-year and 5-year survival rates were 47% and 17%, respectively.[386,390]

In 1963, Morrison et al.[401] reported the results of the only randomized trial comparing surgery with radiation for stage I and II NSCLC. Although the outcome for surgery was superior to that for radiotherapy alone, the trial was severely flawed. This study of patients randomly assigned to radiation alone suffered from small patient numbers, the patients received low radiation doses in the range of 45 Gy, and the study included small cell histology (approximately 30%). Additionally, almost 30% of patients undergoing surgery received adjuvant PORT.[401]

Historical series reporting results with primary radiotherapy alone are often the victims of selection bias. Many of the same medical contraindications that prohibit surgery, such as age, performance status, severe intercurrent medical illness, and poor pulmonary function, are known to be significant prognostic factors for survival.[402,403] Patients referred for radiotherapy are more likely be elderly and to be at greater risk for death from intercurrent diseases. Patients receiving radiotherapy alone generally have also undergone less extensive staging (clinical versus pathologic) than those in surgical series reporting pathologic versus clinical outcome. Some patients discovered on mediastinoscopy to harbor N2 disease may be excluded or separated from outcome analyses in surgical series.[402] Sandler et al.[393] demonstrated the importance of rigorous clinical staging in selecting true stage I NSCLC for primary radiotherapy. In their series of 77 patients with clinical stage I NSCLC treated with primary radiotherapy, treatment in only 2 of 12 patients who underwent "excellent" staging evaluation failed locoregionally at 3 years, in contrast to that in 22 of 24 (87%) and in 30 of 41 (79%) with locoregional failure for "good" or "other" staging, respectively. With the advent of noninvasive assessment of nodal regions through CT and PET, some of this discrepancy might diminish.[402,403]

Tumor size is a prognostic factor in almost every retrospective series reported. For example, Krol et al.[388] found that tumors smaller than 4 cm had a 35% overall survival at 3 years and tumors larger than 4 cm had a 13% 3-year survival. There has also been some evidence that higher doses (>65 Gy) lead to improved survival.[383,394] Jeremic et al.[400] and Morita et al.[397] have reported treating patients with some of the highest doses seen in the literature, 69.6 Gy and 65 Gy, respectively, and report favorable overall survival. These two factors, tumor size and dose, are interrelated, since a very large tumor, technically T2, is often difficult to treat to high doses secondary to pulmonary toxicity. Squamous cell histology has been shown to be a positive prognostic factor, as has younger age.[393,396] The results from many modern series appear in Table 31.2-13. Therefore, patients with smaller tumors treated to higher doses appear to be the best candidates for primary radiotherapy. Treatment of elective nodal regions prophylactically is probably not needed. The best radiotherapy results are still inferior to most surgical series, although there are many confounding factors to account for a portion of this difference. It is hoped that with improved staging and dose delivery, the results with primary radiotherapy will improve.

PRIMARY BRACHYTHERAPY. Hilaris and Martini[404,405] described the use of brachytherapy at MSKCC for medically inoperable NSCLC in the setting of a tumor that was determined to be unresectable intraoperatively. Permanent or temporary implantation was used as a local conformal boost or as primary treatment alone. These authors reported the results of 55 patients with medically unresectable stage I and II NSCLC. Most (44 of 55) patients underwent biopsy only. The remainder underwent subtotal resection. After surgery, 24 patients received additional external-beam irradiation (median dose, 40 Gy). An actuarial 5-year overall survival of 32% was observed, with a local control at 5 years of 65%. Broken down into stages, the local control rates for T1N0, T2N0, and T1–2N0–1 disease were 100%, 70%, and 70%, respectively. The addition of external-beam irradiation for patients with N1 involvement improved the local control (86%), as compared with the local control rate in patients with N1 disease who received no further therapy (57%). These intraoperative situations are less frequent with the advent of better preoperative imaging.

Perol et al.[406] examined the use of high-dose-rate EBB for early-stage NSCLC limited to the endobronchus that was smaller than cm and not visible on CT scan. Nineteen patients were treated with 7 Gy per fraction every week for 3 to 5 weeks. The 2-year overall survival and local control rates were 58% and 75%, respectively.

Tredaniel et al.[407] reported the results of 29 patients with endoluminal localized tumor treated definitively with ^{192}Ir after loading sources prescribed to a depth of 1 cm from the source center. Complete macroscopic regression was seen in 21 of 25 evaluable patients, with histologically complete responses in 18 of 25. At 23-month follow-up, the median survival had not been reached.

"UNRESECTABLE" STAGE IIIA AND IIIB NON–SMALL CELL LUNG CANCER

Whether stage IIIA or IIIB disease is considered unresectable depends, to a large degree, on the experience and attitudes of physicians treating the patient. What one surgeon considers unresectable, another with an aggressive surgical attitude may deem completely resectable. Despite this, when stage IIIA disease is extremely bulky and enlarged lymph nodes surround vital structures in the mediastinum, it is unlikely that any primary surgical approach will allow a complete resection or significant cure. In centers with more aggressive attitudes, these "unresectable" tumors have become eligible for combined-modality programs that include surgery. Despite this, the standard treatment for locoregional unresectable disease does not include surgery.

Patients with unresectable stage IIIA or IIIB NSCLC have traditionally been treated with radiotherapy alone. Since all known macroscopic disease is confined to the chest, therapy is in theory given with curative intent. However, only 5% to 10% of patients survived beyond 5 years. This was frequently owing to distant disease progression (outside the radiation field), which occurs in up to 70% of patients and reflects the presence of systemic micrometastases at the time of initial therapy.[408] Disease in a large proportion of patients also progresses within the irradiated volume, reflecting the inability of radiotherapy to eliminate all macroscopic disease. Efforts to increase cure rates have, therefore, attempted to increase both locoregional and systemic control. In practice, induction chemotherapy or concomitant chemoradiotherapy (or both) has been most frequently studied to achieve these goals.

TABLE 31.2-13. Results for Patients Treated with Radiation Therapy Alone for Early-Stage Non–Small Cell Lung Cancer

Study	No. of Patients	Dose (Gy)	Overall Survival, 3-Y (%)	Overall Survival, 5-Y (%)	Cause-Specific Survival, 3-Y (%)	Cause-Specific Survival, 5-Y (%)	Local Control, 5-Y (%)
Dosoretz[383]	152	60–69	40[a]	10	—	—	—
Jeremic[400]	49	69.6[b]	46	30	—	—	55
Krol[388]	108	60–65	31	15	42	31	~25
Kaskowitz[396]	53	63	19	6	33	13	0
Morita[397]	149	65	34	22	—	—	—
Slotman[450]	31	48 (4-Gy fractions)	42	8	76	—	—
Graham[395]	103	60	35[b]	14	—	—	—
Sandler[393]	77	60	17	—	22	—	44
Sibley[394]	141	55–70	24	13	—	—	—
Zhang[392]	44	55–70	55[c]	32[c]	—	—	—

[a]2-year.
[b]Hyperfractionated.
[c]Crude survival.

Aggressive Surgery

When stage IIIA (N2) disease is bulky, involving mediastinal lymph node stations or extracapsular disease, and is proven by an invasive staging technique, such as mediastinoscopy, the role of the primary surgery has been proven to be of little value with regard to an intent to cure. It is these patients in whom the role of induction therapies combined with surgery or radiotherapy has been intensively investigated. In all these patients, imaging studies must be correlated with invasive staging. Whether PET scanning can replace mediastinoscopy as positive proof of involvement of mediastinal lymph nodes has yet to be defined. At present, even with a positive PET scan, invasive staging is mandatory: Too many inflammatory processes (e.g., sarcoid reactions with concurrent tumors) can produce "positive" PET scan results. All too frequently, disease in some patients is deemed unresectable by imaging studies alone and not considered for a surgical approach because of this. It has been well recognized that imaging studies are in error at least 30% of the time and that confirmation of N2, N3, or T4 disease by invasive staging is mandatory unless there is incontrovertible evidence present.

Stage IIIB disease encompasses patients with a T4 or an N3 lesion, both of which are usually considered unresectable disease. Radiotherapy, chemotherapy, or a combination of both remains the standard treatment for these patients. In general, they are not referred for surgical treatment. Nevertheless, in a large retrospective study, patients with surgically resected stage IIIB disease had an overall 5-year survival rate of 6%.[409] There is a danger of clinically overstaging a tumor as T4 and denying a patient with completely resectable T1–3 disease the opportunity of a curative resection. T4 disease in highly selected patients can be completely resected, and long-term survival can be achieved in some of these patients. In this group of patients as well, combined-modality therapy (including surgery) is being investigated[410,411] (discussed in Induction Chemoradiotherapy).

T4 TUMORS. T4 tumors include those invading mediastinal structures (the carina and trachea, the heart and great vessels, the esophagus or vertebral body) as well as the presence of a malignant pleural effusion. Naruke et al.[409] reported a 5-year survival of 8% in 104 selected patients after resection of such a T4 lesion.

Carinal Invasion. Although primary lung cancer invading the carina is generally considered unresectable, pneumonectomy with tracheal sleeve resection and direct reanastomosis of the trachea to the contralateral main stem bronchus can be accomplished, with reported 5-year survival rates approaching 20%. In most series reported, patients were highly selected, with most long-term survivors having T4N0 tumors.

Anastomotic dehiscence with bronchial fistula formation and postoperative pulmonary insufficiency are major postoperative problems and are the main cause of the high operative mortality rate, which ranges from 11% to 27%. Only highly selected patients without N2 disease should be offered such a resection. For this reason, prior to resection of such a tumor, mediastinoscopy should be considered mandatory. In some patients, "extended" sleeve lobectomies (resecting the carina) can be used to preserve pulmonary function.

Invasion of Superior Vena Cava. Involvement of the superior vena cava has been treated occasionally by *en bloc* resection and graft replacement. Long-term survivors reported in the literature are limited to case reports.[412,413] In a retrospective analysis of 18 patients with superior vena cava invasion at MSKCC, there were no 5-year survivors after resection.[323] Preoperative distinction of superior vena cava invasion by the tumor (T4) or by its involved mediastinal lymph nodes (N2) can be difficult. Reported series include only few cases, and the significance of this finding cannot be assessed. It appears likely, however, that only T4 and not N2 lesions can occasionally be cured with such a radical resection.

Invasion of Myocardium, Aorta, Esophagus, and Vertebral Body. Surgical resection resulting in complete excision of a primary tumor with other mediastinal organ invasion is usually not possible. Palliative incomplete resections have not demonstrated survival or palliation benefit. In the series from MSKCC, although not all patients underwent resection of the primary tumor or part of the invaded organ, there were no 5-year survivors among 19 patients with aorta involvement and 3 patients with atrial invasion, but 1 patient of 7 (14%) with esophageal invasion lived beyond 5 years.[323] Despite these results, a tumor with limited invasion of the atrial wall can occasionally be completely resected with the hope of an occasional cure.

En bloc resection of the lung with part of the involved aorta, esophagus, or vertebral body, not uncommon in the treatment of superior sulcus tumors, may result in long-term survival for selected patients. PORT may be of benefit in these situations to augment local control. An analysis from Japanese investigators suggested that long-term survival is limited to patients with minimal atrial or aortic adventitial involvement in tumors invading great vessels.[414]

Pleural Effusion. Approximately 5% to 10% of patients with lung cancer present with a nonmalignant pleural effusion, a result of atelectasis, obstructive pneumonitis, lymphatic or venous obstruction, or pulmonary embolus. Despite being nonmalignant, an effusion evident on prior chest radiography has a poor prognosis, with a 5-year survival. Investigators at the Mayo Clinic demonstrated that even cytologically negative pleural effusions evident on chest radiographs were predictive of surgical unresectability in 95% of these patients. However, they concluded that in patients with cytologically negative pleural effusions, unresectability must be documented surgically. On the other hand, Naruke et al.[409] reported a 40% 5-year survival rate in 112 patients with nonmalignant effusion, identical to the 5-year survival rate in 1298 patients without effusion.

Even with malignant pleural effusions, occasional 5-year survivals have been documented when all disease has been eradicated.[409,415] In general, however, malignant pleural effusions, cytologically proven, indicate incurable disease by a surgical approach and are usually treated initially with primary chemotherapy. However, one should never consider a pleural effusion malignant without cytologic or histologic proof. A "bloody" pleural effusion may be due to a traumatic thoracentesis or concomitant pulmonary infarction and not indicate T4 disease.

N3 DISEASE. The role of surgery in preoperatively identified N3 disease previously considered totally inoperable has now been reexamined in phase II trials. Hata et al.[416] have investigated the use of two-field lymphadenectomy, including total mediastinal exenteration and supraclavicular node dissection for this group of patients. The exact role of postoperative therapies combined with this has not been discussed. The results of such treatment still await long-term reporting. Also, the induction therapies, especially chemoradiation, have been investigated by the SWOG group and others.[417,418] It does appear that with very intensive induction therapies, some patients survive long term. It does not appear, however, that these survivals are improved by the addition of surgery. In fact, in many phase II trials, no attempt was made to remove the involved N3 lymph nodes. Surgery was directed toward removal of the primary tumor and N2 nodes.

Adjuvant and Neoadjuvant Therapies

After complete resection in patients proven to have T4 or N3 disease, radiotherapy has been usually recommended as adjuvant treatment because of the high incidence of locoregional failure after aggressive surgery for this advanced tumor. Because of the paucity of patients reported to have undergone this treatment, the exact role of adjuvant radiotherapy cannot be assessed. It is in this subset of tumors that neoadjuvant therapies have been investigated in many phase II trials. It does appear that clinically staged T4 tumors (especially T4N0 disease) do reasonably well after this combined-modality approach.[419–421] In one such study,[420] patients with clinically evident T4 tumors, including superior vena caval syndrome, tracheal involvement, and posterior mediastinal invasion, were treated with MVP chemotherapy followed by surgery. Sixty-three percent of patients underwent a complete resection, and overall survival at 4 years was 19.5%. Despite these encouraging results, in most instances T4 and N3 tumors cannot be resected completely and are usually considered for combined-modality therapy, using radiotherapy as the primary control mechanism.

RADIOTHERAPY. The 2-year survival rate for patients with unresectable locally advanced NSCLC receiving supportive care alone is approximately 4%.[422] Historical series examining the ability of thoracic radiotherapy to have an impact on the natural history of locally advanced NSCLC demonstrated mixed results. Higgins and Shields[423] reported the results of a randomized trial by the Veterans Administration in which male patients with a variety of histologic subtypes of lung cancer, including small cell lung cancer, were prospectively randomly assigned to receive supportive care only or external-beam radiotherapy. Two hundred forty-six patients were treated with placebo, and 308 male patients were treated to doses of 40 to 50 Gy. The results of the trial were reported with 1-year minimum follow-up. Most patients had performance status of less than 70. In addition, the radiotherapy was inadequate by modern standards, both in terms of the dose delivered (40 to 50 Gy) and the equipment used (orthovoltage). Radiotherapy alone provided a modest but significant improvement in survival at 1 year, as compared with that in patients who received supportive care only (22% vs. 16%, respectively).[423] Other earlier trials of thoracic radiotherapy for unresectable NSCLC despite inadequate doses also showed a modest but significant improvement in 2-year survival rates in the range of 9% to 18%.[424,425]

Cox et al.[426] analyzed the patterns of failure in locally advanced unresectable NSCLC treated with radiotherapy alone and found that the median survival was increased from 6 to 12 months when the primary tumor was controlled. However, they found that 75% of patients with squamous cell cancer died of complications secondary to intrathoracic tumor progression, as compared with approximately 40% of patients with either large cell cancer or adenocarcinoma. In contrast, Berry et al.,[427] using similar doses of radiotherapy, could find no improvement in survival with the use of thoracic irradiation as compared with chemotherapy alone. A retrospective study from British Columbia that controlled for tumor stage and other prognostic factors reported improved survival of 79 days in patients receiving high-dose palliative radiotherapy and survival of more than a year in patients receiving radical radiotherapy.[428]

In a multiinstitutional cooperative trial, Johnson et al.[429] reported the results of 319 patients with locally advanced unresectable NSCLC without evidence of distant metastases who were randomly assigned prospectively to one of three arms: chemotherapy alone with vindesine, 3 mg/m^2/week; standard thoracic irradiation to a dose of 60 Gy in 6 weeks; or combined vindesine and thoracic radiotherapy. Although the overall response rate was superior in the radiotherapy arms (radiotherapy alone, 30%; radiotherapy plus vindesine, 34%; vindesine alone, 10%; $P = .001$), the intrathoracic progression rates were similar in the vindesine arm (60%) and in the radiotherapy arm (65%), both median survival and overall survival were also comparable in all three arms. This study has been criticized, however, for the large number of patients in the vindesine-alone arm who received radiotherapy and for the number of patients involved, which was inadequate to detect a difference in survival.[430,431] A randomized trial of low-dose thoracic radiotherapy compared to cisplatin and etoposide alone reported a higher response in the radiotherapy arm but similar overall survival.[432]

Although it seems clear that thoracic radiotherapy does offer a survival advantage to patients with disease limited to the thorax, the poor results of these earlier studies led the RTOG to investigate methods of improving outcome with radiation alone by initially concentrating on dose intensification with conventional fractionation and, more recently, using altered fractionation. In addition, they have attempted to identify appropriate selection criteria and prognostic factors for the various approaches and apply the use of innovative treatment planning and technology.

Standard External-Beam Radiotherapy. The earliest trial by the RTOG for unresectable NSCLC focused on dose intensification by attempting to establish the optimal schedule of standard fractionated radiation alone. Protocol 73-01 was limited to 379 patients with either medically inoperable stage I or II or unresectable stage III NSCLC of various histologies. Patients in this trial were randomly selected for one of four dose-escalating arms, including 40-Gy split-course, or 40-Gy, 50-Gy, or 60-Gy continuous-course thoracic radiation delivered in 4, 5, or 6 weeks with a daily fraction size of 2 Gy. Analysis of patterns of failure and survival showed a higher complete response rate (24%) and 3-year survival rate (15%) with 60-Gy continuous-course radiotherapy, in comparison with lower doses of continuous- and split-course irradiation (40 to 50 Gy). The failure rate within the irradiated volume was 53% to 58% for 40 Gy,

49% for 50 Gy, and 35% for 60 Gy. This improvement in local control was still appreciated nearly 5 years later. The median time to any failure increased from 8 to 19 months as dose was increased from 40 to 60 Gy. Overall, patients who achieved a complete tumor response also experienced increased survival, as compared with partial responders or patients with stable disease. The 3-year survival rate in complete responders was 23%, as compared with 10% in partial responders and 15% in patients with stable disease.[424]

By escalating the total dose from 40 to 60 Gy, this trial established a significant dose-response relation between local control and short-term survival. Despite the preliminary local control and survival advantages in patients experiencing a complete response and in patients receiving a dose of 60 Gy, the overall median survival for patients receiving 40 Gy was 9.6 months, as compared with 10.1 months for patients receiving 50 to 60 Gy. In addition, the 5-year survival rate for all patients in this trial was approximately 6%, with no significant differences among the four arms.

Brachytherapy and External-Beam Radiotherapy. Huber et al.[433] randomly assigned 108 patients to either conventional radiotherapy (60 Gy) alone or an EBB boost of 4.8 Gy before and after conventional radiotherapy. There was a trend toward improved local control in patients receiving brachytherapy, although it failed to reach significance. There was no difference in overall survival. Criticisms of the trial include that the majority of patient treatment significantly deviated from the protocol. However, it does suggest that EBB might play a role in the treatment of primary disease.

A pilot study examined the use of Gelfoam radioactive plaques in addition to postoperative external-beam radiation in patients who have had an R1 or R2 resection of stage III NSCLC. In 12 patients, there was a local control rate of 82% and overall survival of 45%. Whether this is an improvement from standard PORT for these patients remains to be examined in further studies.[434]

Three-Dimensional Conformal Radiotherapy. In a dose-escalation protocol using 3D-CRT at the University of Michigan, patients were treated with dose ranges from 69.3 to 102.9 Gy. The researchers have reported a single case of acute grade 3 pneumonitis and five cases of acute grade 2 pneumonitis.[217] Recently, patients with advanced disease have been receiving neoadjuvant chemotherapy in addition to radiotherapy. The median survival in patients with stage III or recurrent disease was 16 months, and 2-year overall survival was 36%.

Graham et al.[216,435] reported the results of 3D-CRT from Washington University. They have treated tumors to a dose of 60 to 74 Gy. Elective nodal irradiation was given to all except those patients with poor pulmonary function. These investigators report a 2-year survival rate of 53% with this technique. The University of Chicago reported a 2-year local control and a survival rate of 23% and 37%, respectively, in patients treated with doses ranging from 60 to 70 Gy.[436] The MSKCC reported a 2-year local control, disease-free survival, and overall survival rates of 36%, 11%, and 22%, respectively, in a group of patients with advanced-stage disease.[218]

Elective Nodal Irradiation. Standard radiotherapy typically involves a dose of 40 Gy to the entire mediastinum, supraclavicular fossa, and ipsilateral hilum, even if there is no evidence of disease in these areas (e.g., T4N0 tumors). It has been shown that this elective treatment can significantly add to the morbidity of radiation.[437,438] Many centers have made the decision to eliminate elective nodal irradiation in an effort to increase the dose to the tumor. When RTOG trials were reviewed to estimate the clinical impact of omitting nodal irradiation, it was found that when the ipsilateral hilum and mediastinum were incorrectly treated, there was an increased risk of progression.[439] The MSKCC reported an elective nodal failure rate of 8% and a local failure rate of 65%,[440] which suggests that until regions of known disease can be better controlled, there is probably no need to treat the entire mediastinum and supraclavicular region electively when T4N0 tumors are being treated. Invasive staging or PET scanning may improve decision making.

ALTERED FRACTIONATION RADIOTHERAPY. Altered fractionation implies any deviation from standard fractionation of 1.8 to 2 Gy delivered once daily, 5 days weekly for 6 to 7 weeks. Several forms of altered fractionation, such as continuous hyperfractionation accelerated radiotherapy (CHART), or variations of these have been investigated.[441] The basic goal of altered fractionation strategies is to deliver higher total doses of radiation to improve the local outcome without increasing late normal tissue toxicity. Altered fractionation schemes exploit the significant differences in the capacity of late-responding and early-responding tissues to repair radiation cellular damage.

Hyperfractionation. Hyperfractionated radiotherapy employs more than 1 fraction per day, using fraction sizes that are smaller than those used with standard fractionation (1.1 to 1.5 Gy per fraction versus 1.8 to 2 Gy per fraction). Thus, hyperfractionation uses multiple small fractions per day to deliver a higher total daily dose and final total dose to improve tumor cell kill without increasing late toxicity and accepting increased but recoverable acute toxicity.[441]

The RTOG initiated a phase I and II trial to evaluate 1.2-Gy twice-daily fractionation for locally advanced unresectable disease. Eight hundred eighty-four patients were randomly picked to receive doses of 60.0, 64.8, and 69.6 Gy, using 1.2 Gy twice daily with a minimum of a 4-hour interfraction interval. After reasonable time had elapsed to evaluate both acute and late effects, which were considered tolerable, patients were further assigned to either 74.4 Gy or 79.2 Gy, with closure of the two lowest dose arms. In a favorable subgroup of patients, the 69.6-Gy dose results appeared significantly better ($P = .002$) than results with standard fractionation in comparable patients from an earlier RTOG study and the other arms of the trial.[382] No increased toxicity was seen in the higher-dose arms to account for the decreased survival as compared to the 69.6-Gy arm.

Based on these results, the RTOG began a phase III trial comparing 69.6 Gy given via hyperfractionation and 60 Gy given via standard fractionation of thirty 2-Gy fractions. The third arm of the trial replicated the study arm of CALGB protocol 8433: induction chemotherapy with cisplatin and vinblastine followed by 60 Gy of irradiation. The 5-year survivals for standard radiotherapy, hyperfractionated radiotherapy, and induction chemotherapy plus radiation were 4%, 5%, and 8%, respectively. The survival in the chemotherapy-plus-radiotherapy arm was significantly higher.[442] As yet, there is no clear survival advantage that can be demonstrated for hyperfractionation as compared to standard radiotherapy. However, many trials continue to use this hyperfractionation regimen of 69.6 Gy. Further studies are needed to find the maximum tolerable dose of radiation with either hyperfractionation or standard fractionation and compare it to 60 Gy.

Accelerated Radiotherapy. RTOG trial 84-07 examined the role of an accelerated concomitant boost of radiotherapy. Patients received 45 Gy over 5 weeks to the primary tumor and mediastinal lymph nodes. Two to three times a week, a concomitant boost of 1.8 Gy would be delivered only to the primary tumor and involved lymph nodes. A dose of 25.2 cGy via concomitant boost (70.2 Gy) was found to be tolerable.[443] Two-year survival was 21% for the higher-dose patients. Another RTOG phase II trial (83-12) demonstrated a 2-year survival rate of 25% and a 3-year survival rate of 18%.[435]

Continuous Radiotherapy. CHART employs many radiobiologic principles in an effort to improve the therapeutic ratio. CHART delivers 54 Gy in three daily doses of 1.5 Gy over 12 continuous days, including weekends. With CHART, treatment is given every day to counteract rapidly proliferating cells. Hyperfractionation with many smaller doses of radiation may reduce long-term toxicity. Accelerating the treatment time from 6 weeks to 2 weeks also may counteract tumor repopulation.

CHART was first examined in a small prospective phase II trial.[444] Some degree of esophageal toxicity was present in all patients. Ten percent of patients developed acute radiation pneumonitis. Two-year survival was 34%.

A phase III randomized study was performed in 13 centers in the United Kingdom. Patients were assigned to either standard radiation of 60 Gy in 30 daily doses of 2 Gy over 6 weeks or CHART. Approximately one-half the patients had stage III disease; the remainder had early-stage disease or unknown staging. No other therapeutic modality was used. Two-year survival significantly increased from 20% to 29% in the CHART arm. In addition, local control significantly improved from 15% to 23%.[445] Severe esophageal toxicity also increased from 3% to 19%, and acute radiation pneumonitis was 19% in the conventional group and 10% in the CHART arm. However, late pulmonary toxicity and fibrosis requiring treatment at 2 years was present in 16% of living patients who received CHART as compared to 4% receiving conventional radiotherapy. The physical and psychological symptoms caused by this aggressive regimen have been shown to be tolerable as well.[446]

The use of CHART has been limited by the need to reorganize radiation departments to accommodate the demanding radiation treatment schedule. In addition, patients are hospitalized during their entire course of radiation, which may significantly increase the cost of treatment. Therefore, trials have been conducted using CHART without treatment on weekends.[447]

An ECOG trial examined the feasibility of hyperfractionated accelerated radiotherapy.[448] Twenty-eight patients received 57.6 Gy over 15 days (12 treatment days) in 1.6-Gy fractions three times daily, 4 hours apart. The need to wait 6 hours was avoided by not treating consecutively those fields containing spinal cord. The investigators found that this regimen was tolerable, with the main toxicity being esophagitis and moist desquamation of the skin. Median survival of 13 months was similar to combined-modality approaches.

A North Central Cancer Treatment Group Trial evaluated standard radiotherapy (60 Gy in 30 daily fractions of 2 Gy over 6 weeks) to an accelerated hyperfractionated approach (60 Gy in 40 fractions of 1.5 Gy twice daily over 4 weeks). A third arm included the accelerated hyperfractionated approach with concomitant cisplatin and etoposide. The two radiation-alone arms were not significantly different, although there was a trend toward improved local control and overall survival when the two hyperfractionated arms were combined.[449]

Hypofractionated Radiotherapy. The reality for most physicians treating unresectable NSCLC is that in many patients, favorable patient parameters are not present. In these patients with unresectable stage III tumors, the results with either radiotherapy alone or combined-modality treatment are poor, and the chance for cure is rare. Studies have examined the use of hypofractionated radiotherapy for unresectable stage III disease and compared the results to those for standard fractionation to 60 Gy in RTOG trials. Depending on one's philosophy, the use of hypofractionated radiotherapy may simply be a palliative approach, or it may be a curative approach with low expectation, based on known results with radiotherapy alone. A study revealed that patients with stage III disease treated with 40-Gy split-course irradiation had longer survival times and lower local relapse rates but higher distant failure rates than those receiving 24 to 32 Gy. Survival rates for patients with stage IIIA disease treated with 40 Gy at 1, 2, and 5 years were 47%, 22%, and 7%, respectively. For stage IIIB disease, the radiation scheme did not correlate with survival and relapse rates. Survival rates at 1, 2, and 5 years were 30%, 9%, and 2%, respectively. The hypofractionated regimen schemes were extremely well tolerated, and no severe complications were observed.[450] Although the data for both schedules of treatment appear comparable, split-course irradiation cannot be routinely recommended based on the available literature for locally advanced NSCLC.

Radiosensitizers. Schaake-Koning et al.[451] demonstrated a survival advantage when weekly or daily cisplatin was added to thoracic radiotherapy. Three-year overall survival improved from 2% to 16% with the addition of daily cisplatin. The benefit was due to increased local control with cisplatin. It is not clear whether cisplatin actually enhances the effect of radiation or whether it is independently cytotoxic, with its effectiveness more dependent on dosing and dose level. Other studies have shown no benefit from the addition of concomitant chemotherapy with thoracic radiation.[452–454]

A CALGB-ECOG study examined induction chemotherapy with cisplatin and vinblastine followed by 60 Gy radiotherapy with or without radiosensitization with carboplatin, 100 mg/m^2.[455] This study differs from those referenced heretofore because it used cytotoxic chemotherapy for induction in both arms and, therefore, was solely testing the value of radiosensitization. There was no difference in overall survival, failure-free survival, or response between the two arms. There was a higher local control in the carboplatin arms, but this did not have an impact on survival.

Radiation Protectors. The radioprotectant amifostine is a sulfhydryl compound the metabolites of which scavenge free radicals that are generated in tissues exposed to radiation.[456] A phase II clinical trial using amifostine with sequential chemotherapy and standard radiation (60 Gy) demonstrated no episodes of grade 3 or worse esophagitis or pneumonitis.[457] There was no evidence of tumor protection, either. Amifostine might allow for the use of higher doses of chemotherapy and radiation with acceptable toxicity. RTOG protocol 98-01 is addressing this issue.

Prophylactic Cranial Irradiation for Locally Advanced Non–Small Cell Lung Cancer

The hypothesis that prophylactic cranial irradiation (PCI) can improve survival is based on the assumption that isolated brain failures occur commonly and lead to death and that these can be effectively prevented by tolerable doses of radiation. PCI has recently been shown on metaanalysis to improve survival in patients with small cell lung cancer.[458] However, isolated brain failures in NSCLC are not common, and it is not possible to predict the patients at risk. Consequently, it is unlikely that survival would be improved to a detectable degree if effective prophylaxis were delivered to the entire population of patients with resected disease. Of 1532 patients treated surgically in prospective trials of the LCSG, only 6.8% (104 of 1532) had first recurrences in the brain. However, 71% of the patients in this series had T1–2N0 tumors. Patients with locally advanced disease treated with thoracic irradiation on the RTOG protocols had an initial brain failure rate of 7% for squamous histology, 19% for adenocarcinoma, and 13% for large cell carcinoma. Even for adenocarcinoma, brain is a less common site of initial failure than are bone (24%) and opposite lung (21%).[286,389]

Four randomized trials of PCI added to chest irradiation (with or without chemotherapy) have been reported for patients with locally advanced NSCLC and have not demonstrated improved survival, although treatment did reduce the rate of development of brain metastasis.[459–462] Thus, until systemic treatment and local therapy are sufficient to render the brain as the main site of clinical failure, PCI cannot be recommended for any stage of NSCLC, and its use remains investigational.

The use of PCI after combined-modality therapy that includes surgery has not been sufficiently investigated. However, a recent report involved 75 patients who had stage IIIA or IIIB NSCLC treated by induction therapy and who were treated with PCI (30 Gy over 3 weeks). In this phase II trial, PCI was started after the end of the final chemotherapy cycle and prior to surgery. In those patients who had partial or complete responses to the induction chemotherapy, there were no relapses in the brain as the first site. Further study is warranted, since brain is the most common site of first relapse in most induction therapy reports.[462]

Combined-Modality Treatments, Including Radiotherapy

SEQUENTIAL CHEMOTHERAPY AND RADIOTHERAPY (INDUCTION OR NEOADJUVANT CHEMOTHERAPY). The use of induction chemotherapy is based on several theoretic considerations.[266,463–465] It has been suggested that the early use of chemotherapy lowers the systemic tumor burden and prevents the growth of microscopic systemic disease, while bulky locoregional macroscopic disease is decreased and addressed more easily by subsequent surgery, radiotherapy, or both.

Several large randomized studies of induction chemotherapy in unresectable NSCLC have been published (Table 31.2-14).[213,266,272,273,463–474] Generally, studies using more intensive chemotherapeutic regimens and entering larger study cohorts have favored the use of chemotherapy. Metaanalyses of chemotherapy in this setting also suggest a significant therapeutic benefit but are compromised by the limitations of this technique, reflecting the poor design or execution of many of the randomized trials.[473,474]

In assessing the role of chemotherapy for unresectable stage III disease, it appears beneficial to concentrate on specific well-designed and -conducted trials. In 1984, the CALGB initiated a randomized study comparing standard radiotherapy to two cycles of induction chemotherapy with cisplatin plus vinblastine followed by radiotherapy.[271,469] Eligible patients had stage III unresectable NSCLC; eligibility was restricted to allow for only 5% weight loss before study entry and a performance status of 0 or 1. Patients with supraclavicular lymph node involvement or cytologically positive pleural effusion were also excluded. Thus, eligible patients were selected to be in a generally favorable state of health and to be treated with curative intent. This study was closed after an interim analysis, with only 155 eligible patients entered, when a survival difference became apparent. The median survival favored chemotherapy (14 vs. 10 months; $P = .0066$). Thus, the addition of 1 month of chemotherapy to radiation resulted in a 4-month prolongation of life. More interestingly, the chemotherapy also resulted in a doubling of long-term survivors. On both study arms, few patients were noted to have recurrences after 2 years of follow-up. Seventeen percent of patients were alive at 5 years' follow-up on the chemotherapy arm, as compared with 7% of patients receiving standard radiotherapy alone.

A confirmatory three-arm intergroup study was subsequently organized.[273,470] In this study, the two study arms of the CALGB trial were repeated; a third arm was added to test the hypothesis that intensified radiotherapy as a single modality might also result in increased survival rates. Eligibility criteria were identical to those spelled out in the CALGB study. This study largely confirms the results of the CALGB study; median survival times for radiotherapy alone, hyperfractionated radiotherapy, and induction chemotherapy were 11, 12, and 14 months, respectively. This difference again favored the addition of chemotherapy to radiotherapy. The use of hyperfractionated radiotherapy alone resulted in no significant benefit. Long-term survival data from this study suggest that 3-year survival rates are similar for induction chemotherapy and hyperfractionated radiotherapy (and superior to standard fractionation radiotherapy).

Given the systemic activity of chemotherapy, it might be expected that the increased survival rate observed with induction chemotherapy would be due to increased systemic control. However, not all studies have included an analysis of the pattern of failure. A European study tested three cycles of induction chemotherapy with vindesine, lomustine, cisplatin, and cyclophosphamide in patients with squamous cell and large cell lung carcinoma and showed a small survival benefit favoring chemotherapy. Increased systemic control due to chemotherapy was also shown in the intergroup trial, while there was no effect on intrathoracic control.[213,272,407]

In summary, induction chemotherapy has been shown in large randomized studies to increase survival rates of patients with unresectable stage III NSCLC. This appears to be due to increased systemic disease control and is, therefore, compatible with the observations of activity for chemotherapy in patients with stage IV disease and the theoretic models sup-

TABLE 31.2-14. Selected Randomized Trials Testing Induction Chemotherapy in Locally Advanced Non–Small Cell Lung Cancer Treated by Radiotherapy

Study	*Radiotherapy (Gy)*	*Design*	*No. of Patients*	*Median Survival (mo)*	*2-Y Survival (%)*	*5-Y Survival (%)*
Mattson[466]	55	XRT vs. CAP/XRT	119/119	10.3/11.0	15/20	NA
Morton[467]	60	XRT vs. MACC/XRT	58/56	9.6/10.4	12/23	7/5
Le Chevalier[272,a]	65	XRT vs. VCPC/XRT	177/176	10.0/12.0	14/21	3/6
Dillman[469]	60	XRT vs. PV/XRT	77/79	9.6/13.7	13/26	6/17
Sause[273] (3 arms)	60 or 69.6 HXRT	XRT vs. HXRT vs. PV/XRT	452/452/452	11.4/12.2/13.7	20/24/31	5/6/8

CAP, cyclophosphamide (Cytoxan), doxorubicin (Adriamycin), and cisplatin (platinum); HXRT, hyperfractionated radiotherapy; MACC, methotrexate, doxorubicin (Adriamycin), cyclophosphamide, lomustine (CCNU); NA, not available; PV, cisplatin (platinum) and vinblastine; VCPC, vindesine, cyclophosphamide (Cytoxan), cisplatin (platinum), and lomustine (CCNU); XRT, radiotherapy.
[a]Improved systemic control.

porting induction chemotherapy. Induction chemotherapy is a current standard therapy for these patients.

CONCOMITANT CHEMORADIOTHERAPY. The simultaneous use of chemotherapy and radiotherapy has also been widely investigated (Table 31.2-15). This approach is based on considerations similar to those for sequential chemoradiotherapy in that chemotherapy may cover systemic disease, while radiotherapy can treat locoregional disease. The concomitant approach provides the additional theoretic benefit of increasing locoregional control through a direct interaction of the two modalities, which is not the case when the two modalities are administered in sequence.[266,270] Clinically, the administration of intensive concomitant chemoradiotherapy is complicated by increased toxicities. This includes esophagitis, a risk of radiation pneumonitis, and increased myelosuppression because the thoracic bone marrow is exposed to the radiation.

As a result, the chemotherapy frequently has been given at suboptimal doses as single-agent chemotherapy instead of combination chemotherapy, or the radiotherapy schedule has been interrupted to allow for recovery of normal tissues. It is known that prolongation of a course of radiotherapy decreases its single-modality efficacy.

Several single-drug chemoradiotherapeutic trials have been published (see Table 31.2-15).[451–455,475] In particular, cisplatin as a single agent has been tested in several randomized clinical trials. A study of weekly cisplatin (15 mg/m^2/week) plus radiotherapy to 50.4 Gy found no survival benefit.[452] Similarly, studies of radiotherapy with low daily doses of cisplatin[453] or cisplatin given every 3 weeks[454] showed no survival benefit. Only one study showed improved local control and survival for daily cisplatin added to radiotherapy; however, the patients on the control arm received protracted radiotherapy.[451] Thus, concomitant chemoradiotherapy using single-agent cisplatin or other drugs has largely failed to improve the survival rates of patients with locoregionally advanced NSCLC, although it may provide a locoregional sensitization effect. This appears to be due to the lack of systemic activity of low-dose single-agent therapy; thus, the predominant site of failure in these patients (distant disease) is inadequately addressed.

Several studies testing combination chemotherapy with concomitant radiotherapy or using hyperfractionated radiotherapy have also been published.[266,475–481] These studies largely have been performed in the phase I and II settings. Results uniformly indicate increased toxicity. Some studies, however, have also suggested therapeutic benefit and encouraging survival data.

The SWOG has published two phase II trials using cisplatin and etoposide with concurrent radiotherapy.[274,482] In the first such trial, concomitant chemoradiotherapy to 45 Gy was administered in the preoperative setting. The response rate to this regimen prior to surgery was 59%, and 71% of patients were able to undergo surgical resection. This study forms the basis for the large current intergroup trial evaluating concomitant chemoradiotherapy plus chemoradiotherapy boost versus surgical resection in patients with marginally resectable stage IIIA NSCLC. The 3-year survival rate was 26%. In a second study, the SWOG evaluated this chemoradiotherapy regimen in patients with unresectable disease. Here patients received two cycles of cisplatin-etoposide with concurrent radiotherapy to 61 Gy followed by an additional two cycles of chemotherapy in the "adjuvant" setting. For 50 patients, the median survival time was 13 months, and 2- and 3-year survival rates were 33% and 26%, respectively. The SWOG has evaluated a similar regimen of carboplatin, etoposide, and concurrent radiotherapy in patients with poor prognostic features.[483] Pilot data in this group of patients indicated similar median and 2-year survival times, indicating the feasibility of chemoradiotherapy for a suboptimal patient population.

Definitive testing of combination chemotherapy with concurrent radiotherapy in the phase III setting has been limited. A three-arm study investigated the combination of carboplatin and etoposide at two dose levels added to hyperfractionated radiotherapy (1.2 Gy twice daily; total dose, 64.8 Gy).[478] Carboplatin, 100 mg/m^2 on days 1 and 2, and etoposide, 100 mg/m^2 on days 1 to 3, of each week of radiotherapy resulted in a significant increase in median survival as compared with hyperfractionated radiotherapy alone (median survival, 8 vs. 18 months). A similar comparison of twice-daily radiotherapy to 69.6 Gy with or without daily intravenous carboplatin (50 mg) and etoposide (50 mg) showed a significant increase in median survival time (22 vs. 14 months) and 4-year survival rates (23% vs. 9%).[479] These studies support the addition of chemotherapy to radiotherapy but do not clarify whether twice-daily radiotherapy is superior to single daily fractions. Intensified radiotherapy schedules are mainly supported by the British CHART study.[445]

TABLE 31.2-15. Randomized Trials of Concomitant Chemoradiotherapy with Single-Agent Cisplatin or Carboplatin in Locally Advanced Non–Small Cell Lung Cancer

Study	*Radiotherapy (Gy)*	*Chemotherapy*	*No. of Pts (RT/ChemoRT)*	*Median Survival (mo) (RT/ChemoRT)*	*2-Y Survival (%) (RT/ChemoRT)*
Soresi[452]	50	CDDP: weekly (15 mg/m^2)	50/45	11.0/16.0	25/40 (NS)
Trovo[453]	45	CDDP: daily (6 mg/m^2)	88/87	10.3/9.9	13/13
Blanke[454]	60	CDDP: q3wk (70 mg/m^2)	111/104	43/46 (weeks)	13/18
Schaake-Koning[451,a]	55	CDDP: Weekly (30 mg/m^2) *or* Daily (6 mg/m^2)	108/98/102	NA	13/19/26
Clamon[455,b]	60	Carboplatin: weekly (100 mg/m^2)	137/146	13/13	14/15

CDDP, cisplatinum; ChemoRT, chemoradiotherapy; NA, not available; NS, not significant; RT, radiotherapy.
[a]Improved local control and survival with cisplatin.
[b]Both arms included induction chemotherapy (cisplatin, vinblastine × 2 cycles).

Since both induction chemotherapy and concomitant chemoradiotherapy prolong survival, it can be asked which of the two approaches is superior. Induction chemotherapy has, indeed, been directly compared with concomitant chemoradiotherapy using the cisplatin-plus-vinblastine regimen in a randomized study by the RTOG. Based on previous pilot studies, patients with stage III NSCLC were randomly chosen to receive induction chemotherapy with cisplatin plus vinblastine (standard), or the same drugs given concomitantly during radiotherapy, or cisplatin with orally administered etoposide and concomitant hyperfractionated radiotherapy.[484,485] Results from this trial are expected in the near future.

A similar study has been reported by Japanese investigators. Furuse et al.[275,486] compared the administration of the MVP regimen as induction chemotherapy to its administration with concurrent radiotherapy. Median survival times were 16 versus 13 months, favoring the concurrent administration of chemoradiotherapy. A pattern-of-failure analysis indicated a higher relapse in the brain for patients treated with concurrent chemoradiotherapy, with the possibility of higher intrathoracic control (Table 31.2-16).

INDUCTION AND CONCOMITANT CHEMORADIATION. An alternative strategy to a direct comparison of induction versus concomitant combined-modality therapy is the administration of both. This strategy is supported by the suggestion that induction chemotherapy and concomitant chemoradiotherapy may exert their favorable influence on survival by different mechanisms. In particular, induction chemotherapy appears to improve systemic disease control, while concomitant chemoradiotherapy leads to higher locoregional control. This hypothesis has been evaluated in several studies. The CALGB compared administration of cisplatin and vinblastine followed by radiotherapy with administration of the same induction chemotherapeutic regimen followed by radiotherapy with weekly doses of concomitant carboplatin.[455] This study showed a median survival time of 13 months on both arms but suggested increased locoregional control for patients receiving carboplatin. This study adds to the evidence that single-agent radiation sensitization with a platinating agent is of clinical benefit.

More recently, similar investigations have focused on the integration of novel chemotherapeutic single agents into the setting. Preclinical and early clinical data support a role as radiation enhancers for the taxanes, gemcitabine, vinorelbine, and topoisomerase I inhibitors.[487–501] Additional trials have evaluated the administration of paclitaxel with or without carboplatin on a weekly schedule with concurrent chest radiotherapy. Phase II trials indicate high response and promising 1- and 2-year survival rates with this approach. Pilot studies using paclitaxel are summarized in Table 31.2-17. A three-arm study by the CALGB evaluating three novel agents (gemcitabine, paclitaxel, or vinorelbine in combination with cisplatin) in the induction and concomitant setting is under way. The radiation dose in this trial is 66 Gy.[499]

To evaluate further the role of induction chemotherapy within the context of concomitant chemoradiotherapy, the CALGB is conducting a randomized trial comparing concom-

TABLE 31.2-16. A Randomized Phase III Study of Concurrent versus Sequential Radiotherapy with MVP in Stage III Non–Small Cell Lung Cancer

Treatment Arm	*No. of Patients*	*Response Rate (%)*	*Survival* Median (mo)	2-Y (%)	3-Y (%)	*P Value*
Concurrent	156	84	16.5	37	27	.0473
Sequential	158	66.4	13.3	25.6	12.5	

MVP = mitomycin, vindesine, cisplatin (platinum).
[Adapted from Furuse K, Fukuoka M, Takada Y, et al. Phase III study of concurrent vs. sequential thoracic radiotherapy (TRT) in combination with mytomycin (M), vindestine (V), and cisplatin (P) in unresectable stage III non-small cell lung cancer: five-year median follow-up results. *Clin Oncol* 1999;18:458(abst 1770).]

TABLE 31.2-17. Selected Phase II Trials of Weekly Paclitaxel-Based Chemotherapy with Concurrent Radiotherapy in Patients with Stage III Unresectable Non–Small Cell Lung Cancer

					Survival	
Author	*No. of Patients*	*Concurrent Chemotherapy*	*Radiotherapy*	*Relative Risk (%)*	1-Y (%)	2-Y (%)
Choy[491]	29	Paclitaxel	60 Gy[a]	86	73	NA
Choy[492]	39	Paclitaxel and carboplatin	66 Gy[a]	75.7	56.3	38.3
Choy[493]	43	Paclitaxel and carboplatin	69.6 Gy[b]	78.6	63	NA
Belani[494]	38	Paclitaxel and carboplatin	60–65 Gy[a]	NA	63	54

NA, not available.
[a]Once-daily radiation.
[b]Twice-daily radiation.

itant chemoradiotherapy with carboplatin, paclitaxel, and concurrent radiotherapy versus two cycles of induction chemotherapy with carboplatin and paclitaxel followed by the same concomitant chemoradiotherapeutic regimen. This trial will evaluate whether induction chemotherapy is of benefit in patients receiving concomitant chemoradiotherapy.

Additional trials are expanding on observations with accelerated radiotherapy. The aforementioned British trial has indicated that administration of accelerated radiotherapy is superior to standard radiotherapy as a single-treatment modality.[445,481] Because accelerated radiotherapy will have an impact on locoregional control only, its administration after induction chemotherapy is being evaluated in a randomized Eastern Oncology Cooperative Group Trial.[502]

In reviewing these studies of combined-modality therapy for unresectable NSCLC, it is clear that induction chemotherapy has led to a significant increase in survival rates; concomitant chemoradiotherapy can also achieve this. The existing data support that patients can be treated with induction chemotherapy or concomitant therapy outside of a clinical trial (as a standard therapy); however, the impact of these strategies in survival is small, and participation in clinical trials is strongly encouraged.

STAGE IV DISEASE

In most instances, stage IV (M1) disease is treated with primary chemotherapy. The goals of therapy are the palliation of symptoms and prolongation of survival time. On occasion, however, when a solitary site of metastasis occurs (e.g., brain), both the primary tumor and the solitary metastatic site can be treated with curative intent either by a surgical or radiotherapeutic approach.

Prolongation of Survival by Chemotherapy

In the 1970s and 1980s, combination chemotherapy, usually cisplatin-based, was demonstrated to result in reproducible response rates of approximately 20% to 30%.[262,265] Although these studies suggested activity of chemotherapy in stage IV NSCLC, they left unanswered what constituted the optimal chemotherapeutic regimen for NSCLC. Furthermore, because overall median survival times were short at 6 to 8 months and few patients survived beyond 1 year, the general value of chemotherapy in the routine management of patients with stage IV NSCLC was questioned.[261,297,503–506]

Some investigators hypothesized that the survival benefits that patients derived from chemotherapy were not sufficient to offset the toxicities and economic costs. A number of randomized studies were initiated to compare directly best supportive care versus chemotherapy plus best supportive care (Table 31.2-18).[408,507,509–516] The first such study was reported by Cormier et al.[507] and supported the use of chemotherapy. However, like most subsequent studies listed in Table 31.2-18, it included insufficient patient numbers to allow for definitive conclusions. The subsequent Canadian study remains the most frequently cited study in this category.[508] Of interest, it demonstrated not only increased survival time with chemotherapy but acceptable treatment costs.[517] Additional studies confirmed the finding of a statistically significant increase in median survival for chemotherapy-treated patients compared with those receiving best supportive care only, and all studies suggested at least a statistical trend for improved outcome favoring chemotherapy.

Since each of these trials comparing the use of chemotherapy with best supportive care can be criticized for methodologic reasons, such as including too few patients or using insufficiently active chemotherapy, metaanalyses of these studies were suggested. Four such metaanalyses have been published and are summarized in Table 31.2-19.[474,518–520] All four metaanalyses support the same conclusion: Chemotherapy prolongs survival time by a modest but statistically significant amount of time and, generally, should be offered to patients. As mentioned, economic analyses support similar conclusions. As a result, many physicians consider the use of chemotherapy a standard therapy approach for most patients with NSCLC.[261–264]

Quality of Life

With the limited survival benefit for patients, quality of life (QOL) has been considered as another relevant end point of chemotherapeutic trials in stage IV NSCLC. Validated questionnaires have been developed to assess QOL accurately. The earlier randomized trials comparing chemotherapy gave indirect evidence that chemotherapy can improve QOL: The reason that chemotherapy reduced health care costs in the Canadian study was that patients receiving chemotherapy had a lower incidence of disease-related complications, leading to fewer hospital admissions.[517] Economic analyses support the use of combined-modality and palliative combination-chemotherapy approaches.[517,521,522]

More recently, improved QOL has been prospectively evaluated as an independent variable.[516,523] Disease-related symp-

TABLE 31.2-18. Randomized Trials

Study	*Chemotherapy*	*No. of Patients BSC/Chemo*	*Median Survival (wk) BSC/Chemo*	*P Value*
Cormier[507]	MACC	19/20	9/31	.0005
Rapp[508]	CAP/VP	50/43/44	17/25/33	.05/.01
Cartei[509]	CCM	50/52	17/37	.0001
Quoix[510]	VP	10/28	17/27	.33
Ganz[511]	VibP	26/22	14/19	.26
Woods[512]	VP	91/97	17/27	.33
Cellerino[513]	CEP/MEC	57/58	21/34	.135
Kassa[514]	VP	43/44	17/22	.28
ELVIS[515]	VNR	81/80	21/28	.03
Cullen[516]	MIC	176/175	21/29	.03

BSC, best supportive care; CAP/VP, cyclophosphamide (Cytoxan), doxorubicin (Adriamycin), cisplatin (platinum)/vinblastine, cisplatin; CCM, cisplatin, cyclophosphamide-mytomycin; CEP/MEC, cyclophosphamide, etoposide + platinum/mito, etoposide + cisplatin; MACC, methotroxate, doxorubicin (Adriamycin), cyclophosphamide, lomustine (CCNU); MIC, mitomycin, ifosfamide, cisplatin; VibP, vinblastine-platinum; VNR, vinorelbine; VP, vindesine-platinum.

toms will improve after chemotherapy, sometimes even in the absence of a measurable tumor response.[516,524,525] QOL scores improved with chemotherapy, whereas they declined over the first 6 weeks with best supportive care. In one study, symptomatic improvement was 70%, whereas the objective response rate was only 35%.[524] Improved survival and QOL were also demonstrated with single-agent chemotherapy in a population of patients exceeding the age of 70 years.[515]

Given the substantial experience with chemotherapy-based clinical trials in stage IV disease, large analyses for prognostic factors have been performed. The SWOG analyzed their database of 2531 patients with advanced NSCLC using Cox modeling, recursive partitioning, and amalgamation to identify prognostic factors in these patients.[144] Good performance status, female gender, age of 70 years or older, low tumor burden, normal lactate dehydrogenase and serum calcium levels, and a hemoglobin level of more than 11 g/dL were favorable factors. The use of cisplatin was an additional significant favorable predictor of survival. A European group conducted a similar analysis in 1052 patients and identified similar favorable prognostic factors of lower tumor burden, good performance status, higher age, and female gender.[526]

Newer Chemotherapeutic Drugs

Randomized phase III trials investigating a new drug in stage IV NSCLC are aimed at demonstrating improved survival when compared with previous standard therapy. The randomized studies of the 1980s established the value of chemotherapy as compared with best supportive care. The combination of cisplatin with etoposide or vinblastine emerged as a standard in the United States, while in Europe, the combination of cisplatin and vindesine was frequently administered. Randomized studies testing a new agent or combination in the 1990s could, therefore, be designed with several possible control arms, including the two combinations noted previously or cisplatin as a single agent.

In the 1990s, reproducible single-agent activity was demonstrated for several new agents. Paclitaxel, docetaxel, vinorelbine, gemcitabine, and irinotecan have been extensively investigated (Table 31.2-20). Their definitive evaluation has frequently included a comparison of the new drug with cisplatin versus cisplatin alone (Table 31.2-21).

Vinorelbine has undergone thorough testing in NSCLC and was the first of the recent drugs to receive approval by the U.S. Food and Drug Administration for use in NSCLC (see Tables 31.2-20 and 31.2-21).[515,527–531] A randomized study conducted in Europe compared a standard of cisplatin and vindesine with cisplatin and vinorelbine and with single-agent vinorelbine.[530] The median survival time was 30 weeks for patients treated with cisplatin and vindesine and for those treated with vinorelbine alone. Patients treated with cisplatin and vinorelbine had a significantly longer median survival time of 40 weeks. An economic evaluation of this study concluded that this chemotherapy had acceptable efficacy and cost-effectiveness as compared with

TABLE 31.2-19. Metaanalysis of Best Supportive Care versus Chemotherapy

Study	*No. of Studies*	*Results*	*Conclusion*
Souquet[513]	7	Reduced mortality at 3 and 6 mo.	CT to be offered
Grilli[519]	6	6-wk gain in survival (24% reduction in probability of death).	CT for selected patients
Marino[519a]	8	Median survival, 3.9 vs. 6.7 mo (20% more at 6 mo).	CT to be offered
NSCLC Collaborative Group[352]	11 (8 cisplatin-based)	Median survival 6 vs. 8 mo; 1-y survival: 16% vs. 26%. Data best for cisplatin-based therapy.	CT improves survival

CT, chemotherapy; NSCLC, non–small cell lung cancer.

TABLE 31.2-20. Single-Agent Activity of New Chemotherapeutic Agents for Non–Small Cell Lung Cancer

Agent	*No. of Studies*[a]	*No. of Patients*	*Total CR + PR*	*Median Survival*[b]	*No. of Studies*[c]	*1-Y Survival (%)*	*No. of Studies*[d]
Paclitaxel[e]	10	317	84 (26%)	37 (24–56)	6	41	7
Docetaxel[f]	8	300	77 (26%)	41 (27–48)	5	52	3
Vinorelbine	6	621	126 (20%)	33 (29–40)	6	24	3
Gemcitabine[g]	9	572	122 (21%)	41 (31–49)	5	39	2
Irinotecan	4	138	37 (27%)	35 (27–42)	2	NR	NR
Topotecan	5	119	15 (13%)	38 (33–40)	4	35	2

CR, complete response; NR, not reported; PR, partial response.
[a]Number of studies reporting results.
[b]Average median survival in weeks (range).
[c]Number of studies with median survival data.
[d]Number of studies with 1-year survival data.
[e]Includes both short (1- to 3-hour) and long (24-hour) infusion schedules. There were no differences in response or survival based on infusion duration.
[f]Includes doses of 60–100 mg/m^2. The response rates were 23% at 60 mg/m^2 and 29% at 100 mg/m^2. Survival data were similar.
[g]Includes doses of 800 mg/m^2 given on days 1, 8, and 15 of a 28-day cycle. At doses >1000 mg/m^2, there were no obvious dose responses.
(Adapted from ref. 262.)

other common medical interventions.[521]

A second study in the United States compared the combination of cisplatin and vinorelbine with single-agent cisplatin. Again, the combination of cisplatin and vinorelbine proved superior to the single agent.[531] Finally, single-agent vinorelbine resulted in superior survival times as compared with 5-fluorouracil plus leucovorin (30 vs. 22 weeks).[532] This study has been criticized for its use of 5-fluorouracil plus leucovorin in the control arm, which is not a commonly used regimen in NSCLC and resulted in a low 6% response rate. An intriguing European study compared vinorelbine with best supportive care in the elderly (70 years). Increased median survival times (6.5 vs./ 4.9 months) and QOL were demonstrated.[515] This study not only supported previous conclusions regarding prolongation of life but specifically indicated that patient age, as an isolated factor, should not be a primary determinant of whether the use of chemotherapy is indicated.

Paclitaxel also showed encouraging single-agent activity (see Table 31.2-20).[533–535] The ECOG performed a three-arm randomized study comparing a regimen of cisplatin plus etoposide with cisplatin plus paclitaxel with a regimen of paclitaxel given either at a low or high dose with granulocyte colony-stimulating factor support. The paclitaxel-plus-cisplatin arms were superior to the etoposide-plus-cisplatin regimen, with no evidence of an increased response rate with a higher paclitaxel dose.[536] This study evaluated paclitaxel as a 24-hour infusion. Shorter infusion duration (3 hours) has been used in most other studies. A European trial showed cisplatin and paclitaxel to result in median survival (10 months) similar to that of cisplatin and teniposide while being better tolerated.[537] Of note, median survival times in both of these studies were better in both arms than historic controls. Other randomized trials confirm the activity of cisplatin or carboplatin-paclitaxel regimens and the favorable toxicity profile of the latter combination (Table 31.2-22).[537–541]

Encouraging data also exist for docetaxel,[542–545] gemcitabine,[546–551] and irinotecan.[552–555] All three have reproducible single-agent activity and have been investigated in combination with a platinating agent. Gemcitabine has been evaluated in random-

TABLE 31.2-21. Cisplatin Alone versus Cisplatin and New Drug Combination

Study	*Regimen*	*No. of Patients*	*Response Rate (%)*	*Median Survival (mo)*	*1-Y Survival (%)*	*P Value*
Wozniak[531]	Cisplatin	209	12	6.0	26	
	Cisplatin + vinorelbine	206	26	8.0	39	.0018
Sandler[556,a]	Cisplatin	(Total 508)	9	7.6	35	
	Cisplatin + gemcitabine		31	8.7	30	.8
Gatzemeier[538,b]	Cisplatin	206	17	8.6	21	
	Cisplatin + paciltaxel	202	26	8.1	33	.0078
Von Pawel[560]	Cisplatin	119	14	6.4	20	
	Cisplatin + tirapazamine	119	28	8.0	36	.078

[a]Survival difference statistically significant.
[b]Survival difference not statistically significant.

TABLE 31.2-22. Comparison of Various Combination Chemotherapy Regimens

Study	Regimen	Response Rate (%)	Median Survival (mo)	1-Y Survival (%)	P Value
Old vs. new combination chemotherapy regimens					
Le Chevalier[530]	Vinorelbine	14	7.2	35	
	Cisplatin + vindesine	19	7.4	35	.04
	Cisplatin + vinorelbine	30	9.3	40	.01
Bonomi[536]	Cisplatin + etoposide	12.5	7.6	32	
	Cisplatin + paclitaxel	25	9.5	37	NA
	Cisplatin + paclitaxel + G-CSF	28	10.1	40	
Giaccome[537]	Cisplatin + teniposide	28	9.9	41	
	Cisplatin + paclitaxel	41	9.7	43	NS
Belani[539]	Cisplatin + etoposide	14	9.9	37	
	Carboplatin + paclitaxel	22	9.5	32	NS
Crino[537a]	Mitomycin, ifosfamide, cisplatin	28	8.8	—	
	Cisplatin + gemcitabine	40	8.1	—	NS
Cardenal[557]	Cisplatin + etoposide	22	7.2	25	
	Cisplatin + gemcitabine	41	8.7	32	.18
New vs. new combination chemotherapy regimens					
Kelly[540]	Cisplatin + vinorelbine	27	8.0	36	
	Carboplatin + paclitaxel	27	8.0	33	NS

NA, not available; NS, not significant.

ized phase II and III trials.[556–559] Equivalence of single-agent gemcitabine with the (more toxic) combination of cisplatin and etoposide was suggested in two small studies. The combination of gemcitabine and cisplatin showed a significant improvement in median survival (7.6 vs. 9.1 months) versus single-agent cisplatin.[556] A smaller European trial compared cisplatin and gemcitabine with cisplatin and etoposide and suggested a favorable impact on median survival.[557] Tirapazamine, a bioreductive alkylating agent, has been shown to increase the cytotoxicity of cisplatin and prolong survival after therapy with that combination.[560]

Docetaxel has been shown to have activity as second-line therapy in patients with cisplatin-refractory disease.[544,545] This is encouraging because second-line activity has rarely been observed with other drugs. Second-line activity has also been described for gemcitabine.[561]

Currently, investigators are focused on comparing some of the recent regimens with one another.[539] A comparison of cisplatin and vinorelbine with carboplatin and paclitaxel has been presented. Identical median survival times of 8 months suggested equivalence of antitumor activity, while the toxicity spectrum of the regimens predictably differed (more nausea and vomiting and myelosuppression with cisplatin, more neurotoxicity with carboplatin). The ECOG is comparing carboplatin-paclitaxel with gemcitabine-cisplatin, docetaxel-cisplatin, and cisplatin-paclitaxel. This is an important study, since it will establish the relative activity and toxicity of several novel cisplatin-based regimens versus the combination of paclitaxel and carboplatin. The CALGB is comparing single-agent paclitaxel therapy with the combination of paclitaxel-carboplatin.[463] Evaluating response, survival, economic, and QOL end points, this study will establish whether a benefit exists for this "doublet" over single-agent paclitaxel. Similarly, three drug regimens using novel drugs are being evaluated. Additional trials are evaluating the weekly administration of paclitaxel,[562] "non-platinum"–containing two-drug regimens,[563,564] three-drug regimens,[275,565] and other new cytoxic agents.[566,567] Of current interest in particular are "cytostatic" molecules inhibiting specific cellular or extracellular targets, including inhibitors of farnesyl transferase, matrix metalloproteinase, or antiangiogenic agents.[568–572]

In summary, chemotherapy for stage IV NSCLC has been shown to prolong survival as compared with best supportive care. The use of chemotherapy can be supported by cost and QOL analyses. Its administration to the elderly has been shown to be of benefit. Based on recent evidence, current standard regimens are the doublets of cisplatin in combination with either vinorelbine, paclitaxel, or gemcitabine or the combination of paclitaxel and carboplatin. In selected cases, administration of second-line chemotherapy should be considered.

Current Clinical Approaches to Stage IV Non–Small Cell Lung Cancer

In the 1990s, most patients with newly diagnosed stage IV NSCLC should undergo treatment with at least one chemotherapeutic regimen. Based on available data from randomized trials, treatment should consist of the combination of cisplatin and vinorelbine, cisplatin and gemcitabine or, alternatively, cisplatin or carboplatin and paclitaxel. Generally, chemotherapy should be restricted to patients with a performance status of 0 to 2, because it is that group of patients in which most phase II and positive phase III studies have been conducted. Available evidence suggests that patients with a performance status of 2 will have, at best, a minor prolongation of survival time by chemotherapy but may experience significant relief of disease-related symptoms. Single-agent therapy in elderly patients should be considered. Patients should understand that the treatment goals are not cure but prolongation of life and palliation of symptoms; additional palliative measures, such as pain relief, radiotherapy, and surgery, should be applied as most beneficial for symptom relief.

In patients with stable or responding disease, the treatment duration has traditionally been six cycles of chemotherapy. Historically, this is largely based on the cumulative toxicity observed with cisplatin, which frequently limits to six or less the total number of cycles. The optimal duration of chemotherapy is undergoing evaluation in randomized trials. It is possible that newer regimens, particularly those not containing cisplatin, might be tolerated (and active) for more than six cycles. In patients with stable or responding disease, it might, therefore, make sense to continue therapy beyond six cycles. The optimal duration of chemotherapy is undergoing evaluation in randomized trials.

Patients who progress on or after first-line chemotherapy but continue to have a good performance status may be offered second-line chemotherapy. Few drugs have undergone formal testing in this setting. Docetaxel has been most extensively evaluated. In phase II studies, the use of docetaxel in patients not previously exposed to another taxane resulted in a response rate of approximately 10%.[542] Two randomized trials have been presented.[544,545] A Canadian trial compared second-line best supportive care with docetaxel (at 75 or 100 mg/m^2).[545] Improvement in survival (7 vs. 5 months) and improved QOL supported the use of docetaxel at the lower dose. In a second study, docetaxel (at two dose levels of 75 or 100 mg/m^2) was compared with vinorelbine or ifosfamide.[544] Median survival times were similar, while 1-year survival was highest at the lower-dose docetaxel arm. QOL analysis also favored docetaxel therapy. Gemcitabine has also had second-line antitumor activity in phase II trials.[561] There is little published information to support the use of other drugs as second-line therapy.

Because novel and more effective or less toxic therapies are still much needed in treating NSCLC, it should be recommended to offer investigational therapies of new drugs or novel combinations of drugs to such patients in prospective phase I and II studies whenever possible. Such an approach holds promise for the intermediate and long-term identification of more active therapies. The empiric use of sequential chemotherapy regimens as second-, third-, or fourth-line therapy cannot be supported using current data. Given the lack of drugs with established activity as second-line therapy, using investigational drugs will not compromise a patient's chance of obtaining benefit from therapy.

Solitary Metastases

METASTASIS (M1) TO LUNG. To differentiate between a second primary lung cancer and a metastasis in synchronous lung lesions or among local recurrence, a new primary lung cancer, and a pulmonary metastasis from a previous resected lung cancer in metachronous lung lesions can be difficult. A second or recurrent lung lesion is considered a metastasis if the histology is identified to the primary tumor and occurs in the opposite lung or a noncontiguous area of the ipsilateral lung.

Deslauriers et al.[572a] found that the presence of satellite nodules discovered at surgery, clearly separated from the primary tumor but with identical histologic characteristics, is a poor prognostic factor. In patients with satellite nodules from all stages of lung cancer, 5-year survival was 21.6%, as compared with 44% if no nodules were present. The mechanism of tumor spread in the lung is not well known, but metastases may develop as a result of a blood-borne or airborne spread from a primary bronchogenic carcinoma. The new TNM staging system fails to classify these synchronous lung lesions specifically.

The same criteria used in selecting patients for surgical resection of a pulmonary metastasis from a primary lung cancer should be used in patients with metastatic carcinoma to the lung from other primary tumors.[572b] If a solitary synchronous lesion is discovered in a different lobe from the primary tumor, both lesions should be resected whenever possible.

METASTASIS (M1) TO BRAIN. Brain metastases constitute more than 25% of all observed recurrences in patients with resected NSCLC and are seen with greater frequency at autopsy.[573] In a review by the LCSG, the brain was the sole site of first recurrence in only 6.4% of patients with completely resected NSCLC but accounted for approximately 20% of all recurrences.[574] Nearly one-half of the patients seen with brain metastases have solitary lesions on CT scan. When these lesions are symptomatic, the median survival without therapy is limited to 1 month. Corticosteroids and whole brain irradiation can offer effective palliation of symptoms but only modestly increase survival up to 6 months.[575]

A synchronous or metachronous solitary brain metastasis can be treated, whenever possible, by surgical resection, with 5-year survival rates of 10% to 20% (Table 31.2-23). Surgical excision of a brain metastasis, no matter the primary site (approximately 75% from NSCLC), followed by radiation has been shown to be superior to whole brain radiotherapy alone in prolonging median survival (9.2 vs. 3.4 months), in preventing local recurrence, and in providing a better QOL.[576]

A resurgence of interest in the use of high-dose 3D-CRT or sterotactic radiosurgery in managing solitary brain metastases has followed early results suggesting equivalence to a surgical approach.[577]

METASTASIS (M1) TO THE ADRENAL GLAND. Adrenal metastases from bronchogenic carcinoma are found in approximately one-third of patients at autopsy. Routine preoperative upper abdominal CT scanning may reveal an adrenal mass in approximately 10% of patients.[578]

A few case reports of adrenalectomy for solitary adrenal metastasis are available, and long-term survival after combined excision of the primary lung tumor and its metastatic lesion has been reported.[579–581] The ultimate role of such an approach has yet to be defined.

METASTASIS (M1) TO LIVER, BONE, OR SKIN. No reports of long-term survival have been made after combined surgical excision of a primary lung cancer with a synchronous solitary liver, bone, or skin metastasis. It is rare that these lesions are truly solitary metastatic foci. However, patients with solitary metachronous sites fare reasonably well after complete surgical excision.

TABLE 31.2-23. Reported Results after Combined Resection for Primary Non–Small Cell Lung Cancer with a Single Brain Metastasis (M1)

Study	*No. of Patients*	*Estimated 5-Y Survival Rate (%)*	*Mortality Rate (%)*
Salerno et al.[631]	23	13	22
Winston et al.[632]	22	9 (2 y)	10
White et al.[633]	38	15 (2 y)	6
Mussi et al.[634]	20	34	0
Ehrenhaft[635]	40	12	2
Magilligan et al.[636]	41	21	2
Read et al.[637]	27	21	0
Macchiarini et al.[638]	37	30	0
Wronski et al.[639]	185	13	3

Palliation

In view of the poor survival rate of patients with locally advanced NSCLC and patients with metastatic disease, effective palliation is an important objective. Carroll et al.[582] followed up 134 inoperable patients and reported that 64% needed immediate local palliation and that, of those with no thoracic symptoms at presentation, one-half required subsequent local treatment. Thus, a watch-and-wait policy is appropriate for only a minority of patients, and it is critical that they be followed up carefully to prevent the development of serious local complications of the disease that may be less easily palliated. It is important to intervene before superior vena cava obstruction, obstructive pneumonia, or lobar collapse develops. The latter two conditions produce a radiographic picture in which tumor and other processes are not easily distinguishable, and large radiation fields may be necessary for effective control.

Radiotherapy

LOCAL DISEASE. *External-Beam Irradiation.* Numerous trials have been conducted in which the palliative benefit of radiotherapy has been documented.[582–585] Various regimens produce a high rate of palliation that often is sustained for a significant proportion of a patient's survival. The randomized trials suggest that certain symptoms, such as hemoptysis and pain, are more effectively palliated, while dyspnea and poor performance status appear to be more refractory. Investigators in Italy used either 5.5 Gy or 8.8 Gy once a week for a total dose of 44 Gy and reported that 80% of 45 patients experienced an average improvement of 20 points on the Karnofsky performance score.[421,586]

The RTOG trial showed that even regimens with larger fraction sizes had a low (8%) incidence of severe complications. An early Medical Research Council trial showed no difference in survival or toxicity between 17 Gy given in two fractions 1 week apart and more conventional palliative fractionation (30 Gy in ten fractions or 27 Gy in six fractions).[583] A follow-up study, however, demonstrated an increase in median survival from 7 months to 9 months when 17 Gy in 2 fractions was compared to 36 to 39 Gy in 12 to 13 fractions.[587] Palliation was quicker and more durable in the hypofractionated arm, however.

A significant number of patients, however, suffer recurrence of symptoms. Few data report on the result of re-treatment with radiation. Jackson and Ball[588] re-treated 22 patients whose disease recurred after radical irradiation and delivered between 20 and 30 Gy in 2-Gy fractions. Symptomatic improvement occurred in 52%, and median survival was 5.4 months.

Superior vena cava syndrome is characterized by venous distention, facial edema, headache, tachypnea, cyanosis, and plethora[589] It is caused by the obstruction of the superior vena cava by compression, invasion, or thrombosis. Approximately 80% of cases are caused by bronchiogenic cancer, most frequently small cell lung cancer, but non–small cell histologies are also very common. Although some have questioned whether emergent radiation treatment is necessary,[589] others report symptomatic relief with palliative radiotherapy in 80% of patients.[590] High dose per fraction (300 cGy or greater) appears to incite faster relief.[590]

Intraluminal Brachytherapy. Intraluminal brachytherapy or EBB is an excellent palliative treatment for symptoms of hemoptysis, obstruction, and dyspnea. It has been shown to work best in tumors that are endoluminal or submucosal.[591] Direct permanent implantation of ^{125}I seeds into endobronchial tumors was developed at MSKCC in the 1960s. Relief of symptoms was achieved in approximately 60% of cases, but there was significant morbidity due to perforation of the airway, hemorrhage, and ventilatory arrest.[592] Subsequent workers avoided direct implantation into tissues and used temporary intraluminal placement of cobalt 60 or ^{192}Ir to deliver one or more large fractions over a few days.[593,594] High-dose-rate fractionated intraluminal therapy was developed to avoid such prolonged treatment times, which were uncomfortable for the patient and required hospitalization with attendant expense and radiation risk to personnel. In a sequential comparison of low- and high-dose rate endobronchial radiation, there was no difference in palliative effect or toxicity.[595] In a population of patients receiving prior radiation, this approach yielded symptomatic improvement in 75% of patients, and there were a few long-term survivors.[425] Similar data were reported by Macha et al.,[596] who obtained a response in 79% (44 of 56) of patients receiving 7.5 Gy 1 cm from the source in four treatments. Radiologic improvement occurred in 88% (22 of 25) of patients with collapse or atelectasis, and improvements in FEV_1 and vital capacity were well documented. Delclos et al.[597] reported an 84% response rate in 81 previously treated patients. The median response duration was 4.5 months. Burt et al.[598] gave 15 to 20 Gy at 1 cm in one fraction of high-dose-rate endoluminal brachytherapy and reported relief of hemoptysis in 86% (24 of 28), dyspnea in 64% (21 of 33), and cough in 50% (9 of 18). Unlike in other series, these authors did not use laser therapy before radiation. Laser treatment provides immediate relief of symptoms, facilitates catheter placement beyond the obstruction, and may increase response rates and duration. Seagren and Harrell[599] reported significantly improved response rates among a population of 36 patients who received laser treatment versus 14 who did not.

The optimum brachytherapy fractionation schedule has yet to be determined. Single large fractions have been associated with a large risk of massive hemoptysis.[258] Huber et al.[600] compared two fractionation schedules of high-dose-rate EBB: 3.8 Gy in four fractions and 7.2 Gy in two fractions. There was no difference in overall survival or complications between the two groups, although there was a trend toward improved survival with the large fraction size. Therefore, doses in the range of 5 to 7.5 Gy prescribed to 1 cm should be considered safe for high-dose-rate endobronchial radiation. EBB has also been given concurrently with chemotherapy safely.[601]

Distant Metastases

NSCLC metastasizes to a variety of organs. For asymptomatic metastatic disease remote from critical locations, the usual approach is expectant management or chemotherapy. Isolated symptomatic lesions, such as bone metastases and spinal cord compression (even if asymptomatic), are managed with palliative courses of radiation (e.g., 30 Gy in ten fractions).

Brain metastases are particularly common in NSCLC and can be debilitating. The standard therapy for multiple brain metastases in NSCLC is whole brain irradiation. This is accompanied by dexamethasone, 4 mg four times daily before and during radiation, and anticonvulsants only if seizures occur.

The RTOG studied a variety of dose and fractionation schemes for 1994 patients with brain metastases arising from several primary sites, including lung (approximately one-half of patients). The schedules used were 20 Gy in 1 week, 30 Gy in 2 weeks, 30 Gy in 3 weeks, 40 Gy in 3 weeks, and 40 Gy in 4 weeks. The shorter schedules tended to give more rapid relief of neurologic symptoms, but otherwise the schedules had comparable palliative effects (50% overall), duration of improvement (9 to 13 weeks), and median survival (15 to 18 weeks).[601,602]

Surgical resection combined with postoperative resection has been advocated for single metastases. At MSKCC, 104 patients with NSCLC were treated with surgery and radiation (n = 35) or radiation alone (n = 69). Median survival was 18 months for the combined-therapy arm versus 4 months for the radiation-alone arm. The patients on the combined-arm had fewer metastases to other organs and tended to have controlled or more aggressively managed primary tumors.[603] Mandell et al.[603] and Patchell et al.[604] randomly assigned 45 patients with resectable single brain metastases (82% NSCLC primary tumors) to receive radiation alone or combined resection and radiation to the entire brain. Median survival (40 weeks vs. 15 weeks) and duration of functional independence (38 weeks vs. 8 weeks) were significantly higher in the combined surgery-plus-radiation arm. The magnitude of the difference in survival documented in the trial has prompted an increasing acceptance of resection and postoperative irradiation for solitary brain metastases arising from NSCLC. A subsequent study from Patchell et al.[605] examined the role of whole brain radiotherapy in patients who underwent surgical resection. They found that whole brain radiotherapy decreased the rate of neurologic death but did not have an effect on overall survival. Stereotactic radiosurgery for solitary brain metastases appears promising as a substitute for surgery.

SURGERY. Even when surgery cannot lead to cure, this approach may be used to afford best palliation of symptoms. Such surgical intervention may include bronchoscopic removal or ablation of tumor to relieve endobronchial obstruction or hemoptysis, pleurodesis to relieve symptomatic malignant pleural effusions, pericardial fenestration for malignant pericardial effusions, endobronchial or endoesophageal stents for relief of obstruction, and (occasionally) surgical resection of primary tumors and lung parenchyma for relief of septic complications or massive hemoptysis. On very rare occasions, *en bloc* resection, albeit incomplete, may be excellent palliation for painful invasion of bony structures, such as vertebrae or ribs.

Relief of Endobronchial Obstruction. Bronchoscopic removal of endobronchial tumor is an efficient way of relieving endobronchial obstruction. Simple mechanical débridement with the use of the bronchoscope is often sufficient. Coagulative techniques, such as CO_2, argon or neodymium–yttrium aluminum garnet laser, electrocautery, and cryotherapy have been used in conjunction with mechanical débridement. There has been an increase in interest in the use of photocoagulation employing hematoporphyrins and argon beam excitation as a method of relieving endobronchial obstructions.[606] All the techniques can be effective. Massive hemorrhage from the lesion is rare but can be avoided by the judicious use of coagulative techniques. In most instances, endobronchial débridement and coagulation are best carried out by rigid bronchoscopy. Frequently, endobronchial stents are employed for long-term palliation.

Hemoptysis. Frequently, hemoptysis can plague the patient with stage IV lung cancer. As with bronchial obstruction, bronchoscopy is often the treatment of choice to control this annoying and sometimes devastating complication. All the coagulative methods discussed for bronchial obstruction can apply. In some patients, the bleeding can be controlled by the use of bronchial artery embolization to obstruct the hypertrophy in the bronchial arteries that have been eroded in the area of the tumor. On rare occasions, massive hemoptysis can be dealt with by a palliative resection.

Pleurodesis of Malignant Pleural Effusions. Malignant pleural effusions associated with lung cancer can be difficult to treat. In most instances, a portion of the ipsilateral lung is atelectatic, making pleurodesis more refractory. Before pleurodesis, a chest tube should be inserted to drain the pleural effusion completely to ensure that the lung is expandable. Occasionally, endobronchial removal of tumor may allow such expansion. After confirmation that the visceral and parietal pleura can be opposed, pleurodesis can be effected using intrapleural tetracycline, bleomycin, or talc. The latter chemical appears to be most effective, especially since tetracycline has become unavailable in the United States.

Pericardial Effusions. Symptomatic pericardial effusion secondary to metastatic disease from lung cancer can be treated by simple pericardial drainage, drainage followed by sclerosis of the pericardium, or the surgical creation of a pericardial window either by the subxiphoid laparotomy approach or anterior thoracotomy approach or using video-assisted thoracoscopic techniques. In all surgical approaches, a pericardial window is created, and a chest tube is inserted to complete the drainage of the pericardium.

Bronchial and Esophageal Obstruction. Extrinsic compression of a major airway or the esophagus sometimes complicates lung cancer that involves mediastinal lymph nodes. When minimal endobronchial disease is present, bronchoscopy or esophagoscopy to relieve such obstruction yields temporary relief. In such instances, insertion of endobronchial or endoesophageal stents may relieve the problem. Because of the proximity of the major airways to the esophagus, these stents may cause compression of the other organ. This is especially true when endoesophageal stenting is used, with resultant major airway compression. Such treatment, however, frequently yields excellent palliation of symptoms.

Palliative Resection. Palliative resection for uncontrolled symptoms rarely is indicated. Endobronchial obstruction with distal uncontrolled pneumonia or lung abscess can be treated by endoscopic removal of tumor or, in the case of lung abscess, percutaneous or transbronchoscopic drainage of the abscess. Massive hemoptysis may not respond to other therapeutic measures. It is rare that a palliative, incomplete surgical resection is required for patients presenting with these complications. In most instances, lesser procedures afford excellent palliation.

Invasion of tumors into vertebral bodies or the spinal canal may, on rare occasions, require surgical resection of all or part of the primary tumor plus the involved vertebral body to relieve uncontrollable pain or impending spinal cord damage. In most instances, such surgery provides palliation for only a short time.

REFERENCES

1. *Cancer facts and figures, 2000.* Atlanta: American Cancer Society, 2000.
2. Parkin DM. Trends in lung cancer worldwide. *Chest* 1989;96:5S.
3. Cullen JW. The National Cancer Institute's smoking, tobacco and cancer program. *Chest* 1989;96:9S.
4. Loeb LA, Ernster VL, Warner KE, et al. Smoking and lung cancer: an overview. *Cancer Res* 1984;44:5940.
5. Minna JD, Higgins GA, Glatstein EJ. Cancer of the lung. In: DeVita VT Jr, Hellman S, Rosenberg SA, eds. *Cancer: principles and practice of oncology,* 3rd ed. Philadelphia: JB Lippincott, 1989:597.
6. Mattson ME, Pollack ES, Cullen JW. What are the odds that smoking will kill you? *Am J Public Health* 1987;77:425.
7. Garfinkel L, Stellman SD. Smoking and lung cancer in women: findings in a prospective study. *Cancer Res* 1988;48:6951.
8. Cullen JW, McKenna JW, Massey MM. International control of smoking and the US experience. *Chest* 1986;89[Suppl 4]:2206.
9. Garfinkel L, Silverberg E. Lung cancer and smoking trends in the United States over the past 25 years. *CA Cancer J Clin* 1991;41:137.
10. Stellman SD, Garfinkel L. Smoking habits and tar levels in a new American Cancer Society prospective study of 1.2 million men and women. *J Natl Cancer Inst* 1986;76:1057.
11. Pierce JP, Fiore MC, Novotny TE. Trends in cigarette smoking in the United States: projections to the year 2000. *JAMA* 1989;261:61.
12. Masironi R, Rothwell K. Trends in and effects of smoking in the world. *World Health Stat Q* 1988;41:228.
13. Liu BQ, Petro R, Chen ZM, et al. Emerging tobacco hazards in China: 1. Retrospective proportional mortality study of one million deaths. *Br Med J* 1998;317:1399.
14. Hoffman D, Haley NJ, Brunnemann KD, et al. Cigarette sidestream smoke: formation, analysis and model studies on the uptake by non-smokers. Presented at the JS-Japan meeting on new etiology of lung cancer, Honolulu, HI, March 1983.
15. Wald NJ, Nanchahal K, Thompson SG, et al. Does breathing other people's smoke cause lung cancer? *Br Med J* 1986;293:1217.
16. Greenberg RA, Haley NJ, Etzel RA, et al. Measuring the exposure of infants to tobacco smoke: nicotine and cotinine in urine and saliva. *N Engl J Med* 1984;310:1075.
17. Janerich DT, Thompson WD, Varela LR, et al. Lung cancer and exposure to tobacco smoke in the household. *N Engl J Med* 1990;323:632.
18. Florin I, Rutberg L, Curvall M, et al. Screening of tobacco smoke constituents for mutagenicity using the Ames' test. *Toxicology* 1980;18:219.
19. Phillips DH, Hewer A, Martin CN, et al. Correlation of DNA adduct levels in human lung with cigarette smoking. *Nature* 1988;336:790.
20. Slebos RJC, Dalesio O, Mooi WJ, et al. Mutational activation of the K-ras oncogene is associated with smoking in adenocarcinoma of the lung. *Proc Am Soc Clin Oncol* 1991;10:244.
21. Slebos RJC, Ruban RH, Dalesio O, et al. Relationship between K-ras oncogene activity and smoking in adenocarcinoma of the human lung. *J Natl Cancer Inst* 1991;83:1024.
22. Westra WH, Slebos RJC, Offerhausg JA, et al. K-ras oncogenic activation in lung adenocarcinomas from former smokers: evidence that K-ras mutations are an early and irreversible event in the development of adenocarcinoma of lung. *Cancer* 1993;72:432.
23. Hecht SS, Hoffman D. Tobacco-specific nitrosamines: an important group of carcinogens in tobacco and tobacco smoke. *Carcinogenesis* 1988;9:875.
24. Castonguay A, Stoner GD, Schut HAJ, et al. Metabolism of tobacco-specific nitrosamines by cultured human tissues. *Proc Natl Acad Sci USA* 1983;80:6694.
25. Fraumeni JF Jr. Carcinogenesis: an epidemiological appraisal. *J Natl Cancer Inst* 1975;55:1039.
26. Fraumeni JF Jr, Blott WJ. Lung and pleura. In: Schottenfeld D, Fraumeni JF Jr, eds. *Cancer epidemiology and prevention.* Philadelphia: WB Saunders, 1982:564.
27. National Academy of Sciences. *Environmental tobacco smoke: measuring exposures and assessing health effects, appendix D.* Washington, DC: National Academy Press, 1986.
28. Seidman H, Selikoff I, Gelb S. Mortality experience of amosite asbestos factory workers: dose-response relationships 5–40 years after onset of short-term work exposure. *Am J Ind Med* 1986;10:479.
29. Kjuus H, Langard S, Skjaerven R. A case-referent study of lung cancer, occupational exposure and smoking: II. Role of asbestos exposure. *Scand J Work Environ Health* 1986;12:203.
30. Kjuus H, Langard S, Skjaerven R. A case-referent study of lung cancer, occupational exposure and smoking: I. Comparison of title-based and exposure-based occupational information. *Scand J Work Environ Health* 1986;12:193.
31. Selikoff IJ, Hammond EC, Seidman H. Mortality experience of insulation workers in the United States and Canada, 1943–76. *Ann N Y Acad Sci* 1979;330:91.
32. Robinson C, Lemen R, Wagoner JK. Mortality patterns, 1940–1975, among workers employed in an asbestos textile friction and packing products manufacturing facility. In: Lemen R, Dement JM, eds. *Dusts and disease.* Park Forest South, IL: Pathatox Publishers, 1979:131.
33. Armstrong BK, de Klerk NH, Musk AW, et al. Mortality in miners and millers of crocidolite in Western Australia. *Br J Ind Med* 1988;45:5.
34. McDonald AD, Fry JS, Woolley AJ, et al. Dust exposure and mortality in American chrysotile abestos friction products plant. *Br J Ind Med* 1984;41:151.
35. Finkelstein MM. Mortality among employees of an Ontario asbestos-cement factory. *Am Rev Respir Dis* 1984;129:754.
36. Talcott JA, Thruber WA, Kantor AF, et al. Asbestos-associated diseases in a cohort of cigarette-filter workers. *N Engl J Med* 1989;321:1220.
37. Omenn G, Merchant J, Boatmann E, et al. Contribution of environmental fibres to respiratory cancer. *Environ Health Perspect* 1986;70:51.
38. Kjuus H, Langard S, Skjaerven R. A case-referent study of lung cancer, occupational exposure and smoking: III. Etiologic fraction of occupational exposures. *Scand J Work Environ Health* 1986;12:210.
39. Weiss W. Asbestosis: a marker for the increased risk of lung cancer among workers exposed to asbestos. *Chest* 1999;115:320.
40. Fabrikant J. Radon and lung cancer: the BEIR IV report. *Health Physics* 1990;59:89.
41. Roscoe R, Steenland K, Halperin W, et al. Lung cancer mortality among nonsmoking uranium miners exposed to radon daughters. *JAMA* 1989;262:629.
42. Schoenberg J, Klotz J, Wilcox H, et al. Case-control study of residential radon and lung cancer among New Jersey women. *Cancer Res* 1990;50:6520.
43. Blot W, Zhao-Yi X, Boice J, et al. Indoor radon and lung cancer in China. *J Natl Cancer Inst* 1990;82:1025.
44. Letourneau EG, Krewski D, Choi MW, et al. Case-control study of residential radon and lung cancer in Winnipeg Manitoba Canada. *Ann J Epidemiol* 1994;140:310.
45. Lippman SM, Benner SE, Hong WK. Cancer chemoprevention. *J Clin Oncol* 1994;12(4):851.
46. Menkes MS, Cornstock GW, Vuilleumier JP, et al. Serum beta-carotene, vitamins A and E, selenium, and the risk of lung cancer. *N Engl J Med* 1986;315:1250.
47. Alpha-Tocopherol, Beta Carotene Cancer Prevention Study Group. The effect of vitamin E and beta carotene on the incidence of lung cancer and other cancers in male smokers. *N Engl J Med* 1994;330(15):1029.
48. Kvale G, Bjelke E, Gart JJ. Dietary habits and lung cancer risks. *Int J Cancer* 1983;31:397.
49. Knekt P, Aromaa A, Maatela J, et al. Serum selenium and subsequent risk of cancer among Finnish men and women. *J Natl Cancer Inst* 1990;82:864.
50. Shekelle R, Lepper M, Liu S. Dietary vitamin A and risk of cancer in the Western Electric Study. *Lancet* 1981;2:1185.
51. Lee JS, Lippman SM, Benner SE, et al. Randomized placebo-controlled trial of isotretinoin in chemoprevention of bronchial squamous metaplasia. *J Clin Oncol* 1994;12(5):937.
52. Hennekens CH, Buring JE, Manson JE, et al. Lack of effect of long-term supplementation with beta carotene on the incidence of malignant neoplasms and cardiovascular disease. *N Engl J Med* 1996;334(18):1145.
53. Omenn GS, Goodman GE, Thornquist MD, et al. Effects of a combination of beta carotene and vitamin A on lung cancer and cardiovascular disease. *N Engl J Med* 1996;334(18):1150.

54. Greenberg ER, Sporn MB. Antioxidant vitamins, cancer, and cardiovascular disease [Editorial]. *N Engl J Med* 1996;334(18):1189.
55. Bolla M, Lefur R, Ton Van J, et al. Prevention of second primary tumours with etretinate in squamous cell carcinoma of the oral cavity and oropharynx. Results of a multicentric double-blind randomised study. *Eur J Cancer* 1994;30A(6):767.
56. Stahelin HB, Gey KF, Eichholzer M, et al. Beta-carotene and cancer prevention: the Basel study. *Am J Clin Nutr* 1991;53[Suppl]:265S.
57. Virtamo J. Vitamins and lung cancer. *Proc Nutr Soc* 1999;58(2):329.
58. Willet WC, Polk BF, Underwood BA. Relation of serum vitamins A and E and carotenoids to the risk of cancer. *N Engl J Med* 1984;310:430.
59. Salonen JT, Alfthan G, Huttenen JK. Association between serum selenium and the risk of cancer. *Am J Epidemiol* 1984;120:342.
60. Clark LC, Combs GF, Turnbull BW, et al. Effects of selenium supplementation for cancer prevention in patients with carcinoma of the skin. *JAMA* 1996;272(24):1957.
61. Law MR, Hetzel Mr, Idel JR. Debrisoquine metabolism and genetic predisposition to lung cancer. *Br J Cancer* 1987;59:686.
62. Caporaso N, Hayes RB, Dosemeci M, et al. Lung cancer risk, occupational exposure, and the debrisoquine metabolic phenotype. *Cancer Res* 1989;49:3675.
63. Spelrs CJ, Murray S, Davies DS, et al. Debrisoquine oxidation phenotype and susceptibility to lung cancer. *Br J Clin Pharmacol* 1990;29:101.
64. Benltez J, Ladero JM, Jara C, et al. Polymorphic oxidation of debrisoquine in lung cancer patients. *Eur J Cancer* 1991;27:158.
65. Nakachi K, Imai K, Hayashi S, et al. Polymorphisms of the CYP1A1 and glutathione S-transferase genes associated with susceptibility to lung cancer in relation to cigarette dose in a Japanese population. *Can Res* 1993;53:2994.
66. Braun MM, Caporaso NE, Page WF, Hoover RN. Genetic component of lung cancer: cohort study of twins. *Lancet* 1994;344:440.
67. Ramalingam S, Pawlish K, Gadgeel S, et al. Lung cancer in young patients: analysis of a surveillance, epidemiology, and end results database. *J Clin Oncol* 1998;16(2):651.
68. Shaw GL, Falk RT, Pickle LW, et al. Lung cancer risk associated with cancer in relatives. *J Clin Epidemiol* 1991;44:429.
69. Heighway J, Thatcher N, Cerny T, et al. Genetic predisposition to human lung cancer. *Br J Cancer* 1986;53:453.
70. Chiba M, Takahashi T, Nau MM, et al. The patients in the p53 gene are frequent in primary resected non–small cell lung cancer. *Oncogene* 1990;5:1603.
71. Rusch V, Baselga J, Cordon-Cardo C, et al. Differential expression of the epidermal growth factor receptor and its ligands in primary non–small cell lung cancers and adjacent benign lung. *Cancer Res* 1993;53:2379.
72. Slebos R, Kibbelaar R, Dalesio O. K-RAS oncogene activation as a prognostic marker in adenocarcinoma of the lung. *N Engl J Med* 1990;323:561.
73. Mills NE, Fishman CL, Rom WN, et al. Increased prevalence of K-ras oncogene mutations in lung adenocarcinoma. *Cancer Res* 1995;55:1444.
74. Ebina M, Steinberg SM, Mulshine JL, et al. Relationship of p53 overexpression and up-regulation of proliferating cell nuclear antigen with the clinical course of non–small cell lung cancer. *Cancer Res* 1994;54:2496.
75. Siu LL, Hidalgo M, Nemunaitis J, et al. Dose and schedule-duration escalation of the epidermal growth factor receptor (EGFR) tyrosine kinase (TK) inhibitor CP-358, 774: a phase I and pharmacokinetic (PK) study. *Proc Am Soc Clin Oncol* 1999;18:388a(abst 1498).
76. Hammond L, Ranson M, Ferry D, et al. ZD 1839, an oral epidermal growth factor receptor (EGFR) tyrosine kinase inhibitor: first phase I, pharmacokinetic (PK) results in patients. *Proc Am Soc Clin Oncol* 1999;18:388a(abst 1500).
77. Roth JA. Molecular events in lung cancer. *Lung Cancer* 1995;12[Suppl 2]:S3.
78. Roth JA, Nguyen D, Lawrence DD, et al. Retrovirus-mediated wild-type p53 gene transfer to tumors of patients with lung cancer. *Nature Med* 1996;2(9):985.
79. Linnoila I. Pathology of non–small cell lung cancer: new diagnostic approaches. *Hematol Oncol Clin North Am* 1990;4(6):1027.
80. Roggli VI, Volmer RB, Greenberg, ST, et al. Lung cancer heterogeneity: a blinded and randomized study of 100 consecutive cases. *Hum Pathol* 1985;16:569.
81. Percy C, Horm JW, Goffman TE. Trends in histologic type of lung cancer, SEER, 1973–1981. In: Mizell M, Korrea P, eds. *Lung causes and prevention.* Deerfield Beach, FL: Verlag, Chemie International, 1984:153.
82. Clayton F. The spectrum and significance of bronchoalveolar carcinomas. *Pathol Annu* 1988;23:361.
83. Hammer SP, Bolan JW, Bockus D, et al. Ultrastructural and immunohistochemical features of common lung tumors: an overview. *Ultrastruct Pathol* 1985;9:283.
84. Souhami RL, Beverly PC, Bobrow LG. Antigens of small–cell lung cancer: first international workshop. *Lancet* 1987;2:325.
85. Matthews MJ. Problems in morphology and behavior of bronchopulmonary malignant disease. In: Israel I, Chahanian P, eds. *Lung cancer: natural history, prognosis and therapy.* New York: Academic Press, 1976:23.
86. Sorenson J, Badsberg J, Olsen J. Prognostic factors in inoperable adenocarcinoma of the lung: a multivariate regression analysis of 259 patients. *Cancer Res* 1989;49:5748.
87. Kris M, Gralla R, Potanovich L, et al. Assessment of pretreatment symptoms and improvement after edam + mitomycin + vinblastine (EMV) in patients (PTS) with inoperable non–small cell lung cancer (NSCLC). *Proc Am Soc Clin Oncol* 1990;9:229.
88. Redman BG, Pazdur R, Zingas AP, et al. Prospective evaluation of adrenal insufficiency in patients with adrenal metastasis. *Cancer* 1987;60:103.
89. Wade JL, Little AG, Vogelzang NJ, et al. Idiopathic pericardial effusions in patients with malignancy. *Proc Am Soc Clin Oncol* 1984;3:15.
90. Posner MR, Cohen AT, Skarin AT. Pericardial disease in patients with cancer. *Am J Med* 1981;71:407.
91. Mountain CF. A new international staging system for lung cancer. *Chest* 1986;89[Suppl]:225.
92. Watanabe Y, Shimizu J, Oda M, et al. Proposals regarding some deficiencies in the new international staging system for non–small cell lung cancer. *Jpn J Clin Oncol* 1991;21:160.
93. Naruke T, Goya T, Tsuchiya R, et al. Prognosis and survival in resected lung carcinoma based on the new international staging system. *J Thorac Cardiovasc Surg* 1988;96:440.
94. Mountain CF. Value of the new TNM staging system for lung cancer. *Chest* 1989;97:935.
95. Tockman MS, Gupa PK, Myers JD, et al. Sensitive and specific monoclonal antibody recognition of human lung cancer antigen on preserved sputum cells. *J Clin Oncol* 1988;6:1685.
96. Tockman MS, Erozan YS, Gupta P, et al. The early detection of second primary lung cancers by sputum immunostaining. *Chest* 1994;106[Suppl]:385S.
97. Tockman MS, Mulshine JL, Piantadosi S, et al. Prospective detection of preclinical lung cancer: results from two studies of heterogeneous nuclear ribonucleoprotein A2/B1 overexpression. *Clin Cancer Res* 1997;3:2237.
98. Melamed MR, Flehinger B, Zaman MB, et al. Detection of true pathologic stage I lung cancer in a screening program and the effect on survival cancer. *Cancer* 1981;47:1182.
99. Vlasbloem H, Schultz Kool LJ. AMBER: a scanning multiple-beam equalization system for chest radiography. *Radiology* 1988;169:29.
100. Wandtke JC, Plewes DB, McFaul JA. Improved pulmonary nodule detection with scanning equalization radiography. *Radiology* 1988;169:23.
101. Jolly PC, Hutchinson CH, Detterbeck F, et al. Routine computed tomographic scans, selective mediastinoscopy and other factors in evaluation of lung cancer. *J Thorac Cardiovasc Surg* 1991;102:226.
102. Dales RE, Stark RM Sankaranarayan AN. Computed tomography to stage lung cancer. *Am Rev Respir Dis* 1990;141:1096.
103. Fontana RS. Metaanalysis of computed tomography for staging non-small cell lung cancer [Editorial]. *Am Rev Respir Dis* 1990;141:1093.
104. Heelan R, Martini N, Westcot JW, et al. Carcinomas involving the hilum and mediastinum: computed tomographic and magnetic resonance evaluation. *Radiology* 1985;156:111.
105. Payne PY, Bronskill MJ, Henkelman RM, et al. Mediastinal lymph node metastases from bronchogenic carcinoma: detection with MR imaging and CT. *Radiology* 1987;162:651.
106. Batra P, Brown K, Collins JD, et al. Evaluation of intrathoracic extent of lung cancer by plain chest radiography, computed tomography and magnetic resonance imaging. *Am Rev Respir Dis* 1988;137:1456.
107. Kies MS, Baker AW, Kennedy PS. Radionuclide scans in staging of carcinoma of lung. *Surg Gynecol Obstet* 1978;147:175.
108. Little AG, DeMeester TR, Ryan JW. The use of radionuclide scans in lung cancer: gallium-67 scanning for preoperative staging. In: Kittle CF, ed. *Current controversies in thoracic surgery.* Philadelphia: WB Saunders, 1986:122.
109. Michel F, Soler M, Imhof E, et al. Initial staging of non–small cell lung cancer: value of routine radioisotope bone scanning. *Thorax* 1991;46:469.
110. Saunders CA, Dussek JE, O'Doherty MJ, et al. Evaluation of fluorine-18-fluorodeoxyglucose whole body positron emission tomography imaging in the staging of lung cancer. *Ann Thorac Surg* 1999;67:790.
111. Gambhir SS, Hoh CK, Phelps ME, et al. Decision tree sensitivity analysis for cost-effectiveness of FDG-PET in the staging and management of non–small cell lung cancer. *J Nucl Med* 1997;38:1173.
112. Rivera-Garcia R, White CS, Templeton PA. Lung cancer: value of various imaging modalities. *Clin Lung Cancer* 1999;1:130.
113. Wescott JL. Direct percutaneous needle aspiration of localized pulmonary lesions: results in 422 patients. *Radiology* 1980;137:31.
113a. Wang JP, Terry PB. Transbronchial needle apiration in the diagnosis of staging of bronchogenic carcinoma. *AM Rev Resp Dis* 1983;127:344.
113b. Harrow EM, Oldenburg FA, Lindenfelter MS, Smith AM. Transbronchial needle aspiration in clinical practice: a five year experience. *Chest* 1989;96:1268
114. Cripp AJ, DiMarco AF, Lankerani M. False-positive transbronchial needle aspiration in bronchogenic carcinoma. *Chest* 1984;85:696.
115. Luke WP, Pearson FG, Todd TRJ, et al. Prospective evaluation of mediastinoscopy for assessment of carcinoma of the lung. *J Thorac Cardiovasc Surg* 1986;91:53.
116. McCaughan JS, William TE Jr, Bethel BH. Photodynamic therapy of endobronchial tumors. *Lasers Surg Med* 1986;6:336.
117. Weigel TL, Meltzer CC, Friedman D, et al. *The role of positron emission tomography in evaluating the mediastinum in patients with non–small cell lung cancer.* Presented at the seventy-ninth annual meeting of the American Association for Thoracic Surgery, New Orleans, LA, April 18–21, 1999 (abst 23).
118. Ginsberg RJ, Rice TW, Goldberg M, et al. Extended cervical mediastinoscopy: a single staging procedure for bronchial carcinoma of the left upper lobe. *J Thorac Cardiovasc Surg* 1987;94:673.
119. McNiel TM, Chamberlain JM. Diagnostic anterior mediastinotomy. *Ann Thorac Surg* 1966;2:523.
120. Patterson GA, Piazza D, Pearson FG, et al. Significance of metastatic disease in subaortic lymph node. *Ann Thorac Surg* 1987;43:155.
121. Landreneau RJ, Mack MJ, Hazelrigg SR, et al. Video-assisted thoracic surgery: a minimally invasive approach to thoracic oncology. *PPO Update* 1994;8:1.
122. Ginsberg RJ. Thoracoscopy: a cautionary note. *Ann Thorac Surg* 1993;56:801.
123. Kirby TJ, Mack MJ, Landreneau RJ, et al. Lobectomy video-assisted thoracic surgery versus muscle-sparing thoracotomy: a randomized trial. *J Thorac Cardiovasc Surg* 1995;109:997.
124. Silvestri GA, Lippenberg B, Collice GL. The clinical evaluation for detecting metastatic lung cancer: a meta analysis. *Am J Respir Crit Care Med* 1995;152:225.
125. Strauss GM, Kwiatkowski DJ, Harpole DH, et al. Molecular and pathologic markers in stage 1 non-small-cell carcinoma of the lung. *J Clin Oncol* 1995;13:1265.
126. Kwiatkowski DJ, Harpole DH Jr, Godleski J, et al. Molecular pathologic substaging in 244 stage I non–small cell lung cancer patients: clinical implications. *J Clin Oncol* 1998;16: 2468.
127. Harpole DH, Herndon JE, Wolfe WG, et al. Prognostic model of recurrence and death in stage I non–small cell lung cancer utilizing presentation, histopathology, and oncoprotein expression. *Cancer Res* 1995;55:51.

128. Harpole DH. Commentary on "Prognostic markers in resected stage I and II non-small-cell lung cancer patients." *Clin Lung Cancer* 1999;1(1):68.
129. Mehdi SA, Tatum AH, Newman NB, et al. Prognostic markers in resected stage I and II non-small-cell lung cancer: an analysis of 260 patients with 5 year follow-up. *Clin Lung Cancer* 1999;1(1):59.
130. Salgia R, Skarin AT. Molecular abnormalities in lung cancer. *J Clin Oncol* 1998;16(3):1207.
131. Mountain CF. Revision in the international system for staging lung cancer. *Chest* 1997;111:1710.
132. Graziano SL. Non–small cell lung cancer: clinical value of new biological predictors. *Lung Cancer* 1997;17:S37.
133. Gall MH, Eagan RT, Feld R, et al. Prognostic factors in patients with resected stage I non–small cell lung cancer. A report from the Lung Cancer Study Group. *Cancer* 1984;54:1802.
134. Yu C, Shun C, Yang P, et al. Sialomucin expression is associated with erbB-2 oncoprotein overexpression, early recurrence, and cancer death in non–small cell lung cancer. *Am J Respir Crit Care Med* 1997;155:1419.
135. Linnoila RI, Piantadosi S, Ruckdeschel JC. Impact of neuroendocrine differentiation in non–small cell lung cancer. The LCSG experience. *Chest* 1994;106:367S.
136. Pastorino U, Andreola S, Tagliabue E, et al. Immunocytochemical markers in stage I lung cancer: relevance to prognosis. *J Clin Oncol* 1997;15:2858.
137. Kubuschok B, Passlick B, Izbicki JR, et al. Disseminated tumor cells in lymph nodes as a determinant for survival in surgically resected non-small-cell lung cancer. *J Clin Oncol* 1999;17(1):19.
138. Pantel K, Izbicki J, Passlick B, et al. Frequency and prognostic significance of isolated tumour cells in bone marrow of patients with non-small-cell lung cancer without overt metastases. *Lancet* 1996;347:649.
139. Green N, Kurohara SS, George FW. Cancer of the lung: an in-depth analysis of prognostic factors. *Cancer* 1971;28:1229.
140. Lanzotti VJ, Thomas DR, Boyle LE, et al. Survival with inoperable lung cancer: an integration of prognostic variables based on simple clinical criteria. *Cancer* 1977;39:303.
141. Stanley KE. Prognostic factors for survival in patients with inoperable lung cancer. *J Natl Cancer Inst* 1980;65:25.
142. Finkelstein DM, Ettinger DS, Ruckdeschel JC. Long-term survivors in metastatic non-small-cell lung cancer: an Eastern Cooperative Oncology Group study. *J Clin Oncol* 1986;4:702.
143. O'Connell JP, Kris MG, Gralla RJ, et al. Frequency and prognostic importance of pretreatment clinical characteristics in patients with advanced non-small-cell lung cancer treated with combination chemotherapy. *J Clin Oncol* 1986;4:1604.
144. Albain KS, Crowley JJ, LeBlanc M, Livingston RB. Survival determinants in extensive-stage non-small-cell lung cancer. The Southwest Oncology Group experience. *J Clin Oncol* 1991;9:1618.
145. Paesmans M, Sculier JP, Libert P, et al. Prognostic factors for survival in advanced non–small cell lung cancer: univariate and multivariate analyses including recursive partitioning and amalgamation algorithms in 1052 patients. *J Clin Oncol* 1995;13:1221.
146. Zimmerman PV, Bint MH, Hawson GAT, et al. Ploidy as a prognostic determinant in surgically treated lung cancer. *Lancet* 1987;2:530.
147. Volm M, Hahn EW, Mattern J, et al. Five-year follow-up study of independent clinical and flow cytometric prognostic factors for the survival of patients with non–small cell lung carcinoma. *Cancer Res* 1988;48:2923.
148. Hittelman WN. Clones and subclones in the lung cancer field. *J Natl Cancer Inst* 1999;91(21):1796.
149. Park I-W, Wistuba II, Maitra A, et al. Multiple clonal abnormalities in the bronchial epithelium of patients with lung cancer. *J Natl Cancer Inst* 1999;91(21):1863.
150. Kern J, Schwartz D, Nordberg J, et al. p185^{neu} expression in human lung adenocarcinomas predicts shortened survival. *Cancer Res* 1990;50:5184.
151. Kern J, Filderman A. Oncogenes and growth factors in human lung cancer. *Clin Chest Med* 1993;14:31.
152. Lee JS, Ro JY, Sahin AA, et al. Expression of blood-group antigen A: a favorable prognostic factor in non-small-cell lung cancer. *N Engl J Med* 1991;324:1084.
153. Rice TW, Tubbs RR, Hoeltge GA, et al. Expression of blood-group antigen A by stage I non–small cell lung carcinomas. *Ann Thorac Surg* 1995;59:568.
154. Dresler CN, Ritter JH, Wick MR, et al. Immunostains for blood-group antigens lack prognostic significance in T1 lung carcinomas. *Ann Thorac Surg* 1995;59:1069.
155. Miyake M, Taki T, Hitomi S, et al. Correlation of expression of H/Ley/Leb antigens with survival in patients with carcinoma of the lung. *N Engl J Med* 1992;327:14.
156. Graziano SL, Tatum AH, Newman NB, et al. The prognostic significance of neuroendocrine markers and carcinoembryonic antigen in patients with resected stage I and II non–small cell lung cancer. *Cancer Res* 1994;54:2908.
157. Graziano SL, Mazid R, Newman N, et al. The use of neuroendocrine immunoperoxidase markers to predict chemotherapy response in patients with non-small-cell lung cancer. *J Clin Oncol* 1989;7:1398.
158. Berendsen HH, de Leij L, Poppema S, et al. Clinical characterization of non-small-cell lung cancer tumors showing neuroendocrine differentiation features. *J Clin Oncol* 1989;7:1614.
159. Rodenhuis S, van de Wetering ML, Mooi WJ, et al. Mutational activation of the K-RAS oncogene: a possible pathogenetic factor in adenocarcinoma of the lung. *N Engl J Med* 1987;317:929.
160. Rosell R, Li S, Mate JL, et al. A prognostic impact of mutated k-ras gene in surgically resected non–small cell lung cancer patients. *Oncogene* 1993;8:2407.
161. Sugio K, Ishida T, Yokoyama H, et al. Ras gene mutations as a prognostic marker in adenocarcinoma of the lung without lymph node metastasis. *Cancer Res* 1992;52:2903.
162. Graziano SL, Gamble GP, Newman NB, et al. The prognostic significance of K-ras-codon 12 mutations in patients with resected stage I and II non–small cell lung cancer. *J Clin Oncol* 1999;17:668.
163. Sulzer MA, Leers MPG, Noord JAV, et al. Reduced E-cadherin expression is associated with increased lymph node metastasis and unfavourable prognosis in non–small cell lung cancer. *Am J Crit Care Med* 1998;157:1319.
164. Schiller JH, Adak S, Feins R, et al. Prognostic significance of p53 and K-RAS mutations in primary resected non–small cell lung cancer: preliminary results from a prospective randomized trial of postoperative adjuvant therapy (Intergroup Trial 0115). *Proc Am Soc Clin Oncol* 1999;18:464a(abst 1789).
165. Rodenhuis S, Boerrigter L, Top B, et al. Mutational activation of the K-ras oncogene and the effect of chemotherapy in advanced adenocarcinoma of the lung: a prospective study. *J Clin Oncol* 1997;15(1):285.
166. Cho JY, Kim JH, Lee YH, et al. Correlation between K-ras gene mutation and prognosis of patients with non–small cell lung carcinoma. *Cancer* 1997;79(3):462.
167. Apolinario RM, van der Valk P, de Jong JS, et al. Prognostic value of the expression of p53, bcl-2, and bax oncoproteins, and neovascularization in patients with radically resected non-small-cell lung cancer. *J Clin Oncol* 1997;15(6):2456.
168. Ohsaki Y, Toyoshima E, Fujiuchi S, et al. P53 protein expression in non–small cell lung cancers: correlation with survival time. *Clin Cancer Res* 1996;2:915.
169. Pantel K, Passlick B, Vogt J, et al. Reduced expression of plakoglobin indicates an unfavorable prognosis in subsets of patients with non-small-cell lung cancer. *J Clin Oncol* 1998;16(4):1407.
170. Pezzella F, Turley H, Kuzu I, et al. Bcl-2 protein in non–small cell lung carcinoma. *N Engl J Med* 1993;329:690.
171. Fontanini G, Vignati S, Bigini JD, et al. BCL-2 protein: a prognostic factor inversely correlated to p53 in non–small cell lung cancer. *Br J Cancer* 1995;71:1003.
172. Uramoto H, Osaki T, Inoue M, et al. Fas expression in non–small cell lung cancer: its prognostic effect in completely resected stage III patients. *Eur J Cancer* 1999;35(10):1462.
173. Weidner N, Semple JP, Welch WR, et al. Tumor angiogenesis and metastatic correlation in invasive breast carcinoma. *N Engl J Med* 1991;324:1.
174. Macchiarini P, Fontanini GM, Hardin MJ, et al. Relation of neovascularization to metastasis of non–small cell lung cancer. *Lancet* 1992;340:145.
175. Harpole DH, Richards WG, Herndon JE, et al. Angiogenesis and molecular biologic substaging in patients with stage I non—small cell lung cancer. *Ann Thorac Surg* 1996;61:1470.
176. Fontanini G, Lucchi M, Vignati S, et al. Angiogenesis as a prognostic indicator of survival in non–small cell lung cancer: a prospective study. *J Natl Cancer Inst* 1997;89:881.
177. Giatromanolaki A, Koukourakis MI, Theodossiou D, et al. Comparative evaluation of angiogenesis assessment with anti-factor-VIII and anti-CD31 immunostaining in non–small cell lung cancer. *Clin Cancer Res* 1997;3:2485.
178. Shibusa T, Shijubo N, Abe S. Tumor angiogenesis and vascular endothelial growth factor expression in stage I lung adenocarcinoma. *Clin Cancer Res* 1998;4:1483.
179. Berlin NI, Buncher CR, Fontana RS, et al. Early lung cancer detection: summary and conclusions. *Am Rev Respir Dis* 1984;30:565.
180. Berlin NI, Buncher CR, Fontana RS, et al. National Cancer Institute Cooperative Lung Cancer Detection Program: results of initial screen (prevalence)—Early Lung Cancer Detection. *Am Rev Respir Dis* 1984;130:545.
181. Strauss GM, Gleason RE, Sugarbaker DJ, et al. Chest x-ray screening improves outcome in lung cancer. A reappraisal of randomized trials on lung cancer screening. *Chest* 1995;107[Suppl 6]:270S.
182. Ohmatsu H, Kakinuma R, Nishiwaki Y, et al. Lung cancer screening with low-dose spiral CT. *Proc Am Soc Clin Oncol* 1999;18:1787(abst).
183. Henschke CI, McCauley DI, Yankelevitz DF, et al. Early lung cancer action project: overall design and findings from baseline screening. *Lancet* 1999;354:99.
184. Smith IE. Screening for lung cancer: time to think positive—a commentary. *Lancet* 1999;354:86.
185. Flehinger BJ. Kimmel M, Melamed MR. The effect of surgical treatment on survival from early lung cancer. Implications for screening. *Chest* 1992;101:1013.
186. Pilotti S, Ralk EF, Gribaudi D, et al. Sputum cytology for the diagnosis of carcinoma of the lung. *Acta Cytol* 1982;26:649.
187. Risse EKJ, Vooigis GP, Van't Hof MA. Diagnostic significance of "severe dysphagia" since sputum cytology. *Acta Cytol* 1988;32:629.
188. Shure D. Fiberoptic bronchoscopy: diagnostic application. *Clin Chest Med* 1987;8:1.
189. Lam S, Palcic D, McLean D, et al. Detection of early lung cancer using low dose Photofrin II. *Chest* 1990;97:333.
190. Kinse JH, Cortese DA. Endoscopic system for simultaneous visual examination and electronic detection of fluorescence. *Rev Sel Instrum* 1987;51:1403.
191. Lam S, Kennedy T, Unger M, et al. Localization of bronchial intraepithelial neoplastic lesions by fluorescence bronchoscopy. *Chest* 1998;113:696.
192. Weigel TL, Kosco PJ, Dacic S, et al. Fluorescence bronchoscopic surveillance in patients with a history of non–small cell lung cancer. *Diag Therap Endosc* 1999;6:1.
193. Cortese DA, Edell ES, Kinsey JH. Photodynamic therapy for early stage squamous cell carcinoma of the lung. *Mayo Clin Proc* 1997;72:595.
194. Hayata Y, Kato H, Komaka C, et al. Photoradiation therapy with hematoporphyrin derivative in early and stage I lung cancer. *Chest* 1984;86:169.
195. Edell ES, Cortese DA. Bronchoscopic localization and treatment of occult lung cancer. *Chest* 1989;96:919.
196. Hong WK, Endicott J, Itri LM. 13-Cis-retinoic acid in the treatment of oral leukoplakia. *N Engl J Med* 1986;315:1501.
197. Hong WK, Lippman SM, Itri LM, et al. Prevention of second primary tumors with isotretinoin in squamous-cell carcinoma of the head and neck. *N Engl J Med* 1990;323:795.
198. Reichl J. Assessment of operative risk of pneumonectomy. *Chest* 1972;62:570.
199. Taube K, Koniezko N. Prediction of postoperative cardiopulmonary function of patients undergoing pneumonectomy. *J Thorac Cardiovasc Surg* 1980;28:348.
200. Putman JB, Lammermeier DE, Colon R, et al. Predicted pulmonary function in survival after pneumonectomy for primary lung cancer. *Ann Thorac Surg* 1990;49:909.
201. Ginsberg RJ. Pre-operative assessment of the thoracic surgical patient: a surgeon's viewpoint. In: Pearson FG, Deslauriers J, Ginsberg RJ, et al., eds. *Thoracic surgery*, vol 1. New York: Churchill Livingstone, 1995:29.
202. Gass GD, Olsen GN. Preoperative pulmonary function testing to predict postoperative morbidity and mortality. *Chest* 1986;89:127.

203. Olsen GN, Block AJ, Swanson EW, et al. Pulmonary function evaluation of a lung resection candidate: a prospective study. *Am Rev Respir Dis* 1975;111:379.

204. Murphy TP, Casey MT. Determination of operability in candidates who undergo lung resection for bronchogenic carcinoma. *Can J Surg* 1990;33:470.

205. Ginsberg RJ, Rubinstein LV, Lung Cancer Study Group. Randomized trial of lobectomy versus limited resection for T1 N0 non–small cell lung cancer. *Ann Thorac Surg* 1995;60:615.

206. Korst RJ, Ginsberg RJ, Ailawadi M, et al. Lobectomy improves ventilatory function in selected patients with severe COPD. *Ann Thorac Surg* 1998;66:898.

207. Graham EA, Sedal JJ. Successful removal of the entire lung for carcinoma of the bronchus. *JAMA* 1933;101:1371.

208. Churchill ED, Sweet RH, Sutter L, et al. The surgical management of carcinoma of the lung: the study of cases treated at the Massachusetts General Hospital from 1930–50. *J Thorac Cardiovasc Surg* 1950;20:349.

209. Jensik RJ, Faber LD, Milloy FJ, et al. Segmental resection for lung cancer: a 15 year experience. *J Thorac Cardiovasc Surg* 1973;66:563.

210. Jensik RJ. The extent of resection for localized lung cancer: segmental resection. In: Kittle CF, ed. *Current controversies in thoracic surgery*. Philadelphia: WB Saunders, 1986:175.

210a. Read RC, Boop WC, Schaeffer RC. Survival after conservative resection for T1 N0 M0 non-small cell lung cancer. *Ann Thoracic Surg* 1990;49:391.

210b. Wain JC, Mathisen DJ, Hilgenberg AD, et al. Wedge and segmental resection for primary lung carcinomas. Proc *Am Assoc Thoracic Surg* 1991;May(abst).

211. Ginsberg RJ, Hill LD, Eagan RT, et al. Modern day operative mortality for surgical resection in lung cancer. *J Thorac Cardiovasc Surg* 1983;86:654.

212. Delauriers J, Ginsberg RJ, Dubois P, et al. Modern operative morbidity for elective surgical resection in lung carcinoma. *Can J Surg* 1989;32:335.

213. Le Chevalier T, Arriagada R, Quoix E, et al. Radiotherapy alone versus combined chemotherapy and radiotherapy in nonresectable non-small-cell lung cancer. First analysis of a randomized trial in 353 patients. *J Natl Cancer Inst* 1991;83:417.

214. Emami B. Three-dimensional conformal radiation therapy in bronchogenic carcinoma. *Semin Radiat Oncol* 1996;6:92.

215. Cox JD, Azarnia N, Byhardt RW, et al. A randomized phase I/II trial of hyperfractionated radiation therapy with total doses of 60.0 Gy to 79.2 Gy: possible survival benefit with greater than or equal to 69.6 Gy in favorable patients with Radiation Therapy Oncology Group stage III non-small-cell lung carcinoma: report of Radiation Therapy Oncology Group 83–11. *J Clin Oncol* 1990;8:1543.

216. Graham MV. Predicting radiation response. *Int J Radiat Oncol Biol Phys* 1997;39:561.

217. Hayman JA, Martel MK, Ten Haken RK, et al. Dose escalation in non–small cell lung cancer (NSCLC) using conformal 3-dimensional radiation therapy (C3DRT): update of a phase I trial. *Proc Am Soc Clin Oncol* 1999;18:459a(abst).

218. Rosenzweig KE, Hanley J, Mychalczak B, et al. Final report of the 70.2 Gy and 75.6 Gy dose levels of a phase I dose escalation study using three dimensional conformal radiotherapy in the treatment of inoperable lung cancer. *Int J Radiat Oncol Biol Phys* 1998;42:165(abst).

219. Munley MT, Marks LB, Scarfone C, et al. Multimodality nuclear medicine imaging in three-dimensional radiation treatment planning for lung cancer: challenges and prospects. *Lung Cancer* 1999;23:105.

220. Dische S, Saunders MI. Continuous, hyperfractionated accelerated radiotherapy (CHART): an interim report upon late morbidity. *Radiother Oncol* 1989;16:65.

221. Evans ML, Graham MM, Mahler PA, et al. Changes in vascular permeability following thoracic irradiation. *Radiat Res* 1986;107:262.

222. Rubin P, McDonald S, Maasilta P, et al. Serum markers for prediction of pulmonary radiation syndromes: I. Surfactant apoprotein. *Int J Radiat Oncol Biol Phys* 1989;17:553.

223. Anscher MS, Murase T, Prescott DM, et al. Changes in plasma TGF-β levels during pulmonary radiotherapy as a predictor of the risk of developing radiation pneumonitis. *Int J Radiat Oncol Biol Phys* 1994;30:671.

224. Marks LB. The pulmonary effects of thoracic radiation. *Oncology* 1994;8:89.

225. Martinet N, Vaillent P, Charles TH, et al. Dexamethasone modulation of tumor necrosis factor-alpha release by activated normal human alveolar macrophages. *Eur Respir J* 1992;5:67.

226. Steel GG. The search for therapeutic gain in the combination of radiotherapy and chemotherapy. *Radiother Oncol* 1988;11:31.

227. Von der Masse H, Overgaard JJ, Vaeth M. Effect of cancer chemotherapeutic drugs on radiation-induced lung damage in mice. *Radiother Oncol* 1986;5:245.

228. Roach M, 3rd, Gandara DR, Yuo HS, et al. Radiation pneumonitis following combined modality therapy for lung cancer: analysis of prognostic factors. *J Clin Oncol* 1995;13:2606.

229. Choy H. Esophagitis in combined modality therapy for locally advanced non–small cell lung cancer. *Semin Radiat Oncol* 1999;9:90.

230. Keller SM, Adak S, Wagner H, et al. Prospective randomized trial of postoperative adjuvant therapy in patients with completely resected stages II and IIIa non–small cell lung cancer: an intergroup trial (E3590). *Proc Am Soc Clin Oncol* 1999;18:465a(abst 1793).

231. Sadeghi A, Payne D, Rubestein L, et al. Combined modality treatment for resected non–small cell lung cancer: local control and recurrence. *Int J Radiat Oncol Biol Phys* 1988;15:89.

232. Eagan RT, Lee RR, Frytak S, et al. Thoracic radiation therapy and adriamycin/cisplatin-containing chemotherapy for locally advanced non–small cell lung cancer. *Cancer Clin Trials* 1981;2:381.

233. Umsawadi T, Valdivieso M, Barkley HT, et al. Esophageal complications from combined chemoradiotherapy (cyclophosphamide + Adriamycin + cisplatin + XRT) in the treatment of non–small cell lung cancer. *Int J Radiat Oncol Biol Phys* 1985;11:511.

234. Ball D, Bishop J, Smith J, et al. A phase III study of accelerated radiotherapy with and without carboplatin in non–small cell lung cancer: an interim toxicity analysis of the first 100 patients. *Int J Radiat Oncol Biol Phys* 1995;31:267.

235. Van Houtte P, Danheir S, Mornex F. Toxicity of combined radiation and chemotherapy in non–small cell lung cancer. *Lung Cancer* 1994;10[Suppl 1]:S271.

236. Sheline GE, William WW, Smith V. Therapeutic irradiation and brain injury. *Oncol Intell* 1980;6:1215.

237. McCunniff AJ, Liang MJ. Radiation tolerance of the cervical spinal cord. *Int J Radiat Oncol Biol Phys* 1989;16:675.

238. Jeremic B, Shibarnoto Y, Milicic B, et al. Absence of thoracic radiation myelitis after hyperfractionated radiation therapy with and without concurrent chemotherapy for stage III non small-cell lung cancer. *Int J Radiat Oncol Biol Phys* 1998;40:343.

239. Emami B, Lyman J, Brown A, et al. Tolerance of normal tissue to therapeutic irradiation. *Int J Radiat Oncol Biol Phys* 1991;21:109.

239a. Armstrong J, Raben A, Zelefsky M, et al. Promising survival with three-dimensional conformal radiation therapy for non–small cell lung cancer. *Radiother Oncol* 1997;44:17.

239b. Robertson JM, Ten Haken RK, Hazuka MB. Dose escalation for non–small cell lung cancer using conformal radiation therapy. *Int J Radiat Oncol Biol Phys* 1997;37:1079.

240. Kwa SL, Lebesque JV, Theuws JC, et al. Radiation pneumonitis as a function of mean lung dose: an analysis of pooled data of 540 patients. *Int J Radiat Oncol Biol Phys* 1998;42:1.

241. Derycke S, De Gersem WR, Van Duyse BB, De Neve WC. Conformal radiotherapy of stage III non–small cell lung cancer: a class solution involving non-coplanar intensity-modulated beams. *Int J Radiat Oncol Biol Phys* 1998;41:771.

242. Ekberg L, Holmberg O, Wiltgren L, Bjelkengren G, Landberg T. What margins should be added to the clinical target volume in radiotherapy treatment planning for lung cancer? *Radiother Oncol* 1998;48:71.

243. Ross CS, Hussey DH, Pennington EC, Stanford W, Doombos JF. Analysis of movement of intrathoracic neoplasms using ultrafast computerized tomography. *Int J Radiat Oncol Biol Phys* 1990;18:671.

244. Kubo HD, Hill BC. Respiration gated radiotherapy treatment: a technical study. *Phys Med Biol* 1996;41:83.

245. Ohara K, Okumura T, Akisada M, et al. Irradiation synchronized with respiration gate. *Int J Radiat Oncol Biol Phys* 1989;17:853.

246. Sontag MR, Merchant TE, Burnham B, Shah AB, Kun LE. Clinical experience with a system for pediatric respiratory gated radiotherapy. *Int J Radiat Oncol Biol Phys* 1998;42:140(abst).

247. Johnson LS, Hadley SW, Pelizzari CA. A video-based technique to gate radiotherapy treatments for respiration. *Int J Radiat Oncol Biol Phys* 1998;42:139(abst).

248. Hanley J, Debois MM, Mah D, et al. Deep inspiration breath-hold technique for lung tumors: the potential value of target immobilization and reduced lung density in dose escalation. *Int J Radiat Oncol Biol Phys* 1999;45:603.

249. Wong JW, Sharpe MB, Jaffray DA, et al. The use of active breathing control (ABC) to reduce margin for breathing motion. *Int J Radiat Oncol Biol Phys* 1999;44:911.

250. Uematsu M, Shioda A, Tahara, K. Focal, high dose, and fractionated modified stereotactic radiation therapy for lung carcinoma patients. *Cancer* 1998;82:1062.

251. Budach V. The role of fast neutrons in radiooncology: a critical reappraisal. *Strahlenther Onkol* 1991;176:677.

252. Koh WJ, Krall JM, Peters LJ, et al. Neutron vs. photon radiation therapy for inoperable regional non–small cell lung cancer: results of a multicenter randomized trial. *Int J Radiat Oncol Biol Phys* 1993;27:499

253. Nori D. Intraoperative brachytherapy in non–small cell lung cancer. *Semin Surg Oncol* 1993;9:99

254. Marchese M, Nori D, Anderson LL, et al. A versatile permanent planar implant technique utilizing I-125 seed embedded in Gelfoam. *Int J Radiat Oncol Biol Phys* 1981;194:747.

255. Nori D. Role of intraoperative brachytherapy in non–small cell lung cancer. In: Nori D, ed. *Proceedings of the International Conference on Thoracic Oncology*. New York: Booth Memorial Medical Center, 1991:43.

256. Raben A, Mychalczak B. Brachytherapy for non–small cell lung cancer and selected neoplasms of the chest. *Chest* 1997;112:276S.

257. Mehta, M, Shahabi S, Jarjour N, et al. Effect of endobronchial radiation therapy on malignant bronchial obstruction. *Chest* 1990;97:662.

258. Langendijk J, Tjwa M, de Jong J, et al. Massive haemoptysis after radiotherapy in inoperable non–small cell lung carcinoma: Is endobronchial brachytherapy really a risk factor? *Radiother Oncol* 1998;49:175.

259. Hennequin C, Tredaniel J, Chevert S, et al. Predictive factors for late toxicity after endobronchial brachytherapy: a multivariate analysis. *Int J Radiat Oncol Biol Phys* 1998;42:21.

260. Abe M, Takahishi M, Yabumoto E, et al. Clinical experiences with intraoperative radiotherapy of locally advanced cancers. *Cancer* 1980;45:40.

261. American Society of Clinical Oncology. Clinical practice guidelines for the treatment of unresectable non-small-cell lung cancer. *J Clin Oncol* 1997;15:2996.

262. Bunn PA, Kelly K. New chemotherapeutic agents prolong survival and improve quality of life in non–small cell lung cancer: a review of the literature and future directions. *Clin Cancer Res* 1998;5:1087.

263. Johnson DH. Treatment strategies for metastatic non-small-cell lung cancer. *Clin Lung Cancer* 1999;1:34.

264. Vokes EE, Bitran JD. Non-small cell lung cancer: towards the next plateau [Editorial]. *Chest* 1994;106:659.

265. Shepherd FA. Treatment of advanced non–small cell lung cancer. *Semin Oncol* 1994;21[Suppl 7]:7.

266. Gordon GS, Vokes EE. Chemoradiation for locally advanced, unresectable NSCLC. New standard of care, emerging strategies. *Oncology* 1999;13(8):1075.

267. Vokes EE. Interactions of chemotherapy and radiation. *Semin Oncol* 1993;20:70.

268. Lilenbaum RC, Green MR. Multimodality therapy for non-small-cell lung cancer. *Oncology* 1994;8:25.

269. Rossenthal DI, Pistenmaa DA, Glatstein E. A review of neoadjuvant chemotherapy for head and neck cancer: partially shrunken tumors may be both leaner and meaner. *Int J Radiat Oncol Biol Phys* 1993;28:315.

270. Vokes EE, Vijayakumar S, Bitran JD, et al. The role of systemic therapy in advanced non–small cell lung cancer: a review. *Am J Med* 1990;89:777.

271. Dillman R, Seagren S, Proprert K, et al. A randomized trial of induction chemotherapy plus high-dose radiation versus radiation alone in stage III non–small cell lung cancer. *N Engl J Med* 1990;323:940.

272. Le Chevalier T, Arriagada R, Lacombe-Terrier M-J, et al. Significant effect of adjuvant chemotherapy on survival in locally advanced non-small-cell lung carcinoma. *J Natl Cancer Inst* 1992;84:58.
273. Sause WT, Scott C, Taylor S, et al. Radiation Therapy Oncology Group (RTOG) 88–08 and Eastern Cooperative Oncology Group (ECOG) 4588: preliminary results of a phase III trial in regionally advanced, unresectable non-small-cell lung cancer. *J Natl Cancer Inst* 1995;87:198.
274. Albain KS, Rusch VW, Crowley JJ, et al. Concurrent cisplatin/etoposide plus chest radiotherapy followed by surgery for stages IIIA (N2) and IIIB non-small-cell lung cancer: mature results of Southwest Oncology Group phase II study 8805. *J Clin Oncol* 1995;13(8):1880.
275. Furuse K, Fukuoka M, Kawahara M, et al. Phase III study of concurrent versus sequential thoracic radiotherapy in combination with mitomycin, vindesine, and cisplatin in unresectable stage III non-small-cell lung cancer. *J Clin Oncol* 1999;17(9):2692.
276. Roth JA, Fosella F, Komaki R, et al. A randomized trial comparing perioperative chemotherapy and surgery with surgery alone in resectable stage IIIa non–small cell lung cancer. *J Natl Cancer Inst* 1994;86:673.
277. Rosell R, Gomez-Codina J, Camps C, et al. A randomized trial comparing preoperative chemotherapy plus surgery with surgery alone in patients with non–small cell lung cancer. *N Engl J Med* 1994;330:153.
278. Joss RA, Cavalli F, Goldhirsch A, et al. New agents in non–small cell lung cancer. *Cancer Treat Rev* 1984;11:205.
279. Robert F, Omura GA, Birch R, et al. Randomized phase III comparison of three doxorubicin-based chemotherapy regimens in advanced non–small cell lung cancer: a Southeastern Cancer Study Group trial. *J Clin Oncol* 1984;2:391.
280. Rosso R, Salvati F, Ardizzoni A, et al. Etoposide versus etoposide plus high-dose cisplatin in the management of advanced non–small cell lung cancer. *Cancer* 1990;66:130.
281. Sorensen JB, Clerici M, Hansen HH. Review: single-agent chemotherapy for advanced adenocarcinoma of the lung. *Cancer Chemother Pharmacol* 1988;21:89.
282. Klastersky J, Sculier J, Ravez P, et al. A randomized study comparing a high and a standard dose of cisplatin in combination with etoposide in the treatment of advanced non–small cell lung carcinoma. *J Clin Oncol* 1986;4:1780.
283. Shepard KV, Golomb HM, Bitran JD, et al. CAMP chemotherapy for metastatic non-oat cell bronchogenic carcinoma. *Cancer* 1985;56:2385.
284. Gandara D, Wold H, Perez E, et al. Cisplatin dose intensity in non–small cell lung cancer: phase II results of a day 1 and day 8 high-dose regimen. *J Natl Cancer Inst* 1989;81:790.
285. Longeval E, Klastersky J. Combination chemotherapy with cisplatin and etoposide in bronchogenic squamous cell carcinoma and adenocarcinoma. *Cancer* 1982;50:2751.
286. Kris M, Gralla R, Wertheim M, et al. Trial of the combination of mitomycin, vindesine, and cisplatin in patients with advanced non–small cell lung cancer. *Cancer Treat Rep* 1986;70:1091.
287. Eguchl K, Etou H, Miyachi S, et al. A study of dose escalation of teniposide (VM-26) plus cisplatin (CDD) with recombinant human granulocyte colony-stimulating factor (rhG-CSF) in patients with advanced small cell lung cancer. *Eur J Cancer* 1994;30A:188.
288. Graziano SL, Herndon JE, Richards F, et al. A phase I trial of ifosfamide, mesna, and cisplatin in advanced non–small cell lung cancer: a Cancer and Acute Leukemia Group B study. *Cancer* 1993;72:62.
289. Krigel RL, Palackdharry CS, Padavic K, et al. Ifosfamide, carboplatin, and etoposide plus granulocyte-macrophage colony-stimulating factor: a phase I study with apparent activity in non-small-cell lung cancer. *J Clin Oncol* 1994;12:1251.
290. Schulman P, Budman DR, Weiselberg L, et al. Phase II trial of mitomycin, vinblastine, and cisplatin (MVP) in non–small cell bronchogenic carcinoma. *Cancer Treat Rep* 1983;67:943.
291. Lynch TJ Jr, Kalish LA, Kass F, et al. Continuous-infusion cisplatin, 5-fluorouracil, and leucovorin for advanced non–small cell lung cancer. *Cancer* 1994;73:1171.
292. Vokes EE, Lyss AP, Herndon JE II, et al. Intravenous 6-thioguanine or cisplatin, fluorouracil and leucovorin for advanced non–small cell lung cancer: a randomized phase II study of the cancer and leukemia group B. *Ann Oncol* 1992;3:727.
293. Jett JR. Current treatment of unresectable lung cancer. *Mayo Clin Proc* 1993;68:603.
294. Gralla R, Casper E, Kelsen D. Cisplatin plus vindesine combination chemotherapy for advanced carcinoma of the lung: a randomized trial investigating two dosage schedules. *Ann Intern Med* 1981;95:414.
295. Gandara DR, Crowley J, Livingston RB, et al. Evaluation of cisplatin intensity in metastatic non-small-cell lung cancer: a phase III study of the Southwest Oncology Group. *J Clin Oncol* 1993;11:873.
296. Ruckdeschel J, Findelstein D, Ettinger D, et al. A randomized trial of the four most active regimens for metastatic non–small cell lung cancer. *J Clin Oncol* 1986;4:14.
297. Bonomi P, Finkelstein D, Ruckdeschel J, et al. Combination chemotherapy versus single agents followed by combination chemotherapy in stage IV non–small cell lung cancer: a study of the Eastern Cooperative Oncology Group. *J Clin Oncol* 1989;7:1602.
298. Fishbein GE. Immunotherapy of lung cancer. *Semin Oncol* 1993;20:351.
299. Ruckdeschel J, Codish S, Stranahan A, et al. Postoperative empyema improves survival in lung cancer: documentation and analysis of a natural experiment. *N Engl J Med* 1972;287:1013.
300. McKneally M, Maver C, Kausel H. Regional immunotherapy of lung cancer with intrapleural B.C.G. *Lancet* 1976;1:377.
301. Ludwig Lung Cancer Study Group. Immunostimulation with intrapleural BCG as adjuvant therapy in resected non-small cell lung cancer. *Cancer* 1986;58:2411.
302. Anthony H. Yorkshire trial of adjuvant therapy with levamisole in surgically treated lung cancer. In: Terry W, Rosenberg S, eds. *Immunotherapy of human cancer.* New York: Elsevier North Holland, 1982:135.
303. Amery W, Cosemans J, Gooszen H, et al. Four year results from double-blind study of adjuvant levamisole treatment in resectable lung cancer. In: Terry W, Rosenberg S, eds. *Immunotherapy of human cancer.* New York: Elsevier North Holland, 1982:123.
304. Holmes E, Gail M. Surgical adjuvant therapy for stage II and stage III adenocarcinoma and large-cell undifferentiated carcinoma. *J Clin Oncol* 1986;4:710.
305. Krown S, Stoopler M, Gralla R, et al. Phase II trial of human leukocyte interferon in non–small cell lung cancer: preliminary results. In: Terry W, Rosenberg S, eds. *Immunotherapy of human cancer.* New York: Elsevier North Holland, 1982:397.
306. Grunberg S, Kempf R, Itri L. Phase II study of recombinant alpha interferon in the treatment of advanced non–small cell lung carcinoma. *Cancer Treat Rep* 1985;69:1031.
307. McDonald S, Chang AY, Rugin P, et al. Combined betaseron R (recombinant human interferon beta) and radiation for inoperable non–small cell lung cancer. *Int J Radiat Oncol Biol Phys* 1993;27:613.
308. Schiller J, Storer B, Dreicer R, et al. Randomized phase II–III trial of combination beta and gamma interferons and etoposide and cisplatin in inoperable non–small cell cancer of the lung. *J Natl Cancer Inst* 1989;81:1739.
309. Wadler S, Schwartz E. Antineoplastic activity of the combination of interferon and cytotoxic agents against experimental and human malignancies: a review. *Cancer Res* 1990;50:3473.
310. Bowman A, Ferguson RJ, Allan SG, et al. Potentiation cis-platinum by alpha-interferon in advanced non–small cell lung cancer: a phase II study. *Ann Oncol* 1990;1:351.
311. Kataja V, Yap A, for the NSCLC Collaborative Study Group. Combination of cisplatin and interferon alpha IIa in patients with non–small cell lung cancer: an open phase II multicentre trial. *Eur J Cancer* 1995;31A:35.
312. Athanasladis I, Kies MS, Miller M, et al. Phase II study of all-*trans*-retinoic acid and α-interferon in patients with advanced non–small cell lung cancer. *Clin Cancer Res* 1995;1:973.
313. Vokes EE, Figlin R, Hochester H, et al. A phase II study of recombinant human interleukin-4 for advanced or recurrent non–small cell lung cancer. *Cancer J Sci Am* 1998;4:46.
314. Martini N, Flehinger BJ. The role of surgery in N2 lung cancer. *Surg Clin North Am* 1987;67:1037.
315. Naruke T, Goya T, Tsuchiya R, et al. The importance of surgery to non–small cell carcinoma of the lung with mediastinal lymph node metastases. *Ann Thorac Surg* 1988;46:603.
316. Izbicki JR, Thetter O, Habekost M, et al. Radical systematic mediastinal lymphadenectomy in non–small cell lung cancer: a randomized controlled trial. *Br J Surg* 1994;81:229.
317. Warren WH, Faber LP. Segmentectomy vs lobectomy in patients with stage I pulmonary carcinoma: five-year survival and patterns of intrathoracic recurrence. *J Cardiovasc Surg* 1994;107:1087.
318. Takizawa T, Haga M, Yagi N, et al. Pulmonary function after segmentectomy for small peripheral carcinoma of the lung. *J Thorac Cardiovasc Surg* 1999;118:536.
319. Downey RJ, Martini N, Rusch VW, et al. Extent of chest wall invasion and survival in patients with lung cancer. *Ann Thorac Surg* 1999;68:188.
320. Hilaris BS, Martini N, Wong GY, et al. Treatment of superior sulcus tumor (Pancoast tumor). *Surg Clin North Am* 1987;67:965.
321. Ginsberg RJ, Martini N, Zaman M, et al. The influence of surgical resection and intraoperative brachytherapy in the management of superior sulcus tumor. *Ann Thorac Surg* 1994;57:1440.
322. Dartevelle P, Macchiarini P. Surgical management of superior sulcus tumors. *Oncologist* 1999;4:398.
323. Burt ME, Pomerantz AH, Bains MS. Results of surgical treatment of stage III lung cancer invading the mediastinum. *Surg Clin North Am* 1987;67:987.
324. Martini N, Yellin A, Ginsberg RJ, et al. Management of non–small cell lung cancer with direct mediastinal involvement. *Ann Thorac Surg* 1994;58:1447.
325. Deslauriers J, Gaulin P, Beaulieu M, et al. Long term clinical and functional results of sleeve lobectomy for primary lung cancer. *J Thorac Cardiovasc Surg* 1986;92:871.
326. Weksler B, Bains MS, Burt ME, et al. Brief communication—resection of lung cancer invading the diaphragm. *J Thorac Cardiovasc Surg* 1997;114:500.
327. Naruke T, Goya T, Tsuchiya R, Suemasu K. The importance of surgery to non–small cell carcinoma of the lung with mediastinal lymph node metastasis. *Ann Thorac Surg* 1988;46:603.
328. Martini N, Flehinger BJ, Zaman MB, Beattie JB. Results of resection in non–oat cell carcinoma of the lung with mediastinal lymph node metastasis. *Ann Surg* 1983;198:386.
329. Martini N, Flehinger BJ. The role of surgery in N2 lung cancer. Surg *Clin North Am* 1987;67:1037.
330. Shields TW. The significance of ipsilateral mediastinal lymph node metastasis (N2 disease) in non–small cell carcinoma of the lung. *J Thorac Cardiovasc Surg* 1990;99:48.
331. Martini N, Flehinger BJ, Nagasaki F, Hart B. Prognostic significance of NI disease in carcinoma of the lung. *J Thorac Cardiovasc Surg* 1983;86:646.
332. Lung Cancer Study Group. Effects of postoperative mediastinal radiation on completely resected stage II and stage III epidermoid carcinoma of the lung. *N Engl J Med* 1986;315:1377.
333. Feld R, Rubinstein L, Weisenberger TH, Lung Cancer Study Group. Sites of recurrence in resected stage I non–small cell lung cancer: a guide for future studies. *J Clin Oncol* 1985;2:1352.
334. Pairolero PC, Williams DE, Bergstralh MS, et al. Post-surgical stage I bronchogenic carcinoma: morbid implications of recurrent disease. *Ann Thorac Surg* 1984;38:331.
335. Bangma P. Post-operative radiotherapy. In: Deeley T, ed. *Carcinoma of the bronchus: modern radiotherapy.* New York: Appleton-Century-Crofts, 1972:163.
336. Paterson R, Russell M. Clinical trials in malignant disease: IV. Lung cancer: value of post-operative radiotherapy. *Clin Radiol* 1962;13:141.
337. Van Houtte P, Rocmans P, Smets P, et al. Postoperative radiation therapy in lung cancer: a controlled trial after resection of curative design. *Int J Radiat Oncol Biol Phys* 1980;6:983.
338. Dautzenberg B, Arriagad R, Chammard A, et al. A controlled study of postoperative radiotherapy for patients with completely resected non–small cell lung carcinoma. *Cancer* 1999;86:265.
339. Stewart L. Postoperative radiotherapy in non–small cell lung cancer: systematic review and meta-analysis of individual patient data from nine randomized controlled trials. *Lancet* 1998;352:257.
340. The Ludwig Cancer Study Group. Patterns of failure in patients with resected stage I and II non-small-cell carcinoma of the lung. *Ann Surg* 1987;205:67.
341. Stephens R, Girling D, Bleehen N, et al. The role of post-operative radiotherapy in non–small cell lung cancer: a multicenter randomized trial in patients with pathologically staged T1–2 N1–2, M0 disease. *Br J Cancer* 1996;74:632.

342. Piehler JM, Pairolero PC, Weiland LH, et al. Bronchogenic carcinoma with chest wall invasion: factors affecting survival following en bloc resection. *Ann Thorac Surg* 1982;34:684.

342a. Paone JF, Spees EK, Newton CG, et al. An appraisal of en bloc resection of peripheral bronchogenic carcinoma involving the Thoracacic wall. *Chest* 1982;81:203.

342b. Patterson GA, Ilves R, Ginsberg RJ, et al. The value of adjuvant radiotherapy in pulmonary and chest wall resection for bronchogenic carcinoma. *Ann Thorac Surg* 1982;34:692.

342c. Van de Wal HJ, Lacquet LK, Jongerius CM. Chirurgische behandeling van longtumoren met doorgroei in de Thoracaxwand. *(Belg) Tijdschr voor Geneeskunde* 1987;43:91.

342d. Allen MS, Mathisen DJ, Grillo HC, et al. Bronchogenic carcinoma with chest wall invasion. *Ann Thorac Surg* 1991;51:948.

343. McCaughan BC. Primary lung cancer invading the chest wall. *Chest Surg Am* 1994;4:17.

344. Gebitekin C, Guipta NK, Satur CM, et al. Fate of patients with residual tumor at the bronchial resection margin. *Eur J Cardiothorac Surg* 1994;8:339.

345. Law MR, Henk JM, Lennox SC, et al. Value of radiotherapy for tumour on the bronchial stump after resection for bronchial carcinoma. *Thorax* 1982;37:496.

346. Kaiser LR, Fleshner P, Keller S, et al. Significance of extramucosal residual tumor at the bronchial resection margin. *Ann Thorac Surg* 1989;47:265.

347. Chen A, Galloway M, Landreneau R, et al. Intraoperative 1251 brachytherapy for high-risk stage I non–small cell lung carcinoma. *Int J Radiat Oncol Biol Phys* 1999;44(5):1057.

348. Vokes EE, Vijayakumar S, Bitran JD, et al. The role of systemic therapy in advanced non–small cell lung cancer: a review. *Am J Med* 1990;89:777.

349. Ihde DC. Is there a place for classical adjuvant treatment? *Lung Cancer* 1994;11[Suppl 3]:S111.

350. Lad T, Rubinstein L, Sadeghi A, et al. The benefit of adjuvant treatment of resected locally advanced non–small cell lung cancer. *J Clin Oncol* 1988;6:9.

351. Niiranen A, Niitamo-Korhonen S, Kouri M, et al. Adjuvant chemotherapy after radical surgery for non–small cell lung cancer: a randomized study. *J Clin Oncol* 1992;10:1927.

352. Non–Small Cell Collaborative Group. Chemotherapy in non–small cell lung cancer: a meta analysis using updated data on individual patients from 52 randomized clinical trials. *Br Med J* 1995;311:899.

353. Wada H, Hitomi S, Teramatsu T, et al. Adjuvant chemotherapy after complete resection in non–small cell lung cancer. *J Clin Oncol* 1996;14:1048.

354. Bromley LL, Szur L. Combined radiotherapy and resection for carcinoma of the bronchus. *Lancet* 1955;5:937.

355. Bloedorn FG, Cowley RA, Cuccia CA, et al. Preoperative irradiation in bronchogenic carcinoma. *Am J Roentgenol Radiat Ther Nucl Med* 1964;92:77.

356. Shields TW, Higgins GA, Lawton R, et al. Preoperative x-ray therapy as an adjuvant in the treatment of bronchogenic carcinoma. *J Thorac Cardiovasc Surg* 1970;59:49.

357. Warram J. Preoperative irradiation of cancer of the lung: final report of the therapeutic trial. *Cancer* 1975;36:914.

358. Takita H, Regal A, Antkowiak J, et al. Chemotherapy followed by lung resection in inoperable non–small cell lung carcinomas due to locally far-advanced disease. *Cancer* 1986;57:630.

359. Raut Y, Huu N, Clavier J, et al. Surgery and chemotherapy: a new method of treatment for squamous cell bronchial carcinoma. *J Thorac Cardiovasc Surg* 1984;88:754.

360. Martini N, Flehinger B, Zaman M, et al. Prospective study of 445 lung carcinomas with mediastinal lymph node metastases. *J Thorac Cardiovasc Surg* 1980;80:390.

361. Martini N, Flehinger B, Zaman M, et al. Results of resection in non–oat cell carcinoma of the lung with mediastinal lymph node metastases. *Ann Surg* 1983;198:386.

362. Pisters K, Kris M, Gralla R, et al. Preoperative chemotherapy in stage IIIA non–small cell lung cancer: an analysis of a trial in patients with clinically apparent mediastinal node involvement. In: Salmin S, ed. *Adjuvant therapy of cancer VI.* Philadelphia: WB Saunders, 1990:133.

363. Burkes R, Ginsberg R, Shepherd F, et al. Neo-adjuvant trial with MVP (mitomycin-C + vindesine + cisplatin) chemotherapy for stage III (T1–3, N2 M0) unresectable non–small cell lung cancer (NSCLC). *Proc Am Soc Clin Oncol* 1989;8:221.

364. Pass HI, Pogrebniak HW, Steinberg SM, et al. Randomized trial of neoadjuvant therapy for lung cancer: interim analysis. *Ann Thorac Surg* 1992;53:992.

365. Depierre A, Milleron B, Moro D, et al. Phase III trial of neoadjuvant chemotherapy (NCT) in resectable stage I (except T1N0), II, IIIa non–small cell lung cancer (NSCLC): the French experience. *Proc Am Soc Clin Oncol* 1999;18:465a(abst 1792).

366. Pisters KMW, Ginsberg RJ, Bunn PA, et al. (for the Bimodality Lung Oncology Team BLOT). Induction chemotherapy prior to surgery for early stage lung cancer-a novel approach. *J Thorac Cardiovasc Surg* 2000;119:429..

367. Faber L, Kittle C, Warren W, et al. Preoperative chemotherapy and irradiation for stage III non–small cell lung cancer. *Ann Thorac Surg* 1989;47:669.

368. Weiden P, Piantadosi S. Preoperative chemoradiotherapy in stage III non–small cell lung cancer (NSCLC): a phase II study of the Lung Cancer Study Group (LCSG). *Proc Am Soc Clin Oncol* 1988;7:197.

369. Eagan R, Ruud C, Lee R, et al. Pilot study of induction therapy with cyclophosphamide, doxorubicin, and cisplatin (CAP) and chest irradiation prior to thoracotomy in initially inoperable stage III M0 non–small cell lung cancer. *Cancer Treat Rep* 1987;71:895.

370. Strauss G, Sherman L, Mathisen D, et al. Concurrent chemotherapy (CT) and radiotherapy (RT) followed by surgery (S) in marginally resectable stage IIIA non–small cell carcinoma of the lung (NSCLC): a cancer and leukemia group B study. *Proc Am Soc Clin Oncol* 1988;7:203.

371. Albain K, Rusch V, Crowley J, et al. Concurrent cisplatin (DDP) VP-16 and chest, irradiation (RT) followed by surgery for stages IIIa and IIIb non–small cell lung cancer (NSCLC): a Southwest Oncology Group (SWOG) study 8805. *Proc Am Soc Clin Oncol* 1991;10:244.

372. Skarin A, Jochelson M, Sheldon T, et al. Neoadjuvant chemotherapy in marginally resectable stage III M0 non–small cell lung cancer: long-term follow-up in 41 patients. *J Surg Oncol* 1989;40:266.

373. Sherman D, Strauss G, Schwartz J, et al. Combined modality therapy for regionally advanced stage III non–small cell carcinoma of the lung (NSCLC) employing neo-adjuvant chemotherapy (CT), radiotherapy (RT), and surgery (S). *Proc Am Soc Clin Oncol* 1978;6:167.

374. Albain KS. Induction therapy followed by definitive local control for stage III non–small cell lung cancer: a review, with focus on recent trimodality trials. *Chest* 1993;103[Suppl]:43S.

375. Choi NC, Carey RW, Daly W, et al. Potential impact on survival of improved tumor downstaging and resection rate by preoperative twice-daily radiation and concurrent chemotherapy in stage IIIa non–small cell lung cancer. *J Clin Oncol* 1997;15:712.

376. Grunenwald D, Le Chavalier T, Arriagada R, et al. Surgical resection of stage IIIb non–small cell lung cancer after concomitant induction chemotherapy: preliminary results of a pilot study. *Proc Am Soc Clin Oncol* 1995;14:349(abst).

377. Eberhardt W, Wilke H, Stamatis G. Preoperative chemotherapy followed by concurrent chemoradiation therapy based on hyperfractionated accelerated radiotherapy and definitive surgery in locally advanced non–small cell lung cancer: mature results of a phase II trial. *J Clin Oncol* 1998;16:622.

378. Bleehen N, Ball D, Belani C, et al. Combined radiation and chemotherapy for unresectable non–small cell lung carcinoma. *Lung Cancer* 1994;10[Suppl 1]:S19.

379. Choi N, Kanarek D. Toxicity of thoracic radiotherapy on pulmonary function in lung cancer. *Lung Cancer* 1994;10[Suppl 1]:S219.

380. Choi N, Kanarek D, Grillo H. Effect of postoperative radiotherapy on changes in pulmonary function in patients with stage II and IIIA lung carcinoma. *Int J Radiat Oncol Biol Phys* 1990;18:95.

381. Marks LB, Munley MT, Bentel GC, et al. Physical and biological predictors of changes in whole-lung function following thoracic irradiation. *Int J Radiat Oncol Biol Phys* 1997;39:563.

382. Cox JD, Azarnia N, Byhardt RW, et al. A randomized phase I/II trial of hyperfractionated radiation therapy with total doses of 60.0 Gy to 79.2 Gy: possible survival benefit with greater than or equal to 69.6 Gy in favorable patients with Radiation Therapy Oncology Group stage III non-small-cell lung carcinoma: report of Radiation Therapy Oncology Group 83–11. *J Clin Oncol* 1990;8:1543.

383. Dosoretz E, Galmanari D, Rubenstein JH, et al. Local control in medically inoperable lung cancer: an analysis of its importance in outcome and factors determining the probability of tumor eradication. *Int J Radiat Oncol Biol Phys* 1993;27:507.

384. Haffty BG. Is radiation therapy a viable alternative to surgery in early stage lung cancer [Editorial]? *Int J Radiat Oncol Biol Phys* 1990;19:223.

385. Haffty BG, Goldberg NB, Gerstley J, et al. Results of radical radiation therapy in clinical stage I, technically operable non–small cell lung cancer. *Int J Radiat Oncol Biol Phys* 1988;15:69.

386. Hilton G. Present position relating to cancer of the lung: results with radiotherapy alone. *Thorax* 1960;15:17.

387. Holsti L, Mattson K. A randomized study of split-course radiotherapy of lung cancer: long-term results. *Int J Radiat Oncol Biol Phys* 1980;6:977.

388. Krol AD, Aussems P, Noordijk EM, et al. Local irradiation alone for peripheral Stage I lung cancer: Could we omit the elective regional nodal irradiation? *Int J Radiat Oncol Biol Phys* 1996;34:297.

389. Perez CA, Pajak TF, Rubin P, et al. Long-term observations of the pattern of failure in patients with unresectable non–oat cell carcinoma of the lung treated with definitive radiotherapy. *Cancer* 1987;59:1874.

390. Smart J. Can lung cancer be cured by irradiation alone? *JAMA* 1965;195:1034.

391. Talton BM, Constable WC, Kersch CR. Curative radiotherapy in non–small cell carcinoma of the lung. *Int J Radiat Oncol Biol Phys* 1990;19:15.

392. Zhang KX, Yin WB, Zhang LJ, et al. Curative radiotherapy of early operable non–small cell lung cancer. *Radiother Oncol* 1989;14:89.

393. Sandler HM, Curran WJ, Turrisi AT. The influence of tumor size and pretreatment staging in outcome following radiation therapy alone for stage I non–small cell lung cancer. *Int J Radiat Oncol Biol Phys* 1990;19:9.

394. Sibley GS, Jamieson TA, Marks LB, Anscher MS, Prosnitz LR. Radiotherapy alone for medically inoperable stage I non-small-cell lung cancer: the Duke experience. *Int J Radiat Oncol Biol Phys* 1998;40:149.

395. Graham PH, Glebski VJ, Stat M. Radical radiotherapy for early non–small cell lung cancer. *Int J Radiat Oncol Biol Phys* 1995;31:261.

396. Kaskowitz L, Graham MV, Emami B, Halverson KJ, Rush C. Radiation therapy alone for stage I non–small cell lung cancer. *Int J Radiat Oncol Biol Phys* 1993;27:517.

397. Morita K, Fuwa N, Suzuki Y, et al. Radical radiotherapy for medically inoperable non–small cell lung cancer in clinical stage I: a retrospective analysis of 149 patients. *Radiother Oncol* 1997;42:31.

398. Gauden S, Ramsey J, Tripcony L. The curative treatment by radiotherapy alone of stage I non–small cell lung cancer of the lung. *Chest* 1995;108:1278.

399. Sawyer TE, Bonner JA, Gould PM, et al. Predictors of subclinical nodal involvement in clinical stages I and II non–small cell lung cancer: implications in the inoperable and three-dimensional dose-escalation settings. *Int J Radiat Oncol Biol Phys* 1999;43:965.

400. Jeremic B, Shibamoto Y, Acimovic L, et al. Hyperfractionated radiotherapy alone for clinical stage I non–small cell lung cancer. *Int J Radiat Oncol Biol Phys* 1997;38:521.

401. Morrison R, Deeley TJ, Cleland WP. The treatment of carcinoma of the bronchus: a clinical trial to compare surgery and supervoltage radiotherapy. *Lancet* 1963;30:683.

402. Armstrong JG, Minsky BD. Primary radiation therapy for stage I and II medically inoperable non–small cell lung cancer. *Cancer Treat Rev* 1989;16:247.

403. Vansteenkiste JF, Stroobants SG, De Leyn PR. Lymph node staging in non–small cell lung cancer with FDG-PET scan: a prospective study on 690 lymph node stations from 68 patients. *J Clin Oncol* 1998;16:2142.

404. Hilaris BS. Lung brachytherapy. *Chest Surg Clin North Am* 1994;4:45.

405. Hilaris BS, Martini N. The current state of intraoperative interstitial brachytherapy in lung cancer. *Int J Radiat Oncol Biol Phys* 1988;15:1347.

406. Perol M, Caliandro R, Pommier P, et al. Curative irradiation of limited endobronchial carcinoma with high-dose rate brachytherapy. *Chest* 1997;111:1417.

407. Tredaniel J, Henneuin C, Zalcman G, et al. Prolonged survival after high-dose rate endobronchial radiation for malignant airway obstruction. *Chest* 1994;105:767.

408. Arriagada R, LeChevalier T, Rekacewicz E, et al. Cisplatin-based chemoradiotherapy (CT) in patients with locally advanced non–small cell lung cancer (NSCLC): late analysis of a French randomized trial. *Proc Am Soc Clin Oncol* 1997;16:446a(abstr 1601).

409. Naruke T, Goya T, Tsuchiya R, et al. Prognosis and survival in resected lung carcinoma based on the new international staging system. *J Thorac Cardiovasc Surg* 1988;96:440.
410. Rusch VW, Albain KS, Crowley JJ. Neoadjuvant therapy: a novel and effective treatment for stage IIIb non–small cell lung cancer. *Ann Thorac Surg* 1994;58:290.
411. Macchiarini P, Chapelier AR, Monnet I, et al. Extended operations after induction therapy for stage IIIb (T4) non–small cell lung cancer. *Ann Thorac Surg* 1994;57:966.
412. Darteville P, Chapelier A, Navajas M, et al. Replacement of superior vena cava with polytetrafluorethylene grafts combined with resection of mediastinal-pulmonary malignant tumors. *J Thorac Cardiovasc Surg* 1987;94:361.
413. Nakahara K, Ohno K, Mastumura A, et al. Extended operation for lung cancer invading the aortic arch and superior vena cava. *J Thorac Cardiovasc Surg* 1989;97:428.
414. Tsuchiya R, Asamura H, Kondo H, et al. Extended resection of left atrium, great vessels or both for lung cancer. *Ann Thorac Surg* 1994;57:960.
415. Reyes L, Parvez Z, Regal AM, et al. Neoadjuvant chemotherapy and operations in the treatment of lung cancer with pleural effusion [Letter]. *J Thorac Cardiovasc Surg* 1991;101:946.
416. Hata E, Miyamoto H, Kohiyama R, et al. Resection of N2/N3 mediastinal disease. In: Motta G, ed. *Lung cancer frontiers in science and treatment.* Genoa, Italy: Grafica L.P. Publishers, 1994:431.
417. Stamatis G, Eberhardt W, Stubent G, et al. Preoperative chemoradiotherapy and surgery for selected non-small cell lung cancer IIIB subgroups: long-term results. *Ann Thorac Surg* 1999;68:1144.
418. Albain KS. Induction chemotherapy with/without radiation followed by surgery in stage III non-small cell lung cancer. *Oncology* 1997;11:(Suppl 9):51.
419. Choi NC, Carey RW, Myojin JC, et al. Preoperative chemo-radiotherapy (CT-RT) using concurrent boost radiation (RT) and resection for good responders in stage IIIb (T4 or N3) non–small cell lung cancer (NSCLC): a feasibility study. *Lung Cancer* 1997;18[Suppl 1]:76(abst 291).
420. Rendina EA, Venuta F, DiGiacomo T, et al. Induction chemotherapy for T4 centrally located non–small cell lung cancer. *J Thorac Cardiovasc Surg* 1999;117:225.
421. Rusch VW, Albain KS, Crowley JJ. Neoadjuvant therapy: a novel and effective treatment for stage IIIb non–small cell lung cancer. *Ann Thorac Surg* 1994;58:290.
422. Cox JD, Komaki R, Byhardt RW. Is immediate radiation therapy indicated for patients with unresectable non–small cell lung cancer? Yes. *Cancer Treat Rep* 1983;67:327.
423. Higgins GA, Shields TW. Experience of the Veterans Administration surgical adjuvant group. In: Muggia F, Rozencweig M, eds. *Lung cancer: progress in therapeutic research.* New York: Raven Press, 1979.
424. Perez CA, Bauer M, Edelstein S, et al. Impact of tumor control on survival in carcinoma of the lung treated with irradiation. *Int J Radiat Oncol Biol Phys* 1986;12:539.
425. Kubota K, Furuse K, Kawahara M, et al. Role of radiotherapy in combined modality treatment of locally advanced non-small-cell lung cancer. *J Clin Oncol* 1994;12:1547.
426. Cox JD, Yesner R, Mietlowski W, et al. Influence of cell type on local failure pattern after irradiation for locally advanced carcinoma of the lung. *Cancer* 1979;44:94.
427. Berry RJ, Liang Ah, Newman CR, Peto J. The role of radiotherapy in the treatment of inoperable lung cancer. *Int J Radiat Oncol Biol Phys* 1977;2:433.
428. Schaafsma J, Coy P. The effect of radiotherapy on the survival of non–small cell lung cancer patients. *Int J Radiat Oncol Biol Phys* 1997;41:291.
429. Johnson DH, Einhorn LH, Bartolucci A, et al. Thoracic radiotherapy does not prolong survival in patients with locally advanced, unresectable, non—small cell lung cancer. *Ann Intern Med* 1990;113:33.
430. Curran W. Effectiveness of treatment for non–small cell lung cancer [Letter]. *Ann Intern Med* 1990;113:637.
431. Prosnitz L. Radiotherapy for lung cancer [Letter]. *Ann Intern Med* 1991;114:95.
432. Kaasa S, Thorud E, Host H. A randomized study evaluating radiotherapy versus chemotherapy in patients with inoperable non–small cell lung cancer. *Radiother Oncol* 1988;11:7.
433. Huber R, Fischer R, Hautmann H, et al. Does additional brachytherapy improve the effect of external irradiation? A prospective randomized study in central lung tumors. *Int J Radiat Oncol Biol Phys* 1997;38:533.
434. Nori D, Li X, Pugkhem T. Intraoperative brachytherapy using Gelfoam radioactive plaque implants for resected stage III non–small cell lung cancer with positive margin: a pilot study. *J Surg Oncol* 1995;60:257.
435. Graham PH, Glebski VJ, Stat M. Radical radiotherapy for early non–small cell lung cancer. *Int J Radiat Oncol Biol Phys* 1995;31:261.
436. Sibley GS, Mundt AJ, Shapiro C, et al. The treatment of stage III non–small cell lung cancer using high dose conformal radiotherapy. *Int J Radiat Oncol Biol Phys* 1995;33:1001.
437. Armstrong J, McGibney C. The impact of 3-dimensional radiation on the treatment of non–small cell lung cancer. *Radiother Oncol* 2000 *(in press).*
438. Pu AT, Harrison AS, Robertson JM. The toxicity of elective nodal irradiation in the definitive treatment of non–small cell carcinoma. *Int J Radiat Oncol Biol Phys* 1997;39(2S):196(abst).
439. Emami B. Three-dimensional conformal radiation therapy in bronchogenic carcinoma. *Semin Radiat Oncol* 1996;6:92.
440. Rosenzweig KE, Sim SE, Mychalczak B. Elective nodal irradiation in the treatment of non–small cell lung cancer with three-dimensional conformal radiation therapy. *Int J Radiat Oncol Biol Phys* 1999;45:23.
441. Byhardt R. The evolution of Radiation Therapy Oncology Group (RTOG) protocols for non–small cell lung cancer. *Int J Radiat Oncol Biol Phys* 1995;32:1513.
442. Sause W, Kolesar P, Taylor S, et al. Five-year results: phase III trial of regionally advanced unresectable non–small cell lung cancer. *Proc Am Soc Clin Oncol* 1998;17:453a(abst).
443. Byhardt RW, Pajak TF, Emami B, et al. A phase I/II study to evaluate accelerated fractionation via concomitant boost for squamous, adeno, and large cell carcinoma of the lung: report of Radiation Therapy Oncology Group 84–07. *Int J Radiat Oncol Biol Phys* 1993;26:459.
444. Saunders M, Dische S. Continuous hyperfractionated accelerated radiotherapy (CHART) in non–small cell lung carcinoma of the bronchus. *Int J Radiat Oncol Biol Phys* 1990;19:1211.
445. Saunders M, Dische S, Barrett A, et al. Continuous hyperfractionated accelerated radiotherapy (CHART) versus conventional radiotherapy in non–small cell lung cancer: a randomized multicenter trial. *Lancet* 1997;350:161.
446. Bailey AJ, Parmar MKB, Stephens RJ, et al. Patient-reported short-term and long-term physical and psychological symptoms: results of the continuous hyperfractionated accelerated radiotherapy (CHART) randomized trial in non–small cell lung cancer. *J Clin Oncol* 1998;16:3082.
447. Saunders MI, Rojas A, Lyn BE, et al. Experience with dose escalation using CHARTWELL (continuous hyperfractionated accelerated radiotherapy weekend less) in non-small-cell lung cancer. *Br J Cancer* 1998;78:1323.
448. Mehta MP, Tannehill SP, Adak S, et al. Phase II trial of hyperfractionated accelerated radiation therapy for nonresectable non–small cell lung cancer: results of Eastern Cooperative Oncology Group 4593. *J Clin Oncol* 1998;16:3518.
449. Bonner JA, McGinnis WL, Stella PJ. The possible advantage of hyperfractionated thoracic radiotherapy in the treatment of locally advanced non–small cell lung carcinoma. *Cancer* 1998;82:1037.
450. Slotman BJ, Njo KH, DeJonge A, et al. Hypofractionated radiation therapy in stage III non–small cell lung cancer. *Cancer* 1993;72:1885.
451. Schaake-Koning C, van den Bogaert W, Dalesio O, et al. Effects of concomitant cisplatin and radiotherapy on inoperable non–small cell lung cancer. *N Engl J Med* 1992;326:524.
452. Soresi E, Clerici M, Grilli R, et al. A randomized clinical trial comparing radiation therapy versus radiation therapy plus cis-dichlorodiammine platinum (II) in the treatment of locally advanced non–small cell lung cancer. *Semin Oncol* 1988;15:20.
453. Trovó MG, Minatel E, Franchin G, et al. Radiotherapy versus radiotherapy enhanced by cisplatin in stage III non–small cell lung cancer. *Int J Radiat Oncol Biol Phys* 1992;24:11.
454. Blanke C, Ansari R, Montravadi R, et al. Phase III trial of thoracic irradiation with or without cisplatin for locally advanced unresectable non-small-cell lung cancer: a Hoosier Oncology Group protocol. *J Clin Oncol* 1995;13:1425.
455. Clamon G, Herndon J, Cooper R, et al. Radiosensitization with carboplatin for patients with unresectable stage III non-small-cell lung cancer: a phase III trial of the Cancer and Leukemia Group B and the Eastern Cooperative Oncology Group. *J Clin Oncol* 1999;17:4.
456. Smoluk GD, Fahey RC, Calabro-Jones PM, Aguilera JA, Ward JF. Radioprotection of cells in culture by WR-2721 and derivatives: form of the drug responsible for protection. *Cancer Res* 1988;48:3641.
457. Tannehill SP, Mehta MP, Larson M, et al. Effect of amifostine on toxicities associated with sequential chemotherapy and radiation therapy for unresectable non-small-cell lung cancer: results of a phase II trial. *J Clin Oncol* 1997;15:2850.
458. Auperin A, Arriagada R, Pignon JP, et al. Prophylactic cranial irradiation for patients with small-cell lung cancer in complete remission. Prophylactic Cranial Irradiation Overview Collaborative Group. *N Engl J Med* 1999;341:476.
459. Cox J, Stanley K, Petrovich Z, et al. Cranial irradiation in cancer of the lung of all cell types. *JAMA* 1981;245:469.
460. Umsawadi T, Valdivieso M, Chen T, et al. Role of elective brain irradiation during combined chemoradiotherapy for limited disease non–small cell lung cancer. *J Neurooncol* 1984;2:253.
461. Mira J, Miller T, Crowley J. Chest irradiation (RT) versus chest RT + chemotherapy +/− prophylactic brain RT in localized non– small cell lung cancer: a Southwest Oncology Group randomized study. *Int J Radiat Oncol Biol Phys* 1990;19[Suppl 1]:145.
462. Stuschke M, Eberhardt W, Pottgen C, et al. Prophylactic cranial irradiation in locally advanced non-small-cell lung cancer after multimodality treatment. *J Clin Oncol* 1997;17:2700.
463. Lilenbaum RC, Langenerg P, Dickersin K. Single agent versus combination chemotherapy in patients with advanced non-small-cell lung carcinoma: a meta-analysis of response, toxicity, and survival. *Cancer* 1998;82:116.
464. Vokes EE, Weichselbaum RR. Concomitant chemoradiotherapy: rationale and clinical experience in patients with solid tumors. *J Clin Oncol* 1990;8:911.
465. Vokes EE, Green MR. Clinical studies in non–small cell lung cancer: the CALGB experience. *Cancer Invest* 1998;16(2):72.
466. Mattson K, Holsti LR, Holsti P, et al. Inoperable non-small-cell lung cancer: radiation with or without chemotherapy. *Eur J Cancer Clin Oncol* 1988;24:477.
467. Morton RF, Jett JR, McGinnis WL, et al. Thoracic radiation therapy alone compared with combined chemoradiotherapy for locally advanced unresectable non-small-cell lung cancer: a randomized phase III trial. *Ann Intern Med* 1991;115:681.
468. Marino P, Preatoni A, Cantoni A. Randomized trials of radiotherapy alone versus combined chemotherapy and radiotherapy in stages IIIa and IIIb non-small-cell lung cancer. *Cancer* 1995;76:593.
469. Dillman RO, Seagren SL, Propert KJ, et al. Improved survival of stage III non-small-cell lung cancer: seven-year follow-up of Cancer and Leukemia Group B (CALGB) 8433 trial. *J Natl Cancer Inst* 1996;88:1210.
470. Komaki R, Scott CB, Sause WT, et al. Induction cisplatin/vinblastine and irradiation vs. irradiation in unresectable squamous cell lung cancer: failure patterns by cell type in RTOG 8808/ECOG 4588. *Int J Radiat Oncol Biol Phys* 1997;39:537.
471. Crino L, Latini P, Meacci M, et al. Induction chemotherapy plus high-dose radiotherapy versus radiotherapy alone in locally advanced unresectable non–small cell lung cancer. *Ann Oncol* 1993;4:847.
472. Planting A, Helle P, Drings P, et al. A randomized study of high-dose split course radiotherapy preceded by high dose chemotherapy versus high-dose radiotherapy only in locally advanced non–small cell lung cancer: the EORTC Lung Cancer Cooperative Group trial. *Ann Oncol* 1996;7:139.
473. Pritchard RS, Anthony SP. Chemotherapy plus radiotherapy compared with radiotherapy alone in the treatment of locally advanced, unresectable, non–small cell lung cancer: a meta-analysis. *Ann Intern Med* 1996;125:723.
474. Non-Small Cell Collaborative Group. Chemotherapy in non–small cell lung cancer: a meta analysis using updated data on individual patients from 52 randomized clinical trials. *Br Med J* 1995;311:899.
475. Mirimanoff RO. Concurrent chemotherapy (CT) and radiotherapy (RT) in locally advanced non–small cell lung cancer (NSCLC): a review. *Lung Cancer* 1994;11[Suppl 3]:S79.
476. Shaw EG, McGinnis WL, Jett JR, et al. Pilot study of accelerated hyperfractionated thoracic radiation therapy plus concomitant etoposide and cisplatin chemotherapy in

patients with unresectable stage III non–small cell carcinoma of the lung. *J Natl Cancer Inst* 1993;85:321.
477. Langer CJ, Curran WJ Jr, Keller SM, et al. Report of phase II trial of concurrent chemoradiotherapy with radical thoracic irradiation (60 Gy), infusional fluorouracil, bolus cisplatin and etoposide for clinical stage IIIB and bulky IIIA non–small cell lung cancer. *Int J Radiat Oncol Biol Phys* 1993;26:469.
478. Jeremic B, Shibamoto Y, Acimovic L, et al. Randomized trial of hyperfractionated radiation therapy with or without concurrent chemotherapy for stage III non-small-cell lung cancer. *J Clin Oncol* 1995;13:452.
479. Jeremic B, Shibamoto Y, Acimovic L, et al. Hyperfractionated radiation therapy with or without concurrent low-dose daily carboplatin/etoposide for stage III non–small cell lung cancer: a randomized study. *J Clin Oncol* 1996;14:1065.
480. Jeremic B, Shibamoto Y, Milicic B, et al. A phase II study of concurrent accelerated hyperfractionated radiotherapy and carboplatin/oral etoposide for elderly patients with stage III non-small-cell lung cancer. *Int J Radiat Oncol Biol Phys* 1999;44(2):343.
481. Bailey AJ, Parmar MKB, Stephens RJ, et al. Patient-reported short-term and long-term physical and psychologic symptoms: results of the continuous hyperfractionated accelerated radiotherapy (CHART) randomized trial in non–small cell lung cancer. *J Clin Oncol* 1998;16:3082.
482. Albain KS, Crowley JJ, Turrisi AT, et al. Concurrent cisplatin/etoposide plus radiotherapy for pathologic stage IIIB non–small cell lung cancer: a Southwest Oncology Group phase II study (S9019). *Proc Am Soc Clin Oncol* 1997;16:446a(abstr 1600).
483. Lau DH, Crowley JJ, Gandara DR, et al. Southwest Oncology Group phase II trial of concurrent carboplatin, etoposide, and radiation for poor-risk stage III non–small cell lung cancer. *J Clin Oncol* 1998;16:3078.
484. Lee JS, Scott C, Komaki R, et al. Concurrent chemoradiation therapy with oral etoposide and cisplatin for locally advanced inoperable non–small cell lung cancer: Radiation Therapy Oncology Group protocol 91–06. *J Clin Oncol* 1996;14:1055.
485. Komaki R, Scott C, Ettinger D, et al. Randomized study of chemotherapy/radiation therapy combinations for favorable patients with locally advanced inoperable non–small cell lung cancer: Radiation Therapy Oncology Group (RTOG) 92–04. *Int J Radiat Oncol Biol Phys* 1997;38:149.
486. Furuse K, Kubota K, Kawahara M, et al. Phase II study of concurrent radiotherapy and chemotherapy for unresectable stage III non-small-cell lung cancer. *J Clin Oncol* 1995;13:869.
487. Vokes EE, Gregor A, Turrisi AT. Gemcitabine and radiation therapy for nonsmall cell lung cancer. *Semin Oncol* 1998;25[Suppl 9]:66.
488. Masters GA, Haraf DJ, Hoffman PC, et al. Phase I study of vinorelbine, cisplatin, and concomitant thoracic radiation in the treatment of advanced chest malignancies. *J Clin Oncol* 1998;16:2157.
489. Mauer AM, Masters GA, Haraf DJ, et al. Phase I study of docetaxel with concomitant thoracic radiation therapy. *J Clin Oncol* 1998;16:159.
490. Choy H, Akerley W, Devore R. Paclitaxel, carboplatin and radiation therapy for non–small cell lung cancer. *Oncology* 1998;12[Suppl 2]:80.
491. Choy H, Akerley W, Safran H, et al. Phase II trial of weekly paclitaxel and concurrent radiation therapy for locally advanced non–small cell lung cancer. *Proc Am Soc Clin Oncol* 1996;15:371(abst 1098).
492. Choy H, Akerley W, Safran S, et al. Multi-institutional phase II trial of paclitaxel, carboplatin, and concurrent radiation therapy for locally advanced non–small cell lung cancer. *J Clin Oncol* 1998;16:3316.
493. Choy H, DeVore RD, Hande KR, et al. Phase II study of paclitaxel, carboplatin, and hyperfractionated radiation therapy for locally advanced inoperable non–small cell lung cancer: A Vanderbilt Cancer Center Affiliate Network (VCCAN) trial. *Proc Am Soc Clin Oncol* 1998;17:467a(abstr 1794).
494. Belani CP, Aisner J, Day R, et al. Weekly paclitaxel and carboplatin with simultaneous thoracic radiotherapy for locally advanced non–small cell lung cancer: three year follow-up. *Proc Am Soc Clin Oncol* 1997;16:448a(abst 1608).
495. Greco FA, Stroup SL, Gray JR, et al. Paclitaxel in combination chemotherapy with radiotherapy in patients with unresectable stage III non–small cell lung cancer. *J Clin Oncol* 1996;14:1642.
496. Wagner H, Antonia S, Shaw G, et al. Induction chemotherapy with carboplatin and paclitaxel followed by hyperfractionated accelerated radiation for patients with unresectable stage IIIA and IIIB non–small cell lung cancer. *Proc Am Soc Clin Oncol* 1998;17:469a(abst 1804).
497. Lau DH, Ryu JK, Gandara DR, et al. Twice-weekly paclitaxel and radiation for stage III non–small cell lung cancer. *Semin Oncol* 1997;24[Suppl 12]:S12-106.
498. Hudes R, Langer C, Movsas B, et al. Induction paclitaxel and carboplatin followed by concurrent chemoradiotherapy in unresectable, locally advanced non–small cell lung carcinoma: report of FCCC 94–001. *Proc Am Soc Clin Oncol* 1997;16:448a(abst 1609).
499. Vokes EE, Leopold KA, Herndon II JE, et al. A randomized phase II study of gemcitabine or paclitaxel or vinorelbine with cisplatin as induction chemotherapy (Ind CT) and concomitant chemoradiotherapy (XRT) for unresectable stage II non–small cell lung cancer (NSCLC) (CALGB Study 9431). *Proc Am Soc Clin Oncol* 1999;18:459a(abst 1771).
500. Saka H, Shimokata K, Yoshida S, et al. Irinotecan (CPT-11) and concurrent radiotherapy in locally advanced non–small cell lung cancer (NCSLC): a phase II study of the Japan Clinical Oncology Group (JCOG9504). *Proc Am Soc Clin Oncol* 1997;16:447a(abst 1607).
501. Niell HB, Kumar P, Miller AA, Griffin JP. Induction paclitaxel and cisplatin followed by concomitant chemoradiation therapy in stage III non-small-cell lung cancer. *Cancer Ther* 1999;2:67.
502. Mehta MP, Tannehill SP, Adak S, et al. Phase II trial of hyperfractionated accelerated radiation therapy for nonresectable non-small-cell lung cancer: results of Eastern Cooperative Oncology Group 4593. *J Clin Oncol* 1998;16:3518.
503. Masters GA, Vokes EE. Should non–small cell carcinoma of the lung be treated with chemotherapy? Pro: chemotherapy is for non–small cell lung cancer [Editorial]. *Am J Respir Crit Care Med* 1995;151:1285.
504. Johnson DH. Chemotherapy for metastatic non-small-cell lung cancer: Can that dog hunt? *J Natl Cancer Inst* 1993;85:766.
505. Slevin ML, Stubbs L, Plant HJ, et al. Attitudes to chemotherapy: comparing views of patients with cancer with those of doctors, nurses, and general public. *Br Med J* 1990;300:1458.
506. Douglas IS, White SR. Therapeutic empiricism: the case against chemotherapy in non–small cell lung cancer. *Am J Respir Crit Care Med* 1995;151:1288.
507. Cormier Y, Bergeron D, LaForge J, et al. Benefits of polychemotherapy in advanced non–small cell bronchogenic carcinoma. *Cancer* 1982;50:845.
508. Rapp E, Pater J, Willan A, et al. Chemotherapy can prolong survival in patients with advanced non–small cell lung cancer: report of a Canadian multicenter randomized trial. *J Clin Oncol* 1988;6:633.
509. Cartei G, Cartei F, Cantone A, et al. Cisplatin-cyclophosphamide-mitomycin combination chemotherapy with supportive care versus supportive care alone for treatment of metastatic non-small-cell lung cancer. *J Natl Cancer Inst* 1993;85:794.
510. Quoix E, Dietemann A, Charbonneau J, et al. La chimiotherapie comportant du cisplatine est-elle utile dans le cancer bronchique non microcellulaire au stade IV? Resultants d'une etude randomise. *Bull Cancer* 1991;78:341.
511. Ganz P, Figlin R, Haskell C, et al. Supportive care versus supportive care and combination chemotherapy in metastatic non–small cell lung cancer: Does chemotherapy make a difference? *Cancer* 1989;63:1271.
512. Woods R, Williams C, Levi J, et al. A randomized trial of cisplatin and vindesine versus supportive care only in advanced non–small cell lung cancer. *Br J Cancer* 1990;61:608.
513. Cellerino R, Tummarello D, Guidi F, et al. A randomized trial of alternating chemotherapy versus best supportive care in advanced non–small cell lung cancer. *J Clin Oncol* 1991;9:1453.
514. Kaasa S, Lund E, Thorud E, et al. Symptomatic treatment versus combination chemotherapy for patients with extensive non–small cell lung cancer. *Cancer* 1991;67:2443.
515. Elderly Lung Cancer Vinorelbine Italian Study Group. Effects of vinorelbine on quality of life and survival of elderly patients with advanced non-small-cell lung cancer. *J Natl Cancer Inst* 1999;91:66.
516. Cullen MH, Billingham KJ, Woodroffe CM, et al. Mitomycin, ifosfamide, and cisplatin in unresectable non-small-cell lung cancer: effects on survival and quality of life. *J Clin Oncol* 1999;17(10):3188.
517. Jaakkimainen L, Goodwin J, Pater J, et al. Counting the costs of chemotherapy in a National Cancer Institute of Canada randomized trial in non–small cell lung cancer. *J Clin Oncol* 1990;8:1301.
518. Souquet PJ, Chauvin F, Boissel JP, et al. Polychemotherapy in advanced non–small cell lung cancer: a meta-analysis. *Lancet* 1993;342:19.
519. Grilli R, Oxman AD, Julian JM. Chemotherapy for advanced non–small cell lung cancer: How much benefit is enough? *J Clin Oncol* 1993;11:1866.
519a. Marino P, Pampallona S, Prestoni A, et al. Chemotherapy versus supportive care in advanced non-small cell lung cancer: results of a meta-analysis of the literature. *Chest* 1994;106:861.
520. Marino P, Preatoni A, Cantoni A. Randomized trials of radiotherapy alone versus combined chemotherapy and radiotherapy in stages IIIa and IIIb non-small-cell lung cancer. *Cancer* 1995;76:593.
521. Smith TJ, Hillner BE, Neighbors DM, et al. Economic evaluation of a randomized clinical trial comparing vinorelbine, vinorelbine plus cisplatin, and vindesine plus cisplatin for non-small-cell lung cancer. *J Clin Oncol* 1995;13:2166.
522. Goodwin PJ, Shepherd FA. Economic issues in lung cancer: a review. *J Clin Oncol* 1998;16(12):3900.
523. Brundage MD, Davidson JR, Mackillop WJ. Trading treatment toxicity for survival in locally advanced non–small cell lung cancer. *J Clin Oncol* 1997;15:330.
524. Ellis PA, Smith IE, Hardy JR, et al. Symptom relief with MVP (mitomycin C, vinblastine and cisplatin) chemotherapy in advanced non-small-cell lung cancer. *Br J Cancer* 1995;71:366.
525. Tummarello D, Graziano F, Isidori P, et al. Symptomatic, stage IV, non-small-cell lung cancer (NSCLC): response, toxicity, performance status change and symptom relief in patients treated with cisplatin, vinblastine and mitomycin-C. *Cancer Chemother Pharmacol* 1995;35:249.
526. Paesmans M, et al. Response to chemotherapy has predictive value for further survival of patients with advanced non–small cell lung cancer: 10 years experience of the European Lung Cancer Working Party. *Eur J Cancer* 1997;33(14):2326.
527. Vokes EE. Integration of vinorelbine into current chemotherapy strategies for advanced non–small cell lung cancer. *Oncology* 1995;9:565.
528. Vokes EE, Rosenberg RK, Jahanzeb M, et al. Multicenter phase II study of weekly oral vinorelbine for stage IV non-small-cell lung cancer. *J Clin Oncol* 1995;13(3):637.
529. Depierre A, Chastang C, Quoix E, et al. Vinorelbine versus vinorelbine plus cisplatin in advanced non–small cell lung cancer: a randomized trial. *Ann Oncol* 1994;5:37.
530. Le Chevalier T, Brisgand D, Douillard J-Y, et al. Randomized study of vinorelbine and cisplatin versus vindesine and cisplatin versus vinorelbine alone in advanced non-small-cell lung cancer: results of a European multicenter trial including 612 patients. *J Clin Oncol* 1994;12:360.
531. Wozniak AJ, Crowley JJ, Balcerzak SP, et al. Randomized trial comparing cisplatin with cisplatin plus vinorelbine in the treatment of advanced non-small-cell lung cancer: a Southwest Oncology Group study. *J Clin Oncol* 1998;16:2459.
532. Crawford J, O'Rourke M, Schiller JH, et al. Randomized trial of vinorelbine compared with fluorouracil plus leucovorin in patients with stage IV non-small-cell lung cancer. *J Clin Oncol* 1996;14(10):2774.
533. Murphy WK, Fossella FV, Winn RJ, et al. Phase II study of Taxol in patients with untreated advanced non-small-cell lung cancer. *J Natl Cancer Inst* 1993;85:384.
534. Chang AY, Kim K, Glick J, et al. Phase II study of Taxol, merbarone, and piroxantrone in stage IV non-small-cell lung cancer: the Eastern Cooperative Oncology Group results. *J Natl Cancer Inst* 1993;85:388.
535. Hainsworth JD, Thompson DS, Greco FA. Paclitaxel by 1 hour infusion: an active drug in metastatic non–small cell lung cancer. *J Clin Oncol* 1995;13:1609.
536. Bonoml P, Kim K, Chang A, et al. Phase III trial comparing etoposide (E) cisplatin (C) versus Taxol (T) with cisplatin-G-CSF (G) versus Taxol-cisplatin in advanced non-small-cell lung cancer. An Eastern Cooperative Oncology Group (ECOG) trial. *Proc Am Soc Clin Oncol* 1996;15:382(abst 1145).

537. Giaccone G, Splinter TAW, Debruyne C, et al. Randomized study of paclitaxel-cisplatin versus cisplatin-teniposide in patients with advanced non-small-cell lung cancer. *J Clin Oncol* 1998;16(6):2133.

537a. Crino L, Mosconi AM, Scagliotti GV, et al. Gemcitabine as second-line treatment for relapsing or refractory advanced non-small cell lung cancer: a phase II trial. *Semin Oncol* 1998;25:23.

538. Gatzemeier U, von Pawel J, Gottfried M, et al. Phase III comparative study of high-dose cisplatin (HD-CIS) versus a combination of paclitaxel (TAX) and cisplatin (CIS) in patients with advanced non-small-cell lung cancer (NSCLC). *Proc Am Soc Clin Oncol* 1998;17:454a(abst 1748).

539. Belani C, Natale R, Lee J, et al. Randomized phase III trial comparing cisplatin/etoposide versus carboplatin/paclitaxel in advanced and metastatic non-small-cell lung cancer (NSCLC). *Proc Am Soc Clin Oncol* 1998;455a(abst 1751).

540. Kelly K, Crowley J, Bunn P, et al. A randomized phase III trial of paclitaxel plus carboplatin (PC) versus vinorelbine plus cisplatin (VC) in untreated advanced non-small cell lung cancer (NSCLC): a Southwest Oncology Group (SWOG) trial. *Proc Am Soc Clin Oncol* 1999;18a(abst 1777).

541. Kosmidis P, Mylonakis N, Skarlos D, et al. A multicenter randomized trial of paclitaxel (175 mg/m^2) plus carboplatin (6 AUC) versus paclitaxel (225 mg/m^2) plus carboplatin (6 AUC) in advanced non-small-cell lung cancer (NSCLC). *Proc Am Soc Clin Oncol* 1999;18a(abst 1785).

542. Fossella FV, Lee J-S, Berille J, et al. Summary of phase II data of docetaxel (Taxotere), an active agent in the first- and second-line treatment of advanced non–small cell lung cancer. *Semin Oncol* 1995;22:22.

543. Francis PA, Rigas JR, Kris MG, et al. Phase II trial of docetaxel in patients with stage III and IV non-small-cell lung cancer. *J Clin Oncol* 1994;12:1232.

544. Fossella FV, DeVore R, Kerr R, et al. Phase II trial of docetaxel 100 mg/m^2 or 75 mg/m^2 vs vinorelbine/ifosfamide for non–small cell lung cancer (NSCLC) previously treated with platinum-based chemotherapy (PBC). *Proc Am Soc Clin Oncol* 1999;18(abst 1776).

545. Shepherd F, Ramlau R, Mattson K, et al. Randomized study of Taxotere (TAX) versus best supportive care (BSC) in non–small cell lung cancer (NSCLC) patients previously treated with platinum-based chemotherapy. *Proc Am Soc Clin Oncol* 1999;18:463a(abst 1784).

546. Abratt RP, Bezwoda WR, Falkson G, et al. Efficacy and safety profile of gemcitabine in non-small-cell lung cancer: a phase II study. *J Clin Oncol* 1994;12:1535.

547. Anderson H, Lund B, Bach F, et al. Single-agent activity of weekly gemcitabine in advanced non-small-cell lung cancer: a phase II study. *J Clin Oncol* 1994;12:1821.

548. Fossella FV, Lippman SM, Shin DM, et al. Maximum tolerated dose defined for single-agent gemcitabine: a phase I dose escalation study in advanced chemotherapy naïve patients with non–small cell lung cancer. *J Clin Oncol* 1997;15:310.

549. Gatzemeler U, Shepherd FA, Le Chevalier T, et al. Activity of gemcitabine in patients with non–small cell lung cancer: a multicenter, extended phase II st ıdy. *Eur J Cancer* 1996;32:243.

550. Iaffaioli RV, Tortoriello A, Facchini G, et al. Phase I–II study of gemcitabine and carboplatin in stage IIIB–IV non-small-cell lung cancer. *J Clin Oncol* 1999;17(3):921.

551. Thatcher N, Jayson G, Bradley B, et al. Gemcitabine: symptomatic benefit in advanced non-small-cell lung cancer. *Semin Oncol* 1997;24[Suppl 8]:S8-6.

552. DeVore RF, Johnson DH, Crawford J, et al. Phase II study of irinotecan plus cisplatin in patients with advanced non-small-cell lung cancer. *J Clin Oncol* 1999;17(9):2710.

553. Fukuoka M, Niitani H, Suzuki A, et al. A phase II study of CPT-11, a new derivative of camptothecin, for previously untreated non–small cell lung cancer. *J Clin Oncol* 1992;10:16.

554. Oshita F, Noda K, Nishiwaki Y, et al. Phase II study of irinotecan and etoposide in patients with metastatic non-small-cell lung cancer. *J Clin Oncol* 1997;15(1):304.

555. Masuda N, Fukuoka M, Kudoh S, et al. Phase I study of irinotecan and cisplatin with granulocyte colony-stimulating factor support for advanced non-small-cell lung cancer. *J Clin Oncol* 1994;12(1):90.

556. Sandler A, Nemunaitis J, Deehnam C, et al. Phase III study of cisplatin (C) with or without gemcitabine (G) in patients with advanced non-small-cell lung cancer (NSCLC). *Proc Am Soc Clin Oncol* 1998;17:454a(abst 1747).

557. Cardenal F, Lopez-Cabreizo M, Anton A, et al. Randomized phase III study of gemcitabine-cisplatin versus etoposide-cisplatin in the treatment of locally advanced or metastatic non-small-cell lung cancer. *J Clin Oncol* 1999;17:12.

558. Perng RP, Chen YM, Ming-Liu J, et al. Gemcitabine versus the combination of cisplatin and etoposide in patients with inoperable non–small cell lung cancer in a phase II randomized study. *J Clin Oncol* 1997;15:2097.

559. Manegold CH, Stahel R, Mattson K, et al. Randomized phase II study of gemcitabine (GEM) monotherapy versus cisplatin plus etoposide (C/E) in patients (pts) with locally advanced or metastatic non–small cell lung cancer (NSCLC). *Proc Am Soc Clin Oncol* 1997;16:1651.

560. Von Pawel J, von Roemeling R. Survival benefit from Triazone (tirapazamine) and cisplatin in advanced non-small-cell lung cancer (NSCLC) patients: final results from the international phase III CATAPULT trial. *Proc Am Soc Clin Oncol* 1998;17:454a(abst 1749).

561. Crino L, Mosconi AM, Scagliotti G, et al. Gemcitabine as second-line treatment for advanced non-small-cell lung cancer: a phase II trial. *J Clin Oncol* 1999;17(7):2081.

562. Akerley W, Hernson J, Egorin MJ, et al. CALGB 9731: phase II trial of weekly paclitaxel for advanced non–small cell lung cancer (NSCLC). *Proc Am Soc Clin Oncol* 1999;18: 463a(abst 1783).

563. Kroep JR, Giaccone G, Voorn DA, et al. Gemcitabine and paclitaxel: pharmacokinetic and pharmacodynamic interactions in patients with non-small-cell lung cancer. *J Clin Oncol* 1999;17(7):2190.

564. Georgoulias V, Kouroussis C, Androulakis N, et al. Front-line treatment of advanced non-small-cell lung cancer with docetaxel and gemcitabine: a multicenter phase II trial. *J Clin Oncol* 1999;17(3):914.

565. Recchia F, De Filippis S, Rosselli M, et al. Ifosfamide, vinorelbine and gemcitabine in advanced non–small cell lung cancer. A phase I study. *Eur J Cancer* 1999;35(10):1457.

566. Thodtmann R, Depenbrock H, Dumez H, et al. Clinical and pharmacokinetic phase I study of multi-targeted antifolate (LY231514) in combination with cisplatin. *J Clin Oncol* 1999;17(10):3009.

567. Rusthoven JJ, Eisenhauer E, Butts C, et al. Multitargeted antifolate LY231514 as first-line chemotherapy for patients with advanced non-small-cell lung cancer: a phase II study. *J Clin Oncol* 1999;17(4):1194.

568. Stetler-Stevenson WG. Matrix metalloproteinase in angiogenesis: a moving target for therapeutic intervention. *J Clin Invest* 1999;103(9):1237.

569. Furuse K, Fukuoka M, Kato H, et al. A prospective phase II study on photodynamic therapy with photofrin II for centrally located early-stage lung cancer: *J Clin Oncol* 1993;11(10):1852.

570. Fujiwara T, Grimm EA, Mukhopadhyay T, et al. Induction of chemosensitivity in human lung cancer cells in vivo by adenovirus-mediated transfer of the wild-type p53 gene. *Cancer Res* 1994;54:2287.

571. Wojtowicz-Praga S, Torri J, Johnson M, et al. Phase I trial of marimastat, a novel matrix metalloproteinase inhibitor, administered orally to patients with advanced lung cancer. *J Clin Oncol* 1998;16:2150.

572. Karp DD, Atkins MB. Adoptive immunotherapy for non–small cell lung carcinoma. *Cancer* 1996;78(2):195.

572a. Deslauriers J, Brisson J, Cartier R, et al. Carcinoma of the lung: Evaluation of satellite nodules as a factor influencing prognosis after resection. *J Thorac Cardiovasc Surg* 1989;97:504.

572b. McCormack P. Surgical resection of pulmonary metastasis. *Semin Surg Oncol* 1990;6:297.

573. Magilligan DJ, Duvernoy C, Malik G, et al. Surgical approach to lung cancer with solitary cerebral metastasis: twenty-five years' experience. *Ann Thorac Surg* 1986;42:360.

574. Figlin RA, Piantadosi S, Feld R, et al. Intracranial recurrence of carcinoma after complete surgical resection of stage I, II and III non–small cell lung cancer. *N Engl J Med* 1988;318:1300.

575. Martini N. Rationale for surgical treatment of brain metastasis in non–small cell lung cancer. *Ann Thorac Surg* 1986;42:357.

576. Patchell RA, Tibbs PA, Walsh JW, et al. A randomized trial of surgery in the treatment of single metastases to the brain. *N Engl J Med* 1990;322:494.

577. Harpole D, Arnos A, Alexander E, et al. Stage of the primary is important when treating isolated brain metastases from lung cancer. *Proc Am Soc Clin Oncol* 1996;15:382.

578. Allard P, Yankaskas BC, Fletcher RH, et al. Sensitivity and specificity of computed tomography for the detection of adrenal metastatic lesions among 91 autopsied lung cancer patients. *Cancer* 1990;66:457.

579. Twomey P, Montgomery C, Clark O. Successful treatment of adrenal metastasis from large-cell carcinoma of the lung. *JAMA* 1982;248:581.

580. Raviv G, Klein E, Yellin A, et al. Surgical treatment of solitary adrenal metastases from lung carcinoma. *J Surg Oncol* 1990;43:123.

581. Reyes L, Parvez Z, Nemoto T, et al. Adrenalectomy for adrenal metastasis from lung carcinoma. *J Surg Oncol* 1990;44:32.

582. Carroll M, Morgan SA, Yarnold JR, et al. Prospective evaluation of a watch policy in patients with inoperable non–small cell lung cancer. *Eur J Cancer Clin Oncol* 1986;22:1353.

583. Bleehan N. Inoperable non–small cell lung cancer (NSCLC): a Medical Research Council randomized trial of palliative radiotherapy with two fractions or ten fractions. *Br J Cancer* 1991;63:265.

584. Teo P, Tal T, Choy D, Tsui K. A randomized study on palliative radiation therapy for inoperable non–small cell carcinoma of the lung. *Int J Radiat Oncol Biol Phys* 1988;14:867.

585. Simpson J, Francis M, Perez-Tamayo R, et al. Palliative radiotherapy for inoperable carcinoma of the lung: final report of the RTOG multi-institutional trial. *Int J Radiat Oncol Biol Phys* 1988;11:751.

586. Bindi M, Tucci E, Pepi F, et al. Changes in performance status in patients with pulmonary carcinoma treated with mono-fractionation radiotherapy once a week. *Giornale Ital Oncol* 1990;10:89.

587. Macbeth FR, Bolger JJ, Hopwood P. Randomized trial of palliative two-fraction versus more intensive 13-fraction radiotherapy for patients with inoperable non–small cell lung cancer and good performance status. *Clin Oncol* 1996;8:167.

588. Jackson M, Ball D. Palliative retreatment of locally recurrent lung cancer after radical radiotherapy. *Med J Aust* 1987;147:391.

589. Ahmann F. A reassessment of the clinical implications of the superior vena caval syndrome. *J Clin Oncol* 1984;2:961.

590. Armstrong B, Perez C, Simpson J, et al. Role of irradiation in the management of superior vena cava syndrome. *Int J Radiat Oncol Biol Phys* 1987;13:531.

591. Ofiara L, Roman T, Schwartzman K, et al. Local determinants of response to endobronchial high-dose rate brachytherapy in bronchogenic carcinoma. *Chest* 1997;112:946.

592. Nori D, Hilaris B, Martini N. Intraluminal irradiation in bronchogenic carcinoma. *Surg Clin North Am* 1987;67:1093.

593. Schray M, McDougall J, Martinez A, et al. Management of malignant airway obstruction: clinical and dosimetric considerations using an iridium-192 afterloading technique in conjunction with the neodymium-YAG laser. *Int J Radiat Oncol Biol Phys* 1985;11:403.

594. Mehta M, Shahabi S, Jarjour N, et al. Endobronchial irradiation for malignant airway obstruction. *Int J Radiat Oncol Biol Phys* 1989;17:847.

595. Mehta M, Petereit D, Chosy L, et al. Sequential comparison of low dose rate and hyperfractionated high dose rate endobronchial radiation for malignant airway occlusion. *Int J Radiat Oncol Biol Phys* 1992;23:133.

596. Macha H, Coch K, Stadler M, et al. New technique for testing occlusive and stenosing tumors of the trachea and main bronchi: endobronchial irradiation by high dose iridium-192 combined with laser utilization. *Thorax* 1987;42:511.

597. Delclos M, Komaki R, Morice R, et al. Endobronchial brachytherapy with high-dose-rate remote afterloading for recurrent endobronchial lesions. *Radiology* 1996;201:279.

598. Burt P, O'Driscoll R, Notley M, et al. Intraluminal irradiation for the palliation of lung cancer with the high dose rate micro-Selectron. *Thorax* 1990;45:765.

599. Seagren S, Harrell J. Prospective trial of palliative high dose rate endobronchial irradiation with or without laser for recurrent non–small cell lung cancer. *Proc Am Soc Clin Oncol* 1990;9:224.
600. Huber R, Fischer R, Hautmann, et al. Palliative endobronchial brachytherapy for central lung tumors. *Chest* 1995;107:463.
601. Lee JS, Komaki R, Morice R, et al. A pilot clinical laboratory trial of paclitaxel and endobronchial brachytherapy in patients with non–small cell lung cancer. *Semin Radiat Oncol* 1999;9:121
602. Borgelt B, Gelber R, Larson M, et al. Ultra-rapid high-dose irradiation schedules for the palliation of brain metastases: final results of the first two studies by the Radiation Therapy Oncology Group. *Int J Radiat Oncol Biol Phys* 1981;7:1633.
603. Mandell L, Hilaris B, Sullivan M, et al. The treatment of single brain metastasis from non–oat cell lung carcinoma: surgery and radiation versus radiation therapy alone. *Cancer* 1986;58:641.
604. Patchell R, Tibbs P, Walsh J, et al. A randomized trial of surgery in the treatment of single metastases to the brain. *N Engl J Med* 1990;322:494.
605. Patchell RA, Tibbs PA, Regine WF, et al. Postoperative radiotherapy in the treatment of single metastases to the brain: a randomized trial. *JAMA* 1998;280:1485.
606. Moghissi K, Dixon K, Stringer M, et al. The place of bronchoscopic photodynamic therapy in advanced unresectable lung cancer: experience of 100 cases. *Eur J Cardiothorac Surg* 1999;15:1.
607. Paulson DL. The "superior sulcus" lesion. In: Delarue NC, Eschapasse H. International trends in general Thoracacic surgery, Vol.1:lung cancer. Philadelphia:W.B. Saunders, 185:121.
608. Anderson TM, Moy PM, Homes EC. Factors affecting survival in superior sulcus tumors. *J Clin Oncol* 1986;4:1598.
609. Devine JW, Mendenhall WM, Million RR, Carmichael MJ. Carcinoma of the superior sulcus treated with surgery and/or radiation therapy. *Cancer* 1986;57:941.
610. Rice TW, Pringle JF, Sinclair JE, et al. Superior sulcus tumors; results of treatment. *Lung Cancer* (abst) 1986;2:156.
611. Miller JI. Discussion of: Shahian DM, Neptune WB, Ellis FH. Pancoast tumors: improved survival with preoperative and postoperative radiotherapy. *Ann Thorac Surg* 1987;43:32.
612. McKneally M. Discussion of: Shahian DM, Neptune WB, Ellis FH. Pancoast tumors: improved survival with preoperative and postoperative radiotherapy. *Ann Thorac Surg* 1987;43:32.
613. Ricci C, Rendina EA, Venuta F. Surgical treatment of superior sulcus tumors (abst). *Lung Cancer* 1988;4:A80.
614. Carrel T, Nachbur B, Bleher A. Is radiotherapy prior to surgical resection indicated for bronchogenic carcinoma with chest wal infiltration and for pancoast tumors? (abst) *Lung Cancer* 1988;4:A80.
615. Komaki R, Mountain CF, Holbert JM, et al. Superior sulcus tumors: treatment selection and results for 85 patients without metastasis (M0) at presentation. *Int J Radiat Oncol Biol Phys* 1000;10:31.
616. Hagan MP, Choi NC, Mathisen DJ, et al. Superior sulcus tumors: impact of local control on survival. *J Thorac Cardiovasc Surg* 1999;117:1086.
617. Attar S, Krasna MJ, Sonett JR, et al. Superior sulcus (Pancoast) tumor: experience with 105 patients. *Ann Thorac Surg* 1998;66:193.
618. Kirschner PA. Lung cancer: preoperative radiation therapy and surgery. *N Y State J Med* 1981;81:339.
619. Sawamura K, Mori T, Hashimoto S, et al. Results of surgical treatment for N2 disease (abst). *Lung Cancer* 1986;2:96.
620. Mastrorilli M, Bragaglia RB, Cipolla G, et al. Surgical management of N2 lung cancer (abst). *Lung Cancer* 1988;4(suppl):A97.
621. Deneffe G, Stalpaert G. Five year survival in resected T3/N2 lung cancer. *Acta Chir Belg* 1989;89:159.
622. Levasseur PH, Regnard JF. Long term results after surgery for N2 non small cell lung cancer. Presented at the IASLC workshop, 17–21 June 1990, Bruges, Belgium.
623. Watanabe Y, Shimizu J, Oda M, et al. Aggressive surgical intervention in N2 non-small cell cancer of the lung. *Ann Thorac Surg* 1991;51:253.
624. Walker WS, Carey F, Cameron EWJ, Lamb D. Results of surgery for N2 status bronchial carcinoma. Presented at the IASLC workshop, 17–21 June 1990, Bruges, Belgium.
625. Mountain CF. The biological operability of stage III non-small cell lung cancer. *Ann Thorac Surg* 1985;40:60.
626. Miller LD, McManus KG, Allen MS, et al. Results of surgical resection in patients with N2 non-small cell lung cancer. *Ann Thorac Surg* 1994;57:1095.
627. Goldstraw P, Mannam GC, Kaplan DK, Michail P. Surgical management of non-small cell lung cancer with ipsilateral mediastinal node metastasis (N2 disease) *J Thorac Cardiovasc Surg* 1994; 107:19.
628. Pearson FG, Delarue NC, Ilves R, et al. Significance of positive superior mediastinal nodes identified at mediastinoscopy in patients with resectable cancer of the lung. *J Thorac Cardiovasc Surg* 1982;83:1.
629. Coughlin M, Deslauriers J, Beaulieu M, et al. Role of mediastinoscopy in pretreatment staging of patients with primary lung cancer. *Ann Thorac Surg* 1985;40:556.
630. Riquet M, Manac'h D, Saab M, LePimpec-Barthes F, et al. Factors determining survival in resected N2 lung cancer. *Eur J CardioThorac Surg* 1995;9:300.
631. Salerno TA, Little JR, Munro DD. Bronchogenic carcinoma with a brain metastasis: a continuing challenge. *Ann Thorac Surg* 1979;27:235–237.
632. Winston KR, Walsh JW, Fischer EG. Results of operative treatment of intracranial metastatic tumors. *Cancer* 1980;45:2639–2645.
633. White KT, Fleming TR, Laws ER. Single metastasis to the brain; surgical treatment in 122 consecutive patients. *Mayo Clin Proc* 1981;56:424–428.
634. Mussi A, Janni A, Pistolesi M, et al. Surgical treatment of primary lung cancer and solitary brain metastasis. *Thoracax* 1985;40:191–193.
635. Ehrenhaft JL. Discussion of: Magilligan DJ, Duvernoy C, Malik G, et al. Surgical approach to lung cancer with solitary cerebral metastasis: twenty-five years' experience. *Ann Thorac Surg* 1986;42:360–364.
636. Magilligan DJ, Duvernoy C, Malik G, et al. Surgical approach to lung cancer with solitary cerebral metastasis: twenty-five years' experience. *Ann Thorac Surg* 1986;42:360–364.
637. Read RC, Boop WC, Yoder G, Schaefer R. Management of nonsmall cell lung carcinoma with solitary brain metastasis. *J Thorac Cardiovasc Surg* 1989;98:884–891.
638. Macchiarini P, Bonaguidi R, Hardin M, Angeletti CA. Results and prognostic factors of surgery in the management of non-small cell lung cancer (NSCLC) with solitary brain metastasis. (SBM) *Proc Am Soc Clin Oncol* 1991;10:253.
639. Wronski N, Arbit E, Burt M, Galicich JH. Survival after surgical treatment of metastases from lung cancer: a follow-up study of 231 patients treated between 1976–1991. *J Neurosurg* 1995;83:605–616.

SECTION 3

JOHN MURREN
ELI GLATSTEIN
HARVEY I. PASS

Small Cell Lung Cancer

EPIDEMIOLOGY AND ETIOLOGY

Small cell lung cancer (SCLC) is the histologic diagnosis in approximately 18% of the more than 171,000 patients diagnosed with lung cancer annually in the United States.[1,2] Across the world, the proportion of lung cancers that are of the small cell histology tends to be between 10% and 20% in male subjects and 10% and 30% in women.[3] The predominant risk factor for lung cancer is tobacco exposure, which is the cause for up to 90% of cases diagnosed.[4] Among the major histologic subtypes of lung cancer, the association between the extent of tobacco exposure and risk is particularly strong for squamous cell and SCLC.[5,6] Thus, the incidence of SCLC has paralleled trends in cigarette smoking after a 20- to 50-year lag period. In the twentieth century, manufactured cigarettes first became popular among men, then among women, and successive generations began smoking at progressively earlier ages. Per capita consumption in the United States increased from approximately 54 cigarettes per adult in 1900, to a peak of 4345 cigarettes per adult in 1963.[7] Between 1965 and 1995, the number of adult men who were active smokers declined from 52% to 27%. For women, smoking prevalence declined from 28% to 23% in this time period. However, smoking prevalence for the adult population has changed little from 1993 to 1997, and during the 1990s there have been increasing trends in tobacco smoking among adolescents, particularly girls.[7–9] In 1997, the prevalence of current cigarette smoking was 36.4% among U.S. secondary school students.[10]

Exposure to other environmental respiratory carcinogens, such as asbestos, benzene, coal tar, and other industrial chemicals may interact with tobacco smoke to increase risk.[11–14] The presence of underlying lung disease and diet have also been implicated.[12,15,16] The risk associated with household exposure to radon gas remains controversial.[12] Pedigree studies and specific metabolic phenotypes have identified familial clusters and populations at increased risk for lung cancer, which is not surprising because several nonrandom genetic defects are associated with this disease.[17–20] Germline mutations of genes such as p53 are not likely to contribute to susceptibility to lung cancer. Rather, genetic polymorphisms in genes involved in the activation and metabolism of the procarcinogens in tobacco smoke probably contribute to risk.[21,22]

These trends in smoking prevalence have important implications for the current and future population demographics of SCLC. Over the next few decades, the incidence of lung cancer should continue to decline in the United States, and as the birth cohorts most heavily exposed to tobacco age, the median age at diagnosis for SCLC will also grow older. Among men, the incidence rates for lung cancer peaked in 1984 and have been declining at a rate of approximately 1.4% per year, with the largest declines noted in the incidence of small cell and squamous cell cancers.[7] Among women, the peak incidence appeared to be in 1994. However, if the increase in popularity of cigarette smoking among adolescents does not change, the declining incidence of lung cancer can be predicted to reverse. Furthermore, female subjects appear to be more susceptible to tobacco smoke carcinogens than male subjects, and racial differences in susceptibility may also exist.[23–25] These factors, along with the changing demographics of the smoking population, will define the patient population who develops SCLC in future generations.

PATHOLOGY

A diagnosis of SCLC is based primarily on light microscopy. In 1981, the World Health Organization proposed a histologic classification that gained wide acceptance.[26] In this classification, SCLC was divided into three subtypes that consist of oat cell, intermediate cell type, and combined oat cell (SCLC combined with squamous or adenocarcinoma). It soon became clear that the morphologic features used to distinguish oat cell from the intermediate cell histology were imprecise, and that even when strict criteria were used, pure SCLC, whether it was classified as oat cell or intermediate cell, behaved identically. Consequently, the International Association for the Study of Lung Cancer proposed a revised classification in 1988 that recognized pure small cell cancer and two less common variants: mixed small cell and large cell carcinoma and combined small cell carcinoma.[27] This classification schema is what is typically used today.

SCLC is composed of neoplastic cells that are typically arranged in clusters, sheets, or trabeculae separated by a delicate fibrovascular stroma. The tumor typically arises in the central airways and initially infiltrates the submucosa, gradually obstructing the lumen by extrinsic or endobronchial spread. The cells are generally 1.5 to 2.5 times the diameter of a small resting lymphocyte.[28] They have scant cytoplasm and a finely granular nuclear chromatin. Nucleoli are absent or inconspicuous. Mitotic rates are high, and necrosis of individual tumor cells within cell clusters is common. Crush artifact, resulting in smearing of nuclear chromatin and hematoxyophilic encrustation of vessel walls is common.[27,29] More than 90% of untreated SCLC falls into this category.

In the mixed small cell and large cell variant, there is a subset of cells that resembles large cell carcinoma. These cells may be larger than, or equivalent in size to, the small cell component. These cells are distinguished by the presence of prominent, frequent nucleoli and a nuclear chromatin pattern that is more coarsely granular or open. There are variable amounts of cytoplasm present. The other subtype recognized in the International Association for the Study of Lung Cancer classification is combined SCLC. In this tumor, small cell carcinoma typically coexists with squamous carcinoma, although adenocarcinoma or one of the less common non–small cell histologies may be present.[27]

In most series, the frequency of the small cell and large cell variant is between 3% and 6%, and for combined SCLC it is 1% to 3%.[27,30–32] There is less concordance among pathologists on the diagnosis of the mixed cell variant than there is for pure SCLC.[30,31] Furthermore, the ability to identify a mixed population is influenced by the size of the biopsied material, with examination of a lymph node more likely to result in identification of a mixed cellular population than a typical bronchial biopsy. It remains unclear whether the presence of a mixed cell or a combined histology confers a different prognosis or response to treatment than pure small cell carcinoma. For the mixed small cell subtype, there are series that have identified survival that is inferior to,[33,34] superior to,[31] or comparable with[30,35] pure SCLC. There is little information regarding the outcome of patients with combined SCLC. A review of 429 patients treated at Vanderbilt University for SCLC identified nine (2%) with combined small cell and non–small cell histologies.[32] Two of these patients were long-term survivors, and both underwent surgical resection in addition to chemotherapy. Thus, surgery may play a role in the management of combined SCLC, and the presence of non–small cell elements, although uncommon, must be considered in patients who might potentially benefit from resection of residual non-SCLC when the initial diagnosis is based on the limited material available by needle or bronchoscopic sampling.

Although the diagnosis of small cell carcinoma rests primarily on morphologic assessment, immunocytochemistry plays a role, and electron microscopy is of occasional value in difficult cases. Virtually all SCLCs are immunoreactive for keratin and epithelial membrane antigen, so that if a tumor does not stain for these markers, other diagnoses should be considered.[36] One or more markers of neuroendocrine differentiation, such as chromogranin, neuron-specific enolase, Leu-7, and synaptophysin, can be detected in approximately 75% of SCLC.[29,36] The presence of these markers, however, is not mandatory for the diagnosis and does not distinguish small cell from non-SCLC, as 10% to 20% of non-SCLC exhibit neuroendocrine differentiation. By electron microscopy, the cells are closely apposed, with a high nuclear to cytoplasmic ratio. Chromatin is finely clumped but uniformly dispersed within the nucleus. Few organelles and only occasional uniformly small dense core granules are located in the cytoplasm. The presence of large granules should raise the diagnosis of a carcinoid tumor.[29]

The major differential diagnostic considerations for a small cell carcinoma are non-SCLC, other small round cell tumors, reserve cell hyperplasia, and a lymphocytic proliferation. Small cell carcinoma composed of larger tumor cells may be difficult to differentiate from a poorly differentiated non-SCLC, particularly if neuroendocrine features are present. Reserve cells are progenitors for bronchial epithelial cells and proliferate in response to chronic irritation of the airways. Features that distinguish reserve cells from small cell carcinoma include retention of cell boundaries within a cell cluster, a lack of the extreme nuclear molding found in small cell carcinoma, and an absence of granularity of the chromatin.[29]

CLINICAL PRESENTATION

In general, the clinical presentation of SCLC is similar to the other histologies of bronchogenic carcinoma. Few patients are asymptomatic at diagnosis. In screening studies, only 4% to 12% of the lung cancers detected as a solitary pulmonary nodule are small cell carcinoma.[37,38] The initial complaints usually reflect the local presence of a tumor. Cough is the most common symptom. Recent acceleration of cough or accompanying hemoptysis increases the likelihood that an underlying cancer is present. Dyspnea and chest pain are reported in 30% to 40% of patients at diagnosis.[1] Because SCLC typically develops in the central airways, hemoptysis, postobstructive pneumonitis, wheezing, or hoarseness due to vocal chord paralysis may be present. Superior vena caval obstruction is present at diagnosis in 10% of patients with SCLC.[39] Chest imaging typically shows hilar and mediastinal invasion and regional adenopathy. One-third of patients have some degree of atelectasis present.[1] A peripheral location or chest wall involvement by the tumor is uncommon. For example, no more than 2% of SCLC present as a superior sulcus tumor.[40,41]

Most patients with SCLC have clinically detectable metastases at diagnosis (Table 31.3-1). Bone involvement is usually characterized by osteolytic lesions, often in the absence of bone pain, or elevations in the serum calcium or alkaline phosphatase.[42–44] However, marked osteoblastic activity is present in a minority of patients. Hepatic and adrenal lesions are typically asymptomatic. Elevations of the serum lactate dehydrogenase (LDH), alkaline phosphatase, or hepatic transaminases are present in the majority of patients in whom liver metastases are identified.[45] In contrast, radiographically confirmed brain metastases are symptomatic in more than 90% of cases. Endovascular metastases (tumor emboli) or lymphangitic spread can be among the underlying causes of dyspnea. Constitutional symptoms, including weight loss, anorexia, and fatigue, are common and correlate with the presence of extensive-stage disease.

The spectrum of paraneoplasia associated with SCLC differs to some degree from the syndromes observed with non-SCLC. Small cell carcinoma is the histology in only 5% of patients with lung cancer diagnosed with hypertrophic pulmonary osteoarthropathy. Humorally mediated hypercalcemia is rare.[46] On the other hand, the vast majority of lung cancer patients who develop the syndrome of inappropriate antidiuretic hormone, Cushing's syndrome, or neurologic paraneoplasia have SCLC. SCLC accounts for approximately 75% of the tumors associated with the syndrome of inappropriate antidiuretic hormone. Although serum concentrations of antidiuretic hormone are elevated in the majority of patients with SCLC, only approximately 10% of patients fulfill the criteria for syndrome of inappropriate antidiuretic hormone, and symptoms are present in no more than 5%. In some cases, ectopic production of atrial natriuretic factor contributes to the disorder in sodium homeostasis. Similarly, increased serum levels of adrenocorticotropic hormone can be detected in up to 50% of patients with lung cancer, but only 5% of patients with SCLC develop Cushing's syndrome. In approximately one-half of these cases, it is present at diagnosis. Some of the cutaneous manifestations of Cushing's syndrome may not be prominent, perhaps because of the rapid growth and clinical course of SCLC. A few studies have demonstrated that a low serum sodium level is an adverse prognostic factor,[47,48] and patients with Cushing's syndrome have a limited survival.[49,50]

Neurologic paraneoplastic syndromes include sensory, sensorimotor, and autoimmune neuropathies and encephalomyelitis. These syndromes are thought to occur through autoimmune mechanisms, and antinuclear antibodies that bind both to SCLC

TABLE 31.3-1. Sites of Involvement of Small Cell Lung Cancer at Diagnosis and Autopsy

	At Presentation		*At Autopsy*
	All Patients (%)	As a Single Site (%)	(*% of Patients*)
Liver	21–27	6–7	69
Bone	27–41	9–13	54
Bone marrow	15–30	2–4	NA
Adrenals	5–31	8–11	35–65
Brain	10–14	4–6	28–50
Retroperitoneal lymph nodes	3–12	NA	29–52
Mediastinal lymph nodes	66–80	80	73–87
Supraclavicular lymph nodes	17	5	42
Contralateral lung	1–12	1–4	8–27
Pleural effusion	16–20	2–7	30
Soft tissues	5	NA	19

NA, not available.
[Modified from Argiris A, Murren J. Staging and prognosis of small cell lung cancer. *Cancer J* 2000 (in press).]

and neuronal tissues have been identified.[51] Symptoms may precede the diagnosis by many months and are often the presenting complaint.[46] They may also be the initial sign of relapse from remission. In contrast to the endocrine syndromes, for which successful treatment of the tumor effectively controls the symptoms, the severity of the neurologic symptoms is unrelated to tumor bulk and often does not improve despite successful antineoplastic therapy. Subacute peripheral neuropathy may be the most frequent neurologic syndrome. The Lambert-Eaton syndrome is characterized by proximal muscle weakness that improves with continued use and hyporeflexia and dysautonomia. Characteristic electromyographic findings confirm the diagnosis. The cause is related to autoantibody impairment of acetylcholine release from the cholinergic nerve terminals.[52] Rare neurologic entities include cerebellar ataxia,[53] retinal degeneration,[51] intestinal dysmotility,[54] limbic encephalomyelitis,[55] and necrotizing myelopathy.[56]

STAGING EVALUATION AND PROGNOSTIC FACTORS

The goal of staging is to establish the prognosis, identify patients with disease confined to the chest who are appropriate for combined modality therapy, and assess whether an individual patient will be at increased risk of mortality if treated with an aggressive chemotherapy program. Surgery plays a minor role in the management of this disease, and less than 10% of patients might be considered candidates for thoracotomy. As a result, the revised TNM system for staging lung cancer is not widely employed.[57] Rather, a simpler system, introduced by the Veterans' Administration Lung Study Group (VALSG) is generally used.[58] In the VALSG system, limited stage is defined as disease confined to one hemithorax that can be encompassed in a tolerable radiation field. These patients are currently treated with a combined modality approach. In all other settings, patients are considered to have extensive-stage disease. At presentation, after appropriate staging procedures are performed, 60% to 70% of patients with SCLC have extensive disease and 30% to 40% have limited-stage disease.[1]

In the VALSG staging system, the appropriate classification of selected sites remains controversial. These sites include an ipsilateral pleural effusion, supraclavicular lymphadenopathy (ipsilateral or contralateral), or contralateral mediastinal lymphadenopathy. Several large series have failed to identify a difference in survival between patients with an isolated ipsilateral pleural effusion compared with other patients with limited SCLC,[59–62] and many groups have included patients with ipsilateral pleural effusions within their definition of limited-stage disease.[63–66] However, only 2% to 7% of all patients with otherwise limited SCLC have an isolated pleural effusion,[61,67] so that small differences in outcome associated with this clinical factor might be missed. In an analysis of two large cooperative group databases, which included in toto more than 4000 patients, the survival of patients with an isolated effusion was similar to patients with one site of extensive disease.[64,67] In one of these analyses, an isolated effusion conferred a poorer survival compared with other patients classified as having limited disease, which was of borderline significance ($P = .051$).[64] In clinical practice, small effusions, usually detected by computed tomography (CT) scan, are sometimes difficult to evaluate. It is assumed that these effusions are malignant, unless the fluid is a transudate, nonhemorrhagic, and cytologically negative on repeated examination results. Clinical judgment in individual cases should be applied for selection of these patients for combined modality therapy until this issue is addressed in a prospective trial.

Although most randomized trials evaluating the role of combined modality therapy in limited-stage SCLC have excluded patients with an ipsilateral pleural effusion, they have usually included patients with ipsilateral, and sometimes contralateral, supraclavicular lymph node metastases. The presence of supraclavicular lymphadenopathy is commonly associated with extensive disease, but when encountered in patients with otherwise limited disease (5% of cases), carries a trend toward poorer survival.[67,68] Contralateral mediastinal involvement is also usually classified as limited-stage disease. However, two randomized studies that evaluated the use of a more aggressive, twice daily, radiation regimen, excluded patients with contralateral hilar disease,[69,70] presumably to reduce the volume of irradiated field and the risk for toxicity. If this form of more intensive radiotherapy becomes a standard of care, the potential prognostic significance of the extent of mediastinal nodal involvement will need to be reexamined. Patients with limited-stage disease who present with superior vena cava syndrome have a similar prognosis to other patients with limited-stage disease[62,71] and have been included in randomized studies investigating the role of combined modality therapy.[72,73]

Several series have identified a more favorable outcome for patients with "very" limited disease, that is a tumor confined to the lung without evidence of spread to the mediastinum.[66,74,75] Retrospective analysis of the University of Toronto database demonstrated that patients without evidence of mediastinal metastases by CT scan or mediastinoscopy who were treated with chemotherapy and radiation had a median survival of almost 16 months and a projected survival at 5 years of 18%.[66] This was significantly better than other patients with limited disease who had more extensive tumor burden. Patients who undergo surgical resection and have an absence of mediastinal metastases have an especially favorable outcome. Survival in this select group is between 50% and 60%. Among the patients with extensive disease, a number of studies have shown that the number of metastatic sites is an important parameter.[59,62,64,67]

OTHER PROGNOSTIC FACTORS

In addition to disease extent based on VALSG stage, multivariate analyses suggest that performance status and the serum LDH are the most reproducible prognostic factors. Performance status reflects both the underlying extent of the disease and partially dictates tolerance for the intensity of treatment. Although patients with a lower performance status are at a higher risk for treatment-related complications, they may still benefit from a combined modality approach.[76]

An elevated LDH is seen in 33% to 57% of all patients with SCLC,[48,64,77] and up to 85% of patients with extensive-stage disease.[64] Biochemical parameters, such as an elevation of the LDH and neuron-specific enolase, are strong predictors of poor outcome in SCLC.[48,61,64,78,79] Male gender is an adverse prognostic factor in some,[80,81] but not all series.[67] Older age has been an independent adverse prognostic factor in limited disease in some series,[67,82,83] but not in others.[48,84] Older age often results in a compromised dose intensity, usually due to treatment delays.[84]

Molecular studies have identified several specific lesions involved in the pathogenesis of SCLC, and the prognostic import of the gain or loss of function of these critical genes and gene products is now being evaluated clinically.[22,85,86] Drug sensitivity testing *in vitro* may be useful to guide selection of a chemotherapy regimen, but with current methodologies it is feasible in only a minority of patients and is labor intensive.[87]

ASSESSMENT OF RISK

In many respects, treatment for SCLC is as demanding as a thoracotomy and pulmonary resection. In some large cooperative group trials, treatment-related mortality has exceeded 10%. Accordingly, a careful assessment of a patient's ability to undergo aggressive therapy, particularly if concurrent chemotherapy and radiation are planned, is warranted. Several retrospective analyses have attempted to identify patients at increased risk for a treatment-related mortality. An analysis of 382 patients treated in a single institution identified age older than 50 years, Karnofsky performance status less than or equal to 50, treatment with a regimen containing three drugs or more, and a prior septic episode during chemotherapy as risk factors for septic complications.[88] In this study, older patients with a poor performance status had a 22-fold greater risk of septic death than patients without those risk factors. In another study involving 610 patients, each one of the 71 fatalities that occurred during the first cycle of VP-16–based chemotherapy was matched to the next patient enrolled on the trial.[89] Patients dying early were more likely to have a poor performance status, clinical hepatomegaly, a low serum albumin, and elevations of the blood urea nitrogen and serum alkaline phosphatase. The Copenhagen Lung Cancer Group compared 937 patients treated in its two most recent studies with 819 patients treated in early clinical studies.[90] The mortality during the first cycle of chemotherapy in the recent studies was threefold higher (12.6% vs. 4.2%) compared with the earlier trials. An algorithm was developed to identify high-risk patients that included age, performance status, and serum LDH. Patients were defined as high risk if they had a poor performance status [Eastern Cooperative Oncology Group (ECOG) 3 or 4], or if they were 65 years old or older and had a serum LDH that was more than twice the upper normal level. Based on this algorithm, 21% of the 937 patients would be considered at high risk. In this high-risk group, the median survival time was 133 days, and the 2-year survival was 4.5%. Mortality during the first chemotherapy cycle was 33%, and among patients treated with etoposide and platinum the frequency was 41%. Of note, more than one-half of these early deaths occurred in older patients with an elevated LDH who had a preserved performance status. For these high-risk patients, therefore, less intensive chemotherapy would be appropriate, and careful monitoring and support during treatment is mandatory.

STAGING PROCEDURES

Autopsy and clinical studies have shown that SCLC commonly disseminates to soft tissue and multiple viscera (see Table 31.3-1). Autopsy studies in patients with lung cancer who were staged without modern imaging methods and died within 1 month of a potentially curative surgical resection but of causes unrelated to the cancer, showed that 12 of 19 patients (63%) with SCLC had distant metastases, in comparison with 14% to 40% for the non-SCLC histologies.[91] Outside of the context of a clinical trial, it is reasonable to discontinue the staging survey once disease outside the chest has been identified. Exceptions would include the presence of additional symptomatic areas that may require prompt therapy, such as symptoms and signs suggestive of metastases to a weight-bearing bone or the neuraxis. In an era of cost containment, algorithms have been proposed that use each diagnostic modality in a stepwise fashion to reduce the costs of the staging workup.[65,92]

History, clinical examination, including neurologic examination, a complete blood cell count, and a biochemical panel, including electrolytes, liver function tests, and LDH determination, and a chest radiographic film make up the first line of pretreatment evaluation in SCLC. Selected biochemical parameters, in particular the serum LDH, have been shown to be predictive of the extent of disease.[48,61,64,77,93,94] Symptoms and abnormalities detected in these tests often direct subsequent testing. CT scanning of the chest is superior to chest radiography in delineating the extension of the primary tumor and detecting mediastinal lymphadenopathy and may up-stage T or N designations in up to 82% of cases.[95] A pericardial effusion is infrequently seen at presentation, but thickening of the pericardium detected on CT scan of the chest is a common finding of unknown significance.[96] A CT is necessary for purposes of planning the radiation portal field and for evaluation of the minority of patients who are candidates for surgical resection. In the pre-CT era, bronchoscopy was found to be helpful as an adjunct to chest radiography findings in assessing a complete response.[97] CT scan is now widely available and is commonly used for pretreatment evaluation and response assessment. However, its capability to assess tumor response is limited in areas of atelectasis and radiation-induced fibrosis where the presence of active tumor cannot be ascertained. The role of positron emission tomography (PET) scanning or somatostatin receptor imaging in distinguishing residual tumor versus benign radiographic abnormalities should be further investigated.

CT scanning detects intraabdominal lesions in approximately 35% of patients with SCLC at presentation.[98,99] By the use of chest and abdominal CT, locally advanced or distant disease is diagnosed in 94% to 96% of patients.[95,98] CT has an accuracy of 85% in detecting liver metastases in SCLC overall,[99,100] and that increases in patients with abnormalities in liver function test results.[100] Involvement of the adrenal glands by metastatic tumor is almost always clinically silent. Clinical studies have implicated the adrenals as the only metastatic site in SCLC in 8% to 11% of patients at presentation; however, the majority of these cases were not biopsy proven. In autopsy series, adrenal metastases are seen in 35% to 65% of patients with SCLC. The accuracy of noninvasive imaging in differentiating between adenomas and adrenal metastases in patients with lung cancer has been suboptimal,[101] although newer magnetic resonance imaging (MRI) techniques, such as chemical shift imaging, may improve the accuracy of MRI in differentiating adenomas from metastatic deposits.[102]

Brain metastases are found in 10% of SCLC patients at the time of diagnosis.[103,104] The cumulative risk for brain metastases increases with survival. Multiple lesions are usually found in autopsy in patients with CNS involvement.[103,105] Leptomeningeal involvement is extremely rare at presentation, but may develop antemortem in 2% to 13% of patients.[103,105,106] The majority of these patients have simultaneous brain metastases.[103,106] The usefulness of a pretreatment brain scan in asymptomatic patients is controversial. Although the yield of brain CT in patients with neurologic abnormalities is high (42% to 88%),[107,108] it is only 3% to 8% in asymptomatic patients with SCLC.[107–109] In a patient in whom metastatic disease has been demonstrated by another test or who is not a potential candidate for thoracic irradiation for other reasons, imaging the brain is probably not a mandatory component of the initial staging evaluation. If asymptomatic brain metastases are present, chemotherapy may be adequate treatment,[110] and the early detection and treatment of asymptomatic brain metastases with radiation therapy has not been shown to significantly improve patient outcome,[107,109] partly due to the effect of systemic failure on survival. If brain metastases are the single site of distant disease, the prognosis may not be significantly altered because the median survival compared with patients with limited disease has been comparable in some series,[111,112] although not in others.[106,107] A CT of the brain is needed in patients considered for prophylactic cranial irradiation, as the presence of clinically occult metastases would affect treatment planning.

Up to 40% of patients with SCLC have a positive radionuclide bone scan at diagnosis; in fewer than 10% of cases this is the only site of metastatic disease.[42,113] Bone involvement shown by bone scan is frequently detected in asymptomatic patients with SCLC and correlates with an elevated alkaline phosphatase level and bone marrow positivity. Further diagnostic evaluation with a plain radiograph and in some cases with a bone CT scan or MRI may be required to investigate areas of equivocal findings that could be due to osteoarthritis or trauma. In assessing response, repeat bone scanning is helpful but not sufficiently reliable.[113] In some cases, patients demonstrate a more intense uptake of metastatic lesions on bone scan, which reflects bone regeneration and is a sign of response to therapy.

The bone marrow is involved in 15% to 30% of patients with SCLC at presentation, but is uncommonly the only site of metastatic disease.[42,61,114–116] As a result, routine bone marrow examinations rarely modify staging. The yield of bone marrow biopsy can be increased by *in vitro* semisolid cultures of bone marrow aspirates or immunostaining with anti-SCLC monoclonal antibodies, which are positive in 10% and 15% to 66% of histologically negative bone marrow, respectively.[117–121] However, the clinical significance of bone marrow involvement demonstrated by these methods has not yet been determined. A leukoerythroblastic picture on the peripheral blood, which is present in 8% to 19% of all cases at presentation, is highly specific for extensive bone marrow infiltration by SCLC.[44,115,116] Severe thrombocytopenia, with a platelet count of less than 50×10^9/L, and an elevated LDH are also suggestive of bone marrow metastases.[44,94,115] Bone marrow involvement usually coincides with bone and liver metastases, but not with CNS involvement.[115] At least one-half of the patients with a positive bone marrow result have bone metastases detected by bone scan.[42,122,123] In patients with a normal bone scan, normal LDH, and no evidence of thrombocytopenia or peripheral blood leukoerythroblastosis, the yield of bone marrow biopsy is extremely low,[123] and it can be omitted.

MRI allows for the noninvasive evaluation of large volumes of bone marrow and is a sensitive method for detecting bone marrow involvement by SCLC. Bone marrow positivity by MRI has been reported in 30% to 60% of patients with SCLC and identifies marrow involvement missed in the initial biopsy in 3% to 19% of patients.[117,124–127] Circulating malignant cells detected by reverse transcriptase polymerase chain reaction for cytokeratin can be found in the peripheral blood of 27% of SCLC patients.[128] The significance of this finding should be investigated.

PET scan has emerged as a promising imaging modality in lung cancer. Most commonly, a radiolabeled glucose analogue, [^{18}F]fluoro-2-deoxy-D-glucose, has been used to demonstrate differences in the metabolism of normal and neoplastic cells. The potential role of PET scan in assessing a solitary lung nodule and mediastinal involvement by tumor has been demonstrated in multiple studies[129–131] and has also proven valuable in the detection of unexpected extrathoracic disease.[132] Thus, as PET continues to technically improve and become more widely available, it may assume an important role in the staging of SCLC.

Technetium-labeled monoclonal antibody imaging has been evaluated as a staging method in SCLC.[133] The accuracy of this imaging modality in staging patients with SCLC is approximately 90%. However, it has limited value in detecting liver metastases or lesions smaller than 2 cm.[133] The presence of somatostatin receptors in SCLC, a neuroendocrine neoplasm, has made possible the use of radiolabeled somatostatin analogues for the imaging of patients with SCLC. Somatostatin receptor imaging is accurate in detecting the primary lesion and mediastinal lymphadenopathy in SCLC, but has not shown sufficient sensitivity (50% or less) in detecting sites of metastatic disease.[134–136]

TREATMENT

Early efforts at the management of SCLC with surgery were characterized by incomplete staging both before and during thoracotomy. Nevertheless, in the 1960s some studies reported 5-year or longer survival in more than 10% of the patients.[137,138] These results, however, were overshadowed by two studies in the 1970s that provided philosophical justification for not using a surgical approach in this disease. The British Medical Research Council published a 144-patient trial (Table 31.3-2) that demonstrated the modest superiority of radiotherapy as primary treatment for "operable" SCLC.[139] Shortly thereafter, an American study[140] compared the survival of 146 operable but nonresected patients with 41 resected patients and found no differences.

The inadequate results with surgery or radiation alone, even in carefully selected patients, highlighted the need for systemic treatment in SCLC, and the primary role of chemotherapy in the management of this disease is now well established. In a study conducted in the late 1960s testing various alkylating

TABLE 31.3-2. Survival in Patients with Operable Small Cell Lung Cancer Randomized to Surgery or Radiotherapy

Group	*Patients*	*Mean Survival (mo)*	*Survival Rate* 1 Y	2 Y	5 Y
Surgery	71	6.5	21	4	1[a]
Radiotherapy	73	10[b]	22	10	4

[a]One patient unable to receive surgery; given irradiation.
[b]Significant survival difference (P = .04) in favor of radiotherapy.
(Modified from ref. 139.)

TABLE 31.3-3. Active Agents in Small Cell Lung Cancer

		No Prior Chemotherapy		*Prior Chemotherapy*	
Drug	*Dose (mg/m²)*[a]	Patient (No.)	Percent Response	Patient (No.)	Percent Response
Cyclophosphamide	1000	112	22	—	—
Ifosfamide	5000–8000	60	57	14	43
Doxorubicin	60–75	16	25	14	29
Epirubicin	85–140	196	48	19	21
Carboplatin	250–450	52	63	54	13
Cisplatin	45–140	—	—	118	14
Vincristine	1.5[b]	10	40	9	44
Vindesine	3–4[b]	—	—	50	24
Vinorelbine	30[b]	47	26	83	14
VP-16	100–300[c]	66	82	151	5
Teniposide	60–100[c]	109	55	80	22
Paclitaxel	250	75	45	24	29
Docetaxel	75–100	58	22	28	25
Irinotecan	100[b]–125[b]	8	50	59	24
	350	—	—	32	16
Topotecan	1.5–2.0[c]	48	39	362	17
Gemcitabine	1000–1250[b]	26	27	36	14

Note: Response rates are weighted averages obtained from selected published trials that administered the chemotherapy drug intravenously in doses and schedules currently used. The duration of drug infusion was variable. Response rates should be regarded as approximate because patient populations were heterogenous.
[a]Cycles repeated every 3 to 4 weeks unless otherwise specified.
[b]Treatment given weekly or biweekly.
[c]Treatment given daily or every other day for 3 to 5 days, repeated every 3 to 4 weeks.
[Modified from Argiris A, Murren J. Advances in the chemotherapy for small cell lung cancer. *Cancer J* 2000 (in press).]

agents, cyclophosphamide was shown to double survival compared with supportive care in patients with extensive disease, and shortly thereafter a combination of cyclophosphamide with radiation was shown to improve survival compared with radiation alone in patients with limited disease.[141,142] An extensive evaluation of the drugs then available demonstrated that anthracyclines and vinca alkaloids, along with certain alkylating drugs, produced single-agent response rates of up to 50%. The antimetabolites appeared to be less active, with response rates reported of 20% to 30%. In the 1980s the epipodophyllotoxins (VP-16 and VM-26) and the platinum analogues were introduced, and their activity ranged from 40% to 60% in previously untreated patients.[143] During the 1990s, two new classes of chemotherapeutic agents, the taxanes and the camptothecins, entered clinical practice and are establishing a role in the management of this disease.

DEFINITIONS OF ACTIVE CHEMOTHERAPY AND STRATEGIES FOR EVALUATING NEW AGENTS

As agents such as cyclophosphamide and doxorubicin became established in the management of this disease, it became clear in the evaluation of new drugs that exposure to prior chemotherapy and response to this therapy were at least as important as other known prognostic factors in predicting response to the new agent. For example, the epipodophyllotoxins produce response rates of 40% to 90% in untreated patients,[144–146] but in relapsed patients the response rate to VP-16 and VM-26 were 5% to 12% and 20%, respectively.[147–149] Based on retrospective analysis of the activity of effective chemotherapy drugs in different populations, response rates greater than or equal to 10% in patients with refractory disease, greater than or equal to 20% in patients in sensitive relapse (typically defined as response to initial therapy and a treatment-free interval of longer than 3 months before disease progression), and greater than or equal to 30% in patients with previously untreated extensive disease have been proposed as the appropriate targets to declare a new chemotherapy drug active.[143,150,151] Because of the biologic aggressiveness of SCLC, the patient population that should be selected to test new drugs remains controversial. Clinical trials that enroll patients with refractory disease, for example, pose the least risk that outcome might be compromised if the new agent turns out to be inactive. However, substantially more patients would need to be evaluated to establish a response rate of greater than or equal to 10% than would be necessary to establish a response rate of greater than or equal to 30% in previously untreated patients. This means that a much larger number of patients would be exposed to the toxicity of a new drug before it was rejected. Thus, the initial testing of new drugs in patients with sensitive relapse has been proposed as a reasonable compromise,[152] although evaluation in previously untreated patients may be reasonable for new drugs of particular promise.[151]

STANDARD CHEMOTHERAPY AGENTS AND ANALOGUES OF STANDARD AGENTS

A number of chemotherapy drugs fulfill the criteria for activity outlined in the previous section. Several of these drugs, such as nitrogen mustard, methotrexate, altretamine, and carmustine, are seldom used today. In the 1990s, five drugs, or analogues of these five drugs, have been used in the management of SCLC (Table 31.3-3). Current treatment recommendations are based on the experience with these agents.

The activity of VP-16 is dependent on the schedule of administration. In randomized trials, bolus administration for 3 or 5 consecutive days repeated every 3 to 4 weeks is superior to one dose by bolus or 24-hour infusion every 3 weeks.[145,153,154] The 5-day bolus schedule is as effective as an 8-day bolus schedule.[146] Two studies that included a pharmacokinetic analysis suggested that the duration of exposure to a threshold concentration of VP-16 was an important determinant of efficacy and toxicity.[145,146] The availability of an oral formulation has led to the development of more prolonged schedules. As a single agent, prolonged oral regimens of VP-16 were tested in previously treated patients and appeared to have activity comparable with the standard 3- to 5-day bolus schedules.[155,156] When included in multidrug regimens, the schedule dependence of activity has not been demonstrated. In a randomized trial comparing cisplatin plus VP-16 given as an intravenous bolus for 3 consecutive days to cisplatin plus VP-16 given as a 21-day oral regimen, there was greater hematologic toxicity with no improvement in response or survival in patients receiving the prolonged oral regimen.[157] Continuous infusion of VP-16 for 72 hours was not superior to a 3-day bolus in combination with cisplatin.[158]

Cisplatin has been evaluated as a single agent, particularly in patients who have had previous treatment, and response rates from these studies approximate 15%. Carboplatin produces a comparable response rate in previously treated patients, and in newly diagnosed patients a 60% response rate has been observed.[159] Ifosfamide is an analogue of cyclophosphamide that appears to be at least as active as cyclophosphamide in the treatment of SCLC. In newly diagnosed patients, response rates of 50% to 65% have been reported. Teniposide is an analogue of VP-16 and, in a randomized trial in newly diagnosed patients with extensive disease, produced a response rate of 43%, compared with a response rate of 49% for ifosfamide and 56% for the standard cyclophosphamide, doxorubicin, and vincristine (CAV) regimen.[160] At the dose tested, hematologic toxicity and life-threatening complications were much more common in the patients treated with CAV. In other phase II studies, the response rate of teniposide has ranged from 38% to 90%, and in one, 5 of 30 patients experienced a toxic death, underlying the importance of patient selection in determining response and toxicity.[161,162] Epirubicin is an anthracycline that in preclinical models was as active as doxorubicin and less cardiotoxic. As a single agent, epirubicin has been shown to produce a response rate of approximately 50% in previously untreated patients with extensive disease.[163]

NEWER CHEMOTHERAPY AGENTS

The taxanes bind microtubules and promote microtubular assembly. This interferes with tubulin depolymerization, resulting in a disruption of cell division. In an ECOG study, paclitaxel at a dose of 250 mg/m^2 infused over 24 hours produced a response rate of 34%.[164] The North Central Cancer Treatment Group used a similar schedule with the addition of granulocyte colony-stimulating factor (G-CSF) support and reported a response rate of 53% with a reduction in the grade IV leukopenia to 14%. Docetaxel at a dose of 100 mg/m^2 has been reported to produce a response rate of 25% in untreated patients and at a dose of 60 mg/m^2 a response rate of 13.5% in previously treated patients.[165,166]

Camptothecin is a plant alkaloid that has the unique mechanism of action of interacting with topoisomerase I, a nuclear enzyme that plays a key role in DNA metabolism. Schiller et al. treated 48 chemotherapy-naive patients with extensive-stage SCLC with intravenous topotecan at 2 mg/m^2/d for 5 days, repeated every 3 weeks. Most patients received G-CSF support. The regimen was active, with a response rate of 40%, 1-year survival of 39%, and median survival of 10 months.[167] In patients progressing or relapsing shortly after completing chemotherapy, the response rate was 6% to 11%.[168,169] Pooled data from three multicenter studies showed a response rate of 18% in 168 patients in sensitive relapse (>3-month interval from previous chemotherapy treatment); the median survival was 30 weeks, and the 1-year survival was 21%.[170] A randomized trial comparing topotecan with CAV in patients in sensitive relapse demonstrated comparable response rates and survival for the two regimens.[171] Topotecan is also available in an oral formulation, and this preparation appears to be at least as active as the intravenous drug.[172] Irinotecan also has activity in SCLC, but has not been as extensively evaluated. In patients previously treated with chemotherapy, response rates of 16% to 47% have been reported.[173–175]

Gemcitabine, a pyrimidine antimetabolite, produced responses in 7 of 26 (27%) previously untreated patients with extensive disease and 12 of 19 (63%) patients resistant to cisplatin and VP-16.[176] Preliminary results in another study enrolling patients with resistant disease identified three brief remissions in 12 evaluable patients, which together with the demonstrated activity of gemcitabine in previously treated non-SCLC suggests that the mechanism of drug resistance may differ between gemcitabine and other agents used to treat lung cancer.[177]

Vinorelbine (Navelbine) is a new vinca alkaloid that in previously treated patients has produced a response rate of 12% to 16%.[178,179] The activity in newly diagnosed patients with extensive disease was 26%.[180] Because vinorelbine is well tolerated in an elderly population, it may be a useful component of palliative combination regimens. In combination with carboplatin, for example, it produced a response rate of 74% (32 of 43 patients) and a median survival of 37 weeks in patients with extensive disease.[180]

COMBINATION CHEMOTHERAPY

After the activity of cyclophosphamide was established in SCLC, multidrug combinations were developed and tested (Table 31.3-4). Randomized trials of these early combinations demonstrated superior activity to single-agent cyclophosphamide. The combination of cyclophosphamide, doxorubicin, and dacarbazine produced a higher response rate and survival when compared with an equally toxic dose of single-agent cyclophosphamide.[181] Hansen et al. demonstrated that the addition of vincristine to the combination of cyclophosphamide, methotrexate, and CCNU improved survival compared with the three-drug combination, highlighting the usefulness of this relatively nonmyelotoxic agent in combination therapy.[182] Livingston et al. developed the CAV combination, and this became a standard.[183]

With the identification of VP-16 as an important new agent, several modifications of the CAV regimen that included VP-16 were tested. In extensive disease, a slight improvement in survival was noted when VP-16 replaced either doxorubicin or vin-

TABLE 31.3-4. Commonly Used Chemotherapy Regimens

Regimen	*Dose (mg/m²)*	*Schedule*
CDE		
Cyclophosphamide	1000	d_1
Doxorubicin	40	d_1
VP-16	120	d_{1-3}
CAV		
Cyclophosphamide	1000	d_1
Doxorubicin	45	d_1
Vincristine	1.4	d_1
EP		
VP-16	100	d_{1-3}
Cisplatin	80	d_1
VIP		
VP-16	75	d_{1-4}
Ifosfamide	1.2	d_{1-4}
Cisplatin	20	d_{1-4}
ICE		
Ifosfamide	5000[a]	d_1
Carboplatin	400	d_1
VP-16	100	d_{1-3}
Carboplatin	AUC = 7[b]	d_1
Paclitaxel	175	d_1

Note: Cycles are repeated every 3 to 4 weeks. Intravenous route of administration is used although the oral formulation of VP-16 has been substituted for the intravenous formulation assuming that it has a bioavailability of 0.50. Mesna also required in regimens that include ifosfamide.
[a]Administered as a 24-hour continuous infusion.
[b]Area under the curve (AUC) dosing according to the formula of Calvert or Chatulet.

cristine, although greater myelosuppression was evident in the cyclophosphamide, doxorubicin, VP-16 (CDE) arm in the latter trial.[184,185] Hong et al. compared intensive CV (with the dose of cyclophosphamide increased from 1000 to 2000 mg/m²) with CAV and cyclophosphamide, VP-16, and vincristine (CEV) and reported that patients treated with CV had a shorter survival and experienced more myelosuppression than patients treated on the other two arms.[184] Substitution of VP-16 for methotrexate in the lomustine, cyclophosphamide, vincristine, and methotrexate regimen also improved survival.[186] Administration of the VP-16 beginning on day 3 produced better survival but more myelosuppression than beginning the VP-16 on day 14 of the cycle, perhaps because this schedule provided greater dose density, or perhaps because it delivered the VP-16 at a point at which more tumor cells were in cell cycle and therefore more susceptible to the drug.[187]

Five randomized trials have evaluated the addition of VP-16 (CAVE) to the CAV regimen.[188–192] In three studies, the doses of CAV were equivalent in each arm.[188–190] Not surprisingly, in these studies the addition of VP-16 resulted in increased hematologic toxicity. Although a better response rate was evident in the arm containing VP-16 in at least some patient subsets in each of these studies, there was an improvement in response duration (of 3 months) and survival (of 6 weeks, $P = .08$) in only one study.[189] Jett et al. compared CAVE with CAV in 231 patients with limited disease.[190] Despite a reduction of the dose of cyclophosphamide by 33%, there was still greater myelosuppression in the CAVE arm. There was a small improvement in median and 2-year survival with CAVE, which was not statistically significant. Two randomized studies intensified components of this regimen: In one the cyclophosphamide was increased from 1000 to 1200 mg/m² and the dose of doxorubicin increased from 40 to 75 mg/m² in the CAV arm compared with the CAVE arm.[192] The regimens produced equivalent myelotoxicity, response rates, and survival. These results were comparable with the outcomes with less intensive CAV regimens in extensive disease.

The VP-16 and cisplatin (EP) regimen was tested in SCLC because this combination produced synergistic activity in preclinical systems and was established as an active regimen in other diseases. Evans et al. reported response rates of 55% in patients previously treated with CAV and 86% in newly diagnosed patients.[193–195] Einhorn et al. reported that two cycles of consolidation with EP added to the treatment of patients with limited disease who were responding to six cycles of CAV had a longer survival than patients randomized to CAV only.[196] Prospective studies comparing these two regimens showed comparable response and survival, with a significant reduction in toxicity with EP.[197,198] There was less myelosuppression with EP, and if given with radiation, patients experienced less esophagitis and interstitial pneumonitis. Consequently, EP became an alternative to CAV as the frontline regimen for SCLC.

Carboplatin can be substituted for cisplatin with no loss of activity and improved tolerance.[199,200] In combination with VP-16, Bishop et al. reported a response rate of 77% and 58% for limited and extensive disease, respectively.[201] Moreover, randomized trials of multiagent regimens in which the two platinum analogues were compared suggested that they were at least equivalent. The Hellenic Cooperative Oncology Group randomized 147 patients to receive VP-16, 100 mg/m², days 1 to 3, and cisplatin, 100 mg/m², or carboplatin, 300 mg/m², along with concurrent radiation.[199] Response and survival were similar in the two arms, although the toxicity, particularly nausea, vomiting, nephrotoxicity, and neurotoxicity, were significantly lower in the patients who received carboplatin. Myelosuppression was also less in the carboplatin arm, but this was not statistically significant. In another large randomized trial, induction with teniposide, vincristine, and either carboplatin or cisplatin produced equivalent activity and toxicity.[200]

Ifosfamide produces less myelosuppression than cyclophosphamide and has significant single-agent activity. Ifosfamide has been substituted for cyclophosphamide in the CAV regimen.[202] Combinations of ifosfamide with cisplatin and with etoposide have also been tested. The three-drug regimen VP-16, ifosfamide, and cisplatin, initially tested in refractory germ cell tumors, has also been evaluated. In patients with SCLC, a population that is older and has more comorbid illness than patients with germ cell tumors, a 20% reduction in dose intensity was necessary to avoid excessive myelosuppression.[203] In a randomized trial comparing VP-16, ifosfamide, and cisplatin with EP, one study, which enrolled only patients with extensive disease, identified a significant, although small, difference in both median survival (9.0 vs. 7.3 months) and 2-year survival rates (13% vs. 5%).[204] Myelosuppression was more severe in the arm treated with ifosfamide. Carboplatin has been substituted for cisplatin in regimens that also include ifosfamide, carboplatin, and VP-16 (ICE), and in single-arm studies impressive response rates and cumulative myelosuppression have been reported.[205,206] Other three-drug regimens that incorporate these agents, such as ifosfamide, doxorubicin, and VP-16[202]; ifosfamide, carboplatin, and oral VP-16[206]; and paclitaxel, cisplatin, and VP-16,[207] have been tested but have not been demonstrated to be superior to either EP or CAV.

Several studies are in progress evaluating camptothecin (topotecan or irinotecan)-based regimens in SCLC. In combination with platinum agents, response rates are between 17% and 29% in previously treated patients and 75% and 84% in newly diagnosed patients.[208–210] Preliminary results of a multicenter randomized trial in Japan found that the combination of irinotecan and cisplatin produced superior survival than the standard VP-16 and cisplatin regimen in patients with extensive stage disease.[211] Combinations of camptothecins with other agents active in SCLC are also being evaluated, and many have shown significant activity, albeit with substantial associated myelosuppression.[212–214] Three-drug regimens, such as paclitaxel, cisplatin, and topotecan,[215] are also being developed.

DURATION OF CHEMOTHERAPY

Through the 1970s, sensitive tumors were often treated with chemotherapy for periods that might extend up to 2 years. This meant that most patients with SCLC received uninterrupted chemotherapy until disease progression or death. In 1984, Feld et al. reported that six cycles of CAV and thoracic irradiation produced survival comparable with the results of a previous treatment program that included 12 months of maintenance therapy.[216] Subsequently, a large number of randomized trials examined whether maintenance chemotherapy prolonged survival.[217–226]

A few studies have suggested that prolonged treatment programs improve survival, at least in certain patient subsets. The CALGB randomized 258 patients to one of four chemotherapy regimens, and 57 patients in complete remission underwent a second randomization to maintenance therapy or observation. Among the 46 patients with limited disease who proceeded to the second randomization, the median survival was improved with maintenance chemotherapy (16.8 vs. 6.8 months).[217] However, the induction regimens utilized in this study might be considered inferior to currently used treatments. The Medical Research Council randomized 265 patients who had responded to six cycles of induction chemotherapy to an additional six cycles of maintenance or observation.[220] Overall, there was no difference in survival between patients treated with six or 12 cycles of chemotherapy, though for patients in complete remission at the time of randomization a subset analysis suggested that maintenance may provide a survival benefit. In a second British study, patients treated with six cycles of CAV were randomized to six additional cycles of the same chemotherapy or observation.[218] Most of the patients treated in this study were in complete or near complete remission. For the patients with extensive disease, the median survival was improved by approximately 4 months with maintenance treatment. An additional trial, organized by the Eastern Cooperative Oncology Group (ECOG), randomized patients to CAV alternating with another three drug combination or CAV alone.[221] After six to eight cycles of induction, patients in complete remission underwent a second randomization to maintenance treatment or observation. Patients assigned to CAV and maintenance therapy had both a longer progression-free survival and overall survival ($P = 0.09$) than patients who received only CAV with no maintenance. For the patients who received the six-drug regimen, those who were given no maintenance survived longer than the patients who received maintenance treatment.

In contrast, four other studies that randomized patients to five or six cycles of chemotherapy or a total of 12 cycles of chemotherapy found no difference in outcome.[219,222,223,225] Among these studies, only one trial evaluated maintenance therapy in complete responders,[222] one study included both complete and partial responders,[225] and two studies randomized all patients without evidence of disease progression following completion of induction chemotherapy.[219,223] In summary, these studies do not exclude the possibility that there is a subset of patients, perhaps those with particularly chemotherapy-sensitive disease treated with moderately intensive chemotherapy, who may derive a benefit from a maintenance program beyond five to eight cycles of standard chemotherapy. In unselected patients, however, treatment programs that extend beyond six cycles of chemotherapy have not demonstrated an advantage in survival and may be associated with inferior quality of life.

A number of additional studies have evaluated whether four cycles of chemotherapy are adequate.[224,227,228] Spiro et al. designed a study that included a double randomization at diagnosis.[227] Patients received four or eight cycles of CEV and on relapse received additional chemotherapy or supportive care. Of the four treatment arms, patients who received four cycles of chemotherapy and only supportive care at relapse had a significantly inferior median survival of 30 weeks. Thus, in this study four cycles of treatment were adequate if chemotherapy was offered to patients appropriate for additional therapy at relapse. Two additional studies also evaluated four cycles of induction with longer treatment programs.[224,228] Both studies found survival with the longer treatment program to be similar to the shorter program. The Medical Research Council randomized a total of 458 patients to treatment with VP-16, cyclophosphamide, methotrexate, and vincristine (ECMV) for three cycles, ECMV for six cycles, or VP-16 and ifosfamide for six cycles.[229,230] The median survival for patients treated for only three cycles was approximately 1 month shorter than for patients who received one of the regimens given for six cycles. Although this difference was not statistically significant, the study was not sufficiently powered to exclude a small advantage with longer treatment programs.[230] Among the more symptomatic patients, palliation of symptoms was slightly better for those treated with the ifosfamide and VP-16 combination, but the differences between the three arms were small.[229]

In summary, four to six cycles of induction chemotherapy appear to be optimal in the management of both limited and extensive SCLC. Maintenance chemotherapy beyond induction is of unproven value but may play a role in selected patients, depending on the sensitivity of their disease to chemotherapy and the induction regimen they received. Treatment at relapse should be considered if clinically appropriate.

GENERAL APPROACH TO PATIENTS WITH LIMITED DISEASE

An overview of the management of patients with limited disease is shown in Figure 31.3-1. An occasional patient has stage I

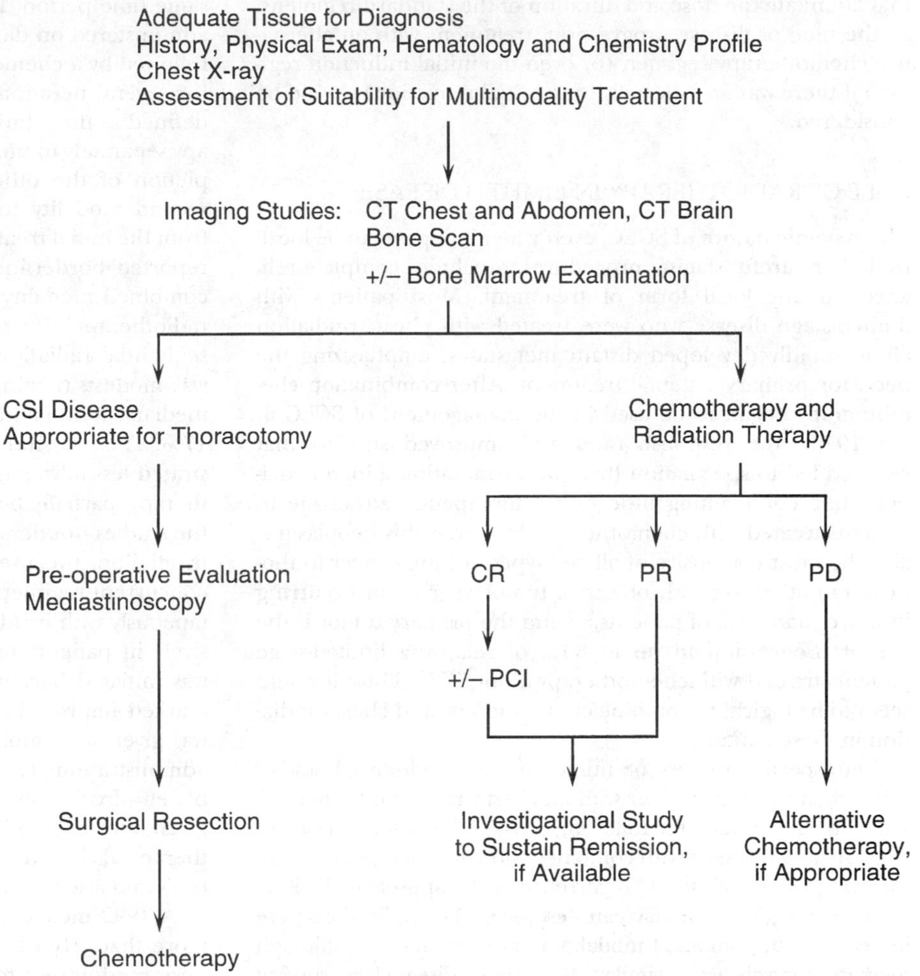

FIGURE 31.3-1. Algorithm outlining management of patients with limited disease. CR, complete response; CSI, clinical stage I; CT, computed tomography; PCI, prophylactic cranial irradiation; PD, progressive disease; PR, partial response.

disease by noninvasive staging; if this patient is a candidate for thoracotomy, a mediastinoscopy should be considered to ensure that mediastinal nodal metastases are not present before thoracotomy is attempted. Adjuvant chemotherapy is indicated in patients whose disease is resected. Other patients with limited disease should be carefully evaluated to determine their capacity to undergo combined modality therapy. Most patients who are not candidates for a clinical protocol should receive four to six cycles of chemotherapy and radiation to the chest. In limited disease, the CAV regimen produces an overall response rate of 80% to 90%, a complete remission rate of 50% to 60%, a median survival time of 12 to 16 months, and a 3-year disease-free survival of 10% to 15%. The VP-16 and cisplatin regimen appears to be at least as active as CAV and is associated with less toxicity if given with concurrent radiation.

Intrathoracic SCLC appears optimally treated with 150 cGy twice a day to a total dose of 4500 cGy in 3 weeks.[69] At least 4 (and preferably 6) hours between treatments are allowed. Customized blocks are used to limit exposure to normal tissues throughout the entire 3-week period. Initial portals are delivered anteriorly and posteriorly each day, switching to a posterior obliqued field to limit direct spinal cord dose to approximately 3600 Gy. Occasionally, a patient's pulmonary function is so marginal that a conscious decision is made not to shift to oblique fields because of fear of expanding total treatment volume and thereby increasing the risk of radiation pneumonitis in high-risk patients. In this setting, it becomes imperative to use a spinal cord block that is suboptimal from the standpoint of tumor control but essential from the standpoint of minimizing the risk of myelopathy. Conformal planning may help in this dilemma, but one must acknowledge that our quantitative knowledge of partial organ tolerance is presently negligible.

Some authors have advocated radiation doses up to 6000 cGy for SCLC.[231] In conjunction with multiagent chemotherapy, the routine need for such doses appears doubtful because of the impressive responsiveness of this neoplasm to both chemotherapy and radiation.

The sequencing of radiation and chemotherapy remains controversial and is more fully discussed later in this chapter (see Sequencing of Radiation with Chemotherapy). Concurrent rather than sequential administration of chemotherapy and radiation has produced superior survival in some but not all studies. Concurrent therapy can produce more toxicity than sequential chemotherapy and radiation, and because there is a broad range among individual patients in their capacity to tolerate aggressive therapy, a challenge in designing a treatment program is to satisfy the need to deliver optimal treatment without exposing patients to unacceptable toxicity. After induction therapy, most centers recommend prophylactic cranial irradiation to patients if they have achieved a complete or near complete remission. Some patients with significant adverse prognostic factors may be best served with treatment programs that attenuate the dose and duration of the standard regimens. At the time of disease progression, treatment with an alternative chemotherapy regimen (or even the initial induction regimen if there was an especially long initial remission) should be considered.

ROLE OF RADIOTHERAPY IN LIMITED DISEASE

The systemic nature of SCLC, even when it appears to be localized after careful staging procedures, precludes complete reliance on any local form of treatment. Most patients with limited-stage disease who were treated with chest irradiation alone rapidly developed distant metastases, emphasizing the need for primary systemic treatment. After combination chemotherapy began to be used in the management of SCLC in the 1970s, the response rates and improved survival that resulted led to speculation that chest irradiation added toxicities while contributing little or no therapeutic advantage in patients treated with chemotherapy. However, this neoplasm is also the most responsive of all cell types of lung cancer to thoracic radiotherapy, with objective tumor regression occurring in more than 90% of patients,[232] and the primary tumor is the site of progression in up to 80% of relapsing limited-stage patients treated with chemotherapy alone.[233,234] Thus, it would seem to be logical to combine chemotherapy and chest irradiation in these patients.

Retrospective reviews of numerous nonrandomized studies using chemotherapy with or without chest irradiation for limited-stage disease revealed the following facts[235,236]: (1) A lower rate of chest relapse was seen with combined modality therapy, although the frequency of local recurrence still approached 33%; (2) hematologic, pulmonary, and esophageal complications were increased with combined modality treatment; and (3) although median survivals were similar, the 2-year disease-free survival appeared superior for combined modality therapy compared with that achieved with chemotherapy alone.

Retrospective data, however, suffer from many deficiencies. Because chemotherapy alone is less toxic than combined modality therapy, there may have been a consistent bias against giving combined modality therapy to poor-risk patients. If the administration of radiotherapy is delayed for several chemotherapy cycles, patients who develop early progression are generally excluded from receiving radiation. An analysis of local relapse may sometimes be misleading because the definition of what constitutes a relapse may be heterogeneous. Variations in dose and schedule of the radiation and specific chemotherapy programs used further complicate comparison of relapse rates from different series. Less effective chemotherapy combined with effective radiation reduces the site of first failure in the chest because distant metastases are more prone to develop, whereas more effective chemotherapy combined with less effective radiation yields the opposite result. All these factors make it difficult to assess the value of adding chest irradiation to combination chemotherapy when reviewing uncontrolled data.

Sequencing of Radiation with Chemotherapy

The problem of how to integrate chemotherapy and radiation therapy remains far from standardized. Concurrent therapy is defined as combined modality treatment in which chemotherapy and radiation therapy are administered throughout the same time period. In alternating therapy, radiation therapy is administered on days during which no chemotherapy is given, followed by a chemotherapy cycle, and the process is repeated for several iterations of interdigitation. Sequential therapy is defined as the administration of chemotherapy and radiotherapy separately in time, with one modality begun only after completion of the other, often associated with a delay for the second modality to allow the patient an adequate recovery from the initial treatment modality. Several randomized studies reported borderline or significantly improved survival using combined modality treatment. Two of these used concurrent radiotherapy[72,237]; one, alternating radiotherapy[238]; and two, sequential radiation.[239,240] The magnitude of survival benefit was modest, ranging from 1 to 4 months in improvement in median survival and increases in the 2-year survival from 7% to 17%. The two studies with the longest follow-up[237,240] demonstrated less advantage beyond 5 years for patients given radiotherapy, partially because of second primary lung cancers. Of the studies not demonstrating improved survival without chest irradiation, two used sequential radiation therapy and one a concurrent regimen in that only a single drug was given simultaneously with irradiation. The negative trial conducted exclusively in patients in complete remission from chemotherapy was initiated because of earlier uncontrolled data suggesting marked improvement in disease-free survival when radiation was given to complete responders at the completion of drug administration. The randomized trial showed a lack of survival benefit from consolidation treatment when irradiation was given after chemotherapy was completed. Combined modality therapy also increased the complete response rate in most of trials and also significantly reduced chest recurrence rates.

A 1992 metaanalysis evaluated randomized trials in which more than 2100 limited-stage small cell lung cancer patients were randomized to receive either chemotherapy alone or in combination with chest irradiation.[76] Patients given combined modality therapy had a 14% reduction in death rate, and an absolute 5.4% improvement in 3-year survival compared with those receiving chemotherapy alone. Both differences were highly significant in this metaanalysis. This study reinforces the results of individual studies that demonstrated modest but statistically significant improvement in survival after combined modality treatment. A second and independent metaanalysis reached similar conclusions.[241]

Whether the variations in the temporal relationships of the radiation therapy and chemotherapy components of combined modality treatment influence the antitumor effects is by no means resolved. Concurrent and alternating combined modality programs that do not incorporate planned delays in chemotherapy for radiotherapy administration may possess superior efficacy. Among the randomized trials, three of four concurrent or alternating programs yielded improved survival, whereas one of three sequential programs produced only marginally significant improvement favoring radiation. However, indirect comparisons from the metaanalysis do not document significant survival advantages for any of the three methods of combining chemotherapy with irradiation.[76]

The dose of thoracic irradiation needed to control local regional SCLC was initially thought to be reduced when chemotherapy was given with irradiation.[242] Because improved drug treatment yielded better control of distant metastases, however, a high frequency of local failures with lower dose schedules such as 3000 cGy in 2 weeks became apparent.[243] Retrospective data in patients given combined modality therapy suggested that doses higher than 5000 cGy were needed for optimal prevention of local regional failure,[244] and one randomized trial demonstrated superior local tumor control with 3750 cGy compared with 2500 cGy.[245] Many authorities recommend higher doses in the range of 4500 to 5000 cGy or more[236,246,247] for optimal local control. Furthermore, simply because a radiotherapy program reduces local recurrences does not mean that it is optimal.

Randomized trials have yielded conflicting results on whether concurrent irradiation is best given early or late in the chemotherapy program. One study by the Cancer and Acute Leukemia Group B found better results with delayed irradiation perhaps because a greater percentage of projected chemotherapy doses were actually administered.[72] The National Cancer Institute of Canada trial came to the opposite conclusion.[73] Indirect comparisons from the metaanalysis could not resolve this issue.[76]

Minimizing the toxicities of combined modality approach without compromising therapeutic efficacy is worthy of further research. The addition of chest irradiation has increased myelosuppressive, pulmonary, and esophageal complications of treatment, particularly with concurrent regimens. In the National Cancer Institute (U.S.) trial[237,248] 26% of combined modality patients developed severe pulmonary toxicity requiring hospitalization within a median of 2 months from the beginning of treatment compared with only 4% of patients given chemotherapy alone; moreover, five combined modality patients in complete remission died of this complication. In patients who responded completely, pulmonary function test results improved in patients given chemotherapy alone, but did not do so in patients receiving combined modality therapy.[237] The Finsen Institute from Denmark, which also used concurrent chemotherapy and irradiation, reported 7% death from pulmonary and pericardial complications in complete responders.[249] This frequency of cardiopulmonary complications among patients given combined modality treatment is clearly higher than what is seen in patients who are given chemotherapy alone.

One study analyzed the frequency of radiation pneumonitis in lung cancer patients treated with chemotherapy and chest irradiation.[250] Almost 80% of the patients in this series had SCLC. In a multivariate analysis, the only factors that significantly correlated with the increased frequency of radiation-related pulmonary injury were individual fraction sizes of more than 2.50 Gy/d, twice daily fractionation as opposed to once-a-day fractions, and the total cumulative dose. Somewhat surprisingly, there were no significant differences among concurrent, alternating, and sequential combined modality treatments. Several trials reported high rates of esophagitis (with occasional strictures) and weight loss in patients given combined modality therapy.[237,249]

Not all concurrent combined modality programs report excessive pulmonary toxicity,[72] suggesting that the selection of drugs combined with irradiation is influential in inducing some of these complications. Platinum and etoposide may be an especially suitable regimen for concurrent treatment in small cell carcinoma of the lung. Two successive trials of sequential combined modality treatment in limited-stage patients produced 4-year survival figures of approximately 10% in the Southwest Oncology Group; a subsequent trial in which a platinum-etoposide combination was given concurrently with chest irradiation beginning on the first day of therapy resulted in 30% 4-year survival, and severe pulmonary toxicity was seen only in one patient.[251]

Although used less often, alternating regimens interdigitating chemotherapy and irradiation appear to have reduced pulmonary toxicity while maintaining the therapeutic advantage of adding radiation therapy.[238,252] In one retrospective study,[253] irradiating only the postchemotherapy tumor volume after several chemotherapy cycles did not appear to increase marginal recurrences and was also associated with a low frequency of radiation injury.

Hyperfractionated Radiation

Delivering chest irradiation in multiple daily fractions was theorized on experimental grounds to reduce long-term pulmonary toxicity while still maintaining antitumor efficacy. SCLC would appear to be an ideal neoplasm for twice-a-day treatment in that it has a high growth fraction, short cell-cycle time, and small to absent shoulder on the *in vitro* cell survival curve. Pilot studies in the late 1980s combining etoposide and platinum plus twice-a-day chest irradiation were promising, with median survivals greater than 2 years and in most series low rates of associated pneumonitis.[254–256] An intergroup study randomized 417 patients with limited-stage SCLC to a program that included cisplatin and etoposide for four cycles and radiation therapy beginning on day 1 of the first cycle.[69] The cumulative dose was 4500 rad in both arms, with one arm receiving the radiation in 180-cGy fractions daily and the other arm receiving 150-cGy fractions on a twice-a-day basis. The daily fractionation scheme required 5 weeks to reach the cumulative dose, whereas the twice-a-day schedule required only 3 weeks. The target volume included the primary tumor plus bilateral mediastinal nodes and the ipsilateral hilum and the supraclavicular nodes when involved. Margins of 1.0 to 1.5 cm were included and cone-downs were prohibited. Local failure was reduced from 52% with the daily schedule to 36% with the twice-a-day schedule ($P = .06$). Patients who failed in both local and distant sites had a frequency of 23% with daily treatment, versus only 6% with the twice-a-day approach ($P = .01$). More important, although statistically significant differences in survival were not seen at 24 months,[255] the curves deviated so that at 5 years the survival was only 16% with once-a-day treatment, as opposed to 26% with the twice-a-day schedule ($P = .04$).[69] Overall morbidities were not significantly different between the two arms, although there was a higher frequency of grade III esophagitis with twice-a-day treatment.

It should be reemphasized that selecting patients for combined modality treatment requires an excellent performance status. Combined modality therapy is a complex undertaking requiring close coordination between both medical and radiation oncologists. Because not all combined modality programs have been shown to increase survival but usually do increase toxicities, chest irradiation need not be considered for all patients, especially those who have impaired pulmonary function or poor performance status. Investigational programs that do not include chest irradiation remain entirely appropriate for many patients because the greater antitumor efficacy of combined modality treatment appears to be at least partially offset by enhanced toxicity. If the results of chemotherapy improve so that most patients have eradication of systemic but not of local disease, then chest radiation therapy could have a survival effect of even greater significance. At present, however, distant metastases remain the predominant cause of failure, and most patients with limited disease who are irradiated still die of their SCLC. Thus, improving systemic treatment currently has a much greater potential for achieving survival gains than does increasing the efficiency of local regional therapy.

Prophylactic Cranial Irradiation

Brain metastases are detected in approximately 10% of SCLC patients at the time of presentation and are subsequently diagnosed during life in another 20% to 25%, with an increasing likelihood of development seen with lengthening survival.[103,104] In the absence of radiation therapy to the CNS, actuarial analysis reveals a probability of brain metastases ranging from 50% to 80% in terms of those patients who survive 2 years.[104,257] At postmortem examination, they are found in up to 65% of patients.[105] Because these metastases are sometimes the sole site of clinical relapse from complete remission and are frequently clinically disabling, prophylactic cranial irradiation has been recommended by many[258] but not all[259] since the mid-1980s to curtail their development. The rationale is essentially an extrapolation from original strategies used in acute lymphocytic leukemia of childhood.

A review of 667 patients entered on several prospective randomized trials assessed the benefit of prophylactic cranial irradiation given at or within a few months of diagnosis in patients who were initially free of CNS involvement.[217,260–269] When these trials were considered together, doses of prophylactic cranial irradiation ranging from 2000 to 4000 cGy reduced the frequency of clinically detectable brain metastases from 24% to 6%.[270] In most of these trials, a significant reduction of intracranial tumor spread was observed. However, no significant effect of prophylactic cranial irradiation on survival was observed in any of those studies. Retrospective analyses suggested that virtually all benefit in preventing intracranial metastases with prophylactic cranial irradiation was confined to patients who achieved a complete remission to their initial treatment.[257,261] In actuarial analysis, partial responders or nonresponders have similar risks of recurrence in the brain regardless of whether prophylactic cranial irradiation was administered.[257] This is not surprising because persisting systemic cancer could readily metastasize to the CNS after completion of prophylactic cranial irradiation.

More recently in a metaanalysis of almost 1000 patients in seven trials between 1977 and 1995, patients were evaluated with and without prophylactic cranial irradiation[271] after initially obtaining a complete response. The primary end point was overall survival, and the analysis was based on intent to treat. Prophylactic cranial irradiation doses ranged from 24 to 40 Gy in most patients, although the metaanalysis did include one series of 25 patients who received only 8 Gy in one fraction. The metaanalysis suggested that there was a significant gain in survival seen with prophylactic cranial irradiation in patients who achieved complete remission, with 3-year survival figures increasing from 15% to almost 21%. Prophylactic cranial irradiation did significantly decrease the probability of brain metastases and increased the likelihood of disease-free survival. Going to higher doses appeared to have no obvious effect on survival, although it did appear to have an increasing effect of eliminating brain metastases. There was also a trend toward a decreased risk of brain metastases when prophylactic cranial irradiation was administered earlier in time. The metaanalysis was not able to assess the effect of prophylactic cranial irradiation on cognitive function, because most of the studies included did not include a baseline assessment. Two studies[272,273] assessed baseline neuropsychological function before treatment and demonstrated that many patients appear to have abnormalities of cognitive function as initial manifestations of their cancer, even when brain metastases were not detected and before any treatment.

Some investigators have proposed forgoing the prophylactic cranial irradiation in favor of therapeutic brain irradiation when metastases are detected.[274] This policy assumes that cranial irradiation can effectively control symptoms from overt brain metastases for a substantial fraction of the patient's remaining life. Because the duration of survival is short in most patients who develop brain metastases during the course of therapy, this assumption is not unreasonable. However, other physicians have questioned the durability of palliation after radiotherapy for overt metastases as well as the difficulty of achieving long-term control in the unusual patient who does survive for a long time.[275–277]

Another factor that produces considerable controversy in recommending prophylactic cranial irradiation to patients who achieve a complete response is the significant risk of toxicity associated with it. Because the 5-year survival appears to have improved, it is evident that some patients have neurologic and intellectual impairment as well as abnormalities on CT scan that may be related to prophylactic cranial irradiation.[277–280] In one study, both CT scan and CNS abnormalities were significantly more frequent in patients who had received prophylactic cranial irradiation or therapeutic brain irradiation than in those who had not.[280] These findings were especially disturbing because complete responders are at greater risk for possible complications. Many deficits on neuropsychological testing have been unsuspected on casual examination, but a few patients have obvious major impairments. CT scan abnormalities continue to worsen for several years after treatment has ended, although the abnormalities may eventually stabilize.[281] Neurologic abnormalities were most prominent in one series of patients who were given prophylactic cranial irradiation concurrently with high-dose chemotherapy or individual radiation fractions of 400 cGy.[278] Some authorities suggest that prophylactic cranial irradiation should be administered only in standard fractions of 200 cGy after completion of chemotherapy.[282]

The neuropsychological and imaging abnormalities may or may not be due to prophylactic cranial irradiation. Chemotherapy, possible paraneoplastic syndromes, and the effects of chronic cigarette and alcohol abuse are some of the factors that may be important contributors. In one study that evaluated cognitive function in patients before and after chemoradiation but before any prophylactic cranial irradiation, deficits were discovered in verbal memory, frontal lobe function, and motor coordination within both groups of patients.[273] Administration of methotrexate, procarbazine, and lomustine has decreased since the 1980s; these particular agents have been incriminated in neuropsychological dysfunction.[280,283]

One of the studies in the metaanalysis included almost 300 patients who were randomized to receive prophylactic cranial irradiation after having achieved a complete remission to initial treatment.[271] Twenty percent of these patients had extensive-stage disease, virtually all of whom are ultimately expected to relapse and die. The mean time between the initiation of treatment and the randomization was 5 months. The actuarial likelihood of isolated brain metastasis as the first site of treatment failure was 19% in patients given prophylactic cranial irradiation and 45% in those who did not receive prophylactic cranial irradiation. Corresponding figures for total brain metastases were 40% and 67%, respectively; both differences were highly significant. However, in this one study, overall survival was not significantly improved. The important observation was that there were no obvious differences in the neuropsychological function between the two groups, but only 33 patients underwent a complete reassessment at 18 months. Inasmuch as neuropsychological abnormalities possibly due to prophylactic cranial irradiation progress over time, these data are insufficient to exclude radiation-associated cognitive damage, but they are nonetheless relevant.

It is important to understand that prophylactic cranial irradiation as opposed to therapeutic irradiation should not require a dose that approaches tissue tolerance. Higher doses may be more successful at eliminating brain metastases but there appears to be prophylactic benefit with relatively modest doses of 24 to 25 Gy. If prophylactic cranial irradiation is administered at a time when no chemotherapeutic agents are being administered, radiation-induced permeability alterations that allow more chemotherapeutic agent into brain parenchyma should be obviated. Our guidelines for prophylactic cranial irradiation, after thorough discussion with the patient of the potential risks and benefits, are (1) prophylactic cranial irradiation is typically not recommended until at least 2 weeks after completion of all chemotherapy and only to complete responders after induction therapy; and (2) radiotherapy fractions of 200 to 300 cGy are given over 2 to 3 weeks to a total dose of 2400 to 3000 cGy.

Large-Field Radiation Therapy

Pilot studies have examined the role of hemibody and total body radiation in radioresponsive tumor. Hemibody irradiation is an active agent in SCLC and can induce some complete clinical responses in patients who achieved only partial response after combination chemotherapy.[284] The initial treatment is usually given to the upper hemibody where the bulk of tumor is located; in some studies treatment of the lower hemibody was administered after hematologic recovery occurred after the upper hemibody dose. A controlled German trial confirmed that chemotherapy produced markedly better survival than hemibody radiation in patients with extensive disease.[285] As an adjunct to combination chemotherapy in both limited and extensive disease, hemibody irradiation yielded substantial toxicity in several pilot studies without any obvious benefit in tumor response or survival.[286,287] There is also no evidence that low doses of total body irradiation are of benefit as an adjuvant to chest irradiation in limited-stage or chemotherapy in extensive-stage disease.[288] In a large randomized trial in patients with limited disease given chemotherapy and chest irradiation, additional hemibody radiation therapy to the upper abdominal sites of potential relapse produced no improvement in response duration or survival.[260] Currently, wide-field irradiation has no proven role in the management of this disease.

ROLE OF SURGERY IN LIMITED DISEASE

Surgery is reserved for selected patients. In contrast to the majority of patients with limited disease, careful TNM staging is important in those patients being considered for surgical resection. The first hint that proper staging would lead to less bias in the interpretation of surgical results came from the subset of SCLC patients described by Higgins et al.[37] in their report of the management of the solitary pulmonary nodule. In a 10-year follow-up of 15 small cell patients with solitary nodules (1% of total cases), 11 who would be presently classified as having stage I tumors[289] had a 5-year survival of 36%. Rejuvenation of interest in surgical resection for this cancer, however, received its greatest support from the recognition that newly available chemotherapeutic agents could possibly provide effective adjunctive therapy. Meyer[290] reported that of ten pathologically staged stage I and II patients resected and given chemotherapy for at least a year, 80% remained well at 30 months. Of greater significance, however, were the carefully designed trials conducted by the Veterans Administration Surgical Oncology Group.[291] Of 148 small cell carcinoma patients entered on four trials, 132 who survived a potentially curative resection were randomized to receive either preoperative adjuvant chemotherapy or surgery alone. A 23% overall 5-year survival was recorded, with survival patterns that were more favorable in less advanced stages: T1 to T2N0, 28% to 60%; T1 to T2N1, 9% to 31%; and T3 or N2, 3.6%. Although survival was marginally better with the addition of postoperative chemotherapy, it was clear that the small group of patients with localized disease after sophisticated surgical staging techniques could enjoy much better survival with surgical resection alone than was previously appreciated.

Several factors have strengthened the rationale for incorporating surgical therapy into the total package of treatment for selected SCLC patients. Despite the high response rate to present chemotherapy regimens, the rate of relapse in the thorax can approach 75% in the absence of properly administered radiotherapy. A gradual shift toward identification of more localized potentially resectable subgroups of limited disease patients with clinical staging occurred, encouraged both by the use of invasive procedures, including Wang needle biopsy, mediastinotomy, and mediastinoscopy, and the recognition that the new international staging system for lung cancer[57] can provide a common language for discussing these issues.

Theoretical justifications for combining surgery with other therapies for SCLC have been enumerated by Meyer.[292]

1. Since local relapse is a problem, could surgical removal offer a better chance for disease control?
2. Surgery used for local control, unlike radiotherapy, would not limit the intensity of chemotherapy that could be delivered.
3. By rendering the patient free of disease in the chest without affecting bone marrow reserves, surgery could possibly make the chemotherapy more effective.
4. Complete surgical staging could identify patients at higher risk of recurrence. Numerous uncontrolled reports, although not definitive, have provided considerable insight into whether these theoretical considerations are valid.

One of the chief theoretical justifications for adding surgery to the treatment regimen for SCLC is the possibility of influencing relapse in the tumor bed or mediastinum. In patients who have had surgery at diagnosis, local recurrences are infrequent,[293,294] possibly because patients with stage I or II disease are overrepresented in this group. Patients who have been pretreated with chemotherapy more often had clinical stage IIIA disease, and their local relapse rate is higher, in the range of 18% to 28%.[295,296] These local relapse rates still appear considerably less than in patients given chemotherapy with or without radiation therapy with no surgical intervention. Patients given initial chemotherapy who have a negative biopsy of the primary tumor site at the time of surgery and therefore do not have resection performed have a high frequency of local recurrence.[297] No cancer is present in the resected specimen in 10% to 20% of cases resected for CT,[30,298–300] and this particular patient subset enjoys a better prognosis.

Only a modest quantity of data exists on how often surgical resection at the diagnosis of SCLC is possible. Prospective studies of the feasibility of initial thoracotomy by their nature cannot include cases discovered only at thoracotomy to have small cell carcinoma. A review of the literature[301] suggests that as many as 16% of patients with SCLC are operative candidates, but this is likely to be an unrealistically high estimate because those patients who are evaluated by a thoracic surgeon constitute a highly selected group.

There does not seem to be a marked increase in mortality in patients who have operative removal of small cell carcinoma. In the few studies that describe operative risks after chemotherapy and radiotherapy, the mortality varies between 0% and 10%,[295–297,302–304] with many studies reporting no operative mortality or increased morbidity compared with expected outcomes in patients undergoing pulmonary resection for other indications. The extent of resection, pneumonectomy or lobectomy, has generally been dictated by the intraoperative findings rather than the original extent of the tumor in patients given preoperative chemotherapy.

Surgery Followed by Chemotherapy

The initial exceedingly poor long-term survival rates with surgery of SCLC were obtained in patients with clinical stages I through III, who for the most part underwent only minimal staging procedures by current standards. Only when results are categorized by tumor stages can the potential curative effects of surgery alone be demonstrated. One report, for example, documents 5-year survival of 35% in stage I and 23% in stage II patients.[304] The only randomized trials of surgery compared with surgery with postoperative chemotherapy were begun approximately 20 years ago and used inferior drug regimens by today's standards.[305–308] Nonetheless, they did in the aggregate reveal a survival advantage from chemotherapy (Table 31.3-5). Suffice it to say that in the 1990s thoracic oncologists never recommend surgery as sole treatment for SCLC.[309]

Statements regarding the efficacy of combined modality approaches for SCLC that include surgical resection can be evaluated only when stratified by the temporal relationships among the different modalities. There have been a number of programs of initial surgery followed by adjunctive chemotherapy after surgery; patients with multiple stages of tumor are included.[75,292,293,303,310–315] In general, modern combination chemotherapy programs, usually including cyclophosphamide, doxorubicin, vincristine, or etoposide, have been used. Survival experience is quite heterogeneous, ranging from 5-year survival of 9% in earlier studies to as high as 83% in more recent studies.

TABLE 31.3-5. Pooled Results from Randomized Surgical Adjuvant Studies in Small Cell Lung Cancer

Adjuvant Therapy	*Patients*	*2-Y Survival Rate (%)*
Chemotherapy	92	26
Placebo	61	8

(Data from refs. 305 through 308.)

Both nodal status and primary tumor or T status have significant effects on the survival of patients whose SCLC is resected. These prognostic factors were addressed directly in a few studies. Angeletti et al.[294] and Shepherd et al.[293] reported increased survival of node-negative compared with N1 and N2 patients after surgical resection and postoperative chemotherapy, while Macchiarini et al.[311] found a decrease in 5-year survival with increasing T category in surgically resected patients without nodal metastases. Retrospective reviews published by Rea et al.[314] and Lucchi et al.[315] have reinforced the importance of surgical staging in evaluating the outcomes for surgery and SCLC. Rea et al. reported that of 51 stage I and II SCLC patients resected and given chemotherapy after resection had 5-year survival rates of 52.2% (stage I) and 30% (stage II). In the review by Lucchi et al.,[315] stage I or II resected SCLC patients having postoperative chemotherapy had 5-year survival rates of 47% and 14.8%, respectively. Stage III patients from this series having surgery followed by adjuvant therapy had a 5-year survival of 14.4%. In general, 5-year survival is rare in patients given postoperative chemotherapy after mediastinal node disease has been documented at initial surgical resection,[303,304] although this observation is not universal.[293]

The largest experience as a cooperative group trial examining the role of surgery followed by adjuvant therapy in SCLC was conducted by the International Society of Chemotherapy Lung Cancer Study Group.[75] Four-year survival rates for completely resected, pathologically staged SCLC patients with N0 (n = 69), N1 (n = 58), and N2 (n = 36) who received postoperative therapy were 60%, 36%, and 33%, respectively. Based on these studies, most authorities believe that any survival benefits of initial surgical resection will likely be confined to patients with pathologic stage I and II disease, and conventional wisdom currently holds that surgical resection at diagnosis in patients with N2 disease is considered experimental.

Because most available data on outcome of patients who receive surgery and postoperative chemotherapy are uncontrolled, one can only observe that the survival of such patients is clearly better than the survival of patients with limited disease who receive chemotherapy alone and better than the reported outcome of all but a few series of patients, most of them more recent, given chemotherapy and chest irradiation. An extremely important point concerning initial surgical resection that remains unresolved is whether the superior outcome of more localized (i.e., stages I and II) disease in patients who undergo complete resection before initiation of chemotherapy is attributable to the resection itself or to an inherently better prognosis in patients with a tumor burden small enough to permit resection.

Because a controlled trial to address this question cannot be done because of the impossibility of randomizing patients whose small cell carcinoma is diagnosed only at the time of thoracotomy to undergo or not undergo surgical extirpation of their cancers, institutional data on patients with similar tumor burden after clinical staging who do and do not proceed to thoracotomy may be relevant. In Denmark, survival of clinically operable patients is similar whether an operation with the intent of completing resecting the tumor is performed,[316] although both these groups live much longer than other limited-stage patients. At the University of Toronto, a similar analysis, evaluating only patients without evidence of mediastinal metastases on chest radiography or mediastinoscopy, produced similar conclusions.[66] At present, one can only conclude that early-stage patients may benefit from surgical resection. Certainly, if a resectable SCLC is documented for the first time at thoracotomy, we recommend the surgeon proceed with the operation if mediastinal node metastases are absent. In patients with a proven pathologic diagnosis, thoracotomy for tumor resection in clinical stage I disease should be considered only after complete staging procedures, including mediastinoscopy or mediastinotomy, reveal no evidence of tumor spread.

The whole question of the SCLC presenting as a solitary pulmonary nodule is somewhat controversial at this time. In a retrospective review of 408 small cell carcinoma patients, Quoix et al.[317] found that solitary pulmonary nodule cases have a median survival of 24 months. The improved prognosis could be explained by a number of factors, not the least of which is simply early diagnosis (lead time bias). Another possibility is that the solitary nodule may represent a fundamentally different category of SCLC or not be small lung cancer at all. Warren et al.[318] reevaluated 50 cases of surgically resected SCLC. Thirty-four were pathologically confirmed to be SCLC, and stage I cases had a surprisingly low 9% 2-year survival. Twelve cases, however, were reclassified as well-differentiated neuroendocrine carcinoma, and 2-year survival of these stage I patients was 75%. The significance of these findings is presently unclear.

Chemotherapy Followed by Surgery

Surgical resection in SCLC might theoretically be more effective if performed after initial chemotherapy rather than at the time of diagnosis. Chemotherapy could be given in an immediate attempt to eradicate occult distant metastatic disease, the major cause of treatment failure. Only patients who respond to the chemotherapy (i.e., those most likely to benefit) would undergo thoracotomy. Comprehensive initial preoperative staging procedures could be avoided, or at least be less rigorous, because chemotherapy would be the first treatment. Finally, after response to chemotherapy, a larger fraction of patients might be surgical candidates.

There has been a steady increase since 1984 in the fraction of cases reported to be resectable after chemotherapy response. Moreover, there is more uniformity in presurgical staging procedures, including mediastinoscopy, used to identify patients who might benefit from postchemotherapy surgery. As shown in Table 31.3-6,[295–297,302,319,320] resection rates in some series can exceed 50%, with estimated 5-year survivals in resected patients of 35% to 65%. Factors that prevent thoracotomy include poor response to chemotherapy, poor pulmonary function or other medical problems, and patient refusal.[296] The selection criteria for potential surgical candidates often exclude those with such adverse prognostic factors as supraclavicular adenopathy, superior vena cava syndrome, bulky mediastinal involvement, and pleural effusions.

The approach of chemotherapy followed by surgery has led to higher survival rates compared with chemotherapy (often with chest irradiation) in patients with stage I disease, with median survival not yet reached in patients from the Toronto study.[293] Stage II and III patients had median survivals of 69 and 52 weeks, respectively, and significant differences in survival were noted in all resected patients compared with 19 eligible patients who did not receive surgery after the chemotherapy. The median survival of stage II and III patients was no different, however, than in otherwise eligible patients not receiving thoracotomy (51 weeks). The best results, not surprisingly, are found in patients with no malignant cells in the surgical specimen.[296] Some[321] but not all[293] authors report absence of long-term survival in patients with initial mediastinal node involvement who undergo postchemotherapy resection.

Whether surgery is best performed before or after chemotherapy in patients with known SCLC who are considered

TABLE 31.3-6. Survival Data with Chemotherapy Followed by Surgical Resection

Investigator	*Patients*	*Stage*	*Response Rate (%)*	*Resected Patients*	*Median Survival*	*Survival (y)*
Prager[320]	40	Limited	85	8 (20%)	NR	50% (1–2)
Holoye[319]	26[a]	Limited	100	17 (65%)	R: 61 mo U: 16 mo	65% (5)
Baker[302]	37	Limited	73	20 (54%)	R: 26 mo U: 12 mo	65% (2–3)
Johnson[297]	24[a]	Limited	100	17 (53%)	R: 20 mo U: 18 mo	NR
Williams[296]	38	Limited	84	21 (55%)	R: 33 mo U: 10 mo	48% (3–5)
Shepherd[322]	72	I, II, IIIa	80	33 (46%)	R: 21 mo U: 12 mo	36% (5)
Lad[323]	70	Limited	66	56 (83%)	R: 12 mo U: 12 mo	20% (2)
Fujimori[324]	22	I, II, IIIa	96	21 (96%)	R: 62 mo	73% (3) I, II 43% (3) IIIA

NR, not reported; R, resected; U, unresectable.
[a]Patients deemed surgical candidates only after response to chemotherapy.

operable at diagnosis is not known. Survival of patients with surgery followed by chemotherapy and with chemotherapy followed by surgery was quite similar in the Toronto study.[322] The more fundamental question, whether postchemotherapy surgery improves survival, also cannot be regarded as settled, although in one institution survival of limited-stage patients who were considered eligible or ineligible for eventual surgical resection should they respond to chemotherapy was similar.[296] A Lung Cancer Study Group trial in which 217 patients who responded to chemotherapy (66% of those beginning chemotherapy) were randomized to undergo or not undergo thoracotomy for attempted surgical resection has matured. This study did not reveal survival differences, and the median survival and 2-year survival were 12 months and 20%, respectively, for both arms.[323] The results of this study, however, are difficult to interpret because only 42% of the registered patients were randomized, 10% did not receive protocol-specified therapy, and the response rate of 65% was low compared with modern response rates with SCLC regimens. This point is emphasized when one considers a more recent pilot study from Japan. Treatment in this pilot study consisted of induction chemotherapy with cisplatin, doxorubicin, vincristine, and etoposide followed by surgical resection. In the 28 patients reported, the response rate was 96% and the resection rate was 95%. The 3-year survival rates were 73% for stage I and II disease and 43% for stage IIIA disease.[324] The majority of patients in the Lung Cancer Study Group (LCSG) study were stage III (N2, T3, or both) tumors, and, not withstanding the previously mentioned data from Japan, the role of surgery in N2 disease is of debate not only in SCLC but in non-SCLC. A trial of similar design that concentrates on patients with early-stage SCLC disease could potentially sort out the role of surgery after induction therapy for SCLC, but as so few patients (less than 10%) fall into this category, it is unlikely that this trial can ever be performed.

GENERAL APPROACH TO PATIENTS WITH EXTENSIVE DISEASE

For more than 90% of patients, extensive SCLC is a fatal disease within 2 years of diagnosis. Nevertheless, compared with supportive care, chemotherapy offers substantial benefit by improving both the quality and quantity of survival within this limited window. Treatment with current chemotherapy produces an overall response rate of 60% to 80%, and the median survival time is 7 to 12 months. Once distant metastases have been identified during staging, further radiographic staging studies are necessary only if dictated by a clinical protocol or as necessary to evaluate a symptomatic complaint (Fig. 31.3-2). Combination chemotherapy is superior to any single agent tested thus far, including oral VP-16.[325,326] Treatment should be administered for a total of four to six cycles. Because many of these patients have poor functional status and other adverse prognostic factors, less aggressive chemotherapy programs are acceptable and may provide comparable palliation with less toxicity. Because relapse invariably occurs, enrollment on an investigational study evaluating new targets designed to impair tumor growth is warranted if available. When disease progression does occur, additional chemotherapy should be offered to most patients with a good functional status.

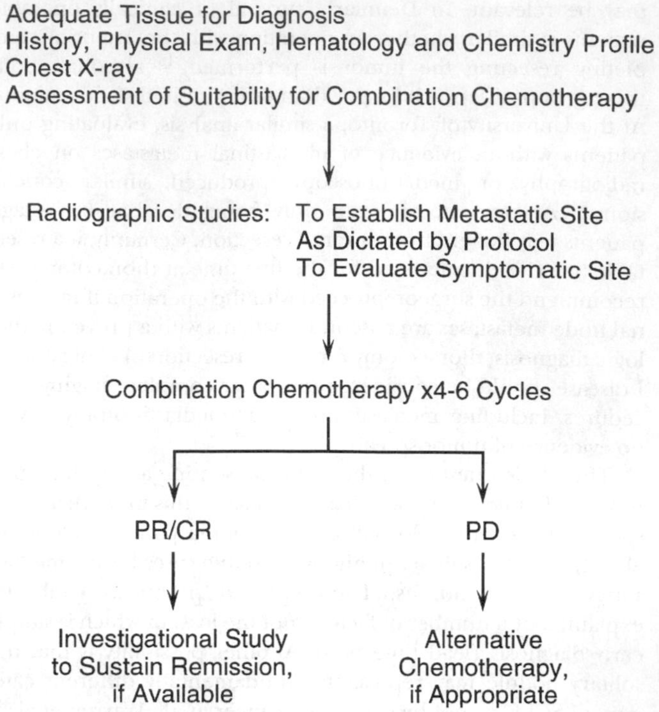

FIGURE 31.3-2. Algorithm outlining management of patients with extensive disease. CR, complete response; PD, progressive disease; PR, partial response.

ROLE OF CHEST IRRADIATION IN EXTENSIVE DISEASE

Retrospective reviews of the literature demonstrate that the addition of chest irradiation plus chemotherapy for patients who have extensive-stage SCLC may reduce the frequency of progressive disease in the thorax, but the overall response rates, median survival, and 2-year disease-free survival figures remain unchanged.[236,327] Because extensive disease patients generally achieve complete response rates of only 20% to 25% with current chemotherapy regimens and frequently relapse in distant metastatic sites, it is logical that an additional localized form of treatment would have minimal effect on survival. Successive large studies by the Southwest Oncology Group also confirm that although thoracic radiotherapy can substantially reduce the frequency of initial relapse at the primary tumor site, there is no apparent effect on survival.[328,329]

There have been several clinical trials that randomize patients with extensive disease to chemotherapy alone or in combination with irradiation to the chest disease as well as to some or all sites of overt distant metastases.[243,329–331] With one more recent exception,[330] no worthwhile advantages in survival have been seen with the addition of radiotherapy for patients with extensive disease. At present, except as part of a clinical trial, there is no indication for chest irradiation in extensive SCLC other than symptomatic palliation.

ROLE OF CHEMOTHERAPY AND RADIATION THERAPY TO THE NEURAXIS

The therapeutic management of overt disease in the CNS with radiation therapy is discussed in detail in Chapter 43.2. For overt metastatic lesions within the CNS, doses of 300 rad daily to doses of 3000 to 3600 Gy typically are used. Overt intracranial metastases appear to be more difficult to sterilize than intrathoracic disease.[332] If there are one or two clinically documented intracranial lesions only, a boost to 5000 cGy may be considered if the patient has an excellent performance status. Stereotactic treatment can also be used.

Chemotherapy is also a therapeutic option for brain metastases, perhaps because the blood–brain barrier is disrupted in the setting of macroscopic metastatic disease. Small series of patients in whom brain metastases were present at diagnosis have been treated with standard chemotherapy regimens without radiation, and the majority have demonstrated both clinical and radiographic improvement.[110] Chemotherapy has also been used at the time of relapse, and response rates of 33% to 43% have been reported.[110,333,334] In previously treated patients, the response to chemotherapy in the brain appears to be comparable with the response rates in other organs, and it is not dissimilar from the activity of irradiation, which in one series produced a partial response rate of 50%, and the median survival was 4.7 months in a series of 22 patients.[335] Thus, while brain irradiation remains the standard for patients who have not been previously irradiated, chemotherapy is a reasonable option for patients who develop recurrent disease after prior brain radiation, particularly if active systemic disease is also present.

STRATEGIES TO OPTIMIZE CHEMOTHERAPY RESPONSE

A number of strategies have been investigated in an attempt to improve treatment outcome using the currently available drugs. These approaches include increasing the number of active agents used in the treatment program, often by the use of cyclic alternation between two combination regimens, increasing the dose intensity, often with the support of hematopoietic growth factors or blood progenitor cells, and weekly chemotherapy regimens, which increase the dose intensity by shortening the interval between treatment rather than increasing the dose.

ALTERNATING CYCLIC COMBINATION CHEMOTHERAPY

The recognition of clonal heterogeneity within a tumor and the inability to develop treatment regimens that included more than four drugs due to overlapping toxicity led to an interest in alternating chemotherapy combinations. The somatic mutation model developed by Goldie and Coldman provided a theoretical underpinning to this approach, as this model predicted that the best probability of cure was achieved by the earliest possible introduction and most rapid alternation of all active agents.[336,337] If two equally effective non–cross-resistant regimens were available, the model predicted that alternating between regimens every other cycle would be more effective than alternating after every three cycles or giving one regimen continuously for five cycles before switching to the second regimen.[337]

A large number of clinical trials have been conducted attempting to evaluate alternating multidrug combinations, particularly in extensive disease.[197,221,328,338–340] The EP regimen was initially tested in patients who had progressed after cyclophosphamide-based chemotherapy, suggesting that these drug combinations were non–cross-resistant.[341] The National Cancer Institute of Canada conducted a study in which 289 patients were randomized to CAV or CAV alternating with EP.[338] Chemotherapy was given for a total of six cycles. Both the response rate (65% vs. 47%), progression-free survival, and median survival time (9.6 vs. 8.0 months) favored the patients who had received alternating therapy. The results could be explained by the inclusion of a more active regimen (EP) within the alternating arm, an advantage due to greater drug diversity with five effective drugs rather than three, or as support of the Goldie and Coldman concept. Roth et al. subsequently evaluated 437 patients with extensive disease in a randomized trial comparing EP for four cycles, CAV for six cycles, or CAV alternating with EP for a total of six cycles.[197] Although there was a slight improvement in progression-free survival ($P = .052$) there was no significant difference in response rate or overall survival between the treatment arms. Nonresponders to CAV crossed over to EP were twice as likely to respond to second-line therapy than nonresponders to EP who crossed over to CAV, although these differences were not statistically significant (28% vs. 14% for induction responders who relapsed, and 15% vs. 8% for patients with primary resistance, respectively). An assumption of the Goldie and Coldman hypothesis is that the alternating regimens are non–cross-resistant, which is not the case with the CAV and EP combinations as demonstrated by the modest activity when nonresponding patients are crossed over from one of these regimens to the other. The European Organization for Research and Treatment of Cancer developed a regimen consisting of vincristine, ifosfamide, mesna, and carboplatin (VIMP) that, in a randomized phase II study, appeared to be as active as CDE.[342] As important, patients who were progressing on, or were within 3 months of stopping either CDE or VIMP, had a greater than 50% likelihood of responding to the alternate combination, indicating that a significant degree of non–cross-resistance existed between these combinations. In a randomized trial, patients with extensive disease were treated with CDE or CDE alternating with VIMP.[339] The study was closed after 143 patients had been registered and demonstrated no significant differences in survival. Although it did not reach its planned accrual, it still had sufficient power to have detected a 2-month increase in median survival time with alternating therapy, had it existed. These studies, therefore, do not support the superiority of an alternating chemotherapy combination in patients with extensive disease.

Alternating non–cross-resistant chemotherapy has also been investigated in patients with limited disease.[198,343–346] The National Cancer Institute of Canada randomized 300 patients with limited disease to either CAV for three cycles followed by EP for three cycles, or CAV alternating with EP for a total of six cycles.[344] No differences were noted in response rates, time to treatment failure, or survival. A Japanese study compared CAV to EP with alternating CAV and EP.[198] Patients with limited disease received four cycles of chemotherapy followed by thoracic irradiation. Patients with extensive disease who responded to chemotherapy continued treatment for 1 year. A total of 288 patients were enrolled. No differences in survival based on treatment were noted in the patients with extensive disease. In patients with limited disease, there was improved survival, even after adjusting for other prognostic factors with the alternating regimen compared with CAV ($P = .058$) or EP ($P = .032$). In contrast, Urban et al. reported inferior survival with an alternating seven-drug regimen compared with a four-drug regimen, although the seven-drug combination was less intensive based on the magnitude of myelosuppression.[346] These results suggest that an equally intensive alternating regimen is a reasonable alternative for patients with limited disease, although the survival advantage noted in the Japanese trial has not been confirmed by another study.

Additional studies have evaluated alternating chemotherapy introduced after achieving a response to an induction regimen.[343,347,348] For example, Wolf et al. randomized 321 patients, 135 of whom had limited disease, to treatment with ifosfamide and VP-16, to response plateau followed by CAV, or ifosfamide and VP-16 alternating with CAV.[343] A total of six cycles of chemotherapy were delivered in each arm. No difference in outcome was noted based on treatment arm in either limited or extensive disease. Other studies have compared alternating regimens that were designed based on the suggestion of *in vitro* synergy[349] or have compared an alternating multidrug combination with a different standard regimen.[350] For example, a German multicenter trial demonstrated that an alternating eight-drug regimen was slightly superior to CAV.[350] In sum, these studies may be viewed as suggesting a modest advantage for regimens that introduce a greater diversity of active drugs into treatment rather than a test of the Goldie-Coldman hypothesis.

DOSE INTENSIFICATION

In experimental models, numerous chemotherapy drugs display log-linear or near linear dose-response curves.[351,352] Increasing the dose of chemotherapy delivered has been demonstrated to improve survival in a number of clinical settings.[353–355] In SCLC, several approaches to increase dose intensity have been evaluated. These include dose intensification without or with hematopoietic growth factor support, dose intensification with marrow or peripheral blood stem cell support, and compression of the time in which chemotherapy is delivered using a weekly schedule.

Hryniuk and Bush developed a methodology that expresses dose intensity as the drug dose administered per meter squared per week.[356] Limitations of this method include the assumption that all drugs and schedules of administration are therapeutically equivalent. Nevertheless, this method has been used to demonstrate a positive correlation between dose intensity and treatment outcome in advanced breast cancer and ovarian cancer.[356,357] In SCLC, a retrospective multivariate analysis of 131 patients suggested that modest increases in the dose intensity of cisplatin and cyclophosphamide in a four-drug regimen produced better survival.[358] In contrast, analysis of 60 clinical trials using this methodology found limited and conflicting correlations between dose intensity, response rates, and median survival.[359]

Several randomized trials have attempted to determine whether a modest increase in dose intensity improves survival in this disease.[360–365] In a small trial comparing different doses of a regimen consisting of cyclophosphamide (500 vs. 1000 mg/m^2), lomustine (50 vs. 100 mg/m^2), and methotrexate (50 vs. 100 mg/m^2), survival was inferior in the lower dose arm.[360] Preliminary findings of a cooperative group study in which the dose of cyclophosphamide was increased from 700 to 1500 mg/m^2 in a regimen that also included lomustine and methotrexate also demonstrated improved survival in the patients treated with the more intensive regimen.[361] These early studies confirm that the use of lower than standard doses of drugs can compromise survival in chemotherapy-sensitive disease.

More recently, several investigators evaluated whether increasing the dose of drugs beyond the dose used in current regimens improves survival. Most of these studies were conducted in patients with extensive disease[364–368] (Table 31.3-7). A trial comparing dose-intensified with standard dose CAV[364] and a study comparing high-dose with standard-dose EP[365] identified increased toxicity without improvement in survival. Neither of these studies used a hematopoietic growth factor in the intensified arm. Standard doses of cyclophosphamide, 4'-epidoxorubicin, etoposide, and cisplatin given for six cycles have been compared with an intensified schedule in which three of the four

TABLE 31.3-7. Randomized Trials Evaluating Dose Intensity in Small Cell Lung Cancer

First Author	*Regimen*	*Patients (No.)*	*Disease Stage*	*Dose Intensity Variable*	*Relative Dose Intensity*[a]	*Toxicity: High versus Standard*	*2-Y Survival: High versus Standard*
Johnson[364]	CAV	247	Extensive	Dose C, A	1.27 cycles 1–3	Increased myelotoxicity, increased nausea	NSD
Figuerado[362]	CAV	103	67% extensive	Dose C, A	1.17 cycles 1–4	Increased myelotoxicity, increased stomatitis	NSD
Arrigada[363]	CAPE	105	Limited	Dose C, P	1.11 cycle 1	NSD	43% vs. 26%
Ihde[365]	EP	90	Extensive	Dose E, P	1.46 cycle 1–2	Increased myelotoxicity, increased weight loss	NSD
Pujol[368]	EpCPE	125	Extensive	Interval	0.9 total	Increased myelotoxicity	8.9 vs. 11.0 mo[b]
Steward[369]	V-ICaE	300	60% limited	Interval	1.26 total	NSD	33% vs. 18%
Woll[380]	V-ICaE	65	92% limited	Interval	1.15 cycle 1	NSD	32% vs. 15%[c]
Thatcher[370]	ACE	403	77% limited	Interval	1.34 total	Increased transfusions	13% vs. 8%

A, doxorubicin; C, cyclophosphamide; Ca, carboplatin; E, VP-16; Ep, 4'-epidoxorubicin; I, ifosfamide; NSD, no significant difference; P, cisplatin; V, vincristine.
[a]Relative dose intensity delivered in high-dose arm, compared with control arm over specified number of cycles or total treatment.
[b]Median survival time.
[c]No significant difference in median survival times.

drugs were given at a 50% higher dose for four cycles.[368] This study demonstrated a shorter response duration and survival in the dose-intensified arm. Although the planned cumulative doses of chemotherapy were equivalent for three of the drugs, the intensified arm actually received a lower total dose because of toxicity. The only study that has suggested that the administration of higher drug doses within a standard regimen was beneficial was conducted in patients with limited disease. This French study randomized 105 patients with limited disease to a higher dose of cisplatin (100 vs. 80 mg/m^2) and cyclophosphamide (1200 vs. 1000 mg/m^2) in a regimen that also included doxorubicin and VP-16.[363] The increased doses of chemotherapy were only given on the first cycle. At 2 years, both the progression-free (28% vs. 8%) and the overall survival (43% vs. 26%) were improved in the higher dose arm. These studies indicate that a modest intensification of the dose of the commonly used agents does not improve outcome for patients with extensive disease and may even compromise survival by producing excessive toxicity. Whether a modest increase in the dose of drugs improves the outcome of patients with limited disease should be confirmed, and this question should probably be addressed in randomized trials that include either growth factor or stem cell support to maximize the delivered dose.

A number of other studies have evaluated whether shortening the interval between chemotherapy cycles improves survival. In patients with extensive disease, delivering CAVE on days 1 and 8 of the first few courses of chemotherapy did not appear promising.[366] A multicenter study randomized 300 patients to six cycles of vincristine, ifosfamide, carboplatin, and VP-16 delivered every 4 weeks or every 3 weeks.[369] Most of the patients included in the study had limited disease. In the group receiving chemotherapy every 3 weeks, the delivered dose intensity was increased by 26% over the entire treatment program compared with the group treated every 4 weeks. Both the median survival (443 vs. 351 days) and the 2-year survival rate (33% vs. 18%) were better in the intensified arm ($P = .0014$), even after adjustment in a multivariate analysis. Another multicenter study also explored the importance of the interval between treatment cycles by randomizing 403 patients, 77% of whom had limited disease, to cyclophosphamide, doxorubicin, and VP-16 delivered on an every-3-week schedule or on an every-2-week schedule. Patients treated every 2 weeks received G-CSF support.[370] The delivered dose intensity was 34% greater on the every-2-week schedule, and both the complete remission rate and the overall survival were better in this group. Improved survival was observed in both patients with limited and extensive-stage disease treated every 2 weeks. These studies suggest that for some standard regimens, compression of the treatment cycle, if this can be accomplished without a significant increase in toxicity, may be an effective means to improve survival.

Hematopoietic Growth Factors

G-CSF and granulocyte-monocyte colony-stimulating factor (GM-CSF) are members of a group of glycoproteins that stimulate the production and maturation of hematopoietic progenitor cells and regulate the function of mature blood cells.[371] Two randomized, placebo-controlled trials demonstrated that the use of G-CSF as an adjuvant to CAE chemotherapy significantly reduced the duration of neutropenia, incidence of febrile neutropenia, and the use of hospital resources.[372,373] A decision analysis based on the results of one of these trials concluded that the routine use of G-CSF led to a net decrease in the total cost per treatment cycle based on billed charges, but was associated with an increased cost based on actual provider costs or payments by the U.S. Medicare system.[374] Moreover, this analysis was extrapolated from the rate of hospitalization due to febrile neutropenia during the first cycle of chemotherapy, which in this study was 55% in the placebo arm and 26% in the group treated with G-CSF. Another decision analysis suggested that from an economic perspective a rate of hospitalization greater than or equal to 40% was necessary to justify the routine inclusion of G-CSF into a chemotherapy regimen.[375] These conclusions are consistent with the 1996 guidelines of the American Society of Clinical Oncology, which recommended primary prophylaxis (G-CSF administration concomitant with the first chemotherapy cycle) only when the expected incidence of febrile neutropenia exceeded 40%.[376] A review by Nichols et al., however, concluded that the incidence of febrile neutropenia after conventional chemotherapy for SCLC was approximately 18%.[377] The differences in the reported rates of febrile neutropenia between studies was related both to the chemotherapy regimen used and also to the diligence with which fever was sought and with how febrile neutropenia was defined. Two analyses that compared the use of G-CSF as secondary prophylaxis (G-CSF administered with all subsequent courses of chemotherapy if febrile neutropenia occurred on the previous cycle) suggested that this approach was more costly than a strategy of reducing the dose of the chemotherapy by 25%.[377,378]

Maintaining the dose of chemotherapy with growth factor support, rather than reducing or delaying the dose because of hematologic toxicity, would be appropriate if this translated into improved treatment efficacy. The results of studies designed to determine whether hematopoietic growth factors can increase the delivered dose intensity have been mixed.[368–370,379–381] A study that randomized a total of 65 patients to vincristine, ifosfamide, carboplatin, and VP-16 demonstrated that the use of G-CSF as an adjunct significantly improved the delivered dose intensity, although there was no difference in the incidence of febrile neutropenia or the days of hospitalization.[380] In this study, there was no difference in median survival between the arms, although there was a suggestion that long-term survival may be improved with the intensified dose delivery. A subsequent larger trial randomized patients to treatment with this regimen at fixed treatment intervals of every 3 or 4 weeks.[369] In a second randomization, patients were given GM-CSF or placebo following each chemotherapy cycle. Survival was improved for patients treated every 3 weeks, but the addition of GM-CSF did not reduce the incidence or the duration of febrile neutropenia, nor was there any difference in survival between the patients who received GM-CSF or placebo. With the use of G-CSF, treatment with standard doses of doxorubicin, cyclophosphamide, and VP-16 are feasible every 2 weeks. A randomized trial comparing doxorubicin, cyclophosphamide, and VP-16 given every 2 weeks with G-CSF or every 3 weeks without the growth factor identified improved survival with the every-2-week schedule.[370] Treatment with intravenous antibiotics was similar in the two arms. Although the intensified group did require more transfusions of red cells and platelets, overall quality of life measured by a symptom scale was comparable between the groups.

Two studies evaluated G-CSF as an adjunct to weekly chemotherapy programs.[379,381] In one trial, G-CSF did not increase the delivered dose intensity,[379] whereas in the other study both dose intensity and survival were improved in the arm that included G-CSF support.[381] A subsequent trial, however, compared this latter regimen with G-CSF support to a standard chemotherapy regimen that was given every 3 weeks and found no survival advantage with the intensified program.[382] An attempt to use G-CSF to increase the dose of three myelotoxic drugs in a four-drug regimen by 50% was not feasible and resulted in increased marrow toxicity, a reduction in cumulative drug dose received, and inferior survival.[368] Inclusion of GM-CSF in a combined modality program that consisted of EP plus concurrent radiation in patients with limited disease demonstrated that although the neutrophil nadirs were increased in the arm receiving GM-CSF, these patients developed more episodes of febrile neutropenia requiring intravenous antibiotics and hospitalization.[383] Serious thrombocytopenia and blood transfusions were also increased in the group receiving GM-CSF.

These data suggest that the inclusion of a hematopoietic growth factor within a chemotherapy regimen may permit a modest escalation in the dose intensity of some regimens, but not others. Whether this dose intensification is clinically meaningful is a separate issue, and broad generalizations are difficult. For example, although it appears that administration of doxorubicin, cyclophosphamide, and VP-16 every 2 weeks rather than every 3 weeks improves survival for patients with favorable prognostic features,[370] a program delivering chemotherapy every week was not better than EP alternating with CAV every 3 weeks in patients with extensive disease.[381] In this latter example, multiple variables (drug doses, drug diversity, patient tolerance) differed between the treatment arms and may have contributed to the observed lack of benefit with the weekly dose-intensive treatment regimen. Another issue that has not been resolved is whether patients who are at higher risk of toxicity due to age or other adverse prognostic factors, and patients who have developed febrile neutropenia on a previous treatment cycle, are better managed by reducing the dose of standard chemotherapy regimens or by adding a myeloid growth factor so that standard regimens can be given at full dose. Thus, dose, treatment interval, drug diversity, and patient selection are all parameters that define clinical outcome. Meaningful improvements in disease control beyond that produced by the programs outlined in Table 31.3-4 using the currently available cytotoxic chemotherapy drugs may still be possible, and this remains an appropriate area of study.

Marrow and Peripheral Blood Stem Cell Transplantation

Dose intensification with high-dose chemotherapy, supported by stem cells collected from the peripheral blood or bone marrow, has provided a survival advantage to select groups of patients with hematologic malignancies.[353–355] In contrast, reviews of the efficacy of high-dose therapy in adult solid tumors have concluded that no role for this approach has been established, even in the diseases most sensitive to chemotherapy and radiation.[384–386] However, the efficacy of high-dose therapy in SCLC has been evaluated in a relatively limited number of patients when compared with other diseases, such as breast cancer. Many of the earliest studies in SCLC enrolled patients with relapsed or chemotherapy-resistant disease. Although response rates were higher than would be anticipated with additional standard doses of chemotherapy, response durations were brief (ranging from 2 to 8 months) and the median survival was often less than 4 months.[387–389]

Some subsequent studies evaluated high-dose therapy as an early component of treatment in newly diagnosed patients.[390–393] With this strategy, patients received little or no induction chemotherapy before the high-dose regimen. It was hoped that by avoiding exposure to multiple cycles of conventional chemotherapy the risk of developing drug resistance in the tumor could be reduced. Response durations and survival, however, were comparable with that achieved with standard chemotherapy.[394]

A more commonly applied approach has been to use high-dose therapy as late intensification after standard treatment.[387,395–401] Theoretic support for this strategy is provided by the mathematical model proposed by Norton and Simon, which predicts that as the tumor volume is reduced relative resistance to chemotherapy develops.[402] These studies differ in the number of cycles and type of regimen used for induction, the extent of tumor response required before high-dose consolidation, the composition of the high-dose regimen, and whether radiation, surgery, or both were included as part of the treatment program.

The only reported phase III trial administered five cycles of induction therapy and then randomized patients who achieved a good response to consolidation with cyclophosphamide, carmustine, and etoposide with bone marrow support, or one additional cycle of conventional doses of these same drugs.[398] A total of 101 patients were registered, and 45 patients were randomized, which included 13 patients who initially had extensive disease. Both the complete remission rate and the median relapse-free survival ($P = .002$) were superior in the high-dose arm. Although the median survival time was improved (68 vs. 55 weeks), this was not statistically significant ($P = .13$), and long-term survival was achieved in only 2 of the 23 patients treated with the high-dose regimen. A criticism of this study has been that thoracic irradiation was not included as part of the treatment plan, and in most patients the site of initial relapse was confined to the chest. Accordingly, many groups that have continued to investigate consolidative high-dose therapy have used a multimodality program. For example, the Southwest Oncology Group treated 58 patients with limited disease with induction chemotherapy and radiation followed by consolidation with high-dose cyclophosphamide and autologous marrow support.[403] Only 21 patients received the consolidation but nine achieved long-term disease-free remissions, and the median survival of the patients receiving consolidation was 27 months.

At the Dana Farber Cancer Institute, patients responding to conventional chemotherapy have been treated with high doses of carmustine, cyclophosphamide, and cisplatin along with stem cell or marrow support followed by thoracic and prophylactic cranial irradiation. The initial report described 19 patients, and this has been updated to include 36 patients.[394,399] With the period of observation after completion of the high-dose therapy ranging from 21 months to 9 years, 52% of these patients with limited disease have remained in remission. The majority of patients (81%) were in complete remission or near complete remission at the time they received high-dose consolidation, and, compared with patients transplanted in a partial remission, maximal cytoreduction with induction therapy appears to have been an important prognostic factor for long-term survival. Despite treatment with 50- to 60-Gy radiation to the chest, approximately one-half of the relapses occurred at the primary site.

Fetscher et al. have described a program whereby patients received two to four cycles of induction chemotherapy followed by dose-intensive VP-16, ifosfamide, carboplatin, and epirubicin along with peripheral blood stem cell support.[401] Additional locoregional therapy consisted of surgical resection or thoracic irradiation. Complete responders received prophylactic cranial irradiation. Over a 6-year period, 100 patients (67 with extensive disease and 32 with limited disease) were treated with this approach. Only 19 of the 33 patients with limited disease proceeded to high-dose therapy. Excluding the favorable subset of patients with early-stage disease in which complete surgical resection was performed, 5-year survival was 33%.[401] Leyvraz et al. have shown that multiple cycles of high-dose therapy can be given within a cooperative group.[404] In this study, treatment consisted of mobilization with epirubicin, collection of stem cells, and then three cycles of dose-intensified ICE given at 4-week intervals. Compared with standard doses of ICE, a two- to threefold escalation of each chemotherapy drug was feasible. The median duration of severe leukopenia was 4 days, and there was no evidence of cumulative toxicity with the multiple cycles of high-dose treatment. This program is now being compared with standard therapy in patients with a favorable prognosis in a randomized trial.

In sum, high-dose consolidative therapy has been evaluated in a selected population that is younger and healthier than the general population of patients with SCLC. Even in this more favorable subset, it is not clear whether survival is better than would have been expected with conventional treatment. Treatment-related complications have been reduced with the substitution of peripheral blood stems cells for bone marrow and with improvements in supportive care, but even the most recent series report treatment-related mortality that exceeds the 2% to 5% mortality currently expected with high-dose therapy. This may be the result of more comorbid illness, even in the best subset of patients with SCLC, or it may simply be due to the small numbers of patients included in the reported series. In addition, among the technical issues that need to be clarified is whether tumor cell contamination of the harvested stem cell product is a significant cause of treatment failure, as marrow involvement can be documented by immunocytochemistry in a substantial minority of patients with limited disease considered to be in a chemotherapy-induced remission by routine histologic examination.[405] Several randomized studies are evaluating the role of high-dose consolidation in SCLC and should help define whether this approach, as currently practiced, is of value in this disease.

WEEKLY DOSE-INTENSIVE CHEMOTHERAPY REGIMENS

Dose intensity is defined both by the dose and the time interval required to deliver the dose.[356] Therefore, shortening the time interval between chemotherapy cycles is an alternative to increasing the dose as a means of achieving greater dose intensity. Some groups have developed weekly regimens that use six or seven drugs.[406–408] For example, the Southwestern Oncology Group developed a six-drug program that included doxorubicin, cyclophosphamide, methotrexate and leucovorin, vincristine, VP-16, and cisplatin.[406] Among the 48 patients with extensive disease, the complete response rate was 38% and the median survival time was 11.4 months. A European group used a fairly comparable six-drug regimen in which the most significant differences were the inclusion of teniposide, a lower dose of methotrexate (30 mg/m^2 instead of 200 mg/m^2), and a shorter treatment interval (12 weeks instead of 16 weeks).[407] In this study, the complete response rate for patients with extensive disease was 9.7%, and the median survival for this group was 7 months. These differences highlighted the importance of patient selection in the resultant outcome and the necessity for randomized trials to evaluate new treatment approaches in SCLC.

Three weekly programs have been tested in randomized multiinstitutional settings.[382,408,409] A multidrug combination developed by Sculier et al., which included seven drugs, was compared with standard treatment of CAV.[408] The planned duration of treatment was 18 weeks in both arms. A total of 215 patients were enrolled that included 120 patients with extensive disease and 95 patients with limited disease. Overall, there was no difference in median survival (49 vs. 43 weeks) or in 2-year survival rates (8.5% vs. 7.9%) between the treatment arms, and analysis by stage of disease failed to identify any difference in outcome based on treatment. A second randomized trial evaluated a regimen consisting of EP alternating on a weekly basis with ifosfamide plus doxorubicin. This was compared with a standard chemotherapy regimen consisting of alternating 3-week cycles of CAV and EP.[409] Patients who achieved at least a partial response to chemotherapy received thoracic irradiation, and some patients also received prophylactic cranial irradiation. Included in this study were 438 patients, the majority of whom had limited disease. No differences in either median or 2-year survival rates were evident. In both of these randomized studies, myelosuppression was a dominant side effect, and the actual dose intensity delivered was a lower percentage of the planned dose in the weekly treatment arms. However, treatment-related mortality was low, and no worse, with weekly treatment than with standard therapy.

A more intensive weekly program that included cisplatin, vincristine, doxorubicin, and VP-16 (CODE) delivered higher doses of chemotherapy by infusing myelosuppressive and relatively nonmyelosuppressive drugs on alternate weeks and by using an aggressive supportive regimen consisting of corticosteroids, gastroprotective agents, and prophylactic antibiotics. In the initial report, 19 of 48 (40%) patients with extensive disease attained a complete remission, and the 2-year survival rate was 30%.[410] In a small randomized trial, a Japanese group reported that G-CSF support improved both the delivered dose intensity and the median survival when CODE was used to treat patients with extensive disease.[381] They subsequently compared CODE plus G-CSF with a standard regimen consisting of alternate 3-week cycles of CAV and EP.[382] There were 220 patients with extensive disease enrolled in this study. Both the overall response rate and the complete remission rate (15%) were similar in the two treatment arms. The median survival time (11.6 vs. 10.9 months) and 2-year survival rates (11.7% vs. 8.5%) were also comparable. The incidence of neutropenic fever was significantly higher, and there were four toxic deaths in the weekly treatment arm. In North America, a randomized intergroup study compared CODE with alternating CAV and EP over 18 weeks.[411] A total of 219 patients with extensive disease with a good performance status were enrolled. Although the response rate was improved (87% vs. 70%) with the weekly program, the response duration and median survival were equivalent between the two treatment arms. Moreover, febrile neutropenia was more common in the patients treated with CODE, and there were more toxic deaths (8.2% vs. 1.0%) compared with the standard treatment arm. In aggregate, these studies demonstrate that weekly chemotherapy programs offer no advantage to standard treatment given every 3 weeks, and if given at the maximum tolerated dose, weekly chemotherapy is significantly more toxic than standard therapy.

MANAGEMENT OF SMALL CELL LUNG CANCER IN THE ELDERLY AND INFIRM

At diagnosis, 25% to 40% of patients with SCLC are 70 years old or older.[412–415] Compared with younger patients, the elderly have a poorer performance status and more comorbidity.[412,413] They are at higher risk for complications from intensive treatment.[88,90,416] As a result, many physicians treat elderly patients less aggressively. For example, one retrospective review management for 20 of 123 (16%) elderly patients consisted only of radiation therapy, and another 23 patients (19%) received only supportive care.[412] Another review of the management of 312 patients diagnosed between 1985 and 1991 showed that in the management of the elderly population, 23% of the patients received only supportive care, and in the subset of patients with limited disease only 43% received both chemotherapy and radiation.[413] In contrast, in patients between the ages of 60 and 69 less than 10% of the patients received supportive care and 65% of the patients with limited disease received combined modality therapy.

When chemotherapy is given to elderly patients, it is usually given at attenuated doses and often for fewer cycles.[84,412,413,415] In one study, the median nadir white blood cell count was 2800/μL and the nadir platelet count was 198,000/μL.[412] Patients who are treated with chemotherapy derive a survival benefit despite attenuation of both the dose and duration of treatment, and in some series the response and survival for the elderly have been comparable with younger patients.[84,412,413]

Few elderly patients have been included in clinical trials, and those who have been enrolled are among a minority with less comorbidity and better functional status.[413,415] As a result, extrapolation of the published data for standard therapies to the general population of elderly patients may be inaccurate. Consequently, several chemotherapy programs have been developed for the elderly and for patients unfit for participation in standard therapy protocols that aim to optimize palliation with acceptable risks. One approach has been to use monotherapy with the epipodophyllotoxins.[144,417,418] VP-16 can be given orally, making it particularly attractive in the palliative setting.[155] In a study of 35 elderly patients, one-third of whom had poor performance status, a 5-day course of oral VP-16 every 4 weeks produced a response rate of 71% and survival comparable with the results with combination treatment in a younger population.[417] The Medical Research Council designed a trial comparing oral VP-16, 50 mg twice daily for 10 days, with standard combination chemotherapy consisting of either VP-16 and vincristine or CAV.[325] In each arm, chemotherapy was repeated every 3 weeks for a total of four cycles. The median age enrolled in this study was 67 years, and 38% of the patients had a performance status equal to 3 to 4. The study was prematurely stopped after an interim analysis that showed inferior survival in the patients treated with VP-16 monotherapy. Hematologic toxicity was also worse with oral VP-16, and there were 17 deaths during the first month of treatment in this arm compared with ten deaths on the control group. A second British trial comparing oral VP-16 given at 100 mg twice daily for 5 days with VP-16 and cisplatin alternating with CAV in poor-prognosis patients was also stopped early because of inferior progression-free and overall survival in the VP-16 monotherapy arm.[326] Moreover, palliation of symptoms and quality of life were better with combination chemotherapy. Based on the results of these two trials, monotherapy with oral VP-16 cannot be recommended as adequate treatment for patients with SCLC.

An alternative approach for providing palliative chemotherapy in Britain was the delivery of chemotherapy as needed to palliate symptoms, rather than at fixed 3- or 4-week treatment intervals. A total of 300 patients were randomized to receive CEV every 3 weeks for a total of eight cycles or to an as-needed treatment program.[419] In this arm, patients were evaluated at 3-week intervals after the first treatment cycle and were retreated only if they were symptomatic or had evidence of tumor growth while not receiving treatment. Patients randomized to receive chemotherapy as needed had a median interval between cycles of 42 days and received only 50% as much total chemotherapy as the patients treated on the fixed schedule. Although the median survival times were equivalent, better symptomatic control was achieved with the fixed interval treatment.

Another investigation of less intensive therapy compared the ECMV regimen with EV.[420] Three cycles were planned for each arm because a prior study comparing three and six cycles of ECMV showed equivalent survival.[230] A total of 310 patients with extensive disease or limited disease and poor performance status were registered. The response rates and survival were comparable between the two arms.[420] There were twice as many early fatalities (death during the first treatment cycle) in patients receiving the four-drug ECMV regimen (37 vs. 18). Nevertheless, ECMV produced better palliation of symptoms than did EV. Another study compared a regimen of EP alternating with CAV every 3 weeks at standard doses with EP alternating with CAV every 10 to 11 days at 50% of the standard dose.[421] Response and survival were comparable with both schedules, and toxicity was not reduced with the more frequent administration of lower doses.

Several other less intensive regimens have been designed for high-risk and elderly patients that use lower doses of chemotherapy than are used in standard regimens and report reasonable response rates and survival with less toxicity.[414,418,422–427] In a study of 75 elderly patients with reasonably good performance status and limited disease, two cycles of carboplatin and prolonged oral VP-16 were given with concurrent hyperfractionated radiation, and a median survival of 15 months and a 5-year survival of 13% were observed.[428] In 55 patients with limited disease unfit for standard treatment, Murray et al. administered one cycle of CAV followed by one cycle of VP-16 and cisplatin along with 20 to 30 Gy of concurrent thoracic irradiation.[414] The complete remission rate was 51%, and 28% of the patients were alive and disease-free at 2 years. This same group of investigators have also reported a series of 66 patients older than 65 years and with a performance status of 3 who were treated with a four-drug regimen consisting of attenuated doses of cisplatin, doxorubicin, vincristine, and VP-16 for a total of four cycles.[427] Concurrent thoracic irradiation was given to patients with limited disease and selected patients with extensive disease. The delivered total dose was 80% of the intended dose. Survival at 2 years was 38% and 18% for patients with limited and extensive disease, respectively. Hospitalization was necessary for 42% of patients receiving combined modality treatment and for 15% of the patients treated with chemotherapy alone. There was just one septic death. Comparison of these single-institution phase II trials with the outcomes observed in controlled cooperative group studies is difficult. Nevertheless, it highlights the importance of developing chemotherapy programs of sufficient intensity to achieve optimal palliation, with manageable toxicity, in elderly and high-risk patients.

BIOLOGIC RESPONSE MODIFIERS AND OTHER TREATMENTS

Although cytotoxic therapy is effective in reducing the disease burden in SCLC, it is rarely curative. The immune response to SCLC appears to be modest, as evidenced by a lack of association with tumor-infiltrating lymphocytes in tumor biopsies. Efforts to augment the immune response have included treatment with nonspecific immunomodulators, therapy with interferons and interleukin-2, and active immunization with antiidiotypic antibodies. Studies that have evaluated bacille Calmette-Guérin, the methanol-extracted residue of bacille Calmette-Guérin, or thymosin fraction V, a soluble product of calf thymus thought to reconstitute immune function, have failed to demonstrate a beneficial effect on response rate, response duration, or survival.[429–433]

The expression of major histocompatability complex antigens is reduced in SCLC, which may play a role in this tumor's ability to escape immune surveillance.[434–436] Interferon has been shown to increase the expression of major histocompatability complex antigens on SCLC cells both *in vitro* and *in vivo*.[437,438] Small studies in newly diagnosed patients, however, treated with either interferon-α or interferon-γ showed a total absence of activity.[439–441] Because immune augmentation may be most effective in patients with low-disease burden, larger studies have evaluated interferons as maintenance treatment in patients responding to chemotherapy. Mattson et al. conducted a study in which patients responding to induction chemotherapy were randomized to a maintenance chemotherapy, natural interferon-α, or observation.[442] Although there were no differences overall, a subset analysis showed improved survival for patients with limited disease who received interferon. Another study that administered interferon-α both along with the induction chemotherapy and as a maintenance reported a higher complete response rate and improved median survival.[443] Due to poor accrual, however, the study was stopped prematurely and only 77 patients were evaluable. Two other randomized trials, one in which interferon-α was included both as part of the induction and maintenance regimen, and a second, cooperative group trial in which interferon-α maintenance was evaluated in patients with limited disease who had responded to induction chemotherapy,[444,445] showed no survival advantage. Interferon-γ maintenance therapy in patients with complete or near complete remissions has also been evaluated in two randomized trials.[446,447] Although the dose and schedule selected from one trial was confirmed to be biologically active as demonstrated by a significant increase in the expression of HLA-DR and Fc receptors on monocytes,[448] neither study produced an effect on survival. In addition to the typical influenza-like side effects and myelosuppression, a few of the studies in lung cancer have suggested that the interferons may enhance radiation-induced lung injury, and there was at least one case of fatal pneumonitis.[447]

High-dose interleukin-2 has also been evaluated in a group of patients with extensive disease who experienced less than a complete remission to induction chemotherapy.[449] The overall response rate was 21%, but the toxicity was severe, and treatment was discontinued in 11 of 24 patients because of life-threatening side effects. These studies indicate that at the present time treatment with cytokine therapy has not established a role in the management of this disease.

SCLC displays a variety of markers of neuroendocrine differentiation that could serve as targets for biologic agents. Neural cell adhesion molecule is one such target to which an immunotoxin, consisting of a murine monoclonal antibody linked to a modified ricin molecule, has been developed. In a dose-escalation trial, 1 of 21 patients had a partial response that lasted 3 months.[450] In an alternate strategy, a monoclonal antibody directed against gastrin-releasing peptide was developed with the intent of interrupting this autocrine growth loop. One of 12 evaluable patients had a complete remission that lasted 6 months.[451] The patients treated with these two biologic agents all had disease resistant to chemotherapy. The activity noted is encouraging for further clinical development.

The variable region of an antibody mirrors its antigen. Therefore, a second antibody raised against this variable region structurally mimics the original antigen. Infusion of this second antiidiotypic antibody often induces a more effective immune response than does infusion of the antigen of interest. Thus, a limitation of monoclonal antibody therapy, the development of a host immune response to the infused mouse protein [human antimouse antibody (HAMA) reaction] can be exploited by infusing a mouse antiidiotypic antibody to augment immunity to antigens preferentially expressed on tumor cells. An antiidiotypic antibody, BEC2, which resembles a ganglioside expressed on SCLC cells, has been tested in 15 patients who had responded to conventional chemotherapy.[452] Side effects of the vaccination were modest and consisted primarily of skin reactions to the bacille Calmette-Guérin adjuvant. The median progression-free survival was 11 months and longer than 47 months for patients with extensive and limited disease, respectively. Comparison with an historic matched control group suggested that both progression-free and overall survival were substantially improved. Antiidiotypic antibodies are being developed that resemble other poorly immunogenetic antigens expressed by SCLC cells. Because the expression of any one of these antigens is variable, a polypeptide vaccine containing multiple immunogenetic antigens will probably be needed to effectively target every SCLC cell.

A potential role of the coagulation system in the propagation of cancer has been recognized for many years. Thrombin is generated *in situ* and may function as a growth factor for the tumor.[453] Tumors produce urokinase-like enzymes that may participate in the degradation of the extracellular matrix.[454] Initial studies evaluating whether the addition of warfarin to

TABLE 31.3-8. Activity of Combination Chemotherapy Regimens at Relapse

First Author	*Evaluable Patients (No.)*	*Previous Chemotherapy*	*Chemotherapy*	*Response (%)*	*Response Duration (wk)*	*Median Survival (wk)*
Evans[193]	34	CAV (23)[a]	EP	44	NR	17
Lopez[459]	30	CAV (23)	EP	27	20	16
Fukuoka,[198] Roth[197]	66	CAV	EP	20	NR	NR
Fukuoka,[198] Roth[197]	26	EP	CAV	8	NR	NR
Shepherd[460]	13	EP	CAV	15	24	15
Smit[468]	22	CDE (13)	JV	36	NR	18
Postmus[342]	25	CDE	VIMP	60	NR	19
Groen[467]	34	CDE (33)	JT	73.5	21	31
Monnet[461]	20	CIV	APE	45	NR	NR
	10	APE	CIV	0	—	—
Postmus[342]	43	JV (22) IMJ (21)	CDE	51	NR	22

APE, doxorubicin, cisplatin, VP-16; CAV, cyclophosphamide, doxorubicin, vincristine; CDE, cyclophosphamide, doxorubicin, VP-16; CIV, carboplatin, ifosfamide, vincristine; EP, VP-16, cisplatin; IMJ, ifosfamide, mesna, carboplatin; JT, carboplatin, paclitaxel; JV, carboplatin, vincristine; VIMP, vincristine, ifosfamide, mesna, cisplatin.
[a]Number treated with specified regimen.

the chemotherapy regimen improved survival yielded mixed results.[455,456] In a randomized trial involving a total of 50 patients, the addition of warfarin significantly improved both progression-free and overall survival.[456] In a larger cooperative group study, patients receiving coumadin with chemotherapy had a higher response rate ($P = .012$) and a 6-week improvement in median progression-free and overall survival, although the difference for the latter two end points was not statistically significant.[457] The addition of 1 g/d of aspirin, a dose sufficient to inhibit platelet aggregation, failed to demonstrate a benefit.[458] A subsequent trial by the same group of investigators demonstrated that the subcutaneous administration of unfractionated heparin at therapeutic doses given during the first 5 weeks of chemotherapy resulted in a higher complete remission rate and improved survival.[453]

TREATMENT AT RELAPSE

The majority of patients with SCLC relapse within a year of initial therapy, and many are candidates for second-line treatment[193,197,198,342,459–461,467,468] (Table 31.3-8). Factors that predict the likelihood of response to subsequent chemotherapy include the interval between completion of induction and relapse, the extent of tumor regression achieved with the induction regimen, and the composition of the induction program.[462] For example, the activity of teniposide in previously treated patients was 53% if the chemotherapy-free interval was greater than 2.6 months, compared with 12% if the treatment-free interval was shorter.[463] As a consequence, sensitive relapse is often, and somewhat arbitrarily, defined as a chemotherapy-free interval of greater than or equal to 3 months. In patients in sensitive relapse, response rates to second-line therapy often exceed 50%, and any chemotherapy regimen active in SCLC appears to be effective, including the drug regimen that was initially used for induction.[152,464–466]

For patients who relapse early, both the regimen used for second-line and the induction regimen may be important in determining the likelihood of a secondary response.[341] For example, in patients treated with CAV as the induction regimen, second-line treatment EP produces a response rate of approximately 35%.[193,459] Only approximately one-half as many patients (15%) who experience early relapse after EP induction respond to CAV as a second-line therapy.[460] In some of the randomized trials that have compared CAV with EP, patients not responding to initial therapy (primarily refractory) and crossed over to the alternative regimen were more likely to respond to EP than to CAV, although in this more resistant group of patients the response rates to second-line treatment overall were lower and were 15% to 23% for EP and approximately 8% for CAV.[197,198]

Drugs that have been reported to be active as second-line agents include carboplatin, ifosfamide, and paclitaxel (Taxol), although the reported response rates have been variable, reflecting the small, heterogeneous populations tested. For example, carboplatin in combination with ifosfamide or paclitaxel has been reported to be active in more than 50% of the patients relapsing early after induction with CDE.[342,467] In contrast, in another study zero of ten patients resistant to cisplatin, doxorubicin, and VP-16 responded to carboplatin, ifosfamide, and vincristine.[461] Furthermore, the survival from the start of second-line therapy is rarely more than 4 to 6 months. More dose-intensive therapy with a weekly regimen has been reported to produce a 30% 1-year survival rate in patients with good performance status in sensitive relapse.[469] These studies indicate that for patients with a reasonable performance status second-line therapy with a moderately intensive drug regimen is appropriate. The likelihood of a secondary response may be better in patients who have not previously been treated with a platinum agent.[470] Symptomatic sites of disease can frequently be managed with radiation.

SURGICAL MANAGEMENT OF PERSISTENT OR RECURRENT LOCAL DISEASE

Histologically mixed disease is a not an uncommon occurrence when SCLC is resected after chemotherapy. Non–small cell lung and mixed small and non–small cell elements occur in 5% to

TABLE 31.3-9. Effect of Treatment on Survival in Small Cell Lung Cancer According to Extent of Disease

Therapy	Median Survival (mo)		2- to 3-Y Survival Rate (%)	
	Limited Disease[a]	Extensive Disease	Limited Disease	Extensive Disease
Supportive care	3	1.5	—	—
Surgery	5–6[a]	—	4–5[a]	—
	11[b]	—	30–35[b]	—
Thoracic radiotherapy	10[a]	—	10[a]	—
	3–9	—	2–7	—
Single-agent chemotherapy	6	4	—	
Combination chemotherapy	10–14	7–11	5–15	1–3
Combination chemotherapy with chest irradiation	15–26	7–11	10–40	1–2

[a]Operable patients in prechemotherapy era.
[b]Selected, carefully evaluated, pathologically staged patients.
(Modified from Morstyn G, Ihde DC, Lichter AS, et al. Small cell lung cancer 1973–1983: early progress and recent obstacles. *Int J Radiat Oncol Biol Phys* 1984;10:51, and from ref. 69, with permission.)

35% of specimens.[296,302,319,471] Whether these pathologic findings may be attributable to selection by chemotherapy of non–small cell elements present in the original tumor, histologic changes induced by chemotherapy, the presence of a second lung cancer, or incorrect initial diagnosis is not resolved. Nevertheless, surgery may prove therapeutically efficacious if the only residual cancer is non–small cell in type. Because of the frequency of mixed histologies at the time of resection after chemotherapy, the Toronto group reported a retrospective analysis of salvage surgery in limited SCLC.[322] Twenty-eight patients underwent thoracotomy after lack of response to induction chemotherapy or relapse after initial response. A resection rate of 82% was possible in this selected group, and ten patients (36%) had mixed elements histologically. Projected 5-year survival is 23%. We believe it is important to verify these findings in other patients who are prospectively identified by specific selection criteria before recommending such an approach.

TREATMENT OUTCOME AND LONG-TERM SURVIVAL

Although current therapy has a significant effect on the natural history of this disease, the number of patients cured remains frustratingly small (Table 31.3-9). Patients are at greatest risk of dying during the first 24 months after diagnosis; this risk declines between years 2 and 3 and is further reduced beyond the third year. In the Surveillance, Epidemiology, and End Results database, overall survival at 2, 3, and 5 years was 11.6%, 7.1%, and 4.6%, respectively.[472] In an analysis of 2196 patients treated on clinical trials in Britain, the hazard fell by a factor of 10 after 3 years but was still approximately seven times that of the general population.[473] Excessive mortality in long-term survivors is due both to late relapse with SCLC and to the development of second primary tumors. Late relapse occurs in approximately 10% of patients who are free of disease at 5 years.[474] Second primary tumors pose an even greater risk than relapse in long-term survivors. Overall, the relative risk of a second primary tumor in survivors beyond 2 years is increased by 3.5-fold.[475] Most of these second primary tumors are non-SCLC or other malignancies of the upper aerodigestive tract, indicating that field cancerization due to tobacco exposure has occurred.[475,476] The risk of a second primary tumor increases significantly over time, and continued smoking after the initial diagnosis of SCLC, radiation to the chest, and treatment with alkylating agents magnifies this risk.[475] For example, the risk of a second lung cancer in patients who continue to smoke was approximately fourfold more than those who stopped before the diagnosis of SCLC and twofold greater in patients who received chest irradiation compared with nonirradiated patients. The cumulative risk of a second lung cancer was 32% at 12 years and continued to increase beyond that time point. Consequently, patients successfully treated for SCLC constitute an extraordinarily high-risk group and deserve close medical follow-up. This population would be appropriate for studies evaluating new screening technologies, such as spiral CT scanning, and are candidates for chemoprevention trials.

Long-term survivors are also at increased risk for noncancer-related morbidity. In a French study of patients surviving beyond 30 months, treatment-related sequelae included neurologic impairment in 13% of the patients, pulmonary fibrosis in 18%, and cardiac disorders in 10%.[477] Return to work was possible in 40% of these patients and was not influenced by the presence of late treatment-related complications. In a Danish analysis of patients surviving 5 years or longer, there was a six-fold increase risk of death from nonneoplastic causes, particularly cardiovascular and pulmonary diseases.[478]

Few patients with extensive disease attain long-term survival. At 2 years after diagnosis no more than 5% of these patients remain alive, and the survival rate at 5 years is only 1%.[472,479] Although the effect of combination chemotherapy on survival is unambiguous, it is not clear whether any of the agents, treatment schedules, or supportive measures introduced since 1980 have improved survival compared with the therapies available in the 1970s. Analysis of 21 phase III trials conducted in North America between 1972 and 1990 showed an improvement in median survival time from 7 months to 8.9 months when studies initiated in the first decade were compared with studies initiated in the second.[480] In contrast, an analysis of 1111 consecutive patients treated in clinical trials in Scandinavia between 1973 and 1992 demonstrated no improvement in survival over those two decades.[481] In this series, severe myelosuppression and febrile neutropenia was significantly more common in patients treated between 1981 and 1992, suggesting that more intensive therapies in a relatively unselective population increase toxicity without improving survival. This study highlights one of the great challenges in the management of SCLC. There is significant heterogeneity among patients in their capacity to tolerate aggressive therapy, and optimal management requires therapy that is tailored to the tolerance of the individual patient.

EXTRAPULMONARY SMALL CELL CARCINOMA

Extrapulmonary small cell anaplastic carcinoma is a clinicopathologic entity distinct from SCLC. It is estimated that approximately 1000 cases are diagnosed in the United States annually.[482] On routine histopathologic examination, pulmonary and extrapulmonary small cell carcinomas are indistinguishable. Mixed tumors, which include a variety of cell types, may occur more frequently, and deletions of chromosome 3p may be less common with extrapulmonary tumors.[483] Primary small cell carcinomas have been identified in virtually every organ site.[484] The most common sites include the esophagus and other gastrointestinal organs, the head and neck region, cervix, and bladder. There appears to be a sex predilection based on the primary site: Most of the small cell carcinomas of the head and neck region, esophagus, and bladder are found in male subjects. With the exception of primary tumors arising in the cervix in which a younger age group is affected, the majority of patients are middle-aged or older.

A history of tobacco use is common, particularly in tumors that occur in the head and neck region and the esophagus, but there is not as strong an association with smoking as there is with pulmonary small cell carcinoma. Paraneoplastic syndromes due to the ectopic production of adrenocorticotropic and antidiuretic hormones also occur with extrapulmonary small cell cancer, and there is at least one case report in which humorally mediated hypercalcemia was identified.[485]

By definition, patients with extrapulmonary small cell cancers must have a normal CT scan of the chest and preferably a normal bronchoscopic examination. Merkel-cell carcinoma is a distinct entity that is primarily found in the skin and can be distinguished by certain immunocytochemical characteristics. Extrapulmonary small cell carcinomas can disseminate widely, and the recommended staging studies are similar for pulmonary small cell carcinoma.[484] A two-stage system is generally used. Limited disease is defined as tumor confined to the organ of origin and the local regional nodes that are encompassable within a radiation protal. Tumors that have spread beyond one radiation portal are defined as extensive. In contrast to SCLC, most patients in whom a primary site is identified have limited disease at the time of diagnosis. In a series of 71 patients from the Mayo Clinic, 76% of the tumors were localized at diagnosis.[486] In this series, the only sites that presented greater than or equal to 50% of the time with extensive disease were primary tumors of the gastrointestinal tract and tumors of unknown primary site.

In many respects, natural history and response to treatment for small cell carcinoma are similar for both pulmonary and extrapulmonary sites. Patients with extensive disease are candidates for treatment with combination chemotherapy. There are several reports in the literature in which a proportion of patients with limited disease managed, with local therapies alone, particularly surgical resection, to achieve a long-term progression-free survival.[482,484,486] Success of local therapy appears to vary depending on the primary site of the small cell carcinoma. For example, Koss et al. reported an approximate 30% 5-year survival in patients with small cell carcinoma of the minor salivary glands managed only with local therapy.[487] Surprisingly, small cell cancers of unknown primary site have been successfully managed by local therapy.[486,488] In contrast, small cell cancer rising in other head and neck sites, such as the larynx and hypopharynx, and primaries of the esophagus, prostate, and bladder recur rapidly despite complete surgical resection.[482,489] Patients with stage I small cell carcinoma of the cervix have been managed successfully by radical hysterectomy, but if the regional lymph nodes are involved local therapy alone is almost never curative.[486,490,491] Although some patients with small-volume disease confined to the organ of origin can be cured with surgery alone, the risk of relapse remains high even in this most favorable subset, and in most patients adjuvant chemotherapy should be strongly considered. For patients with locoregional disease, the combination of chemotherapy and radiation is a reasonable alternative to surgery. Overall, the prognosis for extrapulmonary small cell carcinoma is poor. In the Mayo Clinic series, 3- and 5-year survivals were 38% and 13%, respectively.[486]

REFERENCES

1. Chute CG, Greenberg ER, Baron J, et al. Presenting conditions of 1539 population-based lung cancer patients by cell type and stage in New Hampshire and Vermont. *Cancer* 1985;56:2107.
2. Landes SH, Murray T, Bodden S, et al. Cancer statistics, 1999. *CA Cancer J Clin* 1999;49:8.
3. Parkin DM, Sankaranarayanan R. Overview on small cell lung cancer in the world: industrialized countries, Third World, eastern Europe. *Anticancer Res* 1994;14:277.
4. U.S. Department of Health and Human Services. *Reducing the health consequences of smoking: 25 years of progress.* A report of the Surgeon General. Rockville, MD: Center for Chronic Disease Prevention and Health Promotion, Office on Smoking and Health, 1989.
5. Lubin JH, Blot WJ. Assessment of lung cancer risk factors by histologic category. *J Natl Cancer Inst* 1984;73:383.
6. Morabia A, Wynder EL. Cigarette smoking and lung cancer cell types. *Cancer* 1991;68:2074.
7. Wingo PA, Ries LA, Giovino GA, et al. Annual report to the nation on the status of cancer, 1973–1996, with a special section on lung cancer and tobacco smoking. *J Natl Cancer Inst* 1999;91:675.
8. Cigarette smoking among adults. *MMWR Morb Mortality Wkly Rep* 1997;46:1217.
9. Barrueco M, Cordovilla R, Hernandez Mezquita MA, et al. Sex differences in experimentation and tobacco consumption by children, adolescents and young adults. *Arch Bronconeumol* 1998;34:199.
10. Tobacco use among high school students—United States, 1997. *MMWR Morb Mortality Wkly Rep* 1998;47:229.
11. Saracci R. The interactions of tobacco smoking and other agents in cancer etiology. *Epidemiol Rev* 1987;9:175.
12. Ernster VL. Female lung cancer. *Annu Rev Public Health* 1996;17:97.
13. Hayes RB, Yin SN, Dosemeci M, et al. Mortality among benzene-exposed workers in China. *Environ Health Perspect* 1996;104(Suppl 6):1349.
14. Steenland K, Loomis D, Shy C, et al. Review of occupational lung carcinogens. *Am J Ind Med* 1996;29:474.
15. Alavanja MC, Brownson RC, Boice JD Jr, et al. Preexisting lung disease and lung cancer among nonsmoking women. *Am J Epidemiol* 1992;136:623.
16. Mayne ST, Buenconsejo J, Janerich DT. Previous lung disease and risk of lung cancer among men and women nonsmokers. *Am J Epidemiol* 1999;149:13.
17. Bartsch H, Petruzzelli S, De Flora S, et al. Carcinogen metabolism in human lung tissues and the effect of tobacco smoking: results from a case-control multicenter study on lung cancer patients. *Environ Health Perspect* 1992;98:119.
18. Brownson RC, Alavanja MC, Caporaso N, et al. Family history of cancer and risk of lung cancer in lifetime non-smokers and long-term ex-smokers. *Int J Epidemiol* 1997;26:256.
19. Sellers TA, Bailey-Wilson JE, Elston RC, et al. Evidence for mendelian inheritance in the pathogenesis of lung cancer [see comments]. *J Natl Cancer Inst* 1990;82:1272.
20. Mayne ST, Buenconsejo J, Janerich DT. Familial cancer history and lung cancer risk in United States nonsmoking men and women. *Cancer Epidemiol Biomarker Prev* 1999;8:1065.
21. Bennett WP, Hussain SP, Vahakangas KH, et al. Molecular epidemiology of human cancer risk: gene-environment interactions and p53 mutation spectrum in human lung cancer. *J Pathol* 1999;187:8.
22. Kohno T, Yokota J. How many tumor suppressor genes are involved in human lung carcinogenesis? *Carcinogenesis* 1999;20:1403.
23. Harris RE, Zang EA, Anderson JI, et al. Race and sex differences in lung cancer risk associated with cigarette smoking. *Int J Epidemiol* 1993;22:592.

24. Zang EA, Wynder EL. Differences in lung cancer risk between men and women: examination of the evidence [see comments]. *J Natl Cancer Inst* 1996;88:183.
25. Ramalingam S, Pawlish K, Gadgeel S, et al. Lung cancer in young patients: analysis of a Surveillance, Epidemiology, and End Results database. *J Clin Oncol* 1998;16:651.
26. World Health Organization. *Histologic typing of lung tumors*, 2nd ed. Geneva: World Heath Organization, 1981.
27. Hirsch FR, Matthews MJ, Aisner S, et al. Histopathologic classification of small cell lung cancer. Changing concepts and terminology. *Cancer* 1988;62:973.
28. Carter D, Eggleston JC. Tumors of the lower respiratory tract. In: *Atlas of tumor pathology*, second series, fascicle 17. Washington, DC: Armed Forces Institute of Pathology, 1980.
29. Travis WD, Linder J, Mackay B. Classification, histology, cytology, and electron microscopy. In: Pass HI, Mitchell JB, Johnson DH, et al., eds. *Lung cancer: principles and practice*. Philadelphia: Lippincott–Raven, 1996.
30. Aisner SC, Finkelstein DM, Ettinger DS, et al. The clinical significance of variant-morphology small-cell carcinoma of the lung. *J Clin Oncol* 1990;8:402.
31. Fraire AE, Johnson EH, Yesner R, et al. Prognostic significance of histopathologic subtype and stage in small cell lung cancer. *Hum Pathol* 1992;23:520.
32. Mangum MD, Greco FA, Hainsworth JD, et al. Combined small-cell and non-small-cell lung cancer. *J Clin Oncol* 1989;7:607.
33. Radice PA, Matthews MJ, Ihde DC, et al. The clinical behavior of "mixed" small cell/large cell bronchogenic carcinoma compared with "pure" small cell subtypes. *Cancer* 1982;50:2894.
34. Fushimi H, Kukui M, Morino H, et al. Detection of large cell component in small cell lung carcinoma by combined cytologic and histologic examinations and its clinical implication. *Cancer* 1992;70:599.
35. Bepler G, Neumann K, Holle R, et al. Clinical relevance of histologic subtyping in small cell lung cancer. *Cancer* 1989;64:74.
36. Guinee DG Jr, Fishback NF, Koss MN, et al. The spectrum of immunohistochemical staining of small-cell lung carcinoma in specimens from transbronchial and open-lung biopsies. *Am J Clin Pathol* 1994;102:406.
37. Higgins GA, Shields TW, Keehn RJ. The solitary pulmonary nodule. Ten-year follow-up of Veterans Administration-armed forces cooperative study. *Arch Surg* 1975;110:570.
38. Muhm JR, Miller WE, Fontana RS, et al. Lung cancer detected during a screening program using four-month chest radiographs. *Radiology* 1983;148:609.
39. Sculier JP, Evans WK, Feld R, et al. Superior vena caval obstruction syndrome in small cell lung cancer. *Cancer* 1986;57:847.
40. Paulson DL. Carcinomas in the superior pulmonary sulcus. *J Thorac Cardiovasc Surg* 1975;70:1095.
41. Johnson DH, Hainsworth JD, Greco FA. Pancoast's syndrome and small cell lung cancer. *Chest* 1982;82:602.
42. Levitan N, Byrne RE, Bromer RH, et al. The value of the bone scan and bone marrow biopsy staging small cell lung cancer. *Cancer* 1985;56:652.
43. Michel F, Soler M, Imhof E, et al. Initial staging of non-small cell lung cancer: value of routine radioisotope bone scanning. *Thorax* 1991;46:469.
44. Tritz DB, Doll DC, Ringenberg QS, et al. Bone marrow involvement in small cell lung cancer. Clinical significance and correlation with routine laboratory variables. *Cancer* 1989;63:763.
45. Dombernowsky P, Hirsch F, Hansen HH, et al. Peritoneoscopy in the staging of 190 patients with small-cell anaplastic carcinoma of the lung with special reference to subtyping. *Cancer* 1978;41:2008.
46. Patel AM, Jett JR. Clinical presentation and staging of lung cancer. In: Aisner J, Arriagada R, Green MR, et al., eds. *Comprehensive textbook of thoracic oncology*. Baltimore: Williams & Wilkins, 1996:293.
47. Souhami RL, Bradbury I, Geddes DM, et al. Prognostic significance of laboratory parameters measured at diagnosis in small cell carcinoma of the lung. *Cancer Res* 1985;45:2878.
48. Osterlind K, Andersen PK. Prognostic factors in small cell lung cancer: multivariate model based on 778 patients treated with chemotherapy with or without irradiation. *Cancer Res* 1986;46:4189.
49. Shepherd FA, Laskey J, Evans WK, et al. Cushing's syndrome associated with ectopic corticotropin production and small-cell lung cancer. *J Clin Oncol* 1992;10:21.
50. Dimopoulos MA, Fernandez JF, Samaan NA, et al. Paraneoplastic Cushing's syndrome as an adverse prognostic factor in patients who die early with small cell lung cancer. *Cancer* 1992;69:66.
51. Dalmau J, Furneaux HM, Gralla RJ, et al. Detection of the anti-Hu antibody in the serum of patients with small cell lung cancer—a quantitative western blot analysis. *Ann Neurol* 1990;27:544.
52. O'Neill JH, Murray NM, Newsom-Davis J. The Lambert-Eaton myasthenic syndrome. A review of 50 cases. *Brain* 1988;111:577.
53. Anderson NE, Rosenblum MK, Graus F, et al. Autoantibodies in paraneoplastic syndromes associated with small-cell lung cancer. *Neurology* 1988;38:1391.
54. Lennon VA, Sas DF, Busk MF, et al. Enteric neuronal autoantibodies in pseudoobstruction with small-cell lung carcinoma [see comments]. *Gastroenterology* 1991;100:137.
55. Newman NJ, Bell IR, McKee AC. Paraneoplastic limbic encephalitis: neuropsychiatric presentation. *Biol Psychiatry* 1990;27:529.
56. Ojeda VJ. Necrotizing myelopathy associated with malignancy. A clinicopathologic study of two cases and literature review. *Cancer* 1984;53:1115.
57. Mountain CF. Revisions in the International System for Staging Lung Cancer. *Chest* 1997;111:1710.
58. Zelen M. Keynote address on biostatistics and data retrieval, part 3. *Cancer Chemother Rep* 1973;4:31.
59. Sagman U, Maki E, Evans WK, et al. Small-cell carcinoma of the lung: derivation of a prognostic staging system. *J Clin Oncol* 1991;9:1639.
60. Livingston RB, McCracken JD, Trauth CJ, et al. Isolated pleural effusion in small cell lung carcinoma: favorable prognosis. A review of the Southwest Oncology Group experience. *Chest* 1982;81:208.
61. Dearing MP, Steinberg SM, Phelps R, et al. Outcome of patients with small-cell lung cancer: effect of changes in staging procedures and imaging technology on prognostic factors over 14 years. *J Clin Oncol* 1990;8:1042.
62. Maestu I, Pastor M, Gomez-Codina J, et al. Pretreatment prognostic factors for survival in small-cell lung cancer: a new prognostic index and validation of three known prognostic indices on 341 patients. *Ann Oncol* 1997;8:547.
63. Stahel RA, Ginsberg RJ, Haddad K, et al. Staging and prognostic factors in small cell lung cancer: a consensus report. *Lung Cancer* 1989;5:119.
64. Albain KS, Crowley JJ, LeBlanc M, et al. Determinants of improved outcome in small-cell lung cancer: an analysis of the 2,580-patient Southwest Oncology Group data base. *J Clin Oncol* 1990;8:1563.
65. Chauvin F, Trillet V, Court-Fortune I, et al. Pretreatment staging evaluation in small cell lung carcinoma. A new approach to medical decision making. *Chest* 1992;102:497.
66. Shepherd FA, Ginsberg RJ, Haddad R, et al. Importance of clinical staging in limited small-cell lung cancer: a valuable system to separate prognostic subgroups. The University of Toronto Lung Oncology Group. *J Clin Oncol* 1993;11:1592.
67. Spiegelman D, Maurer LH, Ware JH, et al. Prognostic factors in small-cell carcinoma of the lung: an analysis of 1,521 patients. *J Clin Oncol* 1989;7:344.
68. Urban T, Chastang C, Vaylet F, et al. Prognostic significance of supraclavicular lymph nodes in small cell lung cancer: a study from four consecutive clinical trials, including 1,370 patients. "Petites Cellules" Group. *Chest* 1998;114:1538.
69. Turrisi AT 3rd, Kim K, Blum R, et al. Twice-daily compared with once-daily thoracic radiotherapy in limited small-cell lung cancer treated concurrently with cisplatin and etoposide. *N Engl J Med* 1999;340:265.
70. Bonner JA, Sloan JA, Shanahan TG, et al. Phase III comparison of twice-daily split-course irradiation versus once-daily irradiation for patients with limited stage small-cell lung carcinoma. *J Clin Oncol* 1999;17:2681.
71. Vincent MD, Ashley SE, Smith IE. Prognostic factors in small cell lung cancer: a simple prognostic index is better than conventional staging. *Eur J Cancer Clin Oncol* 1987;23:1589.
72. Perry MC, Eaton WL, Propert KJ, et al. Chemotherapy with or without radiation therapy in limited small-cell carcinoma of the lung. *N Engl J Med* 1987;316:912.
73. Murray N, Coy P, Pater JL, et al. Importance of timing for thoracic irradiation in the combined modality treatment of limited-stage small-cell lung cancer. The National Cancer Institute of Canada Clinical Trials Group. *J Clin Oncol* 1993;11:336.
74. Kreisman H, Wolkove N, Quoix E. Small cell lung cancer presenting as a solitary pulmonary nodule. *Chest* 1992;101:225.
75. Karrer K, Ulsperger E. Surgery for cure followed by chemotherapy in small cell carcinoma of the lung. For the ISC-Lung Cancer Study Group. *Acta Oncol* 1995;34:899.
76. Pignon JP, Arriagada R, Ihde DC, et al. A meta-analysis of thoracic radiotherapy for small-cell lung cancer [see comments]. *N Engl J Med* 1992;327:1618.
77. Byhardt RW, Hartz A, Libnoch JA, et al. Prognostic influence of TNM staging and LDH levels in small cell carcinoma of the lung (SCCL). *Int J Radiat Oncol Biol Phys* 1986;12:771.
78. Fizazi K, Cojean I, Pignon JP, et al. Normal serum neuron specific enolase (NSE) value after the first cycle of chemotherapy: an early predictor of complete response and survival in patients with small cell lung carcinoma. *Cancer* 1998;82:1049.
79. Jorgensen LG, Osterlind K, Genolla J, et al. Serum neuron-specific enolase (S-NSE) and the prognosis in small-cell lung cancer (SCLC): a combined multivariable analysis on data from nine centres [published erratum appears in *Br J Cancer* 1996;74:2043]. *Br J Cancer* 1996;74:463.
80. Wolf M, Holle R, Hans K, et al. Analysis of prognostic factors in 766 patients with small cell lung cancer (SCLC): the role of sex as a predictor for survival. *Br J Cancer* 1991;63:986.
81. Albain KS, Crowley JJ, Livingston RB. Long-term survival and toxicity in small cell lung cancer. Expanded Southwest Oncology Group experience. *Chest* 1991;99:1425.
82. Gronowitz JS, Bergstrom R, Nou E, et al. Clinical and serologic markers of stage and prognosis in small cell lung cancer. A multivariate analysis. *Cancer* 1990;66:722.
83. Rawson NS, Peto J. An overview of prognostic factors in small cell lung cancer. A report from the Subcommittee for the Management of Lung Cancer of the United Kingdom Coordinating Committee on Cancer Research [published erratum appears in *Br J Cancer* 1990;62:550]. *Br J Cancer* 1990;61:597.
84. Siu LL, Shepherd FA, Murray N, et al. Influence of age on the treatment of limited-stage small-cell lung cancer. *J Clin Oncol* 1996;14:821.
85. Young LC, Campling BG, Voskoglou-Nomikos T, et al. Expression of multidrug resistance protein-related genes in lung cancer: correlation with drug response. *Clin Cancer Res* 1999;5:673.
86. Onuki N, Wistuba II, Travis WD, et al. Genetic changes in the spectrum of neuroendocrine lung tumors. *Cancer* 1999;85:600.
87. Gazdar AF, Steinberg SM, Russell EK, et al. Correlation of in vitro drug-sensitivity testing results with response to chemotherapy and survival in extensive-stage small cell lung cancer: a prospective clinical trial [see comments]. *J Natl Cancer Inst* 1990;82:117.
88. Radford JA, Ryder WDJ, Dodwell D, et al. Predicting septic complications from chemotherapy: an analysis of 382 patients treated for small cell lung cancer without dose reduction after major sepsis. *Eur J Cancer* 1993;29A:81.
89. Morittu L, Earl HM, Souhami RL, et al. Patients at risk of chemotherapy-associated toxicity in small cell lung cancer. *Br J Cancer* 1989;59:801.
90. Lassen UN, Osterlind K, Hirsch FR, et al. Early death during chemotherapy in patients with small-cell lung cancer: derivation of a prognostic index for toxic death and progression. *Br J Cancer* 1999;79:515.
91. Matthews MJ, Kanhouwa S, Pickren J, et al. Frequency of residual and metastatic tumor in patients undergoing curative surgical resection for lung cancer. *Cancer Chemother Rep* 1973;4:63.
92. Richardson GE, Venzon DJ, Edison M, et al. Application of an algorithm for staging small-cell lung cancer can save one third of the initial evaluation costs. *Arch Intern Med* 1993;153:329.

93. Sagman U, Feld R, Evans WK, et al. The prognostic significance of pretreatment serum lactate dehydrogenase in patients with small-cell lung cancer. *J Clin Oncol* 1991;9:954.
94. Stokkel MP, van Eck-Smit BL, Zwinderman AH, et al. Pretreatment serum lactate dehydrogenase as additional staging parameter in patients with small-cell lung carcinoma. *J Cancer Res Clin Oncol* 1998;124:215.
95. Norlund JD, Byhardt RW, Foley WD, et al. Computed tomography in the staging of small cell lung cancer: implications for combined modality therapy. *Int J Radiat Oncol Biol Phys* 1985;11:1081.
96. Whitley NO, Fuks JZ, McCrea ES, et al. Computed tomography of the chest in small cell lung cancer: potential new prognostic signs. *AJR Am J Roentgenol* 1984;142:885.
97. Ihde DC, Cohen MH, Bernath AM, et al. Serial fiberoptic bronchoscopy during chemotherapy for small cell carcinoma of the lung: early detection of patients at high risk of relapse. *Chest* 1978;74:531.
98. Harper PG, Houang M, Spiro SG, et al. Computerized axial tomography in the pretreatment assessment of small-cell carcinoma of the bronchus. *Cancer* 1981;47:1775.
99. Ihde DC, Dunnick NR, Johnston-Early A, et al. Abdominal computed tomography in small cell lung cancer: assessment of extent of disease and response to therapy. *Cancer* 1982;49:1485.
100. Mulshine JL, Makuch RW, Johnston-Early A, et al. Diagnosis and significance of liver metastases in small cell carcinoma of the lung. *J Clin Oncol* 1984;2:733.
101. Boland GW, Lee MJ, Gazelle GS, et al. Characterization of adrenal masses using unenhanced CT: an analysis of the CT literature. *AJR Am J Roentgenol* 1998;171:201.
102. Schwartz LH, Ginsberg MS, Burt ME, et al. MRI as an alternative to CT-guided biopsy of adrenal masses in patients with lung cancer. *Ann Thorac Surg* 1998;65:193.
103. Nugent JL, Bunn PA Jr, Matthews MJ, et al. CNS metastases in small cell bronchogenic carcinoma: increasing frequency and changing pattern with lengthening survival. *Cancer* 1979;44:1885.
104. Komaki R, Cox JD, Whitson W. Risk of brain metastasis from small cell carcinoma of the lung related to length of survival and prophylactic irradiation. *Cancer Treat Rep* 1981;65:811.
105. Hirsch FR, Paulson OB, Hansen HH, et al. Intracranial metastases in small cell carcinoma of the lung: correlation of clinical and autopsy findings. *Cancer* 1982;50:2433.
106. van Oosterhout AG, van de Pol M, ten Velde GP, et al. Neurologic disorders in 203 consecutive patients with small cell lung cancer. Results of a longitudinal study. *Cancer* 1996;77:1434.
107. Crane JM, Nelson MJ, Ihde DC, et al. A comparison of computed tomography and radionuclide scanning for detection of brain metastases in small cell lung cancer. *J Clin Oncol* 1984;2:1017.
108. Johnson DH, Windham WW, Allen JH, et al. Limited value of CT brain scans in the staging of small cell lung cancer. *AJR Am J Roentgenol* 1983;140:37.
109. Hardy J, Smith I, Cherryman G, et al. The value of computed tomographic (CT) scan surveillance in the detection and management of brain metastases in patients with small cell lung cancer. *Br J Cancer* 1990;62:684.
110. Kristensen CA, Kristjansen PE, Hansen HH. Systemic chemotherapy of brain metastases from small-cell lung cancer: a review. *J Clin Oncol* 1992;10:1498.
111. van Hazel GA, Scott M, Eagan RT. The effect of CNS metastases on the survival of patients with small cell cancer of the lung. *Cancer* 1983;51:933.
112. Kochhar R, Frytak S, Shaw EG. Survival of patients with extensive small-cell lung cancer who have only brain metastases at initial diagnosis. *Am J Clin Oncol* 1997;20:125.
113. Levenson RM Jr, Sauerbrunn BJ, Ihde DC, et al. Small cell lung cancer: radionuclide bone scans for assessment of tumor extent and response. *AJR Am J Roentgenol* 1981;137:31.
114. Ihde DC, Makuch RW, Carney DN, et al. Prognostic implications of stage of disease and sites of metastases in patients with small cell carcinoma of the lung treated with intensive combination chemotherapy. *Am Rev Respir Dis* 1981;123:500.
115. Campling B, Quirt I, DeBoer G, et al. Is bone marrow examination in small-cell lung cancer really necessary? *Ann Intern Med* 1986;105:508.
116. Bezwoda WR, Lewis D, Livini N. Bone marrow involvement in anaplastic small cell lung cancer. Diagnosis, hematologic features, and prognostic implications. *Cancer* 1986;58:1762.
117. Trillet V, Revel D, Combaret V, et al. Bone marrow metastases in small cell lung cancer: detection with magnetic resonance imaging and monoclonal antibodies. *Br J Cancer* 1989;60:83.
118. Hunter RF, Broadway P, Sun SL, et al. Detection of small cell lung cancer bone marrow involvement by discontinuous gradient sedimentation. *Cancer Res* 1987;47:2737.
119. Pollard EB, Tio F, Myers JW, et al. Utilization of a human tumor cloning system to monitor for marrow involvement with small cell carcinoma of the lung. *Cancer Res* 1981;41:1015.
120. Trillet-Lenoir VN, Arpin D, Brune J. Bone marrow metastases detection in small cell lung cancer. A review. *Anticancer Res* 1994;14:2795.
121. Canon JL, Humblet Y, Lebacq-Verheyden AM, et al. Immunodetection of small cell lung cancer metastases in bone marrow using three monoclonal antibodies. *Eur J Cancer Clin Oncol* 1988;24:147.
122. Muss HB, Jackson DV Jr, Richards FD, et al. Bone marrow evaluation in small cell lung cancer. *Am J Clin Oncol* 1984;7:59.
123. Hamrick RMD, Murgo AJ. Lactate dehydrogenase values and bone scans as predictors of bone marrow involvement in small-cell lung cancer. *Arch Intern Med* 1987;147:1070.
124. Milleron BJ, Le Breton C, Carette MF, et al. Assessment of bone marrow involvement by magnetic resonance imaging in small cell lung cancer. No significant change of staging. *Chest* 1994;106:1030.
125. Hochstenbag MM, Snoep G, Cobben NA, et al. Detection of bone marrow metastases in small cell lung cancer. Comparison of magnetic resonance imaging with standard methods. *Eur J Cancer* 1996;32A:779.
126. Seto T, Imamura F, Kuriyama K, et al. Effect on prognosis of bone marrow infiltration detected by magnetic resonance imaging in small cell lung cancer. *Eur J Cancer* 1997;33:2333.
127. Layer G, Steudel A, Schuller H, et al. Magnetic resonance imaging to detect bone marrow metastases in the initial staging of small cell lung carcinoma and breast carcinoma. *Cancer* 1999;85:1004.
128. Peck K, Sher YP, Shih JY, et al. Detection and quantitation of circulating cancer cells in the peripheral blood of lung cancer patients. *Cancer Res* 1998;58:2761.
129. Wahl RL, Quint LE, Greenough RL, et al. Staging of mediastinal non-small cell lung cancer with FDG PET, CT, and fusion images: preliminary prospective evaluation. *Radiology* 1994;191:371.
130. Kubota K, Matsuzawa T, Fujiwara T, et al. Differential diagnosis of lung tumor with positron emission tomography: a prospective study. *J Nucl Med* 1990;31:1927.
131. Weber W, Young C, Abdel-Dayem HM, et al. Assessment of pulmonary lesions with ^{18}F-fluorodeoxyglucose positron imaging using coincidence mode gamma cameras. *J Nucl Med* 1999;40:574.
132. Weder W, Schmid RA, Bruchhaus H, et al. Detection of extrathoracic metastases by positron emission tomography in lung cancer. *Ann Thorac Surg* 1998;66:886.
133. Balaban EP, Walker BS, Cox JV, et al. Detection and staging of small cell lung carcinoma with a technetium-labeled monoclonal antibody. A comparison with standard staging methods. *Clin Nucl Med* 1992;17:439.
134. Hochstenbag MM, Heidendal GA, Wouters EF, et al. In-111 octreotide imaging in staging of small cell lung cancer. *Clin Nucl Med* 1997;22:811.
135. Berenger N, Moretti JL, Boaziz C, et al. Somatostatin receptor imaging in small cell lung cancer. *Eur J Cancer* 1996;32A:1429.
136. Reisinger I, Bohuslavitzki KH, Brenner W, et al. Somatostatin receptor scintigraphy in small-cell lung cancer: results of a multicenter study [see comments]. *J Nucl Med* 1998;39:224.
137. Taylor AB, Shinton NK, Waterhouse JAH. Histology of bronchial carcinoma in relation to prognosis. *Thorax* 1963;18:178.
138. Lennox SC, Flavell G, Pollock DJ, et al. Results of resection for oat-cell carcinoma of the lung. *Lancet* 1968;2:925.
139. Fox W, Scadding JG. Medical Research Council comparative trial of surgery and radiotherapy for primary treatment of small-celled or oat-celled carcinoma of bronchus. Ten-year follow-up. *Lancet* 1973;2:63.
140. Mountain CF. Clinical biology of small cell lung carcinoma: relationship to surgical therapy. *Semin Oncol* 1978;5:272.
141. Green RA, Humphrey E, Close H. Alkylating agents in bronchogenic carcinoma. *Am J Med* 1969;46:516.
142. Medical Research Council. Radiotherapy alone or with chemotherapy in the treatment of small-cell carcinoma of the lung. *Br J Cancer* 1979;40:1.
143. Grant SC, Gralla RJ, Kris MG, et al. Single-agent chemotherapy trials in small-cell lung cancer, 1970 to 1990: the case for studies in previously treated patients. *J Clin Oncol* 1992;10:484.
144. Bork E, Ersboll J, Dombernowsky P, et al. Teniposide and etoposide in previously untreated small cell lung cancer: a randomized study. *J Clin Oncol* 1991;9:1627.
145. Slevin ML, Clark PI, Joel SP, et al. A randomized trial to evaluate the effect of schedule on the activity of etoposide in small-cell lung cancer. *J Clin Oncol* 1989;7:1333.
146. Clark PI, Slevin ML, Joel SP, et al. A randomized trial of two etoposide schedules in small-cell lung cancer: the influence of pharmacokinetics on efficacy and toxicity. *J Clin Oncol* 1994;12:1427.
147. Wolff SN, Birch R, Sarma P, et al. Randomized dose-response evaluation of etoposide in small cell carcinoma of the lung: a Southeastern Cancer Study Group Trial. *Cancer Treat Rep* 1986;70:583.
148. Issell BF, Einhorn LH, Comis RL, et al. Multicenter phase II trial of etoposide in refractory small cell lung cancer. *Cancer Treat Rep* 1985;69:127.
149. Hansen HH, Dombernowsky P, Hansen M, et al. Teniposide in the treatment of small cell lung cancer: a review. *Semin Oncol* 1992;19:65.
150. Ettinger DS, Finkelstein DM, Abeloff MD, et al. Justification for evaluating new anticancer drugs in selected untreated patients with extensive-stage small-cell lung cancer: an Eastern Cooperative Oncology Group randomized study. *J Natl Cancer Inst* 1992;84:1077.
151. Moore TD, Korn EL. Phase II trial design considerations for small-cell lung cancer. *J Natl Cancer Inst* 1992;84:150.
152. Giaccone G, Ferrati P, Donadio M, et al. Reinduction chemotherapy in small cell lung cancer. *Eur J Cancer Clin Oncol* 1987;23:1697.
153. Cavalli F, Sonntag RW, Jungi F, et al. VP-16-213 monotherapy for remission induction of small cell lung cancer: a randomized trial using three dosage schedules. *Cancer Treat Rep* 1978;62:473.
154. Abratt RP, Willcox PA, de Groot M, et al. Prospective study of etoposide scheduling in combination chemotherapy for limited disease small cell lung carcinoma. *Eur J Cancer* 1991;27:28.
155. Johnson DH, Greco FA, Strupp J, et al. Prolonged administration of oral etoposide in patients with relapsed or refractory small-cell lung cancer: a phase II trial. *J Clin Oncol* 1990;8:1613.
156. Einhorn LH, Pennington K, McClean J. Phase II trial of daily oral VP-16 in refractory small cell lung cancer: a Hoosier Oncology Group study. *Semin Oncol* 1990;17:32.
157. Miller AA, Herndon JE 2nd, Hollis DR, et al. Schedule dependency of 21-day oral versus 3-day intravenous etoposide in combination with intravenous cisplatin in extensive-stage small-cell lung cancer: a randomized phase III study of the Cancer and Leukemia Group B. *J Clin Oncol* 1995;13:1871.
158. Maksymiuk AW, Jett JR, Earle JD, et al. Sequencing and schedule effects of cisplatin plus etoposide in small-cell lung cancer: results of a North Central Cancer Treatment Group randomized clinical trial. *J Clin Oncol* 1994;12:70.
159. Smith IE, Harland SJ, Robinson BA, et al. Carboplatin: a very active new cisplatin analog in the treatment of small cell lung cancer. *Cancer Treat Rep* 1985;69:43.
160. Ettinger DS. The place of ifosfamide in chemotherapy of small cell lung cancer: the Eastern Cooperative Oncology Group experience and a selected literature update. *Semin Oncol* 1995;22(Suppl 2):23.
161. Bork E, Hansen M, Dombernowsky P, et al. Teniposide (VM-26), an overlooked highly active agent in small-cell lung cancer. Results of a phase II trial in untreated patients. *J Clin Oncol* 1986;4:524.

162. Cerny T, Pedrazzini A, Joss RA, et al. Unexpected high toxicity in a phase II study of teniposide (VM-26) in elderly patients with untreated small cell lung cancer (SCLC). *Eur J Cancer Clin Oncol* 1988;24:1791.
163. Blackstein M, Eisenhauer EA, Wierzbicki R, et al. Epirubicin in extensive small-cell lung cancer: a phase II study in previously untreated patients: a National Cancer Institute of Canada Clinical Trials Group Study. *J Clin Oncol* 1990;8:385.
164. Ettinger DS, Finkelstein DM, Sarma RP, et al. Phase II study of paclitaxel in patients with extensive-disease small-cell lung cancer: an Eastern Cooperative Oncology Group study. *J Clin Oncol* 1995;13:1430.
165. Smyth JF, Smith IE, Sessa C, et al. Activity of docetaxel (Taxotere) in small cell lung cancer. The Early Clinical Trials Group of the EORTC. *Eur J Cancer* 1994;8:1058.
166. Hesketh PJ, Crowley JJ, Burris HA 3rd, et al. Evaluation of docetaxel in previously untreated extensive-stage small cell lung cancer: a Southwest Oncology Group phase II trial. *Cancer J Sci Am* 1999;5:237.
167. Schiller JH, Kim K, Johnson D, et al. Phase II study of topotecan in extensive stage small cell lung cancer. *Proc Am Soc Clin Oncol* 1994;13:330(abst 1093).
168. Ardizzoni A, Hansen H, Dombernowsky P, et al. Topotecan, a new active drug in the second-line treatment of small-cell lung cancer: a phase II study in patients with refractory and sensitive disease. The European Organization for Research and Treatment of Cancer Early Clinical Studies Group and New Drug Development Office, and the Lung Cancer Cooperative Group. *J Clin Oncol* 1997;15:2090.
169. Eckardt J, Gralla R, Palmer MC, et al. Topotecan as second-line therapy in patients with small cell lung cancer: a phase II study. *Ann Oncol* 1996;7(Suppl 5; abst 513P).
170. Eckardt J, Depierre A, Ardizzoni A, et al. Pooled analysis of topotecan in the second-line treatment of patients with sensitive small cell lung cancer. *Proc Am Soc Clin Oncol* 1997;16:A1624.
171. von Pawel J, Schiller JH, Shepherd FA, et al. Topotecan versus cyclophosphamide, doxorubicin, and vincristine for the treatment of recurrent small-cell lung cancer. *J Clin Oncol* 1999;17:658.
172. von Pawel J, Gatzemeier U, Harstrick A, et al. A multicentre randomized phase II study of oral topotecan versus IV topotecan for second line therapy in sensitive patients with small cell lung cancer. *Proc Am Soc Clin Oncol* 1999;18:471(abst 1816).
173. Masuda N, Fukuoka M, Kusunoki Y, et al. CPT-11: a new derivative of camptothecin for the treatment of refractory or relapsed small-cell lung cancer. *J Clin Oncol* 1992;10:1225.
174. DeVore RF, Blanke CD, Denham CA, et al. Phase II study of irinotecan (CPT-11) in patients with previously treated small-cell lung cancer (SCLC). *Proc Am Soc Clin Oncol* 1998;17:451(abst 1736).
175. Le Chevalier T, Ibrahim N, Chomy P, et al. A phase II study of irinotecan (CPT-11) in patients (pts) with small cell lung cancer (SCLC) progressing after initial response to first-line treatment. *Proc Am Soc Clin Oncol* 1997;16:450(abst 1617).
176. Cormier Y, Eisenhauer E, Muldal A, et al. Gemcitabine is an active new agent in previously untreated extensive small cell lung cancer (SCLC). A study of the National Cancer Institute of Canada Clinical Trials Group. *Ann Oncol* 1994;5:283.
177. Postmus PE, Schramel FM, Smit EF. Evaluation of new drugs in small cell lung cancer: the activity of gemcitabine. *Semin Oncol* 1998;25:79.
178. Furuse K, Kubota K, Kawahara M, et al. Phase II study of vinorelbine in heavily previously treated small cell lung cancer. Japan Lung Cancer Vinorelbine Study Group. *Oncology* 1996;53:169.
179. Jassem J, Karnicka-Mlodkowska H, van Pottelsberghe C, et al. Phase II study of vinorelbine (Navelbine) in previously treated small cell lung cancer patients. EORTC Lung Cancer Cooperative Group. *Eur J Cancer* 1993;12:1720.
180. Gridelli C, Perrone F, Ianniello GP, et al. Carboplatin plus vinorelbine, a new well-tolerated and active regimen for the treatment of extensive-stage small-cell lung cancer: a phase II study. Gruppo Oncologico Centro-Sud-Isole. *J Clin Oncol* 1998;16:1414.
181. Lowenbraun S, Bartolucci A, Smalley RV, et al. The superiority of combination chemotherapy over single agent chemotherapy in small cell lung carcinoma. *Cancer* 1979;44:406.
182. Hansen HH, Dombernowsky P, Hansen M, et al. Chemotherapy of advanced small-cell anaplastic carcinoma. Superiority of a four-drug combination to a three-drug combination. *Ann Intern Med* 1978;89:177.
183. Livingston RB, Moore TN, Heilbrun L, et al. Small-cell carcinoma of the lung: combined chemotherapy and radiation: a Southwest Oncology Group study. *Ann Intern Med* 1978;88:194.
184. Hong WK, Nicaise C, Lawson R, et al. Etoposide combined with cyclophosphamide plus vincristine compared with doxorubicin plus cyclophosphamide plus vincristine and with high-dose cyclophosphamide plus vincristine in the treatment of small-cell carcinoma of the lung: a randomized trial of the Bristol Lung Cancer Study Group. *J Clin Oncol* 1989;7:450.
185. Bunn PA Jr, Greco FA, Einhorn L. Cyclophosphamide, doxorubicin, and etoposide as first-line therapy in the treatment of small-cell lung cancer. *Semin Oncol* 1986;13:45.
186. Hirsch FR, Hansen HH, Hansen M, et al. The superiority of combination chemotherapy including etoposide based on in vivo cell cycle analysis in the treatment of extensive small-cell lung cancer: a randomized trial of 288 consecutive patients. *J Clin Oncol* 1987;5:585.
187. Vindelov LL, Hansen HH, Gersel A, et al. Treatment of small-cell carcinoma of the lung monitored by sequential flow cytometric DNA analysis. *Cancer Res* 1982;42:2499.
188. Jackson DV Jr, Zekan PJ, Caldwell RD, et al. VP-16-213 in combination chemotherapy with chest irradiation for small-cell lung cancer: a randomized trial of the Piedmont Oncology Association. *J Clin Oncol* 1984;2:1343.
189. Jackson DV Jr, Case LD, Zekan PJ, et al. Improvement of long-term survival in extensive small-cell lung cancer. *J Clin Oncol* 1988;6:1161.
190. Jett JR, Everson L, Therneau TM, et al. Treatment of limited-stage small-cell lung cancer with cyclophosphamide, doxorubicin, and vincristine with or without etoposide: a randomized trial of the North Central Cancer Treatment Group. *J Clin Oncol* 1990;8:33.
191. Messeih AA, Schweitzer JM, Lipton A, et al. Addition of etoposide to cyclophosphamide, doxorubicin, and vincristine for remission induction and survival in patients with small cell lung cancer. *Cancer Treat Rep* 1987;71:61.
192. Lowenbraun S, Birch R, Buchanan R, et al. Combination chemotherapy in small cell lung carcinoma. A randomized study of two intensive regimens. *Cancer* 1984;54:2344.
193. Evans WK, Feld R, Osoba D, et al. VP-16 alone and in combination with cisplatin in previously treated patients with small cell lung cancer. *Cancer* 1984;53:1461.
194. Evans WK, Osoba D, Feld R, et al. Etoposide (VP-16) and cisplatin: an effective treatment for relapse in small-cell lung cancer. *J Clin Oncol* 1985;3:65.
195. Evans WK, Shepherd FA, Feld R, et al. VP-16 and cisplatin as first-line therapy for small-cell lung cancer. *J Clin Oncol* 1985;3:1471.
196. Einhorn LH, Crawford J, Birch R, et al. Cisplatin plus etoposide consolidation following cyclophosphamide, doxorubicin, and vincristine in limited small-cell lung cancer. *J Clin Oncol* 1988;6:451.
197. Roth BJ, Johnson DH, Einhorn LH, et al. Randomized study of cyclophosphamide, doxorubicin, and vincristine versus etoposide and cisplatin versus alternation of these two regimens in extensive small-cell lung cancer: a phase III trial of the Southeastern Cancer Study Group. *J Clin Oncol* 1992;10:282.
198. Fukuoka M, Furuse K, Saijo N, et al. Randomized trial of cyclophosphamide, doxorubicin, and vincristine versus cisplatin and etoposide versus alternation of these regimens in small-cell lung cancer. *J Natl Cancer Inst* 1991;83:855.
199. Skarlos DV, Samantas E, Kosmidis P, et al. Randomized comparison of etoposide-cisplatin vs. etoposide-carboplatin and irradiation in small-cell lung cancer. A Hellenic Co-operative Oncology Group study. *Ann Oncol* 1994;5:601.
200. Lassen U, Kristjansen PE, Osterlind K, et al. Superiority of cisplatin or carboplatin in combination with teniposide and vincristine in the induction chemotherapy of small-cell lung cancer. A randomized trial with 5 years follow up. *Ann Oncol* 1996;7:365.
201. Bishop JF, Raghavan D, Stuart-Harris R, et al. Carboplatin (CBDCA, JM-8) and VP-16-213 in previously untreated patients with small-cell lung cancer. *J Clin Oncol* 1987;5:1574.
202. Kamthan AG, Lind MJ, Thatcher N, et al. Ifosfamide, doxorubicin and etoposide in small cell lung cancer patients with poor prognosis. *Eur J Cancer* 1990;26:691.
203. Loehrer PJ Sr, Rynard S, Ansari R, et al. Etoposide, ifosfamide, and cisplatin in extensive small cell lung cancer. *Cancer* 1992;69:669.
204. Loehrer PJ Sr, Ansari R, Gonin R, et al. Cisplatin plus etoposide with and without ifosfamide in extensive small-cell lung cancer: a Hoosier Oncology Group study. *J Clin Oncol* 1995;13:2594.
205. Thatcher N, Lind M, Stout R, et al. Carboplatin, ifosfamide and etoposide with mid-course vincristine and thoracic radiotherapy for 'limited' stage small cell carcinoma of the bronchus. *Br J Cancer* 1989;60:98.
206. Wolff AC, Ettinger DS, Neuberg D, et al. Phase II study of ifosfamide, carboplatin, and oral etoposide chemotherapy for extensive-disease small-cell lung cancer: an Eastern Cooperative Oncology Group pilot study. *J Clin Oncol* 1995;13:1615.
207. Kelly K, Pan Z, Wood ME, et al. A phase I study of paclitaxel, etoposide, and cisplatin in extensive stage small cell lung cancer. *Clin Cancer Res* 1999;5:3419.
208. Ardizzoni A, Manegold C, Gaafar R, et al. Combination chemotherapy with cisplatin and topotecan as second-line treatment of sensitive (S) and resistant (R) small cell lung cancer (SCLC). *Proc Am Soc Clin Oncol* 1999;18:471(abst 1817).
209. Kudoh S, Fujiwara Y, Takada Y, et al. Phase II study of irinotecan combined with cisplatin in patients with previously untreated small-cell lung cancer. West Japan Lung Cancer Group. *J Clin Oncol* 1998;16:1068.
210. Suigiura S, Saka H, Ando M, et al. Phase II and pharmacokinetic (PK)/pharmacodynamic (PD) study of carboplatin (CBDA) and inrinotecan (CPT-11) in patients with small cell lung cancer (SCLC). *Proc Am Soc Clin Oncol* 1998;17:502(abst 1934).
211. Noda K, Nishiwaki Y, Kawahara M, et al. Randomized phase III study of irinotecan (CPT-11) and cisplatin versus etoposide and cisplatin in extensive-disease small-cell lung cancer. Japan Clinical Oncology Group Study (JCOG9511). *Proc Am Soc Clin Oncol* 2000;19483a(abstr 1887).
212. Murren J, Kraut E, Gams R, et al. Phase II trial of topotecan and cyclophosphamide (Cy) with GCSF in high risk small cell lung cancer. *Proc Am Soc Clin Oncol* 1998;17:495(abst 1907).
213. Nakamura S, Kudoh S, Komuta K, et al. Phase II study of irinotecan (CPT-11) combined with etoposide (VP-16) for previously untreated extensive-disease small-cell lung cancer (ED-SCLC): a study of the West Japan Lung Cancer Group. *Proc Am Soc Clin Oncol* 1998;18:470(abst 1815).
214. Jacobs SA, Jett JR, Belani CP, et al. Topotecan and paclitaxel, and active couplet, in untreated extensive disease small cell lung cancer. *Proc Am Soc Clin Oncol* 1999;18:470(abst 1814).
215. Frasci G, Panza N, Comella P, et al. Cisplatin-topotecan-paclitaxel weekly administration with G-CSF support for ovarian and small-cell lung cancer patients: a dose-finding study. *Ann Oncol* 1999;10:355.
216. Feld R, Evans WK, DeBoer G, et al. Combined modality induction therapy without maintenance chemotherapy for small cell carcinoma of the lung. *J Clin Oncol* 1984; 2:294.
217. Maurer LH, Tulloh M, Weiss RB, et al. A randomized combined modality trial in small cell carcinoma of the lung: comparison of combination chemotherapy-radiation therapy versus cyclophosphamide-radiation therapy effects of maintenance chemotherapy and prophylactive whole brain irradiation. *Cancer* 1980;45:30.
218. Cullen M, Morgan D, Gregory W, et al. Maintenance chemotherapy for anaplastic small cell carcinoma of the bronchus: a randomised, controlled trial. *Cancer Chemother Pharmacol* 1986;17:157.
219. Byrne MJ, van Hazel G, Trotter J, et al. Maintenance chemotherapy in limited small cell lung cancer: a randomised controlled clinical trial. *Br J Cancer* 1989;60:413.
220. Controlled trial of twelve versus six courses of chemotherapy in the treatment of small-cell lung cancer. Report to the Medical Research Council by its Lung Cancer Working Party. *Br J Cancer* 1989;59:584.
221. Ettinger DS, Finkelstein DM, Abeloff MD, et al. A randomized comparison of standard chemotherapy versus alternating chemotherapy and maintenance versus no maintenance therapy for extensive-stage small-cell lung cancer: a phase III study of the Eastern Cooperative Oncology Group. *J Clin Oncol* 1990;8:230.

222. Lebeau B, Chastang C, Allard P, et al. Six vs twelve cycles for complete responders to chemotherapy in small cell lung cancer: definitive results of a randomized clinical trial. The "Petites Cellules" Group. *Eur Respir J* 1992;5:286.
223. Giaccone G, Dalesio O, McVie GJ, et al. Maintenance chemotherapy in small-cell lung cancer: long-term results of a randomized trial. European Organization for Research and Treatment of Cancer Lung Cancer Cooperative Group. *J Clin Oncol* 1993;11:1230.
224. Beith JM, Clarke SJ, Woods RL, et al. Long-term follow-up of a randomised trial of combined chemoradiotherapy induction treatment, with and without maintenance chemotherapy in patients with small cell carcinoma of the lung. *Eur J Cancer* 1996;32A:438.
225. Sculier JP, Paesmans M, Bureau G, et al. Randomized trial comparing induction chemotherapy versus induction chemotherapy followed by maintenance chemotherapy in small-cell lung cancer. European Lung Cancer Working Party. *J Clin Oncol* 1996;14:2337.
226. Sandler AB, Ansari R, Saxman S, et al. Phase III trial of maintainence daily oral VP-16 versus no further therapy following induction chemotherapy with VP-16 (V) plus ifosfamide (I) plus cisplatin (P) (VIP) in extensive small cell lung cancer (SCLC): a Hoosier Oncology Group (HOG) trial (LUN93-2). *Proc Am Soc Clin Oncol* 1999;18:470(abst 1813).
227. Spiro SG, Souhami RL, Geddes DM, et al. Duration of chemotherapy in small cell lung cancer: a Cancer Research Campaign trial. *Br J Cancer* 1989;59:578.
228. Jarry O, Fournel P. A randomized trial of 4 versus 8 courses of chemotherapy with ifosfamide, epirubicin, and etoposide (EVI) in extensive small cell lung cancer. IASLC-SCLC, Denver, CO, 1994 (abst).
229. Bleehen NM, Girling DJ, Machin D, et al. A randomised trial of three or six courses of etoposide cyclophosphamide methotrexate and vincristine or six courses of etoposide and ifosfamide in small cell lung cancer (SCLC). II: Quality of life. Medical Research Council Lung Cancer Working Party. *Br J Cancer* 1993;68:1157.
230. Bleehen NM, Girling DJ, Machin D, et al. A randomised trial of three or six courses of etoposide cyclophosphamide methotrexate and vincristine or six courses of etoposide and ifosfamide in small cell lung cancer (SCLC). I: survival and prognostic factors. Medical Research Council Lung Cancer Working Party. *Br J Cancer* 1993;68:1150.
231. Ajaikumar BS, Barkley HT Jr. The role of radiation therapy in the treatment of small cell undifferentiated bronchogenic cancer. *Int J Radiat Oncol Biol Phys* 1979;5:977.
232. Salazar OM, Rubin P, Brown JC, et al. Predictors of radiation response in lung cancer. A clinico-pathobiological analysis. *Cancer* 1976;37:2636.
233. Cohen MH, Ihde DC, Bunn PA Jr, et al. Cyclic alternating combination chemotherapy for small cell bronchogenic carcinoma. *Cancer Treat Rep* 1979;63:163.
234. Johnson DH, Greco FA. Small cell carcinoma of the lung. *Crit Rev Oncol Hematol* 1986;4:303.
235. Bunn PA, Ihde DC. Small cell bronchogenic carcinoma: a review of therapeutic results. In: Livingston RB, ed. *Lung cancer I*. The Hague: Martinus Nijhoff, 1981.
236. Lichter AS, Bunn PA Jr, Ihde DC, et al. The role of radiation therapy in the treatment of small cell lung cancer. *Cancer* 1985;55:2163.
237. Bunn PA Jr, Lichter AS, Makuch RW, et al. Chemotherapy alone or chemotherapy with chest radiation therapy in limited stage small cell lung cancer. A prospective, randomized trial. *Ann Intern Med* 1987;106:655.
238. Perez CA, Einhorn L, Oldham RK, et al. Randomized trial of radiotherapy to the thorax in limited small-cell carcinoma of the lung treated with multiagent chemotherapy and elective brain irradiation: a preliminary report. *J Clin Oncol* 1984;2:1200.
239. Fox RM, Woods RL, Tattersall MH, et al. A randomized study of adjuvant immunotherapy with levamisole and *Corynebacterium parvum* in operable non-small cell lung cancer. *Int J Radiat Oncol Biol Phys* 1980;6:1043.
240. Rosenthal S, Tattersa MHN, Fox RM, et al. Adjuvant thoracic radiotherapy in small cell lung cancer: ten-year follow-up of a randomized study. *Lung Cancer* 1991;7:235.
241. Warde P, Payne D. Does thoracic irradiation improve survival and local control in limited-stage small-cell carcinoma of the lung? A meta-analysis [see comments]. *J Clin Oncol* 1992;10:890.
242. Cox JD, Byhardt R, Komaki R, et al. Interaction of thoracic irradiation and chemotherapy on local control and survival in small cell carcinoma of the lung. *Cancer Treat Rep* 1979;63:1251.
243. Williams C, Alexander M, Glatstein EJ, et al. Role of radiation therapy in combination with chemotherapy in extensive oat cell cancer of the lung: a randomized study. *Cancer Treat Rep* 1977;61:1427.
244. Choi NC, Carey RW. Importance of radiation dose in achieving improved loco-regional tumor control in limited stage small-cell lung carcinoma: an update. *Int J Radiat Oncol Biol Phys* 1989;17:307.
245. Coy P, Hodson I, Payne DG, et al. The effect of dose of thoracic irradiation on recurrence in patients with limited stage small cell lung cancer. Initial results of a Canadian Multicenter Randomized Trial. *Int J Radiat Oncol Biol Phys* 1988;14:219.
246. Arriagada R, Kramar A, Le Chevalier T, et al. Competing events determining relapse-free survival in limited small-cell lung carcinoma. The French Cancer Centers' Lung Group. *J Clin Oncol* 1992;10:447.
247. Papac RJ, Son Y, Bien R, et al. Improved local control of thoracic disease in small cell lung cancer with higher dose thoracic irradiation and cyclic chemotherapy [published erratum appears in *Int J Radiat Oncol Biol Phys* 1988;14:213]. *Int J Radiat Oncol Biol Phys* 1987;13:993.
248. Brooks BJ Jr, Seifter EJ, Walsh TE, et al. Pulmonary toxicity with combined modality therapy for limited stage small-cell lung cancer. *J Clin Oncol* 1986;4:200.
249. Osterlind K, Hansen HH, Hansen HS, et al. Chemotherapy versus chemotherapy plus irradiation in limited small cell lung cancer. Results of a controlled trial with 5 years follow-up. *Br J Cancer* 1986;54:7.
250. Roach M 3rd, Gandara DR, Yuo HS, et al. Radiation pneumonitis following combined modality therapy for lung cancer: analysis of prognostic factors [see comments]. *J Clin Oncol* 1995;13:2606.
251. McCracken JD, Janaki LM, Crowley JJ, et al. Concurrent chemotherapy/radiotherapy for limited small-cell lung carcinoma: a Southwest Oncology Group Study. *J Clin Oncol* 1990;8:892.
252. Arriagada R, Mouriesse H, Spielmann M, et al. Alternating radiotherapy and chemotherapy in non-metastatic inflammatory breast cancer. *Int J Radiat Oncol Biol Phys* 1990;19:1207.
253. Liengswangwong V, Bonner JA, Shaw EG, et al. Limited-stage small-cell lung cancer: patterns of intrathoracic recurrence and the implications for thoracic radiotherapy. *J Clin Oncol* 1994;12:496.
254. Turrisi ATD, Glover DJ. Thoracic radiotherapy variables: influence on local control in small cell lung cancer limited disease. *Int J Radiat Oncol Biol Phys* 1990;19:1473.
255. Turrisi ATD, Glover DJ, Mason BA. A preliminary report: concurrent twice-daily radiotherapy plus platinum-etoposide chemotherapy for limited small cell lung cancer. *Int J Radiat Oncol Biol Phys* 1988;15:183.
256. Ihde DC, Grayson J, Woods E, et al. Twice daily chest irradiation an adjuvant to etoposide/cisplatin therapy of limited stage small cell lung cancer. In: Salmon S, ed. *Adjuvant therapy of cancer*, 6th ed. Philadelphia: WB Saunders, 1990.
257. Rosen ST, Makuch RW, Lichter AS, et al. Role of prophylactic cranial irradiation in prevention of central nervous system metastases in small cell lung cancer. Potential benefit restricted to patients with complete response. *Am J Med* 1983;74:615.
258. Glantz MJ, Choy H, Yee L. Prophylactic cranial irradiation in small cell lung cancer: rationale, results, and recommendations. *Semin Oncol* 1997;24:477.
259. Einhorn L. The case against prophylactic cranial irradiation in limited small cell lung cancer. *Semin Radiat Oncol* 1995;5:57.
260. Hansen HH, Dombernowsky P, Hirsch FR, et al. Prophylactic irradiation in bronchogenic small cell anaplastic carcinoma. A comparative trial of localized versus extensive radiotherapy including prophylactic brain irradiation in patients receiving combination chemotherapy. *Cancer* 1980;46:279.
261. Aroney RS, Aisner J, Wesley MN, et al. Value of prophylactic cranial irradiation given at complete remission in small cell lung carcinoma. *Cancer Treat Rep* 1983;67:675.
262. Beiler DD, Kane RC, Bernath AM, et al. Low dose elective brain irradiation in small cell carcinoma of the lung. *Int J Radiat Oncol Biol Phys* 1979;5:941.
263. Cox JD, Petrovich Z, Paig C, et al. Prophylactic cranial irradiation in patients with inoperable carcinoma of the lung: preliminary report of a cooperative trial. *Cancer* 1978;42:1135.
264. Eagan RT, Frytak S, Lee RE, et al. A case for preplanned thoracic and prophylactic whole brain radiation therapy in limited small-cell lung cancer. *Cancer Clin Trials* 1981;4:261.
265. Jackson DV Jr, Richards FD, Cooper MR, et al. Prophylactic cranial irradiation in small cell carcinoma of the lung. A randomized study. *JAMA* 1977;237:2730.
266. Katsenis AT, Karpasitis N, Grannakakis D, et al. Elective brain irradiation in patients with small cell carcinoma of the lung. In: *Lung cancer*. Amsterdam: Excerpta Medica, 1982: 558.
267. Seydel HG, Creech R, Pagano M, et al. Prophylactic versus no brain irradiation in regional small cell lung carcinoma. *Am J Clin Oncol* 1985;8:218.
268. Niiranen A, Holsti P, Salmo M. Treatment of small cell lung cancer. Two-drug versus four-drug chemotherapy and loco-regional irradiation with or without prophylactic cranial irradiation. *Acta Oncol* 1989;28:501.
269. Kristjansen PE, Hansen HH. Prophylactic cranial irradiation in small cell lung cancer—an update. *Lung Cancer* 1995;12(Suppl 3):S23.
270. Auperin A, Arriagada R, Pignon JP, et al. Prophylactic cranial irradiation for patients with small-cell lung cancer in complete remission. Prophylactic Cranial Irradiation Overview Collaborative Group [see comments]. *N Engl J Med* 1999;341:476.
271. Arriagada R. Re: Prophylactic cranial irradiation for patients with small-cell lung cancer [letter; comment]. *J Natl Cancer Inst* 1995;87:766; discussion 767.
272. Gregor A, Cull A, Stephens RJ, et al. Prophylactic cranial irradiation is indicated following complete response to induction therapy in small cell lung cancer: results of a multicentre randomised trial. United Kingdom Coordinating Committee for Cancer Research (UKCCCR) and the European Organization for Research and Treatment of Cancer (EORTC) [see comments]. *Eur J Cancer* 1997;33:1752.
273. Meyers CA, Byrne KS, Komaki R. Cognitive deficits in patients with small cell lung cancer before and after chemotherapy. *Lung Cancer* 1995;12:231.
274. Baglan RJ, Marks JE. Comparison of symptomatic and prophylactic irradiation of brain metastases from oat cell carcinoma of the lung. *Cancer* 1981;47:41.
275. Cox JD, Komaki R, Byhardt RW, et al. Results of whole brain irradiation for metastases from small cell carcinoma of the lung. *Cancer Treat Rep* 1980;64:957.
276. Lucas CF, Robinson B, Hoskin PJ, et al. Morbidity of cranial relapse in small cell lung cancer and the impact of radiation therapy. *Cancer Treat Rep* 1986;70:565.
277. Fleck JF, Einhorn LH, Lauer RC, et al. Is prophylactic cranial irradiation indicated in small-cell lung cancer? *J Clin Oncol* 1990;8:209.
278. Johnson BE, Becker B, Goff WB, et al. Neurologic, neuropsychologic, and computed cranial tomography scan abnormalities in 2- to 10-year survivors of small-cell lung cancer. *J Clin Oncol* 1985;3:1659.
279. Laukkanen E, Klonoff H, Allan B, et al. The role of prophylactic brain irradiation in limited stage small cell lung cancer: clinical, neuropsychologic, and CT sequelae. *Int J Radiat Oncol Biol Phys* 1988;14:1109.
280. Lee JS, Umsawasdi T, Lee YY, et al. Neurotoxicity in long-term survivors of small cell lung cancer. *Int J Radiat Oncol Biol Phys* 1986;12:313.
281. Johnson BE, Patronas N, Hayes W, et al. Neurologic, computed cranial tomographic, and magnetic resonance imaging abnormalities in patients with small-cell lung cancer: further follow-up of 6- to 13-year survivors. *J Clin Oncol* 1990;8:48.
282. Turrisi AT. Brain irradiation and systemic chemotherapy for small-cell lung cancer: dangerous liaisons? [see comments]. *J Clin Oncol* 1990;8:196.
283. Frytak S, Shaw JN, O'Neill BP, et al. Leukoencephalopathy in small cell lung cancer patients receiving prophylactic cranial irradiation. *Am J Clin Oncol* 1989;12:27.
284. Urtasun RC, Belch A, Bodnar D, et al. Radiation as a non-cross resistant systemic agent: experience with hemibody and total body irradiation in patients with small cell lung cancer. *Cancer Treat Symp* 1985;2:41.
285. Huttner J, Wiener N, Quadt C, et al. A randomized clinical trial comparing systemic radiotherapy versus chemotherapy versus local radiotherapy in small cell lung cancer. *Eur J Cancer Clin Oncol* 1989;25:933.

286. Byhardt RW, Cox JD, Wilson JF, et al. Total body irradiation vs. chemotherapy as a systemic adjuvant for small cell carcinoma of the lung. *Int J Radiat Oncol Biol Phys* 1979; 5:2043.
287. Powell BL, Jackson DV Jr, Scarantino CW, et al. Sequential hemibody irradiation integrated into a chemotherapy-local radiotherapy program for limited disease small cell lung cancer. *Int J Radiat Oncol Biol Phys* 1986;12:1951.
288. Dillman RO, Seagren SL, Taetle R. Failure of low-dose, total-body irradiation to augment combination chemotherapy in extensive-stage small cell carcinoma of the lung. *J Clin Oncol* 1983;1:242.
289. Cancer AJCO. Lung cancer. In: Beahrs O, Henson D, Hutter R, et al., eds. *Manual for staging cancer*. Philadelphia: Lippincott, 1988:115.
290. Meyer JA. Effect of histologically verified TNM stage on disease control in treated small cell carcinoma. *Cancer* 1985;55:1747.
291. Shields TW, Higgins GA Jr, Matthews MJ, et al. Surgical resection in the management of small cell carcinoma of the lung. *J Thorac Cardiovasc Surg* 1982;84:481.
292. Meyer JA. Indications for surgical treatment in small cell carcinoma of the lung. *Surg Clin North Am* 1987;67:1103.
293. Shepherd FA, Evans WK, Feld R, et al. Adjuvant chemotherapy followed by surgical resection for small cell carcinoma of the lung. *J Clin Oncol* 1988;6:832.
294. Angeletti CA, Macchiarini P, Mussi A, et al. Influence of T and N stages on long-term survival in resectable small cell lung cancer. *Eur J Surg Oncol* 1989;15:337.
295. Shepherd FA, Ginsberg RJ, Patterson GA, et al. A prospective study of adjuvant surgical resection after chemotherapy for limited small cell lung cancer. A University of Toronto Lung Oncology Group study. *J Thorac Cardiovasc Surg* 1989;97:177.
296. Williams CJ, McMillan I, Lea R, et al. Surgery after initial chemotherapy for localized small-cell carcinoma of the lung. *J Clin Oncol* 1987;5:1579.
297. Johnson DH, Einhorn LH, Mandelbaum I, et al. Postchemotherapy resection of residual tumor in limited stage small cell lung cancer. *Chest* 1987;92:241.
298. Gazdar AF, Linnoila RI. The pathology of lung cancer—changing concepts and newer diagnostic techniques. *Semin Oncol* 1988;15:215.
299. Abeloff MD, Eggleston JC, Mendelsohn G, et al. Changes in morphologic and biochemical characteristics of small cell carcinoma of the lung. A clinicopathologic study. *Am J Med* 1979;66:757.
300. Carney DN, Gazdar AF, Bepler G, et al. Establishment and identification of small cell lung cancer cell lines having classic and variant features. *Cancer Res* 1985;45:2913.
301. Sridhar KS, Hussein AM, Thurer RJ. Evolving role of surgical treatment in limited-disease small cell lung carcinoma. *J Surg Oncol* 1989;40:155.
302. Baker RR, Ettinger DS, Ruckdeschel JD, et al. The role of surgery in the management of selected patients with small-cell carcinoma of the lung. *J Clin Oncol* 1987;5:697.
303. Hara N, Ohta M, Ichinose Y, et al. Influence of surgical resection before and after chemotherapy on survival in small cell lung cancer. *J Surg Oncol* 1991;47:53.
304. Prasad US, Naylor AR, Walker WS, et al. Long term survival after pulmonary resection for small cell carcinoma of the lung [see comments]. *Thorax* 1989;44:784.
305. Higgins GA, Shields TW. Experience of the Veterans Administration Surgical Adjuvant Group. In: Muggia FM, Rozencweig M, eds. *Lung cancer: progress in therapeutic research.* New York: Raven, 1979:433.
306. Karrer K, Pridun N, Denck H. Chemotherapy as an adjuvant to surgery in lung cancer. *Cancer Chemother Pharmacol* 1978;1:145.
307. Shields TW, Humphrey EW, Eastridge CE, et al. Adjuvant cancer chemotherapy after resection of carcinoma of the lung. *Cancer* 1977;40:2057.
308. Wingfield HV. Combined surgery and chemotherapy for carcinoma of the bronchus. *Lancet* 1970;1:470.
309. Karrer K, Shields TW, Denck H, et al. The importance of surgical and multimodality treatment for small cell bronchial carcinoma [see comments]. *J Thorac Cardiovasc Surg* 1989;97:168.
310. Friess GG, McCracken JD, Troxell ML, et al. Effect of initial resection of small-cell carcinoma of the lung: a review of Southwest Oncology Group Study 7628. *J Clin Oncol* 1985;3:964.
311. Macchiarini P, Hardin M, Basolo F, et al. Surgery plus adjuvant chemotherapy for T1-3N0M0 small-cell lung cancer. Rationale for current approach [see comments]. *Am J Clin Oncol* 1991;14:218.
312. Hayata Y, Funatsu H, Suemasu K, et al. Surgical indications in small cell carcinoma of the lung. *Jpn J Clin Oncol* 1978;8:93.
313. Osterlind K, Hansen M, Hansen HH, et al. Influence of surgical resection before chemotherapy on the long-term results in small cell lung cancer. A study of 150 operable patients. *Eur J Cancer Clin Oncol* 1986;22:589.
314. Rea F, Callegaro D, Favaretto A, et al. Long term results of surgery and chemotherapy in small cell lung cancer. *Eur J Cardiothorac Surg* 1998;14:398.
315. Lucchi M, Mussi A, Chella A, et al. Surgery in the management of small cell lung cancer. *Eur J Cardiothorac Surg* 1997;12:689.
316. Osterlind K, Hansen M, Hansen HH, et al. Treatment policy of surgery in small cell carcinoma of the lung: retrospective analysis of a series of 874 consecutive patients. *Thorax* 1985;40:272.
317. Quoix E, Fraser R, Wolkove N, et al. Small cell lung cancer presenting as a solitary pulmonary nodule. *Cancer* 1990;66:577.
318. Warren WH, Memoli VA, Jordan AG, et al. Reevaluation of pulmonary neoplasms resected as small cell carcinomas. Significance of distinguishing between well-differentiated and small cell neuroendocrine carcinomas. *Cancer* 1990;65:1003.
319. Holoye PY, Shirinian M. Adjuvant surgery in the multimodality treatment of small-cell lung cancer. *Am J Clin Oncol* 1991;14:251.
320. Prager RL, Foster JM, Hainsworth JD, et al. The feasibility of adjuvant surgery in limited-stage small cell carcinoma: a prospective evaluation. *Ann Thorac Surg* 1984;38:622.
321. Meyer JA, Gullo JJ, Ikins PM, et al. Adverse prognostic effect of N2 disease in treated small cell carcinoma of the lung. *J Thorac Cardiovasc Surg* 1984;88:495.
322. Shepherd FA, Ginsberg R, Patterson GA, et al. Is there ever a role for salvage operations in limited small-cell lung cancer? [see comments]. *J Thorac Cardiovasc Surg* 1991; 101:196.
323. Lad T, Piantadosi S, Thomas P, et al. A prospective randomized trial to determine the benefit of surgical resection of residual disease following response of small cell lung cancer to combination chemotherapy. *Chest* 1994;106(Suppl 6):320S.
324. Fujimori K, Yokoyama A, Kurita Y, et al. A pilot phase 2 study of surgical treatment after induction chemotherapy for resectable stage I to IIIA small cell lung cancer. *Chest* 1997;111:1089.
325. Girling DJ. Comparison of oral etoposide and standard intravenous multidrug chemotherapy for small-cell lung cancer: a stopped multicentre randomised trial. Medical Research Council Lung Cancer Working Party. *Lancet* 1996;348:563.
326. Souhami RL, Spiro SG, Rudd RM, et al. Five-day oral etoposide treatment for advanced small-cell lung cancer: randomized comparison with intravenous chemotherapy. *J Natl Cancer Inst* 1997;89:577.
327. Seifter EJ, Ihde DC. Therapy of small cell lung cancer: a perspective on two decades of clinical research. *Semin Oncol* 1988;15:278.
328. Livingston RB, Mira JG, Chen TT, et al. Combined modality treatment of extensive small cell lung cancer: a Southwest Oncology Group study. *J Clin Oncol* 1984;2:585.
329. Livingston RB, Schulman S, Mira JG, et al. Combined alkylators and multiple-site irradiation for extensive small cell lung cancer: a Southwest Oncology Group Study. *Cancer Treat Rep* 1986;70:1395.
330. Jeremic B, Shibamoto Y, Nikolic N, et al. Role of radiation therapy in the combined-modality treatment of patients with extensive disease small-cell lung cancer: a randomized study. *J Clin Oncol* 1999;17:2092.
331. Wilson HE, Stanley K, Vincent RG, et al. Comparison of chemotherapy alone versus chemotherapy and radiotherapy for extensive small cell carcinoma of the lung. *J Surg Oncol* 1983;23:181.
332. Carmichael J, Crane JM, Bunn PA, et al. Results of therapeutic cranial irradiation in small cell lung cancer. *Int J Radiat Oncol Biol Phys* 1988;14:455.
333. Groen HJ, Smit EF, Haaxma-Reiche H, et al. Carboplatin as second line treatment for recurrent or progressive brain metastases from small cell lung cancer. *Eur J Cancer* 1993;12:1696.
334. Postmus PE, Smit EF, Haaxma-Reiche H, et al. Teniposide for brain metastases of small-cell lung cancer: a phase II study. European Organization for Research and Treatment of Cancer Lung Cancer Cooperative Group. *J Clin Oncol* 1995;13:660.
335. Postmus PE, Haaxma-Reiche H, Gregor A, et al. Brain-only metastases of small cell lung cancer; efficacy of whole brain radiotherapy. An EORTC phase II study. *Radiother Oncol* 1998;46:29.
336. Goldie JH, Coldman AJ. A mathematical model for relating the drug sensitivity of tumors to their spontaneous mutation rate. *Cancer Treat Rep* 1979;63:1727.
337. Goldie JH, Coldman AJ, Gudauskas GA. Rationale for the use of alternating non-cross-resistant chemotherapy. *Cancer Treat Rep* 1982;66:439.
338. Evans WK, Feld R, Murray N, et al. Superiority of alternating non-cross-resistant chemotherapy in extensive small cell lung cancer. A multicenter, randomized clinical trial by the National Cancer Institute of Canada [published erratum appears in *Ann Intern Med* 1988;108:496]. *Ann Intern Med* 1987;107:451.
339. Postmus PE, Scagliotti G, Groen HJ, et al. Standard versus alternating non-cross-resistant chemotherapy in extensive small cell lung cancer: an EORTC Phase III trial. *Eur J Cancer* 1996;32A:1498.
340. Osterlind K, Sorenson S, Hansen HH, et al. Continuous versus alternating combination chemotherapy for advanced small cell carcinoma of the lung. *Cancer Res* 1983;43:6085.
341. Andersen M, Kristjansen PE, Hansen HH. Second-line chemotherapy in small cell lung cancer. *Cancer Treat Rev* 1990;17:427.
342. Postmus PE, Smit EF, Kirkpatrick A, et al. Testing the possible non-cross resistance of two equipotent combination chemotherapy regimens against small-cell lung cancer: a phase II study of the EORTC Lung Cancer Cooperative Group. *Eur J Cancer* 1993;2:204.
343. Wolf M, Pritsch M, Drings P, et al. Cyclic-alternating versus response-oriented chemotherapy in small-cell lung cancer: a German multicenter randomized trial of 321 patients. *J Clin Oncol* 1991;9:614.
344. Feld R, Evans WK, Coy P, et al. Canadian multicenter randomized trial comparing sequential and alternating administration of two non-cross-resistant chemotherapy combinations in patients with limited small-cell carcinoma of the lung. *J Clin Oncol* 1987;5:1401.
345. Goodman GE, Crowley JJ, Blasko JC, et al. Treatment of limited small-cell lung cancer with etoposide and cisplatin alternating with vincristine, doxorubicin, and cyclophosphamide versus concurrent etoposide, vincristine, doxorubicin, and cyclophosphamide and chest radiotherapy: a Southwest Oncology Group Study. *J Clin Oncol* 1990;8:39.
346. Urban T, Baleyte T, Chastang CL, et al. Standard combination versus alternating chemotherapy in small cell lung cancer: a randomised clinical trial including 394 patients. 'Petites Cellules' Group. *Lung Cancer* 1999;25:105.
347. Aisner J, Whitacre M, Van Echo DA, et al. Combination chemotherapy for small cell carcinoma of the lung: continuous versus alternating non-cross-resistant combinations. *Cancer Treat Rep* 1982;66:221.
348. Ettinger DS, Lagakos S. Phase III study of CCNU, cyclophosphamide, adriamycin, vincristine, and VP-16 in small-cell carcinoma of the lung. *Cancer* 1982;49:1544.
349. Osterlind K, Hansen M, Hirsch FR, et al. Combination chemotherapy of limited-stage small-cell lung cancer. A controlled trial on 221 patients comparing two alternating regimens. *Ann Oncol* 1991;2:41.
350. Havemann K, Wolf M, Holle R, et al. Alternating versus sequential chemotherapy in small cell lung cancer. A randomized German multicenter trial. *Cancer* 1987;59:1072.
351. Teicher BA. Preclinical models for high-dose therapy. In: Armitage JO, Antman KH, eds. *High-dose chemotherapy: pharmacology, hematopoietins, stem cells.* Baltimore: Williams & Wilkins, 1992:14.

352. Schabel FM Jr, Griswold DP Jr, Corbett TH, et al. Increasing the therapeutic response rates to anticancer drugs by applying the basic principles of pharmacology. *Cancer* 1984;54:1160.
353. Linch DC, Winfield D, Goldstone AH, et al. Dose intensification with autologous bone-marrow transplantation in relapsed and resistant Hodgkin's disease: results of a BNLI randomised trial. *Lancet* 1993;341:1051.
354. Attal M, Harousseau JL, Stoppa AM, et al. A prospective, randomized trial of autologous bone marrow transplantation and chemotherapy in multiple myeloma. *N Engl J Med* 1996;335:91.
355. Shipp MA, Abeloff MD, Antman KH, et al. International consensus conference on high-dose therapy with hematopoietic stem cell transplantation in aggressive non-Hodgkin's lymphomas: report of the jury. *J Clin Oncol* 1999;17:423.
356. Hryniuk W, Bush H. The importance of dose intensity in chemotherapy of metastatic breast cancer. *J Clin Oncol* 1984;2:1281.
357. Levin L, Hryniuk W. The application of dose intensity to problems in chemotherapy of ovarian and endometrial cancer. *Semin Oncol* 1987;14:12.
358. De Vathaire F, Arriagada R, de The' H, et al. Dose intensity of initial chemotherapy may have an impact on survival in limited small cell lung cancer. *Lung Cancer* 1993;8:301.
359. Klasa RJ, Murray N, Coldman AJ. Dose-intensity meta-analysis of chemotherapy regimens in small-cell carcinoma of the lung. *J Clin Oncol* 1991;9:499.
360. Cohen MH, Creaven PJ, Fossieck BE Jr, et al. Intensive chemotherapy of small cell bronchogenic carcinoma. *Cancer Treat Rep* 1977;61:349.
361. Mehta C, Vogl SE, Farber S, et al. High-dose cyclophosphamide (C) in the induction (IND) chemotherapy (CT) of small cell lung cancer (SCLC)-minor improvements in the rate of remission and survival. *Proc Am Assoc Cancer Res* 1982;23:165(abst).
362. Figueredo AT, Hryniuk WM, Strautmanis I, et al. Co-trimoxazole prophylaxis during high-dose chemotherapy of small-cell lung cancer. *J Clin Oncol* 1985;3:54.
363. Arriagada R, Le Chevalier T, Pignon JP, et al. Initial chemotherapeutic doses and survival in patients with limited small-cell lung cancer. *N Engl J Med* 1993;329:1848.
364. Johnson DH, Einhorn LH, Birch R, et al. A randomized comparison of high-dose versus conventional-dose cyclophosphamide, doxorubicin, and vincristine for extensive-stage small-cell lung cancer: a phase III trial of the Southeastern Cancer Study Group. *J Clin Oncol* 1987;5:1731.
365. Ihde DC, Mulshine JL, Kramer BS, et al. Prospective randomized comparison of high-dose and standard-dose etoposide and cisplatin chemotherapy in patients with extensive-stage small-cell lung cancer. *J Clin Oncol* 1994;12:2022.
366. Brower M, Ihde DC, Johnston-Early A, et al. Treatment of extensive stage small cell bronchogenic carcinoma. Effects of variation in intensity of induction chemotherapy. *Am J Med* 1983;75:993.
367. Gridelli C, Perrone F, D'Aprile M, et al. Phase II study of intensive CEV (carboplatin, epirubicin and VP-16) plus G-CSF (granulocyte-colony stimulating factor) in extensive small cell lung cancer [letter]. *Eur J Cancer* 1995;31A:2424.
368. Pujol JL, Douillard JY, Riviere A, et al. Dose-intensity of a four-drug chemotherapy regimen with or without recombinant human granulocyte-macrophage colony-stimulating factor in extensive-stage small-cell lung cancer: a multicenter randomized phase III study. *J Clin Oncol* 1997;15:2082.
369. Steward WP, von Pawel J, Gatzemeier U, et al. Effects of granulocyte-macrophage colony-stimulating factor and dose intensification of V-ICE chemotherapy in small-cell lung cancer: a prospective randomized study of 300 patients. *J Clin Oncol* 1998;16:642.
370. Thatcher N, Girling DJ, Hopwood P, et al. Improving survival without reducing quality of life in small-cell lung cancer patients by increasing the dose-intensity of chemotherapy with granulocyte colony-stimulating factor support: results of a British Medical Research Council Multicenter Randomized Trial. Medical Research Council Lung Cancer Working Party. *J Clin Oncol* 2000;18:395.
371. Clark SC, Kamen R. The hematopoietic colony-stimulating factors. *Science* 1987;236:1229.
372. Crawford J, Ozer H, Stoller R, et al. Reduction by granulocyte colony-stimulating factor of fever and neutropenia induced by chemotherapy in patients with small-cell lung cancer. *N Engl J Med* 1991;325:164.
373. Trillet-Lenoir V, Green J, Manegold C, et al. Recombinant granulocyte colony stimulating factor reduces the infectious complications of cytotoxic chemotherapy. *Eur J Cancer* 1993;29A:319.
374. Glaspy JA, Bleecker G, Crawford J, et al. The impact of therapy with filgrastim (recombinant granulocyte colony-stimulating factor) on the health care costs associated with cancer chemotherapy. *Eur J Cancer* 1993;29A:S23.
375. Lyman GH, Lyman CG, Sanderson RA, et al. Decision analysis of hematopoietic growth factor use in patients receiving cancer chemotherapy. *J Natl Cancer Inst* 1993;85:488.
376. Update of recommendations for the use of hematopoietic colony-stimulating factors: evidence-based clinical practice guidelines. *J Clin Oncol* 1996;14:1957.
377. Nichols CR, Fox EP, Roth BJ, et al. Incidence of neutropenic fever in patients treated with standard-dose combination chemotherapy for small-cell lung cancer and the cost impact of treatment with granulocyte colony-stimulating factor. *J Clin Oncol* 1994;12:1245.
378. Chouaid C, Bassinet L, Fuhrman C, et al. Routine use of granulocyte colony-stimulating factor is not cost-effective and does not increase patient comfort in the treatment of small-cell lung cancer: an analysis using a Markov model. *J Clin Oncol* 1998;16:2700.
379. Miles DW, Fogarty O, Ash CM, et al. Received dose-intensity: a randomized trial of weekly chemotherapy with and without granulocyte colony-stimulating factor in small-cell lung cancer. *J Clin Oncol* 1994;12:77.
380. Woll PJ, Hodgetts J, Lomax L, et al. Can cytotoxic dose-intensity be increased by using granulocyte colony-stimulating factor? A randomized controlled trial of lenograstim in small-cell lung cancer. *J Clin Oncol* 1995;13:652.
381. Fukuoka M, Masuda N, Negoro S, et al. CODE chemotherapy with and without granulocyte colony-stimulating factor in small-cell lung cancer. *Br J Cancer* 1997;75:306.
382. Furuse K, Fukuoka M, Nishiwaki Y, et al. Phase III study of intensive weekly chemotherapy with recombinant human granulocyte colony-stimulating factor versus standard chemotherapy in extensive-disease small-cell lung cancer. The Japan Clinical Oncology Group. *J Clin Oncol* 1998;16:2126.
383. Bunn PA Jr, Crowley J, Kelly K, et al. Chemoradiotherapy with or without granulocyte-macrophage colony-stimulating factor in the treatment of limited-stage small-cell lung cancer: a prospective phase III randomized study of the Southwest Oncology Group [published erratum appears in *J Clin Oncol* 1995;13:2860]. *J Clin Oncol* 1995;13:1632.
384. Savarese DM, Hsieh C, Stewart FM. Clinical impact of chemotherapy dose escalation in patients with hematologic malignancies and solid tumors. *J Clin Oncol* 1997;15:2981.
385. Antman K, Tiersten A. High-dose chemotherapy for breast cancer: evolving data. *Oncology* 1999;13:1215.
386. McGuire WP. High-dose chemotherapy and autologous bone marrow or stem cell reconstitution for solid tumors. *Curr Probl Cancer* 1998;22:135.
387. Stahel RA, Takvorian RW, Skarin AT, et al. Autologous bone marrow transplantation following high-dose chemotherapy with cyclophosphamide, BCNU and VP-16 in small cell carcinoma of the lung and a review of current literature. *Eur J Cancer Clin Oncol* 1984;20:1233.
388. Eder JP, Antman K, Elias A, et al. Cyclophosphamide and thiotepa with autologous bone marrow transplantation in patients with solid tumors. *J Natl Cancer Inst* 1988;80:1221.
389. Lazarus HM, Spitzer TR, Creger RJ. Phase I trial of high-dose etoposide, high-dose cisplatin, and reinfusion of autologous bone marrow for lung cancer. *Am J Clin Oncol* 1990;13:107.
390. Farha P, Spitzer G, Valdivieso M, et al. High-dose chemotherapy and autologous bone marrow transplantation for the treatment of small cell lung carcinoma. *Cancer* 1983;52:1351.
391. Littlewood TJ, Bentley DP, Smith AP. High-dose etoposide with autologous bone marrow transplantation as initial treatment of small cell lung cancer—a negative report. *Eur J Respir Dis* 1986;68:370.
392. Souhami RL, Hajichristou HT, Miles DW, et al. Intensive chemotherapy with autologous bone marrow transplantation for small-cell lung cancer. *Cancer Chemother Pharmacol* 1989;24:321.
393. Nomura F, Shimokata K, Saito H, et al. High dose chemotherapy with autologous bone marrow transplantation for limited small cell lung cancer. *Jpn J Clin Oncol* 1990;20:94.
394. Elias A. Hematopoietic stem cell transplantation for small cell lung cancer. *Chest* 1999;116(suppl 3):531S.
395. Sculier JP, Klastersky J, Stryckmans P. Late intensification in small-cell lung cancer: a phase I study of high doses of cyclophosphamide and etoposide with autologous bone marrow transplantation. *J Clin Oncol* 1985;3:184.
396. Spitzer G, Farha P, Valdivieso M, et al. High-dose intensification therapy with autologous bone marrow support for limited small-cell bronchogenic carcinoma. *J Clin Oncol* 1986;4:4.
397. Cunningham D, Banham SW, Hutcheon AH, et al. High-dose cyclophosphamide and VP 16 as late dosage intensification therapy for small cell carcinoma of lung. *Cancer Chemother Pharmacol* 1985;15:303.
398. Humblet Y, Symann M, Bosly A, et al. Late intensification chemotherapy with autologous bone marrow transplantation in selected small-cell carcinoma of the lung: a randomized study. *J Clin Oncol* 1987;5:1864.
399. Elias AD, Ayash L, Frei ED, et al. Intensive combined modality therapy for limited-stage small-cell lung cancer. *J Natl Cancer Inst* 1993;85:559.
400. Perey L, Rosti G, Lange A, et al. Sequential high-dose ICE chemotherapy with circulating progenitor cells (CPC) in small cell lung cancer: an EBMT study. *Bone Marrow Transplant* 1996;18(Suppl 1):S40.
401. Fetscher S, Brugger W, Engelhardt R, et al. Standard- and high-dose etoposide, ifosfamide, carboplatin, and epirubicin in 100 patients with small-cell lung cancer: a mature follow-up report. *Ann Oncol* 1999;10:561.
402. Norton L, Simon R. The Norton-Simon hypothesis revisited. *Cancer Treat Rep* 1986;70:163.
403. Goodman GE, Crowley J, Livingston RB, et al. Treatment of limited small-cell lung cancer with concurrent etoposide/cisplatin and radiotherapy followed by intensification with high-dose cyclophosphamide: a Southwest Oncology Group study. *J Clin Oncol* 1991;9:453.
404. Leyvraz S, Perey L, Rosti G, et al. Multiple courses of high-dose ifosfamide, carboplatin, and etoposide with peripheral-blood progenitor cells and filgrastim for small-cell lung cancer: a feasibility study by the European Group for Blood and Marrow Transplantation. *J Clin Oncol* 1999;17:3531.
405. Leonard RC, Duncan LW, Hay FG. Immunocytological detection of residual marrow disease at clinical remission predicts metastatic relapse in small cell lung cancer. *Cancer Res* 1990;50:6545.
406. Taylor CW, Crowley J, Williamson SK, et al. Treatment of small-cell lung cancer with an alternating chemotherapy regimen given at weekly intervals: a Southwest Oncology Group pilot study. *J Clin Oncol* 1990;8:1811.
407. Alba E, Breton JJ, Alonso L, et al. Alternating chemotherapy for small-cell lung cancer. A twelve-week schedule of six drugs. *Ann Oncol* 1992;3:31.
408. Sculier JP, Paesmans M, Bureau G, et al. Multiple-drug weekly chemotherapy versus standard combination regimen in small-cell lung cancer: a phase III randomized study conducted by the European Lung Cancer Working Party. *J Clin Oncol* 1993;11:1858.
409. Souhami RL, Rudd R, Ruiz de Elvira MC, et al. Randomized trial comparing weekly versus 3-week chemotherapy in small-cell lung cancer: a Cancer Research Campaign trial. *J Clin Oncol* 1994;12:1806.
410. Murray N, Shah A, Osoba D, et al. Intensive weekly chemotherapy for the treatment of extensive-stage small-cell lung cancer. *J Clin Oncol* 1991;9:1632.
411. Murray N, Livingston R, Shepherd F, et al. Randomized study of CODE versus alternating CAV/EP for extensive-stage small-cell lung cancer: an intergroup study of the National Cancer Institute of Canada Clinical Trials Group and the Southwest Oncology Group. *J Clin Oncol* 1997;17:2300.
412. Shepherd FA, Amdemichael E, Evans WK, et al. Treatment of small cell lung cancer in the elderly. *J Am Geriatr Soc* 1994;42:64.
413. Dajczman E, Fu LY, Small D, et al. Treatment of small cell lung carcinoma in the elderly. *Cancer* 1996;77:2032.

414. Murray N, Grafton C, Shah A, et al. Abbreviated treatment for elderly, infirm, or noncompliant patients with limited-stage small-cell lung cancer. *J Clin Oncol* 1998;16:3323.
415. Jara C, Gomez-Aldaravi JL, Tirado R, et al. Small-cell lung cancer in the elderly—is age of patient a relevant factor? *Acta Oncol* 1999;38:781.
416. Findlay MP, Griffin AM, Raghavan D, et al. Retrospective review of chemotherapy for small cell lung cancer in the elderly: does the end justify the means? *Eur J Cancer* 1991;27:1597.
417. Smit EF, Carney DN, Harford P, et al. A phase II study of oral etoposide in elderly patients with small cell lung cancer. *Thorax* 1989;44:631.
418. Byrne A, Carney DN. Small cell lung cancer in the elderly. *Semin Oncol* 1994;21:43.
419. Earl HM, Rudd RM, Spiro SG, et al. A randomised trial of planned versus as required chemotherapy in small cell lung cancer: a Cancer Research Campaign trial. *Br J Cancer* 1991;64:566.
420. Randomised trial of four-drug vs less intensive two-drug chemotherapy in the palliative treatment of patients with small-cell lung cancer (SCLC) and poor prognosis. Medical Research Council Lung Cancer Working Party [published erratum appears in *Br J Cancer* 1996;74:997]. *Br J Cancer* 1996;73:406.
421. James LE, Gower NH, Rudd RM, et al. A randomised trial of low-dose/high-frequency chemotherapy as palliative treatment of poor-prognosis small-cell lung cancer: a Cancer Research Campaign trial. *Br J Cancer* 1996;73:1563.
422. Allan SG, Gregor A, Cornbleet MA, et al. Phase II trial of vindesine and VP16-213 in the palliation of poor-prognosis patients and elderly patients with small cell lung cancer. *Cancer Chemother Pharmacol* 1984;13:106.
423. Cerny T, Lind M, Thatcher N, et al. A simple outpatient treatment with oral ifosfamide and oral etoposide for patients with small cell lung cancer (SCLC). *Br J Cancer* 1989;60:258.
424. Michel G, Leyvraz S, Bauer J, et al. Weekly carboplatin and VM-26 for elderly patients with small-cell lung cancer. *Ann Oncol* 1994;5:369.
425. Evans WK, Radwi A, Tomiak E, et al. Oral etoposide and carboplatin. Effective therapy for elderly patients with small cell lung cancer. *Am J Clin Oncol* 1995;18:149.
426. Matsui K, Masuda N, Fukuoka M, et al. Phase II trial of carboplatin plus oral etoposide for elderly patients with small-cell lung cancer. *Br J Cancer* 1998;77:1961.
427. Westeel V, Murray N, Gelmon K, et al. New combination of the old drugs for elderly patients with small-cell lung cancer: a phase II study of the PAVE regimen. *J Clin Oncol* 1998;16:1940.
428. Jeremic B, Shibamoto Y, Acimovic L, et al. Carboplatin, etoposide, and accelerated hyperfractionated radiotherapy for elderly patients with limited small cell lung carcinoma: a phase II study. *Cancer* 1998;82:836.
429. McCracken JD, Heilbrun L, White J, et al. Combination chemotherapy, radiotherapy, and BCG immunotherapy in extensive (metastatic) small cell carcinoma of the lung. A Southwest Oncology Group study. *Cancer* 1980;46:2335.
430. McCracken JD, Chen T, White J, et al. Combination chemotherapy, radiotherapy, and BCG immunotherapy in limited small-cell carcinoma of the lung: a Southwest Oncology Group Study. *Cancer* 1982;49:2252.
431. Jackson DVJ, Paschal BR, Ferree C, et al. Combination chemotherapy-radiotherapy with and without the methanol-extraction residue of Bacillus Calmette-Guerin (MER) in small cell carcinoma of the lung: a prospective randomized trial of the Piedmont Oncology Association. *Cancer* 1982;50:48.
432. Cohen MH, Chretien PB, Ihde DC, et al. Thymosin fraction V and intensive combination chemotherapy. Prolonging the survival of patients with small-cell lung cancer. *JAMA* 1979;241:1813.
433. Scher HI, Shank B, Chapman R, et al. Randomized trial of combined modality therapy with and without thymosin fraction V in the treatment of small cell lung cancer. *Cancer Res* 1988;48:1663.
434. Doyle A, Martin WJ, Funa K, et al. Markedly decreased expression of class I histocompatibility antigens, protein, and mRNA in human small-cell lung cancer. *J Exp Med* 1985;161:1135.
435. Tanio Y, Watanabe M, Osaki T, et al. High sensitivity to peripheral blood lymphocytes and low HLA-class I antigen expression of small cell lung cancer cell lines with diverse chemo-radiosensitivity. *Jpn J Cancer Res* 1992;83:736.
436. Yazawa T, Kamma H, Fujiwara M, et al. Lack of class II transactivator causes severe deficiency of HLA-DR expression in small cell lung cancer. *J Pathol* 1999;187:191.
437. Ball ED, Sorenson GD, Pettengill OS. Expression of myeloid and major histocompatibility antigens in small cell carcinoma of the lung cell lines by cytofluorography: modulation by gamma interferon. *Cancer Res* 1986;46:2335.
438. Funa K, Gazdar AF, Mattson K, et al. Interferon-mediated in vivo induction of beta 2-microglobulin on small-cell lung cancers and mid-gut carcinoids. *Clin Immunol Immunopathol* 1986;41:159.
439. Jones DH, Bleehen NM, Slater AJ, et al. Human lymphoblastoid interferon in the treatment of small cell lung cancer. *Br J Cancer* 1983;47:361.
440. Newman HF, Bleehen NM, Galazka A, et al. Small cell lung carcinoma. A phase II evaluation of r-interferon-gamma. *Cancer* 1987;60:2938.
441. Olesen BK, Ernst P, Nissen MH, et al. Recombinant interferon A (IFL-rA) therapy of small cell and squamous cell carcinoma of the lung. A phase II study. *Eur J Cancer Clin Oncol* 1987;23:987.
442. Mattson K, Niiranen A, Pyrhonen S, et al. Natural interferon alfa as maintenance therapy for small cell lung cancer. *Eur J Cancer* 1992;28A:1387.
443. Prior C, Oroszy S, Oberaigner W, et al. Adjunctive interferon-alpha-2c in stage IIIB/IV small-cell lung cancer: a phase III trial [published erratum appears in *Eur Respir J* 1997;10:963]. *Eur Respir J* 1997;10:392.
444. Ruotsalainen TM, Halme M, Tamminen K, et al. Concomitant chemotherapy and IFN-alpha for small cell lung cancer: a randomized multicenter phase III study. *J Interferon Cytokine Res* 1999;19:253.
445. Kelly K, Crowley JJ, Bunn PA Jr, et al. Role of recombinant interferon alfa-2a maintenance in patients with limited-stage small-cell lung cancer responding to concurrent chemoradiation: a Southwest Oncology Group study. *J Clin Oncol* 1995;13:2924.
446. Jett JR, Maksymiuk AW, Su JQ, et al. Phase III trial of recombinant interferon gamma in complete responders with small-cell lung cancer. *J Clin Oncol* 1994;12:2321.
447. van Zandwijk N, Groen HJ, Postmus PE, et al. Role of recombinant interferon-gamma maintenance in responding patients with small cell lung cancer. A randomised phase III study of the EORTC Lung Cancer Cooperative Group. *Eur J Cancer* 1997;33:1759.
448. Pujol JL, Gibney DJ, Su JQ, et al. Immune response induced in small-cell lung cancer by maintenance therapy with interferon gamma. *J Natl Cancer Inst* 1993;85:1844.
449. Clamon G, Herndon J, Perry MC, et al. Interleukin-2 activity in patients with extensive small-cell lung cancer: a phase II trial of Cancer and Leukemia Group B. *J Natl Cancer Inst* 1993;85:316.
450. Lynch TJ Jr, Lambert JM, Coral F, et al. Immunotoxin therapy of small-cell lung cancer: a phase I study of N901-blocked ricin. *J Clin Oncol* 1997;15:723.
451. Kelley MJ, Linnoila RI, Avis IL, et al. Antitumor activity of a monoclonal antibody directed against gastrin-releasing peptide in patients with small cell lung cancer. *Chest* 1997;112:256.
452. Grant SC, Kris MG, Houghton AN, et al. Long survival of patients with small cell lung cancer after adjuvant treatment with the anti-idiotypic antibody BEC2 plus bacillus Calmette-Guerin. *Clin Cancer Res* 1999;5:1319.
453. Lebeau B, Chastang C, Brechot JM, et al. Subcutaneous heparin treatment increases survival in small cell lung cancer. "Petites Cellules" group. *Cancer* 1994;74:38.
454. Calvo FA, Hidalgo OF, Gonzalez F, et al. Urokinase combination chemotherapy in small cell lung cancer. A phase II study. *Cancer* 1992;70:2624.
455. Stanford CF. Anticoagulants in the treatment of small cell carcinoma of the bronchus. *Thorax* 1979;34:113.
456. Zacharski LR, Henderson WG, Rickles FR, et al. Effect of warfarin on survival in small cell carcinoma of the lung. Veterans Administration study no. 75. *JAMA* 1981;245:831.
457. Chahinian AP, Propert KJ, Ware JH, et al. A randomized trial of anticoagulation with warfarin and of alternating chemotherapy in extensive small-cell lung cancer by the Cancer and Leukemia Group B. *J Clin Oncol* 1989;7:993.
458. Lebeau B, Chastang C, Muir JF, et al. No effect of an antiaggregant treatment with aspirin in small cell lung cancer treated with CCAVP16 chemotherapy. Results from a randomized clinical trial of 303 patients. The "Petites Cellules" group. *Cancer* 1993;71:1741.
459. Lopez JA, Mann J, Grapski RT, et al. Etoposide and cisplatin salvage chemotherapy for small cell lung cancer. *Cancer Treat Rep* 1985;69:369.
460. Shepherd FA, Evans WK, MacCormick R, et al. Cyclophosphamide, doxorubicin, and vincristine in etoposide- and cisplatin-resistant small cell lung cancer. *Cancer Treat Rep* 1987;71:941.
461. Monnet I, Chariot P, Quoix E, et al. Extensive small-cell lung cancer. A randomized comparison of two chemotherapy programs with early crossover in instances of failure. Association pour le Traitement des Tumeurs Intra-Thoraciques (ATTIT). *Ann Oncol* 1992;3:813.
462. Ebi N, Kubota K, Nishiwaki Y, et al. Second-line chemotherapy for relapsed small cell lung cancer. *Jpn J Clin Oncol* 1997;27:166.
463. Giaccone G, Donadio M, Bonardi G, et al. Teniposide in the treatment of small-cell lung cancer: the influence of prior chemotherapy. *J Clin Oncol* 1988;6:1264.
464. Batist G, Ihde DC, Zabell A, et al. Small-cell carcinoma of lung: reinduction therapy after late relapse. *Ann Intern Med* 1983;98:472.
465. Postmus PE, Berendsen HH, van Zandwijk N, et al. Retreatment with the induction regimen in small cell lung cancer relapsing after an initial response to short term chemotherapy. *Eur J Cancer Clin Oncol* 1987;23:1409.
466. Vincent M, Evans B, Smith I. First-line chemotherapy rechallenge after relapse in small cell lung cancer. *Cancer Chemother Pharmacol* 1988;21:45.
467. Groen HJ, Fokkema E, Biesma B, et al. Paclitaxel and carboplatin in the treatment of small-cell lung cancer patients resistant to cyclophosphamide, doxorubicin, and etoposide: a non-cross-resistant schedule. *J Clin Oncol* 1999;17:927.
468. Smit EF, Berendsen HH, de Vries EG, et al. A phase II study of carboplatin and vincristine in previously treated patients with small-cell lung cancer. *Cancer Chemother Pharmacol* 1989;25:202.
469. Kubota K, Nishiwaki Y, Kakinuma R, et al. Dose-intensive weekly chemotherapy for treatment of relapsed small-cell lung cancer. *J Clin Oncol* 1997;15:292.
470. Albain KS, Crowley JJ, Hutchins L, et al. Predictors of survival following relapse or progression of small cell lung cancer. Southwest Oncology Group Study 8605 report and analysis of recurrent disease data base. *Cancer* 1993;72:1184.
471. Shepherd FA, Ginsberg RJ, Feld R, et al. Surgical treatment for limited small-cell lung cancer. The University of Toronto Lung Oncology Group experience. *J Thorac Cardiovasc Surg* 1991;101:385.
472. Merrill RM, Henson DE, Barnes M. Conditional survival among patients with carcinoma of the lung [see comments]. *Chest* 1999;116:697.
473. Stephens RJ, Bailey AJ, Machin D. Long-term survival in small cell lung cancer: the case for a standard definition. Medical Research Council Lung Cancer Working Party. *Lung Cancer* 1996;15:297.
474. Sekine I, Nishiwaki Y, Kakinuma R, et al. Late recurrence of small-cell lung cancer: treatment and outcome. *Oncology* 1996;53:318.
475. Tucker MA, Murray N, Shaw EG, et al. Second primary cancers related to smoking and treatment of small-cell lung cancer. Lung Cancer Working Cadre [see comments]. *J Natl Cancer Inst* 1997;89:1782.
476. Kawahara M, Ushijima S, Kamimori T, et al. Second primary tumours in more than 2-year disease-free survivors of small-cell lung cancer in Japan: the role of smoking cessation. *Br J Cancer* 1998;78:409.
477. Jacoulet P, Depierre A, Moro D, et al. Long-term survivors of small-cell lung cancer (SCLC): a French multicenter study. Groupe d'Oncologie de Langue Francaise. *Ann Oncol* 1997;8:1009.
478. Osterlind K, Hansen HH, Hansen M, et al. Long-term disease-free survival in small-cell carcinoma of the lung: a study of clinical determinants. *J Clin Oncol* 1986;4:1307.
479. Lassen U, Osterlind K, Hansen M, et al. Long-term survival in small-cell lung cancer: posttreatment characteristics in patients surviving 5 to 18+ years—an analysis of 1,714 consecutive patients. *J Clin Oncol* 1995;13:1215.

480. Chute JP, Chen T, Feigal E, et al. Twenty years of phase III trials for patients with extensive-stage small-cell lung cancer: perceptible progress. *J Clin Oncol* 1999;17:1794.
481. Lassen UN, Hirsch FR, Osterlind K, et al. Outcome of combination chemotherapy in extensive stage small-cell lung cancer: any treatment related progress? *Lung Cancer* 1998;20:151.
482. Remick SC, Hafez GR, Carbone PP. Extrapulmonary small-cell carcinoma. A review of the literature with emphasis on therapy and outcome. *Medicine (Baltimore)* 1987;66:457.
483. Johnson BE, Whang-Peng J, Naylor SL, et al. Retention of chromosome 3 in extrapulmonary small cell cancer shown by molecular and cytogenetic studies. *J Natl Cancer Inst* 1989;81:1223.
484. Remick SC, Ruckdeschel JC. Extrapulmonary and pulmonary small-cell carcinoma: tumor biology, therapy, and outcome. *Med Pediatr Oncol* 1992;20:89.
485. Hobbs RD, Stewart AF, Ravin ND, et al. Hypercalcemia in small cell carcinoma of the pancreas. *Cancer* 1984;53:1552.
486. Galanis E, Frytak S, Lloyd RV. Extrapulmonary small cell carcinoma. *Cancer* 1997;79:1729.
487. Koss LG, Spiro RH, Hajdu S. Small cell (oat cell) carcinoma of minor salivary gland origin. *Cancer* 1972;30:737.
488. Kasimis BS, Wuerker RB, Malefatto JP, et al. Prolonged survival of patients with extrapulmonary small cell carcinoma arising in the neck. *Med Pediatr Oncol* 1983;11:27.
489. Casas F, Ferrer F, Farrus B, et al. Primary small cell carcinoma of the esophagus: a review of the literature with emphasis on therapy and prognosis. *Cancer* 1997;80:1366.
490. Yamasaki M, Tateishi R, Hongo J, et al. Argyrophil small cell carcinomas of the uterine cervix. *Int J Gynecol Pathol* 1984;3:146.
491. Randall ME, Kim JA, Mills SE, et al. Uncommon variants of cervical carcinoma treated with radical irradiation. A clinicopathological study of 66 cases. *Cancer* 1986;57:816.

Robert B. Cameron
Patrick J. Loehrer
Charles R. Thomas, Jr.

CHAPTER **32**

Neoplasms of the Mediastinum

Tumors involving the mediastinum may be primary or secondary in nature. Primary neoplasms can originate from any mediastinal organ or tissue but most commonly arise from thymic, neurogenic, lymphatic, germinal, and mesenchymal tissues. All primary mediastinal neoplasms, except those of thymic origin, also occur elsewhere in the body and are discussed in other chapters. Secondary (metastatic) mediastinal tumors are more common than primary neoplasms and most frequently represent lymphatic involvement from primary tumors of the lung or infradiaphragmatic organs, such as pancreatic, gastroesophageal, and testicular cancer. This chapter provides an overview of primary mediastinal neoplasms. Specific tumors are covered in detail, including thymic, primary mediastinal germ cell, mesenchymal, cardiac, and neurogenic tumors. Esophageal cancer and lymphomas are covered elsewhere, in Chapter 33.2 (Cancer of the Esophagus) and Chapter 45 (Lymphomas), respectively.

ANATOMY

The mediastinum occupies the central portion of the thoracic cavity. It is bounded by the pleural cavities laterally, by the thoracic inlet superiorly, by the diaphragm inferiorly, by the sternum anteriorly, and by the chest wall posteriorly. The mediastinum can be divided into three clinically relevant compartments: anterior, middle, and posterior (Fig. 32-1*A*).[1] The anterior mediastinum lies posterior to the sternum and anterior to the pericardium and great vessels, extending from the thoracic inlet to the diaphragm. The middle mediastinum is defined as the space occupied by the heart, pericardium, proximal great vessels, and central airways. The posterior mediastinum is bounded by the heart and great vessels anteriorly, the thoracic inlet superiorly, the diaphragm inferiorly, and the chest wall of the back posteriorly, and it includes the paravertebral gutters. Table 32-1 lists the major anatomic structures within each of the compartments. A thorough understanding of each area's contents helps define the diagnostic possibilities. Other divisions have been proposed, dividing the mediastinum into three or four compartments (Fig. 32-1*B,C*). Heitzman even proposed seven anatomic regions.[1] Although the exact scheme that should be used is still debated, these other schemes have limited clinical utility.

INCIDENCE AND PATHOLOGY

Mediastinal neoplasms are uncommon tumors that can occur at any age but are most common in the third through the fifth decades of life.[2–4] Table 32-2 reviews the classification of mediastinal neoplasms. The incidence of primary mediastinal tumors was documented in a review of 1900 patients (Table 32-3).[2] Additionally, 439 patients (18% of all mediastinal masses) were found to have cystic lesions. The distribution of primary mediastinal neoplasms is shown in Table 32-4. Thymic neoplasms predominate in the anterior mediastinum, followed in frequency by lymphomas, germ cell tumors, and carcinoma. Bronchial, enteric, and pericardial cysts are the most common masses in the middle mediastinum, followed by lymphomas, mesenchymal tumors, and carcinoma.[5] In the posterior mediastinum, neurogenic tumors and esophageal cancers are most common, followed by enteric cysts, mesenchymal tumors, and endocrine neoplasms.[2–4]

The incidence of mediastinal tumors in each anatomic compartment also varies with age. In adults, 54% of mediastinal neoplasms occur in the anterior, 20% in the middle, and 26% in the posterior mediastinum.[2] In pediatric populations, 43%, 18%, and 40% of neoplasms occur in the anterior, middle, and poste-

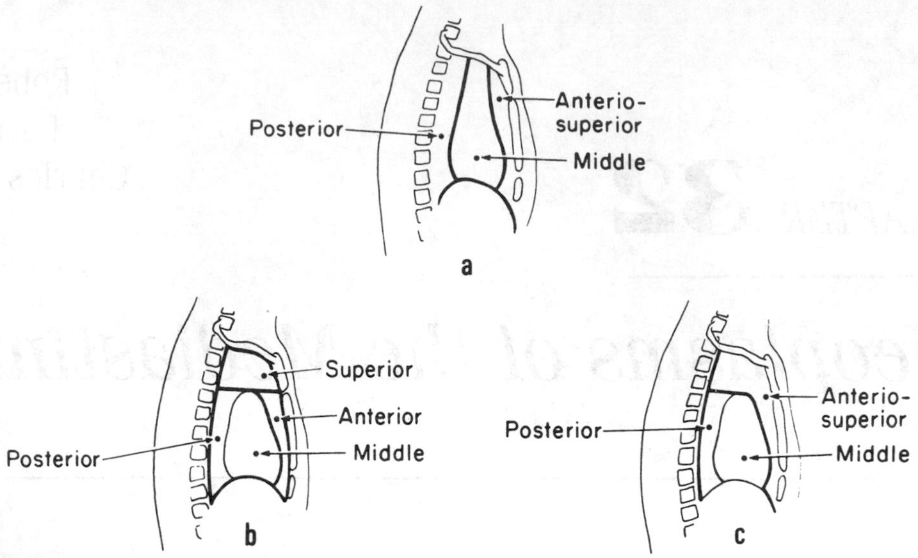

FIGURE 32-1. Mediastinal compartments.

rior mediastinum, respectively.[4,6] A higher incidence of thymic tumors and lymphomas in adults and neurogenic tumors in children account for these differences. Azarow[4] compared mediastinal masses in 195 adult and 62 pediatric patients (Table 32-5). Cysts were not included but accounted for 16% to 18% of adult and 24% of pediatric mediastinal masses.[4] Therefore, age as well as location establishes the probable diagnosis.[2–4,6–9]

TABLE 32-1. Anatomic Structures within the Mediastinum

ANTERIOR MEDIASTINUM
Thymus gland
Internal mammary artery and vein
Lymph nodes
Parathyroid (rarely, if ectopic)
Thyroid (rarely, if ectopic)
MIDDLE MEDIASTINUM
Heart and pericardium
Ascending and transverse aortic arch
Superior and inferior vena cavae
Innominate artery and vein
Main and right pulmonary artery
Pulmonary veins
Trachea and mainstem bronchi
Phrenic nerves
Lymph nodes
POSTERIOR MEDIASTINUM
Esophagus
Descending aorta
Sympathetic chains
Vagus nerves
Azygous and hemiazygous veins
Thoracic duct
Lymph nodes

DIAGNOSTIC CONSIDERATIONS

A meticulous history and physical examination, along with a variety of imaging, serologic, and invasive tests (Table 32-6), often can confirm the suspected diagnosis. With improved imaging, biopsy, and pathologic techniques, the majority of patients no longer require open surgical biopsy before planning definitive therapy.

SYMPTOMS AND SIGNS

Approximately 40% of mediastinal masses are asymptomatic and discovered incidentally on a routine chest radiograph.[2,3] The remaining 60% of cases have symptoms related to compression or direct invasion of surrounding mediastinal structures or to paraneoplastic syndromes. Asymptomatic patients are more likely to have benign lesions, whereas symptomatic patients more often harbor malignancies.[2–4,7,8] Davis found that 85% of patients with a malignancy were symptomatic, but only 46% of patients with benign neoplasms had identifiable complaints. Symptoms and signs of mediastinal neoplasms are shown in Table 32-7. The most commonly described symptoms are chest pain, cough, and dyspnea.[2,3,8] Superior vena cava syndrome, Horner's syndrome, hoarseness, and neurologic deficits more commonly occur with malignancies.[10] Systemic syndromes associated with mediastinal neoplasms are shown in Tables 32-8 and 32-9.

RADIOGRAPHIC IMAGING STUDIES

Radiographic imaging studies initially localize mediastinal neoplasms. The posteroanterior and lateral chest radiographs define the location, size, density, and calcification of a mass, limiting the diagnostic possibilities.[11] After these results, an intravenous contrast-enhanced computed tomography (CT) scan can further assess the nature (cystic vs. solid) of the lesion and detect fat and calcium.[12–17] The relationship to surrounding structures and blood vessels also can be determined.

TABLE 32-2. Classification of Mediastinal Tumors

NEUROGENIC	**ANEURYSMS**
Arising from peripheral nerves	Ascending aortic
Neurofibroma	Transverse arch
Neurilemoma (schwannoma)	Descending aortic
Neurosarcoma	Great vessels
Arising from sympathetic ganglion	
Ganglioneuroblastoma	**MESENCHYMAL TUMORS**
Ganglioneuroma	Fibroma, fibrosarcoma
Neuroblastoma	Lipoma, liposarcoma
Arising from paraganglionic tissue	Myxoma
Pheochromocytoma	Mesothelioma
Chemodectoma (paraganglioma)	Leiomyoma, leiomyosarcoma
	Rhabdomyosarcoma
GERM CELL	Xanthogranuloma
Seminoma	Mesenchymoma
Nonseminomatous	Hemangioma
Pure embryonal cell	Hemangioendothelioma
Mixed embryonal cell	Hemangiopericytoma
With seminomatous elements	Lymphangioma
With trophoblastic elements	Lymphangiopericytoma
With teratoid elements	Lymphangiomyoma
With endodermal sinus elements	
Teratoma, benign	**LYMPHADENOPATHY**
	Inflammatory
HERNIAS	Granulomatous
Hiatal	Sarcoid
Morgagni	
	LYMPHOMA
CYSTS	Hodgkin's disease
Pericardial	Histiocytic lymphoma
Bronchogenic	Undifferentiated
Enteric	
Thymic	**ENDOCRINE**
Thoracic duct	Thyroid
Meningoceles	Parathyroid
THYMIC	
Thymoma	
Carcinoid	
Thymolipoma	
Thymic carcinoma	

Magnetic resonance imaging (MRI) is used less frequently than CT.[18–20] Its advantages include multiplanar imaging and absence of ionizing radiation.[12] MRI scans are superior to CT in defining vascular involvement and in distinguishing recurrent tumor from radiation fibrosis.[20] However, patient claustrophobia, time, and expense limit the use of MRI scanning. Other imaging modalities that may be useful include transthoracic sonography and transesophageal echocardiography.[21,22]

The utility of positron emission tomography in the evaluation of mediastinal masses is yet to be determined, but it may help clarify the nature of such masses and the presence of neoplasm in residual mediastinal tissue after therapy.[23]

SEROLOGY AND CHEMISTRY

Some mediastinal neoplasms release substances into the serum that can be measured by specific radioimmunoassays.

TABLE 32-3. Relative Frequency of Primary Mediastinal Tumors

Tumor	*Incidence (%)*
Neurogenic	25.3
Thymoma	23.3
Lymphoma	15.3
Germ cell neoplasm	12.2
Endocrine tumor	7.8
Mesenchymal tumor	7.3
Primary carcinoma	5.7
Other	2.9

(Adapted from ref. 2, with permission.)

These substances may be used to confirm a diagnosis, evaluate response to therapy, and monitor for tumor recurrence. α-Fetoprotein (AFP), human chorionic gonadotropin-β (β-HCG), and lactate dehydrogenase are elaborated by some germ cell tumors and should be obtained in male patients with anterior mediastinal masses.[1] Also, adrenocorticotropic hormone, thyroid hormone, and parathormone may help differentiate certain mediastinal tumors (see Table 32-9).

INVASIVE DIAGNOSTIC TESTS

The determination of the histologic diagnosis of mediastinal masses often is essential for implementation of appropriate

TABLE 32-4. Distribution of Primary Mediastinal Masses by Anatomic Location

ANTEROSUPERIOR MEDIASTINUM
Thymic neoplasms
Lymphomas
Germ cell tumors
Carcinoma
Cysts
Mesenchymal tumors
Endocrine tumors
Morgagni hernias

MIDDLE MEDIASTINUM
Cysts
Lymphomas
Mesenchymal tumors
Carcinoma
Hiatal hernia
Sarcoidosis

POSTERIOR MEDIASTINUM
Neurogenic tumors
Cysts
Mesenchymal tumors
Endocrine tumors
Esophageal masses
Hiatal hernia
Aortic aneurysms

TABLE 32-5. Relative Frequency of Primary Mediastinal Tumors in Adults and Children

Tumor	Incidence (%) Adults	Children
Thymic	31	28
Neurogenic	15	47
Lymphoma	26	9
Germ cell	15	9
Vascular	1	6
Miscellaneous	13	2

(Adapted from ref. 4, with permission.)

treatment. Previously, most patients underwent surgical procedures to establish the diagnosis of mediastinal neoplasms; however, improvements in less invasive diagnostic and immunohistochemical techniques and in electron microscopy have greatly improved the ability to differentiate the cell types in mediastinal neoplasms.[24–31] CT-guided percutaneous needle biopsy, using either fine-needle aspiration techniques and cytologic assessment or larger-core needle biopsy and histologic evaluation, now are standard in the initial evaluation of most mediastinal masses.[32] Although fine-needle specimens are usually adequate to distinguish carcinomatous lesions, core biopsies are recommended to distinguish most other mediastinal neoplasms, especially lymphoma and thymoma.[26–28] Most series report diagnostic yields for percutaneous needle biopsy of 72% to 100%, and, most recently, that figure is in excess of 90%.[25–27,29] Complications include simple pneumothorax (25%), pneumothorax requiring chest tube placement (5%), and hemoptysis (7% to 15%).[29]

Surgical procedures are still occasionally required in the diagnosis of mediastinal tumors.[24,30] Mediastinoscopy is a relatively simple procedure, accomplished under general anesthesia. It provides access to the middle and a limited portion of the upper posterior mediastinum and has a diagnostic accuracy of more than 90%.[33,34] Anterior parasternal mediastinotomy (Chamberlain procedure) yields a diagnosis in 95% of anterior mediastinal masses.[33,34] Thoracoscopy requires general anesthesia but is minimally invasive and provides a diagnostic accuracy of nearly 100% in most areas of the mediastinum.[34] Thoracoscopy should be reserved, however, for biopsies that cannot be obtained with mediastinoscopy or parasternal mediastinotomy. Thoracotomy is almost never necessary for diagnosis and should be reserved for rare circumstances.

TABLE 32-6. Diagnostic Evaluation of Mediastinal Masses

HISTORY AND PHYSICAL EXAMINATION
RADIOGRAPHY
- Standard chest radiography
- Computed tomographic scanning
- Barium swallow
- Radioisotope scanning
- Angiography
- Myelography
- Ultrasonography
- Magnetic resonance imaging

ENDOSCOPY
SEROLOGY
NEEDLE BIOPSY PROCEDURES
- Computed tomography guided
- Ultrasound guided

SURGICAL PROCEDURES
- Mediastinoscopy
- Mediastinotomy
- Thoracotomy

TABLE 32-7. Symptoms and Signs of Mediastinal Masses

SYMPTOM
- Chest pain
- Dyspnea
- Cough
- Fatigue
- Dysphagia
- Night sweats
- Hemoptysis
- Hoarseness

SIGN
- Weight loss
- Fever
- Adenopathy
- Wheezing, stridor
- Superior vena cava syndrome
- Vocal cord paralysis
- Neurofibromatosis
- Neurologic abnormalities
- Pericardial tamponade
- Arrhythmias

TABLE 32-8. Systemic Syndromes Associated with Mediastinal Neoplasms

Tumor	*Syndrome*
Thymoma	Acute pericarditis, Addison's disease, agranulocytosis, alopecia areata, Cushing's syndrome, hemolytic anemia, hypogammaglobulinemia, limbic encephalopathy, myasthenia gravis, myocarditis, nephrotic syndrome, panhypopituitarism, pernicious anemia, polymyositis, pure red cell aplasia, rheumatoid arthritis, sarcoidosis, scleroderma, sensorimotor radiculopathy, Stiff-person syndrome, thyroiditis, ulcerative colitis
Hodgkin's disease	Alcohol-induced pain, Pel-Ebstein fever
Neurofibroma	von Recklinghausen's disease, osteoarthritis
Thymic carcinoid	Multiple endocrine neoplasia
Neuroblastoma	Opsomyoclonus, erythrocyte abnormalities
Neurilemoma	Peptic ulcer

TABLE 32-9. Systemic Manifestations of Hormone Production by Mediastinal Neoplasms

Symptoms	*Hormone*	*Tumor*
Hypertension	Catecholamines	Pheochromocytoma, chemodectoma, neuroblastoma, ganglioneuroma
Hypercalcemia	Parathyroid hormone	Parathyroid adenoma
Thyrotoxicosis	Thyroxine	Thyroid
Cushing's syndrome	ACTH	Carcinoid tumor
Gynecomastia	HCG	Germ cell tumor
Hypoglycemia	? Insulin	Mesenchymal tumors
Diarrhea	VIP	Ganglioneuroma, neuroblastoma, neurofibroma

ACTH, adrenocorticotropic hormone; HCG, human chorionic gonadotropin; VIP, vasoactive intestinal polypeptide.

THYMIC NEOPLASMS

The thymus is an incompletely understood lymphatic organ functioning in T-lymphocyte maturation. It is composed of an epithelial stroma and lymphocytes. Although lymphomas, carcinoid tumors, and germ cell tumors all may arise within the thymus, only thymomas, thymic carcinomas, and thymolipomas arise from true thymic elements. Epithelial thymic neoplasms have been classified into three proposed categories: (1) thymomas, well-differentiated neoplasms; (2) atypical thymomas, moderately differentiated neoplasms; and (3) thymic carcinomas, poorly differentiated neoplasms. This classification is based on features of glandular differentiation; however, further validation of this system is needed.[35–37]

THYMIC ANATOMY AND PHYSIOLOGY

The thymus develops from a paired epithelial anlage in the ventral portion of the third pharyngeal pouch. It is closely associated with the developing parathyroid glands.[38] The stroma of the thymus consists of epithelial cells, which are likely derived from both ectodermal and endodermal components.[39] During weeks 7 and 8 of development, the thymus elongates and descends caudally and ventromedially into the anterior mediastinum. By week 12, a separate cortex and medulla become evident, and mesenchymal septae develop perivascular spaces that contain blood vessels. Lymphoid cells arrive from the liver and bone marrow during week 9 and are separated from the perivascular space by a flat layer of epithelial cells that create the blood–thymus barrier. Maturation and differentiation occurs in this antigen-free environment. By the fourth fetal month, lymphocytes circulate to peripheral lymphoid tissue.[39]

Six subtypes of epithelial cells have been identified in mature thymus.[39] Four exist primarily in the cortical region and two in the medullary region. Type 6 cells form Hassall's corpuscles that are characteristic of thymus. These cells have an ectodermal origin and are displaced into the thymic medulla, where they hypertrophy and form tonofilaments, finally appearing as concentric cells without nuclei.[38,39]

At maturity, the thymus gland is an irregular, lobulated organ. It attains its greatest relative weight at birth, but its absolute weight increases to 30 to 40 g by puberty. During adulthood, it slowly involutes and is replaced by adipose tissue.[39] Ectopic thymic tissue has been found to be widely distributed throughout the mediastinum and neck, particularly the aortopulmonary window and retrocarinal area, and often is indistinguishable from mediastinal fat.[40,41] This ectopic tissue is the likely explanation for thymomas outside the anterior mediastinum and possibly for failure of thymectomy in some cases to improve myasthenia gravis.[40–42]

THYMOMA

Thymic neoplasms, mostly thymomas, constitute 30% of anterior mediastinal masses in adults.[2–4,8,43,44] Thymomas are less common in children, accounting for only 15% of anterior mediastinal masses.[8] Thymomas exhibit no gender predilection and occur most often in the fifth and sixth decades of life.[45] Nearly one-half of these tumors are asymptomatic and are discovered only on routine radiographs. In symptomatic patients, 40% have myasthenia gravis[35] (diplopia, ptosis, dysphagia, fatigue, etc.), whereas others complain of chest pain and symptoms of hemorrhage or compression of mediastinal structures.[45]

Pathology and Classification

Ninety percent of thymomas occur in the anterior mediastinum, and the remainder are located in the neck or other areas of the mediastinum. Grossly, they are lobulated, firm, tan-pink to gray tumors that may contain cystic spaces, calcification, or hemorrhage. They may be encapsulated, adherent to surrounding structures, or frankly invasive.[46] Microscopically, thymomas arise from thymic epithelial cells, although lymphocytes may predominate histologically.[47] True thymomas contain cytologically bland cells and should be distinguished from thymic carcinomas, which have malignant cytologic characteristics. Confusion exists because of previous "benign" or "malignant" designations. Currently, the terms *noninvasive* and *invasive* are used. Noninvasive thymomas have an intact capsule, are movable, and are easily resected, although they can be adherent to adjacent organs. In contrast, invasive thymomas involve surrounding structures and can be difficult to remove without *en bloc* resection of adjacent structures. Despite this difficulty, their cytologic appearance remains benign.[46] Metastatic disease does occur and is most commonly seen as pleural implants and pulmonary nodules. Metastases to extrathoracic sites are rare.[46]

In 1985, Marino and Muller-Hermelink[48] proposed a histologic classification system determined by the thymic site of origin—that is, tumors arising from epithelial cells of the cortex are termed *cortical thymomas,* those arising from the medullary areas are called *medullary thymomas,* and those with features of both are termed *mixed thymomas.* Spindle-shaped cells predominate in the medullary area and likely correspond to spindle cell thymomas of the traditional classification system. Likewise, the cortex contains predominantly round to oval epithelial cells; thus, cortical thymomas probably correspond to the traditional epithelial thymoma.[49] The Muller-Hermelink classification was later revised and further divided into medullary, mixed, predominantly cortical, and cortical thymomas. Well-differentiated and high-grade thymic carcinoma were also described.[50] Medullary and mixed

TABLE 32-10. World Health Organization Staging System for Thymic Epithelial Tumors

Tumor Type	*Cells*	*Clinicopathologic Classification*	*Histologic Terminology*
A	Spindle or oval	Benign thymoma	Medullary
B	Epithelioid or dendritic	Category I malignant thymoma	Cortical; organoid
B1			Lymphocyte-rich; predominately cortical
B2			Cortical
B3			Well-differentiated thymic carcinoma
AB		Benign thymoma	Mixed
C		Category II malignant thymoma	Nonorganotypic; thymic carcinoma, epidermoid keratinizing and nonkeratinizing carcinoma, lymphoepithelioma-like carcinoma, sarcomatoid carcinoma, clear cell carcinoma, basaloid carcinoma, mucoepidermoid carcinoma, undifferentiated carcinoma

thymomas were considered benign with no risk of recurrence, even with capsular invasion. Predominantly cortical and cortical thymomas exhibited intermediate invasiveness and a low but definite risk of late relapse, regardless of their invasiveness. Well-differentiated thymic carcinomas were always invasive, with a high risk of relapse and death.[51] Some support this revision, claiming that it better correlates pathology with prognosis.[51–53] Others believe that it has no distinct clinicopathologic advantage over the traditional system.[49,50,54–56] This issue has been reexamined,[57,58] and the World Health Organization Committee on the Classification of Thymic Tumors adopted a new classification system for thymic neoplasms based on cytologic similarities between certain normal thymic epithelial cells and neoplastic cells, which is of prognostic significance (Table 32-10).[59]

In 1981, Masaoka et al.[60] developed a staging system based on the previous work of Bergh et al.[61] The four stages are shown in Table 32-11. The Masaoka stage II classification assesses both microscopic invasion (occult in 28%) and gross tumor adherence as determined by surgical findings.[49,54,62] Staging was found to correlate with prognosis, with 5-year survival rates 96% for stage I, 86% for stage II, 69% for stage III, and 50% for stage IV.[60] The Groupe d'Etudes des Tumeurs Thymiques (GETT) staging system is surgery-based and demonstrates 90% concordance with the Masaoka system (Table 32-12).[63,64]

Associated Systemic Syndromes

A wide variety of systemic disorders are associated with 71% of thymomas.[65] The symptoms of these associated disorders often lead to the original discovery of the mediastinal tumor. Autoimmune diseases (systemic lupus erythematosus, polymyositis, myocarditis, Sjögren's syndrome, ulcerative colitis, Hashimoto's thyroiditis, rheumatoid arthritis, sarcoidosis, and scleroderma) and endocrine disorders (hyperthyroidism, hyperparathyroidism, Addison's disease, and panhypopituitarism) are most common.[66]

Blood disorders, such as red cell aplasia, hypogammaglobulinemia, T-cell deficiency syndrome, erythrocytosis, pancytopenia, megakaryocytopenia, T-cell lymphocytosis, and pernicious anemia, also have been noted.[66] Other than myasthenia, neuromuscular syndromes include myotonic dystrophy, myositis, and Eaton-Lambert syndrome.[66] Miscellaneous diseases include hypertrophic osteoarthropathy, nephrotic syndrome, minimal change nephropathy, pemphigus, and chronic mucocutaneous candidiasis.[66] Nearly 15% of patients with thymoma develop a second malignancy, such as Kaposi's sarcoma, chemodectoma, multiple myeloma, acute leukemia, and various carcinomas (e.g., lung, colon).[66]

MYASTHENIA GRAVIS. Myasthenia gravis is the most common autoimmune disorder, occurring in 30% to 50% of patients with thymomas. Younger women and older men usually are affected, with a female to male ratio of 2:1. Myasthenia is a disorder of neuromuscular transmission. Symptoms begin

TABLE 32-11. Thymoma Staging System of Masaoka

Stage	*Description*
I	Macroscopically completely encapsulated and microscopically no capsular invasion
II	Macroscopic invasion into surrounding fatty tissue or mediastinal pleura
	Microscopic invasion into capsule
III	Macroscopic invasion into neighboring organs (pericardium, great vessels, lung)
IVa	Pleural or pericardial dissemination
IVb	Lymphogenous or hematogenous metastasis

(From ref. 60, with permission.)

TABLE 32-12. Thymoma Staging System of Groupe d'Etudes des Tumeurs Thymiques

Stage	*Description*
I	
Ia	Encapsulated tumor, totally resected
Ib	Macroscopically encapsulated tumor, totally resected, but the surgeon suspects mediastinal adhesions and potential capsular invasion
II	Invasive tumor, totally resected
III	
IIIa	Invasive tumor, subtotally resected
IIIb	Invasive tumor, biopsy
IV	
IVa	Supraclavicular metastasis or distant pleural implant
IVb	Distant metastases

(From ref. 63, with permission.)

insidiously and result from the production of antibodies to the postsynaptic nicotinic acetylcholine receptor at the myoneural junction. Ocular symptoms are the most frequent initial complaint, eventually progressing to generalized weakness in 80%. The role of the thymus in myasthenia remains unclear, but autosensitization of T lymphocytes to acetylcholine receptor proteins or an unknown action of thymic hormones remain possibilities.[52,67]

Pathologic changes in the thymus are noted in approximately 70% of patients with myasthenia gravis. Lymphoid hyperplasia, characterized by the proliferation of germinal centers in the medullary and cortical areas, is most commonly seen. Thymomas are identified in only about 15% of patients with myasthenia.

The treatment of myasthenia gravis involves the use of anticholinesterase-mimetic agents [i.e., pyridostigmine bromide (Mestinon)]. In severe cases, plasmapheresis may be required to remove high antibody titers. Thymectomy has become an increasingly accepted procedure in the treatment of myasthenia, although the indications, timing, and surgical approach remain controversial.[42] Some improvement in myasthenic symptoms almost always occurs after thymectomy, but complete remission rates vary from 7% to 63%.[42] Patients with myasthenia gravis and thymomas do not respond as well to thymectomy as those without thymomas. Overall survival for myasthenia patients also is lower for patients with thymomas, but no differences were noted based on the extent of invasion present.[68]

RED CELL APLASIA. Pure red cell aplasia is considered an autoimmune disorder and is found in approximately 5% of patients with thymomas. Of patients with red cell aplasia, 30% to 50% have associated thymomas.[69] Ninety-six percent of the patients affected are older than 40 years of age. Examination of the bone marrow reveals an absence of erythroid precursors and, in 30%, an associated decrease in platelet and leukocyte numbers. Thymectomy has produced remission in 38% of patients. Octreotide and prednisone were effective in one patient with recurrent disease.[70] The pathologic basis of these responses is poorly understood.[69]

HYPOGAMMAGLOBULINEMIA. Hypogammaglobulinemia is seen in 5% to 10% of patients with thymoma, and 10% of patients with hypogammaglobulinemia have been shown to have thymoma. Defects in both cellular and humoral immunity have been described, and many patients also have red cell hypoplasia. Thymectomy has not proven beneficial in this disorder.

Treatment

Thymomas are slow-growing neoplasms that should be considered potentially malignant. Surgery, radiation, and chemotherapy all may play a role in their management.

SURGERY. Complete surgical resection is the mainstay of therapy for thymomas and is the most important predictor of long-term survival.[71–77] Although median sternotomy with a vertical or submammary incision is most commonly used, bilateral anterolateral thoracotomies with transverse sternotomy, or "clamshell procedure," is preferred with advanced or laterally displaced tumors.[45,71,72,76] Video-assisted thoracoscopy also has been reported, but long-term results remain unproven.[78] Because of concern about tumor seeding, biopsy procedures are not routinely performed.[72] During surgery, a careful assessment of areas of possible invasion and adherence should be made by the surgeon, who is the best judge of tumor invasiveness.[62] Extended total thymectomy, including all tissue anterior to the pericardium from the diaphragm to the neck and laterally from phrenic nerve to phrenic nerve, is recommended in all cases. Complete surgical resection is associated with an 82% overall 7-year survival rate, whereas survival with incomplete resection is 71% and with biopsy is only 26%.[71] Survival after complete tumor resection has been similar in patients with noninvasive and invasive thymomas in several studies.[60,72,74,75,79] Patients with myasthenia gravis and thymoma were studied by Crucitti et al.,[84] who reported a 78% 10-year survival rate and a 3% recurrence rate with 4.8% (1.7% since 1980) operative mortality after extended thymectomy. Aggressive resection, including lung, phrenic nerve, pericardium, pleural implants, and pulmonary metastases, is occasionally helpful.[60,71,79]

The role of debulking or subtotal resection in stage III and IV disease remains controversial. Several studies have documented 5-year survival rates from 60% to 75% after subtotal resection and 24% to 40% after biopsy alone.[60,71,76,77,79] More recent studies, however, suggest no survival advantage to debulking followed by radiation when compared to radiation alone.[80,81] The use of surgery in recurrent disease remains to be defined. Maggi et al.[71] reported a 71% 5-year survival rate in 12 surgery patients and a 41% survival rate in 11 patients treated with radiation and chemotherapy alone. Prolonged tumor-free survival also was reported by Kirschner[82] in 23 patients. Urgesi et al.,[83] however, noted a 74% 5-year survival rate in 11 patients undergoing surgery and radiation, compared with 65% in ten patients treated with radiation alone (not statistically different).[83]

RADIATION THERAPY. Thymomas are radiosensitive tumors and, consequently, radiation has been used to treat all tumor stages as well as recurrent disease.[43,45,71,72,74,76,77,79,81,85] In stage I thymomas, adjuvant radiotherapy has been administered but has not improved on the excellent results with surgery alone (more than 80% 10-year survival rate).[71,72,74,77,79] In stage II and III invasive disease, adjuvant radiation can decrease recurrence rates after complete surgical resection from 28% to 5%.[43,76,86,87] In addition, Pollack et al.[76] reported an increase in 5-year disease-free survival for stage II to IVa from 18% to 62% with the addition of adjuvant radiation. Others have documented similar results.[72,79] Stage II patients with cortical tumors[88–90] and microscopic invasion of pleura or pericardium are most likely to benefit from postoperative radiation.[91,92] Preoperative radiotherapy for extensive tumors has been reported in limited studies that suggest a decreased tumor burden and potential for tumor seeding at the time of surgery.[71,77,86]

Radiation therapy has proven beneficial in the treatment of extensive disease.[76,77,80,81,85,86,93] Radiotherapy after incomplete surgical resection produces local control rates of 35% to 74% and 5-year survival rates ranging from 50% to 70% for stage III and 20% to 50% for stage IVa tumors.[72,77,80,83,85,86] In addition, Ciernik et al.[80] and others[81,83] have reported similar survival rates (87% 5-year and 70% 7-year) in patients treated with radiation alone compared with partial surgical resection and adjuvant radiation in small numbers of stage III and IV patients and patients with intrathoracic recurrences. Large variations in the amount of tumor treated and radiation delivered, however, make interpretation of these results difficult.[64,76,77,80,85,94]

Radiation therapy is delivered in doses ranging from 30 to 60 Gy in 1.8 or 2.0 cGy fractions over 3 to 6 weeks.[43,71,73,76,77,79,85,86,94–96] No improvement in local control has been shown with doses exceeding 60 Gy[80]; however, completely resected and microscopic residual disease can be well controlled with only 40 to 45 Gy.[77,80,85] Treatment portals have included single anterior field, unequally weighted (2:1 or 3:2) opposed anterior-posterior fields, wedge-pair, and multifield arrangements.[43,97] The gross tumor volume is defined by visible tumor or surgical clips seen on a treatment-planning CT scan. Areas of possible microscopic disease and a small border to account for daily variability and respiratory motion are added to define the clinical and planning target volumes. Gating techniques to minimize respiratory variation and intensity-modulated radiation therapy are new techniques that can minimize the dose heterogeneity, increase total dose and fraction size, and minimize toxicity.[98–100] Prophylactic supraclavicular and hemithorax fields have been used but are not warranted because of increased risks of pulmonary fibrosis, pericarditis, and myelitis.[43,77,80,81,101,102]

CHEMOTHERAPY. Chemotherapy has been used with increasing frequency in the treatment of invasive thymomas. Both single-agent and combination therapy have demonstrated activity in the adjuvant and neoadjuvant settings. Doxorubicin, cisplatin, ifosfamide, corticosteroids, and cyclophosphamide all have been used as single-agent therapy.[103,104] The most active agents are cisplatin, ifosfamide, and corticosteroids; however, only cisplatin and ifosfamide have undergone phase II testing.[43,104,105] Cisplatin, at doses of 100 mg/m^2, has produced complete responses lasting up to 30 months, but lower doses (50 mg/m^2) have associated response rates of only 11%.[103,104] Ifosfamide (with mesna) at a single dose of 7.5 g/m^2 or as a continuous infusion of 1.5 $g/m^2/d$ for 5 days every 3 weeks has resulted in 50% complete and 57% overall response rates. Duration of complete remission ranged from 6 to 66 months.[105] Varying regimens of corticosteroids have shown effectiveness in the treatment of all histologic subtypes of thymoma (with and without myasthenia), with a 77% overall response rate in limited numbers of patients.[103,106] Corticosteroids also have been effective for patients unsuccessful with chemotherapy[103]; however, the actual impact may only be on the lymphocytic and not the malignant epithelial component of the tumor.

Combination chemotherapy regimens have shown higher response rates and have been used in both adjuvant and neoadjuvant settings in the treatment of advanced invasive, metastatic, and recurrent thymoma. Cisplatin-containing regimens appear to be the most active. Fornasiero et al.[107] reported a 43% complete and 91.8% overall response rate with a median survival of 15 months in 37 previously untreated patients with stage III or IV invasive thymoma treated with monthly (median, 5 months) cisplatin, 50 mg/m^2 on day 1; doxorubicin, 40 mg/m^2 on day 1; vincristine, 0.6 mg/m^2 on day 3; and cyclophosphamide, 700 mg/m^2 on day 4. Loehrer et al.[108] documented 10% complete and 50% overall response rates with a median survival of 37.7 months in 29 patients with metastatic or locally progressive recurrent thymoma treated with cisplatin, 50 mg/m^2; doxorubicin, 50 mg/m^2; and cyclophosphamide, 500 mg/m^2, given every 3 weeks for a maximum of 8 cycles after radiotherapy. Park et al.[109] retrospectively described 35% complete and 64% overall response rates with a median survival of 67 months in responding and 17 months in nonresponding patients in 17 patients with invasive stage II and IV thymoma initially treated after relapse with cyclophosphamide, doxorubicin, and cisplatin, with or without prednisone. The European Organization for Research and Treatment of Cancer noted 31% complete and 56% overall response rates with a median survival of 4.3 years in a small study of 16 patients with advanced thymoma treated with cisplatin and etoposide.[110] The addition of ifosfamide to cisplatin and etoposide had a lower than anticipated response rate (approximately 32%) in patients with thymoma and thymic carcinoma.[111]

COMBINED NODALITY APPROACHES. The use of neoadjuvant chemotherapy as part of a multimodality approach to stage III and IV thymoma was reviewed by Tomiak and Evans.[103] Six combined reports document 31% complete and 89% overall response rates in 61 total patients treated with a variety of neoadjuvant chemotherapy regimens (80% cisplatin-based). Twenty-two patients (36%) underwent surgery, with 11 (18%) achieving a complete resection (all treated with cisplatin). Nineteen patients were treated with radiotherapy, but only five patients had disease-free survivals exceeding 5 years.[103] Rea et al.[112] reported 43% complete and 100% overall response rates with median and 3-year survival rates of 66 months and 70%, respectively, in 16 stage III and IVa patients treated initially with cisplatin, doxorubicin, vincristine, and cyclophosphamide, followed by surgery. At surgery, 69% were completely resected and the other 31% received postoperative radiation. Macchiarini et al.[113] reported similar findings. Twenty-five percent complete and 92% overall response rates with a remarkable 83% 7-year disease-free survival rate were reported in 12 patients at the M. D. Anderson Cancer Center who received cisplatin, doxorubicin, cyclophosphamide, and prednisone induction chemotherapy followed by surgical resection (80% complete) and adjuvant radiotherapy for locally advanced (unresectable) thymoma.[114] The degree of chemotherapy-induced tumor necrosis correlated with Ki-67 expression.

A multiinstitutional prospective trial demonstrated a 22% complete and 70% overall response rate with a median survival of 93 months and a Kaplan-Meier 5-year failure-free survival rate of 54.3% in 23 patients with stage III (22/23) unresectable thymoma (GETT stage IIIA/IIIB) stage IV (1/23) thymoma, and thymic carcinoma (2/23) treated with 2 to 4 cycles of cisplatin, doxorubicin, and cyclophosphamide chemotherapy and sequential radiation therapy (54 Gy).[115,116] Just more than 25% had myasthenia gravis. Although these results compare favorably to those obtained with neoadjuvant therapy followed by surgical resection and radiation, further confirmation is needed.

Results of Treatment

Five- and 10-year survival rates for stage I, III, and IV tumors are reported to be 89% to 95% and 78% to 90%,[65,74,117] 70% to 80% and 21% to 80%,[65,74,117] and 50% to 60% and 30% to

40%,[60,65,74,117] respectively. Disease-free survival rates of 74%, 71%, 50%, and 29% also have been reported for stage I, II, III, and IV disease, respectively.[71] Although Maggi et al.[71] reported a 10% overall recurrence rate in 241 patients, less than 5% of noninvasive thymomas and 20% of invasive thymomas were noted to recur.[65] Although myasthenia gravis was once considered an adverse prognostic factor, this is no longer the case because of improvements in perioperative care. Currently, myasthenia actually may lead to improved survival owing to earlier detection of thymomas.[65,84,118,119]

THYMIC CARCINOMA

Thymic carcinoma is a rare aggressive thymic neoplasm that has a poor prognosis. Like thymoma, it is an epithelial tumor, but cytologically it exhibits malignant features. Extensive local invasion and distant metastases are common. Approximately 150 cases have been reported.[120–125] Suster and Rosai[120] reported the largest single series, which included 60 patients ranging in age from 10 to 76 years and with a slight male predominance. Nearly 70% of patients had symptoms of cough, chest pain, or superior vena cava syndrome. Myasthenia and other thymoma-associated syndromes are rare.[120]

The histologic classification of thymic carcinoma was proposed by Levine and Rosai[126] and revised by Suster and Rosai.[120] The tumors are classified broadly as low or high grade. Low-grade tumors include squamous cell carcinoma, mucoepidermoid carcinoma, and basaloid carcinoma. High-grade neoplasms include lymphoepithelioma-like carcinoma and small cell, undifferentiated, sarcomatoid, and clear cell carcinomas.[120,122,123,127] The classification of thymic carcinoma has prognostic significance, with low-grade tumors following a favorable clinical course (median survival rates of 25.4 months to more than 6.6 years) because of a low incidence of local recurrence and metastasis, and high-grade malignancies exhibiting an aggressive clinical course (median survival of only 11.3 to 15.0 months).[120–122] Although the Masaoka thymoma staging system[120,122,124] and a proposed tumor-node-metastasis classification system[125] have been used in staging thymic carcinoma, their utility is unproven. The histologic grade remains the best prognostic indicator.

The optimal treatment of thymic carcinoma remains undefined, but currently a multimodality approach, including surgical resection, postoperative radiation, and chemotherapy, is recommended. Initial surgical resection followed by radiation has been used in most studies.[47,111,120,122–125] Complete resection should be attempted, but usually is not possible.[122] One analysis noted a 9.5-month median survival after resection and postoperative electron beam radiation therapy,[111] with a trend toward improved survival in other studies.[122,123] Chemotherapy with cisplatin-based regimens similar to those used with thymomas have produced variable responses in small numbers of patients.[120,122–124] Combinations of doxorubicin, cyclophosphamide, and vincristine also have generated partial responses, as has the combination of 5-fluorouracil and leukovorin.[124] Use of neoadjuvant chemotherapy has been reported in a small number of patients.[124]

The prognosis of thymic carcinoma is poor because of early metastatic involvement of pleura; lung; mediastinal, cervical, and axillary lymph nodes; bone; and liver.[120] The overall survival rate at 5 years is approximately 35%.[120,122] Improved survival has been correlated with encapsulated tumors, lobular growth pattern, low mitotic activity, and low histologic grade.[120]

THYMIC CARCINOID

Thymic carcinoid tumors are rare, with fewer than 125 reported cases.[128–131] They occur predominantly in males[129] and originate from normal thymic Kulchitsky's cells, which are part of the amine precursor uptake and decarboxylation (APUD) group. Most have the ability to manufacture peptides, amines, kinins, and prostaglandins. They are aggressive tumors that invade locally and commonly metastasize to regional lymph nodes. Metastases occur in 70% of patients within 8 years of initial diagnosis.[131]

The gross appearance of thymic carcinoids is similar to that of thymomas, but they are rarely encapsulated. Microscopically, the tumors exhibit a ribbon-like growth pattern with rosette formation in a fibrovascular stroma. The cells are small, round, or oval with eosinophilic cytoplasm and uniformly round nuclei.[129] Immunohistochemical studies reveal argyrophilic cells that stain with cytokeratin and neuronal-specific enolase. Electron microscopy reveals the presence of secretory granules.[130] Thymic carcinoids, like other foregut carcinoids, are associated with Cushing's syndrome, multiple endocrine neoplasia and, rarely, the carcinoid syndrome.[129–132]

The diagnosis of thymic carcinoid often requires open surgical biopsy. Complete surgical resection is recommended, although recurrence is common.[129–131] The effectiveness of adjuvant therapy is unproven, but most reports advocate adjuvant radiotherapy for incompletely resected tumors.[129–131] Chemotherapy rarely has been used in cases of metastatic or recurrent disease.[129–131]

Although a 5-year survival rate of 60% has been reported with complete surgical resection,[130] local recurrences are common and distant metastases occur in approximately 30% of patients.[129] The long-term prognosis is generally poor.

THYMOLIPOMA

Thymolipomas are rare benign neoplasms composed of mature adipose and thymic tissue, and they account for 1% to 5% of thymic neoplasms.[133] These tumors are also known as *lipothymomas, mediastinal lipomas with thymic remnants,* and *thymolipomatous hamartomas.*[133,134] In a review of 27 patients, Rosado-de-Christenson et al.[134] noted an equal gender distribution and a mean age of 27 years. Approximately 50% of patients presented with symptoms of vague chest pain, dyspnea, and tachypnea. Others have reported, in adults only, an association with myasthenia gravis, red cell aplasia, hypogammaglobulinemia, lichen planus, and Graves' disease.[133,135]

Thymolipomas are soft, lobulated, encapsulated tumors that originate in the anterior mediastinum. They often attain a large size before becoming symptomatic. They frequently conform to the shape of the cardiac and mediastinal structures and are found in the anterior inferior mediastinum "draped along the diaphragm" and connected to the thymus by a small pedicle.[134] Microscopically, the tumors are composed of thymic tissue, often with calcified Hassall's corpuscles, and more than 50% adipose tissue.[134] Histologically, thymolipomas do not appear malignant, and malignant transformation does not occur.[134] Treatment involves complete resection. Long-term follow-up is not available, but recurrences have not been reported.

GERM CELL TUMORS

The vast majority of germ cell tumors arise within gonadal tissue, but the mediastinum is the most common site for the development of extragonadal germ cell tumors. They are most commonly seen in the anterior mediastinum and account for 10% to 15% of all primary mediastinal tumors.[2] These tumors have generated considerable interest because of their uncertain histogenesis.

ETIOLOGY

Extragonadal germ cell tumors are found along the body's midline from the cranium (pineal gland) to the presacral area. This line corresponds to the embryologic urogenital ridge. It is presumed that these tumors arise from malignant transformation of germ cells that have abnormally migrated during embryonic development.[136,137] Mediastinal germ cell neoplasms account for only 2% to 5% of all germinal tumors, but they constitute 50% to 70% of all extragonadal tumors.[137,138]

CLASSIFICATION

Mediastinal germ cell tumors are broadly classified as benign or malignant. Benign tumors include mature teratomas and mature teratomas with an immature component of less than 50%. Malignant germ cell tumors are divided into seminomas (dysgerminomas) and nonseminomatous tumors. Nonseminomatous tumors include embryonal carcinomas, choriocarcinomas, yolk sac tumors, and immature teratomas.[139] Seminomas may exist in a pure form, but any elevation of AFP indicates the presence of an element of a nonseminomatous tumor. In addition, mediastinal germ cell tumors have a propensity to develop a component of non–germ cell malignancy (e.g., rhabdomyosarcoma, adenocarcinoma, permeative neuroectodermal tumor), which can become the predominant histology.

INCIDENCE AND CLINICAL PRESENTATION

In adults, benign germ cell tumors have no gender predilection, but 90% of malignant germ cell tumors occur in men.[136] In the pediatric population, both benign and malignant extragonadal germ cell tumors occur with equal gender distribution. Mediastinal germ cell tumors are most commonly diagnosed in the third decade of life, but patients as old as 60 years of age have been reported. The incidence of these neoplasms is equal in all races. Many patients with benign tumors, including 50% of teratomas, are asymptomatic; however, 90% to 100% of patients with malignant tumors have symptoms of chest pain, dyspnea, cough, fever, or other findings related to compression or invasion of surrounding mediastinal structures.[140,141]

DIAGNOSIS

Mediastinal germ cell tumors are most often detected on the basis of standard chest radiographs. More than 95% of the chest films are abnormal, with almost all masses noted in the anterior mediastinum. Three percent to 8% of tumors arise within the posterior mediastinum.[136] Chest CT scans demonstrate the extent of disease, relationship to surrounding structures, and presence of cystic areas and calcification within the tumor. Abdominal imaging should be performed to assess for possible liver metastases. Although careful examination of the testes, including a testicular ultrasound, should always be performed, an isolated tumor mass in the anterior mediastinum without retroperitoneal involvement is not consistent with a testicular primary tumor. It is not necessary to perform blind orchiectomy or testicular biopsy in patients with normal physical examinations and unremarkable ultrasound findings.[137]

Determination of serum tumor markers is important in the diagnosis and follow-up of mediastinal germ cell tumors. Immunoassays for β-HCG and AFP should be obtained in all patients possessing mediastinal masses suspicious for germ cell tumors. Elevations of β-HCG and AFP confirm a malignant component to the tumor. AFP or β-HCG, or both, are elevated in 80% to 85% of nonseminomatous germ cell tumors, with AFP being detected in 60% to 80% of these tumors and β-HCG in 30% to 50%.[140] Patients with benign teratomas have normal markers, and patients with pure seminoma may have low levels of β-HCG, but AFP is not detected.

TERATOMAS

Benign teratomas are the most common mediastinal germ cell tumor, accounting for 70% of the mediastinal germ cell tumors in children and 60% of those in adults.[136] They can be seen in any age group but most commonly occur in adults from 20 to 40 years of age. There is no gender predilection.

Teratomas may be solid or cystic in appearance and are often referred to as *dermoid cysts* if unilocular. Teratomas contain elements from all three germ cell layers, with a predominance of the ectodermal component in most tumors, including skin, hair, sweat glands, sebaceous glands, and teeth. Mesoderm is represented by fat, smooth muscle, bone, and cartilage. Respiratory and intestinal epithelium are often seen as the endodermal component. The majority of mediastinal teratomas are composed of mature ectodermal, mesodermal, and endodermal elements and exhibit a benign course. Immature teratomas phenotypically may appear as a malignancy derived from these ectodermal, mesodermal, and endodermal elements. These latter tumors behave aggressively and generally are not responsive to systemic therapy.

Treatment of "benign" mediastinal teratoma includes complete surgical resection, which results in excellent long-term cure rates. Radiotherapy and chemotherapy play no role in the management of this tumor. The tumor may be adherent to surrounding structures, necessitating resection of pericardium, pleura, or lung. Complete resection of teratomas should be the goal of treatment. Resection of mature teratomas has been shown to result in prolonged survival with little chance of recurrence.[139,142] Immature teratomas are potentially malignant tumors; their prognosis is influenced by the anatomic site of the tumor, patient age, and the fraction of the tumor that is immature.[139] In patients younger than 15 years, immature teratomas behave similarly to their mature counterparts. In older patients, they may behave as highly malignant tumors. Currently, a trial of cisplatin-based combination chemotherapy (up to 4 cycles of cisplatin, etoposide, and bleomycin or vinblastine, ifosfamide, and cisplatin, if responding) is frequently administered before attempted surgical resection.[139]

SEMINOMA

Primary pure mediastinal seminoma accounts for approximately 35% of malignant mediastinal germ cell tumors; it is principally seen in men aged 20 to 40 years.[143] Seminomas grow slowly and metastasize later than their nonseminomatous counterparts, and they may have reached a large size by the time of diagnosis. Symptoms are usually related to compression or even invasion of surrounding mediastinal structures. Twenty percent to 30% of mediastinal seminomas are asymptomatic when discovered,[143] but metastases are present in 60% to 70% of patients. Pulmonary and other intrathoracic metastases are most commonly seen. Extrathoracic metastases usually involve bone.[143]

The treatment of mediastinal seminoma has evolved since the early 1970s. Definitive conclusions regarding treatment are difficult, because several potentially curative treatment modalities exist. Seminomas are extremely radiosensitive tumors, and for many years, high-dose mediastinal radiation has been used as initial therapy, resulting in long-term survival rates of 60% to 80%.[144] A review of recommendations for radiation therapy treatment in extragonadal seminoma was reported by Hainsworth and Greco.[143] Thirty-five to 40 Gy are the most commonly used radiation doses. Doses as low as 20 Gy have been reported to be curative, but most reports note a significant local recurrence rate with doses of less than 45 Gy.[143] Radiation portals should include a shaped mediastinal field and both supraclavicular areas.[143]

Mediastinal seminoma often presents as bulky, extensive, and locally invasive disease, requiring large radiotherapy portals. These portals result in excessive irradiation of surrounding normal lung, heart, and other mediastinal structures. Additionally, for 20% to 40% of patients in whom local control is achieved, treatment can be expected to fail at distant sites.[136,143]

Chemotherapy was previously used only in advanced gonadal seminoma, but encouraging results and the abovementioned problems with radiotherapy have led to broadened indications; chemotherapy is now being used as initial therapy in many patients with bulky tumors. Pure mediastinal seminoma falls into the intermediate-risk category of the new International Staging System for Germ Cell Tumors. Even patients with visceral metastases fall into this intermediate category and, as such, have a prognosis with cisplatin-based combination chemotherapy exceeding 75% for 5-year survival. Standard systemic therapy consists of cisplatin-based combination chemotherapy. Lemarie and coworkers[140] reported that 12 of 13 patients treated experienced complete remission, with two recurrences after treatment. Cisplatin-based combination therapy achieved a complete response in three of five patients treated by Giaccone.[145] A collective review of 52 patients was undertaken by Hainsworth and Greco.[143] Fourteen patients had received prior radiation therapy, but all underwent chemotherapy with cisplatin and various combinations of cyclophosphamide, vinblastine, bleomycin, or etoposide. Complete responses to treatment were noted in 85% of patients, and 83% were long-term disease-free survivors.[143] Although chemotherapy appears to be a superior modality in these small series, radiotherapy is less toxic, and the high salvage rate with chemotherapy after radiotherapy failure makes selection difficult. Therefore, the recommended treatment is either supradiaphragmatic radiation or 4 cycles of cisplatin-based combination chemotherapy.

The management of patients with residual radiographic abnormalities after chemotherapy is controversial. Studies have shown that the residual mass is a dense scirrhous reaction in 85% to 90% of patients, and the presence of viable seminoma is rare. Others have shown a 25% incidence of residual viable seminoma in these patients treated with chemotherapy followed by resection of residual masses larger than 3 cm.[146] Close observation without surgery is recommended for residual masses after chemotherapy unless the mass enlarges.[147,148] Empiric radiation therapy is not recommended.[143]

Most authors believe that surgery does not play a role in the definitive treatment of seminoma.[144] In addition, surgical debulking of large tumors has not been shown to be of benefit in improving local control or survival.[143]

All patients with mediastinal seminoma should be treated with curative intent. Isolated mediastinal seminoma without evidence of metastatic disease is most often managed with radiotherapy alone, with an excellent prognosis and long-term survival. Locally advanced and bulky disease may be treated initially with cisplatin-based combination chemotherapy, usually 4 cycles of cisplatin and etoposide, with radiotherapy, and followed by salvage chemotherapy (vinblastine, ifosfamide, and cisplatin) in the event of recurrence.[149] Patients with distant metastases should undergo cisplatin-based combination chemotherapy as initial treatment.

NONSEMINOMATOUS GERM CELL TUMORS

Nonseminomatous germ cell tumors include choriocarcinoma, embryonal carcinoma, teratoma, and endodermal sinus (yolk sac) tumors. They may occur in pure form, but in approximately one-third of cases, multiple cell types are present. Other malignant components, including adenocarcinomas, squamous cell carcinomas, and sarcomas, may be present or even represent the predominant tissue type, as usually occurs in immature teratomas.

Nearly 85% of nonseminomatous germ cell tumors occur in men, with a mean age of 29 years.[136] Karyotypic analyses have been performed on a number of these patients, and the 47,XXY pattern of Klinefelter's syndrome has been found in up to 20% of patients.[136] Mediastinal nonseminomatous germ cell tumors are most commonly found in the anterior mediastinum and appear grossly as lobulated masses with a thin capsule. They are frequently invasive at the time of diagnosis, with almost 90% of patients exhibiting symptoms. They appear on CT scans as large inhomogeneous masses containing areas of hemorrhage and necrosis. Elevated levels of β-HCG are seen in 30% to 50% of patients, and AFP is detected in 60% to 80%.

These tumors carry a poorer prognosis than either pure extragonadal seminoma or their gonadal nonseminomatous counterparts, and all patients with primary mediastinal nonseminomatous germ cell tumors fall into the poor risk category of the new International Germ Cell Consensus Classification.[150] Eighty-five percent to 95% of patients have obvious distant metastases at the time of diagnosis. Common metastatic sites include lung, pleura, lymph nodes, liver, and, less commonly, bone.[143]

A number of non–germ cell malignant processes have been found in association with nonseminomatous germ cell tumors. One of the most interesting is that found in association with acute megakaryocytic leukemia. Other hematologic malignancies, such as acute myeloid leukemia, acute nonlymphocytic leukemia, erythroleukemia, myelodysplastic syndrome, malignant histiocytosis, and thrombocytosis, have all been reported. These malignancies may antedate the discovery of the germ cell tumor or occur synchronously. Solid tumors, such as embryonal rhabdomyosarcoma, small cell undifferentiated carcinoma, neuroblastoma, and adenocarcinoma have been described and occur more frequently in primary mediastinal tumors compared to gonadal germ cell neoplasms.[137]

The diagnosis of nonseminomatous germ cell tumors can often be made without tissue biopsy.[144] In many centers, the presence of an anterior mediastinal mass in a young male with elevated serum tumor markers (AFP and β-HCG) is adequate to initiate treatment. If a tissue diagnosis is deemed necessary, fine-needle guided aspiration with cytologic staining for tumor markers may be used for confirmation. An anterior mediastinotomy provides the best exposure for open biopsy if necessary.[144]

Treatment of nonseminomatous germ cell tumors incorporates cisplatin-based chemotherapy, which has markedly improved the prognosis in these patients. In the past, long-term survival after treatment of nonseminomatous germ cell tumors was very rare; today, however, overall complete remission rates of 40% to 50% are obtained in most series.[139,140,143,145] Treatment is initiated with cisplatin-containing combination chemotherapy, which often includes etoposide and bleomycin. Treatment should be administered every 3 weeks for 4 courses; patients should then be restaged with serum tumor markers and CT scans of the chest and abdomen.[143] In a collective review of 158 patients undergoing a variety of combination chemotherapeutic regimens for the initial treatment of nonseminomatous germ cell tumors, complete responses were noted in 54% of patients, and 42% were long-term disease-free survivors.[143]

Patients with negative tumor markers and no radiographic evidence of residual disease after initial chemotherapy require no further treatment. Persistent elevation of serum tumor markers, particularly if they begin to rise again, usually requires salvage chemotherapy.[143] Patients with normal serum tumor markers but radiographic evidence of residual masses after induction chemotherapy should undergo surgical resection 4 to 6 weeks after completion of chemotherapy.[143,144] Complete resection should be attempted, because debulking procedures provide no benefit. Patients found to have residual viable germ cell tumor undergo 2 additional cycles of chemotherapy. Patients with immature teratoma or non–germ cell malignancies can simply be observed after complete resection. Nichols[136] reports complete remissions in 18 of 31 patients using this regimen, and other series report complete remission rates of 50% to 70%, with long-term survival rates approximating 50%.[136] Equivalent results are obtained in all histologic subtypes.

The treatment of recurrent disease is difficult, because patients with relapsing mediastinal nonseminomatous germ cell tumors do extraordinarily poorly with salvage therapy, such as vinblastine, ifosfamide, and cisplatin[151]; optimal therapy has not been determined. Standard salvage chemotherapy has not proven beneficial, and few patients achieve durable remissions. High-dose chemotherapy with stem cell rescue is effective in only a few selected patients.[152,153] Most patients are candidates for experimental phase I trials.

MESENCHYMAL TUMORS

Mediastinal mesenchymal tumors, or soft tissue tumors, originate from the connective tissue elements of the mediastinum. Smooth and striated muscle, lymphatic tissue, fat, and vascular tissue all give rise to a variety of neoplasms, which may be benign or malignant. Most of these tumors also occur in other parts of the body and are discussed in detail elsewhere in the chapter on soft tissue sarcomas.

Mesenchymal tumors account for approximately 6% of primary mediastinal neoplasms.[2] They are less common in the mediastinum than in other locations. Approximately 55% are malignant, and there is no gender predilection.[10,154] In general, treatment of malignant mesenchymal tumors involves combination therapy, including surgical resection, radiation therapy, and chemotherapy. Benign tumors should be completely excised, after which little chance of recurrence remains.

Lipomas are the most common mesenchymal tumor of the mediastinum, representing 2% of all mediastinal neoplasms.[8] Benign lipomas are most often located in the anterior mediastinum. They may grow to large size without symptoms. Treatment is complete resection, and although local recurrence is possible, it is unusual. Malignant liposarcoma is more commonly found in the posterior mediastinum.

Fibromas are encapsulated asymptomatic tumors that may grow to a very large size. Fibrosarcomas often are symptomatic malignancies associated with hypoglycemia. Fibromas are cured with complete surgical excision, but fibrosarcomas are usually unresectable and respond poorly to radiation and chemotherapy.[10] Leiomyomas, leiomyosarcomas, rhabdomyomas, rhabdomyosarcomas, synovial cell sarcomas, mesotheliomas, and xanthogranulomas also occasionally occur in the mediastinum.[8,154]

Vascular tumors of the mediastinum include hemangiomas, hemangioendotheliomas, and benign and malignant hemangiopericytomas.[8,154] Ten percent to 30% of all vascular tumors are malignant.[10] Mediastinal hemangiomas represent 0.5% of all mediastinal neoplasms but are the most common vascular tumor.[155] They may be cavernous or capillary and are often associated with hemangiomas in other areas of the body.[155,156] Sixty percent occur in the anterior mediastinum, and 25% occur posteriorly.[10] Diagnosis is best accomplished by CT scan or MRI, in which phleboliths may be seen in 30% of these tumors. Angiography is important in identifying and embolizing major feeding vessels before surgery.[156] Total excision is considered the treatment of choice; however, large, incompletely resected hemangiomas usually do not recur.[155]

Lymphangiomas, also known as *cystic hygromas*, often extend into the anterior mediastinum from the cervical area. Seventeen percent are located exclusively in the mediastinum. They tend to enlarge as patients grow, particularly during puberty. Treatment involves surgical resection, but this is often difficult because of adherence to surrounding structures. Response to radiation is variable.[10] Other lymphatic soft tissue tumors include lymphangiosarcoma and lymphangiopericytoma.

NEUROGENIC TUMORS

Thoracic neurogenic tumors occur most commonly in the posterior mediastinum but occasionally are found in the anterior mediastinum and elsewhere. They compose between 19% and 39% of all mediastinal tumors[157,158] and 75% of posterior mediastinal tumors.[159] They originate from peripheral nerves (nerves of the brachial plexus and intercostal nerves), autonomic sympathetic ganglia and, rarely, from the vagus nerve.[160] Neurogenic tumors in the anterior mediastinum originate in chemoreceptor paragangliomas.

Whereas neurogenic tumors in infants and children are frequently malignant and often present with metastatic disease,[161] in adults the majority of these tumors are benign. They occur without gender predilection at any age but are more likely in young adults. Often asymptomatic, they are solitary (except in neurofibromatosis) and found on a routine chest x-ray. Benign tumors can attain a considerable size. They frequently arise in the paravertebral sulcus from the posterior roots of the spinal nerves at the zone of transition between the central and peripheral myelin.[162] They also may arise on the posterior portion of the spinal nerve root in the spinal canal and grow through the intervertebral foramen into the paravertebral area, giving rise to the appearance of a dumbbell- or hourglass-shaped tumor. These tumors must be recognized to plan an appropriate operation in conjunction with a neurosurgeon. Depending on their size and location, lesions may cause spinal cord compression, pain, paresthesias, Horner's syndrome, and muscle atrophy. Superior vena cava syndrome, dyspnea, cough, and bony erosions, which wrongly suggest a malignant process, also have been described.

NEURILEMOMA (SCHWANNOMA)

Neurilemoma (schwannoma) is the most common tumor in the paravertebral sulcus. Arising from the intercostal nerve sheath, the tumor is encapsulated, white or yellowish pink in color, with calcifications and cystic degeneration. Histologically, it is composed of uniform slender biphasic fusiform cells with elongated, twisted nuclei that have a tendency to align in a regimented or palisaded appearance.[163] The tumor may contain large blood vessels and may be a source of considerable blood loss during surgical removal. Schwannoma may be further differentiated into melanotic, adenomatous, or psammomatous tumors (Fig. 32-2).[163]

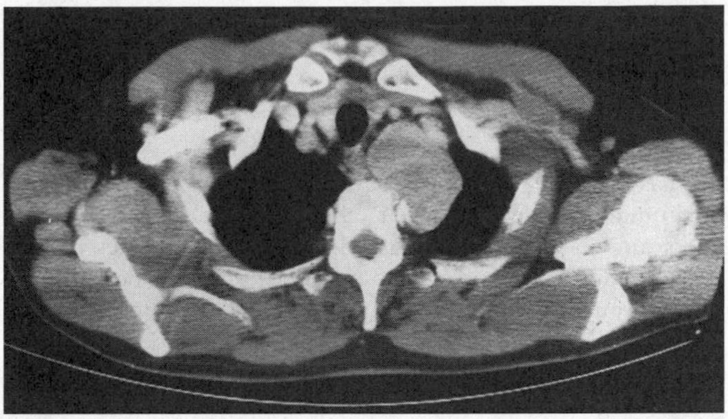

FIGURE 32-2. Schwannoma in the paravertebral area in the apex of the left chest.

NEUROFIBROMA

Neurofibromas are most often benign and asymptomatic. However, they can have an intradural as well as an extradural component and may cause symptoms of cord compression. They are not encapsulated and may have a plexiform appearance.[164] Microscopically, neurofibromas have a heterogeneous cell population, but Schwann cell differentiation is not always present.[157] Neurogenic tumors can be differentiated from leiomyomas, meningiomas, and fibrous histiocytomas by the immunohistochemical identification of S-100 protein. Solitary neurofibromas are cured by surgical excision.

Neurofibromas can occur as multiple lesions in von Recklinghausen's disease.[165] Neurofibromatosis is inherited as an autosomal dominant trait affecting both genders equally; however, approximately one-half of the cases are sporadic.[166,167] The clinical features vary and include hyperpigmented café au lait skin spots, skin and subcutaneous multiple neurofibromas (hamartomas), scoliosis, bowing of long bones, disorders of sexual development, and multiple neurogenic tumors and malignancies, such as malignant schwannomas.[168,169] Mediastinal neurofibromas may be multiple and appear as long plexiform masses. Histologically, they consist of large nerve fibers mixed with connective tissue stroma containing Schwann cells and fibroblasts. Surgical intervention is justified for lesions located in the spinal canal that cause spinal cord or nerve root compression. The prognosis generally is poor.[170]

MALIGNANT SCHWANNOMA

Malignant schwannomas are the malignant counterparts of neurilemmomas and neurofibromas. Ultrastructural studies, however, cannot always document Schwann cells in these tumors derived from nerve sheaths, and therefore the terms *malignant nerve sheath tumor, neurogenic sarcoma,* and *neurofibrosarcoma* are sometimes used.[170] Malignant nerve sheath tumors commonly are large. They are painful and may cause superior vena cava obstruction; Horner's syndrome; dyspnea; dysphagia; hoarseness; and invasion of the lung, bones, and aorta, depending on their location and size.

The diagnostic criteria for malignant nerve sheath tumors are controversial.[166] Origin from a major nerve, presence of Schwann cells and S-100 protein, the diagnosis of neurofibromatosis, and nuclear palisading are important features. Histologic findings include hypercellularity, pleomorphic dense nuclei, multiple and abnormal mitoses, and invasion of the surrounding structures.[160] The malignant nerve sheath tumors are usually large (often larger than 5 cm in diameter), partially encapsulated, soft, and gray, with hemorrhage and necrosis. Histologically, they are composed of spindle cells with comma-shaped, irregular nuclei. Neural and perineural invasion, mature cartilage, bone, striated muscle, squamous differentiation, and mucin-secreting glands also may be seen.[171,172]

Clinically, these tumors are aggressive, locally invasive, and highly metastatic. They often recur after resection, leading to a 75% 5-year survival rate. Patients with neurofibromatosis and a malignant nerve sheath tumor have a 15% to 30% 5-year survival rate. Combination chemotherapy is recommended in stage III and IV disease (Fig. 32-3).

TUMORS OF SYMPATHETIC GANGLIA

Mediastinal ganglioneuromas are found in the posterior mediastinum along the sympathetic chain in children older than 4 years and in adults in the third and fourth decades of life. Occasionally, a neuroblastoma may mature into a benign ganglioneuroma.[173–175] The tumor usually is asymptomatic, but sometimes presents with Horner's syndrome and, rarely, with diarrhea caused by production of vasoactive intestinal polypeptide. Ganglioneuromas have a smooth contour and contain areas of stippled calcification. They may resemble other benign neurogenic tumors, causing rib erosions.[176] Microscopically, spindle cell proliferation is seen that appears identical to that in a neurofibroma, except that ganglioneuromas exhibit the presence of large ganglion cells.[160] Ganglioneuromas are benign tumors, although regional lymph nodes may contain islands of tumor cells attributed to matured neuroblasts.[166] They require complete excision.

NEUROBLASTOMAS

Although neuroblastomas can be found in any location in which embryonic neuroblasts migrated from the neural crest, they usually originate in the adrenal glands and along nerve plexuses. In the chest, they occur along the sympathetic trunk in the paravertebral sulcus. This tumor is the most common malignancy of early childhood, occurring most commonly in the first 2 years of life. Patients with mediastinal neuroblastomas usually are symptomatic and frequently have metastatic disease.[177,178] Symptoms are related to local compression (Horner's syndrome and heterochromia of the iris) or to systemic release of vasoactive peptides, such as catecholamines, vanillylmandelic acid, homovanillic acid, and 3-methoxy-4-hydroxyphenylglycol. Encephalopathy, myasthenia, and Cushing's syndrome may be present.[179] Radiographically, a mass is seen in the posterior mediastinum with stippled calcifications, skeletal erosion, and occasional extension into the spinal canal.

Pathology reveals lobulated gray or red tumors with hemorrhagic areas. Microscopically, small cells with scant cytoplasm and polygonal nuclei exhibit various degrees of differentiation. Intracytoplasmic neurofilaments and neurosecretory granules and extracellular material seen on electron microscopy distinguish neuroblastoma from other childhood tumors, such as lymphoma, Ewing's sarcoma, and rhabdomyosarcoma.[160]

Neuroblastomas are highly aggressive tumors. Survival depends on the age of the patient, the stage of disease, the location of the tumor, and histologic differentiation. The prognosis is better in patients younger than 1 year of age and in patients with limited, well-differentiated tumors. Neuroblastomas may regress spontaneously or undergo maturation into ganglioneuromas. Ganglioneuroblastomas have a better prognosis than neuroblastomas.[180] The staging system for neuroblastoma shown in Table 32-13 was developed to help guide therapy. Treatment for stage I and II disease is simple surgical resection, although adjuvant postoperative radiotherapy is recommended for stage II tumors. For stage III and IV, a combination of chemotherapy and radiation is advised.

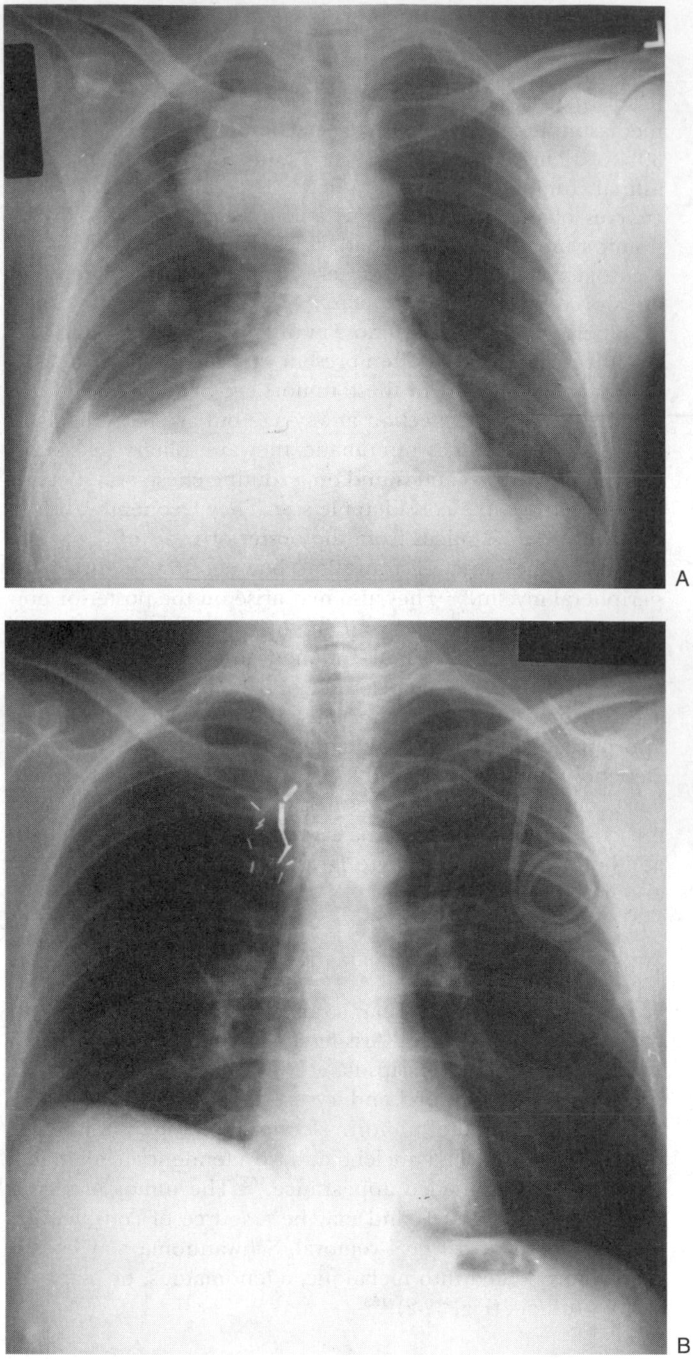

FIGURE 32-3. **A:** Malignant neurofibroma, initially considered to be nonresectable, in a 34-year-old man. **B:** The tumor was resected after a combination of chemotherapy and radiation therapy.

GRANULAR CELL TUMOR

Granular cell tumors (granular cell myoblastomas) are considered benign. They are found in the posterior mediastinum and are derived from Schwann cells. They are soft, gray, and poorly circumscribed tumors consisting of uniform polygonal cells either in nests or strands with eosinophilic granular cytoplasm and a stroma of fibrous connective tissue.[181] Resection is always curative.

TABLE 32-13. Staging System for Neuroblastoma

Stage	*Description*
I	Tumor is limited to site of origin.
II	Tumor extends beyond site of origin, or when limited to site of origin, has metastatic regional lymph nodes present on same side.
III	Tumor extends to contralateral side.
IV	Metastases are present beyond regional lymph nodes.

DIAGNOSIS

Although posterior mediastinal neoplasms are predominately neurogenic, other tumors also must be considered in the differential diagnosis. Goiters, esophageal leiomyomas, solitary fibrous tumors, and bronchial/esophageal duplication cysts all have been reported. Once identified, the nature of these lesions, their relationship to other structures, and the presence of distant metastases can be determined by CT scans. MRI scans can define vascular involvement and provide multiplanar views that are valuable in assessing tumor extension into paravertebral foramina. An iodine 131 nuclear scan may be helpful if a goiter is suspected.

Histologic diagnosis is not necessary before surgery. However, if surgical resection is not contemplated, a definitive diagnosis is required for further treatment planning. This diagnosis generally requires a generous biopsy obtained by an open surgical procedure or a CT-guided core-needle biopsy.

MANAGEMENT

If no contraindication is present, resection of all neurogenic tumors is advised. Neurogenic tumors grow and can cause life-threatening symptoms, depending on their size and location. Therefore, observation of neurogenic tumors may be justified only with a stable, asymptomatic, benign tumor in an otherwise poor surgical candidate. The standard approach uses a posterolateral thoracotomy incision, removing the tumor with normal tissue margins. More recently, thoracscopic resection of small- to moderate-size tumors has been reported. In dumbbell tumors, the intraspinal component should be removed first. The mortality rate for surgical resection is less than 1%. Complications include Horner's syndrome and chylothorax. Surgery on tumors with spinal canal involvement may be complicated by direct spinal cord trauma, ischemia from spinal artery injury and, rarely, an epidural hematoma with spinal cord compression.

PRIMARY CARDIAC MALIGNANCIES

The vast majority of tumors involving the heart and pericardium are metastatic.[182,183] In addition, most primary cardiac tumors are benign myxomas, 75% to 80% of which arise from the left atrium. Other benign primary cardiac neoplasms include rhabdomyoma, fibroma, lipoma, hemangioma, teratoma, and fibroelastoma. Primary malignant cardiac tumors make up one-fourth of all primary cardiac neoplasms and most commonly originate from the atria.[184,185] Most are some variant of sarcomas,[186] including angiosarcoma,[187] rhabdomyosarcoma, leiomyosarcoma,[188] fibrosarcoma,[189] lymphoma, malignant fibrous histiocytoma,[190] and mesothelioma of the pericardium.[191] Pheochromocytomas also occur as primary cardiac neoplasms.

A high index of suspicion is imperative in establishing a diagnosis, because the presenting symptoms often mimic other nonneoplastic cardiac pathology. Whole body gallium scans,[192] echocardiography, CT, and MRI all may serve to localize a primary cardiac neoplasm. Up to 80% of primary cardiac malignancies present with systemic metastases[193] and have clinical evidence of right heart failure, and many develop tamponade. Surgical resection is required for cure; however, negative margins usually are not possible.[194]

Chemotherapy and external-beam radiation can be administered after surgery, although a report of 15 cases treated at the Institut Gustave-Roussy does not support the routine use of adjuvant chemotherapy for primary cardiac sarcomas.[190] There has been a report of a patient receiving neoadjuvant (induction) chemotherapy, which resulted in a response and subsequent surgical resection.[195]

New surgical techniques, including orthotopic and autotransplantation, may be beneficial in carefully selected patients.[196,197] With the advent of "gating" technology and sophisticated treatment planning, more accurate targeting with electron beam radiation therapy may be possible, similar to stereotactic radiosurgery of the brain. At times, a pericardial window may be required to palliate symptoms of pericardial tamponade. Currently, long-term survival is rare.[198,199]

REFERENCES

1. Fraser RS, Pare JAP, Fraser RG, et al. The normal chest. In: *Synopsis of diseases of the chest,* 2nd ed. Philadelphia: WB Saunders, 1994:73.
2. Davis RD, Oldham HN, Sabiston DC. Primary cysts and neoplasms of the mediastinum: recent changes in clinical presentation, methods of diagnosis, management, and results. *Ann Thorac Surg* 1987;44:229.
3. Cohen AJ, Thompson L, Edwards FH, Bellamy RF. Primary cysts and tumors of the mediastinum. *Ann Thorac Surg* 1991;51:378.
4. Azarow KS, Pearl RH, Zurcher R, Edwards FH, Cohen AJ. Primary mediastinal masses: a comparison of adult and pediatric populations. *J Thorac Cardiovasc Surg* 1993;106:67.
5. Strollo DC, Rosado-de-Christenson ML, Jett JR. Primary mediastinal tumors. Part II. Tumors of the middle and posterior mediastinum. *Chest* 1997;112:1344.
6. Grosfeld JL. Primary tumors of the chest wall and mediastinum in children. *Semin Thorac Cardiovasc Surg* 1994;6:235.
7. Adkins RB, Maples MD, Hainsworth JD. Primary malignant mediastinal tumors. *Ann Thorac Surg* 1984;38:648.
8. Mullen B, Richardson JD. Primary anterior mediastinal tumors in children and adults. *Ann Thorac Surg* 1986;42:338.
9. Simpson I, Campbell PE. Mediastinal masses in childhood: a review from a pediatric pathologist's point of view. *Prog Pediatr Surg* 1991;27:93.
10. Davis RD, Oldham HN, Sabiston DC. The mediastinum. In: Sabiston DC, Spencer FC, eds. *Surgery of the chest,* 5th ed. Philadelphia: WB Saunders, 1989.
11. Harris GJ, Harmon PK, Trinkle JK, Grover FL. Standard biplane roentgenography is highly sensitive in documenting mediastinal masses. *Ann Thorac Surg* 1987;44:238.
12. Weisbrod GL, Herman SJ. Mediastinal masses: diagnosis with non-invasive techniques. *Semin Thorac Cardiovasc Surg* 1992;4:3.
13. Tecce PM, Fishman EK, Kuhlman JE. CT evaluation of the anterior mediastinum: spectrum of disease. *Radiography* 1994;14:973.
14. Woodring JH, Johnson PJ. Computed tomography distinction of central thoracic masses. *J Thorac Imaging* 1991;6:32.
15. Waller DA, Rees MR. Computed tomography in the preoperative assessment of mediastinal tumors: does it improve surgical management? *Thorac Cardiovasc Surg* 1991;39:158.
16. Graeber GM, Shriver CD, Albus RA, et al. The use of computed tomography in the evaluation of mediastinal masses. *J Thorac Cardiovasc Surg* 1986;91:662.
17. Naidich DP. Helical computed tomography of the thorax: clinical applications. *Radiol Clin North Am* 1994;32:759.
18. Ikezoe J, Takeuchi N, Johkoh T, et al. MRI of anterior mediastinal tumors. *Radiat Med* 1992;10:176.

19. Batra P, Brown K, Collins JD, et al. Mediastinal masses: magnetic resonance imaging in comparison with computed tomography. *J Natl Med Assoc* 1991;83:969.
20. Mayo JR. Magnetic resonance imaging of the chest: where we stand. *Radiol Clin North Am* 1994;32:795.
21. Wernecke K, Vassallo P, Potter R, Lukener HG, Peters PE. Mediastinal tumors: sensitivity of detection with sonography compared with CT and radiography. *Radiology* 1990;175:137.
22. Faletra F, Ravini M, Moreo A, et al. Transesophageal echocardiography in the evaluation of mediastinal masses. *J Am Soc Echocardiogr* 1992;5:178.
23. Kubota K, Yamada S, Kondo T, et al. PET imaging of primary mediastinal tumours. *Br J Cancer* 1996;73:882.
24. Ferguson MK, Lee E, Skinner DB, Little AG. Selective operative approach for diagnosis and treatment of anterior mediastinal masses. *Ann Thorac Surg* 1987;44:583.
25. Tarver RD, Cances DJ. Interventional chest radiology. *Radiol Clin North Am* 1994;32:689.
26. Morrissey B, Adams H, Gibbs AR, Crane MD. Percutaneous needle biopsy of the mediastinum: review of 94 procedures. *Thorax* 1993;48:632.
27. Herman SJ, Holub RV, Weisbrod GL, Chamberlain DW. Anterior mediastinal masses: utility of transthoracic needle biopsy. *Radiology* 1991;180:167.
28. Heilo A. Tumors in the mediastinum: US-guided histologic core needle biopsy. *Radiology* 1993;189:143.
29. Bressler EL, Kirkham JA. Mediastinal masses: alternative approaches to CT-guided needle biopsy. *Radiology* 1994;191:391.
30. Pearson FG. Mediastinal masses diagnosis: invasive techniques. *Semin Thorac Cardiovasc Surg* 1992;4:23.
31. Yang PC, Cheng DB, Lee YC, et al. Mediastinal malignancy: ultrasound guided biopsy through the supraclavicular approach. *Thorax* 1992;47:377.
32. Kohman LJ. Approach to the diagnosis and staging of mediastinal masses. *Chest* 1993;103:328S.
33. Elia S, Cecera C, Giampaglia F, Ferrante G. Mediastinoscopy vs anterior mediastinotomy in the diagnosis of mediastinal lymphoma. *Eur J Cardiothorac Surg* 1992;6:361.
34. Rendina EA, Venuta F, DeGiacomo T, et al. Comparative merits of thoracoscopy, mediastinoscopy, and mediastinotomy for mediastinal biopsy. *Ann Thorac Surg* 1994;57:992.
35. Kornstein MJ. Thymoma classification: my opinion. *Am J Clin Pathol* 1999;112:304.
36. Harris NL, Muller-Hermelink H-K. Thymoma classification: a siren's song of simplicity. *Am J Clin Pathol* 1999;12:299.
37. Suster S, Moran CA. Thymoma, atypical thymoma, and thymic carcinoma. *Anat Pathol* 1999;111:826.
38. Skandalakis JE, Gray SW, Todd NW. Pharynx and its derivatives. In: Skandalakis JE, Gray SW, eds. *Embryology for surgeons,* 2nd ed. Baltimore: Williams & Wilkins, 1994.
39. VonGaudecker B. Functional histology of the human thymus. *Anat Embryol* 1991;183:1.
40. Jaretski A, Wolff M. "Maximal" thymectomy for myasthenia gravis: surgical anatomy and operative technique. *J Thorac Cardiovasc Surg* 1988;96:711.
41. Fukai I, Funato Y, Mizuno T, Hasimoto T, Masaoka A. Distribution of thymic tissue in the mediastinal adipose tissue. *J Thorac Cardiovasc Surg* 1991;101:1099.
42. Blossom GB, Ernstoff RM, Howells GA, Bendick PJ, Glover JL. Thymectomy for myasthenia gravis. *Arch Surg* 1993;128:855.
43. Thomas CR Jr, Wright CD, Loehrer PJ Sr. Thymoma: state of the art. *J Clin Oncol* 1999;17:2280.
44. Cowen D, Hannoun-Levi JM, Resbeut M, et al. Natural history and treatment of malignant thymoma. *Oncology* 1998;12:1001.
45. Patterson GA. Thymomas. *Semin Thorac Cardiovasc Surg* 1992;4:39.
46. Lewis JE, Wick MR, Scheithauer BW, Bernatz PE, Taylor WF. Thymoma: a clinicopathologic review. *Cancer* 1987;60:2727.
47. Sweeney CJ, Wick MR, Loehrer PJ. Thymoma and thymic carcinoma. In: Raghavan D, Brecher ML, Johnson DH, et al., eds. *Textbook of uncommon cancer,* 2nd ed. New York: John Wiley & Sons, 1999:485.
48. Marino M, Muller-Hermelink HK. Thymoma and thymic carcinoma: relation of thymoma epithelial cells to the cortical and medullary differentiation of thymus. *Virchows Arch A Pathol Anat Histopathol* 1985;407:119.
49. Kornstein MJ. Controversies regarding the pathology of thymomas. *Pathol Ann* 1992;27:1.
50. Kirchner T, Muller-Hermelink H. New approaches to the diagnosis of thymic epithelial tumors. *Prog Surg Pathol* 1989;10:167.
51. Quintanilla-Martinez L, Wilkins EW, Choi N, et al. Thymoma: histologic subclassification is an important prognostic factor. *Cancer* 1994;74:606.
52. Kuo TT, Lo SK. Thymoma: a study of the pathologic classification of 71 cases with evaluation of the Muller-Hermelink system. *Hum Pathol* 1993;24:766.
53. Shimosato Y. Controversies surrounding the subclassification of thymoma. *Cancer* 1994;74:542.
54. Quintanilla-Martinez L, Wilkins EW, Ferry JA, Harris NL. Thymoma-morphologic subclassification correlates with invasiveness and immunohistologic features: a study of 122 cases. *Hum Pathol* 1993;24:958.
55. Pan CC, Wu HP, Yang CF, Chen WYK, Chiang H. The clinicopathological correlation of epithelial subtyping in thymoma: a study of 112 consecutive cases. *Hum Pathol* 1994;25:893.
56. Dawson A, Ibrahim NBN, Gibbs AR. Observer variation in the histopathological classification of thymoma: correlation with prognosis. *J Clin Pathol* 1994;47:519.
57. Suster S, Moran CA. Primary thymic epithelial neoplasms: current concepts and controversies. In: Fechner RE, Rosen PP, eds. *Anatomic pathology 1997,* vol 2. Chicago: ASCP Press, 1997:1.
58. Suster S, Moran CA. Thymoma classification: the ride of the Valkyries? *Am J Clin Pathol* 1999;112:308.
59. Marx A, Muller-Hermelink HK. From basic immunobiology to the upcoming WHO-classification of tumors of the thymus. *Pathol Res Pract* 1999;195:515.
60. Masaoka A, Monden Y, Nakahara K, Tanioka T. Follow-up study of thymomas with special reference to their clinical stages. *Cancer* 1981;48:2485.
61. Bergh NP, Gatzinsky P, Larsson S, Lundin P, Ridell B. Tumors of the thymus and thymic region. I. Clinicopathological studies on thymomas. *Ann Thorac Surg* 1978;25:91.
62. Kornstein MJ, Curran WJ, Turrisi AT, Brooks JJ. Cortical versus medullary thymomas: a useful morphologic distinction? *Hum Pathol* 1988;19:1335.
63. Gamondes JP, Balawi A, Greenland T, et al. Seventeen years of surgical treatment of thymoma: factors influencing survival. *Eur J Cardiothorac Surg* 1991;5:124.
64. Cowen D, Richaud P, Mornex F, et al. Thymoma: results of a multicentric retrospective series of 149 non-metastatic irradiated patients and review of the literature. *Radiother Oncol* 1995;34:9.
65. Souadjian JV, Enriquez P, Silverstein MN, et al. The spectrum of diseases associated with thymoma. *Arch Intern Med* 1974;134:374.
66. Marchevsky AM, Kaneko M. *Surgical pathology of the mediastinum.* New York: Raven Press, 1984:58.
67. Berrih-Akin S, Morel E, Raimond F, et al. The role of the thymus in myasthenia gravis: immunohistological and immunological studies in 115 cases. *Ann N Y Acad Sci* 1987;505:51.
68. Palmisani MT, Evoli A, Batocchi AP, Provenzano C, Torali P. Myasthenia gravis associated with thymoma: clinical characteristics and long term outcome. *Eur Neurol* 1993;34:78.
69. Masaoka A, Hashimoto T, Shibata K, Yamakowa Y, Nakamae K. Thymomas associated with pure red cell aplasia: histology and follow up studies. *Cancer* 1989;64:1872.
70. Palmieri G, Lastoria S, Cala O, et al. Successful treatment of a patient with a thymoma and pure red cell aplasia with octreotide and prednisone. *N Engl J Med* 1997;336:263.
71. Maggi G, Casadio C, Cavallo A, et al. Thymoma: results of 241 operated cases. *Ann Thorac Surg* 1991;51:152.
72. Wilkins EW, Grillo HC, Scannell G, Moncure AC, Mathisen DJ. Role of staging in prognosis and management of thymoma. *Ann Thorac Surg* 1991;51:888.
73. McCart JA, Gaspar L, Inculet R, Casson AG. Predictors of survival following surgical resection of thymoma. *J Surg Oncol* 1993;54:233.
74. Haniuda M, Marimoto M, Nishimura H, et al. Adjuvant radiotherapy after complete resection of thymoma. *Ann Thorac Surg* 1992;54:311.
75. Shimizu N, Moriyama S, Aoe M, et al. The surgical treatment of invasive thymoma: resection with vascular reconstruction. *J Thorac Cardiovasc Surg* 1992;103:414.
76. Pollack A, Komaki R, Cox JD, et al. Thymoma: treatment and prognosis. *Int J Radiol Oncol Biol Phys* 1992;23:1037.
77. Cowen D, Mornex RF, Bachelot T, et al. Thymoma: results of a multicentric retrospective series of 149 non-metastatic irradiated patients and review of the literature. *Radiother Oncol* 1995;34:9.
78. Kaiser LR. Thymoma: the use of minimally invasive resection techniques. *Chest Surg Clin North Am* 1994;4:185.
79. Nakahara K, Ohno K, Hashimoto J, et al. Thymoma: results of complete resection and adjuvant postoperative irradiation in 141 consecutive patients. *J Thorac Cardiovasc Surg* 1988;95:1041.
80. Ciernik IF, Meier U, Lutolf UM. Prognostic factors and outcome of incompletely resected invasive thymoma following radiation therapy. *J Clin Oncol* 1994;12:1484.
81. Ichinose Y, Ohta M, Yano T, et al. Treatment of invasive thymoma with pleural dissemination. *J Surg Oncol* 1993;54:180.
82. Kirschner PA. Reoperation for thymoma: report of 23 cases. *Ann Thorac Surg* 1990;49:550.
83. Urgesi A, Monetti U, Rossi G, et al. Aggressive treatment of intrathoracic recurrences of thymoma. *Radiother Oncol* 1992;24:221.
84. Crucitti F, Daghetto GB, Bellantone R, et al. Effects of surgical treatment in thymoma with myasthenia gravis: our experience in 103 patients. *J Surg Oncol* 1992;50:43.
85. Jackson MA, Ball DL. Postoperative radiotherapy in invasive thymoma. *Radiother Oncol* 1991;21:77.
86. Curran WJ, Kornstein MJ, Brooks JJ, Turrisi AT. Invasive thymoma: the role of mediastinal irradiation following complete or incomplete surgical resection. *J Clin Oncol* 1988;6:1722.
87. Koh WJ, Loehrer PJ Sr, Thomas CR Jr. Thymoma: the role of radiation and chemotherapy. In: Wood DE, Thomas CR Jr, eds. *Mediastinal tumors: update 1995. Medical radiology-diagnostic imaging and radiation oncology volume.* Heidelberg, Germany: Springer-Verlag, 1995:19.
88. Wilkins EW Jr. Thymoma: surgical management. In: Wood DE, Thomas CR Jr, eds. *Mediastinal tumors: update 1995. Medical radiology-diagnostic imaging and radiation oncology volume.* Heidelberg, Germany: Springer-Verlag, 1995:11.
89. Quintanilla-Martinez L, Wilkins EW Jr, Ferry JA, et al. Thymoma: morphologic subclassification correlates with invasiveness and immunohistologic features. A study of 122 cases. *Hum Pathol* 1993;24:958.
90. Harris N. Classification of thymic epithelial neoplasms. In: Marx A, Muller-Hermelink HK, eds. *Epithelial tumors of the thymus. Pathology, biology, treatment.* New York: Plenum Publishing, 1997:1.
91. Haniuda M, Morimoto M, Nishimura H, et al. Adjuvant radiotherapy after complete resection of thymoma. *Ann Thorac Surg* 1992;54:311.
92. Haniuda M, Miyazawa M, Yoshida K, et al. Is postoperative radiotherapy for thymoma effective? *Ann Surg* 1996;224:219.
93. Maggi G, Giaccone G, Donadio M, et al. Thymomas: a review of 169 cases, with particular reference to results of surgical treatment. *Cancer* 1986;58:765.
94. Mornex F, Resbeut M, Richard P, et al. Radiotherapy and chemotherapy for invasive thymomas: a multicentric retrospective review of 90 cases. *Int J Radiat Oncol Biol Phys* 1995;32:651.
95. Latz D, Schraube P, Oppitz U, et al. Invasive thymoma: treatment with postoperative radiation therapy. *Radiology* 1997;204:859.
96. Leung JT. The role of radiotherapy in thymomas. *Aust Radiol* 1996;40:430.
97. Graham MV, Emami B. Mediastinum and trachea. In: Perez CA, Brady LW, eds. *Principles and practice of radiation oncology,* 3rd ed. Philadelphia: Lippincott–Raven Publishers, 1997:1221.

98. Roach M III, Vijayakumar S. The role of three-dimensional conformal radiotherapy in the treatment of mediastinal tumors. In: Wood DE, Thomas CR Jr, eds. *Mediastinal tumors: update 1995. Medical radiology-diagnostic imaging and radiation oncology volume.* Heidelberg, Germany: Springer-Verlag, 1995:117.
99. Marks LB. The impact of organ structure on radiation response. *Int J Radiat Oncol Biol Phys* 1996;34:1165.
100. Thomas CR Jr, Williams TE, Turrisi AT III. Lung toxicity in the treatment of lung cancer: thoughts at the end of the millennium. In: Meyer J, Karger T, eds. *Radiation injury: prevention and treatment. Frontiers of radiation therapy and oncology.* Basel, Switzerland: Karger Medical and Scientific Publishers, 1999.
101. Yoshida H, Yasuda S, Aruga T, et al. [Whole mediastinal irradiation with or without entire hemithoracic irradiation for invasive thymoma]. *Nippon Igaku Hoshasen Gakkai Zasshi* 1995;55:968.
102. Bogart J, Sagerman RH. High-dose hemithorax irradiation in a patient with recurrent thymoma: a study of pulmonary and cardiac radiation tolerance. *Am J Clin Oncol* 1999;22:441.
103. Tomiak EM, Evans WK. The role of chemotherapy in invasive thymoma: a review of the literature and considerations for future clinical trials. *Crit Rev Oncol Hematol* 1993;15:113.
104. Bonami PD, Finkelstein D, Aisner S, Ettinger D. EST 2582 phase II trial of cisplatin in metastatic or recurrent thymoma. *Am J Clin Oncol* 1993;16:342.
105. Harper P, Highly M, Rankin E, et al. The treatment of malignant thymoma with single agent ifosfamide. *Br J Cancer* 1991;63[Suppl 13]:7.
106. Kirkove C, Berghmans J, Noel H, Van de Merckt J. Dramatic response of recurrent invasive thymoma to high dose corticosteroids. *Clin Oncol* 1992;4:64.
107. Fornasiero A, Danilele O, Ghiotto C, et al. Chemotherapy for invasive thymoma: a 13 year experience. *Cancer* 1991;68:30.
108. Loehrer PJ, Kim KM, Aisner SC, et al. Cisplatin plus doxorubicin plus cyclophosphamide in metastatic or recurrent thymoma: final results of an intergroup trial. *J Clin Oncol* 1994;12:1164.
109. Park HS, Shin DM, Lee JS, et al. Thymoma: a retrospective study of 87 cases. *Cancer* 1994;73:2491.
110. Giaccone G, Ardizzoni A, Kirkpatrick A, et al. Cisplatin and etoposide combination chemotherapy for locally advanced or metastatic thymoma: a phase II study of the European Organization for Research and Treatment of Lung Cancer Cooperative Group. *J Clin Oncol* 1996;14:814.
111. Loehrer PJ, Jiroutek M, Aisner S, et al. Phase II trial of etoposide (V), ifosfamide (I), plus cisplatin (P) in patients with advanced thymoma (T) or thymic carcinoma (TC): preliminary results from a ECOG coordinated intergroup trial. *Proc Am Soc Clin Oncol* 1998;17:30(abst 118).
112. Rea F, Sartori F, Lay M, et al. Chemotherapy and operation for invasive thymoma. *J Cardiovasc Surg* 1993;106:543.
113. Macchiarini P, Chella A, Ducci F, et al. Neoadjuvant chemotherapy, surgery and postoperative radiation therapy for invasive thymoma. *Cancer* 1991;68:706.
114. Shin DM, Walsh GL, Komaki R, et al. A multidisciplinary approach to therapy for unresectable malignant thymoma. *Ann Intern Med* 1998;129:100.
115. Loehrer PJ Sr, Chen M, Kim KM, et al. Cisplatin, doxorubicin, and cyclophosphamide plus thoracic radiation therapy for limited-stage unresectable thymoma: an intergroup trial. *J Clin Oncol* 1997;15:3093.
116. Bernatz PE, Harrison EG, Clagget OT. Thymomas: a clinicopathologic study. *J Thorac Cardiovasc Surg* 1961;42:424.
117. Muller-Hermelink HK, Marx A, Gender K, Kirchner T. The pathological basis of thymoma-associated myasthenia gravis. *Ann N Y Acad Sci* 1993;681:56.
118. Tsuchida M, Yamato Y, Souma T, et al. Efficacy and safety of extended thymectomy for elderly patients with myasthenia gravis. *Ann Thorac Surg* 1999;67:1563.
119. Nieto IP, Robledo JP, Pajuelo MC, et al. Prognostic factors for myasthenia gravis treated by thymectomy: review of 61 cases. *Ann Thorac Surg* 1999;67:1568.
120. Suster S, Rosai J. Thymic carcinoma: a clinicopathologic study of 60 cases. *Cancer* 1991;67:1025.
121. Wick MR, Scheithauer BW, Weiland LH, Barnatz PE. Primary thymic carcinomas. *Am J Surg Pathol* 1982;6:613.
122. Hsu CP, Chan CY, Chen CL, et al. Thymic carcinoma: ten years' experience in twenty patients. *J Thorac Cardiovasc Surg* 1994;107:615.
123. Weide LG, Ulbright TM, Loehrer PJ, Williams SD. Thymic carcinoma: a distinct clinical entity responsive to chemotherapy. *Cancer* 1993;71:1219.
124. Yano T, Hara N, Ichinose Y, et al. Treatment and prognosis of primary thymic carcinoma. *J Surg Oncol* 1993;52:255.
125. Shimizu J, Hayashi Y, Monita K, et al. Primary thymic carcinoma: a clinicopathological and immunohistochemical study. *J Surg Oncol* 1994;56:159.
126. Levine GD, Rosai J. Thymic hyperplasia and neoplasia: a review of current concepts. *Hum Pathol* 1978;9:495.
127. Suster S, Moran CA. Spindle cell thymic carcinoma: clinicopathologic and immunohistochemical study of a distinctive variant of primary thymic epithelial neoplasm. *Am J Surg Pathol* 1999;23:681.
128. Rosai J, Higa E. Mediastinal endocrine neoplasm of probable thymic origin related to carcinoid tumors. *Cancer* 1972;29:1061.
129. Wang DY, Chang DB, Kuo SH, et al. Carcinoid tumors of the thymus. *Thorax* 1994;49:33.
130. Vietri F, Illuminati R, Guglielmi R, et al. Carcinoid tumor of the thymus gland. *Eur J Surg* 1994;160:645.
131. Asbun HJ, Calabria RP, Calmes S, Lang AG, Bloch JH. Thymic carcinoid. *Am Surg* 1991;57:442.
132. Zeiger MA, Swartz SE, Macgillivary DC, Linnoila I, Shakir M. Thymic carcinoid in association with MEN syndromes. *Am Surg* 1992;58:430.
133. McManus KG, Allen MS, Trastek VF, et al. Lipothymoma with red cell aplasia, hypogammaglobulinemia and lichen planus. *Ann Thorac Surg* 1994;58:1534.
134. Rosado-de-Christenson ML, Pugatch RD, Moran CA, Galobardes J. Thymolipoma: analysis of 27 cases. *Radiology* 1994;193:121.
135. Litano Y, Yokomari K, Ohkura M, et al. Giant thymolipoma in a child. *J Pediatr Surg* 1993;28:1622.
136. Luna M, Valenzuela-Tamaritz J. Germ cell tumors of the mediastinum: postmortem findings. *Am J Clin Pathol* 1976;65:450.
137. Nichols CR, Fox EP. Extra-gonadal and pediatric germ cell tumors. *Hematol Oncol Clin North Am* 1991;5:1189.
138. Kuhn M, Weissbach L. Localization, incidence, diagnosis and treatment of extratesticular germ cell tumors. *Urol Int* 1985;40:166.
139. Dulmet EM, Macchiarini P, Suc B, Verley J. Germ cell tumors of the mediastinum: a 30 year experience. *Cancer* 1993;72:1994.
140. Lemarie E, Assouline PS, Diot P, et al. Primary mediastinal germ cell tumors: results of a French retrospective study. *Chest* 1992;102:1477.
141. Knapp R, Hurt R, Payne W, et al. Malignant germ cell tumors of the mediastinum. *J Thorac Cardiovasc Surg* 1985;89:82.
142. Lewis BD, Hurt RD, Payne WS, et al. Benign teratomas of the mediastinum. *J Thorac Cardiovasc Surg* 1983;86:727.
143. Hainsworth JD, Greco FA. Extragonadal germ cell tumors and unrecognized germ cell tumors. *Semin Oncol* 1992;19:119.
144. Ginsberg RJ. Mediastinal germ cell tumors: the role of surgery. *Semin Thorac Cardiovasc Surg* 1992;4:51.
145. Giaccone G. Multimodality treatment of malignant germ cell tumors of the mediastinum. *Eur J Cancer* 1991;27:273.
146. Schultz S, Einhorn L, Conces D, et al. Management of residual mass in patients with advanced seminoma: Indiana University experience. *J Clin Oncol* 1989;7:1497.
147. Schultz SM, Einhorn LH, Conces D, et al. Management of postchemotherapy residual mass in patients with advanced seminoma: Indiana University experience. *J Clin Oncol* 1989;7:1497.
148. Horwich A, Paluchowska B, Norman A, et al. Residual mass following chemotherapy of seminoma. *Ann Oncol* 1997;8:37.
149. Miller KD, Loehrer PJ, Gonin R, et al. Salvage chemotherapy with vinblastine, ifosfamide, and cisplatin in recurrent seminoma. *J Clin Oncol* 1997;15:1427.
150. International Germ Cell Collaborative Group. International germ cell consensus classification: a prognostic factor–based staging system for metastatic germ cell cancers. *J Clin Oncol* 1997;15:594.
151. Loehrer PJ, Gonin R, Nichols CR, et al. Vinblastine plus ifosfamide plus cisplatin as initial salvage therapy in recurrent germ cell tumor. *J Clin Oncol* 1998;16:2500.
152. Motzer RJ, Gulati SC, Tang WP, et al. Phase I trial with pharmacokinetic analyses of high dose carboplatin, etoposide and cyclophosphamide with autologous bone marrow transplantation in patients with refractory germ cell tumors. *Cancer Res* 1993;53:3730.
153. Broun ER, Nichols CR, Einhorn LH, Tricot GJK. Salvage therapy with high dose chemotherapy and autologous bone marrow support in the treatment of primary non-seminomatous mediastinal germ cell tumors. *Cancer* 1991;68:1513.
154. Mack TM. Sarcomas and other malignancies of soft tissue, retroperitoneum, peritoneum, pleura, heart, mediastinum, and spleen. *Cancer* 1995;75:211.
155. Cohen AJ, Sbaschnig RJ, Hochholzer L, Cough FC, Albus RA. Mediastinal hemangiomas. *Ann Thorac Surg* 1987;43:656.
156. Worthy SA, Gholkar A, Walls TJ, Todd NV. Case report: multiple thoracic hemangiomas: a rare cause of spinal cord compression. *Br J Radiol* 1995;68:770.
157. Chavez-Espinosa UI, Chavez-Fernandez JA, Hoyer OH, et al. Endothoracic neurogenic neoplasms (analysis of 30 cases). *Rev Int Radiol* 1980;5:49.
158. Davidson KG, Walbaum PR, McCormack RJM. Intrathoracic neural tumors. *Thorax* 1978;33:359.
159. Gale AW, Jelihovsky T, Grant AF, et al. Neurogenic tumors of the mediastinum. *Ann Thorac Surg* 1974;17:434.
160. Marchevsky AM, Kaneko M. Surgical pathology of the mediastinum. New York: Raven Press, 1984:256.
161. Adams GA, Shochat SJ, Smith EL, et al. Thoracic neuroblastoma: a pediatric oncology group study. *J Pediatr Surg* 1993;28:372.
162. Boyd W. *Pathology for the surgeon,* 7th ed. Philadelphia: WB Saunders, 1955:487.
163. Wick MR, Sterenberg SS. *Diagnostic surgical pathology.* New York: Raven Press, 1994:1141.
164. Chalmers AH, Armstrong P. Plexiform mediastinal neurofibromas: a report of two cases. *Br J Radiol* 1977;50:215.
165. Von Recklinghausen FD. Ueber die multiplen fibrome der haut und ihre beziehung zu den multiplen neuromen. Festschrift zur Fierdes Fünfundzwaazigjährigen Bestehens des Pathologischen Instituts za Berlin Herrn Rud. IF Virchow Berlin: A. Hirschwald, 1882 (est. 1982).
166. Enzinger FM, Weiss SW. *Soft tissue tumors.* St. Louis: Mosby, 1983.
167. Crose FW, Schull WJ, Neel JV. *A clinical, pathological, and genetic study of multiple neurofibromatosis.* Springfield, IL: Charles C Thomas Publisher, 1956.
168. Brasfield RD, Das Gupta TK. Von Recklinghausen's disease: a clinical pathologic study. *Ann Surg* 1972;175:1986.
169. Guccion JG, Enzinger FM. Malignant Schwannoma associated with von Recklinghausen's neurofibromatosis. *Virchows Arch A Pathol Anat Histol* 1979;383:43.
170. Akwari OE, Payne WS, Onforio BM, et al. Dumbbell neurogenic tumors of the mediastinum. *Mayo Clin Proc* 1978;53:353.
171. Woodruff JM. Peripheral nerve tumors showing glandular differentiation. *Cancer* 1976;37:2399.
172. MacKay B, Osborne BM. The contribution of electron microscopy to the diagnoses of tumors. *Pathobiology annual,* vol 8. New York: Raven Press, 1978:359.
173. Adam A, Hochholzer L. Ganglioneuroblastoma of the posterior mediastinum: a clinicopathologic review of 80 cases. *Cancer* 1981;47:373.
174. Hamilton JP, Koop CE. Ganglioneuromas in children. *Surg Gynecol Obstet* 1965;121:803.
175. McRae D Jr, Shaw A. Ganglioneuroma, heterochromia iridis, and Horner's syndrome. *J Pediatr Surg* 1979;14:612.

176. Bar-Ziv J, Nogrady MB. Mediastinal neuroblastoma and ganglioneuroma: the differentiation between primary and secondary involvement on the chest roentgenogram. *AJR Am J Roentgenol* 1975;125:380.
177. DeLorimier AA, Bragg KU, Linden G. Neuroblastoma in childhood. *Am J Dis Child* 1969;118:441.
178. Robinson MG, McCorquodale MM. Trisomy 18 and neurogenic neoplasia. *J Pediatr* 1981;99:428.
179. Evans AE, D'Angio GJ, Koop CE. Diagnosis and treatment of neuroblastoma. *Pediatr Clin North Am* 1976;23:161.
180. Fortner J, Nicastri A, Murphy ML. Neuroblastoma: natural history and results of treating 133 cases. *Ann Surg* 1968;167:132.
181. Rosenbloom PM, Barrows GH, Kmetz DR, et al. Granular cell myoblastoma arising from the thoracic sympathetic nerve chain. *J Pediatr Surg* 1975;10:819.
182. Hall RJ, McAllister HA Jr, Cooley DA, et al. Tumors of the heart. In: Cohn J, Willerson JT, eds. *Cardiovascular medicine.* New York: Churchill Livingstone, 1995:1525.
183. Thomas CR Jr, DeVries B, Bitran JD, et al. Cardiac neoplasms. In: Wood DE, Thomas CR Jr, eds. *Mediastinal tumors: update 1995. Medical radiology-diagnostic imaging and radiation oncology volume.* Heidelberg, Germany: Springer-Verlag, 1995:79.
184. Chen HZ, Jiang L, Rong WH, et al. Tumours of the heart. An analysis of 79 cases. *Chin Med J* 1992;105:153.
185. McAllister HA. Primary tumors and cysts of the heart and pericardium. *Curr Probl Cardiol* 1979;4:8.
186. Raaf HN, Raaf JH. Sarcomas related to the heart and vasculature. *Semin Surg Oncol* 1994;10:374.
187. Stein M, Deitling F, Cantor A, et al. Primary cardiac angiosarcoma: a case report and review of therapeutic options. *Med Pediatr Oncol* 1994;23:149.
188. Han P, Drachtman RA, Amenta P, Ettinger LJ. Successful treatment of a primary cardiac leiomyosarcoma with ifosfamide and etoposide. *J Pediatr Hematol Oncol* 1996;18:314.
189. Jyothirmayi R, Jacob R, Nair K, Rajan B. Primary fibrosarcoma of the right ventricle—a case report. *Acta Oncol* 1995;34:972.
190. Llombart-Cussac A, Pivot X, Contesso G, et al. Adjuvant chemotherapy for primary cardiac sarcomas: the IGR experience. *Br J Cancer* 1998;78:1624.
191. Thomason R, Schlegel W, Lucca M, et al. Primary malignant mesothelioma of the pericardium: case report and literature review. *Texas Heart Inst* 1994;21:170.
192. Teramoto N, Hayashi K, Miyatani K, et al. Malignant fibrous histiocytoma of the right ventricle of the heart. *Pathol Int* 1995;45:315.
193. Hermann MA, Shankerman RA, Edwards WD, et al. Primary cardiac angiosarcoma: a clinicopathologic study of six cases. *J Thorac Cardiovasc Surg* 1992;103:655.
194. Thomas CR Jr, Johnson GW Jr, Stoddard MF, et al. Primary malignant cardiac tumors: update 1992. *Med Pediatr Oncol* 1992;20:519.
195. Baat P, Karwande SV, Kushner JP, et al. Successful treatment of a cardiac angiosarcoma with combined modality therapy. *J Heart Lung Transplant* 1994;13:923.
196. Michler RE, Goldstein DJ. Treatment of cardiac tumors by orthotopic cardiac transplantation. *Semin Oncol* 1997; 24:534.
197. Goldstein DJ, Oz MC, Rose EA, et al. Experience with heart transplantation for cardiac tumors. *J Heart Lung Transplant* 1995;14:382.
198. Nakamichi T, Fukuda T, Suzuki T, et al. Primary cardiac angiosarcoma: 53 months' survival after multidisciplinary therapy. *Ann Thorac Surg* 1997;63:1160.
199. Percy RF, Perryman RA, Amornmarn R, et al. Prolonged survival in a patient with primary angiosarcoma of the heart. *Am Heart J* 1987;113:1228.

CHAPTER **33**

Cancers of the Gastrointestinal Tract

SECTION **1** ERIC R. FEARON

Molecular Biology of Gastrointestinal Cancers

The specific etiologic factors and pathogenetic mechanisms underlying the development of cancers of the gastrointestinal tract appear to be complex and heterogeneous. Although likely etiologic factors include environmental and dietary exposures, defining specific agents that influence cancer risk remains a major challenge. Only limited progress has been made in treatment of patients with advanced gastrointestinal cancer. In light of the obstacles that hinder our ability to more effectively prevent and treat gastrointestinal cancers, it is important to recognize that increasingly significant advances have been made in the gastrointestinal cancer field. Arguably, some of the most encouraging advances have been successes in defining the specific genetic defects that underlie inherited forms of gastrointestinal cancer and in gaining new insights into the constellation of molecular alterations present in sporadic tumors. For most gastrointestinal tumor types, the prevalence and nature of mutations in several distinct oncogenes and tumor suppressor genes have been defined. The conversion of cellular protooncogenes into oncogenic variant alleles (gene copies) can result from specific point mutations or rearrangements that alter gene structure and function or from chromosomal rearrangements or gene amplifications that disrupt regulated expression of the protooncogene. Tumor suppressor gene inactivation can result from localized mutations, complete loss of the gene, or via epigenetic alterations that interfere with gene expression. At present, only somatic (arising in nongerm cells during the patient's lifetime) mutations in protooncogenes have been detected in gastrointestinal cancers. Similarly, the vast majority of tumor suppressor gene mutations are also somatic. Nevertheless, germline (constitutional) mutations in tumor suppressor genes do underlie cancer predisposition in several hereditary gastrointestinal cancer syndromes.

It is not possible to present in this chapter an exhaustive summary detailing the molecular alterations present in each gastrointestinal cancer type. Rather, the focus is on molecular defects in colorectal carcinoma. The basis for this focus is several-fold. Colorectal cancer is the most common gastrointestinal cancer type in the United States and several other regions of the world. Understanding of colorectal cancer molecular biology is generally more advanced than that of other gastrointestinal cancer types, although significant progress has been made on the molecular front in esophageal, gastric, pancreatic, and hepatocellular cancer. Some of the frequent genetic alterations in colorectal carcinomas are also common in other gastrointestinal cancers. Furthermore, study of the multiple genetic alterations that accumulate during the adenoma-carcinoma sequence in the colon has nicely illustrated the means by which multiple genetic alterations underlie tumor initiation and progression in other organ sites. Although the focus of this chapter is on colorectal cancer, selected advances in the molecular biology of pancreatic and esophageal cancer also are highlighted. The main objectives of this chapter are to review the following: (1) the genetic basis of two inherited forms of colorectal cancer; (2) some of the frequent molecular abnormalities in colorectal tumors; (3) common molecular abnormalities in pancreatic and esophageal cancer; and (4) the potential clinical utility of genetic alterations in early detection and clinical management of gastrointestinal cancer.

COLORECTAL CANCER AS A MODEL SYSTEM

In 2000, approximately 140,000 U.S. residents will be diagnosed with colorectal cancer, and roughly 55,000 will die from the disease.[1] Males and females have a nearly equal likelihood of being diagnosed, and the cumulative lifetime risk of colorectal cancer in the United States is 6%, with an average age of 66 years at diagnosis. Individuals with a family history of colorectal cancer in a first-degree relative, but who otherwise lack clinical features or a family history consistent with a highly penetrant colorectal cancer syndrome [e.g., familial adenomatous polyposis (FAP) or hereditary nonpolyposis colorectal cancer (HNPCC)], are approximately twice as likely to develop colorectal cancer as those without a family history.[2–5] Other risk factors for colorectal cancer include older age, inflammatory bowel disease, a diet high in fat and animal proteins, and a sedentary lifestyle.[2] Many other exposures, including excess alcohol consumption, smoking, aspirin and nonsteroidal antiinflammatory agent use, and specific dietary components (e.g., micronutrients such as calcium and selenium), have been extensively studied for their effects on colorectal cancer risk.[6–21] However, these exposures remain uncertain risk factors. The reality is that the main dietary and environmental factors that contribute to most colorectal cancers are poorly defined, and perhaps 75% of all incident colorectal cancers arise in people with no well-defined risk factor. On the other hand, many colorectal cancers may be preventable, and improved adoption and implementation of current screening recommendations might save up to 30,000 lives per year.[22]

THE ADENOMA-CARCINOMA SEQUENCE IN THE COLON

A variety of benign gastrointestinal tumors have been identified, but a generic term for a localized lesion projecting above the surrounding mucosa is *polyp.* Most colorectal polyps, particularly small polyps, are of hyperplastic type, and most data indicate hyperplastic polyps are not a precursor to cancer. The adenomatous polyp, or adenoma, is generally thought to be the important precursor lesion to cancer. Adenomas arise from glandular epithelium, and their common features are the dysplastic morphology and abnormal differentiation of the epithelial cells in the lesion. The prevalence of adenomas in the United States is approximately 25% by age 50 years and perhaps 50% by age 70.[22] The notion that most colorectal carcinomas arise from an adenomatous precursor is well supported. First, longitudinal studies have shown a high risk of colorectal cancer development in individuals whose adenomas are not removed,[23,24] and polypectomy decreases colorectal cancer risk.[25] Second, foci of carcinoma can often be detected in adenomatous polyps, and residual regions of adenomatous glands are often noted in carcinoma specimens.[26–28] Third, individuals affected by syndromes that strongly predispose to the development of adenomas, such as FAP (discussed later in Familial Adenomatous Polyposis and the APC Gene), invariably develop colorectal carcinomas by the third to fifth decades of life if their colons are not removed.[29,30] Nevertheless, only a fraction of adenomas progress to cancer, and progression probably occurs over a period measured in years to decades. Adenomas larger than 1 cm in size are estimated to have a 15% chance of progressing to carcinoma over a 10-year period.[31]

Besides adenomatous polyp development, another clinical situation associated with markedly increased colorectal carcinoma risk is ulcerative colitis (UC). Patients with longstanding and severe UC have a 20-fold or greater increase in colorectal cancer risk compared to the general population.[32,33] It is generally thought that carcinomas arise in UC patients as a result of chronic cycles of mucosal injury and subsequent regrowth, a situation that may bear some similarity to processes underlying the development of some esophageal, gastric, and pancreatic cancers. Possible cancer precursors in patients with UC include dysplasia and flat adenomatous plaques.[28] The relationship of these presumptive precursors to one another and to the villous regeneration seen in UC patients as well as the relative risks of progression of the lesion types are less well defined than the adenoma-carcinoma sequence.

INHERITED COLORECTAL CANCER SYNDROMES

Highly penetrant, inherited predisposition syndromes are estimated to account for only approximately 5% of colorectal cancers.[30] Hereditary syndromes predisposing to colorectal cancer include FAP and HNPCC. Other rare syndromes also associated with an increased, but less clearly defined, risk of colorectal or other gastrointestinal cancers include Peutz-Jeghers syndrome, Cowden disease, and juvenile polyposis syndrome. The genes responsible for these inherited syndromes have been identified (Table 33.1-1). Consistent with the Knudson two-hit model for tumor suppressor genes, in all cases, inactivating mutations in both alleles are present in the cancers that arise in affected individuals. However, these other cancer predisposition syndromes are rarer than FAP and HNPCC, and with the exception of the *DPC4* (deleted in pancreatic cancer locus 4) gene, defects in the other familial gastrointestinal cancer genes do not appear to contribute to sporadic cases of colorectal cancer. For these reasons, the discussion here focuses on FAP and HNPCC.

FAMILIAL ADENOMATOUS POLYPOSIS AND THE ADENOMATOUS POLYPOSIS COLI GENE

FAP is an autosomal dominant syndrome affecting approximately 1 in 8000 individuals and accounting for approximately 0.5% of all colorectal cancers.[29,30] Hundreds to thousands of adenomas arise in the colon and rectum of affected individuals by the third to fourth decades of life, and the lifetime incidence of colorectal cancer in untreated FAP patients approaches 100%. Several variants of FAP have been described, including Gardner's syndrome, in which affected individuals may manifest extensive polyposis, epidermoid cysts, desmoid tumors, and osteomas; and Turcot's syndrome, in which polyposis and brain tumors can be seen. Fam-

TABLE 33.1-1. Genetics of Inherited Colorectal Tumor Syndromes

Syndrome	*Features Commonly Seen in Affected Individuals*	*Gene Defect*
Familial adenomatous polyposis	Multiple adenomatous polyps (>100) and carcinomas of the colon and rectum; duodenal polyps and carcinomas; fundic gland polyps in the stomach; congenital hypertrophy of retinal pigment epithelium	*APC*
Gardner's syndrome	Same as familial adenomatous polyposis; also desmoid tumors and mandibular osteomas	*APC*
Turcot's syndrome	Polyposis and colorectal cancer with brain tumors (medulloblastoma)	*APC*
	Colorectal cancer and brain tumors (glioblastoma)	*MLH1, PMS2*
Attenuated adenomatous polyposis coli	Fewer than 100 polyps, although marked variation in polyp number (from ~5 to >1000 polyps) seen in mutation carriers within a single family	*APC* gene (predominantly 5' mutations)
Hereditary nonpolyposis colorectal cancer	Colorectal cancer without extensive polyposis; other cancers include endometrial, ovarian, and stomach cancer; occasionally urothelial, hepatobiliary, and brain tumors	*MSH2, MLH1, PMS1, PMS2, MSH6/GTBP,* ? TGF-β type IIR, other genes
Peutz-Jeghers syndrome	Hamartomatous polyps throughout the gastrointestinal tract; mucocutaneous pigmentation; estimated 9- to 13-fold increased risk of GI and non-GI cancers	*LKB1/STK11*
Cowden disease	Multiple hamartomas involving breast, thyroid, skin, central nervous system, and GI tract; increased risk of breast and thyroid cancer; risk of GI cancer is poorly defined	*PTEN*
Juvenile polyposis syndrome	Multiple hamartomatous/juvenile polyps with predominance in colon and stomach; increase in colorectal and stomach cancer risk is poorly defined	*DPC4; PTEN;* other genes

GI, gastrointestinal; TGF-β type IIR, transforming growth factor-β type II receptor.

ilies with attenuated forms of FAP (termed *attenuated adenomatous polyposis coli*) also have been described in which some affected individuals have only 10 to 20 adenomas by 50 years of age. The gene that, when mutant, underlies FAP, Gardner's syndrome, and other variants is the adenomatous polyposis coli (*APC*) tumor suppressor gene on chromosome 5q.[34]

APC is a large gene encoding a protein of 2843 amino acids, and its last exon is remarkable because it contains a 6579-base-pair open reading frame.[34,35] Although a fraction of germline mutations in FAP patients extinguish *APC* gene expression, more than 95% of the known mutations lead to premature truncation of APC protein synthesis. The mutations are located predominantly in the 5' half of the gene, and two "hot spots" at codons 1061 and 1309 account for approximately 35% of the germline mutations identified (Fig. 33.1-1).[35] Some phenotypic variation among those with FAP appears to be because of the specific mutant *APC* allele present.[34] In spite of the genotype-phenotype associations noted, however, patients with identical *APC* mutations can display distinct clinical features. For instance, some patients with germline mutations between *APC* codons 1403 and 1578 manifest Gardner's syndrome features, whereas others with the identical mutation do not. Similarly, despite the fact FAP patients have a greatly increased risk of medulloblastoma and an elevated risk of hepatoblastoma and thyroid cancers, only a subset of individuals within any one kindred manifests these tumors.

Somatic Adenomatous Polyposis Coli Mutations in Sporadic Tumors

Notwithstanding the *APC* gene's critical role in FAP, the gene has an even more prominent role in sporadic colorectal tumors. Roughly 80% of sporadic colorectal adenomas and carcinomas have somatic mutations inactivating *APC*.[34,35] The nature and distribution of *APC* somatic mutations are similar to the germline mutations in FAP patients (see Fig. 33.1-1), with nearly all somatic mutations leading to premature truncation of the APC protein.[35] The data suggest somatic *APC* mutations are an early and likely rate-limiting event in adenoma development. First, *APC* mutations have essentially the same frequency in small adenomas as advanced adenomas and carcinomas,[34,35] in contrast to other somatically mutated genes in colorectal tumors, such as K-*ras* and *p53*. Second, somatic *APC* mutations are found in the earliest lesions analyzed, including microscopic adenomas composed of only a few dysplastic glands. As predicted by the Knudson model, both *APC* alleles appear to be inactivated in most colorectal adenomas and all colorectal carcinomas. *APC* somatic mutations are infrequent in tumor types other than colorectal carcinomas,[34,35] with the possible exception of ampullary carcinomas and desmoid tumors.[36–38]

Adenomatous Polyposis Coli Protein Function

The APC protein has been suggested to regulate cell-cell adhesion, cell migration, or possibly apoptosis.[34,35,39] Presently, perhaps the best-characterized function of the APC protein is regulation of β-catenin. β-Catenin, an abundant cellular protein, was first identified because of its role in linking the cytoplasmic domain of the E-cadherin cell-cell adhesion molecule to the cortical actin cytoskeleton, via β-catenin's binding to α-catenin. The truncated (mutant) forms of the APC protein present in most colorectal carcinomas lack sequences crucial for binding β-catenin and other cellular proteins (see Fig. 33.1-1).

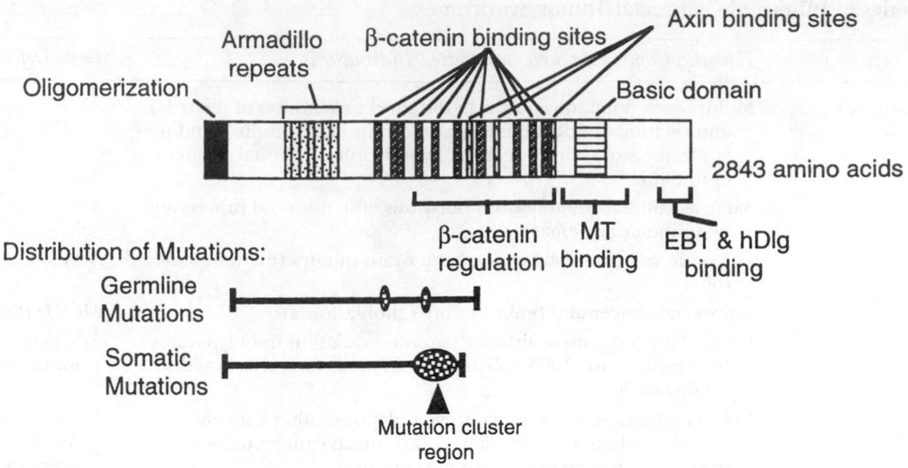

FIGURE 33.1-1. Schematic representation of adenomatous polyposis coli (APC) protein functional domains with respect to germline and somatic mutations. A putative domain involved in homo-oligomerization (?dimerization) of APC is located at the amino-terminus. Also noted are a series of repeats of unknown function with similarity to the *Drosophila* armadillo protein; sequences known to mediate binding to β-catenin and axin and regulate β-catenin's abundance and localization; a basic domain in the carboxy terminal third of the protein that appears to facilitate complexing with microtubules (MT), and sequences near the carboxy terminus of APC that interact with the EB1 protein and the human homologue of the *Drosophila* disc large (hDlg) protein. Germline mutations in the *APC* gene (predominantly chain-terminating) are dispersed throughout the 5' half of the sequence, with two apparent "hot spots" at codons 1061 and 1309. Somatic mutations in the *APC* gene in colorectal cancer appear to cluster in a region termed the *mutation cluster region*, and mutations at codons 1309 and 1450 are most common. (Modified from Fearon ER. Oncogenes and tumor suppressor genes. In: Abeloff MD, Armitage JO, Lichter AS, Niederhuber JE, eds. *Clinical oncology*, 2nd ed. New York: Churchill Livingstone, 2000:77, with permission.)

A model has been developed to explain the significance of APC's interaction with β-catenin and these other proteins (Fig. 33.1-2). The model indicates that, in collaboration with the glycogen synthase kinase-3 (GSK3) and axin proteins, APC regulates β-catenin's abundance in the cytoplasm and nucleus. In 75% to 80% of colorectal cancers, APC is mutated and unable to regulate β-catenin (see Fig. 33.1-2*B*). As a result, β-catenin accumulates in the cytoplasm and nucleus, and complexes with transcription factors of the Tcf (T-cell factor family), such as Tcf-4. On binding to Tcf proteins, β-catenin functions as a transcription co-activator, activating expression of Tcf-regulated genes. The identities and functions of Tcf-regulated target genes are not yet well understood, although they may include powerful stimulators of cell growth and proliferation (e.g., the *c-MYC* and *cyclin D1* genes) and extracellular proteases [e.g., matrix metalloprotease 7 (MMP-7)] that might facilitate invasion and metastasis.[40–43] Further compelling support for the notion that gene activation by the Tcf/β-catenin complex is critical in colorectal tumorigenesis includes the fact that, in a subset of the 20% of colorectal cancers lacking *APC* mutations, somatic mutations in β-catenin have been found.[44–46] These mutations are present in the phosphorylation consensus sequences near β-catenin's amino-terminus, and they appear to render mutant β-catenin proteins resistant to regulation by the APC/GSK3/axin complex. Consequently, β-catenin accumulates and activates Tcf-regulated genes (see Fig. 33.1-2*C*).

Variant Adenomatous Polyposis Coli Alleles and Familial Aggregations of Colorectal Cancer

In the majority of colorectal cancer patients, no definitive hereditary component can be identified. These cases are, therefore, labeled "sporadic." Nonetheless, some of these apparently sporadic cases may well have some hereditary component. The identification of genes that confer weak predisposition to colorectal cancer has been and will continue to be a difficult issue for the colorectal cancer field. One study has, however, provided fascinating insights into familial forms of colorectal cancer that do not manifest as highly penetrant cancer syndromes.[47] The study was initiated because of the identification of eight colorectal adenomas in a 39-year-old patient with a family history of colorectal cancer. The diagnosis of HNPCC was excluded by molecular analyses (the genetics of HNPCC is discussed in the section Hereditary Nonpolyposis Colorectal Cancer). Diagnosis of FAP was unlikely based on clinical findings. Nonetheless, detailed studies of the patient's *APC* alleles were carried out. No germline *APC* mutation of the type predicted to truncate the APC protein was identified. However, a sequence change at codon 1307 was found, resulting in a substitution of lysine (K) for isoleucine (I). Thus, the allele was referred to as the *APC* I1307K allele. The resultant amino acid change was not predicted to alter APC protein function. However, at the DNA sequence level, the variant allele had an extended mononucleotide tract in the coding region of $(A)_8$ instead of (AAATAAAA).

Further studies revealed that the I1307K allele was present only in individuals of Ashkenazi Jewish origin and that those who carried the I1307K allele had a twofold increase in their lifetime risk of colorectal cancer.[47] Moreover, the localized somatic *APC* mutations in colorectal cancers arising in individuals carrying the I1307K allele were nearly always small insertions or deletions in or adjacent to the $(A)_8$ mononucleotide repeat tract. The somatic mutations created frameshifts that lead to truncated APC proteins. Therefore, the I1307K allele appears to be a novel cancer predisposition allele that does not exert its effects by directly altering *APC* function. Rather, the I1307K allele contains a DNA sequence tract that is a more frequent target for somatic mutation in colonic epithelial cells

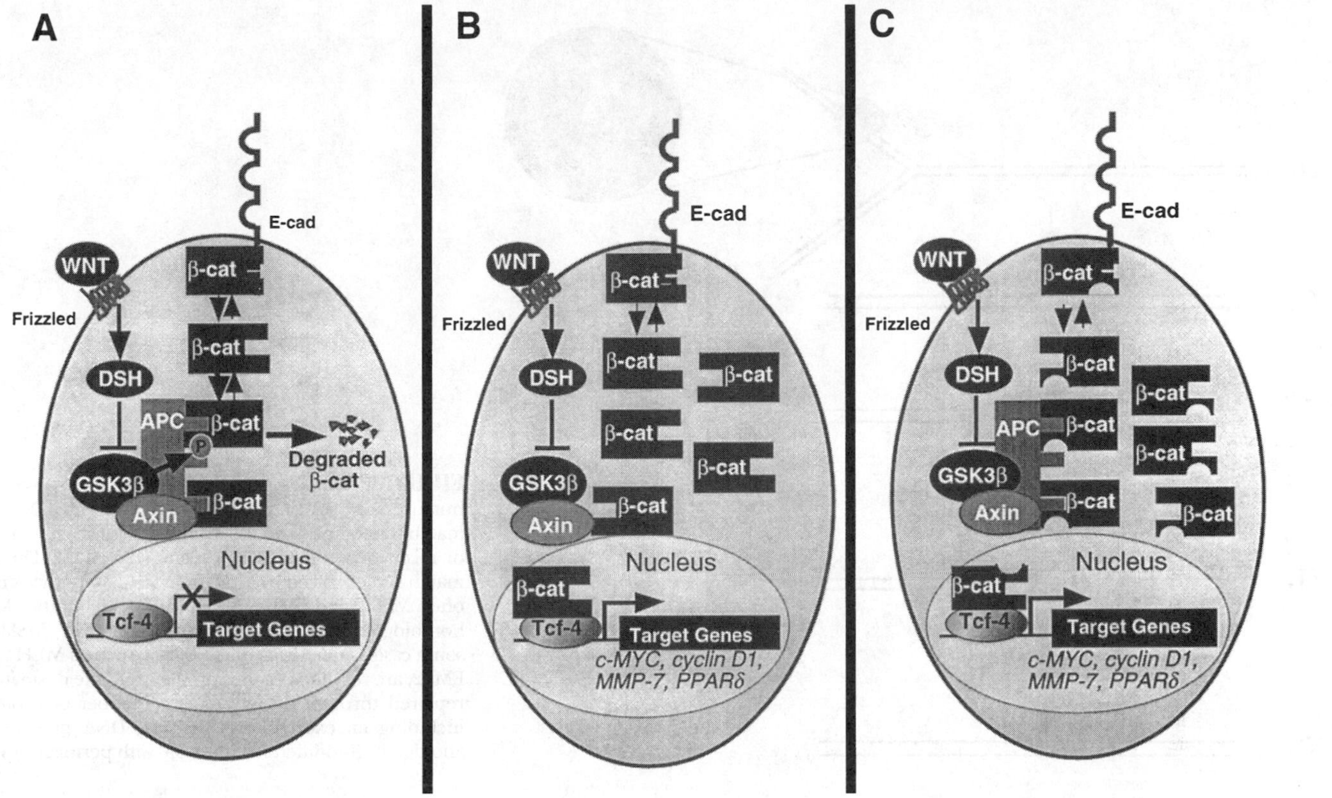

FIGURE 33.1-2. A model indicating the function of the adenomatous polyposis coli (APC), axin, and glycogen synthase kinase 3β (GSK3β) proteins in the regulation of β-catenin (β-cat) in normal cells, and the consequence of APC or β-cat defects in cancer cells. β-cat is an abundant cellular protein, and much of it is often bound to the cytoplasmic domain of the E-cadherin (E-cad) cell-cell adhesion protein. **A:** In normal cells, the proteins GSK3β, APC, and axin function to promote degradation of free cytosolic β-cat, probably as a result of phosphorylation of the N-terminal sequences of β-cat by GSK3β. GSK3β activity and β-cat degradation are inhibited by activation of the wingless (WNT) pathway, as a result of the action of the Frizzled receptor and disheveled (DSH) signaling protein. **B:** Mutation of APC in colorectal and other cancer cells results in accumulation of β-cat, binding to Tcf-4, and transcriptional activation of Tcf-4 target genes, such as *c-MYC*, *cyclin D1*, *MMP-7*, and *PPARδ* (see text). **C:** Point mutations and small deletions in β-cat in cancer cells inhibit phosphorylation and degradation of β-cat by GSK3β and APC, with resultant activation of *c-MYC* and other Tcf-4 target genes. (Modified from Fearon ER. Human cancer syndromes: clues to the origin and nature of cancer. *Science* 1997;278:1043, with permission.)

than the normal *APC* sequence. Future studies may establish that subtle or unconventional mutations in *APC* or other genes also contribute to gastrointestinal cancer predisposition by similar mechanisms.

HEREDITARY NONPOLYPOSIS COLORECTAL CANCER

HNPCC was first described by Warthin in 1913.[48] Roughly half a century later, Lynch and others described kindreds with autosomal dominant patterns of colorectal and other cancers that were not associated with extensive intestinal polyposis.[49,50] Before identification of the specific inherited mutations that underlie HNPCC, clinical criteria useful for ascertaining families most likely to be affected by HNPCC were outlined.[51] These criteria, termed the *Amsterdam* [or *International Collaborative Group* (ICG)] *criteria*, are as follows: (1) FAP must be excluded; (2) at least three affected relatives must have histologically verified colorectal cancer, and at least two of the affected must be first-degree relatives; (3) the affected individuals must be from at least two successive generations; and (4) at least one of the affected individuals must have developed colorectal cancer before age 50 years. Although the ICG criteria do not identify all individuals who are ultimately found to carry HNPCC gene defects, the criteria have proven useful for focusing attention on families most likely to have HNPCC. Based on the criteria, HNPCC cases are estimated to account for 2% to 4% of all colorectal cancer cases. Of note, other cancers often seen in families with HNPCC, including endometrial, ovarian, gastric, and hepatobiliary and urinary tract cancers, are not included in the ICG criteria.

Mutations in DNA Mismatch Repair Genes in Hereditary Nonpolyposis Colorectal Cancer

Unlike FAP, in which the intestinal polyposis phenotype usually permits diagnosis of patients by their late teenage years or early 20s, no distinct clinical features are seen in asymptomatic carriers of HNPCC defects.[30,52] As such, definitively ascertaining the phenotypic status of an individual in an HNPCC kindred who has not yet developed cancer is nearly impossible, thus rendering genetic linkage analyses for mapping predisposition genes very challenging. The initial genetic studies of HNPCC were successful in excluding a role for variant *APC* alleles in cancer predisposition in HNPCC, as well as in excluding a role for several

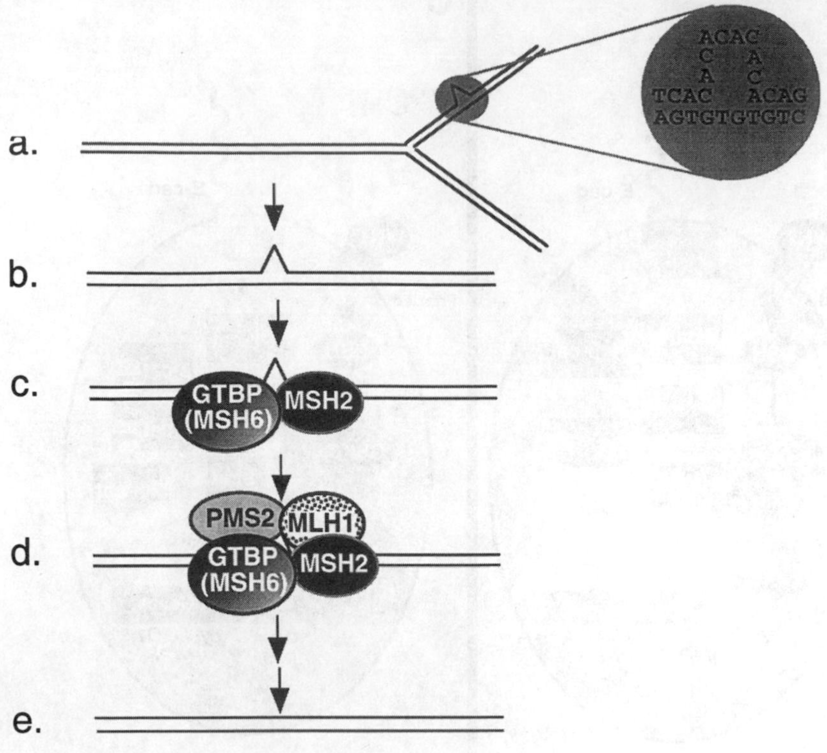

FIGURE 33.1-3. Mismatch repair pathway in human cells. **A,B:** During DNA replication, DNA mismatches may arise, such as from strand slippage (shown) or misincorporation of bases (not shown). **C:** The mismatch is recognized by MutS homologues, perhaps most often MSH2 and GTBP/MSH6, although another MutS homologue, MSH3, may substitute for GTBP/MSH6 in some cases. **D,E:** MutL homologues, such as MLH1 and PMS2, are recruited to the complex, and the mismatch is repaired through the action of a number of proteins, including an exonuclease, helicase, DNA polymerase, and ligase. (Modified from ref. 34, with permission.)

of the genes known to be somatically mutated in sporadic colorectal cancers.[53,54] A subsequent search of the entire genome for linkage to HNPCC was undertaken using microsatellite sequence markers. Microsatellites are short, repetitive DNA sequence tracts, scattered throughout the genome, and many microsatellite tracts show polymorphic length variation among normal individuals. One such search for linkage in several HNPCC kindreds was successful in mapping a cancer predisposition gene to chromosome 2p.[55] In other HNPCC families, a predisposition gene was localized to chromosome 3p.[56] In yet other families with HNPCC, no evidence for linkage to either chromosome 2p or 3p was found. These findings clearly established that HNPCC was a genetically heterogeneous disease.[55,56]

In an attempt to establish the potential relevance of the Knudson two-hit model for HNPCC genes, investigators sought to demonstrate that loss of the wild-type HNPCC allele on chromosome 2p was present in cancers from individuals carrying a defect in that particular predisposition gene. However, not only was there no loss of heterozygosity (LOH) of chromosome 2p sequences in the cancers, but the microsatellite DNA sequences demonstrated marked variation in length in tumor tissue compared to the patient's normal tissue.[57] In fact, in any given cancer from an HNPCC patient, microsatellite sequence alterations were present at many loci scattered throughout the genome. This curious phenotype was termed the *microsatellite instability* (MI) or *replication error–positive* (RER+) phenotype. Independent studies revealed that the MI/RER+ phenotype was present in approximately 15% of apparently sporadic colorectal cancers.[58,59]

The demonstration that the MI/RER+ phenotype was present in all cancers from HNPCC patients and some sporadic cancers piqued the interest of researchers in the DNA mismatch repair field because similar instability phenotypes had previously been seen in yeast strains with defective DNA mismatch repair genes. The prediction that germline mutations in one allele of a DNA mismatch repair gene might underlie HNPCC was quickly borne out. A functional link between MI/RER+ and mutated mismatch repair genes was first provided by the demonstration that cancer cell lines derived from patients with HNPCC have at least a 100-fold increased rate of mutation in repetitive DNA sequence tracts (e.g., microsatellites).[60] Subsequently, a human homologue of the bacterial *mutS* mismatch repair gene, designated *MSH2,* was mapped to chromosome 2p,[61] and one allele was found to be mutated in the germline of some HNPCC patients.[62] As might have been predicted, based on the fact that mismatch repair is dependent on the function of a number of distinct proteins (Fig. 33.1-3), other DNA mismatch repair genes were found to be mutated in subsets of HNPCC patients, including the *MLH1* gene on chromosome 3p, the *PMS1* gene on 2q, the *PMS2* gene on 7q, and the *GTBP/MSH6* gene on chromosome 2p.[63–68] Together, germline mutations in the *MSH2* and *MLH1* genes account for more than 60% of the known mutations present in HNPCC patients (Table 33.1-2).

The prevalence of germline mutations in the DNA mismatch repair genes in colorectal cancer patients not meeting the ICG criteria for HNPCC remains uncertain, although some preliminary findings have emerged. A study of 509 consecutive patients in a Finnish tumor registry found that the MI/RER+ phenotype was present in cancers from 12% of patients.[69] Ten of the 63 patients with MI/RER+ cancers (16%, or roughly 2% of total patients) had a detectable germline mutation in *MLH1* or *MSH2.* Patients with an identifiable germline mutation had either a first-degree relative with endometrial or colorectal cancer, were younger than 50 years, or had a previous colorectal or endometrial cancer. Another study of patients from the Netherlands and Norway found that

TABLE 33.1-2. Germline Mismatch Repair Gene Mutations in Hereditary Nonpolyposis Colorectal Cancer (HNPCC)

Gene	*Chromosome Location*	Escherichia coli *Homologue*	*Estimated Percentage of HNPCC Families with Mutation*
MSH2	2p15-16	MutS	30
MLH1	3p21	MutL	35
PMS1	2q31	MutL	Rare (1 family)
PMS2	7p22	MutL	<5 (2 families)
GTBP/MSH6	2p15-16	MutS	Rare (1 or 2 families)
Other/unknown	?	?	25–30[a]

[a]Estimate is based on the fact that colorectal carcinomas from approximately 95% of patients with a family history meeting the Amsterdam/International Collaborative Group criteria displayed the microsatellite instability/replication error–positive phenotype. (Liu B, Parsons R, Papadopoulos N, et al. Analysis of mismatch repair genes in hereditary non-polyposis colorectal cancer patients. *Nat Med* 1996;2:169.)

26% of the 184 families with clustering of colorectal cancer studied had germline mutations in the *MSH2* or *MLH1* genes.[70] Similar to the Finnish study, germline *MSH2* or *MLH1* mutations were more likely to be found in individuals from families meeting the ICG criteria, individuals whose cancers arose at a particularly young age, or individuals whose families manifested both colorectal and endometrial cancer.

Mechanisms and Mutation Targets in Cancers with Defective Mismatch Repair

In normal cells of a patient with HNPCC, DNA repair is not usually impaired, because the cells have a wild-type copy of the gene. During tumorigenesis, however, and perhaps even at an early stage in that process, the wild-type allele of the gene that is mutant in all of the patient's constitutional cells is inactivated by a somatic mutation. Then, affected cells manifest a mutator phenotype and accumulate mutations in a much more rapid fashion. HNPCC appears, therefore, to be a disease with more rapid tumor progression from a benign, initiated clone to frank malignancy. In HNPCC patients, the transition from a small adenoma to carcinoma has been estimated to take only 3 to 5 years, instead of the 20 to 40 years believed required for development of most sporadic carcinomas.[28,52]

Germline mutations in the known mismatch repair genes have only been detected in 2% to 4% of colorectal cancer patients. However, approximately 15% of all colorectal cancers manifest the MI/RER+ phenotype, implying that germline or somatic mutations in mismatch repair pathway genes may be present in a substantial fraction of colorectal cancers, regardless of the patient's family history. Only a fraction of the 15% of apparently sporadic colorectal cancers with the MI/RER phenotype develop as the result of a germline mutation in a known mismatch repair gene, such as *MSH2* or *MLH1*. Similarly, somatic mutations in *MSH2, MLH1*, or other mismatch repair genes are present in only a small fraction of the apparently sporadic cancers with the MI/RER+ phenotype.[52,71] Although germline or somatic mutation of known mismatch repair genes are infrequent, inactivation of the *MLH1* gene via epigenetic changes, such as DNA hypermethylation of the *MLH1* promoter, appears to be a causal factor in the majority of "sporadic" colorectal cancer cases with the MI/RER+ phenotype.[72,73]

The vast majority of the mutations arising in cells with the MI/RER+ phenotype are likely to have either no effect on cell growth or detrimental effects. Such mutations do not promote the clonal outgrowth and evolution characteristic of colorectal tumor progression. A subset of mutations do, however, activate oncogenes, such as K-*ras*, or inactivate tumor suppressor genes, such as *APC* and *p53*.[57,74,75] Some genes may be more frequent targets for somatic mutations in cancers with MI/RER+. For instance, genes that contain repetitive DNA sequence tracts, such as microsatellites, would appear to be likely targets for mutation in MI/RER+ tumors. A gene containing a mononucleotide repeat tract in its coding sequence and that is frequently inactivated in colorectal cancers with the MI/RER+ phenotype is the transforming growth factor-β (TGF-β) type II receptor (RII).[76,77] The *RII* gene is a likely tumor suppressor gene, because both copies of the gene are inactivated by mutations in more than 90% of MI/RER+ colorectal cancers, and TGF-β is known to be a strong inhibitor of cell proliferation in many normal epithelial tissues, including colonic epithelial cells. Approximately 15% of microsatellite stable colorectal carcinomas also show biallelic inactivation of *RII*, although the mutations are located in regions other than the gene's mononucleotide tract.[78] Other suggested candidates for somatic inactivation in MI/RER colorectal cancers include *bax*, a p53-regulated gene in some cell types and whose protein product functions in promoting apoptosis,[79] and *E2F-4*, a gene encoding a transcription factor that may regulate cell-cycle progression.[80] Moreover, not all genes that appear to be more frequently mutated in MI/RER+ cancers than in microsatellite-stable cancers need themselves be mutated in microsatellite sequence tracts. The *β-catenin* gene appears to be more frequently activated by mutations in MI/RER+ colon cancers than in microsatellite-stable cancers, and the missense mutations seen are not associated with a microsatellite sequence tract.[81,82]

ONCOGENE AND TUMOR SUPPRESSOR GENE MUTATIONS IN COLORECTAL TUMOR PROGRESSION

Somatic mutations in the *APC* gene appear to be an early and, perhaps, rate-limiting event in the development of upwards of

TABLE 33.1-3. Summary of Selected Somatic Mutations in Colorectal Carcinomas

Gene	Estimated Frequency of Mutations	Comments
Oncogenes		
K-RAS	45–50%	Missense mutations (in order of frequency) at codon 12, codon 13, and codon 61; mutations infrequent in adenomas smaller than 1 cm.
N-RAS	<5%	Codon 12 and 13 missense mutations.
HER-2/NEU	<5%	Gene amplification.
β-catenin	2–10%	Exon 3 missense mutations or in-frame deletions alter N-terminal phosphorylation sites regulating β-catenin protein degradation; mutations more common in MI/RER+ carcinomas; mutations mutually exclusive with *APC* mutations.
Tumor suppressor and candidate tumor suppressor genes		
APC	75–80%	Nonsense and frameshift mutations in 5' half of gene leading to protein truncation in >95% of cases; similar mutation frequencies in adenomas and carcinomas; biallelic inactivation in all carcinomas and most adenomas; ? dosage or dominant negative effects in some adenomas with only one mutant allele; mutations less frequent in MI/RER+ cases; mutations mutually exclusive with β-catenin mutations.
p53	60–70%	Missense mutations most frequently at codons 175, 245, 248, 273, 282; mutations in one allele accompanied by LOH of remaining allele.
TGF-β type IIR	25–30%	Approximately 90% of MI/RER+ cancers have mutations in both alleles, most often in the 10-base-pair polyadenine tract; approximately 15% of microsatellite cancers have mutations in both alleles, although not localized to the polyadenine tract.
DPC4/SMAD4	10–15%	Nonsense, frameshift, missense, and deletion mutations; mutations in one allele usually accompanied by LOH of remaining allele on 18q.
SMAD2	<5%	Nonsense, frameshift, missense, and deletion mutations.
DCC	>10%	Majority of mutations reported are expansions of a dinucleotide repeat tract in MI/RER+ cancers; rare homozygous deletions and localized mutations in coding sequences; loss or reduced levels of transcripts and protein in >50% of colorectal carcinomas.

LOH, loss of heterozygosity; MI, microsatellite instability; RER+, replication error–positive; TGF-β type IIR, transforming growth factor-β type II receptor.

75% to 80% of colorectal adenomas and carcinomas. Presumably, mutations in other tumor suppressor genes and oncogenes play an important role in tumor progression. Some of the genes believed critical in colorectal tumor progression are discussed in this chapter and summarized in Table 33.1-3. Another important point already noted is that roughly 15% of colorectal carcinomas display the MI/RER+ phenotype. Although the MI/RER+ cancers have a very elevated rate of localized mutations (e.g., point mutations and small deletions and insertions), they are generally near diploid, with few chromosome losses or gains. In contrast to MI/RER+ cancers, upwards of 85% of colorectal carcinomas display frequent chromosome losses and gains.[83] Defects in genes that regulate formation of the mitotic spindle and proper alignment and segregation of chromosomes at mitosis may underlie the chromosome instability phenotype, although few of the specific defects likely to underlie the chromosome instability phenotype in cancer have been defined.

K-RAS AND OTHER ONCOGENE DEFECTS

The *RAS* genes encode small guanosine triphosphatases with critical roles in signal transduction downstream of growth factor receptors, such as that for epidermal growth factor. *K-RAS* is the most frequently mutated of the three *RAS* genes, with *K-RAS* mutations found in approximately 50% of colorectal adenomas larger than 1 cm in size and a similar fraction of carcinomas.[84–86] The majority of *K-RAS* mutations are at codon 12, but codon 13 is mutated in 15% to 20% of cases, and codon 61 is infrequently affected. *N-RAS* mutations are infrequent, and no *H-RAS* mutations have been reported in colorectal tumors. In adenomatous polyps, *K-RAS* mutations have been associated with features predictive of subsequent progression to cancer—increased size and more severe dysplasia[85,87,88]—although *K-RAS* mutations also have been seen in some colonic lesions with very reduced or no malignant potential (e.g., hyperplastic polyps and aberrant crypt foci lacking dysplasia).[89–92] Notwithstanding these latter observations, inactivation of mutant *K-RAS* activity in advanced colorectal cancer cells abrogates the tumorigenic growth properties of colorectal carcinoma cells.[93] Hence, *RAS* gene mutations in colorectal tumors have a role not only in promoting growth of small adenomas to larger and more clinically significant lesions, but also in maintenance of the fully neoplastic phenotype in advanced carcinomas.

Somatic mutations in other protooncogenes, including amplifications of the *MYC*, *MYB*, *cyclin D1*, and *HER-2/NEU* genes, have been found in only a small percentage of colorectal cancers (see Table 33.1-3).[94,95] Gain of function mutations in the *β-catenin* gene are present in 2% to 8% of colorectal cancers and appear to render the mutant β-catenin protein resistant to regulation by the APC protein.[45,81,82,96,97] Like *APC* mutations, *β-catenin* mutations appear to be an early event in adenoma formation. Finally, some oncogene mutations may vary in their frequency in colorectal carcinomas, depending on whether the tumor has the MI/RER+ phenotype. For example, although *K-RAS* mutations have a roughly similar prevalence in MI/RER+ carcinomas compared with cases with chromosome instability, *β-catenin* mutations appear to be more common in MI/RER+ cases.[82]

THE *p53* GENE

Allelic loss or LOH is believed to be a common mechanism for tumor suppressor gene inactivation in the roughly 85% of colorectal carcinomas that manifest the chromosome instability phenotype. Although allelic loss of chromosome 17p is an infrequent event in adenomas, 17p allelic losses can be detected in nearly 70% to 75% of colorectal carcinomas.[85,98] Wild-type *p53* alleles are presumed to be targeted for inactivation by 17p LOH, because the remaining *p53* allele is mutated in the majority of colorectal tumors with 17p LOH, most often at codons 175, 245, 248, 273, or 282.[99–101] Only a small subset of carcinomas lacking 17p LOH have *p53* mutations, and most adenomas lack 17p LOH and p53 mutation. Hence, mutation and LOH of *p53* appear to arise most frequently during the transition from adenoma to carcinoma. The biologic selection for *p53* inactivation at this point in tumor development is not well understood. However, based on our understanding of the functions of p53 in cell-cycle checkpoints at the G_1/S and G_2/M boundaries and in apoptosis,[102–105] the selection for p53 inactivation may reflect the fact that several distinct stresses on tumor cells activate apoptotic pathways in cells with wild-type *p53* function. Such stresses may include DNA strand breakage, hypoxia, and reduced access to glucose or other nutrients. Loss of *p53* function at the critical juncture between adenoma and carcinoma may facilitate continued growth and the acquisition of invasive properties in the face of stresses that might otherwise severely limit tumor cell growth in the colon and rectum.

CHROMOSOME 18q LOSS OF HETEROZYGOSITY

Chromosome 18q LOH is seen in approximately 60% to 70% of primary colorectal cancers and, rarely, in adenomas, with the exception of large villous adenomas that contain a focus of carcinoma.[85,86] The prevalence of 18q LOH rises to nearly 90% to 100% in liver metastases from colorectal primary tumors.[106] The findings suggest a role for inactivation of a chromosome 18q tumor suppressor gene(s) in the later stages of tumor progression and metastasis. Several studies have reported that patients whose primary colorectal cancers have 18q LOH have an increased likelihood of distant metastasis and death from their disease, independent of stage and perhaps other clinical and histopathologic features.[107–111] In colorectal carcinomas, a common region of LOH includes bands 18q12.3 to 18q21.3, and the *DCC* (deleted in colorectal cancer) gene at 18q21.2 has been suggested to be a candidate tumor suppressor gene.[112,113] In some studies, loss of *DCC* transcripts and protein has been noted in more than 50% of colorectal cancers, although the specific mechanisms accounting for *DCC* inactivation are not well understood.[114] Few specific mutations in the *DCC* gene have been identified, perhaps in part because the *DCC* gene spans more than 1.35 million base pairs.[115] *DCC* encodes a transmembrane protein that functions in transducing signals from netrin chemoattractant and cell guidance factors.[114] Some findings indicate that, in the absence of netrin, the DCC protein may induce apoptosis in epithelial cells,[116] perhaps reconciling why there might be selection for genetic or epigenetic inactivation of *DCC* in colorectal carcinomas.

Although *DCC* remains a candidate tumor suppressor gene in colorectal and other tumors, a well-established tumor suppressor gene, termed *DPC4* (also known as *SMAD4*), is also present in the 18q21 region.[117,118] As is discussed later (see the section Gene Defects in Pancreatic Carcinoma), *DPC4* is mutated in 50% to 55% of pancreatic carcinomas. Furthermore, germline *DPC4* mutations have been seen in a subset of patients affected by juvenile polyposis syndrome.[119] Those with juvenile polyposis syndrome develop benign hamartomatous polyps in the intestinal tract, and they also have an increased risk of colorectal and gastric cancer. Nevertheless, *DPC4* is mutated in only approximately 10% to 15% of colorectal carcinomas and much less frequently in other gastrointestinal tumors, such as gastric and esophageal carcinomas.[120–127] The *DPC4*-related *SMAD2* gene is also located in the region of 18q commonly affected by LOH in colorectal carcinomas. A major role for *SMAD2* in colorectal cancer has been excluded, because *SMAD2* is inactivated in less than 5% of colon carcinomas and *SMAD2* alterations are rare or absent in other gastrointestinal carcinomas.[127–132] Based on the frequencies of mutations in *DPC4* and *MADR2*, neither gene appears to be the primary tumor suppressor gene targeted for inactivation by 18q LOH in colorectal cancer. Nonetheless, inactivation of either of the two genes is likely to have an important role in the tumor process, because each gene encodes a protein that functions to transduce TGF-β growth regulatory signals, and TGF-β has significant growth inhibitory effects on colonic epithelial cells. Whether *DCC* inactivation is associated with 18q LOH in the majority of colorectal carcinomas or whether additional novel tumor suppressor genes are present in the 18q12.3-q21.3 region remains to be determined.

GENE DEFECTS IN PANCREATIC CARCINOMA

Ductal epithelial cells in the pancreas comprise less than 5% of the total cell mass in the organ, yet they are the origin of the most common form of pancreatic carcinoma. The natural history of the progression from normal epithelium to carcinoma in the pancreas is less well understood than in the colon. However, it appears that a flat hyperplastic lesion in which the epithelium changes from its normal cuboidal pattern to columnar may be an early precursor.[118,133] Papillary hyperplasia, in which the mucosa becomes more crowded and folded, arguably represents the next recognizable stage. Papillary hyperplasia can be associated with varying degrees of cellular and nuclear atypia (i.e., dysplasia), and the most advanced premalignant stage is sometimes referred to as *carcinoma in situ.* Bona fide carcinoma is marked by invasion through the duct wall. A major difficulty hindering early molecular analyses of pancreatic carcinoma was the fact that pancreatic carcinoma cells engender a strong host desmoplastic and inflammatory response, and the neoplastic cells only constitute a fraction of the total cells in the cancer specimen. Generation and study of pancreatic carcinoma specimens explanted into the flank of immunocompromised mice (i.e., xenografts) have proven crucial in defining specific genetic alterations in oncogenes and tumor suppressor genes in pancreatic carcinoma, because all human DNA isolated from the xenografts is derived from neoplastic cells.[118,134,135]

As is the case for colorectal carcinomas, accumulation of multiple mutations in oncogenes and tumor suppressor genes is critical in tumor progression (Table 33.1-4). Mutations in *K-RAS* have been found in more than 90% of pancreatic carcino-

TABLE 33.1-4. Summary of Selected Mutations in Pancreatic Carcinoma

Gene	Gene Location	Frequency (%)	Mutation Origin
ONCOGENES			
K-RAS	12p12	95	Somatic
AKT2	19q13.1	10–20	Somatic
MYB	6q24	10	Somatic
TUMOR SUPPRESSOR GENES			
p16^{INK4a}	9p21	>90	Somatic much more frequently than germline
p53	17p13	75	Somatic
DPC4/SMAD4	18q21	55	Somatic
BRCA2	13q13	5–10	Germline more frequently than somatic
DCC	18q21	6	Somatic
LKB1/STK11	19p13	5	Somatic much more frequently than germline
MKK4	17p13	4	Somatic
TGF-β type IIR	3p22	3	Somatic
ALK5	9q21	1	Somatic

(Modified from ref. 118, with permission.)

mas, and the mutations appear to arise early in the natural history of the disease, with more than 50% of flat hyperplasias and the vast majority of papillary hyperplasias exhibiting *K-RAS* mutations.[118] Like colorectal carcinoma, other oncogene defects appear to be much less frequent, with the next most common oncogene changes—amplifications of the *AKT2* and *MYB* genes—present in only 10% to 20% and 10% of carcinomas, respectively.[118]

A number of distinct tumor suppressor gene defects are seen in pancreatic carcinomas, although three tumor suppressor genes stand out because of their frequent inactivation—namely, the *p16*^{INK4a}, *p53*, and *DPC4* genes (see Table 33.1-4). Whereas mutations in the pRb/cyclin D1-cdk4/p16^{INK4a} pathway are uncommon in colorectal carcinoma, mutations inactivating the *p16*^{INK4a} gene are found in roughly 85% of pancreatic carcinomas.[118] A subset of pancreatic carcinomas may epigenetically inactivate *p16*^{INK4a}, perhaps as a result of hypermethylation of *p16*^{INK4} promoter sequences.[136] In another small fraction of cases, rather than *p16*^{INK4a} inactivation, the *RB1* tumor suppressor gene is inactivated,[118] presumably with similar net consequences to *p16*^{INK4a} inactivation, because the pRb protein is functionally inactive when the p16^{INK4a} protein is lacking in a cell (i.e., the cyclin D and cdk4 proteins constitutively phosphorylate pRb in this setting). Mutations in the *p53* gene are found in 50% to 75% of pancreatic carcinomas.[118] Similar to the situation in colorectal carcinomas, the vast majority of the *p53* mutations are missense mutations accompanied by loss of the wild-type *p53* allele. Some alterations inactivating the *p16*^{INK4a} gene, particularly homozygous deletions, also lead to loss of the p14^{ARF} protein, an alternative protein product synthesized in part from sequences shared with those encoding the p16^{INK4a} protein. Because p14^{ARF} inactivation appears to lead to functional inactivation of the p53 protein, the actual frequency of pancreatic carcinomas with p53 inactivation may be higher than the percentage of cases with demonstrable *p53* sequence alterations. As noted earlier in the section Chromosome 18q Loss of Heterozygosity, *DPC4* mutations are found in approximately 50% to 55% of pancreatic carcinomas.[117,118,137] Among other potential effects, the mutations presumably render the cells resistant to the negative growth regulatory effects of TGF-β. Finally, in addition to the frequent alterations of *p16*^{INK4a}, *p53*, and *DPC4*, several other tumor suppressor gene defects are found in a fraction of pancreatic carcinomas, such as *BRCA2* inactivation[118] (see Table 33.1-4). Consistent with the view that *BRCA2* defects have an important role in a subset of pancreatic cancers, in addition to the very elevated risk of breast cancer in those carrying a germline *BRCA2* mutation, the lifetime risk of pancreatic carcinoma for *BRCA2* mutation carriers appears to be increased by three- to fivefold relative to the general population.[138,139]

GENE DEFECTS IN ESOPHAGEAL ADENOCARCINOMA

Esophageal cancers are readily distinguished into squamous and adenocarcinoma types on the basis of their histopathologic appearance. Clear differences exist in the pathogenesis of the two types, as well as differences in their epidemiology and associated risk factors. Not unexpectedly, the genetic alterations detected in the two types appear to be largely distinct. The brief discussion here focuses on esophageal adenocarcinoma because its natural history and genetic alterations are better defined than squamous carcinoma. Moreover, the genetics of esophageal adenocarcinoma has interesting parallels with the genetics of colorectal and pancreatic carcinoma, as well as some interesting differences.

Efforts to define the natural history and likely precursor lesions for esophageal adenocarcinoma have focused on Barrett's esophagus (BE).[140,141] BE is a condition in which the normal squamous epithelium of the esophagus is replaced by a metaplastic columnar epithelium. BE is generally restricted to the lower esophagus, and it is thought to develop in response to the mucosal injury that arises in the setting of chronic gastroesophageal reflux, although only approximately 10% to 12% of patients with reflux develop BE. The important histologic feature that predicts increased adenocarcinoma risk in patients with BE is the development of dysplasia, and increasing grades of dysplasia are associated with increased aneuploidy.[141] Flow cytometry analyses indicate aneuploid cell populations are absent in normal esophageal mucosa from patients with gastroesophageal reflux and no BE. Aneuploidy is rare in metaplasia and low-grade dysplasia. However, aneuploidy is present in biopsy specimens from approximately two-thirds of patients with high-grade dysplasia and nearly 100% of cancers. The flow cytometry studies also have demonstrated clonal heterogeneity in DNA content among the neoplastic cell populations present in distinct dysplastic areas of a single patient with BE,[141] suggesting that a large area of BE is neoplastically transformed and multifocal progression ensues.

Various oncogene defects have been found in esophageal adenocarcinomas, most notably the amplification of several distinct protooncogenes, including the *HER-2/NEU/ErbB2* gene in 22% of cases, the *cathepsin B* and *GATA-4* genes in 14%, the epidermal growth factor receptor (*EGFR*) gene in 13%, and the *K-RAS* gene in 10%.[142–144] Among the tumor suppres-

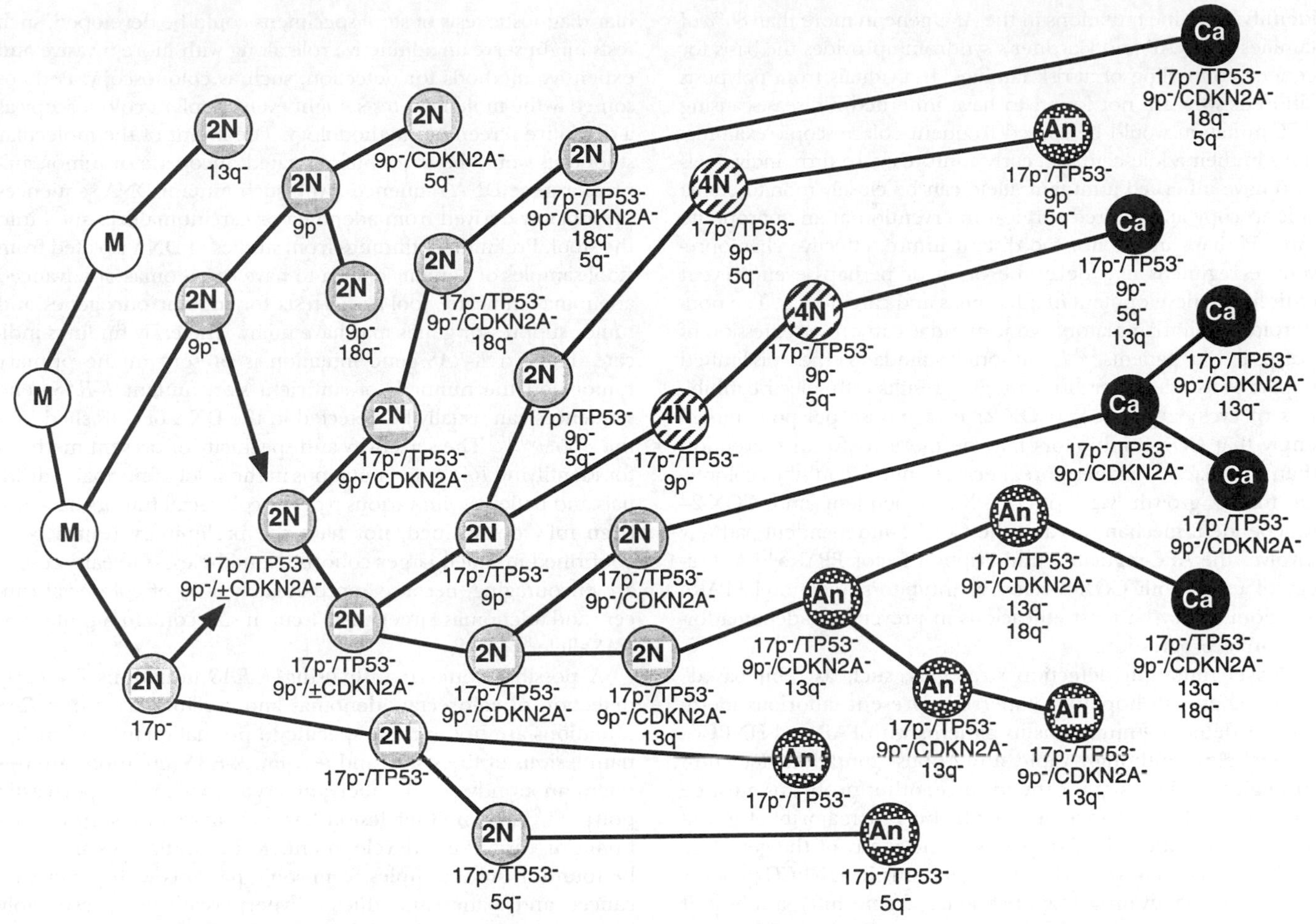

FIGURE 33.1-4. Multiple genetic routes to esophageal adenocarcinoma in the setting of Barrett's esophagus (BE). The clonal progression of cell populations as they progress from the metaplasia (M) seen in BE is illustrated schematically. The figure is not intended to be comprehensive, as there are multiple pathways to cancer. Nevertheless, some general patterns appear to be consistent in studies of progression in many patients. Chromosome losses (i.e., loss of heterozygosity), such as those involving chromosomes 5q, 9p, 13q, 17p, and 18q appear to arise in a diploid, proliferating cell population (2N). Chromosome 17p and 9p losses are both early events and can precede detectable inactivation of the *p53* (*TP53*) or $p16^{INK4a}$ (*CDKN2A*) genes. In some cases, tetraploidy (4N) may precede aneuploidy (An). Progression to cancer (Ca) is shown as an end point, although additional chromosome changes and mutations may contribute to further progression of the cancer. (Modified from ref. 148, with permission.)

sor genes frequently inactivated by genetic and epigenetic alterations in esophageal carcinomas are the *p53* and $p16^{INK4a}$ genes.[141,145–149] Missense mutations in one p53 allele coupled with LOH of chromosome 17p and the remaining p53 allele are found in nearly 100% of esophageal adenocarcinomas. In contrast to the situation in the colon in which p53 mutation and 17p LOH are infrequent in premalignant lesions (i.e., adenomas) but frequent in carcinomas, p53 mutations and 17p LOH are frequently found in high-grade dysplastic regions of premalignant BE. Inactivation of $p16^{INK4a}$ by mutational and epigenetic (e.g., promoter hypermethylation) mechanisms is frequent not only in high-grade dysplasias, but also in low-grade and nondysplastic BE specimens. Hence, $p16^{INK4a}$ inactivation frequently precedes *p53* inactivation in esophageal tumor progression. Nevertheless, as indicated in Figure 33.1-4, there appear to be multiple genetic routes to cancer in BE.[148] Of some note, although several of the chromosome regions frequently affected by LOH in colorectal and pancreatic carcinomas are also frequently affected by LOH in esophageal adenocarcinoma, including chromosomes 5q and 18q,[148,150] the *APC* and *DPC4* tumor suppressor genes appear to be infrequently, if ever, mutated in esophageal adenocarcinoma.[125–127,151] Further work will be needed to define the tumor suppressor genes on chromosomes 5q and 18q that are inactivated in esophageal adenocarcinoma.

POTENTIAL CLINICAL APPLICATIONS OF MOLECULAR ADVANCES

Advances in the understanding of the inherited and somatic genetic alterations in gastrointestinal cancers have made possible several clinical applications that should improve the diagnosis and care of patients and families affected by these cancers. Although many future clinical applications can be envisioned, only a few potential applications in the colorectal cancer area are described here.

RISK ASSESSMENT

Presymptomatic diagnosis of FAP or HNPCC may be of significant value to members of families with these syndromes. The ability to identify germline mutations in the *APC* gene in more than 80% of families with FAP and Gardner's syndrome provides the basis for genetic counseling of at-risk families. Individuals from polyposis kindreds who are not found to have inherited a disease-causing *APC* mutation would be spared frequent colonoscopic examinations in their adolescent and early adult years. In turn, individuals who have inherited a mutant allele can be closely monitored via colonoscopy and offered surgical intervention at an appropriate time. Perhaps in the not too distant future, effective chemopreventive regimens may delay the onset or perhaps even prevent entirely the development of adenomas and carcinomas. The nonsteroidal antiinflammatory agent sulindac can cause regression of polyps in FAP patients,[152–154] although sulindac's efficacy is limited in part by its side effects. Encouraging results with selective inhibitors of cyclooxygenase-2 (COX-2) in a mouse polyposis model imply that COX-2 inhibitors may be more useful in prevention than sulindac.[155] Furthermore, because sulindac inhibits colorectal tumor growth via both COX-2–dependent and COX-2–independent mechanisms and the COX-2–independent pathway involves the APC-regulated transcription factor PPARδ,[156] a strategy of using both COX-2–selective inhibitors and novel PPARδ antagonists may be most efficacious in preventing adenoma formation or progression.

Novel mutation detection strategies, such as "chip-based" approaches, will hopefully supersede present laborious methods for detecting mutations in patients with FAP and HNPCC. Nevertheless, although rapid and robust mutation detection strategies will be a significant advance, other problems must be conquered. For instance, although the vast majority of germline *APC* mutations in FAP patients and many of the germline *MSH2, MLH1, PMS1,* and *PMS2* mutations in HNPCC patients are clearly inactivating (e.g., nonsense, frameshift), a subset of the mutations are missense substitutions. Distinguishing cancer-predisposing missense mutations from benign polymorphic variants is a troublesome issue at present. The development of *in vitro* assays that accurately predict the functional activity of wild type and mutant alleles *in vivo* is critical, particularly if large-scale screening for HNPCC mutations in asymptomatic patients is envisioned. Some progress toward this important goal has been achieved.[157] After identification of novel variant alleles that contribute to modestly increased risk of colorectal cancer, akin to the effects of the I1307K *APC* allele in Ashkenazi Jews,[47] recombinant DNA-based approaches may be used in a more general fashion in the future to estimate an individual's risk of colorectal cancer. The technical and theoretical difficulties of identifying variant alleles that have only subtle effects on colorectal cancer risk are substantial. Moreover, because many uncertainties exist regarding the optimal clinical management of such lower risk patients, as well as legal and ethical issues surrounding presymptomatic genetic testing even in high-risk patients,[158] many challenges lie ahead.

EARLY DETECTION

The results of clinical trials indicate that colonoscopic removal of larger adenomas and early colorectal carcinomas reduces colorectal cancer incidence and most likely decreases mortality.[25,159] Because of the reduced specificity and sensitivity of current noninvasive tests, such as fecal occult blood testing, the development of highly specific and sensitive tests for early detection of colorectal cancer is an important goal. If inexpensive and reliable molecular diagnostic tests of stool specimens could be developed, such tests might serve an adjunctive role along with more invasive and expensive methods for detection, such as colonoscopy. Perhaps someday the molecular tests might even supplant colonoscopy as a definitive screening methodology. The intent of the molecular stool tests would be to identify mutated oncogene or tumor suppressor gene DNA sequences, with such mutant DNA sequences presumably derived from adenoma or carcinoma cells shed into the stool. Preliminary findings from studies of DNA isolated from stool samples of patients known to have carcinomas or advanced adenomas indicate stool-based tests for mutant oncogenes and tumor suppressor genes may have utility. The early findings indicate that if a *K-RAS* gene mutation is present in the primary tumor and the tumor is of sufficient size, mutant *K-RAS* gene sequences can usually be detected in the DNA of cells shed into the stool.[160–163] The sensitivity and specificity of present methods for identifying *RAS* gene mutations in the stool of normal individuals and patients with various types of colorectal tumors have not been fully determined, nor have the preliminary results been confirmed in much larger cohorts. Nonetheless, the early results are encouraging, because approximately 50% of colorectal cancers and adenomas larger than 1 cm in size contain a mutant *K-RAS* allele.[85]

A possible concern with using *K-RAS* mutations for early detection of colorectal adenomas and carcinomas is that *RAS* mutations are not entirely specific to premalignant and malignant lesions of the colon and rectum. *K-RAS* mutations are frequent in nondysplastic aberrant crypt foci and hyperplastic polyps,[89–92] and neither lesion has a clear relationship to adenoma or carcinoma development. *K-RAS* mutations may also be found in stool samples from some patients with pancreatic cancer and pancreatic ductal hyperplasia,[164,165] presumably because the pancreatic duct drains cells from these lesions into the gastrointestinal tract and both lesions have frequent *K-RAS* mutations. Nonetheless, a *K-RAS* mutation test for early detection of colorectal tumors may prove useful because aberrant crypt foci, hyperplastic polyps, and nonneoplastic pancreatic lesions are small lesions that may often shed too few mutant *K-RAS* alleles into the stool to permit their efficient detection. Even if *K-RAS* mutations do not offer a robust stool-based test for colorectal adenomas and carcinomas, similar molecular approaches may be used to detect localized mutations in other oncogenes and tumor suppressor genes, particularly those mutations that are intimately linked to malignant potential in colonic epithelium (e.g., *APC* and *p53* mutations).

PROGNOSTIC MARKERS AND PATIENT STRATIFICATION FOR THERAPY

In addition to presymptomatic diagnosis (risk assessment) and early detection of tumors, several studies indicate characterization of the specific genetic alterations present in a cancer may provide improved or increased prognostic information about the likelihood of local and distant tumor recurrence. Several studies have suggested that chromosome 18q LOH and loss of *DCC* expression in primary colorectal cancer specimens may predict poor outcome in both stage II (lymph node metastases absent) and stage III (lymph node metastases present) patients.[107–111] Molecular analyses of lymph node from patients who do not appear to have metastatic disease on the basis of histologic examination may also be very useful for detecting micrometastases and refining the staging of patients. For instance, carcinoembryonic antigen (CEA) is often highly expressed by colorectal carcinoma cells. Research has shown that *CEA* gene expression may be found in lymph nodes of roughly one-half of stage II patients and that the presence of *CEA* expression in the lymph node predicts poor survival,[166] presumably because *CEA* expression results from occult micrometastases. Molecular studies of lymph nodes for mutant oncogenes or tumor suppressor genes may also prove helpful in refining staging and prognosis.[167,168]

In the future, if differences are noted in the response rates between patients whose tumors have differing constellations of genetic alterations, it may be particularly useful to define the specific mutations in a patient's tumor, so that a patient might receive the particular chemotherapeutic regimen with greatest efficacy on tumors of that genotype. Similarly, analysis of gene expression patterns may also be of clear benefit in predicting response. Finally, some of the oncogene and tumor suppressor gene alterations in colorectal tumors may provide specific targets for novel chemotherapeutic agents. Some of these agents might antagonize or act selectively on the mutated oncogene products or the growth pathways in which they function. Other agents might act to counter loss of tumor suppressor function in affected cells.

REFERENCES

1. Landis SH, Murray T, Bolden S, et al. Cancer statistics, 1999. *CA Cancer J Clin* 1999;49:8.
2. Slattery ML, Kerber RA. Family history of cancer and colon cancer risk: the Utah Population Database [published erratum appears in *J Natl Cancer Inst* 1994;86:1802]. *J Natl Cancer Inst* 1994;86:1618.
3. Potter JD, Slattery ML, Bostick RM, et al. Colon cancer: a review of the epidemiology. *Epidemiol Rev* 1993;15:499.
4. Lovett E. Family studies in cancer of the colon and rectum. *Br J Surg* 1976;63:13.
5. Kerber RA, Slattery ML. Comparison of self-reported and database-linked family history of cancer data in a case-control study. *Am J Epidemiol* 1997;146:244.
6. Longnecker MP, Chen MJ, Probst-Hensch NMH, et al. Alcohol and smoking in relation to the prevalence of adenomatous colorectal polyps detected at sigmoidoscopy. *Epidemiology* 1996;7:275.
7. Baron JA, Sandler RS, Haile RW, et al. Folate intake, alcohol consumption, cigarette smoking, and risk of colorectal adenomas. *J Natl Cancer Inst* 1998;90:57.
8. Thun MJ, Namboodiri MM, Heath CW Jr. Aspirin use and reduced risk of fatal colon cancer. *N Engl J Med* 1991;325:1593.
9. Greenberg ER, Baron JA, Freeman DH Jr, et al. Reduced risk of large-bowel adenomas among aspirin users. The Polyp Prevention Study Group. *J Natl Cancer Inst* 1993;85:912.
10. Giovannucci E, Egan KM, Hunter DJ, et al. Aspirin and the risk of colorectal cancer in women. *N Engl J Med* 1995;333:609.
11. Sturmer T, Glynn RJ, Lee IM, et al. Aspirin use and colorectal cancer: post-trial follow-up data from the Physicians' Health Study. *Ann Intern Med* 1998;128:713.
12. Paganini-Hill A, Chao A, Ross RK, et al. Aspirin use and chronic diseases: a cohort study of the elderly. *BMJ* 1989;299:1247.
13. Gann PH, Manson JE, Glynn RJ, et al. Low-dose aspirin and incidence of colorectal tumors in a randomized trial. *J Natl Cancer Inst* 1993;85:1220.
14. Marincola FM, White DE, Wise AP, et al. Combination therapy with interferon alfa-2a and interleukin-2 for the treatment of metastatic cancer. *J Clin Oncol* 1995;13:1110.
15. Bird CL, Frankl HD, Lee ER, et al. Obesity, weight gain, large weight changes, and adenomatous polyps of the left colon and rectum. *Am J Epidemiol* 1998;147:670.
16. Weiss NS, Daling JR, Chow WH. Incidence of cancer of the large bowel in women in relation to reproductive and hormonal factors. *J Natl Cancer Inst* 1981;67:57.
17. Potter JD, McMichael AJ. Large bowel cancer in women in relation to reproductive and hormonal factors: a case-control study. *J Natl Cancer Inst* 1983;71:703.
18. Grodstein F, Martinez ME, Platz EA, et al. Postmenopausal hormone use and risk for colorectal cancer and adenoma. *Ann Intern Med* 1998;128:705.
19. Chen MJ, Longnecker MP, Morgenstern H, et al. Recent use of hormone replacement therapy and the prevalence of colorectal adenomas. *Cancer Epidemiol Biomarkers Prev* 1998;7:227.
20. Witte JS, Longnecker MP, Lee ER, et al. Relation of vegetable, fruit, and grain consumption to colorectal adenomatous polyps. *Am J Epidemiol* 1996;144:1015.
21. Bird CL, Witte JS, Swendseid ME, et al. Plasma ferritin, iron intake, and the risk of colorectal polyps. *Am J Epidemiol* 1996;144:34.
22. Winawer SJ, Fletcher RH, Miller L, et al. Colorectal cancer screening: clinical guidelines and rationale [published erratum appears in *Gastroenterology* 1997;112:1060]. *Gastroenterology* 1997;112:594.
23. Gilbertson VA. Proctosigmoidoscopy and polypectomy in reducing the incidence of rectal cancer. *Cancer* 1974;34:936.
24. Murakanni R, Tsukuma H, Kanamori S, et al. Natural history of colorectal polyps and the effect of polypectomy on occurrence of subsequent cancer. *Int J Cancer* 1990;46:159.
25. Winawer SJ, Zauber AG, Ho MN, et al. Prevention of colorectal cancer by colonoscopic polypectomy. The National Polyp Study Workgroup. *N Engl J Med* 1993;329:1977.
26. Muto T, Bussey HJ, Morson BC. The evolution of cancer of the colon and rectum. *Cancer* 1975;36:2251.
27. Fenoglio CM, Lane N. The anatomical precursor of colorectal carcinoma. *Cancer* 1974;34[Suppl]:819.
28. Hamilton SR. Pathology and biology of colorectal neoplasia. In: Young GP, Rozen P, Levin B, eds. *Prevention and early detection of colorectal cancer.* London: WB Saunders, 1996:3.
29. Burt RW, Samowitz WS. The adenomatous polyp and the hereditary polyposis syndromes. *Gastroenterol Clin North Am* 1988;17:657.
30. Rustgi AK. Hereditary gastrointestinal polyposis and nonpolyposis syndromes. *N Engl J Med* 1994;331:1694.
31. Stryker SJ, Wolff BG, Culp CE, et al. Natural history of untreated colonic polyps. *Gastroenterology* 1987;93:1009.
32. Ekbom A, Helmick C, Zack M, et al. Ulcerative colitis and colorectal cancer. A population-based study. *N Engl J Med* 1990;323:1228.
33. Lewis JD, Deren JJ, Lichtenstein GR. Cancer risk in patients with inflammatory bowel disease. *Gastroenterol Clin North Am* 1999;28:459.
34. Kinzler KW, Vogelstein B. Lessons from hereditary colorectal cancer. *Cell* 1996;87:159.
35. Polakis P. The adenomatous polyposis coli (APC) tumor suppressor. *Biochim Biophys Acta* 1997;1332:F127.
36. Alman BA, Li C, Pajerski ME, et al. Increased beta-catenin protein and somatic APC mutations in sporadic aggressive fibromatoses (desmoid tumors). *Am J Pathol* 1997;151:329.
37. Achille A, Scupoli MT, Magalini AR, et al. APC gene mutations and allelic losses in sporadic ampullary tumours: evidence of genetic difference from tumours associated with familial adenomatous polyposis. *Int J Cancer* 1996;68:305.
38. Imai Y, Oda H, Tsurutani N, et al. Frequent somatic mutations of the APC and p53 genes in sporadic ampullary carcinomas. *Jpn J Cancer Res* 1997;88:846.
39. Bienz M. APC: the plot thickens. *Curr Opin Genet Dev* 1999;9:595.
40. He TC, Sparks AB, Rago C, et al. Identification of c-MYC as a target of the APC pathway. *Science* 1998;281:1509.
41. Tetsu O, McCormick F. β-catenin regulates expression of cyclin D1 in colon carcinoma cells. *Nature* 1999;398:422.
42. Shtutman M, Zhurinsky J, Simcha I, et al. The cyclin D1 gene is a target of the β-catenin/LEF-1 pathway. *Proc Natl Acad Sci U S A* 1999;96:5522.
43. Crawford HC, Fingleton BM, Rudolph-Owen LA, et al. The metalloproteinase matrilysin is a target of beta-catenin transactivation in intestinal tumors. *Oncogene* 1999;18:2883.
44. Morin PJ, Sparks AB, Korinek V, et al. Activation of β-catenin-Tcf signaling in colon cancer by mutations in β-catenin or APC. *Science* 1997;275:1787.
45. Sparks AB, Morin PJ, Vogelstein B, et al. Mutational analysis of the APC/β-catenin/Tcf pathway in colorectal cancer. *Cancer Res* 1998;58:1130.
46. Polakis P. The oncogenic activation of β-catenin. *Curr Opin Genet Dev* 1999;9:15.
47. Laken SJ, Petersen GM, Gruber SB, et al. Familial colorectal cancer in Ashkenazim due to a hypermutable tract in APC. *Nat Genet* 1997;17:79.
48. Warthin AS. Hereditary with reference to carcinoma. *Arch Intern Med* 1913;12:546.
49. Lynch HT, Shaw MW, Magnuson CW, et al. Hereditary factors in cancer. Study of two large midwestern kindreds. *Arch Intern Med* 1966;117:206.
50. Lynch HT, Krush AJ. Cancer family "G" revisited: 1895–1970. *Cancer* 1971;27:1505.
51. Vasen HF, Mecklin JP, Khan PM. The International Collaborative Group on Hereditary Non-Polyposis Colorectal Cancer (ICG-HNPCC). *Dis Colon Rectum* 1991;34:424.
52. Boland CR. Hereditary nonpolyposis colorectal cancer. In: Vogelstein B, Kinzler KW, eds. *The genetic basis of human cancer.* New York: McGraw-Hill, 1998:333.
53. Peltomaki P, Sistonen P, Mecklin JP, et al. Evidence supporting exclusion of the DCC gene and a portion of chromosome 18q as the locus for susceptibility to hereditary nonpolyposis colorectal carcinoma in five kindreds. *Cancer Res* 1991;51:4135.
54. Peltomaki P, Sistonen P, Mecklin JP, et al. Evidence that the MCC-APC gene region in 5q21 is not the site for susceptibility to hereditary nonpolyposis colorectal carcinoma. *Cancer Res* 1992;52:4530.
55. Peltomaki P, Aaltonen LA, Sistonen P, et al. Genetic mapping of a locus predisposing to human colorectal cancer. *Science* 1993;260:810.
56. Lindblom A, Tannergard P, Werelius B, et al. Genetic mapping of a second locus predisposing to hereditary non-polyposis colon cancer. *Nat Genet* 1993;5:279.
57. Aaltonen LA, Peltomaki P, Sistonen P, et al. Clues to the pathogenesis of familial colorectal cancer. *Science* 1993;260:812.
58. Thibodeau SN, Bren G, Schaid D. Microsatellite instability in cancer of the proximal colon. *Science* 1993;260:816.
59. Ionov Y, Peinado MA, Malkhosyan S, et al. Ubiquitous somatic mutations in simple repeated sequences reveal a new mechanism for colonic carcinogenesis. *Nature* 1993;363:558.
60. Parsons R, Li GM, Longley MJ, et al. Hypermutability and mismatch repair deficiency in RER+ tumor cells. *Cell* 1993;75:1227.
61. Fishel R, Lescoe MK, Rao MR, et al. The human mutator gene homolog MSH2 and its association with hereditary nonpolyposis colon cancer [published erratum appears in *Cell* 1994;77:167]. *Cell* 1993;75:1027.
62. Leach FS, Nicolaides NC, Papadopoulos N, et al. Mutations of a mutS homolog in hereditary nonpolyposis colorectal cancer. *Cell* 1993;75:1215.
63. Bronner CE, Baker SM, Morrison PT, et al. Mutation in the DNA mismatch repair gene homologue hMLH1 is associated with hereditary non-polyposis colon cancer. *Nature* 1994;368:258.
64. Papadopoulos N, Nicolaides NC, Wei YF, et al. Mutation of a mutL homolog in hereditary colon cancer. *Science* 1994;263:1625.

65. Nicolaides NC, Papadopoulos N, Liu B, et al. Mutations of two PMS homologues in hereditary nonpolyposis colon cancer. *Nature* 1994;371:75.
66. Akiyama Y, Sato H, Yamada T, et al. Germ-line mutation of the hMSH6/GTBP gene in an atypical hereditary nonpolyposis colorectal cancer kindred. *Cancer Res* 1997;57:3920.
67. Miyaki M, Konishi M, Tanaka K, et al. Germline mutation of MSH6 as the cause of hereditary nonpolyposis colorectal cancer. *Nat Genet* 1997;17:271.
68. Liu B, Farrington SM, Petersen GM, et al. Genetic instability occurs in the majority of young patients with colorectal cancer. *Nat Med* 1995;1:348.
69. Aaltonen LA, Salovaara R, Kristo P, et al. Incidence of hereditary nonpolyposis colorectal cancer and the feasibility of molecular screening for the disease. *N Engl J Med* 1998;338:1481.
70. Wijnen JT, Vasen HF, Khan PM, et al. Clinical findings with implications for genetic testing in families with clustering of colorectal cancer. *N Engl J Med* 1998;339:511.
71. Liu B, Nicolaides NC, Willson JK, et al. Mismatch repair gene defects in sporadic colorectal cancers with microsatellite instability. *Nat Genet* 1995;9:48.
72. Kane MF, Loda M, Gaida GM, et al. Methylation of the hMLH1 promoter correlates with lack of expression of hMLH1 in sporadic colon tumors and mismatch repair-defective human tumor cell lines. *Cancer Res* 1997;57:808.
73. Herman JG, Umar A, Polyak K, et al. Incidence and functional consequences of hMLH1 promoter hypermethylation in colorectal carcinoma. *Proc Natl Acad Sci U S A* 1998;95:6870.
74. Losi L, Ponz de Leon M, Jiricny J, et al. K-ras and p53 mutations in hereditary non-polyposis colorectal cancers. *Int J Cancer* 1997;74:94.
75. Fujiwara T, Stolker JM, Watanabe T, et al. Accumulated clonal genetic alterations in familial and sporadic colorectal carcinomas with widespread instability in microsatellite sequences. *Am J Pathol* 1998;153:1063.
76. Markowitz S, Wang J, Myeroff L, et al. Inactivation of the type II TGF-β receptor in colon cancer cells with microsatellite instability. *Science* 1995;268:1336.
77. Myeroff LL, Parsons R, Kim SJ, et al. A transforming growth factor beta receptor type II gene mutation common in colon and gastric but rare in endometrial cancers with microsatellite instability. *Cancer Res* 1995;55:5545.
78. Grady WM, Myeroff LL, Swinler SE, et al. Mutational inactivation of transforming growth factor beta receptor type II in microsatellite stable colon cancers. *Cancer Res* 1999;59:320.
79. Rampino N, Yamamoto H, Ionov Y, et al. Somatic frameshift mutations in the BAX gene in colon cancers of the microsatellite mutator phenotype. *Science* 1997;275:967.
80. Souza RF, Yin J, Smolinski KN, et al. Frequent mutation of the E2F-4 cell cycle gene in primary human gastrointestinal tumors. *Cancer Res* 1997;57:2350.
81. Kitaeva MN, Grogan L, Williams JP, et al. Mutations in beta-catenin are uncommon in colorectal cancer occurring in occasional replication error–positive tumors. *Cancer Res* 1997;57:4478.
82. Mirabelli-Primdahl L, Gryfe R, Kim H, et al. β-catenin mutations are specific for colorectal carcinomas with microsatellite instability but occur in endometrial carcinomas irrespective of mutator pathway. *Cancer Res* 1999;59:3346.
83. Lengauer C, Kinzler KW, Vogelstein B. Genetic instabilities in human cancers. *Nature* 1998;396:643.
84. Bos JL. ras oncogenes in human cancer: a review [published erratum appears in *Cancer Res* 1990;50:1352]. *Cancer Res* 1989;49:4682.
85. Vogelstein B, Fearon ER, Hamilton S, et al. Genetic alterations during colorectal-tumor development. *N Engl J Med* 1988;319:525.
86. Rashid A, Zahurak M, Goodman SN, et al. Genetic epidemiology of mutated K-ras proto-oncogene, altered suppressor genes, and microsatellite instability in colorectal adenomas. *Gut* 1999;44:826.
87. Miyaki M, Seki M, Okamoto M, et al. Genetic changes and histopathological types in colorectal tumors from patients with familial adenomatous polyposis. *Cancer Res* 1990;50:7166.
88. Ohnishi T, Tomita N, Monden T, et al. A detailed analysis of the role of K-ras gene mutation in the progression of colorectal adenoma. *Br J Cancer* 1997;75:341.
89. Pretlow TP, Brasitus TA, Fulton NC, et al. K-ras mutations in putative preneoplastic lesions in human colon. *J Natl Cancer Inst* 1993;85:2004.
90. Jen J, Powell SM, Papadopoulos N, et al. Molecular determinants of dysplasia in colorectal lesions. *Cancer Res* 1994;54:5523.
91. Smith AJ, Stern HS, Penner M, et al. Somatic APC and K-ras codon 12 mutations in aberrant crypt foci from human colons. *Cancer Res* 1994;54:5527.
92. Otori K, Oda Y, Sugiyama K, et al. High frequency of K-ras mutations in human colorectal hyperplastic polyps. *Gut* 1997;40:660.
93. Shirasawa S, Furuse M, Yokoyama N, et al. Altered growth of human colon cancer cell lines disrupted at activated Ki-ras. *Science* 1993;260:85.
94. Fearon ER, Vogelstein B. A genetic model for colorectal tumorigenesis. *Cell* 1990;61:759.
95. Leach FS, Elledge SJ, Sherr CJ, et al. Amplification of cyclin genes in colorectal carcinomas. *Cancer Res* 1993;53:1986.
96. Iwao K, Nakamori S, Kameyama M, et al. Activation of the β-catenin gene by interstitial deletions involving exon 3 in primary colorectal carcinomas without adenomatous polyposis coli mutations. *Cancer Res* 1998;58:1021.
97. Samowitz WS, Powers MD, Spirio LN, et al. Beta-catenin mutations are more frequent in small colorectal adenomas than in larger adenomas and invasive carcinomas. *Cancer Res* 1999;59:1442.
98. Boland CR, Sato J, Appelman HD, et al. Microallelotyping defines the sequence and tempo of allelic losses at tumour suppressor gene loci during colorectal cancer progression. *Nat Med* 1995;1:902.
99. Baker S, Fearon ER, Nigro J, et al. Chromosome 17 deletions and p53 gene mutations in colorectal carcinomas. *Science* 1989;244:217.
100. Baker SJ, Preisinger AC, Jessup JM, et al. p53 gene mutations occur in combination with 17p allelic deletions as late events in colorectal tumorigenesis. *Cancer Res* 1990;50:7717.
101. Greenblatt MS, Bennett WP, Hollstein M, et al. Mutations in the p53 tumor suppressor gene: clues to cancer etiology and molecular pathogenesis. *Cancer Res* 1994;54:4855.
102. Levine AJ. p53, the cellular gatekeeper for growth and division. *Cell* 1997;88:323.
103. Burns TF, El-Deiry WS. The p53 pathway and apoptosis. *J Cell Physiol* 1999;181:231.
104. Prives C, Hall PA. The p53 pathway. *J Pathol* 1999;187:112.
105. Brown JM, Wouters BG. Apoptosis, p53, and tumor cell sensitivity to anticancer agents. *Cancer Res* 1999;59:1391.
106. Ookawa K, Sakamoto M, Hirohashi S, et al. Concordant p53 and DCC alterations and allelic losses on chromosomes 13q and 14q associated with liver metastases of colorectal carcinoma. *Int J Cancer* 1993;53:382.
107. Jen J, Kim H, Piantadosi S, et al. Allelic loss of chromosome 18q and prognosis in colorectal cancer. *N Engl J Med* 1994;331:213.
108. Ogunbiyi OA, Goodfellow PJ, Herfarth K, et al. Confirmation that chromosome 18q allelic loss in colon cancer is a prognostic indicator. *J Clin Oncol* 1998;16:427.
109. Lanza G, Matteuzzi M, Gafa R, et al. Chromosome 18q allelic loss and prognosis in stage II and III colon cancer. *Int J Cancer* 1998;79:390.
110. Martinez-Lopez E, Abad A, Font A, et al. Allelic loss on chromosome 18q as a prognostic marker in stage II colorectal cancer. *Gastroenterology* 1998;114:1180.
111. Jernvall P, Makinen MJ, Karttunen TJ, et al. Loss of heterozygosity at 18q21 is indicative of recurrence and therefore poor prognosis in a subset of colorectal cancers. *Br J Cancer* 1999;79:903.
112. Fearon ER, Cho KR, Nigro JM, et al. Identification of a chromosome 18q gene that is altered in colorectal cancers. *Science* 1990;247:49.
113. Cho K, Fearon ER. DCC—linking tumour suppressor genes and altered cell surface interactions in cancer. *Curr Opin Genet Dev* 1995;5:72.
114. Fearon ER. DCC: is there a connection between tumorigenesis and cell guidance molecules? *Biochim Biophys Acta* 1996;1288:M17.
115. Cho KR, Oliner JD, Simons JW, et al. The DCC gene—structural analysis and mutations in colorectal carcinomas. *Genomics* 1994;19:525.
116. Mehlen P, Rabizadeh S, Snipas SJ, et al. The DCC gene product induces apoptosis by a mechanism requiring receptor proteolysis. *Nature* 1998;395:801.
117. Hahn SA, Schutte M, Hoque AT, et al. DPC4, a candidate tumor suppressor gene at human chromosome 18q21.1. *Science* 1996;271:350.
118. Hilgers W, Kern SE. Molecular genetic basis of pancreatic adenocarcinoma. *Genes Chromosomes Cancer* 1999;26:1.
119. Howe JR, Roth S, Ringold JC, et al. Mutations in the SMAD4/DPC4 gene in juvenile polyposis. *Science* 1998;280:1086.
120. Thiagalingam S, Lengauer C, Leach FS, et al. Evaluation of candidate tumour suppressor genes on chromosome 18 in colorectal cancers. *Nat Genet* 1996;13:343.
121. Takagi Y, Kohmura H, Futamura M, et al. Somatic alterations of the DPC4 gene in human colorectal cancers *in vivo*. *Gastroenterology* 1996;111:1369.
122. Koyama M, Ito M, Nagai H, et al. Inactivation of both alleles of the DPC4/SMAD4 gene in advanced colorectal cancers: identification of seven novel somatic mutations in tumors from Japanese patients. *Mutat Res* 1999;406:71.
123. Miyaki M, Iijima T, Konishi M, et al. Higher frequency of Smad4 gene mutation in human colorectal cancer with distant metastasis. *Oncogene* 1999;18:3098.
124. Powell SM, Harper JC, Hamilton SR, et al. Inactivation of Smad4 in gastric carcinomas. *Cancer Res* 1997;57:4221.
125. Barrett MT, Schutte M, Kern SE, et al. Allelic loss and mutational analysis of the DPC4 gene in esophageal adenocarcinoma. *Cancer Res* 1996;56:4351.
126. Lei J, Zou TT, Shi YQ, et al. Infrequent DPC4 gene mutation in esophageal cancer, gastric cancer and ulcerative colitis–associated neoplasms. *Oncogene* 1996;13:2459.
127. Maesawa C, Tamura G, Nishizuka S, et al. *MAD*-related genes on 18q21.1, *Smad2* and *Smad4*, are altered infrequently in esophageal squamous cell carcinoma. *Jpn J Cancer Res* 1997;88:340.
128. Riggins GJ, Thiagalingam S, Rozenblum E, et al. Mad-related genes in the human. *Nat Genet* 1996;13:347.
129. Eppert K, Scherer SW, Ozcelik H, et al. MADR2 maps to 18q21 and encodes a TGFβ-regulated MAD-related protein that is functionally mutated in colorectal carcinoma. *Cell* 1996;86:543.
130. Takenoshita S, Tani M, Mogi A, et al. Mutation analysis of the Smad2 gene in human colon cancers using genomic DNA and intron primers. *Carcinogenesis* 1998;19:803.
131. Takagi Y, Koumura H, Futamura M, et al. Somatic alterations of the SMAD-2 gene in human colorectal cancers. *Br J Cancer* 1998;78:1152.
132. Shitara Y, Yokozaki H, Yasui W, et al. No mutations of the Smad2 gene in human sporadic gastric carcinomas. *Jpn J Clin Oncol* 1999;29:3.
133. Hruban RH, Yeo CJ, Kern SE. Pancreatic cancer. In: Vogelstein B, Kinzler KW, eds. *The genetic basis of human cancer.* New York: McGraw-Hill, 1998:603.
134. Seymour AB, Hruban RH, Redston M, et al. Allelotype of pancreatic adenocarcinoma. *Cancer Res* 1994;54:2761.
135. Hahn SA, Seymour AB, Hoque AT, et al. Allelotype of pancreatic adenocarcinoma using xenograft enrichment. *Cancer Res* 1995;55:4670.
136. Schutte M, Hruban RH, Geradts J, et al. Abrogation of the Rb/p16 tumor-suppressive pathway in virtually all pancreatic carcinomas. *Cancer Res* 1997;57:3126.
137. Wilentz RE, Su GH, Dai JL, et al. Immunohistochemical labeling for dpc4 mirrors genetic status in pancreatic adenocarcinomas: a new marker of DPC4 inactivation. *Am J Pathol* 2000;156:37.
138. Ozcelik H, Schmocker B, Di Nicola N, et al. Germline BRCA2 6174delT mutations in Ashkenazi Jewish pancreatic cancer patients. *Nat Genet* 1997;16:17.
139. Lal G, Liu G, Schmocker B, et al. Inherited predisposition to pancreatic adenocarcinoma: role of family history and germ-line p16, BRCA1, and BRCA2 mutations. *Cancer Res* 2000;60:409.
140. Phillips RW, Wong RK. Barrett's esophagus. Natural history, incidence, etiology, and complications. *Gastroenterol Clin North Am* 1991;20:791.
141. Neshat K, Sanchez CA, Galipeau PC, et al. Barrett's esophagus: a model of human neoplastic progression. Cold Spring Harbor Symposia on Quantitative Biology. Cold Spring Harbor, NY: Cold Spring Harbor Laboratory Press, 1994;59:577.

142. Houldsworth J, Cordon-Cardo C, Ladanyi M, et al. Gene amplification in gastric and esophageal adenocarcinomas. *Cancer Res* 1990;50:6417.
143. Hughes SJ, Glover TW, Zhu XX, et al. A novel amplicon at 8p22-23 results in overexpression of cathepsin B in esophageal adenocarcinoma. *Proc Natl Acad Sci U S A* 1998;95:12410.
144. Lin L, Aggarwal S, Glover TW, et al. A minimal critical region of the 8p22-23 amplicon in esophageal adenocarcinomas defined using sequence tagged site-amplification mapping and quantitative polymerase chain reaction includes the GATA-4 gene. *Cancer Res* 2000;60:1341.
145. Wong DJ, Barrett MT, Stoger R, et al. p16INK4a promoter is hypermethylated at a high frequency in esophageal adenocarcinomas. *Cancer Res* 1997;57:2619.
146. Galipeau PC, Cowan DS, Sanchez CA, et al. 17p (p53) allelic losses, 4N (G2/tetraploid) populations, and progression to aneuploidy in Barrett's esophagus. *Proc Natl Acad Sci U S A* 1996;93:7081.
147. Barrett MT, Sanchez CA, Galipeau PC, et al. Allelic loss of 9p21 and mutation of the CDKN2/p16 gene develop as early lesions during neoplastic progression in Barrett's esophagus. *Oncogene* 1996;13:1867.
148. Barrett MT, Sanchez CA, Prevo LJ, et al. Evolution of neoplastic cell lineages in Barrett oesophagus. *Nat Genet* 1999;22:106.
149. Galipeau PC, Prevo LJ, Sanchez CA, et al. Clonal expansion and loss of heterozygosity at chromosomes 9p and 17p in premalignant esophageal (Barrett's) tissue. *J Natl Cancer Inst* 1999;91:2087.
150. Wu TT, Watanabe T, Heitmiller R, et al. Genetic alterations in Barrett esophagus and adenocarcinomas of the esophagus and esophagogastric junction region. *Am J Pathol* 1998;153:287.
151. Powell SM, Papadopoulos N, Kinzler KW, et al. APC gene mutations in the mutation cluster region are rare in esophageal cancers. *Gastroenterology* 1994;107:1759.
152. Waddell WR, Ganser GF, Cerise EJ, et al. Sulindac for polyposis of the colon. *Am J Surg* 1989;157:175.
153. Giardiello FM, Hamilton SR, Krush AJ, et al. Treatment of colonic and rectal adenomas with sulindac in familial adenomatous polyposis. *N Engl J Med* 1993;328:1313.
154. Giardiello FM. NSAID-induced polyp regression in familial adenomatous polyposis patients. *Gastroenterol Clin North Am* 1996;25:349.
155. Oshima M, Dinchuk JE, Kargman SL, et al. Suppression of intestinal polyposis in Apc delta716 knockout mice by inhibition of cyclooxygenase 2 (COX-2). *Cell* 1996;87:803.
156. He TC, Chan TA, Vogelstein B, et al. PPARδ is an APC-regulated target of nonsteroidal anti-inflammatory drugs. *Cell* 1999;99:335.
157. Shimodaira H, Filosi N, Shibata H, et al. Functional analysis of human MLH1 mutations in *Saccharomyces cerevisiae*. *Nat Genet* 1998;19:384.
158. Petersen GM, Brensinger JD, Johnson KA, et al. Genetic testing and counseling for hereditary forms of colorectal cancer. *Cancer* 1999;86:2540.
159. Markowitz AJ, Winawer SJ. Screening and surveillance for colorectal cancer. *Semin Oncol* 1999;26:485.
160. Sidransky D, Tokino T, Hamilton SR, et al. Identification of RAS oncogene mutations in the stool of patients with curable colorectal tumors. *Science* 1992;256:102.
161. Smith-Ravin J, England J, Talbot IC, et al. Detection of c-Ki-ras mutations in faecal samples from sporadic colorectal cancer patients. *Gut* 1995;36:81.
162. Villa E, Dugani A, Rebecchi AM, et al. Identification of subjects at risk for colorectal carcinoma through a test based on K-ras determination in the stool. *Gastroenterology* 1996;110:1346.
163. Puig P, Urgell E, Capella G, et al. A highly sensitive method for K-ras mutation detection is useful in diagnosis of gastrointestinal cancer. *Int J Cancer* 2000;85:73.
164. Caldas C, Hahn SA, Hruban RH, et al. Detection of K-ras mutations in the stool of patients with pancreatic adenocarcinoma and pancreatic ductal hyperplasia. *Cancer Res* 1994;54:3568.
165. Caldas C. Biliopancreatic malignancy: screening the at risk patient with molecular markers. *Ann Oncol* 1999;10[Suppl 4]:153.
166. Liefers GJ, Cleton-Jansen AM, van de Velde CJ, et al. Micrometastases and survival in stage II colorectal cancer. *N Engl J Med* 1998;339:223.
167. Hayashi N, Ito I, Yanagisawa A, et al. Genetic diagnosis of lymph-node metastasis in colorectal cancer. *Lancet* 1995;345:1257.
168. Sanchez-Cespedes M, Esteller M, Hibi K, et al. Molecular detection of neoplastic cells in lymph nodes of metastatic colorectal cancer patients predicts recurrence. *Clin Cancer Res* 1999;5:2450.

DAVID S. SCHRUMP
NASSER K. ALTORKI
ARLENE A. FORASTIERE
BRUCE D. MINSKY

SECTION **2**

Cancer of the Esophagus

EPIDEMIOLOGY

Esophageal cancer represents the third most common gastrointestinal malignancy and ranks among the ten most common cancers worldwide. The incidence of esophageal cancer varies considerably relative to geographic location; high incidence areas have been identified within the Caspian littoral region of northern Iran, Southern republics of the former Soviet Union, and northern China where the incidence exceeds 100 in 100,000 individuals. The incidence of esophageal cancer ranges from 10 to 50 in 100,000 in Sri Lanka, India, South Africa, France, and Switzerland. This disease is less common (average incidence less than 10 in 100,000) in most areas within Japan, Great Britain, Europe, and Canada.[1,2] Squamous cell carcinomas account for the vast majority of neoplasms observed in these regions.

In the United States, esophageal cancers are relatively uncommon (average incidence less than 5 in 100,000); however, U.S. mortality data from 1990 to 1994 have revealed a steady increase in age-adjusted mortality in male as well as female subjects due to this malignancy.[2] Within the United States, the incidence of esophageal cancer varies with location, with a high frequency of esophageal squamous cell carcinomas being noted in coastal regions in South Carolina and metropolitan areas including New York City, Detroit, Washington, DC, and Los Angeles, where the incidence approximates 30 in 100,000 individuals.[1,3] Squamous cell carcinomas predominate in these high incidence areas within the United States.

In the recent past, the incidence of esophageal adenocarcinomas has risen dramatically, whereas the incidence of squamous cell carcinomas has remained relatively steady in the United States.[2] Before 1980, adenocarcinomas constituted approximately 15% of esophageal malignancies; however, by 1994, nearly 60% of all esophageal malignancies were adenocarcinomas.[2] Rates of adenocarcinoma are highest in white men. The incidence of esophageal carcinoma in women is much lower, although the incidence of adenocarcinomas is also increasing in women. Similar trends have been noted in western European countries.[4–6] The rising incidence of esophageal adenocarcinoma cannot be attributed solely to the increased incidence of carcinomas of the cardia, which now account for approximately one-half of gastric cancers in American men.[4,7] Although the precise etiology of these neoplasms has not been elucidated, considerable data indicate that esophageal adenocarcinomas result from chronic gastroesophageal reflux often in the context of hiatal hernia.[8–11]

Although cultural as well as dietary practices contribute to esophageal cancers in high incidence areas in Asia, South Africa, South America, and the Middle East, tobacco and ethanol exposure are believed to be the primary risk factors associated with esophageal squamous cell carcinomas in the United States and western Europe.[1,2,12,13] Tobacco and ethanol consumption have been identified as individual risk factors for this malignancy, and their effects are multiplicative.[1,14] A five- to tenfold increase in esophageal squamous cell cancers has been noted in smokers relative to nonsmokers, and the risk of esophageal carcinoma correlates with extent of tobacco exposure.[1,15–17] Tobacco abuse may also contribute to the pathogenesis of esophageal adenocarcinomas, although to a much lesser extent; a multicenter study by Gammon et al.[18] as well as additional clinical studies have indi-

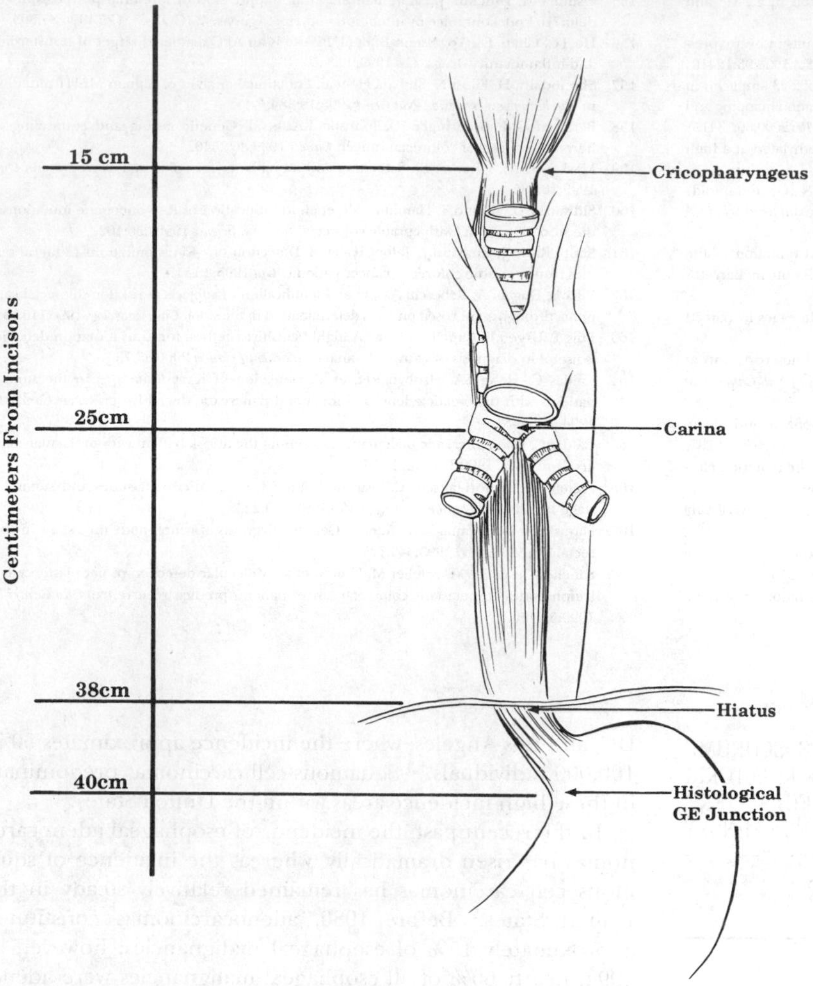

FIGURE 33.2-1. General anatomy of the esophagus with major landmarks identified. GE, gastroesophageal.

cated that the risk of esophageal adenocarcinoma is approximately twofold higher in smokers compared with nonsmokers.[2,14] Interestingly, whereas the risk of esophageal squamous cell cancer decreases significantly following cessation of tobacco abuse, little change is noted in esophageal adenocarcinoma risk following smoking cessation.[18] These data suggest that tobacco-related carcinogens may be influencing different stages of malignant transformation associated with squamous cell cancers relative to adenocarcinomas. Chemicals in tobacco are known to induce p53 mutations,[19] and these mutations appear to be extremely early events during multistep esophageal adenocarcinogenesis.[20,21] The timing of p53 mutations during squamous cell carcinogenesis has not been defined; however, these mutations appear to be relatively late events during pulmonary carcinogenesis.[22,23]

Alcohol abuse has been associated with increased risk of esophageal squamous cell cancers, and risk increases with amount of alcohol consumed.[24,25] Alcohol interacts in a multiplicative manner with tobacco, with nearly a 100-fold increase in the risk of esophageal malignancy observed in individuals with heavy tobacco and ethanol exposure.[1,2] Specific beverages have been implicated in the pathogenesis of squamous cell cancers in Europe, South Africa, South America, and the United States; however, in all likelihood, ethanol is the major component related to the pathogenesis of these cancers.[14] Ethanol consumption appears to have a less significant role in the pathogenesis of esophageal adenocarcinomas.[18,26,27]

Data indicate that obesity may be related to risk of esophageal cancer, particularly adenocarcinomas.[28,29] In general, the risk of esophageal squamous cell cancers decreases, whereas risk of adenocarcinoma increases with enlarging body mass. Esophageal squamous cell cancers have been associated with nutritional deficiencies; a low intake of fruits and vegetables may increase the esophageal cancer risk twofold.[1,30,31] Deficiencies in β-carotene, vitamin E, and selenium may also increase the risk of squamous cell cancer in underdeveloped areas. Dietary practices including drinking of extremely hot beverages or ingestion of fermented vegetables may contribute to increased cancer risk in Asia and South America[32,33]; however, the role of dietary practices in the pathogenesis of esophageal cancers in the United States is unclear. Although several environmental carcinogens, including asbestos, perchlorethylene, and combustion products, may contribute to the pathogenesis of esophageal squamous cell cancers,[34–36] no occupational risk factors have been associated with esophageal adenocarcinomas.

ANATOMY

The esophagus commences at the cricopharyngeus muscle at the level of the cricoid cartilage and extends 5 to 6 cm in the cervical region to enter the thoracic inlet (Fig. 33.2-1). The intrathoracic esophagus extends an additional 20 to 25 cm to the gastroesoph-

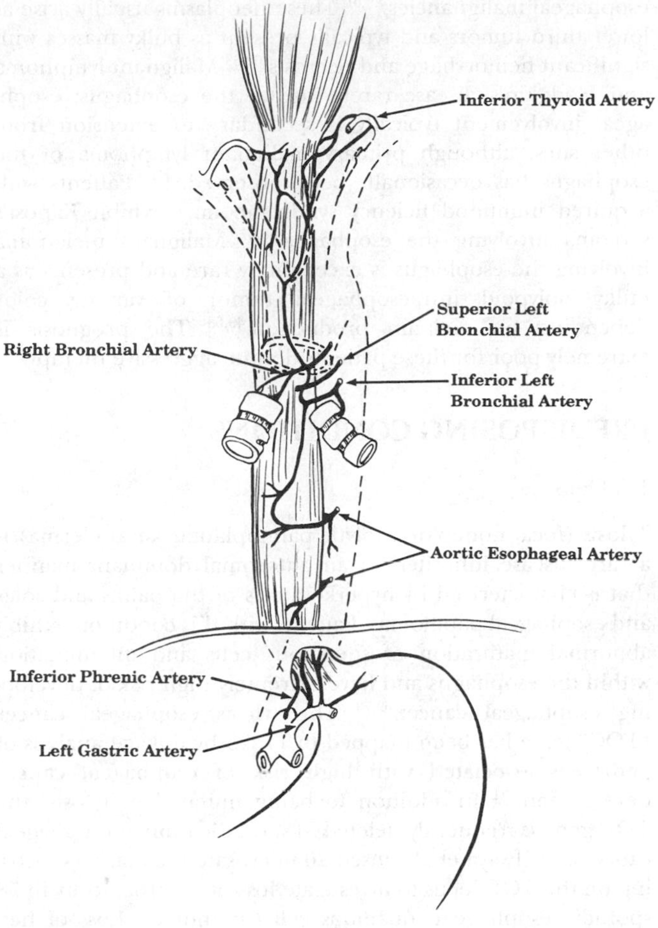

FIGURE 33.2-2. Blood supply of the esophagus.

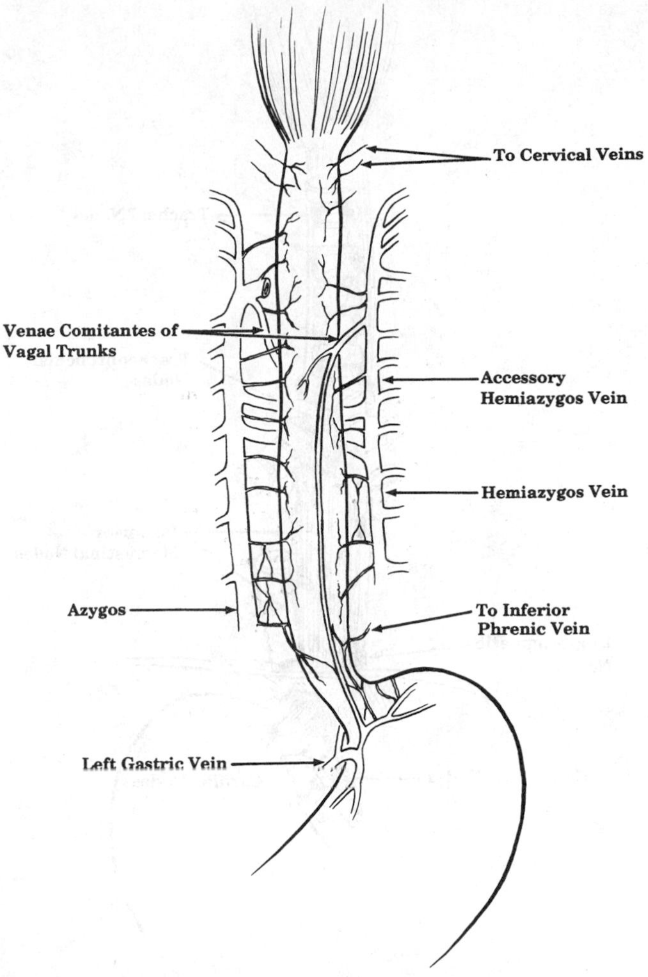

FIGURE 33.2-3. Venous drainage of the esophagus.

ageal junction. Typically, many radiologists and surgeons divide the esophagus into thirds whereby the upper third extends from the cricopharyngeus to the superior portion of the aortic arch, the middle third extends from the aortic arch to the inferior pulmonary veins, and the distal third extends from the level of the inferior pulmonary veins to the gastroesophageal junction.

The blood supply to the esophagus is segmental, with vessels extending into the esophagus to form a submucosal vascular plexus (Fig. 33.2-2). The cervical esophagus is supplied primarily by the superior and inferior thyroid arteries, whereas the thoracic esophagus is supplied by esophageal arteries arising directly from the aorta near the level of the carina; the distal esophagus and gastric cardia are supplied primarily by the left gastric artery. Venous drainage from the esophagus is into the azygous and hemiazygous veins as well as intercostal veins that ultimately drain into the azygous system (Fig. 33.2-3).

The esophagus contains abundant mucosal and submucosal lymphatics that communicate with lymphatic channels in the muscular layers to drain either directly through the esophageal wall to adjacent lymph nodes or to the thoracic duct (Fig. 33.2-4).[37] Lesions in the upper third of the esophagus tend to drain initially to internal jugular, cervical, and supraclavicular nodes; in contrast, middle third lesions drain initially to paratracheal, hilar, subcarinal, paraesophageal, and pericardial nodal regions. Distal third tumors tend to drain to nodes along the lesser curvature, left gastric artery, and celiac axis. However, because the pattern of lymphatic drainage is primarily longitudinal rather than segmental, extensive regional dissemination of cancer cells may occur irrespective of the location of the primary tumor. Celiac nodal metastases have been observed in 10% of patients with upper third carcinomas, and nearly 45% of individuals with middle third lesions; approximately 30% patients with middle or lower third carcinomas have metastatic disease in deep cervical lymph nodes at presentation.[38,39]

HISTOLOGY

The overwhelming majority of esophageal malignancies may be classified as either squamous cell carcinomas or adenocarcinomas. Squamous cell carcinomas account for approximately 40% of esophageal malignancies diagnosed in the United States and the vast majority of cancers arising in high-incidence areas throughout the world.[1,2] Approximately 60% of these neoplasms are located in the middle third of the esophagus, whereas 30% and 10% arise in the distal third or proximal third of the intrathoracic esophagus, respectively.[40,41] Typically, these tumors are moderately well differentiated and often are associated with contiguous or noncontiguous carcinoma *in situ*, as well as widespread submucosal lymphatic dissemination.[42,43]

Adenocarcinomas frequently arise in the context of Barrett's esophagus; as such, these tumors tend to be localized in the dis-

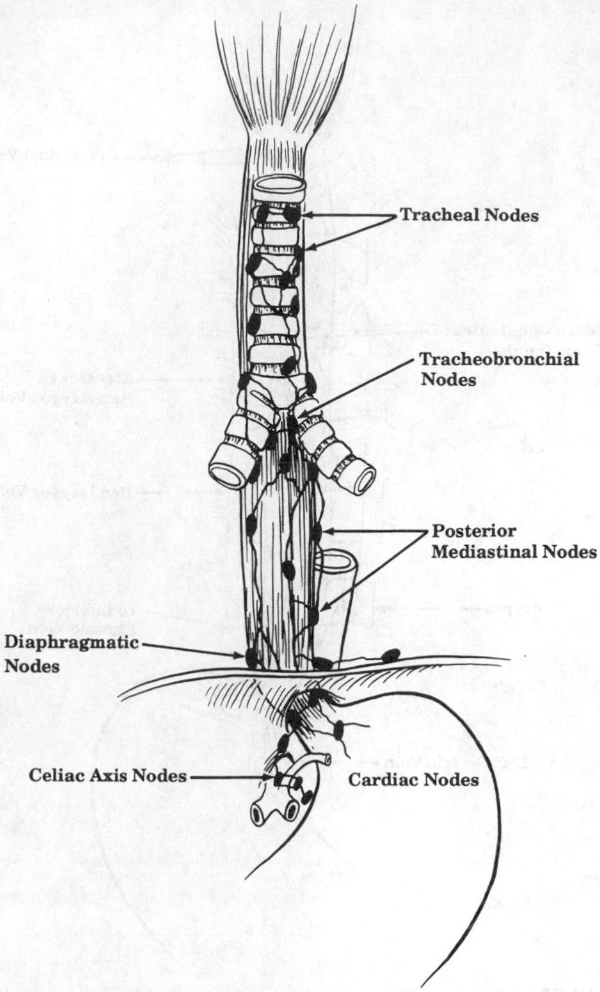

FIGURE 33.2-4. Major lymphatic drainage areas of the esophagus.

tal third of the esophagus and may be fungating or stenotic in appearance.[44,45] Many of these tumors are well-differentiated adenocarcinomas, and the vast majority are associated with intraepithelial neoplasia.[46,47] No significant survival differences have been noted in adenocarcinoma patients compared with similarly staged individuals with squamous cell cancers.[39,48]

Several rare cancers of the esophagus have been described, including squamous cell carcinoma with sarcomatous features, as well as adenoid cystic, and mucoepidermoid carcinomas.[49–53] These neoplasms are indistinguishable clinically and prognostically from the more common types of esophageal carcinomas.

Small cell carcinomas account for approximately 1% of esophageal malignancies and arise from argyrophilic cells in the basal layer of the squamous epithelium.[54,55] These neoplasms are usually located in the middle or lower third of the esophagus and may be associated with ectopic production of a variety of hormones including parathormone, secretin, granulocyte colony-stimulating factor, and gastrin-releasing peptide; individuals with these cancers often present with systemic disease.[56,57] Although small cell carcinomas frequently respond to radiation and chemotherapy, patients with these neoplasms typically succumb to widespread distant metastases.[58–60]

Leiomyosarcoma is the most common mesenchymal tumor affecting the esophagus, accounting for less than 1% of all esophageal malignancies.[49,61] These neoplasms usually arise as lower third tumors and typically present as bulky masses with significant hemorrhage and necrosis.[62,63] Malignant lymphoma and Hodgkin's disease rarely involve the esophagus; esophageal involvement typically is secondary to extension from other sites, although primary malignant lymphoma of the esophagus has occasionally been observed.[64,65] Patients with acquired immunodeficiency syndrome may exhibit Kaposi's sarcoma involving the esophagus.[66,67] Malignant melanoma involving the esophagus is exceedingly rare and presents as a bulky polypoid intraesophageal tumor of varying color depending on melanin production.[49,68] The prognosis is extremely poor for these patients despite aggressive therapy.

PREDISPOSING CONDITIONS

TYLOSIS

Tylosis (focal nonepidermolytic palmoplantar keratoderma) is a rare disease inherited in an autosomal dominant manner that is characterized by hyperkeratosis of the palms and soles and esophageal papillomas. Patients with this condition exhibit abnormal maturation of squamous cells and inflammation within the esophagus and have extremely high risk of developing esophageal cancer.[69,70] The tylosis esophageal cancer (TOC) gene has been mapped to 17q25 by linkage analysis of pedigrees associated with high risk of esophageal cancer development.[71] In addition to being mutated in tylosis, the TOC gene is frequently deleted in sporadic human esophageal cancers.[72,73] Iwaya et al.[73] used 20 microsatellite markers focusing on the TOC locus to investigate loss of heterozygosity in 58 sporadic esophageal squamous cell carcinomas. Loss of heterozygosity was observed in 37 of 52 (71%) informative cases, 80% (33 of 37) of which involved the TOC locus. Envoplakin, encoding a protein component of desmosomes that is expressed in esophageal keratinocytes, has been mapped to the TOC region[74]; however, no tylosis-specific mutations involving this gene have been observed.[75] Further studies are required to define the tumor suppressor gene(s) mapping to 17q25 that are inactivated in tylosis-associated as well as sporadic esophageal carcinomas.

PLUMMER-VINSON/PATERSON-KELLY SYNDROME

Plummer-Vinson/Paterson-Kelly syndrome is characterized by iron-deficiency anemia, glossitis, kelosis, brittle fingernails, splenomegaly, and esophageal webs. Approximately 10% of individuals with Plummer-Vinson/Paterson-Kelly syndrome develop hypopharyngeal or esophageal epidermoid carcinomas.[76] The mechanisms by which these tumors arise have not been fully defined, although nutritional deficiencies as well as chronic mucosal irritation from retained food particles at the level of the webs may contribute to the pathogenesis of these neoplasms.[77]

CAUSTIC INJURY

Squamous cell carcinomas may arise in lye strictures, often developing 40 to 50 years following caustic injury.[78] The majority of these cancers are located in the middle third of the esophagus. The pathogenesis of these neoplasms may be similar to that implicated in esophageal cancers arising in patients with Plummer-Vinson syndrome. These cancers are often diagnosed late due to the fact that chronic dysphagia and pain due to the lye strictures obscure symptoms of esophageal cancer.

ACHALASIA

Achalasia is an idiopathic esophageal motility disorder characterized by increased basal pressure in the lower esophageal sphincter, incomplete relaxation of this sphincter following deglutition, and aperistalsis of the body of the esophagus. A 16- to 30-fold increase in esophageal cancer risk has been noted in achalasia patients.[79,80] In a retrospective analysis, Aggestrup et al.[81] observed the development of esophageal carcinomas in 10 of 147 patients undergoing esophagomyotomy for achalasia. These neoplasms typically are squamous cell carcinomas, believed to result from prolonged irritation from retained foods at the air–fluid interface in the midesophagus, and arise an average of 17 years following onset of achalasia symptoms. The insidious nature of carcinomas arising in the context of chronic dysphagia and pain attributable to megaesophagus contributes to their late diagnosis in achalasia patients.[82]

HELICOBACTER PYLORI INFECTION

Helicobacter infection has been associated with gastritis and peptic ulcer disease. Several studies suggest that the extent of *Helicobacter* gastritis may correlate inversely with diminished gastroesophageal reflux and esophageal cancer.[83,84] Sharma et al.[85] observed no evidence of *Helicobacter pylori* in specialized intestinal metaplasia in 209 esophageal biopsies from 58 patients with columnar-lined epithelium. In another study, El-Serag et al.[86] evaluated the database of the Department of Veterans Affairs and noted that *Helicobacter pylori* infection and atrophic gastritis were associated with diminished acid output and increased risk of gastric carcinoma, but diminished risk of esophageal cancer. These data have been confirmed by Chow et al.,[83] who also noted an inverse relationship between *Helicobacter* infection and risk of gastroesophageal adenocarcinoma. Thus, available data indicate that *Helicobacter* has little, if any, role in the pathogenesis of esophageal cancer.

HUMAN PAPILLOMAVIRUS INFECTION

Several studies suggest that human papillomavirus (HPV) may contribute to the pathogenesis of esophageal squamous cell cancers in high-incidence areas in Asia and South Africa.[87] This oncogenic virus, which has been associated with cervical and oropharyngeal cancers,[88,89] encodes two proteins (E6 and E7) that sequester the Rb and p53 tumor suppressor gene products. Using polymerase chain reaction techniques, de Villiers et al.[90] detected HPV DNA sequences in 17% of esophageal squamous cell cancers from China. In an additional study using similar techniques, Lavergne and de Villiers et al.[91] identified a broad spectrum of HPV in approximately one-third of esophageal cancer specimens obtained from patients living in high-incidence areas in China and South Africa. Shibagaki et al.[92] detected HPV sequences in 15 of 72 (21%) esophageal cancer specimens obtained from Japanese patients. In contrast, HPV sequences have not been observed in cancers arising in low-incidence areas. Poljack et al.[93] observed no evidence of HPV in 121 formalin-fixed, paraffin-embedded esophageal cancer specimens obtained from patients in Slovenia. Similarly, Rugge et al.[94] detected no HPV in 18 carcinomas arising in Italian patients. Turner et al.[95] observed no evidence of HPV in 51 formalin-fixed, paraffin-embedded esophageal cancer specimens obtained from patients in North America. In a large population-based control study, Lagergren et al.[96] compared 121 esophageal squamous cell cancers and 173 adenocarcinoma patients with 302 population-based controls in Sweden. These authors observed no association between HPV infection and risk of esophageal cancer in this low-incidence area. Collectively, these data suggest that HPV may contribute to the pathogenesis of esophageal squamous cancers in high-incidence regions; however, this oncogenic virus appears to have little, if any, role in the pathogenesis of esophageal malignancies arising in low-incidence areas.

PRIOR AERODIGESTIVE TRACT MALIGNANCY

Carcinomas of the aerodigestive tract arise as the consequence of multistep processes in cancerization fields. Patients with upper aerodigestive tract cancers develop second primary cancers at a rate of approximately 4% per year.[97] Nearly 10% of secondary neoplasms arising in patients with prior histories of oropharyngeal carcinoma arise in the esophagus.[97] Levi et al.[98] observed that approximately 10% of second primary cancers in patients with prior histories of lung carcinoma arose in the esophagus. The increased risk of second primary tobacco-related carcinomas[99] warrants close surveillance of patients with histories of aerodigestive tract malignancy.

BARRETT'S ESOPHAGUS

Barrett's esophagus is characterized by the presence of columnar epithelium lining 3 or more cm of the distal tubular esophagus in the presence or absence of hiatal hernia. Short segment Barrett's esophagus is defined as intestinal metaplasia involving less than 3 cm of the distal esophagus at the region of the lower esophageal sphincter.[100–103] The prevalence of Barrett's esophagus ranges between 0.45% and 2.2% among all patients undergoing upper gastrointestinal endoscopy, increasing to 10% to 20% in patients undergoing endoscopy for symptomatic gastroesophageal reflux disease, and 30% to 50% in patients with peptic strictures.[104–108] Barrett's esophagus is twice as prevalent in men compared with women, and increases with age, reaching a plateau in the seventh to ninth decade of life; this disease is infrequently observed in nonwhites.[100,105,109] In all likelihood, the prevalence of Barrett's esophagus exceeds that which has been previously reported given the fact that most individuals with this disease are asymptomatic.[100,110]

Although a congenital etiology has been proposed, considerable data indicate that Barrett's esophagus is primarily an acquired condition resulting from gastroesophageal reflux.[11,100,103] The vast majority of patients diagnosed with Barrett's esophagus have significant gastroesophageal reflux, and Barrett's metaplasia has been observed following esophagogastrectomy or Heller's myotomy presumably as the result of gastroesophageal reflux in the absence of a competent lower esophageal sphincter.[111,112] Three types of columnar metaplasia have been identified in Barrett's esophagus. The fundic type mucosa is characterized by the presence of chief and parietal cells in addition to surface mucus-secreting cells containing neutral sialomucins; junctional type epithelium resembling that of gastric cardia is composed primarily of mucus-secreting cells. Specialized or intestinal type epithelia resemble that of the small bowel, appearing as a villiform surface comprised of mucus-secreting cells as well as goblet cells staining positively for acid nonsulfated mucins. Specialized epithelium is distinctive for Barrett's esophagus, being present in virtually all cases, and is the type most commonly associated with malignant degeneration.[113]

Barrett's esophagus has been associated with a 30- to 40-fold increase in the risk of adenocarcinoma, the incidence of which increased at a rate of 10% per year during the 1980s.[1,7,100] Currently, esophageal adenocarcinomas account for as much as 60% of all esophageal cancers diagnosed in the United States, and nearly 65% of esophageal adenocarcinomas had evidence of metaplastic columnar epithelia adjacent to them.[4,47] Presumably, many other esophageal adenocarcinomas have arisen in and replaced short segment Barrett's esophagus before clinical presentation.[47,114]

Although presumed to arise as the result of malignant transformation in specialized epithelia, the prevalence of adenocarcinoma in Barrett's esophagus has not been conclusively defined; however, estimates range between 0% and 64%.[105] Sharma et al.[115] identified 20 individuals with high-grade dysplasias (nearly one-half of whom would be expected to have invasive carcinomas[10,116]) out of 177 patients with short segment Barrett's esophagus. Hirota et al.[109] prospectively examined the prevalence of adenocarcinoma of the esophagus and gastroesophageal junction in patients with specialized intestinal metaplasia involving long segment Barrett's esophagus, short segment Barrett's esophagus, or esophagogastric junction. Of 833 patients studied by esophagogastroduodenoscopy, the overall prevalence of specialized intestinal metaplasia was 13.2% (1.6% long segment Barrett's esophagus, 6.0% short segment Barrett's esophagus, and 5.6% esophagogastric junction). Dysplasia or cancer was noted in 31% of long segment Barrett's esophagus, 10% of short segment Barrett's esophagus, and 6.4% of esophagogastric junction–specialized intestinal metaplasia patients. Although the prevalence of short segment Barrett's esophagus or esophagogastric junction–specialized intestinal metaplasia was approximately 3.5-fold higher than that of long segment Barrett's esophagus, the prevalence of dysplasia in long segment Barrett's esophagus was two to four times higher than that observed in the two other conditions.

Additional studies have been performed to ascertain the incidence of adenocarcinoma in Barrett's esophagus. Cameron et al.[117] followed 104 patients with Barrett's esophagus for an average of 8.5 years, only two of whom developed carcinoma, for an incidence of 1 in 141 patient-years. In an additional study, Spechler et al.[118] observed the development in carcinoma in 2 of 105 patients followed for an average of 3.3 years. In a prospective study, Robertson et al.[119] observed one case of cancer in Barrett's esophagus in 56 patient-years. In a retrospective study, Katz et al.[120] reported on 102 patients with Barrett's esophagus undergoing surveillance over a 24-year period; during 563 patient-years, three patients developed adenocarcinoma a minimum of 4 years after diagnosis; 23 additional patients progressed to low-grade dysplasia (19) or high-grade dysplasia (4) during the study period. In a large prospective analysis, O'Connor et al.[121] evaluated 136 patients enrolled in an endoscopic surveillance program at the Cleveland Clinic. The average duration of follow-up was 4.2 years, with a total of 570 patient-years. Thirty patients (22%) had short segment Barrett's esophagus. Two patients developed adenocarcinoma (incidence, 1 in 285 patient-years), and four patients progressed to high-grade dysplasia. Low-grade dysplasias developed in an additional 24 patients. In another prospective study, Weston et al.[8] reported that the incidence of high-grade dysplasia or adenocarcinoma in Barrett's esophagus was 1 per 72 patient-years.

Although esophageal adenocarcinomas are frequently preceded by histologically defined stages of metaplasia and progressively severe dysplasia in Barrett's esophagus,[122] the risk of progression to malignancy cannot be predicted by histologic parameters due to significant discordance between histologic, cytogenetic, and flow cytometric abnormalities in this condition. Fennerty et al.[123] analyzed 86 patients with Barrett's esophagus and noted that 23 of 73 patients without dysplasia, and 4 of 13 patients with dysplasia had aneuploidy or increased G_2/tetrapoid fractions evaluated by flow cytometry. Widespread cellular proliferation and aneuploidy occur relatively early in Barrett's esophagus, and progression to malignancy is associated with three well-defined cell-cycle events: (1) mobilization of G_0 cells into G_1; (2) loss of G_1/S regulation and increased S-phase fraction; and (3) accumulation of cells in G_2/M, frequently with significant aneuploidy.[20,124] Evidence of genomic instability has been observed in metaplastic epithelia as well as histologically normal tissues adjacent to Barrett's esophagus, indicating that the histologic alterations underestimate the severity of genetic events during progression to malignancy in Barrett's epithelia.[125–127] Reid et al.[128] prospectively evaluated 62 patients with Barrett's esophagus and observed that 9 of 13 patients with abnormal flow cytometry, including two with Barrett's metaplasia, five with low-grade dysplasias, and two with high-grade dysplasias, progressed to either high-grade dysplasia or invasive carcinoma; none of 49 patients with normal flow cytometry progressed to malignancy during the 34-month study. Interestingly, five patients with low-grade dysplasia who had normal flow cytometry parameters reverted to Barrett's metaplasia during the study. Collectively, these data indicate that histologic changes do not accurately reflect the severity of genomic instability in Barrett's esophagus. Furthermore, 15% to 20% of patients with Barrett's esophagus have columnar-lined epithelia exhibiting aberrant cell-cycle regulation; 70% of these individuals progress to malignancy within a 3-year period. Although the incidence of adenocarcinoma in patients with Barrett's esophagus may be relatively low, use of flow cytometry techniques may help to identify those patients who are at high risk for the development of esophageal cancer.[126,128]

Flow cytometry techniques may enhance the efficiency and optimize expense of screening surveillance programs in patients with Barrett's esophagus, which already appear to identify cancers at earlier stages compared with those detected outside the context of screening programs.[129–134] However, surveillance protocols may have limited effect overall on the incidence of advanced esophageal carcinomas. Bytzer et al.[6] evaluated the incidence of esophageal adenocarcinoma in Denmark over a 20-year period and ascertained the proportion of patients with a prior diagnosis of Barrett's esophagus. A history or diagnosis of reflux was present in 21% of patients, and 23% of individuals had undergone previous endoscopy for reflux or dyspepsia. Interestingly, only 1.3% of 524 esophageal adenocarcinoma patients had a prior diagnosis of Barrett's esophagus. In essence, greater than 98% of patients would not have entered endoscopic surveillance programs. Collectively, those data indicate that endoscopic surveillance may be beneficial in patients with Barrett's esophagus, but the vast majority of esophageal cancer patients have no antecedent symptoms that might enable early detection. Clearly, additional factors other than gastroesophageal reflux contribute to malignant transformation in Barrett's esophagus.

MOLECULAR BIOLOGY

Flow cytometric and molecular analyses of dysplastic squamous and Barrett's epithelia have revealed that esophageal cancers arise via widespread clonal outgrowth of cells exhibiting aberrant cell-cycle regulation.[20,124,135,136] In general, genomic instability precedes the appearance of histologic abnormalities in esophageal mucosa,[125,135] and the extent of cell-cycle derangements influences progression to malignancy in this setting.[128,137,138] Many of the oncogene and tumor suppressor gene mutations frequently observed in esophageal cancers and their precursor lesions perturb cell-cycle regulation by disrupting the G_1 restriction point (Table 33.2-1).

A reciprocal relationship between retinoblastoma (Rb), cyclin D, and p16 expression has been observed in esophageal cancers similar to what has been reported for other solid tumors.[139,140] In general, esophageal cancers that lack Rb expression tend to have normal cyclin D1 and p16 expression, whereas cancers that retain Rb expression typically exhibit overexpression of cyclin D1, p16 inactivation, or both. In the majority of esophageal cancers, restriction point control is circumvented via overexpression of cyclin D1, and inactivation of p16, often in the context of p53 mutations.

The epidermal growth factor receptor (EGFr) is a 170-kD tyrosine kinase receptor that is overexpressed in approximately 30% and 70% of esophageal adenocarcinomas and squamous cell cancers, respectively.[141,142] Approximately 40% of these tumors also express transforming growth factor-α, which binds to EGFr and stimulates proliferation via autocrine mechanisms. Several studies suggest that overexpression of EGFr may have prognostic significance in esophageal cancer patients. Itakura et al.[142] reported that EGFr immunoreactivity correlated significantly with diminished survival of patients undergoing esophagectomy for squamous cell cancer. Iihara et al.[143] noted that expression of transforming growth factor-α, EGFr, or both correlated with reduced survival in patients with node-positive esophageal squamous cell carcinomas. More recently in studies involving a total of 223 patients, Kitagawa et al.[144] and Shimada and coworkers[145] observed that EGFr overexpression significantly enhanced predilection for lymph node metastases, hematogenous recurrence, and diminished survival in patients undergoing potentially curative esophagectomies.

The erbB2 gene product is a 185-kD receptor molecule with intrinsic tyrosine kinase activity, which also regulates expression and function of a variety of other receptors including EGFr; in addition, p185 modulates expression of matrix metalloproteases and vascular endothelial growth factor by cancer cells.[146–149] Overexpression of erbB2 correlates with *in vitro* drug resistance, and abrogation of p185 expression enhances chemosensitivity in cancer cells.[150,151] The prognostic significance of erbB2 overexpression in esophageal cancers is unclear. Polkowski et al.[129]

TABLE 33.2-1. Oncogene and Tumor Suppressor Gene Mutations in Esophageal Cancers and Their Precursor Lesions that Disrupt the G_1 Restriction Point

Oncogenes	*Tumor Suppressors*
EGFr	3p (FHIT)
erbB2	Rb
Cyclin D	p53
	p16
	p14/ARF
	Telomerase

observed overexpression of erbB2 in approximately 25% of adenocarcinomas of the distal esophagus and gastroesophageal junction. Interestingly, 10 of 30 stage III to IV tumors overexpressed erbB2 in contrast to 0 of 11 stage I to II cancers; however, subsequent regression analysis revealed that erbB2 expression was not independent of clinical stage in determining patient survival. Furthermore, Wang and colleagues[152] observed no significant correlation between erbB2 expression and long-term survival in 117 patients undergoing potentially curative resections for esophageal squamous cell carcinoma. In contrast, Brien et al.[153] observed that erbB2 amplification independently correlated with diminished survival in patients with Barrett's adenocarcinomas.

Together with its kinase partners, cdk4 and cdk6, cyclin D1 directly regulates phosphorylation of the Rb protein at the restriction point, thereby facilitating G_1/S transit; abrogation of cyclin D1 expression inhibits the proliferation and tumorigenicity of cancer cells.[154,155] Approximately 40% to 60% of esophageal carcinomas and 30% of premalignant esophageal lesions[156–159] exhibit overexpression of cyclin D1 resulting directly from amplification of the cyclin D1 protooncogene, or indirectly from mutations involving upstream growth factor receptors such as EGFr and p185. Several studies suggest that cyclin D1 overexpression may be prognostically relevant in esophageal cancers. Shimada et al.[145] observed that cyclin D1 overexpression correlated with hematogenous recurrence and diminished survival in esophagectomy patients. In an additional study, Roncalli et al.[160] detected amplification of cyclin D1 in 17 of 55 of esophageal carcinomas, noting that overexpression of cyclin D1 correlated significantly with lymph node metastases, advanced tumor stage, and reduced overall survival in esophageal cancer patients. Takeuchi and colleagues[161] have also observed a significant correlation between cyclin D1 overexpression, and distant metastases as well as diminished survival in esophagectomy patients.

Cytogenetic and molecular analyses have revealed nonrandom patterns of allelic loss in esophageal cancers and their precursor lesions indicative of selective pressure to specifically inactivate tumor suppressor genes in these regions during multistep esophageal carcinogenesis.[136,137,162–164] Deletions involving 3p have been detected in 60% to 100% of esophageal cancers as well as a significant percentage of specimens derived from Barrett's esophagus. Although the tumor suppressor genes that are silenced by 3p mutations have not been identified conclusively, one major target appears to be the fragile histidine triad (FHIT) gene, which modulates cell-cycle progression and apoptosis.[165,166] Point mutations as well as promoter hypermethylation contribute to aberrant expression of FHIT in 50% to 90% of esophageal cancers, and the majority of Barrett's metaplasia specimens examined to date.[167–170] Although FHIT mutations correlate with increased tobacco exposure and diminished survival in lung cancer patients,[171,172] the prognostic significance of these mutations in esophageal cancers has not been defined as yet.

The retinoblastoma (Rb) gene, located on 13q14, encodes a 105-kD nuclear phosphoprotein that governs the G_1 restriction point via complex interactions with a variety of cyclin-dependent kinases, transcription factors, and viral oncoproteins[173,174]; Rb is a critical mediator of cell-cycle arrest after DNA damage.[175] Mutations resulting in the loss of Rb protein expression have been observed in 20% to 60% of esophageal cancers and their precursor lesions[136,139,176]; Rb mutations tend to occur more frequently in tumors that also exhibit mutations involving p53[176] and appear to correlate with advanced disease, nodal metastases, and diminished survival in esophageal cancer patients.[160,176,177]

The p16 tumor suppressor gene product encoded on 9p21 inhibits the activity of cdk4 and cdk6, thereby preventing cyclin D–dependent phosphorylation of the Rb protein at the restriction point.[178] Restoration of p16 expression by gene therapy techniques results in profound cell-cycle arrest in esophageal cancer cells.[140] Allelic deletions or point mutations inactivate p16 in approximately 20% of esophageal cancers, and allelic loss involving 9p21 precedes the onset of aneuploidy in Barrett's esophagus.[179,180] Promoter hypermethylation silences p16 in an additional 30% to 50% of esophageal cancers and adenocarinomas.[179,181] Although not extensively studied, loss of p16 expression appears to correlate with overexpression of cyclin D1 and diminished survival in esophageal cancer patients.[161]

The p14/ARF gene product is encoded by an alternate reading frame in the p16 locus and functions to stabilize p53 by preventing its interaction with MDM2.[182] ARF is critical for initiating p53-mediated apoptosis in response to activated protooncogenes, but appears dispensable for p53-mediated response to genotoxic stress.[183] Inactivation of ARF occurs by allelic deletion as well as methylation mechanisms that may simultaneously inactivate p16.[184] Xing et al.[185] performed a comprehensive analysis of the mechanisms responsible for silencing of p16 and p14/ARF in 40 esophageal cancers. Promoter hypermethylation involving ARF and p16 was observed in 15% and 40% of specimens, respectively. Nearly all of the methylations involving ARF also silenced p16; in contrast, most of the p16 methylations were exclusive. Homozygous deletions involving ARF or p16 were seen in 33% and 18% of specimens, respectively. These data suggest that p14/ARF is a primary target for homozygous deletion, whereas p16 appears to be silenced by hypermethylation in esophageal cancers. The prognostic significance of p14/ARF mutations in established esophageal cancers has not been defined.

The p53 gene product regulates cell-cycle progression, DNA repair, apoptosis, and neovascularization in normal and malignant tissues via highly complex DNA and protein interactions.[186] As previously mentioned, oncogene activation is mediated to p53 via p14/ARF; however, genotoxic stress resulting from DNA damage as well as telomeric shortening directly induces p53 expression.[183,187] In response to aberrant growth signals, p53 mediates either cell-cycle arrest in part via induction of p21 or apoptosis by a variety of transcription-dependent, as well as transcription-independent, mechanisms.[186,188,189] p53 may influence the metastatic potential of tumor cells by inhibiting expression of vascular endothelial growth factor.[190] Additional studies have shown that restoration of p53 expression by gene therapy techniques results in cell-cycle arrest and apoptosis as well as enhanced sensitivity to chemotherapy and ionizing radiation in esophageal cancer cells.[191,192]

Fifty percent to 80% of esophageal cancers exhibit p53 mutations, most of which occur in evolutionarily conserved residues within the sequence-specific DNA binding domain.[164,193,194] p53 mutations precede the development of aneuploidy in Barrett's esophagus,[125] and the frequency of these mutations increases dramatically during histologic progression to malignancy in this condition.[20,195,196] Several studies suggest that p53 mutations correlate with Rb mutations in esophageal cancers, as well as disease-free and overall survival in patients with these neoplasms.[176,177,197]

Malignant transformation not only depends on the inactivation of growth constraints mediated by the Rb and p53 tumor suppressor pathways, but equally important requires activation of telomerase, a ribonucleoprotein that adds hexameric DNA repeats to chromosomal ends to prevent loss of telomere length during DNA replication.[187,198,199] Aberrant expression of telomerase has been observed in the vast majority of esophageal cancers examined to date[200]; Koyanagi et al.[201] detected telomerase expression in 100% of 57 esophageal squamous cell cancers compared with less than 10% of normal tissue samples. In addition, Morales et al.[202] observed high-level telomerase expression in 100% of adenocarcinomas and high-grade Barrett's dysplasias; in contrast, only weak or moderate expression was seen in metaplasia or low-grade dysplasia samples. Similar findings have been noted by Lord et al.,[203] who observed high-level telomerase expression in all stages of Barrett's esophagus, the level of which appeared to increase during histologic progression to cancer. Interestingly, telomerase reverse transcriptase expression in histologically normal esophageal squamous epithelia in cancer patients was significantly higher than that observed in esophageal biopsies obtained from noncancer patients. Although the clinical relevance of telomerase activity in esophageal cancers has not been defined, the fact that telomere length may correlate with chemosensitivity in esophageal cancer cells and that inhibition of telomerase activity induces death in cultured cancer cells[204] strongly suggest that telomerase expression may significantly influence the clinical course of esophageal carcinomas.

CLINICAL PRESENTATION

Because it lacks a serosal coat, the esophagus is able to distend and accommodate considerable intraluminal tumor growth before deglutition is affected; as such, 50% of esophageal cancer patients have locally advanced unresectable disease or distant metastases at presentation. Dysphagia and weight loss are the initial symptoms in approximately 90% of patients presenting with esophageal cancer. Approximately 75% of the esophageal circumference must be involved with tumor before dysphagia is experienced; hence, although many patients relate a vague discomfort with swallowing for several months, dysphagia to solid foods may progress rapidly to total obstruction from circumferential tumor growth. Approximately 20% of patients experience odynophagia (painful swallowing). Although the vast majority of esophageal cancer patients present with weight loss, cachexia is seen in less than 10% of these individuals. Additional presenting symptoms may include dull retrosternal pain resulting from invasion of mediastinal structures, cough, or hoarseness due to paratracheal nodal or recurrent laryngeal nerve involvement. Infrequently, patients may present with pneumonia secondary to tracheoesophageal fistula or exsanguinating hemorrhage due to erosion of the esophageal neoplasm into the aorta.

DIAGNOSIS

Esophageal cancer should be suspected in any patient complaining of dysphagia and weight loss. A thorough history should be ascertained, focusing on preexisting conditions, as well as tobacco and ethanol abuse, which are known to be associated with increased esophageal cancer risk. Aspiration cytology should be performed on palpable cervical lymph nodes to rule out extrathoracic metastases. Chest radiography and barium swallow should be performed; the barium swallow provides an inexpensive and important initial assessment of the extent of the disease within the esophagus and should include the entire esophagus as well as stomach and duodenum; double-contrast studies are preferable because they provide more precise evaluation of mucosal patterns and allow detection of small lesions that may be missed on single-contrast examination. Computed tomography (CT) of the chest and upper abdomen should be obtained to evaluate the extent of disease within the chest and rule out visceral metastases in the abdomen.

Patients who are suspected to have a primary esophageal carcinoma on the basis of history, physical examination, or radiographic studies should undergo esophagoscopy to establish tissue diagnosis and define the extent of the esophageal lesion. At the time of endoscopy, attention should focus on the identification of the neoplasm in relation to cricopharyngeus, the squamocolumnar junction, and the diaphragmatic hiatus; in addition the presence or absence of satellite lesions, Barrett's esophagus, and esophagitis should be noted. Biopsies and brushings should be obtained from suspicious lesions; the combined diagnostic accuracy of these two procedures exceeds 90%.[205] Vital stains including toluidine blue or Lugol's iodine may be useful to guide endoscopic biopsies in situations in which lesions are equivocal. Frequently, strictures are encountered that require dilation to allow passage of the endoscope and provide temporary relief of dysphagia. Occasionally, the esophagus is so strictured it cannot be safely dilated; in these situations, multiple biopsies in four quadrants should be obtained, and the patients treated as if they have esophageal carcinoma irrespective of biopsy results. Bronchoscopy should always be performed in patients with potentially resectable upper and middle third esophageal carcinomas to rule out recurrent laryngeal nerve involvement and to identify and biopsy suspicious areas within the membranous trachea to rule out impending esophagorespiratory fistula.

Once a tissue diagnosis of esophageal cancer has been established, additional studies should be obtained to accurately stage the disease according to American Joint Committee on Cancer criteria (outlined in Tables 33.2-2 and 33.2-3) in order to ascertain prognosis and optimize treatment. Tumor length and the degree of obstruction appear to have less effect than the extent of wall penetration and lymph node metastases in determining survival of esophageal cancer patients. Current noninvasive imaging modalities are imperfect regarding evaluation of local regional disease and detection of distant metastases in these individuals.[206] Conventional CT scans detect the primary tumor in 75% to 80% of cases; however, sensitivity for local regional nodal disease is only 50% to 70%.[207–209] Furthermore, although CT scans may accurately predict resectability in as many as 75% of cases, they have not proven useful for assessing response to induction therapy in esophageal cancer patients.[207,209,210]

Endoscopic ultrasonography (EUS) has been advocated as a means to enhance the accuracy of staging of esophageal cancers.[211] Several studies indicate that in experienced hands, EUS accurately assesses wall involvement in 50% to 90% of tumors and mediastinal lymph node status in 67% to 100% of patients with localized esophageal cancers.[212,213] Reid et al.,[214] as well as Catalano and colleagues,[215] reported that EUS may be a valuable noninvasive means to detect celiac nodal metastases in esophageal cancer patients (sensitivity, 70% to 80%, and specificity, 88% to 98%). However, the accuracy of EUS is highly dependent on the expertise of the ultrasonographer[216]; an incomplete or erroneous assessment of lymph node metastases, invasion of adjacent organs, and poor staging of early carcinomas have been reported.[217] Furthermore, EUS has limited value in staging patients with high-grade obstruction or assessing response to induction therapy in esophageal cancer patients.[218,219]

[^{18}F]fluorodeoxyglucose (FDG) positron emission tomography (PET) scans have been used for staging patients with locally advanced esophageal cancers. Kole et al.[209] prospectively compared FDG PET and CT scans in 26 esophageal cancer patients.

TABLE 33.2-2. Tumor, Node, Metastasis (TNM) System for Esophageal Cancer

Primary tumor	
TX	Primary tumor cannot be assessed
T0	No evidence of primary tumor
Tis	Carcinoma *in situ*
T1	Tumor invades lamina propria or submucosa
T2	Tumor invades muscularis propria
T3	Tumor invades adventitia
T4	Tumor invades adjacent structures
Lymph node	
NX	Regional nodes cannot be assessed
N0	No regional lymph node metastasis
N1	Regional lymph node metastasis
Distant metastasis	
M0	No distant metastasis
M1	Distant metastasis (including positive celiac nodes)

TABLE 33.2-3. Tumor Stages for Esophageal Cancer

Stage 0	Tis	N0	M0
Stage I	T1	N0	M0
Stage IIA	T2	N0	M0
	T3	N0	M0
Stage IIB	T1	N1	M0
	T2	N1	M0
Stage III	T3	N1	M0
	T4	Any N	M0
Stage IV	Any T	Any N	M1

The primary tumor was visualized in 80% of patients by CT scan and 96% by FDG PET; neither modality accurately assessed the extent of wall involvement. Nodal disease was imaged in 62% of patients by CT scan and 90% by PET scan. PET scans detected distant metastases not seen by CT scans in three patients. Although these data suggest that PET scans may improve the staging of esophageal cancer patients, McAteer et al.[220] reported that PET scans do not accurately assess regional lymph node involvement in these individuals. Luketich et al.[208] reported their experience with FDG PET scans in 91 consecutive esophageal cancer patients. Minimally invasive procedures were used to confirm or refute imaging results. FDG PET scans detected metastases in only 27 of 39 cases documented by minimally invasive techniques (sensitivity, 69%; specificity, 97%; accuracy, 84%); CT scans revealed metastases in only 18 of these cases (sensitivity, 46%; specificity, 74%; accuracy, 63%). Although FDG PET scans were more accurate than CT scans in detecting distant metastases, they were only 69% sensitive relative to minimally invasive surgery techniques. Krasna[221] observed greater than 93% diagnostic accuracy using thoracoscopy and laparoscopic techniques to stage esophageal cancers. Collectively, these data indicate that minimally invasive surgery techniques presently represent the most accurate means to stage locally advanced esophageal carcinomas; in addition to enabling pathologic assessment of lymph nodes, thoracoscopy can confirm the presence of unresectable (T4) lesions, which are not accurately assessed by current noninvasive techniques.

Kobori et al.[222] compared ^{11}C-methylcholine PET and ^{18}F-FDG PET in 50 patients with locally advanced esophageal cancer. Methylcholine PET scans were more effective than FDG PET or CT scans in detecting small metastases in the mediastinum, but could not detect metastases in the upper abdomen due to uptake of ^{11}C-choline in the liver. FDG PET scans were superior to CT scans for detection of metastases in the chest and abdomen. When combined, ^{11}C-choline and ^{18}F-FDG PET were 85% sensitive for detecting metastatic nodes in the mediastinum and abdomen. Thus, combination PET scans may enhance the sensitivity for imaging small metastatic deposits in the mediastinum and abdomen. Further refinement may enable the diagnostic accuracy of PET scans to equal that achieved by minimally invasive staging techniques. Furthermore, preliminary data suggest that PET scans may prove to be valuable for assessing response to induction therapy in esophageal cancer patients[223] in contrast to CT scans or EUS, which appear to be unreliable for evaluation of treatment response in these individuals.[207,218,219] Use of these imaging modalities may enhance the accuracy of staging in esophageal cancer patients, thereby improving stratification of individuals for multimodality treatment protocols.

TREATMENT

The treatment of choice for patients with esophageal cancer is controversial. Esophagectomy remains the standard of care; however, its role has been challenged due to the generally poor outcomes following surgical resection alone in patients who typically have locally advanced disease.[224,225] A survey of community care practice patterns between 1988 and 1993 revealed an increase in the use of chemoradiotherapy relative to surgery as primary management of esophageal cancer.[226] Currently, in many institutions, primary resection is deferred in favor of combined modality therapy with or without adjuvant esophagectomy. The routine use of combined modality treatment outside the realms of controlled clinical trials is troublesome since most randomized trials have not shown a survival advantage of various induction regimens compared with esophagectomy alone. Furthermore, there is considerable controversy within the surgical literature as to what represents the appropriate operation for patients with esophageal cancer (Table 33.2-4); the debate focuses primarily on the need for and the extent of lymph node dissection during esophagectomy for cancer. The following discussion summarizes the current status of surgery, chemotherapy, radiation therapy, and combined modality regimens in the treatment of esophageal cancer.

TABLE 33.2-4. Types of Esophageal Resection

TRANSHIATAL ESOPHAGECTOMY
Laparotomy and preparation of gastric conduit with limited upper abdominal and low mediastinal node dissection
Left neck exploration and mobilization of cervical esophagus
Transhiatal resection
Posterior mediastinal placement of conduit
Cervical anastomosis
TRANSTHORACIC (LEWIS) ESOPHAGECTOMY
Laparotomy and preparation of gastric or colon conduit with upper abdominal lymph node dissection
Right thoracotomy for esophageal mobilization and resection with limited mediastinal lymph node dissection
Intrathoracic or cervical anastomosis
EN BLOC ESOPHAGECTOMY (TWO-FIELD DISSECTION)
Laparotomy and preparation of gastric or colon conduit with complete upper abdominal and retroperitoneal lymph node dissection
Thoracotomy with en bloc resection of:
Thoracic esophagus
Mediastinal lymph nodes
Azygous vein
Thoracic duct
Intrathoracic or cervical anastamosis
EN BLOC ESOPHAGECTOMY (THREE-FIELD DISSECTION)
Laparotomy and preparation of gastric or colon conduit with complete upper abdominal and retroperitoneal lymph node dissection
Thoracotomy with en bloc resection of:
Thoracic esophagus
Azygous vein
Thoracic duct
Mediastinal and low cervical lymph nodes
Cervical anastamosis

SURGICAL RESECTION

Transhiatal Esophagectomy

Transhiatal esophagectomy entails extirpation of the intrathoracic esophagus through the esophageal hiatus of the diaphragm without the need for a thoracotomy incision. An upper abdominal incision and a low-neck incision are required to isolate the esophagus at either end. The organ is next carefully stripped from its mediastinal attachments and removed. The prepared esophageal substitute, usually a greater curvature gas-

TABLE 33.2-5. Transhiatal Esophagectomy for Esophageal Cancer

Author	*Year*	*No. of Patients*	*Cell Type*	*Hospital Mortality (%)*	*5-Y Survival (%)*	*Median Survival (mo)*
Orringer[227]	1999	800	A/S	4.5	23	NS
Chu[231,a]	1997	20	S	15	NS	16
Horstmann[232]	1995	46	A/S	15	20	12
Putnam[234]	1994	42	A/S	4.8	18	14
Gertsch[229]	1993	100	A/S	3	23	NS
Vigneswaran[230]	1993	131	A/S	2.3	21	NS
Goldminc[233,a]	1993	32	S	6.25	30 (3 y)	NS
Gelfand[228]	1992	160	A	0.9	21	NS

[a]Randomized trials comparing transhiatal and transthoracic esophagectomy.

tric tube, is advanced across the esophageal bed in the posterior mediastinum, and gastrointestinal continuity is restored by an end-to-side esophagogastrostomy in the neck. No attempt is made to perform a systematic lymph node dissection apart from the few parahiatal nodes removed with the specimen. Occasionally, sampling of readily accessible celiac and periesophageal nodes is performed.[227]

Transhiatal esophagectomy is one of the more commonly used techniques for esophagectomy in North America and Europe. Orringer et al.[227] reported on 800 patients with cancer of the intrathoracic esophagus and cardia treated with transhiatal esophagectomy; adenocarcinoma was present in 69% of these individuals, whereas 28% had epidermoid cancer. Hospital mortality was 4.5% and morbidity was 27%. Major complications included anastomotic leaks (13%), recurrent laryngeal nerve injury (7%), wound infection (3%), pulmonary complications (2%), bleeding (1%), and chylothorax (1%). More than 90% of patients were discharged within 21 days of hospitalization. Overall survivals at 2, 3, and 5 years were 47%, 34%, and 23%, respectively. Five-year survival was 59% for stage I patients and 22% for patients with stage IIA. Patients with stage III disease had 2- and 5-year survival rates of 32% and 10%, respectively. There was an overall statistically significant survival advantage for patients with adenocarcinoma (24% vs. 17%). This study by the University of Michigan group represents the largest experience with transhiatal resections for carcinoma, and the survival rates are quite consistent with those reported by other surgeons who practice a similar approach (Table 33.2-5).[227–234] Gelfand et al.[228] reported on 160 patients who underwent transhiatal esophagectomy for carcinoma of the lower esophagus and cardia. The majority of the tumors were adenocarcinomas, and most were in early stages; survival rates at 2 and 5 years were 40% and 21%, respectively. Gertsch and colleagues[229] described their experience with 100 esophageal cancer patients who were uniformly treated with transhiatal esophagectomy without adjuvant therapy over a 10-year period. Hospital mortality was 3% and morbidity was 68%. The median survival was 18 months and the overall 5-year survival was 23%. Survival was better for T1 and T2 tumors (63% 5-year survival). Vigneswaran et al.[230] reported on 131 patients who underwent transhiatal resection with a 2% operative mortality. Overall 5-year survival was 21%. Patients with stage I disease had a 47.5% 5-year survival compared with patients with stage III disease whose 5-year survival was 5.8%. Patients with adenocarcinoma had a 5-year survival of 27%, whereas none of those with squamous cell cancer were alive at 5 years.

Only two studies have reported local recurrence rates following transhiatal esophagectomy. One of these studies[235] was published in abstract form only as an update of the results of a randomized trial comparing transhiatal esophagectomy alone with transhiatal esophagectomy following induction chemoradiotherapy. A significant reduction in the local recurrence rate without improvement in overall survival was noted in the combined modality arm. Local recurrence as a component of treatment failure was observed in 39% of patients in the surgery alone arm versus 19% of those receiving combined modality treatment. In a prospective study using serial CT scans, Barbier et al.[236] also detected local recurrence in 39% of 50 esophageal cancer patients following transhiatal resection.

In summary, transhiatal esophagectomy can usually be performed with an operative mortality of 5% or less in the hands of experienced esophageal surgeons. Five-year survival rates are generally in the 20% to 25% range. Survival for patients with stage I tumors is in the 60% to 70% range, whereas patients with stage III disease have a 5% to 10% 5-year survival. Finally, the procedure is associated with failure to control or eradicate local disease in nearly 40% of patients.

Standard Transthoracic Esophagectomy

Transthoracic esophagectomy is probably the most widely performed operation for cancer of the esophagus worldwide. The procedure can be carried out through a right or left thoracotomy incision depending on the preference of the surgeon and the location of the tumor within the esophagus. Generally, a right thoracotomy is required for adequate exposure of tumors in the middle or upper third that are anatomically intimately related to the membranous trachea or the arch of the aorta. Tumors located at the gastroesophageal junction or in the lower third of the esophagus can be usually approached through a left thoracotomy incision. A left sixth interspace incision provides excellent exposure of the lower mediastinum, and a semicircular diaphragmatic incision performed 1 inch from the costal arch allows access to the upper abdomen. The esophagus is mobilized from its mediastinal bed along with adjoining periesophageal as well as lesser curvature lymph nodes; no radical mediastinal or upper abdominal lymphadenectomy is performed. Gastrointestinal reconstruction is subsequently achieved by preparation of the esophageal substitute (usually stomach) and advancing it to the neck for a cervical anastomosis. Patients operated on through a right

TABLE 33.2-6. Transthoracic Esophagectomy for Esophageal Cancer

Author	*Year*	*No. of Patients*	*Cell Type*	*Hospital Mortality (%)*	*5-Y Survival (%)*	*Median Survival (mo)*
Ellis[237]	1999	455	A/S	3.3	24.7	NS
Chu[231]	1997	20	S	0	NS	13
Horstmann[232]	1995	41	A/S	10	17	12
Lieberman[238]	1995	258	A/S	5	27	27
Wright[343]	1994	91	A	2	8	NS
Sharpe[240]	1996	562	A/S	9	18	NS
Swisher[241]	1995	316	A/S	5.4	16.4	NS
Adam[242]	1996	597	A/S	6.9	16.3	NS
Putnam[234]	1994	134	A/S	8.2	18	22
Law[243]	1992	467	A/S	6.1	15	NS
Goldminc[233]	1993	35	S	8.5	20 (3 y)	NS

thoracotomy require a laparotomy to prepare the gastric tube and pass it across the posterior mediastinum or retrosternal space for a cervical anastomosis. In patients operated on through a left thoracotomy, the esophagus is mobilized along its course in the supra aortic posterior mediastinum well into the neck. The prepared gastric tube is then passed underneath the aortic arch and attached to the esophageal stump. Following reattachment of the diaphragm and closure of the thoracotomy, a small left cervical incision is performed to retrieve the esophagus and the gastric tube. A cervical incision is then performed and the previously mobilized esophagus and gastric tube are easily delivered to the neck for a cervical anastomosis.

Ellis[237] reported his experience with more than 500 esophageal cancer patients who underwent standard transthoracic esophagectomy. One-third of the patients had squamous cell cancers, whereas the remaining two-thirds had adenocarcinomas of the esophagus or gastroesophageal junction. Hospital mortality was 3.3%. Complications occurred in 34% of patients and resulted in a prolonged hospital stay in 21% of individuals. Overall 5-year survival including operative mortality and noncancer-related deaths was 24.7%. Patients who had a complete (R0) resection had a 5-year survival of 29%, whereas no patients with either residual microscopic (R1) or macroscopic disease (R2) survived 5 years. There was no significant effect of cell type on survival. Five-year survival was 79% for patients with stage I disease, 38% for those with stage IIA, and 27% for those with stage IIB. Patients with stage III disease had 3- and 5-year survival rates of 20% and 13.7%, respectively.

Some of the more pertinent surgical series pertaining to standard transthoracic esophagectomy that have been reported within the last decade from North America and Europe are listed in Table 33.2-6.[231,232,238–243] Resectability rates have ranged from 60% to 90%, and hospital mortality has ranged from 3.2% to 23%. Five-year survival rates have varied between 9% and 24%. The variability in rates of resectability, hospital mortality, and 5-year survival may have been related to differences in patient selection, surgical expertise, and the retrospective nature of most of these studies. More instructive to review are the survival results achieved by the surgical arms of randomized trials comparing various preoperative regimens to surgical resection alone. The most recent of these trials was the North American Intergroup trial that compared chemotherapy followed by surgery with surgery alone.[244] There were 467 eligible patients of whom 227 underwent primary surgical resection, the majority through a transthoracic approach. One hundred six patients had squamous cell cancer (47%) and 121 had adenocarcinoma (53%). Hospital mortality was 6%. Major complications occurred in 26% of patients. Overall survivals at 1, 2, and 3 years were 60%, 37%, and 26%, respectively. Actuarial 5-year survival was 20%. There was no difference in outcome between patients with adenocarcinoma and those with epidermoid cancer. In a separate trial performed by Walsh et al.,[245] 113 patients were randomized to receive either surgery alone or chemoradiation followed by transthoracic esophagectomy. Hospital mortality in the control arm was 2%, and the 3-year survival was 6%. Bossett et al.[246] performed a randomized trial comparing transthoracic esophagectomy alone with radiotherapy followed by esophagectomy. Three- and 5-year survival rates in the surgery alone arm were 38% and 22%, respectively. Finally, Law et al.[247] reported on 147 patients with squamous cell carcinoma randomized to either chemotherapy followed by esophagectomy or esophagectomy alone. There were 73 patients in the control arm, and nearly all underwent resection by a transthoracic approach. Hospital mortality was 8.7%. Survival rates at 2 and 5 years were 31% and 10%, respectively.

Local recurrences following standard transthoracic resections have been reported in 30% to 60% of patients. Most of the data regarding local recurrences have been obtained from surgical control arms of various randomized trials. Gijnoux et al.[248] reported the incidence of local recurrence in a study comparing surgical resection alone with preoperative radiotherapy. Local recurrences were observed in 67% of patients in the surgery alone arm compared with 47% of individuals in the experimental arm. Similarly Nygaard et al.[249] reported a 35% local recurrence rate following resection alone in a four-arm randomized trial comparing resection with preoperative chemotherapy, preoperative radiotherapy, and preoperative chemoradiation. In the Intergroup trial comparing esophagectomy alone with chemotherapy followed by esophagectomy,[244] the local recurrence rate in the control arm was 31% among 135 patients who received a complete (R0) resection. An additional 68 patients had R1 or R2 resections. The overall local failure rate (persistent or recurrent disease) in all 227 patients in the control arm was 61%. In the previously mentioned randomized trial reported by Law et al.,[247] 21% of patients developed local recurrence, while an additional 10% had both local and distant recurrences; thus local recurrence was a component of treatment failure in 31% of patients in this study.

Comparison of Transhiatal and Transthoracic Esophagectomy

Several retrospective studies have shown little difference in the operative mortality and morbidity between transhiatal and transthoracic esophagectomy with limited lymph node dissection. Rindani et al.[250] reviewed the results from 44 series published between 1986 and 1996. Thirty-three articles described results of 2675 patients who underwent transhiatal resection, whereas 29 articles reported results of transthoracic resections performed in 2808 patients. Thirty-day mortality was 6.3% after transhiatal and 9.5% after transthoracic esophagectomy. Major pulmonary and cardiovascular morbidity was similar in both groups. Transhiatal esophagectomy was associated with a higher incidence of anastomotic leaks (16% vs. 10%), anastomotic strictures (28% vs. 16%), and recurrent laryngeal nerve injury (11% vs. 5%). Overall 5-year survival was 24% after transhiatal esophagectomy and 26% following transthoracic resection.

Two randomized trials have compared transthoracic with transhiatal resections. Chu et al.[231] reported on 39 patients with carcinoma of the lower third of the esophagus who were prospectively randomized to receive either a transhiatal (n = 25) or a transthoracic resection (n = 19). There were no significant differences between the groups in terms of blood loss, postoperative ventilatory requirements, cardiopulmonary complication rates, and mean hospital stay. Median survival was 16.0 months after transhiatal esophagectomy and 13.5 months after transthoracic resection. Goldminc et al.[233] prospectively randomized 67 patients to receive either a transhiatal (n = 32) or transthoracic esophagectomy. There were no differences between the two groups with respect to hospital mortality, morbidity, incidence of pulmonary complications, or long-term survival.

In summary, survival rates achieved with the surgical transhiatal esophagectomy are comparable with those reported for standard transthoracic resection. However, radical lymph node dissections have not been performed in any of the aforementioned series; hence the survival results reflect the effect of the surgical incision rather than the extent of lymphadenectomy.

EN BLOC ESOPHAGECTOMY

The deep location of the esophagus within the narrow confines of the mediastinum and the lack of a well-defined mesentery have generally precluded the application of *en bloc* resection to patients with esophageal carcinoma. In 1963, Logan described results pertaining to 250 patients who underwent *en bloc* resection for cancer of the cardia, noting a 16% 5-year survival.[251] Although that survival rate was remarkable at the time, the 21% operative mortality limited a wider adoption of the procedure. Skinner reintroduced the technique in 1969, which was later modified and applied to cancer of the thoracic esophagus.[252] The basic principle of the operation is extirpation of the tumor-bearing esophagus within a wide envelope of adjoining tissues that include both pleural surfaces laterally and the pericardium anteriorly where these structures are intimately related to the esophagus. The lymphatics wedged dorsally between the esophagus and the aorta, and the thoracic duct throughout its mediastinal course, are resected *en bloc* with the specimen. This posterior mediastinectomy necessarily results in a complete mediastinal node dissection from the tracheal bifurcation to the esophageal hiatus. Additionally, an upper abdominal lymphadenectomy is performed including the common hepatic, celiac, left gastric, lesser curvature, parahiatal, and retroperitoneal nodes. The purpose of this extended resection is to maximize locoregional control of the primary tumor; local recurrence rates following *en bloc* esophagectomy are reported to be less than 10%.[253,254] This is a strikingly low local failure rate compared with those observed following transhiatal or standard transthoracic resections, or chemoradiation delivered with curative intent.[255]

Critics have argued that the *en bloc* procedure is associated with a high operative mortality and morbidity without an apparent survival advantage. In fact, in the earliest report by Skinner,[252] the operative mortality for 80 patients with cancer of the cardia treated by *en bloc* resection was 11%, and the 5-year survival was only 18%. However, in more recent series, hospital mortality has ranged between 2% and 7%,[48,256,257] and several investigators have reported survival rates exceeding those achievable by standard resection. Lerut et al.[48] reported their experience with 129 patients who had an R0 resection for cancer of the thoracic esophagus. Approximately two-thirds of patients had squamous cell cancer, and one-third had adenocarcinoma of the esophagus. Resection was accomplished by the *en bloc* technique in 54 patients, with a hospital mortality of 7.5%. Survival was significantly better following *en bloc* resection compared with standard resection (48% vs. 41%; P = .002). Interestingly, multivariate analysis showed that the survival advantage after *en bloc* resection was apparent only in patients with nodal metastasis (P = .005). Furthermore, patients with stage III tumors had a 5-year survival of 22% after *en bloc* resection, compared with 13% after standard resection (P = .05). Hagen et al.[256] reported similar results in a smaller group of patients with adenocarcinoma of the distal esophagus and gastroesophageal junction. *En bloc* resection was performed in 30 patients, and transhiatal resection was done in 16 patients. Overall survival was significantly better after *en bloc* resection (41% vs. 14%; P = .001). A survival advantage was observed in patients with early lesions (T1 and T2) in whom the 5-year survival was 75% versus 21% in favor of *en bloc* resection. Similarly, patients with transmural (T3) tumors and five or fewer positive nodes had a significantly better survival after *en bloc* resection (27% vs. 9%).

An important criticism of most of these studies is the failure to clearly define the criteria used to stratify patients to receive one procedure versus another. For example, in the study by Hagen et al.,[256] patients receiving transhiatal esophagectomies were significantly older or more debilitated than those undergoing *en bloc* resections. Preferential inclusion of early-stage patients into the *en bloc* groups may have biased survival outcomes. Arguably some early-stage patients undergoing *en bloc* resections might have had similarly favorable outcomes following a more limited procedure.

Altorki et al.[257] reported on 155 patients who underwent resection for carcinoma of the esophagus between 1988 and 1998. During the first 4 years of the study, standard transthoracic resections were performed in nearly all patients; thereafter *en bloc* resections were carried out preferentially in nearly all patients. The overall hospital mortality was 5.1% and did not vary significantly by procedure (*en bloc*, 4.8%; standard transthoracic, 5.7%). Overall 5-year survival was 40% in the *en bloc* group. Node-negative patients had 5-year survival rates of 67% following *en bloc* resection and 27% after standard esophagectomy. Interestingly, the mean number of resected nodes per patient in node-negative patients was significantly higher after *en bloc* resection (36 vs. 20 per patient; $P = .03$) suggesting that the extended procedure may improve the accuracy of staging in esophageal cancer patients. Conceivably, some *node-negative* patients were understaged during standard resections, resulting in apparently worse survival relative to similarly staged patients who had undergone *en bloc* resections. Survival was also significantly better after *en bloc* resection in patients with nodal metastases (33% vs. 13%; $P = .002$). Five-year survival was significantly higher in patients with stage III disease treated by *en bloc* resection (34% vs. 11%; $P = .007$). This survival advantage was noted despite an analysis of variance showing no difference between the groups in terms of age, gender, performance status, tumor size, cell type, or number of positive nodes per patient. The 5-year survival rate (11%) in stage III patients undergoing standard resection in this series is similar to those reported in other series following similarly limited resections, suggesting no obvious selection bias in favor of *en bloc* resection. The survival advantage conferred by *en bloc* esophagectomy in patients with stage III disease confirms previous observations by Lerut et al.[48] Furthermore, the 7.8% (8 of 109) local recurrence rate observed following *en bloc* esophagectomy in Altorki's trial is dramatically less than those observed following transhiatal or standard transthoracic resections.

Three-Field Lymphadenectomy

Three-field lymph node dissection for carcinoma of the esophagus has been practiced by Japanese surgeons since the early 1980s. This effort was initially prompted by studies showing that the cervical lymph nodes were the site of tumor recurrence in 30% to 40% of patients in whom a curative resection had been performed.[258] The extended procedure included dissection of the cervical, mediastinal, and upper abdominal nodes in patients with carcinoma of the thoracic and abdominal esophagus. In 1991, Isono et al.[259] reported the results of a nationwide study on three-field dissections performed at 35 institutions throughout Japan. Nearly 1800 patients underwent esophagectomy with three-field lymph node dissection, whereas 2800 underwent two-field dissection. The following observations were made:

- Approximately one-third of patients had previously unsuspected metastases in cervical lymph nodes. The prevalence of cervical nodal metastases was highest for upper third tumors (40%), but even patients with lower third cancers had a 20% probability of metastatic carcinoma involving the cervical lymph nodes.
- The frequency of nodal metastases increased with depth of tumor penetration through the esophageal wall. Patients with intramucosal carcinoma had a 30% probability of nodal metastases, while invasion into the submucosa, muscularis propria, or adventitia signaled a 50%, 60%, and 80% probability of nodal disease, respectively. Interestingly, a statistically higher prevalence of nodal metastases was observed after three-field lymph node dissection in patients with T1 and T2 tumors, but not in those with more advanced disease.
- The cervical lymph nodes most frequently involved with metastatic carcinoma were the nodal chains along the recurrent nerves, as well as the deep cervical nodes along the posterior aspect of the internal jugular vein. Supraclavicular nodal disease was infrequent and was associated with a distinctly poor outcome.

Collectively, these observations indicate that a large number of patients will be inaccurately staged after *en bloc* resection with isolated mediastinal and abdominal lymphadenectomy. Approximately one-third of patients will have their tumor, node, metastasis (TNM) stage upstaged as a result of the extended procedure. Although most surgeons readily concede that extended lymphadenectomy improves tumor staging, many question its effect on the survival of patients with locally advanced esophageal cancer.[260] However, Japanese surgeons have provided a compelling argument for a positive effect of three-field lymph node dissection on survival in these individuals. Akiyama et al.[261] reported their experience with 717 patients in whom an R0 resection was performed using either a two-field (n = 393) or three-field technique (n = 324).[261] Five-year survival in node-negative patients was 84% after the three-field procedure compared with 55% after two-field lymphadenectomy ($P = .004$). Furthermore, in patients with node-positive disease, the 5-year survival rate was 43% in patients receiving three-field dissections, compared with 28% for patients undergoing two-field dissections ($P = .008$), indicating that the improved survival rates observed in patients receiving extended lymphadenectomies were not simply due to stage migration. Similar results have been reported by a number of Japanese surgeons.[262–264] Significantly, most studies have reported 5-year survivals of 25% to 30% in patients with positive cervical lymph nodes. These impressive data suggest that the recurrent laryngeal nodes should be considered a regional (N1) rather than a distant (M1) site of disease for tumors of the intrathoracic and abdominal esophagus. Indeed, lymphoscintigraphy studies using radiolabeled colloid injected into the midthoracic esophagus have routinely demonstrated tracer uptake within the upper mediastinal and cervical nodes as well as the left gastric lymph nodes.[265,266]

In spite of the intriguing results reported by Japanese surgeons, most European and North American oncologists have viewed three-field dissection with skepticism. There are several reasons that might explain the lack of enthusiasm for the procedure:

- There is a prevailing concept among western surgeons that patients with carcinoma of the esophagus have systemic disease at the time of presentation. Cure following resection has often been considered a chance phenomenon dependent more on the biologic behavior of the tumor than on the surgical strategy pursued.
- Three-field lymph node dissection has been associated with a definite, albeit a statistically insignificant, increase in hospital morbidity. Foremost among the potential complications is injury to one or both recurrent nerves, reported in up to 70% of patients, some of whom have required tracheostomy and prolonged mechanical ventilation.[263] Furthermore, at least one study examined the quality of life following esophagectomy with three-field lymph node dissection with particular emphasis on the effect of vocal cord paralysis.[264] Twenty percent of patients reported severe hoarseness, restricted food intake, and reduced exercise tolerance up to 60 months postoperatively.

- Nearly all of the Japanese data are from retrospective studies comparing surgical therapies delivered over two decades. Two randomized studies have been reported.[267,268] Nishihira et al.[267] randomized 62 patients with squamous cell carcinoma of the esophagus to receive a two-field or three-field lymph node dissection. Hospital deaths occurred in 3% after two-field dissection and in 7% after three-field lymphadenectomy. There were no differences between the two groups in 5-year survival or recurrence rates. In another trial, Kato et al.[268] randomized 150 patients to receive transthoracic esophagectomy with either two-field or three-field lymph node dissection. Hospital mortality and morbidity were comparable in both groups; a significantly higher 5-year survival was observed in patients who underwent a three-field dissection (48% vs. 33%).

Altorki et al.[39] reported the only experience with this procedure in North America. Esophagectomy with a three-field node dissection was performed in 34 patients, 10 of whom had adenocarcinomas. Hospital mortality and morbidity were 2.3% and 35%, respectively. Recurrent nerve injury occurred in 6% of patients. An average of 60 nodes were resected per patient; 70% of these individuals had nodal metastases, most of which were within the lesser gastric curve, parahiatal, and recurrent laryngeal nodes. Cervical nodal metastases were present in 30% of patients regardless of cell type or location of the primary tumor within the esophagus. With a median follow-up of 42 months, 3-year and 5-year survival was 46%. Node-negative patients had a 77% 5-year survival, whereas those with nodal metastases had a 5-year survival of 33%. Three of the ten patients with metastases involving cervical or recurrent laryngeal nodes were disease free a minimum of 3 years after operation. Local recurrence was observed in two patients.

Lerut et al.[269] reported the only European experience with esophagectomy and three-field lymph node dissection. Thirty-eight patients underwent the procedure with no hospital mortality. Overall survival rates at 3 and 5 years were 45% and 37%, respectively. Patients with nodal metastases had a 27% 5-year survival; individuals with cervical node disease had a 20% 5-year survival. The patterns of nodal metastases observed by Altorki and Lerut are similar to those reported by Japanese investigators and appear independent of tumor histology. The potential survival advantage offered by three-field dissection in esophageal cancer patients (particularly those with adenocarcinoma) is encouraging given the limited efficacy of chemotherapy and radiation in these individuals.

CHEMOTHERAPY

Five-year survival rates for esophageal cancer patients resected at most major centers in the United States range from 15% to 20%.[270,271] Although radical esophagectomy may salvage some patients with locally advanced carcinomas, the vast majority of individuals succumb to their disease, suggesting that most patients have occult metastases at presentation. Studies of patterns of recurrence, and data from autopsy series confirm the potential for tumor spread to all organs.[41,272–275] These data have provided the rationale for using systemic therapy in conjunction with surgery, radiation, or both in patients with apparently localized disease or as the primary treatment for patients with clinically evident disseminated disease.

Until fairly recently, standard criteria of treatment response required a bidimensional lesion that could be serially measured. For the esophageal cancer patient with metastatic disease, treatment response can be reliably assessed using pulmonary, soft tissue, and liver nodules as indicators. CT, magnetic resonance imaging, and double-contrast barium esophagography, which are typically used to assess response in patients with disease limited to the esophagus, only provide unidimensional measurements of the primary.[276,277] Endoscopy with brushings and biopsy may be performed to confirm a clinical complete response; however, biopsy is subject to sampling error and is not a reliable indicator of complete histologic resolution of disease.

A variety of single agents and combination regimens have been evaluated in patients with recurrent or metastatic carcinoma of the esophagus. These patients often have a high tumor burden and poor performance status with little prospect for prolongation of survival. Phase II clinical trials in this population have identified drugs with activity,[278] and they have been integrated into combined modality regimens for the treatment of earlier stage disease.

The accumulated experience with chemotherapy to date is almost entirely in patients with squamous cell histology. Due to the rising incidence of adenocarcinoma of the esophagus, gastroesophageal junction, and cardia in the United States,[3] patients with this histology now make up two-thirds of referrals for chemotherapy. Only recently have trials with new agents and combined modality regimens included both histologies.

Chemotherapy for Palliation of Recurrent and Metastatic Disease

SINGLE AGENTS. Studies of single agents are summarized in Table 33.2-7.[279–302] The cumulative response rate for any one drug is low (on the order of 15% to 30%), and there is no indication of survival benefit. Symptomatic improvement, if reported, is brief. Response data for many of the older drugs have come from broad phase I and II trials conducted in the early 1970s, which included small numbers of esophageal cancer patients. Bleomycin, 5-fluorouracil (5-FU), mitomycin, and cisplatin (CDDP) have been used most often because of their single-agent activities and their additive or synergistic effects with radiation. Because of the potential for pulmonary toxicity, bleomycin is no longer included in combination regimens, having been replaced by 5-FU. Similarly, mitomycin is less often used because of its toxicity profile, which includes hemolytic-uremic syndrome and cumulative myelosuppression.

5-FU has remained an important drug for the treatment of gastrointestinal malignancies. One study[284] using a protracted infusion schedule for 6 weeks in patients with newly diagnosed esophageal cancer reported an 85% response rate that contrasts with an Eastern Cooperative Oncology Group trial[285] in which a 15% response rate was observed in previously treated patients given intermittent bolus 5-FU.

There are seven trials pertaining to cisplatin as a single agent in esophageal cancer patients,[286,289–294] six of which used doses ranging from 50 to 120 mg/m^2 every 3 to 4 weeks. The cumulative response rate in patients with metastatic or recurrent disease was 21%.[286,289–293] Administration of the drug as a single bolus dose once every 3 weeks or in a divided dose over 5 days every 3 weeks appeared to be equally efficacious. Employ-

TABLE 33.2-7. Trials of Single Agents with Activity in Carcinoma of the Esophagus

Drug	*Dose*	*No. of Patients*	*Histology*	*Percent Complete Response + Partial Response*	*Reference*
Bleomycin	15–30 mg/m²/10–20 mg/m²/day IV or IM	80	S	15	279–283
5-Fluorouracil	300 mg/m² CIVI × 6 wk	13[a]	S	85	284
	500 mg/m² IV daily × 5	26	S	16	285
Mitomycin	20 mg/m² IV q4–5wk	31	S	35	286,287
Doxorubicin	40–60 mg/m² IV q3wk	33	S	18	285,288
Methotrexate	40 mg/m² IV weekly	26	S	12	285
	200 mg/m² q10d	44[a]	S	48	289
Cisplatin	50–120 mg/m² IV q3–4wk	131	S	21	286,289–293
	120 mg/m² IV days 1 and 15	15[a]	S	73	294
Vindesine	3–4 mg/m² IV q2wk	83	S	26	295–297
Mitoguazone	400–700 mg/m² IV weekly	64	S	23	298–300
Venorelbine	20–25 mg/m² IV weekly	30	S	20	301
Paclitaxel	250 mg/m²/24 h IV q3wk	51	S and A	32	302

A, adenocarcinoma; CIVI, continuous intravenous infusion; S, squamous cell carcinoma.
[a]Neoadjuvant therapy.

ing a more dose-intense schedule of cisplatin (120 mg/m² on day 1 and 15), Miller et al.[294] observed a 73% response rate in 15 patients before surgery. Although no complete responses were observed, these data suggest that sensitivity to chemotherapy is greater in the newly diagnosed patient.

A randomized phase II trial of cisplatin alone and cisplatin in combination with 5-FU in 92 patients with metastatic squamous cell carcinoma of the esophagus was reported by the European Organization for Research and Treatment of Cancer (EORTC).[293] An 18% response rate was observed in 45 patients receiving single-agent cisplatin at a dose of 100 mg/m² every 3 weeks. Although the response rate in the combination therapy arm was 36%, survival was similar for both groups. No studies of single-agent cisplatin have been performed in patients with adenocarcinoma of the esophagus.

Two investigational agents have demonstrated moderate activity in squamous cell carcinoma of the esophagus. These are the vinca alkaloid vindesine[295–297] and the polyamine synthesis inhibitor mitoguazone (methyl-GAG).[298–300] Responders included patients previously treated with cisplatin-based combination chemotherapy.

Vinorelbine, a semisynthetic vinca alkaloid that inhibits microtubule assembly, has been approved for use in lung cancer. It has less neurotoxicity compared with vincristine and vinblastine; neutropenia is dose limiting. The EORTC reported a 20% response rate in chemotherapy-naive patients with metastatic squamous cell cancer of the esophagus.[301] In a subsequent trial,[303] vinorelbine was combined with cisplatin in 57 patients with metastatic squamous cell cancer resulting in a 32% response rate and 6-month median duration of response. Vinorelbine has not been evaluated in patients with adenocarcinoma of the esophagus.

The taxane paclitaxel is the first entirely new compound to be tested in both adenocarcinoma and squamous cell carcinoma of the esophagus. Paclitaxel promotes the stabilization of microtubules and is a cycle-specific agent affecting cells in the G_2/M phase. Paclitaxel also enhances radiation effects that may be both concentration and schedule dependent.[304] The only trial of single-agent paclitaxel in esophageal cancer used the maximum tolerable dose of 250 mg/m², derived from initial phase I trials using a 24-hour infusion schedule.[302] A 34% response rate was observed in 33 patients with adenocarcinoma, and a 28% response rate was noted in 18 patients with squamous cell carcinoma of the esophagus. The overall response rate was 32%. All patients had good performance status, were chemotherapy-naive, and had distant metastases. The dose-limiting toxicity of paclitaxel is myelosuppression, primarily neutropenia. There are no completed studies using either shorter or longer infusion schedules such as 1, 3, and 96 hours.

Drugs that have been adequately tested in squamous cell cancer of the esophagus and have response rates of less than 5% are the methotrexate analogues, dichloromethotrexate[305] and trimetrexate,[306,307] and etoposide,[308,309] ifosamide,[310,311] and carboplatin.[312–315] Carboplatin has been studied in both adenocarcinoma and squamous cell carcinoma patients using a fixed dose schedule of 300 to 400 mg/m² in individuals with normal renal function. In contrast to the activity observed in phase II evaluations of cisplatin, responses were observed in only 3 of 59 chemotherapy-naive patients who received carboplatin. Therefore, substitution of carboplatin for cisplatin is not recommended when treating patients with either adenocarcinomas or squamous cell carcinomas of the esophagus.

Combination Chemotherapy

Only in more recent years have combination regimens been evaluated in patients with adenocarcinoma. Older trials (before the mid-1990s) and those from Europe have almost exclusively been limited to patients with squamous cell carcinomas. Because esophageal cancer is a relatively uncommon malignancy, many studies have included patients treated preoperatively as well as those with recurrent or metastatic disease, and some have also included patients with locally advanced, unresectable neoplasms. In addition to the variation in patient populations, more recent trials have often limited eligibility to patients with no prior chemotherapy and performance status of 0 or 1. Thus, it is difficult to compare treatment efficacies reported from these phase II trials.

TABLE 33.2-8. Selected Combination Chemotherapy for Recurrent and Metastatic Carcinoma of the Esophagus

Regimen	*Evaluable Patients*	*Histology*	*Percent Complete Response Plus Partial Response*	*Median Response Duration*	*Reference*
Cisplatin + bleomycin	17	S	17	6 mo	316
Cisplatin + bleomycin + vindesine	51	S	31	5 mo	317,318
Cisplatin + bleomycin + methotrexate	40	S	30	6 mo	319,320
Cisplatin + mitoguazone + vindesine	20	S	40	3 mo	321
Cisplatin + mitoguazone + vinblastine	36	S	11	13 wk	322
Cisplatin + 5-FU	82	S	35		293,323
Carboplatin + vinblastine	16	S	0		324
Cisplatin + vinorelbine	57	S	32	6 mo	303
5-FU + interferon-α_{2a}	57	S and A	26	6.5 mo	325,326
Cisplatin + 5-FU + interferon-α_{2a}	26	S and A	50	29 mo	327
13-*cis* retinoic acid + interferon-α_{2a}	13	A	0		328
Cisplatin + etoposide	65	S	48	7 mo	329
Paclitaxel (24-h) + cisplatin q3wk	32	S and A	44	3.9 mo	331
Paclitaxel (3-h) + cisplatin q2wk	59		52		332
Paclitaxel (3-h) + cisplatin qwk × 6	22	A	50		333
Paclitaxel (3-h) + cisplatin + 5-FU q4wk	60	S and A	48	5.7 mo	331
Irinotecan + cisplatin qwk × 4	35	S and A	57	4.2 mo	335
Irinotecan + cisplatin qwk × 4	25	A	51		336

A, adenocarcinoma; 5-FU, 5-fluorouracil; S, squamous cell carcinoma.

The results of platinum-based combination chemotherapy regimens are detailed in Table 33.2-8.[293,303,316–328] Most series have had small numbers of patients and therefore 95% confidence intervals have been large. Nearly all responses have been partial, with only an occasional clinical complete response. Duration of response has been variable but on average has ranged from 3 to 6 months.

Trials in the 1980s testing three-drug regimens such as cisplatin, bleomycin, and vindesine[317,318] and cisplatin, mitoguazone, and vindesine[321] or vinblastine[322] yielded response rates of 30% to 40% in epidermoid cancer patients. Toxicity was primarily moderate myelosuppression. Bleomycin and mitoguazone were replaced by 5-FU, which has synergistic activity with cisplatin.

The two-drug combination of cisplatin (100 mg/m^2 day 1) and 5-FU (1000 mg/m^2/d continuous infusion for 96 to 120 hours) is the regimen most commonly used to treat patients with either squamous or adenocarcinoma histology. A 35% response rate has been observed in patients with metastatic, recurrent, or locally advanced, incurable squamous cell cancer of the esophagus.[293,323] Higher response rates (in the 40% to 60% range) have been reported from trials administering two to three cycles of cisplatin and 5-FU as neoadjuvant therapy before surgery. The difference in response rates may be related to better performance status, nutrition, and smaller volume disease in the surgical candidates. Attempts to substitute carboplatin for cisplatin have been unsuccessful; in a phase II trial of carboplatin and vinblastine,[324] investigators from Memorial Sloan-Kettering Cancer Center observed no responses in 16 patients even though 11 with advanced, inoperable cancers were previously untreated, and 15 had Karnofsky performance scores of 70% or better.

Three trials using interferon-α_{2a} as a biomodulator of 5-FU suggested possible benefit.[325–327] Preclinical data had indicated synergistic cytolytic activity when interferon was combined with 5-FU, possibly due to interferon-mediated stimulation of thymidine phosphorylase, which increases the conversion of 5-FU to its active metabolite, fluorodeoxyuridylate. Ilson and associates[327] treated 26 incurable esophageal cancer patients with interferon-α_{2a} (3 million U subcutaneously daily), cisplatin (100 mg/m^2 day 1), and continuous infusion 5-FU (750 mg/m^2/d for 5 days) recycled every 28 days; the complete and partial response rates were 50%, and the duration of response ranged from 11 to 74 weeks. Treatment responses were observed in 8 of 11 with squamous cell carcinoma (73%; 95% confidence interval, 47% to 99%) and 5 of 15 adenocarcinoma patients (33%; 95% confidence interval, 9% to 57%). The combination of 13-*cis* retinoic acid and interferon-α_{2a}, however, had no activity.[328]

Despite the lack of single-agent activity for etoposide, the Rotterdam Esophageal Cancer Study Group[329] reported a 48% response rate in patients with unresectable or metastatic squamous cell carcinoma. This experience using cisplatin (80 mg/m^2 day 1) and etoposide (100 mg/m^2 intravenously on days 1 to 2 and 200 mg/m^2 orally on days 3 to 5 every 4 weeks) served as the basis for a phase III evaluation of this regimen in the preoperative setting.[330]

Combination regimens including paclitaxel have been evaluated in esophageal cancer patients. In three phase II trials of paclitaxel and cisplatin, response rates ranged from 44% to 52%; activity was comparable in both histologic types.[331–333] Ilson and associates[331] evaluated paclitaxel administered by 24-hour infusion in doses of 200 to 250 mg/m^2 with growth factor support combined with cisplatin (75 mg/m^2). Toxicity (primarily myelosuppression) was severe, leading to one or more hospitalizations in 50% of patients and five treatment-related deaths; as such, this particular regimen cannot be recommended. Van der Gaast and associates from Rotterdam reported two separate trials.[332,333] The first evaluated escalating doses of 3-hour infusion paclitaxel (100 to 200 mg/m^2) combined with a fixed dose of cisplatin (60 mg/m^2) administered every 2 weeks.[332] A 52% response rate was observed in 59 patients. Doses of paclitaxel above 180 mg/m^2 caused dose-limiting neurotoxicity. The second trial evaluated a weekly regimen of cisplatin (70 mg/m^2) and 3-hour paclitaxel infusion.[333] A preliminary report indicated that the maximum tolerable dose of paclitaxel was 100 mg/m^2/week, and that the response rate in 22 adenocarcinoma patients was 50%. The antitumor activity reported for these three regimens was comparable, but toxicities varied considerably.

The three-drug combination of paclitaxel, 175 mg/m^2 (3-hour infusion), combined with cisplatin (20 mg/m^2/d × 5) and 5-FU (1000 mg/m^2/d continuous infusion × 120 hours) was evaluated in 60 patients at four centers.[331] A 48% response rate was reported (56% in patients with squamous cell cancers and 46% in adenocarcinoma patients); significantly more complete responses were observed in patients with squamous cell carcinomas. Toxicity was severe, resulting in hospitalizations for 48% of patients, primarily for severe stomatitis, fever, and neutropenia. The addition of paclitaxel to the established cisplatin and 5-FU regimen did not raise the response rate sufficiently to warrant further evaluation in a larger comparative trial.

It is clear that the optimal dose and scheduling of paclitaxel in combination with other active drugs remains to be determined. In general, shorter infusion schedules of paclitaxel result in less myelotoxicity, but more neurotoxicity when this taxane is combined with cisplatin. The regimen of paclitaxel and carboplatin has not been tested in esophageal cancer. However, because of the lack of activity of carboplatin as a single agent or in combination with other agents used to treat esophageal cancer, it should not be substituted for cisplatin until appropriate clinical trials have been performed.

A new regimen under evaluation in esophageal cancer patients is the combination of irinotecan and cisplatin administered in low dose on a weekly schedule.[334] *In vitro* studies have demonstrated sequence-dependent synergy for cisplatin followed by irinotecan, which prevents removal of cisplatin-induced DNA-interstrand cross-links. Two trials have yielded encouraging results with a regimen of cisplatin (30 mg/m^2) followed by irinotecan (65 mg/m^2) administered weekly for 4 weeks, repeated every 6 weeks.[335,336] Ilson and associates[335] observed a 57% response rate in 35 patients [12 of 23 (52% response) in adenocarcinoma patients and 8 of 12 (66% response) in patients with squamous cell cancers]; median duration of response was 4.2 months.[335] Dysphagia and global quality of life were improved in the majority of patients. Ajani and associates[336] observed a 51% response rate using the same regimen in 25 adenocarcinoma patients, but recommended reduction of the irinotecan dose to 50 mg/m^2 in previously treated patients. Toxicity in both studies consisted of myelosuppression and diarrhea in a minority of patients. Diarrhea was ameliorated with prophylactic use of antidiarrheal agents, dose reduction, or both.

In summary, more recent trials of combination regimens that have included paclitaxel or irinotecan appear to have higher response rates than previous regimens; however, duration of response remains brief for esophageal cancer patients, and some trials have been reported only in preliminary abstract form and consist of small numbers of evaluable patients. In addition, the toxicities associated with many of these phase II single-institution experiences have been excessive.

Further follow-up of early reports and additional patient trials using the most promising regimens are needed. Based on the available data, the standard regimen of cisplatin and infusional 5-FU remains the recommended first-line treatment for patients with recurrent or metastatic disease of either histology. No specific paclitaxel-based regimen has yet emerged as more efficacious and less toxic than cisplatin/5-FU; however, alternative dosing schedules are currently under investigation.

Preoperative Chemotherapy

Nearly three-fourths of patients in the West present with locally advanced (stages IIB and III) disease, and the poor survival rates achieved with surgery alone have provided the impetus for the evaluation of preoperative chemotherapy in resectable esophageal cancer patients.

The potential benefits of induction chemotherapy include downstaging the disease to facilitate surgical resection, improvement in local control, and eradication of micrometastatic disease. Esophagectomy following induction therapy enables comprehensive pathologic assessment of treatment response, which may be important in selecting patients for postoperative adjuvant therapy. The disadvantages of preoperative chemotherapy include the potential selection of drug-resistant clones and the delay in definitive treatment with the risk of further spread of disease. These are important concerns because approximately 50% of patients do not respond to current chemotherapeutic regimens.

Trials evaluating chemotherapy followed by surgery in esophageal cancer patients have been underway since the late 1970s. Stimulated by the promising results of cisplatin-based induction chemotherapy trials in patients with locally advanced oropharyngeal cancers, phase II trials using similar regimens were conducted in esophageal cancer patients in parallel with studies evaluating concurrent chemoradiation followed by surgery or chemoradiation as definitive therapy. Encouraging results with cisplatin and bleomycin,[316] with or without the addition of a vinca alkaloid[317,337] or mitoguazone,[338] and later with cisplatin and 5-FU,[339–343] led to randomized trials initiated in the 1980s. For squamous histology, the response rate to cisplatin (100 mg/m^2 day 1) and 5-FU (1000 mg/m^2/d for 96 or 120 hours) every 3 weeks ranged between 42% and 66%, with 0% to 10% pathologic complete response rates; curative resection rates ranged from 40% to 80%, and median survival rates ranged from 18 to 28 months.[339–343] In these trials, two or three cycles of chemotherapy were administered before resection. A barium esophagogram and CT scans were used to initially stage patients and to assess response to induction therapy.

Five randomized trials evaluating preoperative chemotherapy in esophageal cancer patients are summarized in Table 33.2-9.[244,249,330,344,345] Four of the trials enrolled only patients with squamous cell carcinoma.[249,330,344,345] The Scandinavian trial reported by Nygaard et al.[249] involved randomization to one of four treatment arms: surgery alone, radiotherapy followed by surgery, two courses of induction cisplatin and bleomycin followed by surgery, and all three modalities in sequence. No improvement in survival was noted in patients in the two treatment arms that included chemotherapy in this study.

In a study performed at the National Cancer Institute, Roth et al.[344] compared the combination of cisplatin, bleomycin, and vindesine for three courses followed by surgery, with surgery alone in 39 esophageal cancer patients. Six months of postoperative adjuvant cisplatin and vindesine were planned for patients

TABLE 33.2-9. Randomized Trials of Preoperative Chemotherapy

Series	Treatment	Histology	No. of Patients	Clinical Response Rate (Pathologic Complete Response)	Median Survival (mo)	Survival (3-Y %)
Nygaard[249]	Cisplatin + bleomycin → surgery	SCC	50			3
	RT → surgery		48			21
	Cisplatin + bleomycin → RT → surgery		47			17
	Surgery		41			9
Roth[344]	Cisplatin + vindesine + bleomycin × 2 → surgery + adjuvant cisplatin + vindesine	SCC	19	47% (6%)	9	25
	Surgery		20		9	5
Schlag[345]	Cisplatin + 5-FU × 3 → surgery	SCC	34	41% (6%)	10	
	Surgery		41		10	
Kelsen[244]	Cisplatin + 5-FU × 3 → surgery + adjuvant[a] cisplatin + 5-FU × 2	SCC/Adenocarcinoma	213	19% (2.5%)	14.9	26
	Surgery		227		16.1	23
Kok[330]	Cisplatin + etoposide × 2–4 → surgery	SCC	81	36%	18.5[b]	
	Surgery		80		11	

RT, radiation therapy; SCC, squamous cell carcinoma.
[a]Adjuvant chemotherapy if curative resection performed and no progression during preoperative chemotherapy.
[b]Significant difference, $P = .002$.

in the preoperative chemotherapy arm. A 47% major response rate including one pathologic complete response was documented using barium esophagogram and CT scans. Resectability rates were similar in the two groups, but a higher percentage of patients in the preoperative chemotherapy group had negative surgical margins. Responders to chemotherapy had significantly longer survival than nonresponders (median, 20 vs. 6.2 months; $P = .008$). However, 3-year survival rates in the two treatment groups were not significantly different. All recurrences included distant metastases; the local recurrence rate was low (6.9%). Weight loss of greater than 10% was associated with poor survival in a multivariate analysis of potential prognostic variables.

A multicenter trial from Germany reported by Schlag et al.[345] compared preoperative cisplatin and 5-FU (three cycles) and surgery with surgery alone. The trial was stopped early after only 46 patients were enrolled because of a substantial increase in operative morbidity and mortality in the chemotherapy group. Response to chemotherapy was documented with serial CT scans, barium esophagogram, and endoscopy before treatment and before surgery. A 41% major response rate was observed, including pathologic complete response in two patients. There was no difference in median survival in the overall comparison; however, responders to preoperative chemotherapy survived longer than nonresponders (13 vs. 5 months).

The small numbers of patients enrolled in these three trials and the lack of prospective randomized controlled data in patients with adenocarcinoma of the esophagus led the U.S. Gastrointestinal Intergroup to mount a multicenter trial. Trial 0113 registered 467 patients with resectable disease to receive either three cycles of cisplatin and 5-FU followed by surgery and then two cycles of the same chemotherapy as adjuvant treatment for those who had a curative resection, or immediate surgery.[244] In contrast to other trials, barium esophagogram was the only test required to assess clinical response to preoperative chemotherapy. Thus, it is not surprising that only a 19% response rate was reported. Survival and patterns of failure were the major study end points. No differences were observed between the surgery control arm and the preoperative cisplatin and 5-FU arm in terms of curative resection rate (59% vs. 62%), treatment mortality (6% vs. 7%), overall median survival (16.1 vs. 14.9 months), or 3-year survival (26% vs. 23%). Furthermore, the median survival of patients who had a curative resection was the same in both treatment groups (27.4 vs. 25.0 months). The patterns of failure were also similar between groups (local recurrence 31% vs. 32%, and distant recurrence 50% vs. 41% in the surgery alone versus chemosurgery arms, respectively). Tumor histology did not influence response to treatment. As reported in the Roth trial,[344] pretreatment weight loss was a significant predictor of poor outcome in this study.

The failure of the large, well-controlled Intergroup 0113 trial to show benefit from the addition of cisplatin and 5-FU to surgery suggests either that this strategy does not work as had been theorized or that the induction chemotherapy agents and surgical techniques have not been optimized. Hence, the efficacy of any preoperative chemotherapy regimen in the treatment of resectable esophageal cancer patients remains unproven; as such, induction chemotherapy should not be routinely considered for these individuals unless administered in the context of well-designed, prospective, randomized clinical trials.

Kok and associates[330] reported preliminary results of a trial involving patients with squamous cell cancers. This study, which represents the only positive randomized trial in the literature, differed from the other trials reviewed previously in that patients in the preoperative chemotherapy arm were evaluated for response after two courses; nonresponders went on to surgery, whereas responding patients received two more courses of chemotherapy before surgery. The regimen consisted of cisplatin (80 mg/m^2 day 1) and etoposide (100 mg/m^2 intravenously on days 1 to 2 and 200 mg/m^2 orally on days 3 to 5). At a median follow-up for surviving patients of 15 months, the median survival of preoperative chemotherapy patients was significantly longer than those randomized to immediate surgery (18.5 vs. 11.0 months; $P = .002$). These data raise the question of possible benefit from more intensive therapy than delivered in other trials and also demonstrate the potential relevance of identifying patients with chemosensitive tumors. A final report with further follow-up is awaited.

In conclusion, although a survival advantage has been demonstrated for definitive chemoradiation compared with radiotherapy alone,[346] four of five randomized trials of chemotherapy followed by surgery versus surgery alone have shown no benefit from this sequence of treatments. As such, more recent trials have focused on the evaluation of preoperative concurrent chemoradiation strategies that may have a greater likelihood of achieving histologic complete response and improving long-term survival in esophageal cancer patients.

Postoperative Adjuvant Chemotherapy

Widespread dissemination of disease is the primary cause of death in esophageal cancer patients. As such, considerable efforts are underway to identify novel chemotherapeutic agents and to intensify exposure to agents with documented activity in this disease. Administering chemotherapy after surgery to patients who have already received chemotherapy or chemoradiation preoperatively has not been easily achieved in phase II[338,339] and phase III trials[244,344]; only 38% of patients who were candidates for adjuvant cisplatin and 5-FU in Intergroup trial 0113 received the two planned courses.[244]

Adjuvant chemotherapy in patients who have had surgery alone as their primary curative treatment is more feasible from the standpoint of patient tolerance, but it remains unclear whether current agents confer a survival advantage. The Japanese Oncology Group has studied this question in three separate randomized trials.[347–349] One study compared postoperative radiotherapy (50 Gy) to postoperative adjuvant chemotherapy (two courses of cisplatin and vindesine) in 258 patients following curative resection.[347] No differences were observed in survival (44% vs. 42% at 5 years), time to recurrence, or site of recurrence. Because these results could be interpreted as showing an equivalent beneficial effect from adjuvant chemotherapy and adjuvant radiotherapy, a second trial of surgery alone compared with surgery followed by two courses of adjuvant cisplatin and vindesine was conducted.[323] A total of 205 resected patients were randomized after stratification for regional node involvement. At a median follow-up of 59.2 months, the 5-year survival rate was 45% in the control arm, and 48% in the adjuvant treatment arm, indicating no survival benefit from this adjuvant chemotherapy regimen.

More recently, these investigators have reported preliminary results of a third trial.[349] The study design was the same as that previously described, except that the chemotherapy was changed to cisplatin and 5-FU for two courses after curative resection. A total of 242 patients were randomized with stratification for N0/1 status. At a median follow-up of 40.4 months, the estimated 5-year disease-free survival rate was 46% for the control group and 58% for chemotherapy patients ($P = .05$); survival rates were 77% versus 82% in node-negative patients ($P = .3$), and 35% versus 53% in node-positive patients ($P = .06$) in the control and adjuvant arms, respectively. Overall survival rates were 51% for controls and 61% for chemotherapy patients ($P = .3$). These data suggest that adjuvant chemotherapy may decrease the rate of development of distant metastases in patients with positive regional nodes. It is unlikely that two courses of chemotherapy would be sufficient to have a major effect on micrometastatic disease; thus, it is not surprising that more significant differences in survival did not emerge from this trial. However, the improvement in disease-free survival that approached statistical significance is intriguing, and further evaluation of adjuvant chemotherapy in both histologic types of esophageal cancer should be performed.

The Eastern Cooperative Oncology Group is currently conducting a phase II trial (E8296) evaluating adjuvant cisplatin and paclitaxel for four courses in patients with resected, node-positive adenocarcinomas of the esophagus, gastroesophageal junction, and cardia. A comparison with matched controls from a contemporary surgical series is planned.

The role of postoperative adjuvant chemotherapy or chemoradiation is currently undefined. There are no clear data indicating that administration of postoperative adjuvant chemotherapy will prolong survival, particularly for patients who have undergone a curative resection and have negative nodes. However, patients who have positive margins of resection should be considered for postoperative radiation. Those who have had R0 resections but have regional nodal metastases (stages IIB and III) should be enrolled in clinical trials evaluating adjuvant treatments.

RADIATION THERAPY

Considerable controversy exists as to the ideal therapeutic approach for esophageal cancer. The Patterns of Care study examined 400 patients treated at 61 academic and nonacademic radiation oncology practices to determine practice patterns in the United States from 1992 to 1994.[350] During that time period, treatment approaches included primary combined modality therapy in 54%, radiation alone in 20%, preoperative combined modality therapy in 13%, postoperative combined modality therapy in 8%, postoperative radiation in 4%, and preoperative radiation in 1%. Various oncology groups have published treatment guidelines; however, there is still no consensus at present.[351] Because the effect of histology has not been adequately assessed, it is reasonable to treat both squamous cell cancers and adenocarcinomas in a similar manner.

Primary Therapy

Primary therapy of esophageal cancer is either surgical or nonsurgical. Although the overall results of these approaches are similar, the patient populations selected for treatment with each modality are usually different, resulting in a potential selection bias against nonsurgical therapy. Patients with poor prognostic features, including those with comorbid conditions, or unresectable or metastatic disease, are more commonly selected for treatment with nonsurgical therapy. Furthermore, surgical series report results based on pathologically staged patients, whereas nonsurgical series express results pertaining to clinically staged individuals. Pathologic staging has the advantage of excluding some patients with metastatic disease.

TABLE 33.2-10. Selected Series of Radiation Therapy Alone for Esophageal Cancer

Series	*Histology*	*Stage*	*Number*	*5-Y Survival (%)*
Sykes[357]	SCC + adeno-carcinoma	<5 cm	101	20
Newaishy[353]	SCC	"Inoperable"	444	9
Okawa[354]	SCC	I	43	20
		II	130	10
		III	92	3
		IV	23	0
		T1	47	18
		T2	147	10
		T3	94	3
		Total	288	9
De-Ren[352]	Various	II	177	22
		III	501	28
		<5 cm	59	25
		5 cm	115	25
		>5 cm	504	6
		Total[a]	678	8
Shi[355]	SCC	<8 cm[b]	43	34

SCC, squamous cell carcinoma.
[a]Includes 184 patients with stage IV disease.
[b]Accelerated fractionation after 41.4 Gy to a total dose of 68.4 Gy.

In addition, because some nonsurgical patients are treated with palliative rather than curative intent, the intensity of chemotherapy and the doses and techniques of radiation therapy may be suboptimal.

Nonsurgical Therapy

RADIATION THERAPY ALONE. Many series have reported results of external-beam radiation therapy alone; most include patients with unfavorable features such as clinical T4 disease and positive lymph nodes (Table 33.2-10). For example, in the series by De-Ren,[352] 184 of the 678 patients had stage IV disease. Overall, the 5-year survival rate for patients treated with conventional doses of radiation therapy alone is 0% to 10%.[352–354] The use of radiation therapy as a potentially curative modality requires doses of at least 50 Gy at 1.8 to 2.0 Gy per fraction. Furthermore, given the large size of many unresectable esophageal cancers, doses of 60 Gy or greater are probably required. Shi and colleagues[355] reported a 33% 5-year survival rate with the use of late-course accelerated fractionation to a total dose of 68.4 Gy. However, in the radiation therapy alone arm of the Radiation Therapy Oncology Group (RTOG) 85-01 trial in which patients received 64 Gy at 2 Gy/d with modern techniques, all patients were dead of disease within 3 years.[255,356]

There is one report of radiation therapy alone for patients with clinically early-stage disease. Sykes et al.[357] evaluated 101 patients (90% with squamous cell carcinoma) with tumors less than 5 cm who received 45.0 to 52.5 Gy in 15 to 16 fractions, noting a 5-year survival of 20%.

Collectively, these data indicate that radiation therapy alone should be reserved for palliation or for patients who are medically unfit to receive chemotherapy. As discussed in the following section, combined modality therapy should be the standard of care.

Combined Modality Therapy

CONVENTIONAL APPROACHES. A number of single-arm, nonrandomized trials have been conducted to evaluate the efficacy of combined modality therapy alone in esophageal cancer patients.[358–362] The series reported by Coia and associates[359] is the only one in which patients with early-stage malignancies (clinical stages I and II) were analyzed separately from those with more advanced disease. Patients received 5-FU and mitomycin C concurrently with 60 Gy. The local failure rate was 25%, the 5-year actuarial local relapse-free survival was 70%, and the 5-year actuarial survival was 30% in early-stage patients.

The Southwest Oncology Group 9060 trial reported by Poplin et al.[363] included 32 patients who received 5-FU and cisplatin concurrently with 50 Gy, followed by two cycles of 5-FU and cisplatin. Since the choice of further management (observation, radiation, chemotherapy, and surgery) was based on the tumor response, this study cannot be considered a pure combined modality therapy trial. Although the median survival was 20 months, the authors concluded that the complexity and toxicity of this treatment regimen precluded its further use.

Six randomized trials have been performed comparing radiation therapy alone with combined modality therapy (Table 33.2-11).[249,255,346,364–368] Five of the six trials used suboptimal doses of radiation, and three used inadequate doses of systemic chemotherapy. For example, in the series from Araujo and colleagues,[364] patients received only one cycle of 5-FU, mitomycin C, and bleomycin. The EORTC trial used subcutaneous methotrexate.[365] In the Scandinavian trial reported by Nygaard and associates,[249] patients received low doses of chemotherapy (cisplatin, 20 mg/m^2, and bleomycin, 10 mg/m^2, for a maximum of two cycles).

In the Eastern Cooperative Oncology Group Esophagal Cancer Trial-1282 trial, patients who received combined modality treatment had a significantly increased median survival compared with those receiving radiation alone (15 vs. 9 months; $P = .04$), but had no improvement in 5-year survival (9% vs. 7%). However, this was not a pure nonsurgical trial since approximately 50% of patients in each arm underwent resection after 40 Gy. Furthermore, the decision to proceed with surgery was left to the discretion of the individual investigator.[368] The operative mortality was 17%. Lastly, the Pretoria trial reported by Slabber et al.[367] was limited to a total of 70 patients with T3 squamous cell cancers and used a low-dose (40 Gy) split-course radiation schedule.

The only trial that was designed to deliver adequate doses of systemic chemotherapy with concurrent radiation therapy was the RTOG 85-01 trial reported by Herskovic et al. (Fig. 33.2-5).[255,346,366] This Intergroup trial primarily included patients with squamous cell carcinoma. Patients received four cycles of 5-FU (1000 mg/m^2/24 hours × 4 days) and cisplatin (75 mg/m^2 on day 1). Radiation therapy (50 Gy at 2 Gy/d) was given concurrently with day 1 of chemotherapy. Curiously, cycles 3 and 4 of chemotherapy were delivered every 3 weeks (weeks 8 and 11) rather than every 4 weeks (weeks 9 and 13). This intensification may explain, in part, why only

TABLE 33.2-11. Randomized Trials of Radiation Therapy versus Combined Modality Therapy for Esophageal Cancer

Series	*Number*	*Overall Survival (%)*	*Median Survival* *Failure (mo)*	*Local (%)*
Herskovic (Radiation Therapy Oncology Group)[346,366]				
Radiation alone	62	0% 5-y[a]	9	68[b]
Combined modality therapy	61	27% 5-y 22% 8-y	14	47[c]
Combined modality therapy	69	NR	17	52
Araujo (National Cancer Institute Brazil)[364]				
Radiation alone	31	6% 5-y		84
Combined modality therapy	28	16%		61
Roussel (European Organization for Research and Treatment of Cancer)[365]				
Radiation alone	69	6% 3-y		
Combined modality therapy	75	12%		
Hattevoll (Scandinavia)[249]				
Radiation alone	51	6% 3-y		
Combined modality therapy	46	0%		
Slabber[d] (Pretoria)[367]				
Radiation alone	36		5	
Combined modality therapy	34		6	
Smith[e] (Eastern Cooperative Oncology Group EST-1282)[368]				
Radiation alone	60	7% 5-y	9[c]	
Combined modality therapy	59	9%	15	

NR, information not reported in the manuscript.
[a]Nonrandomized group treated following early closure of the randomization.
[b]Radiation Therapy Oncology Group reported local failure as local persistence + local recurrence.
[c]Statistically significant difference.
[d]Limited to patients with squamous cell cancer with T3 disease.
[e]Approximately 50% in each arm underwent surgery.

50% of the patients finished all four cycles of the chemotherapy. The control arm was radiation therapy alone, at a higher dose (64 Gy) than that delivered in the combined modality treatment arm.

Patients who were randomized to receive combined modality therapy had a significant improvement in median survival (14 vs. 9 months) and 5-year survival (27% vs. 0%; P <.0001).[366] There was a clear plateau in the survival curve such that with a minimum follow-up of 5years, the 8-year survival was 22%.[346] Histology did not significantly influence the results with 21% of patients with squamous cell carcinomas (n = 107) alive at 5 years compared with 13% of patients with adenocarcinoma (n = 23; P = NS). Although African Americans had larger primary tumors (all of which were squamous cell cancers), there was no difference in their survival compared with whites.[369] The incidence of local failure as the first site of failure (defined as local persistence plus recurrence) was also decreased in the combined modality arm (47% vs. 65%). The protocol was closed early due to the positive results; however, following this early closure, an additional 69 patients were treated with the same combined modality therapy regimen. In this nonrandomized combined modality group, the 5-year survival was 14% and local failure rate was 52%.

Combined modality therapy not only improves the results compared with radiation alone, but is also associated with a higher incidence of toxicity. In the 1997 report of the RTOG 85-01 trial, patients who received combined modality therapy had a higher incidence of acute grade III toxicity (44% vs. 25%) and acute grade IV toxicity (20% vs. 3%) compared with radiation therapy alone. Including the one treatment-related death (2%), the incidence of total acute grade III+ toxicity was 66%.[366] The 1999 report examined late toxicity; the incidence of late grade III+ toxicity was similar in the combined modality arm compared with the radiation alone arm (29% vs. 23%).[346] However, grade IV+ toxicity remained higher (10% vs. 2%, respectively). Interestingly, the nonrandomized combined modality therapy group experienced a similar incidence of late grade III+ toxicity (28%), but a lower incidence of grade IV toxicity (4%), and there were no treatment-related deaths.

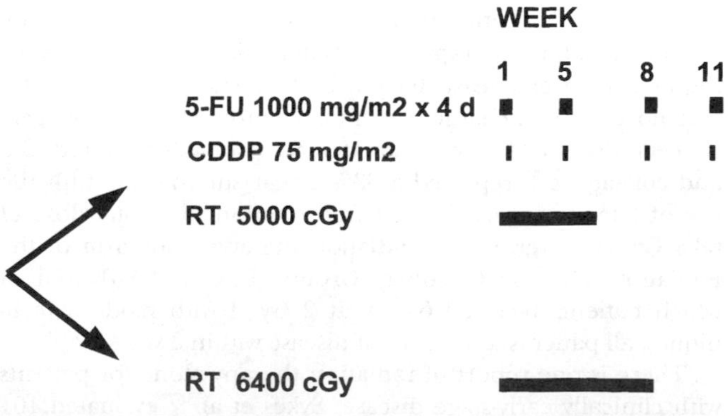

FIGURE 33.2-5. Phase III Intergroup trial Radiation Therapy Oncology Group 85-01 for patients with squamous cell and adenocarcinoma of the esophagus selected for a nonoperative approach. 5-FU, 5-fluorouracil; CDDP, cisplatin; RT, radiation therapy.

Based on the positive results from the RTOG 85-01 trial, the conventional nonsurgical treatment for esophageal carcinoma is combined modality therapy. Notwithstanding, the local failure rate in RTOG 85-01 combined modality therapy arm was 45%; therefore, new approaches such as intensification of combined modality therapy, including escalation of the radiation dose, have been pursued in an attempt to help improve these results.

INTENSIFICATION OF COMBINED MODALITY THERAPY. The phase II Intergroup trial 0122 (Eastern Cooperative Oncology Group PE289/RTOG 90-12) was designed to intensify the RTOG 85-01 combined modality arm.[370] The development of the neoadjuvant chemotherapy approach used in Intergroup 0122 was based, in part, on the results of a randomized trial of preoperative radiation therapy (55 Gy) versus preoperative chemotherapy (5-FU, cisplatin, vindesine) from Memorial Sloan-Kettering Cancer Center. This trial revealed that the resectability (65% vs. 58%), objective response (64% vs. 55%), and local failure (15% vs. 6%) rates with either preoperative radiation therapy or preoperative chemotherapy were similar.[371] Both the chemotherapy and radiation therapy in Intergroup 0122 were intensified as follows: (1) the 5-FU continuous infusion (1000 mg/m^2/24 hours) was increased from 4 days to 5 days; (2) the total number of cycles of chemotherapy was increased from four to five cycles; (3) three cycles of full-dose neoadjuvant 5-FU and cisplatin were delivered before the start of combined modality therapy; and (4) the radiation dose was increased from 50.0 to 64.8 Gy.

The final results of the Intergroup trial 0122 have been reported.[370] For the 38 eligible patients, the primary tumor response rates were 47% complete and 8% partial; 3% had stable disease. The first site of clinical failure was local in 39% of patients and distant in 24% of individuals. For the total patient group, there were six deaths during treatment of which 9% (4 of 45) were treatment related. The median survival was 20 months and the 5-year actuarial survival was 20%. Therefore, this intensive neoadjuvant approach did not appear to offer a benefit compared with conventional doses and techniques of combined modality therapy. However, the higher radiation dose (64.8 Gy) was tolerable and is being further tested in Intergroup trial 0123, which is the replacement trial for RTOG 85-01 (Fig. 33.2-6).

A limited number of phase II trials have tested the use of induction chemotherapy before radiation therapy or combined modality therapy. Valerdi et al.[362] reported the results of 40 patients with clinical stage II and III squamous cell cancers who received two cycles of neoadjuvant cisplatin, vindesine, and bleomycin (days 1 and 29) followed by 60 Gy. In contrast with Intergroup 0122, no chemotherapy was delivered with the radiation therapy. The pathologic complete response rate was 53%. With a median follow-up of 78 months, the local failure rate was 62%, median survival was 11 months, and the 5-year actuarial survival was 15%. These results are similar to those obtained with the RTOG 85-01 combined modality arm, with the exception of the higher treatment-related death rate of 5%.

Using a five-drug neoadjuvant regimen, Roca and colleagues[372] treated 55 patients (54 with squamous cell) with bolus cisplatin, 5-FU, leucovorin, bleomycin, and mitomycin C for 15 days followed by 60 Gy plus concurrent 5-FU, leucovorin, and cisplatin. No maintenance chemotherapy was delivered. All anatomic sites within the esophagus were acceptable, and 53%

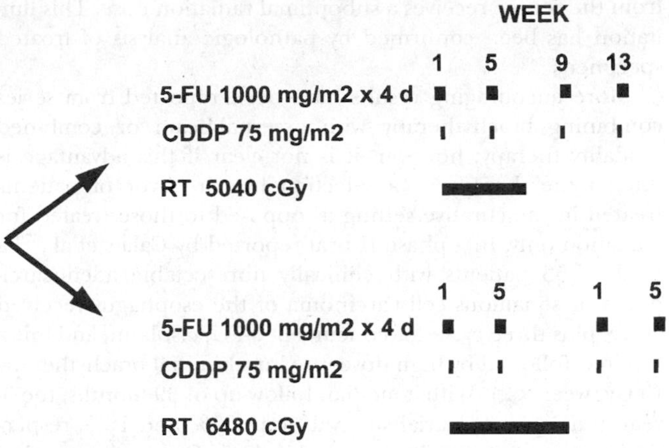

FIGURE 33.2-6. Phase III Intergroup trial 0123 (Radiation Therapy Oncology Group 94-05) for patients with squamous cell or adenocarcinoma of the esophagus. 5-FU, 5-fluorouracil; CDDP, cisplatin; RT, radiation therapy.

of patients had clinical stage III disease. Although the treatment-related mortality was only 4% and the 3-year survival was 35%, the local failure rate was 42%, which was similar to the 45% reported in the RTOG 85-01 combined modality therapy arm.

In summary, neoadjuvant chemotherapy, as delivered in the previously mentioned trials, does not appear to improve the results of combined modality therapy. New trials using paclitaxel (Taxol)-based induction chemotherapy are in progress.[373]

INTENSIFICATION OF THE RADIATION DOSE. Another approach to dose intensification of combined modality therapy involves increasing the radiation dose above 60 Gy. There are two methods by which to increase the radiation dose to the esophagus: brachytherapy and external-beam radiation.

Brachytherapy

Intraluminal brachytherapy allows the escalation of the dose to the primary tumor while protecting the surrounding dose-limiting structures such as the lung, heart, and spinal cord.[374] A radioactive source is placed intraluminally via endoscope or a nasogastric tube. Brachytherapy has been used both as primary therapy (usually as a palliative modality),[375–378] as well as boost following external-beam radiation therapy or combined modality therapy.[375,379–381] It can be delivered by high dose-rate or low dose-rate.[382] Although there are technical and radiobiologic differences between the two dose rates, there are no clear therapeutic advantages.

As a single therapy, brachytherapy is used as a palliative modality and results in a local control rate of 25% to 35% and a median survival of approximately 5 months.[375–378] In the randomized trial from Sur et al.[376] there were no significant differences in local control or survival with high dose-rate brachytherapy compared with external-beam radiation. Jager et al.[377] treated 88 patients with 15 Gy, and 67% had improvement of dysphagia at 4 to 6 weeks and 47% had complete restoration of swallowing.

A major limitation of brachytherapy is the effective treatment distance. The primary isotope is ^{192}Ir, which is usually prescribed to treat to a distance of 1 cm from the source. Therefore, any portion of the tumor that is greater than 1 cm from the source receives a suboptimal radiation dose. This limitation has been confirmed by pathologic analysis of treated specimens.[383]

More encouraging results have been reported from series combining brachytherapy with external-beam or combined modality therapy; however, it is not clear if this advantage is due to the therapy or a selection bias in favor of patients treated in the curative setting as opposed to those treated for palliation only. In a phase II trial reported by Calais et al.,[379] a total of 53 patients with clinically unresectable adenocarcinoma or squamous cell carcinoma of the esophagus received 60 Gy plus three cycles of concurrent 5-FU, cisplatin, and mitomycin C followed by high dose-rate intraluminal brachytherapy (5 Gy/week × 2). With a median follow-up of 39 months, the 3-year and 5-year actuarial survivals were 27% and 18%, respectively. Severe late toxicity occurred in 11%. One patient died of treatment-related toxicity. Two patients (4%) developed a fistula; however, both were due to tumor progression. Swallowing function was reported as *good* in 75%. The local failure rate was 43% (23 of 53).

Other trials of brachytherapy following external-beam radiation or combined modality therapy have reported less favorable results. Schraube and associates[381] treated 54 patients with 60-Gy external-beam radiation followed by a 14-Gy brachytherapy boost, observing a median survival of 8 months and a 2-year overall survival of 10%. Major toxicity was seen in 15%. Using a similar treatment regimen in 35 patients with squamous cell carcinomas, Akagi et al.[380] reported a 26% local failure rate, a 5-year survival of 35%, and a 26% incidence of late complications. Moni et al.[375] reported a 62% local failure rate and 2-year survival of 27% in 21 patients with primary, nonmetastatic disease. However, for the total group of 47 patients there was a 36% grade III+ complication rate including a 17% incidence of fistula.

The trial by Yorozu et al.[384] was limited to a more favorable subset of patients with clinical T1 to T2 disease. A total of 125 patients received 40- to 60-Gy external-beam radiation followed by a 8- to 24-Gy high dose-rate brachytherapy boost. With a median follow-up of 3.1 years, the 5-year survival was 26% and local failure was 44%. Esophageal ulcers occurred in 41% and were fatal in 6% of patients.

In the RTOG 92-07 trial, 75 patients with squamous cell cancers (92%) or adenocarcinomas (8%) of the thoracic esophagus received the RTOG 85-01 combined modality regimen (5-FU, cisplatin × 4 with concurrent 50 Gy) followed by a boost during cycle 3 of chemotherapy with either low dose-rate (19 patients) or high dose-rate (56 patients) intraluminal brachytherapy.[385] The choice of the dose rate was at the discretion of the investigator. Due to low accrual, the low dose-rate option was discontinued and the analysis was limited to patients who received the high dose-rate treatment. High dose-rate brachytherapy was delivered in weekly fractions of 5 Gy during weeks 8, 9, and 10. Following the development of several fistulas, the fraction delivered at week 10 was discontinued. Although the complete response rate was 73%, with a median follow-up of only 11 months, local failure as the first site of failure occurred in 27% of patients. Acute toxicity included 58% grade III, 26% grade IV, and 8% grade V (treatment-related death). The cumulative incidence of fistula was 18% per year and the crude incidence was 14%. Three of the six treatment-related fistulas were fatal. Given the significant toxicity, this treatment approach should be used with caution.

The American Brachytherapy Society has developed guidelines for esophageal brachytherapy.[386] For patients treated in the curative setting, brachytherapy should be limited to tumors less than or equal to 10 cm with no evidence of distant metastasis. Contraindications include tracheal or bronchial involvement, cervical esophagus location, or stenosis that cannot be bypassed. The applicator should have an external diameter of 6 to 10 cm. If combined modality therapy is used (defined as 5-FU–based chemotherapy plus 45 to 50 Gy), the recommended doses of brachytherapy are 10 Gy in 2 weekly fractions of 5 Gy each for high dose-rate, and 20 Gy in a single fraction at 4 to 10 Gy/h for low dose-rate. The doses should be prescribed to 1 cm from the midsource. Lastly, brachytherapy should be delivered after the completion of external-beam radiation, and not concurrently with chemotherapy.

In summary, in the palliative setting, intraluminal brachytherapy is an effective modality for decreasing symptoms such as dysphagia and bleeding. In patients treated in the curative setting, the addition of brachytherapy does not appear to improve results compared with radiation therapy or combined modality therapy alone. Therefore, the benefit of adding intraluminal brachytherapy to radiation or combined modality therapy remains unclear.

External-Beam Therapy

There are limited data examining the tolerance of external-beam doses of greater than or equal to 60 Gy when delivered concurrently with chemotherapy. In a separate toxicity analysis from Coia and associates,[359] the results of 90 patients with clinical stages I to IV squamous and adenocarcinomas of the esophagus were reported; the incidence of grade III toxicity was 22%, and grade IV toxicity was 6%. There were no treatment-related deaths.

Calais et al.[387] reported the results of 53 patients with clinically unresectable disease who received 5-FU, cisplatin, and mitomycin C plus 65 Gy. The full dose of radiation could be delivered in 96% of patients. The incidence of World Health Organization grade III+ toxicity was 30%, and the overall 2-year survival was 42%. It should be noted that the chemotherapy in this trial was not delivered at doses adequate to treat systemic disease.

On the encouraging side, almost all patients in both the Intergroup 0122 and the Calais trials (96% and 94%, respectively) who started radiation therapy were able to complete the full dose (64.8 to 65.0 Gy). Therefore, this higher dose of radiation was considered tolerable and was used in the experimental arm of the Intergroup esophageal trial 0123 (RTOG 94-05). Intergroup 0123 is the follow-up trial to RTOG 85-01. In this trial, patients with either squamous cell or adenocarcinomas who are selected for a nonsurgical approach are randomized to a slightly modified RTOG 85-01 combined modality regimen with 50.4 Gy versus the same chemotherapy with 64.8 Gy (see Fig. 33.2-6).

The modifications to the original RTOG 85-01 combined modality therapy arm include (1) using 1.8 Gy fractions to 50.4 Gy rather than 2 Gy fractions to 50 Gy; (2) treating with 5-cm proximal and distal margins for 50.4 Gy rather than treating the whole esophagus for the first 30 Gy followed by a cone-down with 5-cm margins to 50 Gy; (3) not beginning cycle 3 of 5-FU and cisplatin until 4 weeks following the completion of radiation therapy rather than 3 weeks; and (4) delivering cycles

TABLE 33.2-12. Selected Series of High-Dose Accelerated Fractionation/Hyperfractionated Combined Modality Therapy

Series	*Number*	*Histology*	*Treatment*	*Results*	*Toxicity*
Girinsky[388]	88	NR	65 Gy (2 Gy b.i.d.) ± 5-FU/CDDP	12% 3-y survival; 48% 3-y local control before radiation	13% grade III+
Jeremic[390]	28	SCC	54 Gy (1.5 Gy b.i.d.), 5-FU/CDDP × 4	29% 5-y survival; 71% local control	50% grade III+

CDDP, cisplatin; 5-FU, 5-fluorouracil; NR, information not reported in the manuscript; SCC, squamous cell carcinoma.

3 and 4 of chemotherapy every 4 weeks rather than every 3 weeks. The Intergroup 0123 opened in late 1994 and was closed to accrual in 1999 when an interim analysis revealed that it was unlikely that the high-dose arm would achieve a superior survival compared with the standard-dose arm.

In addition to increasing the total dose, radiation can be intensified by accelerated fractionation or hyperfractionation. Selected series using these approaches are summarized in Table 33.2-12.[355,388–390] Although these approaches are reasonable, most series report an increase in acute toxicity without any clear therapeutic benefit. These regimens remain investigational.

Palliation of Dysphagia with Radiation Therapy

Dysphagia is a common problem in patients with esophageal cancer. Not only is it the most frequently presenting symptom, but it can remain a problem up to the time of the patient's death. Many of the series that have examined palliation are retrospective, and most do not use objective criteria to define and assess this symptom. Some have not reported the number of patients presenting with dysphagia or the percentage who were palliated until the time of death. Furthermore, few series have carefully examined other variables that may have influenced results such as histology, stage, and location of the primary tumor.

As seen in Table 33.2-13, a limited number of series have examined the palliative effects of radiation alone[365,391–394] or combined modality therapy.[360,361,393,395–397] Overall, external-beam radiation therapy alone palliates dysphagia in approximately 70% to 80% of patients.

The most comprehensive and carefully performed analysis of swallowing function in patients receiving combined modality therapy is from Coia et al.[398] Using a swallowing score modified from O'Rourke et al.,[399] Coia et al. analyzed 102 patients treated with three 5-FU–based combined modality regimens. Before the start of therapy, 95% of patients had some degree of dysphagia. Within 2 weeks following the start of treatment, 45% had improvement in dysphagia and by the completion of the 6-week therapy, 83% had improvement. Overall, 88% had an improvement in dysphagia. The median time to maximum improvement was 4 weeks (range, 1 to 21 weeks), and all but two patients were able to swallow at least soft or solid foods at the time of maximum symptomatic improvement.

Variables such as treatment intent, histology, and tumor location were examined. All of the 25 patients treated with curative intent who survived more than 1 year were able to eat soft or solid foods following treatment. The benign stricture rate (defined as a stricture in the absence of recurrent disease) was 12%. Ninety-one percent of patients treated in the noncurative setting had an initial improvement in swallowing, and 67% were palliated until death. Histology and stage had no effect on the rate of palliation; however, patients with distal third lesions had significant improvement in dysphagia compared with individuals with upper or middle third tumors (95% vs. 79%; $P<.05$).

Intraluminal brachytherapy achieves palliation of dysphagia in 40% to 90% of patients.[375–378] Because it is usually prescribed to 1 cm from the source, it may not sufficiently treat gross disease. There is a selection bias against brachytherapy since it is commonly used for patients who have either failed to respond to external-beam radiation or who are medically unfit to travel for daily outpatient treatment. Even accounting for these selection biases, given its limited effective range, brachytherapy has not proven to be as successful as external-beam radiation in treating the entire tumor volume.

In summary, external-beam radiation therapy, either alone or in combination with chemotherapy, palliates dysphagia in approximately 80% of patients, one-half of whom are palliated until death. If a patient requires rapid palliation (within a few days), alternative approaches such as laser or stent are recommended, since external-beam radiation with or without chemotherapy requires at least 2 weeks to obtain palliation. However, palliation achieved by external-beam therapy is more durable

TABLE 33.2-13. Palliation of Dysphagia with External-Beam Radiation Therapy with or without Chemotherapy

		Palliation of Dysphagia[a]	
Series	*Total Number*	At the End of Treatment (%)	Duration of Palliation
RADIATION THERAPY ALONE			
Wara[391]	103	89	6 mo average
Petrovich[392]	133	87	34% ≥ 6 mo 18% ≥ 3 mo 35% ≤ 3 mo
Roussel[365]	69	70	—
Caspers[394]	127	71	54% until death
Whittington[393]	25	—	5% at 9 mo
COMBINED MODALITY THERAPY			
Coia[398]	102	88	67–100% until death
Seitz[361]	35	100[b]	
Whittington[393]	26	—	87% 3-y actuarial
Algan[395]	8	100	
Gill[396]	71	60	
Urba[397]	27	—	59% until death
Izquierdo[360]	25	64	Median 5 mo

[a]See text for the definition and the number of patient presenting with dysphagia.
[b]Patients had dilation or neodymium:yttrium-aluminum-garnet laser at the start of therapy.

than that obtained by other palliative modalities since it treats the problem (the gross tumor mass), not just the symptom. If external-beam radiation is not possible, then brachytherapy should be considered.

Acute and Long-Term Toxicity of Radiation Therapy

The toxicity of radiation therapy is a function of total dose and technique of administration, as well as chemotherapy exposure. There are limited toxicity data in patients who received conventional doses of radiation therapy. Essentially all patients experience lethargy and esophagitis commencing 2 to 3 weeks after the start of radiation; these symptoms begin to resolve 1 week after the completion of therapy.

The most carefully documented acute radiation-related toxicity data are from the control arm of RTOG 85-01 in which patients received radiation therapy alone to a dose of 64 Gy.[255,366] The incidence of acute grade III toxicity was 25%, and grade IV toxicity was 3%; the incidence of long-term grade III+ toxicity was 23% and grade IV+ was 2%.[346] There were no treatment-related deaths.

As with surgery, radiation therapy can produce esophageal strictures. The total incidence of stricture (benign plus malignant) in patients receiving radiation therapy alone or radiation combined with chemotherapy is 20% to 40% in modern studies, and up to 60% in historical series[400]; nearly one-half of these strictures are malignant since they are associated with local recurrence. The incidence of stricture is lower in series in which careful radiation techniques were used. For example, Coia et al.[398] noted that the incidence of benign stricture was 12% in a subset of 25 patients who were locally controlled and survived at least 1 year.

One series examined the functional results in patients who developed benign or malignant strictures.[399] Eighty patients received 45 to 56 Gy and 53% received some form of chemotherapy. Of the 24 patients (30%) who developed a benign stricture, 71% were able to tolerate a full or soft diet and required dilation with a median interval between dilations of 5 months. Therefore, even in the subset of patients who develop a benign stricture, dilation is effective in the majority of patients. In contrast, in the 28% of patients who developed a malignant stricture, dilation was unsuccessful and esophageal intubation was required.

The high incidence of fistulae reported in the RTOG 92-07 trial of combined modality therapy plus intraluminal brachytherapy (18% actuarial, 14% crude) has not been seen in series using radiation therapy or combined modality therapy without intraluminal brachytherapy. The incidence of other long-term grade III+ toxicities such as pneumonitis or pericarditis is 5%. If appropriate radiation doses and techniques are used, spinal cord myelitis should not occur.

TREATMENT-RELATED DEATHS

The issue of treatment-related deaths in patients receiving combined modality therapy is complex. Although the incidence was only 2% in RTOG 85-01, subsequent trials have reported a higher treatment-related mortality (i.e., 9% in Intergroup 0122 and 8% in RTOG 92-07). This mortality is lower than the 10% to 15% incidence reported in the historical surgical series, although only slightly higher than the 6% reported in the surgical control arm of Intergroup 0113.[244] It is interesting to note that as the mortality with surgery has decreased, there has been a corresponding increase in the treatment-related mortality reported in the nonoperative trials. As previously discussed, this may be related, in part, to selection bias against patients treated with the nonoperative approach. Only a randomized trial of surgical versus nonsurgical therapy can address this issue.

COMPARISON OF DEFINITIVE CHEMORADIATION AND SURGERY

Appropriate randomized trials comparing chemoradiation and surgery have not been performed. However, it is an important issue for the practicing oncologist and for the establishment of standards of care. The positive results of RTOG 85-01, demonstrating a 27% 5-year survival rate for patients treated with definitive chemoradiation compared with no survivors after treatment with radiotherapy alone, are a major advance. Without a doubt, this treatment option has influenced the selection of patients for surgical management because it provides an alternative for restoring swallowing function in patients with locally advanced disease for whom resection would likely be palliative.

For patients with earlier stage disease that appears resectable, definitive chemoradiotherapy may also be appropriate treatment; however, prospective trials comparing this approach with surgery, stratified for histology and stage have yet to be performed. Nonetheless, contemporary series suggest that the nonsurgical approach offers a survival rate that is the same or better than that achievable with surgery alone in most medical centers. For example, the median and 5-year survival rates in the surgical control arm of Intergroup 0113 trial were 16 months and 20%, respectively,[244] and in the surgical control arm of the Dutch trial by Kok et al.[330] the median survival rate was 11 months. The incidence of local recurrence (local failure plus local persistence of disease) as the first site of failure was 45% in RTOG 85-01 and 39% in Intergroup 0122. Although local recurrence as the first site of failure in Intergroup 0113 was 31%, this analysis was limited to patients who underwent a complete resection with negative margins (R0 resection). Since an additional 30% of patients had residual local disease, if one was to score these patients as having local persistent disease (as was done in the RTOG 85-01 analysis), the comparable local failure rate with surgery alone was 30% + 31% = 61%. The treatment-related mortality was also similar (2% in RTOG 85-01 and 6% in Intergroup 0113).

In summary, the local failure, survival, and treatment-related mortality of definitive chemoradiation as administered in RTOG 85-01 and those observed following surgery alone appear comparable. Despite these observations, it is clear that both approaches have limited success; as such trials combining all three modalities (surgery plus preoperative chemotherapy and radiotherapy) have been initiated.

TREATMENT IN THE SETTING OF A TRACHEOESOPHAGEAL FISTULA

The presence of a malignant tracheoesophageal fistula is an unfavorable prognostic feature; however, occasionally patients may survive for a prolonged period of time. Historically, radiation therapy was believed to be contraindicated due to con-

TABLE 33.2-14 Randomized Trials of Preoperative Radiation Therapy for Esophageal Cancer

Series	Type	Number	Total Dose (cGy)	Fraction Size (cGy)	Resectable (%)		Local Failure (%)		5-Y Survival (%)	
					Surgery	Radiation Therapy	Surgery	Radiation Therapy	Surgery	Radiation Therapy
Arnott[409]	SCC + adeno-carcinoma	176	2000	200	NR	NR	NR	NR	17	9
Gignoux[248]	SCC	229	3300	330	58	47	67	46[a]	8	10
Nygaard[249]	SCC	186	3500[b]	175	NR	NR	NR	NR	5	18 (3-y)[a]
Launois[408]	SCC	109	4000	NR	70	76	NR	NR	10	10
Huang[410]	NR	160	4000	200	90	92	NR	NR	25	46[c]
Mei[406]	NR	206	4000	NR	85	93	12	13	30	35

NR, information not reported in the manuscript; SCC, squamous cell carcinoma.
[a]$P = .009$.
[b]With or without chemotherapy.
[c]Statistical analysis was not performed.

cerns of exacerbating the fistula as the tumor responded. There have been several reports that challenge these views. In a Mayo Clinic series,[401] ten patients with malignant tracheoesophageal fistula received 30 to 66 Gy external-beam radiation, with a median survival of 5 months. None of these patients experienced an enlarged or more debilitating fistula following radiation. Arlington and Bohorquez[402] described a patient who developed a fistula while receiving external-beam radiation to a total dose of 56.5 Gy, which healed 2 months following the completion of radiation.

Although the experience is limited, data suggest that radiation may not necessarily increase the severity of a malignant tracheoesophageal fistula, and it can be administered safely. Due to the poor prognosis of this group of patients, it is unclear if it improves outcome particularly in individuals who may also be palliated by stents.[403–405]

ADJUVANT THERAPY

Adjuvant Radiation Therapy without Chemotherapy

The rationale of adjuvant radiation therapy is based on the patterns of failure following potentially curative surgery in patients with clinically resectable disease. Unfortunately, few surgical series report these data. The incidence of local failure in the surgical control arms from the preoperative radiation therapy randomized trials from Mei et al.[406] and Gignoux and coworkers[248] was 12% and 67%, respectively. The local failure rate in the surgical control arm from the postoperative radiation therapy randomized trial from Teniere et al.[407] was 35% for patients with negative local regional lymph nodes and 38% for patients with positive local regional lymph nodes. The surgical control arm of Intergroup 0113[244] provides a modern, more relevant baseline for the results of surgery alone. As previously discussed there was a 31% local failure in patients with a R0 resection and a total local failure rate (including the additional 30% of patients with persistent disease) of 61%. Although the majority of patients with esophageal cancer succumb to distant metastases, the incidence of local failure following transhiatal or standard transthoracic resection is high enough to warrant the evaluation of adjuvant radiation therapy.

Preoperative Radiation Therapy

Six randomized trials of preoperative radiation therapy for patients with clinically resectable disease are summarized in Table 33.2-14.[248,249,406,408–410] The series performed by Launois et al.,[408] Gignoux et al.,[248] and Nygaard et al.[249] were limited to patients with squamous cell carcinoma. Patients with both squamous cell carcinoma and adenocarcinoma were included in the series by Arnott et al.[409]; the histologies of the esophageal cancers treated in the series by Huang et al.[410] and Mei et al.[406] were not indicated.

Overall, preoperative radiation therapy did not increase resectability, and only two series reported local failure rates. Although Mei and colleagues[406] reported no difference in local failure, Gignoux et al.[248] observed a significant decrease in local failure in patients who received preoperative radiation therapy compared with those treated by surgery alone (46% vs. 67%, respectively).

Two trials have reported an improvement in survival in patients receiving preoperative radiation therapy, although the significance of these observations is debatable. In a previously described four-arm randomized trial, Nygaard et al.[249] observed that the 48 patients who received preoperative radiation therapy without chemotherapy had a 20% 3-year survival compared with 5% survival in control patients; however, this did not reach statistical significance. Huang et al.[410] also reported improved survival in surgical patients treated with preoperative radiation therapy relative to surgical controls (46% vs. 25%, respectively); however, formal statistical analysis was not performed. Furthermore, metaanalysis from the Oesphageal Cancer Collaborative Group showed no clear evidence of a survival advantage for preoperative radiation therapy.[411]

The aforementioned randomized preoperative radiation therapy trials used suboptimal designs. Conventional radiation therapy doses were not delivered, and some trials used split-course radiation. Furthermore, none of the trials allowed an adequate interval between completion of radiation therapy and surgery (in general, a 4- to 6-week interval is recommended). Consequently, radiation-related morbidity cannot be appropriately assessed in these trials.

The only study that allows analysis of the effect of radiation techniques is a randomized trial from France involving patients

TABLE 33.2-15. Randomized Trials of Postoperative Radiation Therapy for Esophageal Cancer

			Survival (%)		Local Failure (%)			
Series	*Number*	*Median Survival*	Disease-Free Survival (mo)	Overall	Lymph Node–Positive Squamous	Lymph Node Negative	Overall	Distant Failure (%)
Teniere[407]								
Radiation	119		85	19	30	10[a]		
Surgery	102		70	19	38	35		
Fok[417]								
Radiation	30	15					10	40
Surgery	30	21					13	30

[a]Statistically significant.

with squamous cell carcinomas who received combined modality therapy using continuous or split-course radiation.[412] The 95 patients who received continuous-course therapy had a significantly higher local control rate (57% vs. 29%), 2-year event-free survival rate (33% vs. 23%), and a borderline significant 2-year survival rate (37% vs. 23%) relative to patients treated with split-course radiation. Because it is less effective than continuous-course, split-course radiation is not recommended.

In summary, since only two of the six series have reported local failure rates, it is difficult to draw firm conclusions regarding the influence of preoperative radiation therapy on local control. Two series have reported an improvement in survival; one in which half of the patients also received chemotherapy, and in the other a statistical analysis was not performed. Four of the six series have reported no advantage in overall survival. Nonrandomized trials performed by Yadava et al.[413] and Sugimachi and associates[414] have also shown no survival benefit. Based on the available, albeit limited, randomized trials, preoperative radiation therapy does not appear to significantly enhance local control or improve survival in esophageal cancer patients.

Postoperative Radiation Therapy

Several nonrandomized reports of postoperative radiation therapy have suggested that postoperative radiation therapy may be beneficial in esophagectomy patients. Yamamoto and associates[415] reported a 94% 2-year local control rate in node–positive patients. In patients who underwent a three-field dissection, Hosokawa and associates added intraoperative radiation followed by 45 Gy postoperatively; the 5-year survival was 34%.[416] In patients who received the highest dose of intraoperative radiation (25 Gy), 22% developed fatal tracheal ulceration. No treatment-related deaths were seen with doses less than 20 Gy.

There have been only two randomized trials limited to patients treated in the adjuvant setting (Table 33.2-15). Teniere and colleagues[407] reported the results of 221 patients with squamous cell carcinoma randomized to surgery alone versus surgery plus postoperative radiation therapy (45 to 55 Gy at 1.8 Gy per fraction). With a minimum follow-up of 3 years, postoperative radiation therapy had no significant effect on survival. In the series by Fok et al.,[417] patients with squamous cell or adenocarcinomas receiving either curative or palliative resections were evaluated; although the total dose of radiation therapy was conventional, the dose per fraction (3.5 Gy per fraction) was unconventional. No significant decrease in local failure, distant failure, or improvement in median survival was achieved by use of postoperative radiation therapy.

For reasons that are unclear, postoperative radiation therapy has been recommended for patients with positive local regional lymph nodes. Although the data from Teniere et al.[407] support the use of postoperative radiation therapy for decreasing local failure, the benefit was limited to patients with negative lymph nodes in whom postoperative radiation therapy decreased local failure from 35% to 10%. Postoperative radiation therapy had no significant effect in patients with positive nodes.

In summary, although limited data suggest that adjuvant postoperative radiation therapy may decrease local failure in node-negative patients, it appears to have no effect on overall survival. The only role for postoperative radiation therapy is for patients with positive margins. Based on the positive survival results from combined modality therapy trials such as RTOG 85-01, patients selected to receive postoperative radiation therapy should also be considered for systemic chemotherapy.[255,356]

Preoperative Combined Modality Therapy

Given the limited success of single-modality treatment using radiation therapy or surgery for the primary management of esophageal cancer and the absence of survival improvement when radiotherapy is used in the adjuvant setting (preoperatively or postoperatively), efforts have focused on the use of systemic chemotherapy before surgery or in conjunction with preoperative radiation therapy. As previously discussed, the rationale to use chemotherapy before surgery includes the reduction of local and micrometastatic tumor deposits and downstaging the primary tumor by enhanced delivery of cytotoxic agents via intact microvasculature. Furthermore, many of the active agents in esophageal cancer (i.e., 5-FU, cisplatin, mitomycin C, paclitaxel) are known to enhance radiosensitivity in cancer cells. Conceivably, chemotherapy in conjunction with radiotherapy may prevent dissemination of tumor cells during surgery, thus decreasing the rate of distant metastases in patients receiving potentially curative resections.

Combined modality therapy has been used both in the preoperative setting as well as in primary, nonsurgical management of unresectable lesions. In the preoperative trials, patients have had clinically resectable disease, whereas in the nonsurgical trials patients typically have had unresectable neo-

TABLE 33.2-16. Selected Nonrandomized Trials of Planned Preoperative Combined Modality Therapy for Esophageal Cancer

Series	Number	Histology	Number Who Underwent Surgery	Pathologic Complete Response (%)	Survival (%)	Operative Mortality (%)
Le Prise[442]	21	SCC	19	37	18 mo (median)	27
Poplin[425]	113	SCC	71	16	12 mo (median), 16% 3-y	11
Naunheim[468]	47	SCC and Adeno	39	21	23 mo (median), 40% 3-y	5
Forastiere[427,428]	43	SCC and Adeno	39	27	29 mo (median), 46% 3-y	2
Forastiere[435]	50	SCC and Adeno	47	40	31 mo (median), 58% 2-y	0
Urba[426]	24	Adeno	19	10	11 mo (median)	16
Stewart[469]	24	Adeno	23	25	76% 2-y	0
Shahab[429]	24	SCC and Adeno	17	17	9 mo (median)	25[a]
Bates[436]	35	SCC and Adeno	33	51	40% 3-y	9
Malhaire[470]	56	SCC	54	38	37 mo (median), 55% 3-y	11
Chiappori[471]	87	SCC and Adeno	56	27	16 mo (median)	7
Stahl[433]	72	SCC and Adeno	49	33	17 mo (median), 33% 3-y	15
Jones[434]	66	SCC and Adeno	54	41	45% 3-y	7
Adelstein[432]	72	SCC and Adeno	67	27	44% 3-y	18
Posner[423]	44	SCC and Adeno	37	24	52% 2-y	8
Nesbitt[421]	19	SCC and Adeno	10	50	Not reported	0
Safran[422]	33	SCC and Adeno	31	26	Not reported	3[a]
Adelstein[432]	72	SCC and Adeno	67	27	44% 4-y	18
Raoul[431]	32	SCC	29	56	52% 3-y	10
Keller[472]	46	Adeno	33	24	27% 2-y	17

Adeno, adenocarcinoma; SCC, squamous cell carcinoma.
[a]The total treatment-related mortality since the operative mortality was not reported separately.

plasms or have been deemed inoperable on the basis of additional comorbid conditions. Some of the preoperative combined modality regimens have employed accelerated courses of radiation [either twice a day or large fraction sizes (greater than 2 Gy)] plus a short, but intensive course of systemic chemotherapy. Others have used more conventional fractionation (1.8 to 2.0 Gy/d) and moderate total doses of radiation (40 to 50 Gy). In contrast, the nonsurgical combined modality regimens have commonly used conventional fractionation and moderate to high doses of radiation (50.0 to 64.8 Gy) plus longer, but less intensive chemotherapy regimens. Some of these regimens have included neoadjuvant chemotherapy before starting the combined modality therapy.[362,372,418] The differences in patient populations and study designs preclude meaningful comparisons of these trials.

Nonrandomized Trials

In general, the nonrandomized series of preoperative combined modality therapy have used two treatment strategies. Patients have either undergone a planned operation (Table 33.2-16), or for a variety of reasons, were selected for an operation (Table 33.2-17). The results of these two approaches must be analyzed separately since selection factors for surgery may have influenced outcomes. This discussion focuses on series that have been limited to patients with clinically resectable neo-

TABLE 33.2-17. Selected Nonrandomized Series of Preoperative Combined Modality Therapy Plus Surgery for Esophageal Cancer

Series	Number	Local Failure (%)	Distant Failure (%)	Median Survival (mo)		
				Squamous Cell	Adenocarcinoma	Both
Gill[396]						
Surgery	46	25	36	36	14	—
No surgery	36	17	12	26	15	—
Kavanagh[438,a]						
Surgery	72	24	39	—	—	9[b]
No surgery	71	44	38	—	—	15[c]

[a]Results limited to the 103 of 143 patients who had no clinical evidence of metastatic disease at the time of preoperative assessment.
[b]All dead of disease by 5 years.
[c]All dead of disease by 3.5 years.

plasms, thus excluding those with metastatic disease.[419] Most of the trials have used 5-FU and cisplatin–based chemotherapy, although several more recent trials have used Taxol- or docetaxel (Taxotere)-based regimens.[373,420–422] Posner and colleagues[423] added interferon to the regimen, and Nesbitt et al.[421] administered neoadjuvant Taxol before the start of preoperative combined modality therapy.

The results of selected phase II series in which patients have undergone preoperative combined modality therapy followed by a planned operation are summarized in Table 33.2-16. Leichman and colleagues from Wayne State University[424] reported the results of 21 patients with squamous cell carcinomas. Patients received 30 Gy at 2 Gy/d, plus two cycles of concurrent 5-FU and cisplatin. Individuals with residual tumor at surgery received an additional 20 Gy postoperatively. Pathologic complete response rate was 37%, and the median survival was 18 months in the 19 patients who underwent an operation; a 27% operative mortality was observed. Forty-eight percent of patients required hyperalimentation during preoperative therapy. This pilot trial was expanded to a Southwest Oncology Group trial (8037) for patients with squamous cell carcinoma. Of 113 patients evaluated in this trial, only 71 underwent an operation. The pathologic complete response rate was 16%, and the operative mortality was 11%. Despite a 3-year actuarial survival rate of 16%, all patients were dead of disease within 4 years.[425]

Since these initial reports, a variety of treatment approaches have been examined. In most studies, pathologic complete response rates were approximately 25%. Intensive combined modality regimens using hyperfractionated radiation have been evaluated by Urba et al. and Forastiere and associates[426–428] from the University of Michigan, as well as Shahab and colleagues[429] from Ellis Fischel Cancer Center, and Adelstein et al.[430] Some of these regimens achieved higher pathologic complete response and survival rates, usually with corresponding increases in acute toxicity. For example, Raoul et al.[431] reported a 56% complete pathologic response rate and a 52% 3-year survival rate, but a 63% incidence of grade III+ acute toxicity. In the series by Adelestein et al.,[432] patients received preoperative accelerated fractionation (1.5 Gy twice a day to 45 Gy) plus 5-FU and cisplatin. The 27% complete response and 44% 3-year survival rates observed in this trial were comparable with those reported in other series using conventional fractionation; however, the 18% surgical mortality was higher.

In addition to the different treatment schedules, variable surgical techniques have been used in these trials. For instance, investigators from the University of Michigan performed transhiatal resections exclusively, whereas others preferentially did Ivor-Lewis procedures. Transhiatal esophagectomy is thought to be a more conservative operation relative to the Ivor-Lewis procedure, although as previously discussed, both operations appear to be inferior to *en bloc* esophagectomy in terms of achieving local control and improving survival in esophageal cancer patients.

More conventional doses of chemotherapy and radiation therapy techniques have been advocated by Stahl et al.,[433] Jones and colleagues,[434] Forastiere et al.,[435] and Bates and associates.[436] In addition, these investigators have sought to determine if preoperative endoscopy with biopsy can accurately assess response to treatment, and whether achievement of pathologic complete response following chemoradiation improves overall survival. Bates et al.[436] reported a 65% 3-year survival rate in patients who achieved a pathologic complete response, compared with a 25% survival rate in those who did not. Forastiere and associates[435] reported 2-year survival rates of 78% for pathologic complete responders compared with 46% for those having residual tumor in the resected esophagus ($P = .006$); in a previous trial with long-term follow-up,[427] these investigators observed 5-year survival rates of 60% and 32% for pathologic complete responders and those with residual disease following induction therapy, respectively. These nonrandomized data suggest that with aggressive induction chemoradiation therapy, patients who are downstaged to pathology-negative status may have a survival advantage. In addition, the fact that long-term survival was observed in 25% to 30% of patients with residual tumor in the resected specimen suggests that surgery was an important component of the multimodality regimens. Bates et al.[436] noted a 41% false-negative rate with preoperative endoscopy and biopsy, indicating that this technique cannot reliably determine the need for further therapy. Furthermore, Jones and colleagues[437] reported that CT scan had a sensitivity of 65%, specificity of 33%, a positive predictive value of 58%, and a negative predictive value of 41% in evaluating pathologic response following preoperative combined modality therapy in esophageal cancer patients. EUS may have similar limitations,[218,219] although FDG PET may prove to be a useful noninvasive means to assess response to induction therapy.[223] Thus, at present, no methods short of surgical resection accurately determine which patients have achieved pathologic complete response following induction chemoradiation therapy.

In some trials, patients have been selected for surgery based on their overall medical status and response to preoperative therapy (see Table 33.2-17). Gill and colleagues[396] evaluated the role of surgery following combined modality therapy consisting of two cycles of 5-FU and cisplatin and radiation therapy. The study was biased in that only those patients with more favorable prognoses were selected for surgery. Although the differences were not statistically significant, the local failure and distant failure rates were higher in the patients who underwent surgery compared with those who did not. Using a similar approach of limiting surgery to those patients who responded to preoperative therapy and delivering higher radiation doses to nonresponders, Kavanagh and associates[438] reported that patients who underwent surgery had a lower local failure rate (24% vs. 44%); however, there were no differences in distant failure or median survival. The 1992 to 1994 Patterns of Care[439] survey study reported a significant improvement in survival of patients selected to received preoperative combined modality therapy compared with combined modality therapy alone.

Randomized Trials

There have been three randomized trials comparing preoperative combined modality therapy with surgery alone in patients with clinically resectable disease (Table 33.2-18).[245,440,441] The series from Le Prise et al.[442] is not included since patients received sequential rather than concurrent chemotherapy plus radiation.

Urba and associates from the University of Michigan[440] randomized 100 patients (75% with adenocarcinoma) to preoperative cisplatin (20 mg/m^2 days 1 to 5 and 17 to 21), vinblastine (1 mg/m^2 days 1 to 4 and 17 to 20), 5-FU (300 mg/m^2/24 hours

TABLE 33.2-18. Randomized Trials of Preoperative Combined Modality Therapy for Esophageal Cancer

Series	*Number*	*Histology*	*Treatment*	*Pathologic Complete Response (%)*	*Survival* Median	*Survival* 3-Y (%)	*Local Failure (%)*
Urba[440,441]	100	75% adenocarcinoma	Preoperative CMT	28	1.46 y	32[a]	19[b]
		25% SCC	Surgery	0	1.48 y	15	39
Walsh[245]	113	Adenocarcinoma	Preoperative CMT	25	16 mo[b]	32[b]	—
			Surgery	0	11 mo	6	—
Bosset[246]	282	SCC	Preoperative CMT	26	19 mo	36	—
			Surgery	0	19 mo	36	—

CMT, combined modality therapy; SCC, squamous cell carcinoma.
[a]$P = .07$ by univariate analysis and .04 by multivariate analysis.
[b]$P < .05$.

days 1 to 21), and concurrent radiation therapy (1.5 Gy twice a day to 45 Gy), followed on day 42 by a transhiatal esophagectomy versus surgery alone. Preliminary analysis with a median follow-up of 1.82 years in surviving patients revealed no benefit in median survival (1.46 vs. 1.48 years) or estimated 2-year survival (41% vs. 36%) of preoperative combined modality therapy. Subsequent analysis with a median follow-up of 5.2 years in the 19 living patients revealed that preoperative combined modality therapy did not improve median survival (1.41 vs. 1.46 years); however, univariate analysis demonstrated a borderline significant improvement in 3-year survival (32% vs. 15%; $P = .07$). This survival benefit reached statistical significance ($P = .04$) with multivariate analysis. Furthermore, a significant decrease in local recurrence (19% vs. 39%; $P = .04$) was observed in patients receiving combined modality therapy.[441]

In a series from Dublin, Walsh et al.[245] reported a significant survival benefit with preoperative combined modality therapy. In this trial, 113 patients with adenocarcinoma of the midesophagus or distal esophagus (including the cardia) were randomized to two cycles (weeks 1 and 6) of 5-FU (15 mg/kg/24 hours days 1 to 5), cisplatin (75 mg/m^2 day 7), plus concurrent preoperative radiation therapy (2.67 cGy/d to 40 Gy) versus surgery alone. Resection was performed 8 weeks following the start of chemotherapy, and a variety of operations were allowed. Combined modality therapy was well tolerated. The incidence of acute grade III+ toxicity was 15%. The operative mortality was 9% in the multimodality treatment arm compared with 4% in surgery control arm. With a median follow-up in surviving patients of 18 months, a significant improvement in both median survival (16 vs. 11 months; $P = .01$) and 3-year survival (32% vs. 6%; $P = .01$) was observed in patients receiving preoperative therapy compared with those treated with surgery alone. A major criticism of this trial is the high operative mortality (9%) and the low 3-year survival rate (6%) in the surgical control arm. In the Intergroup 0113 (RTOG 89-11) trial the operative mortality and 3-year survival rates were 6% and 25%, respectively, in the surgical control arm.

The third randomized trial of preoperative combined modality therapy was reported by Bosset et al.[246] from the EORTC. A total of 282 patients with clinically resectable (stages I and II) squamous cell carcinomas were randomized to preoperative combined modality therapy versus surgery alone. The preoperative regimen included 3.7 Gy × 5 followed by a 2-week rest and another 3.7 Gy × 5. Chemotherapy was limited to cisplatin, 80 mg/m^2, 0 to 2 days before starting radiation therapy. With a median follow-up of 55 months, patients who received preoperative combined modality therapy had a significantly greater 3-year disease-free survival (40% vs. 28%) and local disease-free survival (relative risk, 0.6), yet had no improvement in median survival (19 months) or overall 3-year survival (36%) compared with patients treated with surgery alone. However, this combined modality therapy regimen was unconventional in design; not only was the radiation split course and delivered with unusually high doses per fraction, but the doses of chemotherapy were not adequate for systemic therapy.

Although two of the three randomized trials demonstrated a survival advantage, they are limited by small numbers of patients and short follow-up, hence their results should be interpreted with caution. To help clarify this controversy, the Intergroup has developed a randomized trial of preoperative combined modality therapy (Cancer and Leukemia Group B C9781), which is the follow-up trial to Intergroup 0113. The preoperative regimen is based on the combined modality arm from RTOG 85-01 and uses conventional 5-FU, cisplatin, and 50.4 Gy; the control arm is surgery alone since preoperative chemotherapy was not beneficial in Intergroup 0113.

Paclitaxel-based regimens have activity in patients with advanced esophageal cancer, and preoperative combined modality regimens using paclitaxel have achieved encouraging results[420–422,443]; however, an increase in acute radiation esophagitis has been seen in initial reports. Safran et al.[422] reported a 9% incidence of radiation esophagitis in patients receiving 3-hour paclitaxel infusion. More protracted infusions appear to be better tolerated; in an ongoing phase I dose escalation trial using 96-hour paclitaxel infusion plus cisplatin and 5040 cGy (reported in abstract form by Kelsen and associates[373]), no patients experienced grade III+ esophagitis at the 80 mg/m^2 dose level of paclitaxel. As with combined modality regimens in other gastrointestinal cancers, development of ideal regimens and schedules remains an active area of clinical investigation.

In summary, the efficacy of preoperative combined modality treatment for resectable esophageal cancer patients remains unclear. Although an apparent benefit has been seen in phase II trials that have used intensive regimens, significant toxicities have been observed. Whereas two of the three randomized trials revealed a survival advantage for combined modality treatment, in the study by Urba et al.[440,441] this advantage reached significance only by multivariate analysis, and the trial by Walsh

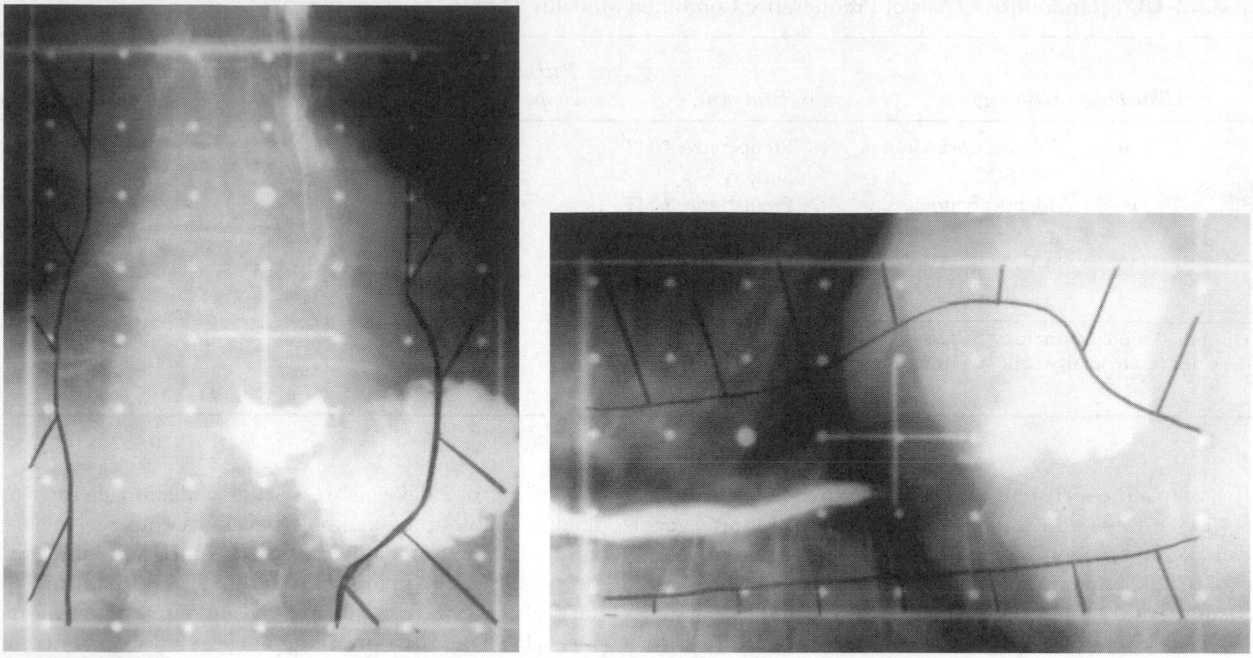

FIGURE 33.2-7. An example of a four-field technique for the treatment of a distal esophageal cancer.

et al.[245] had an unusually low survival rate in the surgical control arm. Both trials had relatively small numbers of patients and limited follow-up. Further maturation of these randomized trials, together with results of the Intergroup trial Cancer and Leukemia Group B C9781, may allow more definitive conclusions regarding the role of preoperative combined modality therapy. In the interim, preoperative combined modality therapy remains an investigational approach, results of which should be compared with the best results achievable by surgery alone in patients who have been optimally staged.

Due to selection bias, it is difficult to determine what is the best treatment for esophageal cancer. The standard of care is either surgery alone or primary combined modality therapy. The results of these two approaches appear similar, although no direct comparative trials have been performed.

Radiation Field Design and Treatment Techniques

Similar to the expert surgical skills required for a successful esophagectomy, radiation field design for esophageal cancer requires careful techniques.[444] There are a number of sensitive organs that, depending on the location of the primary tumor, will be in the radiation field. These include but are not limited to skin, spinal cord, lung, heart, intestine, stomach, kidney, and liver. Minimizing radiation to these structures while delivering an adequate dose to the primary tumor and local regional lymph nodes requires patient immobilization and CT-based treatment planning for organ identification, lung correction, and development of dose-volume histograms.

Although CT can identify adjacent organs and structures, it may be limited in defining the extent of the primary tumor. To assess the consistency of target-volume delineation, Tai and colleagues sent sample cases with CT scans to 48 radiation oncologists throughout Canada and asked them to fill out questionnaires regarding treatment techniques as well as outline the boost target volumes.[445] There was substantial inconsistency in defining the planning target volume, both in the transverse and longitudinal dimensions. Therefore, in addition to a CT scan, barium swallow should be obtained at the time of radiation therapy simulation. The integration of other imaging modalities in radiation treatment planning such as esophageal ultrasound, PET scan, and magnetic resonance imaging are under active investigation.

At present, the standard radiation dose for patients selected for curative nonoperative combined modality therapy approach is 50.4 Gy at 1.8 Gy per fraction. The radiation field should include the primary tumor with 5-cm superior and inferior margins and 2-cm lateral margins. The primary local regional lymph nodes should receive the same dose. For cervical (proximal) primary tumors (defined as at or proximal to the carina), the treatment volume includes the bilateral supraclavicular nodes, and for distal gastroesophageal primaries the celiac axis nodes should be included. An example of a four-field technique for a distal esophageal cancer is seen in Figure 33.2-7.

For cervical primaries, patients are placed supine. Various field designs are possible and their choice depends on the geometry of the primary tumor in relation to the spinal cord. The spinal cord dose should be limited to 45 Gy. Field designs include a three-field technique (two anterior obliques and a posterior) or more commonly anteroposterior and posteroanterior to 39.6 to 41.4 cGy, followed by a left or right opposed oblique pair with photons plus an electron boost to the contralateral supraclavicular area, both to a total dose of 50.4 Gy. For midesophageal primary tumors patients are placed prone to help exclude the spinal cord from the radiation field and receive four fields (anteroposterior and posteroanterior and opposed laterals). For distal primaries patients are treated supine using the same four-field technique. Care should be taken to exclude as much of the normal stomach as possible, especially if the patient is receiving radiation therapy preoperatively. CT-based three-dimensional treatment planning should be performed and all fields treated each day. Dose-volume histograms help guide the radiation oncologist in choosing the radiation plan that minimizes the loss of normal organ function.

A variety of radiation treatment regimens may be used in the palliative setting. Since the goal is rapid amelioration of symptoms, the most common approach is to treat anteroposterior and posteroanterior, including the primary tumor with 2-cm margins with ten 3-Gy fractions to a total dose of 30 Gy.

Tumor Markers and Predictors of Response to Combined Modality Therapy

It would be helpful to predict tumors that have a higher likelihood of responding to radiation or combined modality therapy. In 38 patients with squamous cell carcinoma who received combined modality therapy with or without surgery, Sarbia et al.[446] observed that tumors without p53 expression and those with weak Bcl-XL expression had a higher response to chemotherapy (56% and 53%, respectively) than tumors positive for p53 or those having high-level Bcl-XL expression (30% and 32%, respectively; *P* = NS). Following preoperative combined modality therapy, patients with p53-negative tumors had significantly better mean survivals compared with those whose tumors expressed p53 (31 vs. 11 months; *P* = .0378). There was no prognostic effect of the expression of apoptosis-regulating genes. Using multivariate analysis, Pomp et al.[447] found that overexpression of p53 correlated with diminished survival in 69 patients with squamous or adenocarcinomas treated with radiation alone. In another study, Merchant et al.[448] found a correlation between decreasing phospholipid expression and increasing T stage and grade.

ENDOLUMINAL PALLIATION TECHNIQUES

As previously discussed, surgery remains the standard of care for patients with resectable neoplasms; however, many esophageal cancer patients are inoperable due to locally advanced or distant metastatic disease. Although chemotherapy and radiation therapy are typically used to palliate unresectable disease, many individuals require additional measures to relieve dysphagia and pain. Esophageal dilation frequently can alleviate esophageal obstruction secondary to malignancy; however, results usually are temporary, and patients require repeated treatments. Lundell et al.[449] reported their experience with esophageal dilation in 41 esophageal cancer patients. Although complications were observed in less than 5% of these individuals, dysphagia recurred in all patients, and most dilations had to be repeated every 4 weeks.

Whereas in a strict sense surgery for locally advanced esophageal cancer can be considered palliative in nature, resection of esophageal carcinomas in the context of known distant metastases or the treatment of unresectable obstructing neoplasms using surgical bypass procedures presently cannot be advocated in light of data demonstrating safe and effective palliation by endoluminal stents, laser, or photodynamic therapy (PDT) techniques.[450] Orringer[451] reported results of bypass procedures in 37 patients with unresectable esophageal carcinomas, noting an operative mortality of 24%, an anastomotic leak rate of 19%, and effective palliation in only 25% of individuals. The average survival of patients leaving the hospital following esophageal bypass procedure was less than 6 months. In additional studies, Mannell et al.[452] evaluated 124 patients undergoing esophageal bypass for unresectable disease. Although 82% of patients experienced complete and durable palliation, hospital mortality was approximately 11%, and survival in these individuals was only 5 months. Holting et al.[453] compared results of 26 patients undergoing surgical bypass, with 45 patients undergoing endoscopic laser palliation. Although surgical patients tended to experience more sustained palliation, survival rates were comparable in both patient groups. In a more recent study, Segalin et al.[454] reported an operative mortality of 20% and median survival of 6 months for 49 patients undergoing esophageal resection for advanced metastatic disease. In contrast, 30-day mortality was 10%, and median survival was 4 months for 254 patients treated with intubation procedures. Laser therapy was performed in 50 patients with no operative mortality and a median survival of 4 months.

Although previous studies employing intubation techniques have reported high morbidity and mortality, current data indicate that expandable stents placed by endoscopic methods afford cost-effective and durable palliation in esophageal cancer patients. Raijman et al.[455] evaluated 101 patients with malignant dysphagia, 83 of whom experienced dysphagia secondary to esophageal cancer, and 13 of whom had digestive respiratory tract fistulas. The majority of strictures were in the distal third of the esophagus and most were secondary to exophytic tumors. The mean stricture length was approximately 7 cm. Initial stent placement was successful in 100 patients, and the vast majority experienced significant improvement in their dysphagia. Life-threatening complications were noted in approximately 8%; there were no procedure-related deaths. All digestive respiratory tract fistulas were successfully controlled by endoscopic stents. Ninety-nine patients died of their disease within a mean follow-up of 201 days. In an additional series, Cwikiel et al.[456] reported long-term results of 100 patients with malignant dysphagia treated with self-expanding Nitinol stents. Esophageal strictures were due to squamous cell carcinoma in 43 patients, adenocarcinoma in 18, anastomotic recurrence in 14, or extrinsic compression from mediastinal tumor in 14 individuals. One hundred six stents were placed in 100 patients. Complications included incomplete expansion due to stent twisting (four patients), stent migration (four patients), tumor ingrowth (17 patients), food impaction (five patients), fracture of stent wires (two patients), benign stricture (two patients), and tumor bleeding (four patients). Forty-seven patients experienced transient chest pain following deployment of the stent. Esophageal respiratory fistulas were observed in five patients, three of whom were successfully treated with additional stent placement. Ninety-seven patients experienced significant reduction in dysphagia; at the time of their deaths, 42 patients had no dysphagia, 39 had grade 1 dysphagia, 16 had grade 2 dysphagia, and 3 experienced grade 3 dysphagia.

Cantero et al.[457] compared results of 25 patients undergoing esophageal bypass with 30 patients treated with autoexpandable esophageal stents. Dysphagia was not relieved in 24% of surgical patients, and hospitalization for these patients ranged from 18 to 50 days; the hospital mortality was 24%. Survival in these patients was only 5.4 months. Twenty-eight of 30 individuals treated with esophageal stents experienced significant relief of dysphagia; hospitalization ranged from 5 to 12 days. A 6.6% mortality was observed for these individuals, and no deaths were related to technical difficulties. Mean survival for these patients was 6 months.

Although less commonly used, PDT has been advocated as an additional means to palliate obstructing esophageal carcinomas.[458] Lightdale et al.[459] reported results of a randomized multicenter trial evaluating PDT versus neodymium:yttrium-aluminum-garnet (Nd:YAG) laser treatment for palliation of dysphagia secondary to esophageal carcinomas. Two hundred thirty-six patients were evaluated, of whom 218 patients underwent treatment; 110 individuals received PDT, and 108 patients were treated with YAG laser. Significant improvement in dysphagia was noted in all patients without obvious differences between groups. Objective tumor responses were comparable but slightly improved with PDT. Esophageal perforations occurred in 1% of individuals following PDT treatment versus 7% of individuals treated with laser techniques. These results suggest that PDT and Nd:YAG laser are equally efficacious with regard to palliation of dysphagia, and that PDT may be associated with a relatively lower risk of acute perforations.

Maier et al.[460] reviewed their experience with 119 cases of unresectable esophageal cancers treated with endoluminal palliation techniques. Twenty-one patients required dilation and Nd:YAG laser obliteration before therapy; 44 patients received PDT followed by brachytherapy; 25 of these individuals also received external-beam radiation therapy. Seventy-five patients refused PDT and were treated with high-dose brachytherapy, 17 of whom also received external-beam radiation therapy. PDT was more successful than brachytherapy in relieving stenosis; significant relief of dysphagia was observed. The mean number of PDT treatments was four (range, one to seven); because of concerns regarding stricture formation and perforations, PDT was not repeated within 3 months. Major complications were noted in 9.2% of patients. Four esophageal perforations occurred that were treated by esophageal exclusion and mediastinal drainage techniques. Four esophageal respiratory fistulas were observed, all of which were treated with endoluminal stents. Mean overall survival was 7.7 months; a statistically significant difference in survival was observed for patients receiving PDT and external-beam therapy compared with those receiving brachytherapy alone.

Thus, current data indicate that esophageal stents, laser, or PDT can efficiently palliate obstructing esophageal cancers with far less morbidity and mortality than surgical bypass techniques. Relative contraindications to esophageal stenting include complete obstruction not allowing guidewire placement, noncircumferential tumor not enabling stabilization of the stent, esophageal dilation above the stenosis, or high cervical esophageal lesions. Although laser and PDT require more expertise, these modalities may either be used initially to palliate obstructing esophageal lesions or as an adjunct to treat tumor ingrowth, which occurs in 20% to 30% of stent patients. Endoluminal stenting, YAG laser, and PDT should be viewed as complementary modalities for palliation of unresectable, obstructing esophageal carcinomas.

TREATMENT RECOMMENDATIONS AND FUTURE DIRECTIONS

Although individuals occasionally are diagnosed early due to participation in screening protocols, the vast majority of patients with esophageal cancer present with either locally advanced (stages IIB or III) or inoperable metastatic disease. Esophagectomy remains the standard of care for patients who can tolerate resection. Available data from well-designed prospective randomized trials do not support the routine use of induction chemotherapy in resectable patients. Furthermore, there are no convincing data that justify the routine use of chemotherapy following esophagectomy. Radiation therapy has no proven benefit as the sole modality in the induction setting, and current data indicate a potential benefit of this treatment modality in patients with positive resection margins, but not in completely resected individuals irrespective of nodal status. Limited data suggest that combined chemoradiation therapy may be beneficial in the induction setting in resectable patients, particularly in individuals achieving pathologic complete responses; surgery remains an important component of these aggressive protocols since no other modality enables accurate assessment of response to induction therapy, and no other intervention can enhance local control in this setting. However, further analysis of well-designed, prospective randomized trials is required before multimodality treatment can be considered the standard of care for individuals with resectable cancers. Data from Altorki et al.,[39] Lerut and colleagues,[269] and Akiyama and coworkers[261] indicate that *en bloc* esophagectomy, particularly with three-field lymphadenectomy, enhances the accuracy of staging and appears to improve local control and overall survival in esophageal cancer patients. If confirmed by other expert esophageal cancer surgeons, these results should be considered the standard against which all other treatments are compared. Patients with unresectable cancers should be palliated with chemoradiation therapy in cooperative trials, such that toxicity and survival data can be evaluated in a rigorous manner. Considerable progress must be made in terms of enhancing the accuracy of staging to improve stratification of patients to appropriate prospective trials and minimize stage migration, which may obscure potential benefits of therapeutic interventions.

Although their prognostic significance remains unclear, mutations involving growth factor receptors, cyclin D1, Rb, p16, p53, and telomerase appear to be appropriate targets for intervention in esophageal cancers and their precursor lesions. Several novel compounds have been identified that specifically inhibit the tyrosine kinase activity of EGFr, or erbB2, and enhance the efficacy of conventional cytotoxic agents. Nguyen et al. (manuscript in preparation) observed that 17-allylamino geldanamycin mediated dose-dependent depletion of p185 protein expression and inhibited proliferation of cultured esophageal carcinoma cells overexpressing erbB-2. Interestingly, reduced doses of 17-allylamino geldanamycin that exhibited minimal inhibitory activity synergistically potentiated the effects of paclitaxel in esophageal cancer cells; enhanced paclitaxel sensitivity following 17-allylamino geldanamycin treatment coincided with cell-cycle arrest and apoptosis in these cells. Chemotherapeutic regimens that exploit these observations are currently under evaluation at the National Cancer Institute.

The Rb tumor suppressor pathway is disrupted by a variety of mechanisms in virtually all esophageal cancers, and gene transfer experiments have confirmed that restoration of this pathway significantly inhibits the malignant phenotype of esophageal cancer cells.[140,155] Flavopiridol is a synthetic flavone that inhibits several cyclin-dependent kinases (including cdk4 and cdk6), diminishes cyclin D1 and Bcl-2 expression, and induces cell-cycle arrest and apoptosis in a variety of cancer cells.[461,462] Data indicate that flavopiridol mediates profound cell-cycle arrest and apoptosis in esophageal cancer cells irrespective of histology or genotype; inhibition of cyclin D1, Rb, and p107 expression precedes the onset of apoptosis in these cells.[463] Additional studies have demonstrated that pretreatment of esophageal cancer cells with flavopiridol markedly enhances their sensitivity to paclitaxel, in part, by synchronizing them in G_2/M.[464] In addition to being a novel agent for the treatment of esophageal cancers, flavopiridol may be a potential chemoprevention agent since it effectively targets three mutational events (i.e., cyclin D1 overexpression, as well as Rb and p16 inactivation) that are known to occur early during multistep esophageal carcinogenesis.

Approximately 50% of esophageal cancers exhibit loss of p16 expression due to promoter hypermethylation.[179,181] Studies by Weiser et al.[465] have shown that the demethylating agent, 5 aza-2' deoxycytidine (DAC) at low doses induces p16 expression in cancer cells. Furthermore, these investigators have observed that the novel histone deacetylase inhibitor, depsipeptide FR901228, enhances DAC-mediated growth arrest and apoptosis in esophageal cancer cells irrespective of histology or tumor suppressor gene status. Additional studies have demonstrated that sequential DAC and depsipeptide treatment enhances NY-ESO-1 expression in esophageal cancer cells and enables their recognition by HLA-restricted cytolytic T cells specific for this cancer testis antigen.[466] Clinical trials designed to evaluate the ability of DAC and depsipeptide to mediate target gene induction and apoptosis in esophageal carcinomas and augment antitumor immunity in patients with these malignancies are underway in the Surgery Branch, National Cancer Institute. Evaluation of these agents, as well as other novel compounds targeting p53 mutations and telomerase expression in cancer cells,[246,467] may ultimately enable evolution of more precise and efficacious treatment regimens for highly lethal esophageal neoplasms.

REFERENCES

1. Blot WJ. Epidemiology and genesis of esophageal cancer. In: Roth JA, Ruckdeschel JC, Weisenburger TH, eds. *Thoracic oncology*. Philadelphia: WB Saunders, 1995:278.
2. Blot WJ, McLaughlin JK. The changing epidemiology of esophageal cancer. *Semin Oncol* 1999;26:2.
3. Blot WJ. Esophageal cancer trends and risk factors. *Semin Oncol* 1994;21:403.
4. Devesa SS, Blot WJ, Fraumeni JFJ. Changing patterns in the incidence of esophageal and gastric carcinoma in the United States. *Cancer* 1998;83:2049.
5. Navaratnam RM, Winslet MC. Barrett's oesophagus. *Postgrad Med J* 1998;74:653.
6. Bytzer P, Christensen PB, Damkier P, Vinding K, Seersholm N. Adenocarcinoma of the esophagus and Barrett's esophagus: a population- based study. *Am J Gastroenterol* 1999;94:86.
7. Blot WJ, Devesa SS, Kneller RW, Fraumeni JF Jr. Rising incidence of adenocarcinoma of the esophagus and gastric cardia. *JAMA* 1991;265:1287.
8. Weston AP, Badr AS, Hassanein RS. Prospective multivariate analysis of clinical, endoscopic, and histological factors predictive of the development of Barrett's multifocal high-grade dysplasia or adenocarcinoma [see comments]. *Am J Gastroenterol* 1999;94:3413.
9. Lagergren J, Bergstrom R, Lindgren A, Nyren O. Symptomatic gastroesophageal reflux as a risk factor for esophageal adenocarcinoma [see comments]. *N Engl J Med* 1999;340:825.
10. DeMeester SR, DeMeester TR. The diagnosis and management of Barrett's esophagus. *Adv Surg* 1999;33:29.
11. Cameron AJ. Barrett's esophagus: prevalence and size of hiatal hernia. *Am J Gastroenterol* 1999;94:2054.
12. Kelsen D, Laufer I, Leichman L, et al. Alarming trends in esophageal cancer. *Patient Care* 1992;15:72.
13. Castellsague X, Munoz N, De Stefani E, et al. Independent and joint effects of tobacco smoking and alcohol drinking on the risk of esophageal cancer in men and women. *Int J Cancer* 1999;82:657.
14. Blot WJ. Alcohol and cancer. *Cancer Res* 1992;52:2119s.
15. Hammond EC. Smoking in relation to the death rates of one million men and women. *Natl Cancer Inst Monogr* 1966;19:127.
16. Doll R, Peto R. Mortality in relation to smoking: 20 years' observations on male British doctors. *BMJ* 1976;2:1525.
17. Rogot E, Murray JL. Smoking and causes of death among US veterans: 16 years of observation. *Public Health Rep* 1980;15:213.
18. Gammon MD, Schoenberg JB, Ahsan H, et al. Tobacco, alcohol, and socioeconomic status and adenocarcinomas for the esophagus and gastric cardia. *J Natl Cancer Inst* 1997;89:1277.
19. Denissenko MF, Pao A, Tang M, Pfeifer GP. Preferential formation of benzo[a]pyrene adducts at lung cancer mutational hotspots in p53. *Science* 1996;274:430.
20. Reid BJ, Barrett MT, Galipeau PC, et al. Barrett's esophagus: ordering the events that lead to cancer. *Eur J Cancer Prev* 1996;5(Suppl 2):57.
21. Galipeau PC, Cowan DS, Sanchez CA, et al. 17 p (p53 allelic losses, 4N (G2/tetraploid) populations, and progression to aneuploidy in Barrett's esophagus. *Proc Natl Acad Sci U S A* 1996;93:7081.
22. Horio Y, Chen A, Rice P, et al. Ki-ras and p53 mutations are early and late events, respectively, in urethane-induced pulmonary carcinogenesis in A/J mice. *Mol Carcinogen* 1996;17:217.
23. Rusch V, Klimstra D, Linkov I, Dmitrovsky E. Aberrant expression of p53 or the epidermal growth factor receptor is frequent in early bronchial neoplasia, and coexpression precedes squamous cell carcinoma development. *Cancer Res* 1995;55:1365.
24. Anonymous International Agency for Research on Cancer. *Tobacco smoking, in evaluation of carcinogenic risks to humans*. International Agency for Research on Cancer, 1986:38.
25. Anonymous International Agency for Research on Cancer. *Alcohol drinking, in evaluation of carcinogenic risks to humans*. International Agency for Research on Cancer, 1988:44.
26. Zhang ZF, Kurtz RC, Sun M, et al. Adenocarcinomas of the esophagus and gastric cardia: medical conditions, tobacco, alcohol, and socioeconomic factors. *Cancer Epidemiol Biomarkers Prev* 1996;5:761.
27. Kabat GC, Ng SK, Wynder EL. Tobacco, alcohol intake, and diet in relation to adenocarcinoma of the esophagus and gastric cardia. *Cancer Causes Control* 1993;4:123.
28. Vaughan TL, Davis S, Kristal A, Thomas DB. Obesity, alcohol, and tobacco as risk factors for cancers of the esophagus and gastric cardia: adenocarcinoma versus squamous cell carcinoma. *Cancer Epidemiol Biomarkers Prev* 1995;4:85.
29. Brown LM, Swanson CA, Gridley G, et al. Adenocarcinoma of the esophagus: role of obesity and diet [see comments]. *J Natl Cancer Inst* 1995;87:104.
30. Mettlin C, Graham S, Priore S. Diet and cancer of the esophagus. *Nutr Cancer* 1981;2:143.
31. VanRensburg SJ. Epidemiologic and dietary evidence for a specific nutritional predisposition to esophageal cancer. *J Natl Cancer Inst* 1981;67:243.
32. DeJong UW, Breslow N, Hong JG. Etiological factors in esophageal cancer in Singapore Chinese. *Int J Cancer* 1974;13:291.
33. Victora C, Munoz N, Day NE. Hot beverages and oesophageal cancer in southern Brazil: a case-control study. *Int J Cancer* 1987;39:710.
34. Selikoff IJ, Hammond EC, Seidman H. Mortality experience of insulation workers in the United States and Canada, 1943–1976. *Ann N Y Acad Sci* 1979;330:91.
35. Weiss NS. Cancer in relation to occupational exposure to perchloroethylene. *Cancer Causes Control* 1995;6:257.
36. Gustavisson P, Hogstedt C, Evanoff B. Increased risk of esophageal cancer among workers exposed to combustion products. *Arch Environ Health* 1993;48:243.
37. DeNardi FG, Riddel RH. Esophagus. In: Sternberg SS, ed. *Histology for pathologists*. New York: Raven Press, 1992:515.
38. Guernsey JM, Knudsen DF. Abdominal exploration in the evaluation of patients with carcinoma of the thoracic esophagus. *J Thorac Cardiovasc Surg* 1970;59:62.
39. Altorki NK, Skinner DB. Occult cervical nodal metastasis in esophageal cancer: preliminary results of three-field lymphadenectomy [see comments]. *J Thorac Cardiovasc Surg* 1997;113:540.
40. Sons H, Borchard F. Esophageal cancer: autopsy findings in 171 cases. *Arch Pathol Lab Med* 1984;108:983.
41. Anderson LL, Lad TE. Autopsy findings in squamous-cell carcinoma of the esophagus. *Cancer* 1982;50:1587.
42. Mandard AM, Tourneux J, Gignoux M, et al. In situ carcinoma of the esophagus. Macroscopic study with particular reference to the Lugol test. *Endoscopy* 1980;12:51.
43. Mandard AM, Marnay J, Gignoux M, et al. Cancer of the esophagus and associated lesions: detailed pathologic study of 100 esophagectomy specimens. *Hum Pathol* 1984;15:660.
44. Begin LR. The pathobiology of esophageal cancer. In: Roth JA, Ruckdeschel JC, Weisenburger TH, eds. *Thoracic oncology*. Philadelphia: WB Saunders, 1995:288.
45. Steiger Z, Wilson RF, Leichman L, Busuito MJ, Rosenberg JC. Primary adenocarcinoma of the esophagus. *J Surg Oncol* 1987;36:68.
46. Haggitt RC, Tryzelaar J, Ellis FH, Colcher H. Adenocarcinoma complicating columnar epithelium-lined (Barrett's) esophagus. *Am J Clin Pathol* 1978;70:1.
47. Hamilton SR, Smith RR, Cameron JL. Prevalence and characteristics of Barrett esophagus in patients with adenocarcinoma of the esophagus or esophagogastric junction. *Hum Pathol* 1988;19:942.
48. Lerut T, Devlyn P, Coosemans W. Surgical strategies in esophageal carcinoma with emphasis on radical lymphadenectomy. *Ann Surg* 1992;216:583.
49. Caldwell CB, Bains MS, Burt M. Unusual malignant neoplasms of the esophagus. Oat cell carcinoma, melanoma, and sarcoma. *J Thorac Cardiovasc Surg* 1991;101:100.
50. Osamura RY, Shimamura K, Hata J, et al. Polypoid carcinoma of the esophagus. A unifying term for "carcinosarcoma" and "pseudosarcoma." *Am J Surg Pathol* 1978;2:201.
51. Matsusaka T, Watanabe H, Enjoji M. Pseudosarcoma and carcinosarcoma of the esophagus. *Cancer* 1976;37:1546.
52. Sweeney EC, Cooney T. Adenoid cystic carcinoma of the esophagus: a light and electron microscopic study. *Cancer* 1980;45:1516.
53. Burt M. Unusual malignancies. In: Pearson FG, Deslauriers J, Ginsberg RJ, et al., eds. *Esophageal surgery*. New York: Churchill Livingstone, 1995:629.
54. Reyes CV, Chejfec G, Jao W. Neuroendocrine carcinomas of the esophagus. *Ultrastruct Pathol* 1980;1:367.

55. Tateishi R, Taniguchi H, Wada A. Argyrophil cells and melanocytes in esophageal mucosa. *Arch Pathol* 1974;98:87.
56. Nagashima R, Mabe K, Takahashi T. Esophageal small cell carcinoma with ectopic production of parathyroid hormone-related protein (PTHrp), secretin, and granulocyte colony-stimulating factor (G-CSF). *Dig Dis Sci* 1999;44:1312.
57. Suzuki H, Takayanagi S, Otake T, et al. Primary small cell carcinoma of the esophagus with achalasia in a patient in whom pro-gastrin-releasing peptide and neuron-specific enolase levels reflected the clinical course during chemotherapy. *J Gastroenterol* 1999;34:378.
58. Medgyesy CD, Wolff RA, Putnam JBJ, Ajani JA. Small cell carcinoma of the esophagus: the University of Texas M. D. Anderson Cancer Center experience and literature review. *Cancer* 2000;88:262.
59. Maier A, Woltsche M, Fell B, et al. Local and systemic treatment in small cell carcinoma of the esophagus. *Oncol Rep* 2000;7:187.
60. Kimura H, Konishi K, Maeda K, et al. Highly aggressive behavior and poor prognosis of small-cell carcinoma in the alimentary tract: flow-cytometric analysis and immunohistochemical staining for the p53 protein and proliferating cell nuclear antigen. *Dig Surg* 1999;16:152.
61. Adad SJ, Etchebehere RM, Hayashi EM, et al. Leiomyosarcoma of the esophagus in a patient with chagasic megaesophagus: case report and literature review. *Am J Trop Med Hyg* 1999;60:879.
62. Levine MS, Buck JL, Pantongrag-Brown L, et al. Leiomyosarcoma of the esophagus: radiographic findings in 10 patients. *AJR Am J Roentgenol* 1996;167:27.
63. Rocco G, Trastek VF, Deschamps C, et al. Leiomyosarcoma of the esophagus: results of surgical treatment. *Ann Thorac Surg* 1998;66:894.
64. Herrmann R, Panahon AM, Barcos MP, Walsh D, Stutzman L. Gastrointestinal involvement in non-Hodgkin's lymphoma. *Cancer* 1980;46:215.
65. Agha FP, Schnitzer B. Esophageal involvement in lymphoma. *Am J Gastroenterol* 1985;80:412.
66. Haller JO, Cohen HL. Gastrointestinal manifestations of AIDS in children. *AJR Am J Roentgenol* 1994;162:387.
67. Lim SG, Lipman MC, Squire S, et al. Audit of endoscopic surveillance biopsy specimens in HIV positive patients with gastrointestinal symptoms. *Gut* 1993;34:1429.
68. Chalkiadakis G, Wihlm JM, Morand G, Weill-Bousson M, Witz JP. Primary malignant melanoma of the esophagus. *Ann Thorac Surg* 1985;39:472.
69. Ashworth MT, Nash JR, Ellis A, Day DW. Abnormalities of differentiation and maturation in the oesophageal squamous epithelium of patients with tylosis: morphological features. *Histopathology* 1991;19:303.
70. Risk JM, Mills HS, Garde J, et al. The tylosis esophageal cancer (TOC) locus: more than just a familial cancer gene. *Dis Esophagus* 1999;12:173.
71. Risk JM, Field EA, Field JK, et al. Tylosis oesophageal cancer mapped [letter]. *Nat Genet* 1994;8:319.
72. von Brevern M, Hollstein MC, Risk JM, et al. Loss of heterozygosity in sporadic oesophageal tumors in the tylosis oesophageal cancer (TOC) gene region of chromosome 17q. *Oncogene* 1998;17:2101.
73. Iwaya T, Maesawa C, Ogasawara S, Tamura G. Tylosis esophageal cancer locus on chromosome 17q25.1 is commonly deleted in sporadic human esophageal cancer. *Gastroenterology* 1998;114:1206.
74. Ruhrberg C, Williamson JA, Sheer D, Watt FM. Chromosomal localisation of the human envoplakin gene (EVPL) to the region of the tylosis oesophageal cancer gene (TOCG) on 17q25. *Genomics* 1996;37:381.
75. Risk JM, Ruhrberg C, Hennies H, et al. Envoplakin, a possible candidate gene for focal NEPPK/esophageal cancer (TOC): the integration of genetic and physical maps of the TOC region on 17q25. *Genomics* 1999;59:234.
76. Shamma MH, Benedict EB. Esophageal webs. *N Engl J Med* 1958;259:378.
77. Ribeiro UJ, Posner MC, Safatle-Ribeiro AV, Reynolds JC. Risk factors for squamous cell carcinoma of the oesophagus [see comments]. *Br J Surg* 1996;83:1174.
78. Csikos M, Horvath O, Petri A. Late malignant transformation of chronic corrosive oesophageal strictures. *Langenbecks Arch Chir* 1985;365:231.
79. Sandler RS, Nyren O, Ekbom A, et al. The risk of esophageal cancer in patients with achalasia. A population- based study. *JAMA* 1995;274:1359.
80. Meijssen MA, Tilanus HW, van Blankenstein M, Hop WC, Ong GL. Achalasia complicated by oesophageal squamous cell carcinoma: a prospective study in 195 patients. *Gut* 1992;33:155.
81. Aggestrup S, Holm JC, Sorensen HR. Does achalasia predispose to cancer of the esophagus? *Chest* 1992;102:1013.
82. Loviscek LF, Cenoz MC, Badaloni AE, Agarinakazato O. Early cancer in achalasia. *Dis Esophagus* 1998;11:239.
83. Chow WH, Blaser MJ, Blot WJ, et al. An inverse relation between cagA+ strains of *Helicobacter pylori* infection and risk of esophageal and gastric cardia adenocarcinoma. *Cancer Res* 1998;58:588.
84. Vieth M, Stolte M. Re: Richter, et al. Possibly protective properties of *Helicobacter pylori* in connection with GERD [letter; comment]. *Am J Gastroenterol* 1999;94:3068.
85. Sharma VK, Demian SE, Taillon D, Vasudeva R, Howden CW. Examination of tissue distribution of *Helicobacter pylori* within columnar-lined esophagus. *Dig Dis Sci* 1999;44:1165.
86. El-Serag HB, Sonnenberg A. Ethnic variations in the occurrence of gastroesophageal cancers [see comments]. *J Clin Gastroenterol* 1999;28:135.
87. Sur M, Cooper K. The role of the human papilloma virus in esophageal cancer. *Pathology* 1998;30:348.
88. Stoler MH. Human papillomaviruses and cervical neoplasia: a model for carcinogenesis. *Int J Gynecol Pathol* 2000;19:16.
89. Mineta H, Ogino T, Amano HM, et al. Human papilloma virus (HPV) type 16 and 18 detected in head and neck squamous cell carcinoma. *Anticancer Res* 1998;18:4765.
90. de Villiers EM, Lavergne D, Chang F, et al. An interlaboratory study to determine the presence of human papillomavirus DNA in esophageal carcinoma from China. *Int J Cancer* 1999;81:225.
91. Lavergne D, de Villiers EM. Papillomavirus in esophageal papillomas and carcinomas. *Int J Cancer* 1999;80:681.
92. Shibagaki I, Tanaka H, Shimada Y, et al. p53 mutation, murine double minute 2 amplification, and human papillomavirus infection are frequently involved but not associated with each other in esophageal squamous cell carcinoma. *Clin Cancer Res* 1995;1:769.
93. Poljak M, Cerar A, Seme K. Human papillomavirus infection in esophageal carcinomas: a study of 121 lesions using multiple broad-spectrum polymerase chain reactions and literature review [see comments]. *Hum Pathol* 1998;29:266.
94. Rugge M, Bovo D, Busatto G, et al. p53 alterations but no human papillomavirus infection in preinvasive and advanced squamous esophageal cancer in Italy. *Cancer Epidemiol Biomarkers Prev* 1997;6:171.
95. Turner JR, Shen LH, Crum CP, Dean PJ, Odze RD. Low prevalence of human papillomavirus infection in esophageal squamous cell carcinomas from North America: analysis by a highly sensitive and specific polymerase chain reaction-based approach. *Hum Pathol* 1997;28:174.
96. Lagergren J, Wang Z, Bergstrom R, Dillner J, Nyren O. Human papillomavirus infection and esophageal cancer: a nationwide seroepidemiologic case-control study in Sweden. *J Natl Cancer Inst* 1999;91:156.
97. Leon X, Quer M, Diez S, et al. Second neoplasm in patients with head and neck cancer. *Head Neck* 1999;21:204.
98. Levi F, Randimbison L, Te VC, La Vecchia C. Second primary cancers in patients with lung carcinoma. *Cancer* 1999;86:186.
99. Narayana A, Vaughan AT, Fisher SG, Reddy SP. Second primary tumors in laryngeal cancer: results of long-term follow-up. *Int J Radiat Oncol Biol Phys* 1998;42:557.
100. Spechler SJ. Barrett's esophagus. *Semin Gastrointest Dis* 1996;7:51.
101. Goldblum JR, Rice TW. The columnar-lined esophagus. In: Pearson FG, Deslauriers J, Ginsberg RJ, et al., eds. *Esophageal surgery*. New York: Churchill Livingstone, 1995:273.
102. Wolf C, Timmer R, Breumelhof R, Seldenrijk CA, Smout AJ. Columnar lined oesophagus and intestinal metaplasia: current concepts. *Eur J Gastroenterol Hepatol* 1999;11:793.
103. Nandurkar S, Talley NJ. Barrett's esophagus: the long and the short of it [published erratum appears in *Am J Gastroenterol* 1999;94:1719]. *Am J Gastroenterol* 1999;94:30.
104. Van Asche C, Rahm AEJ, Goldner F, Crumbaker D. Columnar mucosa in the proximal esophagus. *Gastrointest Endosc* 1988;34:324.
105. Altorki NK, Oliveria S, Schrump DS. Epidemiology and molecular biology of Barrett's adenocarcinoma. *Semin Oncol* 1997;13:270.
106. Voutilainen M, Sipponen P, Mecklin J, Juhola M, Farkkila M. Gastroesophageal reflux disease: prevalence, clinical, endoscopic and histopathological findings in 1,128 consecutive patients referred for endoscopy due to dyspeptic and reflux symptoms. *Digestion* 2000;61:6.
107. Spechler SJ, Sperber H, Doos WG, Schimmel EM. The prevalence of Barrett's esophagus in patients with chronic peptic esophageal strictures. *Dig Dis Sci* 1983;28:769.
108. Lundell L. Acid suppression in the long-term treatment of peptic stricture and Barrett's oesophagus. *Digestion* 1992;51(Suppl 1):49.
109. Hirota WK, Loughney TM, Lazas DJ, et al. Specialized intestinal metaplasia, dysplasia, and cancer of the esophagus and esophagogastric junction: prevalence and clinical data. *Gastroenterology* 1999;116:277.
110. Cameron AJ, Zinsmeister AR, Ballard DJ, Carney JA. Prevalence of columnar-lined (Barrett's) esophagus. Comparison of population-based clinical and autopsy findings. *Gastroenterology* 1990;99:918.
111. Meyer WH, Vollmar F, Bar W. Barrett's esophagus following total gastrectomy. *Endoscopy* 1979;202:121.
112. Gallez JF, Berger F, Moulinier B, Partensky C. Esophageal adenocarcinoma following Heller myotomy for achalasia. *Endoscopy* 1987;19:76.
113. Paull A, Trier JS, Dalton MD, et al. The histologic spectrum of Barrett's esophagus. *N Engl J Med* 1976;295:476.
114. de Mas CR, Kramer M, Seifert E, et al. Short Barrett: prevalence and risk factors. *Scand J Gastroenterol* 1999;34:1065.
115. Sharma P, Weston AP, Morales T, et al. Relative risk of dysplasia for patients with intestinal metaplasia in the distal oesophagus and in the gastric cardia. *Gut* 2000;46:9.
116. Falk GW, Rice TW, Goldblum JR, Richter JE. Jumbo biopsy forceps protocol still misses unsuspected cancer in Barrett's esophagus with high-grade dysplasia. *Gastrointest Endosc* 1999;49:170.
117. Cameron AJ, Ott BJ, Payne WS. The incidence of adenocarcinoma in columnar-lined (Barrett's) esophagus. *N Engl J Med* 1985;313:857.
118. Spechler SJ, Robbins AH, Rubins HB, et al. Adenocarcinoma and Barrett's esophagus. An overrated risk? *Gastroenterology* 1984;87:927.
119. Robertson CS, Mayberry JF, Nicholson DA, James PD, Atkinson M. Value of endoscopic surveillance in the detection of neoplastic change in Barrett's oesophagus. *Br J Surg* 1988;75:760.
120. Katz D, Rothstein R, Schned A, et al. The development of dysplasia and adenocarcinoma during endoscopic surveillance of Barrett's esophagus. *Am J Gastroenterol* 1998;93:536.
121. O'Connor JB, Falk GW, Richter JE. The incidence of adenocarcinoma and dysplasia in Barrett's esophagus: report on the Cleveland Clinic Barrett's Esophagus Registry. *Am J Gastroenterol* 1999;94:2037.
122. Reid BJ. Barrett's esophagus and esophageal adenocarcinoma. *Gastroenterol Clin North Am* 1991;20:817.
123. Fennerty MB, Sampliner RE, Way D, et al. Discordance between flow cytometric abnormalities and dysplasia in Barrett's esophagus. *Gastroenterology* 1989;97:815.
124. Reid BJ, Sanchez CA, Blount PL, Levine DS. Barrett's esophagus: cell cycle abnormalities in advancing stages of neoplastic progression. *Gastroenterology* 1993;105:119.
125. Blount PL, Galipeau PC, Sanchez CA, et al. 17p allelic losses in diploid cells of patients with Barretts esophagus who develop aneuploidy. *Cancer Res* 1994;54:2292.
126. Reid BJ, Haggitt RC, Rubin CE, Rabinovitch PS. Barrett's esophagus. Correlation between flow cytometry and histology in detection of patients at risk for adenocarcinoma. *Gastroenterology* 1987;93:1.

127. Prevo LJ, Sanchez CA, Galipeau PC, Reid BJ. p53-mutant clones and field effects in Barrett's esophagus. *Cancer Res* 1999;59:4784.
128. Reid BJ, Blount PL, Rubin CE, et al. Flow-cytometric and histological progression to malignancy in Barrett's esophagus: prospective endoscopic surveillance of a cohort. *Gastroenterology* 1992;102:1212.
129. Polkowski W, van Sandick JW, Offerhaus GJ, et al. Prognostic value of Lauren classification and c-erbB-2 oncogene overexpression in adenocarcinoma of the esophagus and gastroesophageal junction. *Ann Surg Oncol* 1999;6:290.
130. Provenzale D, Schmitt C, Wong JB. Barrett's esophagus: a new look at surveillance based on emerging estimates of cancer risk. *Am J Gastroenterol* 1999;94:2043.
131. Nandurkar S, Talley NJ. Surveillance in Barrett's oesophagus: a need for reassessment? *J Gastroenterol Hepatol* 1998;13:990.
132. Gross CP, Canto MI, Hixson J, Powe NR. Management of Barrett's esophagus: a national study of practice patterns and their cost implications. *Am J Gastroenterol* 1999;94:3440.
133. Atkinson M, Iftikhar SY, James PD, Robertson CS, Steele RJ. The early diagnosis of oesophageal adenocarcinoma by endoscopic screening. *Eur J Cancer Prev* 1992;1:327.
134. Streitz JMJ, Ellis FHJ, Tilden RL, Erickson RV. Endoscopic surveillance of Barrett's esophagus: a cost-effectiveness comparison with mammographic surveillance for breast cancer. *Am J Gastroenterol* 1998;93:911.
135. Barrett MT, Sanchez CA, Galipeau PC, et al. Allelic loss of 9p21 and mutation of the CDKN2/p16 gene develop as early lesions during neoplastic progression in Barrrett's esophagus. *Oncogene* 1996;13:1867.
136. Barrett MT, Galipeau PC, Sanchez CA, Edmond MJ, Reid BJ. Determination of the frequency of loss of heterozygosity in esophageal adenocarcinoma by cell sorting, whole genome amplification and microsatellite polymorphisms. *Oncogene* 1996;12:1873.
137. Barrett MT, Sanchez CA, Prevo LJ, et al. Evolution of neoplastic cell lineages in Barrett oesophagus. *Nat Genet* 1999;22:106.
138. Blount PL, Rabinvitch PS, Haggitt RC, Reid BJ. Early Barrett's adenocarcinoma arises within a single aneuploid population. *Gastrointestinal Oncol* 1990;A273(abst).
139. Jiang W, Zhang Y-J, Kahn SM, et al. Altered expression of the cyclin D1 and retinoblastoma genes in human esophageal cancer. *Proc Natl Acad Sci U S A* 1993;90:9026.
140. Schrump DS, Chen A, Consuli U, Jin X, Roth JA. Inhibition of esophageal cancer proliferation by adenoviral- mediated delivery of p16^{INK4}. *Cancer Gene Ther* 1996;3:357.
141. Al-Kasspooles M, Moore JH, Orringer MB, Beer DG. Amplification and over-expression of the EGFR and erbB-2 genes in human esophageal adenocarcinomas. *Int J Cancer* 1993;54:213.
142. Itakura Y, Sasano H, Shiga C, et al. Epidermal growth factor receptor overexpression in esophageal carcinoma. An immunohistochemical study correlated with clinicopathologic findings and DNA amplification. *Cancer* 1994;74:795.
143. Iihara K, Shiozaki H, Tahara H, et al. Prognostic significance of transforming growth factor-alpha in human esophageal carcinoma. Implication for the autocrine proliferation. *Cancer* 1993;71:2902.
144. Kitagawa Y, Ueda M, Ando N, et al. Further evidence for prognostic significance of epidermal growth factor receptor gene amplification in patients with esophageal squamous cell carcinoma. *Clin Cancer Res* 1996;2:909.
145. Shimada Y, Imamura M, Watanabe G, et al. Prognostic factors of oesophageal squamous cell carcinoma from the perspective of molecular biology. *Br J Cancer* 1999;80:1281.
146. Hung MC, Lau YK. Basic science of HER-2/neu: a review. *Semin Oncol* 1999;26:51.
147. Wiechen K, Karaaslan S, Dietel M. Involvement of the c-erbB-2 oncogene product in the EGF-induced cell motility of SK-OV-3 ovarian cancer cells. *Int J Cancer* 1999;83:409.
148. Roetger A, Merschjann A, Dittmar T, et al. Selection of potentially metastatic subpopulations expressing c-erbB-2 from breast cancer tissue by use of an extravasation model. *Am J Pathol* 1998;153:1797.
149. Petit AM, Rak J, Hung MC, et al. Neutralizing antibodies against epidermal growth factor and ErbB-2/neu receptor tyrosine kinases down-regulate vascular endothelial growth factor production by tumor cells in vitro and in vivo: angiogenic implications for signal transduction therapy of solid tumors. *Am J Pathol* 1997;151:1523.
150. Shi D, He G, Cao S, et al. Overexpression of the c-erbB-2/neu-encoded p185 protein in primary lung cancer. *Carcinogenesis* 1992;5:213.
151. Tsai CM, Levitzki A, Wu LH, et al. Enhancement of chemosensitivity by tyrphostin AG825 in high-p185(neu) expressing non-small cell lung cancer cells. *Cancer Res* 1996;56:1068.
152. Wang LS, Chow KC, Chi KH, et al. Prognosis of esophageal squamous cell carcinoma: analysis of clinicopathological and biological factors. *Am J Gastroenterol* 1999;94:1933.
153. Brien TP, Odze RD, Sheehan CE, McKenna BJ, Ross JS. HER-2/neu gene amplification by FISH predicts poor survival in Barrett's esophagus-associated adenocarcinoma. *Hum Pathol* 2000;31:35.
154. Schrump DS, Chen A, Consoli U. Inhibition of lung cancer proliferation by antisense cyclin D. *Cancer Gene Ther* 1996;3:131.
155. Zhou P, Jiang W, Zhang YJ, et al. Antisense to cyclin D1 inhibits growth and reverses the transformed phenotype of human esophageal cancer cells. *Oncogene* 1995;11:571.
156. Adelaide J, Monges G, Derderian C, Seitz JF, Birnbaum D. Oesophageal cancer and amplification of the human cyclin D gene CCND1/PRAD1. *Br J Cancer* 1995;71:64.
157. Jiang W, Kahn SM, Tomita N, et al. Amplification and expression of the human cyclin D gene in esophageal cancer. *Cancer Res* 1992;52:2980.
158. Yoshida T, Sakamoto H, Terada M. Amplified genes in cancer in upper digestive tract. *Semin Cancer Biol* 1993;4:33.
159. Arber N, Lightdale C, Rotterdam H, et al. Increased expression of the cyclin D1 gene in Barrett's esophagus. *Cancer Epidemiol Biomarkers Prev* 1996;5:457.
160. Roncalli M, Bosari S, Marchetti A, et al. Cell cycle-related gene abnormalities and product expression in esophageal carcinoma. *Lab Invest* 1998;78:1049.
161. Takeuchi H, Ozawa S, Ando N, et al. Altered p16/MTS1/CDKN2 and cyclin D1/PRAD-1 gene expression is associated with the prognosis of squamous cell carcinoma of the esophagus. *Clin Cancer Res* 1997;3:2229.
162. van Dekken H, Geelen E, Dinjens WN, et al. Comparative genomic hybridization of cancer of the gastroesophageal junction: deletion of 14Q31-32.1 discriminates between esophageal (Barrett's) and gastric cardia adenocarcinomas. *Cancer Res* 1999;59:748.
163. Pack SD, Karkera JD, Zhuang Z, et al. Molecular cytogenetic fingerprinting of esophageal squamous cell carcinoma by comparative genomic hybridization reveals a consistent pattern of chromosomal alterations. *Genes Chromosomes Cancer* 1999;25:160.
164. Dolan K, Garde J, Gosney J, et al. Allelotype analysis of oesophageal adenocarcinoma: loss of heterozygosity occurs at multiple sites. *Br J Cancer* 1998;78:950.
165. Brenner C, Bieganowski P, Pace HC, Huebner K. The histidine triad superfamily of nucleotide-binding proteins. *J Cell Physiol* 1999;181:179.
166. Sard L, Accornero P, Tornielli S, et al. The tumor-suppressor gene FHIT is involved in the regulation of apoptosis and in cell cycle control. *Proc Natl Acad Sci U S A* 1999; 96:8489.
167. Ohta M, Inoue H, Cotticelli MG, et al. The FHIT gene, spanning the chromosome 3p14.2 fragile site and renal carcinoma-associated t(3;8) breakpoint, is abnormal in digestive tract cancers. *Cell* 1996;84:587.
168. Tanaka H, Shimada Y, Harada H, et al. Methylation of the 5' CpG island of the FHIT gene is closely associated with transcriptional inactivation in esophageal squamous cell carcinomas. *Cancer Res* 1998;58:3429.
169. Chen YJ, Chen PH, Lee MD, Chang JG. Aberrant FHIT transcripts in cancerous and corresponding non-cancerous lesions of the digestive tract. *Int J Cancer* 1997;72:955.
170. Michael D, Beer DG, Wilke CW, Miller DE, Glover TW. Frequent deletions of FHIT and FRA3B in Barrett's metaplasia and esophageal adenocarcinomas. *Oncogene* 1997;15:1653.
171. Nelson HH, Wiencke JK, Gunn L, et al. Chromosome 3p14 alterations in lung cancer: evidence that FHIT exon deletion is a target of tobacco carcinogens and asbestos. *Cancer Res* 1998;58:1804.
172. Tomizawa Y, Nakajima T, Kohno T, et al. Clinicopathological significance of Fhit protein expression in stage I non-small cell lung carcinoma. *Cancer Res* 1998;58:5478.
173. Ewen ME. The cell cycle and the retinoblastoma protein family. *Cancer Metastasis Rev* 1994;13:45.
174. Chen PL, Riley DJ, Lee WH. The retinoblastoma protein as a fundamental mediator of growth and differentiation signals. *Crit Rev Eukary Gene Exp* 1995;1:79.
175. Harrington EA, Bruce JL, Harlow E, Dyson N. pRB plays an essential role in cell cycle arrest induced by DNA damage. *Proc Natl Acad Sci U S A* 1998;95:11945.
176. Xing EP, Yang GY, Wang LD, Shi ST, Yang CS. Loss of heterozygosity of the Rb gene correlates with pRb protein expression and associates with p53 alteration in human esophageal cancer. *Clin Cancer Res* 1999;5:1231.
177. Hashimoto N, Tachibana M, Dhar DK, Yoshimura H, Nagasue N. Expression of p53 and RB proteins in squamous cell carcinoma of the esophagus: their relationship with clinicopathologic characteristics. *Ann Surg Oncol* 1999;6:489.
178. Grana X, Reddy EP. Cell cycle control in mammalian cells: role of cyclins, cyclin dependent kinases (CDKs), growth suppressor genes and cyclin-dependent kinase inhibitors (CKIs). *Oncogene* 1995;11:211.
179. Xing EP, Nie Y, Wang LD, Yang GY, Yang CS. Aberrant methylation of p16INK4a and deletion of p15INK4b are frequent events in human esophageal cancer in Linxian, China. *Carcinogenesis* 1999;20:77.
180. Esteve A, Martel-Planche G, Sylla BS, et al. Low frequency of p16/CDKN2 gene mutations in esophageal carcinomas. *Int J Cancer* 1996;66:301.
181. Wong DJ, Barrett MT, Stoger R, Emond MJ, Reid BJ. p16INK4a promoter is hypermethylated at a high frequency in esophageal adenocarcinomas. *Cancer Res* 1997;57:2619.
182. Zhang Y, Xiong Y, Yarbrough WG. ARF promotes MDM2 degradation and stabilizes p53: ARF-INK4a locus deletion impairs both the Rb and p53 tumor suppression pathways. *Cell* 1998;92:725.
183. Sherr CJ. Tumor surveillance via the ARF-p53 pathway. *Genes Dev* 1998;12:2984.
184. Robertson KD, Jones PA. The human ARF cell cycle regulatory gene promoter is a CpG island which can be silenced by DNA methylation and down-regulated by wild-type p53. *Mol Cell Biol* 1998;18:6457.
185. Xing EP, Nie Y, Song Y, et al. Mechanisms of inactivation of p14ARF, p15INK4b, and p16INK4a genes in human esophageal squamous cell carcinoma. *Clin Cancer Res* 1999;5:2704.
186. Kastan MB, Canman CE, Leonard CJ. p53, cell cycle control and apoptosis: implications for cancer. *Cancer Metastasis Rev* 1995;14:3.
187. Vaziri H, Benchimol S. Alternative pathways for the extension of cellular life span: inactivation of p53/pRb and expression of telomerase. *Oncogene* 1999;18:7676.
188. El-Deiry WS, Harper JW, O'Connor PM, et al. WAF1/CIP1 is induced in p53-mediated G1 arrest and apoptosis. *Cancer Res* 1994;54:1169.
189. Kastan MB, Onyekwere O, Sidransky D, Vogelstein B, Craig R. Participation of p53 protein in the cellular response to DNA damage. *Cancer Res* 1991;51:6304.
190. Fontanini G, Boldrini L, Vignati S, et al. Bc12 and p53 regulate vascular endothelial growth factor (VEGF)–mediated angiogenesis in non-small cell lung carcinoma. *Int J Cancer* 1998;34:718.
191. Schrump DS, Nguyen DM. Strategies for molecular intervention in esophageal cancers and their precursor lesions. *Dis Esophagus* 1999;12:181.
192. Matsubara H, Kimura M, Sugaya M, et al. Expression of wild-type p53 gene confers increased sensitivity to radiation and chemotherapeutic agents in human esophageal carcinoma cells. *Int J Oncol* 1999;14:1081.
193. Gonzalez MV, Artimez ML, Rodrigo L, et al. Mutation analysis of the p53, APC, and p16 genes in the Barrett's oesophagus, dysplasia, and adenocarcinoma. *J Clin Pathol* 1997;50:212.
194. Hollstein M, Sidransky D, Vogelstein B, Harris CC. p53 mutations in human cancers. *Science* 1991;253:49.
195. Blount PL, Meltzer SJ, Yin J, et al. Clonal ordering of 17p and 5q allelic losses in Barrett dysplasia and adenocarcinoma. *Proc Natl Acad Sci U S A* 1993;90:3221.

196. Wu TT, Watanabe T, Heitmiller R, et al. Genetic alterations in Barrett esophagus and adenocarcinomas of the esophagus and esophagogastric junction region. *Am J Pathol* 1998;153:287.
197. Kobayashi S, Koide Y, Endo M, Isono K, Ochiai T. The p53 gene mutation is of prognostic value in esophageal squamous cell carcinoma patients in unified stages of curability. *Am J Surg* 1999;177:497.
198. Cerni C. Telomeres, telomerase, and myc. An update. *Mutat Res* 2000;462:31.
199. Oulton R, Harrington L. Telomeres, telomerase, and cancer: life on the edge of genomic stability. *Curr Opin Oncol* 2000;12:74.
200. Hiyama T, Yokozaki H, Kitadai Y, et al. Overexpression of human telomerase RNA is an early event in oesophageal carcinogenesis. *Virchows Arch* 1999;434:483.
201. Koyanagi K, Ozawa S, Ando N, et al. Clinical significance of telomerase activity in the non-cancerous epithelial region of oesophageal squamous cell carcinoma [see comments]. *Br J Surg* 1999;86:674.
202. Morales CP, Lee EL, Shay JW. In situ hybridization for the detection of telomerase RNA in the progression from Barrett's esophagus to esophageal adenocarcinoma. *Cancer* 1998;83:652.
203. Lord RV, Salonga D, Danenberg KD, et al. Telomerase reverse transcriptase expression is increased early in the Barrett's metaplasia, dysplasia, adenocarcinoma sequence. *J Gastrointest Surg* 2000;4:135.
204. Hahn WC, Stewart SA, Brooks MW, et al. Inhibition of telomerase limits the growth of human cancer cells [see comments]. *Nat Med* 1999;5:1164.
205. Zargar SA, Khuroo MS, Jan GM, Mahajan R, Shah P. Prospective comparison of the value of brushings before and after biopsy in the endoscopic diagnosis of gastroesophageal malignancy. *Acta Cytol* 1991;35:549.
206. Nishimaki T, Tanaka O, Ando N, et al. Evaluation of the accuracy of preoperative staging in thoracic esophageal cancer. *Ann Thorac Surg* 1999;68:2059.
207. Rankin SC, Taylor H, Cook GJ, Mason R. Computed tomography and positron emission tomography in the pre-operative staging of oesophageal carcinoma. *Clin Radiol* 1998;53:659.
208. Luketich JD, Friedman DM, Weigel TL, et al. Evaluation of distant metastases in esophageal cancer: 100 consecutive positron emission tomography scans. *Ann Thorac Surg* 1999;68:1133.
209. Kole AC, Plukker JT, Nieweg OE, Vaalburg W. Positron emission tomography for staging of oesophageal and gastroesophageal malignancy. *Br J Cancer* 1998;78:521.
210. Griffith JF, Chan AC, Chow LT, et al. Assessing chemotherapy response of squamous cell oesophageal carcinoma with spiral CT. *Br J Radiol* 1999;72:678.
211. Bergman JJ, Fockens P. Endoscopic ultrasonography in patients with gastro-esophageal cancer. *Eur J Ultrasound* 1999;10:127.
212. de Manzoni G, Pedrazzani C, Di Leo A, et al. Experience of endoscopic ultrasound in staging adenocarcinoma of the cardia. *Eur J Surg Oncol* 1999;25:595.
213. Vickers J. Role of endoscopic ultrasound in the preoperative assessment of patients with oesophageal cancer. *Ann R Coll Surg Engl* 1998;80:233.
214. Reed CE, Mishra G, Sahai AV, Hoffman BJ, Hawes RH. Esophageal cancer staging: improved accuracy by endoscopic ultrasound of celiac lymph nodes. *Ann Thorac Surg* 1999;67:319.
215. Catalano MF, Alcocer E, Chak A, et al. Evaluation of metastatic celiac axis lymph nodes in patients with esophageal carcinoma: accuracy of EUS. *Gastrointest Endosc* 1999;50:352.
216. Schlick T, Heintz A, Junginger T. The examiner's learning effect and its influence on the quality of endoscopic ultrasonography in carcinoma of the esophagus and gastric cardia. *Surg Endosc* 1999;13:894.
217. Sozzi M, Nguyen CC, Valentini M. What is the current role of endoscopic ultrasonography in oesophageal cancer? *Ital J Gastroenterol Hepatol* 1999;31:154.
218. Laterza E, de Manzoni G, Guglielmi A, et al. Endoscopic ultrasonography in the staging of esophageal carcinoma after preoperative radiotherapy and chemotherapy. *Ann Thorac Surg* 1999;67:1466.
219. Zuccaro GJ, Rice TW, Goldblum J, et al. Endoscopic ultrasound cannot determine suitability for esophagectomy after aggressive chemoradiotherapy for esophageal cancer. *Am J Gastroenterol* 1999;94:906.
220. McAteer D, Wallis F, Couper G, et al. Evaluation of 18F-FDG positron emission tomography in gastric and oesophageal carcinoma. *Br J Radiol* 1999;72:529.
221. Krasna MJ. Surgical staging and surgical treatment in esophageal cancer. *Semin Oncol* 1999;26:9.
222. Kobori O, Kirihara Y, Kosaka N, Hara T. Positron emission tomography of esophageal carcinoma using (11)C-choline and (18)F-fluorodeoxyglucose: a novel method of preoperative lymph node staging. *Cancer* 1999;86:1638.
223. Couper GW, McAteer D, Wallis F, et al. Detection of response to chemotherapy using positron emission tomography in patients with oesophageal and gastric cancer. *Br J Surg* 1998;85:1403.
224. O'Reilly S, Forastierre AA. Is surgery necessary with multimodality treatment of esophageal cancer. *Ann Oncol* 1995;6:551.
225. Coia LR. Esophageal cancer: is esophagectomy necessary? *Oncology* 1989;3:101.
226. Daly JM, Karnell LH, Menck HR. National Cancer Data Base report on esophageal carcinoma. *Cancer* 1996;78:1820.
227. Orringer MB, Marshall B, Iannettoni MD. Transhiatal esophagectomy: clinical experience and refinements. *Ann Surg* 1999;230:392.
228. Gelfand GA, Finley RJ, Nelems B, et al. Transhiatal esophagectomy for carcinoma of the esophagus and cardia. *Arch Surg* 1992;127:164.
229. Gertsch P, Vauthey JN, Lustenberger AA, Friedlander-Klar H. Long-term results of transhiatal esophagectomy for esophageal carcinoma. A multivariate analysis of prognostic factors. *Cancer* 1993;72:2312.
230. Vigneswaran WT, Trastek VF, Pairolero PC, et al. Transhiatal esophagectomy for carcinoma of the esophagus. *Ann Thorac Surg* 1993;56:838.
231. Chu KM, Law SY, Fok M, Wong J. A prospective randomized comparison of transhiatal and transthoracic resection for lower-third esophageal carcinoma. *Am J Surg* 1997;174:320.
232. Horstmann O, Verreet PR, Becker H, Ohmann C, Roher HD. Transhiatal esophagectomy compared with transthoracic resection and systematic lymphadenectomy for the treatment of esophageal cancer. *Eur J Surg* 1995;161:557.
233. Goldminc M, Maddem G, Le Prise E, et al. Esophagectomy by a transhiatal approach for thoracotomy: a prospective randomized trial. *Br J Surg* 1993;80:367.
234. Putnam JB, Suell DM, McMurtrey MJ, et al. Comparison of three techniques of esophagectomy within a residency training program. *Ann Thorac Surg* 1994;57:319.
235. Urba S, Orringer M, Turrisi A, et al. A randomized trial comparing surgery to preoperative concomittant chemoradiation plus surgery in patients with resectable esophageal cancer. Update analysis. *Proc Am Soc Clin Oncol* 1997;6:227.
236. Barbier PA, Luder PJ, Schupfer G, Becker CD, Wagner HE. Quality of life and patterns of recurrence following transhiatal esophagectomy for cancer: results of a prospective follow-up in 50 patients. *World J Surg* 1988;12:270.
237. Ellis FH Jr. Standard resection for cancer of the esophagus and cardia. *Surg Oncol Clin North Am* 1999;8:279.
238. Lieberman MD, Shriver CD, Bleckner S, Burt M. Carcinoma of the esophagus. Prognostic significance of histologic type. *J Thorac Cardiovasc Surg* 1995;109:130.
239. Wright CD, Mathisen DJ, Wain JC, et al. Evolution of treatment strategies for adenocarcinoma of the esophagus and gastroesophageal junction. *Ann Thorac Surg* 1994;58:1574.
240. Sharpe DA, Moghissi K. Resectional surgery in carcinoma of the esophagus and cardia: what influences long-term survival? *Eur J Cardiothorac Surg* 1996;10:359.
241. Swisher SG, Hunt KK, Holmes EC, Zinner MJ, McFadden DW. Changes in the surgical management of esophageal cancer from 1970 to 1993. *Am J Surg* 1995;169:609.
242. Adam DJ, Craig SR, Sang CT, Walker WS, Cameron EW. Esophagogastrectomy for carcinoma in patients under 50 years of age. *J R Coll Surg Obstet* 1996;41:371.
243. Law SY, Fok M, Cheng SW, Wong J. A comparison of outcome after resection for squamous cell carcinomas and adenocarcinomas of the esophagus and cardia. *Surg Gynecol Obstet* 1992;175:107.
244. Kelsen DP, Ginsberg R, Pajak TF, et al. Chemotherapy followed by surgery compared with surgery alone for localized esophageal cancer [see comments]. *N Engl J Med* 1998;339:1979.
245. Walsh TN, Noonan N, Hollywood D, et al. A comparison of multimodal therapy and surgery for esophageal adenocarcinoma. *N Engl J Med* 1996;335:462.
246. Bosset JF, Gignoux M, Triboulet JP, et al. Chemoradiotherapy followed by surgery compared with surgery alone in squamous cell cancer of the esophagus. *N Engl J Med* 1997;337:161.
247. Law S, Fok M, Chow S, Chu KM, Wong J. Preoperative chemotherapy versus surgical therapy alone for squamous cell carcinoma of the esophagus. A prospective randomized trial. *J Thorac Cardiovasc Surg* 1997;114:203.
248. Gignoux M, Roussel A, Paillot B. The value of preoperative radiotherapy in esophageal cancer: results of a study of the E.O.R.T.C. *World J Surg* 1987;11:426.
249. Nygaard K, Hagen S, Hansen HS, et al. Pre-operative radiotherapy prolongs survival in operable esophageal carcinoma: a randomized, multicenter study of pre- operative radiotherapy and chemotherapy. The second Scandinavian trial in esophageal cancer. *World J Surg* 1992;16:1104.
250. Rindani R, Martin CJ, Cox MR. Transhiatal versus Ivor-Lewis esophagectomy: is there a difference? *Aust N Z J Surg* 1999;69:187.
251. Logan A. The surgical treatment of carcinoma of the esophagus and cardia. *J Thorac Cardiovasc Surg* 1963;46:150.
252. Skinner DB. En-bloc resection for neoplasms of the esophagus and cardia. *J Thorac Cardiovasc Surg* 1983;85:59.
253. Nigro JJ, De Meester SR, Hagen JA, et al. Node status in transmural esophageal adenocarcinoma and outcome after en-bloc esophagectomy. *J Thorac Cardiovasc Surg* 1999;117:960.
254. Altorki NK, Girardi L, Skinner DB. En-bloc esophagectomy improves survival for stage III esophageal cancer. *J Thorac Cardiovasc Surg* 1997;114:948.
255. Herskovic A, Martz K, Al-Sarraf M. Combined chemotherapy and radiotherapy compared with radiotherapy alone in patients with cancer of the esophagus. *N Engl J Med* 1992;326:1593.
256. Hagen JA, Peters JH, De Meester TR. Superiority of extended en bloc esophagogastrectomy for carcinoma of the lower esophagus and cardia. *J Thorac Cardiovasc Surg* 1993;106:850.
257. Altorki NK. The rationale for radical resection. *Surg Oncol Clin North Am* 1999;8:295.
258. Isono K, Onada S, Okuyama K. Recurrence of intrathoracic esophageal cancer. *Jpn J Clin Oncol* 1985;15:49.
259. Isono K, Sato H, Nakayama K. Results of nationwide study of the three-field lymph node dissection of esophageal cancer. *Oncology* 1991;48:411.
260. Orringer MB. Editorial: occult cervical nodal metastases in esophageal cancer: preliminary results of three-field lymphadenectomy. *J Thorac Cardiovasc Surg* 1997;113:538.
261. Akiyama H, Tsurumaru M, Udagawa H. Radical lymph node dissection for cancer of the thoracic esophagus. *Ann Surg* 1994;220:364.
262. Kato H, Tachimore Y, Watanabe H, et al. Recurrent esophageal carcinoma after esophagectomy with three-field lymph node dissection. *J Surg Oncol* 1996;61:267.
263. Fujita H, Kakegawa T, Yamana H, et al. Mortality and morbidity rates, postoperative course, quality of life and prognosis after extended radical lymphadenectomy for esophageal cancer. Comparison of three-field lymphadenectomy with two-field lymphadenectomy. *Ann Surg* 1995;222:654.
264. Baba M, Aikou T, Yoshinaka H, et al. Long-term results of subtotal esophagectomy with three-field lymphadenectomy for carcinoma of the thoracic esophagus. *Ann Surg* 1995;221:432.
265. Tanabe G, Baba M, Kuroshima K. Clinical evaluation of esophageal lymph flow system based on the RI uptake of removed regional lymph nodes following lymphoscintigraphy. *J Jpn Surg Soc* 1986;87:315.
266. Aikou T, Natugoe S, Tenabe G, Baba M, Shimazu H. Lymph drainage originating from the lower esophagus and gastric cardia as measured by radioisotope uptake in the regional lymph nodes following lymphoscintigraphy. *Lymphology* 1987;20:145.
267. Nishihira T, Hirayama K, Mori S. A prospective randomized trial of extended cervical and superior mediastinal lymphadenectomy for carcinoma of the thoracic esophagus. *Am J Surg* 1998;175:47.
268. Kato H, Watanabe H, Tachimori Y, Iizuka T. Evaluation of neck lymph node dissection for thoracic esophageal carcinoma. *Ann Thorac Surg* 1991;51:931.

269. Lerut T, Coosemans W, De Leyn P, et al. Reflections on three field lymphadenectomy in carcinoma of the esophagus and gastroesophageal junction. *Hepto-Gastroenterology* 1999;46:717.
270. Roth JA, Putnam JB. Surgery for cancer of the esophagus. *Semin Oncol* 1994;21:453.
271. Salazar JD, Doty JR, Lin JW, et al. Does cell type influence post-esophagectomy survival in patients with esophageal cancer? *Dis Esophagus* 1998;11:168.
272. Mantravadi R, Ladd T, Briele H, Liebner EJ. Carcinoma of the esophagus: sites of failure. *Int J Radiat Oncol Biol Phys* 1982;8:1897.
273. Mandard AM, Chasle J, Marnay J, et al. Autopsy findings in 111 cases of esophageal cancer. *Cancer* 1981;48:329.
274. Attah E, Hadju S. Benign and malignant tumors of the esophagus at autopsy. *J Thorac Cardiovasc Surg* 1980;55:396.
275. Aisner JA, Forastiere AA, Aaroney R. Patterns of recurrence for cancer of the lung and esophagus. *Cancer Treat Symp* 1983;2:87(abst).
276. Noh HM, Fishman EK, Forastiere AA, et al. CT of the esophagus: spectrum of disease with emphasis on esophageal carcinoma. *RadioGraphics* 1995;15:1113.
277. Ng CS, Husband JE, MacVicar AD, Cunningham DC. Correlation of CT with histopathological finding in patients with gastric and gastro-oesophageal carcinomas following neoadjuvant chemotherapy. *Clin Radiol* 1998;53:422.
278. Flood WA, Forastiere AA. Esophageal cancer. *Curr Opin Oncol* 1995;7:381.
279. Yagoda A, Mukherji B, Young C, et al. Bleomycin, an antitumor antibiotic: clinical experience in 274 patients. *Ann Intern Med* 1972;77:861.
280. Stephens F. Bleomycin: a new approach in cancer chemotherapy. *Med J Aust* 1973;1:1277.
281. Ravry M, Moertel CG, Schutt AJ, et al. Treatment of advanced squamous cell carcinoma of the gastrointestinal tract with bleomycin (NSC 125066). *Cancer Chemother Rep* 1973;57:493.
282. Tancini G, Bejetta E, Bonnadonna G. Therapy with bleomycin alone or in combination with methotrexate in epidermoid carcinoma of the esophagus. *Tumori* 1973;60:65.
283. Kolaric K, Moricic Z, Dujomovic I, Roth A. Therapy of advanced esophageal cancer with bleomycin, irradiation and combination bleomycin and irradiation. *Tumori* 1976;62:255.
284. Lokich J, Shea M, Chaffey J. Sequential infusional 5-fluorouracil followed by concomitant radiation for tumors of the esophagus and the gastroesophageal junction. *Cancer* 1987;60:275.
285. Ezdinli EZ, Gelber R, Desai DV, et al. Chemotherapy of advanced esophageal carcinoma: Eastern Cooperative Oncology Group experience. *Cancer* 1980;46:2149.
286. Engstrom P, Lavin P, Lassen D. Phase II evaluation of mitomycin and cisplatin in advanced esophageal carcinoma. *Cancer Treat Rep* 1983;67:713.
287. Whitington R, Clos H. Clinical experience with mitomycin C. *Cancer Chemother Rep* 1970;54:195.
288. Kolaric K, Maricic Z, Roth A, Qujmovic I. Combination of bleomycin and adriamycin with and without radiation in the treatment of inoperable esophageal cancer. A randomized study. *Cancer* 1980;45:2265.
289. Advani SH, Saikia TK, Swaroop S, et al. Anterior chemotherapy in esophageal cancer. *Cancer* 1985;56:1502.
290. Davis S, Shanmugathasa M, Kessler W. Cis-dichlorodiamminc platinum (11) in the treatment of esophageal carcinoma. *Cancer Treat Rep* 1980;64:709.
291. Ravry M, Moore M. Phase II pilot study of cisplatinum (II) in advanced squamous cell esophageal cancer. *Proc Soc Surg Oncol* 1980;21:353(abst).
292. Panettiere F, Leichman L, Tilchen E, et al. Chemotherapy for advanced epidermoid carcinoma of the esophagus with single agent cisplatin: final report on Southwest Oncology Group study. *Cancer Treat Rep* 1984;68:1023.
293. Bleiberg H, Jacob JH, Bedenne L, et al. Randomized phase II trial of 5-fluorouracil (5-FU) and cisplatin (DDP) versus DDP alone in advanced esophageal cancer. *Proc Soc Clin Oncol* 1991;10:A447(abst).
294. Miller JI, McIntyre B, Hatcher CR. Combined treatment approach in surgical management of carcinoma of the esophagus: a preliminary report. *Ann Thorac Surg* 1985;40:289.
295. Kelsen DP, Bains MS, Cvitkovic E, Golbcy R. Vindesinc in the treatment of esophageal carcinoma: a phase II study. *Cancer Treat Rep* 1979;63:2019.
296. Bedikian AY, Valdivieso M, Bodey GP, Freireich EJ. Phase II evaluation of vindesine in the treatment of colorectal and esophagela tumors. *Cancer Chemother Pharmacol* 1979;2:263.
297. Bezwoda WR, Derman DP, Weaving A, Nissenbaum M. Treatment of esophageal cancer with vindesine: an open trial. *Cancer Treat Rep* 1984;68:783.
298. Kelsen D, Chapman R, Baines M, et al. Phase II study of methyl-GAG in the present treatment of esophageal carcinoma. *Cancer Treat Rep* 1982;66:1427.
299. Ravry MJ, Omura GA, Hill GJ. Phase II evaluation of mitoguazone in cancer of the esophagus, stomach, and pancreas: a Southwestern Cancer Study Group Trial. *Cancer Treat Rep* 1986;70:533.
300. Falkson G. Methyl-GAG (NSC 32946) in the treatment of esophagus cancer. *Cancer Chemother Rep* 1971;55:209.
301. Conroy TC, Etienne PL, Adenis A, et al. Phase II trial of vinorelbine in metastatic squamous cell esophageal carcinoma. *J Clin Oncol* 1996;14:164.
302. Ajani JA, Ilson DH, Daugherty K, et al. Activity of taxol in patients with squamous cell carcinoma and adenocardinoma of the esophagus. *J Natl Cancer Inst* 1994;86:1086.
303. Etienne PL, Conroy T, Adenis A, et al. Vinorelbine and cisplatin in metastatic epidermoid carcinoma of the esophagus (MECE). An EORTC phase II study. *Proc Am Soc Clin Oncol* 1999;18:270a.
304. Milas L, Hunter NR, Mason KA, Kurdoglu B, Peters LJ. Enhancement of tumor radioresponse of a murine mammary carcinoma by paclitaxel. *Cancer Res* 1994;54:3506.
305. Bajorin D, Kelsen D, Heelan R. Phase II trials of dischloromethotrexate in epidermoid carcinoma of the esophagus. *Cancer Treat Rep* 1986;70:1245.
306. Alberts AS, Falkson G, Badata M, Terblanche AP, Schmid EU. Trimetrexate in advanced carcinoma of the esophagus. *Invest New Drugs* 1988;6:319.
307. Brown T, Fleming T, Tangen C, Macdonald J. A phase II trial of trimetrexate in the treatment of esophageal cancer. A Southwest Oncology Group Trial. *Proc Clin Oncol* 1992;11:A479(abst).
308. Coonley C, Bains M, Kelsen DP. VP-16-213 in the treatment of esophageal cancer: a phase II trial. *Cancer Treat Rep* 1983;67:397.
309. Radice P, Bunn P, Ihde D. Therapeutic trials with VP-16 and VM-26. *Cancer Treat Rep* 1979;62:1231.
310. Nanus DM, Kelson DP, Lipperman R, Eisenberger M. Phase II trial of ifosfamide in epidermoid carcinoma of the esophagus: unexpectant severe toxicity. *Invest New Drugs* 1988;6:239.
311. Kok TC, VanDer Gaast A, Splinter TA, Tilanus HW. Ifosfamide in advanced adenocarcinoma of the oesophagus or oesophageal-gastric junction area. *Eur J Cancer* 1991;27:1112.
312. Mannell A, Winters Z. Carboplatin in the treatment of esophageal cancer. *South Afr Med J* 1989;76:213.
313. Queisser W, Preusser P, Mross KB, et al. Phase II evaluation of carboplatin in advanced esophageal carcinoma. A trial of the phase I/II study group of the Association for Medical Oncology of the German Cancer Society. *Onkologie* 1990;13:190.
314. Sternberg C, Kelsen D, Dukeman M, Leichman L, Heelan R. Carboplatin: a new platinum analog in the treatment of epidermoid carcinoma of the esophagus. *Cancer Treat Rep* 1985;69:1305.
315. Steel A, Cullen MH, Robertson PW, Matthews HR. A phase II study of carboplatin in adenocarcinoma of the esophagus. *Br J Cancer* 1988;58:500.
316. Coonley CJ, Bains M, Hilaris B, Chapman R, Kelsen DP. Cisplatin and bleomycin in the treatment of esophageal carcinoma. A final report. *Cancer* 1984;54:2351.
317. Kelsen D, Hilaris B, Coonley C, et al. Cisplatin, vindesine and bleomycin chemotherapy of local regional and advanced esophageal carcinoma. *Am J Med* 1983;75:645.
318. Dinwoodie WR, Bartolucci AA, Lyman GH, et al. Phase II evaluation of cisplatin, bleomycin, and vindesine in advanced squamous cell carcinoma of the esophagus: a south eastern cancer study trail. *Cancer Treat Rep* 1986;70:267.
319. DeBasi P, Salvagno L, Endrizi L, et al. Cisplatin, blcomycin and methotrexate in the treatment of advanced oesophageal cancer. *Eur J Cancer Clin Oncol* 1984;20:743.
320. Vogl SE, Greenwald E, Kaplan BH. Effective chemotherapy for esophageal cancer with methotrexate, bleomycin, and cis-diamminedichloroplatinum II. *Cancer* 1981;48:2555.
321. Kelsen DP, Fein R, Coonley C, Heelan R, Bains M. Cisplatin, vindesine, and mitoguazone in the treatment of esophageal cancer. *Cancer Treat Rep* 1986;70:255.
322. Chapman R, Fleming TR, Van Damme J, Macdonald J. Cisplatin, vinblastine, and mitoguazone in squamous cell carcinoma of the esophagus: a Southwest Oncology Group Study. *Cancer Treat Rep* 1987;71:1185.
323. Lizuka T, Kakegawa T, Ide H, et al. Phase II study of CDDP + 5-FU for squamous esophageal carcinoma: JEOG Co-operative Study results. *Proc Clin Oncol* 1991;10:157(abst).
324. Lovett D, Kelsen D, Eisenberger M, Houston C. A phase II trial of carboplatin and vinblastine in the treatment of advanced squamous cell carcinoma of the esophagus. *Cancer* 1991;67:354.
325. Kelsen D, Lovett D, Wong J, et al. Interferon alfa-2a and fluorouracil in the treatment of patients with advanced esophageal cancer. *J Clin Oncol* 1992;10:269.
326. Wadler S, Fell S, Haynes H, et al. Treatment of carcinoma of the esophagus with 5-fluorouracil and recombinant alfa-2a-interferon. *Cancer* 1993;71:1726.
327. Ilson DH, Sirott M, Saltz L, et al. A phase II trial of interferon alfa-2a, 5-fluorouracil, and cisplatin in patients with advanced esophageal carcinoma. *Cancer* 1995;74:2197.
328. Enzinger PC, Ilson DH, Saltz LB, Martin LK, Kelsen DP. Phase II clinical trial of 13-cisretinoic acid and interferon-alpha-2a in patients with advanced esophageal carcinoma. *Cancer* 1999;85:1213.
329. Kok TC, Van der Gaast A, Dees J, et al. Cisplatin and etoposide in oesophageal cancer: a phase II study. Rotterdam Oesophageal Tumour Study Group. *Br J Cancer* 1996;74:980.
330. Kok TC, Lanschot JV, Siersema PD, Overhagen HV, Tilanus HW. Neoadjuvant chemotherapy in operable esophageal squamous cell cancer: final report of a phase III multicenter randomized trial. *Proc Am Soc Clin Oncol* 1997;16:277.
331. Ilson DH, Ajani J, Bhalla K, et al. Phase II trial of paclitaxel, fluorouracil, and cisplatin in patients with advanced carcinoma of the esophagus. *J Clin Oncol* 1998;16:1826.
332. Van der Gaast A, Kok TC, Kerkhofs L, et al. Phase I study of a biweekly schedule of a fixed dose of cisplatin with increasing doses of paclitaxel in patients with advanced oesophageal cancer. *Br J Cancer* 1999;80:1052.
333. Van der Gaast A, Polee M, Kok TC, Splinter TA. Phase I study with weekly cisplatin and increasing doses of paclitaxel in patients with esophageal cancer. *Proc Am Soc Clin Oncol* 1999;18:303a.
334. Enzinger PC, Ilson DH, Saltz LB, O'Reilly EM, Kelsen DP. Irinotecan and cisplatin in upper gastrointestinal malignancies. *Oncology* 1998;12:110.
335. Ilson DH, Saltz L, Enzinger P, et al. Phase II trial of weekly irinotecan plus cisplatin in advanced esophageal cancer. *J Clin Oncol* 1999;17:3270.
336. Ajani J, Fairweather J, Pisters P, et al. U.T.M.D. Anderson Center: phase II study of CPT-11 plus cisplatin in patients with advanced gastric and GE junction carcinomas. *Proc Am Soc Clin Oncol* 1999;18:241a.
337. Schlag P, Herrmann R, Raeth V, et al. Preoperative chemotherapy in esophageal cancer. A phase II study. *Acta Oncol* 1988;27:811.
338. Forastiere A, Gennis MK, Orringer M, et al. Cisplatin, vinblastine and mitoguazone chemotherapy for epidermoid and adenocarcinoma of the esophagus. *J Clin Oncol* 1987;15:1143.
339. Carey RW, Hilgenberg AD, Wilkins EW. Long-term follow-up of neoadjuvant chemotherapy with 5-fluorouracil and cisplatin with surgical resection and possible postoperative radiotherapy and or chemotherapy in squamous cell carcinoma of the esophagus. *Cancer Invest* 1993;11:99.
340. Kies M, Rosen S, Tsang T, et al. Cisplatin and 5-fluorouracil in primary management of squamous esophageal cancer. *Cancer* 1987;60:2156.
341. Ajani JA, Ryan B, Rich TA, et al. Prolonged chemotherapy for localized squamous carcinoma of the oesophagus. *Eur J Cancer* 1992;28A:880.
342. Vignoud J, Visset J, Paineau J, et al. Preoperative chemotherapy in squamous cell carcinoma of the esopahgus: clincal and pathological analysis, 48 cases. *Ann Oncol* 1990;1:45.

343. Wright CD, Mathisen DJ, Wain JC, et al. Evolution of treatment strategies for adenocarcinoma of the esophagus and gastroesophageal junction. *Ann Thorac Surg* 1994;58:1574.
344. Roth JA, Pass HI, Flanagan MM, et al. Randomized clinical trial of preoperative and postoperative adjuvant chemotherapy with cisplatin, vindesine, and bleomycin for carcinoma of the esophagus. *J Thorac Cardiovasc Surg* 1988;96:242.
345. Schlag PM. Randomized trial of preoperative chemotherapy for squamous cell cancer of the esophagus. The Chirurgische Arbeitsgemeinschaft Fuer Onkologie der Deutschen Gesellschaft Fuer Chirurgie Study Group. *Arch Surg* 1992;127:1446.
346. Cooper JS, Guo MD, Herskovic A, et al. Chemoradiotherapy of locally advanced esophageal cancer: long-term follow-up of a prospective randomized trial (RTOG 85-01). Radiation Therapy Oncology Group. *JAMA* 1999;281:1623.
347. Japanese Esophageal Oncology Group. A comparison of chemotherapy and radiotherapy as adjuvant treatment to surgery for esophageal carcinoma. *Chest* 1993;104:203.
348. Iizuka AT, Isono KK, Watanabe H, et al. A randomized trial comparing surgery to surgery plus postoperative chemotherapy for localized squamous carcinoma of the thoracic esophagus: the Japan clinical oncology study group (JCOG) study. *Proc Am Soc Oncol* 1998;17:282a.
349. Ando N, Iizuka T, Kakegawa T, et al. A randomized trial of surgery with and without chemotherapy for localized squamous carcinoma of the thoracic esophagus: the Japan Clinical Oncology Group Study [see comments]. *J Thorac Cardiovasc Surg* 1997;114:205.
350. Coia LR, Minsky BD, John MJ, et al. The evaluation and treatment of patients receiving radiation therapy for carcinoma of the esophagus. Results of the 1992–1994 Patterns of Care Study. *Cancer* 1999;85:2499.
351. Coia LR, Minsky BD, John MJ, et al. Patterns of care study decision tree and management guidelines for esophageal cancer. *Radiat Med* 1998;16:321.
352. De-Ren S. Ten-year follow-up of esophageal cancer treated by radical radiation therapy: analysis of 869 patients. *Int J Radiat Oncol Biol Phys* 1989;16:334.
353. Newaishy GA, Read GA, Duncan W, Kerr GR. Results of radical radiotherapy of squamous cell carcinoma of the esophagus. *Clin Radiol* 1982;33:347.
354. Okawa T, Kita M, Tanaka M, Ikeda M. Results of radiotherapy for inoperable locally advanced esophageal cancer. *Int J Radiat Oncol Biol Phys* 1989;17:49.
355. Shi X, Yao W, Liu T. Late course accelerated fractionation in radiotherapy of esophageal carcinoma. *Radiother Oncol* 1999;51:21.
356. Al-Sarraf M, Martz K, Herskovic A, et al. Superiority of chemo-radiotherapy (CT-RT) vs radiotherapy (RT) in patients with esophageal cancer. Final report of an Intergroup randomized and confirmed study. *Proc Am Soc Clin Oncol* 1996;15:206(abst).
357. Sykes AJ, Burt PA, Slevin NJ, Stout R, Marrs JE. Radical radiotherapy for carcinoma of the oesophagus: an effective alternative to surgery. *Radiother Oncol* 1998;48:15.
358. John MJ, Flam M, Ager Mowry PA, et al. Radiotherapy alone and chemoradiation for nonmetastatic esophageal carcinoma. *Cancer* 1989;63:2397.
359. Coia LR, Engstrom PF, Paul AR, Stafford PM, Hanks GE. Long-term results of infusional 5-FU, mitomycin-C, and radiation as primary management of esophageal carcinoma. *Int J Radiat Oncol Biol Phys* 1991;20:29.
360. Izquierdo MA, Marcuello E, Gomez de Segura G, et al. Unresectable nonmetastatic squamous cell carcinoma of the esophagus managed by sequential chemotherapy (cisplatin and bleomycin) and radiation therapy. *Cancer* 1993;71:287.
361. Seitz JF, Giovannini M, Padaut-Cesana J, et al. Inoperable nonmetastatic squamous cell carcinoma of the esophagus managed by concomitant chemotherapy (5-flurouracil and cisplatin) and radiation therapy. *Cancer* 1990;66:214.
362. Valerdi JJ, Tejedor M, Illarramendi JJ, et al. Neoadjuvant chemotherapy and radiotherapy in locally advanced esophagus carcinoma: long term results. *Int J Radiat Oncol Biol Phys* 1994;27:843.
363. Poplin EA, Jacobson J, Herskovic A, et al. Evaluation of multimodality treatment of locoregional esophageal carcinoma by Southwest Oncology Group 9060. *Cancer* 1996;78:1851.
364. Araujo CM, Souhami L, Gil RA, et al. A randomized trial comparing radiation therapy versus concomitant radiation therapy and chemotherapy in carcinoma of the thoracic esophagus. *Cancer* 1991;67:2258.
365. Roussel A, Jacob JH, Jung GM. Controlled clinical trial for the treatment of patients with inoperable esophageal carcinoma: a study of the EORTC Gastrointestinal Tract Cancer Cooperative Group. In: Schlag P, Hohenberger P, Metzger U, eds. *Recent Results in Cancer Research.* Berlin: Springer-Verlag, 1988:21.
366. Al-Sarraf M, Martz K, Herskovic A, et al. Progress report of combined chemoradiotherapy versus radiotherapy alone in patients with esophageal cancer: an intergroup study. *J Clin Oncol* 1997;15:277.
367. Slabber CF, Nel JS, Schoeman L, et al. A randomized study of radiotherapy alone versus radiotherapy plus 5 fluorouracil and platinum in patients with inoperable, locally advanced squamous cell cancer of the esophagus. *Am J Clin Oncol* 1998;21:465.
368. Smith TJ, Ryan LM, Douglass HO, et al. Combined chemoradiotherapy vs. radiotherapy alone for early stage squamous cell carcinoma of the esophagus: a study of the Eastern Cooperative Oncology Group. *Oncol Biol Phys* 1998;42:269.
369. Streeter OE, Martz KL, Gaspar LE, et al. Does race influence survival for esophageal cancer patients treated on the radiation and chemotherapy arm of RTOG # 85-01? *Int J Radiat Oncol Biol Phys* 1999;44:1047.
370. Minsky BD, Neuberg D, Kelsen DP. Final report of intergroup trial 0122 (ECOG PE-289, RTOG 90-12): phase II trial of neoadjuvant chemotherapy plus concurrent chemotherapy and high-dose radiation for squamous cell carcinoma of the esophagus. *Int J Radiat Oncol Biol Phys* 1999;43:517.
371. Kelsen DP, Minsky BD, Smith M, et al. Preoperative therapy for esophageal cancer: a randomized comparison of chemotherapy vs. radiation therapy. *J Clin Oncol* 1990;8:1352.
372. Roca E, Pennella E, Sardi M, et al. Combined intensive chemoradiotherapy for organ preservation in patients with resectable and non-resectable oesophageal cancer. *Eur J Cancer* 1996;32A:429.
373. Kelsen D, Ilson D, Lipton R, Baylor L, Minsky B. A phase I trial of radiation therapy (RT) plus concurrent fixed dose cisplatin (C) with escalating doses of paclitaxel (P) as a 96 hour continuous infusion in patients (PTS) with localized esophageal cancer (EC). *Proc Am Soc Clin Oncol* 1999;18:271(abst).
374. Armstrong JG. High dose rate remote afterloading brachytherapy for lung and esophageal cancer. *Semin Radiat Oncol* 1993;4:270.
375. Moni J, Armstrong JG, Minsky BD, Bains MS, Harrison LB. High dose rate intraluminal brachytherapy for carcinoma of the esophagus. *Dis Esophagus* 1996;9:123.
376. Sur RK, Singh DP, Sharma SC. Radiation therapy of esophageal cancer: role of high dose rate brachytherapy. *Int J Radiat Oncol Biol Phys* 1992;22:1043.
377. Jager J, Langendijk H, Pannebakker M, Rijken J, Jong J. A single session of intraluminal brachytherapy in palliation of esophageal cancer. *Radiother Oncol* 1995;37:237.
378. Sur RK, Donde B, Levin VC, Rad FF, Mannell A. Fractionated high dose rate intraluminal brachytherapy in palliation of advanced esophageal cancer. *Int J Radiat Oncol Biol Phys* 1998;40:447.
379. Calais G, Dorval E, Louisot P, et al. Radiotherapy with high dose rate brachytherapy boost and concomitant chemotherapy for stages IIB and III esophageal carcinoma: results of a pilot study. *Int J Radiat Oncol Biol Phys* 1997;38:769.
380. Akagi Y, Hirokawa Y, Kagemoto M, et al. Optimum fractionation for high-dose-rate endoesophageal brachytherapy following external irradiation of early stage esophageal cancer. *Int J Radiat Oncol Biol Phys* 1999;43:525.
381. Schraube P, Fritz P, Wannenmacher MF. Combined endoluminal and external irradiation of inoperable oesophageal carcinoma. *Radiother Oncol* 1997;44:45.
382. Caspers RJL, Zwinderman AH, Griffioen G, et al. Combined external beam and low dose rate intraluminal radiotherapy in oesophageal cancer. *Radiother Oncol* 1993;27:7.
383. Sur M, Sur R, Cooper K, et al. Morphologic alterations in esophageal squamous cell carcinoma after preoperative high dose rate intraluminal brachytherapy. *Cancer* 1996;77:2200.
384. Yorozu A, Dokiya T, Oki Y, Suzuki T. Curative radiotherapy with high-dose-rate brachytherapy boost for localized esophageal carcinoma: dose-effect relationship of brachytherapy with the balloon type applicator system. *Radiother Oncol* 1999;51:133.
385. Gaspar LE, Qian C, Kocha WI, et al. A phase I/II study of external beam radiation, brachytherapy and concurrent chemotherapy in localized cancer of the esophagus (RTOG 92-07): preliminary toxicity report. *Int J Radiat Oncol Biol Phys* 1997;37:593.
386. Gaspar LE, Nag S, Herskovic A, Mantravadi R, Speiser B. American Brachytherapy Society (ABS) consensus guidelines for brachytherapy of esophageal cancer. *Int J Radiat Oncol Biol Phys* 1997;38:127.
387. Calais G, Jadaud E, Chapet S, et al. High dose radiotherapy (RT) and concomitant chemotherapy for nonresectable esophageal cancer. Results of a phase II study. *Proc Am Soc Clin Oncol* 1994;13:197(abst).
388. Girinsky T, Auperin A, Marsiglia H, et al. Accelerated fractionation in esophageal cancers: a multivariate analysis on 88 patients. *Int J Radiat Oncol Biol Phys* 1997;38:1013.
389. Powell MEB, Hoskin PJ, Saunders MT, et al. Continuous hyperfractionated accelerated radiotherapy (CHART) in localized cancer of the esophagus. *Int J Radiat Oncol Biol Phys* 1997;40:1061.
390. Jeremic B, Shibamoto Y, Acimovic L, et al. Accelerated hyperfractionated radiation therapy and concurrent 5-fluorouracil/cisplatin chemotherapy for locoregional squamous cell carcinoma of the thoracic esophagus: a phase II study. *Int J Radiat Oncol Biol Phys* 1998;121:717.
391. Wara WM, Mauch PM, Thomas AN, Phillips TL. Palliation for carcinoma of the esophagus. *Radiology* 1976;121:717.
392. Petrovich Z, Langholz B, Formenti S, Luxton G, Astrahan M. Management of carcinoma of the esophagus: the role of radiotherapy. *Am J Clin Oncol* 1991;14:80.
393. Whittington R, Coia LR, Haller DG, Rubenstein JH, Rosato EF. Adenocarcinoma of the esophagus and esophago-gastric junction: the effects of single and combined modalities on the survival and patterns of failure following treatment. *Int J Radiat Oncol Biol Phys* 1990;19:593.
394. Caspers RJL, Welvaart K, Verkes RJ, Hermans J, Leer JWH. The effect of radiotherapy on dysphagia and survival in patients with esophageal cancer. *Radiother Oncol* 1988;12:15.
395. Algan O, Coia LR, Keller SM, et al. Management of adenocarcinoma of the esophagus with chemoradiation alone or chemoradiation followed by esophagectomy: results of sequential nonrandomized phase II studies. *Int J Radiat Oncol Biol Phys* 1995;32:753.
396. Gill PG, Denham JW, Jamieson GG, et al. Patterns of treatment failure and prognostic factors associated with the treatment of esophageal carcinoma with chemotherapy and radiotherapy either as sole treatment or followed by surgery. *J Clin Oncol* 1992;10:1037.
397. Urba SG, Turrisi AT. Split-course accelerated radiation therapy combined with carboplatin and 5-fluorouracil for palliation of metastatic or unresectable carcinoma of the esophagus. *Cancer* 1995;75:435.
398. Coia LR, Soffen EM, Schultheiss TE, Martin EE, Hanks GE. Swallowing function in patients with esophageal cancer treated with concurrent radiation and chemotherapy. *Cancer* 1993;71:281.
399. O'Rourke IC, Tiver K, Bull C, Gebski V, Langlands AO. Swallowing performance after radiation therapy for carcinoma of the esophagus. *Cancer* 1988;61:2022.
400. Minsky BD. Radiation therapy in the treatment of esophagus cancer. *Chest Surg Clin North Am* 1994;4:285.
401. Gschossmann JM, Bonner JA, Foote RL, et al. Malignant tracheoesophageal fistula in patients with esophageal cancer. *Cancer* 1993;72:1513.
402. Arlington A, Bohorquez J. Irradiation of carcinoma of the esophagus containing a tracheoesophageal fistula. *Cancer* 1993;71:3808.
403. Belleguic C, Lena H, Briens E, et al. Tracheobronchial stenting in patients with esophageal cancer involving the central airways. *Endoscopy* 1999;31:232.
404. Raijman I, Siddique I, Ajani J, Lynch P. Palliation of malignant dysphagia and fistulae with coated expandable metal stents: experience with 101 patients. *Gastrointest Endosc* 1998;48:172.
405. May A, Ell C. Palliative treatment of malignant esophagorespiratory fistulas with Gianturco-Z stents. A prospective clinical trial and review of the literature on covered metal stents [see comments]. *Am J Gastroenterol* 1998;93:532.
406. Mei W, Xian-Zhi G, Weibo Y, et al. Randomized clinical trial on the combination of pre-

operative irradiation and surgery in the treatment of esophageal carcinoma: report on 206 patients. *Int J Radiat Oncol Biol Phys* 1989;16:325.
407. Teniere P, Hay JM, Fingerhut A, Fagniez P-L. Postoperative radiation therapy does not increase survival after curative resection for squamous cell carcinoma of the middle and lower esophagus as shown by a multicenter controlled trial. *Surg Gynecol Obstet* 1991;173:123.
408. Launois B, Delarue D, Campion JP, Kerbaol M. Preoperative radiotherapy for carcinoma of the esophagus. *Surg Gynecol Obstet* 1981;153:690.
409. Arnott SJ, Duncan W, Kerr GR, et al. Low dose preoperative radiotherapy for carcinoma of the oesophagus: results of a randomized clinical trial. *Radiother Oncol* 1993;24:108.
410. Huang GJ, Gu XZ, Wang LJ. Combined preoperative irradiation and surgery for esophageal carcinoma. In: Delarue NC, ed. *International trends in general thoracic surgery.* St. Louis: C.V. Mosby, 1988:315.
411. Arnott SJ, Duncan W, Gignoux M, et al. Preoperative radiotherapy in esophageal carcinoma: a meta-analysis using individual patient data (oesophageal cancer collaboratorive group). *Int J Radiat Oncol Biol Phys* 1998;41:579.
412. Jacob JH, Seitz JF, Langlois C, et al. Definitive concurrent chemo-radiation therapy (CRT) in squamous cell carcinoma of the esophagus (SCCE): preliminary results of a French randomized trial comparing standard vs. split course irradiation (FNCLCC-FFCD 9305). *Proc Am Soc Clin Oncol* 1999;18:270a(abst).
413. Yadava OP, Hodge AJ, Matz LR, Donlon JB. Esophageal malignancies: is preoperative radiotherapy the way to go? *Ann Thorac Surg* 1991;51:189.
414. Sugimachi K, Matsufuji H, Kai H, et al. Preoperative irradiation for carcinoma of the esophagus. *Surg Gynecol Obstet* 1986;162:174.
415. Yamamoto M, Yamashita T, Matsubara T, et al. Reevaluation of postoperative radiotherapy for thoracic esophageal carcinoma. *Int J Radiat Oncol Biol Phys* 1997;37:75.
416. Hosokawa M, Shirato H, Ohara K, et al. Intraoperative radiation therapy to the upper mediastinum and nerve-sparing three-field lymphadenectomy followed by external beam radiotherapy for patients with thoracic esophageal carcinoma. *Cancer* 1999;86:13.
417. Fok M, Sham JST, Choy D, Cheng SWK, Wong JW. Postoperative radiotherapy for carcinoma of the esophagus: a prospective, randomized controlled trial. *Surgery* 1993;113:138.
418. Minsky BD, Neuberg D, Kelsen D, et al. Neoadjuvant chemotherapy plus concurrent chemotherapy and high dose radiation for squamous cell carcinoma of the esophagus—a preliminary analysis of the phase II intergroup trial 0122. *J Clin Oncol* 1996;14:149.
419. Becker M, Adelstein DJ, Rice TW, et al. Concurrent chemotherapy, accelerated hyperfractionated split course radiation therapy and surgery for esophageal cancer. 1996;36(abst).
420. Kelsen D, Ilson D, Minsky B, Lipton R. Phase I trial of combined modality therapy for localized esophageal cancer: radiation therapy + concurrent cisplatin and escalating doses of 96 hour infusional paclitaxel. *Proc Am Soc Clin Oncol* 1998;17:260a(abst).
421. Nesbitt J, Ajani JA, Komaki R, et al. Preoperative taxol-based chemotherapy (CT) followed by chemoradiation therapy (CTRT) in patients (PTS) with potentially resectable esophageal carcinoma (EC). *Proc Am Soc Clin Oncol* 1998;17:282a(abst).
422. Safran H, Gaissert H, Akerman P, et al. Neoadjuvant paclitaxes, cisplatin and radiation for esophageal cancer. *Proc Am Soc Clin Oncol* 1998;17:259a(abst).
423. Posner MC, Gooding WE, Landreneau RJ, et al. Preoperative chemoradiotherapy for carcinoma of the esophagus and gastroesophageal junction. *Cancer J Sci Am* 1998;4:237.
424. Leichman L, Steiger Z, Seydel HG, et al. Preoperative chemotherapy and radiation therapy for patients with cancer of the esophagus: a potentially curative approach. *J Clin Oncol* 1984;2:75.
425. Poplin E, Fleming T, Leichman L, et al. Combined therapies for squamous-cell carcinoma of the esophagus, a Southwest Oncology Group Study (SWOG-8037). *J Clin Oncol* 1987;5:622.
426. Urba SG, Orringer MB, Perez-Tamayo C, Bromberg J, Forastiere A. Concurrent preoperative chemotherapy and radiation therapy in localized esophageal adenocarcinoma. *Cancer* 1992;69:285.
427. Forastiere A. Treatment of locoregional esophageal cancer. *Semin Oncol* 1992;19:57.
428. Forastiere A, Orringer MB, Perez-Tamayo C, et al. Concurrent chemotherapy and radiation therapy followed by transhiatal esophagectomy for local-regional cancer of the esophagus. *J Clin Oncol* 1990;8:119.
429. Shahab N, Wilkes J, Beyer S, et al. Neoadjuvant chemoradiation followed by transhiatal esophagectomy for regional/locally advanced esophageal carcinoma. *Proc Am Soc Clin Oncol* 1996;17:259a(abst).
430. Adelstein DJ, Rice TW, Becker M, et al. Concurrent chemotherapy (CCT), accelerated fractionated radiation (AFR) and surgery for esophageal cancer. *Proc Am Soc Clin Oncol* 1996;15:203(abst).
431. Raoul JL, Le Prise E, Meunier B, et al. Neoadjuvant chemotherapy and hyperfractionated radiotherapy with concurrent low-dose chemotherapy for squamous cell esophageal cardinoma. *Int J Radiat Oncol Biol Phys* 1998;42:29.
432. Adelstein DJ, Rice TW, Becker M, et al. Use of concurrent chemotherapy, accelerated fractionation radiation, and surgery for patients with esophageal cancer. *Cancer* 1997;80:1011.
433. Stahl M, Wilke H, Fink U, et al. Combined preoperative chemotherapy and radiotherapy in patients with locally advanced esophageal cancer: interim analysis of a phase II trial. *J Clin Oncol* 1996;14:829.
434. Jones DR, Detterbeck FC, Egan TM, et al. Induction chemoradiotherapy followed by esophagectomy in patients with carcinoma of the esophagus. *Ann Thorac Surg* 1997; 64:185.
435. Forastierre AA, Heitmiller RF, Lee DJ, et al. Intensive chemoradiation followed by esophagectomy for squamous cell and adenocarcinoma of the esophagus. *Cancer J Sci Am* 1997;3:144.
436. Bates BA, Detterbeck FC, Bernard SA, Qaqish BF, Tepper JE. Concurrent radiation therapy and chemotherapy followed by esophagectomy for localized esophageal carcinoma. *J Clin Oncol* 1996;14:156.
437. Jones DR, Parker LA, Detterbeck FC, Egan TM. Inadequacy of computed tomography in assessing patients with esophageal carcinoma after induction chemoradiotherapy. 1999;85:1032.
438. Kavanagh B, Anscher M, Leopold K, et al. Patterns of failure following combined modality therapy for esophageal cancer, 1984–1990. *Int J Radiat Oncol Biol Phys* 1992;24:633.
439. Coia L, Minsky B, John M, et al. Outcome of patients receiving radiation for cancer of the esophagus: results of the 1992–1994 Patterns of Care study. *Proc Am Soc Clin Oncol* 1998;17:258a(abst).
440. Urba S, Orringer M, Turrisi A, et al. A randomized trial comparing transhiatal esophagectomy (THE) to preoperative concurrent chemoradiation (CT/XRT) followed by esophagectomy in localregional esophageal carcinoma. *Proc Am Soc Clin Oncol* 1995;14:199(abst).
441. Urba S, Orringer M, Turrisi A, et al. A randomized trial comparing surgery (S) to preoperative concomitant chemoradiation plus surgery in patients (pts) with resectable esophageal cancer. *Proc Am Soc Clin Oncol* 1997;16:277(abst).
442. Le Prise E, Etienne PL, Meunier B, et al. A randomized study of chemotherapy, radiation therapy, and surgery versus surgery for localized squamous cell carcinoma of the esophagus. *Cancer* 1994;73:1779.
443. Safran HS, Akerman P, Cioffi W, et al. Paclitaxel and concurrent radiation therapy for locally advanced adenocarcinomas of the pancreas, stomach, and gastroesophageal junction. *Semin Radiat Oncol* 1999;53:57.
444. Phillips TL, Minsky BD, Dicker A. Cancer of the esophagus. In: Leibel S, Phillips TL, eds. *Textbook of radiation oncology.* Philadelphia: WB Saunders, 1998:601.
445. Tai P, van Dyk J, Yu E, et al. Variability of target volume delineation in cervical esophageal cancer. *Int J Radiat Oncol Biol Phys* 1998;42:277.
446. Sarbia M, Stahl M, Fink U, et al. Expression of apoptosis-regulating proteins and outcome of esophageal cancer patients treated by combined therapy modalities. *Clin Cancer Res* 1998;4:2991.
447. Pomp J, Davelaar J, Blom J, et al. Radiotherapy for oesophagus carcinoma: the impact of p53 on treatment outcome. *Radiother Oncol* 1998;46:184.
448. Merchant TE, Minsky BD, Lauwers GY, et al. Esophageal cancer phospholipids correlated with histopathologic findings: a 31P NMR study. *NMR Biomed* 1999;12:184.
449. Lundell L, Leth R, Lind T, et al. Palliative endoscopic dilatation in carcinoma of the esophagus and esophagogastric junction. *Acta Chir Scand* 1989;155:179.
450. Boyce HWJ. Palliation of dysphagia of esophageal cancer by endoscopic lumen restoration techniques. *Cancer Control* 1999;6:73.
451. Orringer MB. Substernal gastric bypass of the excluded esophagus: results of an ill-advised operation. *Surgery* 1984;96:467.
452. Mannell A, Becker PJ, Nissenbaum M. Bypass surgery for unresectable oesophageal cancer: early and late results in 124 cases. *Br J Surg* 1988;75:283.
453. Holting T, Friedl P, Schraube N, et al. Palliation of esophageal cancer—operative resection versus laser and afterloading therapy. *Surg Endosc* 1991;5:4.
454. Segalin A, Little AG, Ruol A, et al. Surgical and endoscopic palliation of esophageal carcinoma. *Ann Thorac Surg* 1989;48:267.
455. Raijman I, Siddique I, Ajani J, Lynch P. Palliation of malignant dysphagia and fistulae with coated expandable metal stents: experience with 101 patients. *Gastrointest Endosc* 1998;48:172.
456. Cwikiel W, Tranberg KG, Cwikiel M, Lillo-Gil R. Malignant dysphagia: palliation with esophageal stents—long-term results with 100 patients. *Gastrointest Endosc* 1998;50:134(abst).
457. Cantero R, Torres AJ, Hernando F, et al. Palliative treatment of esophageal cancer: self-expanding metal stents versus Postlethwait technique. *Hepatogastroenterology* 1999;46:971.
458. Ell C, Gossner L. Photodynamic therapy. *Rec Res Cancer Res* 2000;155:175.
459. Lightdale CJ, Heier SK, Marcon NE, et al. Photodynamic therapy with porfimer sodium versus thermal ablation therapy with Nd:YAG laser for palliation of esophageal cancer: a multicenter randomized trial. *Gastrointest Endosc* 1995;42:507.
460. Maier A, Tomaselli F, Gebhard F, et al. Palliation of advanced esophageal carcinoma by photodynamic therapy and irradiation. *Ann Thorac Surg* 2000;69:1006.
461. Carlson BA, Dubay MM, Sausville EA, Brizuela L, Worland PJ. Flavopiridol induces G_1 arrest with inhibition of cyclin-dependent kinase (CDK) 2 and CDK4 in human breast carcinoma cells. *Cancer Res* 1996;56:2973.
462. Konig A, Schwartz GK, Mohammad RM, Al-Katib A, Gabrilove JL. The novel cyclin-dependent kinase inhibitor flavopiridol downregulates Bcl-2 and induces growth arrest and apoptosis in chronic B-cell leukemia lines. *Blood* 1997;90:4307.
463. Schrump DS, Matthews W, Chen GA, Mixon A, Altorki NK. Flavopiridol mediates cell cycle arrest and apoptosis in esophageal cancer cells. *Clin Cancer Res* 1998;4:2885.
464. Schrump D, Nguyen DM. Strategies for molecular intervention in esophageal cancers and their precursor lesions. *Dis Esophagus* 1999;3:181.
465. Weiser TS, Ohnmacht GA, Guo S, et al. Sequential 5-Aza-2'-deoxycytidine (DAC)/depsipeptide (DP) treatment synergistically enhances MAGE-3 expression and apoptosis in lung and esophageal cancer cells. *Ann Thorac Surg* 2000 *(in press).*
466. Weiser TS, Guo ZS, Ohnmacht GA, et al. Sequential 5-Aza-2'-deoxycytidine (DAC)/depsipeptide FR901228 (DP) treatment induces apoptosis in cancer cells and facilitates their recognition by cytolytic T lymphocytes specific for NY-ESO-1. 2000 *(submitted for publication).*
467. Foster BA, Coffey HA, Morin MJ, Rastinejad F. Pharmacological rescue of mutant p53 conformation and function. *Science* 1999;286:2507.
468. Naunheim KS, Petruska PJ, Roy TS, et al. Preoperative chemotherapy and radiotherapy for esophageal carcinoma. *J Thorac Cardiovasc Surg* 1992;5:887.
469. Stewart JR, Hoff SJ, Johnson DH, et al. Improved survival with neoadjuvant therapy and resection for adenocarcinoma of the esophagus. *Ann Surg* 1993;218:571.
470. Malhaire JP, Labat JP, Lozach P, et al. Preoperative concomitant radiochemotherapy in squamous cell carcinoma of the esophagus: results of a study of 56 patients. *Int J Radiat Oncol Biol Phys* 1996;34:429.
471. Chiappori A, DeVore R, Stewart J, et al. Phase II study of neoadjuvant cisplatin (P), 5-FU, leucovorin (LV), + etoposide (E) & concurrent radiotherapy (RT) in patients with esophageal cancer. *Proc Am Soc Clin Oncol* 1996;15:214(abst).
472. Keller SM, Ryan L, Coia LR, et al. High dose chemoradiotherapy followed by esophagectomy for adenocarcinoma of the esophagus and gastroesophageal junction. Results of a phase II study of the Eastern Cooperative Oncology Group. *Cancer* 1998;83:1908.

MARTIN S. KARPEH
DAVID P. KELSEN
JOEL E. TEPPER

SECTION 3

Cancer of the Stomach

Adenocarcinoma of the stomach has been the leading cause of cancer death worldwide through most of the twentieth century. It now ranks second only to lung cancer with an estimated 755,500 new cases diagnosed annually around the world. The incidence of this disease has gradually decreased in many parts of the world, principally because of changes in diet, food preparation, and other environmental factors. The declining incidence has been dramatic in the United States, where this disease ranks fourteenth as a cause of cancer deaths. It is estimated that 21,900 new cases are diagnosed annually, with approximately 13,500 deaths per year.[1,2] With the exception of just a few countries in the world, the prognosis for this disease remains poor. The overall 5-year survival rate in the United States and most of the Western world ranges from 5% to 15%. The explanations for these poor results are multifactorial. The lack of defined risk factors and specific symptomatology, and the relatively low incidence, have contributed to the late stage of onset seen in most Western countries. In Japan, where gastric cancer is endemic, patients are diagnosed at an early stage, which is reflected in the excellent 50% 5-year survival rate.

Although the incidence of gastric cancer has decreased dramatically over the last century, the decline has been limited to cancers below the gastric cardia. The number of newly diagnosed patients with proximal gastric and gastroesophageal junction adenocarcinomas has increased markedly since the mid-1980s.[3–5] The disturbing fact is that these are thought to be biologically more aggressive than distal tumors and more complex to treat. The only proven, potentially curative treatment is surgical resection of all gross and microscopic disease. Even after a "curative" gastrectomy, disease recurs in both regional and distant sites in at least 80% of patients. Efforts to improve these poor results have focused on developing effective pre- and postoperative systemic and regional adjuvant therapies. It is generally accepted that patients with chemoresponsive tumors are more likely to have a survival advantage. Consequently, a greater emphasis is being placed on predicting chemoresponsiveness in gastric cancer. This chapter details the current thinking regarding the origins, treatment, and prevention of this universal health problem.

EPIDEMIOLOGY

In 1965, Laurén[6] described two distinct histologic types of stomach adenocarcinoma: intestinal and diffuse, which provided a model to better understand the etiology and epidemiology of the disease.[7] The intestinal variant arises from precancerous areas, such as gastric atrophy or intestinal metaplasia within the stomach; occurs more commonly in men than in women; is more frequent in an older population; and represents the dominant histologic type in areas where stomach cancer is epidemic, suggesting a predominantly environmental etiology. The diffuse form does not typically arise from recognizable precancerous lesions. It represents the major histologic type in endemic areas; occurs slightly more frequently in women and in younger patients; and has a higher association with familial occurrence (blood type A), suggesting a genetic etiology.[8] Changes in the incidence of gastric cancer within populations over time or between geographically distinct populations appear to reflect a difference or change in the incidence of the intestinal form.[9–11]

The highest incidences of stomach cancer can be found in Japan, South America, Eastern Europe, and portions of the Middle East. In most countries, the mortality rate approximates the incidence; in Chile and Costa Rica, the mortality rates for gastric cancer exceed 40 per 100,000 population. In contrast, low-incidence areas, such as New Zealand and Australia, have mortality rates of less than 10 per 100,000.[12] In Japan, despite the epidemic incidence of gastric cancer, a decline has been seen in mortality rates since the 1970s as a result of mass screening.[13]

The studies of migrant populations from areas of high to low risk have produced evidence of environmental influences on the development of gastric cancer.[9,14–18] Among Japanese migrating from the highest risk prefectures in Japan to Hawaii, the risk of stomach cancer persisted even when a Western-style diet was adopted. The high risk of stomach cancer also was observed in second-generation offspring who continued to consume a Japanese-style diet but was low in those adopting a Western-style diet.[16] In the population of Polish migrants living in the United States for 10 years or more, the incidence of gastric cancer decreased and became intermediate between the countries of origin and adoption.[15] These studies suggest that environmental exposure in early life is essential in determining risk but that other environmental or cultural factors may be continually influencing the predisposition to cancer.

In the United States, stomach cancer occurs at a higher incidence in men than in women (ratio of approximately 2:1). It is more frequent in black men than in white men (1.5:1). Starting at the fourth decade, the incidence of stomach cancer increases with advancing age and has a peak incidence in the seventh decade in men and a slightly later peak incidence in women.[12,19] The mortality rate for stomach cancer has decreased from 31.5 per 100,000 for white men in 1935 to 7.8 per 100,000 for all U.S. men in 1983. However, this decline in mortality simply reflects the decrease in the incidence of the disease, and relative 5-year survival rates have not changed considerably.

One of the most striking epidemiologic observations has been the increasing incidence of adenocarcinomas involving the proximal stomach and distal esophagus.[3,4,20,21] In 1991, Blot and colleagues,[3] reviewing the National Cancer Institute's Surveillance, Epidemiology, and End Results database, reported that, during the period 1976 to 1987, a shift to proximal gastric lesions was noted. The annual increase in proximal gastric lesions was 4.3% for white men, 4.1% for white women, 3.6% for black men, and 5.6% for black women. This annual rate of increase on a percentage basis is greater than that of lung cancer or melanoma. The incidence of adenocarcinoma elsewhere in the stomach was approximately the same or slightly lower. By 1984 to 1987, cancers of the cardia made up 47% of all gastric cancers in white men. European investigators have reported similar data.[22] This trend is worrisome, because proximal gastric cancers are thought to have a poorer prognosis, stage for stage, compared with distal cancers.[23–26] The etiologic basis for this rising trend is being aggressively pursued. Increasing prevalence of obesity in the United States may be one factor contributing to this trend. Elevated body mass index[27,28] and caloric consumption[29] have been associated with adenocarcinoma of the distal esophagus and gastric cardia. Gastroesophageal reflux disease may be another risk factor. A population-based, case-control study performed in Sweden found that, for persons with recurrent symptoms of reflux, as compared to those without such symptoms, the odds ratio was 7.7 [95% confidence interval (CI), 5.3 to 11.4] for esophageal adenocarcinoma and 2.0 (95% CI, 1.4 to 2.9) for adenocarcinoma of the gastric cardia.[30] Others have found tobacco use to be associated with these tumors at these sites.[31] Gammon et al.[32] observed an increased odds ratio of 2.4 (95% CI, 1.7 to 3.4) for cigarette smokers. Conversely, aspirin and nonsteroidal antiinflammatory drug use has been associated with a lower risk of esophageal and cardia cancers,[33] implicating inflammation in the etiology of this disease.

ETIOLOGY AND PATHOGENESIS

It is generally accepted that the carcinogenic process leading to the intestinal-type cancers takes many years to develop into invasive adenocarcinoma. Many studies have investigated the role of diet in association with the development of stomach cancer, concluding that the consumption of raw (uncooked) vegetables, fruit, citrus fruit, and high fiber are inversely related to stomach cancer risk.[14,18,34,35] Dietary factors that may be associated with an increased risk of stomach cancer are listed in Table 33.3-1. Antioxidants, which can prevent the conversion of nitrates to nitrosamine, appear to be protective. Diets rich in vitamins A and C[14,36] and micronutrients such as selenium, zinc, cooper, iron, and manganese may lower the risk of gastric carcinoma.[37]

The incidence of cancers affecting the gastric body and antrum is inversely related to socioeconomic status, which probably reflects a number of social, occupational, or cultural factors.[18] A higher incidence has been associated with the practice of smoking or salting meat and fish and a low incidence with the use of refrigeration and better food preparation. The use of well water, which may contain high concentrations of nitrates or *Helicobacter pylori*, has been shown to be a risk factor for gastric cancer.[38,39] Smoking has been reported to increase the relative risk, whereas no consistent data have supported that alcohol consumption affects the incidence of stomach cancer.[35]

Correa and colleagues[9] have proposed a model for the pathogenesis of intestinal-type gastric cancer. Normal mucosa, either through environmental or other factors, becomes atrophied in association with impaired gastric acid secretion and an increased gastric pH. Subsequent bacterial overgrowth results in further mucosal injury directly or via the bacterial production of nitrites or N-nitroso compounds from dietary nitrates.[38] In laboratory animals, the ability of chronically administered oral N-nitroso compounds to produce intestinal metaplasia and subsequent carcinoma has been well described.[40,41] In humans, this mechanism is supported by the observation of a high prevalence of chronic atrophic gastritis and intestinal metaplasia in populations with a high incidence of gastric cancer and the association of gastric cancer with pernicious anemia.[10,42–44]

TABLE 33.3-1. Factors Associated with Increased Risk of Developing Stomach Cancer

Acquired factors
Nutritional
High salt consumption
High nitrate consumption
Low dietary vitamin A and C
Poor food preparation (smoked, salt cured)
Lack of refrigeration
Poor drinking water (well water)
Occupational
Rubber workers
Coal workers
Cigarette smoking
Helicobacter pylori infection
Epstein-Barr virus
Radiation exposure
Prior gastric surgery for benign gastric ulcer disease
Genetic factors
Type A blood
Pernicious anemia
Family history
Hereditary nonpolyposis colon cancer
Li-Fraumeni syndrome
Precursor lesions
Adenomatous gastric polyps
Chronic atrophic gastritis
Dysplasia
Intestinal metaplasia
Menetrier's disease

The Epstein-Barr virus genome has been identified in human gastric cancers with lymphoepithelioid features.[45,46] This is an uncommon finding that has been associated with tumors of younger patients (younger than 35 years), tumors located in the cardia, or in stump carcinomas.[47,48] The frequency in Japan is estimated to be approximately three times that of North America.[49]

The data in support of radiation exposure increasing the risk of gastric cancer come from the Japanese atomic bomb reports.[50] An initial analysis of patients irradiated for peptic ulcer disease followed through 1962 showed no significant tumor increase. A subsequent study of 2049 irradiated patients and 763 medically managed patients was undertaken in 1984 to estimate the risk of cancer due to gastric irradiation. A relative risk of 3.7 was found for stomach cancer.[51]

The occurrence of gastric carcinoma clustered in families suggests the existence of a genetic susceptibility to cancer of the stomach. Estimates of familial clustering of gastric cancer range from 1%[52] to 15% of all gastric cancers.[52,53] The most celebrated example of the genetic predisposition toward stomach cancer is illustrated in the Bonaparte family: Napoleon, his father, and his grandfather all died of gastric carcinoma.[54] Gastric cancer occurs with increased frequency in family members diagnosed with hereditary nonpolyposis colorectal cancer and Li-Fraumeni syndrome. In 1998, Guilford et al.[55] identified an E-cadherin germline mutation present in three Maori kindreds with familial gastric cancers in New Zealand. The potential role for this mutated intracellular adhesion protein in the susceptibility of diffuse-type cancers also was documented in non-Maori families of European and Korean dissent.[56] Shinmura et al.[52] studied DNA from 13 proband cases of familial gastric cancer and concluded that DNA mismatch repair, mutated p53, and E-cadherin genes did not contribute to the observed familial clustering.

PRIOR GASTRIC SURGERY AND GASTRIC CANCER

In 1922, Balfour[57] made the original observation that an association existed between the development of gastric cancer and previous partial gastrectomy for benign disease. A gastric stump cancer arises in the gastric remnant no less than 5 years after partial gastrectomy to distinguish a *de novo* gastric stump cancer from a locally recurrent tumor that was not recognized at the original operation.[58] Two metaanalyses have been published that indicate an increased risk of gastric stump cancer in patients with partial gastrectomy.[59,60] The increased risk is observed only after a latency period of at least 15 years, is increased in patients operated on for gastric but not for duodenal ulcer, and is slightly higher in women than in men. The type of reconstruction does not appear to influence the relative risk of developing gastric stump cancer. Baas et al.[48] compared 26 stump carcinomas with 24 conventional stomach cancers and found that RNA *in situ* hybridization for Epstein-Barr virus was positive in nine stump carcinomas versus two carcinomas in the nonoperated stomach, suggesting etiologic differences between stump carcinoma and cancers arising in the intact stomach.

Because histamine-2 receptor antagonists suppress gastric acid secretion, it has been suggested that chronic use of these agents may predispose the gastric epithelium toward malignant degeneration. However, the only increased risk of stomach cancer in histamine-2 receptor antagonist users has been restricted to patients who had started treatment within 5 years before the diagnosis of stomach cancer.[61,62] This suggests that there may have been a misdiagnosis in some patients rather than a causal role for the drug.

HELICOBACTER PYLORI AND GASTRIC CANCER

In 1982, Marshall and Warren first isolated *H pylori* from biopsies of gastric epithelium. The role for *H pylori* in initiating mucosal injury and the subsequent development of chronic atrophic gastritis is well known.[40,63] In patients who had undergone resection for intestinal-type gastric cancer, the presence of *H pylori* has been identified in noncancerous tissue in almost 90% of patients, compared with 32% with the diffuse form of gastric cancer.[64] Several studies have reported a significant association between *H pylori* infection and gastric cancer,[65–67] particularly for tumors in the distal stomach.[68] The risk of developing gastric cancer correlated with increasing *H pylori* immunoglobulin G antibody levels and was higher when the time interval between the diagnosis of *H pylori* infection and gastric cancer was more than 10 years. Parsonnet and colleagues[65] found a particularly strong association between *H pylori* infection and stomach cancer in women and blacks. The intestinal and diffuse types of stomach adenocarcinoma, as well as gastric lymphoma, were associated with *H pylori* infection. However, others have found a significantly higher incidence of *H pylori* infection in patients with intestinal but not diffuse-type gastric cancer.[69] Although *H pylori* has been classified as a class I carcinogen, the incidence of *H pylori* infection in matched controls in these studies was between 61% and 76%, indicating that most people with *H pylori* infection do not develop stomach cancer and that other contributing factors are important in its pathogenesis. It has been shown that *H pylori* isolates that process the cagA gene are more virulent in nature and produce significant amounts of gastritis and epithelial injury. Patients with cagA *H pylori* infection have a slightly higher risk of developing stomach cancer than those with cagA-negative strains.[70] Further research may define whether characteristics of certain subtypes of *H pylori* or unique characteristics of its host promote malignant transformation. At the present time, antibiotic therapy in *H pylori*–positive patients should be reserved for those with proven ulcer disease or nonulcer dyspepsia in whom other measures have been unsuccessful.

ANATOMIC CONSIDERATIONS

The stomach begins at the gastroesophageal junction and ends at the pylorus (Fig. 33.3-1). Above it lie the diaphragm and left lobe of the liver; before it is the abdominal wall; and below it are the transverse colon, mesocolon, and greater omentum. Behind and to the sides are the spleen, pancreas, left adrenal gland, left kidney, and splenic flexure of the colon. Cancers arising from the proximal greater curvature may directly involve the splenic hilum and tail of pancreas, whereas more distal tumors may invade the transverse colon. Proximal cancers may extend into the diaphragm, spleen, or the left lateral segment of the liver.

The blood supply to the stomach is extensive and is based on vessels arising from the celiac axis (see Fig. 33.3-1). The right gastric artery, arising from the hepatic artery, and the left gastric artery, arising from the celiac axis directly, course along the lesser curvature. Along the greater curvature are the right gastroepiploic artery, which originates from the gastroduodenal artery at the inferior border of the proximal duodenum, and the left gastroepiploic artery, branching from the splenic artery laterally. The short gastric arteries (vasa brevia) arise directly from the splenic artery and make a relatively small contribution to the blood supply to the proximal portion of the stomach. The preservation of any of these vessels in the course of a subtotal gastrectomy for carcinoma is not necessary (nor possible if the operation is performed correctly), and the most proximal few centimeters of remaining stomach are well supplied by collateral flow from the lower segmental esophageal arcade. The rich submucosal blood supply of the stomach is an important factor in its ability to heal rapidly and produce a low incidence of anastomotic disruption.

The venous supply of the stomach tends to parallel the arterial supply. The venous efflux ultimately passes the portal venous system and is reflected in the fact that the liver is a primary site for distant metastatic spread.

The lymphatic drainage of the stomach is extensive, and distinct anatomic groups of perigastric lymph nodes have been defined according to their relationship to the stomach and its blood supply. There are six perigastric lymph node groups: along the greater curvature are the subpyloric and gastroepiploic nodes, and along the lesser curvature are the suprapyloric and the lesser curvature lymph nodes. Proximally are found the right and left pericardial nodes. The second echelon (extraperigastric) nodes include the common hepatic, left gastric, splenic hilum, and splenic artery lymphatics, which drain

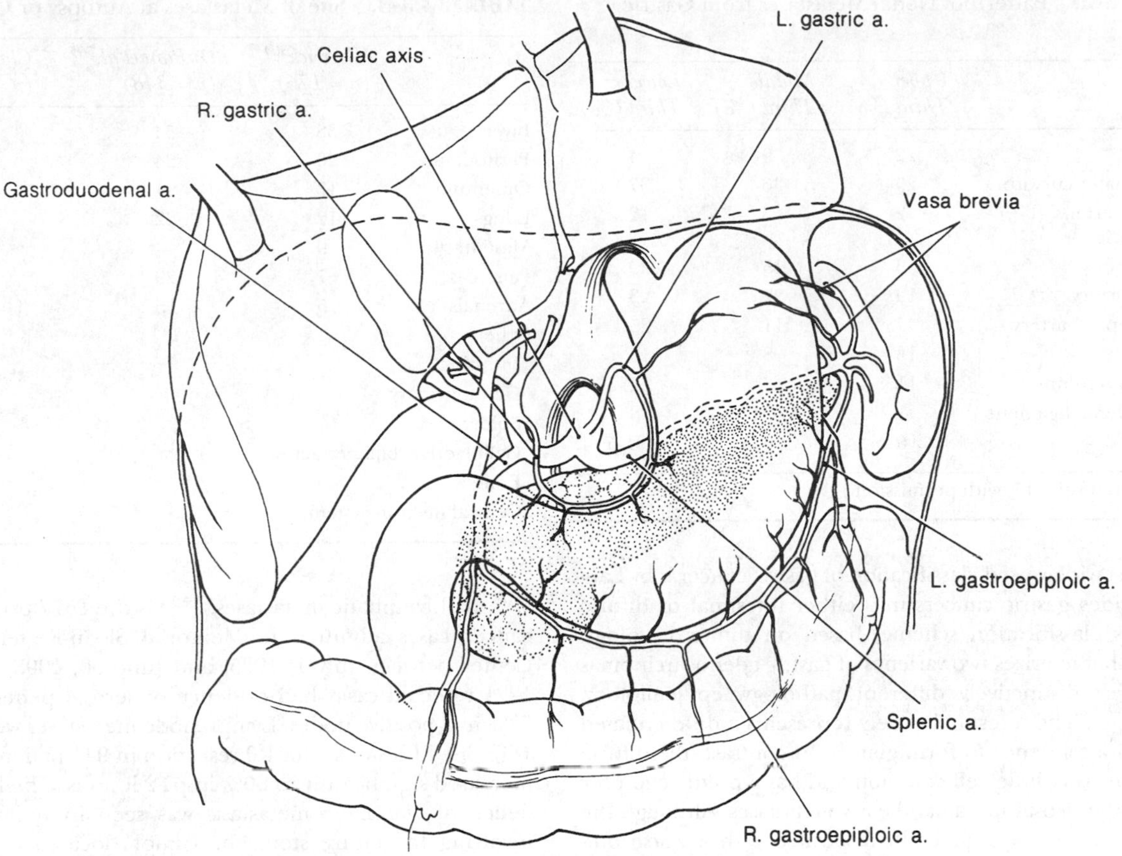

FIGURE 33.3-1. Blood supply to the stomach and anatomic relationships of the stomach with other adjacent organs likely to be involved by direct extension of a large gastric malignancy.

into the celiac and periaortic lymphatics. Proximally are the lower esophageal lymph nodes; extensive spread of gastric cancer along the intrathoracic lymph channels may be manifested clinically by a metastatic lymph node in the left supraclavicular fossa (Virchow's node) or left axilla (Irish's node). As the submucosal lymphatic supply of the stomach becomes extensively involved with tumor, other routes of lymphatic drainage may be recruited. Tumor spread to the lymphatics in the hepatoduodenal ligament can extend along the falciform ligament and result in subcutaneous periumbilical tumor deposits known as *Sister Mary Joseph's nodes.*

PATHOLOGY AND TUMOR BIOLOGY

Approximately 95% of all malignant gastric neoplasms are adenocarcinomas, and in general, the term *gastric cancer* refers to adenocarcinoma of the stomach. Other malignant tumors are very rare and include squamous cell carcinoma, adenoacanthoma, carcinoid tumors, and leiomyosarcoma.[71] Although no normal lymphoid tissue is found in the gastric mucosa, the stomach is the most common site for lymphomas of the gastrointestinal tract. The increased awareness of association between mucosa-associated lymphoid tissue lymphomas and *H pylori* may explain, in part, the rise in incidence.[72] The differentiation between adenocarcinoma and lymphoma can sometimes be difficult but is essential because staging, treatment, and prognosis are different for each disease.[73]

HISTOPATHOLOGY

Several staging schemas have been proposed based on the morphologic features of gastric tumors. The Borrmann classification divides gastric cancer into five types depending on macroscopic appearance. Type I represents polypoid or fungating cancers, type II encompasses ulcerating lesions surrounded by elevated borders, type III represents ulcerated lesions infiltrating the gastric wall, type IV are diffusely infiltrating tumors, and type V are unclassifiable cancers.[74] The gross morphologic appearance of gastric cancer and the degree of histologic differentiation are not independent prognostic variables.[75,76] Ming[76] has proposed a histomorphologic staging system that divides gastric cancer into either a prognostically favorable expansive type or a poor prognosis infiltrating type. Based on an analysis of 171 gastric cancers, the expansive-type tumors were uniformly polypoid or superficial on gross appearance, whereas the infiltrative tumors were almost always diffuse. Grossly ulcerated lesions were equally divided between the expanding or infiltrative forms. Broder's classification of gastric cancer grades tumors histologically from 1 (well differentiated) to 4 (anaplastic). Bearzi and Ranaldi[77] have correlated the degree of histologic differentiation with the gross appearance of 41 primary gastric cancers seen on endoscopy. Ninety percent of protruding or superficial cancers were well differentiated (Broder's grade 1), whereas almost one-half of all ulcerated tumors were poorly differentiated or diffusely infiltrating (Broder's grades 3 and 4).

TABLE 33.3-2. Pattern of Nodal Metastases from Gastric Cancer

	Upper Third (%)	*Middle Third (%)*	*Lower Third (%)*
Paracardia	22	9	4
Lesser or greater curvature	25	36	37
Right gastric artery suprapyloric	2	3	12
Infrapyloric	3	15	49
Left gastric artery	19	22	23
Common hepatic artery	7	11	25
Celiac axis	13	8	13
Splenic artery/hilum	11	3	2
Hepatoduodenal ligament	1	2	8
Others	0–5	0–5	0–5

(Modified from ref. 117, with permission.)

TABLE 33.3-3. Site of Metastases at Autopsy or Operation

	Warwick[304] *(n = 176)*	*DuPont et al.*[305] *(n = 348)*	*Clarke et al.*[306] *(n = 250)*
Liver	38	54	40
Peritoneum	20	24	17
Omentum	13	21	—
Lungs	12	22	19
Mesentery	9	—	—
Pancreas	7	29	—
Adrenals	5	15	12
Others:			
Intestine			
Genitourinary			
Spleen			
Gallbladder/biliary tract			
Bone			
Central nervous system			

The most widely used classification of gastric cancer is by Laurén.[6] It divides gastric cancers into either intestinal or diffuse forms. This classification scheme, based on tumor histology, effectively characterizes two varieties of gastric adenocarcinomas that manifest distinctively different pathology, epidemiology, and etiologies. The intestinal variety represents a differentiated cancer with a tendency to form glands. In contrast, the diffuse form exhibits very little cell cohesion and has a predilection for extensive submucosal spread and early metastases. Although the diffuse-type cancers are generally associated with a worse outcome than the intestinal type, this finding is not independent of tumor, node, metastasis (TNM) stage.

PATTERNS OF SPREAD

Carcinomas of the stomach can spread by local extension to involve adjacent structures and can develop lymphatic metastases, peritoneal metastases, and distant metastases. These extensions can occur by the local invasive properties of the tumor, lymphatic spread, or hematogenous dissemination. The initial growth of the tumor occurs by penetration into the gastric wall, extension through the wall, and involvement of an increasing percentage of the stomach. The two modes of local extension that can have a major therapeutic impact are tumor penetration through the gastric serosa, where the risk of tumor invasion of adjacent structures or peritoneal spread is increased, and involvement of lymphatics. Zinninger[78] has evaluated the spread in the gastric wall and has found a wide variation in its extent. Tumor spread is often through the intramural lymphatics or in the subserosal layers. Local extension can also occur into the esophagus or the duodenum. Duodenal extension is principally through the muscular layer by direct infiltration and through the subserosal lymphatics, but is not generally of great extent. Extension into the esophagus occurs primarily through the submucosal lymphatics.

Local extension does not occur solely by radial intramural spread but also by deep invasion through the wall to involve adjacent structures. Extension can occur through the gastric serosa to involve omentum, spleen, adrenal gland, diaphragm, liver, pancreas, or colon. Data from several large older series indicated that 60% to 90% of patients had primary tumors penetrating the serosa or invading adjacent organs and that at least 50% had lymphatic metastases.[79,80] Of the 1577 primary gastric cancer cases admitted to Memorial Sloan-Kettering Cancer Center between July 1, 1985, and June 30, 1998, 60% of the 1221 resected cases had evidence of serosal penetration, and 68% had positive nodes. Lymph node metastases were found in 18% of pT1 lesions after R0 resection in 941 patients. This rate increased significantly to 60% in pT2 lesions. The highest incidence of lymphatic metastasis was seen in tumors diffusely involving the entire stomach. Tumors located at the gastroesophageal junction also had a high incidence relative to other sites. The pattern of nodal metastases also varies depending on the location of the primary site (Table 33.3-2), with the left gastric artery nodes being consistently at increased risk for nodal metastases regardless of tumor location.

Gastric cancer recurs in multiple sites, both locoregionally and systemically (Table 33.3-3). The literature reveals disagreements over failure patterns (Table 33.3-4); these disagreements are likely related to the patient cohorts accepted for evaluation, the time at which failure was determined, and the method of determination of failure patterns. In two older autopsy series, the rate of locoregional failure [defined as tumor in perigastric tissues (e.g., in the retroperitoneal "gastric bed," perigastric lymph nodes, gastric remnant)] after potentially curative resection was 40% to 80%.[81,82] Many patients had multiple sites of local failure. Shiu and coworkers[79] found a 23% local recurrence rate in 169 patients treated for carcinoma of the body of the stomach.

Gunderson and Sosin[83] reanalyzed the reoperation series performed by Wangensteen at the University of Minnesota, where patients had a second-look laparotomy after resection of the primary tumor. This type of analysis is valuable because it can demonstrate the early (and perhaps most treatable) modes of failure rather than simply showing diffuse metastatic disease at autopsy. Sixty-nine percent of patients had evidence of a locoregional recurrence, and 42% of patients had peritoneal seeding. Most of the local failures were located in the gastric bed (81%), although recurrences also occurred in the anastomosis or stump (39%) or in the regional lymph nodes (63%). A trial from the British Stomach Cancer Group found an incidence of local failure in patients treated with surgery alone to be 37 of 69 (54%).[84] A series evaluating local failure patterns

TABLE 33.3-4. Failure Patterns in Gastric Cancer Patients

Study	Treatment	Evaluation Method	Locoregional	Metastases Peritoneal	Liver	Lung	Total
Clarke et al.[306]	None	Surgery and autopsy	N/A	17%	40%	19%	
Dupont et al.[305]	Surgery	Autopsy	N/A	24%	54%	22%	
Warwick[304]	Surgery	Autopsy	N/A	20%	38%	12%	
Wisbeck et al.[82]	Surgery	Autopsy	94% (15/16)	50% (8/16)	44% (7/16)	13% (2/16)	22% (32/145)
Allum et al.[192]	Surgery	Clinical	27% (39/145)				
Atiq et al.[210]	Surgery + chemotherapy	Clinical	3% (1/35)	26% (9/35)	6% (2/35)		
Bruckner	Surgery	Clinical	14% (10/71)	10% (7/71)	21% (15/71)	10% (7/71)	
Estape et al.[189]	Surgery	Clinical	8% (3/37)	46% (17/37)	30% (11/37)		
Gunderson and Sosin[83]	Surgery	Surgery	69% (74/105)	42% (44/105)			
Landry et al.[85]	Surgery	Clinical	38% (49/130)				52% (68/130)
Wanebo et al.[124]	Surgery	Clinical	41%[a]				59%[a]

N/A, not available.
[a]Percentage of total recurrences; based on 1809 recurrences.

reported by Landry and coworkers[85] showed a total locoregional failure rate of 38%, with most of the local recurrences in the gastric bed, the anastomosis, or the gastric stump. The incidence of local failure increased when the primary disease extended through the gastric wall or when lymph nodes were involved at the initial surgery. Liver metastases occurred in 30% of patients and peritoneal seeding in 23%. Extraabdominal failure was relatively rare and occurred in 13% of patients.

Some newer series suggest a higher incidence of peritoneal seeding as a failure pattern. Wisbeck et al.[82] evaluated autopsy and clinical records of 85 patients who died of gastric cancer. Sixteen patients had a resection with curative intent; 15 of these developed a locoregional recurrence, eight developed peritoneal seeding, and seven developed lung metastases. Of the entire cohort, 40 of 85 (47%) developed peritoneal seeding. Ajani and colleagues[86] treated 25 patients with preoperative chemotherapy. At the time of surgery, eight had peritoneal carcinomatosis, and it developed subsequently in an additional five patients. Because imaging studies were not done routinely postoperatively, they could not accurately determine the risk of locoregional failure. These data suggest that increased attention to methods of controlling local and regional disease as well as systemic disease is needed to improve long-term results.

CLINICAL PRESENTATION

SIGNS AND SYMPTOMS

Most patients with gastric cancer are diagnosed with advanced-stage disease, and this is reflected in the vague, nonspecific symptoms that characterize the disease. Patients may have a combination of signs and symptoms, such as weight loss, anorexia, fatigue, or epigastric discomfort, none of which unequivocally indicates gastric cancer. The clinical significance of weight loss in gastric cancer should not be underestimated. Dewys and colleagues[87] has shown that, in 179 patients with advanced, nonmeasurable gastric cancer, more than 80% of patients had a greater than 10% decrease in body weight. Patients with weight loss had a significantly shorter survival than those without weight loss.

In some patients, symptoms may suggest the presence of a lesion in specific locations. A history of dysphagia may indicate the presence of a tumor in the cardia with extension through the gastroesophageal junction. A complaint of early satiety is actually a very infrequent symptom of gastric cancer, but is indicative of a diffusely infiltrative tumor that has resulted in loss of distensibility of the gastric wall. Persistent vomiting is consistent with an antral carcinoma obstructing the pylorus. Significant gastrointestinal bleeding is uncommon with gastric cancer; however, hematemesis does occur in approximately 10% to 15% of patients. However, many patients are diagnosed after the development of ascites, jaundice, or a palpable mass, indicating extensive and incurable disease.

Because the transverse colon is held in close proximity to the stomach by the gastrocolic ligament, it is a potential site of malignant fistula and large bowel obstruction from a gastric primary. Diffuse peritoneal spread of disease frequently produces other sites of intestinal obstruction. A large ovarian mass (Krukenberg's tumor) or a large peritoneal implant in the pelvis (Blumer's shelf), which can produce symptoms of rectal obstruction, may be felt on pelvic or rectal examination. Nodular metastases in the subcutaneous tissue around the umbilicus or in peripheral lymph nodes represent areas in which tissue diagnosis can be established with minimal morbidity.

SCREENING

Mass screening programs for gastric cancer have been most successful in high-risk areas, especially in Japan.[88] A variety of screening tests have been studied in Japanese patients, with a sensitivity and specificity of approximately 90%.[89] They frequently include the use of double-contrast barium radiographs or upper endoscopy.[89] The yield in screened populations has been substantial; in some Japanese studies, up to 40% of newly diagnosed patients have early gastric cancer, and up to 60% of patients actively participating in routine mass screening programs have the disease.[88] This is clinically important because, as discussed below in Pathologic Staging and Prognosis, early gastric cancer has a very high cure rate when treated surgically. However, the fact that gastric cancer remains the number one cause of death in Japan may reflect the limitations of a mass screening program when the entire population at risk is not effectively screened. Newer studies have verified that a low serum pepsinogen I/II ratio can be used to better select patients at increased risk for atrophic gastritis and gastric cancer.[90]

PRETREATMENT STAGING

TUMOR MARKERS

Carcinoembryonic antigen (CEA) is elevated in approximately one-third of primary gastric cancer patients.[91] The sensitivity of CEA is low, but when elevated, the level does generally correlate with stage. Combining CEA with other markers, such as the sialylated Lewis antigens CA19-9 or CA50, can increase the sensitivity over CEA alone.[92–94] A large study evaluated the prognostic significance of serum levels of CEA (n = 237), α-fetoprotein (n = 164), human chorionic gonadotropin-β (β-HCG) (n = 165), CA19-9 (n = 64), and CA125 (n = 104), as well as tissue staining for C-erb B-2 (n = 160) and β-HCG (n = 160). In a multivariate analysis, only serum β-HCG ≥4 IU/L (hazard ratio, 1.7; 95% CI, 2.8 to 1.1) and CA125 ≥350 U/mL (hazard ratio, 2.2; 95% CI, 4.2 to 1.2) had prognostic significance. Elevated serum β-HCG and CA125 in gastric cancer before chemotherapy may reflect not just tumor burden but aggressive biology, however, these findings must be compared to other known preoperative markers of stage, such as endoscopic ultrasonography (EUS) T and N stage.[95]

ENDOSCOPY

Upper endoscopy is used routinely for the initial diagnosis and staging of gastric adenocarcinoma and should be performed in any patient with localized disease for which surgical treatment is anticipated. Numerous reports have demonstrated diagnostic accuracy of more than 95% for advanced disease.[96,97] The size, location, and morphology of the tumor, including the proximal and distal extent of spread, as well as other mucosal abnormalities, should be carefully evaluated. Decreased distensibility of the stomach, abnormal peristaltic activity, or abnormal pyloric function may indicate extensive submucosal infiltration or extramural extension of tumor into the vagi. The likelihood of a positive yield on biopsy is greater than 95% when six to ten tissue samples are obtained.[96] Detecting the faint mucosal irregularities usually associated with early gastritis-like carcinomas can be enhanced by endoscopic dye spraying with vital dyes, such as 0.1% indigocalmin. This technique has been used extensively in Japan with good success.

EUS has been used extensively to stage the depth of invasion and regional lymph node extent in potentially operable gastric cancer. EUS uses a high-frequency (7.5 or 12 MHz) transducer at the end of an endoscope and allows highly accurate staging of the depth of invasion of the primary tumor (T stage) and is more accurate than a computed tomographic (CT) scan for staging T and N status.[95,98] Although it appears more useful than a CT scan for detecting perigastric lymph node metastases, the overall accuracy of EUS for assessing all regional nodes is less satisfactory. Because CT may identify metastases to distant nodes and sites, such as the liver, ovaries, and peritoneum, CT and EUS are best used as complementary tests. EUS has become an invaluable tool to assess which early gastric cancers are candidates for endomucosal resection, a curative treatment in properly selected patients[99,100] (see Treatment of Local Disease, below).

COMPUTED TOMOGRAPHY

Once gastric cancer is suspected, a barium study or flexible upper endoscopy with biopsy is performed. After the diagnosis is established, staging procedures involve careful physical examination, routine blood screening tests, and abdominal and chest CT scanning.[101] Barium contrast studies have limited accuracy for determining resectability, but by using double-contrast techniques, a positive diagnosis of lesions between 5 and 10 mm can be made in 75% of patients.[102] CT of the chest, abdomen, and pelvis is useful for assessing the lateral extension of the tumor and presence of systemic metastases.[103] However, up to 50% of patients have more extensive disease at laparotomy than was predicted by preoperative CT.[104] With newer triphasic spiral CT scanning methods, greater emphasis has been placed on identifying low-volume disease and predicting the T stage. Takao et al.[105] reported an accuracy for spiral CT of 82% for staging T status in advanced gastric cancer and 15% in early gastric cancer by obtaining images with the stomach filled with water. Few Western centers routinely apply these techniques, and without them the accuracy of T staging is generally poor.

POSITRON EMISSION TOMOGRAPHY

Whole body [^{18}F]fluorodeoxyglucose (FDG) positron emission tomography (PET) is being applied increasingly in the evaluation of gastrointestinal malignancies. The positron-emitting ^{18}F-labeled analogue of 2-deoxyglucose, 2-[^{18}F]-fluoro-2-deoxyglucose is readily transported into cells by either type I or II hexose transporters. Once in the cell, the analogue is phosphorylated into FDG-6-phosphate, which in most tumor tissues is not metabolized further. The preferential accumulation of positron-emitting FDG by tumor cells has been used successfully to image human tumors. Several studies have documented improved efficacy of detecting recurrent colorectal and hepatic (primary and metastatic) tumor sites, with a sensitivity ranging from 92% to 100% and an accuracy of 90% to 96%.[106] Results from a study in esophageal cancer demonstrated that PET could detect 20% of metastases missed by CT.[107] Little information regarding the use of FDG-PET in the management of gastric cancer is available. In a pilot study begun here at Memorial Sloan-Kettering Cancer Center, we set out to assess the feasibility of FDG-PET imaging in gastric cancer patients. Fifteen studies were performed on 14 gastric cancer patients with various stages of disease. One hundred forty-five lesions were imaged with concurrent histologic confirmation. The preliminary results show FDG-PET to have a sensitivity of 60%, specificity of 100%, and an overall accuracy of 94% in identifying gastric cancer. The most consistent finding has been uptake in the primary tumor, indicating a possible role in treatment response assessment as well as for staging.

TABLE 33.3-5. American Joint Committee on Cancer Staging of Gastric Cancer, 1997

DEFINITION OF TNM

Primary tumor (T)

TX	Primary tumor cannot be assessed
T0	No evidence of primary tumor
Tis	Carcinoma *in situ*
T1	Tumor invades lamina propria or submucosa
T2	Tumor invades muscularis propria
T3	Tumor invades adventitia
T4	Tumor invades adjacent structures

Regional lymph nodes (N): a minimum of 15 lymph nodes must be examined

NX	Regional lymph node(s) cannot be assessed
N0	No regional lymph node metastasis
N1	Metastasis in one to six regional lymph node
N2	Metastasis in seven to 15 regional lymph nodes
N3	Metastases in more than 15 regional lymph nodes

Distant metastasis (M)

MX	Presence of distant metastasis cannot be assessed
M0	No distant metastasis
M1	Distant metastasis

STAGE GROUPING

0	Tis	N0	M0
IA	T1	N0	M0
IB	T1	N1	M0
	T2	N0	M0
II	T1	N2	M0
	T2	N1	M0
	T3	N0	M0
IIIA	T2	N2	M0
	T3	N1	M0
	T4	N0	M0
IIIB	T3	N2	M0
IV	T4	N1	M0
	T4	N2	M0
	T1	N3	M0
	T2	N3	M0
	T3	N3	M0
	T4	N2	M0
	Any T	Any N	M1

LAPAROSCOPY

The introduction of fiberoptic, video-assisted laparoscopy in the early 1980s added a means of direct and immediate assessment of the abdominal cavity without the morbidity of a laparotomy. Comparative studies of CT and laparoscopy have consistently shown laparoscopy to provide additional information that was not seen by preoperative CT imaging. In a study of 103 consecutively staged gastric cancer patients, laparoscopy had an accuracy of 94% when compared to what was found at laparotomy. Disease missed by CT was mostly peritoneal metastases. The rate of detecting occult M1 disease by this method ranges from 13% to 37%.[108–113] Patients without clinically significant bleeding or obstruction that are found to have occult metastatic disease are incurable and may benefit from participation in new treatment protocols. Use of induction chemotherapy and selective resection of responding patients is an attractive alternative to immediate resection. Contrary to previously held dogma, most stage IV patients rarely develop significant symptoms from the primary tumor before death. None of the 24 patients with metastatic disease discovered at laparoscopy who were followed until death required subsequent laparotomy for complications of the primary tumor.[109] Because CT may identify metastases to distant sites (liver, adrenal glands, and ovaries), thus avoiding an operation, CT, EUS, and laparoscopy are all considered complementary tests.

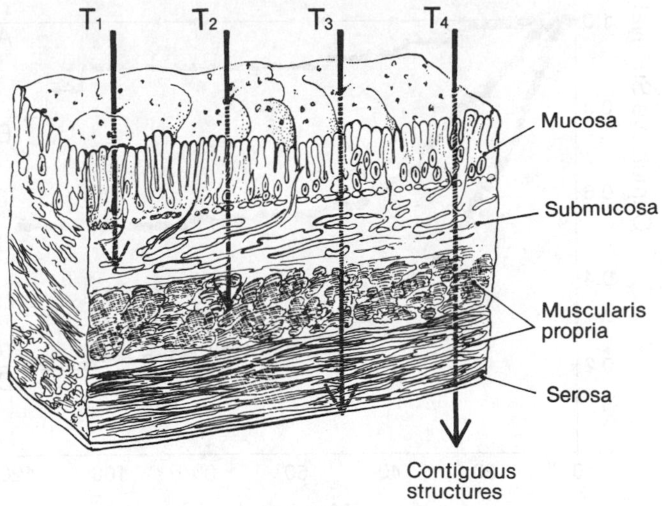

FIGURE 33.3-2. Definition of American Joint Committee on Cancer/International Union Against Cancer T stage based on depth of penetration of the gastric wall.

The development of laparoscopic ultrasonographic probes has added a third dimension to the laparoscopic examination.[114] Laparoscopy with laparoscopic ultrasonography, although more invasive than EUS, is superior in identifying unsuspected metastases to liver and lymph nodes. Considering the low morbidity and significantly shorter hospital stay,[109,112] laparoscopy, whenever feasible, should eliminate the need for patients undergoing laparotomy without resection.

PATHOLOGIC STAGING AND PROGNOSIS

As with other neoplasms, the uniform and accurate staging of gastric cancer is essential to meaningfully predict prognosis and assess response to treatment. The R classification indicates the amount of residual disease left after tumor resection.[115] *R0* indicates no gross or microscopic residual disease; *R1* indicates microscopic residual disease, and *R2* signifies gross residual disease. This is an obvious but most important prognostic factor, but it was not always indicated in the past, making interpretation of survival results difficult.

The International Union Against Cancer (UICC) and American Joint Committee on Cancer (AJCC) TNM classification for stomach cancer is shown in Table 33.3-5. The depth of tumor invasion (Fig. 33.3-2) determines T stage. The relationship between T stage and survival is well defined (Fig. 33.3-3). The General Rules for Gastric Cancer Study in Surgery and Pathology was published in English in 1995 by the Japanese Research Society for Gastric Cancer.[74] The definition of the primary tumor stage based on the depth of invasion and the presence and extent of serosal invasion is shown in Table 33.3-6.

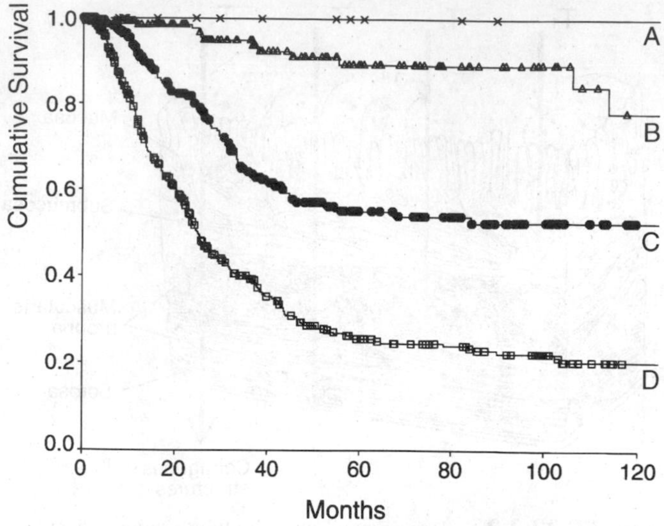

FIGURE 33.3-3. Kaplan-Meier curves of disease-specific survival according to American Joint Committee on Cancer T stage. Tis (tumor *in situ*; n = 16) A; T1 (n = 168) B; T2 (n = 265) C; T3 (n = 464) D; T4 (*not shown*), n = 28. (From the Memorial Sloan-Kettering Cancer Center Department of Surgery Prospective Gastric Cancer Database.)

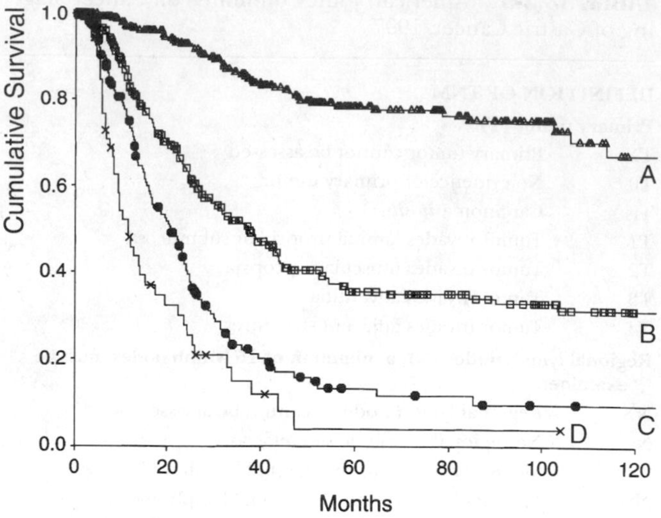

FIGURE 33.3-4. Kaplan-Meier curves of disease-specific survival according to the 1997 American Joint Committee on Cancer N stage. N0 (no positive nodes; n = 355) A; N1 (one to six positive nodes; n = 354) B; N2 (7 to 15 positive nodes; n = 164) C; N3 (>15 positive nodes; n = 60) D. (From the Memorial Sloan-Kettering Cancer Center Department of Surgery Prospective Gastric Cancer Database.)

T stage is further divided into mucosa (m), submucosa (sm), and muscularis propria (pm). The subserosa (ss) and S1 tumors have been reclassified to further stratify the degree and type of serosal invasion. INFα is a subserosal tumor with expansive growth, INFβ is a subserosal tumor with intermediate-type growth, and INFγ is a subserosal tumor with infiltrating growth. S2 and S3 are now defined as either se (cancer cells exposed to the peritoneal cavity), si (cancer cells infiltrating neighboring tissue), or sei (the coexistence of se and si).[74] Survival results based on T stage are fairly consistent among Japan, Europe, and the United States[116–121] (see Table 33.3-6).

The AJCC/UICC N stage was changed in 1997 to reflect the number of involved lymph nodes. Tumors with one to six involved nodes are classified as pN1; 7 to 15 involved nodes are pN2, and more than 15 involved nodes is N3. Survival decreases dramatically as the number of metastatic lymph nodes increase. The N stage survival rate based on the number of nodes involved is shown in Figure 33.3-4 for 941 R0 gastric cancer patients treated at Memorial Sloan-Kettering Cancer Center. The previous classification was based on the localization of lymph node metastases. An analysis of 477 R0 resected node-positive cases from the German Gastric Cancer Study compared survival using both staging systems. This new 1997 AJCC further separated the survival of patients categorized by the old N definition (Fig. 33.3-5). Survival was significantly changed in the old N2 group by applying the new N stage classification.[122] Differences between the two staging systems were not as great for N1 patients. Within the groups with one to six, 7 to 15, and more than 15 involved nodes, the location of metastatic lymph nodes did not significantly alter the prognosis. The new classification can now be applied in surgical trials with fewer methodologic problems, and it seems more reproducible provided that a minimum of at least 15 lymph nodes are examined. Several studies

TABLE 33.3-6. Survival after Curative Resection for Gastric Cancer with Respect to Depth of Invasion

		5-Y Survival (%)					
		T1		*T2*		*T3*	*T4*
Study	*Number of Patients*	M	SM	PM	SS	SE	SI/SEI
Noguchi et al.[146] (Japan)	3143	94	87	75	51	23 (S2)	5
Maruyama et al.[136] (Japan)	3176	95	87	82	65	34 (S2)	14
Boku et al.[118] (Japan)	238	—	—	90	—	42 (S2)	29
Baba et al.[119] (Japan)	142	—	—	55	—	34	32
Hermanek[120] (Germany)	977	84	75	73	40	24	25
Shiu et al.[121] (United States)	246	—	—	--------56--------		32	—
Bozzetti et al.[307] (Italy)	361	82	69	--------38--------		—	—
MSKCC (United States)[310]	944	--------91--------		--------56--------		26	—

M, mucosa; MSKCC, Memorial Sloan-Kettering Cancer Center; PM, muscularis propria; S2, serosal invasion; SE, cancer cells exposed to the peritoneal cavity; SEI, the coexistence of SE and SI; SI, cancer cells infiltrating neighboring tissue; SM, submucosa; SS, subserosa.

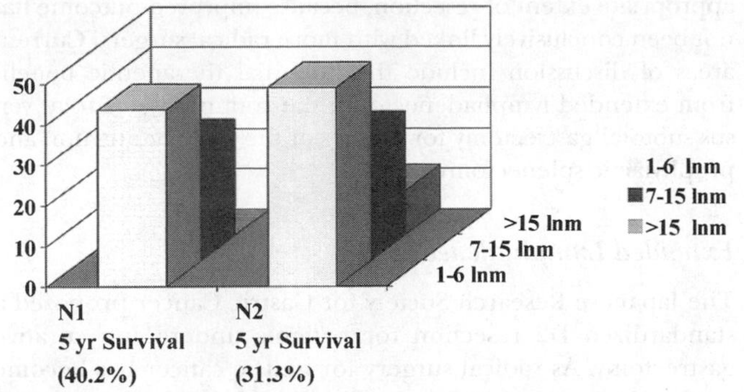

FIGURE 33.3-5. This graph demonstrates the range in 5-year survival rates according to the 1997 American Joint Committee on Cancer/International Union Against Cancer N stage within two groups of patients classified by the 1992 N1 and N2 staging. lnm, lymph node metastases. (Data modified from ref. 122.)

have assessed quantitative involvement of lymph nodes and survival after resection for gastric cancer and found that survival with up to three to four metastatic lymph nodes is better than with more extensive lymph node involvement.[121,123] Once nodal metastases are found, Japanese survival statistics are better than those seen in Western patients[123] (Table 33.3-7). Possible explanations for this observation include a potential difference in the biology of the tumor between the two patient populations or that the Japanese are removing and analyzing more lymph nodes, resulting in stage migration. The new AJCC/UICC requirement that a minimum of 15 nodes be removed and analyzed may minimize these differences.

Under the current staging system, the presence of more than 15 perigastric lymph node metastases is classified as N3 disease, which is staged as M1. The Japanese staging system extensively classifies 18 lymph node regions into four N categories depending on their relationship to the primary tumor as well as anatomic location. The careful and complete prosection of the operative specimen may often be performed by the attending surgeon or designated surgical resident. Involvement with N1 and N2 lymph node groups represent regional disease, which is encompassed by the D2 lymphadenectomy, whereas N3 and N4

TABLE 33.3-7. Survival after Resection for Gastric Cancer with Respect to Lymph Node Status

Study	Number of Patients	*5-Y Survival (%) by 1988 AJCC N Stage*				
		N0	N1	N2	N3	N4
Noguchi et al.[146] (Japan)	3145	80	53	26	10	3
Maruyama et al.[117] (Japan)	3176	85	61	31	10	2
Bozzetti et al.[307] (Italy)	361	57	-------	43	-------	—
Hermanek[120] (Germany)	977	74	36	20	10	—
MSKCC[310] (United States)	961	78	29	18	—	—

AJCC, American Joint Committee on Cancer; MSKCC, Memorial Sloan-Kettering Cancer Center.

TABLE 33.3-8. Japanese Surgical Staging System for Gastric Cancer

S0	No serosal invasion
S1	Suspected serosal invasion
S2	Definite serosal invasion
S3	Adjacent organ involvement
N1	Perigastric lymph nodes
N2	Lymph nodes around the left gastric artery, common hepatic artery, splenic artery, and celiac axis
N3	Lymph nodes in the hepatoduodenal ligament, posterior aspect of pancreas, and root of mesentery
N4	Paraaortic and middle colic lymph nodes
P0	No peritoneal metastases
P1	Adjacent peritoneal involvement
P2	A few scattered metastases to distant peritoneum
P3	Many distant peritoneal metastases
H0	No liver metastases
H1	Metastases limited to one lobe
H2	A few bilateral metastases
H3	Numerous bilateral metastases
Stage grouping	
I	S0, N0, P0, H0
II	S1, N0–1, P0, H0
III	S2, N0–2, P0, H0
IV	S3, N3–4, P1–3, H1–3

lymph nodes are considered distant metastases. In addition, the presence and extent of intraabdominal metastases to the peritoneum and liver are categorized (Table 33.3-8).

Stage for stage, considerable disparity exists between the survival of patients with stomach cancer in Japanese and Western series. Wanebo and coworkers[124] have reported on the results of a tumor registry survey in 1982 and 1987 of 18,365 U.S. patients. In the entire cohort, 18% of patients were stage I, 16% stage II, 36% stage III, and 30% stage IV. Although early diagnosis, a higher incidence of intestinal-type tumors, and the use of radical surgery in Japan may explain these differences, in part, a major contributing factor may be the extensive and meticulous surgical and pathologic staging of gastric cancer in Japan. Several reports from the United States, Japan, and Europe have demonstrated similar survival results by applying more similar surgical and pathologic staging techniques.[125–127] The 1997 AJCC TNM survival curves are shown in Figure 33.3-6 for R0-resected patients.

Although not a formal component of stage grouping, the histopathologic grade and type and, when available, the peritoneal lavage cytology status should be recorded. The presence of free peritoneal cancer cells has been shown by a number of investigators to be an M1 equivalent.[128–131] Burke et al.[132] found no survivors beyond 18 months among stage III patients with positive peritoneal lavage.

TREATMENT OF LOCALIZED DISEASE

ENDOSCOPIC MUCOSAL RESECTION

It has been shown that a subset of early gastric cancers can undergo an R0 resection without lymphadenectomy or gastrectomy. The Japanese have popularized endoscopic mucosal resection of early gastric cancers that meet specific criteria.

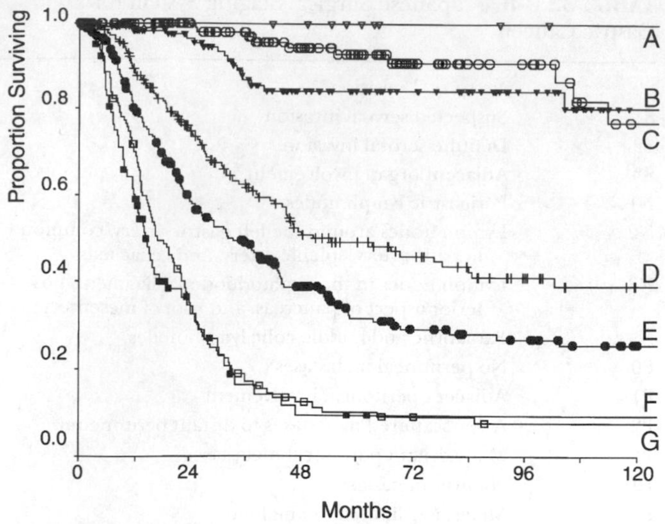

FIGURE 33.3-6. Kaplan-Meier curves of disease-specific survival according to the 1997 American Joint Committee on Cancer system. Stage 0 (n = 16) A; IA (n = 139) B; IB (n = 133) C; II (n = 206) D; IIIA (n = 239) E; IIIB (n = 130) F; IV (n = 81) G. (From the Memorial Sloan-Kettering Cancer Center Department of Surgery Prospective Gastric Cancer Database.)

This approach involves the submucosal injection of fluid to elevate the lesion to facilitate complete mucosal resection. The technique is suitable for lesions that have a low metastatic potential.[133] These include well-differentiated, superficial type IIa or IIc lesions that are generally smaller than 3 cm in diameter and located in an easily manipulated area. Tumors invading the submucosa are at increased risk for metastasizing to lymph nodes and are not appropriate for endoscopic resection. Takekoshi et al.[134] reported a series of 308 endoscopic resections for early cancer. Forty-four patients had residual or recurrent lesions after endoscopic mucosal resection. All recurrences were resected, and no patients died of gastric cancer. In experienced hands, endoscopic mucosal resection is a suitable alternative to gastrectomy for favorable early gastric cancer.

SURGERY

The only potentially curative treatment for localized gastric cancer is complete surgical resection. The principles that guide operative management are based on the Halstedian belief that gastric cancer progresses from mucosa to submucosa where it then invades into lymphatics. From there, lymph node involvement occurs but before the disease reaches the systemic circulation. Clearly this is an oversimplified view of tumor progression; however, support for this theory comes from the strong correlation between depth of invasion and the extent and number of lymph node metastases. Others have argued that epithelial cancers can metastasize directly into the systemic circulation, thus bypassing lymph nodes.[20] Molecular factors, which govern invasion and metastases, differ from one tumor to the next, such that even some early gastric cancers do recur and are fatal after curative surgery.[135] In general, the success of an R0 resection is directly dependent on stage as determined by the TNM system. It is well accepted that surgery carries a high cure rate for stage IA and IB cancers and much poorer results for stages IIIA and IIIB. Disagreement exists among surgeons with respect to the appropriate extent of resection, because improved outcome has not been conclusively linked with more radical surgery. Current areas of discussion include the potential therapeutic benefit from extended lymphadenectomy, the routine use of total versus subtotal gastrectomy for tumors of the body or antrum, and prophylactic splenectomy.

Extended Lymphadenectomy

The Japanese Research Society for Gastric Cancer proposed a standardized D2 resection for patients undergoing curative gastrectomy. As radical surgery for gastric cancer has become uniformly accepted in Japan, the operative mortality rate for D2 resection has declined and 5-year survival after curative resection has improved. Many large retrospective reports from Japan, other Asian countries, and specialty centers in the West advocate a D2 lymphadenectomy for patients with resectable gastric cancer.[136] Maruyama and colleagues[117] have reported results from more than 20,000 cases from a nationwide registry in Japan for three periods: 1963 to 1966, 1969 to 1973, and 1971 to 1985. The 30-day operative mortality rate declined from 3.8% in the first period to 1.0% in the latest. When patients were compared with respect to stage, depth of tumor invasion, presence of serosal invasion, and N1 or N2 nodal metastases, improved survival was noted in the most recent period compared to the first. However, radical (D2) resection did not improve survival for patients with extranodal disease, such as peritoneal metastases, distant lymph node metastases (N3–4), or diffusely infiltrating carcinomas (linitis plastica). Takeda and coworkers[137] also have reported that 5-year survival improved from 21% to 46% in 166 patients undergoing total gastrectomy with curative intent for tumors with positive serosal invasion when a D2 lymphadenectomy was performed compared with 62 patients in whom no systematic lymphadenectomy was performed. Kodama and colleagues[138] have compared survival in 254 patients undergoing simple resection with 454 patients undergoing extensive regional lymph node dissection (ELD) for gastric carcinoma. The therapeutic effect of ELD was greatest in patients with serosal invasion (T3) or with positive lymph node metastases; patients with T1, T2, T4, or N0 disease did not show a benefit from ELD. In all of these studies, outcomes of patients operated on in different periods were compared, and it is possible that other factors could have influenced survival. In a series of 486 patients who underwent curative (D2) resection for gastric cancer, Sowa and coworkers[139] demonstrated that tumor size and depth of penetration were directly related to the incidence of lymph node metastases in gastric cancer and that the rate of skip metastases was less than 1%. In this study, as well as in others,[140] T1–2 lesions had metastases limited to perigastric lymph nodes in 15% to 40% of patients, suggesting that, in cases of less-advanced cancers, a systematic lymphadenectomy may be needed to clear all nodal disease.

Reports have also come from the United States and Europe that are mostly retrospective series advocating D2 lymphadenectomy for gastric cancer.[141] Keller and colleagues,[142] reporting for the German Stomach Cancer TNM Study Group, recommended systematic lymphadenectomy for resectable gastric cancer because occult lymph node metastases were pathologically identified two to three times more frequently than when no systematic lymphadenectomy was performed. Roder et al.[143] reported the results of the German Gastric Carcinoma Study, in which the treatment of 1999 patients was prospectively recorded and assessed in a systematic, uniform manner. They demonstrated a survival advantage after D2 lymphadenectomy for stage II and IIIA tumors. The issue of stage migration was dismissed on the basis that both the standard and extended lymph node dissection groups had far more than the recommended 15 lymph nodes examined. In a retrospective analysis of 210 patients, Shiu et al.[121] found that, if their lymphadenectomy encompassed one echelon of pathologically uninvolved nodes beyond the level of nodal metastases, survival was significantly improved over those with a less extensive lymphadenectomy (60% vs. 25%, respectively). Irvin and Bridger[144] have reported a similar 60% 5-year survival rate in 22 patients undergoing curative D1 resection, but all 22 had pathologically negative nodes (T1–3,N0).

Because of the technical difficulty of an extended lymphadenectomy, some authors have addressed the possibility of using selective lymph node dissection in gastric cancer with macroscopically suspicious nodes. In one series, however, the mean size of metastatic lymph nodes in 370 patients undergoing D2 gastrectomy was 7 mm,[145] and others have reported that surgeons could correctly diagnose metastatic involvement by intraoperative macroscopic examination in only 20% of patients.[142,145] Noguchi and colleagues[146] have reported that, although a direct correlation exists between lymph node size and the frequency of metastases, 30% of all metastases to lymph nodes occur in nodes smaller than 3 mm in size. Therefore, it is unlikely that selective lymphadenectomy based on gross appearance of lymph nodes is feasible or appropriate.

The need for and extent of lymphadenectomy necessary for patients with early gastric cancer, defined as primary tumors limited to the mucosa or submucosa, is controversial.[147–151] Risk factors for lymph node metastases have been identified for intramucosal tumors[133,152] in early gastric cancer. Some have advocated selective lymphadenectomy, particularly when other favorable factors exist, such as a primary tumor of small size (less than 1.5 cm), protruded-type tumor (Borrmann type I), and tumors confined to the mucosa.[145] Hochwald et al.[152] analyzed 165 early gastric cancers for clinical and pathologic factors associated with a low incidence of lymph node metastases. Tumor size [relative risk (RR), 4.8; 95% CI, 4.0 to 5.5], depth of invasion (RR, 3.4; 95% CI, 2.9 to 4.0), and the presence of venous invasion (RR, 3.3; 95% CI, 2.8 to 3.8) were all independently associated with having positive nodes. However, of the 47 tumors smaller than 4.5 cm in size and limited to the mucosa only, 4% had lymph node metastases. Kurihara et al.[153] found that when submucosal carcinomas were classified into three categories according to depth of invasion by dividing the submucosal (sm) layer into three equal parts—sm1, sm2, and sm3—the incidence of lymph node metastasis increased from 2% to 12% and 20%, respectively. With the availability of EUS and mucosal strip biopsy techniques such as endoscopic mucosal resection, informed decisions can be made regarding the risk of lymph node metastases and need for lymphadenectomy. The approach to early gastric cancer is evolving into one of selective management. The favorable long-term results of endoscopic mucosal resection suggest that lymphadenectomy is not needed in properly selected cases.[134]

For advanced cancers, considerable debate continues as to whether the routine use of an extensive *en bloc* resection of second-echelon lymph nodes (D2 resection) is superior to a more limited lymphadenectomy of the perigastric lymph nodes (D1 resection). Four prospective randomized trials have now been completed on this subject. Dent et al.[154] reported the first prospective randomized trial of D1 versus D2 gastrectomy from Cape Town, South Africa (Table 33.3-9). At surgery, only 43 patients of 403 explored were randomized to receive either D2 or D1 gastrectomy. They found no difference in 5-year survival rates.[155] Patients undergoing D2 resection had a significantly longer operating time, greater transfusion requirement, and longer hospital stay. A second single-institution, prospective, randomized trial comparing D1 subtotal gastrectomy to D3 total gastrectomy (omentectomy, splenectomy, distal pancreatectomy, lymphadenectomy of celiac axis, and porta hepatis) in 55 patients with antral cancer was reported from Hong Kong.[156] The length of hospitalization and morbidity was significantly increased in the D3 group. Median survival was significantly shorter than for D1 resection patients. In Japan and in specialty centers in the West, however, where extended D2 resection is performed routinely, operative mortality is minimal and does not appear to be related to the extent of lymphadenectomy.[117,157,158] Given the small sample sizes, these trials lacked the statistical power needed for meaningful interpretation of survival results.

In 1989, two major randomized trials were conducted to further address the D2 controversy. In the United Kingdom, the Medical Research Council (MRC) conducted a trial that accrued 737 patients, with 400 patients randomized into two equal arms at the time of laparotomy. Postoperative morbidity was significantly greater in the D2 group (46% vs. 28%; $P < .001$). Hospital mortality was an alarming 13% for the D2 group and 6% for D1 ($P < .04$; 95% CI for D2, 4% to 11%).[159] The excess morbidity and mortality seen in the D2 group was associated with the routine use of distal pancreatectomy and splenectomy, which proponents of the D2 lymphadenectomy would point out is not required for adequate lymph node clearance. In a follow-up publication, Cuschieri et al.[160] reported that the 5-year survival rates were 35% for D1 resection and 33% for D2 resection (difference, –2%; 95% CI, –12% to 8%). Both overall and recurrence-free survival were the same. The authors concluded that their findings indicated that the classic Japanese D2 lymphadenectomy offered no survival advantage over the D1. The question of whether D2 resection without pancreaticosplenectomy is better than standard D1 resection could not be dismissed by the results of this trial.

The Dutch Gastric Cancer Group conducted a subsequent larger and rigorously monitored trial. In this study, 996 patients were entered and 711 were randomized (380 in the D1 group and 331 in the D2 group). In an effort to assure quality control, all operations were monitored. Initially, this oversight was done by a Japanese surgeon who trained a group of Dutch surgeons who, in turn, acted as supervisors during surgery at any one of the 80 participating centers. A number of observations were made from this trial. Despite the extraordinary efforts made to ensure quality control of the two types of lymph node dissection, both noncompliance (not removing all lymph node stations) and contamination (removing more than was indicated) occurred, thus blurring the distinction between the two operations.[161] The postoperative morbidity was again higher in the D2 group (43% vs. 25%, $P < .001$). The mortality rate also was significantly higher in the D2 group (10% vs. 4%, $P = .004$), and these patients required a longer hospitaliza-

TABLE 33.3-9. Prospective Randomized Trial Comparing D1 versus D2–3 Resection for Potentially Curable Gastric Carcinoma

	Extent of Lymphadenectomy		
	D1	D2	*P Value*
Groote Schuur Hospital, Cape Town			
Number of patients	22	21	—
Length of operation (hr)	1.7 ± 0.6	2.33 ± 0.7	<.005
Transfusions (units/group)	4	25	<.05
Postoperative stay (d)	9.3 ± 4.7	13.9 ± 9.7	<.05
5-Y survival (log rank test)	0.69	0.67	NS
Prince of Wales Hospital, Hong Kong			
Number of patients	25	29	—
Length of operation (hr)	140	260	<.05
Operative blood loss (mL)	300	600	<.05
Postoperative stay	8	16	<.05
Median survival (d)	1511	922	<.05
Medical Research Council Trial, United Kingdom			
Number of patients	200	200	—
Operative mortality (%)	6.5	13	<.04
Postoperative complications (%)	28	46	<.001
5-Y survival (%)	35	33	NS
Dutch Gastric Cancer Trial, The Netherlands			
Number of patients	380	331	—
Operative mortality rate (%)	4	10	.004
Postoperative complications (%)	25	43	<.001
Postoperative stay (d)	18	25	<.001
5-Y survival (%)	42	47	NS

NS, not stated.

tion.[162] Pancreaticosplenectomy also was performed *en passant* in the D2 group as part of the classic operation.

In summary, the D2 operation is a systematic approach toward the removal of high-risk perigastric lymph nodes. Most retrospective single-center reports indicate that the routine use of extended lymphadenectomy for potentially curable gastric cancer can be performed safely. Four published prospective randomized trials have not shown a survival advantage for the D2 lymph node dissection and do not support the routine use of extended D2 gastrectomy. A modified D2 operation avoiding pancreaticosplenectomy will provide superior staging information and may avoid the added morbidity and mortality associated with the additional organ resection. The advanced stage of disease at surgery in most patients remains the key determinant of survival. If there is a survival benefit from the D2 lymphadenectomy, it is limited to those with few lymph node metastases.

Total versus Subtotal Gastrectomy

Ideally, the extent of gastric resection should provide the optimal cancer procedure with the minimal attendant morbidity. The rationale for the routine use of total gastrectomy is presumably based on the appreciation that extensive intramural extension of tumor may be present and that simultaneous multiple gastric cancers have been reported.[163] Although older retrospective data do suggest that survival is improved with total gastrectomy compared with subtotal gastrectomy,[81] current evidence does not support this finding.[164] Three prospective randomized trials have addressed this question for the treatment of distal gastric cancers.[156,164,165] A French cooperative prospectively randomized trial of total gastrectomy versus subtotal gastrectomy has reported data on postoperative morbidity, mortality, and 5-year survival. One hundred sixty-nine patients with adenocarcinoma of the antrum who were operated on with curative intent were included for analysis.[164] The groups were well matched for the usual prognostic variables. The overall complication rate and postoperative mortality rate was 32% and 1.3% for total gastrectomy and 34% and 3.2% for subtotal gastrectomy, respectively. No difference was found in cumulative 5-year survival between groups. The second single institution prospective randomized trial, as reported above in the Extended Lymphadenectomy section, compared subtotal gastrectomy and D1 lymphadenectomy with total gastrectomy and D3 lymphadenectomy in 55 patients with antral cancers from Hong Kong.[156] No survival advantage was found after the more extensive resection. Bozzetti et al.[166] reported the 5-year survival rates from a multicenter randomized Italian trial conducted by the Italian Gastrointestinal Tumor Study Group. The median follow-up was 72 months after subtotal gastrectomy (range, 2 to 125 months) and 75 months after total gastrectomy (range, 7 to 113 months). The 5-year survival rate was 65.3% after subtotal gastrectomy and 62.4% after total gastrectomy for gastric cancer. The data support the use of subtotal gastrectomy for the treatment of advanced distal tumors, provided a 5-cm gross negative margin can be achieved.

Other series have reported an operative mortality after total gastrectomy, ranging from 4% to 18%, and that anastomotic leak is responsible for up to 50% of these operative deaths.[167–169] Others have argued that the functional results after total gastrectomy may be slightly worse than with distal subtotal gastrectomy.[170–172] Moreover, the ability to completely dissect paracardial lymph nodes is not related to the extent of gastric resection.[173] Therefore, although routinely used by many, total gastrectomy should not be considered the initial option in patients in whom a 5-cm gross proximal margin can be obtained with a subtotal resection.

Carcinomas arising in the proximal one-third of the stomach have a worse prognosis than distal gastric lesions.[24,25,121] Total gastrectomy has traditionally been the procedure of choice for proximal tumors. Review of the prospective gastric database at Memorial Sloan-Kettering Cancer Center from July 1985 to August 1995 identified 391 patients with proximal gastric cancers. Ninety-eight of these patients underwent either a total or proximal gastrectomy exclusively through an abdominal approach. Patients undergoing esophagogastrectomy were excluded. Patients were matched for clinical and pathologic factors. The length of hospital stay was the same for patients undergoing resection for proximal gastrectomy (16.5 days; range, 8 to 55 days) and for total gastrectomy (18 days; range, 8 to 48). Postoperative mortality for proximal gastrectomy (6.0%) and total gastrectomy (3.0%) were not significantly different. The overall 5-year survival rate for proximal gastric cancer was 43% and was 41% for total gastrectomy. Total and proximal gastrectomy have similar time to first recurrence, and the pattern of recurrence was the same. As was found for distal tumors, the extent of resection for proximal gastric cancer does not affect long-term outcome.

The functional sequelae and postoperative mortality of proximal gastric resection are considered to be worse than for total gastrectomy. In a series of 89 patients reported by Buhl and associates[174] who were treated with total gastrectomy, distal gastric resection, or proximal gastric resection, the latter group had a higher incidence of dumping, heartburn, and reduced appetite. In addition, quality of life and capacity to work were reduced in patients with proximal gastric resection. The Norwegian Stomach Cancer Trial has prospectively studied the incidence of postoperative complications and mortality in more than 1000 consecutive patients undergoing surgery for gastric cancer.[175] The postoperative mortality rate in more than 760 patients undergoing resection was 8.3% and was highest in patients undergoing proximal resection (16%) compared with total gastrectomy (8%), subtotal gastrectomy (10%), or distal resection (7%). Factors significantly related to the incidence of postoperative complications included advancing age, male gender, no antibiotic prophylaxis, and splenectomy. Similar to the postoperative mortality, the complication rate was highest for proximal resections (52%), followed by total gastrectomy (38%), subtotal resection (28%), and distal resection (19%). Therefore, for proximal lesions, it appears that total gastrectomy using a variety of reconstructive options may provide better functional results, but this observation has not been tested in a prospective randomized fashion.[175a] There appear to be fewer complications and a lower operative mortality after total gastrectomy for the treatment of proximal gastric cancers.

Prophylactic Splenectomy

Several authors have critically evaluated the value of routine splenectomy during gastric resection for tumors not adjacent to or invading the spleen.[175–180] In a multivariate analysis of more than 250 patients who underwent total gastrectomy with curative intent, no correlation was found between splenectomy and survival.[177] The Norwegian Stomach Cancer Trial has demonstrated a higher complication rate with the use of splenectomy in their prospective trial (42% vs. 27%).[175] In Sasako's analysis of potential risk factors in patients from the Dutch multicenter randomized study of D1 versus D2 lymphadenectomy, splenectomy was the most important risk factor for developing a complication (RR, 2.13; 95% CI, 1.44 to 3.16).[175b] The consensus from the literature is that prophylactic splenectomy increases morbidity and mortality without an apparent survival benefit.[177,179–182]

TECHNIQUE OF OPERATION

Beginning with laparoscopy allows for careful intraoperative staging of disease. Inspection for the presence of ascites; hepatic metastases; peritoneal seeding; disease in the pelvis, such as a "drop" metastasis; or ovarian involvement should be performed. Once distant metastases have been ruled out depending on the location of the lesion, a bilateral subcostal incision or a midline abdominal incision can be used to gain adequate exposure to the upper abdomen. The stomach should be inspected to assess the location and extent of tumor. The size and location of the primary tumor dictates the extent of gastric resection. A D2 lymphadenectomy sparing the spleen and pancreas can be done safely and provides an excellent specimen for surgical and pathologic staging, but this procedure should only be performed by or with an experienced surgeon.

The D2 subtotal gastrectomy commences with mobilization of the greater omentum from the transverse colon. After the omentum is mobilized, the anterior peritoneal leaf of the transverse mesocolon is incised along the lower border of the colon, and a plane is developed down to the head of the pancreas. The infrapyloric lymph nodes are dissected, and the origin of the right gastroepiploic artery and vein are ligated. With a combination of blunt and sharp dissection, the plane of dissection continues on to the anterior surface of the pancreas, extending to the level of the common hepatic and splenic arteries. This maneuver can be tedious, but theoretically it provides additional protection against serosal spread of tumor to the local peritoneal surface.

The right gastric artery is ligated. At this point, the duodenum is divided distal to the pylorus. The stomach and omentum are then reflected cephalad. The gastrohepatic ligament is divided close to the liver up to the gastroesophageal junction. Dissection is then continued on the hepatic artery toward the celiac axis. Once near the celiac axis, the lymph node–bearing tissue is dissected until the left gastric artery is visualized and can be divided at its origin. The proximal peritoneal attachments of the stomach and distal esophagus can then be incised, and the proximal extent of resection is chosen.

For tumors of the mid- and proximal stomach, dissection of the lymph nodes along the splenic artery and splenic hilum is important. This technique is not indicated for antral tumors, given the low rate of splenic hilar nodal metastases seen with these tumors. The stomach is then divided 5 cm proximal to the tumor, which dictates the extent of gastric resection. Despite the fact that the entire blood supply of the stomach has been interrupted, a cuff of proximal stomach invariably shows good vascularization from the feeding distal esophageal arcade. When feasible, most surgeons prefer to anastomose jejunum to stomach versus esophagus because of the technical ease and excellent healing. Reconstruction using a variety of techniques has been described and is a matter of personal choice (Fig. 33.3-7).

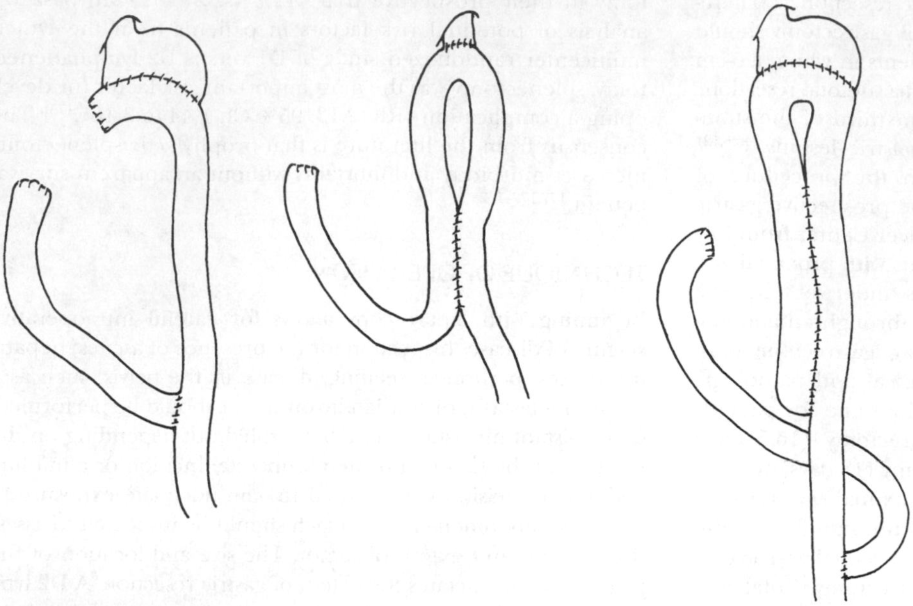

FIGURE 33.3-7. Variations in types of reconstruction after total or subtotal gastrectomy include (*left to right*) the Roux-en-Y, Braun, and Lawrence techniques.

ADJUVANT THERAPY

RATIONALE FOR ADJUVANT THERAPY

As already mentioned, the prognosis for patients with gastric cancer is, to a large extent, dependent on the stage of the disease at the time of diagnosis. Patients with early-stage gastric cancer (Tis; T1N0M0; or shallow penetrating T2N0M0) have a good to excellent prognosis, with cure rates exceeding 70% to 80% after operation alone. After curative surgery, however, patients with locally advanced cancers without nodal metastases (T3N0 gastric cancers) have an at least 50% chance of dying within 5 years; lymph node metastases have an even more ominous prognosis. Although 80% to 90% of American patients fall in the high-risk group, preoperative identification of patients at low risk for recurrence is difficult. Newer preoperative staging techniques, such as laparoscopy, have been demonstrated to be highly sensitive and specific in identifying patients with intraabdominal metastatic tumor, particularly in the peritoneal cavity. However, these techniques still have a relatively low sensitivity for separating deeply penetrating T2 from T3 tumors, as well as a low sensitivity for identifying metastatic lymphadenopathy. Therefore, for patients who have more than early-stage gastric cancer (deeply penetrating T2 or T3 tumors and patients with lymph node metastasis), the use of systemic therapy early in the treatment plan is rational in a disease in which a high propensity is seen for systemic failure with or without local recurrence. Neoadjuvant chemotherapy (also known as *preoperative* or *primary chemotherapy*) is an attractive concept in diseases such as gastric cancer for which complete resection of the primary tumor is often difficult or impossible, and because systemic dissemination at the time of diagnosis is common. A more traditional approach to adjuvant therapy is the use of postoperative treatment.

POSTOPERATIVE TREATMENT

Table 33.3-10 summarizes the results of a number of prospective randomized trials of postoperative chemotherapy in gastric cancer. These studies date back to the 1960s. Two early trials from the Veterans Administration Surgical Oncology Group investigated the use of thiotepa or 5-fluorodeoxyuridine (FUDR) after surgical resection.[183,184] Both were negative.

Nitrosourea-Containing Regimens

Four studies have used a combination of 5-fluorouracil (5-FU) and the nitrosourea methyl chloroethylcyclohexylnitrosourea (CCNU) as adjuvant therapy after gastric resection. It should be noted that, in advanced disease, 5-FU and methyl CCNU had only modest effectiveness, and this combination was an inferior arm in a randomized trial in patients with advanced disease (see Table 33.3-10). The Gastrointestinal Tumor Study Group randomly assigned patients to either no additional treatment or to 18 months (originally 2 years) of methyl CCNU and 5-FU.[185] At a final analysis, the survival curves reached statistical significance in favor of the chemotherapy arm. However, an identical study using 5-FU and methyl CCNU performed during the same period by the Eastern Cooperative Oncology Group using the same dose and schedule and including a group of 180 patients (89 controls, 91 treated) demonstrated no difference in disease-free or overall survival rate (median survival, 32.7 and 36.6 months; 2-year survival rate, 57% for both groups)[186] (see Table 33.3-10). A third study by the Veterans Administration Surgical Oncology Group using the same agents on a different schedule was also negative.[187]

Estrada and colleagues[188] studied the use of 12 to 18 months of methyl CCNU, 5-FU, and doxorubicin or observation in a small group of 66 evaluable patients after resection. At 5 years, no difference was noted in disease-free survival (29% treated vs. 34% observed) or overall survival (29% vs. 37%). Two treatment-related deaths were reported. Most current adjuvant or neoadjuvant studies do not include a nitrosourea.

Mitomycin-Containing Regimens

A series of trials have involved the use of mitomycin (see Table 33.3-10). One Spanish trial investigated the use of high-dose mitomycin C alone after surgical resection. In this study, only 33 patients received chemotherapy; 37 patients were in a control group. A striking difference in survival was noted (seven

TABLE 33.3-10. Intravenous Adjuvant Therapy for Gastric Cancer: Selected Phase III Trials

Study	*Regimen*	*Patients*	*Median Survival*	*5-Y Survival (%) Rate*	*P Value*
GITSG[311]	Methyl CCNU–FU	71	56 mo	50	.06
	Control	71	33 mo	31	
ECOG	Methyl CCNU–FU	91	33 mo	57	.73
	Control	89	37 mo	57	
VASOG	Methyl CCNU–FU	66	2.1 y	39	.88
	Control	68	2.1 y	38	
Estape	Mitomycin C	33	Not reached	76	<.001
	Control	37	12 mo	30	
Carrato et al.[191]	Mitomycin C–UFT	69	2.3 y	NS	NS
	Control	75	2.6 y	NS	
Allum et al.[192]	Mitomycin C–FU	141	16 mo	28	.98
	Mitomycin C–FU-CMFV	140	16 mo	10	
	Control	130	15 mo	18	
Nakajima et al.[193]	Mitomycin C–FU-araC	81	>5 y	68	.09
	Mitomycin C–UFT-araC	83	>5 y	63	
	Control	79	>5 y	51	
MacDonald[197]	FAM	83	32 mo	NS	.52
	Control	93	28 mo	NS	
Coombes et al.[196]	FAM	133	36 mo	46	.17
	Control	130	15 mo	18	
Krook et al.[198]	FA	61	36 mo	32	.88
	Control	64	34 mo	33	
Nakajima et al.[194]	Mitomycin C–FU-UFT	288	>5 y	86	.17
	Control	285	>5 y	83	
Italian GITSG[312]	Control	69	NS	~50	.9
	MaCCNU-FU	75	NS	~50	
	MaCCNU-FU-levamisole	69	NS	~50	
Neri et al.[199]	Control	55	13.9 mo	13	.01
	FU-leucovorin-epirubicin	48	20.4 mo	25	
Hallissey et al.[246]	Control	145	14.7	20	.14
	RT, 4500 cGy	153	12.9	12	
	FAM	138	17.3	19	
EORTC	Control	159	NS	~43	.3
	FAM	155	NS	~43	
MacDonald[197]	Control	100	NS	31	.45
	FAM	93	NS	33	
Grau	Control	66	NS	26	.025
	Mitomycin	68	NS	41	
Tsavaris et al.[200]	FU-epirubicin-mitomycin	42	NS	64	NS
	Control	42	NS	81	

araC, arabinosylcytosine (cytarabine); CCNU, chloroethylcyclohexylnitrosourea; CMFV, cyclophosphamide, methotrexate, fluorouracil, vincristine; ECOG, Eastern Cooperative Oncology Group; EORTC, European Organization for Research and Treatment of Cancer; FAM, fluorouracil, doxorubicin (Adriamycin), and mitomycin; FU, fluorouracil; GITSG, Gastrointestinal Tumor Study Group; NS, not stated; RT, radiation therapy; UFT, uracil and ftorafur; VASOG, Veterans Administration Surgical Oncology Group.

relapses in the treatment arm, 23 in the control arm; $P<.001$). The chemotherapy dose schedule was mitomycin C, 20 mg/m^2 once every 6 weeks for four doses. An update continues to show a significant survival advantage for the mitomycin-treated group.[189] However, this study has not been confirmed by other mitomycin-containing trials.

In a larger study,[190] evaluable patients were randomized after gastrectomy to receive (within 7 days of surgery) mitomycin C, 10 mg/m^2 monthly for six doses, plus oral uracil and ftorafur (UFT) or to expectant observation. With a median follow-up of 3.1 years, no difference was noted in disease-free or overall survival between treatment and control groups (median survival for patients receiving chemotherapy, 2.3 years; for observation, 2.6 years). This study does not confirm the role of mitomycin C in the adjuvant setting. However, although the total dose was similar (80 mg/m^2 vs. 60 mg/m^2), the dose intensity was different.[191] Allum and coworkers[192] reported the results of a three-arm randomized trial comparing postoperative 5-FU and mitomycin C with or without cyclophosphamide, 5-FU, vincristine, and methotrexate induction compared with surgery only. The study allowed entrance up to 12 weeks after surgery. The surgery-only group received saline every 3 weeks; 140 patients received 5-FU and mitomycin C plus a 5-day induction course of cyclophosphamide, 5-FU, vincristine, and methotrexate; 141 patients received 5-FU and mitomycin C alone. Therapy was continued for 2 years. With a median follow-up of 100 months, the median survival was 15.5 months; no significant difference was noted between the treated or control groups.

Japanese studies involving mitomycin also have been reported. Nakajima et al.[193] treated a group of 243 patients who received either mitomycin C, 5-FU, plus cytosine arabinoside or a similar regimen in which 5-FU was replaced by ftorafur, with the control patients having surgery only. No statistical differences in survival were seen at 5 years, although 5-year survival for the chemotherapy patients was somewhat better than for the control group ($P = .09$). Subgroup analyses indicated significant differences in survival for those with earlier stage disease (stages I and II), but these were retrospective and unplanned. More recently, Nakajima and colleagues[194] have reported the results of another, larger trial performed in Japan. Five hundred seventy-nine patients with early-stage gastric cancer (T1 or T2 lesions) were stratified and randomized to receive postoperative chemotherapy or observation. The treatment plan involved mitomycin C, 1.4 mg/m^2, twice weekly for 3 weeks after surgery in conjunction with FU, 167.7 mg/m^2, also given twice weekly for 3 weeks. This was followed by 18 months of oral UFT given 300 mg daily. The primary end point was survival. Two hundred eighty-eight patients received treatment and 285 were followed expectantly. Slightly more than one-half of the patients had lymph node–negative tumors. With a median follow-up of 72 months, the overall 5-year survival rate was 82.9% for those in the control group and 85.8% for those in the treatment group ($P = .17$; hazard ratio, 0.738). The authors of this study concluded that this regimen has no survival benefit in patients with serosa-negative, surgically resected gastric cancer.

A preliminary report in patients with advanced gastric cancer has compared a cisplatin, epirubicin, and FU combination to a combination of mitomycin, epirubicin, and FU. Although the initial report indicated an advantage to the mitomycin-containing arm, at the presentation itself no advantage was reported.[195] Most current adjuvant or neoadjuvant studies do not include mitomycin.

Anthracycline-Containing Regimens

The uses of several doxorubicin-containing combination chemotherapy adjuvant regimens have been reported (see Table 33.3-10). Coombes and colleagues[196] studied 315 patients with curatively resected gastric cancer who were randomized to receive FU, doxorubicin (Adriamycin), and mitomycin (FAM) or no postoperative therapy. Two hundred eighty-one patients were evaluable for analysis. Chemotherapy could be started as late as 6 weeks from surgery. Twenty-six percent of patients in the control arm had N2 disease versus 18% in the treated group, but this difference was not statistically significant. With a median follow-up of 68 months, 56% of patients in the treated arm and 61% of those in the control arm had a recurrence in disease. No significant difference was reported in disease-free survival or overall survival (FAM, 45.7%; control, 35.4%). A number of subgroup analyses were performed, the most positive of which was an effect for patients with T3 or T4 tumors who had positive lymph nodes ($P = .07$ in favor of the FAM group). This, however, was an unplanned subgroup analysis. Three FAM patients died from suspected treatment-related complications. In a second FAM study, the Southwest Oncology Group also failed to note an improvement in survival for the treated group.[197] Both groups of investigators concluded that chemotherapy, including FAM, when given in the adjuvant setting, should be used only in an investigational setting.

Krook and colleagues[198] used a different doxorubicin-containing combination in the adjuvant setting. After curative resection, 125 evaluable patients were randomized to either observation alone or to three cycles of 5-FU, 250 mg/m^2/d, for 5 days plus doxorubicin, 40 mg/m^2, on day 1. Treatment began between 4 and 6 weeks after resection. No differences were noted in overall survival between the two groups (median survival of observation group, 31 months; treatment group, 36 months). The 5-year survival rate was almost identical (33% vs. 32%). Two treatment-related deaths, both related to sepsis during leukopenia, were reported.

The FU, doxorubicin (Adriamycin), and methotrexate (FAMTX) regimen has been extensively studied in patients with advanced metastatic disease, and in randomized trials it was superior to regimens such as FAM.[198] There is one random assignment trial from the Netherlands comparing neoadjuvant FAMTX to surgery alone. Fifty-six eligible and evaluable patients were entered: 27 were randomized to receive FAMTX before surgery and 29 to undergo surgery only. In the FAMTX plus surgery treatment group, 15 of 27 (56%) had curative resections versus 18 of 29 (62%) in the surgery-only arm. Forty-four percent of treated patients could not complete the planned four courses of FAMTX due to disease progression or toxicity. Response evaluation after chemotherapy was possible in 25 patients: two complete responses, six partial responses. The difference in curative resectability rate was 6.5% (95% confidence interval –32% to +19%) in favor of surgery only. The authors concluded that more active regimens than FAMTX will be required for future randomized trials.

Neri et al.[199] used a regimen containing epirubicin, FU, and leucovorin for patients with stage III disease. Chemotherapy was given for 7 months. Fifty-five patients were followed expectantly, and 48 received chemotherapy. The median survival rate for patients receiving therapy (20.4 months) was superior to those undergoing observation (13.6 months; $P = .01$). At an average of 36 months of follow-up, 25% of patients receiving adjuvant therapy were alive compared to 13% of those being followed expectantly. Although these results are encouraging, they are at odds with the study by Krook et al.[198] in a similar number of patients. Use of this regimen should still be considered experimental, and it requires a larger confirmatory trial.

Tsavaris et al.[200] performed a small randomized trial in which epirubicin was substituted for doxorubicin to create the FU, epirubicin, and mitomycin (FEM) regimen. Eighty-four patients were randomized to receive three cycles of FEM or no treatment. Recurrence or death occurred in 64% of patients receiving FEM versus 81% of the control group; however, this difference was not statistically significant.

Cisplatin-Containing Regimens

Although cisplatin-containing combinations have undergone extensive studies in patients with advanced metastatic disease, as discussed below (see Palliative Treatment of Gastric Cancer), currently no randomized trials are available in which patients with curative resections of gastric cancer were postoperatively and randomly assigned to receive or not receive a cisplatin-based regimen.

METAANALYSIS OF ADJUVANT CHEMOTHERAPY TRIALS

Earle and Maroun[201] presented the preliminary results of a metaanalysis involving 12 trials performed in Western countries. It was not clear that individual patient data was obtained. In this analysis, the crude odds ratio for death for patients receiving adjuvant therapy was 0.81 (0.67 to 0.98) with a relative risk of 0.94 (0.88 to 1.01). These authors concluded that the survival benefit from these trials in patients undergoing curative resections was small. In an earlier analysis, Hermans et al.[202] reviewed 11 trials reported since 1980. In these studies, surgery was followed by postoperative chemotherapy or by observation alone. A total of 2096 patients were studied. The odds ratio was 0.88 (0.78 to 1.08), which was not statistically significantly superior to observation alone. In a later brief report by the same authors, two additional trials were added to this database that indicated a slight benefit to postoperative adjuvant therapy.

In both cases, the metaanalysis performed involved a variety of chemotherapy regimens, most of which had FU in common. They were a review of the literature, rather than a pooled analysis of individual patient data. Furthermore, the number of patients involved is relatively small in comparison to the metaanalysis in breast cancer, for example. Gastric cancer overviews to date suggest a modest benefit for older chemotherapeutic regimens. Almost all of these trials are seriously handicapped by their statistical design: With a small number of patients accrued, only very large differences could be expected to show a statistical benefit. Particularly as newer, potentially more effective chemotherapy regimens are developed, a high priority should be placed on designing trials that have adequate numbers of patients who are carefully staged so that the trials have appropriate power to allow an assessment of benefit.

INTRAPERITONEAL CHEMOTHERAPY

The rationale for the use of intraperitoneal therapy after resection of primary gastric cancer is based on the high risk of peritoneal metastasis as a component of first failure. Autopsy series and second-look laparotomy series have reported that up to 50% of patients have clinically evident peritoneal carcinomatosis as a site (sometimes the only site) of failure. The pharmacokinetic rationale for intraperitoneal therapy has been well described. Drug concentrations within the peritoneal cavity are severalfold to one to two logs higher than concentrations that can be achieved after oral or intravenous treatment. Clinical support for the use of intraperitoneal chemotherapy also comes from other tumors. For example, a decrease of all sites of failure in patients receiving adjuvant colon cancer treatment using intravenous FU plus oral levamisole was reported; the only exception was peritoneal recurrence. In ovarian cancer, a large randomized trial demonstrated a small but statistical and clinically significant survival advantage for women receiving a portion of their therapy intraperitoneally. Thus, as is the case for many abdominal malignancies, a strong rationale exists for maximizing the effectiveness of currently available antineoplastic agents by using intraperitoneal treatment as a portion of the adjuvant therapy.

During the 1990s, an increasing number of reports have summarized data on the use of immediate postoperative intraperitoneal therapy for patients with gastric cancer. Interpretation of this data is hampered, however, by the retrospective nature of some of these trials. In addition, most prospective studies are pilot or phase II, involving small numbers of patients and testing feasibility. Last, even the small number of phase III trials reported to date are severely underpowered, making definitive conclusions regarding the use of intraperitoneal therapy, at this point, impossible. Table 33.3-11 lists selected reports involving intraperitoneal chemotherapy given as adjuvant treatment in the postoperative setting. Although the database is limited, several themes are clear. The technique most commonly used is to administer intraperitoneal treatment (with or without hyperthermia) at the end of resection of all gross disease. Intraperitoneal chemotherapy is delivered in the operating room or recovery room or, at the latest, within several days of resection. In the latter case, this involves placement of an intraperitoneal catheter with therapy started soon after operation and given for repeated courses. No randomized comparative studies of the two techniques are available. The theoretical advantage of immediate intraoperative treatment is better distribution, whereas the theoretical advantage of intraperitoneal therapy via an implanted catheter is the ability to give repeated courses. Both techniques also have been used with established peritoneal carcinomatosis, but it is even harder to draw conclusions regarding this patient population. A fluorinated pyrimidine (FU or FUDR) or mitomycin C is usually part of the treatment plan.

In preclinical studies, Archer and Grey[203] used a rat model to demonstrate that intraperitoneal chemotherapy is capable of treating both peritoneal and liver micrometastasis. In a second study, Murthy and coworkers[204] demonstrated in a mouse model that the frequency of tumor formation at sites of surgical trauma in the peritoneum ranged from 28% to 82%, depending on the type of incisions made in the peritoneal cavity, as

TABLE 33.3-11. Intraperitoneal Therapy for Gastric Cancer: Phase III Trials

Study	*Regimen*	*Number of Patients*	*Median Survival*	*2-Y Survival Rate (%)*	*P Value*
Hajiwara et al.[308]	Mitomycin C	24	>3 y	69	.01
	Control	25	1.2 y	27	
Rosen et al.[208]	Mitomycin C	46	738 d	NS	.44
	Control	45	515 d	NS	
Schiessel et al.[309]	Cisplatin	31	15 mo	38	NS
	Control	33	12 mo	36	
Sautner et al.[185]	Cisplatin	33	17	33	.6
	Control	34	16	30	
Yu et al.[211]	Mitomycin-FU	125	NS	38.7[a]	.2
	Control	123	NS	29.3[a]	

FU, fluorouracil; NS, not stated.
[a]Five-year survival.

opposed to a 33% rate of peritoneal tumors in nonoperated mice. Data from several animal models indicate that the risks of peritoneal implantation and intraabdominal tumor spread immediately after laparotomy are high.[205,206] Clinically, a randomized trial in colon cancer by Sugarbaker and colleagues[207] demonstrated a marked decrease in peritoneal metastasis with intraperitoneal chemotherapy when compared with intravenous treatment, but showed no change in survival.

During the late 1980s and early 1990s, one of the most extensively used intraperitoneal agents in gastric cancer was mitomycin C. As is the case for all intraperitoneal therapy in gastric cancer, however, the small number patients involved hamper interpretation of this data. The initial promising study of Hajiwara and colleagues[308] indicated a marked improvement in survival for patients randomized to intraperitoneal therapy compared to those receiving no postoperative treatment. Mitomycin was adsorbed to a carbon-containing solution and infused immediately after the end of the operative procedure. In this study, 24 patients received treatment with mitomycin and 25 were observed after operation. A highly significant difference in favor of the intraperitoneally treated group was found (2-year survival, 68.6% vs. 26.9%; the difference was maintained at 3 years). This study sparked a number of reports, some of which are included in Table 33.3-11. Retrospective reviews using higher-dose mitomycin with or without activated charcoal raised concerns regarding toxicity, with some studies indicating a high risk of intraabdominal toxicity leading to an increase in perioperative mortality. To more definitively test the hypothesis that intraperitoneal mitomycin offered benefit, Rosen and colleagues[208] reported their results using a similar technique. Ninety-one patients were randomly assigned to resection followed by observation or resection followed by carbon-adsorbed mitomycin C, 50 mg, given intraperitoneally. The study was stopped prematurely when an interim analysis revealed a marked increase in postoperative complications (25% vs. 16%) and an increased perioperative mortality (11% for patients receiving intraperitoneal therapy vs. 2% for the control arm). No survival advantage was noted at the time of the interim analysis, and the trial was closed. This randomized trial, plus the phase II and retrospective data, indicate that intraperitoneal mitomycin C, particularly in higher dosages of 25 to 50 mg, given with or without activated charcoal and with or without hyperthermia may be associated with a marked increase in toxicity with only questionable improvement in survival.

Regimens that do not contain mitomycin C also have been studied. These primarily involve the use of fluorinated pyrimidines (either FU or floxuridine), usually given with leucovorin or other agents (e.g., cisplatin) or both. Mitomycin in lower doses also has been used with FU. Phase II studies performed in the United States at single institutions by Crookes et al.[209] and Atiq et al.[210] indicated that postoperative intraperitoneal therapy using fluorinated pyrimidines could be given with safety. However, unusual toxicity has occasionally been noted. Atiq and colleagues[210] from Memorial Sloan-Kettering Cancer Center reported the results of a phase II study involving intraperitoneal cisplatin and FU plus systemic FU in high-risk patients having undergone potentially curative resections with gastric cancer. Thirty-five patients (most with stage IIIA or IIIB tumors) received intraperitoneal cisplatin, 25 mg/m^2, on days 1 to 4 and FU, 750 mg/m^2, as a single dose. Each drug was given daily for 4 days in a row for up to five cycles on a once a month basis. FU systemically as a continuous 24-hour infusion was given simultaneously. With a median follow-up of 24 months, 51% of patients remained alive and free of disease. Toxicity was acceptable. An unusual side effect of sclerosing encapsulating peritonitis was noted in 15% of patients. Further investigation revealed that solutions containing FU had a pH of greater than 8.5. The authors speculated that this resulted in hydrolysis of cisplatin to a reactive alkylating species. To avoid further sclerosing encapsulating peritonitis, the authors subsequently avoided mixing cisplatin and FU together before administration. No further episodes of sclerosing encapsulating peritonitis were seen. In a further update of this trial with a minimum follow-up of 42 months, 40% of patients remain alive and free of disease.

Yu et al.[211] reported the results of a randomized trial in which 248 patients were randomly assigned to receive intraperitoneal therapy or to observation. Patients receiving intraperitoneal chemotherapy were given mitomycin C on postoperative day 1 and FU on postoperative days 2 to 5. The study included patients with all stages of disease (I to IV). As is the case in other mitomycin-containing trials, morbidity and mortality were higher in the experimental arm (postoperative mortality, 5.6% vs. 0.8%). No statistical difference was noted in overall survival for the investigation arm (38.7% vs. 29.3%; $P = .219$), although an unplanned subset analysis showed a benefit for patients with stage II or III disease.

Similarly, Sautner and colleagues[185] performed a small, randomized phase III trial using intraperitoneal cisplatin as a single agent. Cisplatin, 90 mg/m^2, was given intraperitoneally once a month. Therapy began 2 to 4 weeks after surgery. This study also allowed entrance of patients with documented peritoneal metastasis so that not all those treated were in the adjuvant setting. No difference was reported in survival for patients receiving or not receiving additional treatment. The authors concluded that intraperitoneal cisplatin as a single agent had no significant impact on recurrence.

CONTINUOUS HYPERTHERMIC PERITONEAL PERFUSION

Continuous hyperthermic peritoneal perfusion (CHPP) for the treatment or prophylaxis of peritoneal carcinomatosis usually is administered during exploratory laparotomy after a primary tumor resection in patients who have established carcinomatosis or who are considered at high risk for developing peritoneal disease. CHPP takes advantage of the favorable pharmacokinetics that can be achieved with intraperitoneal chemotherapy[212] and the established synergistic cytotoxicity of hyperthermia and chemotherapy.[213,214]

Most of the initial clinical experiences came from Japanese investigators who administered CHPP to patients in whom peritoneal seeding was identified at the time of gastric resection for cancer.[215–218] The therapeutic agent administered into the perfusate was usually mitomycin C (10 mg/mL). Steady-state concentrations of mitomycin C were approximately tenfold higher in the perfusate compared with serum. With the significant hyperthermia, a mild increase in hepatic transaminases was noted after treatment. However, the studies did confirm that CHPP could be safely administered after a major extirpative procedure.

Fujimoto and coworkers[219] and Gilly and colleagues[220] reported that malignant ascites could be palliated effectively with CHPP. Fujimoto's group reported that five of six patients with malignant ascites secondary to recurrent gastrointestinal cancer had resolution of the ascites after undergoing tumor

TABLE 33.3-12. Clinical Results of Multiarm Studies Evaluating the Efficiency of Prophylactic or Therapeutic Continuous Hyperthermic Peritoneal Perfusion (CHPP) after Resection for Gastric Cancer

Study	*Number of Patients*	*Treatment Arm*	*Agents*	*Dose*	*Duration (min)*	*Temperature (°C)*	*Follow-Up (y)*	*Survival Rate (%)*	*P Value*
Koga et al.[221]	26	CHPP	Mitomycin C	8–10 mg/L	60	44–45	2.5	83	NS
	21	Control	—	—	—	—		67	
Koga	38	CHPP	Mitomycin C	8–10 mg/L	60	44–45	3	74	<.04
	55	Control[a]	—	—	—	—		53	
Fujimoto et al.[222]	30	CHPP	Mitomycin C	10 mg/L	120	45–47	1	80	<.001
	29	Control	—	—	—	—		34	
Fujimura et al.[218]	22	CHPP	Mitomycin C	30 mg	60	41–42	3	68	<.01[b]
	18	CNPP[c]	Cisplatin	300 mg	60	37–38		51	
	18	Control	—	—	—	—		23	
Hamazoe et al.[223]	42	CHPP	Mitomycin C	10 mg/L	60	48–50	5	64	NS
	40	Control	—	—	—	—		53	

CNPP, continuous normothermic peritoneal perfusion; NS, not significant.
[a]Historical control group.
[b]CHPP or CNPP versus control.
[c]Continuous normothermic peritoneal perfusion.

resection and CHPP; all five patients were without evidence of recurrent disease at a mean follow-up of 12.8 ± 5 months. Gilly's group reported that nine of ten patients had no evidence of recurrent ascites on ultrasound obtained 2 months after CHPP. Fujimura and colleagues[218] treated 31 patients with peritoneal carcinomatosis secondary to recurrent gastric cancer with cisplatin and mitomycin C administered via CHPP. In 12 of 31 patients who underwent a second-look operation, four had a complete response and one had a partial response to treatment. However, it is important to appreciate that CHPP is only effective in treating small-volume peritoneal disease. Yonemura and coworkers[216] introduced CHPP with 30 mg mitomycin C and 300 mg cisplatin as prophylactic treatment for peritoneal recurrence after curative resection of 79 advanced gastric cancers. Survival was compared to that of 81 patients treated during the same period. Prolonged survival was reported in the subgroup of patients with tumors that penetrated the serosa. No increase in morbidity or mortality was reported between the two groups.[216]

Several multiarm studies have evaluated the efficacy of prophylactic or therapeutic CHPP administered immediately after resection for gastric cancer reported primarily from centers in Japan[218,221] (Table 33.3-12). In a report by Koga and coworkers[221] of a subset of 47 patients who had histopathologic evidence of serosal invasion, the 3-year survival rate in the CHPP-treated group was better than in the control group, but not significantly. In the same study, a larger CHPP-treated cohort did have a significantly better 5-year survival rate compared with historically matched controls. In patients who underwent major gastric resection, the incidence of an anastomotic leak or the length of postoperative ileus was affected by CHPP treatment. Fujimoto and colleagues[222] reported that overall survival was significantly longer in patients treated with CHPP; in the subgroup analysis, the beneficial effect was observed in patients with and without documented peritoneal seeding. Peritoneal disease was the major contributing cause of death in patients who did not receive CHPP. In a three-arm randomized trial reported by Fujimura and colleagues,[218] the efficacy of CHPP was compared with continuous normothermic peritoneal perfusion and surgery alone in patients with gastric cancer and serosal invasion undergoing resection with curative intent. In the two perfusion groups, survival was significantly better compared with the group receiving surgery alone. Hamazoe and colleagues[223] reported that survival was slightly better in 42 patients treated prophylactically with CHPP compared with 40 untreated control patients. Several centers in the United States and Europe are currently evaluating the feasibility of CHPP for patients with peritoneal carcinomatosis.[224–228]

In summary, intraperitoneal chemotherapy given with curative intent is a rational strategy to pursue until such time as more highly effective systemic agents can be developed. Future studies will probably require intergroup or international trials to accrue adequate numbers of patients in a timely fashion.

IMMUNOCHEMOTHERAPY

Japanese and Korean investigators have performed a number of trials investigating the use of immunochemotherapy as adjuvant treatment after curative resection of gastric cancer. Many of these trials involve using a protein-bound polysaccharide (PSK) alone or combined with chemotherapy after gastrectomy. PSK is a polysaccharide extracted from *Coriolis versicolor*, whose mechanism of action is not fully understood. The control arm in most of these studies, however, also received chemotherapy. Nakazato and coworkers[229] reported the results of a study involving[230] patients who were randomly assigned to receive mitomycin plus FU (given by mouth) or the same chemotherapy plus PSK. The experimental arm received treatment with PSK for 36 months after surgery. As part of the eligibility process, patients had to have a positive purified protein derivative of tuberculin (PPD) test. Both groups received ten cycles of chemotherapy. With a minimum follow-up of 5 years, a significant survival advantage was seen for the PSK group; 70.7% of the PSK group versus 59.4% of the standard treatment group were alive and disease-free at 5 years. Ochiai and colleagues[231] compared chemotherapy versus chemoimmunotherapy after resection. The immunotherapy used was a *Nocardia rubra* cell wall skeleton extract. No surgery-only control group was established; both groups received mitomycin, FU, and cytosine arabinoside chemotherapy. In this study, therapy was started perioperatively: Patients received mitomycin during surgery and on day 1, and then began weekly mitomycin, FU, and cytosine arabinoside. The chemotherapy group had 90 patients, and the chemotherapy immunotherapy group had 97 patients. No difference in survival for patients having curative resections was seen. A subgroup of 71 patients did not undergo a curative resection and were analyzed separately. A survival advantage for those receiving immunochemotherapy was seen.

In other trials, Korean investigators have studied the use of chemotherapy plus immunostimulants after potentially curative resection. In one trial, chemotherapy with mitomycin, FU, and cytosine arabinoside plus OK432 (a *Streptococcus pyrogenes* preparation) was given to 74 patients, whereas a control group of 64 patients underwent surgery alone.[232] Of the group receiving postoperative treatment, 44.6% were alive at 5 years compared to 23.4% of those randomized to surgery only. In a follow-up three-arm trial, patients were randomized to receive immunotherapy with OK432 plus chemotherapy with mitomycin and FU. A second group received chemotherapy alone, whereas the third arm was a control arm of observation after surgery. At 5 years, 45.3% of the immunochemotherapy group were alive compared to 29.8% of the chemotherapy group and 24.4% of the surgery group. Kim and colleagues[233] performed a similar trial using FAM chemotherapy with or without OK-432. Fifty patients received chemotherapy alone, and 49 patients received chemotherapy plus OK-432. These authors reported a significant improvement in survival for chemotherapy plus immunotherapy versus chemotherapy alone (62% vs. 52%, $P = .04$).

In summary, data from Japanese and Korean investigators suggest that immunotherapy may improve outcome for patients undergoing potentially curative resection. The number of patients in any given trial is small, however, and the power of the observation therefore relatively weak. Large-scale confirmatory trials are necessary before accepting immunochemotherapy as a standard of care.

RANITIDINE

Preliminary data had suggested that ranitidine or cimetidine might be useful in preventing recurrence of resected gastric cancer. Primrose et al.[234] performed a double-blind placebo-controlled trial of ranitidine, 150 mg twice daily, versus placebo taken for up to 5 years. No other adjuvant therapy was allowed. Patients with resectable gross disease, including those with stage IV tumors, were allowed entrance into this trial. The study, as is the case with other adjuvant trials, has only a small number of patients (41 in one arm and 46 in the other). No difference was seen in overall outcome, although a trend to benefit in stage IV patients was noted. In a second trial with a similar design using cimetidine, a similar lack of benefit was noted. Thus, to date, therapy using histamine-2 blockers has not shown benefit in preventing recurrence in patients with resected gastric tumors.

TAMOXIFEN

Using a hormonal approach, Harrison and colleagues[235] treated 100 patients in a randomized trial with tamoxifen as a single agent. This study allowed entrance of patients who had residual gross disease, and thus the study was not evaluating truly adjuvant chemotherapy. Slightly more than one-half (55.8%) of tumors were estrogen receptor–positive. Tamoxifen had no effect on survival outcome; in fact, the control group did slightly better than the treated group.

NEOADJUVANT CHEMOTHERAPY

A strong rationale exists for the use of neoadjuvant chemotherapy before attempted resection in high-risk gastric cancer patients. For patients with locally advanced gastric cancers, performing a potentially curative resection (R0) frequently is difficult; the risk of distant failure, even with resection, is high. Locally advanced localized gastric cancers usually are defined as those with potentially resectable T3 or T4 tumors without distant metastases. Because assessment of lymph node involvement is difficult with the preoperative staging techniques currently available, T2 lesions, particularly those with suspicious lymph nodes, also are frequently included in these studies. Many pilot and formal phase II trials have been reported, either in complete or abstract form during the last 3 to 5 years. Results from selected trials are shown in Table 33.3-13. Almost all of these trials have involved the use of systemic chemotherapeutic regimens, which have demonstrated moderate response rates in patients with metastatic measurable gastric cancer. However, assessing response in patients with localized tumors is difficult. The overall accuracy of repeat endoscopy after induc-

TABLE 33.3-13. Neoadjuvant Therapy for Locally Advanced Gastric Cancer: Selected Phase II and Phase III Trials

Study	*Regimen*	*Number of Patients*	*Operable*	*Resectable*	*Median Survival*	*2-Y Survival Rate (%)*
Wilke	EAP	34	19 (56%)	10 (29%)	18 mo	26
Ajani[86]	EAP	48	41 (85%)	37 (77%)	16 mo	42
Ajani[313]	EFP	25	12 (100%)	18 (72%)	15 mo	44
Crookes et al.[209]	Cisplatin-FU-LV IP FUDR-cisplatin	59	(95%)	(71%)	>4 y	64
Siewert et al.[125]	Cisplatin-FU-LV	41	(88%)	(73%)	NS	56[a]
Kang et al.[244]	Cisplatin-etoposide-FU	53	(89%)	(71%)	33 mo	55
	Control	54	(100%)	(61%)	32 mo	55
Kelsen[236]	FAMTX-IP FP	56	50 (89%)	34 (61%)	15 mo	40
Alexander[243]	FU/LV IFN	22	20 (90%)	18 (82%)	18 mo	52

EAP, etoposide, doxorubicin (Adriamycin), and cisplatin; FAMTX, fluorouracil, doxorubicin (Adriamycin), and methotrexate; EFP, etoposide, fluorouracil, cisplatin; FU, fluorouracil; FUDR, 5-fluorodeoxyuridine; IFN, interferon; IP, intraperitoneal; LV, leucovorin; NS, not stated.
[a]Median follow-up, 18 months.

tion chemotherapy has been poor.[236] Reports indicate that even CT scans performed carefully after induction chemotherapy have a low overall sensitivity and accuracy, primarily because their negative predictive value is so limited.[237] Kelsen et al.[236] and others have investigated the use of EUS and CT scans in predicting pathologic stage in patients undergoing induction chemotherapy. In these trials, preoperative EUS stage before and after neoadjuvant chemotherapy was compared to pathologic T, N, and M stage. Postchemotherapy EUS was inaccurate in separating T2 from T3 tumors and in assessing lymph node status.[236] Therefore, data from phase II trials indicating down-staging should be interpreted with caution.

Another technique for predicting outcome early in the treatment course involves the use of PET scanning. A decrease in F-18 fluorodeoxyglucose uptake has been proposed as an early marker for objective regression in patients receiving systemic chemotherapy for locally advanced or metastatic disease.[238] Although preliminary studies with PET in gastric cancer have now been reported, definitive, large-scale trials correlating survival outcome with change in PET scan are still awaited.

Although assessing the degree of tumor regression is difficult, phase II studies of neoadjuvant chemotherapy have demonstrated that such treatment can be given with acceptable toxicity and with no apparent increase in operative morbidity or mortality. Several phase II pilot studies have been reported using this approach (see Table 33.3-13). Ajani and colleagues[239] at the M. D. Anderson Cancer Center performed a single-arm phase II trial involving 48 patients who had gastric cancers that were potentially operable. Etoposide, doxorubicin, and cisplatin chemotherapy was given for three courses before operation followed by two planned postoperative courses. Eighty-five percent of patients underwent operation, and 77% had potentially curative resections. Toxicity, primarily due to neutropenia, was substantial but generally manageable. One chemotherapy-related death was reported. In a second study, Ajani and colleagues[86] used a similar regimen of cisplatin, FU, and etoposide for two preoperative and three postoperative courses. One postoperative death was reported. All patients underwent operation, and 72% had potentially curative resections. The most common site for recurrent disease was peritoneal carcinomatosis either found at surgery or developing subsequently. Lowy et al.[240] summarized the long-term results of these and a third sequential phase II trial. A total of 83 patients were treated. All the studies involved the use of cisplatin-based therapy. Seventy-three percent of patients underwent R0 resections. Although response to therapy can be difficult to interpret, 4% of patients had pathologic complete remissions. Response to chemotherapy as assessed clinically was thought to be an independent predictor of survival.

Leichman and colleagues[241] reported the initial results of a trial in which 38 patients with resectable gastric tumors received two cycles of a preoperative chemotherapy regimen involving 5-FU, 200 $mg/m^2/d$, given over 3 weeks with weekly intravenous leucovorin, 20 mg/m^2, and monthly cisplatin, 100 mg/m^2. Postoperative intraperitoneal therapy involved FUDR, 3000 mg total dose, daily for 3 days plus cisplatin, 200 mg/m^2, with intravenous sodium thiosulfate. Ninety-two percent of patients underwent laparotomy; 87% of patients had resection. Postoperative intraperitoneal therapy was possible in 68% of study patients. One treatment-related death was reported. Prestudy clinical tumor staging (by CT and endoscopy) was not provided. Postoperative staging showed 14 patients with either stage 0 (one patient) or stage I disease. An additional seven patients had stage II tumors. Crookes et al.[209] reported the long-term results of this phase II study. In the final report, a total of 59 patients were included. A 71% R0 resection rate was noted. The operative mortality was 5%. Median survival of this group of patients was estimated to exceed 4 years. Because these patients did not undergo preoperative laparoscopy or EUS, however, they may have included patients with both locally advanced and earlier-stage tumors.

Kelsen and coworkers[236] performed two trials involving preoperative chemotherapy followed by postoperative intraperitoneal treatment. The first study used the FAMTX regimen preoperatively and gave postoperative intraperitoneal FU and cisplatin.[236] Fifty-six evaluable patients were identified by EUS as having advanced disease; most had stage IIIA or IIIB tumors. Toxicity was tolerable, the major side effect was myelosuppression leading to hospitalization for neutropenic fever on at least one occasion in 60% of patients. Down-staging occurred in 51% of patients. The operability rate was 89%, and the resectability rate was 74% (61% curative, 20% palliative). With a median follow-up of 28 months, the median duration of survival for all patients was 15.3 months.

In a follow-up study, the same group of investigators treated a group of 35 patients with preoperative cisplatin and FU chemotherapy for two cycles followed by postoperative intraperitoneal floxuridine plus leucovorin. All patients underwent pretreatment laparoscopy and EUS, and all had T3 or lymph node–positive tumors. Preoperative toxicity was tolerable, without any increase in operative morbidity or mortality. The R0 resection rate was 82%, and the estimated medial duration of survival was 22.5 months. Fink and colleagues[242] treated a group of 49 patients with preoperative cisplatin, FU, and leucovorin (PLF). The R0 resection rate was 76%. Median duration of survival for all patients was 36 months, and at a median follow-up of 28 months, the median survival for the R0-resected patients had not been reached.[242]

Alexander and coworkers[243] treated 22 patients with locally advanced gastric cancer with three cycles of 5-FU, leucovorin, and interferon followed by resection and three cycles of postoperative consolidation therapy. The response rate to neoadjuvant therapy was 38%, and 18 patients (82%) underwent resection with curative intent. Endoscopic tumor biopsies were obtained in 13 patients before and during cycle two of neoadjuvant chemotherapy, and thymidylate synthase (TS) levels were quantitated by Western blot. Pretreatment TS levels in tumor were significantly higher in responders versus nonresponders. After exposure to 5-FU, levels of free TS were significantly lower, and the percentage of TS complexed with 5-FU was significantly higher in responders. These preliminary data indicate that quantification of TS in tumor may provide a method to select patients most likely to respond to 5-FU–based chemotherapy.

Kang et al.[244] reported the preliminary results of a small randomized trial of neoadjuvant cisplatin, etoposide, and FU therapy versus surgery alone. Fifty-three patients received preoperative chemotherapy, and 54 underwent immediate operation. No significant difference was noted in operability rate (89% vs. 100%), resection rate (71% vs. 61%), or in median survival (33 vs. 32 months). All of these trials have demonstrated that preoperative chemotherapy can be given safely without an increase in operative morbidity or mortality when experienced surgeons perform the operation. Most studies are single-institution trials, and all investigators have emphasized the need for multiinstitutional pro spective studies to test the hypothesis that preoperative treatment will improve outcome as measured by overall survival. Although it is unclear as to whether one chemotherapy regimen, including cisplatin-based treatment, is markedly superior to another (as discussed in Palliative Treatment of Gastric Cancer, below), almost all preoperative regimens do involve this agent. The identification of the taxanes docetaxel and paclitaxel and, more recently, of the camptothecan irinotecan as active agents in the treatment of this disease has led to the introduction of these agents into newer neoadjuvant regimens.

Larger-scale phase III trials with a surgery-only control arm are now under way, and additional studies are in the advanced planning stage. A European group, led by the United Kingdom MRC, is currently performing a randomized trial with a projected accrual of 500 patients. The investigational arm involves preoperative chemotherapy with epirubicin, cisplatin, and FU (ECF) followed by operation versus operation alone. Three preoperative courses are delivered, followed by operation within 6 weeks of completing chemotherapy. An additional three courses of postoperative ECF is planned. This study is still accruing patients. Phase II pilot trials are nearing completion in the United States preliminary to a large-scale randomized study. These pilot trials include neoadjuvant chemotherapy using cisplatin, taxotere, and FU followed by surgery followed by intraperitoneal chemotherapy; a second study uses neoadjuvant chemoradiation with cisplatin, FU, and taxotere plus concurrent radiation followed by resection. Last, the Eastern Gastric Oncology Group is performing a study of cisplatin and taxotere therapy followed by surgery followed by postoperative chemoradiation therapy. It is anticipated that the control arm in the next intergroup trial will be the best arm of the Intergroup 116 study (discussed later, in Adjuvant Radiation and Chemoradiation Therapy), in which patients having undergone curative resection for gastric cancer were randomized to observation or chemoradiation therapy using FU and leucovorin as the chemotherapeutic agents.

In summary, neoadjuvant approaches involving preoperative chemotherapy with or without postoperative intraperitoneal treatment are now under way in the United States and in Europe. To date, the data indicate no increase in operative morbidity or mortality. Because evaluating the primary tumor is difficult, down-staging can only be estimated. The approach, although promising, requires definitive randomized phase III trials before firm conclusions regarding the value of this technique are established.

ADJUVANT RADIATION AND CHEMORADIATION THERAPY

Few studies have evaluated radiation therapy alone (with no concomitant chemotherapy) as an adjuvant to surgical resection of gastric cancer. Most of the studies that have evaluated radiation therapy as an adjuvant have used concomitant 5-FU chemotherapy.

Some of the earliest data on radiation therapy of gastric cancer comes from the Mayo Clinic, where studies were performed in the 1960s on the use of radiation therapy and 5-FU in a variety of gastrointestinal malignancies. Although these reports were based on patients with locally advanced tumors, they laid the groundwork for the subsequent adjuvant studies. Childs and colleagues[245] reported a study of patients with advanced gastric cancer who were randomized to either radiation therapy alone to a dose of approximately 4000 cGy or radiation therapy combined with 5-FU as a radiation sensitizer (bolus 5-FU for 3 days, 15 mg/kg/d). This study showed a significant improvement in survival with the combination of 5-FU and radiation compared with radiation alone. Because the dose of 5-FU was extremely low, most people have interpreted these data as showing an advantage to 5-FU as a radiation sensitizer. This observation also is consistent with the data that have been obtained in other gastrointestinal sites, such as rectal and pancreatic cancer, for which 5-FU has improved survival when combined with radiation therapy. The British Stomach Cancer Group study randomized patients to postoperative radiation therapy; postoperative chemotherapy with FAM; or surgery alone. At 5-year follow-up, no significant difference was seen among any of the three arms, but the local recurrence rate was decreased by the use of radiation therapy (54% with surgery alone vs. 32% with radiation therapy, $P<.01$).[246]

Two studies used chemotherapy plus concurrent radiation. In one study, however, incompletely resected patients were included. Dent and colleagues[247] treated 142 patients who were randomly assigned to no additional therapy or to 2000 cGy given in eight treatments over 10 days plus FU, 12.5 mg/kg, daily for 4 days immediately before the beginning of radiation. A second cycle was given on day 28. Patients in "division one" had no residual gross disease but may have had incomplete resection. The control group had 31 patients, and the chemotherapy/radiation group had 35 patients. No difference in survival between the two groups was reported. Moertel and coworkers[247a] from the Mayo Clinic have reported the results of a randomized trial of radiation therapy (3750 cGy in 24 fractions) plus 5-FU (15 mg/kg × 3) versus surgery alone for poor prognosis patients, including those with scirrhous carcinomas, metastases to regional lymph nodes, invasion of adjacent structures, or tumors originating in the cardia. Eighty percent of patients had positive nodal disease, and approximately 25% had invasion of adjacent structures. The treated patients had a 5-year survival rate of 20% versus a 4% 5-year survival rate in the surgery-only controls. However, the issue is confused by the fact that ten patients who were randomized to adjuvant treatment refused therapy. In this small cohort of patients, the 5-year survival rate was 30%. Locoregional recurrence was decreased from 54% in the surgery-alone arm to 39% in the combined modality arm. The survival results in these studies are also similar to those reported in nonrandomized series, such as that by Slot and colleagues,[248] in which 57 patients with poor prognostic factors received postoperative radiation therapy to a dose of 30 to 50 Gy combined with 5-FU. The 5-year survival rate was 26%, with 16 patients having a locoregional recurrence as their first sign of relapse.

Although others have evaluated other combinations of chemotherapy with radiation therapy,[249,250] no advantage has been shown to date with any drug regimen besides 5-FU when combined with chemotherapy. The data suggest that, for patients with nodal positivity, serosal involvement, or close or positive surgical resection margins, postoperative radiation therapy may be of value. This approach has been studied in the United States in a national intergroup trial (INT 116) evaluating two cycles of chemotherapy with 5-FU and leucovorin followed by radiation therapy to a dose of 4500 cGy with concurrent chemotherapy. Intergroup 116 involved a total of 556 evaluable patients, 275 of whom were followed expectantly after operation, and 281 who were randomly assigned to receive postoperative chemoradiation therapy. All patients had undergone an R0 resection. The type of lymphadenectomy was not mandated by the study protocol. Postoperative chemoradiation therapy involved the use of FU and leucovorin chemotherapy and 45 Gy of external-beam radiation therapy. One cycle using the Mayo Clinic regimen of FU, 425 mg/m^2, and leucovorin, 20 mg/M^2, for 5 consecutive days was followed by concurrent chemoradiation. Doses were decreased during radiation to FU, 400 mg/M^2, and leucovorin, 20 mg/M^2, daily for 4 days during week 1 of radiation, and for 3 days at the end of radiation. One month after the completion of radiation, additional chemotherapy using FU, 425 mg/M^2, and leucovorin, 20 mg/M^2, daily for 5 days was given for two additional cycles. This data has been presented in abstract form. The two arms were well balanced for important prognostic indicators. Eighty-five percent of patients had lymph node metastases. With close attention to detail, especially to radiation therapy treatment planning, toxicity was tolerable, although three (1%) toxic deaths on the experimental arm were reported. Postoperative adjuvant chemoradiation therapy resulted in a significant improvement in both disease-free and overall 3-year survival rates. The median survival was improved from 26 months for the surgery-only group to 40 months for those receiving chemoradiation. Three-year survival was 41% for surgery only and 52% for postoperative chemoradiation (P = .03; hazard ratio, 1.28) (J. McDonald, personal communication). If the final report confirms these initial data, postoperative chemoradiation using FU and leucovorin will become the standard of care for resected R0 patients able to tolerate such treatment.

To try to increase the total radiation dose that can safely be delivered, newer radiation approaches have been tried. An approach that has been investigated at a few centers is intraoperative electron-beam radiation therapy. In this technique, pioneered by Abe and Takahashi,[251] patients receive a single dose of high-energy electrons delivered to the tumor bed at the time of gastrectomy. Because most of the radiosensitive normal structures can be moved from the radiation beam, the risk of producing significant bowel complications is reduced. In a nonrandomized trial, Abe has demonstrated an improved 5-year survival rate in patients with locally advanced disease (usually because of posterior infiltration) who were treated with intraoperative radiation therapy (20%).[251a] A small randomized trial of a similar approach at the National Cancer Institute[252] did not demonstrate any significant survival advantage, although it did demonstrate an improvement in local control compared with surgery alone. A number of phase II trials have been performed that demonstrate the feasibility of this approach in a large number of centers, but these trials do not allow any conclusions regarding efficacy[251–254] (Table 33.3-14).

TABLE 33.3-14. Gastric Cancer: Surgery Alone versus Surgery and Intraoperative Radiation Therapy (IORT), Japan

	5-Y Survival			
	Surgery		*Surgery + IORT*	
Stage	Number of Patients	%	Number of Patients	%
I	43	93	20	88.1
II	11	54.5	18	77.6
III	38	36.8	19	44.6
IV (no distant metastases)	18	0	27	19.5

(Modified from ref. 251, with permission.)

TECHNIQUE OF RADIATION THERAPY

In general, the presence of normal tissues close to the tumor mass limits the radiation dose that can be delivered safely. The spinal cord, kidneys, small bowel, and liver are all in close proximity and cannot be entirely avoided. In addition, the stomach itself is a radiation-sensitive tissue, and high doses (more than 5000 cGy) to a functional stomach produce a significant incidence of ulceration and bleeding.

When irradiating the upper abdomen, a number of acute side effects from therapy may occur, including nausea, weight loss, and fatigue. With properly planned radiation fields, the nausea is not generally severe, but given the prolonged course of radiation, if careful attention is not given to the patient's nutritional status, the therapy can end up producing more harm than good. Usually, a combination of antiemetics, multiple small feedings, and nutritional supplements are sufficient to control the side effects of treatment, but on occasion, feeding tubes are useful. If patients cannot maintain their weight before the initiation of radiation therapy, they usually have difficulty with the therapy. The other acute side effects are relatively minor and easily managed. The possible late side effects that must be considered include damage to spinal cord, liver, kidney, and stomach.

Late liver and renal failure or radiation-induced spinal cord transection are all possible complications from excess irradiation, but if proper attention is paid to these structures during treatment planning, a clinical problem should rarely develop. The tolerance dose of the stomach itself is on the order of 5000 cGy, so those doses above this level have a real risk of producing gastric ulceration.

It is common for at least one kidney to be required in the radiation field to a high dose (more than 3000 cGy), which produces a very high chance of significant renal injury, usually to the left kidney. Studies have demonstrated[255] that, for a patient with baseline renal function that is within normal range, treating one kidney to high dose has a very low likelihood of producing renal injury that adversely effects the patient's quality of life. The compensatory hypertrophy of the unirradiated kidney results in adequate renal function, and the risk of renovascular hypertension is very low. If the equivalent of one kidney can be eliminated from the radiation field and the patient starts with a relatively normal creatinine clearance, then the patient should tolerate the radiation course adequately in regard to the kidneys. Standard radiation tolerance doses should be observed for the other normal tissues mentioned previously.

If radiation therapy is being used as an adjuvant or with curative intent, the patterns of spread of the tumor must be considered in planning the radiation field. In contrast to many other tumor sites, a standard radiation field is often inappropriate in treatment of gastric cancer because the spread patterns relate to the site of origin and the extension that is found on preoperative imaging studies and at surgery. The lymphatic pattern of spread has already been discussed, and this pattern greatly influences the radiation fields that are appropriate.

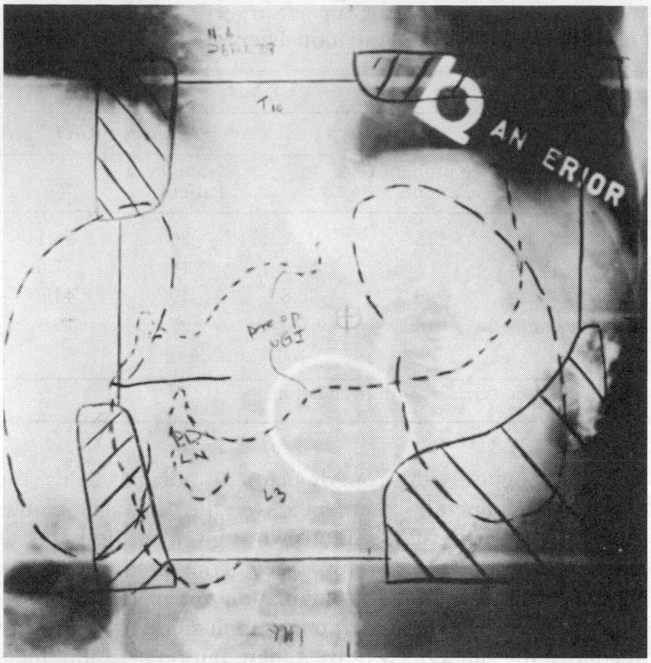

FIGURE 33.3-8. Typical treatment field for postoperative radiation therapy of a tumor of the body of the pancreas. This field encompasses the entire tumor bed and virtually all regional lymphatic sites. For tumors that are located more proximally or distally in the stomach, the fields can be shaped to avoid regions at lower risk (see text).

Although one usually wishes to encompass much of the stomach (or the gastric bed), for tumors that originated and remained limited to the gastric antrum, it is not necessary to irradiate the entire cardia of the stomach and to extend the radiation field to encompass the lower esophagus, but it is necessary to treat the periduodenal lymph nodes. Similarly, for tumors originating in the cardia, it is essential that the field extend up into the esophagus and that there is full coverage of the bed of the gastric cardia and fundus, but one can safely avoid irradiating the periduodenal nodes. Often, a local failure from gastric cancer occurs from posterior extension of the primary tumor onto the pancreas and into other retroperitoneal tissues. Therefore, full coverage of these areas of posterior invasion is essential. An example of a typical radiation field is shown in Figure 33.3-8. The radiation fields are primarily anteroposterior fields, although lateral and oblique fields can be very useful for the final boost. If lateral fields are used for a substantial portion of the large-field treatment, then care must be taken to avoid treating large segments of the liver to doses higher than 2000 or 2500 cGy.

The total radiation dose to be used is determined primarily by the tolerance of the normal tissues mentioned above. Generally, a dose of 4500 cGy given at 180 cGy/d has a minimal chance of producing significant late complications. At doses higher than 5000 cGy, the risk of late complications increases, and doses greater than this should be limited to very small volumes. As mentioned above, the data strongly suggest that the combination of 5-FU and radiation is more effective than radiation alone. Although the optimal method of drug administration is not known, it is appropriate to use, as a minimum, 3 days of bolus 5-FU during the first and last week of radiation therapy.

TABLE 33.3-15. Chemotherapeutic Agents

Drug	*Number of Patients*	*Response Rates (%)*
Antimetabolites		
5-Fluorouracil	416	21
Methotrexate	28	11
Trimetrexate	26	19
Triazinate	26	15
Gemcitabine	15	0
Oral antimetabolites		
UFT	188	28
S-1	51	49
Hydroxurea (oral)	31	19
Carmofur (oral)	31	27
Ftorafur (oral)	19	19
Antibiotics		
Mitomycin C	211	30
Doxorubicin	141	17
Epirubicin	80	19
Heavy metals		
Cisplatin	139	19
Carboplatin	41	5
Taxanes		
Paclitaxel	98	17
Docetaxel	123	21
Camptothecans		
Irinotecan	66	23
Topotecan	33	6

UFT, uracil and ftorafur.

PALLIATIVE TREATMENT OF GASTRIC CANCER

Since the late 1970s, many chemotherapeutic agents have been studied in gastric cancer. Although reports of very high response rates with some of the newer combination chemotherapy regimens have been published, the median survival of patients with advanced cancer continues to be dismal.

SINGLE-AGENT CHEMOTHERAPY

The objective response rates reported for single agents in patients with gastric cancer are shown in Table 33.3-15. FU is the most extensively studied single agent in this disease, with an overall objective response rate of 21%.[256,257] The two most commonly used schedules for administering 5-FU as a single agent are daily intravenous injections for 5 consecutive days, repeated every 4 to 5 weeks, and weekly intravenous injections. Both schedules have similar response rates and toxicity profiles. The major side effects of 5-FU are mucositis, diarrhea, myelosuppression, and (using a continuous infusion) the hand-foot syndrome. 5-FU has been a common element in most combination chemotherapy regimens for gastric cancer.

Mitomycin C, an antitumor antibiotic, also has been extensively used in the treatment of gastric cancer, especially in Japan. The overall objective response rate for mitomycin C has been approximately 30%.[258–260] Its greatest toxicity is delayed and cumulative myelosuppression, so the drug is usually given on an intermittent basis every 4 to 8 weeks.

Doxorubicin (Adriamycin), an anthracycline antibiotic, also has been studied. In 141 evaluable patients with advanced disease, it had an overall response rate of 17%.[258,259,261] Doxorubicin is a potent agent with significant but manageable early side effects. Its most critical toxicity is irreversible myocardial damage. Several groups have studied cisplatin. As a single agent, it is reported to produce major responses in 19% of patients, including those previously treated.[262–264]

Several new agents have been identified as having substantial activity in advanced gastric cancer. As shown in Table 33.3-15, the taxanes paclitaxel and docetaxel have both undergone phase II trials. For paclitaxel, both 3-hour and 24-hour infusions given every 3 weeks have been studied. Overall, approximately 20% of patients have had major objective regressions, primarily partial remissions. It is unclear as to whether a substantial difference exists between the two schedules. Response also has been seen in patients who have received prior chemotherapy. Similar data exists for docetaxel. The overall response rate is approximately 20% to 25%, with most studies having used an every 3-week dosing schedule. The two taxanes have not yet been compared in prospective randomized studies. Irinotecan, a new agent in the treatment of patients with colorectal cancer, also has single-agent activity in gastric cancer. Responses have been reported in both previously treated and untreated patients.

Both of these new classes of agents have now been used in multidrug combinations as described in the following sections. In addition to the identification of the taxanes and irinotecan, interest is increasing in oral fluorinated pyrimidine therapy. In this case, although the agents being studied are not of a new class but rather are FU prodrugs, ease of administration and the mimicking of chronic infusional therapy is of interest. UFT has been the most well-studied oral fluorinated pyrimidine. Responses in 20% to 30% of patients have been reported. Fewer data are available for S1, although in one study, an unusually high response rate of 49% was reported. Also shown in Table 33.3-15 are newer agents studied since 1996 that have not demonstrated antineoplastic activity.

COMBINATION CHEMOTHERAPY

Numerous attempts have been made to develop more effective combination chemotherapy regimens using known active drugs; some trials also have included other agents that did not have substantiated activity. Both phase II and prospective randomized phase III trials have been reported (Tables 33.3-16 and 33.3-17). In general, results from multicenter phase III trials have had lower response rates than single-institution phase II studies for the same drug regimens.[230,261,265–272a] Several combination chemotherapy regimens have shown response rates in the range of 30% to 50%, usually in phase II studies.

FAM and FAM Variants

The FAM combination was widely used in the 1980s (see Table 33.3-16). In the initial report of this regimen, 26 of 62 patients (42%) achieved a partial response; no complete responses were reported.[273] The median duration of response was 9 months; the median survival for the whole group was 5.5 months, although the median survival for responding patients was 12.5 months. Results using FAM have since been reported in more than 650 patients in various dose schedules with a cumulative response rate of 30%; the complete remission rate has been 2%.[260] The median remission duration is 5 to 10 months. Other studies have used variants of the FAM regimen (e.g., increased doxorubicin dose). The overall response rate of 28% for such modified regimens is similar to the response rate reported in patients treated with the original FAM combination. The median survival of patients treated on FAM variants was also identical to those treated on the original FAM regimen.[260]

In a review of Japanese studies, Ogawa[274] reported a cumulative response rate of 36% in 356 patients with a combination of 5-FU, mitomycin C, and cytarabine. The mean survival was

TABLE 33.3-16. Combination Chemotherapy

Drugs	*Evaluable Patients*	*Response Rate (%)*	*95% Confidence Limits*	*Median Survival (mo)*
FU-doxo-mito (FAM)	656	30	27–33%	6–9+
FAM (variants)	310	28	23–33%	—
FU-doxo–methyl CCNU (FAMe)	141	25	18–32%	5.5–8.5
FU-doxo-BCNU (FAB)	194	41	34–48%	6–8
FU-doxo-CDDP (FAP)	234	34	28–40%	6–13
FU-epirub-mito (FEM)	123	32	23–40%	5–6
FU-epirub-BCNU (FEB)	45	42	28–57%	9
FU-epirub-CDDP (FEP)	66	44	32–56%	NS
FU–methyl CCNU	224	19	14–24%	3.5–5.5
FAM-BCNU	41	22	9–35%	6.0
FU-mito-araC	356	36	31–41%	16–20 (mean)
Etop-CDDP	79	18	9–26%	4.5
Etop-doxo-CDDP (EAP)	173	53	46–61%	6–9
FU-etop-leucovorin (ELF)	51	53	39–67%	11.0
FU-doxo-MTX (FAMTX)	364	41	36–46%	3.5–10.5

araC, arabinosylcytosine (cytarabine); BCNU, bischloroethylnitrosourea (carmustine); CCNU, chloroethylcyclohexylnitrosourea; CDDP, cisplatin; doxo, doxorubicin (Adriamycin); epirub, epirubicin; etop, etoposide; FU, fluorouracil; mito, mitomycin; MTX, methotrexate; NS, not stated.
[From Kelsen D, Atiq O. Cancer of the upper gastrointestinal tract. *Curr Concepts Cancer* (*in press*), with permission.]

TABLE 33.3-17. Prospective Randomized Trials of Combination Chemotherapy in Advanced Gastric Cancer

Drugs	*Evaluable Patients*	*Response Rate (%)*	*Median Survival (mo)*
FU vs.	51	18	7 (NS)
FU-dox vs.	49	27	7
FAM	51	38	7
FU-dox vs.	78	5	6.3 (NS)
FAM vs.	78	17	6.4
FAMe	76	25	7.1
DOX vs.	37	22	4 (NS)
FU-mito	53	43	4.5
FAMTX vs.	30	33	7 (NS)
EAP	30	20	6
FAM vs.	103	9	7.2 ($P = .004$)
FAMTX	105	41	10.5
FAMTX[a] vs.	45	20	7 (NS)
ELF vs.	42	21	7
Cisplatin-FU	44	27	8
Cisplatin-FU vs.	103	51	9 (NS)
FAM vs.	98	25	7
FU	94	26	7.5
ECF vs.	126	46	8.7 ($P = .0005$)
FAMTX	130	21	6.1

dox, doxorubicin; EAP, etoposide, doxorubicin, and cisplatin; ECF, epirubicin, cisplatin, and fluorouracil; ELF, etoposide, leucovorin, fluorouracil; FAM, fluorouracil, doxorubicin (Adriamycin), mitomycin; FAMe, fluorouracil, doxorubicin (Adriamycin), methyl CCNU (chloroethylcyclohexylnitrosourea); FAMTX, fluorouracil, doxorubicin (Adriamycin), methotrexate; FU, fluorouracil; mito, mitomycin; NS, not significant.
[a]Analysis of patients with measurable disease.

reported as 16 to 20 months. In a randomized trial of 5-FU alone versus 5-FU, mitomycin, and cytarabine, however, Cocconi and colleagues[257] found no statistical difference among the response rate, duration of response, or median survival in the two arms.

In a phase III trial, the North Central Cancer Treatment Group compared single-agent 5-FU to 5-FU plus doxorubicin and to FAM[275] (see Table 33.3-17). The primary end point of this study was survival. The median survival of all patients was 29 weeks. The investigators also did not notice any significant differences in the palliative effect among these three treatment regimens.

Cisplatin-Based Chemotherapy

Although many phase II studies have been performed during the 1990s involving a variety of cisplatin-containing and non–cisplatin-containing combinations, only a few phase III randomized studies have been reported. Most of these trials involve relatively small numbers of patients, so that the ability to make definitive statements of superiority of one treatment over the other is limited.

The *in vitro* synergy between cisplatin and 5-FU, the activity of cisplatin as a single agent in gastric cancer, and the bone marrow toxicity of mitomycin led several investigators to replace mitomycin in the FAM combination with cisplatin. The cumulative overall response rate for this FAP regimen was 34%, with 5% of the patients achieving complete remission.[260,268,276] Cisplatin and doxorubicin were given in doses of 60 to 100 and 30 to 60 mg/m^2 per cycle, respectively. 5-FU dose and schedule also varied in individual trials.

To assess the individual contribution of cisplatin, methyl CCNU, and triazinate in combination with 5-FU and doxorubicin, the Gastrointestinal Tumor Study Group performed a prospective randomized trial comparing FAP, FAMe [FU, doxorubicin (Adriamycin), and methyl CCNU], and FAT [5-FU, doxorubicin (Adriamycin), triazinate].[276] The primary end point was survival. Of 249 patients studied, 38% had measurable disease and were evaluable for response. The response rates for FAP, FAMe, and FAT were 19%, 15%, and 20%, respectively. Median survival rates were 31 weeks (FAP), 24 weeks (FAMe), and 30 weeks (FAT). Severe toxicity was seen in 69% of patients treated with FAP, 62% on FAMe, and 42% on FAT.

Cunningham and coworkers[277] substituted epirubicin, an analogue of doxorubicin that, in preclinical studies, has less cardiac toxicity with equivalent tumor activity to doxorubicin, for doxorubicin in the ECF regimen in one report. Ten of 14 evaluable patients (71%) achieved an objective response. In a second trial involving 52 evaluable patients, the response rate was 37%, with a 17% complete remission rate.[278] Median durations of survival were not reported. The Italian Oncology Group for clinical research performed a randomized phase III trial comparing the FAM regimen to a cisplatin, epirubicin, leucovorin, and FU (PELF) regimen.[279] Nonhematologic toxicity was significantly more frequent with PELF compared with FAM, including two treatment-related deaths. PELF had a significantly higher response rate (43%) than did FAM (15%). The median duration of survival was not significantly different. Waters et al.[279a] reported the long-term results of a randomized trial in which ECF was compared to the FAMTX combination. This is one of the largest phase III trials in advanced gastric cancer reported.

In phase II studies led by Cunningham and colleagues,[277] ECF had a high response rate with acceptable toxicity. FAMTX had been shown in earlier trials to be superior to FAM, which was one of the standards of the early 1980s. In the randomized MRC study,[279a] 126 patients received ECF and 130 patients received FAMTX. The overall response rate for ECF was significantly higher than that of FAMTX (46% vs. 21%). Median survival was also longer for ECF (8.7 vs. 6.1 months). In the update, long-term survival was presented. At 2 years, 14% of patients receiving ECF were alive versus 5% of FAMTX patients. In an earlier trial, Kim and colleagues[279b] compared FU and cisplatin to FU alone and to the FAM regimen. This smaller trial had 54 to 57 patients per arm. The response rate to the cisplatin-containing combination was 51%, significantly better than the 25% to 26% for the non–cisplatin-containing arms. The median duration of survival of 8.5 months was almost identical to the median duration of survival for ECF.

Barone and colleagues[279c] compared a cisplatin, epirubicin, and etoposide combination to FU plus leucovorin. In this small study, 32 patients received cisplatin-containing therapy and 33 received FU plus leucovorin. Response rates were similar (22% vs. 18%, respectively), as was median survival. The 2-year survival rate was 14% for patients receiving cisplatin, epirubicin, and etoposide compared to 3% of those receiving 5-FU plus leucovorin. The Turkish Oncology Group[279d] compared two cisplatin-containing combinations: etoposide, epirubicin, cisplatin versus FU, epirubicin, and cisplatin; 20% of patients responded to the etoposide, epirubicin, and cisplatin regimen versus 15% to FU, epirubicin, and cisplatin. Median survival rates were short (6 vs. 5 months). Thus, to date, epirubicin- and cisplatin-containing combinations have been reported to have higher response rates and, in some trials, a survival advantage.

Cisplatin-Etoposide Variants

Because of evidence that etoposide and cisplatin may be synergistic and that the combination of the two may be helpful in overcoming multidrug resistance,[280,281] these drugs have been combined in many tumors. Two phase II trials of etoposide and cisplatin in advanced gastric cancer (including gastroesophageal junction adenocarcinoma) showed an 18% response rate in 79 evaluable patients. Kelsen and colleagues[282] reported only one major objective regression in 33 evaluable patients. Cisplatin at a dose of 60 mg/m^2 was given on days 1 and 29 and every 6 weeks thereafter, with etoposide given at a dose of 100 mg/m^2 on days 3, 5, 7, and 31, 33, and 35. Toxicity was generally tolerable. In the second trial, Elliott and coworkers[283] saw 13 responses in 46 evaluable patients. Etoposide was given at a dose of 130 mg/m^2/d × 3 plus cisplatin, 45 mg/m^2/d, on days 2 and 3. Both drugs were given by continuous intravenous infusion, and the cycles were repeated every 4 weeks. Most patients experienced severe toxicity. The median duration of response was 4 months.

Preusser and colleagues[284] used the combination of etoposide, doxorubicin, and cisplatin (EAP) and reported a 64% response rate in 67 patients, with a complete remission rate of 21%. Including patients with locoregional tumor treated in a separate trial, Wilke and colleagues[285] treated 145 patients with EAP, resulting in a cumulative response rate of 57%. Analyzing response as a function of extent of disease, patients with locoregional tumor had a response rate of 73%, with a 29% complete remission rate, as opposed to those with metastatic disease who had a response rate of 49% with a complete remission rate of 8%. Similarly, the median survival time for patients with locally advanced disease was 17 months in comparison with 8.5 months for those with metastatic disease. In four subsequent phase II trials of EAP involving 173 evaluable patients, a cumulative response rate of 53% and a complete remission rate of 6% has been seen.[286,287] However, in each of the subsequent trials after the initial study reported by Preusser, a treatment-related death rate of 10% to 14% with EAP was noted.

In part because EAP caused severe toxicity in older patients, Wilke and colleagues,[288] devised a combination chemotherapy regimen of etoposide, leucovorin, and FU (ELF) for patients older than 65 years with advanced gastric cancer. The rationale for this combination was that 5-FU and etoposide are active agents in gastric cancer that are well tolerated and have no cumulative organ toxicity, the dose limiting toxicity being overlapping myelosuppression; etoposide and 5-FU are synergistic and are not cross-resistant; and leucovorin enhances the cytotoxicity of FU in other tumors. Fifty-one patients older than 65 years of age or with cardiac disease were treated. The overall response rate was 53%, including 12% complete remissions. The response rate in patients with locally advanced disease was 70% compared with 49% in patients with distant metastases. The median duration of response was 9.5 months. Twenty percent of patients experienced grade 3 or 4 myelosuppression; however, nonhematologic toxicity was generally mild. The authors recommended ELF as a suitable regimen for high-risk patients (advanced age or cardiac risk factors).

Fluorouracil, Doxorubicin (Adriamycin), and Methotrexate

The concept of biochemical modulation of 5-FU involves the use of agents designed to increase the pool of phosphoribosylpyrophosphate in tumor cells, resulting in increased 5-FU ribonucleotide metabolites, thereby increasing the effectiveness of 5-FU–directed tumor kill. This approach led Klein[289] to study sequential high-dose methotrexate followed by 5-FU in combination with doxorubicin (Adriamycin) (the FAMTX regimen) in advanced gastric cancer. The interval between methotrexate and 5-FU is 1 hour in the original FAMTX regimen. Klein reported a response rate of 59% in 100 evaluable patients, with a complete remission rate of 12% and a treatment-related mortality rate of 3%. In a review of his experience,[289] Klein noted a 6% long-term (more than 5 years) survival rate for patients receiving FAMTX.

Kelsen and colleagues[290] reported the results of a randomized trial comparing EAP to FAMTX in advanced gastric cancer. The response rates were similar. Three patients (10%) had complete remission rates in the FAMTX arm; no complete remissions were seen with EAP. Although no significant differences were reported in the response rate, EAP was significantly more toxic than FAMTX for neutropenia, anemia, and thrombocytopenia. Most important, four treatment-related deaths (13%) were noted on the EAP arm as opposed to none on the FAMTX arm (P = .04). In view of the significant toxicity difference, the study was closed. The median durations of survival of all patients was similar (FAMTX, 7 months; EAP, 6 months). The authors concluded that FAMTX was at least as active as EAP but was significantly less toxic.

The European Organization for Research and Treatment of Cancer published the results of a multicenter prospective randomized trial comparing FAMTX with FAM[291] (see Table 33.3-17). The response rate of 41% for FAMTX was significantly superior to the 9% response rate for FAM (P<.0001). Five complete responders were reported in the FAMTX arm compared with none on the FAM regimen. Survival among FAMTX patients was also superior (42 weeks compared with 29 weeks for FAM; P = .004). The toxic death rate of the two combinations was similar (FAMTX, 4%; FAM, 3%). At 1 year, 41% of FAMTX versus 22% of FAM patients were alive. None were surviving at the 2-year mark on FAM, whereas 9% of the patients survived on the FAMTX arm. Severe hematologic toxicity was seen in more patients on FAM than on the FAMTX regimen. As noted previously, in a randomized trial performed by Cunningham and colleagues,[277] ECF was superior to FAMTX in terms of response rate, quality of life, and survival.

The European Organization for Research and Treatment of Cancer has performed a randomized trial of FAMTX versus ELF versus cisplatin and 5-FU. In a preliminary result of this study, 274 eligible patients were randomized.[291] No significant difference was found in severe toxicity (World Health Organization scale 3 or 4+) between the three arms. The response rates in the subgroups of patients with measurable disease in the preliminary report also showed no significant difference. Median survival was 7 to 8 months. The analysis was preliminary because not all patients had been fully assessed.[292]

In summary, as is the case for adjuvant trials, few adequately powered, large-scale phase III studies have been performed comparing one regimen with another. From the point of view of median survival, little substantial difference exists between one regimen and another, particularly in those in which both arms include cisplatin. However, it is of note that 2-year survival rates of 10% to 15% have been reported in several series reporting longer-term data, indicating that at least some patients have substantial palliative benefit. Although some investigators have proposed that one regimen be considered the standard of care, as yet no convincing data shows that one cisplatin and FU–containing combination is markedly better than another.

The identification of several new classes of agents with substantial single-agent activity (the taxanes and irinotecan) and new modalities of treatment (including newer approaches, such as immunotherapy, angiogenesis blockade, monoclonal antibody chemotherapy combinations, and manipulation of molecular biologic targets) should be vigorously pursued. Their inclusion in multidrug combinations may lead to further improvements in palliation, and eventually to cure, when these agents are used in the multimodality setting. Several large-scale randomized trials are currently under way comparing, for example, docetaxel and cisplatin–containing treatment to "standard" cisplatin and FU or, alternatively, irinotecan and cisplatin–containing therapy to cisplatin and FU.

PREDICTING RESPONSE

The development of techniques that will allow physicians to choose those individual chemotherapeutic agents that are most likely to work in the individual patient is a high priority. It is particularly important because currently available cytotoxic chemotherapy for gastric cancer has only modest to moderate effectiveness, with objective regressions in 25% to 40% of all patients treated, and toxicities can be substantial. Earlier *in vitro* assays have not proven to have adequate sensitivity; however, several studies suggest that molecular analysis of tumor tissue might be a more accurate measure to predict outcome. The hypothesis is that levels of expression of target molecules, or of molecules associated with the mechanism of action of an individual agent, are associated with response or resistance.

Several new techniques for molecular analysis are being studied to allow individualization of therapy. These include immunohistochemical stains for expression of the molecular marker of interest (such as TS) or use of reverse transcriptase-polymerase chain reaction technology to measure relative gene expression. In gastric cancer, a substantial amount of data involves the use of relative gene expression of messenger RNA. For example, in trials from the University of Southern California and Memorial Sloan-Kettering Cancer Center, studies have been performed in patients with locally advanced but not metastatic gastric cancer. Although response has been used in the outcome analysis in several of these trials, it should be recognized that response assessment in locoregional gastric cancer can be difficult; survival is a firmer end point. Lenz and colleagues[293] and Metzger et al.[294] from the same group reported an analysis of a subgroup of patients receiving neoadjuvant cisplatin and FU chemotherapy followed by resection and intraperitoneal FUDR chemotherapy. Response and survival were correlated with molecular markers in 38 evaluable patients. Those with low levels of relative TS and ERCC1 (excision repair cross complementing gene; a marker for cisplatin sensitivity) had a significantly longer median and long-term survival than did patients with high levels of expression. Fata and colleagues[294a] evaluated the predictive value of TS, thymidylate phosphorylase, dihydropyrimidine dehydrogenase, and ERCC1 in inoperable gastric cancer patients undergoing surgery, without pre- or postoperative chemotherapy. This study addressed the question as to whether levels of expression of a molecular marker were independent predictors of outcome, or whether levels of gene expression were only important in the context of chemotherapy. In a preliminary assessment, patients with low relative gene expression of TS, TP, or ERCC1 did not have an improved outcome (either disease-free or overall survival). They noted that surgery-only patients with high TS gene expression, a marker that would predict resistance to chemotherapy, had a better survival compared to patients with low TS. This finding was persistent even in a multivariant analysis adjusting for stage. Conversely, patients receiving cisplatin and FU preoperative chemotherapy with low TS were more likely to have better outcome. Several other groups also have investigated the use of similar molecular markers. Boku and colleagues[295] used immunohistochemistry to measure TS, p53, vascular endothelial growth factor, and glutathione S-transferase. Thirty-nine patients in this study had unresectable disease and received cisplatin plus FU. Patients with immunohistochemistry negative for TS (indicating low expression) had a higher response rate and survived longer than patients with positive stains, as did those negative for p53, BCL2, and glutathione S-transferase. Conversely, patients with vascular endothelial growth factor–positive tumors had a higher response rate. A multivariant analysis indicated that a combination of favorable molecular phenotypes had a greater impact on survival than did performance status or other clinical parameters.

Resistance to chemotherapy has been reported by many investigators to be associated with mutations of the p53 oncogene. Several such studies have been performed in gastric cancer. Cascinu and colleagues[296] performed immunohistochemistry on pretreatment endoscopic biopsies in 30 patients with locally advanced but not metastatic disease. As is the case in other studies in this group of patients, assessing response can be difficult. With this caveat, 16 of 30 patients had high levels of p53 expression by immunohistochemistry. Ten of 12 responding patents had p53-negative tumors. These authors concluded that mutation of p53 oncogene confers resistance to chemotherapy. On the other hand, Ikeguchi et al.[297] found no relationship between p53 status and intraperitoneal chemotherapy, nor did Yeh and colleagues.[298] A definitive study in which adequate numbers of patients with advanced gastric cancer receive the same chemotherapy irrespective of their molecular marker profile and are followed prospectively has not yet been performed. Such studies have been proposed for other tumors (such as colorectal cancer). The identification of molecular markers measured by immunohistochemistry, by reverse transcriptase-polymerase chain reaction, or by other techniques that could predict outcome would be a substantial improvement in directing therapy.

CHEMOTHERAPY VERSUS BEST SUPPORTIVE CARE

During the late 1980s and early 1990s, considerable debate occurred over whether chemotherapy for patients with advanced gastric cancer had any advantages over best supportive care. This issue is of importance, not only in addressing the options for stan-

TABLE 33.3-18. Chemotherapy for Advanced Gastric Cancer: Treatment versus Best Supportive Care

Regimen	*Number of Patients*	*Median Survival (mo)*	*Survival Rate (%)* 1 Y	2 Y
FAMTX	30	10	40	6
BSC	10	3	10	0
FEMTX	17	12	—	—
BSC	19	3	—	—
EtopLF	10	10	—	—
BSC	8	4	—	—
ELF	52	10.2	34.6	9.6
BSC	51	5	7.8	0

A, doxorubicin (Adriamycin); BSC, best supportive care; E, epirubicin; etop, etoposide; F, fluorouracil; L, leucovorin; MTX, methotrexate. (Modified from Wils J. The treatment of advanced gastric cancer. *Semin Oncol* 1996;23:397, with permission.)

dard care treatment for patients with advanced disease, but in the implication that effective systemic therapy given in the palliative setting may lead to an increase in cure rate for patients with localized, high-risk, potentially curable tumors. Four randomized trials have been reported in which patients were assigned to either chemotherapy and best supportive care or best supportive care alone. In all of these trials, the option for the initiation of chemotherapy at the time of symptomatic or objective progression was at the discretion of the treating physician. Although these studies have relatively small numbers of patients (recognizing the difficulty of performing such studies and that, in several cases, the study was stopped when benefit was seen in the chemotherapy-receiving arm), the data are fairly consistent. Patients randomized to receive best supportive care alone, even when allowed to receive chemotherapy at a later date, have a median survival of 3 to 5 months. Patients randomized to immediate chemotherapy had a median survival of 9 to 11 months. More impressive is 1- and 2-year survival when reported. As shown in Table 33.3-18, the 1-year survival rate is 35% to 40% for patients receiving chemotherapy versus approximately 10% for those randomized to best supportive care. The 2-year survival rate is 6% to 10% for patients receiving chemotherapy versus 0% of patients with initial observation. These data strongly support the conclusion similar to that of other malignancies, such as colorectal and breast cancer, that systemic chemotherapy has a real although modest affect on survival in patients with advanced disease. Furthermore, the results support the use of systemic cytotoxic chemotherapy as part of multimodality therapy in patients with less-advanced but high-risk cancers. None of the regimens used in the best supportive care trials included cisplatin nor, of course, the more recently identified active agents paclitaxel, docetaxel, and irinotecan. As already discussed, however, reports on longer-term follow-up of randomized chemotherapy trials also show 5% to 15% of patients living for longer than 2 years.

SURGERY FOR PALLIATION

Because the survival for patients with advanced gastric cancer is so poor, any proposed operation should have a good chance of providing sustained symptomatic relief while minimizing the attendant morbidity and need for prolonged hospitalization. Ekbom and Gleysteen[299] have reviewed the results of palliative resection versus intestinal bypass (gastrojejunostomy) in 75 patients with advanced gastric cancer. The most frequent symptoms for which patients underwent operation included pain, hemorrhage, nausea, dysphagia, or obstruction. Operative mortality was 25% for gastrojejunostomy, 20% for palliative partial or subtotal gastrectomy, and 27% for total or proximal palliative gastrectomy. The most common and often fatal complication was anastomotic leak. After gastrojejunostomy, 80% of patients had relief of symptoms for a mean of 5.9 months compared with palliative resection, which provided relief of symptoms in 88% of patients for a mean of 14.6 months. Although the duration of palliation was significantly longer after resection (P <.01), the selection criteria for resection versus bypass were not controlled, and some bias against performing a palliative resection in high-risk patients with more advanced disease may have occurred. Meijer and colleagues[300] also have reported a retrospective analysis of 51 patients undergoing either palliative intestinal bypass or resection. In 20 of 26 patients (77%) undergoing resection, palliation was considered moderate to good with a mean survival of 9.5 months. After gastroenterostomy, some palliation was noted in 8 of 25 patients (30%), and survival was 4.2 months. Butler and colleagues[167] have presented the results of total gastrectomy for palliation in 27 patients with advanced gastric cancer. Operative mortality was only 4%, whereas morbidity occurred in 48% of patients. Median survival was 15 months, with a survival rate of 38% at 2 years. This substantial survival rate at 2 years reflects the fact that, although all patients were symptomatic before surgery, only one-half had stage IV disease. Patients with linitis plastica present a very difficult therapeutic challenge. Resection may provide palliation of symptoms; however, survival after total gastrectomy is exceedingly poor, ranging from 3 months to 1 year.[301]

Bozzetti and colleagues[302] have reviewed the outcomes of 246 patients with advanced gastric cancer who underwent simple exploratory laparotomy alone, gastrointestinal bypass, or palliative resection at the National Cancer Institute of Milan. When survival was compared in patients with similar type and extent of disease, a consistent trend was seen for improved median survival with palliative resection in patients with local spread (4.4 vs. 8 months) and distant spread of disease (3 vs. 8 months). Boddie et al.[303] has reported similar results in 45 patients undergoing palliative resection at the M. D. Anderson Cancer Center for advanced gastric cancer. Operative mortality for resection was 22%. In 21 patients who had undergone a palliative bypass procedure, survival was significantly shorter than for those undergoing resection (P<.01).

In select patients with symptomatic advanced gastric cancer, resection of the primary disease appears to provide symptomatic relief with acceptable morbidity and mortality, even in the presence of macroscopic residual disease. The criteria for deciding which patients may benefit from palliative operation have not been established, and the data available represent retrospective analyses of patients selected for operation. The choice of procedure in these studies may have been influenced by differences in opinion regarding the value of palliative surgery in patients with such a grave prognosis.

RADIATION FOR PALLIATION

To date, no studies have evaluated the use of radiation therapy in patients with locally recurrent or metastatic carcinoma of the stomach. Its use is likely to be limited to palliation of symptoms, such as bleeding or controlling pain secondary to local tumor infiltration. Although minimal data are available, radiation therapy seems to be fairly effective (from anecdotal experience) in controlling bleeding, as is true in other sites. This can often be accomplished at relatively low radiation doses. Pain from local tumor invasion can also be palliated, although the doses required are higher (4000 cGy). On rare occasions, a case may arise of a patient with a focal local recurrence without metastases who would be amenable to relatively high-dose radiation therapy to try to prolong survival or in whom radiation therapy would be given as an adjuvant to surgical resection. At present, however, no data support such an approach.

REFERENCES

1. Landis SH, Murray T, Bolden S, Wingo PA. Cancer statistics, 1999. *CA Cancer J Clin* 1999;49:8.
2. Boring C, Squires T, Tong J. Cancer statistics. *CA Cancer J Clin* 1991;41:28.
3. Blot WJ, Devesa SS, Kneller RW, Fraumeni JF Jr. Rising incidence of adenocarcinoma of the esophagus and gastric cardia. *JAMA* 1991;265:1287.
4. Meyers WC, Damiano RJ Jr, Rotolo FS, Postlethwait RW. Adenocarcinoma of the stomach. Changing patterns over the last 4 decades. *Ann Surg* 1987;205:1.
5. Salvon-Harman JC, Cady B, Nikulasson S, et al. Shifting proportions of gastric adenocarcinomas. *Arch Surg* 1994;129:381, discussion 388.
6. Laurén P. The two histological main types of gastric carcinoma: diffuse and so-called intestinal-type carcinoma. *Acta Pathol* 1965;64:31.
7. Holtz J, Goebell H. Epidemiology and pathogenesis of gastric carcinoma. In: Meyer HJ, Schmoll HJ, Holtz J, eds. *Gastric carcinoma.* New York: Springer-Verlag New York, 1989:3.
8. Aird I, Bentall H. A relationship between cancer of the stomach and the ABO blood group. *BMJ* 1953:799.
9. Correa P, Cuello C, Duque E. Carcinoma and intestinal metaplasia in the stomach in Colombian migrants. *J Natl Cancer Inst* 1970;44:297.
10. Imai T, Kubo T, Watanabe H. Chronic gastritis in Japanese with reference to high incidence of gastric carcinoma. *J Natl Cancer Inst* 1971;47:179.
11. Fortner JG, Lauwers GY, Thaler HT, et al. Nativity, complications, and pathology are determinants of surgical results for gastric cancer. *Cancer* 1994;73:8.
12. Mettlin C. Epidemiologic studies in gastric adenocarcinoma. In: Douglass HJ, ed. *Gastric cancer.* New York: Churchill Livingstone, 1988:1.
13. Murakami R, Tsukuma H, Ubukata T, et al. Estimation of validity of mass screening program for gastric cancer in Osaka, Japan. *Cancer* 1990;65:1255.
14. Hotz J, Goebell H. Epidemiology and pathogenesis of gastric carcinoma. In: Meyer H, Schmoll HJ, Hotz J, eds. *Gastric carcinoma.* New York: Springer-Verlag New York, 1989:3.
15. Staszewski J. Migrant studies in alimentary tract cancer. *Recent Results Cancer Res* 1972;39:85.
16. Haenszel W, Kurihara M, Segi M, Lee RK. Stomach cancer among Japanese in Hawaii. *J Natl Cancer Inst* 1972;49:969.
17. Correa P. Clinical implications of recent developments in gastric cancer pathology and epidemiology. *Semin Oncol* 1985;12:2.
18. Boeing H. Epidemiological research in stomach cancer: progress over the last ten years [Editorial] [published erratum appears in *J Cancer Res Clin Oncol* 1991;117:273]. *J Cancer Res Clin Oncol* 1991;117:133.
19. Nagayo T. Background data to study of advanced gastric cancer. In: *Histogenesis and precursors of human gastric cancer.* New York: Springer-Verlag New York, 1986:17.
20. Cady B, Rossi RL, Silverman ML, et al. Gastric adenocarcinoma. A disease in transition. *Arch Surg* 1989;124:303.
21. Powell J, McConkey CC. The rising trend in oesophageal adenocarcinoma and gastric cardia. *Eur J Cancer Prev* 1992;1:265.
22. Powell J, McConkey CC. Increasing incidence of adenocarcinoma of the gastric cardia and adjacent sites. *Br J Cancer* 1990;62:440.
23. Rohde H, Bauer P, Stutzer H, et al. Proximal compared with distal adenocarcinoma of the stomach: differences and consequences. German Gastric Cancer TNM Study Group. *Br J Surgery* 1991;78:1242.
24. Harrison LE, Karpeh MS, Brennan MF. Proximal gastric cancers resected via a transabdominal-only approach. Results and comparisons to distal adenocarcinoma of the stomach. *Ann Surg* 1997;225:678, discussion 683.
25. Maehara Y, Moriguchi S, Kakeji Y, et al. Prognostic factors in adenocarcinoma in the upper one-third of the stomach. *Surg Gynecol Obstet* 1991;173:223.
26. Ohno S, Tomisaki S, Oiwa H, et al. Clinicopathologic characteristics and outcome of adenocarcinoma of the human gastric cardia in comparison with carcinoma of other regions of the stomach. *J Am Coll Surg* 1995;180:577.
27. Chow WH, Blot WJ, Vaughan TL, et al. Body mass index and risk of adenocarcinomas of the esophagus and gastric cardia. *J Natl Cancer Inst* 1998;90:150.
28. Lagergren J, Bergstrom R, Nyren O. Association between body mass and adenocarcinoma of the esophagus and gastric cardia. *Ann Intern Med* 1999;130:883.
29. Zhang ZF, Kurtz RC, Yu GP, et al. Adenocarcinomas of the esophagus and gastric cardia: the role of diet. *Nutr Cancer* 1997;27:298.
30. Lagergren J, Bergstrom R, Lindgren A, Nyren O. Symptomatic gastroesophageal reflux as a risk factor for esophageal adenocarcinoma. *N Engl J Med* 1999;340:825.
31. Zhang ZF, Kurtz RC, Sun M, et al. Adenocarcinomas of the esophagus and gastric cardia: medical conditions, tobacco, alcohol, and socioeconomic factors. *Cancer Epidemiol Biomarkers Prev* 1996;5:761.
32. Gammon MD, Schoenberg JB, Ahsan H, et al. Tobacco, alcohol, and socioeconomic status and adenocarcinomas of the esophagus and gastric cardia. *J Natl Cancer Inst* 1997;89:1277.
33. Farrow DC, Vaughan TL, Hansten PD, et al. Use of aspirin and other nonsteroidal anti-inflammatory drugs and risk of esophageal and gastric cancer. *Cancer Epidemiol Biomarkers Prev* 1998;7:97.
34. Chyou PH, Nomura AM, Hankin JH, Stemmermann GN. A case-cohort study of diet and stomach cancer. *Cancer Res* 1990;50:7501.
35. Nomura A, Grove JS, Stemmermann GN, Severson RK. A prospective study of stomach cancer and its relation to diet, cigarettes, and alcohol consumption [See comments]. *Cancer Res* 1990;50:627.
36. Weisburger JH, Marquardt H, Mower HF, et al. Inhibition of carcinogenesis: vitamin C and the prevention of gastric cancer. *Prev Med* 1980;9:352.
37. Dorgan JF, Schatzkin A. Antioxidant micronutrients in cancer prevention. *Hematol Oncol Clin North Am* 1991;5:43.
38. Forman D. Are nitrates a significant risk factor in human cancer? *Cancer Surv* 1989;8:443.
39. Burstein M, Monge E, Leon-Barua R, et al. Low peptic ulcer and high gastric cancer prevalence in a developing country with a high prevalence of infection by *Helicobacter pylori. J Clin Gastroenterol* 1991;13:154.
40. Matsukura N, Kawachi T, Sasajima K, et al. Induction of intestinal metaplasia in the stomachs of rats by N-methyl-N'-nitro-N-nitrosoguanidine. *J Natl Cancer Inst* 1978;61:141.
41. Sasajima K, Kawachi T, Matsukura N, et al. Intestinal metaplasia and adenocarcinoma induced in the stomach of rats by N-propyl-N'-nitro-N-nitrosoguanidine. *J Cancer Res Clin Oncol* 1979;94:201.
42. Morson B. Carcinoma arising from areas of intestinal metaplasia in the gastric mucosa. *Br J Cancer* 1955;9:377.
43. Hoffman NR. The relationship between pernicious anemia and cancer of the stomach. *Geriatrics* 1970;25:90.
44. Correa P, Haenszel W, Cuello C, et al. Gastric precancerous process in a high risk population: cross-sectional studies. *Cancer Res* 1990;50:4731.
45. Selves J, Bibeau F, Brousset P, et al. Epstein-Barr virus latent and replicative gene expression in gastric carcinoma. *Histopathology* 1996;28:121.
46. Adachi Y, Yoh R, Konishi J, et al. Epstein-Barr virus–associated gastric carcinoma. *J Clin Gastroenterol* 1996;23:207.
47. Tokunaga M, Land CE, Uemura Y, et al. Epstein-Barr virus in gastric carcinoma. *Am J Pathol* 1993;143:1250.
48. Baas IO, van Rees BP, Musler A, et al. *Helicobacter pylori* and Epstein-Barr virus infection and the p53 tumour suppressor pathway in gastric stump cancer compared with carcinoma in the non-operated stomach. *J Clin Pathol* 1998;51:662.
49. Watanabe S, Tsugane S, Ohno Y. Etiology. In: Sugimura T, Sasako M, eds. *Gastric cancer.* Tokyo: Oxford, 1997:33.
50. Kato H, Schull WJ. Studies of the mortality of A-bomb survivors. 7. Mortality, 1950–1978: Part I. Cancer mortality. *Radiat Res* 1982;90:395.
51. Griem ML, Justman J, Weiss L. The neoplastic potential of gastric irradiation. IV. Risk estimates. *Am J Clin Oncol* 1984;7:675.
52. Shinmura K, Kohno T, Takahashi M, et al. Familial gastric cancer: clinicopathological characteristics, RER phenotype and germline p53 and E-cadherin mutations. *Carcinogenesis* 1999;20:1127.
53. Zanghieri G, Di Gregorio C, Sacchetti C, et al. Familial occurrence of gastric cancer in the 2-year experience of a population-based registry. *Cancer* 1990;66:2047.
54. Sokoloff B. Predisposition to cancer in the Bonaparte family. *Am J Surg* 1938;40:673.
55. Guilford P, Hopkins J, Harraway J, et al. E-cadherin germline mutations in familial gastric cancer. *Nature* 1998;392:402.
56. Richards FM, McKee SA, Rajpar MH, et al. Germline E-cadherin gene (CDH1) mutations predispose to familial gastric cancer and colorectal cancer. *Hum Mol Genet* 1999;8:607.
57. Balfour DC. Factors influencing the life expectancy of patients operated on for gastric surgery. *Ann Surg* 1922;76:405.
58. Lygidakis NJ. Gastric stump carcinoma after surgery for gastroduodenal ulcer. *Ann R Coll Surg Engl* 1981;63:203.
59. Stalnikowicz R, Benbassat J. Risk of gastric cancer after gastric surgery for benign disorders. *Arch Intern Med* 1990;150:2022.
60. Tersmette AC, Offerhaus GJ, Tersmette KW, et al. Meta-analysis of the risk of gastric stump cancer: detection of high risk patient subsets for stomach cancer after remote partial gastrectomy for benign conditions. *Cancer Res* 1990;50:6486.
61. La Vecchia C, Negri E, Franceschi S, D'Avanzo B. Histamine-2-receptor antagonists and gastric cancer: update and note on latency and covariates. *Nutrition* 1992;8:177.
62. Schumacher MC, Jick SS, Jick H, Feld AD. Cimetidine use and gastric cancer. *Epidemiology* 1990;1:251.
63. Dooley CP, Cohen H, Fitzgibbons PL, et al. Prevalence of *Helicobacter pylori* infection and histologic gastritis in asymptomatic persons. *N Engl J Med* 1989;321:1562.
64. Parsonnet J, Vandersteen D, Goates J, et al. *Helicobacter pylori* infection in intestinal- and diffuse-type gastric adenocarcinomas [published erratum appears in *J Natl Cancer Inst* 1991;83:881]. *J Natl Cancer Inst* 1991;83:640.
65. Parsonnet J, Friedman GD, Vandersteen DP, et al. *Helicobacter pylori* infection and the risk of gastric carcinoma [See comments]. *N Engl J Med* 1991;325:1127.
66. Nomura A, Stemmermann GN, Chyou PH, et al. *Helicobacter pylori* infection and gastric carcinoma among Japanese Americans in Hawaii [See comments]. *N Engl J Med* 1991;325:1132.
67. Lin JT, Lee WC, Wu MS, et al. Diagnosis of gastric adenocarcinoma using a scoring system: combined assay of serological markers of *Helicobacter pylori* infection, pepsinogen I and gastrin. *J Gastroenterol* 1995;30:156.
68. Hansson LE, Engstrand L, Nyren O, et al. *Helicobacter pylori* infection: independent risk indicator of gastric adenocarcinoma [See comments]. *Gastroenterology* 1993;105:1098.
69. Endo S, Ohkusa T, Saito Y, et al. Detection of *Helicobacter pylori* infection in early stage gastric cancer. A comparison between intestinal- and diffuse-type gastric adenocarcinomas. *Cancer* 1995;75:2203.
70. Blaser MJ, Perez-Perez GI, Kleanthous H, et al. Infection with *Helicobacter pylori* strains possessing cagA is associated with an increased risk of developing adenocarcinoma of the stomach. *Cancer Res* 1995;55:2111.

71. Lewin JK, Appelman HD. Carcinoma of the stomach. In: Rosai J, Sobin LH, eds. *Tumors of the esophagus and stomach,* vol 18. Washington, DC: Armed Forces Institute of Pathology, 1995:245.
72. Isaacson PG. Gastric MALT lymphoma: from concept to cure. *Ann Oncol* 1999;10:637.
73. Haber DA, Mayer RJ. Primary gastrointestinal lymphoma. *Semin Oncol* 1988;15:154.
74. Japanese Research Society for Gastric Cancer. *Japanese classification of gastric cancer.* Tokyo: Kanehara & Co, 1995.
75. Kitamura K, Beppu R, Anai H, et al. Clinicopathologic study of patients with Borrmann type IV gastric carcinoma. *J Surg Oncol* 1995;58:112.
76. Ming SC. Gastric carcinoma. A pathobiological classification. *Cancer* 1977;39:2475.
77. Bearzi I, Ranaldi R. Early gastric cancer: a morphologic study of 41 cases. *Tumori* 1982;68:223.
78. Zinninger M. Extension of gastric cancer in the intramural lymphatics and its relation to gastrectomy. *Am Surg* 1954;20:920.
79. Shiu MH, Papacristou DN, Kosloff C, Eliopoulos G. Selection of operative procedure for adenocarcinoma of the midstomach. Twenty years' experience with implications for future treatment strategy. *Ann Surg* 1980;192:730.
80. Papachristou DN, Shiu MH. Management by *en bloc* multiple organ resection of carcinoma of the stomach invading adjacent organs. *Surg Gynecol Obstet* 1981;152:483.
81. McNeer G, Bowden L, Booner RJ, McPeak CJ. Elective total gastrectomy for cancer of the stomach: end results. *Ann Surg* 1974;180:252.
82. Wisbeck W, Becher E, Russel A. Adenocarcinoma of the stomach: autopsy observations with therapeutic implications for the radiation oncologist. *Radiother Oncol* 1986;7:13.
83. Gunderson L, Sosin H. Adenocarcinoma of the stomach: areas of failure in a reoperative series (second or symptomatic look) clinicopathologic correlation and implications for adjuvant therapy. *Int J Radiat Oncol Biol Phys* 1982;8:1.
84. Allum WH, Hallissey MT, Ward LC, Hockey MS. A controlled, prospective, randomised trial of adjuvant chemotherapy or radiotherapy in resectable gastric cancer: interim report. British Stomach Cancer Group. *Br J Cancer* 1989;60:739.
85. Landry J, Tepper JE, Wood WC, et al. Patterns of failure following curative resection of gastric carcinoma. *Int J Radiat Oncol Biol Phys* 1990;19:1357.
86. Ajani JA, Ota DM, Jessup JM, et al. Resectable gastric carcinoma. An evaluation of preoperative and postoperative chemotherapy. *Cancer* 1991;68:1501.
87. Dewys WD, Begg C, Lavin PT, et al. Prognostic effect of weight loss prior to chemotherapy in cancer patients. Eastern Cooperative Oncology Group. *Am J Med* 1980;69:491.
88. Kaneko E, Nakamura T, Umeda N, et al. Outcome of gastric carcinoma detected by gastric mass survey in Japan. *Gut* 1977;18:626.
89. Murakami R, Tsukuma H, Ubukata T, et al. Estimation of validity of mass screening program for gastric cancer in Osaka, Japan. *Cancer* 1990;65:1255.
90. Yoshihara M, Sumii K, Haruma K, et al. Correlation of ratio of serum pepsinogen I and II with prevalence of gastric cancer and adenoma in Japanese subjects. *Am J Gastroenterol* 1998;93:1090.
91. Nakane Y, Okamura S, Akehira K, et al. Correlation of preoperative carcinoembryonic antigen levels and prognosis of gastric cancer patients. *Cancer* 1994;73:2703.
92. Ikeda Y, Oomori H, Koyanagi N, et al. Prognostic value of combination assays for CEA and CA 19-9 in gastric cancer. *Oncology* 1995;52:483.
93. Kodera Y, Yamamura Y, Torii A, et al. The prognostic value of preoperative serum levels of CEA and CA19-9 in patients with gastric cancer. *Am J Gastroenterol* 1996;91:49.
94. Pectasides D, Mylonakis A, Kostopoulou M, et al. CEA, CA 19-9, and CA-50 in monitoring gastric carcinoma. *Am J Clin Oncol* 1997;20:348.
95. Botet JF, Lightdale CJ, Zauber AG, et al. Preoperative staging of gastric cancer: comparison of endoscopic US and dynamic CT. *Radiology* 1991;181:426.
96. Graham DY, Schwartz JT, Cain GD, Gyorkey F. Prospective evaluation of biopsy number in the diagnosis of esophageal and gastric carcinoma. *Gastroenterology* 1982;82:228.
97. Kurtz RC, Sherlock P. The diagnosis of gastric cancer. *Semin Oncol* 1985;12:11.
98. Grimm H, Binmoeller KF, Hamper K, et al. Endosonography for preoperative locoregional staging of esophageal and gastric cancer. *Endoscopy* 1993;25:224.
99. Akahoshi K, Chijiiwa Y, Hamada S, et al. Endoscopic ultrasonography: a promising method for assessing the prospects of endoscopic mucosal resection in early gastric cancer. *Endoscopy* 1997;29:614.
100. Yanai H, Matsumoto Y, Harada T, et al. Endoscopic ultrasonography and endoscopy for staging depth of invasion in early gastric cancer: a pilot study. *Gastrointest Endosc* 1997;46:212.
101. Karpeh M, Brennan M. Gastric carcinoma: counterpoints. In: Johnson F, Virgo K, eds. *Cancer patient follow-up.* St. Louis: Mosby, 1997:100.
102. Kurihara M, Shirakabe H, Yarita T, et al. Diagnosis of small early gastric cancer by x-ray, endoscopy, and biopsy. *Cancer Detect Prev* 1981;4:377.
103. Miller FH, Kochman ML, Talamonti MS, et al. Gastric cancer. Radiologic staging. *Radiol Clin North Am* 1997;35:331.
104. Cook AO, Levine BA, Sirinek KR, Gaskill HV. Evaluation of gastric adenocarcinoma. Abdominal computed tomography does not replace celiotomy. *Arch Surg* 1986;121:603.
105. Takao M, Fukuda T, Iwanaga S, et al. Gastric cancer: evaluation of triphasic spiral CT and radiologic-pathologic correlation. *J Comput Assist Tomogr* 1998;22:288.
106. Gupta N, Bradfield H. Role of positron emission tomography scanning in evaluating gastrointestinal neoplasms. *Semin Nucl Med* 1996;26:65.
107. Luketich JD, Schauer PR, Meltzer CC, et al. Role of positron emission tomography in staging esophageal cancer. *Ann Thorac Surg* 1997;64:765.
108. Asencio F, Aguilo J, Salvador JL, et al. Video-laparoscopic staging of gastric cancer. A prospective multicenter comparison with noninvasive techniques. *Surg Endosc* 1997;11:1153.
109. Burke EC, Karpeh MS, Conlon KC, Brennan MF. Laparoscopy in the management of gastric adenocarcinoma. *Ann Surg* 1997;225:262.
110. Stell DA, Carter CR, Stewart I, Anderson JR. Prospective comparison of laparoscopy, ultrasonography and computed tomography in the staging of gastric cancer [See comments]. *Br J Surg* 1996;83:1260.
111. Stell DA, Carter CR, Stewart I, Anderson JR. Prospective comparison of laparoscopy, ultrasonography and computed tomography in the staging of gastric cancer. *Br J Surg* 1996;83:1260.
112. Lowy AM, Mansfield PF, Leach SD, Ajani J. Laparoscopic staging for gastric cancer. *Surgery* 1996;119:611.
113. Possik RA, Franco EL, Pires DR, et al. Sensitivity, specificity, and predictive value of laparoscopy for the staging of gastric cancer and for the detection of liver metastases. *Cancer* 1986;58:1.
114. Bartlett DL, Conlon KC, Gerdes H, Karpeh MS Jr. Laparoscopic ultrasonography: the best pretreatment staging modality in gastric adenocarcinoma? Case report. *Surgery* 1995;118:562.
115. Hermanek P, Wittekind C. Residual tumor (R) classification and prognosis. *Semin Surg Oncol* 1994;10:12.
116. Lisborg PH, Jatzko GR, Denk H, et al. Long-term survival analysis of gastric cancer limited to the subserosa. *Zeitschrift fur Gastroenterologie* 1997;35:663.
117. Maruyama K, Okabayashi K, Kinoshita T. Progress in gastric cancer surgery in Japan and its limits of radicality. *World J Surg* 1987;11:418.
118. Boku T, Nakane Y, Minoura T, et al. Prognostic significance of serosal invasion and free intraperitoneal cancer cells in gastric cancer. *Br J Surg* 1990;77:436.
119. Baba H, Korenaga D, Okamura T, et al. Prognostic factors in gastric cancer with serosal invasion. Univariate and multivariate analyses. *Arch Surg* 1989;124:1061.
120. Hermanek P. Prognostic factors in stomach cancer surgery. *Eur J Surg Oncol* 1986;12:241.
121. Shiu MH, Perrotti M, Brennan MF. Adenocarcinoma of the stomach: a multivariate analysis of clinical, pathologic and treatment factors. *Hepatogastroenterology* 1989;36:7.
122. Roder JD, Bottcher K, Busch R, et al. Classification of regional lymph node metastasis from gastric carcinoma. German Gastric Cancer Study Group. *Cancer* 1998;82:621.
123. Adachi Y, Kamakura T, Mori M, et al. Prognostic significance of the number of positive lymph nodes in gastric carcinoma. *Br J Surg* 1994;81:414.
124. Wanebo HJ, Kennedy BJ, Winchester DP, et al. Gastric carcinoma: does lymph node dissection alter survival? *J Am Coll Surg* 1996;183:616.
125. Siewert JR, Bottcher K, Roder JD, et al. Prognostic relevance of systematic lymph node dissection in gastric carcinoma. German Gastric Carcinoma Study Group [See comments]. *Br J Surg* 1993;80:1015.
126. Brennan MF, Karpeh MS Jr. Surgery for gastric cancer: the American view. *Semin Oncol* 1996;23:352.
127. Sue-Ling HM, Johnston D, Martin IG, et al. Gastric cancer: a curable disease in Britain. *BMJ* 1993;307:591.
128. Murphy PD, Wadhera V, Griffin SM, et al. Free peritoneal tumour cell identification in patients with gastric and colorectal cancer. *J R Coll Surg Edinb* 1993;38:28.
129. Nekarda H, Gess C, Stark M, et al. Immunocytochemically detected free peritoneal tumour cells (FPTC) are a strong prognostic factor in gastric carcinoma. *Br J Cancer* 1999;79(3–4):611.
130. Ribeiro U Jr, Gama-Rodrigues JJ, Safatle-Ribeiro AV, et al. Prognostic significance of intraperitoneal free cancer cells obtained by laparoscopic peritoneal lavage in patients with gastric cancer. *J Gastrointest Surg* 1998;2:244.
131. Ikeguchi M, Oka A, Tsujitani S, et al. Relationship between area of serosal invasion and intraperitoneal free cancer cells in patients with gastric cancer. *Anticancer Res* 1994;14(5B):2131.
132. Burke EC, Karpeh MS Jr, Conlon KC, Brennan MF. Peritoneal lavage cytology in gastric cancer: an independent predictor of outcome. *Ann Surg Oncol* 1998;5:411.
133. Yamao T, Shirao K, Ono H, et al. Risk factors for lymph node metastasis from intramucosal gastric carcinoma. *Cancer* 1996;77:602.
134. Takekoshi T, Baba Y, Ota H, et al. Endoscopic resection of early gastric carcinoma: results of a retrospective analysis of 308 cases. *Endoscopy* 1994;26:352.
135. Ishigami S, Hokita S, Natsugoe S, et al. Carcinomatous infiltration into the submucosa as a predictor of lymph node involvement in early gastric cancer. *World J Surg* 1998;22:1056, discussion 1059.
136. Maruyama K, Gunven P, Okabayashi K, et al. Lymph node metastases of gastric cancer. General pattern in 1931 patients. *Ann Surg* 1989;210:596.
137. Takeda J, Koufuji K, Kodama I, et al. Total gastrectomy for gastric cancer: 12-year data and review of the effect of performing lymphadenectomy. *Kurume Med J* 1994;41:15.
138. Kodama Y, Sugimachi K, Soejima K, et al. Evaluation of extensive lymph node dissection for carcinoma of the stomach. *World J Surg* 1981;5:241.
139. Sowa M, Kato Y, Nishimura M, et al. Surgical approach to early gastric cancer with lymph node metastasis. *World J Surg* 1989;13:630.
140. Boku T, Nakane Y, Okusa T, et al. Strategy for lymphadenectomy of gastric cancer. *Surgery* 1989;105:585.
141. Jatzko G, Lisborg PH, Klimpfinger M, Denk H. Extended radical surgery against gastric cancer: low complication and high survival rates. *Jpn J Clin Oncol* 1992;22:102.
142. Keller E, Stutzer H, Heitmann K, et al. Lymph node staging in 872 patients with carcinoma of the stomach and the presumed benefit of lymphadenectomy. German Stomach Cancer TNM Study Group. *J Am Coll Surg* 1994;178:38.
143. Roder JD, Bottcher K, Siewert JR, et al. Prognostic factors in gastric carcinoma. Results of the German Gastric Carcinoma Study 1992. *Cancer* 1993;72:2089.
144. Irvin TT, Bridger JE. Gastric cancer: an audit of 122 consecutive cases and the results of R1 gastrectomy. *Br J Surg* 1988;75:106.
145. Okamura T, Tsujitani S, Korenaga D, et al. Lymphadenectomy for cure in patients with early gastric cancer and lymph node metastasis. *Am J Surg* 1988;155:476.
146. Noguchi Y, Imada T, Matsumoto A, et al. Radical surgery for gastric cancer. A review of the Japanese experience. *Cancer* 1989;64:2053.
147. Sue-Ling HM, Martin I, Griffith J, et al. Early gastric cancer: 46 cases treated in one surgical department. *Gut* 1992;33:1318.
148. Iriyama K, Asakawa T, Koike H, et al. Is extensive lymphadenectomy necessary for surgical treatment of intramucosal carcinoma of the stomach? *Arch Surg* 1989;124:309.
149. Farley DR, Donohue JH, Nagorney DM, et al. Early gastric cancer. *Br J Surg* 1992;79:539.
150. Maehara Y, Orita H, Moriguchi S, et al. Lower survival rate for patients under 30 years of age and surgically treated for gastric carcinoma. *Br J Cancer* 1991;63:1015.
151. Lawrence M, Shiu MH. Early gastric cancer. Twenty-eight-year experience. *Ann Surg* 1991;213:327

152. Hochwald S, Brennan M, Klimstra D, et al. Is lymphadenectomy necessary for early gastric cancer? *Ann Surg Oncol* 1999;6:664.
153. Kurihara N, Kubota T, Otani Y, et al. Lymph node metastasis of early gastric cancer with submucosal invasion. *Br J Surg* 1998;85:835.
154. Dent DM, Madden MV, Price SK. Randomized comparison of R1 and R2 gastrectomy for gastric carcinoma. *Br J Surg* 1988;75:110.
155. Dent DM, Madden MV, Price SK. Controlled trials and the R1/R2 controversy in the management of gastric carcinoma. *Surg Oncol Clin North Am* 1993;2:433.
156. Robertson CS, Chung SC, Woods SD, et al. A prospective randomized trial comparing R1 subtotal gastrectomy with R3 total gastrectomy for antral cancer [See comments]. *Ann Surg* 1994;220:176.
157. Smith JW, Shiu MH, Kelsey L, Brennan MF. Morbidity of radical lymphadenectomy in the curative resection of gastric carcinoma. *Arch Surg* 1991;126:1469.
158. Roder JD, Bonenkamp JJ, Craven J, et al. Lymphadenectomy for gastric cancer in clinical trials: update. *World J Surg* 1995;19:546.
159. Cuschieri A, Fayers P, Fielding J, et al. Postoperative morbidity and mortality after D1 and D2 resections for gastric cancer: preliminary results of the MRC randomised controlled surgical trial. The Surgical Cooperative Group. *Lancet* 1996;347:995.
160. Cuschieri A, Weeden S, Fielding J, et al. Patient survival after D1 and D2 resections for gastric cancer: long-term results of the MRC randomized surgical trial. Surgical Co-operative Group. *Br J Cancer* 1999;79(9–10):1522.
161. Bunt TM, Bonenkamp HJ, Hermans J, et al. Factors influencing noncompliance and contamination in a randomized trial of "Western" (r1) versus "Japanese" (r2) type surgery in gastric cancer. *Cancer* 1994;73:1544.
162. Bonenkamp JJ, Songun I, Hermans J, et al. Randomised comparison of morbidity after D1 and D2 dissection for gastric cancer in 996 Dutch patients. *Lancet* 1995;345:745.
163. Isozaki H, Okajima K, Hu X, et al. Multiple early gastric carcinomas. Clinicopathologic features and histogenesis. *Cancer* 1996;78:2078.
164. Gouzi JL, Huguier M, Fagniez PL, et al. Total versus subtotal gastrectomy for adenocarcinoma of the gastric antrum. A French prospective controlled study. *Ann Surg* 1989;209:162.
165. Bozzetti F, Marubini E, Bonfanti G, et al. Subtotal versus total gastrectomy for gastric cancer: five-year survival rates in a multicenter randomized Italian trial. Italian Gastrointestinal Tumor Study Group. *Ann Surg* 1999;230:170.
166. Bozzetti F, Marubini E, Bonfanti G, et al. Total versus subtotal gastrectomy: surgical morbidity and mortality rates in a multicenter Italian randomized trial. The Italian Gastrointestinal Tumor Study Group. *Ann Surg* 1997;226:613.
167. Butler JA, Dubrow TJ, Trezona T, et al. Total gastrectomy in the treatment of advanced gastric cancer. *Am J Surg* 1989;158:602, discussion 604.
168. Kawaura Y, Mori Y, Nakajima H, Iwa T. Total gastrectomy with left oblique abdominothoracic approach for gastric cancer involving the esophagus. *Arch Surg* 1988;123:514.
169. Paolini A, Tosato F, Cassese M, et al. Total gastrectomy in the treatment of adenocarcinoma of the cardia. Review of the results in 73 resected patients. *Am J Surg* 1986;151:238.
170. Anderson ID, MacIntyre IM. Symptomatic outcome following resection of gastric cancer. *Surg Oncol* 1995;4:35.
171. Santoro E, Garofalo A, Carlini M, et al. Early and late results of 100 consecutive total gastrectomies for cancer. *Hepatogastroenterology* 1994;41:489.
172. Bozzetti F. Total versus subtotal gastrectomy in cancer of the distal stomach: facts and fantasy. *Eur J Surg Oncol* 1992;18:572.
173. Huscher C, Chiodini S, Freni V, et al. Adequacy of paracardial dissection in subtotal versus total gastrectomy. *Br J Surg* 1992;79:942.
174. Buhl K, Schlag P, Herfarth C. Quality of life and functional results following different types of resection for gastric carcinoma. *Eur J Surg Oncol* 1990;16:404.
175. Viste A, Haugstvedt T, Eide GE, Soreide O. Postoperative complications and mortality after surgery for gastric cancer. *Ann Surg* 1988;207:7.
175a. Harrison LE, Karpeh MS, Brennan MF. Total gastrectomy is not necessary for proximal gastric cancer. *Surgery* 1998;123(2):127.
175b. Sasako M. Risk factors for surgical treatment in the Dutch Gastric Cancer Trial. *Br J Surg* 1997;84(11):1567.
176. Sugimachi K, Kodama Y, Kumashiro R, et al. Critical evaluation of prophylactic splenectomy in total gastrectomy for the stomach cancer. *Gann* 1980;71:704.
177. Brady MS, Rogatko A, Dent LL, Shiu MH. Effect of splenectomy on morbidity and survival following curative gastrectomy for carcinoma. *Arch Surg* 1991;126:359.
178. Maehara Y, Moriguchi S, Yoshida M, et al. Splenectomy does not correlate with length of survival in patients undergoing curative total gastrectomy for gastric carcinoma. Univariate and multivariate analyses. *Cancer* 1991;67:3006.
179. Adachi Y, Kamakura T, Mori M, et al. Role of lymph node dissection and splenectomy in node-positive gastric carcinoma. *Surgery* 1994;116:837.
180. Griffith JP, Sue-Ling HM, Martin I, et al. Preservation of the spleen improves survival after radical surgery for gastric cancer. *Gut* 1995;36:684.
181. Otsuji E, Yamaguchi T, Sawai K, et al. End results of simultaneous splenectomy in patients undergoing total gastrectomy for gastric carcinoma. *Surgery* 1996;120:40.
182. Wanebo HJ, Kennedy BJ, Winchester DP, et al. Role of splenectomy in gastric cancer surgery: adverse effect of elective splenectomy on long-term survival. *J Am Coll Surg* 1997;185:177.
183. Group VCSAS. Use of thiotepa as an adjuvant to the surgical management of carcinoma of the stomach. *Cancer* 1965;18:291.
184. Serlin O, Wolkoff JS, Amadeo JM, Keehn RJ. Use of 5-fluorodeoxyuridine (FUDR) as an adjuvant to the surgical management of carcinoma of the stomach. *Cancer* 1969;24:223.
185. Sautner T, Hofbauer F, Depisch D, et al. Adjuvant intraperitoneal cisplatin chemotherapy does not improve long-term survival after surgery for advanced gastric cancer. *J Clin Oncol* 1994;12:970.
186. Engstrom P, Labin P, Douglas H. Postoperative adjuvant 5 fluorouracil plus methyl CCNU therapy for gastric cancer. *Cancer* 1985;55:1868.
187. Higgins GA, Amadeo JH, Smith DE, et al. Efficacy of prolonged intermittent therapy with combined 5-FU and methyl-CCNU following resection for gastric carcinoma. A Veterans Administration Surgical Oncology Group report. *Cancer* 1983;52:1105.
188. Estrada E, Lacave L, Valle M, et al. Methyl CCNU 5 fluorouracil, and Adriamycin (MeFA) as adjuvant chemotherapy in gastric cancer. *Proc ASCO* 1988;7:94.
189. Estape J, Grau JJ, Alcobendas F, et al. Mitomycin C as an adjuvant treatment to resected gastric cancer. A 10-year follow-up. *Ann Surg* 1991;213:219.
190. Endo M, Habu H. Clinical studies of early gastric cancer. *Hepatogastroenterology* 1990;37:408.
191. Carrato A, Diaz-Rubio E, Medrano J, et al. Phase III trial of surgery versus adjuvant chemotherapy with mitomycin C and tegafur plus uracil, starting within the first week after surgery, for gastric adenocarcinoma. *Proc ASCO* 1995;14:198.
192. Allum WH, Hallissey MT, Kelly KA. Adjuvant chemotherapy in operable gastric cancer: 5 year follow-up of first British Stomach Cancer Group trial. *Lancet* 1989;1:571.
193. Nakajima T, Takahashi T, Takagi K, et al. Comparison of 5-fluorouracil with ftorafur in adjuvant chemotherapies with combined inductive and maintenance therapies for gastric cancer. *J Clin Oncol* 1984;2:1366.
194. Nakajima T, Nashimoto A, Kitamura M, et al. Adjuvant mitomycin and fluorouracil followed by oral uracil plus tegafur in serosa-negative gastric cancer: a randomised trial. Gastric Cancer Surgical Study Group. *Lancet* 1999;354:273.
195. Ross P, Cunningham D, Scarffe H, et al. Results of a randomised trial comparing ECF with MCF in advanced oesophago-gastric cancer. In: Perry MC, ed. *American Society of Clinical Oncology Thirty-Fifth Annual Meeting*, vol 18. Atlanta: American Society of Clinical Oncology, 1999:272a.
196. Coombes RC, Schein PS, Chilvers CE, et al. A randomized trial comparing adjuvant fluorouracil, doxorubicin, and mitomycin with no treatment in operable gastric cancer. International Collaborative Cancer Group. *J Clin Oncol* 1990;8:1362.
197. Macdonald JS, Fleming TR, Peterson RF, et al. Adjuvant chemotherapy with 5-FU, Adriamycin, and mitomycin-C (FAM) versus surgery alone for patients with locally advanced gastric adenocarcinoma: a Southwest Oncology Group study. *Ann Surg Oncol* 1995;2:488.
198. Krook JE, O'Connell MJ, Wieand HS, et al. A prospective, randomized evaluation of intensive-course 5-fluorouracil plus doxorubicin as surgical adjuvant chemotherapy for resected gastric cancer. *Cancer* 1991;67:2454.
198a. Klein HO, Wils J, Bleiberg H, et al. An EORTC gastrointestinal group randomized evaluation of the toxicity of sequential high-dose methotrexate and 5-fluorouracil combined with adriamycin (FAMTX) vs. 5-fluorouracil, adriamycin, and mitomycin (FAM) in advanced gastric cancer. *Med Oncol Tumor Pharmacol* 1989;6(2):171.
198b. Songun I, Keizer HJ, Hermans J, et al. Chemotherapy for operable gastric cancer: results of the Dutch randomised FAMTX trial. The Dutch Gastric Cancer Group (DGCG). *Eur J Cancer* 1999;35(4):558.
199. Neri B, de Leonardis V, Romano S, et al. Adjuvant chemotherapy after gastric resection in node-positive cancer patients: a multicentre randomised study. *Br J Cancer* 1996;73:549.
200. Tsavaris N, Tentas K, Kosmidis P, et al. A randomized trial comparing adjuvant fluorouracil, epirubicin, and mitomycin with no treatment in operable gastric cancer. *Chemotherapy* 1996;42:220.
201. Earle CC, Maroun JA. Adjuvant chemotherapy after curative resection for gastric cancer in non-Asian patients: revisiting a meta-analysis of randomised trials. *Eur J Cancer* 1999;35:1059.
202. Hermans J, Bonenkamp JJ, Boon MC, et al. Adjuvant therapy after curative resection for gastric cancer: meta-analysis of randomized trials. *J Clin Oncol* 1993;11:1441.
203. Archer S, Grey B. Intraperitoneal 5-fluorouracil infusion for treatment of both peritoneal and liver micro-metastasis. *Surgery* 1990;108:502.
204. Murthy SM, Goldschmidt RA, Rao LN, et al. The influence of surgical trauma on experimental metastasis. *Cancer* 1989;64:2035.
205. Gunduz N, Fisher B, Saffer EA. Effect of surgical removal on the growth and kinetics of residual tumor. *Cancer Res* 1979;39:3861.
206. Eggermont A, Steller E, Sugarbaker P. Laparotomy enhances intraperitoneal tumor growth and abrogates the antitumor effects of interleukin-2 and lymphokine-activated killer cells. *Surgery* 1987;102:71.
207. Sugarbaker PH, Cunliffe WJ, Belliveau J, et al. Rationale for integrating early postoperative intraperitoneal chemotherapy into the surgical treatment of gastrointestinal cancer. *Semin Oncol* 1989;16:83.
208. Rosen HR, Jatzko G, Repse S, et al. Adjuvant intraperitoneal chemotherapy with carbon-absorbed mitomycin in patients with gastric cancer: results of a randomized multicenter trial of the Austrian Working Group for Surgical Oncology. *J Clin Oncol* 1998;16:2733.
209. Crookes P, Leichman CG, Leichman L, et al. Systemic chemotherapy for gastric carcinoma followed by postoperative intraperitoneal therapy: a final report. *Cancer* 1997;79:1767.
210. Atiq OT, Kelsen DP, Shiu MH, et al. Phase II trial of postoperative adjuvant intraperitoneal cisplatin and fluorouracil and systemic fluorouracil chemotherapy in patients with resected gastric cancer. *J Clin Oncol* 1993;11:425.
211. Yu W, Whang I, Suh I, et al. Prospective randomized trial of early postoperative intraperitoneal chemotherapy as an adjuvant to resectable gastric cancer. *Ann Surg* 1998;228:347.
212. Dedrick RL. Theoretical and experimental bases of intraperitoneal chemotherapy. *Semin Oncol* 1985;XII:1.
213. Kitamura K, Kuwano H, Matsuda H, et al. Synergistic effects of intratumor administration of *cis*-diamminedichloroplatinum(II) combined with local hyperthermia in melanoma bearing mice. *J Surg Oncol* 1992;51:188.
214. Los G, Smals OA, van Vugt MJ, et al. A rationale for carboplatin treatment and abdominal hyperthermia in cancers restricted to the peritoneal cavity. *Cancer Res* 1992;52:1252.
215. Fujimoto S, Shrestha RD, Kokubun M, et al. Clinical trial with surgery and intraperitoneal hyperthermic perfusion for peritoneal recurrence of gastrointestinal cancer. *Cancer* 1989;64:154.
216. Yonemura Y, Ninomiya I, Kaji M, et al. Prophylaxis with intraoperative chemohyperthermia against peritoneal recurrence of serosal invasion-positive gastric cancer. *World J Surg* 1995;19:450.
217. Yonemura Y, Fujimura T, Fushida S, et al. Hyperthermo-chemotherapy combined with cytoreductive surgery for the treatment of gastric cancer with peritoneal dissemination. *World J Surg* 1991;15:530.

218. Fujimura T, Yonemura Y, Fushida S, et al. Continuous hyperthermic peritoneal perfusion for the treatment of peritoneal dissemination in gastric cancers and subsequent second-look operation. *Cancer* 1990;65:65.
219. Fujimoto S, Shrestha R, Kokubun M, et al. [Pharmacokinetic analysis in intraperitoneal hyperthermic perfusion using mitomycin C in far-advanced gastric cancer]. *Gan To Kagaku Ryoho* 1989;16:2411.
220. Gilly FN, Sayag AC, Carry PY, et al. Intra-peritoneal chemo-hyperthermia (CHIP): a new therapy in the treatment of the peritoneal seedings. Preliminary report. *Int Surg* 1991;76:164.
221. Koga S, Hamazoe R, Maeta M, et al. Prophylactic therapy for peritoneal recurrence of gastric cancer by continuous hyperthermic peritoneal perfusion with mitomycin C. *Cancer* 1988;61:232.
222. Fujimoto S, Shrestha RD, Kokubun M, et al. Positive results of combined therapy of surgery and intraperitoneal hyperthermic perfusion for far-advanced gastric cancer. *Ann Surg* 1990;212:592.
223. Hamazoe R, Maeta M, Kaibara N. Intraperitoneal thermochemotherapy for prevention of peritoneal recurrence of gastric cancer. *Cancer* 1994;73:2048.
224. Alexander HR, Buell JF, Fraker DL. Rationale and clinical status of continuous hyperthermic peritoneal perfusion (CHPP) for the treatment of peritoneal carcinomatosis. In: DeVita VT, Hellman S, Rosenberg SA, eds. *Principles and practices of oncology updates.* Philadelphia: JB Lippincott, 1995.
225. Alexander HR, Fraker DL. Continuous hyperthermic peritoneal perfusion with cisplatin in the treatment of peritoneal carcinomatosis. 1995;8:2.
226. Gilly GN, Carry PY, Brachet A, et al. Treatment of malignant peritoneal effusion in digestive and ovarian cancer. *Med Oncol Tumor Pharmacother* 1992;9:177.
227. Gilly FN, Carry PY, Sayag AC, et al. Regional chemotherapy (with mitomycin C) and intraoperative hyperthermia for digestive cancers with peritoneal carcinomatosis. *Hepatogastroenterology* 1994;41:124.
228. Yamaguchi A, Tsukioka Y, Fushida S, et al. Intraperitoneal hyperthermic treatment for peritoneal dissemination of colorectal cancers. *Dis Colon Rectum* 1992;35:964.
229. Nakazato H, Koike A, Saji S, Ogawa N, Sakamoto J. Efficacy of immunochemotherapy as adjuvant treatment after curative resection of gastric cancer. *Lancet* 1994;343:1122.
230. Douglass H Jr, Lavin P, Goudsmit A, et al. An Eastern Cooperative Oncology Group evaluation of combination of methyl-CCNU, mitomycin-C, Adriamycin, and 5-fluorouracil in advanced measurable gastric cancer. *J Clin Oncol* 1984;2:1372.
231. Ochiai T, Sato H, Hayashi R, et al. Randomly controlled study of chemotherapy versus chemoimmunotherapy in postoperative gastric cancer patients. *Cancer Res* 1983;43:3001.
232. Kim JP, Kwon OJ, Oh ST, Yang HK. Results of surgery on 6589 gastric cancer patients and immunochemosurgery as the best treatment of advanced gastric cancer. *Ann Surg* 1992;216:269, discussion 278.
233. Kim SY, Park HC, Yoon C, et al. OK-432 and 5-fluorouracil, doxorubicin, and mitomycin C (FAM-P) versus FAM chemotherapy in patients with curatively resected gastric carcinoma: a randomized phase III trial. *Cancer* 1998;83:2054.
234. Primrose JN, Miller GV, Preston SR, et al. A prospective randomised controlled study of the use of ranitidine in patients with gastric cancer. Yorkshire GI Tumour Group [See comments]. *Gut* 1998;42:17.
235. Harrison JD, Morris DL, Ellis IO, et al. The effect of tamoxifen and estrogen receptor status on survival in gastric carcinoma. *Cancer* 1989;64:1007.
236. Kelsen D, Karpeh M, Schwartz G, et al. Neoadjuvant therapy of high-risk gastric cancer: a phase II trial of preoperative FAMTX and postoperative intraperitoneal fluorouracil-cisplatin plus intravenous fluorouracil. *J Clin Oncol* 1996;14:1818.
237. Ng CS, Husband JE, MacVicar AD, et al. Correlation of CT with histopathological findings in patients with gastric and gastro-oesophageal carcinomas following neoadjuvant chemotherapy. *Clin Radiol* 1998;53:422.
238. Ichiya Y, Kuwabara Y, Sasaki M, et al. A clinical evaluation of FDG-PET to assess the response in radiation therapy for bronchogenic carcinoma. *Ann Nucl Med* 1996;10:193.
239. Ajani JA, Mayer RJ, Ota DM, et al. Preoperative and postoperative combination chemotherapy for potentially resectable gastric carcinoma. *J Natl Cancer Inst* 1993;85:1839.
240. Lowy AM, Mansfield PF, Leach SD, et al. Response to neoadjuvant chemotherapy best predicts survival after curative resection of gastric cancer. *Ann Surg* 1999;229:303.
241. Leichman L, Silberman H, Leichman CG, et al. Preoperative systemic chemotherapy followed by adjuvant postoperative intraperitoneal therapy for gastric cancer: a University of Southern California pilot program. *J Clin Oncol* 1992;10:1933.
242. Fink U, Ott K, Dittler HJ, et al. Neoadjuvant cisplatin leucovorin and fluorouracil (PLF) in adequately staged patients with locally advancer gastric carcinoma. In: Perry MC, ed. *American Society of Clinical Oncology Thirty-Fifth Annual Meeting,* vol 18. Atlanta: American Society of Clinical Oncology, 1999:272a.
243. Alexander HR, Grem JL, Hamilton JM, et al. Thymidylate synthase protein expression association with response to neoadjuvant chemotherapy and resection for locally advanced gastric and gastroesophageal adenocarcinoma. *Cancer J Sci Am* 1995;1:49.
244. Kang YK, Choi DW, Im YH, et al. A phase III randomized comparison of neoadjuvant chemotherapy followed by surgery versus surgery for locally advanced stomach cancer. *Proc ASCO* 1996;15:215.
245. Childs D, Moertel C, Holbrook M, et al. Treatment of unresectable adenocarcinomas of the stomach with a combination of 5-fluorouracil and radiation. *Am J Roentgenol Radium Ther Nucl Med* 1968;102:541.
246. Hallissey MT, Dunn JA, Ward LC, Allum WH. The second British Stomach Cancer Group trial of adjuvant radiotherapy or chemotherapy in resectable gastric cancer: five-year follow-up. *Lancet* 1994;343:1309.
247. Dent DM, Werner ID, Novis B, et al. Prospective randomized trial of combined oncological therapy for gastric carcinoma. *Cancer* 1979;44:385.
247a. Moertel CG, Childs DS, O'Fallon JR, et al. Combined 5-fluorouracil and radiation therapy as a surgical adjuvant for poor prognosis gastric carcinoma. *J Clin Oncol* 1984;2(11)1249.
248. Slot A, Meerwaldt J, van Putten W, Treurniet-Donker A. Adjuvant postoperative radiotherapy for gastric carcinoma with poor prognostic signs. *Radiother Oncol* 1989;16:269.
249. Gunderson LL, Hoskins RB, Cohen AC, et al. Combined modality treatment of gastric cancer. *Int J Radiat Oncol Biol Phys* 1983;9:965.
250. Caudry M, Escarmant P, Maire J, et al. Radiotherapy of gastric cancer with a three field combination: feasibility, tolerance, and survival. *Int J Radiat Oncol Biol Phys* 1987;13:1821.
251. Abe M, Takahashi M. Intraoperative radiotherapy: the Japanese experience. *Int J Radiat Oncol Biol Phys* 1981;7:863.
251a. Abe M, Nishimura Y, Shibamoto Y. Intraoperative radiation therapy for gastric cancer. *World J Surg* 1995;19(4):544.
252. Sindelar WF, Kinsella TJ, Tepper JE, et al. Randomized trial of intraoperative radiotherapy in carcinoma of the stomach. *Am J Surg* 1993;165:178, discussion 186.
253. Ogata T, Araki K, Matsuura K, et al. A 10-year experience of intraoperative radiotherapy for gastric carcinoma and a new surgical method of creating a wider irradiation field for cases of total gastrectomy patients. *Int J Radiat Oncol Biol Phys* 1995;32:341.
254. Calvo FA, Aristu JJ, Azinovic I, et al. Intraoperative and external radiotherapy in resected gastric cancer: updated report of a phase II trial. *Int J Radiat Oncol Biol Phys* 1992;24:729.
255. Willett C, Tepper J, Orlow E, Shipley W. Renal complications secondary to radiation treatment of upper abdominal malignancies. *Int J Radiat Oncol Biol Phys* 1986;12:1601.
256. Comis S. Integration of chemotherapy into combined modality treatment of solid tumors. *Cancer Treat Rep* 1974;1:221.
257. Cocconi G, DeLisi V, DiBlasio B. Randomized comparison of 5-FU alone or combined with mitomycin and cytarabine (MFC) in the treatment of advanced gastric cancer. *Cancer Treat Rep* 1982;66:1263.
258. The Gastrointestinal Tumor Study Group. Phase II/III chemotherapy studies in advanced gastric cancer. *Cancer Treat Rep* 1979;63:1871.
259. Moertel CG, Lavin PT. Phase II–III chemotherapy studies in advanced gastric cancer. *Cancer Treat Rep* 1979;63:1863.
260. Preusser P, Achterrath W, Wilke H, et al. Chemotherapy of gastric cancer [Review]. *Cancer Treat Rev* 1988;15:257.
261. Levi J, Fox R, Tattersall M, et al. Analysis of a prospectively randomized comparison of doxorubicin versus 5-fluorouracil, doxorubicin, and BCNYU in advanced gastric cancer: implications for future studies. *J Clin Oncol* 1986;4:1348.
262. Lacave AJ, Wils J, Diaz-Rubio E, et al. Cisplatinum as second-line chemotherapy in advanced gastric adenocarcinoma: a phase II study of the EORTC gastrointestinal tract cancer cooperative group. *Eur J Cancer Clin Oncol* 1985;21:1321.
263. Aabo K, Pedersen H, Rorth M. Cisplatin in the treatment of advanced gastric carcinoma: a phase II study. *Cancer Treat Rep* 1985;69:449.
264. Perry MC, Green MR, Mick R, et al. Cisplatin in patients with gastric cancer: a cancer and leukemia group B phase II study. *Cancer Treat Rep* 1986;70:415.
265. The Gastrointestinal Tumor Study Group. A comparative clinical assessment of combination chemotherapy in the management of advanced gastric carcinoma. *Cancer* 1982;49:1362.
266. The Gastrointestinal Tumor Study Group. Randomized study of combination chemotherapy in unresectable gastric cancer. *Cancer* 1984;53:13.
267. Lacave A, Wils J, Bleiberg H, et al. An EORTC Gastrointestinal Group phase III evaluation of combinations of methyl-CCNU, 5-fluorouracil, and Adriamycin in advanced gastric cancer. *J Clin Oncol* 1987;5:1387.
268. Epelbaum R, Haim N, Stein M, et al. Treatment of advanced gastric cancer with DDP (cisplatin), Adriamycin, and 5-fluorouracil (DAF). *Oncology* 1987;44:201.
269. Schnitzler G, Queisser W, Heim ME, et al. Phase III study of 5-FU and carmustine versus 5-FU, carmustine, and doxorubicin in advanced gastric cancer. *Cancer Treat Rep* 1986;70:477.
270. Lopez M, Di Lauro L, Papaldo P, Conti EM. Treatment of advanced measurable gastric carcinoma with 5-fluorouracil, Adriamycin, and BCNU. *Oncology* 1986;43:288.
271. Janieson G, Gill P. A prospective trial of 5-FU and BCNU in the treatment of advanced gastric cancer. *Aust N Z J Surg* 1985;5:16.
272. Levi J, Dalley D, Aroney R. Improved combination chemotherapy in advanced gastric cancer. *BMJ* 1979;2:1471.
272a. Gastrointestinal Tumor Study Group. Triazinate and platinum efficacy in combination with 5-fluorouracil and doxorubicin: results of a three-arm randomized trial in metastatic gastric cancer. *J Natl Cancer Inst* 1988;80:1011.
273. Macdonald JS, Schein PS, Woolley PV, et al. 5-Fluorouracil, mitomycin-C, and Adriamycin (FAM): a new combination chemotherapy program for advanced gastric carcinoma. *Ann Intern Med* 1980;93:533.
274. Ogawa M. A recent overview of chemotherapy for advanced stomach cancer in Japan. *Appl Cancer Chemother* 1978;24:149.
275. Cullinan SA, Moertel CG, Fleming TR, et al. A comparison of three chemotherapeutic regimens in the treatment of advanced pancreatic and gastric carcinoma. *JAMA* 1985; 253:2061.
276. Group GTS. Triazinate and platinum efficacy in combination with 5-fluorouracil and doxorubicin: results of a three-arm randomized trial in metastatic gastric cancer. *J Natl Cancer Inst* 1988;80:1011.
277. Cunningham D, Cahn A, Menzies-Gow N. Cisplatin, epirubicin and 5-fluorouracil (CEF) has significant activity in advanced gastric cancer. *Proc ASCO* 1990;9:123.
278. Caccia G, Alasino C, Fein L. 5-Fluorouracil + epirubicin + cisplatin in patients with advanced gastric cancer. 1990;9:123.
279. Cocconi G, Bella M, Zironi S, et al. Fluorouracil, doxorubicin, and mitomycin combination versus PELF chemotherapy in advanced gastric cancer: a prospective randomized trial of the Italian oncology group for clinical research. *J Clin Oncol* 1994;12:2687.
279a. Waters JS, Norman A, Cunningham D, et al. Long-term survival after epirubicin, cisplatin and fluorouracil for gastric cancer: results of a randomized trial. *Br J Cancer* 1999;80:269.
279b. Kim NK, Park YS, Heo DS, et al. A phase III randomized study of 5-fluorouracil alone in the treatment of advanced gastric cancer. *Cancer* 1993;71(12):3813.
279c. Barone C, Cassano A, Astone A, et al. Association of epirubicin, etoposide and cisplatin in gastric cancer. A phase II study. *Oncology* 1991;48(5):353.
279d. Turkish Oncology Group. A randomized phase III trial of etoposide, epirubicin, and cis-

platin versus 5-fluorouracil, epirubicin, and cisplatin in the treatment of patients with advanced gastric carcinoma. *Cancer* 1998;83:2475.
280. Mabel JA, Little AD. Therapeutic synergism in murine tumors for combinations of *cis*-dichlorodiammine platinum with VP-16-213 or BCNU. *Proc AACR ASCO* 1979;20:230.
281. Seeber S, Osieka R, Schmidt CG, et al. *In vivo* resistance towards anthracyclines, etoposide, and *cis*-diamminedichloroplatinum (II). *Cancer Res* 1982;67:4719.
282. Kelsen DP, Buckner J, Einzig A, et al. Phase II trial of cisplatin and etoposide in adenocarcinomas of the upper gastrointestinal tract. *Cancer Treat Rep* 1987;71:329.
283. Elliott T, Moertel C, Wieand H, et al. A phase II study of the combination of etoposide and cisplatin in the therapy of advanced gastric cancer. *Cancer* 1990;65:1491.
284. Preusser P, Wilke H, Achterrath W, et al. Phase II study with the combination etoposide, doxorubicin, and cisplatin in advanced measurable gastric cancer. *J Clin Oncol* 1989;7:1310.
285. Wilke H, Preusser P, Fink U, et al. Preoperative chemotherapy in locally advanced and nonresectable gastric cancer: a phase II study with etoposide, doxorubicin, and cisplatin. *J Clin Oncol* 1989;7:1318.
286. Katz A, Gansl R, Simon S. Phase II trial of VP-16, Adriamycin, and cisplatinum in patients with advanced gastric cancer. *Proc ASCO* 1989;8:98.
287. Lerner A, Steele GD, Mayer RJ. Etoposide, doxorubicin, cisplatin for advanced gastric adenocarcinoma: results of a phase II trial. *Proc ASCO* 1990;9:103.
288. Wilke H, Preusser P, Fink U, et al. New developments in the treatment of gastric carcinoma. *Semin Oncol* 1990;17[Suppl 2]:61.
289. Klein HO. Long-term results with FAMTX (5-fluorouracil, Adriamycin, methotrexate) in advanced gastric cancer. *Anticancer Res* 1989;9:1025.
290. Kelsen D, Atiq O, Saltz L, et al. FAMTX (fluorouracil, methotrexate, Adriamycin) is as effective and less toxic than EAP (etoposide, Adriamycin, cisplatin): a random assignment trial in gastric cancer. *Proc ASCO* 1991;10:137.
291. Wils JA, Klein HO, Wagener DJ, et al. Sequential high-dose methotrexate and fluorouracil combined with doxorubicin—a step ahead in the treatment of advanced gastric cancer: a trial of the European Organization for Research and Treatment of Cancer Gastrointestinal Tract Cooperative Group [See comments]. *J Clin Oncol* 1991;9:827.
292. Wilke H, Wils J, Rougier P, et al. Preliminary analysis of a randomized phase III trial of FAMTX versus ELF versus cisplatin/FU in advanced gastric cancer: a trial of the EORTC Gastrointestinal Tract Cancer Cooperative Group and the AIO. *Proc ASCO* 1995;14:206.
293. Lenz HJ, Leichman CG, Danenberg KD, et al. Thymidylate synthase mRNA level in adenocarcinoma of the stomach: a predictor for primary tumor response and overall survival. *J Clin Oncol* 1996;14:176.
294. Metzger R, Leichman CG, Danenberg KD, et al. ERCC1 mRNA levels complement thymidylate synthase mRNA levels in predicting response and survival for gastric cancer patients receiving combination cisplatin and fluorouracil chemotherapy. *J Clin Oncol* 1998;16:309.
294a. Fata F, Baylor L, Karpeh M, et al. Thymidylate symthase (TS) is not an independent predictor of outcome in patients with operable gastric cancer. *Proc ASCO* 1998;17:280a.
295. Boku N, Chin K, Hosokawa K, et al. Biological markers as a predictor for response and prognosis of unresectable gastric cancer patients treated with 5-fluorouracil and *cis*-platinum. *Clin Cancer Res* 1998;4:1469.
296. Cascinu S, Graziano F, Del Ferro E, et al. Expression of p53 protein and resistance to preoperative chemotherapy in locally advanced gastric carcinoma. *Cancer* 1998;83:1917.
297. Ikeguchi M, Saito H, Katano K, et al. Relationship between the long-term effects of intraperitoneal chemotherapy and the expression of p53 and p21 in patients with gastric carcinoma at stage IIIa and stage IIIb. *Int Surg* 1997;82:170.
298. Yeh KH, Shun CT, Chen CL, et al. High expression of thymidylate synthase is associated with the drug resistance of gastric carcinoma to high dose 5-fluorouracil–based systemic chemotherapy. *Cancer* 1998;82:1626.
299. Ekbom GA, Gleysteen JJ. Gastric malignancy: resection for palliation. *Surgery* 1980;88:476.
300. Meijer S, De Bakker OJ, Hoitsma HF. Palliative resection in gastric cancer. *J Surg Oncol* 1983;23:77.
301. Aranha GV, Georgen R. Gastric linitis plastica is not a surgical disease. *Surgery* 1989;106:758, discussion 762.
302. Bozzetti F, Bonfanti G, Audisio RA, et al. Prognosis of patients after palliative surgical procedures for carcinoma of the stomach. *Surg Gynecol Obstet* 1987;164:151.
303. Boddie A Jr, McMurtrey M, Diacco G, McBride C. Palliative total gastrectomy and esophagogastrectomy. *Cancer* 1983;51:1195.
304. Warwick M. Analysis of one hundred and seventy-six cases of carcinoma of the stomach submitted to autopsy. *Ann Surg* 1928;88:216.
305. Dupont JB Jr, Lee JR, Burton GR, Cohn I Jr. Adenocarcinoma of the stomach: review of 1,497 cases. *Cancer* 1978;41:941.
306. Clarke JS, Cruze K, El Farra S. The natural history and results of surgical therapy for carcinoma of the stomach: an analysis of 250 cases. *Am J Surg* 1961;102:143.
307. Bozzetti F, Bonfanti G, Morabito A, et al. A multifactorial approach for the prognosis of patients with carcinoma of the stomach after curative resection. *Surg Gynecol Obstet* 1986;162:229.
308. Hajiwara A, Takahashi T, Kojima O, et al. Prophylaxis with carbon-adsorbed mitomycin against peritoneal recurrence of gastric cancer [See comments]. 1992;339:629.
309. Schiessel R, Funovics J, Schick B, et al. Adjuvant intraperitoneal cisplatin therapy in patients with operated gastric carcinoma: results of a randomized trial. *Acta Med Aust* 1989;16:68.
310. Karpeh MS, Leon L, Klimstra D, and Brennan MF. Lymph node staging in gastric cancer: Is location more important than number? An analysis of 1,038 patients. *Ann Surg* 2000;232(3):362.
311. Gastrointestinal Tumor Study Group. The concept of locally advanced gastric cancer. *Cancer* 1990;66:2324.
312. The Italian Gastrointestinal Tumor Study Group. Adjuvant treatments following curative resection of gastric cancer. *Br J Surg* 1988;75:1100.
313. Ajani JA, Roth JA, Putnam JB, et al. Feasibility of five courses of pre-operative chemotherapy in patients with resectable adenocarcinoma of the oesophagus or gastrointestinal junction. *Eur J Cancer* 1995;31A:665.

DOUGLAS B. EVANS
JAMES L. ABBRUZZESE
CHRISTOPHER G. WILLETT

SECTION 4

Cancer of the Pancreas

Cancer of the exocrine pancreas continues to be a major unsolved health problem, with approximately 28,200 deaths per year in the United States and 50,000 deaths per year in Europe (excluding the former USSR).[1,2] In the United States in the year 2000, pancreatic cancer is expected to be the fourth leading cause of cancer-related death for both men and women and to be responsible for close to 5% of all cancer-related deaths.[1] Because of difficulties in diagnosis, the aggressiveness of pancreatic cancers, and the lack of effective systemic therapies, generally fewer than 5% of patients with adenocarcinoma of the pancreas survive 5 years after diagnosis.[3,4] Thus, incidence rates and mortality rates are virtually identical.

EPIDEMIOLOGY

In the United States, the incidence of pancreatic cancer steadily increased for several decades but has leveled off since the late 1970s, with 28,300 new cases (2% of all cancer diagnoses) estimated in the year 2000.[1] Studies evaluating this trend suggest that the decreased incidence is due to a steady decline in the rate for white men, which peaked during the period of 1970 to 1974. By contrast, rates for white women, African American men, and African American women have not fallen and may have increased slightly.[4] In Japan, the incidence of pancreatic cancer increased sharply from 1.8 per 100,000 in 1960 to 5.3 per 100,000 in 1985.[5,6]

Overall, pancreatic cancer incidence and mortality statistics are similar for the United States and Western Europe. Between 1989 and 1991, mortality rates for pancreatic cancer in the United States were 10 per 100,000 for men and 7.2 per 100,000 for women.[7] Although the overall mortality rates in industrialized societies appear similar, geographically and ethnically dissimilar populations show considerable differences in mortality rates from pancreatic cancer. In Europe, for the time period of 1985 to 1989, mortality rates ranged from 5.3 per 100,000 in Spain to 10.3 per 100,000 in Hungary and Czechoslovakia.[2] Spain, Portugal, and Greece recorded an extremely low mortality rate of 3 per 100,000 among men.[2] The reasons for these regional differences and the changing incidence of pancreatic cancer remain obscure, but they might possibly be related to the trend of a declining smoking rate.[8]

ETIOLOGIC FACTORS

Investigations have identified a number of factors that may contribute to the pathogenesis of pancreatic cancer. Current estimates suggest that approximately 30% of pancreatic cancer cases are due to cigarette smoking.[9,10] Studies that have explored the dose-response relationship have shown that the risk of pancreatic cancer increases as the amount and duration of smoking increase and that long-term smoking cessation (more than 10 years) reduces risk by approximately 30% relative to the risk of current smokers.[9,11] Application of molecular epidemiologic techniques that are being developed for lung cancer may provide greater specificity in linking tobacco exposure with the development of pancreatic cancer[12,13] and may facilitate the study of chemopreventive strategies.[14]

Data regarding the effect of coffee consumption and excessive alcohol consumption appear to be conflicting. For each of these factors, a few studies have suggested an increased risk of pancreatic cancer,[11,15–18] but the majority of studies conducted during the 1990s have failed to consistently demonstrate such a risk.[11,17,19–23] In some cases, significant methodologic problems may have confounded interpretation of the data, leading to erroneous conclusions.[20]

Diabetes mellitus has been long associated with pancreatic cancer; however, not all studies have supported such a relationship,[24] and the precise mechanism has yet to be defined. Diabetes mellitus has been implicated as both an early manifestation of pancreatic carcinoma[25–28] and a predisposing factor.[22,29–32] It is known that pancreatic cancer can induce peripheral insulin resistance,[33–35] and the argument that long-standing diabetes mellitus is also a risk factor for pancreatic cancer is supported by a cohort study showing that, after an initial hospitalization for diabetes, patients had an increased risk of developing pancreatic cancer and that this risk persisted for more than a decade.[30] However, the increased risk was limited to patients with non–insulin-dependent diabetes or patients whose diabetes was diagnosed after 40 years of age.[30] Metaanalysis of studies published between 1975 and 1994 showed that pancreatic cancer occurred with increased frequency in patients with long-standing diabetes.[36] The mechanisms underlying the association between pancreatic cancer and diabetes are obscure; however, the diabetic state seems to enhance the growth of pancreatic cancer in animal models.[37]

A series of reports have validated the epidemiologic association between chronic pancreatitis and pancreatic cancer,[38–42] but the magnitude of the risk of pancreatic cancer attributable to pancreatitis remains controversial.[43] Pathologic and molecular biologic studies have begun to explore the relationship between both hereditary and nonhereditary chronic pancreatitis and pancreatic cancer.[44] Pathologic examination of lesions along the pancreatic duct has revealed a spectrum of mucous cell hyperplasias (papillary and nonpapillary hyperplastic lesions and atypical hyperplastic lesions currently termed *pancreatic intraepithelial neoplasia*) in patients with chronic pancreatitis and patients with pancreatic cancer.[45] The identification of mutations in the K-*ras* oncogene, a mutation found almost universally in established pancreatic cancers, in regions of mucous cell hyperplasia in patients with chronic pancreatitis provided the first molecular link between chronic inflammation and the initiation of multistep pancreatic carcinogenesis.[46] Calculation of a general estimate of population-attributable risk has suggested that chronic pancreatitis may explain as many as 5% of pancreatic cancer cases.[47]

The emergence of the importance of inherited genetic syndromes in gastrointestinal tract neoplasia has led to closer investigation of the potential role for heritable factors in pancreatic cancer. Considerable progress in our understanding of familial pancreatic cancer has been made since the late 1990s.[48,49] Currently, it is estimated that possibly as many as 5% to 8% of pancreatic cancer cases are associated with a familial predisposition.[32,50] Several hereditary disorders predispose persons to both endocrine and exocrine pancreatic cancer. These include the multiple endocrine neoplasia type 1 syndrome,[51,52] hereditary pancreatitis,[44,53] hereditary nonpolyposis colon cancer/Lynch syndrome II,[54] von Hippel-Lindau syndrome,[55] ataxia-telangiectasia,[56] and the familial atypical multiple mole melanoma syndrome.[57–59] In addition, case reports and formal epidemiologic studies have suggested the possibility of familial aggregations of pancreatic cancer outside the context of these rare familial syndromes.[60–62]

Through the establishment of large familial pancreatic cancer registries,[48,53] progress has been made in understanding the specific genetic alterations responsible for the familial aggregation of pancreatic cancer in some families. Genetic testing of kindreds with increased rates of pancreatic cancer has revealed germline mutations in genes known to be important in pancreatic carcinogenesis: *p16* (*CDKN2*),[58,59] *BRCA2*,[63] and *STK11/LKB1*,[64] but not *Smad4*.[65] Evaluation of approximately 30 extended families with presumed familial pancreatic cancer has suggested that transmission is consistent with an autosomal dominant pattern[66] and that even second-degree relatives of patients from these families are at increased risk.[48] Interestingly, unlike for other familial gastrointestinal cancers (e.g., colon cancer in familial polyposis coli), the age at onset, tumor histopathology, and overall survival for patients with familial pancreatic cancer are often the same as those for patients with sporadic cancers.[49,54,63]

Presently, the management of individuals documented to be at increased risk of pancreatic cancer is extremely controversial.[67] Options range from close observation to aggressive surgical intervention[68]; the optimal surveillance and surgical strategies have yet to be defined. However, continued study of patients with familial pancreatic cancer and their families is expected to provide insight into the critical molecular genetic abnormalities leading to familial pancreatic cancer. These genetic abnormalities may then provide new perspectives on the process of pancreatic carcinogenesis for patients with sporadic pancreatic cancer and provide opportunities for early detection and chemoprevention.[69,70]

PATHOLOGY AND MOLECULAR PATHOGENESIS

CELLULAR PATHOLOGY

The normal pancreatic architecture is characteristic of a secretory gland: A background of acinar cells accounts for approximately 80% of the cell number and volume of the gland; 1% to 2% is clusters of islet cells; 10% to 15% is single-layered, cuboidal ductal cells; and a sparse interlacing network of blood vessels, lymphatics, nerves, and collagenous stroma is present. This architecture is markedly altered in carcinoma, in which the predominant histologic feature is a dense collagenous stroma with atrophic acini, remarkably preserved islet cell clusters, and a slight to moderate increase in the number of ducts, both of normal appearance and cancerous. The diagnosis of ductal adenocarcinoma rests on the identification of mitoses; nuclear and cellular pleomorphism; discontinuity of ductal epithelium; and evidence of perineural, vascular, or lymphatic invasion.[71]

TABLE 33.4-1. Histologic Classification of Epithelial Tumors of the Exocrine Pancreas

Malignant
Ductal adenocarcinoma[a]
Mucinous cystadenocarcinoma
Acinar carcinoma
Unclassified large cell carcinoma
Small cell carcinoma
Pancreatoblastoma
Uncertain malignant potential
Intraductal papillary mucinous tumor
Mucinous cystadenoma
Papillary cystic neoplasm
Benign
Serous cystadenoma[b]

[a]Variants include adenosquamous carcinoma, pleomorphic giant cell carcinoma, mucinous adenocarcinoma, and osteoclast-like giant cell carcinoma.
[b]May exhibit uncontrolled local tumor growth, causing the designation *benign* to be questioned.

Ninety-five percent of malignant neoplasms of pancreatic origin arise from the exocrine portion of the gland and have light-microscopic features consistent with those of adenocarcinomas.[71] Much more infrequent are tumors arising from the islets of Langerhans' (endocrine) cells of the pancreas. Primary nonepithelial tumors of the pancreas (e.g., lymphomas or sarcomas) are extremely rare. A current view of the histologic classification of exocrine pancreatic neoplasms is presented in Table 33.4-1.

Extensive "preneoplastic" lesions have been demonstrated in the pancreatic ducts adjacent to frankly invasive cancers with a higher frequency than was seen in a matched control population without pancreatic cancer.[72] Furthermore, clinical studies have documented progression of lesions from mild dysplasia to high-grade dysplasia[73] and from high-grade dysplasia to infiltrating ductal adenocarcinoma.[74] Finally, the identification of mutated K-*ras*, a genetic change found in the majority of patients with invasive pancreatic cancer,[75–77] in papillary and dysplastic papillary ductal lesions has provided further evidence that these hyperproliferative states are the precursors of infiltrative ductal carcinoma. Current evidence supports the general hypothesis that progression of the ductal lesions is characterized by the accumulation of additional genetic and biochemical changes. For example, preneoplastic ductal lesions can be shown to harbor mutations in genes that are typically altered in invasive pancreatic carcinoma, including *p16* and *p53*.[78–80] Activated telomerases can also be found.[81,82] Interestingly, other malignancies that can masquerade as pancreatic cancer, such as carcinoma of the ampulla of Vater, only infrequently contain a mutated K-*ras* oncogene.[83] At present, however, accurate identification of high-risk patient subsets who are destined to develop invasive cancer and thus are candidates for intervention is not possible.

ONCOGENES AND TUMOR SUPPRESSOR GENES

Studies using archival human pancreatic tumor tissue and human pancreatic cancer cell lines have identified a number of characteristic genetic abnormalities associated with pancreatic cancer. As described previously, these studies have revealed specific point mutations at codon 12 of the K-*ras* oncogene in 75% to 90% of pancreatic adenocarcinoma specimens.[75–77] The ras protein is an important signal-transduction mediator for receptor protein tyrosine kinases. Signaling is initiated by the recruitment of guanine nucleotide exchange proteins that promote hydrolysis of guanosine triphosphate (GTP) to guanosine diphosphate (GDP). Ras bound to GTP is maintained in an active configuration that triggers other enzymatic second messengers, such as the raf, phosphatidylinositol, and protein kinase C pathways, which leads to nuclear signals resulting in cellular division and proliferation. The mutated *ras* oncogene is not able to convert GTP to inactive GDP, resulting in a constitutively active ras protein product, unregulated cellular proliferation signals, and susceptibility to transformation.[84] The K-*ras* mutation in pancreatic carcinogenesis is proposed to be an early event in pancreatic tumor progression.[85]

Data suggest that up-regulation of vascular endothelial growth factor (VEGF) occurs as a result of the activation of mutations of the *ras* oncogene.[86] VEGF is an endothelial cell–specific mitogen that promotes angiogenesis in solid tumors. Angiogenesis is essential for tumors to grow larger than 1 mm^3, and angiogenesis must occur for metastasis formation and growth. Overexpression of VEGF has been demonstrated in several tumors, and VEGF messenger RNA has been shown to be overexpressed in a Syrian hamster pancreatic cancer cell line.[87,88] Therefore, *ras* mutations may contribute to pancreatic carcinogenesis not only by promoting tumor cell proliferation but also indirectly by stimulating tumor angiogenesis. The available data also suggest that *ras* and *src* oncogenes mediate their effects on gene expression partly by activating the transcription factors AP-1 and Rel/NF-κB. These transcription factors have been shown to up-regulate a number of genes whose protein products play important roles in tumor invasion, angiogenesis, and metastasis[89,90] and are relevant to pancreatic cancer carcinogenesis.[91,92] Other proangiogenic factors, such as interleukin-8, are also up-regulated by AP-1 and NF-κB.[93,94] In addition, the tumor suppressor genes *p53* and *p16* have been shown to regulate the expression of VEGF.[95,96] Numerous agents that inhibit angiogenesis are currently undergoing testing in phase I and II clinical trials in patients with various types of cancer in the United States.[97,98]

Additional genetic alterations in human pancreatic cancer have been described, many by Kern and colleagues[99–103] at Johns Hopkins University. Their studies have been facilitated by xenograft enrichment of human tumors obtained at the time of surgical resection.[99] Pieces of the fresh human tumors are implanted subcutaneously in athymic nude mice, and the resulting tumors are harvested when they have grown to 1 cm in diameter. This allows the neoplastic cells to expand while preventing similar expansion of contaminating stromal cells. Subsequent molecular studies can then be performed on a population of pure tumor cells. Using this technology, three chromosomal loci with homozygous deletions have been identified in pancreatic ductal carcinomas. They are appropriately termed *DPC* (deleted in pancreatic cancer) 1/2, 3, and 4. *DPC1/2* is located on chromosome 13q12 (the region of the *BRCA2* gene),[100] *DPC3* (*p16/MTS-1*) on chromosome 9q21,[101] and *DPC4* on chromosome 18q21.1.[102,103] *DPC4* (*Smad4*), the most recently discovered tumor suppressor gene, is an important component of the transforming growth factor-β signaling pathway that normally down-regulates the growth of epithelial cells, stimulates differentiation, and promotes apoptosis.[104,105] Loss of this important growth regulatory pathway contributes to unregulated cell growth.[106,107] *DPC4* was found to be homozygously deleted in 30% of pancreatic carcinomas and inactivated through loss of heterozygosity and intragenic mutation in another 20% of the cases studied.[108]

The p16 protein belongs to a class of cyclin-dependent kinase (CDK)–inhibitory proteins (including p21/WAF1/Cip1) and inhibits the cyclin D1/CDK-4 complex that normally acts to phosphorylate the retinoblastoma (Rb) protein. Inactivation of *p16* leads to hyperphosphorylated Rb, loss of cell-cycle control, and unregulated cell growth. Allelic deletions involving *p16* have been found in 85% of human pancreatic tumor xenografts.[101] The second p16 allele is inactivated by three mechanisms: point mutations in 40% of cases,[101,109] deletion of the second allele in 40%,[110] and promoter silencing through hypermethylation of the p16 promoter in 15%.[111] Interestingly, *p16* mutations also have been detected in 30% to 50% of melanoma-prone kindreds. A report of 19 families with a history of melanoma in at least two first-degree relatives found pancreatic cancer only in families with germline *p16* mutations.[58] Patients with malignant melanoma in the cancer registries of the Surveillance, Epidemiology, and End Results program were followed to determine the incidence of pancreatic cancer in this cohort. Nearly twice as many pancreatic cancers as expected were found in patients diagnosed with malignant melanoma before age 50, and the pancreatic cancer incidence was more than twice that expected in female melanoma patients younger than 50 years.[112]

The tumor suppressor gene *p53* is critical to normal cellular function, and its amino acid sequence is highly conserved among many species. After DNA damage, p53 protein levels increase because of posttranslational changes in protein stability. The normal p53 response to DNA damage leads to both cell-cycle arrest and apoptosis. The *p53* gene is the most commonly mutated gene in human cancer. Seventy percent of pancreatic adenocarcinomas have loss of *p53* function.[56,108] Inactivation of *p53* function occurs through loss of one p53 allele and mutational inactivation of the other. Mutations in the *p53* sequence are more frequently seen in poorly differentiated tumors, and patients whose tumors have a *p53* intragenic frameshift deletion experience a significantly reduced disease-free survival (compared to those with other mutations or wild-type *p53*).[113] However, this type of relationship has not been documented in all studies.[114]

Based on the frequency with which mutations in K-*ras*, *p53*, and *p16* are found, a model of pancreatic carcinogenesis has been suggested whereby the malignant clone evolves from cells driven by a dominant oncogene (K-*ras*) with subsequent deregulation of cell growth precipitated by abnormal cell-cycle control resulting from mutations in *p53*, *p16*, or both.[115,116]

Exactly how the increasingly complex molecular alterations described thus far in human pancreatic cancer interact during pancreatic carcinogenesis is still unclear. However, *in vitro* studies designed to correct these alterations may lead to novel treatment strategies and improve our understanding of the relative roles of these changes in pancreatic cancer biology.

CLINICAL SIGNS AND SYMPTOMS

The lack of obvious clinical signs and symptoms delays diagnosis in most patients with pancreatic cancer. Jaundice, due to extrahepatic biliary obstruction, is present in approximately 50% of patients at diagnosis and is associated with a less advanced stage of disease than are other signs or symptoms.[117] Small tumors of the pancreatic head may obstruct the intrapancreatic portion of the bile duct and cause the patient to seek medical attention when the tumor is still localized and potentially resectable. In the absence of extrahepatic biliary obstruction, few patients present with potentially resectable disease.

The pain typical of locally advanced pancreatic cancer is a dull, fairly constant pain of visceral origin localized to the region of the middle and upper back. The pain is due to tumor invasion of the celiac and mesenteric plexus. Vague, intermittent epigastric pain occurs in some patients; its etiology is less clear. Fatigue, weight loss, and anorexia are common, even in the absence of mechanical gastric outlet obstruction. Pancreatic exocrine insufficiency due to obstruction of the pancreatic duct may result in malabsorption and steatorrhea. Although malabsorption and mild changes in stool frequency are common, diarrhea occurs infrequently.

Glucose intolerance is present in the majority of patients with pancreatic cancer.[118–120] Although the exact mechanism of hyperglycemia remains unclear, both altered β-cell function and impaired tissue insulin sensitivity are present.[118,121] The importance of islet cell function to the development of exocrine cancer is suggested by the work of Bell and Stayer,[122] who demonstrated that pretreatment of hamsters with streptozocin and the resulting destruction of islet cells prevented the induction of pancreatic cancer in these animals by the carcinogen N-nitrosobis-(2-oxopropyl) amine. This work was substantiated by studies in Chinese hamsters, which demonstrated that only genetically diabetic animals did not develop cancers in response to this carcinogen.[123]

In the absence of jaundice, patient complaints are nonspecific, as are clinical signs on physical examination. However, important staging information with direct implications for therapy can be obtained from the physical examination. This information includes performance status, cardiopulmonary function, and the presence or absence of left supraclavicular adenopathy and ascites.

NATURAL HISTORY AND PATTERNS OF TREATMENT FAILURE

Rational anticancer therapy for solid malignancies is based on accurate knowledge of the natural history and patterns of treatment failure for each tumor type. Pancreatic cancer spreads early to regional lymph nodes, and subclinical liver metastases are present in the majority of patients at the time of diagnosis, even when findings from imaging studies are normal. Patient survival depends on the extent of disease and performance status at diagnosis.[124] The extent of disease is best categorized as resectable, locally advanced, or metastatic. Patients who undergo surgical resection for localized nonmetastatic adenocarcinoma of the pancreatic head have a long-term survival rate of approximately 20% and a median survival of 13 to 20 months (Table 33.4-2).[125–139] As is discussed later (see Treatment of Potentially Resectable Disease), survival is clearly maximized by combining surgery with either preoperative or postoperative 5-fluorouracil (5-FU)-based chemotherapy and radiation therapy (chemoradiation). However, disease recur-

TABLE 33.4-2. Survival in Patients with Localized Adenocarcinoma of the Pancreas Who Underwent Surgical Resection of the Primary Tumor (with or without Adjuvant Therapy)

Study	*Number of Patients*	*Follow-Up (mo)*	*Median Survival (mo)*	*Estimated 4- or 5-Y Survival (%)*
Trede et al.[131] (1990)	133	NA	NA	24
Cameron et al.[127] (1991)	81	NA	12.7	21
Whittington et al.[133] (1991)	72	NA	15–16	NA
Roder et al.[130] (1992)	53	24[a]	12	6
Bakkevold and Kambestad[126] (1993)	83	NA	11.4	NA
Geer and Brennan[128] (1993)	146	28[a]	18	24
Willett et al.[134] (1993)	72	11[a]	NA	13
Tsao et al.[132] (1994)	27	30[a]	18	6.6
Zerbi et al.[136] (1994)	90	16[a]	12/19[b]	NA
Allema et al.[125] (1995)	67	NA	NA	15
Nitecki et al.[129] (1995)	174	22[c]	17.5	6.8
Yeo et al.[138] (1997)	282	12[a]	18	NA
Spitz et al.[139] (1997)	60	19[a]	20.2	NA

NA, not available.
[a]Median.
[b]Received adjuvant intraoperative radiation therapy.
[c]Mean.

rence after a potentially curative pancreaticoduodenectomy remains common, as illustrated in Table 33.4-3.[133–135,137,140–149] Local recurrence occurs in up to 86% of patients who undergo surgery alone; local-regional tumor control is maximized with combined-modality therapy in the form of chemoradiation and surgery.[124] With improved local-regional disease control, liver metastases become the dominant form of tumor recurrence and occur in 25% to 53% of patients after potentially curative combined-modality treatment.[124]

Patients with locally advanced, nonmetastatic disease have a median survival of 6 to 10 months. A survival advantage has been demonstrated for patients with locally advanced disease treated

TABLE 33.4-3. Incidence of Subsequent Local Recurrence and Peritoneal and Liver Metastases in Patients with Adenocarcinoma of the Pancreas Who Underwent a Potentially Curative Resection of the Primary Tumor

				Incidence of Metastases (%)			
Study	*Number of Patients*	*Adjuvant EBRT Dose (Gy)*	*Chemotherapy*	Local	Peritoneal	Liver	*Method of Follow-Up*
Tepper et al.[146] (1976)	26	NA	No	13 (50)	NA	NA	Patient records
GITSG[141] (1987)	35	40	Yes	18 (51)	NA	15 (43)	Patient records
	21	NA	No	7 (33)	NA	11 (52)	
Splinter et al.[145] (1989)	15	NA	Yes	5 (33)	NA	NA	Patient records
Griffin et al.[142] (1990)	36	45–60 (10/36)	Yes (8/36)	19 (53)	11 (31)	16 (44)	CT/autopsy
Whittington et al.[133] (1991)	26	NA	No	22 (85)	6 (23)	6 (23)	CT
	19	45	Yes (8/19)	9 (47)	4 (21)	8 (42)	
	20	45	Yes	5 (25)	3 (15)	5 (25)	
Bossett et al.[137] (1992)	14	54	No	7 (50)	2 (14)	5 (36)	CT
Ozaki[144] (1992)	14	NA	No	12 (86)	5 (36)	11 (79)	Autopsy
Foo et al.[140] (1993)	28	54	Yes	2 (7)	12 (43)	12 (43)	CT/reoperation/autopsy
Johnstone et al.[143] (1993)	4	45–55	No	3 (75)	1 (25)	3 (75)	Autopsy/reoperation
	11	IORT (7/11)	No	4 (36)	4 (36)	3 (27)	
Westerdahl et al.[147] (1993)	74	NA	No	64 (86)	NA	68 (92)	Reoperation/autopsy/CT
Willett et al.[134] (1993)	72	40–50 (39/72)	Yes (39/72)	48 (67)	NA	NA	Patient records
Staley et al.[148] (1996)	38	30.0–50.4	Yes	4 (11)	4 (11)	20 (53)	CT
Pisters et al.[149] (1998)	20	30	Yes	1 (5)	1 (5)	10 (50)	CT
Total	473			243/473 (51)	53/230 (23)	193/360 (54)	

CT, computed tomography; EBRT, external-beam radiation therapy; GITSG, Gastrointestinal Tumor Study Group; IORT, intraoperative radiation therapy; NA, not available.

with 5-FU–based chemoradiation compared to no treatment or radiation therapy alone.[150–154] Patients with metastatic disease have a short survival (3 to 6 months), the length of which depends on the extent of disease and performance status.

Knowledge of the prognosis and patterns of treatment failure associated with adenocarcinoma of the pancreas leads to the following basic treatment principles: (1) The treatment must not be worse than the disease. The low cure rate and modest median survival after pancreatectomy mandate that treatment-related morbidity be low and treatment-related death be rare. (2) Improvements in patient survival and quality of life will result from the development of innovative treatment strategies directed at the known sites of tumor recurrence. To date, the data have clearly demonstrated that, as local-regional treatment has become more effective, the dominant site of failure has shifted to hepatic metastases.[124] Therefore, future improvements in survival duration will result either from effective systemic or regional therapy directed at subclinical liver metastases or from strategies for screening and early diagnosis directed at increasing the number of patients eligible for potentially curative surgery. Future improvements in the quality of patient survival will result from the application of innovative multimodality therapy to carefully selected (staged) patients and the avoidance of unnecessary patient morbidity due to the inappropriate use of surgery, radiation, and chemotherapy in poorly selected (advanced disease) patients.

CLINICAL AND PATHOLOGIC (SURGICAL) STAGING

A standardized system for the clinical and pathologic staging of pancreatic cancer does not currently exist in the United States. The system of the American Joint Committee on Cancer in cooperation with the TNM Committee of the International Union Against Cancer appears in Table 33.4-4.[155] However, this TNM (tumor, node, metastasis) staging system provides only one system for both clinical (radiographic) and pathologic staging. Pathologic staging can be applied only to patients who undergo pancreatectomy; in all other patients, only clinical staging, based on radiographic examinations, can be done. Without surgery, the histologic status of regional lymph nodes cannot be determined. In addition, treatment and prognosis are based on whether the tumor is potentially resectable, locally advanced, or metastatic, definitions that may not directly correlate with TNM status.[156] For example, both potentially resectable and locally advanced tumors may be categorized as T4; isolated involvement of the superior mesenteric vein (SMV) would be considered T4 disease but does not preclude resection in the absence of arterial encasement.

Tumors of the pancreas are unlike other solid tumors of the gastrointestinal tract in that accurate diagnosis, clinical staging, and pathologic evaluation of resected specimens require extensive interaction and cooperation among physicians of different specialties. Accurate clinical staging requires high-quality computed tomography (CT) to accurately define the relationship of the tumor to the celiac axis and superior mesenteric vessels. The use of standardized, objective radiologic criteria for preoperative tumor staging allows physicians to develop detailed treatment plans for their patients, avoid unnecessary laparotomy in

TABLE 33.4-4. TNM Staging System for Pancreatic Cancer

DEFINITIONS

Primary tumor (T)	
TX	Primary tumor cannot be assessed
T0	No evidence of primary tumor
Tis	*In situ* carcinoma
T1	Tumor 2 cm or less in greatest dimension
T2	Tumor more than 2 cm in greatest dimension
T3	Tumor extends directly to any of the following: duodenum, bile duct, or peripancreatic tissues
T4	Tumor extends directly to any of the following: stomach, spleen, colon, or adjacent large vessels
Regional lymph nodes (N)	
NX	Regional lymph nodes cannot be assessed
N0	No regional lymph node metastasis
N1	Regional lymph node metastasis
	pN1a: metastasis in a single regional lymph node
	pN1b: metastasis in multiple regional lymph nodes
Distant metastasis (M)	
MX	Distant metastasis cannot be assessed
M0	No distant metastasis
M1	Distant metastasis

STAGE GROUPING

0	Tis	N0	M0
I	T1–2	N0	M0
II	T3	N0	M0
III	T1–3	N1	M0
IVA	T4	Any N	M0
IVB	Any T	Any N	M1

(Adapted from ref. 155.)

patients with locally advanced or metastatic disease, and improve rates of resectability at laparotomy.[157] Therefore, a system for clinical staging like the one illustrated in Table 33.4-5 is useful to practicing medical oncologists, surgeons, and radiation oncologists.

Standardized criteria also are needed for the pathologic analysis of pancreaticoduodenectomy specimens to allow accurate interpretation of reported survival statistics. Retrospective pathologic analysis of archival material does not allow accurate assessment of margins of resection or number of lymph nodes retrieved. However, these are the most accurate predictors of outcome. In studies by Yeo et al.,[135,138] positive resection margin status, lymph node metastases, poorly differentiated tumor histology, and tumor size of 3 cm or greater were the tumor characteristics that most strongly predicted disease recurrence and short survival duration. To determine which patient subsets may benefit from the most aggressive treatment strategies, accurate pathologic staging and histologic assessment of response are mandatory.

At the University of Texas M. D. Anderson Cancer Center, the surgeon and pathologist evaluate each specimen first by frozen-section examination of the common bile duct transection margin and the pancreatic transection margin.[156] The retroperitoneal margin, defined as the soft tissue margin directly adjacent to the proximal 3 to 4 cm of the superior mesenteric artery (SMA),[157] is evaluated by permanent-section examination. This

TABLE 33.4-5. Clinical (Radiologic) Staging of Pancreatic Cancer

Stage	*Clinical/Radiologic Criteria*
I	Resectable (T1–3, selected T4,[a] NX, M0)
	No encasement of the celiac axis or SMA
	Patent SMPV confluence
	No extrapancreatic disease
II	Locally advanced (T4, NX–1, M0)
	Tumor extension to involve the celiac axis or SMA, or venous occlusion (SMV or SMPV confluence)
	No extrapancreatic disease
III	Metastatic (T1–4, NX–1, M1)
	Metastatic disease (typically to liver and peritoneum and occasionally to lung)

SMA, superior mesenteric artery; SMPV, superior mesenteric–portal vein.
[a]Resectable T4 tumors include those with isolated involvement of the superior mesenteric vein, portal vein or, rarely, hepatic artery without tumor extension to involve the celiac axis or SMA.

can be done either by taking a 2- to 3-mm full-face (*en face*) section of the margin or by inking the margin and sectioning the tumor perpendicular to the margin. The retroperitoneal margin must be evaluated or accurately inked at the time of tumor resection by the pathologist and surgeon; identification of the retroperitoneal margin is not possible later. A positive bile duct or pancreatic transection margin is treated with re-resection; however, this is not possible in the retroperitoneum, where the aorta and SMA origin limit the extent of surgical resection.

Samples of multiple areas of each tumor, including the interface between the tumor and adjacent uninvolved tissue, are submitted for paraffin-embedded histologic examination (five to ten blocks). Sections 4-μm thick are cut and stained with hematoxylin and eosin. Final pathologic evaluation of permanent sections includes a description of tumor histology and differentiation; gross and microscopic evaluation of the tissue of origin (pancreas, bile duct, ampulla of Vater, or duodenum); and assessments of maximum transverse tumor diameter, lymph node status, and the presence or absence of perineural, lymphatic, and vascular invasion. When segmental resection of the SMV is required, the area of presumed tumor invasion of the vein wall is serially sectioned and examined in an attempt to discriminate benign fibrous attachment from direct tumor invasion. In patients who received preoperative chemoradiation, the grade of treatment effect is assessed on permanent sections using the grading schema developed by Cleary and reported by Evans et al.[158]

The method for classifying subsets of regional lymph nodes in pancreaticoduodenectomy specimens[156] is based on the work of Cubilla et al.[159] The soft fibrofatty tissue containing regional lymph nodes is divided into six regions as outlined on an anatomic pathology dissection board.[156] If lymph nodes are not identified, fat or other potentially neoplastic tissue is submitted for microscopic examination. Staley and colleagues[156] have demonstrated that the number of lymph nodes identified in the surgical specimen is increased by the use of a standardized system of specimen analysis. The dissection board used at our institution provides a simple means of improving lymph node identification and documenting the location of histologically confirmed lymph node metastases.[156] The Japanese staging system involves extremely detailed analysis of margins and lymph node groups but is not a practical system for widespread application.[160] As the use of multimodality treatment strategies for pancreatic cancer becomes more common, it will be even more important to standardize pathologic assessment of tumor specimens.

Maintaining an active pancreatic tumor banking program is critical to the ongoing success of translational research programs. Only through the coordinated efforts of such interdisciplinary programs will new treatments advance from the laboratory to clinical practice. Pathologists should routinely bank tumors for collaborative research efforts. At the M. D. Anderson Cancer Center, small sections of normal pancreas (when possible) and tumor are collected immediately for RNA extraction, and additional samples are snap frozen in liquid nitrogen and stored at –80°C. A representative section of tumor and normal tissue is routinely fixed in 70% ethyl alcohol for paraffin block processing, and a hematoxylin and eosin–stained slide is made.

PRETREATMENT DIAGNOSTIC STUDIES

TUMORS OF THE PANCREATIC HEAD AND PERIAMPULLARY REGION

Few anatomic regions in the human body cause greater confusion and controversy regarding appropriate diagnostic evaluation and treatment than does the periampullary region. The reasons for this are unclear because the differential diagnosis of extrahepatic biliary obstruction is limited to a malignant neoplasm (of the pancreas, bile duct, ampulla of Vater, or duodenum), a benign stricture (usually due to pancreatitis), and choledocholithiasis. Benign tumors of the periampullary region are exceedingly rare and therefore need not be considered in this differential diagnosis. Unlike for tumors in other parts of the gastrointestinal tract, the diagnostic algorithm cannot be separated from the treatment plan—diagnosis and treatment represent a continuum. Patients often receive diagnostic studies and treatment based more on established lines of physician referral than on sound knowledge of the natural history and current therapies for periampullary cancer. This fact is largely responsible for the variability in diagnostic and treatment recommendations: Typically, surgeons favor surgery, gastroenterologists favor endoscopically placed stents, and radiologists favor transhepatic stents.

General Principles

The recommended diagnostic evaluation for a patient with extrahepatic biliary obstruction and presumed cancer of the head of the pancreas is based on the following three principles.

LAPAROTOMY SHOULD BE THERAPEUTIC, NOT DIAGNOSTIC. If the primary tumor cannot be resected completely, surgery (pancreaticoduodenectomy) for pancreatic cancer offers no survival advantage. However, only 30% to 50% of patients who undergo operation with curative intent have their tumors successfully removed; the remaining patients are found to have unsuspected liver or peritoneal metastases or local tumor extension to the mesenteric vessels.[128,161,162] Therefore, the majority of patients who undergo surgical exploration for

TABLE 33.4-6. Median Survival for Patients Who Underwent Surgical Resection for Adenocarcinoma of the Pancreas and Were Found to Have a Positive Margin of Resection

Study	*Number of Patients*	*Margin*	*Median Survival (mo)*
Trede et al.[131] (1990)	54	G/M	10
Willett et al.[134] (1993)	37	G/M	11
Nitecki et al.[129] (1995)	28	G	9
Yeo et al.[135] (1995)	58	G/M	10
Sperti et al.[168] (1996)	19	G/M	7
Nishimura et al.[166] (1997)	70	G/M	6
Yeo et al.[167] (1997)	39	G/M	18[a]
Surgery alone	11	G/M	5
Millikan et al.[165] (1999)	22	M	8

G, grossly positive margin; M, microscopically positive margin.
[a]Received postoperative 5-fluorouracil–based chemoradiation.

presumed cancer of the pancreatic head receive no survival benefit; however, the laparotomy results in a perioperative morbidity rate of 20% to 30%, a mean hospital stay of 1 to 2 weeks, and a median survival after surgery of only 6 months.[161,163,164] Furthermore, in patients whose tumors are resected with positive margins (Table 33.4-6),[129,131,133–135,146,165–168] the survival duration is less than 1 year and is no different from the survival duration achieved with palliative chemotherapy and irradiation in patients who have locally advanced, unresectable disease.[150,153] Therefore, in contrast to the case for selected patients with colorectal or gastric cancer, no data support palliative (positive-margin) resection for adenocarcinoma of the pancreas.

RESECTABILITY SHOULD BE DETERMINED PREOPERATIVELY. Accurate preoperative assessment of resectability increases resectability rates and minimizes positive-margin resections. A common misconception in pancreatic tumor surgery is that resectability is determined best at laparotomy. In fact, however, resectability is most accurately determined preoperatively by imaging studies, not at the time of "exploratory" laparotomy.[124,139,157,169] Surgeons declare a tumor to be unresectable at the time of laparotomy when unsuspected liver metastases, peritoneal implants or, most commonly, locally advanced disease is found. The term *locally advanced* is often poorly defined, leaving the patient, the medical oncologist, and the radiation oncologist without a clear understanding of why the primary tumor was not resected.[170] At the time of surgical exploration for pancreatic head cancer, a Kocher maneuver (mobilization of the pancreatic head and duodenum from their retroperitoneal attachments) is the first procedure performed to assess the relationship of the tumor to the SMA by palpation. However, the presumed accuracy of this maneuver to assess SMA involvement evolved before the development of contrast-enhanced CT, and no anatomic basis exists for the maneuver's use as a determinant of resectability. Direct intraoperative assessment of the extent of retroperitoneal tumor growth in relation to the SMA origin is not completed until the final step in tumor resection, after gastric and pancreatic transection, when the surgeon is committed to resection even if all of the tumor cannot be safely removed.

Data from the M. D. Anderson Cancer Center have demonstrated improved rates of resectability and low rates of margin positivity when high-quality CT is combined with the use of objective preoperative criteria for resectability.[139,149,157] The CT criteria for resectability are (1) the absence of extrapancreatic disease, (2) a patent superior mesenteric–portal vein (SMPV) confluence (assuming the technical ability to resect isolated involvement of the SMV or SMPV confluence), and (3) no direct tumor extension to the celiac axis or SMA. Patients whose tumors are deemed unresectable by these radiologic criteria are not considered candidates for a potentially curative resection.

Fuhrman and colleagues[157] studied 145 consecutive patients referred for pancreaticoduodenectomy because of a presumed or biopsy-proven periampullary cancer. Thin-section, contrast-enhanced CT was performed on all patients, and only 42 patients fulfilled the criteria for resectability. Thirty-seven of the 42 patients were able to undergo pancreaticoduodenectomy, for a resectability rate of 88%. Final pathologic evaluation of the retroperitoneal margin was used to confirm the accuracy of the CT criteria in predicting resectability. No patient had a grossly positive margin of resection, and only 5 of 25 patients with adenocarcinoma of pancreatic head origin were found to have a microscopic focus of adenocarcinoma at the retroperitoneal margin. This was despite the fact that many patients had undergone a previous nontherapeutic laparotomy before referral and that nine patients required resection of the SMV or SMPV confluence. In contrast, the intraoperative use of the Kocher maneuver is much less effective in determining resectability. Robinson and colleagues[170] studied 29 patients who underwent a successful pancreaticoduodenectomy after a previous unsuccessful laparotomy during which the pancreatic tumor was judged to be unresectable. Incorrect assessment of resectability (at the time of the Kocher maneuver) was the reason why 17 of the 29 patients did not undergo resection at their first laparotomy. The data thus demonstrate that, unlike intraoperative palpation, contrast-enhanced CT can accurately assess the relationship of the tumor to the SMA and celiac axis; this tumor-vessel relationship should be the main focus of the staging (preoperative) radiologic evaluation.

PALLIATIVE LAPAROTOMY SHOULD BE AVOIDED WHEN POSSIBLE. In patients with locally advanced or metastatic pancreatic cancer, operation for palliation is rarely needed. Multiple studies have compared operative biliary decompression and endoscopic stent placement in patients with jaundice due to malignant obstruction of the intrapancreatic portion of the common bile duct.[171–173] The higher initial morbidity and mortality rates and longer hospital stay associated with operative biliary bypass are countered by the higher frequency of hospital readmission for stent occlusion and cholangitis with endoscopic stent placement. Physicians typically advocate either surgery or endoscopic stenting; however, a selective approach based on the patient's extent of disease and performance status is more appropriate. Patients with liver metastases or ascites have a median survival of less than 6 months, making endoscopic stent placement an obvious choice. Patients with locally advanced disease treated with chemoradiation have a median survival of 10 to 12 months, with 20% surviving 2 years.[152,153] Patients with a superior performance status at diagnosis often survive longer, yet it is difficult in most patients to predict, at diagnosis, the tempo of disease progression. Clearly, one would like to avoid operation (with its morbidity and often lengthy recovery period) in patients with rapidly progressive disease. Similarly, one would like to have a durable means of biliary decompression in patients who are expected to survive longer than 6 to 9 months. Therefore, in patients with locally advanced nonmetastatic disease, it is reasonable to proceed with endoscopic stent placement and reserve operative biliary bypass for patients who survive long enough to experience stent occlusion. As is discussed later (see the section Palliative Methods of Biliary and Gastric Decompression), innovations in stent construction and the development of the expandable 10-mm metal stent have improved patency rates and resulted in more widespread application of stenting. Data from Raikar and colleagues[174] at the Mayo Clinic have demonstrated that endoscopic stenting for unresectable pancreatic cancer provides an equivalent duration of survival with a reduced cost and shorter hospital stay than operative biliary decompression, despite the need for subsequent stent exchanges.

Computed Tomography and Endoscopic Retrograde Cholangiopancreatography

Improved CT technology has resulted in CT being the study of choice to determine the extent of disease and resectability status in patients with pancreatic cancer. Image resolution has improved considerably with the use of dynamic scanning, whereby intravenous contrast material is delivered by an automatic injector. The development of helical or spiral scanning has improved scan speed through continuous rotation of the x-ray tube around the gantry. This allows the entire pancreas to be imaged during the bolus phase of contrast enhancement. In addition, scan data can be processed to display images in three-dimensional and multiplanar formats. Helical CT performed with contrast enhancement and a thin-section technique can accurately assess the relationship of the low-density tumor to the celiac axis, SMA, and SMPV confluence. However, design of the scanning protocol and interpretation of scans must be done by experienced radiologists who understand the clinical importance of accurate staging and assessment of resectability in patients with pancreatic cancer. A completed CT scan report should contain the following information necessary to determine resectability: (1) the presence or absence of extrapancreatic metastatic disease, (2) the patency of the SMV and SMPV confluence and their relationship to the tumor, and (3) the relationship of the tumor to the celiac axis and SMA. If such information is not apparent from review of the scans or the report, the study should be repeated.

Our diagnostic schema, based on high-quality CT, appears in Figure 33.4-1. A patient is deemed to have locally advanced, unresectable disease when clear evidence on the CT scans shows encasement of the SMA or celiac axis or occlusion of the SMPV confluence. The accuracy of CT in predicting unresectability is well established; current technology has eliminated the use of laparotomy to assess local tumor resectability.[175–177] If a low-density mass is not seen on CT scans, patients with extrahepatic biliary obstruction undergo diagnostic and therapeutic endoscopic retrograde cholangiopancreatography (ERCP). A malignant obstruction of the intrapancreatic portion of the common bile duct is characterized by the double-duct sign (proximal obstruction of the common bile and pancreatic ducts), which can often be accurately differentiated from choledocholithiasis and the long, smooth tapering bile duct stricture seen with chronic pancreatitis. To prevent cholangitis in patients who undergo diagnostic ERCP in the setting of extrahepatic biliary obstruction, endoscopic stents are routinely placed. Endoscopic stent placement also is done in patients with elevated bilirubin levels who are enrolled in preoperative chemoradiation protocols.

Endoscopic Ultrasonography and the Role for Pancreatic Biopsy

Accurate staging and biliary decompression are achieved with CT and ERCP in the majority of patients. Endoscopic ultrasonography (EUS)–guided fine-needle aspiration (FNA) is currently the procedure of choice for obtaining a cytologic diagnosis of malignancy. Pretreatment confirmation of malignancy is mandatory in all patients with locally advanced or metastatic disease before treatment with systemic therapy or external-beam radiation therapy (EBRT) and is being considered more commonly in patients with localized, potentially resectable disease because of the growing popularity of neoadjuvant therapy. Reports of EUS-guided FNA of the pancreas have demonstrated its accuracy and safety.[178–180] When biopsy material is interpreted by an experienced cytopathologist, false-positive results should not occur. However, false-negative results may be common, resulting in negative predictive values as low as 40%.[178] In a patient who presents with extrahepatic biliary obstruction, has a malignant-appearing stricture of the intrapancreatic portion of the common bile duct, and has no history of recurrent pancreatitis or alcohol abuse, the absence of a mass on CT or EUS should not exclude the possibility of a carcinoma of the pancreas or bile duct. Similarly, negative results of EUS-guided FNA should not be interpreted as definitive proof that a malignancy does not exist. The results of EUS, with or without FNA, should be considered in the context of the clinical situation and as a complement to CT and ERCP findings.

Although pretreatment pancreatic biopsy is frequently used, physicians should be cautioned about the use of intraoperative pancreatic biopsy. In patients with resectable disease, there is no indication for routine intraoperative pancreatic biopsy, and as stated, the use of preoperative EUS-guided FNA should be limited to those patients receiving preoperative chemoradiation in whom cytologic confirmation of malignancy is needed. In contrast to the minimal risk of FNA, a risk of peritoneal dissemination of tumor cells resulting from surgical manipulation and intraoperative large-needle biopsy is supported by data from Staley et al.[148] Having undergone a previous laparotomy with tumor biopsy before definitive pancreaticoduodenectomy was the only factor associated with an increased risk of local-regional tumor recurrence in their study. Furthermore, intraoperative pancreatic biopsy has been associated with significant complications, such as pancreatitis, pancreatic fistula, and hemorrhage.[170] Nevertheless, because of the perceived risk of tumor dissemination due to preoperative FNA (a common concern when CT-guided FNA was popular), patients with presumed periampullary or pancreatic neoplasms are often brought to the operating room for planned intraoperative diagnostic biopsy before extirpative surgery. If the frozen-section findings are negative, many surgeons do not proceed with tumor resection

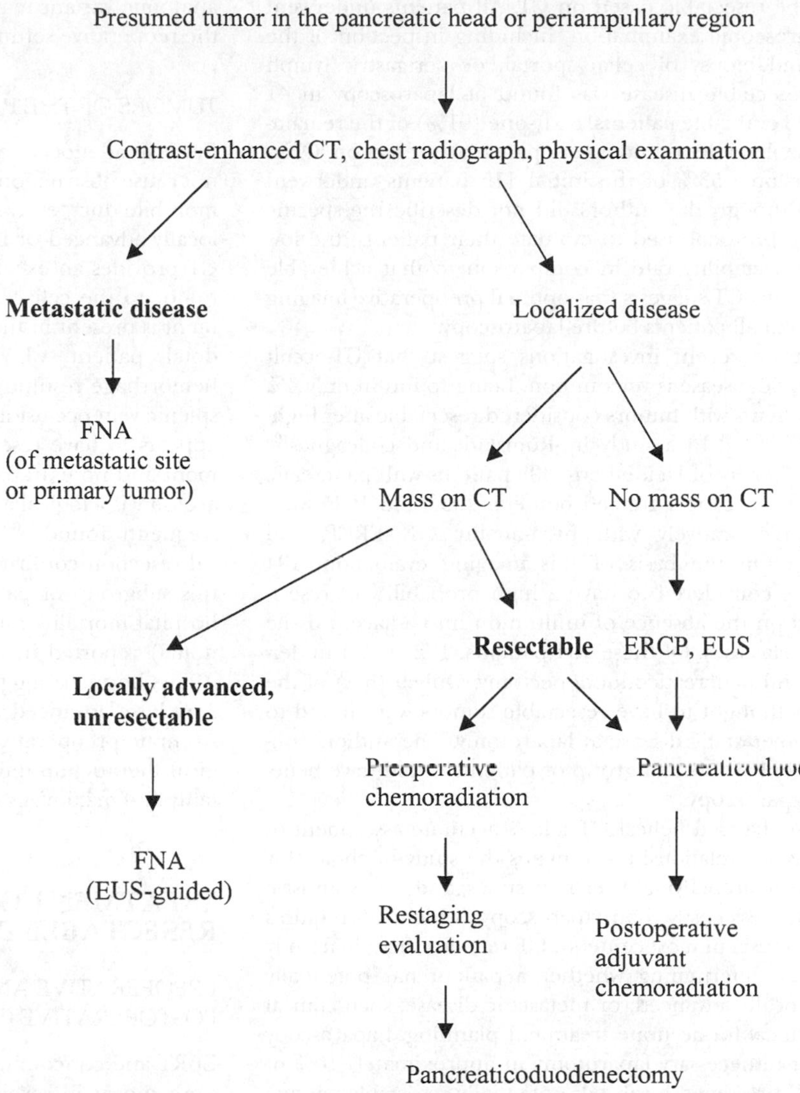

FIGURE 33.4-1. Management algorithm used at the M. D. Anderson Cancer Center for patients with suspected or biopsy-proven (from previous laparotomy before referral) adenocarcinoma of the pancreatic head. Accurate radiographic imaging allows patients to be staged as having resectable, locally advanced, or metastatic disease (see text). In patients with locally advanced or metastatic disease, biopsy confirmation of malignancy is mandatory before the initiation of specific anticancer therapy. Similarly, before initiation of neoadjuvant chemoradiation, cytologic confirmation of malignancy is required. The development of endoscopic ultrasonography (EUS)-guided fine-needle aspiration (FNA) has greatly simplified tissue acquisition in patients with localized, nonmetastatic pancreatic cancer. Angiography is performed selectively and is largely limited to patients who have undergone a previous biliary bypass involving the common bile duct to define hepatic arterial anatomy before reoperative pancreaticoduodenectomy. Laparoscopy should be considered before opening the abdomen in patients with potentially resectable disease. CT, computed tomography; ERCP, endoscopic retrograde cholangiopancreatography.

because of concerns about performing such an extensive operation for benign disease.[170,181] In contrast, most experienced pancreatic surgeons believe that preoperative or intraoperative pancreatic biopsy is unnecessary, because a negative biopsy in the appropriate clinical setting is likely due to sampling error and therefore should not influence the decision to proceed with pancreaticoduodenectomy.[182–185] In the absence of choledocholithiasis found at ERCP or a history of pancreatitis, obstruction of the intrapancreatic portion of the common bile duct is almost always secondary to malignancy. If the decision to perform pancreaticoduodenectomy is based on high-quality images obtained by CT and ERCP and on an accurate clinical history, it is extremely unlikely that pancreaticoduodenectomy will be performed for benign disease. Furthermore, if the preoperative FNA result is benign or nondiagnostic, it is a mistake to assume that the patient does not have cancer or that a tissue diagnosis can be obtained at surgery before complete tumor resection. The diagnosis of a malignant obstruction of the intrapancreatic portion of the common bile duct should be accurately established by high-quality images obtained by CT, ERCP, and EUS; unnecessary and preventable patient morbidity occurs when laparotomy, pancreatic biopsy, or both are used as diagnostic studies because of the physician's failure to obtain state-of-the-art pretreatment imaging.

Laparoscopy and Angiography

During the 1990s, laparoscopy has been used in patients with radiologic evidence of localized disease to detect extrapancreatic tumor not seen on CT scans, thereby allowing laparotomy to be limited to patients with localized disease. Studies by Cusheri[186] and Warshaw et al.[187] have demonstrated the value of laparoscopy in detecting liver and peritoneal metastases not seen on CT scans. This favorable initial experience with laparoscopy in the identification of subclinical metastatic disease has led to a policy of routine laparoscopy in the staging of pancreatic adenocarcinoma in many centers.[188–190] However, it is important to remember that 70% to 80% of patients with pancreatic cancer present with locally advanced or metastatic disease; if laparoscopy is done early in the diagnostic sequence, it will have a very high yield of positive findings. If laparoscopy is performed after high-quality contrast-enhanced CT, the yield will likely be much lower. For example, Conlon and colleagues[188] evaluated 115 patients with periampullary tumors thought to be resectable based on CT. All patients underwent careful laparoscopic examination, including inspection of the lesser sac and biopsy of celiac, portal, or perigastric lymph nodes. Unresectable disease was found at laparoscopy in 41 (38%) of 108 evaluable patients. Sixty-one (91%) of the remaining 67 evaluable patients underwent pancreatic resection. Overall, however, only 53% of the initial 115 patients underwent resection. Although the authors did not describe the specific CT scanning protocol used to evaluate their patients, the low radiologic resectability rate in comparison to that achievable with high-quality CT suggests that optimal preoperative imaging was not used in all patients before laparoscopy.

Other, more recent investigations suggest that CT-occult extrapancreatic disease is uncommon, being found in only 4% to 15% of patients with tumors considered resectable after high-quality CT.[139,191–194] In a study by Rumstadt and colleagues[192] from the University of Heidelberg, 398 patients with pancreatic or periampullary cancer treated between 1990 and 1995 were evaluated preoperatively with high-quality CT, ERCP, and angiography. On the basis of this imaging evaluation, 194 patients were considered to have a high probability of resectability based on the absence of infiltration into adjacent tissue or distant metastases. Of these 194 patients, 172 (89%) underwent successful pancreaticoduodenectomy. Only 9 (5%) of the 194 patients thought to have resectable tumors were found to have occult metastatic disease at laparotomy. The authors concluded that only this small group of patients would have benefited from laparoscopy.

Contrast-enhanced helical CT allows accurate assessment of vital tumor-vessel relationships, remains the study of choice for detecting intraparenchymal liver metastases, and is less invasive and therefore less costly than laparoscopy (which still requires general anesthesia in most centers). CT remains the initial study of choice for determining whether a patient has potentially resectable, locally advanced, or metastatic disease; such clinical staging is critical for accurate treatment planning. Laparoscopy may prevent unnecessary laparotomy in approximately 10% of patients with presumed localized, potentially resectable pancreatic cancer. Laparoscopy before laparotomy (during a single anesthesia induction) is a reasonable approach in patients with biopsy-proven or suspected potentially resectable pancreatic cancer in whom a decision has been made to proceed with pancreaticoduodenectomy. However, data are not available to support the cost-effectiveness of laparoscopy's routine use as a staging procedure under a separate anesthesia induction before treatment planning. Furthermore, laparoscopy should not be used to compensate for inadequate CT imaging.

Contrast-enhanced helical CT also has reduced the role of preoperative angiography. Angiography does not provide the detail that is needed to determine the anatomic relationship between the tumor and the SMA that is provided by high-quality contrast-enhanced CT. Angiography allows contrast enhancement of only the vessel lumen; the surrounding tumor and soft tissue cannot be evaluated. We limit the use of angiography to reoperative cases, in which identification of aberrant hepatic arterial anatomy may prevent iatrogenic injury during portal dissection when there is extensive scarring from a previous biliary procedure.[195] Tyler and Evans[181] reported a replaced or accessory right hepatic artery arising from the SMA in 26% of patients who underwent reoperative pancreaticoduodenectomy. Preoperative knowledge of this common anatomic variant may help prevent operative misadventure in the reoperative setting.

TUMORS OF THE PANCREATIC BODY AND TAIL

Because adenocarcinomas of the pancreatic body and tail do not cause obstruction of the intrapancreatic portion of the common bile duct, early diagnosis is rare; virtually all patients have locally advanced or metastatic disease at the time of diagnosis. CT provides an excellent assessment of the relationship of the tumor to the celiac axis and the SMA origin. Arterial encasement is present in the majority of patients, except for the anecdotal patient who presents with upper gastrointestinal hemorrhage resulting from sinistral hypertension secondary to splenic vein occlusion by a small tumor. In the rare patient who appears to have resectable disease on CT (no arterial encasement and no extrapancreatic disease), laparoscopy before laparotomy is a logical approach because peritoneal metastases are frequently found.[196,197] The scant data available regarding surgical resection confirm the short survival and poor prognosis in this subgroup of patients.[198,199] Furthermore, the high 30-day hospital mortality rate (43%; 6 of 14 patients with adenocarcinoma) reported in a study from the Department of Veterans Affairs hospitals suggests that many of the patients taken to surgery have advanced disease and a poor performance status.[200] Accurate preoperative imaging and a selective approach to surgical therapy minimizes treatment-related morbidity and mortality and maximizes the length and quality of patient survival.

TREATMENT OF POTENTIALLY RESECTABLE DISEASE

PREOPERATIVE AND POSTOPERATIVE CHEMORADIATION

EBRT and concomitant 5-FU chemotherapy (chemoradiation) were shown in several studies to prolong survival in patients with locally advanced adenocarcinoma of the pancreas.[150,151,201] Those data were the foundation for a prospective randomized study of adjuvant chemoradiation (500 mg/m^2/d of 5-FU for 6 days and 40 Gy of radiation) after pancreaticoduodenectomy conducted by the Gastrointestinal Tumor Study Group (GITSG); that trial also demonstrated a survival advantage from multimodality therapy compared with resection alone (20 months vs. 11 months).[141,202] However, owing to a prolonged recovery, 5 (24%) of the 21 patients in the adjuvant chemoradiation arm could not begin chemoradiation until more than 10 weeks after pancreaticoduodenectomy, despite the fact that the only patients likely to be considered for protocol entry were those who recovered rapidly from surgery and had a good performance status. Similar findings have been reported from the European Organization for Research and Treatment of Cancer (EORTC).[203–205] In 1987, the EORTC initiated trial 40891 comparing adjuvant 5-FU–based chemoradiation after pancreatectomy with surgery alone. Between 1987 and 1995, 218 patients were randomized to receive either chemoradiation (40 Gy in a split course and 5-FU given as a continuous infusion at a dose of 25 mg/kg/d during EBRT) or no further treatment after pancreaticoduodenectomy for adenocarcinoma of the pancreas or periampullary region. Patients were recruited from 29 centers in Europe, one in France, and three in the Netherlands. Analysis was performed on 207 of the patients, 114 (55%) of whom had pancreatic cancer. Eleven patients were deemed ineligible for analysis because of extensive local disease with incomplete resection. The median survival duration was 24.5 months for those who received adjuvant therapy and 19 months for those who received surgery alone ($P = .2$); for patients with pancreatic cancer, the median survival was 17.1 months for those who received adjuvant therapy compared with 12.6 months for those who received surgery alone ($P = .099$). Concerns over trial design, methodology, and data interpretation include the following:

1. The precise anatomic (pathologic) distinction between pancreatic and periampullary adenocarcinoma was not defined, and the high proportion of periampullary (nonpancreatic) tumors is unexplained.
2. Patients were considered for enrollment in this trial after recovery from pancreaticoduodenectomy; despite this selection bias, 21 (20%) of 104 evaluable patients randomized to receive chemoradiation did not receive intended therapy owing to patient refusal, medical comorbidities, or rapid tumor progression.
3. No assessment of the retroperitoneal margin of resection was performed, and therefore no mechanism to assess the completeness of surgical resection was available. Furthermore, although the method of follow-up was not defined (raising the concern that sites of recurrent disease were underestimated), tumor recurrence in the pancreatic bed was a site of first progression in 20% of patients. This finding, combined with the short survival in the observation arm (12 months for patients with pancreatic adenocarcinoma), suggests that many patients underwent incomplete resection.
4. Although the survival differences for the subset of patients with pancreatic cancer were not significant ($P = .099$), the wide confidence interval (relative risk, 0.7; 95% confidence interval, 0.5–1.1) does not exclude the possibility of a clinically meaningful improvement in survival in the chemoradiation arm that was not apparent because of the small sample size.

Despite these concerns, the authors concluded that postoperative adjuvant chemoradiation should not be considered standard therapy after pancreaticoduodenectomy for cancer.[204]

Two additional trials of postoperative adjuvant therapy after pancreaticoduodenectomy are ongoing: the European Study Group of Pancreatic Cancer (ESPAC)-1 trial and a Radiation Therapy Oncology Group (RTOG) trial. The ESPAC-1 trial is a four-arm study incorporating a two-by-two factorial design to compare adjuvant chemoradiation (40 Gy in a split course and 5-FU), adjuvant chemotherapy (5-FU and folinic acid), chemoradiation followed by chemotherapy, and observation alone after pancreaticoduodenectomy for pancreatic and periampullary carcinomas.[206,207] More than 40 centers in nine countries are participating in this study, which began accrual in 1994. In July 1998, the RTOG activated the first American phase III cooperative group study of postoperative adjuvant therapy for resected pancreatic adenocarcinoma since the GITSG trial.[208] Patients are randomized to receive either gemcitabine or 5-FU to be given before and after 5-FU–based chemoradiation.

Despite the selection bias involved in the enrollment of patients into postoperative adjuvant therapy studies, prospective and retrospective data suggest an improved survival duration with the addition of postoperative adjuvant chemoradiation after pancreaticoduodenectomy (Table 33.4-7).[133,139–141,149,167,202,209–213] The most compelling data reported of late come from Yeo and colleagues[167] at Johns Hopkins University, who reviewed all

TABLE 33.4-7. Chemoradiation Studies in Patients with Resectable Pancreatic Cancer

Study	*Number of Patients*[a]	*EBRT Dose (Gy)*	*Chemotherapy Agent(s)*	*Median Survival (mo)*
Postoperative (adjuvant)				
Kalser and Ellenberg[202] (1985)	21	40	5-FU	20
Surgery alone	22	—	—	11
GITSG[141] (1987)	30	40	5-FU	18
Whittington et al.[133] (1991)	28	45–63	5-FU	16
Foo et al.[140] (1993)	29	35–60	5-FU	23
Davis et al.[209] (1996)	34	50.4	5-FU	16
Spitz et al.[139] (1997)	19	50.4	5-FU	22
Yeo et al.[167] (1997)	120	40.0–57.6	5-FU	19.5
Surgery alone	53	—	—	13.5
Demeure et al.[210] (1998)	30	50.4–54.0	5-FU	24.2
Surgery alone	31	—	—	16.9
Abrams et al.[211] (1999)	23	50.4–57.6	5-FU + LV	15.9
Klinkenbijl et al.[204] (1999)	60	40	5-FU	17.1
Surgery alone	54	—	—	12.6
Preoperative (neoadjuvant)				
Hoffman et al.[212] (1995)	11	50.4	5-FU + Mito-C	45
Hoffman et al.[213] (1998)	24	50.4	5-FU + Mito-C	15.7
Spitz et al.[139] (1997)	41	30.0–50.4	5-FU	19.2
Pisters et al.[149] (1998)	20	30	5-FU	25

5-FU, 5-fluorouracil; EBRT, external-beam radiation therapy; GITSG, Gastrointestinal Tumor Study Group; LV, leucovorin; Mito-C, mitomycin C.
[a]All patients underwent a pancreatectomy with curative intent.

patients who underwent pancreaticoduodenectomy for adenocarcinoma of the pancreatic head during a 4-year period. One hundred twenty patients received adjuvant chemoradiation, and 53 underwent pancreaticoduodenectomy alone. The median survival for those who received adjuvant therapy was 19.5 months, compared with 13.5 months for the group who received surgery alone.

A survival advantage was also demonstrated for patients treated with adjuvant combination chemotherapy (5-FU, doxorubicin, and mitomycin C) after pancreatectomy.[214] The median survival was 23 months in the 30 patients randomized to receive adjuvant therapy, compared to 11 months in the 31 patients treated with surgery alone. Forty-six additional patients were ineligible after surgery, attesting to the difficulty in performing multiinstitutional protocol-based research involving as complex a surgical procedure as pancreaticoduodenectomy. The toxicity of the surgery and chemotherapy was significant; only 24 of 30 patients received chemotherapy, and only 13 of those received all six planned courses of chemotherapy. A previous pilot study of adjuvant 5-FU, doxorubicin, and mitomycin C using a different schedule of administration found similar toxicity and therefore questioned the use of adjuvant combination chemotherapy, even of moderate toxicity, after pancreatectomy.[145]

The risk of delaying or not receiving postoperative adjuvant therapy,[167,203,214,215] combined with small published experiences of successful pancreatic resection after EBRT,[216–218] prompted many institutions to initiate studies in which chemoradiation was given preoperatively.[158,219] Results of these and other studies have suggested specific advantages of preoperative versus postoperative chemoradiation, including the following considerations[124]: (1) Because chemotherapy and radiation are given first, delayed postoperative recovery has no effect on the delivery of multimodality therapy[139,149]; (2) pancreaticojejunal anastomotic leaks, the most common major complication after pancreaticoduodenectomy, are decreased in patients who receive preoperative chemoradiation[220]; (3) the high frequency of positive-margin resections that have been reported supports the concern that the retroperitoneal margin of excision, even when negative, may be only a few millimeters—surgery alone is thus inadequate local therapy for most patients[134,167]; and (4) patients with disseminated disease evident on restaging studies after chemoradiation are not subjected to laparotomy.[149]

In patients who receive chemoradiation before planned pancreaticoduodenectomy, repeat staging CT after chemoradiation reveals liver metastases in approximately 25%.[139,149] If these patients had undergone pancreaticoduodenectomy at the time of diagnosis, it is probable that the liver metastases would have already been present subclinically; these patients would therefore have undergone a major surgical procedure only to have liver metastases found soon after surgery. In the M. D. Anderson Cancer Center trials, patients who were found to have disease progression at the time of restaging had a median survival of only 7 months.[124] The avoidance of a lengthy recovery period and the potential morbidity of pancreaticoduodenectomy in patients with such a short expected survival duration represents a distinct advantage of preoperative over postoperative chemoradiation. Furthermore, when delivering multimodality therapy for any disease, it is beneficial, when possible, to deliver the most toxic therapy last, thereby avoiding morbidity in patients who experience rapid disease progression not amenable to currently available therapies.

The survival advantage for the combination of chemoradiation and surgery compared with surgery alone (see Table 33.4-7) likely results from improved local-regional tumor control. Because of the poor rates of response to 5-FU–based systemic therapy in patients with measurable metastatic disease, it is unlikely that 5-FU–based chemoradiation regimens significantly impact the development of distant metastatic disease. Data from the M. D. Anderson Cancer Center support this belief.[148,149] Staley and colleagues[148] reported on 39 consecutive patients who underwent pancreaticoduodenectomy and intraoperative electron-beam radiation therapy (IOERT; 10 Gy) for adenocarcinoma of the pancreatic head after preoperative infusional 5-FU (300 mg/m^2/d, 5 days per week) and EBRT (50.4 Gy). Thirty-eight patients were evaluable for analysis of patterns of treatment failure; one perioperative death occurred. Overall, 38 recurrences were found in 29 patients; eight recurrences (21%) were local-regional (pancreatic bed, peritoneal cavity, or both), and 30 (79%) were distant (lung, liver, bone). The liver was the most frequent site of tumor recurrence, and liver metastases were a component of treatment failure in 53% of patients (69% of all patients who had recurrences). Fourteen patients (37% of all patients; 48% of patients who had recurrences) had liver metastases as their only site of recurrence. Isolated local or peritoneal recurrences were documented in only four patients (11%). In contrast, previous reports of pancreaticoduodenectomy alone for adenocarcinoma of the pancreas documented local recurrence in 50% to 80% of patients.[134,142,147] The improvement in local-regional control with preoperative chemoradiation was seen despite the fact that 14 of 38 evaluable patients had undergone laparotomy with tumor manipulation and biopsy before referral for chemoradiation and reoperation. If these 14 patients are excluded, only two patients (8%) experienced local or peritoneal recurrence as any component of treatment failure. However, the chemoradiation program was associated with gastrointestinal toxic effects (nausea, vomiting, and dehydration) that required hospital admission in one-third of patients.[148] In addition, the multicenter Eastern Cooperative Oncology Group trial documented the need for hospital admission in 51% of patients during or within 4 weeks of completing chemoradiation.[213] These findings led to a change in the delivery of radiation therapy and 5-FU at the M. D. Anderson Cancer Center. A rapid-fractionation program of chemoradiation was designed to avoid the gastrointestinal toxicity seen with standard-fractionation chemoradiation (5.5 weeks) while attempting to maintain the excellent local tumor control achieved with multimodality therapy.[149] In a study of the revised regimen, rapid-fractionation chemoradiation was delivered over 2 weeks with 18-MeV photons using a four-field technique to a total dose of 30 Gy (3 Gy per fraction for ten fractions, 5 days per week). 5-FU was given concurrently by continuous infusion at a dosage of 300 mg/m^2/d, 5 days per week. Restaging with chest radiography and abdominal CT was performed 4 weeks after completion of chemoradiation in preparation for pancreaticoduodenectomy. Thirty-five patients received this treatment, 27 were taken to surgery, and 20 (74%) underwent successful pancreaticoduodenectomy. Local tumor control and patient survival were equal to the results reported above with standard-fractionation (5.5 weeks) chemoradiation: Local-regional recurrence developed in only 2 (10%) of the 20 patients who underwent resection, and the median survival for all 20 patients was 25 months.[149]

Because of the large percentage of patients who develop distant metastatic disease, predominantly in the liver, the improved local-regional tumor control achieved with combined-modality therapy (chemoradiation and surgery) translates into only a small improvement in median survival. Therefore, more effective systemic agents are needed to both maximize radiation sensitization and treat microscopic extrapancreatic metastatic disease. One such potential agent is gemcitabine (2'-deoxy-2',2'-difluorocytidine; Gemzar), a deoxycytidine analogue capable of inhibiting DNA replication and repair. After a phase I study,[221] gemcitabine was evaluated in a multicenter trial of 44 patients with advanced pancreatic cancer.[222] Although only five objective responses were documented, the investigators noted frequent subjective symptomatic benefits, often in the absence of an objective tumor response. Toxicity appeared to be minor and included myelosuppression, particularly thrombocytopenia, as well as a flu-like syndrome and mild hemolytic-uremic syndrome. Based on these observations, gemcitabine was compared to 5-FU in previously untreated patients with advanced pancreatic cancer.[223] Patients treated with gemcitabine had a median survival of 5.65 months, compared to 4.41 months ($P = .0025$) in those treated with 5-FU. Twenty-four percent of patients treated with gemcitabine were alive at 9 months, compared to 6% of patients treated with 5-FU. In addition, more clinically meaningful effects on disease-related symptoms (pain control, performance status, and weight gain) were seen with gemcitabine (24% of patients) than with 5-FU (5% of patients). Similar systemic effects and demonstrable disease responses were documented in patients who were treated with gemcitabine after experiencing disease progression while receiving 5-FU.[224]

Gemcitabine is also a potent radiation sensitizer of human pancreatic cancer cells *in vitro*, supporting studies examining its use *in vivo*. Laboratory studies suggest that the inhibitory effect of gemcitabine on DNA synthesis (when combined with irradiation) is prolonged in tumor compared to normal tissues.[225] This may provide a window of opportunity for the combination of gemcitabine and EBRT when delivered in a fractionated schedule. Such data provide the basis for the ongoing phase I studies of this drug-radiation combination in patients with locally advanced pancreatic cancer; gemcitabine (combined with EBRT) is being given in escalating doses weekly as a single agent,[226] in combination with 5-FU,[227] in combination with cisplatin,[228] at a fixed dose with escalating doses of EBRT,[229] and as a twice-weekly infusion with either standard-fractionation EBRT[230] or split-course EBRT.[231] Wolff and colleagues[226] from the M. D. Anderson Cancer Center have reported a phase I study of rapid-fractionation EBRT (30 Gy over 2 weeks, 3 Gy per fraction) and concomitant weekly gemcitabine in patients with locally advanced adenocarcinoma of the pancreatic head. Gemcitabine was given during the first 2 weeks of irradiation and continued weekly to complete a 7-week course of systemic therapy. The maximum tolerated dose of gemcitabine using this treatment schedule was 350 mg/m^2/week. Dose-limiting toxicities included fatigue, anorexia, nausea, vomiting, and dehydration; febrile neutropenia occurred in only one patient. Future studies of gemcitabine-based chemoradiation will likely incorporate a fixed dose-rate schedule of administration because current data suggest an improved response rate with such a schedule.[232]

The results with gemcitabine for locally advanced and metastatic pancreatic cancer suggest that gemcitabine may be useful in patients with potentially resectable disease. Hoffman and colleagues[233] have reported a phase I study of preoperative standard-fractionation EBRT (50.4 Gy) and escalating weekly doses of gemcitabine (300 mg/m^2, 400 mg/m^2, 500 mg/m^2) for potentially resectable pancreatic cancer. Eight (53%) of 15 patients required hospitalization after chemoradiation. Pancreaticoduodenectomy was completed in eight patients; so far, the histologic response to the preoperative therapy appears to be superior to that with prior chemoradiation combinations. No experience with adjuvant gemcitabine-based chemoradiation after pancreaticoduodenectomy has been published; acute and late toxic effects of this drug-radiation combination may be more significant than when it is used in the preoperative setting.

The evolution of multimodality therapy for patients with potentially resectable pancreatic cancer appears in Figure 33.4-2. Future regimens will likely emphasize neoadjuvant therapy and capitalize on our expanding understanding of the molecular basis of metastasis, allowing conventional chemoradiation and surgery to be combined with systemic or regional delivery of novel agents that inhibit essential steps in tumor cell growth.

PANCREATICODUODENECTOMY

Background

Current surgical treatment is based on the procedure of pancreaticoduodenectomy as described in 1935 by Whipple et al.[234] Their two-stage pancreaticoduodenectomy consisted of biliary diversion and gastrojejunostomy during a first operation and, after the patient recovered (approximately 3 weeks later), resection of the duodenum and pancreatic head. By 1941, the world experience totaled 41 cases, and the perioperative mortality rate was 30%.[235] Before 1940, the pancreatic remnant was not reanastomosed to the small bowel, and the high mortality rate was largely due to pancreatic fistula from the oversewn pancreatic remnant. In 1941, Whipple modified his reconstruction to include a pancreaticojejunostomy, with the entire procedure done in one operation. In 1946, Waugh and Clagett[236] from the Mayo Clinic described their modification of the one-stage procedure to its current form. The goals of surgical therapy outlined by Waugh and Clagett have not changed since that date: (1) there should be reasonable opportunity for cure, (2) the risk of death should not outweigh the prospects for cure, and (3) the patient should be left in as normal a condition as possible.[236]

Surgical Mortality Rates

Advances in operative technique, anesthesia, and critical care have resulted in a 30-day in-hospital mortality rate of less than 2% for pancreaticoduodenectomy when performed at major referral centers by experienced surgeons.[138,220,237] At such centers, mortality rates remain less than 2% despite the use of multimodality therapy, the frequent need for complex vascular resection and reconstruction, and the referral of many patients after an initial unsuccessful attempt at tumor resection.[238,239] Mortality rates from other institutions, including university centers and the Department of Veterans Affairs hospitals, have been reported in the range from 7.8% to more than 10%.[240–243] Data from New York State have demonstrated that hospitals performing fewer than nine pancreatic resections per year have an unacceptably high perioperative mortality rate of 12%.[244] Data from Maryland and Ontario, Canada, also have demonstrated that increased patient volume is associated with lower surgery-related mortality.[245–247] The most compelling data on the relationship of hospital volume

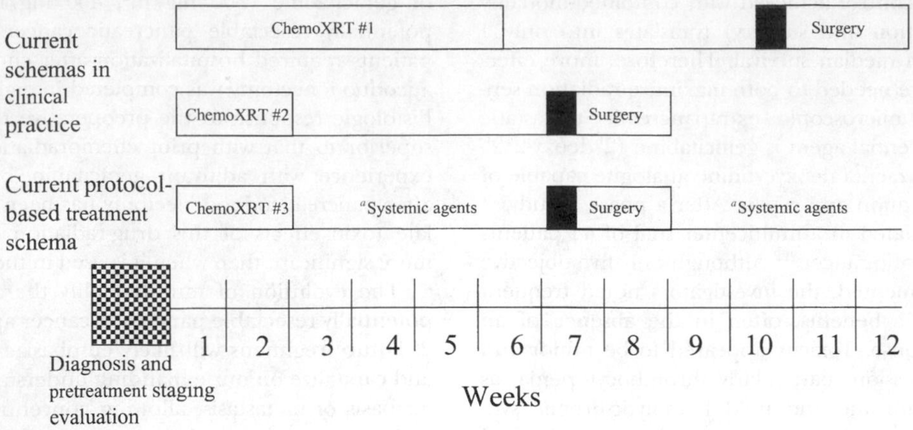

FIGURE 33.4-2. The evolution of multimodality neoadjuvant (preoperative) therapy for patients with potentially resectable adenocarcinoma of the pancreatic head. Current treatment schemas combine 5-fluorouracil (5-FU) chemoradiation (ChemoXRT) and pancreaticoduodenectomy. Short-course rapid-fractionation chemoradiation avoids the gastrointestinal toxicity of standard-fractionation chemoradiation and reduces overall treatment time. Future treatment schemas (currently being studied in the protocol setting) emphasize the importance of improving local and systemic disease control with more potent radiation-sensitizing agents and novel systemic therapies. ■, restaging evaluation; ChemoXRT #1, 50.4 Gy, 1.8 Gy per fraction: 5-FU 300 mg/m^{2}d, M–F; ChemoXRT #2, 30 Gy, 3.0 Gy per fraction: 5-FU 300 mg/m^{2}d, M–F; ChemoXRT #3, 30 Gy, 3.0 Gy per fraction: with improved radiation-sensitizing agents (gemcitabine). [a]Systemic agents: novel systemic agents, such as inhibitors of angiogenesis, farnesyl-protein transferase, epidermal growth factor, and so forth.

to perioperative mortality and long-term survival after pancreaticoduodenectomy come from the Center for the Evaluative Clinical Sciences at Dartmouth Medical School.[248,249] Birkmeyer et al.[248] studied 7229 Medicare patients older than 65 years of age who underwent pancreaticoduodenectomy at 1772 hospitals between 1992 and 1995. The study population was divided into quartiles according to hospital volume, with high-volume centers defined as those that performed five or more pancreaticoduodenectomies per year. Forty high-volume hospitals (2%) performed 1541 (21%) of the 7229 pancreaticoduodenectomies. In-hospital mortality was 11% overall, 4% in high-volume hospitals, and 10% to 16% in medium-volume (two to five pancreaticoduodenectomies per year) and very low-volume (fewer than one pancreaticoduodenectomy per year) hospitals. These data suggest a linear relationship between surgical volume and outcome. Birkmeyer and colleagues suggested that more that 100 deaths per year could potentially be prevented by the referral of pancreatic cancer patients to high-volume hospitals. Furthermore, in an analysis of survival duration, after exclusion of perioperative deaths and adjustment for case mix, patients who underwent surgery at high-volume hospitals were less likely to experience late mortality.[249] The authors concluded that patients considering pancreaticoduodenectomy at low-volume hospitals should be given the option of referral to a high-volume center.

Patient outcome is optimized and costs minimized by the referral of patients requiring major pancreatic resections for malignant disease to centers with active multidisciplinary treatment programs.[250] However, because surgical resection benefits only patients who undergo a complete resection, it is essential that surgery be done only on patients with localized, potentially resectable pancreatic cancer. In the absence of significant innovations in systemic therapy, the only potential for major improvements in the quality of life of patients with pancreatic cancer lies in our ability to limit surgery-related morbidity to those patients most likely to benefit from surgical intervention (i.e., to avoid laparotomy in patients with unresectable disease). Therein lies the importance of determining resectability using strict CT criteria (see Pretreatment Diagnostic Studies, earlier in this chapter).

Technique

Pancreaticoduodenectomy as currently performed in the United States incorporates selected aspects of the traditional Whipple procedure and emphasizes the importance of removing all soft tissue to the right of the SMA.[251] The surgical resection is divided into six clearly defined steps,[181,251] the most important of which is step 6, during which the pancreas is divided and the specimen is removed from the SMPV confluence and the right lateral border of the SMA. This is performed by completely mobilizing the SMV and portal vein medially; the uncinate process is then dissected off of the SMV and its posteriorly located first jejunal branch. Only after full medial mobilization of the SMV can one identify the SMA (lateral to the SMV). The pancreatic head and all soft tissue to the right of the SMA are then removed with direct ligation of the inferior pancreaticoduodenal artery or arteries.

The high incidence of local recurrence after standard pancreaticoduodenectomy (see Table 33.4-3) mandates that close attention be paid to the retroperitoneal margin. The retroperitoneal margin is the soft tissue margin along the right lateral border of the proximal SMA. This margin contains the lateral portion of the mesenteric neural plexus that surrounds the artery. Importantly, perineural invasion involving the mesenteric plexus at the SMA origin and tumor cell infiltration of lymphatic vessels and connective tissue may extend beyond the confines of the palpable tumor in the pancreatic head and result in a microscopically positive retroperitoneal margin, even when all gross disease is easily resected.[252–254] A more extensive retroperitoneal dissection to the right of the SMA is not associated with greater operative morbidity and is necessary to obtain a negative retroperitoneal margin.[124,157,238] This important margin of resection is often confused with the soft tissue posterior to the pancreatic head and duodenum and anterior to the inferior vena cava (posterior pancreaticoduodenal region). Direct invasion of the inferior vena cava is uncommon, and removal of all tissue anterior to this vessel is easily accomplished. As is true for other solid tumors, adequate local-regional control of pancreatic cancer requires negative margins of excision, and the margin of greatest importance at the time of pancreaticoduodenectomy is the soft tissue margin along the proximal SMA (retroperitoneal margin). In addition, clear identification of the SMA avoids the potential for iatrogenic injury.

Segmental resection of the SMPV confluence is performed when the tumor is inseparable from the lateral wall of the SMV or portal vein.[239] Although an occasional patient may have such a small area of venous involvement that a saphenous vein patch is an obvious choice, the majority of patients with involvement of the SMPV confluence require segmental venous resection. The technical feasibility of portal vein resection was first reported by Fortner[255] in his large series of type I regional pancreatectomies that included routine portal vein resection. More recently, surgeons have reported the safety of pancreatectomy with *en bloc* resection of the SMPV confluence.[256,257] Fuhrman and colleagues[238] have demonstrated that invasion of the SMV or portal vein is not associated with histopathologic variables (margin and lymph node positivity) that suggest a poor prognosis. Their data imply that venous involvement is a function of tumor location rather than an indicator of aggressive tumor biology. Additional data from the M. D. Anderson Cancer Center have confirmed that patient survival is not affected by the need for venous resection at the time of pancreaticoduodenectomy.[258] In contrast to previous reports on venous resection, the preferred technique for resection of the SMPV confluence at M. D. Anderson involves preservation of the splenic vein–portal vein junction and use of an internal jugular vein interposition graft placed between the SMV and portal vein.[195,239,257]

It is important to emphasize the distinction between regional pancreatectomy and pancreaticoduodenectomy with segmental resection of the SMV or SMPV confluence. Venous resection is not an attempt to improve *en bloc* lymphatic and soft tissue clearance, as is performed in regional pancreatectomy. It is unlikely that larger local-regional resections (to the left of the SMA and celiac axis) in poorly selected patients with advanced disease will impact survival.[195,258] Venous resection should be performed only in carefully selected patients who have tumor adherence to the SMV or SMPV confluence but no evidence of tumor extension to the SMA or celiac axis. The rationale for venous resection and the anatomic difference between tumor invasion of venous and arterial structures have been reviewed.[238,239,258] Because the need for venous resection is unexpected in many patients and is discovered only after gastric and pancreatic transection, when nonresectional procedures are no longer an option, surgeons who perform pancreaticoduodenectomies should be familiar with standard vascular techniques for resection and reconstruction of the SMPV confluence.

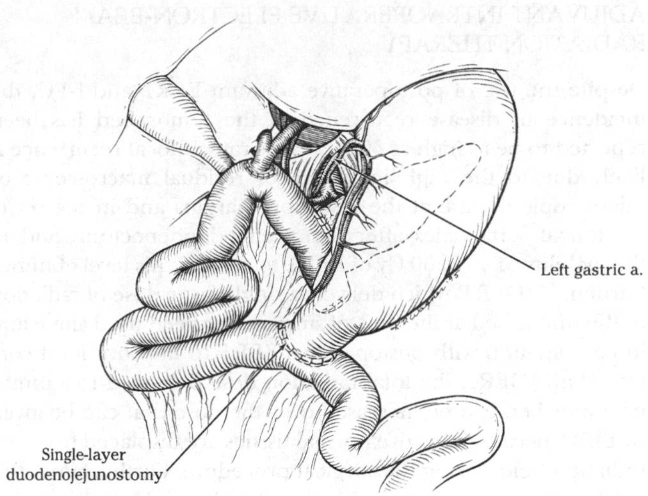

FIGURE 33.4-3. Illustration of the completed reconstruction after pylorus-preserving pancreaticoduodenectomy.

PYLORUS PRESERVATION

Preservation of the antropyloroduodenal segment in combination with pancreaticoduodenectomy (Fig. 33.4-3) was first described by Traverso and Longmire in 1978.[259] Since then, increasing numbers of pancreatic surgeons have used this modification of the procedure, particularly for patients with benign disease or small periampullary lesions. Proponents of the technique argue that preservation of the antropyloric pump mechanism results in improved long-term upper gastrointestinal tract function with associated salutary nutritional sequelae.[132,135,260] Physiologic studies suggest that pylorus preservation decreases intestinal transit time, lessens diarrhea (steatorrhea), normalizes glucose metabolism, and improves postoperative weight gain.[261,262] Detractors of pylorus-preserving pancreaticoduodenectomy counter that the reported improvements in gastrointestinal tract function and nutrition are small, if any, and that they come at the expense of an increased incidence of delayed gastric emptying during the early postoperative period.[263,264] Clinically significant long-term gastrointestinal dysfunction occurs in very few patients after standard pancreaticoduodenectomy with distal gastric resection.[261] Additionally, leaving the distal stomach and duodenum may compromise margins of excision, prevent adequate peripyloric lymphadenectomy, and negatively impact patient survival.[130,263,265] Published data to date involve retrospective comparisons that have yielded mixed results. Most investigators would agree that pylorus preservation should not be performed in patients with bulky tumors of the pancreatic head or with duodenal tumors involving the first or second portions of the duodenum.

However, a far greater body of literature exists on the use of pylorus preservation than on innovative, multimodality therapies for patients with localized pancreatic cancer. The resection or retention of the pylorus is of much less significance than the proper selection of patients for pancreaticoduodenectomy and the status of the retroperitoneal margin after tumor resection. For example, three reports advocating pylorus preservation for malignant pancreatic and periampullary cancers reported positive resection margins in 25%, 29%, and 37% of patients.[132,135,266] In the presence of a positive margin of resection, patients do not survive long enough to receive a potential nutritional benefit (if one exists) from pylorus preservation.

ADJUVANT INTRAOPERATIVE ELECTRON-BEAM RADIATION THERAPY

Despite the use of postoperative adjuvant EBRT and 5-FU, the incidence of disease recurrence in the tumor bed has been reported to be as high as 50%.[267] This rate of local recurrence is likely due to the high incidence of residual macroscopic or microscopic disease at the resection margins and in the retroperitoneal soft tissues after pancreaticoduodenectomy and to the inability of 40 to 50 Gy of EBRT to control this level of tumor burden.[134] IOERT, which delivers a single large dose of radiation to the tumor bed at the time of surgery, has been used alone and in combination with postoperative EBRT to improve local control. With IOERT, the total radiation dose delivered to a tumor or tumor bed can be increased over the dose that can be given by EBRT because sensitive normal tissues are displaced from the radiation field during the surgical procedure. Furthermore, this single intraoperative dose is believed to be biologically equivalent to an external-beam radiation dose at least two to three times greater given by means of conventional fractionation.

The data on the efficacy of pancreatic resection with IOERT alone or in combination with preoperative or postoperative EBRT are limited to retrospective or prospective single-institution studies and one small randomized trial.[136,268-272] The only reported prospective, randomized, controlled clinical trial of IOERT for resectable pancreatic cancer was performed at the U.S. National Cancer Institute beginning in 1980.[272] Twenty-four patients who underwent resection for pancreatic adenocarcinoma were randomized to receive IOERT (20 Gy) to the bed of the resected pancreas or observation. Patients in the IOERT group who had extrapancreatic tumor extension also received postoperative EBRT (45 to 55 Gy). Most patients had locally advanced disease that would be considered unresectable by conventional criteria. Patients underwent extensive extirpative surgery to remove all gross evidence of the primary tumor; the procedures frequently required vascular and adjacent organ resections, and this extent of surgical therapy resulted in considerable morbidity. The overall perioperative mortality rate was 27%, and the morbidity rate was 71%; the mortality and morbidity did not differ significantly between the IOERT and observation groups. The median survival of patients who received IOERT was 18 months, compared to 12 months for the observation group. Local recurrences occurred in all 12 patients (100%) in the observation group but in only 4 (33%) of 12 patients who received IOERT. One patient who received IOERT remained disease-free more than 15 years after therapy. Because of the small patient numbers, statistically significant survival differences were not reached between the IOERT and control groups.

More recently, investigators from the M. D. Anderson Cancer Center studied a regimen that included preoperative chemoradiation and IOERT. Patients with potentially resectable pancreatic cancer received preoperative EBRT (50.4 Gy in 28 fractions or 30 Gy in ten fractions) and concomitant protracted-infusion 5-FU (300 mg/m^2/d) followed by pancreaticoduodenectomy and IOERT (10 to 20 Gy) to the resection bed.[139,149] Based on this group's experience, it appears that IOERT can be delivered with minimal morbidity after preoperative chemoradiation and pancreaticoduodenectomy. The median survival duration in their most recent study was 25 months.[149] Disease recurrence occurred in 70% of patients at a median follow-up of 37 months; 86% of recurrences were distant, and only 14% were local-regional.

The results of these studies show that IOERT can be combined safely with pancreaticoduodenectomy and contemporary chemoradiation protocols. Although local control appears improved by IOERT, marked improvements in survival have not been demonstrated. At present, IOERT should be limited to investigative protocols.

RECONSTRUCTION

After pancreaticoduodenectomy with or without IOERT, gastrointestinal reconstruction is performed in a counterclockwise direction (Fig. 33.4-4).[251,273] The transected jejunum is brought through a small incision in the transverse mesocolon to the right or left of the middle colic vessels, and a two-layer, end-to-side, duct-to-mucosa pancreaticojejunostomy is performed over a small Silastic stent (if the pancreatic duct is not dilated). A two-layer anastomosis that invaginates the cut end of the pancreas into the jejunum can be performed if the pancreatic duct is not suitable for a duct-to-mucosa anastomosis. However, we prefer a duct-to-mucosa anastomosis. A single-layer biliary anastomosis is then completed, followed by an antecolic, end-to-

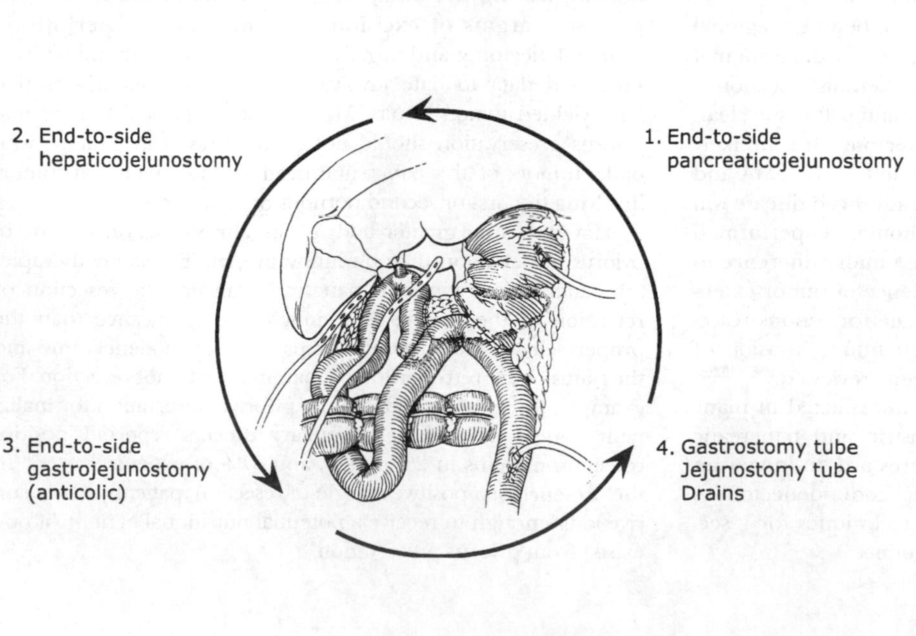

FIGURE 33.4-4. Illustration of pancreatic, biliary, and gastric reconstruction after standard pancreaticoduodenectomy. The remaining pancreas is anastomosed to the jejunum; we prefer a direct duct-to-mucosa anastomosis of the pancreatic duct.

side gastrojejunostomy constructed in two layers. Gastrostomy and feeding jejunostomy tubes are placed using the Witzel technique, and two closed-suction drains are placed.

Gastrointestinal reconstruction after pancreaticoduodenectomy is associated with two recognized complications: leak at the pancreaticojejunostomy and delayed gastric emptying. Anastomotic leak from the biliary and gastric anastomoses should be very uncommon. Initial techniques for gastrointestinal reconstruction after pancreaticoduodenectomy involved simple closure of the pancreatic stump. Because of a high rate of pancreatic fistula formation, surgeons quickly switched to implantation of the pancreatic remnant into the jejunum.[274] A more recent alternative is implantation of the pancreatic remnant into the posterior wall of the stomach.[275–277] Regardless of the technique used, results appear dependent on the experience of the surgeon. With greater experience, the incidence of complications decreases.

Delayed gastric emptying is common after standard pancreaticoduodenectomy and may be more frequent with pylorus preservation.[278] The cause is multifactorial but largely related to denervation of the upper gastrointestinal tract during resection of the pancreatic head and attached soft tissues and nerves to the right of the SMA. Symptoms of nausea, vomiting, and postprandial fullness resolve in 4 to 12 weeks in virtually all patients. The routine placement of gastrostomy and jejunostomy tubes at the time of surgery avoids needless patient morbidity due to temporary gastric emptying dysfunction. Patients can be discharged while receiving enteral feeding (via the jejunostomy tube) and allowed to advance their oral diet as tolerated. In addition, such tube placement prevents the expense and potential complications associated with intravenous hyperalimentation in patients who require prolonged hospitalization because of perioperative or postoperative complications. Poor gastric emptying in the absence of other concomitant intraabdominal pathologic conditions should not be the cause of prolonged hospitalization.

TREATMENT DECISIONS: POTENTIALLY RESECTABLE DISEASE

The use of contrast-enhanced helical CT allows accurate assessment of local tumor resectability. High-quality CT with objective CT criteria for resectability has replaced exploratory laparotomy as a means of assessing resectability. Pancreaticoduodenectomy should be considered only in patients with a good performance status (Karnofsky scale, 70% or higher) and as part of a multimodality treatment program that includes either preoperative or postoperative chemoradiation. The modest survival rates seen with current treatments (see Table 33.4-2) argue strongly for enrollment of all patients into clinical trials of new combinations of surgery, chemoradiation, and newly developed systemic agents. Published perioperative mortality rates support the referral of patients with potentially resectable disease to centers that are experienced with the operative management of pancreatic cancer and that perform at least nine major pancreatic resections per year.[244,248,249]

PALLIATIVE METHODS OF BILIARY AND GASTRIC DECOMPRESSION

Debate over the best method of biliary decompression (surgical bypass or endoscopic stent) in patients with terminal pancreatic cancer stimulated a series of prospective randomized trials.[171–173] These studies demonstrated that both methods are effective in relieving jaundice. Stenting is associated with lower initial morbidity and mortality rates and shorter hospital stays than operative bypass, but stent occlusion often results in the need for readmission to the hospital. Surgical biliary bypass provides a durable means of biliary decompression, but with greater initial morbidity. It is reasonable to assume that surgical complications are higher in patients with advanced disease and a poor performance status. In contrast, stent occlusion is more likely in patients with locally advanced or low-volume metastatic disease who survive long enough to experience this complication. Logic argues strongly for a selective approach to biliary decompression based on an accurate assessment of performance status and tumor burden.[279]

Patients with unresectable pancreatic cancer due to locally advanced or metastatic disease have a median survival of 6 months[280]; this duration of survival can be quite variable, ranging from 3 to 14 months depending on performance status and extent of disease. Laparotomy in this patient group is associated with a mortality rate of 2.5% to 5.0%, a morbidity rate of 20% to 30%, and a mean hospital stay of 10 to 14 days.[161,280–282] If one assumes that satisfactory recovery requires an additional 2 to 4 weeks, the patient with unresectable disease has invested 10% to 20% of overall survival time in achieving biliary drainage. Therefore, the incentive for the development of a less invasive method of biliary decompression is obvious. Technological advances in stent construction have now made endoscopic stent placement the procedure of choice in patients with advanced pancreatic cancer.[174,283,284] In patients with metastatic disease, whose survival duration is rarely longer than 6 to 9 months, biliary obstruction should be managed with outpatient endobiliary stent placement; this avoids the morbidity, hospital stay, and prolonged recovery period associated with operative biliary bypass. Stent occlusion is minimized with the use of large-caliber polyethylene stents (10.0 or 11.5 Fr.) without side holes; these stents reduce sludge and improve patency compared with smaller stents. Expandable 10-mm metal stents further decrease bacterial colonization and biofilm formation, resulting in improved patency compared with polyethylene stents[285,286]; however, that improved patency comes at a higher initial cost.

Patients with locally advanced, nonmetastatic pancreatic cancer have a median survival of 10 to 14 months (with current chemotherapy and chemoradiation regimens); endoscopic biliary decompression (even with an expandable metal stent) is associated with an increased incidence of stent occlusion as survival duration increases. Currently consensus has not been reached on how to manage an obstructed bile duct in patients with locally advanced, unresectable, nonmetastatic pancreatic cancer who have a good performance status. The desire to avoid palliative surgery (biliary bypass) that provides no anticancer therapy is balanced by the need for durable biliary decompression without the risk of recurrent cholangitis secondary to stent occlusion. This controversy is best illustrated by two publications from the same institution: one supports endobiliary stenting,[174] whereas the other supports operative bypass.[279]

We use a selective approach to biliary decompression. Outpatient endoscopic stenting is performed in all patients who are not candidates for pancreaticoduodenectomy. In patients with a life expectancy of 3 to 5 months (i.e., those with poor performance status or liver or peritoneal metastases), an 11.5-Fr. polyethylene stent is placed. In patients with a life expectancy of 6 to 12 months (i.e., those with locally advanced, nonmetastatic disease), a self-expanding metal stent is preferred. However, patients who develop early stent occlusion or migration or who by clinical criteria appear to do poorly with endoscopic biliary decompression are quickly referred for operative biliary bypass. A multidisciplinary approach to these patients is critical—the medical oncologist, gastroenterologist, and surgeon must communicate and avoid overly dogmatic approaches to palliative care.

Operative biliary bypass is routinely performed in patients who are brought to the operating room for planned pancreaticoduodenectomy and are found to have locally advanced or extrapancreatic metastatic disease. In such patients, a biliary-enteric bypass is performed. Previous studies have demonstrated no difference in outcome between cholecystojejunostomy and choledochojejunostomy.[161] However, the gallbladder should not be used for biliary decompression in the setting of acute or chronic gallbladder disease, cephalad tumor extension, or prolonged stent placement before surgery. In patients with a previous endoscopic stent, hypertrophy and fibrosis of the wall of the bile duct may make the cystic duct–common bile duct junction unsuitable for biliary decompression. Our choice for biliary bypass at the time of surgery is a Roux-en-Y choledochojejunostomy. The gallbladder is removed and the common bile duct transected. The endoscopic stent (if present) is removed, the distal bile duct is closed, and an end-to-side choledochojejunostomy is created with a single layer of interrupted monofilament sutures.

In patients with unresectable disease, laparoscopic cholecystojejunostomy represents another alternative for biliary decompression.[287–290] We use this technique in patients with locally advanced, nonmetastatic disease in whom attempted endoscopic stenting has been unsuccessful. Tumors of the uncinate process or the inferior aspect of the pancreatic head that extend to the root of the mesentery often deform the ampulla of Vater, making endoscopic cannulation difficult. Laparoscopic biliary decompression is an attractive option in these patients. Because laparoscopically assisted cholecystojejunostomy depends on a patent cystic duct–common bile duct junction, it is important not to consider this form of biliary decompression in patients with large tumors that extend cephalad to the porta hepatis.

Patients with symptomatic jaundice and ascites present a unique technical challenge. A subset of these patients have such advanced disease (and poor performance status) that pain control and hospice care are all that is indicated. For the occasional patient who presents with jaundice and the rapid onset of ascites and requires palliative treatment, we prefer endoscopic stent placement followed by early peritoneovenous shunting if an initial attempt at diuretic therapy is unsuccessful. If endoscopic stenting is not technically possible, laparoscopic cholecystojejunostomy is a reasonable alternative in the absence of high-volume carcinomatosis. Transhepatic biliary drainage with an internal-external catheter is not advised in patients with ascites because the ascitic fluid leaks around the catheter at the skin entrance site. In patients with malignant ascites, the surgeon should avoid using transabdominal catheters and making large abdominal incisions because of the risk of ascitic leak.

The subject of prophylactic gastrojejunostomy is not as relevant to the current surgical management of patients with pancreatic cancer as it was before the 1990s. Accurate preoperative imaging has increased resectability rates so that fewer patients are found to have unresectable disease at surgery. Advocates of prophylactic gastrojejunostomy state that the procedure can be performed safely, is not associated with postoperative delayed gastric emptying, and prevents subsequent gastric outlet obstruction in 10% to 20% of patients.[161,280] Detractors argue that concomitant gastric bypass at the time of therapeutic biliary bypass significantly increases operative morbidity, that the incidence of subsequent gastric outlet obstruction (in patients who receive only a biliary bypass) is much less than 10%, and that, if clinically evident gastric outlet obstruction does occur, it is usually a manifestation of end-stage disease.[281,291–293] Lillemoe et al.[294] from Johns Hopkins University reported on a prospective randomized trial of prophylactic gastrojejunostomy in patients with adenocarcinoma of the pancreatic head and periampullary region. Patients found to have unresectable disease and not to have intraoperative evidence of impending gastric outlet obstruction (such patients were excluded from analysis) at the time of laparotomy were randomly assigned to receive either a prophylactic gastrojejunostomy or no further surgery. Subsequent gastric outlet obstruction developed in 8 (19%) of the 43 patients who did not receive a gastric bypass, compared to 0 of 44 patients who received a gastrojejunostomy. Postoperative delayed gastric emptying occurred in 2% of patients in both groups, and the mean survival duration (8.3 months) was identical in both groups. Furthermore, no perioperative deaths occurred, and the mean hospital stay was approximately 8 days; again, no difference was noted between groups. The authors concluded that a retrocolic gastrojejunostomy should be performed routinely when a patient with pancreatic or periampullary cancer is found at operation to have unresectable disease. It appears that high-volume referral centers can perform palliative surgical biliary and gastric bypass procedures with low morbidity and mortality; however, these results may not be easily translated to low-volume centers with less experience. For example, a review of patients at 74 Department of Veterans Affairs hospitals from 1987 to 1991 concluded that prophylactic gastric bypass should be performed in patients with locally advanced, nonmetastatic pancreatic cancer, but the 30-day operative mortality rate (15% to 20%) was unacceptably high for palliative surgery in patients with such a short anticipated survival.[295]

In contrast to the data from Johns Hopkins University, Espat et al.[296] from Memorial Sloan-Kettering Cancer Center reported a low incidence of gastric outlet obstruction in patients with advanced pancreatic cancer. These investigators reported the longitudinal follow-up of 155 patients with pancreatic adenocarcinoma who were found to have locally advanced or metastatic disease at the time of staging laparoscopy (for presumed localized disease by CT). The median survival was 6.2 months for those with metastatic disease and 7.8 months for those with locally advanced disease; these survival durations support the authors' contention that the patients did not have high-volume metastatic disease at the time of laparoscopy. At a median follow-up of 6 months (81% of patients had died of disease), only 3 (2%) of 155 patients had undergone a subsequent open surgical procedure. Gastrojejunostomy for symptomatic gastric outlet obstruction was performed in two of these three patients. Two additional patients underwent elective gastric bypass (one was performed laparoscopically) at the time of biliary bypass. One additional patient required a percutaneous gastrostomy tube for poor gastric emptying during the terminal phase of his disease. Raikar et al.[174] from the Mayo Clinic also reported a low incidence of subsequent gastric outlet obstruc-

TABLE 33.4-8. Prospective Randomized Studies of Radiation Therapy and Chemotherapy for Locally Advanced Unresectable Pancreatic Cancer

Study	*Number of Patients*	*Median Survival (mo)*	*Local Failure in Evaluable Patients (%)*	*2-Y Survival Rate (%)*
Mayo Clinic[151]				
EBRT (35.0–37.5 Gy in 4 wk) only	32	6.3	NA	NA
EBRT (35.0–37.5 Gy in 4 wk) + 5-FU	32	10.4	NA	NA
GITSG[201]				
EBRT (60 Gy in 10 wk) only	25	5.2	24	5
EBRT (40 Gy in 6 wk) + 5-FU	83	9.6	26	10
EBRT (60 Gy in 10 wk) + 5-FU	86	9.2	27	10
GITSG[297]				
EBRT (60 Gy in 10 wk) + 5-FU	73	8.4	58	12
EBRT (60 Gy in 10 wk) + doxorubicin	72	7.5	51	6
GITSG[298]				
EBRT (54 Gy in 6 wk) + 5-FU/SMF	31	6.5	38	41 (1 y)
SMF only	26	5.1	29	19 (1 y)

5-FU, 5-fluorouracil; EBRT, external-beam radiation therapy; GITSG, Gastrointestinal Tumor Study Group; NA, not available; SMF, streptozocin, mitomycin C, and 5-FU.

tion in patients with unresectable pancreatic cancer who had endoscopic biliary decompression. In their study, only 1 (3%) of 34 patients treated with endoscopic biliary decompression required surgical bypass for gastric outlet obstruction. These two nonrandomized studies do not support the practice of routine prophylactic gastric bypass.

The apparent differences in the incidences of gastric outlet obstruction in the above studies are not readily explained. In general, we do not perform prophylactic surgery in patients with pancreatic cancer. If a patient is found to have unresectable disease during surgery for planned pancreaticoduodenectomy, we consider gastrojejunostomy when clinical symptoms or anatomic findings suggest impending obstruction. However, in patients with locally advanced or limited metastatic disease with good performance status, the Johns Hopkins data[294] (based on a prospective randomized trial) would support the creation of a retrocolic gastrojejunostomy.

TREATMENT OF LOCALLY ADVANCED DISEASE

Approximately 40% of the 28,600 patients diagnosed with ductal adenocarcinoma of the pancreas in 1999 presented with unresectable but nonmetastatic disease. Because these patients' tumors are unresectable by a Whipple procedure or total pancreatectomy owing to invasion of the portal or mesenteric vessels and they have no clinically demonstrable metastases, radiotherapeutic approaches frequently have been used. These approaches have included EBRT, with and without 5-FU chemotherapy; IOERT; and, more recently, EBRT with new chemotherapeutic (radiosensitizing) agents.

EXTERNAL-BEAM IRRADIATION WITH OR WITHOUT 5-FLUOROURACIL

In all except one study, conventional EBRT combined with 5-FU chemotherapy has been shown to improve survival in patients with locally advanced unresectable pancreatic cancer compared to irradiation alone or chemotherapy alone (Table 33.4-8).[151,201,297,298] The most favorable median survival duration and 2-year survival rate for EBRT plus 5-FU were approximately 10 months and 12%, respectively. When interpreting the GITSG trials of this combination, it is important to remember that all patients were entered in the GITSG studies after laparotomy, at which time the disease was deemed unresectable by the operating surgeon. The significant morbidity reported with palliative pancreatic surgery[295] suggests that only patients with a high performance status could have recovered rapidly enough to be eligible for these studies. Thus, although surgical staging provided a more uniform study population, it also introduced significant selection bias: Only rapidly recovering patients were considered for treatment. Comparison of future findings to these data must take into account this selection bias.

Because of the limited tolerance of normal tissue in the upper abdomen (liver, kidney, spinal cord, and bowel) to EBRT, total doses of only 45 to 54 Gy, in 25 to 30 fractions, have usually been given. For an unresectable lesion, this dose of radiation is inadequate, as demonstrated by the high rates of tumor progression and poor survival seen in both prospective and retrospective studies. For example, the Mayo Clinic reported a local failure rate of 72% for 122 patients with unresectable pancreatic cancer treated with an EBRT dose of 40 to 60 Gy.[299]

Because surgical resection of the primary tumor remains the only potentially curative treatment for pancreatic cancer, preoperative irradiation has been studied to assess its ability to convert locally unresectable pancreatic cancer to resectable disease (Table 33.4-9).[230,300–305] In a study from the New England Deaconess Hospital,[304] 16 patients with locally advanced unresectable pancreatic cancer were treated with 45 Gy of EBRT and infusional 5-FU to enhance resectability. Of these 16 patients, only two (13%) were able to undergo resection. Similarly, investigators from Duke University reported that only 2 (8%) of 25 patients with locally advanced pancreatic cancer treated with 45 Gy of EBRT and 5-FU (with or without cisplatin or mitomycin C) subsequently underwent

TABLE 33.4-9. Surgical Resection after Chemoradiation for Locally Advanced Pancreatic Cancer

Study	*Number of Patients*	*EBRT Dose (Gy)*	*Chemotherapy*	*Radiographic Response*	*Number of Surgically Resected*	*Median Survival (mo)*
White et al.[300] (1999)	25	45	5-FU + Mito (12) or CDDP (10)	6/22 had decrease >1 cm	5[a] (CR,[b] 1)	NA
Blackstock et al.[230] (1999)	17	50.4	Gem	PR, 3/15	0	Phase I study
Todd et al.[301] (1998)	38	0	5-FU + LV + Mito + dipyridamole	PR, 14; CR, 1	4 (CR,[b] 1)	15.5
Kamthan et al.[302] (1997)	35	54	5-FU + STZ + CDDP	PR, 9; CR, 6	5 (CR,[b] 2)	15
Safran et al.[303] (1997)	14	50	Paclitaxel	PR, 4/13	1	Phase I study
Jessup et al.[304] (1993)	16	45	5-FU	NA	2	9.6[c]
Jeekel and Treurniet-Donker[305] (1991)	20	50	5-FU	NA	2	10

5-FU, 5-fluorouracil; CDDP, cisplatin; CR, complete response; EBRT, external-beam radiation therapy; Gem, gemcitabine; LV, leucovorin; Mito, mitomycin C; NA, not available; PR, partial response; STZ, streptozocin.
[a]Three of five had positive margins of resection.
[b]Histologic CR.
[c]Mean.

complete resection with negative margins.[300] These and other studies (see Table 33.4-9) indicate that it is unlikely that neoadjuvant chemoradiation can convert unresectable lesions to resectable ones and thereby increase the number of patients potentially cured with combined-modality therapy. It is important to remember that as one loosens the definition of a locally advanced pancreatic cancer, results appear more optimistic. If, however, one maintains a strict (CT) definition of locally advanced pancreatic cancer that includes only arterial involvement (low-density tumor inseparable from the SMA or celiac axis on contrast-enhanced CT) or SMV or SMPV confluence occlusion, successful down-staging to allow complete surgical resection will be rare with currently available chemotherapy or chemoradiation techniques.

INTRAOPERATIVE ELECTRON-BEAM RADIATION THERAPY

To enhance the local-regional tumor control achieved by conventional EBRT and chemotherapy, specialized radiation therapy techniques that increase the dose of radiation to the desired tumor volume have been used in an attempt to improve local tumor control without increasing normal tissue morbidity. These include iodine 125 implants or intraoperative electrons as a boost dose in combination with EBRT and chemotherapy. A lower incidence of local failure in most series and improved median survival in some have been reported with these techniques when compared with conventional EBRT (Table 33.4-10),[299,306–309] but it is uncertain whether the differences are due to superior treatment or to case selection.

In the Massachusetts General Hospital[308] and Mayo Clinic studies[308] combining EBRT and IOERT for locally advanced pancreatic cancer, local tumor control was improved; however, the median survival was only approximately 12 months, and the 2-year survival rate remained approximately 20%. Most patients developed liver metastases, peritoneal seeding, or both. Although slight gains in survival may be achieved by improving local tumor control, the high incidence of distant metastases precludes significant improvements in long-term survival duration with IOERT.

NEW AGENTS COMBINED WITH RADIATION THERAPY

Because of the high incidence of hepatic and peritoneal metastases and the poor results with standard chemotherapy, current and future research efforts include evaluation of EBRT

TABLE 33.4-10. External-Beam and Intraoperative Radiation Therapy for Locally Advanced Unresectable Pancreatic Cancer

Study	*Number of Patients*	*Median Survival (mo)*	*2-Y Actuarial Local Failure Rate (%)*	*2-Y Actuarial Survival Rate (%)*
RTOG[306]	51	9	NA	9 (18 mo)
MGH[307,308]				
^{125}I + EBRT (40–45 Gy in 5 wk) ± Chemo	12	12	33	20
EBRT (45–50 Gy in 6 wk) ± Chemo/IOERT (15–25 Gy)	41	12	55	20
Mayo Clinic[299,309]				
EBRT (40–60 Gy in 6 wk) ± Chemo	122	12.6	80	16
Preoperative EBRT (50.4–54 Gy) ± Chemo/IOERT (20 Gy)	27	14.9	32	27
Postoperative EBRT (45–55 Gy in 6 wk) ± Chemo/IOERT (20 Gy)	56	10.5	35	6

Chemo, chemotherapy; EBRT, external-beam radiation therapy; IOERT, intraoperative electron-beam radiation therapy; MGH, Massachusetts General Hospital; NA, not available; RTOG, Radiation Therapy Oncology Group.

with new radiosensitizing agents (paclitaxel and gemcitabine). Interest in these agents is based on both their systemic cytotoxic effects and their radiosensitizing properties. In radiobiologic models, paclitaxel results in enhanced radiosensitization through tumor reoxygenation after apoptotic clearance of paclitaxel-damaged cells. In a phase I trial at Brown University[303] evaluating paclitaxel and 50 Gy of EBRT for patients with unresectable pancreatic and gastric cancers, the maximum tolerated dose of weekly paclitaxel with conventional irradiation was 50 mg/m^2. The response rate was 31% among 13 evaluable pancreatic cancer patients. In the Brown University phase II study,[310] which administered 50 Gy of EBRT with 50 mg/m^2/week of paclitaxel, 6 (33%) of 18 evaluable pancreatic cancer patients have had a partial response; stable disease has been observed in seven patients (39%); only one patient (6%) has had local tumor progression after completion of treatment; and four (22%) have developed distant metastases. These data have led to the initiation of an RTOG phase II study evaluating paclitaxel with EBRT for patients with unresectable pancreatic cancer.

Gemcitabine also has been the focus of an investigation in patients with advanced pancreatic cancer. Burris and colleagues[223] randomized 160 previously untreated patients with advanced and metastatic pancreatic cancer to receive either gemcitabine or 5-FU. Patients who received gemcitabine had a statistically improved median survival, 1-year survival rate, and clinical benefit compared to patients who received 5-FU. In radiobiologic models, gemcitabine also has been observed to be a potent radiosensitizer, likely because it depletes intracellular deoxynucleoside triphosphates. At present, numerous investigators are pursuing phase I and II studies combining EBRT with gemcitabine. Investigators from Wake Forest University and the University of North Carolina have reported the results of a phase I trial[230] of twice-weekly gemcitabine and 50.4 Gy of concurrent upper abdominal EBRT in 19 patients with unresectable pancreatic cancer. In this study, the maximum tolerated dose of gemcitabine was 40 mg/m^2. At this dose level, gemcitabine was well tolerated. Of eight patients with a minimum follow-up of 12 months, three remain alive, and one of the three has no evidence of disease progression. On the basis of these data, a phase II Cancer and Leukemia Group B study of EBRT and twice-weekly gemcitabine is currently accruing patients with locally advanced pancreatic cancer. At the Massachusetts General Hospital, Dana-Farber Cancer Institute, and Brigham and Women's Hospital, a phase I/II study (unpublished) is under way examining preoperative EBRT (50.4 Gy) to the pancreas with continuous-infusion 5-FU and weekly gemcitabine for locally advanced pancreatic cancer. If no evidence of distant metastases is found at the time of restaging after completion of chemoradiation, patients proceed to laparotomy and IOERT to the primary tumor.

RADIATION THERAPY TECHNIQUES

For patients undergoing surgery, clips should be placed to mark the extent of the lesion for postoperative EBRT. Used sparingly (e.g., a single small vascular clip placed in each location to mark superior, inferior, lateral, and medial margins), small clips produce only minimal interference on CT scans. Titanium clips produce less CT interference but sometimes cannot be located on lateral simulation x-ray films because of their lesser density. During simulation and treatment, the patient should be supine. An initial set of anteroposterior and cross-table lateral x-ray films is obtained after injection of renal contrast medium to identify operative clips and renal position relative to the field center. Additional films can be obtained with contrast medium in the stomach and duodenal loop.

Radiation therapy for locally advanced pancreatic cancer generally involves multiple-field, fractionated, external-beam techniques with high-energy photons to deliver 45 to 54 Gy in 1.8-Gy fractions to unresected or residual tumor (as defined by CT and clips) and to at-risk nodal areas. For lesions in the head of the pancreas, major at-risk lymph node groups include the pancreaticoduodenal, porta hepatis, celiac, and suprapancreatic nodes. The suprapancreatic lymph node group is included with the body of the pancreas in the radiation field to encompass a 3- to 5-cm margin beyond gross disease; however, more than two-thirds of the left kidney is excluded from the anteroposterior-posteroanterior field because at least 50% of the right kidney needs to be included in this field to treat the entire pancreatic head and duodenum. The entire duodenal loop with a margin of grossly uninvolved tissue is included because pancreatic head lesions may invade the medial wall of the duodenum and place the entire circumference at risk.

For pancreatic body or tail lesions, at least 50% of the left kidney may need to be included in the radiation field to achieve adequate margins and to include lymph node groups at risk (i.e., lateral suprapancreatic and splenic hilum nodes). Because inclusion of the entire duodenal loop is not indicated with body or tail lesions, at least two-thirds of the right kidney can be preserved; with tailored blocks, it is usually possible to do this and still cover the pancreaticoduodenal and porta hepatis nodes adequately.

For pancreatic head lesions, the superior field extent is at the middle or upper portion of the T11 vertebral body to achieve adequate margins along the celiac vessels (T12-L1). The superior field extent is occasionally more superior for pancreatic body lesions to obtain an adequate margin around the primary lesion.

For the lateral fields, the anterior field margin is 1.5 to 2.0 cm beyond gross disease. The posterior margin is at least 1.5 cm behind the anterior portion of the vertebral body to allow adequate margins around paraaortic nodes, which are at risk for posterior tumor extension of head or body lesions. The dose to the lateral fields is usually limited to 18 to 20 Gy because a moderate volume of kidney or liver may be in the fields.

After resection, anteroposterior-posteroanterior and lateral fields are designed on the basis of preresection CT tumor volumes, operative clip placement, and postoperative CT lymph node volumes. The only border that can be reduced is the anterior border of the lateral fields, because the primary tumor has been resected. This border is determined by vascular or nodal boundaries (porta hepatis, superior mesenteric, and celiac arteries) as demonstrated on CT.

Three-dimensional conformal therapy is currently being investigated in patients with pancreatic cancer. Figure 33.4-5 illustrates a multifield technique and composite isodose distribution for a patient with an unresectable pancreatic head cancer. Preliminary studies indicate that five or six conformal fields can be designed to improve dose-volume characteristics over those achieved with conventional four-field treatment designs, but the posterior wall of the stomach and the medial wall of the duodenum cannot be excluded from the high-dose volume.[311]

A

B

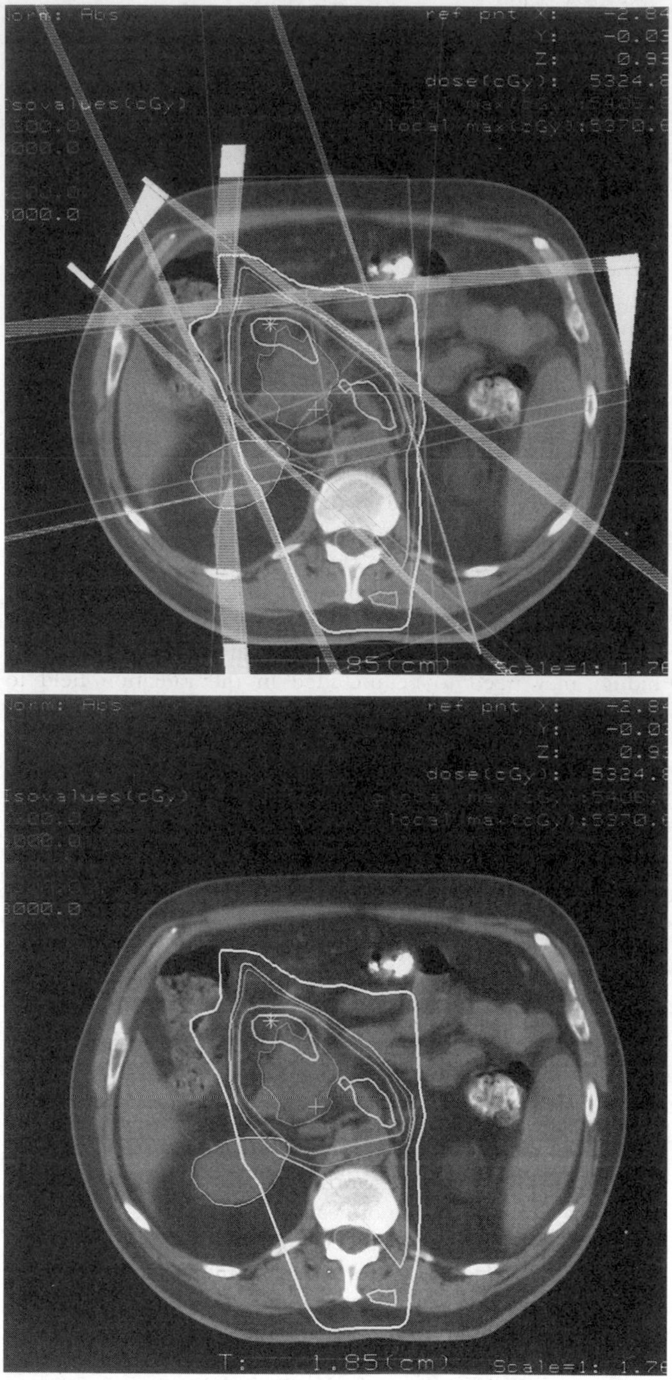

FIGURE 33.4-5. A multifield radiation technique **(A)** and composite isodose distributions **(B)** for a patient with an unresectable adenocarcinoma of the pancreatic head. (See Color Fig. 33.4-10 in the CD-ROM and on the Web at www.LWWoncology.com.)

TREATMENT DECISIONS: LOCALLY ADVANCED, NONMETASTATIC DISEASE

Patients with clear evidence of encasement of the celiac axis or SMA or occlusion of the SMPV confluence on contrast-enhanced helical CT do not require laparotomy to confirm that the tumor is unresectable; cytologic confirmation of malignancy can be achieved with EUS- or CT-guided FNA. This fundamental advance in the pretreatment diagnosis of pancreatic tumors can improve the quality of patient survival and reduce health care costs by avoiding the morbidity and prolonged recovery associated with palliative pancreatic cancer surgery. Published data have suggested an increased survival duration for patients treated with chemoradiation, but this benefit is limited largely to patients with higher performance status. In selected patients, aggressive treatment programs consisting of EBRT and chemotherapy may result in a median survival of approximately 12 months and a 2-year survival rate of 20%, although long-term survivors are rare. A program of chemoradiation is justified in fully ambulatory patients with locally advanced disease who have minimal symptoms. Systemic therapy with gemcitabine also represents a reasonable alternative in these patients. For patients with poor performance status, chemoradiation is probably not indicated. Current pharmacologic and interventional techniques for pain control, including percutaneous injection of alcohol into the celiac plexus, have proven highly successful in patients with pancreatic cancer.[312] Furthermore, adequate pain control improves performance status and quality of life, which may translate into increased length of life.[313] The limited therapeutic options available for patients with locally advanced disease and the modest impact of current treatments on survival rates provide the rationale for the entry of these patients into trials examining novel systemic agents.

TREATMENT OF METASTATIC AND RECURRENT DISEASE

The early emergence of metastatic disease in patients with exocrine pancreatic cancer suggests that systemic therapy (chemotherapy) should play a major role in the management of this disease. However, only marginal success has been achieved in identifying effective systemic therapies for pancreatic cancer. Most studies of single-agent or combination chemotherapy in patients with advanced adenocarcinoma of the pancreas have documented low response rates and little reproducible impact on patient survival or quality of life. Response rates as high as 15% to 30% occasionally seen in pilot studies of novel agents or combinations have generally been difficult to reproduce in larger trials, suggesting that patient selection often accounts for apparent differences between study results. The inherent difficulty in accurately applying bidimensional measurements to local pancreatic masses and the problem of interobserver variations in the measurement of metastatic disease may also contribute to the poor reproducibility of clinical trial findings in patients with locally advanced or metastatic pancreatic cancer.[314,315]

Because of the large volume of published material on this disease, we have chosen to present the results of important new studies and approaches to therapy; comprehensive reviews of the results of chemotherapy for pancreatic cancer are available,[316–320] and a previous edition of this text provides a comprehensive review of past chemotherapy trials.[321]

SINGLE-AGENT CHEMOTHERAPY

The thymidylate synthase inhibitor 5-FU remains the most extensively evaluated chemotherapeutic agent for pancreatic cancer. In 212 cases collected from the literature in the pre-CT era, the response rate to 5-FU was 28%.[322] However, despite numerous trials, the optimal dose and schedule of 5-FU have not been clearly defined. Two of the most commonly used schedules

TABLE 33.4-11. Single-Agent Chemotherapy Trials in Patients with Advanced Pancreatic Cancer

Study	*Agent*	*Objective Responses/ Total Patients (%)*	*Median Survival (mo)*
Hubbard et al.[328] (1992)	Iproplatin	3/32 (9)	NA
Carlson et al.[329] (1990)	Trimetrexate	0/14 (0)	3.3
Casper et al.[330] (1992)	Edatrexate	0/17 (0)	3.0
	Fazarabine	0/14 (0)	NA
Bukowski et al.[332] (1993)	Diaziquone	0/21 (0)	1.3
	Mitoguazone	2/32 (6)	7.6
Linke et al.[333] (1991)	Amonafide	0/14 (0)	2.8
Rougier et al.[334] (1994)	Docetaxel	5/29 (17)	NA
Okada et al.[335] (1999)	Docetaxel	0/21 (0)	3.9
Whitehead et al.[336] (1997)	Paclitaxel	3/39 (8)	5.0
O'Reilly et al.[337] (1996)	Topotecan	0/27 (0)	4.4
Scher et al.[338] (1996)	Topotecan	3/30 (10)	4.8
Wagener et al.[339] (1995)	Irinotecan	3/34 (9)	5.2
Casper et al.[222] (1994)	Gemcitabine	5/44 (11)	5.6

NA, not available.

are continuous infusion of 1000 $mg/m^2/d$ for 5 days or bolus infusion of 400 to 500 $mg/m^2/d$ for 5 days.[318,323,324] A highly potent and specific thymidylate synthase inhibitor, Tomudex, has been evaluated in patients with advanced pancreatic cancer. However, despite its potent inhibition of thymidylate synthase and other biochemical advantages over 5-FU, clinical trial results have been disappointing, with only 2 of 42 patients achieving an objective response.[325] Additional regimens based on protracted infusions of 5-FU continue to be explored but have not demonstrated any major effect on the outcome of the disease.[326,327] The new oral 5-FU prodrugs (capecitabine, uracil-tegafur, and S-1) have not yet been comprehensively tested in pancreatic cancer, but given the limited impact of intravenous 5-FU on this disease, expectations for these agents are low.

Most of the cytotoxic chemotherapeutic agents studied during the 1990s have demonstrated little objective evidence of significant activity against advanced pancreatic cancer (Table 33.4-11).[222,328–339] Inactive drugs that have undergone evaluation during this period include iproplatin,[328] trimetrexate,[329] edatrexate,[330] fazarabine,[331] diaziquone,[332] mitoguazone,[332] and amonafide.[333] Ifosfamide, evaluated in the 1980s, showed initial promise, with six partial responses in 29 patients with advanced disease.[340] A subsequent phase II trial that used ifosfamide as a continuous infusion with mesna yielded three partial responses, one complete response, and six minor responses in 25 evaluable patients.[341] However, a follow-up study did not confirm these favorable results.[342]

More recently, the semisynthetic taxanes paclitaxel and docetaxel have been studied in patients with locally advanced and metastatic pancreatic cancer. *In vitro*, docetaxel demonstrated significant activity against human pancreatic cancer cell lines.[343] In a subsequent clinical trial, Rougier and coworkers[334] at the Institut Gustave-Roussy reported five objective responses (29%) in 17 patients with hepatic metastases. However, toxic effects were substantial and included grade 3 or 4 neutropenia in all patients and severe edema in 13%. In three patients, the edema was so severe that therapy had to be discontinued. Three confirmatory phase II trials failed to confirm the initial response findings.[335,344,345] Similarly, paclitaxel, even when administered using an aggressive schedule with granulocyte colony-stimulating factor, had only minimal efficacy against advanced pancreatic cancer.[315]

Novel analogues of the topoisomerase I inhibitor camptothecin also have undergone evaluation in patients with advanced pancreatic cancer. Topotecan, administered once daily for 5 days or using a 21-day continuous infusion schedule, was ineffective.[337,338,346,347] Irinotecan (CPT-11) was evaluated in 34 patients by the EORTC Early Clinical Trials group.[339] Irinotecan was administered intravenously over 30 minutes at a dose of 350 mg/m^2 every 3 weeks; objective partial responses were documented in only three patients, with a median survival for the entire group of 5 months.

Gemcitabine is a deoxycytidine analogue with structural and metabolic similarities to cytarabine.[348] As a prodrug, gemcitabine must be phosphorylated to its active metabolites gemcitabine diphosphate and gemcitabine triphosphate (dFdCTP). In both preclinical and clinical testing, gemcitabine demonstrated activity in solid tumors greater than that of cytarabine.[349] These observations can be potentially explained by the following properties of gemcitabine: (1) It is three to four times more lipophilic than cytarabine, resulting in greater membrane permeability and cellular uptake; (2) it has higher affinity for deoxycytidine kinase; and (3) the intracellular retention of dFdCTP is long.[350] In the initial multicenter trial,[222] objective responses to gemcitabine were documented in only 5 (11%) of 44 patients with advanced pancreatic cancer, but the investigators noted frequent subjective symptomatic benefits, often in the absence of an objective tumor response. Based on these observations, two subsequent trials of gemcitabine in patients with advanced pancreatic cancer have been completed. In one randomized trial,[223] gemcitabine was compared to 5-FU in previously untreated patients. Patients treated with gemcitabine had a median survival of 5.65 months, compared to 4.41 months ($P = .0025$) in those treated with 5-FU. Twenty-four percent of patients treated with gemcitabine were alive at 9 months, compared to 6% of patients treated with 5-FU. In addition, more clinically meaningful effects on disease-related symptoms (pain control, performance status, weight gain) were seen with gemcit-

TABLE 33.4-12. Gemcitabine-Based Combination Chemotherapy Trials in Patients with Advanced Pancreatic Cancer

Study	*Agents*	*Objective Responses/Total Patients (%)*	*Median Survival (mo)*	*Clinical Benefit[a] (%)*
Cascinu et al.[361] (1999)	Gem/5-FU	2/54 (4)	7	51
Hidalgo et al.[362] (1999)	Gem/5-FU	5/26 (19)	7.4	38
Heinemann et al.[363] (1999)	Gem/cisplatin	4/41 (10)	8.3	NA
Colucci et al.[364] (1999)	Gem/cisplatin	10/32 (31)	NA	38
Scheithauer et al.[369] (1999)	Gem/epirubicin	14/66 (21)	7.8	43

5-FU, 5-fluorouracil; Gem, gemcitabine; NA, not available.
[a]Includes improvements in performance status and pain intensity, and weight gain.

abine (23.8% of patients) than with 5-FU (4.8% of patients). Similar systemic effects and demonstrable disease responses were documented in patients who were treated with gemcitabine after experiencing disease progression while receiving 5-FU.[351] These results have helped gemcitabine to become the accepted first-line therapy for patients with advanced pancreatic adenocarcinoma in the United States, although this approach is not necessarily shared worldwide.[352]

During the early phase II trials of weekly gemcitabine in chemotherapy-naive patients, it became clear that much higher doses could be safely administered (using 30-minute bolus infusions) than were tolerated in patients who had received multiple prior chemotherapies. However, previous cellular pharmacologic studies of this agent suggested that simply increasing the dose administered over 30 minutes may not increase cytotoxicity or improve gemcitabine's therapeutic index. During the early clinical experience in patients with solid tumors, dFdCTP levels were measured in peripheral blood mononuclear cells and showed that the rate of gemcitabine phosphorylation, like that of cytarabine, was subject to saturation kinetics.[221,353] The concentration of dFdCTP in the circulating mononuclear cells increased in proportion to the gemcitabine dose between 35 and 250 mg/m^2, but further increments in cellular dFdCTP were not observed at higher doses (350 to 1000 mg/m^2); instead, the plasma gemcitabine concentrations rose to more than 20 nmol/L, suggesting saturation of gemcitabine 5'-phosphate accumulation. The rate of dFdCTP accumulation and the peak cellular concentration were highest at a dose rate of 350 mg/m^2 per 30 minutes (approximately 10 mg/m^2/min), during which steady-state gemcitabine levels of 15 to 20 nmol/L were achieved in plasma.[353] Similar results were found in a pilot trial of gemcitabine in leukemia patients in which dFdCTP levels were measured in circulating malignant cells.[354] A more comprehensive phase I trial[355] in leukemia patients showed that a gemcitabine dose rate of 10 mg/m^2/min achieved a mean steady-state gemcitabine level of 26.5 nmol/L and was sufficient to maximize the rate of dFdCTP accumulation in circulating leukemic cells.

The most commonly applied approach to dose intensification in phase II studies of gemcitabine was to maintain the weekly schedule and increase the dose administered over 30 minutes.[356] However, because the plasma levels of gemcitabine achieved using this approach are well above 20 nmol/L, this strategy is not likely to increase intracellular levels of the active metabolite dFdCTP or improve efficacy. The pharmacodynamic relationships documented through the studies just described suggest that increasing the infusion time while holding the dose rate constant increases intracellular levels of the active metabolites gemcitabine diphosphate and dFdCTP and thus achieves the goal of dose intensification. To establish the feasibility of this approach, a phase I study[357,358] of gemcitabine was conducted in patients with advanced solid tumors whereby dose escalation was achieved by increasing the duration of the weekly gemcitabine infusions while maintaining the dose rate at 10 mg/m^2/min. A subsequent randomized phase II trial[232] in patients with metastatic pancreatic cancer suggested that short infusions (10 mg/m^2/min) of gemcitabine may be more effective than the standard 30-minute bolus technique.

Given gemcitabine's manageable toxicity profile and favorable intracellular pharmacology, gemcitabine-based combinations are also under active evaluation.[359,360] Early trials have combined gemcitabine with 5-FU,[361,362] cisplatin,[363,364] docetaxel,[365–367] paclitaxel,[368] epirubicin,[369] and marimastat[370] (Table 33.4-12).

Despite the encouraging results with gemcitabine and gemcitabine-based combinations, the median survival for patients with metastatic disease continues to be less than 6 months, with very few patients achieving long-term disease stabilization. Although two trials have supported the superiority of chemotherapy over supportive care,[371,372] some of the effects attributed to chemotherapy may not be substantially different from what can be achieved with aggressive supportive care alone. The study of novel chemotherapeutic agents based on the evolving understanding of the pathobiology of pancreatic cancer must continue.

MODULATION OF 5-FLUOROURACIL

Interest remains in the possibility of increasing the activity and therapeutic index of 5-FU by the use of biochemical modulators. N-(Phosphonoacetyl)-L-aspartate disodium (PALA) depletes uridine nucleotide pools by inhibiting aspartate transcarbamoylase, favoring incorporation of 5-FU nucleotide metabolites into RNA and thereby potentiating the antitumor activity of 5-FU. Administering methotrexate before PALA and 5-FU results in increased formation of fluorouridine monophosphate. A study by Morrell et al.[373] using a weekly schedule of PALA at a dose of 250 mg/m^2 followed 24 hours later by a 24-hour continuous infusion of 5-FU (2600 mg/m^2) in patients with advanced pancreatic cancer was associated with severe toxicity, including one death, and only one response. A similar study demonstrated less toxicity but also no benefit from the use of PALA plus 5-FU compared with 5-FU alone.[374] The addition of methotrexate or 6-methylmercaptopurine riboside also provided no benefit over 5-FU alone.[375,376]

Regimens that rely on the modulation of 5-FU and prolong inhibition of thymidylate synthase have demonstrated efficacy against colon cancer but have shown little activity against pancreatic cancer. Prospective clinical trials in patients with advanced pancreatic cancer have evaluated high-dose leucovorin (500 mg/m^2), administered daily or as a continuous infusion for 6 days, in combination with 5-FU.[377,378] The daily dose of 5-FU ranged from 375 mg/m^2 to 600 mg/m^2. Objective response rates averaged less than 10%, and toxicity was often significant. The substitution of 5-methyltetrahydrofolate for leucovorin also failed to demonstrate clinically meaningful biochemical modulation of 5-FU.[379] Thus, despite some evidence to the contrary,[371,380] the current consensus is that the addition of leucovorin to 5-FU provides no therapeutic advantage over single-agent 5-FU in advanced pancreatic cancer.

Another potential modulator of 5-FU is interferon-α, with or without leucovorin.[381–384] Scheithauer et al.[385] combined 5-FU (20 mg/kg on day 3) with interferon-α (10×10^6 U/d for 3 days) and leucovorin (200 mg on day 3). The observed response rate (4 of 32) and median duration of survival (5.5 months) were no different than with 5-FU alone. Gattani et al.[386] used three potential biomodulators—cisplatin, leucovorin, and methotrexate—in an effort to enhance the cytotoxicity of 5-FU. Six responses were seen in 24 patients with advanced pancreatic cancer, but mucositis occurred in more than one-half of the study population. Thus, the results from clinical trials to date have not demonstrated any reproducible benefit of 5-FU modulation in patients with pancreatic cancer.

HORMONAL THERAPY

Johnson and Corbishley[387] were the first to note that pancreatic tumors contain sex steroid hormone receptors, stimulating interest in a hormonal approach to the management of pancreatic cancer. This interest continues as investigators refine their understanding of the hormonally controlled signal transduction pathways that control cellular proliferation.[388–390] Early research in this area demonstrated that serum testosterone concentrations were lower in both men and women with pancreatic cancer than in patients with other cancers or healthy controls.[391–393] Laboratory evidence that exocrine pancreatic cancers are sensitive to gastrointestinal hormones, sex steroids, and growth factors led to the use of hormonal manipulation in patients with pancreatic cancer.[394–397] Cyproterone acetate, an antiandrogen, inhibited the growth of human pancreatic xenografts in nude mice,[398] and a luteinizing hormone–releasing hormone (LHRH) analogue, D-trp-6-LHRH, induced regression of nitrosamine-induced pancreatic cancers in hamsters.[399] When this analogue was combined with RC-160, an experimental somatostatin analogue, the same growth inhibition was observed.[400] Another somatostatin analogue, SMS-201-995, also demonstrated *in vivo* inhibition of human adenocarcinoma cell lines.[401] These laboratory observations stimulated clinical trials evaluating LHRH agonists, growth factor inhibitors (octreotide),[402–404] tamoxifen, and more recently, flutamide[405,406] in patients with advanced pancreatic cancer. Consistent with the cytostatic effect of hormonal therapy, objective responses were not seen; median survival duration ranged from 3 to 8 months.[405,407–418] The potential cytostatic effects of tamoxifen continue to be studied in the laboratory.[419]

Several uncontrolled clinical studies have suggested improved survival in patients with pancreatic cancer treated with tamoxifen,[407,408,420,421] yet other studies have not confirm this observation.[414–416] A case-control study involving 80 patients did suggest a survival advantage for patients treated with tamoxifen.[409] However, in a prospective, randomized, double-blind trial, pancreatic cancer patients receiving tamoxifen had a median survival of 115 days compared to 122 days for the placebo-treated patients; 8% of patients were alive at 1 year in both groups.[415] A small trial reported by Crowson et al.[410] using CT to evaluate tumor response also demonstrated no benefit with tamoxifen. Studies with octreotide,[417] steroids, and LHRH agonists,[411,422] as well as combinations of these agents,[403,412,413] have not shown an increase in survival for patients with pancreatic cancer. Likewise, a pilot study of MK329, a cholecystokinin antagonist, in 18 patients with pancreatic cancer demonstrated no antitumor activity.[423] Nevertheless, despite the lack of a clear effect of currently available hormonal therapies on exocrine pancreatic carcinoma, research in this area continues.

COMBINATION CHEMOTHERAPY

In general, combination chemotherapy has not been a successful approach to the management of pancreatic cancer. However, the results of prior studies of combination chemotherapy are presented here for historical purposes.

5-Fluorouracil, Doxorubicin (Adriamycin), and Mitomycin C Regimen

The combination of 5-FU, doxorubicin (Adriamycin), and mitomycin C (FAM) for metastatic pancreatic adenocarcinoma was first described by Smith et al.[424] in 1980, based on previous work demonstrating a 13% partial response rate with doxorubicin in previously untreated patients.[425] Twenty-seven of 39 patients had measurable disease; ten (37%) of these achieved a partial response.[424] These ten patients had a median survival of 12 months, compared with 3.5 months in nonresponders. Bitran et al.[426] reported similar results. An earlier report of streptozocin, mitomycin C, and 5-FU (SMF) for advanced pancreatic cancer suggested a response rate of 43%, although many patients experienced severe gastrointestinal and renal toxicity.[427] Therefore, several cooperative groups compared FAM and SMF. The Cancer and Leukemia Group B studied 184 patients and found response rates of 14% for FAM and 4% for SMF (not significantly different), both of which were much lower than suggested by previous reports.[428] Comparison of FAM to two schedules of SMF,[429] to 5-FU alone, and to 5-FU and doxorubicin[430] confirmed these low response rates. More recently, FAM was combined with aminoglutethimide without benefit.[431] Despite these negative trials, a randomized study of a modified FAM regimen compared to no treatment demonstrated an improved median survival for FAM-treated patients.[432] However, this was a small study involving only 44 patients, and the pancreatic cancer was pathologically confirmed in only 31. Based on the results to date, the use of FAM chemotherapy in the management of advanced pancreatic cancer cannot be recommended.

Mallinson Regimen

In 1980, Mallinson et al.[433] first reported on a regimen of induction therapy with 5-FU, cyclophosphamide, methotrexate, and vincristine followed by maintenance treatment with 5-

FU and mitomycin C for advanced pancreatic cancer. A median survival of 44 weeks was reported for patients who received therapy, compared with 9 weeks for patients offered only supportive care. However, a phase III trial comparing the Mallinson regimen to 5-FU alone and to 5-FU, doxorubicin, and cisplatin was unable to confirm these results; the median survival was only 4.5 months in patients who received the Mallinson regimen.[434]

Cisplatin-Containing Regimens

After a trial that showed significant activity of cisplatin administered at a dose of 100 mg/m^2 every 4 weeks,[435] cisplatin was combined with continuous-infusion 5-FU. However, poor results have been seen with low-dose schedules,[436] and toxic effects have been seen in a high percentage of patients.[437] Somewhat better results have been observed with higher doses of cisplatin (100 mg/m^2) combined with 5-FU (1000 mg/m^2/d) administered by continuous infusion. In a study of 40 pancreatic cancer patients,[438] 13 of whom were previously treated and 36 of whom had metastatic disease, one complete and nine partial remissions (response rate, 26.5%) were documented; the median survival rate was 7 months. This high-dose regimen was associated with one treatment-related death and the occurrence of grade 4 granulocytopenia in 27% of patients. The most recent report of cisplatin and 5-FU comes from Japan.[439] These investigators used a lower dose of both agents (5-FU, 500 mg/m^2/d; cisplatin, 80 mg/m^2) based on phase I studies in their country. In 37 previously untreated patients with pancreatic adenocarcinoma, the response rate was only 8%.

Other Combinations

A combination regimen of 5-FU, leucovorin, mitomycin C, and dipyridamole produced 12 responses in 16 patients with locally advanced pancreatic cancer.[440] Five of these were objective complete responses documented by CT and tumor marker measurements. At the time of this report, median survival had not yet been reached but was projected to be greater than 1 year. Five patients had received EBRT, but this was not believed to have affected overall survival. In a subsequent report from the same group, this regimen achieved an overall response rate of 39% in patients with locally advanced pancreatic cancer, with six patients achieving sufficient improvement in their tumor status on CT scans to justify surgical exploration.[301]

Based on laboratory data suggesting synergy of this drug combination, Dougherty et al.[441] reported on a phase I/II study of cisplatin, high-dose cytarabine, and caffeine (CAC) in 28 patients with advanced pancreatic cancer. A partial response was documented in 7 of 18 evaluable patients. This finding prompted a phase III study by Kelsen et al.[442] comparing CAC to SMF. Eighty-two patients were randomized, and 90% were evaluable; objective responses were seen in two patients who received CAC and four patients who received SMF.

The question of the benefit gained by multiagent chemotherapy compared with single-agent therapy also has been examined. The Southwest Oncology Group performed a series of phase II trials comparing single-agent chemotherapy with combination chemotherapy (5-FU, doxorubicin, mitomycin C, and streptozocin).[332] The single agents studied included mitoguazone, dihydroxyanthracenedione, and diaziquone. Eighty-two patients received single-agent therapy, and 71 received combination chemotherapy; the median survival durations were 3.4 and 4.8 months, respectively, indicating no significant benefit from combination chemotherapy.

In sum, these results confirm the ineffectiveness of conventional combination chemotherapy and support clinical studies evaluating novel single agents in previously untreated patients with advanced pancreatic cancer.

REGIONAL CHEMOTHERAPY

The high incidence of liver metastases and local tumor recurrence in the pancreatic bed has prompted investigation of regional chemotherapy. Regional approaches to chemotherapy for pancreatic cancer have included infusion of the SMA or celiac axis,[443,444] combined intraarterial and SMV infusion,[445,446] and isolated perfusion with extracorporeal chemofiltration.[447,448] One report includes a phase II study from the Puget Sound Oncology Consortium of combined intraarterial cisplatin, intravenous infusional 5-FU, and EBRT in 16 patients with locally advanced pancreatic adenocarcinoma.[443] No treatment-related deaths occurred, five patients achieved a minor response, and the median survival was 9 months. The authors thus concluded that this regimen was not superior to more standard chemoradiation regimens.

Maurer et al.[444] treated 12 patients with locally advanced, recurrent, or metastatic pancreatic cancer with intraarterial chemotherapy (mitoxantrone, folinic acid, 5-FU, and cisplatin). Only one patient achieved a partial response, and the median survival was 6 months. However, an improvement in tumor-related pain was achieved in 9 of 11 evaluable patients.

Researchers at Tulane University combined intraarterial chemotherapy (mitomycin C, 5-FU, and mitoxantrone) with hemofiltration.[449] They reported two complete responses and ten partial responses in 32 patients with advanced pancreatic cancer. Although these results demonstrate the feasibility of the regional chemotherapy approach to pancreatic cancer, future pilot studies aimed at achieving local control of disease in the pancreas or at decreasing the growth or development of liver metastases will require more sophisticated therapeutic agents to achieve meaningful anticancer effects.

Regional chemotherapy infusion may be more applicable to patients who have undergone pancreaticoduodenectomy and in whom liver metastases are the dominant site of disease recurrence. Ishikawa and colleagues[445] treated 21 patients with continuous-infusion 5-FU (125 mg/d) delivered through the hepatic artery and portal vein for the first 4 to 5 weeks after pancreaticoduodenectomy. No chemotherapy-related complications were reported; one patient died of surgery-related complications. Survival in the 20 evaluable patients was superior to that of historical controls, and liver metastases were the cause of death in only 8% of patients at 3 years of follow-up. Updated results from Ishikawa et al.[446] with 27 patients who received postoperative adjuvant intraarterial and portal venous 5-FU demonstrated a 5-year survival rate of 39%; this high survival rate was thought to be secondary to a marked decrease in hepatic metastases. Reported experiences from both Lygidakis and Stringaris[450] (intraarterial immunochemotherapy) and Beger et al.[451] (intraarterial chemotherapy) support the potential benefit of adjuvant intraarterial therapy after pancreaticoduodenectomy. These results come from highly talented and very experienced physicians; similar results will be difficult to produce outside of specialty centers because of the complexity of treatment delivery. However, the concept of postoperative, adjuvant, liver-directed regional therapy will likely receive greater attention because of improved local tumor control with contemporary forms of chemoradiation and surgery.

NEW APPROACHES TO SYSTEMIC DISEASE

Despite advances in the understanding of the molecular biology of pancreatic cancer, the systemic treatment of metastatic disease remains unsatisfactory. Chemotherapy and the administration of biologically active molecules, such as tumor necrosis factor[452,453] or interferons,[381,453] have not resulted in significant improvements in response rates or patient survival. The study of novel chemotherapeutic agents based on the evolving understanding of the molecular biology of pancreatic cancer must receive the highest priority.

A number of general areas of clinical investigation may yield favorable results. These include interruption or modulation of known growth factors and signal transduction pathways involved with cell growth, invasion, and angiogenesis. Some of the systemic agents undergoing clinical investigation are described in this section, with an emphasis on therapies that are intended to inhibit specific signals required for cell growth and metastasis.

Farnesyl Transferase Inhibition

Because the *ras* oncogene is mutated and thereby constitutively activated in the majority of pancreatic cancers, inhibition of *ras* signaling has been postulated as a possible target for therapy. A particularly attractive approach under active development is the inhibition of ras protein function through interruption of essential posttranslational processing (farnesylation) necessary to localize ras proteins to the cytoplasmic side of the plasma membrane. This effort involved the discovery and synthesis of specific small molecules that inhibit the protein farnesyl transferase.[454–456] The functional consequence of this inhibitory effect is that the ras oncoprotein cannot localize to the cell membrane and is rendered inactive. A number of these small molecules are under investigation and include drugs that are administered orally and intravenously. Phase I and II trials of these agents are under way.[457]

Other approaches are also under investigation. The monoterpene limonene and its more potent metabolite perillyl alcohol decrease farnesylated ras levels, probably through a different mechanism than lovastatin (which acts via hepatic hydroxymethylglutaryl coenzyme A reductase inhibition, thereby lowering plasma levels of farnesyl pyrophosphate).[458] Orally administered perillyl alcohol demonstrated significant *in vivo* activity against pancreatic cancer in a Syrian golden hamster model.[459] A phase I clinical trial of orally administered perillyl alcohol has been reported.[460] Perillyl alcohol also holds promise as a potential chemopreventive agent for pancreatic cancer.[461]

Somatostatin Analogues

Overexpression of the somatostatin receptor occurs in both ductal adenocarcinomas and neuroendocrine tumors. Physiologically, somatostatin is an antitrophic hormone that inhibits the trophic effects of cholecystokinin and other factors. Binding the somatostatin receptor with the octapeptide somatostatin analogue octreotide has been demonstrated to inhibit cell growth *in vitro*. Initial animal studies were encouraging, but early clinical trials have proved disappointing.[462–464] Two large multicenter phase III clinical trials have been conducted comparing a long-acting octreotide analogue with a placebo in the treatment of advanced pancreatic cancer. In one trial,[417] patients received either a placebo or a long-acting octreotide analogue (SMS-201-995 pa LAR; octreotide pamoate LAR) alone. No objective responses were observed, and the median survival times for patients receiving the octreotide analogue or the placebo were equivalent (16 weeks). In the other trial,[418] all patients received 5-FU infusions with either an octreotide analogue (SMS-201-995 pa LAR) or a placebo. The addition of the octreotide analogue to 5-FU provided no advantage in terms of objective response or survival.

A novel variation of this approach used an octapeptide analogue of somatostatin containing methotrexate attached to the α-amino group of D-phenylalanine in position 1 of the octapeptide. Subsequent experiments with this agent against the MIA PaCa-2 human pancreatic cancer cell line in nude mice demonstrated significant inhibition of tumor growth.[465] Further preclinical trials investigating the efficacy of such an approach continue.

Another strategy being explored is binding somatostatin analogues, such as octreotide, with radioisotopes, specifically yttrium 90, to selectively deliver therapeutic doses of radiation.[466]

Receptor Tyrosine Kinase Inhibition

TRASTUZUMAB (HERCEPTIN). Binding the HER2/neu oncoprotein with specific antibodies leads to growth-inhibitory signaling and promotes apoptosis. Trastuzumab (Herceptin) is a humanized monoclonal antibody developed in mice that specifically binds the HER-2 receptor. Preclinical studies have shown that Herceptin leads to growth inhibition in cell lines that overexpress *HER2/neu*. Clinical trials in patients with metastatic breast cancer whose tumors overexpress *HER2/neu* have demonstrated that Herceptin has activity as a single agent, with objective response rates of 11% to 26%.[467,468] Preclinical studies also have suggested synergy between Herceptin and cytotoxic agents.[469] In a clinical trial,[470] response rates and survival were both improved in women receiving Herceptin and chemotherapy compared to chemotherapy alone for metastatic breast cancer (all patients had tumors that overexpressed *HER2/neu*.) Side effects were generally mild, but it should be noted that, when Herceptin was delivered in combination with an anthracycline, class III or IV heart failure (by New York Heart Association criteria) was observed in 19% of patients, compared to only 3% of patients receiving anthracycline-based chemotherapy without herceptin.[470]

In pancreatic cancer, 30% to 40% of human tumors overexpress *HER2/neu*; however, the role of Herceptin has not yet been defined. A phase II trial is now under way to assess the combination of Herceptin and gemcitabine in patients with advanced pancreatic cancer.

EPIDERMAL GROWTH FACTOR RECEPTOR MONOCLONAL ANTIBODY (C225). Antibodies to the epidermal growth factor receptor have been shown to compete with the growth stimulatory ligands for binding to this receptor. Binding with specific antibodies leads to growth inhibition and in some cases to apoptosis. A humanized monoclonal antibody to epidermal growth factor receptor (C225) has demonstrated potent competitive binding to the receptor, leading to growth inhibition. *In vitro* studies suggest an additive effect of C225 with cytotoxic agents.[471] Data from laboratories at the M. D. Anderson Cancer Center suggest a synergistic interaction in animal models of metastasis when gemcitabine and C225 are combined.[472] The exact mechanisms of this synergy are being investigated, including effects on growth inhibition, apoptotic cell death, and angiogenesis. Clinical trials are under way with C225 in head and neck cancer patients; a clinical trial studying the toxicity and efficacy of gemcitabine combined with C225 is planned for patients with advanced pancreatic cancer.

Matrix Metalloproteinase Inhibitors

Matrix metalloproteinase inhibitors (MMPIs) occur as both endogenous factors that tightly regulate the activity of proteases in the extracellular milieu and as exogenous synthetic molecules. The two primary endogenous inhibitors are tissue metalloproteinase inhibitors 1 and 2. Both are fairly large proteins (28 kD and 21 kD, respectively) and unlikely to be clinically relevant because of their poor pharmacologic properties.[473]

A number of synthetic MMPIs have been developed, including batimastat, marimastat, and BAY 12-9566. Marimastat is an orally bioavailable agent that has been studied clinically in patients with advanced prostate cancer, colorectal cancer, ovarian cancer, and pancreatic cancer. Interestingly, the dose-limiting toxicity is often musculoskeletal pain with arthralgias and myalgias.[474] BAY 12-9566 is another orally bioavailable MMPI. Both marimastat and BAY 12-9566 are under investigation in multicenter phase III trials. In one randomized trial, marimastat is being compared with gemcitabine as a treatment for advanced pancreatic cancer; the results from this trial will be available soon. Marimastat is also being investigated in a randomized, double-blind, placebo-controlled trial designed to evaluate whether this agent can delay or prevent the onset of metastatic disease after pancreaticoduodenectomy in patients undergoing surgery with curative intent. In yet another clinical trial, patients with advanced pancreatic cancer are being randomized to receive gemcitabine with marimastat or gemcitabine alone; the primary end point of this trial is survival (data unpublished).

Antiangiogenic Agents

Tumor vascularity is an important requirement for tumor growth beyond a few millimeters, and it is now accepted that specific endogenous angiogenic factors exist that allow for endothelial cell growth and migration into tumor nodules. One such factor is VEGF, which is up-regulated in pancreatic cancer. Strategies have been developed to inhibit the effects of VEGF, including monoclonal antibodies to VEGF. In addition, a specific inhibitor to the receptor tyrosine kinase for VEGF has been discovered (SU5416).[475] Phase I and early phase II clinical trials of SU5416 are currently under way.

Another antiangiogenic agent being studied is TNP-470, an analogue of fumagillin. Fumagillin is derived from the fungus *Aspergillus fumigatus fresenius* and was found to inhibit angiogenesis in an *in vitro* angiogenesis model. Pharmacokinetic studies of TNP-470 have demonstrated that it has a half-life of only 1 hour, suggesting that prolonged or frequent infusions of the agent may be required for activity.[476] Nevertheless, as a single agent, TNP-470 produced a complete response in one patient with metastatic cervical cancer, with other study subjects achieving disease stabilization.[477]

Two other antiangiogenic molecules that have been isolated from tumor-bearing animals are angiostatin, which is a peptide fragment of plasminogen, and endostatin, a fragment from collagenase XVIII.[478] Both angiostatin and endostatin have shown significant antitumor activity in animal models, and angiostatin has induced tumor dormancy in mice.[479,480] Endostatin entered clinical trials in the latter part of 1999.

Gene Therapy

Given the large number of somatic mutations in pancreatic cancer, gene therapy represents a potentially powerful approach to this disease. Generally, gene therapy for pancreatic cancer includes approaches designed to replace the function of inactivated tumor suppressor genes such as *p53*, *p16*, and *SMAD4/DPC4*. Correcting loss of functional cellular changes is more challenging than inhibiting overexpressed proteins or a mutated oncogene. However, *in vitro* reintroduction of genetic information into cells has been shown to be an effective way to alter cellular growth, induce apoptosis, and sensitize pancreatic cancer cells to chemotherapy and radiation.[481–483] Other approaches use genetic strategies to inhibit dominant oncogene function. The high frequency with which K-*ras* is altered in exocrine pancreatic cancer and its central function in signal transduction suggest that inhibiting production of the K-ras protein could lead to significant growth-inhibitory effects. This strategy has been used successfully in lung adenocarcinoma cells using retroviral constructs coding for K-ras antisense RNA.[484] In addition, evolving ribozyme technologies offer the possibility of improved inhibition compared with traditional antisense approaches.[485] A particularly interesting gene-therapy approach uses an oncolytic adenovirus that is genetically modified to replicate only in *p53*-deficient cells.[486] Direct injection of this oncolytic virus has been shown to be feasible.[487] The challenge in gene therapy for pancreatic cancer will be to develop delivery strategies that are capable of targeting both the local and metastatic components of this neoplasm.

TREATMENT DECISIONS: METASTATIC DISEASE

The complex pathophysiologic abnormalities accompanying metastatic pancreatic cancer often make specific treatment decisions extremely difficult. Many patients present to the medical oncologist or surgeon with profound debilitation, severe pain, and extensive metastatic disease. For these patients, chemotherapy is unlikely to result in significant improvements in quality of life or survival, and the toxic effects of chemotherapy may create additional complications. Management with supportive care or nontoxic hormonal approaches may be the optimal strategies for these patients.

For patients with metastatic pancreatic cancer who present with a good performance status, systemic chemotherapy is appropriate. In view of the limited impact of the currently available agents on survival, continued enrollment of patients in phase II trials of new agents or combinations is essential. In the absence of access to a phase II trial, treatment with gemcitabine appears to be the standard in the United States. However, it must be recognized that the primary impact of gemcitabine is on quality of life; therefore, continued evaluation of novel agents, especially those targeted against specific molecular events important in the pathogenesis of pancreatic cancer, is crucial. With the expansion of our understanding of the molecular and biochemical basis of pancreatic cancer, we are entering an era in which treatments may be tailored to interact with specific molecular and biochemical targets thought to be important in the development or maintenance of neoplasia.

REFERENCES

1. Greenlee RT, Murray T, Bolden S, et al. Cancer statistics, 2000. *CA Cancer J Clin* 2000;50:12.
2. Fernandez E, La Vecchia C, Porta M, et al. Trends in pancreatic cancer mortality in Europe, 1955–1989. *Int J Cancer* 1994;57:786.
3. Williamson RCN. Pancreatic cancer: the greatest oncological challenge. *BMJ* 1991;296:445.
4. Gold EB, Goldin SB. Epidemiology of and risk factors for pancreatic cancer. *Surg Oncol Clin North Am* 1998;7:67.
5. Hirayama T. Epidemiology of pancreatic cancer in Japan. *Jpn J Clin Oncol* 1989;19:208.
6. Oomi K, Amano M. The epidemiology of pancreatic diseases in Japan. *Pancreas* 1998;16:233.
7. American Cancer Society. *Cancer facts and figures—1995.* Atlanta: American Cancer Society, 1990.
8. Tominaga S, Kuroishi T. Epidemiology of pancreatic cancer. *Semin Surg Oncol* 1998;15:3.
9. Silverman DT, Dunn JA, Hoover RN, et al. Cigarette smoking and pancreas cancer: a case-control study based on direct interviews. *J Natl Cancer Inst* 1994;86:1510.
10. La Vecchia C, Boyle P, Franceschi S, et al. Smoking and cancer with emphasis on Europe. *Eur J Cancer* 1991;27:94.
11. Zheng W, McLaughlin JK, Gridley G, et al. A cohort study of smoking, alcohol consumption, and dietary factors for pancreatic cancer (United States). *Cancer Causes Control* 1993;4:477.
12. Hecht SS. Environmental tobacco smoke and lung cancer: the emerging role of carcinogen biomarkers and molecular epidemiology. *J Natl Cancer Inst* 1994;86:1369.
13. Wang M, Abbruzzese JL, Friess H, et al. DNA adducts in human pancreatic tissues and their potential role in carcinogenesis. *Cancer Res* 1998;58:38.
14. Perera FP, Tang D, Grinberg-Funes RA, et al. Molecular epidemiology of lung cancer and the modulation of markers of chronic carcinogen exposure by chemopreventive agents. *J Cell Biochem Suppl* 1993;17F:119.
15. MacMahon B, Yen S, Trichopoulos D, et al. Coffee and cancer of the pancreas. *N Engl J Med* 1981;304:630.
16. Lin RS, Kessler IL. A multifactorial model for pancreatic cancer in man. *JAMA* 1981;245:147.
17. Olsen GW, Mandel JS, Gibson RW, et al. A case-control study of pancreatic cancer and cigarettes, alcohol, coffee, and diet. *Am J Public Health* 1989;79:1016.
18. Hakulinen T, Lehtimaki L, Lehtonen M, et al. Cancer morbidity among two male cohorts with increased alcohol consumption in Finland. *J Natl Cancer Inst* 1974;52:1711.
19. Friedman GD, van den Eeden SK. Risk factors for pancreatic cancer: an exploratory study. *Int J Epidemiol* 1993;22:30.
20. Feinstein AR, Horwitz RI, Stitzer WO, et al. Coffee and pancreatic cancer. The problems of etiologic science and epidemiologic research. *JAMA* 1981;246:957.
21. Gordis L. Consumption of methylxanthine-containing beverages and risk of pancreatic cancer. *Cancer Lett* 1990;52:1.
22. Shibata A, Mack TM, Paganini-Hill A, et al. A prospective study of pancreatic cancer in the elderly. *Int J Cancer* 1994;58:46.
23. Velema JP, Walker AM, Gold EB. Alcohol and pancreatic cancer. Insufficient epidemiologic evidence for a causal relationship. *Epidemiol Rev* 1986;8:28.
24. Gullo L. Diabetes and the risk of pancreatic cancer. *Ann Oncol* 1999;10[Suppl 4]:79.
25. Mack TM, Yu MC, Hanisch R, et al. Pancreas cancer and smoking, beverage consumption, and past medical history. *J Natl Cancer Inst* 1986;76:49.
26. Gullo L, Pezzilli R, Morselli-Labate AM. Diabetes and the risk of pancreatic cancer. *N Engl J Med* 1994;331:81.
27. La Vecchia C, Negri E, Franceschi S, et al. A case-control study of diabetes mellitus and cancer risk. *Br J Cancer* 1994;70:950.
28. Permert J, Larsson J, Westermark GT, et al. Islet amyloid polypeptide in patients with pancreatic cancer and diabetes. *N Engl J Med* 1994;330:313.
29. Kalapothaki V, Tzonou A, Hsieh CC, et al. Tobacco, ethanol, coffee, pancreatitis, diabetes mellitus, and cholelithiasis as risk factors for pancreatic carcinoma. *Cancer Causes Control* 1993;4:375.
30. Chow WH, Gridley G, Nyrén O, et al. Risk of pancreatic cancer following diabetes mellitus: a nationwide cohort study in Sweden. *J Natl Cancer Inst* 1995;87:930.
31. Wideroff L, Gridley G, Mellemkjaer L, et al. Cancer incidence in a population-based cohort of patients hospitalized with diabetes mellitus in Denmark. *J Natl Cancer Inst* 1997;89:1360.
32. Silverman DT, Schiffman M, Everhart J, et al. Diabetes mellitus, other medical conditions and familial history of cancer as risk factors for pancreatic cancer. *Br J Cancer* 1999;80:1830.
33. Permert J, Ihse I, Jorfeldt L, et al. Improved glucose metabolism after subtotal pancreatectomy for pancreatic cancer. *Br J Surg* 1993;80:1047.
34. Fogar P, Basso D, Pasquali C, et al. Portal but not peripheral serum levels of interleukin 6 could interfere with glucose metabolism in patients with pancreatic cancer. *Clin Chim Acta* 1998;277:181.
35. Valerio A, Basso D, Brigato L, et al. Glucose metabolic alterations in isolated and perfused rat hepatocytes induced by pancreatic cancer conditioned medium: a low molecular weight factor possibly involved. *Biochem Biophys Res Commun* 1999;257:622.
36. Everhart J, Wright D. Diabetes mellitus as a risk factor for pancreatic cancer. A meta-analysis. *JAMA* 1995;273:1605.
37. Fisher WE, Boros LG, O'Dorisio TM, et al. GI hormonal changes in diabetes influence pancreatic cancer growth. *J Surg Res* 1995;58:754.
38. Talamini G, Bassi C, Falconi M, et al. Alcohol and smoking as risk factors in chronic pancreatitis and pancreatic cancer. *Dig Dis Sci* 1999;44:1303.
39. Lowenfels AB, Maisonneuve P, Cavallini G, et al. Pancreatitis and the risk of pancreatic cancer. *N Engl J Med* 1993;328:1433.
40. Ekbom A, McLaughlin JK, Karlsson BM, et al. Pancreatitis and pancreatic cancer: a population-based study. *J Natl Cancer Inst* 1994;86:625.
41. Bansal P, Sonnenberg A. Pancreatitis is a risk factor for pancreatic cancer. *Gastroenterology* 1995;109:247.
42. Lowenfels AB, Maisonneuve P, Lankisch PG. Chronic pancreatitis and other risk factors for pancreatic cancer. *Gastroenterol Clin North Am* 1999;28:673.
43. Gold EB, Cameron JL. Chronic pancreatitis and pancreatic cancer [Editorial]. *N Engl J Med* 1993;328:1485.
44. Gates LK Jr, Ulrich CD II, Whitcomb DC. Hereditary pancreatitis. Gene defects and their implications. *Surg Clin North Am* 1999;79:711.
45. Kozuka S, Sassa R, Taki T, et al. Relation of pancreatic duct hyperplasia to carcinoma. *Cancer* 1979;43:1418.
46. Yanagisawa A, Ohtake K, Ohashi K, et al. Frequent c-Ki-ras oncogene activation in mucous cell hyperplasias of pancreas suffering from chronic inflammation. *Cancer Res* 1993;53:953.
47. Fernandez E, La Vecchia C, Porta M, et al. Pancreatitis and the risk of pancreatic cancer. *Pancreas* 1995;11:185.
48. Hruban RH, Petersen GM, Goggins M, et al. Familial pancreatic cancer. *Ann Oncol* 1999;10[Suppl 4]:69.
49. Kern SE. Advances from genetic clues in pancreatic cancer. *Curr Opin Oncol* 1998;10:74.
50. Lynch HT, Smyrk T, Kern SE, et al. Familial pancreatic cancer: a review. *Semin Oncol* 1996;23:251.
51. Marx S, Spiegel A, Allen M, et al. Multiple endocrine neoplasia type 1: clinical and genetic topics. *Ann Intern Med* 1998;129:484.
52. Bordi C, Brandi ML. Ductal adenocarcinoma of the pancreas in Men-1 patients. *Virchows Arch* 1998:432;385.
53. Finch MD, Howes N, Ellis I, et al. Hereditary pancreatitis and familial pancreatic cancer. *Digestion* 1997;58:564.
54. Lynch HT, Voorhees GJ, Lanspa SJ, et al. Pancreatic carcinoma and hereditary nonpolyposis colorectal cancer: a family study. *Br J Cancer* 1985;52:271.
55. Neumann HP, Dinkel E, Brambs H, et al. Pancreatic lesions in the von Hippel-Lindau syndrome. *Gastroenterology* 1991;101:465.
56. Swift M, Sholman L, Perry M, et al. Malignant neoplasms in the families of patients with ataxia telangiectasia. *Cancer Res* 1976;36:209.
57. Lynch HT, Fusaro RM. Pancreatic cancer and the familial atypical multiple mole (FAMMM) syndrome. *Pancreas* 1991;6:127.
58. Goldstein AM, Fraser MC, Struewing JP, et al. Increased risk of pancreatic cancer in melanoma-prone kindreds with p16INK4 mutations. *N Engl J Med* 1995;333:970.
59. Whelan AJ, Bartsch D, Goodfellow PJ. Brief report: a familial syndrome of pancreatic cancer and melanoma with a mutation in the CDKN2 tumor-suppressor gene. *N Engl J Med* 1995;333:975.
60. Ghadirian P, Boyle P, Simard A, et al. Reported family aggregation of pancreatic cancer within a population-based case-control study in the Francophone community in Montreal, Canada. *Int J Pancreatol* 1991;10:183.
61. Lynch HT, Fitzsimmons ML, Smyrk TC, et al. Familial pancreatic cancer: clinicopathologic study of 18 nuclear families. *Am J Gastroenterol* 1990;85:54.
62. Friedman JM, Fialkow PJ. Familial carcinoma of the pancreas. *Clin Genet* 1976;9:463.
63. Goggins M, Schutte M, Lu J, et al. Germline BRCA2 gene mutations in patients with apparently sporadic pancreatic carcinomas. *Cancer Res* 1996;56:5360.
64. Su GH, Hruban RH, Bansal RK, et al. Germline and somatic mutations of the STK11/LKB1 Peutz-Jeghers gene in pancreatic and biliary cancers. *Am J Pathol* 1999;154:1835.
65. Moskaluk CA, Hruban RH, Schutte M, et al. Genomic sequencing of DPC4 in the analysis of familial pancreatic carcinoma. *Diagn Mol Pathol* 1997;6:85.
66. Lynch HT. Genetics and pancreatic cancer. *Arch Surg* 1994;129:266.
67. Steinberg WM, Barkin J, Bradley EL III, et al. Workup of a patient with familial pancreatic cancer. *Pancreas* 1999;18:219.
68. Brentnall TA, Bronner MP, Byrd DR, et al. Early diagnosis and treatment of pancreatic dysplasia in patients with a family history of pancreatic cancer. *Ann Intern Med* 1999;131:247.
69. Ji BT, Chow WH, Hsing AW, et al. Green tea consumption and the risk of pancreatic and colorectal cancers. *Int J Cancer* 1997;70:255.
70. Levin B. An overview of preventive strategies for pancreatic cancer. *Ann Oncol* 1999;10[Suppl 4]:193.
71. Cubilla AL, Fitzgerald PJ. *Tumors of the exocrine pancreas.* Washington, DC: Armed Forces Institute of Pathology, 1984.
72. Cubilla AL, Fitzgerald PJ. Morphological lesions associated with human primary invasive nonendocrine pancreas cancer. *Cancer Res* 1976;36:2690.
73. Furukawa T, Chiba R, Kobari M, et al. Varying grades of epithelial atypia in the pancreatic ducts of humans. Classification based on morphometry and multivariate analysis and correlated with positive reactions of carcinoembryonic antigen. *Arch Pathol Lab Med* 1994;118:227.
74. Brat DJ, Lillemoe KD, Yeo CJ, et al. Progression of pancreatic intraductal neoplasias to infiltrating adenocarcinoma of the pancreas. *Am J Surg Pathol* 1998;22:163.
75. Almoguera C, Shibata D, Forrester K, et al. Most human carcinomas of the exocrine pancreas contain mutant c-K-ras genes. *Cell* 1988;53:549.

76. Smit VT, Boot AJ, Smits AM, et al. KRAS codon 12 mutations occur very frequently in pancreatic adenocarcinomas. *Nucleic Acids Res* 1988;16:7773.
77. Pellegata NS, Losekoot M, Foddie R, et al. Detection of K-ras mutations by denaturing gradient gel electrophoresis (DGGE): a study on pancreatic cancer. *Anticancer Res* 1992;12:1731.
78. Boschman CR, Stryker S, Reddy JK, et al. Expression of p53 protein in precursor lesions and adenocarcinoma of human pancreas. *Am J Pathol* 1994;145:1291.
79. DiGuseppe JA, Hruban RH, Goodman SN, et al. Overexpression of p53 protein in adenocarcinoma of the pancreas. *Am J Clin Pathol* 1994;101:684.
80. Moskaluk CA, Hruban RH, Kern SE. p16 and K-ras gene mutations in the intraductal precursors of human pancreatic adenocarcinoma. *Cancer Res* 1997;57:2140.
81. Uehara H, Nakaizumi A, Tatsuta M, et al. Diagnosis of pancreatic cancer by detecting telomerase activity in pancreatic juice: comparison with K-ras mutations. *Am J Gastroenterol* 1999;94:2513.
82. Suehara N, Mizumoto K, Muta T, et al. Telomerase elevation in pancreatic ductal carcinoma compared to nonmalignant pathological states. *Clin Cancer Res* 1997;3:993.
83. Motojima K, Tsunoda T, Kanematsu T, et al. Distinguishing pancreatic carcinoma from other periampullary carcinomas by analysis of mutations in the Kirsten-ras oncogene. *Ann Surg* 1991;214:657.
84. Bos JL. Ras oncogenes in human cancer: a review. *Cancer Res* 1989;49:4682.
85. Pellegata NS, Sessa F, Renault B, et al. K-ras and p53 gene mutations in pancreatic cancer: ductal and nonductal tumors progress through different genetic lesions. *Cancer Res* 1994;54:1556.
86. Rak J, Mitsuhashi Y, Bayko L. Mutant ras oncogenes upregulate VEGF/VPF expression: implications for induction and inhibition of tumor angiogenesis. *Cancer Res* 1995;55:4575.
87. Brown LF, Berse B, Jackman RW, et al. Expression of vascular permeability factor (vascular endothelial growth factor) and its receptors in adenocarcinomas of the gastrointestinal tract. *Cancer Res* 1993;53:4727.
88. Egawa S, Tsutsumi M, Konishi Y, et al. The role of angiogenesis in the tumor growth of Syrian hamster pancreatic cancer cell line HPD-NR. *Gastroenterology* 1995;108:1526.
89. Bours V, Dejardin E, Goujon-Letawe F, Merville M, Castronovo V. The NF-κB transcription factor and cancer: high expression of NF-κB- and IκB-related proteins in tumor cell lines. *Biochem Pharmacol* 1994;47:145.
90. Grilli M, Chiu JJS, Lenardo MJ. NF-κB and Rel: participants in a multiform transcriptional regulatory system. *Int Rev Cytol* 1993;143:1.
91. Wang W, Abbruzzese JL, Evans DB, et al. The nuclear factor-κB RelA transcription factor is constitutively activated in human pancreatic adenocarcinoma cells. *Clin Cancer Res* 1999;5:119.
92. Wang W, Abbruzzese JL, Evans DB, Chiao PJ. Overexpression of urokinase-type plasminogen activator in pancreatic adenocarcinoma is regulated by constitutively activated RelA. *Oncogene* 1999;18:4554.
93. Shi Q, Abbruzzese JL, Huang S, et al. Constitutive and inducible interleukin 8 expression by hypoxia and acidosis renders human pancreatic cancer cells more tumorigenic and metastatic. *Clin Cancer Res* 1999;5:3711.
94. Shi Q, Le X, Abbruzzese JL, et al. Cooperation between transcription factor AP-1 and NF-κB in the induction of interleukin-8 in human pancreatic adenocarcinoma cells by hypoxia. *J Interferon Cytokine Res* 1999;19:1363.
95. Bouvet M, Ellis LM, Nishizaki M, et al. Adenovirus-mediated wild-type p53 gene transfer down-regulates vascular endothelial growth factor expression and inhibits angiogenesis in human colon cancer. *Cancer Res* 1998;58:2288.
96. Harada H, Nakagawa K, Iwata S, et al. Restoration of wild-type p16 down-regulates vascular endothelial growth factor expression and inhibits angiogenesis in human gliomas. *Cancer Res* 1999;59:3783.
97. Brower V. Tumor angiogenesis—new drugs on the block. *Nat Biotechnol* 1999;17:963.
98. Pluda JM. Tumor-associated angiogenesis: mechanisms, clinical implications, and therapeutic strategies. *Semin Oncol* 1997;24:203.
99. Hahn SA, Seymour AB, Hoque ATM, et al. Allelotype of pancreatic adenocarcinoma using xenograft enrichment. *Cancer Res* 1995;55:4670.
100. Schutte M, Da Costa LT, Hahn SA, et al. Identification by representational difference analysis of a homozygous deletion in pancreatic carcinoma that lies within the BRCA2 region. *Proc Natl Acad Sci U S A* 1995;92:5950.
101. Caldas C, Hahn SA, da Costa LT, et al. Frequent somatic mutations and homozygous deletions of the p16 (MTS1) gene in pancreatic adenocarcinoma. *Nat Genet* 1994;8:27.
102. Hahn SA, Hoque ATM, Moskaluk CA, et al. Homozygous deletion map at 18q21.1 in pancreatic cancer. *Cancer Res* 1996;56:490.
103. Hahn SA, Schutte M, Hoque ATM, et al. DPC4, a candidate tumor suppressor gene at human chromosome 18q21.1. *Science* 1996;271:350.
104. Lagna G, Hata A, Hemmati Brivanlou A, et al. Partnership between DPC4 and SMAD proteins in TGF-beta signalling pathways. *Nature* 1996;383:832.
105. Derynck R, Zhang Y, Feng XH. Smads: transcriptional activators of TGF-beta responses. *Cell* 1998;95:737.
106. Grau AM, Zhang L, Wang W, et al. Induction of $p21^{waf1}$ expression and growth inhibition by transforming growth factor-β is mediated by the tumor suppressor gene DPC-4 in human pancreatic adenocarcinoma cells. *Cancer Res* 1997;57:3929.
107. Hunt KK, Fleming JB, Abramian A, et al. Overexpression of the tumor suppressor gene Smad4/DPC4 induces p21waf1 expression and growth inhibition in human carcinoma cells. *Cancer Res* 1998;58:5656.
108. Hruban RH, Petersen GM, Ha PK, et al. Genetics of pancreatic cancer. *Surg Clin North Am* 1998;7:1.
109. Bartsch D, Shevlin DW, Tung WS, et al. Frequent mutations of CDKN2 in primary pancreatic adenocarcinomas. *Genes Chromosomes Cancer* 1995;14:189.
110. Naumann M, Savitskaia N, Eilert C, et al. Frequent codeletion of p16/MTS1 and p15/MTS2 and genetic alterations in p16/MTS1 in pancreatic tumors. *Gastroenterology* 1996;110:1215.
111. Merlo A, Herman JG, Mao L, et al. 5' CpG island methylation is associated with transcriptional silencing of the tumour suppressor p16/CDKN2/MTS1 in human cancers. *Nat Med* 1995;1:686.
112. Schenk M, Severson RK, Pawlish KS. The risk of subsequent primary carcinoma of the pancreas in patients with cutaneous malignant melanoma. *Cancer* 1998;82:1672.
113. Redston MS, Caldas C, Seymour AB, et al. p53 mutations in pancreatic carcinoma and evidence of common involvement of homocopolymer tracts in DNA microdeletions. *Cancer Res* 1994;54:3025.
114. Bold RJ, Hess KR, Pearson AS, et al. Prognostic factors in resectable pancreatic cancer: p53 and Bcl-2. *J Gastrointest Surg* 1999;3:263.
115. Schutte M, Hruban RH, Geradts J, et al. Abrogation of the Rb/p16 tumor-suppressive pathway in virtually all pancreatic carcinomas. *Cancer Res* 1997;57:3126.
116. Moskaluk CA, Hruban RH, Kern SE. p16 and K-ras mutations in the intraductal precursors of human pancreatic adenocarcinoma. *Cancer Res* 1997;57:2140.
117. Bakkevold KE, Arnesjø B, Kambestad B. Carcinoma of the pancreas and papilla of Vater: presenting symptoms, signs, and diagnosis related to stage and tumour site. *Scand J Gastroenterol* 1992;27:317.
118. Permert J, Ihse I, Jorfeldt L, et al. Pancreatic cancer is associated with impaired glucose metabolism. *Eur J Surg* 1993;159:101.
119. Permert J, Larsson J, Fruin AB, et al. Islet hormone secretion in pancreatic cancer patients with diabetes. *Pancreas* 1997;15:60.
120. Pour PM. The role of Langerhans islets in exocrine pancreatic cancer. *Int J Pancreatol* 1995;17:217.
121. Basso D, Plebani M, Fogar J, et al. β-Cell function in pancreatic adenocarcinoma. *Pancreas* 1994;3:332.
122. Bell RH, Stayer DS. Streptozotocin prevents development of nitrosamine-induced pancreatic cancer in the Syrian hamster. *J Surg Oncol* 1983;24:258.
123. Bell RH, Pour PM. Induction of pancreatic tumors in genetically non-diabetic but not in diabetic Chinese hamsters. *Cancer Lett* 1987;34:221.
124. Evans DB, Pisters PWT, Lee JE, et al. Preoperative chemoradiation strategies for localized adenocarcinoma of the pancreas. *J Hepatobiliary Pancreat Surg* 1998;5:242.
125. Allema JH, Reinders ME, vanGulik TM, et al. Prognostic factors for survival after pancreaticoduodenectomy for patients with carcinoma of the pancreatic head region. *Cancer* 1995;75:2069.
126. Bakkevold KE, Kambestad B. Long-term survival following radical and palliative treatment of patients with carcinoma of the pancreas and papilla of Vater—the prognostic factors influencing the long-term results: a prospective multicentre study. *Eur J Surg Oncol* 1993;19:147.
127. Cameron JL, Crist DW, Sitzmann JV, et al. Factors influencing survival after pancreaticoduodenectomy for pancreatic cancer. *Am J Surg* 1991;161:120.
128. Geer RJ, Brennan MF. Prognostic indicators for survival after resection of pancreatic adenocarcinoma. *Am J Surg* 1993;165:68.
129. Nitecki SS, Sarr MG, Colby TV, vanHeerden JA. Long-term survival after resection for ductal adenocarcinoma of the pancreas. Is it really improving? *Ann Surg* 1995;221:59.
130. Roder JD, Stein HJ, Hüttl W, Siewert JR. Pylorus-preserving versus standard pancreaticoduodenectomy: an analysis of 110 pancreatic and periampullary carcinomas. *Br J Surg* 1992;79:152.
131. Trede M, Chir B, Schwall G, Saeger H. Survival after pancreaticoduodenectomy: 118 consecutive resections without an operative mortality. *Ann Surg* 1990;211:447.
132. Tsao JI, Rossi RL, Lowell JA. Pylorus-preserving pancreaticoduodenectomy. *Arch Surg* 1994;129:405.
133. Whittington R, Bryer MP, Haller DG, Solin LJ, Rosato EF. Adjuvant therapy of resected adenocarcinoma of the pancreas. *Int J Radiat Oncol Biol Phys* 1991;21:1137.
134. Willett CG, Lewandrowski K, Warshaw AL, et al. Resection margins in carcinoma of the head of the pancreas: implications for radiation therapy. *Ann Surg* 1993;217:144.
135. Yeo CJ, Cameron JL, Lillemore KD, et al. Pancreaticoduodenectomy for cancer of the head of the pancreas: 201 patients. *Ann Surg* 1995;221:721.
136. Zerbi A, Fossati V, Parolini D, et al. Intraoperative radiation therapy adjuvant to resection in the treatment of pancreatic cancer. *Cancer* 1994;73:2930.
137. Bossett JF, Pavy JJ, Gillet M, et al. Conventional external irradiation alone as adjuvant treatment in resectable pancreatic cancer: results of a prospective study. *Radiother Oncol* 1992;24:191.
138. Yeo CJ, Cameron JL, Sohn TA, et al. Six hundred fifty consecutive pancreaticoduodenectomies in the 1990s. *Ann Surg* 1997;226:248.
139. Spitz FR, Abbruzzese JL, Lee JE, et al. Preoperative and postoperative chemoradiation strategies in patients treated with pancreaticoduodenectomy for adenocarcinoma of the pancreas. *J Clin Oncol* 1997;15:928.
140. Foo ML, Gunderson LL, Nagorney DM, et al. Patterns of failure in grossly resected pancreatic ductal adenocarcinoma treated with adjuvant irradiation ± 5-fluorouracil. *Int J Radiat Oncol Biol Phys* 1993;26:483.
141. Gastrointestinal Tumor Study Group. Further evidence of effective adjuvant combined radiation and chemotherapy following curative resection of pancreatic cancer. *Cancer* 1987;59:2006.
142. Griffin JF, Smalley SR, Jewell W. Patterns of failure after curative resection of pancreatic carcinoma. *Cancer* 1990;66:56.
143. Johnstone PA, Sindelar WF. Patterns of disease recurrence following definitive therapy of adenocarcinoma of the pancreas using surgery and adjuvant radiotherapy: correlations of a clinical trial. *Int J Radiat Oncol Biol Phys* 1993;27:831.
144. Ozaki H. Improvement of pancreatic cancer treatment from the Japanese experience in the 1980s. *Int J Pancreatol* 1992;12:5.
145. Splinter TAW, Obertop H, Kok TC, et al. Adjuvant chemotherapy after resection of adenocarcinoma of the periampullary region and the head of the pancreas. *J Cancer Res Clin Oncol* 1989;115:200.

146. Tepper J, Nardi G, Suit H. Carcinoma of the pancreas: review of MGH experience from 1963–1973. *Cancer* 1976;37:1519.
147. Westerdahl J, Andrén-Sandeberg Å, Ihse I. Recurrence of exocrine pancreatic cancer—local or hepatic? *Hepatogastroenterology* 1993;40:384.
148. Staley CA, Lee JE, Cleary KA, et al. Preoperative chemoradiation, pancreaticoduodenectomy, and intraoperative radiation therapy for adenocarcinoma of the pancreatic head. *Am J Surg* 1996;171:118.
149. Pisters PWT, Abbruzzese JL, Janjan NA, et al. Rapid-fractionation preoperative chemoradiation, pancreaticoduodenectomy, and intraoperative radiation therapy for resectable pancreatic adenocarcinoma. *J Clin Oncol* 1998;16:3843.
150. Gastrointestinal Tumor Study Group. A multi-institutional comparative trial of radiation therapy alone and in combination with 5-fluorouracil for locally unresectable pancreatic carcinoma. *Ann Surg* 1979;189:205.
151. Moertel CG, Childs DS, Reitemeier RJ, et al. Combined 5-fluorouracil and supervoltage radiation therapy of locally unresectable gastrointestinal cancer. *Lancet* 1969;2:865.
152. Mohiuddin M, Cantor RJ, Biermann W, et al. Combined modality treatment of localized unresectable adenocarcinoma of the pancreas. *Int J Radiat Oncol Biol Phys* 1988;14:79.
153. Whittington R, Neuberg D, Tester WJ, et al. Protracted intravenous fluorouracil infusion with radiation therapy in the management of localized pancreaticobiliary carcinoma: a phase I Eastern Cooperative Oncology Group trial. *J Clin Oncol* 1995;13:227.
154. Treurniet-Donker AD, Van Mierlo MJM, Van Putten WLJ. Localized unresectable pancreatic cancer. *Int J Radiat Oncol Biol Phys* 1990;18:592.
155. Exocrine pancreas. In: Fleming ID, Cooper JS, Henson DE, et al., eds. *American Joint Committee on Cancer manual for staging of cancer*, 5th ed. Philadelphia: Lippincott–Raven, 1997:122.
156. Staley CA, Cleary KR, Abbruzzese JL, et al. Need for standardized pathologic staging of pancreaticoduodenectomy specimens. *Pancreas* 1996;12:373.
157. Fuhrman GM, Charnsangavej C, Abbruzzese JL, et al. Thin-section contrast enhanced computed tomography accurately predicts resectability of malignant pancreatic neoplasms. *Am J Surg* 1994;167:104.
158. Evans DB, Rich TA, Byrd DR, et al. Preoperative chemoradiation and pancreaticoduodenectomy for adenocarcinoma of the pancreas. *Arch Surg* 1992;127:1335.
159. Cubilla AL, Fortner J, Fitzgerald PJ. Lymph node involvement in carcinoma of the head of the pancreas area. *Cancer* 1978;41:880.
160. International Pancreatic Cancer Study Group. Staging for carcinoma of the pancreas: Japanese stage classification compared to UICC stage classification. In: Pour PM, Konishi Y, Klöppel G, Longnecker DS, eds. *Atlas of exocrine pancreatic tumors.* Hong Kong: Springer-Verlag Tokyo, 1994:247.
161. Lillemoe KD, Sauter PK, Pitt HA, et al. Current status of surgical palliation of periampullary carcinoma. *Surg Gynecol Obstet* 1993;176:1.
162. Kelsen DP, Portenoy R, Thaler H, Tao Y, Brennan M. Pain as a predictor of outcome in patients with operable pancreatic carcinoma. *Surgery* 1997;122:53.
163. de Rooij PD, Rogatko A, Brennan MF. Evaluation of palliative surgical procedures in unresectable pancreatic cancer. *Br J Surg* 1991;78:1053.
164. DiFronzo LA, Egrari S, O'Connell TX. Choledochoduodenostomy for palliation in unresectable pancreatic cancer. *Arch Surg* 1998;133:820.
165. Millikan KW, Deziel DJ, Silverstein JC, et al. Prognostic factors associated with resectable adenocarcinoma of the head of the pancreas. *Am Surg* 1999;65:618.
166. Nishimura Y, Hosotani R, Shibamoto Y, et al. External and intraoperative radiotherapy for resectable and unresectable pancreatic cancer: analysis of survival rates and complications. *Int J Radiat Oncol Biol Phys* 1997;39:39.
167. Yeo CJ, Abrams RA, Grochow LB, et al. Pancreaticoduodenectomy for pancreatic adenocarcinoma: postoperative adjuvant chemoradiation improves survival. *Ann Surg* 1997;225:621.
168. Sperti C, Pasquali C, Piccoli A, Pedrazzoli S. Survival after resection for ductal adenocarcinoma of the pancreas. *Br J Surg* 1996;83:625.
169. McGrath PC, Sloan DA, Kenady DE. Surgical management of pancreatic carcinoma. *Semin Oncol* 1996;23:200.
170. Robinson EK, Lee JE, Lowy AM, et al. Reoperative pancreaticoduodenectomy for periampullary carcinoma. *Am J Surg* 1996;172:432.
171. Andersen JR, Soren SM, Kruse A, et al. Randomized trial of endoscopic endoprosthesis versus operative bypass in malignant obstructive jaundice. *Gut* 1989;30:1132.
172. Shepherd HA, Royle G, Ross AP, et al. Endoscopic biliary endoprosthesis in the palliation of malignant obstruction of the distal common bile duct: a randomized trial. *Br J Surg* 1988;75:1166.
173. Smith AC, Dowsett JF, Hatfield ARW, et al. Prospective randomised trial of bypass surgery versus endoscopic stenting in patients with malignant obstructive jaundice. *Gut* 1989;30:A1513.
174. Raikar GV, Melin MM, Ress A, et al. Cost-effective analysis of surgical palliation versus endoscopic stenting in the management of unresectable pancreatic cancer. *Ann Surg Oncol* 1996;3:470.
175. Freeny PC, Traverso LW, Ryan JA. Diagnosis and staging of pancreatic adenocarcinoma with dynamic computed tomography. *Am J Surg* 1993;165:600.
176. Yeung RS, Weese JL, Hoffman JP, et al. Neoadjuvant chemoradiation in pancreatic and duodenal carcinoma. *Cancer* 1993;72:2124.
177. Warshaw AL, Gu Z, Wittenberg J, et al. Preoperative staging and assessment of resectability of pancreatic cancer. *Arch Surg* 1990;125:230.
178. Baron PL, Aabakken LE, Cole DJ, et al. Differentiation of benign from malignant pancreatic masses by endoscopic ultrasound. *Ann Surg Oncol* 1997;4:639.
179. Faigel DO, Ginsberg GG, Bentz JS, et al. Endoscopic ultrasound-guided real-time fine-needle aspiration biopsy of the pancreas in cancer patients with pancreatic lesions. *J Clin Oncol* 1997;15:1439.
180. Suits J, Frazee R, Erickson RA. Endoscopic ultrasound and fine needle aspiration for the valuation of pancreatic masses. *Arch Surg* 1999;134:639.
181. Tyler DS, Evans DB. Reoperative pancreaticoduodenectomy. *Ann Surg* 1994;2:211.
182. Smith CD, Behrns E, vanHeerden JA, Sarr MG. Radical pancreaticoduodenectomy for misdiagnosed pancreatic mass. *Br J Surg* 1994;81:585.
183. vanHeerden JA. Invited commentary. *Arch Surg* 1994;129:642.
184. Warshaw AL. Implications of peritoneal cytology for staging of early pancreatic cancer. *Am J Surg* 1991;161:26.
185. Temudom T, Sarr MG, Douglas MG, Farnell MB. An argument against routine percutaneous biopsy, ERCP, or biliary stent placement in patients with clinically resectable periampullary masses: a surgical perspective. *Pancreas* 1995;11:283.
186. Cusheri A. Laparoscopy for pancreatic cancer: does it benefit the patient? *Eur J Surg Oncol* 1988;14:41.
187. Warshaw AL, Tepper JE, Shipley WU. Laparoscopy in the staging and planning of therapy for pancreatic cancer. *Am J Surg* 1985;151:76.
188. Conlon KC, Dougherty E, Klimstra DS, et al. The value of minimal access surgery in the staging of patients with potentially resectable peripancreatic malignancy. *Ann Surg* 1996;223:134.
189. Fernandez-delCastillo C, Rattner DW, Warshaw AL. Further experience with laparoscopy and peritoneal cytology in the staging of pancreatic cancer. *Br J Surg* 1995;82:1127.
190. Bemelman WA, de Wit LT, van Delden OM, et al. Diagnostic laparoscopy combined with laparoscopic ultrasonography in staging of cancer of the pancreatic head region. *Br J Surg* 1995;82:820.
191. Gloor B, Todd KE, Reber HA. Diagnostic workup of patients with suspected pancreatic carcinoma: the University of California–Los Angeles approach. *Cancer* 1997;79:1780.
192. Rumstadt B, Schwab M, Schuster K, Hagmiller E, Trede M. The role of laparoscopy in the preoperative staging of pancreatic carcinoma. *J Gastrointest Surg* 1997;1:245.
193. Holzman MD, Reintgen KL, Tyler DS, Pappas TN. The role of laparoscopy in the management of suspected pancreatic and periampullary malignancies. *J Gastrointest Surg* 1997;1:236.
194. Friess H, Kleeff J, Silva JC, et al. The role of diagnostic laparoscopy in pancreatic and periampullary malignancies. *J Am Coll Surg* 1998;186:675.
195. Evans DB, Lee JE, Leach SD, et al. Vascular resection and intraoperative radiation therapy during pancreaticoduodenectomy: rationale and technique. *Adv Surg* 1995;29:235.
196. Fernandez-delCastillo C, Warshaw AL. Laparoscopy for staging in pancreatic carcinoma. *Surg Oncol* 1993;2:25.
197. Fernandez-delCastillo C, Warshaw A. Peritoneal metastases in pancreatic carcinoma. *Hepatogastroenterology* 1993;40:430.
198. Dalton RR, Sarr MG, van Heerden JA, et al. Carcinoma of the body and tail of the pancreas: is curative resection justified? *Surgery* 1992;111:489.
199. Johnson CD, Schwall G, Flechtenmacher J, Trede M. Resection for adenocarcinoma of the body and tail of the pancreas. *Br J Surg* 1993;80:1177.
200. Wade TP, Virgo KS, Johnson FE. Distal pancreatectomy for cancer: results in US Department of Veterans Affairs Hospitals, 1987–1991. *Pancreas* 1995;11:341.
201. Moertel CG, Frytak S, Hahn RG, et al. Therapy of locally unresectable pancreatic carcinoma: a randomized comparison of high dose (6000 rads) radiation alone, moderate dose radiation (4000 rads + 5-fluorouracil), and high dose radiation + 5-fluorouracil. The Gastrointestinal Tumor Study Group. *Cancer* 1981;48:1705.
202. Kalser MH, Ellenberg SS. Pancreatic cancer: adjuvant combined radiation and chemotherapy following curative resection. *Arch Surg* 1985;120:899.
203. Jeekel J. Adjuvant or neoadjuvant therapy for pancreatic carcinoma? *Digestion* 1997;58:533.
204. Klinkenbijl JH, Jeekel J, Sahmoud T, et al. Adjuvant radiotherapy and 5-fluorouracil after curative resection for the cancer of the pancreas and peri-ampullary region. Phase III trial of the EORTC Gastrointestinal Tract Cancer Cooperative Group. *Ann Surg* 1999;230:776.
205. van Eijck CHJ, Link KH, van Rossen MEE, Jeekel J. (Neo)adjuvant treatment in pancreatic cancer—the need for future trials. *Eur J Surg* 1999;25:132.
206. Neoptolemos JP, Baker P, Berger H, et al. A randomized multicenter European study vs no-adjuvant treatment in resectable pancreatic cancer (ESPAC-1). *Int J Pancreatol* 1997;21:97.
207. Neoptolemos JP, Kerr DJ, Beger H, et al. ESPAC-1 trial progress report: the European randomized adjuvant study comparing radiochemotherapy, 6 months chemotherapy and combination therapy versus observation in pancreatic cancer. *Digestion* 1997;58:570.
208. Regine WF, John WJ, Mohiuddin M. Evolving trends in combined modality therapy for pancreatic cancer. *J Hepatobiliary Pancreat Surg* 1998;5:227.
209. Davis BJ, Raben A, Casper E, Minsky BD. Acute toxicity and efficacy of postoperative combined modality therapy for adenocarcinoma of the pancreas. Proceedings of the 38th Annual ASTRO Meeting 1996:2039.
210. Demeure MJ, Doffek KM, Komorowski RA, et al. Molecular metastases in stage I pancreatic cancer: improved survival with adjuvant chemoradiation. *Surgery* 1998;124:663.
211. Abrams RA, Grochow LB, Chakravarthy A, et al. Intensified adjuvant therapy for pancreatic and periampullary adenocarcinoma: survival results and observations regarding patterns of failure, radiotherapy dose and CA19-9 levels. *Int J Radiat Oncol Biol Phys* 1999;44:1039.
212. Hoffman JP, Weese JL, Solin LJ, et al. A pilot study of preoperative chemoradiation for patients with localized adenocarcinoma of the pancreas. *Am J Surg* 1995;169:71.
213. Hoffman JP, Lipsitz S, Pisansky T, et al. Phase II trial of preoperative radiation therapy and chemotherapy for patients with localized, resectable adenocarcinoma of the pancreas: an Eastern Cooperative Oncology Group study. *J Clin Oncol* 1998;16:317.
214. Bakkevold KE, Arnesjo B, Dahl O, Kambestad B. Adjuvant combination chemotherapy (AMF) following radical resection of carcinoma of the pancreas and papilla of Vater—results of a controlled, prospective, randomized multicentre study. *Eur J Cancer* 1995;29A:698.
215. Crucitti F, Doglietto GB, Frontera D, et al. Integrated radiosurgical treatment of resectable pancreatic head carcinoma. *Pancreas* 1998;16:31.
216. Ishikawa O, Ohhigashi H, Teshima T. Clinical and histopathological appraisal of preoperative irradiation for adenocarcinoma of the pancreaticoduodenal region. *J Surg Oncol* 1989;40:143.
217. Pilepich MV, Miller HH. Preoperative irradiation in carcinoma of the pancreas. *Cancer* 1980;46:1945.
218. Kopelson G. Curative surgery for adenocarcinoma of the pancreas/ampulla of Vater: the role of adjuvant pre- or postoperative radiation therapy. *Int J Radiat Oncol Biol Phys* 1983;9:911.

219. Hoffman JP, Weese JL, Solin LJ. A single institutional experience with preoperative chemoradiation for stage I–III pancreatic adenocarcinoma. *Am Surg* 1993;59:772.
220. Lowy AM, Lee, JE, Pisters PWT, et al. Prospective, randomized trial of octreotide to prevent pancreatic fistula after pancreaticoduodenectomy for malignant disease. *Ann Surg* 1997;226:632.
221. Abbruzzese JL, Grunewald R, Weeks EA, et al. A phase I clinical, plasma and cellular pharmacology study of gemcitabine. *J Clin Oncol* 1991;9:491.
222. Casper ES, Green MR, Kelsen DP, et al. Phase II trial of gemcitabine (2',2'-difluorodeoxycytidine) in patients with adenocarcinoma of the pancreas. *Invest New Drugs* 1994;12:29.
223. Burris HA III, Moore MJ, Andersen J, et al. Improvements in survival and clinical benefit with gemcitabine as first-line therapy for patients with advanced pancreas cancer: a randomized trial. *J Clin Oncol* 1997;15:2403.
224. Rothenberg ML, Burris HA III, Andersen JS, et al. Gemcitabine: effective palliative therapy for pancreas cancer patients failing 5-FU. *Proc Am Soc Clin Oncol* 1995;14:198(abst).
225. Lawrence TS, Chang EY, Hahn TM, Hertel LW, Shewach DS. Radiosensitization of pancreatic cancer cells by 2',2'-difluoro-2'-deoxycytidine. *Int J Radiat Oncol Biol Phys* 1996;34:867.
226. Wolff RA, Evans DB, Gravel DM, et al. Phase I trial of gemcitabine (GEM) combined with radiation (XRT) for the treatment of locally advanced pancreatic adenocarcinoma. *Proc Am Soc Clin Oncol* 1998;17:1091(abst).
227. Osteen RT, Zinner MJ, Fuchs CS, et al. Phase I trial of concurrent gemcitabine (GEM), infusional 5-fluorouracil (FU) and radiation therapy (RT) in patients with localized, unresectable pancreatic adenocarcinoma (PAC). *Proc Am Soc Clin Oncol* 1999;18:1091(abst).
228. Safar AM, Altamira PS, Recht A, Stevenson M, Stuart K. Phase I trial of gemcitabine, cisplatin (CDDP) and external beam radiation therapy (EBRT) for pancreatic cancer. *Proc Am Soc Clin Oncol* 1999;18:873(abst).
229. McGinn CJ, Shureiqi I, Robertson JM, et al. A phase I trial of radiation dose escalation with full dose gemcitabine (GEM) in patients (pts) with pancreatic cancer. *Proc Am Soc Clin Oncol* 1999;18:1051(abst).
230. Blackstock AW, Bernard SA, Richards F, et al. Phase I trial of twice-weekly gemcitabine and concurrent radiation in patients with advanced pancreatic cancer. *J Clin Oncol* 1999;17:2208.
231. Brierley J, Oza A, Patnaik A, et al. A phase I study of radiation therapy and gemcitabine in patients with locally advanced pancreatic carcinoma. *Proc Am Soc Clin Oncol* 1999;18:713(abst).
232. Tempero M, Plunkett W, van Haperen VR, et al. Randomized phase II trial of dose intense gemcitabine by standard infusion vs. fixed dose rate in metastatic pancreatic adenocarcinoma. *Proc Am Soc Clin Oncol* 1999;18:1048(abst).
233. Hoffman JP, McGinn CJ, Szarka CE, et al. A phase I study of preoperative gemcitabine with radiation therapy followed by postoperative gemcitabine for patients with localized, resectable pancreatic adenocarcinoma. *Proc Am Soc Clin Oncol* 1998;17:1090(abst).
234. Whipple AO, Parson WV, Mullin CR. Treatment of carcinoma of the ampulla of Vater. *Ann Surg* 1935;102:763.
235. Whipple AO. The rationale of radical surgery for cancer of the pancreas and ampullary region. *Ann Surg* 1941;114:612.
236. Waugh JM, Clagett OT. Resection of the duodenum and head of the pancreas for carcinoma. *Surgery* 1946;20:224.
237. Fernandez-delCastillo C, Rattner DW, Warshaw AL. Standards for pancreatic resection in the 1990s. *Arch Surg* 1995;130:295.
238. Fuhrman G, Leach SD, Staley CA, et al. Rationale for *en-bloc* vein resection in the treatment of pancreatic adenocarcinoma adherent to the superior mesenteric–portal venous confluence. *Ann Surg* 1996;223:154.
239. Bold RJ, Charnsangavej C, Cleary KR, et al. Major vascular resection as part of pancreaticoduodenectomy for cancer: radiologic, intraoperative, and pathologic analysis. *J Gastrointest Surg* 1999;3:233.
240. Doerr RJ, Yildiz I, Flint LM. Pancreaticoduodenectomy: university experience and resident education. *Arch Surg* 1990;125:463.
241. Edge SB, Schmieg RE, Rosenlof LK, et al. Pancreas cancer resection outcome in American university centers. *Cancer* 1993;71:3502.
242. Wade TP, Kraybill WG, Virgo KS, et al. Pancreatic cancer treatment in the U.S. veteran from 1987 to 1991: effect of tumor stage on survival. *J Surg Oncol* 1995;58:104.
243. Wade TP, Radford DM, Virgo KS, et al. Complications and outcomes in the treatment of pancreatic adenocarcinoma in the United States veteran. *J Am Coll Surg* 1994;179:38.
244. Lieberman MD, Kilburn H, Lindsey M, Brennan MF. Relation of perioperative deaths to hospital volume among patients undergoing pancreatic resection for malignancy. *Ann Surg* 1995;222:638.
245. Sosa JA, Bowman HM, Gordon TA, et al. Importance of hospital volume in the overall management of pancreatic cancer. *Ann Surg* 1998;228:429.
246. Gordon TA, Bowman HM, Tielsch JM, et al. Statewide regionalization of pancreaticoduodenectomy and its effect on in-hospital mortality. *Ann Surg* 1998;228.71.
247. Simunovic M, To T, Theriault M, Langer B. Relation between hospital surgical volume and outcome for pancreatic resection for neoplasm in a publicly funded health care system. *CMAJ* 1999;160:643.
248. Birkmeyer JD, Finlayson SR, Tosteson AN, et al. Effect of hospital volume on in-hospital mortality with pancreaticoduodenectomy. *Surgery* 1999;125:250.
249. Birkmeyer JD, Warshaw AL, Finlayson SR, Grove MR, Tosteson AN. Relationship between hospital volume and late survival after pancreaticoduodenectomy. *Surgery* 1999;126:178.
250. Gordon TA, Burleyson GP, Tielsch JM, et al. The effects of regionalization on cost and outcome for one general high-risk surgical procedure. *Ann Surg* 1995;221:43.
251. Evans DB, Lee JE, Pisters PWT. Pancreaticoduodenectomy (Whipple operation) and total pancreatectomy for cancer. In: Nyhus LM, Baker RJ, Fishcer JF, eds. *Mastery of surgery*, 3rd ed. Boston: Little, Brown and Company, 1997:1233.
252. Kayahara M, Nagakawa T, Konishi I, et al. Clinicopathological study of pancreatic carcinoma with particular reference to the invasion of the extrapancreatic neural plexus. *Int J Pancreatol* 1991;10:105.
253. Nagakawa T, Kayahara M, Ohta T, et al. Patterns of neural and plexus invasion of human pancreatic cancer and experimental cancer. *Int J Pancreatol* 1991;10:113.
254. Nagakawa T, Mori K, Nakano T, et al. Perineural invasion of carcinoma of the pancreas and biliary tract. *Br J Surg* 1994;80:619.
255. Fortner J. Technique of regional subtotal and total pancreatectomy. *Am J Surg* 1985;150:593.
256. Ishikawa O, Ohigashi H, Imaoka S, et al. Preoperative indications for extended pancreatectomy for locally advanced pancreas cancer involving the portal vein. *Ann Surg* 1992;215:231.
257. Cusack JC, Fuhrman GM, Lee JE, et al. Management of unsuspected tumor invasion of the superior mesenteric–portal venous confluence at the time of pancreaticoduodenectomy. *Am J Surg* 1994;168:352.
258. Leach SD, Lee JE, Charnsangavej C, et al. Survival following pancreaticoduodenectomy with resection of the superior mesenteric–portal vein confluence for adenocarcinoma of the pancreatic head. *Br J Surg* 1998;85:611.
259. Traverso LW, Longmire WP. Preservation of the pylorus in pancreaticoduodenectomy. *Surg Gynecol Obstet* 1978;146:959.
260. Grace PA, Pitt HA, Longmire WP. Pylorus preserving pancreaticoduodenectomy: an overview. *Br J Surg* 1990;77:968.
261. Crucitti F, Doglietto G, Bellantone R, et al. Digestive and nutritional consequences of pancreatic resections. *Int J Pancreatol* 1995;17:37.
262. Kozuschek W, Reith HB, Waleczek H, et al. A comparison of long term results of the standard Whipple procedure and the pylorus preserving pancreaticoduodenectomy. *J Am Coll Surg* 1994;178:443.
263. Patel AG, Toyama MT, Kusske AM, et al. Pylorus-preserving Whipple resection for pancreatic cancer. Is it any better? *Arch Surg* 1995;130:838.
264. Lin PW, Lin YJ. Prospective randomized comparison between pylorus preserving and standard pancreaticoduodenectomy. *Br J Surg* 1999;86:603.
265. Sharp KW, Ross CB, Halter SA, et al. Pancreaticoduodenectomy with pyloric preservation for carcinoma of the pancreas: a cautionary note. *Surgery* 1988;105:645.
266. Zerbi A, Balzano G, Patuzzo R, et al. Comparison between pylorus-preserving and Whipple pancreaticoduodenectomy. *Br J Surg* 1995;82:975.
267. Gunderson LL, Willett CG. Pancreas and hepatobiliary tract. In: Perez C, Brady L, eds. *Principles and practice of radiation oncology*, 3rd ed. Philadelphia: Lippincott–Raven, 1997:1467.
268. Manabe T, Baba N, Ono K, et al. Radical pancreatectomy with intraoperative radiation therapy for pancreatic head cancer. In: Abe M, Takahashi M, eds. *Intraoperative radiation therapy*. Proceedings of the Third International Symposium on Intraoperative Radiation Therapy. New York: Pergamon Press, 1991:249.
269. Hiraoka T, Watanabe E, Mochinaga M, et al. Intraoperative irradiation combined with radical resection for cancer of the head of the pancreas. *World J Surg* 1984;8:766.
270. Hiraoka T. Extended radical resection of cancer of the pancreas with intraoperative radiotherapy. *Ballieres Clin Gastroenterol* 1990;4:985.
271. Coquard R, Ayzac L, Gilly N, et al. Intraoperative radiotherapy in resected pancreatic cancer: feasibility and results. *Radiother Oncol* 1997;44:271.
272. Sindelar WF, Kinsella TJ. Studies of intraoperative radiotherapy in carcinoma of the pancreas. *Ann Oncol* 1999;10[Suppl 4]:S226.
273. Evans DB, Roh M. Pancreaticoduodenectomy. In: Roh M, Ames FC, eds. *Atlas of advanced surgical oncology*. London: Mosby–Year Book, 1994:4.2.
274. Whipple AO. Observations on radical surgery for lesions of the pancreas. *Surg Gynecol Obstet* 1946;82:623.
275. Mason GR, Freeark RJ. Current experience with pancreatogastrostomy. *Am J Surg* 1995;169:217.
276. Park CD, Mackie JA, Rhoads J. Pancreaticogastrostomy. *Am J Surg* 1967;113:85.
277. Yeo CJ, Cameron JL, Maher MM, et al. A prospective randomized trial of pancreaticogastrostomy versus pancreaticojejunostomy after pancreaticoduodenectomy. *Ann Surg* 1995;222:580.
278. Warshaw AL, Torchiana DL. Delayed gastric emptying after pylorus-preserving pancreaticoduodenectomy. *Surg Gynecol Obstet* 1985;160:1.
279. Luque-de Leon E, Tsiotos GG, Balsiger B, et al. Staging laparoscopy for pancreatic cancer should be used to select the best means of palliation and not only to maximize the resectability rate. *J Gastrointest Surg* 1999;3:111.
280. Sohn TA, Lillemoe KD, Cameron JL, et al. Surgical palliation of unresectable periampullary adenocarcinoma in the 1990s. *J Am Coll Surg* 1999;188:658.
281. de Rooij PD, Rogatko A, Brennan MF. Evaluation of palliative surgical procedures in unresectable pancreatic cancer. *Br J Surg* 1991;78:1053.
282. Glazer G, Coulter C, Crofton ME, et al. Controversial issues in the management of pancreatic cancer. Part One. A debate held at St. Mary's Hospital, London on 18 November 1993. *Ann R Coll Surg Engl* 1995;77:111.
283. Sung JJY, Chung S. Endoscopic stenting for palliation of malignant biliary obstruction. A review of progress in the last 15 years. *Dig Dis Sci* 1995;40:1167.
284. Consensus statement. Management of unresectable pancreatic ductal cancer. *J Gastrointest Surg* 1999;3:331.
285. Born P, Rosch T, Bruhl K, et al. Long-term results of endoscopic treatment of biliary duct obstruction due to pancreatic disease. *Hepatogastroenterology* 1998;45:833.
286. Brugge WR, VanDam J. Pancreatic and biliary endoscopy. *N Engl J Med* 1999;341:1808.
287. Evans DB, Winchester DJ, Lee JE. Laparoscopic cholecystojejunostomy. In: MacFadyen BV, Ponsky JL, eds. *Operative laparoscopy and thorascopy*. New York: Raven Press, 1996.
288. Fletcher DR, Jones RM. Laparoscopic cholecystojejunostomy as palliation for obstructive jaundice in inoperable carcinoma of pancreas. *Surg Endosc* 1992;6:147.
289. Nathanson LK. Laparoscopic cholecyst-jejunostomy and gastroenterostomy for malignant disease. *Surg Oncol* 1993;2:19.
290. Park A, Schwartz R, Tandan V, Anvari M. Laparoscopic pancreatic surgery. *Am J Surg* 1999;177:158.
291. Egrari S, O'Connell TX. Role of prophylactic gastroenterostomy for unresectable pancreatic carcinoma. *Am Surg* 1995;61:862.

292. van der Schelling GP, van den Bosch R, Klinkenbij JHG, et al. Is there a place for gastroenterostomy in patients with advanced cancer of the head of the pancreas? *World J Surg* 1993;17:128.
293. Weaver DW, Wiencek RG, Bouwman DL, Walt AJ. Gastrojejunostomy: is it helpful for patients with pancreatic cancer? *Surgery* 1987;102:608.
294. Lillemoe KD, Cameron JL, Hardacre JM, et al. Is prophylactic gastrojejunostomy indicated for unresectable periampullary cancer? A prospective randomized trial. *Ann Surg* 1999;230:322.
295. Wade TP, Neuberger TJ, Swope TJ, et al. Pancreatic cancer palliation: using tumor stage to select appropriate operation. *Am J Surg* 1994;167:208.
296. Espat NJ, Brennan MF, Conlon KC. Patients with laparoscopically staged unresectable pancreatic carcinoma do not require subsequent surgical biliary or gastric bypass. *J Am Coll Surg* 1999;188:649.
297. Gastrointestinal Tumor Study Group. Radiation therapy combined with Adriamycin or 5-fluorouracil for the treatment of locally unresectable pancreatic carcinoma. *Cancer* 1985;56:2563.
298. Gastrointestinal Tumor Study Group. Treatment of locally unresectable carcinoma of the pancreas: comparison of combined-modality therapy (chemotherapy plus radiotherapy) to chemotherapy alone. *J Natl Cancer Inst* 1988;80:751.
299. Roldan GE, Gunderson LL, Nagorney DM, et al. External beam versus intraoperative and external beam irradiation for locally advanced pancreatic cancer. *Cancer* 1988;61:1110.
300. White R, Lee C, Anscher M, et al. Preoperative chemoradiation for patients with locally advanced adenocarcinoma of the pancreas. *Ann Surg Oncol* 1999;6:38.
301. Todd KE, Gloor B, Lane JS, Isacoff WH, Reber HA. Resection of locally advanced pancreatic cancer after downstaging with continuous-infusion 5-fluorouracil, mitomycin-C, leucovorin, and dipyridamole. *J Gastrointest Surg* 1998;2:159.
302. Kamthan AG, Morris JC, Dalton J, et al. Combined modality therapy for stage II and stage III pancreatic carcinoma. *J Clin Oncol* 1997;15:2920.
303. Safran H, King T, Choy H, et al. Paclitaxel and concurrent radiation for locally advanced pancreatic and gastric cancer: a phase I study. *J Clin Oncol* 1997;15:901.
304. Jessup JM, Steele G, Mayer RJ, et al. Neoadjuvant therapy for unresectable pancreatic adenocarcinoma. *Arch Surg* 1993;128:559.
305. Jeekel J, Treurniet-Donker AD. Treatment perspectives in locally advanced unresectable pancreatic cancer. *Br J Surg* 1991;78:1332.
306. Tepper JE, Moyes D, Krall JM, et al. Intraoperative radiation therapy of pancreatic carcinoma: a report of RTOG-8505. *Int J Radiat Oncol Biol Phys* 1991;21:1145.
307. Shipley WU, Nardi GL, Cohen AM. Iodine-125 implant and external beam irradiation in patients with localized pancreatic carcinoma: a comparative study to surgical resection. *Cancer* 1980;45:709.
308. Tepper JE, Shipley WU, Warshaw AL, et al. The role of misonidazole combined with intraoperative radiation therapy in the treatment of pancreatic carcinoma. *J Clin Oncol* 1987;5:579.
309. Garton GR, Gunderson LL, Nagorney DM, et al. High-dose preoperative external beam and intraoperative irradiation for locally advanced pancreatic cancer. *Int J Radiat Oncol Biol Phys* 1993;28:1153.
310. Safran H, Akerman P, Cioffi W, et al. Paclitaxel and concurrent radiation therapy for locally advanced adenocarcinomas of the pancreas, stomach, and gastroesophageal junction. *Semin Radiat Oncol* 1999;9:53.
311. Higgins PD, Sohn JW, Fine RM, et al. Three-dimensional conformal pancreas treatment: comparison of four- to six-field techniques. *Int J Radiat Oncol Biol Phys* 1995;31:605.
312. Lee MJ, Mueller PR, vonSonnenberg E, et al. CT-guided celiac ganglion block with alcohol. *AJR Am J Roentgenol* 1993;161:633.
313. Lillemoe KD, Cameron JL, Kaufman HS, et al. Chemical splanchnicectomy in patients with unresectable pancreatic cancer. *Ann Surg* 1993;217:447.
314. Rothenberg ML. New developments in chemotherapy for patients with advanced pancreatic cancer. *Oncology* 1996;10[Suppl]:18.
315. Rothenberg ML, Abbruzzese JL, Moore M, et al. A rationale for expanding the endpoints for clinical trials in advanced pancreatic carcinoma. *Cancer* 1996;78[Suppl]:627.
316. Abbruzzese JL. Novel diagnostic and therapeutic approaches to pancreatic cancer. *Cancer Bull* 1994;46:525.
317. Kelsen D. The use of chemotherapy in the treatment of advanced gastric and pancreatic cancer. *Semin Oncol* 1994;21:58.
318. Bukowski RM. Role of chemotherapy in patients with adenocarcinoma of the pancreas. *Adv Oncol* 1995;11:25.
319. Glimelius BJ. Chemotherapy in the treatment of cancer of the pancreas. *J Hepato-Biliary-Pancreatic Surg* 1998;5:235.
320. Cascinu S, Graziano F, Catalano G. Chemotherapy for advanced pancreatic cancer: it may no longer be ignored. *Ann Oncol* 1999;10:105.
321. Brennan MR, Kinsella TJ, Casper ES. Cancer of the pancreas. In: DeVita VT Jr, Hellman S, Rosenberg SA, eds. *Cancer: principles and practice of oncology,* 4th ed. Philadelphia: JB Lippincott, 1993:849.
322. Carter SK. The integration of chemotherapy into a combined modality approach for cancer treatment. VI. Pancreatic adenocarcinoma. *Cancer Treat Rev* 1975;3:193.
323. Hansen R, Quebbeman E, Ritch P, et al. Continuous 5-fluorouracil infusion in carcinoma of the pancreas: a phase II study. *Am J Med Sci* 1988;295:91.
324. Tajiri H, Yashimori M, Okazaki N, et al. Phase II study of continuous infusion of 5-fluorouracil in advanced pancreatic cancer. *Oncology* 1991;48:18.
325. Pazdur R, Meropol NJ, Casper E, et al. Phase II trial of ZD1694 (Tomudex) in patients with advanced pancreatic cancer. *Ann Oncol* 1996;13:355.
326. Auerbach M, Wampler GL, Lokich JJ, et al. Treatment of advanced pancreatic carcinoma with a combination of protracted infusional 5-fluorouracil and weekly carboplatin: a Mid-Atlantic Oncology Program study. *Ann Oncol* 1997;8:439.
327. John WJ, Flett MQ. Continuous venous infusion 5-fluorouracil and interferon-alpha in pancreatic carcinoma. *Am J Clin Oncol* 1998;21:147.
328. Hubbard KP, Pazdur R, Ajani JA, et al. Phase II evaluation of iproplatin in patients with advanced gastric and pancreatic cancer. *Am J Clin Oncol* 1992;15:524.
329. Carlson RW, Doroshow JH, Odujinrin OO, et al. Trimetrexate in locally advanced or metastatic adenocarcinoma of the pancreas: a phase II study of the Northern California Oncology Group. *Invest New Drugs* 1990;8:387.
330. Casper ES, Schwartz GK, Johnson B, et al. Phase II trial of edatrexate in patients with advanced pancreatic cancer. *Invest New Drugs* 1992;10:313.
331. Casper ES, Schwartz GK, Kelsen DP. Phase II trial of fazarabine (arabinofuranosyl-5-azacytidine) in patients with advanced pancreatic adenocarcinoma. *Invest New Drugs* 1992;10:205.
332. Bukowski RM, Fleming TR, MacDonald JS, et al. Evaluation of combination chemotherapy and phase II agents in pancreatic adenocarcinoma: a Southwest Oncology Group study. *Cancer* 1993;71:322.
333. Linke K, Pazdur R, Abbruzzese J, et al. Phase II study of amonafide in advanced pancreatic adenocarcinoma. *Invest New Drugs* 1991;9:353.
334. Rougier P, De Forni M, Adenis A, et al. Phase II study of Taxotere (RP56976, docetaxel) in pancreatic adenocarcinoma. Proc Am Soc Clin Oncol 1994;13:200(abst).
335. Okada S, Sakata Y, Matsuno S, et al. Phase II study of docetaxel in patients with metastatic pancreatic cancer: a Japanese cooperative study. Cooperative Group of Docetaxel for Pancreatic Cancer in Japan. *Br J Cancer* 1999;80:438.
336. Whitehead RP, Jacobson J, Brown TD, et al. Phase II trial of paclitaxel and granulocyte colony-stimulating factor in patients with pancreatic carcinoma: a Southwest Oncology Group study. *J Clin Oncol* 1997;15:2414.
337. O'Reilly S, Donehower RC, Rowinsky EK, et al. A phase II trial of topotecan in patients with previously untreated pancreatic cancer. *Anticancer Drugs* 1996;7:410.
338. Scher RM, Kosierowski R, Lusch C, et al. Phase II trial of topotecan in advanced or metastatic adenocarcinoma of the pancreas. *Invest New Drugs* 1996;13:347.
339. Wagener DJT, Verdonk HER, Dirix LY, et al. Phase II trial of CPT-11 in patients with advanced pancreatic cancer. An EORTC Early Clinical Trials Group study. *Ann Oncol* 1995;6:129.
340. Loehrer PJ Sr, Williams SD, Einhorn LH, et al. Ifosfamide: an active drug in treatment of adenocarcinoma of the pancreas. *J Clin Oncol* 1985;3:367.
341. Cerny T, Martinelli G, Goldhirsch A, et al. Continuous 5 day infusion of ifosfamide and mesna in inoperable pancreatic cancer patients: a phase II study. *J Cancer Res Clin Oncol* 1991;117:135.
342. Ajani JA, Abbruzzese JL, Goudeau P, et al. Ifosfamide and mesna: marginally active in patients with advanced carcinoma of the pancreas. *J Clin Oncol* 1988;6:1703.
343. Bissery MC, Guenard D, Gueritte-Voegelein F, et al. Experimental antitumor activity of Taxotere (RP 56976, NSC 628503), a Taxol analogue. *Cancer Res* 1991;51:4845.
344. Abbruzzese JL, Evans D, Markowitz A, et al. Docetaxel, a potentially active agent for patients with pancreatic adenocarcinomas . *Proc Am Soc Clin Oncol* 1995;14:221(abst).
345. Androulakis N, Kourousis C, Dimopoulos MA, et al. Treatment of pancreatic cancer with docetaxel and granulocyte colony-stimulating factor: a multicenter phase II study. *J Clin Oncol* 1999;17:1779.
346. Sugarman SM, Pazdur R, Daugherty K, et al. A phase II trial of topotecan for the treatment of unresectable pancreatic cancer. *Proc Am Soc Clin Oncol* 1994;13:224(abst).
347. Stevenson JP, Scher RM, Kosierowski R, et al. Phase II trial of topotecan as a 21-day continuous infusion in patients with advanced or metastatic adenocarcinoma of the pancreas. *Eur J Cancer* 1998;34:1358.
348. Hertel LW, Kroin JS, Misner JW, Tustin JM. Synthesis of 2-deoxy-2',2'difluoro-D-ribose and 2-deoxy-2',2'difluoro-D-fibofuranosyl nucleosides. *J Organic Chem* 1988;53:2406.
349. Hertel LW, Boder GB, Kroin JS, et al. Evaluation of the antitumor activity of gemcitabine (2',2'-difluoro-2'-deoxycytidine). *Cancer Res* 1990;50:4417.
350. Heinemann V, Hertel LW, Grindey GB, Plunkett W. Comparison of the cellular pharmacokinetics and toxicity of 2',2'-difluorodeoxycytidine and 1-β-D-arabinofuranosylcytosine. *Cancer Res* 1988;48:4024.
351. Rothenberg ML, Moore MJ, Cripps MC, et al. A phase II trial of gemcitabine in patients with 5-FU-refractory pancreas cancer. *Ann Oncol* 1996;7:347.
352. Ragnarson-Tennvall G, Wilking N. Treatment of locally advanced pancreatic carcinoma in Sweden. A health economic comparison of palliative treatment with best supportive care versus palliative treatment with gemcitabine in combination with best supportive care. *Pharmacoeconomics* 1999;15:377.
353. Grunewald R, Abbruzzese JL, Tarassoff P, et al. Saturation of 2',2'-difluorodeoxycytidine 5'-triphosphate accumulation by mononuclear cells during a phase I trial of gemcitabine. *Cancer Chemother Pharmacol* 1991;27:258.
354. Grunewald R, Kantarjian H, Keating MJ, et al. Pharmacologically directed design of the dose rate and schedule of 2',2'-difluorodeoxycytidine (gemcitabine) administration in leukemia. *Cancer Res* 1990;50:6823.
355. Grunewald R, Kantarjian H, Du M, et al. Gemcitabine in leukemia: a phase I clinical, plasma, and cellular pharmacology study. *J Clin Oncol* 1992;10:406.
356. Fossella FV, Lippman SM, Shin DM, et al. Maximum-tolerated dose defined for single-agent gemcitabine: a phase I dose-escalation study in chemotherapy-naive patients with advanced non–small-cell lung cancer. *J Clin Oncol* 1997;15:310.
357. Touroutoglou N, Gravel D, Raber MN, et al. Clinical results of a pharmacodynamically-based strategy for higher dosing of gemcitabine in patients with solid tumors. *Ann Oncol* 1998;9:1003.
358. Brand R, Capadano M, Tempero M. A phase I trial of weekly gemcitabine administered as a prolonged infusion in patients with pancreatic cancer and other solid tumors. *Invest New Drugs* 1997;15:331.
359. van Moorsel CJ, Peters GJ, Pinedo HM. Gemcitabine: future prospects of single-agent and combination studies. *Oncologist* 1997;2:127.
360. van Moorsel CJ, Veerman G, Bergman AM, et al. Combination chemotherapy studies with gemcitabine. *Semin Oncol* 1997;24[Suppl 7]:S7-17.
361. Cascinu S, Silva RR, Barni S, et al. A combination of gemcitabine and 5-fluorouracil in advanced pancreatic cancer, a report from the Italian Group for the Study of Digestive Tract Cancer (GISCAD). *Br J Cancer* 1999;80:1595.

362. Hidalgo M, Castellano D, Paz-Ares L, et al. Phase I–II study of gemcitabine and fluorouracil as a continuous infusion in patients with pancreatic cancer. *J Clin Oncol* 1999;17:585.
363. Heinemann V, Wilke H, Possinger K, et al. Gemcitabine and cisplatin in the treatment of advanced and metastatic pancreatic cancer. Final results of a phase II study. *Proc Am Soc Clin Oncol* 1999;18:274a(abst).
364. Colucci G, Riccardi F, Giuliani F. et al. Randomized trial of gemcitabine alone or with cisplatin in advanced pancreatic cancer: a phase II multicenter study of the Southern Italy Oncology Group. *Proc Am Soc Clin Oncol* 1999;18:250a(abst).
365. Spiridonidis CH, Laufman LR, Jones J, et al. Phase I study of docetaxel dose escalation in combination with fixed weekly gemcitabine in patients with advanced malignancies. *J Clin Oncol* 1998;16:3866.
366. Rizvi NA. Docetaxel (Taxotere) and gemcitabine in combination therapy. *Semin Oncol* 1999;26[Suppl 11]:19.
367. Lueck A, Ridwelski K, Lippert H. Phase I study of a treatment of gemcitabine and docetaxel weekly in advanced pancreatic cancer. *Ann Oncol* 1998;9[Suppl 4]:52(abst).
368. Rothenberg ML, Sharma A, Weiss GR, et al. Phase I trial of paclitaxel and gemcitabine administered every two weeks in patients with refractory solid tumors. *Ann Oncol* 1998;9:733.
369. Scheithauer W, Kornek GV, Raderer M, et al. Phase II trial of gemcitabine, epirubicin and granulocyte colony-stimulating factor in patients with advanced pancreatic adenocarcinoma. *Br J Cancer* 1999;80:1797.
370. Carmichael J, Lederman JA, Woll PJ, et al. Phase 1B study of concurrent administration of marimastat and gemcitabine in non-resectable pancreatic cancer. *Proc Am Soc Clin Oncol* 1998;17:232a(abst).
371. Glimelius B, Hoffman K, Sjoden PO, et al. Chemotherapy improves survival and quality of life in advanced pancreatic and biliary cancer. *Ann Oncol* 1996;7:593.
372. Palmer KR, Kerr M, Knowles G, et al. Chemotherapy prolongs survival in inoperable pancreatic carcinoma. *Br J Surg* 1994;81:882.
373. Morrell LM, Bach A, Richman SP, et al. A phase II multi-institutional trial of low-dose N-phosphonoacetyl-L-aspartate and high dose 5-fluorouracil as a short-term infusion in the treatment of adenocarcinoma of the pancreas. A Southwest Oncology Group study. *Cancer* 1991;67:363.
374. Rosvold E, Schilder R, Walczak J, et al. Phase II trial of PALA in combination with 5-fluorouracil in advanced pancreatic cancer. *Cancer Chemother Pharmacol* 1992;29:305.
375. Harstrick A, Kohne-Wompner CH, Preusser P, et al. A phase II study of the combination of PALA, methotrexate and 5-FU in advanced pancreatic carcinoma. *Proc Am Soc Clin Oncol* 1993;12:219(abst).
376. Redei I, Green F, Hoffman JP, et al. Phase II trial of PALA and 6-methylmercaptopurine riboside (MMPR) in combination with 5-fluorouracil in advanced pancreatic cancer. *Invest New Drugs* 1994;12:319.
377. Crown J, Casper ES, Botet J, et al. Lack of efficacy of high dose leucovorin and fluorouracil in patients with advanced pancreatic adenocarcinoma. *J Clin Oncol* 1991;9:1682.
378. DeCaprio JA, Mayer RJ, Gonin R, et al. Fluorouracil and high dose leucovorin in previously untreated patients with advanced adenocarcinoma of the pancreas. Results of a phase II trial. *J Clin Oncol* 1991;9:2128.
379. Bolli E, Saccomanno S, Mondini G, et al. 5-Fluorouracil plus 5-methyltetrahydrofolate in advanced pancreatic cancer. *Cancer Chemother Pharmacol* 1995;35:339.
380. Weinerman BH, MacCormick RE. A phase II survival comparison of patients with adenocarcinoma of the pancreas treated with 5-fluorouracil and calcium leucovorin versus a matched tumor registry control population. *Am J Clin Oncol* 1994;17:467.
381. Pazdur R, Ajani JA, Abbruzzese JL, et al. Phase II evaluation of fluorouracil and recombinant α-2a-interferon in previously untreated patients with pancreatic adenocarcinoma. *Cancer* 1992;70:2073.
382. Moore MJ, Erlichman C, Kaizer L, et al. A phase II study of 5-fluorouracil, leucovorin and interferon-alpha in advanced pancreatic cancer. *Anticancer Drugs* 1993;4:555.
383. Knuth A, Bernhard H, Klein O, et al. Combination fluorouracil, folinic acid, and interferon alfa-2a: an active regimen in advanced pancreatic adenocarcinoma. *Semin Oncol* 1992;19:211.
384. Bernhard H, Jèger-Arand E, Bernhard G, et al. Treatment of advanced pancreatic cancer with 5-fluorouracil, folinic acid and interferon alpha-2A: results of a phase II trial. *Br J Cancer* 1995;71:102.
385. Scheithauer W, Pfeffel F, Komek G, et al. A phase II trial of PALA in combination with 5-fluorouracil, leucovorin and recombinant alpha-2B interferon in advanced adenocarcinoma of the pancreas. *Cancer* 1992;70:1864.
386. Gattani A, Mandeli J, Chesser MR, et al. An active biochemical modulation regimen for advanced adenocarcinoma of the pancreas. *Proc Am Soc Clin Oncol* 1992;11:193(abst).
387. Johnson PJ, Corbishley TP. Sex steroid receptors and antisteroid agents in the treatment of pancreatic adenocarcinoma. Monograph Series. European Organization for Research and Treatment of Cancer 1987;18:99.
388. Fisher WE, Muscarella P, Boros LG, et al. Gastrointestinal hormones as potential adjuvant treatment of exocrine pancreatic adenocarcinoma. *Int J Pancreatol* 1998;24:169.
389. Andren-Sandberg A, Hoem D, Backman PL. Other risk factors for pancreatic cancer: hormonal aspects. *Ann Oncol* 1999;10[Suppl 4]:131.
390. Yamashita J, Abe M, Ogawa M. Endocrine therapy in pancreatic carcinoma. *Oncology* 1998;55[Suppl 1]:17.
391. Greenway B, Iqbal MJ, Johnson PJ, Williams R. Oestrogen receptor proteins in malignant and fetal pancreas. *BMJ* 1981;283:751.
392. Iqbal MJ, Greenway BA, Wilkinson ML, et al. Sex steroid enzymes, aromatase and 5-alpha-reductase in the pancreas: a comparison of normal adult, foetal and malignant tissue. *Clin Sci* 1983;65:71.
393. Greenway B, Iqbal MJ, Johnson PJ, Williams R. Low serum testosterone concentrations in patients with carcinoma of the pancreas. *BMJ* 1983;286:93.
394. Siu TO, Kwan WB. Hormones in chemotherapy for pancreatic cancer, chemoagents or carriers? *In Vivo* 1989;3:255.
395. Comaru-Schally AM, Schally AV. LHRH agonists as adjuncts to somatostatin analogs in the treatment of pancreatic cancer. *Hum Reprod* 1990;3:203.
396. Klijn JG, Setyono-Han B, Bakker GH, et al. Effects of somatostatin analog (Sandostatin) treatment in experimental and human cancer. Monograph Series, European Organization for Research and Treatment of Cancer 1987;18:459.
397. Schally AV, Redding TW, Cal RZ, et al. Somatostatin analogs in the treatment of various experimental tumors. Monograph Series, European Organization for Research and Treatment of Cancer 1987;18:431.
398. Greenway B, Duke D, Pym B, et al. The control of human pancreatic adenocarcinoma xenografts in nude mice by hormone therapy. *Br J Surg* 1982;69:595.
399. Szende B, Srkalovic G, Schally AV, et al. Inhibitory effects of analogs of luteinising hormone-releasing hormone and somatostatin on pancreatic cancer in hamsters. *Cancer* 1990;65:2279.
400. Zalatnai A, Schally AV. Treatment of N-nitrosobis(2-oxopropyl)amine–induced pancreatic cancer in Syrian golden hamsters with D-Trp-6-LH-RH and somatostatin analogue RC-160 microcapsules. *Cancer Res* 1989;49:1810.
401. Upp JR Jr, Olson D, Poston DJ, et al. Inhibition of growth of two human pancreatic adenocarcinomas *in vivo* by somatostatin analog SMS 201-995. *Ann Surg* 1988;155:29.
402. Helle SI, Geisler J, Poulsen JP, et al. Microencapsulated octreotide pamoate in advanced gastrointestinal and pancreatic cancer: a phase I study. *Br J Cancer* 1998;78:14.
403. Fazeny B, Baur M, Prohaska M, et al. Octreotide combined with goserelin in the therapy of advanced pancreatic cancer—results of a pilot study and review of the literature. *J Cancer Res Clin Oncol* 1997;123:45.
404. Weckbecker G, Raulf F, Tolcsvai L, et al. Potentiation of the anti-proliferative effects of anti-cancer drugs by octreotide *in vitro* and *in vivo*. *Digestion* 1996;57[Suppl 1]:22.
405. Greenway BA. Effect of flutamide on survival in patients with pancreatic cancer: results of a prospective, randomised, double blind, placebo controlled trial. *BMJ* 1998;316:1935.
406. Sharma JJ, Razvillas B, Stephens CD, et al. Phase II study of flutamide as second line chemotherapy in patients with advanced pancreatic cancer. *Invest New Drugs* 1997;15:361.
407. Theve NO, Pousette A, Carlstrom K. Adenocarcinoma of the pancreas—a hormone sensitive tumor? A preliminary report on Nolvadex treatment. *Clin Oncol* 1983;9:193.
408. Tonnesen K, Kamp-Jensen M. Antiestrogen therapy in pancreatic carcinoma: a preliminary report. *Eur J Surg Oncol* 1986;12:69.
409. Wong A, Chan A. Survival benefit of tamoxifen therapy in adenocarcinoma of the pancreas. A case-control study. *Cancer* 1993;71:2200.
410. Crowson MC, Dorrell A, Rolfe EB, et al. A phase II study to evaluate tamoxifen in pancreatic adenocarcinoma. *Eur J Surg Oncol* 1986;12:335.
411. Allegretti A, Lionetto R, Saccomanno S, et al. LH-RH analogue treatment in adenocarcinoma of the pancreas: a phase II study. *Oncology* 1993;50:77.
412. Philip PA, Carmichael J, Tonkin K, et al. Hormonal treatment of pancreatic carcinoma: a phase II study of LHRH agonist goserelin plus hydrocortisone. *Br J Cancer* 1993;67:379.
413. Swarovsky B, Wolf M, Havemann K, et al. Tamoxifen or cytoproterone acetate in combination with buserelin is ineffective in patients with pancreatic adenocarcinoma. *Oncology* 1993;50:226.
414. Taylor OM, Benson IA, McMahon MJ. Clinical trial of tamoxifen in patients with irresectable pancreatic adenocarcinoma. The Yorkshire Gastrointestinal Tumor Group. *Br J Surg* 1993;80:384.
415. Bakkevold KE, Pattersen A, Ames JB, et al. Tamoxifen therapy in unresectable adenocarcinoma of the pancreas and the papilla of Vater. *Br J Surg* 1990;77:725.
416. Keating JJ, Johnson PJ, Cochrane AM, et al. A prospective randomized trial of tamoxifen and cytoproterone acetate in pancreatic carcinoma. *Br J Cancer* 1989;60:789.
417. Pederzoli P, Maurer U, Vollmer K, et al. Phase 3 trial of SMS 201-995pa LAR vs. placebo in unresectable stage II, III, and IV pancreatic cancer. *Proc Am Soc Clin Oncol* 1998;17:257a(abst).
418. Roy A, Jacobs A, Bukowski R, et al. Phase 3 trial of SMS 201-995 pa LAR (SMS PA LAR) and continuous infusion (CI) 5-FU in unresectable stage II, III, and IV pancreatic cancer. *Proc Am Soc Clin Oncol* 1998;17:257a(abst 987).
419. Robinson EK, Grau AM, Evans DB, et al. Cell cycle regulation of human pancreatic cancer by tamoxifen. *Ann Surg Oncol* 1998;5:342.
420. Wong A, Chan A, Arthur K. Tamoxifen therapy in unresectable adenocarcinoma of the pancreas. *Cancer Treat Rep* 1987;71:7.
421. Horimi T, Takasaki M, Toki A, et al. The beneficial effect of tamoxifen therapy in patients with resected adenocarcinoma of the pancreas. *Hepatogastroenterology* 1996;43:1225.
422. Andren-Sandberg A. Treatment with an LH-RH analogue in patients with advanced pancreatic cancer. A preliminary report. *Acta Chir Scand* 1990;156:540.
423. Abbruzzese JL, Gholson CF, Daugherty K, et al. A pilot clinical trial of the cholecystokinin receptor antagonist MK 329 in patients with advanced pancreatic cancer. *Pancreas* 1992;7:165.
424. Smith FP, Hoth DF, Levin B, et al. 5-Fluorouracil, Adriamycin, and mitomycin-C (FAM) chemotherapy for advanced adenocarcinoma of the pancreas. *Cancer* 1980;46:2014.
425. Schein PS, Lavin PT, Moetel CG, et al. Randomized phase II trial of Adriamycin, methotrexate, and actinomycin-D in advanced measurable pancreatic carcinoma. *Cancer* 1978;42:19.
426. Bitran JD, Desser RR, Kozloff MF, et al. Treatment of metastatic pancreatic and gastric adenocarcinoma with 5-FU, Adriamycin and mitomycin (FAM). *Cancer Treat Rep* 1979;63:2049.
427. Wiggans RG, Woolley PV, MacDonald JS, et al. Phase II trial of streptozotocin, mitomycin C, and 5-fluorouracil (SMF) in the treatment of advanced pancreatic cancer. *Cancer* 1978;41:387.
428. Oster MW, Gray R, Panasci L, et al. Chemotherapy for advanced pancreatic cancer. A comparison of 5-fluorouracil, Adriamycin, and mitomycin (FAM) with 5-fluorouracil, streptozotocin, and mitomycin (FSM). *Cancer* 1986;57:29.
429. Gastrointestinal Tumor Study Group. Phase II studies of drug combinations in advanced pancreatic carcinoma: fluorouracil plus doxorubicin plus mitomycin C and two regimens of streptozotocin plus mitomycin C plus fluorouracil. *J Clin Oncol* 1986;4:1794.
430. Cullinan SA, Moertel CG, Fleming TR, et al. A comparison of three chemotherapeutic regimens in the treatment of advanced pancreatic and gastric carcinoma. *JAMA* 1985;253:2061.

431. Lipton A, Harvey HA, Santen RJ, et al. FAM chemotherapy ± aminoglutethimide in the treatment of pancreatic carcinoma. *Eur J Surg Oncol* 1990;16:12.
432. Palmer KR, Kerr M, Knowles G, et al. Chemotherapy prolongs survival in inoperable pancreatic carcinoma. *Br J Surg* 1994;81:882.
433. Mallinson CN, Rake MO, Cocking JB. Chemotherapy in pancreas cancer. *BMJ* 1980;281:1589.
434. Cullinan S, Moertel CG, Wieand HS, et al. A phase III trial. On the therapy of advanced pancreatic carcinoma. Evaluations of the Mallinson regimen and combined 5-fluorouracil, doxorubicin and cisplatin. *Cancer* 1990;65:2207.
435. Wils JA, Kok T, Wagener DJ, et al. Activity of cisplatin in adenocarcinoma of the pancreas. *Eur J Cancer* 1993;29:203.
436. Rothman H, Cantrell JE Jr, Lokich J, et al. Continuous infusion of 5-fluorouracil plus weekly cisplatin for pancreatic carcinoma. A Mid-Atlantic Oncology Program study. *Cancer* 1991;68:264.
437. Lokich JJ, Ahlgren JD, Cantrell J, et al. A prospective randomized comparison of protracted infusional 5-fluorouracil with or without weekly bolus cisplatin in metastatic colorectal carcinoma. A Mid-Atlantic Oncology Program study. *Cancer* 1991;67:14.
438. Rougier P, Zarba JJ, Ducreux M, et al. Phase II study of cisplatin and 120 hour continuous infusion of 5-fluorouracil in patients with advanced pancreatic adenocarcinoma. *Ann Oncol* 1993;4:333.
439. Nose H, Shuichi O, Okusaka T, et al. 5-fluorouracil continuous infusion combined with cisplatin for advanced pancreatic cancer: a Japanese cooperative study. *Hepatogastroenterology* 1999;46:3244.
440. Isacoff WH, Botnick L, Rose C, et al. Treatment of patients with locally advanced pancreatic carcinoma with continuous infusion 5-fluorouracil, calcium leucovorin, mitomycin-C and dipyridamole. *Proc Am Soc Clin Oncol* 1993;12;225(abst).
441. Dougherty JB, Kelsen D, Kemeny N, et al. Advanced pancreatic cancer: a phase I–II trial of cisplatin, high-dose cytarabine and caffeine. *J Natl Cancer Inst* 1989;81:1735.
442. Kelsen D, Hudis C, Nredwiecki D, et al. A phase III comparison of streptozotocin, mitomycin and 5-fluorouracil with cisplatin, cytosine arabinoside and caffeine in patients with advanced pancreatic cancer. *Cancer* 1991;68:965.
443. Thomas CR, Weiden PL, Traverso LW, Thompson T. Concomitant intraarterial cisplatin, intravenous 5-fluorouracil, and split-course radiation therapy for locally advanced unresectable pancreatic adenocarcinoma: a phase II study of the Puget Sound Oncology Consortium (PSOC-703). *Am J Clin Oncol* 1997;20:161.
444. Maurer CA, Borner MM, Lauffer J, et al. Celiac axis infusion chemotherapy in advanced nonresectable pancreatic cancer. *Int J Pancreatol* 1998;23:181.
445. Ishikawa O, Ohigashi H, Sasaki Y, et al. Liver perfusion chemotherapy via both the hepatic artery and portal vein to prevent hepatic metastasis after extended pancreatectomy for adenocarcinoma of the pancreas. *Am J Surg* 1994;168:361.
446. Ishikawa O, Ohigashi H, Sasaki Y, et al. Adjuvant therapies in extended pancreatectomy for ductal adenocarcinoma of the pancreas. *Hepatogastroenterology* 1998;45:644.
447. Crist KA, Arredondo MA, Chaudhuri B, et al. Pharmacokinetics and toxicity of isolated perfusion of human pancreas-duodenum with mitomycin-C. *Reg Cancer Treat* 1991;3:305.
448. Lorenz M, Petrowsky H, Heinrich S, et al. Isolated hypoxic perfusion with mitomycin C in patients with advanced pancreatic cancer. *Eur J Surg Oncol* 1998;24:542.
449. Muchmore JH, Carter RD, Preslan JE, George WJ. Regional chemotherapy with hemofiltration: a rationale for a different treatment approach to advanced pancreatic cancer. *Hepatogastroenterology* 1996;43:346.
450. Lygidakis NJ, Stringaris K. Adjuvant therapy following pancreatic resection for pancreatic duct carcinoma: a prospective randomized study. *Hepatogastroenterology* 1996;43:671.
451. Beger HG, Gansauge F, Buchler MW, Link KH. Intraarterial adjuvant chemotherapy after pancreaticoduodenectomy for pancreatic cancer: significant reduction in occurrence of liver metastasis. *World J Surg* 1999;23:946.
452. Abbruzzese JL, Levin B, Ajani JA, et al. A phase I trial of recombinant human interferon-gamma and recombinant human tumor necrosis factor in patients with gastrointestinal cancer. *Cancer Res* 1989;49:4057.
453. Abbruzzese JL, Levin B, Ajani JA, et al. A phase II trial of recombinant human interferon-gamma and recombinant tumor necrosis factor in patients with advanced gastrointestinal malignancies: Results of a trial terminated by excessive toxicity. *J Biol Response Mod* 1990;9:522.
454. Gibbs JB, Oliff A, Kohl NE. Farnesyltransferase inhibitors: *ras* research yields a potential cancer therapeutic. *Cell* 1994;77:175.
455. Gibbs JB, Oliff A. Pharmaceutical research in molecular oncology. *Cell* 1994;79:193.
456. Sun J, Qian Y, Hamilton AD, Sebti SM. Ras CAAX peptidomimetic FTI 276 selectively blocks tumor growth in nude mice of a human lung carcinoma with K-*Ras* mutation and *p53* deletion. *Cancer Res* 1995;55:4243.
457. Rowinsky EK, Windle JJ, Von Hoff DD. Ras protein farnesyltransferase: a strategic target for anticancer therapeutic development. *J Clin Oncol* 1999;17:3631.
458. Hohl RJ, Lewis K. Differential effects of monoterpenes and lovastatin on *RAS* processing. *J Biol Chem* 1995;270:17508.
459. Stark MJ, Burke YD, McKinzie JH, Ayoubi AS, Crowell PL. Chemotherapy of pancreatic cancer with the monoterpene perillyl alcohol. *Cancer Lett* 1995;96:15.
460. Ripple GH, Gould MN, Stewart JA, et al. Phase I clinical trial of perillyl alcohol administered daily. *Clin Cancer Res* 1998;4:1159.
461. Montoya RG, Velasco MA, Price RE, Abbruzzese JL, Wargovich MJ. Pilot study on the chemoprevention of N-nitrosobis(2-oxopropyl)amine–induced cancers of the pancreas in Syrian golden hamsters by the monoterpene perillyl alcohol. *Proc Am Assoc Cancer Res* 1996;37:274(abst 1872).
462. Klijn JG, Hoff AM, Planting AS, et al. Treatment of patients with metastatic pancreatic and gastrointestinal tumors with the somatostatin analogue Sandostatin: a phase II study including endocrine effects. *Br J Cancer* 1990;62:627.
463. Savage AP, Calam J, Wood CB, Bloom SR. SMS 201-995 treatment and advanced intestinal cancer: a pilot study. *Aliment Pharmacol Ther* 1987;1:133.
464. Canobbio L, Boccardo F, Cannota D, Gallotti P, Epis R. Treatment of advanced pancreatic carcinoma with the somatostatin analogue BIM 23014. Preliminary results of a pilot study. *Cancer* 1992;69:648.
465. Radulovic S, Nagy A, Szoke B, Schally AV. Cytotoxic analog of somatostatin containing methotrexate inhibits growth of MIA PaCa-2 human pancreatic cancer xenografts in nude mice. *Cancer Lett* 1992;62:263.
466. Smith-Jones PM, Stolz B, Albert R, et al. Synthesis and characterisation of [^{90}Y]-Bz-DTPA-oct: a yttrium-90–labelled octreotide analogue for radiotherapy of somatostatin receptor–positive tumours. *Nucl Med Biol* 1998;25:181.
467. Cobleigh MA, Vogel CL, Tripathy D. Multinational study of the efficacy and safety of humanized anti-HER2 monoclonal antibody in women who have HER2-overexpressing metastatic breast cancer that has progressed after chemotherapy for metastatic disease. *J Clin Oncol* 1999;17:2639.
468. Baselga J, Tripathy D, Mendelsohn J, et al. Phase II study of weekly intravenous recombinant humanized anti-p185HER2 monoclonal antibody in patients with *HER2/neu*-overexpressing metastatic breast cancer. *J Clin Oncol* 1996;14:737.
469. Baselga J, Norton L, Albanell J, Kim YM, Mendelsohn J. Recombinant humanized anti-HER2 antibody (Herceptin) enhances the antitumor activity of paclitaxel and doxorubicin against *HER2/neu* overexpressing human breast cancer xenografts. *Cancer Res* 1998;58:2825.
470. Norton L, Slamon D, Leyland-Jones B, et al., for the Multinational Herceptin Investigator Group. Overall survival advantage to simultaneous chemotherapy plus the humanized anti-HER2 monoclonal antibody Herceptin in HER2-overexpressing metastatic breast cancer. *Proc Am Soc Clin Oncol* 1998;18:127a(abst).
471. Mendelsohn J. Epidermal growth factor receptor inhibition by a monoclonal antibody as anticancer therapy. *Clin Cancer Res* 1997;3:2703.
472. Bruns CJ, Portera CA, Tsan R, Hicklin DJ, Radinsky R. Regression of human pancreatic carcinoma growing orthotopically in athymic nude mide by blockade of epidermal growth factor receptor (EGF-R) signaling in combination with gemcitabine. *Proc Am Assoc Cancer Res* 1999;40:23(abst 154).
473. Bramhall SR. The matrix metalloproteinases and their inhibitors in pancreatic cancer. From molecular science to a clinical application. *Int J Pancreatol* 1997;21:1.
474. Rasmussen H, Rugg T, Brown P, Baillet M, Millar A. A 371 patient meta-analysis of studies of marimastat in patients with advanced cancer. *Proc Am Soc Clin Oncol* 1997;16:429a(abst 1538).
475. Fong TA, Shawver LK, Sun L, et al. SU5416 is a potent and selective inhibitor of the vascular endothelial growth factor receptor (Flk-1/KDR) that inhibits tyrosine kinase catalysis, tumor vascularization, and growth of multiple tumor types. *Cancer Res* 1999;59:99.
476. Figg WD, Pluda JM, Lush RM, et al. The pharmacokinetics of TNP-470, a new angiogenesis inhibitor. *Pharmacotherapy* 1997;17:91.
477. Kudelka AP, Levy T, Verschraegen CF, et al. A phase I study of TNP-470 administered to patients with advanced squamous cell cancer of the cervix. *Clin Cancer Res* 1997;3:1501.
478. O'Reilly MS. The preclinical evaluation of angiogenesis inhibitors. *Invest New Drugs* 1997;15:5.
479. O'Reilly MS, Holmgren L, Chen C, et al. Angiostatin induces and sustains dormancy of human primary tumors in mice. *Nat Med* 1996;2:689.
480. Cao Y, O'Reilly MS, Marshall B, et al. Expression of angiostatin cDNA in a murine fibrosarcoma suppresses primary tumor growth and produces long-term dormancy of metastases. *J Clin Invest* 1998;101:1055.
481. Bouvet M, Bold RJ, Lee J, et al. Adenovirus-mediated wild-type *p53* tumor suppressor gene therapy induces apoptosis and suppresses growth of human pancreatic cancer. *Ann Surg Oncol* 1998;5:681.
482. Joshi US, Dergham ST, Chen YQ, et al. Inhibition of pancreatic tumor cell growth in culture by p21WAF1 recombinant adenovirus. *Pancreas* 1998;16:107.
483. Hwang RF, Gordon EM, Anderson WF, et al. Gene therapy for primary and metastatic pancreatic cancer with intraperitoneal retroviral vector bearing the wild-type *p53* gene. *Surgery* 1998;124:143.
484. Mukhopadhyay T, Tainsky M, Cavender AC, Roth JA. Specific inhibition of K-*ras* expression and tumorgenicity of lung cancer cells by anti-sense RNA. *Cancer Res* 1991;51:1744.
485. Feng M, Cabrera G, Deshane J, Scanlon KJ, Curiel DT. Neoplastic reversion accomplished by high efficiency adenoviral-mediated delivery of an anti-*ras* ribozyme. *Cancer Res* 1995;55:2024.
486. Mulvihill SJ, Warren RS, Fell S, et al. A phase I trial of intratumoral injection with an E1B-attenuated adenovirus, ONYX-015, into unresectable carcinomas of the exocrine pancreas. *Proc Am Soc Clin Oncol* 1998;17:211a(abst 815).
487. Hecht JR, Abbruzzese JL, Lahoti S, et al. Feasibility of multiple direct injections of Onyx-015 adenovirus into pancreatic carcinomas under endoscopic ultrasound guidance. *Proc Am Soc Clin Oncol* 1999;18:186a(abst 715).

SECTION 5

YUMAN FONG
NANCY KEMENY
THEODORE S. LAWRENCE

Cancer of the Liver and Biliary Tree

Primary hepatobiliary malignancies are the most common of solid-organ cancers, and include hepatocellular carcinomas (HCCs), cholangiocarcinomas, and gallbladder cancers. As a group, these tumors represent both major diagnostic and therapeutic challenges. Though surgery can be potentially curative for these tumors, until recently, most cases of hepatobiliary cancers were discovered at a stage far too advanced for complete excision. These tumors also are highly resistant to chemotherapy, limiting options for palliative treatment. However, the last two decades have seen great advances in the diagnosis of and therapy for these tumors. Advances in imaging have allowed for earlier detection and more accurate staging of disease. The safety of surgical therapy has improved and, as a consequence of increased understanding of the biology of these diseases, favorable short- and long-term results are increasingly achieved by extensive but rational resection. Palliative measures such as radiotherapy and ablative therapy have extended the limits of tumor eradication and treatment. In this chapter, a discussion of the current therapy for these hepatobiliary tumors will be presented, emphasizing the recent major advances as well as the most important areas of ongoing and future studies.

HEPATOCELLULAR CARCINOMA

HCC is the most common solid-organ tumor worldwide, being responsible for more than 1 million deaths annually. The difficulties in treating HCC and the high mortality associated with it are attributable to a number of factors. First, this cancer usually is associated with cirrhosis, which is not only a cause of morbidity but also limits treatment options for the cancer. Second, HCC is usually asymptomatic at early stages and has a great propensity for intravascular or intrabiliary extension, even when the primary tumor is small. As a result, the carcinoma is usually at an advanced stage when discovered. This tumor is, therefore, usually beyond curative therapy at presentation and, indeed, often beyond any useful therapy.

EPIDEMIOLOGY AND ETIOLOGY

At least 1 million new cases of HCC occur yearly.[1] The incidence of HCC increases with age and is four to eight times more common in men than in women.[2] This cancer is clearly associated with chronic liver injury and, therefore, geographic distribution of HCC closely mirrors that of viral hepatitis (Table 33.5-1). Countries with a high incidence of hepatitis B virus (HBV) infection—namely Taiwan, Korea, Thailand, Hong Kong, Singapore, Malaysia, China, and countries of tropical Africa—have the highest incidence of HCC.[3–5] Areas in which hepatitis C virus (HCV) infections are endemic, such as Japan and Italy, also experience an increased rate of HCC.[3,6–10] In these areas, incidence varies from a high of 150 per 100,000 in Taiwan[3] to 28 per 100,000 in Singapore.[4] Comparatively, in low-incidence areas such as Australia, North America, and Europe, HCC occurs in only 1 to 3 per 100,000 population. In high-incidence areas, HCC also occurs in younger individuals as compared to its occurrence in low incidence areas. In Mozambique, one of the areas of highest incidence of HCC, 50% of patients with the tumor are younger than 30 years. In fact, the incidence of HCC among men aged 25 to 34 years is more than 500-fold that of the same age group in Western countries.[11]

TABLE 33.5-1. Conditions Predisposing to or Associated with Development of Hepatocellular Carcinoma

INFECTIONS
Hepatitis B virus
Hepatitis C virus
CIRRHOSIS
Alcohol
Autoimmune hepatitis
Primary biliary cirrhosis
Cryptogenic cirrhosis
ENVIRONMENT
Androgenic steroid
Aflatoxins
Tobacco
N-nitrosylated compounds
Pyrrolizidine alkaloids
Thorotrast
METABOLIC DISEASES
Hemochromatosis
α_1-Antitrypsin deficiency
Wilson's disease
Porphyria cutanea tarda
Types 1 and 3 glycogen storage disease
Galactosemia
Citrullinemia
Hereditary tyrosinemia
Familial cholestatic cirrhosis

This etiologic association between HBV infection and HCC is well established. In a landmark study examining HBV infection and HCC, Beasley et al.[12] followed 22,707 male subjects in Taiwan, 15.2% of whom were HBV chronic carriers, as exhibited by detection of hepatitis B surface antigen (HB_sAg) in the serum. Of the 116 cases of HCC that occurred during a mean follow-up period of 7 years, 113 occurred in patients positive for HB_sAg. This study demonstrated that HCC was related not simply to a history of HBV infection but to the chronic carrier states and that the relative risk of developing HCC was 200-fold greater in individuals with evidence of HBV infection than in noninfected individuals.[12]

Epidemiologic evidence has also clearly linked HCV infection with HCC. Antibodies to HCV have been found in as many as 76% of patients with HCC in Japan, Italy, and Spain[13] and in

36% in the United States.[14] In contrast to HBV-associated HCC, however, HCC rarely occurs in HCV carriers before the development of cirrhosis. In addition, the incidence of HCC in cirrhotic carriers of HCV is estimated to be as high as 5% per year, as compared to 0.5% per year for HBV carriers.[15]

Chemical carcinogens also have been linked to primary liver cancers. Chemicals such as nitrites, hydrocarbons, solvents, organochlorine pesticides, primary metals, and polychlorinated biphenyls have been implicated in the development of HCC.[16] Colloidal thorium dioxide (Thorotrast), which emits high level α, β, and γ radiation and was used as an angiographic agent in the 1930s, has been linked to angiosarcoma, cholangiocarcinoma, and HCC.[1]

Of all the chemicals linked to development of HCC, the most important is ethanol. Alcohol abuse has been linked to the development of not only HCC but also carcinomas in the larynx, mouth, and esophagus. Ethanol is thought to produce HCC through development of hepatic cirrhosis or as a cocarcinogen with other agents such as HBV, HCV, hepatotoxins, and tobacco,[17–22] rather than through direct effect on the hepatocytes.

Aflatoxins produced by the fungi *Aspergillus flavus* and *Aspergillus parasiticus* have also been linked to HCC. These are fungi that grow on grains, peanuts, and other food products and are the most common cause of food spoilage in the tropics. These fungi produce aflatoxins designated as B_1, B_2, G_1, and G_2. Aflatoxin B_1 is the most hepatotoxic, and chronic exposure to these mycotoxins leads to development of HCC.[23]

Some congenital conditions also lead to development of HCC. Genetic diseases such as hemochromatosis, Wilson's disease, hereditary tyrosinemia, type 1 glycogen storage disease, hepatic porphyria of both intermittent and cutanea tarda types, familial polyposis coli, ataxia telangiectasia, familial cholestatic cirrhosis, biliary atresia, congenital hepatic fibrosis, neurofibromatosis, situs inversus, fetal alcohol syndrome, α-antitrypsin deficiency, and the Budd-Chiari syndrome[11] have all been linked to a higher incidence of HCC. Ultimately, though, the unifying etiology of HCC may be chronic injury and inflammation.

PATHOLOGIC FEATURES

HCC has been graded as well differentiated, moderately well differentiated, and poorly differentiated. The well-differentiated variety may be difficult to distinguish from a regenerating nodule on fine-needle biopsy. No firm correlation of grade to prognosis has been established. HCC can be classified generally into three different growth patterns, and these growth patterns have a much greater influence than does histologic grade on resectability and, therefore, greater influence on long-term outcome. The hanging type of tumor is attached to the normal liver by a small vascular stalk, even if the tumor is large. This type is easily excised with little loss in functional parenchyma. The pushing type generally is well demarcated and often encapsulated by a fibrous capsule. This type of tumor displaces normal vasculature rather than infiltrates and invades the major vessels. It is often resectable, even when tumor bulk is substantial. Finally, the infiltrative variety has a very indistinct tumor-liver interface and tends to exhibit a much greater degree of vascular infiltration and invasion, even when the tumor is small. Excising the infiltrative variety often is complicated by positive margins. The practical nature of this gross pathologic classification is reinforced by the distinctive radiologic appearance of these three different growth patterns on imaging.

TABLE 33.5-2. Comparison of Standard Hepatocellular Carcinoma with the Fibrolamellar Variant

Characteristic	*HCC*	*Fibrolamellar HCC*
Male-female ratio	4:1–8:1	1:1
Median age	55	25
Tumor	Invasive	Well circumscribed
Resectability	<25%	50–75%
Cirrhosis	90%	5%
AFP+	80%	5%
HepB+	65%	5%

AFP+, α-fetoprotein–positive; HCC, hepatocellular carcinoma; HepB+, hepatitis B–positive.

The most important pathologic issue is the distinct appearance and clinical behavior of the fibrolamellar variant of HCC. The contrast in clinical behavior is summarized in Table 33.5-2. On gross and radiologic inspection, fibrolamellar HCC is generally well demarcated and often encapsulated, with a central fibrotic area. It is a variant that generally occurs in young patients who lack underlying cirrhosis. α-Fetoprotein (AFP), which is commonly elevated in the usual case of HCC, is not elevated in fibrolamellar HCC. Other serum markers that often are elevated in fibrolamellar HCC include neurotensin[24] and vitamin B_{12} binding protein. The fibrolamellar variant of HCC is associated with a prolonged survival as compared with typical HCC, likely owing to the well-demarcated nature of the tumor and the greater range in treatment options for patients without underlying cirrhosis.[25]

HCC can also appear with mixed or combined features of HCC and cholangiocarcinoma. The two components of this tumor may be separate, adjacent to each other, or intimately mixed.[1,26] Biliary differentiation in HCC is associated with a poor prognosis, because such tumors are more rapidly growing and less vascular and, therefore, are more resistant to embolic therapy.[27] In the clear-cell variant of HCC, the cells have an abundant, pale, finely granular or vacuolated cytoplasm as a result of abundant glycogen, fat, or water. The prognostic importance of finding the clear-cell variant has been debated, but this subtype may be associated with a better prognosis.[28,29]

CLINICAL PRESENTATION

Even though it is generally a slow-growing tumor, the majority of HCCs present at an advanced stage, when most are beyond curative treatment. Because the liver is relatively hidden behind the right costal cartilages, tumors must reach substantial size before they are palpable. Furthermore, the large functional reserve of the liver masks any small impairment produced by local parenchymal disturbances. Therefore, small tumors are most often asymptomatic and are usually discovered during screening programs[30–32] or incidentally during imaging performed for other abdominal conditions.

Most cases of HCC are detected only when tumors are large, at a stage when local symptoms are common. Patients usually complain of a dull, right upper quadrant ache, sometimes referred to the shoulder. Hepatomegaly is a frequent accompanying finding. The liver edge is hard and irregular, due both to tumor and the usual accompanying cirrhosis. A vascular bruit can be heard in approximately 25% of cases.[33] General symptoms of malignancy, including anorexia, nausea, lethargy, and weight loss, are common. The most common clinical presentation is the triad of right upper quadrant pain, mass, and weight loss.[34–36] Central necrosis of large tumors can also lead to fever, and HCC can present as pyrexia of unknown origin. For most patients, the presentation of HCC will also be the first presentation of the underlying cirrhosis. In one study, although 90% of patients were eventually found to have cirrhosis, fewer than 10% were thought, at first evaluation for HCC, to have chronic liver disease on the basis of history and clinical examination.[35]

Hepatic decompensation is another common presentation of HCC, with patients seeking medical attention owing to typical symptoms of liver failure such as ascites, jaundice, or encephalopathy. This decompensation of liver function is most often attributable to bulk replacement of functional parenchyma in a patient with previously compensated cirrhosis. HCC has a great propensity for vascular invasion and intravascular growth. Therefore, hepatic failure may also be due to portal vein occlusion secondary to intravascular tumor thrombus.[37–39] A much rarer cause of liver failure is Budd-Chiari syndrome, resulting from direct invasion and occlusion of the hepatic vein and inferior vena cava by tumor and tumor thrombus.

Gastrointestinal bleeding often complicates the clinical course of patients with HCC and, in 10% of patients, is the presenting finding.[39] In approximately one-half of these cases, bleeding is from esophageal varices,[39] which can result from portal hypertension due to cirrhosis alone or with an added contribution of intraportal thrombus. Patients with gastrointestinal bleeding from esophageal varices have an extraordinarily poor prognosis, with a median survival measurable in weeks.[38] The particularly poor prognosis of variceal bleeding complicating HCC is due to the common finding of intraportal thrombus, which further increases the portal pressure and makes control of bleeding varices more difficult. In fact, in one study, nearly one-fourth of patients with HCC died from massive variceal hemorrhage.[37] Gastrointestinal bleeding can occur from other causes as well, such as benign peptic ulcer or direct invasion of the gastrointestinal tract by tumor.[39]

The most dramatic presentation of HCC is tumor rupture, which is the initial presentation in 2% to 5% of patients with HCC.[40–45] Patients present with acute abdominal pain and swelling and are found to have, in addition to swelling, guarding, rebound tenderness, and ileus. Patients also commonly have signs of hemodynamic instability or overt hypovolemic shock. Diagnosis is confirmed by findings of either tumor mass or peritoneal blood through imaging, laparotomy, or paracentesis.[44,46,47]

Jaundice as a presenting symptom of HCC occurs in up to one-half of all patients. The most common cause of the jaundice is hepatic parenchymal insufficiency.[34,48–50] On rare occasions (<10% of jaundiced patients), jaundice associated with HCC results from biliary obstruction.[34,51–56] The biliary obstruction can occur from intraluminal tumor, from hemobilia, or from extraluminal bile duct obstruction. In the clinical evaluation of jaundice in a patient with HCC, it is enormously important to distinguish hepatocellular failure from obstruction. The former usually indicates that the patient is beyond any therapeutic benefit, whereas the latter can be treated, often with good palliation and even potential cure.[53,54,57–61]

Rarely (<5% of cases), HCC can present with paraneoplastic syndromes owing to hormonal or immune effects of the tumors.[62] The most important of these syndromes are hypoglycemia, erythrocytosis, hypercalcemia, and hypercholesterolemia. Porphyria cutanea tarda, virilization and feminization syndromes, carcinoid syndrome, hypertrophic osteoarthropathy, hyperthyroidism, and osteoporosis can also occur.[63–65]

DIAGNOSTIC INVESTIGATIONS

For patients suspected of suffering from HCC, the aims of diagnostic investigations are (1) verification of diagnosis, (2) determination of extent of disease, (3) determination of functional liver reserve, and (4) assessment of biologic determinants that affect long-term prognosis.

Verification of Diagnosis

Diagnosis of HCC can usually be positively established noninvasively by a combination of history, physical assessment, imaging, and blood tests. There is little diagnostic doubt in a patient with a liver mass consistent with an HCC visible on computed tomography (CT) or magnetic resonance imaging (MRI) and a serum AFP of more than 500 ng/dL. This combination is diagnostic, and treatment can be instituted without tissue diagnosis. The presence of cirrhosis or hepatitis infection, as documented by presence of HB_sAg or HCV virus in the blood, is further confirmation.

In the patient with a space-occupying lesion on ultrasonography (US) or CT and a nondiagnostic AFP level, the role of a percutaneous needle biopsy often is debated. There is no doubt that needle biopsy is diagnostic for HCC. However, complications are also not infrequent. Hemorrhage or tumor rupture can occur. Furthermore, there is also a small but finite risk of tumor spillage and seeding of the needle biopsy tract.[66] In cases of potentially resectable HCC, where the diagnostic certainty is high, we would proceed to surgical exploration without tumor biopsy. Indeed, in this clinical scenario, the histologic appearance of the nonneoplastic liver may have a greater impact on surgical planning. If advanced cirrhosis will preclude safe resection, we often perform a biopsy the portion of the liver that does not contain tumor, for histologic evaluation.

In patients with a nondiagnostic AFP level who are not surgical candidates and, therefore, are not candidates for curative therapy, tumor biopsy is performed if the patients are candidates for palliative therapy. In that case, fine-needle aspiration for cytologic evaluation is usually performed in preference to core-needle biopsy for histology, as comparative studies indicate that smear cytology yielded a much higher percentage of correct diagnoses as compared to microhistology (86% vs. 66%).[67] Patients who are not candidates for palliative therapy do not need a definitive diagnosis, and biopsy is discouraged.

Determination of Extent of Disease

The two issues to be resolved by the extent-of-disease evaluation are whether the disease is isolated to the liver and whether distribution of tumor in the liver is amenable to surgical excision. The most common sites of metastases of HCC include lung, peritoneum, adrenal gland, and bone. Hence, chest radiography is mandatory. Cross-sectional imaging, such as CT or

MRI, of the abdomen should be scrutinized for peritoneal and adrenal sites of disease. Many centers consider bone scans mandatory prior to liver resection. Certainly, in patients with pain attributable to bony metastases, a bone scan should be performed. A finding of extrahepatic disease changes the prognosis of the patients greatly, as such a finding precludes the possibility of hepatectomy as curative therapy.

The extent of liver involvement usually is determined by CT scanning. This diagnostic imaging modality is widely available and relatively inexpensive. In interpreting any cross-sectional imaging modality for the patient with HCC, the number and distribution of liver tumors must be determined, as well as the degree of vascular invasion. In this regard, triple-phase (non–contrast-enhanced, arterial phase, and portal phase) CT images should be obtained. HCCs are generally highly vascular tumors, and tumors on images with contrast enhancement may become isodense with the surrounding liver. Tumors sometimes are visible only during the non–contrast-enhanced phase. Because HCC has a great propensity for vascular invasion and extension, tumor thrombus in the portal vein, hepatic vein, or vena cava is not unusual. Scans should therefore be scrutinized for evidence of such invasion, as therapy and prognosis can be altered significantly by such findings. If such invasion is suspected but not proven by CT, Doppler US or MRI is indicated.

At some centers, hepatic angiography is standard.[68,69] Some have even advocated routine use of iodized oil (Lipiodol) injected angiographically to delineate hepatic extent of disease further.[70] This lipid is preferentially retained in HCC because of the particle size. These angiographic methods are highly sensitive for the presence of tumor. Nonetheless, with current helical CT or MRI, there is only minor incremental yield. We rely on angiography only when we suspect small tumors not visible by conventional cross-sectional imaging, such as for a patient with small amounts of disease seen on CT who has a very high AFP level.

Assessment of the Patient's General Condition and Hepatic Functional Reserve

In the evaluation of patients for possible hepatectomy, cardiopulmonary assessment should be conducted as for any major procedure. Patients older than 65 years or patients with a history or symptoms consistent with cardiopulmonary disease should be referred for formal medical preoperative evaluation.

Assessment of baseline liver function and assessment of complications of cirrhosis are paramount in the process of determining the optimal treatment option for each patient. Recovery from liver resection is reliant on the capacity of the liver to regenerate. The cirrhotic liver often has a reduced capacity for regeneration. In addition, cirrhosis and portal hypertension often are associated with derangements in hepatic production of coagulation factors and with thrombocytopenia, which explains the increased risk of liver failure and bleeding after resection for HCC. Indeed, the complication rate after ablative therapies is increased proportionate to the degree of liver dysfunction.[71,72] Consequently, many clinical and laboratory methods have been devised for determining the level of risk for various therapies.

SERUM LIVER FUNCTION TESTS AND CLINICAL ASSESSMENT. Various liver function tests, alone or in combination, have been touted as useful for predicting risks of liver resection and other treatments for HCC. Various single serum measures of liver function have been suggested to be useful predictors of perioperative outcome, including serum bilirubin[73] and serum alanine aminotransferase.[74] A doubling of bilirubin has been suggested as a contraindication for liver resection.[73] Other investigators have deemed a platelet count of fewer than 50,000 or a prolonged prothrombin time (>4 seconds over control) as a relative contraindication for hepatic resection.[75] Most investigators, however, have not relied on a single parameter but rather have used a combination of clinical and biochemical parameters to gauge safety of hepatectomy and other treatments. In this regard, the most clinically useful system is the Pugh-Child's classification, which is a point-scoring system for evaluation of liver function based on the levels of serum bilirubin, coagulation profile, serum albumin, presence or absence of ascites and encephalopathy, and nutritional status (Table 33.5-3).[76,77] Functionally well-compensated cirrhosis is classified as Pugh-Child's classification grade A; decompensating cirrhosis is grade B; and decompensated cirrhosis is grade C. Generally, partial hepatectomy is offered only to patients who are Pugh-Child's grade A and to the most favorable grade B patients.[78] In general, Pugh-Child's grade C patients are offered only supportive care, as even nonsurgical ablative methods, such as embolization, are associated with procedure-related mortality in one-third of patients.[71]

TABLE 33.5-3. Pugh's Modification of Child's Grading of Cirrhosis

Measurement	*1 Point*	*2 Points*	*3 Points*
Bilirubin (mg/dL)	1–1.9	2–2.9	>2.9
Prothrombin time prolongation (sec)	1–3	4–6	>6
Albumin (g/dL)	>3.5	2.8–3.4	<2.8
Ascites	None	Mild	Moderate to severe
Encephalopathy	None	Grade 1 or 2	Grade 3 or 4

Note: Pugh-Child's grade A, 5–6 points; B, 7–9 points; C, 10–15 points.

DYNAMIC TESTS. Many sophisticated dynamic measures of liver function have also been used in attempts to quantitate hepatic function. Investigators have attempted to use elimination of certain dyes that are exclusively cleared by the liver, such as bromsulfophthalein or indocyanine green, as measures of hepatic function. Galactose clearance or [^{14}C]aminopyrine clearance has also been used to evaluate the specific metabolic capacity of the liver. Of these, the most commonly used evaluative modalities in clinical practice are indocyanine green retention at 15 minutes[79] and the [^{14}C]aminopyrine breath test,[80] though controversy still exists concerning their usefulness.[81] We do not use these tests on a routine basis in our care of the patient with HCC but have found the clinical Pugh-Child's classification sufficiently discriminatory for selecting patients for therapies.

PORTAL PRESSURES AND BLOOD FLOW. Another relatively simple test that may be predictive of perioperative outcome is the hepatic venous wedge pressure. By passing a venous catheter through the vena cava into the hepatic vein, the hepatic venous pressure can be directly ascertained. By balloon occlusion of the hepatic vein, the hepatic venous wedge pressure, which is a reflec-

TABLE 33.5-4. Treatment Options for Hepatocellular Carcinoma

POTENTIALLY CURATIVE OPTIONS
Partial hepatectomy
Total hepatectomy with orthotopic liver transplantation
PALLIATIVE TREATMENTS
Regional therapies
Ablative therapies: cytoreductive therapies
Palliative resection
Cryosurgery
Microwave ablation
Ethanol injection
Acetic acid injection
Hepatic artery transcatheter treatments
Transarterial chemotherapy
Transarterial embolization
Transarterial chemoembolization
Transarterial radioembolization
^{90}Y microspheres
Lipiodol ^{131}I
Conformal radiation
Systemic therapies
Chemotherapy
Immunotherapy
Hormonal therapy
SUPPORTIVE CARE

tion of the portal pressure, can be determined. These measurements have been touted as useful in segregating Pugh-Child's grade B patients who may have favorable results from resection from those likely to experience major complications.[82]

POTENTIALLY CURATIVE TREATMENTS

Therapies for HCC can be separated into resection, ablation, radiotherapy, systemic chemotherapy or immunotherapy, and supportive care (Table 33.5-4). Resectional therapy represents the only potentially curative option.

Partial Hepatectomy

Partial hepatectomy represents the most common procedure for treatment of HCC performed with curative intent. The liver is normally a very resilient organ with remarkable regenerative capacity. In a noncirrhotic liver, routine recovery can be expected even after resection of more than two-thirds of the functional parenchyma.[83] In the United States, nearly one-half the patients with HCC will have no associated cirrhosis.[84] For patients with no cirrhosis, operative mortality at most major centers is generally less than 5%, and very extensive procedures are justified by the low risk and the potential for long-term survival and cure. Resection is associated with a 5-year survival in more than 30% of patients.[85–89] For a patient without cirrhosis, partial hepatectomy is a relatively safe procedure and is the treatment of choice for eradication of HCC (Table 33.5-5).

Worldwide, however, most cases of HCC are associated with cirrhosis, which greatly increases the risk for partial hepatectomy (see Table 33.5-5). This increase in risk is due in part to intraoperative factors. These patients will usually have rigid and hard parenchyma and established varices that are difficult to manipulate and are prone to bleeding. In addition, such patients will have thrombocytopenia and coagulation defects that further exacerbate the risk of hemorrhage. Postoperatively, the liver may not regenerate, resulting in liver failure. Furthermore, postoperative exaggeration of portal hypertension may lead to ascites and variceal bleeds. It is understandable, therefore, that resection is associated with increased morbidity and mortality in these patients. Even for a cirrhotic patient with well-compensated liver function, we are reluctant to remove more than 20% to 25% of the functional parenchyma.[81,89–92] Until recently, even at centers with a low mortality for partial hepatectomy in the noncirrhotic population, partial hepatectomy for patients with cirrhosis was associated with a 10% mortality or higher (see Table 33.5-5).[85,86,93–95] This explains the nihilistic view adopted by some for this disease, as well as the interest in treating this disease by total hepatectomy and liver transplantation. Nevertheless, even now, cirrhotic patients who survive the operation have a 5-year survival of approximately 30% (Table 33.5-6).[85–89,93–95] Over the last decade, a number of series have demonstrated increasing safety of partial hepatectomy in cirrhotic patients (see Table 33.5-5). The mortality at most major centers treating HCC has been reduced to the 5% level, owing to improvements in patient selection, perioperative support, and surgical technique.[84,96–98]

Patient selection for surgery depends first and foremost on hepatic function. As discussed earlier, in Serum Liver Function Tests and Clinical Assessment, the most commonly used clinical selection criteria for patient's fitness for surgery relies on the Pugh-Child's score. Few surgeons are willing to perform hepatic resection for patients with a Pugh-Child's grade C liver status. Most surgeons will consider resection only for patients with Pugh-Child's grade A liver functional reserve and the best Pugh-Child's grade B patients.

The major changes in operative conduct that have improved perioperative outcome include a willingness to use inflow occlusion during resection and a willingness to accept nonanatomic resection. Temporary occlusion of the hepatic artery and portal vein during liver resection by clamping the gastrohepatic ligament has been a useful technique for reducing blood loss during hepatectomy for patients with no cirrhosis.[99] In the past, surgeons have been reluctant to use such inflow occlusion, called the *Pringle maneuver*, in cirrhotic patients because of fears that cirrhotic parenchyma will not tolerate the transient ischemia. Recent studies have indicated that the reluctance to use this technique was largely unfounded and that cirrhotic liver can tolerate a Pringle maneuver for more than 30 minutes.[100,101] The most important change in operative technique, however, is a willingness to use limited, nonanatomic resections. For patients with no cirrhosis, most major centers adhere to the anatomic boundaries of the various segments during liver resection for cancer. Lobectomies, sectorectomies, and segmentectomies are preferred over wedge and other nonanatomic resections because limited resections are more likely to result in a positive microscopical margin.[102] In the cirrhotic liver, however, a smaller resection margin is acceptable if it will reduce the chance of postoperative liver failure. The smallest resection that will remove all gross tumor is generally used at most centers.

TABLE 33.5-5. Operative Mortality as Related to Liver Cirrhosis

Study	*No. of Cases*	*Cirrhosis (%)*	*Mortality (%)*	*Comments*
Noncirrhotic patients				
Mnegchao et al., 1980[85]	55	0	2	—
Tsuzuki et al., 1990[86]	39	0	3	—
Chen et al., 1989[87]	65	0	2	—
Bagasue et al., 1993[88]	52	0	6	—
Vauthey et al., 1995[89]	70	0	1	—
Bismuth et al., 1995[503]	68	0	3	—
Mixed patients				
Kishi et al., 1983[504]	57	39.4	11	—
Lee et al., 1986[505]	109	40.4	3	—
Kanematsu et al., 1988[506]	121	80	12	—
Lai et al., 1991[507]	39	84.6	8	Small HCC
Nagasue et al., 1993[91]	229	77	7	—
Hemming et al., 1993[79,508]	50	26	0.5	Segmental resection
Fan et al., 1994[509]	124	31.5	11	—
Chen et al., 1994[510]	205	49.8	4	Large HCC
Lai et al., 1995[511]	149	69	22	Before 1987
	128	78	15	1987–1991
	66	74	6	1992–1995
Kawasaki et al., 1995[98]	112	67.9	1	—
Takenaka et al., 1996[512]	280	52	2	—
Nadig et al., 1997[513]	71	24	21	—
Cirrhotic patients				
Liver Study Group of Japan, 1980[93]	153	100	30	—
Nagao et al., 1987[94]	72	100	19	—
Mnegchao et al., 1980[85]	126	100	12	—
Kanematsu et al., 1984[95]	50	100	12	—
Franco et al., 1990[514]	72	100	7	—
Tsuzuki et al., 1990[86]	119	100	13	—
Chen et al., 1989[87]	55	100	7	—
Bagasue et al., 1993[88]	177	100	12	—
Capussotti et al., 1994[97]	33	100	6	—
Vauthey et al., 1995[89]	30	100	14	—
Fuster et al., 1996[96]	48	100	4	—

HCC, hepatocellular carcinoma.

As safety of resections has improved, reports of increasingly large experiences in the treatment of HCC provide long-term results that allow for analysis of prognostic factors that influence long-term outcome. Many factors that previously were thought to be contraindications to surgical resection have not been substantiated by data. It is now clear that multiple lesions do not preclude surgical resection[88,89]: Five-year survival in patients resected of multiple tumors is expected to be between 24%[89] and 28%.[88] Presentation with intraductal tumor and obstructive jaundice also does not preclude long-term survival after surgical resection.[86] Therefore, distinguishing biliary obstruction from hepatic insufficiency as the cause for jaundice is very important in a patient who presents with HCC and jaundice. Finally, synchronous direct invasion of adjacent organs such as the diaphragm by HCC is not an absolute contraindication to resectional surgery.[103,104]

One group that has a particularly poor prognosis is patients with major intravascular extension of tumor. Even though tumor thrombus can be treated with liver resection and thrombus extraction, the risk of disseminated disease is extremely high in these patients.[105] If the tumor thrombus involves the vena cava or main portal vein, liver resections accompanied by venous tumor thrombectomies are unlikely to result in long-term survival.

Neoadjuvant Treatment of Tumors

Many groups have attempted to treat HCC with local or systemic therapies prior to attempts at surgical resection. The rationale for such neoadjuvant therapies is that large primary tumors may be sufficiently reduced in bulk to make resection safer and that local and systemic microscopic disease may be reduced or eradicated, thereby improving long-term outcome. In this regard, methods that have been employed to achieve these goals include transarterial chemoembolization,[106,107] combined chemotherapy [doxorubicin (Adriamycin) and 5-fluorouracil (5-FU)] and radiotherapy (2100 cGy),[103] hepatic artery infusion of chemotherapeutic agents, radioimmunotherapy, fractionated regional radiotherapy,[108] and transarterial ^{90}Y microspheres.[109]

TABLE 33.5-6. Survival Rates after Liver Resection for Hepatocellular Carcinoma

Study	No. of Cases	Survival (%) 1-Y	2-Y	3-Y	5-Y	10-Y	Comments
Kanematsu et al., 1984[95]	37	80	60	—	33	—	Limited resection
	13	79	68	—	23	—	Major resection
Okuda et al., 1984[516]	98	62	43	34	—	—	—
Hsu et al., 1985[517]	49	96	91	—	—	—	HCC <5 cm
	49	63	51	—	—	—	HCC >5 cm
Lee et al., 1986[505]	109	84	72	—	—	—	—
Nagao et al., 1987[94]	94	58	—	33	20	—	—
Kanematsu et al., 1988[506]	107	83	—	51	26	—	—
Franco et al., 1990[514]	72	68	55	51	—	—	100% cirrhosis
Yamanaka et al., 1990[519]	295	76	—	44	31	—	—
LCSG, Japan 1990[93]	2174	67	—	40	29	—	—
Ringe et al., 1991[521]	131	68	54	42	36	—	—
Lai et al., 1991[507]	39	59	—	28	11	—	HCC <5 cm
Sasaki et al., 1992[522]	186	—	—	—	44	—	Cirrhotic
	57	—	—	—	68	—	Noncirrhotic
Nagasue et al., 1993[91]	229	80	—	51.3	26	19	—
Ouchi et al., 1993[523]	47	89	—	65	43	—	—
Takenaka et al., 1994[524]	229	89	—	76	76	—	<70 y
	39	87	—	70	52	—	>70 y
Suenaga et al., 1994[525]	134	100	—	88	68	—	—
Capussotti et al., 1994[97]	33	66	43	37	—	—	Large HCC
Bismuth et al., 1995[503]	68	74	—	52	40	26	Noncirrhotic
Lai et al., 1995[511]	343	60	—	33	24	—	1987–1991
Vauthey et al., 1995[89]	106	—	—	—	41	—	—
Kawasaki et al., 1995[98]	112	92	—	79	—	—	—
Fuster et al., 1996[96]	48	—	—	64	—	—	—
Takenaka et al., 1996[512]	280	88	—	70	50	—	—
Nadig et al., 1997[513]	71	—	—	—	20	—	—
Fong et al., 1999[84]	154	80	—	51	39	—	67% cirrhosis

HCC, hepatocellular carcinoma; LCSG, Liver Cancer Study Group.

Another form of preoperative treatment is immunoembolization. Neoadjuvant transarterial immmunoembolization (TIE) was tested with OK-432, a *Streptococcus* preparation. In a comparison of 22 patients who underwent TIE versus transarterial embolization (TAE) alone, the 1- and 2-year disease-free survival rates after resection were 85% and 85% for TIE and 62% and 56% for TAE, respectively.[110] Lygidakis and Tsiliakos[111] randomized 91 patients with HCC to resection alone or to resection with neoadjuvant chemoembolization and immunotherapy. Of 20 patients, 2 had preoperative complete necrosis of tumor as a consequence of preoperative therapy. Overall, survival was 18 months for resection alone and 36 months for the group receiving chemoembolization.

Promising data have recently emerged from studies of neoadjuvant use of systemic chemoimmunotherapy consisting of cisplatin, 5-FU, Adriamycin, and interferon-α (IFN-α).[112] In a regimen modified from that initially suggested by Patt et al.,[113] Leung et al.[112] were able to produce objective response in tumors believed not to be resectable and converted one-fourth of these tumors to resectability. Whether preoperative use of this regimen by Leung et al.[112] would help to select the patients most favorably treated with resection and whether continuing such chemotherapy as adjuvant therapy after resection will improve long-term outcome await prospective studies. Overall, though, each of these studies consisted of only a few patients and, though such neoadjuvant therapy seems promising, a definitive role for any of these treatments in a neoadjuvant setting has not been unequivocally demonstrated.

An alterative neoadjuvant approach that attempts to improve outcome of resections involves embolization of the portal vein nourishing the side of the liver to be removed. Compensatory preoperative hypertrophy of the side of the liver not involved by the tumor will ensue and potentially allows a safer hepatic resection.[114] Whether such theoretic advantage is sustained by clinical data awaits prospective randomized trials.

Adjuvant Therapy

Though up to one-third of patients can expect to remain disease-free long after hepatectomy for HCC, the majority will experience recurrence, indicating the presence of microscopic residual disease at the time of liver resection.[115–117] This explains the keen interest in developing adjuvant therapy directed at microscopic residual disease.

In a study from China, 61 patients with resected HCC were randomized to no further therapy or postoperative hepatic infusion of Lipiodol and cisplatin with systemic epirubicin. The treated group seemed to have a higher extrahepatic recurrence and a worse outcome.[118] Another study of 57 patients with resected HCC randomized to hepatic arterial infusion and systemic epirubicin versus no further treatment again demonstrated no difference in overall and disease-free survival.[119]

Though transarterial chemoembolization is used extensively for the treatment of unresectable disease, randomized studies have not supported the use of this modality in the adjuvant setting. In fact, in three different studies, survival has been worse for those treated with chemoembolization after resection.[120–122] To date, no study has demonstrated that any systemic chemotherapy or immunotherapy improves survival after hepatectomy for HCC.

Two positive randomized trials of adjuvant therapy after resection for HCC have been reported. The first involves the use of the retinoid derivative polyprenoic acid, which had been shown to inhibit hepatocarcinogenesis in rodents.[123] In a study randomizing patients, after curative resection or PEI for HCC, to receiving either polyprenoic acid or placebo, significantly higher numbers of patients receiving placebo developed additional HCC. Currently, polyprenoic acid is not available in the United States, but these data encourage further study of this and other retinoid derivatives in adjuvant treatment for HCC and in chemoprevention for patients at high risk for developing HCC.

The other positive adjuvant study involved the use of radioembolization employing transarterial delivery of ^{131}I-labeled Lipiodol. This compound has demonstrated significant activity against small HCCs, but problems with dosimetry have limited its use for patients with bulky unresectable disease. In a prospective, randomized study, Lau et al.[124] compared 21 patients who received 50 mCi of transarterial ^{131}I-Lipiodol within 6 weeks of liver resection for HCC with 22 patients receiving no adjuvant therapy. The 3-year survival rates for the treated group and the control group were 85% and 46%, respectively. These results await multicenter studies to confirm with bigger numbers not only the long-term cancer results but also the feasibility of using such radioembolization methods in diverse centers.

Total Hepatectomy and Liver Transplantation

From a theoretic standpoint, total hepatectomy and liver transplantation is the most attractive treatment for HCC. This treatment allows for removal of the liver cancer with the widest margin possible. It also allows for removal of diseased parenchyma that may contain microscopic metastatic disease as well as parenchyma that may be predisposed to formation of second primary tumors. A number of studies have attempted to define the biologic parameters predicting good long-term outcome after liver transplantation. The best results are seen in patients with fibrolamellar histology and in patients with small incidental tumors found unexpectedly within the explanted liver. Characteristics associated with poor long-term outcome include advanced stage, the presence of a margin involved by tumor, large tumors, multiple tumors, microscopic or macroscopic vascular invasion, and bilobar disease.[125,126] Patients with tumors smaller than 5 cm have a mean survival of 55 months,

TABLE 33.5-7. Results of Liver Transplantation for Hepatocellular Carcinoma

Study	*No. of Cases*	*Operative Mortality (%)*	*Survival (%)* 1-Y	3-Y	5-Y
O'Grady et al., 1988[129]	50	23	40	—	—
Ringe et al., 1989[526]	52	15	—	37	—
Yokoyama et al., 1990[127]	80	13	64	45	45
Iwatsuki et al., 1991[527]	71	NR	—	43	—
Pichlmayr et al., 1992[528]	87	24	—	—	20
Haug et al., 1992[128]	24	17	71	42	—
Moreno-Gonzalez et al., 1992[529]	12	0	80	16	—
Bismuth et al., 1993[530]	60	5	—	49	—
Romani et al., 1994[531]	27	11	82	71	—
Chung et al., 1994[532]	29	14	61	46	—
Dalgic et al., 1994[533]	39	NR	56	32	26
Farmer et al., 1994[139]	44	17	71	42	—
Tan et al., 1995[132]	15	7	—	63	—
Selby et al., 1995[125]	105	NR	66	39	36
Pichlmayr et al., 1995[528]	36	19	57	31	27
Schwartz et al., 1995[130]	57	0	72	57	—
Mazzaferro et al., 1996[131]	48	6%	75 at 4 y	—	—

NR, not reported.

whereas those with tumors larger than 5 cm have a mean survival of only 24 months.[127,128] Therefore, most transplantation centers will not consider patients with tumors larger than 5 cm for transplantation. Currently, at most centers, only patients with fewer than three tumors, all smaller than 5 cm, and with no main portal vein or vena caval involvement are considered for liver transplantation.

In clinical practice, however, biology of the cancer is not the most important determinant of the usefulness of transplantation. Liver transplantation is associated with substantial morbidity and mortality (Table 33.5-7). Series from the 1980s and early 1990s often report mortality rates as high as 10% to 20%.[129] Though some recent series have reported much-improved perioperative mortality (see Table 33.5-7),[130–132] the morbidity is still substantial. In patients with liver dysfunction in either the Pugh-Child's grade B or C categories, however, total hepatectomy with liver transplantation represents the only potentially curative option.

The greatest obstacle is the limited availability of livers for transplantation. Even in the United States, where active public campaigns have resulted in comparatively high rates of organ donations for transplantation, only 3000 to 4000 livers are available each year. This would explain the limited numbers of livers used in transplantation for treatment of liver cancers. Only approximately 100 transplantations are performed each year for this indication (Fig. 33.5-1). In countries in the Far East, where organ donation goes against social and religious beliefs, the shortage of donated organs is even greater. Living-relative liver transplants offer a potential source of organs for such use.[133,134] However, the morbidity associated with donation of a lobe of liver is substantial, and mortality is not only a

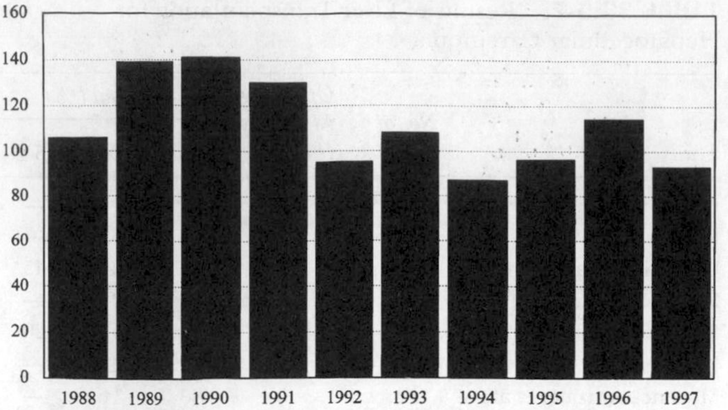

FIGURE 33.5-1. Number of liver transplantations performed each year in the United States for cancer. Use of liver transplantation for this indication is greatly limited by the shortage of organs. (Data from UNOS.)

theoretic but a documented actual complication. For patients with cancer, the likelihood of recurrence brings into question the ethics of endangering a donor's life.

In addition, the costs of liver transplantation are substantial. Certainly, it is much more cost-effective to use available livers for the treatment of benign diseases. In many parts of the world, however, the high costs completely rule out transplantation for any indication. Because of these obstacles, liver transplantation is not likely to make an important impact on the worldwide treatment of cancer in the near future.

Comparing results of partial hepatectomy with results of liver transplantation for HCC has been difficult, primarily because patients with very distinct clinical characteristics are usually selected for each treatment. Patients selected for partial hepatectomy generally have good liver function and may have enormous tumors. Patients selected for transplantation almost always have small tumors but may have advanced liver failure. In the past, the reported 1-, 3-, and 5-year survival rates of liver transplantation for HCC were 40% to 82%, 16% to 71%, and 19.6% to 36%, respectively, rates that were highly comparable to those achieved with partial hepatectomy (see Table 33.5-7). This indicated not so much that these two techniques were equivalent as that the right patients were being selected for each treatment.

Recently, two series of studies have encouraged a renewed comparison of these two treatment options. In a series from the transplantation literature, operative mortality appears to have been dramatically reduced to a current low of less than 5%.[126,130–132] With such low operative mortality, Mazzaferro et al.[131] are reporting 3-year survival after transplantation of 85% for small HCC. This has fueled enthusiasm for liver transplantation in this clinical setting. At the same time, a number of articles examining partial hepatectomy for HCC have been published that include sufficient data in the subset of patients with small tumors to allow comparison.[84,135] It appears that partial hepatectomy for patients with small tumors also results in very favorable outcomes. For a patient with a tumor that is less than 5 cm in diameter, the 5-year survival can be expected to be 45% to 57%.[84,135,136] In fact, disease-free survival can be expected in 44% of patients (Fig. 33.5-2).[84] These results are comparable to the best results for liver transplantation. Therefore, given the organ shortage and costs of liver transplantation, partial hepatectomy should still be regarded as the

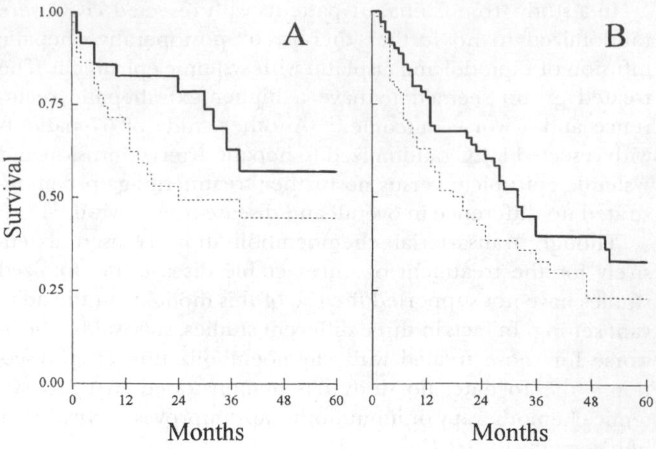

FIGURE 33.5-2. Survival (*solid line*) and disease-free survival (*dotted line*) after resection of **(A)** small (<5 cm) or **(B)** large (>10 cm) hepatocellular carcinoma. Results of resection for these small tumors are highly favorable and comparable to liver transplantation. (From ref. 84, with permission.)

curative treatment of choice. For patients without cirrhosis or with Pugh-Child's grade A cirrhosis, partial hepatectomy should be considered first. Total hepatectomy with transplantation may be necessary in this group if removal of tumor requires extensive resection of nonneoplastic liver. For patients with severe liver dysfunction, total hepatectomy and transplantation is a better option and may be the only viable option.

Because the incidence of recurrence of HCC after liver transplantation is high, many investigators have attempted to improve long-term results by use of adjuvant therapies. Cherqui et al.[137] used an adjuvant regimen combining neoadjuvant chemoembolization and radiotherapy with posttransplantation chemotherapy. Stone et al.[138] used a regimen of aggressive neoadjuvant, intraoperative, and postoperative chemotherapy. Farmer et al.[139] used an adjuvant chemotherapeutic regimen combining 5-FU, cisplatin, and doxorubicin. These are all small studies based on a sound understanding of HCC and represent promising approaches. All use neoadjuvant therapy because patients often spend a considerable amount of time awaiting availability of a liver for transplantation. However, given the small number of transplantations performed yearly for HCC, the role, timing, and regimens to be used are far from decided.

PALLIATIVE TREATMENT MODALITIES

Most patients presenting with HCC will have disease that is not treatable by partial hepatectomy. Even if the disease is confined to the liver, the likelihood of treatment with total hepatectomy and transplantation is low for reasons outlined in the preceding section, Total Hepatectomy and Liver Transplantation. Nevertheless, if the disease is confined completely or largely to the liver, local tumor ablative therapies can be performed and result in good local control of disease. The ablative methods with the longest track record include ethanol injection, embolization, and cryotherapy. These will be discussed with specific emphasis on technical limitations, morbidity, and their likely role in patient clinical management. Other more investigative modalities, such as radiotherapy, radiofrequency ablation, and laser heat ablation, also are discussed.

TABLE 33.5-8. Systemic Chemotherapy for Hepatocellular Carcinoma

Study	*No.*	*Treatment*	*Partial Response (%)*	*Stable Disease (%)*
Leung[534]	50	Cisplatin, doxorubicin, 5-FU + IFN	13 (26)	10 (20)
O'Reilly[535]	7	CPT-11	1	2 (29)
Umsawasdi[536]	13	5-FU, mitomycin C	5 (38)	NR
Vogel[537]	41	Doxorubicin	7 (17)	9 (29)
Baker[538]	38	Doxorubicin + 5-FU	5 (13)	NR
Ravey[539]	26	Doxorubicin + bleomycin	5 (19)	8 (31)
Okada[540]	27	Cisplatin, mitoxantrone, CI + 5-FU	9 (33)	16 (59)
Patt[113]	20	Cisplatin, doxorubicin, 5-FU + IFN	2 (10)	10 (50)
Zanibone[541]	14	Vitamin K	0	4 (29)
Noy[542]	20	FUDR, doxorubicin + IFN	4 (10)	NR
Benson[543]	25	Eniluracil + 5-FU	0	6 (24)
Cheng[168]	33	Etoposide + tamoxifen	8 (24)	NS
Bobbio-Pallavicini[169]	36	Epirubicin + etoposide	14 (39)	11 (30)
Strumberg[544]	16	Paclitaxel	1 (6)	9 (56)
Chao[545]	20	Paclitaxel	0	5 (25)
Stuart[546]	10	5-FU + IFN	0	NR
Mani[547]	16	UFT + LV	0	3 (19)
Gebbia[548]	50	5-FU + LV + hydroxyurea	5 (10)	15 (30)
Chlebowski[549]	157	Doxorubicin	17 (11)	NR
Falkson[550]	25	Neocarzinostatin	2 (8)	NR
Melia[551]	44	VP-16	7 (16)	NR
Falkson[552]	35	Cisplatin	6 (17)	NR
Ji[553]	30	Cisplatin + IFN	4 (13)	NR
Falkson[552]	35	Mitoxantrone	0	NR

CI, continuous infusion; CPT-11, irinotecan; 5-FU, 5-fluorouracil; FUDR, fluorouridine; IFN, interferon; NR, not reported; NS, not significant; LV, leucovorin; UFT, uracil + tegafur; VP-16, etoposide.

Systemic Therapies

When a patient has widely disseminated disease, only systemic therapies make sense. However, the results of chemotherapeutic therapy or other systemic therapies for HCC have been dismal.

SYSTEMIC CHEMOTHERAPY. Numerous chemotherapeutic regimens have been tested for use against HCC (Table 33.5-8). HCC is, however, highly resistant to chemotherapy, owing to multiple factors: Tissue analysis has revealed that HCC harbors high levels of dehydropyrimidine dehydronase (DPD), and it is known that cells high in DPD are generally resistant to 5-FU.[140] In addition, HCC exhibits overexpression of the MDR1 (multidrug resistance) gene[141,142] and the gene product P glycoprotein.[141] This would explain the modest effects of 5-FU on HCC. In an Eastern Cooperative Oncology Group (ECOG) study of eniluracil (a DPD inhibitor) and 5-FU, 5 of 35 patients with HCC developed stable disease but no responses.

Doxorubicin is the most popular drug studied, though published data from 13 studies indicate that administration of this drug either alone or in combinations results in less than a 20% response and a median survival of less than 4 months.[143,144] Response to either single agent or multiagent systemic chemotherapy occurs in only 10% to 20% of patients (see Table 33.5-8). Furthermore, even the objective responses are short-lasting. In a systemic review[145] and metaanalysis[146] of the published randomized studies on HCC, neither doxorubicin nor any chemotherapeutic agent used singly or in combination has been shown to have any survival benefit for HCC patients. It is generally acknowledged that systemic chemotherapy has minimal impact on survival of patients with this disease. At our institution, systemic chemotherapy is offered mostly in the context of clinical trials. Moreover, most patients with unresectable disease are jaundiced or have a poor performance status because of extensive liver disease, making use of chemotherapeutic drugs virtually impossible.

HEPATIC ARTERIAL INFUSION. Because the results with systemic chemotherapy are far from optimal, regional delivery of chemotherapy has been attempted. Such regional approaches rely on the dual nutrient blood supply of the liver, portal vein, and hepatic artery. Hepatic tumors, however, derive their blood supply mainly from the hepatic artery.[147,148] Infusion of chemotherapy directly into the hepatic artery may allow increased effective dose at the tumor with fewer systemic side effects.

Hepatic arterial infusion (HAI) chemotherapy can be accomplished through a percutaneously placed angiographic catheter, through an implantable arterial port inserted at open operation and connected to an external infusion pump, or using self-contained subcutaneous infusion pumps implanted at surgery. Drugs with high liver extraction rates and short plasma half-lives are particularly well suited for HAI chemotherapy.[149] The fluoropyrimidines [5-FU and 5-fluorodeoxyuridine (5-FUDR)], cisplatin, doxorubicin, and 4'-epidoxorubicin are chemotherapeutic agents that have been tested in this mode of delivery.

TABLE 33.5-9. Hepatic Arterial Chemotherapy for Hepatocellular Carcinoma and Other Hepatobiliary Tumors

Study	*No.*	*Treatment*	*PR (%)*
Ansfield, 1971[554]	11	5-FU	27
Misra, 1977[555]	13	5-FU, mitomycin C	69
Kinami, 1978[556]	14	Mitomycin C	50
Wellwood, 1979[557]	28	FUDR	54
Olweny, 1980[558]	10	Doxorubicin	60
Cheng, 1982[559]	16	Cisplatin	19
Urist and Balch, 1984[560]	13	Doxorubicin	47
Shildt, 1984[561]	30	FUDR, doxorubicin, streptozotocin	10
Atiq, 1992[153]	10	FUDR, mitomycin C, IFN	50
Patt, 1994[151]	29	FUDR, leucovorin, doxorubicin, cisplatin	41
Carr, 1998[562]	26	Cisplatin	42
Urabe, 1998[563]	15	Methotrexate, 5-FU, cisplatin, IFN	47
Okuda, 1999[194]	31	Cisplatin, 5-FU	29

5-FU, 5-fluorouracil; FUDR, fluorouridine; IFN, interferon; PR, partial response.

Most data for treatment of HCC by HAI chemotherapy are gleaned from various phase II clinical trials (Table 33.5-9). Intraarterial doxorubicin seems to be more active than intravenous treatment.[150,151] The highest response rates have been obtained with the drug FUDR. This drug has a high hepatic extraction ratio and short serum half-life, making it ideal for regional therapy. Warren et al.[152] reported a response rate of 60% in 15 patients. Atiq et al.[153] reported a 50% response rate in ten patients using an HAI regimen of mitomycin C, FUDR, and subcutaneous IFN. Makela and Kairaluoma[154] reported a 48% response rate with HAI mitomycin, with a median survival of 14 months. HAI of cisplatin has produced responses between 20% and 40%. In a small study comparing HAI of doxorubicin with systemic administration of doxorubicin, the response rate was greatly increased with HAI.[155]

Though these results are encouraging, this route of chemotherapy is unlikely to make a great impact on the treatment of HCC. Significant toxicity, including cholangitis and bone marrow suppression, can still be encountered. Furthermore, the studies with the most encouraging results used surgically implanted infusion pumps or ports. Most patients with unresectable disease are not in sufficiently fit condition for surgery and pump implantation, as any operation in patients with underlying cirrhosis of the liver carries significant morbidity.

SYSTEMIC IMMUNOTHERAPY. Most studies of immunotherapy for HCC have involved the use of IFN-α or IFN-β. In a randomized controlled trial, high-dose IFN-α (18 to 50 mU/m^2 three times weekly) was found to be superior to doxorubicin in inducing more tumor regression (10% partial response), less toxicity, and fewer fatalities.[156] The same group also compared high-dose IFN-α (50 mU/m^2 three times weekly) to supportive treatment and found better survival and tumor regression for the patients treated with IFN. However, the median survival was only 14.5 weeks for patients so treated.[157] In another study comparing IFN-β with the chemotherapeutic agent menogaril, a slightly longer 1-year but shorter 2-year survival was found for the patients treated with IFN-β.[158] These modest results certainly do not support the use of IFN as a single agent. Furthermore, all these studies used relatively high doses of IFN, and therefore toxicities requiring dose reduction were not uncommon.

Most current studies of immunotherapies, therefore, involve use of lower doses of IFN in combination with chemotherapeutic agents. The most promising combination is a regimen of cisplatin, doxorubicin, 5-FU, and IFN-α. Using this combination, Leung and Lau[112] achieved a partial response rate of 26% in 50 patients with unresectable HCC. Six of these patients experienced sufficient regression of tumor to allow subsequent surgical resection. Two of these six patients had a complete response as confirmed by pathologic analysis. This regimen incites significant toxicity, as demonstrated by a 4% treatment-related mortality.[112] Future randomized multicenter trials must be performed to define completely the clinical role for this regimen.

SYSTEMIC HORMONAL THERAPY. HCC has long been observed to be more common in men. Subsequently, it was noted that these tumors also express receptors for estrogens and androgens.[159] Therefore, hormonal manipulation has been the basis of a number of trials directed at HCC. Of the antiestrogen compounds, tamoxifen has undergone the most extensive testing. This drug inhibits growth of HCC *in vitro.* The mechanisms of action against HCC, however, may not be related to its antiestrogen effects. Hepatocellular tumors express a high level of the MDR gene product P glycoprotein.[160] Tamoxifen is a potential MDR-reversing agent.[161] Overall, results of clinical trials using tamoxifen have been mixed. Three small, randomized studies comparing tamoxifen to no treatment or placebo showed that tamoxifen significantly prolonged survival.[162–164] A large study involving 120 patients showed no benefit of tamoxifen over placebo in terms of tumor progression or survival.[165,166] Another recent randomized study of 496 patients with HCC showed no difference in survival in patients receiving tamoxifen or no tamoxifen.[167] Tamoxifen is not believed to be clinically useful as a single agent.

A number of trials have also attempted to combine tamoxifen with other therapeutic agents. There were encouraging results in phase II trials. In 33 patients with HCC who were receiving tamoxifen and etoposide (VP-16), 8 (24%) had a partial response, with a median survival of 8 months in the responders.[168] Combining epirubicin and VP-16 produced a 36% response rate in 36 patients.[169] However, a randomized study of 59 patients with inoperable HCC showed no difference in response rates or survival between patients who received doxorubicin and those who received doxorubicin plus tamoxifen.[170] Further larger-scale randomized trials are required to define tamoxifen's exact role in the management of HCC in combination with chemotherapeutic agents.

Antiandrogenic treatment has also been attempted using agents such as ketoconazole and cyproterone acetate. The experience is, however, still too preliminary to permit firm conclusions.[171] Overall, hormonal manipulation in the treatment of HCC has a good theoretic basis but has not yet been upheld by clinical data.

Ablative Therapies

PERCUTANEOUS ETHANOL INJECTION. Percutaneous ethanol injection (PEI) was first advocated by Sugiura[171a] in 1983 for ablation of liver tumors. Tumor cells are killed by a combination of cellular dehydration, coagulative necrosis, and vascular thrombosis. Direct injections can be easily performed during open surgery or laparoscopy or percutaneously using ultrasound guidance. This ablative procedure is most often performed percutaneously and is very effective and safe for treating small HCCs. Ethanol injections are usually very well tolerated by patients, side effects being primarily pain, fever, and a transient rise in liver enzymes. Though other side effects, including bleeding, tumor rupture, needle tract tumor implantation,[172] and death, can occur, these are uncommon complications. HCC is well suited for such injections also because these tumors are most often soft and lie in a hard, cirrhotic liver. The injected alcohol tends to diffuse well within the soft tumors for good coverage of the cancerous tissues.

Because of technical limitations, only tumors smaller than 3 cm are generally treatable by PEI.[173] In addition, most clinicians are unwilling to treat more than three tumors by this method. Tumors at the dome of the liver are difficult to treat because of overlying lung and the risk of pneumothorax. Patients with ascites are poor candidates for such injections, as the risk of bleeding is higher in these patients because the abdominal wall is not directly against the liver and cannot act to tamponade the sites of injection.

When tumors are within the limits for injection, results are very good. Nonrandomized studies have demonstrated a 3-year survival rate of 55% to 77% after PEI.[172,174–176] In one large phase II trial that included 210 patients, the 5-year survival was found to be 33%.[177] These treatments are unlikely to be curative, however. Patients should be followed up closely by imaging, and repeated treatments should be given when appropriate.

In a nonrandomized case study comparing liver resection (n = 33) with PEI (n = 30) in the treatment of small (<4-cm) HCCs, the recurrence rate was higher with PEI, but 1- and 4-year survival rates were similar for both treatment modalities.[175] Two randomized, controlled trials have been performed, one comparing PEI to no treatment[178] and the other comparing PEI plus transarterial chemotherapy to transarterial chemotherapy alone.[179] No definitive differences were found, but this may be due to small sample size.[146]

Currently, we use PEI as the ablative method of choice for small (<3 cm) HCCs of limited number (<3) in Pugh-Child's grade A or B cirrhotics in whom resection is not possible. The procedure is well tolerated and the risks minimal. Patients are followed up closely, and treatments are repeated when viable tumor is again demonstrated. Larger trials comparing this technique with supportive care and other ablative techniques are sorely needed for patients with unresectable small tumors. In addition, for patients with resectable small tumors, a comparative study of resection versus PEI is important. The greatest limitation to PEI, however, is that few patients in the Western world present with tumors of sufficiently small size for such treatments.

Tumor ablation can also be accomplished by injection of other agents. Agents so tested have included acetic acid, hot saline, glass microspheres containing ^{90}Y, and various chemotherapeutic drugs.[180] Partial and complete destruction of tumors has been documented with each of these. However, an advantage of any of these agents over ethanol has not been demonstrated to date. Ethanol is so well tolerated and the procedure so simple, particularly as compared to injections of radioactive isotopes, that until results from future comparative trials demonstrate a better alternative, PEI remains the treatment of choice for small, locally limited HCC.

CRYOSURGERY. Repeated freezing and thawing of tissues also produces tissue destruction. Recent technologic advancements have allowed for design and mass marketing of vacuum-sealed probes that are cooled by liquid nitrogen or argon. These probes can be introduced into tumors, and freezing can be performed under ultrasound guidance until the ice ball is more than 2 cm beyond the tumor margin. The tumor then is thawed and frozen again to produce effective cryoablation. The major advantage of this method over ethanol injection is the relatively larger size of tumor that can be treated effectively by cryoablation. Using probes of a diameter of 2 to 3 mm, a 5- to 6-cm ice ball can be produced. By placing multiple probes in proximity to one another, ice balls of up to 10 cm can be produced.

The major disadvantage is the need for general anesthesia and laparoscopy or laparotomy. Furthermore, not only is freezing of tumors near major vascular channels difficult because of the risks of bleeding, but complete freezing is virtually impossible because warm blood circulates in the vessels.

A number of series have been published that clearly demonstrate the safety of such an ablative approach in experienced hands.[181,182] Recently, as smaller and smaller cryoprobes have become available, some investigators have also attempted to perform the cryoablation percutaneously. Whether this will represent an advance is not yet known. Certainly, comparative studies of cryoablation to nonsurgical ablative methods such as ethanol injection or embolization are needed.[174,183,184]

In our practice, we are prepared to perform cryoablation whenever an operation is performed to attempt resection. If a tumor is found to be unresectable at the time of surgery, and the patient has already incurred the risks of anesthesia and laparotomy, we will proceed with cryoablation if it is technically feasible. We will also perform cryoablation for patients with clearly unresectable cancers in whom nonsurgical forms of ablative therapy fail.

RADIOFREQUENCY ABLATION. An ablation technique that is becoming increasingly popular is radiofrequency ablation (RFA). In this ablative modality, heat as generated by a radiofrequency electrode is used to kill tumors. The radiofrequency electrode is passed under radiologic guidance into the tumor of interest and tumor is ablated by thermal energy. The major advantage of RFA results from the small diameter of the electrodes, which allows routine percutaneous and laparoscopic ablation.[185–187] RFA equipment is also much less expensive than is cryotherapy equipment and is more portable and easier to maintain. However, RFA is limited by the small size of tumors that can be completely ablated by current radiofrequency instruments. As heat is generated within the tumor, charring of tissues occurs, decreasing the conduction of heat. The result is that tumors of only 3-cm diameter or smaller can currently be ablated reliably. In addition, in contrast to cryoablation, wherein the ice ball appears unequivocally as a homogeneous, hypoechoic lesion on US, the RFA lesion is much more difficult to follow radiographically.

The published experience to date on use of RFA is meager.[186,188] It is already clear, however, that patients tolerate RFA well. The tumors treatable by RFA are currently being treated by PEI. RFA carries a theoretically lower risk of bleeding, as the needle track can be coagulated during withdrawal of the radiofrequency electrode. PEI however, is simpler, less expensive, and has a longer track record. A direct trial comparing these two techniques is essential. For now, PEI represents the standard ablative modality for unresectable, small HCC, though RFA is a promising investigational treatment for this same population.

HEPATIC ARTERIAL EMBOLIZATION. The liver has a dual nutrient blood supply consisting of the hepatic artery and the portal vein. Under normal conditions, the hepatic parenchyma derives most of its nutrients from the portal vein, and complete occlusion of the hepatic artery does not render the liver ischemic. In contrast, hepatic tumors derive most of their nutrients from the hepatic artery. To induce ischemia and death of unresectable tumors, surgical hepatic arterial ligation was at one time the treatment of choice but has largely been abandoned for two main reasons. First, long-term clinical efficacy is poor, probably owing to the rapid development of collateral vessels after ligation of the main vessels.[189] Second, in patients with cirrhosis and portal hypertension, a high percentage of nutrient blood supplying functional noncancerous parenchyma is derived from the hepatic artery. Ligation of the main hepatic artery therefore was associated with a high procedure-related mortality, as high as 13%. Hence, this procedure has largely been abandoned as a treatment mode for HCC in the cirrhotic patient.[118,190]

Percutaneous selective TAE is a much safer method for treating liver tumors when vascular interruption is desired and has largely replaced surgical arterial ligation. In this method, a catheter is introduced through a percutaneous femoral approach and is threaded under fluoroscopic guidance to the hepatic artery. The branch feeding each tumor can then be cannulated selectively and occluded with degradable or nondegradable particles, coils, or oils. Such selective embolization maintains patency of the main hepatic arteries, thus sparing normal functional liver parenchyma. In addition, it allows repeated treatments through the same arteries. Possible adverse effects include pain, fever, nausea, and transient increase in liver enzymes.[191] Hepatic insufficiency and infected necrotic tumor are rare complications but may be a cause of treatment-related mortality. The risk of complications is clearly related to the degree of hepatic dysfunction. Treatment-related mortality is as high as 30% in patients with Pugh-Child's grade C hepatic function.[71] Therefore, embolization generally is performed only for patients with Pugh-Child's grade A or B liver function. In addition, patients with portal vein occlusion tolerate arterial interruption very poorly, and presence of tumor thrombus in the main portal vein is considered a relative contraindication to embolization.

There is no doubt that such embolization produces objective responses in approximately one-half the patients (Table 33.5-10).[192–196] For patients with painful, unresectable tumors, embolization is effective therapy. It can also be life-saving therapy for patients with ruptured HCC.[197] Documenting the benefits of embolization in other settings has been more difficult. Randomized studies comparing TAE to chemotherapy[198] or to supportive care[199–201] have been unable to document an improvement in survival. However, most studies are plagued by difficulties and

TABLE 33.5-10. Embolization and Chemoembolization for Hepatocellular Carcinoma

Study	*No. of Cases*	*Survival* 1-Y	2-Y	3-Y	*Embolic Agent*	*Chemotherapy*	*Response (%)*
Kanematsu et al., 1989[193]	149	56	29	17	O	D	47
Nakamura, 1989[564]	100	53.8	33.3	17.6	G, O	D	—
	104	45.2	16.3	3.8	G	D, M	—
Shibata et al., 1989[564a]	71	55	—	—	O	C	47
Pelletier et al., 1990[565]	42	24	—	—	G	D	17
Venook et al., 1990[566]	50	—	—	—	G	D, M, C	24
Yamada, 1990[567]	793	51	24	NR	G	D, M	—
Nakao, 1991[568]	66	88	57	42	G, O	D, M	—
Bismuth, 1992[72]	291	62	26	NR	G, O	D	—
Rougier et al., 1993[395]	232	—	—	—	G, O	D	41
Stuart et al., 1993[569]	52	—	—	—	G, O	D	43
Uchida, 1993[570]	863	60.7	37.7	22.4	G, O	D	—
	57	93.2	71.6	49	O	D	—
	212	48.6	24.9	13.7	G	None	—
Carr et al., 1994[195]	56	—	—	—	O	D, C	57
Carr et al., 1995[571]	26	—	—	—	G	D, C	58
Chung, 1995[572]	110	30	18	9	G, O	D, M	31
Ryder et al. 1996[206]	67	—	—	—	O	D	22
Ngan et al., 1996[196]	132	55	33	25	G, O	C	56
Brown, 1997[192]	46	50	32	~29	PVA	None	—

C, cisplatin; D, doxorubicin; G, Gelfoam; M, mitomycin; O, oils (Lipiodol-Ethiodol); PVA, polyvinyl alcohol.

flaws, including small sample size. More important, treatment in these studies has usually involved embolization of the main hepatic arteries rather than the safer and more effective selective embolization performed at major centers.

To improve on the efficacy of embolization, investigators have attempted to soak the embolization particles, such as Gelfoam, with chemotherapeutic agents prior to delivery by chemoembolization. In two randomized studies of chemoembolization versus embolization alone, however, there were no differences in survival.[202,203]

In other attempts to improve the results of TAE, investigators have used Lipiodol or ethiodized oil (Ethiodol). Each of these agents is a lymphangiogram dye derived from poppy seed oil that selectively wedges within HCC when administered via the hepatic artery.[204,205] Embolization of tumors using these oils was originally developed to enhance visualization of HCC. It then was discovered that these oils can be used to deliver and concentrate chemotherapeutic agents at sites of tumor. By mixing hydrophilic drugs with Lipiodol, an emulsion is produced that can be administered intraarterially to produce Lipiodol chemoembolization.

Phase I and II studies and small phase III studies have demonstrated a significant tumor response rate after such treatment. Treatment with doxorubicin and Lipiodol produced responses in 10 of 18 patients with small HCCs (<4 cm) and in 5 of 49 patients with large tumors.[206] Yoshikawa et al.[207] randomized 19 patients to receive Lipiodol-epirubicin and compared them with 17 patients who received epirubicin alone through the hepatic artery. Lipiodol-epirubicin gave a higher tumor response rate as compared with epirubicin alone (42% vs. 12%, respectively).

Larger, randomized trials have been unable to substantiate a survival benefit for such Lipiodol chemoembolizations, however. Madden et al.[208] randomized 136 HCC patients to receive intraarterial Lipiodol-epirubicin versus supportive care and found no survival benefit. Instead, there was an increased morbidity for the treatment arm. A randomized study comparing treatment using Lipiodol plus Adriamycin to Lipiodol alone showed a trend toward a better response at 1 and 2 years with the combination of Lipiodol and Adriamycin, but the difference was not statistically significant.[202]

A further modification of this same theme involved the intraarterial administration of hydrophilic drugs mixed with Lipiodol in an emulsion, followed by temporary or permanent occlusion of the hepatic artery by embolization using a Gelfoam pellet, Ivalon particles, or starch particles. Okuda et al.[194] treated 52 patients with HCC using HAI 5-FU plus cisplatin followed by particle embolization and Lipiodol injections. They reported a response rate of 71% and a 5-year survival of 46%.[194] In another study comparing particle embolization with epirubicin and Lipiodol versus chemotherapy alone in 38 patients, the 1- and 2-year survivals were 73 and 35 versus 43 and 0 in the two groups, respectively.[207] A randomized study comparing intraarterial Lipiodol-cisplatin and Gelfoam embolization to supportive care showed no improvement in survival among the treated group, though this is likely attributable to the high incidence of liver failure in the treated patients.[200] Another randomized study comparing treatment with Lipiodol-cisplatin plus Gelfoam embolization to Lipiodol and Gelfoam in patients with HCC showed a worse outcome in the group using cisplatin.[203] The case for chemoembolization with or without Lipiodol administration is, therefore, far from proven. Because of the small size of individual studies, metaanalyses of the published randomized studies have been performed[146] but have failed to show any clear benefit of transarterial chemoembolization over no treatment.

Particle embolization clearly produces responses in the majority of tumors. At times, the response can be very dramatic, resulting in impressive relief of symptoms. Hence, these treatments may be useful in a patient with ruptured tumors or tumors that are symptomatic in pain or paraneoplastic syndromes. In addition, it is our bias (though not yet supported by randomized trials) that, for the subset of patients with good liver function, tumors of less than 10 cm in diameter, less than 50% liver replacement by tumors, and no portal vein thrombus, selective embolization may be beneficial. It is in this favorable subset of patients that future clinical trials should be directed, examining the utility of embolization. We believe that current data do not support the use of chemoembolization or Lipiodol mixtures but rather indicate that these complex mixtures may merely add cost and complications without improving efficacy. At present, we prefer to use simple particle embolization for treatment of symptomatic or favorable tumors. It is likely that effective palliative therapy will be a combination of local therapy by embolization and an as-yet unidentified systemic treatment.

Radiotherapy

Initial attempts to use whole liver radiation in the treatment of primary hepatobiliary cancer were unsuccessful.[209,210] For instance, in the series by El-Domeiri et al.[209] and Phillips and Murikami,[210] only 1 of 31 patients with unresectable disease who underwent radiation survived more than 1 year. The most important reason for this lack of success is the low tolerance of the liver to whole organ radiation. Indeed, the radiation tolerance of the whole liver in patients with primary HCC may tend to be lower than in those with metastatic cancer to the liver, as many patients with primary disease have some degree of underlying cirrhosis.

Attempts have been made to increase the effectiveness of whole liver irradiation in the treatment of patients with unresectable hepatoma by the addition of intravenous chemotherapy[211,212] and ^{131}I antiferritin monoclonal antibody therapy.[213,214] Radiation Therapy Oncology Group (RTOG) trial RTOG 83-19 was a randomized trial assessing the benefit of adding ^{131}I antiferritin monoclonal antibody therapy to doxorubicin and 5-FU for patients who had received initial treatment with doxorubicin plus 5-FU and whole liver irradiation (21 Gy in seven fractions).[214] RTOG 88-23 measured the benefit of combining antibody with hepatic artery cisplatin for patients who had received induction treatment with whole liver irradiation (21 Gy in seven fractions) and intravenous cisplatin. The conclusions from these and other studies[215] are that ^{131}I antiferritin increased toxicity without benefit and that hepatic arterial cisplatin may be superior to either intravenous[211] or hepatic arterial[212] doxorubicin and 5-FU when combined with irradiation. The finding that hepatic arterial cisplatin and radiation can produce an objective response rate of 43% and a median survival of 7.5 months in a relatively large group of patients[76] suggests that these combinations have some activity.[215]

In contrast to the relative ineffectiveness of whole liver irradiation (when used alone), focal liver irradiation can produce regression of primary hepatobiliary cancers (Fig. 33.5-3). At

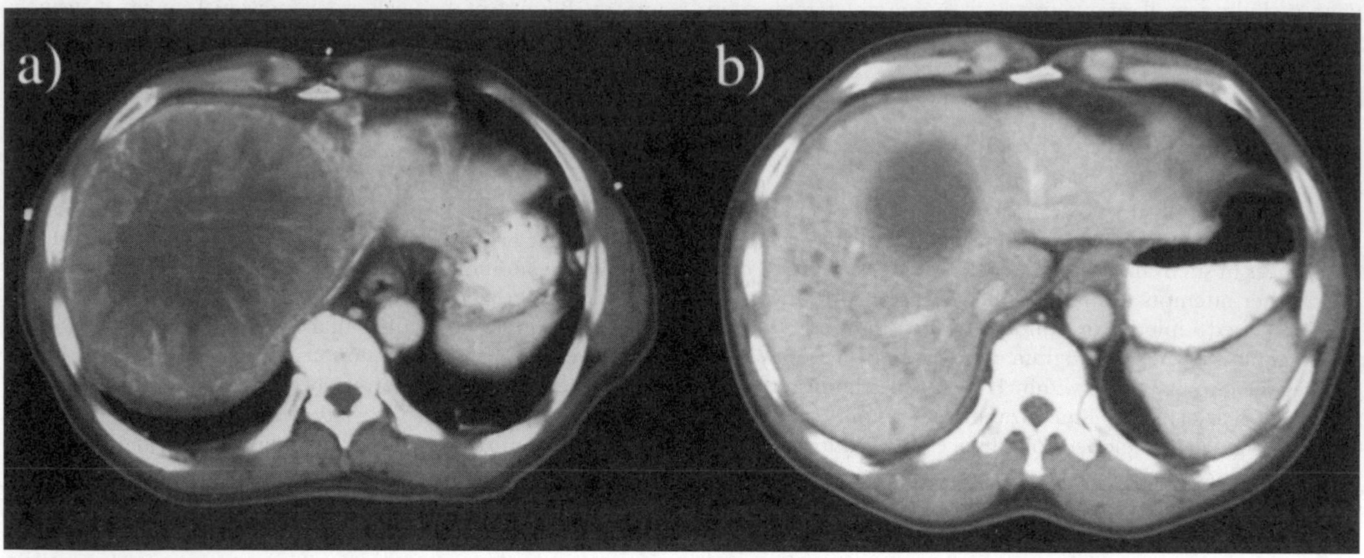

FIGURE 33.5-3. Treatment of hepatocellular carcinoma (HCC) by conformal radiation. The large HCC in the right lobe of the liver **(A)** has had a dramatic response **(B)** to such treatment.

least four techniques have been assessed: ^{90}Y microspheres, ^{131}I-labeled ethiodized oil, and external-beam radiotherapy with either protons or photons. In ^{90}Y therapy, ^{89}Y oxide is incorporated into a stable glass matrix. When bombarded with neutrons, ^{89}Y is converted to ^{90}Y, a pure beta emitter with a half-life of 64.5 hours and average electron energy of 2.23 MeV, which produces an electron range of approximately 2.5 cm. The microspheres have been infused into the hepatic artery as a form of regional therapy for well-vascularized tumors, producing objective response rates ranging from 0% to 25%[109,216–218] (for review, see Ho et al.[219]). Note that ^{90}Y doses (50 to 150 Gy) cannot be compared directly to the more familiar external-beam doses, as the former are calculated by assuming full decay with all radiation homogeneously deposited within the liver. More important, low dose-rate irradiation (<0.2 Gy/h) delivered by ^{90}Y has far less effect than the same physical dose delivered by standard external-beam treatment (>2 Gy/min). A better understanding of the dosimetry of this technique[220] as well as of the technical factors (such as pulmonary shunting, which can lead to radiation pneumonitis,[221] or variant arterial supply to the stomach, which can produce gastric ulcers) is required before the application of microspheres can become routine. ^{90}Y microspheres are not available for clinical use in the United States currently.

Another method of delivering focal liver irradiation involves hepatic arterial administration of ^{131}I ethiodized oil. Ethiodized oil has been used extensively for chemoembolization for HCC (discussed earlier in the section Hepatic Arterial Embolization); in this approach it is formulated with radioactive iodine in an attempt to deliver localized irradiation using the beta (electron) component of the ^{131}I emissions.[222,223] Randomized trials led by French investigators compared ^{131}I-labeled ethiodized oil to chemoembolization[224] and ^{131}I-labeled ethiodized oil to supportive care for patients with portal vein thrombosis.[225] In the former study, 129 patients were randomized to receive either 60 mCi of ^{131}I-labeled ethiodized oil or chemoembolization with cisplatin (70 mg). There was no difference in overall survival between the two groups (median survival, approximately 40 weeks), but the toxicity of the ethiodized oil arm was significantly less. In the latter study, 27 patients were randomized to receive either 60 mCi of ^{131}I-labeled ethiodized oil or control treatment (such as tamoxifen). The ethiodized oil group showed a statistically significantly greater median survival (approximately 6 months as compared to 2 months). Although these findings suggest that ^{131}I-labeled ethiodized oil has activity in HCC, this small study does not permit a firm conclusion to be drawn. Furthermore, as is the case for ^{90}Y, little is known about the tumor and normal tissue dosimetry. ^{131}I-labeled ethiodized oil is not available for use in the United States.

Traditional external-beam photon techniques, either alone[226] or in combination with chemoembolization,[227] have produced objective responses in patients with unresectable HCC. However, standard photon techniques often require the treatment of large volumes of normal liver. In contrast, three-dimensional conformal radiotherapy (3D-CRT) planning using beams not confined to the axial plane can substantially reduce irradiation of normal liver.[228,229] Phase I and II trials for patients using 3D conformal external-beam irradiation combined with hepatic arterial FUDR have demonstrated that high-dose focal irradiation can produce a 60% response rate (see Fig. 33.5-3).[230,231] Recent results support the hypothesis that the dose delivered is an important prognostic factor in both local control and survival for patients with primary hepatobiliary cancers. In this study, dose is prescribed (to a maximum of 90 Gy) according to the fraction of normal liver that is spared, based on a normal tissue complication probability (NTCP) model. Patients who can receive more than 70 Gy have a median survival in excess of 17 months, which approaches that achieved by surgical resection. In a multivariate analysis, dose is a prognostic factor independent of tumor size.[232]

Although 3D techniques permit parts of the liver to be treated with doses of radiation far higher than the entire liver can tolerate, it is possible that both higher doses and larger volumes than have been used in the current studies could be used safely. A first step in defining these limits is to develop an NTCP model to describe the dependence of liver tolerance on the combination of dose and volume. A number of theoretic models (all of which require knowledge of the 3D dose distribution) have been proposed to estimate the volume dependence of normal tissue tolerance.[233,234] Initial investigations have suggested that it will be possible to derive a quantitative model to predict radiation-induced liver disease.[235] More recently, an NTCP model with parameters calculated from patient data has been used prospectively to prescribe a dose that would subject each patient to a predetermined complication risk. Twenty-one patients have completed treatment on such a protocol. The mean dose delivered was 56.6 ± 2.3 Gy (range: 40.5 to 81 Gy). One of 21 patients developed radiation-induced liver disease. The observed complication rate of 4.8% (95% confidence interval, 0% to 23.8%) did not differ significantly from the predicted 8.8% NTCP (based on dose delivered). These results suggest that an NTCP model can be used prospectively to deliver safely far higher doses of radiation to patients with intrahepatic cancer than were possible using previous approaches.[236] The widespread adoption of 3D conformal planning systems should permit these concepts to be tested in multiinstitutional trials.

Another method of delivering highly conformal radiation is with protons. Investigators at the Proton Medical Research Center in Japan have demonstrated response rates similar to those just reported using 3D-CRT.[237,238] Interestingly, high-dose focal irradiation using either photons[239] or protons[240] can produce hypertrophy in the nonirradiated liver, resembling the effect of partial hepatectomy.

In summary, whole liver irradiation alone has little efficacy in the treatment of HCC. The addition of hepatic arterial cisplatin may increase the efficacy somewhat. High-dose focal irradiation, especially using external-beam photons or protons, can produce objective responses in the majority of patients, although the relative merit of these techniques as compared to other nonsurgical approaches described in this chapter has not been assessed in randomized trials.

SCREENING FOR HEPATOCELLULAR CARCINOMA

Patients found to have small (<5-cm) HCC have a much better prognosis than do those presenting with larger tumors. The size of a tumor is a significant risk factor for intrahepatic and extrahepatic spread.[241–243] The frequency of intrahepatic metastases rose by almost one-third between HCCs smaller and larger than 5 cm (60% to 90%), and the rate of portal vein tumor thrombosis almost doubled (40% to 75%).[242,243] Many more treatment options are also available for patients with small tumors. Tumors smaller than 3 cm can be treated by PEI, RFA, resection, or transplantation, whereas tumors smaller than 5 cm can be treated by cryoablation, resection, or transplantation. Hence, smaller tumors are not only biologically more favorable but are technically more easily treated. Because symptomatic tumors are usually large, widely disseminated, and beyond therapeutic option, the rationale for screening patients at risk for HCC is clear.

Whole population screening, even in areas where HBV is endemic, is almost certainly not a financially viable option. In epidemiologic studies, it is apparent that the incidence of HCC in HB_sAg-positive patients is approximately 0.5% annually.[244] Therefore, the yield for screening programs is low. Hepatitis occurs mainly in developing countries, where the cost of any population screening program will also be too prohibitive.

In the presence of HCV, however, the risk of HCC in a patient with established cirrhosis is estimated to be as high as 5% per year.[15] Also, HCV occurs more often in industrialized nations. Hence, it is much more justifiable and likely that screening programs will be developed for detection of HCC in patients with cirrhosis due to HCV infection.

As a clinician striving to deliver optimal care for individual patients, screening high-risk patients for HCC is justifiable. Patients with established cirrhosis or chronic HCV infection are clearly important candidates for screening. Patients with chronic HBV infection should also be considered for screening. Furthermore, only patients with Pugh-Child's grade A or B liver functional status should be screened, as patients with Pugh-Child's grade C disease will generally be too sick for therapeutic interventions and early detection of HCC will only cause anxiety and detrimentally affect the patient's likelihood for liver transplantation. Screening protocols are largely based on the biases of each major center. Some have advocated frequent testing, including ultrasound examination every 3 months[245] and serum AFP testing once every 2 months.[246] Because HCC is slow-growing, however, with a documented median doubling time of 4 to 5 months for small HCCs,[245] we advocate AFP and liver function tests every 3 months and liver imaging every 6 months.

OTHER PRIMARY TUMORS OF THE LIVER

HEPATOBLASTOMA

Hepatoblastoma affects approximately 1 in 100,000 children and is the most common primary malignant liver tumor in children.[247,248] It is usually diagnosed before the age of 3 years, with a 2:1 male predominance. Patients usually present with abdominal swelling[247,248] and elevated serum AFP (>75% of patients).[249] CT scans will reveal a vascular mass that often (50%) is speckled with calcifications.[249] The Children's Cancer Study Group staging system is shown in Table 33.5-11.[250] Overall long-term survival varies between 15% and 37%.[249,251–253] Poor prognosis is associated with unresectable tumors and tumors demonstrating aneuploidy and anaplastic characteristics.[251,254,255]

Complete resection is possible in 50% to 65% of children with hepatoblastoma and is associated with cure rates between 30% and 70%.[247,248] Unlike adult primary liver tumors, chemotherapy may produce response in a significant number of patients with hepatoblastomas. Preoperative chemotherapy has been used with some success in converting unresectable tumors to resectable

TABLE 33.5-11. Children's Cancer Study Group Staging for Hepatoblastoma

Group I	Complete resection of tumor by wedge, lobectomy, or extended lobectomy as initial treatment
Group IIA	Tumor rendered completely resectable by initial irradiation and chemotherapy
Group IIB	Residual tumor confined to one lobe
Group IIIA	Tumor involving both lobes of the liver
Group IIIB	Regional lymph node involvement with tumor
Group IV	Distant metastases of tumor regardless of the extent of liver involvement

lesions.[256,257] Adjuvant chemotherapy has also been used after resection of hepatoblastoma.[250] Evans et al.[250] reported that 20% of 24 patients with hepatoblastoma were relapse-free 8 to 42 months after surgical resection coupled with adjuvant vincristine, doxorubicin, 5-FU, and cyclophosphamide.

Radiotherapy has been used in the treatment of unresectable hepatoblastomas, but its utility is far from proven.[256,258] Orthotopic liver transplantation should be considered in children with unresectable hepatoblastoma if the tumor does not become resectable after preoperative chemotherapy. Penn[259] reported on 18 patients undergoing liver transplantation for unresectable hepatoblastoma. Though tumors recurred in six patients, five have survived disease-free for more than 2 years, with actuarial survival rates of approximately 50%.

ANGIOSARCOMA

Angiosarcomas are malignant mesenchymal tumors of the liver that are also referred to as *hemangiosarcomas*. Only approximately 25 cases occur in the United States each year.[260] Peak incidence is in the sixth and seventh decades, with a predominance in men (85%).[261] Abdominal pain, abdominal swelling (usually due to liver enlargement), liver failure, nausea, anorexia, vomiting, and jaundice are seen. These malignant tumors have been associated with exposure to thorotrast, arsenic, or vinyl chloride.

Angiosarcomas are aggressive neoplasms. Partial hepatectomy can result in long-term survival, but most patients present with advanced tumors that cannot be treated by excision. Distant metastases are found at initial presentation in one-half of patients. Most patients die within 6 months of diagnosis. Even with surgical excision, few patients survive more than 1 to 3 years after complete resection because of metastatic disease. Results of radiotherapy and chemotherapy or both have been disappointing.[261] The results of orthotopic liver transplantation for treatment of angiosarcoma have also been poor. Penn et al. reported development of tumor recurrences in 9 of 14 transplant patients with tumors classified as either angiosarcomas or epithelioid tissue sarcomas. The 2-year survival rate was 15%, and no patient survived more than 28 months postoperatively.[259]

The liver can occasionally be the primary site for rhabdomyosarcoma,[262] though this is more common in children than in adults. Hepatic metastases from a gastrointestinal or uterine primary tumor must be ruled out before the diagnosis of primary leiomyosarcoma of the liver can be made. Surgical resection is the treatment of choice for these primary hepatic sarcomas.[262] Unresectable disease carries an unfavorable prognosis.

Undifferentiated sarcomas of the liver are very rare and usually occur in children between the ages of 6 and 15 years.[263,264] Most undifferentiated sarcomas of the liver are found at an advanced stage, when surgical resection is not possible. The patient with such a tumor rapidly succumbs to the sarcoma, as such tumors usually are not responsive to radiotherapy or chemotherapy.[263]

EPITHELIOID HEMANGIOENDOTHELIOMA

Epithelioid hemangioma is another malignant soft tissue tumor of endothelial cell origin.[260,262,265] Factor VII staining differentiates hemangioendothelioma from other nonvascular tumors. Infantile hemangioendothelioma, which is benign, is unlikely; the adult variety is malignant and highly aggressive. Average age at presentation is 50 years, and the usual presenting signs and symptoms consist generally of nonspecific complaints, including pain, and an abdominal mass. In contrast to angiosarcoma, there is a female predominance (63% of patients).[262] Epithelioid hemangioendothelioma has also been related to vinyl chloride exposure in some patients.[265]

Weiss and Enzinger[260] recommended radical surgery, if possible. However, these tumors are almost always diffuse and multifocal and, therefore, are unlikely to be cured by partial hepatectomy. If hemangioendothelioma is suspected, a percutaneous biopsy is performed for diagnosis. Frozen-section analysis is not usually helpful at open surgery because special stains are required for diagnosis of this tumor. Patients with hemangioendotheliomas should be considered for total hepatectomy and liver transplantation. Penn[259] reported a series of 21 patients who underwent orthotopic liver transplantation for treatment of epithelioid hemangioendotheliomas; 7 of 21 patients experienced tumor recurrence. The actuarial survival rate was 82% at 2 years and 43% at 5 years.

CHOLANGIOCARCINOMA

Cancers of the bile ducts are rare tumors, with only approximately 4000 cases presenting in the United States annually. Because of the proximity of the bile duct to the liver, the pancreas, and major vascular structures, surgical excision of these tumors usually requires a major hepatic or pancreatic resection or both. Major vascular reconstructions may also be necessary. The technical demands of such resections and the lack of effective alternative therapies for cholangiocarcinomas explain the nihilistic attitude that generally surrounds this disease. Advances in imaging over the last two decades now allow for earlier diagnosis of bile duct cancer and better surgical planning. Recent improvements in operative technique have substantially improved the outlook of patients presenting with this cancer.

EPIDEMIOLOGY AND ETIOLOGY

Cholangiocarcinoma is an uncommon cancer, with an incidence of 1 to 2 cases per 100,000 population in the United States[266] and constituting approximately 2% of all reported cancers.[267] It is a disease of the elderly, with the majority of such lesions occurring in patients older than 65 years and the peak incidence occurring in the eighth decade of life.[266] Untreated, bile duct cancers are rapidly fatal diseases, and the majority of patients will die within 6 months to a year of diagnosis. Death usually results from liver failure or biliary sepsis.[267–270] Long-term survival is highly dependent on the effectiveness of surgical therapy. Indeed, it has been shown that tumor location within the biliary tree has no impact on survival, provided that complete resection is achieved.[271] Nonetheless, it is more likely that distal bile duct cancer will be resected with curative intent, which explains the relatively more favorable prognosis of distal tumors.

A number of conditions are associated with an increased incidence of cholangiocarcinomas, including PSC, choledochal cysts or Caroli's disease, and pyogenic cholangiohepatitis and other hepatic infections. In addition, environmental agents may influence the incidence of cholangiocarcinomas.

Primary Sclerosing Cholangitis

In Western nations, the disease most often associated with development of cholangiocarcinoma is primary sclerosing cholangitis (PSC). This is an autoimmune disease characterized by inflammation of the periductal tissues and, at advanced stages, is characterized by multifocal strictures of the intrahepatic and extrahepatic bile ducts.[272–274] The majority (70% to 80%) of patients with PSC also have associated inflammatory bowel disease in the form of ulcerative colitis.[272] In a longitudinal study of patients with PSC, 8% of patients developed clinically apparent cholangiocarcinoma over a 5-year period.[272] This explains the high incidence (30% to 40%) of occult cholangiocarcinoma found in autopsy or explant specimens from patients with PSC.[272–274] Cholangiocarcinomas presenting in patients with PSC are often multifocal and not amenable to treatment by partial hepatectomy. Liver transplantation is often the only treatment possible for these patients, not only because of multifocal cancer but also because of the baseline hepatic insufficiency from the underlying inflammatory disease.

Choledochal Cysts or Caroli's Disease

The increased risk of cholangiocarcinoma in patients with congenital cystic disease of the biliary tree is well recognized.[275,276] The reason for the malignant transformation is thought to be related to chronic inflammation and bacterial contamination within the cystic areas.[276–279] Early excision of the choledochal cyst significantly reduces the risk of cancer.[276,277] Fifteen to twenty percent of adult patients with unexcised choledochal cysts or cysts previously treated with bypass will be found to have a cholangiocarcinoma.[276,277]

Pyogenic Cholangiohepatitis and Other Hepatic Infections

In the Orient, chronic infections of the liver can predispose to development of cholangiocarcinoma. Pyogenic cholangiohepatitis or Oriental cholangiohepatitis results from chronic portal bacteremia and portal phlebitis, which gives rise to intrahepatic pigment stone formation. This hepatolithiasis leads to recurrent episodes of cholangitis and stricture formation.[280–283] Those patients who do not succumb to sepsis will have approximately a 10% chance of developing cholangiocarcinoma.[281–283] In Southeast Asia, biliary parasites (*Clonorchis sinensis, Opisthorchis viverrini*) are also associated with an increased risk of cholangiocarcinoma.[273] In areas where these parasites are endemic, the incidence of cholangiocarcinoma is as high as 87 per 100,000.[284]

Influence of Environmental Agents

Several radionuclides and chemical carcinogens, including thorium, radon, nitrosamines, dioxin, and asbestos, have also been implicated in the development of cholangiocarcinomas.

PATHOLOGY AND CLASSIFICATION

Cholangiocarcinoma can arise anywhere within the biliary tree. Approximately 10% of cholangiocarcinoma cases arise within the intrahepatic bile ducts.[285–289] These usually present as hepatic masses that are thought at first to be HCCs or metastatic tumor of unknown origin. The extrahepatic variety is more common and can occur along the entire length of the bile duct from the confluence of the hepatic ducts to the ampulla. Some have classified these extrahepatic tumors into proximal (hilar), middle, and distal bile duct tumors. Nakeeb et al.[290] proposed a more practical division of cholangiocarcinomas into intrahepatic, perihilar, and distal subgroups, thus eliminating the midduct group. Those lesions that are proximal to the cystic duct–common duct junction usually require a liver resection for extirpation. These represent approximately 40% to 60% of cases of cholangiocarcinoma and include the hilar cholangiocarcinomas or Klatskin tumors.[270,290–296] Those tumors distal to the cystic duct usually require pancreatectomy for treatment. Fewer than 10% of patients will present with multifocal or diffuse involvement of the biliary tree.[297]

Cholangiocarcinomas are characterized by early invasion of adjacent organs.[298] Nodal metastases are also common and occur in up to one-third of cases.[270,299] In addition to lymphatic involvement, these tumors are also characterized by neural, perineural, and subepithelial extension.[298]

Cholangiocarcinomas can be separated into three distinct macroscopic subtypes: sclerosing, nodular, and papillary.[298] Most are *sclerosing* tumors, which are very firm and are seen as annular thickening of the bile duct, often with diffuse infiltration and fibrosis of the periductal tissues. *Nodular* tumors are firm tumors that project into the lumen of the duct. Frequently, features of both sclerosing and nodular tumors are found, and the tumor is described as *nodular-sclerosing*. *Papillary* tumors are soft and friable and often demonstrate little transmural invasion. These tumors have a more favorable prognosis than do the others,[273] are more common in the distal bile duct, and account for approximately 10% of all cholangiocarcinomas.[298]

The overwhelming majority (>90%) of cholangiocarcinomas are adenocarcinomas, often well differentiated and mucin-producing.[266,298,300] Rarely, malignant obstruction of the bile duct may be due to other cell types, such as carcinoid tumors, arising primarily in the biliary tree or to tumors metastatic to the biliary tree.[301–303]

DISTAL BILE DUCT CANCERS

Distal bile duct cancers are rare cancers that usually are reported as part of a series of periampullary tumors or as a series describing all bile duct cancers. Distal bile duct tumors represent approximately 20% to 30% of all cholangiocarcinomas or 5% to 10% of all periampullary tumors.[290,293,294,304] Approximately 2000 new cases of distal bile duct cancer are diagnosed in the United States each year.[293] They are almost always adenocarcinomas. The papillary variety is also more common in this location than in other parts of the bile duct.[292]

Clinical Presentation and Diagnosis

On the practical level, patients with distal bile duct cancers usually present with jaundice and a mass at the head of the pancreas. Except in the case of the papillary variety of this cancer, patients are brought to the operating room with the diagnosis of periampullary cancer, and it is in the final pathologic analysis that the anatomic site of origin of the tumor becomes clear. The importance of distinguishing distal bile duct cancer from the other periampullary tumors is in the prognostic implications, as distal bile duct cancer has a much more favorable outcome than does the more common adenocarcinoma of the pancreas.

Jaundice is the presenting symptom in up to 90% of patients with distal bile duct cancer. Abdominal pain, weight loss, fever, or pruritus are also common symptoms, though these occur in one-third of cases or fewer.[290,293] If the patient reports that the jaundice is intermittent, a papillary bile duct cancer should be suspected. Most often, however, the symptoms and signs will be indistinguishable from adenocarcinoma of the pancreatic head or other periampullary malignancies.

US will demonstrate a dilated extrahepatic and intrahepatic biliary tree. Cross-sectional imaging by CT scanning will usually then demonstrate a mass in the region of the head of the pancreas. Endoscopic retrograde cholangiopancreatography (ERCP) may be diagnostic if it demonstrates an obstruction in the bile duct that does not involve the pancreatic duct. Most often, however, ERCP will demonstrate distal biliary obstruction without diagnostic information on the cell origin of the malignancy. In fact, we tend not to perform ERCP if the patient is a surgical candidate, preferring to operate on the patient without direct biliary manipulation, as this decreases the risk of biliary sepsis.[305]

If surgical resection is planned, a preoperative tissue diagnosis of cancer is not necessary and often is not possible. Endoscopic brush biopsy has a low sensitivity, making a negative result virtually useless.[306] Performing a percutaneous needle biopsy is difficult because of the small size of these tumors. Therefore, preoperative diagnosis is usually based on clinical impression. In patients with a stricture of the distal bile duct and a clinical presentation consistent with cholangiocarcinoma, cross-sectional imaging studies are scrutinized for signs of unresectable cancer. In this regard, a contrast-enhanced helical CT scan with overlapping 5-mm sections through the area of the pancreas is the most useful. This test allows for evaluation for vascular involvement or metastatic disease. Magnetic resonance cholangiopancreatography (MRCP) may also be used for evaluation of these periampullary tumors.[307]

If the tumor is judged unresectable by radiologic criteria, it is usually of sufficient size for diagnosis by percutaneous needle biopsy. Biliary obstruction then can also be treated by endoscopic stenting or, if necessary, through percutaneous transhepatic stenting to avoid surgery.

Treatment Options

Complete resection is the only effective and potentially curative therapy for cancers of the lower bile duct.[271,290,292–294,304] Resection usually requires a pancreaticoduodenectomy.[293,304] In comparison to pancreatic cancer, distal bile duct cancer is more often amenable to resection and patients less often have microscopic disease at the resection margin and less frequently demonstrate spread of tumor to adjacent lymph nodes.[290,293,294] Completeness of resection, presence of lymphatic metastases,[293,304] and tumor differentiation[290] are the prognostic factors that most strongly influence long-term outcome. Fong et al.[293] found that lymph node status was the only independent predictor of long-term survival in patients who have undergone resection, with positive nodes conferring a 6.7 times greater likelihood of recurrence and death.

The results of resection for distal bile duct cancer as compared to the other periampullary tumors are demonstrated in Figure 33.5-4. The results are similar to those for duodenal can-

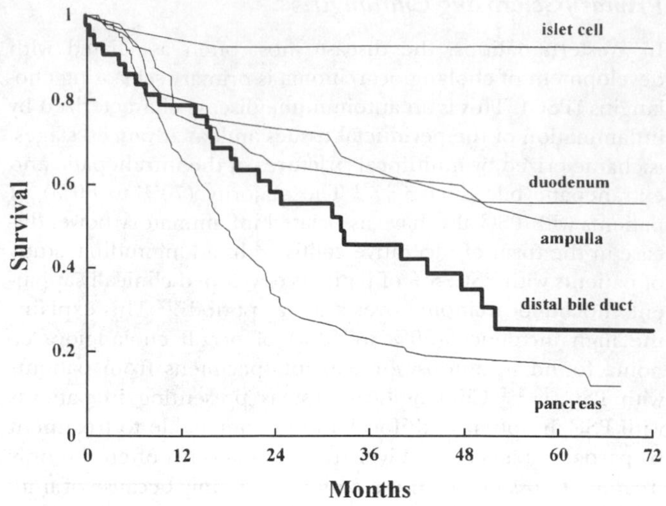

FIGURE 33.5-4. Survival for patients with various peripancreatic tumors.

cer, more favorable than those for adenocarcinoma of the pancreas,[293,304] and less favorable than those for neuroendocrine or ampullary tumors. Five-year survival rates of up to 40% have been reported after complete resection (Table 33.5-12). It has long been assumed that survival after resection of distal bile duct tumors is more favorable than after resection of hilar cholangiocarcinomas,[292] but this commonly held belief has been refuted by data. Though it is true that resectability rates are higher for distal bile duct cancers and the likelihood of achieving a negative margin during resection is greater, the survival rates of the various bile duct tumors, if adjusted for stage and completeness of resection, appear to be comparable.[271]

Because of the rarity of distal cholangiocarcinoma, no prospective data are available to guide the use of adjuvant therapy after resection.[290] We tend not to use adjuvant therapy if resection margins are clear of tumor, though many other practitioners use regimens of chemoradiation originally developed for adenocarcinoma of the pancreas.

In patients with nonresectable cancers, palliation for biliary obstruction can be achieved with a surgical bypass or biliary endoprostheses. Endoprostheses for distal biliary obstruction are usually placed endoscopically and provide more durable palliation than does an endoprosthesis placed for hilar obstruction.[277] Surgical bypasses also provide excellent relief of jaundice and can be achieved with an acceptably low morbidity and mortality. In our practice, patients found to have unresectable disease at laparotomy are subjected to surgical bypasses, as they will already have incurred the risk of anesthesia and laparotomy. Furthermore, patients expected to survive longer than 6 months are also considered for surgical bypass.[308] All other patients are treated with biliary endoprostheses.

Chemotherapy or radiotherapy or both have offered generally poor results as palliative treatment for unresectable cases. Survival beyond 1 year is uncommon in patients subjected to palliative therapies.[290,292,293,304]

PROXIMAL OR HILAR CHOLANGIOCARCINOMA

Proximal or hilar cholangiocarcinomas were first described by Altemeier[341] in 1957 and subsequently by Klatskin[309] in 1965.

TABLE 33.5-12. Survival after Resection of Distal Cholangiocarcinoma

Study	*Years*	*No. of Institutions*	*Total No. of Patients*	*No. Resected*	*Operative Mortality (%)*	*Median Survival (mo)*	*3-Y Survival (%)*	*5-Y Survival (%)*
Warren, 1975[573]	30	1	—	47	21	—	32	25
Nakase, 1975[574]	25	57	309	161	22	17	8	5
Tompkins, 1981[292]	25	1	18	12	8	18	28	28
Alexander, 1983[575]	13	1	14	14	21	16	20	18
Lerut, 1983[576]	15	1	—	5	—	11	0	0
Tarazi, 1986[577]	35	1	—	11	0	—	—	17
Nagorney, 1994[271]	10	1	39	22	—	24	40	40
Fong, 1996[293]	10	1	104	45	4	33	46	27
Wade, 1997[304]	4	159	156	34	—	22[a]	—	14
Yeo, 1997[294]	6	1	—	65	—	20	16	—

[a]Mean survival.

Of the hepatobiliary tumors, these cholangiocarcinomas represent the greatest diagnostic and therapeutic challenge because of the vast number of vital structures that can be involved by even a small hilar cholangiocarcinoma. Proximal or hilar cholangiocarcinomas require the most extensive of liver resections and vascular reconstruction for extirpation.

Clinical Presentation and Diagnosis

CLINICAL FINDINGS. Most patients with cholangiocarcinoma come to medical attention because of jaundice or abnormal liver function tests. Other associated symptoms are nonspecific. Abdominal pain or discomfort, anorexia, weight loss, and pruritus are the most common symptoms but are seen in only approximately one-third of patients. Fever usually is seen only after biliary manipulation.[273,274,283,290,310,311] In some patients, pruritus precedes jaundice by some weeks, and this symptom should prompt an evaluation, especially if associated with abnormal liver function tests. Intermittent jaundice may be seen with papillary tumors and is usually due to intermittent detachment of pieces of friable tumors from the right or left hepatic duct that pass into and occlude the common hepatic duct. The serum bilirubin level is usually greater than 10 mg/dL and averages 18 mg/dL, whereas bilirubin levels of 2 to 4 mg/dL are the norm in patients with obstruction from choledocholithiasis.[312] Malignancy should be strongly suspected in patients with deep, painless jaundice who present with no fever or other signs of infection.

On physical examination, jaundice is usually obvious. Patients with pruritus may have multiple excoriations of the skin. Proximal biliary obstruction is usually associated with a decompressed and nonpalpable gallbladder. Thus, a palpable gallbladder would suggest a more distal obstruction or gallbladder cancer. Signs of portal hypertension are rare but would be an ominous indication of advanced vascular involvement or the alternative diagnosis of cirrhosis and HCC.

Medical history and family history should be scrutinized for conditions such as PSC or Oriental cholangiohepatitis that may predispose to cholangiocarcinoma. Many tumors express carcinoembryonic antigen (CEA) and the carbohydrate antigen CA 19-9. The diagnostic value of these serum markers is, however, debated.[273] It has been suggested that CEA levels in hepatic bile may help to distinguish between benign and malignant strictures in patients with premalignant conditions.[313] Diagnosis of cholangiocarcinoma is usually made radiologically.

RADIOGRAPHIC EVALUATION. Radiologic imaging is central to the diagnosis and treatment planning for patients with cholangiocarcinomas. The importance of imaging studies results from the difficulties in obtaining a positive tissue diagnosis by biopsy, particularly when the tumors are small and in the potentially curable stages. Relying on the results of percutaneous needle biopsy or biliary brush cytology is dangerous, as the results of these tests are often misleading and one may miss the opportunity to resect an early cancer.[314,315] Therefore, the preoperative and, often, operative diagnoses are based mainly on the history and radiologic appearance of the tumors.

The differential diagnosis must include gallbladder carcinoma, Mirizzi syndrome, idiopathic benign focal stenosis (malignant masquerade), or sclerosing cholangitis. Unless there is a large intraluminal mass in the gallbladder, distinguishing gallbladder carcinoma from hilar cholangiocarcinoma can be difficult. Mirizzi syndrome is caused by a large gallstone impacted in the neck of the gallbladder, resulting in biliary obstruction from periductal inflammation.[316–318] Benign focal strictures (malignant masquerade) can also occur at the hepatic duct confluence but are uncommon.[319–322]

Beyond diagnosis, the radiologic evaluation is aimed at determining resectability, as surgical resection is the most effective and only potentially curative therapy. Imaging may locate occult distant metastases and thereby spare patients from nontherapeutic surgery. In defining the degree of invasion of adjacent organs and vasculature, imaging is also essential for planning the surgical procedure and directing major vascular reconstructions when necessary.

Most patients will present to the surgeon having already been subjected to a sonogram and CT. US is usually the first investigation performed because it is noninvasive, readily available, and provides important diagnostic information regarding the jaundiced patient. Generally, intrahepatic biliary dilatation will be seen without evidence of extrahepatic bile duct abnormality and without evidence of stones. In experienced hands, the tumor will often be clearly defined by US, as will information important for planning of surgery such as delineation of the biliary extent of disease, vascular involvement, presence of lymph node metastases in the porta hepatis, and presence of noncontiguous liver metastases. US not only may demonstrate the level of biliary ductal obstruction but can also provide information regarding tumor extension within the bile duct and in the periductal tissues.[323–325] In centers specializing in treatment of cholangiocarcinomas, a good Doppler US may indeed provide diagnostic information equivalent to that provided by a combination of angiography and CT and is highly accurate in predicting resectability.[325,326] However, US is more operator-dependent than is most cross-sectional imaging. Therefore, in most circumstances, other cross-sectional imaging is necessary.

Most patients will present to a tertiary care center having already been imaged by CT. CT remains an important study for evaluating patients and is less dependent than US on the skills of the operator. Important information regarding level of biliary obstruction, vascular involvement, and presence of nodal or noncontiguous metastases can be assessed. One of the most important findings to be gleaned from a CT scan, however, is the presence of hepatic lobar atrophy, which is usually indicative of portal venous occlusion.[327]

In years past, most patients also were subjected to direct angiography and cholangiography. Angiography allows for determination of arterial or portal venous vascular encasement. Cholangiography demonstrates the location of the tumor and the biliary extent of disease. Recently, however, MRCP has emerged as a noninvasive substitute for direct cholangiography.[328–331] MRCP not only may identify the tumor and the level of biliary obstruction but also may reveal obstructed and isolated ducts not appreciated at endoscopic or percutaneous study. Magnetic resonance angiography (MRA) or CT angiography has become a substitute for direct angiography. Today, the need to perform invasive tests is moot. When direct cholangiography is needed, percutaneous transhepatic cholangiography (PTC) is preferred over ERCP because it is more likely to provide the details of the intrahepatic biliary tree necessary for surgical planning.

For patients presenting with proximal cholangiocarcinomas, a Doppler US, helical CT, and chest radiograph may suffice as preoperative radiologic evaluation. In patients in whom further delineation of biliary or vascular involvement may be necessary, MRCP and MRA are the next tests of choice. This noninvasive approach prevents biliary instrumentation and bacterbilia and the associated increased perioperative morbidity.[305,332] When necessary, direct cholangiography or angiography is used.

Staging

The most commonly used staging systems are the modified Bismuth-Corlette and the American Joint Committee on Cancer (AJCC) TNM (tumor, node, metastasis) staging system. The former classifies patients based on the extent of biliary duct involvement by tumor,[333] whereas the latter is based largely on pathologic criteria (Table 33.5-13). These staging systems do not distinguish between extensive unilateral disease and bilateral disease because, before surgical resections became commonplace, such distinctions had little value. Thus, a patient with tumor extension into third-order biliary ducts on one side of the liver accompanied by ipsilateral portal vein occlusion will be classified as having very advanced disease, though this patient may now be treatable with potentially curative resection as disease is confined to one side.

TABLE 33.5-13. American Joint Committee on Cancer TNM Staging System for Proximal (Hilar) Cholangiocarcinoma and Cancer of the Extrahepatic Bile Ducts

TUMOR (T)	
Tis	Carcinoma *in situ*
T1	Tumor invades subepithelial connective tissue or fibromuscular layer
T2	Tumor invades perifibromuscular connective tissue
T3	Tumor invades adjacent organs (liver, pancreas, duodenum, gallbladder, colon, stomach)
NODE (N)	
N0	No regional lymph node metastases
N1	Metastasis to lymph nodes within the hepatoduodenal ligament (cystic duct, pericholedochal and/or hilar lymph nodes)
N2	Metastasis to peripancreatic, periduodenal, periportal, celiac, superior mesenteric, and/or posterior pancreaticoduodenal lymph nodes
METASTASIS (M)	
M0	No distant metastasis
M1	Distant metastasis

STAGE GROUPING			
Stage 0	Tis	N0	M0
Stage I	T1	N0	M0
Stage II	T2	N0	M0
Stage III	T1 or T2	N1 or N2	M0
Stage IVA	T3	Any N	M0
Stage IVB	Any T	Any N	M1

We recently proposed a staging system, using preoperative imaging and taking into account the extent of biliary ductal involvement, vascular involvement, and lobar atrophy, that may be more applicable than the other systems, given modern surgical therapies (Table 33.5-14).[270] In the era of effective surgical therapy for cholangiocarcinomas, this staging system is a better predictor of resectability and outcome than is the AJCC classification.

Treatment with Curative Intent

The only curative option is complete surgical excision of the cholangiocarcinoma. Until the last decade, such surgical resections were rarely accomplished, because complete excision usually requires a major liver resection, biliary resection and reconstruction and, often, a major vascular resection and reconstruction.[270,334,335] As advances in diagnostic imaging have been made, earlier detection of cholangiocarcinoma and improved operative planning are possible. As surgical techniques have evolved to make major hepatectomies routine, increasing numbers of resections have been accomplished. The results generated over the last decades has firmly established resection as safe and effective treatment and have helped to define patient selection and operative conduct.

RESECTION. It has become clear over the last three decades that curative treatment of tumors involving the upper third of the bile duct very much depends on aggressive surgical excision. Until as recently as one decade ago, surgical treatment of hilar cholangiocarcinomas was associated with a mortality as high as

TABLE 33.5-14. Proposed Staging System for Proximal (Hilar) Cholangiocarcinoma in the Era of Effective Surgical Therapy

T Stage	*Biliary Involvement*	*Ipsilateral Lobar Atrophy*	*Ipsilateral Portal Vein Involvement*	*Main Portal Vein Involvement*
T1	Hilus and/or right or left hepatic duct	No	No	No
T2	Hilus and/or right or left hepatic duct	Yes	No	No
T3	Hilus and/or right or left hepatic duct	Yes/No	Yes	No
T4	Secondary biliary radicles bilaterally	Yes/No	Yes/No	Yes

(Data from ref. 270.)

30%.[333,336–340] Before the 1990s, most surgical series were small, operative mortalities were high, and only a handful of 5-year survivors were reported.[578–583] That this entire disease was regarded with pessimism was understandable.[309,341,342] It is not surprising, therefore, that until recently, the surgical therapy for proximal biliary malignancies consisted mainly of biliary-enteric bypass as palliation for jaundice and cholangitis. Results reported over the last decade, however, have indicated a major improvement in safety of these operations such that resections of hilar tumors can be accomplished (even when liver resections are required) with a mortality of less than 10% (Table 33.5-15).[271,333,337,343] Increasingly large series have been reported that have firmly documented the curative potential of such major resections (see Table 33.5-15). Given that unresected disease is uniformly fatal, usually within 6 to 12 months, surgical resection has become the treatment of choice when possible.

The goals of surgical management for cholangiocarcinomas are eradication of tumor and establishment of adequate biliary drainage. For tumors of the hepatic ducts and the biliary confluence, symptoms often appear late in the course of disease when the lesion has already involved adjacent structures, including the portal vein or adjacent hepatic parenchyma. Complete resection, therefore, usually requires not only biliary resection but also major liver resection and, often, major vascular and biliary reconstruction.

Discussion of the fine details of resections for hilar cholangiocarcinomas is beyond the scope of this chapter. The reader is referred to standard texts of surgical techniques for detailed technical discussions.[126,344,345] Nonetheless, some major points and principles warrant emphasis.

Laparoscopic evaluation should be considered before a formal laparotomy is performed. Metastatic disease is common in patients with hilar cholangiocarcinoma. One-half or more of the patients will have metastatic disease found at surgery.[270,343,346,347] Recent studies suggest that staging laparoscopy combined with laparoscopic US may be useful in hepatobiliary malignancies to find such metastatic disease and thereby prevent unnecessary laparotomies.[318] In our recent series, 50% of unresectable cases were identified as such by laparoscopy.[347] Of the causes of unresectability, laparoscopy was best at identifying peritoneal metastases and noncontiguous liver metastases and was poor at identifying vascular invasion and nodal metastases.[347] Hence, we would recommend a laparoscopic evaluation immediately before laparotomy. We also recommend that the examination concentrate on peritoneal and liver disease and not perseverate on the biliary or nodal extent of disease in the porta hepatis because of low yield and risk of violation and spread of tumor.

Laparotomy then commences with a thorough exploration of the abdomen. The lymph nodes in the porta hepatis and celiac and retropancreatic area are carefully assessed. If there is spread to celiac or retropancreatic nodes, the chance of long-term survival is sufficiently low that resection is ill-advised. Though a segmental bile duct resection and biliary reconstruction are possible in some patients, most require partial hepatectomy to achieve complete tumor clearance. The extent of liver resection should be tailored to achieve tumor clearance. Some patients with small tumors and low bifurcation of the hepatic ducts may be treatable with a central liver resection. Most patients will, however, require either a lobectomy or a trisegmentectomy for resection of tumor. A subset of patients

TABLE 33.5-15. Results of Resection for Proximal (Hilar) Cholangiocarcinoma after 1990

				Survival			
	No. of Cases	*No. Resected*	*Mortality (%)*	Median (mo)	1-Y (%)	3-Y (%)	5-Y (%)
Cameron, 1990[343]	96	53 (41%)	2	24	66	21	12
Nimura, 1990[352]	NR	55	6	—	—	55	41
Hadjis, 1990[339]	131	27 (21%)	7	25	76	26	22
Bismuth, 1991[333]	122	23 (19%)	0	24	87	25	—
Baer, 1993[337]	48	21 (44%)	5	36	72	50	—
Guthrie, 1993[584]	69	10 (14%)	10	16	—	—	—
Washburn, 1995[585]	88	59 (67%)	10	23	69	40	11
Su, 1996[586]	162	49 (30%)	10	19	—	—	35
Nakeeb, 1996[290]	196	109 (55%)	4	18	68	30	11
Klempnauer, 1997[362]	339	151 (55%)	10	24	72	40	29
Burke, 1997[270]	90	30 (33%)	6	40	—	—	56

NR, not reported.

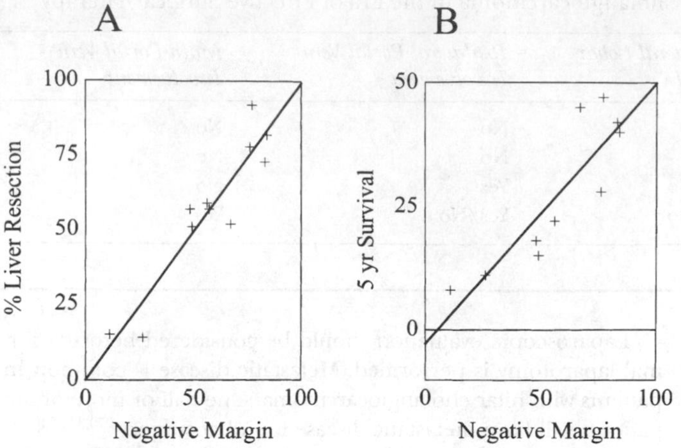

FIGURE 33.5-5. **A:** Relationship of percentage of liver resection to percentage of margin-negative cases for proximal (hilar) cholangiocarcinomas. Willingness to resect liver is essential for complete excision of cholangiocarcinomas and for achieving negative surgical margins. **B:** Relationship of percentage of margin-negative cases to percentage of 5-year survivors for proximal (hilar) cholangiocarcinomas. Achieving a negative margin is essential for favorable long-term outcome.

will also require excision of the caudate lobe (segment 1) to clear tumor completely.[348,349]

The factors most influential in predicting recurrence are a margin-positive resection,[350] node-positive tumor,[351] and vascular involvement by tumor. Of these, the only factor over which the surgeon can routinely have influence is the surgical margin. There is now substantial evidence that partial hepatectomy is usually required to achieve a surgical margin clear of tumor. Bile duct excision and partial hepatectomy, often with *en bloc* caudate lobectomy,[352] are frequently necessary to achieve negative margins. Indeed, several recent studies show a parallel between the number of patients undergoing partial hepatectomy and the number of patients with negative margins (Fig. 33.5-5*A*).[270,339,353–355] Furthermore, there is a direct correlation between negative margins and long-term survival (see Fig. 33.5-5*B*). Clearance of tumor is essential for potential cure.[270]

In the era when surgeons were unwilling to perform major liver resections to clear tumor, only the smallest of hilar cholangiocarcinomas could be resected. Given that extensive liver resections are now routine at many major centers, extensive unilobar disease is commonly resected with curative intent. In a recent study, of the 30 patients subjected to resections of cholangiocarcinoma, including 25 (83%) with negative histologic margins, 15 patients had tumor involvement of secondary biliary radicals, 11 had unilateral lobar liver atrophy, and 8 had encasement or occlusion of a major portal vein branch.[270] In the past, these findings would have been considered technically insurmountable.

The entire extrahepatic bile duct should be removed, as this assists in resection of the lymphatic tissues in the porta hepatis. Lymphatic metastases are common,[270] and a complete portal lymphadenectomy is essential. Biliary continuity is then reestablished using a jejunal reconstruction.[356,357] Portal vein invasion by tumor does not rule out resection, long-term survival, or potential cure,[270] provided that the portal vein involvement is unilobar and on the side of the dominant biliary involvement. Bilateral portal venous involvement or unilobar invasion contralateral to extensive biliary invasion usually denotes unresectable disease and, consequently, poor prognosis.

Recent results of resection have shown great improvement over previous results. Median survival is longer than 24 months.[271,333,337] Five-year survival is accomplished in nearly 30% of patients (see Table 33.5-15). Such long-term survival can be achieved with an acceptable operative mortality.[187,270,271,295,313,316,339,352–355,358–362] For those surviving the operative procedure, surgical resection provides not only improved survival but also improved quality of survival.[363]

ADJUVANT THERAPY. To date, no chemotherapeutic regimen has consistently shown activity in cholangiocarcinoma.[364] Although chemotherapy based on 5-FU often is offered to patients with nonresectable disease, the likelihood of response is less than 10% (see later in Chemotherapy and Immunotherapy). There is certainly no proven role for adjuvant chemotherapy in the treatment of cholangiocarcinoma.

The role of radiotherapy in the treatment of resected extrahepatic bile duct cancer is controversial. Given the poor prognosis of patients who have undergone a complete resection (median survival range, 1.5 to 2.0 years) and the fact that many resections leave microscopically positive margins, many practitioners have advocated postoperative irradiation with or without systemic chemotherapy (Table 33.5-16). External-beam doses in the range of 45 to 60 Gy (with the latter doses for positive margins) are usually administered. In addition to external-beam radiation, boost doses can be administered using intraluminal brachytherapy (ILB). In this approach, a wire or string of radioactive seeds (typically ^{192}Ir) is introduced into the bile duct, which delivers 20 to 30 Gy at a 0.5- to 1.0-cm depth. Traditionally, this has been performed using low dose-rate radiation (<1 Gy/h); more recently, high dose-rate radiation (approximately 2 Gy/min) has been administered.[365] The advantage of ILB is the potential to deliver a high dose of radiation to the duct itself with minimal damage to surrounding liver.[366,367] The disadvantage is that disease more than 1 cm from the duct tends to be underdosed. In addition, ILB may be associated with an increased risk of infection.

In two separate reports from Johns Hopkins, no benefit of adjuvant external-beam and intraluminal radiotherapy was demonstrated.[343,368] In contrast, Kamada et al.[369] suggested that radiation may improve survival in patients with histologically positive hepatic duct margins. Additionally, in a small series of patients (five with hilar cholangiocarcinoma) from Louisville, resectability was reportedly greater in patients given neoadjuvant radiotherapy prior to exploration.[370] In a series of 23 patients with cholangiocarcinoma, Urego et al.[371] used a chemoradiation regimen for adjuvant therapy, consisting of postoperative irradiation, 5-FU, leucovorin, and IFN. The 5-year survival was 53%.[371] These results certainly encourage further study of radiotherapy with or without chemosensitization in the adjuvant treatment of cholangiocarcinoma. Given the small size of the studies and lack of randomized trials, the utility of radiotherapy, and particularly ILB, is far from proven. In our practice, adjuvant therapy is generally used only if there is a positive margin or in the setting of metastases to lymph nodes. Other patients are not offered adjuvant therapy.

LIVER TRANSPLANTATION. Orthotopic liver transplantation has been attempted for unresectable hilar tumors. Klempnauer et al.[372] reported 4 long-term survivors of 32 patients submitted to transplantation for hilar cholangiocarcinoma.

TABLE 33.5-16. Results of Adjuvant Radiotherapy in Patients with Resected Cholangiocarcinoma

		Radiotherapy			
Study	*Schedule*	Dose	No. of Patients	*Chemotherapy*	*Median Survival (mo)*
Pitt[213]	Postop (includes positive margins)	40–60 Gy ± ILB (2–18 Gy)	14	None	20
		None	17	None	20
Urego[371]	Preop[a] (complete resection)	49.5 Gy (median)	23	Chiefly 5-FU	NA[d]
Gonzalez[407]	Postop[b] (includes positive margins)	50 Gy (mean)	30	None	24
		45 Gy (mean) + 22–25 Gy ILB	41		24
Kurosaki[587]	IO + Postop	40 Gy + 20 Gy IO (median)	35	None[c]	19
McMasters[370]	Preop	45–50.4 Gy	9	5-FU by infusion	22
	Postop	45–50.4 Gy	20	5-FU by infusion	22
		None	11	5-FU by infusion	22

5-FU, 5-fluorouracil; ILB, intraluminal brachytherapy; IO, intraoperatively; NA, not available; Postop, postoperatively; Preop, preoperatively.
[a]Orthotopic liver transplantation in 17 patients.
[b]Nineteen patients received 10.5 Gy preoperatively.
[c]Four patients received unspecified chemotherapy.
[d]Five-year survival, 54%.

Comparable results were reported by Iwatsuki et al.[373] These results do not justify the use of precious organs when many patients with benign disease are dying awaiting liver transplantation. Therefore, most centers do not currently perform liver transplantation for cholangiocarcinoma.

Palliative Treatments

Patients with hilar cholangiocarcinoma most often die from liver failure due to tumor progression or from sepsis due to biliary infection. If resection is not feasible, then palliative treatment must be directed first and foremost at preventing or relieving biliary infection. Secondarily, palliative antitumor treatments such as radiotherapy or chemotherapy should be considered, though neither of these modalities has been clearly proven to prolong survival significantly.

BILIARY DRAINAGE. The important concept in the prevention of biliary sepsis is the understanding that jaundice alone is not necessarily an indication for biliary decompression. Unlike biliary obstruction in the lower bile duct, where a single stent usually effectively relieves the biliary obstruction, biliary obstruction near the hilus is much more difficult to relieve. Even with a small tumor, a single stent likely will drain only one-half of the liver. When the tumors are large and involve second- or third-order bile ducts, many stents may be required to provide effective biliary decompression; it is also possible that effective biliary decompression cannot be achieved in such cases. Biliary manipulation of any kind may therefore introduce bacteria into the biliary tree and cause sepsis that may not subsequently be fixable.

Good indication for biliary drainage must exist before attempts are made. Our current indications for biliary decompression in inoperable patients are intractable pruritus, cholangitis, the need for access for intraluminal radiotherapy, or the need for drainage for administration of chemotherapeutic agents. When none of these indications exists, the patient is probably better served by avoiding biliary manipulation. Supportive care alone is probably the best approach, particularly for elderly patients with significant comorbid conditions.

Unfortunately, most patients present to a tertiary care center already having undergone manipulation of the biliary tree. Most of these patients, therefore, have bacterbilia and, possibly, overt sepsis, and drainage of the biliary tree is an essential part of the therapy to prevent immediate life-threatening complications.

Biliary drainage can be accomplished nonsurgically or surgically. Nonsurgical drainage is preferred if the patient has significant comorbid conditions or if the tumor as evaluated by preoperative imaging is clearly not resectable for cure. Though biliary decompression can theoretically be accomplished either by percutaneous transhepatic puncture or by endoscopic stent placement, hilar tumors are notoriously difficult to traverse with the endoscopic technique. Moreover, the failure rates and incidence of subsequent cholangitis are high.[374] Thus, most patients with unresectable hilar tumors are not candidates for endoscopic biliary drainage. Percutaneous transhepatic biliary drainage and subsequent placement of a self-expandable metallic endoprosthesis (Wallstent, Boston Scientific, Boston, MA) is the palliative procedure of choice for these patients. However, as mentioned, satisfactory results are more difficult to achieve in patients with hilar tumors than in those with distal biliary obstruction.[277,375,376] Frequently, hilar tumors isolate the liver into multiple obstructed biliary units, and two or more stents must be placed for adequate drainage.[377] Portal venous involvement and consequent hepatic lobar atrophy may also complicate drainage procedures, as drainage through an atrophic lobe usually does not relieve jaundice. Furthermore, a stent placed for a hilar obstruction is associated with a substantially higher rate of occlusion than that placed in the distal duct.[277,378] Therefore, most patients will require multiple manipulations of their stents placed for hilar obstruction.[277,377–382] These difficulties also explain the high periprocedural mortality in this patient population: 14% at 30 days.[380]

Biliary enteric bypass is a surgical alternative to percutaneous placement of an endobiliary prosthesis. Certainly, patients whose tumors are found to be unresectable at operation should be con-

TABLE 33.5-17. Results of Chemotherapy for Biliary Tract Tumors (Cholangiocarcinomas or Gallbladder Cancers)

Study	*No. of Cases*	*Treatment*	*PR*	*Stable Disease*
Davis, 1974[589]	23	5-FU	3 (13%)	NR
Haskell, 1980[590]	17	5-FU	2 (11%)	NR
Falkson, 1985[386]	30	5-FU	3 (10%)	NR
Crooke, 1976[592]	15	Mitomycin C	7 (47%)	NR
Taal, 1993[484]	30	Mitomycin C	3 (10%)	NR
Okada, 1994[593]	13	Cisplatin	1 (8%)	NR
Jones, 1996[390]	14	Paclitaxel	0	2
Mezger, 1997[396]	11	Gemcitabine	0	6 (54%)
Raderer, 1999[594]	19	Gemcitabine	3 (16%)	4 (21%)
Falkson, 1985[386]	26	5-FU + streptozotocin	2 (8%)	NR
Falkson, 1985[386]	31	5-FU + MeCCNU	3 (10%)	NR
Patt, 1996[389]	18	5-FU + IFN	6 (34%)	NR
Chen, 1998[595]	18	5-FU (high-dose) + LV	6 (33%)	7 (39%)
DeGusmao, 1998[397]	14	5-FU + gemcitabine	6 (43%)	NR
Rougier, 1995[596]	18	5-FU, cisplatin, CI	6 (24%)	NR
Di Lauro, 1997[393]	15	5-FU, cisplatin, epirubicin	5 (33%)	5 (33%)
Harvey, 1984[391]	13	5-FU, mitomycin C, doxorubicin	4 (31%)	7 (53%)
Sanz-Altamira, 1998[394]	14	5-FU, LV, carboplatin	3 (21%)	4 (28%)
Raderer, 1999[594]	20	5-FU, LV, mitomycin C	5 (25%)	6 (30%)
Hall, 1979[597]	8	Doxorubicin + BCNU + tegafur	3 (38%)	1 (13%)
Isacoff, 1993[598]	7	5-FU, mitomycin C, doxorubicin, CI	3 (43%)	NR
Kajanti, 1994[599]	22	5-FU, LV, methotrexate, epirubicin	0	NR

CI, continuous infusion; 5-FU, 5-fluorouracil; IFN, interferon; LV, leucovorin; MeCCNU, semustine; NR, not reported; PR, partial response.

sidered for such bypasses,[270] because they will have already incurred the morbidity of laparotomy. Patients with small, unresectable, but well-localized disease are particularly good candidates for biliary enteric bypass, as this allows access to the biliary tree for ILB.[383] Typically, segment III bypass is used.[384] Relief of jaundice will be achieved if at least one-third of the functioning hepatic parenchyma is adequately drained. Additional percutaneous stenting to reestablish biliary continuity of the two sides of the liver is required if the bypass is to an atrophic or a small lobe or if infection has occurred in the contralateral lobe of liver.[385] In our recent report of 55 consecutive bypasses in patients with malignant hilar obstruction, segment III bypass yielded a 1-year bypass patency of 80%, and there were no perioperative deaths.[384]

CHEMOTHERAPY AND IMMUNOTHERAPY. Many different chemotherapeutic regimens have been investigated in small uncontrolled studies, with generally poor results (Table 33.5-17). A study by the European Organization for Research and Treatment of Cancer testing mitomycin C on patients with gallbladder and biliary carcinomas showed a response rate of 10% (3 of 30). The group also compared oral 5-FU to 5-FU with either streptozotocin or MeCCNU in patients with gallbladder or biliary duct cancer and demonstrated a similarly low response rate of 9%, with no differences in the types of drugs used.[386] Some of the newer drugs have also not demonstrated significant efficacy as single-agent therapy. Paclitaxel demonstrated no activity in 15 patients with biliary carcinoma,[387] and a phase II study of docetaxel likewise demonstrated no activity.[388]

Combinations of various chemotherapeutic agents have been tested, with mixed and conflicting results. Patt et al.[389] used 5-FU and IFN as combined therapy for patients with cholangiocarcinoma. Of 32 patients, 11 (34%) had a partial response, with a median time to disease progression of 9.5 months and a median survival of 12 months.[389] However, another phase II study analyzing the effect of 5-FU combined with IFN-α_{2b} and paclitaxel failed to show any benefit.[390] In one study combining 5-FU, mitomycin, and doxorubicin, 31% of patients responded,[391] whereas in another trial, there were no responses among 18 patients.[392] The combination of 5-FU, cisplatin, and epirubicin produced a 33% response rate in 15 patients with biliary tract carcinoma in an Italian study,[393] and 5-FU, leucovorin, and carboplatin produced a 21% response rate among 14 patients.[394] Rougier et al.,[395] using continuous-infusion 5-FU and cisplatin, produced a 33% response rate in 18 patients. Gemcitabine[396] and 5-FU plus gemcitabine[397] have also been tested and, in one study involving 14 patients, 42% responded.[397] At present, either 5-FU and cisplatin or 5-FU and gemcitabine must be considered the regimens of greatest promise in the palliative treatment of unresectable cholangiocarcinoma. We tend to use the latter combination because of its lower toxicity as compared to the former.

The blood supply to the biliary tree is derived primarily from the hepatic artery. Therefore, attempts have been directed at delivering chemotherapeutic treatment via hepatic arterial infusion to patients with cholangiocarcinoma. In one study of 11 patients (4 with cholangiocarcinomas and 7 with gallbladder cancers), hepatic infusion of 5-FU and mitomycin produced 7 responses but a median duration of response of only 3 months and a median survival of 12.5 months.[398] Reed et al.[399] reported seven significant regressions in nine patients with biliary carcinoma treated with intraarterial FUDR. This approach is far from proven and, at present, operative intervention to implant an arterial infusion pump for delivery of regional chemotherapy should be performed only in the investigational setting.

Tamoxifen is a potential MDR-reversing agent[161] and has been shown to inhibit human cholangiocarcinoma cell lines.[400] No clinical data exist, however, to indicate whether this may be a reasonable therapeutic modality for patients with unresectable cholangiocarcinomas.

PALLIATIVE RADIOTHERAPY. External-beam irradiation with or without ILB has also been used for palliation of patients with unresectable perihilar bile duct cancer. External-beam irradiation is usually delivered to a dose of 5000 to 6000 cGy. ILB most often uses ^{192}Ir (2000 cGy) delivered percutaneously. Several authors have demonstrated the feasibility of radiotherapy in small, nonrandomized trials.[343,383,401–404] However, to date, no study has clearly demonstrated efficacy for this modality. In a group of 12 patients treated with a combination of endoluminal and external-beam radiotherapy, the median survival was 15 months. Though episodes of cholangitis and intermittent jaundice were relatively common, the incidence of serious complications was low, and there were no treatment-related deaths.[383] Cameron et al.[343] reported improved survival in irradiated patients as compared to a group of patients who were not irradiated; however, the median survival in both groups was less than 1 year. Others have reported no benefit of radiotherapy in this setting and question its routine use, given the increased incidence of complications and the greater time spent in hospital.[401] Certainly, radiotherapy has not been shown to produce improved survival as compared with biliary decompression in randomized, controlled trials. Though anecdotal reports of long-term survivors after external-beam radiotherapy show that some individuals may benefit from such treatment, such potential benefit must be weighed against the possible complications, such as duodenal or bile duct stenosis and duodenitis.

Evidence in the literature supports using fluoropyrimidines as radiosensitizers, and chemoradiotherapy is used as standard therapy for a number of other tumor types. For bile duct cancers in particular, however, evidence supporting the use of chemoradiotherapy is sparse. In a study conducted by the Eastern Cooperative Oncology Group, 16 patients with pancreatic carcinoma and 9 with bile duct cancers were treated with a combination of 5-FU (200 mg/m^2/d) and concurrent radiotherapy (59.4 Gy). The entire group had a median survival time of 11.9 months. Unfortunately, 15 of the 25 patients had clinical or radiographic evidence of progression of disease at the site of the primary tumor, which was in the radiotherapy port.[405] Moreover, median survival for the patients with locally advanced, unresectable disease that was treated with radiotherapy with or without systemic chemotherapy tends to be less than 1 year.[273,370,371,401,406–408] Our current practice is to use combined interstitial irradiation and external-beam irradiation in patients with very limited, locally unresectable disease, when there are no indications of distant spread. Multicenter, randomized trials are in order for this subpopulation. Radiotherapy is clearly inappropriate in patients with widespread disease.

PERIPHERAL CHOLANGIOCARCINOMA

Peripheral or intrahepatic cholangiocarcinoma is another rare disease, accounting for 1000 to 2000 cases per year in the United States.[409] Clinical presentation is similar to that for HCC, with the most common symptoms being right upper quadrant pain, epigastric pain, and weight loss.[287,409] Jaundice occurs in only 24% of patients with peripheral cholangiocarcinoma as compared with 71% of patients with hilar or Klatskin tumors.[409] Because the tumor is usually asymptomatic in its early stages, most patients have advanced disease at presentation. On cross-sectional imaging by CT or MRI, the peripheral cholangiocarcinoma usually is confused with HCC or metastatic tumor from an unknown primary source. Unlike HCC, AFP levels will be normal. A search for alternative primary cancers that may have produced a liver metastases will not be fruitful. A solitary lesion not associated with the gallbladder in a patient with no cirrhosis and no other primary cancer and with a normal serum AFP should raise suspicion of a peripheral cholangiocarcinoma. However, intrahepatic metastases and tumor growth along the biliary tract frequently occur. When multiple tumors are found, it is even more difficult to distinguish these tumors from metastatic disease originating from a distant site.

Lymph node involvement is more common with peripheral cholangiocarcinoma with hilar bile duct tumors. In a series of 65 peripheral and 27 hilar cholangiocarcinomas, Nakajima et al.[410] found lymph node involvement in 86% of peripheral tumors as compared with 33% of hilar tumors. Intrahepatic and systemic metastases were found in 68% and 71%, respectively. The TNM staging of intrahepatic or peripheral cholangiocarcinoma is the same as that for HCC.

Conventional surgical resection, when possible, is the treatment of choice. In a series of 42 patients with peripheral cholangiocarcinoma, Altaee et al.[336] reported that survival was indistinguishable from that of 70 patients with hilar cholangiocarcinomas. The median survival was 12 months, and no patient survived more than 42 months. Others have reported more favorable results. Chen et al.[409] reported on 20 patients with peripheral cholangiocarcinoma undergoing surgery over a 10-year period who had a median survival of 21 months. Four patients lived more than 3 years, and one patient was alive 5 years after resection. In our own report of 32 cases of resected peripheral cholangiocarcinoma, median survival was 59 months, with an actuarial 5-year survival of 42%. Vascular invasion and intrahepatic satellite lesions were predictors of worse survival (P<.05).[287]

The few data available concerning results of liver transplantation for this disease have not been encouraging. Penn[259] reported a 17% actuarial 5-year survival rate for 109 intrahepatic and extrahepatic cholangiocarcinoma patients who received liver transplants at various centers throughout the world. In this series also, there was no significant difference between the recurrence rates of hilar and peripheral tumors.

Data for chemotherapy or radiotherapy in treating this disease is even more sketchy. Stillwagon et al.[411] reported a 5% complete response and 46% partial response for the treatment of peripheral cholangiocarcinoma with a regimen of initial whole liver irradiation to 2100 cGy in seven fractions and doxorubicin, cisplatin, and ^{131}I anti-CEA antibody.[411] Although the median survival was 14 months from diagnosis and 10 months from treatment, no patient survived more than 2 years from the start of therapy.

TUMORS OF THE GALLBLADDER

Alfred Blalock recommended in 1924 that ". . . in malignancy of the gallbladder when a diagnosis can be made without exploration, no operation should be performed, inasmuch as it only shortens the patient's life."[412] This nihilistic view of gallbladder cancer is understandable because this rapidly growing tumor has a propensity for early dissemination by direct invasion of liver, by lymphatic spread, by hematogenous spread, and by production of peritoneal "drop" metastases. In addition, because of the proximity of the liver and major vasculature, extensive hepatic resections often are required to eradicate local disease. Until recently, therefore, most cases in which patients were cured of gallbladder cancer occurred "accidentally" when early-stage disease was completely excised by simple cholecystectomy for suspected stone disease. With improving safety of liver resections and biliary reconstructions, major resections are increasingly performed for gallbladder cancer and have demonstrated a curative potential even for advanced disease. Given that gallbladder cancer treated by any method other than complete excision is associated with a median survival of less than 6 months, surgery, when possible, is standard treatment.

EPIDEMIOLOGY AND ETIOLOGY

Gallbladder cancer is a relatively rare disease in the United States, with an incidence of approximately 1.2 cases per 100,000 population per year.[266] Even though this would still make gallbladder cancer the most common biliary tract malignancy in this country and the fifth most common gastrointestinal malignancy, only 2000 to 3000 cases occur in the United States annually. Certain geographic regions and racial or ethnic groups demonstrate a much higher incidence, which can be 25 times higher than the national figure.[413] The highest incidences are reported in Chileans, northeastern Europeans, Israelis, American Indians, and Americans of Mexican origin. In fact, gallbladder cancer is the main cause of death from cancer among women in Chile.[414] Within the United States and the United Kingdom, urban areas show higher incidences than rural regions.[413,415] This cancer affects women two to six times more often than it does men.[416,417] The incidence steadily increases with age, reaching its maximum in the seventh decade of life.[418]

The epidemiology of gallbladder cancer is similar to the epidemiology of gallbladder stones,[415] though there is still no general agreement as to whether this represents cause and effect or common risk factors. Seventy-five to ninety-eight percent of all patients with carcinoma of the gallbladder have cholelithiasis.[419] Gallbladder cancer is usually associated with cholesterol-type gallstones. Other risk factors include the presence of an anomalous pancreaticobiliary duct junction,[420] chronic typhoid infection,[421] and inflammatory bowel disease.[422] Calcification of the gallbladder (porcelain gallbladder), signifying long-standing inflammation, is associated with gallbladder cancer in 10% to 25% of cases.[423] These conditions suggest that chronic inflammation may play an important role in the development of gallbladder cancer. Though reports of family clusters of gallbladder cancer exist in the literature,[424] congenital predisposition is not believed to play a major role in the development of this cancer.

Exposure to a number of chemicals has been suggested to play a role in carcinogenesis in the gallbladder, including methyldopa,[425] oral contraceptives,[426] isoniazid,[427] and chemicals used in the rubber industry.[428] None of these associations have been definitively proven, however. It may be that chronic inflammation acts as a promoter for some other carcinogenic exposure. This is suggested by the studies of Kowalewski and Todd,[429] in which carcinoma of the gallbladder was induced in 68% of hamsters in whom cholesterol pellets were inserted into the gallbladder and the carcinogen dimethylnitrosamine was administered, as compared to only 6% of control hamsters who received the carcinogen only.

PATHOLOGIC FEATURES

In general, gallbladder cancers can be categorized by growth pattern into infiltrative, nodular, papillary, or combined forms.[430] Most common are the infiltrative and combined nodular-infiltrative forms. The infiltrative tumors cause thickening and induration of the gallbladder wall, sometimes extending to involve the entire gallbladder. These infiltrative tumors often are difficult to distinguish from a chronically inflamed but benign gallbladder. Because the spread of tumor is often along the subserosal plane, which, incidentally, is the plane of dissection during cholecystectomy for gallstone disease, it is not uncommon for tumor to go recognized and for tumor to be disseminated by cholecystectomy.

Nodular types of gallbladder cancer are more distinctive and can show early invasion through the gallbladder wall into the liver or neighboring structures. Despite this invasiveness, nodular disease may be easier to control surgically than the infiltrative form, wherein the margins are less defined.

Papillary carcinomas exhibit a polypoid appearance. This variety has a much better prognosis than the other types owing to its relatively low invasiveness. A papillary tumor may be sufficiently large to fill the entire lumen of the gallbladder and still show minimal invasion of the gallbladder wall.

Most gallbladder cancers (99%) are of epithelial cell origin[431] and can be separated histologically into adenocarcinoma, squamous, adenosquamous,[432] and oat cell[433] subtypes. Most are adenocarcinomas. Rarely, tumors can be of mesenchymal cell origin and result in embryonal rhabdomyosarcoma, leiomyosarcoma, malignant fibrous histiocytoma, angiosarcoma, and Kaposi's sarcoma. Even more rarely, carcinosarcoma, carcinoid, lymphoma, and melanoma can occur at this site. In addition, the gallbladder can be involved with metastatic cancers. While classification is academically interesting, the only primary histologic type having clear prognostic significance is the papillary adenocarcinoma, for which the outlook is comparatively favorable.[266] Grading of tumors is also performed and may have prognostic significance.[433] However, it is extent of dissemination and resectability that has the greatest influence on outcome.

PATTERN OF SPREAD AND STAGING

Gallbladder cancer generally disseminates by all four routes of tumor spread: direct adjacent organ invasion, lymphatic spread, hematogenous spread, and peritoneal drop metastases. The gallbladder is attached to the undersurface of the liver along segments IVb and V. The organ has a thin wall, a narrow lamina propria, and only a single muscle layer. Direct invasion of the liver is therefore common. In addition, the infundibulum and the cystic duct abut the common bile duct and are in proximity of the major vasculature of the porta hepatis. Tumors of the infundibulum or the cystic duct may occlude the hepatic arteries, portal veins, and bile ducts, making tumor unresectable at an early stage or dictating an extensive resection and vascular reconstruction. Whereas tumors of the fundus may be resected by a limited liver resection, tumors of the infundibulum most often will require a major liver resection for extirpation.

Once gallbladder cancer penetrates the thin muscle layer, it has access to major lymphatic and vascular channels. Lymph node metastases and hematogenous metastases are therefore common. An autopsy study revealed a 94% incidence of lymphatic metastasis and 65% incidence of hematogenous dissemination.[434] In general, lymphatic spread of tumor descends around the bile duct and involves cystic and pericholedochal nodes first and subsequently descends to portacaval and celiac nodes. Further spread will lead tumor to nodes in the retropancreatic, interaortocaval, and superior mesenteric artery lymph nodes. Therefore, it is essential that full mobilization of the duodenum and head of the pancreas be performed for full evaluation of the extent of lymphatic spread of disease. Though autopsy studies demonstrate as high a rate of distant metastases as 32% in lung and 5% in brain,[435] such spread is clinically apparent only late in the disease. Metastasis to the lung is rare, however, in the absence of advanced locoregional disease.

Gallbladder cancer has a great propensity for peritoneal spread and for seeding incisions and laparoscopic port sites.[436,437] At postmortem examination, Perpetuo et al.[435] reported that 60% of gallbladder cancer patients had peritoneal spread. This reflects a predilection for transserosal tumor both to shed and to implant and grow. In addition, a large proportion of patients present after previous cholecystectomy for presumed gallstone disease, when violation of tumor is likely.

Multiple staging systems have been advocated for the classification of gallbladder cancer. The most popular systems are listed in Table 33.5-18. Most useful are the modified Nevin system[438,439] and the AJCC–Union Internationale Contre le Cancer TNM staging system.[440] The Japanese Biliary Surgical Society system[441] is included because of the extensive literature on gallbladder cancer originating in Japan. Understanding the Japanese system is essential for interpreting this literature.

Nevin et al.[439] originally classified patients into five stages, based primarily on the thickness of invasion, and combined patients with direct liver extension or distant metastasis into stage V. This staging system was later modified by Donohue et al.[438] such that tumors with contiguous liver invasion were reclassified as stage 3 and noncontiguous liver involvement as stage 5. Stage 4 continued to include lymph node metastasis. The disadvantage of this system is that it does not differentiate between tumors that invade through muscle without invading the liver and tumors with minimal (<2 cm) or extensive (>2 cm) invasion of the liver, factors that seem to have significant prognostic significance.

In the TNM staging system, T1 tumors are those involving only the mucosa or muscle layer. T2 tumors involve perimuscular connective tissue. T3 tumors extend beyond the serosa but involve less than 2 cm of liver. T4 tumors invade beyond 2 cm of liver. T1 or T2 tumors with no lymph node metastases are stage I and II, respectively. T3 of N1 (perihilar) nodal involvement is classified as stage III. T4 tumors with no lymph node or distant metastasis constitute stage IVA, while distant nodal or other metastases are classified as stage IVB. We agree with Donohue et al.[438] that direct liver invasion is less ominous than nodal metastases, which in turn are less ominous than distant metastases. Included in Table 33.5-18 is a proposed revision of the TNM staging system that we believe more closely segregates patients according to biologic features of the disease.

CLINICAL PRESENTATION

Distinguishing the clinical presentation of gallbladder cancer from gallstone disease is usually difficult. Pain is the most common symptom, occurring in 60% to 95% of cases. Symptoms are often mistaken for biliary colic or chronic cholecystitis. Jaundice occurs in one-fourth to one-half of patients and usually denotes far-advanced disease[442,443] or an infundibular tumor. Gallbladder cancer can also cause obstructive jaundice by direct invasion of the common hepatic duct or by compression and involvement of the common hepatic duct by pericholedochal lymph nodes. A high correlation between Mirizzi syndrome and gallbladder cancer exists.[444] Anorexia, weight loss, and anemia are other nonspecific symptoms that often accompany this cancer. Obstruction of the cystic duct or the neck of the gallbladder may lead to hydrops of the gallbladder, which manifests as a mass in the right upper quadrant. A firm, fixed mass, however, would be an ominous sign and usually denotes extensive local invasion. In a review from Thorbjarnarson and Glenn,[443] the presence of a right upper quadrant mass in association with gallbladder cancer reflected unresectability in 23 of 25 patients.

Laboratory examination usually reveals nonspecific liver function abnormalities. Increased alkaline phosphatase or

TABLE 33.5-18. Summary of Most Commonly Used Staging Systems for Gallbladder Cancer

Stage	*TNM System*	*Modified Nevin System*	*Japanese Biliary Surgical Society System*	*Proposed New Staging System*
I	Mucosal or muscular invasion (T1N0M0)	*In situ* carcinoma	Confined to gallbladder capsule	Mucosal or muscular invasion
II	Transmural invasion (T2N0M0)	Mucosal or muscular invasion	N1 lymph nodes; minimal liver or bile duct invasion	Transmural invasion
III	Liver invasion <2 cm; lymph node metastases (T3N1M0)	Transmural direct liver invasion	N2 lymph nodes; marked liver or bile duct invasion	A: liver invasion <2 cm (T3N0M0) B: liver invasion >2 cm (T4N0M0)
IV	A: liver invasion >2 cm (T4N0M0, TXN1M0) B: distant metastasis (TXN2M0, TXNXM1)	Lymph node metastasis	Distant metastasis	A: N1 disease (TXN1M0) B: distant metastases (TXNXM1)
V	—	Distant metastasis	—	—

TNM, tumor, node, metastasis.

bilirubin levels are found commonly in cases of advanced tumors. CEA and CA 19-9 are tumor markers that may be useful in the diagnosis and treatment of this cancer. A CEA level greater than 4 ng/mL is 93% specific for the diagnosis of gallbladder cancer, as compared to controls undergoing cholecystectomy or upper abdominal surgery for benign conditions, though it is only 50% sensitive.[445] Serum CA 19-9 levels greater than 20 units/mL have a 79.4% sensitivity and 79.2% specificity.[446] These markers may be useful when radiologic imaging is ambiguous or indeterminate.

RADIOLOGIC EVALUATION

Before the routine use of CT and US, the preoperative diagnosis rate for gallbladder carcinoma was generally less than 10%, which, in part, explains the dismal outcomes of surgical therapy in the era prior to sophisticated cross-sectional imaging, as many patients with incurable disease were subjected to exploration. With the routine use of CT scanning and real-time US in the 1980s, preoperative diagnosis was achieved in 75% to 88% of patients.[447] Beyond diagnosis, the goals of imaging also include accurate staging. The goal of imaging is to determine extent of liver invasion, invasion of other adjacent organs, vascular involvement, extent of biliary involvement, presence of nodal metastases, and presence of peritoneal metastases.

Because the majority of patients will present with symptoms suggestive of biliary colic or chronic cholecystitis, the diagnostic workup will usually begin with abdominal US. Discontinuous gallbladder mucosa, echogenic mucosa, submucosal echolucency, or a mass greater than 1 cm should arouse suspicion of gallbladder cancer.[448] The finding most convincing of a gallbladder malignancy is an inhomogeneous mass replacing all or part of the gallbladder.[449,450] The index of suspicion should be high for elderly patients, patients with atypical symptoms, and patients with suspicious laboratory findings such as anemia, hypoalbuminemia, and abnormal liver function tests. US can also delineate the degree of biliary involvement and can define the presence of arterial or portal venous involvement by tumor. In experienced hands, US will provide diagnostic information equivalent to that provided by much more expensive cross-sectional imaging.

CT scanning is usually the next imaging examination performed because of its wide availability, low cost, low risk, and high yield. On CT, gallbladder cancer can appear as a mass almost filling the gallbladder lumen in 42% of cases, a polypoid mass in 26%, and diffuse wall thickening in 6% of gallbladder cancer patients.[451] CT is better than US in demonstrating liver atrophy, which usually is indicative of ipsilateral portal vein involvement by tumor. CT is also better at detecting lymphadenopathy,[452] particularly for retropancreatic nodal disease, which would rule out the potential for cure, though only 38% of pathologically positive nodes were identified preoperatively by CT scan.[452]

In years past, jaundice or radiologic signs of biliary obstruction would lead to direct cholangiography via ERCP or PTC. Indeed, direct cholangiography may provide a diagnosis. A long stricture at the mid–common bile duct is more likely to be a gallbladder cancer than any other malignancy. Direct cholangiography also allows brush sampling of the area of tumor invasion for diagnosis by cytology. Such cholangiography, however, carries the risk of introducing bacteria into an obstructed biliary tree and may cause infection and sepsis.[332] In addition, the presence of a biliary catheter or stent may produce sufficient inflammation to obscure margins between tumor and normal ductal epithelium. This may, in turn, compromise surgical resection.

Angiography was another common test for assessing vascular invasion when the mass encroached on the porta hepatis, but this invasive method of examination carries finite risks. Cholangiography and angiography remain important tests in certain settings, but Doppler US, magnetic resonance cholangiography, and MRA have largely replaced these invasive procedures in the majority of cases.[307,453]

Magnetic resonance procedures have long been accepted as invaluable for characterizing hepatic tumors. Such procedures may also identify and characterize lymph node metastases with greater precision than can other cross-sectional imaging techniques.[454] With recent advances in hardware and software, the extent of biliary involvement can now be determined through MRCP.[455] MRA allows for assessment of vascular invasion to determine resectability and can demonstrate anomalous anatomic findings to assist in surgical planning.

If a patient presents with a clinical picture and ultrasound scans suspicious for gallbladder cancer, a CT scan of the abdomen and a chest radiograph usually are obtained. Findings of pulmonary metastases, peritoneal metastases, vascular or biliary involvement not amenable to reconstruction, discontiguous liver metastases, or distant nodal disease indicate unresectability. Tissue confirmation of diagnosis can be obtained by needle biopsy, and the patient can be sent for alternative therapy.

Barring signs of unresectability, medically fit and nonjaundiced patients may proceed directly to surgical exploration. For those with jaundice or equivocal CT findings, MRCP represents the next least invasive test that may have utility. In patients with medical contraindications to immediate surgery, particularly those with renal insufficiency or sepsis, a PTC should be performed to delineate extent of biliary involvement and to treat the jaundice. At times, arteriography is still needed to demonstrate clearly unresectable vascular involvement. On rare occasions, the gallbladder cancer can erode into the transverse colon and produce a colonic fistula as a source of sepsis. In patients in whom this condition is suspected, a colonoscopy should be performed and full bowel preparation should be undertaken prior to surgical exploration.

ROLE FOR NEEDLE BIOPSY

Generally, needle biopsy is contraindicated if a patient is thought to have a resectable gallbladder cancer. This cancer has a great propensity to spread in needle tracts, a laparoscopic port site, surgical wounds, and the peritoneal cavity.[456,457] Therefore, needle biopsy is not indicated if surgical exploration is otherwise appropriate. However, if radiologic studies demonstrate an unresectable tumor, percutaneous fine-needle aspiration cytology is highly accurate[458] and may avoid an unnecessary laparotomy in many patients. If the tumor is clearly unresectable and the patient is jaundiced, direct cholangiography allows for placement of stents to relieve jaundice and allows diagnosis to be established by either bile cytology or brush biopsy.[458–460] Yield can be expected in 50% to 75% of cases, and the false-positive rate is less than 1%.

TABLE 33.5-19. Morbidity and Mortality of Resection for Gallbladder Cancer

Author	*Year*	*No. of Cases*	*Procedure*	*Morbidity (%)*	*Mortality (%)*
Ouchi, 1987[467]	1987	12	Extended procedures	—	21
Nakamura, 1989[418]	1989	13	Extended procedures	46	0
Donohue, 1991[438]	1990	17	Extended procedures	5	0
Todoroki, 1991[492]	1991	27	Extended cholecystectomy + IORT	—	7
Nimura, 1991[461]	1991	14	Hepatopancreaticoduodenectomy	—	21
Gall, 1991[476]	1991	8	Extended procedures	—	0
Ogura, 1991[463]	1991	659	Extended procedures	22	2
		302	Hepatic lobectomy	48	18
		150	Hepatopancreatoduodenectomy	54	15
de Aretxabala, 1994[414]	1992	25	Extended procedures	—	0
Matsumoto, 1992[475]	1992	35	Extended procedures	15	4
Chijiiwa, 1994[603]	1994	30	Extended procedures	—	3
Bartlett, 1996[473]	1996	23	Extended procedures	26	0

IORT, intraoperative radiotherapy.
Note: Extended procedures include common bile duct resection and liver resection.

TREATMENT

Surgical Management

Much controversy exists as to the extent of surgery required for treatment of gallbladder cancer. Recommendations have ranged from simple cholecystectomy to ultraaggressive resections consisting of combined major liver resection and pancreaticoduodenectomy.[461] This controversy exists because, until recently, the operations required for complete resection of cancer were associated with prohibitive morbidity and mortality.[462,463] The majority of patients undergoing treatment for gallbladder cancer are in their seventh or eighth decade of life and may be at increased risk for radical surgery as a consequence of concomitant medical problems. The major morbidity after resection for gallbladder cancer has ranged from 5% to 54% and mortality from 0% to 21% (Table 33.5-19). In a multiinstitutional review of 1686 gallbladder cancer resections from Japan, a comparison of morbidity by procedure was made.[463] The review reports 12.8% morbidity for cholecystectomy, 21.9% for extended cholecystectomy, and 48.3% for hepatic lobectomy. The mortality rates were 2.9%, 2.3%, and 17.9%, respectively.[463] The morbidity and mortality rates of major liver resections have decreased in recent reports, even in the aged population.[464,465] Most recent series report a mortality rate of 5% or less even with extensive liver resections. With these improvements in perioperative outcome, radical resections are increasingly accepted.

Controversy concerning the extent of resection is also based on the dismal results of treatment in decades past. Until the last decade, the results of treatment for gallbladder cancer in general, including surgical treatment, were dismal. Piehler and Crichlow[466] reviewed 5836 cases in the world's literature from 1960 to 1978. The overall 5-year survival rate was consistently less than 5%, with a median survival of 5 to 8 months. Even for the 25% who were treated by resections with curative intent, only 16.5% survived 5 years. In fact, the only long-term survivors were among the group in which the tumor was small enough not to be recognized at the time of cholecystectomy. Perpetuo et al.[435] reviewed a 36-year experience with gallbladder cancer from the M. D. Anderson Cancer Center and reported a 5-year survival rate of less than 5% and median survival of 5.2 months. Cubertafond et al.[467] recently reported the results of a French Surgical Association survey of 724 carcinomas of the gallbladder. These investigators reported a median survival of 3 months, a 5-year survival rate of 5%, and a 1-year survival rate of 14%. They observed no differences among the various surgical procedures adopted and concluded that no progress had been made in the treatment of gallbladder cancer. A review of gallbladder cancer from Australia revealed a 12% 5-year survival rate, with all survivors having stage I or II disease. The median survival for patients with stage III or IV disease was only 46 days.[468] These miserable results sowed the seeds of nihilism that surrounded this disease in the past.

Over the last decade, many reports have demonstrated the utility of aggressive therapy. As a result, a more reasoned approach based on the biology of the disease is now advocated. The following recommendations are based on the goal of complete resection of tumor. To achieve this goal, surgery must remove the cancerous gallbladder, remove any adjacent organ invaded by tumor, remove involved lymph glands, and provide biliary continuity if resection of the bile duct is necessary. Surgical strategy is best directed by the suspected T stage of disease.

T1 DISEASE. Patients with T1 stage tumor (tumor confined within the mucosa or muscular layers of the gallbladder) most often present after the gallbladder has already been removed by simple cholecystectomy for presumed gallstone disease. Ample literature reports that patients with T1 tumors may be cured by simple cholecystectomy alone. The 5-year survival rate is expected to be 85% to 100% (Table 33.5-20).[469–472] Therefore, when patients present after simple cholecystectomy, the pathologic findings are reviewed to ensure that margins are negative. Particular attention is paid to the cystic duct margin. If all margins are negative, no other therapy is undertaken. If the cystic duct margin is positive, patients should be subjected to a common bile duct excision and biliary reconstruction.

Alternatively, the early-stage tumor may be discovered radiographically by a vigilant radiologist. If a T1 cancerous lesion is suspected, an open simple cholecystectomy should be performed and the diagnosis and stage confirmed immediately by

TABLE 33.5-20. Survival after Resection of Stage I Gallbladder Cancers

Study	*No. of Cases*	*Procedure*	*3-Y Survival (%)*	*5-Y Survival (%)*
Ouchi, 1987[462]	14	Not specified	78	71.4
Yamaguchi, 1988[432]	11	Not specified	100	NR
Donohue, 1990[438]	6	83% Simple cholecystectomy	100	100
Gall, 1991[476]	7	Simple cholecystectomy	86	86
Ogura, 1991[463,a]	366	Not specified	87	78
Shirai, 1992[600]	39	Simple cholecystectomy	100	100
Yamaguchi, 1992[470]	6	Simple cholecystectomy	100	100
Shirai, 1992[474]	56	Simple cholecystectomy	100	100
	38	Extended cholecystectomy	100	100
Matsumoto, 1992[475]	4	Extended cholecystectomy	100	100
Oertli, 1993[442]	6	Simple cholecystectomy	100	100
de Aretxabala, 1997[601]	32	69% Simple cholecystectomy	94	94

NR, not reported.
[a]Multiinstitutional survey.

frozen-section pathology. If a benign lesion or a T1 tumor is confirmed, simple cholecystectomy is all that is necessary. If deeper invasion is found, further resection according to stage should be performed, as outlined next.

T2 DISEASE. T2 tumors remain subserosal but have invaded through the muscular layer. It would at first seem logical that a simple cholecystectomy may be adequate for T2 tumors. However, there are two good reasons for performing more extensive resection. First, the plane that is generally taken between the liver and gallbladder is subserosal and may violate T2 tumors along the liver interphase. In the review by Yamaguchi and Tsuneyoshi,[470] 25 patients had tumor extending into the subserosal layer and 11 of these had positive microscopic margins after simple cholecystectomy. Second, T2 tumors are associated with a high incidence of regional nodal metastases (Table 33.5-21). Therefore, the most reasonable primary operation for T2 gallbladder cancer is the radical cholecystectomy that was first advocated by Thorbjarnarson and Glenn.[443] This includes a wedge resection of the gallbladder bed and regional lymphadenectomy of the hepatoduodenal ligament. Except for the thinnest of patients, total nodal clearance in the porta hepatis is difficult without removal of the common bile duct. In addition, adequate lymph node dissection of the porta hepatis has a good chance of devascularizing the common bile duct, and subsequent benign structure is a possible late consequence. For both reasons, we prefer to resect the common bile duct as part of the clearance of lymphatic tissue in this region. A hepaticojejunostomy using a Roux-en-Y loop of jejunum is the preferred method of reestablishing biliary continuity.

A large number of patients will present for definitive therapy after simple cholecystectomy. Good evidence supports a repeat exploration for a more definitive resection. Data from many series have demonstrated that simple cholecystectomy results in 30% to 40% 5-year survival, while radical cholecystectomy or a more extensive liver resection results in a 5-year survival of 80% to 90% (Table 33.5-22). This could be explained by the possibility of residual tumor in the gallbladder bed or the 30% to 50% chance of regional lymph node involvement in cases of T2 gallbladder cancer.[469,473] In an article by Shirai et al.,[471] the 5-year survival rate after radical re-resection for stage II tumors was 90%, as compared to 40% 5-year survival for simple cholecystectomy alone. In a study comparing 20 patients treated by radical re-resection for T2 tumors with 18 patients treated by simple cholecystectomy, de Aretxabala[472] demonstrated a 50% improved 5-year survival rate for the more aggressive approach (70% vs. 20%).

TABLE 33.5-21. Incidence of Nodal and Peritoneal Metastases from Gallbladder Cancer According to T Stage of Disease

Stage	*Definition*	*Total No. of Cases*	*Peritoneal Metastases (%)*	*Nodal Metastases (%)*
T2	Submucosal invasion	9	12	50
T3	Full-thickness invasion through gallbladder wall with <2-cm extension into liver	16	43	50
T4	More than 2-cm extension into liver	16	68	66

(From ref. 436, with permission.)

T3 AND T4 CANCERS. The greatest controversy in surgical management of gallbladder cancer lies in the treatment of advanced tumors. The debate centers on whether radical surgery is ever justified for such advanced disease, given the perceived poor long-term prognosis. The literature from the last decade has provided much support for an aggressive approach by confirming a possibility for long-term survival after resection of locally advanced disease (Table 33.5-23). Onoyama et al.[441] recently reported a 63.6% 5-year survival for patients with Japanese Biliary Surgical Society stage II disease and a 44.4% 5-year survival for stage III disease after extended cholecystectomy (these stages combined represent AJCC stage III). Similarly, Nakamura et al.[418] reported 13 radical resections for tumors of Nevin's stage V, with 54% alive at 1 year and 15% (two patients) alive for longer than 7 years.[474] Similar results were recently reported from the Memorial Sloan-Kettering Cancer Center,

TABLE 33.5-22. Survival after Resection of Stage II (T2) Gallbladder Cancers

Study	*No. of Cases*	*Procedure*	*3-Y Survival (%)*	*5-Y Survival (%)*
Yamaguchi, 1988[432]	73	Not specified	40.1	NR
Donohue, 1990[438]	12	67% Extended cholecystectomy	58	22
Ogura, 1991[463,a]	499	Not specified	53	37
Gall, 1991[476]	7	86% Simple cholecystectomy	86	86
Shirai, 1992[600]	35	Simple cholecystectomy	57	40.5
	10	Extended cholecystectomy	90	90
Yamaguchi, 1992[470]	25	Simple cholecystectomy	36	36
Matsumoto, 1992[475]	9	Extended cholecystectomy	100	100
Oertli, 1993[442]	17	Simple cholecystectomy	29	24
Cubertafond, 1994[467,a]	52	88% Simple cholecystectomy	20	NR
Bartlett, 1996[473]	8	Extended cholecystectomy	100	88
Paquet, 1998[602]	5	Extended cholecystectomy	100	80

NR, not reported.
[a]Multiinstitutional survey.

where a 67% 5-year survival was achieved for patients with completely resected stage III disease and a 33% 5-year survival was noted for patients with completely resected stage IV tumors.[473] It is clear from these results that an aggressive approach to locally advanced disease is justified.

POSITIVE RETROPERITONEAL NODES. Metastases to cystic, portal, and portacaval lymph nodes may be curable by regional lymphadenectomy. Onoyama et al.[441] reported a 5-year survival rate of 60% for patients having metastatic disease to N1 nodes. Shirai et al.[474] reported a 45% 5-year survival for patients with positive regional nodes, documenting nine patients surviving for more than 5 years after radical resection. Such findings support radical lymphadenectomy for gallbladder cancer.

Some researchers have advocated even more radical lymphadenectomies. The next nodal area for extension of tumor includes the retropancreatic and aortocaval nodes, which explains the recommendation of some investigators to perform a pancreaticoduodenectomy for patients with suspicious retropancreatic nodes.[461,475] It is assumed that nodal clearance is improved with pancreaticoduodenectomy. One multicenter series of 150 hepatopancreaticoduodenectomies for gallbladder cancer reported a 54% morbidity and 15.3% mortality rate.[463] Most other series report higher mortality rates. Such high morbidity and mortality of combined hepatectomy and pancreaticoduodenectomy is not justified by the long-term outcome. Long-term survival is extremely rare, even after such radical resection, when N2 nodes contain metastatic disease.

RE-RESECTION AFTER LAPAROSCOPIC CHOLECYSTECTOMY. A significant number of gallbladder cancers will present for definitive therapy after prior cholecystectomy. This is particularly common for early-stage tumors, which account for most cancers diagnosed at pathologic analysis. For patients treated ini-

TABLE 33.5-23. Survival after Extended Resection of Stage III and IV Gallbladder Cancers

Study	*No. of Cases*	*Stage*	*3-Y Survival (%)*	*5-Y Survival (%)*	*Comments*
Matsumoto, 1992[475]	8	III	38	—	Majority with common bile duct resection
Chijiiwa, 1994[603]	12	III	80	—	Extended resections only
Onoyama, 1995[441]	12	III	44	44	Extended resections only
Bartlett, 1996[473]	8	III	63	63	Extended resections only
Ouchi, 1987[462]	12	III/IV	17	—	Extended resections only
Nakamura, 1989[418]	13	III/IV	16	16	Includes 5 HPD, 10 extended hepatectomies
Donohue, 1990[438]	17	III/IV	50	29	Extended resections only
Gall, 1991[476]	8	III/IV	50	—	Includes only curative resection at initial surgery
Shirai, 1992[600]	20	III/IV	—	45	All patients have lymph node metastases
Ogura, 1991[463]	453	IV	18	8	Multiinstitutional series with 25% simple cholecystectomy
Todoroki, 1991[492]	27	IV	7	—	All patients underwent IORT
Nimura, 1991[461]	14	IV	10	—	All patients underwent HPD
Matsumoto, 1992[475]	27	IV	25	—	Includes 3 HPD, 6 extended hepatectomies, 11 CBD resections
Chijiiwa, 1994[603]	11	IV	11	—	Extended resections only
Onoyama, 1995[441]	14	IV	8	8	Japanese staging
Bartlett, 1996[473]	7	IV	25	25	Long-term survivors with no lymph node metastases

CBD, common bile duct; HPD, hepatopancreaticoduodenectomy; IORT, intraoperative radiotherapy.

tially with open cholecystectomy, data clearly indicate that a radical re-resection is justified for tumors with a depth of penetration equal to or greater than T2.[471] As would be expected, however, prognosis for patients subjected to two operations is less favorable than for patients treated with a single procedure. Gall et al.[476] reported a median survival of 42 months for patients undergoing a curative resection at the first operation as compared to 13 months for those requiring two operations.

Laparoscopic cholecystectomy has given birth to an entirely new clinical entity since 1989—namely, laparoscopically discovered gallbladder cancer. To date, few data have addressed the utility of radical re-resection after gallbladder cancer has been discovered laparoscopically. We recently reported a series of 42 gallbladder cancers discovered at laparoscopy.[436] One patient with T1 gallbladder cancer was advised that his laparoscopic cholecystectomy was a definitive procedure, and no additional therapy was undertaken. All other patients underwent extent-of-disease evaluation and re-resection as appropriate. Of the 41 patients with T2, T3, or T4 disease, 5 were not offered further surgery because disease was determined on imaging to be unresectable. The remaining 36 patients were subjected to surgical exploration, which revealed that an additional 17 patients had unresectable disease. The survival of the 19 re-resected patients was significantly different from that of the patients whose disease was found to be unresectable. Only 3 of these 19 patients subjected to re-resection have died, and the median survival has not been reached, whereas 14 of the 17 patients whose disease was deemed unresectable have died, with a median survival of 4 months. These data would indicate that such reexploration and re-resection are justified and useful.

Gallbladder cancer has a great potential for peritoneal dissemination. This propensity for abdominal seeding is further enhanced by laparoscopic exploration. Data indicate that the incidence of peritoneal metastases is higher now than that reported in the prelaparoscopy age.[475] During reexploration, therefore, care must be taken to perform a full abdominal inspection to rule out peritoneal disease.

Special consideration should also be extended for the laparoscopic port sites: A number of studies have demonstrated the propensity of tumor to recur in the laparoscopic port sites.[437,456,477–483] It has become our standard practice to excise laparoscopic port sites at reexploration. Whether such excision of port sites is useful will be proven only by future follow-up, but it is known that the procedure adds little morbidity.

Chemotherapy, Radiotherapy, and Adjuvant Therapy

In general, chemotherapy and radiotherapy have offered poor results in the treatment of gallbladder cancer. A European Organization for Research and Treatment of Cancer cooperative study examined bolus mitomycin C in advanced gallbladder and biliary tree carcinoma, with no significant activity identified.[484] Other regimens based on 5-FU, Adriamycin, or nitrosoureas alone and in combination for gallbladder cancer result in only minimal responses.[435] In a study that treated 30 patients with advanced gallbladder carcinoma with 5-FU, leucovorin, and hydroxyurea, 9 had a partial response. However, the median duration of response was only 6.5 months, and the median survival was only 8 months.[485] Regional therapy has recently been examined using intraarterial mitomycin C for gallbladder cancer. A 48% overall response rate and a prolongation of median survival from 5 months to 14 months as compared to historic controls was reported.[486] However, a regional approach is rarely indicated, since the major reasons for unresectability usually are disseminated disease and extensive involvement of the porta hepatis.

The results for radiotherapy have also been poor, because the mode of spread of gallbladder cancer does not lend itself well to radiotherapy. Although Houry et al.[487] suggest that radiotherapy may increase survival after no resection or palliative resection of gallbladder carcinoma, the suggested benefit is small, with a median survival of only 6 to 8 months. However, because it does appear to be well tolerated, radiotherapy with or without chemosensitization is the most common palliative modality used.

Because of the rarity of this disease in general and the rarity of completely resected gallbladder cancers, it is not surprising that there are no prospective, randomized studies examining the utility of adjuvant therapy. Nonetheless, as part of many retrospective studies, the issue of adjuvant therapy has been addressed. Chao and Greager[488] compared 15 patients who received some form of chemotherapy or radiotherapy (or both) after resection for gallbladder cancer to 7 patients who did not receive any adjuvant therapy and found no significant difference in outcome. Oswalt and Cruz[489] reported a median survival of 20 weeks in 13 patients treated with adjuvant chemotherapy, as compared to 8 weeks in patients treated with surgery alone. Morrow et al.[490] from the University of Minnesota reported a median survival of 4.5 months for those receiving adjuvant chemotherapy or radiotherapy versus 3 months for those treated with surgery alone. With such small sample sizes and the generally dismal results in these series, it is difficult to draw firm conclusions from these data.

Definitive data for adjuvant radiotherapy also are lacking, but the existing data are a bit more encouraging than are those for chemotherapy.[491] Todoroki et al.[492] examined intraoperative radiotherapy after complete resection for stage IV gallbladder cancer and reported a 10% 3-year survival for patients receiving intraoperative radiotherapy versus 0% for surgery alone. Hanna and Rider[493] reviewed results for 51 patients with gallbladder cancer and found survival to be significantly longer in patients receiving postoperative radiotherapy as compared with those who underwent only surgery. In another retrospective study, the median survival of patients receiving postoperative irradiation was 63 months, as compared with 29 months for patients undergoing surgery alone.[494] Though the data are encouraging, firm support for such adjuvant therapy awaits confirmation by prospective trials. Nevertheless, given the high incidence of local recurrence of gallbladder carcinoma and the low morbidity of radiotherapy, it is not unreasonable to recommend some form of radiotherapy, particularly for patients with advanced-stage disease.

Other Palliative Management

Palliative management for gallbladder cancer usually is directed at relief of jaundice, treatment of sepsis, and palliation for pain and bowel obstruction. Decisions on palliative treatment should take into account the short survival of patients with nonresectable gallbladder cancer. The median survival for patients presenting with unresectable disease is generally 2 to 4 months, with a 1-year survival rate of less than 5%.[413,442] All palliative treatments should, therefore, be kept as simple as possible, given the aggressive nature of this disease. For jaundiced patients, for example, procedures to achieve relief of jaundice should be attempted only if patients are symptomatic (itching or experiencing biliary sepsis) or require a normal bilirubin level for chemotherapy. This is because any attempt to relieve the jaundice can result in introduction of bacteria into the biliary tree, which subsequently becomes a source of biliary sepsis. If the patient is experiencing pruritus or biliary sepsis, percutaneous drainage of the biliary tree is preferred. Surgical bypass often is difficult because of advanced disease in the porta hepatis. Even though a segment III bypass is possible[495] and can be performed at the time of laparotomy for attempted resection, it is unreasonable to perform exploratory surgery on patients with the sole goal of achieving biliary bypass. Kapoor et al.[496] report a 12% 30-day mortality rate for segment III bypasses. In addition, subjecting a patient with an anticipated 4-month survival to a palliative procedure that requires a 1- to 2-month recovery period is unwise. In the event of a preoperative diagnosis of advanced, unresectable gallbladder cancer in the jaundiced patient, a noninvasive radiologic approach to biliary drainage is justified. This disease is rapidly progressive, and so it is preferable to avoid the morbidity and recovery time of a laparotomy and surgical bypass.

GALLBLADDER POLYPS

A section on gallbladder cancer must include a discussion of gallbladder polyps, as polyps are found in up to 5% of patients in the general population.[497,498] The majority of polyps are benign and can be classified as epithelial tumors (adenoma), mesenchymal tumors (fibroma, lipoma, hemangioma), or pseudotumors (cholesterol polyps, inflammatory polyps, and adenomyoma). Most polyps are cholesterol polyps,[499] which histologically are submucosal deposits of lipid-laden macrophages. Of the various types of polyps, the only type believed to be precancerous is the adenoma.[500]

Distinguishing benign from malignant or premalignant lesions is essential in the patient presenting with a polyp. US is the most practical test for evaluating polypoid lesions of the gallbladder and has a sensitivity of 90.1% and a specificity of 93.9% in making the diagnosis.[501] In general, malignant lesions were significantly more likely to be found in patients older than 50 years and more likely to be present as a solitary lesion, to be sessile in character, and to measure greater than 1.0 cm in diameter. Conversely, cholesterol polyps, which account for more than 90% of benign lesions, are more likely to occur as multiple lesions (more than three), to be small, and to retain an intact mucosa. Because of the poor prognosis of gallbladder cancer and the low morbidity of a cholecystectomy, most investigators recommend open cholecystectomy for any solitary polyp greater than 1.0 cm. Some investigators have advocated an even more aggressive approach. Shinkai et al.[499] recommend cholecystectomy for patients with fewer than three polyps, regardless of size.

Figure 33.5-6 is our recommended algorithm for the treatment of gallbladder polyps. It is based on the recommendations of Boulton and Adams[498] and on the findings in longitudinal follow-up studies in which small (<1-cm) gallbladder polyps were followed by imaging, demonstrating a low rate of subsequent diagnosis of cancer.[502] For symptomatic polyps, cholecystectomy should be performed. For patients with gallbladder polyps and other conditions that warrant cholecystectomy (e.g., cholelithiasis), cholecystectomy should be performed. Likewise, for patients with characteristics suspicious for cancer—namely, a lesion larger than 1 cm, fewer than three lesions, and eroded mucosa—cholecystectomy should be performed. Other patients should be followed by US every 6 months, and any suspicious findings should prompt cholecystectomy.

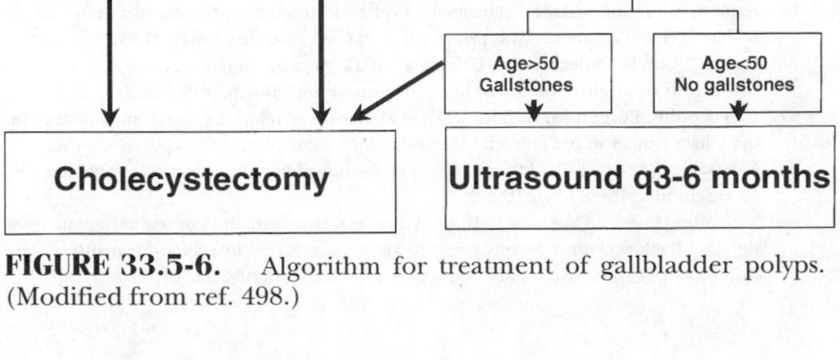

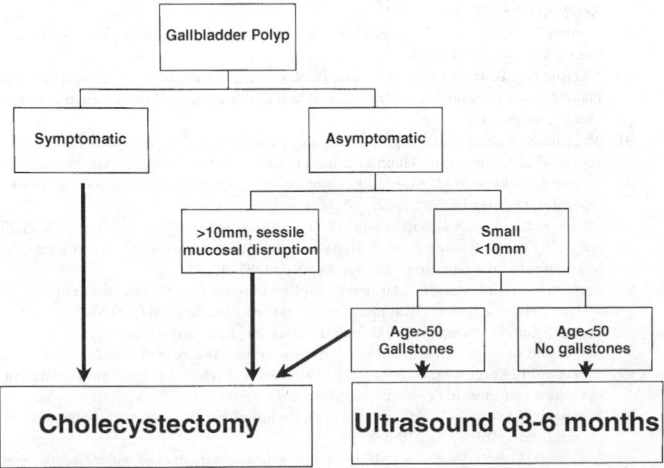

FIGURE 33.5-6. Algorithm for treatment of gallbladder polyps. (Modified from ref. 498.)

REFERENCES

1. Okuda K, Kojiro M. Neoplasms of the liver. In: Schiff L, Schiff ER, eds. *Diseases of the liver,* 7th ed. Philadelphia: JB Lippincott Co, 1993:1236.
2. Grasso P. Experimental liver tumors in animals. In: Johnson PJ, ed. *Bailliere's Clinical Gastroenterology* 1987;183.
3. Rustgi V. Epidemiology of hepatocellular carcinoma. *Gastroenterol Clin North Am* 1987;16:545.
4. Oon C, Rauff A, Tan LK. Treatment of primary liver cancer in Singapore. A review of 3,200 cases seen between January 1, 1977, and July 31, 1987. *Cancer Chemother Pharmacol* 1989;23:S13.
5. Benveniste R, Bixler D, Conneally PM. Periodontal disease in diabetics. *J Periodontol* 1967;38:271.
6. Munoz N, Linsell A. Epidemiology of primary liver cancer. In: Correa P, Haenzel W, eds. *Epidemiology of cancer in the digestive tract.* The Hague: Nijoff, 1982:161.
7. Munoz N, Bosch X. Epidemiology of hepatocellular carcinoma. In: Okuda K, Ishak KG, eds. *Neoplasms of the liver.* Berlin: Springer, 1988:3.
8. Bosch X, Muñoz N. Epidemiology of hepatocellular carcinoma. In: Bannasch P, Keppler D, Weber C, eds. *Liver cell carcinoma. Falk Symposium No. 15.* Dordrecht: Kluwer Academic Publishers, 1989:3.
9. Lau JYN, Lai CL. Hepatocarcinogenesis. *Trop Gastroenterol* 1990;11:9.
10. Simonetti RG, Camma C, Fiorello Fea. Hepatocellular carcinoma: a worldwide problem and the major risk factors. *Dig Dis Sci* 1991;36:962.
11. Leong ASY, Liew CT. Epidemiology, risk factors, etiology, premalignant lesions and carcinogenesis. In: Leong ASY, Liew CT, Lau JWY, Johnson PJ, eds. *Hepatocellular carcinoma, diagnosis, investigation and management.* London: Arnold, 1999:1.
12. Beasley RP, Hwang LY. Epidemiology of hepatocellular carcinoma. In: Vyas GH, Dienstag JL, Hoofnagle JH, eds. *Viral hepatitis and liver disease.* New York: Grune & Stratton, 1984:209.
13. Simonetti RG. Prevalence of antibodies to hepatitis C virus in hepatocellular carcinoma. *Lancet* 1989;2:1338.
14. Hasan F, Jeffers ZJ, DeMedina M, et al. Hepatitis C–associated hepatocellular carcinoma. *Hepatology* 1990;12:589.
15. Di Bisceglie AM. Hepatitis C and hepatocellular carcinoma. *Semin Liver Dis* 1995;15:64.
16. Forman D. Ames, the Ames test and the causes of cancer [editorial]. *Br Med J* 1991;303:428.
17. Saunder J, Latt W. Epidemiology of alcoholic liver disease. *Baillieres Clin Gastroenterol* 1993;7:555.
18. Nalpas B, Pol S, Theopot V, et al. Hepatocellular carcinoma in alcoholics. *Alcohol* 1995;12:117.
19. Schiff ER. Hepatitis C and alcohol. *Hepatology* 1997;26[Suppl 1]:S39.
20. Austin H, Delzell E, Grufferman S, et al. A case-control study of hepatocellular carcinoma and the hepatitis B virus, cigarette smoking and alcohol consumption. *Cancer Res* 1986;46:962.

21. Trichopoulos D, Day NE, Kaklamani E, et al. Hepatitis B virus, tobacco smoking and ethanol consumption in the etiology of hepatocellular carcinoma. *Int J Cancer* 1987;39:45.
22. Naccarato R, Farinati F. Hepatocellular carcinoma, alcohol and cirrhosis: facts and hypothesis. *Dig Dis Sci* 1991;36:1137.
23. Yu SZ. Primary prevention of hepatocellular carcinoma. *J Gastroenterol Hepatol* 1995;10:674.
24. Collier NA, Bloom SR, Hodgson HJF, et al. Neurotensin secretion by fibrolamellar carcinoma of the liver. *Lancet* 1984;1:538.
25. Craig JR. Fibrolamellar carcinoma: clinical and pathological features. In: Okuda K, Tabor E, eds. *Liver cancer.* New York: Churchill Livingstone, 1999:255.
26. Taguchi J, Nakashima O, Tanaka M, et al. A clinicopathological study on combined hepatocellular and cholangiocarcinoma. *J Gastroenterol Hepatol* 1996;11:758.
27. Wu PC, Fang JWS, Lar VKT, et al. Classification of hepatocellular carcinoma according to hepatocellular and biliary differentiation markers. Clinical and biological implications. *Am J Pathol* 1996;149:1167.
28. Lai CL, Wu PC, Lam KC, Todd D. Histologic prognostic indicators in hepatocellular carcinoma. *Cancer* 1979;44:1677
29. Yang SH, Watanabe J, Nakashima O, et al. Clinicopathologic study on clear cell hepatocellular carcinoma. *Pathol Int* 1996;46:503.
30. Heyward W, Lanier A, McMahon B, et al. Early detection of primary hepatocellular carcinoma. *JAMA* 1985;254:791.
31. Lok ASF, Lai CL. Alpha-fetaprotein monitoring in Chinese patients with chronic hepatitis B virus infection: role in early detection of hepatocellular carcinoma. *Hepatology* 1989;9:110.
32. Johnson PJ, Leung N, Cheng P, et al. "Hepatoma-specific" alphafetoprotein may permit preclinical diagnosis of malignant change in patients with chronic liver disease. *Br J Cancer* 1997;75:236.
33. Sherman H, Hardison J. The importance of a coexistent hepatic rub and bruit. *JAMA* 1979;241:1495.
34. Ihde DC, Sherlock P, Winawer SJ, et al. Clinical manifestations of hepatoma. A review of 6 years experience at a cancer hospital. *Am J Med* 1974;56:83.
35. Lai CL, Wu PC, Chan GC, et al. Clinical features of hepatocellular carcinoma review of 211 patients in Hong Kong. *Cancer* 1988;47:2746.
36. Shiu W, Dewar G, Leung N, et al. Hepatocellular carcinoma in Hong Kong: clinical study on 340 cases. *Oncology* 1990;47:241.
37. Ho J, Wu PC, Kung TM. An autopsy study of hepatocellular carcinoma in Hong Kong. *Pathology* 1981;13:409.
38. Ng WD, Chan YT, Ho KK, et al. Injection sclerotherapy for bleeding esophageal varices in cirrhotic patients with hepatocellular carcinoma. *Gastrointest Endosc* 1989;35:69.
39. Yeo W, Surg JY, Ward SC, et al. A prospective study of upper gastrointestinal haemorrhage in patients with hepatocellular carcinoma. *Dig Dis Sci* 1995;40:2516.
40. Spontaneous rupture of the liver [editorial]. *Br Med J* 1976;2:1278.
41. Nagasue N, Inokuchi K. Spontaneous and traumatic rupture of hepatoma. *Br J Surg* 1979;66:248.
42. Chearanai O, Plengvanit UAC, Asavanich C, et al. Spontaneous rupture of primary hepatoma; report of 63 cases with particular reference to the pathogenesis and rationale treatment by hepatic artery ligation. *Cancer* 1983;51:1532.
43. Chen MF, Hwang TL, Jeng LB, et al. Surgical treatment for spontaneous rupture of hepatocellular carcinoma. *Surg Gynecol Obstet* 1988;167:99.
44. Dewar GA, Griffin SM, Ku KW, Lau WY, Li AK. Management of bleeding liver tumours in Hong Kong. *Br J Surg* 1991;78:463.
45. Kew MC, Dos Santos HA, Sherlock S. Diagnosis of primary liver cancer of the liver. *Br Med J* 1971;4:408.
46. Ong GB, Taw J. Spontaneous rupture of hepatocellular carcinoma. *Br Med J* 1972;4:146.
47. Miyamoto M, Sudo T, Kuyama T. Spontaneous rupture of hepatocellular carcinoma: a review of 172 Japanese cases. *Am J Gastroenterol* 1991;86:68.
48. Edmondson HA, Steiner PE. Primary carcinoma of the liver: a study of 100 cases. *Cancer* 1954;7(462):503.
49. Kappel DA, Miller DR. Primary hepatic carcinoma. A review of thirty-seven patients. *Am J Surg* 1972;124:798.
50. Kew MC, Geddes EW. Hepatocellular carcinoma in rural Southern African blacks. *Medicine* 1982;61:98.
51. Lin TY. Tumors of the liver: I. Primary malignant tumors. In: Bockus HL, ed. *Gastroenterology,* 3rd ed. Philadelphia: WB Saunders, 1976:522.
52. Okuda K. Clinical aspects of hepatocellular carcinoma—analysis of 134 cases. In: Okuda K, Peters F, eds. *Hepatocellular carcinoma.* New York: John Wiley and Sons, 1976:387.
53. Kojiro M, Kawabaata K, Kawano Y, et al. Hepatocellular carcinoma presenting as intrabile duct tumor growth. A clinicopathologic study of 24 cases. *Cancer* 1982;49:2144.
54. Lee NW, Wong KP, Siu KF, et al. Cholangiography in hepatocellular carcinoma with obstructive jaundice. *Clin Radiol* 1984;35(119):123.
55. Lai ECS, Ng IOL, Ng MMT, et al. Long-term results of resection for large hepatocellular carcinoma: a multivariate analysis of clinicopathological features. *Hepatology* 1990;11:815.
56. Lau WY, Leung KL, Leung TW, et al. Obstructive jaundice secondary to hepatocellular carcinoma. *Surg Oncol* 1995;4:303.
57. Afroudakis AP, Bhuta SM, Ranganath KA, et al. Obstructive jaundice caused by hepatocellular carcinoma. Report of three cases. *Dig Dis* 1978;23:609.
58. Van Sonnenberg E, Ferucci J. Bile duct obstruction in hepatocellular carcinoma (hepatoma)—clinical and cholangiographical characteristics. Report of 6 cases and review of the literature. *Radiology* 1979;130:7.
59. Roslyn JJ, Kuchenbecker S, Longmire WP, Tompkins RK. Floating tumor debris. A cause of intermittent biliary obstruction. *Arch Surg* 1984;119:1312.
60. Wu CS, Wu SS, Chen PC, et al. Cholangiography of icteric type hepatoma. *Am J Gastroenterol* 1994;89:774.
61. Lau WY, Leow CK, Li AKC. A logical approach to hepatocellular carcinoma presenting with jaundice. *Ann Surg* 1997;225:281.
62. Kew MC, Dusheiko GM. Paraneoplastic manifestations of hepatocellular carcinoma. In: Berk PD, Chalmers TC, eds. *Frontiers of liver and disease.* New York: Thieme-Stratton, 1981:305.
63. Shapiro E, Bell GI, Polonsky K, et al. Tumor hypoglycemia: relationship to high molecular weight insulin-like growth factor II. *J Clin Invest* 1990;85:1672.
64. McFrazean AJS, Yeung RRT. Further observations on hypoglycaemia in hepatocellular carcinoma. *Am J Med* 1969;47:220.
65. Helzberg JH, McPhee MS, Zarling EJ, et al. Hepatocellular carcinoma: an unusual course with hyperthyroidism and inappropriate thryoid-stimulating hormone production. *Gastroenterology* 1985;88:181.
66. Lau JWY, Leow CK. Surgical management (including liver transplantation). In: Leong ASY, Leiw CT, Lau JWY, Johnson PJ, eds. *Hepatocellular carcinoma. Diagnosis, investigation and management.* London: Arnold, 1999:147.
67. Caturelli E, Bisceglia M, Fusilli S, et al. Cytology versus microhistological diagnosis of hepatocellular carcinoma. Comparative accuracies in the same fine-needle biopsy specimen. *Dig Dis Sci* 1996;41:2326.
68. Williamson BW, Blumgart LH, McKellar NJ. Combined use of arteriography and venography in the assessment of resectability especially in hilar tumours. *Am J Surg* 1980;139:210.
69. Voyles CR, Bowley NJ, Allison DJ, Benjamin IS, Blumgart LH. Carcinoma of the proximal extrahepatic biliary tree radiologic assessment and therapeutic alternatives. *Ann Surg* 1983;197:188.
70. Lau WY, Arnold M, Leung NW, et al. Hepatic intraarterial lipiodol ultrasound guided biopsy in the management of hepatocellular carcinoma. *Surg Oncol* 1993;2:119.
71. Bismuth H, Chiche L, Adam R, et al. Liver resection versus transplantation for hepatocellular carcinoma in cirrhotic patients. *Ann Surg* 1993;218(2):145.
72. Bismuth H, Morino M, Sherlock D, et al. Primary treatment of hepatocellular carcinoma by arterial chemoembolization. *Am J Surg* 1992;163:387.
73. Hasegawa H, Yamazaki S, Makuuchi M, et al. Hepatectomies pour hepatocarcinome sur goie cirrhotique: schemes desionnels et principes de reanimation peri-operatoir. Experience de 204 cas. *J Chirurg* 1987;124:425.
74. Noun R, Jagot P, Farges O, Sauvanet A, Belghiti J. High preoperative serum alanine transferase levels: effect on the risk of liver resection in child grade A cirrhotic patients. *World J Surg* 1997;21:390.
75. Lau WY, Leow CK, Li AKC. Hepatocellular carcinoma—current management and treatment. *GI Cancer* 1996;2:35.
76. Child CG, Turcotte JG. Surgery and portal hypertension. In: Child CG, ed. *The liver and portal hypertension.* Philadelphia: WB Saunders, 1964:50.
77. Pugh R, Murray-Lyon IM, Dawson JL, et al. Transection of the oesophagus for bleeding oesophageal varices. *Br J Surg* 1973;60:646.
78. Franco D, Borgonovo G. Liver resection in cirrhosis of the liver. In: Blumgart LH, ed. *Surgery of the liver and biliary tract.* Edinburgh: Churchill Livingstone, 1994:1539.
79. Hemming AW, Scudamore CH, Shackleton CR, Pudek M, Erb SR. Indocyanine green clearance as a predictor of successful hepatic resection in cirrhotic patients. *Am J Surg* 1992;163:515.
80. Gill RA, Goodman MW, Golfus GR, et al. Aminopyrine breath test predicts surgical risk for patients with liver disease. *Ann Surg* 1983;198:701.
81. Takenaka K, Kanematsu T, Fukuzawa K, Sugimachi K. Can hepatic failure after surgery for hepatocellular carcinoma in cirrhotic patients be prevented? *World J Surg* 1990;14:123.
82. Bruix J, Castells A, Bosch J, et al. Surgical resection of hepatocellular carcinoma in cirrhotic patients: prognostic value of preoperative portal pressure. *Gastroenterology* 1996;111(4):1018.
83. Bismuth H, Houssin D, Mazmanian G. Postoperative liver insufficiency: prevention and management. *World J Surg* 1983;7:505.
84. Fong Y, Sun RL, Jarnagin W, Blumgart LH. An analysis of 412 cases of hepatocellular carcinoma at a Western center. *Ann Surg* 1999;229(6):790.
85. Mnegchao W, Han C, Xiaohua Z, Xiaoping Y, Jiamei Y. Primary hepatic carcinoma resection over 18 years. *Chin Med J* 1980;93:723.
86. Tsuzuki T, Sugoika A, Ueda M, et al. Hepatic resection for heaptocellular carcinoma. *Surgery* 1990;107:511.
87. Chen MF, Hwang TL, Jeng LBB, et al. Hepatic resection in 120 patients with hepatocellular carcinoma. *Arch Surg* 1989;124:1025.
88. Bagasue N, Kohno H, Chang YC, et al. Liver resection for hepatocellualr carcinoma. *Ann Surg* 1993;217:375.
89. Vauthey JN, Klimstra D, Franceschi D, et al. Hepatic resection for hepatocellular carcinoma. *Am J Surg* 1995;169:28.
90. Nagasue N, Yukaya H, Ogawa Y, Kohno H, Nakamura T. Human liver regeneration after major hepatic resection. A study of normal liver and livers with chronic hepatitis and cirrhosis. *Ann Surg* 1987;206:30.
91. Nagasue N, Kohno H, Chang YC, et al. Liver resection for hepatocellular carcinoma: results of 229 consecutive patients during 11 years. *Ann Surg* 1993;217(4):375.
92. Tanabe G, Sakamoto M, Akazawa K. Intraoperative risk factors associated with hepatic resection. *Br J Surg* 1995;82:1262.
93. Okuda K, Liver Study Group of Japan. Primary liver cancer in Japan. *Cancer* 1980;71:19.
94. Nagao T, Goto S, Kawano N, et al. Hepatic resection for hepatocellular carcinoma: clinical features and long-term prognosis. *Ann Surg* 1987;205:33.
95. Kanematsu T, Takenaka K, Matsumata T, et al. Limited hepatic resection effective for selected cirrhotic patients with primary liver cancer. *Ann Surg* 1984;199:51.
96. Fuster J, Garcia-Valdecasas JC, Grande L, et al. Hepatocellular carcinoma and cirrhosis—results of surgical treatment in a European series. *Ann Surg* 1996;223(3):297.
97. Capussotti L, Borgonovo G, Bouzari H, et al. Results of major hepatectomy for large primary liver cancer in patients with cirrhosis. *Br J Surg* 1994;81:427.
98. Kawasaki S, Makuuchi M, Miyagawa S, et al. Results of hepatic resection for hepatocellular carcinoma. *World J Surg* 1995;19:31.
99. Melendez JA, Arslan V, Fischer ME, et al. Perioperative outcomes of major hepatic resections under low central venous pressure anesthesia: blood loss, blood transfusion, and the risk of postoperative renal dysfunction. *J Am Coll Surg* 1998;187(6):620.

100. Kim YI, Nakashima K, Tada I, Kawano K, Kobayashi M. Prolonged normothermic ischaemia of human cirrhotic liver during hepatectomy: a preliminary report. *Br J Surg* 1993;80:1566.
101. Man K, Fan ST, Ng IO, et al. Prospective evaluation of Pringle maneuver in hepatectomy for liver tumors by a randomized study. *Ann Surg* 1997;226(6):704.
102. DeMatteo RP, Palese C, Jarnagin WR, et al. Anatomic segmental hepatic resection is superior to wedge resection as an oncologic operation for colorectal liver metastases. *J Gastrointest Surg* 2000;4(2):178.
103. Sitzmann JV, Abrams R. Improved survival for hepatocellular cancer with combination surgery and multimodality treatment. *Ann Surg* 1993;217:149.
104. Lau WY, Leung KL, Leung TW, et al. Resection of hepatocellular carcinoma with diaphragmatic invasion. *Surg Oncol* 1995;82:264.
105. Yamanaka N, Okamoto E, Fujihara S, et al. Do the tumor cells of hepatocellular carcinomas dislodge into the portal venous system during hepatic resection? *Cancer* 1992;70:2263.
106. Harada T, Matsuo K, Inoue T. Is preoperative hepatic arterial chemoembolisation safe and effective for hepatocellular carcinoma? *Ann Surg* 1996;224:4.
107. Fan J, Tang ZY, Yu YQ, et al. Improved survival with resection after transcatheter arterial chemoembolisation (TACE) for unresectable hepatocellular carcinoma. *Dig Surg* 1998;15:674.
108. Tang ZY, Yu YQ, Zhou XD, et al. Cytoreduction and sequential resection for surgically verified unresectable hepatocellular carcinoma: evaluation with analysis of 72 patients. *World J Surg* 1995;19:784.
109. Lau WY, Ho S, Leung TW, et al. Selective internal radiation therapy for nonresectable hepatocellular carcinoma with intraarterial infusion of 90 yttrium microspheres. *Int J Radiat Oncol Biol Phys* 1998;40:583.
110. Sakon M, Yoshida T, Kanai T, et al. Transcatheter arterial immunoembolization for hepatocellular carcinoma. *Proc Am Soc Clin Oncol* 1999;18:456a(abst).
111. Lygidakis NJ, Tsiliakos S. Multidisciplinary management of hepatocellular carcinoma. *Hepatogastroenterology* 1996;43(12):1611.
112. Leung TW, Lau WY, Ho SK, et al. Final report on a pahse II study of combination cisplatin, interferon alpha, doxorubicin and 5-fluorouracil for inoperable hepatocellular carcinoma. *Hepatology* 1998;28:227A.
113. Patt YZ, Hoque A, Lozano R, et al. Systemic therapy with platinol, interferon α 2B, doxorubicin and 5-fluorouracil (5-FU) (PIAF) for treatment of non-resectable hepatocellular carcinoma (HCC). *Proc Am Soc Clin Oncol* 1998;17[Suppl]:301a(abst).
114. Borzutzky CA, Turbiner EH. The predictive value of hepatic artery perfusion scintigraphy. *J Nucl Med* 1985;26:1153.
115. Friedman M. Primary hepatocellular cancer: present results and future prospects. *Int J Radiat Oncol Biol Phys* 1983;9:1841.
116. Okuda K, Ohtsuki T, Obata H, et al. Natural history of hepatocellular carcinoma and prognosis in relation to treatment. *Cancer* 1985;56:918.
117. Dewar GA, Griffin SM, Ku KW, et al. Hepatocellular carcinoma. *Ann Intern Med* 1991;108:390.
118. Lai E, Choi T, Tong S, et al. Treatment of unresectable hepatocellular carcinoma: results of a randomised controlled trial. *World J Surg* 1986;10:501.
119. Carr BI, Zajko A, Bron K, et al. Phase II study of Spherex (degradable starch microspheres) injected into the hepatic artery in conjunction with doxorubicin and cisplatin in the treatment of advanced-stage hepatocellular carcinoma: interim analysis. *Semin Oncol* 1997;24[Suppl 6]:S6.
120. Lai EC, Lo CM, Fan ST, et al. Postoperative adjuvant chemotherapy after curative resection of hepatocellular carcinoma: a randomized controlled trial. *Arch Surg* 1998;133:183.
121. Izumi R, Shimizu K, Iyobe T, et al. Postoperative adjuvant arterial infusion of lipiodol containing anticancer drugs in patients with hepatocellular carcinoma. *Hepatology* 1994;20:295.
122. Wu CC, Ho YZ, Ho WL, et al. Preoperative transcatheter arterial chemoembolisation for resectable large hepatocellular carcinoma. A reappraisal. *Br J Surg* 1995;82:122.
123. Muto Y, Moriwaki H, Ninomiya M, et al. Prevention of second primary tumors by an acyclic retinoid, polyprenoic acid, in patients with hepatocellular carcinoma. *N Engl J Med* 1996;334:1561.
124. Lau WY, Leung TW, Ho SK, et al. Adjuvant intra-arterial iodine-131-labeled lipiodol for resectable hepatocellular carcinoma: a prospective randomised trial. *Lancet* 1999; 353(9155):797.
125. Selby R, Kadry Z, Carr B, et al. Liver transplantation for hepatocellular carcinoma. *World J Surg* 1995;19:53.
126. Blumgart LH. Liver resection—liver and biliary tumours. In: Blumgart LH, ed. *Surgery of the liver and biliary tract.* New York: Churchill Livingstone, 1988:1251.
127. Yokoyama I, Todo S, Iwatsuki S, Starzl TE. Liver transplantation in the treatment of primary liver cancer. *Hepatogastroenterology* 1990;37:188.
128. Haug CE, Jenkins RL, Rohrer RJ, et al. Liver transplantation for primary hepatic cancer. *Transplantation* 1992;53:376.
129. O'Grady JG, Polson RJ, Rolles K, Calne RY, Williams R. Liver transplantation for malignant disease. *Ann Surg* 1988;207:373.
130. Schwartz ME, Sung M, Mor E, et al. A multidisciplinary approach to hepatocellular carcinoma in patients with cirrhosis. *J Am Coll Surg* 1995;180:596.
131. Mazzaferro V, Regalia E, Doci R, et al. Liver transplantation for the treatment of small hepatocellular carcinomas in patients with cirrhosis. *N Engl J Med* 1996;334(11):693.
132. Tan K, Rela M, Ryder S. Experience of orthotopic liver transplantation and hepatic resection for hepatocellular carcinoma of less than 8 cm in patients with cirrhosis. *Br J Surg* 1995;82:253.
133. Emond JC, Leib M. The living-related liver transplant evaluation: linking risk factors and outcome. *Liver Transpl Surg* 1996;2[Suppl 1]:57.
134. Wadstrom J, Rogiers X, Malago M, et al. Experience from the first 30 living related liver transplants in Hamburg. *Transplant Proc* 1995;27(1):1173.
135. Livraghi T, Bolondi L, Buscarini L, et al. No treatment, resection and ethanol injection in hepatocellular carcinoma: a retrospective analysis of survival in 391 patients with cirrhosis. Italian Cooperative HCC Study Group. *J Hepatol* 1995;22(5):522.
136. Nonami T, Harada A, Kurokawa T, Nakao A, Takagi H. Hepatic resection for hepatocellular carcinoma. *Am J Surg* 1997;173(4):288.
137. Cherqui D, Piedbois P, Pierga J, et al. Multimodal adjuvant treatment and liver transplantation for advanced hepatocellular carcinoma. A pilot study. *Cancer* 1994;73:2721.
138. Stone M, Goran B, Klintmalm G, et al. Neoadjuvant chemotherapy and liver transplantation for hepatocellular carcinoma: a pilot study in 20 patients. *Gastroenterology* 1993;104:196.
139. Farmer DG, Rosove MH, Shaked A, Busuttil RW. Treatment of hepatocellular carcinoma. *Ann Surg* 1994;219:236.
140. Jiang W, Lu Z, He Y, Diasio RB. Dihydropyrimidine dehydrogenase activity in hepatocellular carcinoma: implication in 5-fluorouracil-based chemotherapy. *Clin Cancer Res* 1997;3(3):395.
141. Soini Y, Virkajarvi N, Raunio H, et al. Expression of P-glycoprotein in hepatocellular carcinoma: a potential marker of prognosis. *J Clin Pathol* 1996;49:470.
142. Chenivesse X, Franco D, Brechot C. MDRI (multiple resistance) gene expression in human primary liver cancer and cirrhosis. *J Hepatol* 1993;18:168.
143. Nerenstone SR, Ihde DC, Friedman MA. Clinical trials in primary hepatocellular carcinoma: current status and future directions. *Cancer Treat Rev* 1988;15:1.
144. Lai CL, Wu PC, Chan GC, et al. Doxorubicin vs. no antitumor therapy in an inoperable hepatocellular carcinoma: a prospective randomized trial. *Cancer* 1988;62:479.
145. Simonetti RG, Liberati A, Angiolini C, et al. Treatment of hepatocellular carcinoma: a systemic review of randomised controlled trials. *Ann Oncol* 1997;8:117.
146. Mathurin P, Rixe O, Carbonell N, et al. Review article: overview of medical treatments in unresectable hepatocellular carcinoma—an impossible meta-analysis. *Aliment Pharmacol Ther* 1998;12:111.
147. Breedis C, Young C. The blood supply of neoplasms in the liver. *Am J Pathol* 1954;30:969.
148. Ackerman NB. Experimental studies on the circulatory dynamics of intrahepatics tumor blood flow supply. *Cancer* 1972;29:435.
149. Civalleri D. Methods to enhance the efficacy of regional chemotherapeutic treatment of liver malignancies. In: Civalleri D, ed. *An update on regional treatment of liver cancer.* London: Wells Medical Press, 1992:17.
150. Carr BI, Starlz T, Iwatsuki S, et al. Aggressive treatment for advanced hepatocellular carcinoma (HCC). High response rate and prolonged survival. *Hepatology* 1991;14:243.
151. Patt Y, Charnsangavej C, Yoffe B, et al. Hepatic arterial infusion of fluorouridine, leucovorin, doxorubicin and cisplatin for hepatocellular carcinoma: effects of hepatitis B and C viral infection on drug toxicity and patient survival. *J Clin Oncol* 1994;12:1204.
152. Warren KW, Mountain JC, Lloyd-Jones W. Malignant tumours of the bile-ducts. *Br J Surg* 1972;59(7):501.
153. Atiq OT, Kemeny N, Niedzwiecki D, Botet J. Treatment of unresectable primary liver cancer with intrahepatic fluorodeoxyuridine and mitomycin C through an implantable pump. *Cancer* 1992;69(4):920.
154. Makela JT, Kairaluoma MI. Superselective intra-arterial chemotherapy with mitomycin for gallbladder cancer. *Br J Surg* 1993;80(7):912.
155. Tzoracoleftherakis EE, Spiliotis JD, Kyriakopoulou T, Kakkos SK. Intra-arterial versus systemic chemotherapy for non-operable hepatocellular carcinoma. *Hepatogastroenterology* 1999;46(26):1122.
156. Lehner K, Reiser M, Gebhardt U, Heuck A, Schaff J. DSA—control of implanted devices for arterial hepatic perfusion. *Cardiovasc Intervent Radiol* 1987;10:71.
157. Krahenbuhl L, Feodorovici M, Renzulli P, et al. Laparoscopic partial hepatectomy in the rat: a new resectional technique. *Dig Surg* 1998;15(2):140.
158. Falkson G, Lipsitz S, Borden E, et al. Hepatocellular carcinoma. An ECOG randomised phase II study of beta-interferon and menagoril. *Am J Clin Oncol* 1995;18:287.
159. Nagasue N, Yu L, Yukaya H, Kohno H, Nakamura T. Androgen and oestrogen receptors in hepatocellular carcinoma and surrounding liver parenchyma: impact on intrahepatic recurrence after hepatic resection. *Br J Surg* 1995;82(4):542.
160. Huang CC, Wu MC, Xu GW, et al. Overexpression of the MDR1 gene and P-glycoprotein in human hepatocellular carcinoma. *J Natl Cancer Inst* 1992;84(4):262.
161. Berman E, Adams M, Duigou-Osterndorf R, et al. Effect of tamoxifen on cell lines displaying the multidrug-resistant phenotype. *Blood* 1991;77(4):818.
162. Farinati F, De Maria N, Fornasiero A, et al. Prospective controlled trial with anti-estrogen drug tamoxifen in patients with unresectable hepatocellular carcinoma. *Dig Sci* 1992;37:659.
163. Martinez-Cerezo FJ, Tomas A, Donoso L, et al. Controlled trial of tamoxifen in patients with advanced hepatocellular carcinoma. *J Hepatol* 1994;20:702.
164. Manesis EK, Giannoulis G, Zoumboulis P, et al. Treatment of hepatocellular carcinoma with combined suppression and inhibition of sex hormones: a randomised controlled trial. *Hepatology* 1995;21:1535.
165. Paliard P, Clement G, Saez S, et al. Traitment du carcinome hepato-cellulaire par le tamoxifene. *Gastroenterol Clin Biol* 1984;8:680.
166. Castells A, Bruix J, Bru C, et al. Treatment of hepatocellular carcinoma with tamoxifen: a double-blind placebo-controlled trial in 120 patients. *Gastroenterology* 1995;109:917.
167. Pignata S, Izzo F, Farinati F, et al. Role of tamoxifen (TM) in the treatment of hepatocellular carcinoma (HCC). Results from the Clip-01 randomized trial.*Proc Am Soc Clin Oncol* 1998;17[Suppl]:257a(abst).
168. Cheng AL, Chen YC, Yeh KH, et al. Chronic oral etoposide and tamoxifen in the treatment of far-advanced hepatocellular carcinoma. *Cancer* 1996;77(5):872.
169. Bobbio-Pallavicini E, Porta C, Moroni M, et al. Epirubicin and etoposide combination chemotherapy to treat hepatocellular carcinoma patients: a phase II study. *Eur J Cancer* 1997;33(11):1784.
170. Melia WM, Johnson PJ, Williams R. Controlled clinical trial of doxorubicin and tamoxifen versus doxorubicin alone in hepatocellular carcinoma. *Cancer Treat Rep* 1987;71:1213.
171. Forbes A, Wilkinson ML, Iqbal MJ, et al. Response to cyproterone acetate treatment in primary hepatocellular carcinoma is related to fall in free 5a-dihydrotestosterone. *J Cancer Res Clin Oncol* 1987;23:1659.

171a. Sugiura N, Takara K, Ohto M, et al. Treatment of small hepatocellular carcinoma by percutaneous injection of ethanol into tumor with real-time ultrasound monitoring. *Acta Hepatology Japan* 1983;24:920.
172. Ebara M, Ohto M, Sugiura N, et al. Percutaneous ethanol injection for the treatment of small hepatocellular carcinoma. Study of 95 patients. *J Gastroenterol Hepatol* 1990;5:616.
173. Vilana R, Bruix N, Bru C, et al. Tumor size determines the efficacy of percutaneous ethanol injection for the treatment of small hepatocellular carcinoma. *Hepatology* 1992;16:354.
174. Livraghi T, Bolondi L, Lazzaroni S, et al. Percutaneous ethanol injection in the treatment of hepatocellular carcinoma in cirrhosis. A study on 207 patients. *Cancer* 1992;69:925.
175. Yu JS, Burwick JA, Dranoff G, Breakefield XO. Gene therapy for metastatic brain tumors by vaccination with granulocyte-macrophage colony-stimulating factor-transduced tumor cells. *Hum Gene Ther* 1997;8(9):1065.
176. Isobe H, Sakai H, Imari Y, et al. Intratumor ethanol injection therapy for solitary minute hepatocellular carcinoma. A study of 37 patients. *J Clin Gastroenterol* 1994;18:122.
177. Livraghi T, Lazzaroni S, Meloni F, et al. Intralesional ethanol in the treatment of unresectable liver cancer. *World J Surg* 1995;19:801.
178. Karin SK, Sreenivas DV, Saraya A, et al. Improved survival with percutaneous ethanol injection in patients with large hepatocellular carcinoma. *Eur J Gastroenterol Hepatol* 1994;6:999.
179. Bartolozzi C, Lencioni R, Caramella D, et al. Treatment of large HCC: transcatheter arterial chemoembolization combined with percutaneous ethanol injection versus repeated transcatheter arterial chemoembolization. *Radiology* 1995;197(3):812.
180. Tian J, Xu BX, Zhang J, et al. Ultrasound guided internal radiotherapy using yttrium-90 glass microspheres for liver malignancies. *J Nucl Med* 1996;37:958.
181. Zhou XD. Improved cryosurgery for primary liver cancer [in Chinese]. *Chung Hua Chung Liu Tsa Chih* 1992;14:61.
182. Tang ZY, Yu YQ, Zhou XD, et al. Cytoreduction and sequential resection: a hope for unresectable primary liver cancer. *J Surg Oncol* 1991;47:27.
183. Shiina S, Tagawa K, Unuma T, et al. Percutaneous ethanol injection therapy for hepatocellular carcinoma. A histopathologic study. *Cancer* 1991;68:1524.
184. Sironi S, Livraghi T, DelMaschio A. Small hepatocellular carcinoma treated with percutaneous ethanol injection: MR imaging findings. *Radiology* 1991;180:333.
185. Siperstein AE, Rogers SJ, Hansen PD, Gitomirsky A. Laparoscopic thermal ablation of hepatic neuroendocrine tumor metastases. *Surgery* 1997;122(6):1147.
186. Goldberg SN, Hahn PF, Tanabe KK, et al. Percutaneous radiofrequency tissue ablation: does perfusion-mediated tissue cooling limit coagulation necrosis? *J Vasc Interv Radiol* 1998;9(1):101.
187. Nagata Y, Hiraoka M, Akuta K, et al. Radiofrequency thermotherapy for malignant liver tumors. *Cancer* 1990;65:1730.
188. Livraghi T, Goldberg SN, Monti F, et al. Saline-enhanced radio-frequency tissue ablation in the treatment of liver metastases. *Radiology* 1997;202(1):205.
189. Plengvanit U, Chearanai O, Sindhvananda K, et al. Collateral arterial blood supply of the liver after hepatic artery ligation. Angiographic study of 20 patients. *Ann Surg* 1972;175:105.
190. Mooka REM, Larmi TKI, Huttunen R, Kairaluoma MI. Evaluation of the ligation of the hepatic artery and regional arterial chemotherapy in the treatment of primary and secondary cancer of the liver. *Ann Chir Gynaecol* 1975;64:347.
191. Hickman MA, Bruss ML, Morris JG, Rogers QR. Dietary protein source (soybean vs. casein) and taurine status affect kinetics of the enterohepatic circulation of taurocholic acid in cats. *J Nutr* 1992;122(4):1019.
192. Brown KT, Nevins AB, Getrajdman GI, et al. Particle embolization for hepatocellular carcinoma. *J Vasc Interv Radiol* 1998;9(5):822.
193. Kanematsu T, Furuta T, Takenaka K, et al. A 5-year experience of lipiodolisation: selective regional chemotherapy for 200 patients with hepatocellular carcinoma. *Hepatology* 1989;10:98.
194. Okuda K, Tanaka M, Shibata J, et al. Hepatic arterial infusion chemotherapy with continuous low dose administration of cisplatin and 5-fluorouracil for multiple recurrence of hepatocellular carcinoma after surgical treatment. *Oncol Rep* 1999;6(3):587.
195. Carr B, Orons P, Zajko A, et al. Prolonged survival with chemotherapy alone for hepatocellular carcinoma (HCC) with intra-arterial chemotherapy. In: *Proceedings of the Annual Meeting of the American Society of Clinical Oncology*, vol 13. 1994:A606(abst).
196. Ngan H, Lai CL, Fan ST. Transcatheter arterial chemoembolisation in inoperable hepatocellular carcinoma: four-year follow-up. *J Vasc Interv Radiol* 1996;7:419.
197. Corr P, Chan M, Lau WY, et al. The role of hepatic arterial embolisation in the management of ruptured hepatocellular carcinoma. *Clin Radiol* 1993;48:163.
198. Lin DY, Liaw YF, Lee TY, et al. Hepatic arterial embolisation in patients with unresectable hepatocellular carcinoma. A randomised controlled trial. *Gastroenterology* 1988;109:917.
199. Pelletier G, Roche A, Ink O, et al. A randomized trial of hepatic arterial chemoembolization in patients with unresectable hepatocellular carcinoma. *J Hepatol* 1990;11:181.
200. Groupe D'Etude et de Traitement du Carcinome Hepatocellulaire. A comparison of lipiodol chemoembolization and conservative treatment for unresectable hepatocellular carcinoma. *N Engl J Med* 1995;332:1256.
201. Bruix J, Llovet J, Castellas A, et al. Transarterial embolisation versus symptomatic treatment in patients with advanced hepatocellular carcinoma: results of a randomised controlled trial in a single institution. *Hepatology* 1998;27:1578.
202. Kawai S, Okamura J, Ogawa M, et al. Prospective and randomised clinical trial for the treatment of hepatocellular carcinoma—a comparison lipiodol transcatheter embolisation with and without adriamycin (first cooperative study). *Cancer Chemother Pharmacol* 1992;31[Suppl]:S1.
203. Chang JM, Tzeng WS, Pan HB, Yang CF, Lai KH. Transcatheter arterial embolization with or without cisplatin treatment of hepatocellular carcinoma. *Cancer* 1994;74:2449.
204. Yumoto Y, Jinno K, Tokuyama K, et al. Hepatocellular carcinoma detected by iodized oil. *Radiology* 1985;154:19.
205. Okayasu I, Hatakeyama S, Yoshida T, et al. Selective and persistent deposition and gradual drainage of iodized oil, Lipiodol in the hepatocellular carcinoma after injection into the feeding hepatic artery. *Cancer* 1988;90:536.
206. Ryder S, Rissi P, Metivier E, et al. Chemoembolisation with lipiodol and doxorubicin: applicability in British patients with hepatocellular carcinoma. *Gut* 1996;38:125.
207. Yoshikawa M, Saisho H, Ebara M, et al. A randomised trial of intrahepatic aterial infusion of 4'-epidoxorubicin with Lipiodol versus 4'-epidoxorubicin alone in the treatment of hepatocellular carcinoma. *Cancer Chemother Pharmacol* 1994;33[Suppl]:149.
208. Madden MV, Krige JE, Bailey S. Randomised trial of targeted chemotherapy with lipiodol and 5-epidoxorubicin compared with symptomatic treatment of hepatoma. *Gut* 1993;34:1598.
209. El-Domeiri AA, Huvos AG, Goldsmith HS, Foote FW. Primary malignant tumors of the liver. *Cancer* 1971;27:7.
210. Phillips R, Murikami K. Primary neoplasms of the liver. *Cancer* 1960;13:714.
211. Cochrane AMD, Murray-Lyon IM, Brinkley DM, Williams R. Quadruple chemotherapy versus radiotherapy in treatment of primary hepatocellular carcinoma. *Cancer* 1977;40:609.
212. Friedman MA, Volberding PA, Cassidy MJ, et al. Therapy for hepatocellular cancer with intrahepatic arterial Adriamycin and 5-fluorouracil combined with whole-liver irradiation: a Northern California Oncology Group Study. *Cancer Treat Rep* 1979;63(11):1885.
213. Abrams R, Pajak TF, Haulk TL, Flam M, Asbell SO. Survival results among patients with a-fetoprotein-positive, unresectable hepatocellular carcinoma: analysis of three sequential treatments of the RTOG and Johns Hopkins Oncology Center. *Cancer J* 1998;4:178.
214. Order SE, Pajak T, Leibel S, et al. A randomized prospective trial comparing full dose chemotherapy to I131 antiferritin: an RTOG study. *Int J Radiat Oncol Biol Phys* 1991;1:953.
215. Abrams RA, Cardinale RM, Enger C, et al. Influence of prognostic groupings and treatment results in the management of unresectable hepatoma: experience with cisplatinum-based chemoradiotherapy in 76 patients. *Int J Radiat Oncol Biol Phys* 1997;39:1077.
216. Shepherd FA, Rotstein LE, Houle S, et al. A phase I dose escalation trial of Yttrium-90 microspheres in the treatment of primary hepatocellular carcinoma. *Cancer* 1992;70:2250.
217. Houle S, Yip TK, Shepherd FA, et al. Hepatocellular carcinoma: pilot trial of treatment with Y-90 microspheres. *Radiology* 1989;172:857.
218. Tain JH, Xu BX, Zhang JM, et al. Ultrasound-guided internal radiotherapy using yttrium-90-glass microspheres for liver malignancies. *J Nucl Med* 1996;37:958.
219. Ho S, Lau WY, Leung TW, Johnson PJ. Internal radiation therapy for patients with primary or metastatic hepatic cancer: a review. *Cancer* 1998;83(9):1894.
220. Ho S, Lau WY, Leung TW, et al. Clinical evaluation of the partition model for estimating radiation doses from yttrium-90 microspheres in the treatment of hepatic cancer. *Eur J Nucl Med* 1997;24(3):293.
221. Leung WT, Lau WY, Ho SK, et al. Radiation pneumonitis after selective internal radiation treatment with intra-arterial 90-yttrium-microspheres for inoperable hepatic tumors. *Int J Radiat Oncol Biol Phys* 1995;33:919.
222. Leung WT, Lau WY, Ho S, et al. Selective internal radiation therapy with intra-arterial iodine-131-Lipiodol in inoperable hepatocellular carcinoma. *J Nucl Med* 1994;35(8):1313.
223. Raoul JI, Bretagne JF, Caucanas JP, et al. Internal radiation therapy for hepatocellular carcinoma. Results of a French multicenter phase II trial of transarterial injection of iodine 131-labeled Lipiodol. *Cancer* 1992;69(2):346.
224. Raoul JL, Guyader D, Bretagne JF, et al. Randomized controlled trial for hepatocellular carcinoma with portal vein thrombosis: intra-arterial iodine-131-iodized oil versus medical support. *J Nucl Med* 1994;35(11):1782.
225. Raoul JL, Guyader D, Bretagne JF, et al. Prospective randomized trial of chemoembolization versus intra-arterial injection of 131 I-labeled-iodized oil in the treatment of hepatocellular carcinoma. *Hepatology* 1997;26(5):1156.
226. Matsuura M, Nakajima N, Arai K, Ito K. The usefulness of radiation therapy for hepatocellular carcinoma. *Hepatogastroenterology* 1998;45(21):791.
227. Seong J, Keum KC, Han KH, et al. Combined transcatheter arterial chemoembolization and local radiotherapy of unresectable hepatocellular carcinoma. *Int J Radiat Oncol Biol Phys* 1999;43(2):393.
228. Ten Haken RK, Lawrence TS, McShan DL, et al. Technical considerations in the use of 3-D beam arrangements in the abdomen. *Radiother Oncol* 1991;22:19.
229. Lawrence TS, Tesser RJ, Ten Haken RK. An application of dose volume histograms to the treatment of intrahepatic malignancies with radiation therapy. *Int J Radiat Oncol Biol Phys* 1990;19(4):1041.
230. Lawrence TS, Dworzanin LM, Walker-Andrews SC, et al. Treatment of cancers involving the liver and porta hepatis with external beam irradiation and intraarterial hepatic fluorodeoxyuridine. *Int J Radiat Oncol Biol Phys* 1991;20:555.
231. Robertson JM, Lawrence TS, Andrews JC, et al. Long-term results of hepatic artery fluorodeoxyuridine and conformal radiation therapy for primary hepatobiliary cancers. *Int J Radiat Oncol Biol Phys* 1997;37(2):325.
232. Dawson LA, McGinn NJ, Ensminger W, et al. Preliminary results of escalated focal liver radiation and hepatic artery floxuridine for unresectable liver malignancies. *Proc Am Soc Clin Oncol* 1999;18[Suppl]:86a(abst).
233. Lyman JT. Complication probability as assessed from dose-volume histograms. *Radiat Res* 1985;8:13.
234. Jackson A, Ten Haken RK, Robertson JM, et al. Analysis of clinical complication data for radiation hepatitis using a parallel architecture model. *Int J Radiat Oncol Biol Phys* 1995;31(4):883.
235. Lawrence TS, Ten Haken RK, Kessler ML, et al. The use of 3-D dose volume analysis to predict radiation hepatitis. *Int J Radiat Oncol Biol Phys* 1992;23:781.
236. McGinn CJ, Ten Haken RK, Ensminger WD, et al. Treatment of intrahepatic cancers with radiation doses based on a normal tissue complication probability model. *J Clin Oncol* 1998;16(6):2246.

237. Tusjii H, Inada T, Maruhashi A, et al. Clinical results of fractionated proton therapy. *Int J Radiat Oncol Biol Phys* 1992;25:49.
238. Matsuzaki Y, Osuga T, Saito Y, et al. A new, effective, and safe therapeutic option using proton irradiation for hepatocellular carcinoma. *Gastroenterology* 1994;106(4):1032.
239. Yamasaki SA, Marn CS, Francis IR, Robertson JM, Lawrence TS. High-dose localized radiation therapy for treatment of hepatic malignant tumors: CT findings and their relation to radiation hepatitis. *AJR Am J Roentgenol* 1995;165(1):79.
240. Ohara K, Okumura T, Tsuji H, et al. Radiation tolerance of cirrhotic livers in relation to the preserved functional capacity: analysis of patients with hepatocellular carcinoma treated by focused proton beam radiotherapy. *Int J Radiat Oncol Biol Phys* 1997;38(2):367.
241. The Liver Cancer Study Group of Japan, et al. The general rules of the clinical and pathological study of primary liver cancer. *Jpn J Surg* 1989;19:98.
242. Yuki K, Hirohashi S, Sakamoto M, et al. Growth and spread of hepatocellular carcinoma: a review of 240 consecutive autopsy cases. *Cancer* 1990;66:2174.
243. Adachi E, Maeda T, Kajiyama K, et al. Factors correlated with portal venous invasion by hepatocellular carcinoma: univariate and multivariate analyses of 232 resected cases without preoperative treatments. *Cancer* 1996;77(10):2022.
244. Beasley RP. Hepatitis B virus: the major etiology of hepatocellular carcinoma. *Cancer* 1988;61:1942.
245. Ebara M, Ohto M, Shinagawa T, et al. Natural history of minute hepatocellular carcinoma smaller than three centimeters complicating cirrhosis. *Gastroenterology* 1986;90:289.
246. Kaneko S, Unoura M, Kobayashi K. Early detection of hepatocellular carcinoma. In: Okuda K, Tabor E, eds. *Liver cancer.* New York: Churchill Livingstone, 1997:393.
247. Halpern E, Kun LE, Constine LS, et al. *Pediatric radiation oncology.* New York: Raven Press, 1989:280.
248. Stocker JT, Ishak KG. Hepatoblastoma. In: Okuda K, Ihak KG, eds. *Neoplasms of the liver.* New York: Springer-Verlag, 1987.
249. Lack EE, Neave C, Vawter GF. Hepatoblastoma. A clinical and pathologic study of 54 cases. *Am J Surg Pathol* 1982;6(8):693.
250. Evans AE, Land VJ, Newton WA, et al. Combination chemotherapy (vincristine, Adriamycin, cyclophosphamide, and 5-fluorouracil) in the treatment of children with malignant hepatoma. *Cancer* 1982;50(5):821.
251. Mahour GH, Wogu GU, Siegel SE, Isaacs H. Improved survival in infants and children with primary malignant liver tumors. *Am J Surg* 1983;146(2):236.
252. Weinberg AG, Finegold MJ. Primary hepatic tumors of childhood. *Hum Pathol* 1983;14(6):512.
253. Schmidt D, Harms D, Lang W. Primary malignant tumors in childhood. *Virchows Arch* 1985;407:387.
254. Stevens WR, Johnson CD, Stephens DH, Nagorney DM. Fibrolamellar hepatocellular carcinoma: stage at presentation and results of aggressive surgical management. *AJR Am J Roentgenol* 1995;164:1153.
255. Hata Y, Ishizu H, Ohmori K, et al. Flow cytometric analysis of the nuclear DNA content of hepatoblastoma. *Cancer* 1991;68(12):2566.
256. Filler RM, Ehrlich PF, Greenberg ML, Babyn PS. Preoperative chemotherapy in hepatoblastoma. *Surgery* 1991;110(4):591.
257. Ninane J, Perilongo G, Stalens JP, et al. Effectiveness and toxicity of cisplatin and doxorubicin (PLADO) in childhood hepatoblastoma and hepatocellular carcinoma: a SIOP pilot study. *J Med Pediatr Oncol* 1991;19:199.
258. Habrand JL, Pritchard J. Role of radiotherapy in hepatoblastoma and hepatocellular carcinoma in children and adolescents: results of a survey conducted by the SIOP Liver Tumour Study Group. *J Med Pediatr Oncol* 1991;19:208.
259. Penn I. Hepatic transplantation for primary and metastatic cancers of the liver. *Surgery* 1991;110:726.
260. Weiss SW, Enzinger FM. Epithelioid hemangioendothelioma: a vascular tumor often mistaken for a carcinoma. *Cancer* 1982;50(5):970.
261. Makk L, Delmore F, Creech JL, et al. Clinical and morphological features of hepatic angiosarcoma in vinyl chloride workers. *Cancer* 1976;37:149.
262. Ishak KG, Sesterhenn IA, Goodman ZD, Rabin L, Stromeyer FW. Epithelioid hemangioendothelioma of the liver: a clinicopathologic and follow-up study of 32 cases. *Hum Pathol* 1984;15(9):839.
263. Stocker JT, Ishak KG. Undifferentiated (embryonal) sarcoma of the liver. *Ann Surg* 1955;141:246.
264. Leuschner I, Schmidt D, Harms D. Undifferentiated sarcoma of the liver in childhood: morphology, flow cytometry, and literature review. *Hum Pathol* 1990;21(1):68.
265. Shin MS, Carpenter JT Jr, Ho KJ. Epithelioid hemangioendothelioma: CT manifestations and possible linkage to vinyl chloride exposure 45. *J Comput Assist Tomogr* 1991;15(3):505.
266. Carriaga MT, Henson DE. Liver, gallbladder, extrahepatic bile ducts, and pancreas. *Cancer* 1995;75[Suppl]:171.
267. Kuwayti K, Baggenstoss AH, Stauffer MH, Priestly JI. Carcinoma of the major intrahepatic and extrahepatic bile ducts exclusive of the papilla of Vater. *Surg Gynecol Obstet* 1957;104:357.
268. Sako S, Seitzinger GL, Garside E. Carcinoma of the extrahepatic ducts. Review of the literature and report of six cases. *Surgery* 1957;41:416.
269. Okuda K, Kubo Y, Okazaki N, et al. Clinical aspects of intrahepatic bile duct carcinoma including hilar carcinoma. A study of 57 autopsy proven cases. *Cancer* 1977;39:232.
270. Burke EC, Jarnagin WR, Hochwald SN, et al. Hilar cholangiocarcinoma: patterns of spread, the importance of hepatic resection for curative operation, and a presurgical clinical staging system. *Ann Surg* 1998;228(3):385.
271. Nagorney DM, Donohue JH, Farnell MB, Schleck CD, Ilstrup DM. Outcomes after curative resections of cholangiocarcinoma. *Arch Surg* 1993;128:871.
272. Broome U, Olsson R, Loof L, et al. Natural history and prognostic factors in 305 Swedish patients with primary sclerosing cholangitis. *Gut* 1996;38:610.
273. Pitt HA, Nakeeb A, Abrams RA, et al. Perihilar cholangiocarcinoma. Postoperative radiotherapy does not improve survival. *Ann Surg* 1995;221:788.
274. Katoh H, Shinbo T, Otagiri H, et al. Character of a human cholangiocarcinoma CHGS, serially transplanted to nude mice. *Hum Cell* 1988;1:101.
275. Hewitt PM, Krige JE, Bornman PC, Terblanche J. Choledochal cyst in pregnancy: a therapeutic dilemma. *J Am Coll Surg* 1995;181:237.
276. Vogt DP. Current management of cholangiocarcinoma. *Oncology* 1988;2:37.
277. Becker CD, Glattli A, Maibach R, Baer HU. Percutaneous palliation of malignant obstructive jaundice with the Wallstent endoprosthesis: follow-up and reintervention in patients with hilar and non-hilar obstruction. *J Vasc Interv Radiol* 1993;4:597.
278. Tanaka K, Ikoma A, Hamada N, et al. Biliary tract cancer accompanied by anomalous junction of pancreaticobiliary ductal system in adults. *Am J Surg* 1998;175:218.
279. Jeng KS, Ohta I, Yang FS, et al. Coexisting sharp ductal angulation with intrahepatic biliary strictures in right hepatolithiasis. *Arch Surg* 1994;129:1097.
280. Chu KM, Lo CM, Liu CL, Fan ST. Malignancy associated with hepatolithiasis. *Hepatogastroenterology* 1997;44:352.
281. Kubo S, Kinoshita H, Hirohashi K, Hamba H. Hepatolithiasis associated with cholangiocarcinoma. *World J Surg* 1995;19:637.
282. Winslet MC, Bramhall S, Neoptolemos JP, Harding LK, Hesslewood RS. Diffuse increase in renal uptake of technetium 99m methylene diphosphonate in association with disseminated cholangiocarcinoma. *Eur J Nucl Med* 1990;17:372.
283. Meade CJ, Birke F, Metcalfe S, et al. Serum PAF-acetylhydrolase in severe renal or hepatic disease in man: relationship to circulating levels of PAF and effects of nephrectomy or transplantation. *J Lipid Mediat Cell Signal* 1994;9:205.
284. Wantanapa P. Cholangiocarcinoma in patients with opisthorchiasis. *Br J Surg* 1996;83:1062.
285. Berdah SV, Delpero JR, Garcia S, Hardwigsen J, Le Treut YP. A western surgical experience of peripheral cholangiocarcinoma. *Br J Surg* 1996;83:1517.
286. Chu KM, Lai EC, al-Hadeedi SY, et al. Intrahepatic cholangiocarcinoma. *World J Surg* 1997;21:301.
287. Harrison LE, Fong Y, Klimstra DS, Zee SY, Blumgart LH. Surgical treatment of 32 patients with peripheral intrahepatic cholangiocarcinoma. *Br J Surg* 1998;85(8):1068.
288. Shimizu Y, Iwatsuki S, Herberman RB, Whiteside TL. Effects of cytokines in in vitro growth of tumor-infiltrating lymphocytes obtained from human primary and metastatic liver tumors. *Cancer Immunol Immunother* 1991;32:280.
289. Severini A, Belloni M, Cozzi G, Pizzetti P, Spinelli P. Lymphomatous involvement of intrahepatic and extrahepatic biliary ducts. PTC and ERCP findings. *Acta Radiol Diagn* 1981;22:159.
290. Nakeeb A, Pitt HA, Sohn TA, et al. Cholangiocarcinoma: a spectrum of intrahepatic perihilar, and distal tumors. *Ann Surg* 1996;224:463.
291. Ahmed T, Wuest D, Ciavarella D. Peripheral blood stem cell mobilization by cytokines. *J Clin Apheresis* 1992;7:129.
292. Tompkins RK, Thomas D, Wile A, Longmire WP. Prognostic factors in bile duct carcinoma. Analysis of 96 cases. *Ann Surg* 1981;194:447.
293. Fong Y, Blumgart LH, Lin E, Fortner JG, Brennan MF. Outcome of treatment for distal bile duct cancer. *Br J Surg* 1996;83(12):1712.
294. Yeo CJ, Sohn TA, Lillemoe KD, et al. Six hundred fifty consecutive pancreaticoduodenectomies in the 1990s: pathology, complications and outcomes. *Ann Surg* 1997;226:248.
295. Haswell-Elkins MR, Sithithaworn P, Mairiang E, et al. Immune responsiveness and parasite-specific antibody levels in human hepatobiliary disease associated with *Opisthorchis viverrini* infection. *Clin Exp Immunol* 1991;84:213.
296. Kuo YC, Wu CS. Spontaneous cutaneous biliary fistula: a rare complication of cholangiocarcinoma. *J Clin Gastroenterol* 1990;12:451.
297. Saunders K, Longmire WP Jr, Tompkins R, et al. Diffuse bile duct tumors: guidelines for management. *Am Surg* 1991;57:816.
298. Weinbren K, Mutum SS. Pathological aspects of cholangiocarcinoma. *J Pathol* 1983;139:217.
299. Tsuzuki T, Ogata Y, Iida S, et al. Carcinoma of the bifurcation of the hepatic ducts. *Arch Surg* 1983;118:1147.
300. Rodgers CM, Adams JT, Schwartz SI. Carcinoma of the extrahepatic bile ducts. *Surgery* 1981;90:596.
301. Jutte DL, Bell RHJ, Penn I, Powers J, Kolinjivadi J. Carcinoid tumor of the biliary system. Case report and literature review. *Dig Dis Sci* 1987;32(7):763.
302. Rugge M, Sonego F, Militello C, Guido M, Ninfo V. Primary carcinoid tumor of the cystic and common bile ducts. *Am J Surg Pathol* 1992;16(8):802.
303. Sankary HN, Foster P, Frye E, Williams JW. Carcinoid tumors of the extrahepatic bile duct: an unusual cause of bile duct obstruction. *Liver Transplant Surg* 1995;1:122.
304. Wade TP, Prasad CN, Virgo KS, Johnson FE. Experience with distal bile duct cancers in U.S. Veterans Affairs hospitals. *J Surg Oncol* 1997;64:242.
305. Heslin MJ, Brooks AD, Hochwald SN, et al. A preoperative biliary stent is associated with increased complications after pancreaticoduodenectomy. *Arch Surg* 1998;133:149.
306. Ryan ME. Cytologic brushings of ductal lesions during ERCP. *Gastrointest Endosc* 1991;37:139.
307. Georgopoulso SK, Schwartz LH, Jarnagin WR, et al. A comparison of magnetic resonance cholangiopancreatography (MRCP) and endoscopic retrograde cholangiopancreatography (ERCP) in malignant pancreaticobiliary obstruction. *Arch Surg* 1999.
308. van den Bosch RP, van der Schelling GP, Klinkenbijl JHG, et al. Guidelines for the application of surgery and endoprostheses in the palliation of obstructive jaundice in advanced cancer of the pancreas. *Ann Surg* 1994;219:18.
309. Klatskin G. Adenocarcinoma of the hepatic duct at its bifurcation within the porta hepatis. *Am J Med* 1965;38:241.
310. Farley DR, Weaver AL, Nagorney DM. "Natural history" of unresected cholangiocarcinoma: patient outcome after noncurative intervention. *Mayo Clin Proc* 1995;70:425.
311. Vatanasapt V, Tangvoraphonkchai V, Titapant V, et al. A high incidence of liver cancer in Khon Kaen Province, Thailand. *Southeast Asian J Trop Med Public Health* 1990;21:489.

312. Way LW. *Current surgical diagnosis and treatment: biliary tract,* 10th ed. Norwalk: Appleton & Lange, 1994:537.
313. Nakeeb A, Lipsett PA, Lillemoe KD, et al. Biliary carcinoembryonic antigen levels are a marker for cholangiocarcinoma. *J Surg Oncol* 1996;171:147.
314. Rabinovitz M, Zajko AB, Hassanein T, et al. Diagnostic value of brush cytology in the diagnosis of bile duct carcinoma: a study in 65 patients with bile duct stricture. *Hepatology* 1990;12:747.
315. Enjoji M, Sakai H, Nakashima M, Nawata H. Integrins: utility as cell type- and stage-specific markers for hepatocellular carcinoma and cholangiocarcinoma. *In Vitro Cell Dev Biol Anim* 1998;34:25.
316. Baer HU, Matthews JB, Schweizer WP, Gertsch P, Blumgart LH. Management of the Mirizzi syndrome and the surgical implications of cholecystcholedochal fistula. *Br J Surg* 1990;77:743.
317. Cabooter M, Sas S, Laukens P. Mirrizi syndrome. *Ned Tijdschr Geneeskd* 1990;134:708.
318. Callery MP, Strasberg SM, Doherty GM, Soper NJ, Norton JA. Staging laparoscopy with laparoscopic ultrasonography: optimizing resectability in hepatobiliary and pancreatic malignancy. *J Am Coll Surg* 1997;185:33.
319. Wetter LA, Ring EJ, Pellegrini CA, Way LW. Differential diagnosis of sclerosing chlangiocarcinomas of the common hepatic duct (Klatskin tumors). *Am J Surg* 1991;161:57.
320. Hadjis NS, Collier NA, Blumgart LH. Malignant masquerade at the hilum of the liver. *Br J Surg* 1985;72:659.
321. Verbeek PC, Van Leeuwen DJ, de Wit LT, et al. Benign fibrosing disease at the hepatic confluence mimicking Klatskin tumors. *Surgery* 1992;112:866.
322. Saldinger PF, Blumgart LH. Resection of hilar cholangiocarcinoma—a European and United States experience. *J Hepatobil Pancreat Surg* 2000;7:111.
323. Gibson RN, Yeung E, Thompson JN, et al. Bile duct obstruction: radiologic evaluation of level, cause and tumor resectability. *Radiology* 1986;160:43.
324. Okuda K, Ohto M, Tsuchiya Y. The role of ultrasound, percutaneous transhepatic cholangiography, computed tomographic scanning, and magnetic resonance imaging in the preoperative assessment of bile duct cancer. *World J Surg* 1988;12:18.
325. Hann LE, Greatrex KV, Bach AM, Fong Y, Blumgart LH. Cholangiocarcinoma at the hepatic hilus: sonographic findings. *AJR Am J Roentgenol* 1997;168(4):985.
326. Bach AM, Hann LE, Brown KT, et al. Portal vein evaluation with US: comparison to angiography combined with CT arterial portography. *Radiology* 1996;201(1):149.
327. Hadjis NS, Blumgart LH. Role of liver atrophy, hepatic resection and hepatocyte hyperplasia in the development of portal hypertension in biliary disease. *Gut* 1987;28:1022.
328. Itoh K, Fujita N, Kubo K, et al. MR imaging of hilar cholangiocarcinoma—comparative study with CT. *Nippon Igaku Hoshasen Gakkai Zasshi* 1992;52:443.
329. Guthrie JA, Ward J, Robinson PJ. Hilar cholangiocarcinomas: T2-weighted spin-echo and gadolinium-enhanced FLASH MR imaging. *Radiology* 1996;201:347.
330. Lee MG, Lee HJ, Kim MH, et al. Extrahepatic biliary diseases: 3D MR cholangiopancreatography compared with endoscopic retrograde cholangiopancreatography. *Radiology* 1997;202:663.
331. Wei MX, Tamiya T, Chase M, et al. Experimental tumor therapy in mice using the cyclophosphamide-activating cytochrome P450 2B1 gene. *Hum Gene Ther* 1994;5(8):969.
332. Hochwald SN, Burke EC, Jarnagin WR, Fong Y, Blumgart LH. Association of preoperative biliary stenting with increased postoperative infectious complications in proximal cholangiocarcinoma. *Arch Surg* 1999;134(3):261.
333. Bismuth H, Nakache R, Diamond T. Management strategies in resection for hilar cholangiocarcinoma. *Ann Surg* 1992;215:31.
334. Blumgart LH, Hadjis NS, Benjamin IS, Beazley R. Surgical approaches to cholangiocarcinoma at confluence of hepatic ducts. *Lancet* 1984;1:66.
335. Nimura Y, Hayakawa N, Kamiya J, et al. Combined portal vein and liver resection for carcinoma of the biliary tract. *Br J Surg* 1991;78:727.
336. Altaee MY, Johnson PJ, Farrant JM, Williams R. Etiologic and clinical characteristics of peripheral and hilar cholangiocarcinoma. *Cancer* 1991;68:2051.
337. Baer HU, Stain SC, Dennison AR, Eggers B, Blumgart LH. Improvements in survival by aggressive resections of hilar cholangiocarcinoma. *Ann Surg* 1993;217:20.
338. Bengmark S, Ekberg H, Evander A, Klofver Stahl B, Tranberg KG. Major liver resection for hilar cholangiocarcinoma. *Ann Surg* 1988;207:120.
339. Hadjis NS, Blenkharn JI, Alexander N, Benjamin IS, Blumgart LH. Outcome of radical surgery in hilar cholangiocarcinoma. *Surgery* 1990;107:597.
340. Launois B, Campion J-P, Brissot P, Gosselin M. Carcinoma of the hepatic hilus: surgical management and the case for resection. *Ann Surg* 1978;190:151.
341. Altermeier WA, Gall EA, Zinninger MM, Hoxworth PI. Sclerosing carcinoma of the major intrahepatic bile ducts. *Arch Surg* 1957;75:450.
342. Longmire WP, McArthur MS, Bastounis EA, Hiatt J. Carcinoma of the extrahepatic biliary tract. *Ann Surg* 1973;178:333.
343. Cameron JL, Pitt HA, Zinner MJ, Kaufman SL, Coleman J. Management of proximal cholangiocarcinomas by surgical resection and radiotherapy. *Am J Surg* 1990;159:91.
344. Fong Y, Blumgart LH. Resection for bile duct carcinoma: technical considerations. In: Terblanche J, ed. *Hepatobiliary malignancy—its multidisciplinary management.* London: Edward Arnold, 1994:571.
345. Blumgart LH, Benjamin IS. Liver resection for bile duct cancer. *Surg Clin North Am* 1989;69:323.
346. Lai EC, Tompkins RK, Mann LL, Roslyn JJ. Proximal bile duct cancer. Quality of survival. *Ann Surg* 1987;205:111.
347. Jarnagin WR, Bodniewicz J, Dougherty E, et al. A prospective analysis of staging laparoscopy in patients with primary and secondary hepatobiliary malignancies. *J Gastrointest Surg* 1999 (*in press*).
348. Mizumoto R, Kawarada Y, Suzuki H. Surgical treatment of hilar carcinoma of the bile duct. *Surg Gynecol Obstet* 1996;162:153.
349. Mizumoto R, Suzuki H. Surgical anatomy of the hepatic hilum with special reference to the caudate lobe. *World J Surg* 1988;12:2.
350. Yeo CJ, Pitt HA, Cameron JL. Cholangiocarcinoma. *Surg Clin North Am* 1990;70:1429.
351. Reding R, Buard JL, Lebeau G, Launois B. Surgical management of 552 carcinomas of the extrahepatic bile ducts (gallbladder and periampullary tumors excluded). Results of the French Surgical Association Survey. *Ann Surg* 1991;213:236.
352. Nimura Y, Hayakawa N, Kamiya J, Kondo S, Shionoya S. Hepatic segmentectomy with caudate lobe resection for bile duct carcinoma of the hepatic hilus. *World J Surg* 1990;14:535.
353. Lupi L, Bighi S, Cervi PM, Marzola A. The CT and US aspects in hepatic cholangiocarcinoma due to thorum dioxide (Thorotrast). A case report and review of the literature. *Radiol Med Torino* 1990;79:399.
354. Pichlmayr R, Weimann A, Klempnauer J, et al. Surgical treatment in proximal bile duct cancer. A single-center experience. *Ann Surg* 1996;224:628.
355. Ahrendt SA, Pitt HA, Kalloo AN, et al. Primary sclerosing cholangitis: resect, dilate, or transplant? *Ann Surg* 1998;227:412.
356. Blumgart LH, Kelley CJ. Hepaticojejunostomy in benign and malignant high bile duct stricture: approaches to the left hepatic ducts. *Br J Surg* 1984;71:257.
357. Voyles CR, Blumgart LH. A technique for the construction of high biliary-enteric anastomoses. *Surg Gynecol Obstet* 1982;154:885.
358. Olthoff KM, Millis JM, Rosove MH, et al. Is liver transplantation justified for the treatment of hepatic malignancies? *Arch Surg* 1990;125:1261.
359. Rosen CB, Nagorney DM. Cholangiocarcinoma complicating primary sclerosing cholangitis. *Semin Liver Dis* 1991;11:26.
360. Wolber RA, Greene CA, Dupuis BA. Polyclonal carcinoembryonic antigen staining in the cytologic differential diagnosis of primary and metastatic hepatic malignancies. *Acta Cytol* 1991;35:215.
361. Parc Y, Frileux P, Balladur P, et al. Surgical strategy for the management of hilar bile duct cancer. *Br J Surg* 1997;84:1675.
362. Klempnauer J, Ridder GJ, von Wasielewski R, et al. Resectional surgery of hilar cholangiocarcinoma: a multivariate analysis of prognostic factors. *J Clin Oncol* 1997;15:947.
363. Blumgart LH, Hadjis NS, Benjamin IS, Beazley R. Surgical approaches to cholangiocarcinoma at confluence of hepatic ducts. *Lancet* 1984;1:66.
364. Ottow RT, August DA, Sugarbaker PH. Treatment of proximal biliary tract carcinoma: an overview of techniques and results. *Surgery* 1985;97:251.
365. Erickson BA, Nag S. Biliary tree malignancies. *J Surg Oncol* 1998;67(3):203.
366. Picus J, Myerson R, Drebin J, et al. A phase II trial of continuous infusion (CIVI) 5-FU with 3-D conformal radiation in the adjuvant treatment of pancreatic, ampullary and biliary cancers. *Proc Am Soc Clin Oncol* 1998;17:266a(abst).
367. Chakravarthy A, Yeo CJ, Cameron JL, et al. Preliminary results of a phase II study of adjuvant combined modality therapy for resected pancreatic and periampullary adenocarninoma using local irradiation, R-FU, Leucovorin, Dipyridamole, and Mitomycin-C. *Proc Am Soc Clin Oncol* 1998;17[Suppl]:266a(abst).
368. Pitt HA, Dooley WC, Yeo CJ, Cameron JL. Malignancies of the biliary tree. *Curr Probl Surg* 1995;32(1):1.
369. Kamada T, Saitou H, Takamura A, Nojima T, Okushiba SI. The role of radiotherapy in the management of extrahepatic bile duct cancer: an analysis of 145 consecutive patients treated with intraluminal and/or external beam radiotherapy. *Int J Radiat Oncol Biol Phys* 1996;34:767.
370. McMaster KM, Tuttle TM, Leach SD, et al. Neoadjuvant chemoradiation for extrahepatic cholangiocarcinoma. *Am J Surg* 1997;174:605.
371. Urego M, Flickinger JC, Carr BI. Radiotherapy and multimodality management of cholangiocarcinoma. *Int J Radiat Oncol Biol Phys* 1999;44(1):121.
372. Klempnauer J, Ridder GJ, Werner M, Weimann A, Pichlmayr R. What constitutes long-term survival after surgery for hilar cholangiocarcinoma? *Cancer* 1997;79:26.
373. Iwatsuki S, Todo S, Marsh JW, et al. Treatment of hilar cholangiocarcinoma (Klatskin tumors) with hepatic resection or transplantation. *J Am Coll Surg* 1998;187:358.
374. Liu CL, Lo CM, Lai EC, Fan ST. Endoscopic retrograde cholangiopancreatography and endoscopic endoprosthesis insertion in patients with Klatskin tumors. *Arch Surg* 1998;133:293.
375. Cheung KL, Lai EC. Endoscopic stenting for malignant biliary obstruction. *Arch Surg* 1995;130:204.
376. Miyazaki M, Ito H, Nakagawa K, et al. Aggressive surgical approaches to hilar cholangiocarcinoma: hepatic or local resection? *Surgery* 1998;123:131.
377. Schima W, Prokesch R, Osterreicher C, et al. Biliary Wallstent endoprosthesis in malignant hilar obstruction: long-term results with regard to the type of obstruction. *Clin Radiol* 1997;52:213.
378. Stoker J, Lameris JS. Complications of percutaneously inserted biliary Wallstents. *Interv Radiol* 1993;4:767.
379. Rossi P, Bezzi M, Adam A, et al. Metallic stents in malignant biliary obstruction: results of multicenter European study of 240 patients. *J Vasc Interv Radiol* 1994;5:279.
380. Glattli A, Stain SC, Baer HU, et al. Unresectable malignant biliary obstruction: treatment by self-expandable biliary endoprostheses. *HPB Surg* 1993;6:175.
381. Bergquist A, Glaumann H, Persson B, Broome U. Risk factors and clinical presentation of hepatobiliary carcinoma in patients with primary sclerosing cholangitis: a case-control study. *Hepatology* 1998;27:311.
382. Hurlimann J, Gardiol D. Immunohistochemistry in the differential diagnosis of liver carcinomas. *Am J Surg Pathol* 1991;15:280.
383. Kuvshinoff BW, Armstrong JG, Fong Y, et al. Palliation of irresectable hilar cholangiocarcinoma with biliary drainage and radiotherapy. *Br J Surg* 1995;82(11):1522.
384. Jarnagin WR, Burke E, Powers C, Fong Y, Blumgart LH. Intrahepatic biliary enteric bypass provides effective palliation in selected patients with malignant obstruction at the hepatic duct confluence. *Am J Surg* 1998;175(6):453.
385. Baer HU, Rhyner M, Stain SC, et al. The effect of communication between the right and left liver on the outcome of surgical drainage for jaundice due to malignant obstruction at the hilus of the liver. *HPB Surg* 1994;8:27.

386. Falkson G, MacIntyre JM, Moertel CG. Eastern Cooperative Oncology Group experience with chemotherapy for inoperable gallbladder and bile duct cancer. *Cancer* 1984;54(6):965.
387. Jones DV, Lozano R, Hoque A, Markowitz A, Patt Y. Phase II study of paclitaxel therapy for unresectable biliary tree carcinomas. *J Clin Oncol* 1996;14:2306.
388. Pazdur R, Royce ME, Rodriguez GI, et al. Phase II trial of docetaxel for cholangiocarcinoma. *Am J Clin Oncol* 1999;22(1):78.
389. Patt YZ, Jones DVJ, Hoque A, et al. Phase II trial of intravenous fluorouracil and subcutaneous interferon alfa-2b for biliary tract cancer. *J Clin Oncol* 1996;14(8):2311.
390. Jones DVJ, Lozano R, Hoque A, Markowitz A, Patt YZ. Phase II study of paclitaxel therapy for unresectable biliary tree carcinomas. *J Clin Oncol* 1996;14(8):2306.
391. Harvey JH, Smith FP, Schein PS. 5-Fluorouracil, mitomycin, and doxorubicin (FAM) in carcinoma of the biliary tract. *J Clin Oncol* 1984;2:1245.
392. Takada T, Kato H, Matsushiro T, et al. Comparison of 5-fluorouracil, doxorubicin, and mitomycin C with 5-fluorouracil alone in the treatment of pancreatic-biliary carcinomas. *Oncology* 1994;51:396.
393. Di Lauro L, Carpano S, Campomolla E, et al. Cisplatin, epirubicin, and fluorouracil (PEF) for advanced biliary tract carcinoma. *Proc Am Soc Clin Oncol* 1997;16:287a(abst).
394. Sanz-Altamira PM, Ferrante K, Jenkins RL, et al. A phase II trial of 5-fluorouracil, leucovorin and carboplatin in patients with unresectable biliary tree carcinoma. *Cancer* 1998;82(12):2321.
395. Rougier P, Roche A, Pelletier G, et al. Efficacy of chemoembolisation for hepatocellular carcinomas: experience from the Gustave Roussy Institute and the Bicentre Hospital. *J Surg Oncol Suppl* 1993;3:94.
396. Mezger J, Sauerbruch T, Ko Y, Wolter H, Funk C. Phase II trial of gemcitabine in biliary tract cancers. *Proc Am Soc Clin Oncol* 1997;16:297a.
397. DeGusmao CBRA, Murad AM. Phase II trial of the use of gemcitabine (G) and 5-fluorouracil (5-FU) in the treament of advanced pancreatic (APC) and biliary tract (ABTC) adenocarcinoma. *Proc Am Soc Clin Oncol* 1998;17[Suppl]:290a(abst).
398. Smith GW, Bukowski RM, Hewlett JS, Groppe CW. Hepatic artery infusion of 5-fluorouracil and mitomycin C in cholangiocarcinoma and gallbladder carcinoma. *Cancer* 1984;54(8):1513.
399. Reed ML, Vaitkevicius VK, Al-Sarraf M, et al. The practicality of chronic hepatic artery infusion therapy of primary and metastatic hepatic malignancies: ten-year results of 124 patients in a prospective protocol. *Cancer* 1981;47:402.
400. Sampson LK, Vickers SM, Ying W, Phillips JO. Tamoxifen-mediated growth inhibition of human cholangiocarcinoma. *Cancer Res* 1997;57(9):1743.
401. Bowling TE, Galbraith SM, Hatfield AR, Solano J, Spittle MF. A retrospective comparison of endoscopic stenting alone and with stenting and radiotherapy in non-resectable cholangiocarcinoma. *Gut* 1996;39:852.
402. Vallis KA, Benjamin IS, Munor AJ, et al. External beam and intraluminal radiotherapy for locally advanced bile duct cancer: role and tolerability. *Radiother Oncol* 1996;41:61.
403. Vatanasapt V, Uttaravichien T, Mairiang EO, et al. Cholangiocarcinoma in north-east Thailand. *Lancet* 1990;335:116.
404. Nagano H, Sasaki Y, Imaoka S, et al. Intraarterial and intraportal chemotherapy combined with decollateralization for cholangiocellular carcinoma and metastic liver cancer. *Jpn J Cancer Chemother* 1990;17:1758.
405. Whittington R, Neuberg D, Tester WJ, Benson III AB, Haller DG. Protracted intravenous fluorouracil infusion with radiation therapy in the management of localized pancreaticobiliary carcinoma: a phase I Eastern Cooperative Oncology Group trial. *J Clin Oncol* 1995;13:227.
406. Ohnishi H, Asada M, Shichijo Y, et al. External radiotherapy for biliary decompression of hilar cholangiocarcinoma. *Hepatogastroenterology* 1995;42(3):265.
407. Gonzalez DG, Gouma DJ, Rauws EAJ, et al. Role of radiotherapy, in particular intraluminal brachytherapy, in the treament of proximal bile duct carcinoma. *Ann Oncol* 1997;4:s215.
408. Foo ML, Gunderson LL, Bender CE, Buskirk SJ. External radiation therapy and transcatheter iridium in the treatment of extrahepatic bile duct carcinoma. *Int J Radiat Oncol Biol Phys* 1997;39(4):929.
409. Chen MF, Jan YY, Wang CS, Jeng LB, Hwang TL. Clinical experience in 20 hepatic resections for peripheral cholangiocarcinoma. *Cancer* 1989;64:2226.
410. Nakajima T, Kondo Y, Miyazaki M, Okui K. A histopathologic study of 102 cases of intrahepatic cholangiocarcinoma: histologic classification and modes of spreading. *Hum Pathol* 1988;19(10):1228.
411. Stillwagon GB, Order SE, Haulk T, et al. Variable low dose rate irradiation (131I-anti-CEA) and integrated low dose chemotherapy in the treatment of nonresectable primary intrahepatic cholangiocarcinoma. *Int J Radiat Oncol Biol Phys* 1991;21(6):1601.
412. Blalock AA. A statistical study of 888 cases of biliary tract disease. *Johns Hopkins Hosp Bull* 1924;35:391.
413. Wanebo HJ, Castle WN, Fechner RE. Is carcinoma of the gallbladder a curable lesion? *Ann Surg* 1982;196:624.
414. de Aretxabala X, Roa I, Araya JC, et al. Gallbladder cancer in patients less than 40 years old. *Br J Surg* 1994;81(1):111
415. Zatonski WA, Lowenfels AB, Boyle P, et al. Epidemiologic aspects of gallbladder cancer: a case-control study of the SEARCH Program of the International Agency for Research on Cancer. *J Natl Cancer Inst* 1997;89(15):1132.
416. Ghadirian P, Simard A, Baillargeon J. A population-based case-control study of cancer of the bile ducts and gallbladder in Quebec, Canada. *Rev Epidemiol Sante Publ* 1993;41(2):107.
417. Kodama M, Kodama T. Epidemiological peculiarities of cancers of the gall-bladder and larynx that distinguish them from other human neoplasias. *Anticancer Res* 1994;14(5B):2205.
418. Nakamura S, Sakaguchi S, Suzuki S, Muro H. Aggressive surgery for carcinoma of the gallbladder. *Surgery* 1989;106:467.
419. Wanebo HJ, Vezeridis MP. Treatment of gallbladder cancer. *Cancer Treat Res* 1994;69:97.
420. Chijiiwa K, Tanaka M, Nakayama F. Adenocarcinoma of the gallbladder associated with anomalous pancreaticobiliary ductal junction. *Am Surg* 1993;59(7):430.
421. Welton JC, Marr JS, Friedman SM. Association between hepatobiliary cancer and typhoid carrier state. *Lancet* 1979;1(8120):791.
422. Joffe N, Antonioli DA. Primary carcinoma of the gallbladder associated with chronic inflammatory bowel disease. *Clin Radiol* 1981;32(3):319.
423. Berk RN, Armbuster TG, Saltzstein SL. Carcinoma in the porcelain gallbladder. *Radiology* 1973;106(1):29.
424. Trajber HJ, Szego T, de Camargo HS Jr, et al. Adenocarcinoma of the gallbladder in two siblings. *Cancer* 1982;50(6):1200.
425. Broden G, Bengtsson L. Biliary carcinoma associated with methyldopa therapy. *Acta Chir Scand* 1980;500:7.
426. Ellis EF, Gordon PR, Gottlieb LS. Oral contraceptives and cholangiocarcinoma. *Lancet* 1978;1:207.
427. Lowenfels AB, Norman J. Isoniazid and bile duct cancer. *JAMA* 1999;240:434.
428. Mancuso TF, Brennan MJ. Epidemiological considerations of cancer of the gallbladder, bile ducts and salivary glands in the rubber industry. *J Occup Med* 1970;12(9):333.
429. Kowalewski K, Todd EF. Carcinoma of the gallbladder induced in hamsters by insertion of cholesterol pellets and feeding dimethylnitrosamine. *Proc Soc Exp Biol Med* 1971;136:482.
430. Sumiyoshi K, Nagai E, Chijiiwa K, Nakayama F. Pathology of carcinoma of the gallbladder. *World J Surg* 1991;15(3):315.
431. Santi L, Civalleri D, Conte PF, Fraschini G, Sertoli MR. Regional intra-arterial chemotherapy of metastatic liver cancer. *Chemioterapia* 1985;4:359.
432. Yamaguchi K, Enjoji M. Carcinoma of the gallbladder—a clinicopathology of 103 patients and a newly proposed staging. *Cancer* 1988;62:1425.
433. Henson DE, Albores-Saavedra J, Corle D. Carcinoma of the gallbladder. Histologic types, stage of disease, grade, and survival rates. *Cancer* 1992;70(6):1493.
434. Kimura W, Nagai H, Kuroda A, Morioka Y. Clinicopathologic study of asymptomatic gallbladder carcinoma found at autopsy. *Cancer* 1989;64:98.
435. Perpetuo MD, Valdivieso M, Heilbrun LK, et al. Natural history study of gallbladder cancer: a review of 36 years experience at M.D. Anderson Hospital and Tumor Institute. *Cancer* 1978;42(1):330.
436. Fong Y, Heffernan N, Blumgart LH. Gallbladder carcinoma discovered during laparoscopic cholecystectomy: aggressive reresection is beneficial. *Cancer* 1998;83(3):423.
437. Winston CB, Chen JW, Fong Y, Schwartz LH, Panicek DM. Recurrent gallbladder carcinoma along laparoscopic cholecystectomy port tracks: CT demonstration. *Radiology* 1999;212(2):439.
438. Donohue JH, Nagorney DM, Grant CS, et al. Carcinoma of the gallbladder. Does radical resection improve outcome? *Arch Surg* 1990;125:237.
439. Nevin JE, Moran TJ, Kay S, King R. Carcinoma of the gallbladder: staging, treatment, and prognosis. *Cancer* 1976;37:141.
440. Bears OH, Henderson DE, Hutter RV, et al., eds. *AJCC Cancer Staging Manual.* Philadelphia: JB Lippincott Co, 1988:93.
441. Onoyama H, Yamamoto M, Tseng A, Ajiki T, Saitoh Y. Extended cholecystectomy for carcinoma of the gallbladder. *World J Surg* 1995;19(5):758.
442. Oertli D, Herzog U, Tondelli P. Primary carcinoma of the gallbladder: operative experience during a 16 year period. *Eur J Surg* 1993;159(8):415.
443. Thorbjarnarson B, Glenn F. Carcinoma of the gallbladder. *Cancer* 1959;12:1009.
444. Redaelli CA, Buchler MW, Schilling MK, et al. High coincidence of Mirizzi syndrome and gallbladder carcinoma. *Surgery* 1997;121:58.
445. Strom BL, Maislin G, West SL, et al. Serum CEA and CA 19-9: potential future diagnostic or screening tests for gallbladder cancer? *Int J Cancer* 1990;45(5):821.
446. Ritts RE, Nagorney DM, Jacobson DJ, Talbot RW, Zurawski VR Jr. Comparison of preoperative serum CA19-9 levels with results of diagnostic imaging modalities in patients undergoing laparotomy for suspected pancreatic or gallbladder disease. *Pancreas* 1999;9:707.
447. Chijiiwa K, Sumiyoshi K, Nakayama F. Impact of recent advances in hepatobiliary imaging techniques on the preoperative diagnosis of carcinoma of the gallbladder. *World J Surg* 1991;15(3):322.
448. Wibbenmeyer LA, Sharafuddin MJ, Wolverson MK, et al. Sonographic diagnosis of unsuspected gallbladder cancer: imaging findings in comparison with benign gallbladder conditions. *AJR Am J Roentgenol* 1995;165(5):1169.
449. Franquet T, Montes M, Ruiz DA, Jimenez FJ, Cozcolluela R. Primary gallbladder carcinoma: imaging findings in 50 patients with pathologic correlation. *Gastrointest Radiol* 1991;16(2):143.
450. Bach AM, Loring LA, Hann LE, et al. Gallbladder cancer: can ultrasonography evaluate extent of disease? *J Ultrasound Med* 1998;17(5):303.
451. Kumar A, Aggarwal S. Carcinoma of the gallbladder: CT findings in 50 cases. *Abdom Imaging* 1994;19(4):304.
452. Ohtani T, Shirai Y, Tsukada K, Hatakeyama K, Muto T. Carcinoma of the gallbladder: CT evaluation of lymphatic spread. *Radiology* 1993;189(3):875.
453. Soto JA, Yucel EK, Barish MA, Chuttani R, Ferrucci JT. MR cholangiopancreatography after unsuccessful or incomplete ERCP. *Radiology* 1996;199(1):91.
454. Wilbur AC, Gyi B, Renigers SA. High-field MRI of primary gallbladder carcinoma. *Gastrointest Radiol* 1988;13(2):142.
455. Schwartz LH, Coakley FV, Sun Y, et al. Neoplastic pancreaticobiliary duct obstruction: evaluation with breath-hold MR cholangiopancreatography. *AJR Am J Roentgenol* 1998;170(6):1491.
456. Fong Y, Brennan MF, Turnbull A, Coit DG, Blumgart LH. Gallbladder cancers discovered during laparoscopic surgery: potential for iatrogenic tumor dissemination. *Arch Surg* 1993;128:1054.
457. Merz BJ, Dodge GG, Abellera RM, Kisken WA. Implant metastasis of gallbladder carcinoma in situ in a cholecystectomy scar: a case report. *Surgery* 1993;114(1):120.
458. Akosa AB, Barker F, Desa L, Benjamin I, Krausz T. Cytologic diagnosis in the management of gallbladder carcinoma. *Acta Cytol* 1995;39(3):494.

459. Harada H, Sasaki T, Yamamoto N, Tanaka J, Tomiyama Y. Assessment of endoscopic aspiration cytology and endoscopic retrograde cholangio-pancreatography in patients with cancer of the hepato-biliary tract: II. *Gastroenterol Jpn* 1977;12(1):59.
460. Mohiuddin M, Chen E, Ahmad N. Combined liver radiation and chemotherapy for palliation of hepatic metastases from colorectal cancer. *J Clin Oncol* 1996;14(3):722.
461. Nimura Y, Hayakawa N, Kamiya J, et al. Hepatopancreatoduodenectomy for advanced carcinoma of the biliary tract. *Hepatogastroenterology* 1991;38(2):170.
462. Ouchi K, Owada Y, Matsuno S, Sato T. Prognostic factors in the surgical treatment of gallbladder carcinoma. *Surgery* 1987;101:731.
463. Ogura Y, Mizumoto R, Isaji S, et al. Radical operations for carcinoma of the gallbladder: present status in Japan. *World J Surg* 1991;15:337.
464. Fong Y, Blumgart LH, Fortner JG, Brennan MF. Pancreatic or liver resection for malignancy is safe and effective in the elderly. *Ann Surg* 1995;222(4):426.
465. Tsau JJ, Loftus JP, Nagorney DM, Adson MA, Ilstrup DM. Trends in morbidity and mortality of hepatic resection for malignancy—a matched comparative analysis. *Ann Surg* 1993;220(2):199.
466. Piehler JM, Crichlow RW. Primary carcinoma of the gallbladder. *Surg Gynecol Obstet* 1978;147:929.
467. Cubertafond P, Gainant A, Cucchiaro G. Surgical treatment of 724 carcinomas of the gallbladder. Results of the French Surgical Association Survey. *Ann Surg* 1994;219(3):275.
468. Wilkinson DS. Carcinoma of the gall-bladder: an experience and review of the literature. *Aust N Z J Surg* 1995;65(10):724.
469. Tsukada K, Kurosaki I, Uchida K, et al. Lymph node spread from carcinoma of the gallbladder. *Cancer* 1997;80(4):661.
470. Yamaguchi K, Tsuneyoshi M. Subclinical gallbladder carcinoma. *Am J Surg* 1992;163:382.
471. Shirai Y, Yoshida K, Tsukada K, Muto T. Inapparent carcinoma of the gallbladder—an appraisal of a radical second operation after simple cholecystectomy. *Cancer* 1988;62(Oct):1422.
472. de Aretxabala X, Roa IS, Burgos LA, et al. Curative resection in potentially resectable tumours of the gallbladder. *Eur J Surg* 1997;163(6):419.
473. Bartlett DL, Fong Y, Fortner JG, Brennan MF, Blumgart LH. Long-term results after resection for gallbladder cancer. *Ann Surg* 1996;224(5):639.
474. Shirai Y, Yoshida K, Tsukada K, Muto T, Watanabe H. Radical surgery for gallbladder carcinoma—long-term results. *Ann Surg* 1992;216(5):565.
475. Matsumoto Y, Fujii H, Aoyama H, et al. Surgical treatment of primary carcinoma of the gallbladder based on the histologic analysis of 48 surgical specimens. *Am J Surg* 1992;163:239.
476. Gall FP, Kockerling F, Scheele J, Schneider C, Hohenberger W. Radical operations for carcinoma of the gallbladder: present status in Germany. *World J Surg* 1991;15:328.
477. Drouard F, Delamarre J, Capron J. Cutaneous seeding of gallbladder cancer after laparoscopic cholecystectomy. *N Engl J Med* 1991;325:1316.
478. Clair DG, Lautz DB, Brooks DC. Rapid development of umbilical metastases after laparoscopic cholecystectomy for unsuspected gallbladder carcinoma. *Surgery* 1993;113(3):355.
479. Landen SM. Laparoscopic surgery and tumor seeding [letter]. *Surgery* 1993;114(1):131.
480. Fligelstone L, Rhodes M, Flook D, Puntis M, Crosby D. Tumour inoculation during laparoscopy [letter]. *Lancet* 1993;342(8867):368.
481. Nduka CC, Monson JRT, Menzies-Gow N, Darzi A. Abdominal wall metastases following laparoscopy. *Br J Surg* 1994;81:648.
482. Nally C, Preshaw RM. Tumour implantation at umbilicus after laparoscopic cholecystectomy for unsuspected gallbladder carcinoma. *Can J Surg* 1994;37(3):243.
483. Kim HJ, Roy T. Unexpected gallbladder cancer with cutaneous seeding after laparoscopic cholecystectomy. *South Med J* 1994;87(8):817.
484. Taal BG, Audisio RA, Bleiberg H, et al. Phase II trial of mitomycin C (MMC) in advanced gallbladder and biliary tree carcinoma. An EORTC gastrointestinal tract cancer cooperative group study. *Ann Oncol* 1993;607.
485. Gebbia V, Majello E, Testa A, et al. Treatment of advanced adenocarcinomas of the exocrine pancreas and the gallbladder with 5-fluorouracil, high dose levofolinic acid and oral hydroxyurea on a weekly schedule. Results of a multicenter study of the Southern Italy Oncology Group (G.O.I.M.). *Cancer* 1996;78(6):1300.
486. Makela J, Tikkakoski T, Leinonen A, et al. Superselective intra-arterial chemotherapy with mitomycin C in hepatic neoplasms. *Eur J Surg Oncol* 1993;19(4):348.
487. Houry S, Schlienger M, Huguier M, et al. Gallbladder carcinoma: role of radiation therapy. *Br J Surg* 1989;76:448.
488. Chao TC, Greager JA. Primary carcinoma of the gallbladder. *J Surg Oncol* 1995;46:215.
489. Oswalt CE, Cruz AB Jr. Effectiveness of chemotherapy in addition to surgery in treating carcinoma of the gallbladder. *Rev Surg* 1977;34(6):436.
490. Morrow CE, Sutherland DE, Florack G, Eisenberg MM, Grage TB. Primary gallbladder carcinoma: significance of subserosal lesions and results of aggressive surgical treatment and adjuvant chemotherapy. *Surgery* 1983;94(4):709.
491. Todoroki T. Radiation therapy for primary gallbladder cancer. *Hepatogastroenterology* 1997;44(17):1229.
492. Todoroki T, Iwasaki Y, Orii K, et al. Resection combined with intraoperative radiation therapy (IORT) for stage IV (TNM) gallbladder carcinoma. *World J Surg* 1991;15:357.
493. Hanna SS, Rider WD. Carcinoma of the gallbladder or extrahepatic bile ducts: the role of radiotherapy. *Can Med Assoc J* 1978;118(1):59.
494. Vaittinen E. Carcinoma of the gall-bladder. A study of 390 cases diagnosed in Finland 1953–1967. *Ann Chir Gynaecol* 1970;168:1.
495. Bismuth H, Corlett MB. Intrahepatic cholangioenteric anastomosis in carcinoma of the hilus of the liver. *Surg Gynecol Obstet* 1975;140:170.
496. Kapoor VK, Pradeep R, Haribhakti SP, et al. Intrahepatic segment III cholangiojejunostomy in advanced carcinoma of the gallbladder. *Br J Surg* 1996;83(12):1709.
497. Ozmen MM, Patankar RV, Hengirmen S, Terzi MC. Epidemiology of gallbladder polyps [letter]. *Scand J Gastroenterol* 1994;29(5):480
498. Boulton RA, Adams DH. Gallbladder polyps: when to wait and when to act. *Lancet* 1997;349(9055):817.
499. Shinkai H, Kimura W, Muto T. Surgical indications for small polypoid lesions of the gallbladder. *Am J Surg* 1998;175(2):114.
500. Kozuka S, Tsubone N, Yasui A, Hachisuka K. Relation of adenoma to carcinoma in the gallbladder. *Cancer* 1982;50(10):2226.
501. Yang HL, Sun YG, Wang Z. Polypoid lesions of the gallbladder: diagnosis and indications for surgery. *Br J Surg* 1992;79(3):227.
502. Furukawa H, Kosuge T, Shimada K, et al. Small polypoid lesions of the gallbladder: differential diagnosis and surgical indications by helical computed tomography. *Arch Surg* 1998;133(7):735.
503. Bismuth H, Chiche L, Castaing D. Surgical treatment of hepatocellular carcinomas in noncirrhotic liver: experience with 68 liver resections. *World J Surg* 1995;19:35.
504. Kishi K, Shikata T, Hirohashi S, et al. Hepatocellur carcinoma. A clinical and pathologic analysis of 57 hepatectomy cases. *Cancer* 1983;51:542.
505. Lee CS, Sung JL, Hwang LY, et al. Surgical treatment of 109 patients wth symptomatic and asymptomatic hepatocellular carcinoma. *Surgery* 1986;99:481.
506. Kanematsu T, Matsumata T, Takenaka K, et al. Clinical management of recurrent hepatocellular carcinoma after primary resection. *Br J Surg* 1988;75:203.
507. Lai ECS, Ng IOL, You KT, et al. Hepatic resection for small hepatocellular carcinoma: the Queen Mary Hospital Experience. *World J Surg* 1991;15:654.
508. Hemming AW, Scudamore CH, Davidson A, et al. Evaluation of 50 consecutive segmental hepatic resections. *Am J Surg* 1993;165:621.
509. Fan ST, Lo CM, Lai EC, et al. Perioperative nutritional support in patients undergoing hepatectomy for hepatocellular carcinoma. *N Engl J Med* 1994;331:1547.
510. Chen MF, Hwang TL, Jeng LB, et al. Postoperative recurrence of hepatocellular carcinoma. Two hundred five consecutive patients who underwent hepatic resection in 15 years. *Arch Surg* 1994;129:738.
511. Lai EC, Fan ST, Lo CM, et al. Hepatic resection for hepatocellular carcinoma. An audit of 343 patients. *Ann Surg* 1995;221(3):291.
512. Takenaka K, Kawahara N, Yamamoto K, et al. Results of 280 liver resections for hepatocellular carcinoma. *Arch Surg* 1996;131(1):71.
513. Nadig DE, Wade JP, Fairchild RB, et al. Major hepatic resection. Indications and results in a national hospital system from 1988 to 1992. *Arch Surg* 1997;132:115.
514. Franco D, Capussotti L, Smadja C, et al. Resection of hepatocellular carcinomas: results in 72 European patients with cirrhosis. *Gastroenterology* 1990;98:733.
515. Honjo I, Mizumoto R. Primary carcinoma of the liver. *Am J Surg* 1974;128:31.
516. Okuda K, Obata H, Nakajima Y, et al. Prognosis of primary hepatocellular carcinoma. *Hepatology* 1984;4:S3.
517. Hsu HC, Sheu JC, Lin YH, et al. Prognostic histologic features of resected small hepatocellular carcinoma (HCC) in Taiwan. A comparison with resected large HCC. *Cancer* 1985;56:672.
518. Stukart MJ, Rijnsent A. Induction of tumoricidal activity in isolated rat liver macrophages by liposomes containing recombinant rat G-IFN supplemented with lipopolysaccharide or muramyldipeptide. *Cancer Res* 1987;47:3880.
519. Yamanaka N, Okamoto E, Toyosaka A, et al. Prognostic factors after hepatectomy for hepatocellular carcinoma. A univariate and multivariate analysis. *Cancer* 1990;65:1104.
520. Fong Y, Blumgart LS. Liver resection for cancer. In: Zakim D, Boyer T, eds. *Hepatology*. Philadelphia: WB Saunders, 1996.
521. Ringe B, Pichlmayr R, Wittekind C, Tusch G. Surgical treatment of hepatocellular carcinoma: experience with liver resection and transplantation in 198 patients. *World J Surg* 1991;15:270.
522. Sasaki Y, Imaoka S, Masutani S, et al. Influence of coexisting cirrhosis on long-term prognosis after surgery in patients with hepatocellular carcinoma. *Surgery* 1992;112:515.
523. Ouchi K, Matsubara S, Fukuhara K, et al. Recurrence of hepatocellular carcinoma in the liver remnant after hepatic resection. *Am J Surg* 1993;166:270.
524. Takenaka K, Shimada M, Higahi H, et al. Liver resection for hepatocellular carcinoma in the elderly. *Arch Surg* 1994;129:846.
525. Suenaga M, Sugiura H, Kokuba Y, Uehara S, Kurumiya T. Repeated hepatic resection for recurrent hepatocellular carcinoma in eighteen cases. *Surgery* 1994;115:452.
526. Ringe B, Wittekind C, Bechstein WO, et al. The role of liver transplantation in hepatobiliary malignancy: a retrospective analysis of 95 patients with particular regard to tumor stage and recurrence. *Ann Surg* 1989;209:88.
527. Iwatsuki S, Starzl TE, Sheahan DG, et al. Hepatic resection versus transplantation for hepatocellular carcinoma. *Ann Surg* 1991;214:221.
528. Pichlmayr R, Weimann A, Steinhoff G, Ringe B. Liver transplantation for hepatocellular carcinoma: clinical results and future aspects. *Cancer Chemother Pharmacol* 1992;21[Suppl 1]:S157.
529. Moreno-Gonzalez EM, Comez R, Garcia I, et al. Liver transplantation in malignant hepatic neoplasms. *Am J Surg* 1992;163:395.
530. Bismuth H, Chiche L, Adam R, et al. Liver resection versus transplantation for hepatocellular carcinoma in cirrhotic patients. *Ann Surg* 1993;218:145.
531. Romani F, Belli LS, Rondinara GF, et al. The role of transplantation in small hepatocellular carcinoma complicating cirrhosis of the liver. *J Am Coll Surg* 1994;178:379.
532. Chung SW, Toth JL, Rezieg M, et al. Liver transplantation for hepatocellular carcinoma. *Am J Surg* 1994;167:317.
533. Dalgic A, Mirza DF, Gunson BK, et al. Role of total hepatectomy and transplantation in hepatocellular carcinoma. *Transplant Proc* 1994;26:3564.
534. Leung TW, Patt YZ, Lau WY, et al. Complete pathological remission is possible with systemic combination chemotherapy for inoperable hepatocellular carcinoma. *Clin Cancer Res* 1999;5(7):1676.
535. O'Reilly E, Stuart K, Kemeny N, et al. A phase II trial of irinotecan (CPT-11) in patients with advanced hepatocellular carcinomas (HCC). *Proc Am Soc Clin Oncol* 1998;17[Suppl]: 267a(abst).

536. Umsawasdi T, Chainuvati T, Viranuvatti V. Combination chemotherapy of hepatocellular carcinoma with fluorouracil and mytomycin-C. *Proc Am Soc Clin Oncol* 1978;19:193(abst).
537. Vogel CL, Bayley AC, Brocker RJ, et al. A phase II study of adriamycin in patients with hepatocellular carcinoma from Zambia and the United States. *Cancer* 1977;39:1936(abst).
538. Baker HL, Kaiki J, Jones S, et al. Adriamycin and 5-fluorouracil in the treatment of advanced hepatoma: a Southwest Oncology Study. *Cancer Treat Rep* 1977;61:1595.
539. Ravey M, Omura G, Bartolucci A. Phase II evaluation of doxorubicin plus bleomycin in hepatocellular carcinoma: a Southeastern Cancer Study Group trial. *Cancer Treat Rep* 1984;68:1517.
540. Okada S, Okusaka T, Ueno H, et al. Phase II trial of cisplatin, mitoxantrone and continuous-infusion 5-fluorouracil (5-FU) (FMP therapy) for hepatocellular carcinoma (HCC). *Proc Am Soc Clin Oncol* 1999;18[Suppl]:248a(abst).
541. Zaniboni A, Biasi L, Graffeo M, et al. Phase II study of high-dose vitamin K_1 in hepatocellular carcinoma: a Giscad study. *Proc Am Soc Clin Oncol* 1998;17[Suppl]:307a(abst).
542. Noy L, Feun L, Marini A, et al. A phase II trial of recombinant leukocyte interferon (IFN), doxorubicin, and 5FUDR in patients with hepatocellular carcinoma. *Proc Am Soc Clin Oncol* 1999;18[Suppl]:295a(abst).
543. Benson AB, Mitchell E, Abramson N, et al. A multicenter, phase II trial of oral eniluracil plus 5-FU in patients with inoperable hepatocellular carcinoma. *Proc Am Soc Clin Oncol* 1999;18[Suppl]:256a(abst).
544. Strumberg D, Erhard J, Harstrick A, et al. Phase I study of a weekly 1-h infusion of paclitaxel in patients with unresectable hepatocellular carcinoma. *Eur J Cancer* 1998;34(8):1290.
545. Chao Y, Chan WK, Birkhofer MJ, et al. Phase II and pharmacokinetic study of paclitaxel therapy for unresectable hepatocellular carcinoma patients. *Br J Cancer* 1998;78(1):34.
546. Stuart K, Tessitore J, Huberman M. 5-Fluorouracil and alpha-interferon in hepatocellular carcinoma. *Am J Clin Oncol* 1996;19(2):136.
547. Mani S, Schiano T, Garcia JC, et al. Phase II trial of uracil/tegafur (UFT) plus leucovorin in patients with advanced hepatocellular carcinoma. *Invest New Drugs* 1998;16(3):279.
548. Gebbia V, Maiello E, Serravezza G, et al. 5-Fluorouracil plus high dose levofolinic acid and oral hydroxyurea for the treatment of primary hepatocellular carcinomas: results of a phase II multicenter study of the Southern Italy Oncology Group (G.O.I.M.). *Anticancer Res* 1999;19(2B):1407.
549. Chlebowski RT, Brzechwa-Adjukiewicz A, Cowden A, et al. Doxorubicin (75 mg/m^2) for hepatocellular carcinoma: clinical and pharmacokinetic results. *Cancer Treat Rep* 1984;68(3):487.
550. Falkson G, MacIntyre J, Schutt A, et al. Neocarzinostatin versus m-AMSA or doxorubicin in hepatocellular carcinoma. *J Clin Oncol* 1984;2:581.
551. Melia WM, Johnson P, Williams R. Induction of remission in hepatocellular carcinoma. A comparison of VP16 with adriamycin. *Cancer* 1983;51:206.
552. Falkson G, Ryan LM, Johnson LA, et al. A random phase II study of mitoxantrone and cisplatin in patients with hepatocellular carcinoma. An ECOG study. *Cancer* 1987;60:2141.
553. Ji SK, Park NH, Choi HM, et al. Combined cis-platinum and alpha interferon therapy of advanced hepatocellular carcinoma. *Korean J Intern Med* 1996;11(1):58.
554. Ansfield FJ, Ramirez G, Davis HL Jr, et al. The treatment of metastatic carcinoma of the liver by percutaneous selective hepatic artery infusion of 5-fluorouracil. *Cancer* 1975;36:2413.
555. Misra NC, Jaiswal MS, Singh RV, Das B. Intrahepatic arterial infusion of combination of mitomycin-C and 5-fluorouracil in treatment of primary and metastatic liver carcinoma. *Cancer* 1977;39(4):1425.
556. Kinami Y, Shinmura K, Miyazaki I. The super-selective and the selective one-shot methods for treatment of inoperable cancer of the liver. *Cancer* 1978;41:1720.
557. Wellwood J, Cady B, Oberfield R. Treatment of primary liver cancer: response to regional chemotherapy. *Clin Oncol* 1979;5:25.
558. Olweny CLM, Katongole-Mbidde E, Bahendeka S, et al. Further experiences in treating patients with hepatocellular carcinoma in Uganda. *Cancer* 1980;46:2717.
559. Cheng E, Watson R, Fortner J, et al. Regional intra-arterial infusion of cisplatin in primary liver cancer: a phase II trial. *Proc Am Soc Clin Oncol* 1982;2:179(abst).
560. Urist M, Balch C. Intra-arterial chemotherapy for hepatoma using adriamycin administered via an implantable infusion pump. *Proc Am Soc Clin Oncol* 1984;3:148
561. Shildt R, Baker L, Stuckey W. Hepatic artery infusion (HAI) with 5-FUDR, Adriamycin (A) and streptozotocin (St) in unresectable hepatoma. A Southwest Oncology Group Study. *Proc Am Soc Clin Oncol* 1984;3:150(abst).
562. Carr BI, Dvorchik I. Effects of cisplatin (DDP) intensity on hepatocellular carcinoma (HCC) responses and survival in 57 patients. *Proc Am Soc Clin Oncol* 1998;17[Suppl]:288a(abst).
563. Urabe T, Kaneko S, Matsushita E, Unoura M, Kobayashi K. Clinical pilot study of intrahepatic arterial chemotherapy with methotrexate, 5-fluorouracil, cisplatin and subcutaneous interferon-alpha-2b for patients with locally advanced hepatocellular carcinoma. *Oncology* 1998;55(1):39.
564. Nakamura H, Hashimoto T, Oi H, et al. Transcatheter oily chemoembolization of hepatocellular carcinoma. *Radiology* 1989;170:783.
564a. Shibata J, Fujiyama S, Sata T, et al. Hepatic arterial injection chemotherapy with cisplatin suspended in an oily lymphographic agent for hepatocellular carcinoma. *Cancer* 1989;64:1586.
565. Pelletier C, Roche A, Ink O. A randomised trial of hepatic aterial chemoembolisation in patients with unresectable hepatocellular carcinoma. *J Hepatol* 1990;11:181.
566. Venook A, Stagg R, Lewis B, et al. Chemoembolization for hepatocellular carcinoma. *J Clin Oncol* 1990;8:1108.
567. Yamada R, Kishi K, Sonomura T, et al. Transcatheter arterial embolization in unresectable hepatocellular carcinoma. *Cardiovasc Interv Radiol* 1990;13(3):135.
568. Nakao N, Kamino K, Miura K, et al. Recurrent hepatocellular carcinoma after partial hepatectomy: value of treatment with transcatheter arterial chemoembolization. *AJR Am J Roentgenol* 1991;156:1177.
569. Stuart K, Stokes K, Jenkins R, et al. Treatment of hepatocellular carcinoma using doxorubicin/ethiodized oil/gelatin powder chemoembolisation. *Cancer* 1993;72:3202.
570. Uchida H, Matsuo N, Nishimine K, et al. Transcatheter arterial embolization for hepatoma with lipiodol: hepatic arterial and segmental use. *Semin Interv Radiol* 1993;10:19.
571. Carr B, Orons P, Zajko A, et al. Phase II study of intra-hepatic arterial (I/A) cisplatinum, doxorubicin and Spherex for advanced stage hepatocellular carcinoma (HCC). In: *Proceedings of the Annual Meeting of the American Society of Clinical Oncology.* 1995:A451(abst).
572. Chung J, Park J, Han J, et al. Hepatocellular carcinoma and portal vein invasion: results of treatment with transcatheter oily chemoembolization. *AJR Am J Roentgenol* 1995;(165):315.
573. Warren KW, Choe DS, Plaza J, Relihan M. Results of radical resection for periampullary cancer. *Ann Surg* 1975;181:534.
574. Nakase A, Matsumoto Y, Uchida K, Honjo I. Surgical treatment of cancer of the pancreas and the periampullary region. *Ann Surg* 1977;185:52.
575. Alexander F, Rossi RL, O'Bryan M, et al. Biliary carcinoma. A review of 109 cases. *Am J Surg* 1984;147:503.
576. Lerut JP, Gianello PR, Otte JB, Kestens PJ. Pancreaticoduodenal resection. Surgical experience and evaluation of risk factors in 103 patients. *Ann Surg* 1984;199:432.
577. Tarazi RY, Hermann RE, Vogt D, et al. Results of surgical treatment of periampullary tumors: a thirty-five-year experience. *Surgery* 1986;100:716.
578. Fortner JG, Kallum BO, Kim DK. Surgical management of carcinoma of the junction of the main hepatic ducts. *Ann Surg* 1976;184:68.
579. Akwari OE, Kelly KA. Surgical treatment of adenocarcinoma. Location: junction of the right, left, and common hepatic ducts. *Arch Surg* 1979;114:22.
580. Cameron JL, Broe P, Zuidema GD. Proximal bile duct tumors. Surgical management with silastic transhepatic biliary stents. *Ann Surg* 1982;196:412.
581. Beazley RM, Hadjis N, Benjamin IS, Blumgart LH. Clinicopathological aspects of high bile duct cancer. Experience with resection and bypass surgical treatment. *Ann Surg* 1984;199:623.
582. Iwasaki Y, Okamura T, Ozaki A, et al. Surgical treatment for carcinoma at the confluence of the major hepatic ducts. *Surg Gynecol Obstet* 1986;162:457.
583. Iida S, Tsuzuki T, Ogata Y, et al. The long-term survival of patients with carcinoma of the main hepatic duct junction. *Cancer* 1987;60:1612.
584. Guthrie CM, Haddock G, De Beaux AC, Garden OJ, Carter DC. Changing trends in the management of extrahepatic cholangiocarcinoma. *Br J Surg* 1993;80:1434.
585. Washburn WK, Lewis WD, Jenkins RL. Aggressive surgical resection for cholangiocarcinoma. *Arch Surg* 1995;130(3):270.
586. Su CH, Tsay SH, Wu CC, et al. Factors influencing postoperative morbidity, mortality, and survival after resection for hilar cholangiocarcinoma. *Ann Surg* 1996;223:384.
587. Kurosaki H, Karasawa K, Kaizu T, et al. Intraoperative radiotherapy for resectable extrahepatic bile duct cancer. *Int J Radiat Oncol Biol Phys* 1999;45:634.
588. Brayman KL, Dafoe DC, Smythe WR, et al. Prophylaxis of serious cytomegalovirus infection in renal transplant candidates using live human cytomegalovirus vaccine. Interim results of a randomized controlled trial. *Arch Surg* 1988;123(12):1502.
589. Davis HLJ, Ramirez G, Ansfield FJ. Adenocarcinomas of stomach, pancreas, liver, and biliary tracts. Survival of 328 patients treated with fluoropyrimidine therapy. *Cancer* 1974;33(1):193.
590. Haskell CM. Cancer in the liver. In: Haskell CM, ed. *Cancer treatment.* Philadelphia: WB Saunders, 1980:319.
591. Sons HU, Borchard F, Joel BS. Carcinoma of the gallbladder: autopsy findings in 287 cases and review of the literature. *J Surg Oncol* 1985;28(3):199.
592. Crooke ST, Bradner WT. Mitomycin C: a review. *Cancer Treat Rev* 1976;3:131.
593. Okada S, Ishii H, Nose H, et al. A phase II study of cisplatin in patients with biliary tract carcinoma. *Oncology* 1994;51:515.
594. Raderer M, Hejna MH, Valencak JB, et al. Two consecutive phase II studies of 5-fluorouracil/leucovorin/mitomycin C and of gemcitabine in patients with advanced biliary cancer. *Oncology* 1999;56(3):177.
595. Chen JS, Jan YY, Lin YC, et al. Weekly 24 h infusion of high-dose 5-fluorouracil and leucovorin in patients with biliary tract carcinomas. *Anticancer Drugs* 1998;9(5):393.
596. Rougier P, Fandi A, Ducreux M, et al. Demonstrated efficiency of 5- fluorouracil continuous infusion and cisplatin in patients with advanced biliary tract carcinoma. *Proc Am Soc Clin Oncol* 1995;14:205.
597. Hall SW, Benjamin RS, Murphy WK, Valdivieso M, Bodey GP. Adriamycin, BCNU, ftorafur chemotherapy of pancreatic and biliary tract cancer. *Cancer* 1979;44(6):2008.
598. Isacoff WH, Botnick L, Tompkins R, et al. Treatment of patients with advanced tumors of the bile ducts with continuous infusion 5-fluorouracil in conjuction with calcium, leucovorin, mitomycin C, and dipyridamole. *Proc Am Soc Clin Oncol* 1993;12:225(abst).
599. Kajanti M, Pyrhonen S. Epirubicin-sequential methotrexate-5-fluorouracil-leucovorin treatment in advanced cancer of the extrahepatic biliary system: a phase II study. *Am J Clin Oncol* 1994;17:223.
600. Shirai Y, Yoshida K, Tsukada K, Muto T, Watanabe H. Early carcinoma of the gallbladder. *Eur J Surg* 1992;158(10):545.
601. de Aretxabala X, Roa I, Burgos L, et al. Gallbladder cancer in Chile. A report on 54 potentially resectable tumors. *Cancer* 1992;69:60.
602. Paquet KJ. Appraisal of surgical resection of gallbladder carcinoma with special reference to hepatic resection. *J Hepatobil Pancreat Surg* 1998;5(2):200.
603. Chijiiwa K, Tanaka M. Carcinoma of the gallbladder: an appraisal of surgical resection. *Surgery* 1994;115:751.

SECTION **6**

DANIEL G. COIT

Cancer of the Small Intestine

HISTORY

The first small bowel tumor, a perforated duodenal carcinoma, was described by Hamberger in 1746.[1] The first small bowel leiomyoma was described by Foerster in 1858,[2] and the first small bowel leiomyosarcoma was described by Wesener in 1883.[3] An early review of malignant small bowel tumors was published by Leichtenstern in 1876,[4] and Heurtaux published a review of benign small bowel tumors in 1899.[5] Many of the earlier reviews were weighted heavily by the autopsy incidence of tumors. Most of the current information we have about the presentation, diagnosis, management, and outcome of bowel tumors is derived either from small single-center series or larger collective reviews.

INCIDENCE

Small bowel tumors, both benign and malignant, are exceedingly unusual. It has been estimated that small bowel tumors constitute fewer than 10% of all gastrointestinal tumors,[6] although the incidence varies significantly depending on whether autopsy data are included. Approximately 64% of all small bowel tumors are malignant. These account for 0.1% to 0.3% of all malignancies.[7–9] Some 2100 to 2400 new cases of small bowel malignancies occur each year in the United States,[10,11] approximately 0.4 to 1 case per 100,000 population,[12–14] with a slight male predominance.[15–20] Fewer than 1000 deaths are due to primary malignant small bowel tumors annually in the United States, which is approximately 0.5 deaths per 100,000 population.[21] By contrast, approximately 36% of small bowel tumors are benign, with roughly equal gender incidence.

In a review of the Surveillance, Epidemiology, and End Results program registries from 1973 to 1982, Weiss and Yang[14] showed the incidence of malignant small bowel tumors to be low in patients younger than 30 years of age, with a steady increase in incidence with age for adenocarcinoma, carcinoid, and lymphoma. The incidence of sarcoma levels off after the seventh decade.[14]

ETIOLOGY

CHARACTERISTICS OF THE SMALL BOWEL

The small bowel constitutes approximately 75% of the length of the gastrointestinal tract and provides 90% of the absorptive surface. Despite this predominance in length and surface area, however, it appears to be resistant to the development of malignancy. Small bowel malignancies account for only 1% to 3% of all gastrointestinal malignancies,[7,10–13,22,23] and they are estimated at 36 to 60 times less frequent than malignancies of the colon.[9,15,24–26] A number of hypotheses have been formulated to explain this finding. Transit through the small bowel is relatively rapid compared with the colon, resulting in less contact of the mucosa with potential carcinogens. Any potential carcinogens would be diluted by the large volume of secretions, which create liquid small bowel contents. This liquid in turn may be less mechanically irritating to the small bowel mucosa than solid stool would be to the colonic mucosa. The small bowel contains a small, metabolically inactive bacterial population, one that may not be capable of transforming potential procarcinogens to their active component.[9] The contribution of the alkaline pH to the resistance of small bowel neoplasms is unknown. The proximal small bowel contains a number of microsomal enzyme systems known to detoxify carcinogens, particularly benzopyrene hydroxylase.[27,28] Finally, high numbers of lymphocytes and B cells secrete immunoglobulin A in the distal ileum, which may contribute to a local immunosurveillance system that prevents the development of malignancies. Evidence in support of this supposition is derived from immunocompromised patients, either those with acquired immunodeficiency syndrome or those on chronic immunosuppression, who seem more prone to the development of malignancies, both lymphoma and Kaposi's sarcoma, in the distal small bowel.

The small intestine does appear to be susceptible to carcinogens. It is of interest that, as is shown later, adenocarcinomas in the small intestine occur proximally, in much the same distribution as azoxymethane-induced adenocarcinoma in rats.[29,30] This distribution of small bowel adenocarcinomas also correlates with the length of contact of the small bowel mucosa with pancreaticobiliary secretions, implicating bile as a possible carcinogen.[31] Diversion of the bile in animals has been shown to decrease the incidence of experimentally induced small bowel malignancy.[32]

Chow and colleagues[33] looked at risk factors in 430 patients with small bowel cancer, who they compared with 921 case-control patients dying of other causes. They found that weekly or more frequent consumption of red meat and monthly or more frequent consumption of salt-cured smoked foods was associated with a two- to threefold increase in risk. Tobacco use and alcohol consumption were not associated with increased risk of small bowel cancer in the study.[33] Lowenfels and Sonni[34] showed an excellent correlation between dietary fat intake and the incidence of small bowel carcinoma in various countries around the world. Pollard[34a] showed that the incidence of methylazoxymethanol acetate–induced intestinal carcinoma in rats could be markedly reduced by dietary restriction, further implicating oral intake as a possible promoter of intestinal malignancy.

Other factors that predispose patients to development of large bowel adenocarcinoma may also play a role in the development of small bowel adenocarcinoma. Neugut and Santos[16] looked at the incidence of second cancers among 2581 cases of small bowel malignancy from a Surveillance, Epidemiology, and End Results program cohort collected from 1973 to 1988. They found an increased probability of subsequent colorectal carcinoma after small bowel carcinoma (relative risk, 3.6 to 5.0) and an increased risk of small bowel carcinoma after colorectal carcinoma (relative risk, 7.1 to 9.0).

PREMALIGNANT LESIONS

A number of small bowel lesions are thought to predispose patients to the development of small bowel malignancy. The adenoma-carcinoma sequence has been well described.[29,35]

Perzin and Bridge[36] observed that 25% of primary small bowel carcinomas demonstrated adenomatous epithelium in the same lesion. This finding has particular significance in patients with familial adenomatous polyps, in whom polyps of the upper gastrointestinal tract are being recognized with increasing frequency.[37–42]

Patients with chronic Crohn's disease are at increased risk for the development of small bowel carcinoma.[43–46] These patients usually exhibit malignancy by the appearance of dysplasia.[47,48] However, distinguishing clinically between distal small bowel malignancy and Crohn's disease without histologic confirmation can be exceedingly difficult.[49–53]

Patients with adult celiac disease (nontropical sprue), particularly those who are unresponsive to dietary gluten withdrawal, are also at significantly increased risk for development of small bowel malignancy, particularly lymphoma, although adenocarcinomas also have been reported.[54–57]

Patients with Peutz-Jeghers syndrome have been reported to develop primary carcinoma of the gastrointestinal tract.[58–61] The primary polyp of Peutz-Jeghers is a hamartoma, and the *in situ* transformation of a hamartomatous polyp to adenocarcinoma has not been clearly demonstrated. Because these patients often have an adenomatous component in their primarily hyperplastic and hamartomatous polyps, the development of malignancy more likely represents malignant evolution of that adenomatous component rather than transformation of the other hamartomatous elements.[60,61]

Patients with von Recklinghausen's neurofibromatosis also have been reported to have gastrointestinal involvement, both benign and malignant.[62–65] Although most of these small bowel tumors are benign neurofibromas and leiomyomas, malignant tumors of nerve tissue origin have been reported.[66] Case reports of a proximal small bowel adenocarcinoma and carcinoid tumor occurring in association with neurofibromatosis have also appeared.[67,68]

ANATOMY

Grossly, the small bowel extends from the pylorus to the iliosacral valve. It is estimated to measure 625 cm in length but may vary from 300 to 850 cm.[69] The duodenum, measuring approximately 25 cm, forms a C loop; the first portion extends 5 cm horizontally from the pylorus before turning inferiorly into the second portion. The second, or descending, portion of the duodenum is approximately 10 cm long, just anterior to the hilus of the right kidney. Typically, the ampulla of Vater, through which pancreaticobiliary secretions pass into the small bowel, is found midway down the descending second portion of the duodenum medially. The third portion of the duodenum travels transversely in close relationship to the uncinate process of the pancreas, anterior to the ureter, inferior vena cava, vertebral column, and aorta. This leads to the fourth portion of the duodenum, which measures approximately 2.5 cm in diameter, ascends to join with the proximal jejunum, and is suspended on the right cross of the diaphragm by the ligament of Treitz at the level of the second lumbar vertebra.

The jejunum, comprising the proximal 250 cm of the small bowel distal to the duodenum, and the ileum, the remaining 350 cm of small bowel, are supported on a fan-shaped mesentery that measures approximately 15 cm in length. More distally, this mesentery becomes progressively longer, with arterial blood supply, venous and lymphatic drainage, and small bowel innervation traversing between its two leaves. Grossly, the duodenum tends to be the largest in diameter and the ileum the smallest.

The arterial blood supply for the duodenum is derived from the gastroduodenal branch of the hepatic artery as well as the inferior pancreaticoduodenal branch of the superior mesenteric artery. The blood supply for the remaining small bowel is derived from intestinal branches of this superior mesenteric artery. Venous return from the entire small intestine is into the portal vein. Lymphatic drainage of the duodenum is to peripancreatic nodes. The remainder of the small bowel drains into the abundant lymph nodes through channels that parallel the course of the mesenteric blood vessels. Autonomic innervation of the small bowel is by means of the celiac and superior mesenteric plexus. Sensory fibers are responsive to distention but not to other painful stimuli.

Microscopically, the intestine is a hollow muscular tube composed of four layers: serosa, muscularis, submucosa, and mucosa. The muscular layer consists of an outer longitudinal layer and an inner circular layer. Immediately beneath the mucosa is the lamina propria. The absorptive surface of the intestine is increased manifold by the presence of dense glandular villi covered by an epithelium of mucus-secreting goblet cells and absorptive cells, secretory Paneth's cells, and rare argentaffin cells. Mucus-secreting Brunner's glands are found in the duodenum but not in the distal small bowel. The myenteric plexus of Auerbach is located between the two muscular layers of the intestine; Meissner's plexus is located in the small bowel submucosa. Lymphatic tissue is found in the lamina propria of the submucosa; this tissue increases as one progresses distally, becoming quite abundant in the distal ileum, where it is seen as Peyer's patches.

PATHOLOGY

More than 35 histologic variants of small bowel neoplasms have been described. For practical purposes, they can be subdivided as benign and malignant and further classified according to their cell of origin (Table 33.6-1). Thirty-six percent of all small bowel tumors are benign.

A number of authors have commented on the inordinately high incidence of second primary malignant tumors in patients with primary small bowel malignancy.[16,18] The reason for this high incidence is not clear, although many have linked it to a defect in the individual patient's immune surveillance system. The clinical implications of these observations are clear. Any patient who has had a primary small bowel malignancy should be watched closely for the development of a second malignant tumor.

PRESENTATION

Although no specific symptom complex is diagnostic of small bowel tumors, either benign or malignant, a few generalizations can be made. Presentation depends on the location of the tumor and its growth pattern. Malignant lesions are more often symptomatic than are benign lesions, and for a shorter duration.[15,70–76] Furthermore, in large part because of the nonspecific nature of the symptoms, the delay between the onset of symptoms and the

TABLE 33.6-1. Pathology of Primary Small Bowel Tumors by Cell of Origin

Cell of Origin	*Benign*	*Malignant*
Epithelium	Adenoma	Adenocarcinoma
Connective tissue	Fibroma	Fibrosarcoma
Smooth muscle	Leiomyoma	Leiomyosarcoma
Fat	Lipoma	Liposarcoma
Vascular endothelium	Hemangioma	Angiosarcoma
Lymphatics	Lymphangioma	Lymphangiosarcoma
Lymphoid tissue	Pseudolymphoma	Lymphoma
Nerve	Neurofibroma	Neurofibrosarcoma
	Ganglioneuroma	GAN tumor
Argentaffin cell	—	Carcinoid
Mixed	Hamartoma	—

GAN, giant axonal neuropathy.
(Modified from Sindelar WF. Cancer of the small intestine. In: DeVita VT Jr, Hellman S, Rosenberg SA, eds. *Cancer: principles and practice of oncology*, 3rd ed. Philadelphia: JB Lippincott, 1989:878, with permission.)

final diagnosis is often significant, averaging 6 to 8 months.[71,77–80] The average age at presentation of patients with small bowel tumors is the seventh decade and is slightly younger for patients with malignant tumors than for patients with benign tumors.[15]

Although fewer than 50% of patients with benign small bowel tumors develop symptoms,[15] more than 90% of patients with malignant tumors of the small bowel have symptoms before diagnosis.[11,24,81,82] These symptoms can be subdivided into four general categories: mass, obstruction, bleeding, and perforation.

In patients with benign tumors, pain from obstruction is the most common symptom, occurring in 42% to 70% of cases. Bleeding, usually chronic, is seen in 20% to 53% of patients.[15,79,83] The most common cause of adult intussusception is a benign small bowel tumor. A palpable mass or perforation is rare.

In patients with malignant tumors, the most common symptoms are pain (not always associated with obstruction) in 32% to 86% and weight loss in 32% to 67% of cases.[15,70,79,83] Bleeding occurs somewhat less frequently than in patients with benign small bowel tumors.[25] Perforation, usually localized, is seen in roughly 10% of patients, usually those with lymphomas or sarcomas. A mass that may represent dilated bowel proximal to an obstructing tumor is palpable in fewer than 25% of patients with malignant small bowel tumors.

DIAGNOSIS

The diagnosis of small bowel tumors is rarely made preoperatively. In fact, the diagnosis of small bowel malignancy is frequently delayed, not necessarily because of delay in presentation to the physician. Maglinte and colleagues,[80] in a review of 77 patients with small bowel malignancy, reported the average delay between onset of symptoms and presentation to the physician as 1 month, whereas the average interval from seeing the physician to final diagnosis was 7.8 months.

With the exception of an elevated 5-hydroxyindole acetic acid level in the presence of carcinoid syndrome, all the presenting signs and symptoms of small bowel tumors are nonspecific. Laboratory examination may reveal a mild anemia in the presence of chronic blood loss. Hyperbilirubinemia may be seen in the presence of periampullary duodenal tumors. Mild to moderate elevations of liver function tests may be seen in the presence of hepatic metastases, occasionally associated with an elevation in carcinoembryonic antigen.

Radiologic studies may be more suggestive of the diagnosis. Plain abdominal films that reveal signs of partial or complete bowel obstruction in the absence of prior laparotomy are suggestive of primary small bowel neoplasm, although nonspecific as to the diagnosis. Upper gastrointestinal series with small bowel follow-through is abnormal in 53% to 83% of patients and delineates small bowel tumor in 30% to 44% of patients.[84,85] A number of investigators have suggested that this diagnostic accuracy can be improved to in excess of 90% using enteroclysis, with particular attention to the distensibility of the small bowel.[85–87] Barium enema can be useful in the diagnosis of small bowel disease, particularly lymphoma, in which thickening of the distal ileum can be seen on refluxing contrast material into the distal small bowel. This finding, however, is nonspecific and can be identical to the appearance of regional ileitis. Hyams and associates[49] suggested that a rectal biopsy revealing granulomatous disease can reliably distinguish between inflammatory and neoplastic changes in the terminal ileum.

Computed tomography (CT) is thought to be somewhat more accurate in detecting small bowel tumors.[88–93] In a review of 35 patients with small bowel tumors, Laurent and colleagues[89] found the CT scan to be abnormal in 97%, predicting tumor in 80%. CT was predictive of the tumor histology 69% of the time and of the tumor stage in 61% of patients. Of 18 malignant tumors, the CT predicted extramural invasion and liver metastases correctly 75% of the time; CT was accurate in predicting regional lymph node status only 25% of the time. Laurent and colleagues described characteristic CT findings for the following[89]:

- Adenocarcinoma: partially obstructing concentric narrowing in the proximal small bowel, best detected with tumors more than 3 cm in diameter
- Lymphoma: thickened distal small bowel, best seen with tumors larger than 2 cm
- Leiomyosarcoma: eccentric tumor of the mid- or distal small bowel, with malignancy suggested by the presence of necrosis, ulceration, and size greater than 5 cm
- Carcinoid: homogeneous mesenteric mass, often associated with stranding of the mesentery
- Lipoma: small homogeneous fat density; small bowel or mesenteric nodule

Dudiak and coworkers,[91] in a review of 63 patients with small bowel tumors, found that CT was able to detect a tumor in 73% of patients and to correctly predict the diagnosis in 43%. Radiologic criteria similar to those of Laurent and associates were described.[91]

Other investigators have focused on small bowel thickness as measured by CT scanning to predict enteric disease.[88,93] However, although small bowel wall thickness is predictive of disease, it is not predictive of malignancy.

Angiography is rarely helpful in the diagnosis of small bowel tumors. Angiograms may be distinctly abnormal in vascular smooth muscle tumors of the small bowel[84] and may help to define the source of occult but active upper gastrointestinal bleeding in patients with a small bowel hemangioma. Alfidi and colleagues[94] reported angiography as being helpful in patients with small bowel arteriovenous malformations, identifying lesions in nine patients after negative laparotomy. In addition, angiography may on occasion demonstrate occlusion of the peripheral branches of the mesenteric circulation that is responsible for a syndrome of mesenteric ischemia seen occasionally in the carcinoid syndrome.

Nuclear medicine scans using technetium-labeled red blood cells may be helpful, again to delineate an occult source of chronic gastrointestinal blood loss in the presence of a normal colonic and upper gastrointestinal endoscopy. It can be difficult to localize the site of bleeding with this test, however, and Oliver and coworkers[95] suggested that if technetium-labeled red blood cell scanning is used, the sensitivity of the examination improves if more frequent images are obtained.

With more sophisticated instrumentation, endoscopy is being more frequently used in the investigation of small bowel disease. Clearly, upper gastrointestinal endoscopy with total duodenoscopy is the mainstay for detection, diagnosis and, occasionally, treatment of more proximal neoplasms. Interest has been renewed in perioral enteroscopy.[96] With new instrumentation, and some experience, total small bowel enteroscopy can be achieved. Enteroscopy can be helpful in diagnosing both focal lesions[97] and more diffuse lesions, such as Mediterranean lymphoma.[98] It may be most useful in localizing the source of occult nongastric, noncolonic gastrointestinal bleeding.[99] Lida and associates[100] described the use of intraoperative enteroscopy to increase the detection of polyps in familial adenomatous polyposis syndrome. In addition, intraoperative enteroscopy with trans–illumination of the bowel wall has been useful in patients with identified arteriovenous malformations that cannot be otherwise localized at the time of operation.[96,101]

Colonoscopy with retrograde ileoscopy has been described as useful in the diagnosis of primary lymphoma of the ileum.[102] In experienced hands, the small bowel can be visualized by retrograde ileoscopy in up to 30% of patients.[83]

MANAGEMENT

BENIGN TUMORS OF THE SMALL BOWEL

The distribution of benign small bowel tumors by diagnosis and anatomic location is shown in Table 33.6-2. Most common are leiomyomas, followed by adenomas, lipomas, vascular lesions, and fibrous lesions.

Leiomyomas

Leiomyomas of the small bowel account for 20% to 40% of all benign small bowel tumors and are the most common small bowel tumor according to a review by Wilson and associates.[103] These tumors may grow within or outside the bowel lumen, and the growth pattern determines the presenting symptoms. Perforation is unusual. It can be difficult to distinguish benign from malignant smooth muscle tumors of the gastrointestinal tract intraoperatively, even with histologic evaluation by frozen section. According to the comprehensive review by Skandalakis and Gray,[104] malignancy in lesions less than 4 cm in diameter is distinctly unusual. Histologic criteria of malignancy include necrosis, nuclear pleomorphism, and frequent mitotic activity. Surgical management of small bowel leiomyomas includes adequate segmental resection with grossly negative serosal margins. Because lymph node metastases are unusual, even for malignant leiomyosarcomas of the small bowel, extensive mesenteric lymphadenectomy is not required.

Small bowel polyps can be divided into three broad categories based on principles of management: villous adenomas of the duodenum, adenomas of the distal small bowel, and Peutz-Jeghers hamartomas.

VILLOUS ADENOMAS OF THE DUODENUM. Although villous adenomas of the duodenum are unusual, the duodenum is the most common small bowel location for these lesions. Their most common presenting sign is obstructive jaundice, and diagnosis is straightforward with upper gastrointestinal endoscopy. Most lesions are located in the second portion of the duodenum, usually on the medial wall, surrounding the ampulla of Vater. They are being increasingly recognized as a component of the familial adenomatous polyposis syndrome.[37–42] A number of reports of villous tumors of the duodenum have appeared since the late 1980s. These tumors have a high propensity for malignant degeneration, averaging 45%. Risk factors associated with malignancy include size greater than 5 cm,[105] age over 50 years,[106] and more distally situated polyps.[106] This propensity toward malignant degeneration, together with their location around the ampulla of Vater, combine to make management decisions difficult. Although a number of experts have advocated local excision for benign lesions,[107,108] one cannot always be certain of the benign nature of a tumor before complete histologic examination. Furthermore, local recurrence rates of 17% to 75% have been reported after local excision of these tumors,[109–113] occasionally with malignant degeneration. Certainly, close ongoing endoscopic surveillance is mandatory after local excision of these lesions. Lesions in the third and fourth portion of the duodenum should be managed with wedge or sleeve resection. Lesions in the first or second portion of the duodenum should be managed with pancreaticoduodenectomy, particularly if any question remains about the diagnosis.

TABLE 33.6-2. Distribution of Benign Tumors of the Small Bowel by Site in 13 Series

Tumor	*Duodenum*	*Jejunum*	*Ileum*	*Total*
Leiomyoma	24	64	47	135 (37%)
Polyp, adenoma	34	17	17	68 (19%)
Lipoma	11	13	30	54 (15%)
Hemangioma	1	10	26	37 (10%)
Fibroma	4	7	12	23 (6%)
Other	27	8	13	48 (13%)
Total	101 (27%)	119 (33%)	145 (40%)	365 (100%)

TABLE 33.6-3. Distribution of Malignant Tumors of the Small Bowel by Site in 27 Series

Tumor	*Duodenum*	*Jejunum*	*Ileum*	*Total*
Adenocarcinoma	634	454	301	1389 (44%)
Carcinoid	60	92	781	933 (29%)
Lymphoma	34	183	276	493 (15%)
Sarcoma	61	159	148	368 (12%)
Total	789 (25%)	888 (28%)	1506 (47%)	3183 (100%)

Survival after complete excision is excellent in patients with both benign villous adenomas and carcinoma *in situ*. Patients with invasive carcinoma fare comparably to those with periampullary adenocarcinoma.

SMALL BOWEL ADENOMAS. Adenomas in the remainder of the small intestine are distinctly unusual. These tend to be distributed more proximally, and case reports of malignant degeneration have appeared.[114] These tumors should be managed with segmental resection.

PEUTZ-JEGHERS HAMARTOMAS. Peutz-Jeghers hamartomas are always multifocal and occur primarily in the small intestine.[115,116] Symptoms of low-grade obstruction with chronic recurrent intussusception usually become apparent in the second decade of life and frequently warrant repeated surgical intervention.

Appropriate surgical management of these tumors includes enterotomy and polypectomy. If bowel resection is required, an absolute minimum length of bowel should be sacrificed, because this is a chronic problem, and frequent reoperation can be anticipated. It is important to verify the status of both the stomach and colon before laparotomy, because intraoperative palpation of these structures can be notoriously unreliable. Furthermore, gastrointestinal malignancy occurs in these patients with increased frequency, probably because of malignant generation of adenomatous polyps.

Other Benign Lesions

Angiomas of the small bowel are less common and may be multifocal. They are usually discrete and well circumscribed, presenting most often as occult gastrointestinal bleeding. Management consists of segmental resection of the small bowel.[103,117,118]

Lipomas of the small intestine are distinctly unusual. Patients usually present with symptoms of abdominal pain consistent with partial bowel obstruction.[119] The difficulty in managing these lesions is that they may involve the small bowel diffusely.[120] Surgical management involves resection of the symptomatic segment of bowel.

Brunner's gland hamartomas are extremely rare, with fewer than 100 reports in the world literature. Symptoms at presentation depend on the size of the tumor and range from a lack of symptoms to chronic upper gastrointestinal bleeding and duodenal or biliary obstruction. Because these are submucosal tumors, preoperative diagnosis is rarely possible. Treatment involves either endoscopic removal of pedunculated lesions or surgical resection of larger lesions.[121–123]

Upper digestive tract involvement has been estimated to occur in 2% to 25% of patients with systemic neurofibromatosis (von Recklinghausen's disease).[63] This range may well represent an underestimate, because much of the involvement is asymptomatic and detected only on postmortem examination. Typically, the involvement is characterized by submucosal neurofibromas, originating in the submucosal nerve plexus. Duodenal paragangliomas have been reported to occur in association with von Recklinghausen's disease.[64,65] Although these lesions are generally considered benign, Inai and colleagues[66] reported a case of duodenal paraganglioma with regional lymph node metastases.

Inflammatory polyps may occur at any point within the small bowel, from the duodenum through the ileum, and occasionally are reported in association with preexisting Crohn's disease.[124–127] These are uniformly benign lesions arising from the submucosa, are usually solitary, and present with symptoms of obstruction. Management consists of polypectomy or segmental small bowel resection.

MALIGNANT TUMORS OF THE SMALL BOWEL

The distribution of malignant small bowel tumors by anatomic location and diagnosis is shown in Table 33.6-3.

Adenocarcinoma

Adenocarcinomas constitute 25% of all small bowel tumors and 39% of all malignant small bowel tumors. These tumors are distributed proximally in the small bowel, with nearly 80% located in the duodenum or jejunum. For purposes of analyzing mode of presentation, diagnosis, management, and outcome, these tumors can be separated into two categories: those of the duodenum and those of the jejunum and ileum.

DUODENUM. Approximately 45% of all adenocarcinomas of the small bowel arise within the duodenum. In general, approximately 15% of these are in the first portion of the duodenum, 40% are in the second portion of the duodenum, and 45% are in the distal duodenum,[128–133] a distribution pattern that parallels the relative lengths of each portion. The median age of these patients is 60 years. Symptoms relate primarily to the size and site of the tumor. The most common symptom is upper abdominal pain related to partial duodenal obstruction.[129,132] Series that include periampullary tumors also report an incidence of biliary obstruction.[130] Anemia with Hemoccult-positive stools is frequent, although frank upper gastrointestinal hemorrhage is unusual.[132]

Diagnosis is usually suspected from an upper gastrointestinal series. Hypotonic duodenography may improve the accuracy of this test.[134] Histologic confirmation can be obtained preoperatively in most patients by upper gastrointestinal endoscopy with total duodenoscopy.

TABLE 33.6-4. Duodenal Adenocarcinoma

Author	*Year*	*Tumors*	*Explored*	*Operative Mortality Rate*[a] *(%)*	*Resected*[b]	*5-Y Survival Rate (%)*
Awlmark et al.[133]	1980	66	49 (74%)	24	49 (100%)	33
Lillemoe and Imbembo[222]	1980	12	11 (92%)	36	6 (55%)	33
Joesting et al.[132]	1981	104	104 (100%)	18	53 (51%)	46
Cohen et al.[223]	1982	40	—	—	—	38
Herter et al.[224]	1982	38	—	—	—	27
Williamson et al.[30]	1983	26	26 (100%)	—	18 (69%)	17
Kellum et al.[225]	1983	3	—	0	—	33
Ouriel and Adams[128]	1984	34	32 (94%)	—	19 (54%)	25
Gaddy and Max[226]	1985	5	5 (100%)	0	2 (40%)	0
Jones et al.[227]	1985	12	12 (100%)	0	12 (100%)	18
Grace et al.[136]	1986	5	—	—	—	60
Tarazi et al.[228]	1986	17	—	—	—	28
Gonzalez and Evans[229]	1987	3	3 (100%)	0	2 (67%)	0
Sarma and Weilbaecher[230]	1987	3	2 (67%)	0	1 (50%)	33
Crist et al.[137]	1987	9	—	—	—	33
Lai et al.[129]	1988	24	24 (100%)	8	24 (100%)	8
Michelassi et al.[231]	1989	16	10 (63%)	10	10 (100%)	10
Brennan[135]	1990	32	29 (91%)	0	18 (62%)	60

[a]Mortality rate as a percentage of those explored.
[b]Resected rate as a percentage of those explored.

As can be seen from Table 33.6-4, most patients who present with duodenal carcinoma undergo exploration; in these patients, resectability rates tend to be high. In general, patients with tumors of the first and second portions of the duodenum require pancreaticoduodenectomy; patients with tumors of the third and fourth portions of the duodenum often can undergo complete resection with segmental duodenectomy and primary anastomosis. Because 22% to 71% of patients with duodenal adenocarcinoma have positive nodes at presentation[129–133,135] and a finite 5-year survival rate is seen in the presence of regional nodal involvement,[129,135] curative resection of duodenal carcinomas should always include a systemic regional lymphadenectomy regardless of the primary tumor location.

A number of authors have commented on the steady decrease in operative mortality after pancreaticoduodenectomy; this procedure can now be performed with an operative mortality rate of less than 5%.[132,135–137] Outcome in duodenal carcinoma patients is determined by resectability, lymph node involvement and, in some series, histologic grade.[129–133] No clear-cut evidence has established that pancreaticoduodenectomy results in superior survival to that with segmental resection when the latter is technically feasible.[136,138]

The role of postoperative adjuvant therapy has not been clearly defined in this group of patients. In patients with advanced unresectable disease, it may be that palliative radiation therapy can be of some benefit in controlling chronic blood loss. Because these tumors clinically appear to behave more like gastric cancer than pancreatic cancer,[135] participation in an investigational chemotherapy program with a 5-fluorouracil (5-FU)-based regimen may be warranted.

JEJUNUM AND ILEUM. Tumors of the jejunum and ileum account for the remaining 55% of small bowel adenocarcinoma. As can be seen in Table 33.6-5, much of the information about these tumors is derived from small series collected over a number of years. The report by Adler and associates[53] is a collected series based on several large tumor registries. In general, most reports are from institutions that see fewer than one patient with small bowel adenocarcinoma per year.

These patients present with signs or symptoms of obstruction in 50% to 74%, or occult gastrointestinal bleeding in 33%

TABLE 33.6-5. Survival of Patients with Adenocarcinoma of the Small Intestine

Author	*Year*	*Number of Patients*	*Period (y)*	*5-Y Survival Rate (%)*
Awrich et al.[81]	1980	26	25	26
Mittal and Bodzin[219]	1980	10	21	62
Norberg and Emas[72]	1981	11	34	0
Waterhouse et al.[74]	1981	24	28	18
Adler et al.[53]	1982	338	43	17
Lanzafame et al.[232]	1982	29	40	35
Barclay and Schapira[13]	1983	74	30	22
Williamson et al.[30]	1983	68	64	14
Ouriel and Adams[128]	1984	65	31	30
Cooper et al.[29]	1985	25	15	0
Johnson et al.[12]	1985	16	28	6
Zollinger et al.[79]	1986	18	20	17
Martin[23]	1986	87	38	21
Ciccarelli et al.[10]	1987	17	14	12
Brophy and Cahow[82]	1989	18	14	36
Lioe and Biggart[140]	1990	25	34	16
Desa et al.[76]	1991	7	15	20
Bauer et al.[233]	1994	38	21	23
DiSario et al.[17]	1994	80	25	25
Frost et al.[18]	1994	18	30	30
Garcia Marcilla et al.[19]	1994	26	15	34

to 64%.[30,53,139] Although adenocarcinoma of the small bowel may be suspected based on a small bowel follow-through series or CT scan, neither examination is specific, and the diagnosis is frequently not made until laparotomy.[30]

At the time of operation, 77% to 100% of distal small bowel adenocarcinomas are resectable,[30,128,139] although regional lymph node metastases are frequent.[128,140,141] The principles of surgical resection include attainment of negative surgical margins and wide resection of the corresponding mesentery of the involved segment of small bowel.

Survival in these patients is generally poor, with most series reporting only 20% to 30% of patients alive at 5 years (see Table 33.6-5). Prognostic factors in these patients include depth of tumor penetration and the presence of nodal or systemic metastases. Histologic grade of the tumor also has been shown to be predictive of outcome.[128] Survival rates of 45% to 70% have been reported in patients with negative nodes after curative resection; these rates fall to 12% to 14% in patients with positive nodes.[53,128] Radiation therapy is difficult in these patients given the mobile nature of the small bowel mesentery and the inability to localize the target field. Because these tumors are rare, any meaningful comment on the impact of chemotherapy in their management is difficult. Jigyasu and associates[142] reported one partial response in 14 patients treated with 5-FU–based combination chemotherapy accrued over 30 years.

Carcinoid Tumors

Carcinoid tumors represent 29% of all small bowel malignancies and 19% of all small bowel tumors; they are second only to adenocarcinoma in frequency. The small bowel is the second most common site of carcinoid tumors after the appendix. Ninety percent of all small bowel carcinoids arise in the ileum. These tumors are often silent, with many series including otherwise asymptomatic tumors discovered incidentally, either at laparotomy or autopsy. When present, the most common presenting symptom is vague, nonspecific abdominal pain.[143–145] This pain may be due to a number of causes. Frequently, an intense desmoplastic fibrous reaction occurs around the primary tumor, with shortening of the small bowel mesentery, which is thought to be induced in some way by the biochemical products of the tumor. This reaction induces foreshortening of the mesentery with kinking of the bowel and either ileus or partial bowel obstruction. Partial bowel obstruction may also occur from the tumor itself, although this appears less often. In addition, a syndrome of chronic mesenteric ischemia has been described in these patients, associated with a mesenteric angiopathy described as *elastic vascular sclerosis.*[146] On angiography, this condition is manifest by occlusion of the peripheral small vessels of the mesenteric arcade.

Although only 10% to 17% of patients with small bowel carcinoid present with carcinoid syndrome,[147,148] up to 67% develop features of the syndrome at some point during the course of the disease.[149] Symptoms include flushing of the head, neck, and upper chest in 84% to 94% of patients and a watery secretory diarrhea in 70% to 86% of patients; both symptoms are present in 58% of patients. Right-sided valvular heart disease is present in 37% to 50% of patients, and bronchial asthma is manifest in 17% to 23% of patients.[147,149–151] These symptoms are often prompted by emotion, alcohol intake, or the ingestion of tyramine-containing foods, such as blue cheese or chocolate.[150] Virtually all patients with evidence of carcinoid syndrome have bulky liver metastases and elevated urinary 5-hydroxyindole acetic acid levels.

In the absence of the classic carcinoid syndrome, preoperative diagnosis of these tumors is unusual. Radiologic findings, even with small bowel follow-through studies, are inconclusive, revealing only an ileus-like or partial obstruction picture. CT scanning may reveal a mass infiltrating the mesentery with or without liver metastases, but this finding is nonspecific.[152] Mesenteric angiography may reveal occlusion of the peripheral mesenteric vessels, but this finding is unusual.

At laparotomy, carcinoid tumors appear as firm, tan, submucosal nodules, usually in the distal small bowel. Invariably, symptomatic tumors are larger than those found incidentally or at autopsy.[144] The frequency of metastatic disease to regional lymph nodes and liver is directly related to the size of the tumor. Nodal metastases are unusual with tumors less than 1 cm in diameter but are present in 33% to 67% of tumors 1 to 3 cm in size and in 75% to 90% of tumors larger than 3 cm.[143,147,150,153–155] The majority of patients presenting with symptomatic carcinoids of the small intestine have metastatic disease at the time of operation.

Approximately 30% of small bowel carcinoids are multiple,[143–145,148,151,153] mandating a careful search of the remainder of the small bowel for other primary lesions before definitive surgical management.

Surgical management of the primary tumor includes wide resection of all visible disease, together with complete resection of the supporting mesentery. Although the likelihood of regional lymph node metastases is known to increase with tumor size, metastases have been reported in carcinoids smaller than 1 cm.[147,156]

Management of carcinoid tumors metastatic to liver is aimed primarily at controlling the symptoms of the carcinoid syndrome. Prolonged remission of symptoms has been observed with resection of bulk liver metastases, even if incomplete.[147,154,157,158] For unresectable disease, short-term remission of symptoms has been observed with hepatic dearterialization.[147,158] Hepatic arterial infusion chemotherapy has been attempted without convincing reports of success.[149,154]

Medical management of the symptoms of carcinoid syndrome has included a long list of drugs, all with limited success. The most effective drug in controlling these symptoms is the long-acting somatostatin analogue SMS-201. Given as a subcutaneous injection, this drug controls symptoms in nearly all patients.[150]

Systemic chemotherapy has been disappointing in carcinoid syndrome. Active agents include 5-FU, streptozotocin, mitomycin C, cyclophosphamide, methotrexate, interferon-α, and doxorubicin (Adriamycin). The most active single agents are 5-FU and doxorubicin, and the most effective combination regimens are methotrexate with cyclophosphamide, 5-FU with streptozotocin, and streptozotocin with doxorubicin.[147] Although response rates of 30% to 55% are reported, none of these drugs, either alone or in combination, has clearly demonstrated any impact on the generally indolent natural history of carcinoid tumors.

The prognosis in patients with carcinoid tumors of the small intestine is generally better than that for adenocarcinoma and depends on a number of factors, including tumor size, depth of invasion, presence of lymph node, and liver metastases.[143–145,147,159] Other factors identified as prognostically significant by univariate analysis are lack of symptoms, complete resectability,[143] and histologic growth pattern.[160] In advanced disease, two groups have looked at the association of DNA ploidy and prognosis, with both finding a trend toward better prognosis in patients with solely diploid tumors.[161,162] In general, however, this tumor can be characterized as one of indolent growth. In the absence of metastatic disease, complete resection of localized carcinoid tumors results in a 75% to 94% 5-year survival rate.[150,159] With regional lymph node involvement, 5-year survival rates of 45% to 90% have been reported.[145,147,149,154,159] Five-year survival rates of 19% to 54% have been reported in the presence of liver metastases.[145,147,149–151,159]

Lymphoma

Lymphoma may involve the gastrointestinal tract either primarily or as a manifestation of extensively disseminated systemic disease. Primary small bowel lymphoma constitutes 1% to 4% of all gastrointestinal malignancies and, in a review of series, 15% of all small bowel malignancies (see Table 33.6-3). The gastrointestinal tract is the most frequent site of extranodal lymphoma, the stomach being the most frequent site, followed by the small bowel and colon, respectively.[163] Within the small bowel, the incidence of lymphoma increases as one progresses distally, the most frequent site being the ileum. The incidence parallels the relative amount of lymphatic tissue in the wall of the small bowel at these locations.

The incidence of primary intestinal lymphoma in the United States nearly doubled in the period from 1985 to 1990.[164] Factors implicated in this increase include the increasing number of immunocompromised patients (acquired immunodeficiency syndrome patients, transplantation recipients) and the increasing number of immigrants from Third World countries.

For the diagnosis of primary small bowel lymphoma, one must satisfy the criteria specified by Dawson and coworkers[165]: (1) There must be no peripheral or mediastinal lymphadenopathy, (2) the peripheral blood smear must display a normal white blood cell count and differential, and (3) tumor involvement must be predominantly in the gastrointestinal tract.

Most authors think that there should be no evidence of liver or spleen involvement.[166,167] Antecedent conditions reported to be associated with the development of primary small bowel lymphoma include nontropical sprue and Crohn's disease.[56,138,166]

Patients with gastrointestinal lymphoma have been traditionally staged using a modification of the Ann Arbor staging system.[168] Because this was not a staging system originally designed for lymphomas of the gastrointestinal tract, Blackledge and colleagues[169] described a staging system to incorporate the prognostic significance of perforation (Table 33.6-6). Another clinically relevant modification of the Ann Arbor staging system, by Mussoff and Schmidt-Vollmer,[164] recognizes the prognostic significance of regional (stage II_1E), as opposed to extraregional (stage II_2E), lymph node involvement.

Five clinically distinct subtypes of primary small intestinal lymphoma have been described: the adult Western type; the pediatric type; the immunoproliferative small intestinal disease, or Mediterranean, type; enteropathy-associated T-cell lymphoma; and Hodgkin's lymphoma.[164]

The most common lymphoma of the small intestine, the Western type, occurs primarily in adults at a median age of 54 to 61 years and has a distinct male predominance.[170–172] These lesions are usually focal and are found in the distal small bowel. The most common presenting symptom is abdominal pain related to partial bowel obstruction. The most common physical finding is a mass. Anemia occurs in approximately 20% of these patients, and approximately 10% of patients present with perforation.[138,170,172–174]

TABLE 33.6-6. Staging Systems for Small Bowel Lymphoma

Stage	*Description*
ANN ARBOR STAGING SYSTEM	
I	Involvement of a single nodal group or single nodal site (IE)
II	Involvement of more than one nodal group on the same side of the diaphragm or involvement of a single extranodal site with one or more nodal groups on the same side of the diaphragm (IIE)
III	Involvement of nodes on both sides of the diaphragm, with or without involvement of extranodal sites (IIIE), spleen (IIIS), or both (IIIES)
IV	Diffuse involvement of viscera or bone marrow
BLACKLEDGE STAGING SYSTEM	
I	Tumor confined to the gastrointestinal tract
II	Tumor with local mesenteric nodal involvement
III	Tumor with perforation
IV	Tumor with distant (paraaortic and beyond) nodal involvement
V	Tumor with visceral or bone marrow involvement

The diagnosis of Western-type lymphoma is often made only at laparotomy. Radiologic findings suggestive of this diagnosis include a diffuse segment of thickened distal small bowel on follow-through examination. This finding can often be even better demonstrated by CT scan. However, radiologically, the diagnosis is easily confused with other segmental disease of the distal small intestine, such as Crohn's disease.[175]

Several systems have been described to classify the pathology of small bowel lymphomas. Using the Rappaport system, approximately 60% of non-Hodgkin's lymphomas are diffuse histiocytic (40% diffuse large cell and 20% immunoblastic), 25% are lymphocytic, and the remainder are of mixed type. The more recently described Kiel system uses both morphology and cell surface markers to classify lymphomas. Although histologic staging systems remain in evolution, the grade of the lymphoma remains most predictive of outcome. Most small bowel lymphomas are intermediate or high grade.[166,171,176,177]

Management of these patients usually entails surgical exploration with resection of the affected segment of small bowel together with its subjacent mesentery. Fifty percent to 78% of patients who present with this type of lymphoma undergo complete surgical resection.[30,138,170,171]

The role of adjuvant therapy in patients who undergo complete resection is debated. Most authors agree that any patient with evidence of incompletely resected disease or regional nodal metastases can benefit from systemic chemotherapy.[170] Some believe that adjuvant chemotherapy is warranted after complete resection of all high-grade lymphomas, even if they are stage IE.[178,179] Auger and Allan[171] reported on 16 patients undergoing complete surgical resection of intestinal lymphomas. The median survival in patients who underwent complete resection with chemotherapy was 34 months, compared with 14 months in patients who underwent complete surgical resection without adjuvant chemotherapy.[171] These 16 patients were not broken down by the presence or absence of nodal metastases, and as such, the issue of adjuvant chemotherapy remains unresolved in patients with lymphoma localized to the bowel.

Adjuvant radiation therapy had been advocated by some investigators,[138,170] although the permanent long-term side effects of abdominal radiation therapy, together with the efficacy of contemporary combination chemotherapy, make this option less attractive.[178]

Most of the larger more recent series report 5-year survival rates in excess of 50% with aggressive multimodality therapy. Prognostic factors include tumor grade, stage at presentation, complete response to therapy, complete resectability, histologic subtype, and the use of multimodality therapy.[163,166,170,171,175,177,178,180] Patients with B-cell lymphomas tend to have better median survival than those with T-cell lymphomas.[57,181] In contrast to the indolent course of patients with carcinoid tumors, most deaths in patients with small bowel lymphoma occur within 2 years of diagnosis.[173,182,183]

The second major type of lymphoma is childhood lymphoma. This disease typically occurs in patients younger than 15 years of age and presents with symptoms of pain and physical findings of a mass in the right lower quadrant, often with associated intussusception. Histologically, nearly one-half of these lymphomas resemble a Burkitt's-type lymphoma.[184] These patients often require resection before systemic therapy, because perforation while on treatment is not uncommon. The prognosis for these children is improving in the era of combined-modality therapy, with a survival rate of 76% reported by Fleming and colleagues[184]; all deaths in this series occurred within 10 months of diagnosis. Outcome depends on stage at presentation and resectability.[166,185,186]

A third clinically distinct type of intestinal lymphoma is immunoproliferative small intestinal disease, or Mediterranean lymphoma. This is the most common lymphoma encountered in Middle Eastern and African populations, occurring with equal gender predilection in young adults, with a median age of 30.[183,185,186] Typically, these patients present with the triad of pain, malabsorption (manifest by weight loss and diarrhea), and nail clubbing.[185] Approximately 50% of these patients present with a mass. Mediterranean lymphoma generally involves the entire small bowel and is manifested histologically by villous atrophy and an intense lymphoplasmacytoid infiltrate in the lamina propria of the small bowel. As such, diagnosis can often be made by peroral jejunal biopsy. Surgery is reserved for cases in which the diagnosis is unclear or for complications such as obstruction or perforation. Grossly, the bowel appears to be involved by a diffuse thickening with some nodularity. Lymph nodes are involved in 85% of patients. As a biologic curiosity, approximately 30% of patients with Mediterranean lymphoma have free α heavy-chain protein in their serum and jejunal fluid. This finding, however, is neither specific nor diagnostic in this disease.

Treatment of patients with Mediterranean lymphoma consists primarily of systemic chemotherapy, although reports of whole abdominal radiation therapy have appeared.[178] The use of tetracycline in the management of this lymphoma supports the role of an infectious etiology.[187,188] Prognosis is variable, with Al-Bahrani and associates[185] reporting a 23% 5-year survival rate; El Saghir and colleagues[187] reported an overall 5-year survival rate of 58% after aggressive therapy.

Enteropathy-associated T-cell lymphoma is an unusual variant of intestinal lymphoma, most often seen in the Middle East and often associated with an antecedent history of malabsorption or frank celiac disease. The malignancy is believed to arise from unrestricted proliferation of T-cell clones from the reactive T-cell population in the enteropathic bowel.[189] It is usually disseminated at presentation and is often associated with significant malnutrition. Prognosis is generally poor despite multiagent chemotherapy.[57]

Primary Hodgkin's lymphoma of the small bowel is extremely unusual, accounting for fewer than 3% of all small bowel lymphomas.[166,176] In many cases, this diagnosis may represent impingement of mesenteric lymphadenopathy on the small bowel rather than primary visceral involvement.[190] Management consists of diagnostic and palliative surgery followed by definitive systemic chemotherapy.

Sarcoma

Sarcomas of the small intestine are extremely unusual, constituting only approximately 9% of all small bowel tumors and 14% of all small bowel malignancies (see Table 33.6-2). Most are of smooth muscle origin (leiomyosarcomas and leiomyoblastomas), although case reports of other histologies have appeared. More recent reports have grouped these tumors under the category of gastrointestinal stromal tumors, from which another variant, gastrointestinal autonomic nerve tumors, can be distinguished based on immunohistochemistry and electron microscopy.[191,192] From a clinical and prognostic viewpoint, however, these tumors can be discussed together.

Sarcomas of the small intestine can present with a number of symptoms, depending on their growth pattern. Endoenteric lesions can present as either bleeding or obstruction. Exoenteric lesions can present as an abdominal mass or perforation before any sense of obstruction is evident. Although the diagnosis may be suggested by upper gastrointestinal series with small bowel follow-through or enteroclysis, with or without abdominal CT scan, it is rarely made with certainty preoperatively. These tumors also tend to be highly vascular, with a plethora of tumor vessels seen with arteriography. Intraoperatively, these tumors have a variety of appearances, but they are usually appreciated as firm, encapsulated masses that arise in relation to the bowel. It is difficult both clinically and by frozen-section examination to distinguish a small leiomyosarcoma from its benign counterpart, the leiomyoma.

The principles of surgical management include wide resection of the primary tumor, including any adjacent structures that may be invaded. Duodenal tumors often require pancreaticoduodenectomy if the medial wall of the second portion of the duodenum is involved. Smaller leiomyosarcomas of the duodenum may be treated with wedge or sleeve resection. For sarcomas of the jejunum and ileum, the involved segment of intestine is resected together with its supporting mesentery. Deliberate or extended lymphadenectomy is unnecessary, because these tumors involve regional lymph nodes in fewer than 15% of cases.[104]

The overall 5-year survival rate for patients with small bowel sarcoma is approximately 20% and depends on tumor size, histologic grade, local invasiveness, and resectability.[193–200] In a review of patients at Memorial Sloan-Kettering Cancer Center, all of nine patients with high-grade sarcomas of the small bowel had experienced recurrences, whereas none of four patients with low-grade sarcomas had recurrences.[201]

Peritoneal and liver metastases are the most common causes of treatment failure. No evidence suggests that adjuvant chemotherapy or radiation therapy after complete resection diminishes the risk of subsequent recurrence.

Standard treatment of symptomatic metastatic disease usually involves doxorubicin-based combination chemotherapy, with or without high-dose ifosfamide. Although response rates of up to 40% have been reported with these regimens, no convincing impact on the survival of patients with advanced metastatic gastrointestinal sarcoma has been demonstrated.

Metastatic Disease

The small bowel is not infrequently involved by metastatic disease. The most common tumor metastasizing to the gastrointestinal tract is melanoma, with 60% of patients who die of melanoma having autopsy evidence of metastatic disease involving the gastrointestinal tract.[202] Other extraabdominal tumors known to metastasize to the small intestine include those of the lung,[203,204] breast,[205,206] cervix,[207,208] and kidney.[209,210] Case reports of small bowel metastases from other tumors, including tumors of the thyroid,[211] Merkel cell carcinoma,[212] and hepatoma,[213] have appeared. Intraabdominal tumors that may involve the small bowel by transperitoneal spread include colorectal carcinoma, ovarian carcinoma, gastric carcinoma, pancreatic carcinoma, and transitional cell carcinoma of the genitourinary system. The small bowel may also be involved by direct extension from any intraabdominal malignancy.

Symptoms of small bowel metastases most commonly include bleeding and obstruction; rarely, perforation is seen. Although surgical treatment of patients with local small bowel invasion can often be performed with curative intent, it is almost always palliative in patients with hematogenous or peritoneal metastases. Identification of an obstructing metastatic lesion is usually possible, although these lesions are rarely solitary. Identification of a bleeding metastasis among multiple small bowel lesions can be difficult.

The outcome in patients undergoing small bowel resection for metastatic melanoma has been summarized by a number of authors. Median survival rates of 4.5 to 8.5 months have been reported, with few, if any, long-term survivors.[202,214–217] Caputy and colleagues[215] were able to identify small bowel involvement as an independent adverse prognostic indicator in patients with melanoma metastatic to the gastrointestinal tract. Branum and Seigler[216] found a mean survival of 31 months in patients who underwent complete resection, compared with 10 months in patients who underwent noncurative procedures, which is more likely a reflection of the extent of tumor rather than the impact of therapy. Ricaniadis and colleagues[218] reported a 28% 5-year survival rate in 12 patients with no other site of metastatic melanoma who underwent complete surgical resection; these patients were selected from a group of 68 patients with involvement of the gastrointestinal tract by recurrent melanoma.

REFERENCES

1. Hamberger GE. *Proempticum auspicale quo dissertantionem solemnen: indicit et de ruptura intestini duodeni disserit.* Jena: Litteris Ritterianis, 1746:1.
2. Foerster G. Fibroid der muscularis des ileum. *Virchows Arch Pathol Anat* 1858;13:270.
3. Wesener F. Geirtrage zur casuistil der geschwulste i uebe Telangiectatisches myom des Duodenum von Ungewohnlichen. *Virchows Arch Pathol Anat* 1833;93:377.
4. Leichtenstern O. Handbuch des speciellen Pathologie und Therapie. In: Vogel FCW, ed. *Handbuch des speciellen Pathologie und Therapie.* Leipzig: Vogel FCW, 1876:523.
5. Heurtaux A. Note sur les tumeurs benignes de l'intestin. *Arch Prov Chir* 1899;8:701.
6. Ellis H. Tumours of the small intestine. *Semin Surg Oncol* 1987;3:12.
7. Sager GF. Primary malignant tumors of the small intestine. *Am J Surg* 1978;135:601.
8. Coutsoftides T, Shibata HR. Primary malignant tumors of the small intestine. *Dis Colon Rectum* 1979;22:24.
9. Lowenfels AB. Why are small-bowel tumours so rare? *Lancet* 1973;1:24.
10. Ciccarelli O, Welch JP, Kent G. Primary malignant tumors of the small bowel: the Hartford Hospital experience 1969–1983. *Am J Surg* 1987;153:350.
11. Collin CF, Amerson JR, Fulenwider JT, et al. Primary malignant small bowel tumors: clinical imitators of benign disease. *Surg Gastroenterol* 1982;1:203.
12. Johnson AM, Harman PK, Hanks JB. Primary small bowel malignancies. *Am Surg* 1985;51:31.
13. Barclay THC, Schapira DV. Malignant tumors of the small intestine. *Cancer* 1983;51:878.
14. Weiss NS, Yang C. Incidence of histologic types of cancer of the small intestine. *J Natl Cancer Inst* 1987;78:653.
15. Herbsman H, Western L, Rosen Y, et al. Tumors of the small intestine. *Curr Probl Surg* 1980;17:123.
16. Neugut AI, Santos J. The association between cancers of the small and large bowel. *Cancer Epidemiol Biol Prev* 1993;2:551.
17. DiSario JA, Vargas H, McWhorter WP. Small bowel cancer: epidemiological and clinical characteristics from a population based registry. *Am J Gastroenterol* 1994;89:699.
18. Frost DB, Mercado PD, Tyrell JS. Small bowel cancer: a 30 year review. *Ann Surg Oncol* 1994;1:290.
19. Garcia Marcilla JA, Sanchez Bueno F, Aguilar J, et al. Primary small bowel malignant tumors. *Eur J Surg Oncol* 1994;20:630.
20. Baillie CT, Williams A. Small bowel tumors: a diagnostic challenge. *J R Coll Surg Edinb* 1994;39:8.
21. Laws H, Han SY, Aldrete J. Malignant tumors of the small bowel. *South Med J* 1984;77:1087.
22. Goel JP, Didolkar MS, Elias EG. Primary malignant tumors of the small intestine. *Surg Gynecol Obstet* 1976;143:717.
23. Martin RG. Malignant tumors of the small intestine. *Surg Clin North Am* 1986;66:779.
24. Wilson JM, Melvin DB, Gray GF, Thorbjarnarson B. Primary malignancies of the small bowel: a report of 96 cases and review of the literature. *Ann Surg* 1974;180:175.
25. Miles RM, Crawford D, Duras S. The small bowel tumor problem. *Ann Surg* 1979;189:732.
26. Reyes EL, Talley RW. Primary malignant tumors of the small intestine. *Am J Gastroenterol* 1970;54:30.
27. Wattenberg LW. Carcinogen-detoxifying mechanisms in the gastrointestinal tract. *Gastroenterology* 1966;51:932.
28. Wattenberg LW. Studies of polycyclic hydrocarbon hydroxylases of the intestine possibly related to cancer effect of diet on benzpyrene hydroxylase activity. *Cancer* 1971;28:99.
29. Cooper MJ, Williamson RCN, Chir M. Enteric adenoma and adenocarcinoma. *World J Surg* 1985;9:914.
30. Williamson RC, Welch CE, Malt RA. Adenocarcinoma and lymphoma of the small intestine. *Ann Surg* 1983;197:171.
31. Ross RK, Hartnett NM, Bernstein L, Henderson BE. Epidemiology of adenocarcinomas of the small intestine: is bile a small bowel carcinogen? *Br J Cancer* 1991;63:143.
32. Scudamore CH, Freeman HJ. Effects of small bowel transection, resection, or bypass in 1,2-dimethylhydrazine-induced rat intestinal neoplasia. *Gastroenterology* 1983;84:725.
33. Chow WH, Linet MS, McLaughlin JK, et al. Risk factors for small intestine cancer. *Cancer Cause Control* 1993;4:163.
34. Lowenfels AB, Sonni A. Distribution of small bowel tumors. *Cancer Lett* 1977;3:83.

34a. Pollard M, Luckert PM. Tumorigenic effect of direct and indirect acting chemical carcinogens in rats on a restricted diet. *J Natl Cancer Inst* 1985;74:1347.

35. Sellner F. Investigations on the significance of the adenoma-carcinoma sequence in the small bowel. *Cancer* 1990;66:702.
36. Perzin KH, Bridge MF. Adenomas of the small intestine: a clinicopathologic review of 51 cases and a study of their relationship to carcinoma. *Cancer* 1981;48:799.
37. Gahtan V, Nochomovitz LE, Robinson AM, et al. Gastroduodenal polyps in familial polyposis coli. *Am Surg* 1989;55:278.
38. Bulow S, Lauritsen KB, Johannsen A, et al. Gastroduodenal polyps in familial polyposis coli. *Dis Colon Rectum* 1985;28:90.
39. Jarvinen HJ, Sipponen P. Gastroduodenal polyps in familial adenomatosis and juvenile polyposis. *Endoscopy* 1986;18:230.
40. Iida M, Yao T, Watanabe H, et al. Natural history of duodenal lesions in Japanese patients with familial adenomatosis coli (Gardner's syndrome). *Gastroenterology* 1989;96:1301.
41. Domizio P, Talbot IC, Spigelman AD, et al. Upper gastrointestinal pathology in familial adenomatous polyposis: results from a prospective trial of 102 patients. *J Clin Pathol* 1990;43:738.
42. Kurtz RC, Sternberg SS, Miller HH, Decosse JJ. Upper gastrointestinal neoplasia in familial polyposis. *Dig Dis Sci* 1987;32:459.
43. Hawker PC, Glyde SN, Thompson H, Allan RN. Adenocarcinoma of the small intestine complicating Crohn's disease. *Gut* 1982;23:188.
44. Frank JD, Shorey BA. Adenocarcinoma of the small bowel as a complication of Crohn's disease. *Gut* 1973;14:120.
45. Morowitz DA, Block GE, Kirsner JB. Adenocarcinoma of the ileum complicating chronic regional enteritis. *Gastroenterology* 1968;55:397.
46. Michelassi F, Testa G, Pomidor WJ, et al. Adenocarcinoma complicating Crohn's disease. *Dis Colon Rectum* 1993;36:654.
47. Petras RE, Mir-Madjlessi SH, Farmer RG. Crohn's disease and intestinal carcinoma: a report of 11 cases with emphasis on associated epithelial dysplasia. *Gastroenterology* 1987;93:1307.
48. Simpson S, Traube J, Riddell RH. The histologic appearance of dysplasia (precarcinomatous change) in Crohn's disease of the small and large intestine. *Gastroenterology* 1981;81:492.
49. Hyams JS, Goldman H, Katz AJ. Differentiating small bowel Crohn's disease from lymphoma: role of rectal biopsy. *Gastroenterology* 1980;79:340.

50. Ribeiro MB, Greenstein AJ, Heiman TM, et al. Adenocarcinoma of the small intestine in Crohn's disease. *Surg Gynecol Obstet* 1991;173:343.
51. Bonacina E, Barbano PR, Barberis M, Rossi MV. Primary adenocarcinoma of terminal ileum with clinical and gross morphologic features simulating Crohn's disease: a case report. *Tumori* 1985;71:513.
52. Keller RJ, Hertz I, Zimmerman M, Geller S. Carcinoma of the ileum simulating Crohn disease. *AJR Am J Roentgenol* 1982;138:151.
53. Adler SN, Lyon DT, Sullivan PD. Adenocarcinoma of the small bowel clinical features, similarity to regional enteritis, and analysis of 338 documented cases. *Am J Gastroenterol* 1982;77:326.
54. Swinson CM, Coles EC, Slavin G, Booth CC. Coeliac disease and malignancy. *Lancet* 1983;1:111.
55. Holmes GKT, Dunn GI, Cockel R, Brookes VS. Adenocarcinoma of the upper small bowel complicating coeliac disease. *Gut* 1980;21:1010.
56. Trier JS. Celiac sprue. *N Engl J Med* 1991;325:1709.
57. Domizio P, Owen RA, Shepherd NA, et al. Primary lymphoma of the small intestine: a clinicopathological study of 119 cases. *Am J Surg Pathol* 1993;17:429.
58. Giardiello FM, Welsh SB, Hamilton SD, et al. Increased risk of cancer in the Peutz-Jeghers syndrome. *N Engl J Med* 1987;316:1511.
59. Konishi F, Wyse NE, Muto T, et al. Peutz-Jeghers polyposis associated with carcinoma of the digestive organs. *Dis Colon Rectum* 1989;30:790.
60. Spigelman AD, Murday V, Phillips RKS. Cancer and the Peutz-Jeghers syndrome. *Gut* 1990;30:1588.
61. Linos DA, Dozois RR, Dahlin DC, Bartholomew LG. Does Peutz-Jeghers syndrome predispose gastrointestinal malignancy? *Arch Surg* 1981;116:1182.
62. Hochberg FH, Dasilva AB, Galdabini J, Richardson EP. Gastrointestinal involvement in von Recklinghausen's neurofibromatosis. *Neurology* 1974;24:1144.
63. Rutgeerts P, Hendrick H, Geboes K, et al. Involvement of the upper digestive tract by systemic neurofibromatosis. *Gastrointest Endosc* 1981;27:22.
64. Williams SJ, Lucas RJ, McCaughey RS. Paraganglioma of the duodenum: a case report. *Surgery* 1980;87:454.
65. Kheir SM, Halpern NB. Paraganglioma of the duodenum in association with congenital neurofibromatosis. *Cancer* 1984;53:2491.
66. Inai K, Kobuke T, Yonehara S, Tokuoka S. Duodenal gangliocytic paraganglioma with lymph node metastasis in a 17-year-old boy. *Cancer* 1989;63:2540.
67. Kingston RD. Neurofibromatosis and small bowel adenocarcinoma: an unrecognized association. *Gut* 1988;29:134.
68. Wheeler MH, Curley IR, Williams ED. The association of neurofibromatosis pheochromocytoma, and somatostatin-rich duodenal carcinoid tumor. *Surgery* 1986;100:1163.
69. Adkins RB, Davies J. Gross and microscopic anatomy of the stomach and small intestine. In: Scott HW, Sawyers JL, eds. *Surgery of the stomach, duodenum, and small intestine.* Oxford: Blackwell Scientific, 1987:45.
70. Silberman H, Crichlow RW, Caplan HS. Neoplasms of the small bowel. *Am Surg* 1974;180:157.
71. Treadwell TA, White R. Primary tumors of the small bowel. *Am J Surg* 1975;130:749.
72. Norberg K, Emas S. Primary tumors of the small intestine. *Am J Surg* 1981;142:569.
73. Ahlman H, Kjellstrom T. Clinically diagnosed small intestinal tumors in an urban Swedish area. *Acta Chir Scand* 1981;147:371.
74. Waterhouse G, Skudlarick J, Adkins RB. A clinical review of small bowel neoplasms. *South Med J* 1981;74:1202.
75. Gupta S. Primary tumors of the small bowel: a clinicopathological study of 58 cases. *J Surg Oncol* 1982;20:161.
76. Desa L, Bridger F, Grace PA, Krausz T, Spencer J. Primary jejunoileal tumors: a review of 45 cases. *World J Surg* 1991;15:81.
77. Croom RD, Newsome JF. Tumors of the small intestine. *Am Surg* 1975;41:160.
78. Freund H, Lavi A, Pfefferman R, Durst AL. Primary neoplasms of the small bowel. *Am J Surg* 1978;135:757.
79. Zollinger RM, Sternfeld W, Schreiber H. Primary neoplasms of the small intestine. *Am J Surg* 1986;151:654.
80. Maglinte DDT, O'Connor K, Bessette J, et al. The role of the physician in the late diagnosis of primary malignant tumors of the small intestine. *Am J Gastroenterol* 1991;86:304.
81. Awrich AE, Irish CE, Vetto RM, Fletcher WS. A twenty-five year experience with primary malignant tumors of the small intestine. *Surg Gynecol Obstet* 1980;151:9.
82. Brophy C, Cahow CE. Primary small bowel malignant tumors. Unrecognized until emergent laparotomy. *Am Surg* 1989;55:408.
83. Ashley SW, Wells SA. Tumors of the small intestine. *Semin Oncol* 1988;15:116.
84. Ekberg O, Ekholm S. Radiography in primary tumors of the small bowel. *Acta Radiol Diagn (Stockh)* 1980;21:79.
85. Bessette J, Maglinte DDT, Kelvin FM, Chernish SM. Primary malignant tumors in the small bowel: a comparison of the small-bowel enema and conventional follow-through examination. *AJR Am J Roentgenol* 1989;153:741.
86. Maglinte DDT, Hall R, Miller RE, et al. Detection of surgical lesions of the small bowel by enteroclysis. *Am J Surg* 1984;147:225.
87. Cohen ME, Barkin JS. Enteroscopy and enteroclysis: the combined procedure. *Am J Gastroenterol* 1989;84:1413.
88. Schnyder PA, Candardjis G. CT detection of benign and malignant abnormalities of the small bowel. *Eur J Radiol* 1983;3:33.
89. Laurent F, Raynaud M, Biset JM, et al. Diagnosis and categorization of small bowel neoplasms: role of computed tomography. *Gastrointest Radiol* 1991;16:115.
90. James S, Balfe DM, Lee JKT, Picus D. Small bowel disease: categorization by CT examination. *AJR Am J Roentgenol* 1987;148:863.
91. Dudiak KM, Johnson CD, Stephens DH. Primary tumors of the small intestine: CT evaluation. *AJR Am J Roentgenol* 1989;152:995.
92. Scatairge JC, Allen HA, Fishman EK. Computed tomography of the small bowel. *Semin Ultrasound CT MR* 1987;8:403.
93. Siegel MJ, Evans SJ, Balfe DM. Small bowel disease in children: diagnosis with CT. *Radiology* 1988;169:127.
94. Alfidi RJ, Esselstyn CD, Tarar R, et al. Recognition and angio-surgical detection of arteriovenous malformations of the bowel. *Ann Surg* 1971;174:573.
95. Oliver GC, Rubin RJ, Park YH, Ashton JK. Preoperative localization of intermittently bleeding small intestinal tumors using Tc-99m labeled red blood cell scanning report of two cases. *Dis Colon Rectum* 1987;30:715.
96. Bowden TA. Endoscopy of the small intestine. *Surg Clin North Am* 1989;69:1237.
97. Foutch PG, Sanowski RA, Kelly S. Endoscopy: a method for detection of small bowel tumors. *Am J Gastroenterol* 1985;80:887.
98. Halphen M, Najjar T, Jaafoura H, et al. Diagnostic value of upper intestinal fiber endoscopy in primary small intestinal lymphoma. *Cancer* 1986;58:2140.
99. Gilbert DA, Buelow RG, Chung RSK, et al. Status evaluation: enteroscopy. *Gastrointest Endosc* 1991;37:673.
100. Iida M, Yao T, Ohsato K, et al. Diagnostic value of intraoperative fiberscopy for small-intestinal polyps in familial adenomatosis coli. *Endoscopy* 1980;12:161.
101. Frucht J, Norton JA, London JF, et al. Detection of duodenal gastrinomas by operative endoscopic transillumination. *Gastroenterology* 1990;99:1622.
102. Estrin HM, Farhy DC, Ament AA, Yang P. Ileoscopic diagnosis of malignant lymphoma of the small bowel in acquired immunodeficiency syndrome. *Gastrointest Endosc* 1987;33:390.
103. Wilson JM, Melvin DB, Gray G, Thorbjornson B. Benign small bowel tumors. *Ann Surg* 1975;181:247.
104. Skandalakis JE, Gray SW. Smooth muscle tumors of the small intestine. In: *Smooth muscle tumors of the alimentary tract: leiomyomas and leiomyosarcomas, a review of 2525 cases.* Springfield, IL: Charles C Thomas Publisher, 1962:112.
105. Delpy JC, Bruneton JN, Drouillard J, Leconte P. Non-vaterian duodenal adenomas: report of 24 cases and review of the literature. *Gastrointest Radiol* 1983;8:135.
106. Kutin ND, Ranson JHC, Gouge TH, Localio SA. Villous tumors of the duodenum. *Ann Surg* 1975;181:164.
107. Everett GD, Shirazi SS, Mitros FA. Villous tumors of the duodenum. *Am J Gastroenterol* 1981;75:376.
108. Schulten MF, Oyasu R, Beal JM. Villous adenoma of the duodenum: a case report and review of the literature. *Am J Surg* 1976;132:90.
109. Reddy RR, Schuman BM, Priest RJ. Duodenal polyps: diagnosis and management. *J Clin Gastroenterol* 1981;3:139.
110. Haglund U, Fork FT, Genell S, Rehnberg O. Villous adenomas in the duodenum. *Br J Surg* 1985;72:26.
111. Galandiuk S, Hermann RE, Jagelman DG, et al. Villous tumors of the duodenum. *Ann Surg* 1988;207:234.
112. Chappuis CW, Divincenti FC, Cohn I Jr. Villous tumors of the duodenum. *Ann Surg* 1989;209:593.
113. Bjork KJ, Davis CJ, Nagorney DM, Mucha P Jr. Duodenal villous tumors. *Arch Surg* 1990;125:961.
114. Steinberg LS, Shieber W. Villous adenomas of the small intestine. *Surgery* 1972;71:423.
115. Dormandy TL. Gastrointestinal polyposis with mucocutaneous pigmentation (Peutz-Jeghers syndrome). *N Engl J Med* 1957;256:1186.
116. Dormandy TL. Gastrointestinal polyposis with mucocutaneous pigmentation (Peutz-Jeghers syndrome). *N Engl J Med* 1957;256:1093.
117. Bilton JL, Riahl M. Hemangioma of the small intestine. *Am J Gastroenterol* 1967;48:120.
118. Sivula A. Intestinal hemangioma. *Acta Chir Scand* 1966;131:485.
119. Brzezinski W, Bailey RJ, Besney M, Turner G. Small-bowel lipoma: an uncommon cause of obstruction. *Can J Surg* 1990;33:423.
120. Climie ARW, Wylin RF. Small-intestinal lipomatosis. *Arch Pathol Lab Med* 1981;105:40.
121. Silverman L, Waugh JM, Huizenga KA, Harrison EG. Large adenomatous polyp of Brunner's glands. *Am J Clin Pathol* 1961;36:438.
122. DeSilva S, Chandrasoma P. Giant duodenal hematoma consisting mainly of Brunner's glands. *Am J Surg* 1977;133:240.
123. Maglinte DDT, Mayes SL, Ng AC, Pickett RD. Brunner's gland adenoma: diagnostic considerations. *J Clin Gastroenterol* 1982;4:127.
124. Shimer GR, Helwig EB. Inflammatory fibroid polyps of the intestine. *Am J Clin Pathol* 1984;81:708.
125. Manning RJ, Lewis C. Inflammatory ileal polyps in Crohn's disease presenting as refractory iron deficiency anemia. *Gastrointest Endosc* 1986;32:122.
126. Ott DJ, Wu WC, Shiflett DW, Pennell TC. Inflammatory fibroid polyp of the duodenum. *Am J Gastroenterol* 1980;73:62.
127. Assarian GS, Sundareson A. Inflammatory fibroid polyp of the ileum. *Hum Pathol* 1985;16:311.
128. Ouriel K, Adams J. Adenocarcinoma of the small intestine. *Am J Surg* 1984;147:66.
129. Lai ECS, Doty JE, Irving C, Tompkins RK. Primary adenocarcinoma of the duodenum: analysis survival. *World J Surg* 1988;12:695.
130. Kerremans RP, Lerut J, Penninck FM. Primary malignant duodenal tumors. *Ann Surg* 1979;190:179.
131. Spira IA, Ghazi A, Wolff WI. Primary adenocarcinoma of the duodenum. *Cancer* 1977;39:1721.
132. Joesting DR, Beart RW, VanHeerden JA, Weiland LH. Improving survival in adenocarcinoma of the duodenum. *Am J Surg* 1981;141:228.
133. Awlmark A, Andersson A, Lasson A. Primary carcinoma of the duodenum. *Ann Surg* 1980;191:13.
134. Chernish SM, Miller RE, Rosenak B, Scholz NE. Hypotonic duodenography with the use of glucagon. *Gastroenterology* 1972;62:392.
135. Brennan MF. Duodenal cancer. *Asian J Surg* 1990;13:204.
136. Grace PA, Pitt HA, Tompkins RK, et al. Decreased morbidity and mortality after pancreatoduodenectomy. *Am J Surg* 1986;151:141.

137. Crist DW, Sitzmann JV, Cameron JL. Improved hospital morbidity, mortality, and survival after the Whipple procedure. *Ann Surg* 1987;206:358.
138. O'Rourke MGE, Lancashire RP, Vattoune JR. Lymphoma of the small intestine. *Aust N Z J Surg* 1986;56:351.
139. Morgan DF, Busuttil RW. Primary adenocarcinoma of the small intestine. *Am J Surg* 1977;134:331.
140. Lioe TF, Biggart JD. Primary adenocarcinoma of the jejunum and ileum: clinicopathological review of 25 cases. *J Clin Pathol* 1990;43:533.
141. Koretz MJ, Graham R. Primary adenocarcinoma of the jejunum. *Am Surg* 1989;55:539.
142. Jigyasu D, Bedikian AY, Stroehlein JR. Chemotherapy for primary adenocarcinoma of the small bowel. *Cancer* 1984;53:23.
143. Strodel WE, Talpos G, Eckhauser F, Thompson N. Surgical therapy for small-bowel carcinoid tumors. *Arch Surg* 1983;118:391.
144. Peck JJ, Shields AB, Boyden AM, et al. Carcinoid tumors of the ileum. *Am J Surg* 1983;146:124.
145. Sjoblom SM. Clinical presentation and prognosis of gastrointestinal carcinoid tumors. *Scand J Gastroenterol* 1988;23:779.
146. Makridis C, Oberg K, Juhlin C, et al. Surgical treatment of mid-gut carcinoid tumors. *World J Surg* 1990;14:377.
147. Moertel CG. Treatment of the carcinoid tumor and the malignant carcinoid syndrome. *J Clin Oncol* 1983;1:727.
148. Olney JR, Urdaneta LF, Al-Jurf AS, et al. Carcinoid tumors of the gastrointestinal tract. *Am Surg* 1985;51:37.
149. Tilson MD. Carcinoid syndrome. *Surg Clin North Am* 1974;54:409.
150. Vinich AI, McLeod MK, Fig LM, et al. Clinical features, diagnosis, and localization of carcinoid tumors and their management. *Gastrointest Clin North Am* 1989;18:865.
151. Thompson GB, VanHeerden JA, Martin JK Jr, et al. Carcinoid tumors of the gastrointestinal tract: presentation, management and prognosis. *Surgery* 1985;98:1054.
152. Woodard PK, Feldman JM, Paine SS, Baker ME. Midgut carcinoid tumors: CT findings and biochemical profiles. *J Comput Assist Tomogr* 1995;19:400.
153. Woods HF, Bax NDS, Smith JAR. Small bowel carcinoid tumors. *World J Surg* 1985;9:921.
154. Dawes L, Schulte WJ, Condon RE. Carcinoid tumors. *Arch Surg* 1984;119:375.
155. Nwiloh JO, Pillarisetty S, Moscovic EA, Freeman HP. Carcinoid tumors. *J Surg Oncol* 1990;45:261.
156. O'Rourke MGE, Lancashire RP, Vattoune JR. Carcinoid of the small intestine. *Aust N Z J Surg* 1986;56:405.
157. Moertel CG, Sauer WG, Dockerty MB, Baggenstoss AH. Life history of the carcinoid tumor of the small intestine. *Cancer* 1961;14:901.
158. Martin JK Jr, Moertel CG, Adson MA, Schutt AJ. Surgical treatment of functioning metastatic carcinoid tumors. *Arch Surg* 1983;118:537.
159. Godwin JD. Carcinoid tumors: an analysis of 2837 cases. *Cancer* 1975;36:560.
160. Johnson LA, Lavin P, Moertel CG, et al. Carcinoids: the association of histologic growth pattern and survival. *Cancer* 1983;51:882.
161. Nobin AP, Erhardt K, Auer G, et al. Nuclear DNA patterns and survival in metastasizing ileal carcinoids. *World J Surg* 1987;11:372.
162. Tsushima K, Nagorney DM, Weiland LH, Lieber MM. The relationship of flow cytometric DNA analysis and clinicopathology in small-intestinal carcinoids. *Surgery* 1989;105:366.
163. Rosenfelt F, Rosenberg SA. Diffuse histiocytic lymphoma presenting with gastrointestinal tract lesions: the Stanford experience. *Cancer* 1980;45:2188.
164. Turowski GA, Basson MD. Primary malignant lymphoma of the intestine. *Am J Surg* 1995;169:433.
165. Dawson IM, Cornes JS, Morson BC. Primary malignant lymphoid tumors of the intestinal tract: report of 37 cases with a study of factors influencing prognosis. *Br J Surg* 1961;40:80.
166. Cooper BT, Read AE. Small intestinal lymphoma. *World J Surg* 1985;9:930.
167. Sweetenhaus JW, Mead GM, Wright DH, et al. Involvement of the ileocaecal region by non-Hodgkin's lymphoma in adults: clinical features and results of treatment. *Br J Cancer* 1989;60:366.
168. Carbone PP, Kaplan HS, Mussoff K, et al. Report of the committee on Hodgkin's disease staging classification. *Cancer Res* 1971;31:1860.
169. Blackledge G, Bush H, Dodge OG, Crowther D. A study of gastrointestinal lymphoma. *Clin Oncol* 1979;5:209.
170. Contreary K, Nance FC, Becker WF. Primary lymphoma of the gastrointestinal tract. *Ann Surg* 1980;191:593.
171. Auger MJ, Allan NC. Primary ileocecal lymphoma. *Cancer* 1990;65:358.
172. Gray GM, Rosenberg SA, Cooper AD, et al. Lymphomas involving the gastrointestinal tract. *Gastroenterology* 1982;82:143.
173. Rao AR, Kagan AR, Potyk D, et al. Management of gastrointestinal lymphoma. *Am J Clin Oncol* 1984;7:213.
174. ReMine SG, Braasch JW. Gastric and small bowel lymphoma. *Surg Clin North Am* 1986;66:713.
175. Sartoris DJ, Harell GS, Anderson MF, Zboralske FF. Small bowel lymphoma and regional enteritis: radiographic similarities. *Radiology* 1984;152:291.
176. Morgan DR, Holgate CS, Dixon MF, Bird CC. Primary small intestinal lymphoma: a study of 39 cases. *J Pathol* 1985;147:211.
177. Weingrad DN, Decosse JJ, Sherlock P, et al. Primary gastrointestinal lymphoma: a 30-year review. *Cancer* 1982;49:1258.
178. Shepherd FA, Evans WK, Kutas G, et al. Chemotherapy following surgery for stages IE and IIE non-Hodgkin's lymphoma of the gastrointestinal tract. *J Clin Oncol* 1988;6:253.
179. Steward WP, Harris M, Wagstaff J, et al. A prospective study of the treatment of high grade histology non-Hodgkin's lymphoma involving the gastrointestinal tract. *Eur J Cancer Clin Oncol* 1985;21:1195.
180. Aozasa K, Ueda T, Kurata A, et al. Prognostic value of histologic and clinical factors in 56 patients with gastrointestinal lymphomas. *Cancer* 1988;61:309.
181. Li G, Ouyang Q, Liu K, et al. Primary non-Hodgkin's lymphoma of the intestine: a morphological, immunohistochemical and clinical study of 31 Chinese cases. *Histopathology* 1994;25:113.
182. Skudder PA Jr, Schwartz SI. Primary lymphoma of the gastrointestinal tract. *Surg Gynecol Obstet* 1985;160:5.
183. Chandran RR, Hemanth E, Chaturvedi HK. Primary gastrointestinal lymphoma: 30-year experience at the Cancer Institute, Madras, India. *J Surg Oncol* 1995;60:41.
184. Fleming ID, Turk PS, Murphy SB, et al. Surgical implications of primary gastrointestinal lymphoma of childhood. *Arch Surg* 1990;125:252.
185. Al-Bahrani ZR, Al-Mondhiry H, Bakir F, Al-Saleem T. Clinical and pathologic subtypes of primary intestinal lymphoma. *Cancer* 1983;52:1666.
186. Haghigi P, Nasr K. Primary upper small intestinal lymphoma (so-called Mediterranean lymphoma). *Pathol Annu* 1973;8:231.
187. El Saghir NS, Jessen K, Mass RE, et al. Combination chemotherapy for primary small intestinal lymphoma of the Middle East. *Eur J Cancer Clin Oncol* 1989;5:851.
188. El Saghir NS. Combination chemotherapy with tetracycline and aggressive supportive care for immunoproliferative small intestinal disease lymphoma [Letter]. *J Clin Oncol* 1995;13:794.
189. Murray A, Cuevas EC, Jones DB, Wright DH. Study of the immunohistochemistry and T cell clonality of enteropathy-associated T cell lymphoma. *Am J Pathol* 1995;146:509.
190. Monco A, Sartori C. Hodgkin's primary lymphoma of the small intestine. *Haematologica* 1984;69:568.
191. Antonioli DA. Gastrointestinal autonomic nerve tumors: expanding the spectrum of gastrointestinal stromal tumors. *Arch Pathol Lab Med* 1989;113:831.
192. Herrera GA, Cerezo L, Jones JE, et al. Gastrointestinal autonomic nerve tumors: plexosarcomas. *Arch Pathol Lab Med* 1989;113:846.
193. Chiotasso PJP, Fazio VW. Prognostic factors of 28 leiomyosarcomas of the small intestine. *Surg Gynecol Obstet* 1982;155:197.
194. Shiu MH, Farr GH, Egeli RA, et al. Myosarcomas of the small and large intestine: a clinicopathological study. *J Surg Oncol* 1983;24:67.
195. McGrath PC, Neifeld JP, Lawrence W, et al. Gastrointestinal sarcomas: analysis of prognostic factors. *Ann Surg* 1987;206:706.
196. Kimura H, Yonemura Y, Kadoya N, et al. Prognostic factors in primary gastrointestinal leiomyosarcoma: a retrospective study. *World J Surg* 1991;15:771.
197. Dougherty MJ, Compton C, Talbert M, Wood WJ. Sarcomas of the gastrointestinal tract: separation into favorable and unfavorable prognostic groups by mitotic count. *Ann Surg* 1991;214:569.
198. Conlon KC, Casper ES, Brennan MF. Primary gastrointestinal sarcomas: analysis of prognostic variables. *Ann Surg Oncol* 1995;2:26.
199. Horowitz J, Spellman JE, Driscoll DL, et al. An institutional review of sarcomas of the large and small intestine. *J Am Coll Surg* 1995;180:465.
200. Chou FF, Eng HL, Sheen-Chen SM. Smooth muscle tumors of the gastrointestinal tract: analysis of prognostic factors. *Surgery* 1996;119:171.
201. Shiu MH, Brennan MF. Soft tissue sarcoma of the gastrointestinal tract. In: Shiu MH, Brennan MF, eds. *Surgical management of soft tissue sarcomas.* Philadelphia: Lea & Febiger, 1989:170.
202. Ihde JK, Coit DG. Melanoma metastatic to the stomach, small bowel and colon. *Am J Surg* 1991;162:208.
203. McNeill PM, Wagman LD, Neifeld JP. Small bowel metastases from primary carcinoma of the lung. *Cancer* 1987;59:1486.
204. Leidich RB, Rudolf LE. Small bowel perforation secondary to metastatic lung carcinoma. *Ann Surg* 1981;193:67.
205. Koos L, Field RE. Metastatic carcinoma of breast simulating Crohn's disease. *Int Surg* 1980;65:359.
206. Nyberg B, Sonnenfeld T. Metastatic breast carcinoma causing intestinal obstruction. *Acta Chir Scand Suppl* 1986;530:95.
207. Farmer RG, Hawk WA. Metastatic tumors of the small bowel. *Gastroenterology* 1964;47:496.
208. Ngan H. Involvement of the duodenum by metastases from tumours of the genital tract. *Br J Radiol* 1970;43:701.
209. Haynes IG, Wolverson RL, O'Brien JM. Small bowel intussusception due to metastatic renal carcinoma. *Br J Urol* 1986;58:460.
210. Lawson LJ, Holt LP, Rooke HWP. Recurrent duodenal haemorrhage from renal carcinoma. *Br J Urol* 1966;38:133.
211. Phillips DL, Benner KG, Keefe EB, Traweek ST. Isolated metastasis to small bowel from anaplastic thyroid carcinoma. *J Clin Gastroenterol* 1987;9:563.
212. Naunton Morgan TC, Henderson RG. Small bowel metastases from a Merkel cell tumor. *Br J Radiol* 1985;58:1212.
213. Yang PM, Sheu JC, Yang TH, et al. Metastasis of hepatocellular carcinoma to the jejunum manifested by occult gastrointestinal bleeding. *Am J Gastroenterol* 1987;82:165.
214. Reintgen DS, Thompson W, Garbutt J, Seigler HF. Radiologic, endoscopic and surgical consideration of malignant melanoma metastatic to the small intestine. *Curr Surg* 1984;41:87.
215. Caputy G, Donohue JH, Goellner JH, Ilstrup DM. Metastatic melanoma of the gastrointestinal tract: the results of surgical management. *Arch Surg* 1991;126:1353.
216. Branum GD, Seigler HF. Role of surgical intervention in the management of intestinal metastases from malignant melanoma. *Am J Surg* 1991;162:428.
217. Wilson BG, Anderson JR. Malignant melanoma involving the small bowel. *Postgrad Med J* 1986;62:355.
218. Ricaniadis N, Konstadoulakis MM, Walsh D, Karakousis CP. Gastrointestinal metastases from malignant melanoma. *Surg Oncol* 1995;4:105.
219. Mittal VK, Bodzin JH. Primary malignant tumors of the small bowel. *Am J Surg* 1980;140:396.
220. Giuliani A, Caporale A, Teneriello F, et al. Primary tumors of the small intestine. *Int Surg* 1985:331.
221. Matsuo S, Eto T, Tsunoda T, et al. Small bowel tumors: an analysis of tumor-like lesions, benign and malignant neoplasms. *Eur J Surg Oncol* 1994;20:47.

222. Lillemoe K, Imbembo AL. Malignant neoplasms of the duodenum. *Surg Gynecol Obstet* 1980;150:822.
223. Cohen JR, Kuchta N, Geller N, et al. Pancreaticoduodenectomy. *Ann Surg* 1982;195:608.
224. Herter FP, Cooperman AM, Ahinorn TN, Antinori C. Surgical experience with pancreatic and periampullary cancer. *Ann Surg* 1982;195:274.
225. Kellum JM, Clark J, Miller HH. Pancreatoduodenectomy for resectable malignant periampullary tumors. *Surg Gynecol Obstet* 1983;157:362.
226. Gaddy M, Max MH. Carcinoma of the duodenum. *South Med J* 1985;78:150.
227. Jones BA, Langer B, Taylor BR, Girotti M. Periampullary tumors: which ones should be resected? *Am J Surg* 1985;149:46.
228. Tarazi RY, Hermann RE, Vogt DP, et al. Results of surgical treatment of periampullary tumors: a thirty-five-year experience. *Surgery* 1986;100:716.
229. Gonzalez CD, Evans EC. Primary adenocarcinoma of the duodenum. *Am Surg* 1987;53:174.
230. Sarma DP, Weilbaecher TG. Adenocarcinoma of the duodenum. *J Surg Oncol* 1987;34:262.
231. Michelassi F, Erroi F, Dawson PJ, et al. Experience with 647 consecutive tumors of the duodenum, ampulla, head of the pancreas, and distal common bile duct. *Ann Surg* 1989;210:544.
232. Lanzafame RJ, Long JE, Hinshaw JR. Primary cancer of the small bowel. *N Y State J Med* 1982;82:1325.
233. Bauer RL, Palmer ML, Bauer AM, et al. Adenocarcinoma of the small intestine: 21 year review of diagnosis, treatment, and prognosis. *Ann Surg Oncol* 1994;1:183.
234. Zeitels J, Naunheim K, Kaplan EL, Straus F. Carcinoid tumors: a 37 year experience. *Arch Surg* 1982;117:732.
235. Dragosics B, Bauer P, Radaszkiewicz T. Primary gastrointestinal non-Hodgkin's lymphoma: a retrospective clinicopathologic study of 150 cases. *Cancer* 1985;55:1060.
236. Conlon KC, Casper ES, Brennan MF. Primary gastrointestinal sarcomas: analysis of prognostic variables. *Ann Surg Oncol* 1995;2:26.
237. Horowitz J, Spellman JE, Driscoll DL, et al. An institutional review of sarcomas of the large and small intestine. *J Am Coll Surg* 1995;180:465.

JOHN M. SKIBBER
BRUCE D. MINSKY
PAULO M. HOFF

SECTION 7
Cancer of the Colon

Colorectal cancer represents a major public health problem, especially in developed countries. As such, it has attracted the efforts of researchers from a wide variety of disciplines, including epidemiologists, molecular biologists, nutritionists, gastroenterologists, prevention experts, surgeons, radiation therapists, nurses, medical oncologists, and outcomes researchers. This chapter section and Chapter 33.8 present some of the exciting information that has been generated about this common malignancy.

ANATOMY

GROSS ANATOMY

The large bowel is divided into the colon and the rectum. Segments of both may be intraperitoneal or extraperitoneal. The treatment and pattern of recurrence of colon and rectal cancer are affected by the location of the tumor in these organs and its relationship to the peritoneal cavity and surrounding structures. Treatment failures in large bowel tumors involving extraperitoneal segments often occur because of a locoregional recurrence.[1] This is especially true of rectal cancers, which usually have no serosal covering and are surrounded by fat, bone, nerves, blood vessels, and viscera within the confines of the pelvis. The colon has segments that are largely intraperitoneal, and the relationship of certain aspects of the colon to the retroperitoneum and its structures are important factors in tumor spread. The cecum, transverse colon, and sigmoid loop are the intraperitoneal portions of the colon. The ascending colon, descending colon, splenic and hepatic flexures, and beginning and end of the sigmoid colon have their posterior surface in the retroperitoneum.

The large bowel is immediately recognized by its large diameter, haustra, and presence of appendices epiploicae and tenia coli. The tenia consist of condensations of longitudinal muscle fibers starting near the base of the appendix and continuing throughout the abdominal colon to form a continuous longitudinal muscle coat in the upper rectum. Haustra are outpouchings of bowel wall separated by folds that give a classic appearance on radiography or barium enema.

The first part of the colon is the cecum, with the appendix lying at the lower pole. The ascending colon lies on the right aspect of the retroperitoneum and extends up to the hepatic flexure. The hepatic flexure lies near the gallbladder fossa and porta hepatis and overlies the lower portion of the right kidney and the duodenum. The transverse colon is variable in its length. The splenic flexure lies just beneath the left diaphragm and abuts the hilum of the spleen and tail of the pancreas. The descending colon lies along the left retroperitoneum and terminates in the sigmoid colon. The descending colon is of variable length. The sigmoid colon is the narrowest portion of the large bowel, and it terminates at its junction with the upper rectum just below the sacral promontory.

VASCULAR SUPPLY

In general, the artery and vein supplying and draining each segment of the colon accompany each other in the mesocolon. The mesocolon contains vessels, lymph nodes, nerves, and lymphatic trunks. The marginal artery and vein form an arcade along the mesocolic side of the colon. The presence of collateral circulation allows performance of mesenteric resection to the level of the principal nodes found at the origin of the major vessels supplying segments of the colon.

The superior mesenteric artery (SMA) and the inferior mesenteric artery (IMA) contribute to the arterial supply of the colon (Fig. 33.7-1).[2] Shortly after its origin, the SMA divides into the middle colic artery and the trunk of the SMA. The middle colic artery immediately forms two to three large arcades in the transverse mesocolon. The SMA ileocolic arterial branches then extend from the SMA. The right colic artery arises as a separate branch from the SMA in 10.7% of cases.[3] The ileocolic artery gives off a right colic artery to the upper ascending colon and forms an anastomosis with branches from the middle colic artery. The ileal branch of the ileocolic artery gives off branches to the distal small bowel and cecum, whereas the colic branch supplies the ascending colon. An anastomosis occurs between the distal SMA and the ileal branch of the ileocolic artery at the junction of the terminal ileum and cecum.

The arterial supply to the left side of the colon comes from the IMA, which arises from the aorta. The IMA gives off the left colic artery. It also gives off three to four sigmoidal arteries. The anastomosis between the vessels of the middle colic artery and those of the left colic artery occurs at the splenic flexure.

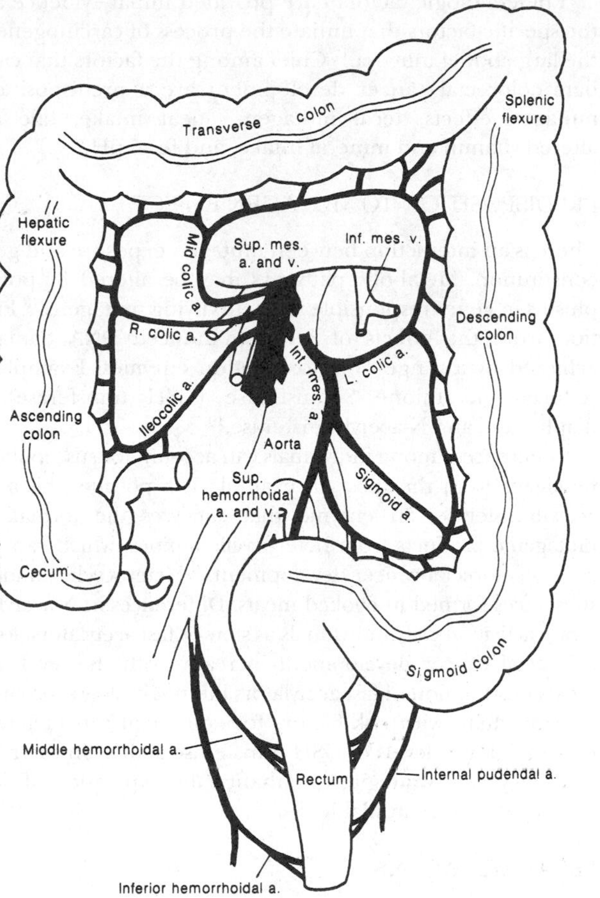

FIGURE 33.7-1. Anatomic segments and vascular supply to the colon and rectum. a, artery; Inf, inferior; Int, internal; L, left; mes, mesenteric; R, right; Sup, superior; v, vein. (From Jones T, Shepard WC, *A manual of surgical anatomy.* Philadelphia: WB Saunders, 1945, with permission.)

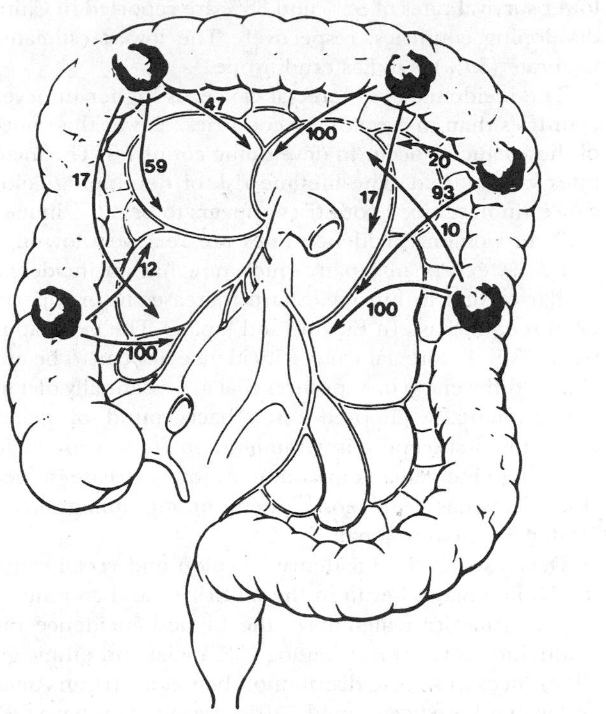

FIGURE 33.7-2. For tumors that lie between two pedicles, lymphatic flow may drain in either or both directions. From a study of cleared specimens, it was possible to determine the preferential route by the location of lymphatic metastases. The numbers signify the percentage of metastasizing carcinomas in the indicated locations that have demonstrated positive nodes along a given vascular route. For example, node-positive tumors lying between the ileocolic and right colic arcades metastasize along the ileocolic pedicle in 100% of cases and along the right colon in 12% of cases. (From Hertzer FP, Slanetz CA, Patterns and significance of lymphatic spread from cancer of the colon and rectum. In: Weiss L, Gilbert HA, Ballon SC, eds, *Lymphatic system metastasis.* Boston: GK Hall, 1980:283, with permission.)

This vessel parallels the course of the colon between the middle colic artery and the branches of the IMA. This is critical in surgical reconstruction of the left colon and rectum.

The venous drainage of the colon parallels that of the arterial supply. The drainage of the superior and inferior mesenteric veins is to the portal vein. This enhances the production of liver metastases. The venous drainage of the lower rectum is also into the vena cava and, therefore, rectal cancers are more likely to produce isolated pulmonary metastases than are cancers at other large bowel sites.

LYMPHATIC DRAINAGE

Curative surgical resection and staging of large bowel cancer requires resection of the lymph nodes that drain the primary tumor site. The relationship between the blood vessels supplying the affected segment of colon and the draining lymphatics determines the extent of bowel resection to be done.

Lymphatic drainage of the large bowel follows its arterial supply in the mesocolon (Fig. 33.7-2). Invasive carcinoma of the large bowel is identified by spread beyond the muscularis mucosa into the submucosa, where it gains access to lymphatic channels through open junctions formed by the destruction of lymphatic endothelial cells.[4] The efferent lymphatic channels pass from the submucosa to the intramuscular and subserosal plexus of the bowel to the first tier of lymph nodes lying adjacent to the large intestine and known as *epicolic nodes. Paracolic nodes* lie on the marginal vessels along the mesenteric side of the colon and are frequently involved in metastases. *Intermediate nodes* are found along the major arterial branches of the SMA and IMA in the mesocolon. The *principal nodes* are found around the origin of these vessels from the aorta, and they drain into retroperitoneal nodes.

EPIDEMIOLOGY

Colorectal cancers rank third in frequency in men and second in women. Male incidence rates, adjusted for age and race, appear greater than female rates for both proximal and distal cancers [odds ratio (OR), 1.32 for proximal cancers and 1.68 for distal cancers, respectively]. The mortality rate is similar in men and women, the ratio being 1.05:1.00. Colorectal cancer is the fourth leading cause of cancer mortality because it has a better prognosis than more common cancers. A 5-year survival rate of 61% is reported by the U.S. Surveillance, Epidemiology, and End Results program,[6,7] as compared with a 5-year survival rate of 41% to 42% in European and Indian registries.[5] Slightly lower survival rates of 32% and 38% are reported in China and developing countries, respectively. The lowest estimated survival rate (30%) is in Eastern Europe.

The incidence of colorectal cancer is higher in developed countries than in developing countries.[7] Fewer than one-third of these cancers occur in developing countries. The incidence rates vary tenfold. The lifetime risk of developing colorectal cancer in developed countries appears to be 4.6% in men and 3.2% in women. Incidence rates are relatively low in Africa and Asia, except in Japan, which now has an incidence rate similar to that in Europe. Sharp increases in incidence have been seen in Eastern Europe and Japan.[8] The geographic differences in colorectal cancer incidence appear to be attributable to differences in exposures that are essentially dietary and environmentally imposed on a background of genetically determined susceptibility. Immigration from a low-incidence to a high-incidence environment will increase a person's risk.[11] This has been most evident among immigrants to the United States from Japan.

Decreases in the incidence of colon and rectal cancers in the United States began in the mid-1980s and continue today. African American men have the highest incidence rates of colon and rectal cancer among U.S. racial and ethnic groups. Differences in subsite distribution between African Americans and whites have been noted.[9] African Americans have the highest mortality rates for colon and rectal cancer among ethnic and racial groups. Studies have postulated that these differences are not due to biologic aggressiveness of the tumors but rather to access to care.[10] U.S. colorectal cancer mortality and incidence rates continue to decline, with age-adjusted rates dropping to 16.8 and 42.7 per 100,000 population, respectively, in 1996.[11] An analysis of data from population studies that included the National Cancer Institute's Surveillance, Epidemiology, and End Results program reports that changes in the use of endoscopic polypectomy, dietary factors, energy intake, physical activity, serum cholesterol, cigarette smoking, and obesity contributed to this fall in incidence after 1986.[12]

Recent epidemiologic studies have suggested that the anatomic distribution of colorectal cancer may have undergone a distal to proximal shift over several decades. The U.S. National Cancer Database has reported that cecal and ascending colon tumors increased in incidence from 33.9% to 36.1%, tumors of the transverse colon increased from 15.8% to 17.2%, and tumors of the sigmoid colon decreased from 36.0% to 33.4%. These changes occurred between 1986 and 1992.[13] Reports suggest that the apparent distal to proximal shift may be a result of preventive measures and improved diagnostic techniques used in developed, high-incidence countries but that these have not had an impact in less developed nations.[14] In an analysis of improvements in survival over time by anatomic subsites of colon cancer, it was found that 5-year survival rates improved significantly for patients with left colon and transverse colon cancers, owing to advances in treatment and diagnostic techniques, whereas survival rates from right colon cancer did not improve.[15]

ETIOLOGY

The essential element of the etiology of colorectal cancer is a process of genetic change in the epithelial cells of the colonic mucosa.[16] These changes are discussed more fully in the Chapter 33.1 that address the molecular biology of this disease.

Epidemiologic factors have provided initial evidence about the specific factors that initiate the process of carcinogenesis in the large bowel mucosa.[17] Chief among the factors that can initiate colorectal cancer development are a predisposition to mutagen effects, fecal mutagens, meat intake, bile acids, altered vitamin and mineral intake, and fecal pH.

PREDISPOSITION TO MUTAGEN EFFECTS

There is an interaction between mutagen exposure and genetic constitution. Metabolic pathways may be altered by polymorphisms in genes responsible for detoxifying mutagens.[18] Protection from the effects of mutagen-induced DNA damage is achieved by a range of detoxification enzymes. Examples are reduced glutathione S-transferase (GSH transferase), DT-diaphorase, and N-acetyltransferase.[19]

Differences among individuals can account for susceptibility to mutagens from the diet. An example is a polymorphism in N-acetyltransferase, an enzyme that catalyzes the formation of mutagenic products from heterocyclic amines, which can play a role in colorectal cancer development.[20] Heterocyclic amines are substances formed in cooked meats. Differences in N-acetyltransferase activity classify individuals as slow or fast acetylators. Risk for colorectal cancer development increases with the level of red meat consumption in fast acetylators but not in slow acetylators.[21]

Individuals with risk factors for colorectal cancer have significantly lower levels of GSH transferase activity in their blood lymphocytes.[22] Strategies to enhance the expression of detoxifying enzymes are available.[23]

FECAL MUTAGENS

Mutagenic compounds such as fecapentaenes, 3-ketosteroids, and heterocyclic amines in the stool may be produced by the interaction of digestion and food products.[24] These compounds produce reactive molecules that may form bulky adducts to DNA. One of the chief influences of diet is the production of fecal mutagens by certain diets. Changes in the fecal microflora indicate that changes in diet may alter mutagenic activity by altering extracellular superoxide formation.[25] For instance, a change in a lactovegetarian diet to a diet with increased fiber intake caused a dilution of mitogenic activity within the stool.[26] Other factors may moderate the effects of fecal mutagens. Intake of antioxidants reduces the mutagenicity of compounds in the stool. Changes in intestinal transit time owing to fiber intake affects the exposure of the mucosa to mutagens.

In addition to mutagenic compounds such as fecapentaenes, the presence of other products of digestion such as 3-ketosteroids, which are products of cholesterol metabolism, may act as tumor promoters or initiators.

MEAT INTAKE

Armstrong and Doll (1975) described the high correlation of meat intake and mortality from colorectal cancer. Among the risk factors are the intake of red meats and the compounds that result from cooking meats at high temperatures.[27] In a study of meat preparation, it was observed that the association between red meat and colorectal cancer could be due to heterocyclic amines present in cooked meat.[28] This mechanism has been implicated in the high incidence of colorectal cancer in New Zealand.[29] The method of red meat preparation and frequency of intake can be correlated with the prevalence of distal colorectal adenomas. Subjects who ate browned, fried red meat more than once per week had an OR of 2.2 for distal colorectal adenomas, as compared with those who ate lightly browned red meat one time or less per week.[30] In Western countries, fried meat is the main source of exposure to heterocyclic amines. Nurses who consumed the highest ratio of red meat to white meat had a higher relative risk (RR) of colon cancer (OR 2.49, $P<.001$).[31]

BILE ACIDS

Normal bile acids that are related to the digestion of fat can induce intestinal mucosal hyperproliferation, which acts as a marker for neoplasia risk.[32] The presence of bile acids correlates with fat consumption, which is a known risk factor for colorectal cancer.[33] Bile acids have been shown to activate AP-1, a transcription factor associated with the promotion of neoplastic transformation in colonic cells.[34] They are also able to induce apoptosis, and variations in the epithelial apoptotic response to bile acids may correlate with risk.[35] Cholecystectomy can result in high levels of bile acids in the cecum and ascending colon and appears to increase the frequency of right-sided carcinoma. In a retrospective study of colorectal cancer patients, it was found that levels of the secondary bile acid deoxycholic acid were higher than normal and that the ratio between deoxycholic acid and cholic acid may be an indicator of risk.[36]

VITAMIN AND MINERAL INTAKE

Calcium can alter colonic mucosal proliferation by binding fatty acids and bile acids in the stool, resulting in insoluble complexes that are less likely to affect the mucosa. It can also decrease proliferation of the mucosa directly.[37] These effects of calcium may be site-specific within the colon.[38] In a large study of U.S. health professionals, the risk reduction from high calcium intake appeared modest after adjusting for confounding variables.[39] Two case-control studies suggest that any protective effect of calcium may occur only at low levels of fat intake.[40] The National Polyp Prevention Trial indicated that supplemental calcium intake reduced adenoma formation by 19%.[41] A similar effect has been seen in patients with hereditary nonpolyposis colon cancer (HNPCC) syndrome.[38]

In case-control studies, the use of multivitamins has been shown to reduce the risk of adenoma formation in high-risk patients.[42] In an update of the Nurses' Health Study, Giovannucci et al.[43] found a reduced risk of colon cancer [OR, 0.25; confidence interval (CI), 0.13 to 0.51] after 15 years of use of folate-containing multivitamins. The contribution of dietary folate appeared to be modest.

That folate is a potentially protective agent has been demonstrated also by other studies. Experimental tumor studies have shown that folate depletion increases the risk of tumor formation and that it also reduces methyl group availability for DNA methylation. Individuals with different forms of the 5,10-methylenetetrahydrofolate reductase gene may demonstrate different risks for colorectal cancer, which may account for differences in the effectiveness of folate supplementation on colorectal cancer risk.[48] Administration of a folate agent may interact with alcohol consumption as a risk factor because demands for folate are raised by alcohol consumption.[49] Low folate intake has been implicated in increased colorectal cancer risk, especially when combined with alcohol and a low-protein diet.[50]

Populations with increased vitamin D intake have been noted to be at reduced risk for colon carcinoma.[44] The effects of dihydroxyvitamin D_3 on differentiation are mediated through protein kinase C and its activation by dihydroxyvitamin D_3. Total vitamin D intake was inversely related to colorectal cancer incidence in the Nurses' Health Study (RR, 0.33; CI, 0.16 to 0.70).[45]

A reduced risk of colon cancer is associated with the use of vitamin C.[46] Antioxidants such as vitamin E have been given in conjunction with vitamins C and A in studies indicating some protection against colorectal cancer risks.[47]

There is a weak association between high iron exposure and colorectal polyps (OR, 1.5; CI, 1.0 to 2.3).[51] Low levels of selenium correlated with the presence of adenomas, whereas increased levels were associated with reduced risk of adenomas (OR, 0.58; CI, 0.31 to 1.08).[52] Intervention trials have found a beneficial effect of selenium supplementation.[53]

FECAL PH

Another aspect of the interaction between the intestinal milieu and the genome of the intestinal mucosa is the fact that alkaline environments in the stool support higher concentrations of free bile acids and other potential carcinogens.[54] This pH may affect the solubility of bile acid and carcinogens and make them more damaging to the DNA of the intestinal mucosal cells. Epidemiologic studies show that higher rates of colon carcinoma are found in subjects with a higher stool pH.[55]

PRIMARY PREVENTION

Primary prevention of colorectal carcinoma is defined as the identification and eradication of etiologic factors responsible for this disease. Dietary factors, energy intake, nonsteroidal antiinflammatory drug (NSAID) use, and such lifestyle factors as hormone use in women, tobacco and alcohol use, parity, and exercise, will be discussed. These issues are addressed extensively in Chapters 22, 23.1, 23.2, 23.3, 23.4, 23.5, 23.6, and 23.7.

DIETARY FACTORS

Fiber

The term *fiber* refers to a diverse group of complex carbohydrates. Numerous epidemiologic studies suggest that fiber exerts a protective effect, whereas other epidemiologic studies report no protective activity of fiber in relation to colorectal carcinoma.[56] High fiber intake may be associated with other dietary habits that also decrease cancer risk.[57]

Certain types of fiber appear to be more effective than others in reducing the risk of carcinogenesis. Cellulose and bran are specific examples of fibers that have demonstrated increased effectiveness.[58] In an epidemiologic study of 16,448 health professionals, a trend toward a reduced risk of distal colorectal adenomas from fruit fiber ingestion but not from cereals or vegetables was seen. When data from this study were adjusted for incidents of polyp development, the risk reduction associated with soluble fiber intake was stronger (RR, 0.27; CI, 0.11 to 0.66).[59] Fiber may not reduce rectal cancer risk as much as it reduces colon cancer risk.[59] Intervention trials involving fiber are appealing because of fiber's ready availability and low cost.[60] However, the effect of fiber may not be independent of meat intake.[31] A recent long-term analysis of this issue failed to demonstrate a significant reduction in risk for colorectal cancer or adenomas (OR, 0.95; CI, 0.73 to 1.25) attributable to dietary fiber.[56]

Dietary Fat

Epidemiologic data suggest a direct relationship between total fat intake and increased cancer risk in the colon and rectum, and migrant studies show that changes toward a low-fat, low-fiber Western diet result in a rise in colorectal cancer incidence.[61] Type of dietary fat may be important in the risk for colorectal cancer, as studies appear to link animal fat and red meat to colon cancer risk but do not support an association between colon cancer and vegetable fat.[31] However, fish oils may have protective effects.[62] Elevated levels of serum triglycerides have been associated with a higher risk of adenomatous polyps (OR, 1.5).[63] Interestingly, lower cholesterol levels have been demonstrated in patients in whom colorectal cancer is diagnosed.[64]

ALCOHOL AND TOBACCO INTAKE

Daily alcohol intake has been associated with a twofold increase in colon carcinoma.[65] A more moderate risk is likely when a number of studies are considered.[66] Genetic polymorphisms in metabolic pathways may modify this risk. In addition, current and past smoking habits are independent factors that increase risk. Among Japanese men and women, it was found that long-term smoking conveyed a 1.6 to 4.54 RR for adenoma formation.[67]

HORMONE REPLACEMENT IN WOMEN

In a review of 59,002 postmenopausal participants in the Nurses' Health Study, self-reported data were used to study the relationship between postmenopausal hormone therapy and colorectal carcinomas and adenomas.[68] Current use of postmenopausal hormones was associated with decreased risk of colorectal cancer (RR, 0.65; CI, 0.50 to 0.83). The protective effect of hormonal replacement disappeared within 5 years after hormone use was discontinued. Similar protective effects were noted in a Minnesota study.[69,70] In the Nurses' Health Study, oral contraceptive use has been implicated in reducing the risk of colorectal cancer development by 40% (OR, 0.60; CI, 0.40 to 0.89).[71] A higher parity was found to increase risk in those women with a family history of colorectal cancer.[72]

ENERGY INTAKE, PHYSICAL ACTIVITY, AND OBESITY

Multiple studies have correlated factors such as energy intake, physical activity, and other lifestyle factors with colorectal cancer risk.[73] In animal models, restricted energy intake has reduced the development of colonic tumors.[74] The interaction between obesity and reduced physical activity was demonstrated by an alteration in intestinal prostaglandin activity, which can correlate with colon cancer risk.[75] The Nurses' Health Study showed an inverse relationship between physical activity and adenomas. In this same study, obesity was associated with an increased risk.[76] A similar protective effect from physical activity in men was noted in a population-based cohort study conducted in Norway.[77]

Excessive weight and abdominal obesity were found to be risk indicators in men and women.[78] An exploration of the relationship among obesity, energy intake, and insulin as a growth factor indicated an increased risk of colorectal cancer in the face of a high fasting glucose level, high insulin levels, and obesity.[79,80] Epidemiologic studies in the United States and Italy have shown a similar association between diabetes mellitus and colorectal cancer risk.[81]

NONSTEROIDAL ANTIINFLAMMATORY DRUGS

Experimental, epidemiologic, and intervention trails address the role of aspirin and NSAIDs in colorectal cancer biology.[82] Human and experimental animal colon tumors contain increased amounts of prostaglandin E_2, and this compound is thought to participate in colon cancer carcinogenesis.[83] Formation of prostaglandins requires the action of cyclooxygenase (COX), which exists in two isoforms. COX-2 appears to be responsible for increased prostaglandin E_2 in response to growth factors in human and animal colonic tumors.[84] COX-2 inhibition, therefore, may play a role in colon cancer prevention.

Aspirin, a relatively nonspecific COX-2 inhibitor, has been associated with lower-than-expected rates of colorectal adenomas and carcinomas in epidemiologic studies.[85–87] However, in a large aspirin intervention trial involving more than 22,000 U.S. male physicians, a secondary analysis did not confirm a reduced incidence of colorectal cancer.[88]

In a Wisconsin study, regular NSAID use conferred a lower risk of a colorectal cancer diagnosis than did nonuse (OR, 0.65; CI, 0.40 to 1.03).[89] Importantly, the risk reduction was greater for those using nonaspirin compounds (OR, 0.43; 95% CI, 0.20 to 0.89) as compared with users of aspirin compounds (OR, 0.79; CI, 0.46 to 1.36). The NSAID sulindac has been studied in the setting of familial adenomatous polyposis (FAP), where it achieved a 56% reduction in polyps.[90] The long-term use of nonselective COX inhibitors can be associated with increased toxicity.[91] Use of more selective COX-2 inhibitors may be beneficial in preventing toxicity with long-term use while maintaining the agents' preventive effects.[92]

SECONDARY PREVENTION

Secondary prevention focuses on the identification of high-risk populations and interventions that can prevent the development of colorectal carcinoma. It involves identifying those persons at increased risk of death from colorectal cancer owing to the presence of premalignant lesions or early cancers. Examples of secondary prevention strategies are screening for adenomas, treatment of adenomatous polyps by endoscopic polypectomy, or excision of the large bowel in FAP. High-risk states can be identified by an individuals' age, genetic makeup, and predisposing diseases such as previous cancer or inflammatory bowel disease. In addition, previous medical treatments can have an impact on a patient's risk (Table 33.7-1). In nearly three-fourths of colorectal cancer cases, no predisposing factors will be identifiable.[93]

CLINICAL RISK FACTOR: AGE

Age is the most relevant factor affecting colorectal cancer risk in most general populations (Fig. 33.7-3). The peak onset of col-

TABLE 33.7-1. Risk Factors for Colorectal Cancer

Average risk
Age ≥50 y
Increased risk
Adenomatous polyposis syndromes
Familial adenomatous polyposis
Attenuated familial adenomatous polyposis
I 1307K mutation
Hamartomatous polyposis syndromes
Peutz-Jeghers syndrome
Juvenile adenomatous polyposis
Hereditary nonpolyposis colon cancer
Family history of polyps or colorectal cancer
Inflammatory bowel disease
Chronic ulcerative colitis
Chronic granulomatous colitis
Medical history
Colorectal carcinoma
Colorectal polyps
Pelvic irradiation
Noncancer surgery (cholecystectomy and ureterosigmoidostomy)

orectal cancer in the United States is at age 65 years. People older than 40 years are the largest increased-risk group. Fewer than 10% of cancers of the colorectum occur in people younger than 40 years. The increase in incidence occurs into the eighth decade of life, when a decline begins. The most common risk factor for polyp development is age greater than 50 years.[94]

GENETIC RISK FACTORS

FAMILIAL POLYPOSIS SYNDROMES

FAP syndromes are a group of syndromes characterized by the early onset of multiple polyps and a virtually 100% risk of colorectal cancer development.[95] FAP represents but a small percentage of the overall number of colorectal cancer cases. Its importance as a model for sporadic colorectal cancer development far outweighs its importance as a problem in public health.[96] It affects from 1 in 8000 to 1 in 10,000 persons. These syndromes have autosomal dominant inheritance with high but variable penetrance. The phenotype may vary by mutation site.[97] Synchronous cancers are common in FAP patients.

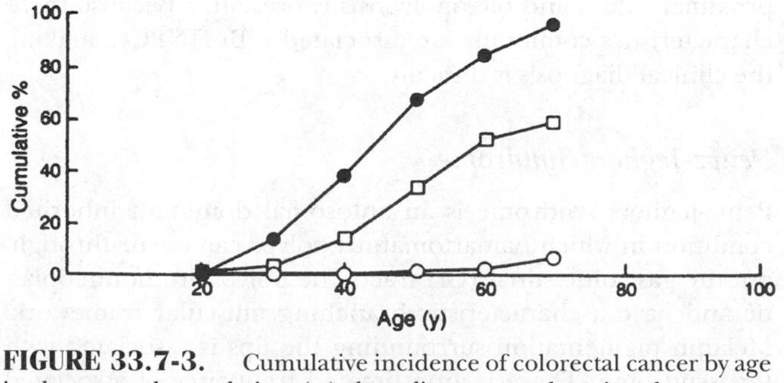

FIGURE 33.7-3. Cumulative incidence of colorectal cancer by age in the general population (○), hereditary nonpolyposis colon cancer population (□), and familial adenomatous polyposis population (●).

There is an association between FAP and periampullary, thyroid, and specific cancers or nonneoplastic growth such as osteomas, sebaceous cysts, and gastric fundic gland polyps. It is important to realize that 10% to 20% of the cases are *de novo* mutations with no apparent family history. After the colorectal cancer risk has been controlled by surgery, other neoplasms such as periampullary tumors are prominent causes of death among people with FAP.[98]

A subset of polyposis patients have Gardner's syndrome, which is characterized by colonic adenomatous polyposis associated with the presence of mesenteric or abdominal wall desmoid tumors, lipomas, and fibromas.[99] The presence of a mesenteric desmoid tumor is a cause of great morbidity in these patients. Other diseases included under the category of polyposis syndromes are Turcot's syndrome and Oldfield's syndrome. Hamilton[96a] has described the presence of two germline defects in Turcot's syndrome that are seen with both polyposis and HNPCC syndromes. There can often be considerable overlap between these adenomatous polyposis syndromes, and they are best characterized on the basis of their common genetic abnormality in the adenomatosis polyposis coli (*APC*) gene.

The basic genetic defect in FAP is a mutation in the *APC* gene. The genetic locus for the *APC* gene has been identified at 5q21.[100] The most common abnormality is an alteration in the genetic sequence resulting in the generation of a stop codon, which in turn results in the production of a truncated nonfunctional protein.[101] This is the basis for a commonly used screening procedure in which the truncated protein is synthesized *in vitro* and is identified. Since the introduction of genetic testing into the medical armamentarium, it is important that patients have access to appropriate genetic counseling and proper interpretation of test results.[102]

HEREDITARY NONPOLYPOSIS COLON CANCER

The HNPCC syndrome is inherited as an autosomal dominant trait with high penetrance. Its phenotypic features are early-onset colorectal cancer (mean age, 46 years), multiple (synchronous or metachronous) colorectal cancers (35%), and colorectal cancers usually (but not always) located in the proximal colon.[103] There is an associated early onset of adenocarcinoma of the colon, ovary, pancreas, breast, bile duct, endometrium, stomach, genitourinary tract, and small bowel.[104] In addition, sebaceous gland adenomas and carcinomas are seen in the Muir-Torre syndrome, a variant of HNPCC.[105] A high rate of colorectal cancer is seen in first-degree relatives of patients with HNPCC.[106] Approximately 1% to 6% of colorectal cancers fit the criteria for HNPCC.[107]

The phenomenon of microsatellite instability is present in the tumor of patients (90%) with HNPCC and in 12% to 15% of sporadic colorectal cancer cases. The genes responsible for this are *hMSH2, hMLH1, PMS1, PMS2,* and *hMSH6.*[108] Germline mutations in these genetic loci produce the DNA mismatch repair phenomenon, causing the development of colorectal cancer in patients with HNPCC. Though the results of genetic testing depend on criteria used for instituting testing, the overall mutation detection rate appears to be greater than 50% in suspected cases.[109]

HNPCC cancers are more likely to be signet-ring cancers and poorly differentiated, with extensive inflammatory infiltrates.[110,111] There may be a more rapid time course for the

TABLE 33.7-2. Amsterdam II Criteria

There should be at least three relatives with an HNPCC-associated cancer (CRC, endometrium, small bowel, ureter, or renal pelvis).
One affected relative should be a first-degree relative of the other two.
At least two successive generations should be affected.
At least one relative should receive diagnosis before age 50 years.
Familial adenomatous polyposis should be excluded.
Tumors should be verified by pathologic examination.

CRC, colorectal carcinoma; HNPCC, hereditary nonpolyposis colon cancer.

development of cancers in this syndrome.[107] The adenomas tend to have a villous component and to be more dysplastic than in sporadic cases.[112] In general, on a stage-for-stage basis, survival for colorectal cancer patients with HNPCC is better than for patients with sporadic cases.[104]

The Amsterdam criteria, developed in 1991, are helpful in identifying and categorizing patients with a familial history of colorectal cancer.[113] The initial Amsterdam criteria—Criteria I—require first that at least three relatives have colorectal cancer. In addition, one of the three relatives must be a first-degree relative of the other two; the colorectal cancer must involve at least two successive generations; at least one family member who developed colorectal cancer must be younger than 50 years; and FAP must by excluded and tumors must be verified by pathologic examination.[113] These criteria may underestimate the true incidence of HNPCC as pedigree analysis is uninformative for some families.[110] Because the initial Amsterdam criteria were established to be specific and to define criteria for HNPCC recognition strictly, families with more subtle histories or extracolonic cancers may be missed. Therefore, newer criteria were established to address these concerns.[112]

Amsterdam Criteria II (Table 33.7-2) include consideration of extracolonic tumors and eliminate the requirement that one of the index cancers be a colorectal cancer. The HNPCC cancers accepted are colorectal, endometrial, small bowel, ureteral, or renal pelvic. This less exclusionary set of criteria will reduce the number of families in which colorectal cancer is suspected but that fail to receive genetic counseling and mutation analysis. Counseling is critical for appropriate management.[114]

Aaltonen et al.[115] examined the feasibility of screening for HNPCC mutations in patients with colorectal carcinoma. They prospectively screened tumor specimens from patients with colorectal adenocarcinomas for microsatellite instability. DNA from the normal tissues of patients with tumors demonstrating replication errors was screened for germline mutations in the mismatched repair genes *MLH1* and *MSH2*. Sixteen percent of patients with replication errors had detectable germline mutations. All the patients in whom germline mutations were detected had a family history of colorectal cancer or were younger than 50 years. In patients with replication errors, further testing should be carried out for germline mutations in known DNA mismatch repair genes.

Because successful strategies for identifying patients suspected of harboring HNPCC have been terminated, the Bethesda guidelines for testing colorectal tumors for microsatellite instability have been developed (Table 33.7-3). These guidelines are expected to apply to 15% to 20% of colorectal cancer patients in the United States.

TABLE 33.7-3. Bethesda Guidelines for Testing Colorectal Tumors for Microsatellite Instability

1. Individuals with cancer in families that meet the Amsterdam Criteria
2. Individuals with two HNPCC-related cancers, including synchronous and metachronous colorectal cancer or associated extracolonic cancers
3. Individuals with colorectal cancer and a first-degree relative with colorectal cancer or HNPCC-related extracolonic cancer (or both) or a colorectal adenoma (one of the cancers diagnosed at age <46 y and the adenoma diagnosed at age <40 y)
4. Individuals with colorectal cancer or endometrial cancer diagnosed at age <45 y
5. Individuals with right-sided colorectal cancer with an undifferentiated pattern (solid, cribriform) on histopathology in whom diagnosis is made at age <45 y
6. Individuals with signet-ring type colorectal cancer diagnosed at age <45 y
7. Individuals with adenomas diagnosed at age <40 y

HNPCC, hereditary nonpolyposis colon cancer.

INHERITED COLORECTAL CANCER IN ASHKENAZI JEWS

Israeli Jews of European birth have the highest colorectal cancer incidence of any Israeli ethnic group. There are reports of a missense mutation (I 1307 K) in the *APC* gene found in 6% of unselected Ashkenazi Jews and 28% of this population who have a family history of colorectal cancer. Colorectal cancer is found in 13% of those with polyps.[116,117] This condition lacks the florid polyposis seen in FAP. These polymorphisms of the *APC* gene create a hypermutable region of the *APC* gene that causes a predisposition to colorectal cancer.[118] There do not appear to be any differences in clinical presentation or family history between carriers of the mutation and noncarriers, so genetic testing in this population may be required to identify high-risk individuals for screening. This mutation appears to be unique to Ashkenazi Jews.[116]

ATTENUATED FAMILIAL ADENOMATOUS POLYPOSIS SYNDROME

Attenuated FAP syndrome is characterized by the development of flat adenomas that are precursor lesions to carcinoma.[67] Genetic linkage studies identify abnormalities on chromosome 5Q, and this may be a variant of FAP, with the mutation being more proximal or distal in the gene than common mutations with classic FAP. In patients with attenuated FAP syndrome, disease onset is later than usual for FAP, neoplasms appear in the proximal colon, and oligopolyposis is present.[97] Because these characteristics commonly are associated with HNPCC, making the clinical diagnosis is difficult.

Peutz-Jeghers Syndrome

Peutz-Jeghers syndrome is an autosomal dominant inherited condition in which hamartomatous polyps can occur throughout the gastrointestinal (GI) tract. The polyps are nonneoplastic and have a characteristic branching muscular framework. Melanin pigmentation surrounding the lips is associated with this syndrome. There is an estimated frequency of associated GI cancer of 2% to 3%. Although these patients may develop a variety of cancers throughout life, their polyps should be managed symptomatically. Prophylactic colectomy is not recommended. Germline mutations in a chromosome 19 gene have been found in Peutz-Jeghers syndrome families. This gene may act as a tumor suppressor gene.[119] Inactivating mutations in the responsible gene act on a protein kinase.[119]

Juvenile Polyposis

In juvenile polyposis, multiple hamartomatous polyps occur in the colorectum, although they may also be found in the small bowel and stomach. Jass et al.[120] defined this syndrome as the presence of more than five juvenile polyps, which differs from the solitary juvenile polyp seen in children. These investigators found colorectal cancer in 18 of 80 cases.[120] Neoplasia can occur in the index polyps or in a separate adenoma. Colonoscopic control of polyps appears appropriate, whereas colectomy may be used for large numbers of polyps, symptomatic polyps, or cancers.[121]

A subset of patients with juvenile polyposis has been identified to carry germline mutations in the *SMAD4* gene,[122] which causes a defect in growth factor control. The risk of colorectal cancer has been estimated at 38%. There is a 21% risk of upper GI cancers.[123]

FAMILY HISTORY OF COLON CARCINOMA OR POLYPS

Even among populations that do not exhibit any of the well-characterized familial cancer syndromes, there is an increased risk among those who have first-degree relatives with colorectal cancer. This group accounts for most of the increased risk population (15% to 20% of patients).[124] An autosomal dominant mode of inheritance has been suggested. Depending on the age at onset of the cancer and the number of relatives involved, lifetime risk can increase from 1.8-to 8-fold.[125] It appears that the age-adjusted risk for those with one affected first-degree relative is approximately 1.72 (CI, 1.34 to 2.19).[126] For those with two or more affected first-degree relatives, the risk is 2.75 (CI, 1.34 to 5.63). The age at onset of the colorectal cancer in the affected relative is an important factor: Risk can be increased 5.37-fold (CI, 1.98 to 14.6) in those who have an affected first-degree relative whose colorectal cancer occurred at less than 45 years of age.[127] When the age at onset is 60 years or older, there is little increased risk, beyond that of having an affected first-degree relative.[126] People with first-degree relatives having colorectal cancer have an 8% risk of developing large adenomas, and colonoscopy appears to be the most appropriate screening technique for these lesions.[128]

In the review of data from participants in the National Polyp Study who had a newly diagnosed adenomatous polyp, information was gathered on the history of colorectal cancer in their parents and siblings.[129] The RR of colorectal cancer was 1.78 for parents and siblings of patients with adenomas as compared with controls. The RR for colorectal cancer in siblings of patients in whom adenomas were diagnosed before 60 years of age was 2.59 (CI, 1.46 to 4.58). When this group was compared with the siblings of patients 60 years of age or older at the time of diagnosis, a decrease in the risk for colorectal cancer was associated with an increase in age at the time of diagnosis of the adenoma. First-degree relatives of patients with adenomatous polyps are at increased risk for developing colorectal cancer, particularly when an adenoma is diagnosed before the age of 60 or, in the case of siblings, when a parent has had colorectal cancer. The subsequent familial risk of colon cancer is independent of the size and histologic features of the polyp.

PREDISPOSING MEDICAL CONDITIONS

INFLAMMATORY BOWEL DISEASE

There is an increased colorectal cancer risk in patients with inflammatory bowel disease.[131] Specifically, patients with ulcerative colitis demonstrate a high risk of colorectal cancer that is related to the duration and extent of disease and dysplasia.[132] The risk of colorectal cancer in people with ulcerative colitis is estimated to be 5% or 10% at 20 years after diagnosis of ulcerative colitis and 12% to 20% at 30 years.[133] This justifies the intensive surveillance that is carried out in patients with longstanding disease, especially those who demonstrate pancolitis. Synchronous cancers are seen in 10% to 20% of cases.[134]

Genetic alterations associated with inflammatory bowel disease suggest that there are accumulated genetic defects similar to those of sporadic carcinomas.[135] The pattern of progressive genetic abnormalities has been confirmed by analysis of p53 abnormalities found in both active colitis and dysplasia. The RR for patients with proctitis alone is 1.7 (CI, 4.6 to 7.0); patients with left-sided colitis have an RR of 2.8 (CI, 1.6 to 4.4); and a 14.8-fold RR (the highest risk of colorectal cancer) is seen in those suffering from pancolitis (CI, 11.4 to 18.9). The mean age at onset of cancer has been found to be 48 years. The value of assessment of cancer risk based totally on the presence of dysplasia has been questioned.[136] Ulcerative colitis patients operated on for colorectal cancer may not have a preoperative diagnosis of dysplasia. Other researchers have found that screening for high-grade dysplasia is a useful marker of the risk of coexistent cancer mandating colectomy.

GRANULOMATOUS COLITIS

Crohn's disease can affect the ileocolic area or may be limited to portions of the colon. In the absence of colonic involvement, there is no increased risk of colorectal cancer. The RR for ileocolic involvement was 3.2 and, for colonic involvement, was 5.6. The RR for those with colonic involvement in whom diagnosis was made before age 30 was 20.9.[137] In addition to being at increased risk for large bowel cancer, all patients with Crohn's disease also have an increased risk of small bowel carcinomas.[138] In studies of specimens of intestinal adenocarcinoma complicating Crohn's disease, an early age at onset for adenocarcinomas (49 years) was noted.[138] The carcinomas are associated with the site of the Crohn's disease. Seventy-three percent of the intestinal cancers in patients with Crohn's disease are found in the colon or rectum. Most carcinomas were found to be poorly differentiated. Dysplasia was found adjacent to carcinoma in 87% of the cases. Mucinous adenocarcinomas accounted for one-third of the carcinomas affecting Crohn's disease.[139]

HISTORY OF COLORECTAL CARCINOMA OR POLYPS

The incidence of metachronous colorectal cancer often is reported to be between 0.5% and 3%.[140] In an analysis that takes into account the number of patients remaining at each time point during follow-up, the incidence at 18 years was

6.3%.[141] In this study of 5476 patients, it was also demonstrated that metachronous colorectal cancers were diagnosed at earlier stages than were index lesions. Metachronous tumors occur four times more often in patients with HNPCC.[142] An Italian study of patients with multiple tumors of the large bowel demonstrated that the interval between first and second malignancies was 8.7 years. The recommendations for colonoscopic follow-up and complete colonic evaluation at the time of colorectal cancer diagnosis are based on these risks.

A personal history of colonic polyps is important in the risk assessment of patients for colon carcinoma. The presence of adenomatous polyps within the colon carries a risk of carcinoma in the index polyp as well as for additional sites within the colon. The risk of carcinoma in the individual polyp is related to the size and the histology of the polyp. Tubular adenomas are less likely to carry a risk of carcinoma as compared with villous polyps. In general, approximately half of the polyps larger than 2 cm will harbor a carcinoma. The greater the number of adenomas, the more likely it is that a cancer will develop. If these multiple polyps harbor advanced characteristics, the incidence of colon cancer development increases sixfold (OR, 6.6; CI, 3.3 to 11.8).[143]

In studies of patients with colon polyps identified on flexible sigmoidoscopy, it was found that at complete colonoscopy, 20% had advanced lesions such as adenomas greater than 1 cm with a villous component, severe dysplasia, or invasive cancer.[144] The risk of proximal colonic neoplasia was increased with sessile lesions in the distal colorectum.[145] In a multicenter, prospective study of colonoscopic findings in patients with proximal colon cancer, 116 patients were found to have cancer proximal to the splenic flexure, and 34% had neoplasia distal to the splenic flexure.[145] Most average-risk patients with proximal colon cancer will have normal results on flexible sigmoidoscopy.

After the removal of rectal or sigmoid polyps with villous or tubulovillous histology or size greater than 1 cm, the rate of colon cancer incidence was increased threefold over the general population (OR, 3.6; CI, 2.4 to 5.0).[143] The cumulative incidence of colon cancer appears to be approximately 4% at 5 years and 14% at 10 years in patients with an untreated rectosigmoid polyp. Sixty-six percent of these cancers are in the index polyp, and 34% are at other sites.[146] These findings help to demonstrate the effectiveness of polypectomy in preventing colon cancer.[147]

PELVIC IRRADIATION

The data implicating irradiation as a cause of colorectal cancer are controversial.[148] Such reports imply that patients are followed up for extremely long periods, because the interval between pelvic irradiation and the onset of a radiation therapy–induced GI tract malignancy appears to be 15 to 28 years.[149] The radiation doses and techniques may have an impact on the overall incidence of GI tract cancers induced by pelvic radiation therapy. Second cancers are increased in patients with previous malignancies. The risk of colorectal cancer in this population is small and should not alter plans for curative treatment for pelvic malignancies.

NONCANCER SURGERY

Some studies suggest that cholecystectomy increases the incidence of colorectal cancer. The etiology for the relationship between cholecystectomy and colorectal carcinoma is controversial.[150] In a study conducted in the United Kingdom, a metaanalysis of 35 studies was conducted.[151] The OR for a positive association between cholecystectomy and colorectal cancer was found to be only 1.11 (95% CI, 1.02 to 1.21). For women, the OR was 1.14 (95% CI, 1.01 to 1.28) and, for right-sided cancers, the ratio was 1.86 (95% CI, 1.31 to 2.65). It appeared from this that any additional risk was quite small. Data from case-control studies have shown an increased risk for proximal colon cancers after cholecystectomy. However, there was no indication that there was an increased risk for distal colorectal cancer.[152] The risk of colorectal cancer after cholecystectomy cannot be separated from the presence of cholelithiasis as a possible marker for dietary changes that affect colorectal cancer risk.[153] The risks associated with ureterosigmoidostomy may be related to the presence of mutagens within the stool or urine. An additional factor is that patients subjected to such operations may have confounding factors such as previous pelvic irradiation.

SCREENING

Screening involves testing asymptomatic individuals to assess the likelihood that they may have colorectal cancer or precursors. For a screening technique to be practical, it must be a risk-based approach to the assessment of asymptomatic patients. Colorectal cancer lends itself to screening because of the long period between the development of early mucosal abnormalities and the development of invasive carcinoma.[143–146] Adenomatous polyps are the well-described precursor lesions of invasive colorectal cancer and can be effectively managed by endoscopic intervention.[147] In the general population, the risk of development of a colorectal adenoma is approximately 19%, and it is estimated that 2% to 5% of these sporadic polyps will develop into an invasive carcinoma.[154]

Screening tests are available that detect early curable disease and are well-established aspects of medical practice.[155] The screening techniques do not involve excessive risk.[156] The benefits of early diagnosis are improvements in treatment effectiveness and survival.

SCREENING OF HIGH-RISK GROUPS

Familial Adenomatous Polyposis

Once an average-risk person reaches the fourth decade of life, his or her risk of developing colorectal cancer increases almost 100%. Screening is not an effective management tool. On establishment of a diagnosis of FAP, patients should be considered for colectomy to reduce the risk of colorectal cancer development. In cases in which there is a remaining rectal stump that has been cleared of polyps, the patient should undergo annual screening to assess for polyp development and the need for proctectomy or fulguration of polyps. The usual recommendation is to start annual screening for FAP during early adolescence. If no polyps are found after age 24, the screening schedule can be modified to every 2 years until age 34, then every 3 years until age 44, when screening reverts to that of an average-risk individual. Molecular testing for genetic mutations is appropriate in screening at-risk family members when the mutation is known.

Hereditary Nonpolyposis Colon Cancer

Patients affected by HNPCC have cancers that develop from adenomatous polyps that are commonly proximal to the splenic flexure. The risk of colorectal cancer in HNPCC patients begins to increase by age 20 and is very high by age 45.[157] The risk for colorectal cancer by age 60 is estimated to be 57% to 80%.[158] Colonoscopy is the preferred method of surveillance because it allows complete examination of the colon. Its yields are high in HNPCC because of the high risk of cancer. Metachronous cancers are common in people who have an intact colon after an initial cancer; the annual rate of metachronous colorectal cancer appears to be 2.1% to 1.7%.

There is a concern of rapid *de novo* development of carcinomas from flat lesions that may be inapparent during endoscopy. Therefore, intervals between screening for HNPCC patients should probably be shorter than for average-risk persons. Because of a higher 5-year survival of colorectal cancer in many patients with HNPCC as compared to patients with sporadic colorectal cancer, it may be even more beneficial to screen these patients than average-risk patients. The Cancer Genetic Studies Consortium reviewed the literature on cancer surveillance and risk reduction for individuals with HNPCC and concluded that the efficacy of cancer surveillance in reducing risk in these individuals is unknown. However, on the basis of observational studies, the Consortium recommended colonoscopy every 1 to 3 years starting at age 25 for individuals known to have HNPCC-associated mutations.

Jarvinen et al.[159] described the effects of screening on colorectal cancer rates in families with HNPCC. They evaluated the effectiveness of long-term screening in 22 families with HNPCC. The incidence of colorectal cancer and colorectal cancer mortality between those who were screened at 3-year intervals by colonoscopy or barium enema sigmoidoscopy and those who did not undergo screening were compared. Colorectal cancer occurred in 4.5% of the screened subjects and 11.9% of the unscreened group. No deaths due to colorectal cancer occurred in the screened group, as compared with colorectal cancer death in 5 of the 14 cases in the control group.[159] This provides strong evidence that increased screenings reduce the colorectal cancer death rate in members of families with a history of HNPCC.

Syngal et al.[160] conducted a decision analysis study of the benefits of colonoscopic surveillance and subsequent colectomy on mortality and quality of life for patients with HNPCC mutations. They assessed risk for colorectal cancer in the study to be 31.5% by 40 years, 54.5% by 50 years, 63% by 60 years, and 87.5% by 75 years of age. The cumulative lifetime risk for colorectal cancer was 88.2%. The risk of metachronous colorectal cancer was estimated at 45% in those not undergoing a prophylactic total colectomy. Endoscopic surveillance would reduce lifetime risk by 52%. Mortality from endoscopic surveillance was estimated to be approximately 0.02%. These investigators found a life expectancy benefit of 2.1 years associated with prophylactic colectomy as compared with surveillance.[160] However, when estimates of health-related quality of life were incorporated into the analysis, surveillance became the preferred cancer prevention mode.

In a study using data from the International Collaborative Group on HNPCC, rectal cancers were found to have developed in 11% of patients at a median of 158 months from the time of their abdominal colectomy.[161] Adenomas were found to have developed in the rectal mucosa in five of eight of the patients who developed rectal carcinoma and hence were deemed a marker of risk. The risk of developing rectal cancer was estimated to be 3% for every 3 years after abdominal colectomy for the first 12 years of follow-up. The authors recommended endoscopic surveillance of the rectum after abdominal colectomy. Lin et al. (1998) estimated that rectal cancer was more common in *MSH2* kindreds.

Family History of Colorectal Cancer or Adenomatous Polyps

Specialty organizations recommend that people with first-degree relatives who have had colorectal cancer or adenomatous polyps should be screened on a schedule similar to that for average-risk persons but beginning at age 40 instead of 50.[157] Individuals who have a relative with early-onset disease should begin surveillance 3 to 10 years prior to the age of onset in the index individual. Owing to the overlap between patients who have been affected by an HNPCC mutation and an otherwise genetically undefined familial colorectal cancer risk, it is prudent to consider complete examination of the colon in these patients as opposed to flexible sigmoidoscopy.[162]

Personal History of Colorectal Cancer or Adenomatous Polyps

Patients who have had a previous colorectal cancer are at increased risk for polyp formation and development of second primary cancers. It is recommended that patients in whom a colorectal cancer has been resected undergo complete examination of the colon within 1 year after resection. This surveillance schedule is similar to that recommended for patients with a previous polypectomy. If the results of this examination are otherwise normal, then the patient can undergo evaluation in 3 years, with subsequent examinations dependent on the findings at that initial examination. Any subsequent cancers often are preceded by polyps, in the same adenoma-to-carcinoma sequence seen in sporadic colorectal cancer. Because of the effectiveness of polypectomy, the follow-up procedure should be colonoscopy.[162]

Patients who have undergone previous removal of an adenomatous polyp should undergo colonoscopy during follow-up. The rate of metachronous adenoma formation is 3.3% over 3 years.[147] The Polyp Prevention Study did not demonstrate any increase in risk of developing advanced polyps when subsequent screening was deferred for 3 years.[163] No direct evidence supports a recommendation for the cessation of screening.[164]

Inflammatory Bowel Disease

Because the rate of colorectal cancer development in patients with inflammatory bowel disease is related to dysplasia and duration and extent of disease, surveillance colonoscopy is an important consideration in the management of these patients.[165] Colonoscopic surveillance should begin annually after 8 years of disease in patients with pancolitis or after 15 years of disease in those with colitis involving the left side of the colon.[166] Random biopsy should be performed to detect dysplasia, which is a marker for the presence of colorectal cancer.[167] However, there is no direct evidence that this practice is more effective than colectomy performed on the basis of extent and duration of disease.

SCREENING OF AVERAGE-RISK GROUPS: THE GENERAL POPULATION

Subjects who are healthy and have an average risk of colon cancer represent the largest population appropriate for screening. There is a relatively high risk of colorectal cancer in the United States, and the screening can be targeted to older individuals in whom colorectal cancer is much more common. For average-risk groups, the screening techniques consist primarily of digital rectal examination, fecal occult blood testing, and endoscopic examination. It is hoped that less invasive but sensitive tests such as virtual colonoscopy may be useful in screening in the future.[168]

Any discussion of screening techniques must be analyzed in terms of the effectiveness and cost of such programs for asymptomatic individuals. These considerations and evolving clinical practice have generated recommendations that asymptomatic patients with no family history of colorectal cancer begin screening at 50 years of age with digital rectal examination and fecal occult blood assessment annually and flexible sigmoidoscopy every 5 years.[157] Alternative approaches may be total colonoscopy every 10 years or a double-contrast barium enema every 5 to 10 years.[169]

Digital Rectal Examination

The digital rectal examination is part of the routine physical examination. Approximately 5% to 10% of colorectal cancers may be palpable.

Fecal Occult Blood Testing

Fecal occult blood testing relies on the presence of blood in the stool to indicate a neoplastic lesion in the large bowel. Testing for the presence of fecal occult blood using guaiac-impregnated paper slides is a relatively low-cost examination that is based on the ability of heme to catalyze a reaction involving the oxidation of guaiac in the presence of hydrogen peroxide, which produces a blue stain.[170] Other techniques rely on the detection of hemoglobin by its conversion to porphyrin or the detection of human hemoglobin by immunochemical approaches.

The advantages of this test are ease, low cost, and low risk to the patient. The use of this test has been criticized, however, for its relatively low ability to predict the presence or absence of disease, leading to missed lesions (owing to poor sensitivity) and unnecessary invasive workups in patients without colorectal neoplasia. Nonetheless, studies have demonstrated a decline in mortality from colorectal cancer in patients screened annually with fecal occult blood testing as compared with control groups. This improvement is attributable to the fact that cancers detected by fecal occult blood testing were at an earlier stage of disease at diagnosis, resulting in a decrease in the proportion of patients who had metastatic disease at the time of cancer discovery. These findings support the use of this method of cancer screening.[171]

Not all rectal cancers bleed and not all blood in the GI tract is due to cancer. Some cancers may bleed intermittently. False-negative fecal occult blood test results have been reported in 20% to 30% of patients with known colorectal cancers.[172] The ability to detect polyps in the colon and rectum by testing for fecal occult blood is even less successful.[172] Yearly testing for fecal occult blood has been recommended, because randomized trials show that yearly testing is more effective than testing every 2 years.

Fecal occult blood testing provides only a suspicion of colorectal cancer or polyps. The consequences of a positive test are that the patient requires a complete colon examination, usually in the form of a barium enema and sigmoidoscopy or colonoscopy.[173] The costs and effectiveness of fecal occult blood testing as a screening modality must be evaluated in the context of these additional tests resulting from a positive examination. Elements of an ordinary diet, including red meat and certain vegetables that may have peroxidase activity, can cause false-positive reactions in guaiac-based tests. The use of salicylates and vitamin C can cause either false-positive or false-negative examinations, respectively.[174] Because of these factors, the best results for fecal occult blood testing in screening for colorectal cancer are from studies that use rehydrated tests on two samples from each of three consecutive stools in individuals who were adhering to a restricted diet and who were abstaining from compounds that could alter test results. Fecal occult blood testing is limited by the fact that the testing is aimed mainly at detecting cancer, owing to the low incidence of bleeding in small adenomatous polyps. An additional drawback of such testing is that the false-positive rate commits large groups of patients to undergoing the cost and inconvenience of testing with colonoscopy or barium enema when no colorectal pathologic process is present.[175]

In a randomized trial of 46,551 asymptomatic people between the ages of 50 and 80 years, fecal occult blood testing was studied. Patients were evaluated with colonoscopy after fecal occult blood tests proved positive. The 13-year cumulative mortality rate per 1000 from colorectal cancer was 5.88% in the annually screened group, 8.33% in the biannually screened group, and 8.83% in the control group.[86] A randomized, controlled trial was performed in England with patients aged 45 to 74 years who were offered either fecal occult blood testing every 2 years or routine medical management. Again, colonoscopy was used to evaluate positive tests, which resulted in a 15% reduction in mortality in the screened group.[172] Some practitioners have expressed concern that the improvement in mortality seen is these studies could be related to chance selection for colonoscopy and its effects.[176]

Flexible Sigmoidoscopy

Flexible sigmoidoscopy can be used to evaluate the region from the anal verge to approximately 60 cm of the distal large intestine. This can allow detection of up to one-half to two-thirds of colorectal adenomas and cancers.[177] Because distal adenomas and cancers are an indicator of more proximal neoplasia, a patient with findings of neoplastic polyp on flexible sigmoidoscopy should undergo complete colonic examination.

Flexible sigmoidoscopy screening programs can be expected to detect neoplasms in the distal colon and rectum in up to 8% of asymptomatic persons older than 40 years. Reductions in sigmoid and rectal cancer risk with rigid proctosigmoidoscopy of 70% were seen in a case-control study.[178,179] It has been proposed that once-only sigmoidoscopy would be a cost-effective method of screening and subsequently assigning patients to low- or high-risk groups.[180] Its use is a recommended part of screening for low- and average-risk patients older than 50 years in the Untied States.[157]

DIAGNOSIS

WORKUP OF A SYMPTOMATIC PATIENT

The diagnosis of colorectal cancer can be made either by the workup of a symptomatic patient or by discovery of cancer by screening in an asymptomatic patient. Most Americans are not currently screened for colorectal cancer. In a survey of the general population, it was found that only approximately 17.3% of people aged 50 years or older had undergone fecal occult blood testing in the previous year and that only 9.4% had undergone sigmoidoscopy in the previous 3 years. The majority of patients will be found to have colorectal cancer on investigation of symptoms or signs.

Patients who present with symptoms are not appropriate candidates for a screening examination (i.e., less than a total colonic examination). Those in whom symptoms are compatible with the diagnosis of colorectal cancer, such as those with rectal bleeding, iron-deficiency anemia, obstruction, or alteration in bowel habits, should undergo total colonic examination. Colonoscopy will allow biopsy of colonic masses as well as removal of polyps; however, a mass in the colon should not be managed conservatively, even in the case of an equivocal biopsy. Those individuals with obstructive tumors should undergo examination of the whole colon as soon as is practical after management of the obstructing tumor.

A wide variety of abdominal symptoms and signs are consistent with colorectal cancer. These include rectal bleeding, discovery of occult blood in the stool, abdominal pain, change in bowel habits, nausea, vomiting, distention, weight loss, fatigue, and anemia. Rectal bleeding is more commonly associated with rectal cancer than colon cancer. Because it can be such an obvious symptom, patients who develop rectal bleeding come to medical attention sooner than those who do not have obvious rectal bleeding. Patients who present with rectal bleeding must not be managed for hemorrhoids without workup, even though many more patients will have benign causes for rectal bleeding as compared to the number who will have rectal carcinoma.

Abdominal pain in colorectal cancer may be caused by partial obstruction, which is commonly a cramping type of pain. A more diffuse type of abdominal pain may occur with the development of perforations, leading to signs of generalized peritonitis. Other pain syndromes that may be present in colorectal carcinoma can develop from involvement of the pelvic floor by rectal cancer–caused tenesmus. Locally advanced rectal cancer may be associated with involvement of the sciatic nerve or obturator nerve, producing a neuropathic pain syndrome.

Partial or complete obstruction may occur in 2% to 16% of newly diagnosed cases of rectal cancer. The presence of obstruction has been found to reduce the 5-year survival rate to 31%, as compared with 72% for patients without obstruction.[181]

Malignancy of the colon can result in a free perforation with peritonitis or a contained perforation and fistula formation. Approximately half of perforations caused by colorectal cancer are into the free abdominal cavity. Contained perforation with involvement of adjacent organs is most commonly seen in cecal or sigmoid carcinomas. Either type of carcinoma may involve loops of small bowel, bladder, abdominal wall, or the retroperitoneum. When there is such involvement in the setting of a sigmoid colon carcinoma, the condition may mimic diverticulitis. Diagnosis in these circumstances can be difficult. It is justifiable to pursue surgery in such patients to clarify the diagnosis as well as to treat. Radiologic signs indicating diverticulitis include the presence or absence of intramural fistulas and the degree of mucosal abnormality. Tumor perforation can occur either at the site of a primary tumor or in the cecum when it is dilated because of obstruction. Perforation is a bad prognostic factor, not only because it heralds an increased risk of cancer spread but also because of the mortality associated with peritonitis.

In the 10% to 15% of patients who present with metastatic disease, signs and symptoms are usually present. Pain in the right upper quadrant, especially when accompanied by palpable hepatomegaly or a mass, often will indicate the presence of liver metastases. This finding should prompt investigation with imaging as well as endoscopy. Fever without an overt cause may also be a manifestation of metastatic disease. Patients with diffuse liver involvement or carcinomatosis may manifest ascites with signs of abdominal distention or symptoms of early satiety or bowel obstruction. Development of umbilical nodules may occur as a sign of intraperitoneal disease. In patients with advanced colorectal cancer, supraclavicular adenopathy may be present. Inguinal adenopathy may develop in patients with an advanced low rectal carcinoma.

PATHOLOGIC FEATURES

Gross Appearance

Size alone is not a reliable predictor of outcome from colorectal cancer because of the predominance of biologic behavior in predicting outcome. A 1-cm, clinically detectable colorectal neoplasm may contain 30 or more successive generations of malignant cells prior to detection. Colorectal cancers can be exophytic or fungating, or tumors may be ulcerated. In general, ulcerated tumors predominate. Annular tumors produce obstructive symptoms and have the classic appearance of an apple-core lesion on barium enema. Tumors of the right colon often are fungating masses that grow into the lumen and for which the symptom is occult bleeding as opposed to obstruction; they often present with a palpable mass. Left-sided tumors tend to be more annular and cause obstructive symptoms.

Residual adenomas can often be found in addition to invasive cancer. Assessment of the colon specimen for synchronous lesions is important. In 3% to 5% of primary colorectal cancers, a synchronous carcinoma will be found. The number and type of neoplastic lesions, polyps, or invasive carcinomas in a colorectal specimen are important in identifying associated inherited colorectal cancer syndromes.

Histologic Types

Adenocarcinoma represents 90% to 95% of all colorectal tumors. Tumors can be further classified by grade and histologic subtypes (Table 33.7-4).

The vast majority of colorectal cancers are moderately differentiated, gland-forming adenocarcinomas. Less common

TABLE 33.7-4. World Health Organization Classification of Malignant Primary Tumors of the Large Intestine: Histopathologic Variants of Colorectal Carcinoma

Mucinous adenocarcinoma
Signet-ring adenocarcinoma
Adenosquamous carcinoma
Squamous carcinoma
Small cell carcinoma
Choriocarcinoma
Medullary carcinoma

variants are classified on the basis of the predominance of an unusual pattern as compared with the usual adenocarcinoma of the colon. Mucinous or colloid carcinomas exhibit the majority of tumor in mucin pools, which are often of low cellularity.[182] Signet-ring tumors display a large amount of intracellular mucus pushing the nucleus to the side of the cell. These often are associated with diffuse intramural spread beyond the obvious mucosal lesion. In poorly differentiated cancers, features of neuroendocrine differentiation may appear.

Approximately 4% to 17% of carcinoid tumors appear in the rectum, and 2% to 7% are found in the colon.[183] They often present as submucosal masses with normal colonic mucosa overlying lesions. Sarcomas may account for 0.1% to 0.3% of all colorectal malignancies. These are chiefly leiomyosarcomas.

DEGREE OF DIFFERENTIATION. Broders (1925) designated four grades of differentiation based on the percentage of differentiated tumor cells found in the overall tumor specimen. The degree of differentiation for colonic adenocarcinoma commonly refers to the degree to which there are well-formed glands. There is a spectrum of histopathologic findings used to assess differentiation in typical cancers of the colon and rectum. Glands may range from large and dilated to small and compact. Gland formation is usually associated with tumors that are well or moderately differentiated. At the other extreme of differentiation, glandular architecture may form sheets of infiltrating individual cells, which characterize a poorly differentiated tumor.

Dukes' (1932) grading system was based on cytologic characteristics as well as glandular formation and nuclear polymorphism. the system ranges from stage A through stage D, the latter stage being the most poorly differentiated, with only occasional gland formation and markedly pleomorphic cells marked by a high incidence of mitoses. Jass et al. (1986) provided a system of classifying differentiation based on histologic type, overall differentiation, nuclear polarity, tubal configuration, pattern of growth, lymphocytic infiltration, and amount of desmoplastic reaction. Other aspects of the histopathologic evaluation of a colorectal tumor include assessments for vascular or lymphatic invasion. Extramural venous invasion is considered an indicator of worsening prognosis. Invasion of perineural spaces can be identified.

The degree of fibrosis present in tumors will vary widely. The pattern of infiltration at the edge of tumors can be pushing, expansile, or infiltrative. The host inflammatory response at the periphery of tumors can be composed of lymphocytes, neutrophils, mast cells, and macrophages. Angiogenesis may be noted at a tumor's periphery.

The inclusion of lymphoid nodules and germinal centers at the periphery of infiltrating carcinomas is termed a *Crohn's-like lymphoid reaction.* This is sometimes considered to be associated with HNPCC or with a high incidence of microsatellite instability.[184] Many of these adjunctive characteristics of the histopathologic assessment of a tumor are subject to considerable intraobserver and interobserver variability in reporting.

DEGREE OF LOCAL INVASION. Invasion into the submucosa is the hallmark of the development of the potential for metastatic spread and is the key histopathologic characteristic of colorectal cancer. It is best assessed by histopathologic assessment. In colon carcinoma, the mesentery and serosal surfaces are at greatest risk for violation by tumor penetration. In rectal cancer, perirectal fat and adjacent organs are most commonly involved by direct invasion through the bowel wall. Gross assessment of local extent can be misleading in some cases due to desmoplastic response, the effect of neoadjuvant therapies, or infection surrounding tumor perforation. Locally recurrent tumors are characterized by the predominance of the tumor mass in or around the bowel wall or an anastomotic site rather than in the mucosa itself.

Lymph Node Pathology

Gross pathologic evaluation of lymph nodes in colorectal cancer specimens is unreliable. Large nodes may show only lymphoid hyperplasia, whereas smaller nodes may harbor micrometastases detectable only by histologic examination, immunohistochemistry, or molecular techniques. This factor is important in understanding the inaccuracy of imaging techniques that typically rely on the size of lymph nodes as criteria for determining nodal involvement with tumor.

The number of lymph nodes found directly influences the accuracy and frequency of findings of Dukes' grade C cases.[185] By using more intensive methods of lymph node assessment such as fat clearance, fewer false-negative lymph node stagings occur.[186]

Goldstein et al.[187] showed an increase in the percentage of patients with at least one lymph node metastasis when 12 to 20 lymph nodes were recovered from each specimen, as compared with specimens in which fewer lymph nodes were found. Wong et al.[188] found, in a sample of patients statistically similar to a sample in the National Cancer Database Report, that examination of at least 14 T2 or T3 carcinoma colorectal cancer specimens was required to stage patients accurately.

Molecular Detection of Micrometastases

Owing to the effective use of adjuvant therapies for node-positive colorectal cancer, there is a theoretic advantage to the use of a more intensive method of detecting cancer cells in the lymph nodes of resected specimens. This improved detection is necessary of the approximately 20% rate of distant metastases in patients with resected stage II colon carcinoma who could theoretically benefit from systemic adjuvant chemotherapy. An increase in the detection of micrometastases has been demonstrated with fat-clearing techniques, serial sectioning, and immunohistochemistry, detection of epithelial antigens, and molecular screening with polymerase chain reaction–based (PCR-based) methods to detect tumor-specific RNA.[189] The detection of micrometastases in regional lymph nodes by PCR technique has been demonstrated to have prognostic value in stage II colon carcinoma.[189] Though the potential for the use of these techniques is great, currently gross pathology and histopathology are the mainstays of pathologic staging of colorectal carcinoma.

SPREAD OF COLORECTAL CANCER

The capability of a tumor to invade and metastasize is not only the most visible hallmark of cancer but also the leading cause of death in cancer patients. Colorectal cancers can spread locally or distantly via the lymphatic and venous systems. In addition to unregulated tumor growth, imbalances in regulation of motility and proteolysis are required for those events to occur.[190] We owe much of our current knowledge in this area to the pioneering work of Dukes et al. in the early 1930s involving careful analyses of rectal cancer cases. Although Dukes's work helped to explain the natural history of colorectal cancer and this information remains largely current, it hypothesized a very rigid pattern of spread. Dukes believed that lymph node invasion and distant metastasis could occur only after the tumor had extended through the bowel wall. Although years earlier, Miles had described metastasis with earlier-stage primaries, Dukes considered these rare events. Dukes hypothesis could not explain why a large number of patients with complete surgical resection eventually die of tumor recurrence.

LOCAL SPREAD

Percival Cole, in 1913, was the first to report that colorectal cancers usually grow preferentially in the transverse direction rather than in the horizontal direction. After reviewing 20 rectal cancer specimens, he made the important observation that the long axis of the ulcerating tumor was always transverse, with the lesion tending to involve the bowel circularly rather than longitudinally. Therefore, the tumors tended to narrow and constrict the bowel wall. Contrary to the previously held belief, Cole theorized that recurrences were due to extramural deposits of tumor cells that were not removed by local excision and not to persistence of tumor along the bowel wall. Several authors corroborated Cole's findings.

One notable exception to this common pattern of circumferential growth is seen in tumors showing perineural invasion. Tumor cells may reach as far as 10 cm from the primary tumor when spreading through the perineural spaces, and local recurrences are 2.5 times more frequent in patients who present with perineural invasion than in patients who do not. This preferential mural growth, the importance of which was recognized early, may result in local failure and peritoneal seeding. Staging systems from the initial work by Dukes to the tumor, node, metastasis (TNM) system used today have included degree of mural invasion as one of the most important prognostic factors.

LYMPHATIC EXTENSION

As early as 1925, Miles described cases of early rectal cancers presenting with lymph node involvement. Although Dukes initially incorrectly considered these events to be rare, he and Bussey (1958) demonstrated the direct relationship of the extent of local spread to the incidence of lymphatic metastasis. Grinnell (1964) was able to demonstrate that tumor limited to the submucosa and muscularis propria metastasized to lymph nodes in 13% of patients. More recent studies have corroborated these findings, with a 10% to 20% incidence of lymph node metastasis for tumors limited to the bowel wall.[191]

In 1935, Gabriel et al. analyzed 62 specimens with lymphatic metastasis and described the orderly and predictable course of lymphatic spread in rectal cancer. One-half of the patients studied had three fewer glands involved, and half had four or more. Dukes hypothesized that if the spread from gland to gland had been rapid, patients would either have no lymph node involvement or multiple glands at the time of diagnoses. Hence, he concluded that the lymphatic spread was a slow process. The first glands to be involved were situated in the perirectal tissues at the level of the primary tumor or immediately above it, followed by the chain along the superior hemorrhoidal vessels. In an advanced case, the involved lymph nodes extended to the ligature of the inferior mesentery vessels. The same orderly progression was demonstrated by Gilchrist and David.[192]

Exceptions to this orderly spread are possible and have been well-documented by Gabriel et al. (1935). Atypical presentations could be due to spread through aberrant lymphatic routes, which were described as early as 1925. Several authors have documented the existence of these discontinuous or skip metastases. Wood and Wilkie (1933) found them in 6 of 51 specimens, Gabriel et al. (1935) in 1 of 62, and Grinnell (1939) in 4 of 118 specimens.

A second exception to the usual mode of lymphatic spread is seen when the lymphatics are blocked by tumor. When this occurs, the natural interconnection of lymphatic channels allows lymph nodes at a great distance from the relevant chain to be affected. Lymphatic obstructions are responsible for the retrograde extension of tumor below the primary lesion.[193] In a review of 913 specimens from patients with colorectal cancer, Grinnell (1966) found 34 (3.7%) to have this type of spread. In colon carcinoma, the lymphatic flow follows the major arteries, with three levels of lymph nodes: pericolic, intermediate, and principal. Tumors located between more than one major vessel may metastasize in any direction.

Dukes divided 985 rectal cancers into four different categories depending on the tumor grade. Stage A tumors were very well differentiated, whereas stage D tumors were anaplastic. There was a close correlation between the tumor grade and the incidence of local spread, lymph node involvement, and venous spread. The same correlation between tumor grade and lymphatic involvement has been demonstrated by other researchers.

With the advent of advanced staging techniques such as sentinel node biopsy and molecular analysis of lymph nodes, the existence of discontinuous or skip metastases needs to be taken into consideration when planning changes in current surgical techniques.

HEMATOGENOUS SPREAD

Despite our continuous efforts toward early detection, approximately 10% to 15% of colorectal cancer patients have evidence of distant metastasis at the time of the initial diagnosis. The liver is by far the most commonly involved organ. The colon is drained by the portal venous system. The rectum is drained by two different systems: The superior hemorrhoidal veins enter the portal system to the liver, whereas the middle and inferior hemorrhoidal veins drain to the inferior vena cava and spread to the lungs via the systemic circulation. This dual venous drainage system has important implications in the pattern of hematogenous spread. Brown and Warren[194] retrospectively analyzed the results of 70 autopsies in patients with rectal cancer. They identified 23 patients (33%) with metastasis to the liver only and 6 patients (9%) with metastasis to the lung only. Metastasis to other sites without liver or lung involvement were rare, seen in only three patients (4%). The patients with lung metastasis only were found to have lower primary lesions. In a larger study involving 506 patients, Dionne (1965) described rectal cancer patients with upper rectal lesions and lung metastasis only. However, because metastasis was determined in routine clinical examinations, liver metastasis may have been missed in those patients.

Brown and Warren reported that 14% of the patients they analyzed had vertebral involvement. In his larger series, Dionne (1965) described 6% of the patients with spread to the pelvis and lumbosacral spine. Even though some (or even most) of those lesions were the result of direct extension or were present in patients with widespread metastases, at least some patients have isolated metastases to the spine. Although the vertebral venous plexus is a high-pressure system, it may open during special circumstances, such as defecation. This would allow tumor cells to invade vertebral bones and the central nervous system using communications between the portal system and the paravertebral veins.

IMPLANTATION

Implantation refers to the capability of cancer cells to deposit and grow on another surface after being released from the primary tumor. Most normal human cells, regardless of their origin, are in constant contact with an extracellular matrix and cannot survive for long when away from it, undergoing apoptosis or cell-cycle arrest.[195] However, cancer cells have been known to be able to survive without interaction with an extracellular matrix. The ability of cancer cells to detach from the primary tumor and either to penetrate into the circulation or to implant in a different surface away from their original extracellular matrix is most likely related to changes in the cell adhesion molecules.[195]

Implantation may occur when cancer cells are shed intraluminally, from the serosal surface, and by surgical manipulation.[196] Umpleby and Williamson (1987) determined the viability of tumor cells shed into the intestinal lumen in 49 patients. Viable exfoliated tumor cells were demonstrated in 52 of 74 specimens collected (70%).[197] The number of viable tumor cells recovered from the distal resection margin was inversely related to the distance of the tumor from that margin, confirming earlier observations made by McGrew et al. (1954). Zeng et al.[196] prospectively scraped the serosa overlying the primary tumor mass in 65 patients who underwent surgery for colon cancer. Malignant cells were present in the cytologic analysis of 23% of all patients and 26% of those with tumors invading through the muscularis propria but not through serosa. After reviewing clinical, reoperation, and autopsy series, Brodsky and Cohen[198] determined the incidence of peritoneal seeding followed by peritoneal failure to be fairly frequent among patients who experience recurrence of colorectal cancer. The risk of colorectal cancer spread caused by surgical manipulation is well recognized, and the improvement of surgical technique has been considered a way of preventing recurrences since the early decades of the twentieth century.

STAGING AND PROGNOSTIC FEATURES

The most reliable prognostic factor identified to date in colorectal cancer is the staging of disease at the time that treatment is initiated.[199] The staging of colorectal cancer has been an evolving field since the beginning of the twentieth century, with multiple authors attempting to develop a reliable and reproducible system. The first widely used system was introduced by Dukes in the 1930s and, like the majority of staging systems developed to date, relied on information obtained during surgery. Imaging techniques used preoperatively have not been successful in reliably staging colorectal cancer.[200] Both conventional computed tomography (CT) scanning and conventional magnetic resonance imaging have an unacceptably low accuracy for identifying the early stages of primary colorectal cancers.[200] The low staging accuracy of these imaging techniques is related to the fact that neither method can assess the depth of tumor infiltration within the bowel wall, and both have difficulty in diagnosing lymph node involvement. For colorectal cancer patients evaluated with CT scans or magnetic resonance imaging, the overall accuracy of primary tumor staging is approximately 70%, with sensitivity for lymph node detection of only approximately 45%. The sensitivity for positive lymph nodes is higher for rectal tumors.[200] The development of new imaging techniques such as positron emission tomography (PET)[201] and endoscopic ultrasonography[202,203] may enhance the usefulness of imaging studies in the staging of colorectal cancer. These imaging techniques would be especially important in rectal cancer, wherein preoperative treatment with chemotherapy and radiation therapy is a viable therapeutic option.[204]

Besides the pathologic staging determined by depth of penetration through the bowel wall and involvement of lymph nodes, distant organs, or both, several other potential independent factors for survival have been identified. The number of factors reported to have an impact on the overall survival of patients with colorectal cancer continues to grow, but the prognostic value of few of these factors has been confirmed in larger trials. The presence of obstruction or perforation,[205] vascular or lymphatic invasion (or both), perineural invasion,[206] peritumoral lymphocytic invasion,[207] the character of invasive margin and tumor type,[208] presence and number of mast cells,[209] age and gender, tumor grade,[210] DNA content,[211] increased mitosis and low *Bcl-2* expression, low apoptosis rate,[212] vascular endothelial growth factor (VEGF) levels, and allelic loss of chromosome 18q[213,214] are among the growing number of prognostic factors used in the analysis of colorectal cancer. The rapidly evolving field of molecular biology holds the promise of accurate staging and, it is hoped, individualized prognosis and treatment tailoring in the not-so-distant future.

DUKES' CLASSIFICATION

At the beginning of the twentieth century, surgery became routine for the treatment of colorectal cancers, including those arising in the colon and rectum. Almost immediately, the need arose for a staging system that allowed for comparisons among different surgical experiences and for determination of prognosis. A number of authors have tackled this challenge, with varying results. Based partially on earlier experiences, Dukes[315] developed the first practical system in the early 1930s. The initial Dukes' system was directed to rectal cancers and was remarkable for its simplicity and ability to give adequate prognostic information. The tumors were classified from A to C, with stage A indicating penetration restricted to the bowel wall, stage B indicating penetration through the bowel wall, and stage C indicating lymph node involvement. Over the years, several authors have attempted to make improvements on the initial work by Dukes, and the system has been extended to include both colon and rectal cancers. Dukes himself made a few changes in his system, first dividing stage C into C1 (local lymph nodes involved) and C2 (lymph nodes at the point of ligature involved) and later adding a fourth stage for distant metastasis, which was denoted as stage D by subsequent authors.

Kirklin et al. (1949) divided Dukes' stage A into a more restricted stage A (mucosa and submucosa involvement only) and a new B1, which involved the muscularis propria (but not penetration through it). The old stage B became B2. One problem seen with the earlier version of the Dukes' system was its inability to separate the depth of wall penetration and the involvement of lymph nodes. The revision by Astler and Coller in 1954 changed that feature, introducing the concept of stages C1 and C2, which are used commonly today. Gunderson and Sosin further modified the Astler-Coller system, subdividing the patients based on the presence of microscopic (B2m or C2m) and gross penetration (B2m + g, and C2m + g) through the bowel wall.

One of the problems not addressed by any of the commonly used variations of the Dukes' system is its inability to classify patients further based on the extent of their lymph node involvement. After the initial revision by Gabriel and Dukes in 1935 in which the location of the affected lymph nodes was considered, the issue was left unaddressed. The ideal number of lymph nodes that should be evaluated before the specimen can be considered negative for lymph node involvement remains controversial. It is well-known that up to 70% of affected lymph nodes in colorectal cancer are less than 5 mm in diameter, making them easy to overlook.[215,216] In 1994, Hernanz et al.[185] analyzed 193 specimens and suggested that at least six nodes had to be identified before the specimen could be called negative. Wong et al.[217] recently readdressed the same question and, after analyzing 196 cases, concluded that at least 14 nodes should be evaluated in each specimen. The advent of improved pathologic techniques and sensitive methods such as PCR may have an impact on the number of positive lymph nodes detected.[186] However, the prognostic value of these positive lymph nodes, which otherwise would not be detected, is still undetermined.

The National Surgical Adjuvant Breast and Bowel Program (NSABP) carried out an analysis of the prognostic variables in 844 patients with Dukes' stage C lesions.[218] The level of positive nodes provided little information over and above that provided by the two most important prognostic factors, depth of tumor penetration and the number of positive nodes. The subset of patients with one to four positive nodes fared remarkably better than did patients with larger numbers of involved nodes, and the number of positive nodes appeared to be the single most important prognostic factor.[218] The newer classifications of colorectal cancer have incorporated the number of involved lymph nodes as an important prognostic factor.

The size of the primary tumor in colorectal cancer, contrary to most solid tumors, does not seem to influence prognosis. A review of 391 patients treated surgically at the University of Texas M. D. Anderson Cancer Center from 1955 to 1975 demonstrated that the mean diameter of Dukes' stage B2 tumors was actually greater than the mean diameter of stage C2 tumors ($P < .001$) and D tumors ($P < .05$). The size of the primary tumor showed no relationship to 5-year adjusted survival. These results were confirmed by the NSABP experience.

Even though the modified Dukes' staging still is commonly used worldwide, the number of applied variations makes correlation of different studies less than ideal. Therefore, use of the TNM staging has been encouraged. This system is compatible with and is gradually replacing the Dukes' system.

THE JASS SYSTEM

The traditional Dukes system was primarily anatomic; the influence of the tumor grade and other pathologic features remained largely ignored. After analyzing 447 patients treated surgically for rectal cancer, Jass et al. (1986) were able to assess a number of histopathologic factors using the Cox regression model. The important variables included lymphocytic infiltration, tubule configuration, and pattern of growth. Subsequently, the authors compared the grade-related parameters with the established stage-related parameters. The best prognostic model included the number of affected lymph nodes, the presence of lymphocytic infiltration, and extent of spread through the bowel wall. The model was tested on a second data set comprising 331 patients, and similar results were derived. The authors concluded that their classification was simple to use and was superior to staging by the method of Dukes. The NSABP compared the Jass classification with the traditional Dukes system and validated its results.[219] However, the criteria used in the Jass prognostic system for colorectal cancer have been found to be less than optimal in routine practice and are not readily reproducible.[220]

Others have also questioned the superiority of the Jass system over the conventional Dukes' system. In a retrospective study of 312 colorectal carcinomas, Deans' et al.[221] found the Dukes classification to be of greater prognostic value and more reproducible than the components of Jass's classification. The simplicity and reproducibility of the new TNM staging system has discouraged further use of the Jass system by the major clinical groups.

TUMOR, NODE, METASTASIS (TNM) CLASSIFICATION

Despite its initial shortcomings, the TNM classification is the preferred system for colorectal cancer patients (Table 33.7-5). Starting in the late 1970s, both the American Joint Committee on Cancer (AJCC) and the Union Internationale Contre le Cancer (UICC) made attempts to unify the staging system for colorectal cancer with a simple classification similar to the TNM system used for most solid tumors. However, the initial TNM classifications were complicated and failed to provide adequate prognostic information for the different stages. The survival for patients with stage II disease was the same as or worse than that for patients with stage III cancer.[222–224] One of

TABLE 33.7-5. Tumor, Node, Metastasis Stage Grouping

Stage	*Tumor (T)*	*Lymph Nodes (N)*	*Metastasis (M1)*
0	Tis	N0	M0
I	T1	N0	M0
	T2	N0	M0
II	T3	N0	M0
	T4	N0	M0
III	Any T	N1	M0
	Any T	N2	M0
IV	Any T	Any N	M1

the main problems with those initial classifications was the fact that the number of positive lymph nodes was ignored.

Eventually, the AJCC and the UICC unified their TNM systems, creating a simpler system with greater prognostic value. The 1988 and 1994 revised systems included the number of affected lymph nodes as an important variable, and the newest system was found to have greater prognostic accuracy.

The rules for classification of colorectal cancer are relatively simple.[225] Colorectal cancers are commonly staged after surgical exploration and pathologic evaluation of the resected specimen. Tumors invading the stalk of polyps are classified according to the same definitions adopted for colorectal cancers. Carcinoma *in situ* (Tis) includes cancers confined to the glandular basement membrane or lamina propria. T1 tumors invade the submucosa, T2 tumors invade the muscularis propria, and T3 tumors invade through the muscularis propria into the subserosa or into nonperitonealized pericolic or perirectal tissue. T4 tumors invade other organs or structures or perforate the visceral peritoneum. Tumors invading other colorectal segments by way of the serosa (i.e., carcinoma of the cecum invading the sigmoid) are classified as T4.[225] Recurrent tumors at the site of surgery are assigned to the proximal segment of the anastomosis.[225]

The new TNM classification calls for at least 12 lymph nodes to be analyzed. N0 denotes that all nodes are negative. N1 includes tumors with metastasis in one to three regional lymph nodes. N2 indicates metastasis in four or more regional lymph nodes. Metastatic nodules or foci found in the pericolic, perirectal, or adjacent mesentery without evidence of residual lymph node tissue are equivalent to regional node metastasis. Involvement of the external iliac or common iliac lymph nodes is classified as metastatic disease (M1).[225] The concept of distant metastasis is virtually self-explanatory.

The TNM system also classifies a tumor based on its histologic grade, including four levels from well-differentiated to undifferentiated, and should not be used for sarcomas, lymphomas, and carcinoids arising in the colorectum. Additional independent prognostic factors worthy of attention include the histologic type, carcinoembryonic antigen (CEA) level, and vascular invasion.[225] The authors strongly recommend that the TNM staging system be used routinely (Table 33.7-6).

TABLE 33.7-6. American Joint Committee on Cancer–Union Internationale Contre le Cancer Tumor, Node, Metastasis Staging of Colon and Rectal Cancer

PRIMARY TUMOR (T)	
TX	Primary tumor cannot be assessed
T0	No evidence of primary tumor
Tis	Carcinoma *in situ*: intraepithelial or invasion of lamina propria[a]
T1	Tumor invades submucosa
T2	Tumor invades muscularis propria
T3	Tumor invades through muscularis propria into subserosa, or into nonperitonealized pericolic or perirectal tissues
T4	Tumor directly invades other organs or structures, and/or perforates visceral peritoneum[b]
REGIONAL LYMPH NODES (N)	
NX	Regional lymph nodes cannot be assessed
N0	No regional lymph node metastasis
N1	Metastasis in 1 to 3 regional lymph nodes
N2	Metastasis in 4 or more regional lymph nodes
DISTANT METASTASIS (M)	
MX	Distant metastasis cannot be assessed
M0	No distant metastasis
M1	Distant metastasis

[a]Tis includes cancer cells confined within the glandular basement membrane (intraepithelial) or lamina propria (intramucosal), with no extension through the muscularis mucosae into the submucosa.
[b]Direct invasion in T4 includes invasion of other segments of the colorectum by way of the serosa (e.g., invasion of the sigmoid colon by a carcinoma of the cecum).
(From ref. 225, with permission.)

ADDITIONAL PROGNOSTIC FEATURES

Clinical Features

AGE. Although colorectal cancer is a disease that occurs predominantly in older adults, it also affects a significant number of younger patients. Starting with the 1958 article by Hoerner, several investigators have reported more aggressive tumor behavior and a worse overall survival rate for patients with colorectal cancer whose disease was diagnosed before the patient had reached the age of 40. Several explanations for this finding have been explored, including the notion that younger patients are more prone to delayed diagnoses. They seem to have a higher frequency of high-grade tumors, and their disease is more commonly diagnosed at an advanced stage. Recio and Bussey (1965) noted an increased percentage of mucinous tumors in younger patients. In their study, high-grade tumors accounted for 53% of all tumors in the young group and only 20% in the older group. The most common histologic pattern in young patients is an aggressive, mucin-producing adenocarcinoma,[226] particularly in patients younger than 20 years old. When comparing patients with colorectal cancer who were younger than 40 years with older patients, Behbehani et al. (1985) found both a higher incidence of poorly differentiated tumors (21% vs. 8%, respectively) and a more advanced stage at presentation in the young patients. The survival rate for young patients was 23% versus 61%, respectively, for the general population. Stage III patients had a survival rate of 56% in the general population, as compared with 34% in young adults. Data compiled by the Commission on Cancer Data from the National Cancer Database from hospital cancer registries across the United States showed that the very elderly tended to present with an earlier stage of disease than younger patients.[227] Others have supported the notion that young patients tend to present with more advanced disease,[228] reflecting a more aggressive tumor or a delay in diagnosis; however, most analyses have failed to show a significant difference in prognosis when stage-adjusted survival is analyzed.

The prognosis for elderly patients with colorectal cancer is less well studied. Patients older than 80 years submitted for curative surgery have similar operative mortality when compared with patients in their fifties to seventies.[229] Data supplied by cancer registries in 17 countries in Europe on patients in whom colorectal cancer was diagnosed between 1978 and 1989 showed a possible decreased survival rate with increasing age.[230] Additional data on the prognosis for very elderly patients affected by colorectal cancer is greatly needed in view of the expected rapid growth of this segment of society.

GENDER. Several older analyses have shown a survival advantage for women (as compared to men) with colorectal cancer. Among known associations with reduced colorectal cancer risk, women appear to ingest more dietary fiber, to benefit more from physical activity and body mass, and to consume less alcohol. Hormonal characteristics may also affect a woman's risk of developing colorectal cancer.[231] However, others have failed to demonstrate a significant difference in prognosis based on gender alone.[232,233]

An inverse association has been detected between the number of pregnancies and the risk of colon cancer.[234] Parity appears to exert its predominant effect on risk of cancer of the right colon.[235] The use of oral contraceptives has also been linked to lower risk of colon and rectal cancer.[236] However, some investigators have recently questioned the true effect of reproductive events or oral contraceptives. Interestingly, parity could have no effect on the absolute risk of colorectal cancer but appears to have led to a decrease in proximal and an increase in distal colon cancer. Increasingly, the use of estrogen replacement therapy in postmenopausal women has been linked with a decrease in risk of subsequent colorectal cancer.[237] The confirmation of this finding would have far-reaching implications in public health.

Although the risk of colon cancer is similar in men and women, women frequently have the perception that colorectal cancer is a male disease and so they underestimate their true risk.[238] Partially in consequence, women are less likely than men to undergo screening studies.[239] This represents a true public health problem.

SYMPTOMS. As the natural history of colorectal cancer becomes better understood,[240] we are compelled to believe that the length of time required for the development and growth of colorectal cancer allows a window of opportunity for early detection and an increase in cures for colorectal cancer.[241] Indeed, screening efforts have been proven to reduce mortality from colorectal cancer.[242] Cancers detected by routine screening are less likely to have spread to lymph nodes or adjacent organs and, consequently, are less likely to be symptomatic. Beahrs and Sanfelippo (1971) reported that the 5-year survival for symptomatic colorectal cancer patients was 49%, as compared with 71% for asymptomatic patients, confirming that patients who present with symptoms from their tumors are more likely to have advanced disease and less likely to have a favorable outcome.

The duration of symptoms has not been conclusively proven as a prognostic factor. Contrary to what could be expected, several large studies have failed to demonstrate a direct relation between the duration of symptoms prior to diagnosis and pathologic stage at the time of surgery for colorectal cancer.[243] Patients in whom disease is diagnosed and treated prior to the development of any symptoms do tend to have early-stage colorectal cancer and improved survival.[243] However, patients with a short symptomatic history of colon cancer do not have a better prognosis than patients with a long history.[437] Pescatori et al.[436] found that, in a relatively small study, those patients with symptoms lasting more than 6 months actually had a significantly lower postoperative mortality and a higher 5-year survival rate than patients with symptoms lasting for less than 6 months. Copeland et al.,[438] in a much larger trial (1084 patients), reported a slightly worse 5-year survival rate for patients with symptoms lasting longer than 6 months. The available data support the notion that patients in whom colorectal cancer is diagnosed prior to the development of any symptoms tend to have a better prognosis than do symptomatic patients. The duration of symptoms does not seem to yield any significant prognostic value.[372]

OBSTRUCTION AND PERFORATION. Carcinoma of the colon that is complicated by obstruction or perforation has been recognized as having a poorer prognosis.[205] Data obtained from 1021 patients with Dukes stage B and C colorectal cancer who were entered into randomized clinical trials of the NSABP showed that the presence of bowel obstruction strongly influenced the prognostic outcome. The effect of bowel obstruction was more pronounced when the obstruction was located in the right colon. The larger-sized tumor needed to block the ascending colon completely might allow a longer time for these tumors to grow and spread when compared with tumors located in the descending colon.

A review of the Massachusetts General Hospital records compared patients presenting with obstruction or perforation with a control group undergoing curative resection. The actuarial 5-year survival rate seen in patients presenting with obstruction was 31%, in contrast to 59% in control patients. For patients with localized perforation, the 5-year actuarial survival rate was 44%.

According to a study involving 709 patients who underwent resection for colorectal carcinoma, stage was the strongest prognostic variable. However, obstruction had an independent effect in the same multivariate analysis. The Gastrointestinal Tumor Study Group (GITSG) multivariate analysis concluded that obstruction was an important indicator of prognosis, independent of Dukes stage. Bowel perforation was a poor prognostic factor only for disease-free survival.

HEMORRHAGE OR RECTAL BLEEDING. Cancers characterized by erosion are believed to manifest earlier than those characterized by invasion. Therefore, tumors presenting with bleeding are thought to be found earlier and to be associated with a better prognosis. This belief has not been confirmed in other studies. In the GITSG multivariate analysis, the presence of melena or rectal bleeding showed a trend as a prognostic factor for prolonged survival but failed to reach statistical significance ($P = .08$). Chapuis et al. (1985) demonstrated by univariate analysis in a large study conducted in Australia that the presence of rectal bleeding predicted longer survival; however, the significance of this symptom disappeared on multivariate analysis.

PRIMARY TUMOR LOCATION. Multiple analyses have shown that cancers arising at or below the peritoneal reflection (rectosigmoid and rectum) have a worse 5-year survival rate than those arising above the reflection.[232] With regard to colon primary tumors, different authors have reached different conclusions. Some, including Wolmark et al. (1967, 1983) in a large retrospective review of data from the NSABP, reported that lesions in the right side carry a worse prognosis. Poorer prognosis for patients with disease in the left colon has been reported. Several investigators report no difference based on the location of the primary tumor. The large GITSG colon cancer experience showed that tumor location (left, right, and rectosigmoid or sigmoid) was of low prognostic value.

PRIMARY TUMOR SIZE. In contrast to most solid tumors, the size of the primary tumor is not considered in the staging of colorectal cancer, reflecting the unusual nature of these cancers. Even though some authors have shown improved survival with smaller tumors, most studies have failed to demonstrate a significant prognostic value for the size of the primary tumor at the time of diagnosis.[191] Data collected by the NSABP also underscore the lack of a relation between tumor size and lymph node metastasis. Indeed, an M. D. Anderson Cancer Center review demonstrated that patients with Dukes B2 tumors frequently had larger primary lesions than did patients with Dukes stage C and D tumors.

PRIMARY TUMOR CONFIGURATION. When compared with ulcerating tumors, exophytic tumors tend to penetrate the bowel wall less frequently (24% vs. 39%, respectively) and have less frequent nodal metastases and fewer hematogenous metastases (23% vs. 31%, respectively). Analysis of a GITSG colon adjuvant study revealed that the presence of an exophytic lesion had a beneficial effect on survival when compared with ulcerating lesions.

BLOOD TRANSFUSION. Considerable controversy has surrounded the association of perioperative blood transfusions and the recurrence rate of colorectal cancer.[244] Some investigators have reported worse disease-free survival in patients who require transfusions.[245] The reason for this outcome would be a transfusion-related form of immunosuppression.[246] However, when differences in confounding background variables are accounted for, the significance of transfusion seems less evident,[247] and several authors believe it to have no direct relation to prognosis.[248] By multivariate analysis in a prospective study, no negative influence of transfusion on survival could be detected.[249]

A retrospective analysis evaluating 1051 patients treated with curative surgery for stage II or III colorectal adenocarcinoma at the Mayo Clinic demonstrated that the use of blood components probably had no impact on disease recurrence, and the documented adverse impact of transfusions is more likely due to other variables or to the underlying illness necessitating the transfusion.[250] This was confirmed in a study in which patients were randomized to receive, when needed, perioperative transfusions with either allogeneic or autologous blood.[251] There were no differences in disease-free survival between the two groups. Disease-free and cancer-specific survivals were increased in the group that donated but did not receive any transfusions, as opposed to those who received the transfusions, suggesting that the conditions that necessitate transfusion may be more important than the transfusion itself.[251]

Pathologic Features

VASCULAR ENDOTHELIAL GROWTH FACTOR. VEGF is an important factor in the angiogenic process. Several studies have demonstrated a correlation between the expression of VEGF and vessel count in the tumor specimen, and a combination of vessel count and expression of VEGF may be useful for predicting distant recurrence in patients with node-negative colon cancer.[252] VEGF is being evaluated as a possible prognostic marker and also is currently an important new target for novel therapeutic agents in the treatment of cancer.[253]

LYMPH NODE MICROMETASTASIS. Lymph node status has long been recognized as one of the best prognostic markers in patients with colorectal cancer. To minimize false-negative results, a minimum number of lymph nodes should be evaluated, though there is no clear consensus on the ideal number. The TNM classification calls for at least 12 nodes to be examined,[225] whereas a recent review suggested that 14 nodes may be a better target.[217] New techniques directed at increasing the number of lymph nodes available for analysis are being developed, including new staining procedures[254] and sentinel lymph node mapping.[255] Unfortunately, despite all efforts, a significant number of patients with grossly negative lymph nodes eventually experience disease recurrence, and many of those patients who experience recurrence are believed to have had microscopic involvement of their lymph nodes.

Determining the actual lymph node status of patients who received potentially curative surgery would be a valuable tool in the treatment of colorectal cancer. This is especially true for those patients with stage II disease in whom the need for adjuvant therapy remains an intensely debated topic. Several different techniques are being explored, including immunohistochemistry,[256] radioimmunologically guided surgery,[257] and histochemical detection of micrometastatic deposits in bone marrow aspirates.[258] An area of intensive research is the use of reverse transcriptase–PCR (RT-PCR) targeting different primers in blood, bone marrow, and lymph nodes. Primers used thus far with varying degrees of success have included matrilysin (matrix metalloproteinase 7), cytokeratin, and guanylyl cyclase C.[259–261]

Perhaps no other primer has been sought and studied as much as CEA.[262] Mori et al.[263] performed both histologic and molecular examination of CEA-specific RT-PCR in 406 lymph nodes obtained from 65 patients with breast or GI carcinomas. Patients were followed prospectively for 2 years, and the positive detection rate increased from 20% by histologic examination to 60% by RT-PCR. The recurrence rate was 40% in 15 cases showing positive results in the histologic and molecular examinations, 14% in 29 cases showing histologically negative but RT-PCR-positive results, and 0% in 21 cases showing negative results in both examinations. The positive detection rate in peripheral blood samples increased with advancing stage of disease. With respect to 62 cases in which curative surgery was performed, CEA was detected in 12 cases. In 4 of these 12 cases, metastatic disease developed after surgery, whereas, at the time of the study's publication, metastasis had failed to develop in any of 50 cases that were negative by RT-PCR.[263] Novel potential targets for diagnostic PCR and RT-PCR are constantly being sought.

ADJACENT ORGAN INVOLVEMENT. Involvement of adjacent organs has long been considered an important adverse prognostic factor. Furthermore, the surgical removal of the affected organ did not seem to alter overall survival for such patients. The prognostic value of adjacent organ invasion seems to be more pronounced in node-negative patients, and the type and duration of presenting symptoms had no effect on the survival in a series reported by Eldar et al.[264] The presence of pathologically confirmed organ invasion had a significant impact on overall survival when compared with clinical involvement only in a series of colon cancer patients reported by Minsky et al.[199] The 5-year survival for stage B3 patients with pathologic involvement was only 27% versus 88% for the others. Interestingly, the same authors failed to demonstrate this difference in patients with stage B3 tumors of the rectum.[191]

RADIAL (LATERAL) MARGINS. Whether the proximal and distal margins are involved in colorectal cancer has traditionally been emphasized in pathologic reports. However, the fact that penetration of the primary tumor carries significant prognostic value should be carefully considered. Quirke et al.[265] reported an 85% incidence of local failure in patients with rectal cancer and positive lateral margins, versus only 3% in the patients with completely negative margins. Some reports have found up to an impressive 33% positive lateral margins in patients with negative proximal and distal margins.[266] A large review of 325 patients who underwent curative surgery for rectal or rectosigmoid cancer demonstrated 29% local recurrence for patients with positive radial margins versus 8% local recurrence for those with negative radial margins.[267] Radial margins seem to be particularly important in rectal cancer, and the concept of total mesorectal excision explores the idea that clean lateral margins improve local control.

DEGREE OF DIFFERENTIATION (GRADE). The degree of tumor differentiation, also known as *tumor grading*, has long been suspected to be a prognostic factor in colorectal cancer. Several recent metaanalyses and multivariate analyses confirm the importance of tumor grading as an independent prognostic factor for survival.[205] Grade has been associated with several other prognostic factors, and most patients with poorly differentiated tumors will have multiple poor prognostic factors. Interestingly, patients with lower-grade tumors at the initial diagnosis may be more likely to undergo a second curative surgery for recurrences than patients whose original tumors were of a higher grade.[268]

COLLOID (MUCINOUS) CANCER. Colonic mucins are high-molecular-weight glycoproteins produced by goblet cells of colonic epithelium. Some studies have indicated that colon cancers that produce high amounts of mucin have a poorer prognosis and are frequently diagnosed at advanced stages[269] and in younger patients.[270] In animal models, mucin-producing cancer cells form tumors larger than those of low-mucin variants and seem to have increased metastatic potential.[271] In humans, mucinous tumors are associated with a clear, gelatinous fluid, present either within or outside the cancer cells. The variant in which the mucin remains inside the cell is commonly referred to as signet-ring carcinoma. This rare variant of colorectal cancer accounts for only 1% to 2% of all colorectal cancers but is well-known for its aggressiveness.[271a]

Initial reports emphasized the fact that signet-ring carcinoma is capable of growing and spreading intramurally, sparing the mucosa and forming a linitis plastica appearance. This presentation is uncommon and is seen in fewer than 20% of the signet-ring carcinoma cases but has important implications for diagnosis, as the cancer may not be easily detected on a routine colonoscopy. Despite a few reports indicating otherwise, most authors report a worse prognosis for signet-ring carcinomas than for common adenocarcinomas and even the conventional mucinous carcinoma. The 5-year overall survival rate is poor and varies from 0% to 36%, with most series falling toward the lower value.[271a] Signet-ring carcinoma patients tend to have a higher rate of peritoneal seeding, and several series have demonstrated that peritoneal carcinomatosis is more frequently seen than liver metastasis.[271a]

The extracellular variant, commonly termed *mucinous carcinoma*, is considerably more common. In a series of 352 patients with colorectal cancer, Secco et al.[272] identified 39 cases (11%). The same incidence had been reported previously.[273] Mucinous carcinomas seem to have a predilection for the rectum and the sigmoid colon.[272] Several series have indicated that the prognosis for mucinous carcinoma is intermediate between that for signet-ring carcinoma and the prognosis for regular adenocarcinoma.[272] Some authors have argued that the worse outcome for these patients is due to the more advanced stage at presentation.[269]

Recent reports showing a reduced incidence of the K-ras mutation in patients with signet-ring and poorly differentiated carcinomas in relation to ordinary colorectal carcinoma suggest that these types of carcinomas may have a different genetic background than well- or moderately differentiated colorectal carcinoma.[271] Mucinous carcinomas seems to exhibit less apoptotic activity than does regular colorectal cancer (19% vs. 51%, respectively; $P = .01$).[275]

CELL-CYCLE PARAMETERS AND PLOIDY. Aneuploidy is an abnormal balance of chromosomes, and recent evidence seems to indicate that it may cause genetic instability, leading to the karyotypic and phenotypic heterogeneity commonly seen in cancer cells.[276] Even though the results of DNA analysis of colorectal adenocarcinomas varies greatly depending on study methodology,[277] aneuploidy is commonly observed in colorectal cancer cells, especially in advanced stages.[211] In a series of 51 cases analyzed by Saccani et al.,[211] normal mucosa adjacent to aneuploid tumors showed only a 7% incidence of aneuploidy, whereas the mucosa adjacent to diploid cancers demonstrated only diploid characteristics.

Despite the controversies, there is enough evidence to suggest that a greater proportion of the higher-stage tumors are aneuploid and that aneuploid tumors tend to have a higher growth rate and poorer survival than diploid tumors.[278] When various prognostic factors are analyzed, aneuploid tumors are associated with factors that are indicative of a poor prognosis.[278] The prognostic value of the tumor's ploidy is especially important in stage II patients. In a small study by Nori et al. (1995), the DNA content of colon cancers in 20 stage II patients with evidence of disease relapse was measured and compared with 20 stage II patients in whom there was no evidence of relapse. Aneuploidy occurred in 16 patients (80%) with recurrence, as compared to only 8 patients (40%) in the control group. Aneuploidy was associated with significantly higher tumor recurrence rate ($P = .024$) and a shorter overall survival ($P < .002$). These results are consistent with an earlier North Central Cancer Treatment Group (NCCTG) analysis of 694 patients with stage II or III colorectal cancer enrolled in some of their adjuvant trials. Patients with diploid tumors had a higher survival rate than did those with aneuploid tumors (P <.001). The proliferation index (the sum of the percentage of cells in S phase plus those in G_2/M phase) was also a strong prognostic factor (P <.001). When the ploidy and proliferation data were combined, the patients in the favorable group had a 5-year survival rate of 74%, as compared with 54% for the unfavorable group (P <.001).[279] Despite some negative reports,[280,281] most series and multivariate analyses have confirmed that the DNA content is an important independent prognostic factor for survival in colorectal cancer.[279,280,282–284]

BLOOD VESSEL INVASION. Vascular invasion can be divided into blood vessel and lymphatic invasion. *Blood vessel invasion* generally refers to venous invasion, as arterial invasion is considered a rare phenomenon. *Intramural* blood vessel invasion refers to the involvement of vessels located within the bowel wall, whereas *extramural* invasion refers to the involvement of vessels located outside the bowel wall. The incidence of blood vessel invasion in colorectal cancer varies from as low as 17% to as high as 81%, depending on the series reported and on whether special elastic tissue stains were used.[285] The prognostic value of the presence of blood vessel invasion for overall survival remains controversial. Whereas some researchers have found it to be an independent prognostic factor,[286] others have not been able to confirm this finding.[285]

Minsky et al. (1988) have evaluated the prognostic value of blood vessel invasion independently in colon and in rectal cancers. Analysis of 294 patients who had curative surgery for colon cancer showed that blood vessel involvement resulted in a significant decrease in the 5-year actuarial survival rate. However, when examined by proportional hazards analysis, blood vessel invasion was not an independent prognostic variable. The same group retrospectively reviewed 168 patients who had curative surgery for rectal cancer. A significant decrease in 5-year actuarial survival was seen in patients with extramural blood vessel involvement as compared with patients who had tumors with intramural or no blood vessel involvement. When the intramural and extramural types of involvement were combined, no significant impact was noted on the patterns of failure or survival.[287]

Krasna et al.[288] and Inoue et al. have used elastic tissue stains and evaluated the prognostic value of blood vessel invasion independently from lymphatic vessel involvement. In the first series, metastases were seen in 60% of patients with vascular invasion as opposed to 17% of those with no vascular invasion (P <.0001). Survival in these patients was 29.7% and 62.2%, respectively (P <.003). In the second series, a higher incidence of vascular invasion was seen in patients who died of cancer within 2 years of surgery. These differences were not evident with the use of routine hematoxylin and eosin staining.

LYMPHATIC VESSEL INVASION. In contrast to blood vessel invasion, the presence of lymphatic vessel involvement has been almost uniformly reported as a poor prognostic factor. Minsky et al.[289] retrospectively reviewed 61 patients with colorectal carcinoma who were found to have lymphatic vessel invasion and compared them with 401 patients who had tumors without such invasion. In patients with lymphatic vessel invasion, the incidence of positive lymph nodes was 59% as opposed to 25% for the control group (P = .0004). The 5-year survival rate also was statistically lower for the patients with lymphatic vessel invasion. Proportional hazards analysis confirmed that lymphatic vessel invasion is an independent prognostic factor for survival.[289] Other authors have reached a similar conclusion in their own reviews, suggesting that the presence of lymphatic vessel invasion should be considered a useful prognostic factor for survival in colorectal cancer.[290]

PERINEURAL INVASION. The ability of colorectal cancers to invade perineural spaces as far as 10 cm from the primary tumor was first reported in 1943 by Seefeld and Bargen. This was also the first work in which the presence of perineural invasion was demonstrated to be associated with increased disease recurrences and worse 5-year survival. This conclusion has been confirmed by others. Krasna et al.[288] reported a 73% incidence of metastasis in patients with perineural invasion, as compared with 27% in those without such invasion (P <.01) and a 30% survival rate versus 58%, respectively (P<.003). Several other authors have confirmed that perineural invasion can be considered an independent prognostic factor for survival,[206] whereas Bouvet et al.[291] failed to demonstrate that perineural invasion is a significant prognostic factor for recurrence in treated rectal cancer. Investigators from the M. D. Anderson Cancer Center found by univariate analysis (but not by multivariate analysis) that the presence of perineural invasion was a significant prognostic factor for time to cancer recurrence.[252]

CARCINOEMBRYONIC ANTIGEN. Since it was first described in 1965, CEA has become the most reliable tumor marker for use in the detection of colorectal cancer. It is recommended as a monitoring tool for patients who have been treated with curative intent. Further, it is a poor prognostic factor for cancer recurrence in patients in whom the CEA level is elevated preoperatively and who failed to normalize after a potentially curative operation.[54] The prognostic potential of the preoperative CEA level remains unclear, and even the value above which the CEA is considered significantly elevated has varied from as low as 2.5 ng/dL to as high as 10 ng/mL, depending on the series reported.

Since the 1970s, several authors have presented evidence indicating that CEA is an independent prognostic factor.[292] In one of the largest reports, Harrison et al.[293] reviewed 572 patients who underwent curative resection for node-negative colon cancer at the Memorial Sloan-Kettering Cancer Center. The preoperative CEA level and the stage of disease predicted survival by both univariate and multivariate analysis.

However, Chapman et al.[294] reported that, although the 5-year survival rate for patients with an elevated CEA was 39% as compared with 57% for patients with a normal CEA level (P = .001), the proportion of patients with an elevated CEA level increased with more advanced tumor stage and a poorly differentiated tumor grade. Once controls were in place for the variable of stage, CEA was not a predictor of survival. This study confirmed the work by other authors that failed to demonstrate a significant independent prognostic value for preoperative CEA level.[295] An elevated CEA level may be a reflection of a more advanced colorectal carcinoma.

IMMUNE RESPONSE TO THE PRIMARY TUMOR. Careful pathologic evaluation of the primary tumor site has demonstrated that a significant number of tumors exhibit evidence of local inflammation and that this reaction is a positive prognostic factor. Jass et al.[207] demonstrated that the presence of lymphocytic infiltration was a very important independent prognostic factor in colorectal cancer. This finding led to the development of the Jass staging system.[207] By univariate analysis, the presence of lymphocytic infiltration has been demonstrated to have prognostic importance for survival in colon cancer,[208] and lymphatic stroma reaction has been demonstrated to be of prognostic value for local failure in rectal cancer.[296] NSABP protocol R-01 showed that survival was significantly decreased with increasing numbers of eosinophils and mast cells present at the tumor border.[297] Recent work by Diederichsen et al.[298] using flow cytometry to study the phenotype of tumor-infiltrating lymphocytes in 41 cases of colorectal cancer showed that expression of class II human leukocyte antigens (HLA) did not correlate with any lymphocyte surface markers. Because tumor-infiltrating lymphocytes are "turned off" rather than stimulated when tumor cells express HLA class II but not CD80, the lack of correlations could be due to anergy.

DELETIONS IN COLORECTAL CANCER. Allelic deletions involving chromosome 18q occur in more than 70% of colorectal cancers. In colorectal cancer, the *DCC* gene was cloned from a region of chromosome 18q, and whereas the *DCC* gene was expressed in most normal tissues, including colonic mucosa, its expression was greatly reduced or absent in most colorectal carcinomas tested.[299] The mechanism of action of *DCC* is unknown. It may function as a tumor suppressor gene by inducing apoptosis.[300] Experimentally, *DCC* induces apoptosis in the absence of ligand binding and blocks apoptosis when engaged by netrin-1. It is a caspase substrate, and mutation of the site at which caspase 3 cleaves *DCC* suppresses the proapoptotic effect of *DCC* completely.[300]

In a series of 118 patients who had undergone curative surgery for stage II or III colon cancer, those patients whose tumor exhibited no evidence of chromosome 18q allelic loss showed a better disease-free and overall survival than did those whose tumor demonstrated 18q allelic loss. When patients were stratified by tumor stage, a significant survival advantage for patients whose tumor had no allelic loss on chromosome 18q was observed in stage II and in stage III disease. In particular, patients with stage II disease whose tumor had no chromosome 18q allelic loss demonstrated an excellent clinical outcome, with a 5-year disease-free survival rate of 96%. In contrast, the 5-year disease-free survival rate of patients with stage II disease and chromosome 18q allelic loss was only 54%. In a multivariate analysis, the status of chromosome 18q was a significant independent prognostic factor for both disease-free and overall survival.[213] Several investigators have shown that not only deletion of and lowered messenger RNA expression of the *DCC* gene but also marked reduction of DCC protein occurred in colon cancer tissues.[301] In addition, colon cancer patients with liver metastases expressed significantly lower levels of *DCC* as compared to patients without such metastases.

Additional Tumor Biologic Features

ONCOGENES AND MOLECULAR MARKERS. Oncogenes and molecular markers are discussed extensively in Chapter 33.1. However, the study of molecular markers has enormously advanced our understanding of the development and treatment of colorectal cancer. Molecular markers have the potential to revolutionize the way such cancers are treated. Some of the areas of intensive research currently are thymidylate synthase,[302] dihydropyrimidine dehydrogenase (DPD),[303] and the presence of microsatellite instability.[304]

p53 GENE. The *p53* gene located on chromosome 17p is a well-known tumor suppressor gene. Attallah et al.[305] reported no significant difference in *p53* overexpression between patients with stage II and III colorectal cancer; however, flow cytometric analysis revealed a slightly higher incidence of DNA aneuploidy in 75% of *p53*-positive cases as compared with 64.3% *p53* positivity in diploid tumors.

The abnormal *p53* appears to be a late phenomenon in colorectal carcinogenesis. This mutation may allow the growing tumor with multiple genetic alterations to evade cell-cycle arrest and apoptosis.[306] In a retrospective review of 141 patients with resected stage II and stage III colon carcinoma, the presence of a *p53* mutation was the single most important risk factor associated with poorer survival in patients with either stage of disease (stage II, $P = .02$; stage III, $P = .006$).[307] A *p53* mutation increased the risk of death by 2.82 times in patients with stage II disease and by 2.39 times in patients with stage III colon carcinoma.[307]

The Southwest Oncology Group (SWOG) assessed the prognostic value of *p53* in 66 stage II and 163 stage III colon cancer patients in adjuvant intergroup trial 0035.[308] *p53* expression was found in 63% of cancers and was associated with favorable survival in stage III but not stage II disease. Seven-year survival with stage III disease was 56% with *p53* expression versus 43% with no *p53* expression ($P = .012$).[308] The true independent prognostic value of *p53* remains to be defined.

IMMUNOLOGY AND MARKERS. The most frequently used tumor marker in colorectal cancer continues to be CEA, though several other markers have been evaluated in this disease. For example, many investigators have demonstrated that the blood group antigens ABH and Lewis, which are normally expressed only in the proximal colon, can be reexpressed in distal colon cancers. Also, an antigen that is incompatible with the individual's blood type can be expressed.[309] Similar alterations occur in adenomatous polyps, but with reduced frequency. ABH antigens are not commonly expressed in hyperplastic polyps but are seen in neoplastic polyps.[309]

CA 19-9 is a carbohydrate cell surface antigen, a sialylated lacto-N-fucopentose related to the Lewis blood group substance. CA 19-9 does not appear to be as sensitive as CEA but does have some value as a prognostic factor, especially if combined with CEA.[310] However, currently available data do not justify the routine use of CA 19-9 in colorectal cancer outside of an investigational trial. Several other antigens have been defined with the use of monoclonal antibodies, but their use remains restricted and has not been adopted in clinical practice because these antibodies seem to add little to the currently available markers.

ADDITIONAL FACTORS. A comprehensive review of every prognostic factor studied in colorectal cancer is beyond the scope of this chapter. Extensive review of such factors as the amount of collagen type IV present in the tumor matrix,[311] the presence of reactive lymph nodes, and the morphometric measurements of the tumor cell (nuclear morphology) have yielded conflicting results.[181] Such other factors as proliferating cell nuclear antigen expression,[312] sucrase isomaltase,[313] helix pomatia agglutinin,[314] microacinar growth pattern,[210] autocrine motility factor,[315] ornithine decarboxylase,[316] fibronectin, and tumor-associated glycoprotein DF3[317] have shown some prognostic value, but the true value of many of these factors continues to be explored in colorectal cancer.[318]

TREATMENT OF PRECANCEROUS CONDITIONS

NEOPLASTIC POLYPS (ADENOMAS)

Adenomas are the most common neoplasms in the large bowel. They are classified into three types—tubular, tubulovillous, and villous—according to their histologic appearance. Tubular adenomas account for 75% of polyps found, tubulovillous adenomas account for 15% of all neoplastic polyps, and villous adenomas account for 10%. The malignancy rate of tubular adenomas is 5%, but it rises to 40% in villous adenomas. The malignancy rate for tubulovillous adenomas is 22%, suggesting that these tumors behave more like villous than like tubular adenomas. The entire colon must be examined if a histologically proven adenoma has been removed from the colon or is found on endoscopic biopsy.[164] Endoscopic removal of polyps should be performed to confirm the diagnosis of a benign or malignant polyp. Polyps with a stalk can be removed by endoscopic snare polypectomy. Sessile lesions can be removed in a piecemeal fashion; however, there is an increased risk of complications, and judgment must be used to assess this risk and the practicality of attempting piecemeal removal of tumors, especially in the relatively thin-walled abdominal colon.

The National Polyp Study demonstrated a synchronous polyp detection rate of 29% to 35% at colonoscopic follow-up for patients in whom an adenomatous polyp has been demonstrated.[164] This detection rate depends on the number of interventions and the time intervals from the last colonoscopy. Approximately 15% of patients will have evidence of small adenomas after the colon is considered cleared of polyps at colonoscopy.

Further management and timing of surveillance depends on the characteristics of the adenomas removed initially, as well as on their number and the clinical status of the patient. Follow-up of adenomas containing *in situ* carcinoma or severe dysplasia that have been completely removed is the same as that for benign adenomas: routine follow-up colonoscopy at 3-year intervals once the colon is cleared.[164] Individuals in whom the colon is not cleared of all polyps will require an earlier examination. In addition, patients having multiple adenomas are at a higher risk for oversight of synchronous adenomas and, therefore, these patients should be examined at 1 year. A large sessile adenoma that cannot be removed endoscopically will often require surgery.

Large villous adenomas (i.e., >2 cm in diameter) have a malignant potential that is significantly greater than that for other adenomatous polyps. Even small villous adenomas have a greater malignant potential than do adenomatous polyps of the same size. They are sessile, in most cases, and grossly appear velvety owing to frond-like glands. Villous adenomas require complete excision for histologic examination. Random biopsies of villous adenomas are unreliable and only contribute to difficulties in management. If such adenomas can be palpated in the rectum, they are more likely to be benign if they are soft. However, excision is still required.

Surgical resection should be performed. This is due to the high risk of recurrence, complications from endoscopic polypectomy, and presence of invasive cancer. When located in the rectum, such lesions can often be treated by local excision. Submucosal techniques of transanal excision or the Kraske approach, which are used for large lesions that otherwise cannot be approached by transanal excision, are appropriate in the complete excision of rectal villous adenomas.[319] Circumferential villous adenomas of the lower rectum can be removed in three to four longitudinal strips and have subsequent mucosal advancement. Alternatively, low anterior resection or proctectomy with coloanal anastomosis can be used to manage large circumferential villous adenomas of the lower rectum. Laser ablation of the lesion has the disadvantage of destroying tissue before pathologic examination is carried out. Nonetheless, this may be reasonable when an operative approach is prohibited.

MANAGEMENT OF FAMILIAL ADENOMATOUS POLYPOSIS

Because the risk of development of colorectal carcinoma in patients with FAP is virtually 100% when the colon and rectum are left intact, resection is the only therapeutic intervention known to alter the natural history of this disease.[98] Owing to the high rate of development of carcinomas before the age of 40, this surgical intervention usually is performed relatively early in life (15 to 20 years of age). Surgery should not be delayed once the diagnosis is established.[320] Surgical procedures in these patients range from total abdominal colectomy and ileorectal anastomosis to total proctocolectomy with ileoanal anastomosis.[321] Total proctocolectomy and end ileostomy are rarely used for these patients except in the presence of a failed ileoanal reservoir, in patients older than 50 years, in the face of poor medical condition, or in patients with poor sphincter tone. An alternative to end ileostomy in these patients may be the use of a Kock pouch to act as a continent ileostomy.

Removal of the entire abdominal colon with a small bowel anastomosis performed to the upper rectum is the procedure selected for many patients with polyposis. It carries a relatively low mortality rate and low morbidity rate.[322] Advantages to this procedure include the avoidance of a stoma, relatively normal bowel habits, and avoidance of bladder and sexual dysfunction.[323] Selection of this procedure requires that the surgeon be able to remove or fulgurate any rectal polyps and necessitates continued endoscopic surveillance of the rectum. Risk of subsequent carcinoma in the rectal stump increases with age, the presence of malignancy in the original colectomy specimen, the length of the rectal stump, and the number of rectal polyps present preoperatively (Fig. 33.7-4).[324] Patients with a rectal stump greater than 10–15 cm long appear to be at greater risk of rectal cancer.[325] In a review of 11 member registries from the Leads Castle Polyposis Group, the cumulative incidence of rectal carcinoma was found to be 13% at 25 years.

Total proctocolectomy with ileoanal anastomosis is commonly used in patients who are unable to accept the risk of sub-

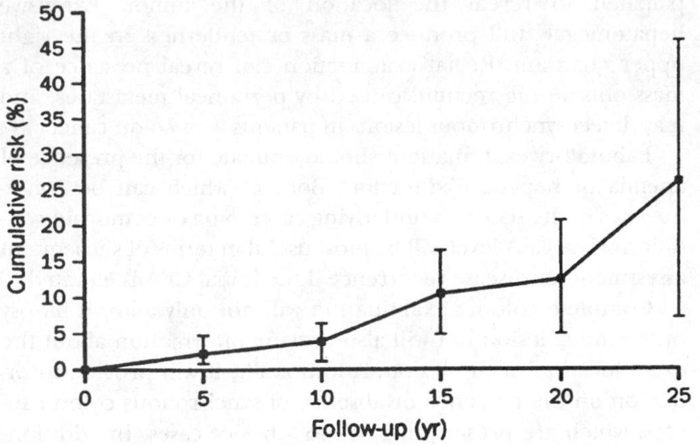

FIGURE 33.7-4. Cumulative risk of rectal cancer after ileorectal anastomosis over 25 years of follow-up.

sequent rectal carcinoma, those with extensive rectal polyps, or those who develop large numbers of rectal polyps after ileorectal anastomosis. The advantages of this procedure are virtual elimination of rectal cancer risk and avoidance of a permanent stoma. Patients Total proctocolectomy with ileoanal anastomosis does carry a higher complication rate than does abdominal colectomy. Morbidity rates vary from 10% to 24.[326] Stool frequency varies from three to six bowel movements per day, with occasional nocturnal stooling; however, quality of life is similar to that of patients with ileorectal anastomosis.[327] Continence and bowel habits improve with time, and most patients are free of antidiarrheal agents by 1 year after surgery. Satisfaction for patients undergoing total proctocolectomy and ileoanal anastomosis can be quite high. This operation can be performed in selected patients with FAP and coexistent cancer without compromising oncologic or functional outcomes.[328] It also can be performed after a previous ileorectal anastomosis.

Vasen et al. (1996) and Wu et al.[329] have described a correlation between specific sites of mutations within the *APC* gene and the subsequent development of rectal carcinoma after ileorectal anastomosis. Vasen's group noted that the risk of secondary surgery for cancer or polyps is higher in patients with a mutation after codon 1250 (RR, 2.7; $P<.05$). Wu's group[329] reported that *APC* gene mutations at codons 1309 and 1328 were associated with severe polyposis and should be treated with total proctocolectomy. The utility of this technique in selecting patients for the appropriate surgical procedure requires further investigation.[330] A thorough discussion between patient and physician, taking into account the patient's medical characteristics, history, and wishes, will help in the decision making about management techniques for FAP.[331,332] Referral to an established registry will lower the stage of disease at which cancer is diagnosed in relatives of the proband and thereby will improve survival.

Colorectal carcinoma is but one component of the overall syndrome of FAP. Additional tumors of the GI tract (e.g., periampullary cancer) as well as thyroid, brain, or hepatic tumors can complicate this disease.[333] A difficult problem that occurs in approximately 3.5% to 38.0% of patients with FAP is desmoid tumor. Specific mutations can be associated with severe desmoid disease.[330] These tumors frequently occur in the mesentery of the small bowel and extend into the retroperitoneum. Mesenteric desmoid tumors often are unresectable because of involvement of the superior mesenteric vessels. Even if resected, there is a very high recurrence rate and a very high surgical morbidity rate.[334] Because of the poor results of surgical resection of mesenteric desmoid tumors, a variety of medical treatments, as well as radiation therapy, have been described. In an FAP patient who has been protected from colorectal cancer by surgery, upper GI tract tumors and desmoids become more frequent causes of mortality.[98]

ULCERATIVE COLITIS

The process of screening and selection of patients for surgery based on biopsy-proven, high-grade dysplasia of the colon in patients with ulcerative colitis was presented earlier, in Screening. As described, patients can be observed, with surgery performed only for those with high cancer risk or invasive carcinoma. This discussion of the indications for surgery related to the risk of colorectal cancer is not relevant to the indications for surgery related to complications of inflammatory bowel disease itself.

Commonly, the timing of colectomy is related to findings of dysplasia on random biopsy of the colon. Some studies have emphasized the development of cancer in patients with ulcerative colitis in whom dysplastic changes were seen in the colon on biopsy. Such findings have generated screening strategies based on the presence of dysplasia.[335] The disadvantages to this approach are the need for life-long screening even in the presence of quiescent disease and the requirement that experienced pathologists perform the evaluation for dysplasia.[329] The appeal of this technique is that it can provide indications for resection of the large bowel before the presence of a colorectal carcinoma becomes obvious by symptoms or gross appearance.

Duration of disease is another factor in timing surgery. Identifying neoplastic lesions at colonoscopy can be difficult because of the marked distortion of the mucosa and the flat appearance of many cancers associated with ulcerative colitis. The presence of a mass is an indication for surgery even in the absence of a biopsy specimen that exhibits dysplasia or cancer.

The options for a patient who has indications for surgery due to cancer risk in ulcerative colitis include total proctocolectomy with end ileostomy, total proctocolectomy with Kock pouch, total abdominal colectomy with ileorectal anastomosis, and total proctocolectomy with ileoanal anastomosis.[336] Each of these procedures has advantages and disadvantages that should be considered in light of each patient's individual circumstances. Total proctocolectomy with end ileostomy is most suitable for elderly patients, those with impaired sphincter function, and those in whom an ileoanal pouch is technically impossible or has failed. It is a single-stage procedure with a lower rate of complications than the alternative procedures. Total abdominal colectomy with ileorectal anastomosis is a relatively simple procedure that avoids any of the risks of proctectomy and the need for ileostomy. However, it does appear to carry the risks of recurrence of symptoms in the retained rectum as well as a small risk of carcinoma in the retained rectal segment. It should not be used in patients with preexisting large bowel cancer or rectal dysplasia, because of an approximately 70% risk of subsequent development of rectal carcinoma or dysplasia. Close endoscopic follow-up is required for any patient with a retained rectum who undergoes ileorectal anastomosis for chronic ulcerative colitis. Rectal cancer risk has been estimated to be 0% to 22%.[336]

In selected cases, restorative proctocolectomy can be performed for patients with cancer in the setting of ulcerative colitis.[328] Multicentricity is seen in 25% of such patients.[328] A complication with this procedure can be pouchitis, which occurs in 7% to 42% of patients. Pouch failure occurs in a small number of patients because of either technical difficulties at the time of surgery or pelvic sepsis. Problems of early age at onset of colorectal cancer, multiple neoplasms, and need for surveillance are similar to those encountered by patients with Crohn's disease.[337]

HEREDITARY NONPOLYPOSIS COLON CANCER

The development of molecular genetic techniques to establish a presymptomatic diagnosis of HNPCC and the increasing clinical recognition of families with this syndrome have made the consideration of prophylactic colectomy realistic. Total abdominal colectomy appears to be appropriate, even though there is still a small but cumulative risk of rectal carcinoma development in patients with HNPCC who have undergone abdominal colectomy.[334] Because the majority of such patients will be adequately treated by an abdominal colectomy, it could be considered as prophylactic management of their colorectal cancer risk.[338] It is appropriate to perform total abdominal colectomy at the time of operation for colorectal cancer or endoscopically untreatable colorectal polyps in patients with HNPCC, because of the high risk of synchronous and metachronous colorectal cancer.

Experience with this operation for FAP demonstrates that abdominal colectomy has low complication rates and good functional outcomes that are acceptable for such a prophylactic procedure. Some have recommended that patients with proven germline mutations be given the option of prophylactic abdominal colectomy. The Cancer Genetics Consortium, however, has not found adequate evidence to make a recommendation for prophylactic abdominal colectomy in patients with HNPCC.[329]

MANAGEMENT OF POTENTIALLY CURABLE COLON CANCER

PRETREATMENT EVALUATION

After colorectal carcinoma has been diagnosed, the pretreatment assessment is conducted to determine the most appropriate form of treatment. Whereas surgical management is required for most patients with a diagnosis of colon carcinoma, the appropriateness of a surgical resection will be determined by the extent of disease and comorbidities. Even in cases of metastatic colorectal carcinoma, surgery may be required for palliation. Some authors have recently documented an ability to manage colon cancer patients nonoperatively in the presence of metastatic disease without significant complications from bleeding, perforation, or obstruction.[339]

A well-conducted history and physical examination will provide a great deal of information about the patient's extent of disease and suitability for treatment. Specific aspects of the history taking should focus on a personal history of cancer or polyps and family history of colorectal cancer or polyps. Physical examination will reveal the patient's general suitability for anesthesia and extent of disease. Supraclavicular adenopathy can indicate advanced disease. The abdominal examination can reveal distention due to ascites or obstruction. An abdominal mass may be palpated to reveal the location of the tumor. Extensive hepatomegaly will produce a mass or tenderness in the right upper quadrant. Rectal examination can reveal presence of a mass outside the rectum, caused by peritoneal metastases, and may detect synchronous lesions in patients with colon cancer.

Laboratory examinations should evaluate for the presence of anemia or hepatic dysfunction. Both of which can be consequences of the patient's underlying carcinoma or comorbid conditions. The CEA level will be most useful in terms of subsequent assessment for disease recurrence if the initial CEA is elevated.

Complete colonic examination will not only allow a biopsy of the index lesion but will also provide information about the exact location of the lesion. Additionally, it will provide information on the presence or absence of synchronous colon cancers, which are present in 1.5% to 7.6% of cases. In addition, significant synchronous polyps can occur in 25% to 40% of patients.[129] The colon should be endoscopically cleared of these lesions. If polyps cannot be removed endoscopically, they should be included in the planned resection.

Chest radiography may reveal the presence of metastases or preexisting severe pulmonary disease that might contraindicate laparotomy. CT scanning is used to reveal clinically inapparent liver metastases or the extent of local spread of a colon carcinoma. Intraoperative ultrasonography is another useful technique that will be more sensitive in the detection of liver metastases.

SURGICAL MANAGEMENT OF CARCINOMA OF THE COLON

Radical resection with curative intent is appropriate for 80% to 90% of patients with colon carcinoma. The surgical principles of elective colonic resection include the appropriate use of outpatient bowel preparation to reduce the fecal and bacterial load of the colon. This, along with the use of parenteral antibiotics and appropriate anastomotic techniques, will reduce the risk of postoperative sepsis and morbidity. In patients with partially obstructing lesions, modification of the bowel preparation or the use of hydration along with the bowel preparation may be required preoperatively. It is important to use prophylaxis for deep venous thrombosis to reduce the subsequent risks of deep venous thrombosis and pulmonary embolism. Measures such as early ambulation and the use of intermittent compression devices and consideration of the use of low-dose heparin or low-molecular-weight heparin in the perioperative period reduce the incidence of venous thrombosis.

Surgical management must include the assessment of liver metastases. Although this is commonly accomplished by palpation and inspection, intraoperative ultrasonography of the liver has increased the rate of detection of small metastases.[340–342] The Doppler perfusion index has also been found to predict liver failure, because occult disease alters liver blood flow.[343] However, liver metastases still occur in 13% to 21% of patients who have negative results on intraoperative ultrasonography.[344]

Extent of Resection

The extent of colonic resection is determined by the blood vessels that must be divided to remove the lymphatic drainage of the tumor-bearing portion of the colon with tumor-free margins (Fig. 33.7-5). This is the primary treatment approach in patients with colon carcinoma.[345] Segmental resections without

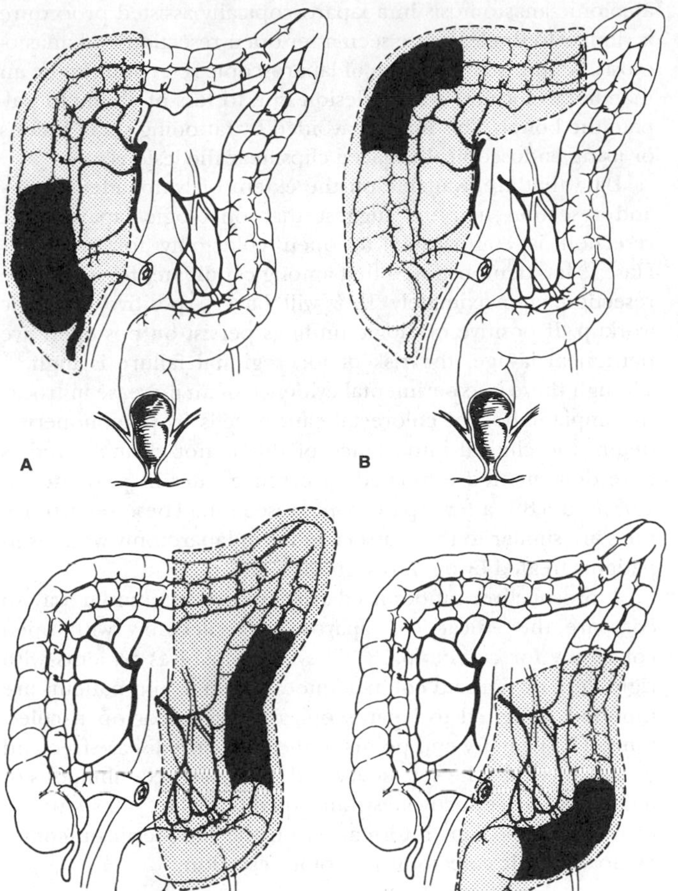

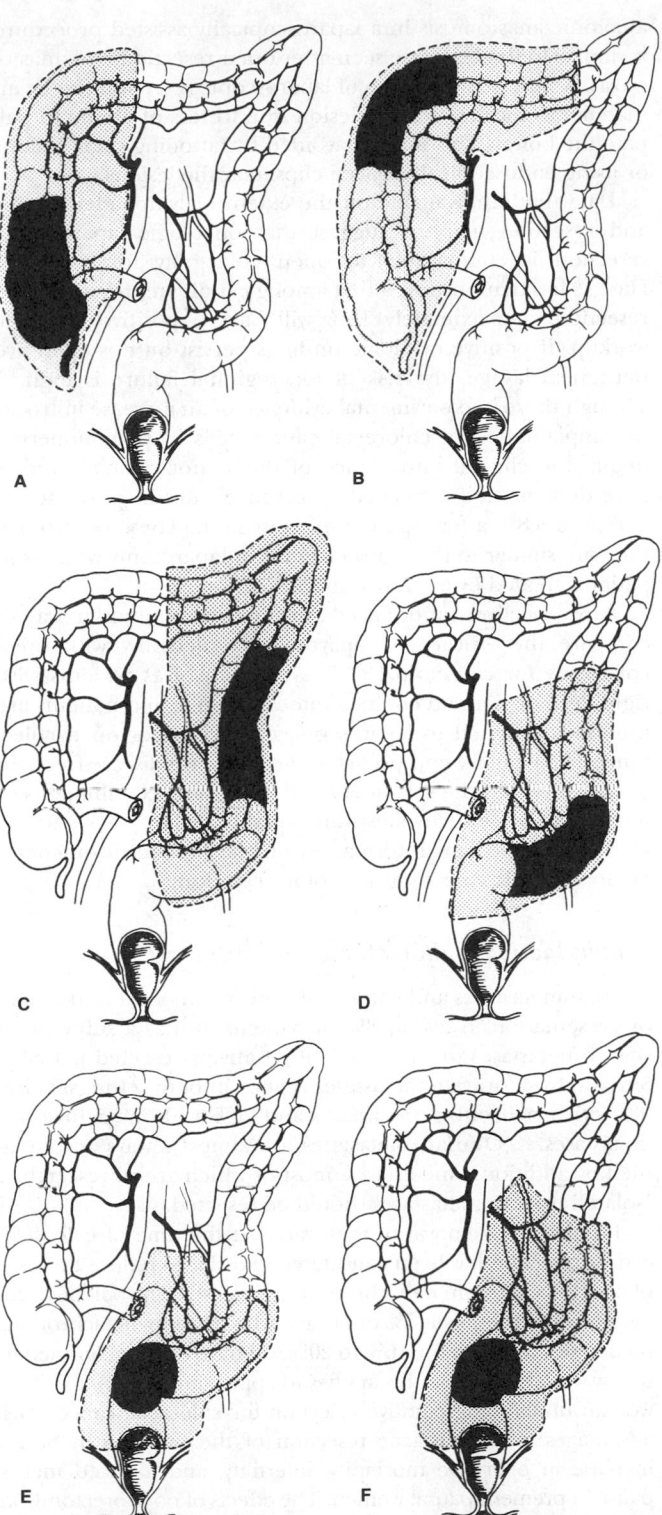

FIGURE 33.7-5. **A:** Surgical resection for a cecal or ascending colon cancer. **B:** Surgical resection for a cancer at the hepatic flexure. **C:** Surgical resection for a descending colon cancer. **D:** Preferred surgical procedure for cancer of the middle and proximal sigmoid colon. In poor-risk patients, the inferior mesenteric artery and the left colic artery may be preserved. **E:** Surgical resection for cancer of the retrosigmoid. **F:** A more radical surgical resection for cancer of the rectosigmoid. (Modified from Enker WE, Surgical treatment of large bowel cancer. In: Enker WE, *Cancer of the colon and rectum.* Chicago: Year Book, 1978:73.)

extensive mesenteric resection sometimes are performed in palliative situations. Resection of intermediate and principal nodes requires ligation and division of the main vascular trunks to the affected colon segment. Tumor-free margins usually are accomplished by resection of at least 5 cm of normal bowel proximal and distal to the tumor. However, in very aggressive tumors with lymphatic submucosal spread, this may be inadequate. In general, spread beyond the gross limits of the tumor of more than 1.2 cm occurs only in rare cases.

Tumors of the right colon include those of the cecum, ascending colon, hepatic flexure, and proximal half of the transverse colon. The ileocolic artery, right colic artery, and right branches of the middle colic artery usually are divided, and resection of the distal 10 cm of ileum is carried out along with resection of the cecum, ascending colon, and proximal transverse colon. If the main branch of the middle colic artery is taken near the origin from the superior mesenteric vessels, the bowel resection is extended to the distal third of the transverse colon to ensure that there is viable bowel for anastomosis. Uncontrolled data exist to demonstrate improvement in outcomes from extending this resection.

For tumors of the left colon, which includes the descending and upper sigmoid colon, the IMA is ligated near its origin at the aorta, and the splenic flexure of the colon is anastomosed to the upper rectum. In more limited resections for tumors in the left half of the transverse colon and splenic flexure, the resection may be limited to the ascending and descending left colic arteries and left branch of the middle colic artery. Anastomosis then is constructed between the proximal transverse colon and proximal sigmoid colon. Tumors of the distal sigmoid colon are usually resected along with the IMA near its origin at the aorta and the vessels that supply the sigmoid colon. The anastomosis is created between the area of the splenic flexure and the upper rectum. Growths between the hepatic flexure and splenic flexure may require a transverse colectomy or an extended right colectomy. The aim of transverse colectomy is removal of the transverse colon, the attached greater omentum, and the lymphatics lying in the drainage of the middle colic artery. For all these procedures, anastomosis may be created by either hand-sewn techniques or the use of stapling devices, with a low rate of anastomotic leak.

Extent of Lymph Node Resection

Some patients with node-positive colon carcinoma may be cured by surgical resection alone. Therefore, adequate lymphadenectomy is critical. In addition to its therapeutic benefits of preventing local progression and subsequent development of symptoms due to mesenteric recurrence, lymphadenectomy is critical in the staging of patients with colon carcinoma.[329] In colon cancer, recovery of lymph nodes is the parameter used for adjuvant therapy recommendations in the United States.

Controversy exists over the curative efficacy of extensive lymphadenectomy in patients with colon carcinoma. Excellent results have been obtained with wide mesenteric resection, whereas other studies have found patients with principle node involvement to be incurable. In a recent update regarding this issue, Slanetz and Grimson[346] reviewed 2409 cases of curative resections. They found that specific groups of patients benefited from high ligation of the vascular pedicle. These were patients with transmural node-negative tumors and those with limited nodal spread. Those in whom the highest nodes were involved did not appear to benefit.

Contiguous Organ Involvement

For tumors that are adherent to adjacent organs, adhesions should not be divided. In one-half of cases, the adherence may be caused by invasion of these adjacent organs by a transmural bulky colon carcinoma.[347] Separation of sites of adherence can disrupt the tumor, increase recurrence, and reduce survival rates. The organs commonly involved with transverse colon tumors are the stomach and omentum. Tumors of the splenic flexure may involve the spleen, tail of pancreas, left kidney, or diaphragm. Tumors of the right colon or cecum may involve the duodenum or right kidney. Tumors anywhere in the colon may involve the abdominal wall or may have adherent loops of small intestine. Occasionally, tumors of the cecum or sigmoid may involve the bladder at its dome or, in female patients, the uterus. Adjacent organ involvement should be resected in continuity with the colon and primary tumor. Radical resection may still be curative in 20% to 50% of patients, even if adjacent tissues are invaded by malignant infiltration.[347]

No-Touch Technique

Manipulation of a tumor-bearing colon during mobilization has been shown to release tumor cells into the circulation. This fact provides a theoretic basis for using a no-touch technique consisting of early vascular ligation prior to mobilization, to prevent subsequent development of distant metastases due to seeding. Molecular techniques have enhanced the ability to detect cancer cells released into the circulation during operative manipulation.[348] A prospective, randomized trial by Wiggers et al.[349] showed that in patients who underwent preliminary ligation of vessels, liver metastases appeared later than in patients who did not undergo this procedure. However, no overall survival benefit was demonstrated. The small benefit seen in this study occurred only in the subset of patients with sigmoid colon cancer and histologic evidence of venous invasion.

Laparoscopic Colectomy

Laparoscopic techniques have become widely used in the management of benign and malignant colorectal conditions.[350] These techniques are able to be carried out safely and successfully, especially in the hands of an experienced laparoscopic surgeon. Even assessment of the liver is carried out by laparoscopic intraoperative ultrasonography.[351,352] With laparoscopic colectomies, there is a theoretic advantages of a shortened hospital stay and a more rapid recovery.[353] The shortened stay associated with laparoscopic colectomy, attributable to early postoperative feeding, has also translated to a change in the management of colon resection patients who are treated by open techniques.[354]

The overall complications of laparoscopic colorectal surgery are comparable to those of open resection in a large randomized trial of laparoscopic and open colectomy in the United States.[355] However, the intraabdominal complications with laparoscopic surgery may be somewhat different from those seen with open surgery and include cauterization injury to the bowel, hypercapnia, ureteric injury, and development of hernia at the port site.[356] The risk of an anastomotic leak from a colonic anastomosis in a laparoscopically assisted procedure is similar to the leak rate seen after open resection and anastomosis. An unusual problem of laparoscopic resection can be an inability to localize a small lesion due to loss of ability to palpate the bowel. This may be avoided by tattooing small lesions or using endoscopically placed clips near the lesions.

Data that are available on the extent of lymphadenectomy and resection margins suggest that oncologic laparoscopic resection is comparable to open colectomy for cancer.[357] Hase[358] has demonstrated that among candidates for a curative resection, approximately 10% will have a positive cytologic workup. If positive cytologic findings persist on postoperative peritoneal lavage, the risk of locoregional failure is high.[358] Though there is experimental evidence of an increase in trocar site implantation of colorectal cancer cells by pneumoperitoneum, the clinical importance of this is not clear.[359] Studies have documented estimated recurrence rates in port sites of 1.08% to 3.8% after laparoscopic resection. These recurrence rates are similar to those associated with laparotomy wounds in patients treated by open resection.[355]

A prospective, randomized trial is currently under way to compare the efficacy of laparoscopic colectomy with open colectomy for carcinoma.[355] The study involves patients with right, left, or sigmoid colon adenocarcinoma, and patients are randomly assigned to laparoscopically assisted or open colectomy. The primary end points of the study are disease-free and overall survival. The secondary end points are examinations of morbidity, cost-effectiveness, and quality of life. This study is providing important information on the long-term outcomes of laparoscopic colectomy for colon resection.

Prophylactic Oophorectomy

Ovarian metastases and colorectal cancer can occur at the time of presentation in 2% to 8% of patients and as a subsequent site of metastases in 1% to 7% of curatively resected patients. Survival from ovarian metastases is poor in both settings, being 9% with synchronous metastases and 20% with metachronous metastases.[360] Ovarian metastases are almost always accompanied by additional metastases, most of which are unresectable. Isolated ovarian metastases should be resected.

Prophylactic removal of the ovaries at the time of colorectal cancer resection has been considered in order to reduce the risks of poor survival from metachronous metastases. This will be pertinent for only the 1% to 7% of women who develop metachronous metastases, of whom only 6% to 20% will have disease confined to the ovaries. Ultimately, this applies to approximately 1% to 4% of women undergoing curative resection for colorectal cancer. Disadvantages to prophylactic resection of the ovaries can be an increase in operative morbidity, infertility, and induced menopause in premenopausal women. The effects of oophorectomy on cardiovascular risk and bone density are important considerations in the quality of life of long-term survivors. A policy of prophylactic oophorectomy in postmenopausal women has been proposed owing to the risk of ovarian metastases or subsequent development of an ovarian primary cancer.

In a study of prophylactic oophorectomy in postmenopausal women by Sielezneff et al.,[361] the incidence of occult ovarian metastases was 2.4%. The 5-year survival rates in this study were equal, whether or not a prophylactic oophorectomy was performed.[362] In a preliminary report of a randomized trial of prophylactic oophorectomy in patients with Dukes stage B and C colorectal cancer treated at the Mayo Clinic, no incidence of gross or microscopic ovarian metastases was found in 77 patients randomized to oophorectomy. No differences were seen in overall survival, whether or not patients were randomized to oophorectomy. A trend was noted toward an improved recurrence-free survival with prophylactic oophorectomy. No selection criteria based on tumor size, grade, or other characteristics exist at this time.[363]

In clinical practice, isolated synchronous ovarian metastases should be resected by oophorectomy. In premenopausal women, there is no substantial proof of benefit of this procedure, though the potential for harm by prophylactic oophorectomy does exist. In postmenopausal women, prophylactic oophorectomy can be considered after careful explanation to the patient of the risks and potential benefits.

Oncologic Results of Surgical Management

For patients undergoing curative resection for colon cancer, overall survival rates vary between 55% and 75%, with most recurrences seen in the first 2 years of follow-up. Survival after curative resection is markedly affected by the presence of nodal metastases. For node-negative patients, survival with surgery alone varies between 75% and 90%.[364] Even in these cancers, such factors as depth of penetration, contiguous organ involvement, lymphatic and vascular invasion, differentiation, and perineural invasion, as well as molecular and cellular characteristics, will affect survival.[365]

Important issues in surgically resected apparently node-negative colon cancer are the methods of lymph node evaluation and the detection of occult metastatic disease. Standardizing node evaluation and using immunohistochemical techniques can identify occult nodal metastases in up to 26% of those whose nodes test negatively by routine techniques.[366] In addition, radioimmunologically guided surgical evaluation of apparently node-negative patients after resection is highly predictive of occult metastatic disease causing recurrence.[367] However, convincing data on survival improvement based on these techniques are lacking. Some have even questioned the relevance of occult micrometastatic disease in patients who have undergone curative resection.[368] In a group of surgically resected patients with micrometastases in resected nodes and original Dukes' stage A or B colorectal cancer, survival time was 48 months, which mimicked the survival time for patients without micrometastases.

Among patients with node-positive cancers, survival can be affected by the number of positive nodes. Patients with one positive node may have survival rates in the 69% to 75% range, whereas 5-year survival for those with four or more positive nodes or metastases along a named vascular trunk will be in the 27% to 40% range.[364] Overall, survival rates for patients with node-positive cancers appear to be approximately 40% to 50%. The analysis by Cohen et al. (1991) of node-positive colon cancer patients treated with resection alone showed a significant difference in survival for patients having one to three positive nodes (66% 5 year survival) and those with four or more positive nodes (37% 5-year survival).

Patterns of Recurrence

Locoregional failure in colon cancer occurs in adjacent soft tissues, regional and retroperitoneal nodes, and the peritoneum. The major pattern of recurrence in colon cancer is disseminated disease with liver metastasis in two-thirds of patients in whom treatment fails. Few patients will have isolated recurrence. There is a 6% rate of anastomosis recurrence.[369] As mentioned, the abdominal colon consists of portions that are intraperitoneal (e.g., the cecum, transverse colon, and sigmoid colon) and portions that are less mobile and lie against the retroperitoneum (e.g., the ascending and descending colon and hepatic and splenic flexures). The portions lying against the retroperitoneum are at higher risk for minimal radial margins at the time of surgical resection and therefore are at higher risk for local recurrence. Gunderson demonstrated that local failure increased in these areas of immobility and with extension of tumor through the bowel. In patients with transmural node-positive disease, areas of mobile bowel had a 13% local failure rate, whereas areas of immobile bowel had a 29% local failure rate. Local recurrence rates were even higher when there was gross extension into pericolonic fat. Retroperitoneal nodal failures can be seen in up to two-thirds of patients in whom resection of transmural tumors fails. Patients with node-positive disease exhibit locoregional failure more commonly than do those with negative nodes.

In lesions that occur in areas of the bowel covered by serosa, extension through the bowel wall will increase the risk for peritoneal spread. In the autopsy series reported from the University of Washington, treatment failure manifested as peritoneal seeding in 36% of patients who died from colon cancer. This is chiefly a component of multiple sites of recurrence. In a series of 533 patients studied at the Massachusetts General Hospital, peritoneal failure rates varied from 0% to 4% for stage A and B lesions, whereas for stage C lesions, rates of peritoneal failure ranged from 14% to 16%.

SPECIFIC MANAGEMENT PROBLEMS

Synchronous Cancer

Synchronous cancers are relatively uncommon, having an incidence of 3.4%, as described by Finan et al.[370] In addition to the presence of another malignancy, there can be up to a 30% to 40% incidence of synchronous neoplastic polyps in the colon of a patient with a large bowel carcinoma.[371] These facts emphasize the need for complete colonic examination at the time of diagnosis of a colon carcinoma.

Most synchronous neoplastic polyps can be removed at the time of preoperative colonoscopy. If this cannot be accomplished owing to obstructing lesions or an emergency operation for perforation, the index lesion should be addressed at the time of surgery and subsequent complete colonoscopic examination should be carried out in the early postoperative period.[372] If the synchronous lesions are in the same colonic segment, they can be included in the resection, which should maintain the principles of wide anatomic resection and lymphadenectomy.

When lesions are in widely disparate parts of the colon and cannot otherwise be cleared by endoscopic polypectomy, then consideration should be given to either two segmental resections or subtotal colectomy. Partial colectomies will require subsequent intensive colonic surveillance. However, they may be the most appropriate alternative for an elderly patient. Subtotal colectomy may be the treatment of choice for a younger patient with synchronous lesions.[373] Passman et al.[373] conducted an 18-year, multiinstitutional database study of 4878 patients with colon cancer. They found a 3.3% incidence of synchronous tumors. They also found that patients with synchronous colon cancers have the same survival rate as patients with solitary colon tumors when the highest stage of the synchronous tumor is considered.[373]

Obstructing Cancers

Intestinal obstruction is the most common emergency presentation of colorectal carcinoma.[374] Poor prognosis is associated with this presentation, even when analyzed stage for stage, with an overall survival of 31% at 5 years. Patients who present with this problem are frequently elderly or in poor condition because of dehydration, and operative mortality can approach 28%.[374] Operative approaches in such patients have included a three-stage operation with an initial diverting colostomy followed by resection and then colostomy closure. An alternative approach is the use of a two-stage Hartmann procedure in which the resection is performed and an end colostomy is created while the distal colon is closed. The second operation then reestablishes continuity.

Staged resection is most useful in elderly persons with multiple comorbidities.[374] As techniques of preoperative resuscitation and perioperative care have advanced, further alternatives for obstructing lesions distal to the splenic flexure have been studied. The first is subtotal colectomy, the second is an extended right colectomy to include the obstructing lesion without colonic decompression, and a third is the use of intraoperative colonic lavage and segmental resection. Nyam et al.[362] reported on a series of 103 patients with obstructing left-side colon carcinomas undergoing an extended right colectomy without colonic decompression or a segmental left colectomy with intraoperative lavage. They found that both procedures had an acceptably low anastomotic leak rate and mortality. Poon et al.[375] studied emergency primary resection and anastomosis with intraoperative colonic lavage for left-sided obstruction. Hospital mortality rate was 5% to 9%. The anastomotic leak rate with this approach was 4%.

The alternative approach of subtotal colectomy with ileorectal anastomosis has been compared with intraoperative lavage in primary colonic anastomosis in a randomized trial.[376] This trial showed no difference in mortality or morbidity rates. However, patients with subtotal colectomy had a higher postoperative frequency of bowel movements.[376]

Patients with right-sided obstructing lesions should undergo a radical right hemicolectomy with primary anastomosis.

Perforating Cancers

Perforation of the colon due to carcinoma can occur either at the site of the colon tumor itself (in approximately 65% to 82% of patients with perforation) or in the bowel proximal to an obstructing tumor (in 18% to 35% of patients).[377] Many of these patients will have local or regionally advanced disease at the time of the discovery of perforation, and approximately one-third of these patients will have metastatic disease at the time of laparotomy. Overall 5-year survival for patients with localized perforation is approximately 44%. This complication occurs in 2% to 8% of all patients with colorectal cancer. These patients can present with diffuse peritonitis and require emergency management. Some contained perforations will extend into adjacent bowel loops or viscera and therefore cause a fistula that should be resected *en bloc* with the tumor at the time of resection.

The presence of a perforation or fistula will increase cancer recurrence rates. Local recurrence rates of 23% have been reported by Carraro et al.[377] in a study of 83 patients with large bowel perforation and colorectal cancer. This compares with figures of 28% to 44% reported in the literature. Peritoneal seeding is a particularly common failure in patients with perforated colorectal cancers, with carcinomatosis rates of 17% to 18%.

Malignant Polyps

The management of neoplastic polyps that are benign has already been addressed. In this section, we will consider the management of a malignant polyp in which the invasive component has perforated the muscularis mucosae and therefore has the potential for metastatic spread. The rationale for colon resection for a malignant colorectal polyp after endoscopic removal is minimization of the risk of residual carcinoma at the site of the polypectomy, the risk of metastatic spread to regional lymph nodes, and the risk of disease dissemination.

The risks and benefits of resection must be weighed against the patient's potential for morbidity and mortality from either the cancer or a surgical resection.[378] The risks of mortality from elective colorectal surgery are approximately 1% to 2%. However, in a given individual, age and the presence or absence of comorbidity will dictate surgical mortality.

Malignant colorectal polyps may be pedunculated or sessile. Endoscopic removal will be more successful in managing malignant pedunculated polyps. Critical factors in determining the need for surgery after colonoscopic removal of a malignant polyp are the differentiation features of the carcinoma (well or moderately differentiated), the presence of vascular or lymphatic invasion, the presence of a clear polyp resection margin, and assessment that the polyp has been completely removed.[378] Most commonly, the issue dictating surgical resection will be an inadequate or questionable margin.[379]

Haggitt et al. (1985) have described various levels of invasion of carcinoma into pedunculated polyps (Fig. 33.7-6). They noted that, in a pedunculated polyp, an invasive component in the head of the polyp may be a substantial distance from the submucosa and therefore may be resected endoscopically with a significant margin. In a sessile polyp, the invasive component has early access to the submucosa and therefore has an earlier opportunity for dissemination. Sessile polyps will have a higher incidence of lymph node metastases than pedunculated polyps with invasive cancer.[380] When the invasive cancer is limited to the head of a pedunculated polyp, lymph node metastasis rates appear to be approximately 3%, in contrast to 10% to 25% for sessile polyps (Table 33.7-7). The incremental improvement related to extensive surgery in patients with cancers limited to the head of the polyp is low. Patients with favorable risk criteria and a cancer limited to the head of a pedunculated polyp will be treated best by colonoscopic polypectomy alone. Sessile polyps are best treated by surgical resection,[381] though some investigators have disputed this.[382]

After colonoscopic removal of the malignant polyp, it is important to document carefully the site of polypectomy in the event that surgical resection is warranted. We commonly perform this procedure using endoscopically placed clips, which are both pal-

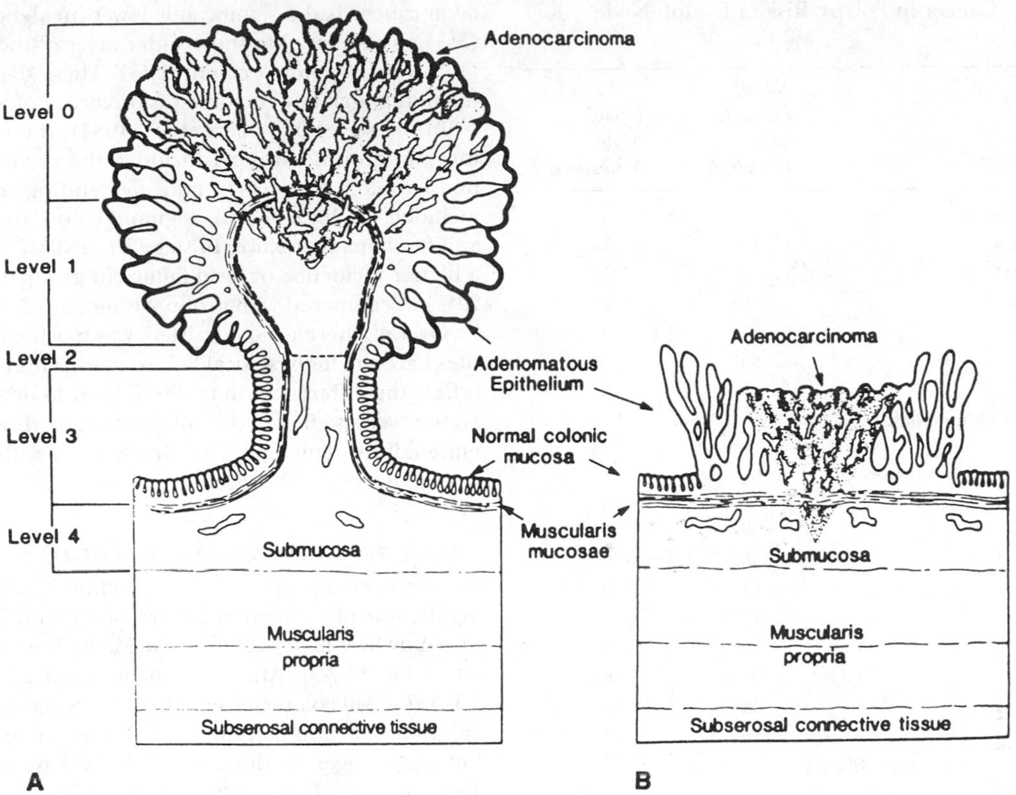

FIGURE 33.7-6. Levels of invasion in a pedunculated adenoma **(A)** and a sessile adenoma **(B)**. The stippled areas represent zones of carcinoma. Any invasion below the muscularis mucosae in a sessile lesion represents level 4 invasion (submucosa). In contrast, invasive carcinoma in a pedunculated adenoma must traverse a considerable distance before it reaches the submucosa of the underlying bowel wall. However, any cancer that penetrates the muscularis mucosae is at risk for dissemination.

pable and evident on abdominal radiographs. Follow-up colonoscopy is generally performed 3 to 6 months after removal of a malignant polyp, to assess the polypectomy site for any residual mass. Presence of a mass is an indication for surgical resection. In patients in whom there is no further evidence of residual carcinoma, colonoscopic follow-up can be carried out at 1 year.[154]

Whitlow et al.[379] studied a group of 59 patients who underwent treatment for malignant colonic polyps. Sixty-three percent of the patients were managed with polypectomy and surveillance. The remainder underwent colectomy. The most common indications for colectomy were Haggitt level 3 or 4 invasion, inadequate margins, patient preference, or poor differentiation, in that order. Residual disease was found in 3 of the 22 patients undergoing colectomy. Importantly, there were no cancer-related deaths in either treatment group. None of the patients in Whitlow's group had evidence of lymph node involvement at the time of colectomy.

Netzer et al.[380] studied the outcomes in 32 patients with endoscopically removed low-risk malignant polyps versus the outcomes of 38 patients with high-risk polyps. High-risk malignant polyps were defined as having an incomplete polypectomy, a margin that was not clearly cancer-free, lymphatic or vascular invasion, or grade 3 carcinoma. In this series, 73% of the patients had pedunculated malignant polyps and, of these, 8.5% had adverse outcomes. Of the 27% of patients with sessile malignant polyps, 58% had had adverse outcomes defined as residual disease at colectomy or cancer recurrence during the follow-up period.[380] Large sessile lesions in the colon often require surgical resection as the safest approach. Biopsy and observation alone is usually not the best approach, unless operative morbidity is expected to be excessive.

ADJUVANT THERAPIES

Adjuvant Radiation Therapy for Colon Cancer

PATTERNS OF FAILURE OF AND THE RATIONALE FOR RADIATION THERAPY. The role of adjuvant radiation therapy in colon cancer is less well defined than in rectal cancer. This is due to differences in the natural history of colon cancer as compared with rectal cancer. As seen in Table 33.7-8, the most common failure site after potentially curative surgery in colon cancer is abdominal rather than local. Furthermore, because most local failures in colon cancer are extrapelvic, local failure usually does not result in the same degree of debilitating pelvic pain as that seen in rectal cancer.

Although the overall incidence of local failure is relatively low in colon cancer, data suggest that, on the basis of anatomic location and selected pathologic features, certain subsets of patients have a higher incidence of local failure. However, there is not uniform agreement as to how to define these subsets. For example, Gunderson et al. (1985) divided the colon into two regions. The "anatomically immobile" (or mainly retroperitoneal) region included the ascending colon, hepatic flexure, splenic flexure, and descending colon. The "anatomically mobile" (or mainly intraperitoneal) region included the cecum and transverse

TABLE 33.7-7. Cancer in Polyps: Risk of Lymph Node Metastases

	No. of Patients with Resection	*Lymph Node Metastases*
Sessile polyps with invasive cancer		
Grinnell and Lane	13	3
Waye and Frankel	9	1
Wolff and Shyna	5	2
Locke et al.	12	4
Kodaira et al.	34	2
Nivatvong	25	3
Lymph nodes with metastases, 15%		
Pedunculated polyps with invasive cancer		
Grinnell and Lane	39	3
Waye and Frankel	8	0
Wolff and Shinya	11	0
Shatney et al.	23	1
Locke et al.	15	1
Colachio et al.	24	6
Kodaira et al.	64	3
Shatney et al	16	3
Lymph nodes with metastases, 8%		
Pedunculated polyps with invasive cancer limited to head of polyp		
Grinnell and Lane	28	0
Shatney et al.	14	0
Nivatvong	12	0
Colachio et al.	11	2
Lymph nodes with metastases, 3%		

(Modified from Nivatong S. Management of polyps containing invasive carcinoma. In: Codner IJ, et al. *Colon, rectal and anal surgery*. St. Louis, Mosby, 1985:183, with permission.)

colon. The highest incidence of local failure occurred in the cecum (30%), whereas the other intraperitoneal site, the transverse colon, had one of the lowest rates of local failure (13%).

In contrast, Minsky et al. (1988) reported a general trend of increased local failure with more distal colon sites. Patients with cecal cancer had a significantly lower incidence of local failure (3%), as compared to those with cancer of the transverse colon (15%) or descending colon (25%). These data do not support the notion that bowel mobility is predictive of local failure.

In the series by Willett et al. (1984), the colon was divided into two groups. Group 1 included the cecum and ascending, midsigmoid, transverse, and descending colon. Group 2 included the high and low sigmoid colon, the splenic flexure, and the hepatic flexure. In stage T1–2N0M0 disease, there was a higher incidence of local failure in group 1 tumors (16% to 24%) as compared with group 2 tumors (0% to 11%).

Overall, there is no consistency as to which anatomic site or sites have the highest local failure rates. This inconsistency may reflect the differences in methods used to detect failure (reoperation versus clinical or radiographic methods) and to determine failure (cumulative vs. first failure) rather than the true natural history of the disease.

LOCOREGIONAL RADIATION THERAPY. Although all the series are retrospective, the most comprehensive series examining the role of locoregional radiation therapy in colon cancer is the study by Willett et al.[383] at the Massachusetts General Hospital (Table 33.7-9). After potentially curative surgery for stages T3–4N0–2M0 colon cancer, 203 patients received postoperative adjuvant radiation therapy. Eligibility included patients with the following stages of disease: T4N0–2M0 tumors regardless of anatomic site, T3N1–2M0 tumors excluding midsigmoid and transverse colon, and selected high-risk T3N0M0 tumors with close margins. Patients received 45 Gy to the primary tumor bed with a 5-cm margin and inclusive of the primary draining lymph nodes. This was followed by a shrinking-field technique to 50.4 to 55.0 Gy depending on the volume of small bowel that could be excluded from the high-dose field. Of the 203 patients, 173 were treated in the adjuvant setting and 30 after a subtotal resection. Sixty-three received bolus 5-fluorouracil (5-FU) with a variety of doses and schedules.

The results were compared with a historical control group of 395 patients who underwent surgery only. Three patient groups appeared to benefit from postoperative radiation therapy. There was a significant improvement in local control and disease-free survival for patients with stage T4N0M0 or T4N1–2M0 disease. Also, patients with stage T4N0 disease with a perforation or fistula had improved local control and disease-free survival. Finally,

TABLE 33.7-8. Patterns of Failure after Potentially Curative Surgery for Colon Cancer (All Stages)[a]

Series	*Detection and Definition of Failure*	*Stage*	*No.*	*No. Experiencing Local Failure (%)*		*No. Experiencing Abdominal Failure (%)*		*No. Experiencing Distant Failure*	
				Only	Component	Only	Component	Only	Component
Gunderson (1985)	Reoperation, cumulative failure	All stages	91	22 (0–30)	48 (0–64)	4 (0–9)	21 (0–36)	7 (0–16)	30 (0–38)
		T3–4 and/or N1–2	72	17	49	6	26	7	35
Willett[383]	Clinical, cumulative failure	All stages	533	6 (0–12)	19 (0–49)	11 (2–24)	21 (3–43)	4 (0–10)	13 (0–25)
		T3–4 and/or N1–2	395	8	26	14	25	5	16
Minksy (1988)	Clinical, first failure	All stages	284	6 (0–8)	9 (0–25)	8 (0–29)	13 (0–57)	3 (0–11)	6 (0–25)
		T3–4 and/or N1–2	229	4	10	10	15	5	6

[a]In the Gunderson series, liver metastasis are considered distant failure, whereas in the series by Willett and by Minsky, liver metastases are considered abdominal failure.

TABLE 33.7-9. Local Adjuvant Radiation Therapy in Colon Cancer

		Locoregional Failure				*5-Y Disease-Free Survival*	
Group	*Stage*	No.	Surgery (%)	No.	Surgery + Radiation (%)	Surgery (%)	Surgery + Radiation (%)
Adjuvant therapy	T3N0	163	10	23	9[a]	70	72
	T4N0	83	31	54	7	63	79
	T3N1–2	100	35	55	30	44	47
	T4N1–2	49	53	39	28	37	53
Residual disease	All stages	—	—	30	47	—	37
Perforation or fistula	T4N0	21	48	23	6	43	91

[a]Actuarial component of total failure.
(From Willett, Massachusetts General Hospital.)

radiation therapy salvaged some patients with residual disease after subtotal resection, resulting in a 37% 5-year disease-free survival. There was no benefit in local control or disease-free survival in patients with stage T3N0M0 or T3N1–2M0 disease.

For the total patient group, the incidence of grade 3+ acute bowel toxicity was 8%. The incidence was lower in the patients who received radiation therapy plus chemotherapy (4% vs. 16%, respectively). Grade 3+ long-term bowel toxicity was 4.5%. Therefore, with careful treatment techniques, the acute and long-term bowel toxicities of postoperative locoregional radiation therapy (with or without chemotherapy) for colon cancer are comparable with those reported for rectal cancer.

Other reports of adjuvant locoregional radiation therapy are limited by small numbers of patients and short follow-up.[384] Most have been limited to cecal cancers.

Based on the retrospective data from the Massachusetts General Hospital, a randomized phase III intergroup trial coordinated by the Mayo Clinic and NCCTG (INT 0130) was developed. Patients with T4 or selected T3N1–2 colon tumors were randomized to 12 cycles of bolus 5-FU plus levamisole with or without locoregional radiation therapy (45.0 to 50.4 Gy in 25 to 28 fractions) beginning with cycle two of chemotherapy. The trial was closed early due to poor accrual, with only 222 of the anticipated 400 patients randomized, leaving 189 eligible patients.[385] Grade 3+ toxicity was modestly higher in the combined-modality therapy arm (43% vs. 35%). With a median follow-up of 35 months, there was no significant difference in survival between the two arms. The patterns of failure data have not been reported.

In a phase I trial of 21 patients (4 with colon cancers) who received upper abdominal radiation plus continuous-infusion 5-FU at 150 mg/m^2, Martenson et al.[386] reported a 40% grade 3+ toxicity rate. In contrast, the recommended dose of continuous-infusion 5-FU plus concurrent radiation for patients with rectal cancer who receive adjuvant therapy is 225 mg/m^2.[387] These data suggest that the dose of continuous-infusion 5-FU needs to be attenuated in patients receiving combined-modality therapy for upper abdominal malignancies. This is most likely related to the larger radiation field.

In summary, the retrospective data from the Massachusetts General Hospital suggest that there are subsets of colon cancer patients with high local failure rates in whom the addition of postoperative locoregional radiation therapy may improve local control and disease-free survival. The randomized INT 0130 trial did not show a survival advantage with combined-modality therapy versus chemotherapy alone. It must be emphasized, however, that the INT 0130 trial was closed prior to meeting its accrual goals and has not yet reported local control results. Although postoperative locoregional radiation therapy in colon cancer remains investigational, two clinical situations exist in which its use is reasonable: in a patient with close or positive resection margins and in a patient who has undergone a resection of a T4 colon cancer adherent to pelvic structures. These cancers (most commonly sigmoid or cecal primary lesions) have local failure rates similar to rectal cancers, and it is reasonable to treat them as such with adjuvant combined-modality therapy, including six cycles of 5-FU–based chemotherapy plus concurrent pelvic radiation.[388]

WHOLE ABDOMEN RADIATION THERAPY. The use of whole abdomen radiation therapy is limited by dose considerations. To treat the volume at risk with a potentially curative dose of radiation required for microscopic disease, the whole abdomen would need to receive 45 Gy. Although limited portions of the abdomen can tolerate this dose, the tolerance of the whole abdomen with conventional fractionation is 30 Gy. Based on the high incidence of abdominal failure in some colon cancers, a number of phase II adjuvant trials were designed to examine the efficacy of whole abdomen radiation therapy (Table 33.7-10).[389,390]

In general, patients received 20 to 30 Gy to the whole abdomen with or without a boost to the primary tumor bed. In three of the series, 5-FU was delivered with a variety of doses and schedules. The combined results revealed an in-field (abdominal) failure rate of 12% to 50%. Significant toxicity varied from 5% to 38%. Although the initial phase II results appeared promising, three of the series have never been updated.

The most encouraging data have been reported by Fabian et al.[389] from the SWOG 8572 study. In this phase II adjuvant pilot trial, 41 patients with T3N1–2M0 disease received whole abdomen radiation therapy plus continuous-infusion 5-FU (200 mg/m^2/24 h) followed by 9 monthly cycles of maintenance continuous-infusion 5-FU (1000 mg/m^2/24 h × 4 days). Due to unacceptable toxicity in the first six patients, the protocol was modified such that the 5-FU was started on day 1 and radiation began concurrently on day 8 *and* a 1-week treatment break from both the 5-FU and radiation was required at day 42. The tumor bed boost (1.6 Gy × 10 days) was delivered first, followed by whole abdomen radiation therapy (1 Gy/d × 30 days) for a total dose of 30 Gy to the whole abdomen and 46 Gy to the tumor bed.

TABLE 33.7-10. Whole Abdomen Adjuvant Radiation Therapy for Colon Cancer

Series	*No.*	*Stage*	*Abdominal Chemotherapy*	*In-Field RT Dose*[a]	*Failure (%)*	*Survival*	*Toxicity*
Brenner (1983)	21	T1–4N2M0	5-FU	20	14	65% at 5 y (1 at risk)	10% SBO
Meek (1983)	8	T3N0–2M0	None	30 Gy + a 10- to 16-Gy boost	50	50% NED at 10–35 mo	38% unable to complete treatment
Wong (1984)	30	T1–4N0–2M0	7 had 5-FU	14–22.5 Gy ± a 15- to 30-Gy boost	27	55% at 5 y	2% SBO, 5% severe diarrhea
Fabian (1988)	41	T3N1–2M0	CI 5-FU + maintenance	30 Gy + a 16-Gy boost	12–22	67% at 5 y	17% grade 3, 4% grade 4
Ben-Josef (1995)	18	T1–3NO–2	14 had CI 5-FU	30 Gy ± a 9.6- to 16-G boost	28 (22 liver)	78% at 5 y	17% acute grade 3+A,[b] 11% late grade 3+

CI, continuous infusion; 5-FU, 5-fluorouracil; NED, no evidence of disease; RT, radiation therapy; SBO, small bowel obstruction.
[a]In-field failure includes the tumor bed and the peritoneal cavity.
[b]"A"does not include patients who had an unplanned treatment break; therefore, the true incidence is higher.

With a median follow-up of 5 years, the 5-year disease-free and overall survival rates were 58% and 67%, respectively.[389] Limiting the analysis to the 20 patients with more than four positive nodes, the 5-year disease-free and overall survival rates were 55% and 74%, respectively. For the total patient group, the patterns of failure included local failure (12%), liver failure (22%), and peritoneal and other abdominal failure (15%). In contrast with other whole abdomen radiation therapy trials, toxicity during the combined-modality segment was tolerable (17%, grade 3; 7%, grade 4). The toxicity during the maintenance chemotherapy was also acceptable (25%, grade 3; 3%, grade 4). These results are encouraging, but further follow-up is needed. Currently, whole abdomen radiation therapy remains investigational.

Adjuvant Systemic Therapy for Colon Cancer

SINGLE-AGENT STUDIES. The fact that a substantial number of patients treated surgically with curative intent eventually die of metastatic disease was understood early. Once the natural history of the disease became better defined, subsets of patients with a higher risk of recurrence could be identified. The next logical step was the development of adjuvant treatments attempting to improve the long-term disease-free and overall survival rates. The first trials were conducted in the 1950s,[391,392,393] and a partial summary of these first-generation studies is provided in Table 33.7-11. The chemotherapeutic agents available were restricted to thiotepa, floxuridine (FUDR), and 5-FU, and they were commonly used with suboptimal intensity.

Even though these early trials are generally considered negative because no dramatic benefit could be elicited, some studies with the fluoropyrimidines did demonstrate a 5% to 10% benefit in 5-year survival. The results were intriguing enough to justify continuous efforts with novel agents and combinations of the available agents in the same setting.

INITIAL COMBINATION CHEMOTHERAPY STUDIES. The combinations explored in the 1970s included chemotherapy and, occasionally, nonspecific immunotherapy with bacille Calmette-Guérin (BCG), BCG variations, and levamisole. These drugs are well represented in six large studies published in peer-reviewed journals and are summarized in Table 33.7-12. Methyl-CCNU plus 5-FU (MF) and MF plus vincristine (Oncovin; MOF) were commonly used, because at that time, they were believed to be more active in advanced disease than 5-FU alone. With more than 3700 patients entered in these six trials, a trend favoring the chemotherapy-treated groups was noted. However, the only trials to achieve statistical significance were NSABP C-01 and NCCTG 78-48-52.

TABLE 33.7-11. First-Generation Randomized Trials of Adjuvant Therapy for Large Bowel Cancer

Study	*Study Period*	*Treatment Regimen*	*Duration*	*Total Accrual*
Dixon et al.[393]	1957–1960	Thiotepa	2 d	695
Dwight et al.[391]	1957–1961	Thiotepa	2 d	1064
Dwight et al.[392]	1961–1964	FUDR	7 wk	548
Higgins et al.[509]	1965–1969	5-FU	6 wk	308
	1969–1973	5-FU	18 mo	518
Grage and Moss (1981)	1971–1976	5-FU	12 mo	233

5-FU, 5-fluorouracil; FUDR, floxuridine.
Note: All studies had a surgery-only control group.

TABLE 33.7-12. Second-Generation Colon Cancer Adjuvant Trials

Study	*Total Accrual*	*Chemotherapy*	*Immunotherapy*	*Chemoimmunotherapy*	*Results*
VASOG 5[510]	654	5-FU, 9 mg/kg on d 1 + methyl-CCNU, 120 mg/m^2 on d 1, every 7 wk for 12 cycles	—	—	MF results in survival benefit for Dukes' stage C1
GITSG 6175[511]	621	5-FU, 325 mg/m^2 on d 1–5, 375 mg/m^2 on d 36–40, + methyl-CCNU, 130 mg/m^2 on d 1, every 10 wk for 7 cycles	BCG-MER, 1 mg ID on d 1 and 0.5 mg ID once weekly at wk 1, 5, 10, 15, 20, 25, 40, 55, 70	MF + BCG-MER	Apparent overall improved survival compared to historical controls
ECOG 2276[512]	866	5-FU + methyl-CCNU, same as GITSG 6175, for 8 cycles, or 5-FU, 450 mg/m^2/d × 5 d, every 5 wk for 15 cycles	—	—	No significant differences in overall survival
NSABP C-O1[394]	1166	MF, same as in GITSG 6175 protocol, + VCR, 1 mg/m^2 on d 1, every 10 wk for 8 cycles	BCG, 6 × 10^8 organisms/wk for scarification for 12 wk, then every other week for 33 wk	—	MOF results in 67% 5-year survival vs. 58% for control
SWOG 7510[394,416]	626	5-FU, 400 mg/m^2 on d 1, 8, 15, methyl-CCNU, 175 mg/m^2 on d 1, every 8 wk for 7 cycles		MF + BCG (6 × 10^8 organisms PO) every other week for 26 wk	Superior disease-free survival for MF ± BCG
Abali et al.[513]	253	—	BCG, 120 mg po monthly × 5 y	BCG + methyl-CCNU, 130 mg/m^2 d 1, + 5-FU, 325 mg/m^2/d d 1–5 and 375 mg/m^2/d d 36–40 for 8 cycles	No survival advantage for either treatment compared to untreated control
NCCTG 78-48-52[514]	398	—	Levamisole, 150 mg d 1–3 every 3 wk	Levamisole + 5-FU, 450 mg/m^2/wk for 52 wk	5-FU ± levamisole results in superior disease-free survival

BCG, bacille Calmette-Guérin; ECOG, Eastern Cooperative Oncology Group; 5-FU, 5-fluorouracil; GITSG, Gastrointestinal Tumor Study Group; ID, intradermally; MER, methanol extraction residue of BCG; MF, methyl-CCNU + 5-FU; MOF, MF plus vincristine (Oncovin); NCCTG, North Central Cancer Treatment Group; NSABP, National Surgical Adjuvant Breast and Bowel Project; SWOG, Southwest Oncology Group; VASOG, Veterans Administration Surgical Oncology Group; VCR, vincristine.

The NSABP C-01 study randomly assigned 1166 patients with Dukes stage B and C colon carcinoma to receive chemotherapy or immunotherapy or to be observed only. When compared with the control group, the patients treated with MOF had statistically superior disease-free survival (P = .02) and overall survival (P= .05). At 5-year follow-up, the group treated with MOF had an 8% survival improvement over the control group. There was no significant difference between the BCG and control groups (P = .40).[394] This was the first randomized trial to demonstrate a benefit in disease-free and overall survival for patients treated with chemotherapy. The toxicity of the MOF regimen is significant, and five patients in the NSABP C-01 trial developed acute leukemia or myelodysplasia. This particular toxicity was evaluated by Boice et al., who found 19 cases of leukemia or myelodysplasia among 2067 patients treated with regimens containing MF, with an estimated risk of 2.3 cases per 1000 patients per year.

Levamisole. Levamisole is a synthetic, orally active agent with antihelmintic and immunomodulatory properties. The observation that levamisole enhances the immune response of mice vaccinated against *Brucella* bacteria led to its investigation in cancer. The drug is well absorbed from the GI tract after oral administration and is extensively metabolized by the liver.[395]

Levamisole was initially evaluated in the treatment of advanced colorectal cancer in combination with 5-FU. More than 400 patients were enrolled in three randomized trials evaluating the addition of levamisole to 5-FU chemotherapy. The results were disappointing, with no improvement in response rate, time to progression, or survival in favor of the levamisole-treated groups.[396]

Since 1974, levamisole has been investigated as a single agent in the adjuvant treatment of colorectal cancer.[397] Despite the good results seen initially, two large, prospective, randomized, placebo-controlled trials reported subsequently have failed to demonstrate a significant benefit for levamisole administered as a single agent.[398] Eventually, levamisole was combined with 5-FU in the adjuvant setting. Small trials comparing 5-FU-based chemotherapy with or without levamisole did not demonstrate a benefit for the levamisole-treated group. In a larger trial, after curative surgery for colorectal cancer, 141 patients were randomized to receive a 6-month course of 5-FU with or without levamisole or supportive treatment only.[399] After 5 years of follow-up, a significant survival advantage was detected in the patients receiving levamisole as compared with patients treated with 5-FU alone.

The true turning point in the adjuvant treatment of colorectal cancer came with the results of two well-known randomized trials (Table 33.7-13). In one, conducted by the NCCTG and the

TABLE 33.7-13. Adjuvant Studies of Levamisole plus 5-Fluorouracil

Study	No. of Patients	Dukes' Stage	Treatment Regimen 5-FU[a]	Levamisole	Survival Rate (%) Stage C	Comment
Laurie et al.[514]	401	B and C	A: 450 mg/m²/d × 5, then weekly × 1 y	50 mg t.i.d. PO d 1–3 every other week	5-y DFS, 60; 5-y OS, 64	OS for arm A: *P* = .05
			B: None	As above	5-y DFS, 60; 5-y OS, 60	—
			C: None	None	5-y DFS, 50; 5-y OS, 58	—
Moertel et al.[400]	929	C	A: 450 mg/m²/d × 5, then weekly	50 mg t.i.d. PO d 1–3 every other week × 1 y	5-y DFS, 61; 5-y OS, 60	OS for arm A: *P*<.0007
			B: None	As above	5-y DFS, 44; 5-y OS, 49	—
			C: None	None	5-y DFS, 44; 5-y OS, 47	—

DFS, disease-free survival; 5-FU, 5-fluorouracil; OS, overall survival.
[a]Administered by intravenous push except when marked PO.

Mayo Clinic, 401 eligible patients with Dukes stage B and C colorectal cancer after curative surgery were randomized to receive no further treatment, levamisole alone, or 5-FU plus levamisole.[364] Levamisole plus 5-FU (*P* = .003) and, to a lesser extent, levamisole alone (*P* = .05) reduced cancer recurrence in comparison with no adjuvant therapy. Whereas both treatment regimens were associated with overall improvements in survival, these improvements reached borderline significance only for patients with stage C disease treated with levamisole plus 5-FU (*P* = .03).[364] These promising results led to a large national intergroup confirmatory trial involving the NCCTG, the Eastern Cooperative Oncology Group, and SWOG, which changed dramatically the way oncologists approached and treated colon cancer.[400] Twelve hundred and ninety-six patients with Dukes stage B2 or C resected colon cancer were randomly assigned to observation or to treatment for 1 year with levamisole combined with 5-FU or with levamisole alone. Therapy with levamisole plus 5-FU reduced the risk of cancer recurrence among patients with stage C disease by 41% (*P*<.0001) after a median follow-up of 3 years. The overall death rate was reduced by 33% (*P* = .006). Treatment with levamisole alone had no detectable effect. The results in patients with stage B2 disease were equivocal, and no treatment recommendation could be made.[400] In 1995, Moertel et al.[401] updated the results of this trial. With the 929 patients with stage C disease followed for a median of 6.5 years, 5-FU plus levamisole reduced the recurrence rate by 40% (*P*<.0001) and the death rate by 33% (*P* = .0007). Levamisole alone reduced the recurrence rate by only 2% and the death rate by only 6%.[401]

Toxic effects of levamisole alone were infrequent, usually consisting of mild nausea with occasional metallic taste, fatigue, dermatitis, or leukopenia, and those of levamisole plus 5-FU were essentially the same as those of 5-FU alone, including nausea, vomiting, stomatitis, diarrhea, dermatitis, and leukopenia. The cost-effectiveness of this treatment for a typical patient has been calculated as a very reasonable $2094 per year of life saved. Even after using a variety of less favorable assumptions, cost-effectiveness remains less than $5000 per year of life saved.[402] The NCCTG and the National Cancer Institute of Canada attempted to compare 5-FU plus conventional-dose levamisole with a 5-FU plus high-dose levamisole regimen. Accrual was stopped owing to the significant toxicity seen in the high-dose levamisole group.

Combinations of 5-Fluorouracil and Leucovorin. The relative success of combinations of 5-FU with leucovorin in the treatment of advanced colorectal cancer[403] led several investigators to explore this combination in the adjuvant setting. Combinations of 5-FU and leucovorin were tested against different control groups (Table 33.7-14). The NSABP C-03 randomized 1081 patients with Dukes stage B and C colon cancer to receive either MOF or 5-FU plus leucovorin.[404] A comparison of these

TABLE 33.7-14. Adjuvant Trials with 5-FU plus Leucovorin for Colon Cancer

Study	Total Accrual	Regimen	3-Y Disease-Free Survival (%)	3-Y Survival (%)	Estimated 5-Y Survival
NSABP C-03[515]	519	5-FU/LV	73	84	—
	522	MOF	64	77	—
			P = .0004	*P* = .003	—
NCCTG[406]	158	5-FU/LV	77	75	—
	151	Surgery alone	64	71	—
			P = .004	*P* = .13	—
IMPACT[516]	754	5-FU/LV	71	83	—
	772	Surgery alone	62	78	—
			P = .0001	*P* = .018	—
Francini et al.[517]	118	5-FU/LV	81[a]	—	69
	121	Surgery alone	64[a]	—	43
			P = .00016	—	*P* = .0025

5-FU/LV, 5-fluorouracil plus leucovorin; IMPACT, International Multicentre Pooled Analyses of Colon Cancer Trials; MOF, methyl-CCNU, 5-fluorouracil, and vincristine; NCCTG, North Central Cancer Treatment Group; NSABP, National Surgical Adjuvant Breast and Bowel Project.
[a]Stage C patients.

two groups indicated a disease-free survival advantage for patients treated with 5-FU plus leucovorin ($P = .0004$). The 3-year disease-free survival rate for patients in this group was 73%, as compared with 64% for patients receiving MOF. The overall survival at 3 years was 84% for those randomized to receive 5-FU plus leucovorin and 77% for the MOF-treated cohort ($P = .003$). Patients treated with postoperative 5-FU plus leucovorin had a 30% reduction in the risk of developing a treatment failure and a 32% reduction in mortality risk as compared with similar patients treated with MOF.[404]

In the International Multicentre Pooled Analyses of Colon Cancer Trials (IMPACT), three randomized trials conducted to investigate the efficacy of 5-FU and high-dose leucovorin after surgery for stage II and III colon cancer were pooled for combined analysis. All included trials using the same treatment regimen: 5-FU, 370 to 400 mg/m^2/d, plus leucovorin, 200 mg/m^2/d, 5 days every 28 days for six cycles. A pooled analysis of the results was performed, including 1493 eligible patients with resected stage II and III carcinoma of the colon. 5-FU plus leucovorin significantly reduced mortality by 22% and adverse events by 35%, increasing 3-year event-free survival from 62% to 71% and overall survival from 78% to 83%.[405]

In an Italian study reported by Francini et al.,[517] 239 patients with surgically resected Dukes stage B2 or C colon cancer were randomly assigned to chemotherapy with 5-FU and leucovorin or to observation alone. In stage B2, no significant difference between the adjuvant arm and the observation arm was noted. In stage C, adjuvant chemotherapy produced an advantage over observation in terms of a reduction in cancer recurrence rate, with a 3-year disease-free survival of 81% versus 64% and an improvement in overall survival ($P = .0025$).

An intergroup study was planned to compare 5-FU plus leucovorin to control only, but the study was closed prematurely in September 1989 after 309 patients had been enrolled, when reports of the positive results of 5-FU plus levamisole adjuvant therapy precluded randomization to an untreated control group. Patients were randomized to observation or 5-FU plus low-dose leucovorin daily for 5 days every 28 days for six cycles. Preliminary results released after a median follow-up of 3.5 years showed a significant advantage in recurrences in favor of the 5-FU plus leucovorin group ($P = .001$).[406]

5-Fluorouracil plus Levamisole versus 5-Fluorouracil plus Leucovorin. Both 5-FU plus levamisole and 5-FU plus leucovorin regimens have been found to be successful in prolonging disease-free and overall survival. The similar results obtained with the use of either levamisole or leucovorin as 5-FU modulators made necessary a direct comparison between the two modalities (Table 33.7-15). When these two regimens were directly compared in randomized clinical trials, it appeared that a small disease-free survival and overall survival advantage had emerged in favor of 5-FU plus leucovorin.[407]

The intergroup study INT 0089 was the largest trial to address this question. Starting in 1989, 3759 patients with stage II (20%) and stage III (80%) colon cancer were randomly assigned to receive 5-FU plus low-dose leucovorin, 5-FU plus high-dose leucovorin, or 5-FU plus both levamisole and leucovorin for 6 to 7 months, or 5-FU plus levamisole for 12 months. The results are summarized in Table 33.7-16. The leucovorin-containing arms demonstrated a trend toward better results than the 5-FU plus levamisole only arm. Additionally, the toxicity profile was different among the regimens. Patients in the 5-FU plus low-dose leucovorin or the 5-FU plus levamisole arms experienced a greater incidence of stomatitis and neutropenia, whereas patients in the 5-FU plus high-dose leucovorin arm had a greater incidence of diarrhea.[408] The addition of levamisole to 5-FU plus leucovorin did increase toxicity, with no significant increase in disease-free or overall survival.[408]

The NSABP C-04 study, also summarized in Table 33.7-16, compared 5-FU plus levamisole to 5-FU plus high-dose leucovorin and to a combination of the three agents.[409] A total of 2152 patients with Dukes B (41%) or Dukes C (59%) colon cancer were randomized into one of the three treatment arms. At 5 years, there was an advantage for the leucovorin-containing arms, with 69% of the patients treated with 5-FU plus levamisole alive as compared to 74% of the patients receiving 5-FU plus leucovorin and 72% of those receiving 5-FU, leucovorin, and levamisole.[409]

The NCCTG joined with the National Cancer Institute of Canada to examine the effectiveness of a regimen of 5-FU plus levamisole plus leucovorin as adjuvant therapy for patients with high-risk colon cancer and evaluated 6 months versus 12 months of chemotherapy in the same setting.[410] A total of 891 eligible patients with stage II or III colon cancer were randomly assigned to receive adjuvant chemotherapy with 5-FU and leucovorin combined with levamisole or a standard regimen of 5-FU plus levamisole. Patients also were randomly assigned to receive either 12 months or 6 months of chemotherapy. After a median follow-up of 5.1 years, there was no significant improvement in patient survival when chemotherapy was given for 12 months as compared with 6 months. When chemotherapy was given for 6 months, standard 5-FU plus levamisole was associated with inferior patient survival ($P < .01$). These data suggest that a 6-month regimen of 5-FU plus levamisole should not be used in clinical practice, whereas 6 months of treatment with 5-FU plus leucovorin plus levamisole is effective.[410]

An analysis of the available randomized trials indicates that whereas 5-FU with levamisole given for 1 year could still be considered an acceptable regimen, 5-FU plus leucovorin for 6 months is clearly superior in terms of convenience and, possibly, efficacy. 5-FU plus leucovorin should be considered the new standard against which new therapies should be tested.

FUTURE ADJUVANT CHEMOTHERAPY TRIALS. The NSABP C-06 trial compared intravenous 5-FU plus leucovorin to a combination of the oral 5-FU prodrug UFT (uracil, 5-FU, and tegafur) with oral leucovorin. More than 1500 patients with stage II and III colon cancer were eligible to participate in this study. Accrual was completed in early 1999, and final results are not expected for at least a few years. Preliminary analysis of toxicity findings among 473 evaluated patients indicate that both regimens are well tolerated and have similar toxicity profiles.[411]

The availability of newer regimens with higher response rates than traditional 5-FU-based regimens has led to different strategies that attempt to maximize the benefit of adjuvant chemotherapy (Table 33.7-17). The NSABP has focused on the impressive response rates reported with the use of oxaliplatin. This diaminocyclohexane platinum derivative has synergistic activity with 5-FU in advanced colorectal cancer. The NSABP C-07 study is being planned to compare 5-FU plus leucovorin against a regimen containing 5-FU, leucovorin, and oxaliplatin in patients with stage II and III colon cancer. Similarly, the impressive response rates reported with the use of 5-FU, leuco-

TABLE 33.7-15. Summary of Randomized Trials of 5-FU plus LV as Compared with 5-FU for the Treatment of Advanced Colorectal Cancer

Study	*No. of Patients*	*5-FU*	*LV*	*Comment*
Roswell Park Memorial Institute[521]	74	A: 450 mg/m^2 IVP	500 mg/m^2, 2-h infusion	No statistically significant difference in overall survival; 5-FU and leucovorin statistically superior (P = .0009).
		B: 600 mg/m^2 IVP	—	—
		C: 600 mg/m^2 IVP		
GITSG[455,522]	343	A: 500 mg/m^2 IVP	500 mg/m^2, 2-h infusion	A trend toward longer survival in arm B. High-dose LV (arm B) has a response rate of 30.3%, which is significantly greater than 5-FU alone (P<.01).
		B: 600 mg/m^2/IVP	—	—
		C: 600 mg/m^2 IVP	25 mg/m^2, 10-min infusion	—
NCCTG–Mayo Clinic[403]	429	A: 500 mg/m^2 IVP	—	Significant survival advantage of the low- and high-dose LV over 5-FU alone; P£.05. Only 5-FU + low-dose LV associated with benefit in quality-of-life parameters.
		B: 370 mg/m^2 IVP	200 mg/m^2 IVP	—
		C: 425 mg/m^2 IVP	20 μm/m^2 IVP	—
Nordic combination[523]		A: 600 mg/m^2 IVP	—	Superior objective responses and slight survival benefit in the treatment arm (8.5 mo vs. 6 mo; P<.02).
		B: 500 mg/m^2 IVP^a	15 mg	—
Northern California Oncology Group[524]	249	A: 12 mg/kg/d IVP	—	No difference in response rates (NS).
		B: 400 mg/m^2, 15-min infusion	200 mg/m^2 IVP; 10 mg/m^2 PO	—
		C: 500 mg/m^2 IVP	—	—
City of Hope[525]	79	A: 370 mg/m^2 IVP	—	Superior response rates for combined treatment (P = .0019); no overall survival differences.
		B: 370 mg/m^2 IVP	500 mg/m^2 continuous infusion	—
Princess Margaret Hospital[526]	130	A: 370 mg/m^2 IVP	200 mg/m^2 IVP	Statistically significant difference in response rates (33% vs. 7%) in favor of 5-FU + LV; P = .05. Overall survival longer in the 5-FU + LV arm.
		B: 370 mg/m^2 IVP	—	—
Italian Oncology Group[527]	181	A: 540 mg/m^2 IVP	—	No difference in response rates or survival.
		B: 400 mg/m^2 IVP	200 mg/m^2 IVP	—

5-FU, 5-fluorouracil; GITSG, Gastrointestinal Tumor Study Group; IVP, intravenous push; NCCTG, North Central Cancer Treatment Group; NS, not significant.
^{a}Methotrexate, 250 mg/m^2, given before 5-FU.

vorin, and irinotecan in the treatment of advanced colorectal cancer[412] led to an intergroup trial randomizing patients to two arms: intravenous 5-FU plus leucovorin versus a combination of 5-FU, leucovorin, and irinotecan. The results of those trials are eagerly awaited.

LOCOREGIONAL THERAPY. The liver is a major site of recurrence in patients with colorectal cancer and is frequently the only site of metastasis. Even though established liver metastasis is primarily fed by the hepatic arteries, micrometastasis still is dependent on portal venous blood, and animal models have demonstrated the potential benefit for intrahepatic delivery of chemotherapy immediately after surgery for the primary tumor.[413] Chemotherapy delivered by means of continuous portal vein infusion into the liver during the immediate postoperative period may improve therapeutic efficacy.

In 1975, a randomized trial of adjuvant portal vein infusion with 5-FU at 1 g/d and heparin at 5000 U/d for 7 days was initiated in patients undergoing surgery for Dukes' stage A, B, and C colorectal cancer. A total of 117 patients received the infusion, and 127 were enrolled in the control arm. There were fewer liver metastases in the perfusion group, and a statistically important overall survival improvement was noted in Dukes' stage B and C patients.[179] Several other trials have followed the same basic design.

The Swiss Group for Clinical Cancer Research investigated the efficacy of a perioperative intraportal cytotoxic regimen in a randomized trial of 533 patients with operable colorectal carcinoma. Patients were randomly assigned to either a single course of portal infusion with mitomycin (one dose of 10 mg/m^2) plus 5-FU (500 mg/m^2 every 24 hours for 7 days) starting immediately after surgery or to no adjuvant treatment. Five hundred and five patients were evaluated. At a median follow-up of 8 years, adjuvant therapy reduced the risk of recurrence by 21% and the risk of death by 26%. The benefit obtained with a single course of adjuvant chemotherapy via the portal

TABLE 33.7-16. Recently Reported Adjuvant Colon Cancer Trials

Study	*No. of Patients*	*Dukes' Stage*	*Study Design*	*4-Y DFS Rate (%)*	*4-Y OS Rate (%)*	*5-Y DFS Rate (%)*	*5-Y OS Rate (%)*	*Comment*
NSABP C-04[518]	2151	B2, C	A: 5-FU/LV	—	—	65	74	5-FU/LV for 6 mo. superior to 5-FU/lev for 1 y $P = .04$
			B: 5-FU/lev	—	—	60	70	—
			C: 5-FU/LV/lev	—	—	64	73	—
INT 0089[519]	3759	B2, C	A: 5-FU/lev 12 mo	—	—	56		No statistical difference among arms except for 5-FU/LV/lev superior to 5-FU/lev $P = .04$
			B: 5-FU/HDLV 8 mo			59		
			C: 5-FU/LDLV 8 mo	—	—	59	—	—
			D: 5-FU/LV/lev	—	—	60	—	—
NSABP C-05 (1983)	2176	B2, C	A: 5-FU/LV	69, $P = .34$	80, $P = .41$	—	—	IFN increased toxicity without survival benefit
			B: 5-FU/LV/IFN	70	81	—	—	—
NCCTG[520]	915	B2, C	A: 5-FU/LV/lev 12 mo	—	—	—	—	Treatment given for 12 mo compared with 6 mo did not result in significant improvement in survival
			B: 5-FU/lev 12 mo	—	—	—	—	—
			C: 5-FU/LV/lev 6 mo	—	—	—	—	—
			D: 5-FU/lev 6 mo	—	—	—	60, $P = .01$	—

DFS, disease-free survival; 5-FU, fluorouracil; HDLV, high-dose LV; IFN, interferon-α_{2a}; INT, intergroup study; LDLV, low-dose LV; lev, levamisole; LV, leucovorin; NCCTG, North Central Cancer Treatment Group; NSABP, National Surgical Adjuvant Breast and Bowel Project; OS, overall survival.

vein for patients with operable colorectal carcinoma might be due to the systemic effects of the portal chemotherapy.[414]

Between March 1984 and July 1988, in the largest randomized trial to date, the NSABP explored the use of chemotherapy and heparin administered by portal vein infusion versus no further treatment. A total of 1158 patients with Dukes' stage A, B, and C carcinoma of the colon were entered into the NSABP C-02 protocol. Therapy began on the day of operation and consisted of 5-FU, 600 mg/m^2/d, with 5000 U/d by constant infusion for 7 successive days. Randomization was assigned prior to

TABLE 33.7-17. Recently Completed or Ongoing Randomized Adjuvant Colon Cancer Trials

Study	*No. of Patients*	*Accrual Status*	*Stage*	*Study Design*
NSABP C-06	1500	Completed	II, III	Intravenous 5-FU/LV weekly for 6 wk every 8 wk for 3 courses or oral UFT and LV d 1–28; repeated every 5 wk for 5 courses
GW-157-001	1800	Completed	III	MOAB 17-1A plus 5-FU and LV or Lev[a] or 5-FU and LV or Lev[a]
(INT) CALGB-9581	2100	Ongoing	II	MOAB 17-1A every 28 d for 4 courses or MOAB 17-1A every 28 d for 4 courses plus observation at 3 and 6 mo after randomization or observation only at 3 and 6 mo after randomization
(INT) CALGB-89803	1260	Ongoing	III	5-FU/LV weekly for 6 wk every 8 wk for 4 courses or irinotecan, 5-FU/LV weekly for 4 wk every 6 wk for 5 courses
NSABP C-07	2472	Ongoing	II, III	5-FU/LV weekly for 6 wk every 8 wk for 3 courses or 5-FU/LV (as above) and oxaliplatin on d 1, 15, 29 of each course
EFC 3313 (MOSAIC)	1500	Ongoing	II, III	5-FU/LV d1 + 2 every 2 wk for 12 cycles (de Gramont) or 5-FU/LV (as above) and oxaliplatin d 1 every 2 weeks
V307	1794	Ongoing	III	5-FU/LV AIO schedule (weekly) or de Gramont schedule (every 6 wk) vs. CPT-11 plus AIO schedule or de Gramont schedule

AIO, Arbeitsgemeinschaft Internistische Onkologie; CALGB, Cancer and Leukemia Group B; 5-FU, fluorouracil; INT, intergroup study; Lev, levamisole; LV, leucovorin; MOAB, monoclonal antibody; NSABP, National Surgical Adjuvant Breast and Bowel Project; UFT, uracil, 5-FU, and tegafur.

[a]Each participating center prospectively determines whether levamisole or leucovorin is used.

surgery, and 23% of patients were later found to be ineligible, primarily because of metastatic disease. A comparison at 4 years involving 901 eligible patients distributed between the two groups indicated both an improvement in disease-free survival, from 64% to 74% ($P = .02$), and a borderline improvement in overall survival, from 73% to 81% ($P = .07$) in favor of the chemotherapy-treated group. When compared with the treated group, patients who received no further treatment had 1.26 times the risk of developing a treatment failure and 1.25 times the likelihood of dying after 4 years. However, the incidence of hepatic metastasis was not significantly altered, and the benefits observed could potentially be explained by the systemic effect of the chemotherapy.

A large metaanalysis has been conducted to assess the effects on recurrence and survival of administering 5-FU-based chemotherapy by portal infusion after colorectal cancer surgery.[415] Data from ten trials involving approximately 4000 patients were available for analysis. The final result showed that portal infusion of 5-FU for approximately 1 week after surgery in patients with colorectal cancer may produce a small absolute improvement in 5-year survival.[415] This result is somewhat disappointing, and it is possible that the reason for the survival benefit is the systemic exposure to chemotherapy. The use of portal vein infusion cannot be considered routine in the adjuvant treatment of colorectal cancer.

The use of hepatic arterial infusion in the adjuvant setting has been controversial. However, recent data published by the Memorial Sloan-Kettering Cancer Center group demonstrated that patients who had liver resections did benefit from the addition of hepatic arterial infusion to their adjuvant regimen.[194] Further studies are necessary to confirm this.

ADJUVANT IMMUNOTHERAPY. The use of immunotherapy in the fight against cancer has been a goal of cancer research for decades. Despite initial encouraging results with the use of BCG and other agents such as levamisole, nonspecific stimulation of the immune system has not been proven effective in the adjuvant treatment of colon cancer.[416]

The combination of traditional chemotherapy with immunotherapeutic agents is an interesting field of research. At least one combination was proven effective in a large, randomized trial. In fact, until recently the combination of 5-FU plus levamisole was considered the standard adjuvant treatment for stage III colorectal cancer.[401] Preclinical[417] and early clinical data[418] have suggested that interferon-α_{2a} (INF-α_{2a}) enhances the efficacy of 5-FU therapy in colorectal cancer. In an attempt to improve on the results obtained with the use of 5-FU and leucovorin in the adjuvant setting, the NSABP C-05 protocol evaluated the addition of recombinant IFN to 5-FU plus leucovorin in a randomized trial including 2176 patients with Dukes stage B or C colon cancer. The results showed no statistically significant difference in either disease-free survival or overall survival at 4 years of follow-up. Toxicity was more pronounced in the 5-FU, leucovorin, and IFN arm as compared with 5-FU plus leucovorin alone.[419]

The use of vaccines has been explored extensively as well. Hoover and Hanna[420] randomized 98 colorectal patients with Dukes stage B2 and C disease into groups treated by resection alone or resection plus a vaccine made with irradiated autologous tumor cells plus BCG. After 6.5 years, no statistically significant differences were detected in survival or disease-free survival for the 80 eligible patients. However, there was a significant improvement in survival ($P = .02$) and disease-free survival ($P = .039$) in the colon cancer group, although no benefits were seen in patients with rectal cancer. The potential negative impact of the radiation therapy in the immune system of the rectal patients has been postulated as a reason for this difference.[421]

The Eastern Cooperative Oncology Group conducted a larger trial that enrolled a total of 412 patients with Dukes' stage B2 and C colon cancer and randomized them to observation or to vaccination with autologous irradiated tumor cells in combination with BCG and with irradiated tumor cells alone.[422] When the results were analyzed, there were no significant differences in time to relapse or overall survival among the two groups.

A more recent study involving 254 patients presented by a group of Dutch investigators showed that in patients with stage II colon cancer, there was a 32% relative reduction in mortality when a tumor vaccine was compared with observation only.[423]

The use of vaccines for the treatment of colorectal cancer remains an interesting and active field of research. However, no conclusive evidence of benefit has emerged to this date, and it continues to be an experimental treatment reserved for clinical trials.

The use of passive-specific immunotherapy has met with more success. The monoclonal antibody 17-1A is specific for an antigen expressed on cells of human GI malignancies. It was originally developed in mice and later produced in a chimeric version.[424] The chimeric version of the monoclonal antibody 17-1A exhibits molecular characteristics of normal human immunoglobulin G (IgG) but retains the specificity and binding affinity of the native 17-1A murine monoclonal antibody.[424] Reithmuller et al.[425] recently published a 7-year analysis of their randomized trial comparing the use of the monoclonal antibody 17-1A to controls in 189 patients with resected stage III colorectal cancer. The monoclonal antibody was administered as a 500-mg infusion postoperatively followed by 4 monthly doses of 100 mg each.[386] After 7 years of follow-up, treatment had reduced overall mortality by 32% ($P < .01$) and had decreased the recurrence rate by 23% ($P < .04$). The reduction in recurrence and mortality is similar to that seen with the use of 5-FU plus levamisole or leucovorin.

In the United States, two large trials are evaluating the use of the monoclonal antibody 17-1A in the adjuvant setting. The first study randomized patients with stage III colon cancer to receive either modulated 5-FU or a combination of modulated 5-FU plus the antibody. The second study randomized stage II colon cancer patients to receive the antibody or no further treatment. In the next few years, the results of these trials will help to determine the role of the monoclonal antibody in the adjuvant treatment of colorectal cancer.

TREATMENT OF INITIALLY ADVANCED COLON CANCER

SYNCHRONOUS METASTATIC DISEASE

From 10% to 15% of patients with primary colorectal cancer will present with synchronous metastatic cancer disease. Scroggins et al.[339] have presented data on a series of patients presenting with stage IV disease. They found that only 8.7% of a selected asymptomatic group of patients managed nonoperatively required surgical intervention. None of the nonoperatively managed group required surgery for hemorrhage or perforation. These data challenge the traditional teaching that in patients with colon cancer who have metastatic disease at presentation the primary tumor should always be resected. Survivals were on the order of 14 to 16 months in this group of patients with asymptomatic intact primary tumors.

Patients with symptomatic primary colon tumors should have appropriate resections unless their medical condition does not allow it. Whereas palliative surgery in colorectal cancer patients with synchronous metastases is a reasonable method to control perforation, obstruction, hemorrhage, and bleeding, it can carry substantial morbidity and mortality. In a series presented by Liu et al., patients with colon cancer underwent resection as palliation. As compared with standard operative mortality for elective colon resection, 3% of patients in this group had an operative mortality of 10%, whereas in those in whom more than 50% of the liver was replaced, mortality was significantly higher.

Patients with synchronous metastases that are potentially resectable should undergo definitive surgical resection of the primary tumor.

LOCALLY UNRESECTABLE COLON CANCER

Unresectable primary tumor in the absence of peritoneal metastases or unresectable visceral metastases is uncommon. The areas commonly involved with advanced colon tumors are the abdominal wall, retroperitoneum, kidney, duodenum, pancreas, and bladder. Fixation to major nerves or great vessels may confer unresectability based on local spread. Consideration should be given to preoperative irradiation. In such cases, conversion to resectability has been seen in up to 75% of cases. Extensive nodal disease is common with locally advanced primary tumors and can extend into the retroperitoneum and along the SMA. Perforated tumors can produce a profound inflammatory reaction around the site of perforation. After resolution of sepsis, such tumors can be reassessed for resectability, preoperative therapy, or both. Palliative ostomies and bypass procedures may improve quality of life for some patients.

FOLLOW-UP AFTER POTENTIALLY CURATIVE TREATMENT

Follow-up is carried out to find potentially curable recurrences, to palliate symptomatic recurrences, and to identify and resolve treatment-related problems. The biology of colorectal cancer works both for and against the effectiveness of follow-up after the curative resection of colorectal cancer. Solitary liver and lung metastases can be resected and result in long-term survivals in a significant number of patients. Local recurrences of rectal cancer can also be resected with curative intent. Detection of these recurrences can be worthwhile in terms of survival. However, the reality is that most recurrences will represent the outgrowth of multiple occult metastatic sites that were unresponsive to initial surgery and adjuvant therapy. These are unlikely to respond to subsequent therapy, and so they prevent any survival advantage that might have resulted from earlier therapies. Most colorectal cancers that recur or metastasize are biologically determined to be incurable.

FOLLOW-UP STRATEGIES

Critical factors in carrying out and designing follow-up protocols for colorectal cancer patients are the cost-effectiveness of such follow-up and the effects of follow-up on survival. An important study was carried out by Schoemaker et al. in a university hospital setting in South Australia. These researchers conducted a randomized controlled trial with 5-year follow-up in patients who had undergone curative resections for colorectal cancer. Patients were followed by either an intensive follow-up regimen or a standard follow-up regimen. The study group encompassed Dukes stage A, B, and C cancer patients. Standard follow-up consisted of history and physical examination, blood counts, and liver function tests that were carried out every 3 months for 2 years and every 6 months thereafter. The intensive follow-up consisted of the standard follow-up plus annual chest radiography, CT of the liver, and colonoscopy. The results of this study demonstrated no difference in the survival rate at 5 years between patients who received intensive follow-up and those who received standard follow-up.

In a prospective, randomized study of follow-up after radical surgery for colorectal cancer, Kjeldsen et al.[426] made similar findings. The differences between the randomized groups in this study were based on the frequency of follow-up. The intensively followed group had examinations at 6 and 12 months after treatment, whereas the other group had examinations at 5 and 10 years. It was found that recurrences were detected with the same frequency in both groups, but the diagnosis of recurrence was made earlier in the intensively followed group. There was no overall improvement in survival by the intensive follow-up regimen.

The pattern of recurrence of rectal cancer as opposed to colon cancer is an important factor in evaluating the role of follow-up strategies. The role of follow-up in detection and management of local recurrences of colorectal cancer was studied by Pietra et al.[427] Patients were randomly assigned to either a conventional follow-up or to intensive follow-up after resection of primary colorectal carcinoma. In the intensively followed group, local recurrence of rectal carcinoma was more frequently detected. More than 90% of these recurrences in the intensively followed group were detected at scheduled visits. Again, local recurrences were detected earlier in the intensively followed group, and curative re-resection was more frequently carried out in this group. In this study, patients in the intensive follow-up group had an improved 5-year survival, mainly due to the re-resection of local recurrences of rectal carcinoma. The usefulness of CEA determination in detecting luminal recurrences of colorectal cancer was also supported, because it initiated workup for recurrence in asymptomatic patients who were most likely to undergo a curative reoperation.[428]

Other studies have disputed the value of CEA in the follow-up of patients with colorectal carcinoma, on the basis of a lack of detectable increase in survival. In a study of second-look operations for recurrent colorectal cancer initiated by an elevation of CEA level, it was found that nearly half of the colorectal cancer patients who developed recurrence underwent second-look operations and that approximately half of these patients underwent resection.[429] As determined by modern imaging techniques, 1 patient in 72 who underwent exploration for recurrence had no detectable disease at the second-look operation. The group who underwent resection at a second-look operation had a 5-year survival rate of 41%. It appears that when modern imaging techniques are used to evaluate an elevated CEA level, patients can be more appropriately selected for surgery.

The issue of cost in the postsurgical surveillance of patients with colon cancer is addressed by Graham et al.[430] In a cooperative group study of 421 patients who underwent surgical resection for Dukes stage B2 and C colon carcinoma, patients were treated with surgery and adjuvant therapy. Patients underwent physical examination every 3 months, along with CEA determination, chest radiography, and colonoscopy every 6 months in year 1, physical examination and CEA level determination every 6 months in years 2 through 5, and colonoscopy every 1 to 2 years during this period. Costs were estimated on the basis of Medicare reimbursement guidelines. It was found that of the 421 patients in whom recurrent disease was found, 96 underwent surgical resection with curative intent. CEA level determination was the most cost-effective way to identify patients with recurrence that could be surgically treated. CEA monitoring is controversial but has been adopted for routine surveillance by national groups in the United States.[431]

Rosen[432] conducted a metaanalysis evaluating two randomized and three comparative cohort studies examining more than 2000 patients. The analysis looked at the outcomes of curative resection rates, survival after re-resection, length of survival after recurrence, and cumulative 5-year survival in these patients. Fourteen single-cohort studies were also included in the analysis, and a study of these additional patients supported the findings of the metaanalysis. The metaanalysis indicated that the cumulative 5-year survival rate was 1.16 times higher in the intensively followed group ($P = .003$). Furthermore, 2.5 times more curative re-resections were performed for patients undergoing intensive follow-up, and those in the intensive follow-up group had a higher survival rate than did those followed less intensively.

EXTENT OF DISEASE WORKUP AFTER RECURRENCE

Certain groups of patients with proven or suspected recurrence may benefit from a more extensive workup to identify occult metastatic disease. Examples of this situation are patients with potentially resectable hepatic metastases or patients with locally recurrent rectal cancer. Another group that may benefit are those patients with a rising CEA level in whom the source has not been identified on conventional evaluation with physical examination, endoscopy, chest radiography, and CT scan.[433] Two such tests are 18-fluorodeoxyglucose PET and scanning after the injection of radiolabeled antibodies that bind to CEA.

Studies of patients with recurrent or metastatic colorectal cancer have demonstrated high sensitivity (91% to 93%) and specificity (98% to 100%) of these tests in identifying sites of recurrence.[434] In patients with solitary hepatic metastases on conventional imagery, PET found additional inoperable disease in 11%. PET was able to identify additional unsuspected sites of tumor in 21% of patients. Overall, approximately 20% to 30% of patients with a potentially resectable recurrence have been found by PET to have additional disease.[434] The positive predictive value of elevated CEA determinations in patients with an equivocal or negative conventional workup was 89%.[435] This group of patients appeared to benefit most from the additional information provided by PET.[436] It appears, however, that PET will be limited in detecting certain variances due to small size or the presence of necrotic low metabolically acting tumors.

The use of injectable radiolabeled antibodies demonstrated the presence of occult metastatic sites in many patients believed to have a localized primary lesion or recurrent disease.[437] This technique appears to be especially adept at identifying microscopic disease in celiac or extraperitoneal nodes that usually are not evaluated by traditional surgical exploration.[438] When imaging techniques were used to identify antibody uptake, there was a significant increase over the use of CT alone in the ability to detect unresectability.[439]

CHEMOTHERAPY FOR METASTATIC COLORECTAL CANCER

Metastatic colorectal cancer is a resistant disease, and the dismal 5-year survival reflects this difficulty extremely well. Both *MDR1* and GSH S-transferase gene expression are thought to be increased in colon cancer cells.[440] However, this belief has not been confirmed universally.[441] The human mdr1 P glycoprotein is overexpressed in multidrug resistant tumor cells and is believed to play a role in the elimination of certain cytotoxic drugs used in the chemotherapy of colorectal cancer.[442] GSH S-transferases are thought to impart resistance to different chemotherapeutic agents, especially alkylating agents.[443] The mean GSH S-transferase level is significantly increased in colon cancer as compared with the level in adjacent normal tissue.[444] The paucity of chemotherapeutic agents with activity in colorectal cancer reflects the intrinsic resistance demonstrated in those cells.

5-FLUOROURACIL

Since its introduction by Heidelberger et al. (1957) in 1957, 5-FU has become firmly established as the most important antineoplastic drug in the treatment of colorectal cancer. Early trials demonstrated that 5-FU's bioavailability when administered orally is erratic, with less than 75% of a dose reaching the systemic circulation and marked variability in plasma levels observed among patients. This pharmacologic observation led to the development of 5-FU as an intravenous agent. The variability in oral absorption might be associated with varying levels of DPD, the first catabolic enzyme in 5-FU metabolism in the GI tract. 5-FU has been used in a variety of schedules, and determining the best dose, method, and duration of its administration has been the object of intense investigation.[403,445]

The overall response rate for single-agent 5-FU has been reported to be as high as 30% but, realistically, it is closer to 20%. Median survival for patients responding to 5-FU treatment is believed to be in the 12- to 18-month range. Accumulated clinical evidence suggests that the use of protracted intravenous infusion of 5-FU may be superior and better tolerated than intravenous bolus dosing[446] and that modulation of 5-FU may yield higher response rates.[403,447]

Continuous Infusion

Lokich et al.[448] demonstrated clearly the feasibility of a continuous infusion of 5-FU as a treatment for colorectal cancer. When administered for protracted periods, the major toxicity of 5-FU is mucositis. Additionally, hand-foot syndrome is seen in approximately 5% to 25% of patients.[446] The lack of significant hematologic toxicity makes continuous-infusion regimens very attractive. The results from larger randomized trials are encouraging. Despite a response rate and overall survival that are statistically equivalent to those of bolus regimens, as shown in the SWOG experience, the single-agent infusion regimens demonstrated a favorable toxicity profile and a trend toward longer survival.[449] A metaanalysis involving 1219 patients treated in six randomized trials confirmed the superiority of continuous infusion 5-FU over bolus regimens regarding response rates and toxicity. Even though the overall survival was superior for the continuous-infusion group, the medians were very similar.[450] The need for a central venous catheter, with its inherent problems (e.g., infection, thrombus, and slippage) and for a portable pump and the cost and inconvenience for the patients are the major problems associated with continuous-infusion regimens. However, they are acceptable alternatives in the treatment of colorectal cancer patients.

Biochemical Modulation of 5-Fluorouracil

The relatively disappointing results of single-agent 5-FU led many investigators to explore the use of agents that could modulate its activity. One approach to improve the activity of 5-FU has been the addition of biochemical modulators to 5-FU regimens. Several modulators have been studied, among them leucovorin, methotrexate, trimetrexate, and IFN-α.[451] Of these biochemical modulators, leucovorin is without doubt the most successful.[452] This agent, also known as folinic acid, is a tetrahydrofolic acid derivative that can enhance the therapeutic and toxic effects of fluoropyrimidines such as 5-FU.[403] The reduction in DNA synthesis by 5-FU involves the formation of a complex of FdUMP, thymidylate synthetase (TS), and a cofactor designated 5'10 methylene tetrahydrofolate (Me-THP). The enzyme TS is essential to DNA synthesis because it is the only source of thymidylate in the cell, converting dUMP to dTMP. If the enzyme becomes trapped in a complex with FdUMP and Me-THP, it is no longer available to convert dUMP to dTMP, and DNA synthesis is reduced. DNA synthesis is not completely inhibited because there is turnover of the FdUMP/TS/Me-THP complex, freeing up the TS to convert dUMP to dTMP, although in reduced quantities. Leucovorin enhances the inhibition of DNA synthesis by stabilizing the FdUMP/TS/Me-THP complex.[453]

In a metaanalysis of nine randomized clinical trials of advanced colorectal cancer comparing 5-FU alone with 5-FU plus leucovorin, significant improvement in response rate was seen in patients receiving 5-FU and leucovorin as compared with those receiving 5-FU alone.[454] This improvement in response did not result in a significant survival advantage in most studies.[454,455] However, Poon et al.[403,447] were able to demonstrate a statistically significant survival advantage for the combination of 5-FU with leucovorin over 5-FU alone or in combination with methotrexate. The leucovorin dose and schedule required for optimal modulation of 5-FU has not been clearly defined. Doses ranging from 20 to 500 mg/m^2/d of leucovorin have been administered on daily or weekly schedules.

In an attempt to determine the best regimen of 5-FU, the SWOG randomly allocated 626 patients to receive one of seven regimens: (1) 5-FU alone, (2) 5-FU with low-dose leucovorin, (3) 5-FU with high-dose leucovorin, (4) 5-FU by continuous infusion, (5) 5-FU by continuous infusion plus weekly leucovorin, (6) 5-FU by 24-hour infusion, and (7) 5-FU by 24-hour infusion plus PALA.[449] There was no statistical difference in the response rates, which ranged between 15% and 29%, with a median survival for the entire group of 14 months. Despite the statistically equivalent efficacy, the single-agent infusion regimens demonstrated encouraging results, with a favorable toxicity profile trend toward longer survival.[449]

A metaanalysis involving 1219 patients treated in six randomized trials confirmed the superiority of continuous-infusion 5-FU over bolus regimens in terms of response rates and toxicity. Even though the overall survival was superior for the continuous-infusion group, the medians were very similar.[450]

A bimonthly regimen combining bolus with 24-hour infusion of 5-FU plus high-dose leucovorin has been extensively examined in France. A study comparing bimonthly with monthly 5-FU plus leucovorin noted a higher response and more favorable toxicity profile for the bimonthly schedule but no statistically significant improvement in overall survival.[456]

INTERFERON. The combination of IFN-α and 5-FU has demonstrated synergistic cytotoxicity against human colon cancer cell lines in preclinical studies.[157,158] The exact mechanism of action of IFN when combined with 5-FU is unknown. IFN has been shown to enhance conversion of 5-FU to FdUMP,[459] to reduce TS,[460] to inhibit thymidine salvage pathways,[459] and to potentiate 5-FU-induced DNA strand breaks. The addition of IFN also seemed to increase the 5-FU exposure by decreasing its clearance.[461]

Wadler et al.[457] initially reported a response rate of 63% for the combination of 5-FU and IFN. Based on this promising result, multiple trials were conducted using IFN as a 5-FU modulator, showing response rates in the range of 25% to 40%.[418] The toxic effects were significant and included leukopenia, mucositis, diarrhea, fever, chills, myalgia, and neurotoxicity. A group of researchers at the Royal Marsden Hospital randomized patients to receive 5-FU, 750 mg/m^2/d by continuous infusion for 5 consecutive days, followed by weekly bolus 5-FU, 750 mg/m^2 either with or without IFN (10 MU subcutaneously three times weekly). Objective response was observed in 19% of the patients who received 5-FU plus IFN and in 30% of those who received 5-FU only. Patients who received IFN did experience significantly more toxicity.[462] The NSABP C-05 protocol compared 5-FU plus leucovorin with the same combination plus IFN. With 2176 patients evaluated, there was no statistically significant difference in either disease-free survival or overall survival. Toxic effects were observed in 61.8% of patients in the 5-FU plus leucovorin group and in 72.1% of patients in the IFN group.[419] These results indicate that the use of IFN as a 5-FU modulator added to the toxicity of the regimen without affecting efficacy. This regimen has been largely abandoned and should not be used outside an investigational trial.

TRIMETREXATE. Trimetrexate, a dihydrofolate reductase inhibitor, potentiates the cytotoxicity of 5-FU.[463] Phase II studies demonstrated objective responses with trimetrexate plus 5-FU and leucovorin in patients previously treated with and without 5-FU.[402] However, severe diarrhea and hypersensitivity were observed with this combination regimen. Blanke et al.[464] reported the results of a phase II study combining trimetrexate, 5-FU, and leucovorin in patients with advanced colorectal cancer. Thirty-six patients received trimetrexate, 110 mg/m^2 on day 1, leucovorin, 200 mg/m^2 on day 2, and 5-FU, 500 mg/m^2 on day 2 immediately after leucovorin. Oral leucovorin, 15 mg, was given every 6 hours for seven doses. This regimen was repeated weekly for six courses every 8 weeks. Two patients achieved a complete response, and the overall response rate was 50%. Diarrhea was the most common toxicity. A phase II trial involving patients with previously treated colorectal cancer disclosed a disappointing 4% overall response rate.[465] A randomized phase III trial comparing 5-FU plus leucovorin against a combination of 5-FU, leucovorin, and trimetrexate has completed accrual. Final results have not been reported.

ORAL FLUOROPYRIMIDINES

Oral fluoropyrimidines are thought to provide prolonged exposure to 5-FU with lower peak concentrations than those observed with bolus schedules of intravenous 5-FU. This may reduce the occurrence of toxic effects associated with a high plasma concentration of 5-FU, such as neutropenia and stomatitis. 5-FU has been studied in several different dosing schedules, and clinical trials suggest the importance of constant exposure to 5-FU.[450] The toxicity profile of 5-FU is schedule-dependent and, whereas bolus schedules produce mainly neutropenia, protracted infusions produce mainly stomatitis and hand-foot syndrome.[446] Additionally, cancer patients seem to prefer the convenience of oral instead of intravenous medications, as long as the efficacy remains at least equal for both modalities.[466]

In the last decade, several oral agents have been introduced for the treatment of colorectal cancer in the Western world (Table 33.7-18). The erratic bioavailability of oral 5-FU caused by the varying GI levels of DPD, the primary catabolic enzyme of 5-FU,[467,468] was overcome by the development of 5-FU prodrugs that are well absorbed enterally and then are enzymatically converted to 5-FU or by the coadministration of DPD inactivators.[303]

Uracil, 5-Fluorouracil, and Tegafur

Tegafur is a prodrug of 5-FU originally studied in the United States as an intravenous medication. The agent was believed to be too toxic, and so its development as an intravenous medication was discontinued. In the early 1980s, tegafur was tested as an oral medication at the M. D. Anderson Cancer Center, and it was shown to have antitumor activity when administered this way. At the same time, Japanese investigators began to study and use tegafur as an oral medication.[469] Uracil, a competitive inhibitor of DPD, was later combined with tegafur to provide sustained levels of 5-FU.[470] The combination of uracil, 5-FU, and tegafur is known as *UFT*. The previously demonstrated activity and favorable toxicity profile of UFT led to its development as an oral alternative to intravenous 5-FU for the treatment of solid tumors, especially colorectal cancer.[471]

Two large, multinational phase III trials comparing the oral regimen of UFT plus leucovorin to intravenous 5-FU and leucovorin as the initial treatment for patients with metastatic colorectal cancer have been reported.[472,473] In the first trial, 816 patients were randomly allocated to intravenous 5-FU plus leucovorin or to oral UFT and leucovorin.[472] UFT was taken at a dose of 300 mg/m^2/d in three divided doses for 28 days followed by 1 week of rest. Oral leucovorin was administered at 90 mg/d, with the UFT administered at the same frequency daily. The intravenous 5-FU and leucovorin were administered for 5 consecutive days, with cycles repeated every 28 days. The study demonstrated statistical equivalence between the treatment arms, with a median survival of 12.4 months for the UFT plus leucovorin arm and 13.4 months for the intravenous arm. No statistical difference was seen for the two treatment arms regarding response (12% for UFT plus

TABLE 33.7-18. Summary of Recent Randomized Trials Comparing Intravenous 5-FU/LV versus Oral Fluorinated Pyrimidines for the Treatment of Advanced Colorectal Cancer

Investigator	*No. of Patients*	*Regimens*	*Response Rate (%)*	*Median PFS*	*Median OS*
Pazdur et al[472]	816	Oral UFT, 300 mg/m^2/d, and oral LV, 75 or 90 mg/d, d 1–28 every 35 d	12	NA	NA
		or IV 5-FU, 425 mg/m^2/d, and IV LV, 20 mg/m^2/d, d 1–5 every 28 d	15 $P = .232$	NA	NA
Carmichael et al.[473]	380	Oral UFT, 300 mg/m^2/d, and oral LV, 90 mg/d, d 1–28 every 35 d	11	3.4 mo	12.2 mo
		or IV 5-FU, 425 mg/m^2/d, and IV LV, 20 mg/m^2/d, d 1–5 every 35 d	9 $P = .593$	3.3 mo $P = .591$	11.9 mo $P = .682$
Cox et al.[528]	605	Capecitabine, 2500 mg/m^2/d × 14 every 3 wk	23.2	4.4 mo	NA
		or IV 5-FU, 425 mg/m^2/d, and IV LV, 20 mg/m^2/d, d 1–5 every 28 d	15.5 $P = .02$	5.1 mo	NA
Twelves et al.[529]	602	Capecitabine, 2500 mg/m^2/d × 14 every 3 wk	26.6	5.3 mo	NA
		or IV 5-FU, 425 mg/m^2/d, and IV LV, 20 mg/m^2/d, d 1–5 every 28 d	17.9 $P = .013$	4.8 mo	NA

5-FU, 5-fluorouracil; IV, intravenous; LV, leucovorin; NA, not available; OS, overall survival; PFS, progression-free survival; UFT, uracil, 5-FU, and tegafur.

leucovorin and 15% for intravenous 5-FU plus leucovorin). Severe neutropenia and stomatitis were less common in the oral regimen.[472]

The second trial compared time to progression between patients receiving an intravenous 5-FU plus leucovorin regimen or UFT plus leucovorin.[473] Three hundred and eighty patients were randomized to two treatment groups that were identical to those described in the first study except that the intravenous 5-FU plus leucovorin was repeated every 35 days. The treatment arms were equivalent in terms of time to progression, with a median of 3.4 months in the UFT plus leucovorin group and 3.3 months in the intravenous 5-FU plus leucovorin group. The median survival times were 12.2 and 11.9 months, respectively.[473]

Capecitabine

Capecitabine, a fluoropyrimidine carbamate, was developed as an oral alternative to intravenous 5-FU.[474] Capecitabine is absorbed through the intestinal mucosa as an intact molecule, not being affected by the thymidine phosphorylase present in the intestines. It then is metabolized in the liver by carboxylesterase to 5'-deoxy-5-fluorocytidine (5'DFCR), which is converted by cytidine deaminase to 5'DFUR mainly in the liver and tumor tissues. Finally, 5'DFUR is metabolized by thymidine phosphorylase to 5-FU at the tumor site.[475] Preclinical studies demonstrated capecitabine's activity in 5-FU-sensitive and -resistant cell lines.[476] Colorectal cancers, like many other solid tumors, tend to have high levels of thymidine phosphorylase, which is known for its angiogenic properties.[477]

In phase I trials, diarrhea, vomiting, and hand-foot syndrome (palmar-plantar erythrodysesthesia) were dose-limiting toxic effects.[478] A large multinational, randomized, open-label phase II trial evaluated three schedules of capecitabine (i.e., continuous, intermittent, and intermittent with leucovorin) in metastatic colorectal cancer. The response rates for the three groups ranged from 21% to 24%. The median time to disease progression ranged from 127 to 230 days, with the best time to disease progression seen in patients treated in the intermittent capecitabine arm, without leucovorin.[479] The addition of leucovorin seemed to increase the incidence of toxic effects, without improving therapeutic activity.

Results of two phase III trials comparing capecitabine, 2500 mg/m^2/d for 2 weeks every 3 weeks, to bolus 5-FU, 425 mg/m^2/d, plus leucovorin, 20 mg/m^2/d, daily for 5 days every 4 weeks, as first-line treatment for metastatic colorectal cancer, were recently reported at the 1999 American Society of Clinical Oncologists' meeting. The first trial enrolled 602 patients, and the second trial enrolled 605 patients. Both trials demonstrated a higher response rate with capecitabine as compared with bolus 5-FU plus leucovorin. Taking into account all randomized patients using intention-to-treat analysis, investigator response rates were 26.6% versus 17.9% (95% CI , 1.9% to 15.1%) in the first trial and 24.8% versus 15.5% (95% CI, 2.8% to 15.5%) in the second trial. The median survival duration was 54 versus 57.1 weeks (P = .2363), respectively. The toxicity profile of capecitabine was favorable, with fewer treatment-related serious adverse events and hospitalizations in the capecitabine arm as compared with the 5-FU plus leucovorin arm. The most common adverse events with capecitabine were palmar-plantar erythrodysesthesia (hand-foot syndrome) and diarrhea.

Eniluracil

Eniluracil, also known as *776C85* and *ethynyluracil,* is a potent irreversible inactivator of DPD, the first enzyme in the degradative pathway of 5-FU.[480] When it is used in combination with an oral formulation of 5-FU, eniluracil makes the absorption and bioavailability of 5-FU more reliable,[481] and the 5-FU bioavailability and half-life are increased.

Phase I trials have demonstrated that a dose ranging from 10 to 40 mg/d of eniluracil inactivates DPD maximally. The concentration of 5-FU obtained with a 28-day oral dosing regimen of this agent plus eniluracil is similar to steady-state concentrations from protracted intravenous infusions of 5-FU.[481] Main toxic effects included fatigue and diarrhea. Nausea, vomiting, mucositis, pain, dehydration, and constipation were relatively uncommon.

Based on these results, a phase II trial of 5-FU, 1.0 mg/m^2, plus eniluracil, 10 mg/m^2, orally twice daily for 28 days followed by a 7-day rest period was conducted in patients with previously untreated colorectal cancer.[482] However, after approximately one-third of the patients had been treated, the doses of both agents were increased because of the unexpectedly low toxicity observed. The doses were increased to 5-FU, 1.15 mg/m^2, and eniluracil, 11.5 mg/m^2, twice daily for 28 days. The objective response rate was 29%.[482] This dose and schedule is currently being used in two pivotal trials comparing this oral combination with intravenous 5-FU plus leucovorin and with a protracted intravenous schedule of 5-FU in metastatic colorectal cancer patients.

IRINOTECAN

Camptothecin is an agent derived from the Chinese ornamental tree *Camptotheca acuminata.* Its clinical development began in the United States in the late 1960s but was eventually halted due to excessive toxicity. In the late 1980s, irinotecan, also known as *CPT-11,* an analogue of camptothecin, was developed in Japan.[483] Pivotal phase II studies of irinotecan in advanced colorectal carcinoma were conducted in the United States, including patients who had received prior chemotherapy with 5-FU and had progressed while on treatment within the last 6 months. The dose of irinotecan ranged from 100 to 150 mg/m^2 given weekly for 4 weeks, followed by 2 weeks of rest. The overall response rate ranged from 12.5% to 23%. Grade 3 and 4 toxicities were noted in 30% of patients, with a 20% hospitalization rate for management of toxicity-related events. The principle toxicities included diarrhea, nausea, vomiting, and neutropenia. Severe diarrhea was seen in up to 23% of patients and was not well controlled by standard therapy but was limited by use of an intensive loperamide regimen and appropriate dose modification.[484]

The real value of irinotecan in the treatment of metastatic colorectal cancer refractory to 5-FU was determined by two randomized clinical trials conducted in Europe. In the first one, Cunningham et al.[479] randomly assigned patients in whom 5-FU therapy had failed to receive either 300 to 350 mg/m^2 of irinotecan every 3 weeks or supportive care alone (Fig. 33.7-7). A total of 189 patients were randomized to the irinotecan arm

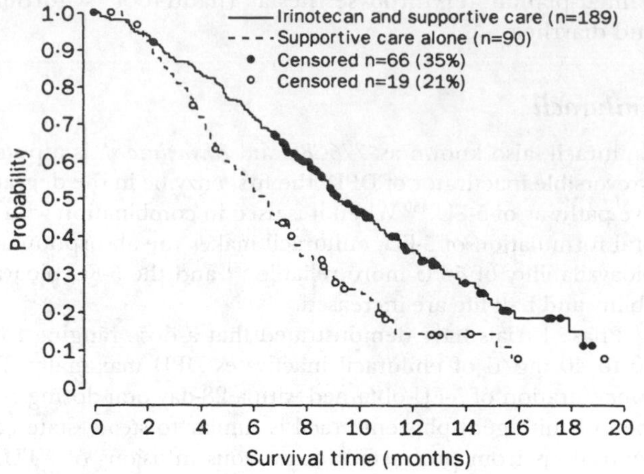

FIGURE 33.7-7. Probability of survival of the 279 patients enrolled in a trial of irinotecan versus supportive care for metastatic colorectal cancer refractory to 5-fluorouracil. (From ref. 479, with permission.)

and 90 to the supportive-care alone arm. The mean age of the participants was 58.8 years; performance status was 0 in 79 patients (42%), 1 in 77 patients (41%), and 2 in 32 patients (17%). After a median follow-up of 13 months, the overall survival was significantly better in the irinotecan group (P = .0001), with a 36.2% 1-year survival rate in the irinotecan group versus 13.8% in the supportive-care group. In a quality-of-life analysis, all significant differences except diarrhea favored the irinotecan group.[479]

Rougier et al.[485] reported the results of the second trial, in which 267 patients with advanced colorectal cancer in whom 5-FU therapy had failed received either second-line fluorouracil by continuous infusion or irinotecan, 300 to 350 mg/m^2 infused once every 3 weeks. Patients treated with irinotecan lived longer than patients receiving second-line infusional 5-FU (P = .035). Median survival duration was 10.8 months in the irinotecan group and 8.5 months in the 5-FU group (Fig. 33.7-8).[485]

A randomized phase III trial compared the combinations of irinotecan plus 5-FU and leucovorin with 5-FU plus leucovorin and single-agent irinotecan as first-line treatment of patients with advanced colorectal cancer (Table 33.7-19).[412] Approximately 220 patients were enrolled in each of the three treatment groups. Objective responses were noted in 51% of patients receiving the three-drug combination, 29% of patients receiving 5-FU with leucovorin, and 30% of patients receiving single-agent irinotecan (P <.001). The median time to treatment failure for each of the three treatment groups was 5.4, 3.9, and 3.2 months, respectively. The median survival duration, however, did not achieve a statistical difference, with a median survival of 14.4 months for the triple combination, 12.6 months for 5-FU plus leucovorin, and 12.0 months for the group receiving irinotecan (P= .173). A new analysis is planned when the data mature further.

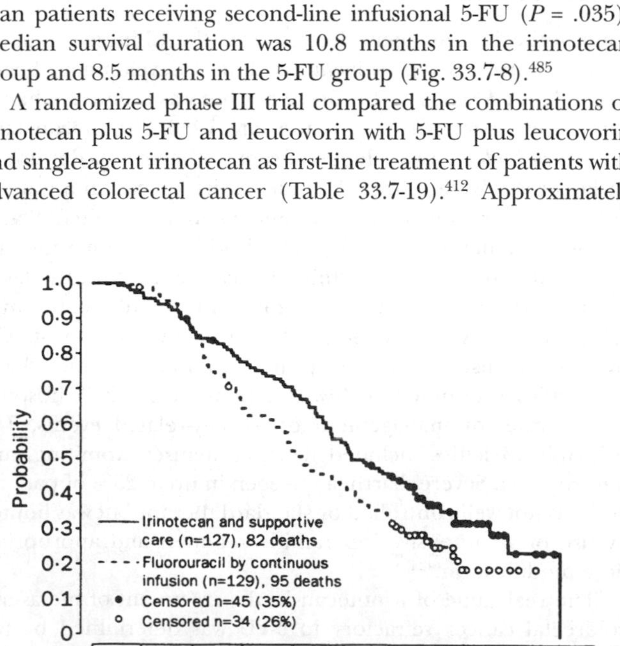

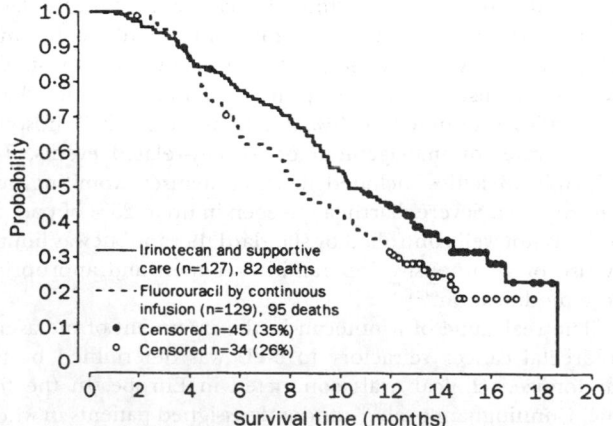

FIGURE 33.7-8. Survival curve in patients on irinotecan or infused 5-fluorouracil for advanced colorectal cancer refractory to first-line 5-fluorouracil. (From ref. 485, with permission.)

A second phase III trial, conducted primarily in Europe, examined the role of irinotecan plus 5-FU and leucovorin in the first-line setting. This trial randomized 387 patients to receive either of two commonly used 5-FU plus leucovorin regimens with or without irinotecan. Response rates were significantly improved with the use of irinotecan (49% vs. 23%). Additionally, the median survival was statistically superior for the group receiving irinotecan with the 5-FU plus leucovorin (16.8 vs. 14 months). The combination of irinotecan with 5-FU and leucovorin is being investigated against other promising combinations and against standard 5-FU plus leucovorin in a large intergroup trial in the United States.

OXALIPLATIN

Oxaliplatin is a novel diaminocyclohexane platinum agent that acts mainly by causing interstrand and intrastrand cross-links in DNA.[481] It has been investigated as a single agent in colorectal cancer both in previously treated and untreated patients. In chemotherapy-naive patients with advanced colorectal cancer, two phase II trials assessed the activity of oxaliplatin, 130 mg/m^2 given over 2 hours every 3 weeks.[486] Response rates ranged from 20% to 24%, with a median response duration of 6 to 7 months and a median progression-free survival of approximately 4 months. Peripheral neuropathy and laryngopharyngeal dysesthesia were the main toxicities reported. In previously treated patients, the overall response rate was considerably lower (≈10%), and the median survival duration was 8.5 months.[481]

Preclinical models demonstrated synergy between oxaliplatin and 5-FU, and this was subsequently confirmed in clinical trials.[487] A phase II trial involving 90 patients with advanced colorectal cancer evaluated the combination of chronomodulated 5-FU, 700 mg/m^2/d, leucovorin, 300 mg/m^2/d, and oxaliplatin, 25 mg/m^2/d, given for 4 days every 2 weeks. The response rate was 58%, and the median survival duration was 15 months.[488]

The potential benefits of oxaliplatin when added to 5-FU and leucovorin as first-line therapy for patients with advanced colorectal cancer were subsequently evaluated in phase III randomized trials (see Table 33.7-19). A study with 200 patients compared chronomodulated 5-FU plus leucovorin administered every 3 weeks with or without oxaliplatin at 125 mg/m^2 given over 6 hours on day 1. The overall response rates were 53% versus 16% (P<.001) for the combinations with and without oxaliplatin, respectively. However, the overall survival duration was equivalent in both arms (19.4 vs. 17.6 months, respectively). This survival equivalence was attributed to crossover and surgery after chemotherapy.

A second study reported by De Gramont et al. randomized 420 patients to receive 5-FU plus leucovorin on days 1 and 14

TABLE 33.7-19 Summary of Recent Randomized Trials Comparing 5-FU/LV versus Irinotecan or Oxaliplatin for the Treatment of Advanced Colorectal Cancer

Study	*No. of Patients*	*Regimens*	*Response Rate (%)*	*Median PFS*	*Median OS*
Saltz et al.[530]	666	CPT-11, 125 mg/m^2; LV, 20 mg/m^2; 5-FU, 500 mg/m^2/wk × 4 every 6 wk	39.4[a]	7 mo	14.5
		or			
		5-FU, 425 mg/m^2/d; LV, 20 mg/m^2/d × 5 d every 28 d	20.8[a]	4.3 mo	12.6
		or			
		CPT-11, 125 mg/m^2/wk × 4 every 6 wk	18.1[a] P<.001	4.2 mo P<.004	12 P= .173
Douillard et al.[531,532]	387	5-FU/LV regimen of choice	23[a]	4.4 mo	14 mo
		or			
		5-FU/LV regimen of choice with CPT-11	41[a] P<.001	6.7 mo P<.001	16.8 mo P= .03
de Gramont et al.[533]	420	LV, 200 mg/m^2 d 1; 5-FU, 400 mg/m^2 bolus and 600 mg/m^2 d 1 + 2 every 2 wk	26	27.8 wk	NA
		or			
		As above, with oxaliplatin, 85 mg/m^2 d 1	57 P<.05[b]	39.6 wk	
Giacchetti et al.[531]	200	Chronomodulated 5-FU, 700 mg/m^2, and LV, 300 mg/m^2/d d 1–5 every 21 d	12[a]	6.1 mo	19.9 mo
		or			
		As above, with oxaliplatin, 125 mg/m^2 d 1	34[a] P<.0001	8.7 mo P= .048	19.4 mo NS

5-FU, fluorouracil; LV, leucovorin; NS, not significant; OS, overall survival; PFS, progression-free survival.
[a]Confirmed response rate.
[b]Analysis of first 200 patients.

of a 28-day schedule with or without oxaliplatin, 85 mg/m^2. The response rates in the first 200 patients were 57% versus 26% in patients treated with and without oxaliplatin, respectively. The corresponding median progression-free survival duration for the treatment groups were 39.6 versus 27.8 weeks. Once more, however, no significant impact on overall survival has been demonstrated (P = .12).

As second-line therapy, oxaliplatin in combination with 5-FU and leucovorin has also shown promising results. In one trial, 46 patients with 5-FU-refractory colorectal cancer were treated with oxaliplatin administered as a 2-hour infusion on day 1, followed by leucovorin on days 1 and 2, and 5-FU as a 24-hour infusion for 2 consecutive days. Treatment was repeated every 2 weeks. The overall response rate was 46%, and median survival duration was 17 months. Limiting toxicities were neutropenia and peripheral neuropathy. A second trial involving the addition of oxaliplatin, 85 mg/m^2 every 2 weeks, to the same 5-FU plus leucovorin regimen under which patients had progressed produced an overall response rate of 20%, a median response duration of 37 weeks, and a median survival duration of 57 weeks.[489]

The combination of oxaliplatin and irinotecan in patients with 5-FU-refractory colorectal cancer was recently reported. The overall response rate among the 34 treated patients was 44%, with stable disease in another 35% and a median time to progression of 7.5 months.

RALTITREXED

Raltitrexed is transported into cells by the reduced folate carrier, metabolized to a polyglutamate species, and retained intracellularly, resulting in prolonged TS inhibition.[490] It is the first of the specific TS inhibitors to have undergone extensive clinical evaluation,[490] and it is currently approved for treatment of colorectal cancer by regulatory agencies in Europe, Canada, Australia, and South America.

The efficacy of raltitrexed as monotherapy for patients with advanced colorectal cancer was evaluated in three phase III clinical trials.[491] Two international trials, one with 439 patients[492] and the other with 495 patients,[493] compared intravenous bolus raltitrexed, 3 mg/m^2 repeated every 3 weeks, to daily intravenous bolus 5-FU, 425 mg/m^2/d, plus leucovorin, 20 mg/m^2/d for 5 days (Mayo regimen), or to 5-FU, 400 mg/m^2/d, plus leucovorin, 200 mg/m^2/d (Machover regimen) repeated every 4 weeks. The third trial was conducted in the United States[494] and compared two raltitrexed dosages (3 mg/m^2 and 4 mg/m^2 every 3 weeks) with the Mayo regimen. However, because of the unacceptable toxicities seen with the 4 mg/m^2 dose, subsequent analyses were based on a two-treatment comparison with 427 patients. All three trials produced similar response rates ranging from 14% to 19% for the raltitrexed group and from 15% to 18% for the 5-FU plus leucovorin group. In all three trials, survival duration ranged from 10 to 12 months. The study conducted in the United States showed a significant difference in survival duration (9.7 vs. 12.7 months; P = .01) between the two treatment groups, favoring the 5-FU with leucovorin group. The main advantage of raltitrexed is its easy schedule, allowing a single intravenous treatment every 3 weeks.

Several studies have been conducted using hepatic arterial infusion in patients with advanced colorectal cancer with liver metastasis. Response rates have been consistently superior for the arms using hepatic arterial infusion; however, a convincing survival advantage has never been shown (Table 33.7-20). The use of hepatic arterial infusion for treatment of advanced colorectal cancer still must be considered investigational.

TABLE 33.7-20. Hepatic Intraarterial Fluoropyrimidine Therapy for Liver Metastases in Colorectal Cancer

Study	*Treatment-Drug*	*Mode*	*No. of Patients*	*Dosage*	*Objective Response Rate (%)*	*Median Survival Rate (mo)*
Kemeny et al.[534]	FUDR	IV	51	0.15 mg/kg/d × 14 d every 28 d	20	12
		IA	48	0.3 mg/kg/d × 14 d every 28 d	50	17
					P = .001	*P*=.424
Hohn et al.[535]	FUDR	IV	72	0.075 mg/kg/d × 14 d every 28 d	10	16.1
		IA	64	0.20 mg/kg/d × 14 d every 28 d	42	16.7
					P = .0001	NS
Chang et al.[536]	FUDR	IV	32	0.125 mg/kg/d × 14 d every 28 d	17	12
		IA	32	0.3 mg/kg/d × 14 d every 28 d	62	17
					P = .003	
Martin et al.[537]	5-FU	IV	33	500 mg/m²/d × 5 d every 5 wk	21	10.5
	FUDR	IA	36	0.3 mg/kg/d × 14 d every 28 d	48	12.6
					P = .02	*P* = .53
Rougier et al.[538]	5-FU/obs	IV	82	500 mg/m²/d × 5 d every 4 wk	9	11
	FUDR	IA	81	0.3 mg/kg/d × 14 every 28 d	43	15

5-FU, 5-fluorouracil; FUDR, floxuridine; IA, intraarterial; IV, intravenous; obs, observation.

SUMMARY

After four decades, 5-FU remains the mainstay of treatment for colorectal cancer. However, the advent of newer agents has introduced new options for the treatment of this disease. Ongoing trials are determining which agent, or combination of agents, should be considered the gold standard in treatment of advanced colorectal cancer. The increased response rates and prolonged progression-free survival seen with the combinations of 5-FU, leucovorin, and either irinotecan or oxaliplatin are very exciting and warrant their consideration as front-line therapy. The use of agents that are able to maintain the same efficacy as older regimens with improved convenience and less toxicity may have a positive impact in the quality of life of patients as well. However, an improvement in survival will be needed for the establishment of a clear new standard. For now, whenever possible, patients should be encouraged to participate in well-designed clinical trials involving new regimens, because despite the impressive advances seen in the last few years, advanced colorectal cancer remains a highly lethal disease.

MISCELLANEOUS COLORECTAL TUMORS

CARCINOIDS

Carcinoid tumors of the GI tract, although characteristically indolent, are also quite heterogeneous with respect both to histologic and endocrine features and to clinical presentation and behavior. Because they are relatively uncommon, most reports do not have a significant number of patients for a detailed analysis. For decades, a series including 2837 cases published in 1975 remained the largest available reference. Modlin and Sandor recently evaluated an impressive 8305 cases. The most frequent sites for carcinoids were the GI tract (74% of cases) and the bronchopulmonary system (25% of cases). Within the GI tract, 29% of cases occurred in the small bowel, 19% in the appendix, and 13% in the rectum. The highest incidence rates were seen among African American men (2.12 per 100,000 per year). This large analysis indicates that metastases are already evident at the time of diagnosis in 45% of the patients and that the overall 5-year survival rate of all carcinoid tumors, regardless of site, is 50%. The 5-year survival rate for carcinoid tumors of the GI tract varied markedly. It was considerably lower for pancreatic (34%), colonic (41%), and small intestinal tumors (55%) and better for appendiceal (86%), bronchopulmonary (76.6%), and rectal carcinoids (72.2%).[495] These improved 5-year survival rates were associated with a lower incidence of invasive growth or metastatic spread. A search for additional tumors is generally advised, because multiple carcinoids and second neoplasms are not uncommon.[496]

Most carcinoid tumors are clinically silent, and the diagnosis is not made before surgery. Surgical treatment depends on the localization and size of the tumor. Small bowel carcinoid tumors metastasize in 20% to 30% of the cases if the tumor is smaller than 1 cm. Therefore, the primary tumor should always be resected widely, including the regional lymph nodes. Carcinoid tumors of the appendix measuring less than 1 cm usually do not metastasize. For such patients, an appendectomy is the treatment of choice. For tumors larger than 2 cm, a right hemicolectomy should be performed. If the tumor is between 1 and 2 cm, surgical treatment depends on the presence of positive lymph nodes, extension of the tumor into the mesoappendix or subserosal lymphatic invasion, and age of the patient.[497] Carcinoid tumors of the colon and rectum measuring less than 2 cm rarely metastasize. Surgical treatment for patients with such small tumors is local excision, whereas for patients with tumors larger than 2 cm, wide resection is advocated.[497]

SARCOMAS

Rarely, tumors may arise directly from the stromal and smooth muscle elements in the colon or rectum. These tumors are known as *smooth muscle tumors* or *stromal tumors* of the colon and rectum. These mesodermal tumors are essentially leiomyosarcomas. The true incidence of leiomyosarcomas in the colon and rectum is unknown. Only small numbers of patients have been reported to date, all in small series.[498]

The most common anatomic location of leiomyosarcoma is the stomach (47%), followed by small intestine (24%), rectum (11%), colon (7%), duodenum (5%), and esophagus (5%). Symptoms and physical findings are nonspecific, with pain, palpable masses, and melena being the most common. Patients frequently present with GI bleeding and significant anemia. The only therapy with accepted value is surgery with wide margins. Chemotherapy is of unproven value as an adjuvant and as treatment for this type of tumor. The tumor grade is an important prognostic factor. In patients resected with curative intent who have low-grade lesions, disease-free survival at 8 years exceeds 80%, as compared with a mean disease-free interval of only 18 months for patients with high-grade lesions.[499]

Other authors have confirmed that the stage of the tumors and the presence of high-grade features are the main independent factors that affect survival. DNA ploidy is not an independent prognostic factor for survival in patients with leiomyosarcomas.[500] Recurrences are noted at regional and distant sites.[501] The prognosis for patients with leiomyosarcoma is guarded, and almost two-thirds of the patients die within 1 year. The use of adjuvant radiation therapy in patients with resected leiomyosarcomas of the rectum may improve local control and allow for sphincter preservation.[501] It is unlikely that large randomized trials for the treatment of colorectal leiomyosarcomas will ever be conducted owing to the rarity of this disease. Patients with advanced cases should be encouraged to participate in trials designed for GI leiomyosarcomas in general.

LYMPHOMA

Colorectal lymphomas account for fewer than 1% of all colorectal cancers but account for 15% of all GI lymphomas.[502] Most cases involve the cecum and the rectum.[503] Virtually all colorectal lymphomas are non-Hodgkin's type, including both B- and T-cell types of low-, intermediate-, and high-grade histologies. Immunohistochemical studies usually show a preponderance of B-cell phenotype. Colorectal non-Hodgkin's lymphoma is a disease that affects both the pediatric and adult population and, although pediatric patients have an excellent prognosis, long-term survival can be expected in only approximately 50% of adult patients.

The diagnosis of colorectal lymphoma must be confirmed histologically and by the absence of evidence of primary lymphoma elsewhere by imaging studies or clinical examination (i.e., evidence of splenomegaly, or palpable lymphadenopathy). In addition, both the peripheral smear and the bone marrow must be determined to be normal. Colorectal lymphomas usually present with a mass, symptoms of obstruction, or signs of bleeding.[502] The clinical presentation is usually indistinguishable from that of colorectal adenocarcinoma, and most patients are symptomatic at the time of diagnosis.[503]

Patients with colon lymphoma often are treated initially with surgery. The lack of well-designed trials makes any recommendation extremely difficult. The use of combined-modality treatment, including surgery and chemotherapy, seems to yield superior results.[504] Several authors have recommended the use of radiation therapy, especially in cases involving low-grade lymphomas, bulky disease, positive lymph nodes, or incomplete resection. The true role of radiation therapy in colon lymphomas is still uncertain.

Radiation therapy is more attractive in cases involving the rectum. However, patients treated with radiation therapy alone have a very poor long-term survival.[502] Whenever possible, combined-modality surgery and radiation therapy should be considered. The use of chemotherapy in earlier disease stages is controversial but should be considered for patients with advanced-stage disease or more aggressive histologic types. Because of the rarity of this cancer, patients should be encouraged to be treated in larger centers where there is experience in the management of lymphomas.

SMALL CELL CARCINOMA

Extrapulmonary small cell cancers are very uncommon, accounting for fewer than 1000 cases annually.[505] Histologically, small cell cancers arising from different organs are indistinguishable, and a lung primary should always be ruled out.[506] Fewer than 100 cases have been reported since 1961, the most frequent site being the rectum, followed by the cecum and sigmoid.[506]

The presentation is similar to that of adenocarcinomas and includes weight loss, bleeding, abdominal pain, and change in bowel habits.[507] Metastasis is common, affecting 85% of the patients at the time of diagnosis.[506] The liver is the organ most frequently involved by metastasis, but almost any organ may be affected. Patients with localized disease should be treated aggressively with a multimodality approach, including local therapy with surgery or radiation therapy (or both) and chemotherapy. Patients with advanced disease should receive chemotherapy.[508] The chemotherapy should be based on accepted treatment regimens used in the treatment of small cell lung carcinomas.[506]

REFERENCES

1. Tepper JE. Reflections in rectosigmoid: retro-peritoneal vs. intra-peritoneal. *Int J Radiat Oncol Biol Phys* 1988;14(5):1043.
2. Van Damme J. *The superior mesenteric artery.* New York: Thieme Medical Publishers, 1990:48.
3. Garcia-Ruiz A, Milsom JW, Ludwig K, Marchesa P. Right colonic arterial anatomy: implications for laparoscopic surgery. *Dis Colon Rectum* 1996;39(8):906.
4. Chen Y, Liu ZY, Li RX, Guo Z. Structural studies of initial lymphatics adjacent to gastric and colonic malignant neoplasms. *Lymphology* 1999;32:70.
5. Parkin DM, Pisani P, Ferlay J. Global cancer statistics. *CA Cancer J Clin* 1999;49:33.
6. Ries L, Kosary CL, Hankey BF, et al. SEER cancer statistics review 1973–1995. Bethesda: National Cancer Institute, 1998.
7. Parkin DM, Pisani P, Ferlay J. Estimates of worldwide incidence of eighteen major cancers in 1985. *Int J Cancer* 1993;54(4):594.
8. Chu KC, Tarone RE, Chow W, et al. Temporal patterns in colorectal cancer incidence, survival, and mortality from 1950 through 1990. *J Natl Cancer Inst* 1994;86(13):997.
9. Nelson RL, Dollear T, Freels SPV. The relation of age, race, and gender to the subsite location of colorectal carcinoma. *Cancer* 1997;80:1408.
10. Akerley WL, Moritz TE, Ryan LS, et al. Racial comparison of outcomes of male Department of Veterans Affairs patients with lung and colon cancer. *Arch Intern Med* 1993; 153:1681.
11. Garfinkel L, Mushinski M. U.S. cancer incidence, mortality and survival: 1973–1996. *Stat Bull Metrop Insur Co* 1999;80:23.
12. Nelson RL, Persky V, Turyk M. Determination of factors responsible for the declining incidence of colorectal cancer. *Dis Colon Rectum* 1999;42:741.
13. Steele GD, Jessup JM, Winchester DP, et al. Colorectal cancer. National cancer data base. *Annu Rev Patient Care* 1995;67:66.
14. Huang J, Seow A, Shi CY, Lee HP. Colorectal carcinoma among ethnic Chinese in Singapore: trends in incidence rate by anatomic subsite from 1968 to 1992. *Cancer* 1999;85:2519.
15. Kawazuma Y, Tanaka H, Tsukuma H, et al. Improvement of survival over time for colon cancer patients by anatomical sub-sites. *Jpn J Cancer Res* 1999;90:705.

16. Vogelstein B, Fearon ER, Hamilton SR, et al. Genetic alterations during colorectal-tumor development. *N Engl J Med* 1988;319:525.
17. Winawer SJ, Shike M. Dietary factors in colorectal cancer and their possible effects on earlier stages of hyperproliferation and adenoma formation. *J Natl Cancer Inst* 1992;84(2):74.
18. Potter JD. Colorectal cancer: molecules and populations. *J Natl Cancer Inst* 1999;91:916.
19. Gertig DM, Hunter DJ. Genes and environment in the etiology of colorectal cancer. *Semin Cancer Biol* 1998;8:285.
20. Roberts-Thomson IC, Ryan P, Khoo KK, et al. Diet, acetylator phenotype, and risk of colorectal neoplasia. *Lancet* 1996;347:1372.
21. Welfare MR, Cooper J, Bassendine MF, Daly AK. Relationship between acetylator status, smoking, and diet and colorectal cancer risk in the north-east of England. *Carcinogenesis* 1997;18:1351.
22. Szarka CE, Pfeiffer GR, Hum ST, et al. Glutathione S-transferase activity and glutathione S-transferase mu expression in subjects with risk for colorectal cancer. *Cancer Res* 1995;55:2789.
23. O'Dwyer PJ, Szarka CE, Yao KS, et al. Modulation of gene expression in subjects at risk for colorectal cancer by the chemopreventive dithiolethione oltipraz. *J Clin Invest* 1996;98:1210.
24. Reddy B, Engle A, Katsifis S, et al. Biochemical epidemiology of colon cancer: effect of types of dietary fiber of fecal mutagens, acid and neutral sterols in healthy subjects. Stockholm Rectal Cancer Study Group. Short-term preoperative radiotherapy for adenocarcinoma of the rectum. *Am J Clin Oncol* 1987;10:369.
25. Winters MD, Schlinke TL, Joyce WA, et al. Prospective case-cohort study of intestinal colonization with enterococci that produce extracellular superoxide and the risk for colorectal adenomas or cancer. *Am J Gastroenterol* 1998;93:2491.
26. Johansson G, Holmen A, Persson L, et al. Dietary influence on some proposed risk factors for colon cancer: fecal and urinary mutagenic activity and the activity of some intestinal bacterial enzymes. *Cancer Detect Prev* 1997;21:258.
27. de Meester C, Gerber GB. The role of cooked food mutagens as possible etiological agents in human cancer: a critical appraisal of recent epidemiological investigations. *Rev Epidemiol Sante Publique* 1995;43(2):147.
28. Gerhardsson de Verdier M, Hagman U, Peters RK, et al. Meat, cooking methods and colorectal cancer: a case-referent study in Stockholm. *Int J Cancer* 1991;49:520.
29. Thomson B. Heterocyclic amine levels in cooked meat and the implication for New Zealanders. *Eur J Cancer Prev* 1999;8:201.
30. Probst-Hensch NM, Sinha R, Longnecker MP, et al. Meat preparation and colorectal adenomas in a large sigmoidoscopy-based case-control study in California (United States). *Cancer Causes Control* 1997;8:175.
31. Willett WC, Stampfer MJ, Colditz GA, et al. Relation of meat, fat and fiber intake to the risk of colon cancer in a prospective study among women. *N Engl J Med* 1990;323:1664.
32. Suzuki K, Bruce WR. Increase by deoxycholic acid of the colonic nuclear damage induced by known carcinogens in C57BL/6J mice. *J Natl Cancer Inst* 1986;76:1129.
33. Minsky BD, Conti JA, Huang Y, Knopf K. The relationship of acute gastrointestinal toxicity and the volume of irradiated small bowel in patients receiving combined modality therapy for rectal cancer. *J Clin Oncol* 1995;13:1409.
34. Glinghammar B, Holmberg K, Rafter J. Effects of colonic lumenal components on AP-1-dependent gene transcription in cultured human colon carcinoma cells. *Carcinogenesis* 1999;20:969.
35. Bernstein C, Bernstein H, Garewal H, et al. A bile acid-induced apoptosis assay for colon cancer risk and associated quality control studies. *Cancer Res* 1999;59:2353.
36. Kamano T, Mikami Y, Kurasawa T, et al. Ratio of primary and secondary bile acids in feces: possible marker for colorectal cancer? *Dis Colon Rectum* 1999;42:668.
37. Rozen P, Fireman E, Fine N, et al. Oral calcium suppresses increased rectal epithelial proliferation of persons at risk of colorectal cancer. *Gut* 1989;30:650.
38. Cats A, Kleibeuker JH, van der Meer R, et al. Randomized, double-blinded, placebo-controlled intervention study with supplemental calcium in families with hereditary nonpolyposis colorectal cancer. *J Natl Cancer Inst* 1995;87:598.
39. Kearney J, Giovannucci E, Rimm EB, et al. Calcium, vitamin D, and dairy foods and the occurrence of colon cancer in men. *Am J Epidemiol* 1996;143:907.
40. De S, Mendilaharsu M, Deneo-Pellegrini H, Ronco A. Influence of dietary levels of fat, cholesterol, and calcium on colorectal cancer. *Nutr Cancer* 1997;29:83.
41. Baron JA, Beach M, Mandel JS, et al. Calcium supplements for the prevention of colorectal adenomas. Calcium Polyp Prevention Study Group. *N Engl J Med* 1999;340(2):101.
42. Whelan RL, Horvath KD, Gleason NR, et al. Vitamin and calcium supplement use is associated with decreased adenoma recurrence in patients with a previous history of neoplasia. *Dis Colon Rectum* 1999;42:212.
43. Giovannucci E, Stampfer MJ, Colditz GA, et al. Multivitamin use, folate, and colon cancer in women in the Nurses' Health Study. *Ann Med* 1998;129:517.
44. Garland CF, Comstock GW, Garland FC, et al. Serum 25-hydroxyvitamin D and colon cancer: eight-year prospective study. *Lancet* 1989;2(8673):1176.
45. Martinez ME, Giovannucci EL, Colditz GA, et al. Calcium, vitamin D, and the occurrence of colorectal cancer among women. *J Natl Cancer Inst* 1996;88:1375.
46. Howe GR, Benito E, Castelleto R, et al. Dietary intake of fiber and decreased risk of cancers of the colon and rectum: evidence from the combined analysis of 13 case-control studies. *J Natl Cancer Inst* 1992;84:1887.
47. Newberne PM, Bueche D, Riengropitak S, Schrager TF. The influence of dietary levels of vitamin A and fat on colon cancer. *Nutr Cancer* 1990;13:235.
48. Slattery ML, Potter JD, Samowitz W, et al. Methylenetetrahydrofolate reductase, diet, and risk of colon cancer. *Cancer Epidemiol Biomarkers Prev* 1999;8:513.
49. Baron JA, Sandler RSHRW, Mandel JS, et al. Folate intake, alcohol consumption, cigarette smoking, and risk of colorectal adenomas. *J Natl Cancer Inst* 1998;90:57.
50. Kato I, Dnistrian AM, Schwartz M, et al. Serum folate, homocysteine and colorectal cancer risk in women: a nested case-control study. *Br J Cancer* 1999;79:1917.
51. Bird CL, Witte JS, Swendseid ME, et al. Plasma ferritin, iron intake, and the risk of colorectal polyps. *Am J Epidemiol* 1996;144:34.
52. Russo MW, Murray SC, Wurzelmann JI, et al. Plasma selenium levels and the risk of colorectal adenomas. *Nutr Cancer* 1997;28:125.
53. Lippman SM, Lee JJ, Sabichi AL. Cancer chemoprevention: progress and promise. *J Natl Cancer Inst* 1998;90:1514.
54. McKeown-Eyssen GE, Bright-See E. Dietary prevention of recurrences of adenomatous polyps in the colon and rectum. In: *Proceedings of the UICC cancer congress, Budapest.* Geneva: Union Internationale Contre le Cancer, 1986.
55. Mikhailowski R, Shpitz B, Polak-Charcon S, et al. Controlled release of TGF-beta1 impedes rat colon carcinogenesis in vivo. *Int J Cancer* 1998;78:618.
56. Fuchs CS, Giovannucci EL, Colditz GA, et al. Dietary fiber and the risk of colorectal cancer and adenoma in women. *N Engl J Med* 1999;340:169.
57. Lubin F, Rozen P, Arieli B, et al. Nutritional and lifestyle habits and water-fiber interaction in colorectal adenoma etiology. *Cancer Epidemiol Biomarkers Prev* 1997;6:79.
58. Greenwald P, Lanza E. Role of dietary fiber in the prevention of cancer. In: DeVita VT Jr, Hellman S, Rosenberg SA, eds. *Important advances in oncology.* Philadelphia: JB Lippincott Co, 1986:37.
59. Platz EA, Giovannucci E, Rimm EB, et al. Dietary fiber and distal colorectal adenoma in men. *Cancer Epidemiol Biomarkers Prev* 1997;6:661.
60. Faivre J, Giascosa A. Primary prevention of colorectal cancer through fibre supplementation. *Eur J Cancer* 1998;7:S29.
61. Reddy BS, Ekelund G, Bohe M, et al. Metabolic epidemiology of colon cancer: dietary pattern and fecal sterol concentrations of three populations. *Nutr Cancer* 1978;5:34.
62. Schloss I, Kidd MS, Tichelaar HY, et al. Dietary factors associated with a low risk of colon cancer in coloured west coast fishermen. *S Afr Med J* 1997;87:152.
63. Bird CL, Ingles SA, Frankl HD, et al. Serum lipids and adenomas of the left colon and rectum. *Cancer Epidemiol Biomarkers Prev* 1996;5:607.
64. Forones NM, Falcao JB, Mattos D, Barone B. Cholesterolemia in colorectal cancer. *Hepatogastroenterology* 1998;45:1531.
65. Giovannucci E, Rimm EB, Ascherio A, et al. Alcohol, low-methionine-low-folate diets, and risk of colon cancer in men. *J Natl Cancer Inst* 1995;87:265.
66. Franceschi S, La V. Alcohol and the risk of cancers of the stomach and colon-rectum. *Dig Dis* 1994;12:276.
67. Nagata C, Shimizu H, Kametani M, et al. Cigarette smoking, alcohol use, and colorectal adenoma in Japanese men and women. *Dis Colon Rectum* 1999;42:337.
68. Grodstein F, Martinez ME, Platz EA, et al. Postmenopausal hormone use and risk for colorectal cancer and adenoma. *Ann Med* 1998;128:705.
69. Newcomb PA, Storer BE. Postmenopausal hormone use and risk of large-bowel cancer. *J Natl Cancer Inst* 1995;87:1067.
70. Potter JD, Bostick RM, Grandits GA, et al. Hormone replacement therapy is associated with lower risk of adenomatous polyps of the large bowel: the Minnesota Cancer Prevention Research Unit Case-Control Study. *Cancer Epidemiol Biomarkers Prev* 1996;5:779.
71. Martinez ME, Grodstein F, Giovannucci E, et al. A prospective study of reproductive factors, oral contraceptive use, and risk of colorectal cancer. *Cancer Epidemiol Biomarkers Prev* 1997;6:1.
72. Platz EA, Martinez ME, Grodstein F, et al. Parity and other reproductive factors and risk of adenomatous polyps of the distal colorectum (United States). *Cancer Causes Control* 1997;8:894.
73. Shike M. Diet and lifestyle in the prevention of colorectal cancer: an overview. *Am J Med* 1999;106:11S.
74. Lasko CM, Good CK, Adam J, Bird RP. Energy restriction modulates the development of advanced preneoplastic lesions depending on the level of fat in the diet. *Nutr Cancer* 1999;33:69.
75. Martinez ME, Heddens D, Earnest DL, et al. Physical activity, body mass index, and prostaglandin E2 levels in rectal mucosa. *J Natl Cancer Inst* 1999;91:950.
76. Giovannucci E, Colditz GA, Stampfer MJ, Willett WC. Physical activity, obesity, and risk of colorectal adenoma in women (United States). *Cancer Causes Control* 1996;7:253.
77. Thune I, Lund E. Physical activity and risk of colorectal cancer in men and women. *Br J Cancer* 1996;73:1134.
78. Russo A, Franceschi S, La V, et al. Body size and colorectal-cancer risk. *Int J Cancer* 1998;78:161.
79. Ma J, Giovannucci E, Pollak M, Stampfer M. Response: re: prospective study of colorectal cancer risk in men and plasma levels of insulin-like growth factor (IGF)-I and IGF-binding protein-3. *J Natl Cancer Inst* 1999;91:2052.
80. Schoen RE, Tangen CM, Kuller LH, et al. Increased blood glucose and insulin, body size, and incident colorectal cancer. *J Natl Cancer Inst* 1999;91:1147.
81. Will JC, Galuska DA, Vinicor F, Calle EE. Colorectal cancer: another complication of diabetes mellitus? *Am J Epidemiol* 1998;147:816.
82. Muscat JE, Stellman SD, Wynder EL. Nonsteroidal antiinflammatory drugs and colorectal cancer. *Cancer* 1994;74:1847.
83. Rigas B, Goldman IS, Levine L. Altered eicosanoid levels in human colon cancer. *J Lab Clin Med* 1993;122:518.
84. Sheehan KM, Sheahan K, O'Donoghue DP, et al. The relationship between cyclooxygenase-2 expression and colorectal cancer. *JAMA* 1999;282:1254.
85. Giovannucci E, Egan KM, Hunter DJ, et al. Aspiran and the risk of colorectal cancer in women. *N Engl J Med* 1995;333(10):609.
86. Greenberg ER, Baron JA, Freeman DHJ, et al. Reduced risk of large-bowel adenomas among aspirin users. The Polyp Prevention Study Group. *J Natl Cancer Inst* 1993;85:912.
87. Marnett LJ. Aspirin and the potential role of prostaglandins in colon cancer. *Cancer Res* 1992;52:5575.
88. Sturmer T, Glynn RJ, Lee IM, et al. Aspirin use and colorectal cancer: post-trial follow-up data from the Physicians' Health Study. *Ann Intern Med* 1998;128(9):713.
89. Reeves MJ, Newcomb PA, Trentham-Dietz A, et al. Nonsteroidal anti-inflammatory drug use and protection against colorectal cancer in women. *Cancer Epidemiol Biomarkers Prev* 1996;5:955.
90. Giardiello FM, Hamilton SR, Krush AJ, et al. Treatment of colonic and rectal adenomas with sulindac in familial adenomatous polyposis. *N Engl J Med* 1993;328:1313.

91. Hong WK, Sporn MB. Recent advances in chemoprevention of cancer. *Science* 1997;278:1073.
92. Tsujii M, Kawano S, Tsuji S, et al. Cyclooxygenase regulates angiogenesis induced by colon cancer cells. *Cell* 1998;93:705.
93. Burt RW, Bishop DT, Lynch HT, et al. Risk and surveillance of individuals with heritable factors for colorectal cancer. WHO Collaborating Centre for the Prevention of Colorectal Cancer. *Bull World Health Organ* 1990;68:655.
94. Foutch PG, Mai H, Pardy K, et al. Flexible sigmoidoscopy may be ineffective for secondary prevention of colorectal cancer in asymptomatic, average risk men. *Dig Dis Sci* 1991;36(7):924.
95. Bussey HJR. Historical familial polyposis. In: Herrera L, ed. *Familial adenomatous polyposis*. New York: Alan R. Liss, 1990:1.
96. Fearon ER, Vogelstein B. A genetic model for colorectal tumorigenesis. *Cell* 1990;61:759.
96a. Hamilton RS, Lin B, Parsons RE, et al. The molecular basis of Turcot's Syndrome. *N Engl J Med* 1995;332:839.
97. Bresinger JD, Laken SJ, Luce MC, et al. Variable phenotype of familial adenomatous polyposis in pedigrees with 3' mutation in the APC gene. *Gut* 1998;43:548.
98. Nugent KP, Spigelman AD, Phillips RK. Life expectancy after colectomy and ileorectal anastomosis for familial adenomatous polyposis. *Dis Colon Rectum* 1993;36:1059.
99. Arvanitis ML, Jagelman DG, Fazio VW, et al. Mortality in patients with familial adenomatous polyposis. *Dis Colon Rectum* 1990;33:639.
100. Kinzler KW, Nilbert MC, Su LK, et al. Identification of FAP locus genes from chromosome 5q21. *Science* 1991;253:661.
101. Powell SM, Petersen GM, Krush AJ, et al. Molecular diagnosis of familial adenomatous polyposis. *N Engl J Med* 1993;329(27):1982.
102. Cromwell DM, Moore RD, Brensinger JD, et al. Cost analysis of alternative approaches to colorectal screening in familial adenomatous polyposis. *Gastroenterology* 1998;114:893.
103. Peltomaki P, de la Chapelle A. Mutations predisposing to hereditary nonpolyposis colorectal cancer. *Adv Cancer Res* 1997;71:93.
104. Aarnio M, Sankila R, Pukkala E, et al. Cancer risk in mutation carriers of DNA-mismatch-repair genes. *Int J Cancer* 1999;81:214.
105. Muir EG, Bell AJ, Barlow KA. Multiple primary carcinomata of the colon, duodenum, and larynx associated with kerato-acanthomata of the face. *Br J Surg* 1967;54:191.
106. Voskuil D, Vasen H, Kampman E, van't Veer P. Colorectal cancer risk in HNPCC families: development during lifetime and in successive generations. National Collaborative Group on HNPCC. *Int J Cancer* 1997;72:205.
107. Marra G, Boland CR. Hereditary nonpolyposis colorectal cancer: the syndrome, the genes, and historical perspectives. *J Natl Cancer Inst* 1995;87:1114.
108. Akiyama Y, Sato H, Yamada T, et al. Germ-line mutation of the hMSH6/GTBP gene in an atypical hereditary nonpolyposis colorectal cancer kindred. *Cancer Res* 1997;57(18):3920.
109. Park JG, Vasen HF, Park KJ, et al. Suspected hereditary nonpolyposis colorectal cancer: International Collaborative Group on Hereditary Non-Polyposis Colorectal Cancer (ICG-HNPCC) criteria and results of genetic diagnosis. *Dis Colon Rectum* 1999;42:710.
110. Lynch HT, Smyrk TC, Watson P, et al. Genetics, natural history, tumor spectrum, and pathology of hereditary nonpolyposis colorectal cancer: an updated review. *Gastroenterology* 1993;104:1535.
111. Shashidharan M, Smyrk T, Lin KM, et al. Histologic comparison of hereditary nonpolyposis colorectal cancer associated with MSH2 and MLH1 and colorectal cancer from the general population. *Dis Colon Rectum* 1999;42:722.
112. Vasen HF, Watson P, Mecklin JP, Lynch HT. New clinical criteria for hereditary nonpolyposis colorectal cancer (HNPCC, Lynch syndrome) proposed by the International Collaborative group on HNPCC. *Gastroenterology* 1999;116:1453.
113. Vasen HF, Mecklin JP, Khan PM, Lynch HT. The International Collaborative Group on Hereditary Non-Polyposis Colorectal Cancer (ICG-HNPCC). *Dis Colon Rectum* 1991;34:424.
114. Menko FH, Wijnen JT, Khan PM, et al. Genetic counseling in hereditary nonpolyposis colorectal cancer. *Oncology (Huntingt)* 1996;10:71.
115. Aaltonen LA, Salovaara R, Kristo P, et al. Incidence of hereditary nonpolyposis colorectal cancer and the feasibility of molecular screening for the disease. *N Engl J Med* 1998;338:1481.
116. Prior TW, Chadwick RB, Papp AC, et al. The I1307K polymorphism of the APC gene in colorectal cancer. *Gastroenterology* 1999;116:58.
117. Rozen P, Shomrat R, Strul H, et al. Prevalence of the I1307K APC gene variant in Israeli Jews of differing ethnic origin and risk for colorectal cancer. *Gastroenterology* 1999;116:54.
118. Laken SJ, Petersen GM, Gruber SB, et al. Familial colorectal cancer in Ashkenazim due to a hypermutable tract in APC. *Nat Genet* 1997;17:79.
119. Hemminki A, Markie D, Tomlinson I, et al. A serine/threonine kinase gene defective in Peutz-Jeghers syndrome. *Nature* 1998;391:184.
120. Jass JR, Williams CB, Bussey HJ, Morson BC. Juvenile polyposis—a precancerous condition. *Histopathology* 1988;13:619.
121. Church JM. Other polyposis syndromes. *Semin Colon Rectal Surg* 1995;6:61.
122. Howe JR, Mitros FA, Summers RW. The risk of gastrointestinal carcinoma in familial juvenile polyposis. *Ann Surg Oncol* 1998;5:751.
123. Howe JR, Roth S, Ringold JC, et al. Mutations in the SMAD4/DPC4 gene in juvenile polyposis. *Science* 1998;280:1086.
124. Boutron MC, Faivre J, Quipourt V, et al. Family history of colorectal tumours and implications for the adenoma-carcinoma sequence: a case control study. *Gut* 1995;37:830.
125. St John D, McDermott F, Hopper J, et al. Cancer risk in relatives of patients with common colorectal cancer. *Ann Med* 1993;118:785.
126. Fuchs CS, Giovannucci EL, Colditz GA, et al. A prospective study of family history and the risk of colorectal cancer. *N Engl J Med* 1994;331:1669.
127. Pariente A, Milan C, Lafon J, Faivre J. Colonoscopic screening in first-degree relatives of patients with "sporadic" colorectal cancer: a case-control study. The Association Nationale des Gastroenterologues des Hopitaux and Registre Bourguignon des Cancers Digestifs (INSERM CRI 9505). *Gastroenterology* 1998;115:7.
128. Hunt LM, Rooney PS, Hardcastle JD, Armitage NC. Endoscopic screening of relatives of patients with colorectal cancer. *Gut* 1998;42:71.
129. Winawer SJ, Zauber AG, Gerdes H, et al. Risk of colorectal cancer in the families of patients with adenomatous polyps. National Polyp Study Workgroup. *N Engl J Med* 1996;334:82.
130. Winawer SJ, Zauber AG, Gerdes H. Risk of colorectal cancer in the families of patients with adenomatous polyps. *N Engl J Med* 1996;334(2):82.
131. Karlen P, Lofberg R, Brostrom O, et al. Increased risk of cancer in ulcerative colitis: a population-based cohort study. *Am J Gastroenterol* 1999;94:1047.
132. Mir-Modjlessi SH, Farmer RG, Easley KA, Beck CJ. Colorectal and extracolonic malignancy in ulcerative colitis. *Cancer* 1986;58(7):1569.
133. Solomon MJ, Schnitzler M. Cancer and inflammatory bowel disease: bias, epidemiology, surveillance, and treatment. *World J Surg* 1998;22:352.
134. Levin B. Inflammatory bowel disease and colon cancer. *Cancer* 1992;70:1313.
135. Fogt F, Alsaigh N. Polypoid dysplasias in ulcerative colitis and sporadic adenomas: genetic approach to the differential diagnosis [Review]. *Oncol Rep* 1999;6:721.
136. Taylor BA, Pemberton JH, Carpenter HA, et al. Dysplasia in chronic ulcerative colitis: implications for colonoscopic surveillance. *Dis Colon Rectum* 1992;35:950.
137. Ekbom A, Helmick C, Zack M, Adami HO. Increased risk of large-bowel cancer in Crohn's disease with colonic involvement. *Lancet* 1990;336:357.
138. Sigel JE, Petras RE, Lashner BA, et al. Intestinal adenocarcinoma in Crohn's disease: a report of 30 cases with a focus on coexisting dysplasia. *Am J Surg Pathol* 1999;23:651.
139. Rubio CA, Befrits R. Colorectal adenocarcinoma in Crohn's disease: a retrospective histologic study. *Dis Colon Rectum* 1997;40:1072.
140. Heald RJ. Synchronous and metachronous carcinoma of the colon and rectum. *Ann R Coll Surg Engl* 1990;72:172.
141. Cali RL, Pitsch RM, Thorson AG, et al. Cumulative incidence of metachronous colorectal cancer. *Dis Colon Rectum* 1993;36:388.
142. Fante R, Roncucci L, Di G, et al. Frequency and clinical features of multiple tumors of the large bowel in the general population and in patients with hereditary colorectal carcinoma. *Cancer* 1996;77:2013.
143. Atkin WS, Morson BC, Cuzick J. Long-term risk of colorectal cancer after excision of rectosigmoid adenomas. *N Engl J Med* 1992;326:658.
144. Collett JA, Platell C, Fletcher DR, et al. Distal colonic neoplasms predict proximal neoplasia in average-risk, asymptomatic subjects. *J Gastroenterol Hepatol* 1999;14:67.
145. Rex DK, Chak A, Vasudeva R, et al. Prospective determination of distal colon findings in average-risk patients with proximal colon cancer. *Gastrointest Endosc* 1999;49:727.
146. Stryker SJ, Wolff BG, Culp CE, et al. Natural history of untreated colonic polyps. *Gastroenterology* 1987;93:1009.
147. Winawer SJ, Zauber AG, Ho MN, et al. Prevention of colorectal cancer by colonscopic polypectomy. *N Engl J Med* 1993;329:1977.
148. Levitt MD, Millar DM, Stewart JO. Rectal cancer after pelvic irradiation. *J R Soc Med* 1990;83:152.
149. Tsunoda A, Shibusawa M, Kawamura M, et al. Colorectal cancer after pelvic irradiation: case reports. *Anticancer Res* 1997;17:729.
150. Neugut AI, Murray TI, Garbowski GC, et al. Cholecystectomy as a risk factor for colorectal adenomatous polyps and carcinoma. *Cancer* 1991;68:1644.
151. Reid FD, Mercer PM, Harrison M, Bates T. Cholecystectomy as a risk factor for colorectal cancer: a meta-analysis. *Scand J Gastroenterol* 1996;31:160.
152. Anonymous. Cholecystectomy and the risk for colorectal cancer: a meta-analysis. *ACP Journal Club* 1994;120:25.
153. Jorgensen T, Rafaelsen S. Gallstones and colorectal cancer—There is a relationship, but it is hardly due to cholecystectomy. *Dis Colon Rectum* 1992;35:24.
154. Markowitz AJ, Winawer SJ. Management of colorectal polyps. *CA Cancer J Clin* 1997;47:93.
155. Ransohoff DF, Lang CA. Screening for colorectal cancer. *N Engl J Med* 1991;325:37.
156. Byrd U, Boggs HW, Slagle GW, Cole PA. Reliability of colonoscopy. *Dis Colon Rectum* 1989;32:1023.
157. Simmang CL, Senatore P. Practice parameters for detection of colorectal neoplasms. *Dis Colon Rectum* 1999;42:1123.
158. Froggatt NJ, Green J, Brassett C, et al. A common MSH2 mutation in English and North American HNPCC families: origin, phenotypic expression, and sex specific differences in colorectal cancer. *J Med Genet* 1999;36:97.
159. Jarvinen HJ, Mecklin JP, Sistonen P. Screening reduces colorectal cancer rate in families with hereditary nonpolyposis colorectal cancer. *Gastroenterology* 1995;108:1405.
160. Syngal S, Weeks JC, Schrag D, et al. Benefits of colonoscopic surveillance and prophylactic colectomy in patients with hereditary nonpolyposis colorectal cancer mutations. *Ann Med* 1998;129:787.
161. Rodriguez-Bigas MA, Vasen HF, Pekka-Mecklin J, et al. Rectal cancer risk in hereditary nonpolyposis colorectal cancer after abdominal colectomy. International Collaborative Group on HNPCC. *Ann Surg* 1997;225:202.
162. Winawer SJ, O'Brien MJ, Waye JD, et al. Risk and surveillance of individuals with colorectal polyps. Who Collaborating Centre for the Prevention of Colorectal Cancer. *Bull World Health Organ* 1990;68:789.
163. Van Stolk RU, Beck GJ, Aaltonen L, et al. Adenoma characteristics at first colonscopy as predictors of adenoma recurrence and characteristics at follow-up. *Gastrenterology* 1998;115:13.
164. Winawer SJ, Zauber AG, O'Brien MJ. Randomized comparison of surveillance intervals after colonscopic removal of newly diagnosed adenomatous polyps. *N Engl J Med* 1993;328:901.
165. Provenzale D, Kowdley KV, Arora S, Wong JB. Prophylactic colectomy or surveillance for chronic ulcerative colitis? A decision analysis. *Gastroenterology* 1995;109:1188.
166. Manning AP, Bulgim OR, Dixon MF, Axon AT. Screening by colonoscopy for colonic epithelial dysplasia in inflammatory bowel disease. *Gut* 1987;28:1489.
167. Leonard-Jones JE, Mellville DM, Morson BC, et al. Precancer and cancer in extensive ulceration colitis: fndings among 401 patients over 22 years. *Gut* 1990;31:800.
168. Fenlon HM, Nunes DP, Schroy PC III, et al. A comparison of virtual and conventional colonoscopy for the detection of colorectal polyps. *N Engl J Med* 1999;341:1496.
169. Byers T, Levin B, Rothenberger D, et al. American Cancer Society guidelines for screening and surveillance for early detection of colorectal polyps and cancer: update 1997. American Cancer Society Detection and Treatment Advisory Group on Colorectal Cancer. *CA Cancer J Clin* 1997;47:154.

170. Morris JB, Stellato TA, Guy BB, et al. A critical analysis of the largest reported mass fecal occult blood screening program in the United States. *Am J Surg* 1991;161:101.
171. Kewenter J, Brevinge H, Engaras B, et al. Results of screening, rescreening, and follow-up in a prospective randomized study for detection of colorectal cancer by fecal occult blood testing. Results for 68,308 subjects. *Scand J Gastroenterol* 1994;29:468.
172. Hardcastle JD, Armitage NC, Chamberlin J, et al. Fecal occult blood screening for colorectal cancer in the general population. *Cancer* 1986;58:397.
173. Barry MJ, Mulley AG, Richter JM. Effect of workup strategy of the cost-effectiveness of fecal occult blood screening for colorectal cancer. *Gastroenterology* 1987;93:301.
174. Fleisher M, Winawer SJ, Zauber AG, et al. Accuracy of fecal occult blood test interpretation. National Polyp Study Work Group. *Ann Med* 1991;114:875.
175. Fletcher RH. Clinical debate: Should all people over the age of 50 have regular fecal occult-blood tests? *N Engl J Med* 1998;338:1151.
176. Lang CA, Ransohoff DF. Fecal occult blood screening for colorectal cancer. Is mortality reduced by chance selection for screening colonoscopy? *JAMA* 1994;271:1011.
177. Wilking N, Petrelli NJ, Herrera L, et al. A comparison of the 25 cm rigid proctosigmoidoscope with the 65 cm flexible endoscope in the screening of patients for colorectal carcinoma. *Cancer* 1986;57:669.
178. Selby JV, Friedman GD, Quesenberry CP Jr, Weiss NS. A case-control study of screening sigmoidoscopy and mortality from colorectal cancer. *N Engl J Med* 1992;326:653.
179. Kavanagh AM, Giovannucci EL, Fuchs CS, Colditz GA. Screening endoscopy and risk of colorectal cancer in United States men. *Cancer Causes Control* 1998;9:455.
180. Atkin WS, Cuzick J, Northover JM, Whynes DK. Prevention of colorectal cancer by once-only sigmoidoscopy. *Lancet* 1993;341:736.
181. Mitmaker B, Begin LR, Gordon PH. Nuclear shape as a prognostic discriminant in colorectal carcinoma. *Dis Colon Rectum* 1991;34:249.
182. Minsky BD. Clinicopathologic impact of colloid in colorectal carcinoma. *Dis Colon Rectum* 1990;33:714.
183. DiSario JA, Burt RW, Kendrick ML, McWhorter WP. Colorectal cancers of rare histologic types compared with adenocarcinomas. *Dis Colon Rectum* 1994;37:1277.
184. Jass JR. Diagnosis of hereditary non-polyposis colorectal cancer. *Histopathology* 1998;32:491.
185. Hernanz F, Revuelta S, Redonodo C, et al. Colorectal adenocarcinoma: quality of the assessment of lymph node metastases. *Dis Colon Rectum* 1994;37:373.
186. Scott KW, Grace RH, Gibbons P. Five-year follow-up study of the fat clearance technique in colorectal carcinoma. *Dis Colon Rectum* 1994;37:126.
187. Goldstein N, Hart J. Histologic features associated with lymph node metastasis in stage T1 and superficial T2 rectal adenocarcinomas in abdominoperineal resection specimens. Identifiying a subset of patients for whom treatment with adjuvant therapy or completion abdominoperineal resection should be considered after local excision. *Am J Clin Pathol* 1999;111(1):51.
188. Wong JH, Severino R, Honnebier MB, et al. Number of nodes examined and staging accuracy in colorectal carcinoma. *J Clin Oncol* 1999;17:2896.
189. Leifers GJ, Cleton-Jansen AM, van de Velde CJ, et al. Micrometastases and micro-survival in stage II colorectal cancer. *N Engl J Med* 1998;339:223.
190. Liotta L. Cancer cell invasion and metastasis. *Sci Am* 1992;266:54.
191. Minsky BD, Mies C, Recht A, et al. Resectable adenocarcinoma of the rectosigmoid and rectum: 1. Patterns of failure and survival. *Cancer* 1988;61:1408.
192. Gilchrist R, David D. Lymphatic spread of carcinoma of the rectum. *Ann Surg* 1948;38(108):621.
193. Rigau J, Pique JM, Rubio E, et al. Effects of long-term sulindac therapy on colonic polyposis. *Ann Med* 1991;115:952.
194. Brown C, Warren S. Visceral metastasis from carcinoma. *Surg Gynecol Obstet* 1938;66:611.
195. Dedhar S, Hannigan GE, Rak J, Kerbel RS. The extracellular environment and cancer. In: Tannock IF, Hill RP, eds. *The basic science of oncology.* New York: McGraw-Hill, 1998:197.
196. Zeng Z, Cohen AM, Hajdu S. Serosal cytologic study to determine free mesothelial penetration of intraperitoneal colon cancer. *Cancer* 1992;70:737.
197. Umpleby HC, Williamson RCN. Anastomotic recurrence in large bowel cancer. *Br J Surg* 1987;74:873.
198. Brodsky JT, Cohen AM. Peritoneal seeding following potentially curative resection of colonic carcinoma: implications for adjuvant therapy. *Dis Colon Rectum* 1991;34:723.
199. Minsky BD, Mies C, Rich TA, et al. Potentially curative surgery of colon cancer. The influence of blood vessel invasion. *J Clin Oncol* 1988;6:119.
200. Thoeni RF. Colorectal cancer. Radiologic staging. *Radiol Clin North Am* 1997;35:457.
201. Alauddin MM, Shahinian A, Kundu RK, et al. Evaluation of 9-[(3-18F-fluoro-1-hydroxy-2-propoxy)methyl]guanine ([18F]-FHPG) in vitro and in vivo as a probe for PET imaging of gene incorporation and expression in tumors. *Nucl Med Biol* 1999;26:371.
202. Isern AM, Fernandez C, Salamanca M, et al. Ultrasonido transrectal en la estadificacion preoperatoria del adenocarcinoma de recto. Estudio transversal 1991–1994. *GEN* 1995;49(2):104.
203. Waizer A, Zitron S, Ben-Baruch D, et al. Comparative study for preoperative staging of rectal cancer. *Dis Colon Rectum* 1989;32:53.
204. Hoff P, Brito R, Slaughter M, et al. Preoperative UFT, oral leucovorin (LV) and radiotherapy (RT) for patients (pts) with resectable rectal carcinoma: an oral regimen with complete pathological responses. *Proc Am Soc Clin Oncol* 1998;17:223a.
205. Griffin MR, Bergstralh EJ, Coffey RJ, et al. Predictors of survival after curative resection of carcinoma of the colon and rectum. *Cancer* 1987;60:2318.
206. Bognel C, Rekacewicz C, Mankarios H, et al. Prognostic value of neural invasion in rectal carcinoma: a multivariate analysis on 339 patients with curative resection. *Eur J Cancer* 1995;31A:894.
207. Jass JR. The pathological grading and staging of rectal cancer. *Scand J Gastroenterol Suppl* 1988;149:21.
208. Shepherd NA, Saraga EP, Love SB, Jass JR. Prognostic factors in colonic cancer. *Histopathology* 1989;14:613.
209. Fisher ER, Pail SM, Rockette H, et al. Prognostic significance of eosinophils and mast cells in rectal cancer: Findings from the National Surgical Adjuvant Breast and Bowel Project (Protocol R-01). *Hum Pathol* 1989;20:159.
210. Gagliardi G, Stepniewska KA, Hershman MJ, et al. New grade-related prognostic variable for rectal cancer. *Br J Surg* 1995;82:599.
211. Saccani Jotti G, Fontanesi M, Orsi N, et al. DNA content in human colon cancer and non-neoplastic adjacent mucosa. *Int J Biol Markers* 1995;10:11.
212. Sinicrope FA, Hart J, Hsu HA, et al. Apoptotic and mitotic indices predict survival rates in lymph node-negative colon carcinomas. *Clin Cancer Res* 1999;5:1793.
213. Lanza G, Matteuzzi M, Gafa R, et al. Chromosome 18q allelic loss and prognosis in stage II and III colon cancer. *Int J Cancer* 1998;79:390.
214. Ogunbiyi OA, Goodfellow PJ, Herfarth K, et al. Confirmation that chromosome 18q allelic loss in colon cancer is a prognostic indicator. *J Clin Oncol* 1998;16(2):427.
215. Kotanagi H, Fukuoka T, Shibata Y, et al. The size of regional lymph nodes does not correlate with the presence or absence of metastasis in lymph nodes in rectal cancer. *J Surg Oncol* 1993;54:252.
216. Herrera-Ornelas L, Justiniano J, Castillo N, et al. Metastases in small lymph nodes from colon cancer. *Arch Surg* 1987;122(11):1253.
217. Wong JH, Severino R, Honnebier MB, et al. Number of nodes examined and staging accuracy in colorectal carcinoma. *J Clin Oncol* 1999;17:2896.
218. Wolmark N, Fisher B, Wieand HS. The prognostic value of the modifications of the Dukes' C class of colorectal cancer. *Ann Surg* 1986;203:115.
219. Fisher ER, Robinsky B, Sass R, Fisher B. Relative prognostic value of the dukes and the jass systems in rectal cancer: findings from the National Surgical Adjuvant Breast and Bowel Projects (Protocol R-01). *Dis Colon Rectum* 1989;32:944.
220. Jass JR, Ajioka Y, Allen JP, et al. Assessment of invasive growth pattern and lymphocytic infiltration in colorectal cancer. *Histopathology* 1996;28:543.
221. Deans GT, Heatley M, Anderson N, et al. Jass' classification revisited. *J Am Coll Surg* 1994;179:11.
222. Chapuis PH, Dent OF, Newland RC, et al. An evaluation of the American Joint Committee (pTNM) staging method for cancer of the colon and rectum. *Dis Colon Rectum* 1986;29:6.
223. Enderlin F, Gloor F. Colorectal cancer: the relationship of staging to survival. A cancer registry study of 800 cases in St. Gallen-Appenzell. *Prev Med* 1986;31:85.
224. Hermanek P. Problems of pTNM classification of carcinoma of the stomach, colorectum and anal margin. *Pathol Res Pract* 1986;181:296.
225. American Joint Committee on Cancer. Colon and rectum. In: *AJCC Cancer Staging Manual.* Philadelphia: Lippincott-Raven Publishers, 1997:83.
226. Sebbag G, Lantsberg L, Arish A, et al. Colon carcinoma in the adolescent. *Pediatr Surg Int* 1997;12:446.
227. Jacobs LR. Relationship between dietary fiber and cancer: metabolic, physiologic, and cellular mechanisms. *Proc Soc Exp Biol Med* 1986;183:299.
228. Minardi AJ, Sittig KM, Zibari GB, McDonald JC. Colorectal cancer in the young patient. *Am Surg* 1998;64:849.
229. Coburn MC, Pricolo VE, Soderberg CH. Factors affecting prognosis and management of carcinoma of the colon and rectum in patients more than eighty years of age. *J Am Coll Surg* 1994;179:65.
230. Gatta G, Faivre J, Capocaccia R, Ponz de Leon M. Survival of colorectal cancer patients in Europe during the period 1978–1989. EUROCARE Working Group. *Eur J Cancer* 1998;34:2176.
231. DeCosse JJ, Ngoi SS, Jacobson JS, Cennerazzo WJ. Gender and colorectal cancer. *Eur J Cancer Prev* 1993;2:105.
232. Corman J, Arnoux R, Peloquin A, et al. Blood transfusions and survival after colectomy for colorectal cancer. *Can J Surg* 1986;29:325.
233. Fielding LP, Phillips RKS, Fry JS, Hittinger R. Prediction of outcome after curative resection for large bowel cancer. *Lancet* 1986;2:904.
234. Ghadirian P, Maisonneuve P, Perret C, et al. Epidemiology of sociodemographic characteristics, lifestyle, medical history, and colon cancer: a case-control study among French Canadians in Montreal. *Cancer Detect Prev* 1998;22:396.
235. Peter RK, Pike MC, Chang WWL, et al. Reproductive factors and colon cancers. *Br J Cancer* 1990;61:741.
236. Fernandez E, La Vecchia C, Franceschi S, et al. Oral contraceptive use and risk of colorectal cancer. *Epidemiology* 1998;9:295.
237. Calle EE, Miracle-McMahill HL, Thun MJ, Heath CW Jr. Estrogen replacement therapy and risk of fatal colon cancer in a prospective cohort of postmenopausal women. *J Natl Cancer Inst* 1995;87:517.
238. Wilcox S, Stefanick ML. Knowledge and perceived risk of major diseases in middle-aged and older women. *Health Psychology* 1999;18:346.
239. Donovan JM, Syngal S. Colorectal cancer in women: an underappreciated but preventable risk. *J Womens Health* 1998;7:45.
240. Winawer SJ. Natural history of colorectal cancer. *Am J Med* 1999;106:3S.
241. Winawer SJ. Can mortality from colorectal cancer be reduced? *Ann N Y Acad Sci* 1995;768:60.
242. Mandel JS, Church TR, Ederer F, Bond JH. Colorectal cancer mortality: effectiveness of biennial screening for fecal occult blood. *J Natl Cancer Inst* 1999;91:434.
243. Barillari P, de Angelis R, Valabrega S, et al. Relationship of symptom duration and survival in patients with colorectal carcinoma. *Eur J Surg Oncol* 1989;15:441.
244. Marquet RL, Busch OR, Jeekel J, et al. Are allogeneic blood transfusions acceptable in elective surgery in colorectal carcinoma? *Eur J Cancer* 1999;35:352.
245. Voogt PJ, van de Velde CJ, Brand A, et al. Perioperative blood transfusion and cancer prognosis. Different effects of blood transfusion on prognosis of colon and breast cancer patients. *Cancer* 1987;59:836.
246. Busch OR, Marquet RL, Hop WC, Jeekel J. Colorectal cancer recurrence and perioperative blood transfusions: a critical reappraisal. *Semin Surg Oncol* 1994;10:195.

247. Tang R, Wang JY, Chien CR, et al. The association between perioperative blood transfusion and survival of patients with colorectal cancer. *Cancer* 1993;72:341.
248. Weiden PL, Bean MA, Schultz P. Perioperative blood transfusion does not increase the risk of colorectal cancer. *Cancer* 1987;60:870.
249. Sibbering DM, Locker AP, Hardcastle JD, Armitage NC. Blood transfusion and survival in colorectal cancer. *Dis Colon Rectum* 1994;37:358.
250. Donohue JH, Williams S, Cha S, et al. Perioperative blood transfusions do not affect disease recurrence of patients undergoing curative resection of colorectal carcinoma: a Mayo/North Central Cancer Treatment Group study. *J Clin Oncol* 1995;13:1671.
251. Busch OR, Hop WC, Marquet RL, Jeekel J. The effect of blood transfusions on survival after surgery for colorectal cancer. *Eur J Cancer* 1995;31A:1226.
252. Takahashi Y, Tucker SL, Kitadai Y, et al. Vessel counts and expression of vascular endothelial growth factor as prognostic factors in node-negative colon cancer. *Arch Surg* 1997;132:541.
253. Siemeister G, Martiny-Baron G, Marme D. The pivotal role of VEGF in tumor angiogenesis: molecular facts and therapeutic opportunities. *Cancer Metastasis Rev* 1998;17:241.
254. Koren R, Siegal A, Klein B, et al. Lymph node-revealing solution: simple new method for detecting minute lymph nodes in colon carcinoma. *Dis Colon Rectum* 1997;40:407.
255. Schneebaum S, Even-Sapir E, Cohen M, et al. Clinical applications of gamma-detection probes-radioguided surgery. *Eur J Nucl Med* 1999;26:S26.
256. Greenson JK, Isenhart CE, Rice R, et al. Identification of occult micrometastases in pericolic lymph nodes of Duke's B colorectal cancer patients using monoclonal antibodies against cytokeratin and CC49. Correlation with long-term survival. *Cancer* 1994;73:563.
257. Cote RJ, Houchens DP, Hitchcock CL, et al. Intraoperative detection of occult colon cancer micrometastases using 125 I–radiolabled monoclonal antibody CC49. *Cancer* 1996;77:613.
258. Calaluce R, Miedema BW, Yesus YW. Micrometastasis in colorectal carcinoma: a review. *J Surg Oncol* 1998;67:194.
259. Ichikawa Y, Ishikawa T, Momiyama N, et al. Detection of regional lymph node metastases in colon cancer by using RT-PCR for matrix metalloproteinase 7, matrilysin. *Clin Exp Metastasis* 1998;16:3.
260. Waldman SA, Cagir B, Rakinic J, et al. Use of guanylyl cyclase C for detecting micrometastasis in lymph nodes of patients with colon cancer. *Dis Colon Rectum* 1998;41:310.
261. Nakamori S, Kameyama M, Furukawa H, et al. Genetic detection of colorectal cancer cells in circulation and lymph nodes. *Dis Colon Rectum* 1997;40:S29.
262. Jonas S, Windeatt S, A O-Boateng A, et al. Identification of carcinoembryonic antigen-producing cells circulating in the blood of patients with colorectal carcinoma by reverse transcriptase polymerase chain reaction. *Gut* 1996;39:717.
263. Mori K, Yamaguchi T, Maeda M. Mechanism of 201 thallium-chloride uptake in tumor cells and its relationship to potassium channels. *Neurol Res* 1998;20:19.
264. Eldar S, Kemeny MM, Terz JJ. Extended resections for carcinoma of the colon and rectum. *Surg Gynecol Obstet* 1985;161:319.
265. Quirke P, Durdey P, Dixon MF, Williams NS. Local recurrence of rectal adenocarcinoma due to inadequate surgical resection. Histopathological study of lateral tumor spread and surgical excision. *Lancet* 1986;1:996.
266. Adam IJ, Mohamdee MO, Martin IG, et al. Role of circumferential margin involvement in the local recurrence of rectal cancer. *Lancet* 1994;344:707.
267. Haas-Kock DFM, Baeten CGMI, Jager JJ, et al. Prognostic significance of radial margins of clearance in rectal cancer. *Br J Surg* 1996;83:781.
268. Peethambaram P, Weiss M, Loprinzi CL, et al. An evaluation of postoperative follow-up tests in colon cancer patients treated for cure. *Oncology* 1997;54:287.
269. Green JB, Timmcke AE, Mitchell WT, et al. Mucinous carcinoma—just another colon cancer? *Dis Colon Rectum* 1993;36:49.
270. Parramore JB, Wei JP, Yeh KA. Colorectal cancer in patients under forty: presentation and outcome. *Am Surg* 1998;64:563.
271. Schwartz B, Bresalier RS, Kim YS. The role of mucin in colon-cancer metastasis. *Int J Cancer* 1992;52:60.
271a. Nissan A, Guillem JG, Paty PB, et al. Signet-ring cell carcinoma of the colon and rectum: a matched control study. *Dis Colon Rectum* 1999;42:1176.
272. Secco GB, Fardelli R, Campora E, et al. Primary mucinous adenocarcinomas and signet-ring cell carcinomas of colon and rectum. *Oncology* 1994;51:30.
273. Minsky BD, Mies C, Rich TA, et al. Colloid carcinoma of the colon and rectum. *Cancer* 1987;60:3103.
274. Kawabata Y, Tomita N, Monden T, et al. Molecular characteristics of poorly differentiated adenocarcinoma and signet-ring-cell carcinoma of colorectum. *Int J Cancer* 1999;84:33.
275. Zhang H, Evertsson S, Sun X. Clinicopathological and genetic characteristics of mucinous carcinomas in the colorectum. *Intl J Cancer* 1999;14:1057.
276. Duesberg P, Rausch C, Rasnick D, Hehlmann R. Genetic instability of cancer cells is proportional to their degree of aneuploidy. *Proc Natl Acad Sci U S A* 1998;95:13692.
277. Deans GT, Williamson K, Heatley M, et al. The role of flow cytometry in carcinoma of the colon and rectum. *Surg Gynecol Obstet* 1993;177:377.
278. Crissman JD, Zarbo RJ, Ma CK, Visscher D.W. Histopathologic parameters and DNA analysis in colorectal adenocarcinomas 24. *Pathol Annu* 1989;24(2):103.
279. Witzig TE, Loprinzi CL, Gonchoroff NJ, et al. DNA ploidy and cell kinetic measurements as predictors of recurrence and survival in stages B2 and colorectal adenocarcinoma. *Cancer* 1991;68:879.
280. Schillaci A, Tirindelli DD, Freei M, et al. Flow cytometric analysis in colorectal carcinoma: prognostic significance of cellular DNA content. *Int J Colorectal Dis* 1990;5:223.
281. Rognum TO, Thorud E, Lund E. Survival of large bowel carcinoma patients with different DNA ploidy. *Br J Cancer* 1987;56:633.
282. Tomoda H, Kakeji Y, Furusawa M. Prognostic significance of flow cytometric analysis of DNA content in colorectal cancer: a prospective study. *J Surg Oncol* 1993;53:144.
283. Heimann TM, Martinelli G, Szporn A, et al. Prognostic significance of DNA content abnormalities in young patients with colorectal cancer. *Ann Surg* 1989;210:792.
284. Kokal WA, Gardine RL, Sheibani K, et al. Tumor DNA content in resectable, primary colorectal carcinoma. *Ann Surg* 1989;209:188.
285. Wiggers T, Arends JW, Schutte B, et al. A multivariate analysis of pathologic prognostic indicators in large bowel cancer. *Cancer* 1988;61:386.
286. Shirouzu K, Isomoto H, Kakegawa T, Morimatsu M. A prospective clinicopathologic study of venous invasion in colorectal cancer. *Am J Surg* 1991;162:216.
287. Minsky BD, Mies C, Recht A, et al. Resectable adenocarcinoma of the rectosigmoid and rectum: 2. The influence of blood vessel invasion. *Cancer* 1988;61:1417.
288. Krasna MJ, Flancbaum L, Cody RP, et al. Vascular and neural invasion in colorectal carcinoma. Incidence and prognostic significance. *Cancer* 1988;61:1018.
289. Minsky BD, Mies C, Rich TA, Recht A. Lymphatic vessel invasion is an independent prognostic factor for survival in colorectal cancer. *Int J Radiat Oncol Biol Phys* 1989;17:311.
290. Shirouzu K, Isomoto H, Morodomi T, Kakegawa T. Carcinomatous lymphatic permeation. Prognostic significance in patients with rectal carcinoma—a long term prospective study. *Cancer* 1995;75:4.
291. Bouvet M, Milas M, Giacco GG, et al. Predictors of recurrence after local excision and postoperative chemoradiation therapy of adenocarcinoma of the rectum. *Ann Surg Oncol* 1999;6:26.
292. Forones NM, Tanaka M, Falcao JB. CEA as a prognostic index in colorectal cancer. *Rev Paul Med* 1997;115:1589.
293. Harrison LE, Guillem JG, Paty P, Cohen AM. Preoperative carcinoembryonic antigen predicts outcomes in node-negative colon cancer patients: a multivariate analysis of 572 patients. *J Am Coll Surg* 1997;185:55.
294. Chapman MA, Buckley D, Henson DB, Armitage NC. Preoperative carcinoembryonic antigen is related to tumour stage and long-term survival in colorectal cancer. *Br J Cancer* 1998;78:1346.
295. Filella X, Molina R, Pique JM, et al. CEA as a prognostic factor in colorectal cancer. *Anticancer Res* 1994;14:705.
296. Feil W, Wunderlich M, Neuhild N, et al. Rectal cancer: factors influencing the development of local recurrence after radical anterior resection. *Int J Colorectal Dis* 1988;3:195.
297. Fisher B, Wolmark N, Rockette H, et al. Postoperative adjuvant chemotherapy or radiation therapy for rectal cancer: results from NSABP protocol R-01. *J Natl Cancer Inst* 1988;80:21.
298. Diederichsen AC, Zeuthen J, Christensen PB, Kristensen T. Characterisation of tumour infiltrating lymphocytes and correlations with immunological surface molecules in colorectal cancer. *Eur J Cancer* 1999;35:721.
299. Fearon ER, Cho KR, Nigro JM, et al. Identification of a chromosome 18q gene that is altered in colorectal cancers. *Science* 1990;247:49.
300. Mehlen P, Rabizadeh S, Snipas SJ, et al. The DCC gene product induces apoptosis by a mechanism requiring receptor proteolysis. *Nature* 1998;395:801.
301. Saito M, Yamaguchi A, Goi T, et al. Expression of DCC protein in colorectal tumors and its relationship to tumor progression and metastasis. *Oncology* 1999;56:134.
302. van Triest B, Pinedo HM, van Hensbergen Y, et al. Thymidylate synthase level as the main predictive parameter for sensitivity to 5-fluorouracil, but not for folate-based thymidylate synthase inhibitors, in 13 nonselected colon cancer cell lines. *Clin Cancer Res* 1999;5:643.
303. Diasio RB. Clinical implications of dihydropyrimidine dehydrogenase inhibition. *Oncology* 1999;13:17.
304. Genuardi M, Viel A, Bonora D, et al. Characterization of MLH1 and MSH2 alternative splicing and its relevance to molecular testing of colorectal cancer susceptibility. *Hum Genet* 1998;102:15.
305. Attallah AM, Elhak NG, Nasif WA, et al. Detection of p53 protein overexpression and DNA ploidy analysis in colon cancer. *Hepatogastroenterology* 1997;44:1595.
306. Gryfe R, Swallow C, Bapat B, et al. Molecular biology of colorectal cancer. *Curr Probl Cancer* 1997;21:233.
307. Pricolo VE, Finkelstein SD, Hansen K, et al. Mutated p53 gene is an independent adverse predictor of survival in colon carcinoma. *Arch Surg* 1997;132:371.
308. Ahnen DJ, Feigl P, Quan G, et al. Ki-ras mutation and p53 overexpression predict the clinical behavior of colorectal cancer: a Southwest Oncology Group study. *Cancer Res* 1998;58:1149.
309. Itzkowitz SH. Blood group-related carbohydrate antigen expression in malignant and premalignant colonic neoplasms. *J Cell Biochem Suppl* 1992;16G:97.
310. Griesenberg D, Nurnberg R, Bahlo M, Klapdor R. CEA, TPS, CA 19-9 and CA 72-4 and the fecal occult blood test in the preoperative diagnosis and follow-up after resective surgery of colorectal cancer. *Anticancer Res* 1999;19:2443.
311. Offerhaus GJ, Giardiello FM, Bruijn JA, et al. The value of immunohistochemistry for collagen IV expression in colorectal carcinomas. *Cancer* 1991;67:99.
312. Cayrol C, Knibiehler M, Ducommun B. p21 binding to PCNA causes G1 and G2 cell cycle arrest in p53-deficient cells. *Oncogene* 1998;16:311.
313. Jessup JM, Lavin PT, Andrews CW, et al. Sucrase-Isomaltase is an independent prognostic marker for colorectal cancer. *Dis Colon Rectum* 1995;38:1257.
314. Ikeda Y, Mori M, Adachi Y, et al. Prognostic value of the histochemical expression of helix pomatia agglutinin in advanced colorectal cancer. A univariate and multivariate analysis. *Dis Colon Rectum* 1994;37:181.
315. Nakamori S, Watanabe H, Kameyama M, et al. Expression of autocrine motility factor receptor in colorectal cancer as a predictor for disease recurrence. *Cancer* 1994;74:1855.
316. Matsubara N, Hietala OA, Gilmour SK, et al. Association between high levels of ornithine decarboxylase activity and favorable prognosis in human colorectal carcinoma. *Clin Cancer Res* 1995;1:665.
317. Andrews CW Jr, Jessup JM, Goldman H, et al. Localization of tumor-associated glycoprotein DF3 in normal, inflammatory, and neoplastic lesions of the colon. *Cancer* 1993;72:3185.
318. Nakamori S, Kameyama M, Imaoka S, et al. Involvement of carbohydrate antigen sialyl Lewis(x) in colorectal cancer metastasis. *Dis Colon Rectum* 1997;40:420.
319. Pello MJ. Transanal excision of large sessile villous adenomas using an endorectal traction flap. *Surg Gynecol Obstet* 1987;164:281.
320. Phillips RK, Spigelman AD. For debate: Can we safely delay or avoid prophylctic colectomy in familial adenomatous polyposis? *Br J Surg* 1996;83:769.

321. Phillips RKS. Familial adenomatous polyposis: the surgical treatment of the colorectum. *Semin Colon Rectal Surg* 1995;6:33.
322. Sarre RG, Jagelman DG, Beck GJ, et.al. Colectomy with ileorectal anastomosis for familial adenomatous polyposis: the risk of rectal cancer. *Surgery* 1986;101:20.
323. Church JM, Fazio VW, Lavery IC, et al. Quality of life after prophylactic colectomy and illeo-rectal anastomosis in patients with familial adenomatous polyposis. *Dis Colon Rectum* 1996;39:1404.
324. DeCosse JJ, Cennerazzo W. Treatment options for the patient with colorectal cancer. *Cancer* 1992;70:1342.
325. Iwama T, Mishima Y. Factors affecting the risk of rectal cancer following rectum-preserving surgery in patients with familial adenomatous polyposis. *Dis Colon Rectum* 1994;37:1024.
326. Fazio VW, O'Riordain MG, Lavery IC, et al. Long term functional outcome and quality of life after stapled restorative proctocolectomy. *Ann Surg* 1999;230:575.
327. Hojo K, Vernava AM, III, Sugihara K, Katumata K. Preservation of urine voiding and sexual function after rectal cancer surgery. *Dis Colon Rectum* 1991;34:532.
328. Ziv Y, Church JM, Oakley JR, et al. Results after restorative proctocolectomy and ileal pouch anal anastomosis in patients with familial adenomatous polyposis and coexisting colorectal cancer. *Br J Surg* 1996;83:1578.
329. Wu J, Paul P, McGannon EA, Church JM. APC genotype, polyp number, and surgical options in familial adenomatous polyposis. *Ann Surg* 1998;227:57.
330. Gebert JF, Dupon C, Kadmon M, et al. Combined molecular and clinical approaches for the identification of families with familial adenomatous polyposis coli. *Ann Surg* 1999;229:350.
331. Evans DG, Hill J, Dudding T, et al. Molecular genetic tests in surgical management of familial adenomatous polyposis. *Lancet* 1997;350:1777.
332. Setti-Carraro P, Nicholls RJ. Choice of prophylactic surgery for the large bowel component of familial adenomatous polyposis. *Br J Surg* 1996;83:885.
333. Short note: risk of extracolonic cancer in familial adenomatous polyposis. *Br J Surg* 1996;83:1121.
334. Rodriguez-Bigas MA, Mahoney MC, Karakousis CP, Petrelli NJ. Desmoid tumors in patients with familial adenomatous polyposis. *Cancer* 1994;74:1270.
335. Morson BC, Pang LSC. Rectal biopsy as an aid to cancer control and ulcerative colitis. *Gut* 1987;8:423.
336. Cohen A, Winawer SJ, Madoff R, Goldberg S. Operative approaches to patients with inflammatory bowel disease. In: Cohen AM, Winawer SJ, Friedman MA, eds. *Cancer of the colon, rectum, and anus.* New York: McGraw Hill, 1995:379.
337. Ribeiro MB, Greenstein AJ, Sachar DB, et al. Colorectal adenocarcinoma in Crohn's disease. *Ann Surg* 1996;223:186.
338. Church JM. Prophylactic colectomy in patients with hereditary nonpolyposis in colorectal cancer. *Ann Med* 1996;28:479.
339. Scroggins CR, Mesyaely IM, Blansee CD, et al. Nonoperative management of primary colorectal cancer in patients with stage IV disease. *Ann Surg Oncol* 1999;6:651.
340. Charnely RM, Morris DL, Dennison AR, et al. Detection of colorectal metastases using intraoperative ultrasonography. *Br J Surg* 1991;78:45.
341. Rafaelson SR, Kronborg O, Larsen C, Fenger C. Intraoperative ultrasonography in detection of hepatic metastases from colorectal cancer. *Dis Colon Rectum* 1995;38:355.
342. Nagorney DM. Diagnosis of liver metastases in colorectal cancer. *World J Surg* 1991;15:557.
343. Leen E, Angerson WJ, Wotherspoon H, et al. Comparison of the Doppler perfusion index and intraoperative ultrasonograpy in diagnosing colorectal liver metastases. *Ann Surg* 1994;220:663.
344. Paul MA, Blomjous JG, Cuesta MA, Meijer S. Prognostic value of negative intraoperative ultrasonography in primary colorectal cancer. *Br J Surg* 1996;83:1741.
345. Fazio VW, Tjandra JJ. Primary therapy of carcinoma of the large bowel. *World J Surg* 1991;15:568.
346. Slanetz CA, Grimson R. Effect of high and intermediate ligation on survival and recurrence rates following curative resection of colorectal cancer. *Dis Colon Rectum* 1997; 40:1205.
347. Gall FP, Tonak J, Altendorf A. Multivisceral resections in colorectal cancer. *Dis Colon Rectum* 1987;30:337.
348. Sales JP, Wind P, Douard R, et al. Blood dissemination of colonic epithelial cells during no-touch surgery for rectosigmoid cancer. *Lancet* 1999;354:392.
349. Wiggers T, Jeekel J, Arends JW, et al. No-touch isolation technique in colon cancer: a controlled prospective trial. *Br J Surg* 1988;75:409.
350. Ota DM. Laparoscopic resection for colon cancer: a favorable view. *Important Adv Oncol* 1996;227.
351. Marchesa P, Milsom JW, Hale JC, et al. Intraoperative laparoscopic liver ultrasonography for staging of colorectal cancer: initial experience. *Dis Colon Rectum* 1996;39:S73.
352. Foley EF, Kolecki RV, Schirmer BD. The accuracy of laparoscopic ultrasound in the detection of colorectal cancer liver metastases. *Am J Surg* 1998;176(3):262.
353. Schwenk W, Bohm B, Witt C, et al. Pulmonary function following laparoscopic or conventional colorectal resection: a randomized controlled evaluation. *Arch Surg* 1999;134:6.
354. Khalili T, Fleshner PR, Hiatt JR, et al. Colorectal cancer: comparison of laparoscopic with open approaches. *Dis Colon Rectum* 1998;41:832.
355. Cost Group 1996. Early results of laparoscopic surgery for colorectal cancer: retrospective analysis of 372 patients treated by clinical outcomes of surgical therapy. *Dis Colon Rectum* 2000;39:S53.
356. Bokey EL, Moore JWE, Keating JP, et al. Laparoscopic resection of the colon and rectum for cancer. *Br J Surg* 1997;84:822.
357. Ockerling F, Reymond M, Schneider C, et al. Prospective multicenter study of the quality of oncologic resections in patients undergoing laparoscopic colorectal surgery for cancer. *Dis Colon Rectum* 1998;41:936.
358. Hase K, Ueno H, Kuranaga N, et al. Intraperitoneal exfoliated cancer cells in patients with colorectal cancer. *Dis Colon Rectum* 1998;41:1134.
359. Kim SH, Milsom JW, Gramlich TL, et al. Does laparoscopic vs conventional surgery increase exfoliated cancer cells in the peritoneal cavity during resection of colorectal cancer? *Dis Colon Rectum* 1998;41:971.
360. Huang PP, Weber TK, Mendoza C, et al. Long term survival in patients with ovarian metastasis from colorectal cancer. *Ann Surg Oncol* 1998;5:695.
361. Sielezneff I, Salle E, Antoine K, et al. Simultaneous bilateral oopherectomy does not improve prognosis of postmenopausal women undergoing colorectal resection for cancer. *Dis Colon Rectum* 1997;40:1299.
362. Nyam DC, Leong AF, Ho YH, Seow-Choen F. Comparison between segmental left and extended right colectomies for obstructing left-sided colonic carcinomas. *Dis Colon Rectum* 1996;39:1000.
363. Young-Fadok TM, Wolff BG, Nivatvongs S, et al. Prophylactic oophorectomy in colorectal carcinoma. Preliminary results of a randomized prospective trial. *Dis Colon Rectum* 1998;41:277.
364. Laurie J, Moertel C, Flemming T, et al. Surgical adjuvant therapy of poor prognosis colorectal cancer with levamisole alone or combined levamisole and 5-fluorouracil: a North Central Cancer Treatment Group and Mayo Clinic Study. *Proc Am Soc Clin Oncol* 1986;5:81(abst).
365. Mulcahy HE, Toner M, Patchett SE, et al. Identifying stage B colorectal cancer patients at high risk of tumor recurrence and death. *Dis Colon Rectum* 1997;40:326.
366. Mainprize KS, Hewavisinthe J, Savage A, et al. How many lymph nodes to stage colorectal carcinoma? *J Clin Pathol* 1998;51:165.
367. Tartter PI. Perioperative blood transfusion and colorectal cancer recurrence: a review. *J Surg Oncol* 1988;39:197.
368. Oberg A, Stenling R, Tavelin B, Lindmark G. Are lymph node micrometastasis of any clinical significance in Dukes stages A and B colorectal cancer? *Dis Colon Rectum* 1998;41:1244.
369. Obrand DI, Gordon PH. Incidence and patterns of recurrence following curative resection for colorectal carcinoma. *Dis Colon Rectum* 1997;40:15.
370. Finan PJ, Ritchie JK, Hawley PR. Synchronous and early metachronous carcinomas of the colon and rectum. *Br J Surg* 1987;74:945.
371. Isler JJ, Brown PC, Lewis FG. The role of preoperative colonoscopy in colorectal cancer. *Dis Colon Rectum* 1987;30:435.
372. Tate JJ, Rawlinson J, Royle GT, et al. Pre-operative or postoperative colonic examination. *Br J Surg* 1988;75:1016.
373. Passman MA, Pommier RF, Vetto Jt. Synchronous colon primaries have the same prognosis as solitary colon cancers. *Dis Colon Rectum* 1996;39:329.
374. Koperna T, Kisser M, Schulz F. Emergency surgery for colon cancer in the aged. *Arch Surg* 1997;132:1032.
375. Poon RTP, Law WL, Chu KW, Wong J. Emergency resection and primary anastomosis for left sided obstructing colorectal carcinoma in the elderly. *Br J Surg* 1998;85:1539.
376. The Scotia Study Group. Single stage treatment for malignant left sided colonic obstruction: a prospective randomized clinical trial comparing subtotal colectomy with segmental resection following intraoperative irrigation. *Br J Surg* 1995;82:1622.
377. Carraro P, Segala M, Orlotti C, Tiberio G. Outcomes of large bowel perforation in patients with colorectal cancer. *Dis Colon Rectum* 1998;41:1421.
378. Gordon MS, Cohen AM. Management of invasive carcinoma in pedunculated colorectal polyps. *Oncology* 1989;3:99.
379. Whitlow C, Gathright JB, Hebert S, et al. Long term survival after treatment of malignant colonic polyps. *Dis Colon Rectum* 1997;40:929.
380. Netzer P, Forster C, Biral R, et al. Risk factor assessment of endoscopically removed malignant colorectal polyps. *Gut* 1998;43:669.
381. Wilcox GM, Beck JR. Early invasive cancer in adenomatous colonic polyps: evaluation of the therapeutic options by decision analysis. *Gastroenterology* 1987;92:1159.
382. Ehrinpreis MN, Kinzie JL, Jaszewski R, Peleman RL. Management of the malignant polyp. *Gastroenterol Clin North Am* 1988;17:837.
383. Willett CG, Fung CY, Kaufman DS, et al. Postoperative radiation therapy for high-risk colon cancer. *J Clin Oncol* 1993;11:1112.
384. Shehata WM, Meyer RL, Jazy FK, et al. Regional adjuvant irradiation for adenocarcinoma of the cecum. *Int J Radiat Oncol Biol Phys* 1987;13:843.
385. Martenson J, Willett C, Sargent D, et al. A phase III study of adjuvant radiation therapy (RT), 5-fluorouracil (5-FU) and levamisole (LEV) vs. 5-FU and LEV in selected patients with resected high risk colon cancer: initial results of INT 0130. *Proc Am Soc Clin Oncol* 1999;18:235a(abst).
386. Martenson JA, Swaminathan R, Burch PA, et al. Pilot study of continuous-infusion 5-fluorouracil, oral leucovorin, and upper-abdominal radiation therapy in patients with locally advanced residual or recurrent upper gastrointestinal or extrapelvic colon cancer. *Int J Radiat Oncol Biol Phys* 1997;37:615-618.
387. O'Connell MJ, Martenson JA, Weiand HS, et al. Improving adjuvant therapy for rectal cancer by combining protracted infusion fluorouracil with radiation therapy after curative surgery. *N Engl J Med* 1994;331:502.
388. Tepper JE, O'Connell MJ, Petroni GR, et al. Adjuvant postoperative fluorouracil-modulated chemotherapy combined with pelvic radiation therapy for rectal cancer: initial results of Intergroup 0114. *J Clin Oncol* 1997;15:2030.
389. Fabian C, Shankar S, Estes N, et al. Adjuvant continuous infusion 5-FU, whole-abdominal radiation, and tumor bed boost in high-risk stage III colon carcinoma: a Southwest Oncology Group pilot study. *Int J Radiat Oncol Biol Phys* 1995;32:457.
390. Ben-Joseph E, Court WS. Whole abdominal radiotherapy and concomitant 5-fluorouracil as adjuvant therapy in advanced colon cancer. *Dis Colon Rectum* 1995;38:1088.
391. Dwight RW, Higgins GA, Keehan RJ. Factors influencing survival after resection in cancer of the colon and rectum. *Am J Surg* 1969;117:512.
392. Dwight RW, Humphrey EW, Higgins GA, Keehn RJ. FUDR as an adjuvant to surgery in cancer of the large bowel. *J Surg Oncol* 1973;5:243.
393. Dixon WJ, Longmire WP Jr, Holden WD. Use of triethylenethiophosphomamide as adjuvant to the surgical treatment of gastric and colorectal cancer: ten year follow-up. *Ann Surg* 1971;173:26.

394. Wolmark N, Fisher B, Rockette H, et al. Postoperative adjuvant chemotherapy or BCG for colon cancer: results from NSABP Protocol C-01. *J Natl Cancer Inst* 1988;80:30.
395. Stevenson HC, Green I, Hamilton JM, et al. Levamisole: known effects on the immune system, clinical results and future applications to the treatment of cancer. *J Clin Oncol* 1991;9:2052.
396. Mansour EG, Cnaan A, Davis T, et al. Combined modality therapy following resection of colorectal carcinoma in patients with non-measurable intra-abdominal metastases. An ECOG study 3282. *Proc Am Soc Clin Oncol* 1990;9:107.
397. Amery WK, Bruynseels JP. Levamisole, the story and the lessons. *Intl J Immunopharmacol* 1992;14:481.
398. Arnaud JP, Buyse M, Nordlinger B, et al. Adjuvant therapy of poor prognosis colon cancer with levamisole: results of an EORTC double-blind randomized clinical trial. *Br J Surg* 1989;76:284.
399. Windle R, Bell PRF, Shaw D. Five year results of a randomized trial of adjuvant 5-fluorouracil and levamisole in colorectal cancer. *Br J Surg* 1987;74:569.
400. Moertel CG, Fleming TR, Macdonald JS, et al. Levamisole and fluorouracil for adjuvant therapy of resected colon carcinoma. *N Engl J Med* 1990;322:352.
401. Moertel CG, Fleming TR, Macdonald JS, et al. Fluorouracil plus levamisole as effective adjuvant therapy after resection of stage III colon carcinoma: a final report. *Ann Med* 1995;122:321.
402. Blanke CD, Messenger M, Taplin SC. Trimetrexate: review and current clinical experience in advanced colorectal cancer. *Semin Oncol* 1997;24:S18.
403. Poon MA, O'Connell MJ, Moertel CG, et al. Biochemical modulation of fluorouracil: evidence of significant improvement of survival and quality of life in patients with advanced colorectal carcinoma. *J Clin Oncol* 1989;7:1407.
404. Wolmark N, Rockette H, Petrelli N, et al. Long-term results of the efficacy of perioperative portal vein infusion of 5-FU for treatment of colon cancer: NSABP C-02. *Proc Am Soc Clin Oncol* 1994;A561(abst).
405. IMPACT. Efficacy of adjuvant fluorouracil and folinic acid in colon cancer. International Multicentre Pooled Analysis of Colon Cancer Trials (IMPACT) investigators. *Lancet* 1995;345:939.
406. O'Connell M, Mailliard J, Macdonald J, et al. An intergroup trial of intensive course 5FU and low dose leucovorin as surgical adjuvant therapy for high risk colon cancer. *Proc Am Soc Clin Oncol* 1993;12:190.
407. Mamounas EP, Wieand HS, Jones J, et al. Future directions in the adjuvant treatment of colon cancer. *Oncology* 1997;11:44.
408. Peeters M, Haller DG. Therapy for early-stage colorectal cancer. *Oncology* 1999;13:307.
409. Wolmark N, Rockette H, Mamounas EP, et al. The relative efficacy of 5-FU+ leucovorin (FU-LV), 5-FU + levamisole (FU-LEV), and 5-FU + leucovorin + levamisole (FU-LV-LEV) in patients with Dukes' B and C carcinoma of the colon: first report of NSABP C-04. *Proc Am Soc Clin Oncol* 1996;15:205.
410. O'Connel MJ, Laurie JA, Kahn M, et al. Prospectively randomized trial of postoperative adjuvant chemotherapy in patients with high-risk colon cancer. *J Clin Oncol* 1998;16:295.
411. Smith R, Wickerham DL, Wieand HS, et al. UFT plus calcium folinate vs 5-FU plus calcium folinate in colon cancer. *Oncology* 1999;13:44.
412. Saltz LB, Locker PK, Pirotta N, et al. Weekly irinotecan (CPT-11), leucovorin, (LV), and fluorouracil (FU) is superior to daily X 5 LV/FU in patients (pts) with previously untreated metastatic colorectal cancer. *Proc Am Soc Clin Oncol* 1999;18:233a(abst).
413. Sutanto-Ward E, Sigurdson ER, Tremiterra S, et al. Adjuvant chemotherapy for colorectal hepatic metastases: role of route of administration and timing. *Surg Oncol* 1992;1:87.
414. Swiss Group for Clinical Cancer Research. Long-term results of single course of adjuvant intraportal chemotherapy for colorectal cancer. Swiss Group for Clinical Cancer Research (SAKK). *Lancet* 1995;345:349.
415. Portal vein chemotherapy for colorectal cancer: a meta-analysis of 4000 patients in 10 studies. Liver Infusion Meta-analysis Group. *J Natl Cancer Inst* 1997;89:497.
416. Panettiere FJ, Goodman PJ, Costanzi JJ, et al. Adjuvant therapy in large bowel adenocarcinoma: long-term results of a Southwest Oncology Group study. *J Clin Oncol* 1988;6:947.
417. Ijzermans JN, Marquet RL, Bouwman E, et al. Successful treatment of colon cancer in rats with recombinant interferon-gamma. *Br J Cancer* 1987;56:795.
418. Pazdur R, Ajani JA, Winn R, et al. A phase II trial of 5-fluorouracil and recombinant alpha-2a-interferon in previously untreated metastatic gastric carcinoma. *Cancer* 1992;69:878.
419. Wolmark N, Bryant J, Smith R, et al. Adjuvant 5-fluorouracil and leucovorin with or without interferon alfa-2a in colon carcinoma: National Surgical Adjuvant Breast and Bowel Project protocol C-05. *J Natl Cancer Inst* 1998;90:1810.
420. Hoover HC Jr, Hanna MG Jr. Tumor-specific BCG therapy in colon cancer. *Cancer Invest* 1990;8:281.
421. Hoover HC Jr, Brandhorst JS, Peters LC, et al. Adjuvant active specific immunotherapy for human colorectal cancer: 6.5-year median follow-up of a phase III prospectively randomized trial. *J Clin Oncol* 1993;11:390.
422. Harris J, Ryan L, Adams G, et al. Survival and relapse in adjuvant autologous tumor vaccine therapy for Dukes B and C colon cancer-EST 5283. *Proc Am Soc Clin Oncol* 1994;A955(abst).
423. Vermorken J, Classen A, Gall H. Randomized phase III trial of active specific immunotherapy (ASI) vs control in patients with Dukes' B2, B3 or C colon cancer. *Eur J Cancer* 1997;33:5162.
424. Shaw DR, Khazaeli MB, LoBuglio AF. Mouse/human chimeric antibodies to a tumor-associated antigen: biologic activity of the four human IgG subclasses. *J Natl Cancer Inst* 1988;80:1553.
425. Riethmuller G, Holz E, Schlimok G, et al. Monoclonal antibody therapy for resected Dukes' C colorectal cancer: seven-year outcome of a multicenter randomized trial. *J Clin Oncol* 1998;16:1788.
426. Kjeldsen BJ, Kronborg O, Fenger C, Jorgensen OD. A prospective randomized study of follow-up after radical surgery for colorectal cancer. *Br J Surg* 1997;84:666.
427. Pietra N, Sarli L, Costi R, et al. Role of follow-up in management of local recurrences of colorectal cancer: a prospective, randomized study. *Dis Colon Rectum* 1998;41:1127.
428. Barillari P, Ramacciato GMG, Bovino A, et al. Surveillance of colorectal cancer: effectiveness of early detection of intraluminal recurrences on prognosis and survival of patients treated for cure. *Dis Colon Rectum* 1996;39:388.
429. Hida JI, Yasutomi M, Shindoh K, et al. Second look operation for recurrent colorectal cancer based on carcinoembryonic antigen and imaging techniques. *Dis Colon Rectum* 1996;39:74.
430. Graham RA, Wang S, Catalano PJ, Haller DG. Postsurgical surveillance of colon cancer: preliminary cost analysis of physician examination, carcinoembryonic antigen testing, chest x-ray, and colonoscopy. *Ann Surg* 1998;228:59.
431. Desch CE, Benson AB III, Smith TJ, et al. Recommended colorectal cancer surveillance guidelines by the American Society of Clinical Oncology. *J Clin Oncol* 1999;17:1312.
432. Rosen LS. Irinotecan in lymphoma, leukemia, and breast, pancreatic, ovarian, and small-cell lung cancers. *Oncology* 1998;12:103.
433. Cohen AM. Comparison of positron emission tomography and computed tomography in detection of recurrent and metastatic colorectal cancer. *Ann Surg Oncol* 1997;4:610.
434. Valk PE, Abella-Columna-E., Haseman MK, et al. Whole body PET imaging with (^{18})F Fluorodeoxyglucose in managment of recurrent colorectal cancer. *Arch Surg* 1999;134:503.
435. Flanagan FL, Dehdashti F, Ogunbiyi OA, et al. Utility of FDG-PET for investigating unexplained plasma CEA elevation in patients with colorectal cancer. *Ann Surg* 1998;227:319.
436. Flamen P, Stroobants S, van Cutsem E, et al. Additional value of whole-body positron emission tomography with fluorine-18-2-fluoro-2-deoxy-d-glucose in recurrent colorectal cancer. *J Clin Oncol* 1999;17:894.
437. Arnold MW, Young DM, Hitchcock CL, et al. Staging of colorectal cancer: Biology vs morphology. *Dis Colon Rectum* 1998;41:1482.
438. Manayan RC, Hart MJ, Friend WG. Radioimmunoguided surgery for colorectal cancer. *Am J Surg* 1997;173:386.
439. Serafini AN, Klein JL, Wolff BG, et al. Radioimmunoscintigraphy of recurrent, metastatic, or occult colorectal cancer with technetium 99m-labeled totally human monoclonal antibody 88BV59: results of pivotal, phase III multicenter studies. *J Clin Oncol* 1998;16:1777.
440. Shen H, Kauvar L, Tew KD. Importance of glutathione and associated enzymes in drug response. *Oncol Res* 1997;9:295.
441. Beaumont PO, Moore MJ, Ahmad K, et al. Role of glutathione S-transferases in the resistance of human colon cancer cell lines to doxorubicin. *Cancer Res* 1998;58:947.
442. Danova M, Giordano M, Erba E, et al. Flow cytometric analysis of multidrug-resistance-associated antigen (P-glycoprotein) and DNA ploidy in human colon cancer. *J Cancer Res Clin Oncol* 1992;118:575.
443. Butler RN, Butler WJ, Moraby Z, et al. Glutathione concentrations and glutathione S-transferase activity in human colonic neoplasms. *J Gastroenterol Hepatol* 1994;9:60.
444. Hengstler JG, Bottger T, Tanner B, et al. Resistance factors in colon cancer tissue and the adjacent normal colon tissue: glutathione S-transferases alpha and pi, glutathione and aldehyde dehydrogenase. *Cancer Lett* 1998;128:105.
445. O'Connell MJ. A Phase III trial of 5-fluorouracil and leucovorin in the treatment of advanced colorectal cancer. A Mayo Clinic/North Central Cancer Treatment Group Study. *Cancer* 1989;63:1026.
446. *Cancer* TMA. Toxicity of fluorouracil in patients with advanced colorectal cancer: effect of administration schedule and prognostic factors. Meta-Analysis Group in Cancer. *J Clin Oncol* 1998;16:3537.
447. Poon MA, O'Connell MJ, Wieand HS, et al. Biochemical modulation of fluorouracil with leucovorin: confirmatory evidence of improved therapeutic efficacy in advanced colorectal cancer. *J Clin Oncol* 1991;9:1967.
448. Lokich J. Infusional 5-FU for advanced colorectal cancer. *J Infusion Chemother* 1995;5:208.
449. Leichman CG, Fleming TR, Muggia FM, et al. Phase II study of fluorouracil and its modulation in advanced colorectal cancer: a Southwest Oncology Group study. *J Clin Oncol* 1995;13:1303.
450. Meta-Analysis Group in Cancer. Efficacy of intravenous continuous infusion of fluorouracil compared with bolus administration in advanced colorectal cancer. *J Clin Oncol* 1998;16:301.
451. Ardalan B, Luis R, Jaime M, Franceschi D. Biomodulation of fluorouracil in colorectal cancer. *Cancer Invest* 1998;16:237.
452. Rustum YM, Cao S, Zhang Z. Rationale for treatment design: biochemical modulation of 5-fluorouracil by leucovorin. *Cancer J Sci Am* 1998;4:12.
453. Asbury RF, Boros L, Brower M, et al. 5-Fluorouracil and high-dose folic acid treatment for metastatic colon cancer. *Am J Clin Oncol* 1987;10:47.
454. Project ACCM. Modulation of fluorouracil by leucovorin in patients with advanced colorectal cancer: evidence in terms of response rate. Advanced Colorectal Cancer Meta-Analysis Project. *J Clin Oncol* 1992;10:896.
455. Petrelli N, Douglass HO Jr, Herrera L, et al. The modulation of fluorouracil with leucovorin in metastatic colorectal carcinoma: a prospective randomized phase III trial. *J Clin Oncol* 1989;7:1419.
456. de Gramont A, Bosset JF, Milan C, et al. Randomized trial comparing monthly low-dose leucovorin and fluorouracil bolus with bimonthly high-dose leucovorin and fluorouracil bolus plus continuous infusion for advanced colorectal cancer: a French intergroup study. *J Clin Oncol* 1997;15:808.
457. Wadler S, Schwartz EL, Goldman M, et al. 5-Fluorouracil and recombinant alpha-2a-interferon: an active regimen against advanced colorectal cancer. *J Clin Oncol* 1989;7:1769.
458. Wadler S, Wersto R, Weinberg V, et al. Interaction of fluorouracil and interferon in human colon cancer cell lines: cytotoxic and cytokinetic effects. *Cancer Res* 1990;50:5735.
459. Elias L, Crissman HA. Interferon effects upon the adenocarcinoma 38 and HL-60 cell lines: antiproliferative responses and synergistic interactions with halogenated pyrimidine antimetabolites. *Cancer Res* 1988;48:4868.
460. Chu E, Allegra CJ. Regulation of thymidylate synthase in human colon cancer cells treated with 5-fluorouracil and interferon-gamma. *Adv Exp Med Biol* 1993;339:143.
461. Grem JL, Chu E, Boarman D, et al. Biochemical modulation of fluorouracil with leucovorin and interferon: preclinical and clinical investigations. *Semin Oncol* 1992;19:36.

462. Hill M, Norman A, Cunningham D, et al. Royal Marsden phase III trial of fluorouracil with or without interferon alfa-2b in advanced colorectal cancer. *J Clin Oncol* 1995;13:1297.
463. Romanini A, Li WW, Colofiore JR, Bertino JR. Leucovorin enhances cytotoxicity of trimetrexate/fluorouracil, but not methotrexate/fluorouracil, in CCRF-CEM cells. *J Natl Cancer Inst* 1992;84:1033.
464. Blanke CD, Kasimis B, Schein P, et al. Phase II study of trimetrexate, fluorouracil, and leucovorin for advanced colorectal cancer. *J Clin Oncol* 1997;15:915.
465. Blanke C, Cassidy J, Gerhartz H, et al. A phase II trial of trimetrexate (TMTX), 5-fluorouracil (5-FU), and leucovorin (LCV) in patients (PTS) with previously treated unresectable or metastatic colorectal cancer (CRC). *Proc Am Soc Clin Oncol* 1999;18:246a(abst).
466. Liu G, Franssen E, Fitch MI, Warner E. Patient preferences for oral versus intravenous palliative chemotherapy. *J Clin Oncol* 1997;15:110.
467. Diasio RB, Lu Z. Dihydropyrimidine dehydrogenase activity and fluorouracil chemotherapy [Editorial]. *J Clin Oncol* 1994;12:2239.
468. Diasio RB. The role of dihydropyrimidine dehydrogenase (DPD) modulation in 5-FU pharmacology. *Oncology* 1998;12:23.
469. Taguchi T. Development of fluorinated pyrimidines in Japan. *Gan To Kagaku Ryoho* 1993;20:10.
470. Hoff PM, Pazdur R, Benner SE, Canetta R. UFT and leucovorin: a review of its clinical development and therapeutic potential in the oral treatment of cancer. *Anticancer Drugs* 1998;9:479.
471. Hoff PM, Pazdur R. UFT plus oral leucovorin: a new oral treatment for colorectal cancer. *Oncologist* 1998;3:155.
472. Pazdur R, Douillard JY, Skillings J, et al. Multicenter phase III study of 5-fluorouracil (5-FU) or UFT in combination with leucovorin (LV) in patients with metastatic colorectal cancer. *Proc Am Soc Clin Oncol* 1999;18:263a(abst).
473. Carmichael J, Popiela T, Radstone D, et al. Randomized comparative study of Orzel (oral uracil/tegafur (UFT) plus leucovorin (LV)) versus parenteral 5-fluorouracil (5-FU) plus LV in patients with metastatic colorectal cancer. *Proc Am Soc Clin Oncol* 1999;18:264a(abst).
474. Miwa M, Ura M, Nishida M, et al. Design of a novel oral fluoropyrimidine carbamate, capecitabine, which generates 5-fluorouracil selectively in tumours by enzymes concentrated in human liver and cancer tissue. *Eur J Cancer* 1998;34:1274.
475. Ishikawa T, Sawada N, Sekiguchi F, et al. Xeloda (capecitabine), a new oral fluoropyrimidine carbamate with an improved efficacy profile over other fluoropyrimidines. *Proc Am Soc Clin Oncol* 1997;A79:6(abst).
476. Cao S, Rustum YM. 5-Fluorouracil prodrug, ftorafur, modulated by uracil (UFT): preclinical and clinical prospective. *Tumori* 1997;83:S90.
477. Ishikawa T, Utoh M, Sawada N, et al. Tumor selective delivery of 5-fluorouracil by capecitabine, a new oral fluoropyrimidine carbamate, in human cancer xenografts. *Biochem Pharmacol* 1998;55:1091.
478. Meropol NJ, Creaven PJ, Petrelli NJ, et al. A Phase I and pharmacokinetic study of oral UFT and leucovorin (LV). *Proc Am Soc Clin Oncol* 1994;A433.
479. Cunningham D, Pyrhonen S, James RD, et al. Randomised trial of irinotecan plus supportive care versus supportive care alone after fluorouracil failure for patients with metastatic colorectal cancer. *Lancet* 1998;352:1413.
480. Porter DJ, Chestnut WG, Merrill BM, Spector T. Mechanism-based inactivation of dihydropyrimidine dehydrogenase by 5-ethynyluracil. *J Biol Chem* 1992;267:5236.
481. Wiseman LR, Adkins JC, Plosker GL, Goa KL. Oxaliplatin: a review of its use in the management of metastatic colorectal cancer. *Drugs Aging* 1999;14:459.
482. Brito RA, Medgyesy D, Zukowski TH, et al. Fluoropyrimidines: a critical evaluation. *Oncology* 1999;57[Suppl 1]:2.
483. Fukuoka M, Negoro S, Niitani H, et al. A phase I study of weekly administration of CPT-11 in lung cancer. *Gan to Kagaku Ryoho* 1990;17:993.
484. Pitot HC. US pivotal studies of irinotecan in colorectal carcinoma. *Oncology* 1998;12:48.
485. Rougier P, van Cutsem E, Bajetta E, et al. Randomised trial of irinotecan versus fluorouracil by continuous infusion after fluorouracil failure in patients with metastatic colorectal cancer. *Lancet* 1998;352:1407.
486. Becouarn Y, Ychou M, Ducreux M, et al. Phase II trial of oxaliplatin as first line chemotherapy in metastatic colorectal cancer patients. *J Clin Oncol* 1998;16:2739.
487. de Gramont A, Vignoud J, Tournigand C, et al. Oxaliplatin with high-dose leucovorin and 5-fluorouracil 48-hour continuous infusion in pretreated metastatic colorectal cancer. *Eur J Cancer* 1997;33:214.
488. Levi F, Misset JL, Brienza S, et al. A chronopharmacologic phase II clinical trial with 5-fluorouracil, folinic acid, and oxaliplatin using an ambulatory multichannel programmable pump. High antitumor effectiveness against metastatic colorectal cancer. *Cancer* 1992;69:893.
489. Andre T, Louvet C, Raymond E, et al. Bimonthly high-dose leucovorin, 5-fluorouracil infusion and oxaliplatin (FOLFOX3) for metastatic colorectal cancer resistant to the same leucovorin and 5-fluorouracil regimen. *Ann Oncol* 1998;9:1251.
490. Judson IR. "Tomudex" (raltitrexed) development: preclinical, phase I and II studies. *Anticancer Drugs* 1997;8[Suppl 2]:S5.
491. Cunningham D. Mature results from three large controlled studies with raltitrexed ("tomudex"). *Br J Cancer* 1998;77(S2):15.
492. Cunningham D, Zalcberg JR, Rath U, et al. Final results of a randomised trial comparing "Tomudex" (raltitrexed) with 5-fluorouracil plus leucovorin in advanced colorectal cancer. "Tomudex" Colorectal Cancer Study Group. *Ann Oncol* 1996;7:961.
493. Cocconi G, Cunningham D, van Cutsem E, et al. Open, randomized, multicenter trial of raltitrexed versus fluorouracil plus high-dose leucovorin in patients with advanced colorectal cancer. Tomudex Colorectal Cancer Study Group. *J Clin Oncol* 1998;16:2943.
494. Pazdur R, Vincent M. Raltitrexed (Tomudex) versus 5-fluorouracil and leucovorin (5-FU + LV) in patients with advanced colorectal cancer (ACC): results of a randomized, multicenter, North American trial. *Proc Am Soc Clin Oncol* 1997;A801(abst).
495. Shebani KO, Souba WW, Finkelstein DM, et al. Prognosis and survival in patients with gastrointestinal tract carcinoid tumors. *Ann Surg* 1999;229:815.
496. Memon MA, Nelson H. Gastrointestinal carcinoid tumors: current management strategies. *Dis Colon Rectum* 1997;40:1101.
497. Rothmund M, Kisker O. Surgical treatment of carcinoid tumors of the small bowel, appendix, colon and rectum. *Digestion* 1994;55[Suppl 3]:86.
498. Iwasa K, Taniguchi K, Noguchi M, et al. Leiomyosarcoma of the colon presenting as acute suppurative peritonitis. *Surg Today* 1997;27:337.
499. Moertel CG, O'Fallon JR, Go VL, et al. The preoperative carcinoembryonic antigen test in the diagnosis, staging, and prognosis of colorectal cancer. *Cancer* 1986;58:603.
500. Chou FF, Eng HL, Sheen-Chen SM. Smooth muscle tumors of the gastrointestinal tract: analysis of prognostic factors. *Surgery* 1996;119:171.
501. Luna-Perez P, Rodriguez DF, Lujan L, et al. Colorectal sarcoma: analysis of failure patterns. *J Surg Oncol* 1998;69:36.
502. Shepherd NA, Hall PA, Coates PJ, Levison DA. Primary malignant lymphoma of the colon and rectum. A histopathological and immunohistochemical analysis of 45 cases with clinicopathological correlations. *Histopathology* 1988;12:235.
503. Cheng P, Saltz L. Unusual tumors of the colon, rectum and anus. In: Raghavan D, Brecher M, Johnson D, et al., eds. *Textbook of uncommon cancer.* Chichester, UK: John Wiley and Sons, 1999:439.
504. Hwang WS, Yao JC, Cheng SS, Tseng HH. Primary colorectal lymphoma in Taiwan. *Cancer* 1992;70:575.
505. Remick SC, Hafez GR, Carbone PP. Extrapulmonary small-cell carcinoma. A review of the literature with emphasis on therapy and outcome. *Medicine* 1987;66:457.
506. Hoff PM, Pazdur R. Small cell carcinomas of the gastrointestinal tract. In: Raghavan D, Brecher M, Johnson D, et al., eds. *Textbook of uncommon cancer.* Chichester, UK: John Wiley and Sons, 1999:463.
507. Wick MR, Weatherby RP, Weiland LH. Small cell neuroendocrine carcinoma of the colon and rectum: clinical, histologic, and ultrastructural study and immunohistochemical comparison with cloacogenic carcinoma. *Hum Pathol* 1987;18:9.
508. Burke AB, Shekitka KM, Sobin LH. Small cell carcinomas of the large intestine. *Am J Clin Pathol* 1991;95:315.
509. Higgins GA, Lee LE, Dwight RW, et al. The case for adjuvant 5-fluorouracil in colorectal cancer. *CCT* 1978;1:35.
510. Higgins GA Jr, Amadeo JH, McElhinney J, et al. Efficacy of prolonged intermittent therapy with combined 5-fluorouracil and methyl-CCNU following resection for carcinoma of the large bowel. A Veterans Administration Surgical Oncology Group report. *Cancer* 1984;53:1.
511. Gastrointestinal Tumor Study Group. Adjuvant therapy of colon cancer: results of a prospectively randomized trial. *N Engl J Med* 1984;310:737.
512. Mansour EG, MacIntyre JW, Johnson R, et al. Adjuvant studies in colorectal carcinoma: experience of the Eastern Cooperative Oncology Group (ECOG)-preliminary report. In: Gerard A, ed. *Progress and perspectives in the treatment of gastrointestinal tumors.* New York: Pergamon Press, 1981:68.
513. Abdi E, Harbora D, Hanson J, McPherson T. Adjuvant chemoimmuno-and immunotherapy in stage B2 and C colorectal cancer. *Proc Am Soc Clin Oncol* 1987;6:93.
514. Laurie JA, Moertel CG, Fleming TR, et al. Surgical adjuvant therapy of large-bowel carcinoma: an evaluation of levamisole and the combination of levamisole and fluorouracil. *J Clin Oncol* 1989;7(10):1447.
515. Wolmark N, Rockette H, Fisher B, et al. The benefit of leucovorin-modulated fluorouracil as postoperative adjuvant therapy for primary colon cancer: results from National Surgical Adjuvant Breast and Bowel Project protocol C-03. *J Clin Oncol* 1993;11:1879.
516. Efficacy of adjuvant fluorouracil and folinic acid in colon cancer. International multicentre pooled analysis of colon cancer trials (impact) investigators. *Lancet* 2000; 345(8955):939.
517. Francini G, Petrioli R, Lorenzini L, et al. Folinic acid and 5-fluorouracil as adjuvant chemotherapy in colon cancer. *Gastroenterology* 1994;106:899.
518. Wolmark N, Rockette H, Mamounas E, et al. Clinical trial to assess the relative efficacy of fluorouracil and leucovorin, fluorouracil and leucovorin, fluorouracil and levamisole, and fluorouracil, leucovorin, and levamisole in patients with Dukes' B and C carcinoma of the colon: results from National Surgical Adjuvant Breast and Bowel Project C-04. *J Clin Oncol* 1999;17(11):3553.
519. Haller D, Catalano P, Macdonald J. Fluorouracil (FU), leucovorin (LV) and levamisole (LEV) adjuvant therapy for colon cancer: five-year final report of INT-0089. *Proc Am Soc Clin Oncol* 1998;17:256a(abst).
520. O'Connell MJ, Laurie JA, Kahn M, et al. Prospectively randomized trial of postoperative adjuvant chemotherapy in patients with high-risk colon cancer. *J Clin Oncol* 1998;16:295.
521. Petrelli N, Herrera L, Rustum Y. A prospective randomized trial of 5-fluorouracil versus 5-fluorouracil and high-dose leucovorin versus 5-fluorouracil and methotrexate in previously untreated patients with advanced colorectal cancer. *J Clin Oncol* 1987;5:1559.
522. Coller FA, Kay EB, MacIntyre RS. Regional lymphatic metastasis in carcinoma of the colon. *Ann Surg* 1941;114:56.
523. Nordic Gastrointestinal Tumor Adjuvant Therapy Group. Superiority of sequential methotrexate, fluorouracil and leucovorin to fluorouracil alone in advanced symptomatic colorectal carcinoma: a randomized trial. *J Clin Oncol* 1989;7:1437.
524. Valone FH, Friedman MA, Wittlinger PS, et al. Treatment of patients with advanced colorectal carcinomas with fluorouracil alone, high-dose leucovorin plus fluorouracil, or sequential methotrexate, fluorouracil and leucovorin: a randomized trial of the Northern California oncology group. *J Clin Oncol* 1989;7:1427.
525. Doroshaw JH, Multhauf P, Leong L, et al. Prospective randomized comparison of fluorouracil versus fluorouracil and high dose continuous infusion leucovorin calcium for the treatment of advanced measurable colorectal cancer in patients previously unexposed to chemotherapy. *J Clin Oncol* 1990;8:491.
526. Erlichman C, Fine S, Wong A, Elhakim T. A randomized trial of fluorouracil and folinic acid in patients with metastatic colorectal carcinoma. *J Clin Oncol* 1988;6:469.
527. DiCostanzo F, Bartolucci R, Calabresi F, et al. Fluorouracil-alone versus high dose folinic

acid and fluorouracil in advanced colorectal cancer: a randomized trial of the Italian Oncology Group for Clinical Research (GOIRC). *Ann Oncol* 1992;3:371.
528. Cox J, Pazdur R, Thibault A, et al. A phase III trial of XELODA (capecitabine) in previously untreated advanced/metastic colorectal cancer. *Proc Am Soc Clin Oncol* 1999;18:265a(abst 1016).
529. Twelves C, Harper P, Van Cutsem E, et al. A phase III Trial (SO14796) of Xeloda (capecitabine) in previously untreated advanced/metastatic colorectal cancer. *Proc Am Soc Clin Oncol* 1999;18:263a(abst 1010).
530. Saltz L, Locker P, Pirotta N, et al. Weekly irinotecan (CPT-11), leucovorin (LV), and fluorouracil (FU) is superior to daily x 5 LV/FU in patients (PTS) with previously untreated metastatic colorectal cancer (CRC). *Proc Am Soc Clin Oncol* 1999;18:233(abst).
531. Giacchetti S, Perpoint B, Zidani R, et al. Phase III multicenter randomized trial of oxaliplatin added to chronomodulated fluorouracil-leucovorin as first-line treatment of metastatic colorectal cancer. *J Clin Oncol* 2000;18(1):136.
532. Douillard J, Cunningham D, Roth A, et al. A randomized phase III trial comparing irinotecan +5-fluorouracil (5FU) with or without oxaliplatin in advanced colorectal cancer (CRC). ASCO Virtual Meeting. *Proc Am Soc Clin Oncol* 1999;18:233a(abst 899).
533. de Gramont A, Figer A, Seymour M, et al. A randomized trial of leucovorin (LV) and 5-fluorouracil (5FU) with or without oxaliplatin in advanced colorectal cancer (CRC). *Proc Am Soc Clin Oncol* 1998;17:257a(abst 985).
534. Kemeny N, Daly J, Reichman B, et al. Intrahepatic or systemic infusion of fluorodeoxyuridine in patients with liver metastases from colorectal carcinoma—a randomized trial. *Ann Med* 1987;107:459.
535. Hohn DC, Stagg RJ, Friedman MA, et al. A randomized trial of continuous intravenous versus hepatic intraarterial floxuridine in patients with colorectal cancer metastatic to the liver: the Northern California oncology group trial. *J Clin Oncol* 1989;7:1646.
536. Chang AE, Schneider PD, Sugarbaker PH, et al. A prospective randomized trial of regional vs. systemic continuous 5-FU chemotherapy in the treatment of colorectal metastases. *Ann Surg* 1987;206:685.
537. Martin JK, O'Connell MJ, Wieand HS, et al. Intra-arterial floxuridine vs systemic fluorouracil for hepatic metastases from colorectal cancer. *Arch Surg* 1990;125:1022.
538. Rougier P, Laplanche A, Huguier M, et al. Hepatic arterial infusion of floxurdine in patients with liver metastases from colorectal carcinoma: long-term results of a prospective randomized trial. *J Clin Oncol* 1992;10(7):1112.

SECTION **8**

JOHN M. SKIBBER
PAULO M. HOFF
BRUCE D. MINSKY

Cancer of the Rectum

Many overlapping issues in the management, biology, pathology, and staging of colon and rectal cancer are discussed in Chapter 33.7. Issues of sphincter preservation, locoregional recurrence, and the application of multidisciplinary management in rectal cancer are the focus of this chapter.

ANATOMY

The rectum is usually divided into three portions (Fig. 33.8-1). The lower rectum is the area 3 to 6 cm from the anal verge. The midrectum is 6 to 10 cm, and the upper rectum extends approximately 10 to 15 cm, from the anal verge. The rectum usually reaches its upper limit at approximately 12 cm from the anal verge. Externally, its upper extent can be identified where the tenia spread to form a longitudinal coat of muscle. The upper third of the rectum is surrounded by peritoneum on its anterior and lateral surfaces. At the rectovesical or rectouterine pouch, the rectum becomes completely extraperitoneal. The rectum follows the curve of the sacrum in its lower two-thirds. It enters the anal canal at the level of the levator ani. The anorectal ring is at the level of the puborectalis sling portion of the levator muscles. The location of a rectal tumor is usually indicated by the distance between the anal verge, dentate line, or anorectal ring and the lower edge of the tumor. These points of reference are all different. Also, these measurements differ depending on the use of a rigid or flexible endoscope.

LYMPHATIC DRAINAGE

The majority of the lymphatic drainage of the rectum passes upward along the superior hemorrhoidal artery toward the inferior mesenteric artery. Perirectal nodes above the midrectum drain along the superior hemorrhoidal artery. Below 7 to 8 centimeters from the anal verge, they drain laterally along the middle hemorrhoidal artery and the iliac nodes and the obturator fossa. Hypogastric and iliac node drainage is along the aorta. Lymphatics are common in the rectovaginal septum in women, which is analogous to the Denonvilliers' fascia in men.

BOWEL FUNCTION

Mechanisms of fecal continence include both sphincter control and creation of the neorectal angle where the rectum sweeps anteriorly and then enters the anal canal. The floor of the pelvis is formed by the levator ani muscles, which separate the pelvis from the perineum and ischiorectal fossa. The urethra, vagina, and anus pass through the levators.

Surgical procedures for rectal carcinoma can have marked impact on rectal function. The degree of this alteration depends on the extent of rectal resection. Other factors affecting bowel function include postoperative radiation therapy or pelvic sepsis. These may reduce the compliance of the newly constructed rectal reservoir.[1] Although overall sphincter function usually is maintained after sphincter-preserving surgery and adjuvant therapy, subtle changes in function can be observed that reduce discrimination between gas, liquid, or formed stool.

AUTONOMIC NERVES

An understanding of the autonomic nerve supply to pelvic organs is critical in preservation of sexual and bladder function after rectal cancer surgery.[2] The sympathetic trunks converge over the sacral promontory to form the hypogastric plexus. These trunks run underneath the pelvic peritoneum laterally to the sidewall or the pelvis. These trunks are lateral to the mesorectum. The fibers from these nerves follow arteries supplying the pelvic viscera. Parasympathetic fibers to the pelvic viscera emerge from the second, third, and fourth sacral nerve roots overlying the piriformis muscle. The parasympathetic fibers proceed laterally as the nervi erigentes to join the sympathetic fibers at the site of the pelvic plexus that is just lateral and somewhat anterior to the tips of the seminal vesicle in men.[3] Sharp section of the mesorectum preserves these structures.[4]

DIAGNOSIS

Compared to more proximal colon cancers, tumors arising in the rectosigmoid area are much more prone to present with

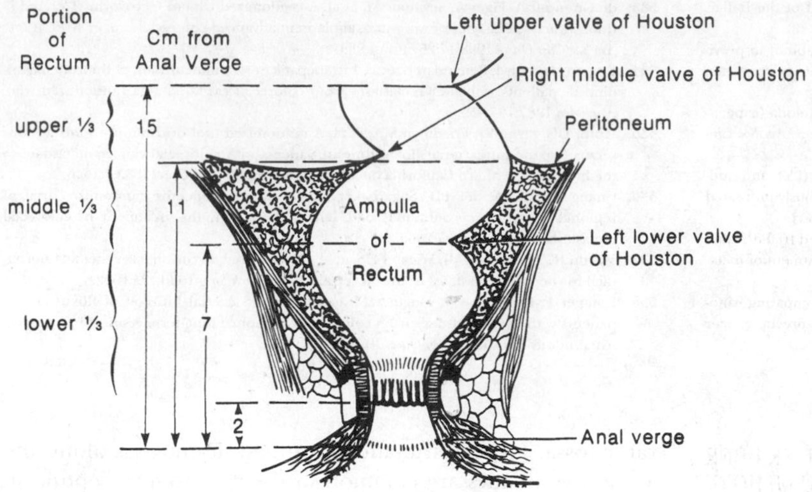

FIGURE 33.8-1. Division of the rectum into upper, middle, and lower thirds.

symptoms. Although all colorectal cancers have a high rate of occult blood in the stools, and the right-sided colon cancers are associated with a higher incidence of anemia, left colon and rectal cancers have a higher incidence of gross bleeding.[5] Cheung and colleagues[6] evaluated prospectively 337 patients presenting with frank rectal bleeding. After making a clinical diagnosis, flexible sigmoidoscopy followed by barium enema was performed. Excluding seven digitally palpable rectal cancers, 30 cancers (9.5%), 34 polyps (10%), 7 cases of proctocolitis (2%), and 25 cases of bleeding diverticula (7%) were detected. The authors concluded that patients with frank rectal bleeding should be screened routinely for left colon cancer irrespective of the clinical diagnosis.[6] This recommendation highlights the fact that hemorrhoids should be considered a diagnosis of exclusion. Patients should have a total colon examination by either a combination of flexible sigmoidoscopy and barium enema, or by a colonoscopy. Barium enema may miss a distal cancer and should not be used alone.

Changes in the bowel habits are a common presenting feature for rectal cancers. Although the incidence of bowel obstruction appears to be lower for the rectal lesions,[5] compromise of the rectal reservoir by tumor makes symptoms common. Unexplained constipation, frequently alternating with diarrhea, and changes in the caliber of stools are classic presenting symptoms for rectal cancer and should be promptly investigated. The entire colon should be carefully evaluated, with particular attention to the rectosigmoid area.

Another common symptom from rectal cancer is tenesmus. This sensation results from the circumferential growth and transmural penetration by the primary tumor. It is characterized by a sensation of urgency and inadequate emptying of the rectum. Even though some degree of tenesmus may be seen with less extensive tumors located distally in the rectum, it is usually a sign of advanced disease. Additional symptoms of local invasion are seen with tumors that have invaded the prostate or bladder or that have destroyed the high sacral nerve roots, causing urinary symptoms. Tumors invading posteriorly may cause buttock or perineal pain. These symptoms imply a locally advanced tumor and poor overall prognosis.

Besides the obvious benefits from early diagnosis of colorectal cancer, appropriate staging in rectal cancer is of particular importance. Increased emphasis has been placed on conservative surgical techniques as an alternative to radical surgery for selected patients. The goals of conservative management are to select patients with low risk for nodal metastases and achieve local tumor control while preserving anal sphincter function. Patient selection is critical to obtain results comparable to patients treated with radical surgery.[7] Alternatively, interest has been increasing in the use of neoadjuvant combinations of chemotherapy and radiotherapy in the treatment of more advanced rectal cancers.[8]

RADIOLOGIC EVALUATION

Computed Tomography

The intravenous pyelography that was obtained preoperatively in the past has fallen out of favor[9] and has been replaced by the use of other imaging techniques, such as the computed tomographic (CT) scan. Although conventional CT scanners and experienced radiologists are now widely available, this test remains of limited value in the staging of rectal cancer. It is very useful to evaluate the presence of distant metastasis,[10] to evaluate gross invasion of adjacent organs, and as a follow-up tool. However, it still lacks sufficient accuracy to be used for preoperative staging as a single test.

Netri and colleagues (1985) preoperatively evaluated 78 patients with rectal adenocarcinoma with digital rectal examination, proctoscopy, double-contrast barium enema, pelvic CT scan, liver ultrasound, and chest x-ray. Data obtained by each diagnostic procedure were compared with the pathologic data. CT scan had an accuracy of 100% for detecting infiltration of the muscularis of the rectum. However, it was less accurate in identifying extrarectal tumor invasion, with an accuracy of 72%. In the evaluation of lymph node involvement, accuracy was 77%, specificity was 74%, and sensitivity was 80%. Liver metastases were detected with 94% accuracy, 97% specificity, and 50% sensitivity. Similarly, Zheng and colleagues (1984) assessed the extent of local spread in 85 patients with rectal carcinoma. In 37 patients with carcinoma of the rectum who were scanned before surgery, good correlation was found between the extent of local invasion assessed by scanning and by postoperative histologic assessment. Scanning was not a reliable method for assessing regional lymph node involvement.

Hundt and colleagues[11] evaluated the use of a subsecond spiral-CT scanner using two contrast medium phases in staging of 37 patients with proven colorectal cancer (14 patients with rectal primaries). The results were compared with the findings of pathologic examination after surgery. The spiral CT had a sensitivity of 97% in the arterial phase and 89% in the venous phase in detecting the carcinoma. The staging results were in accordance with the pathology in 30 of 37 cases (81%) during the arterial phase and in 24 of 37 cases (65%) in the venous phase. Lymph nodes were detected in 27 of 32 patients (84%) during the venous phase. The correct classification of the N stage was possible in 23 of 34 cases (68%). The authors concluded that the arterial phase is superior compared with the venous phase for local tumor staging, and the venous phase is used for lymph node assessment.[11] These results are not dramatically better than the ones previously reported with conventional CT.[12] The role of conventional CT in assessing patients with colorectal tumors is well established. However, the low accuracy of CT for identifying early stages of primary colorectal cancers prevents its routine use for preoperative clinical staging.[13]

Magnetic Resonance Imaging

Magnetic resonance imaging (MRI) remains a relatively expensive imaging method and is not as widely used as CT scanning. However, it has been extensively studied in the diagnosis and staging of rectal cancer.[14,15] Kusunoki and colleagues (1994) used MRI to evaluate preoperatively the local extension of rectal cancer in 33 patients. The sensitivity rate was 84.2% and the specificity rate was 92.9%. In a series including 61 patients, MRI was reported to have an accuracy of 79% for extent of local involvement, but only 58% for extent of lymph node involvement. These results were inferior to the ones obtained with the use of ultrasound in the same population.[16]

MRI using an endorectal coil allows for an excellent anatomic detail of the three rectal wall layers and a very high spatial resolution. Regular MRI has been compared with endorectal MRI and with endorectal ultrasound (EUS) for preoperative staging of rectal carcinoma.[17] In a small series, the results of the preoperative staging were correlated with the histopathologic findings in 15 patients. MRI correctly staged 10 of 15 patients. Without the endorectal surface coil, only three of six were correct, and with the endorectal surface coil, seven of nine were correct. The authors of this study suggested that endorectal surface coil MRI use may lead to better staging results than with other MRI techniques and that the results with endorectal MRI could equal those of EUS for staging small tumors in the rectal wall. Another study[17] evaluated 23 patients with rectal carcinoma using endorectal MRI. The diagnostic accuracy in the evaluation of tumor extent and nodal involvement as compared to surgical pathology was 78.2% and 78.9%, respectively. The major problem was a tendency to overstage parietal infiltration and lymph node involvement.[17]

Although not widely used in the initial staging of rectal cancer, MRI has gained respect for its results in the evaluation of local recurrences. In a small study[18] comparing the relative values of MRI versus CT in diagnosing local recurrence for rectosigmoid cancer, MRI showed superior sensitivity, specificity, and accuracy to CT and better definition of the extent of tumor. At the time of the initial imaging, ten patients had recurrent tumor and four of the remaining eight patients later demonstrated local recurrence. MRI demonstrated 91% sensitivity and 100% specificity, with an accuracy of 95%. CT demonstrated a sensitivity of 82% and a specificity of 50%, with an accuracy of 68%. In four cases, MRI revealed tumor involving the sacrum and sacral nerves not apparent on CT.[18] MRI is also useful to distinguish recurrent rectosigmoid carcinoma from benign postoperative fibrosis.[19]

ENDORECTAL ULTRASOUND

The interest in developing endoscopic ultrasound as an accurate imaging technique for rectal cancer is not recent. In rectal cancer, the depth of tumor infiltration and metastatic involvement of lymph nodes are important prognostic factors, and EUS of the rectum combines the advantages of both endoscopy and sonography, providing information not available from other imaging diagnostic techniques (Fig. 33.8-2). Early animal models using dogs demonstrated its superiority against conventional CT scans, and its potential in predicting pathologic stage.[20] The superiority of EUS against CT scan has been confirmed in studies involving human patients,[21] and it has become the preferred method of preoperative local tumor staging.[7] Hildebrandt and Feifel (1985) even proposed an

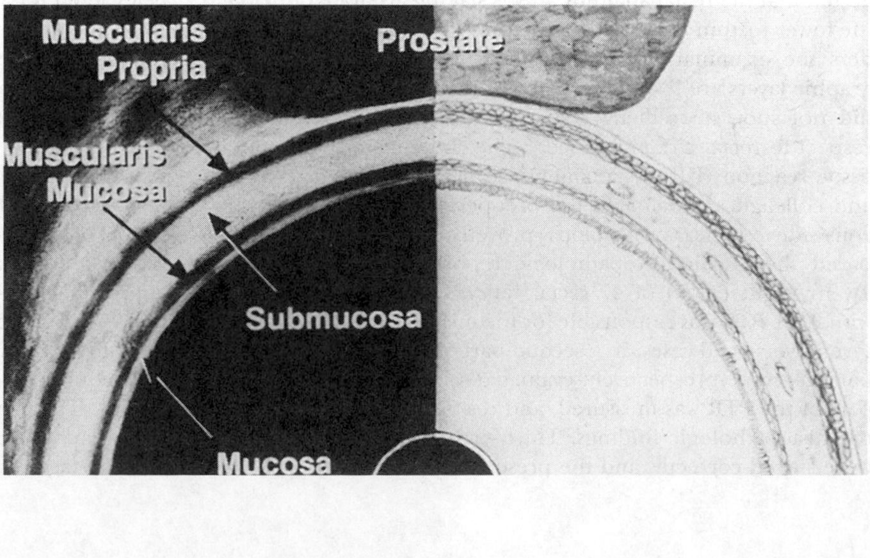

FIGURE 33.8-2. Layers of the rectal wall on endorectal ultrasound.

ultrasonic staging system, which corresponded to the standard pathologic staging systems (e.g., uT for ultrasound T stage, uN for ultrasound N stage).

Detry and colleagues[22] suggested that a low percentage of affected lymph nodes were detected by EUS and that lymph node size was the most reliable parameter to determine tumor involvement. The group at the University Hospital of Wurzburg examined the value of EUS in the preoperative staging of 160 potentially locally resectable tumors. The sensitivity for adenomas and T1 tumors was 81% and the specificity was 98%. For T2 tumors, the sensitivity was only 41% and the specificity, 92%. The majority of T2 tumors were overstaged. The overall staging accuracy for all tumors was 77.5%. The accuracy for lymph node staging was 83%. The authors concluded that adenomas and T1 tumors could be assessed with a high degree of accuracy using EUS. However, T2 carcinomas tended to be overstaged.[23] Similarly, Bernini and colleagues (1996) found that EUS after adjuvant therapy for rectal cancer is of a lesser predictive value, chiefly because of overstaging. However, a more recent report by Massari and colleagues[24] that included 85 patients affected by rectal carcinoma showed an overall accuracy in staging depth of infiltration of 91%. Overstaging occurred in only 4% of patients, whereas understaging occurred in 5%. The overall accuracy in staging lymph node involvement was 76%, sensitivity was 69.8%, specificity was 84.4%, positive predictive value was 85.7%, and negative predictive value was 67.5%. The authors concluded that EUS is a safe and accurate diagnostic method for staging both tumor invasion and lymph node metastatic involvement, and for selecting an appropriate surgical strategy in patients affected by rectal cancer.[24]

It is interesting to note that the accuracy of EUS is improving in more recent series, indicating that experience and new knowledge may have an impact on the staging inaccuracies resulting from over- or underestimation of tumor depth and misinterpretation of lymph node involvement. Technical pitfalls in EUS of the rectal wall include difficulty locating the lesion, improper balloon inflation, improper imaging plane, shadowing artifacts due to air or stool, reverberation artifacts, refraction artifacts, and inappropriate transducer setting. Sources of error in tumor staging with EUS include interpretation differences, operator bias, tumor stenosis, peritumoral inflammation, postbiopsy and postsurgical changes, postirradiation changes, hemorrhage, and pedunculated or villous tumors.[25] Sailer and colleagues[26] suggested that the rectal anatomy affects staging accuracy of EUS in the lower rectum because the structure of the ampulla recti renders the examination more difficult and that the endosonographic layers are less well defined at this level. The same study did not show a predictive value for the tumor position with respect to rectal circumference.[26] The presence of peritumoral tissue reaction (PTR) is a common cause of overstaging. Maier and colleagues[27] evaluated the preoperative EUS results in 40 consecutive patients with biopsy-proven rectal cancer and compared them with histopathologic reports on the specimens. Twenty-eight (70%) of 40 rectal cancers were staged correctly with EUS. PTR was responsible for the misinterpretation in six of seven overstaged cases. In a second part of the study, another 40 patients were prospectively evaluated with EUS. The thickest part of the PTR was measured, and results were compared with the histopathologic findings. Thirty-eight (95%) of 40 cancers were staged correctly, and the presence or absence of PTR was described in 39 cases (98%). A statistically significant positive correlation was noted between histopathologic classification of PTR and its thickness measured with EUS ($P = .0001$).[27]

Despite the increased use of preoperative radiotherapy alone or in combination with chemotherapy for the treatment of stages II and III rectal cancers, our ability to assess local eradication of rectal cancer after radiation therapy remains poor. Conventional imaging and clinical examination techniques are unable to safely predict which patients do not require surgical excision after curative radiation therapy for rectal cancer.[28] The postradiation preoperative staging results of 25 patients with rectal cancer who were found to have stage T0N0 lesions after surgery were examined. All 25 patients were staged by digital rectal examination. In addition, 13 patients were assessed using CT, six by EUS, and one by MRI. Radiologic assessment and physical examination overstaged most irradiated lesions. No technique could reliably distinguish between postradiation fibrosis and residual cancer.[28]

CLINICAL STAGING SYSTEM

The same pathologic staging systems extensively described in Chapter 33.7 are used for rectal tumors. However, the pathologic staging systems cannot be used for making preoperative treatment decisions. Furthermore, patients treated with local modalities, such as transanal resection, do not have a lymph node pathologic evaluation. A reliable and reproducible clinical staging system would be very useful.

Several authors have proposed innovative ways of clinically staging rectal cancer patients. Abrams (1980), for example, evaluated the gross and microscopic pathologic features of 167 rectal cancers. He demonstrated that 63% of nonulcerated tumors were limited to the bowel wall versus only 28% of the ulcerated ones. Zorzitto and colleagues (1982) retrospectively evaluated six clinical variables: the presence or absence of metastatic disease; whether the rectal tumor was fixed; an annular rectal tumor; and the systemic symptoms of weight loss or anorexia, weakness, and anemia. They were able to classify patients in four clinical stages, with substantial gradients in survival among them. However, the correlation between the clinical stage and Dukes' stage was not reliable. Several authors have devised clinical staging systems centered in the degree of mobility of the primary tumor. However, correlation with the pathologic stage was at best 67% to 83%, being lower for less-experienced physicians.

At the University of Texas M. D. Anderson Cancer Center, preoperative treatment of rectal cancers with chemotherapy and radiotherapy has become common. Patients are routinely staged by physical examination, proctoscopy, and conventional imaging studies (i.e., chest x-ray, CT scans of abdomen and pelvis). The degree of rectal wall involvement and the presence of involved lymph nodes are determined by EUS. Based on the results of these studies, patients are clinically classified according to a "clinical" TNM stage. The main problem with this approach is the risk of overstaging,[29,30] especially if the EUS is done by inexperienced physicians, because this imaging modality is highly operator-dependent. Prospective studies are still required to determine the best clinical staging for rectal cancer. The new molecular markers and positron emission tomography (PET) should be added and explored in future clinical staging systems.

TREATMENT OF RESECTABLE RECTAL CANCER

Goals in the treatment of rectal carcinoma are local control of disease and cure, with maintenance of an acceptable quality of life. The biology of a particular patient's tumor is the most important factor in overall outcome. Adequate surgical removal of the tumor is the major treatment factor affecting local control and cure. The principles of the surgical management of rectal cancer are (1) removal of the primary tumor with adequate margins of normal tissue, (2) treatment of the draining lymphatics, and (3) restoration of function. Appropriate adjuvant therapies can enhance local control, reduce systemic recurrence, and increase organ preservation. Clinical staging by history, physical examination, proctoscopy, and imaging is appropriate for establishing resectability and proper sequencing of adjunctive therapies. The management of rectal cancer is best planned by clinical staging that takes into account the extent and location of the primary tumor, its locoregional spread, and presence or absence of metastatic sites.

In patients with low rectal cancer, abdominoperineal resection (APR) has been the standard of management. However, APR requires a permanent colostomy, which adversely affects the patient's quality of life. The majority of patients with rectal cancer do not require a permanent colostomy for curative therapy. Curative excisions can extend from endoscopic removal of malignant polyps to local excision, radical resection, or multivisceral resections.

SITE-SPECIFIC TREATMENT OPTIONS

For purposes of surgical management, the rectum is usually divided into thirds. The middle and lower thirds are extraperitoneal, whereas the upper third may be covered on its anterior or lateral surfaces by peritoneum. The selection of an appropriate surgical technique takes into account not only the extent and location of the tumor, but also the biologic characteristics of the tumor and the patient's overall condition (Table 33.8-1).

Upper Third

Recurrence patterns and cure rates for tumors in the upper third of the rectum are similar to those for the colon. Advanced tumors in this location may involve the retroperitoneal structures (i.e., ureters, bladder, muscle) or major vessels. The lowermost edge of these tumors is usually 10 to 12 cm from the anal verge. Extirpation of these tumors should include resection of the bowel segment containing the tumor along with the mesorectum to approximately 5 cm below the lower edge of the tumor (Lopez-Kostner, [1998]). It is usually inappropriate to attempt local excision techniques in this area because of the relationship between the upper rectum and peritoneal cavity and because of the poor exposure due to the distance from the anal verge.

Middle Third

The appropriate procedure for radical resection of most rectal carcinomas is a low anterior resection (LAR). This procedure encompasses the sigmoid colon, a segment of the rectum containing the tumor with a margin of tissue below the tumor, and the mesorectum. Reconstruction is performed between the left colon and the rectal stump. Most tumors in the middle rectum are not amenable to local excision because of the proximal extension of the tumor. APR does not reduce local recurrence rates compared to appropriate sphincter-preservation surgery for patients with midrectal tumors.

TABLE 33.8-1. Surgical Procedures for Rectal Cancer

Abdominoperineal resection
Low anterior resection
Proctectomy and coloanal anastomosis
Local excision
Transanal excision
Posterior proctotomy
Transanal endoscopic microsurgery
Ablative procedures
Endoscopic laser
Fulguration

Lower Third

Cancers in the distal rectum can require APR for adequate radial and distal margins. The entire mesorectum is included in this resection. Management of these tumors has been most clearly affected by multidisciplinary treatment strategies that allow for adequate oncologic resection and preservation of the anal canal. Important techniques have been proctectomy and coloanal anastomosis (CAA), as well as local excision.[31] Both of these treatments are commonly combined with either preoperative or postoperative radiation therapy.[32]

The use of staplers has evolved to make an anastomosis easier when there is a short rectal stump deep within the pelvis. The double-staple technique of Knight and Griffin is most commonly used to restore intestinal continuity after resections in which a short rectal stump remains (Griffin, 1990). Alternative forms of local therapy for low rectal cancers include transanal endoscopic microsurgery (TEM), endocavitary radiation, fulguration, and laser ablation.

SURGICAL ISSUES IN RESECTABLE RECTAL CANCER

This section discusses the major issues that are common to surgical procedures for rectal cancer.

Mucosal Margins

Attaining tumor-free margins at the edges of a rectal cancer resection specimen is the hallmark of curative surgical therapy. The purpose of obtaining such a margin is to prevent local failure and effect cure.

Spread beyond the lower edge of a rectal cancer may occur by submucosal spread in intramural lymphatics. Fewer than 5% of rectal cancers show distal mucosal spread beyond the edge of the tumor, and only 2.5% have histologic evidence of spread beyond 2 cm. These tumors commonly show aggressive biologic characteristics. Margins may need to be increased in locally aggressive tumors, such as those showing poor differentiation or vascular and lymphatic invasion. In these cases, the spread may be discontinuous. It does not appear that a mural mucosal margin of 5 cm is necessary to prevent local recur-

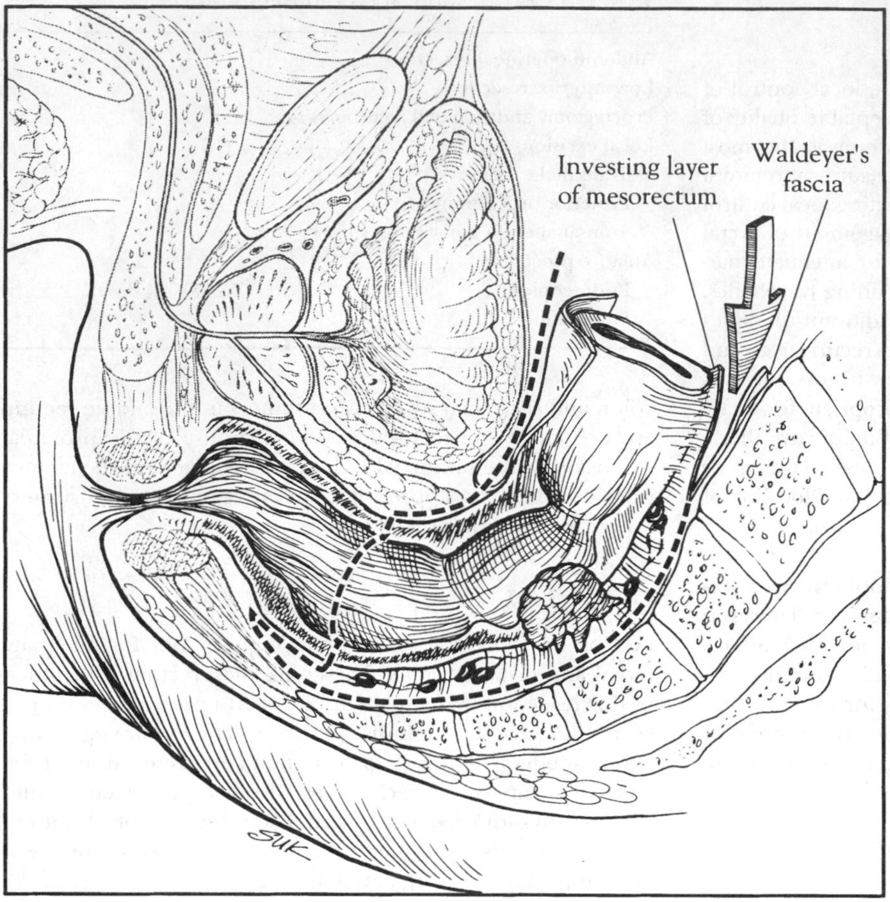

FIGURE 33.8-3. Total mesorectal excision.

rence. Even margins of 1 cm have been demonstrated to provide adequate protection from local recurrence in the absence of aggressive histologic features.[33] Distal margins of more than 2 cm do not reduce the risk of anastomotic recurrence.[34]

The impact of neoadjuvant therapies on the suitability of margins is unclear at this time. However, some have proposed that distal margins may be reduced in the face of preoperative chemoradiation. These concepts have allowed for an increase in sphincter-preserving procedures without detracting from local control and survival. However, clinical response at the primary site can be misleading. Many patients have residual microscopic disease within the bowel wall, despite a complete response at the mucosal surface.[35] Complete excision of the primary site with margins of normal tissue is recommended.

The difference between margins reported in the literature and margins *in situ* at surgery can be significant. This fact is due to contraction of the specimen after its excision and the stretching of the rectal wall. Therefore, generous gross margins can be required to assure adequate resection. A microscopically involved margin is unacceptable for a curative resection and will not be salvaged by radiation and chemotherapy. The need for negative mural margins also applies to local excision specimens for which a 1-cm margin of grossly normal bowel wall around the tumor is recommended for satisfactory resection.[36]

Proximal Lymph Node Dissection

The lymphatic spread of rectal cancer is upward as well as lateral and distal. The proximal extent of the mesorectum and the rectosigmoid mesentery should be included in the resection. Lymph node excision at the base of the inferior mesenteric artery does not enhance survival compared with lymph node excision just distal to the origin of the left colon. This is particularly true for low rectal cancers in which positive nodes between the left colic origin and the inferior mesenteric artery origin are found in fewer than 6% of resectable cases.[37] For low rectal resections or CAA, however, ligation of the inferior mesenteric artery just above its origin at the aorta is required to eliminate tension on the anastomosis. Retroperitoneal adenopathy above the level of the inferior mesenteric artery is frequently a harbinger of occult systemic spread that is not amenable to cure by surgery alone.

Total Mesorectal Excision

The mesentery of the rectum contains its blood supply and lymphatics in a bilobed fat packet situated immediately posterior and lateral to the thick-walled rectum. Both are contained in the visceral layer of the endopelvic fascia. The majority of resectable primary rectal tumors and involved lymph nodes in rectal cancer specimens are found within this structure. Nodes are involved in T1 cancers in 5.7% of cases; T2 tumors have positive nodes in 19.6%, and T3 and T4 cancers have positive nodes in 65% and 78% of cases, respectively.[38] Involvement of the radial or circumferential margin correlates with subsequent local recurrence and poor survival.[39] Resection of the mesorectum should extend farther distally than the acceptable margin for rectal wall transection (Fig. 33.8-3). Because the

TABLE 33.8-2. Distal Mesorectal Spread in Producing an Involved Radial Margin

Curative Resection Specimens (N = 20)	*Distal Mesorectal Spread*	*Involvement of Radial Margin*
16	Negative	2 (13%)
4	Positive	2 (50%)

[From Adam IJ, Mohamdee MO, Martin IG, et al. Role of circumferential involvement in the local recurrence of rectal cancer. *Lancet* 1994;344(8924):707, with permission.]

mesorectum tapers as it proceeds distally, it is totally excised for most middle and lower rectal cancers. More proximal rectal tumors can be treated by a mesorectal excision extending 5 cm beyond the lower tumor edge. Total mesorectal excision has been associated with a high rate of anastomotic leak when used for upper rectal tumors.[40]

The work of Quirke and others (1986) has dramatically demonstrated the importance of lateral tumor spread in the local recurrence of resected rectal cancers (Table 33.8-2). Among patients with local recurrence, tumor involvement at the circumferential margin of resection has been found in 85% of cases. Because of difficulty in obtaining adequate exposure in the low pelvis and the surrounding structures, circumferential margins around rectal cancer can be highly variable and minimal. Surgical experience and surgical technique have demonstrated their key role in the prevention of local recurrence by controlled sharp dissection done with attention to these margins.[41] The mechanism for involvement of the circumferential margins can be direct spread, mesenteric implants, vascular or lymphatic invasion, or cancer-bearing lymph nodes. Up to 23% of patients can have mesorectal tumor implants aside from discrete nodes.[42] Tumor involvement of the circumferential margins of resection is frequently due to spread in the mesorectum distal to the tumor that can be violated by blunt dissection.[43] It has been implied that a positive circumferential margin after mesorectal excision is a prognostic factor for distant metastases also.[44]

Circumferential clearance of rectal tumors by total mesorectal excision has become the accepted surgical procedure for the management of most rectal cancer. Total mesorectal excision by full mobilization of the rectum along anatomic planes has been demonstrated to be effective in the surgical management of rectal cancer.[45,46] Dissection is carried out along areolar planes that allow for hemostasis, identification of important nerves, and prevention of violation of the visceral fascia investing the mesorectum.[47] This type of surgical resection for rectal cancer produces a negative surgical margin in more than 90% of resectable rectal cancers and reduces the possibility of local recurrence.

Lateral Pelvic Lymph Node Dissection

Lymphatic drainage of the rectum not only flows proximally along the inferior mesenteric vessels, but also follows the middle rectal vessels to the lateral pelvic sidewall and into internal iliac nodes. These nodes may be a source of recurrence. The incidence varies from 1% to 7% in resectable cases. Wide pelvic lymphadenectomy including lateral pelvic lymph nodes has been proposed for the treatment of rectal cancer. Although there is little doubt that the presence of metastases in such lymph nodes is a significant negative prognostic factor, no evidence supports a therapeutic benefit of the routine addition of extensive lymphadenectomy to standard locoregional procedures.[48] Gross disease can be resected when this procedure would provide a negative margin of resection.[47] The morbidity of this procedure is significant, with the majority of patients developing urinary dysfunction and impotence.

RADICAL SURGICAL TREATMENT OPTIONS

Patients with stage II and III rectal cancer (60% to 80% of patients with rectal cancer) have tumors that are large and biologically aggressive. They are at higher risk of local and systemic recurrence after treatment. Accordingly, strategies have been developed to address these issues through locoregional resection and multimodality therapy. However, adequate surgical resection and technique are the most critical treatment factors determining patient outcome.

The surgical management of stage II and III tumors is based on several issues: (1) the importance of the lateral spread of rectal cancer in local tumor recurrence; (2) the need for total mesorectal excision to minimize pelvic recurrence; (3) restoration of function by CAA after resection of low rectal cancers; and (4) optimization of bowel function and quality of life after low rectal anastomosis. Oncologic results of radical resection and patterns of failure are discussed later in this chapter.

Selection of Radical Excision Procedures

The surgical procedure chosen for radical excision is determined largely by tumor location. Three different operative procedures can be performed, all with adherence to the principles of total mesorectal excision: LAR, APR, and total proctectomy with CAA. For rectal cancer patients, a major component of quality of life is sphincter preservation. This is simple to accomplish in middle and upper rectal cancers where LAR achieves adequate removal of the tumor and surrounding lymphatics and end-to-end anastomosis. In patients with low rectal cancers that do not involve the levators or sphincters, the anus may still be spared by proctectomy and CAA.[49] Preoperative chemoradiation may facilitate this. However, patients with levator or sphincter involvement are best managed by APR and permanent colostomy.

Abdominoperineal Resection

Preoperative planning of the stoma site and counseling about the consequences of a colostomy are critical to a successful outcome. Proper selection of a site must be planned preoperatively with attention to belt lines, scars, and body habitus. APR involves a combined transabdominal and perineal approach to complete resection of the rectum, mesorectum, levator muscles, and anus, with formation of a permanent colostomy. The rectum and mesorectum are mobilized via an abdominal approach down to the levator muscles. A perineal approach is used to widely resect the levator complex and anus along with an appropriate margin of perianal skin. A permanent end colostomy is done. As sphincter preservation (LAR and proctectomy plus CAA) has advanced, the overall proportion of rectal cancer patients undergoing APR has decreased.[50] However,

APR remains the only surgical option for some patients with rectal cancer, specifically in those patients with sphincter complex involvement or levator muscle involvement.

Low Anterior Resection

LAR involves the transabdominal resection of a portion of the rectum as well as the mesorectum. After complete mobilization of the rectum *en bloc* with the mesorectum, the rectum is divided at least 2 cm below the distal edge of the tumor (see Fig. 33.8-3). Although the length of mesorectal excision will exceed this, evidence indicates that total mesorectal excision is not required for upper rectal cancers. Reconstruction of the rectum is then carried out between the completely mobilized left colon and the remaining rectal stump. The use of LAR in midrectal and selected low rectal cancer has increased for two main reasons. First, the double-stapled technique has permitted a simpler and lower anastomosis, with leak rates (clinical or radiographic) similar or better than with handsewn techniques. Second, although 5 cm was previously felt to be the minimum acceptable distal margin, the acceptance of a 2-cm distal margin has enabled lower tumors to be resected by LAR.[51] The timing of sphincter-preserving surgery after preoperative radiation has been demonstrated to influence sphincter preservation. A 6- to 8-week interval increases the sphincter preservation rate from 68% for a 2-week interval to 76%.[52]

Proctectomy and Coloanal Anastomosis

Although LAR and APR are the traditional methods of locoregional resection in rectal cancer, proctectomy with CAA has emerged as a well-accepted surgical option in carefully selected patients. This procedure spares patients a permanent colostomy while obtaining good functional and cancer-related outcomes.[49] A review of 117 patients from the Mayo and Cleveland Clinics provides a perspective on the current utility of proctectomy and CAA in patients with low rectal cancer.[53] The patients were treated over a 10-year period (1981 to 1991). The median distance of the tumor from the anal verge was 6 to 7 cm. The technique used required complete mobilization of the rectum to the levators, transanal transection of the rectum, complete mobilization of the left colon, and endoanal anastomosis (Fig. 33.8-4). The authors recommend loop ileostomy. The effectiveness of the procedure in preventing local recurrence was demonstrated by the low local recurrence rate of 7%. Fecal continence was satisfactory in 78%, and overall bowel function appeared to be improved in patients who had a colonic J pouch reservoir created for the CAA. No surgery-related deaths were reported. Early and late complications were related mainly to the anastomosis leaking and healing with a stricture.

The mobilization of the rectum is extended down to the level of the upper anal canal and levators. Lateral ligaments are divided with attention to obtaining an adequate radial margin and to preserving the pelvic autonomic nerves. This dissection results in the complete exposure of the pelvic floor and complete excision of the mesorectum. The fully mobilized rectum can be amputated by a transanal technique or by transection at the upper end of the anal canal with a stapler. The reconstruction consists of delivering the mobilized left colon to the anal canal and performing an anastomosis. A hand-sewn anastomosis can be performed with full-thickness sutures through the colon and internal sphincter. Alternatively, a stapled anastomosis may be done. A diverting stoma is then usually created.

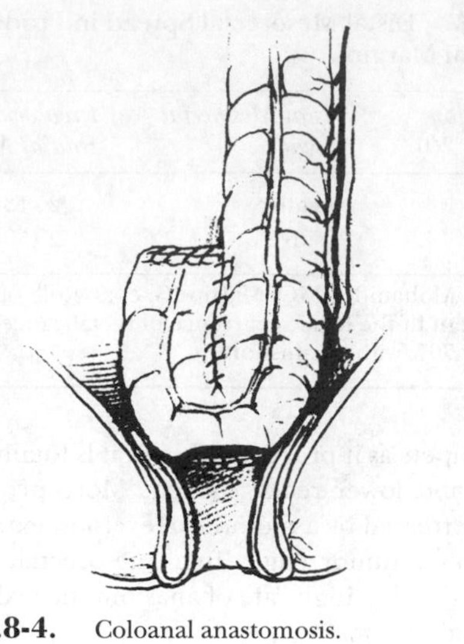

FIGURE 33.8-4. Coloanal anastomosis.

Several groups have reported on patients who have a 6- to 10-cm colonic J pouch reservoir constructed with no additional risk or compromise of the anastomosis.[54] The formation of the colonic pouch has been compared to the straight CAA in a randomized clinical trial. Hallbook and colleagues (1996) demonstrated a reduction in the frequency and urgency of bowel movements in the first year after pouch formation. Physiologic measures and short-term outcomes appear to be improved with the pouch. However, these differences may disappear with time.[55] It has been suggested that lower leak rates with a colonic J pouch may be obtained because of improved vascular supply to the apex of the pouch and the side-to-end anastomosis.[56] Postoperative problems after CAA are related to rectal capacitance and compliance. These manifest as the problems of urgency and frequency in bowel movements. This gradually improves over the 9 to 10 months after temporary stoma closure. Complete fecal continence usually is achieved in 85% to 100% of patients. In a series from the Mayo Clinic by Drake et al.,[57] patients who had a CAA for malignancies had a stool frequency of 2.6 per 24 hours, and only 1 of 19 patients had any incontinence. The Mayo and Cleveland Clinics study is similar to the reports of others in describing proctectomy and CAA for rectal cancer.[58]

Multivisceral Resection for Locally Advanced Rectal Cancer

Approximately 6% to 10% of rectal cancers are locally advanced in, and require extensive surgery for, complete tumor extirpation. Pelvic exenteration involving *en bloc* removal of the rectum, bladder, distal ureters, and other pelvic organs can be required to obtain negative margins of resection.[59] A number of studies have demonstrated 5-year survival rates ranging from 33% to 50% for these selected patients with locally advanced rectal cancer. Despite the ability to achieve long-range survival rates in selected patients, the operation remains a formidable one, with significant morbidity and a mortality up to 6%.[60] Patients who undergo such resections for primary tumors have better survival rates than those with recurrence.

Meterissian et al.[35] reported a series of 40 patients undergoing pelvic exenteration for rectal carcinoma in which tumor-free margins were obtained. The 5-year overall survival rate was 49%, with a median survival of 56 months. Adjuvant chemoradiation appeared to provide a reduction in risk of recurrence. In the series, five patients experienced local failure. Comparable results have been recorded by Lopez and associates (1987). Long-term local control is obtained in approximately 70% of the patients who undergo resection with tumor-free margins. The results of such surgery cannot be separated from the benefits of adjuvant chemoradiation in this high-risk population.

Results from surgical procedures for rectal cancer requiring multivisceral resection have improved.[61] This finding may be related to improvements in perioperative care, patient selection, and surgical techniques. Of major importance in the management of such patients, who are often heavily radiated, is the use of vascularized tissue flaps to accomplish healing of pelvic and perineal wounds.[62]

Morbidity and Mortality from Radical Resection

The major cause of infection in procedures in which reconstruction has been done is anastomotic leak. Anastomotic leaks can occur in 2% to 5% of cases, and they may result in subsequent stricture.[63] The consequences of pelvic sepsis can be a major cause of mortality from resection of rectal cancer. Use of a diverting stoma for a low rectal anastomosis will not prevent anastomotic leak, but it will reduce the clinical manifestations of sepsis, the need for reoperation, and mortality.

Bladder dysfunction can be a complication of extensive pelvic dissection, especially if disruption of autonomic nerve trunks occurs. Sacral parasympathetic nerve injuries result in loss of the awareness of the need to void. Management by intermittent catheterization, medications, or transurethral resection may be required.

Resection of the rectum for carcinoma has been associated with a high rate of erectile dysfunction or retrograde ejaculation in men. This sexual dysfunction is caused by injury to pelvic autonomic nerves and is especially frequent in cases in which extensive lateral dissection has been done. Pelvic dissection to preserve the hypogastric sympathetic nerve trunks arising from the preaortic plexus and the parasympathetic trunks arising from the sacral nerve roots can reduce this morbidity.[64] It is also important to realize that erectile dysfunction is not uncommon in the age group of individuals who develop sporadic rectal cancer and that factors other than an intact autonomic nervous system can impact on a patient's sexual function after the diagnosis and management of rectal carcinoma.

With sharp nerve-sparing dissection, impotence has been reduced to a rate of 10% to 28%, or lower, in many series with resection of rectal carcinoma.[2]

Creation of a stoma can produce complications requiring reoperation in 15% to 20% of patients.[65] Reconstruction of the rectum avoids a permanent colostomy. However, bowel movements and urgency may be frequent because of the smaller neorectum.[66] The reconstructed rectum usually is composed of a more proximal segment of left colon, which is brought down to a rectal stump of varying lengths. Improving the rectal reservoir function by construction of a colonic J pouch improves short-term functional results.[67] Function does improve with time. The use of fiber supplements may enhance this improvement. Episodic clustering of bowel movements is also a prominent symptom in patients with a small rectal pouch after reconstruction. Anal sphincter tone and local reflexes regulating sphincter function are generally preserved after resection. Actual sphincter function usually is maintained in the majority of patients. Function is diminished by the presence of postoperative pelvic sepsis or the use of postoperative radiotherapy. Operative mortality for radical resections ranges from 0.6% to 3.0%.[46,63]

TABLE 33.8-3. Indications for the Local Excision of Rectal Cancer

Tumor >3 cm in greatest dimension
Invades only the submucosa or superficial muscularis
Favorable pathologic grade

(From ref. 73, with permission.)

TREATMENT OF INVASIVE CANCER BY NONRADICAL APPROACHES

SELECTION OF PATIENTS

The criteria used to select patients for local excision are intended to make a negative-margin, full-thickness local excision technically feasible and to ensure a low risk of lymph node metastases (Table 33.8-3). Physical assessment, CT, and EUS are helpful in the preoperative evaluation of these rectal cancer patients. Imaging findings can be used to select patients for local excision procedures by determining the depth of tumor penetration into the rectal wall and the presence of enlarged lymph nodes in the mesorectum. Ninety percent of rectal cancers do not meet the criteria for treatment by local excision alone because of the size or extent of the tumor.[68] Factors that can help identify patients who are at low risk for lymphatic metastases include small tumor size, absence of lymphatic and vascular invasion, well or moderate tumor differentiation ploidy, and absence of clinical or radiologic evidence of enlarged lymph nodes.[69]

The major factor predicting patient survival and perirectal lymph node metastases is the depth of penetration of the primary tumor. Morson (1966) has reported that lymphatic metastases occur with 10% of tumors confined to the submucosa, 12% of tumors invading the muscularis propria, and 58% of tumors extending beyond the bowel wall. A study of T1 and T2 tumors treated by radical resection showed an incidence of lymphatic metastasis of 12% for T1 tumors and 22% for T2 tumors. The incidence of lymphatic metastasis was increased by lymphatic or blood vessel invasion (BVI) and in poorly differentiated tumors.[70] Nelson et al.[71] reported that 29% of patients with lesions smaller than 2 cm in diameter had evidence of lymph node metastasis. Thus, selection for local excision based on the classic indications fails to adequately treat a significant number of patients with lymphatic involvement. This makes the addition of adjuvant therapy to local excision a logical choice.

LOCAL EXCISION TECHNIQUES

Full-thickness local excision is effective in the treatment of selected early, low rectal cancers. Local excision is used as curative therapy for patients who have superficial tumors, and it is used as alternative therapy in medically compromised patients and in those who refuse standard therapy. Patient selection is paramount to using these techniques successfully, which requires an understanding of the limitations of the techniques and an appreciation of the biology of T1–2 rectal cancer. The oncologic results of local treatment with and without adjuvant treatment are described in Adjuvant Radiation Therapy for Resectable Rectal Cancer, later in this chapter.

The choice of technique for local excision is dictated by tumor characteristics and the surgeon's ability to have adequate exposure and control of the margins of excision. In general, the transanal approach has less morbidity. Posterior approaches can offer the advantage of better exposure for larger lesions. However, posterior approaches entail a higher rate of fistula formation and the potential for tumor seeding of the posterior wound. Whichever method is selected, the surgeon must perform a full-thickness excision with at least 1-cm margins of normal tissue surrounding the tumor. An inadequate margin is a predictor of failure.[72] Piecemeal or submucosal excision is not considered adequate surgical treatment of invasive rectal cancer. Fragmentation of the tumor is associated with an increased incidence of local recurrence. If the lesion cannot be adequately resected by local excision, then a more standard locoregional operative approach should be used. In a curative case, the patients should be counseled to consider local excision as a form of definitive biopsy. This is especially true when transmural penetration or adverse histologic characteristics are found in the local excision specimen. In most instances, these patients should undergo more extensive surgical therapy.

Transanal Excision

Transanal excision is the most common method used for local excision. Size and degree of circumferential involvement predict the potential for a technically successful transanal excision. Both adequate dilatation of the anus and a good light source are essential, and exposure is aided by the use of specialized retractors.[73] The excision is begun by marking a margin of normal tissue around the lesion, which must be greater than 1 cm.[74] The local excision is performed in a full-thickness manner, meaning that the deep plane of dissection includes the perirectal fat. The defect usually is closed to avoid subsequent scarring. Proper orientation of the specimen is required for pathologic assessment of the margins. Lymph nodes are usually not recovered by this technique.

Posterior Proctotomy

A posterior proctotomy is useful for large posterior lesions and provides better access to more proximal lesions. Otherwise known as a *Kraske's procedure*, a posterior longitudinal incision is made just above the anus to the inferior border of the gluteus maximus. The coccyx is removed and the underlying levator muscles are divided in a longitudinal fashion in the midline. This permits excellent exposure for mobilization of the rectum and allows for a full-thickness local excision or, alternatively, a sleeve resection. A transsphincteric excision (Bevan's or York-Mason) involves a similar approach as the posterior proctotomy, except the entire anal sphincter is divided posteriorly in the midline. It is critical to identify, mark, and reconstruct each portion of the sphincter complex, but if this is done, minimal functional problems are observed.[75]

Transanal Endoscopic Microsurgery

TEM, in which either submucosal (for adenomas) or full-thickness (for invasive carcinomas) excision is performed though an operating rectoscope, has emerged as an option for the local treatment of rectal cancer.[76] It allows improved exposure compared to the transanal approach and does not carry the risk of fecal fistula or sphincter dysfunction associated with posterior or transsphincteric proctotomy. In one series, local recurrence occurred in 2 of 16 (13%) patients with T1 lesions undergoing TEM.[76] The authors of this series believe that TEM alone is not an appropriate treatment for T2 lesions. Further follow-up and experience is required to establish the role for TEM.

Fulguration

Fulguration can be used in highly selected patients to treat lower rectal carcinomas.[77] Chin and Eiserstat[78] have reported good results with rectal coagulation for rectal cancers less than 4 cm in diameter that are well or moderately differentiated and less than 7.5 cm from the anal verge. Eighty-one of 114 patients with low rectal cancers were treated primarily by electrocoagulation with curative intent, and a 65% 5-year survival rate is achieved in highly selected individuals. Stahl et al.[79] reported similar results in 33 patients treated with electrocoagulation. This is carried out through an operating proctoscope. Bipolar coagulating current is used to coagulate the lesion along with a 1-cm margin of normal mucosa. This procedure is followed by débridement of the coagulated tissue, and the process is repeated until no residual tumor is noted. This technique can be carried out through the entire bowel wall for posterior and lateral lesions. Although it is used for anterior lesions, it should be carried out with caution because of the proximity of the rectovaginal septum or prostate. Complications of this procedure can include bleeding, stricture, abscess, or perforation. The overall complication rate is 21%, and a mortality rate of 2.7% was reported.

Endoscopic Laser

Endoscopic laser may be used for palliative purposes in patients with extensive metastases for rectal obstruction or hemorrhage. It may be used as definitive therapy in those who refuse surgery or are a poor surgical risk, as a bridge to neoadjuvant therapy, or to allow bowel preparation. It is most useful for noncircumferential lesions that are less than 7 cm in diameter and have limited invasion. It may be combined with external-beam radiotherapy after successful recanalization.[80] Highly selected patients with small tumors who undergo complete local destruction of the tumor with subsequent negative biopsies can occasionally be treated definitively. A mean survival of 50 months has been achieved by Brunetaud et al.[81] in a series of patients treated by such techniques. Laser treatment can be combined with photosensitizing agents to achieve more efficient tumor oblation. This technique of photodynamic therapy is especially useful in patients being managed for obstruction who are otherwise unresectable.

Endocavitary Irradiation

Radiation has been used as a single modality with curative intent for selected early rectal cancers. Most investigators have used intracavitary irradiation alone for early, noninvasive tumors. For more advanced tumors, it is combined with a temporary iridium 192 implant or external-beam radiation, or both.[82] Before delivery, the anus is dilated and a 4-cm proctoscope is introduced. A low-energy x-ray unit is placed through the scope almost against the tumor. Generally, 50-kV x-rays, in doses of 30 Gy per treatment, are given using this "contact" approach. Three or four such treatments over 1 month are required. Bulky tumors may require additional irradiation with an ^{192}Ir implant or external beam to reach the deeper pararectal tissues.

RESULTS OF TREATMENT OF RECTAL CANCER

This section presents the results after potentially curative surgery alone for clinically resectable rectal cancer. Overall, cure rates for cancers in the lower third of the rectum are lower than those for cancers in the upper two-thirds.

ONCOLOGIC RESULTS OF RADICAL SURGICAL RESECTION ALONE

Numerous studies have compared the oncologic results of APR with those of sphincter-preserving procedures (LAR or proctectomy plus CAA). In a randomized clinical trial intended to examine the benefit of adjuvant therapy in rectal cancer, patients who underwent APR had a higher recurrence rate than patients undergoing LAR (P <.05).[83] However, this finding was likely reflective of the larger, more advanced tumors seen in the patients undergoing APR. Several other studies involving large numbers of rectal cancer patients have shown no significant differences in local recurrence or survival between patients undergoing APR and those undergoing sphincter preservation.[63] Survival does not appear to be compromised.

Outstanding surgical results have indicated that total mesorectal excision is the optimal technique for the radical resection of rectal cancer (Table 33.8-4). McAnena et al.[84] have described the long-term outcome of 57 patients treated by this approach. The mean follow-up was 4.8 years. Local recurrences were seen in only 3.5% of the patients, and the overall 5-year survival rate was 81%. In a report by MacFarlane and coworkers[85] on patients undergoing operation exclusively, 135 patients with Dukes' B and C rectal cancers were treated over a 13-year period with a mean follow-up of 7.5 years. None of these patients received adjuvant radiation or chemotherapy. Despite this fact, only a 5% local recurrence rate was reported.

TABLE 33.8-4. Local Recurrence Rates after Surgery Alone

Series	*n*	*Stage*	*Local Recurrence Rate (%)*
Enker et al.[46] 1999	156	I, II, III	7
Arbman et al.[334] 1996	128	I, II, III	7
Pocard et al.[335] 1998	118	I, II, III	15
Zaheer et al.[63] 1998	514	I, II, III	7

Further long-term follow-up of a larger group of patients confirmed these findings, specifically with a 10-year local recurrence rate of 4% and a 10-year disease-free survival rate of 78%.[73] Heald (1986) reported his group's experience between 1978 and 1997 with 380 patients who underwent curative resection with a 10-year local recurrence rate of 8%. This reduction in local recurrence rate has been reported as the reason for a high survival rate for these patients.[45] This compares favorably with the results from the North Central Cancer Treatment Group (NCCTG) study that forms the basis for current recommendations for adjuvant therapy in the United States in which chemotherapy and radiation were used for high-risk rectal cancers in addition to surgical resection.

In North America, similar results have been obtained with high rates of local recurrence-free survival when a total mesorectal excision is done by meticulous sharp dissection along the pelvic sidewalls. Enker's report on this subject called for full rectal mobilization along anatomic planes to obtain complete mesorectal excision. In a series of 42 men who underwent sphincter-preserving surgery for low rectal cancer using this technique, only one local recurrence was noted (median follow-up, 20 months).[2] This result was accomplished with preservation of potency in 86.7% of patients. In 156 stage I and II rectal cancer patients treated without adjuvant therapy between 1987 and 1995 at Memorial Sloan-Kettering Cancer Center, local recurrences rates were reduced to 8.3% by using mesorectal excision without radiotherapy.[86] Zaheer (1998) reported the Mayo Clinic experience in 514 patients with surgical resection of stage I, II, and III rectal cancer. Two hundred seventy-two of these patients had stage I disease, and 173 had stage II or III rectal cancer. The local recurrence rate for all stages was 7%, whereas the local recurrence rate for node-positive cancers was 13%.[63]

SURGEON-RELATED OUTCOMES

The frequency of local recurrence varies greatly for individual surgeons, from less than 10% to more than 50%. Norwegian surgeons have removed rectal cancer surgery from routine surgical teaching and concentrate training in total mesorectal excision among specialized surgeons. They propose that the surgical specimens obtained by such surgeons be audited. Where regionalization of all rectal cancer surgery has occurred, survival appears to have improved and local recurrence rates have dropped to 7% after the addition of total mesorectal excision from historical controls, with a local recurrence rate of 23%.[50]

Several studies have suggested that the surgeon is an important prognostic factor in rectal cancer. In a population-based study of 683 patients, Porter et al. (1998) found a significant local recurrence and survival advantage in patients of both surgeons with colorectal surgery fellowship training and surgeons with a higher caseload. In addition, a greater rate of sphincter preservation for low rectal cancer also was found to be associated with higher case loads. Other studies suggest that hospital volume, hospital type (university vs. community), and surgeon experience improve survival and recurrence outcomes.[87]

ONCOLOGIC RESULTS OF NONRADICAL APPROACHES

The incidence of lymph node metastases in patients with T1 tumors approximate the recurrence rate for T1 cancer treated by local excision alone. Studies describe a 3% to 10% rate of

TABLE 33.8-5. Patterns of Local Recurrence after Local Excision Alone

Series	*n*	*Local Recurrence*
Chakravarti et al.[117]	52	10 (19%)
Bailey et al.[336]	28	2 (7%)
Willett et al.[110]	40	6 (15%)
Biggers et al.[31]	141	36 (25%)

local recurrence after excision alone.[88] Survival rates in patients with T1 rectal carcinomas treated with local excision alone or radical resection are 90% to 100%.

In patients with T2 rectal carcinomas, the risk of lymph node metastasis is 10% to 30%. Recurrence rates may be 17% to 24% in patients with T2 tumors after local excision alone. Survival rates are 78% to 82% with excision alone.

Many studies, mostly retrospective and single institutional studies, examine the results of local excision alone in the management of T1–2 rectal cancer (Table 33.8-5). In a review of all published series with reasonable follow-up describing this approach, Graham et al.[88] found the combined local recurrence rate for T1 lesions was 5% (range, 0% to 12%) and for T2 lesions was 18% (range, 8% to 27%). Lower local recurrence rates in similar patients treated by APR (0% to 10%)[89] have brought into question the use of local excision alone for early rectal cancer.[90]

Papillon and colleagues (1992) in Lyon, France, pioneered the treatment of selected patients with rectal cancers using endocavitary irradiation. Exophytic, superficial, well to moderately differentiated tumors without colloid histology with a maximum diameter less than 4.5 cm were treated. If the tumor was felt to invade muscle, an interstitial ^{192}Ir implant was added. In 245 patients, the 5-year disease-free survival rate was 76%, and the local failure rate was only 5%. Sischy and associates (1984) have reported similar results. The local failure rate in 94 patients treated with endocavitary irradiation alone was 5%. Hull et al. (1994) reported a 71% disease-free survival rate in 126 patients. With a median follow-up of 55 months, Schild and associates[91] reported 10% local failure and 76% 5-year survival. In 102 patients treated by Maingon et al.,[82] the local failure rate was 15% and the 5-year survival was 81%. In 22 patients who were stage T1,N0 by rectal ultrasound, none developed local failure.[92]

Five-year survival rates with local treatment options vary from 50% to 90%, with many deaths secondary to intercurrent disease and not related to cancer. In selected patients, a 10% cancer-related 5-year mortality can be expected with local excision, fulguration, or primary irradiation. For clinically staged T1 and early T2 cancers, our treatment preference it to perform a full-thickness local excision when possible. This allows an assessment of margins and other pathologic features, thereby providing the best determination of whether any additional therapy is needed.

In an attempt to help select the ideal combination of radiotherapeutic and surgical approaches for sphincter preservation, the Dijon clinical staging system has been proposed. The staging system takes into account the tumor size and depth of penetration of the rectal wall. Briefly, T1A tumors are defined as superficial, exophytic, and smaller than 3 cm; CS T1B tumors have a limited infiltrative component and are smaller than 3 cm; CS T2A tumors are superficial, exophytic, and are 3 to 5 cm in size; CS T2B tumors have a limited infiltrative component and are 3 to 5 cm; and CS T3 tumors are deeply infiltrative or fixed, regardless of size. High-grade and colloid tumors are excluded. The rationale for the different T stages is based on the technical parameters of endocavitary radiation. Tumors smaller than 3 cm are easily covered with the intracavitary cone, whereas tumors 3 cm or larger require overlapping of fields and therefore a higher level of technical expertise. The radiotherapeutic doses and techniques of Papillon (1992) were used.

According to the Dijon guidelines, patients with CS T1A tumors can be adequately treated with endocavitary radiation alone. Stages CS T1B and T2A require the combination of endocavitary radiation and interstitial ^{192}Ir brachytherapy, and CS T2B tumors should receive preoperative external-beam therapy followed by, depending on the tumor response, either surgery or endocavitary radiation.

In an update from Maingon et al.[82] of 151 patients treated with this approach, the incidence of initial local control and ultimate local control by stage was 78% and 87% for T1, 58% and 79% for T2, and 54% and 69% for T3, respectively. For the Dijon stage T1 tumors (treated by endocavitary radiation alone), local failure increased with tumor size (13% for 3 cm or smaller vs. 28% for larger than 3 cm).

Nonradical Approaches: Advanced Rectal Cancers

Patients with extensive T2 or transmural (T3) disease are not adequately treated with conservative measures such as local excision, fulguration, cryosurgery, or endocavitary radiation alone. Those selected for radiation therapy alone are usually medically inoperable or have such advanced local disease that resection would compromise a vital structure. In the nonradical setting, a variety of techniques have been used, including various combinations of external-beam, ^{192}Ir interstitial brachytherapy, and endocavitary radiation. Papillon and Berard (1992) have treated 67 patients with T2–3 rectal cancers with pelvic radiation (3 Gy × 10) followed by endocavitary radiation. The 5-year disease free survival rate was 60%. A similar approach was reported by Kodner et al. (1993). Twenty-eight patients with invasive but favorable tumors received 45 Gy followed 6 weeks later by 60 Gy with endocavitary radiation. Favorable tumors were defined as smaller than 3 cm, mobile, well to moderately differentiated, and clinically confined to the rectal wall. No local failures were reported, and the cure rate was 82%. As already discussed, Maingon et al.[82] have recommended the addition of preoperative external-beam radiation or ^{192}Ir brachytherapy for these more advanced tumors.[82]

Although the best results are seen in patients who are able to have radical surgery as a component of their therapy, some patients do not undergo surgery because they are medically inoperable, present with extensive unresectable disease grossly invading bone, have received prior pelvic radiation, or refuse surgery. In general, they have been treated with external-beam radiation with or without chemotherapy. The largest series is from the Princess Margaret Hospital, which reports a 14-month median survival rate and 5% 5-year survival rate in 519 patients.[93] In the subset of patients in whom high doses of radiation are delivered (50 Gy or more), the median survival is 24 months and is 13% at 5 years. Other series report similar results (14% at 3 years[94] and 31% at 2 years[95]); however, they have shorter follow-up and a smaller number of patients. Selected series are seen in Table 33.8-6. In a subset of patients without metastatic disease who received more than 46 Gy, Overgaard and colleagues (1984) reported a 30% 2-year survival rate. A 30% 3-year survival rate was reported by Minsky and associates (1991).

TABLE 33.8-6. Palliative Radiotherapeutic Options (Nonsurgical)

Series	Treatment	Number of Patients	Subset	Median F/U	% Local Failure	% Survival	Definition of Palliation	% Palliation of Those Patients with Symptoms at Presentation					
								Pain	Bleeding	Neurologic	Mass	Discharge	Total
Princess Margaret Hospital[93]	20–60 Gy ± 5-FU	519	Total	—	93% 5-y	5% 5-y	6–8 wk after EBRT	78	68	27	53	44	—
	>45 Gy ± 5-FU	84		—	—	—	6–8 wk after EBRT	89	79	52	71	50	—
	≥50 Gy ± 5-FU	74		—	85% 5-y	13% 5-y		—	—	—	—	—	—
	≥50 Gy ± 5-FU	42	Resectable but refused	—	—	21% 5-y		—	—	—	—	—	—
Thomas Jefferson University[94]	Reirradiation with 30.6 Gy ± %-FU (failed EBRT)	52	Total	16 mo	—	14% 3-y	Complete	65	100	—	24	—	—
							Partial	28	—	—	64	—	—
							Total	93	100	—	88	—	—
							Duration	9 mo	10 mo	—	8 mo	—	—
							Until death	33	100	—	20	—	—
Peter McCallum Cancer Institute[95]	50–60 Gy	39	Radically treated	49 mo	—	31% 2-y	Complete	—	—	—	—	—	33
							Partial	—	—	—	—	—	52
							Total	—	—	—	—	—	85
Centre Hospitalier Lyon Sud[105]	Intracavitary + 39-Gy accelerated EBRT ± brachytherapy	29	Total	46 mo	38%	68% 5-y	—	—	—	—	—	—	—

EBRT, external-beam radiation therapy; 5-FU, 5-fluorouracil; F/U, follow-up.

Pelvic radiation also provides very effective palliation. In the subset of 84 patients who received more than 45 Gy in the series from the Princess Margaret Hospital, the following presenting symptoms were palliated by 6 to 8 weeks after the completion of radiation: pain (89%), bleeding (79%), neurologic (52%), mass effect (71%), discharge (50%), urologic (22%), and other (42%).[93] In the Thomas Jefferson University series, symptomatic relief was achieved in the following categories: pain (65% complete, 28% partial), bleeding (100% complete), and mass effect (24% complete, 64% partial).[94] The duration of palliation was 8 to 10 months.

Even in elderly patients, pelvic radiation offers effective palliation. Valentini et al.[96] delivered combined modality therapy [38 to 45 Gy plus mitomycin C and continuous infusion 5-fluorouracil (5-FU)] to a group of 17 patients with a median age of 79 (range, 75 to 90). Symptomatic relief was obtained in four of four patients with pelvic pain and five of six patients with rectal bleeding. The 18% incidence of grade 3+ toxicity was similar to that reported for the general population who receive preoperative combined modality therapy.

These data suggest that patients with advanced rectal cancers who are medically inoperable should be treated aggressively with pelvic radiation therapy as a component of their therapy. It offers not only a defined cure rate but a high degree of palliation of symptoms.

PATTERNS OF RECURRENCE AFTER RADICAL SURGERY

Despite radical surgery, local-regional failure occurs frequently in patients with transmural or node-positive rectal cancers. The incidence of treatment failure in the pelvis is directly related to the extent of transmural penetration (microscopic vs. gross) and the additive risks of lymph node metastases. Local failure rates as a function of stage are listed in Table 33.8-7. Wound recurrence is rare (0.6%); however, it is a harbinger of metastatic disease.[97]

A major limitation in assessing the true incidence and patterns of failure is the heterogeneity of the series. This is due to variables such as the diagnosis by clinical, surgical, or autopsy criteria; reporting failure as the first site or as total (cumulative) failure; whether local failure includes extrapelvic disease; whether crude or actuarial calculations are used; the technical expertise of the surgeon[98]; and whether patients have received adjuvant therapy. For example, in a series from the Netherlands,[99] 36% of patients received radiation therapy.

Based on a compilation of selected series, the incidence of local failure (as a component of failure) is less than 10% in stage T1–2N0M0; this rate increases to 15% to 35% in stages T3N0M0 and T1N1M0 and is as high as 45% to 65% in stage T3–4N1–2M0.[100–103] When local failure does occur, it is severely debilitating and salvage has been of limited success. Therefore, decreasing local failure is, by itself, an important end point in the treatment of rectal cancer.

TABLE 33.8-7. Local Failure after Surgery Alone for Resectable Rectal Cancer: Selected Single Institution Series

Series	*Definition of Failure*	*Number of Patients*	*Stage*	*Local Failure (%)*[a]
Gunderson and Sosin[102]	Cumulative by reoperation	74	AC B2/C	65 (crude)[b]
Rich et al.[100]	Cumulative by clinical examination and surgery	39	MAC A/B1	8 (crude)
		12	MAC B2m	17
		32	MAC B2m+g	25
		15	MAC B3	53
		4	MAC C1	50
		7	MAC C2m	28
		27	MAC C2m+g	52
		6	MAC C3	67
		142	Total	30
Minsky et al.[101]	First failure by clinical examination and surgery	11	MAC A	11 (5-y actuarial)
		36	MAC B1	3
		60	MAC B2	23
		9	MAC B3	11
		11	MAC C1	14
		31	MAC C2	25
		10	MAC C3	22
		168	Total	15

AC, Astler Coller; MAC, modified Astler Coller.
[a]Includes paraaortic lymph node metastasis.
[b]Local recurrence as a component of failure.

RADIATION THERAPY ALONE FOR RESECTABLE RECTAL CANCER

In most cases, radiation therapy without surgery is limited to patients who are medically inoperable. This section excludes patients amenable to a local excision and adjuvant radiation therapy.

A variety of techniques have been used, including various combinations of external-beam irradiation, ^{192}Ir interstitial brachytherapy, and intracavitary irradiation. In a report from Papillon,[104] 71 patients with clinical T2 or T3 rectal cancers received 3 Gy × 10 to the pelvis. Eight weeks later, an additional 25 Gy was delivered by intracavitary irradiation and 20 to 30 Gy by ^{192}Ir interstitial brachytherapy. The 5-year disease-free survival rate was 65%, and 62% of patients retained normal sphincter function. Although 7% developed anal necrosis, they all healed.

In a report from the Princess Margaret Hospital,[93] 42 patients with early-stage, potentially resectable (T2–3) disease who were either medically inoperable or refused surgery received 50 Gy or more with or without 5-FU and achieved a 5-year survival rate of 21% (see Table 33.8-6). At the Centre Hospitalier Lyon Sud, 29 patients received endocavitary radiation plus 39 Gy of accelerated pelvic radiation with or without brachytherapy.[105] With a median follow-up of 46 months, the local failure rate was 38% and the 5-year survival rate was 68%.

A similar approach was reported by Myerson and coworkers (1989). Thirty patients received 45 Gy followed 6 weeks later by 30 to 90 Gy with intracavitary irradiation. Their tumors were defined as larger than 3 cm, nonmobile, well- or moderately well-differentiated, and clinical stage T2 or pathologic stage

T3. Deeply ulcerated or infiltrating tumors were excluded. With a median follow-up of 2 years, the local failure rate was 30%, and the 2-year disease-free survival rate was 42% (55% with salvage). Minor proctitis occurred in 17%.

As recommended for patients with advanced disease, patients with clinically resectable but medically inoperable disease should be treated aggressively with radiation therapy as a component of their therapy.

ADJUVANT THERAPY AND SPHINCTER-SAVING OPERATIONS AS AN ALTERNATIVE TO ABDOMINOPERINEAL RESECTION

Conservative management (sphincter preservation) has been used in two broad groups of patients with distal rectal cancer as an alternative to APR. The first are early localized tumors. In general, these include small, exophytic, mobile tumors without adverse pathologic factors [i.e., high grade, BVI, lymphatic vessel invasion (LVI), colloid histology, or the penetration of tumor into or through the bowel wall].[106] These selected tumors comprise 3% to 5% of all rectal cancers and are adequately treated with a variety of local therapies alone.

The second group of patients includes those tumors that otherwise would be suitable for one of the above local therapies except for (1) invasion of tumor into or through the muscularis propria, (2) positive lymph nodes, or (3) the presence of one or more adverse clinical or pathologic factors. In the context of conservative management, these tumors are considered unfavorable, because local therapy alone is not adequate treatment.

LOCAL EXCISION AND POSTOPERATIVE RADIATION THERAPY

The standard surgical treatment for resectable, transmural, or node-positive rectal cancer is an LAR or APR. If the pathology confirms that the tumor penetrates through the bowel wall or involves the mesorectal or pelvic lymph nodes, adjuvant combined modality therapy consisting of six cycles of 5-FU–based chemotherapy plus concurrent pelvic radiation therapy is recommended.[107]

Given the morbidity of standard surgery as well as the frequent need for adjuvant therapy, the use of a more conservative approach, such as local excision plus adjuvant therapy (radiation therapy with or without chemotherapy), as primary therapy for selected cases of rectal cancer is appealing. This approach has been successful in other anatomic sites, such as in breast cancer and sarcomas of the extremities. In the rectum, it offers an opportunity for sphincter preservation.

The results of local excision and postoperative therapy depend on a number of factors, such as the type of surgery (full-thickness vs. piecemeal excision), and clinicopathologic factors, such as tumor size, T stage, grade, margins, and LVI. Most series include some patients who have undergone suboptimal surgery, such as a piecemeal excision, or have positive or unassessable margins.[108] Because few of the published series have adequate numbers to perform a meaningful multivariate analysis, it is difficult to determine the influence of these selected clinicopathologic features on one another. Until more complete data are available, a patient should not be excluded from treatment with local excision and radiation therapy based solely on these clinicopathologic features.

Local excision has been performed both before and after radiation therapy. The advantage of performing a local excision before radiation is that pathologic details, such as margins, depth of bowel wall penetration, and histologic features, can be well characterized.[108,109] Knowledge of these details are useful in the development of selection criteria.

SELECTION CRITERIA

To determine which tumors have a high enough incidence of local failure or positive mesorectal or pelvic lymph nodes to require adjuvant pelvic radiation, it first must be determined which tumors are adequately treated with local therapy alone. The selection of tumors for local therapy is based on both clinical and pathologic factors. Clinical information such as tumor size, mobility, location, and circumference can be obtained at the time of physical examination. Accurate pathologic information is more difficult to obtain from a biopsy. Of the available local therapies, only a full-thickness local excision provides accurate pathologic information.

Clinical

A major limitation of the series that examine local excision alone is that the analyses are univariate rather than multivariate. Therefore, clinical and pathologic factors are not examined as independent variables. Furthermore, variation is seen in patient selection, the definition of clinical and pathologic features, and the length of follow-up among the series. Because of these differences, it is difficult to make firm recommendations for the selection of patients for conservative management based solely on clinical criteria. The most reasonable approach is to determine whether a local excision can be performed adequately (i.e., full thickness, nonfragmented, and with negative margins). If so, then the clinical criteria for a local excision have been met.

Pathologic

Pathologic criteria are more objective. Patients with T1 tumors without adverse pathologic factors have a low enough incidence of local failure (5% to 10%) and positive nodes (less than 10%) that they do not require adjuvant therapy. However, once adverse pathologic factors are present (high grade, BVI, LVI, colloid histology, signet-ring cell).[110,111] or the tumor invades into or through the muscularis propria,[31,110] the local failure rate is at least 17% and the incidence of positive mesorectal or pelvic nodes is at least 10% to 15%. Biggers et al.[31] reported the results of 141 patients with T2 rectal cancers who underwent local excision alone at the Mayo Clinic. Blumberg and associates[112] found positive nodes in 10% of T1 and 17% of T2 cancers. In the combined group of 159 patients, the incidence increased with the presence of LVI (14% for LVI vs. 33% for LVI-positive). Even in the 42 patients with the most favorable characteristics (well or moderately differentiated, LVI-negative, T1 cancers), 7% had positive nodes. The 5-year survival rate was 65% and the local failure rate was 27%. Hager and colleagues (1983) performed a local excision on 20 patients with T2 rectal cancers that were otherwise "low risk" (nonmucinous, well to moderately differentiated, no LVI, with negative margins). The incidence of local failure was still 17%. Other series have reported local failure rates as high as 43% in patients with T2 cancers after either local excision or transanal excision.[113]

Willett et al.[110] reported a group of 40 patients who underwent local excision alone at the Massachusetts General Hospital (MGH). In this series, a separate analysis was performed on those patients whose tumors had unfavorable clinical and pathologic factors. Factors including tumor size larger than 3 cm, high grade, T2 stage or higher, vascular invasion (BVI and/or LVI), moderate or marked stromal fibrosis, a fragmented resection, and positive margins were associated with a local failure rate of at least 20% as well as an increase in distant metastasis. Therefore, local therapy alone is inadequate for tumors with these adverse pathologic factors.

An alternative approach to pathologically determine the incidence of positive pararectal lymph nodes is ultrasound-guided biopsy. Milsom and colleagues[114] from the Cleveland Clinic performed biopsies on 26 patients and reported an accuracy rate of 77%, with a sensitivity of 71%, a specificity of 89%, a positive predictive value of 92%, and a negative predictive value of 62%.

RESULTS

Results Compared with Radical Surgery

Because the pelvic lymph nodes are not pathologically examined at the time of a local excision, it is not possible to accurately compare, stage for stage, the results of this approach with radical surgery.

Although data exist to help predict the incidence of positive pelvic nodes based on the clinical and pathologic features of the primary tumor,[69,115] an accurate comparison of this approach with standard surgery requires a randomized trial. Most series select patients for adjuvant therapy based on the presence of unfavorable clinical or pathologic features, or both. In the series from the University of Florida,[116] for example, patients had at least one or more of the following adverse features: equivocal, close, or positive margins; T2–3 disease; perineural invasion; and had undergone a fragmented excision. Likewise in the MGH series,[117] 38 of the 47 patients had T2 or high-risk T1 cancers (poorly differentiated and/or LVI).

Survival

As seen in Table 33.8-8, the 5-year actuarial survival in these selected series is approximately 80% (range, 70% to 94%).[32,116–124] In most series, patients had T1–3 tumors and underwent a local excision followed 4 to 6 weeks later by 45 to 50 Gy to the pelvis. Some patients received an external-beam or brachytherapy boost. In most series, a limited number of patients received 5-FU. Although not randomized, these survival data appear comparable with the results of radical surgery alone for stage T1–2N0 disease.

The Intergroup Cancer and Leukemia Group B 8984 trial is the only prospective, multiinstitutional phase II trial. Patients underwent a local excision with careful assessment of negative margins and, depending on T stage, received postoperative combined modality therapy.[125] A total of 110 eligible patients (all with negative margins) were entered. The 51 patients with T2 disease received postoperative combined modality therapy.

TABLE 33.8-8. Local Excision plus Postoperative Therapy: Survival, Salvage, and Functional Results: Selected Series

Series	*Number of Patients*	*% T3*	*% 5-FU*	*Survival*	*Function*	*Local Failures Salvaged with APR*
University of Florida[116]	45	2	4	88% cause specific	—	One of five salvaged
Beth Israel Deaconess Medical Center[116]	48	10	54	94% crude	—	Three of four salvaged
M. D. Anderson Cancer Center[119]	46	33	17	—	All continent	—
University of Pennsylvania[32]	16	32	0	94% 3-y actuarial; 77% 3-y colostomy free	92% satisfactory	Two of two salvaged
Massachusetts General Hospital[117]	47	0	55	74% 5-y disease free	—	Of 14 failures, five of nine salvaged
Catholic University[123]	21	0	0	81% 5-y actuarial	100% good to excellent[a]	One of two salvaged
Fox Chase[124]	21	19	10	77% 5-y actuarial	82% good to excellent	Three of four salvaged
CALGB[125]	51[b]	0	100	85% 6-y actuarial	—	Four of seven salvaged
Memorial Sloan-Kettering Cancer Center[120]	39	21	51	70% 5-y actuarial; 87% colostomy free	94% good to excellent[a]	Of eight failures, five of eight salvaged
Vancouver[122]	23	9	0	81% 5-y disease free; 77% cause specific	—	Three of seven salvaged

APR, abdominoperineal resection; CALGB, Cancer and Leukemia Group B; 5-FU, 5-fluorouracil.
[a]Memorial Sloan-Kettering Cancer Center Sphincter Function Scale.
[b]Analysis is limited to the 51 of 110 patients (all with T2 disease) who underwent a local excision and received postoperative radiation therapy plus chemotherapy.

TABLE 33.8-9. Local Excision plus Postoperative Therapy: Local Recurrence by T Stage: Selected Series

		Local Failure by T Stage			
Series	*Follow-Up (mo)*	T1	T2	T3	Total
University of Florida[116]	24 minimum	—	—	—	11% (5/45) crude[a]; 14% 5-y actuarial
Beth Israel Deaconess Medical Center[118]	41 mean		0% (0/21)	—	0% (0/21)
M. D. Anderson Cancer Center[119]	36 median	0% (0/16)	7% (1/15)	20% (3/15)	9% (4/46)
University of Pennsylvania[32]	33 median	0% (0/2)	22% (2/9)	0% (0/5)	13% (2/16)
Massachusetts General Hospital[117]	51 median	0% (0/14)	15% (5/33) crude; 15% 5-y actuarial	—	11% (5/47) crude; 10% 5-y actuarial
Catholic University[123]	54 median	11% (1/9)	17% (2/12)	—	14% (3/21)
Fox Chase[124]	56 median	50% (1/2)	13% (2/15)	25% (1/4)	19% (4/21)
CALGB[125]	48 median	—	14% (7/51)	—	14% (7/51)[b]
Memorial Sloan-Kettering Cancer Center[120]	41 median	0% (0/6)	24% (6/25); 31% 5-y actuarial	25% (2/8)	21% (8/39); 27% 5-y actuarial
Vancouver[122]	52 median	8% (1/12)	11% (1/9)	50% (1/2)	13% (3/23)
Total	—	5% (3/61)	14% (26/190)	22% (8/37)	12% (41/330)

CALGB, Cancer and Leukemia Group B.
[a]Data were not reported by T stage.
[b]Analysis is limited to the 51 patients who underwent a local excision and received postoperative radiation therapy plus chemotherapy.

With a median follow-up of 48 months, the crude local failure rate was 14%, the 6-year failure-free survival rate was 71%, and overall survival was 85%. This approach is feasible in a multiinstitutional, cooperative group setting.

Local Failure

When the series are combined, the average crude local failure rate increases with T stage: 5% for T1, 14% for T2, and 22% for T3 (Table 33.8-9). When the series are combined, the crude incidence is 12% and increases with the percentage of T3 cancers included in each series.

Actuarial analysis is an alternative method of determining the risk of local failure. The actuarial method, which accounts for the different length of follow-up for each patient, offers the most accurate method of risk analysis. As with crude failure, the incidence of actuarial failure increases with increasing T stage. It was 10% in the series of T1–2 cancers from the MGH,[117] 14% from the University of Florida series in which only 2% of patients had T3 cancers,[116] and 27% in the Memorial Sloan-Kettering Cancer Center series in which 21% of patients had T3 cancers.[120]

The impact of positive margins on local failure is unclear. In the Memorial Sloan-Kettering series, for the total patient group, 5-year actuarial local failure was higher in patients with positive versus negative margins (35% vs. 23%).[120] A similar increase in crude local failure rates was reported in the Vancouver series (40% vs. 6%).[122] In contrast, no significant differences were reported in the series from Fox Chase Cancer Center[124] or the MGH.[117] In the MGH series, this lack of difference may have been related to a higher radiation dose delivered to that subset. Of the six patients with positive margins (none of whom developed local failure), five of the six received doses of more than 60 Gy.

A full-thickness local excision is recommended because patients who undergo a piecemeal excision usually have higher local failure rates.[126]

In those patients who do undergo a full-thickness excision, the impact of positive margins is unclear. Most investigators would recommend that negative margins be obtained if technically feasible and a reexcision performed if needed, providing that it does not compromise sphincter function. If this is not possible, doses of more than 50.4 Gy, if the small bowel is excluded from the high-dose field, are probably necessary.

In patients who undergo radical surgery for rectal cancer, 80% of local recurrences occur within the first 2 years. In contrast, the Memorial Sloan-Kettering series[120] has reported local failures at 48 months, and the MGH series[117] has reported local failures as late as 64, 72, 86, and 91 months. Furthermore, in the MGH series the median time to local recurrence was 55 months compared with 14 months in a group of 52 patients with more favorable prognostic factors who underwent local excision alone. Therefore, patients who are treated with local excision and postoperative adjuvant therapy require close follow-up beyond 5 years.

On a positive note, most local failures occur at the anastomotic site and not in pelvic lymph nodes. Of the 18 local failures reported in the MGH series, only one involved the pelvic nodes. None were seen in the series from the University of Pennsylvania[32] and Catholic University.[123] Furthermore, salvage of local failures is possible. With the exception of the University of Florida experience, in which only one of five local failures could be salvaged with an APR, most series report that at least one-half of the patients who undergo a salvage APR can be cured: Beth Israel Deaconess Medical Center reported three cures out of four[118]; University of Pennsylvania, two of two[32]; Memorial Sloan-Kettering Cancer Center, five of eight[120]; Vancouver, three of seven[122]; Catholic University, one of two[123]; Fox Chase, three of four[124]; Intergroup trial, four of seven[125]; and MGH, five of nine.[117]

Sphincter Function

However, a few series prospectively assess functional results. As seen in Table 33.8-8, the five series that do measure sphincter function report favorable outcomes. Both the Memorial Sloan-Kettering[120] and Catholic University[123] series use the previously published Memorial Sloan-Kettering Sphincter Function Scale.[127] They report 94% and 100% good to excellent function, respectively. Using a different scale, investigators from Fox Chase Cancer Center[124] reported 82% good to excellent function, the University of Pennsylvania[32] reported 92% satisfactory function,[32] and the M. D. Anderson Cancer Center[119] reported that all patients were continent.

Chemotherapy

Limited data are available on the use of chemotherapy in patients who undergo local excision and postoperative radiation therapy. In most series, 5-FU was delivered as a radiosensitizer rather than in the adjuvant setting. In a subgroup analysis, the MGH reported a lower 5-year actuarial local failure rate (4% vs. 19%, *P* = NS) but at the same time a lower relapse-free survival rate (67% vs. 81%, *P* = NS) in patients receiving 5-FU–based combined modality therapy versus radiation alone.[117] Because the numbers are limited and the data are not stratified by T stage, the impact of chemotherapy is unclear. However, given the positive impact of chemotherapy on local control and survival in patients with resectable rectal cancer reported in the randomized postoperative rectal adjuvant trials,[128] all patients should receive two cycles of 5-FU–based therapy concurrently with radiation. For patients with T2–3 disease in whom the incidence of pelvic lymph nodes is at least 20%, an additional four cycles of adjuvant chemotherapy for a total of six cycles is recommended.

Summary

The data suggest that the approach of local excision and postoperative radiation is a reasonable alternative to radical surgery in selected patients. It should be limited to patients with either T2 tumors, or T1 tumors with adverse pathologic factors (poorly differentiated and/or LVI). Although the local failure rates are approximately double those reported with radical surgery, one-half of the failures can be salvaged with an APR without an apparent detriment to overall survival. Functional results are generally good to excellent. Transmural (T3) tumors have a 25% local failure rate and are treated more effectively with radical surgery and pre- or postoperative therapy. The results of local excision and postoperative radiation therapy are encouraging; however, randomized trials are needed to determine if this approach ultimately has similar local control and survival rates as radical surgery.

PREOPERATIVE RADIATION THERAPY FOLLOWED BY SURGERY

Sphincter preservation is a major goal of preoperative therapy. A number of preoperative treatment approaches have been used, and their selection depends on factors such as tumor histology, size, location, mobility, and anatomic constraints, and the technical expertise of the surgical, radiation, and medical oncologists.

An analysis of 1316 patients treated in two previously published Scandinavian trials of intensive short course radiation reveals that down-staging is most pronounced when the interval between the completion of radiation and surgery is at least 10 days.[129] However, none of the randomized trials of intensive short course preoperative radiation address whether the degree of down-staging is adequate to enhance sphincter preservation.

From the viewpoint of sphincter preservation, the advantage of preoperative therapy is to decrease the volume of the primary tumor. When the tumor is located in close proximity to the dentate line, this decrease in tumor volume may allow the surgeon to perform a sphincter-preserving procedure that would not otherwise be possible. However, patients whose tumors directly invade the anal sphincter are unlikely to undergo sphincter preservation, even after a complete response to radiation therapy.

In general, when sphincter preservation is the goal of therapy, the use of preoperative therapy should be limited to patients who are not technically able to undergo a local excision because of tumor size or anatomic constraints. For example, if the tumor is close to the anal sphincter, a full-thickness local excision with negative margins may require partial removal of the sphincter, resulting in compromised sphincter function.

Two surgical approaches have been used after preoperative pelvic radiation: local excision and LAR plus CAA. To assist in the choice of the surgical procedure, some investigators have used transrectal ultrasound for restaging after the completion of preoperative therapy. However, most series reveal that post-treatment staging is only of modest accuracy. Williamson and colleagues[130] reported that, in 15 patients who completed preoperative combined modality therapy, 38% were down-staged by transrectal ultrasound. At pathology, T stage was down-staged in 47% and N stage in 88%. Another series found that, in 25 patients who received preoperative radiation, digital rectal examination, CT, and transrectal ultrasound accurately staged only 24%, 23%, and 17%, respectively, of the primary tumors that were stage T0 at pathology.[28] Bernini and associates[30] found transrectal ultrasound correctly predicted the T and N stage in 62% and 76%, respectively. In another series, the accuracy of transrectal ultrasound was 93% for T stage, but only 61% for N stage.[131] Newer techniques, such as color Doppler flow[132] and intracavitary MRI coils[133] and PET,[134–136] are being investigated. In a comparative study of 89 patients, the accuracy of predicting T stage and N stage preoperatively was 81% and 84% with transrectal ultrasound, 65% and 57% with CT, and 81% and 63% with an MRI endorectal coil, respectively.[137]

LOCAL EXCISION

The results of 25 patients who received 34.95 Gy at 2.33 Gy per fraction to a partial pelvic field followed in 6 to 8 weeks by a transanal or transsphincteric local excision and a 20- to 25-Gy boost with afterloading ^{192}Ir was reported by Otmezguine et al.[138] The median tumor size was 4 cm, 80% were exophytic, 72% were well to moderately differentiated, and all were mobile. With a mean follow-up of 41 months, the local failure rate was 20%, and three of the five failures were salvaged with an APR. Of the six patients with positive margins, two developed local failure. The 20 patients with local control had "normal" sphincter function.

In a report by Mohiuddin et al.,[139] 48 selected patients who met specific criteria [group I, T3 and medically unsuitable for a LAR (n = 15); group II, <T2 and <3 cm suitable for a local excision (n = 18); or group III, T3 or >3 cm down-staged with preoperative radiation to <T2 and <3 cm] underwent a local

TABLE 33.8-10. Results of Preoperative Therapy in Patients Prospectively Declared to Require an Abdominoperineal Resection (APR)

	Wagman et al.[145] *(MSKCC)*	*Grann et al.*[146] *(MSKCC)*	*Rouanet et al.*[147] *(Montpellier)*	*Hyams et al.*[141] *(NSABP R-03)*	*Maghfoor et al.*[148] *(Ellis Fischel)*	*Valentini et al.*[149] *(Catholic University)*	*Francois et al.*[52] *(Lyon R90-01)*
Number of patients enrolled	36	32	37	59	29	83	201
Number declared to need an APR	36	20	37	22	29	47	34[a]
Number who underwent surgery	35	20	27	22	29	81	34
Number with T3 disease	31 (86%)	20 (100%)	12 (32%)	22 (100%)	25 (86%)	83 (100%)	62%
Number who underwent LAR ± coloanal anastomosis	27 (77%)	17 (85%)	17 (63%)[b]	16 (23%)	22 (76%)	31 (66%)	15 (44%)
% Local failure	17	0	8	NA	3	10	12
% Survival	64 5-y	100 2-y	83 2-y	NA	87[c]	72 5-y	75 3-y
Number evaluable for sphincter Function analysis	27 (77%)	NA	14 (52%)	NA	NA	63	82[d]
Sphincter function	85% good to excellent	NA	71% perfect	NA	NA	6% moderate soilage	78% normal

LAR, low anterior resection; MSKCC, Memorial Sloan-Kettering Cancer Center; NA, data not reported in the manuscript; NSABP, National Surgical Adjuvant Breast Project.
[a]Limited to the subset of 34 patients (out of a total of 201) randomized to either arm who were declared to need an APR.
[b]Fifteen percent underwent a local excision; therefore, 78% had sphincter preservation.
[c]Disease-free survival with a median follow-up of 12 months.
[d]Includes all patients in the trial who underwent sphincter preservation.

excision after 45 to 55 Gy. With a median follow-up of 40 months, the 5-year actuarial survival rate was 84% and the local failure rate was 10%. Local failure by group was 20% for group I, 11% for group II, and 0% for group III. Postoperative wound complications were seen in 10%, and four patients required a subsequent colostomy (three for local failure). Sphincter function was good to excellent in 88% of patients with an intact rectum. In an update of 44 patients with tumors of 3 cm or smaller from the dentate line selected to undergo a local excision after preoperative radiation therapy, the local failure rate was 14% and the 5-year survival rate was 90%.[140]

LOW ANTERIOR RESECTION AND COLOANAL ANASTOMOSIS

PREOPERATIVE PROSPECTIVE CLINICAL ASSESSMENT

The most accurate method by which to determine if preoperative therapy has contributed to sphincter preservation is to perform a prospective clinical assessment. This requires that the operating surgeon examines the patient before the start of preoperative therapy and declares the type of operation required. It should be noted that this assessment is based on an office examination and may not accurately reflect the assessment when the patient is relaxed under general anesthesia. The only method by which to account for this potential bias is a randomized trial of preoperative versus postoperative therapy. With this randomized design, the accuracy of the assessment could be determined, because one-half of the patients are randomized to undergo surgery before postoperative therapy.

An interval analysis of the first 116 patients enrolled on the National Surgical Adjuvant Breast Project (NSABP) R-03 randomized trial of preoperative versus postoperative combined modality therapy has been reported by Hyams and colleagues[141] (Table 33.8-10). Because one-half of the patients were randomized to undergo surgery before the postoperative therapy, the accuracy of the office assessment to predict the type of operation required could be determined. Of the 57 patients randomized to the postoperative combined modality arm, 26 were declared clinically to require an APR and all 26 patients underwent the procedure. Therefore, the data suggest that the office assessment is an accurate method by which to predict the type of operation required. The incidence of postoperative complications was similar in the preoperative and postoperative arms (33% and 30%, respectively). The results from this report should be considered preliminary, because the trial was still open to accrual at the time of the analysis.

SURGICAL ISSUES IN COLOANAL ANASTOMOSIS

Careful surgical techniques must be used when performing a CAA after preoperative therapy. To perform the anastomosis with unirradiated bowel, the splenic flexure must be mobilized. To enhance anastomotic healing, a diverting colostomy should be performed and is closed 2 to 4 months postoperatively. For example, in the R90-01 trial of preoperative radiation therapy, patients received 3 Gy × 13 and were randomized to either a short interval (2 weeks) or a long interval (6 to 8 weeks) between the end of radiation and surgery.[52] Of the total of 144 patients who underwent a sphincter-preserving operation, 57 had a temporary diverting colostomy. The incidence of anastomotic complications requiring surgery was 5% in that group compared with 23% in the 87 patients who did not undergo the temporary diverting colostomy.

TECHNICAL ASPECTS OF PREOPERATIVE RADIATION THERAPY

If the goal of preoperative therapy is sphincter preservation, conventional doses and techniques of radiation are recommended. These include multiple-field techniques to a total dose of 45.0 to 50.4 Gy at 1.8 Gy per fraction. Surgery should be performed 4 to 6 weeks after the completion of radiation. This design allows for recovery from the acute side effects of radiation and enhances tumor down-staging.

Since the publication of the Swedish Rectal Cancer Trial,[142] which revealed a significant improvement in survival with intensive short course preoperative radiation, some physicians have advocated this alternative approach. Typically, the intensive short course includes 25 Gy in five fractions followed by surgery 1 week later. Not only are these treatment programs associated with increased surgical morbidity and mortality,[143,144] but by virtue of their design, they do not enhance sphincter preservation. Therefore, they should be used with great caution.

CLINICAL EXPERIENCE

A total of seven series have reported results in patients with clinically resectable, invasive rectal cancer (T2–3 or T4 tethered to the vagina) who underwent a prospective clinical assessment by their surgeon before the start of preoperative therapy and were declared to need an APR (see Table 33.8-10). All use conventional radiation techniques and, with the exception of the R90-01 trial which used 3-Gy fractions, the remainder used standard radiation doses (1.8 to 2.0 Gy per fraction). Two of the series are from Memorial Sloan-Kettering Cancer Center. The initial approach to sphincter preservation at Memorial Sloan-Kettering was preoperative radiation therapy alone, and the results of this prospective phase I/II trial have been reported by Wagman et al.[145] The current approach at Memorial Sloan-Kettering is preoperative combined modality therapy, which has been reported by Grann and associates.[146] Preoperative radiation therapy (without chemotherapy) was reported by Rouanet et al.[147] from the Montpellier Cancer Institute and by Francois and associates[52] from the Lyon R90-01 trial. The other three trials used combined modality therapy. Hyams and colleagues[141] reported an interval analysis of the ongoing NSABP R-03 phase III randomized trial of preoperative versus postoperative combined modality therapy. The remaining trials were reported by Maghfoor and colleagues[148] from Ellis Fischel Cancer Center and Valentini et al.[149] from the Catholic University in Rome.

Other series have been conducted in which patients receive preoperative radiation therapy followed by sphincter preservation. In the series from Papillon and Gerard[150] from the Centre Leon Berard, patients did not undergo a prospective clinical assessment by their surgeon, and therefore, the impact of preoperative radiation therapy on enhancing sphincter preservation cannot be determined. Thomas Jefferson University[151] has a large experience with preoperative radiation therapy. In tumors located in the distal 2 cm of the rectum, preoperative radiation therapy allowed sphincter preservation in 91% of patients, 86% of whom had "satisfactory" functional results. Because this trial included patients with early (T1) as well as unresectable (T4) disease, the results are not comparable to the other series.

As seen in Table 33.8-10, sphincter-preservation rates were only 23% in the interim analysis of the NSABP R-03 trial and 44% in the R90-01 trial, whereas the other five trials report that approximately 75% of patients are able to undergo sphincter preservation after preoperative therapy. Local failure rates vary from 0% to 17%, and survival rates range from 100% at 2 years to 72% at 5 years. Four series report functional outcome. Wagman et al. and Valentini et al. both use the Memorial Sloan-Kettering Cancer Center Sphincter Function Scale.[152] The R90-01 trial defines normal function as a patient without soiling or requiring pads. The Montpellier series does not define "perfect" function.

One series has reported that the detrimental effect on sphincter function associated with postoperative therapy[153,154] may not be as problematic with preoperative therapy. The short-term[155] and long-term[156] impact of preoperative radiation therapy on sphincter function has been examined by Birnbaum and colleagues. Patients received conventional doses and techniques of radiation and were assessed objectively by anal manometry with or without transrectal ultrasound. In the 20 patients assessed for short-term results and the ten patients assessed for long-term results, radiation therapy had a "minimal" effect on sphincter function.

The results of the R90-01 trial support the advantage of a longer interval (at least 4 weeks) between the completion of radiation and surgery.[52] A total of 201 eligible patients were randomized to either a short interval (2 weeks) or a long interval (6 to 8 weeks). Patients randomized to the long interval had a significantly higher incidence of clinical complete response (pathologic complete response and/or a few residual foci of cells; 26% vs. 10%, respectively; $P = .0054$), with no increase in operative morbidity.

In summary, five of the seven trials suggest that preoperative therapy allows sphincter preservation in approximately 75% of patients judged clinically to require an APR. The majority have good to excellent functional results. Given the suggestion of decreased acute toxicity and enhanced sphincter preservation with preoperative radiation therapy, three randomized trials of conventional dose preoperative versus postoperative combined modality therapy for clinically resectable, T3 rectal cancer have been developed. Two are from the United States (INT 0147, NSABP R-03) and one from Germany (CAO/ARO/AIO 94). All three use conventional doses and techniques of radiation therapy and concurrent 5-FU–based chemotherapy, and they require a preoperative clinical assessment declaring the type of operation required. However, low accrual resulted in the early closure of the INT 0147 trial and may jeopardize the NSABP R-03 trial as well. The German trial continues to accrue patients and should help provide an answer to the relative effectiveness of preoperative versus postoperative therapy and its ability to enhance sphincter preservation.

TREATMENT RECOMMENDATIONS

For patients with clinically resectable disease, the preoperative approach should be used in situations in which sphincter-preserving surgery is not technically possible at initial presentation. The decision of whether to use preoperative radiation therapy or preoperative combined modality therapy is based on the results of transrectal ultrasound. If a transrectal ultrasound reveals T2 disease, the patient may have pathologic T2N0M0 disease; therefore, the sole reason for the preoperative therapy is to convert the operation from an APR to an LAR plus CAA. In this setting, preoperative radiation therapy alone is recommended. If positive mesorectal or pelvic lymph nodes are identified at the time of surgery, the patient should receive 6 months of adjuvant postoperative 5-FU–based chemotherapy. Two potential disadvantages are associated with this approach. First, the ultrasound may under-stage approximately 10% of patients who have pathologic stage T3 disease. Second, because preoperative radiation down-stages pelvic lymph nodes by approximately 50%, the true incidence of node-positive disease is unknown, and some node-positive patients may not receive chemotherapy. Obviously, these disadvantages need to be weighed against the risk of overtreating these patients with combined modality therapy.

For patients with transrectal ultrasound stage T3 disease, preoperative combined modality therapy followed by surgery and postoperative 5-FU–based chemotherapy is recommended. This approach is based on extrapolation of the significant improvement in local control and survival in patients with T3 or N1–3 disease who receive adjuvant postoperative combined modality therapy. Whether preoperative combined modality therapy is more effective than preoperative radiation therapy is unknown. An ongoing randomized trial from the European Organization for Research and Treatment of Cancer (EORTC) will address this question.

At the present time, the most common preoperative combined modality therapy regimens include 45.0 to 50.4 Gy of pelvic radiation at 1.8 Gy per fraction plus concurrent bolus 5-FU plus leucovorin[146,157] or continuous infusion 5-FU.[158,159] Some have advocated 5-FU plus mitomycin C, which is more commonly used in the treatment of anal cancer.[149] One trial using neoadjuvant 5-FU plus methotrexate followed by continuous infusion 5-FU plus concurrent radiation did not report a benefit compared with conventional 5-FU plus leucovorin.[160] Phase I/II trials are in progress combining new systemic chemotherapeutic agents, such as raltitrexed (Tomudex),[161,162] Orzel (oral tegafur, uracil, and 5-fluorouracil plus leucovorin),[163] CPT-11,[164,165] and oxaliplatin, with preoperative radiation therapy. Whether any of these combinations will be more effective than 5-FU–based therapy remains to be determined.

ADJUVANT RADIATION THERAPY FOR RESECTABLE RECTAL CANCER

The rationale of radiation therapy is based on the patterns of failure after potentially curative surgery (see Table 33.8-7). The incidence of local failure as a component of failure is less than 10% in stages T1–2N0M0; the incidence increases to 15% to 35% in stage T3N0M0 and is as high as 45% to 65% in stages T3–4N1–2M0.[100–102] When local failure does occur, it is severely debilitating and salvage has been of limited success. In 1936, Daland et al. (1936) stated that the morbidity associated with local failure is often devastating, and as many as 68% of patients have one or more pelvic symptoms, including infection, ulceration, obstruction, and intractable pain for 9 to 12 months before death. The same holds true today. Therefore, even

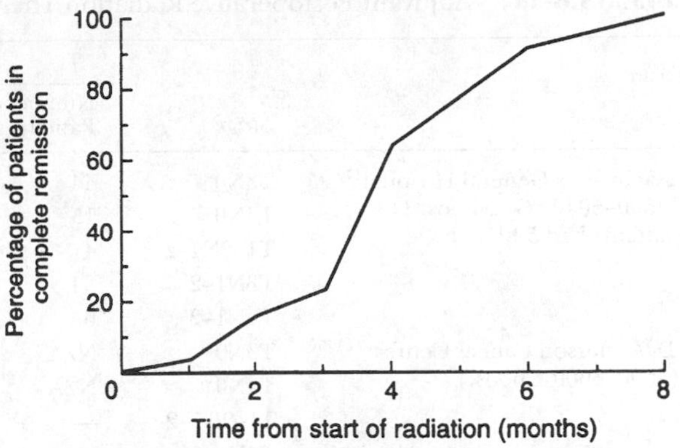

FIGURE 33.8-5. Time to a complete response from the start of treatment for 66 patients with inoperable rectal cancer who received radiation therapy alone and achieved a clinical complete response. (From Brierley JD, Cummings BJ, Wong CS, et al. Adenocarcinoma of the rectum treated by radical external radiation therapy. *Int J Radiat Oncol Biol Phys* 1995:31:255, with permission.)

though it does not increase survival, the ability of radiation therapy to decrease local failure is, by itself, an important end point.

For unsubstantiated reasons, some consider colorectal adenocarcinomas to be radioresistant. This assumption has been based on the observation that these tumors do not respond as rapidly to radiation as other histologies. The radioresistant theory was disproved in 1965 by Suit et al. (1965), who showed that the rapidity of tumor response to radiation is not an accurate reflection of their curability. Brierley et al. (1995) reported the results of 66 patients with rectal cancer treated with radiation therapy alone. As seen in Figure 33.8-5, of the patients who achieved a complete response to radiation therapy, only 60% had achieved the complete response by 4 months.

Some physicians contend that adjuvant therapy is not necessary if patients undergo resection with a total mesorectal excision. In one series, total mesorectal excision, which involves sharp dissection around the integral mesentery of the hindgut, decreased the local recurrence rate to 5%.[85] These data must be interpreted with caution for a number of reasons. First is selection bias. This operation allows the identification and exclusion of patients with more advanced disease as compared with patients treated in the adjuvant trials in which more conventional surgery is performed. Second, some patients with T3 or N1–2 disease received radiation therapy with or without chemotherapy (i.e., 18% in the series by Haas-Kock et al.,[166] 28% in the series from Enker and associates,[86] and 58% in the series from Arenas et al.[167]). In a combined analysis of 1411 patients from five international centers, an undisclosed number received adjuvant radiation or combined modality therapy.[47] Third, some series (i.e., Aitken et al.[168]) exclude operative deaths. Lastly, total mesorectal excision may also be associated with higher complication rates. In the Basingstoke Hospital experience reported by Carlsen and colleagues,[169] the anastomotic leak rate was 16% in patients who underwent total mesorectal excision (all of whom required hospitalization) compared with a leak rate of 8% in a similar group of patients who underwent conventional surgery (with only 25% requiring hospitalization). Poon and colleagues[170] recommend the creation of a diverting stoma to decrease the high leak rate with total mesorectal excision.

TABLE 33.8-11. Adjuvant Postoperative Radiation Therapy for Resectable Rectal Cancer: Selected Nonrandomized Trials

		Local Failure (%)[a]				*5-Y Survival (%)*	
Series	*Stage*	Number of Patients	Surgery	Number of Patients	Surgery + Radiation	Surgery	Surgery + Radiation
Massachusetts General Hospital[172] [4500–5040 cGy ± boost (14 patients had 5-FU)]	T3N0	44	23	53	9	47	76 (NED)
	T4N0	15	53	7	0	27	69
	T1–2N1–2	4	50	10	20	25	69
	T3N1–2	34	17	77	21	27	34
	T4N1–2	6	67	15	53	0	1
M. D. Anderson Cancer Center[174,175] (4000–5000 ± boost)	T3N0	N/A	13	24	4	—	65
	T4N0	N/A	26	13	21	—	48
	T1–2N1–2	—	—	12	8	—	65
	T3N1–2	N/A	30	45	18	—	48
	T4N1–2	N/A	49	5	20	—	60

5-FU, 5-fluorouracil; N/A, data not available in the manuscript; NED, no evidence of disease.
[a]Cumulative local failure as a component of failure.

The Dutch CKVO 95-04 trial examines the role of intensive short course preoperative radiation therapy in patients who undergo a total mesorectal excision. Patients are randomized to an intensive short course of radiation (5 Gy × 5) versus surgery alone. Postoperative radiation, which is performed with conventional doses, is reserved for patients in the surgery-only arm who do not undergo a curative resection. Investigator participation is limited to surgeons who have demonstrated proficiency in performing a total mesorectal excision. The trial is open to accrual.

Dahlberg and colleagues[50] report a 3% local failure rate in patients with resectable rectal cancer with the combination of total mesorectal excision and intensive short course preoperative radiation. Because patients with clinical stage T1–3 disease were included, it is difficult to compare these results with series that are limited to T3 disease.

The use of total mesorectal excision has increased awareness of the importance of surgical technique. Careful surgical techniques are central to the successful management of rectal cancer. However, they should be considered a valuable component of therapy, not competitive with adjuvant therapy. Given the selection bias, higher complication rates in some series, and the fact that adjuvant therapy is used in some series, the benefits and risks of total mesorectal excision must be more carefully documented. The total mesorectal excision series need to focus on all end points, such as local control, survival, sphincter preservation and function, surgical morbidity and mortality, and quality of life.

Radiation therapy has been used in three major approaches to the adjuvant treatment of resectable rectal cancer. These include postoperative, preoperative, and pre- plus postoperative radiation therapy.

ADJUVANT POSTOPERATIVE RADIATION THERAPY

Most patients in the United States undergo surgery and, if needed, receive postoperative therapy. The primary advantage with this approach is pathologic staging. Despite advances in preoperative imaging techniques, which allow more accurate patient selection, postoperative therapy remains the most common approach. The primary disadvantages include an increased amount of small bowel in the radiation field[171] and a potentially hypoxic postsurgical bed, and if the patient has undergone an APR, the radiation field must be extended to include the perineal scar.

Nonrandomized Trials

Nonrandomized data from the MGH[172,173] and the M. D. Anderson Cancer Center[174,175] reveal crude local failure rates of 4% to 31% in patients with stage T3–4N0M0 disease and 8% to 53% in patients with stage T3–4N1–2M0 disease who received 4500 to 5500 cGy (Table 33.8-11). The MGH series is the largest reported experience from a single institution in which careful radiation techniques were used and long follow-up is available. The MGH results were compared with a historical control group of 142 patients who underwent surgery only. Stage for stage, an improvement was seen in both local control and survival in those patients who received postoperative radiation therapy. The MGH results of 261 patients who received postoperative radiation therapy have been updated, providing 5-year actuarial local control data.[173] Actuarial local control by stage include 87% for T3N0M0, 83% for T4N0M0, 76% for T1–2N1–2M0, 77% for T3N1–2M0, and 23% for T4N1–2M0.

Wiggenraad and associates[176] treated 123 patients with postoperative radiation and correlated results with p53 status as determined by immunohistochemistry. With a median follow-up of 40 months, no significant difference was noted in local failure or survival by p53 status.

Randomized Trials

Five randomized trials have examined the use of adjuvant postoperative radiation therapy alone in stages T3 or N1–2 rectal cancer.[83,177–179] None have shown an improvement in overall survival. The series from Odense University is a two-arm trial comparing postoperative radiation therapy with surgery alone. In two of the series, one of the arms included radiation plus chemotherapy [Gastrointestinal Tumor Study Group (GITSG)][83,177] or chemotherapy alone (NSABP R-01).[178] In the Mayo Clinic/ NCCTG trial 79-47-51, there was no surgery-only control arm.

Two trials reveal a decrease in local failure: NSABP R-01 (16% vs. 25%, *P* = .06) and the Medical Research Council (21% vs. 34%, *P* = .001).[179] These trials are discussed at length in the section on combined modality therapy of resectable rectal cancer (see Radical Surgery and Adjuvant Postoperative Combined Modality Therapy for Resectable Rectal Cancer, earlier in this chapter). In this section, the discussion is limited to the comparison of the radiation therapy arm compared with the surgical control arm.

As discussed in the section on patterns of failure (see Patterns of Recurrence after Radical Surgery, earlier in this chapter), local failure rates depend on whether they are reported as first or cumulative failure. The randomized trials usually express failure as first site of failure as opposed to the nonrandomized trials, which express failure as cumulative failure. For example, in the Mayo Clinic/NCCTG trial, the incidence of local failure in node-positive patients was 25% when expressed as first failure compared with 63% when expressed as cumulative failure. More favorable local failure results (local failure as the first site of failure) were reported from the GITSG (18%)[83,177] and the NSABP (15%).[178]

In the GITSG series, 58 patients underwent surgery alone and 50 received postoperative radiation therapy (40 to 48 Gy). No significant differences were noted in either local failure or survival between these two arms.[83,177] Many criticisms have been leveled at the radiation therapy techniques used in the GITSG series. First, 39% of the patients treated with radiation therapy varied from the protocol specifications. Second, the radiation dose was chosen by the individual investigator (patients could receive 40 or 48 Gy). The issue of radiation dose is important, because dose response in radiation therapy follows a sigmoidal distribution. Therefore, a small decrease in dose can result in a large difference in local control. For example, in the Mayo Clinic/NCCTG trial 79-47-51, patients in the postoperative radiation-alone arm who received 50.4 Gy had a slightly lower local failure rate compared with those who received 45 Gy (18% vs. 24%). Although no difference in overall survival was reported, patients who received adjuvant radiation therapy in the NSABP trial had a borderline significant decrease in local failure compared with surgery alone (16% vs. 25%, *P* = .06).[178]

In the series from Odense University, 494 patients were randomized to postoperative radiation therapy (45 to 50 Gy) versus surgery alone. In patients with stage T2–3N0 disease, no difference was noted in the incidence (6%) or mean time to local failure between the arms. In patients with stage T1–3N1–2 disease, no difference was reported in local failure (6% vs. 9%); however, the mean time to local failure was significantly longer in patients who received radiation therapy compared with the surgical control arm (19 months vs. 6 months, *P* = .01). This series also has raised many criticisms. These include a short median follow-up (3 years) and that 43% of the patients were not randomized, the radiation therapy was split course, 20 patients in the radiation arm received less than 45 Gy, and the incidence of local failure in the surgery control arm was unusually low for node-positive cancers (9%).

The EORTC randomized 172 patients with T3 or N1–2 disease to 46 Gy versus observation.[180] No significant difference was seen in local failure or survival. An increase was noted in chronic diarrhea and cystitis in the radiation arm; however, it must be emphasized that patients were treated with only two fields per day. As discussed in the section on toxicity of pelvic radiation (see Complications of Pelvic Radiation Therapy, later in this chapter), this two-field technique is associated with an increase in radiation associated toxicity.

In summary, the retrospective data suggest that postoperative radiation therapy decreases local failure. The only randomized trial, which confirms this finding (with borderline significance), is from the NSABP. It should be noted that, of the randomized trials that compare radiation therapy to a surgical control arm, the NSABP is the only trial in which the radiation therapy was delivered with a continuous course, in full doses, and with "modern" techniques.

ADJUVANT PREOPERATIVE THERAPY

Preoperative adjuvant therapy (most commonly radiation therapy combined with systemic chemotherapy) is an alternative to postoperative therapy.[52,141,145–149,181–184] The primary advantages of preoperative therapy are sphincter preservation and a lower incidence of acute toxicity.

The disadvantage of preoperative radiation therapy is the potential of overtreating patients with either early (pathologic stage T1–2N0) or metastatic disease. With improved imaging techniques, such as EUS,[185] ultrasound-guided pararectal lymph node biopsy,[114] CT, MRI with a phased-array[186] or an endorectal coil,[187] and PET,[188] the number of patients who are overtreated is decreased. Experienced investigators report the accuracy of EUS in predicting T stage preoperatively as high as 90%.[189]

Results of Adjuvant Preoperative Therapy

Nonrandomized trials of preoperative radiation therapy with or without chemotherapy have reported decreased local recurrence and, possibly, improved survival.[151] Some trials include patients with early-stage or metastatic disease. Because these patients are excluded from the postoperative adjuvant therapy trials, a randomized trial is necessary to accurately compare the results of preoperative and postoperative therapy. The phase I/ II trials in which preoperative radiation or combined modality therapy is used to enhance sphincter preservation have been discussed in the section on sphincter preservation (see Adjuvant Therapy and Sphincter-Saving Operations as an Alternative to Abdominoperineal Resection, earlier in this chapter) and are reviewed in Table 33.8-10.

The only randomized trial comparing preoperative versus postoperative radiation therapy (without chemotherapy) is the Uppsala trial, in which 471 patients were randomized to receive either intensive short course preoperative radiation (25.5 Gy in five fractions) or, for patients with T3 or N1–2 disease, 60 Gy postoperatively.[190] A significant decrease was noted in local recurrence with preoperative radiation (13% vs. 22%, *P* = .02); however, no difference was found in 5-year survival (42% vs. 38%). Although a significant increase of perineal wound sepsis was seen in the preoperative group (33% vs. 18%, *P* <.01), other short- and long-term side effects were decreased. For example, the incidence of small bowel obstruction (5% vs. 11%) and total grade 3+ toxicity (20% vs. 41%) was lower in the preoperative group compared with the postoperative group. The increase in the incidence of perineal wound sepsis in the preoperative arm may have been related to the antiquated radiation techniques and high dose per fraction delivered. It should be emphasized that this increase has not been reported in the series that use conventional radiation doses and block the perineal skin in the lateral fields.

Given the advantage of the addition of concurrent chemotherapy to radiation therapy in the postoperative setting, a variety of preoperative combined modality treatment programs have been developed. Retrospective studies suggest that preoperative combined modality therapy increases pathologic down-staging compared with preoperative radiation therapy[191] and is associated with a lower incidence of acute toxicity compared with postoperative combined modality therapy. Most trials of preoperative combined modality therapy primarily include patients with unresectable disease. These are discussed in the section on locally advanced and unresectable rectal cancer (see Treatment of Locally Advanced and Unresectable Rectal Cancer, later in this chapter). Most preoperative combined modality therapy trials for patients with clinically resectable disease have used either bolus[146] or continuous infusion 5-FU–based chemotherapy.[192]

Combining the results of the published series, grade 3+ toxicity during the combined modality segment is 15% to 25%, the pathologic complete response rates are 9% to 29%, and the incidence of local failure is 0% to 10%. The limited data do not allow a valid comparison of the results of bolus versus continuous infusion 5-FU.

Whether preoperative combined modality therapy is more effective than preoperative radiation therapy is being addressed in an ongoing randomized trial from the EORTC. This trial will determine if bolus 5-FU plus leucovorin, either preoperatively or postoperatively, or both, is superior to preoperative radiation therapy alone.

Eleven modern randomized trials of preoperative radiation therapy (without chemotherapy) for resectable rectal cancer are ongoing.[107] All use low to moderate doses of radiation. The Second Medical Research Trial, which revealed a significant improvement in local control, distant control, and disease-free survival is excluded from this discussion because patients had fixed or partially fixed disease.[193]

Some of the trials show a decrease in local recurrence, and in five of the trials, this difference reached statistical significance. An analysis of the trials reported before 1988 suggests that a dose-response effect may favor preoperative radiation compared with postoperative radiation.[194] Although in some trials a subset analysis has revealed a significant improvement in survival,[195] until the Swedish Rectal Cancer Trial[142] none had reported a survival advantage for the total treatment group.

Intensive Short Course Preoperative Radiation

The first randomized trial of preoperative radiation therapy to reveal a significant improvement in survival by intent to treat was the Swedish Rectal Cancer Trial.[142] A total of 1168 patients with clinically resectable rectal cancer were randomized to 25 Gy in five fractions, followed by surgery 1 week later versus surgery alone. With a median follow-up of 75 months, patients randomized to the preoperative arm had a significant decrease in local failure (12% vs. 27%, $P<.001$) and an improvement in 5-year survival (58% vs. 48%, $P = .004$). A separate analysis of 798 patients from Sweden who underwent surgery alone during the same period but were not enrolled in the randomized trial revealed a 5-year survival rate (48%) and incidence of local failure (27%) identical to the surgical control arm, providing further validation of the surgical control arm.[196]

Although the results are intriguing, these data need to be confirmed by additional studies, because the other ten randomized trials of preoperative radiation therapy have been negative. Even if future trials confirm this survival advantage, other equally important end points in rectal cancer need to be addressed. These include acute toxicity, sphincter preservation and function, and quality of life. Radiation fraction sizes and techniques have a major impact on these end points.

Conventional radiation techniques include the use of multiple fields rather than simple anteroposterior fields, computerized treatment planning, and customized blocking. These techniques allow the delivery of high doses of radiation while sparing the surrounding normal tissues, such as the small bowel. The simple anteroposterior radiation techniques commonly used with the other intensive short course radiation therapy trials, such as the Uppsala trial,[190] are associated with an increase in toxicity.

Although prior trials of intensive short course radiation have revealed a significant increase in mortality,[143] these differences were not reported in the Swedish Rectal Cancer Trial. This may have been related to the use of multiple-field techniques. In the Swedish Trial, patients who received radiation with multiple-field techniques had a significant decrease in postoperative mortality compared with those who received treatment with anteroposterior techniques (3% vs. 15%, $P<.001$). The postoperative mortality with surgery alone was 12%. However, the incidence of postoperative morbidity for the total group of patients receiving radiation (regardless of the technique) was still significantly higher when compared with the surgery control arm (44% vs. 34%, $P = .001$). This increase is consistent with other trials of intensive short course preoperative radiation.[144]

The absence of an increase in mortality in the Swedish trial may have been related to the fact that 91% of patients received radiation using the more sophisticated multiple-field radiation techniques. In patients who receive conventional doses and techniques of preoperative combined modality therapy, the volume of small bowel in the radiation field may be the dose-limiting organ with radiation therapy.[197]

It should be noted that even when multiple-field techniques are used, data from the Stockholm I and II trials[143] report a significant increase in postoperative mortality when patients receive intensive short course radiation compared with surgery alone (4% vs. 1%). These high complication rates with intensive short course radiation have not been reported in patients who receive conventional doses and techniques of preoperative radiation. In the R90-01 trial,[52] patients were treated with multiple-field techniques but with 3-Gy fractions. The anastomotic complication rate was 17%.

Another criticism of the intensive short course preoperative radiation trials is the lack of preoperative staging. Myerson et al.[198] treated 83 patients with this approach, and only 20 had transrectal ultrasound staging.

In summary, even with suboptimal radiation techniques, the more recent randomized preoperative trials reveal a significant decrease in local failure. Although the intensive short course (25 Gy) of preoperative radiation therapy is used in some European countries, it is not favored in North America because (1) it is unlikely that it could be combined with adequate doses of sys-

TABLE 33.8-12. Prognostic Predictors of Response to Preoperative Therapy in Rectal Cancer

Series	*Number of Patients*	*Clinical Stage*	*Preoperative Therapy*	*% CR*	*Findings*
Scott[337]	24	T3–4	CMT	25	↑ apoptotic index with CR. No relationship to p53 or bcl-2.
Tannapfel et al.[338]	32	T3–4	CMT	—	↑ apoptotic index after preoperative CMT. ↓ proliferative capacity (Ki67, PCNA) after CMT but did not predict the CR rate.
Luna-Perez et al.[339]	26	T3–4	CMT	15	↑ CR with normal p53 vs. mutated p53.
Desai[340]	23	T3–4	RT	9	↑ downstaging with normal p53 and/or PCNA-negative.
Fu et al.[341]	49	T1–3	RT	4	↑ downstaging, ↑ local failure, and ↓ survival with mutated p53 and normal p21.
Sakakura et al.[342]	28	T3–4	CMT + hyper-thermia	—	↑ downstaging with ↑ apoptotic index; highest correlation with wild-type p53.
Willett et al.[202]	153	T3–4	RT ± CMT	12	↑ downstaging with ↑ growth fraction (↑ mitotic count and Ki-67 and PCNA).
Nehls et al.[343]	100	T1–3	RT	—	No change in p53 expression pre-RT vs. post-RT.
Adell et al.[344]	148	T1–4	RT	—	In p53-negative patients, preoperative RT decreased local failure, whereas p53-positive patients had no benefit from preoperative RT.

CMT, combined modality therapy (radiation + chemotherapy); CR, pathologic complete response; PCNA, proliferating cell nuclear antigen; RT, radiation therapy; ↑, increased; ↓, decreased.
All analyses were performed by immunohistochemistry on paraffin-fixed tissues.

temic chemotherapy; (2) it is not designed to enhance sphincter preservation; and (3) regardless of the technique, it is still associated with a significant increase in postoperative morbidity.

PREOPERATIVE AND POSTOPERATIVE RADIATION THERAPY

The approach of using both preoperative and postoperative therapy, also known as the *sandwich technique*, includes a short preoperative course of radiation (5 to 15 Gy), followed by surgery, and in patients with T3N1M0 disease, an additional 40 to 45 Gy postoperatively. This approach was designed to combine the theoretical advantages of low-dose preoperative radiation therapy (decreased tumor seeding) while reserving postoperative radiation therapy for those patients with T3 or N1–2M0 disease. The results of this approach have been reported by a number of investigators.[199]

The Radiation Therapy Oncology Group (RTOG) presented the results of a randomized trial of 350 patients (87% with rectal cancer) who were randomized to 5 Gy preoperative therapy versus surgery alone (RTOG 81-15). Patients with a pathologic stage T3 or N1–2 disease received a minimum of 45 Gy postoperatively. No chemotherapy was delivered. With a minimum follow-up of 5 years, no differences were found in local failure, distant failure, or overall survival between the arms. A retrospective analysis of 155 patients treated at the Institut Gustave Roussy also revealed no advantage of the sandwich technique compared with preoperative radiation.[199] Because the randomized trials of postoperative combined modality therapy reveal a significant improvement in survival, the benefits of preoperative therapy, including down-staging and sphincter preservation, require a standard dose rather than low to intermediate doses of radiation, and because the RTOG randomized trial was negative, the sandwich approach should be abandoned.

SELECTED CONTROVERSIES IN THE ROLE OF PREOPERATIVE THERAPY

PREDICTION OF RESPONSE WITH TUMOR MARKERS

A variety of tumor markers have been identified that may help predict those tumors that will respond favorably to preoperative therapy (Table 33.8-12). Based on the experience that rapidly dividing cells are more sensitive to radiation, Willett et al.[200] analyzed the proliferative index in patients with locally advanced or unresectable disease who received preoperative radiation therapy with or without 5-FU.[200] Tumors with a higher proliferation index had a higher response rate to preoperative therapy and, after radiation, a corresponding reduction was noted in the proliferative index.[201] In a follow-up study, the authors reported that the addition of 5-FU to preoperative radiation decreased three markers of proliferation [mitotic counts, Ki-67, and proliferating cell nuclear antigen (PCNA)] compared with radiation therapy alone.[202]

Desai and colleagues[203] reported a higher incidence of recurrence but less down-staging in PCNA-positive rectal cancers. By multivariate analysis, Neoptolemos and associates[204] showed that this index did not add to the prognostic value of the Dukes' staging system. The proliferative index may be useful in predicting the response to preoperative therapy. However, given the conflicting data, additional experience is needed.

In the series reported by Rich[192] of 50 patients treated with preoperative combined modality therapy, tumors with a low spontaneous apoptosis index and positive BCL-2 staining had lower rates of down-staging. In 167 patients treated with preoperative radiation, a significant increase in down-staging in well-differentiated cancers was reported.[205] Using residual tumor cell density rather than stage as a measure, this difference did not reach statistical significance. By univariate analysis, patients with a pathologic complete response had a nonsignificant improvement in survival. Berger and associates[206] found that well-differentiated tumors had a greater degree of down-staging compared with moderately or poorly differentiated tumors.

In conclusion, although some tumor markers may be predictive of response, the decision to use preoperative therapy should not be made solely on their presence or absence. The development of tumor markers to predict response and prognosis remains an active area of investigation.[207]

DOES THE RESPONSE OF THE PRIMARY TUMOR PREDICT OUTCOME?

Most studies suggest that sphincter preservation is increased with a corresponding increase in the response rate of the primary tumor. It is more controversial as to whether the response rate predicts outcome and if the subset of patients who achieve a complete response still require radical surgery.

In an analysis of 88 patients with clinical T3–4 rectal cancers who received preoperative radiation with or without 5-FU plus leucovorin, a decrease was noted in local failure (4% vs. 15%) and a significant increase was noted in 5-year cancer-specific survival (100% vs. 45%, $P = .01$) in patients who achieved a complete or near-complete response (pathologic stage T0–2N0 disease) compared with those with less of a response (pathologic stage T3–4 or N1–2).[181] Ahmad and colleagues[182] reported a 5-year actuarial local control rate of 96% and a 91% survival rate in the subset of 49 of a total of 315 patients with clinical T3–4 disease who achieved a complete response after preoperative radiation.

Two studies have examined whether surgery is still necessary after a complete response, and the reported results have been conflicting. Habr-Gama and colleagues[183] treated 118 patients with clinical T1–3 rectal cancers with preoperative 50.4-Gy radiation plus 5-FU plus leucovorin. Of the 36 patients who achieved a biopsy-proven complete response, 30 did not undergo surgery. With a median follow-up of 36 months, 28 (93%) remained without evidence of disease. In a smaller series from Rossi et al.,[184] 16 patients (13 with tethered disease) received similar preoperative treatment. If they achieved a biopsy-proven complete response, they received an additional boost of 20 to 30 Gy with brachytherapy. Of the six patients (38%) who had a complete response, they remained without evidence of disease for a median of only 11 months.

Although the results from Habr-Gama and colleagues[183] are intriguing, radical surgery after preoperative adjuvant therapy remains the standard of care. In the subset of patients who are either medically inoperable or refuse radical surgery, local excision may be an alternative.[140]

RADICAL SURGERY AND ADJUVANT POSTOPERATIVE COMBINED MODALITY THERAPY FOR RESECTABLE RECTAL CANCER

The anatomy and natural history of rectal adenocarcinoma require attention to issues of local and systemic tumor control. Despite many clinical trials, until 1990 there was considerable controversy about whether adjuvant therapy improved the survival rate of patients undergoing surgical resection of their primary tumors. Even a metaanalysis of the worldwide published experience, which demonstrated a statistically significant benefit for adjuvant chemotherapy in rectal cancer patients (38% decrease in the mortality rate), was not completely convincing for many physicians. However, a Consensus Development Conference sponsored by the National Institutes of Health in 1990 concluded that effective adjuvant therapy exists for stages II and III (Modified Astler Coller stages B2 and C or TNM stage T3 or N1–2) rectal cancers. This conclusion was based on the clinical data derived over the preceding 20 years. Especially important were the results of some of the randomized studies summarized in Table 33.8-13. Two of the studies included a surgery-only control group, and four studies used surgery plus postoperative pelvic irradiation as the means for achieving definitive local control.[83,177,208]

The majority of U.S. patients undergo surgery and, if they have stage T3 or N1–2 disease, receive postoperative adjuvant combined modality therapy. The most compelling advantage to this approach is pathologic staging. Although advances in preoperative imaging techniques allow more accurate patient selection, it still remains the most common approach. The primary disadvantages of the postoperative approach include an increased amount of small bowel in the radiation field[171] and a potentially hypoxic postsurgical bed, and if the patient has undergone an APR, the radiation field must be extended to include the perineal scar.

RESULTS OF POSTOPERATIVE THERAPY

After the publication of the randomized trials from the GITSG[83,177] and Mayo/NCCTG (79-47-51), which revealed a significant improvement in local control (Mayo/NCCTG) and survival (GITSG and Mayo/NCCTG) with postoperative radiation plus bolus 5-FU plus methyl chloroethylcyclohexylnitrosourea (CCNU; lomustine), the National Cancer Institute Consensus Conference concluded in 1990 that combined modality therapy was the standard postoperative adjuvant treatment for patients with T3 or N1–2 disease. Although radiation therapy decreases local recurrence in one-half of patients, it is the addition of 5-FU–based chemotherapy that further decreases local recurrence to approximately 10% to 12% and is the agent responsible for increasing overall 5-year survival rates by approximately 10% to 15% (from 50% up to 60% to 65%).

With this increase in local control and survival with the addition of chemotherapy comes an increase in acute toxicity. The incidence of grade 3+ toxicity in the combined modality arms of the GITSG and Mayo/NCCTG 79-47-51 trials was 25% to 50%. Furthermore, the percentage of patients finishing six cycles of chemotherapy in those trials was only 65% and 50%, respectively. Miller and colleagues[209] reported that patients who received combined modality therapy versus radiation therapy alone in the Mayo/NCCTG 79-47-51 trial had a higher rate of severe and life-threatening diarrhea, both during radiation (20% vs. 4%, $P = .001$) and at any time during treatment (22% vs. 4%, $P = .001$). As previously discussed, the acute toxicity with preoperative combined modality therapy may be less than in the postoperative setting.

The majority of combined modality therapy regimens include six cycles of 5-FU–based chemotherapy plus concurrent pelvic radiation. Six cycles of chemotherapy are thought to be necessary to treat systemic disease. However, in a randomized trial from Norway, 144 patients were randomized to postoperative radiation plus bolus 5-FU (500 to 750 mg/m^2 limited

TABLE 33.8-13. Stage T3,N1–2,M0 Rectal Cancer: Selected Completed Adjuvant Trials

Trial	*Total Accruals*	*Treatment*	*Results*
GITSG 7175[83,177]	227	Control MF RT + MF RT	RT + MF results in 59% 5-y survival vs. 43% in controls (*P*<.01).
Mayo/NCCTG 79-47-51	204	MF → RT + 5-FU → MF RT	RT + MF resulted in 63% 7-y survival vs. 48% for RT alone (*P* = .04).
NSABP R-01[178]	555	Control Pelvic RT MOF	MOF resulted in 52% 5-y survival vs. 42% in controls (and RT) and significantly superior disease-free survival.
GITSG 7189[228]	210	RT + 5-FU → 5-FU RT + MF → MF	3-y DFS was 45% for MF and 69% for 5-FU.
Mayo/NCCTG 86-47-51[128,213]	453	MF → RT + 5-FU → MF 5-FU → RT + 5-FU → 5-FU (Infusion vs. bolus for 5-FU)	With 46-mo median follow-up, MF is not superior to 5-FU; 5-FU infusion superior to bolus in time to relapse and survival.
INT 0114[216]	1792	5-FU → RT + 5-FU → 5-FU 5-FU + LV → RT + 5-FU + LV → 5-FU + LV 5-FU + LEV → RT + 5-FU → 5-FU + LEV 5-FU + LEV → RT + 5-FU + LV → 5-FU + LV + LEV (5-FU was bolus)	No significant difference in 3-y local control, survival, or total toxicity between the arms.

→, sequential therapy; CCNU, chloroethylcyclohexylnitrosourea (lomustine); DFS, disease-free survival; 5-FU, 5-fluorouracil; GITSG, Gastrointestinal Tumor Study Group; INT, Intergroup; LEV, levamisole; LV, leucovorin; Mayo/NCCTG, Mayo Clinic/North Central Cancer Treatment Group; MF, methyl CCNU + 5-FU; MOF, methyl-CCNU + vincristine (Oncovin) + 5-FU; NSABP, National Surgical Adjuvant Breast Project; RT, pelvic radiation therapy, 50.4–54.0 Gy.
All patients undergo complete surgical resections.

to days 1 and 2 of weeks 1, 2, and 3 of radiation) versus surgery alone.[210] Despite the fact that 5-FU was delivered with radiosensitizing doses rather than doses adequate to treat systemic disease, this combined modality therapy regimen significantly decreased local recurrence (12% vs. 30%, *P* = .01) and improved 5-year survival (64% vs. 50%, *P* = .05). Although these results with limited-dose 5-FU are encouraging, additional experience with this approach is needed before modifying the standard recommendation of six cycles of systemic chemotherapy.

Retrospective data suggest that there may be subsets of patients with T3N0 disease who may not require adjuvant therapy and that there may be patients with stage I disease who should be considered for adjuvant therapy. In a review of 117 patients with T3N0 disease, Willett et al.[211] identified a favorable subset of patients with well- or moderately differentiated cancers invading less than 2 mm into the perirectal fat who, after surgery alone, had a 10-year actuarial local failure rate of only 5% compared with 29% in T3N0 patients without those favorable features. In a separate analysis, they identified a subset of patients with stage I disease who have an increased incidence of local failure after an APR.[212] These results must be confirmed in a randomized trial before a change in the standard of care of combined modality therapy can be recommended.

Since the 1990 National Cancer Institute Consensus Conference, the focus of the intergroup postoperative trials has been the identification of the optimal chemotherapeutic agents and their method of administration. In the follow-up trial to the 79-47-51 trial, the Mayo/NCCTG designed a four-arm trial (86-47-51) to determine if methyl CCNU was necessary, as well as to compare the relative effectiveness of 5-FU when delivered as a bolus versus a continuous infusion.[128] Because methyl CCNU did not improve either local control or survival, it is no longer recommended for use in the adjuvant treatment of rectal cancer.[213]

When compared with bolus 5-FU (with or without methyl CCNU), patients who received continuous infusion 5-FU (also known as *prolonged venous infusion*) had a significant decrease in the overall rate of tumor relapse (37% vs. 47%, *P* = .01), distant metastasis (31% vs. 40%, *P* = .03), as well as an improvement in 4-year survival (70% vs. 60%, *P* = .005). These data suggest that, when 5-FU is used as a single agent with radiation therapy, it is more effective as a continuous infusion compared with a bolus.

Differences were also found in the individual acute toxicities of continuous infusion and bolus 5-FU regimens. For example, during the combined modality segment, patients who received continuous infusion 5-FU had a significant increase in grade 3+ diarrhea (24% vs. 14%, *P* <.01), whereas they had a significant decrease in grade 3+ leukopenia (2% vs. 11%, *P* <.01) compared with bolus 5-FU.

Building on the positive results of continuous infusion 5-FU reported in the Mayo/NCCTG 86-47-51 trial, the replacement postoperative Intergroup trial INT 0114 was designed. The primary end point of this trial is to determine whether a benefit exists to continuous infusion 5-FU throughout the entire chemotherapy course (six cycles) as compared with continuous infusion only during the combined modality segment (two cycles) and bolus 5-FU during the remaining four cycles. The control arm is arm 4 (bolus 5-FU, leucovorin, and levamisole). The trial opened to accrual in 1993 and is actively accruing.

The NSABP R-01 three-arm trial of comparing the postoperative methyl-CCNU, vincristine (Oncovin), and 5-FU (MOF) regimen vs. radiation therapy vs. surgery alone revealed a significant improvement in 5-year disease-free survival (42% vs. 30%, $P = .006$) and overall survival (53% vs. 43%, $P = .05$) with postoperative MOF chemotherapy compared with surgery.[178] The advantage in overall survival of the chemotherapy arm was most evident in males (60% vs. 37%) and in males younger than 65 years of age (44% vs. 26%). In contrast, females who received chemotherapy experienced a lower survival (37% vs. 54%). It should be emphasized that the trial was not stratified by gender. Additional studies revealed that overexpression of thymidylate synthase in the primary tumor was associated with a worse prognosis[214] and that such patients derived the greatest benefit from adjuvant MOF chemotherapy.

As a follow-up to the R-01 trial, the NSABP designed a four-arm trial (R-02) in which patients were randomized, depending on gender, to either MOF with or without radiation or 5-FU plus leucovorin with or without radiation.[215] A preliminary analysis revealed a significant decrease in local failure in the two combined modality therapy arms compared with the two that included chemotherapy alone (7% vs. 11%, $P = .045$).[215] However, this decrease in local failure did not result in an increase in median survival. Other results are pending.

The most recent Intergroup postoperative trial to report results was INT 0114 (see Table 33.8-13).[216] This was a four-arm trial in which all patients received six cycles of postoperative chemotherapy plus concurrent radiation therapy during cycles three and four. The goal of this trial was to determine if combinations of bolus 5-FU–based chemotherapy (5-FU plus low-dose leucovorin vs. 5-FU plus levamisole vs. 5-FU and leucovorin and levamisole) were superior to single-agent 5-FU.

With a median follow-up of 4 years, no significant differences were found between the four arms (5-FU alone, 5-FU plus leucovorin, 5-FU plus levamisole, or 5-FU and leucovorin and levamisole) in terms of local failure (12%, 9%, 13%, 9%, respectively) or 3-year survival (78%, 80%, 79%, 79%, respectively).[216] Although the total incidence of acute grade 3+ toxicity was similar for the four arms (76%, 72%, 70%, 75%, respectively), differences were noted between the regimens. For example, the 5-FU alone arm had a higher incidence of hematologic toxicity, whereas the 5-FU plus levamisole arm had a higher incidence of diarrhea. A subset analysis revealed that, in all four arms, women had a significantly greater incidence of acute grade 3+ toxicity compared with men. The reason for this difference in toxicity by gender is unclear.

The choice of which postoperative adjuvant regimen to recommend in the nonprotocol setting remains controversial. Given that the Mayo/NCCTG 86-47-51 trial revealed that continuous infusion 5-FU is more effective than bolus 5-FU and because modulation with leucovorin, levamisole, or both did not improve the results of bolus 5-FU alone in the INT 0114 trial, one could argue that continuous infusion 5-FU is the regimen of choice. INT 0114 directly compares continuous infusion 5-FU with bolus 5-FU, leucovorin, and levamisole; however, the results are not yet available. Therefore, for patients not enrolled in a clinical trial, acceptable regimens at this time include either continuous infusion 5-FU (225 mg/m^2 days 1 to 7, or 300 mg/m^2 days 1 to 5) or bolus 5-FU plus modulation with leucovorin (5-FU, 325 mg/m^2, plus leucovorin, 20 mg/m^2 bolus daily $\times$ 5), levamisole, or both. However, because the colon adjuvant trials reveal that six cycles of 5-FU plus leucovorin is as effective as 12 cycles of 5-FU plus levamisole,[217,218] most physicians no longer use levamisole in the adjuvant treatment of either colon or rectal cancer. When a 7-day continuous infusion of 5-FU is combined with oral leucovorin and pelvic radiation, the recommended 5-FU dose is decreased to 150 mg/m^2.[219] In summary, bolus or continuous infusion 5-FU, when combined with radiation in the treatment of rectal cancer, probably have equal efficacy, and the choice of a regimen should be based on factors such as their acute toxicity profiles and patient compliance.

FUTURE OF ADJUVANT THERAPY

Given the increased morbidity and marginal benefits seen in the randomized trials of low- or moderate-dose adjuvant preoperative radiation, interest in treating resectable rectal cancer with preoperative therapy was limited until the 1990s. The primary focus of clinical research in the adjuvant treatment of resectable rectal cancer had involved the use of postoperative combined modality therapy. However, there are three reasons why the postoperative approach may not be the most innovative one: increased toxicity, less chance of sphincter preservation, and lower chemotherapy doses.

Despite the survival advantage of postoperative combined modality therapy, it is associated with substantial toxicity. For example, the incidence of grade 3+ toxicity in patients who received combined modality therapy in the GITSG trial was 26% for hematologic toxicity and 35% nonhematologic toxicity.[83,177] In the Mayo Clinic/NCCTG 79-47-51 trial, the most significant grade 3+ toxicities included diarrhea (41%) and leukopenia (33%). The only grade 3+ toxicity in patients receiving radiation therapy alone was diarrhea (5%). In the GITSG and Mayo Clinic/NCCTG trials, 35% to 50% of the patients never finished all the planned cycles of chemotherapy. The total incidence of grade 3+ toxicity in the INT 0114 trial of postoperative radiation with 5-FU with or without leucovorin and/or levamisole modulation was 72% to 76%.[216]

Preoperative radiation therapy increases the chance of sphincter preservation. By down-staging the primary tumor, preoperative irradiation allows the surgeon to change the planned operation from an APR to a LAR and CAA.[107]

Higher initial doses of chemotherapy can be delivered with preoperative than with postoperative irradiation. This difference was observed in comparing two phase I trials of combined bolus 5-FU, high-dose leucovorin, and radiation therapy (50.4 Gy) reported from Memorial Sloan-Kettering Cancer Center.[220] Patients with unresectable disease received preoperative radiation therapy and two cycles of concurrent 5-FU plus leucovorin followed by surgery and postoperative 5-FU plus leucovorin. Patients with resectable disease received the same chemotherapy and radiation therapy in the postoperative setting. The dose of radiation and leucovorin remained constant while the 5-FU dose was escalated. The maximal tolerated dose of 5-FU was higher with preoperative versus postoperative therapy.

Based on its toxicity, increased chance of sphincter preservation, and higher chemotherapy doses, preoperative combined modality therapy, if delivered with appropriate doses and techniques, is an attractive approach and is a standard of care for clinical T3 disease. The NSABP R-03 and the German CAO/ARO/AIO 94 randomized trials will help determine the relative effectiveness of preoperative versus postoperative combined modality therapy.

COMPLICATIONS OF PELVIC RADIATION THERAPY

ETIOLOGY AND MANIFESTATIONS

As seen with other cancer therapies, pelvic radiation is associated with acute and long-term toxicity. Complications of pelvic radiation therapy are a function of the volume of the radiation field, overall treatment time, fraction size, radiation energy, total dose, and technique.[221] Large field sizes, a short overall treatment time, large fraction sizes (more than 2 Gy per fraction), orthovoltage or low-energy megavoltage radiation (cobalt 60), doses of more than 50.4 Gy when small bowel is in the high dose field, the use of a two-field [anteroposterior (AP)/posteroposterior (PA)] technique, treatment of only one field per day, the use of a direct perineal boost field, and the lack of computerized dosimetry all contribute to an increased incidence of radiation complications.

Risk factors unrelated to radiation techniques include patients with pelvic inflammatory disease, hypertension, diabetes mellitus, inflammatory bowel disease, or obesity, and patients who have had prior pelvic surgery or receive concurrent chemotherapy.

Most studies describing the tolerance of patients with inflammatory bowel disease have been limited to case reports.[222] Furthermore, most do not indicate whether the disease is active, requiring antiinflammatory therapy, or if the patient had undergone a total proctocolectomy.[223] This factor is important because the issue of toxicity may not be relevant for patients with ulcerative colitis who have undergone a total proctocolectomy. The most comprehensive analysis of the tolerance of patients with inflammatory bowel disease was reported by Willett and colleagues.[224] They examined the records of 28 patients (17 colorectal patients and 11 who received concurrent 5-FU) who were treated with 40 Gy or more of pelvic or abdominal radiation therapy. Of the 28 patients, 18 had ulcerative colitis and 10 had Crohn's disease. Overall, 43% of patients had active disease requiring antiinflammatory therapy.

The total incidence of severe toxicity was 46%, which caused 22% of patients to stop radiation and 29% to undergo surgery for complications. Acute toxicity was similar in ulcerative colitis and Crohn's disease; however, late toxicity was limited to patients with ulcerative colitis. In the 16 patients treated with specialized radiation techniques to reduce total dose to or exclude the small and large bowel from the radiation field, the 5-year actuarial incidence of late toxicity was 23% compared with 73% in the 12 patients who were not treated with these specialized techniques ($P = .02$). Unless the large bowel can be excluded from the radiation field in patients with ulcerative colitis and the large and small bowel is excluded from the radiation field in patients with Crohn's disease, the use of radiation in patients with inflammatory bowel disease is contraindicated.

Radiation complications also are increased in patients with collagen vascular disease. However, a report of six patients with systemic lupus erythematosus who received chest wall radiation for breast cancer or Hodgkin's disease suggests that it is not an absolute contraindication to radiation therapy.[225]

Acute (short-term) and long-term complications of pelvic radiation occur with distinct clinical courses and pathologic manifestations.[226] The most frequent serious complication of pelvic radiation is small bowel damage. In animals, transforming growth factor-β and mast cell hyperplasia may be involved in the molecular pathogenesis of radiation enteritis.[227]

ACUTE COMPLICATIONS

Acute complications occur in all patients during treatment and include thrombocytopenia, leukopenia, dysuria, and effects on the small bowel (diarrhea, abdominal cramping, and increased bowel frequency) and large bowel (acute proctitis, tenesmus, bloody or mucus discharge). Proctoscopic examination of the rectal mucosa normally reveals an inflamed, edematous, and friable rectal mucosa consistent with acute radiation proctitis and should be discouraged while patients are receiving radiation therapy. These symptoms usually are transient and resolve within a few weeks after the completion of radiation therapy. They appear to be a function of the dose rate and fraction size more than of the total dose of radiation. The mechanism is primarily the depletion of actively dividing cells in what is otherwise a stable cell renewal system. In the small bowel, loss of the mucosal cells results in malabsorption of various substances, including fat, carbohydrate, protein, and bile salts. The management of bowel-related complications usually involves the use of diphenoxylate, narcotics, or both. The bowel mucosa usually recovers in 1 to 3 months after the completion of radiation.

Dysuria occurs in 10% to 15% of patients and is usually controlled with phenazopyridine hydrochloride (Pyridium). Skin erythema most commonly occurs in skin folds and is treated prophylactically with nonmetallic skin creams. If grade 3+ toxicity develops, a 3-day to 1-week treatment break commonly is required.

Although concurrent chemotherapy significantly improves the local control rate of radiation therapy, it increases the acute toxicity. The incidence of grade 3+ toxicity with postoperative radiation therapy is approximately 5%, whereas in some reports it is increased to as high as 25% to 50% in patients receiving postoperative combined modality therapy.[228] In the INT 0114 trial of postoperative combined modality therapy using 50.4 Gy plus bolus 5-FU with or without leucovorin and/or levamisole, the total incidence of grade 3+ toxicity was 72% to 76%.[216] An analysis of 204 patients who received the postoperative combined modality therapy arm of the Mayo/NCCTG 79-47-51 trial showed the incidence of acute grade 3+ diarrhea was 22% compared with 4% who received radiation therapy alone ($P = .001$).[229] The acute toxicity of preoperative combined modality therapy appears to be lower than postoperative combined modality therapy.[107,171,230]

LONG-TERM COMPLICATIONS

Long-term complications occur less frequently but are substantially more serious. The initial symptoms commonly occur 6 to 18 months after completion of radiation. Complications may include persistent diarrhea, increased bowel frequency, proctitis, small bowel obstruction, perineal and scrotal tenderness, delayed perineal wound healing, urinary incontinence, and bladder atrophy and bleeding. Injury to the vascular and supporting stromal tissues of the bowel is the presumed pathophysiology. Schuster et al.[231] found that bile acid malabsorption due to ileal dysfunction was not an inevitable late complication of pelvic radiation, and it is not the major determinant in the pathophysiology of chronic radiation-induced diarrhea.

The most common long-term complications are due to small bowel damage and include enteritis, adhesions, and small bowel obstruction requiring surgical intervention.[221,232] At the MGH, 165 patients received 45 Gy postoperatively to the pelvis with a boost to the tumor bed to 50.4 Gy.[172] The incidence of long-term mild to moderate complications was 8% [2% proctitis, 2% perineal and scrotal tenderness (resolved), 1% delayed perineal wound healing, 1% small bowel obstruction (resolved), 1% urinary incontinence, and 1% bladder atrophy and bleeding (resolved)]. The incidence of small bowel obstruction requiring surgery was similar in the patients who received radiation (6%) compared to a historical group of patients who were treated with surgery alone (5%).

A retrospective review of 304 patients treated with a median of 50.84 Gy of postoperative pelvic radiation at the Mayo Clinic was presented by Miller et al.[232] The median follow-up was 5.3 years; 65% of patients received chemotherapy; and the small bowel was excluded after 50.4 Gy. The crude incidence of complications included 4% acute enteritis, 6% chronic enteritis, and 12% chronic proctitis. The actuarial incidence of complications at 5 years included 14% proctitis and 7% enteritis. The mean time from diagnosis to complications was 2.1 years. By multivariate analysis, the two independent factors associated with an increase in complications were increasing age (median age, 67 years vs. 62 years) and radiation dose (median, 54 Gy vs. 50.4 Gy).

Other long-term complications, such as pelvic fractures[233,234] and lumbosacral plexopathy,[235,236] are very rare occurrences and may be caused by factors unrelated to the radiation, such as osteoporosis or disease progression.

Overall, the incidence of small bowel obstruction requiring surgery after postoperative pelvic radiation for rectal cancer is 4% to 12% in most series and as high as 17.5% in earlier series.[172,174,175] In patients treated with surgery only, 2% to 15% may develop similar complications. Small bowel–related late complications are directly proportional to the volume of small bowel in the radiation field. Late radiation proctitis, similar to small bowel injury, is related to the treatment volume and dose of radiation.

SPHINCTER FUNCTION

Radiation therapy can adversely effect sphincter function; however, most series are retrospective, nonrandomized, nonblinded, retrospective telephone surveys. Furthermore, sphincter function is affected by other factors, such as the type of operation, the functional scale used, and whether patients received conventional radiation techniques as opposed to intensive short course radiation.

Using a retrospective telephone survey, Kollmorgen et al.[153] from the Mayo Clinic assessed the impact of postoperative combined modality therapy delivered with conventional doses and techniques of pelvic radiation and 5-FU–based chemotherapy on bowel function and compared it with a matched group of patients who underwent surgery alone. The 41 patients who received combined modality therapy had a significant increase in the number of bowel movements, clustering of bowel movements, nighttime bowel movements, occasional incontinence, urgency, and wore pads more often compared with 59 patients who underwent surgery alone. Sphincter function after a CAA was retrospectively assessed by Paty and associates.[154] The 40 patients who received pre- or postoperative radiation therapy, or both (with or without chemotherapy) after a CAA had increased stool frequency and difficulty with evacuation compared with 41 patients who underwent surgery alone. Unconventional radiation doses and techniques were used in 43% of patients.

In contrast with the previous studies, Birnbaum and colleagues have prospectively examined the short-term[155] and long-term[156] impact of preoperative radiation therapy on sphincter function. Patients received conventional doses and techniques of radiation and were assessed objectively by anal manometry with or without transrectal ultrasound. In the 20 patients assessed for short-term and ten patients assessed for long-term results, radiation therapy had a minimal effect on sphincter function. As one would predict, patients who receive preoperative radiation with intensive short course radiation have inferior function results. Patients who received 5 Gy × 5 in the Swedish Rectal Cancer Trial had a significant increase in bowel frequency, incontinence, urgency, and emptying difficulty.[237] This impaired the patient's social life 30% of the time compared with 10% of the time with surgery alone. In another analysis of patients who received 5.1 Gy per fraction, a significant increase in bowel frequency was found.[238]

SEXUAL FUNCTION

In addition to the previously discussed variables that can effect assessment of sphincter function, series examining sexual function using subjective methods have the additional shortcoming of bias due to the sensitive nature of the questions. Answers to such questions are subjective and may be influenced by the interaction between the patient and interviewer. Age and psychological factors, such as depression and anxiety about the diagnosis of cancer, can further influence the results. Furthermore, it should be emphasized that both the surgery required for an APR and the psychological impact of a permanent colostomy can have an adverse impact on sexual function.

A retrospective analysis of sexual function in men and women by Havenga and associates[3] found that radiation therapy with or without 5-FU had a negative impact after total mesorectal excision for rectal cancer. In a review of 18 males with a median age of 70 who received 52.5 Gy with an unconventional fraction size of 2.63 Gy per fraction for bladder cancer, 56% were able to attain an erection sufficient for intercourse compared with 72% of patients in the 6 months before the start of radiation therapy.[239] Because the patients did not undergo surgery, receive hormonal therapy, or have prostate cancer, this study is a better indication of the impact of radiation therapy alone.

In conclusion, although radiation can adversely affect sphincter and sexual function, the ultimate functional results are a result of a combination of therapies, including radiation, surgery, and chemotherapy. The risk of dysfunction must be evaluated in the context of the benefit of adjuvant therapy, which includes decreased local failure, improved survival, and, in selected patients, the ability to perform sphincter-preserving surgery as an alternative to an APR.

MINIMIZING TOXICITY OF RADIATION THERAPY

RADIATION TREATMENT TECHNIQUES

Small bowel–related complications are directly proportional to the volume of small bowel in the radiation field.[197] In patients receiving combined modality therapy, the volume of small bowel in the radiation field limits the ability to escalate the dose of 5-FU.[171] A number of simple radiotherapeutic techniques are available to decrease radiation-related small bowel toxicity (Table 33.8-14). First, small bowel contrast allows identification of the location of the small bowel. The use of multiple-field techniques (preferably a three-field technique) permits a larger volume of small bowel to be blocked from the pelvis compared with an AP/PA (two field) technique. In one series, the small bowel obstruction rate in patients with rectal cancer who received pelvic radiation therapy was higher with a single-field (21%) as compared with a multiple-field technique (9%).[240] The small bowel obstruction rate increased to 30% when an extended-field radiation was used.

TABLE 33.8-14. Techniques to Minimize the Acute Toxicity to the Small Bowel from Radiation Therapy

Surgical techniques
Pelvic reconstruction to exclude small bowel from the pelvis
Reperitonealize pelvic floor
Retrovert the uterus
Construct an omental sling
Absorbable mesh
Pelvic clips to delineate high-risk areas
Radiation therapy techniques
Treatment simulation and planning
Small bowel contrast
Prone position
Multiple-field techniques (three-field preferred)
Wire perineum and block if an abdominoperineal resection has not been performed
Use high-energy (≥6 MeV) linear accelerators
Shaped blocks
Computerized dosimetry
Do not exceed 50.4 Gy to the small bowel
Standard fraction sizes (1.8–2.0 Gy/fraction)
Bladder distention and belly board—providing it does not make the patient uncomfortable, thereby causing movement
During treatment
Treatment of all fields each day
Low-fiber, low-fat diet

The treatment of all fields each day results in a lower integral dose and more homogeneous dose distribution. A study by Sigmon et al.[241] suggests that patients with endometrial or rectal cancer who receive pelvic radiation by a continuous course as compared with a planned split course have fewer chronic bowel complications. The use of lateral fields for the boost as well as positioning the patient in the prone position further decreases the volume of small bowel in the lateral radiation fields.

The treatment should be designed with the use of computerized radiation dosimetry and be delivered by high-energy linear accelerators, which, by nature of their depth dose characteristics, deliver a higher dose to the tumor volume while sparing the surrounding normal structures. When the perineal scar must be treated, it should be included in the pelvic radiation fields. The use of a separate perineal field is associated with an increased risk of overlap of the radiation fields and should be avoided.

Even in expert hands, daily variations occur in patient positioning for pelvic radiation ranging from 3.4 to 9.0 mm.[242,243] Using electronic portal imaging, Tinger et al.[244] found that errors exceeding 5 mm or 10 mm are significantly more frequent intertreatment (40% to 51%, and 3% to 23%, respectively) compared with intratreatment (1% to 7%, and 0%, respectively). In national clinical trials, pretreatment quality control review can decrease the error rate in radiation field design.[245]

The advantage to the combination of a multiple-field technique, high-energy photons, and computerized dosimetry is illustrated in Figure 33.8-6. With this combination, a homogenous dose distribution is maintained throughout the target volume such that prescribing to the 98% isodose line covers the volume at risk and gives only 35% to 55% of the dose to the small bowel. In contrast, when the same patient receives ^{60}Co with an AP/PA arrangement, an inhomogeneous dose distribution is provided throughout the target volume such that the dose must be prescribed to the 90% isodose line to cover the volume at risk, thereby giving 110% to 130% of the dose to the small bowel. Furthermore, if computerized treatment planning was not performed and the dose was prescribed to the midplane, parts of the tumor volume would be underdosed by 10%.

After pelvic surgery, the small bowel commonly fills the pelvis. Adhesions can form, resulting in fixed loops of small bowel in the radiation fields. In this situation, despite treatment of the patient in the prone position, the use of multiple-field techniques may be of limited value (Fig. 33.8-7). In contrast, when radiation therapy is delivered preoperatively to a patient who has not undergone prior pelvic surgery, the small bowel is usually mobile. As illustrated in Figure 33.8-8, when no small bowel fixation is present, treatment in the prone position was successful in excluding most of the small bowel from the posteroanterior field and completely from the lateral fields.

Figure 33.8-8 also illustrates the technique of placing a wire on the perineum to allow blocking in the lateral preoperative radiation fields. This technique not only decreases acute grade 3+ skin toxicity (reported as high as 94% by Rossi et al.[184] when this techniques is not used) but decreases the high incidence of perineal wound sepsis in those patients who have an APR (reported as high as 33% in the Uppsala trial[190]). A more comprehensive review of techniques for the delivery of pelvic radiation has been published.[221]

Clinical series document the importance of field size and technique in minimizing the toxicity of pelvic radiation. In the

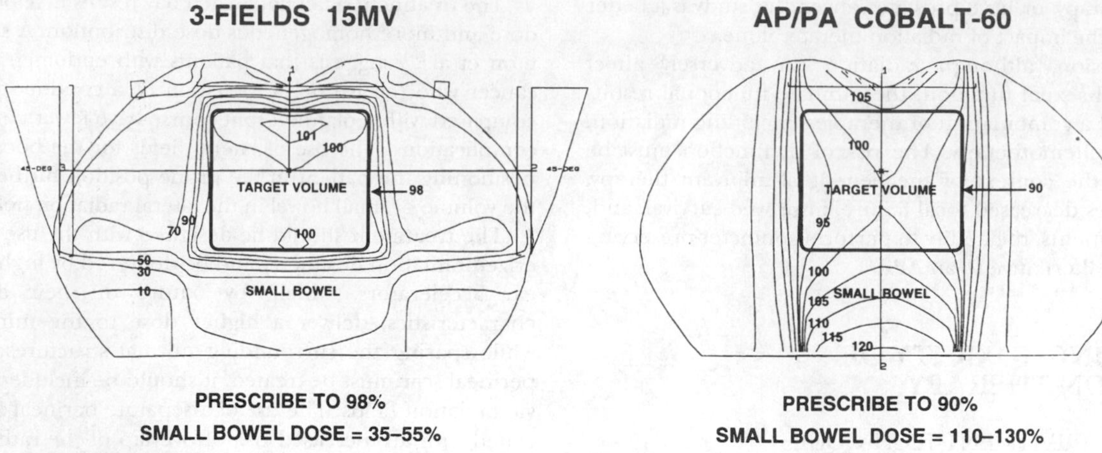

FIGURE 33.8-6. Small bowel sparing using high-energy linear accelerator radiation combined with prone three-field treatment. AP/PA, anteroposterior/posteroanterior.

series from the M. D. Anderson Cancer Center, 62 patients received postoperative pelvic radiation (40 to 50 Gy plus 6- to 10-Gy boost).[174,175] Some patients received the radiation by a combination of AP/PA and a boost with opposed laterals or a direct perineal field. In selected patients, the superior border of the field was at L2-3 and the incidence of small bowel obstruction requiring surgery was 17.5%. When the superior border of the field was decreased to L5, the incidence of small bowel obstruction decreased to 10% to 12%. The incidence of small bowel obstruction after surgery alone was 5%.

Various physical maneuvers to exclude the small bowel from the pelvis have been examined. Gallagher et al.[246] determined the volume, distribution, and mobility of small bowel in the pelvis after a variety of maneuvers. Regardless of the prior surgical history, a significant decrease was seen in the average small bowel volume when the patients were treated in the prone position with the combination of abdominal wall compression and bladder distention compared with the supine position. Use of a four-field technique further decreased the volume of small bowel. Treatment in the prone position without abdominal wall compression was not consistently effective in displacing small bowel and, in some patients (most commonly obese), the volume of small bowel increased.

Caspers and Hop (1983) performed a similar study in 50 patients who received pelvic radiation for bladder or prostate cancer. The use of the Trendelenburg or inclined procubitis positions were helpful in excluding small bowel from the pelvic radiation fields, especially for obese patients. Although the prone position was less effective than these inclined positions, it was superior to the supine position.

SMALL BOWEL CONTRAST

Small bowel contrast is essential to determine the position of small bowel during radiation simulation. It should be used routinely in patients receiving curative pelvic radiation therapy. Herbert et al.[247] found that, in patients with endometrial and rectal cancer who had small bowel contrast used at the time of radia-

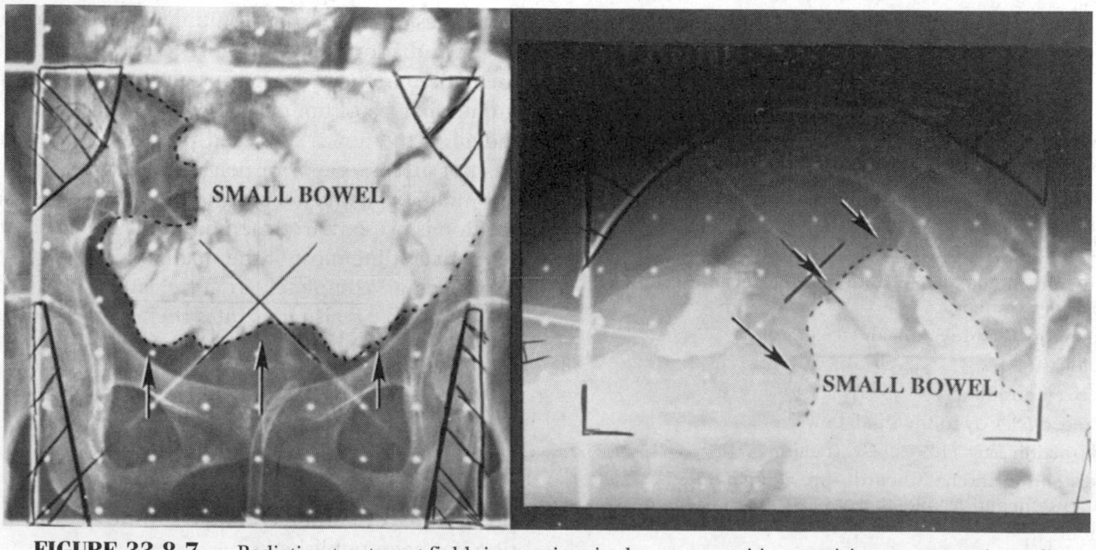

FIGURE 33.8-7. Radiation treatment fields in a patient in the prone position receiving postoperative radiation therapy using a three-field technique. Despite the prone position, the small bowel (*arrows*) remains fixed in the pelvis, and it cannot be excluded from the lateral fields.

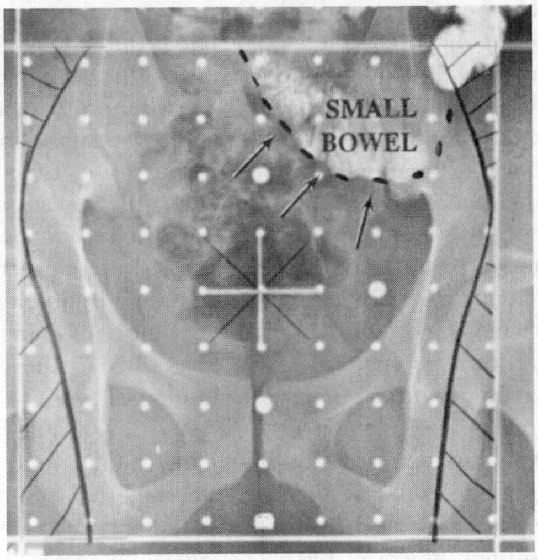

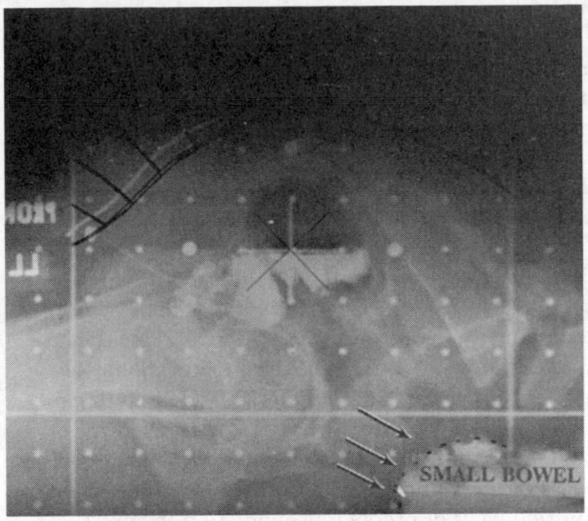

FIGURE 33.8-8. Radiation treatment fields in a patient in the prone position receiving preoperative radiation therapy using a three-field technique. The small bowel (*arrows*) is excluded from the lateral fields.

tion simulation, there was a change in the treatment field as well as a lower incidence of overall and chronic complications.[247] A multivariate analysis revealed that both the use of small bowel contrast and a lower superior border of the treatment field were predictive for decreased radiation toxicity. Visualization of small bowel contributed to an adjustment in the radiation field, resulting in a decrease in the incidence of toxicity.

IMMOBILIZATION MOLDS AND TISSUE EXPANDERS

The effectiveness of custom bowel immobilization molds (belly board) in 30 patients with pelvic malignancies has been analyzed by Shanahan et al.[248] Using a CT-based volumetric analysis, the combination of the prone position and immobilization molds decreased the mean small bowel volume in the radiation field by 66% compared with patients treated in the supine position without the immobilization mold. Fu and colleagues[249] reported that, when patients with pelvic malignancies were treated in the prone position, a belly board reduced the volume of small bowel by 28% to 50%, depending on the type of prior surgery. A similar benefit using dose volume histogram analysis in 12 patients was reported by Das and associates.[250]

Pelvic tissue expanders are also effective in decreasing the volume of small bowel in the radiation field. Herbert and colleagues[251] reported a significant decrease in small bowel volume in 14 patients who had a tissue expander compared with 63 who did not (25 cm^3 vs. 239 cm^3, P <.0001). The decrease of small bowel volume was associated with a decrease in acute toxicity. Hoffman and colleagues[252] recommended their use when native tissue is not available for small bowel exclusion. To examine the effectiveness of a silicone rubber–molded balloon during pelvis radiation, Sezeur et al.[253] measured stool weight, steatorrhea, and α_1-antitrypsine clearance. The tests remained stable, suggesting that the tissue expander was effective throughout the course of radiation.

It must be emphasized that any physical maneuver beyond the use of the prone position may be associated with patient discomfort, thereby leading to increased movement and daily setup errors. For example, Brierley and associates[254] analyzed the variation of small bowel volume in the pelvis before and during adjuvant pelvic radiation therapy for rectal cancer. They found that the displacement of small bowel from the posterior pelvis by bladder distention was not reliably maintained throughout the treatment course. Therefore, the previously described physical maneuvers and techniques, such as abdominal wall compression and belly boards, may not be beneficial. The use of such techniques should be tailored to the individual patient.

Likewise, uncertainties exist with the use of small bowel contrast. Gallagher et al.[246] reported a 20% average increase in small bowel volume after full doses of pelvic radiation when patients were reexamined after the completion of treatment.

THREE-DIMENSIONAL RADIATION TREATMENT PLANNING

Innovative techniques using three-dimensional treatment planning are being investigated. In a report from the Photon Treatment Planning Collaborative Working Group, it was found that the most important contribution of three-dimensional treatment planning in rectal cancer was the ability to plan and localize the target and normal tissues at all levels of the treatment volume rather than using the traditional method of planning with only a single central transverse slice and simulation films. A slight improvement also was noted when no constraints were placed on the type of plans (i.e., when non-coplanar beams were used). A randomized trial of conformal versus conventional radiation therapy in 266 evaluable patients with pelvic malignancies has been reported by Tait et al.[255] Although a decrease in the volume of normal tissue volumes in the radiation field was seen with conformal versus conventional treatment (689 cm^3 vs. 792 cm^3), no difference was noted in the level of symptoms or in medication prescribed.

Investigators in Uppsala examined six patients with rectal cancer who underwent both proton and conventional photon treatment planning.[256] By dose-volume histogram analysis, protons offered only a marginal benefit in sparing normal tissues.

RADIATION THERAPY AND SURGERY SEQUENCING

The major disadvantage of delivering radiation therapy in the postoperative setting is the increased incidence of fixed loops of small bowel in the pelvis. The potential merits of the use of preoperative compared with postoperative radiation therapy have been previously discussed. From the issue of toxicity, the primary advantages of preoperative radiation are decreased volume of small bowel in the radiation field and the absence of a perineal scar to be treated.

Some of the randomized trials of preoperative radiation therapy report an increased incidence of complications compared with surgery alone. However, as previously discussed, the radiation therapy in these trials was commonly delivered with inferior techniques, such as AP/PA ^{60}Co using large fields and fraction sizes. These techniques all contribute to an increased incidence of radiation complications. For example, in the Stockholm Rectal Cancer Study Group, the radiation therapy was delivered in 5-Gy fractions, the superior border was at L2, the majority of patients received ^{60}Co with an AP/PA technique, and surgery was within 7 days of the completion of radiation.[257] In contrast, the nonrandomized trials of preoperative radiation therapy that use higher doses with smaller fraction and field sizes reveal that, when preoperative radiation therapy is delivered with careful radiation techniques, the toxicity is minimized.

SURGICAL TECHNIQUES

Surgical techniques to minimize small bowel injury include reperitonealization of the pelvic floor[258]; construction of an omental pedicle flap[259]; retroversion of the uterus; placement of clips in the high-risk areas to better define the tumor volume; and the use of absorbable mesh, which temporarily removes the small bowel from the pelvis.[260] Rodier and colleagues[261] reported their experience with polyglycolic acid mesh in 60 patients. The mesh was effective in excluding the small bowel from the pelvis in 93% of patients with various pelvic malignancies. It was completely resorbed in 3 to 5 months, and the complication rate related to the mesh was 8%. Thom and associates[260] used a similar approach in 52 patients. They noted a prolonged postoperative ileus (median, 8.5 days), but no other unusual postoperative compilations. In 20 patients who underwent placement of mesh, Beitler et al.[262] reported postoperative complications possibly related to mesh in five patients and a mild postoperative ileus in 17. Because pelvic radiation therapy does not begin until approximately 4 months postoperatively, the mesh may be resorbed by that time.

DIETARY SUPPLEMENTS AND RADIOPROTECTORS

The benefit of dietary supplements and radioprotectors is controversial. Five randomized trials have examined the efficacy of various compounds to decrease bowel toxicity. These trials have included such compounds as butyric acid to decrease chronic radiation proctitis,[263] sucralfate enemas to decrease acute radiation proctitis,[264] olsalazine to decrease acute enteritis, and mesalazine (5-aminosalicylic acid) to decrease acute radiation enteritis.[265] All of these randomized trials have been negative. In another randomized trial of 73 patients with pelvic malignancies, the addition of 5-aminosalicylic acid increased rather than decreased acute radiation toxicity. Diarrhea was more frequent in the radiation plus 5-aminosalicylic acid arm compared with radiation alone (91% vs. 74%, $P = .07$).

In a phase II trial using an elemental diet, Craighead and Young[266] reported a decrease in acute enteritis in 17 patients with gynecologic cancer, but only 77% of the patients complied with the diet. McArdle et al. (1986) compared the results of an elemental diet in 24 patients with bladder cancer who received 4 Gy × 5 before cystectomy with a similar historical group of 32 patients who received a regular diet or total parenteral nutrition with the same therapy. A significant decrease was reported in the incidence and severity of diarrhea, nausea and vomiting, abdominal cramps, and the time to the recovery of small bowel function in the patients who received the elemental diet. The mechanism of protection of the mucosa by an elemental diet is unclear. Theories include a reduction of pancreaticobiliary secretion, the removal of abrasive bulk in the chyme, and a decrease in the rate of crypt cell turnover.

In a phase I/II study of 13 patients with chronic radiation proctitis, oral sodium pentosanpolysulfate resulted in a complete resolution of symptoms in 82% and a partial resolution in 9%. Although patients receiving pelvic radiation have reduced lactose absorption, the available data suggest that lactose-restricted diets do not prevent radiation-induced diarrhea. Stryker and Bartholomew[267] examined 64 patients undergoing pelvic radiation for various malignancies who were randomized to a regular diet, a regular diet including lactase enzyme, or a lactose-restricted diet. No significant differences were found in stool frequency or diphenoxylate usage among the three dietary groups.

Liu et al.[268] performed a randomized trial of pelvic radiation therapy (2.25 Gy per fraction to 45 Gy) with or without the radioprotector WR-2721 in patients with inoperable or unresectable rectal cancer. The incidence of RTOG long-term grade 3+ gastrointestinal, genitourinary, and skin toxicity was 3% in the radiation therapy alone arm compared with 0% in the radiation therapy plus WR-2721 arm. A separate trial by Montana and colleagues (1992) showed no benefit with a topical application of WR-2721 to the rectal mucosa. Based on these data, WR-2721 does not offer radioprotection in patients with rectal cancer who receive pelvic radiation therapy.

Patients with gynecologic malignancies who receive pelvic radiation therapy may have a lower long-term incidence of severe toxicity with increased caffeine consumption. One study suggested that sucralfate may decrease acute and long-term small bowel toxicity in patients receiving pelvic radiation therapy for prostate and bladder cancer.

In summary, all cancer therapies have associated toxicities. It must be emphasized that all patients receiving pelvic radiation therapy have acute treatment-related toxicity, and despite the use of careful treatment techniques, approximately 1% have severe long-term toxicity. These toxicities must be examined in perspective, because the benefits of radiation therapy include significantly decreasing local failure and, in the preoperative setting, sphincter preservation. This is all the more reason to pay careful attention to techniques, which help to decrease the acute and long-term toxicities of pelvic radiation.

The exclusion of small bowel from the treatment field is the most important factor in decreasing the toxicity. With the use of careful radiation techniques as well as physical and surgical methods, the toxicity can be reduced to an acceptable level. In patients who have not had prior pelvic surgery, preoperative radiation therapy (when delivered with conventional fractionation and multiple-field techniques) may have less toxicity compared with postoperative radiation therapy.[220] The results of the ongoing randomized trials of preoperative versus postoperative combined modality therapy for resectable rectal cancer (NSABP R-03 and CAO/ARO/AIO 94) will provide a more definitive answer. Unless a contraindication exists, the most simple techniques to decrease radiation toxicity, such as the use of small bowel contrast, multiple-field techniques, high-energy linear accelerators, custom blocks, avoiding a direct perineal boost, and treatment in the prone position, should be part of the standard treatment of patients receiving curative adjuvant radiation therapy.

TREATMENT OF LOCALLY ADVANCED AND UNRESECTABLE RECTAL CANCER

A significant improvement in local control and survival can be achieved for patients with primary resectable (T3) rectal cancer with the use of combined modality therapy.[83,177] It is more difficult to obtain these results for locally advanced or unresectable cancers. For locally advanced or unresectable rectal cancers, collectively defined as T4 disease, no uniform determination of resectability has been established. Depending on the series, T4 disease can vary from a tethered or "marginally resectable" cancer to a fixed cancer with adherence or direct invasion of adjacent organs or vital structures. This definition has prognostic implications, because patients with gross invasion of tumor into vital pelvic structures may be approached in a palliative rather than a curative fashion. The definition of resectability also depends on whether the assessment is made by radiographic criteria, a clinical office examination, examination under anesthesia, or at the time of surgery. For example, tumors thought to be unresectable at the time of clinical or radiographic examination may be found to be more mobile when the patient is relaxed under anesthesia. Prognostic differences also exist between primary and recurrent tumors, and many series do not report the results separately. The heterogeneity of the disease and absence of a uniform definition of resectability may explain some of the variation in results seen among the series.

TUMORS AMENABLE TO POTENTIALLY CURATIVE RADICAL SURGERY

Selected patients with primary unresectable disease may be cured with radical surgery, such as a pelvic exenteration. These include tumors invading the prostate, the base of the bladder, or the uterus, where the disease can be resected *en bloc* with negative margins.

MULTIVISCERAL RESECTION FOR LOCALLY ADVANCED RECTAL CANCER

Approximately 6% to 10% of rectal cancers are locally advanced and require extensive surgery for complete tumor extirpation. Pelvic exenteration involving *en bloc* removal of the rectum, bladder, distal ureters, and reproductive organs can be required to obtain negative margins of resection.[146] A number of studies have demonstrated 5-year survival rates ranging from 33% to 50% for these selected patients with locally advanced rectal cancer. Despite the ability to achieve long-range survival rates in selected patients, the operation remains a formidable one, with significant morbidity and a mortality of up to 6%.[60] Patients who undergo such resections for primary tumors have better survival rates than those with recurrence.

In a report by Meterissian et al.,[35] a series of 40 patients undergoing pelvic exenteration for rectal carcinoma obtained tumor-free margins. The 5-year overall survival rate was 49% with a median survival of 56 months. Adjuvant chemoradiation appeared to provide a reduction in risk of recurrence. In the series, five patients developed local failure. Comparable results have been recorded by Lopez et al. (1987), Kraybill et al. (1988), and Boey et al. (1982). Long-term local control is obtained in approximately 70% of the patients who undergo resection with tumor-free margins. The results of such surgery cannot be separated from the benefits of adjuvant chemoradiation in this high-risk population.

Improved results from surgical procedures for rectal cancer requiring multivisceral resection have occurred in more recent years.[61] This finding may be related to improvements in perioperative care, patient selection, and surgical techniques. Of major importance in the management of such patients, who are often heavily radiated, is the use of vascularized tissue flaps to accomplish healing of pelvic and perineal wounds.[62]

Physical examination, CT scan, MRI, and cystoscopy all play a role in staging patients with locally advanced rectal cancer. Involvement of the sciatic notch indicated by symptoms or scans predicts a situation unlikely to be helped by surgery. With CT or MRI imaging, recurrent pelvic tumor, especially following an APR, is difficult to differentiate from scar. PET may offer a more accurate assessment.[136]

RADIATION THERAPY

Preoperative Pelvic Radiation Therapy

Because surgery commonly leaves residual disease in the pelvis in patients with locally advanced or unresectable disease, the standard approach has been to use preoperative pelvic radiation therapy. Given the increased complete response[269] and resection[157] rates when 5-FU–based chemotherapy is added to radiation in the preoperative setting, as well as the improvement in local control in the postoperative setting, most patients receive combined modality therapy. The goals of preoperative therapy are to convert an unresectable cancer to a resectable status and decrease the incidence of local failure.

The optimal use of preoperative radiation therapy requires full doses (45 Gy or more) and, to achieve optimal down-staging, a 4- to 6-week delay between the completion of radiation and surgery. This discussion is limited to those series that meet these criteria.

In a seminal report from the MGH of 25 patients with recurrent or primary unresectable cancer, a complete resection with negative margins was possible in 64% of patients after preoperative radiation therapy. Despite negative margins, the incidence of local failure was 38%. The nine patients who were unable to undergo a complete resection were dead of disease within 28 months.

The British Medical Research Council completed a randomized trial of preoperative radiation therapy (40 Gy in 20 fractions) versus surgery alone for 279 patients with clinical T4 primary rectal cancer.[193] Patients who received preoperative radiation had a significant decrease in local failure (36% vs. 46%, $P = .04$) and distant failure (35% vs. 48%, $P = .02$). An improvement was noted in median survival (31 months vs. 24 months, $P =$ NS), but no difference in survival was reported (32% vs. 28%). The 36% local failure rate after preoperative radiation is consistent with the MGH data and supports the need for additional treatment, such as intraoperative radiation therapy (IORT).

As one would predict, the results of the patients with primary disease are more favorable than those with recurrent disease. In the MGH series, the rate of complete resection with negative margins was 59% for patients with primary cancers[270] compared with 44% of those with recurrent cancers.[271] Limiting the analysis to the most favorable group of patients with primary cancers and negative margins, the 5-year actuarial local failure rate was 29%, and the disease-free survival rate was 60%. Therefore, even in the most favorable group of patients (primary cancer and negative margins), local failure is still almost 30%. At the University of Florida, in the 48% of patients who were able to undergo a complete resection with negative margins, the local failure rate was 55% and the 5-year determinate survival rate was 20%.[272,273] Tobin and colleagues[274] reported a local failure rate of 20% and a 5-year survival rate of 60% in 85 patients treated with preoperative radiation. At Memorial Sloan-Kettering Cancer Center, 58% of patients underwent a complete resection with negative margins after preoperative radiation, and the local failure rate was 25%.

Tethered cancers have the most favorable outcome of all T4 cancers. In a separate report from the MGH, the results of 28 patients with tethered rectal cancers treated with preoperative radiation were presented.[275] Tethered was defined as the sensation on the examining finger of partial tumor mobility consistent with extensive perirectal spread and adherence but not fixation to unresectable structures. Although a complete resection with negative margins was possible in 93%, the local failure rate was 24%. Tobin et al.[274] report a local failure rate of 14% and 5-year survival rate of 68% in 49 patients with tethered cancers treated with preoperative radiation.

In summary, after full-dose preoperative radiation, most series report that 48% to 64% of patients are converted to a resectable status. However, despite a complete resection and negative margins, the local failure rate varies, depending on the degree of tumor fixation, from 24% to 55%.

IMPROVING THE RESULTS OF PREOPERATIVE RADIATION THERAPY

A major limitation of pelvic radiation therapy is that the dose required to achieve an adequate level of local control, in many cases, exceeds the tolerance of the surrounding normal tissues. In an attempt to improve the results of preoperative radiation, a number of approaches have been used. The most promising have included IORT and the addition of systemic chemotherapy.

Intraoperative Radiation Therapy

The primary advantage of IORT is that radiation can be delivered at the time of surgery to the site with the highest risk of local failure (the tumor bed) while decreasing the dose to the surrounding normal tissues. IORT can be delivered by two techniques: electron beam and brachytherapy. With the electron-beam technique, the radiation is delivered by a linear accelerator and, with the use of a cone, is directed to the tumor bed. When the IORT is finished, the cone is removed and the surgery is completed.

Brachytherapy is delivered with both low-dose and high-dose techniques. The low-dose method involves implantation of radioactive sources, with either removable ^{192}Ir-afterloading catheters or iodine 125 or palladium 103 permanent seeds.[276] The permanent seeds can be sutured or implanted directly into the tumor. As an alternative, they can be placed in a Dexon mesh that is then sutured to the tumor bed.[277] Most of the low-dose brachytherapy experience has been in patients with gross residual disease. It also has been used as an alternative to electron-beam IORT in patients with negative margins.[278] High dose-rate brachytherapy uses a flexible multichannel applicator that conforms to the tumor bed. The applicator is positioned, and an ^{192}Ir source is programmed to deliver a uniform dose to the area at risk using a similar dose rate to electron-beam IORT.[278,279]

The results of IORT depend on whether the patient has primary unresectable or recurrent disease and whether the margins of resection are negative or whether microscopic or gross residual disease is present. This discussion is limited to patients who, in general, receive preoperative pelvic radiation with or without 5-FU–based chemotherapy. Most receive 45.0 to 50.4 Gy to the pelvis and 10 to 20 Gy IORT with either electrons or high dose-rate with a flexible applicator. The lower IORT dose is used for patients with negative margins, and the higher doses are used for patients with microscopic or gross residual disease.

Primary Unresectable Disease

The largest experience and longest median follow-up in preoperative therapy followed by IORT has been reported from the MGH.[280] As seen in Table 33.8-15, for patients with negative margins, local failure is decreased from 18% without IORT to 11% with IORT. In patients with positive margins, local failure is decreased from 83% without IORT to 43% with IORT if gross residual disease is present and to 32% with IORT if microscopic residual disease is present. For the total patient group (with or without IORT), the 5-year disease-free survival rate was 63% for patients with negative margins and 32% for patients with positive margins. These results underscore the importance of delivering preoperative therapy to help achieve the most complete resection possible. If negative margins cannot be obtained, then microscopic residual is still preferable to gross residual. Series from the Mayo Clinic[281] and Memorial Sloan-Kettering Cancer Center[278] report similar local failure rates in patients with negative margins (7% and 8%, respectively). The results of other series from Munich,[279] Heidelberg,[282] and the Beth Israel Deaconess Medical Center[283] are seen in Table 33.8-15.

Recurrent Disease

In the setting of recurrent disease, the largest experience with IORT is from the Mayo Clinic.[284] In contrast with the series of patients treated for primary unresectable disease, those with recurrent disease have less uniform treatment programs, including some who have received prior pelvic radiation[284,285] and some treated with IORT alone.[278] Selected series in which all patients received IORT are seen in Table 33.8-16.

At the Mayo Clinic, 119 patients received, in general, 50.4 to 54.0 Gy preoperatively followed by 7.5 to 20.0 Gy electron-beam IORT.[284] The higher IORT doses were used for patients with residual disease. For patient with negative margins, the crude local failure rate was 6%, which increased to 18% for micro-

TABLE 33.8-15. Primary Locally Advanced or Unresectable Rectal Cancer with and without Intraoperative Radiation (IORT): Selected Series

					Local Failure Margins					*Survival Margins*		
Series	*Number of Patients*	*F/U (mo)*	*Preoperative Treatment[a]*	*IORT*	No.	Negative	No.	Positive	Total	Negative	Positive	Total
Massachusetts General Hospital[280]	145	41 median	45.0–50.4 Gy ± 5-FU	Yes	45	11% 5-y	21 microscopic	32% 5-y		63% 5-y	32% 5-y	
			± 10–20 Gy IORT				7 gross	43% 5-y		DFS	DFS	
							28 total	35% 5-y				
				No	66	18% 5-y	6 total	83% 5-y				
Mayo[295]	61	18 minimum	45–55 Gy ± 5-FU	Yes	18	6% crude	19 microscopic	5% crude	13% crude		Gross 21% 5-y	46% 5-y
			10–20 Gy IORT			7% 5-y		14% 5-y	16% 5-y			
							16 gross	25% crude				
								27% 5-y				
Munich[279]	19	—	39.6 Gy b.i.d. + 5-FU	Yes					10% crude			
			15 Gy HDR IORT									
Heidelberg[282]	40	18 median	41.4 Gy + 5-FU	Yes						91% DFS		
			10–18 Gy IORT									
Memorial Sloan-Kettering Cancer Center[278]	18	18 median	50.4 Gy + 5-FU/LV	Yes		8% 2-y		62% 2-y	19% 2-y	77% 2-y	38% 2-y	69% 2-y
			10–20 Gy HDR IORT							DFS	DFS	
Beth Israel Deaconess Medical Center[283]	27	24 median	50.4 Gy ± 5-FU	Yes					27% crude			41% NED
			12.5–17.0 Gy Orthovoltage IORT									

DFS, disease-free survival; 5-FU, 5-fluorouracil; F/U, follow-up; HDR, high dose-rate intraoperative radiation; LV, leucovorin; NED, no evidence of disease.
[a]In most patients.

TABLE 33.8-16. Role of Intraoperative Radiation (IORT) in Recurrent Rectal Cancer: Selected Series

Series	Number of Patients	F/U (mo)	Preoperative Treatment[a]	Local Failure Margins					Survival Margins		
				No.	Negative	No.	Positive	Total	Negative	Positive	Total
Massachusetts General Hospital[285]	41	31 median	50.4 Gy ± 5-FU	27	58% 5-y (or micro-scopic+)	14	89% 5-y (gross)	70% 5-y	21% 5-y	7% 5-y	16% 5-y
			10–20 Gy IORT						DFS	DFS	
			Some prior EBRT								
Mayo[284]	119	—	50.4–54.0 Gy	17	6% crude	40 micro-scopic	18% crude	20% crude			20% 5-y
			7.5–20.0 Gy IORT				27% 5-y	37% 5-y			
			Some postoperative EBRT			65 gross	25% crude				
							40% 5-y				
Heidelberg[288]	31	28 median	41.4 Gy (22 preoperative)	14	21% crude	9 micro-scopic	33% crude	29% crude	71% 4-y	29% 4-y	48% 4-y (DFS)
			Mean 13.7 Gy IORT		22% 4-y		39% 4-y		DFS	DFS	58% 4-y
						8 gross	37% crude				
							40% 4-y				
M. D. Anderson Cancer Center[286]	43[b]	26 median	45 Gy + 5-FU ± CDDP					36%			37% 5-y (DFS)
			10–20 Gy IORT								58% 5-y
Memorial Sloan-Kettering Cancer Center[278]	46	18 median	(16) 50.4 Gy ± 5-FU/LV		18% 2-y		81% 2-y	37% 2-y	71% 2-y	0% 2-y	47% 2-y
			10–20 Gy HDR IORT						DFS	DFS	
			(25) 10–20 Gy IORT alone								
Beth Israel Deaconess Medical Center[283]	13	24 median	50.4 Gy ± 5-FU					73%			27% NED
			12.5–17.0 Gy								
			Orthovoltage IORT								
French IORT Group[300]	73	30 median	(30) 39 Gy ± 5-FU					31% 3-y (57% margins negative)			31% 3-y
			10–15 Gy IORT								
			(43) 10–15 Gy IORT alone								

CDDP, *cis*-diamminedichloroplatinum; DFS, disease-free survival; EBRT, external-beam pelvic radiation therapy; 5-FU, 5-fluorouracil; F/U, follow-up; HDR, high dose-rate intraoperative radiation; LV, leucovorin; NED, no evidence of disease.

[a]In most patients.

[b]Excluding ten patients with multifocal or extrapelvic disease.

scopic and 25% for gross residual disease. The 5-year actuarial local failure rates were 27% for microscopic disease and 45% for gross residual disease. For the total patient group, overall 5-year survival was 20%. The M. D. Anderson Cancer Center,[286] Memorial Sloan-Kettering Cancer Center,[278] and the French IORT group reported similar local failure rates for the total patient group (36%, 37%, and 31%, respectively). In one series of 25 patients selected to receive IORT, the 5-year survival rate was 21%.[287] In contrast, the results from the MGH were not as favorable.[285] They reported an 89% 5-year actuarial local failure rate for patients with gross residual disease and 70% for the total patient group. The 5-year disease-free survival rate was 21% for patients with negative margins and only 7% for those with positive margins. Memorial Sloan-Kettering reported no survivors at 2 years with positive margins,[278] whereas in the Heidelberg series, the 4-year disease-free survival rate was 29%.[288] In contrast to patients with recurrent disease who have negative or microscopic positive margins, it is unclear if those with positive margins benefit from aggressive therapy.

Complications of Electron-Beam Intraoperative Radiation Therapy

Initial reports of neuropathy, vasculitis, bone necrosis, and ureteral injury in dogs who received IORT have been described.[164,165] In two series, hyperthermia increased the neurologic complication of IORT.[200] In canines, IORT-induced secondary malignancies are seen in 15%, with most occurring with doses of more than 25 Gy.[290]

As the IORT data have matured, similar morbidity has been reported in humans. The incidence of toxicity depends on whether the patient has primary or recurrent cancer. In the MGH IORT experience, the incidence of complications was higher in those with recurrent disease (10%, soft tissue or sacral injury; 10%, pelvic neuropathy) compared with primary disease (2%, sacral necrosis or ureteral obstruction).[270,271]

Higher complication rates have been reported from the Mayo Clinic.[291] In patients with primary or recurrent colorectal cancer, the incidence of peripheral neuropathy was 32%. The symptoms of pain, numbness, and tingling resolved in 40% of patients, but only 13% had resolution of weakness. Ureteral obstruction or hydronephrosis were seen in 63% of patients who did not have evidence of ureteral obstruction at presentation. Although no relationship was found between the incidence of complications and the external-beam dose, the incidence of complications increased with the IORT dose.

In contrast to patients who undergo adjuvant therapy for resectable rectal cancers, it is difficult to clearly separate treatment-related complications from disease-related complications in patients with recurrent rectal cancers. Complications such as delayed healing, infection, fistula, and neuropathy may be the result of recurrent tumor, aggressive surgery, radiation, or a combination of these. The 2-year actuarial risk of significant complications in the 42 patients with advanced or recurrent rectal cancer who received IORT as a component of their therapy in the RTOG 85-08 trial was 16%.[292] However, compared with a nonrandomized group who underwent surgery without IORT, no significant increase was found in acute surgical complications in the IORT patients.[293]

In summary, the phase I/II data suggest that the addition of IORT to preoperative radiation therapy improves local control compared with preoperative radiation therapy alone. The results in the subset of patients with recurrent cancer or residual disease are not optimal. No phase III trials of IORT are in progress.

Preoperative Combined Modality Therapy

The encouraging results seen in patients with resectable rectal cancer who receive adjuvant postoperative combined modality therapy[83,177] have resulted in a shift to preoperative combined modality therapy. A number of potential advantages to such therapy exist. First, nonrandomized data from Minsky et al. (1992) suggest that the patients are able to tolerate higher chemotherapy doses and experience significantly lower acute toxicity compared with postoperative combined modality therapy.

Second, in patients with unresectable disease, the addition of chemotherapy to preoperative radiation therapy increases the down-staging and resectability rates.[269] Frykholm et al.[294] reported an enhanced resectability rate in patients with unresectable rectal cancer who received preoperative radiation therapy, 5-FU, methotrexate, and leucovorin rescue compared with 38 patients who received radiation alone (71% vs. 34%). Enhanced resectability is important, because patients with initially unresectable rectal cancer who have microscopic or gross residual disease have higher local failure rates and lower survival rates compared with those patients who undergo a complete resection.[280,284,295]

The third advantage is that the start of systemic therapy is not delayed, the metastatic burden is the smallest, and few drug-resistant cells are likely to be present.[296] The fourth advantage is sphincter preservation.

A number of phase I/II trials of preoperative combined modality therapy for patients with T4 disease have been conducted.[279,280,282–286,288,295,297–300] Some include patients with T3 disease, thereby making interpretation of the local control and survival results difficult.[151,159,273] The majority have used 45.0 to 50.4 Gy plus two cycles of concurrent 5-FU–based chemotherapy, with bolus 5-FU plus leucovorin or continuous infusion 5-FU, followed by surgery and an additional four cycles of postoperative chemotherapy. Some have used methotrexate[160] or interferon.[301] Marsh et al.[273] have combined chronobiologically shaped 5-FU infusion with preoperative radiation therapy. Trials examining the use of newer chemotherapeutic agents, such as raltitrexed (Tomudex),[161,162,302] Orzel (oral tegafur, uracil, and 5-fluorouracil plus leucovorin),[163] CPT-11,[164,165] and oxaliplatin, with preoperative radiation therapy are in progress.

INTRAOPERATIVE OR POSTOPERATIVE RADIATION THERAPY FOR RESIDUAL DISEASE

For a variety of reasons, some patients with locally advanced or unresectable cancer do not receive preoperative radiation therapy or, despite a preoperative assessment of resectability, are not able to undergo a complete resection. In this setting, does IORT or postoperative pelvic radiation therapy have any benefit? As previously discussed, the interpretation of treatment results is complicated, because many studies combine patients with primary and recurrent cancers as well as those with gross

TABLE 33.8-17. Failure after External Beam Radiation: Aggressive Surgical and Radiotherapeutic Options

Series	*Number of Patients*	*Treatment*	*Median F/U (mo)*	*Margins*	*% Local Failure*	*Survival*
Thomas Jefferson University[94]	39	Preoperative 36 Gy (reirradiation) + surgery	36	—	55 5-y	24% 5-y; 45 mo median
USC/Mayo[345]	30	Surgery and brachytherapy	27	20 gross+ 8 microscopic+ 2 negative	62 34 0	23% NED
Mayo[130]	16	Sacral resection + IORT	18		25	48% 2-y
Ohio State[346]	26[a]	Surgery and IORT	28	—	77 4-y	36% 4-y; 23 mo median
Memorial Sloan-Kettering Cancer Center[276]	36	Surgery and brachytherapy	24	Gross+	44	25% 4-y
Memorial Sloan-Kettering Cancer Center[278]	46	HDR IORT[b] + surgery	17.5	—	37 2-y	47% 2-y

EBRT, external-beam radiation therapy; F/U, follow-up; HDR, high dose-rate intraoperative radiation; IORT, intraoperative radiation therapy; NED, no evidence of disease; USC, University of Southern California.
[a]Only 69% with prior EBRT.
[b]Includes 16 patients who received preoperative radiation who did not receive prior pelvic radiation.

and microscopic residual disease. Patients are randomly selected to receive chemotherapy, and some series include patients with metastatic disease. This discussion is limited to those series in which patients have disease limited to the pelvis.

Likewise, for patients who have been unsuccessful with prior pelvic radiation, the options are limited. The standard therapy is usually palliative surgery or systemic chemotherapy. The response rate with chemotherapy may be reduced in a pelvis that has received full-dose radiation. Is there a role for more aggressive treatment? A variety of radiotherapeutic options for patients who have been unsuccessful with prior pelvic radiation are available and are listed in Table 33.8-17. Although these are investigational approaches in selected patients, they may offer an improvement in local control.

SUBTOTAL RESECTION AND POSTOPERATIVE RADIATION THERAPY

At the Mayo Clinic, 17 patients with rectal cancer received postoperative radiation therapy (40 to 60 Gy).[303] Six received concurrent 5-FU–based systemic chemotherapy. For the total patient group, local failure was 76% and 5-year actuarial survival was 24%. The seven patients with gross residual disease had higher local failure (86% vs. 70%) and lower survival (14% vs. 30%) compared with the ten patients with microscopic residual disease. No clear dose-response curve emerged, but only one patient received 56 Gy or more.

In a separate report from the Mayo Clinic, the results of 106 patients who underwent a palliative (subtotal) resection for locally recurrent rectal cancer were presented.[304] 5-FU was delivered in 48%. In the subset of 34 patients with gross residual disease who received IORT and postoperative therapy, the 3-year survival rate was 44%. However, despite the encouraging survival rate, 40% developed local failure and 60% developed distant failure. Univariate analysis revealed a significant improvement in survival in those patients with microscopic compared with gross residual disease, the use of IORT, a limited number of sites of tumor fixation, and higher performance status. These data suggest that, even in patients with locally recurrent residual disease, an aggressive approach should be considered.

Other reports have included patients with both rectal and colon cancers as well as patients with both primary and recurrent disease. At the MGH, patients received somewhat higher doses of radiation (60 to 70 Gy) compared with the Mayo Clinic external-beam therapy alone series.[305] Seven patients received electron-beam IORT. For the total group, local failure was 42% and the 5-year disease-free survival rate was 18%. The 23 patients with gross residual disease had a higher local failure rate (57% vs. 30%) and a significant decrease in survival (4% vs. 42%) compared with the 30 patients with microscopic residual disease. The improvement in local control compared with the Mayo Clinic external-beam therapy alone series may have been related to the higher radiation doses. No clear dose-response curve was noted in patients with gross disease, but patients with microscopic residual disease who received less than 60 Gy did have a higher incidence of local failure compared with those who received 60 Gy or more (38% vs. 26%).

Another factor that may have an impact on the local failure rate is the volume of gross residual disease. As seen in Tables 33.8-15 and 33.8-16, this is consistent with the experience from the MGH[280,285] and the Mayo Clinic[284,295] IORT series, in which patients with gross residual disease had lower survival and higher local failure rates compared with patients with microscopic residual disease.

The dose of radiation needed to treat potential microscopic disease (after a complete resection) is 45.0 to 50.4 Gy, which is within the tolerance of the surrounding normal tissues. However, when microscopic or gross biopsy-proven residual disease is present (after a subtotal resection), the dose of required radiation is higher. Even in situations in which the small bowel can be excluded from the external-beam radiation field, other surrounding normal tissues limit the dose to 60 to 65 Gy, which may be inadequate to control large volumes of gross residual tumor. Therefore, it is not surprising that the results for patients with residual disease who receive postoperative radiation therapy are disappointing. The obvious advantage of preoperative therapy is that it decreases the primary tumor volume, thereby allowing maximum surgery and IORT.

REIRRADIATION FOLLOWED BY SURGERY

In patients with a local recurrence who have received prior pelvic radiation, Lingareddy et al.[94] reported the use of reirradiation in a selected group of 39 patients. They received a median dose of 36 Gy using limited lateral fields plus continuous infusion 5-FU. The whole pelvis was not treated, and the bladder and small bowel were excluded as much as possible from the radiation field. With a median follow-up of 3 years, the 5-year actuarial local failure rate was 55% and survival was 24%. In highly selected patients, retreatment with limited fields may be an option; however, this approach should be considered experimental.

EXTERNAL-BEAM RADIATION THERAPY ALONE

Patients selected for radiation therapy alone are usually medically inoperable or have very advanced local disease such that resection would compromise a vital structure. This approach has been previously discussed in the section Radiotherapy Alone for Rectal Cancer[93–95,105] (see Table 33.8-6).

POSTOPERATIVE RADIATION THERAPY AND CHEMOTHERAPY

Two randomized trials of postoperative combined modality therapy versus radiation alone have been conducted in patients with medically inoperable or advanced local disease. In the RTOG trial, 129 patients with residual, primary unresectable, or recurrent rectal cancer were randomized to radiation therapy plus concurrent 5-FU followed by maintenance 5-FU plus methyl CCNU versus radiation therapy alone. Some patients received IORT. No significant difference was reported in the estimated actuarial 2-year survival rate in patients who received combined modality therapy compared with radiation therapy alone (44% vs. 36%). Of the patients with gross residual disease (in either arm), 25% were without evidence of disease, 6% were locally controlled, and 50% died with a component of local failure.

The Eastern Cooperative Oncology Group randomized 30 patients with recurrent, residual, or primary inoperable rectal cancer to postoperative continuous course radiation therapy versus split course radiation therapy plus 5-FU followed by maintenance 5-FU plus methyl CCNU. The median survival in both arms was 17 months. The five patients with primary inoperable cancer (considered gross residual) had the shortest 2-year survival rate (0%), compared with the 16 patients with recurrent disease (25%) or the nine with residual disease (54%).

Therefore, postoperative combined modality therapy, as delivered in these two randomized trials, did not have a significant impact on survival compared with postoperative radiation therapy alone in this subset of patients. Other chemotherapeutic agents and schedules are being investigated.

INTRAOPERATIVE RADIATION THERAPY ALONE FOR GROSS RESIDUAL DISEASE

A subset of patients with recurrent rectal cancer have clinically unresectable gross residual pelvic disease and, because of prior full-dose pelvic radiation therapy, would require an attempt at resection without the benefit of pre- or postoperative radiation therapy, or both. Furthermore, when IORT is not available, this group of patients is commonly approached in a palliative fashion, because surgery alone cannot control gross residual disease.

The results of 36 patients with recurrent rectal cancer who had gross residual disease remaining in the pelvis after biopsy alone or subtotal resection were reported by Minsky et al.[276] from the Memorial Sloan-Kettering Cancer Center. With a median follow-up of 24 months, the local failure rate was 44% and the 4-year actuarial survival rate was 25%. The local control rate was dependent on the volume of residual disease. With brachytherapy, the tumor volume is proportional to the volume of the implant. The local failure rate was lower in those patients who underwent subtotal resection compared with a biopsy alone (33% vs. 66%), and in those with an ^{125}I implant volume of less than 40 cm^3 compared to 40 cm^3 or more (39% vs. 100%). Severe treatment-related complications were seen in 11% of locally controlled patients.

The experience with electron-beam IORT in this group of patients is more limited. Calvo et al.[306] reported a subgroup of five patients with gross residual or recurrent colorectal cancer who received 10- to 80-Gy electron-beam IORT. All tumors were larger than 4 cm. With a median follow-up of 11 months, the incidence of local failure was 40%. Complications included pelvic abscess (in one patient), pelvic pain (in two), and lower extremity neuropathy (in one). The more recent trial by Martinez-Monge and associates[137] included patients with extrapelvic disease; therefore, it is not discussed.

In summary, the limited data suggest that IORT with electrons or brachytherapy does not improve the ultimate survival rate in this group of patients. However, it does offer reasonable local control (56% to 60%) with acceptable morbidity. Because local control, in and of itself, is an important end point in the treatment of rectal cancer, it is appropriate to continue to evaluate IORT as part of an overall aggressive approach in patients with residual disease who are unable to receive pelvic radiation therapy.

INVESTIGATIONAL RADIATION THERAPY APPROACHES

A number of investigational radiation therapy approaches have been used in an attempt to enhance the treatment results in patients with both resectable and unresectable rectal cancers and other pelvic malignancies. These include neutron beam radiation, hyperthermia, radiosensitizers, and altered radiation fractionation schemes. Radioprotectors[263–265,268] (discussed earlier in Dietary Supplements and Radioprotectors) and three-dimensional treatment planning[255] (discussed earlier in Three-Dimensional Radiation Treatment Planning) already have been described.

NEUTRON BEAM RADIATION THERAPY

The theoretical advantages of neutrons compared with more conventional radiation include increased sensitivity of hypoxic cells and more advantageous radiation repair and sensitivity characteristics of normal tissues. The results of two randomized trials that have compared neutrons and photons in patients with unresectable and recurrent rectal cancers were reported by Duncan et al.[307] A total of 35 patients received neutrons using a variety of techniques and doses. Not only were no significant differences in local control or survival detected, but patients who received neutrons experienced higher acute and long-term grade 3+ skin toxicity. The preferential absorption in fat of neutrons may have contributed to the complications seen in the skin and subcutaneous tissues. Similar severe and fatal complications were reported in a series of 25 patients with advanced rectal cancer treated by Battermann et al. (1982). Despite the theoretical advantages, little interest has been shown in the treatment of rectal cancer with neutrons.

HYPERTHERMIA

Hyperthermia, in conjunction with radiation, has been mostly used as a palliative modality in rectal cancer.[308–312] Its rationale is based on an *in vitro* synergistic interaction of radiation and hyperthermia. The results of this combination in patients with various pelvic and abdominal malignancies has been reported in a phase I/II trial by the RTOG.[313] The acute and long-term toxicities were acceptable; however, in 68% of the patients, the hyperthermia had to be discontinued because of discomfort. Final results are pending. Hyperthermia has been reported to increase the neurologic complications of patients receiving IORT.[289]

RADIOSENSITIZERS

Randomized clinical trials in rectal cancer have clearly shown that 5-FU is a radiosensitizer. When combined with adjuvant postoperative radiation therapy, it significantly decreases local failure compared with radiation therapy alone.[83,177] Various mechanisms for 5-FU–mediated radiosensitization have been proposed, but none alone explain all the interactions.[314] Nonrandomized data from Rhomberg et al.[315] suggest that razoxane may improve local control and median survival in patients who receive radiation for inoperable recurrent rectal cancer. Other trials of radiosensitizers have not revealed a clear benefit.

ALTERED RADIATION FRACTIONATION SCHEMAS

Various fractionation programs have evolved with the goal of enhancing tumor cell damage by radiation without increasing normal tissue injury. The repair of subcellular injury, regeneration, cell-cycle redistribution, and reoxygenation are all factors at the cellular level contributing to differences in how various normal tissues and tumors respond to fractionated radiation. The use of hyperfractionation and accelerated fractionation schemes take advantage of some of these factors. The late effects should be the same as or, more likely, less than conventional fractionation schemes. A phase I trial from Lausanne of postoperative accelerated hyperfractionation (1.6 Gy twice a day to 48 Gy) reported acceptable acute toxicity.[316] Updated data from this group suggests that twice daily radiation is better tolerated when delivered preoperatively rather than postoperatively.[317] Bozzetti et al.[318] reported a pathologic complete response rate of 9% in 59 patients with ultrasound stage T2–3 disease who preoperatively received 1.5 Gy twice a day to 45 Gy. This rate was lower than the 14% pathologic complete response rate in 36 patients with ultrasound stage T2–3 disease who received 50.4 Gy with conventional 1.8-Gy fractions at the Memorial Sloan-Kettering Cancer Center.

The major limitation of accelerated hyperfractionation is acute normal tissue toxicity. Because it is unlikely that these altered fractionation schemes can be combined with adequate doses of systemic chemotherapy, Movsas and colleagues[298] have limited the hyperfractionated portion to the boost. In their phase I trial of preoperative combined modality therapy, patients receive conventional pelvic radiation plus continuous infusion 5-FU followed by a boost with escalating doses of hyperfractionated radiation (1.2 Gy twice a day).[298] Providing that the small bowel was excluded after 52.3 Gy, the recommended dose level with this approach was 61.8 Gy.

In a randomized trial of patients receiving radiation therapy for pelvic malignancies, three-dimensional conformal radiation therapy decreased the volume of normal tissue in the field, but did not decrease acute toxicity.[255] Other techniques, such as neutron beam radiation, hyperthermia, radiosensitizers, radioprotectors, altered radiation fractionation schemes, and proton and three-dimensional treatment planning, are encouraging but remain experimental.[107]

TREATMENT OF PATIENTS WITH SYNCHRONOUS METASTATIC DISEASE

A subset of patients present with unresectable pelvic disease and synchronous extrapelvic disease. Because the natural history of these patients is dependent on a variety of factors, such as the volume and site(s) of metastatic disease and, in those with recurrent disease, the disease-free interval, treatment recommendations are individualized and no standard of care has been established. The management of these patients is discussed in greater detail in Chapter 52. At Memorial Sloan-Kettering, the general approach is to deliver preoperative combined modality therapy both as a therapeutic measure and to help identify those who may benefit from an aggressive surgical approach. If after the completion of therapy a response has been seen in both the primary and metastatic site(s), then the patient is evaluated, on a case by case basis, for surgery of the primary and metastasis.

FOLLOW-UP AFTER POTENTIALLY CURATIVE TREATMENT

Patients should follow up with their primary treatment team after curative treatment for many reasons. An important aspect of this follow-up is management of treatment-related problems and assessment for local-regional recurrences. These may have an impact on quality of life that is not apparent from survival statistics. Dietary modifications, including the use of a fiber supplement, may be necessary for management of bowel function. Antidiarrheal agents frequently are required. This management can occur on an ongoing basis during follow-up, because these symptoms are most profound during the initial year after treatment and tend to abate during the latter part of the follow-up period. In addition, patients who undergo creation of ostomies for their colorectal cancer management benefit from consultation with an enterostomal therapist. Counseling and appropriate referral for the management of sexual or bowel dysfunction can occur during follow-up visits.

TREATMENT OF RECURRENCE

Management of recurrent disease is individualized. The treatment is based on the extent of recurrence as well as the patient's overall potential for curative therapy and their medical condition. In most patients, recurrent disease is multifocal and treated with systemic chemotherapy. Highly selected patients can be considered for operative therapy. Others with an unresectable recurrence may need palliation. A chief symptom requiring palliation in patients with recurrent rectal carcinoma is obstruction. The use of salvage surgery for recurrence after local excision is presented in Recurrent Disease, earlier in this chapter. The use of surgery for lung metastases or hepatic metastases is discussed in Chapters 52.2 and 52.3, respectively.

PALLIATION OF OBSTRUCTION DUE TO LOCALLY RECURRENT RECTAL CANCER

In patients with synchronous metastatic disease, the management of rectal obstruction can make use of a number of techniques that can help avoid palliative colostomy. Frequently, patients in this circumstance are markedly debilitated and very poor surgical risks. These circumstances often make the risks of surgical intervention prohibitive, especially in light of the limited potential for survival. Palliative pelvic irradiation is a useful technique in patients who have not undergone previous radiotherapy. Palliative endoscopic placement of self-expanding metallic stents has also been used as an alternative to palliative colostomy. Success rates can be high with stenting. In a majority of patients, this technique results in the successful placement of the stent. Many have no further complications from their obstruction for a period of 1 to 7 months after stent placement.[319] For those in whom stent placement is unsuccessful, palliative colostomy can be performed. Neodymium:yttrium-aluminum garnet laser treatment also can be highly successful in relieving obstruction.[320]

SURGERY FOR LOCALLY RECURRENT RECTAL CANCER

Among patients with failure after curative treatment of rectal carcinoma, between 10% and 30% of recurrences are confined to the pelvis. The absence of metastatic disease is one of the key factors in determining a patient's potential for curative surgical resection for locally recurrent disease. Local recurrences of rectal cancer tend to be highly symptomatic, with pelvic pain, rectal obstruction, bleeding, urinary tract dysfunction, and fistulas.

LOCATION OF RECURRENCE

Localized pelvic recurrences may be classified based on the tumor location within the pelvis. Recurrences can be heterogeneous, and the pattern of extension of local recurrence is much more infiltrative within the previous operative bed than primary rectal cancers. They tend to be in perianastatomotic tissues and more frequently involve adjacent organs.[321] Axial recurrences appear centrally in the pelvis. These may include anastomotic recurrences after local or radical surgery. Anteriorly based recurrences in the pelvis chiefly involve the seminal vesicles and prostate in men and the vagina and uterus or bladder in women. Posterior recurrences tend to predominantly involve the sacrum and may extend into the pyriformis muscle, the sciatic notch, and sciatic nerve. Lateral recurrences can involve the soft tissues of the pelvic sidewall and the iliac blood vessels and lymph nodes, as well as the obturator internus muscles and the pyriformis muscles. Recurrences may extend into the bony sidewalls of the pelvis.

EVALUATION OF THE PATIENT WITH LOCALLY RECURRENT RECTAL CANCER

The preoperative workup of a patient with a suspected local rectal cancer recurrence involves assessment of both the presence of extrapelvic metastatic disease and a determination of the extent of the local recurrence. Under certain circumstances, intraoperative exploration may be required to reveal an unresectable recurrence; however, it is best to avoid this procedure because of morbidity without improvement in survival.

When patients present with locally recurrent rectal cancer, they usually are symptomatic. These symptoms may range from cramping or constipation from bowel obstruction to pelvic or sciatic pain to dysuria and urinary tract dysfunction. Important examinations are pelvic examination in females, digital rectal examination, proctoscopy, and cystoscopy. Examination of the inguinal lymph nodes in patients with a previous low rectal cancer can detect lymph node recurrence.

IMAGING PATIENTS WITH LOCAL RECURRENCE

When presented with a patient having locally recurrent rectal carcinoma, staging of the abdomen and pelvis, either with CT or MRI, and imaging of the pulmonary fields with chest x-ray is required. These tests do an excellent job of identifying patients with visceral metastases; however, peritoneal implants may be missed until surgery is done.

The operative approach is determined by the extent and location of the recurrence. Specific questions can be asked from pelvic imaging studies, such as MRI or CT, that help to determine resectability and the procedure required. These questions pertain to (1) sacral nerve root involvement and the level at which this involvement occurs; (2) invasion of the sciatic nerve or lumbosacral plexus; (3) extension outside the pelvis through the sciatic notch or levators; and (4) involvement of seminal vesicles or prostate and bladder in men and involvement of vagina, cervix, and bladder in women. Although EUS can aid in the assessment of local recurrence, it is limited because of the postoperative changes seen around a rectal anastomosis. CT scan identifies distant metastases as well as the extent of pelvic involvement. However, postoperative or postradiation chemotherapy changes may lead to fibrosis, making it indistinguishable from recurrence. CT scanning sensitivity for detecting pelvic recurrences is between 70% and 82%.[322–324] CT scans can also identify potential sites for fine-needle aspiration biopsies of suspected areas of recurrence. MRI studies can be useful in evaluating the extent of local recurrence and in planning operative therapy. MRI appears to be especially useful in determining neurologic and sacral involvement and planning for the resections of these structures.

Nuclear imaging has been reported to be useful in the pretreatment evaluation of patients with recurrent colorectal cancer. It can identify sites of occult metastatic disease that would make pursuit of an extensive resection fruitless. Although nuclear imaging studies frequently lack the anatomic definition necessary to enhance the determination of the local extent of disease, their ability to exclude patients with clinically undetectable metastatic disease may be of value.[325] A further discussion of this topic is found in Chapter 33.7.

PET is a technique that has been used in conjunction with the glucose analogue [^{18}F]fluorodeoxyglucose to image colorectal cancers. Accuracy in detecting sites of recurrent colorectal cancer has been reported to approach 83% in patients with recurrent colorectal cancer.[188] PET whole body scanning has provided additional information beyond conventional imaging.[326]

SURGERY FOR RECURRENT DISEASE

In patients taken to the operating room for locally recurrent rectal cancer, cystoscopy and bilateral ureteral stent placement should be performed to facilitate subsequent evaluation and to allow the operation to proceed with alacrity. Thorough exploration of the abdominal cavity should be carried out to assess for evidence of metastatic disease. Specific sites to be examined are the peritoneal surface, omentum, retroperitoneal lymph nodes, and liver. If metastatic sites are found, then consideration can be given to palliative management, such as colostomy or urologic diversion.[327] Patients with perianastomotic recurrence should undergo resection to achieve negative margins. In most cases, this involves an APR. In perineal recurrences after APR, patients should undergo wide excision. It should be noted, however, that the tumor presenting at the level of the perineal skin is often a small component of the overall pelvic recurrence. Most of these cases require extensive soft tissue reconstruction for adequate closure of the excision site. Recurrences that involve adjacent structures may require pelvic exenteration to achieve negative margins. Multiple organs may be adherent to the site of the recurrence, and these should be resected *en bloc* to avoid violation of the recurrent tumor. This requires development of planes outside the normal anatomic planes used for resectable lesions. Removal of nodal disease along the internal iliac artery and wide excision of the pelvic floor is required.

In patients with a posterior extension of pelvic recurrence, sacrectomy can be required in combination with the pelvic visceral resection. When there is limited distal sacral and coccyx involvement, this can be resected *en bloc* with the pelvic viscera resected through an abdominal and perineal approach. If more extensive sacral involvement is present, the patient can undergo a combined abdominal, perineal, and posterior approach for formal sacrectomy.[328,329] Vascular ligations of the internal iliac vessels and nodal resection below this level are carried out through the abdominal approach as well as the division of any remaining rectal segment and division of the ureters and construction of an ileal conduit.[330] The patient can then be turned into a prone position for subsequent resection of the perineal soft tissues, laminectomy, and ligation of the dural sac followed by *en bloc* removal of the pelvic tissues.[331] Patients with extensive pelvic sidewall involvement can undergo extended lateral resections to include obturator and internal iliac nodes as well as surrounding pelvic soft tissues. Areas of close margins can be treated with IORT or brachytherapy techniques.[300,332] Patients who undergo such extensive soft tissue resections in the irradiated pelvis require soft tissue reconstruction with a rectus abdominus myocutaneous flap or gracilis flap to provide for an adequately healed or vaginal reconstruction wound and to minimize complications of pelvic sepsis and bowel obstruction.[333]

REFERENCES

1. Kollmorgen CF, Meagher AP, Wolff BG, et al. The long-term effect of adjuvant postoperative chemoradiotherapy for rectal carcinoma on bowel function. *Ann Surg* 1994;220:676.
2. Enker WE. Potency, cure, and local control in the operative treatment of rectal cancer. *Arch Surg* 1992;127:1396.
3. Havenga K, Enker WE, McDermott K, et al. Male and female sexual and urinary function after total mesorectal excision with autonomic nerve preservation for carcinoma of the rectum. *J Am Coll Surg* 1996;182:495.
4. Enker WE. Operative considerations in rectal cancer. In: Cohen AM, Winawer SJ, eds. *Cancer of the colon, rectum, and anus.* New York: McGraw-Hill, 1995:561.
5. Vanek VW, Whitt CL, Abdu RA, Kennedy WR. Comparison of right colon, left colon, and rectal carcinoma. *Am Surg* 1986;52:504.
6. Cheung PS, Wong SK, Boey J, Lai CK. Frank rectal bleeding: a prospective study of causes in patients over the age of 40. *Postgrad Med J* 1988;64:364.
7. Kim DG, Madoff RD. Transanal treatment of rectal cancer: ablative methods and open resection. *Semin Surg Oncol* 1998;15:101.
8. Hoff PM, Lassere Y, Pazdur R, et al. Preoperative UFT and calcium folinate and radiotherapy in rectal cancer. *Oncology (Huntingt)* 1999;13:129.
9. Tartter PI, Steinberg BM. The role of preoperative intravenous pyelogram in operations performed for carcinoma of the colon and rectum. *Surg Gynecol Obstet* 1986;163:65.
10. Degen L, Beglinger C. Preoperative approach to rectal carcinoma. *Swiss Surg* 1997;3:240.
11. Hundt W, Braunschweig R, Reiser M. Evaluation of spiral CT in staging of colon and rectum carcinoma. *Eur Radiol* 1999;9:78.
12. Williams MP, Husband JE. CT scanning in carcinoma of the rectum: a review. *J R Soc Med* 1987;80:701.
13. Thoeni RF, Rogalla P. CT for the evaluation of carcinomas in the colon and rectum. *Semin Ultrasound CT MR* 1995;16:112.
14. Debatin JF, Patak MA. MRI of the small and large bowel. *Eur Radiol* 1999;9:1523.
15. Stoker J, Rociu E. Endoluminal MR imaging of diseases of the anus and rectum. *Semin Ultrasound CT MR* 1999;20:47.
16. Barbaro B, Savastano M, Sallustio G. Combined modality staging of low risk rectal cancer. *Rays* 1995;20:145.
17. Indinnimeo M, Grasso RF, Cicchini C, et al. Endorectal magnetic resonance imaging in the preoperative staging of rectal tumors. *Int Surg* 1996;81:419.
18. Pema PJ, Bennett WF, Bova JG, Warman P. CT vs MRI in diagnosis of recurrent rectosigmoid carcinoma. *J Comput Assist Tomogr* 1994;18:256.
19. Markus J, Morrissey B, deGara C, Tarulli G. MRI of recurrent rectosigmoid carcinoma [See comments]. *Abdom Imaging* 1997;22:338.
20. Senagore A, Milsom JW, Senagore P, et al. A comparison between intrarectal ultrasound and CT scanning in staging of experimental rectal tumors. *J Surg Res* 1988;44:522.
21. Niederhuber JE. Colon and rectum cancer. Patterns of spread and implications for workup. *Cancer* 1993;71:4187.
22. Detry RJ, Kartheuser AH, Lagneaux G, Rahier J. Preoperative lymph node staging in rectal cancer: a difficult challenge. *Int J Colorectal Dis* 1996;11:217.
23. Sailer M, Leppert R, Kraemer M, et al. The value of endorectal ultrasound in the assessment of adenomas, T1- and T2-carcinomas. *Int J Colorectal Dis* 1997;12:214.
24. Massari M, De S, Cioffi U, et al. Value and limits of endorectal ultrasonography for preoperative staging of rectal carcinoma. *Surg Laparosc Endosc* 1998;8:438.
25. Kruskal JB, Kane RA, Sentovich SM, Longmaid HE. Pitfalls and sources of error in staging rectal cancer with endorectal US. *Radiographics* 1997;17:609.
26. Sailer M, Leppert R, Bussen D, et al. Influence of tumor position on accuracy of endorectal ultrasound staging. *Dis Colon Rectum* 1997;40:1180.
27. Maier AG, Barton PP, Neuhold NR, et al. Peritumoral tissue reaction at transrectal US as a possible cause of overstaging in rectal cancer: histopathologic correlation. *Radiology* 1997;203:785.
28. Kahn H, Alexander A, Rakinic J, et al. Preoperative staging of irradiated rectal cancers using digital rectal examination, computed tomography, endorectal ultrasound, and magnetic resonance imaging does not accurately predict T0,N0 pathology. *Dis Colon Rectum* 1997;40:140.
29. Nielsen MB, Qvitzau S, Pedersen JF, Christiansen J. Endosonography for preoperative staging of rectal tumours. *Acta Radiol* 1996;37:799.
30. Bernini A, Deen KI, Madoff RD, Wong WD. Preoperative adjuvant radiation with chemotherapy for rectal cancer: its impact on stage of disease and the role of endorectal ultrasound. *Ann Surg Oncol* 1996;3:131.
31. Biggers OR, Beart RW Jr, Ilstrup DM. Local excision of rectal cancer. *Dis Colon Rectum* 1986;29:374.
32. Rosenthal SA, Yeung RS, Weese JL, et al. Conservative management of extensive low-lying rectal carcinomas with transanal local excision and combined preoperative and postoperative radiation therapy: report of a phase I/II trial. *Cancer* 1992;69:335.
33. Andreola S, Leo E, Belli F, et al. Distal intramural spread in adenocarcinoma of the lower third of the rectum treated with total rectal resection and coloanal anastomosis. *Dis Colon Rectum* 1997;40:25.
34. Hojo K. Anastomotic recurrence after sphincter-saving resection for rectal cancer: length of distal clearance of the bowel. *Dis Colon Rectum* 1986;29:11.
35. Meterissian S, Skibber J, Rich T, et al. Patterns of residual disease after preoperative chemoradiation in ultrasound T3 rectal carcinoma. *Ann Surg Oncol* 1994;1:111.
36. Nagle D. Full thickness local excision of favorable rectal cancer. In: Fry RD, ed. *Seminars in colon and rectal surgery.* Philadelphia: WB Saunders 1996;7:215.
37. Hida J, Yasutomi M, Fujimoto K, et al. Analysis of regional lymph node metastases from rectal carcinoma by the clearing method: justification of the use of sigmoid in J-pouch construction after low anterior resection. *Dis Colon Rectum* 1996;39:1282.
38. Sitzler PJ, Seow-Choen F, Ho YH, Leong AP. Lymph node involvement and tumor depth in rectal cancers: an analysis of 805 patients. *Dis Colon Rectum* 1997;40:1472.
39. Hall NR, Finan PJ, al Jaberi T, et al. Circumferential margin involvement after mesorectal excision of rectal cancer with curative intent. Predictor of survival but not local recurrence? *Dis Colon Rectum* 1998;41:979.
40. Hainsworth PJ, Egan MJ, Cunliffe WJ. Evaluation of a policy of total mesorectal excision for rectal and rectosigmoid cancers [See comments]. *Br J Surg* 1997;84:652.
41. Heald RJ. Rectal cancer: the surgical options. *Eur J Cancer* 1995;31A:1189.
42. Reynolds JV, Joyce WP, Dolan J, et al. Pathological evidence in support of total mesorectal excision in the management of rectal cancer. *Br J Surg* 1996;83:1112.
43. Scott N, Jackson P, Al-Jaberi T, et al. Total mesorectal excision and local recurrences: a study of tumour spread in the mesorectum distal to rectal cancer. *Br J Surg* 1995;82:1031.

44. de Haas-Kock DF, Baeten CG, Jager JJ, et al. Prognostic significance of radial margins of clearance in rectal cancer [See comments]. *Br J Surg* 1996;83:781.
45. Heald RJ, Moran BJ, Ryall RD, et al. Rectal cancer: the Basingstoke experience of total mesorectal excision, 1978–1997. *Arch Surg* 1998;133:894.
46. Enker WE, Merchant N, Cohen AM, et al. Safety and efficacy of low anterior resection for rectal cancer. *Ann Surg* 1999;230:544.
47. Havenga K, Enker WE, Norstein J, et al. Improved survival and local control after total mesorectal excision or D3 lymphadenectomy in the treatment of primary rectal cancer: an international analysis of 1411 patients. *Eur J Surg Oncol* 1999;25:368.
48. Moreira LF, Hizuta A, Iwagaki H, et al. Lateral lymph node dissection for rectal carcinoma below the peritoneal reflection. *Br J Surg* 1994;81:293.
49. Cohen AM. Colon J-pouch reconstruction after total or subtotal proctectomy. *World J Surg* 1993;17:267.
50. Dahlberg M, Glimelius B, Pahlman L. Changing strategy for rectal cancer is associated with improved outcome. *Br J Surg* 1999;86:379.
51. Wolmark N, Fisher B. An analysis of survival and treatment failure following abdominoperineal and sphincter-saving resection in Dukes' B and C rectal carcinoma. *Ann Surg* 1986;204:480.
52. Francois Y, Nemoz CJ, Baulieux J, et al. Influence of the interval between preoperative radiation therapy and surgery on downstaging and on the rate of sphincter-sparing surgery for rectal cancer: the Lyon R90-01 randomized trial. *J Clin Oncol* 1999;17:2396.
53. Cavaliere F, Pemberton JH, Cosimelli M, et al. Coloanal anastomosis for rectal cancer. Long-term results at the Mayo and Cleveland Clinics. *Dis Colon Rectum* 1995;38:807.
54. Lazorthes F, Fages P, Chiotasso P, et al. Resection of the rectum with construction of a colonic reservoir and colo-anal anastomosis for carcinoma of the rectum. *Br J Surg* 1986;73:136.
55. Dehni N, Tiret E, Singland JD, et al. Long-term functional outcome after low anterior resection: comparison of low colorectal anastomosis and colonic J-pouch-anal anastomosis. *Dis Colon Rectum* 1998;41:817.
56. Hallbook O, Johansson K, Sjodahl R. Laser Doppler blood flow measurement in rectal resection for carcinoma—comparison between the straight and colonic J pouch reconstruction. *Br J Surg* 1996;83:389.
57. Drake DB, Pemberton JH, Beart RW, et al. Coloanal anastomosis in the management of benign and malignant rectal disease. *Ann Surg* 1987;206:600.
58. Minsky B, Cohen A, Enker W, et al. Phase I trial of postoperative 5-FU, radiation therapy, and high dose leucovorin for resectable rectal cancer. *Int J Radiat Oncol Biol Phys* 1992;22:139.
59. Cohen AM, Minsky BD. Aggressive surgical management of locally advanced primary and recurrent rectal cancer. *Dis Colon Rectum* 1990;33:432.
60. Law WL, Chu KW, Choi HK. Total pelvic exenteration for locally advanced rectal cancer. *J Am Coll Surg* 2000;190:78.
61. Goldberg JM, Piver MS, Hempling RE, et al. Improvements in pelvic exenteration: factors responsible for reducing morbidity and mortality. *Ann Surg Oncol* 1998;5:399.
62. de Hass WG, Miller MJ, Kroll WJ, et al. Perineal wound closure with the rectus abdominous flap following tumor ablation. *Ann Surg Oncol* 1995;2:400.
63. Zaheer S, Pemberton JH, Farouk R, et al. Surgical treatment of adenocarcinoma of the rectum. *Ann Surg* 1998;227:800.
64. Banerjee AK. Sexual dysfunction after surgery for rectal cancer [See comments]. *Lancet* 1999;353:1900.
65. Shellito PC. Complications of abdominal stoma surgery. *Dis Colon Rectum* 1998;41:1562.
66. Camilleri-Brennan J, Steele RJ. Quality of life after treatment for rectal cancer. *Br J Surg* 1998;85:1036.
67. Hallbook O, Sjodahl R. Comparison between the colonic J pouch-anal anastomosis and healthy rectum: clinical and physiological function. *Br J Surg* 1997;84:1437.
68. Beart RW Jr. Predictors of recurrence after local excision. *Ann Surg Oncol* 1999;6:2.
69. Zenni GC, Abraham K, Harford FJ, et al. Characteristics of rectal carcinomas that predict the presence of lymph node metastases: implications for patient selection for local therapy. *J Surg Oncol* 1998;67:99.
70. Huddy SP, Husband EM, Cook MG, et al. Lymph node metastases in early rectal cancer. *Br J Surg* 1993;80:1457.
71. Nelson JC, Nimr AF, Thomford NR. Criteria for the selection of "early" carcinomas of the rectum. Are they valid? *Arch Surg* 1987;122:533.
72. Bouvet M, Milas M, Giacco G, et al. Predictors of recurrence after local excision and postoperative chemoradiation therapy of adenocarcinoma of the rectum. *Ann Surg Oncol* 1999;6:26.
73. Nivatvongs S, Wolff BG. Technique of per anal excision for carcinoma of the low rectum. *World J Surg* 1992;16:447.
74. Guillem JG, Paty PB, Cohen AM. Surgical treatment of colorectal cancer. *CA Cancer J Clin* 1997;47:113.
75. Bevan AD. Carcinoma of the rectum: treatment by local excision. *Dis Colon Rectum* 1986;29:906.
76. Saclarides TJ. Transanal endoscopic microsurgery: a single surgeon's experience. *Arch Surg* 1998;133:595.
77. National Institutes of Health. Adjuvant therapy for patients with colon and rectum cancer. *NIH Consens Statement* 1991;8:1.
78. Chin BT, Eiserstat TE. Electrocoagulation of selected adenomacarcinoma of the distal rectum. In: *Seminars in Colon and Rectal Surgery.* WB Saunders 1996:7.
79. Stahl T, Murray JJ, Coller JA, et al. Sphincter-saving alternatives in the management of adenocarcinoma involving the distal rectum. *Arch Surg* 1993;128:545.
80. Kodner IJ, Shemesh EI, Fry RD, et al. Preoperative irradiation for rectal cancer: improved local control and long-term survival. *Ann Surg* 1989;209:194.
81. Brunetaud JM, Maundoudry V, Cochelard D. Laser in rectosigmoid tumors. *Semin Surg Oncol* 1995;11:319.
82. Maingon P, Guerif S, Darsouni R, et al. Conservative management of rectal adenocarcinoma by radiotherapy. *Int J Radiat Oncol Biol Phys* 1998;40:1077.
83. Gastrointestinal Tumor Study Group. Prolongation of the disease-free interval in surgically treated rectal carcinoma. *N Engl J Med* 1985;312:1465.
84. McAnena OJ, Heald RJ, Lockhart-Mummery HE. Operative and functional results of total mesorectal excision with ultra-low anterior resection in the management of carcinoma of the lower one-third of the rectum. *Surg Gynecol Obstet* 1990;170:517.
85. MacFarlane JK, Ryall RD, Heald RJ. Mesorectal excision for rectal cancer. *Lancet* 1993;341:457.
86. Enker WE, Thaler HT, Cranor ML, Polyak T. Total mesorectal excision in the operative treatment of carcinoma of the rectum. *J Am Coll Surg* 1995;181:335.
87. Simons AJ, Ker R, Groshen S, et al. Variations in the treatment of rectal cancer: the influence of hospital type and caseload. *Dis Colon Rectum* 1997;40:641.
88. Graham RA, Garnsey L, Jessup JM. Local excision of rectal carcinoma. *Am J Surg* 1990;160:306.
89. Sticca RP, Rodriguez-Bibas M, Penetrante RB, Petrelli NJ. Curative resection for stage I rectal cancer: natural history, prognostic factors, and recurrence patterns. *Cancer Invest* 1996;14:491.
90. Weber TK, Petrelli NJ. Local excision for rectal cancer: an uncertain future. *Oncology (Huntingt)* 1998;12:933.
91. Schild SE, Martenson JA, Gunderson LL. Endocavitary radiotherapy of rectal cancer. *Int J Radiat Oncol Biol Phys* 1996;3:677.
92. Gerard JP, Ayzac L, Coquard R, et al. Endocavitary irradiation for early rectal carcinomas T1 (T2). A series of 101 patients treated with the Papillon's technique. *Int J Radiat Oncol Biol Phys* 1996;34:775.
93. Wong CS, Cummings BJ, Brierley JD, et al. Treatment of locally recurrent rectal carcinoma—results and prognostic factors. *Int J Radiat Oncol Biol Phys* 1998;40:427.
94. Lingareddy V, Ahmad NR, Mohiuddin M. Palliative reirradiation for recurrent rectal cancer. *Int J Radiat Oncol Biol Phys* 1997;38:785.
95. Guiney MJ, Smith JG, Worotniuk V, et al. Radiotherapy treatment for isolated locoregional recurrence of rectosigmoid cancer following definitive surgery: Peter McCallum Cancer Institute experience: 1981–1990. *Int J Radiat Oncol Biol Phys* 1997;38:1019.
96. Valentini V, Morganti AG, Luzi S, et al. Is chemoradiation feasible in elderly patients? A study of 17 patients with anorectal carcinoma. *Cancer* 1997;80:1387.
97. Merchant TE, Diamantis PA, Lauwers G, et al. Characterization of malignant colon tumors with 31P nuclear magnetic resonance phospholipid and phosphatic metabolite profiles. *Cancer* 1995;76:1715.
98. Stocchi L, Nelson H, Sargent D, et al. Impact of individual surgeon on rectal cancer outcome within 3 North Central Cancer Treatment Group (NCCTG) protocols. *Proc ASCO* 1999;18:234.
99. Kapiteijn E, Marijnen CAM, Colenbrander AC, et al. Local recurrence in patients with rectal cancer diagnosed between 1988 and 1992: a population based study in the west Netherlands. *Eur J Surg Oncol* 1998;24:528.
100. Rich T, Gunderson LL, Lew R, et al. Patterns of recurrence of rectal cancer after potentially curative surgery. *Cancer* 1983;52:1317.
101. Minsky BD, Mies C, Recht A, et al. Resectable adenocarcinoma of the rectosigmoid and rectum. 1. Patterns of failure and survival. *Cancer* 1988;61:1408.
102. Gunderson LL, Sosin H. Areas of failure found at reoperation (second or symptomatic look) following "curative surgery" for adenocarcinoma of the rectum: clinicopathologic correlation and implications for adjuvant therapy. *Cancer* 1974;34:1278.
103. Zaheer S, Pemberton JH, Farouk R, et al. Surgical treatment of adenocarcinoma of the rectum. *Ann Surg* 1998;227:800.
104. Papillon J. Present status of radiation therapy in the conservative management of rectal cancer. *Radiother Oncol* 1990;17:275.
105. Gerard JP, Roy P, Coquard R, et al. Combined curative radiation therapy alone in (T1) T2-3 rectal adenocarcinoma: a pilot study of 29 patients. *Radiother Oncol* 1996;38:131.
106. Minsky BD, Cohen AM. Conservative management of invasive rectal cancer: alternative to abdominoperineal resection. *Oncology* 1989;3:137.
107. Minsky BD. Adjuvant therapy for rectal cancer: results and controversies. *Oncology* 1998;12:1129.
108. Minsky BD. Conservative management of rectal cancer with local excision and postoperative radiation therapy. *Eur J Cancer* 1995;31A:1343.
109. Minsky BD. Clinical experience with local excision and postoperative radiation therapy for rectal cancer. *Dis Colon Rectum* 1993;36:405.
110. Willett CG, Tepper JE, Donnely S, et al. Patterns of failure following local excision and local excision and postoperative radiation therapy for invasive rectal adenocarcinoma. *J Clin Oncol* 1989;7:1003.
111. Willett CG, Compton CC, Shellito PC, Efird JT. Selection factors for local excision or abdominoperineal resection of early stage rectal cancer. *Cancer* 1994;73:2716.
112. Blumberg D, Paty PB, Guillem JG, et al. All patients with small intramural rectal cancers are at risk for lymph node metastasis. *Dis Colon Rectum* 1999;42:881.
113. Horn A, Halvorsen JF, Morild I. Transanal extirpation for early rectal cancer. *Dis Colon Rectum* 1989;32:769.
114. Milsom JW, Czyrko C, Hull TL, et al. Preoperative biopsy of pararectal lymph nodes in rectal cancer using endoluminal ultrasonography. *Dis Colon Rectum* 1994;37:364.
115. Jessup JM, Loda M, Bleday R. Clinical and molecular prognostic factors in sphincter-preserving surgery for rectal cancer. *Semin Radiat Oncol* 1998;8:54.
116. Mendenhall WM, Rout WR, Vauthey JN, et al. Conservative treatment of rectal adenocarcinoma with endocavitary irradiation or wide local excision and post-operative irradiation. *J Clin Oncol* 1997;15:3241.
117. Chakravarti A, Compton CC, Shellito PC, et al. Long-term follow-up of patients with rectal cancer managed by local excision with and without adjuvant irradiation. *Ann Surg* 1999;230:49.
118. Bleday R, Breen E, Jessup JM, et al. Prospective evaluation of local excision for small rectal cancers. *Dis Colon Rectum* 1997;40:388.
119. Ota DM, Skibber J, Rich TA. M. D. Anderson Cancer Center experience with local excision and multimodality therapy for rectal cancer. *Surg Oncol Clin North Am* 1992;1:147.

120. Wagman R, Minsky BD, Cohen AM, et al. Conservative management of rectal cancer with local excision and post-op radiation ± chemotherapy. *Int J Radiat Oncol Biol Phys* 1999;44:841.
121. Steele G, Tepper J, Herndon J, Mayer R. Failure and salvage after sphincter sparing treatment for distal rectal adenocarcinoma—a CALGB coordinated intergroup study. *Proc ASCO* 1999;18:235a.
122. Taylor RH, Hay JH, Larsson SN. Transanal local excision of selected low rectal cancers. *Am J Surg* 1998;175:360.
123. Valentini V, Morganti AG, De Santis M, et al. Local excision and external beam radiotherapy in early rectal cancer. *Int J Radiat Oncol Biol Phys* 1996;35:759.
124. Fortunato L, Ahmad NR, Yeung RS, et al. Long-term follow-up of local excision and radiation therapy for invasive rectal cancer. *Dis Colon Rectum* 1995;38:1193.
125. Steele GD, Herndon JE, Bleday R, et al. Sphincter-sparing treatment for distal rectal adenocarcinoma. *Ann Surg Oncol* 1999;6:433.
126. Willett CG. Local excision followed by postoperative radiation therapy. *Semin Radiat Oncol* 1998;8:24.
127. Minsky BD, Cohen AM, Enker WE, Sigurdson E. Phase I/II trial of pre-operative radiation therapy and coloanal anastomosis in distal invasive resectable rectal cancer. *Int J Radiat Oncol Biol Phys* 1992;23:387.
128. O'Connell MJ, Martenson JA, Weiand HS, et al. Improving adjuvant therapy for rectal cancer by combining protracted infusion fluorouracil with radiation therapy after curative surgery. *N Engl J Med* 1994;331:502.
129. Graf W, Dahlberg M, Osman MM, et al. Short-term preoperative radiotherapy results in down-staging of rectal cancer: a study of 1316 patients. *Radiother Oncol* 1997;43:133.
130. Williamson PR, Hellinger MD, Larach SW, Ferrara A. Endorectal ultrasound of T3 and T4 rectal tumor after preoperative chemoradiation. *Dis Colon Rectum* 1996;39:45.
131. Barbaro B, Schulsinger A, Valentini V, et al. The accuracy of transrectal ultrasound in predicting the pathological stage of low-lying rectal cancer after preoperative chemoradiation therapy. *Int J Radiat Oncol Biol Phys* 1999;43:1043.
132. Alexander AA, Palazzo JP, Ahmad NR, et al. Endosonographic and color Doppler flow imaging alterations observed within irradiated rectal cancer. *Int J Radiat Oncol Biol Phys* 1996;35:369.
133. Merchant TE, Ballon D, Koutcher JA, et al. A birdcage resonator for intracavitary MR imaging. *Magn Reson Imaging* 1993;11:1119.
134. Kim NK, Kim MJ, Yun SH, et al. Comparative study of transrectal ultrasonography, pelvic computerized tomography, and magnetic resonance imaging in preoperative staging of rectal cancer. *Dis Colon Rectum* 1999;42:770.
135. Flamen P, Stroobants S, van Cutsem E, et al. Additional value of whole-body positron emission tomography with fluorine-18-2-fluoro-2-deoxy-D-glucose in recurrent colorectal cancer. *J Clin Oncol* 1999;17:894.
136. Takeuchi O, Saito N, Koda K, et al. Clinical assessment of positron emission tomography for the diagnosis of local recurrence in colorectal cancer. *Br J Surg* 1999;86:932.
137. Martinez-Monge R, Nag S, Martin EW. Three different intraoperative radiation modalities (electron beam, high-dose-rate brachytherapy, and iodine-125 brachytherapy) in the adjuvant treatment of patients with recurrent colorectal adenocarcinoma. *Cancer* 1999;86:236.
138. Otmezguine Y, Grimard L, Calitchi E, et al. A new combined approach in the conservative management of rectal cancer. *Int J Radiat Oncol Biol Phys* 1989;17:539.
139. Mohiuddin M, Marks J, Bannon J. High-dose preoperative radiation and full thickness local excision: a new option for selected T3 distal rectal cancer. *Int J Radiat Oncol Biol Phys* 1994;30:845.
140. Ahmad NR, Nagle DA. Preoperative radiation therapy followed by local excision. *Semin Radiat Oncol* 1998;8:36.
141. Hyams DM, Mamounas EP, Petrelli N, et al. A clinical trial to evaluate the worth of preoperative multimodality therapy in patients with operable carcinoma of the rectum. A progress report of the National Surgical Adjuvant Breast and Bowel Project protocol R0-3. *Dis Colon Rectum* 1997;40:131.
142. Swedish Rectal Cancer Trial. Improved survival with preoperative radiotherapy in resectable rectal cancer. *N Engl J Med* 1997;336:980.
143. Holm T, Rutqvist LE, Johansson H, Cedermark B. Postoperative mortality in rectal cancer treated with or without preoperative radiotherapy: causes and risk factors. *Br J Surg* 1996;83:964.
144. Holm T, Singnomklao T, Rutqvist LE, Cedermark B. Adjuvant preoperative radiotherapy in patients with rectal carcinoma. Adverse effects during long term follow-up of two randomized trials. *Cancer* 1996;78:968.
145. Wagman R, Minsky BD, Cohen AM, et al. Sphincter preservation with preoperative radiation therapy and coloanal anastomosis: long term follow-up. *Int J Radiat Oncol Biol Phys* 1998;42:51.
146. Grann A, Minsky BD, Cohen AM, et al. Preliminary results of pre-operative 5-fluorouracil (5-FU), low dose leucovorin, and concurrent radiation therapy for resectable T3 rectal cancer. *Dis Colon Rectum* 1997;40:515.
147. Rouanet P, Fabre JM, Dubois JB, et al. Conservative surgery for low rectal carcinoma after high-dose radiation. Functional and oncologic results. *Ann Surg* 1995;221:67.
148. Maghfoor I, Wilkes J, Kuvshinoff B, et al. Neoadjuvant chemoradiotherapy with sphincter-sparing surgery for low lying rectal cancer. *Proc ASCO* 1997;16:274.
149. Valentini V, Coco C, Cellini N, et al. Preoperative chemoradiation for extraperitoneal T3 rectal cancer: acute toxicity, tumor response, and sphincter preservation. *Int J Radiat Oncol Biol Phys* 1998;40:1067.
150. Papillon J, Gerard JP. Role of radiotherapy in anal preservation for cancers of the lower third of the rectum. *Int J Radiat Oncol Biol Phys* 1990;19:1219.
151. Mohiuddin M, Regine WF, Marks GJ, Marks JW. High-dose preoperative radiation and the challenge of sphincter-preservation surgery for cancer of the distal 2 cm of the rectum. *Int J Radiat Oncol Biol Phys* 1998;40:569.
152. Minsky BD, Cohen AM, Enker WE, Paty P. Sphincter preservation with preoperative radiation therapy and coloanal anastomosis. *Int J Radiat Oncol Biol Phys* 1995;31:553.
153. Kollmorgen CF, Meagher AP, Pemberton JH, et al. The long term effect of adjuvant postoperative chemoradiotherapy for rectal cancer on bowel function. *Ann Surg* 1994;220:676.
154. Paty PB, Enker WE, Cohen AM, et al. Long-term functional results of coloanal anastomosis for rectal cancer. *Am J Surg* 1994;167:90.
155. Birnbaum EH, Dreznik Z, Myerson RJ, et al. Early effect of external beam radiation on anal sphincter: a study using anal manometry and transrectal ultrasound. *Dis Colon Rectum* 1992;35:757.
156. Birnbaum EH, Meyerson RJ, Fry RD, et al. Chronic effects of pelvic radiation therapy on anorectal function. *Dis Colon Rectum* 1994;37:909.
157. Minsky BD, Cohen A, Enker W, et al. Pre-operative 5-FU, low dose leucovorin, and concurrent radiation therapy for rectal cancer. *Cancer* 1994;73:273.
158. Janjan NA, Khoo VS, Abbruzzese J, et al. Tumor downstaging and sphincter preservation with preoperative chemoradiation in locally advanced rectal cancer: the M. D. Anderson Cancer Center experience. *Int J Radiat Oncol Biol Phys* 1999;44:1027.
159. Janjan NA, Abbruzzese J, Pazdur R, et al. Prognostic implications of response to preoperative infusional chemoradiation in locally advanced rectal cancer. *Radiother Oncol* 1999;51:153.
160. Minsky BD, Conti J, Cohen AM, et al. Acute toxicity of neoadjuvant bolus 5-FU/methotrexate and leucovorin rescue followed by continuous infusion 5-FU plus pre-operative radiation therapy for rectal cancer. *Radiat Oncol Invest* 1996;4:90.
161. James RD, Price P, Valentini V. Raltitrexed (Tomudex) concomitant with radiotherapy as adjuvant treatment for patients with rectal cancer: preliminary results of phase I studies. *Eur J Cancer* 1999;35:s19.
162. Valentini V, Morganti AG, Fiorentino G, et al. Chemoradiation with raltitrexed (Tomudex) and concomitant preoperative radiotherapy has potential in the treatment od stage II/III resectable rectal cancer. *Proc ASCO* 1999;18:257a.
163. Feliu J, Calvillo J, Escribano A, et al. Neoadjuvant therapy of rectal carcinoma with UFT-folonic acid (LV) plus radiotherapy. *Proc ASCO* 1999;18:239a.
164. Mitchell E, Ahmad N, Fry RD, et al. Combined modality therapy of locally advanced or recurrent adenocarcinoma of the rectum: preliminary report of a phase I trial of chemotherapy (CT) with CPT-11, 5-FU, and concomitant irradiation (RT). *Proc ASCO* 1999;18:247a.
165. Minsky BD, O'Reilly E, Wong D, et al. Daily low-dose irinotecan (CPT-11) plus pelvic irradiation as preoperative treatment of locally advanced rectal cancer. *Proc ASCO* 1999;18:266a.
166. Haas-Kock DFM, Baeten CGMI, Jager JJ, et al. Prognostic significance of radial margins of clearance in rectal cancer. *Br J Surg* 1996;83:781.
167. Arenas RB, Fichera A, Mhoon D, Michelassi F. Total mesenteric excision in the surgical treatment of rectal cancer. A prospective study. *Arch Surg* 1998;133:608.
168. Aitken RJ. Mesorectal excision for rectal cancer. *Br J Surg* 1996;83:214.
169. Carlsen E, Schlichting E, Guldvog I, et al. Effect of the introduction of total mesorectal excision for the treatment of rectal cancer. *Br J Surg* 1998;85:526.
170. Poon RTP, Chu KW, Ho JWC, et al. Prospective evaluation of selective defunctioning stoma for low anterior resection with total mesorectal excision. *World J Surg* 1999;23:463.
171. Minsky BD, Conti JA, Huang Y, Knopf K. The relationship of acute gastrointestinal toxicity and the volume of irradiated small bowel in patients receiving combined modality therapy for rectal cancer. *J Clin Oncol* 1995;13:1409.
172. Tepper JE, Cohen AM, Wood WC, et al. Postoperative radiation therapy of rectal cancer. *Int J Radiat Oncol Biol Phys* 1987;13:5.
173. Willett CG, Tepper JE, Kaufman DS, et al. Adjuvant postoperative radiation therapy for rectal adenocarcinoma. *Am J Clin Oncol* 1992;15:371.
174. Romsdahl MM, Withers HR. Radiotherapy combined with curative surgery: its use as therapy for carcinomas of the sigmoid colon and rectum. *Arch Surg* 1978;113:446.
175. Vigliotti A, Rich TA, Romsdahl MM, et al. Postoperative adjuvant radiotherapy for adenocarcinoma of the rectum and rectosigmoid. *Int J Radiat Oncol Biol Phys* 1987;13:999.
176. Wiggenraad R, Tamminga R, Blok P, et al. The prognostic significance of P53 expression for survival and local control in rectal carcinoma treated with surgery and postoperative radiotherapy. *Int J Radiat Oncol Biol Phys* 1998;41:29.
177. Gastrointestinal Tumor Study Group. Adjuvant therapy of colon cancer: results of a prospectively randomized trial. *N Engl J Med* 1984;310:737.
178. Fisher B, Wolmark N, Rockette H, et al. Postoperative adjuvant chemotherapy or radiation therapy for rectal cancer: results from NSABP protocol R-01. *J Natl Cancer Inst* 1988;80:21.
179. Medical Research Council Rectal Cancer Working Party. Randomized trial of surgery alone versus surgery followed by post-operative radiotherapy for mobile cancer of the rectum. *Lancet* 1996;348:1610.
180. Arnaud JP, Nordlinger B, Bosset JF, et al. Radical surgery and postoperative radiotherapy as combined treatment in rectal cancer. Final results of a phase III study of the European Organization for Research and Treatment of Cancer. *Br J Surg* 1997;84:352.
181. Kaminsky-Forrett MC, Conroy T, Luporsi E, et al. Prognostic implications of downstaging following preoperative radiation therapy for operable T3-T4 rectal cancer. *Int J Radiat Oncol Biol Phys* 1998;42:935.
182. Ahmad NR, Nagle DA, Topham A. Pathologic complete response predicts long-term survival following preoperative radiation therapy for rectal cancer. *Int J Radiat Oncol Biol Phys* 1997;39:284.
183. Habr-Gama A, Santinho B, de Souza PM, et al. Low rectal cancer. Impact of radiation and chemotherapy on surgical treatment. *Dis Colon Rectum* 1998;41:1087.
184. Rossi BM, Nakagawa WT, Novaes PE, et al. Radiation and chemotherapy instead of surgery for low infiltrative rectal adenocarcinoma: a prospective trial. *Ann Surg Oncol* 1998;5:113.
185. Hunerbein M, Schlag PM. Three-dimensional endosonography for staging of rectal cancer. *Ann Surg* 1997;25:432.
186. Hadfield MB, Nicholson AA, MacDonald AW, et al. Preoperative staging of rectal carcinoma by magnetic resonance imaging with a pelvic phased-array coil. *Br J Surg* 1997;84:529.
187. deSouza NM, Hall AS, Puni R, et al. High resolution magnetic resonance imaging of the anal sphincter using a dedicated endoanal coil. Comparison of magnetic resonance imaging with surgical findings. *Dis Colon Rectum* 1996;39:926.

188. Falk PM, Gupta NC, Thorson AG, et al. Positron emission tomography for preoperative staging of colorectal carcinoma. *Dis Colon Rectum* 1994;37:153.
189. Herzog U, von Flue M, Tondelli P, Schuppisser JP. How accurate is endorectal ultrasound in the preoperative staging of rectal cancer? *Dis Colon Rectum* 1993;36:127.
190. Frykholm GJ, Glimelius B, Pahlman L. Preoperative or postoperative irradiation in adenocarcinoma of the rectum: final treatment results of a randomized trial and an evaluation of late secondary effects. *Dis Colon Rectum* 1993;36:564.
191. Minsky BD. Multidisciplinary management of resectable rectal cancer. *Oncology* 1996;10:1701.
192. Rich TA. Infusional chemoradiation for operable rectal cancer: post-, pre-, or nonoperative management? *Oncology* 1997;11:295.
193. Medical Research Council Rectal Cancer Working Party. Randomized trial of surgery alone versus radiotherapy followed by surgery for potentially operable, locally advanced rectal cancer. *Lancet* 1996;348:1605.
194. Glimelius B, Isacson U, Jung B, Pahlman L. Radiotherapy in addition to radical surgery in rectal cancer: evidence for a dose-response effect favoring preoperative treatment. *Int J Radiat Oncol Biol Phys* 1997;37:281.
195. Cedermark B, Johansson H, Rutqvist LE, Wilking N. The Stockholm I trial of preoperative short term radiotherapy in operable rectal carcinoma. *Cancer* 1995;75:2269.
196. Dahlberg M, Glimelius B, Pahlman L. Improved survival and reduction in local failure rates after preoperative radiotherapy. Evidence for the generalizability of the results of Swedish Rectal Cancer Trial. *Ann Surg* 1999;229:493.
197. Frykholm GJ, Isacsson U, Nygard K, et al. Preoperative radiotherapy in rectal carcinoma—aspects of acute adverse effects and radiation technique. *Int J Radiat Oncol Biol Phys* 1996;35:1039.
198. Myerson RJ, Genovesi D, Lockett MA, et al. Five fractions of preoperative radiotherapy for selected cases of rectal carcinoma: long-term tumor control and tolerance to treatment. *Int J Radiat Oncol Biol Phys* 1999;43:537.
199. Lusinchi A, Wibault P, Lasser P, et al. Abdominoperineal resection combined with pre- and postoperative radiation therapy in the treatment of low-lying rectal carcinoma. *Int J Radiat Oncol Biol Phys* 1997;37:59.
200. Willett CG, Warland G, Coen J, et al. Rectal cancer: the influence of tumor proliferation on response to preoperative irradiation. *Int J Radiat Oncol Biol Phys* 1995;32:57.
201. Willett CG, Warland G, Hagan MP, et al. Tumor proliferation in rectal cancer following preoperative irradiation. *J Clin Oncol* 1995;13:1417.
202. Willett CG, Hagan M, Daley W, et al. Changes in tumor proliferation of rectal cancer induced by preoperative 5-fluorouracil and irradiation. *Dis Colon Rectum* 1998;41:62.
203. Desai GR, Meyerson RJ, Higashikubo R, et al. Carcinoma of the rectum: possible cellular predictors of metastatic potential and response to radiation therapy. *Dis Colon Rectum* 1996;39:1090.
204. Neoptolemos JP, Oates GD, Newbold KM, et al. Cyclin/proliferation cell nuclear antigen immunohistochemistry does not improve the prognostic power of Dukes' or Jass' classifications for colorectal cancer. *Br J Surg* 1995;82:184.
205. Rich TA, Sinicrope F, Stephens C, et al. Downstaging of T3 rectal cancer after preoperative infusional chemoradiation is correlated with spontaneous apoptosis index and BCL-2 staining. *Int J Radiat Oncol Biol Phys* 1996;36:259.
206. Berger C, de Muret A, Garaud P, et al. Preoperative radiotherapy (RT) for rectal cancer: predictive factors of tumor downstaging and residual tumor density (RTCD): prognostic implications. *Int J Radiat Oncol Biol Phys* 1997;37:619.
207. Nicholl ID, Dunlop MG. Molecular markers of prognosis in colorectal cancer. *J Natl Cancer Inst* 1999;91:1267.
208. Fisher B, Wolmark N, Rockette HE, et al. Adjuvant chemotherapy or postoperative radiation for rectal cancer: five year results of NSABP R01. In: Salmon SE, ed. *Adjuvant therapy of cancer V.* New York: Grune & Stratton, 1987:547.
209. Miller RC, Martenson JA, Sargent DJ, et al. Acute diarrhea during rectal adjuvant postoperative pelvic radiation therapy (RT) with or without 5-fluorouracil: a detailed analysis of toxicity from a randomized North Central Cancer Treatment Group study. *Proc ASCO* 1998;17:279a.
210. Tveit KM, Guldvog I, Hagen S, et al. Randomized controlled trial of post-operative radiotherapy and short-term time-scheduled 5-fluorouracil against surgery alone in the treatment of Dukes B and C rectal cancer. *Br J Surg* 1997;84:1130.
211. Willett CG, Badizadegan K, Ancukiewicz M, Shellito PC. Prognostic factors in stage T3N0 rectal cancer. Do all patients require post-operative pelvic irradiation and chemotherapy? *Dis Colon Rectum* 1999;42:167.
212. Willett CG, Lewandrowski K, Donnelly S, et al. Are there patients with stage I rectal carcinoma at risk for failure after abdominoperineal resection? *Cancer* 1992;69:1651.
213. O'Connell M, Wieand H, Krook J, et al. Lack of value for methyl CCNU as a component of effective rectal cancer surgical adjuvant therapy. Interim analysis of intergroup protocol 86-47-51. *Proc ASCO* 1991;10:134.
214. Elwell A, Xoing YP, Chang M, et al. p53, p21 and thymidylate synthase (TS) protein expression: associations with recurrence in stage II and III rectal cancer. *Proc ASCO* 1997;16:258.
215. Rockette H, Deutsch M, Petrelli N, et al. Effect of postoperative radiation therapy (RTX) when used with adjuvant chemotherapy in Dukes' B and C rectal cancer: results from NSABP-R02. *Proc ASCO* 1994;13:193.
216. Tepper JE, O'Connell MJ, Petroni GR, et al. Adjuvant postoperative fluorouracil-modulated chemotherapy combined with pelvic radiation therapy for rectal cancer: initial results of Intergroup 0114. *J Clin Oncol* 1997;15:2030.
217. O'Connel MJ, Laurie JA, Kahn M, et al. Prospectively randomized trial of postoperative adjuvant chemotherapy in patients with high-risk colon cancer. *J Clin Oncol* 1998;16:295.
218. Haller DG, Catalano PJ, Macdonald JS, Mayer RJ. Fluorouracil (FU), leucovorin (LV) and levamisole (LEV) adjuvant therapy for colon cancer: preliminary results of INT-0089. *Proc ASCO* 1996;15:211.
219. Martenson JA, Shanahan TG, O'Connell MJ, et al. Phase I study of 5-fluorouracil administered by protracted venous infusion, leucovorin, and pelvic radiation therapy. *Cancer* 1999;86:710.
220. Minsky BD, Cohen AM, Enker WE, et al. Efficacy of post-operative 5-FU, high dose leucovorin and sequential radiation therapy for clinically resectable rectal cancer. *Cancer Invest* 1995;13:1.
221. Minsky BD. Pelvic radiation therapy in rectal cancer: technical considerations. *Semin Radiat Oncol* 1993;3:42.
222. Grann A, Wallner K. Prostate brachytherapy in patients with inflammatory bowel disease. *Int J Radiat Oncol Biol Phys* 1998;40:135.
223. Green S, Stock RG, Greenstein AJ. Rectal cancer and inflammatory bowel disease: natural history and implications for radiation therapy. *Int J Radiat Oncol Biol Phys* 1999;44:835.
224. Willett CG, Ooi CJ, Zeitman AL, et al. Acute and late toxicity of patients with inflammatory bowel disease undergoing irradiation for abdominal and pelvic neoplasms. *Int J Radiat Oncol Biol Phys* 2000;46:995.
225. Rakfal SM, Deutsch M. Radiotherapy for malignancies associated with lupus. Case reports of acute and late complications. *Am J Clin Oncol* 1998;21:54.
226. Coia L, Myerson R, Tepper JE. Late effects of radiation therapy on the gastrointestinal tract. *Int J Radiat Oncol Biol Phys* 1995;31:1213.
227. Richter KK, Langberg CW, Sung CC, Hauer-Jensen M. Increased transforming growth factor β (TGF-β) immunoreactivity is independently associated with chronic injury in both consequential and primary enteropathy. *Int J Radiat Oncol Biol Phys* 1997;39:187.
228. Gastrointestinal Tumor Study Group. Radiation therapy and fluorouracil with or without semustine for the treatment of patients with surgical adjuvant adenocarcinoma of the rectum. *J Clin Oncol* 1992;10:549.
229. Miller RC, Martenson JA Jr, Sargent DJ, et al. Acute treatment-related diarrhea during postoperative adjuvant therapy for high-risk rectal carcinoma. *Int J Radiat Oncol Biol Phys* 1998;41:593.
230. Grann A, Minsky BD, Cohen AM, et al. Preliminary results of pre-operative 5-FU, low dose leucovorin, and concurrent radiation therapy for resectable T3 rectal cancer. *Int J Radiat Oncol Biol Phys* 1996;36:260.
231. Schuster JJ, Stryker JA, Demers LM, Mortel R. Absence of bile acid malabsorption as a late effect of pelvic radiation. *Int J Radiat Oncol Biol Phys* 1986;12:1605.
232. Miller AR, Martenson JA Jr, Nelson H, et al. The incidence and clinical consequences of treatment-related bowel injury. *Int J Radiat Oncol Biol Phys* 1999;43:817.
233. Carmichael J, Popiela T, Radstone D, et al. Randomized comparative study of Orzel [oral uracil/tegafur (UFT) plus leucovorin (LV)] versus parenteral 5-fluorouracil (5-FU) plus LV in patients with metastatic colorectal cancer. *Proc ASCO* 1999;18:264a.
234. Konski A, Sowers M. Pelvic fractures following irradiation for endometrial carcinoma. *Int J Radiat Oncol Biol Phys* 1996;35:361.
235. Iglicki F, Coffin B, Ille O, et al. Fecal incontinence after pelvic radiotherapy: evidence for a lumbosacral plexopathy. *Dis Colon Rectum* 1996;39:465.
236. Frykholm GJ, Sintorn K, Montelius A, et al. Acute lumbosacral plexopathy after preoperative radiotherapy in rectal cancer. *Radiother Oncol* 1996;38:121.
237. Dahlberg M, Glimelius B, Graf W, Pahlman L. Preoperative irradiation affects functional results after surgery for rectal cancer. *Dis Colon Rectum* 1998;41:543.
238. Graf W, Ekstrom K, Glimelius B, Pahlman L. A pilot study of factors influencing bowel function after colorectal anastomosis. *Dis Colon Rectum* 1996;39:744.
239. Little FA, Howard GCW. Sexual function following radical radiotherapy for bladder cancer. *Radiother Oncol* 1998;49:157.
240. Mak AC, Rich TA, Schultheiss TE, et al. Late complications of postoperative radiation therapy for cancer of the rectum and rectosigmoid. *Int J Radiat Oncol Biol Phys* 1994;28:597.
241. Sigmon WR, Randall ME, Olds WE, et al. Increased chronic bowel complications with split-course pelvic irradiation. *Int J Radiat Oncol Biol Phys* 1993;28:349.
242. Huddart RA, Nahum A, Neal A, et al. Accuracy of pelvic radiotherapy: prospective analysis of 90 patients in a randomised trial of blocked versus standard radiotherapy. *Radiother Oncol* 1996;39:19.
243. Creutzberg CL, Althof VGM, de Hoog M, et al. A quality control study of the accuracy of patient positioning in irradiation of pelvic fields. *Int J Radiat Oncol Biol Phys* 1996;34:697.
244. Tinger A, Michalski JM, Bosch WR, et al. An analysis of intratreatment and intertreatment displacements in pelvic radiotherapy using electronic portal imaging. *Int J Radiat Oncol Biol Phys* 1996;34:683.
245. Martenson JA Jr, Urias RE, Smalley SR, et al. Radiation therapy quality control in a clinical trial of adjuvant postoperative treatment for rectal cancer. *Int J Radiat Oncol Biol Phys* 1999;32:51.
246. Gallagher MJ, Brereton HD, Rostock RA, et al. A prospective study of treatment techniques to minimize the volume of pelvic small bowel with reduction of acute and late effects associated with pelvic irradiation. *Int J Radiat Oncol Biol Phys* 1986;12:1565.
247. Herbert SH, Curran WJ, Solin LJ, et al. Decreasing gastrointestinal morbidity with the use of small bowel contrast during treatment planing for pelvic radiation. *Int J Radiat Oncol Biol Phys* 1991;20:835.
248. Shanahan TG, Mehta MP, Bertelrud KL, et al. Minimization of small bowel volume within treatment fields utilizing customized "belly boards." *Int J Radiat Oncol Biol Phys* 1990;19:469.
249. Fu YT, Lam JC, Tze JMY. Measurement of irradiated small bowel volume in pelvic irradiation and the effect of a bellyboard. *Clin Oncol* 1995;7:188.
250. Das IJ, Lanciano RM, Movsas B, et al. Efficacy of a belly board device with CT-simulation in reducing small bowel volume within pelvic irradiation fields. *Int J Radiat Oncol Biol Phys* 1997;39:67.
251. Herbert SH, Solin LJ, Hoffman JP, et al. Volumetric analysis of small bowel displacement from radiation portals with the use of a pelvic tissue expander. *Int J Radiat Oncol Biol Phys* 1993;25:885.
252. Hoffman JP, Sigurdson ER, Eisenberg BL. Use of saline-filled expanders to protect the small bowel from radiation. *Oncology* 1998;12:51.
253. Sezeur A, Martella L, Abbou C, et al. Small intestine protection from radiation by means of a removable adapted prosthesis. *Am J Surg* 1999;178:22.

254. Brierley JD, Cummings BJ, Wong CS, et al. The variation of small bowel volume within the pelvis before and during adjuvant radiation for rectal cancer. *Radiother Oncol* 1994;31:110.
255. Tait DM, Nahum AE, Meyer LC, et al. Acute toxicity in pelvic radiotherapy; a randomised trial of conformal versus conventional treatment. *Radiother Oncol* 1997;42:121.
256. Isacsson U, Montelius A, Jung B, Glimelius B. Comparative treatment planning between proton and X-ray therapy in locally advanced rectal cancer. *Radiother Oncol* 1997;41:263.
257. Stockholm Rectal Cancer Study Group. Preoperative short-term preoperative radiation therapy in operable rectal cancer: a randomized trial. *Cancer* 1990;66:49.
258. Chen JS, Chang Chien CR, Wang JY, Fan HA. Pelvic peritoneal reconstruction to prevent radiation enteritis in rectal carcinoma. *Dis Colon Rectum* 1992;35:897.
259. Lechner P, Cesnik H. Abdominopelvic omentopexy: preparatory procedure for radiotherapy for rectal cancer. *Dis Colon Rectum* 1992;35:1157.
260. Thom A, Baumann J, Chandler JJ, Devereux DF. Experience with high-dose radiation therapy and the intestinal sling procedure in patients with rectal carcinoma. *Cancer* 1992;70:581.
261. Rodier JF, Janser JC, Rodier D, et al. Prevention of radiation enteritis by an absorbable polyglycolic acid mesh sling. A 60-case multicentric study. *Cancer* 1991;68:2545.
262. Beitler A, Rodriguez-Bigas MA, Weber TK, et al. Complications of absorbable pelvic mesh slings following surgery for rectal carcinoma. *Dis Colon Rectum* 1997;40:1336.
263. Talley NA, Chen F, King D, et al. Short-chain fatty acid in the treatment of radiation proctitis. A randomized, double-blind, placebo-controlled, cross-over pilot trial. *Dis Colon Rectum* 1997;40:1046.
264. O'Brien PC, Franklin CI, Dear KBG, et al. A phase III double-blind randomised study of rectal sucralfate suspension in the prevention of acute radiation proctitis. *Radiother Oncol* 1997;45:117.
265. Resbeut M, Marteau P, Cowen D, et al. A randomized double blind placebo controlled multicenter study of mesalazine for the prevention of acute radiation enteritis. *Radiother Oncol* 1997;44:59.
266. Craighead PS, Young S. Phase II study assessing the feasibility of using elemental supplements to reduce acute enteritis in patients receiving radical pelvic radiotherapy. *Am J Clin Oncol* 1998;21:573.
267. Stryker JA, Bartholomew M. Failure of lactose-restricted diets to prevent radiation-induced diarrhea in patients undergoing whole pelvic irradiation. *Int J Radiat Oncol Biol Phys* 1986;12:789.
268. Liu T, Liu Y, He S, et al. Use of radiation with or without WR-2721 in advanced rectal cancer. *Cancer* 1992;69:2820.
269. Minsky BD, Cohen AM, Kemeny N, et al. Enhancement of radiation induced downstaging of rectal cancer by 5-FU and high dose leucovorin chemotherapy. *J Clin Oncol* 1992;10:79.
270. Willett CG, Shellito PC, Tepper JE, et al. Intraoperative electron beam radiation therapy for primary locally advanced rectal and rectosigmoid carcinoma. *J Clin Oncol* 1991;9:843.
271. Willett CG, Shellito PC, Tepper JE, et al. Intraoperative electron beam radiation therapy for recurrent locally advanced rectal or rectosigmoid carcinoma. *Cancer* 1991;67:1504.
272. Mendenhall WM, Bland KI, Pfaff WW, et al. Initially unresectable rectal adenocarcinoma treated with preoperative irradiation and surgery. *Ann Surg* 1986;205:41.
273. Marsh RW, Chu NM, Vauthey JN, et al. Preoperative treatment of patients with locally advanced unresectable rectal adenocarcinoma utilizing continuous chronobiologically shaped 5-fluorouracil infusion and radiation therapy. *Cancer* 1996;78:217.
274. Tobin RL, Mohiuddin M, Marks G. Preoperative irradiation for cancer of the rectum with extrarectal fixation. *Int J Radiat Oncol Biol Phys* 1991;21:1127.
275. Willett CG, Shellito PC, Rodkey GV, Wood WC. Preoperative irradiation for tethered rectal carcinoma. *Radiother Oncol* 1991;21:141.
276. Minsky BD, Cohen AM, Enker WE, et al. Intraoperative brachytherapy alone in incompletely resected recurrent rectal cancer. *Radiother Oncol* 1991;21:115.
277. Dibiase SJ, Rosenstock JG, Shabason L, Corn BW. Tumor bed brachytherapy with a mesh template: an accessible alternative to intraoperative radiotherapy. *J Surg Oncol* 1997;66:104.
278. Harrison LB, Minsky BD, Enker WE, et al. High dose rate intraoperative radiation therapy (HDR-IORT) as part of the management strategy for locally advanced primary and recurrent rectal cancer. *Int J Radiat Oncol Biol Phys* 1998;42:325.
279. Huber FT, Stepan R, Zimmermann F, et al. Locally advanced rectal cancer: resection and intraoperative radiotherapy using the flab method combined with preoperative or postoperative radiochemotherapy. *Dis Colon Rectum* 1996;39:774.
280. Nakfoor BM, Willett CG, Shellito PC, et al. The impact of 5-fluorouracil and intraoperative electron beam radiation therapy on the outcome of patients with locally advanced primary rectal and rectosigmoid cancer. *Ann Surg* 1998;228:194.
281. Saltz LB, Locker PK, Pirotta N, et al. Weekly irinotecan (CPT-11), leucovorin (LV), and fluorouracil (FU) is superior to daily × 5 LV/FU in patients (pts) with previously untreated metastatic colorectal cancer. *Proc ASCO* 1999;18:233a.
282. Kallinowski F, Eble MJ, Buhr HJ, et al. Intraoperative radiotherapy for primary and recurrent rectal cancers. *Eur J Surg Oncol* 1995;21:191.
283. Kim HK, Jessup JM, Beard CJ, et al. Locally advanced rectal carcinoma: pelvic control and morbidity following preoperative radiation therapy, resection, and intraoperative radiation therapy. *Int J Radiat Oncol Biol Phys* 1997;38:777.
284. Gunderson LL, Nelson H, Martenson JA, et al. Intraoperative electron and external beam irradiation with or without 5-fluorouracil and maximum surgical resection for previously unirradiated, locally recurrent colorectal cancer. *Dis Colon Rectum* 1996;39:1379.
285. Wallace JH, Willett CG, Shellito PC, et al. Intraoperative radiation therapy for locally advanced recurrent rectal or rectosigmoid cancer. *J Surg Oncol* 1995;60:122.
286. Lowy AM, Rich TA, Skibber JM, et al. Preoperative infusional chemoradiation, selective intraoperative radiation, and resection for locally advanced pelvic recurrence of colorectal adenocarcinoma. *Ann Surg* 1996;223:177.
287. Hashiguchi Y, Sekine T, Sakamoto H, et al. Intraoperative irradiation after surgery for locally recurrent rectal cancer. *Dis Colon Rectum* 1999;42:886.
288. Eble MJ, Lehnert T, Treiber M, et al. Moderate dose intraoperative and external beam radiotherapy for locally recurrent rectal carcinoma. *Radiother Oncol* 1998;49:169.
289. Vujaskovic Z, Powers BE, Paardekoper G, et al. Effects of intraoperative irradiation (IORT) and intraoperative hyperthermia (IOHT) on canine sciatic nerve: histopathological and morphometric studies. *Int J Radiat Oncol Biol Phys* 1999;43:1103.
290. Johnstone PAS, Laskin WB, DeLuca AM, et al. Tumors in dogs exposed to experimental intraoperative radiotherapy. *Int J Radiat Oncol Biol Phys* 1996;34:853.
291. Gunderson LL, O'Connell MJ, Dozois RR. The role of intraoperative irradiation in locally advanced primary and recurrent rectal adenocarcinoma. *World J Surg* 1992;16:495.
292. Lanciano RM, Calkins AR, Wolkov HB, et al. A phase I/II study of intraoperative radiotherapy in advanced unresectable or recurrent carcinoma of the rectum: a radiation therapy oncology group (RTOG) study. *J Surg Oncol* 1993;53:20.
293. Noyes RD, Weiss SM, Krall JM, et al. Surgical complications of intraoperative radiation therapy: the Radiation Therapy Oncology Group experience. *J Surg Oncol* 1993;50:209.
294. Frykholm G, Glimelius B, Pahlman L. Preoperative irradiation with and without chemotherapy (MFL) in the treatment of primary non-resectable adenocarcinoma of the rectum. Results from two consecutive studies. *Eur J Clin Oncol* 1989;11:1535.
295. Gunderson LL, Nelson H, Martenson JA, et al. Locally advanced primary colorectal cancer: intraoperative electron and external beam irradiation + 5-FU. *Int J Radiat Oncol Biol Phys* 1997;37:601.
296. Kelsen DP, Hilaris B, Martini N. Neoadjuvant chemotherapy and surgery of cancer of the esophagus. *Semin Surg Oncol* 1986;2:170.
297. Chen ET, Mohiuddin M, Brodovsky H, et al. Downstaging of advanced rectal cancer following combined preoperative chemotherapy and high dose radiation. *Int J Radiat Oncol Biol Phys* 1994;30:169.
298. Movsas B, Hanlon A, Lanciano R, et al. Phase I dose escalating trial of hyperfractionated preoperative chemoradiation for locally advanced rectal cancer. *Int J Radiat Oncol Biol Phys* 1998;42:43.
299. Videtic GMM, Fischer BJ, Perera FE, et al. Preoperative radiation with concurrent 5-fluorouracil continuous for locally advanced unresectable rectal cancer. *Int J Radiat Oncol Biol Phys* 1998;42:319.
300. Bussieres E, Gilly FN, Rouanet P, et al. Recurrences of rectal cancers: results of a multimodal approach with intraoperative radiation therapy. *Int J Radiat Oncol Biol Phys* 1995;34:49.
301. Perera F, Fisher B, Kocha W, et al. A phase I pilot study of pelvic radiation and alpha-2A interferon in patients with locally advanced or recurrent rectal cancer. *Int J Radiat Oncol Biol Phys* 1997;37:297.
302. James RD, Price P, Smith M. Raltitrexed (Tomudex) plus radiotherapy is well tolerated and warrants further investigation in patients with advanced inoperable/recurrent rectal cancer. *Proc ASCO* 1999;18:288a.
303. Schild SE, Martenson JA, Gunderson LL, Dozois RR. Long-term survival and patterns of failure after postoperative radiation therapy for subtotally resected rectal adenocarcinoma. *Int J Radiat Oncol Biol Phys* 1989;16:459.
304. Suzuki K, Gunderson LL, Devine RM, et al. Intraoperative irradiation after palliative surgery for locally recurrent rectal cancer. *Cancer* 1995;75:939.
305. Allee PE, Tepper JE, Gunderson LL, Munzenrider JE. Postoperative radiation therapy for incompletely resected colorectal carcinoma. *Int J Radiat Oncol Biol Phys* 1989;17:1171.
306. Calvo FA, Algarra SM, Azinovic I, et al. Intraoperative radiotherapy for recurrent and/or residual colorectal cancer. *Radiother Oncol* 1989;15:133.
307. Duncan W, Arnott SJ, Jack WJL, et al. Results of two randomized trials of neutron therapy in rectal adenocarcinoma. *Radiother Oncol* 1987;8:191.
308. Nishimura Y, Hiraoka M, Akuta K, et al. Hyperthermia combined with radiation therapy for primarily unresectable and recurrent colorectal cancer. *Int J Radiat Oncol Biol Phys* 1992;23:759.
309. Graf R, Wust P, Gellermann J, et al. Phase II trial of radiation therapy with 45 Gy, 5-fluorouracil (5-FU), and mitomycin-C (MMC) in patients with anal cancer—a rationale to add regional hyperthermia. *Int J Radiat Oncol Biol Phys* 1996;36:296.
310. Furuta K, Konishi F, Kanazawa K, et al. Synergistic effects of hyperthermia in preoperative radiochemotherapy for rectal carcinoma. *Dis Colon Rectum* 1997;40:1303.
311. Ohno S, Tomoda M, Tomisaki S, et al. Improved surgical results after combining preoperative hyperthermia with chemotherapy and radiotherapy for patients with carcinoma of the rectum. *Dis Colon Rectum* 1997;40:401.
312. Ichikawa D, Yamaguchi T, Yoshioka Y, et al. Prognostic evaluation of preoperative combined treatment for advanced cancer in the lower rectum with radiation, intraluminal hyperthermia, and 5-fluorouracil suppository. *Am J Surg* 1996;171:346.
313. Emami B, Myerson RJ, Scott C, et al. Phase I/II study, combination of radiotherapy and hyperthermia in patients with deep-seated malignant tumors: report of a pilot study by the Radiation Therapy Oncology Group. *Int J Radiat Oncol Biol Phys* 1991;20:73.
314. Pu AT, Robertson JM, Lawrence TS. Current status of radiation sensitization by fluoropyrimidines. *Oncology* 1995;9:707.
315. Rhomberg W, Eiter H, Hergan K, Schneider B. Inoperable recurrent rectal cancer: results of a prospective trial with radiation therapy and razoxane. *Int J Radiat Oncol Biol Phys* 1994;30:419.
316. Coucke PA, Cuttat JF, Mirimanoff RO. Adjuvant postoperative accelerated hyperfractionated radiotherapy in rectal cancer: a feasibility study. *Int J Radiat Oncol Biol Phys* 1993;27:885.
317. Coucke PA, Sartorelli B, Cuttat JF, et al. The rationale to switch from postoperative hyperfractionated accelerated radiotherapy to preoperative hyperfractionated accelerated radiotherapy in rectal cancer. *Int J Radiat Oncol Biol Phys* 1995;32:181.
318. Bozzetti F, Baratti D, Andreola S, et al. Preoperative radiation therapy for patients with T2-T3 carcinoma of the middle-to-lower rectum. *Cancer* 1999;86:398.
319. Turegano-Fuentes F, Echenagusia-Belda A, Simo-Muerza G, et al. Transanal self-expanding metal stents as an alternative to palliative colostomy in selected patients with malignant obstruction of the left colon. *Br J Surg* 1998;85:232.
320. Eckhauser ML, Imbembo AL, Mansour EG. The role of pre-resectional laser recanalization for obstructing carcinomas of the colon and rectum. *Surgery* 1989;106:710.

321. Sagar PM, Pemberton JH. Surgical management of locally recurrent rectal cancer. *Br J Surg* 1996;83:293.
322. Romano G, Esercizio L, Santangelo M, et al. Impact of computed tomography vs. intrarectal ultrasound on the diagnosis, resectability, and prognosis of locally recurrent rectal cancer. *Dis Colon Rectum* 1993;36:261.
323. Freeny PC, Marks WM, Ryan JA, Bolen JW. Colorectal carcinoma evaluation with CT: preoperative staging and detection of postoperative recurrence. *Radiology* 1986;158:347.
324. Farouk R, Nelson H, Radice E, et al. Accuracy of computed tomography in determining resectability for locally advanced primary or recurrent colorectal cancers. *Am J Surg* 1998;175:283.
325. Cohen AM, Martin EW, Lavery I, et al. Radioimmunoguided surgery using iodine 125 B72.3 in patients with colorectal cancer. *Arch Surg* 1991;126:349.
326. Beets G, Penninck F, Schiepers C. Clinical value of whole-body positron emission tomography with [^{18}F]fluorodeoxyglucose in recurrent colorectal cancer. *Br J Surg* 1994;81:1666.
327. Donat SM, Russo P. Ureteral decompression in advanced nonurologic malignancies. *Ann Surg Oncol* 1996;3:393.
328. Pearlman NW, Donohue RE, Stiegmann GV, et al. Pelvic and sacropelvic exenteration for locally advanced or recurrent anorectal cancer. *Arch Surg* 1987;122:537.
329. Wanebo HJ, Gaker DL, Whitehill R, et al. Pelvic recurrence of rectal cancer. *Ann Surg* 1987;205:482.
330. Temple WJ, Ketcham AC. Sacral resection for control of pelvic tumors. *Am J Surg* 1992;163:370.
331. Zacherl J, Schiessel R, Windhager R, et al. Abdominosacral resection of recurrent rectal cancer in the sacrum. *Dis Colon Rectum* 1999;42:1035.
332. Mohiuddin M, Marks GM, Lingareddy V, Marks J. Curative surgical resection following reirradiation for recurrent rectal cancer. *Int J Radiat Oncol Biol Phys* 1997;39:643.
333. Yeh KA, Hoffman JP, Kusiak JE, et al. Reconstruction with myocutaneous flaps following total resection of locally recurrent rectal cancer. *Am Surg* 1995;61:581.
334. Arbman G, Nilsson E, Hallbook O, Sjodahl R. Local recurrence following mesorectal excision for rectal cancer. *Br J Surg* 1996;83:375.
335. Pocard M, Panis Y, Malassagne B, et al. Assessing the effectiveness of mesorectal excision in rectal cancer. Prognostic value of the number of lymph nodes found in resected specimens. *Dis Colon Rectum* 1998;41:839.
336. Bailey HR, Huval WV, Max E, et al. Local excision of carcinoma of the rectum for cure. *Surgery* 1992;111:555.
337. Scott N, Hale A, Deakin M, et al. A histopathologic assessment of the response of rectal adenocarcinoma to combination chemo-radiotherapy. *Eur J Surg Oncol* 1998;24:169.
338. Tannapfel A, Nusslein S, Fietkau R, et al. Apoptosis, proliferation, bax, bcl-2, and p53 status prior to and after preoperative radiochemotherapy for locally advanced rectal cancer. *Int J Radiat Oncol Biol Phys* 1998;41:585.
339. Luna-Perez P, Arriola EL, Cuadra Y, et al. p53 protein overexpression and response to induction chemoradiation therapy in patients with locally advanced rectal adenocarcinoma. *Ann Surg Oncol* 1998;5:203.
340. Desai GR, Meyerson RJ, Higashikubo R, et al. Carcinoma of the rectum. Possible cellular predictors of metastatic potential and response to radiation therapy. *Dis Colon Rectum* 1996;39:1090.
341. Fu CG, Tominaga O, Nagawa H, et al. Role of p53 and p21/WAF1 detection in patient selection for preoperative radiotherapy in rectal cancer patients. *Dis Colon Rectum* 1998; 41:58.
342. Sakakura C, Koide K, Ichikawa D, et al. Analysis of histological therapeutic effect, apoptosis rate and p53 status after combined treatment with radiation, hyperthermia, and 5-fluorouracil suppositories for advanced rectal cancers. *Br J Cancer* 1998;77:159.
343. Nehls O, Klump B, Holzmann K, et al. Influence of p53 status on prognosis in preoperatively irradiated rectal carcinoma. *Cancer* 1999;85:2541.
344. Adell G, Sun XF, Olle S, et al. p53 status: an indicator for the effect of preoperative radiotherapy of rectal cancer. *Radiother Oncol* 1999;51:169.
345. Goes RN, Beart RW, Simons AJ, et al. Use of brachytherapy in management of locally recurrent rectal cancer. *Dis Colon Rectum* 1997;40:1177.
346. Nag S, Martinez-Monge R, Mills J, et al. Intraoperative high dose rate brachytherapy in recurrent metastatic colorectal carcinoma. *Ann Surg Oncol* 1998;5:16.

BRUCE D. MINSKY
JOHN P. HOFFMAN
DAVID P. KELSEN

SECTION 9

Cancer of the Anal Region

Anal cancers, while still uncommon tumors, have increased substantially in incidence since the 1980s.[1] As discussed in this chapter, it is possible that this increase in incidence is due to sexual transmission of human papilloma virus (HPV). Thus, in theory at least, anal squamous cell (epidermoid) tumors may represent a preventable disease. For almost two decades, combined modality treatment involving radiation and chemotherapy has resulted in 5-year survival rates of approximately 80% and in sphincter preservation for most patients with squamous cell carcinomas of the anal canal. Surgical resection involving an abdominal perineal resection (APR) is reserved for patients with local failure or progression. This approach has served as a model for other cancers of the successful use of curative nonoperative combined modality therapy.

EPIDEMIOLOGY AND ETIOLOGY

INCIDENCE, AGE, AND GENDER

In the United States, cancers of the anal region account for 1% to 2% of all large bowel cancers and 3.9% of all anorectal carcinomas. The majority of these patients (75% to 80%) have squamous cell carcinomas.[2] Approximately 15% have adenocarcinomas. In 1998, a total of 3300 cases of cancers of the anal region were reported in the United States, including 1400 men and 1900 women.[1] It is estimated that there will be 500 deaths per year.

The U.S. National Cancer Database provided data to examine the epidemiology of patients with anal canal cancer. In this analysis, a total of 2339 cases of anal carcinoma diagnosed in 1988 and 1993 were compared. There was little difference in mean age or in the male to female ratio during the 5-year period. Two-thirds of newly diagnosed patients were women, indicating that both in the United States and in Europe, women are substantially more likely to develop anal canal cancers than are men. Most patients were white. The proportion of patients with squamous cell carcinoma increased slightly, compromising between 75% and 80% of newly diagnosed patients. Seventy-five percent of patients have stage I or II tumors. In this analysis, no comment was made regarding the incidence of disease in homosexual or bisexual men.

HUMAN PAPILLOMA VIRUS INFECTION AND ANAL CANCER

HPV infection is closely correlated with squamous cell carcinoma. Frisch et al. conducted a population-based case-control study in Denmark and Sweden for patients with anal canal cancers.[3] Two control groups (patients with adenocarcinoma of the rectum and healthy persons from the general population) were included. A variety of behavioral factors, such as sexual activity and venereal infection, tobacco consumption, and anal inflammatory lesions, were examined. In this large study involving 417 patients with anal cancer, 534 controls with adenocarcinoma of the rectum, and 554 general population controls, a strong positive correlation was found both in univariate and multivariate analysis for the amount of sexual activity and the risk of anal cancer. An additional association between venereal infection in both men and women was noted. The authors concluded that sexual activity was strongly associated with the development of anal canal cancer and that HPV infection was the presumed etiologic cause.

Anal intraepithelial neoplasia (AIN) is rare in heterosexual men, whereas the incidence is 5% to 30% in human immunodeficiency virus (HIV)–negative homosexual men. Similarly, such changes are rare among HIV-negative women. High-grade anal lesions that almost always contain HPV have been reported, primarily among HIV-positive individuals. It is suspected that, similar to cervical carcinoma in which HPV is strongly associated and may be a necessary factor for development of the disease, high-grade AIN lesions are the immediate precursors to anal cancer.[4–6]

ANAL CANCER AND ACQUIRED IMMUNODEFICIENCY SYNDROME

An association between acquired immunodeficiency syndrome (AIDS) and an increased risk for anal canal cancer has been noted for some time. Treatment of the HIV-positive patient is discussed later in this chapter (see Treatment of the Human Immunodeficiency Virus–Positive Patient). Melbye et al. linked databases for AIDS and those for cancer in American patients.[7] The relative risk (RR) of anal cancer at the time of or after AIDS diagnosis was 84.1 among homosexual men. The relative risk of anal cancer for up to 5 years before AIDS diagnosis was 13.9. This marked increased risk of anal cancer in patients with AIDS is presumably because of immunodeficiency, perhaps increasing susceptibility to HPV infection. A similar increase in risk has been noted for renal transplant patients undergoing immunosuppression.[8]

Although earlier studies suggested that anal-receptive intercourse was directly linked to an increased risk of anal cancer, this finding has not been confirmed in more recent larger scale trials. Particularly in women, most patients did not report sexual activity involving anal intercourse.

Goldie et al. reviewed the clinical outcome and cost effectiveness of screening for premalignant (squamous intraepithelial lesions) or malignant anal lesions in homosexual and bisexual HIV-positive men.[9] Their analysis indicated that screening of homosexual and bisexual men who were HIV-positive, no matter what the stage of their HIV status, prolongs quality-adjusted life expectancy.

Anal canal carcinoma has also been associated with condylomata in both the general population and in male homosexuals.[10–12] Pfister and Fuchs also noted that HPV-16 infection has a strong association with high-grade AIN and a risk of anogenital malignancy. HPV infection alone may be insufficient for malignant transformation, however, as many persons with HPV-positive cytology do not develop either AIN or anal carcinoma.[13]

In women without a history of genital warts, anal cancer was associated with seropositivity for herpes simplex virus type 1 (RR, 4.1) and *Chlamydia trachomatis* (RR, 2.3).[14] In men without a history of warts, there was an association with gonorrhea (RR, 17.2). Among individuals with AIDS, an increased risk of anal cancer has been found.[7,15]

MOLECULAR AND CHROMOSOMAL ABNORMALITIES

The E6 oncoprotein of HPV inactivates the growth-controlling p53 suppressor gene product, which may play an important role in the pathogenesis of anal cancer.[16,17] Overexpression of p53 protein has been studied in patients receiving combined modality therapy. In an analysis involving approximately 20% of patients entered into Radiation Therapy Oncology Group (RTOG) protocol 87-04, in whom 5-fluorouracil (5-FU) plus radiation with or without mitomycin C was given, immunohistochemistry for p53 overexpression was performed. Although there was a trend toward worse outcome (decreased local control and survival) in patients overexpressing p53, this did not reach statistical significance.[18]

Other investigators have studied MIB-1 in patients with anal canal carcinomas receiving radiation therapy alone or combined modality therapy. In a group of 55 patients, MIB-1 murine monoclonal antibody measuring Ki-67, used as an index of cellular proliferation, failed to predict outcome for patients treated with radiation with or without chemotherapy.[19]

OTHER ASSOCIATIONS

Anal canal carcinomas have been associated with anal fistulas and other benign conditions. In one study, 41% of anal canal carcinomas were preceded by benign anorectal disease for at least 5 years.[20] However, two studies have now shown only a temporal relationship but no evidence of causation.[21,22] There is a high risk of anal cancer in the first year after diagnosis of the benign lesion and a rapid decline in risk thereafter. In a study from California, however, homosexual men had an elevated risk of anorectal squamous cell carcinoma with a history of anal fissure or fistula (RR, 9.1).[23] Anal canal cancers have been reported in patients with Crohn's disease, but the incidence appears low.[24]

Frisch et al. studied the relationship between anal canal cancers and smoking in Danish and Swedish patients.[25] A positive correlation for an increased risk of anal canal cancer in premenopausal women who smoked versus lifelong nonsmokers was noted [odds ratio (OR), 5.6). Smoking was not statistically significantly related to anal canal cancers in men or postmenopausal women. They suggested that suppression of estrogen may play a role for anal carcinogenesis in premenopausal women. In the case-control study reported by Daling and colleagues, current cigarette smoking was a major risk factor in both sexes (RR, 7.7 in women and 9.4 in men).[14] This is similar to the report by Daniell, who noted that 54% of 13 women with anal cancer were current smokers, compared with only 26% of 202 age-matched patients with colon cancer.[26] In a matched controlled study of 56 women with anal carcinoma, there were strong associations with herpes simplex virus titer, cigarette smoking, and increasing numbers of sexual partners. In a multivariate analysis, cigarette smoking was an independent variable.[27]

Prior radiation therapy may play a role in the development of anal carcinoma, as may immunosuppression.[28–30] Immunosuppressed renal transplant patients have a 100-fold increase in anogenital tumors compared with the general population.[8] As noted previously, increasing immunosuppression in HIV-positive patients is correlated with increased risk for anal canal cancer.

Several general conclusions with regard to etiology can be made. Anal canal carcinoma is highly correlated with HPV infection, especially HPV-16. Immunosuppression, whether by HIV infection or iatrogenically (e.g., in the setting of renal transplantation), increases the relative risk of precursor high-grade AIN and anal carcinoma. Increasingly severe immunodeficiency (e.g., CD4 counts less than 200/μL) also increases the risk of developing anal cancer.

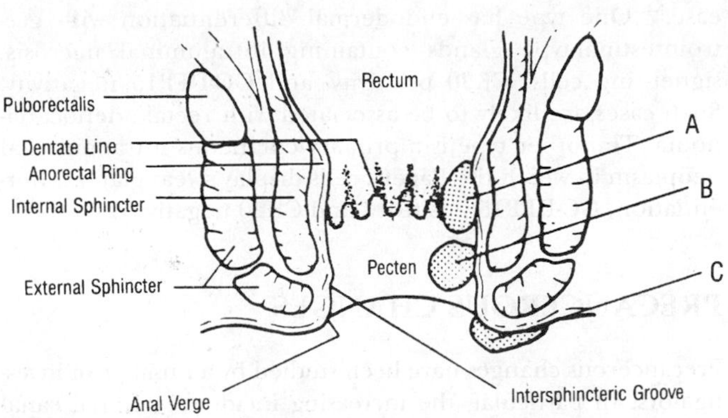

FIGURE 33.9-1. Anatomy of the anal canal. A tumor in location A is always considered anal canal cancer; in location C, it is anal margin cancer. A tumor in location B has been called *canal* or *margin cancer,* depending on institutional preference, but now should be called *anal canal cancer* by the American Joint Committee on Cancer and the Union Internationale Contra le Cancer definition.

ANIMAL STUDIES

Animal studies offer some clues to the genesis of anal tumors. In mice, anal carcinomas may be induced by chemical carcinogens.[31,32] In a study by Kingsnorth and colleagues, the induction of anal squamous cell carcinomas (but not colon tumors) was promoted by epidermal growth factor (EGF).[32] The frequency of anal squamous cell carcinomas induced by dimethylhydrazine alone was only 10%, whereas in mice treated with both dimethylhydrazine and EGF, the frequency was 33% ($P < .05$). It was postulated that this potentiation was a result of EGF-stimulated squamous cell hyperplasia, with the EGF thus acting as a cocarcinogen.

ANATOMY

A clear anatomic distinction between the anal canal and the anal margin is needed because of the different natural histories of cancers that arise in these two distinct anatomic areas. Considerable confusion exists when comparing series in the literature because of the use of different definitions of the anal canal and the anal margin. The anatomic components of the anal canal and anal margin are illustrated in Figure 33.9-1.

The upper or proximal limit of the anal canal is accepted as commencing at the anorectal ring. The anorectal ring is defined as the muscle bundle formed by the junction of the upper portion of the internal sphincter, the distal portion of the longitudinal muscle, the puborectalis, and the deep portion of the external sphincter. This ring can be identified on digital examination. The epithelium lining the anal canal at this level is columnar. The anal columns, vertical folds of mucous membranes lined by cuboidal epithelium, start just distal to the anorectal ring and extend to the dentate line. The dentate line is defined as the demarcation between the columnar epithelium of the proximal canal and the stratified squamous epithelium of the lower canal and is the site where the anal glands empty. The junction is not an abrupt histologic change but rather a transition zone that extends for 6 to 12 mm and contains columnar, cuboidal, squamous, and transitional epithelia. The stratified squamous epithelium extends from just below the dentate line to the anal verge, which is defined as the junction of the squamous epithelium with the perianal skin, which is a keratinized squamous epithelium containing hair follicles.

Definitions of the proximal and distal extent of the anal canal have varied among authors. A number of authors have defined the distal limit of the anal canal as the dentate line and all tumors below this as anal margin cancers.[33–36] Some have defined the distal extent of the anal canal to reach to the anal verge.[37–39] Others refer to anal margin tumors as tumors that arise within 5 cm of the anal verge.[37,40] The anatomic boundary used for distinguishing anal canal from anal margin tumors alters their incidence. When the anal verge is used as the distal margin of the anal canal, 15% of tumors arise from the anal margin, but this number climbs to 30% when the dentate line is used as the distal limit. To clarify this issue, the American Joint Committee on Cancer (AJCC) and the Union Internationale Contra le Cancer (UICC) have formed a consensus that the anal canal extends from the anorectal ring (dentate line) to the anal verge.[41,42] This is an important distinction, as these two governing bodies agree that anal margin tumors behave in a similar fashion to skin cancers and therefore are to be classified as skin tumors and treated as such.

The arterial supply to the distal rectum and anal canal is supplied by the superior, middle, and inferior hemorrhoidal arteries, which arise from the inferior mesenteric, hypogastric, and internal pudendal arteries, respectively. Venous drainage follows the inflow patterns. The internal rectal sphincter motor innervation is supplied by sympathetic fibers, whereas the sacral parasympathetics mediate the sensation of distention. The external rectal sphincter is innervated by the inferior hemorrhoidal nerve, which is derived from the internal pudendal nerve. The lower rectal wall is supplied by the rectal plexus composed of the pelvic sympathetic and parasympathetic nerves. The sensory component of the hair-bearing skin beyond the anal verge is innervated by the inferior hemorrhoidal branches of the internal pudendal nerve.

The anal canal has a rich supply of lymphatics, which drain via three main routes, including the inguinal, pelvic visceral, and hypogastric nodes.[43] The lymphatics of the anal margin drain into the inguinal-femoral nodes, which subsequently drain into the external iliac to the common iliac nodes. The lymphatic drainage of the anal canal is primarily to the perirectal and superior rectal lymphatics, which drain to the inferior mesenteric nodes and eventually to the paraaortic nodes. Lymphatic drainage may also drain laterally into the obturator and hypogastric nodes. Extensive interconnections exist between the lymphatic channels, which explains why patients with distal lesions may have mesenteric nodal involvement.

Squamous tumors may arise from the entire length of the anal canal as well as develop from the anal margin. Basaloid carcinomas, which are a variant of squamous carcinoma, arise from the epithelium just above the dentate line and are commonly referred to as *cloacogenic carcinomas.* The adenocarcinomas in this region arise from the glands at the dentate line. Small cell carcinomas in this region are of neuroendocrine origin and are rare. Tumors of the anal margin include squamous carcinoma, basal cell carcinoma, Bowen's disease, Paget's disease, verrucous carcinoma, and Kaposi's sarcoma. Malignant melanomas may arise from either location, but more commonly from below the dentate line.

TABLE 33.9-1. Distribution of Histologic Types in Patients with Anal Carcinoma (Surveillance, Epidemiology, and End Results Data)

Type	*Percentage of Patients*
Squamous cell carcinoma	47
Transitional (cloacogenic) carcinoma	27
Adenocarcinoma	15
Carcinoma, not otherwise specified	3
Papillary villous (adeno) carcinoma	3
Mucinous adenocarcinoma	2
Melanoma	1
Other	2

(Adapted from Young JL, Percy CCL, Asire AJ. Surveillance, epidemiology, and end results: incidence and mortality data, 1973–77. *Natl Cancer Inst Mongr* 1981;57.)

PATHOLOGY

Many different histologic cell types may occur in the anal area.[44] In addition to the more common types seen in Table 33.9-1, other rare histologic entities can arise, such as small cell carcinomas similar to those in lung,[45] and lymphoma. Melanomas constitute 1% to 2% of all anal cancers.[46]

Some pathologists divide anal canal tumors into those that exhibit keratinization and those that do not[33] and further subdivide nonkeratinizing tumors into basosquamous, basaloid, and cloacogenic carcinomas. Other investigators have found no difference in clinical outcome with such subdivisions and believe that all histologic varieties are subsets of squamous cell carcinoma.[47,48] Most investigators currently believe that, with the exception of melanoma and sarcoma, prognosis is much more dependent on stage than on histology.[49]

An interesting difference in the presence of HPV DNA between cloacogenic and squamous carcinomas has been found.[50] When studied by *in situ* hybridization, all 14 cloacogenic carcinomas were HPV-negative, whereas two-thirds of the 21 squamous carcinomas were HPV-positive (mostly for types 16 to 18). In another study,[51] however, there was no difference in the percentage of HPV RNA positivity (approximately 75%) between cloacogenic and squamous carcinomas.

In the anal margin, histologies other than squamous cell carcinoma include basal cell carcinoma identical with that in skin in other areas, Bowen's disease, and Paget's disease.[52] Patients with Bowen's disease usually present with long-standing perianal pruritus. Raised irregular eczematous-appearing plaques are seen. Biopsy of this intraepithelial neoplasm is diagnostic with large periodic acid–Schiff-negative cells. As with Bowen's disease, patients with perianal Paget's disease frequently present with pruritus, although they may be asymptomatic or, at the other extreme, have a bleeding erythematous or eczematoid plaque.[53] The histologic appearance reveals characteristic periodic acid–Schiff-positive large vacuolated cells. In the absence of an underlying anal canal cancer, the origin of the cells is likely from the apocrine glands. An associated anorectal carcinoma should be excluded. Goldblum and Hart studied immunohistochemical features of specimens from 11 patients with Paget's disease and were able to distinguish two types of perianal Paget's disease.[54] One type has endodermal differentiation with gastrointestinal-type glands containing intraluminal necrosis, signet-ring cells, CK20 positivity, and GC-DFP15 negativity. Such cases are likely to be associated with rectal adenocarcinoma. The other type is a primary cutaneous intraepithelial neoplasm in which the Paget's cells display sweat gland differentiation, GC-DFP15 positivity, and CK20 negativity.

PRECANCEROUS CHANGES

Precancerous changes have been studied by a number of investigators. In particular, the increasing incidence of anal canal carcinomas among certain populations (e.g., homosexual or bisexual men who are HIV-positive) has led to scrutiny of the role of AIN and dysplasia (see Epidemiology and Etiology, earlier in this chapter).

Fenger and Nielsen studied the incidence of precancerous changes in the anal canal epithelium.[55,56] Of 306 specimens of the anal transition zone, seven (2.3%) showed squamous cell dysplasia, which was severe in only one. With an average follow-up of 27 months, no case of dysplasia had progressed to carcinoma. In a group of 139 patients who underwent APR (most with carcinomas of the rectum but some with anal canal tumors), 15 (10.8%) had dysplasia that was thought to be precancerous or to represent carcinoma *in situ*. Severe dysplasia or carcinoma *in situ* was seen in 13 of the 16 patients (81%) with squamous cell carcinoma of the anal canal. They concluded that most anal canal tumors arising in the anal transition zone are preceded by multicentric areas of dysplasia.

Palefsky and colleagues[57] studied the incidence of the premalignant condition, AIN, and its relationship to anal HPV infection among homosexual men who were HIV-positive. Infection with multiple subtypes of HPV was seen in 12% of patients; these patients had a markedly increased risk for cytologic abnormalities (RR, 39.0). In addition, patients who had abnormal cytology were significantly more likely to have lower median T4 counts. They concluded that immunosuppressed male homosexuals may be at significant risk for the development of anal canal neoplasia, related to the presence of HPV.

Surawicz and colleagues found that in 90 homosexual men with an abnormal examination result of the anal canal, 89% had HPV-associated changes.[58] In a prospective study of 37 homosexual men, Palefsky and associates found a substantial increase over time in the percentage of patients with cytologic abnormalities of the anal canal (27% to 65% over an average 17-month period).[59] There was also an increase in the presence of AIN and of identifiable HPV infection.

Flow cytometric analysis of normal epithelium along the anal transition zone and, in smaller groups of patients, of anal canal tumors has been performed in fresh specimens by Fenger and Bichel.[60] A normal diploid population was seen in normal squamous epithelium in the anal transition zone, along with a small hyperdiploid peak, the relevance of which was unclear. Three patients with squamous cell carcinoma of the anal canal were studied. They had a high proliferative index but near diploid peaks. In contrast, Goldman and coworkers found that most anal tumors had an aneuploid pattern.[61] Scott and colleagues studied flow cytometry in 235 patients with resected tumors of the anal canal and perianal skin.[62] In a multivariate analysis, depth of penetration, inguinal node involvement, and DNA ploidy were of independent prognostic significance.

SQUAMOUS CELL CANCER

NATURAL HISTORY

Anal canal carcinomas often spread by local extension, extending cephalad to involve other organs in the pelvis. Local extension to adjacent structures and into the sphincteric muscles is common on initial presentation. Extension to the vaginal septum was seen in 9 of 76 (12%) women in the Memorial Sloan-Kettering series.[43] Although it is often stated that these tumors can invade the prostate, urethra, bladder, and seminal vesicles in male subjects, in this series the tumors approached these organs but did not invade them.[43]

Hematogenous spread appears to occur more often from tumors that arise at the dentate line or above.[63] This pattern of spread allows tumor cells into the portal system, and liver metastases also involve the lung in 5% to 8% of patients.[43,63,64] Hematogenous metastases also involve the lung in 2% to 4% of cases[43,63,64] and bone in 2% of cases.[64] Distant metastases occur with equal frequency independent of the histologic cell type involved. Distant metastases rarely, if ever, are seen with anal margin tumors.

Lymphatic spread can occur via the inguinal, pelvic, and mesenteric nodes (see Anatomy, earlier in this chapter). Because routine lymphadenectomy is no longer performed in anal cancers, the data pertaining to lymph node involvement are from historic surgical series. Many interconnections exist between these lymphatic channels, and tumors arising above or below the dentate line may have mesenteric nodal involvement. Of 33 anal canal tumors arising below the dentate line, six had mesenteric nodal involvement in their abdominoperineal specimens, confirming these interconnections.[43]

Inguinal lymph nodes are involved in 15% to 63% of cases of anal canal tumors.[43,64–67] In one series, 17 of the 115 patients (15%) had inguinal nodes involved at the time of presentation, similar to the incidence reported in other series.[43,63,64,68] Metachronous inguinal nodes appeared in 24 of 96 patients (25%), with a median time to presentation of 12 months. Pelvic nodes are not as commonly involved, whereas mesenteric nodes are more likely to be involved if the tumors are proximal (50%) compared with distal (14%).[43] Anal margin tumors rarely spread to the mesenteric nodes.

Survival after lymph node dissection with positive nodes at presentation ranged from 0% to 20%.[63,64,68–71] However, modern combined modality therapy has greatly affected this result. Patients who have lymph node dissection for metachronous lesions have a better long-term survival, with rates up to 83%.[37,63,70,72] The majority of these recurrences occur by 2 years but may take up to 8 years to present.[43]

DIAGNOSIS

Although anal cancers are located in one of the most accessible sites of the digestive tract, these tumors are frequently misdiagnosed and a delay in treatment often results. The initial and most common symptom is bleeding, and this occurs in more than one-half of the patients.[43,66,67,73–76] The bleeding is rarely substantial and is usually attributed to hemorrhoids. Other common symptoms include pain, tenesmus, pruritus, change in bowel habits, abnormal discharge, and infrequently, inguinal lymphadenopathy.[43,64,73,74,76] Most of these symptoms are associated with benign conditions of the anus, including fissure, fistula in ano, hemorrhoids, anal pruritus, and anal condyloma, which results in a delay of diagnosis. The diagnosis may be further confounded because benign perianal conditions may coexist in 60% of anal margin tumors and in 6% of anal canal tumors.[76] Patients often treat themselves for extended periods before seeking medical attention.[74] The duration of symptoms varies from 2 weeks to longer than 4 years, with a mean of 6 months.[37,47,64,67,70,74,75]

Proper treatment for these tumors is often delayed due to inappropriate diagnosis at the initial evaluation in up to one-third of patients.[37,43,47,67,74,77] It has been generally accepted that the delay in diagnosis has an adverse effect on the outcome, but this has been challenged.[43,64,78] The diagnosis may also be made indirectly in tissues examined routinely after minor anorectal procedures. The patients with these incidental tumors have the most favorable outcomes.[39,43,79–82] Screening of high-risk populations (i.e., HIV-positive homosexual men) may increase the percent of patients diagnosed with earlier stage tumors.

Diagnosis can be made on rectal examination, but anoscopy, proctoscopy, and transrectal ultrasound are important in the evaluation of these tumors. The most common physical finding is an intraluminal mass.[64,66] The physical examination should describe the location, extent, and size of the tumor and the relationship of the tumor to the dentate line. On palpation, the characteristically hard, indurated, inelastic quality of the tumor is detected, which may or may not be ulcerated. Endoscopically, the tumors may appear as flat or slightly raised lesions, as raised lesions with indurated borders, or as polypoid lesions. As the tumor enlarges, it may become fixed to adjacent structures. The use of transrectal ultrasound allows for the determination of depth of penetration and involvement of adjacent organs.[83] In women, the vagina may be infiltrated with tumor and, although it is commonly thought in men that the prostate and seminal vesicles are involved, this is not often confirmed pathologically.[43,69]

Any suspicious lesion in the anal canal should have a biopsy taken, and this can frequently be done in an outpatient procedure. If the patient has pain or spasm precluding this, then an examination under anesthesia is performed. An incisional biopsy is used to make the diagnosis. The lesion should be excised only if it is a small superficial lesion. Inguinal lymphadenopathy should be aspirated to determine tumor involvement to accurately stage the patient. Inguinal lymph node dissection is not warranted due to the associated morbidity, failure to have an effect on outcome, and the adequate control with combined modality therapy (radiation therapy plus concurrent chemotherapy).

An extent of disease workup should include computed tomography of the abdomen and pelvis to evaluate the primary tumor and to detect liver metastases. Chest radiography is performed to determine if pulmonary metastases are present.

STAGING

In 1997 the AJCC[41] and UICC[42] developed a common staging system. This current staging system takes into account the fact that anal canal carcinoma is primarily treated by combined

TABLE 33.9-2. American Joint Committee on Cancer 1998 and the Union Internationale Contra le Cancer 1997 Joint Staging System for Anal Canal Cancer

PRIMARY TUMOR (T)			
Tx	Primary tumor cannot be assessed		
T0	No evidence of primary tumor		
Tis	Carcinoma *in situ*		
T1	Tumor 2 cm or smaller in greatest dimension		
T2	Tumor larger than 2 cm but not larger than 5 cm in greatest dimension		
T3	Tumor larger than 5 cm in greatest dimension		
T4	Tumor of any size invades adjacent organ(s) [e.g., vagina, urethra, bladder (involvement of sphincter muscle[s] alone is not classified as T4)]		
REGIONAL LYMPH NODES (N)			
Nx	Regional lymph nodes cannot be assessed		
N0	No regional lymph node metastasis		
N1	Metastasis in perirectal lymph node(s)		
N2	Metastasis in unilateral internal iliac, inguinal lymph node(s), or both		
N3	Metastasis in perirectal and inguinal lymph nodes, bilateral internal iliac, inguinal lymph nodes, or all three		
DISTANT METASTASIS (M)			
Mx	Distant metastasis cannot be assessed		
M0	No distant metastasis		
M1	Distant metastasis		
STAGE GROUPING			
0	Tis	N0	M0
I	T1	N0	M0
II	T2	N0	M0
	T3	N0	M0
IIIA	T1	N1	M0
	T2	N1	M0
	T3	N1	M0
	T4	N0	M0
IIIB	T4	N1	M0
	Any T	N2	M0
	Any T	N3	M0
IV	Any T	Any N	M1

(Data from refs. 41 and 42.)

modality therapy (or in selected cases by radiation alone). APR is reserved for patients who fail to respond to initial treatment. Thus, the TNM classification for anal canal cancers is primarily clinical. The primary tumor is assessed for size and, for T4 tumors, invasion of local structures such as the vagina, urethra, or bladder. The TNM classification is seen in Table 33.9-2. Nodal status is based on distance from the primary site rather than number of lymph nodes involved. This staging system applies to carcinomas, including cloacogenic carcinomas. Melanomas and sarcomas are not included in this staging system.

PROGNOSTIC FACTORS

The most important prognostic factors in anal cancer are T stage and lymph node status. As seen in Table 33.9-2, these two factors, as well as the presence or absence of metastatic disease, define the stage. The most striking difference in results is seen when comparing T1 and 2 primary cancers (smaller than or equal to 5 cm) versus T3 and 4 primary cancers (larger than 5 cm) (Tables 33.9-3, 33.9-4, and 33.9-5). The local failure rates with T3 to 4 primary cancers are approximately 50% after combined modality therapy. Because prognostic factors such as tumor size and lymph node status may be interrelated, a multivariate analysis is required to determine if they are independent prognostic variables.

T Stage: Univariate Analysis

Salmon and colleagues found that size was significantly related to survival in a study in which radiation therapy alone was the primary treatment.[49] In another radiation therapy alone series, size was prognostic for 5-year survival but not for primary tumor control.[84]

In a series of 118 patients treated by external-beam and brachytherapy by Peiffert et al., there was an increase in local failure with T stage (T1, 11%; T2, 24%; T3, 45%; and T4, 43%) and a corresponding decrease in 5-year survival (T1, 94%; T2, 79%; T3, 53%; and T4, 19%) (Table 33.9-6).[85] Similar data were reported by Gerard and colleagues. In 95 patients treated with combined modality therapy plus brachytherapy there was an increase in 5-year colostomy-free survival with T1 and T2 tumors versus T3 and T4 tumors (T1, 83% and T2, 89%, vs. T3, 50% and T4, 54%).[86] Doci and associates treated 35 patients with 5-FU, cisplatin, and external-beam radiation and reported a complete response rate of 100% for T1 and T2 cancers versus 60% for T3 cancers (see Table 33.9-4).[87] The Intergroup randomized phase III trial of radiation, 5-FU with or without mitomycin C, reported a significantly higher complete response rate by tumor size (smaller than 5 cm, 93%, vs. larger than or equal to 5 cm, 83%; $P = .02$) (see Table 33.9-5).[88] Similar findings were reported by univariate analysis in the European Organization for Research and Treatment of Cancer (EORTC) randomized trial of 45 Gy with or without 5-FU/mitomycin C.[89]

In a series from the Princess Margaret Hospital, tumor size did not appear to have a significant effect on local failure, providing the patients received the combination of 5-FU, mitomycin C, and external-beam radiation (smaller than 4 cm, 95% vs. larger than 4 cm, 86%).[90]

N Stage: Univariate Analysis

In contrast to T stage, the effect of positive lymph nodes is less clear. Furthermore, although the 1997 AJCC/UICC staging system differentiates between positive inguinal and pelvic lymph nodes, most series do not report the data separately. It must be emphasized that, unlike rectal cancer, inguinal lymph nodes in anal cancer are considered nodal metastasis rather than distant metastasis, and patients should be treated in a potentially curative fashion. In the historic literature, synchronous metastases to inguinal lymph nodes have been considered an indicator of a poor prognosis.[49,70,91] However, the use of combined modality therapy has altered the poor prognosis previously reported with positive inguinal nodes.

In a series by Cummings et al. from the Princess Margaret Hospital (see Table 33.9-3), patients with negative nodes who received combined modality therapy had a higher 5-year cause-specific survival compared with those with positive nodes (81%

TABLE 33.9-3. Mitomycin C–Based Phase II Combined Modality Therapy Trials for Anal Cancer: Selected Series[a]

								Percentage Survival	
Series	*Number*	*Percentage T3 or T4*	*Percentage Lymph Node Positive*	*Months Follow-Up*	*Treatment*	*Percentage Complete Response*	*Percentage Local Control*	Colostomy-Free Survival	Overall
Cummings,[92] 1991	69	55	19	>36 median	40–50 Gy EBRT pelvis (16 continuous, 53 split course), 5-FU/MMC × 2	—	—	—	75% (5-y) cancer specific
Tanum,[206] 1991	86[b]	62	26	—	50 Gy EBRT pelvis, 5-FU/MMC × 1	—	86	—	72% (5-y)
Miller,[126] 1991	42	26	21	71 median	30 Gy EBRT pelvis, 5-FU/MMC × 2	45			82% (5-y)
Doci,[93] 1992	56	30	14	—	36 Gy EBRT pelvis + 18 Gy perineum, 5-FU/MMC q6wk	87	64		81% (5-y)
John,[207] 1995	34	41	29	98 median	Median 41.4 Gy EBRT pelvis, 5-FU/MMC × 2	—	—	—	92% (5-y)
John,[129] 1996 (RTOG 92-08)	47	49	7	21 median	36 Gy EBRT pelvis + 23.4 Gy boost (to 59.4 Gy), 5-FU/MMC × 2	81	—	70	75% (2-y)
Constantinou,[98] 1997	50	32	22	43 median	Median 54 Gy EBRT pelvis, all had chemotherapy, 84% 5-FU/MMC	—	70 (5-y)		66% (5-y)

	Toxicity	
	Grade 3+	
Type	Continuous	Split course
Acute	75%	40%
Late	63%	17%

EBRT, external-beam radiation therapy; 5-FU, 5-fluorouracil; MMC, mitomycin C.
[a]Limited to series in which all patients received chemotherapy.
[b]Limited to primary disease only.

vs. 57%).[92] The incidence of local failure was only 13% in patients with positive nodes. Doci et al. found no significant difference in the complete response rate after 5-FU, cisplatin, and external-beam radiation in patients with node-positive compared with node-negative cancers (100% vs. 92%).[87] In a separate report of 56 patients who received 5-FU, mitomycin C, and radiation, the eight patients who had node-positive disease all achieved a complete response.[93] By univariate analysis, Allal and colleagues reported a significant increase in local failure in patients with positive versus negative nodes who received 5-FU, mitomycin C, and radiation (36% vs. 19%; $P = .03$); however, this difference was not found to be significant by multivariate analysis.[94] In patients treated with 5-FU, cisplatin, and external-beam and brachytherapy, Gerard et al. also reported no significant differences in 5-year colostomy-free and overall survival in patients with node-positive compared with node-negative disease.[86]

The Intergroup randomized phase III trial of radiation and 5-FU, with or without mitomycin C, reported a higher colostomy rate (which is an indirect measurement of local failure) in N1 versus N0 patients (28% vs. 13%).[88] In node-negative patients, and possibly node-positive patients, the addition of mitomycin C decreased the overall colostomy rates. The EORTC randomized trial of 45 Gy with or without 5-FU/mitomycin C also reported that patients with positive nodes experienced significantly higher local failure ($P = .035$) and lower survival ($P = .038$) rates compared with node-negative patients.[89] However, there was no difference in prognosis between N1 versus N2 and N3 disease.

Multivariate Analysis

In the series from Allal and associates, factors by univariate analysis associated with a significant increase in local failure included age younger than 66 years, male gender, tumor extent more than one-third circumference, lymph node involvement, overall treatment time 75 days or greater, and the use of external-beam radiation for the boost treatment.[94] By multivariate analysis, however, the only variable for which there was a possible effect was overall treatment time ($P = .09$). In the EORTC randomized trial of 45 Gy with or without 5-FU/mitomycin C, multivariate analysis identified that positive nodes, skin ulceration, and male gender were independent negative prognostic factors for local control and survival.[89] Goldman and coworkers also reported by multivariate analysis that gender was also important, with women faring better than men.[95] In a multivariate analysis of 242 patients by Schlienger et al., T stage was the only significant prognostic factor.[96] In a further update with 286 patients analyzed by multivariate analysis, tumor size, clinically

TABLE 33.9-4. Cisplatin-Based Phase II Combined Modality Therapy Trials for Anal Cancer: Selected Series

Series	*Number*	*Percentage T3 or T4*	*Percentage Lymph Node Positive*	*Months Follow-Up*	*Treatment*	*Percentage Complete Response*	*Percentage Local Control*	*Percentage Survival* Colostomy-Free Survival	*Percentage Survival* Overall	*Toxicity*
Doci,[87] 1996	35	14	26	37 median	36–38 Gy EBRT pelvis + perineal boost to 54–62 Gy, 5-FU/CDDP × 2–3	94	94	86	94 (5-y no evidence of disease)	—
Martenson,[130] 1996 (ECOG 4292)	19	68	32	33 maximum	36 Gy EBRT pelvis + 23.4 Gy boost (to 59.4 Gy), 5-FU/CDDP × 2	68	—	—	—	79% grade 3+
Pieffert,[131] 1997	30	43	63	—	30–45 Gy EBRT pelvis + 15–20 Gy boost with brachytherapy or EBRT perineal, 5-FU/CDDP induction × 2, 5-FU/CDDP concurrent × 2	96	—	—	—	67% grade 3+
Gerard,[86] 1998	95	44	44	64 median	30–48 Gy EBRT pelvis or perineal; 89% had 19 Gy brachytherapy boost, 5-FU/CDDP × 1	89	80 (93 with salvage)	72	84 (5-y)	—
Meropol,[127] 1999 (Cancer and Leukemia Group B)	45	100	22	21 median	45 Gy EBRT pelvis ± 9-Gy boost, 5-FU/CDDP induction × 2, 5-FU/CDDP concurrent × 2	80 (18% after induction)	—	56	78% crude	—

CDDP, cisplatin; EBRT, external-beam radiation therapy; 5-FU, 5-fluorouracil; MMC, mitomycin C.

abnormal lymph nodes, and total irradiation dose influenced prognosis.[97] Constantinou and colleagues (see Table 33.9-3) reviewed 50 patients who received combined modality therapy and found that radiation dose and percent hemoglobin were independent prognostic factors for local control; radiation dose was an independent prognostic factor for disease-free survival; and radiation dose, percent hemoglobin, and T stage were independent prognostic factors for survival.[98]

Other Prognostic Features

Histologic cell type for squamous cancers of the anal canal (squamous vs. cloacogenic) has not been found to be of major prognostic relevance. Cloacogenic carcinomas have been considered to have a slightly better prognosis in some series[49,99]; however, in 243 patients with resectable anal canal tumors, Papillon and Montbarbon reported a worse prognosis for patients with nonkeratinizing and basaloid carcinoma than for patients with keratinizing lesions.[84] Small cell carcinomas of the anus are rare and, similar to extrapulmonary small cell cancers in other parts of the body, appear to have a worse prognosis, with a high propensity for systemic dissemination.[45,100]

Asymptomatic patients have a better prognosis than symptomatic patients, but this may be directly related to the size of the tumor.[39] Location may be of modest prognostic importance, with anal margin tumors having a better outcome than those in the anal canal (see Treatment, later in this chapter).

Three studies have examined DNA content (i.e., whether tumors were diploid or nondiploid); two found no prognostic effect of this factor,[61,62] whereas in one large multivariate analysis,[100] DNA ploidy was an independent prognostic factor in the 184 patients whose tumors were analyzed for DNA. In one study,[61] grade was a significant prognostic factor, with low-grade tumors resulting in a 5-year survival of 75% compared with only 24% for high-grade tumors. Data from the Princess Margaret Hospital suggest the DT-diaphorase mutation is not a strong determinant of treatment outcome in patients who fail combined modality therapy.[101]

Tanum and Holm reported p53 expression in 34% of patients with anal carcinoma.[102] Pretreatment biopsies from 80 patients treated on the combined modality therapy arm of the Intergroup randomized trial were examined by immunohistochemistry for p53 expression.[103] For the total group, p53 protein was overexpressed in 47% of tumors. By multivariate analysis, the 4-year local disease-free survival was significantly decreased in those patients whose tumors overexpressed p53 (64% vs. 88%; $P = .027$). However, significant differences were not seen in disease-free or overall survival.

In a retrospective analysis from the Princess Margaret Hospital, p53 was measured by immunohistochemistry in 49 patients

TABLE 33.9-5. Randomized Trials of Combined Modality Therapy for Anal Cancer

Trial	Number	Initial Treatment	*Assessment/ Treatment of Residual at 6 Weeks*		Arm	*Percentage Complete Response*	*Percentage with Colostomy*	*Percentage Local Control*		*Percentage Survival*		*Percentage Grade 4+ Toxicity*	
								Crude	Actuarial	Colostomy-Free Survival	Overall	Early	Late
Intergroup[88]	291	45 Gy EBRT pelvis	Residual	Boost	RT/5-FU	85	22	—	—	59	70 (4-y)	7	—
RTOG 87-04	(47% T3)	5-FU: 1000/mg^2 × 96 h, weeks 1 + 5	Positive	9 Gy + 5-FU			[a]			[a]		[a]	
ECOG 1289	(17% LN+)			Cisplatin	RT/5-FU/MMC	92	9	—	—	71	75 (4-y)	23	—
			Negative	Observe									
		VERSUS											
		45 Gy pelvis; 5-FU, 1000 mg/m^2 × 96 h, weeks 1 + 5; MMC, 10 mg/m^2, bolus day 1											
UKCCCR[107,b]	585	45 Gy EBRT pelvis	≥50% CR	15–20 Gy EBRT or brachytherapy	RT	—	—	41	39 (3-y)	—	58 (4-y)	39	38
	(51% T3)							[a]	[a]			[a]	
	(20% LN+)				RT/5-FU/MMC	—	—	64	61 (3-y)	—	65 (4-y)	48	42
		VERSUS	<50% CR	Salvage surgery									
		45 Gy EBRT pelvis; 5-FU: 750–1000 mg/m^2 × 96–120 h, weeks 1 + 5; MMC, 12 mg/m^2, bolus day 1											
EORTC[89]	110	45 Gy EBRT pelvis	PR/CR	15–20 Gy EBRT or brachytherapy	RT	54	—	55	50 (5-y)	40 (5-y)	52 (5-y)	—	—
	(85% T3)							[a]	[a]	[a]			
	(48% LN+)	VERSUS			RT/5-FU/MMC	80	—	73	68 (5-y)	72 (5-y)	57 (5-y)	Increased ulceration	
			<PR	Salvage surgery									
		45 Gy EBRT pelvis weeks 1 + 5; 5-FU: 750 mg/m^2 × 120 h; MMC, 15 mg/m^2, bolus day 1											

CR, complete response; EBRT, external-beam radiation therapy; EORTC, European Organization for Research and Treatment of Cancer; 5-FU, 5-fluorouracil; LN+, lymph node positive; MMC, mitomycin C; PR, partial response; RT, radiation therapy; UKCCCR, United Kingdom Coordinating Committee on Cancer Research.
[a]Statistically significant ($P \leq .05$).
[b]The UKCCCR trial includes 23% anal margin cancers.

TABLE 33.9-6. Brachytherapy as a Component of Treatment for Anal Cancer: Selected Series

Series	*Number*	*Percentage T3 or T4*	*Percentage Lymph Node Positive*	*Months Follow-Up*	*Treatment*	*Percentage Complete Response*	*Percentage Local Control*	*Percentage Colostomy-Free Survival*	*Percentage Survival*	*Comments*
Sandhu,[135] 1998	79	39	15	37 median	40–50 Gy pelvis or perineal EBRT, 20–25 Gy ^{192}Ir implant, 15% had 5-FU/MMC	91	78	71	75% 3-y	14% adenocarcinoma; 8% required abdominal perineal resection for complications
Gerard,[86] 1998	95	44	44	64 median	30–48 Gy pelvis or perineal EBRT, 5-FU/CDDP × 1, 89% had 19 Gy ^{192}Ir implant	89	80	72	84% 5-y	15% anal necrosis
Papillon,[84] 1987	276	70[a]	21	—	30–39 Gy pelvis or perineal EBRT, 15–20 Gy ^{192}Ir implant	—	—	—	64% 5-y no evidence of disease	2% anal necrosis
Roed,[134] 1996	17	53	—	—	46 Gy pelvis EBRT, 25.2 Gy HDR ^{192}Ir	—	—	—	—	76% anal necrosis
Lohnert,[138] 1998	18	33	17	24 median	45 Gy pelvis EBRT, 4–6 Gy HDR ^{192}Ir, 50% had 5-FU/MMC	—	89	—	—	63% who had >4 Gy had severe complications
Allal,[137] 1997	144	38	—	82	55 Gy pelvis or perineal EBRT, 83% had 20 Gy ^{192}Ir, 62% had 5-FU/MMC or CDDP	78	—	—	72% 5-y	12% toxicity at 5 y
Peiffert,[85] 1997	118	25	20	72 median	36–45 Gy pelvis or perineal EBRT, 86% had 20 Gy ^{192}Ir	—	73	—	60% 5-y	25% anal necrosis (16% grade IV)
Wagner,[136] 1994	108	36	28	—	30 Gy perineal EBRT, 88% mean 20 Gy ^{192}Ir, 55% 5-FU/MMC or CDDP	73	83	85	64% 5-y	9% grade III late toxicity

CDDP, cisplatinum; EBRT, external-beam radiation therapy; 5-FU, 5-fluorouracil; HDR, high dose rate; MMC, mitomycin C.
[a]Centre Leon Berard Staging System.

who received combined modality therapy.[104] The incidence of p53 expression was 82%. By univariate analysis, p53 expression of 5% or greater was a poor prognostic factor for 5-year survival (78% vs. 90%) compared with less than 5%. It was an independent poor prognostic factor for disease-free survival (P = .01).

TREATMENT

Anal Margin

Cancers of the anal margin are uncommon, accounting for approximately 15% of all tumors of the anal region. They account for 15% to 25% of all squamous cell cancers of the anus and, in general, have a different natural history and more favorable prognosis than squamous cell carcinomas of the anal canal.[105] The average age of onset is 60 to 70 years, with a wide range.[106] Most are well to moderately differentiated, with fewer than 10% being poorly differentiated. The 1997 AJCC/UICC staging system defines the anal margin as a cancer arising at the junction of the hair-bearing skin and the mucous membrane of the anal canal.[41,42] It must be emphasized that these tumors are staged as skin cancers rather than anal canal cancers. There is confusion in the literature as a variety of other definitions has been used, the most common being an area of skin measuring from 5 cm to as wide as 10 cm centered on the anal orifice.[37] To further confuse the issue, some series do not report results of anal canal and margin separately.[107]

The lymphatic drainage of anal margin cancers is different from anal canal cancers. Cancers of the anal margin drain primarily to the inguinal lymph nodes, whereas cancers of the anal canal drain primarily to the inguinal as well as the internal iliac and superior hemorrhoidal nodes.

SURGERY. Squamous cell carcinoma of the anal margin, as in skin elsewhere, has a favorable prognosis and rarely requires radical surgery. Wide local excision of these lesions is an attractive approach because it can be performed with primary closure and infrequently requires a split-thickness skin graft. The use of a wide local excision implies that an adequate margin of normal tissue (1 cm) can be secured beyond the tumor without anal incontinence. If the tumor encompasses more than one-half of the circumference of the anus, local excision should be abandoned due to poor anal control; combined modality therapy or APR are advocated.[34,37]

Most authors recommend wide local excision for squamous cell carcinomas of the anal margin,[34,36,37,65,108,109] Bowen's disease,[110] and Paget's disease.[77,111] Wide excision results in control of local disease in the majority of patients.[33,34,37,112,113] Anal margin tumors rarely metastasize to visceral organs or regional lymph nodes, and this represents an important difference between anal margin tumors and anal canal tumors.[34,68,114] High-grade intraepithelial tumors (AIN III or carcinoma *in situ*) may be surgically treated.[115] Other options may include laser ablation[116] or combined modality therapy for extensive lesions that would otherwise require an APR.

Local recurrence after primary treatment of anal margin cancers is routinely treated by repeat local excision. APR or combined modality therapy is reserved for patients with extensive disease. Of the 11 local recurrences treated at Memorial Sloan-Kettering,[43] ten had a local excision and one had an APR.[114] Of the nine patients who survived longer than 5 years, two required a second procedure to control disease. In the same study, four patients had an inguinal node recurrence as the only site of failure, and all underwent inguinal lymphadenectomy. Two of these patients were long-term survivors, one died of disease, and one was lost to follow-up. The median survival exceeded 5 years. The authors concluded that few patients die from anal margin tumors.

An APR or combined modality therapy should be performed when anal margin cancers invade into deep muscle or have vascular, lymphatic, or perineural involvement. A number of series have shown no benefit to the routine use of APR for anal margin tumors, but the small number of patients in these studies combined with patient selection bias makes interpretation of these data difficult.[37,74,109,117]

RADIATION THERAPY. Squamous cell carcinoma of the anal margin tends to be early or only moderately advanced at the time of diagnosis.[117,118] Lymph nodes are rarely involved (0% to 15%).[72,118] Although early cancers of the anal margin are successfully treated by local excision, nonoperative treatment should be considered for some patients. Papillon suggested that radiation therapy should be used for patients with anal margin carcinomas that are considered unresectable or patients who have extensive or recurrent lesions; in addition, patients who are medically inoperable may be able to have radiation therapy.

Early studies of therapy for anal margin cancers used interstitial radium needle implants; however, the high incidence of radionecrosis and the relatively poor geometry suggested that external-beam therapy was better tolerated.[118,119] Although photons are most the frequent radiation treatment, electron-beam therapy may also be successfully used for early perianal epidermoid carcinomas.[120] Results of radiation therapy for perianal lesions, stage for stage, are similar to results for anal canal lesions, with more extensive lesions requiring more aggressive therapy.[117,121] Some authors have recommended APR for extensive lesions.[117] Radiation therapy with or without chemotherapy, however, appears to be an excellent alternative that yields a similar cure rate while offering sphincter preservation.

Selected series reporting the use of primary nonoperative therapy for anal margin cancers are seen in Table 33.9-7. Patients received radiation therapy (external beam with or without brachytherapy) or combined modality therapy. The numbers of patients in each series are small, making it difficult to make definitive conclusions. Combining the series, the overall local control rate is approximately 75% and the 5-year survival is 65% to 70%. In a retrospective analysis from Cummings, local control with T1 and T2 disease was 100% compared with 60% for patients with T3 disease.[90] Likewise, patients who received combined modality therapy had an 88% local control rate compared with 64% local control in patients who received external-beam radiation alone. Peiffert and associates reported the results of 32 patients who were treated with external-beam radiation, brachytherapy, or both. Patients with node-negative disease had a 100% 5-year survival compared with 40% 5-year survival in patients with node-positive disease.[122]

In a retrospective comparison of 54 patients with anal margin cancers with 216 patients with anal canal cancers treated with 40-Gy external-beam radiation plus bleomycin, Friberg et al. reported better results in patients with cancers of the anal margin versus anal canal.[212] There was an improvement in 5-year survival (74% vs. 57%), tumor-specific survival (90% vs. 68%), relapse-free survival (83% vs. 54%), and the incidence of an intact sphincter (91% vs. 58%), respectively.

In summary, squamous cell carcinoma of the anal margin is uncommon, and the literature is limited by small numbers and the lack of a standard anatomic definition. A reasonable approach is to recommend a local excision for smaller tumors (smaller than or equal to 4 cm) that are not in direct contact with the anal verge. If the patient requires an APR due to anatomic constraints or if a local excision would compromise sphincter function, or if the tumor is larger than 4 cm, node positive, or both, then nonoperative treatment is an appropriate alternative. Based on the randomized trials from the EORTC or United Kingdom Coordinating Committee on Cancer Research (UKCCCR) revealing an advantage of combined modality therapy compared with radiation therapy alone in patients with anal canal cancers (EORTC)[89] or anal canal and margin cancers (UKCCCR),[107] combined modality therapy rather than radiation therapy alone is recommended.

Anal Canal

LOCAL EXCISION. Local treatment of epidermoid tumors of the anal canal is reserved for selected patients with tumors that are smaller than 2 cm in diameter, well-differentiated tumors, or tumors found incidentally at the time of hemorrhoidectomy.[36,45,70,123] Local excision may also be performed

TABLE 33.9-7. Treatment of Anal Margin Cancer: Selected Series

Series	*Number*	*Treatment*	*Percentage 5-Y Survival*	*Percentage Local Control*	*Comments*
Cuttuli,[208] 1988	21	EBRT with or without brachytherapy	52	67	—
Cheung,[209] 1989	16	EBRT with or without brachytherapy	—	75	—
Papillon,[106] 1992	26	EBRT with or without brachytherapy	59	67	—
	10	EBRT + chemotherapy	—	—	—
Svennson,[210] 1993	15	EBRT + chemotherapy (bleomycin only)	57	70	—
Cummings,[90] 1993	11	EBRT alone	—	79	Local control: T1–2 = 100%, T3 = 60%, EBRT = 64%, EBRT + chemotherapy = 88%
	18	EBRT + chemotherapy	—	—	—
Touboul,[211] 1995	17	EBRT with or without brachytherapy	86	87	Nine patients with prior local excision
Mendenhall,[105] 1996	7	EBRT alone	75	100	—
	3	EBRT + chemotherapy	—	—	—
Peiffert,[122] 1997	16	EBRT + brachytherapy			Node negative, 100% 5-y survival; node positive, 40% 5-y survival; 6 had prior local excision; 26% grade 3+ complications; 58% colostomy-free survival
	12	Brachytherapy alone	67	67	—
	4	EBRT alone	—	—	—
Friberg,[212] 1998	54	EBRT + chemotherapy (bleomycin)	74	—	—

EBRT, external-beam radiation therapy.

for patients who are medically inoperable or who refuse a permanent colostomy.

Of 188 patients with anal canal carcinoma treated at the Mayo Clinic, 19 were treated with local excision.[45] For the 12 patients with tumors confined to the epithelium and subepithelial connective tissues, 11 had tumors smaller than 2 cm in size and one patient had two lesions. Overall survival for these patients was 100%. One of 12 patients had a recurrence, and this patient was without evidence of disease 5 years after an APR. Patients with tumors penetrating into muscle who refused a colostomy had a higher recurrence rate. These patients' disease often can be salvaged with an APR or combined modality therapy.

Results of local treatment for tumors smaller than 2 cm were not as favorable at Memorial Sloan-Kettering: Only three of eight patients with local excisions had prolonged survival.[70] For more advanced lesions, high local recurrence rates and poor overall survival mitigate against the use of local excision.[37,64,66,70,75]

COMBINED MODALITY THERAPY

Biopsy. With the advent of combined modality therapy, surgery for the initial diagnosis and staging of anal canal tumors should be limited to a biopsy of the primary tumor and evaluation of the inguinal lymph nodes. For most distal lesions, the biopsy is performed under local anesthesia. A punch or incisional biopsy obtains adequate tissue to make a histologic diagnosis. For patients with more proximal tumors or significant pain and spasm, the biopsy may require spinal or general anesthesia. Clinically enlarged lymph nodes should be aspirated. If the cytology is nondiagnostic or demonstrates only benign disease, an open excisional biopsy of one or two lymph nodes should be performed. Under no circumstances should a formal lymph node dissection be performed for the initial evaluation of suspicious nodes.

Therapy. Until the late 1970s, the conventional treatment for anal canal cancer was an APR. The landmark publication that challenged this practice was a report from Nigro et al. of three patients with squamous cell cancer of the anal canal who, after preoperative 30 Gy plus concurrent 5-FU and mitomycin C, were found to have a pathologic complete response at the time of surgery.[124]

Since that time, increasing evidence from single-arm phase II studies has indicated that initial combined modality therapy (chemotherapy plus concurrent external-beam radiation therapy) yields a high rate of tumor regression (including a complete response rate of approximately 80% to 90%) in most patients with squamous cell cancers of the anal canal. Surgery, most commonly an APR, is reserved for salvage. Even in patients with relatively large (larger than or equal to 5 cm) primary cancers, although the complete response rates are lower (50% to 75%), the majority of patients may be spared a colostomy and has an excellent overall survival.

Given that anal canal tumors are uncommon, and because the results of phase II trials using combined modality therapy are impressive, there has been, until relatively recently, no prospective controlled randomized trials of combined modality therapy versus radiation alone or surgery alone. Results of two prospective randomized trials from Europe of combined modality therapy versus radiation alone (EORTC[89] and UKCCCR[107]) support the use of combined modality therapy. In the United States, combined modality therapy has been well established, and randomized trials focus on defining the ideal combined modality therapy regimen. For example, the Intergroup trial

(RTOG 87-04/ECOG 1289)[88] examined the role of adding mitomycin C to radiation plus 5-FU. It is unlikely that a prospective trial of surgery versus nonoperative therapy (combined modality therapy or radiation alone) will be performed. Combined modality therapy has an acceptable toxicity profile as well as a high disease-free and overall survival and is considered the standard of care for squamous cell carcinoma of the anal canal.

The results of two randomized trials that confirm an advantage for combined modality therapy using 45-Gy external-beam pelvic radiation plus continuous infusion 5-FU and bolus mitomycin C versus radiation alone are seen in Table 33.9-5. The UKCCCR trial randomized a total of 585 patients of whom 51% had T3 disease, 20% had positive nodes, and 23% had anal margin cancers.[107] At 6 weeks after treatment, patients with 50% or greater response had additional radiation, whereas those with less than 50% response had salvage surgery. Although the improvement in 4-year survival with combined modality therapy did not reach statistical significance (65% vs. 58%), the improvement in crude (64% vs. 41%) and 3-year actuarial local control (61% vs. 29%) was significant. The early grade 4+ toxicity was significantly higher (48% vs. 39%); however, the incidence of late toxicity was similar (42% vs. 38%).

In the EORTC trial, 110 patients, of whom 85% had T3 disease and 48% had positive nodes, underwent a similar randomization.[89] At 6 weeks after treatment, patients with a partial or complete response had additional radiation, whereas those with less than a partial response had salvage surgery. Patients who received combined modality therapy had a higher complete response rate (80% vs. 54%) and a significantly higher 5-year actuarial local control rate (68% vs. 50%) and colostomy-free survival rate (72% vs. 40%). The overall survival rate was not significantly different (57% vs. 52%). Patients receiving combined modality therapy had a higher incidence of ulceration.

Although neither of the randomized trials revealed a significant advantage in overall survival with combined modality therapy, given the advantage in local control and colostomy-free survival, they helped to establish combined modality therapy as the standard of care in squamous cell cancers of the anal canal.

The Intergroup trial has established that mitomycin C is an important component of combined modality therapy.[88] A total of 291 patients (47% with T3 disease and 17% with positive nodes) were randomized to 45 Gy plus continuous infusion 5-FU with or without mitomycin C. At 6 weeks after the completion of treatment, patients with less than a complete response had an additional 9 Gy to the primary tumor plus concurrent 5-FU and cisplatin. If there was still less than a complete response 6 weeks after the completion of this salvage therapy, an APR was performed. Patients who received mitomycin C had a higher complete response rate (92% vs. 85%) and a significantly lower colostomy rate (9% vs. 22%) and a corresponding significant increase in colostomy-free survival (71% vs. 59%). There was little difference in overall 4-year survival (75% vs. 70%). Early grade 4+ toxicity was significantly increased in the mitomycin C arm (23% vs. 7%). Although overall survival was not significantly increased given the advantage in colostomy-free survival, mitomycin C is considered a necessary component of combined modality therapy.

The combined modality therapy arm using radiation, 5-FU, and mitomycin C from the Intergroup trial is the most common treatment approach in the United States. Details are seen in Table 33.9-5. Patients received continuous course pelvic radiation to a total dose of 45 Gy (30 Gy to the whole pelvis followed by 15 Gy to the true pelvis) and two cycles (weeks 1 and 5) of concurrent continuous infusion 5-FU (1000 mg/m^2 days 1 through 4) and bolus mitomycin C (10 mg/m^2 bolus day 1). If 6 weeks following completion of the initial treatment there was persistent disease, patients received 1 week of salvage therapy. Salvage therapy involved one cycle of chemotherapy (continuous infusion 5-FU, 1000 mg/m^2/d 1–4; bolus cisplatin, 100 mg/m^2 day 2) and concurrent 900 cGy (limited to the primary tumor). If there was residual disease on biopsy 6 weeks after the salvage therapy, then an APR was recommended.

There is considerable controversy as to the need for the first biopsy at 6 weeks after initial treatment. Data from the Princess Margaret Hospital suggest that squamous cell cancers of the anus regress slowly and continue to decrease in size for 3 to 12 months after the completion of combined modality treatment.[92] Based on these data, an increasing number of investigators advocate a more conservative approach and do not recommend a posttreatment biopsy. In the Intergroup trial, of the 25 patients with biopsy residual disease after 45 Gy and 5-FU and mitomycin C who then received salvage therapy with 9 Gy plus 5-FU and cisplatin, 55% achieved a complete response 6 weeks later (a total of 12 weeks after the completion of the initial 45 Gy).[88] It is unclear if the complete response was a result of the salvage therapy or was due to an additional 6 weeks of tumor regression after initial therapy.

At the Princess Margaret Hospital, Memorial Sloan-Kettering, and other centers, if there is residual disease at the 6-week posttreatment evaluation patients do not receive the 1 week of salvage therapy. The patients are examined every 6 weeks, and providing the tumor continues to decrease in size, no salvage therapy is performed. If there is progression of disease or no response at 6 weeks after initial therapy, however, APR is necessary. In addition to careful physical examination, anal ultrasound may be helpful in following the tumor. In the current Intergroup phase III anal canal cancer protocol (RTOG 98-11) (Fig. 33.9-2), biopsy at 6 weeks after the initial 45 Gy is optional.

There are a subset of patients who, for a variety of reasons, undergo an excisional biopsy, such as a hemorrhoidectomy, polypectomy, or local excision, first and then are referred for definitive combined modality therapy. Because the margins may be either negative or at most microscopically positive, is full-dose radiation (45 Gy) necessary? Hu and colleagues treated eight patients after excision biopsy with 30 to 34 Gy plus 5-FU and mitomycin C.[82] With a median follow-up of 81 months, the

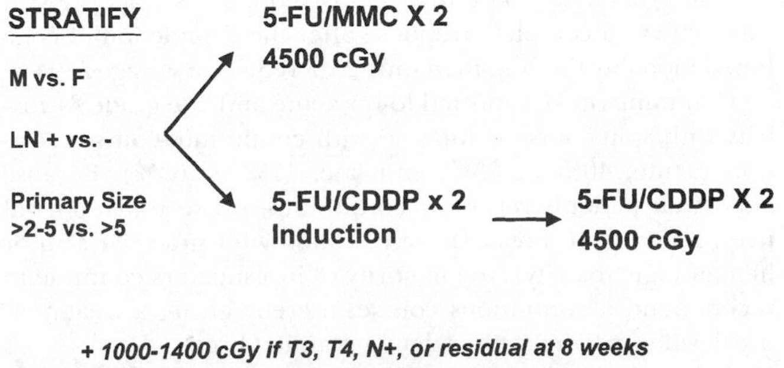

FIGURE 33.9-2. Intergroup phase III anal canal cancer protocol (RTOG 98-11). CDDP, cisplatinum; 5-FU, 5-fluorouracil; LN + and –, lymph node positive and negative; MMC, mitomycin C.

5-year actuarial local control rate was 100% and the overall survival was 88%. Although the data are limited, they do suggest that combined modality therapy with 30 Gy as opposed to 45 Gy may be an adequate dose in this select group of patients.

There are a number of phase II trials of combined modality therapy with external-beam pelvic radiation plus concurrent chemotherapy. The treatment design usually involves the use of one or two cycles of 5-FU by continuous 24-hour infusion (750 to 1000 mg/m^2) for 4 to 5 days plus a bolus dose of mitomycin C (10 to 15 mg/m^2) given on day 1 or 2 of each cycle. If given, the second chemotherapy cycle usually begins on day 28. In those trials using cisplatin, it is substituted for mitomycin C at a bolus dose of 75 mg/m^2. The group from Humbolt University in Berlin has added regional hyperthermia to combined modality therapy.[125] However, this approach remains investigational.

Combined modality therapy can be delivered concurrently or sequentially. In the concurrent regimen, radiation therapy and chemotherapy are initiated on the same day. In the sequential regimen, chemotherapy is given before the start of radiation therapy. Since the report from Miller et al. that reported a complete response rate of only 45% with sequential 5-FU, mitomycin C, and 30 Gy, almost all combined modality therapy trials have used concurrent chemotherapy plus radiation.[126] Although concurrent therapy is favored because the need for salvage APR appears lower, there are no randomized comparison trials. For certain subgroups of high-risk patients (e.g., large T4 tumors), induction chemotherapy followed by concurrent chemotherapy and radiation to higher doses may prove to be a useful option. This is currently being tested in a single-arm Cancer and Leukemia Group B trial for advanced anal canal tumors.[127] Combined modality therapy trials can be broadly divided into those that use either 5-FU and mitomycin C chemotherapy or, more recently, 5-FU and cisplatin chemotherapy.

Mitomycin C versus Cisplatin. Mitomycin C–based trials are shown in Table 33.9-3. When comparing the results, it is important to consider the percentage of patients with T3 disease, node-positive disease, or both. With the exception of the series by Miller et al., which used sequential chemotherapy, the mean (average) results include a complete response rate of 84% (81% to 87%), a local control rate of 73% (64% to 86%), and a 5-year survival rate of 77% (66% to 92%). These results are comparable with the 5-FU and mitomycin C–containing combined modality arms of the three randomized trials seen in Table 33.9-5. For patients with T1 and T2 disease, the complete response rates are in excess of 90%, with ultimate local control rates after surgical salvage of 80% to 90%. In patients with T3 and T4 disease, approximately 50% of patients require a salvage APR. If they achieve a complete response after the completion of combined modality therapy, then only 25% require a salvage APR.

Cummings et al. reported lower acute and late grade 3+ toxicity with split-course compared with continuous-course radiation (acute, 40% vs. 75%, and late, 17% vs. 63%). Because almost all patients receiving continuous-course radiation will need a treatment break (most commonly for grade 3+ skin or hematologic toxicity), the majority of investigators continue to recommend a continuous course, thereby giving a treatment break when needed rather than a planned break.

Although the results of 5-FU, mitomycin C, and concurrent 45 Gy are impressive, there is room for improvement, especially in patients with T3 and T4 disease. A variety of treatment approaches have been tested. These include the use of 5-FU and cisplatin (as induction therapy or concurrently with radiation) and intensifying the radiation dose beyond 45 Gy using external-beam or brachytherapy. The combination of 5-FU plus cisplatin is an attractive regimen because (1) patients who have failed 5-FU and mitomycin C still respond to 5-FU and cisplatin and (2) cisplatin is an active radiation sensitizer.

Selected trials using cisplatin-based therapy are seen in Table 33.9-4. Most also use higher radiation doses compared with the mitomycin C–based trials seen in Table 33.9-3. Although the numbers are small, with the exception of a similar average complete response rate (85%; range, 80% to 96%), the data suggest that the average rates of local control (87%; range, 80% to 94%), colostomy-free survival (71%; range, 56% to 86%), and overall 5-year survival (89%; range, 84% to 94%) may be higher than the mitomycin C–based regimens. It must be emphasized, however, that these differences may be due to other factors such as patient selection bias and higher radiation doses.

The Cancer and Leukemia Group B pilot trial reported by Meropol et al. was limited to patients with T3 and T4 disease. With induction 5-FU and cisplatin and concurrent 5-FU and cisplatin plus radiation, the complete response rate was 80%, colostomy-free survival was 56%, and crude survival was 78%.[127] The Intergroup has developed a randomized trial (RTOG 98-11) to compare this approach with conventional 5-FU, mitomycin C, and 45 Gy (see Fig. 33.9-2).

Intensification of the Radiation Dose: External Beam. Retrospective data from the Massachusetts General Hospital,[98] M. D. Anderson Hospital,[128] and others suggest improved local control with increased radiation dose. In an attempt to improve local control and survival, two parallel pilot trials of radiation-dose intensification were designed. In both trials, patients received 36 Gy to the pelvis (30.6 to the whole pelvis plus 5.4 Gy to the true pelvis), and, after a 2-week break, received an additional 23.4 Gy to the primary tumor with a 2- to 3-cm margin for a total dose of 59.4 Gy. The main differences between the two trials was the type of chemotherapy. The RTOG 92-08 trial[129] (see Table 33.9-3) used concurrent 5-FU and mitomycin C, whereas the ECOG 4292 trial[130] (see Table 33.9-4) used 5-FU and cisplatin.

The RTOG 92-08 trial included 47 patients, 49% with T3 and T4 and 89% with node-positive disease.[129] With a median follow-up of 21 months, the local failure rate was 19%, 4-year colostomy-free survival was 71%, and overall survival was 73%. Although the incidence of grade 3 to 4 toxicity (26%) was similar to a standard regimen of 45 Gy plus 5-FU and mitomycin C used in RTOG 89-04, the 2-year colostomy rate was higher (30% vs. 7%). The reason for the increase is unclear. The investigators postulate that it may be related to the higher percentage of patients requiring a treatment break of longer than 2 weeks (96% vs. 12%). The ECOG 4292 trial entered 19 patients and reported a 68% complete response rate 8 weeks after the completion of 59.4 Gy and a 79% grade 3+ toxicity rate.[130] In contrast, Pieffert et al.[131] and Gerard and colleagues[86] treated patients with similar doses (the boost given with either external-beam or brachytherapy) and reported higher complete response rates (96% and 89%, respectively).

Intensification of the Radiation Dose: Brachytherapy. Brachytherapy is an ideal method by which to deliver conformal radiation for anal cancer while sparing the surrounding normal structures such as small intestine and bladder. Much of the initial experience with brachytherapy in anal cancer was from investigators in England and France who used radium needles.[132] Due to radiation protection concerns and a high anal necrosis rate, afterloading ^{192}Ir catheters have replaced radium needles. However, it is not clear that ^{192}Ir has a lower rate of complications.

Selected series that use brachytherapy as a component of treatment of anal cancer are shown in Table 33.9-6. In most series, patients received 30 to 55 Gy of pelvic radiation with or without 5-FU and mitomycin C or cisplatin followed by a 15- to 25-Gy boost with ^{192}Ir afterloading catheters. Most use low dose-rate; however, some investigators have advocated high dose-rate.[133,134] There are biologic differences between low dose- and high dose-rate brachytherapy; however, at the present time there does not appear to be a difference in efficacy.

Combining the series, the mean results include a complete response rate of 83% (73% to 91%), local control rates of 81% (73% to 89%), and a 5-year survival rate of 70% (60% to 84%). The average complete response and local control rates appear similar to those achieved with external-beam–based combined modality therapy. Furthermore, the 5-year survival rates appear lower. Of equal concern is the increased incidence of anal necrosis. Reports of anal necrosis rates include those of Papillon et al. (2%),[84] Gerard et al. (15%),[86] Peiffert et al. (25%),[85] and Roed et al. (76%).[134] The incidence of severe complications included those of Sandhu et al. (8%),[135] Wagner et al. (9%),[136] and Allal et al. (12%).[137]

A new technique of ultrasound-guided three-dimensional tumor reconstruction and brachytherapy has been reported by Lohnert and colleagues.[138] In patients receiving more than 4-Gy fractions, the incidence of severe complications was 63%; however, none were seen when the dose was limited to less than 4-Gy fractions.

In summary, it is unclear if increasing the radiation dose in patients receiving combined modality therapy improves the results compared with conventional doses of 45 to 50 Gy. Although there are no randomized data, the phase II trials suggest that even in experienced hands, brachytherapy is associated with higher complication rates than external-beam therapy.

The ideal combined modality therapy regimen and the most appropriate radiation dose to use for patients with anal canal tumors limited to the primary site have not yet been defined. At the present time in the United States, combined modality therapy with the RTOG combined modality therapy regimen of continuous-course radiation (45 Gy in 1.8-Gy fractions) plus two cycles of concurrent continuous infusion 5-FU on weeks 1 and 5, plus mitomycin C bolus on days 1 and 29, remains the standard of care. This is the control arm of RTOG 98-11 seen in Figure 33.9-2. For patients with T3 and T4 disease (primary tumors larger than 5 cm) it is reasonable to boost with an additional 5.4 to 9.0 Gy. In RTOG 98-11 the experimental arm uses the same design except it adds two cycles of induction 5-FU and cisplatin as well as 5-FU and cisplatinum (CDDP) during the radiation. The posttreatment biopsy at 8 weeks is now optional.

Radical Surgery. With the advent of multimodality therapy for the primary treatment of patients with anal canal tumors, the role of surgery is important mostly from an historic perspective. Because of the high propensity of anal canal tumors to recur locally, a wide perineal resection was initially proposed for treatment.[64,74,139,140] If necessary, gluteal or perineal flaps were raised to cover the residual defect.[139] Some authors advocated the resection of the posterior vaginal wall to obtain clear surgical margins,[30,64,66,69] whereas others thought this to be unnecessary unless the rectovaginal septum was involved.[43] Bilateral inguinal lymph node dissection was performed in patients undergoing radical surgical resection of their primary tumor[47,63,64,71,141,142] until it was shown that prophylactic inguinal lymph node dissections were beneficial in only 6% of patients.[34] The high morbidity with little gain led others to quickly condemn the use of this procedure.[34,37,64,65,69] Combined modality therapy controls more than 90% of inguinal nodal disease.[92,143]

Recurrence develops in up to 40% of patients having an APR for primary treatment of anal canal tumors.[45,63,66,70] The median time to recurrence is 12 to 15 months. Local recurrence is the rule, with the majority in the pelvis and the remainder in the inguinal or pelvic nodes.[45,69,70,126] Distant metastases are less common but can be seen in up to 31% of patients. Greenall and colleagues observed a median survival of 10 months for patients with pelvic recurrence and 7 months with visceral metastases.[70]

Overall survival did not improve dramatically after the advent of radical surgery. Five-year survival rates after APR for primary treatment range from 55% to 71%.[37,45,64,70,75,108,110,112,117] Survival was adversely affected by the size of the primary tumor. In patients treated at Memorial Sloan-Kettering Cancer Center, 60% of patients with tumors smaller than 5 cm were alive at 5 years, whereas only 40% of those with tumors larger than 5 cm were alive at 5 years.[70] Miller et al. improved overall survival from 55% in historic controls to 82% for patients treated with a preoperative combined modality therapy regimen.[126] Of equal significance was the preservation of anal function in the majority of patients treated with combined modality therapy.

Radiation Therapy Alone. There is a subset of patients who have been treated with radiation therapy alone. Because both the UKCCCR[107] and EORTC[89] randomized trials have shown a significant advantage to the combined modality arm for local control (UKCCCR) and local control and colostomy-free survival (EORTC), combined modality therapy is standard of care. However, external irradiation alone is a reasonable alternative for patients who cannot tolerate chemotherapy due to medical contraindications.

Age alone is not a contraindication to combined modality therapy. Although some elderly patients may not tolerate chemotherapy well, less aggressive treatment in patients older than 65 years old appeared to jeopardize their outcome in a Canadian retrospective study.[144] Studies of combined modality therapy in patients 75 years old or older have been reported from both Valentini and colleagues[145] and Allal et al.[146] Rates of complete response, local control, and acute and long-term toxicity were similar to those reported for the general population. Although some chemotherapy dose attenuation and radiation field modifications may be needed, combined modality therapy in selected patients 75 years old and older should be considered.

Radiation Alone: External Beam. The results of major studies using external-beam radiation alone are seen in Table 33.9-8. The mean results include a local control rate of 74% (61% to 100%) and a 5-year survival rate of 63% (50% to 94%). Although the series of 18 patients from Martenson and Gun-

TABLE 33.9-8. Radiation Therapy Alone: Selected Series

Series	*Number*	*Dose (Gy)*	*Stage*	*Percentage 5-Y Survival*	*Percentage Local Control*	*Percentage Complications Requiring Surgery*
Eschwege,[213] 1985	64	60–65	—	50	81	14
Doggett,[214] 1988	39	65	—	79	80	10
Schlienger,[96] 1989	193	55–65	—	—	66	10
Cummings,[92] 1991	57	45–60	—	68 (cancer specific)	56	8
Dubois,[149] 1991	28	60–65	T1	86	71	—
			T2	92	67	—
			T3	75	57	—
			Total	85	61	4
Touboul,[143] 1994	270[a]	55–65	—	76 (cancer specific)	71	10
Martenson,[147] 1993	18	45–67	—	94	100	17
Newman,[215] 1992	72	50	T1	—	89	3
			T2	—	79	—
			T3	—	75	—
			T4	—	50	—
			Total	66	76	—

[a]Fourteen patients had brachytherapy and five received chemotherapy.

derson from the Mayo Clinic had the highest survival and local control rate, they also had a high rate of complications requiring surgery (17%).[147] In most series, local control and survival decrease with increasing T stage. Overall, these results are comparable with those of patients who receive combined modality therapy with 45 Gy plus 5-FU and mitomycin C. However, the mean incidence of complications requiring surgery is 10% (range, 3% to 17%), which probably reflects the high radiation doses that must be delivered to the primary site to control this disease if radiation therapy is the sole treatment modality. Therefore, unless there is a compelling reason to avoid systemic chemotherapy in an individual patient, combined modality therapy should remain the standard of care.

Radiation Alone: Brachytherapy with or without External Beam. Brachytherapy (interstitial radiation) alone has the potential of curing only early lesions that are unlikely to have spread to the lymph nodes. Historically, radium needles have been used, although interstitial implants with ^{192}Ir are most common in modern series. Radium needles have been used for many years at the Christie Hospital in Manchester, England, for early anal cancers.[118,121] Radium needles were the exclusive treatment modality in 74 patients, 43 with anal canal lesions and 31 with anal margin lesions.[121] Of the 68 evaluable patients with minimum follow-up of 5 years, there were 35 locoregional failures, of which only seven were salvaged by surgery. Local control was achieved in only 64% of tumors smaller than 5 cm in diameter and in only 23% of tumors larger than 5 cm.

Radium needle implantation has also been used extensively by Papillon, but he has abandoned this technique because of painful local reactions and inability to achieve lymph node control because of the small target volume.[84,119] Early studies with radium needles yielded a severe necrosis rate of approximately 25%.[148]

Several studies with small numbers of patients have been reported in which external-beam radiation is combined with brachytherapy (^{137}Cs, ^{192}Ir, or radium needles).[72,120,132,149–151] Good local control was achieved, but there was a relatively high rate of complications requiring surgery or leading to death.

The largest experience is from the Centre Leon Berard in which 221 patients with anal carcinoma were treated over a 15-year period with external-beam radiation therapy (^{60}Co) to a dose of 35 Gy, followed 2 months later by an additional 15 to 20 Gy with ^{192}Ir implant.[84,132] The investigators reported only a 3% rate of serious complications and achieved a 65% 5-year disease-free survival and a 79% locoregional control rate. Combined brachytherapy and external irradiation may be useful in treating extensive lesions.[152–154]

Another study from France confirmed a high 5-year survival rate (61%) and good local control (75%), but a 6% rate of complications requiring surgery.[151] The importance of treating the inguinal nodes prophylactically was illustrated in this study. In 28 N0 patients, two had an inguinal recurrence, neither of whom had received inguinal irradiation. Both developed distant metastases and died of disease.

In summary, radiation therapy alone with either external-beam or combined with brachytherapy may yield comparable local control and survival rates with combined modality therapy. However, it is associated with increased complication rates. In contrast to combined modality therapy in which the complications are commonly acute (i.e., diarrhea, hematologic, skin, and nadir fever), the complications with radiation therapy alone usually involve anal necrosis requiring surgery. As seen in Table 33.9-6, similar toxicity has been reported in patients receiving combined modality therapy plus brachytherapy. Even in experienced hands, brachytherapy is associated with a moderate degree of anal necrosis and should be used with caution.

RADIATION THERAPY TREATMENT TECHNIQUES

A comprehensive discussion of techniques to decrease the toxicity of pelvic radiation, such as physical maneuvers, immobilization molds, dietary supplements and radioprotectors, three-dimensional treatment planning, and other investigational approaches, is presented in Chapter 33.8 and is not discussed

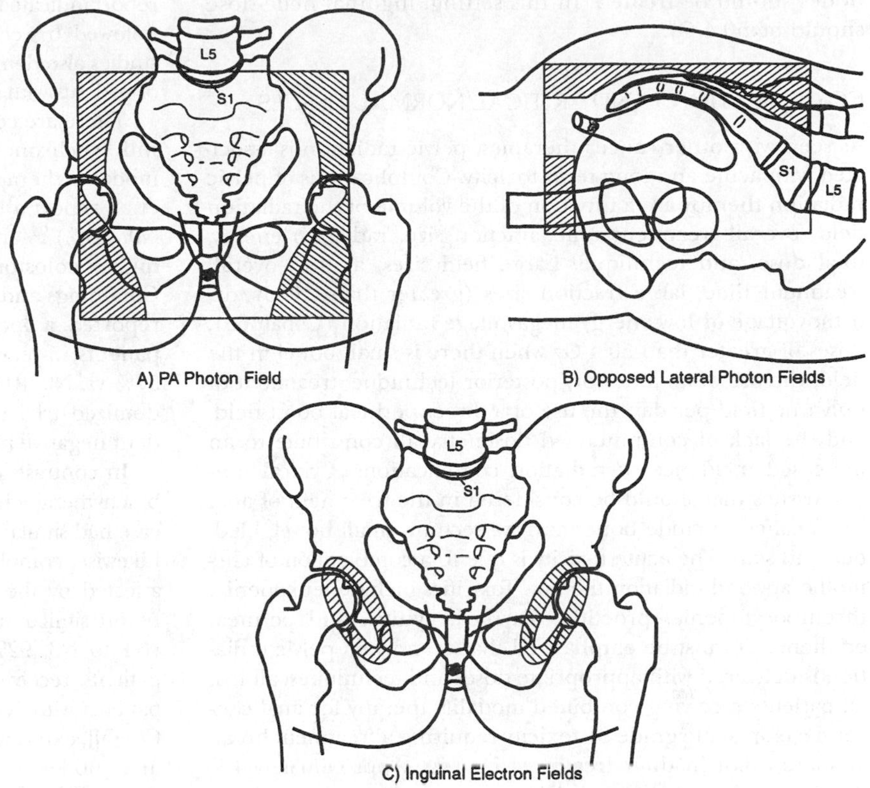

FIGURE 33.9-3. Idealized treatment fields for a clinical T2N0M0 squamous cell carcinoma of the anal canal. The inguinal nodes are included in the posteroanterior (PA) field and are supplemented with electrons.

here. However, there are some general principles specific to the design and delivery of radiation for anal cancer that are presented in this chapter. Last, a caveat: Technique recommendations should be interpreted with caution. Radiation oncology, as with other medical specialties, is both an art and a science. Therefore, the recommendations made in this chapter should serve as a guide rather than a *cookbook*.

The design of pelvic radiation therapy fields for anal cancer is based on knowledge of the natural history of the disease and the primary nodal drainage. Because the internal iliac and presacral nodes are posterior in reference to the external iliac nodes, many of the normal structures in the anterior pelvis can be spared with the use of lateral fields. As this approach underdoses the inguinal nodes, they should be supplemented with electrons. Examples of field arrangements are seen in Figure 33.9-3.

PELVIC FIELD

A prone three-field technique (posterior plus opposed laterals) is recommended. This arrangement results in the lowest dose to the anterior structures such as the genitalia and bladder. The underdosed inguinal nodes are then treated concurrently with electrons to bring the dose up to 100% of the prescription dose. An alternative method is to use an anterior/posterior technique. Although this technique treats the pelvic and inguinal nodes in the same field, it results in the highest dose to the anterior pelvic structures and skin, thereby increasing toxicity. An electron boost for the perineum is not recommended as there will be overlap between the electron and photon fields. The portion of the perineum that needs to be treated should be included in the photon fields. The whole pelvis receives 30.6 Gy followed by a 14.4-Gy cone down to the true pelvis for a total dose of 45 Gy.

PRIMARY TUMOR BOOST FIELD FOR COMBINED MODALITY THERAPY SALVAGE AT 6 WEEKS

If the RTOG recommendations for combined modality therapy salvage are followed, then an additional 9 Gy (concurrent with 5-FU and cisplatin) are delivered. Using opposed laterals, the field includes the primary tumor plus a 2- to 3-cm margin in all directions. As an alternative, patients with T3 tumors can receive an additional 5.4 Gy to the primary tumor plus a 2- to 3-cm margin to a total dose of 50.4 Gy, which is delivered immediately after the 45 Gy of pelvic radiation.

MEDIAL AND LATERAL INGUINAL LYMPH NODES

After treatment of the pelvis in the prone position, the patient is treated in the supine position with electrons for inguinal nodes. The medial and lateral inguinal nodes are outlined with a 2-cm margin in all directions. The inguinal nodes are included in the posterior pelvic photon field. They receive only exit dose from this field, usually approximately 30% to 40% of the pelvic field prescription. This is determined from the treatment plan. Because they need to receive a total of 1.8 Gy/d, the remaining dose should be given concurrently with electrons. The depth of the inguinal nodes can be determined from a computed tomographic scan.[155,156] If this is not available, then a clinical estimate may be used. If the inguinal lymph nodes are positive by biopsy, a four-field technique (anterior/posterior plus opposed laterals) is recommended as the external iliac nodes should be treated. In this setting, inguinal node dose should be 50.4 Gy.

COMPLICATIONS AND CRITICAL NORMAL TISSUES

As seen with other cancer therapies, pelvic radiation is associated with acute and long-term toxicity. Complications of pelvic radiation therapy are a function of the volume of the radiation field, overall treatment time, fraction size, radiation energy, total dose, and technique. Large field sizes, a short overall treatment time, large fraction sizes (greater than 2.0 Gy/d), orthovoltage or low-energy megavoltage radiation (Cobalt 60), doses of greater than 50.4 Gy when there is small bowel in the field, the use of an anterior/posterior technique, treatment of only one field per day, the use of a direct perineal boost field, and the lack of computerized dosimetry all contribute to an increased incidence of radiation complications. Critical normal tissues that should be considered in the treatment of anal canal cancer include bone marrow, rectum, small bowel, bladder, and skin. The acute toxicity is due to a combination of chemotherapy and radiation therapy. Toxicities include leukopenia, thrombocytopenia, proctitis, diarrhea, cystitis, and perineal erythema. It must be emphasized that even when pelvic radiation is delivered with appropriate doses and techniques, almost all patients receiving combined modality therapy for anal cancer develop acute grade 3+ toxicity requiring a treatment break at some point in their treatment courses. Approximately 1% develop long-term severe toxicity.

Unless there is a contraindication, the most simple techniques to decrease radiation toxicity, such as the use of small bowel contrast, multiple field techniques, high-energy linear accelerators, custom blocks, avoiding a direct perineal boost, and treatment in the prone position, should be part of the standard treatment of patients receiving curative pelvic radiation therapy. Any physical maneuver beyond the use of the prone position, such as a belly board, abdominal wall compression, or a full bladder, may be associated with patient discomfort, thereby leading to increased movement and daily setup errors.

Radiation therapy can affect sphincter function. There is an increasing body of literature reporting the effect of radiation therapy on functional results in rectal cancer.[157] However, it is not directly applicable to anal cancer as patients do not undergo pelvic surgery. There are limited reports of functional outcome in the anal cancer literature. One series reports that full function was maintained in 93% of patients,[158] and a second series that used anorectal manometry reported complete continence in 56%.[159] Both series used brachytherapy as a component of therapy. It is hoped that new trials will include a functional analysis.

INGUINAL NODE INVOLVEMENT

When examining the effect of positive lymph nodes on local control and survival, it is important to differentiate the site of nodal disease as well as synchronous versus metachronous nodal disease. Most series do not separate N1 versus N2 versus N3 disease. However, there are data examining synchronous versus metachronous nodal disease.

Early experience from the 1950s from Stearns et al. suggested that patients with grossly positive inguinal lymph nodes synchronous with the primary tumor were incurable.[47] A subsequent report indicated that 2 of 13 patients survived 5 years after an APR followed 6 weeks later by inguinal lymphadenectomy.[76] Older studies also demonstrated a small cure rate for surgical treatment of patients with synchronous unilateral inguinal nodes.[37,65]

There are conflicting reports as to the prognosis of patients with synchronous nodal disease who are treated with combined modality therapy. Compared with node-negative patients, Allal et al. report a higher rate of local failure (N1 to N3, 36%, vs. N0, 19%),[94] and the Intergroup randomized trial reports a higher colostomy rate (N1, 28%, vs. N0, 13%).[85] Although Cummings and associates from the Princess Margaret Hospital reported a local failure rate of only 13% in node-positive patients, 5-year cause-specific survival was lower (N1 to N3, 57% vs. N0, 81%).[92] By multivariate analysis, the EORTC randomized trial reported that positive nodes were an independent negative prognostic factor for local failure and survival.[89]

In contrast, in the series of combined modality therapy plus brachytherapy from Gerard et al., patients with N1 versus N0 disease had similar 5-year disease-specific and overall survival rates.[86] Likewise, complete response rates in the primary tumor are not affected by the presence of nodal disease. Doci and associates report similar rates in patients receiving cisplatin-based therapy (N1 to N3, 92%, vs. N0, 100%)[87] and in a separate series of patients receiving mitomycin C–based therapy, eight of eight patients with N1 to N3 disease achieved a complete response.[93] Overall, external-beam radiation alone[90,96,119,151] can control positive nodes in 65% of patients, and combined modality therapy[88–90,107] can achieve nodal control in approximately 90% of patients.

The current treatment recommendations for patients with positive inguinal nodes include biopsy followed by combined modality therapy with a boost of 45.0 to 50.4 Gy to the involved groin. Because the external iliac nodes should be treated in the pelvic radiation field, a four-field technique is recommended. Inguinal node dissection should not be performed as part of the initial therapy; however, it may be done for isolated inguinal recurrence.

The development of unilateral metachronous inguinal lymph nodes does not carry such an ominous prognosis. After therapeutic groin dissection, the 5- to 7-year survival rates exceeded 50% in two series,[68,114] but it was 0% in a small series reported from the Mayo Clinic.[37] Current strategies in patients with metachronous isolated inguinal node metastases after combined modality therapy include a formal groin dissection followed by chemotherapy. The use of radiation under these circumstances depends on prior dose and fields.

RESIDUAL OR RECURRENT CANCER

ANAL MARGIN

Locally recurrent anal margin cancers are more successfully controlled by local excision than are recurrences of anal canal cancer.[105,160] The largest reported series of recurrent tumors included 16 of 48 patients who, after a local excision, had local recurrences (11), in the inguinal nodes (4), or both (1).[114] There were no visceral failures. The median time to recurrence was 26 months. Ten of the patients with local recurrences underwent repeat local excision, and only one required an APR. Nine of these patients survived longer than 5 years. All four patients with inguinal node recurrences had inguinal lymphadenectomies, and two were long-term survivors. Although there is little reported experience with radiation therapy or combined modality therapy for patients with local recurrence after a local excision, it is a reasonable for those who would otherwise require an APR.

ANAL CANAL

After primary treatment of anal canal tumors with combined modality therapy, patients should be evaluated for response to therapy. This is usually done 4 to 6 weeks after the completion of therapy, but Nigro[161] recommended waiting for 8 weeks and Cummings et al. recommended at least 8 to 12 weeks.[92] Depending on the initial T stage and how soon the biopsy is performed after the completion of combined modality therapy, persistent disease is found in 10% to 25% of patients.[161–164]

Controversy exists concerning the appropriate definition and management of patients with residual disease after combined modality therapy. Whether one waits 6 or 30 weeks after the completion of therapy, if the tumor continues to decrease in size, it has been hypothesized that the cancer is in the process of responding to the therapy and therefore is not a *treatment failure.*[92] Selected patients with microscopic foci of tumor may undergo local excision of persistent disease. Therefore, patients who undergo salvage APR or further combined modality therapy within 8 weeks after the completion of initial therapy may be treated unnecessarily. Patients with progressive residual microscopic or gross disease are candidates for either an APR or additional combined modality therapy. There are no randomized trials to suggest which of these two alternatives are superior. APR is the most frequently reported salvage therapy, with 5-year survival rates of 30% to 58%. However, there are also reports of successful long-term salvage with combined modality therapy.[88,165] Because there is a maximum radiation dose that pelvic structures can safely tolerate, the decision to give additional radiation depends on careful review of the radiation fields and dosimetry.

A retrospective, nonrandomized study of patients from all of the Veterans Administration hospitals suggested that salvage surgery was superior to salvage with chemotherapy either with or without radiation therapy, with a 53% salvage rate with surgery compared with only 19% for the conservative attempts.[166] Nigro and others recommend a second course of combined modality therapy for patients with macroscopic disease, and several have been salvaged with this therapy.[161] If local failure occurs after a second course of combined modality therapy and there is no evidence of extrapelvic disease, then an APR should be done.

In the RTOG randomized study, discussed in the section Combined Modality Therapy, biopsy was performed on most patients after their initial therapy.[88] For those with positive biopsy results, salvage chemotherapy using cisplatin and 5-FU and localized boost radiation were given. Of the 27 patients who received this salvage regimen, 24 underwent biopsy after its completion. Of these, 12 (50%) had a negative biopsy result, and five of these had no further surgery after a minimum of 3 years of follow-up. This indicates that at least some patients can have sphincter-sparing treatment despite failure to achieve a complete remission with first-line therapy.

In a French study, local failure after radiation therapy alone occurred in 50 patients of whom 26 subsequently underwent salvage APR.[143] Local tumor control was obtained in 12 of 26 patients (46%), and the 5-year survival was 56%. Similar local control rates and overall survival were found in 24 patients treated with APR after failure with combined modality therapy at Memorial Sloan-Kettering Cancer Center.[91] Others have not had such good results with salvage APR.[167]

The literature is confusing as investigators have used varying definitions of persistent and recurrent disease. Two series from France used different definitions of persistent versus recurrent disease and reported conflicting results.[168,169] When *persistent disease* was defined as a recurrence up to 6 months after combined modality therapy, surgical salvage with APR improved survival.[168] In contrast, when *recurrent disease* was defined as any recurrence after a clinical complete response, regardless of the disease-free interval, patients with recurrent disease had survival rates superior to those with persistent disease.[169] In this series, of the 27 patients who underwent salvage surgery for local failure after combined modality therapy, only 44% died of disease.[169]

It must be emphasized that patients should be followed closely by digital rectal examination and anoscopy (every 6 to 12 weeks) until a complete clinical response is documented. Any local progression of disease should be defined and treated as early as possible.

METASTATIC DISEASE

Because primary combined modality therapy has been so effective, the number of patients with this uncommon malignancy who developed advanced metastatic disease is small. Perhaps as a result, the number of chemotherapeutic agents that have been tested in patients with advanced anal canal cancer is small and the reports are anecdotal.

Single-agent trials of doxorubicin (Adriamycin) and of cisplatin have been reported by several investigators. Fischer and colleagues reported a response to both doxorubicin as a single agent and cisplatin at a dosage of 2 mg/kg in an elderly man with advanced disease.[170] Salem and coworkers studied cisplatin as a single agent in three patients: One achieved a complete response and the other two had partial responses.[171] Earlier trials with 5-FU and vinblastine in small groups of patients were ineffective. Bleomycin and vincristine were used by Livingston and colleagues in a single patient, and a partial regression was observed.[172] Combination chemotherapy with cisplatin and 5-FU in patients with advanced disease has now been reported in small groups of patients. Responses have been reported using both systemic and regional (hepatic-arterial) routes. Of a total of six patients described in three reports, three complete and three partial responses were noted.[173–175] In a study from France using this combination and involving seven patients with local recurrence alone and 13 patients with metastasis, there were two complete and nine partial responses.[176] In one study, three of eight patients achieved a complete clinical response with cisplatin and fluorouracil, of whom two were 5-year survivors.[177]

A noncisplatin regimen was used by Wilking and colleagues.[178a] A total of 15 patients with advanced disease received bleomycin, vincristine, and high-dose methotrexate. Major objective regressions were seen in 3 of 12 patients with measurable tumors, but their duration of response was only 1 to 5 months. Toxicity was severe, with four patients having probable treatment-related deaths. McGill and Quan treated 24 patients using cisplatin, bleomycin, and alkaloid. Six of 21 evaluable patients (29%) responded.[179] Carboplatin has also been reported to have activity in this disease.[178]

Although response rates in patients with metastatic disease are difficult to evaluate in view of the paucity of data, the use of neoadjuvant (induction) therapy has allowed an assessment of the effectiveness of chemotherapy alone without the confounding variable of concurrent radiation in larger groups of patients. Most more recent regimens involve the use of a platinum compound with 5-FU. Peiffert et al. reported the preliminary results of a trial involving induction cisplatin plus 5-FU chemotherapy for two cycles followed by combined modality therapy. In a group of 28 evaluable patients, 72% had complete or partial responses from neoadjuvant chemotherapy alone. The regimen used was cisplatin, 80 mg/m^2 on day 1, followed by a 4-day continuous intravenous infusion of 5-FU at 800 mg/m^2. Other investigators have reported similar findings.

At the present time, therefore, cisplatin plus 5-FU–containing combinations appear to have a high degree of activity in patients with anal canal tumors whether used in metastatic disease or as part of induction therapy for advanced local regional disease. The high cure rate seen with primary combined modality therapy may slow the identification of newer agents. The use of agents with high degrees of activity in other squamous cell malignancies as part of a neoadjuvant approach may be a strategy to identify newer agents in this disease.[180]

FOLLOW-UP

Close observation of patients after treatment of anal cancer is essential, because patients with local failure are amenable to resection and may be salvaged with long-term survival. The majority of recurrences occur within the first 3 years, and patients should be examined by physical examination and anoscopy every 6 to 12 weeks until a complete response is achieved, then every 3 months for a total of 2 years. Follow-up examinations can then be decreased to every 6 months for the next 3 years and then yearly after 5 years. The usefulness of computed tomography of the abdomen and pelvis for follow-up is unclear. Transrectal ultrasound may be of value. It must be emphasized that because the most common site of failure is at the primary tumor site, there is no substitute for physical examination. In a limited series of 33 patients, Petrelli and colleagues report a 76% sensitivity, 86% specificity, and a 62% positive predictive value of squamous cell carcinoma tumor–associated antigen.[181]

ANORECTAL MELANOMA

Anorectal melanomas are relatively rare, accounting for less than 1% of all anal canal tumors. The patients present with nonspecific complaints, which are often attributed to benign anal conditions, and the correct diagnosis is seldom made accurately at the initial examination. This delay may be responsible for the advanced stage seen in most at diagnosis. The stage (tumor thickness and nodal status) at presentation is the primary determinant of survival, and distant metastasis is common.[182–187]

CLINICAL PRESENTATION AND PATHOLOGIC FEATURES

Anorectal melanomas are slightly more common in women, and the median age at presentation is in the sixth decade. Most patients present with bleeding as the initial complaint, which is often attributed to hemorrhoids. Symptoms are often present for 1 to 3 months before evaluation and also include pain, tenesmus, pruritus, change in bowel habits, and weight loss. An initial error in diagnosis has been reported in up to 80% of patients who subsequently were diagnosed with anorectal melanoma.[182,188] The most common physical finding is a mass felt on rectal examination or seen extruding from the anus. It may appear pigmented in only one-third of patients.[188] The tumors measure 3 to 5 cm in diameter in most cases and can be as large as 12 cm. Inguinal lymph nodes are frequently positive. The primary tumor may arise from the skin of the anal verge, mucocutaneous junction, transitional epithelium of the anal canal, or rectal mucosa, but is seldom found more than 5 cm from the dentate line. The diagnosis can also be made by finding an incidental melanoma in a hemorrhoid specimen. The morphologic characteristics of anorectal melanomas are the same as for cutaneous melanomas.

PATTERNS OF SPREAD

Anorectal melanomas spread locally by direct extension upward in the submucosal plane of the rectum, but they seldom invade bladder, vagina, sacrum, or prostate. Regional spread via the lymphatic channels is superiorly to the mesenteric system or laterally to the inguinal system. Inguinal nodes are present in 20% of patients, and mesenteric nodes are involved in up to 65% of patients undergoing radical surgery.[188–192] Hematogenous spread is found in up to 29% of patients at diagnosis[187,190,192] and overall in up to 69% of patients.[191] Distant metastasis is most common in the lungs, liver, and bone.

TREATMENT AND OUTCOME

The classic surgical approach for the treatment of anorectal melanoma was APR with pelvic lymph node dissection and bilateral groin dissection.[189] Because those with inguinal metastases uniformly died of disease, this part of the procedure is no longer performed.[189,193] Because of the high systemic failure rate, several authors have questioned the wisdom of radical surgery and have advocated wide local excision for treatment of this disease.[182,190,191,194] In the early reports from Memorial Sloan-Kettering Cancer Center,[189,195,196] the only long-term survivors were patients who had undergone an APR with or without lymphadenectomy. Similar results were found at the Mayo Clinic.[193] Siegel and colleagues[182] had two long-term survivors treated with local excision and chemotherapy, and the M. D. Anderson group[191] had one survivor at 5 years who was treated with wide local excision alone. Despite a better local control rate with APR, no series has shown a survival advantage for patients who have had an APR compared with patients having wide local excision.[182,183,190–192,197] However, none of these studies was randomized, thus lending potential bias in favor of local excision, which was usually performed for smaller lesions.

Several factors have been analyzed to determine their effect on outcome. Age and race are the only factors that have consistently been shown not to affect overall survival. Size was not an important factor in the results from the study by Quan et al.[189] but had a direct effect on survival in the study by Goldman and colleagues.[190] Tumor thickness is the most important factor in determining outcome for cutaneous melanomas. Wanebo and colleagues noted three survivors at 5 years; all had tumors less than 2 mm thick, and all were treated with an APR.[195] Of the patients with tumors larger than 2 mm, none lived 5 years, and 85% were dead by 2 years. Another study noted three long-term survivors who had anorectal melanoma discovered incidentally at the time of hemorrhoidectomy.[192] Of the 18 patients with mesenteric lymph node metastases, there was only one long-term survivor.[192] Female gender is associated with a better prognosis.

The inability of several authors to show a survival benefit for APR compared with wide local excision can be entirely attributed to the small numbers of patients involved in the studies, selection bias, and the lack of the scientific method. Any relative advantage of adjuvant immunotherapies, chemotherapy, and radiation therapy is similarly obscured and difficult to interpret. Treatment recommendations must therefore be less than absolute. A histologic margin of at least 3 mm should be obtained if local excision is to be used. In view of probably higher local control rates, APR can still be recommended.[183–186,190,191] There is a clear need for studies of sentinel node mapping and adjuvant therapies.[183,190,191]

ADENOCARCINOMA

Primary adenocarcinoma of the anal canal arising from the anal glands is a rare tumor. Most adenocarcinomas in the canal represent rectal cancer with downward spread. In general, they should be treated like adenocarcinomas of the rectum, including APR, and if T3 disease, node-positive disease, or both exist, six cycles of adjuvant combined modality therapy with 5-FU–based chemotherapy plus preoperative or postoperative concurrent radiation therapy are given. However, the radiation fields should include the inguinal nodes. Basik and colleagues treated ten patients with surgery and reported a median survival of 29 months.[198] Adenosquamous cancers of the anus are also rare and have an equally poor prognosis.[199] Given the squamous component, it is reasonable to treat these patients with combined 5-FU and mitomycin C and concurrent radiation therapy. If there is residual disease, this would be followed by a salvage APR.

SARCOMA

Leiomyosarcomas of the large intestine are unusual neoplasms, accounting for less than 0.1% of all malignancies of the colon and rectum. Few cases of leiomyosarcoma of the anus have been reported. The optimal treatment for this neoplasm is not known. The standard surgical approach is APR. Using a technique well established for management for sarcomas of the extremities, Minsky et al. have treated several patients using local excision and ^{192}Ir brachytherapy in an attempt to preserve the anal sphincter.[200–202] This technique may be an alternative to APR in selected patients.

TREATMENT OF THE HUMAN IMMUNODEFICIENCY VIRUS–POSITIVE PATIENT

Given the 40- to 80-fold increase of anal cancer in the HIV-positive population compared with the general population, HIV-positive patients have received lower doses of radiation and chemotherapy due to a concern that standard therapy may not be tolerated.[7] With a better understanding of the immunologic deficiencies seen in HIV-positive patients, more recent reports have recommended therapy based on clinical and immunologic parameters such as a history of prior opportunistic infections and CD4 counts.

Hoffman and associates treated 17 HIV-positive patients with a median of 51.8 Gy plus concurrent 5-FU and mitomycin C.[203] With a median follow-up of 17 months, the nine patients with CD4 counts greater than 200 μL were all without evidence of disease with acceptable toxicity. In contrast, of the eight patients with a CD4 count less than 200 μL, four had grade 4 toxicity and four required a colostomy for toxicity or local failure. Despite the increase in morbidity, the disease of seven (88%) was locally controlled after salvage surgery. They recommend treating HIV-positive patients with standard doses of combined modality therapy but minimizing the radiation fields in patients with CD4 counts less than 200 μL. Similar results were reported from Peddada et al., who treated eight HIV-positive patients with 30 Gy plus concurrent 5-FU and mitomycin C.[204] Of the four with a CD4 count less than 200 μL, three of four developed grade 4 toxicities, whereas one of the four with a CD4 count greater than 200 μL had grade 4 toxicity. However, all achieved a complete response. With a median follow-up of 38 months, four are alive without evidence of disease, and of the four who died of HIV-related complications, all had no evidence of anal cancer at the time of death. In another report, four HIV-positive patients without evidence of other HIV-related diseases received combined modality therapy.[205] Only one patient required a treatment break.

Management of the HIV-positive patient is complex and requires careful attention to all aspects of the patient's medical history, coexisting medical conditions, and personal wishes. The limited experience suggests that in patients with a CD4 count greater than 200 μL who do not have signs or symptoms of other HIV-related diseases, aggressive combined modality therapy is appropriate. They should be followed carefully, however, and frequent modifications during therapy will likely be necessary. For those patients with a CD4 count less than 200 μL or who have signs or symptoms of other HIV-related diseases, attenuated doses of radiation, chemotherapy, or both are recommended at the start of treatment.

FUTURE DIRECTIONS

PREVENTION AND EARLY DETECTION

Accumulating evidence has implicated HPV as a causative and perhaps necessary factor in the development of squamous cell carcinoma of the anus. Because this is the most common histology, anal cancer may represent a preventable disease as is the case for cervical carcinoma. Both in women and in men (particularly homosexual men) increasing use of measures for *safe sex*, initiated to stem the spread of AIDS, may also affect the incidence of anal cancer. Early detection and screening in high-risk individuals (such as the use of anal cytology in male homosexuals and immunosuppressed patients) should be encouraged to diagnose the tumor at the earliest possible stage. The use of antiviral agents in patients with HPV infection may be another method for decreasing incidence of this disease. If the tumor is not diagnosed at a stage early enough to allow cure by surgical resection alone (the minority of cases), new approaches involving combined modality therapy have clearly been demonstrated to offer equivalent or better results when compared with an APR. APR should be reserved for patients failing to respond to combined modality therapy. New efforts aimed at finding better chemotherapeutic regimens for the higher risk patients (T4 and node-positive tumors) are under way. In addition, the identification of new noncytotoxic agents capable of curative therapy without the toxicities of chemoradiation therapy should be explored.

REFERENCES

1. Landis SH, Murray T, Bolden S. Cancer statistics, 1999. *CA Cancer J Clin* 1999;49:8.
2. Myerson RJ, Karnell LH, Menck HR. The National Cancer Data Base report on carcinoma of the anus. *Cancer* 1997;80:805.
3. Frisch M, Fenger C, van den Brule AJ, et al. Variants of squamous cell carcinoma of the anal canal and perianal skin and their relation to human papillomaviruses. *Cancer Res* 1999;59:753.
4. Freidman HB, Saah AJ, Sherman ME, et al. Human papillomavirus, anal squamous intraepithelial lesions, and human immunodeficiency virus in a cohort of gay men. *J Infect Dis* 1998;178:45.
5. Palefsky JM, Holly EA, Ralston ML, et al. High incidence of anal high-grade squamous intra-epithelial lesions among HIV-positive and HIV-negative homosexual and bisexual men. *AIDS* 1998;12:495.
6. Scholefield JH, Hickson WGE, Smith JHF, et al. Anal intraepithelial neoplasia: part of a multifocal disease process. *Lancet* 1992;340:1271.
7. Melbye M, Cote T, Kessler L, et al. AIDS/Cancer Working Group. High incidence of anal cancer among AIDS patients. *Lancet* 1994;343:636.
8. Penn I. Cancers of the anogenital region in renal transplant recipients. *Cancer* 1986;58:611.
9. Goldie SJ, Kuntz KM, Weinstein MC, et al. The clinical effectiveness and cost-effectiveness of screening for anal squamous intraepithelial lesions in homosexual and bisexual HIV-positive men. *JAMA* 1999;281:1822.
10. Prasad ML, Abcarian H. Malignant potential of perianal condyloma acuminatum. *Dis Colon Rectum* 1980;23:191.
11. Chuang TY, Perry HO, Kurland LT, et al. Condyloma acuminatum in Rochester, Minnesota, 1950–1978. *Arch Dermatol* 1984;120:476.
12. Zaki SR, Judd R, Coffield LM, et al. Human papillomavirus infection and anal carcinoma: retrospective analysis by in situ hybridization and the polymerase chain reaction. *Am J Pathol* 1992;140:1345.
13. Pfister H, Fuchs PG. Relation of papillomaviruses to anogenital cancer. *Dermatol Clin* 1991;9:267.
14. Daling JR, Weiss NS, Hislop TG. Sexual practices, sexually transmitted diseases, and the incidence of anal cancer. *N Engl J Med* 1987;317:973.
15. Caussey D, Goedert JJ, Palefsky J, et al. Interaction of human immunodeficiency and papilloma viruses: association with anal epithelial abnormality in homosexual men. *Int J Cancer* 1990;46:214.
16. Jakate SM, Saclarides TJ. Immunohistochemical detection of mutant p53 protein and human papillomavirus-related E6 protein in anal cancers. *Dis Colon Rectum* 1993;36:1026.
17. Ogunbuyi OA, Scholefield JH, Smith JHF, et al. Immunohistochemical analysis of p53 expression in anal squamous neoplasia. *J Clin Pathol* 1993;46:507.
18. Bonin SR, Pajak TJ, Russell AH, et al. Overexpression of p53 protein and outcome of patients with chemoradiation for carcinoma of the anal canal: a report of the randomized trial RTOG 87-04. Radiation Therapy Oncology Group. *Cancer* 1999;85:1226.
19. Allal AS, Alonso Pentzke L, Remadi S. Apparent lack of prognostic value of MIB-1 index in anal carcinomas treated by radiotherapy. *Br J Cancer* 1998;77:1333.
20. Buckwalter JA, Jurayj MN. Relationship of chronic anorectal disease to carcinoma. *Arch Surg* 1957;75:352.
21. Frisch M, Olsen JH, Bautz A, et al. Benign anal lesions and the risk of anal cancer. *N Engl J Med* 1994;331:300.
22. Lin AY, Gridley G, Tucker M. Benign anal lesions and cancer. *N Engl J Med* 1995;332:190.
23. Holly EA, Whittemore AS, Aston DA, et al. Anal cancer incidence: genital warts, anal fissure, hemorrhoids, and smoking. *J Natl Cancer Inst* 1989;81:1726.
24. Ky A, Sohn N, Weinstein MA, Korelitz BI. Carcinoma arising in anorectal fistulas of Crohn's disease. *Dis Colon Rectum* 1998;41:992.
25. Frisch M, Glimelius B, Wohlfahrt J, et al. Tobacco smoking as a risk factor in anal carcinoma: an antiestrogenic mechanism? *J Natl Cancer Inst* 1999;91:708.
26. Daniell HW. Causes of anal carcinoma. *JAMA* 1985;254:358.
27. Holmes F, Borek D, Medge OK, et al. Anal cancer in women. *Gastroenterology* 1988;95:107.
28. Wolfe HRI, Bussey HJR. Squamous cell carcinoma of the anus. *Br J Surg* 1968;55:295.
29. Cabrera A, Tsukada Y, Pickren JW, et al. Development of lower genital carcinomas in patients with anal carcinoma: a more than casual relationship. *Cancer* 1966;19:470.
30. Goligher JC, ed. *Surgery of the anus, rectum, and colon.* London: Bailliere, Tindall, and Cassell, 1975:815.
31. Kawaura A, Kumagai H, Shibata M, et al. Tumors of the anal region induced in mice painted with methylazoxymethanol acetate. *Gann* 1981;72:886.
32. Kingsnorth AN, Abu-Khalaf M, Ross JS, et al. Potentiation of 1,2-dimethylhydrazine-induced anal carcinoma by epidermal growth factor in mice. *Surgery* 1985;97:696.
33. Morson BC. The pathology and results of treatment of squamous cell carcinoma of the anal canal and anal margin. *Proc R Soc Med* 1960;53:414.
34. Greenall MJ, Quan SHQ, Stearns MW, et al. Epidermoid cancer of the anal margin. *Am J Surg* 1985;149:95.
35. Hardy KJ, Hughes ESR, Cuthbertson AM. Squamous cell carcinoma of the anal canal and anal margin. *Aust NZ J Surg* 1969;38:301.
36. Al-Jurf AS, Turnbull RB, Fazio VW. Local treatment of squamous cell carcinoma of the anus. *Surg Gynecol Obstet* 1979;148:576.
37. Beahrs O, Wilson S. Carcinoma of the anus. *Ann Surg* 1976;184:422.
38. Kuehn PG, Beckett R, Eisenberg H. Hematogenous metastasis from epidermoid carcinoma of the anal canal. *Am J Surg* 1965;109:445.
39. Grodsky L. Unsuspected anal cancer discovered after minor anorectal surgery. *Dis Colon Rectum* 1967;10:471.
40. Cummings BJ. The treatment of anal cancer. *Int J Radiat Oncol Biol Phys* 1989;17:1359.
41. American Joint Committee on Cancer. Anal canal. In: Fleming ID, Cooper JS, Henson DE, et al., eds. *AJCC cancer staging manual.* Philadelphia: Lippincott–Raven, 1998:91.
42. Anal canal. In: Sobin LH, Wittekind CH, eds. *TNM classification of malignant tumors.* New York: Wiley-Liss, 1997:70.
43. Stearns MW, Urmacher C, Sternberg SS. Cancer of the anal canal. *Curr Probl Cancer* 1980;4:1.
44. Wood DA. Tumors of the intestines. In: *Atlas of tumor pathology.* Washington, DC: Armed Forces Institute of Pathology, 1967:200.
45. Boman BM, Moertel C, O'Connell M, et al. Carcinoma of the anal canal, a clinical and pathologic study of 188 cases. *Cancer* 1984;54:114.
46. Remigio PA, Der BK, Forsberg RT. Anorectal melanoma: report of two cases. *Dis Colon Rectum* 1976;19:350.
47. Stearns MW. Epidermoid carcinoma of the anal region. *Surg Gynecol Obstet* 1958;106:92.
48. Dougherty B, Evans H. Carcinoma of the anal canal: a study of 79 cases. *Am J Clin Pathol* 1985;83:159.
49. Salmon RJ, Zafrani B, Habib A, et al. Prognosis of cloacogenic and squamous cancers of the anal canal. *Dis Colon Rectum* 1986;29:336.
50. Wolber R, Dupuis B, Thiyagaratnam P, et al. Anal cloacogenic and squamous cell carcinomas. Comparative histologic analysis using in situ hybridization for human papillomavirus DNA. *Am J Surg Pathol* 1990;14:176.
51. Higgins GD, Uzelin DM, Phillips GE. Differing characteristics of human papillomavirus RNA-positive and RNA-negative anal carcinomas. *Cancer* 1991;68:561.
52. Ordonez NG, Awalt H, Mackay B. Mammary and extramammary Paget's disease: an immunocytochemical and ultrastructural study. *Cancer* 1987;59:1173.
53. Tjandra J. Perianal Paget's disease: report of 3 cases. *Dis Colon Rectum* 1988;31:112.
54. Goldblum JR, Hart WR. Perianal Paget's disease: a histologic and immunohistochemical study of 11 cases with and without associated rectal adenocarcinoma. *Am J Surg Pathol* 1998;22:170.
55. Fenger C, Nielsen VT. Precancerous changes in anal canal epithelium in resection specimens. *Acta Pathol Microbiol Immunobiol Scand (A)* 1986;94:63.
56. Fenger C, Nielsen VT. Dysplastic changes in the anal canal epithelium in minor surgical specimens. *Acta Pathol Microbiol Immunobiol Scand (A)* 1981;89:463.
57. Palefsky J, Gonzalez J, Greenblatt R, et al. Anal intraepithelial neoplasia and anal papillomavirus infection among homosexual males with group IV HIV disease. *JAMA* 1990;263:1911.
58. Surawicz CM, Kirby P, Critchlow C, et al. Anal dysplasia in homosexual men: role of anoscopy and biopsy. *Gastroenterology* 1993;105:658.
59. Palefsky JM, Holly EA, Gonzales J, et al. Natural history of anal cytologic abnormalities and papillomavirus infection among homosexual men with group IV HIV disease. *J Acquir Immune Defic Syndr* 1992;5:1258.
60. Fenger C, Bichel P. Flow cytometric DNA analysis of anal canal epithelium and ano-rectal tumors. *Pathol Microbiol Immunobiol Scand (A)* 1981;89:351.
61. Goldman S, Auer G, Erhardt K, et al. Prognostic significance of clinical stage, histologic grade, and nuclear DNA content in squamous cell carcinoma of the anus. *Dis Colon Rectum* 1987;30:444.
62. Scott NA, Beart RW, Weiland LH, et al. Carcinoma of the anal canal and flow cytometric DNA analysis. *Br J Cancer* 1989;60:450.
63. Kuehn PG, Eisenberg H, Reed JF. Epidermoid carcinoma of the perianal skin and anal canal. *Cancer* 1968;22:932.
64. Klotz R, Pamukcoglu T, Souilliard D. Transitional cloacogenic carcinoma of the anal canal. *Cancer* 1967;20:1727.
65. Dillard BM, Spratt JS, Ackerman LV. Epidermoid carcinoma of the anal margin and canal. *Arch Surg* 1963;86:772.
66. Clark J, Petrelli N, Herrera L, et al. Epidermoid carcinoma of the anal canal. *Cancer* 1986;57:400.
67. Pyper PC, Parks TG. The results of surgery for epidermoid carcinoma of the anus. *Br J Surg* 1985;72:712.
68. Wolfe HRI. The management of metastatic inguinal adenitis in epidermoid cancer of the anus. *Proc R Soc Med* 1961;61:626.
69. Welch JP, Malt RA. Appraisal of treatment of carcinoma of the anus and anal canal. *Surg Gynecol Obstet* 1977;145:837.
70. Greenall M, Quan SHQ, Urmacher C, et al. Treatment of epidermoid carcinoma of the anal canal. *Surg Gynecol Obstet* 1985;161:509.
71. Pack GT, Oropeza R. A comparative study of melanoma and epidermoid carcinoma of the anal canal: a review of 20 melanomas and 29 epidermoid carcinomas. *Dis Colon Rectum* 1967;10:161.

72. Frost DB, Richards PC, Montague ED, et al. Epidermoid cancer of the anorectum. *Cancer* 1984;53:1285.
73. Richards JC, Beahrs OH, Woolner LB. Squamous cell carcinoma of the anus, anal canal, and rectum in 109 patients. *Surg Gynecol Obstet* 1962;114:475.
74. Sawyers JL, Herrington JL, Main FB. Surgical considerations in the treatment of epidermoid carcinoma of the anus. *Ann Surg* 1963;157:817.
75. Singh R, Nime F, Mittelman A. Malignant epithelial tumors of the anal canal. *Cancer* 1981;48:411.
76. Greenall MJ, Quan SHQ, DeCosse J. Epidermoid cancer of the anus. *Br J Surg* 1985;72:S97.
77. Berardi R, Lee S, Chen HP. Perianal extramammmary Paget's disease. *Surg Gynecol Obstet* 1988;167:359.
78. McDermott F, Hughes E, Pihl E. Symptoms, duration, and survival prospects in cancer of the rectum. *Surg Gynecol Obstet* 1931;52:350.
79. Binkley GE, Derrick WA. The association of squamous cell cancer with anal manifestations of lymphogranuloma venerum. *Am J Dig Dis* 1945;12:46.
80. Kuehn PG, Beckett R, Eisenberg H, et al. Epidermoid carcinoma of the perianal skin and anal canal. *N Engl J Med* 1964;270:614.
81. Gordon BS. Unsuspected lesions in anal tissue removed for minor conditions. *Ann Surg* 1956;73:741.
82. Hu K, Minsky BD, Cohen AM, et al. 30 Gy may be an adequate dose in patients with anal cancer treated with excisional biopsy followed by combined-modality therapy. *J Surg Oncol* 1999;70:77.
83. Goldman S, Glimelius B, Norming U, et al. Transanorectal ultrasonography in anal carcinoma: a prospective study of 21 patients. *Acta Radiol* 1988;29:337.
84. Papillon J, Montbarbon JF. Epidermoid carcinoma of the anal canal. *Dis Colon Rectum* 1987;30:324.
85. Peiffert D, Bey P, Pernot M, et al. Conservative management by irradiation of epidermoid cancers of the anal canal: prognostic factors of tumor control and complications. *Int J Radiat Oncol Biol Phys* 1997;37:313.
86. Gerard JP, Ayzac L, Hun D, et al. Treatment of anal canal carcinoma with high dose radiation therapy and concomitant fluorouracil-cisplatinum. Long term results in 95 patients. *Radiother Oncol* 1998;46:249.
87. Doci R, Zucali R, La Monica G, et al. Primary chemoradiation therapy with fluorouracil and cisplatin for cancer of the anus: results in 35 consecutive patients. *J Clin Oncol* 1996;14:3121.
88. Flam M, John M, Pajak T, et al. Role of mitomycin in combination with fluorouracil and radiotherapy, and salvage chemoradiation in the definitive nonsurgical treatment of epidermoid carcinoma of the anal canal: results of a phase III randomized intergroup study. *J Clin Oncol* 1996;14:2537.
89. Bartelink H, Roelofsen F, Eschwege F, et al. Concomitant radiotherapy and chemotherapy is superior to radiotherapy alone in the treatment of locally advanced anal cancer: results of a phase III randomized trial of the European Organization for Research and Treatment of Cancer radiotherapy and gastrointestinal cooperative groups. *J Clin Oncol* 1997;15:2040.
90. Cummings BJ. Anal canal. In: Perez C, Brady L, eds. *Principles and practice of radiation oncology*. Philadelphia: Lippincott, 1993:1015.
91. Ellenhorn JDI, Enker WE, Quan SHW. Salvage abdominoperineal resection following combined chemotherapy and radiotherapy for epidermoid carcinoma of the anus. *Ann Surg Oncol* 1994;1:105.
92. Cummings BJ, Keane TJ, O'Sullivan B, et al. Epidermoid anal cancer: treatment by radiation alone or by radiation and 5-fluorouracil with and without mitomycin-C. *Int J Radiat Oncol Biol Phys* 1991;21:1115.
93. Doci R, Zucali R, Bombelli L, et al. Combined chemoradiation therapy for anal cancer. *Ann Surg* 1992;215:150.
94. Allal AS, Mermillod B, Roth AD, et al. The impact of treatment factors on local control in T2-T3 anal carcinomas treated by radiotherapy with or without chemotherapy. *Cancer* 1997;79:2329.
95. Goldman S, Glimelius B, Glas U, et al. Management of anal epidermoid carcinoma: an evaluation of treatment results in two population-based series. *Int J Colorect Dis* 1989;4:234.
96. Schlienger M, Krzisch C, Pene F, et al. Epidermoid carcinoma of the anal canal treatment results and prognostic variables in a series of 242 cases. *Int J Radiat Oncol Biol Phys* 1989;17:1141.
97. Schlienger M, Touboul E, Mauban S, et al. Resultats du traitement de 286 cas de cancers epidermoides du canal anal dont 236 par irradiation a visee conservatrice. *Lyon Chir* 1991;87:61.
98. Constantinou EC, Daly W, Fung CY, et al. Time-dose considerations in the treatment of anal cancer. *Int J Radiat Oncol Biol Phys* 1997;39:651.
99. Serota AI, Weil M, Williams RA. Anal cloacogenic carcinoma. *Arch Surg* 1981;116:456.
100. Shepherd NA, Scholefield JH, Love SB, et al. Prognostic factors in anal squamous carcinoma: a multivariate analysis of clinical, pathological, and flow cytometric parameters in 235 cases. *Histopathology* 1990;16:545.
101. Goldberg ZI, Cummings BJ, Chapman WB, et al. Role of a DT-diaphorase mutation in the response of anal canal carcinoma to radiation, 5-fluorouracil, and mitomycin c. *Int J Radiat Oncol Biol Phys* 1998;42:331.
102. Tanum G, Holm R. Anal carcinoma: a clinical approach to p53 and RB gene proteins. *Oncology* 1996;53:369.
103. Bonin SR, Qian C, Russell AH, et al. Overexpression of p53 protein is associated with decreased local disease-free survival in patients treated with chemoradiation for anal canal cancer: a report of RTOG 87-04. *Int J Radiat Oncol Biol Phys* 1996;36:210.
104. Wong CS, Tsao MS, Sharma V, et al. Prognostic role of p53 protein expression in epidermoid carcinoma of the anal canal. *Int J Radiat Oncol Biol Phys* 1999;45:309.
105. Mendenhall WM, Zlotecki RA, Vauthey JN, et al. Squamous cell carcinoma of the anal margin. *Oncology* 1996;10:1843.
106. Papillon J, Chassard JL. Respective roles of radiotherapy and surgery in the management of epidermoid carcinoma of the anal margin. *Dis Colon Rectum* 1992;35:422.
107. UKCCCR Anal Cancer Trial Working Party. Epidermoid anal cancer: results from the UKCCCR randomised trial of radiotherapy alone versus radiotherapy, 5-fluorouracil, and mitomycin. *Lancet* 1997;348:1049.
108. Grinnell RS. An analysis of forty-nine cases of squamous cell carcinoma of the anus. *Surg Gynecol Obstet* 1954;98:29.
109. McConnell EM. Squamous cell carcinoma of the anus: a review of 96 cases. *Surg Gynecol Obstet* 1970;141:411.
110. Beck DE, Fazio VW, Jagelman DG, et al. Perianal Bowen's disease. *Dis Colon Rectum* 1988;31:419.
111. Beck DE, Fazio VW. Perianal Paget's disease. *Dis Colon Rectum* 1987;30:263.
112. Hardcastle JD, Bussey HJR. Results of surgical treatment of squamous cell carcinoma of the anal canal and anal margin seen at St. Mark's Hospital. *Proc R Soc Med* 1968;61:629.
113. Turell R. Epidermoid squamous cell cancer of the perianus and anal canal. *Surg Clin North Am* 1962;42:1235.
114. Greenall MJ, Magill G, Quan SHQ. Recurrent epidermoid carcinoma of the anus. *Cancer* 1986;57:1437.
115. Scholefield JH, Ogunbuyi OA, Smith JHF, et al. Treatment of intraepithelial neoplasia. *Br J Surg* 1994;81:1238.
116. Brittain PC, Carlson JW, Hawley-Bowlnd C. Laser ablation of squamous cell carcinoma in situ of the anal canal: a case report. *J Reprod Med* 1994;39:913.
117. Schraut WH, Wang CH, Dawson PJ, et al. Depth of invasion, location, and size of cancer of the anus dictate operative treatment. *Cancer* 1983;51:1291.
118. Dalby JF, Pointon RS. The treatment of anal carcinoma by interstitial irradiation. *Am J Radiol* 1961;85:515.
119. Papillon J. *Rectal and anal cancers*. New York: Springer-Verlag, 1982.
120. Hintz BL, Charyulu KKN, Sudarsanam A. Anal carcinoma: basic concepts and management. *J Surg Oncol* 1978;10:141.
121. James RD, Pointon RS, Martin S. Local radiotherapy in the management of squamous carcinoma of the anus. *Br J Surg* 1985;72:282.
122. Peiffert D, Bey P, Pernot M, et al. Conservative treatment by irradiation of epidermoid carcinomas of the anal margin. *Int J Radiat Oncol Biol Phys* 1997;39:57.
123. Gordon PH. Current status—perianal and anal canal neoplasms. *Dis Colon Rectum* 1990;33:799.
124. Nigro ND, Vaitkevicius VK, Considine B. Combined therapy for cancer of the anal canal: a preliminary report. *Dis Colon Rectum* 1974;17:354.
125. Graf R, Wust P, Gellermann J, et al. Phase II trial of radiation therapy with 45 Gy, 5-fluorouracil (5-FU), and mitomycin-C (MMC) in patients with anal cancer—a rationale to add regional hyperthermia. *Int J Radiat Oncol Biol Phys* 1996;36:296.
126. Miller EJ, Quan SHQ, Thaler HT. Treatment of squamous cell carcinoma of the anal canal. *Cancer* 1991;67:2038.
127. Meropol NJ, Niedzwiecki D, Shank B, et al. Combined-modality therapy of poor risk anal canal carcinoma; a phase II study of the Cancer and Leukemia Group B (CALGB). *Proc Am Soc Clin Oncol* 1999;18:245.
128. Hughes LL, Rich TA, Delclos L, et al. Radiotherapy for anal cancer: experience from 1979–1987. *Int J Radiat Oncol Biol Phys* 1989;17:1153.
129. John M, Pajak T, Flam M, et al. Dose escalation in chemoradiation for anal cancer: preliminary results of RTOG 92-08. *Cancer J Sci Am* 1996;2:205.
130. Martenson JA, Lipsitz SR, Wagner H, et al. Initial results of a phase II trial of high dose radiation therapy, 5-fluorouracil, and cisplatin for patients with anal cancer (E4292): an Eastern Cooperative Oncology Group study. *Int J Radiat Oncol Biol Phys* 1996;35:745.
131. Pieffert D, Seitz JF, Rougier P, et al. Preliminary results of a phase II study of high-dose radiation therapy and neoadjuvant plus concomitant 5-fluorouracil with CDDP chemotherapy for patients with anal canal cancer: a French cooperative study. *Ann Oncol* 1997;8:575.
132. Papillon J, Montbarbon JF, Gerard JP, et al. Interstitial curietherapy in the conservative treatment of anal and rectal cancers. *Int J Radiat Oncol Biol Phys* 1989;17:1161.
133. Gerard JP, Mauro F, Thomas L, et al. Treatment of squamous cell anal canal carcinoma with pulsed dose rate brachytherapy. Feasibility study of a French cooperative group. *Radiother Oncol* 1999;51:131.
134. Roed H, Engelholm SA, Svendsen LB, et al. Pulsed dose rate (PDR) brachytherapy of anal carcinoma. *Radiother Oncol* 1996;41:131.
135. Sandhu APS, Symonds RP, Robertson AG, et al. Interstitial iridium-192 implantation combined with external radiotherapy in anal cancer: ten years experience. *Int J Radiat Oncol Biol Phys* 1998;40:575.
136. Wagner JP, Mahe MA, Romestaing P, et al. Radiation therapy in the conservative treatment of carcinoma of the anal canal. *Int J Radiat Oncol Biol Phys* 1994;29:17.
137. Allal A, Mermillod B, Roth AD, et al. Impact of clinical and therapeutic factors on major late complications after radiotherapy with or without concomitant chemotherapy for anal carcinoma. *Int J Radiat Oncol Biol Phys* 1997;39:1099.
138. Lohnert M, Doniec JM, Kovacs G, et al. New method of radiotherapy for anal cancer with three-dimensional tumor reconstruction based on endoanal ultrasound and ultrasound-guided afterloading therapy. *Dis Colon Rectum* 1998;41:169.
139. Michaelson RA, Magill G, Quan SHQ, et al. Pre-operative chemotherapy and radiation therapy in the management of anal epidermoid carcinoma. *Cancer* 1983;51:390.
140. Sischy B, Doggett S, Krall J, et al. Definitive irradiation and chemotherapy for radiosensitization in management of anal carcinoma: interim report on radiation therapy oncology group study no. 8314. *J Natl Cancer Inst* 1989;81:850.
141. Buxton RW. Squamous cell anal carcinoma. *Ann Surg* 1953;67:821.
142. Cattell RB, Williams AC. Epidermoid carcinoma of the anus and rectum. *Ann Surg* 1943;46:336.
143. Touboul E, Schlienger M, Buffat L, et al. Epidermoid carcinoma of the anal canal. Results of curative-intent radiation therapy in a series of 270 patients. *Cancer* 1994;73:1569.
144. deGara CJ, Basrur V, Figueredo A, et al. The influence of age on the management of anal cancer. *Hepato-Gastroenterology* 1995;42:73.

145. Valentini V, Morganti AG, Luzi S, et al. Is chemoradiation feasible in elderly patients? A study of 17 patients with anorectal carcinoma. *Cancer* 1997;80:1387.
146. Allal A, Obradovic M, Laurencet F, et al. Treatment of anal canal carcinoma in the elderly. Feasibility and outcome of radical radiotherapy with or without concomitant chemotherapy. *Cancer* 1999;85:26.
147. Martenson JA, Gunderson LL. External radiation therapy without chemotherapy in the management of anal cancer. *Cancer* 1993;71:1736.
148. Keiling R, Grunewald JM, Achille E. Radiotherapie des cancers malpighiens de l'anus. *J Radiol Electrol Med Nucl* 1973;54:634.
149. Dubois JB, Garrigues JM, Pujol H. Cancer of the anal canal: report on the experience of 61 patients. *Int J Radiat Oncol Biol Phys* 1991;20:575.
150. Ager P, Samala E, Bosworth J, et al. The conservative management of anorectal cancer by radiotherapy. *Am J Surg* 1979;137:228.
151. Ng Ying Kin KNY, Pigneux J, Auvray H, et al. Our experience of conservative treatment of anal canal carcinoma combining external irradiation and interstitial implants: 32 cases treated between 1973 and 1982. *Int J Radiat Oncol Biol Phys* 1988;14:253.
152. Martinez A, Edmundson GK, Cox RS, et al. Combination of external beam irradiation and multiple-site perineal applicator (MUPIT) for treatment of locally advanced or recurrent prostatic, anorectal, and gynecologic malignancies. *Int J Radiat Oncol Biol Phys* 1985;11:256.
153. Puthawala AA, Syed N, Gates TC, et al. Definitive treatment of extensive anorectal carcinoma by external and interstitial irradiation. *Cancer* 1982;50:1746.
154. Papillon J. Effectiveness of combined radio-chemotherapy in the management of epidermoid carcinoma of the anal canal. *Int J Radiat Oncol Biol Phys* 1990;19:1217.
155. Koh WJ, Chiu M, Stelzer KJ, et al. Femoral vessel depth and the implications for groin node radiation. *Int J Radiat Oncol Biol Phys* 1993;27:969.
156. Wang CJ, Chin YY, Leung SW, et al. Topographic distribution of inguinal lymph nodes metastasis: significance in determination of treatment margin for elective inguinal lymph nodes irradiation of low pelvic tumors. *Int J Radiat Oncol Biol Phys* 1996;35:133.
157. Kollmorgen CF, Meagher AP, Pemberton JH, et al. The long term effect of adjuvant postoperative chemoradiotherapy for rectal cancer on bowel function. *Ann Surg* 1994;220:676.
158. Kapp KS, Geyer E, Gebhart FH, et al. Evaluation of sphincter function after external beam irradiation and Ir-192 high-dose-rate (HDR) brachytherapy +/- chemotherapy in patients with carcinoma of the anal canal. *Int J Radiat Oncol Biol Phys* 1999;45s:339.
159. Vodermark D, Sailer M, Flentje M, et al. Continence and anorectal manometry after curative-intent radiation therapy for anal carcinoma. *Int J Radiat Oncol Biol Phys* 1999;45s:340.
160. Mendenhall WM, Zlotecki RA, Vauthey JN, et al. Squamous cell carcinoma of the anal margin treated with radiotherapy. *Surg Oncol* 1996;5:29.
161. Nigro ND. The force of change in the management of squamous-cell cancer of the anal canal. *Dis Colon Rectum* 1991;34:482.
162. Leichman LP, Nigro N, Vaitkevicius V, et al. Cancer of the anal canal: model for preoperative adjuvant combined modality therapy. *Am J Med* 1985;78:211.
163. Habr-Gama A, da Silva e Sousa Jr. AH, Nadalin W, et al. Epidermoid carcinoma of the anal canal: results of treatment by combined chemotherapy and radiation therapy. *Dis Colon Rectum* 1989;32:773.
164. Cummings B. Concomitant radiotherapy and chemotherapy for anal cancer. *Semin Radiat Oncol* 1992;19:102.
165. Flam M, John M, Mowry P, et al. Definitive combined modality therapy of carcinoma of the anus: a report of 30 cases including results of salvage therapy in patients with residual disease. *Dis Colon Rectum* 1987;30:495.
166. Longo WE, Vernava AM, Wade TP, et al. Recurrent squamous cell carcinoma of the anal canal. Predictors of initial treatment failure and results of salvage therapy. *Ann Surg* 1994;220:40.
167. Zelnick RS, Haas PA, Ajlouni M, et al. Results of abdominoperineal resections for failures after combination chemotherapy and radiation therapy for anal canal cancers. *Dis Colon Rectum* 1992;35:574.
168. Pocard M, Tiret E, Nugent K, et al. Results of salvage abdominoperineal resection for anal cancer after radiotherapy. *Dis Colon Rectum* 1998;41:1493.
169. Allal AS, Laurencet FM, Reymond MA, et al. Effectiveness of surgical salvage therapy for patients with locally uncontrolled anal carcinoma after sphincter-conserving treatment. *Cancer* 1999;86:409.
170. Fisher W, Herbst K, Sims J, et al. Metastatic cloacogenic carcinoma of the anus: sequential responses to Adriamycin and cis-dichlorodiamineplatinum (III). *Cancer Treat Rep* 1978;62:91.
171. Salem P, Habboubi N, Naanasissie E, et al. Effectiveness of cisplatin in the treatment of anal squamous cell carcinoma. *Cancer Treat Rep* 1985;69:891.
172. Livingston R, Bodey G, Gottlieb J, et al. Kinetic scheduling of vincristine and bleomycin in patients with lung cancer and other malignant tumors. *Cancer Treat Rep* 1973;57:219.
173. Khater R, Frenay M, Bourry J, et al. Cisplatin plus 5-fluorouracil in the treatment of metastatic squamous cell carcinoma: a report of 2 cases. *Cancer Treat Rep* 1986,70:1345.
174. Ajani JA, Carrasco H, Jackson D, et al. Combination of cisplatin plus fluoropyrimidine chemotherapy effective against liver metastasis from carcinoma of the anal canal. *Am J Med* 1989;87:221.
175. Jaiyesimi IA, Pazdur R. Cisplatin and 5-fluorouracil as salvage therapy for recurrent metastatic squamous cell carcinoma of the anal canal. *Am J Clin Pathol* 1993;16:536.
176. Mahjoubi M, Sadek H, Francois E, et al. Epidermoid anal canal carcinoma (EACC): activity of cisplatin (P) and continuous 5 fluorouracil (5-FU) in metastatic (M) and/or local recurrent (LR) disease. *Proc Am Soc Clin Oncol* 1990;9:114.
177. Tanum G. Treatment of relapsing anal carcinoma. *Acta Oncol* 1993;32:33.
178. Evans TRJ, Mansi JL, Glees JP. Case report: response of metastatic anal carcinoma to single agent carboplatin. *Clin Oncol* 1993;5:57.
178a. Wilking N, Petrelli N, Herrera L, Mittleman A. Phase II study of combination belomycin, vincristine, and high dose methotrexate (BOM) with leucovorin rescue in advanced squamous cell carcinoma of the anal canal. *Cancer Chemother Pharmacol* 1985;15(3):300.
179. Magill G, Quan S. Salvage chemotherapy of anal epidermoid carcinoma with cisplatin based protocols. *Proc Am Soc Clin Oncol* 1989;8:117.
180. Peiffert D, Seitz JF, Rougier P, et al. Preliminary results of a phase II study of high-dose radiation therapy and neoadjuvant plus concomitant 5-fluorouracil with CDDP chemotherapy for patients with anal canal cancer: a French cooperative study. *Ann Oncol* 1997;8:575.
181. Petrelli NJ, Palmer M, Herrera L, et al. The utility of squamous cell carcinoma antigen for the follow-up of patients with squamous cell carcinoma of the anal canal. *Cancer* 1992;70:35.
182. Siegel B, Cohen D, Jacob ET. Surgical treatment of anorectal melanomas. *Am J Surg* 1983;146:336.
183. Slingluff CL, Vollmer RT, Seigler HF. Anorectal melanoma: clinical characteristics and results of surgical management in twenty-four patients. *Surgery* 1990;107:1.
184. Wong JH, Cagle LA, Storm FK, et al. Natural history of surgically treated mucosal melanoma. *Am J Surg* 1987;154:54.
185. Whooley BP, Astrow AB, Toth IR, et al. Long term survival after locally aggressive anorectal melanoma. *Am Surg* 1998;64:245.
186. DeMatos P, Tyler DS, Siegler HF. Malignant melanoma of the mucous membranes: a review of 119 cases. *Ann Surg Oncol* 1998;5:733.
187. Weinstock MA. Epidemiology and prognosis of anorectal melanoma. *Gastroenterology* 1993;104:174.
188. Morson BC, Volkstadt H. Malignant melanoma of the anal canal. *J Clin Pathol* 1963;16:126.
189. Quan SHQ, White JE, Deddish MR. Malignant melanoma of the anorectum. *Dis Colon Rectum* 1959;2:275.
190. Goldman S, Glimelius B, Pahlman L. Anorectal malignant melanoma in Sweden—report of 49 patients. *Dis Colon Rectum* 1990;33:874.
191. Ross M, Pezzi C, Pezzi T, et al. Patterns of failure in anorectal melanoma: a guide to surgical therapy. *Arch Surg* 1990;125:313.
192. Brady MS, Kavolius JP, Quan SHQ. Anorectal melanoma: a 64-year experience at Memorial Sloan-Kettering Cancer Center. *Dis Colon Rectum* 1995;38:146.
193. Chiu YS, Unni KK, Beart RW. Malignant melanoma of the anorectum. *Dis Colon Rectum* 1980;23:122.
194. Garnick M, Lokich JJ. Primary malignant melanoma of the rectum: rationale for conservative surgical management. *J Surg Oncol* 1978;10:529.
195. Wanebo HJ, Woodruff JM, Farr GH, Quan SHQ. Anorectal melanoma. *Cancer* 1981;47:1891.
196. Pack GT, Martins FG. Treatment of anorectal malignant melanoma. *Dis Colon Rectum* 1960;3:15.
197. Ward MW, Romano G, Nicholls R. The surgical treatment of anorectal malignant melanoma. *Br J Surg* 1986;73:68.
198. Basik M, Rodriguez-Bigas MA, Penetrante R, et al. Prognosis and recurrence patterns of anal adenocarcinoma. *Am J Surg* 1995;169:233.
199. Cagir B, Nagy MW, Topham A, et al. Adenosquamous carcinoma of the colon, rectum, and anus. Epidemiology, distribution, and survival characteristics. *Dis Colon Rectum* 1999;42:263.
200. Minsky BD, Mies C, Rich TA. Leiomyosarcoma of the anus treated with sphincter preserving surgery and radiation therapy. *J Surg Oncol* 1986;32:91.
201. Minsky BD, Cohen AM, Hajdu SI. Conservative management of anal leiomyosarcoma. *Cancer* 1991;68:1643.
202. Grann A, Paty PB, Guillem JG, et al. Sphincter preservation of leiomyosarcoma of the rectum and anus with local excision and brachytherapy. *Dis Colon Rectum* 1999;42:1296.
203. Hoffman R, Welton ML, Klencke B, et al. The significance of pretreatment CD4 count on the outcome and treatment tolerance of HIV-positive patients with anal cancer. *Int J Radiat Oncol Biol Phys* 1999;44:131.
204. Peddada AV, Smith DE, Rao AR, et al. Chemotherapy and low dose radiotherapy in the treatment of HIV-infected patients with carcinoma of the anal canal. *Int J Radiat Oncol Biol Phys* 1997;37:1101.
205. Hocht S, Weigel T, Kroesen AJ, et al. Low acute toxicity of radiotherapy and radiochemotherapy in patients with cancer of the anal canal and HIV infection. *Acta Oncol* 1997;36:799.
206. Tanum G, Tveit K, Karlsen K, et al. Chemotherapy and radiation therapy for anal carcinoma. *Cancer* 1991;67:2462.
207. John M, Flam M, Palma N. Ten-year results of chemoradiation for anal cancer: focus on late morbidity. *Int J Radiat Oncol Biol Phys* 1996;34:65.
208. Cutuli B, Fenton J, Labib A, et al. Anal margin carcinoma: 21 cases treated at the Institut Curie by exclusive conservative radiotherapy. *Radiother Oncol* 1988;11:6.
209. Cheung ACY. The place of interstitial irradiation in epidermoid carcinoma of the anal margin. *Endocurie Hypertherm Oncol* 1989;5:140.
210. Svensson C, Goldman S, Friberg B. Radiation treatment of epidermoid cancer of the anus. *Int J Radiat Oncol Biol Phys* 1993;27:73.
211. Touboul E, Schlienger M, Buffat L, et al. Epidermoid carcinoma of the anal margin: 17 cases treated with curative-intent radiation therapy. *Radiother Oncol* 1995;34:195.
212. Friberg B, Svensson C, Goldman S, et al. The Swedish national care programme for anal carcinoma—implementation and overall results. *Acta Oncol* 1998;37:25.
213. Eschwege F, Lasser P, Chavy A, et al. Squamous cell carcinoma of the anal canal: treatment by external beam irradiation. *Radiother Oncol* 1985;3:145.
214. Doggett SW, Green JP, Cantril ST. Efficacy of radiation therapy alone for limited squamous cell carcinoma of the anal canal. *Int J Radiat Oncol Biol Phys* 1988;15:1069.
215. Newman G, Calverley DC, Acker BD, et al. The management of carcinoma of the anal canal by external beam radiotherapy, experience in Vancouver 1971–1988. *Radiother Oncol* 1992;25:196.

CHAPTER 34

Cancers of the Genitourinary System

W. MARSTON LINEHAN
BERTON ZBAR
FREDRICK LEACH
CARLOS CORDON-CARDO
WILLIAM ISAACS

SECTION 1
Molecular Biology of Genitourinary Cancers

KIDNEY CANCER

Kidney cancer, or renal carcinoma, affects more than 30,000 Americans annually and is responsible for nearly 12,000 deaths in the United States each year. Renal carcinoma occurs most commonly in adults between 50 and 70 years of age, although it has been reported in children as young as 3 years.[1,2] Renal carcinoma is responsible for approximately 3% of adult malignancies, and the male to female ratio is 1.5:1.[3,4] Leatherworkers and workers exposed to asbestos have an increased incidence of renal carcinoma. A strong correlation exists between cigarette smoking and the development renal carcinoma.[5,6] Up to 85% of renal carcinomas are of the clear cell type; 5% to 15% of renal carcinomas are a papillary histologic variant.[7,8] An increased incidence of renal carcinoma is seen in dialysis patients with acquired cystic disease, in which a rate 30 times higher than normal has been estimated.[9] A family history of this malignancy has been associated with an increased risk of developing of renal carcinoma.[2]

Like colon cancer, breast cancer, and retinoblastoma, renal carcinoma occurs in both a familial (hereditary) and sporadic (nonhereditary) form. It has been estimated that up to 4% of renal carcinomas may have a hereditary basis.[2] At least four types of hereditary renal carcinoma have been categorized: renal carcinoma associated with von Hippel-Lindau disease (VHL), hereditary papillary renal carcinoma (HPRC), hereditary renal carcinoma associated with Birt-Hogg-Dubé syndrome,[10] and hereditary clear cell renal carcinoma. VHL disease is a hereditary cancer syndrome with an autosomal dominant inheritance pattern in which affected individuals develop tumors in a number of organs, including the kidney. HPRC is a newly described form of inherited renal carcinoma in which affected individuals develop multifocal, bilateral, early-onset papillary renal carcinoma. Birt-Hogg-Dubé syndrome is a dominantly inherited cancer syndrome in which affected individuals are at risk to develop cutaneous, renal, and other manifestations. The cutaneous manifestation involves fibrofolliculomas; the kidney tumors can be chromophobe renal carcinoma, oncocytoma, or papillary renal carcinoma.[10] In the fourth, but less well understood form of inherited renal carcinoma, hereditary clear cell renal carcinoma, patients have a predisposition to develop bilateral, multifocal clear cell renal carcinoma.

LOCATION OF A RENAL CARCINOMA GENE

The initial studies to provide information with reference to a potential location for a renal carcinoma gene came from the

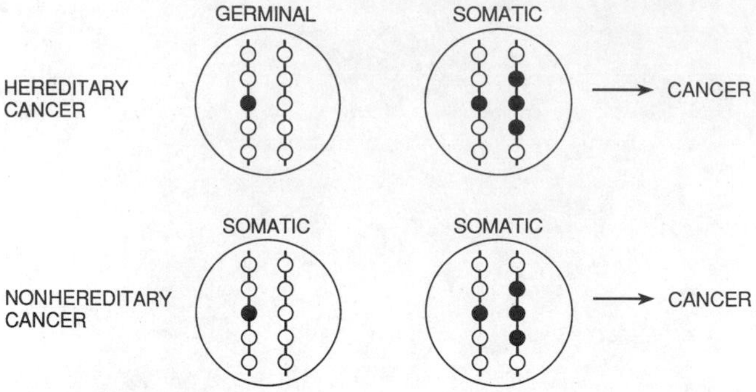

FIGURE 34.1-1. Knudson's two-hit model was the model for scientists searching for the clear cell renal carcinoma gene. In accord with Knudson's model, both copies of the gene for the hereditary form of renal carcinoma associated with von Hippel-Lindau (VHL) disease are inactivated in renal carcinomas from VHL patients (germinal inactivation of the VHL gene plus a somatic inactivation of the VHL gene).[317,318] In sporadic (nonhereditary) clear cell renal carcinoma somatic inactivation of both copies of the VHL gene has been detected in the majority of tumors.[44] (From ref. 319, with permission.)

work of Cohen and coworkers,[11] who in 1979 reported a kindred in which affected individuals developed early-onset, bilateral, multifocal clear cell renal carcinoma. In this family, every member who developed kidney cancer had a germline abnormality detectable on karyotypic analysis, a balanced translocation from the short arm of chromosome 3 to the long arm of chromosome 8. Every patient who was found to have early-onset kidney cancer in this kindred had this abnormality; no patient who did not have this translocation was found to have kidney cancer.[11] Subsequently, Pathak and coworkers[12] identified another family with a chromosome 3 to chromosome 11 translocation, and Kovaks and colleagues[13] reported a family with a chromosome 3 to chromosome 6 translocation. In both studies, the common abnormality was on the short arm of chromosome 3 (Fig. 34.1-1).

ABNORMALITIES IN SPORADIC CLEAR CELL RENAL CARCINOMA

These mutations in hereditary renal carcinoma led scientists to study nonhereditary renal carcinoma to determine if changes on chromosome 3 were also present in sporadic cases. When Zbar et al.[14] studied tumor tissue from 18 patients with sporadic, nonhereditary renal carcinoma by restriction fragment polymorphism analysis, loss of heterozygosity (LOH) on the short arm of chromosome 3 was detected in tumor tissue from 11 of 11 evaluable patients. LOH was detected in tumor tissue from patients with localized as well as advanced disease, suggesting the presence of a gene involved in the earliest development of this neoplasm. To more precisely define the prevalence of chromosome 3p LOH in sporadic renal carcinoma, as well as the location of a candidate gene for renal carcinoma, Anglard et al.[15] analyzed DNA from normal and tumor tissue from 60 patients with various stages of renal carcinoma for losses of alleles at different chromosomal loci. LOH that was independent of tumor stage was detected at one or more of ten loci tested on chromosome 3 in tumor tissue from nearly 90% of patients.[15] LOH was detected in clear cell renal carcinoma but not in papillary renal carcinoma. These findings and those of others showed deletion of a segment of chromosome 3p to be a consistent finding in clear cell renal carcinoma.[16–20]

Although these findings pointed to the presence of a renal carcinoma gene on the short arm of chromosome 3, the chromosome 3p area of minimal deletion in the renal tumors was too large to search by conventional cloning strategies available at the time. This then led investigators to initiate studies of the familial form of renal carcinoma associated with VHL disease, with the supposition that the gene for VHL may be involved in the sporadic form of renal carcinoma.

HEREDITARY RENAL CARCINOMA (VON HIPPEL-LINDAU DISEASE)

VHL disease is a familial cancer syndrome in which affected individuals develop tumors in a number of organs, including kidney, cerebellum, spine, eyes, pancreas, adrenal glands, inner ear, and epididymis.[1,2] Patients with VHL disease often develop early-onset, bilateral, multifocal renal carcinoma and multiple renal cysts. Frequently, renal tumors are found growing inside the renal cysts. The renal carcinoma in VHL patients is uniformly clear cell renal carcinoma.[21] It has been estimated that up to 600 clear cell renal carcinomas and 1100 benign or atypical cysts may be found per kidney in an affected VHL patient.[22] These kidney cancers are malignant and have been reported to metastasize in up to 40% of untreated patients. The cerebellar and spinal hemangioblastomas are multifocal and marked by extreme vascularity. Although these central nervous system tumors are benign, they can cause significant morbidity. The retinal angiomas can be the first clinical manifestation of VHL. These benign, hypervascular retinal tumors can be detected as early as 1 year of age. One identified manifestation of VHL is a tumor that develops in the endolymphatic sac of the inner ear.[23] These papillary tumors are low-grade malignancies that rarely metastasize but can invade locally. VHL patients can develop islet cell tumors of the pancreas and pancreatic cysts. The islet cell tumors are rarely functional; however, they can be malignant and can spread.[24,25] Eighteen percent to 20% of VHL patients develop pheochromocytomas.[26–28] These tumors can be bilateral or extraadrenal and can be malignant. The epididymal cystadenomas that VHL patients develop are frequently bilateral and are uniformly benign[2,29] (Fig. 34.1-2).

Localization of the von Hippel-Lindau Gene to Chromosome 3

To identify the VHL gene, studies were carried out to perform genetic linkage analysis on chromosome 3p. The VHL gene was initially mapped to a 6- to 8-centimorgan (cM) region of chromosome 3 at 3p25-26.[30–32] Subsequent multipoint linkage analysis localized the VHL gene to a 4-cM interval at 3p26 between RAF1 and the anonymous marker D3S18.[33] No evidence for genetic heterogeneity was identified.[31,32,34] However, early evidence was found for clinical heterogeneity; kindreds with different tumor phenotypes were identified.[34] The VHL gene was found to have characteristics of a tumor suppressor gene. Tory et al.[35] studied VHL renal carcinomas and showed loss of the chromosome 3p, which carried the wild-type allele of the VHL gene. Knudson's model[36] and the finding of frequent LOH in sporadic renal carcinoma[14–17] suggested that

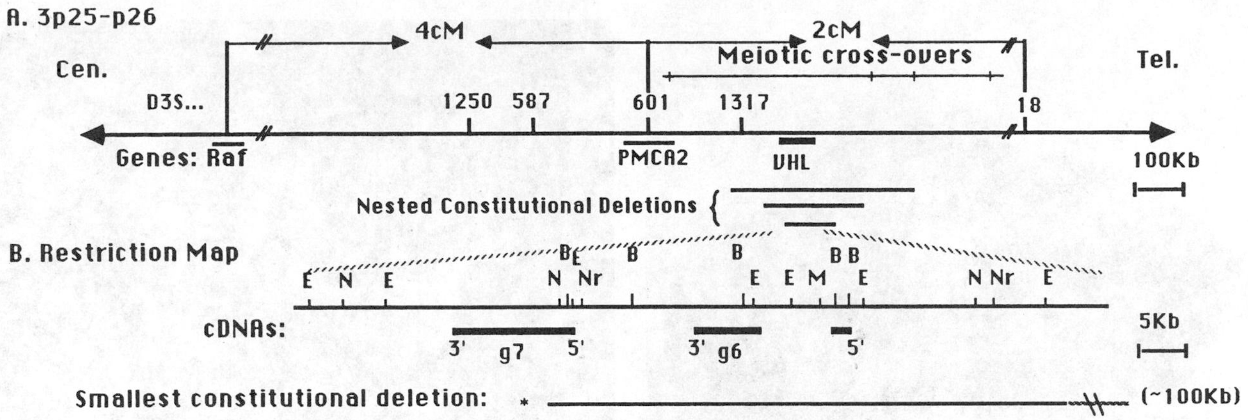

FIGURE 34.1-2. Physical **(A)** and genetic **(B)** map of the von Hippel-Lindau (VHL) region which was used to identify the VHL gene. cDNAs, complementary DNAs; Cen., centromere; Tel., telomere. (From ref. 39, with permission.)

inactivation of both copies of the VHL gene was an early step in renal carcinogenesis (Fig. 34.1-3).

Identification of the von Hippel-Lindau Gene

A critical step in identification of the VHL gene was the finding by Yao et al.[37] and Richards et al.[38] of overlapping germline deletions in unrelated VHL kindreds. The detection of these nested germline deletions in the VHL kindreds was crucial for detection of candidate complementary DNAs for the VHL gene. In 1993, Latif et al.[39] reported the identification of the VHL gene. In the initial report, rearrangements of the VHL gene were detected in 28 of 221 VHL kindreds. Eighteen of the rearrangements were due to deletions of the VHL gene, including three nonoverlapping deletions. Intragenic mutations that segregated with the disease were detected in three VHL kindreds.[39] The initial sequence of the VHL complementary DNA revealed a short open reading frame encoding only 284 amino acids, the remainder representing a large 3' untranslated region of the gene. Neither the predicted amino acid nor the nucleotide sequences showed any significant homology to proteins or genes in the databases.[39]

Genotype and Phenotype Correlations: von Hippel-Lindau Subtype Classification

In the initial studies, Chen et al.[40] detected mutations in 85 of 114 families (75%). Stolle et al.[41] developed an improved method for detection of germline mutations in the VHL gene and reported detection of germline mutations in the VHL gene in 99% of VHL families tested. Striking correlations were noted between the germline mutations and the clinical phenotype. VHL families are classified as VHL type 1 (families without pheochromocytoma) and VHL type 2 (families with

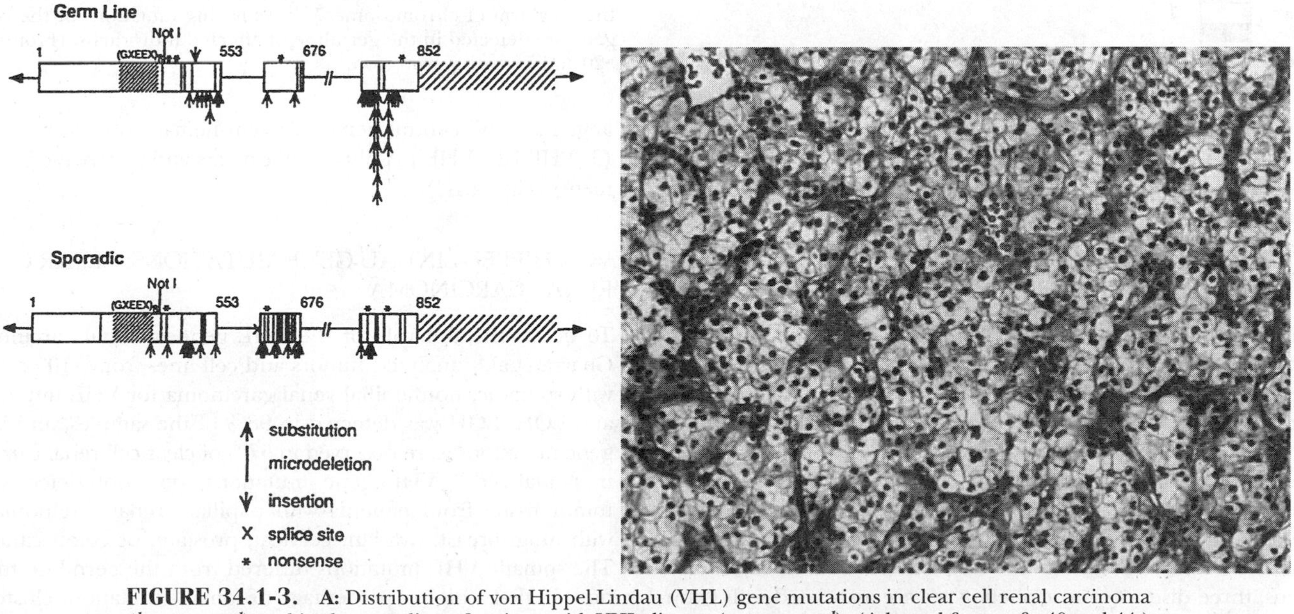

FIGURE 34.1-3. **A:** Distribution of von Hippel-Lindau (VHL) gene mutations in clear cell renal carcinoma (*lower panel*) and in the germline of patients with VHL disease (*upper panel*). (Adapted from refs. 40 and 44.) **B:** Clear cell renal carcinoma is characterized by mutation of the VHL gene. (See Color Fig. 34.1-3*B* in the CD-ROM and on the Web at www.LWWoncology.com.)

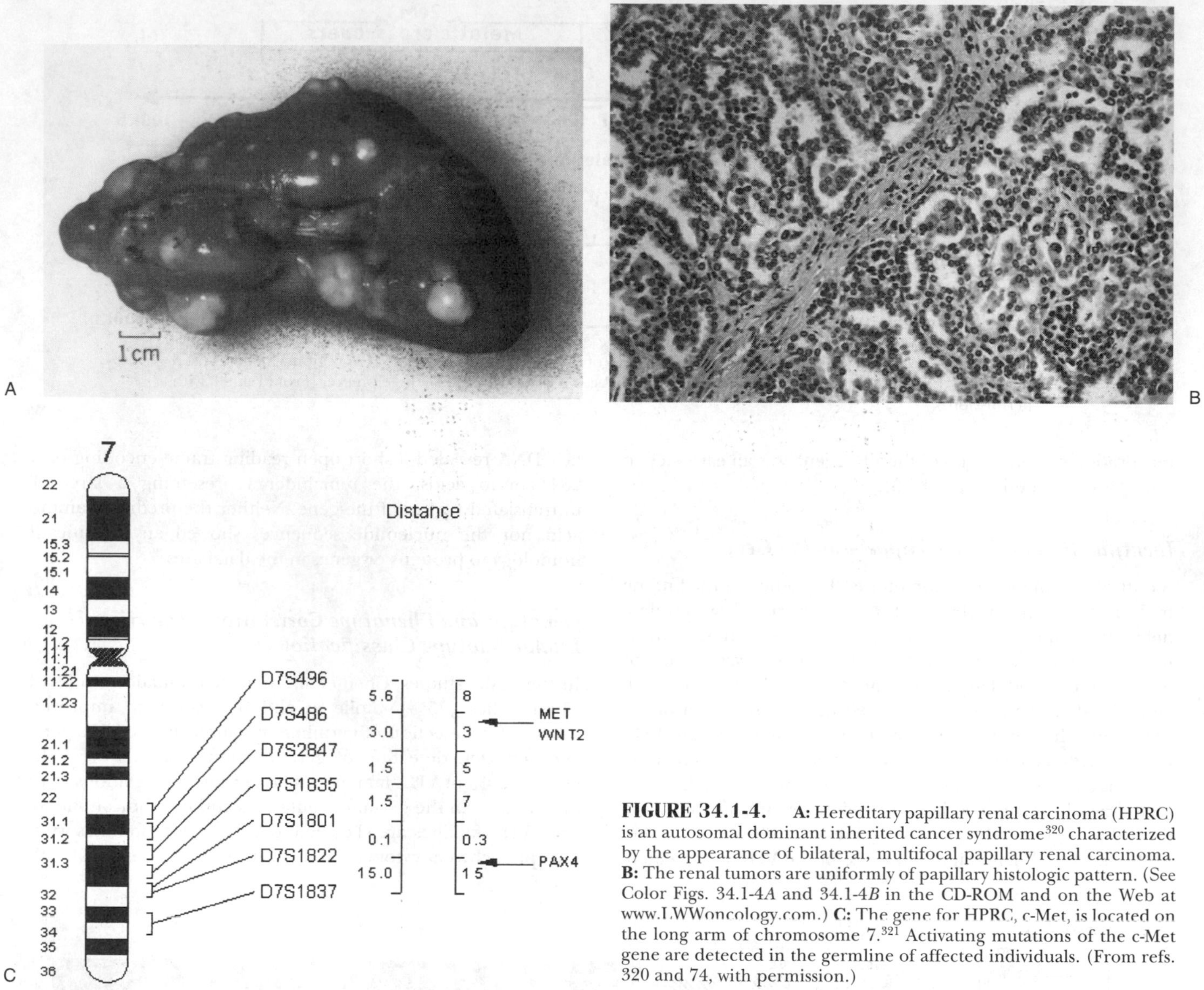

FIGURE 34.1-4. **A:** Hereditary papillary renal carcinoma (HPRC) is an autosomal dominant inherited cancer syndrome[320] characterized by the appearance of bilateral, multifocal papillary renal carcinoma. **B:** The renal tumors are uniformly of papillary histologic pattern. (See Color Figs. 34.1-4*A* and 34.1-4*B* in the CD-ROM and on the Web at www.LWWoncology.com.) **C:** The gene for HPRC, c-Met, is located on the long arm of chromosome 7.[321] Activating mutations of the c-Met gene are detected in the germline of affected individuals. (From refs. 320 and 74, with permission.)

pheochromocytoma). Whereas 56% of the mutations associated with VHL type 1 were insertions or microdeletions, nonsense mutations, or length mutations, 96% of the mutations associated with VHL type 2 were missense mutations. Crossey et al.[42] detected missense VHL gene mutations in 9 of 11 families with pheochromocytoma, and large deletions or mutations predicted to cause a truncated protein in 36 of 53 families without pheochromocytoma. When Zbar et al.[43] analyzed mutations in 473 families from North America, Europe, and Japan, germline mutations were detected in 299 of 473 families (63%) tested. Mutations predicted to produce full length, mutant VHL proteins were detected in 89% of VHL families with pheochromocytoma with mutations detected. A mutation hot spot was identified at a CpG island in codon 167, where 12% of the mutations were found. The codon 167 mutations were associated with a phenotype characterized by few to no renal carcinomas and frequent pheochromocytomas.[43] Thus, three distinct cancer phenotypes are associated with germline VHL gene mutations: (1) VHL type 1 (VHL without pheochromocytoma), (2) VHL IIA (pheochromocytomas, retinal angiomas, and central nervous system hemangioblastomas), and (3) VHL IIB (VHL IIA plus renal cancers and pancreatic involvement) (Fig. 34.1-4).

VON HIPPEL-LINDAU GENE MUTATIONS: CLEAR CELL RENAL CARCINOMA

To determine the role of the VHL gene in renal carcinoma, Gnarra et al.[44] analyzed tumors and cell lines from 110 patients with sporadic, nonfamilial renal carcinoma for VHL mutations and LOH. LOH was detected in 98% of the samples, and VHL gene mutations were observed in 57% of clear cell renal carcinomas analyzed.[44] VHL gene mutations were not detected in tumor tissue from patients with papillary renal carcinoma or with lung, breast, ovarian, cervical, prostate, or colon cancers. The somatic VHL mutations differed from the germline mutations in that a higher percentage of somatic mutations clustered in exon 2 than were detected in the germlines. VHL gene mutations were found in early- and late-stage clear cell renal carcinomas, and when multiple samples were tested from the same patient, the identical mutation was found. Shuin et al.[45] detected somatic mutations in 56% of primary renal carcinomas and an 84% LOH of the VHL gene. Whaley et al.[46] detected somatic VHL in renal carcinoma and no mutations in more than180 sporadic tumors of other types. VHL gene mutations have been identified in clear cell renal carcinomas in Europe,[42,47–51] Japan,[45] and North America.[44,52,53] VHL gene mutations also have been detected in tumor tissue from patients from the 3;8 translocation family described by Cohen et al.[11,44,54] and from tumor tissue from patients with 2;3 translocations,[55,56] further supporting the conclusion that the VHL gene has an important and specific role in clear cell renal carcinoma.

Silencing of the von Hippel-Lindau Gene by DNA Methylation in Renal Carcinoma

Herman et al.[57] demonstrated that hypermethylation of a normally unmethylated CpG island in the 5' region of the VHL gene provides another important mechanism for inactivation of the VHL gene in a significant portion of clear cell renal carcinomas. In 5 of 27 (19%) of the renal tumors evaluated, hypermethylation of the VHL gene was found. The VHL gene is expressed normally in both nonneoplastic kidney and in renal carcinomas with inactivating VHL gene mutations. However, as would be predicted as a consequence of methylation of a 5' CpG island, none of the five renal tumors expressed the VHL gene.[57] When one of the renal carcinoma cell lines with a hypermethylated (and silent) VHL gene was treated with the hypomethylating agent (5-aza-2'deoxycytidine), the VHL transcript was reexpressed, revealing that methylation of the gene was associated with nonexpression. Further studies are needed to determine the prevalence of hypermethylation of the VHL gene in sporadic clear cell renal carcinomas and the potential role of such hypomethylating agents as 5-aza-2'deoxycytidine.[2,57]

The VHL Gene Has the Characteristics of a Tumor Suppressor Gene

Studies of the genetics of VHL and the VHL gene in sporadic renal cell carcinoma have determined that this kidney cancer gene fits Knudson's two-hit model for a tumor suppressor gene.[58] In tumors from VHL patients and from patients with sporadic renal cell carcinoma, a frequent loss of the nonmutant allele is noted, demonstrating that both copies of the VHL gene are inactivated in these tumors.[35,44,59]

CHARACTERISTICS OF THE VON HIPPEL-LINDAU TUMOR SUPPRESSOR GENE PRODUCT

The von Hippel-Lindau Product Is Part of a Multiprotein Complex

When the VHL gene was identified, no significant homology was identified with any known genes. The rat homologue is 88% identical to human VHL; however, it lacks the human protein's NH_2-terminus acidic pentamer repeat.[60] Duan et al.[60] determined that the rat and human VHL proteins formed oligomeric complexes with a number of unidentified proteins in cultured mammalian cells. A complex containing proteins of apparent molecular masses of 9 and 16 kD and VHL was the most consistently observed.[60] When certain naturally occurring VHL missense mutations were introduced into the VHL gene in COS-7 cells, complete or partial loss of the p16-p9 complex was observed. When the p16 and p9 proteins were purified and sequenced, they were found to be part of the elongin (SIII) complex. Elongin (SIII) is a heterotrimer consisting of two regulatory subunits (B and C) and a transcriptionally active subunit (A) that activate transcription elongation by RNA polymerase II.[61] The VHL protein binds specifically and tightly to elongin B and C *in vitro*. Kibel et al.[62] demonstrated that the region of binding of the VHL protein to elongin B and C is in a short, colinear region of the VHL protein that is frequently mutated in renal carcinomas. These studies suggest that the tumor suppression function of the VHL protein may be associated with its ability to bind to elongin B and C.[62]

Cul-2 is a Component of the von Hippel-Lindau Complex

A series of studies have been performed to determine that Cul-2 is a part of the VHL complex.[63,64] Cul-2 is from a family of proteins called *cullins*, which are highly homologous to the *Saccharomyces cerevisiae* protein Cdc53p.[65] Based on the apparent similarity of members of the VHL multiprotein complex with yeast proteins (e.g., elongin C and Cul2 to Skp1 and Cdc53, respectively), a model for the regulation of hypoxia-inducible messenger RNAs (mRNAs) has been developed.

Regulation of Vascular Endothelial Growth Factor Messenger RNA by the von Hippel-Lindau Product

Angiogenesis is a marked feature in the clinical manifestation of VHL and sporadic clear cell renal carcinoma. A number of growth factors have been implicated in angiogenesis, including vascular endothelial growth factor (VEGF). VEGF is markedly elevated in renal carcinomas and in VHL-associated tumors.[66–69] The VHL gene product has been found to regulate the stability of VEGF mRNA,[66,70] potentially explaining the increased VEGF levels in these tumors and providing an explanation for the angiogenesis associated with their development. This fact may provide unique opportunities for treatment of patients with these tumors.[53]

Nuclear and Cytoplasmic Localization of the von Hippel-Lindau Gene Product

Duan et al.[60] demonstrated that the VHL protein can be found both in the nucleus and the cytosol of transiently transfected cells. To define the determinants of VHL localization, Lee et al.[71] showed that nuclear transport of VHL is tightly regulated and that it is determined by the density at which the cells are cultured.[71] When the cells in culture are sparse, the VHL protein is found predominantly in the nucleus. When the cells in culture were grown to confluence, the VHL protein is found in the cytoplasm. Deletion mutation analysis revealed that a putative nuclear localization signal is located in the N-terminal region of the VHL gene. This study suggests that VHL nuclear transport is regulated by density of the cells. Understanding this novel physiologic control mechanism could provide unique insights into the role of this multifunctional tumor suppressor gene.

HEREDITARY PAPILLARY RENAL CARCINOMA

Papillary renal carcinoma is a histologic variant of renal carcinoma that is distinct from clear cell renal carcinoma. Whereas clear cell renal carcinoma is characterized by LOH on the short arm of chromosome 3 and mutation of the chromosome 3p VHL gene, neither chromosome 3 LOH nor VHL gene mutation are detected in tumor tissue from patients with papillary renal carcinoma. HPRC, a distinct form of hereditary renal carcinoma, has been described.[72,73] HPRC is an autosomal dominant form of inherited renal carcinoma that is characterized by the appearance of bilateral, multifocal papillary renal carcinoma (i.e., HPRC is distinct from VHL disease or other inherited forms of renal carcinoma).

Hereditary Papillary Renal Carcinoma Is Characterized by Germline Mutation of the MET Gene

Genetic linkage analysis localized the HPRC gene to a 27-cM interval at chromosome 7q31.1-34. Missense mutations were identified in the tyrosine kinase domain of the MET gene in the germline of affected members of HPRC families.[74] Subsequent studies identified MET mutations in two other large North American HPRC families, confirming that the mutation in the MET protooncogene is the basis for HPRC.[75] Activating mutations of the MET gene have been shown to cause malignant transformation *in vitro* and *in vivo*, implicating this gene in both hereditary and sporadic forms of papillary renal carcinoma.[74–76]

These findings support the molecular genetic classification of renal carcinoma between clear cell and papillary renal carcinoma, with clear cell renal carcinoma being characterized by VHL gene mutation. HPRC is characterized by a germline mutation of the Met protooncogene. Understanding of the fundamental genetic basis of these forms of kidney cancer will hopefully lead to better methods for diagnosis, prevention, and therapy of patients with kidney cancer.

PROSTATE CANCER

In 1990, prostate cancer became the most common form of cancer (other than skin cancer) diagnosed in U.S. men, surpassing lung cancer. In 1999, an estimated 200,000 new prostate cancer cases were diagnosed, accounting for more than 35% of all cancers affecting men, and more than 40,000 deaths will result from this disease.[77] Despite these figures, our understanding of the molecular genetics of prostate cancer is still in an embryonic stage. This section provides an overview of the efforts to define and characterize genetic alteration responsible for the initiation and progression of prostate cancer. The first part of this section describes familial prostate cancer and reviews the evidence supporting the existence of a hereditary form of the disease. The second part reviews aspects of somatic alterations found in prostate cancer cells, and the potential role of these genetic changes in the progression of prostate cancer.

MULTISTEP CARCINOGENESIS AND PROSTATE CANCER PROGRESSION

The process of carcinogenesis is complex, requiring a number of steps. In the case of prostate cancer, evidence for this multistep requirement is readily demonstrated in the studies of experimental carcinogenesis in rodent models. In the pioneering studies of Thompson et al.,[78] expression of a single oncogene (ras) in normal prostate cells of the mouse is insufficient for transformation; the overexpression of a second oncogene (myc) is necessary before transformation becomes a frequent event. Even in the case of two oncogenes, not every cell expressing these becomes transformed, suggesting that further steps are necessary, presumably including inactivation of tumor suppressor genes. Although in clinical specimens of human cancers the requirement for multiple steps is less easily demonstrated, the finding of multiple genetic alterations as a common characteristic of human tumors supports this concept.[79]

Application of the multistep concept to carcinogenesis in the human prostate would suggest that incidental or latent cancers (i.e., clinically undetected prostate cancers found in most aged men dying from non–prostate cancer causes at autopsy) as well as putative precursor lesions [i.e., prostatic intraepithelial neoplasia (PIN)][80] have undergone only a subset of the steps, "hits," or mutations necessary for the emergence of the fully malignant phenotype. Furthermore, this hypothesis would suggest that specific and discrete genetic alterations may be associated with different stages and even grades of prostate cancer. Although such a hypothesis is attractive, no definite proof has been provided to suggest that this is the case, although certain specific mutations (e.g., in the p53 gene) have been shown to be strongly associated with progression of prostate cancer.[81–85]

What are the molecular events responsible for the progression of prostate cancer, or, in other words, why and how does prostate cancer evolve from an indolent to a life-threatening disease? Is this evolution inevitable, or are some prostate cancers destined never to progress to advanced disease, let alone clinically detectable disease, regardless of the time frame provided? Conversely, are some prostate cancers capable of metastasis very early in their natural history? A critical issue for addressing these questions effectively is to understand the mechanisms of prostate cancer progression in molecular genetic terms, particularly if therapeutic approaches aimed at blocking this progression are to be other than empirically based.

PROSTATE CANCER INITIATION AND PROGRESSION: GENETICS VERSUS ENVIRONMENT

The *initiation* of prostate cancer (i.e., the formation of a histologically identifiable lesion) appears to be a very frequent event, occurring in one-third of men older than 45 years.[86] Geographically, this rate of histologic cancer incidence is roughly the same worldwide.[87,88] The number of clinically manifest cases and the mortality rates, however, differ widely among various populations, strongly suggesting important environmental factors in modulating the transition between tumor initiation and progression.[89] This feature of prostate cancer is emphasized by studies demonstrating large increases in prostate cancer incidence in Japanese men (a low-risk population) when they move to the United States.[90]

On the other hand, studies of familial aggregation of this disease have suggested that between 5% and 10% of prostate cancers may be directly attributable to the inheritance of dominant prostate cancer susceptibility alleles, which may act as genetic factors driving this progression independent of environmental exposure. Thus, as with numerous other cancers, strong evidence indicates both genetic and environmental factors in the etiology of prostate cancer, with the majority of disease most likely being a result of the interaction the two.[91]

HEREDITARY PROSTATE CANCER

Although not widely recognized as having a strong familial component until more recently, evidence demonstrating familial clustering of prostate cancer has been available as early as 1960 from studies of the Utah Mormon population,[92] and multiple subsequent studies have confirmed this observation.[93–98] Two large studies are of particular interest in answering the question of whether prostate cancer clusters in families. Cannon et al.[99] published a genetic epidemiologic study on prostate cancer in the Utah Mormon population. Notably, prostate cancer showed the fourth strongest degree of familial clustering after lip cancer, skin melanoma, and ovarian cancer. Prostate cancer had a higher familiality than both colon and breast carcinoma, two solid tumors that are well recognized as having a genetic or familial component.

A case-control study of patients treated for prostate cancer at Johns Hopkins University School of Medicine was carried out to assess the extent of familial aggregation in prostate cancer.[100] Extensive cancer pedigrees were obtained for 691 men with prostate cancer and 640 spouse controls. A positive family history of prostate cancer was the only consistent risk factor found in this study. Men with a father or brother affected were twice as likely to develop prostate cancer as men with no relatives affected. In addition, a trend of increasing risk was found with increasing number of affected family members, such that men with two or three first-degree relatives affected had a five- and 11-fold increased risk of developing prostate cancer. Cox proportional hazards analysis in the case relatives revealed that risk was particularly increased to relatives of younger probands (younger than 55 years).

These studies suggest a familial clustering in risk to prostate cancer but do not directly address the underlying etiologic mechanism. It is important to note that familial clustering could as easily reflect a shared environmental risk factor as a genetic mechanism. To directly address this question and to test whether a Mendelian form of prostate cancer could explain the observed clustering of this disease, segregation analyses have been carried out. Carter et al.[101] suggested that familial clustering of prostate cancer was best explained by dominant inheritance of a rare (estimated population frequency = 0.003) high-risk allele. The estimated cumulative risk of clinically evident prostate cancer revealed that the allele was highly penetrant: By 85 years of age, 88% of the carriers are projected to be affected with prostate cancer, compared with only 5% of the noncarriers. This model suggests that the inherited form of prostate cancer may account for a significant portion (43%) of early-onset disease (disease onset before 55 years of age), although it represents only a small proportion (9% by age 85) of all prostate cancer occurrences. Furthermore, these analyses demonstrate that families with multiple affected members and early onset of disease are most likely to have a Mendelian form of prostate cancer, and thus are most appropriate for linkage analysis. Additional segregation analyses by Gronberg at al.[102] and Schaid et al.[103] provide further support for the existence of dominantly acting prostate cancer susceptibility alleles.

These results emphasize that the genetics of prostate cancer are likely similar to those of colon and breast cancer, in which a subset of the disease occurs in persons who inherit defective copies of one of a series of critical, rate-limiting steps required for neoplastic transformation. Just as linkage studies in families with multiple members affected with these diseases were critical to the identification of colon and breast cancer susceptibility genes (e.g., APC, hMSH2, BRCA1, BRCA2), linkage analyses in prostate cancer families are an active area of study. As of 1999, four separate loci suspected of harboring hereditary prostate cancer genes have been reported (Table 34.1-1). Three of these loci are on chromosome 1, and the fourth is on the X chromosome. The finding of multiple distinct loci, along with the high likelihood that multiple additional loci will be identified, emphasizes the extensive and potentially complex genetic heterogeneity that characterizes hereditary prostate cancer. Only when these genes are cloned and characterized will their contributions to the underlying pathogenesis of this disease be assessable.

TABLE 34.1-1. Prostate Cancer Susceptibility Loci Identified by Linkage Studies

Locus	*Chromosomal Location*	*Reference*
HPC1	1q24-25	Smith et al. (1996)[104]
HPCX	Xq27-28	Xu et al. (1998)[105]
PCAP	1q42-43	Berthon et al. (1998)[106]
CAPB	1p36	Gibbs et al. (1999)[107]

SOMATIC ALTERATIONS IN PROSTATE CANCER

Role of Oncogenes

A number of oncogenes have been examined in prostate cancer tissue and cell lines, primarily at the expression level, including ras, myc, sis, fos, EGFR, and ERBB2 (reviewed by Strohmeyer and Slamon[108]). Expression of each of these genes and, in some cases, overexpression when compared to normal genes has been detected in prostate cancer cells, but at widely varying frequencies. None of these genes have been observed to undergo mutational activation in a majority of prostate cancers, and the mechanisms responsible for their overexpression, when present, remain largely undefined. Of particular interest in this regard is the study by Bubendorf et al.,[109] which demonstrated that, whereas gene amplifications of ERBB2 and NMYC were never observed in any stage prostate cancer, the androgen receptor gene, myc, and cyclin D1 were observed to be amplified in 22%, 11%, and 5% of hormone-refractory, metastatic prostate cancers, respectively.

RAS. Several studies provided early evidence of a potentially important role for activated ras genes in prostate cancer, particularly in rodent models.[78,110] Peehl et al.,[111] using DNA transfection experiments, were the first to demonstrate the presence of an activated K-ras gene in a human prostate cancer specimen. Subsequent studies found low frequencies of ras gene mutations in both localized and metastatic prostate cancer (less than 4%).[112–115] These results, all obtained in North American patients, demonstrate that activation of ras oncogenes via point mutation is not a common event in either the initiation or progression of prostatic neoplasia.

In contrast to these studies, other reports examining prostate tissue from Japanese men suggest that ras gene mutations *do* occur at significant frequencies (approximately 25%) in prostate cancer, both in latent carcinoma[116] and clinically manifest disease.[117] These studies raise the interesting possibility that significant differences may exist in the genetic events associated with prostate cancer in American men compared with Japanese men (wherein the latter have an approximately fivefold lower incidence rate of clinically manifest disease).

Additionally, in this latter study,[117] human papillomavirus DNA was detected in more than 40% of the prostate cancer samples analyzed. The detection of human papillomavirus DNA in prostate cancer from North American men is controversial, but the most recent evidence[118–120] suggests that this family of viruses is not commonly found in prostate cancer, at least not at levels comparable to those found in cervical cancer, in which a definitive etiologic link has been established.

C-MYC. The c-myc gene has been implicated in prostate cancer since the experimental carcinogenesis studies of Thompson et al.[78] A role for c-myc overexpression as an important aspect of prostate cancer has been suggested by the frequent finding of increased copy number of the portion of 8q containing the c-myc gene in clinical prostate cancer specimens, particularly advanced cases. Sato et al.[121] observed that cases of prostate cancer characterized by fluorescence *in situ* hybridization (FISH) as having more copies of c-myc than copies of chromosome 8 centromere were highly associated with poor outcomes.

bcl-2: An Inhibitor of Apoptosis

The bcl-2 gene is located on chromosome 18q21. It was identified because of its involvement at the breakpoint of the t(14;18) interchromosomal translocation occurring in human follicular B-cell lymphomas.[122] This translocation results in enhanced expression of the bcl-2 gene.[123,124] The bcl-2 gene encodes for a membrane-bound 26-kD protein.[125] bcl-2 has been demonstrated to be an oncogene, in that its induced overexpression can lead to malignant transformation.[123] bcl-2 is unique among oncogenes, however, in that its expression does not enhance the rate of cell proliferation, but instead decreases the rate of cell death.[123,124] The role of bcl-2 in the development and progression of carcinoma of the prostate has been examined by McDonnell et al.[125] Using immunohistochemical (IHC) techniques, bcl-2 is not usually expressed in androgen-dependent prostatic cancer cells, whereas it is expressed in androgen-independent prostatic cancer cells.[125] This observation has been confirmed by Colombel et al.[126] These findings suggest that enhanced expression of bcl-2 protein in carcinomas of the prostate is associated with the transition to androgen independence.

Androgen Receptor

The role of androgen in normal prostate physiology is unquestioned, because these hormones are strictly required for normal development and maintenance of prostate growth and function. However, the role of androgens and androgen receptors (*AR*) in prostate cancer is much less clear. Studies have generated a great deal of renewed interest in this pathway and its role in the critical progression of prostate cancer to androgen independence. An initial hypothesis that loss of *AR* gene expression may be important in androgen-independent disease was not supported by several studies that showed continued or even elevated *AR* gene expression in androgen-independent tumors.[127,128] Newmark et al.[129] were the first to report a mutated androgen receptor in a clinical specimen of prostate cancer; curiously, it was found in a localized cancer before any hormonal therapy. This and other findings of mutations before hormonal therapy[141] would suggest that mutant *AR* might provide a growth advantage, even in the presence of normal androgen levels. Kelly et al.[130] and Sartor et al.[131] described a number of patients who experienced a paradoxical response to withdrawal of the antiandrogen, flutamide, in that a number of clinical parameters (e.g., prostate-specific antigen levels, bone pain) improved on cessation of drug treatment. One explanation proposed for this response is that such patients harbor *AR* gene mutations similar to those found in the prostate cancer cell line LNCaP (Thr to Ala change at codon 868), which alters the ligand specificity of the receptor such that both estrogens and antiandrogens, as well as androgens, act as agonists.[132,133] The frequency of such mutations in prostate cancer patients is unknown, but a study by Taplin et al.[134] found five of ten samples of hormone-refractory prostate cancer metastatic to bone had mutations of the *AR* gene, and at least two of these mutations resulted in a shift in hormone specificity of *AR*. Visakorpi et al.[135] demonstrated that up to 30% of prostate cancer specimens from men unsuccessful with hormonal therapy are characterized by increases in copy number of the X chromosomal region (q11-q13) containing the androgen receptor. These results suggest that instead of being insensitive to androgen, such tumors may become supersensitive to androgen by an as yet undetermined mechanism, or perhaps sensitive to a different nonandrogen steroid hormone. Furthermore, a number of studies suggest that via novel interaction with other growth factor or signaling pathways, the requirement for androgen binding to the receptor may be bypassed.[136,137] Thus, although the precise role of androgen and the androgen receptor is still being defined, it is possible that altered regulation of the pathway plays a fundamental role in prostate cancer progression to androgen-independent disease.

Chromosomal Deletions in Prostate Cancer

Unlike other solid tumors, such as renal cell carcinoma, cytogenetic analyses of prostate cancer specimens have revealed few consistent chromosomal deletions.[138,139] An early cytogenetic study by Atkin and Baker,[140] however, suggested chromosomes 7q and 10q as the sites of frequent chromosomal losses in prostate cancer. Early studies of allelic loss by Carter et al.[141] and Kunimi et al.[142] confirmed frequent LOH on chromosome 10 and also highlighted portions of chromosomes 16 and 8 as being frequently deleted in clinical specimens of prostate cancer. Deletion mapping studies by Bergerheim et al.[143] suggested that the critical regions resided between pter and the plasminogen activator, tissue type locus at p12-q11.2 on chromosome 8 and q22.1 and qter on chromosome 16. Interestingly, loss of chromosome 8p in prostate cancer had been previously observed in a study by Konig et al.,[145] who found cytogenetic evidence of chromosome 8p deletions in a number of prostate cancer xenografts, and suggested a correlation existed between loss of this region and the development of androgen independence.

Of the chromosomal regions analyzed in prostate cancer, the short arm of chromosome 8 has received the most attention, because it appears to be the most frequent site of LOH, occurring in the majority of cases of prostate cancer examined. Two or possibly three distinct regions of LOH occur on this chromosomal arm, with the region 8p21-12 being deleted in the majority of prostate cancer precursor lesions (PIN). More distally, 8p22 is deleted in most adenocarcinomas.[145–150] In this latter region, a homozygous deletion of approximately 1 megabase has been observed.[151] Subregional deletion analysis of chromosome 8p in prostate cancer has been performed using a variety of molecular methods, all of which have confirmed a high frequency of loss in this region, especially, but not exclusively, within chromosome band 8p22.[143–148,152–157] The rate of 8p22 loss reported in these regions varies from 32% to 65% in primary tumors and from 65% to 100% in DNA derived from metastases.

Separate discrete regions of loss in more proximal regions, including 8p21[147,150] and 8p12,[148,150] have been described. Frequent loss (63%) of portions of 8p21-p12 have been identified in PIN lesions,[149] suggesting that a gene in this area may become frequently inactivated at a relatively early stage in prostate tumorigenesis. Evidence of heterogeneity of 8p LOH among different PIN lesions within the same gland was observed.[149] A combined comparative genomic hybridization (CGH), Southern, and microsatellite study has shown loss of chromosome 8p22-p12 in 80% of prostate cancer lymph node metastases.[158] Microcell transfer of human chromosome 8 into a rat prostate cancer cell line has been reported to suppress metastatic ability.[159] An association of chromosome 8p loss and higher stage has been reported.[148]

Several 8p candidate tumor suppressor genes have been identified, including N33, which is located in a homozygously deleted region of 8p22. This novel gene is expressed in many normal tissues but not in some cancers, most notably those of the colon.[160] Other candidate genes identified on this chromosomal arm include the putative transcription factor FEZ1[161] and an androgen-regulated homeobox gene, NKX3.1.[162]

The frequent loss of sequences on chromosome 8p provides a marker to determine the similarity or difference between primary prostate cancers and their metastases. This approach has been used to determine the concordance rates for 8p loss in a series of PIN, primary, and metastatic lesions obtained from the same patient.[153] Cases were observed in which there was a complete concordance in that all samples of cancer had retained or lost the same 8p marker, but cases also were noted in which the PIN sample would show loss, but not the primary tumor or the lymph node tumor samples. In addition, some cases showed differences among the multiple primary lesions within the prostate. These data and similar findings[163] demonstrate the complex genetic relationship that exists between primary and metastatic lesions and suggest that the primary prostate cancer that gives rise to a given metastatic deposit is not easily predicted on the basis of morphologic characteristics.

Concomitant with deletion of sequences from the short arm, chromosome 8 is frequently affected by gain of sequences on the long arm. First observed by Southern analysis,[145] a CGH study of lymph node metastases indicated that 85% of such tumors showed evidence of 8q gain, making this the most common numerical alteration observed in this study.[158] Van den Berg et al.[164] reported that gain of 8q sequences in prostate cancer was highly correlated with disease progression. Similarly, in the CGH study of Visakorpi et al.,[157] gain of 8q sequences was seen in 89% of tumor recurrences after hormonal therapy, whereas only 6% of primary tumors showed this alteration. An obvious candidate gene that may be the target of these amplification events in prostate cancer is the oncogene *c-myc*, which is located at 8q24, although most of the amplification events on 8q are large, suggesting that many genes are affected. In this respect, two other 8q genes, PSCA and the p40 subunit of translation initiation factor 3, are found to be frequently included in the gained regions of chromosome 8 and show increased expression in a subset of prostate cancers.[165,166]

Comparative Genomic Hybridization Analysis of Prostate Cancer

Visakorpi et al.[157] used CGH to survey the genome of a series of both untreated, localized prostate cancers and tumors from patients unsuccessful on hormonal therapy. This important study found chromosome 8p to be the most frequently deleted, followed by 13q, 6q, 16q, 18q, and 9p. In a series of nine advanced prostate cancers from men unsuccessful with hormonal therapy, a significant increase was found in deletions of chromosome 5q and gains of chromosomes 7p, 8q, and X, when compared to untreated primary tumor samples. Evidence has been found that the androgen receptor gene may be the target of gene amplification events on this latter chromosome.[167] Thus, these studies confirm previous studies of allelic loss in prostate cancer and, at the same time, expand the chromosomal regions implicated as harboring "prostate cancer genes."

Specific Gene Alterations in Prostate Cancer

A number of genes have been found to be mutated in prostate cancer, including *p53, PTEN, Rb, ras, CDKN2, AR, MXI1,* and *POLB,* although the latter two, located on chromosomes 10q25 and 8p11.2, respectively, remain to be confirmed. *ras* mutations are uncommon (fewer than 5% of cases),[112,114,115] as are point mutations of *Rb*,[168] although loss of one copy of *Rb* readily occurs. To date, the most consistently observed site of point mutations is the *p53* gene, and these mutations are common only in advanced disease. Microsatellite instability is uncommon but detectable in prostate cancer,[169] and the hPMS2 gene has been found to be mutated in a prostate cancer cell line that exhibits this phenotype.[170]

P53. *p53* mutations are uncommon in localized disease but become frequent in deposits of metastatic prostate cancer, particularly those to bone.[81–83,171–174] Observed heterogeneity of *p53* mutations within different tumors in the same gland, and within different regions of the same gland, appears to be a somewhat unique feature of prostate cancer.[175,176] Furthermore, LOH and point mutation of *p53* do not appear to be tightly coupled in this disease.[177] A large number of studies have examined the prognostic significance of nuclear p53 protein immunostaining in both localized and advanced prostate cancer,[178–191] and although the results are somewhat disparate, two conclusions can be drawn: (1) p53 staining tends to be very heterogeneous, resulting in problems for scoring and interpretation of staining results and in inconsistencies due to sampling biases; and (2) in general, tumors with positive p53 staining are associated with a worse prognosis.

PTEN. A series of studies have examined prostate cancer specimens for alterations in the dual function phosphatase gene *PTEN* and found that this gene is inactivated by a combination of mechanisms, including hemi- and homozygous deletion,[192–197] point mutation,[192,193,196] and promoter methylation.[197] These changes are observed most commonly in advanced disease, and they may play a role in the acquisition of metastatic potential. However, McMenamin et al.[198] demonstrated that the majority of clinically localized prostate cancers had abnormal PTEN protein expression, with one in five cases being completely negative.

Wu et al.[199] demonstrated that, in prostate cancer cells lines with inactivated PTEN, the AKT/phosphoinositide 3 kinase pathway is constitutively activated due to increased accumulation of the PTEN substrate PIP3. Activation of this pathway results in suppression of apoptosis and increased cell survival. These findings have stimulated extensive interest in these pathways as novel therapeutic targets in advanced prostate cancer.

Rb. The importance of *Rb* gene inactivation in prostate cancer was initially suggested by the studies of Bookstein et al.,[200,201] who demonstrated the presence of inactivating mutations in the *Rb* gene in clinical specimens of prostate cancer, as well as the ability of reintroduction of a cloned copy of *Rb* to suppress the tumorigenicity of DU145 prostate cancer cells, which had been shown to produce a nonfunctional truncated *Rb* protein. Combined CGH and LOH studies reveal that one copy of *Rb* is lost in advanced prostate cancer at rates approaching 80%,[158] although limited sequencing studies suggest that point mutations are present in fewer than 20% of clinical samples.[168] IHC studies of *Rb* expression demonstrate lack of expression in 10% to 22% of tumors, with a questionable correlation between tumor LOH of *Rb* and lack of expression.[202,203] These data, together with LOH events on 13q that do not include *Rb*, suggest the presence of an additional or alternative prostate tumor suppressor gene near the *Rb* locus.[203]

CDKN2. Much attention has been focused on the *p16/CDKN2* gene, a negative regulator of cell-cycle progression located at chromosome 9p21, since the finding of frequent homozygous deletions in a wide variety of cancer cell lines.[204] A relatively high frequency of homozygous (approximately 20%)[205] and hemizygous losses of *CDKN2* have been observed in clinical specimens of prostate cancer.[206] In the latter case, loss events in the vicinity of the *CDKN2* gene are more common in metastatic deposits of prostate cancer (43% vs. 20% in primary tumors). In a small but detectable fraction of tumors (approximately 15%), the *CDKN2* gene shows evidence of inactivation by promoter methylation.[206] Whether all of the allelic loss events at 9p21 in prostate cancer are associated with *CDKN2* inactivation or whether they reflect inactivation of a neighboring gene (e.g., *p15*) has not been determined.

P27 (CDKN1B). A number of studies that reduced levels of the cyclin kinase inhibitor *p27* are associated with a more aggressive prostate cancer phenotype,[207–209] although the mechanism of this down-regulation is not clear. Interestingly, Kibel et al.[210] described a homozygous deletion of the *p27* gene in a lethal case of prostate cancer, and in a high frequency of LOH of *p27* in advanced prostate cancers in general. Thus, it is possible that, in prostate cancer, in addition to increased ubiquitin-mediated p27 protein degradation, which has been demonstrated in colon and other cancers, at least a subset of lesions may inactivate this gene via deletion.

E-CADHERIN AND KAI-1. Genes whose down-regulation has been implicated in prostate cancer progression include the cell adhesion molecule genes E-cadherin and KAI-1, which are located at chromosomes 16q22.1 (a frequent site of LOH) and 11p11.2, respectively.[211] E-cadherin protein levels are frequently reduced in high-grade prostate cancers, and this finding has prognostic significance.[212–214] KAI-1 was identified by its ability to suppress metastasis in experimental animal studies.[211,215] Although the predominate mechanism for down-regulation of these genes has not been determined, in the case of E-cadherin, gene inactivation via promoter methylation has been found in prostate cancer cell lines and at a low but detectable rate in clinical specimens of prostate cancer.[216]

GSTΠ. Similarly, the gene for the phase II detoxification enzyme glutathione S-transferase π, has also been found to be extensively methylated in the promoter region, in a completely cancer-specific fashion, with concomitant absence of expression.[217] In fact, this methylation event, being found in more than 90% of all prostate cancers and in PIN lesions, is the most common genomic alteration yet observed in prostate cancer. The mechanism by which this region becomes specifically methylated in prostate cancer and the basis for its apparent selection in the carcinogenic pathway is unclear at present. Because this enzyme is a key part of an important cellular pathway to prevent damage from a wide range of carcinogens, the inactivation of this activity may result in increased susceptibility of prostate tissue to both tumor initiation and progression resulting from an increased rate of accumulated DNA damage. Indeed, reactivation of this or a similar cellular defense pathway, perhaps by dietary intervention, has been proposed as a treatment strategy aimed at blocking the progression of initiated prostate cancer foci.

BLADDER CANCER

Approximately 90% of malignant tumors arising in the urinary bladder are of epithelial origin, the vast majority being transitional cell carcinomas.[218,219] Based on morphologic evaluation and natural history, urothelial neoplasms have been classified into two groups having distinct behavior and prognosis: low-grade tumors (always papillary and usually superficial) and high-grade tumors (either papillary or nonpapillary, and often invasive).[220] Clinically, superficial bladder tumors (stage pTa, pTis, and pT1) account for 75% to 85% of neoplasms, whereas the remaining 15% to 25% are invasive (pT2, pT3, pT4) or metastatic (N+, M+) lesions at the time of initial presentation.[221] More than 70% of patients affected with superficial tumors have one or more recurrences after initial treatment, and approximately one-third of those patients progress and eventually succumb to their disease.[222,223] Because clinical staging and morphologic evaluation determine the therapeutic modality, the pathologic assessment of tumor specimens carries significant consequences. However, it is well known that two morphologically similar tumors presenting in any assigned stage may behave in different fashions, a fact that seriously hampers the ability to accurately predict clinical outcome. For these reasons, biologic markers and new detection methods are being developed to monitor and identify recurrence and progression in patients treated for superficial disease.[224] The important issues in patients presenting with muscle-invasive carcinomas include metastatic potential and response to neoadjuvant regimens. The implementation of objective predictive assays will enhance our ability to assess tumor biologic activities and to design effective treatment regimens.

CYTOGENETICS AND INTERPHASE CYTOGENETICS OF BLADDER TUMORS

Cytogenetic studies of bladder cancer cells by karyotyping have revealed a variety of chromosomal abnormalities. Nonrandom chromosomal changes consisting of monosomy of chromosome 9[225,226] and interstitial deletions of chromosome 13[225] have been observed. Other common abnormalities include trisomy of chromosome 7, deletions of chromosomes 11p and 3p, and chromosome 1 alterations.[227–229] However, most of these analyses were performed using small cohorts, lacking clinicopathologic correlations, and combining superficial and muscle-invasive lesions. In one study, Tyrkus et al.[230] karyotyped 17 carcinomas *in situ* of the urinary bladder and found no chromosome 9 alterations, but identified nonrandom chromosomal changes involving chromosomes 1, 5, 8, and 11.

More recent interphase cytogenetic studies have been conducted, mainly using centromeric probes, in a search for numerical alterations in bladder cancer. In addition, new telomeric and locus-specific probes are being used to identify genetic aberrations using nonisotopic detection methods. Podighe and collaborators[231] reported chromosomal alterations at 1q12, as well as numerical abnormalities of chromosomes 1, 7, 9, 11, and 18.[232] Waldman et al.[233] also reported numerical aberration of chromosomes 7, 9, and 11 in 27 bladder tumors.

FISH has been used to assess erbB-2 (17q21) gene amplification and c-myc (8q24) copy number gains in bladder cancer.[234,235] Sauter et al.[234] reported amplification of erbB-2 in 10 of 141 bladder tumors using a dual labeling hybridization assay. Gene amplification was associated with protein overexpression and was found only in tumors with aneusomy of chromosome 17, and more frequently in muscle-invasive lesions.[234] A similar approach was used for the analysis of c-myc gene copy number on 87 bladder tumors. Obvious amplification was found in three cases, whereas 32 of the remaining 84 tumors showed a low-level c-myc copy number increase. No association was found between low-level copy number increase and protein overexpression. However, strong association was demonstrated between c-myc gains and tumor grade, stage, and Ki-67 labeling index, consistent with a role of chromosome 8 alterations in bladder cancer progression.[235] FISH assays also have been used for analyses of specific gene losses. Physical p53 gene deletion (at 17p13) was examined by FISH in 151 bladder tumors.[236] 17p deletion was found to be highly correlated with tumor stage and grade ($P < .01$). FISH has been used more recently to assay bladder irrigation specimens.[237] Labeled probes to centromeric sequences for chromosomes 1, 7, 9, 11, 15, and 17 were used on samples from 76 patients monitored for recurrent bladder tumors. Significantly, 24% of patients with history of bladder cancer but no clinical evidence of disease exhibited monosomy of chromosome 9.[237]

ONCOGENES: MOLECULAR AND IMMUNOPATHOLOGY ANALYSES OF BLADDER TUMORS

The first mutation of the RAS family of oncogenes, a point mutation in codon 12 of the H-RAS gene (11p15.1), was identified in the bladder cancer cell line T24[238] and subsequently identified in bladder cancers.[239] There has been controversy regarding the mutation frequency of RAS genes in bladder tumors. Before the advent of polymerase chain reaction (PCR)-mediated DNA amplification, it was estimated that the rate of point mutations in RAS oncogenes ranged from 10% to 16% of samples analyzed.[240–242] The predominant alteration identified was codon 12 substitutions of the H-RAS gene, with a few cases presenting K-RAS mutations and no mutations detected affecting N-RAS. However, two reports by Czerniak and colleagues,[243,244] using a PCR-based method, revealed that approximately 40% of bladder tumors harbor H-RAS codon 12 mutations. Several studies have confirmed this high frequency of H-RAS point mutations. Ooi et al.[245] studied a cohort of 124 patients affected with pTa or pT1 transitional cell carcinomas. The codon 12 G to T substitution was found in nonrecurring and recurring primary tumors, as well as in initial pTa/T1 lesions from patients who had disease progression. More recently, a prospective study by Fitzgerald et al.[246] reported the detection of mutations in exon 1 of the H-RAS gene in urine sediments from 44 of 100 patients presenting with bladder neoplasms. It should be noted that different members of the RAS family are mutated in distinct tumor types. The frequency of K-RAS mutations in colorectal cancer is approximately 40%,[247,248] whereas mutations of N-RAS are commonly found in hematopoietic neoplasms.[249] Moreover, evidence indicates that mutant RAS alleles are involved in the earlier phases of neoplastic transformation of colorectal carcinomas.[250] Further studies in well-characterized cohorts of patients, using tissue microdissection techniques, are required to delineate the potential role of H-RAS mutations in bladder cancer.

Overexpression and amplification of particular growth factor receptors have been reported in bladder cancer. Neal and coworkers[251] observed increased expression of epidermal growth factor receptors (EGFR) in invasive versus superficial bladder tumors. This group of investigators also reported that overexpression of EGFR was associated with high-grade, high-stage bladder cancer and was an independent prognostic factor.[252] Messing[253] noticed that EGFR was expressed at detectable levels in the basal layer of the normal urothelium, whereas increased expression in basal and suprabasal layers was identified in transitional cell carcinomas. Rao et al.[254] also found increased expression of EGFR in urothelial samples with dysplastic changes, postulating that overexpression of EGFR may be an early event in bladder carcinogenesis. In a more recent study, Nguyen et al.[255] reported that overexpression of EGFR was not an independent prognostic marker in patients with advanced bladder cancer.

Amplification of the c-erbB-2 gene was found in 1 of 14 bladder tumors in a study by Wood and collaborators.[256] This case also displayed overexpression when analyzed for mRNA and protein levels. In addition, five cases displayed high levels of mRNA with no signs of gene amplification, and only three of these five cases had protein overexpression. Sato et al.[257] observed c-erbB-2 protein (p185) overexpression in 23 of 88 bladder tumors analyzed and found a significant association with overexpression and poor clinical outcome, which is an independent prognostic factor. More recently, Underwood et al.[258] studied c-erbB-2 status in 236 bladder tumors. Sixteen of 89 patients with recurrent disease had evidence of c-erbB-2 amplification; however, gene amplification was not observed in the nonrecurrent tumors. A strong association with disease progression and c-erbB-2 amplification was reported. Nevertheless, protein overexpression could not be linked to disease progression. C-erbB-2 amplification was of predictive value in multivariate analysis for overall bladder cancer death; however, stage and grade remained the most significant independent prognostic parameters.[258]

A cellular protooncogene product, mdm2, has been shown to bind to p53 and act as a negative regulator, inhibiting its transcriptional transactivation activity[259] and targeting p53 for ubiquinin-mediated degradation.[260,261] The MDM2 gene is located on the long arm of chromosome 12 (12q13-14) and encodes a 90-kD nuclear protein.[262] Lianes et al.[263] undertook a study to determine the frequency and clinical relevance of identifying MDM2 and TP53 alterations in patients affected with bladder neoplasms. These investigators analyzed a cohort of 87 patients and observed that 26 of 87 cases had abnormally high levels of mdm2 protein; however, only one case showed MDM2 amplification. A striking association was noted between mdm2 overexpression and low-stage/low-grade bladder tumors ($P < .01$). Based on these results, it was concluded that aberrant mdm2 phenotypes are frequent events in bladder cancer and may be involved in tumorigenesis or early tumor progression in urothelial neoplasms. In an independent study, Barbareschi et al.[264] reported mdm2 nuclear overexpression in 5 of 25 bladder tumors analyzed, but this survey lacked clinicopathologic correlations.

TUMOR SUPPRESSOR GENES: MOLECULAR AND IMMUNOPATHOLOGY ANALYSIS OF BLADDER TUMORS

Molecular genetic studies of bladder cancer have identified abnormalities of tumor suppressor genes involved in tumor development and progression. Confirming initial cytogenetic observations, LOH on the short arm of chromosome 11 and 9q allelic losses were reported as frequent events in bladder tumors.[265,266] It was also observed that 17p LOH was a common event[266,267] in high-grade bladder cancer.[267]

In an attempt to define the role of molecular abnormalities of tumor suppressor genes in the pathogenesis and progression of human bladder cancer, a combined molecular genetics and immunopathology approach was undertaken by Presti et al.[268] In a survey of 34 unselected patients, five suspected or known tumor suppressor gene regions (3p21-25, 11p15, 13q14, 17p11-13, and 18q21) were studied. An IHC assay was also used for the analysis of the retinoblastoma gene product (pRB). This study demonstrated that tumor grade correlated with deletions of 3p ($P = .004$) and 17p ($P = .063$). Tumor stage was correlated with deletions of 3p ($P = .010$), 17p ($P = .015$), and altered pRB expression ($P = .054$). Vascular invasion correlated only with deletions of 17p ($P = .038$). This study also revealed that deletions of 17p (TP53 locus) and 18q (DCC gene locus) occur only in invasive tumors, whereas deletions of 3p and 11p occur in both superficial and invasive tumors.[268] Dalbagni et al.[269] followed this study by analyzing 60 paired normal and bladder tumor tissues using polymorphic DNA markers on 18 different chromosomal arms. Allelic deletions were correlated with clinicopathologic parameters. Distinct genotypic patterns were associated with early and late stages of bladder cancer. Correlation of genetic alterations with clinicopathologic data suggested the existence of two different genetic pathways for the evolution of superficial bladder tumors. Briefly, 9q deletions were found in 60% of the informative cases, confirming previous reports. Superficial papillary tumors confined to the mucosa (pTa) and almost all tumors invading the lamina propria (pT1) showed 9q alterations. In contrast, only 10 of 23 muscle-invasive tumors (pT2–4 or pT2+) had 9q deletions. A statistically significant difference was observed when comparing 9q LOH between pT1 versus pT2+ tumors ($P = .021$). Moreover, 9q deletions were the sole abnormality found in some of the bladder lesions studied, suggesting the presence of a candidate tumor suppressor gene on chromosome 9q important in a subset of superficial bladder tumors. None of the pTa lesions showed 5q alterations; however, three of ten T1 tumors and 8 of 26 T2+ tumors presented with 5q LOH, indicating that 5q deletions may be involved in the transition from papillary superficial (pTa) to early invasive (pT1) tumors. Allelic loss of 17p was detected in 21 of 47 informative cases. Deletions were not identified among pTa lesions, whereas 21 of 38 invasive tumors exhibited 17p LOH. These findings support the involvement of 17p in the progression of bladder cancer. Allelic deletion of 3p was not present in any of the informative pTa neoplasms; however, 18 of 33 invasive tumors had such alterations. A statistically significant association was reported with the various pathologic parameters of poor outcome and 3p LOH. Allelic losses of 11p, 6q, and 18q were frequently detected in the corresponding informative bladder tumors analyzed. However, statistically significant differences were not observed between these abnormalities and clinical pathologic parameters of poor outcome, suggesting late involvement in bladder cancer progression. Other bona fide and putative suppressor loci analyzed in the Dalbagni et al. study showed a lower rate of LOH and lacked association with clinicopathologic parameters.[269]

In a subsequent allelotyping study, Habuchi et al.[270] investigated the role of allelic losses of seven chromosomal arms (1p, 3p, 9q, 10q, 11p, 13q, and 17p) in 49 urothelial cancers. They found 9q LOH as a common event in bladder tumors, and invasive tumors showed higher frequencies of 17p and 13q losses when compared to noninvasive lesions. Deletions of the long arm of chromosome 13, including the RB locus on 13ql4, were independently reported by two groups.[95,96] In one of these studies, Cairns et al.[271] used intragenic RB probes and found 28 of 94 informative cases with LOH at the RB locus, with 26 of these 28 lesions being muscle-invasive tumors.

The relevance of RB alterations in bladder cancer was disclosed in two independent studies.[272,273] Using a mouse monoclonal antibody (mAB) and IHC in frozen tissue sections of 48 primary bladder tumors, Cordon-Cardo and collaborators[272] found normal levels of pRB expression in 34 cases. However, a spectrum of altered patterns of expression, from undetectable pRB levels to heterogeneous expression of pRB, was observed in 14 patients. Thirteen of the 38 patients diagnosed with muscle-invasive tumors were categorized as pRB altered, whereas only

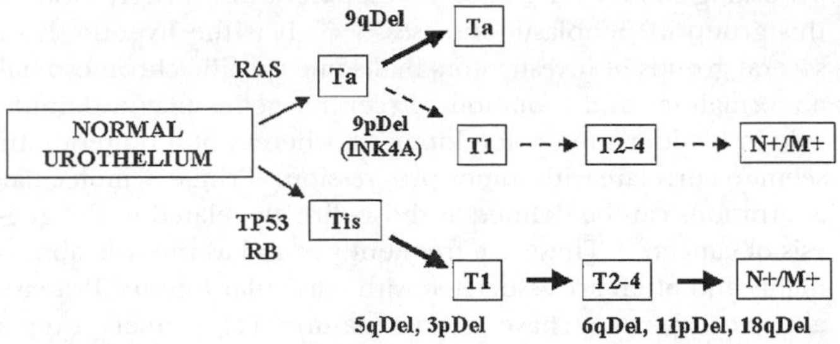

FIGURE 34.1-5. Schematic representation of the proposed model of bladder cancer progression as it may relate to the pathologic staging of this cancer.

one of the ten superficial carcinomas had the altered pRB phenotype. The survival rate was significantly decreased in pRB altered patients compared to those with normal pRB expression (P <.001).[272] Similarly, Logothetis et al.[273] found altered pRB expression in locally advanced bladder cancer. Forty-three patients were evaluated using the Rb-WL-1 polyclonal antiserum and IHC. These investigators reported altered pRB expression in 37% of the tumor specimens analyzed. A significant decrease in disease-free survival rate was reported for patients with documented abnormal pRB levels. Taken together, these data suggest that altered pRB expression occurred in all grades and stages of bladder cancer but was more commonly associated with muscle-invasive tumors. Moreover, altered patterns of pRB may become an important prognostic variable in patients presenting with invasive bladder cancer (Fig. 34.1-5).

The clinical implications of detecting TP53 mutations and altered patterns of its encoded product (p53) in bladder tumors has been the focus of a series of investigations.[274–282] Early studies revealed that TP53 mutations were common events in bladder cancer and associated with tumor stage and grade.[274,275] Dalbagni et al.[276] correlated alterations of chromosome 17 with p53 nuclear overexpression in a cohort of 60 bladder tumors. Deletion of 17p correlated with grade (P = .039) and stage (P = .004), whereas p53 nuclear overexpression correlated with grade (P = .027), stage (P = .008), vascular invasion (P = .021), and the presence of nodal metastases (P = .007). A strong correlation was observed between the p53 overexpression and TP53 deletions (P<.001). Following this study, Cordon-Cardo et al.[277] designed a study to evaluate the sensitivity and specificity of different laboratory assays directed to the identification of TP53 mutations, including IHC with mAB PAb1801, restriction fragment length polymorphism, PCR-SSCP (single-strand confirmation polymorphism), and sequencing.[277] Using this approach, they also tested the hypothesis that p53 nuclear overexpression detected by IHC can reliably identify the presence of mutant TP53 products in bladder neoplasms. Nuclear immunoreactivities were observed in 26 of 42 bladder tumors analyzed. Abnormal shifts in mobility were noted in 14 of the 42 cases in distinct exons. A strong association was noted between p53 nuclear overexpression and 17p LOH (P <.001), as well as p53 nuclear overexpression and detection of TP53 mutations by SSCP and sequencing (P<.001). Using receiver operating curve (ROC) statistical analysis, the accuracy of detecting TP53 mutations by IHC was estimated to be 90.3%. In addition, this study defined as an appropriate cutoff point for IHC 20% tumor cells displaying nuclear immunoreactivities (p53-positive phenotype).

The aim of three analyses[105,278,279] was to investigate altered patterns of p53 expression with tumor progression in patients with superficial bladder tumors. Detection of p53 nuclear overexpression was evaluated by IHC using mAB PAb1801 on deparaffinized tissue sections in tumors from 43 patients with pT1 bladder cancer,[278] 54 patients with pTa neoplasms,[279] and 33 patients affected with pure pTis.[105] Nuclear p53 overexpression was correlated with clinicopathologic variables, and results were submitted to Fisher exact test, as well as univariate and multivariate analyses.[105,278,279] The median follow-up for these cohorts of patients was 119, 110, and 124 months, respectively. Patients in each stage were stratified into two groups, using the cutoff point identified through the ROC analysis previously conducted (20% nuclear-positive tumor cells).[277] A strong association was found between tumor progression and p53-positive phenotype in the three studies (P <.01). Moreover, nuclear overexpression of p53 was an independent variable associated with disease progression and death due to bladder cancer.

Two studies dealing with p53 nuclear overexpression conducted in unselected bladder cancer patients have been reported. Lipponen[280] analyzed 212 bladder tumors, using IHC and 20% positive nuclear staining as the cutoff value. However, the primary antibody used was a purified rabbit polyserum (NCL-CM1, 1:150 dilution). The mean follow-up time was more than 10 years. Nuclear overexpression of p53 was associated with tumor grade and disease progression. In univariate analysis, p53 overexpression predicted poor outcome in the entire cohort. However, in a multivariant survival analysis, overexpression of p53 had no independent prognostic value over clinical stage and mitotic index. Esrig et al.[281] determined the relation between nuclear accumulation of p53 and tumor progression in a cohort of 243 patients treated by radical cystectomy using IHC and antibody PAb1801. These investigators noticed that detection of nuclear p53 was significantly associated with an increased risk of recurrence (P <.001) and decreased overall survival (P <.001). Moreover, p53-positive phenotype was an independent predictor of recurrence and survival.

The neoadjuvant use of chemotherapy offers the advantages of bladder preservation and early treatment of micrometastases in patients diagnosed with invasive bladder cancer. However, despite the chemosensitivity of invasive urothelial neoplasms, complete pathologic response in the primary lesion occurs in only 20% to 30% of patients. To determine whether aberrant p53 expression has independent significance for response, relapse, and survival in patients with muscle-invasive bladder cancer treated with neoadjuvant M-VAC [methotrexate, vinblastine, Adriamycin (doxorubicin), and cisplatin] chemotherapy, Sarkis et al.[108a] evaluated 90 patients who received this regimen with a median follow-up of 5.8 years. Patients whose tumors had p53-positive phenotype (n = 47) had a significantly higher proportion of cancer deaths. Multivariate analysis revealed that p53 overexpression had independent significance for long-term survival (P<.001).[108]

As already discussed, loss of genetic material on chromosome 9 is an early abnormality detected in bladder tumors.[225,266,269,270,282] More recently, the existence of two altered loci, one in each of the chromosome 9 arms, was postulated.[283,284] A detailed analysis conducted by Orlow et al.[285] on 73 bladder tumors showed that two regions, one on 9p at the IFN cluster (9p21) and the other on 9q associated with the q34.1-2 bands, had the highest frequencies of allelic losses. The 9p21 region has been found to be mutated frequently in a wide variety of human tumor cell lines, and the search for a putative tumor suppressor gene in this region led to the characterization of the so-called multiple tumor suppressor 1 (MTS1) gene.[286] It was confirmed that the MTS1 gene was the previously identified p16/INK4A/CDKN2 (p16) gene.[287] In addition to the p16 gene, the p15/INK4B/MTS2 (p15) gene is found in tandem at 9p21.[288] These genes encode members of negative cell-cycle regulators, called *cyclin-dependent kinase* (cdk) *inhibitory molecules*.[287–289] The initial enthusiasm over the high frequency of mutations of these genes in cell lines has been confirmed by genetic alterations mainly of p16, as well as deletions of p15, in human primary tumors, including bladder cancer.[290–295] Moreover, it has been shown that genetic alterations of p16 are independent of TP53 mutations, suggesting that p16 and p53 function in separate pathways of tumor suppression.[294]

Identification of the p14 ARF gene within the same locus as p16 and p15 links the p16/pRB and p53 pathways of tumor suppression. p16 inhibits the ability of cyclin D1 and its associated cdk to phosphorylate pRB. Unphosphorylated pRB sequesters the transcription factor E2F1, a transcription factor necessary for cell-cycle progression.[296] Absence of p16 (as in a homozygous deletion at chromosome 9p) allows unregulated phosphorylation of pRB and increased free E2F1. The p14ARF gene shares a portion of the p16 transcription unit and encodes a novel protein product that interacts with and causes destabilization of the mdm-2 protein.[297,298] Decreased mdm-2 results in increased p53 availability; increased p53 can mediate cell-cycle arrest at G_1 or induce apoptosis. E2F1 causes increased expression of the p14ARF gene, causing a negative feedback for cell-cycle progression. Lack of p14 ARF due to alterations at the p16 locus results in uninhibited mdm-2 and decreased p53 function. Although p16 and p53 are independent, the p16 locus encodes a gene that links the p53 and pRB pathways. Therefore, genetic alterations of the p16/p15/p14ARF locus can affect both p53 and pRB tumor suppressor function. However, it should be kept in mind that the p14ARF pathway can only modulate p53 activity via mdm-2, and mutations of the p53 or amplification of MDM2 may be more important in complete inactivation of p53 as previously discussed. Alternatively, genetic alterations that affect p16 and p15 may not affect p14ARF.

Orlow et al.[295] have reported an overall frequency of deletions and rearrangements for the p16 and p15 genes in bladder cancer of 19% and 18%, respectively. Moreover, this study revealed that p16 and p15 alterations were associated with low-stage, low-grade bladder tumors. It should be emphasized that only pTa and pT1, but not pTis, lesions showed deletions of either p16 or p15. Because p16 alterations occur independently of p53 mutations[294] and p53 mutations are frequent events in Tis bladder tumors,[105] data from that report further support the hypothesis that bladder carcinogenesis may develop through two distinct molecular pathways.[269,299] Taken together, the results suggest that p16 and p15 alterations confer selective growth advantage to urothelial tumor cells, but mutations in other genes are required to produce an overt malignant phenotype.

BLADDER CANCER AS A MODEL FOR THE STUDY OF TUMOR PROGRESSION AND FUTURE DIRECTIONS

The molecular abnormalities reported to date, as well as the natural history of bladder cancer, have allowed the proposal of a working model for tumor development and progression of this group of neoplastic diseases.[269,299] It is the hypothesis of several groups of investigators that some specific chromosomal abnormalities and mutations of certain genes play a definite role in bladder tumor development, whereas other alterations seem to correlate with tumor progression. "Primary" molecular aberrations can be defined as those directly related to the genesis of cancer.[300] These are frequently found as the sole abnormality and often are associated with particular tumors. Primary abnormalities may have a dual nature: (1) primary events involved in the production of low-grade/well-differentiated neoplasms that destabilize cellular proliferation, but have minimal or no effects on cellular "social" interactions or differentiation, as well as rate of cell death or apoptosis; and (2) primary events leading to high-grade/poorly differentiated tumors that disrupt growth control, including cell-cycle and apoptosis regulators, and have a major impact on cellular differentiation. There are evidence and data to support the idea that a target site(s) for primary event(s) in low-grade papillary superficial bladder tumors may reside on chromosome 9. However, a candidate for the initiation of high-grade, flat carcinoma *in situ* lesions has not been yet elucidated. Novel approaches using tissue microdissection techniques and molecular genetic assays are needed to shed light on this subject. Conversely, "secondary" abnormalities may be fortuitous or may determine the biologic behavior of the tumor.[300] Multiple molecular abnormalities are identified in most human cancers studied, including bladder neoplasms, with the accumulation rather than the order of these genetic alterations being important and probably acting synergistically. In this regard, it is noteworthy that most of the identified genes involved in late stages of tumor progression act as major regulators of the cell cycle and apoptosis programs, such as TP53 and RB.

HEREDITARY PREDISPOSITIONS AND UROTHELIAL CANCER

In 1993, one of the genes responsible for a hereditary cancer predisposition syndrome known as *hereditary nonpolyposis colon cancer* (HNPCC) was identified.[301–303] Although colon cancer is the predominant malignancy in this syndrome, Lynch and colleagues[304] previously described an increased incidence of upper tract transitional cell carcinoma (TCC) in a subset of HNPCC families. The genes responsible for HNPCC are highly conserved DNA repair genes involved in the correction of misincorporated deoxyribonucleotides formed during DNA replication known as *mismatch repair* (MMR).[305] Tumors deficient for MMR display a characteristic pattern of genetic alterations termed *microsatellite instability* (MSI) or *replication errors*.[306–308] MSI is caused by slippage of the DNA polymerase at mono-, di-, and trinucleotide tracts normally repaired by MMR proteins.[309] Almost all tumors from HNPCC patients display MSI, because the normal MMR allele is lost in these tumors. The instability that results can cause mutations in other genes, which leads to tumorigenesis.

Subsequent studies in sporadic bladder tumors demonstrate MSI in 6% of superficial tumors,[1] and immunohistochemical analysis of one of the MMR genes (hMSH2) revealed lack of expression in only two.[311] However, decreased expression of hMSH2 was observed in 25% of tumors, and this finding correlated with high-grade and recurrent disease. Analysis of expression of MMR genes in bladder tumors from HNPCC patients has not been reported, and it will be interesting to determine if these tumors display MSI. The investigation of MMR genes in urothelial malignancies may be important in management of patients with bladder cancer, because HNPCC is the only cancer syndrome that predisposes affected individuals to TCC. Also, tumors with MMR deficiency are resistant to alkylating agents[312] sometimes used in treatment of superficial TCC, such as thiotepa. Further investigation of these genes in urothelial malignancies seems warranted.

Are other protooncogenes involved in cell-cycle control, such as cyclin D1 and Cdk4, altered in bladder tumors? Is the genetic instability observed in some uroepithelial carcinomas due to mutations of MMR genes? Is the deficiency in apoptotic signals responsible for lack of response to adjuvant therapy? Are unconstrained transcription factors, such the E2F family members in the advent of RB alterations, accountable in part for the clinical phenomenon of the resistant phenotype? To what extent do other drug resistance mechanisms, such as P glycoprotein, play a role in treatment failure? Which are the genes involved in the phenotype of metastatic bladder cancer? These clinically relevant questions await further studies. The current need is to translate newly developed scientific knowledge into diagnostic and therapeutic strategies, using well-characterized cohorts of patients and novel approaches to the analysis of available tissue samples.

POTENTIAL CLINICAL APPLICATIONS

Inherent in the study of the fundamental genetic events leading to bladder cancer is the hope that the understanding of the molecular mechanisms of transformation in this malignancy may lead to insights for new treatment strategies for this disease. Another potential application of studies on molecular genetics of bladder cancer is that detection of alterations in certain genes may lead to improved methods for early diagnosis of uroepithelial tumors. Sidransky et al.[274] have shown that identification of alterations, such as p53 gene mutations in bladder tumors and urine samples, can provide a potentially extremely sensitive method for detection of bladder cancer. In one instance, genetic abnormalities could be detected years before the disease was clinically apparent.[313] In a series of studies, these scientists have demonstrated that microsatellite instability is associated with some bladder tumors and can occur early in bladder tumorigenesis.[310,314] In a blinded study in which urine samples from 25 patients with suspicious bladder lesions were analyzed by conventional cytology and genomic instability analysis, microsatellite changes identical to those in the tumors were detected in the urine sediment of 19 of 20 patients (95%) who were found to have bladder cancer.[315] Cytology detected cancer cells in only 9 of 18 cases (50%).[316] These studies suggest that molecular genetic analysis for disease gene alterations and microsatellite instability may become useful additions to current screening methods for detecting bladder cancer and may provide improved methods for prediction of clinical course in individual patients.

REFERENCES

1. Linehan WM, Klausner RD. Renal carcinoma. In: Vogelstein B, Kinzler K, eds. *The genetic basis of human cancer.* New York: McGraw-Hill, 1998:455.
2. Linehan WM, Lerman MI, Zbar B. Identification of the VHL gene: its role in renal carcinoma. *JAMA* 1995;273:564.
3. Wingo PA, Tong T, Bolden S. Cancer statistics, 1995. *CA Cancer J Clin* 1995;45:8.
4. Linehan WM, Shipley W, Parkinson D. Cancer of the kidney and ureter. In: DeVita VT, Hellman S, Rosenberg SA, eds. *Cancer: principles and practices of oncology.* Philadelphia: JB Lippincott Co, 1993:1023.
5. La Vecchia C, Negri E, D'Avanzo B, Franceschi S. Smoking and renal cell carcinoma. *Cancer Res* 1990;50:5231.
6. Yu MC, Mack TM, Hanisch R, Cicioni C, Henderson BE. Cigarette smoking, obesity, diuretic use, and coffee consumption as risk factors for renal cell carcinoma. *J Natl Cancer Inst* 1986;77:351.
7. Kovacs G, Ishikawa I. High incidence of papillary renal cell tumours in patients on chronic haemodialysis. *Histopathology* 1993;22:135.
8. Bard RH, Lord B, Fromowitz F. Papillary adenocarcinoma of kidney. *Urology* 1982;19:16.
9. Brennan JF, Stilmant MM, Babayan RK, Siroky MB. Acquired renal cystic disease: implications for the urologist. *Br J Urol* 1991;67:342.
10. Toro J, Duray PH, Glenn GM, et al. Birt-Hogg-Dube syndrome: a novel marker of kidney neoplasia. *Arch Dermatol* 1999;135:1195.
11. Cohen AJ, Li FP, Berg S, et al. Hereditary renal-cell carcinoma associated with a chromosomal translocation. *N Engl J Med* 1979;301:592.
12. Pathak S, Strong LC, Ferrell RE, Trindade A. Familial renal cell carcinoma with a 3:11 chromosome translocation limited to tumor cells. *Science* 1982;217:939.
13. Kovacs G, Brusa P, de Riese W. Tissue-specific expression of a constitutional 3;6 translocation: development of multiple bilateral renal-cell carcinomas. *Int J Cancer* 1989;43:422.
14. Zbar B, Brauch H, Talmadge C, Linehan WM. Loss of alleles of loci on the short arm of chromosome 3 in renal cell carcinoma. *Nature* 1987;327:721.
15. Anglard P, Brauch TH, Weiss GH, et al. Molecular analysis of genetic changes in the origin and development of renal cell carcinoma. *Cancer Res* 1991;51:1071.
16. Carroll PR, Murty VVS, Reuter V, et al. Abnormalities of chromosome region 3p12-14 characterize clear cell renal carcinoma. *Cancer Genet Cytogenet* 1987;26:253.
17. Szucs S, Muller-Brechlin R, DeRiese W, Kovacs G. Deletion 3p: the only chromosome loss in a primary renal cell carcinoma. *Cancer Genet Cytogenet* 1987;26:369.
18. Kovacs G, Erlandsson R, Boldog F, et al. Consistent chromosome 3p deletion and loss of heterozygosity in renal cell carcinoma. *Proc Natl Acad Sci U S A* 1988;85:1571.
19. Presti JC, Rao PH, Chen Q, et al. Histopathological, cytogenetic, and molecular characterization of renal cortical tumors. *Cancer Res* 1991;51:1544.
20. Ogawa O, Kakehi Y, Ogawa K, et al. Allelic loss at chromosome 3p characterizes clear cell phenotype of renal cell carcinoma. *Cancer Res* 1991;51:949.
21. Poston CD, Jaffe GS, Lubensky IA, et al. Characterization of the renal pathology of a familial form of renal cell carcinoma associated with von Hippel-Lindau disease: clinical and molecular genetic implications. *J Urol* 1995;153:22.
22. Walther MM, Lubensky IA, Venzon D, Zbar B, Linehan WM. Prevalence of microscopic lesions in grossly normal renal parenchyma from patients with von Hippel-Lindau disease, sporadic renal cell carcinoma and no renal disease: clinical implications. *J Urol* 1995;154:2010.
23. Manski TJ, Heffner DK, Glenn GM, et al. Endolymphatic sac tumors: a source of morbid hearing loss in von Hippel-Lindau disease. *JAMA* 1997;277:1461.
24. Lubensky IA, Pack S, Ault D, et al. Multiple neuroendocrine tumors of the pancreas in VHL patients: histopathological and molecular genetic analysis. *Am J Pathol* 1998;153:223.
25. Libutti SK, Choyke PL, Bartlett DL, et al. Pancreatic neuroendocrine tumors associated with von Hippel Lindau: diagnostic and management recommendations. *Surgery* 1998;124:1153.
26. Eisenhofer G, Lenders JWM, Linehan WM, et al. Plasma normetanephrine and metanephrine for detecting pheochromocytomas in von Hippel-Lindau disease and multiple endocrine neoplasia type 2. *N Engl J Med* 1999;340:1872.
27. Walther MM, Keiser HR, Linehan WM. Management of hereditary pheochromocytoma in von Hippel Lindau kindreds with partial adrenalectomy. *J Urol* 1999;161:395.
28. Walther MM, Reiter R, Keiser HR, et al. Clinical and genetic characterization of pheochromocytoma in von Hippel-Lindau families. Comparison with sporadic pheochromocytoma gives insight into natural history of pheochromocytoma. *J Urol* 1999;162:659.
29. Glenn GM, Choyke PL, Zbar B, Linehan WM. Von Hippel-Lindau disease: clinical review and molecular genetics. In: Anderson EE, ed. *Problems in urologic surgery: benign and malignant tumors of the kidney.* Philadelphia: JB Lippincott Co, 1990:312.
30. Seizinger BR, Rouleau GA, Ozelius LJ, et al. Von Hippel-Lindau disease maps to the region of chromosome 3 associated with renal cell carcinoma. *Nature* 1988;332:268.
31. Hosoe S, Brauch H, Latif F, et al. Localization of the von Hippel-Lindau disease gene to a small region of chromosome 3. *Genomics* 1990;8:634.
32. Maher ER, Bentley E, Yates JRW, et al. Mapping of the von Hippel Lindau disease gene to a small region of chromosome 3p by genetic linkage analysis. *Genomics* 1991;10:957.
33. Richards FM, Maher ER, Latif F, et al. Detailed genetic mapping of the von Hippel-Lindau disease tumour suppressor gene. *J Med Genet* 1993;30:104.
34. Glenn GM, Daniel LN, Choyke P, et al. Von Hippel-Lindau disease: distinct phenotypes suggest more than one mutant allele at the VHL locus. *Hum Genet* 1991;87:207.
35. Tory K, Brauch H, Linehan WM, et al. Specific genetic change in tumors associated with von Hippel-Lindau disease. *J Natl Cancer Inst* 1989;81:1097.
36. Knudson AG. Genetics of human cancer. *Ann Rev Genet* 1986;20:231.
37. Yao M, Latif F, Kuzmin I, et al. Von Hippel-Lindau disease: identification of deletion mutations by pulsed field gel electrophoresis. *Hum Genet* 1993;92:605.
38. Richards FM, Phipps ME, Latif F, et al. Mapping the von Hippel-Lindau disease tumor suppressor gene: identification of germline deletions by pulsed field gel electrophoresis. *Hum Mol Genet* 1993;2:879.
39. Latif F, Tory K, Gnarra JR, et al. Identification of the von Hippel-Lindau disease tumor suppressor gene. *Science* 1993;260:1317.
40. Chen F, Kishida T, Yao M, et al. Germline mutations in the von Hippel-Lindau disease tumor suppressor gene: correlation with phenotype. *Hum Mutat* 1995;5:66.
41. Stolle CA, Glenn G, Zbar B, et al. Improved detection of germline mutations in the von Hippel-Lindau disease tumor suppressor gene. *Hum Mutat* 1998;12:417.

42. Crossey PA, Richards FM, Foster K, et al. Identification of intragenic mutations in the von Hippel-Lindau disease tumor suppressor gene and correlation with disease phenotype. *Hum Mol Genet* 1994;3:1303.
43. Zbar B, Kishida T, Chen F, et al. Germline mutations in the von Hippel-Lindau disease (VHL) gene in families from North America, Europe and Japan. *Hum Mutat* 1996;8:348.
44. Gnarra JR, Tory K, Weng Y, et al. Mutation of the VHL tumour suppressor gene in renal carcinoma. *Nat Genet* 1994;7:85.
45. Shuin T, Kondo K, Torigoe S, et al. Frequent somatic mutations and loss of heterozygosity of the von Hippel-Lindau tumor suppressor gene in primary human renal cell carcinomas. *Cancer Res* 1994;54:2852.
46. Whaley JM, Naglich J, Gelbert L, et al. Germ-line mutations in the von Hippel-Lindau tumor-suppressor gene are similar to von Hippel-Lindau aberrations in sporadic renal cell carcinoma. *Am J Hum Genet* 1994;55:1092.
47. Foster K, Prowse A, van den Berg A, et al. Somatic mutations of the von Hippel-Lindau disease tumour suppressor gene in non-familial clear cell renal carcinoma. *Hum Mol Genet* 1994;3:2169.
48. Bailly M, Bain C, Favrot MC, Ozturk M. Somatic mutations of von Hippel-Lindau (VHL) tumor-suppressor gene in European kidney cancers. *Int J Cancer* 1995;63:660.
49. Brauch H, Weirich G, Hornauer MA, et al. Trichloroethylene exposure and specific somatic mutations in patients with renal cell carcinoma. *J Natl Cancer Inst* 1999;91:854.
50. Brauch H, Weirich G, Hornauer M, et al. Trichloroethylene is a potential mutagen of the VHL tumor suppressor gene in renal cell cancer. *N Engl J Med* 2002 (*submitted*).
51. Kenck C, Wilhelm M, Bugert P, Staehler G, Kovacs G. Mutation of the VHL gene is associated exclusively with the development of non-papillary renal cell carcinomas. *J Pathol* 1996;179:157.
52. Zhuang Z, Gnarra JR, Dudley CF, et al. Detection of von Hippel-Lindau disease gene mutations in paraffin-embedded sporadic renal cell carcinoma specimens. *Mod Pathol* 1996;9:838.
53. Linehan WM, Zbar B, Klausner RD. Renal carcinoma. In: Scriver CR, Beaudet AL, Sly WS, Valle D, eds. *The metabolic and molecular bases of inherited disease.* New York: McGraw-Hill, 2001.
54. Schmidt L, Li F, Brown RS, et al. Somatic mutations of the von Hippel-Lindau disease tumor suppressor gene in renal carcinomas of patients with an inherited t(3;8) balanced translocation. *Amer Assoc Cancer Res* 1995;36:582(abst).
55. Koolen MI, van der Meyden AP, Bodmer D, et al. A familial case of renal cell carcinoma and a t(2;3) chromosome translocation. *Kidney Int* 1998;53:273.
56. Bodmer D, Eleveld MJ, Ligtenberg MJ, et al. An alternative route for multistep tumorigenesis in a novel case of hereditary renal cell cancer and a t(2;3)(q35;q21) chromosome translocation. *Am J Hum Genet* 1998;62:1475.
57. Herman JG, Latif F, Weng Y, et al. Silencing of the VHL tumor suppressor gene by DNA methylation in renal carcinoma. *Proc Natl Acad Sci U S A* 1994;91:9700.
58. Knudson AG. VHL gene mutation and clear-cell renal carcinomas. *Cancer J* 1995;1:180.
59. Lubensky IA, Gnarra JR, Bertheau P, et al. Allelic deletions of the VHL gene detected in multiple microscopic clear cell renal lesions in von Hippel-Lindau disease patients. *Am J Pathol* 1996;149:2089.
60. Duan DR, Humphrey JS, Chen DYT, et al. Characterization of the VHL tumor suppressor gene product: localization, complex formation, and the effect of natural inactivating mutations. *Proc Natl Acad Sci U S A* 1995;92:6459.
61. Duan DR, Pause A, Burgess WH, et al. Inhibition of transcription elongation by the VHL tumor suppressor protein. *Science* 1995;269:1402.
62. Kibel A, Iliopoulos O, DeCaprio JA, Kaelin WG. Binding of the von Hippel-Lindau tumor suppressor protein to elongin B and C. *Science* 1995;269:1444.
63. Pause A, Lee S, Worrell RA, et al. The von Hippel-Lindau tumor-suppressor gene product forms a stable complex with human CUL-2, a member of the Cdc53 family of proteins. *Proc Natl Acad Sci U S A* 1997;94:2156.
64. Lonergan KM, Iliopoulos O, Ohh M, et al. Regulation of hypoxia-inducible mRNAs by the von Hippel-Lindau tumor suppressor protein requires binding to complexes containing elongins B/C and Cul2. *Mol Cell Biol* 1998;18:732.
65. Elledge SJ, Harper JW. The role of protein stability in the cell cycle and cancer. *Biochim Biophys Acta* 1998;1377:M61.
66. Gnarra JR, Zhou S, Merrill MJ, et al. Post-transcriptional regulation of vascular endothelial growth factor mRNA by the product of the VHL tumor suppressor gene. *Proc Natl Acad Sci U S A* 1996;93:10589.
67. Siemeister G, Weindel K, Mohrs K, et al. Reversion of deregulated expression of vascular endothelial growth factor in human renal carcinoma cells by von Hippel-Lindau tumor suppressor protein. *Cancer Res* 1996;56:2299.
68. Berger DP, Herbstritt L, Dengler WA, et al. Vascular endothelial growth factor (VEGF) mRNA expression in human tumor models of different histologies. *Ann Oncol* 1995;6:817.
69. Takahashi A, Sasaki H, Kim SJ, et al. Markedly increased amounts of messenger RNAs for vascular endothelial growth factor and placenta growth factor in renal cell carcinoma associated with angiogenesis. *Cancer Res* 1994;54:4233.
70. Iliopoulos O, Jiang C, Levy AP, Kaelin WG, Goldberg MA. Negative regulation of hypoxia-inducible genes by the von Hippel-Lindau protein. *Proc Natl Acad Sci U S A* 1996;93:10595.
71. Lee S, Chen DYT, Humphrey JS, et al. Nuclear/cytoplasmic localization of the VHL tumor suppressor gene product is determined by cell density. *Proc Natl Acad Sci U S A* 1996;93:1770.
72. Zbar B, Tory K, Merino M, et al. Hereditary papillary renal cell carcinoma. *J Urol* 1994; 151:561.
73. Zbar B, Glenn G, Lubensky IA, et al. Hereditary papillary renal cell carcinoma: clinical studies in 10 families. *J Urol* 1995;153:907.
74. Schmidt L, Duh FM, Chen F, et al. Germline and somatic mutations in the tyrosine kinase domain of the MET proto-oncogene in papillary renal carcinomas. *Nat Genet* 1997;16:68.
75. Schmidt L, Junker K, Weirich G, et al. Two North American families with hereditary papillary renal carcinoma and identical novel mutations in the MET proto-oncogene. *Cancer Res* 1998;58:1719.
76. Jeffers M, Schmidt L, Nakaigawa N, et al. Activating mutations for the met tyrosine kinase receptor in human cancer. *Proc Natl Acad Sci U S A* 1997;94:11445.
77. Landis SH, Murray T, Bolden S, Wingo PA. Cancer statistics, 1998 [published errata appear in *CA Cancer J Clin* 1998;48:192 and 1998;48:329]. *CA Cancer J Clin* 1998;48:6.
78. Thompson TC, Southgate J, Kitchener G, Land H. Multistage carcinogenesis induced by ras and myc oncogenes in a reconstituted organ. *Cell* 1989;56:917.
79. Fearon ER, Vogelstein B. A genetic model for colorectal tumorigenesis. *Cell* 1990;61:759.
80. Bostwick DG, Montironi R. Prostatic intraepithelial neoplasia and the origins of prostatic carcinoma. *Pathol Res Pract* 1995;191:828.
81. Aprikian AG, Sarkis AS, Fair WR, et al. Immunohistochemical determination of p53 protein nuclear accumulation in prostatic adenocarcinoma. *J Urol* 1994;151:1276.
82. Navone NM, Troncoso P, Pisters LL, et al. p53 protein accumulation and gene mutation in the progression of human prostate carcinoma. *J Natl Cancer Inst* 1993;85:1657.
83. Bookstein R, MacGrogan D, Hilsenbeck SG, Sharkey F, Allred DC. p53 is mutated in a subset of advanced-stage prostate cancers. *Cancer Res* 1993;53:3369.
84. Lewis WH, Yeger H, Bonetta L, et al. Homozygous deletion of a DNA marker from chromosome 11p13 in sporadic Wilms tumor. *Genomics* 1988;3:25.
85. Koivisto PA, Rantala I. Amplification of the androgen receptor gene is associated with P53 mutation in hormone-refractory recurrent prostate cancer. *J Pathol* 1999;187:237.
86. Dhom G. Epidemiologic aspects of latent and clinically manifest carcinoma of the prostate. *J Clin Res Clin Oncol* 1983;106:210.
87. Lee EY, To H, Shew JY, et al. Inactivation of the retinoblastoma susceptibility gene in human breast cancers. *Science* 1988;241:218.
88. Diaz MO, Ziemin S, Le Beau MM, et al. Homozygous deletion of the alpha- and beta 1-interferon genes in human leukemia and derived cell lines. *Proc Natl Acad Sci U S A* 1988;85:5259.
89. Carter BS, Carter HB, Issacs JT. Epidemiologic evidence regarding predisposing factors to prostate cancer [Review]. *Prostate* 1990;16:187.
90. Haenszel W, Kurihara M. Studies of Japanese migrants. I. Mortality from cancer and other diseases among Japanese in the United States. *J Natl Cancer Inst* 1968;40:43.
91. Taylor JA. Epidemiologic evidence of genetic susceptibility to cancer [Review]. *Birth Defects* 1990;26:113.
92. Woolf CM. An investigation of familial aspects of carcinoma of the prostate. *Cancer* 1960;13:739.
93. Morganti G, Cianferrari L, Cresseri A, Arrigoni G, Lovati F. Recherches clinico-statistiques et genetiques sur les neoplasies de la prostate. *Acat Genet Statis* 1956;6:304.
94. Schuman LM, Mandel J, Blackard C, et al. Epidemiologic study of prostate cancer: preliminary report. *Cancer Treat Rep* 1971;61:181.
95. Krain LS. Some epidemiologic variables in prostatic carcinoma in California. *Prev Med* 1974;3:154.
96. Meikle AW, Smith JA, West DW. Familial factors affecting prostatic cancer risk and plasma sex-steroid levels. *Prostate* 1985;6:121.
97. Spitz MR, Currier RD, Fueger JJ, Babaian RJ, Newell GR. Familial patterns of prostate cancer: a case-control analysis. *J Urol* 1991;146:1305.
98. Gronberg H, Wiklund F, Damber JE. Age specific risks of familial prostate carcinoma: a basis for screening recommendations in high risk populations. *Cancer* 1999;86:477.
99. Cannon L, Bishop DT, Skolnick M. Genetic epidemiology of prostate cancer in the Utah Mormon genealogy. *Cancer Surv* 1982;1:47.
100. Steinberg GD, Carter BS, Beaty TH, Childs B, Walsh PC. Family history and the risk of prostate cancer. *Prostate* 1990;17:337.
101. Carter BS, Beaty TH, Steinberg GD, Childs B, Walsh PC. Mendelian inheritance of familial prostate cancer. *Proc Natl Acad Sci U S A* 1992;89:3367.
102. Gronberg H, Damber L, Damber JE, Iselius L. Segregation analysis of prostate cancer in Sweden: support for dominant inheritance. *Am J Epidemiol* 1997;146:552.
103. Schaid DJ, McDonnell SK, Blute ML, Thibodeau SN. Evidence for autosomal dominant inheritance of prostate cancer. *Am J Hum Genet* 1998;62:1425.
104. Smith JR, Freije D, Carpten JD, et al. Major susceptibility locus for prostate cancer on chromosome 1 suggested by a genome-wide search [see comments]. *Science* 1996;274:1371.
105. Xu J, Meyers D, Freije D, et al. Evidence for a prostate cancer susceptibility locus on the X chromosome. *Nat Genet* 1998;20:175.
106. Berthon P, Valeri A, Cohen-Akenine A, et al. Predisposing gene for early-onset prostate cancer, localized on chromosome 1q42.2-43. *Am J Hum Genet* 1998;62:1416.
107. Gibbs M, Stanford JL, McIndoe RA, et al. Evidence for a rare prostate cancer–susceptibility locus at chromosome 1p36. *Am J Hum Genet* 1999;64:776.
108. Strohmeyer TG, Slamon DJ. Proto–oncogenes and tumor suppressor genes in human urological malignancies. [Review]. *J Urol* 1994;151:1479.
108a. Sarkis AS, Bajorin DF, Reuter VE. Prognostic value of p53 nuclear overexpression in patients with invasive bladder cancer treated with neoadjuvant MVAC. *J Clin Oncol* 1995;13:1384.
109. Bubendorf L, Kononen J, Koivisto P, et al. Survey of gene amplifications during prostate cancer progression by high-throughput fluorescence *in situ* hybridization on tissue microarrays [published erratum appears in *Cancer Res* 1999;59:1388]. *Cancer Res* 1999; 59:803.
110. Treiger B, Issacs J. Expression of a transfected v-Harvey-ras oncogene in a Dunning rat prostate adenocarcinoma and the development of high metastatic ability. *J Urol* 1988;140:1580.
111. Peehl DM, Wehner N, Stamey TA. Activated Ki–ras oncogene in human prostatic adenocarcinoma. *Prostate* 1987;10:281.
112. Carter BS, Epstein JL, Issacs WB. ras gene mutations in human prostate cancer. *Cancer Res* 1990;50:6830.
113. Isaacs WB, Carter BS. Genetic changes associated with prostate cancer in humans. *Cancer Surv* 1991;11:15.
114. Gumerlock PH, Poonamallee UR, Meyers FJ, deVere White RW. Activated ras alleles in human carcinoma of the prostate are rare. *Cancer Res* 1991;51:1632.
115. Moul JW, Friedrichs PA, Lance RS, Theune SM, Chang EH. Infrequent RAS oncogene mutations in human prostate cancer. *Prostate* 1992;20:327.
116. Konishi N, Enomoto T, Buzard G, et al. K-ras activation and ras p21 expression in latent prostatic carcinoma in Japanese men. *Cancer* 1992;20:327.

117. Anwar K, Nakakuki K, Shiraishi T, et al. Presence of ras oncogene mutations and human papillomavirus DNA in human prostate carcinomas. *Cancer Res* 1992;52:5991.
118. Serth J, Panitz F, Paeslack U, Kuczyk MA, Jonas U. Increased levels of human papillomavirus type 16 DNA in a subset of prostate cancers. *Cancer Res* 1999;59:823.
119. Noda T, Sasagawa T, Dong Y, et al. Detection of human papillomavirus (HPV) DNA in archival specimens of benign prostatic hyperplasia and prostatic cancer using a highly sensitive nested PCR method. *Urol Res* 1998;26:165.
120. Strickler HD, Burk R, Shah K, et al. A multifaceted study of human papillomavirus and prostate carcinoma. *Cancer* 1998;82:1118.
121. Sato K, Qian J, Slezak JM, et al. Clinical significance of alterations of chromosome 8 in high-grade, advanced, nonmetastatic prostate carcinoma. *J Natl Cancer Inst* 1999;91:1574.
122. Hockenbery DM. The bcl–2 oncogene and apoptosis. [Review]. *Semin Immunol* 1992;4:413.
123. Reed JC, Cuddy M, Slabiak T, et al. Oncogenic potential of bcl–2 demonstrated by gene transfer. *Nature* 1988;336:259.
124. Liu J, Johnson RM, Traweek ST. Rearrangement of the BCL-2 gene in follicular lymphoma. Detection by PCR in both fresh and fixed tissue samples. *Diagn Mol Pathol* 1993; 2:241.
125. McDonnell TJ, Troncoso P, Brisbay SM, et al. Expression of the protooncogene bcl–2 in the prostate and its association with emergence of androgen–independent prostate cancer. Cancer Res 1992;52:6940.
126. Colombel M, Symmans F, Gil S, et al. Detection of the apoptosis–supressing oncoprotein bcl–2 in hormone–refractory human prostate cancers. Am J Pathol 1993;143:390.
127. Anderson DM, Johnson L, Glaccum MB, et al. Chromosomal assignment and genomic structure of IL15. *Genomics* 1995;25:701.
128. Hortnagel K, Mautner J, Strobl LJ, et al. The role of immunoglobulin kappa elements in c-myc activation. *Oncogene* 1995;10:1393.
129. Newmark JR, Hardy DO, Tonb DC, et al. Androgen receptor gene mutations in human prostate cancer. *Proc Natl Acad Sci U S A* 1992;89:6319.
130. Kelly WK, Slovin S, Scher HI. Steroid hormone withdrawal syndromes. Pathophysiology and clinical significance. *Urol Clin North Am* 1997;24:421.
131. Sartor O, Cooper M, Weinberger M, et al. Surprising activity of flutamide withdrawal when combined with aminoglutethimide in treatment of "hormone-refractory" prostate cancer. *J Natl Cancer Inst* 1994;86:222.
132. Harris SE, Rong Z, Harris MA, Lubahn DD. Androgen receptor in human prostate adenocarcinoma LNCaP/ADEP cells contains a mutation which alters the specificity of the steroid-dependent transcriptional activation region. *Endocrinology* 1990;126:93.
133. Veldscholte J, Berrevoets CA, Ris-Stalpers C, et al. The androgen receptor in LNCaP cells contains a mutation in the ligand binding domain which affects steroid binding characteristics and response to antiandrogens [Review]. *J Steroid Biochem Mol Biol* 1992;41:665.
134. Taplin ME, Bubley GJ, Shuster TD, et al. Mutation of the androgen-receptor gene in metastatic androgen-independent prostate cancer. *N Engl J Med* 1995;332:1393.
135. Visakorpi T, Hyytinen E, Koivisto P, et al. *In vivo* amplification of the androgen receptor gene and progression of human prostate cancer. *Nat Genet* 1995;9:401.
136. Culig Z, Hobisch A, Hittmair A, et al. Expression, structure, and function of androgen receptor in advanced prostatic carcinoma. *Prostate* 1998;35:63.
137. Craft N, Shostak Y, Carey M, Sawyers CH. A mechanism for hormone-independent prostate cancer through modulation of androgen receptor signaling by the HER-2/neu tyrosine kinase. *Nat Med* 1999;5:280.
138. Brothman AR, Peehl DM, Patel AM, McNeal JE. Frequency and pattern of karyotypic abnormalities in human prostate cancer. *Cancer Res* 1990;50:3795.
139. Lundgren R, Mandahl N, Heim S, et al. Cytogenetic analysis of 57 primary prostatic adenocarcinomas. *Genes Chromosomes Cancer* 1992;4:16.
140. Atkin NB, Baker MC. Chromosome study of five cancers of the prostate. *Hum Genet* 1985;70:359.
141. Carter BS, Ewing CM, Ward WS, et al. Allelic loss of chromosomes 16q and 10q in human prostate cancer. *Proc Natl Acad Sci U S A* 1990;87:8751.
142. Kunimi K, Bergerheim US, Larsson IL, Ekman P, Collins VP. Allelotyping of human prostatic adenocarcinoma. *Genomics* 1991;11:530.
143. Bergerheim US, Kunimi K, Collins VP, Ekman P. Deletion mapping of chromosomes 8, 10, and 16 in human prostatic carcinoma. *Genes Chromosomes Cancer* 1991;3:215.
144. Macoska JA, Trybus TM, Sakr WA, et al. Fluorescence *in situ* hybridization analysis of 8p allelic loss and chromosome 8 instability in human prostate cancer. *Cancer Res* 1994;54:3824.
145. Konig JJ, Kamst E, Hagemeijer A, et al. Cytogenetic characterization of several androgen responsive and unresponsive sublines of the human prostatic carcinoma cell line LNCaP. *Urol Res* 1989;17:79.
146. MacGrogan D, Levy A, Bostwick D, et al. Loss of chromosome arm 8p loci in prostate cancer: mapping by quantitative allelic imbalance. *Genes Chromosomes Cancer* 1994;10:151.
147. Trapman J, Sleddens HFBM, van der Weiden MM, et al. Loss of heterozygosity of chromosome 8 microsatellite loci implicates a candidate tumor suppressor gene between the loci D8S87 and D8S133 in human prostate cancer. *Cancer Res* 1994;54:6061.
148. Suzuki H, Emi M, Komiya A, et al. Localization of a tumor suppressor gene associated with progression of human prostate cancer within a 1.2 Mb region of 8p22-p21.3. *Genes Chromosomes Cancer* 1995;13:168.
149. Emmert-Buck MR, Vocke CD, Pozzatti RO, et al. Allelic loss on chromosome 8p12-21 in microdissected prostatic intraepithelial neoplasia (PIN). *Cancer Res* 1997;1995:2959.
150. Macoska JA, Trybus TM, Benson PD, et al. Evidence for three tumor suppressor gene loci on chromosome 8p in human prostate cancer. *Cancer Res* 1995;55:5390.
151. Bova GS, MacGrogan D, Levy A, et al. Physical mapping of chromosome 8p22 markers and their homozygous deletion in a metastatic prostate cancer. *Genomics* 1996;35:46.
152. Latil A, Baron JC, Cussenot O, et al. Genetic alterations in localized prostate cancer: identification of a common region of deletion on chromosome arm 18q. *Genes Chromosomes Cancer* 1994;11:119.
153. Sakr WA, Macoska JA, Benson P, et al. Allelic loss in locally metastatic, multisampled prostate cancer. *Cancer Res* 1994;54:3273.
154. Cher ML, MacGrogan D, Bookstein R, et al. Comparative genomic hybridization allelic imbalance and fluorescence *in situ* hybridization on chromosome 8 in prostate cancer. *Genes Chromosomes Cancer* 1995;11:153.
155. Matsuyama H, Pan Y, Skoog L, et al. Deletion mapping of chromosome 8p in prostate cancer by fluorescence *in situ* hybridization. *Oncogene* 1994;9:3071.
156. Massenkeil G, Oberhuber H, Hailemariam S, et al. P53 mutations and loss of heterozygosity on chromosomes 8p, 16q, 17p, and 18q are confined to advanced prostate cancer. *Anticancer Res* 1994;14:2785.
157. Visakorpi T, Kallioniemi A, Syvanen AC, et al. Genetic changes in primary and recurrent prostate cancer by comparative genomic hybridization. *Cancer Res* 1995;55:342.
158. Cher ML, Bova GS, Moore DH, et al. Genetic alterations in untreated metastases and androgen-independent prostate cancer detected by comparative genomic hybridization and allelotyping. *Cancer Res* 1996;56:3091.
159. Ichikawa T, Nihei N, Suzuki H, et al. Suppression of metastasis of rat prostatic cancer by introducing human chromosome 8. *Cancer Res* 1994;54:2299.
160. MacGrogan D, Levy A, Bova GS, et al. Structure and methylation-associated silencing of a gene within a homozygously deleted region of human chromosome band 8p22. *Genomics* 1996;35:55.
161. Ishii H, Baffa R, Numata SI, et al. The FEZ1 gene at chromosome 8p22 encodes a leucine-zipper protein, and its expression is altered in multiple human tumors. *Proc Natl Acad Sci U S A* 1999;96:3928.
162. He WW, Sciavolino PJ, Wing J, et al. A novel human prostate-specific, androgen-regulated homeobox gene (NKX3.1) that maps to 8p21, a region frequently deleted in prostate cancer. *Genomics* 1997;43:69.
163. Qian J, Bostwick DG, Takahashi S, et al. Chromosomal anomalies in prostatic intraepithelial neoplasia and carcinoma detected by fluorescence *in situ* hybridization. *Cancer Res* 1995;55:5408.
164. Van den Berg C, Guan XY, Von Hoff D, et al. DNA sequence amplification in human prostate cancer identified by chromosome microdissection: potential prognostic implications. *Clin Cancer Res* 1995;1:11.
165. Reiter RE, Sato I, Thomas G, et al. Coamplification of prostate stem cell antigen (PSCA) and MYC in locally advanced prostate cancer. *Genes Chromosomes Cancer* 2000;27:95.
166. Nupponen NN, Porkka K, Kakkola L, et al. Amplification and overexpression of p40 subunit of eukaryotic translation initiation factor 3 in breast and prostate cancer. *Am J Pathol* 1999;154:1777.
167. Raskind WH, Conrad EU, Chansky H, Matsushita M. Loss of heterozygosity in chondrosarcomas for markers linked to hereditary multiple exostoses loci on chromosomes 8 and 11. *Am J Hum Genet* 1995;56:1132.
168. Kubota Y, Fujinami K, Uemura H, et al. Retinoblastoma gene mutations in primary human prostate cancer. *Prostate* 1995;27:314.
169. Bussemakers MJG, Bova GS, Schoenberg MP, et al. Microsatellite instability in human prostate cancer. *J Urol* 1995;151:469A.
170. Boyer JC, Umar A, Risinger JI, et al. Microsatellite instability, mismatch repair deficiency, and genetic defects in human cancer cell lines. *Cancer Res* 1995;55:6063.
171. Visakorpi T, Kallioniemi O, Heikkinen A, Koivula T, Isola J. Small subgroup of aggressive, highly proliferative prostatic carcinomas defined by p53 accumulation. *J Natl Cancer Inst* 1991;84:883.
172. Scher HI, Kelly WK. Flutamide withdrawal syndrome: its impact on clinical trials in hormone-refractory prostate cancer. *J Clin Oncol* 1993;11:1566.
173. Ruprecht RM, Rossoni LD, Haseltine WA, Broder S. Suppression of retroviral propagation and disease by suramin in murine systems. *Proc Natl Acad Sci U S A* 1985;82:7733.
174. Chi SG, deVere White RW, Meyers FJ, et al. p53 in prostate cancer: frequent expressed transition mutations. *J Natl Cancer Inst* 1994:86:926.
175. Mirchandani D, Zheng J, Miller GJ, et al. Heterogeneity in intratumor distribution of p53 mutations in human prostate cancer. *Am J Pathol* 1995;147:92.
176. Roy-Burman P, Zheng J, Miller GJ. Molecular heterogeneity in prostate cancer: can TP53 mutation unravel tumorigenesis? *Mol Med Today* 1997;3:476.
177. Brooks JD, Bova GS, Ewing CM, et al. An uncertain role for p53 gene alterations in human prostate cancers. *Cancer Res* 1996;56:3814.
178. Osman I, Drobnjak M, Fazzari M, et al. Inactivation of the p53 pathway in prostate cancer: impact on tumor progression. *Clin Cancer Res* 1999;5:2082.
179. Scherr DS, Vaughan EDJ, Wei J, et al. BCL-2 and p53 expression in clinically localized prostate cancer predicts response to external beam radiotherapy [published erratum appears in *J Urol* 1999;162:503]. *J Urol* 1999;162:12.
180. Moul JW. Angiogenesis, p53, bcl-2 and Ki-67 in the progression of prostate cancer after radical prostatectomy. *Eur Urol* 1999;35:399.
181. Matsushima H, Sasaki T, Goto T, et al. Immunohistochemical study of p21WAF1 and p53 proteins in prostatic cancer and their prognostic significance. *Hum Pathol* 1998;29:778.
182. Kuczyk MA, Serth J, Bokemeyer C, et al. The prognostic value of p53 for long-term and recurrence-free survival following radical prostatectomy. *Eur J Cancer* 1998;34:679.
183. Ruijter E, van de Kaa C, Aalders T, et al. Heterogeneous expression of E-cadherin and p53 in prostate cancer: clinical implications. BIOMED-II Markers for Prostate Cancer Study Group. *Mod Pathol* 1998;11:276.
184. Uzoaru I, Rubenstein M, Mirochnik Y, et al. An evaluation of the markers p53 and Ki-67 for their predictive value in prostate cancer. *J Surg Oncol* 1998;67:33.
185. Stapleton AM, Zbell P, Kattan MW, et al. Assessment of the biologic markers p53, Ki-67, and apoptotic index as predictive indicators of prostate carcinoma recurrence after surgery. *Cancer* 1998;82:168.
186. Matsushima H, Kitamura T, Goto T, et al. Combined analysis with Bcl-2 and P53 immunostaining predicts poorer prognosis in prostatic carcinoma. *J Urol* 1997;158:2278.

187. Theodorescu D, Broder SR, Boyd JC, Mills SE, Frierson HFJ. p53, bcl-2 and retinoblastoma proteins as long-term prognostic markers in localized carcinoma of the prostate. *J Urol* 1997;158:131.
188. Grignon DJ, Caplan R, Sarkar FH, et al. p53 status and prognosis of locally advanced prostatic adenocarcinoma: a study based on RTOG 8610. *J Natl Cancer Inst* 1997;89:158.
189. Stricker HJ, Jay JK, Linden MD, Tamboli P, Amin MB. Determining prognosis of clinically localized prostate cancer by immunohistochemical detection of mutant p53. *Urology* 1996;47:366.
190. Shurbaji MS, Kalbfleisch JH, Thurmond TS. Immunohistochemical detection of p53 protein as a prognostic indicator in prostate cancer. *Hum Pathol* 1995;26:106.
191. Thomas DJ, Robinson M, King P, et al. p53 expression and clinical outcome in prostate cancer. *Br J Urol* 1993;72:778.
192. Cairns P, Okami K, Halachmi S, et al. Frequent inactivation of PTEN/MMAC1 in primary prostate cancer. *Cancer Res* 1997;57:4997.
193. Suzuki H, Freije D, Nusskern DR, et al. Interfocal heterogeneity of PTEN/MMSC1 gene alterations in multiple metastatic prostate cancer tissues. *Cancer Res* 1998;58:204.
194. Wang SI, Parsons R, Ittmann M. Homozygous deletion of the PTEN tumor suppressor gene in a subset of prostate adenocarcinomas. *Clin Cancer Res* 1998;4:811.
195. Gray IC, Stewart LM, Phillips SM, et al. Mutation and expression analysis of the putative prostate tumour-suppressor gene PTEN. *Br J Cancer* 1998;78:1296.
196. Vlietstra R, van Alewijk D, Hermans K, van Stratum P, Trapman J. Frequent inactivation of PTEN in prostate cancer cell lines and xenografts. *Cancer Res* 1998;58:2720.
197. McNeal JE, Redwine EA, Freiha FS, Stamey TA. Zonal distribution of prostatic adenocarcinoma. Correlation with histologic pattern and direction of spread. *Am J Surg Pathol* 1988;12:897.
198. McMenamin ME, Soung P, Perera S, et al. Loss of PTEN expression in paraffin-embedded primary prostate cancer correlates with high Gleason score and advanced stage. *Cancer Res* 1999;59:4291.
199. Wu X, Senechal K, Neshat MS, Whang YE, Sawyers CL. The PTEN/MMAC1 tumor suppressor phosphatase functions as a negative regulator of the phosphoinositide 3-kinase/Akt pathway. *Proc Natl Acad Sci U S A* 1998;95:15587.
200. Bookstein R, Shew JY, Chen PL, Scully P, Lee WH. Suppression of tumorigenicity of human prostate carcinoma cells by replacing a mutated RB gene. *Science* 1990;247:712.
201. Bookstein R, Rio P, Madreperla SA, et al. Promoter deletion and loss of retinoblastoma gene expression in human prostate carcinoma. *Proc Natl Acad Sci U S A* 1990;87:7762.
202. Ittmann MM, Wieczorek R. Alterations of the retinoblastoma gene in clinically localized, stage B prostate adenocarcinomas. *Hum Pathol* 1996;27:28.
203. Cooney KA, Wetzel JC, Merajver SD, et al. Distinct regions of allelic loss on 13q in prostate cancer. *Cancer Res* 1996;56:1142.
204. Kamb A, Gruis NA, Weaver-Feldhaus J, et al. A cell cycle regulator potentially involved in genesis of many tumor types. *Science* 1994;264:436.
205. Cairns P, Polascik TJ, Eby Y, et al. Frequency of homozygous deletion at p16/CDKN2 in primary human tumours. *Nat Genet* 1995;11:210.
206. Jarrard D, Bova GS, Ewing CM, et al. Deletional, mutational, and methylation analyses of CDKN2 (p16/MTS1) in primary and metastatic prostate cancer. *Genes Chromosomes Cancer* 1997;19:90.
207. Guo Y, Sklar GN, Borkowski A, Kyprianou N. Loss of the cyclin-dependent kinase inhibitor p27(Kip1) protein in human prostate cancer correlates with tumor grade. *Clin Cancer Res* 1997;3:2269.
208. Yang RM, Naitoh J, Murphy M, et al. Low p27 expression predicts poor disease-free survival in patients with prostate cancer. *J Urol* 1998;159:941.
209. Cote RJ, Shi Y, Groshen S, et al. Association of p27Kip1 levels with recurrence and survival in patients with stage C prostate carcinoma. *J Natl Cancer Inst* 1998;90:916.
210. Kibel AS, Schutte M, Kern SE, Isaacs WB, Bova GS. Identification of 12p as a region of frequent deletion in advanced prostate cancer. *Cancer Res* 1998;58:5652.
211. Dong JT, Lamb PW, Rinker-Schaeffer CW, et al. KAI1, a metastasis suppressor gene for prostate cancer on human chromosome 11p11.2. *Science* 1995;268:884.
212. Morton RA, Ewing CM, Nagafuchi A, Tsukita S, Issacs WB. Reduction of E-cadherin levels and deletion of the alpha-catenin gene in human prostate cancer cells. *Cancer Res* 1993;53:3585.
213. Umbas R, Issacs WB, Bringuier PP, et al. Decreased E-cadherin expression is associated with poor prognosis in patients with prostate cancer. *Cancer Res* 1994;54:3929.
214. Umbas R, Schalken JA, Aalders TW, et al. Expression of the cellular adhesion molecular E-cadherin is reduced or absent in high-grade prostate cancer. *Cancer Res* 1992;52:5104.
215. Ichikawa T, Ichikawa Y, Dong J, et al. Localization of metastasis suppressor gene(s) for prostatic cancer to the short arm of human chromosome 11. *Cancer Res* 1992;52:3486.
216. Graff JR, Herman JG, Lapidus RG, et al. E-cadherin expression is silenced by DNA hypermethylation in human breast and prostate carcinomas. *Cancer Res* 1995;55:5195.
217. Lee WH, Morton RA, Epstein JI, et al. Cytidine methylation of regulatory sequences near the class glutathione-S-transferase gene accompanies human prostatic carcinogenesis. *Proc Natl Acad Sci U S A* 1994;91:11733.
218. Mostofi FK, Sobin LH, Torloni H. Histologic typing of urinary bladder tumours. In: *International histological classification of tumors.* Geneva: The World Health Organization, 1973.
219. Koss LG. Atlas of tumor pathology. In: *Tumors of the urinary bladder,* fascicle 11. Washington, DC: Armed Forces Institute of Pathology, 1975.
220. Tumors of the urinary tract and prostate in urinary sediment. In: Koss L, ed. *Diagnostic cytology and its histopathologic basis,* 4th ed. Philadelphia: JB Lippincott Co, 1992.
221. Prout GR. Bladder carcinoma and a TNM system of classification. *J Urol* 1997;117:583.
222. Altausen AF, Prout GR, Daly JJ. Non-invasive papillary carcinoma of the bladder associated with carcinoma *in situ. J Urol* 1976;116:575.
223. Reuter VE, Melamed MR. The lower urinary tract. In: Sternberg SS, ed. *Diagnostic surgical pathology.* New York: Raven Press, 1989.
224. Stein JP, Grossfeld GD, Ginsberg DA, et al. Prognostic markers in bladder cancer: a contemporary review of the literature. *J Urol* 1998;160:645.
225. Gibas Z, Prout GR, Connolly JG, Pontes JE, Sandberg AA. Nonrandom chromosomal changes in transitional cell carcinoma of the bladder. *Cancer Res* 1984;44:1257.
226. Smeets W, Pauwels R, Laarakkers L, Debruyne F, Geraedts J. Chromosomal analysis of bladder cancer. III. Nonrandom alterations. *Cancer Genet Cytogenet* 1987;29:29.
227. Atkin NB, Baker MC. Cytogenetic study of ten carcinomas of the bladder: involvement of chromosomes 1 and 11. *Cancer Genet Cytogenet* 1985;15:253.
228. Babu VR, Lutz MD, Miles BJ, et al. Tumor behavior in transitional cell carcinoma of the bladder in relation to chromosomal markers and histopathology. *Cancer Res* 1987;47:6800.
229. Vanni R, Scarpa RM, Nieddu M, Usai E. Cytogenetic investigation on 30 bladder carcinomas. *Cancer Genet Cytogenet* 1988;30:35.
230. Tyrkus M, Powell I, Fakr W. Cytogenetic studies of carcinoma *in situ* of the bladder: prognostic implications. *J Urol* 1992;148:44.
231. Poddighe PJ, Ramaekers FCS, Smeets WGB, Vooijs GP, Hopman AHN. Structural chromosome 1 aberrations in transitional cell carcinoma of the bladder: interphase cytogenetics combining a centromeric, telomeric, and library DNA probe. *Cancer Res* 1992; 52:4929.
232. Hopman AHN, Moesker O, Smeets W, et al. Numerical chromosome 1, 7, 9, and 11 aberrations in bladder cancer detected by *in situ* hybridization. *Cancer Res* 1991;51:644.
233. Waldman FM, Carroll PR, Kerschmann R, et al. Centromeric copy number of chromosome 7 is strongly correlated with tumor grade and labeling index in human bladder cancer. *Cancer Res* 1991;51:3807.
234. Sauter G, Moch H, Moore D, et al. Heterogeneity of erbB-2 gene amplification in bladder cancer. *Cancer Res* 1993;53:2199.
235. Sauter G, Carroll P, Moch H, et al. c-myc copy number gains in bladder cancer detected by fluorescence *in situ* hybridization. *Am J Pathol* 1995;146:1131.
236. Sauter G, Deng G, Moch H, et al. Physical deletion of the p53 gene in bladder cancer. *Am J Pathol* 1994;144:756.
237. Wheeless LL, Reeder JE, Han R, et al. Bladder irrigation specimens assayed by fluorescence *in situ* hybridization to interphase nuclei. *Cytometry* 1994;17:319.
238. Reddy EP, Reynolds RK, Santos E, Barbacid M. A point mutation is responsible for the acquisition of transforming properties by the T24 bladder carcinoma oncogene. *Nature* 1982;300:149.
239. Feinberg AP, Vogelstein B, Droller MJ, Baylin SB, Nelkin BD. Mutation affecting the 12th amino acid of the c-Ha-ras oncogene product occurs infrequently in human cancer. *Science* 1983;220:1175.
240. Fujita J, Srivastava SK, Kraus MH. Frequency of molecular alterations affecting ras protooncogenes in human urinary tract tumors. *Proc Natl Acad Sci U S A* 1985;82:3849.
241. Visvanathan KV, Pocock RD, Summerhayes IC. Preferential and novel activation of Haras in human bladder carcinoma. *Oncogene Res* 1988;3:77.
242. Nagatava Y, Abe M, Kobayashi K, et al. Point mutations of c-ras genes in human bladder cancer and kidney cancer. *Jpn J Cancer Res* 1990;81:22.
243. Czerniak B, Deitch D, Simmons H, et al. Ha-ras gene codon 12 mutations and DNA ploidy in urinary bladder carcinomas. *Br J Cancer* 1990;62:762.
244. Czerniak B, Cohen GL, Etkind P, et al. Concurrent mutations of coding and regulatory sequences of the Ha-ras gene in urinary bladder carcinomas. *Hum Pathol* 1992;23:1199.
245. Ooi A, Herz F, Setsuko I, et al. Ha-ras codon 12 mutation in papillary tumors of the urinary bladder. A retrospective study. *Int J Oncol* 1994;4:85.
246. Fitzgerald JM, Ramchurren N, Rieger K, et al. Identification of H-ras mutations in urine sediments complements cytology in the detection of bladder tumors. *J Natl Cancer Inst* 1995;87:129.
247. Vogelstein B, Fearon ER, Hamilton SR, et al. Genetic alterations during colorectal tumor development. *N Engl J Med* 1988;319:525.
248. Burmer GC, Loeb LA. Mutations of the KRAS2 oncogene during progressive stages of human colon carcinomas. *Proc Natl Acad Sci U S A* 1989;86:2403.
249. Bos JL. Ras oncogene in human cancer: a review. *Cancer Res* 1989;49:4682.
250. Jen J, Powel SM, Papadopoulos N, et al. Molecular determinants of dysplasia in colorectal lesions. *Cancer Res* 1994;54:5523.
251. Neal DE, Sharples L, Smith K, et al. Epidermal growth-factor receptors in human bladder cancer: comparison of invasive and superficial tumors. *Lancet* 1985;1:366.
252. Neal DE, Sharples L, Smith K, et al. The epidermal growth factor receptor and the prognosis of bladder cancer. *Cancer* 1990;65:1619.
253. Messing EM. Clinical implications of the expression growth factor receptors in human transitional cell carcinomas. *Cancer Res* 1990;50:2530.
254. Rao JY, Hemstreet GP, Hurst RE, et al. Alterations in phenotypic biochemical markers in bladder epithelium during tumorigenesis. *Proc Natl Acad Sci U S A* 1993;90:8287.
255. Nguyen PL, Swanson PE, Jaszcz W, et al. Expression of epidermal growth factor receptor in invasive transitional cell carcinoma of the urinary bladder: a multivariate survival analysis. *Am J Clin Pathol* 1994,101:166.
256. Wood D, Wartinger DD, Reuter V, et al. DNA, RNA and immunohistochemical characterization of the HER-2/neu oncogene in transitional cell carcinoma of the bladder. *J Urol* 1991;146:1398.
257. Sato K, Moriyama M, Mori S, et al. An immunohistologic evaluation of c-erbB-2 gene product in patients with urinary bladder carcinoma. *Cancer* 1992;70:2493.
258. Underwood M, Barlett J, Reeves J, et al. C-erbB-2 gene amplification: a molecular marker in recurrent bladder tumors? *Cancer Res* 1995;55:2422.
259. Oliner JD, Kinzler KW, Metlzer PS, et al. Amplification of a gene encoding a p53 associated protein in human sarcomas. *Nature* 1992;358:80.
260. Kubbutat MH, Jones SN, Vousden KH. Regulation of p53 stability by Mdm2. *Nature* 1997;387:299.
261. Haupt Y, Maya R, Kazaz A, Oren M. Mdm2 promotes the rapid degradation of p53. *Nature* 1997;387:296.
262. Momand J, Zambetti G, Olson D, et al. The mdm-2 oncogene product forms a complex with the p-53 protein and inhibits TP53-mediated transactivation. *Cell* 1992;69:1237.

263. Lianes P, Orlow I, Zhang ZZ, et al. Altered patterns of MDM2 and TP53 expression in human bladder cancer. *J Natl Cancer Inst* 1994;86:1325.
264. Barbareschi M, Girlando S, Fellin G, et al. Expression of mdm2 and p53 proteins in transitional cell carcinoma. *Urol Res* 1995;22:349.
265. Fearon ER, Feinberg AP, Hamilton SH, Vogelstein B. Loss of genes on the short arm of chromosome 11 in bladder cancer. *Nature* 1985;318:377.
266. Tsai YC, Nichols PW, Hiti AL, et al. Allelic losses of chromosomes 9, 11, and 17 in human bladder cancer. *Cancer Res* 1990;50:44.
267. Olumi AF, Tsai YC, Nichols PW, et al. Allelic loss of chromosomes 17p distinguishes high grade from low grade transitional cell carcinoma of the bladder. *Cancer Res* 1990;50:7081.
268. Presti JC, Reuter VE, Galan T, et al. Molecular genetic alterations in superficial and locally advanced human bladder cancer. *Cancer Res* 1991;51:5405.
269. Dalbagni G, Presti J, Reuter V, Fair WR, Cardo-Cardo C. Genetic alterations in bladder cancer. *Lancet* 1993;324:469.
270. Habuchi T, Ogawa O, Kakehi Y, et al. Accumulated allelic losses in the development of invasive urothelial cancer. *Int J Cancer* 1993;53:579.
271. Cairns P, Proctor AJ, Knowles MA. Loss of heterozygosity at the RB locus in frequent and correlates with muscle invasion in bladder carcinoma. *Oncogene* 1991;6:2305.
272. Cordon-Cardo C, Wartinger D, Petrylak D, et al. Altered expression of the retinoblastoma gene product is a prognostic indicator in bladder caner. *J Natl Cancer Inst* 1992; 84:1251.
273. Logothetis CJ, Xu HJ, Ro JY, et al. Altered retinoblastoma protein expression and known prognostic variables in locally advanced bladder cancer. *J Natl Cancer Inst* 1992;84:1257.
274. Sidransky D, Von Eschenbach A, Tsai YC, et al. Identification of p53 gene mutations in bladder cancer and urine samples. *Science* 1991;252:706.
275. Fujimoto K, Yamada Y, Okajima E, et al. Frequent association of p53 gene mutations in invasive bladder cancer. *Cancer Res* 1992;52:1393.
276. Dalbagni G, Presti JC, Reuter VE, et al. Molecular genetic alterations of chromosome 17 and p53 nuclear overexpression in human bladder cancer. *Diagn Mol Pathol* 1993;2:4.
277. Cordon-Cardo C, Dalbagni D, Saez GT, et al. TP53 mutations in human bladder cancer: genotypic versus phenotypic patterns. *Int J Cancer* 1994;56:347.
278. Sarkis AS, Dalbagni G, Cordon-Cardo C, et al. Nuclear overexpression of p53 protein in transitional cell bladder carcinoma: a marker for disease progression. *J Natl Cancer Inst* 1993;85:53.
279. Sarkis AS, Zhang ZF, Cordon-Cardo C, et al. p53 nuclear overexpression and disease progression in Ta bladder carcinoma. *Int J Oncol* 1993;3:355.
280. Lipponen PK. Over-expression of p53 nuclear oncoprotein in transitional cell bladder cancer and its prognostic value. *Int J Cancer* 1993;53:365.
281. Esrig D, Elmajian D, Groshen S, et al. Accumulation of nuclear p53 and tumor progression in bladder cancer. *N Engl J Med* 1994;331:1259.
282. Miyao N, Tsai YC, Lerner SP, et al. Role of chromosome 9 in human bladder cancer. *Cancer Res* 1993;53:4066.
283. Cairns P, Shaw ME, Knowles MA. Preliminary mapping of the deleted region of chromosome 9 in bladder cancer. *Cancer Res* 1993;53:1230.
284. Ruppert JM, Tokino K, Sidransky D. Evidence for two bladder cancer suppressor loci on human chromosome 9. *Cancer Res* 199453:5093.
285. Orlow I, Lianes P, Lacombe L, et al. Chromosome 9 deletions and microsatellite alterations in human bladder tumors. *Cancer Res* 1994;54:2848.
286. Kamb A, Gruis NA, Weaver-Feldhaus J, et al. A cell cycle regulator potentially involved in genesis of many tumor types. *Science* 1994;264:436.
287. Serrano M, Hannon GJ, Beach D. A new regulatory motif in cell-cycle control causing specific inhibition of cyclin D/CDK4. *Nature* 1993;366:704.
288. Hannon GJ, Beach D. p15ink4B is a potential effector of TGF-β-induced cell cycle arrest. *Nature* 1994;371:257.
289. Cordon-Cardo C. Mutation of cell cycle regulators: biological and clinical implications for human neoplasias. *Am J Pathol* 1995;147:545.
290. Kamb A, Lui Q, Harshman K, et al. Rates of p16 (MTS1) mutations in primary tumors with 9p loss. *Science* 1994;265:416.
291. Spruck CH, Gonzalez-Zulueta M, Shibata A, et al. p16 gene in uncultured tumours. *Nature* 1994;370:183.
292. Williamson M, Elder PA, Shaw ME, Devlin J, Knowles M. P16 (CDKN2) is a major deletions target at 9p21 in bladder cancer. *Hum Mol Genet* 1995;4:1569.
293. Cairns P, Polascik TJ, Eby Y, et al. Frequency of homozygous deletion at p16/CDKN2 in primary human tumours. *Nat Genet* 1995;11:210.
294. Gruis NA, Weaver-Feldhaus J, Liu Q, et al. Genetic evidence in melanoma and bladder cancers that p16 and p53 function in separate pathways of tumor suppression. *Am J Pathol* 1995;146:1199.
295. Orlow I, Lacombe L, Hannon GJ, et al. Deletion of the p16 and p15 genes in human bladder tumors. *J Natl Cancer Inst* 1995;87:1524.
296. Johnson DG, Schwarz JK, Cress WD, Nevins JR. Expression of transcription factor E2F1 induces quiescent cells to enter S phase. *Nature* 1993;365:349.
297. Pomerantz J, Schreiber-Agus N, Liegeois NJ, et al. The Ink4a tumor suppressor gene product, p19Arf, interacts with MDM2 and neutralizes MDM2's inhibition of p53. *Cell* 1998;92:713.
298. Zhang Y, Xiong Y, Yarbrough WG. ARF promotes MDM2 degradation and stabilizes p53: ARF-INK4a locus deletion impairs both the Rb and p53 tumor suppression pathways. *Cell* 1998;92:725.
299. Spruck CH, Ohneseit PE, Gonzalez-Zulueta M, et al. Two molecular pathways to transitional cell carcinoma of the bladder. *Cancer Res* 1994;54:784.
300. Cordon-Cardo C, Dalbagni D, Sarkis A, Reuter VE. Genetics alterations associated with bladder cancer. In: DeVita VT, Hellman S, Rosenberg SA, eds. *Important advances in oncology*. Philadelphia: Lippincott Company, 1994.
301. Peltomaki P, Aaltonen LA, Sistonen P, et al. Genetic mapping of a locus predisposing to human colorectal cancer. *Science* 1993;260:810.
302. Fishel R, Lescoe MK, Rao MRS, et al. The human mutator gene homolog MSH2 and its association with hereditary nonpolyposis colon cancer. *Cell* 1993;75:1027.
303. Leach FS, Nicolaides NC, Papadopoulos N, et al. Mutations of a mutS homolog in hereditary nonpolyposis colorectal cancer. *Cell* 1993;75:1215.
304. Lynch HT, Ens JA, Lynch JF. The Lynch syndrome II and urological malignancies. *J Urol* 1990;143:24.
305. Modrich P, Lahue R. Mismatch repair in replication fidelity, genetic recombination, and cancer biology. *Annu Rev Biochem* 1996;65:101.
306. Aaltonen LA, Peltomaki P, Leach FS, et al. Clues to the pathogenesis of familial colorectal cancer. *Science* 1993;260:812.
307. Thibodeau SN, Bren G, Schaid D. Microsatellite instability in cancer of the proximal colon. *Science* 1993;260:816.
308. Ionov Y, Peinado MA, Malkhosyan S, Shibata D, Perucho M. Ubiquitous somatic mutations in simple repeated sequences reveal a new mechanism for colonic carcinogenesis. *Nature* 1993;363:558.
309. Strand M, Prolla TA, Liskay RM, Petes TD. Destabilization of tracts of simple repetitive DNA in yeast by mutations affecting DNA mismatch repair [see comments; published erratum appears in *Nature* 1994;368;569]. *Nature* 1993;365:274.
310. Gonzalez-Zulueta M, Ruppert JM, Tokino K, et al. Microsatellite instability in bladder cancer. *Cancer Res* 1993;53:5620.
311. Jin TX, Furihata M, Yamasaki I, et al. Human mismatch repair gene (hMSH2) product expression in relation to recurrence of transitional cell carcinoma of the urinary bladder. *Cancer* 1999;85:478.
312. Humbert O, Fiumicino S, Aquilina G, et al. Mismatch repair and differential sensitivity of mouse and human cells to methylating agents. *Carcinogenesis* 1999;20:205.
313. Caldas C, Hahn SA, da Costa LT, et al. Frequent somatic mutations and homozygous deletions of the p16 (MTS1) gene in pancreatic adenocarcinoma. *Nat Genet* 1994;8:27.
314. Mao LDJ, Tockman MS, Erozan YS, Askin F, Sidransky D. Microsatellite alterations as clonal markers for the detection of human cancer. *Proc Natl Acad Sci U S A* 1994;91:9871.
315. Bova GS, Fox WM, Epstein JI. Methods of radical prostatectomy specimen processing: a novel technique for harvesting fresh prostate cancer tissue and review of processing techniques. *Mod Pathol* 1993;6:201.
316. Mao L, Schoenberg MP, Scicchitano M, et al. Molecular detection of primary bladder cancer by microsatellite analysis. *Science* 1996;271:659.
317. Edwards A, Hammond HA, Jin K, Caskey CT, Chakrabority R. Genetic variation at five trimeric and tetrameric tandem repeat loci in four human population groups. *Genomics* 1992;12:241.
318. Lokeshwar BL, Block NL. Isolation of a prostate carcinoma cell proliferation-inhibiting factor from human seminal plasma and its similarity to transforming growth factor B. *Cancer Res* 1992;52:5821.
319. Zbar B. Chromosomal deletions in lung cancer and renal cancer. In: DeVita VT, Hellman S, Rosenberg SA, eds. *Important advances in oncology*. Philadelphia: JB Lippincott Co, 1989:41.
320. Zbar B, Tory K, Merino M, et al. Hereditary papillary renal cell carcinoma. *J Urol* 1994;151:561.
321. Mahul AB, Crotty TB, Tickoo SK, Farrow GM. Renal oncocytoma: a reappraisal of morphologic features with clinicopathologic findings in 80 cases. *Am J Surg Pathol* 1997;21:1.

W. MARSTON LINEHAN
BERTON ZBAR
SUSAN E. BATES
MICHAEL J. ZELEFSKY
JAMES C. YANG

SECTION 2

Cancer of the Kidney and Ureter

RENAL CARCINOMA

Each year in the United States, approximately 31,000 cases of kidney and upper urinary tract cancer occur, resulting in more than 11,900 deaths.[1] These tumors account for approximately 3% of adult malignancies and occur in a male-female ratio of 1.5:1. They are more common among urban than rural residents. Although most cases occur in persons aged 50 to 70 years, renal carcinoma has been observed in children as young as 6 months. Between 1975 and 1995, a steady and significant increase in the incidence of renal carcinoma was seen, from 2% to 4% per year, an increase of 43% since 1973.[2–5]

Renal carcinoma was first described by Konig in 1826. As early as 1855, Robin concluded that the renal tubular epithelium was the most probable tissue of origin of the cancer, an observation that was confirmed by Waldeyer in 1867. In 1883, Grawitz, noting that the fatty content of the cancer cells was similar to that of adrenal cells, concluded that the tumors arose from adrenal rests within the kidney and introduced the term *stroma lipomatodes aberrata renis* for these clear cell tumors. The term *hypernephroid tumors* was introduced in 1984 by Birch-Hirschfeld. Since then the conceptually incorrect term *hypernephroma* has frequently been applied to renal tumors.[6,7]

Renal carcinoma occurs in both a sporadic and a hereditary form. There are four main forms of hereditary renal carcinoma (HRC). The most studied form of HRC is von Hippel-Lindau (VHL) syndrome. VHL syndrome is a hereditary cancer syndrome in which affected individuals are at risk to develop tumors in a number of organs, including the kidney.[2,8] A recently described form of HRC is hereditary papillary renal carcinoma (HPRC).[9,10] Another recently described form of hereditary kidney cancer is familial renal oncocytoma (FRO),[11] which has been found to be associated with the cutaneous condition Birt-Hogg-Dubé syndrome.[12] Hereditary clear cell renal carcinoma is a rare condition that is inherited in an autosomal dominant fashion in which patients develop clear cell variant renal carcinoma. In the hereditary syndromes, the kidney cancer is often bilateral and tends to occur in a younger age group.[8] An increased incidence of renal carcinoma has also been observed in patients with autosomal dominant polycystic kidney disease and tuberous sclerosis.[13]

ETIOLOGY

A number of environmental, hormonal, cellular, and genetic factors have been studied as possible causal factors in the development of renal carcinoma. In studies of risk of renal carcinoma, cigarette smoking has been found to be a definite risk factor.[14–16] A statistically significant dose response has been observed in both genders for pack-years of cigarette use.[17] It has been estimated that 30% of renal carcinomas in men and 24% in women may be directly due to smoking.[18] Obesity is associated with an increased risk of development of renal carcinoma, particularly in women.[19] Analgesic abuse, which is known to be associated with renal pelvis cancer, is also associated with an increased incidence of kidney cancer. The increased risk for the development of renal carcinoma is observed primarily in patients who abuse phenacetin-containing analgesics and develop analgesic nephropathy.[5,16,20]

Environmental and occupational factors have also been associated with the development of kidney cancer. Brauch et al.[21] demonstrated an association between the development of renal carcinoma and long-term exposure to high levels of the industrial solvent trichloroethylene. There is an increased incidence of renal carcinoma among leather tanners, shoe workers, and workers exposed to asbestos.[22] Exposure to cadmium is associated with an increased incidence of kidney cancer, particularly in men who smoke.[23] An association between gasoline exposure and kidney cancer has been observed in animal studies. Although there is an increased incidence of renal carcinoma reported with exposure to petroleum, tar, and pitch products, studies of oil refinery workers and petroleum products distribution workers do not identify a definite relationship between gasoline exposure and renal cancer. There may be an increased risk of kidney cancer in older workers or in workers exposed to gasoline for prolonged periods.[24]

An increased incidence (100-fold) of renal carcinoma has been noted in patients with end-stage renal disease who develop acquired cystic disease of the kidneys.[25] Acquired cystic disease is a recently described phenomenon in which patients on long-term dialysis for renal failure develop cysts in their native kidneys. Renal carcinoma has been found in association with the papillary hyperplasia observed in the cyst epithelium of these kidneys. The risk of developing kidney cancer has been estimated to be greater than 30 times higher in dialysis patients with cystic changes in their kidney than in the general population.[26] It is estimated that 35% to 47% of patients on long-term dialysis will develop acquired cystic disease and that nearly 5.8% of the patients with acquired cystic disease will develop renal cancer. Kidney cancer can develop at any time in patients with end-stage renal disease, and it can occur in kidney transplant recipients as well. It can develop in patients with end-stage renal disease who are undergoing either hemodialysis or chronic ambulatory dialysis, but it also has been reported to occur in patients with end-stage renal disease who are not being dialyzed.[25] Although many of these cancers are clinically insignificant and are found incidentally at autopsy or after bilateral nephrectomy, some will follow an aggressive course.[27] Careful surveillance of patients with end-stage renal disease with ultrasonography and computed tomography (CT) is recommended.[14]

HEREDITARY FORMS OF RENAL CARCINOMA

Like breast cancer, colon cancer, and retinoblastoma, renal cancer occurs in both a sporadic (nonhereditary) and a hereditary form. At least four forms of HRC are recognized: VHL, HPRC, FRO, and HRC (Table 34.2-1).[224–227]

von Hippel-Lindau Syndrome

The VHL syndrome, which is predicted to occur in 1 in 36,000 live births, is a familial cancer syndrome in which affected individuals have a predisposition to develop tumors in a number of organs, including the kidneys, brain, spine, eyes, adrenal

TABLE 34.2-1. Hereditary Forms of Renal Carcinoma

Form of Carcinoma	*Abbreviation*	*Studies*
Renal carcinoma associated with von Hippel-Lindau disease	VHL	8,224,225
Hereditary papillary renal carcinoma	HPRC	9,10
Hereditary renal carcinoma associated with Birt-Hogg-Dubé syndrome	BHDS	12
Hereditary renal carcinoma (clear cell)	HCRC	226,227

glands, pancreas, inner ear, and epididymis.[2,8,28] Forty percent of VHL patients develop multiple, bilateral tumors or cysts in the kidneys. The renal carcinoma acquired by VHL patients is clear cell renal carcinoma.[29] These patients can have hundreds of small clear cell tumors and cysts in their kidneys. The tumors, which tend to occur early in life, can metastasize, and the affected individual may succumb to the malignancy. VHL patients can also develop pheochromocytoma, pancreatic cysts and islet cell tumors, retinal angiomas, central nervous system hemangioblastomas, inner ear tumors (endolymphatic sac tumors), and epididymal cystadenomas (Table 34.2-2).[8]

THE VHL GENE. Identification of the VHL gene by Latif et al.[30] in 1993 was an important step for physicians managing patients with VHL disease. Critical to management of VHL patients is the knowledge of who is affected and who is not. Early identification of at-risk individuals is essential for initiation of early intervention with the potential to prevent of life-threatening complications of the disease, such as metastatic kidney cancer.[2,8]

VHL GERMLINE MUTATION TESTING. Identification of the VHL gene has allowed the detection of germline mutation in nearly 100% of VHL families.[31,32] The VHL clinical features can be heterogeneous, and manifestations such as kidney cancer occult. In some families, VHL syndrome can be confused with other hereditary cancer syndromes, such as multiple endocrine neoplasia type 2. The availability of germline mutation screening can aid the physician in making the correct diagnosis as well as in performing presymptomatic screening in at-risk individuals. (See Chapter 34.1.)

ROLE OF THE VHL GENE IN CLEAR CELL RENAL CANCER. The VHL gene has been found to be mutated in a high percentage of tumors and cell lines from patients with sporadic (nonhereditary) clear cell renal carcinoma.[33,34] VHL gene mutations have not been detected in either tumors from patients with papillary renal carcinoma or from the germline of patients with HPRC. This has led to the development of a molecular genetic

TABLE 34.2-2. Classification of von Hippel-Lindau (VHL) Syndrome

Type	*Description*
I	VHL syndrome without pheochromocytomas
II	VHL syndrome with pheochromocytomas
IIA	Pheochromocytomas, retinal angiomas, and central nervous system hemangioblastomas
IIB	VHL IIA syndrome plus renal cancers and pancreatic involvement

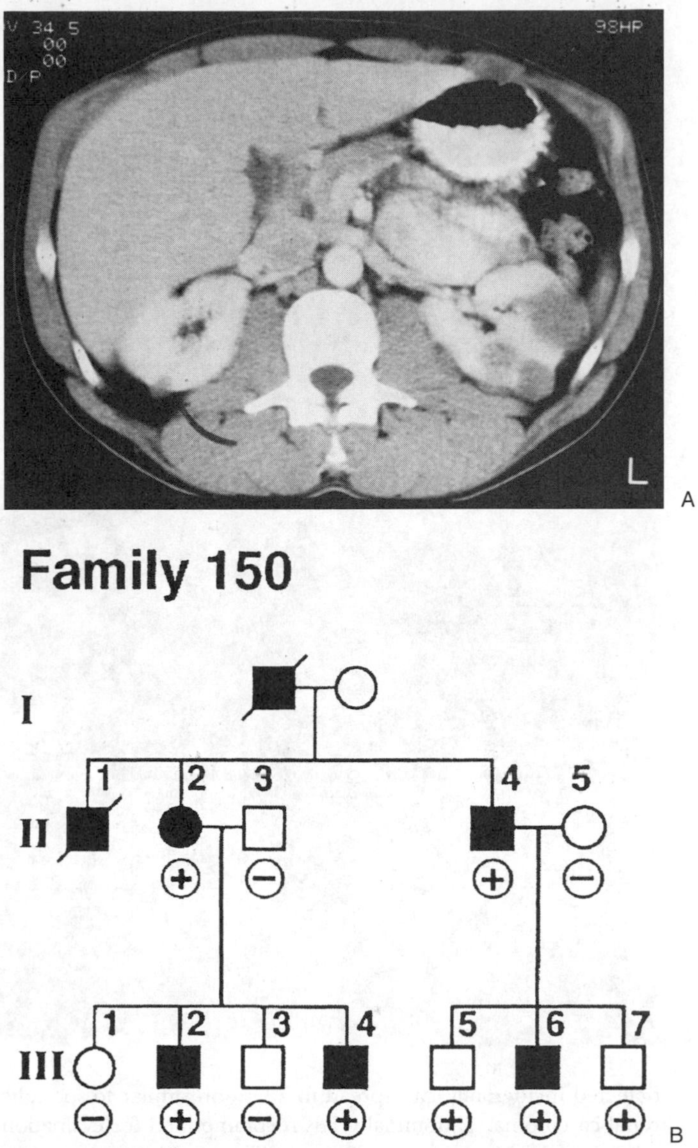

FIGURE 34.2-1. **A:** Abdominal computed tomography scan of a patient with hereditary papillary renal carcinoma, demonstrating bilateral, multifocal papillary renal carcinoma.[9,10] **B:** Hereditary papillary renal carcinoma kindred. The black boxes and circles represent individuals found to have kidney cancer. The circles below these represent the result of germline testing for the c-Met mutation. (From ref. 39, with permission.)

classification of renal carcinoma of papillary versus clear cell (nonpapillary) renal carcinoma,[8,35] with clear cell renal carcinoma being characterized by inactivation of the VHL gene.[33,34] The determination that VHL gene mutations can be detected in formalin-fixed tissue from patients with clear cell renal carcinoma provides a potential method for significantly improving clinicians' ability to diagnose this disease, by analysis of either tissue blocks or tissue aspirates from patients suspected of having this disease.[36]

Hereditary Papillary Renal Carcinoma

HPRC is a recently described form of HRC.[9,10] HPRC is an inherited disorder with an autosomal dominant inheritance pattern in which affected individuals develop bilateral, multifocal papillary renal carcinoma (Fig. 34.2-1). These tumors, which are often

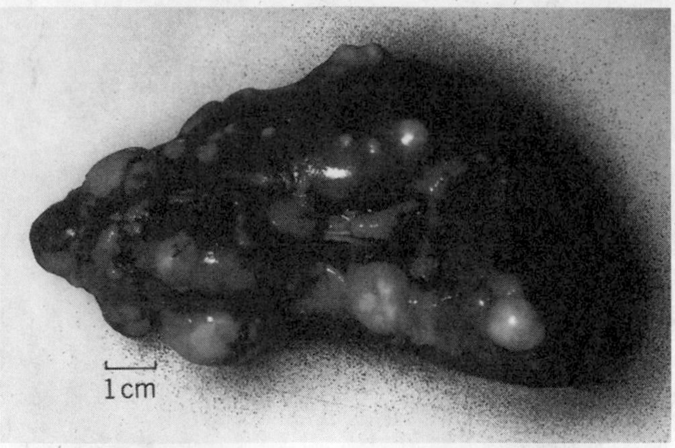

A

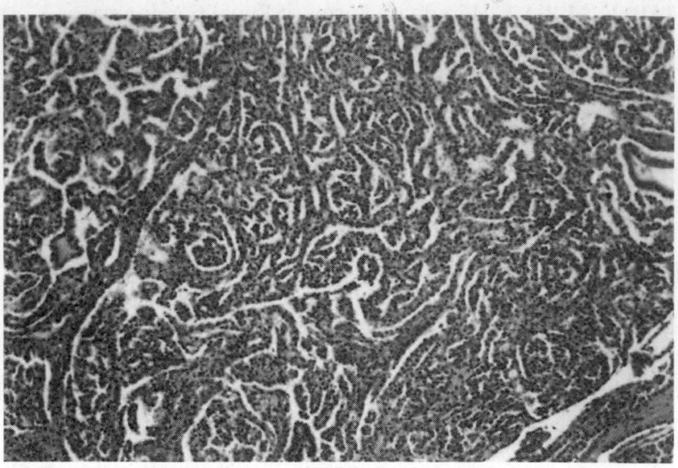

B

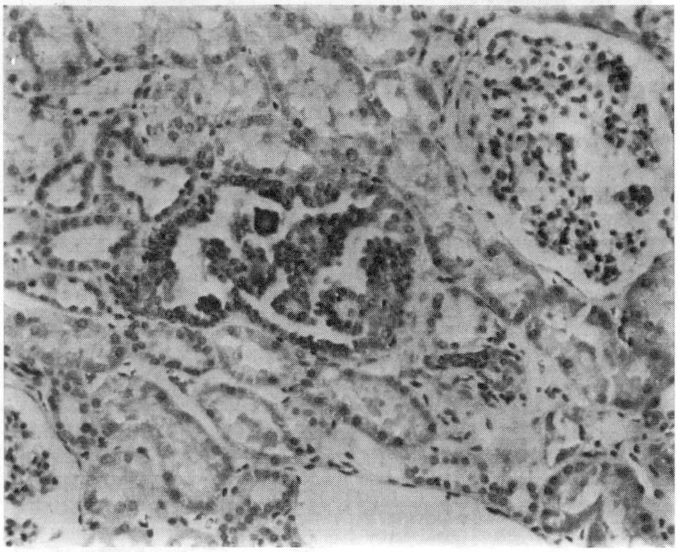

C

FIGURE 34.2-2. **A:** A kidney from an asymptomatic man who was found to have hereditary papillary renal carcinoma (HPRC), demonstrating multifocal papillary renal carcinoma. HPRC is a hereditary cancer syndrome in which affected individuals are at risk to develop multifocal papillary renal carcinoma. **B:** The histology of HPRC renal tumors is uniformly papillary. **C:** Hundreds of small tumors and adenomas may be present in each kidney. HPRC is characterized by a germline mutation of the c-Met gene, and germline testing is recommended for at-risk individuals. (From ref. 9, with permission.)

detected incidentally, can spread in a fashion similar to sporadic renal carcinoma. Abdominal CT is recommended for evaluation of at-risk individuals, as even large papillary renal tumors are frequently undetectable by renal ultrasound evaluation.[37]

THE HPRC GENE: MET. Genetic linkage studies in HPRC kindreds localized the HPRC gene and led to the identification of the c-Met protooncogene as the gene responsible for HPRC.[38] Germline mutations in the tyrosine kinase domain of the MET gene have been found in affected individuals in HPRC kindreds.

HPRC GERMLINE TESTING. Germline MET mutation testing is recommended for patients at risk for HPRC. Individuals in HPRC kindreds, those with bilateral, multifocal papillary renal carcinoma (Fig. 34.2-2), or those with a family history of papillary kidney cancer are considered candidates for germline testing.[39]

Familial Renal Oncocytoma and Birt-Hogg-Dubé Syndrome

A new, recently described form of HRC is FRO.[11] Affected individuals can develop bilateral, multifocal oncocytoma or oncocytic neoplasms in the kidney. Similar renal manifestations have been found to occur in patients with a hereditary cutaneous syndrome, Birt-Hogg-Dubé syndrome (BHDS). BHDS patients have a dominantly inherited predisposition to develop fibrofolliculomas, benign tumors of the hair follicle that appear predominantly on the face, neck, and upper trunk. Affected BHDS individuals are at risk to develop fibrofolliculomas, renal tumors, colon polyps or tumors, and pulmonary cysts.[12] Individuals in BHDS kindreds are at risk to develop renal tumors. The renal tumors that occur in BHDS can be clear, papillary, chromophobe, or oncocytomas and are malignant and can metastasize if not detected and treated. Studies are currently under way to identify the gene for this hereditary cancer syndrome and to develop a test for germline testing of at-risk individuals.

PATHOLOGY

Immunohistologic and ultrastructural analysis has established that the proximal renal tubular epithelium is the true tissue of origin of renal carcinoma. Renal tumors tend to be spherical but may vary widely in size. The average diameter is approximately 7 cm; however, renal tumors can often grow to fill the entire retroperitoneum. Previously, renal lesions 2 cm or less in diameter were considered to be renal adenomas, while lesions 2 cm or more in diameter were considered to be carcinomas. The distinction between benign and malignant tumors is no longer made on the basis of size but on the basis of classic histologic criteria.[40] Although renal carcinoma tends to arise in the cortex of the kidney, it can originate in the interior of the kidney. Often a pseudocapsule is formed around the tumor by compression of surrounding tissue. Hemorrhage and necrosis may be present and, frequently, large areas of sclerosis and fibrosis are found within the tumor. Calcification and single or multiple fluid-filled cysts may be seen within the tumor also. Sporadic renal carcinoma appears in either kidney with equal frequency; it is most often solitary and unilateral.

Renal tumors can be of five main cellular types: clear cell, papillary, chromophobe, oncocytoma, and collecting duct (for review, see Zambrano et al.[40]). Clear cell carcinomas contain lightly staining cells with vacuolated cytoplasm containing cholesterol-like substances, neutral lipids, phospholipids, and glycogen; these constitute 85% of kidney cancers.[40,41] Papillary renal carcinoma makes up approximately 10% of all kidney cancers,[42] with the remainder being chromophobe, collecting duct, and miscellaneous histologic types. Papillary renal carcinoma has been divided into two morphologic subtypes, types 1 and 2.[42] Collecting duct carcinoma is an unusual variant of renal cell carcinoma (RCC) that is characterized by a very aggressive clinical course. It is not uncommon for a patient with collecting duct carcinoma to present with locally or widespread advanced disease.[43] Chromophobe carcinoma, described by Thoenes et al.[44] in 1985, is characterized by large polygonal cells with pale reticular cytoplasm. Renal oncocytoma, which consists predominantly of eosinophilic cells in a characteristic nested or organoid pattern, is considered to be predominantly a benign lesion.[45] Whether oncocytoma can occur in a malignant form or whether so-called malignant oncocytoma is actually a variant of chromophobe renal carcinoma is not completely understood.[40,46]

The sarcomatoid variant, which can occur with any histologic subtype,[47] is associated with a significantly poorer prognosis than are nonsarcomatous renal carcinomas.[48] A median survival of only 6.6 months is reported for patients with sarcomatoid-type renal carcinoma, as compared to a 19.0-month median survival for patients with nonsarcomatous renal carcinoma.[49] Although infrequently used in renal carcinoma, tumor grading may correlate with survival, particularly in patients with nonmetastatic cancer.

CLINICAL PRESENTATION

Renal carcinoma may remain clinically occult for most of its course. The classic presentation of pain, hematuria, and flank mass occurs in only 9% of patients and often is indicative of advanced disease.[50] A tumor in the kidney can progress unnoticed to a large size in the retroperitoneum until a metastasis appears. Approximately 30% of patients with renal carcinoma present with metastatic disease, 25% with locally advanced renal carcinoma, and 45% with localized disease. Some 75% of patients with metastatic renal carcinoma have metastases to the lung, 36% to soft tissues, 20% to bone, 18% to liver, 8% to cutaneous sites, and 8% to the central nervous system.[51]

A considerable number of patients with renal carcinoma develop systemic symptoms of this disease (Table 34.2-3).[52] Hypochromic anemia, due to either hematuria or hemolysis, has been observed in 29% to 88% of patients with renal carcinoma. Pyrexia is observed in 20% and cachexia, fatigue, and weight loss in 33%. Nonmetastatic hepatic dysfunction, initially described by Stauffer in 1961, is a reversible syndrome associated with renal carcinoma that tends to occur in association with fever, fatigue, and weight loss and resolves when the primary tumor is removed. Nonmetastatic hepatic dysfunction, which is usually associated with poor long-term prognosis, occurs in up to 7% of patients with renal carcinoma. Abnormal hepatic function is observed in up to 40%.[53]

TABLE 34.2-3. Presenting Symptoms, Laboratory Abnormalities, or Abnormalities on Physical Examination and Their Relation to Survival Rate in 309 Consecutive Patients Undergoing Nephrectomy for Renal Carcinoma

Presenting Symptom, Abnormal Laboratory Findings, or Abnormalities on Physical Examination	*Patients (n = 309)*	*Patients Surviving 5 Y*
Classic triad (gross hematuria, abnormal mass, pain)	29 (9%)	9/29 (31%)
Hematuria	183 (59%)	74/183 (40%)
Pain	127 (41%)	56/127 (44%)
Abdominal mass	139 (45%)	49/139 (35%)
Fever	21 (7%)	8/21 (38%)
Weight loss	85 (28%)	29/85 (34%)
Anemia	64 (21%)	24/64 (38%)
Erythrocytosis	10 (3%)	4/10 (40%)
Hypercalcemia	11 (4%)	4/11 (36%)
Acute varicocele	7 (2%)	3/7 (43%)
Tumor calcification on x-ray film	39 (13%)	18/39 (46%)
Symptoms of metastases	31 (10%)	1/31 (3%)
Cancer, incidental finding	20 (6%)	13/20 (65%)

(Modified from ref. 228.)

One to five percent of patients with kidney cancer have polycythemia.[54] Renin levels often are elevated in patients with renal carcinoma but tend to return to normal after the kidney is removed. Whether the tumor itself produces renin or whether it induces renin production by compression of adjacent tissue is unclear. Immunocytochemical studies suggest that renal carcinoma may produce renin, which, however, may be biologically inactive.[55] Plasma fibrinogen levels may be elevated in patients with renal carcinoma and may correlate with tumor stage, disease activity, and response to therapy. Acquired dysfibrinogenemia has also been reported in association with renal carcinoma and can be a sensitive plasma marker for the disease and for tumor progression.[56]

SYSTEMICALLY ACTIVE TUMOR-PRODUCED FACTORS

In many patients with RCC, there is evidence of tumor-produced factors that have systemic effects. Pyrexia, cachexia, abnormal liver function, increased alkaline phosphatase levels, hypercalcemia, polycythemia, neuromyopathy, and amyloidosis have all been reported in association with RCC.[57]

Humoral hypercalcemia of malignancy, frequently observed in patients with advanced RCC, is believed to be caused by a tumor-produced, systemically active bone-resorbing factor. A number of investigators have demonstrated that kidney cancer produces a factor with parathyroid hormone–like bioactivity.[58] A parathyroid hormone–related protein that has been implicated in malignant hypercalcemia has been cloned from a human lung cancer cell

TABLE 34.2-4. Underlying Pathologic Conditions in 940 Asymptomatic Space-Occupying Lesions of the Kidney

Type of Lesion	*No. of Lesions*	*% of Total No. of Lesions*
Cystic lesions		58
Benign cysts	515	
Benign hemorrhagic cysts	4	
Hydronephrosis	8	
Cystic dysplastic kidney	3	
Polycystic kidney	17	
Malignant neoplasms		5.5
Hypernephromas	21	
Other malignant neoplasms	31	
Benign neoplasms	40	4.2
Inflammatory lesions (pyelonephritis, abscess)	213	23
Intrarenal hematoma	7	0.7
Pseudotumors	81	8.6

(Modified from EK Lang. Asymptomatic space-occupying lesions of the kidney: a programmed sequential approach and its impact on quality and cost of health care. *South Med J* 1977;70:277.)

line and is expressed in mammalian cells.[59] Whether the parathyroid hormone–like factor induces paracrine or endocrine effects, such as bone resorption or hypercalcemia of malignancy, in patients with RCC is currently being studied (Table 34.2-4).

RADIOGRAPHIC EVALUATION

Determining whether a space-occupying renal mass is benign or malignant can be difficult. A number of diagnostic modalities are used to evaluate and stage renal masses, including excretory urography, CT, arteriography, venography, ultrasonography, and magnetic resonance imaging (MRI). Excretory urography is infrequently used in the initial evaluation of renal masses but, because it is neither sensitive nor specific in RCC, a small to medium-sized tumor may be present when the excretory urogram appears normal. Excretory urography does provide important information about the location and function of the contralateral kidney and, while this is particularly useful when surgery is being considered, CT has replaced excretory urography in the evaluation of renal masses.[60–62]

Ultrasound examination provides excellent staging and diagnostic information and can provide accurate anatomic detail of extrarenal extension of tumor, adrenal involvement, involvement of lymph nodes, and infiltration of adjacent viscera.[60,63]

Renal arteriography is infrequently used in the evaluation of patients with a suspicious renal mass (Fig. 34.2-3). In a renal carcinoma, the arteriogram often will show neovascularity, arteriovenous fistulas, pooling of contrast medium, and accentuation of capsular vessels. Epinephrine may be used as an aid in the diagnosis of an equivocal renal mass. When epinephrine is infused into a normal kidney during arteriography, the renal vessels constrict; in contrast, the vessels in a renal carcinoma do not constrict, owing to lack of musculature in the tumor vessels.[64] A renal arteriogram may be useful in evaluating an indeterminate small renal mass and as an aid to the surgeon in defining the vasculature during the surgical removal of a large tumor.[65,66] Although renal arteriography can be performed with minimal risk, false aneurysms, arterial emboli, hemorrhage, and decreased renal function secondary to contrast agent injection have been reported.[67] Dual-phase three-dimensional magnetic resonance angiography can be a useful technique in depicting renal vessels before surgical therapy. This technique is very accurate for the detection of the renal arteries, renal vein involvement, and extension into the inferior vena cava.[61]

CT is a useful imaging technique for renal carcinoma (Fig. 34.2-4).[37,60] CT and ultrasonography have become the main modalities used to characterize renal masses.[63,68] Although arteriography and CT are equivalent in depicting renal vein involvement, CT is better for demonstrating local nodal involvement. The use of contrast agent enhancement has greatly increased the sensitivity of CT for abnormal renal masses.[37] Contrast-enhanced CT allows the clinician to detect very small changes in the density of a renal lesion that might indicate the presence of an early neoplastic lesion. In a comparison study, dynamic CT was superior to standard CT arteriography, ultrasonography, and radionuclide scanning. Dynamic CT correctly demonstrated tumor involvement of the kidney, involvement of the renal fascia, or extension into adjacent organs in all of the 22 patients studied (see Fig. 34.2-4).[69]

Inferior venacavography may be performed when a large renal tumor is present or when there is uncertainty about tumor involvement of the vena cava. Ultrasonography, CT, and MRI can provide information about tumor involvement of the vena cava (Fig. 34.2-5)[61,63]; however, the inferior venacavogram is the most reliable means of accurately determining the precise extent of vena caval involvement by tumor. This information is important to the surgeon in planning the vascular aspect of the operative procedure. MRI is very useful for staging renal carcinoma.[70,71] MRI can produce a unique three-dimensional picture of the tumor, which, in the case of a large lesion, may be an invaluable aid to the surgeon in planning the operative approach. In patients with tumor involving the inferior vena cava, transesophageal echocardiography has been shown to be an accurate diagnostic technique for tumor imaging to document the extent of involvement of the vena cava (see Fig. 34.2-5).

No single imaging technique is best for all patients with renal carcinoma. Depending on the size of the primary tumor and the extent of extrarenal disease, excretory urography, CT, ultrasonography, arteriography, venography, and MRI each can provide unique information in an individual case. Because CT, MRI, and ultrasonography are outpatient procedures and are less invasive than arteriography, arteriography now is infrequently used. Multiple imaging modalities often are combined to provide the most complete information, particularly when surgical removal of a large tumor is being considered.

STAGING AND PROGNOSIS

Robson Classification

The staging system used in the past by most physicians in the United States is the Robson modification of the system of Flocks and Kadesky (Table 34.2-5).[72] In the Robson classification, stage I renal carcinoma is confined to the kidney. Stage II carcinoma extends through the renal capsule but is confined to Gerota's fascia, and stage III carcinoma involves the renal vein or inferior vena cava (IIIA) or the local hilar lymph nodes (IIIB). In stage IV renal carcinoma, the tumor has spread to local, adjacent organs (other than the adrenal gland) or to dis-

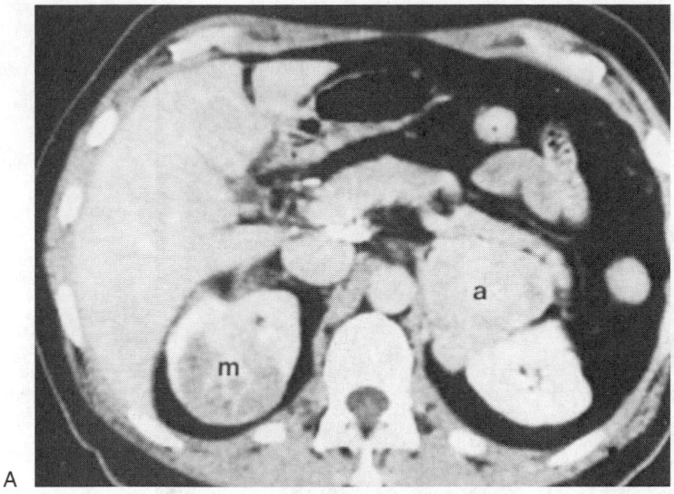

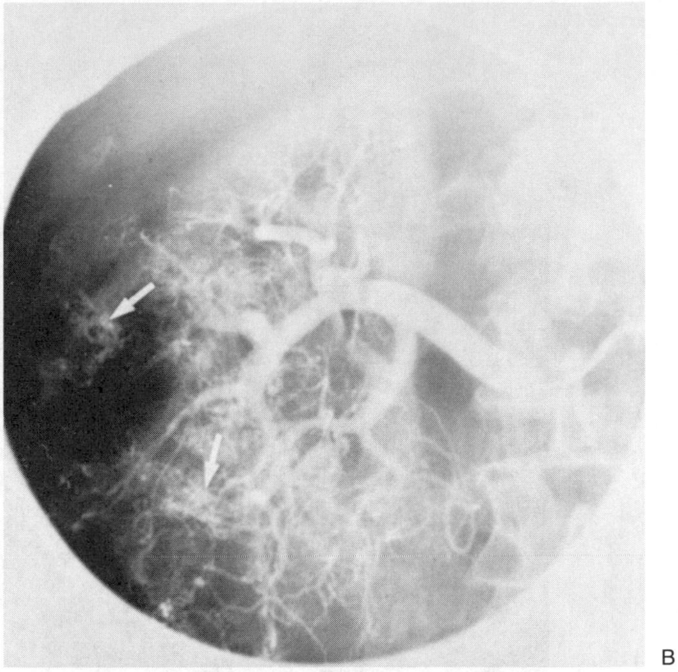

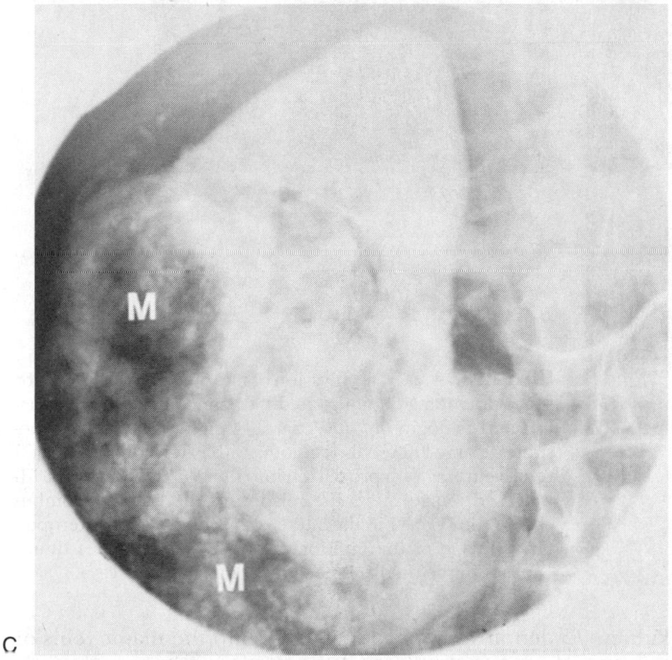

FIGURE 34.2-3. Angiographic appearance of a renal carcinoma. **A:** Computed tomography demonstrates a right renal carcinoma (m) with a large contralateral adrenal metastasis (a). **B:** Early phase of the arteriogram demonstrates vascular changes indicative of a malignancy, with puddling and tortuosity (*arrows*). **C:** Late phase of the arteriogram demonstrates that the tumor (M) is relatively avascular despite its early appearance.

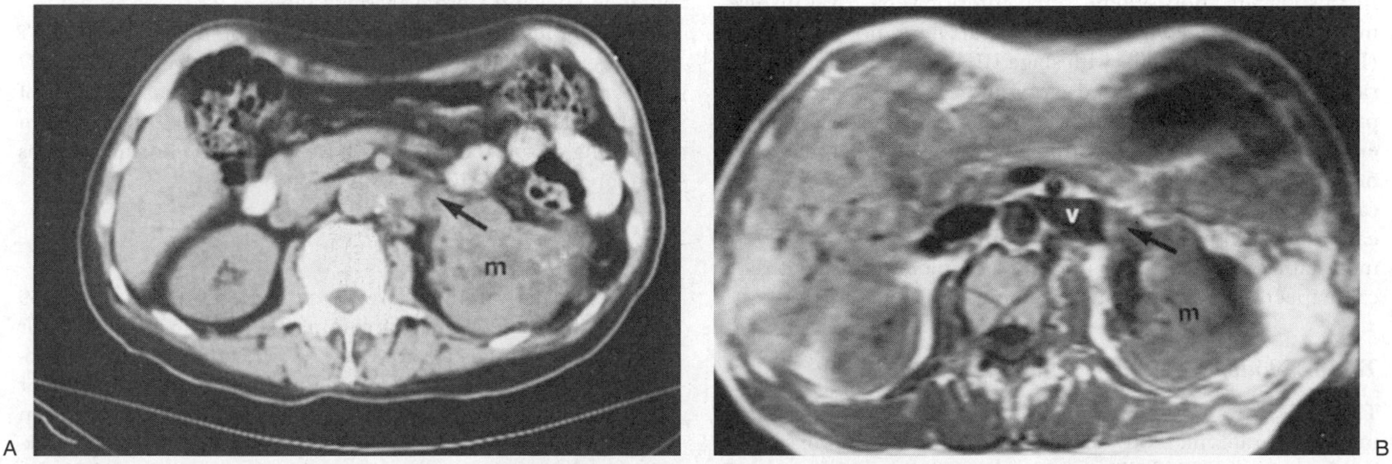

FIGURE 34.2-4. Renal vein invasion by a renal carcinoma as shown by computed tomography (CT) and magnetic resonance imaging. **A:** Nonenhanced CT scan shows large left renal mass with calcification (m) invading the left renal vein (*arrow*). **B:** T1-weighted magnetic resonance image demonstrates tumor (m) and vascular invasion (*arrow*). Flowing blood (v) in the left renal vein is black on this scan.

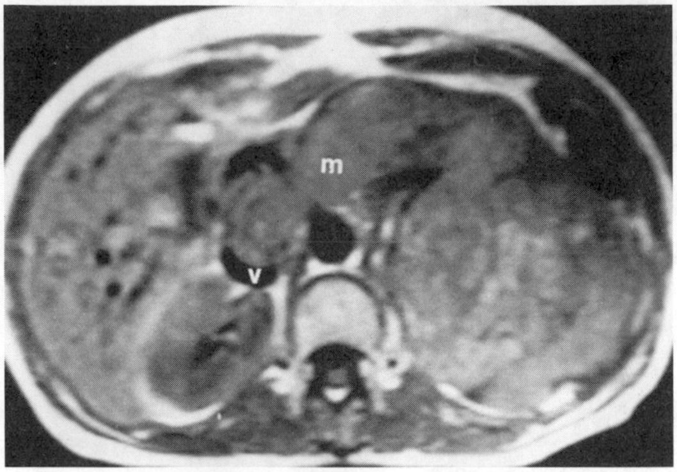

A

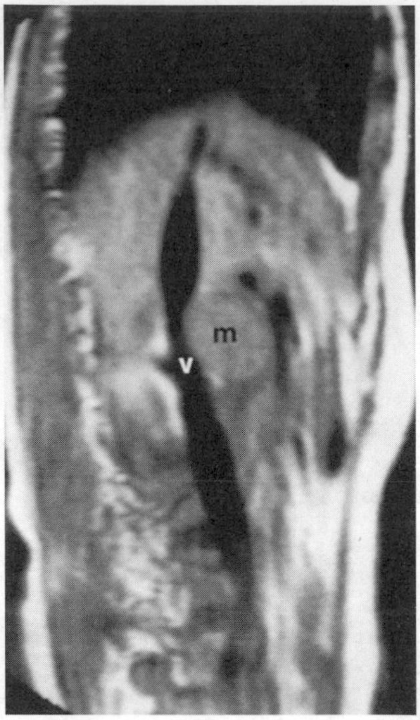

B

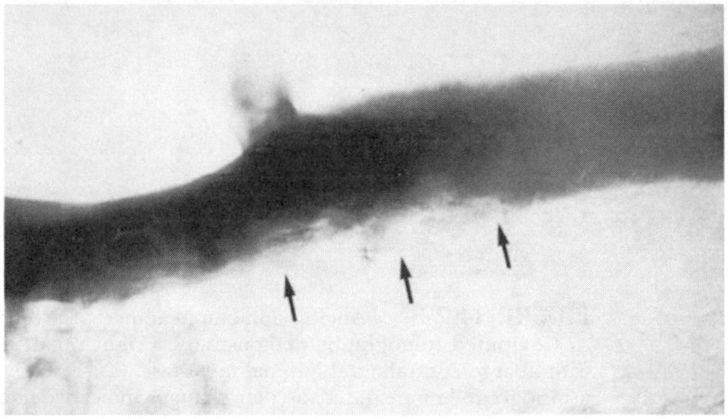

C

FIGURE 34.2-5. Invasion of inferior vena cava (IVC) by renal carcinoma demonstrated by magnetic resonance imaging and venography. **A:** Axial T1-weighted image demonstrates a large left renal carcinoma with extension into the left renal vein (m) with protrusion into the IVC (v). **B:** Sagittal T1-weighted image shows the relation of the tumor thrombus (m) to the IVC (v) in the lateral projection. **C:** An anteroposterior image of the interior cavogram demonstrates tumor (*arrows*) in the medial aspect of the inferior vena cava.

tant sites. The Robson staging system is uncomplicated and widely used. A disadvantage of this system is that it combines stages that may have significantly different survival prognoses. In this classification system, renal inferior vena caval involvement (IIIA) is staged the same as is local lymph node metastasis (IIIB). Although patients with stage IIIB renal carcinoma experience a greatly decreased survival,[73,74] the prognosis for patients with stage IIIA renal carcinoma is not markedly different from that for patients with stage I or stage II renal carcinoma. Patients who have disease that involves the inferior vena cava often have either locally advanced or micrometastatic disease. However, patients who are found to have no evidence of metastatic disease and who undergo complete surgical excision can expect to have a reasonable chance for 5-year survival.

Tumor, Node, Metastasis Classification

The TNM (tumor, node, metastasis) classification proves a more accurate method for classifying the extent of tumor involvement. In the TNM classification, *T1* denotes a tumor 7 cm or less confined to the kidney, *T2* denotes a tumor more than 7 cm in greatest dimension but that is still confined to the kidney, *T3* denotes tumor that extends into the major veins or invades the adrenal gland or perinephric tissues but not beyond Gerota's fascia, and *T4* denotes tumor that has extended beyond Gerota's fascia (Table 34.2-6).

N1 denotes metastasis in a single regional lymph node; *N2* denotes metastasis in more than one regional lymph node. *M1* indicates distant metastasis.[75] The 1997 TNM classification of renal carcinoma appears to provide improved stratification according to survival and may have enhanced clinical utility as compared with previous classification systems.[76]

SURVIVAL

The 5-year survival initially reported by Robson et al.[72] in 1969 was 66% for stage I renal carcinoma, 64% for stage II, 42% for stage III, and only 11% for stage IV. Except for stage I carcinoma, these survival statistics remained essentially the same for a number of years (Table 34.2-7). However, it has since been noted that while renal vein involvement does not have a markedly negative effect on prognosis, the 5-year survival for patients with stage IIIB RCC is only 18%. Recent studies have reported better survival for patients with tumor confined to the

TABLE 34.2-5. Comparison of the Two Classification Systems for Staging of Renal Carcinoma

Findings	*TNM Classification (1997)*	*Robson Classification*
Small tumor, no enlargement of kidney	T1	A (I)
Large tumor, cortex not broken	T2	A (I)
Perinephric or hilar extension	T3a	B (II)
Renal vein involved	T3b	C (III)
Vena cava involved	T3b,c	C (III)
Extension to neighboring organs	T4	D
Nodal invasion	N+	C (III)
Distant metastases	M+	D

TNM, tumor, node, metastasis.
(From ref. 76, with permission.)

kidney: approximately 95% 5- and 10-year disease-specific survival for T1 renal carcinoma and an 88% 5-year and an 81% 10-year disease-specific survival for stage T2 disease.[76] Patients with T3 renal carcinoma had a 59% 5-year survival, and those with T4 disease, a 20% 5-year disease-specific survival.[76]

In patients with N0M0 tumors, studies have detected no statistically significant difference in survival in relationship to the T stage of the disease.[77] The 5-year survival for patients with metastatic renal carcinoma continues to be low, from 0% to 20%.[77]

With the expanded use of CT scans and ultrasonography, the rate of incidentally found carcinomas of the kidney has increased. The prognosis for patients whose tumor was diagnosed incidentally is more favorable than that for patients who present with symptoms, as the former group consists of patients with smaller tumors that usually tend to be confined to the kidney.[78] Patients with metastatic renal carcinoma who present with humoral hypercalcemia of malignancy have a poor prognosis. Fahn et al.[79] reported the median survival of patients with stage IV kidney cancer to be fewer than 50 days. Most studies show increased survival in patients in whom metastatic disease has been diagnosed and in whom the following conditions obtain: (1) a long disease-free interval between initial nephrectomy and the appearance of metastases, (2) presence of only pulmonary metastases, (3) good performance status, and (4) removal of the primary tumor.[51]

TABLE 34.2-6. TNM Classification of Kidney Cancer

PRIMARY TUMOR (T)	
TX	Minimum requirements cannot be met
T0	No evidence of primary tumor
T1	Tumor confined to kidney, <7.0 cm in greatest diameter
T2	Tumor confined to kidney, >7.0 cm in greatest diameter
T3a	Tumor involving perinephric tissues, inside Gerota's fascia
T3b	Tumor involving renal vein or vena cava below the diaphragm
T3c	Tumor involving vena cava and extending above the diaphragm
T4	Tumor invasion of neighboring structures (e.g., muscle, bowel)
NODAL INVOLVEMENT (N)	
TX	Minimum requirements cannot be met
N0	No evidence of involvement of regional nodes
N1	Single, homolateral regional nodal involvement
N2	Metastasis in more than one regional lymph node
DISTANT METASTASIS (M)	
MX	Not assessed
M0	No (known) distant metastasis
M1	Distant metastasis

(From ref. 76, with permission.)

TABLE 34.2-7. Summary of Published Survival Rates in Renal Carcinoma Demonstrating Improvement in Survival Over Time

Study	*Survival (y)*	*Survival Rate by Stage (%)* I	II	III	IV
Robson et al.[72]	5	66	64	42	11
	10	60	67	38	0
Skinner et al.[228]	5	65	47	51	8
	10	56	20	37	7
Boxer et al.[53]	5	56	100	50	8
	10	20	66	25	0
McNichols et al.[229]	5	67	51	34	14
	10	56	28	20	3
Cherrie et al.[230]	5	—	—	0–53	0
	10	—	—	—	—
Selli et al.[231]	5	93	63	80	13
	10	—	—	—	—
Bassil et al.[232]	5	91–100	—	—	18
	10	—	—	—	—
Golimbu et al.[233]	5	88	67	40	2
	10	66	35	15	—
Javidan et al.[76]	5	95	88	59	20
	10	95	81	43	14

SURGICAL TREATMENT

Surgery is the only known effective therapy for localized renal carcinoma. The first nephrectomy was performed by Eratus B. Walcott in Milwaukee on June 4, 1861, on a 58-year-old man with a kidney tumor who died 15 days after surgery.[80] Professor Gustave Simon, after completing a number of experimental nephrectomies on dogs, undertook the first deliberate, planned, and successful nephrectomy in Heidelberg on August 2, 1889, in a patient with a persistent ureteral fistula. The first successful nephrectomy in a patient with kidney cancer was performed in 1883 by Grawitz.[80] The standard procedure today for treatment of localized renal carcinoma is radical nephrectomy (Fig. 34.2-6). Radical nephrectomy involves complete removal of Gerota's fascia and its contents, including the kidney and the adrenal gland, and provides a better surgical margin than simple removal of the kidney.[81] Owing to the rarity of ipsilateral adrenal metastasis and the potential morbidity associated with adrenalectomy, many surgeons believe that a macroscopically normal ipsilateral adrenal gland should not be removed with the kidney (see Fig. 34.2-6).[82,83]

A number of different surgical approaches have been described for removal of kidney cancer. Common approaches are the anterior transperitoneal approach, the flank approach, and the thoracoabdominal approach. The choice of surgical

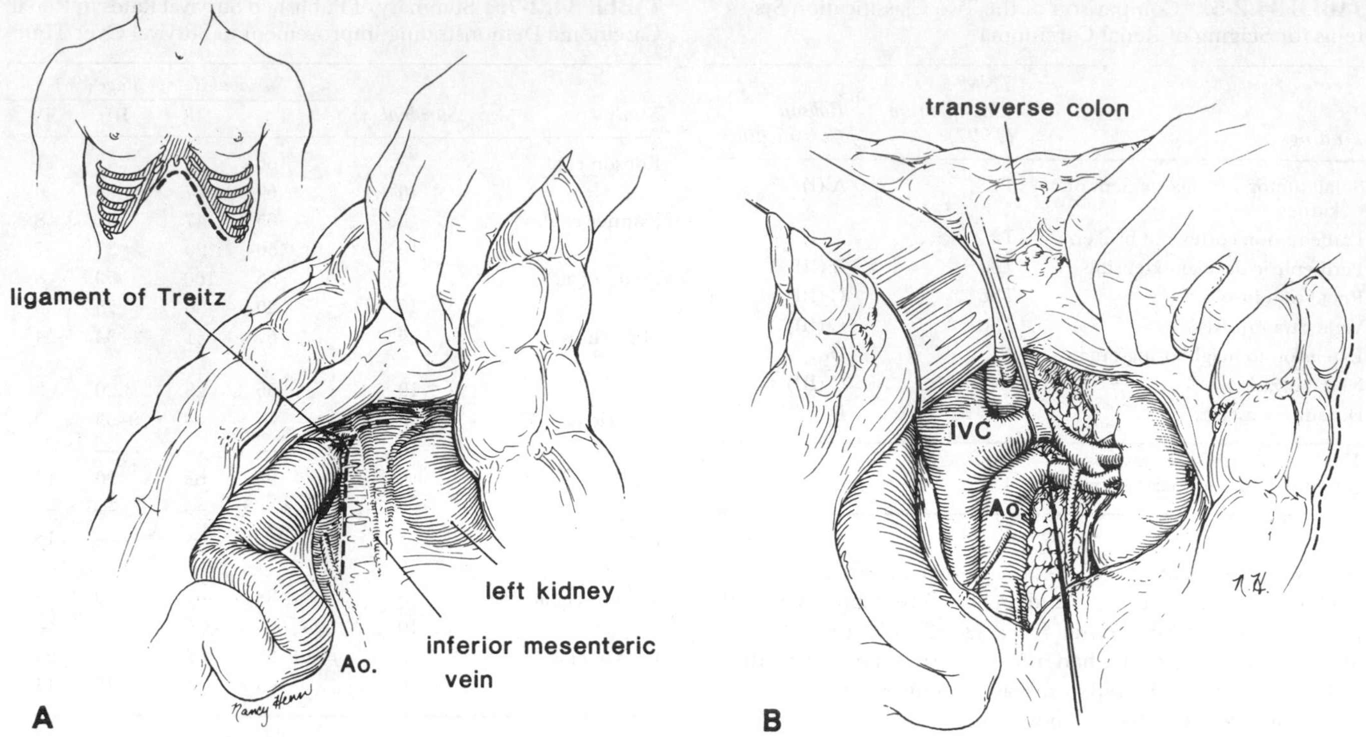

FIGURE 34.2-6. **A:** Area of lymph node dissection for radical nephroureterectomy should be from the superior mesenteric artery to the level of the inferior mesenteric artery, with the anatomic structures identified. **B:** The left colon can be reflected from the anterior surface of Gerota's fascia with exposure of the renal artery before ligation and division. The dotted line to the right of the descending colon indicates a line of incision on the left pericolic gutter that should extend superiorly to include division of the splenocolic attachments. Ao, aorta; IVC, inferior vena cava. (From ref. 262, with permission.)

approach depends on the location and size of the tumor and the body habitus of the patient. The type of incision is chosen to ensure that the tumor may safely be removed. A flank incision, with or without removal of a portion of the tenth or eleventh rib, often is used for small tumors without venous involvement. A subcostal transabdominal incision may be used when a large tumor occupies the middle or lower aspect of the kidney or when vascular involvement is anticipated and access to the major vessels is essential. A thoracoabdominal incision often is required when a large middle or upper pole tumor is present.

In a thoracoabdominal incision, a rib is removed, the thoracic cavity is opened, and the diaphragm is incised. The incision then is carried down transabdominally to allow maximal exposure of the upper abdominal region and the great vessels. In removal of a right-sided tumor, the hepatic flexure of the colon is mobilized toward the midline away from the kidney and duodenum. The duodenum is also dissected up anteriorly and medially to the great vessels, and the renal artery and vein are identified. The renal vessels are divided and ligated early in the surgical procedure to decrease the vascularity of the tumor so that it may be removed with a minimum of blood loss. Following ligation of the vessels, Gerota's fascia is incised away from the posterior abdominal wall, diaphragm, and liver (pancreas and spleen on a left-sided tumor) (see Fig. 34.2-6). Once Gerota's fascia and its contents have been dissected away from the surrounding structures and the vasculature has been ligated with nonabsorbable suture, the specimen can be lifted out of the retroperitoneum. When there is tumor in the renal vein, the renal vein can be ligated distal to the tumor thrombus. If there is tumor extension into the vena cava, the vena cava may need to be partially resected. If the tumor has grown into the sidewall of the vena cava or if the vena caval involvement is too extensive for a simple partial wall resection, a portion of the vena cava itself may be resected. When the tumor is in the right kidney, the adjacent vena cava can often be resected safely. If, however, the tumor in the left kidney and the adjacent vena cava are resected, vascular reconstruction of the right renal vein may be needed to establish adequate venous drainage. If the suprahepatic caval extension of a renal tumor thrombus extends up to the right atrium, cardiopulmonary bypass may be required for tumor removal (Fig. 34.2-7).

Laparoscopic nephrectomy has been evaluated as a less invasive procedure for the removal of kidneys with a small volume of RCC.[84,85] Walther et al.[86] have also evaluated the use of laparoscopic cytoreductive nephrectomy in patients with advanced RCC as preparation for interleukin-2 (IL-2) treatment.

Regional lymphadenectomy often is performed at the time of radical nephrectomy, although its role in prolonging survival has not been demonstrated. In a regional lymphadenectomy, ipsilateral nodal tissue from the diaphragm to the bifurcation of the aorta as well as nodal tissue in the interaortocaval region at the hilum of the kidney is removed. Proponents of regional lymphadenectomy point out that 5-year survival in patients with node-positive renal carcinoma is greatly decreased, and there is no known effective therapy for metastatic renal carcinoma. If local nodes were the first site of metastasis, resection of microscopic disease might be of benefit. Long-term survival in patients with node-positive disease

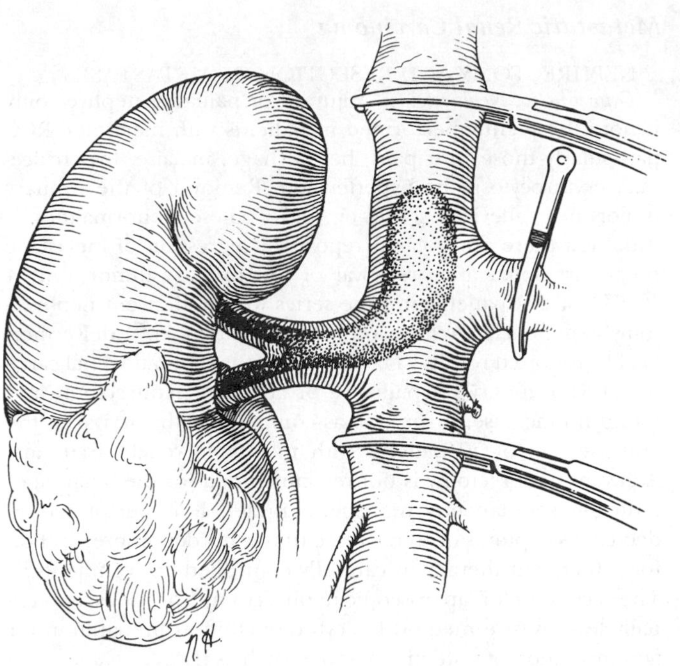

FIGURE 34.2-7. Surgical removal of a kidney tumor in which there is tumor extension through the renal vein into the inferior vena cava.

who underwent lymphadenectomy has been reported.[87] The ultimate role of regional lymphadenectomy remains to be determined in further randomized trials. In patients with locally advanced RCC (node-positive), no evidence to date supports the theory that adjuvant, postsurgical treatment of patients with an agent such as IL-2 or interferon-α (IFN-α) increases survival. In patients in whom all visible disease has been resected surgically, most physicians recommend treatment when residual or recurrent disease becomes detectable.

Bilateral Renal Carcinoma or Tumors in Solitary Kidneys

The treatment of patients with either bilateral renal carcinoma or renal carcinoma in a solitary kidney is challenging. Patients with tumor in a solitary kidney may be treated by either partial nephrectomy or nephrectomy followed by dialysis or transplantation (or both). In selected patients, nephron-sparing surgery may be recommended for patients with sporadic renal cell cancer, particularly those with a small tumor (≤4 cm) or a tumor in a solitary kidney.[88,89] Extracorporeal partial nephrectomy plus autotransplantation is an infrequently used technique that allows the surgeon accurately to remove large tumors from the center of a solitary kidney. This *ex vivo* procedure entails radical excision of the kidney and division of the ureter. The kidney then is placed on a table and is intermittently perfused with a chilled solution to enhance viability. Under optical magnification, the tumor is carefully dissected from the surrounding renal parenchyma. Care is taken to preserve the vasculature of the normal kidney, which has been defined by preoperative arteriography. A small rim of normal tissue is removed along with the tumor to provide a tumor-free margin of resection. After the kidney has been surgically reconstructed, it is autotransplanted back into the iliac space. Vascular anastomosis of the renal artery and vein to the iliac vessels and ureteroureterostomy are performed.

Surgical Management of Patients with Hereditary Forms of Renal Carcinoma

Patients with hereditary forms of renal carcinoma are often challenging to manage. Individuals with VHL syndrome or HPRC can have widespread renal involvement.[29,90,91] Surgical management in these patients involves careful parenchyma-sparing surgery, which is recommended when the renal tumors reach a certain size threshold, generally 3 cm. The use of parenchyma-sparing surgery in these patients is based on a strategy designed to maintain the patient's renal function as long as possible while decreasing the risk for metastasis.[92]

Radiotherapy as an Adjuvant to Nephrectomy

The value of adjuvant external-beam radiotherapy for patients with RCC remains unclear. Previous reports have demonstrated increased complication rates using conventional radiotherapeutic techniques.[93–98] In addition, several randomized studies performed 20 to 30 years ago showed no apparent survival benefit with adjuvant therapy.[93,94] These considerations led to an overall lack of enthusiasm for using radiotherapy in this disease. However, recent studies have suggested that the use of more sophisticated radiation techniques is less likely to result in treatment-related complications.[99,100] In addition, previous trials testing preoperative or postoperative radiotherapy for this disease may not have been designed in an optimal fashion to evaluate its potential benefit fully for improving outcome in high-risk patients.

Though some retrospective reports have indicated an improvement in local tumor control or overall survival with the addition of postoperative radiotherapy,[95,101,102] subsequent randomized prospective trials could not confirm any benefit. In one randomized study reported by Finney et al.,[93] the incidence of local recurrence was 7% in both the adjuvant radiotherapy and control arms. In addition, no survival advantage was detected in the radiotherapy arm. In fact, a trend for an inferior 5-year survival outcome was observed for the adjuvant radiotherapy group (36% as compared to 47% for patients with nephrectomy), owing to a higher complication rate observed in these patients. Ten years later, a second randomized prospective trial comparing nephrectomy and postoperative radiotherapy to nephrectomy alone demonstrated identical results.[94] In that study, the incidence of local recurrence was reduced from 25% to 3% with adjuvant local radiotherapy. Further, the incidence of treatment-related morbidity in these two randomized trials was unacceptably high. Severe complications were experienced in 20% to 44% of treated patients, with an associated increased mortality rate due to radiation-related toxicities. The potential value of preoperative radiotherapy has also been tested in two randomized trials,[97,98] neither of which could demonstrate any advantage for improved local control or survival with adjuvant radiotherapy.

However, it is difficult to draw any meaningful conclusions about the safety and value of adjuvant therapy for patients with RCC who are at increased risk for local recurrence. Previously published postoperative studies used relatively crude radiation techniques, and the radiation dose per fraction of 250 cGy to cumulative doses of 5000 to 5500 cGy used in some reports likely directly contributed to the high gastrointestinal and liver-related toxicities observed. In addition, a significant percentage of patients treated in these trials did not have prognostic features indicating a high risk for local recurrence for which adjuvant radiotherapy may have been potentially beneficial. Based on patterns-of-failure studies after nephrectomy alone,[103,104] the overall local recurrence rate is low, and routine administration of adjuvant local therapy for all patients on the basis of advanced stage only would not be expected to improve outcome. Rabinovitch et al.[103] reported on 172 patients treated with nephrectomy alone to identify patterns of failure and risk factors for local recurrence. In that report, the 7-year actuarial local failure rate was 5%. However, among patients with positive surgical margins or positive lymph nodes, the incidence of local recurrence was 21%. Advanced T-stage disease in the absence of these prognostic features did not predict for local recurrence and thus is not necessarily an indication for local adjuvant therapy.

More recent reports have demonstrated that with the application of more sophisticated radiotherapeutic planning techniques, the incidence of treatment-related complications has been minimal. Using CT-based treatment planning, Kao et al.[99] at the University of Pennsylvania retrospectively reported the outcome of postoperative radiotherapy for selected patients with positive surgical margins or perinephric disease extension. Doses ranged from 4140 cGy to 6300 cGy using conventional fractionation. The overall local failure and survival rates were 100% and 75%, respectively, as compared to 30% and 62%, respectively, for similar patients at the University of Pennsylvania who underwent nephrectomy alone. Despite the higher radiation doses used, no late complications were observed.

An additional limitation of prior studies is the relatively low postoperative doses used secondary to concerns of late radiation sequelae. Several reports have suggested that higher doses may be necessary in this disease to overcome the relative radioresistance of the renal cell histology.[105,106] With the introduction of three-dimensional conformal radiotherapy and intensity-modulated treatment delivery systems, it now is possible to deliver higher radiation doses in the adjuvant setting with less potential toxicity. The use of intraoperative radiation for high-risk patients may prove to be an effective approach for the delivery of high radiation doses, with the ability to easily shield the adjacent normal gastrointestinal structures. Eble et al.[107] and Frydenberg[108] reported the results of a phase I study in 11 patients with advanced-stage or locally recurrent RCC that incorporated intraoperative radiotherapy (15 to 20 Gy) in combination with fractionated external-beam radiotherapy. The 4-year survival outcome was 75%, and no local relapses or complications were noted. In a limited number of patients with recurrent RCC, other investigators have reported the feasibility of postoperative, hyperfractionated, high-dose-rate brachytherapy using iridium 192 as a means of effectively delivering a high radiation dose to the postoperative bed.[109]

The aforementioned studies would suggest that adjuvant radiotherapy may be of benefit for selected patients with high-risk features predicting for local recurrence after nephrectomy. Using modern external-beam and brachytherapy techniques, higher radiation doses can now be delivered more safely and may further improve the efficacy of radiotherapy for selected patients. Nevertheless, randomized trials limited to high-risk patients will be required to assess fully the local control benefit of postoperative radiotherapy in this clinical setting.

Metastatic Renal Carcinoma

NEPHRECTOMY AND RESECTION OF METASTASES

Cytoreductive Nephrectomy. Adjuvant or palliative nephrectomy is not infrequently performed in patients with metastatic RCC particularly those with pain, hemorrhage, malaise, hypercalcemia, erythrocytosis, or hypertension. Removal of the primary tumor may alleviate some or all of these abnormalities.[110] Although there are isolated reports of regression of metastatic renal carcinoma after removal of the primary tumor, only 4 (0.8%) of 474 patients in nine series who underwent nephrectomy experienced "regression" of metastatic foci.[111] deKernion et al.[112] reported results in 26 patients with metastatic renal carcinoma who underwent palliative or adjuvant nephrectomy and found no increase in survival, as compared with survival in the entire group of 79 patients with metastatic renal carcinoma. Adjuvant nephrectomy is not recommended for the purpose of inducing spontaneous regression; rather, it is performed to decrease symptoms or to decrease tumor burden in preparation for subsequent therapy in carefully controlled environments.[113] The recent use of laparoscopic nephrectomy[86] provides a potentially less invasive method for cytoreduction as preparation for administration of systemic therapies such as IL-2.

Resection of Metastases. Of the approximately 30% of patients with RCC who present with metastases, fewer than 4% have solitary metastases.[114] Patients with a solitary metastasis synchronous with a primary lesion experience decreased survival when compared with patients who develop metastasis after the primary tumor is removed.[115] Surgical resection is recommended in selected patients with metastatic renal carcinoma. In a study of 59 patients with renal carcinoma who underwent surgical resection for a solitary metastasis, 45% had a 3-year survival, and 34% survived 5 years.[114] O'Dea et al.[115] reported on patients who presented with primary tumor in place and a solitary metastasis. Of the patients who underwent nephrectomy and who later developed metastasis, 23% lived more than 5 years after removal of the metastatic lesions. Three of the 26 patients were alive 58, 94, and 245 months after resection of the metastatic lesions.[115] Nephrectomy and resection of metastases will render few cures but frequently will produce some long-term survivors.

ROLE OF RADIOTHERAPY. Palliative radiotherapy for patients with symptomatic metastatic osseous lesions can be effective. Previous reports have noted response rates of 50% to 70% after local palliative radiotherapy for patients with metastatic RCC.[105,116] In a randomized trial assessing various fractionation schemes for the palliation of symptomatic bone metastases, renal cell histology was found to respond less favorably to standard palliative radiation regimens as compared to metastatic breast and prostate cancers.[117] In light of the relative radioresistance of this histology, higher radiation doses are critical to achieve adequate palliation. In general, doses of at least 50 Gy are required to achieve durable palliation. To deliver these higher doses safely, complex treatment planning often is necessary to minimize treatment-related toxicity. Investigators from the Jefferson College of Medicine have shown that higher radiation doses were associated with an improved palliative response.[106] In a multivariate analysis, a higher baseline performance status and the use of higher radiation doses predicted for a greater likelihood for significant pain relief after radiotherapy for painful osseous lesions. Large-volume metastatic lesions such as those found within the renal bed require higher radiation doses to achieve palliation and, in general, this therapy is successful in fewer than 50% of treated patients.

Brain metastases from RCC are often hemorrhagic in nature, and the rapid initiation of palliative radiotherapy may be necessary to halt potential neurologic progression. Surgery should be considered for solitary lesions of the brain or spine, followed by postoperative radiotherapy. The results of routine administration of short-course whole brain radiotherapy using the conventional fractionation program of 3000 cGy in ten fractions has been disappointing.[118,119] Investigators from the M. D. Anderson Cancer Center have reported that, in the majority of treated patients with short-course whole brain radiotherapy, the cause of death was neurologic deterioration.[119] For selected patients with good performance status or solitary lesions, radiosurgery alone or in combination with whole brain radiotherapy provides an opportunity to deliver higher doses and should be considered.[120,121] Pomer et al.[120] have shown that for patients with metastatic RCC, radiosurgery was more effective among those with a Karnofsky performance score in excess of 70 and among those with a greater than 1-year interval from diagnosis to manifestation of central nervous system metastases.

Osseous lesions in weight-bearing areas such as the femora should be considered for initial orthopedic stabilization, followed by postoperative radiotherapy. Treatment with radiotherapy alone should be exercised with some caution owing to the potential for posttreatment fracture.

SYSTEMIC CHEMOTHERAPY FOR RENAL CELL CARCINOMA

Limited options are available for the systemic therapy of RCC, and no hormonal or chemotherapeutic regimen is accepted as a standard of care. Reviews surveying phase II clinical trials for RCC have appeared at intervals (1967, 1973, 1983, 1995, and 2000),[263–268] without a change in the final conclusion: No systemic chemotherapeutic or hormonal approach has provided a reasonable level of activity.

A comprehensive review by Yagoda et al.[267] encompassed 4542 patients enrolled in 83 clinical trials published from 1983 through 1993. Among 4093 evaluable patients, a 6.0% response rate was recorded, with 53 complete responses (CRs; 1.3%) and 192 partial responses (PRs; 4.7%). Response rates in excess of 25% were noted in eleven trials; in each case another trial incorporating the same or a comparable treatment regimen reported lower or zero response rates.

Three agents warrant particular mention: floxuridine, 5-fluorouracil (5-FU), and vinblastine. One of the most intensively studied agents has been infusional floxuridine, which, studied in both standard and circadian schedules, appears to have a level of activity above the background. Fourteen trials yielded response rates ranging from 0% to 43%, with an average rate of 12%. Seven trials had response rates of less than 10%, and four had response rates exceeding 20%. For 5-FU, which has been primarily used in combination with immunotherapy, responses were somewhat fewer, with an overall response rate of 10% for infusional 5-FU alone and 19% for 5-FU in combination with interferon. Similar results were reported for vinblastine, an agent initially thought to have activity in RCC. In the Yagoda series,[267] seven trials incorporating infusional vinblastine yielded an overall response rate of 7%, whereas three trials reported no responses. Since 1993, further results with vinblastine have been equally discouraging. As the control arm for a multidrug resistance modulator trial, vinblastine produced one PR in 80 patients; as the control arm for an interferon trial, vinblastine produced one complete and one PR among 81 patients.[269,270]

The 83 trials reported in the review by Yagoda[267] included compounds from every class of anticancer agent: antimitotics (paclitaxel and docetaxel); vinca alkaloids (vinblastine, vindesine, and vinorelbine); anthracyclines (epirubicin, doxorubicin, and idarubicin); anthracenediones (mitoxantrone, bisantrene); alkylating agents (both nitrosoureas and sulfonylureas, as well as ifosfamide and melphalan); metals (carboplatinum and gallium nitrate); pyrimidines (floxuridine, 5-FU, and gemcitabine); and purines (6-thioguanine, fludarabine, and 2-deoxycoforomycin). Yagoda et al.[267] concluded that the responses may be mediated by an indirect effect on the immune system. Considering that the response rates in these trials are higher than the frequency of spontaneous remissions, and observing the occasional complete remission, one could speculate that the responses involve an effect triggered by the chemotherapy but mediated by the immune system. However, scientific evidence to support this thesis is lacking. Although the majority of patients experiencing a complete remission were noted in trials including cimetidine, vinblastine, 5-FU, and floxuridine, the CR rate ranges between 2% and 4%, which is not very different from the 1.3% CR rate noted in the entire series. These considerations favor a conclusion that little, if any, cytotoxic activity has been exerted in renal cell cancer. It can be concluded that the best recommendation for patients with this disease, after immunotherapy, is participation in clinical trials studying new agents or new approaches.[271,268]

Hormonal Therapy in Renal Cell Cancer

Hormonal agents have also been used in systemic therapy. This strategy had its origins in studies showing that progesterone could inhibit the development of estrogen-induced renal cell cancers in Syrian hamsters[272] and in the observation that both estrogen and progesterone receptors could be found in a portion of human kidney cancers.[273] Subsequently, medroxyprogesterone acetate (Megace) became conventional treatment for renal cell cancer. However, multiple studies have concluded that hormonal therapy is of no definite benefit. A series of studies collected from 1967 through 1976, using progestins or androgens included 644 patients.[265] Response rates were highest (17%) in the earliest studies. With more stringent response criteria used in the studies conducted after 1971, an overall rate of 2% was observed. Except for its value in appetite stimulation, the use of Megace cannot be recommended in the treatment of renal cell cancer today.

Studies with antiestrogens in more recent years have yielded similar results. An overall response rate of 7% (three patients with CR) was identified in four studies treating 146 patients with high-dose tamoxifen (100 mg/m^2/d or more).[121a] More recently, two CRs (3%) were reported in 63 patients receiving 40 mg of oral tamoxifen daily in the control arm of a randomized study.[275] Similar activity was suggested also in a pilot study of high-dose toremifene (300 mg/d), a novel anti-

TABLE 34.2-8. Phase II Studies in Renal Cell Cancer: 1993–1999

Investigator	*Agent*	*Enter.*	*Eval.*	*No. CR*	*No. PR*	*RR (%)*	*Regimen*
Mahjoubi et al.[350]	LY186641	16	16	1	0	6.3	700 mg/m²/d PO × 14 q21d
Walpole et al.[351]	Paclitaxel	17	12	0	0	0	250 mg/m² CIVI × 24 h q21d
Mertens et al.[352]	Docetaxel	20	18	0	0	0	100 mg/m² × 1 q21d
Chang et al.[234]	Echinomycin	17	13	0	0	0	1200 mg/m²/wk × 4 q42d
Flanigan et al.[353]	Merbarone	41	36	0	1	3	1000 mg/m² CIVI × 96 h q21d
Kish et al.[235]	Infusional 5-FU	61	58	1	2	5.2	300 mg/m²/d CIVI
Law et al.[354]	Topotecan	15	14	0	0	0	1.5 mg/m²/d × 5 q28d
Law et al.[355]	Lipodox, LED	14	14	0	0	0	75 mg/m²/d × 1 q21d
Shevrin et al.[356]	6-Thioguanine	41	39	0	3	8	55 mg/m²/d × 5 q35d
De Mulder et al.[236]	Gemcitabine	39	37	1	2	8.1	800 mg/m²/wk × 3 q28d
Witte et al.[357]	Amonafide	19	17	0	0	0	300 mg/m²/d × 5 q21d
Witte et al.[357]	Caracemide	18	17	0	0	0	550 mg/m²/d × 5 q21d
Witte et al.[357]	Homoharringtonine	15	14	0	0	0	4 mg/m²/d CIVI × 120h q28d
Berg et al.[358]	13-*cis* Retinoic acid	26	25	0	0	0	1 mg/kg/d PO
Dreicer et al.[359]	Edatrexate	44	37	0	2	5.4	80 mg/m²/wk × 5 q35d
Lummen et al.[360]	Titanocene dichloride	14	11	0	0	0	270 mg/m² × 1 q21d
Vogelzang et al.[361]	Pyrazine diazohydroxide	15	14	0	0	0	100 mg/m²/d × 5 q42d
Rigos et al.[362]	Treosulfan	15	10	0	0	0	10 g/m² × 1 q28d
Berg et al.[363]	Pyrazoloacridine	12	12	0	0	0	750 mg/m² × 1 q21d
Stadler et al.[364]	TNP-470	33	33	0	1	3	60 mg/m² t.i.w.
Stadler et al.[237]	Flavopiridol	35	34	0	2	6	50 mg/m²/d CIVI × 72 h q14d
Dreicer et al.[365]	Suramin	14	13	0	0	0	Fixed dose[a]
Rini et al.[121b]	Gemcitabine +5-FU	41	39	0	7	17	600 mg/m²/wk × 3 q28d; 150 mg/m²/d CIVI × 21 days q28d
1998–1999 ABSTRACTS							
Di Palma et al.[366]	Temozolomide	12	12	0	0	0	200 mg/m²/d PO × 5 q28d
Dumas et al.[367]	Onconase	14	14	0	0	0	480 µg/m²/wk
Fishkin et al.[368]	CI-980	12	12	0	0	0	4.5 mg/m²/d CIVI × 72 h
Pennington et al.[369]	Doxil	32	28	0	1	3.5	50 mg/m² × 1 q28d
Sauter et al.[370]	LY231514	22	16	0	1	6	600 mg/m² × 1 q21d
Gunnett et al.[371]	Anti-EGFR antibody	54	—	0	1	—	400 mg/m² × 1; 250 mg/m²/wk × 7
O'Shaughnessy et al.[372]	CI-994	48	45	0	0	0	8 mg/m²/d PO
Redman et al.[373]	Diethylnorspermine	22	20	0	0	0[b]	100 mg/m²/d × 5 q21d
Rubins et al.[374]	rHuEPO	14	14	0	0	0	150 µg/kg SC t.i.w.

CIVI, continuous intravenous infusion; CR, complete responders; EGFR, epidermal growth factor receptor; Enter., number of patients entered in study; Eval., number of patients assessable for response; 5-FU, 5-fluorouracil; LED, liposomal encapsulated doxorubicin; PR, partial responders; rHuEPO, recombinant human erythropoietin; RR, response rate.
[a]Suramin dose: days 1–5: 1000, 400, 300, 250, 200 mg/m²; then 275 mg/m² on days 11, 15, 19, and 22, and then once weekly.
[b]Seven (35%) minor responses were observed.

estrogen with activity in breast cancer.[276] Thus, reported responses to treatment with hormonal therapy most likely mimic the same level of inactivity identified with most chemotherapeutic agents.

Recent Chemotherapy Trials in Renal Cell Cancer

More recently, an effort has been made to identify new treatment targets in cancer. A limited search for phase II single agents examined in renal cell cancer and reported since 1993 (and thus not included in earlier reviews) identified 23 published studies. These compounds, shown in Table 34.2-8, are from various pharmaceutical classes, including taxanes, camptothecins, anthracyclines, antifolates, and alkylating agents. In recent abstracts from the American Society of Clinical Oncology, an additional nine new agents were tested. Once again, the refractory nature of renal cell cancer is observed. One new study—the combination of gemcitabine and 5-FU—warrants mention. In a study reported by Vogelzang at the University of Chicago, 7 PRs (17%) were observed among 39 patients receiving gemcitabine at 600 mg/m² on days 1, 8, and 15 and continuous-infusion 5-FU at 150 mg/m²/d for 21 days in 28-day cycles.[121b]

To some extent, the refractory nature of renal cell cancer highlights a general problem with anticancer agents developed over the last three decades. A review of cytotoxic drugs introduced into clinical trial by the National Cancer Institute between 1970 and 1985 found that half of the 47 new agents adequately studied in phase II trials could be rated as having anticancer activity.[277] Among these active compounds, 74% were active in lymphoma, 35% in leukemia, 22% in breast cancer, and 18% in ovarian cancer. Only one drug was active in colon cancer; no activity was reported with any of the 25 drugs

TABLE 34.2-9. Randomized Phase III Trials with Interferon and Chemotherapy

Studies		*No. of Patients*	*% Responses*	*Response Duration (mo)*	*Median Survival (mo)*	*Survival Benefit for Combination*
Kriegmair et al.[375]	Interferon + vinblastine	41	20.5	—	16	No
	Medroxyprogesterone	35	0	—	10	
Pyrhonen et al.[376]	Interferon + vinblastine	79	16.5	3.25	17	Yes
	Vinblastine	81	2.5	2.25	10	
Fossa et al.[238]	Interferon + vinblastine	66	24	6.0	—	No
	Interferon	53	11	8.6	—	
Neidhart et al.[239]	Interferon + vinblastine	83	8	—	—	No
	Interferon	82	12	—	—	
Sagaster et al.[240]	Interferon + coumarin + cimetidine	70	17.1	10	9	No
	Interferon	67	20.8	7.5	8	
Motzer et al.[377]	Interferon + *cis*-retinoic acid	139	11	—	15	No
	Interferon	145	6	—	15	

(Adapted from ref. 122.)

properly tested in renal cell cancer. These data suggested that the prevailing screening strategies for anticancer agents were biased toward agents active in leukemia and lymphoma and were not likely to identify agents active in solid tumors.[278] Thus, the drug screen was reorganized and a 60–cell line *in vitro* screen was established in 1990 with cell lines derived from solid tumors including RCC.[279] It is hoped that this effort, along with compounds under development for defined intracellular and extracellular targets, will identify agents with activity in those tumors that are most difficult to treat. The antiangiogenesis agents currently being developed are examples of compounds with a novel approach to this difficult problem.

Chemotherapy Combined with Interferon in Renal Cell Cancer

Interferon, one of two immunotherapeutic agents widely used in the treatment of renal cell cancer (as discussed later, in Biologic Therapy), has a modest response rate and confers a survival advantage as a single agent.[122,122a,123] Numerous trials have been conducted combining interferon with cytotoxic chemotherapy in the hope that the immunologic benefit from interferon would improve the response to chemotherapy. Wirth[280] identified response rates ranging from 0% to 45% among 315 patients in 11 trials combining vinblastine with IFN-α. The response rates were highest in the oldest trials, where less stringent response criteria were used. Randomized studies have failed to provide any evidence for combining interferon with vinblastine (Table 34.2-9).

Interferon has also been combined with floxuridine or 5-FU in multiple studies, with several reporting higher response rates than usually reported with either agent alone.[281] However, more recent, nonrandomized, multiinstitutional studies have been disappointing, suggesting little or no benefit from combining interferon with floxuridine given over 14 days[282] or with 5-FU.[283,284]

A similar evolution occurred with the combination of interferon and *cis*-retinoic acid; Motzer et al.[285] originally observed a 30% response rate for the combination. However, when this trial was taken forward to a combination with IL-2, only 8 of 47 patients (17%) responded.[286] Preliminary results of a randomized trial comparing IFN-α plus *cis*-retinoic acid with IFN-α alone suggest no significant difference between the two arms.[287]

One potential confounding factor in all these trials may be the inclusion of patients with varying prognoses. In future studies, evaluation of data taking into account clinical prognostic factors may help to eliminate the variation in results long observed in renal carcinoma trials.[288] To date, there is no convincing evidence that chemotherapy adds to the effectiveness of single-agent IFN-α.[122] The combination of interferon with a cytotoxic agent in patients whose disease progressed after treatment with IL-2 must be considered unproven, and enrollment in clinical trials is the most logical alternative.

Drug Resistance in Renal Cell Cancer

The ineffectiveness of chemotherapy can be ascribed to the primary, or intrinsic, resistance to chemotherapy, which, although poorly understood, is a hallmark of RCC. Overexpression of the 170-kD drug transporter P glycoprotein (P-gp) and its encoding gene, *MDR-1*, has been most frequently cited as a mechanism of resistance. Expression of P-gp in RCC is related to its normal tissue expression in the cell of origin, the renal proximal tubule; and the level of expression correlates with differentiation.[289–291] Fojo et al.[292] reported high levels of expression of this transporter in kidney cancer and *in vitro* sensitization of kidney cancer cell lines to vinblastine with the antagonists verapamil and quinidine. Chemosensitivity studies with fresh tumor specimens demonstrated high levels of resistance in 30 of 35 samples, and overexpression of P-gp in 70% of cases.[293] Together, these findings suggest that P-gp expression could explain, at least in part, the notorious resistance of RCC.

However, efforts to modulate P-gp by treating patients with antagonists have met with disappointing results to date. Except for a single phase I study with doxorubicin,[294] most of the trials have attempted modulation of vinblastine (Table 34.2-10). Though the studies, at face value, suggest no role for P-gp in RCC, it can be argued that this question is not fully resolved.[295] Most of the reversal agents used in the trials were first-generation agents with low potency, selected because they were already in clinical use for other indications. Most of the trials incorporated vinblastine. Although vinblastine is a substrate for P-gp, renal cell cancers may have other mechanisms of resistance to vinblastine that were not addressed by these studies. P-gp may represent an avenue to increase intracellular concentrations of

TABLE 34.2-10. Trials Testing the Reversal of P-glycoprotein–Mediated Resistance

Study	*N*[a]	*Modulator*	*Vinblastine Schedule*	*No. CR/ No. PR*
Schwartsmann et al.[378]	14	Nifedipine 20 mg PO q6h d1–5	5 mg/m² IV d3 q14d	0/0
Murphy et al.[379]	15	Dipyridamole 75 mg PO qid d1–4	0.2 mg/kg IV d3 q21d	0/0
Motzer et al.[380]	23	Dexverapamil[b] 120 mg/m² PO q6h d0–2	0.11 mg/kg IV d1&2 q21d	0/0
Warner et al.[381]	15	Cyclosporin A 5 mg/kg PO × 1; 10–17 mg/kg PO qid d1 –3	6–10 mg/m² IV d3 q28d	0/0
Agarwala et al.[382]	12[c]	Quinidine 200–400 mg PO qid	5 mg/m² IV q7d	1/0
Samuels et al.[269]				
Regimen A	33	Cyclosporin A CIVI; 12.5 mg/kg/d d1–5	1.2 mg/m²/d CIVI d2–6 q28d[d]	0/0
Regimen B	35	Tamoxifen 400 mg/m² × 1; 300 mg/m²/d PO d1–13	1.5 mg/m²/d CIVI d8–13 q28d[d]	1/0

CIVI, continuous intravenous infusion; CR, complete responses; PR, partial responses.
[a]Number assessable for response.
[b]Dexverapamil initiated 18 hours before day 1.
[c]Twelve patients treated at doses of 200 mg or more of quinidine.
[d]A 5-day infusion is tolerable for vinblastine in combination with tamoxifen, whereas only a 4-day infusion is tolerable in combination with cyclosporin A.

an agent, but that agent must have intrinsic activity for successful resistance reversal.

ABC TRANSPORTERS. The broad nature of clinical resistance in renal cell cancer suggests that P-gp may be one of multiple resistance mechanisms. Recent studies have identified the existence of an increasing number of ATP-binding cassette (ABC) transporters, of which P-gp is the prototype.[296] These include the family of multidrug resistance–associated proteins (MRP1 through MRP6), which have organic anion transport activity[297–302] and a half-ABC transporter designated *MXR/BCRP/ABCP1*,[303–305] which confers mitoxantrone and camptothecin resistance, bringing to three the number of transporter families expressed in renal cell cancer and potentially linked to drug resistance. If these transporters are confirmed as being active in renal cell cancer, their inhibition offers a future strategy for increasing drug accumulation in kidney cancer cells.

INTRACELLULAR MECHANISMS. While drug transporters would directly affect intracellular concentrations of drug, other mechanisms of drug resistance have been identified that confer resistance at the levels of cell survival pathways, drug metabolism, and the drug target. Many of these have been examined in renal cell cancer, but the findings are preliminary and must be validated. Cell survival in RCC may be linked to the frequently observed overexpression of the epidermal growth factor receptor and its homologue, ErbB2[306–310] or to overexpression of the antiapoptosis protein, Bcl-2.[124,311] Alternatively, increased metabolism of anticancer agents may be promoted by higher levels of enzymes of the cytochrome P-450 family in concert with glutathione and glutathione transferases.[312,313] Finally, decreased levels of topoisomerase II have been observed in RCC, which could confer resistance to agents that impair cell division through inhibition of topoisomerase II.[314,315] Thus, ample evidence for intracellular mechanisms of resistance exists in RCC. The challenge is to determine the importance of such mechanisms and to identify strategies for their circumvention.

DRUG DELIVERY. To some, the generalized resistance just described supports an argument that drug resistance in RCC is not based primarily on cellular mechanisms. Although investigators have worked principally in other model systems, studies evaluating tumor drug delivery may cast light on the problem of drug resistance in kidney cancer. Factors that influence drug delivery include blood flow, permeability of tumor vasculature, and drug diffusion into the interstitium, which is affected both by properties of the drug and by interstitial pressure within the tumor.[316–319] Strategies aimed at identifying and reducing these physiologic barriers to drug delivery are under investigation and could have a particular relevance to the very large tumor masses seen in renal cell cancer.

Prognostic Factors

Clinical prognostic factors relating to survival after nephrectomy have been well defined. Molecular prognostic factors that may reflect chemosensitivity have been examined but, without reliable and effective therapy for RCC, their value cannot be determined. It could be predicted from experience in other cancers that correlations obtained for good and poor prognosis would generally relate to the inherent biology of the tumor cell in the absence of effective therapy. Thus, markers of differentiation and indolent biology will confer a better prognosis at the present time because of the limitations of current therapy. A frequently identified poor prognostic factor is expression of PCNA [proliferating cell nuclear antigen] or MIB-1/Ki-67, antigens associated with cell proliferation. Disease-free and prolonged survival is more likely in tumors with a low proliferation index.[320–324] Patients with diploid tumors are more likely to have longer disease-free intervals.[125] Interestingly, response to interferon treatment is also more likely to occur in patients whose tumors manifest a more indolent biology.[322] That finding is in contrast to laboratory observations with chemotherapy in which a slower growth rate is associated with increased drug resistance. When effective treatment for renal cell cancer is identified, tumor markers relevant to response to treatment can then be identified.

Although patients who have stage IV disease experience a reported median survival of 12 to 24 months, the range of survival times in this group of patients is very broad. A variety of studies have looked at the parameters that predict survival in patients with metastatic renal cancer, and performance status is the most commonly identified predictive parameter. Other factors that have been identified in some studies as predictors of poorer survival of patients with stage IV disease are a short interval from initial diagnosis, multiple organ involvement, recent weight loss, previous chemotherapy, anemia, and an elevated serum lactate dehydrogenase level.[288,325] Such factors should be considered in evaluating survival in nonrandomized studies.

Summary

In conclusion, RCC is a remarkably refractory solid tumor. More resistant than most other cancers, new phase II agents have failed time and again. The explanation for this drug resistance may lie within the tumor as an entity or within the individual cells. The broad spectrum of drugs to which RCCs are resistant suggests tumor-based mechanisms, while resistance in even the tiniest pulmonary nodule suggests cellular mechanisms. A detailed understanding of drug resistance in renal cell cancer is a major challenge for the new millennium. It is most likely that new agents directed against novel targets will be subject to the same mechanisms of resistance that have plagued treatment of this disease for decades.

BIOLOGIC THERAPY

The primary therapies for widespread metastatic RCC involve the use of biologic agents. IFN-α and IL-2 are the predominant agents used, yet several major questions remain about their application. The optimal dose and schedule have not been determined for either agent, the relative efficacy of combination therapy versus single-agent therapy is not known, and the factors that predict or produce dramatic, durable responses in a minority of patients have not been elucidated. There has even been debate as to whether these agents truly have benefit for patients with metastatic renal cell cancer or whether long-term survival results from chance or spontaneous tumor regression. The experience from two decades of biologic therapy for renal cancer has clarified this latter issue, made biologic agent administration safer, and defined the role of a number of cellular agents used in renal cancer therapy. The principle that immunotherapy can cause the complete and durable regression of large burdens of metastatic renal cancer and melanoma in some patients has been conclusively established. The most significant goal not yet accomplished is to increase significantly the percentage of patients who achieve these regressions. This objective will require improvements in our understanding of current agents as well as the development of new modalities that target different biologic mechanisms.

Spontaneous Tumor Regression

Although it does not represent a bona fide treatment modality, much has been made of the phenomenon of spontaneous tumor regression in patients with advanced renal cancer, and the mechanism is presumed to be immunologic. The practice of nephrectomy in patients with metastatic disease in the hope of inducing a spontaneous regression has been largely abandoned owing to the disappointingly low incidence of success of this method.[126] In reviews of spontaneous tumor regression, another striking feature is that the majority of regressions are short-lived. In one randomized study of IFN-α in patients with RCC, the placebo control population demonstrated a singularly high response rate of 6%, but the duration of these regressions were 2 to 13 months with only one ongoing response of 9 months at the time of publication.[127] Other larger reviews show that the true incidence of this phenomenon is probably less than 1% and that the vast majority of documented spontaneous regressions will relapse with progressive metastatic disease and require other therapy.[128,129] In addition, the few well-documented cases of durable regressions often occurred in patients in whom life-threatening infectious or inflammatory events were possible instigators of their regression.[130] These data indicate that spontaneous regression of RCC often is transient and is not a phenomenon that should be relied on as therapy. Furthermore, spontaneous regression clearly cannot account for the consistent fraction of patients who achieve complete and durable regressions with some immunotherapies.

Interferons

Early studies of leukocyte interferon in the treatment of cancer reported sporadic responses in patients with RCC.[131] Subsequently, increased dosages and larger studies were possible using recombinant IFN-α, and this experience was repeated and confirmed. The response rates in the largest studies ranged from 0% to 29% (Table 34.2-11), with few CRs and few long-term survival data.[132,133] In a review of the literature in 1989, Quesada[134] reported an overall response rate of 16% for 654 patients. Factors that seemed to increase the likelihood of responding included good performance status, prior nephrectomy, and metastases confined to the lungs. Nevertheless, these factors could not be used to identify patients without a significant possibility of response, and so they should serve only as general guidelines. Few data exist on the long-term results from interferon therapy but, from the very small number of completely responding patients, it is safe to conclude that interferon has no significant curative potential in RCC.

Recently, randomized prospective studies have been performed to measure the benefit of IFN-α in patients with advanced renal cancer. A randomized comparison of IFN-α versus medroxyprogesterone acetate in 335 patients demonstrated a significant prolongation of median survival (6 months for medroxyprogesterone acetate and 8.5 months for IFN-α).[135] This modest, albeit statistically significant, prolongation of survival was offset by greater symptoms and lesser quality of life in patients receiving IFN-α. In addition, responses did not appear durable, with estimated progression-free survival at 2 years of 5% or less for both groups.

Many different types and preparations of interferons have been used in clinical trials. Early trials with "natural" interferon produced from donor leukocytes and subsequent trials with several different subtypes of recombinant IFN-α have not suggested a difference in efficacy among these preparations. Recent trials using IFN-β and IFN-γ have indicated that these agents have either similar or less activity than IFN-α.[136] A randomized comparison of IFN-α and placebo showed no difference in response rates or survival.[127]

TABLE 34.2-11. Treatment of Metastatic Renal Cell Cancer with Interferon

Study	*IFN*	*Route and Schedule*	*N*	*RR (%)*	*CR (%)*
deKernion et al.[241]	IFN-α	6 MU/d IM	48	15	2
Quesada et al.[242]	IFN-α	3 MU/d IM	50	26	6[a]
Quesada et al.[132]	IFN-α	2 MU/d IM	15	0	0
		20 MU/d IM	41	29	2
Umeda and Niijima[243]	IFN-α	3–36 MU/d IM	153	15	2
	Lymphoblastoid	5 MU 2–7 doses/wk	73	23	1
Muss et al.[244]	IFN-α_{2b}	2–10 MU; 3 doses/wk SC	58	9	2
		30–50 MU/d IV	54	6	2
Minasian et al.[245]	IFN-α_{2a}	50 MU/wk IM	42	17	0
		3–36 MU/d SC	117	8	2

IFN, interferon; MU, million units; RR, response rate.
[a]Duration of complete responses all less than or equal to 10 months.

Interferon is one of the few biologic agents that has been tested in a randomized adjuvant study after nephrectomy. Two hundred and ninety-four patients with completely resected T3 or T4a or N1, N2, or N3 disease were randomized to observation or to 9 months of subcutaneous lymphoblastoid interferon.[137] With a median follow-up of 4.4 years, patients receiving interferon had similar recurrence rates and significantly worse survival than patients randomized to observation only. In view of the limited response rate to biologic therapy and the absence of any indication that responses are related to lesser tumor burdens, there is currently no rationale for recommending adjuvant biotherapy outside of a protocol setting.

One important consideration in evaluating interferon therapy is that the optimal dose, schedule and route of interferon administration is not yet known. Although refinement of schedules may have the potential of increasing response rates somewhat, in view of the small benefit demonstrated to this point, it is unlikely that randomized studies will ever be done to effectively optimize these parameters. In summary, disseminated renal cell cancer shows a small but consistent response rate to interferon (primarily IFN-α), but these benefits must be weighed against the toxicity of chronic therapy and the lack of documented long-term benefit.

Interleukin-2

After its discovery in 1976 and the demonstration of its activities as a T-cell growth factor and activator of T cells and natural killer cells, IL-2 was used in clinical trials against a variety of malignancies. From the first trials in 1984, renal cell cancer was identified as a tumor that could respond to IL-2 (Figs. 34.2-8, 34.2-9, and 34.2-10).[138,139] These early trials rapidly escalated the dose of IL-2 to the maximum tolerated dose and then added lymphokine-activated killer (LAK) cells to the therapy, based on preclinical results. These trials initially reported response rates of 33% in RCC and, in a subsequent multicenter experience, the response rate was 16%.[140] The remarkable feature of many of these responses is that they appear complete and durable. Median follow-up of greater than 10 years is available from those early studies, and a review of the follow-up data indicates that 7% to 9% of all patients (nearly half of all those responding) had a CR and the majority of those completely responding patients have never relapsed (see Fig. 34.2-8).[141–143] This constitutes the most convincing evidence that IL-2 has clinical benefit in the treatment of metastatic renal cell cancer and led to the approval of IL-2 by the U.S. Food and Drug Administration as the only currently approved therapy for this disease in the United States. It should be emphasized that it is the curative potential of these responses and not their frequency that is of value (Fig. 34.2-11).[254,255]

Since those early studies, several developments have occurred. The use of LAK cells with IL-2 has been critically examined in randomized studies, and many investigators have explored the use of lower-dose IL-2 regimens to avoid the toxicity of high-dose IL-2. Although murine models predicted that the addition of LAK cells to IL-2 would substantially increase therapeutic efficacy, this has not proved to be true in clinical studies. A randomized comparison of high-dose intravenous bolus IL-2 with and without LAK cells showed an insignificant difference in response rate (21% for IL-2 and 31% for IL-2 combined with LAK cells) with no difference in survival.[144] Other studies have confirmed this[145] and, currently, there is no evidence to support the use of LAK cells in patients with RCC.

The initial rapid escalation of IL-2 to its maximum tolerated dose identified as the maximum tolerated dose 600,000 to 720,000 IU/kg by intravenous bolus given every 8 hours. On that schedule, patients tolerated approximately seven to nine consecutive doses before treatment had to be stopped for vascular leak syndrome, hypotension, multiorgan dysfunction, and a variety of other toxicities.[146] These effects rapidly reversed after therapy was stopped but, with hypotension requiring vasopressor support, pulmonary edema, and potential infectious complications, a 2% to 4% treatment-related mortality was initially encountered (see Fig. 34.2-10). Since then, increased experience with IL-2, prophylactic antibiotics (when indicated), and patient screening for occult coronary disease have dramatically decreased this mortality rate. A recent report cites 809 consecutive patients who received high-dose bolus IL-2 without a treatment-related mortality,[147] a statistic unattainable with most multiagent chemotherapeutic regimens.

Nevertheless, the expense of intensive care unit care and the precipitous nature of toxicities on high-dose IL-2 led many investigators to try lower-dose regimens. In particular, daily subcutaneous self-administration was adopted as a convenient and inexpensive route. In a scenario that has been replayed many times during the development of IL-2, a multitude of small phase

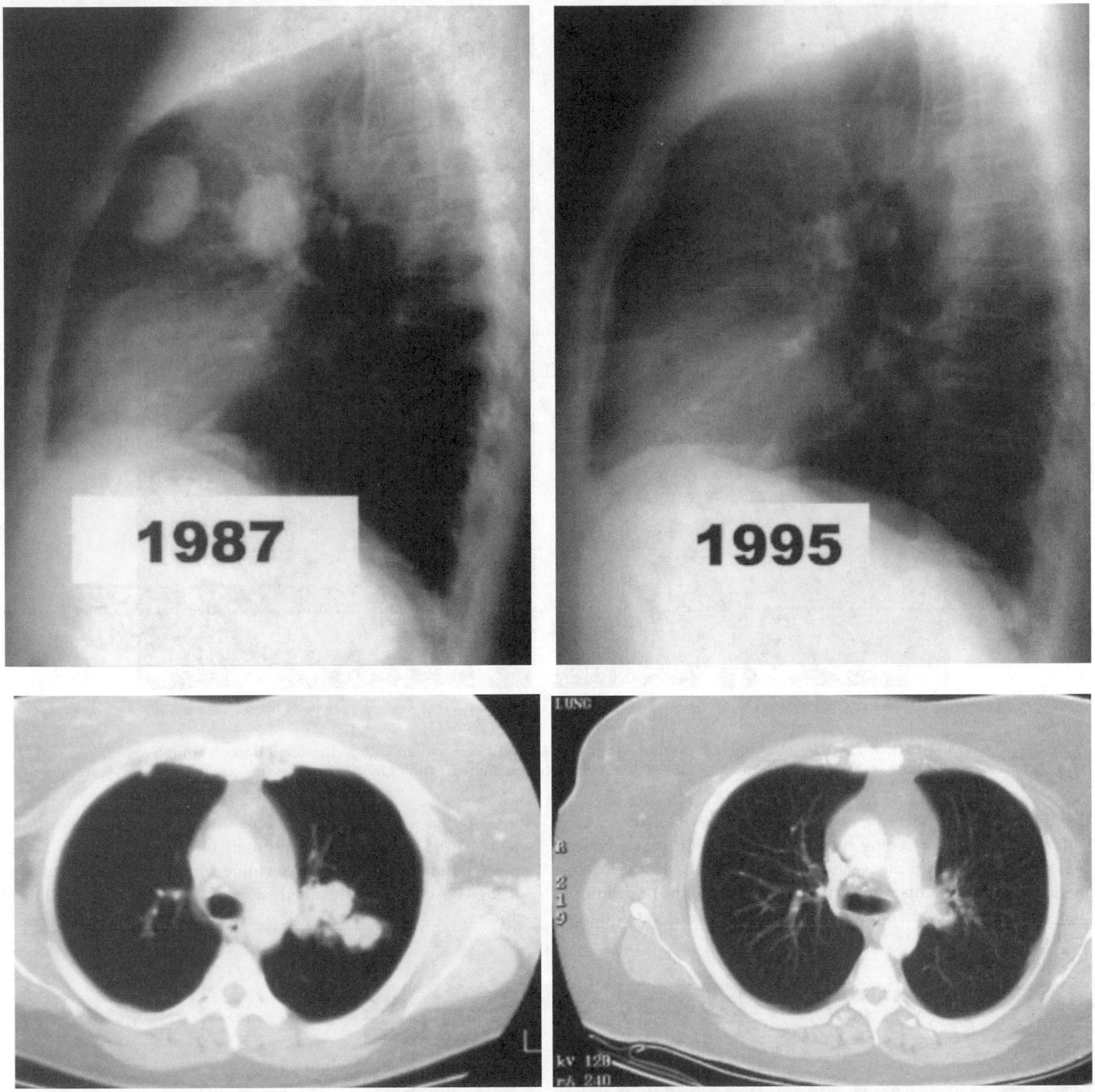

1992 **1999**

FIGURE 34.2-8. Radiographs of two patients with long-term complete regressions of pulmonary metastases from renal cancer in response to high-dose therapy with interleukin-2 alone. In most studies, patients with only pulmonary metastases appear to have a slightly higher probability of response.

II studies were performed that reported short-term response rates similar to those seen with high-dose IL-2. An outpatient, daily, self-administered regimen using an initial week (Monday through Friday) of 18 million IU (fixed dose) followed by 5 weeks at half that dose was well tolerated and produced a response rate of 23% in 26 evaluable patients.[148] Later, continued experience with a modification of this regimen showed a 20% overall response rate, with one ongoing CR in 47 patients[149]; another group of investigators achieved an 18% response rate with a similar regimen.[150] Others reported on the use of continuous-infusion IL-2, describing a similar response rate with less toxicity (and less overall IL-2 given over the same period).[151] A review of the literature (Table 34.2-12) shows response rates to IL-2 monotherapy or IL-2 and LAK cells, delivered on many different schedules and at different doses, ranging from 8% to 35%, and it is clear that smaller, nonrandomized studies cannot discern whether one schedule is more effec-

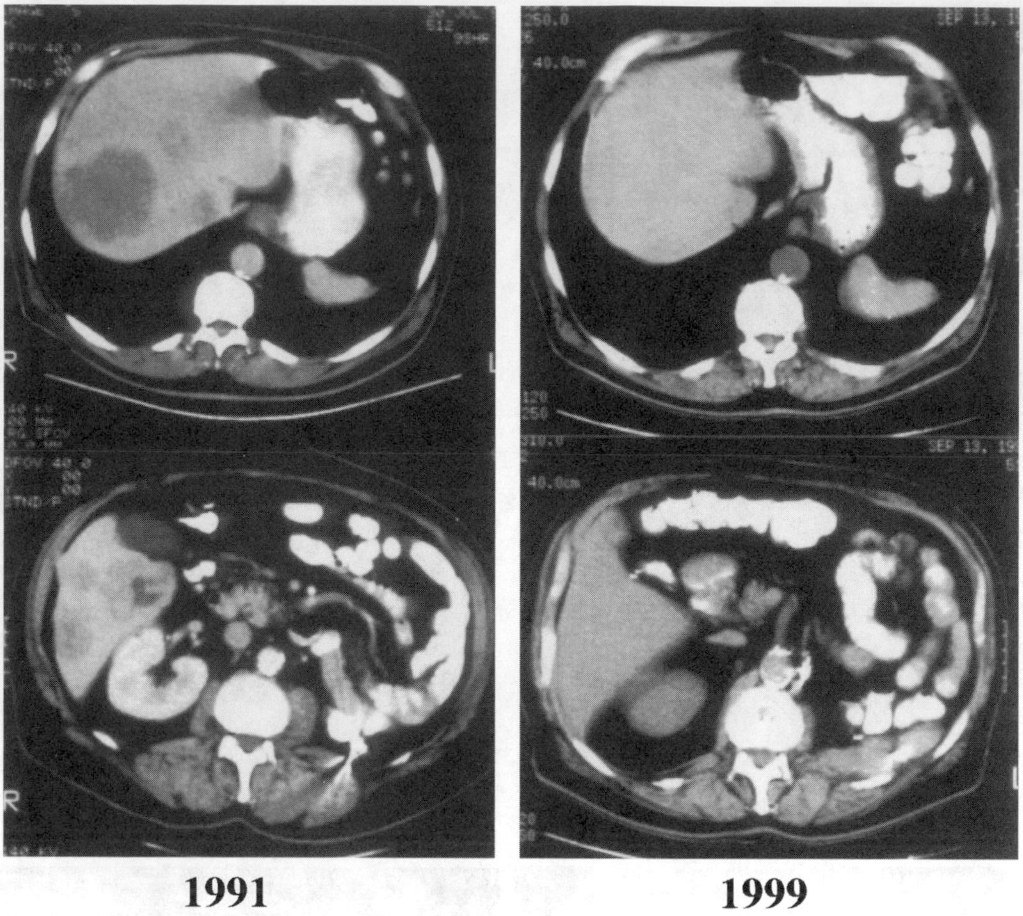

FIGURE 34.2-9. Abdominal computed tomography scans of a patient with a durable, ongoing complete response to high-dose interleukin-2 therapy, which included the regression of extensive liver metastases.

tive than another. Nevertheless, lower-dose schedules have been widely adopted before being critically evaluated. There is no question that patients with metastatic RCC can respond to these regimens and that patients with other significant medical conditions may not be able to tolerate high-dose IL-2. In these cases, lower-dose options represent a reasonable therapeutic choice. For those patients who are able to tolerate any of the published IL-2 regimens, it remains crucial to determine whether the added toxicity of high-dose IL-2 is associated with any improvement in clinical efficacy.

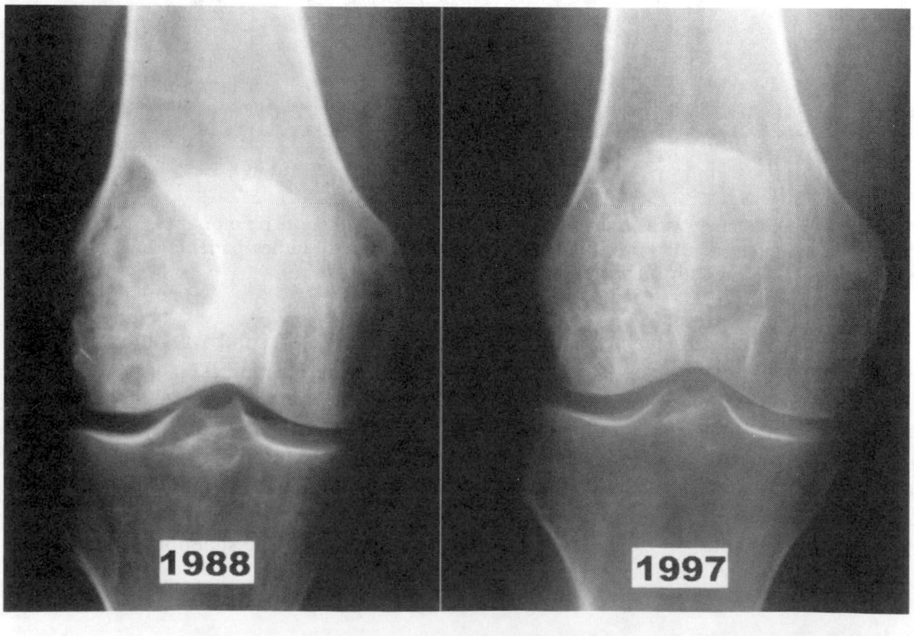

FIGURE 34.2-10. Regression and recalcification of a large lytic metastasis of the lateral femoral condyle in a patient with widely metastatic renal cell cancer. This patient also had a durable complete response of all soft tissue metastases with interleukin-2–based immunotherapy.

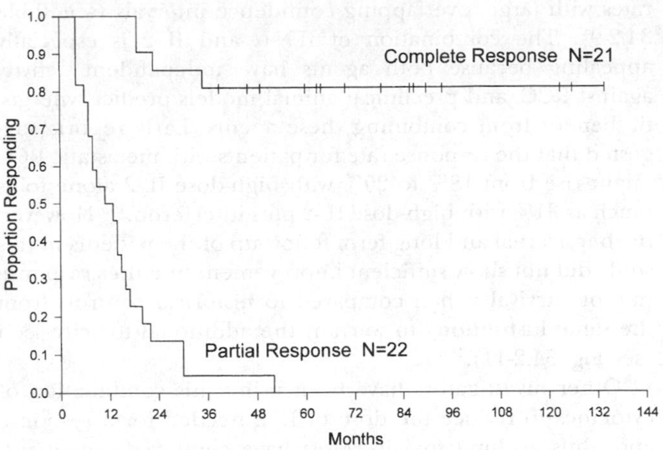

FIGURE 34.2-11. Complete responses to high-dose interleukin-2 in patients with metastatic renal carcinoma are typically durable. An actuarial curve of response duration for patients with metastatic renal cell carcinoma responding to high-dose bolus interleukin-2 is shown. Among completely responding patients, 81% have not experienced relapse (median follow-up, 7 years), and no patients have experienced relapse beyond 3 years. Partial responses can be sustained for years but, in this study, all partially responding patients eventually experienced relapse. (Adapted from ref. 143.)

Such a study is under way, and an interim analysis is available.[152] This study randomized patients to receive IL-2 at either 720,000 IU/kg or 72,000 IU/kg every 8 hours by intravenous bolus to maximum tolerance (up to 15 consecutive doses). The lower dose was selected as the maximum dose that still resulted in a well-tolerated regimen not requiring intensive care unit care and vasopressor support. This two-arm comparison constitutes the most precise determination of whether the dose of IL-2 is important. Subsequently, a third arm was added to the trial to evaluate the widely used subcutaneous route of administration. This arm delivered 250,000 IU/kg/d for 5 days in the first week and then half that dose 5 days per week for the subsequent 5 weeks. Of course, only concurrently randomized patients are compared in this two-phase trial. With 228 randomized patients of a projected study population of 400, it is evident that the two lower-dose regimens are associated with lower toxicity, especially in the areas of hypotension requiring pressors (43% of courses of high-dose intravenous IL-2 vs. 4% of courses of low-dose intravenous IL-2 and 0% with subcutaneous IL-2), thrombocytopenia, pulmonary distress, and disorientation. It is important to note that there have been no deaths in any of the treatment arms. The interim response rates are shown in Table 34.2-13. In the two-arm comparison of high- and low-dose intravenous bolus IL-2, the respective response rates are 19% and 10% ($P = .06$). The durations of the responses bear watching, as seven of nine patients completely responding to high-dose IL-2 remain in CR beyond 2 years, whereas two of five patients completely responding to low-dose IL-2 maintained their response at 2 years. The three-arm comparison including subcutaneous IL-2 is still preliminary, with response rates of only 16%, 4%, and 11% for high-dose intravenous, low-dose intravenous, and subcutaneous IL-2 reported.[152]

Because the clinical benefit of IL-2 resides in the long-term CRs achieved, any interpretation of this study will require pro-

TABLE 34.2-12. Therapy with IL-2 Alone or with LAK Cells

Study	*IL-2 Dose Range*[a]	*Route and Schedule*	*N*	*RR (%)*	*CR (%)*
IL-2 alone					
Rosenberg et al.[143]	High	IV bolus q8h	227	19	9
Cytokine Working Group[141,159]	High	IV bolus q8h	71	17	7
Yang and Rosenberg[152]	Low	IV bolus q8h	112	10	4
Bukowski et al.[246]	Moderate	IV 3 times/wk	41	12	2
Gold et al.[154]	High	IV continuous	47	13	6
von der Maase et al.[247]	High	IV continuous	51	16	4
Escudier et al.[248]	Moderate	IV continuous	104	19	4
Negrier et al.[158]	High	IV continuous	138	7	1
Lissoni et al.[249]	Low	SC daily	91	23	2
Buter et al.[149]	Low	SC daily	47	19	4
Tourani et al.[150]	Low	SC 1–2/d	39	18	3
Yang and Rosenberg[152]	Low	SC daily	53	11	6
Total			1021	15.5	4.8
IL-2 and LAK cells					
Rosenberg[250a]	High	IV bolus q8h	72	35	11
Fisher et al.[140]	High	IV bolus q8h	35	14	6
Weiss et al.[153]	High	IV bolus q8h	46	20	7
Parkinson et al.[251]	High	IV continuous	47	9	4
Negrier et al.[252]	High	IV continuous	51	27	10
Dillman et al.[250,253]	High	IV continuous	46	15	NA
Thompson et al.[254]	High	IV continuous	76	22	8
Weiss et al.[153]	High	IV continuous	48	15	4
Total			421	20.9	7.5

CR, complete response; IL-2, interleukin-2; LAK, lymphokine-activated killer; RR, response rate.
[a]*High-dose* indicates significant multiorgan toxicity and vasopressors, with intensive care unit support needed in more than one-fourth of treatments. *Moderate-dose* indicates occasional multiorgan toxicity or significant single-organ toxicity with occasional intensive care unit support. *Low-dose* indicates rare or mild multiorgan toxicity and rare intensive care unit support; typically given in the outpatient setting.
(Adapted from ref. 225.)

TABLE 34.2-13. A Randomized Study of High-Dose versus Low-Dose Interleukin-2 in Patients with Metastatic Renal Cell Cancer

	High-Dose IV Bolus	*Low-Dose IV Bolus*	*Outpatient SC Daily*
Two-arm comparison			
No. of patients	115	112	—
Response rate (% PR + CR)	19	10	—
CR (%)	8	4	—
CR durations (mo)	19, 23, 24+, 38+, 48+, 52+, 53+, 54+, 61+	3, 19, 20, 53+, 61+	
PR (%)	11	5	—
PR durations (mo)	4, 4, 4+, 6, 7, 8, 9, 13, 13,14, 16, 17, 21	4, 7, 7, 11,22, 23	
Three-arm comparison			
No. of patients	56[a]	55[a]	53
Response rate (% PR + CR)	16	4	11
CR (%)	7	0	4

CR, complete recovery; PR, partial recovery.
[a]A concurrently randomized subset of the patients analyzed in two-arm comparison.

longed follow-up and survival analyses after full accrual. As a drug that conveys great benefit to a minority of patients (who happen to possess the unidentified tumor or immune system qualities that allow them to respond), IL-2 is unlikely to affect the median survival of patients in randomized studies, and study design must take this into account.

Other studies have addressed the issue of continuous-infusion IL-2 versus bolus IL-2. The initial nonrandomized studies using continuous-infusion IL-2 reported response rates similar to those for bolus IL-2 but with lesser toxicities.[151] In a subsequent randomized study in which all patients received LAK cells, there was a randomization to receive either continuous-infusion IL-2 at 18 to 22.5 million IU/m^2/d or 600,000 IU/kg/dose by bolus every 8 hours (the cumulative daily dose by bolus was more than three times the dose by continuous infusion).[153] Both of these doses represented the respective maximally tolerated doses for these regimens, and the few significant differences in toxicities did not favor either regimen. In this study, patients receiving LAK cells and bolus IL-2 had a 20% major response rate, as compared to a 15% response rate for patients given LAK cells and continuous-infusion IL-2; the difference was not significant. Fortunately, it has been established that the CRs to high-dose continuous-infusion IL-2 can be of long duration. A single-institution study of 123 patients (some also receiving LAK cells) with follow-up of 1 to 109 months reported an overall response rate of 19%, with 7% CRs and 78% of those patients sustaining their CRs at 42 to more than 109 months.[154]

A more complex issue is whether any combination of cytokine or chemotherapy added to IL-2 is superior to IL-2 alone. Here again, small, nonrandomized phase II studies have clouded this issue. Innumerable small studies have combined IL-2 with interferon and chemotherapy, and sometimes both agents, and reported improved short-term response rates with large, overlapping confidence intervals (see Table 34.2-9). The combination of IFN-α and IL-2 is especially appealing because both agents have independent activity against RCC, and preclinical animal models predict synergistic benefit from combining these agents. Early reports suggested that the response rate for patients with metastatic RCC might rise from 18% to 20% with high-dose IL-2 alone to as much as 31% with high-dose IL-2 plus interferon.[155] However, further accrual and long-term follow-up of the patients in this study did not show sufficient improvement in either response rate or survival (when compared to historical controls from the same institution) to warrant the additional toxicity seen (see Fig. 34.2-11).[156]

Other investigators have been using this combination of cytokines to reduce the dose of IL-2 needed for a response and, thus, to limit toxicity. Most have employed outpatient, subcutaneous schedules, as widely described by Atzpodien et al.[157] The initial nonrandomized reports on this regimen emphasized lesser toxicities but similar response rates to high-dose IL-2 monotherapy. Yet when others have tried the same or similar regimens, their response rates as well as their toxicity profiles have not been as favorable. Without randomized studies, it is impossible to reconcile these disparate results.

Some experience in randomized evaluations of IL-2 and interferon is available. Negrier et al.[158] randomized 425 patients to receive continuous-infusion, high-dose IL-2 alone, subcutaneous IFN-α three times weekly, or both agents simultaneously. There was a significantly higher response rate to the combination (18.6%) than to only IL-2 (6.5%) or interferon (7.5%), but this increased response rate did not translate into improved survival. This study demonstrated an unusually low response rate to IL-2 alone, and patients with tumor progression crossed over between therapy arms. Other small randomized studies of IL-2 and interferon have also failed to demonstrate an advantage to combination therapy, but these studies are largely underpowered.[159,160]

In a further effort to enhance the efficacy of IL-2 by adding other agents, investigators have tried to exploit the reported synergy between 5-FU (which has a low single-agent response rate against RCC) and interferon by adding this agent to IL-2 and interferon. Again, early phase II studies reported major increases in response rates,[161] but later studies did not always substantiate these findings.[162] In fact, an attempt to reproduce the initial studies exactly with 5-FU, IFN, and IL-2 (which had a reported response rate of 49%) resulted in a PR and CR rate of 16%—exactly the same as with IL-2 alone.[163]

One issue rarely addressed in evaluating these combinations is the durability of the responses. Long-term follow-up with sufficient patients to evaluate response durations in the minority of patients showing regression is crucial to evaluating IL-2 therapies. Dutcher et al.[163] have raised a possible red flag by reviewing their sequential use of IL-2, IL-2 plus interferon, and IL-2 plus interferon plus 5-FU. Not only did they fail to see an increased response rate as the dose of IL-2 was moderated and other agents were added to IL-2, but their percentage of patients attaining durable CRs seemed to decrease. Although their numbers still are small and patients were not randomized, this is a potentially important issue. If IL-2's durable responses are indeed forfeited by these combinations, then these regimens are indistinguishable from the many ineffective chemotherapeutic agents with 15% to 25% partial or transient responses and should not be advocated.

Vaccines and Cellular Therapy

An effort to identify immune cells with reactivity to renal cancer is ongoing. The use of nonspecific activated killer cells (natural killer or LAK cells) has largely been ineffective, but current efforts have concentrated on T cells and the induction of a T-cell response via vaccination. After the lead of melanoma research, tumor-infiltrating lymphocytes (TIL) isolated from renal cancer specimens and cells from mixed lymphocyte-tumor reactions were examined for antitumor reactivity. With some notable exceptions,[164–167] little specific tumor reactivity was seen.[168] Attempts to use TIL clinically have showed some promising early results (usually combined with IL-2 and IFN-α),[169] but a randomized trial of IL-2 with and without CD8-enriched TIL was fraught with technical difficulties and showed no augmentation in response rate or survival with cell transfer.[170] Another study of the use of peripheral blood cells nonspecifically activated by anti-CD3-stimulated mononuclear cell supernatant (autolymphocyte therapy) appeared to be beneficial in a small randomized trial[171] but, despite the undertaking of a large multicenter trial, no confirmatory data for this approach have been produced since that trial.

Because of the relative scarcity of tumor-reactive specific T cells against renal cancer, another approach has been the use of vaccines. Typically, whole tumor preparations have been used because of the failure to identify broadly applicable, common tumor antigens expressed by RCC. In one study, the gene for granulocyte-macrophage colony-stimulating factor (GM-CSF) was introduced into autologous cultured renal cell cancer lines by retroviral transduction in a concept based on preclinical studies.[172] Patients then were immunized with irradiated tumor cells secreting large amounts of GM-CSF (or control nontransduced cells) and were evaluated for immune responses and clinical tumor regression. One PR was seen in 16 evaluable patients, and evidence was seen of cutaneous delayed-type hypersensitivity responses generated against tumor as well as an antitumor T-cell response in the responding patient. This approach is limited by the requirement for an autologous cultured tumor line. Other approaches are investigating the use of tumor lysates and whole tumor cells co-incubated with autologous dendritic cells to vaccinate patients. Data on the clinical and laboratory responses generated by dendritic cell vaccines should be forthcoming soon.

Another recent early-phase trial has used a nonmyeloablative allogeneic peripheral blood stem cell transplant, hypothesizing that a graft-versus-tumor response may lead to regression of metastatic renal cancer. It appears, in the single patient presented, that tumor regression did not occur until the onset of complete donor chimerism, tapering of immunosuppression, and the appearance of mild graft-versus-host disease, supporting an immunological mechanism of action related to the allograft.[173] Still not clear is whether there is specific recognition of tumor-associated antigens by the matched sibling allograft or whether generalized graft-versus-host disease is leading to *in situ* production of cytokines, which then can treat an intrinsically cytokine-sensitive tumor (i.e., renal cancer). This is an interesting approach, given the magnitude of the few responses seen thus far, but it remains to be confirmed by a larger experience, and the mechanism of action requires further investigation.

Antiangiogenic Agents

The field of angiogenesis and its role as a target for cancer therapy has burgeoned in the last decade. New inhibitors of angiogenesis such as endostatin and angiostatin have been discovered,[174] and old compounds such as thalidomide have found new life as antiangiogenic agents. RCC presents an attractive target for these agents for two reasons. First, it is a tremendously vascular tumor consisting largely of capillaries and blood sinuses surrounded by malignant clear cells. In addition, there appears to be a highly angiogenic environment within clear cell cancers, driven by tumor-elaborated vascular endothelial growth factor (VEGF). As described in Chapter 34.1, the elaboration of VEGF by RCC in response to a variety of stimuli appears to be linked to the functional mutation of the VHL protein found in nearly all clear cell renal cancers. Thus, the common genetic event that leads to clear cell RCC involves a deregulation of the VEGF pathway and, presumably, angiogenesis is a consequence. One ongoing randomized trial is studying the use of a neutralizing antibody to human VEGF that is highly effective in slowing the growth of VEGF-secreting human tumors implanted into nude mice.[175] The clinical trial is a blinded, placebo-controlled trial designed to determine whether survival or time to progression are altered by the chronic administration of this antibody. A small trial of thalidomide (the highly teratogenic sedative now thought to cause deformities via an *in utero* antiangiogenic mechanism) in patients with metastatic renal cancer was recently reported to produce tumor regression in some patients (R. Amato, unpublished data). Another agent, endostatin, which showed broad preclinical activity in mice, has also just been entered into highly anticipated clinical trials. Although this is a field of intense activity and interest, it is not yet clear whether a single antiangiogenic agent will be sufficient to interrupt the vascular supply of a tumor. It may be that tumors use a variety of angiogenic pathways and that only with carefully combined multiagent therapy will clinically significant tumor arrest or regression be accomplished.

Summary

In the last two decades, a burgeoning supply of new biologic agents has been made available in amounts sufficient for clinical trials by recombinant gene technology. Most of these proteins did not meet the unrealistic expectations generated by preclinical work and entrepreneurial publicity. In the face of these disappointments, several important principles were established in the treatment of renal cell cancer and melanoma that should not be overlooked. It has been established that purely immunologic therapy, which has no direct, intrinsic antitumor activity, was able to cause the regression of large, metastatic tumors by stimulating host immune cells. Even more crucial was the demonstration that some of these regressions were potentially curative, with a small but consistent fraction of patients maintaining their CRs to IL-2 beyond 10 years. These results argue effectively that predicted pitfalls to immunotherapy such as tumor heterogeneity and antigen loss, immunosuppression by the cancer-bearing state or tumor microenvironment, and a lack of tumor-specific antigens in human cancers are not insurmountable problems. To increase the frequency of successful immune attack on renal cell cancer, it will be important to understand the mechanisms and cellular elements that are responsible for these few dramatic responses. Both immune effector factors as well as tumor characteristics are likely to be involved in the successful interplay that occurs in responding patients. The treatment of patients with renal cell cancer is likely to contribute to our future understanding of these factors and to continue at the forefront of progress in biologic therapies for cancer.

CARCINOMA OF THE RENAL PELVIS AND URETER

CARCINOMA OF THE RENAL PELVIS

Carcinoma of the renal pelvis is a relatively rare tumor that accounts for 5% of all renal tumors. It occurs more frequently in men than in women (2:1 to 3:1). Upper urinary tract carcinoma is a multifocal process; patients with cancer at one site in the upper urinary tract are at greater risk of developing tumors elsewhere.[256–258] The probability of multifocal occurrence is greater in patients with larger lesions and in those with carcinoma *in situ*. A patient with one upper tract urothelial tumor has a 30% to 50% chance of developing a bladder tumor as well. Some 2% to 4% of patients with an upper tract urothelial tumor develop bilateral renal pelvic tumors. If a patient has both a renal pelvic tumor and a ureteral tumor simultaneously, there is a 75% chance that a bladder tumor will develop in this patient. Alternatively, a patient with a bladder tumor initially has a 2% to 3% chance of developing an upper tract tumor.[176]

Etiologic Features and Genetics

Recent studies have demonstrated that the major cause of cancer of the renal pelvis is smoking and that cessation of smoking can eliminate a large number of these tumors.[177] A significant increase in risk for upper genitourinary (GU) tract urothelial cancer is found in smokers, the risk being highest among the heaviest smokers.[22] In 1965, Hultengren et al.[178] first identified a connection between epithelial tumors of the renal pelvis and abuse of compound analgesics. Since then, a number of other reports[179–181] from Sweden,[182] Australia,[183] the Netherlands,[184] Denmark,[185] Italy,[186] Germany,[187] and the United States[22] have demonstrated an association between analgesic abuse and renal pelvic tumors.[188] Most of the patients ingested a significant amount (5 kg) of compound analgesic, usually containing phenacetin, phenazone, and caffeine.[189,190] Typically, upper GU tract tumors occur in patients in whom prolonged and heavy analgesic ingestion is followed by renal papillary necrosis.[190]

There is also an association between cancer of the renal pelvis and danubian endemic familial nephropathy (Balkan nephropathy). Balkan nephropathy is a slowly progressive inflammation of the interstitium of the kidney that ultimately results in renal failure.[191] This disorder, which is prevalent in the Balkan countries (Yugoslavia, Romania, Bulgaria, and Greece), is associated with multifocal, slow-growing, superficial, low-grade tumors of the renal pelvis. The cause of Balkan nephropathy is unclear; however, a number of potential etiologic agents such as fungal toxins, viruses, silicates, and heavy metals have been studied.[192]

TABLE 34.2-14. Classification of Tumors of the Ureter

PRIMARY TUMORS
Epithelial
Malignant
Transitional cell carcinoma (71%)
Transitional cell carcinoma with differentiation (20%)
Squamous differentiation
Glandular differentiation
Mixed
Squamous cell carcinoma (pure) (8%)
Adenocarcinoma (1%)
Undifferentiated carcinoma (1%)
Benign
Papilloma
Mesodermal
Malignant
Leiomyosarcoma
Benign
Fibroepithelial polyp
Leiomyoma
Neurilemmoma
Angioma
SECONDARY TUMORS (ALL MALIGNANT)
Drop metastases
Metastases via blood or lymph
Direct extension

(Modified from ref. 256.)

An association has been observed between renal pelvic tumors and urban residence as well as occupation in the aniline dye, textile, plastics, and rubber industries.[189,192] Chronic inflammation and irritation are associated with the development of renal pelvic tumors, particularly in patients who have upper urinary tract stones.

There are reports of kindreds exhibiting a hereditary pattern in the development of transitional cell carcinoma of the urinary tract.[193,194] Of the affected family members, 22% had upper GU tract tumors, 59% had bladder cancer, and 18% had both upper and lower GU tract tumors.[193] Upper GU tract urothelial tumors are found in patients with hereditary nonpolyposis colorectal cancer, which is associated with a germline abnormality in DNA mismatch repair genes.[195] Studies of the molecular and cellular aspects of urothelial transformation should provide further insight into the etiology and mechanisms of progression and metastasis of this disease.

Pathology

Transitional cell carcinoma accounts for 90% of the tumors of the renal pelvis and can be *in situ*, papillary, or planar (Table 34.2-14). Squamous cell carcinoma, which usually is associated with chronic inflammation or infection of the renal pelvis, accounts for 7% of renal pelvic tumors.[196] Squamous cell cancer of the renal pelvis often is deeply invasive and is associated with a worse prognosis than is transitional cell carcinoma. Adenocarcinoma of the renal pelvis has been reported in few patients and occurs in association with inflammation, infection, or calculi.[197]

Diagnosis and Staging

Hematuria is the initial pelvic presenting symptom in the majority of patients with renal pelvic carcinoma. Gross hematuria is present in 62% to 75%, and microscopic hematuria is seen in 10%. The triad of flank mass, pain, and hematuria is encountered infrequently, in 20% or fewer cases, and often is associated with advanced disease. Excretory urography frequently is used in the initial evaluation of patients with renal pelvic tumors and will often reveal a filling defect in the collecting system. There may also be either a hydronephrotic or a nonfunctional kidney due to obstruction by a blood clot or mass. Retrograde pyelography (in which contrast medium is injected into the ureter through an endoscope) accurately delineates upper GU tract filling defects. If there is uncertainty about the nature of a renal pelvic lesion, CT performed before and after administration of intravenous contrast material will differentiate a tumor from another radiolucent mass such as a stone.[198–200] Angiography is not used often in the diagnostic evaluation of a suspected renal pelvic tumor. However, a renal mass that lacks the characteristic neovascularity of a renal carcinoma may be the first indication of a renal pelvic tumor invading the renal parenchyma.

Urine cytology is useful in evaluating a renal pelvis mass, and endoscopically obtained barbotage specimens allow an accurate diagnosis to be made in approximately 80% of cases.[201,202] Tissue can also be obtained by introducing a biopsy brush into the ureter and removing a specimen for cytologic or histologic examination. Brush biopsy increases diagnostic accuracy to between 80% and 90%. Endoscopic ureteroscopy and percutaneous nephroscopy are techniques that have dramatically improved the diagnosis of upper tract tumors.[203–205] Endoluminal sonographic evaluation may also be useful for diagnosis and staging.[206,207] With currently available endoscopic instruments, the renal pelvis can be inspected visually in more than 90% of patients.

The most significant prognostic factors for survival of patients with renal pelvic carcinoma are stage and grade of tumor. Renal pelvic upper urinary tract cancer is divided into four stages by the TNM classification (Table 34.2-15). The primary tumor is classified as low-stage (Ta, limited to mucosa; T1, lamina propria invasion) and high-stage (T2, muscularis involvement; T3, tumor beyond the muscularis).[75] Renal pelvic tumors are graded from 1 to 3. The median survival for patients with high-grade tumors is 14 to 16 months as compared with 67 months for patients with low-grade tumors. Median survival for patients with high-stage tumors is 13 months, whereas median survival for patients with low-stage tumors is 91 months.[176] Invasion of the renal hilum occurs in 95% of patients who ultimately develop metastases.[208]

TABLE 34.2-15. Staging of Ureteral and Pelvic Tumors

Stage	*Description*
TUMOR	
Ta (stage O/I)	Limited to mucosa
T1 (stage A/II)	Lamina propria invasion
T2 (stage B/III)	Confined to the muscularis propria
T3 (stage C/IV)	Invasion of periureteral or peripelvic tissue or renal parenchyma
T4 (stage D/IV)	Invasion of contiguous structures
NODE	
N1	Single node ≤ 2 cm
N2	Multiple nodes ≤ 5 cm
N3	Multiple nodes > 5 cm
METASTASIS	
M	Hematogenous or distant nodal metastasis

Surgical Treatment

Carcinoma of the renal pelvis may be treated with a radical nephrectomy that includes removal of Gerota's fascia and its contents, total removal of the ipsilateral ureter, and removal of a cuff of bladder.[209,210] When transitional cell carcinoma of the renal pelvis invades the renal vein or vena cava, an extensive surgical procedure including thrombus extraction or partial vena cava resection may be required.[211]

More conservative endourologic surgical excision is advocated by some who note that renal pelvic carcinoma can be bilateral and that survival of patients with low-stage, low-grade renal pelvic carcinoma treated with a conservative surgical procedure is approximately the same as in patients treated with more radical surgery.[203,212] The incidence of low-grade, low-stage renal pelvic carcinoma is approximately 8%, and that of bilateral disease is 2%. Often there is also a long latent period prior to recurrence. Papillary, low-grade, low-stage tumors of the upper urinary tract often are considered amenable to endoscopic resection. However, most clinicians offer radical surgery to patients with high-grade endoscopically defined lesions.[203] Currently, most clinicians consider that local, partial excision is potentially appropriate for patients with a solitary kidney, with bilateral renal pelvic carcinoma, or with renal insufficiency. Treatment strategies involving percutaneous or ureteroscopic resection of renal pelvic tumors followed by either laser irradiation or supplemental intracavitary therapy are currently being evaluated.[213–215]

Follow-Up

Conscientious follow-up after surgery for renal pelvic carcinoma is essential. Urinalysis, urine cytology, and cystourethroscopy are performed every 3 months for 2 to 3 years and then less frequently. For patients who undergo a conservative upper tract procedure, periodic retrograde pyelography and ureteroscopy also are performed.[203]

URETERAL CARCINOMA

Ureteral carcinoma is an uncommon neoplasm that accounts for only 1% of all malignancies of the upper GU tract. Ureteral carcinoma was first described by the French pathologist Rayer in 1841; the first ureteral carcinoma to be removed by nephroureterectomy was reported by Vorphl in 1905. Ureteral carcinoma tends to occur in the older age groups, predominantly in the sixth, seventh, and eighth decades of life. The male-female ratio is 2:1. The most common site for the occurrence of a ureteral tumor is in the lower one-third of the ureter, with a lesser incidence higher up.

Histology and Etiology

Ninety percent of malignant tumors of the ureter are transitional cell carcinomas; 20% have squamous or glandular differentiation.

Eight percent of the tumors are pure squamous cell carcinomas, and 1% are adenocarcinomas. Tumors of the ureter share embryologic, morphologic, and etiologic characteristics with renal pelvic tumors. As with renal pelvic tumors, there is an increased incidence of ureteral carcinoma associated with Balkan nephropathy, prolonged exposure to phenacetin, or prolonged exposure to environmental agents such as aniline dyes.[216]

Clinical Presentation: Grade and Stage

Hematuria is the most common presenting symptom and is present in 75% of patients with ureteral carcinoma. The hematuria is usually painless; however, colicky pain due to obstruction by clot or by tumor occurs in up to 35%. Urinary frequency or dysuria, present in only 10% of patients with renal pelvic carcinoma, occurs in up to 50% of patients with ureteral carcinoma.[216]

As in pelvic carcinoma, the primary ureteral carcinoma is classified as grades 1 through 3 and stage Ta (limited to the mucosa), T1 (lamina propria invasion), T2 (muscularis involvement), or T3 (invasion beyond the muscularis).[75] Although up to 100% of grade 1 tumors and 85% of grade 2 tumors may be noninvasive, only 30% of grade 3 and 8% of grade 4 tumors are noninvasive.[176,216]

Diagnosis

Excretory urography is an initial part of the evaluation of a suspected ureteral mass lesion. On excretory urography, the upper tract above the tumor may be completely normal or there may be hydronephrosis or complete nonfunction. Retrograde pyelography may be performed to delineate accurately the precise location of the ureteral lesion. Urine is collected for cytologic examination, and brush biopsy may be performed to obtain tissue for histologic examination. Advances in ureteroscopic techniques have revolutionized the diagnosis and treatment of upper tract transitional carcinomas.[217] The flexible endoscope has greatly improved the surgeon's ability to visualize and perform a biopsy of ureteral lesions, and its use is now part of the standard management of this disease.[217,218] Abdominal CT also provides useful staging information, particularly with regard to extension of the tumor outside the ureter.

Treatment

Carcinoma of the ureter has historically been treated by either nephroureterectomy or partial ureterectomy. The advantage of a partial ureterectomy is that the more conservative procedure preserves the kidney. However, mapping studies of the urothelium have demonstrated that carcinoma of the upper urinary tract is a multifocal disease. Often atypia and carcinoma *in situ* are noted in multiple areas of the urothelium, particularly in high-grade, high-stage carcinomas. Small, solitary, low-grade tumors are most often treated by endoscopic resection, fulguration, or laser photocoagulation, which allows acceptable survival and renal preservation, particularly in patients with a solitary kidney, bilateral tumors, a poor operative risk, or impaired renal function.[203,217,218] Nephroureterectomy is recommended for patients with high-grade or high-stage tumor and for those with disease at an unresectable location.

The surgical procedure of radical nephrectomy plus ureterectomy entails removal of the kidney and the entire contents of

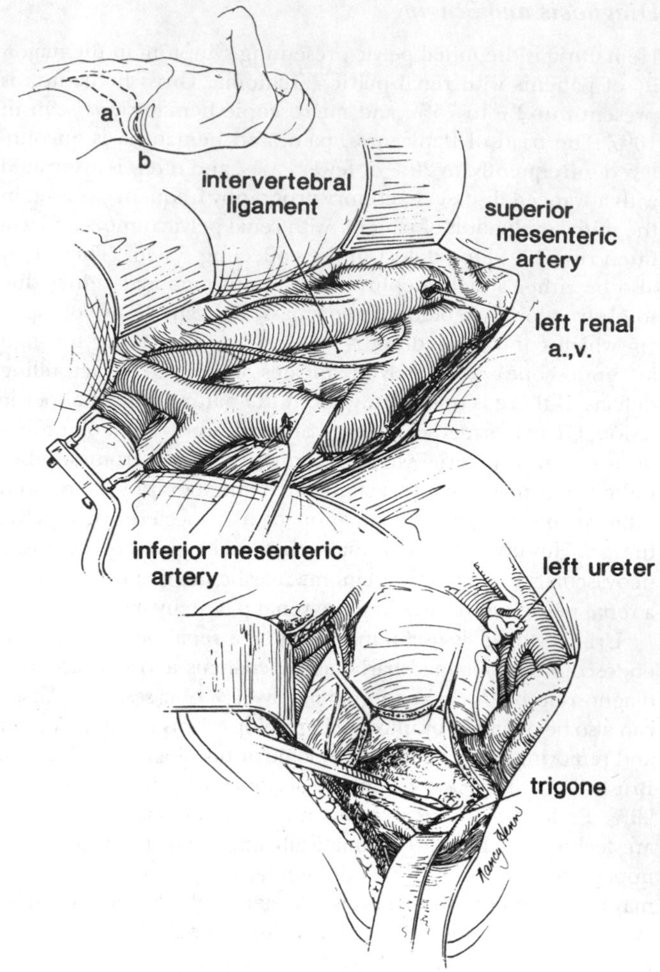

FIGURE 34.2-12. The patient who will undergo a nephroureterectomy with lymph node dissection should be placed in a modified flank position and an incision made through either line a or line b. The area of dissection is as indicated in the middle panel, being divested from the superior mesenteric artery to the bifurcation. The ureter is removed by opening the bladder, circumscribing the orifice, and sharply dissecting the ureter from the surrounding detrusor muscle. The defect in the bladder then is closed appropriately. (From ref. 262, with permission.)

Gerota's fascia, the ureter, and a cuff of bladder including the ureteral orifice and intramural ureter (Fig. 34.2-12). Regional lymph nodes may be removed, particularly if there is indication that they are involved. This surgical procedure may be performed using one or two incisions, depending on the patient's body habitus and the surgeon's preference. When partial ureterectomy is performed, urinary tract continuity is reestablished with either ureteroureterostomy or ureteroneocystostomy.

Results of Therapy

The 5-year survival of patients with ureteral carcinoma is determined primarily by the grade and stage of the disease. Thorough endoscopic follow-up is essential at regular intervals to rule out recurrences.[205] Endourologic techniques combined with conservative treatment of ureteral transitional cell carcinoma can be effectively and safely used as first-line therapy for selected individuals.[212] Patients with Ta or T1 ureteral carci-

TABLE 34.2-16. Correlation of Survival Rate with Stage of Ureteral and Pelvic Tumors

Tumor Stage	*5-Y Survival Rate (%)*
T1 (stage A/II)	92
T2 (stage B/III)	40–70
T3 (stage C/IV)	23–43
T4 (stage D/IV)	0

(From refs. 257 and 258, with permission.)

noma can experience a 90% to 100% 5-year survival rate; those with T2 disease, a 45% to 85% 5-year survival rate; and patients with T3 disease, a 25% to 30% 5-year survival rate. The 5-year survival for patients with metastatic disease is currently 0% to 5% (Table 34.2-16).

ADJUVANT RADIOTHERAPY FOR CARCINOMA OF THE RENAL PELVIS AND URETER

In the absence of randomized prospective data, there is no consensus regarding the need for adjuvant radiotherapy for patients with renal pelvis or ureteral cancers. Brookland and Richter[219] reported on 23 patients with stage III to IV transitional cancers of the upper GU tract. Postoperative radiotherapy (45 to 50 Gy) was given to 11 patients. Among these 11, 5 patients (45%) developed a local recurrence, as compared to 1 of 9 patients (11%) treated with a nephroureterectomy alone ($P = .23$). Cozal et al.[220] reported on 67 patients with stage I through IV upper tract transitional cell tumors. Though the authors demonstrated a reduction in the crude local relapse rate with the administration of 45 to 50 Gy of postoperative radiotherapy as compared to patients who did not receive adjuvant therapy (26% vs. 10%), these differences were not significant ($P = .42$). Other recent retrospective reports could not demonstrate a significant benefit for adjuvant therapy for advanced-stage disease.[221–223] These authors have highlighted the systemic nature of stage III and IV disease—namely, the high risk of distant metastases and the relative infrequent incidence of isolated local recurrences after initial local aggressive surgical therapy, which likely explain the lack of conclusive evidence that adjuvant radiotherapy is of any benefit. Nevertheless, as most patients in these reports were followed without the benefit of routine CT evaluations, the true incidence of a local failure for advanced-stage patients remains unclear. Until more effective systemic regimens are available for patients with locally advanced disease, distant metastasis appears to be the predominant mode of failure, and routine administration of adjuvant local radiotherapy is not recommended.

CHEMOTHERAPY FOR METASTATIC CARCINOMAS OF THE RENAL PELVIS AND URETER

Except for its role in the conservation and preservation of the bladder, considerations for systemic treatment of cancer of the ureter and renal pelvis are identical to those of bladder cancer. It is believed that the biology of transitional cell carcinomas of the renal pelvis, ureter, and bladder is the same, with comparable etiology, pathology, and pattern of spread. This paradigm is supported by the frequent occurrence of multifocal neoplastic sites in the transitional epithelium. Systemic chemotherapy for upper urinary tract cancers mirrors that for bladder cancer and has been administered in the metastatic, adjuvant, and neoadjuvant setting. Indeed, patients with carcinomas of the renal pelvis and ureter usually are included in clinical trials for bladder cancer, because the chemoresponsiveness of both upper and lower urothelial cancers is considered to be comparable. A retrospective review of 203 patients in five trials of methotrexate, vinblastine, doxorubicin (Adriamycin), and cisplatin (M-VAC) from the Memorial Sloan-Kettering Cancer Center could identify no difference in response or survival between patients with bladder and nonbladder primary sites (Table 34.2-17).[326] Because the incidence of cancer of the upper urinary tract is a fraction of that of cancer of the bladder, chemotherapeutic trials do not address the upper urothelium separately. Hence, this section will briefly outline the issues relating to systemic treatment of upper urinary tract cancer, drawing from the bladder cancer literature. For a more extensive discussion, the reader is referred to Chapter 34.3.

TABLE 34.2-17. Effect of Nonbladder Primary Site of Transitional Cell Carcinoma on Response to M-VAC

Primary Site	*No. of Pts.*	*CR (%)*	*CR+PR (%)*	*Median Survival (mo)*	*5-Y Survival*
Renal pelvis	21			19.7	10
Ureter	12			17.7	25
Urethra	10			17.5	20
Nonbladder	43	31	67	17.8[a]	16
Bladder	160	22	66	13.1[a]	13

CR, complete responders; M-VAC, methotrexate, vinblastine, doxorubicin (Adriamycin), and cisplatin; PR, partial responders.
[a] $P = .56$.
Note: Data from 203 patients with unresectable or metastatic transitional cell cancer in five previously reported trials of M-VAC chemotherapy from Memorial Sloan-Kettering Cancer Center, New York, was retrospectively reviewed to determine whether primary site adversely affects response or survival (D. F. Bajorin, personal communication, 2000). There was no significant difference in response to M-VAC, in median survival ($P = .56$) or in 5-year survival when the outcome for patients with bladder or nonbladder primary site were compared.

CHEMOTHERAPY FOR ADVANCED CANCER OF THE RENAL PELVIS AND URETER

Urothelial cancers are highly responsive to chemotherapy. After local recurrence or metastasis has developed, systemic chemotherapy is indicated. While combination chemotherapeutic regimens, including cisplatin, are most widely used, the single-agent activity for a variety of agents is solid. Response rates ranging from 25% to 35% have been reported for cisplatin, methotrexate, cyclophosphamide, and paclitaxel.[327] Most recently, single-agent activity of 28% for gemcitabine has been reported.[328] Table 34.2-18 includes results from both combined and single-agent chemotherapy trials.

As with other cancers that are responsive to chemotherapy, combination regimens elicit a higher response rate than do single-agent regimens. Although others have been described, the most widely accepted regimen for bladder and other urothelial cancers has been M-VAC (methotrexate, 30 mg/m^2 on days 1, 15,

TABLE 34.2-18. M-VAC and New Agents for Urothelial Cancer

Study	*Agent*	*Prior Chemotherapy*	*No. of Pts.*[a]	*No. of Pts. with UTC*	*No. CR*	*No. PR*	*RR (%)*	*Median Survival (mo)*
M-VAC								
Sternberg et al.[383]	M-VAC	Yes (10%)	121	11% RP 6% Ur	44[b] (36%)	43 (36%)	72	13.4 mo
Logothetis et al.[331]	M-VAC (vs. CISCA)	No	54 (37)	14 RP[c] 6 Ur	(35%)	(30%)	65	11.3 mo
Loehrer et al.[332]	M-VAC (vs. cisplatin)	No	126 (112)	10%[d]	17(13%)	32 (25%)	39	12.5 mo
Phase I/II single-agent trials								
Seidman et al.[384]	Gallium nitrate	Yes	22[e]	5 RP	1	3	17.4	—
Moore et al.[385]	Gemcitabine	Adj or Neo[f]	37	—	3	6	24	8 mo
Stadler et al.[328]	Gemcitabine	Adj or Neo[f]	39	—	4	7	28	12.6 mo
Lorusso et al.[386]	Gemcitabine	Yes	31	—	4	3	22.5	5 mo
Roth et al.[387]	Paclitaxel	No	26 (25)	2 RP	7	4	42	8.4 mo
Papamichael et al.[388]	Paclitaxel	Yes	14	—	0	1	7	—
de Wit et al.[389]	Docetaxel	No	29	—	4	5	31	—
McCaffrey et al.[390]	Docetaxel	Yes	30	5 RP	0	4	13.3	9 mo
Witte et al.[391]	Topotecan	Yes	44 (41)	—	0	4	9.1	6.3 mo
Phase II combined trials								
Einhorn et al.[392]	Vinblastine Ifosfamide Gallium	Adj or Neo[f]	27 (19)	4 RP	5	13	67	10 mo
Sengelov et al.[393]	Methotrexate Carboplatin Cisplatin	No	51	9 RP/Ur[g]	8	13	41	8.4 mo
Kosmidis et al.[259]	5-FU Interferon Cisplatin	No	32	4 RP 2 Ur	6	16	65	15.3 mo
McCaffrey et al.[394]	Gallium nitrate 5-FU[h]	No	17	2 RP 1 Ur	0	2	12	19 mo
Oh et al.[337c]	Methotrexate Cisplatin 5-FU/Leuc	No	21 (20)	1 RP	9	6	71	17 mo
Bajorin et al.[395]	Paclitaxel Cisplatin Ifosfamide	No	44	7 RP 1 Ur	10	20	68	20 mo
Bellmunt et al.[396,i]	Paclitaxel Cisplatin Gemcitabine	Adj or Neo[f]	40	—	10	22	80	—
Sengelov et al.[397]	Docetaxel Cisplatin	No	25	3 RP 2 Ur	7	8	60	13.6 mo
Dimopoulos et al.[260]	Docetaxel Cisplatin	Adj or Neo[f]	66 (58)	12 RP/Ur	8	26	52	8 mo
Zielinski et al.[398]	Paclitaxel Carboplatin	No	20	—	8	5	65	82.5% survived 9.1 mo
Otto et al.[261,j]	Paclitaxel Carboplatin	Yes	18[k]	—	2	2	22.2	—
Redman et al.[399]	Paclitaxel Carboplatin	Adj or Neo[f]	35 (32)	2 RP 5 Ur	7	11	51.5	9.5 mo
Vaughn et al.[400]	Paclitaxel Carboplatin	Adj or Neo[f]	33 (32)	6 RP/Ur	4	13	50	8.5 mo
Moore et al.[401]	Gemcitabine Cisplatin	Adj or Neo[f]	28	—	6	10	57	13.2 mo
Kaufman et al.[402]	Gemcitabine Cisplatin	No	46	—	10	9	41	14.3 mo

Adj, adjuvant therapy; CISCA, cisplatin, cyclosphosphamide, and doxorubicin (Adriamycin); CR, complete responders; 5-FU, 5-fluorouracil; Leuc, leucovoran; M-VAC, methotrexate, vinblastine, doxorubicin (Adriamycin), and cisplatin; Neo, neoadjuvant therapy; PR, partial responders; RP, cancer of renal pelvis; RR, response rate; TCC, transitional cell histology; Ur, cancer of ureter; UTC, upper tract cancer.

[a] All patients had TCC histologies unless otherwise noted in parentheses.

[b] 36% CR including patients rendered free of disease by surgery.

[c] Among 102 patients randomized.

[d] 10% of patients treated with M-VAC had extravesical primaries.

[e] 23 of 40 patients in Phase I/II trial received doses above 350 $mg/m^2/d$ continuous intravenous infusion × 5 d.

[f] Adjuvant or Neoadjuvant therapy allowed if >6–12 months have elapsed.

[g] Nine patients with nephroureterectomy; primary site not designated.

[h] Experimental arm of randomized Phase II against M-VAC; 16/17 patients responded on the M-VAC arm.

[i] Preliminary report.

[j] Treatment also included an antimotility factor, acellular pertussis vaccine.

[k] Histology not identified.

Note: No. indicates number of patients assessable for response.

and 22; vinblastine, 3 mg/m^2 on days 2, 15, and 22; Adriamycin, 30 mg/m^2 on day 2; and cisplatin, 70 mg/m^2 on day 2, in a 28-day cycle), originally described in 1985 with a 70% overall response rate.[329,330] A single-institution randomized trial comparing M-VAC with cisplatin, cyclophosphamide, and Adriamycin (CISCA) confirmed a 65% response rate for M-VAC, including 35% of patients with a complete remission.[331] Among 110 patients enrolled in the study, 81 had a primary bladder tumor, 14 had cancer of the renal pelvis, and 6 had cancer of the ureter. The site of origin of the tumor had no influence on response rate. A randomized intergroup study comparing M-VAC with cisplatin monotherapy also demonstrated M-VAC to be significantly superior with regard to both response rate (39% vs. 12%) and survival (median 12.5 vs. 8.2 months).[332] Long-term follow-up of this trial at 6 years confirmed the superiority of M-VAC over cisplatin alone.[333] Escalation of methotrexate to 1000 mg/m^2 failed to improve response rate or median survival.[334] M-VAC is associated with significant hematologic toxicity, and studies aimed at ameliorating the toxicity or supporting dose escalation with GM-CSF or granulocyte colony-stimulating factor have shown little benefit.[335,336]

Patients experiencing a CR survive longer[337] but, despite the regular occurrence of CRs, there is a high relapse rate. In the intergroup study, only 5 of 17 patients with CR remained disease-free from 8.5 to 39.5 months.[332] Similarly, Igawa et al.[337a] reported that among 51 patients who received M-VAC, 10 patients experienced CRs, but 8 relapsed, with a median duration of response of 11.9 months. These considerations have urged the pursuit of treatment that would provide more durable benefit with less toxicity.

For patients whose tumors progress after treatment with M-VAC, several newer agents have shown single-agent activity in urothelial cancer (see Table 34.2-18). Both paclitaxel and gemcitabine have response rates in the 20% to 30% range. Phase II combination studies of paclitaxel with carboplatin or gemcitabine with cisplatin have shown reproducible response rates, generally 50% to 60% in previously untreated (or adjuvant-only treated) patients.[337b] Although the response rates are lower than those seen in the original M-VAC trials,[330,331] the results are comparable to the findings of the large intergroup trial of M-VAC, which demonstrated a 39% response rate and improved survival.[332] A recently reported phase I trial incorporated a sequential approach: doxorubicin plus gemcitabine for six 2-week cycles followed by ifosfamide, paclitaxel, and cisplatin in four 3-week cycles.[223a] A sequential approach such as this may allow the use of multiple known active agents without compromising doses, while minimizing toxicity.

Enrollment has been completed in a large randomized study comparing gemcitabine plus cisplatin with M-VAC in metastatic transitional cell carcinoma.[337c] A second randomized study conducted by the Eastern Cooperative Oncology Group is ongoing, comparing M-VAC with carboplatin and paclitaxel.[337d] Patients must be previously untreated and have advanced or metastatic urothelial cancer (from the renal pelvis, ureter, bladder, or urethra). This study should help to determine whether M-VAC can be challenged as front-line therapy in urothelial cancer.

PROGNOSTIC FACTORS IN UROTHELIAL CANCER

The randomized trial comparing M-VAC with cisplatin alone, encompassing 255 patients, was examined for prognostic factors.[333] Factors that predicted a poor outcome included nontransitional cell histology, poor performance status, and liver or bone metastases. Overall, fewer than 4% of patients treated with M-VAC for advanced urothelial cancer were alive and disease-free at 6 years. Among 99 patients treated with M-VAC or CMV [cisplatin, methotrexate, and vinblastine], good performance status, low metallothionein expression, and high tumor grade were significant predictors of response to chemotherapy.[337e] Molecular factors important in tumor progression—p53, the retinoblastoma gene product (Rb), E-cadherin, and epidermal growth factor receptor—have also been identified in urothelial cancer.[338] It is not known whether, beyond tumor progression, these factors may play a role in determining chemosensitivity.

ADJUVANT AND NEOADJUVANT CHEMOTHERAPY FOR CANCER OF THE RENAL PELVIS AND URETER

The responsiveness of urothelial cancer to chemotherapy offered the possibility that adjuvant or neoadjuvant chemotherapy could improve survival in patients undergoing curative resections. However, evidence for benefit of either strategy is limited, in part because of the large trial size that would be required to prove it. As in advanced disease, it is believed that upper urinary tract cancers have the same responsiveness to chemotherapy as do bladder cancers. A small adjuvant trial supporting this included 18 patients with bladder cancer and 10 patients with upper urinary tract cancer treated postoperatively with a combination of methotrexate, vincristine, cisplatin, cyclophosphamide, Adriamycin, and bleomycin.[339] Disease-free survivals were comparable for both groups of patients.

Randomized adjuvant chemotherapy trials in bladder cancer have not provided clear support for the benefit of adjuvant treatment.[340–343] Several factors can be cited for the failure of some trials to show benefit, including use of weaker chemotherapeutic regimens such as single-agent cisplatin,[340] treatment of node-negative populations,[343] and small trial size. Neoadjuvant chemotherapy before cystectomy has also been studied in bladder cancer. A study from the M. D. Anderson Cancer Center compared neoadjuvant M-VAC (two cycles before cystectomy and three cycles afterward) with adjuvant M-VAC (five cycles after cystectomy).[344] Randomizing 98 patients, no survival difference (60% vs. 63%) between the two strategies could be seen when the study was analyzed at 31.7 months. Neoadjuvant trials in bladder cancer have also failed to provide conclusive evidence for the benefit of chemotherapy,[327,345] including a recently reported study from an international collaboration of trialists in which 976 patients were randomized between no chemotherapy and neoadjuvant chemotherapy consisting of three cycles of cisplatin, methotrexate, and vinblastine prior to curative local therapy.[346] Median survival in the no-chemotherapy group was 37.5 months and, in the chemotherapy group, was 44 months. The absolute difference in 3-year survival was 5.5% (50% vs. 55.5%), an insufficient number to allow a broad recommendation for the inclusion of chemotherapy in the initial treatment of patients with urothelial cancer. One goal of neoadjuvant therapy is the downstaging of tumor size, potentially allowing bladder preservation. In this regard, neoadjuvant therapy seldom is applicable to patients with upper urinary tract cancer, as the only candidates for conservative surgery are patients with low-grade, superficial, noninvasive tumors in whom the prognosis is better (85% at 5 years) and the likelihood of benefit from chemotherapy is difficult to prove.[347–349]

Most authors conclude that further randomized studies are required to prove a survival benefit for adjuvant or neoadjuvant chemotherapy in urothelial cancer. However, some clinicians administer adjuvant chemotherapy in the absence of convincing data because of the responsiveness to chemotherapy that has been observed in advanced disease and the incurability of recurrent or metastatic disease. Indeed, the current Eastern Cooperative Oncology Group trial for adjuvant chemotherapy in bladder cancer is not a randomization with or without chemotherapy but rather an assignment to treatment with M-VAC or carboplatin and paclitaxel.[337d] In the absence of randomized data and specific data from upper urinary tract cancers, a decision in favor of adjuvant chemotherapy seems reasonable, particularly in patients in whom the risk of relapse is high, in whom tumors are invasive, nodal metastases are present, or the tumor grade suggests an aggressive biology.

SUMMARY

Cancer of the renal pelvis and ureter most frequently is a transitional cell carcinoma, as in carcinoma of the bladder. Because the biology of these urothelial cancers is considered to be identical, treatment recommendations have followed those for bladder cancer. At present, M-VAC is the mainstay of systemic chemotherapy for urothelial cancer; however, hematologic toxicity is significant and often results in reduced dosing. Thus, regimens with equal efficacy and less toxicity have been pursued, and several randomized trials are currently being evaluated. Insufficient data are available to define clearly subgroups of patients who will or will not benefit from adjuvant chemotherapy; many physicians opt for adjuvant treatment in the absence of randomized data because of the poor survival that results from tumor recurrence.

REFERENCES

1. Greenlee RT, Murray T, Bolden S, Wingo PA. Cancer statistics 2000. *CA Cancer J Clin* 2000;50:7.
2. Linehan WM, Klausner RD. Renal carcinoma. In: Vogelstein B, Kinzler K, eds. *The genetic basis of human cancer.* New York: McGraw-Hill, 1998:455.
3. Chow W, Devesa S, Warren JL, Fraumeni JF. Rising incidence of renal cell cancer in the United States. *JAMA* 1999;281:1628.
4. Wingo PA, Tong T, Bolden S. Cancer statistics 1995. *CA Cancer J Clin* 1995;45:8.
5. Vogelzang NJ, Scardino PT, Shipley WU, Coffey DS. Epidemiology of renal cell carcinoma In: Vogelzang NJ, ed. *Comprehensive textbook of genitourinary oncology.* Philadelphia: Lippincott Williams & Wilkins, 1998.
6. Grawitz VP. Die sogenannten lipome der niere. *Pathol Anat* 1883;93:39.
7. Doderlein A, Birch-Hirschfeld FV. Embryonale drusengeschwulst der nierengegend im kindesalter. *Sex Organe* 1894;3:88.
8. Linehan WM, Lerman MI, Zbar B. Identification of the VHL gene: its role in renal carcinoma. *JAMA* 1995;273:564.
9. Zbar B, Tory K, Merino M, et al. Hereditary papillary renal cell carcinoma. *J Urol* 1994;151:561.
10. Zbar B, Glenn G, Lubensky IA, et al. Hereditary papillary renal cell carcinoma: clinical studies in 10 families. *J Urol* 1995;153:907.
11. Weirich G, Glenn G, Junker K, et al. Familial renal oncocytoma: clinicopathologic study of 5 families. *J Urol* 1998;160:335.
12. Toro J, Duray PH, Glenn GM, et al. Birt-Hogg-Dube syndrome: a novel marker of kidney neoplasia. *Arch Dermatol* 1999;135:1195.
13. Washecka R, Hanna M. Malignant renal tumors in tuberous sclerosis. *Urology* 1991;37:340.
14. Mellemgaard A, Engholm G, McLaughlin JK, Olsen JH. Risk factors for renal cell carcinoma in Denmark: I. Role of socioeconomic status tobacco use beverages and family history. *Cancer Causes Control* 1994;5:105.
15. Moore MA, Park CB, Tsuda H. European registry comparisons provide evidence of shared risk factors for renal colon and gallbladder cancer development. *Eur J Cancer Prev* 1999;8:137.
16. Tavani A, La Vecchia C. Epidemiology of renal-cell carcinoma. *J Nephrol* 1997;10:93.
17. Maclure M, Willett W. A case-control study of diet and risk of renal adenocarcinoma. *Epidemiology* 1990;1:430.
18. McLaughlin JK, Mandel JS, Blot WJ, et al. A population-based case control study of renal cell carcinoma. *J Natl Cancer Inst* 1984;72:275.
19. Shapiro JA, Williams MA, Weiss NS. Body mass index and risk of renal cell carcinoma. *Epidemiology* 1999;10:188.
20. Gago-Dominguez M, Yuan JM, Castelao JE, Ross RK, Yu MC. Regular use of analgesics is a risk factor for renal cell carcinoma. *Br J Cancer* 1999;81:542.
21. Brauch H, Weirich G, Hornauer MA, et al. Trichloroethylene exposure and specific somatic mutations in patients with renal cell carcinoma. *J Natl Cancer Inst* 1999;91:854.
22. Ross RK, Paganini-Hill A, Landolph J, Gerkins V, Henderson BE. Analgesics cigarette smoking and other risk factors for cancer of the renal pelvis and ureter. *Cancer Res* 1989;49:1045.
23. deKernion JB, Smith RB. The kidney and adrenal glands. In: Paulson DF, ed. *Genitourinary surgery.* New York: Churchill Livingstone, 1984:1.
24. McLaughlin JK, Blot WJ, Mehl ES, et al. Petroleum-related employment and renal cell cancer. *J Occup Med* 1985;27(9):672.
25. Doublet JD, Peraldi MN, Gattegno B, Thibault P, Sraer JD. Renal cell carcinoma of native kidneys: prospective study of 129 renal transplant patients. *J Urol* 1997;158:42.
26. Brennan JF, Stilmant MM, Babayan RK, Siroky MB. Acquired renal cystic disease: implications for the urologist. *Br J Urol* 1991;67:342.
27. MacDougall ML, Welling LW, Wiegmann TB. Renal adenocarcinoma and acquired cystic disease in chronic hemodialysis patients. *Am J Kidney Dis* 1987;9:166.
28. Glenn GM, Linehan WM, Hosoe S, et al. Screening for von Hippel-Lindau disease by DNA-polymorphism analysis. *JAMA* 1992;267:1226.
29. Walther MM, Lubensky IA, Venzon D, Zbar B, Linehan WM. Prevalence of microscopic lesions in grossly normal renal parenchyma from patients with von Hippel-Lindau disease, sporadic renal cell carcinoma and no renal disease: clinical implications. *J Urol* 1995;154:2010.
30. Latif F, Tory K, Gnarra JR, et al. Identification of the von Hippel-Lindau disease tumor suppressor gene. *Science* 1993;260:1317.
31. Chen F, Kishida T, Yao M, et al. Germline mutations in the von Hippel-Lindau disease tumor suppressor gene: correlation with phenotype. *Hum Mutat* 1995;5:66.
32. Stolle CA, Glenn G, Zbar B, et al. Improved detection of germline mutations in the von Hippel-Lindau disease tumor suppressor gene. *Hum Mutat* 1998;12:417.
33. Gnarra JR, Tory K, Weng Y, et al. Mutation of the VHL tumour suppressor gene in renal carcinoma. *Nat Genet* 1994;7:85.
34. Shuin T, Kondo K, Torigoe S, et al. Frequent somatic mutations and loss of heterozygosity of the von Hippel-Lindau tumor suppressor gene in primary human renal cell carcinomas. *Cancer Res* 1994;54:2852.
35. Kovacs G, Wilkens L, Papp T, de Riese W. Differentiation between papillary and nonpapillary renal cell carcinomas by DNA analysis. *J Natl Cancer Inst* 1989;81:527.
36. Zhuang Z, Gnarra JR, Zbar B, Linehan WM, Lubensky IA. Detection of the von Hippel-Lindau disease gene mutation by PCR and SSCP in sporadic renal cell carcinoma in paraffin-embedded tissue. *Mod Pathol* 1994;7:86A.
37. Choyke PL, Walther MM, Glenn GM, et al. Imaging features of hereditary papillary renal cancers. *J Comput Assist Tomogr* 1997;21:737.
38. Schmidt L, Duh F-M, Chen F, et al. Germline and somatic mutations in the tyrosine kinase domain of the MET proto-oncogene in papillary renal carcinomas. *Nat Genet* 1997;16:68.
39. Schmidt L, Junker K, Weirich G, et al. Two North American families with hereditary papillary renal carcinoma and identical novel mutations in the MET proto-oncogene. *Cancer Res* 1998;58:1719.
40. Zambrano NR, Lubensky IA, Merino MJ, Linehan WM, Walther MM. Histopathology and molecular genetics of renal tumors: toward unification of a classification system. *J Urol* 1999;162:1246.
41. Walther MM, Jennings SB, Gnarra JR, Zbar B, Linehan WM. Molecular genetics of renal cell carcinoma. In: Vogelzang NJ, Scardino PT, Shipley WU, Coffey DS, eds. *Comprehensive textbook of genitourinary oncology.* Baltimore: Williams & Wilkins, 1996:160.
42. Delahunt B, Eble JN. Papillary renal cell carcinoma: a clinicopathologic and immunohistochemical study of 105 tumors. *Mod Pathol* 1997;10:537.
43. Kirkali Z, Celebi I, Akan G, Yorukoglu K. Bellini duct (collecting duct) carcinoma of the kidney. *Urology* 1996;47:921.
44. Thoenes W, Storkel S, Rumpelt HJ. Human chromophobe renal cell carcinoma. *Virchows Arch B Cell Pathol* 1985;48:207.
45. Amin M, Crotty TB, Tickoo SK, Farrow GM. Renal oncocytoma: a reappraisal of morphologic features with clinicopathologic findings in 80 cases. *Am J Surg Pathol* 1998;21:1.
46. Noguchi S, Nagashima Y, Shuin T, et al. Renal oncocytoma containing "chromophobe" cells. *Int J Urol* 1995;2:279.
47. Delahunt B. Sarcomatoid renal carcinoma: the final common dedifferentiation pathway of renal epithelial malignancies. *Pathology* 1999;31:185.
48. Cangiano T, Liao J, Naitoh J, et al. Sarcomatoid renal cell carcinoma: biologic behavior, prognosis, and response to combined surgical resection and immunotherapy. *J Clin Oncol* 1999;17:523.
49. Ro JY, Ayala AG, Sella A, Samuels ML, Swanson DA. Sarcomatoid renal cell carcinoma: clinicopathologic. A study of 42 cases. *Cancer* 1987;59:516.
50. Jennings S, Linehan WM. Renal perirenal and ureteral neoplasms. In: Gillenwater JY, Grayhack JT, Howards SS, Duckett JW, eds. *Adult and pediatric urology.* St Louis: Mosby, 1997:643.

51. Maldazys JD, deKernion JB. Prognostic factors in metastatic renal carcinoma. *J Urol* 1986;136:376.
52. Samaan NA. Paraneoplastic syndromes associated with renal carcinoma: a pilot study. *J Clin Oncol* 1987;6:862.
53. Boxer RJ, Waisman J, Lieber MM, Mampaso FM, Skinner DG. Renal carcinoma: computer analysis of 96 patients treated by nephrectomy. *J Urol* 1979;122:598.
54. Da Silva JL, Lacombe C, Bruneval P, et al. Tumor cells are the site of erythropoietin synthesis in human renal cancers associated with polycythemia. *Blood* 1990;75:577.
55. Lindop GBM, Leckie B, Winearls CG. Malignant hypertension due to a renin-secreting renal cell carcinoma: an ultrastructural immunocytochemical study. *Histopathology* 1986;10:1077.
56. Dawson NA, Barr CF, Alving BM. Acquired dysfibrinogenemia. *Am J Med* 1985;78:682.
57. Evans BK, Fagan C, Arnold T, Dropcho EJ, Oh SJ. Paraneoplastic motor neuron disease and renal cell carcinoma: improvement after nephrectomy. *Neurology* 1990;40:960.
58. Thiede MA, Strewler GJ, Nissenson RA, Rosenblatt M, Rodan GA. Human renal carcinoma expresses two messages encoding a parathyroid hormone–like peptide: evidence for the alternative splicing of a single-copy gene. *Proc Natl Acad Sci U S A* 1988;85:4605.
59. Suva LJ, Winslow GA, Wettenhall REH, et al. A parathyroid hormone–related protein implicated in malignant hypercalcemia: cloning and expression. *Science* 1987;237:893.
60. Jamis-Dow CA, Choyke PL, Jennings SB, et al. Small (<3-cm) renal masses: detection with CT versus US and pathologic correlation. *Radiology* 1996;198:785.
61. Choyke P, Walther MM, Wagner JR, et al. Renal cancer: preoperative evaluation with dual-phase three-dimensional MR angiography. *Radiology* 1997;205:767.
62. Bechtold RE, Zagoria RJ. Imaging approach to staging of renal cell carcinoma. *Urol Clin North Am* 1997;24:507.
63. Habboub HK, Abu-Yousef MM, Williams RD, See WA, Schweiger GD. Accuracy of color Doppler sonography in assessing venous thrombus extension in renal cell carcinoma. *AJR Am J Roentgenol* 1997;168:267.
64. Sokoloff MH, deKernion JB, Figlin RA, Belldegrun A. Current management of renal cell carcinoma. *CA Cancer J Clin* 1996;46:284.
65. Karp W, Ekelung L, Olafsson G, Olsson A. Computed tomography angiography and ultrasound in staging of renal carcinoma. *Acta Radiol* 1981;22:625.
66. Mauro MA, Wadsworth DE, Stanley RJ, McClenna BL. Renal cell carcinoma: angiography in the CT era. *AJR Am J Roentgenol* 1982;139:1135.
67. deKernion JB. Renal tumors. In: Walsh PC, Gittes RF, Perlmutter AD, eds. *Campbell's urology*. Philadelphia: WB Saunders, 1986:1291.
68. Narumi Y, Hricak H, Presti JCJ, et al. MR imaging evaluation of renal cell carcinoma. *Abdom Imaging* 1997;22:216.
69. Lang EK. Comparison of dynamic and conventional computed tomography angiography and ultrasonography in the staging of renal cell carcinoma. *Cancer* 1984;54:2205.
70. Choyke PL. Detection and staging of renal cancer. *Magn Reson Imaging Clin N Am* 1997;5:29.
71. Gilfeather M, Woodward PJ. MR imaging of the adrenal glands and kidneys. *Semin Ultrasound CT MR* 1998;19:53.
72. Robson CJ, Churchill BM, Anderson W. The results of radical nephrectomy for renal cell carcinoma. *J Urol* 1969;101:297.
73. Peters PC, Brown GL. The role of lymphadenectomy in the management of renal cell carcinoma. *Urol Clin North Am* 1991;10:705.
74. Siminovitch JMP, Montie JE, Straffon RA. Prognostic indicators in renal adenocarcinoma. *J Urol* 1983;130:20.
75. Guinan P, Sobin LH, Algaba F, et al. TNM staging of renal cell carcinoma: Workgroup No. 3, Union International Contre le Cancer (UICC) and the American Joint Committee on Cancer (AJCC). *Cancer* 1997;80:992.
76. Javidan J, Stricker HJ, Tamboli P, et al. Prognostic significance of the 1997 TNM classification of renal cell carcinoma. *J Urol* 1999;162:1277.
77. Giuliani L, Giberti C, Martorana G, Rovida S. Radical extensive surgery for renal cell carcinoma: long-term results and prognostic factors. *J Urol* 1990;143:468.
78. Tsukamoto T, Kumamoto Y, Yamazaki K, et al. Clinical analysis of incidentally found renal cell carcinomas. *Eur Urol* 1991;19:109.
79. Fahn HJ, Lee YH, Chen MT, et al. The incidence and prognostic significance of humoral hypercalcemia in renal cell carcinoma. *J Urol* 1991;145:248.
80. Gilbert JB. Diagnosis and treatment of malignant renal tumors. *J Urol* 1937;39:223.
81. von Knobloch R, Seseke F, Riedmiller H, et al. Radical nephrectomy for renal cell carcinoma: is adrenalectomy necessary? *Eur Urol* 1999;36:303.
82. Wunderlich H, Schlichter A, Reichelt O, et al. Real indications for adrenalectomy in renal cell carcinoma. *Eur Urol* 1999;35:272.
83. Kardar AH, Arafa M, Al Suhaibani H, et al. Feasibility of adrenalectomy with radical nephrectomy. *Urology* 1998;52:35.
84. Ono Y, Katoh N, Kinukawa T, Matsuura O, Ohshima S. Laparoscopic radical nephrectomy: the Nagoya experience. *J Urol* 1997;158(3):719.
85. Higashihara E, Baba S, Murai M, et al. Learning curve and conversion to open surgery in cases of laparoscopic adrenalectomy and nephrectomy. *J Urol* 1998;159:650.
86. Walther MM, Lyne JC, Libutti SK, Linehan WM. Laparoscopic cytoreductive nephrectomy as preparation for administration of systemic interleukin-2 in the treatment of metastatic renal cell carcinoma: a pilot study. *Urology* 1999;53:496.
87. Schafhauser W, Ebert A, Brod J, Petsch S, Schrott KM. Lymph node involvement in renal cell carcinoma and survival chance by systematic lymphadenectomy. *Anticancer Res* 1999;19:1573.
88. Hafez KS, Novick AC, Campbell SC. Patterns of tumor recurrence and guidelines for followup after nephron sparing surgery for sporadic renal cell carcinoma. *J Urol* 1997;157:2067.
89. Wunderlich H, Reichelt O, Schumann S, et al. Nephron sparing surgery for renal cell carcinoma 4 cm or less in diameter: indicated or undertreated? *J Urol* 1998;159:465.
90. Choyke PL, Glenn G, Walther MM, et al. The natural history of renal lesions in von Hippel-Lindau disease: a serial CT study in 28 patients. *AJR Am J Roentgenol* 1992;159:1229.
91. Ornstein DK, Lubensky IA, Venzon D, et al. Prevalence of microscopic tumors in normal appearing renal parenchyma from patients with hereditary papillary renal cancer. *J Urol* 2000;163:431.
92. Walther MM, Choyke PL, Weiss G, et al. Parenchymal sparing surgery in patients with hereditary renal cell carcinoma. *J Urol* 1995;153:913.
93. Finney R. Radiotherapy in the treatment of hypernephroma: a clinical trial. *Br J Urol* 1973;45:26.
94. Kjaer M, Frederiksen PL, Engelholm SA. Postoperative radiotherapy in stage II and III renal adenocarcinoma. A randomized trial by the Copenhagen renal cancer study group. *Int J Radiat Oncol Biol Phys* 1987;13:665.
95. Rafla S. Renal cell carcinoma: natural history and results of treatment. *Cancer* 1970;25:26.
96. Stein M, Kuten A, Halpern J, et al. The value of postoperative irradiation in renal cell cancer. *Radiother Oncol* 1992;24:41.
97. van der Werf-Messing B, van der Heul RO, Ledeboer RCH. Renal cell carcinoma trial. *Cancer Clin Trials* 1978;1:13.
98. Juusela H, Malmio K, Alfthan D. Preoperative irradiation in the treatment of renal adenocarcinoma. *Scand J Urol Nephrol* 1977;11:277.
99. Kao GD, Malkowicz SB, Whittington R, D'Amico AV, Wein AJ. Locally advanced renal cell carcinoma: low complication rate and efficacy of postnephrectomy radiation therapy planned with CT. *Radiology* 1994;193:725.
100. Kortmann RD, Becker G, Classen J, Bamberg M. Future strategies in external radiation therapy of renal cell carcinoma. *Anticancer Res* 1999;19:1601.
101. Bloom HJ. Adjuvant therapy for adenocarcinoma of the kidney: present position and prospects. *Br J Urol* 1973;45:237.
102. Riches EW, Griffiths IH, Thackray AC. New growths of the kidney and ureter. *Urology* 1951;12:297.
103. Rabinovitch RA, Zelefsky MJ, Gaynor JJ, Fuks Z. Patterns of failure following surgical resection of renal cell carcinoma: implications for adjuvant local and systemic therapy. *J Clin Oncol* 1994;12:206.
104. Schmieder RE, Delles C. Renal cell carcinoma and diuretics—should one restrict the use of diuretics? [Editorial]. *Nephrol Dial Transplant* 1999;14:1621.
105. Onufrey V, Mohiuddin M. Radiation therapy in the treatment of metastatic renal cell carcinoma. *Int J Radiat Oncol Biol Phys* 1985;11:2007.
106. DiBiase SJ, Valicenti RK, Schultz D, et al. Palliative irradiation for focally symptomatic metastatic renal cell carcinoma: support for dose escalation based on a biological model. *J Urol* 1997;158:746.
107. Eble MJ, Staehler G, Wannenmacher M. [The intraoperative radiotherapy (IORT) of locally spread and recurrent renal-cell carcinomas.] *Strahlenther Onkol* 1998;174:30.
108. Frydenberg M, Gunderson L, Hahn G, Fieck J, Zincke H. Preoperative external beam radiotherapy followed by cytoreductive surgery and intraoperative radiotherapy for locally advanced primary or recurrent renal malignancies. *J Urol* 1994;152:15.
109. Kwiatkowski J, Schmidt B, Merkle P, Keller K. Perioperative brachytherapy as an additional therapeutic option in patients with renal cell carcinoma (RCC), either inoperable or after completed percutaneous radiotherapy. *Anticancer Res* 1999;19:1597.
110. Walther MM, Patel B, Choyke PL, et al. Hypercalcemia in patients with metastatic renal cell carcinoma: effect of nephrectomy and metabolic evaluation. *J Urol* 1997;158:733.
111. Montie JE, Stewart BH, Straffon RA, et al. The role of adjunctive nephrectomy in patients with metastatic renal cell carcinoma. *J Urol* 1977;117:272.
112. deKernion JB, Ramming KP, Smith RB. The natural history of metastatic renal cell carcinoma: a computer analysis. *J Urol* 1978;120:148.
113. Walther MM, Yang JC, Pass HI, Linehan WM, Rosenberg SA. Cytoreductive surgery before high dose interleukin-2 based therapy in patients with metastatic renal cell carcinoma. *J Urol* 1997;158:1675.
114. Middleton RG. Surgery for metastatic renal cell carcinoma. *J Urol* 1967;97:973.
115. O'Dea MJ, Zincke H, Utz DC. The treatment of renal cell carcinoma with solitary metastasis. *J Urol* 1978;120:540.
116. Halperin EC, Harisiadis L. The role of radiation therapy in the management of metastatic renal cell carcinoma. *Cancer* 1983;51:614.
117. Tong D, Gillick L, Hendrickson FR. The palliation of symptomatic osseous metastases: final results of the study by the Radiation Therapy Oncology Group. *Cancer* 1982;50:893.
118. Maor MH, Frias AE, Oswald MJ. Palliative radiotherapy for brain metastases in renal carcinoma. *Cancer* 1988;62:1912.
119. Wronski M, Maor MH, Davis BJ, Sawaya R, Levin VA. External radiation of brain metastases from renal carcinoma: a retrospective study of 119 patients from the M D Anderson Cancer Center. *Int J Radiat Oncol Biol Phys* 1997;37:753.
120. Pomer S, Klopp M, Steiner HH, et al. [Brain metastases in renal cell carcinoma. Results of treatment and prognosis.] *Urologe A* 1997;36:117.
121. Becker G, Duffner F, Kortmann R, et al. Radiosurgery for the treatment of brain metastases in renal cell carcinoma. *Anticancer Res* 1999;19:1611.
121a. Rini BL, Vogelzang NJ, Dumas MC, et al. Phase II trial of weekly intravenous gemcitabine with continuous infusion fluorouracil in patients with metastatic renal cell cancer. *J Clin Oncol* 2000;18(12):2419.
122. Motzer RJ, Russo P. Systemic therapy for renal cell carcinoma. *J Urol* 2000;163(2):408.
122a. [No authors listed]. Interferon-alpha and survival in metastatic renal carcinoma: early results of a randomised controlled trial. Medical Research Council Renal Cancer Collaborators. *Lancet* 1999;353(9146):14.
123. Motzer RJ, Mazumdar M, Bacik J, et al. Effect of cytokine therapy on survival for patients with advanced renal cell carcinoma. *J Clin Oncol* 2000;18(9):1928.
124. Sejima T, Miyagawa I. Expression of bcl-2, p53 oncoprotein, and proliferating cell nuclear antigen in renal cell carcinoma. *Eur Urol* 1999;35:242.

125. Di Silverio F, Casale P, Colella D, et al. Independent value of tumor size and DNA ploidy for the prediction of disease progression in patients with organ-confined renal cell carcinoma. *Cancer* 2000;88(4):835.
126. Middleton AWJ. Indications for and results of nephrectomy for metastatic renal cell carcinoma. *Urol Clin North Am* 1980;7:711.
127. Gleave ME, Elhilali M, Fradet Y, et al. Interferon gamma-1b compared with placebo in metastatic renal-cell carcinoma. Canadian Urology and Oncology Group [see comments]. *N Engl J Med* 1998;338:1265.
128. Bloom HJG. Hormone-induced and spontaneous regression of metastatic renal cancer. *Cancer* 1973;32:1066.
129. Snow RM, Schellhammer PF. Spontaneous regression of metastatic renal cell carcinoma. *Urology* 1982;20:177.
130. Marcus SG, Choyke PL, Reiter R, et al. Regression of metastatic renal cell carcinoma after cytoreductive nephrectomy. *J Urol* 1993;150:463.
131. Quesada JR, Swanson DA, Trindade A, Gutterman JU. Renal cell carcinoma: antitumor effects of leukocyte interferon. *Cancer Res* 1983;43:940.
132. Quesada JR, Rios A, Swanson D, et al. Antitumor activity of recombinant-derived interferon alpha in metastatic renal cell carcinoma. *J Clin Oncol* 1985;3:1522.
133. Moss HB. Interferon therapy for renal cell carcinoma. *Semin Oncol* 1987;14:36.
134. Quesada JR. Role of interferons in the therapy of metastatic renal cell carcinoma. *Urology* 1989;34:80.
135. Medical Research Council Renal Cancer Collaborators. Interferon-α and survival in metastatic renal carcinoma: early results of a randomized controlled trial. *Lancet* 1999;353:14.
136. Small EJ, Weiss GR, Malik UK, et al. The treatment of metastatic renal cell carcinoma patients with recombinant human gamma interferon. *Cancer J Sci Am* 1998;4:162.
137. Trump DL, Elson P, Propert K, et al. Randomized controlled trial of adjuvant therapy with lymphoblastoid interferon (L-IFN) in resected high-risk renal cell carcinoma (HR-RCC). *Proc Am Soc Clin Oncol* 1996;15:253(abst).
138. Rosenberg SA, Lotze MT, Muul LM, et al. A progress report on the treatment of 157 patients with advanced cancer using lymphokine-activated killer cells and interleukin-2 or high-dose interleukin-2 alone. *N Engl J Med* 1987;316:889.
139. Lotze MT, Chang AE, Seipp CA, et al. High-dose recombinant interleukin 2 in the treatment of patients with disseminated cancer: responses, treatment-related morbidity, and histologic findings. *JAMA* 1986;256:3117.
140. Fisher RI, Coltman CA, Doroshow JH, et al. Metastatic renal cancer treated with interleukin-2 and lymphokine-activated killer cells. *Ann Intern Med* 1988;108:518.
141. Fisher RI, Rosenberg SA, Sznol M, Parkinson DR, Fyfe G. High-dose aldesleukin in renal cell carcinoma: long-term survival update. *Cancer J Sci Am* 1997;3:S70.
142. Rosenberg SA, Yang JC, Topalian SL, et al. Treatment of 283 consecutive patients with metastatic melanoma or renal cell cancer using high-dose bolus interleukin-2. *JAMA* 1994;271:907.
143. Rosenberg SA, Yang JC, White DE, Steinberg SM. Durability of complete responses in patients with metastatic cancer treated with high-dose interleukin-2. *Ann Surg* 1998;228:319.
144. Rosenberg SA, Lotze MT, Yang JC, et al. Prospective randomized trial of high-dose interleukin-2 alone or with lymphokine activated killer cells for the treatment of patients with advanced cancer. *J Natl Cancer Inst* 1993;85:622.
145. Law TM, Motzer R, Mazumdar M, et al. Phase III randomized trial of interleukin-2 with or without lymphokine activated killer cells in the treatment of patients with advanced renal cell carcinoma. *Cancer* 1995;76:824.
146. Margolin KA, Raynor MJ, Hawkins MB, et al. Interleukin-2 and lymphokine-activated killer cell therapy of solid tumors: analysis of toxicity and management guidelines. *J Clin Oncol* 1989;7:486.
147. Kammula US, White DE, Rosenberg SA. Trends in the safety of high dose bolus interleukin-2 administration in patients with metastatic cancer. *Cancer* 1998;83:797.
148. Sleijfer DT, Janssen RA, Buter J, et al. Phase II study of subcutaneous interleukin-2 in unselected patients with advanced renal cell cancer on an outpatient basis. *J Clin Oncol* 1992;10:1119.
149. Buter J, Sleijfer DT, Winette TA, et al. A progress report on the outpatient treatment of patients with advanced renal cell carcinoma using subcutaneous recombinant interleukin-2. *Semin Oncol* 1993;20:16.
150. Tourani JM, Lucas V, Mayeur D, et al. Subcutaneous recombinant interleukin-2 (rIL-2) in outpatients with metastatic renal cell carcinoma. Results of a multicenter SCAPP1 trial. *Ann Oncol* 1996;7:525.
151. West WH, Tayer KW, Yannelli JR, et al. Constant-infusion recombinant interleukin-2 plus lymphokine-activated killer cells in metastatic renal cancer. *N Engl J Med* 1987;316:898.
152. Yang JC, Rosenberg SA. An ongoing prospective randomized comparison of interleukin-2 regimens for the treatment of metastatic renal cell cancer. *Cancer J Sci Am* 1997;3:S79.
153. Weiss GR, Margolin KA, Aronson FR, et al. A randomized phase II trial of continuous infusion interleukin-2 or bolus injection interleukin 2 plus lymphokine activated killer cells for advanced renal cell carcinoma. *J Clin Oncol* 1992;10:275.
154. Gold PJ, Thompson JA, Markowitz DR, Neumann S, Fefer A. Metastatic renal cell carcinoma: long-term survival after therapy with high-dose continuous-infusion interleukin-2 [see comments]. *Cancer J Sci Am* 1997;3[Suppl 1]:S85.
155. Rosenberg SA, Lotze MT, Yang JC, et al. Combination therapy with interleukin-2 and alpha-interferon for the treatment of patients with advanced cancer. *J Clin Oncol* 1989;7:1863.
156. Marincola FM, White DE, Wise AP, Rosenberg SA. Combination therapy with interferon alfa-2a and interleukin-2 for the treatment of metastatic cancer. *J Clin Oncol* 1995;13:1110.
157. Atzpodien J, Hanninen EL, Kirchner H, et al. Multiinstitutional home-therapy trial of recombinant human interleukin-2 and interferon alfa-2 in progressive metastatic renal cell carcinoma. *J Clin Oncol* 1995;13:497.
158. Negrier S, Escudier B, Lasset C, et al. Recombinant human interleukin-2, recombinant human interferon alfa-2a, or both in metastatic renal-cell carcinoma. Groupe Francais d'Immunotherapie [see comments]. *N Engl J Med* 1998;338:1272.
159. Atkins MB, Sparano J, Fisher RI. Randomized phase II trial of high-dose interleukin-2 either alone or in combination with interferon alfa-2b in advanced renal cell carcinoma. *J Clin Oncol* 1993;11:661.
160. Jayson GC, Middleton M, Lee SM, et al. A randomized phase II trial of interleukin 2 and interleukin 2–interferon alpha in advanced renal cancer. *Br J Cancer* 1998;78:366.
161. Atzpodien J, Kirchner H, Hanninen EL, et al. Interleukin-2 in combination with interferon-alpha and 5-fluorouracil for metastatic renal cell cancer. *Eur J Cancer* 1993;29A[Suppl 5]:S6.
162. Ravaud A, Audhuy B, Gomez F, et al. Subcutaneous interleukin-2, interferon alfa-2a, and continuous infusion of fluorouracil in metastatic renal cell carcinoma: a multicenter phase II trial. Groupe Francais d'Immunotherapie. *J Clin Oncol* 1998;16:2728.
163. Dutcher JP, Atkins M, Fisher R, et al. Interleukin-2-based therapy for metastatic renal cell cancer: the Cytokine Working Group experience 1989–1997. *Cancer J Sci Am* 1997;3[Suppl 1]:S73.
164. Brandle D, Brasseur F, Weynants P, Boon T, Van den Eynde B. A mutated HLA-A2 molecule recognized by autologous cytotoxic T lymphocytes on a human renal cell carcinoma. *J Exp Med* 1996;183:2501.
165. Gaudin C, Kremer F, Angevin E, Scott V, Triebel F. A hsp70-2 mutation recognized by CTL on a human renal cell carcinoma. *J Immunol* 1999;162:1730.
166. Gaugler B, Brouwenstijn N, Vantomme V, et al. A new gene coding for an antigen recognized by autologous cytolytic T lymphocytes on a human renal carcinoma. *Immunogenetics* 1996;44:323.
167. Ronsin C, Chung-Scott V, Poullion I, et al. F A non-AUG-defined alternative open reading frame of the intestinal carboxyl esterase mRNA generates an epitope recognized by renal cell carcinoma–reactive tumor-infiltrating lymphocytes in situ. *J Immunol* 1999;163:483.
168. Belldegrun A, Muul LM, Rosenberg SA. Interleukin 2 expanded tumor-infiltrating lymphocytes in human renal cell cancer: isolation, characterization, and antitumor activity. *Cancer Res* 1988;48:206.
169. Figlin RA, Pierce WC, Kaboo R, et al. Treatment of metastatic renal cell carcinoma with nephrectomy, interleukin-2, and cytokine-primed or CD8(+) selected tumor infiltrating lymphocytes from primary tumor. *J Urol* 1997;158:740.
170. Figlin RA, Thompson JA, Bukowski RM, et al. Multicenter randomized phase III trial of CD8(+) tumor-infiltrating lymphocytes in combination with recombinant interleukin-2 in metastatic renal cell carcinoma. *J Clin Oncol* 1999;17:2521.
171. Osband ME, Lavin PT, Babayan RK, et al. Effect of autolymphocyte therapy on survival and quality of life in patients with metastatic renal-cell carcinoma. *Lancet* 1990;335:994.
172. Simons JW, Jaffee EM, Weber CE, et al. Bioactivity of autologous irradiated renal cell carcinoma vaccines generated by ex vivo granulocyte-macrophage colony-stimulating factor gene transfer. *Cancer Res* 1997;57:1537.
173. Childs RW, Clave E, Tisdale J, et al. Successful treatment of metastatic renal cell carcinoma with a nonmyeloablative allogeneic peripheral-blood progenitor-cell transplant: evidence for a graft-versus-tumor effect. *J Clin Oncol* 1999;17:2044.
174. O'Reilly MS, Boehm T, Shing Y, et al. Endostatin: an endogenous inhibitor of angiogenesis and tumor growth. *Cell* 1997;88:277.
175. Kim KJ, Li B, Winer J, et al. Inhibition of vascular endothelial growth factor–induced angiogenesis suppresses tumour growth in vivo. *Nature* 1993;362:841.
176. Huben RP, Mounzer AM, Murphy GP. Tumor grade and stage as prognostic variables in upper tract urothelial tumors. *Cancer* 1988;62:2016.
177. McLaughlin JK, Silverman DT, Hsing AW, et al. Cigarette smoking and cancers of the renal pelvis and ureter. *Cancer Res* 1992;52:254.
178. Hultengren N, Lagergren C, Ljungqvist A. Carcinoma of the renal pelvis in renal papillary necrosis. *Acta Chir Scand* 1985;130:314.
179. Gago-Dominguez M, Yuan JM, Castelao JE, Ross RK, Yu MC. Regular use of analgesics is a risk factor for renal cell carcinoma. *Br J Cancer* 1999;81:542.
180. Stewart JH, Hobbs JB, McCredie MR. Morphologic evidence that analgesic-induced kidney pathology contributes to the progression of tumors of the renal pelvis. *Cancer* 1999;86:1576.
181. McCredie M, Stewart J, Smith D, Supramaniam R, Williams S. Observations on the effect of abolishing analgesic abuse and reducing smoking on cancers of the kidney and bladder in New South Wales, Australia, 1972–1995. *Cancer Causes Control* 1999;10:303.
182. Bengtsson U, Johansson S, Angervall L. Malignancies of the urinary tract and their relation to analgesic abuse. *Kidney Int* 1978;13:107.
183. McCredie M, Stewart JH, Carter JJ, Turner J, Mahony JF. Phenacetin and papillary necrosis: independent risk factors for renal pelvic cancer. *Kidney Int* 1986;30:81.
184. Gaakeer HA, Ruiter HJ. Carcinoma of the renal pelvis following the abuse of phenacetin-containing analgesic drugs. *Br J Urol* 1979;51:188.
185. Jensen OM, Knudsen JB, Tomasson H, Sorensen BL. The Copenhagen case-control study of renal pelvis and ureter cancer: role of analgesics. *Int J Cancer* 1989;44:965.
186. Campo B, Zanitzer L, Torelli T, et al. Renal cell carcinoma and transitional cell carcinomas of the pelvis and bladder in a patient affected by chronic renal failure due to abuse of phenacetin. *Tumori* 1986;72:215.
187. Rathert P, Melchior H, Lutzeyer W. Phenacetin: a carcinogen for the urinary tract? *J Urol* 1975;113:653.
188. Palvio DHB, Andersen JC, Falk E. Transitional cell tumors of the renal pelvis and ureter associated with capillary sclerosis indicating analgesic abuse. *Cancer* 1987;59:972.
189. Droller MJ. Transitional cell cancer: upper tracts and bladder. In: Walsh PC, Gittes RF, Perlmutter AD, Stamey TA, eds. *Urology*. Philadelphia: WB Saunders, 1986:1343.
190. Mahony JF, Storey BG, Ibanez RC, Stewart JH. Analgesic abuse, renal parenchymal disease, and carcinoma of the kidney or ureter. *Aust NZ J Med* 1977;7:463.
191. Stefanovic V. Balkan endemic nephropathy: a need for novel aetiological approaches. *Q J Med* 1998;91:457.
192. Clayman RV, Lange PH, Fraley EE. Cancer of the upper urinary tract. In: Javadpour N, ed. In *Principles and management of urologic cancer.* Baltimore: Williams & Wilkins, 1983: 544.

193. Orphali SLJ, Shols GW, Hagewood J, Tesluk H, Palmer JM. Familial transitional cell carcinoma of renal pelvis and upper ureter. *Urology* 1986;27:394.
194. Frischer Z, Waltzer WC, Gonder MJ. Bilateral transitional cell carcinoma of the renal pelvis in the cancer family syndrome. *J Urol* 1985;134:1197.
195. Lynch HT, Smyrk T. Hereditary nonpolyposis colorectal cancer (Lynch syndrome). An updated review. *Cancer* 1996;78:1149.
196. Oh SJ, Lim DJ, Cho JY, Kim SH, Lee SE. Squamous cell carcinoma of the renal pelvis with invasion of the infradiaphragmatic inferior vena cava. *Br J Urol* 1998;82:918.
197. Blacher EJ, Johnson DE, Abdul-Karim FW, Ayala AG. Squamous cell carcinoma of renal pelvis. *Urology* 1985;25:124.
198. Takebayashi S, Hosaka M, Takase K, et al. Computerized tomography nephroscopic images of renal pelvic carcinoma. *J Urol* 1999;162:315.
199. Urban BA, Buckley J, Soyer P, Scherrer A, Fishman EK. CT appearance of transitional cell carcinoma of the renal pelvis: 2. Advanced-stage disease. *AJR Am J Roentgenol* 1997;169:163.
200. Urban BA, Buckley J, Soyer P, Scherrer A, Fishman EK. CT appearance of transitional cell carcinoma of the renal pelvis: 1. Early-stage disease. *AJR Am J Roentgenol* 1997;169:157.
201. Aslan P, Fitzgerald KB, Preminger GM. Muscle-invasive transitional cell carcinoma of the renal pelvis visualized and biopsied via semirigid ureteroscopy. *Urology* 1998;52:888.
202. Sadek S, Soloway MS, Hook S, Civantos F. The value of upper tract cytology after transurethral resection of bladder tumor in patients with bladder transitional cell cancer. *J Urol* 1999;161:77.
203. Grasso M, Fraiman M, Levine M. Ureteropyeloscopic diagnosis and treatment of upper urinary tract urothelial malignancies. *Urology* 1999;54:240.
204. Wong YCJ, Wagner BJ, Davis CJJ. Transitional cell carcinoma of the urinary tract: radiologic-pathologic correlation. *Radiographics* 1998;18:123.
205. Keeley FXJ, Bibbo M, Bagley DH. Ureteroscopic treatment and surveillance of upper urinary tract transitional cell carcinoma. *J Urol* 1997;157:1560.
206. Goldman SM. Endoluminal sonographic evaluation of ureteral and renal pelvic neoplasms. *J Urol* 1998;159:318.
207. Liu JB, Bagley DH, Conlin MJ, et al. Endoluminal sonographic evaluation of ureteral and renal pelvic neoplasms. *J Ultrasound Med* 1997;16:515.
208. Ozsahin M, Zouhair A, Villa S, et al. Prognostic factors in urothelial renal pelvis and ureter tumours: a multicentre Rare Cancer Network study. *Eur J Cancer* 1999;35:738.
209. Salomon L, Hoznek A, Cicco A, et al. Retroperitoneoscopic nephroureterectomy for renal pelvic tumors with a single iliac incision. *J Urol* 1999;161:541.
210. Zubac DP, Kihl B. One or two incisions for nephroureterectomy in transitional cell renal pelvis tumours. *Scand J Urol Nephrol* 1997;31:431.
211. Oba K, Suga A, Shimizu Y, et al. Transitional cell carcinoma of the renal pelvis with vena caval tumor thrombus. *Int J Urol* 1997;4:307.
212. Elliott DS, Blute ML, Patterson DE, Bergstralh EJ, Segura JW. Long-term follow-up of endoscopically treated upper urinary tract transitional cell carcinoma. *Urology* 1996;47:819.
213. Wong AK, Lupu AN, Shanberg AM. Laser ablation of renal pelvic transitional cell carcinoma in a solitary kidney: a 9-year follow-up. *Urology* 1996;48:298.
214. Patel A, Fuchs GJ. New techniques for the administration of topical adjuvant therapy after endoscopic ablation of upper urinary tract transitional cell carcinoma. *J Urol* 1998;159:71.
215. Okada H, Eto H, Hara I, et al. Percutaneous treatment of transitional cell carcinoma of the upper urinary tract. *Int J Urol* 1997;4:130.
216. Richie JP. Management of ureteral tumors. In: Skinner DG, deKernion JB, eds. *Genitourinary cancer.* Philadelphia: WB Saunders, 1978:150.
217. Tawfiek ER, Bagley DH. Upper-tract transitional cell carcinoma. *Urology* 1997;50:321.
218. Keeley FX, Kulp DA, Bibbo M, McCue PA, Bagley DH. Diagnostic accuracy of ureteroscopic biopsy in upper tract transitional cell carcinoma [see comments]. *J Urol* 1997;157:33.
219. Brookland RK, Richter MP. Postoperative irradiation of transitional cell carcinoma of the renal pelvis and ureter. *J Urol* 1985;133:952.
220. Cozal SC, Smalley SR, Austenfeld M, et al. Transitional cell carcinoma of the renal pelvis or ureter: patterns of failure. *Urology* 1995;46:796(abst).
221. Maulard-Durdux C, Dufour B, Hennequin C, et al. Postoperative radiation therapy in 26 patients with invasive transitional cell carcinoma of the upper urinary tract: no impact on survival? [see comments]. *J Urol* 1996;155:115.
222. Hall MC, Womack JS, Roehrborn CG, Carmody T, Sagalowsky AI. Advanced transitional cell carcinoma of the upper urinary tract: patterns of failure survival and impact of postoperative adjuvant radiotherapy. *J Urol* 1998;160:703.
223. Catton CN, Warde P, Gospodarowicz MK, et al. Transitional cell carcinoma of the renal pelvis and ureter: outcome and patterns in patients treated with postoperative radiation. *Urol Oncol* 1996;2:171.
223a. Dodd PM, McCaffrey JA, Hilton S, et al. Phase I evaluation of sequential doxorubicin gemcitabine then ifosfamide paclitaxel cisplatin for patients with unresectable or metastatic transitional-cell carcinoma of the urothelial tract. *J Clin Oncol* 2000;18(4):840.
224. Glenn GM, Choyke PL, Zbar B, Linehan WM. Von Hippel-Lindau disease: clinical review and molecular genetics. In: Anderson EE, ed. *Problems in urologic surgery: benign and malignant tumors of the kidney.* Philadelphia: JB Lippincott Co, 1990:312.
225. Melmon KL, Rosen SW. Lindau's disease: review of the literature and study of a large kindred. *Am J Med* 1964;36:595.
226. Cohen AJ, Li FP, Berg S, et al. Hereditary renal-cell carcinoma associated with a chromosomal translocation. *N Engl J Med* 1979;301:592.
227. Kovacs G, Brusa P, de Riese W. Tissue-specific expression of a constitutional 3;6 translocation: development of multiple bilateral renal-cell carcinomas. *Int J Cancer* 1989;43:422.
228. Skinner DG, Calvin RB, Vermillion CD, Pfister RC, Leadbetter WF. Diagnosis and management of renal cell carcinoma. *Cancer* 1971;28:1165.
229. McNichols DW, Segura JW, Deweerd JH. Renal cell carcinoma: long-term survival and late recurrence. *J Urol* 1981;126:17.
230. Cherrie RJ, Goldman DG, Lindner A, deKernion JB. Prognostic implications of vena caval extension of renal cell carcinoma. *J Urol* 1982;128:910.
231. Selli C, Hinshaw WM, Woodard BH, Paulson DF. Stratification of risk factors in renal cell carcinoma. *Cancer* 1983;52:899.
232. Bassil B, Dosoretz DE, Prout GR. Validation of the tumor nodes and metastasis classification of renal cell carcinoma. *J Urol* 1985;134:450.
233. Golimbu M, Joshi P, Sperber A, et al. Renal cell carcinoma: survival and prognostic factors. *Urology* 1986;27:291.
234. Chang AY, Tu ZN, Bryan GT, et al. Phase II study of echinomycin in the treatment of renal cell carcinoma. ECOG study E2885. *Invest New Drugs* 1994;12:151.
235. Kish JA, Wolf M, Crawford ED, et al. Evaluation of low dose continuous infusion 5-fluorouracil in patients with advanced and recurrent renal cell carcinoma. A Southwest Oncology Group Study. *Cancer* 1994;74:916.
236. De Mulder PH, Weissbach L, Jakse G, et al. Gemcitabine: a phase II study in patients with advanced renal cancer. *Cancer Chemother Pharmacol* 1996;37:491.
237. Stadler WM, Vogelzang NJ, Amato R, et al. Flavopiridol, a novel cyclin-dependent kinase inhibitor in metastatic renal cancer: a University of Chicago Phase II Consortium study. *J Clin Oncol* 2000;18(2):371.
238. Fossa SD, Martinelli G, Otto U, et al. Recombinant interferon alfa-2a with or without vinblastine in metastatic renal cell carcinoma: results of a European multi-center phase III study. *Ann Oncol* 1992;3:301.
239. Neidhart JA, Anderson SA, Harris JE, et al. Vinblastine fails to improve response of renal cancer to interferon alfa-n1: high response rate in patients with pulmonary metastases. *J Clin Oncol* 1991;9:832.
240. Sagaster P, Micksche M, Flamm J, Ludwig H. Randomised study using IFN-alpha versus IFN-alpha plus coumarin and cimetidine for treatment of advanced renal cell cancer. *Ann Oncol* 1995;6:999.
241. deKernion JB, Sarna G, Figlin R, Lindner A, Smith RB. The treatment of renal cell carcinoma with human leukocyte alpha-interferon. *J Urol* 1983;130:1063.
242. Quesada JR, Swanson DA, Gutterman JU. Phase II study of interferon alpha in metastatic renal-cell carcinoma: a progress report. *J Clin Oncol* 1985;3:1086.
243. Umeda T, Niijima T. Phase II study of alpha interferon on renal cell carcinoma. Summary of three collaborative trials. *Cancer* 1986;58:1231.
244. Muss HB, Costanzi JJ, Leavitt R, et al. Recombinant alfa interferon in renal cell carcinoma: a randomized trial of two routes of administration. *J Clin Oncol* 1987;5:286.
245. Minasian LM, Motzer RJ, Gluck L, et al. Interferon alfa-2a in advanced renal cell carcinoma: treatment results and survival in 159 patients with long-term follow-up. *J Clin Oncol* 1993;11:1368.
246. Bukowski RM, Goodman P, Crawford ED, et al. Phase II trial of high-dose intermittent interleukin-2 in metastatic renal cell carcinoma: a Southwest Oncology Group study. *J Natl Cancer Inst* 1990;82:143.
247. von der Maase H, Geertsen P, Thatcher N, et al. Recombinant interleukin-2 in metastatic renal cell carcinoma—a European multicentre phase II study. *Eur J Cancer* 1991;27:1583.
248. Escudier B, Ravaud A, Fabbro M, et al. High-dose interleukin-2 two days a week for metastatic renal cell carcinoma: a FNCLCC multicenter study. *J Immunother Emphasis Tumor Immunol* 1994;16:306.
249. Lissoni P, Barni S, Tancini G, et al. Clinical response and survival in metastatic renal carcinoma during subcutaneous administration of interleukin-2 alone. *Arch Ital Urol Androl* 1997;69:41.
250. Dillman RO, Oldham RK, Tauer KW, et al. Continuous interleukin-2 and lymphokine-activated killer cells for advanced cancer: a national biotherapy study group. *J Clin Oncol* 1991;9:1233.
250a. Rosenberg SA, Lotze MT, Yang JC, et al. Experience with the use of high-dose interleukin-2 in the treatment of 652 cancer patients. *Ann Surg* 1989;210:474.
251. Parkinson DR, Fisher RI, Rayner AA, et al. Therapy of renal cell carcinoma with interleukin-2 and lymphokine-activated killer cells: phase II experience with a hybrid bolus and continuous infusion interleukin-2 regimen. *J Clin Oncol* 1990;8:1630.
252. Negrier S, Philip T, Stoter G, et al. Interleukin-2 with or without LAK cells in metastatic renal cell carcinoma: a report of a European multicentre study. *Eur J Cancer Clin Oncol* 1989;25[Suppl 3]:S21.
253. Dillman RO, Church C, Oldham RK, et al. Inpatient continuous-infusion interleukin-2 in 788 patients with cancer. *Cancer* 1993;71:2358.
254. Thompson JA, Shulman KL, Benyunes MC, et al. Prolonged continuous intravenous infusion interleukin-2 and lymphokine-activated killer-cell therapy for metastatic renal cell carcinoma. *J Clin Oncol* 1992;10:960.
255. Yang JC. Interleukin-2: clinical applications, renal carcinoma. In: Rosenberg S, DeVita V Jr, Hellman S, eds. *Biologic therapy of cancer.* Philadelphia: Lippincott Williams & Wilkins, 2000.
256. Bennington JL, et al. Armed Forces Institute of Pathology. *Tumors of the kidney, renal pelvis, and ureter.* Washington, DC: Armed Forces Institute of Pathology, 1975.
257. Batata MA, Whitmore WF, Hilaris BS, Tokita N, Grabstald H. Primary carcinoma of the ureter: a prognostic study. *Cancer* 1975;35:1626.
258. Hall MC, Womack S, Sagalowsky AI, et al. Prognostic factors, recurrence, and survival in transitional cell carcinoma of the upper urinary tract: a 30-year experience in 252 patients. *Urology* 1998;52:594.
259. Kosmidis PA, Bacoyiannis C, Fountzilas G, et al. 5-Fluorouracil, interferon-alpha-2b, and cisplatin (FAP) for advanced urothelial cancer. A phase II study, Hellenic Cooperative Oncology Group. *Ann Oncol* 1997;8:373.
260. Dimopoulos MA, Bakoyannis C, Georgoulias V, et al. Docetaxel and cisplatin combination chemotherapy in advanced carcinoma of the urothelium: a multicenter phase II study of the Hellenic Cooperative Oncology Group. *Ann Oncol* 1999;10:1385.
261. Otto T, Bex A, Krege S, Walz PH, Rubben H. Paclitaxel-based second-line therapy for patients with advanced chemotherapy-resistant bladder carcinoma (M1): a clinical phase II study. *Cancer* 1997;80:465.
262. Paulson DF, Perez CA, Anderson T. Cancer of the kidney and ureter. In: DeVita VT Jr,

Hellman S, Rosenberg SA, eds. *Cancer: principles and practice of oncology*, 2nd ed. Philadelphia: JB Lippincott Co, 1985:907.

263. Woodruff MW, Wagle D, Gailani SD, et al. The current status of chemotherapy for advanced renal carcinoma. *J Urol* 1967;97:611.
264. Talley RW. Proceedings: chemotherapy of adenocarcinoma of the kidney. *Cancer* 1973; 32:1062.
265. Hrushesky WJ, Murphy GP. Current status of the therapy of advanced renal carcinoma. *J Surg Oncol* 1977;9:277.
266. Harris DT. Hormonal therapy and chemotherapy of renal-cell carcinoma. *Semin Oncol* 1983;10:422.
267. Yagoda A, Abi-Bached B, Petrylak D. Chemotherapy for advanced renal cell carcinoma: 1983-1993. *Semin Oncol* 1995;22:42.
268. Motzer RJ, Russo P. Systemic therapy for renal cell carcinoma. *J Urol* 2000;163(2):408.
269. Samuels BL, Hollis DR, Rosner GL, et al. Modulation of vinblastine resistance in metastatic renal cell carcinoma with cyclosporine A or tamoxifen: a Cancer and Leukemia Group B study. *Clin Cancer Res* 1997;3:1977.
270. Pyrhonen S, Salminen E, Ruutu M, et al. Prospective randomized trial of interferon alfa-2a plus vinblastine versus vinblastine alone in patients with advanced renal cell cancer. *J Clin Oncol* 1999;17:2859.
271. Motzer RJ, Bander NH, Nanus DM. Renal-cell carcinoma [see comments]. *N Engl J Med* 1996;335:865.
272. Bloom HJG, Baker WH, Dukes CE, Mitchley BCV. The oestrogen-induced renal tumour of the Syrian hamster. Hormone treatment and possible relationship to carcinoma of the kidney in man. *Br J Cancer* 1963;17:611.
273. Karr JP, Pontes JE, Schneider S, Sandberg AA, Murphy GP. Clinical aspects of steroid hormone receptors in human renal cell carcinoma. *J Surg Oncol* 1983;23:117.
274. Concolino G, Marocchi A, Conti C, et al. Human renal cell carcinoma as a hormone-dependent tumor. *Cancer Res* 1978;38:4340.
275. Henriksson R, Nilsson S, Colleen S, et al. Survival in renal cell carcinoma—a randomized evaluation of tamoxifen vs interleukin 2, alpha-interferon (leucocyte) and tamoxifen [see comments]. *Br J Cancer* 1998;77:1311.
276. Gershanovich MM, Moiseyenko VM, Vorobjev AV, et al. High-dose toremifene in advanced renal-cell carcinoma. *Cancer Chemother Pharmacol* 1997;39:547.
277. Marsoni S, Hoth D, Simon R, et al. Clinical drug development: an analysis of phase II trials, 1970-1985. *Cancer Treat Rep* 1987;71:71.
278. Muggia FM. Closing the loop: providing feedback on drug development [editorial]. *Cancer Treat Rep* 1987;71:1.
279. Boyd MR, Paull KD. Some practical considerations and applications of the National Cancer Institute in vitro anticancer drug discovery screen. *Drug Dev Res* 1995;34:91.
280. Wirth MP. Immunotherapy for metastatic renal cell carcinoma. *Urol Clin North Am* 1993;20:283.
281. Motzer RJ, Vogelzang NJ. Chemotherapy for renal cell carcinoma. In: D Raghavan, HI Scher, SA Leibel, PH Lange, eds. *Principles and practice of genitourinary oncology*. Philadelphia: Lippincott-Raven, 1999;889.
282. Soori GS, Schulof RS, Stark JJ, et al. Continuous-infusion floxuridine and alpha interferon in metastatic renal cancer: a national biotherapy study group phase II study [see comments]. *Cancer Invest* 1999;17:379.
283. Elias L, Blumenstein BA, Kish J, et al. A phase II trial of interferon-alpha and 5-fluorouracil in patients with advanced renal cell carcinoma. A Southwest Oncology Group study. *Cancer* 1996;78:1085.
284. Igarashi T, Marumo K, Onishi T, et al. Interferon-alpha and 5-fluorouracil therapy in patients with metastatic renal cell cancer: an open multicenter trial. The Japanese Study Group Against Renal Cancer. *Urology* 1999;53:53.
285. Motzer RJ, Schwartz L, Law TM, et al. Interferon alpha-2a and 13-cis-retinoic acid in renal cell carcinoma: antitumor activity in a phase II trial and interactions in vitro. *J Clin Oncol* 1995;13:1950.
286. Stadler WM, Kuzel T, Dumas M, Vogelzang NJ. Multicenter phase II trial of interleukin-2, interferon-alpha, and 13-cis-retinoic acid in patients with metastatic renal-cell carcinoma. *J Clin Oncol* 1998;16:1820.
287. Motzer RJ, Murphy BA, Mazumdar M, et al. Randomized phase III trial of interferon alpha-2a (IFN) versus IFN plus 13-cis-retinoic acid (CRA) in patients (pts) with advanced renal cell carcinoma (RCC). *Proceedings of the Thirty-Fifth Annual Meeting of the American Society of Clinical Oncology*; 18:330a. 1999.
288. Motzer RJ, Mazumdar M, Bacik J, et al. Survival and prognostic stratification of 670 patients with advanced renal cell carcinoma. *J Clin Oncol* 1999;17:2530.
289. Nishiyama K, Shirahama T, Yoshimura A, et al. Expression of the multidrug transporter, P-glycoprotein, in renal and transitional cell carcinomas. *Cancer* 1993;71:3611.
290. Kanamaru H, Kakehi Y, Yoshida O, et al. MDR1 RNA levels in human renal cell carcinomas: correlation with grade and prediction of reversal of doxorubicin resistance by quinidine in tumor explants. *J Natl Cancer Inst* 1989;81:844.
291. Rochlitz CF, Lobeck H, Peter S, et al. Multiple drug resistance gene expression in human renal cell cancer is associated with the histologic subtype. *Cancer* 1992;69:2993.
292. Fojo AT, Shen DW, Mickley LA, Pastan I, Gottesman MM. Intrinsic drug resistance in kidney cancers is associated with expression of a human multidrug resistance gene. *J Clin Oncol* 1987;5:1922.
293. Mickisch GH, Roehrich K, Koessig J, et al. Mechanisms and modulation of multidrug resistance in primary human renal cell carcinoma. *J Urol* 1990;144:755.
294. Punt CJ, Voest EE, Tueni E, et al. Phase IB study of doxorubicin in combination with the multidrug resistance reversing agent S9788 in advanced colorectal and renal cell cancer. *Br J Cancer* 1997;76: 1376.
295. Sandor V, Fojo T, Bates SE. Future perspectives for the development of P-glycoprotein modulators. *Drug Resistance Updates* 1998;1:190.
296. Dean M, Allikmets R. Evolution of ATP-binding cassette transporter genes. *Curr Opin Genet Dev* 1995;5:779.
297. Borst P, Kool M, Evers R. Do cMOAT (MRP2), other MRP homologues, and LRP play a role in MDR? *Semin Cancer Biol* 1997;8:205.
298. Nooter K, Westerman AM, Flens MJ, et al. Expression of the multidrug resistance-associated protein (MRP) gene in human cancers. *Clin Cancer Res* 1995;1:1301.
299. Schaub TP, Kartenbeck J, Konig J, et al. Expression of the MRP2 gene-encoded conjugate export pump in human kidney proximal tubules and in renal cell carcinoma. *J Am Soc Nephrol* 1999;10:1159.
300. Kool M, van der Linden M, de Haas M, et al. MRP3, an organic anion transporter able to transport anti-cancer drugs. *Proc Natl Acad Sci U S A* 1999;96:6914.
301. Cole SF, Deeley RG. Multidrug resistance mediated by the ATP-binding cassette transporter protein MRP. *Bioessays* 1998;20:931.
302. Belinsky MG, Kruh GD. MOAT-E (ARA) is a full-length MRP/cMOAT subfamily transporter expressed in kidney and liver. *Br J Cancer* 1999;80:1342.
303. Doyle LA, Yang W, Abruzzo LV, et al. A multidrug resistance transporter from human MCF-7 breast cancer cells [published erratum appears in *Proc Natl Acad Sci U S A* 1999;96(5):2569]. *Proc Natl Acad Sci U S A* 1998;95:15665.
304. Miyake K, Mickley L, Litman T, et al. Molecular cloning of cDNAs which are highly overexpressed in mitoxantrone-resistant cells: demonstration of homology to ABC transport genes. *Cancer Res* 1999;59:8.
305. Allikmets R, Schriml LM, Hutchinson A, Romano-Spica V, Dean M. A human placenta-specific ATP-binding cassette gene (ABCP) on chromosome 4q22 that is involved in multidrug resistance. *Cancer Res* 1998;58:5337.
306. Freeman MR, Washecka R, Chung LWK. Aberrant expression of epidermal growth factor receptor and HER2 messenger RNAs in human renal cancers. *Cancer Res* 1989;49:6221.
307. Ishikawa J, Maeda S, Umezu K, Sugiyama T, Kamidono S. Amplification and overexpression of the epidermal growth factor receptor gene in human renal-cell carcinoma. *Int J Cancer* 1990;45:1018.
308. Danova M, Giordano M, Torelli F, et al. HER-2/neu oncogene expression and DNA ploidy in normal human kidney and renal cell carcinoma. *Eur J Histochem* 1992;36:279.
309. Yoshida K, Tosaka A, Takeuchi S, Kobayashi N. Epidermal growth factor receptor content in human renal cell carcinomas. *Cancer* 1994;73:1913.
310. Stumm G, Eberwein S, Rostock-Wolf S, et al. Concomitant overexpression of the EGFR and erbB-2 genes in renal cell carcinoma (RCC) is correlated with dedifferentiation and metastasis. *Int J Cancer* 1996;69:17.
311. Tomita Y, Bilim V, Kawasaki T, et al. Frequent expression of Bcl-2 in renal-cell carcinomas carrying wild-type p53. *Int J Cancer* 1996;66:322.
312. Murray GI, McFadyen MC, Mitchell RT, et al. Cytochrome P450 CYP3A in human renal cell cancer. *Br J Cancer* 1999;79:1836.
313. Ahn H, Lee E, Kim K, Lee C. Effect of glutathione and its related enzymes on chemosensitivity of renal cell carcinoma and bladder carcinoma cell lines. *J Urol* 1994;151:263.
314. Volm M, Kastel M, Mattern J, Efferth T. Expression of resistance factors (P-glycoprotein, glutathione S-transferase-pi, and topoisomerase II) and their interrelationship to proto-oncogene products in renal cell carcinomas. *Cancer* 1993;71:3981.
315. Scheltema JM, Romijn JC, van Steenbrugge GJ, et al. Decreased levels of topoisomerase II alpha in human renal cell carcinoma lines resistant to etoposide. *J Cancer Res Clin Oncol* 1997;123:546.
316. Curti BD. Physical barriers to drug delivery in tumors. *Crit Rev Oncol Hematol* 1993;14:29.
317. Jain RK. Understanding barriers to drug delivery: high resolution in vivo imaging is key [editorial; comment]. *Clin Cancer Res* 1999;5:1605.
318. Jain RK. The next frontier of molecular medicine: delivery of therapeutics. *Nat Med* 1998;4:655.
319. Less JR, Posner MC, Boucher Y, et al. Interstitial hypertension in human breast and colorectal tumors. *Cancer Res* 1992;52:6371.
320. Aaltomaa S, Lipponen P, Ala-Opas M, et al. Expression of cyclins A and D and p21(waf1/cip1) proteins in renal cell cancer and their relation to clinicopathological variables and patient survival. *Br J Cancer* 1999;80:2001.
321. Lipponen P, Eskelinen M, Hietala K, Syrjanen K, Gambetta RA. Expression of proliferating cell nuclear antigen (PC10), p53 protein and c-erbB-2 in renal adenocarcinoma. *Int J Cancer* 1994;57:275.
322. Papadopoulos I, Rudolph P, Weichert-Jacobsen K, Thiemann O, Papadopoulous D. Prognostic indicators for response to therapy and survival in patients with metastatic renal cell cancer treated with interferon alpha-2 beta and vinblastine. *Urology* 1996;48:373.
323. Tannapfel A, Hahn HA, Katalinic A, et al. Prognostic value of ploidy and proliferation markers in renal cell carcinoma. *Cancer* 1996;77:164.
324. de Riese WT, Crabtree WN, Allhoff EP, et al. Prognostic significance of Ki-67 immunostaining in nonmetastatic renal cell carcinoma. *J Clin Oncol* 1993;11:1804.
325. Elson PJ, Witte RS, Trump DL. Prognostic factors for survival in patients with recurrent or metastatic renal cell carcinoma. *Cancer Res* 1988;48:7310.
326. McCaffrey JA, Dodd PM, Herr H, et al. Nonbladder primary site of transitional cell carcinoma (TCC) does not affect probablility of response to M-VAC or survival. *Proceedings of the Thirty-Fourth Annual Meeting of American Sociey of Clinical Oncology*;17:337a. 1998.
327. McCaffrey JA, Herr HW. Adjuvant and neoadjuvant chemotherapy for urothelial carcinoma. *Surg Oncol Clin N Am* 1997;6:667.
328. Stadler WM, Kuzel T, Roth B, Raghavan D, Dorr FA. Phase II study of single-agent gemcitabine in previously untreated patients with metastatic urothelial cancer. *J Clin Oncol* 1997;15:3394.
329. Sternberg CN, Yagoda A, Scher HI, et al. Preliminary results of M-VAC (methotrexate, vinblastine, doxorubicin and cisplatin) for transitional cell carcinoma of the urothelium. *J Urol* 1985;133:403.
330. Sternberg CN, Yagoda A, Scher HI, et al. Methotrexate, vinblastine, doxorubicin, and cisplatin for advanced transitional cell carcinoma of the urothelium. Efficacy and patterns of response and relapse. *Cancer* 1989;64:2448.

331. Logothetis CJ, Dexeus FH, Finn L, et al. A prospective randomized trial comparing MVAC and CISCA chemotherapy for patients with metastatic urothelial tumors. *J Clin Oncol* 1990;8:1050.
332. Loehrer PJS, Einhorn LH, Elson PJ, et al. A randomized comparison of cisplatin alone or in combination with methotrexate, vinblastine, and doxorubicin in patients with metastatic urothelial carcinoma: a cooperative group study [published erratum appears in *J Clin Oncol* 1993;11(2):384]. *J Clin Oncol* 1992;10:1066.
333. Saxman SB, Propert KJ, Einhorn LH, et al. Long-term follow-up of a phase III intergroup study of cisplatin alone or in combination with methotrexate, vinblastine, and doxorubicin in patients with metastatic urothelial carcinoma: a cooperative group study. *J Clin Oncol* 1997;5:2564.
334. Dodd PM, McCaffrey JA, Mazumdar M, et al. Phase II trial of intermediate dose methotrexate in combination with vinblastine, doxorubicin, and cisplatin in patients with unresectable or metastatic transitional cell carcinoma. *Cancer* 1999;85:1145.
335. Seidman AD, Scher HI, Gabrilove JL, et al. Dose-intensification of MVAC with recombinant granulocyte colony-stimulating factor as initial therapy in advanced urothelial cancer [see comments]. *J Clin Oncol* 1993;11:408.
336. Logothetis CJ, Finn LD, Smith T, et al. Escalated MVAC with or without recombinant human granulocyte-macrophage colony-stimulating factor for the initial treatment of advanced malignant urothelial tumors: results of a randomized trial. *J Clin Oncol* 1995;13:2272.
337. Dodd PM, McCaffrey JA, Herr H, et al. Outcome of postchemotherapy surgery after treatment with methotrexate, vinblastine, doxorubicin, and cisplatin in patients with unresectable or metastatic transitional cell carcinoma. *J Clin Oncol* 1999;17:2546.
337a. Igawa M, Urakami S, Shiina H, et al. Long-term results with MVAC for advanced urothelial cancer: high relapse rate and low survival in patients with a complete response. *Br J Urol* 1995;76:321.
337b. Vogelzang NJ, Stadler WM. Gemcitabine and other new chemotherapeutic agents for the treatment of metastatic bladder cancer. *Urology* 1999;53:243.
337c. Oh WK, Manola J, Richie JP, et al. A phase II trial of methotrexate, cisplatin, 5-fluorouracil, and leucovorin in the treatment of invasive and metastatic urothelial carcinoma. *Cancer* 1999;86:1329.
337d. PDQ Summary. World Wide Web URLs: http://cancernet.nci.nih.gov/pdq.html and http://cancernet.nci.nih.gov/trialsrch.shtml.
337e. Siu LL, Banerjee D, Khurana RJ, et al. The prognostic role of p53, metallothionein, P-glycoprotein, and MIB-1 in muscle-invasive urothelial transitional cell carcinoma. *Clin Cancer Res* 1998;4:559.
338. Van Brussel JP, Mickisch GH. Prognostic factors in renal cell and bladder cancer. *BJU Int* 1999;83:902.
339. Gohji K, Higuchi A, Maruyama S, et al. Adjuvant chemotherapy for invasive urothelial cancer: experience with a methotrexate, vincristine, cisplatin, cyclophosphamide, adriamycin and bleomycin (MVP-CAB) regimen: a preliminary report. *Jpn J Clin Oncol* 1993;23:291.
340. Studer UE, Bacchi M, Biedermann C, et al. Adjuvant cisplatin chemotherapy following cystectomy for bladder cancer: results of a prospective randomized trial. *J Urol* 1994;52:81.
341. Stockle M, Meyenburg W, Wellek S, et al. Adjuvant polychemotherapy of nonorgan-confined bladder cancer after radical cystectomy revisited: long-term results of a controlled prospective study and further clinical experience. *J Urol* 1995;153:47.
342. Freiha F, Reese J, Torti FM. A randomized trial of radical cystectomy versus radical cystectomy plus cisplatin, vinblastine and methotrexate chemotherapy for muscle invasive bladder cancer [see comments]. *J Urol* 1996;155:495.
343. Bono A, Benvenuti C, Gibba A. Adjuvant chemotherapy in locally advanced bladder cancer: final analysis of a controlled multicentre study. *Acta Urol Ital* 1997;11:1241.
344. Logothetis C, Swanson D, Amato R, et al. Optimal delivery of perioperative chemotherapy: preliminary results of a randomized, prospective, comparative trial of preoperative and postoperative chemotherapy for invasive bladder carcinoma. *J Urol* 1996;155:1241.
345. Does neoadjuvant cisplatin-based chemotherapy improve the survival of patients with locally advanced bladder cancer: a meta-analysis of individual patient data from randomized clinical trials. Advanced Bladder Cancer Overview Collaboration. *Br J Urol* 1995;75:206.
346. Neoadjuvant cisplatin, methotrexate, and vinblastine chemotherapy for muscle-invasive bladder cancer: a randomised controlled trial. International collaboration of trialists [see comments]. *Lancet* 1999;354:533.
347. McCarron JP, Mills C, Vaughn EDJ. Tumors of the renal pelvis and ureter: current concepts and management. *Semin Urol* 1983;1:75.
348. Seaman EK, Slawin KM, Benson MC. Treatment options for upper tract transitional-cell carcinoma. *Urol Clin North Am* 1993;20:349.
349. Tawfiek ER, Bagley DH. Upper-tract transitional cell carcinoma. *Urology* 1997;50:321.
350. Mahjoubi M, Kattan J, Bonnay M, Schmitt H, Droz JP. Phase II trial of LY 186641 in advanced renal cancer. *Invest New Drugs* 1993;11:323.
351. Walpole ET, Dutcher JP, Sparano J, et al. Survival after phase II treatment of advanced renal cell carcinoma with taxol or high-dose interleukin-2. *J Immunother* 1993;13:275.
352. Mertens WC, Eisenhauer EA, Jolivet J, et al. Docetaxel in advanced renal carcinoma. A phase II trial of the National Cancer Institute of Canada Clinical Trials Group. *Ann Oncol* 1994;5:185.
353. Flanigan RC, Saiers JH, Wolf M, et al. Phase II evaluation of merbarone in renal cell carcinoma. *Invest New Drugs* 1994;12:147.
354. Law TM, Ilson DH, Motzer RJ. Phase II trial of topotecan in patients with advanced renal cell carcinoma. *Invest New Drugs* 1994;12:143.
355. Law TM, Mencel P, Motzer RJ. Phase II trial of liposomal encapsulated doxorubicin in patients with advanced renal cell carcinoma. *Invest New Drugs* 1994;12:323.
356. Shevrin DH, Kilton LJ, Lad TE, et al. Phase II trial of 6-thioguanine in advanced renal cell carcinoma. An Illinois Cancer Center study. *Invest New Drugs* 1994;12:345.
357. Witte RS, Hsieh P, Elson P, Oken MM, Trump DL. A phase II trial of amonafide, caracemide, and homoharringtonine in the treatment of patients with advanced renal cell cancer. *Invest New Drugs* 1996;14:409.
358. Berg WJ, Schwartz LH, Amsterdam A, et al. A phase II study of 13-cis-retinoic acid in patients with advanced renal cell carcinoma. *Invest New Drugs* 1997;15:353.
359. Dreicer R, Propert KJ, Kuzel T, et al. A phase II trial of edatrexate in patients with advanced renal cell carcinoma. An Eastern Cooperative Oncology Group study. *Am J Clin Oncol* 1997;20:251.
360. Lummen G, Sperling H, Luboldt H, Otto T, Rubben H. Phase II trial of titanocene dichloride in advanced renal-cell carcinoma. *Cancer Chemother Pharmacol* 1998;42:415.
361. Vogelzang, NJ, Mani S, Schilsky RL, et al. Phase II and pharmacodynamic studies of pyrazine diazohydroxide (NSC 361456) in patients with advanced renal and colorectal cancer. *Clin Cancer Res* 1998;4:929.
362. Rigos D, Weschel HW, Bichler KH. Treosulfan in the treatment of metastatic renal cell carcinoma. *Anticancer Res* 1999;19(2c):1549.
363. Berg WJ, McCaffrey J, Schwartz LH, et al. A phase II study of pyrazoloacridine in patients with advanced renal cell carcinoma. *Invest New Drugs* 1998;16:337.
364. Stadler WM, Kuzel T, Shapiro C, et al. Multi-institutional study of the angiogenesis inhibitor TNP-470 in metastatic renal carcinoma [In Process Citation]. *J Clin Oncol* 1999;17:2541.
365. Dreicer R, Smith DC, Williams RD, See WA. Phase II trial of suramin in patients with metastatic renal cell carcinoma. *Invest New Drugs* 1999;17:183.
366. di Palma M, Vannetzel JM, Bansadoun G, et al. Phase II study of temozolomide (TEM) in metastatic renal cell carcinoma (MRCC). *Proceedings of the Thirty-Fourth Annual Meeting of the American Society of Clinical Oncology,* 17:330a. 1998.
367. Dumas MC, Stadler W, Mikulski S, Vogelzang NJ. Phase II clinical trial of intravenous onconase (ONC) in patients (pts) with metastatic renal cell carcinoma (MRCC). *Proceedings of the Thirty-Fourth Annual Meeting of the American Society of Clinical Oncology,* 17:330a. 1998.
368. Fishkin P, Stadler WM, Gibbons J, Vogelzang NJ, Vokes EE. A University of Chicago phase II consortium study (UCPC) of CI-980 in patients (PTS) metastatic renal cell carcinoma (RCC). *Proceedings of the Thirty-Fourth Annual Meeting of the American Society of Clinical Oncology,* 17:330a. 1998.
369. Pennington K, Gordon M, Picus JA. A phase II trial of liposomal doxorubicin (DOXIL) in the treatment of advanced renal cell cancer: a Hoosier Oncology Group (HOG) Study. *Proceedings of the Thirty-Fourth Annual Meeting of the American Society of Clinical Oncology,* 17:339a. 1998.
370. Sauter T, Boucsein R, Thoedtmann R, et al. Multicenter phase II trial of MTA (multi-targeted antifolate, LY231514) in chemonaive patients with metastatic renal cancer (MRCC). *Proceedings of the Thirty-Fourth Annual Meeting of the American Society of Clinical Oncology,* 17:342a. 1998.
371. Gunnett K, Motzer R, Amato R, et al. Phase II study of anti-epidermal growth factor receptor (EGFr) antibody C225 alone in patients (pts) with metastatic renal cell carcinoma (MRCC). *Proceedings of the Thirty-Fifth Annual Meeting of the American Society of Clinical Oncology,*18:340a. 1999.
372. O'Shaughnessy J, Flaherty L, Fiorica J, Grove W. Phase II trial of CI-994 in patients (pts) with metastatic renal cell carcinoma (RCC). *Proceedings of the Thirty-Fifth Annual Meeting of the American Society of Clinical Oncology,*18:349a. 1999.
373. Redman BG, Streiff RR, Nemunaitis J, et al. A phase II trial of diethylnorspermine (DENSPM) on renal cell carcinoma. *Proceedings of the Thirty-Fifth Annual Meeting of the American Society of Clinical Oncology,*18:351a. 1999.
374. Rubins J, Chang A, Asbury R, Boros L, Navone L. Recombinant Human Erythropoietin (rHuEPO) in advanced renal cell carcinoma (RCC). *Proceedings of the Thirty-Fifth Annual Meeting of the American Society of Clinical Oncology,*18:352a. 1999.
375. Kriegmair M, Oberneder R, Hofstetter A. Interferon alfa and vinblastine versus medroxyprogesterone acetate in the treatment of metastatic renal cell carcinoma. *Urology* 1995; 45:758.
376. Pyrhonen S, Salminen E, Ruutu M, et al. Prospective randomized trial of interferon alfa-2a plus vinblastine versus vinblastine alone in patients with advanced renal cell cancer. *J Clin Oncol* 1999;17:2859.
377. Motzer RJ, Murphy BA, Mazumdar M, et al. Randomized phase III trial of interferon alpha-2a (IFN) versus IFN plus 13-cis-retinoic acid (CRA) in patients (pts) with advanced renal cell carcinoma (RCC). *Proceedings of the Thirty-Fifth Annual Meeting of the American Society of Clinical Oncology,*18:330a. 1999.
378. Schwartsmann G, Medina DC, Silveira LA, et al. Phase II trial of vinblastine plus nifedipine (VN) in patients with advanced renal cell carcinoma (RCC). Brazilian Oncology Trials Group [letter]. *Ann Oncol* 1991;2:443.
379. Murphy BR, Rynard SM, Pennington KL, Grosh W, Loehrer PJ. A phase II trial of vinblastine plus dipyridamole in advanced renal cell carcinoma. A Hoosier Oncology Group Study. *Am J Clin Oncol* 1994;17:10.
380. Motzer RJ, Lyn P, Fischer P, et al. Phase I/II trial of dexverapamil plus vinblastine for patients with advanced renal cell carcinoma. *J Clin Oncol* 1995;13:1958.
381. Warner E, Tobe SW, Andrulis IL, et al. Phase I-II study of vinblastine and oral cyclosporin A in metastatic renal cell carcinoma. *Am J Clin Oncol* 1995;18:251.
382. Agarwala SS, Bahnson RR, Wilson JW, Szumowski J, Ernstoff MS. Evaluation of the combination of vinblastine and quinidine in patients with metastatic renal cell carcinoma. A phase I study. *Am J Clin Oncol* 1995;18:211.
383. Sternberg CN, Yagoda A, Scher HI, et al. Methotrexate, vinblastine, doxorubicin, and cisplatin for advanced transitional cell carcinoma of the urothelium. Efficacy and patterns of response and relapse. *Cancer* 1989;64:2448.
384. Seidman AD, Scher HI, Heinemann MH, et al. Continuous infusion gallium nitrate for patients with advanced refractory urothelial tract tumors. *Cancer* 1991;68:2561.
385. Moore MJ, Tannock IF, Ernst DS, Huan S, Murray N. Gemcitabine: a promising new agent in the treatment of advanced urothelial cancer. *J Clin Oncol* 1997;15:3441.
386. Lorusso V, Pollera CF, Antimi M, et al. A phase II study of gemcitabine in patients with transitional cell carcinoma of the urinary tract previously treated with platinum. Italian Co-operative Group on Bladder Cancer. *Eur J Cancer* 1998;34:1208.

387. Roth BJ, Dreicer R, Einhorn LH, et al. Significant activity of paclitaxel in advanced transitional-cell carcinoma of the urothelium: a phase II trial of the Eastern Cooperative Oncology Group. *J Clin Oncol* 1994;12:2264.
388. Papamichael D, Gallagher CJ, Oliver RT, Johnson PW, Waxman J. Phase II study of paclitaxel in pretreated patients with locally advanced/metastatic cancer of the bladder and ureter. *Br J Cancer* 1997;75:606.
389. de Wit R, Kruit WH, Stoter G, et al. Docetaxel (Taxotere): an active agent in metastatic urothelial cancer; results of a phase II study in non–chemotherapy-pretreated patients. *Br J Cancer* 1998;78:1342.
390. McCaffrey JA, Hilton S, Mazumdar M, et al. Phase II trial of docetaxel in patients with advanced or metastatic transitional-cell carcinoma. *J Clin Oncol* 1997;15:1853.
391. Witte RS, Manola J, Burch PA, et al. Topotecan in previously treated advanced urothelial carcinoma: an ECOG phase II trial. *Invest New Drugs* 1998;16:191.
392. Einhorn LH, Roth BJ, Ansari R, et al. Phase II trial of vinblastine, ifosfamide, and gallium combination chemotherapy in metastatic urothelial carcinoma. *J Clin Oncol* 1994;12:2271.
393. Sengelov L, Nielsen OS, Kamby C, von der M. Platinum analogue combination chemotherapy: cisplatin, carboplatin, and methotrexate in patients with metastatic urothelial tract tumors. A phase II trial with evaluation of prognostic factors. *Cancer* 1995;76:1797.
394. McCaffrey JA, Hilton S, Mazumdar M, et al. Phase II randomized trial of gallium nitrate plus fluorouracil versus methotrexate, vinblastine, doxorubicin, and cisplatin in patients with advanced transitional-cell carcinoma. *J Clin Oncol* 1997;15:2449.
395. Bajorin DF, McCaffrey JA, Dodd PM, et al. Ifosfamide, paclitaxel, and cisplatin for patients with advanced transitional cell carcinoma of the urothelial tract: final report of a phase II trial evaluating two dosing schedules. *Cancer* 2000;88(7):1671.
396. Bellmunt J, Guillem V, Paz-Ares L, et al. Gemcitabine/paclitaxel-based three-drug regimens in advanced urothelial cancer. *Eur J Cancer* 2000;36:S17.
397. Sengelov L, Kamby C, Lund B, Engelholm SA. Docetaxel and cisplatin in metastatic urothelial cancer: a phase II study. *J Clin Oncol* 1998;16:3392.
398. Zielinski CC, Schnack B, Grbovic M, et al. Paclitaxel and carboplatin in patients with metastatic urothelial cancer: results of a phase II trial. *Br J Cancer* 1998;78:370.
399. Redman BG, Smith DC, Flaherty L, Du W, Hussain M. Phase II trial of paclitaxel and carboplatin in the treatment of advanced urothelial carcinoma. *J Clin Oncol* 1998;16:1844.
400. Vaughn DJ, Malkowicz SB, Zoltik B, et al. Paclitaxel plus carboplatin in advanced carcinoma of the urothelium: an active and tolerable outpatient regimen. *J Clin Oncol* 1998;16:255.
401. Moore MJ, Winquist EW, Murray N, et al. Gemcitabine plus cisplatin, an active regimen in advanced urothelial cancer: a phase II trial of the National Cancer Institute of Canada Clinical Trials Group. *J Clin Oncol* 1999;17:2876.
402. Kaufman D, Raghavan D, Carducci M, et al. Phase II trial of gemcitabine plus cisplatin in patients with metastatic urothelial cancer. *J Clin Oncol* 2000;18(9):1921.

HARRY W. HERR
WILLIAM U. SHIPLEY
DEAN F. BAJORIN

SECTION 3

Cancer of the Bladder

Urinary bladder cancers represent a spectrum of neoplasms that can be grouped into three general categories: superficial, invasive, and metastatic. Each differs in clinical behavior, prognosis, and primary management. For treating superficial tumors, the aim is to prevent recurrences and progression to an incurable stage. For treating invasive disease, the issue becomes how to determine which tumors can be cured with single-modality therapies (e.g., surgery), which can be treated without surgical removal of the bladder, and which, by virtue of a high metastatic potential, require an integrated systemic approach to achieve cure. For treating metastatic disease, combination chemotherapy is the standard; yet, despite responses in more than 50% of cases, overall cure rates remain low. Recent progress with evolving chemotherapeutic regimens suggest that cure rates may improve in the future.

A unique aspect of bladder cancer treatment is that repeated surgical biopsy is an integral part of routine patient management, thus permitting molecular genetic studies of tumors from specific stages of the disease. The results of these studies suggest that bladder cancers develop and progress along at least two discrete pathways, which may account for differences in invasiveness and metastatic potential.[1] It may also explain why some tumors recur on the surface, without invasion, while others metastasize with minimal infiltration below the epithelial layers. These considerations, along with identifying several chemotherapeutic agents active in patients who have progressed on cisplatin-based combinations, have led to clinical trials seeking to define new standards of care. It is hoped that incorporating molecular genetic factors into the currently used staging systems will change the paradigm of treatment so that the probability of cure is optimized and the quality of life maintained.

EPIDEMIOLOGY

Bladder cancer is the fourth most common cancer in men and the seventh most common in women. More than 54,000 cases (in 29,500 men and 14,900 women) were diagnosed in 1999, and 12,500 individuals (8400 male and 4100 female) succumbed.[2] Bladder cancer, primarily a disease of men older than age 65, is rarely diagnosed before the age of 40. White men receive diagnoses twice as often as black men. Additionally, the diagnosis rate is higher in urban than in rural areas. Bladder cancer death rates declined substantially for both whites and blacks of both genders from 1973 to 1996, approximately 24% overall.[3] This decrease is likely to be the result of more cases being diagnosed at a noninvasive stage and more effective therapies.

Cigarette smoking is the most important risk factor, although work in the dye, rubber, or leather industries is also strongly associated with bladder cancer.[4] The latency period from initial exposure to the development of a urothelial tumor is a median of 18 years. Cigarette smoking is believed to contribute to upward of 50% of the cancers in men and 33% of the cancers in women.[5] Overall, smokers have a two- to fourfold higher relative risk of bladder cancer than nonsmokers. Smoking contributes to the field change of the urothelium, because the urothelium from individuals who "never smoked" shows atypia in only 4% of cases versus up to 50% in "smokers."[5] Discontinuing smoking decreases risk, although a higher risk than nonsmokers remains for up to 10 years after smoking cessation. A high fluid intake is associated with a decreased incidence of bladder cancer in men, and lesser intake of daily fluids proportionally increases the risk of bladder cancer.[6]

Dietary components consumed in high quantities, such as fried meats and fats, are associated with bladder cancer. Vitamin A supplements appear to be protective.[7] Coffee consumption and artificial sweeteners confer little or no risk.[8] Several drugs (e.g., phenacetin) are implicated in the development of urothelial tumors, and cyclophosphamide, used as an oncolytic or immunosuppressive agent, can increase risk ninefold.[9]

Exposure to *Schistosoma haematobium*, a parasite found in many developing countries, is associated with an increased risk of both squamous and transitional cell carcinomas of the bladder.[8] A link between a history of urinary tract infection and squamous cell carcinoma of the urinary bladder has been shown,[10] particularly in paraplegics and those with bladder stones or indwelling Foley catheters. An association is not identified between infection and transitional cell tumors.

CLINICAL PRESENTATION AND DIAGNOSIS

The frequencies of a specific symptom at diagnosis parallel the occurrence of the three clinical subtypes. At presentation, 75% of tumors are superficial, 20% are invasive, and up to 5% have *de novo* metastases. Although hematuria is the presenting sign in 80% to 90% of cases, urinary frequency, the result of irritative symptoms or a reduction in overall bladder capacity, is common. Depending on a lesion's location and depth of invasion, ureteral obstruction may develop, resulting in flank pain, discomfort, and overall reduced renal function. In rare cases, pain from a metastatic bone lesion or local progression of disease is the presenting sign.

Individuals older than 40 years of age who develop hematuria should have a urine specimen for cytology and undergo cystoscopy and imaging of the urinary tract with an intravenous pyelogram or computed tomographic (CT) scan. Screening of asymptomatic subjects for hematuria has not been shown to affect overall survival, although it does increase the probability of diagnosing the disease at an earlier stage.[11] Prospective studies are ongoing to assess the role of screening in high-risk populations. Other urine assays have been used to diagnose disease and to follow up patients, including flow cytometry, blood group antigens (i.e., Lewis X), cytokeratins, the bladder tumor–associated test, and tests for nuclear matrix protein, fibrin degradation product, and telomerase. None is sensitive or specific enough to replace cystoscopy and urine cytology.

CYSTOSCOPY

The cystoscopic evaluation forms the mainstay of diagnosis and staging. It begins with an examination under anesthesia to determine whether a palpable mass is present and, if present, whether it is movable. A cystoscope is then inserted into the bladder, and urine is obtained to determine the presence or absence of malignant cells. The bladder is inspected visually, and a detailed notation of the size, number, location, and growth pattern (papillary or solid) of all lesions is recorded. The status of uninvolved mucosa is also noted. These data are recorded on a detailed bladder map for future reference (Fig. 34.3-1). Biopsy specimens are taken from visible tumors or resected in stages to determine the histologic subtype and depth of invasion into the submucosa and muscle layers of the bladder. In cases where there is suspected or minimal tumor invasion, a repeat biopsy is advised to ensure that all visible tumor is completely resected and to detect the presence of muscle invasion.[12]

Selected biopsy specimens from the "apparently" normal transitional cell epithelium and prostatic urethra are also performed to assess whether a field change has occurred. The presence of carcinoma *in situ* (CIS) provides important information if organ preservation is being considered because it portends frequent tumor recurrences. For patients with a positive cytology and no apparent tumor within the bladder, selective catheterization of the ureters is required, with retrograde studies to evaluate for the presence of upper urinary tract disease.

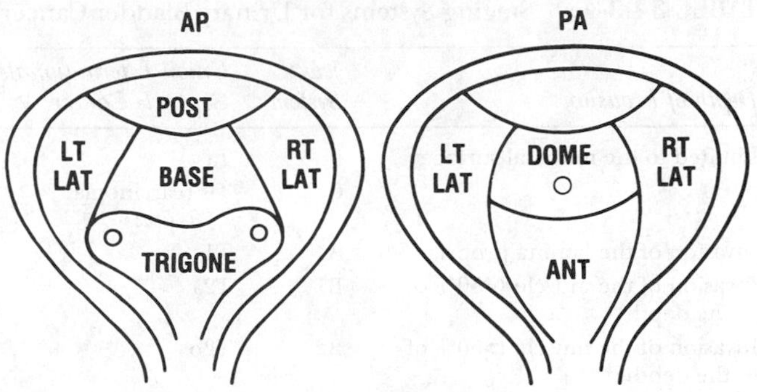

FIGURE 34.3-1. Bladder cancer map. AP, anteroposterior; ANT, anterior; LT LAT, left lateral; RT LAT, right lateral; PA, posteroanterior; post, posterior.

The cystoscopic evaluation is also used after treatment to assess the response to therapeutic intervention. For an invasive tumor, cystoscopic biopsy is considered *clinical* (T) evaluation and does not constitute *pathologic* (P) staging because of the recognized inability of cystoscopy to predict with certainty residual disease in the bladder after treatment. The results of the posttreatment cystoscopy are, nevertheless, being used with increasing frequency to help to select the type of treatment required to eradicate disease within the bladder and to determine the feasibility of bladder preservation.

The decision whether to perform additional diagnostic studies is based on the results of the cystoscopy and the pathologic studies of the tumor. An intravenous pyelogram or CT scan is used to evaluate the upper urinary tracts. A CT scan or magnetic resonance imaging assists in distinguishing between a tumor that is confined to the bladder (stage T2) and one that extends into perivesical fat (stage T3) and documents whether regional lymph nodes are involved (N+). None of these can precisely predict the depth of invasion within the bladder wall.[13] The presence or absence of distal metastases can be documented with physical examination, CT, a chest radiogram, and a radionuclide bone scan. Because bladder tumors occur in elderly individuals, a general medical evaluation is essential to document significant comorbid conditions.

PATHOLOGY AND NATURAL HISTORY

Transitional cell carcinomas (TCCs) constitute 90% to 95% of the urothelial tumors in the United States.[14] They occur anywhere along the urinary tract from the renal pelvis to the ureter, bladder, and proximal two-thirds of the urethra, at which point a squamous epithelium predominates. More than 90% of tumors originate in the urinary bladder and 8% in the renal pelvis; primary tumors of the ureter and urethra constitute the remaining 2% of tumors in these locations. Pure squamous cell tumors, defined by the presence of keratinization in the pathologic specimen, comprise 3%, adenocarcinomas 2%, and small cell carcinoma fewer than 1% of tumors that develop in this region. Tumors of mixed histology, consisting of transitional cell and squamous or adenocarcinomatous elements, can also be identified. These are considered variants of the transitional cell lesion, and they do not portend a worse prognosis. Adenocarcinomas may occur in the embryonal remnant of the urachus on the bladder dome or in the periurethral tissues, or they may assume a signet cell histology. In rare cases, a lymphoma or melanoma develops in the bladder.

TABLE 34.3-1. Staging Systems for Urinary Bladder Cancer

Depth of Invasion	*Jewett System*	*Union Internationale Contre le Cancer*
Limited to the mucosal surface	0	Ta
	0	Tis (carcinoma *in situ*)
Invasion of the lamina propria	A	T1
Invasion of the muscle (<50% of the depth)	B1	T2a
Invasion of the muscle (>50% of the depth)	B2	T2b
Perivesical fat	C	T3
Growth into adjacent structures (prostate, uterus, vagina, bowel) but still mobile	C	T4a
Tumor is fixed to the pelvic wall	C	T4b
Nodal metastases	D1	N+
Distant metastases	D2	M+

Approximately 70% of newly diagnosed cases have exophytic papillary tumors that are confined to the mucosa (stage Ta) or invade the submucosa (stage T1). They tend to be friable, with a high propensity to bleed. These tumors may recur at the same part or in other portions of the bladder and at the same or at a more advanced stage and grade. They are generally managed endoscopically by complete resection. An estimated 50% to 70% of patients with a tumor confined to the mucosa have a recurrence or a new occurrence of a TCC within 5 years, whereas 5% to 20% of superficial tumors progress to a more advanced stage. An important area of research is determining which tumors will recur, which will progress to a higher stage, and which will metastasize.

GRADING

Bladder tumors are classified as low-grade (G1) or high-grade (G2, G3).[15] Grading is more important for noninvasive tumors because almost all invasive neoplasms (T1 or greater) are high-grade. The epithelium has a thickness of less than five to seven layers, normal polarity of nuclei, and no pleomorphism. Papillary carcinomas of low grade are considered to be relatively benign tumors that closely resemble the normal urothelium. They have more than seven layers of urothelium, normal nuclear polarity in more than 95% of the tumor, and no or only slight pleomorphism. More important, they rarely progress to a higher stage.[15] High-grade papillary tumors show loss of polarization of the nuclei and moderate or prominent pleomorphism. Progression to higher-stage lesions is frequent. For invasive tumors, stage is the most important independent prognostic variable for progression and overall survival.

Primary CIS (Tis), without a concurrent exophytic tumor, constitutes 1% to 2% of newly detected cases of bladder cancer.[16] CIS is found in more than one-half the bladders with multiple papillary tumors, either adjacent to or involving mucosal sites remote from papillary lesions. CIS is, by definition, high-grade and believed to be a predominant precursor of invasive tumors.[17] Left untreated, CIS will develop invasive disease in 5 years in more than 50% of patients.

TABLE 34.3-2. TNM Staging System for Bladder Cancer

DEFINITIONS	
Primary tumor	
TX	Primary tumor cannot be assessed
T0	No evidence of primary tumor
Ta	Noninvasive papillary carcinoma
Tis	Carcinoma *in situ*: "flat tumor"
T1	Tumor invades lamina propria
T2	Tumor invades muscle
T2a	Tumor invades superficial muscle
T2b	Tumor invades deep muscle (outer half)
T3	Tumor invades perivesical fat
	T3a Microscopically
	T3b Macroscopically (extravesical mass)
T4	Tumor invades prostate, uterus, vagina, pelvic wall, or abdominal wall
T4a	Tumor invades prostate, uterus, vagina
T4b	Tumor invades pelvic or abdominal wall
Lymph node	
NX	Regional lymph nodes cannot be assessed
N0	No regional lymph node metastasis
N1	Metastasis in a single lymph node, 2 cm or less in greatest dimension
N2	Metastasis in a single lymph node, more than 2 cm, but not more than 5 cm, in greatest dimension, or multiple lymph nodes, none more than 5 cm in greatest dimension
N3	Metastasis in a lymph node more than 5 cm in greatest dimension
Distant metastasis	
MX	Presence of distant metastasis cannot be assessed
M0	No distant metastasis
M1	Distant metastasis
STAGE GROUPING	
0a	Ta, N0, M0
0is	Tis, N0, M0
I	T1, N0, M0
II	T2, N0, M0
	T3a, N0, M0
III	T3b, N0, M0
	T4a, N0, M0
IV	T4b, N0, M0
	Any T, N1, M0
	Any T, N2, M0
	Any T, N3, M0
	Any T, Any N, M1

STAGING

The most commonly used staging systems are the Jewett-Strong-Marshall and TNM (tumor-node-metastasis) systems.[18,19] They were developed from pathologic studies of cystectomy specimens in which the association between depth of invasion and clinical course was first identified. They are contrasted in Tables 34.3-1 and 34.3-2. The major difference is that the TNM system provides for the two patterns of growth and clinical behavior of superficial lesions and delineates more clearly the extent of extravesical spread. Because of this, it is more widely used.

TABLE 34.3-3. Treatment Options for Muscle-Infiltrating Disease

Bladder sparing	
TUR alone	
Nd:YAG laser	
Radiotherapy alone	
	External beam
	Implantation
	Intraoperative
Partial cystectomy	
Chemotherapy alone	
Chemotherapy + radiation	
	Concurrent
	Alternating
	Sequential
Non–bladder-sparing	
Radical surgery	
Chemotherapy + surgery	
Radiation + surgery	
Chemotherapy + radiation + surgery	

Nd:YAG, neodymium:yttrium-aluminum garnet; TUR, transurethral resection.

Ta lesions grow as exophytic lesions and tend to recur but generally do not invade. If a tumor invades the layer below the mucosa, the submucosa, or lamina propria, it is a T1 tumor. A breakpoint in both classifications is invasion into muscle, at which point surgical removal of the bladder is considered standard therapy (Table 34.3-3). Once invasion into the muscle layer is documented, the risk of nodal and subsequent distant metastases increases. The TNM system divides muscle-infiltrating (T2) disease into superficial (T2a) or deep (T2b) invasion but confined within the bladder. In clinical practice, the accuracy of determining the degree of muscle infiltration is modest, at best. Even in experienced hands, the correlation between depth of invasion, based on the cystoscopic evaluation, and the final bladder removed by cystectomy is only 70%. As treatment outcomes are further evaluated, it is becoming apparent that the most important determination is whether the tumor is organ-confined (T2 or less) or non–organ-confined (T3 or greater).[20] The T3 category includes tumors that extend to the perivesical fat. In some cases, surgeons take specimens from deep in the bladder wall, rendering it possible for the pathologist to determine the boundary between muscle and perivesical fat. CT scans or magnetic resonance imaging may help to identify disease that has spread outside the bladder.

The TNM system differentiates tumors extending into adjacent organs from those extending into perivesical fat. A tumor that grows into the prostate, vagina, uterus, or bowel is classified as T4a, and a tumor fixed to the abdominal wall, pelvic wall, or other organs is a T4b lesion. Urothelial tumors may also grow into the prostate, along the prostatic ducts—noninvasive lesions with a good prognosis when resected—or directly invade the prostatic stroma, which harbors a worse prognosis.[21] The TNM system categorizes nodal disease based on the number and size of involvement. It also accounts for metastases to specific sites. Once invasion outside the bladder[20] or nodal disease[22] is documented, outcomes without systemic therapy are poor, with overall survival rates ranging from 4% to 35% at 5 years (Tables 34.3-4 and 34.3-5).[20,22] A similar bleak prognosis is also apparent for patients with metastases, whose median survival rates range from 6 to 9 months; few patients survive 5 years.

TABLE 34.3-4. Survival Based on Pathologic Stage

Series	*Year*	*No. of Patients*	*5-Y Survival Rate (%)* P2	P3	P4
Richie	1975	134	39	40	—
Whitmore	1980	174	50	25	18
Mather	1981	58	70	33	29
Skinner	1982	130	47	39	25
Skinner	1984	197	69	29	22
Montie	1984	99	63	57	—
Giuliani	1991	202	56	19	—
Roehrborn	1991	280	61	36	27
Pagano	1991	261	50	15	21
Wishnow	1992	71	75	48	—
Waehre	1997	227	60	31	29
Herr	1999	686	58	22	15
Totals		2519	57	31	24

Note: Replaces previous T4.
(From ref. 20 with permission.)

PATHOGENESIS

The natural history of a urothelial tumor is recurrence. Recurrences may develop at any time, at the same or separate site of the urothelial tract, and at the same or a more advanced stage. This is termed *polychronotopism* and has led investigators to postulate that a field defect occurs in the urothelial tract, resulting in a genetically unstable urothelium that facilitates the continued development of new lesions. The observation of atypia in the urothelial lining of smokers is consistent with this view. An area of controversy is whether tumors that occur in separate sites in the urothelial tract are derived from the same clone or are polyclonal in origin. Reports by Sidransky et al.,[23] demonstrating the clonality of multiple bladder tumors from different sites, and by Miyao et al.,[24] showing concordant genetic alterations in asynchronous tumors from individual patients, suggest that disparate urothelial tumors are derived from the same neoplastic clone.

Studies of different stages and grades of bladder cancer have shown a higher frequency of genetic abnormalities in advanced-stage lesions. The changes are classified as primary chromosomal

TABLE 34.3-5. Survival of Patients with Node-Positive Bladder Cancer

Series	*Year*	*Patients*	*5-Y Survival Rate (%)*
Whitmore	1981	134	7
Smith	1983	230	4
Skinner	1984	36	35
Vieweg	1991	229	19
Pagano	1991	26	4
Herr	1999	193	22

Note: Replaces previous T5.
(Adapted from ref. 22.)

aberrations if they are associated with the development of the disease or as secondary if they are associated with progression to a more advanced stage.[1] These changes represent the activation of protooncogenes by point mutation, amplification, or translocation that results in a gain of function and the inactivation of tumor suppressor genes, primarily by allelic deletion and point mutation of the contralateral allele, which results in a "negative" event. In general, deletions of *17p* (the TP53 locus) and the *RB* gene locus are seen in patients with invasive disease, whereas aberrations of *9q* occur predominantly in superficial tumors.[25]

Several studies report associations between specific pathologic and molecular markers and prognosis.[26] More significantly, tumor markers are beginning to be incorporated into clinical practice. Caution is advised when interpreting the results of different studies because of the different sensitivities of the technique used, the specific stage of the tumor included, the number of patients, and the follow-up interval on which the conclusions are based. An example of the differences is provided by the reported results evaluating *p53* alterations. These have variably been assessed by immunohistochemical staining, single-strand conformational polymorphism analysis, and direct sequencing of different gene exons. With a panel of antibodies that recognize the mutated *p53* protein, nuclear overexpression correlated with grade, stage, vascular invasion, and the presence of nodal metastases. Multivariate analyses showed that *p53* mutation is associated with a higher frequency of progression to a more advanced stage and a higher rate of death from bladder cancer.[27–29] The status of p53 is currently being used to stratify patients for risk of metastasis, probability of nonmetastasis, and response to specific chemotherapeutic regimens. Whether determinations of *p53* can provide more information than staging and grade for the choice between different treatment modalities remains to be investigated in comparative trials.

TREATMENT

Treatment selection is based on the extent or stage of disease. For certain patients, one therapeutic modality is sufficient. For others, a combined-modality approach is required. For superficial tumors, cystoscopic resection with and without intravesical therapy is preferred. Once invasion into muscle is documented, the standard treatment is surgical removal of the bladder. After cystectomy, and depending on whether disease is documented outside the bladder, systemic therapies may be advised. Developing standards of care beyond single-modality approaches has been hampered by inconclusive clinical trials. Demonstrating the superiority of one treatment approach over another requires large numbers of patients and long follow-up to be clinically meaningful. Furthermore, the higher the morbidity of the "new" approach, the greater the reluctance to offer it to patients.

SUPERFICIAL DISEASE

The standard initial treatment of superficial bladder tumors is a complete cystoscopic resection. The majority of patients develop new tumors over time, 30% of which progress to a higher stage. As a result, vigilant follow-up with cystoscopy, urine cytology, and repeat transurethral resections (TURs) as needed are performed every 3 to 6 months, at least for the first 5 years of follow-up. Depending on the number of lesions, the size, the depth of invasion, and the number of prior tumors in that individual, intravesical therapy may or may not be recommended. Intravesical treatment is rarely advised for the first Ta tumor that is low-grade, although it is recommended for high-grade Ta, Tis, and T1 lesions.

Intravesical therapies are used for two indications: therapeutic and adjuvant or prophylactic. The former refers to the clinical situation in which residual disease remains in the bladder despite an attempt at a complete endoscopic resection. This is relatively infrequent except in cases with CIS. Prophylactic or adjuvant therapy is applied when a patient has shown a repeated tendency to develop new lesions in the bladder. The recurrences may represent new papillary lesions, CIS, or a combination of both.

Intravesical instillations have been performed with chemotherapeutic agents, such as thiotepa, doxorubicin (Adriamycin), and mitomycin C; immunologic agents, such as bacille Calmette-Guérin (BCG); and cytokines, such as interferon and interleukin.[30–32] For all agents, the mechanism of action is debated. Although the rationale for instilling chemotherapeutic agents initially was a postulated direct toxic effect on the tumor cells, a nonspecific inflammatory reaction is also believed to be contributory. Side effects include the local toxicities based on the instillation itself and whether the drug is systemically absorbed. The latter depends partly on the size of the molecule, the pH at the time of instillation, and the timing of the instillation relative to the diagnostic and therapeutic cystoscopy. All intravesical treatments have some side effects in common, especially those related to bladder irritation, such as dysuria and frequency, but also other unique side effects specific to a particular drug, such as myelosuppression or contact dermatitis. BCG differs in one important aspect from the chemotherapeutic agents: A small proportion of patients develop a systemic "BCGosis" requiring treatment with tuberculostatic agents and steroids. Deaths have been reported. Allowing 2 to 3 weeks for healing after the endoscopic resection has been performed and before chemotherapy or BCG is administered reduces the chance of severe local or systemic toxicities.

Indications for intravesical instillations vary. Generally, the indications for adjuvant therapy include two or more tumor recurrences in a given year, the presence of diffuse Tis or multiple papillary tumors, or the identification of T1 disease that carries a high risk of stage progression. The risk of tumor recurrence and progression is associated with tumor type (Ta, T1, or Tis), tumor grade (low vs. high), length of follow-up (5 or more years), and treatment (TUR alone or TUR plus chemotherapy or BCG). The majority of papillomas and TaG1 tumors recur within 5 years, but they rarely invade or cause a cancer death. Recurrent tumors are treated with TUR or fulguration (as outpatient procedures) and are a low biologic risk. On the other hand, almost all high-grade (G3) Ta tumors recur within 2 to 3 years, 20% progress in stage within 5 years, and 30% to 40% progress by 10 years. All adjuvant treatments using thiotepa, doxorubicin, mitomycin C, or BCG decrease the probability of tumor recurrences over TUR alone. BCG has been shown to delay tumor progression to a more advanced stage, to decrease the need for cystectomy, and to improve survival.[33–35]

Tis is generally treated by a combination of endoscopic resection followed by the intravesical instillation of BCG.[36] This recommendation is based on the results of large-scale randomized comparisons showing its proven superiority relative to doxorubicin[37] and mitomycin C.[38] In the past, thiotepa was the most widely used agent, but it is now used less frequently because of limited efficacy and high frequency of myelosuppression. BCG is typically instilled weekly for 6 weeks. BCG eradicates Tis for more than 1 year in 70% of cases and prevents subsequent disease for 5 years in 60% of cases and for up to 10 years in 40% of cases.[36]

Treatment-predictive information is provided by follow-up evaluation after 3 and 6 months and whether the bladder has been rendered tumor free, both endoscopically and cytologically.[35] If it is not, some urologists recommend a repeat course of treatment. The maintenance role of BCG treatments has been debated. Some feel that regular treatment beyond the initial 6-week course further delays tumor recurrence and progression. Others believe that continued BCG not only increases the frequency of complications but fails to reduce tumor progression.[39] Patients who have recurrent or persistent tumors after one or two cycles of intravesical therapy are often considered for cystectomy.

TUR alone is generally sufficient for noninvasive papillary (Ta) tumors. In some patients, the disease does not recur and, if no disease is documented after several sequential 3-month evaluations, the follow-up can be restricted to a yearly examination. In other cases in which recurrences are documented, more frequent and longer follow-up is essential. In these cases, intravesical therapy has been shown to diminish both the probability of recurrences and the number of tumors documented at a given recurrence.[40] Because the probability of progression to a more advanced stage is low, however, no definitive benefit of delayed progression or improved survival has been shown. The decision to administer such therapy must be balanced by the adverse effects and potential benefit of therapy. Intravesical therapy is commonly recommended if the number of recurrent episodes during a 24-month period exceeds two[41] and if a large part of the urinary bladder wall is covered with tumors. Repeat cystoscopic examinations are generally advised at 3- to 6-month intervals, depending on the number of tumor recurrences, for the first 5 years, and annually thereafter in the absence of tumor recurrence.[42]

Were it possible to determine which tumors were destined to progress to an invasive stage, early cystectomy would be preferred. Currently, no single factor or combination of factors has been useful in guiding treatment selection for patients with superficial disease. Some surgeons suggest radical surgery in patients with multiple tumors and frequent recurrences, especially if such tumors recur despite BCG therapy. Other agents undergoing clinical trials for BCG-refractory bladder tumors include gemcitabine, taxanes, broperimine, and valrubicine (AD 32).

Recurrences after intravesical treatment can develop anywhere that transitional epithelium exists, including the renal pelvis, ureters, and urethra. In fact, one consequence of the "successful" treatment of tumors in the bladder is an increase in the frequency of extravesical recurrences.[43] In patients with multifocal CIS, the risk of developing an upper tract tumor is 15% at 5 years, 25% at 10 years, and 33% with 15-year follow-up. Tumor involvement of the prostatic urethra and ducts may be detected in 10% to 15% of cases in 5 years and in 20% to 40% within 10 years. Patients with a positive cytology and no obvious tumor in the bladder need careful monitoring of the upper tracts.[44] Tumors of the upper tract are particularly difficult to manage, because contact between a topical therapeutic agent and the diseased urothelium is limited. The development of tumors in extravesical sites is cited as evidence of the "field change" theory of carcinogenesis. Selected tumors in the ureter or renal pelvis may be managed by ureteroscopic resection or, in some cases, by instilling BCG through the renal pelvis. Tumors of the prostatic urethra are frequently managed by cystectomy, particularly if a complete resection cannot be accomplished.

The prevalence of panurothelial tumor diathesis suggests that chemoprevention strategies will be needed as an adjunct to active therapy directed against the primary bladder tumors. Broperimine, an interferon inducer, and fenretinide (4-HPR), a synthetic retinoid, are being investigated as oral chemoprevention agents, but neither appears to be effective (National Cancer Institute and Bladder Cancer Italian Trial Group [BLINST], unpublished data, 1999).

T1 DISEASE

The T1 tumor is an invasive (lamina propria) neoplasm. Virtually all are high-grade, and one-half the cases have associated Tis. Recurrence rates are 50% by 1 year, 80% by 3 years, and 90% within 5 years.[45] Considering progression, 50% of T1G3 cases develop invasive disease within 5 years; this number rises to 80% if associated Tis is in the pathologic specimen. Because of the high risk of progression, T1 tumors are generally treated with intravesical therapy. BCG reduces tumor recurrence in 50% of patients and reduces the progression rate to 15% at 5 years and 50% at 10 years. These rates mean that 50% of patients with T1 tumors will develop a muscle-invasive cancer in 10 years, despite the best available conservative therapy. Each present and recurrent T1 tumor has a 5% to 10% probability of distant metastasis. The survival rate is 70% at 5 years with BCG therapy and resembles that achieved after immediate radical cystectomy. On the other hand, patients who relapse with recurrent T1 tumors within 6 months to 1 year after an adequate trial of TUR and BCG (one or two courses) are best treated currently with cystectomy.[46]

MUSCLE-INVADING TUMORS

Therapies for muscle-infiltrating disease can be divided into bladder-sparing and non–bladder-sparing (see Table 34.3-3). The standard treatment is surgical removal of the entire organ by radical cystectomy. In appropriately selected cases, an aggressive TUR may be adequate, although this is controversial.[47] In other cases, a resection is combined with radiation or chemotherapy. These combined-modality approaches are limited to selected cases. End points include time to recurrence, in either the primary or a distant site, disease-free status, and overall survival.

Radical cystectomy achieves the best local control of invasive bladder cancer. The exact indications vary between institutions. Most physicians recommend cystectomy for (1) muscle-invading tumors unsuitable for segmental resection, (2) low-stage tumors unsuitable for conservative management (i.e., because of multicentric and frequent recurrences resistant to intravesical instillations), (3) high-grade tumors (T1G3) associated with Tis, or (4) bladder symptoms, such as frequency or hemorrhage, rendering the patient a "bladder cripple." Survival distributions are expected to vary for patients who undergo treatment for these indications.

SURGICAL APPROACHES

Radical cystectomy in men involves the *en bloc* removal of the bladder, prostate, seminal vesicles, and proximal urethra, with a wide margin of pelvic adipose tissue and peritoneum. Loss of sexual

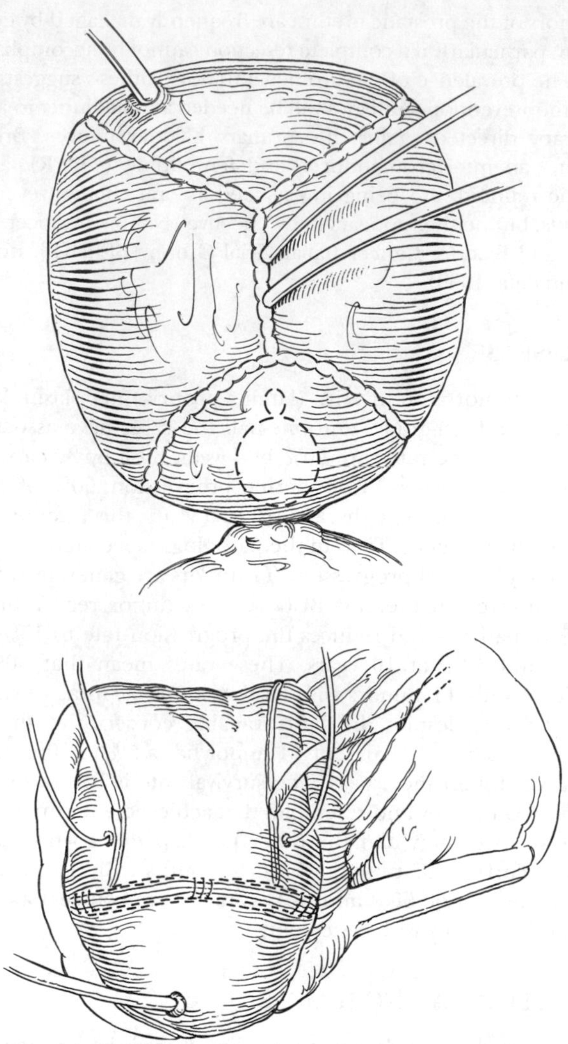
A
B

FIGURE 34.3-2. The ileoneobladder (**A**) and the Indiana reservoir (**B**).

function is often a consequence of the operation. In women, the procedure involves an anterior exenteration to remove the bladder, urethra, uterus, fallopian tubes, ovaries, anterior vaginal wall, and surrounding fascia. Pelvic lymph nodes are also removed.

Urinary flow is directed through a conduit diversion or a continent reservoir, a bladder substitute. In the standard ileal conduit, urine drains directly from the ureters through a segment of ileum to the skin surface, where it is collected. No internal reservoir is created. A few patients with this form of diversion develop hypochloremic acidosis, hyperkalemia, hyponatremia, and uremia. Ureteral obstruction and urinary tract infection are also relatively common.

Continent reservoirs are becoming increasingly popular and include external continent stomas, which the patient self-catheterizes at regular intervals, and internal, orthotopic neobladders that can be fashioned in both men and women. All involve the creation of a low-pressure reservoir from a detubularized segment of bowel that is then anastomosed to either abdominal wall (Indiana pouch) or the urethra (neobladder) (Fig. 34.3-2).[48,49] When an anastomosis to the urethra is created, primarily in men without urethral disease, the patient can void in the natural position. Complication rates are acceptable and most patients achieve urinary continence. An indication for urethrectomy precludes the creation of a urethral anastomosis, such as documented CIS or exophytic tumor in the urethra but also tumors that involve the bladder neck, rendering spread to the urethra likely. In addition, elderly or infirm patients or those with locally extensive tumors who are at high risk of local recurrence are better served with an ileal conduit. An ileal stoma has fewer complications than continent diversions and is less demanding on the patient for daily care.

Medical clearance before cystectomy is essential and includes optimizing cardiac medication and nutritional status. Complications of the operation include those typical for major surgery and those specific to the cystectomy. Among the former are adverse reactions to the agents used during anesthesia, blood loss and complications secondary to blood transfusions, pulmonary depression, myocardial damage secondary to prolonged anesthesia time or blood loss, and wound infection. Complications specific to cystectomy include rectal perforation and pelvic abscesses. Early and late complications associated with the urinary diversion procedure include intestinal obstruction, acute pyelonephritis, ureteral obstruction, stomal stenosis, intestinal fistula, renal calculus, and ureteroileal urinary leakage. Outcomes are usually reported on the basis of 5-year survival rates. As Tables 34.3-4 and 34.3-5 show,[20,22] survival rates vary inversely with depth of invasion and lymph node status. In most cases, patients succumb to distant disease, believed to be the result of the continued growth of micrometastases present at the time of surgery. This, in turn, has led to the integration of systemic chemotherapy to manage these tumors. Survival is also improved and complications are minimized in patients who undergo cystectomy by experienced surgeons in centers that treat a high volume of bladder cancer.[50]

RADIOTHERAPY AS DEFINITIVE TREATMENT

In some countries, external-beam radiotherapy is considered standard but not in the United States. It is also recommended for patients deemed unfit for cystectomy, based on either comorbid conditions or disease extent. In most series, despite negative selection, results are inferior to those observed with radical surgery. These results are partially because of the difficulty of rendering the bladder tumor-free by external-beam radiation alone and the continued risk for developing new tumors in the retained bladder.

In most cases, treatments are delivered in five daily fractions a week, ranging from 2.0 to 2.5 Gy to a total treatment dosage of 55 to 65 Gy without interruptions. In designing the radiation fields to treat a patient with bladder cancer, the target is best defined by information from the planning cystogram, the CT scan, the cystoscopic and bimanual examinations, and having the bladder empty to assist setup reproducibility and adequate coverage of the tumor at each treatment. Even with these efforts, a prospective CT study from Manchester reported significant movement in the bladder target volume, with possible underdosing of the tumor in one-third of the evaluated patients.[51] Thus, care must be taken to ensure that the target volume is well defined and adequate margins are included, especially posteriorly.[52,53]

The initial complete response (CR) rate (T0), based on clinical restaging with a cystoscopy and biopsy after conventional radiation, is 40% to 52% (Table 34.3-6).[54–58] For patients who do not respond completely or whose disease progresses locally without metastases and who are medically fit, a salvage cystectomy is performed. When radiation is used in patients with T2 to T4 disease,

TABLE 34.3-6. Local Control Based on Clinical Staging Radiotherapy Alone

Series	*Patients*	*Stage*	*5-Y Survival Rate (%)*	*5-Y Rate of Local Control in the Bladder (%)*
London Hospital[54]	182	T2–T3	40	41
UK Cooperative Group[55]	157	T3	23	45
Princess Margaret Hospital[56]	121	T2–T4a	40	35
Sydney, Prince of Wales[57]	342	T1–T4b	—	45
Belgium-Netherlands Group[58]	147	T2, T3	31	35

the probability of keeping the bladder free of disease at 5 years ranges from 35% to 45%; overall survival is from 23% to 40%. Toxicities are classified as acute or chronic, with radiation delivery to the rectum and bladder being dose-limiting, and include symptoms of an irritated bowel and bladder, inflammation of the skin, and fatigue. A persistent proctitis, with bleeding and secretion of mucus, is rare but does occur, and bowel obstruction may be severe enough to require a colostomy. A markedly reduced bladder capacity resulting from fibrosis may render a cystectomy or urinary diversion necessary. Sexual function can also be impaired. Occurrence of secondary tumors in the urinary bladder or the surrounding tissue is a potential late complication. Radiation techniques have evolved with surgical techniques, encouraging the therapeutic index to improve in both increased radiation dosage to tumor and decreased exposure of normal tissue with three-dimensional treatment planning.

EVOLVING STANDARDS OF CARE FOR MUSCLE-INVASIVE DISEASE: COMBINED-MODALITY APPROACHES

Developing treatment guidelines for tumors of a specific stage is easier than applying guidelines to an individual patient. For example, although the standard treatment of an invasive bladder tumor is radical cystectomy, numerous reports in the literature of selected series of patients treated by TUR alone, partial cystectomy, external-beam radiotherapy, chemotherapy, or combinations of these appear to have comparable survival rates. Given the choice, most patients prefer a bladder-sparing approach, yet cumulative results suggest that some of these alternatives produce inferior survival rates as compared to radical surgery if salvage cystectomy for local recurrence is not done promptly. Refining the choice of treatment to optimize quality of life without compromising cure is difficult, because preservation of a tumor-free bladder still has some risk of the subsequent development of a superficial or an invasive tumor.

In the 1970s and 1980s, four randomized phase III trials compared preoperative irradiation and immediate cystectomy to external-beam radiotherapy with cystectomy deferred for recurrence. Three of the four trials (involving a total of 442 patients from the United Kingdom, Denmark, and the United States National Bladder Cancer Group) found no significant difference in survival.[59–61] However, a trial of 67 patients from the M. D. Anderson Cancer Center (MDACC) is the only phase III study, to our knowledge, that shows a statistically significant survival advantage to immediate versus deferred cystectomy.[62] Combined-modality treatment with bladder preservation as an alternative to cystectomy is still investigational, and we recommend that such therapy be administered by dedicated multimodality teams. This treatment may be considered a reasonable alternative, if careful cystoscopic surveillance is conducted, in patients who are deemed unfit for cystectomy and for those definitely seeking an alternative to radical cystectomy.

Strong inferential data also suggest improved outcomes for which randomized trials are not truly definitive. The role of postoperative or adjuvant chemotherapy is one such scenario. Difficulties are encountered in interpreting both negative and positive outcomes. In a negative-outcomes trial designed in 1980 with the best available therapy at the time, for example, only 19% of patients enrolled actually received full doses of the planned chemotherapy.[63] Not administering treatment virtually guarantees failure. Furthermore, instead of being representative of the population of bladder cancer patients as a whole, many trials enroll only highly selected patients. This situation is illustrated in a study in which only 17 of 41 randomly selected patients completed therapy in a specific treatment program; these patients were derived from 453 patients with invasive disease seen at the treating institution over the same interval.[64] Extrapolating these results to all patients can be misleading. If a treatment is associated with significant morbidity or may increase mortality, the question becomes: What is the level of benefit a physician requires to adopt the approach as a standard? Considering the difficulties encountered in completing clinical trials in this disease, a more effective developmental strategy might be conducting trials in populations who have specific high-risk factors for developing metastatic disease and in whom treatment effects can be discerned rapidly.

Preoperative Radiotherapy

In the 1970s, moderate-dose preoperative radiation, either 20 Gy by accelerated fractionation or 40 to 50 Gy with conventional fractionation, was the standard. The results showed that radiotherapy alone could eradicate disease in the resected specimen and the regional lymph nodes in a small but definite proportion of patients.[65,66] The technique was largely abandoned when no survival benefit was observed in randomized comparisons.[67]

A recent trial at the MDACC identified a clinical subset for whom radiotherapy might be beneficial. The trial included 135 patients with clinical stage T3 tumors who were treated by either preoperative radiotherapy and cystectomy (92 patients) or cystectomy without irradiation (43 patients), using modern-day surgical techniques and adjunctive multiagent chemotherapy.[68] Although no survival benefit was observed, the results showed a significant decrease in pelvic recurrence rates from 28% to 9% at 5 years for patients with T3 disease who received radiation. No difference was observed for patients with T2 disease. Because the true rate of pelvic recurrences after radical surgery is not known, as disease in most patients who experience relapse systemically is

TABLE 34.3-7. Randomized Trials of Irradiation Plus Cystectomy versus Radiation and Deferred (Salvage) Cystectomy

Series	*Treatment*	*No. of Patients*	*Stage*	*5-Y Survival Rate (%)*	*Distant Metastases (%)*
M. D. Anderson Cancer Center[62]	50 Gy + cystectomy	35	T3	46	—
	60 Gy + salvage cystectomy	32		22	—
U.K. Cooperative Group[60]	40 Gy + radical cystectomy	98	T3	39	—
	60 Gy + salvage cystectomy	91		28	—
National Danish Trial[59]	40 Gy + radical cystectomy	88	T3	29	34
	60 Gy + salvage cystectomy	95		23	32
National Bladder Cancer Group (1983)[a]	50 Gy + radical cystectomy	37	T2–4a	27	38
	60–68 Gy + salvage cystectomy	35		40	31

[a]S. D. Cutler, personal communication, 1983.

not restaged locally, the study raises the question whether precystectomy radiation might be an option for patients who present with extravesical tumors. With drawbacks including the potential effect on the ability to create internal urinary reservoirs with irradiated bowel, the question requires prospective evaluation.

Postoperative Radiotherapy

When a positive surgical margin is documented after cystectomy, local recurrence rates are high with or without chemotherapy. However, no randomized trial has evaluated the use of postoperative radiation for patients with transitional cell tumors. A Radiation Therapy Oncology Group (RTOG) phase II trial of postoperative irradiation reported the incidence of small bowel obstruction or fistula in 30% of patients.[69] Recently, investigators using multivariate analysis in a retrospective study of 92 patients from Milan reported that patients without evidence of nodal metastases receiving 50.4 Gy after radical cystectomy had significantly improved cancer-specific and disease-specific survival rates.[70] With a median follow-up of 36 months, one of 32 irradiated patients has required reoperation for bowel toxicity. While encouraging, this result requires longer follow-up to be considered for further prospective evaluation. One randomized trial evaluating postoperative radiotherapy has been completed in Egypt for patients with squamous cell carcinomas.[71] In this trial, the rate of pelvic recurrences was reduced from 50% to 10% in the irradiated patients. It must be noted that squamous cell tumors seen in the Middle East tend to recur locally and have a low metastatic rate as compared to the transitional cell tumors that occur in North America, which have a high metastatic rate.

Deferred Cystectomy: Treatment with External-Beam Radiation and Salvage Cystectomy

Four randomized trials have addressed the question of whether a regimen of preoperative radiation and immediate cystectomy compares with one of external-beam radiotherapy followed by a salvage cystectomy for radiation failures. A small trial with 67 patients showed a difference in survival at 5 years,[62] and a second showed a lower frequency of pelvic recurrence but no survival difference with combined modality therapy.[59] Based on the sample sizes, a 25% difference, either negative or positive, could not be excluded (Table 34.3-7; S. D. Cutler, personal communication, 1983).[59,60,62] Nevertheless, the trials do suggest that deferring a cystectomy until local progression is documented does not appear to affect adversely the rate of metastases or to compromise overall survival.

INTEGRATING SYSTEMIC CHEMOTHERAPY

The major cause of death in patients with invasive bladder cancer is metastatic disease. In most cases, the course of tumor relapse supports the concept that micrometastases are present at the time of initial therapy. The primary role for chemotherapy in the perioperative setting is to increase survival. Additionally, a substantial number of studies address the use of chemotherapy alone and concurrent with radiotherapy to preserve the native bladder. Specific considerations in evaluating chemotherapy's role in patients presenting with invasive disease include the activity of the various combinations of multiagent therapy—as judged by the proportion of patients with known metabolic diseases who achieve complete remissions and are ultimately cured—and the number of patients needed to prove the benefit of currently available therapies. Reviewing the activity of chemotherapy in metastatic disease provides insight into the studies exploring perioperative chemotherapy.

Chemotherapy

Urothelial cancer is a chemotherapy-sensitive neoplasm. A broad number of single agents with different mechanisms of action are effective (Table 34.3-8).[61,72–78] Complete responses using older agents are rare; most produce partial responses, with response durations of approximately 3 to 4 months. Recently, several agents were identified as active in phase I and II studies, including docetaxel, paclitaxel, gemcitabine, piritrexim, and ifosfamide. Observations distinguishing these new, active agents from older drugs are moderate activity as both first- and second-line therapy[79,80]; favorable toxicity profiles[73,76]; drug metabolism independent of renal excretion[61]; and CR in metastatic disease to a single agent.[73,76]

Combination Chemotherapy: Randomized Trial Results

Clinical outcomes (i.e., response and survival) are better for multiagent therapy than those observed with single-agent treatment in advanced TCC. The regimens most extensively studied in the 1980s were cisplatin, cyclophosphamide, and Adriamycin (CISCA); cisplatin, methotrexate, and vinblastine (CMV); and

TABLE 34.3-8. Cumulative Results with Single-Agent Chemotherapy Used in Metastatic or Unresectable Disease

Agent	*No. of Patients*	*Response (%)*	*95% Confidence Intervals*
Cisplatin	522	24	20–28
Carboplatin	327	14	10–18
Methotrexate	293	29	24–34
Doxorubicin	274	17	13–22
Vinblastine	38	16	4–28
Cyclophosphamide	98	31	22–40
5-Fluorouracil	141	17	11–25
Mitomycin C	42	13	2–22
Ifosfamide	101	28	19–37
Docetaxel	29	31	17–50
Paclitaxel	35	46	29–63
Gemcitabine	112	22	15–30

Note: Data are compiled irrespective of trial design (i.e., phase II or phase III dose and schedule).
(Data compiled from refs. 61 and 72–78.)

methotrexate, vinblastine, Adriamycin, and cisplatin (M-VAC; Table 34.3-9).[74,81–105] These regimens demonstrate strikingly similar CR and overall response proportions in 20% to 22% and 50% to 60% of patients, respectively. The comparable efficacy and toxicity of the various regimens were discerned by randomized trial results. The CMV combination was superior to methotrexate and vinblastine without cisplatin; CMV was associated with significantly longer progression-free survival (4.5 months vs. 2.5 months) and 1-year survival (28% vs. 16%).[83] M-VAC was superior to single-agent cisplatin in both response and survival.[84] In the only direct comparison of cisplatin-based combinations, M-VAC was superior to CISCA.[85] Despite the popularity of the CMV regimen, median survival in one randomized trial was only 7 months; CMV has not been directly compared with M-VAC. It is concluded from these studies that cisplatin-based therapy should be the primary consideration for all patients requiring chemotherapy, and that M-VAC should be the regimen of choice.

Undermining the favorable response data for M-VAC in advanced TCC are the toxicity of the regimen and the disappointing long-term survival. Approximately 20% to 30% of patients develop neutropenia and fever, and 10% to 20% experience mucositis.[84] Diminished renal function, a decrease in auditory acuity, and peripheral neuropathy may also be seen. Death as a complication of M-VAC therapy occurs in 3% to 4% of patients.[81,84] Despite promising overall response proportions, the median survival for patients receiving M-VAC is consistently reported to be approximately 1 year,[81,84,85] and follow-up of the intergroup trial reported that only 3.7% of M-VAC patients remained continuously relapse-free at 6 years.[106]

Impact of Pretreatment Prognostic Factors and Postchemotherapy Surgery

Several analyses demonstrated that pretreatment prognostic features affect the outcome of patients treated with M-VAC chemotherapy for metastatic TCC.[84,106,107] Prognostic factors predicting poor response and survival are bone or liver metastases (determined either by radiographic abnormality or by an elevated baseline alkaline phosphatase) and poor performance status. The intergroup study by Loehrer et al.[84] reported a median survival of 18.2 months for patients with the most favorable combination of prognostic features, compared with only 4.4 months for patients with the least favorable combination; none of the patients with liver or bone metastasis and only one patient with Karnofsky performance score (KPS) of less than 80% survived for 6 years.[106] The impact of prognostic features on survival was further emphasized in an analysis of more than 200 patients with metastatic or unresectable disease treated with M-VAC in Memorial Sloan-Kettering Cancer Center (MSKCC) phase I and II trials. The median survival was 14.8 months at a median follow-up of 40 months, and 5-year survival was 17%; at the time of the report, 19 of the 203 patients (9%) were alive. Three strata with distinctly different long-term survival rates were developed using the presence of any visceral metastasis and a KPS of less than 80.[108] No patient with both a poor KPS and visceral metastases experienced long-term survival, in contrast to an 11% 5-year survival in patients with either a poor KPS or visceral disease and a 33% likelihood of 5-year survival in patients with none of these poor-risk features.

Several studies show that postchemotherapy resection of persistent viable cancer in selected patients after M-VAC and CMV chemotherapy for unresectable or metastatic disease enhances long-term survival in patients who would have otherwise succumbed to their disease.[109–111] Criteria to select the optimal candidates are not uniform. However, retrospective analysis from MSKCC suggests that benefit is greatest in patients who have had a major response to chemotherapy and have persistent disease restricted to the primary lesion or a single site of metastatic disease in a lymph node or lung.[111]

Dose-Intensity Studies

One strategy for improving therapeutic response is to increase drug delivery (or dose intensity in milligrams per square meter per week). This approach appeared promising because of a dose-response relationship suggested for cisplatin and doxorubicin and evidence of benefit in patients failing standard-dose therapy when hematopoietic growth factors were given to increase drug dose in the salvage setting.[112] Trials have reported dose-intensive therapy with M-VAC using either recombinant human granulocyte-macrophage colony-stimulating factor or human granulocyte colony-stimulating factor.[113–116] These studies demonstrated that it is possible to increase drug delivery by as much as 60% over standard-dose M-VAC either by increasing the doses of the individual agents or decreasing the cycling intervals (or both). Toxicities seen with the dose-intense regimens range from side effects that resemble standard-dose M-VAC to substantially increased toxicity and an increased toxic death rate.[113,116] Despite more intensive chemotherapy, the CR proportions for these studies still approximate 20%, suggesting no meaningful impact on survival. A randomized trial in the European Organization for Research and Treatment of Cancer (EORTC) is evaluating whether dose-intense M-VAC improves survival over standard-dose therapy.

NEW CHEMOTHERAPEUTIC REGIMENS. Developing new agents and combining agents is necessary if improvement in long-term survival or reduction of chemotherapy-associated toxicity (or both) is to be achieved. In combination chemotherapy trials, several cytotoxic agents introduced in this

TABLE 34.3-9. Cisplatin- and Carboplatin-Containing Regimens Used to Treat Urothelial Carcinoma

Regimen	Agents	Schedule	Composite No. of Assessable Patients (with Studies)	Response (%) CR	Response (%) OR	Median Survival (mo)	Comments
Randomized trials							
M-VAC	Methotrexate	30 mg/m² days 1, 15, 22	180[84,85]	13–35	39–65	12.5–12.6	M-VAC superior to cisplatin and to CISCA regimen
	Vinblastine	3 mg/m² days 2, 15, 22					
	Doxorubicin (Adriamycin)	30 mg/m² day 2					
	Cisplatin	70 mg/m² day 2					
CMV	Methotrexate	30 mg/m² days 1, 8	104[83,a]	10	36	7	CMV superior to methotrexate and vinblastine
	Vinblastine	4 mg/m² days 1, 8					
	Cisplatin	70 mg/m² day 2					
Phase II trials	Cisplatin	70–75 mg/m² day 1	76[86–88]	10–34	62–72	13	—
	Paclitaxel	135–175 mg/m² over 3 hr					
GC	Cisplatin	70–100 mg/m² day 1	75[99,100]	21–28	57–66	14	—
	Gemcitabine	1000 mg/m² days 1, 8, 15					
	Docetaxel	75 mg/m² day 1	25[89]	26	60	13.6	
	Cisplatin	75 mg/m² day 1					
TCG	Cisplatin	70 mg/m² day 1	29[104]	21	79	NS	—
	Paclitaxel	80 mg/m² days 1, 8					
	Gemcitabine	100 mg/m² days 1,8					
ITP	Ifosfamide	1500 mg/m² days 1–3	44[102,103]	23	68	20	—
	Paclitaxel	200 mg/m² day 1					
	Cisplatin	70 mg/m² day 1					
	Paclitaxel	150–225 mg/m² day 1	210[91–97]	8–40	14–65	8.5–9.5	
	Carboplatin	AUC = 5–6 day 1					
	Gemcitabine	800 mg/m² days 1, 8	19[105]	26	58	NS	
	Paclitaxel	200 mg/m² day 1					
	Carboplatin	AUC = 5, day 1					

AUC, plasma concentration time-curve (area under the curve) of the drug; CISCA, cisplatin, cyclophosphamide, and doxorubicin (Adriamycin); CR, complete response; NS, not stated; OR, overall response.
[a]104 patients assessable for survival and 88 assessable for response.
Note: Studies selected are phase II studies and randomized trials published in either abstracts or articles.

decade are undergoing evaluation for treating urothelial tumors. The most extensively studied agents are gemcitabine, a deoxycytidine analog with structural similarities to cytarabine, and the taxanes: paclitaxel and docetaxel.

Most combination regimens include a platinum analog, either cisplatin or carboplatin, in part because of the reported complementary or synergistic actions of these new agents with platinum analogs. The single-agent activity of carboplatin in urothelial cancer appears less than that observed with cisplatin (see Table 34.3-8).[61,72–78] Controversy exists as to whether the efficacy of carboplatin combinations compares favorably with cisplatin combinations. A small, randomized phase II trial compared M-VAC with the carboplatin-based regimen of methotrexate, carboplatin, and vinblastine.[117] Relative to M-VAC, the carboplatin-containing regimen produced a lower response proportion (52% vs. 39%) and shorter median survival (16 vs. 9 months). Criticisms of the trial included the phase II nature of the study (i.e., a small number of patients) and the lack of doxorubicin in the carboplatin arm.

Cisplatin combinations are associated with greater renal, neurologic, and auditory toxicity; they are more difficult to administer to patients who have renal impairment or other medical comorbidities. In contrast, carboplatin is not only more feasible in the patient with impaired renal function or medical comorbidities, it is more easily administered in the outpatient setting. Although carboplatin has greater myelosuppression, this toxicity is easily managed by adjusting the dose according to the patient's creatinine clearance to provide a predetermined area under the plasma concentration–time curve (AUC) of the drug. The controversy surrounding the efficacy of carboplatin- versus cisplatin-containing therapy in phase II trials is being addressed by ongoing and planned randomized phase III trials.

NEW TWO- AND THREE-DRUG COMBINATIONS AS FIRST-LINE THERAPY. The combinations of either paclitaxel (42% to 55% single-agent activity)[61,76] or docetaxel (31% activity)[78,118] with cisplatin (at 70 to 75 mg/m²/course) have been evaluated in four phase II trials.[86–89] Three trials evaluating paclitaxel at 135 to 175 mg/m² over 3 hours in combination with cisplatin produced overall response rates ranging from 62% to 72% and CR rates ranging from 10% to 34%.[86–88] Responses were predominantly in lymph node and lung metastases; however, some patients with liver or adrenal metastases also responded.[87] A median survival of 13 months was reported in one of the trials.[86] Myelosuppression and neurotoxicity were the most common toxicities. This two-drug combination is active, generally well tolerated, and can be given in the outpatient setting. Docetaxel (75 mg/m²) and cisplatin had a major response in 60% of patients; 7 of 25 (28%) patients achieved CR, with a median survival rate of 13.6 months.[89] The most predominant toxicity was granulocytopenia, but fluid retention, neuropathy, and mucositis were also observed. No plans exist to compare further either the paclitaxel-cisplatin or the docetaxel-cisplatin doublet to standard therapy.

The paclitaxel-carboplatin doublet has been evaluated in numerous phase II trials. The initial phase I–phase II trial exploring paclitaxel doses of 150 to 225 mg/m² in a 3-hour infusion plus carboplatin at an AUC of 6 every 3 weeks reported an overall response rate of 51%.[90] Trials 90 through 97 of more than 200 patients treated with paclitaxel (150 to 225 mg/m²) and carboplatin (AUC of 5 to 6) have provided several important observations. The regimen is well tolerated; myelosuppression is the most common toxicity, but granulocytopenic fever and cycling delays for hematologic toxicity are uncommon. Neurotoxicity is commonly observed but is not severe. Response rates vary, ranging from 14% to 65%, with CR rates ranging from 0% to 40%. Efficacy is highest among patients with lymph node metastases, but patients with lung and liver metastases also respond. No clear dose-response correlations exist for either paclitaxel or carboplatin. Mature results are not available for all studies, but the survival rate ranges from 8.5 to 9.5 months in the three trials reporting survival data.[95–97] It is as yet unclear whether this doublet has survival inferior to the approximately 1-year survival seen with M-VAC or that the reported phase II results are affected by pretreatment prognostic factors,[88] the small number of patients resulting in wide confidence intervals of efficacy parameters, or the inclusion of previously treated patients.[95–97]

Gemcitabine (single-agent activity of 22% to 28%)[73–75,79] has been examined in combination with cisplatin. Von der Maase et al.[98] reported on 37 assessable patients using a weekly regimen of both gemcitabine and cisplatin. Although the response rate was 41%, toxicity was severe, with granulocytopenia of at least grade 3 in 46% and thrombocytopenia of at least grade 3 in 71% of patients. The schedule of gemcitabine at 1000 mg/m² on days 1, 8, and 15 and cisplatin on day 1 was explored in two separate trials conducted in the United States and Canada.[99,100] Kaufman et al.[99] explored this schedule with an initial cisplatin dose of 100 mg/m². Toxicity was excessive, so the dose of cisplatin was reduced to 75 mg/m², resulting in better patient tolerance. The overall response proportion in 38 assessable patients was 59%. Moore et al.[100] reported a 57% overall response rate with a 21% CR proportion using the same dose and schedule of gemcitabine and a cisplatin dose of 70 mg/m². This regimen is well tolerated, with predominantly hematologic toxicity and a reported median survival of 14 months. The gemcitabine-carboplatin combination is also active, with a 68% overall response proportion.[101]

The three-drug combination of ifosfamide, paclitaxel (Taxol), and cisplatin (platinum) (ITP) recycled every 4 weeks was reported by MSKCC investigators to be effective and tolerable in previously untreated patients with advanced TCC.[102,103] Thirty of 44 (68%) assessable patients (95% confidence interval, 52% to 81%) demonstrated a major response (10 complete [23%], 20 partial [45%]), with durations of response ranging from 4 to 36 months. At a median follow-up of 28 months, the median survival was 20 months.[103] Eleven (25%) patients are disease-free. The median survival of 20 months in this trial is the best reported result for unresectable or metastatic TCC patients receiving chemotherapy and is greater than previously observed experiences with M-VAC (median survival, 12 to 13 months).[81] The possibility exists that adding ifosfamide to a cisplatin-based combination may enhance survival; alternatively, the improved survival may be a consequence of favorable pretreatment prognostic factors and aggressive postchemotherapy surgery.

The combinations of gemcitabine, paclitaxel, and either cisplatin or carboplatin have been reported in two separate trials.[104,105] The cisplatin-containing triplet, reported for 29 assessable patients, demonstrated a 79% response proportion.[104] Myelosuppression and asthenia were the predominant toxicities. Investigators at Wayne State University explored the paclitaxel-gemcitabine-carboplatin regimen, building on prior experience with the paclitaxel-carboplatin regimen. In 19 assessable patients, 11 (58%) had a major response.[105]

Tu et al.[119] evaluated paclitaxel, cisplatin, and methotrexate every 3 weeks in 25 previously treated patients. Partial responses lasting from 2 to more than 9 months were achieved in ten patients (40%), including three of seven patients with liver metastases. The primary toxicity was hematologic, with 9 of 25 patients experiencing severe neutropenia, resulting in six episodes of neutropenic fever requiring hospitalization. Severe thrombocytopenia, defined as grade 3 or greater, occurred in 8 of 25 patients. Meyers et al.[120] evaluated the triplet of paclitaxel-carboplatin-methotrexate in 23 assessable patients. Adjunctive care included leucovorin and granulocyte colony-stimulating factor (G-CSF). Fourteen of 23 patients (61%) responded, including four complete responses, resulting in a median survival of 16 months. The primary toxicities were neutropenia and neurotoxicity. Leucovorin was subsequently eliminated from the regimen, and reduction of the carboplatin dose to AUC 5 allowed deletion of G-CSF.[121]

Gallium nitrate as second-line therapy sponsored first-line combinations. The initial report of the three-drug regimen of vinblastine, ifosfamide, and gallium nitrate had a 67% major response rate.[122] Activity was confirmed in the Eastern Cooperative Oncology Group (ECOG) trial, with 44% of patients responding.[123] Toxicity was substantial; ocular blindness, arrhythmias, and myelosuppression were reported. A separate randomized phase II study examined the efficacy of gallium nitrate plus fluorouracil versus dose-intense M-VAC, finding only marginal activity for the gallium combination (12% major response proportion).[124] The toxicity profile and the cost of administering gallium nitrate on a 5-day inpatient schedule limit further study. Seven of 15 (47%) patients obtained a major response to the combination of paclitaxel, vinblastine, and cisplatin.[125] Calvo et al.[126] evaluated the paclitaxel-cisplatin-fluorouracil triplet in both chemotherapy-naïve and previously treated patients. Among 12 patients, eight partial (67%) responses were observed, for an overall response rate of 75%. Grade 3 or 4 toxicity included neutropenia, thrombocytopenia, mucositis, diarrhea and vomiting, and paralytic ileus.

SECOND-LINE THERAPY AND FIRST-LINE REGIMENS WITHOUT PLATINUM ANALOGS. Regimens devoid of a platinum analog have not been extensively studied. Sweeney et al.[80] reported the combination of ifosfamide, 1000 mg/m^2 days 1 to 4, plus paclitaxel, 135 mg/m^2 by 24-hour infusion on day 4 of a 3-week cycle, using G-CSF support. Twenty-six patients were evaluable for response: Two of 13 patients (15%) treated in a second-line setting responded with CR, as did 4 (1 CR, 3 partial responses) of 13 (31%) previously untreated patients. The authors concluded that ifosfamide did not add to paclitaxel activity as first-line therapy and that paclitaxel did not increase the second-line activity of ifosfamide. The ECOG is currently exploring the combination of docetaxel and gemcitabine in chemotherapy-naïve patients, and the Hoosier Oncology Group is evaluating the combination of paclitaxel and gemcitabine.

Limited experience exists for the paclitaxel-carboplatin combination in patients with prior therapy or preexisting renal impairment. Otto et al.[127] performed a phase II trial of this doublet in combination with an antimotility agent (acellular pertussis vaccine) in 18 patients with cisplatin- and methotrexate-resistant metastatic cancer; 4 (22%) patients responded, including 2 CR (11%). It is implied from these studies that multiple-agent regimens offer no advantage over single-agent therapy in patients eligible for second-line therapy.

Randomized Trials: Developing a New Standard of Chemotherapy for Advanced Disease

Initiatives to develop a new standard of therapy with greater efficacy, better tolerance, or both are essential to improve conventional therapy. Randomized comparison to M-VAC is a critical step in this process, and two randomized comparisons to M-VAC recently have been reported. Preliminary data for improved drug delivery with dose-intense M-VAC prompted a large, prospective trial conducted by the EORTC that compares dose-intense M-VAC with conventional M-VAC to evaluate response and survival differences. A preliminary analysis demonstrated that the response rate was slightly higher in the high-dose M-VAC arm, but no statistical differences in the median survival were observed, suggesting no substantial benefit by increasing drug delivery of all four drugs simultaneously.[128] Longer follow-up is necessary to determine whether dose-intense M-VAC results in any meaningful impact on long-term survival. The second international, multicenter randomized trial compared the gemcitabine-cisplatin doublet, a combination with identified activity and good patient tolerance, to the M-VAC combination. Preliminary analysis in this trial with more than 400 patients demonstrated that the complete and overall response proportions were similar, with no statistical differences.[129] The survival distributions with early follow-up were also comparable, but long-term survival rates were not available. Drug tolerance and toxicity profiles favored the gemcitabine-cisplatin doublet. The two-drug combination was associated with delivery of a greater number of chemotherapy cycles, a smaller incidence of treatment-related death, and a lower incidence of infectious complications. Based on the results of this randomized trial, gemcitabine and cisplatin should be considered a conventional chemotherapy standard for TCC.

Two randomized trials are ongoing. 5-Fluorouracil (5-FU) combined with interferon-α alone and together with cisplatin has been reported to be active.[130] A randomized comparison of the 5-FU, interferon-α, and cisplatin combination and M-VAC regimens in chemotherapy-naïve patients is ongoing at the MDACC. The second trial ongoing in the ECOG compares the paclitaxel-carboplatin regimen with M-VAC. Carboplatin and paclitaxel is a regimen that has a favorable toxicity profile; it is easy to administer, has activity in phase II studies, and is frequently used in clinical practice. However, questions remain regarding the efficacy of this regimen in relation to M-VAC; this controversy is being addressed by comparing the paclitaxel-carboplatin regimen to standard M-VAC to determine whether this new doublet has similar efficacy with less toxicity. The phase II data for combination of gemcitabine, paclitaxel, and cisplatin have been encouraging.[104] An international randomized trial has been proposed to compare this triplet to standard therapy.

A chemotherapy hypothesis novel to urothelial cancer is being tested at MSKCC. The Norton-Simon model, a mathematical prediction of chemotherapy sensitivity based on gompertzian growth rates displayed by malignant tumors, predicts that efficacy is increased with sequenced "dose-dense" therapy using either single agents or combination regimens compared to either alternating chemotherapeutic regimens or combination chemotherapy in which maximal doses of each agent are limited by overlapping toxicity.[131,132] The sequence of Adriamycin plus gemcitabine (AG) followed by the ITP combination is under evaluation for treating unresectable or metastatic TCC. A phase I study explored the feasibility of doxorubicin at 30 to 50 mg/m^2 plus gemcitabine at 1000 to 2000 mg/m^2 every 2 weeks for six treatment cycles with G-CSF in the AG/ITP sequence.[133] Among the 14 patients assessable for response to the entire sequence, complete regression was observed in 3 (21%), and more than 50% regression occurred in 6 (43%), for an overall response rate of 64%. All six patients at the highest dose levels responded. The most common grade 3 and grade 4 toxicities were anemia and neutropenia. A preliminary report of an MSKCC phase II trial of AG at a doxorubicin dose of 50 mg/m^2 and gemcitabine dose of 2000 mg/m^2 followed by ITP is associated with an encouraging CR proportion of more than 30%.[134] An attempt to confirm the high CR proportion of this sequenced approach has been proposed in the cancer and leukemia group B.

NEOADJUVANT AND ADJUVANT CHEMOTHERAPY ROLES IN MUSCLE-INVASIVE DISEASE. Given the chemosensitivity of urothelial cancer, attempts to improve the survival of patients with muscle-invasive disease have focused on administering chemotherapy at the time of definitive treatment of the primary tumor, most commonly in the perioperative setting. This approach attempts to enhance cure based on the putative advantages of greater efficacy in a smaller volume of disease and greater cure rate in patients whose disease is restricted to nodal sites rather than visceral sites.[84,108]

Several considerations arise in analyzing the trial data. First, the odds of reducing mortality by perioperative chemotherapy are independent of the absolute odds of that event occurring in the absence of chemotherapy. For example, a group of pT4 or N+ patients (or both) would be expected to have an 80% death rate. A hypothetical 20% chemotherapy benefit in mortality will reduce the actual mortality from 80% to 64% (i.e., survival improves from 20% to 36%). However, the same 20% chemotherapeutic benefit would reduce mortality of pT2 patients from the expected 25% to only 20% (i.e., survival improves from 75% to 80%). Therefore, the heterogeneity of patient accrual will significantly affect the number of patients necessary to prove efficacy. Second, the trials should be large enough to detect important differences. A trial of adequate power and acceptable false-positive rate to detect a 10% survival advantage of one approach over the other (i.e., the demonstration of a 60% survival rate for patients receiving chemotherapy as compared to a 50% survival in those who receive local therapy alone) requires randomly selecting 1000 patients. Four hundred patients are required to detect a 15% difference and 200 to detect a 20% difference. Studies that are substantially underpowered but detect a survival difference must be reviewed with caution, since the demonstration of survival benefit may reflect a false-positive result. Third, optimal trial design requires studying optimal chemotherapy to assess survival benefit.

DILEMMA: ADJUVANT OR NEOADJUVANT CHEMOTHERAPY? If a survival benefit is conferred by perioperative chemotherapy, that benefit should be evident whether the chemotherapy is administered in an adjuvant or neoadjuvant setting. Lessons learned in treating other malignancies show that if chemotherapy is effective, survival benefit is conferred in either setting. However, such data do not exist for urothelial cancer, and advantages and disadvantages of each approach exist.

Adjuvant Chemotherapy. The major advantages for adjuvant chemotherapy are the following: (1) The risk of relapse is best predicted by pathologic stage, (2) the removal of the bladder eliminates the risk for new tumors, and (3) any potential risk of delay in surgery that may compromise cure is reduced. Radical cystectomy allows the treatment decision regarding chemotherapy to be based on the pathologic risk of recurrence, restricting chemotherapy to patient subsets most likely to benefit from chemotherapy, such as patients with pT3 to pT4 or positive lymph node (N+) disease. In addition to removing the bladder and reducing the risk of new tumor formation, repeated cystoscopy is not needed to evaluate for recurrent tumor.

The major disadvantages are that (1) drug delivery may be more difficult after surgery and (2) response to chemotherapy cannot be objectively measured. Clinical trials evaluating adjuvant therapy do not have a surrogate end point for response; therefore, long patient follow-up is necessary to determine disease recurrence and survival. Historically, patients have had more difficulty in tolerating adjuvant chemotherapy after a radical cystectomy, so drug delivery, particularly cisplatin-based therapy, may be more difficult to give in the adjuvant setting.

Nonrandomized data suggest a survival benefit for adjuvant chemotherapy.[135] In a study performed at MDACC, patients who did not receive adjuvant chemotherapy (not referred for chemotherapy, refused chemotherapy, or were considered medically unfit) were subdivided into a high-risk subgroup (defined as having resected nodal metastases, extravesical involvement of tumor, lymph-vascular permeation of the primary tumor, or pelvic visceral invasion) and low-risk subgroup (having none of the above). These untreated patients were compared to those in a second high-risk group that received adjuvant chemotherapy with cisplatin, doxorubicin, and cyclophosphamide. The 5-year, disease-free survival for the treated high-risk group was twice that of the untreated high-risk group and equaled that observed for the low-risk group. These data imply that adjuvant chemotherapy is beneficial for high-risk treated patients, but the absence of randomization and patient selection may have biased the results.

Five randomized trials have examined adjuvant therapy in muscle-invasive disease (Table 34.3-10).[64,136–139] Three trials have not shown benefit of single-agent cisplatin; the combination of cisplatin, vinblastine, and methotrexate; or a regimen of 5-FU and doxorubicin. Two trials suggest a benefit for chemotherapy over observation alone after cystectomy.[64,139] In a University of Southern California (USC) trial, patients with pT3 or pT4 or node-positive disease were randomly assigned to either observation or four cycles of cyclophosphamide, doxorubicin, and cisplatin.[64] A significant delay in time to progression was observed for patients who received chemotherapy (70% compared to 46% disease-free survival at 3 years; $P = .001$), and the improvement in survival (4.3 years vs. 2.4 years) was also statistically significant ($P = .0062$). Flaws in this trial include (1) low numbers of patients, (2) premature termination of the study, (3) the statistical methodology, and (4) the use of nonstandardized chemotherapy. Investigators in the Mainz trial[139] studied 49 patients

TABLE 34.3-10. Randomized Trials of Adjuvant Chemotherapy versus Observation in Patients with Muscle-Invasive Urothelial Cancer

Trial Organization or Country	*No. of Patients*	*Investigational Arm Therapy and Primary Tumor Management*	*Investigational Arm Survival*	*Control Arm Therapy*	*Control Arm Survival*	*Chemotherapy Benefit*
United Kingdom[136]	129	Radiation plus 5-FU-doxorubicin	35%	Radiation	37%	No
Stanford University[137]	55	Cystectomy and CMV	40%	Cystectomy	38%	No
Swiss Group for Clinical Cancer Research[138]	77	Cystectomy and cisplatin	57%	Cystectomy	54%	No
University of Mainz[139]	49	Cystectomy and M-VAC/MVEC	80%[a]	Cystectomy	10%[a]	Yes
University of Southern California[64]	91	Cystectomy and CAP	70%	Cystectomy	46%	Yes

CAP, cyclophosphamide, doxorubicin (Adriamycin), and cisplatin (platinum); CMV, cisplatin, methotrexate, vinblastine; 5-FU, 5-fluorouracil; M-VAC, methotrexate, vinblastine, Adriamycin, and cisplatin; MVEC, methotrexate, vinblastine, epirubicin, and cisplatin.
[a]Estimated survival from published survival distributions when proportions are not provided.

with pT2 to pT4 or node-positive TCC who were randomly chosen to receive M-VAC or CMV and either doxorubicin or epirubicin or to undergo observation. However, patients in the observation arm did not routinely receive chemotherapy at relapse. A significant reduction in the risk of tumor recurrence was observed in the adjuvant chemotherapy arm: 3 of 18 (17%) patients who received chemotherapy experienced relapse as compared to 18 of 23 (78%) untreated patients ($P = .0007$). A survival benefit was reported in a follow-up report with additional patients entered into the study.[140]

Collectively, these trials fail to prove definitively that adjuvant chemotherapy provides a survival benefit in muscle-invasive TCC. The trials performed to date are substantially flawed. Problems encountered in the interpretation of results include (1) insufficient numbers of patients, raising the possibility of false interpretation, (2) inadequate chemotherapy, or (3) premature closure. Despite the reported activity of cisplatin-based chemotherapy in more advanced disease over the last 15 years, the hypothesis that multiagent chemotherapy may be beneficial after cystectomy for muscle-invasive disease has not been adequately tested.

Both nonrandomized and randomized data suggest that adjuvant chemotherapy delays tumor progression; however, a survival benefit has not been definitively proven. The MSKCC approach for nonprotocol patients with muscle-invasive disease is to consider four cycles of adjuvant M-VAC for patients with at least T3,N0 primary tumors and any patients with node-positive disease provided that they can tolerate aggressive chemotherapy. If such patients cannot tolerate M-VAC therapy, surveillance is recommended. These treatment recommendations are based on the following data: (1) Cure can be achieved in patients with node-positive disease treated with chemotherapy followed by cystectomy[111]; (2) M-VAC must be considered the most efficacious regimen based on randomized comparisons to single-agent cisplatin and to the combination of cisplatin, doxorubicin, and cyclophosphamide[84,85]; and (3) independent prognostic factors for survival in the advanced disease setting are a good performance status (reflecting lower tumor burden) and disease restricted to lymph nodes; cure is greatest in patients with both features.[108]

Neoadjuvant Chemotherapy. The major advantages of the neoadjuvant approach are the response of the primary lesion, which has prognostic importance, and the degree of response, which can be used to recommend further treatment.[141,142] Response of a primary lesion to combination therapy is associated with improved long-term survival. In a report of 125 patients on multiple trials of cisplatin-based therapy followed by definitive surgery, 91% of the responders (≤pT1 at cystectomy) were disease-free, in contrast to only 37% of nonresponders (≥pT2 at cystectomy).[143] A major response to neochemotherapy can also result in preservation of the bladder by repeated and aggressive transurethral resections or by a partial cystectomy.[144,145] Patients whose disease is not responding appropriately can be referred for definitive cystectomy.

Major disadvantages of neoadjuvant chemotherapy include a marked discordance between the clinical and pathologic response to chemotherapy and persistent risk of new bladder tumor formation in the preserved bladder. Approximately 30% of bladder tumors staged as T0 after completing neoadjuvant chemotherapy will have persistent muscle-invasive disease if a cystectomy is performed.[146] Second, even in the patient whose tumor is in complete pathologic response after chemotherapy, the bladder remains at risk for new muscle-invasive bladder tumors that may result in the need for cystectomy. Herr et al.[147] reported a 56% incidence of new bladder tumors in patients 10 years after bladder preservation with neoadjuvant M-VAC and conservative surgery; 30% of the patients had invasive disease requiring a cystectomy.

Studies evaluating chemotherapy in the neoadjuvant setting include both phase III trials examining survival advantage and phase II studies examining response or potential bladder preservation (or both). The latter studies are not controlled for patient selection, cystoscopic resection, staging and restaging techniques, and chemotherapeutic regimens. Most randomized studies of neoadjuvant chemotherapy failed to show a survival benefit for chemotherapy (Table 34.3-11).[55,148–159] Similar to the adjuvant trials, these studies suffer from suboptimal regimens of chemotherapy or small sample size. The only reported trial with enough power to detect a 10% difference in survival is the intergroup trial performed by the Medical Research Council and the EORTC evaluating CMV for three cycles followed by the participating institutions' recommended management of the primary lesion versus similar primary tumor management without neoadjuvant chemotherapy.[159] Primary tumor management in this trial included cystectomy, radiotherapy, or both. With an accrual of 976 patients, a 5.5% advantage in 3-year survival for patients receiving neoadjuvant CMV was observed. The survival advantage was not statistically significant, because the trial was powered to detect a 10% survival advantage, the minimal benefit discerned by these collaborating investigators to substantiate the routine use of chemotherapy. Trial interpretation is difficult, as not all patients underwent similar treatment of the primary tumor; it is possible that benefit might be different in patients treated with cystectomy versus those treated with radiotherapy.

A Nordic Cooperative Bladder Cancer Study Group trial explored neoadjuvant doxorubicin plus cisplatin, and the ongoing Southwest Oncology Group (SWOG) trial is evaluating neoadjuvant M-VAC.[152] The Scandinavian trial explored doxorubicin and cisplatin prior to low-dose preoperative radiotherapy and cystectomy. This trial with 325 patients reported nonsignificant survival differences in patients treated with adjuvant chemotherapy [59% in the chemotherapy arm vs. 51% in the control arm ($P = .1$), with cancer-specific survival rates of 64% and 54%, respectively]. The authors reported a 15% survival benefit in the subset of patients with T3 and T4 disease ($P = .03$) but no differences in patients with T1 and T2 disease. A multivariate analysis revealed that chemotherapy and T stage were independent prognostic factors for survival and that the relative death risk for patients who received chemotherapy was 0.69 as compared to the control group. Results from the SWOG trial of neoadjuvant chemotherapy are awaited with great interest. This neoadjuvant trial evaluates the use of M-VAC chemotherapy, a regimen that many feel is the optimal conventional standard, for three cycles followed by cystectomy versus cystectomy alone. The accrual goal was reached in 1998, and results should be available in the year 2001.

Ongoing Clinical Trials Evaluating Adjuvant and Neoadjuvant Chemotherapy. The combination of paclitaxel and carboplatin is active in urothelial cancer and well tolerated when carboplatin is dosed to a predetermined AUC according to the patient's renal function. The activity and tolerance of this regimen are the basis

TABLE 34.3-11. Results of Randomized Trials of Neoadjuvant Chemotherapy in Patients with Muscle-Invasive Urothelial Cancer

Trial Organization or Country	*No. of Patients*	*Investigational Arm Therapy Primary Tumor Management*	*Investigational Arm Survival (%)*	*Standard Arm Therapy*	*Survival Results (%)*	*Chemotherapy Benefit*
United Kingdom[55]	376	Methotrexate; radiation, cystectomy, or both	39%	Radiation, cystectomy, or both	37%	No
MRC/EORTC/ABCSG/NCIC/NBCSG/CUETO[159]	976	CMV; radiation or cystectomy	62%	Radiation or cystectomy	60%	No
NCIC[148]	99	Cisplatin and concurrent RT or RT-cystectomy	47%	RT or RT-cystectomy	33%	No
Australia[149]	225	Cisplatin, radiation	39%	Radiation	40%	No
Italy (GISTV)[150]	171	MVEC, cystectomy	85%	Cystectomy	74%	No
Nordic I[151,152]	325	Cisplatin-doxorubicin, radiation and cystectomy	59%	Radiation and cystectomy	51%	Trend for T3–T4 disease
Spain (CUETO)[153]	122	Cisplatin, cystectomy	41%	Cystectomy	41%	No
Italy (Genoa)[154]	184	Cisplatin, 5-fluorouracil, RT; cystectomy	NA	Cystectomy	NA	No
MDACC[155]	100	Neo-M-VAC × 2; cystectomy; adjuvant M-VAC × 3	49%	Cystectomy, adjuvant M-VAC × 5	52%	No
RTOG[156]	123	CMV, cisplatin-RT	48%	Cisplatin-RT	49%	No
Ongoing trials pending publication						
Nordic II	NA	Cisplatin-methotrexate, cystectomy	NA	Cystectomy	NA	Results pending
SWOG/ECOG[157]	300	M-VAC, cystectomy	NA	Cystectomy	NA	Results pending
Italy (Guone)[158]	230	M-VAC, cystectomy	NA	Cystectomy	NA	No

ABCSG, Australian Bladder Cancer Study Group; CUETO, Club Urologico Espag ol de Tratimieneto Oncologico; ECOG, Eastern Cooperative Oncology Group; EORTC, European Organization for Research and Treatment of Cancer; GISTV, Gruppo Italiano per lo Studio dei Tumori de la Vesicula; CMV, cisplatin, methotrexate, and vinblastine; MDACC, M. D. Anderson Cancer Center; MRC, Medical Research Council; M-VAC, methotrexate, vinblastine, doxorubicin (Adriamycin), and cisplatin; MVEC, methotrexate, vinblastine, epidoxorubicin, and cisplatin; NA, not available from published data; NBCSG, Nordic Cooperative Bladder Cancer Study Group; NCIC, National Cancer Institute of Canada; NS, not stated in published data; RT, radiotherapy; RTOG, Radiation Therapy Oncology Group; SWOG, Southwest Oncology Group.

of a randomized adjuvant trial designed by the ECOG. This proposed trial will randomly choose approximately 330 patients with either pT4N0M0 or pT(any)N+M0 tumors after cystectomy and pelvic lymph node dissection to receive either four cycles of M-VAC or four cycles of paclitaxel plus carboplatin.

Current MSKCC trials are testing the hypothesis of maximizing individual drugs or combinations of agents devoid of overlapping toxicities according to the model originally proposed by Norton and Simon.[132] After local control surgery, enrolled patients receive sequential, dose-intensive gemcitabine and doxorubicin, then either paclitaxel and cisplatin or paclitaxel and carboplatin, depending on renal function. The studies are designed to determine the feasibility, drug delivery, specific toxicity, and the noncomparative efficacy of a dose-intensive sequential chemotherapeutic regimen for high-risk resectable transitional cell urothelial cancer (extravesical, extraureter, extrapelvic disease or positive regional lymph nodes).

BLADDER PRESERVATION

Evolving data show that the categorical recommendation of surgically removing the bladder in all cases with invasive disease is outdated. It is nevertheless important to stress that the primary goal of treatment is survival, and sparing the bladder is justified only when (1) it has a high likelihood of eradicating the tumor in the bladder, (2) the risk of recurrence is low, and (3) bladder function is not compromised. A patient who has had multiple recurrences before an invasive tumor developed may not be an appropriate candidate for such an approach because of the potential risk of future recurrences. Thus, for patients with invasive bladder cancer after multiple prior superficial tumors or for those with poor bladder capacity, surgical removal of the bladder and creation of an internal urinary reservoir, if possible, is preferable.

Many groups have reported favorable cure rates with bladder-preserving methods in selected patients with tumors who met certain criteria, with cystectomy reserved for those who do not meet the criteria. Because it is uncertain which factors predict a favorable outcome if the bladder is left *in situ*, any approach inevitably requires both physician judgment (selection) and some patient risk. With these caveats in mind, factors that have been associated with a favorable outcome include tumor size (≤4 cm), confined to the bladder (stage T2), and a CR to initial therapy as judged by a cystoscopy and biopsy performed after induction therapy. Selection by tumor response allows for prompt cystectomy, if the disease is persistent, and minimizes the risk of metastatic dissemination from failed initial local therapy. Importantly, any patient in whom the bladder is left in place must be monitored continually for recurrent disease in the bladder, because virtually all series show new tumors, both superficial and invasive, developing after successful bladder-sparing treatments.

MONOTHERAPIES

Transurethral Resection Alone

Three studies suggest that a maximal or aggressive TUR alone may control some muscle-invasive bladder tumors.[47,160–162] One study evaluated 466 consecutively referred patients with muscle-invasive disease by a repeat TUR. Twenty-five percent (118 patients) were followed up conservatively after the second TUR failed to document residual muscle invasion. Of these 118 patients, 77 (65%) remained free of invasive tumor beyond 5 years with an intact bladder. The overall 5-year survival rate of these 77 patients was 83%. Tumors most amenable to TUR alone tended to be papillary, solitary, 2 cm or less in size, minimally invasive into muscle, and not associated with Tis, a palpable mass, or hydronephrosis.[161,162] These are the same tumor characteristics that are most favorable for bladder preservation in general.[163]

Partial Cystectomy

Approximately 5% to 10% of invasive tumors develop in a location where a curative resection by partial cystectomy is possible. This is most frequently accomplished when a lesion develops on the dome of the bladder, where a 2-cm margin of resection can be obtained, no association with CIS in other bladder sites exists, and bladder capacity is adequate once the tumors are removed. Tumors in the bladder neck and trigone are relative contraindications to the procedure.[164,165] A wide segmental resection of the bladder's dome is the recommended surgical procedure for urachal carcinoma.

Radiotherapy Alone

Several series of patients treated with radiotherapy alone provide the benchmark against which new treatment approaches are judged. As noted, responses based on clinical grounds alone range from 40% to 52%, of which 30% to 40% are durable (see Table 34.3-6).[54–58] The most consistently reported factors predictive for a successful outcome are clinical stage (T2), tumor size (<5 cm maximum diameter), and the absence of ureteral obstruction.[163,166]

Recent data suggest that the proportion of complete responses may be improved with accelerated fractionation schemes. In an older randomized trial with 168 patients unsuited for cystectomy with T2 to T4 tumors, hyperfractionated (not accelerated) external-beam irradiation alone (i.e., 1.0 Gy three times daily to a total dose of 84 Gy) was shown to be superior to conventional treatment (e.g., 2.0 Gy daily to 64 Gy) with respect to survival at 5 years (27% vs. 18%) and CR rate (41% vs. 25%), without a significant increase in toxicities.[167] In a series at the Royal Marsden Hospital, 66% (56 of 85) of patients were found to be tumor-free after a cystoscopic examination was performed 3 to 6 months after treatment of twice-daily fractions of 1.8 to 2.0 Gy, 5 days per week, to a dosage of 57.6 to 64 Gy.[168] Prospective trials are ongoing, and the published results of a phase III trial from the United Kingdom are expected in 2000.[169]

Interstitial Brachytherapy

Interstitial brachytherapy combined with external-beam irradiation and conservative surgery has been used successfully in some European centers in highly selected cases. The approach requires close cooperation between urologists and radiation oncologists. Candidates include patients with solitary, nonrecurrent, or clinical stage T2 and T3a tumors less than 5 cm in diameter, with adequate bladder capacity. Local control rates are 75% to 80%, with 5-year survival rates of 50% to 76%.[170–173] The approach has not been widely adopted in the United States because it is judged more invasive than transurethral surgery followed by chemotherapy and radiotherapy.

Results with Chemotherapy Alone

The demonstration of CRs in advanced disease led to subsequent trials evaluating preoperative or neoadjuvant chemotherapy in patients with invasive disease in the 1980s.[174] A prerequisite for safe bladder preservation is eradicating the tumor in the bladder. Published reports based on clinical (cystoscopic) staging showed CRs in up to 50% of cases; however, when the same reports are evaluated for the proportion of tumors free of disease at cystectomy, a more modest 20% to 30% rate based on pathologic grounds alone, pathologic complete response (PCR) is observed.[173,174] Of equal concern is that the ability to predict which bladders clinically free of tumor by cystoscopic staging (T0) will actually be pathologically free of tumor at cystectomy (P0). Understaging in up to 30% to 40% of cases has been observed in selected series.[174] Thus, cumulative data show that chemotherapy alone is inadequate therapy to control the primary tumor for most patients. Analyses also show that the proportion of bladders rendered free of tumor varies inversely with T stage.[175] PCR rates are less than 10% in patients with pT3 to pT4 disease or a palpable mass at presentation. Cumulatively, the data show that chemotherapy alone is inadequate as monotherapy if the primary goal is to preserve bladder function.

Bladder Sparing: Combined-Modality Approaches

The 20% to 40% success rates achieved with single-modality approaches are, when used nonselectively, inferior to contemporary cystectomy series in which local control rates for pelvic disease approach 90%. The evolution of combined-modality approaches aimed at bladder preservation began with reports suggesting that the combination of an aggressive TUR followed by radiation alone or in combination with multidrug systemic chemotherapy could increase the proportion of bladders that are rendered tumor-free. These strategies are based on the principle that final treatment of the bladder is determined by the response to initial therapy, whether unimodality or multimodality.[141,148,163,174,176–181]

Table 34.3-12[142,144,178,179,182–187] shows results of combined-modality therapies for survival and survival with a bladder preserved.[181–192] The ideal candidate for bladder preservation has clinical stage T2 primary tumor, no associated ureteral obstruction, visibly complete TUR, and a documented CR after induction by chemotherapy or chemoradiation. Combined-modality treatment as an alternative to cystectomy is still investigative; it is recommended that such therapy be administered by dedicated multimodality teams.

Chemotherapy Followed by Partial Cystectomy

Only 5% to 10% of invasive tumors present in a location amenable to a curative resection by partial cystectomy at diagnosis.[165] In appropriately selected cases, the approach has the advantage of surgically removing the diseased portion of the bladder, with definitive staging of the bladder and lymph nodes. After a response to chemotherapy, less extensive surgery may be necessary to achieve control. The proportion of tumors that could be removed by partial—as opposed to radical—cystectomy increased to 27% after M-VAC was used.[178] Early results, confirmed by Sternberg et al.,[179] were excellent for this highly selected patient group. However, the long-term risk of recurrent disease is substantial. Herr et al.[147] reported that salvage cystectomy was necessary in one-third of the patients, owing to new muscle-invasive neoplasms.

Chemotherapy Combined with Radiotherapy

The strategy of combining chemotherapy and radiotherapy evolved from clinical trials performed in the 1980s, which showed the importance of a complete endoscopic resection of the tumor within the bladder before radiation[163] and, in a randomized comparison, a higher rate of local control in the bladder using concurrent cisplatin and radiotherapy versus radiotherapy alone.[148] At the same time, laboratory studies demonstrated that several cytotoxic agents, particularly cisplatin and 5-FU, could sensitize tumor tissue to radiation and increase the killing of tumor cells in a synergistic fashion.[180]

Chemotherapy has been combined with radiotherapy in concurrent, sequential, and alternating fashions.[181] No optimal schedule has been defined. Nevertheless, several reports[182–184,186–190] show that radiation adds to TUR and systemic chemotherapy to maintain the bladder free of tumor. These reports suggest a higher response rate after TUR and chemoradiation therapy (74%) than after TUR and chemotherapy (20% to 30%) as well as 5-year survival rates *with* the bladder (range, 36% to 44%), which are within the limits of comparing nonrandomized series. These survival rates appear to be superior to those reported with conservative surgery and chemotherapy alone [20% at 5 years and 33% at 30 months (median follow-up)]. When the results are analyzed, the number of patients with tumor-free bladders must be considered in the context of the total number of patients entered into a study, as was done in the previously mentioned series (see Table 34.3-12).[142,144,178,179,182–187] Considering the number of retained bladders relative to the number of patients who complete therapy artificially inflates the outcome. Finally, it must be remembered that the results of contemporary trials, though encouraging, do not exclude the possibility that a bladder-sparing approach may result in reduced survival compared to radical surgery.[147]

The highly selective nature of patients treated with combined modality approaches the limits of comparisons of survival distributions between these patients and those treated by more conventional means. These caveats notwithstanding, in contemporary combined-modality series, 5-year survival rates in the range of 45% to 52% have been reported.[182,184,190,191] Three included radiation with a cisplatin-based regimen. Perhaps a reason why the survival rates with complete TUR of the bladder and chemoradiation are higher than those of other reported experiences is that patients who are at high risk for local failure are identified early and are referred for immediate cystectomy. At what point the patient is designated to have experienced failure of treatment and is referred for cystectomy is controversial. For example, in the Massachusetts General Hospital (MGH) series, patients first undergo an aggressive TUR followed by two cycles of CMV chemotherapy. A cystoscopy is performed 8 weeks from the initial TUR, and the response is assessed. All patients then receive radiation to a maximum of 40 Gy and two concurrent doses of cisplatin. A third cystoscopy is performed and, if residual disease is documented, the patient is referred for cystectomy. In this series, 41% of the patients without a CR (T0) after TUR and chemotherapy at cystoscopy were rendered tumor-free by concurrent radiation of 40 Gy.[175] The policy of referring nonresponding patients for surgery before definitive radiation doses has been effective and used successfully by other groups.[182,184,191] No increase in surgical complications has been observed. In any case, it is unlikely that the "window of surgical curability" would be closed with monitoring at these frequent time intervals.

TABLE 34.3-12. Recent Results of Various Combined-Modality Therapies for Survival and Survival with Bladder Preserved

Series	*Therapy*	*No. of Patients*	*5-Y Survival Rate (%)*	*5-Y Survival Rate with Bladder Preservation (%)*
Tester[182,a]	Concurrent DDP/RT	42	52	41
Dunst[183]	TURB plus concurrent DDP/RT	79	52	41
Tester[184,a]	CMV plus concurrent DDP/RT	91	62[b]	44
Kahnic[185,a]	TURB plus CMV plus concurrent DDP-radiotherapy	106	52	43
Given[186]	TUR plus CMV plus concurrent DDP-radiotherapy in 49 patients	93	51	18
Srougi[187,a]	M-VAC plus partial cystectomy	30	53	20
Sternberg[179,a]	M-VAC plus TUR	66	—[c]	33[c]
MSKCC[142,144,178,a]	M-VAC plus conservative surgery	111	48	30

DDP, cisplatin; CMV, cisplatin, methotrexate, and vinblastine; M-VAC, methotrexate, vinblastine, doxorubicin (Adriamycin), cisplatin; TUR, transurethral resection of tumor; RT, external-beam irradiation.

[a]Bladder preservation performed selectively, based on initial tumor response and suitability for cystectomy.

[b]Based on 4-year follow-up.

[c]Median follow-up of 30 months at time of report.

This practice differs from a treatment policy of salvage cystectomy, in that tumor regrowth is not required before a patient is referred for surgery.

Evidence that the optimal dose and schedule of chemoradiation have not been developed is provided by a nevertheless encouraging report from Paris evaluating cisplatin and 5-FU with concomitant twice-daily high-dose-fraction pelvic irradiation.[191] To evaluate the efficacy and safety of the regimen, initially all patients were restaged both clinically and pathologically. All 18 patients who were clinically T0 proved to have no tumor at cystectomy (P0). As a result of this experience, the group changed their treatment policy to focus more on selective bladder preservation. This high rate (100%) of PCR in patients who were CRs (T0) appears to be a marked improvement over the experience of others using neoadjuvant chemotherapy, in which approximately 50% of patients judged to be clinically T0 after induction are confirmed pathologically at cystectomy.[141] In an update of the Parisian experience, 74% of referred patients have retained their bladders. Equally encouraging is that only 10% of these have developed new tumors within the preserved bladder. In the MGH, RTOG, and Erlangen studies, CR rates at cystoscopic rebiopsy after induction range from 70% to 80%, of which 83% to 89% (representing 58% to 72% of all referred patients) remain free from invasive recurrence. The RTOG has recently evaluated the Paris approach in 34 patients and found a 65% clinical CR (T0) rate.[193]

The concern that a conserved, irradiated bladder functions poorly has also been answered by recent reports after modern radiation techniques. In the Erlangen experience, only three cystectomies were necessary for bladder shrinkage among 192 preserved bladders, for an incidence of 1.6%.[183] An analysis of bladder function in 72 patients successfully treated with 60 Gy in 30 fractions found no differences in urinary and rectal function as compared with an age- and gender-matched control group. Similarly, the MGH reported excellent tolerance in 21 women treated by bladder conservation using chemoradiation.[192] With a median follow-up of 56 months, all patients were continent and free of dysuria and hematuria. Bladder function improved or was unchanged after treatment in 91% of the patients, and no patients reported a compromise in bowel or sexual function. In an update of 106 consecutively entered patients on prospective protocols at the MGH, including induction by TUR of tumor, two cycles of methotrexate, cisplatin, and vinblastine chemotherapy followed by 64.8-Gy irradiation with concomitant cisplatin, none of the 76 patients whose bladders were preserved had to undergo a cystectomy for shrinkage or bleeding. The median follow-up of the 76 patients who had no cystectomy for tumor was 59 months.

After multimodality organ-preserving therapy, 20% to 30% of patients may subsequently develop superficial tumors. These tumors are usually amenable to standard management with TUR and intravesical agents. Of 18 patients (24%) who developed either Ta or CIS among the 76 patients with initial bladder presentation at MGH, 14 have been maintained in remission by TUR and intravesical drug therapy, with 15 to 49 months of follow-up after development of their new superficial tumor.[181] Obviously, all patients treated by multimodality bladder-preserving therapies must be willing to return to the urologist for regular cystoscopic follow-up so that TUR, intravesical chemotherapy, or cystectomy can be used at the earliest opportunity, if necessary.

CASE SELECTION

Developing a coherent strategy for treating invasive bladder tumors will ultimately require designing and completing comparative trials. The Medical Research Council–EORTC international study, involving almost 1000 patients, was a landmark trial in that it was the first study with a sufficient number of patients to detect a survival difference for chemotherapy. Similarly, the SWOG intergroup trial evaluating neoadjuvant chemotherapy is also important because it tests M-VAC, shown to be the most active chemotherapeutic regimen, with a sufficient number of patients to detect a survival difference.

A novel approach in selecting patients for perioperative chemotherapy is incorporating prognostic markers of the primary tumor to allow a more precise definition of metastatic risk. Clinical prognostic factors predicting adverse outcome include depth of invasion, presence or absence of a palpable mass, and presence or absence of hydronephrosis. Several molecular markers have also been investigated.[190] Invasive bladder tumors that have a dysfunctional retinoblastoma (*Rb*) gene product or mutant p53,[29,194–196] implied by immunohistochemistry assays,[197,198] are at increased risk of metastatic disease. These molecular markers must be validated in clinical trials of appropriate sample sizes to determine their clinical utility.

Two ongoing investigational trials explore the use of p53 mutations in urothelial cancer. Studies at USC determined that patients whose tumors had mutant p53 were more likely to have disease recurrence and death ($P<.0001$) than patients whose primary tumor had wild-type p53.[29] At MSKCC, the p53 status of the tumors in patients treated with neoadjuvant chemotherapy showed similar results. Patients whose primary tumors had nuclear staining of p53 protein by immunohistochemistry, which implied mutant p53, were three times more likely to die from disease than were those patients whose tumor staining was consistent with wild-type p53.[195] In the latter study, the use of both clinical stage and p53 status could predict patients with a favorable outcome. Patients with good prognostic features [i.e., wild-type p53 and low stage of disease (T2 tumors)], had a 77% survival at 5 years after neoadjuvant chemotherapy; bladder preservation and survival were more frequent in patients whose tumors had wild-type p53.[199] A prospective trial attempts bladder preservation in patients with wild-type p53 tumors. USC investigators are testing a different hypothesis; preliminary retrospective data from their center suggest that adjuvant chemotherapy enhances survival in patients whose tumors have mutant p53.[200] Based on these data, patients with mutant p53 tumors are randomly assigned to receive either adjuvant M-VAC chemotherapy or observation after cystectomy to assess a survival advantage associated with adjuvant chemotherapy.

SUMMARY

Urinary bladder cancer is a common disease, with increasing incidence but a decreasing mortality. Several carcinogens of the urothelium and risk groups have been identified, such as aromatic amines, combustible gases, a dietary component in meat or fat, the drug phenacetin, and tobacco smoking. An understanding of the pathogenesis of the disease is evolving, and at least two pathways lead to urinary bladder cancer. Mutations in *p53, Rb*, and as yet uncharacterized genes on chromosome 9 are common and probably important. Urinary bladder cancers typically present with macroscopic hematuria. The clinical course of the disease is strongly heterogeneous. Superficial TaG1 lesions almost never progress and can easily be handled with an endoscopic resection. Recurrent and high-grade superficial bladder tumors can be controlled in most cases with repeated TURs and intravesical BCG, with cystectomy reserved for refractory tumors.

Muscle-invasive disease may require both a locally aggressive therapy and systemic therapy of micrometastases for cure. Metastatic urinary bladder cancer is a fast-growing and often lethal malignancy. In the latter stage, only a small proportion of patients are currently cured with chemotherapy. Newer chemotherapeutic regimens may improve survival of patients with advanced disease. Current refinements in therapy include identifying subgroups of patients with superficial disease in whom the intensity of follow-up can be reduced or intravesical therapy is needed. For muscle-invasive disease, efforts are being made to identify patients for whom organ preservation is possible without compromising overall survival, as well as those with subclinical micrometastases for whom systemic therapy is needed for cure. Efforts to improve therapy include better surgical techniques, computed three-dimensional treatment planning for more precise delivery of external-beam radiotherapy, and the incorporation of newly identified chemotherapeutic agents into combination regimens.

For most patients, combined-modality approaches are essential to optimal management. It is likely that the improved overall survival observed during the last two decades will continue. With the increasing focus on preventive measures, such as the cessation of smoking[201] and reducing exposure to known carcinogens, the incidence of the disease is likely to decrease, and the current trend of reduced bladder cancer mortality is likely to continue.

REFERENCES

1. Cordon-Cardo C, Dalbagni G, Sarkis AS, Reuter VE. Genetic alterations associated with bladder cancer. In: DeVita VT, Hellman S, Rosenberg SA, eds. *Important advances in oncology*. Philadelphia: JB Lippincott Co, 1994:71.
2. Landis SH, Murray T, Bolden S, Wingo PA. Cancer statistics, 1999. *CA Cancer J Clin* 1999;49(8):1.
3. Hankey BF, Silverman DT. SEER cancer statistics review, 1973–1996. *J Natl Cancer Inst* 1999;91:1362.
4. Silverman DT, Levin LI, Hoover RN, Hartge P. Occupational risks of bladder cancer in the United States: I. White men. *J Natl Cancer Inst* 1989;81:1472.
5. International Agency for Cancer Research. *Overall evaluations of carcinogenicity: an updating of IARC monographs, volumes 1 to 42. IARC Monographs on the Evaluation of the Carcinogenic Risk of Chemicals to Humans, Supplement 7.* Lyon, France: IARC, 1987.
6. Michaud DS, Spiegelman D, Clinton SK, et al. Fluid intake and the risk of bladder cancer in men. *N Engl J Med* 1999;340:1390.
7. Steineck G, Hagman U, Gerhardsson M, Norell SE. Vitamin A supplements, fried foods, fat and urothelial cancer. A case-referent study in Stockholm in 1985–87. *Int J Cancer* 1990;45:1006.
8. Silverman DT, Hartge P, Morrison AS, Devesa SS. Epidemiology of bladder cancer. *Hematol Oncol Clin North Am* 1992;6:1.
9. Levine LA, Richie JP. Urological complications of cyclophosphamide. *J Urol* 1989;141:1063.
10. Kantor AF, Hartge P, Hoover RN, Fraumeni JF Jr. Epidemiological characteristics of squamous cell carcinoma and adenocarcinoma of the bladder. *Cancer Res* 1988;48:3853.
11. Messing EM, Young TB, Hunt VB, Wehbie JM, Rust P. Urinary tract cancers found by homescreening with hematuria dipsticks in healthy men over 50 years of age. *Cancer* 1989;64:2361.
12. Herr HW. The value of a second transurethral resection in evaluating patients with bladder tumors. *J Urol* 1999;162:74.
13. Herr HW. Routine CT scan in cystectomy patients: does it change management? *Urology* 1996;47:324.
14. Reuter VE. Pathology of bladder cancer: assessment of prognostic variables and response to therapy. *Semin Oncol* 1990;17:524.
15. Epstein JI, Amin MB, Reuter VR, Mostofi FK. The World Health Organization/International Society of Urological Pathology consensus classification of urothelial (transitional cell) neoplasms of the urinary bladder. Bladder Consensus Conference Committee. *Am J Surg Pathol* 1998;22:1435.
16. Norming U, Nyman CR, Tribukait B. Comparative flow cytometric deoxyribonucleic acid studies on exophytic tumor and random mucosal biopsies in untreated carcinoma of the bladder. *J Urol* 1989;142:1442.
17. Farrow GM. Pathology of carcinoma in situ of the urinary bladder and related lesions. *J Cell Biochem Suppl* 1992:39.
18. Jewett HJ, Strong GH. Infiltrating carcinoma of the bladder: relation of depth of penetration of the bladder wall to incidence of local extension in metastases. *J Urol* 1946;55:366.
19. American Joint Committee on Cancer. Urinary bladder. In: Fleming ID, ed. *AJCC cancer staging manual.* Philadelphia: Lippincott Williams & Wilkins, 1997:241.
20. Herr HW. Uncertainty and outcome of invasive bladder tumors. *Urol Oncol* 1996;2:92.
21. Herr HW, Donat SM. Prostatic tumor relapse in patients with superficial bladder tumors: 15-year outcome. *J Urol* 1999;161:1854.
22. Vieweg J, Gschwend JE, Herr HW, Fair WR. Pelvic lymph node dissection can be curative in patients with node positive bladder cancer. *J Urol* 1999;161:449.
23. Sidransky D, Frost P, von Eschenbach A, et al. Clonal origin bladder cancer. *N Engl J Med* 1992;326:737.
24. Miyao N, Tsai YC, Lerner SP, et al. Role of chromosome 9 in human bladder cancer. *Cancer Res* 1993;53:4066.
25. Cairns P, Shaw ME, Knowles MA. Initiation of bladder cancer may involve deletion of a tumour-suppressor gene on chromosome 9. *Oncogene* 1993;8:1083.
26. Cordon-Cardo C, Dalbagni G, Saez GT, et al. p53 mutations in human bladder cancer: genotypic versus phenotypic patterns. *Int J Cancer* 1994;56:347.
27. Sarkis AS, Dalbagni G, Cordon-Cardo C, et al. Detection of p53 mutations in superficial (T1) bladder carcinomas as a marker for disease progression. *J Natl Cancer Inst* 1993;85:53.
28. Sarkis AS, Dalbagni G, Cordon-Cardo C, et al. Association of p53 nuclear overexpression and tumor progression in carcinoma in situ of the bladder. *J Urol* 1994;52:388.
29. Esrig D, Elmajian D, Groshen S, et al. Accumulation of nuclear p53 and tumor progression in bladder cancer. *N Engl J Med* 1994;331:1259.
30. Lamm DL, Griffith JG. Intravesical therapy: does it affect the natural history of superficial bladder cancer? *Semin Urol* 1992;10:39.
31. Herr HW. Intravesical therapy. *Hematol Oncol Clin North Am* 1992;6:117.
32. Kilbridge KL, Kantoff P. Intravesical therapy for superficial bladder cancer: is it a wash? *J Clin Oncol* 1994;12:1.
33. Herr HW, Schwalb DM, Zhang ZF, et al. Intravesical bacille Calmette-Guérin therapy prevents tumor progression and death from superficial bladder cancer: ten-year follow-up of a prospective randomized trial. *J Clin Oncol* 1995;13:1404.
34. Cookson MS, Herr HW, Zhang ZF, et al. The treated natural history of high risk superficial bladder cancer: 15- year outcome. *J Urol* 1997;158:62.
35. Herr HW, Badalament RA, Amato DA, et al. Superficial bladder cancer treated with bacille Calmette-Guérin: a multivariate analysis of factors affecting tumor progression. *J Urol* 1989;141:22.
36. Hudson MA, Herr HW. Carcinoma in situ of the bladder. *J Urol* 1995;153:564.
37. Lamm DL, Blumenstein BA, Crawford ED, et al. A randomized trial of intravesical doxorubicin and immunotherapy with bacille Calmette-Guérin for transitional-cell carcinoma of the bladder. *N Engl J Med* 1991;325:1205.
38. Lamm DL, Crawford ED, Blumenstein BA, et al. A randomized comparison of BCG and mitomycin-C prophylaxis in stage Ta and T1 transitional cell carcinoma of the bladder. *J Urol* 1993;149:282.
39. Badalament RA, Herr HW, Wong GY, et al. A prospective randomized trial of maintenance versus nonmaintenance intravesical bacille Calmette-Guérin therapy of superficial bladder cancer. *J Clin Oncol* 1987;5:441.
40. Oosterlinck W, Kurth KH, Schroder F, et al. A prospective European Organization for Research and Treatment of Cancer Genitourinary Group randomized trial comparing transurethral resection followed by a single intravesical instillation of epirubicin or water in single stage Ta, T1 papillary carcinoma of the bladder. *J Urol* 1993;149:749.
41. Holmang S, Hedelin H, Anderstrom C, et al. Recurrence and progression in low grade papillary urothelial tumors. *J Urol* 1999;162:702.
42. Hall RR, Parmar MK, Richards AB, Smith PH. Proposal for changes in cystoscopic follow up of patients with bladder cancer and adjuvant intravesical chemotherapy. *Br Med J* 1994;308:257.
43. Herr HW. Extravesical tumor relapse in patients with superficial bladder tumors. *J Clin Oncol* 1998;16:1099.
44. Schwalb MD, Herr HW, Sogani PC, et al. Positive urinary cytology following a complete response to intravesical bacille Calmette-Guérin therapy: pattern of recurrence. *J Urol* 1994;152:382.
45. Herr HW, Jakse G, Sheinfeld J. The T1 bladder tumor. *Semin Urol* 1990;8:254.
46. Herr HW. Tumour progression and survival in patients with T1G3 bladder tumours: 15-year outcome. *Br J Urol* 1997;80:762.
47. Solsona E, Iborra I, Ricos JV, Monros JL, Dumont R. Feasibility of transurethral resection for muscle-infiltrating carcinoma of the bladder: prospective study. *J Urol* 1992;147:1513.
48. Kock NG, Nilson AE, Norlen L, et al. Urinary diversion via a continent ileum reservoir: clinical experience. *Scand J Urol Nephrol* 1978;49[Suppl]:23.
49. Hautmann RE, Miller K, Steiner U, Wenderoth U. The ileal neobladder: 6 years of experience with more than 200 patients. *J Urol* 1993;150:40.
50. Begg CB, Cramer LD, Hoskins WJ, Brennan MF. Impact of hospital volume on operative mortality for major cancer surgery. *JAMA* 1998;280:1747.
51. Turner S, Swindell R, Bowl N, et al. Bladder movement during radiation therapy for bladder cancer: implication for treatment planning. *Int J Radiat Oncol Biol Phys* 1994;30:199.
52. Marks LB, Shipley WU. Techniques for external beam irradiation of patients with invasive carcinoma of the urinary bladder. In: Levitt SH, Khan FM, Potish RA, eds. *Levitt & Tapley's technological basis of radiation therapy: practical clinical application*, 2nd ed. Philadelphia: Lea & Febiger, 1992:335.

53. Sur RK, Clinkard J, Jones WG, et al. Changes in target volume during radiotherapy treatment of invasive bladder carcinoma. *Clin Oncol* 1993;5:30.
54. Jenkins BJ, Caulfield MJ, Fowler CG, et al. Reappraisal of the role of radical radiotherapy and salvage cystectomy in the treatment of invasive (T2/T3) bladder cancer. *Br J Urol* 1988;62:343.
55. Shearer RJ, Chilvers CF, Bloom HJ, et al. Adjuvant chemotherapy in T3 carcinoma of the bladder. A prospective trial: preliminary report. *Br J Urol* 1988;62:558.
56. Gospodarowicz MK, Hawkins NV, Rawlings GA, et al. Radical radiotherapy for muscle invasive transitional cell carcinoma of the bladder: failure analysis. *J Urol* 1989;142:1448.
57. Mameghan H, Fisher R, Mameghan J, et al. Analysis of failure following definitive radiotherapy for invasive transitional cell carcioma of the bladder. *Int J Radiat Oncol Biol Phys* 1995;31:247.
58. De Neve W, Lybeert ML, Goor C, Crommelin MA, Ribot JG. Radiotherapy for T2 and T3 carcinoma of the bladder: the influence of overall treatment time. *Radiother Oncol* 1995;36:183.
59. Sell A, Jakobsen A, Nerstrom B, et al. Treatment of advanced bladder cancer category T2, T3 and T4a. A randomized multicenter study of preoperative irradiation and cystectomy versus radical irradiation and early salvage cystectomy for residual tumor. DAVECA protocol 8201. Danish Vesical Cancer Group. *Scand J Urol Nephrol Suppl* 1991;138:193.
60. Bloom HJ, Hendry WF, Wallace DM, Skeet RG. Treatment of T3 bladder cancer: controlled trial of pre-operative radiotherapy and radical cystectomy versus radical radiotherapy. *Br J Urol* 1982;54:136.
61. Dreicer R, Gustin DM, See WA, Williams RD. Paclitaxel in advanced urothelial carcinoma: its role in patients with renal insufficiency and as salvage therapy. *J Urol* 1996;156:1606.
62. Miller LS. Bladder cancer: superiority of preoperative irradiation and cystectomy in clinical stages B2 and C. *Cancer* 1977;39:973.
63. Einstein AB, Coombs J, Pearse H, et al. Cisplatin (CP) adjuvant therapy following preoperative radiotherapy plus radical cystectomy (RT+RCy) for invasive bladder carcinoma: a randomized trial of the National Bladder Cancer Group (NBCG). *J Urol* 1985;133:222.
64. Skinner DG, Daniels JR, Russell CA, et al. The role of adjuvant chemotherapy following cystectomy for invasive bladder cancer: a prospective comparative trial. *J Urol* 1991; 145:459.
65. Whitmore WF Jr, Batata MA, Ghoneim MA, Grabstald H, Unal A. Radical cystectomy with or without prior irradiation in the treatment of bladder cancer. *J Urol* 1977;118:184.
66. Shipley WU, Cummings KB, Coombs LJ, et al. 4,000 RAD preoperative irradiation followed by prompt radical cystectomy for invasive bladder carcinoma: a prospective study of patient tolerance and pathologic downstaging. *J Urol* 1982;127:48.
67. Crawford ED, Das S, Smith JA Jr. Preoperative radiation therapy in the treatment of bladder cancer. *Urol Clin North Am* 1987;14:781.
68. Cole CJ, Pollack A, Zagars GK, et al. Local control of muscle-invasive bladder cancer: preoperative radiotherapy and cystectomy versus cystectomy alone. *Int J Radiat Oncol Biol Phys* 1995;32:331.
69. Reisinger SA, Mohiuddin M, Mulholland SG. Combined pre- and postoperative adjuvant radiation therapy for bladder cancer—a ten year experience. *Int J Radiat Oncol Biol Phys* 1992;24:463.
70. Cozzarini C, Pelegrini D, Fallini M, et al. Reappraisal of the role of adjuvant radiotherapy in muscle-invasive transitional cell carcinoma of the bladder. *Int J Radiat Oncol Biol Phys* 1999;45:221(abst 144).
71. Zaghloul MS, Awwad HK, Akoush HH, et al. Postoperative radiotherapy of carcinoma in bilharzial bladder: improved disease free survival through improving local control. *Int J Radiat Oncol Biol Phys* 1992;23:511.
72. Mottet-Auselo N, Bons-Rosset F, Costa P, Louis JF, Navratil H. Carboplatin and urothelial tumors. *Oncology* 1993;50[Suppl 1]:28.
73. Moore MJ, Tannock IF, Ernst DS, Huan S, Murray N. Gemcitabine: a promising new agent in the treatment of advanced urothelial cancer. *J Clin Oncol* 1997;15:3441.
74. Stadler WM, Kuzel T, Roth B, Raghavan D, Dorr FA. Phase II study of single-agent gemcitabine in previously untreated patients with metastatic urothelial cancer. *J Clin Oncol* 1997;15:3394.
75. Lorusso V, Pollera CF, Antimi M, et al. A phase II study of gemcitabine in patients with transitional cell carcinoma of the urinary tract previously treated with platinum. Italian Co-operative Group on Bladder Cancer. *Eur J Cancer* 1998;34:1208.
76. Roth BJ, Dercer R, Einhorn LH, et al. Significant activity of paclitaxel in advanced transitional cell caricnoma of the urothelium: a Phase II trial of the Eastern Cooperative Oncology Group. *J Clin Oncol* 1994;12:2264.
77. Bajorin DF, Scher HI. Chemotherapy for urothelial cancer. In: Ernstoff MS, Heaney JA, Peschel RE, eds. *Urologic cancer.* Cambridge, MA: Blackwell Science, 1997:321.
78. de Wit R, Kruit WH, Stoter G, et al. Docetaxel (Taxotere): an active agent in metastatic urothelial cancer; results of a phase II study in non-chemotherapy-pretreated patients. *Br J Cancer* 1998;78:1342.
79. De Lena M, Gridelli C, Lorusso V, et al. Gemcitabine activity (objective responses and symptom improvement) in resistant stage IV bladder cancer. *Proc Am Soc Clin Oncol* 1996;15:246.
80. Sweeney CJ, Williams SD, Finch DE, et al. A Phase II study of paclitaxel and ifosfamide for patients with advanced refractory carcinoma of the urothelium. *Cancer* 1999;86:514.
81. Sternberg C, Yagoda A, Scher HI, et al. Methotrexate, vinblastine, doxorubicin and cisplatinum for advanced transitional cell carcinoma of the urothelium: efficacy and patterns of response and relapse. *Cancer* 1989;64:2448.
82. Harker W, Meyers FJ, Freiha FS, et al. Cisplatin, methotrexate, and vinblastine (CMV): an effective chemotherapy regimen for metastatic transitional cell carcinoma of the urinary tract. A Northern California Oncology Group study. *J Clin Oncol* 1985;3:1463.
83. Mead GM, Russel K, Clark P, et al. A randomized trial comparing methotrexate and vinblastine (MV) with cisplatin, methotrexate and vinblastine (CMV) in advanced transitional cell carcinoma: results and a report on prognostic factors in a Medical Research Council study. *Br J Cancer* 1998;78:1067.
84. Loehrer P, Einhorn LH, Elson PJ, et al. A randomized comparison of cisplatin alone or in combination with methotrexate, vinblastine, and doxorubicin in patients with metastatic urothelial carcinoma: a Cooperative Group Study. *J Clin Oncol* 1992;10:1066.
85. Logothetis CJ, Dexeus F, Sella A, et al. A prospective randomized trial comparing CISCA to MVAC chemotherapy in advanced metastatic urothelial tumors. *J Clin Oncol* 1990;8:1050.
86. Burch PA, Richardson RL, Cha SS, et al. Combination paclitaxel and cisplatin is active in advanced urothelial carcinoma (UC). *Proc Am Soc Clin Oncol* 1997;16:329a(abst).
87. Dreicer R, Roth B, Lipsitz S, et al. Cisplatin and paclitaxel in advanced carcinoma of the urothelium: a Phase II trial of the Eastern Cooperative Oncology Group (ECOG). *Proc Am Soc Clin Oncol* 1998;17:320a(abst 1233).
88. Murphy BA, Johnson DR, Smith J, et al. Phase II trial of paclitaxel (P) and cisplatin (C) for metastatic or locally unresectable urothelial cancer. *Proc Am Soc Clin Oncol* 1996;15:245(abst 617).
89. Sengelov L, Kamby C, Lund B, Engelholm SA. Docetaxel and cisplatin in metastatic urothelial cancer: a phase II study. *J Clin Oncol* 1998;16:3392.
90. Vaughn D, Malkowicz S, Zlotick B, et al. Phase I trial of paclitaxel/carboplatin in advanced carcinoma of the urothelium. *Semin Oncol* 1997;24:S2.
91. Vaughn DJ. Review and outlook for the role of paclitaxel in urothelial carcinoma. *Semin Oncol* 1999;26:117.
92. Redman BG, Smith DC, Flaherty L, Du W, Hussain M. Phase II trial of paclitaxel and carboplatin in the treatment of advanced urothelial carcinoma. *J Clin Oncol* 1998;16:1844.
93. Zielinski CC, Schnack B, Grbovic M, et al. Paclitaxel and carboplatin in patients with metastatic urothelial cancer: results of a phase II trial. *Br J Cancer* 1998;78:370.
94. Bauer J, Stalder M, Roth A, et al. Phase II trial of paclitaxel (P) plus carboplatin (C) in advanced urothelial tract cancer (UTC). *Proc Am Soc Clin Oncol* 1998;17:326a(abst).
95. Droz JP, Mottet N, Prapotrich D, et al. Phase II study of paclitaxel and carboplatin in patients with advanced transitional cell carcinoma of the urothelium: preliminary results. *Proc Am Soc Clin Oncol* 1998;17:316a(abst).
96. Vaughn DJ, Malkowitcz SB, Zotlick B, et al. Paclitaxel plus carboplatin in advanced carcinoma of the urothelium: an active and tolerable outpatient regimen. *J Clin Oncol* 1998;16:255.
97. Small E, Lew D, Petrylak D, Crawford ED. Carboplatin and paclitaxel (Carbo/Tax) for advanced transitional cell carcinoma (TCC) of the urothelium. *Proc Am Soc Clin Oncol* 1999;18:333a(abst).
98. von der Maase H, Anderson L, Crino L, Weissbach L, Dogliotti L. A phase II study of gemcitabine and cisplatin in patients with transitional cell carcinoma (TCC) of the urothelium. *Proc Am Soc Clin Oncol* 1997;16:324a(abst).
99. Kaufman D, Stadler W, Carducci M, et al. Gemcitabine (Gem) plus cisplatin (CDDP) in metastatic transitional cell carcinoma (TCC): final results of a phase II study. *Proc Am Soc Clin Oncol* 1998;17:320a(abst).
100. Moore MJ, Winquist EW, Murray N, et al. Gemcitabine plus cisplatin, an active regimen in urothelial cancer: a phase II trial of the National Institute of Canada Clinical Trials Group. *J Clin Oncol* 1999;17:2876.
101. Santoro A, Santoro M, Maiorino L, Forestieri V, Forestieri P. Phase II trial of gemcitabine plus carboplatin for urothelial transitional cell carcinoma in advanced or metastatic stage. *Ann Oncol* 1998;9[Suppl 2]:647.
102. Bajorin DF, McCaffrey JA, Hilton S, et al. Treatment of patients with transitional cell carcinoma of the urothelial tract with ifosfamide, paclitaxel, and cisplatin: a phase II trial. *J Clin Oncol* 1998;16.
103. McCaffrey JA, Dodd PM, Hilton S, et al. Ifosfamide + paclitaxel + cisplatin (ITP) chemotherapy for patients (pts) with unresectable or metastatic transitional cell carcinoma (TCC). *Proc Am Soc Clin Oncol* 1999;18:329a(abst 1267).
104. Bellmunt J, Guillem V, Paz-Ares L, et al. A phase II trial of paclitaxel, cisplatin and gemcitabine (TCG) in patients (pts) with advanced transitional cell carcinoma (TCC) of the urothelium. *Proc Am Soc Clin Oncol* 1999;18:332a(abst).
105. Vaishampayan U, Smith D, Redman B, et al. Phase II evaluation of carboplatin, paclitaxel, and gemcitabine in advanced urothelial carcinoma. *Proc Am Soc Clin Oncol* 1999;18:333a(abst).
106. Saxman S, Propert K, Einhorn L, et al. Long term follow-up of a phase III intergroup study of cisplatin alone or in combination with methotrexate, vinblastine and doxorubicin in patients with metastatic urothelial cancer: a cooperative group study. *J Clin Oncol* 1997;15:2564.
107. Geller NL, Sternberg CN, Penenberg D, Scher H, Yagoda A. Prognostic factors for survival of patients with advanced urothelial tumors treated with methotrexate, vinblastine, doxorubicin, and cisplatin chemotherapy. *Cancer* 1991;67:1525.
108. Bajorin DF, Dodd PM, Mazumdar M, et al. Long-term survival in metastatic transitional cell carcinoma and prognostic factors predicting outcome to chemotherapy. *J Clin Oncol* 1999;17:3173.
109. Donat SM, Herr HW, Bajorin DF, et al. Methotrexate, vinblastine, doxorubicin and cisplatin chemotherapy and cystectomy for unresectable bladder cancer. *J Urol* 1996;156:368.
110. Miller R, Freiha F, Reese J, Ozen H, Torti F. Surgical restaging of patients with advanced transitional cell carcinoma of the urothelium treated with cisplatin, methotrexate, and vinblastine: update of the Stanford University experience. *Proc Am Soc Clin Oncol* 1992;10:167.
111. Dodd PM, McCaffrey JA, Herr H, et al. Outcome of post-chemotherapy surgery after treatment with methotrexate, vinblastine, doxorubicin, and cisplatin in patients with unresectable or metastatic transitional cell carcinoma. *J Clin Oncol* 1999;17:2546.
112. Logothetis CJ, Dexeus FH, Sella A, et al. Escalated therapy for refractory urothelial tumors: methotrexate-vinblastine-doxorubicin-cisplatin plus unglycosylated recombinant human granulocyte-macrophage colony-stimulating factor. *J Natl Cancer Inst* 1990;82:667.
113. Loehrer PJ, Elson P, Dreicer R, et al. A phase I–II study: escalated dosages of methotrexate (M), vinblastine (V), doxorubicin (A), and cisplatin (C) plus rhG-CSF in advanced urothelial carcinoma: an ECOG trial. *Proc Am Soc Clin Oncol* 1992;11:201.
114. Logothetis C, Finn L, Amato R, Hossan E, Sella A. Escalated (ESC) MVAC ± rhGM-CSF (Schering-Plough) in metastatic transitional cell carcinoma (TCC): preliminary results of a randomized trial. *Proc Am Soc Clin Oncol* 1992;11:202.

115. Seidman AD, Scher HI, Gabrilove JL, et al. Dose-intensification of methotrexate, vinblastine, doxorubicin, and cisplatin with recombinant granulocyte-colony stimulating factor as initial therapy in advanced urothelial cancer. *J Clin Oncol* 1992;11:414.
116. Sternberg C, de Mulder P, van Oosterom AT, Fossa S, Chemotherapy Committee of the EORTC GU Group. Intensified M-VAC chemotherapy and recombinant human granulocyte-macrophage colony stimulating factor (GM-CSF) in patients with advanced urothelial tract tumors. *Proc Am Soc Clin Oncol* 1992;11:210.
117. Bellmunt J, Ribas A, Eres N, et al. Carboplatin-based versus cisplatin-based chemotherapy in the treatment of surgically incurable advanced bladder cancer. *Cancer* 1997;80:1966.
118. McCaffrey JA, Hilton S, Mazumdar M, et al. Phase II trial of docetaxel in patients with advanced or metastatic transitional-cell carcinoma. *J Clin Oncol* 1997;15:1853.
119. Tu S-M, Hossan E, Amato R, Kilbourn R, Logothetis CJ. Paclitaxel, cisplatin and methotrexate combination chemotherapy is active in the treatment of refractory urothelial malignancies. *J Urol* 1995;154:1719.
120. Meyers FJ, Miller TR, Williams SG, et al. Response to a taxol based chemotherapy regimen in advanced transitional cell carcinoma is independent of p53 expression. *Proc Am Soc Clin Oncol* 1999;18:333a(abst).
121. Meyers FJ, Edelman MJ, Houston J, Lauder I. Phase I/II trial of paclitaxel, carboplatin and methotrexate in advanced transitional cell carcinoma. *Proc Am Soc Clin Oncol* 1998; 17:317a(abst).
122. Einhorn LH, Roth BJ, Ansari R, et al. Phase II trial of gallium nitrate, vinblastine and ifosfamide in metastatic urothelial cancer. *J Clin Oncol* 1994;12:2271.
123. Dreicer R, Propert KJ, Roth BJ, Einhorn LH, Loehrer PJ. Vinblastine, ifosfamide, and gallium nitrate—an active regimen in patients with advanced carcinoma of the urothelium. A phase II trial of the Eastern Cooperative Oncology Group (E5892). *Cancer* 1997;79:110.
124. McCaffrey JA, Hilton S, Mazumdar M, et al. Phase II randomized trial of gallium nitrate plus fluorouracil versus methotrexate, vinblastine, doxorubicin, and cisplatin in patients with advanced transitional-cell carcinoma. *J Clin Oncol* 1997;15:2449.
125. McLaren B, Gallagher CJ, Mason M, Melesi G, Oliver RTD. Paclitaxel, vinblastine, cisplatin (PVC) in patients with advanced transitional cell cancer. *Proc Am Soc Clin Oncol* 1997;16:337a(abst).
126. Calvo E, Aramendia JM, Garcia-Foncillas J, et al. Paclitaxel (T) combination chemotherapy in untreated and in resistant stage IV transitional cell carcinoma (TCC) of the urinary bladder: a retrospective study. *Proc Am Soc Clin Oncol* 1997;16:330a(abst).
127. Otto T, Bex A, Krege S, Walz PH, Rubben H. Paclitaxel-based second-line therapy for patients with advanced chemotherapy-resistant bladder carcinoma (M1): a clinical Phase II study. *Cancer* 1997;80:465.
128. Sternberg CN, De Mulder P, Fossa S, et al. Interim toxicity analysis of a randomized trial in advanced urothelial tract tumors of high-intensity MVAC chemotherapy (HD-MVAC) and recombinant human granulocyte colony-stimulating factor (G-CSF) versus classic MVAC chemotherapy(EORTC 30924). *Proc Am Soc Clin Oncol* 2000 (*in press*).
129. von der Masse H, Hansen SW, Roberts JT, et al. Gemcitabine and cisplatin (GC) versus methotrexate, vinblastine, adrimycin and cisplatin (MVAC) chemotherapy in advanced or metastatic transitional cell carcinoma (TCC) of the urothelium: a large randomized, multicenter, multinational phase III study. *Proc Am Soc Clin Oncol* 2000 (*in press*).
130. Logothetis CJ, Hossan E, Sella A, Dexeus FH, Amato RJ. Fluorouracil and recombinant human interferon alfa-2a in the treatment of metastatic chemotherapy-refractory urothelial tumors. *J Natl Cancer Inst* 1991;83:285.
131. Norton L, Simon R, Brereton HD, et al. Predicting the course of Gompertzian growth. *Nature* 1976;264:542.
132. Norton L, Simon R. The Norton-Simon hypothesis revisited. *Cancer Treat Rep* 1986;70:163.
133. Dodd PM, McCaffrey JA, Hilton S, et al. Phase I evaluation of sequential doxorubicin + gemcitabine (AG) then ifosfamide + paclitaxel + cisplatin (ITP) for patients (pts) with unresectable or metastatic transitional cell carcinoma (TCC). *Proc Am Soc Clin Oncol* 1999;18:330a(abst).
134. Maluf F, Bajorin DF. Preliminary analysis of a phase II study of doxorubicin and gemcitabine (AG) followed by ifosfamide, paclitaxel and cisplatin (ITP) sequenced therapy in transitional cell carcinoma (TCC). *Proc Am Soc Clin Oncol* 2000 (*in press*).
135. Logothetis CJ, Johnson DE, Chong C, et al. Adjuvant cyclophosphamide, doxorubicin, and cisplatin chemotherapy for bladder cancer: an update. *J Clin Oncol* 1988;6:1590.
136. Richards B, Bastable JR, Freedman L, et al. Adjuvant chemotherapy with doxorubicin (Adriamycin) and 5-fluorouracil in T3, NX, MO bladder cancer treated with radiotherapy. *Br J Urol* 1983;55:386.
137. Freiha F, Reese J, Torti F. A randomized tral of radical cystectomy versus radical cystectomy plus cisplatin, vinblastine and methotrexate chemotherapy for muscle-invasive bladder cancer. *J Urol* 1996;155:495.
138. Studer U, Bacchi M, Biederman C, et al. Adjuvant cisplatin chemotherapy following cystectomy for bladder cancer: results of a prospective randomized trial. *J Urol* 1994;152:81.
139. Stockle M, Meyenburg W, Wellek S, et al. Non organ-confined bladder cancer: improved survival after radical cystectomy by three adjuvant cycles of M-VAC/M-VEC. *J Urol* 1992;147:446A.
140. Stockle M, Meyenburg W, Wellek S, et al. Adjuvant polychemotherapy of nonorgan-confined bladder cancer after radical cystectomy revisited: long-term results of a controlled prospective study and further experience. *J Urol* 1995;153:47.
141. Scher H, Herr H, Sternberg C, et al. Neo-adjuvant chemotherapy for invasive bladder cancer: experience with the M-VAC regimen. *Br J Urol* 1989;64:250.
142. Schultz P, Herr HW, Zhang ZF, et al. Neoadjuvant chemotherapy for invasive bladder cancer: prognostic factors for survival of patients treated with M-VAC with 5-year follow-up. *J Clin Oncol* 1994;12:1394.
143. Splinter TA, Scher HI, Denis L, et al. The prognostic value of the pathological response to combination chemotherapy before cystectomy in patients with invasive bladder cancer. European Organization for Research on Treatment of Cancer—Genitourinary Group. *J Urol* 1992;147:606.
144. Herr HW, Scher HI. Neoadjuvant chemotherapy and partial cystectomy for invasive bladder cancer. *Cancer Treat Res* 1992;59:99.
145. Sternberg CN, Arena MG, Calabresi F, et al. Neoadjuvant M-VAC (methotrexate, methotrexate, adriamycin and cisplatin) for infiltrating transitional cell carcinoma of the bladder. *Cancer* 1993;72:1975.
146. Scher HI, Kantoff PW. Chemotherapy for muscle-infiltrating bladder cancer. *Hematol Oncol Clin North Am* 1992;6:169.
147. Herr HW, Bajorin DF, Scher HI. Neoadjuvant chemotherapy and bladder-sparing surgery for invasive bladder cancer: ten-year outcome. *J Clin Oncol* 1998;16:1298.
148. Coppin CM, Gospodarowicz MK, James K, et al. Improved local control of invasive bladder cancer by concurrent cisplatin and preoperative or definitive radiation. The National Cancer Institute of Canada Clinical Trials Group. *J Clin Oncol* 1996;14:2901.
149. Wallace DM, Raghavan D, Kelly KA, et al. Neo-adjuvant (pre-emptive) cisplatin therapy in invasive transitional cell carcinoma of the bladder. *Br J Urol* 1991;67:608.
150. Cortesi E. Neoadjuvant treatment for locally advanced bladder cancer: a prospective randomized clinical trial. *Proc Am Soc Clin Oncol* 1995;14:237.
151. Rintala E, Hannisdahl E, Fossa SD, Hellsten S, Sander S. Neoadjuvant chemotherapy in bladder cancer: a randomized study. Nordic Cystectomy Trial I. *Scand J Urol Nephrol* 1993;27:355.
152. Malmstrom PU, Rintala E, Wahlqvist R, et al. Five-year followup of a prospective trial of radical cystectomy and neoadjuvant chemotherapy: Nordic Cystectomy Trial I. The Nordic Cooperative Bladder Cancer Study Group. *J Urol* 1996;155:1903.
153. Martinez Pineiro JA, de la Pena JJ, Hidalgo L, et al. Aggressive preoperative chemotherapy in infiltrating bladder carcinoma with a combination of cisplatin, cyclophosphamide and adriamycin. Preliminary report. *Arch Esp Urol* 1986;39:33.
154. Curotto A, Canobbio C, Orsatti M, et al. Chemo-radiotherapy in locally advanced bladder cancer: neo-adjuvant treatment. In: Giuliani LS, Boccardo F, Pescatore D, eds. Vol. 3. Munchen, FRG: Sympomed, 1994:433.
155. Logothetis C, Swanson D, Amato R, et al. Optimal delivery of perioperative chemotherapy: preliminary results of a randomized, prospective, comparative trial of preoperative and postoperative chemotherapy for invasive bladder carcinoma. *J Urol* 1996;155:1241.
156. Shipley WU, Winter KA, Kaufman DS, et al. An RTOG phase III trial (89-03) of neo-adjuvant chemotherapy in patients with invasive bladder cancer treated with selective bladder preservation by combined radiation therapy and chemotherapy. *Proc Am Soc Clin Oncol* 1998;17:311a.
157. Crawford ED, Natale RB, Burton H. Southwest Oncology Group Study (8710): trial of cystectomy alone versus neo-adjuvant M-VAC and cystectomy in patients with locally advanced bladder cancer (Intergroup Trial 0080). *Prog Clin Biol Res* 1991;353:111.
158. Sternberg CN. Neoadjuvant and adjuvant chemotherapy in locally advanced bladder cancer. *Semin Oncol* 1996;23:621.
159. Neoadjuvant cisplatin, methotrexate, and vinblastine chemotherapy for muscle-invasive bladder cancer: a randomised controlled trial. *Lancet* 1999;354:533.
160. Henry K, Miller J, Mori M, Loening S, Fallon B. Comparison of transurethral resection to radical therapies for stage B bladder tumors. *J Urol* 1988;140:964.
161. Herr HW. Conservative management of muscle-infiltrating bladder cancer: prospective experience. *J Urol* 1987;138:1162.
162. Kata EJ, Herr HW. The role of transurethral resection for muscle invasive bladder carcinoma. *J Urol* 1993;149:316.
163. Shipley WU, Prout GR Jr, Kaufman SD, Perrone TL. Invasive bladder carcinoma. The importance of initial transurethral surgery and other significant prognostic factors for improved survival with full-dose irradiation. *Cancer* 1987;60:514.
164. Dandekar NP, Tongaonkar HB, Dalal AV, Kulkarni JN, Kamat MR. Partial cystectomy for invasive bladder cancer. *J Surg Oncol* 1995;60:24.
165. Sweeney P, Kursh ED, Resnick MI. Partial cystectomy. *Urol Clin North Am* 1993;19:701.
166. Shipley WU, Rose MA. Bladder cancer. The selection of patients for treatment by full-dose irradiation. *Cancer* 1985;55:2278.
167. Naslund I, Nilsson B, Littbrand B. Hyperfractionated radiotherapy of bladder cancer. A ten-year follow-up of a randomized clinical trial. *Acta Oncol* 1994;33:397.
168. Cole DJ, Durrant KR, Roberts JT, et al. A pilot study of accelerated fractionation in the radiotherapy of invasive carcinoma of the bladder. *Br J Radiol* 1992;65:792.
169. Horwich A, Pendlebury S, Dernaley DP. Organ conservation in bladder cancer. *Eur J Cancer* 1995;31:208.
170. Van der Werf-Messing BHP, Menon RS, Hop WCJ. Cancer of the urinary bladder category T2, T3 treated by interstitial radium implant: second report. *Int J Radiat Oncol Biol Phys* 1993;9:481.
171. Wijnmalen A, Van der Werf-Messing BHP. Factors influencing the prognosis in bladder cancer. *Int J Radiat Oncol Biol Phys* 1986;12:559.
172. Moonen LM, Horenblas S, van der Voet JC, Nuyten MJ, Bartelink H. Bladder conservation in selected T1G3 and muscle-invasive T2-T3a bladder carcinoma using combination therapy of surgery and iridium-192 implantation. *Br J Urol* 1994;74:322.
173. Steineck G, Scher HI. Integrated therapy for advanced bladder cancer. *Curr Opin Urol* 1994;4:281.
174. Scher HI. Chemotherapy for invasive bladder cancer: neoadjuvant versus adjuvant. *Semin Oncol* 1990;17:555.
175. Scher HI, Yagoda A, Herr HW, et al. Neoadjuvant M-VAC (methotrexate, vinblastine, doxorubicin and cisplatin) effect on the primary bladder lesion. *J Urol* 1988;139:470.
176. Shipley WU, Prout GR Jr, Einstein AB, et al. Treatment of invasive bladder cancer by cisplatin and radiation in patients unsuited for surgery. *JAMA* 1987;258:931.
177. Hall RR. Bladder preserving treatment: the role of transurethral surgery alone and with combined modality therapy. In: Vogelzang NJ, Scardino PT, Shipley WU, Coffey DS, eds. *Comprehensive textbook of genitourinary oncology.* Baltimore: Williams & Wilkins, 1995:509.
178. Herr HW, Scher HI. Neoadjuvant chemotherapy and partial cystectomy for invasive bladder cancer. *J Clin Oncol* 1994;12:975.

179. Sternberg CN, Pansodoro V, Lauretti S, et al. Neoadjuvant M-VAC (methotrexate, vinblastine, adriamycin, and cisplatin) chemotherapy and bladder preservation for muscle-infiltrating transitional cell carcinoma of the bladder. *Urol Oncol* 1995;1:127.
180. Sauer R, Dunst J, Altendorf-Hofmann A, et al. Radiotherapy with and without cisplatin in bladder cancer. *Int J Radiat Oncol Biol Phys* 1990;19:687.
181. Shipley WU, Kaufman DS, Heney NM, et al. An update of combined modality therapy for patients with muscle invading bladder cancer using selective bladder preservation or cystectomy. *J Urol* 1999;162:445.
182. Tester W, Porter A, Asbell S, et al. Combined modality program with possible organ preservation for invasive bladder carcinoma: results of RTOG protocol 85-12. *Int J Radiat Oncol Biol Phys* 1993;25:783.
183. Dunst J, Sauer R, Schrott KM, et al. Organ-sparing treatment of advanced bladder cancer: a 10-year experience. *Int J Radiat Oncol Biol Phys* 1994;30:261.
184. Tester W, Caplan R, Heaney J, et al. Neoadjuvant combined modality program with selective organ preservation for invasive bladder cancer: results of Radiation Therapy Oncology Group phase II trial 8802. *J Clin Oncol* 1996;14:119.
185. Kachnic LA, Kaufman DS, Zietman AL, et al. Selective bladder preservation by combined modality therapy for invasive bladder cancer. *Int J Radiat Oncol Biol Phys* 1995;1:271 (abst).
186. Given RW, Parsons JT, McCarley D, Wajsman Z. Bladder-sparing multimodality treatment of muscle-invasive bladder cancer: a five-year follow-up. *Urology* 1995;46:499.
187. Srougi M, Simon SD. Primary methotrexate, vinblastine, doxorubicin and cisplatin chemotherapy and bladder preservation in locally invasive bladder cancer: a 5-year followup. *J Urol* 1994;151:593.
188. Geller NL, Scher HI, Parmar MK, Dalesio O, Kaye S. Can we combine available data to evaluate the effects of neoadjuvant chemotherapy for invasive bladder cancer? *Semin Oncol* 1990;17:628.
189. Sternberg CN, Raghaven D, Ohi Y, et al. Neoadjuvant and adjuvant chemotherapy in advanced disease—what are the effects on survival and prognosis? *Int J Urol* 1995;2[Suppl]:76.
190. Kaufman DS, Shipley WU, Griffin PP, et al. Selective bladder preservation by combination treatment of invasive bladder cancer. *N Engl J Med* 1993;329:1377.
191. Housset M, Maulard C, Chretien Y, et al. Combined radiation and chemotherapy for invasive transitional-cell carcinoma of the bladder: a prospective study. *J Clin Oncol* 1993;11:2150.
192. Kachnic LA, Shipley WU, Griffin PP, et al. Combined modality treatment with selective bladder conservation for invasive bladder cancer: long-term tolerance in the female patient. *Cancer J Sci Am* 1996;2:79.
193. Shipley WU, Winter KA, Kaufman DS, et al. Initial results of RTOG 95-06: a phase I/II trial of transurethral surgery and fractionated twice-daily radiation with concurrent cisplatin and 5-fluorouracil followed either by selective bladder preservation or cystectomy for patients with muscle-invading bladder cancer. *Int J Radiat Oncol Biol Phys* 1999;45:222 (abst 145).
194. Lipponen PK. Over-expression of p53 nuclear oncoprotein in transitional-cell bladder cancer and its prognostic value. *Int J Cancer* 1993;53:365.
195. Sarkis AS, Bajorin DF, Reuter VE, et al. Prognostic value of p53 nuclear overexpression in patients with invasive bladder cancer treated with neoadjuvant MVAC. *J Clin Oncol* 1995;13:1384.
196. Wu CS, Pollack A, Czerniak B, et al. Prognostic value of p53 in muscle-invasive bladder cancer treated with preoperative radiotherapy. *Urology* 1996;47:305.
197. Cordon-Cardo C, Wartinger D, Petrylak D, et al. Altered expression of the retinoblastoma gene product: prognostic indicator in bladder cancer. *J Natl Cancer Inst* 1992;84:1251.
198. Logothetis CJ, Xu H, Ro JY, et al. Altered expression of retinoblastoma protein and known prognostic variables in locally advanced bladder cancer. *J Natl Cancer Inst* 1992;84:1256.
199. Herr HW, Bajorin DF, Scher HI, Cordon-Cardo C, Reuter VE. Can p53 help select patients with invasive bladder cancer for bladder preservation? *J Urol* 1999;161:20.
200. Cote RJ, Esrig D, Groshen S, Jones PA, Skinner DG. p53 and the treatment of bladder cancer. *Nature* 1997;385:123.
201. Fleshner N, Garland J, Moadel A, et al. Influence of smoking status on the disease-related outcomes of patients with tobacco-associated superficial transitional cell carcinoma of the bladder. *Cancer* 1999;86:2337.

SECTION 4

PETER R. CARROLL
KEITH L. LEE
ZVI Y. FUKS
PHILIP W. KANTOFF

Cancer of the Prostate

Prostate cancer is a significant health care problem in the United States due to its high incidence and mortality, the costs associated with its detection and treatment, and the fact that no consensus exists on what constitutes the best form of treatment for any stage of this disease. Excluding superficial skin cancers, prostate cancer is the most common malignancy afflicting American men.

Since the advent in the late 1980s of prostate-specific antigen (PSA) level as an effective screening test, the medical community has witnessed a dramatic increase in the incidence of prostate cancer cases. Between 1985 and 1992, the age-adjusted incidence in the United States more than doubled, reaching a peak of more than 190 cases per 100,000 in 1992.[1] Perhaps reflecting stage migration or more effective treatment for localized disease, 5-year cancer survival rates have increased from approximately 70% in the early 1980s to more than 90% a decade later.[1] Since 1992, the incidence rate has steadily declined.

To date, no conclusive data confirm that screening reduces disease morbidity and mortality. Observations that support screening and early detection include the following: PSA screening improves detection of clinically important tumors without significantly increasing the detection of unimportant tumors; the disease is more burdensome at later stages; most PSA-detected tumors are curable using current techniques; and there is no cure for metastatic disease. However, until properly conducted trials of screening are completed, the benefits and risks of prostate cancer's early detection and the associated treatment methods should be discussed carefully with patients.

NORMAL PROSTATE ANATOMY AND HISTOLOGY

The prostate is an ovoid structure located between the urinary bladder superiorly and the pelvic floor inferiorly (Fig. 34.4-1). The urethra traverses this gland, entering its base below the bladder neck and exiting at the narrowed apex at the level of the urogenital diaphragm. The anterior surface of the prostate is attached to the pubis, and the posterior surface is flattened with a midline depression that lies against the rectal ampulla. The lateral and inferior surfaces of the gland are in contact with the levator ani muscles. The levator ani muscles have an almost vertical orientation, funneling inferiorly to surround the rectum and bracket the striated urethral sphincter and middle and apical portions of the prostate.[2] The ejaculatory ducts enter the posterior surface laterally and pass obliquely toward the midline, where they end at the verumontanum on the posterior surface of the prostatic urethra. Because of the gland's location deep within the pelvis behind the pubic bone, surgical as well as radiation-based approaches to expose and target the prostate and protect surrounding structures may be challenging.

The prostate's anterior surface and the adjacent lateral pelvic floor are covered by the periprostatic fascia, which is formed by the prostatic and levator fasciae. Lateral to the gland, this layer is called the *endopelvic fascia,* and it covers both the pelvic floor and important underlying neurovascular structures. The prostatic venous plexus (of Santorini), a rich network of tributary veins that serve as the primary penile drainage, is seen within this fascial covering. Erectile nerves to the corpora cavernosa travel outside the prostatic capsule in the lateral pelvic fascia between the prostate and the rectum

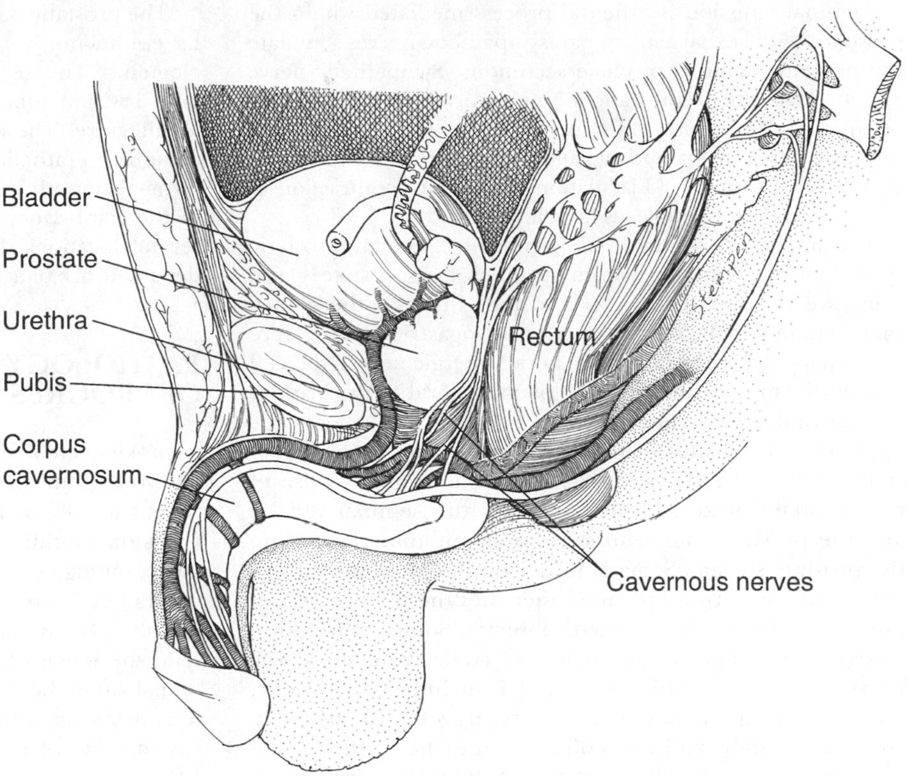

FIGURE 34.4-1. Prostate and regional anatomy.

(see Fig. 34.4-1). The cavernous nerves arise from the pelvic plexus, contain both sympathetic and parasympathetic fibers, and pass beneath the arch of the pubis to supply the corpora cavernosa and the corpus spongiosum. These end in a network of nerve fibers around the cavernous vessels at the penile hilum. Appreciating these anatomic relationships intraoperatively is essential to avoid unnecessary injury and bleeding.[3] The prostatic capsule, composed of condensed smooth muscle and connective tissue, blends with the prostatic sheath on the anterior and anterolateral surfaces of the gland and with the anterior lamella of Denonvilliers' fascia on the posterior gland surface.[4] The puboprostatic ligaments extend anterolaterally from the surface of the gland to fix the apex of the prostate to the pubis.[5] At both the apex and base, no clear capsule separates the prostate from the striated urethral sphincter or bladder neck, respectively. Prostatic glands can be seen in the substance of the urethral sphincter, and smooth muscle fibers from the detrusor blend with the muscular coat of the prostate. Separating the prostate from the rectum is a layer of fascia, Denonvilliers' fascia, derived from two layers of pelvic peritoneum in the retrovesical space.

While voluntary control of voiding begins with relaxation of the striated sphincter in the membranous urethra, smooth muscle components of the bladder neck and prostate contribute to continence in men.[6] The preprostatic sphincter is composed of muscle elements from the bladder. These muscles encircle the urethra and travel along and insert into the urethra more distally. The preprostatic sphincter provides resistance to urine leakage and retrograde seminal ejaculation. A passive prostatic sphincter is located distal to the verumontanum and is related closely to the striated muscle elements of the prostatomembranous sphincter.[7]

The prostatic striated sphincter forms a thick muscle layer over the anterior surface of the gland. Distally, these fibers almost completely surround the gland, except for a posterior gap at the apex, and merge with muscles of the membranous urethral sphincter. Fibers of the membranous striated sphincter encircle the urethra, originating at the anterior decussation of the prostatic sphincter and inserting at the perineal body at the level of the perineal membrane. These sphincteric fibers insert broadly over the surface of the prostatic fascia near the apex and play an important role in regaining continence after radical prostatectomy.[8–10]

The primary arterial supply to the prostate comes from the prostatovesical artery that descends inferiorly along the bladder base. The origin of this artery is variable, but it usually comes from the anterior division of the internal iliac artery. The prostatic artery divides at the base of the prostate into the large posterolateral branch and the smaller anterior branch. The superolateral gland may receive arterial supply from the middle and superior rectal arteries. Urethral branches from the prostatic artery enter the capsule posterolaterally below the bladder neck to supply the transitional zone and periurethral glands. Capsular branches, traveling in the neurovascular bundle posterolaterally to the gland, enter the capsule more distally and laterally, to supply the central and peripheral zones. Prostate parenchymal veins, as well as veins draining all deep pelvic structures, intercommunicate with the prostatic venous plexus lying within the periprostatic fascia on the anterior surface of the gland.[11] The deep dorsal vein of the penis emerges beneath the symphysis pubis between the puboprostatic ligaments to join this plexus. The majority of venous blood drains directly into the prostatic and inferior vesical veins to the internal iliac veins.

Seminal emission is a neural process mediated within the prostate. With sexual activity, parasympathetic nerves stimulate the prostatic acini to produce secretions. Sympathetic nerve activity closes the preprostatic sphincter, preventing retrograde ejaculation, and increases smooth muscle tone in both the prostatic parenchyma and capsule to deposit secretions in the urethra (emission).[12,13] Ejaculation occurs with contraction of the striated bulbospongiosus muscle.

Preganglionic sympathetic nerves to the preprostatic sphincter and smooth musculature of the prostate gland originate at spinal level L2-3 and pass through the sympathetic chain ganglia to the superior hypogastric plexus. Here they synapse with postganglionic noradrenergic nerves, the cell bodies of which lie in the pelvic plexus lateral to the bladder and prostate. Parasympathetic innervation to the prostatic epithelium originates in the pelvic splanchnic nerves from spinal levels S2-4. These preganglionic neurons synapse in the prostatic plexus, located between the seminal vesicles and the prostate, and send short postganglionic fibers into the prostate stroma. Somatic motor output from the pudendal nerve arises from S1-3 and innervates the pubococcygeus muscle of the external striated sphincter. Some contribution to external sphincter tone may also come from the pelvic nerve.[14–17] The prostatic nerve, which includes sympathetic, parasympathetic, and somatic fibers, travels with the neurovascular bundle and sends off main branches at the level of the prostate base. This nerve continues posterolaterally along the prostate and divides into apical branches and a branch to the ejaculatory duct. The main branches pierce the prostatic capsule, then travel along the fibromuscular trabeculae as acinar branches before reaching their terminals at muscular and glandular cells. Afferent nerves from the prostate travel through the pelvic plexus to reach sensory tracts in the spinal cord.

Lymph capillaries emerge from the fibrous stroma and anastomose to form a lobular network of channels. The major route of lymphatic drainage occurs along the prostatic artery to the obturator and internal iliac nodes. Secondary lymphatic drainage originates at the base of the prostate, where lymphatic trunks travel along the medial border of the seminal vesicles to drain into the external iliac nodes. Two more minor routes are along capsular lymphatics on the posterior surface of the gland to the sacral and internal iliac lymph nodes.

The internal structure of the prostate has been organized into *lobes* or *zones*. Early descriptions of five lobes were based on the embryologic concept of the prostate beginning as five groups of epithelial buds that branch off of the urogenital sinus between gestational weeks 11 and 16. By successively branching and rebranching, a complex system of ducts is formed circumferentially around the urethra, forming anterior, posterior, median, and two lateral lobes. However, the zonal description of prostate structure is more commonly used in clinical practice today.[18] According to this scheme, the prostate consists of two primary areas: the peripheral zone and the central zone. In the normal gland of young adults, these two zones make up 95% of the prostate mass. The remaining 5% of the gland is made up of the transitional zone, an anterior fibromuscular segment, and a preprostatic sphincter zone. It is well recognized that prostate cancer occurs primarily in the peripheral zone, while the adenomatous growth of benign prostatic hypertrophy occurs primarily in the transitional zone.

The prostatic parenchyma is composed primarily of glandular epithelium, yet 30% of its mass is composed of muscular elements. The secretory epithelium of the prostate is contained within tubuloalveolar glands with a simple branching architecture. These glands are lined with simple cuboidal or columnar epithelium under which lie flattened basal cells. Stromal smooth muscle and connective tissue surround most of the acini. Ducts draining each gland enter the urethra in several locations. Periurethral glands, not connected to the deep network of acini, drain into the urethra.

PATHOLOGY AND PATTERNS OF PROGRESSION OF PROSTATE CANCER

Approximately 75% of prostate cancers will arise in the peripheral zone of the gland. Another 15% may occur in the central zone, and 10% to 15% will be located in the transitional zone. Carcinoma within the peripheral zone of the gland may be palpable, on digital rectal examination (DRE), as firm nodules or induration. However, it is not uncommon for cancers to be nonpalpable. Gross examination of cancerous tissue in prostatectomy specimens often reveals a similarly firm and gritty texture on palpation; however, lesions can be extremely difficult to differentiate visually from the surrounding normal prostatic parenchyma.[19] Histologically, 95% of prostate cancers or more are adenocarcinomas derived from prostatic acinar cells. Carcinomas tend to be multifocal and show heterogeneous glandular patterns of malignant growth.[20] The glands are typically small or medium-sized, lined with a single layer of cuboidal or low columnar epithelium. The outer basal layer, found in normal and hyperplastic glands, usually is absent in carcinoma. In suspicious lesions, immunohistochemical staining for basal cells can assist in diagnosis.[21] Cancerous acini are irregularly shaped and packed closely together with varying amounts of stroma. In some poorly differentiated tumors, cells in cords or sheets may replace the glandular pattern. Perineurial, lymphatic, and vascular invasions are common and are reliable signs of malignancy. The mechanism of transformation from benign to malignant adenocarcinomas is unclear; however, androgen stimulation appears to play an important role in pathogenesis.[22]

Similar to other cancers, prostate adenocarcinomas are graded histologically. Pathologic interpretation of needle biopsy and prostatectomy specimens focuses on the degree of glandular differentiation, cytologic atypia, and nuclear abnormalities. Several grading systems have been proposed, of which the Gleason system is the most commonly used.[23,24] This grading system recognizes the fact that prostate cancer is a multifocal disease with heterogeneous glandular patterns. Thus, two individual scores, each ranging from 1 to 5, are given to the two most predominant histologic patterns of prostate cancer. The two scores are added together to give the Gleason sum. Sums of 2 to 4 represent well-differentiated disease; 5 to 7, moderately differentiated disease; and 8 to 10, poorly differentiated disease (Fig. 34.4-2). In well-differentiated cancers, groups of small acini are spaced closely "back to back," with little intervening stroma and a loss of the normal myoepithelium that surrounds the glandular elements. Histologically, glands may show luminal distention with mucin (so-called colloid carcinoma) or may take on a cribriform or papillary organization.[25,26] Moderately differentiated cancers are characterized by more haphazardly organized acini,

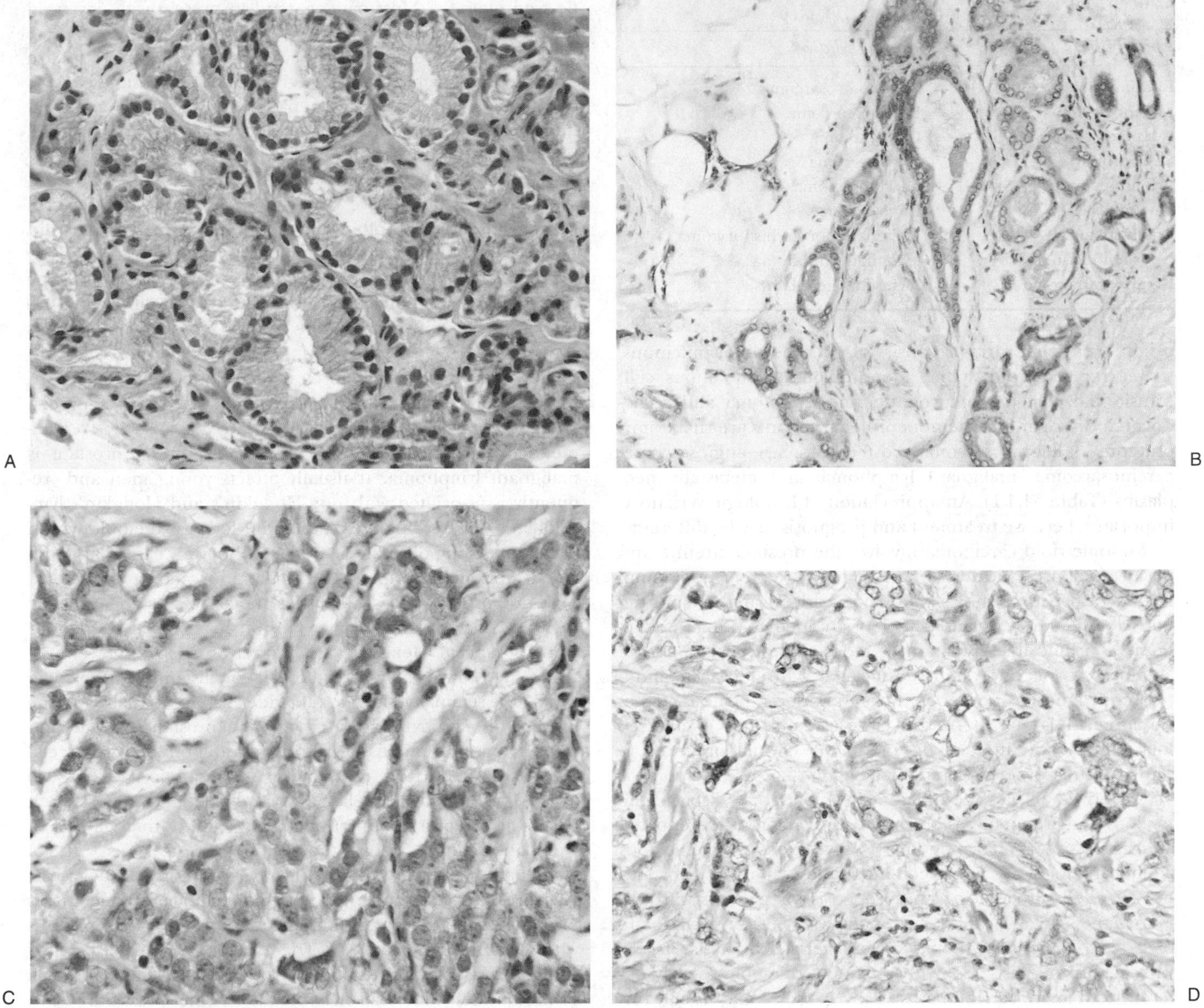

FIGURE 34.4-2. Prostate cancer histology. **A:** Gleason grade 2 (200×). Glands are medium-sized and well developed, with only mild variation in gland size and shape, luminal blue mucin, and no basal cell layer. The glands are tightly packed with minimal intervening stroma and grow in circumscribed nodules, with a minimal peripheral infiltrative pattern. Nuclear features of malignancy include mild nuclear enlargement, granular chromatin, and nucleoli. **B:** Gleason grade 3 (200×). Glands are well developed, with more profound variation in contour and morphology. The glands grow in an infiltrative pattern as seen here, with extension into extra-prostatic tissues. **C:** Gleason grade 4 (200×). Malignant cells have trabecular and glandular growth pattern, forming small solid nests and abortive, fused glandular lumens. This tumor has a highly infiltrative pattern with scattered small angulated nests. Malignant nuclear features include marked nuclear enlargement and macro-nucleoli. **D:** Gleason grade 5 (200×). Highly infiltrative growth pattern with single cells and small nests of malignant epithelial cells. Cytologic features include marked nuclear pleomorphism and anisonucleosis with irregular contours, coarse irregular chromatin distribution, and macronucleoli.

more pronounced nuclear anaplasia, and infiltration of surrounding normal glands. In poorly differentiated adenocarcinoma, cells appear to be in sheets or cords, and glandular components may not be discernible. There is pronounced nuclear anaplasia, and invasion of surrounding tissue may be seen. When comparing patients with similar Gleason sums, it is important to note that the major Gleason pattern score may have additional prognostic value. For instance, patients with 3+4 disease tend to do better than those with 4+3 disease. In our experience, 3-year actuarial PSA failure–free survival rates in patients treated with prostatectomy are approximately 82% for the former group and 77% for the latter.

The histology of the remaining 5% of prostate cancers is heterogeneous, arising from stromal, epithelial, or ectopic cells. Nonadenocarcinoma variants can be categorized into two groups—epithelial and nonepithelial—based on the cellular

TABLE 34.4-1. Examples of Nonadenocarcinoma Prostate Cancer Cell Types

Epithelial	*Nonepithelial*
Endometrioid	Rhabdomyosarcoma
Mucinous	Leiomyosarcoma
Adenoid cystic	Osteosarcoma
Signet-ring	Angiosarcoma
Adenosquamous	Carcinosarcoma
Squamous cell	Fibrosarcoma
Transitional cell	Malignant fibrous histiocytoma
Neuroendocrine	Malignant lymphoma
Comedocarcinoma	Metastatic neoplasms

origin. Epithelial variants consist of endometrioid, mucinous, signet-ring, adenoid cystic, adenosquamous, squamous cell, transitional cell, and neuroendocrine carcinoma and comedocarcinoma. Among the nonepithelial variants are rhabdomyosarcoma, leiomyosarcoma, osteosarcoma, angiosarcoma, carcinosarcoma, malignant lymphoma, and metastatic neoplasms (Table 34.4-1). An appreciation of histologic variants is important, because treatment and prognosis may be different.

Endometrioid carcinoma involves the prostatic urethra and periurethral prostatic ducts in the region of the verumontanum. Histologically, it resembles endometrial adenocarcinoma of the uterus with complex glands lined by stratified columnar epithelium.[27,28] Clinically, this variant is more aggressive than simple adenocarcinoma and often is associated with metastases and a poorer prognosis. Another epithelial variant is mucinous adenocarcinoma. It is characterized by large accumulations of extracellular mucin and luminal distention.[26,29] Overall prognosis is similar to that of adenocarcinoma. Signet-ring cell carcinoma is characterized by large cytoplasmic vacuoles that displace the nucleus and frequently is associated with poorly differentiated and aggressive adenocarcinoma.[30] Associations with mucinous adenocarcinoma are not uncommon, and vacuoles may or may not be filled with mucin. The prognosis for patients with primary signet-ring cell carcinoma is poor, with a 3-year survival rate of 27%.[31] Comedocarcinoma is characterized by nests of cells with central necrosis. Comedocarcinoma resembles poorly differentiated adenocarcinoma (Gleason grade 5) and usually carries a poor prognosis.[32] A rare variant with a better prognosis is adenoid cystic carcinoma. Histologically, lesions resemble basal cell hyperplasia, and disease usually is organ-confined.[33,34]

Squamous cell carcinoma of the prostate accounts for 0.5% to 1% of all prostate cancers and sometimes is difficult to differentiate from disease originating from the bladder and urethra.[35] Such histologic features as keratinization and intercellular bridging are seen, as is the lack of glandular differentiation. Clinically, patients present in fashions similar to those with adenocarcinoma; however, serum tumor markers such as acid phosphatase and PSA will remain normal.[35–38] This epithelial variant is more aggressive than adenocarcinoma, with an average survival after diagnosis of approximately 14 months.[39] Primary transitional cell carcinoma (TCC) of the prostate has also been reported, although secondary spread from the bladder is much more common.[40] Primary prostatic TCC does not respond to hormonal therapy but has been shown to respond to combination therapy.[41] Prognosis is variable, and TCC is best treated with primary surgery or combinations of chemotherapy, radiation therapy, and surgery. Neuroendocrine tumors of the prostate are rare and can present with paraneoplastic syndromes.[42,43] Most patients tend to present with advanced disease at the time of diagnosis.[44]

Nonepithelial nonadenocarcinomas of the prostate are rare. Sarcomas represent fewer than 0.1% of prostate cancers and tend to occur in younger patients.[45] The two most common types are rhabdomyosarcoma and leiomyosarcoma. The former is the most common prostatic tumor in the pediatric age group, whereas the latter tends to occur in adults.[46] Both are extremely aggressive and tend to invade locally and hematogenously. Pathologically, rhabdomyosarcomas are solid neoplasms, with a histologic appearance that ranges from primitive mesenchyma to well-differentiated, myofiber-type cells.[47] Leiomyosarcomas tend to be bulky, with diffuse infiltration into the periprostatic soft tissues. Histologically, lesions show interlacing spindle cells, eosinophilic cytoplasm, and nuclear atypia accompanied by necrosis and hemorrhage.[48] A multidisciplinary approach to treatment, including surgery, chemotherapy, and radiation therapy, is usually recommended.[44] A third nonepithelial cancer of the prostate is malignant lymphoma. It usually affects young men and frequently is associated with non-Hodgkin's and Hodgkin's lymphoma.[49] On histologic examination, lesions resemble lymph nodes consisting of small-cleaved lymphocytic cells or large diffuse lymphomas. Prognosis is usually poor, and prostatectomy may not prolong survival. Other metastases to the prostate include leukemia and local extension from rectal or bladder primary cancers. Metastases from other organs are rare.[45]

Prostate cancer may spread locally or distantly. Cancers can invade the seminal vesicles and bladder base proximally and the urethra distally. Extension through the prostatic capsule and into the periprostatic tissues is not uncommon; however, rectal invasion posteriorly is rare, owing to separation of the two organs by Denonvilliers' fascia. Lymphatic spread most often occurs in a stepwise manner and follows the normal pattern of lymphatic drainage. The obturator nodes are the primary sites of lymphatic metastases, followed by the perivesical, hypogastric, iliac, presacral, and paraaortic nodes. Hematogenous metastases primarily affect the bones and occur in up to 85% of patients who die of prostate cancer.[50] The axial skeleton is particularly vulnerable, as the preprostatic and periprostatic venous complex communicates with Batson's plexus of the presacral veins. Osseous sites of involvement, in decreasing order of frequency, include the lumbar spine, proximal femur, pelvis, thoracic spine, ribs, sternum, and skull. Bone metastases are typically osteoblastic (80%). Osteolytic (5%) and mixed osteoblastic-osteolytic (15%) lesions are less common. Hematogenous spread to viscera can occur, but widespread visceral dissemination is rare. Lung and liver metastases are seen in approximately 25% and 20% of patients, respectively, with end-stage prostate cancer. The current tumor, node, and metastasis (TNM) staging system for prostate cancer is presented in Table 34.4-2.

PREMALIGNANT LESIONS (PROSTATIC INTRAEPITHELIAL NEOPLASIA)

Prostate carcinoma often is accompanied by atypical lesions such as intraductal dysplasia or prostatic intraepithelial neoplasia (PIN). It has been estimated that approximately 70% of prostate tissue ultimately removed for carcinoma will also harbor

TABLE 34.4-2. Prostate Cancer Staging

TNM Staging System		*Jewett Staging System (Modified)*	
TUMOR			
TX	Tumor cannot be assessed		
T0	No evidence of tumor		
Tis	Carcinoma *in situ* (PIN)		
T1a	Incidental, tumor ≤5%	Stage A1	Tumor ≤5%, Gleason score ≤4
T1b	Incidental, tumor >5%	Stage A2	Tumor >5%, Gleason score >4
T1c	Identified by biopsy (PSA screening)		
T2a	Palpable or seen on TRUS; one lobe	Stage B1	Palpable, <one lobe, ≤1.5 cm
T2b	Palpable or seen on TRUS; both lobes	Stage B2	Palpable, both lobes, >1.5 cm
T3a	Extracapsular extension	Stage C1	ECE, negative margins
		Stage C2	ECE, positive margins
T3b	Seminal vesicle involvement	Stage C3	Seminal vesicle involvement
T4	Bladder neck, external sphincter, rectal, levator muscles, or pelvic side wall involvement		
NODE			
NX	Lymph nodes cannot be assessed	Stage D1	Microscopic pelvic lymph node involved
N0	No regional lymph node involved		
N1	Metastases, regional lymph node(s)		
METASTASIS			
MX	Distant metastases cannot be assessed		
M0	No distant metastases		
M1a	Nonregional lymph node involvement	Stage D2	Disease outside pelvis
M1b	Bone involvement		
M1c	Other sites involved		

ECE, extracapsular extension; M, metastasis; N, node; PIN, prostatic intraepithelial neoplasia; PSA, prostate-specific antigen; T, tumor; TRUS, transrectal ultrasonography.

PIN.[19,51,52] A presumptive precursor lesion to prostate cancer, PIN is characterized by large glands separated by modest amounts of stroma with an overall normal-appearing architecture.[53,54] Glandular cells appear basophilic with enlarged nuclei, hyperchromatism, and anaplasia. Categorized into low- and high-grade PIN, the latter is associated with significant epithelial hyperplasia. Unlike carcinoma, however, the basal cell layer surrounding the dysplastic cells remains intact. Moreover, an intact basement membrane has been demonstrated in PIN, in contrast to moderately and poorly differentiated adenocarcinoma.[55] High-grade PIN has a zonal distribution similar to that of adenocarcinoma and appears to be directly associated with cancer grade and stage.[52] In our experience, roughly 50% of patients with an initial diagnosis of high-grade PIN alone will later demonstrate carcinoma on repeat biopsy.[56] Moreover, high-grade PIN may be associated with aggressive disease and a poorer prognosis.[57] However, its true prognostic value requires further research, as cancers in the transitional zone seldom are accompanied by PIN and as many as 70% of early carcinomas may lack any high-grade PIN.[51]

The DNA content (ploidy) of cancerous lesions may correlate with patient outcomes. Patients with diploid cancers generally have better survival outcomes than do those with aneuploid cancers.[58,59] In a study of nearly 900 patients with pathologically non–organ-confined disease (pT3), Hawkins et al.[60] showed that DNA ploidy was a significant prognostic factor for both clinical and biochemical failure–free survival. Others have reported that immunohistochemical staining for p27, a nuclear protein inhibitor of the cell cycle, may be of value. Decreased p27 expression is seen with more aggressive disease. Cheville et al.[61] showed that patients with low p27 expression had higher-grade tumors, increased tumor aneuploidy, and higher incidences of seminal vesicle and nodal invasion than did men with normal p27 expression.

STAGING

In addition to histologic examination, staging is also important in patient risk assessment and prognosis. The two most commonly used staging systems are the tumor, node, and metastasis TNM system and the Jewett staging system (see Table 34.4-2).[19,62] In the Jewett staging system are four stages of prostate cancer, A to D, with subclassifications within each stage. Stage A disease is clinically nonpalpable disease found incidentally during surgery for benign prostatic hyperplasia (BPH). Stage A1 disease is well differentiated and involves less than 5% of a pathologic specimen. Stage A2 involves more than 5% of a specimen or is moderate to poorly differentiated. Stage B (T2) cancers are clinically palpable but confined to the prostate. Stage B1 cancers are 1.5 cm in diameter or smaller and involve only one lobe of the prostate. Stage B2 involves either several nodules in both lobes or a lesion larger than 1.5 cm. Stage C (T3 and T4) tumors are non–organ-confined with invasion of soft tissue outside the prostate. Stage C1 tumors invade through the prostatic capsule but have a negative surgical margin. Margins are positive for stage C2 tumors, and C3 tumors invade the seminal vesicles. Stage D cancer is metastatic, with *D1* referring to microscopical pelvic lymph node involvement and *D2* to disease involving bones or distant organs (or both). Most clinicians use the TNM system.

Given that autopsy studies show a high prevalence of histologic evidence of prostate cancer in men (>30%) who die of other diseases, there is some concern that many cancers currently detected may be "insignificant" or of such low biologic potential that treatment is not necessary and possibly harmful.[63] Cancer grade, cancer stage, serum PSA level, and the age and health of the patient most often define the risk associated with a prostate cancer. Tumor volume also correlates with risk, although it cannot be determined *in vivo* with precise accuracy as yet. Generally, those cancers that exceed 0.5 mL are more likely to be associated with extraprostatic disease as compared to smaller cancers.[64] Approximately 20% of autopsy or incidental cancers exceed this size. Similarly, higher-grade cancers (Gleason score 4 or 5) are also more likely to be associated with extracapsular disease and cancer progression as compared to lower-grade cancers. According to criteria of cancer size, grade, and stage, the vast majority of cancers currently identified by early detection efforts appear to be clinically significant. Indeed, at least one-third have adverse features, including extracapsular extension (ECE), seminal vesicle invasion, lymph node metastases, or very high-grade histology, all of which are associated with a significant risk of cancer progression, certainly without treatment and often with treatment.

EPIDEMIOLOGY

Excluding superficial skin cancers, prostate cancer is the most common malignancy afflicting American men. In 1999, some 179,300 new cases were diagnosed, and an estimated 37,000 prostate cancer deaths occurred, making it the second most common cause of cancer death, after lung cancer, in American men.[1]

Beginning in the late 1980s, PSA screening became a common practice, and the incidence of prostate cancer cases increased dramatically as a direct result. Between 1985 and 1992, the age-adjusted incidence in the United States more than doubled, reaching a peak of more than 190 cases per 100,000 in 1992.[1] This increase was not unanticipated, as the introduction of any effective screening test should lead to detection of earlier-stage disease in more patients (i.e., stage migration).[65,66] Stage migration has, in fact, occurred in the United States, and approximately three-fourths of prostate cancer cases diagnosed now are recognized while the disease is still clinically organ-confined, as compared to only one-fourth prior to the introduction of PSA screening.[67,68] Perhaps reflecting patients' earlier disease stage at presentation and more effective treatment for localized disease, 5-year cancer survival rates have increased from approximately 70% in the early 1980s to more than 90% a decade later.[1] Since 1992, the incidence rate has declined steadily as the pool of men with no previous diagnosis of lower-staged disease became slowly exhausted. Incidence rates today are approaching those before PSA screening.

Worldwide, prostate cancer ranks third in cancer incidence and sixth in cancer mortality among men. There is, however, a notable variability in incidence and mortality among world regions. The incidence per 100,000 is low in Japan and China at 8.51 and 1.08, respectively, and is intermediate in regions of Central America (24.77) and Western Africa (23.85). In North American countries, where PSA screening is widely adopted (e.g., in the United States), the incidence may be as high as 95.1 per 100,000.[69] Although less variable than incidence, there remains a 30-fold difference in the age-standardized mortality rate between global regions, ranging from 0.7 per 100,000 in China, to 18.5 per 100,000 in North America, to 22.2 per 100,000 in the Caribbean.[69] The basis for this difference is multifactorial and has been attributed to more aggressive screening and diagnosis in aging populations, genetic predisposition, and environmental causes.

Predominantly a disease of elderly men, the clinical diagnosis of prostate cancer is rare before age 40 but increases steadily thereafter. Autopsy studies worldwide have shown that histologic disease increases with age and that roughly three-fourths of men older than 80 years will have some evidence of latent disease.[70–75] In parallel, more than 80% of clinically apparent disease occurs in men older than 65 years.[1] In the United States, it is estimated that 1 in 55 men between the ages of 40 and 59 will develop clinically apparent disease. This incidence climbs almost exponentially to 1 in 7 for men between 60 and 79. This association is also reflected in mortality rates, as prostate cancer accounts for 10.8% of cancer-related deaths in men between 60 and 79 years of age and 24.6% in those older than 80. As the proportion of older men increases in our population, the impact of prostate cancer will continue to grow. In fact, the doubling of age-adjusted mortality rates in Taiwan over the past three decades has been attributed mainly to aging of the population.[76]

Ethnic and racial differences are also seen in disease incidence and mortality. African Americans are in the highest-risk group, with an incidence of 224.3 cases per 100,000 for the period between 1990 and 1995. The incidence in white and Asian counterparts during that same period was considerably lower at 150.3 and 82.2 (per 100,000), respectively.[1] In addition, African Americans tend to present with more advanced disease and may have poorer overall prognosis than their white counterparts. It has been reported that African Americans are 1.3 to 1.8 times more likely to present with distant disease and, stage for stage, African Americans have lower survival rates.[77,78] The underlying cause for this difference has been attributed to social, economic, educational, hereditary, and dietary differences.[78–82] Conlisk et al.[83] reported that among African Americans, disease stage at presentation was inversely correlated with income and health insurance status. When one controls for access to medical care, the difference in disease stage at presentation and survival persists.[77,84,85] Recent reports from nations with a large concentration of black patients demonstrate a high incidence of the disease nationally, suggesting a genetic association.[86,87] Several investigators have shown that differences in testosterone levels or androgen receptor gene activity may contribute to the racial differences observed in prostate cancer.[88–91]

Migrant studies, particularly of Asian men, also suggest an environmental, social, or dietary etiology in prostate cancer. When migrants from a low-risk country such as Japan move to the United States, a high-risk nation, their prostate cancer incidence and mortality become severalfold higher than native Japanese counterparts.[92,93] Other investigators have found a positive correlation between the number of years since migration to the United States and cancer risk.[80] Although diagnostic biases exist between countries, the upward shift in risk nevertheless seems real. This rise in clinically detectable disease may be related to differences in diet. High fat intake has been positively associated with increased risk in these studies and may, in part, explain the rising incidence of prostate cancer in Japan, as dietary habits become more Westernized.[94]

Family history of prostate cancer also contributes to risk. It has been reported that men with prostate cancer are two to three times more likely than controls to have at least one first- or second-degree relative with prostate cancer.[95–97] Keetch et al.[95] reported that a patient with prostate cancer is 3.1 and 4.3 times more likely than a control to give a history of prostate cancer in his father and brother, respectively. Together with the observation that clustering of prostate cancer cases exists in some high-risk families, a hereditary component clearly exists.[98,99] However, the role of specific gene activity and molecular mechanisms of disease remains largely unsolved and continues to be an area of active research. A word of caution is warranted in interpreting family history studies, however, as they are subject to recall, self-selection, and socioeconomic biases.[100–102]

The role of vasectomy and prostate cancer risk remains controversial. Retrospective and prospective cohort epidemiologic studies have demonstrated a relative risk of approximately 1.6 in men who underwent vasectomy.[103–106] However, others could not confirm these findings and suggest that earlier studies were flawed by detection, control selection, and publication biases.[95,107–110] In a recent metaanalysis that included five cohort and nine case-control studies, no causal association was found.[108]

In summary, prostate cancer is a disease of older men worldwide. It is more common in Westernized countries, in those with a family history of the disease, and in African Americans. The cause is likely multifaceted, with genetic, dietary, and social modifiers. Further investigation is necessary to elucidate the role and significance of each factor in prostate cancer induction and progression.

CHEMOPREVENTION AND DIET

Chemoprevention is the administration of medicines or other agents to prevent, slow, or reverse cancer progression. The concept of primary chemoprevention for prostate cancer has gained much interest in the 1990s because of the disease's high prevalence, slowly progressive nature, and long latency period.[111–113] The ideal therapeutic intervention would arrest disease progression during this latency period and decrease the incidence of clinical disease. The success of chemoprevention, however, depends on consideration of several important factors. First, because "healthy" men are treated, the therapeutic agent must offer low to no toxicity and no side effects and must require a simple dosing regimen. Second, epidemiologic and laboratory evidence should support the agent's efficacy. Finally, the ideal patient is one at high risk for developing clinical disease and motivated to adhere to chronic dosing of chemopreventive agents.[114]

To date, several promising chemopreventive agents have been identified and are under laboratory and clinical investigation.[115–120] Finasteride is among the agents now being tested in a large, phase III, randomized clinical trial, the Prostate Cancer Prevention Trial (PCPT).[115,121,122] A joint effort of the Southwest Oncology Group (SWOG), the Eastern Cooperative Oncology Group (ECOG), and the Cancer and Leukemia Group B (CALGB), the PCPT is a 10-year study of 18,882 men, aged 55 or older, with normal DRE and a PSA level of less than 3.0 ng/mL, who have been randomized to either placebo or the 5α-reductase inhibitor finasteride (5 mg/d).[123] Given prostate cancer's slowly progressive nature, the end point of prostate cancer mortality will not be pursued because of long study duration and large sample size requirements. Instead, the primary end point of prostate cancer period prevalence, as determined by sextant prostate biopsy, is used. The PCPT is designed to have greater than 90% power in detecting a 25% reduction in period prevalence of biopsy-proven disease when it reaches its end point in mid-2004.

The use of finasteride to prevent disease seems rational, given that prostate cancer is androgen-responsive.[124–127] An inhibitor of 5α-reductase, finasteride blocks the conversion of testosterone to its active metabolite dihydrotestosterone (DHT) and lowers the prostatic androgen levels.[128] Bologna et al.[124,129] have shown that finasteride can attenuate *in vitro* prostate cancer cell growth in a dose-dependent manner, and others suggest that the lower incidence of prostate cancer among Japanese men may be associated with lower 5α-reductase activity. In addition, as a chemopreventive agent taken chronically, finasteride is well absorbed orally and does not appear to have any clinically relevant drug interactions or toxicity.[130] The frequency of side effects is low and includes decreased libido, impotence, and decreased ejaculate volume.[123,128]

Dietary manipulations have also gained much interest.[131–133] Epidemiologic studies have shown that the incidence of clinically significant prostate cancer is much lower in parts of the world where people eat a predominantly low-fat, plant-based diet.[69,134] In addition, migrant studies demonstrate that when men from a low-risk country move to the United States and begin eating a Westernized diet, their rates of prostate cancer increase severalfold and approach that of the host country.[92] However, which component of a certain diet increases prostate cancer risk remains unclear. Researchers have suggested fat, soy, green tea, lycopene, selenium, and vitamins, among others, as modifiers of prostate cancer risk.

Dietary fat intake is positively associated with prostate cancer risk and may be a rational target for chemoprevention. In a case-control study from the Physicians' Health Study, those who had higher plasma α-linolenic acid levels (a fatty acid found in animal fat) had a two- to threefold increase in prostate cancer risk as compared to those with lower α-linolenic acid levels.[135] Similarly, in a prospective cohort study of more than 47,000 men, Giovannucci et al.[136] found that fat intake was directly correlated with risk of advanced disease and, specifically, animal fat, red meat, and α-linolenic acid were associated with the greatest risk [relative risk (RR) = 1.63, 2.64, and 3.43, respectively].[136] Others have studied saturated fat and reported an attributable risk of 13% for saturated fat intake in excess of 26 g/d as compared to diets with less than 13 g/d. This suggests that 13% of prostate cancer cases may be preventable by reducing saturated fat intake to less than 13 g/d.[137] In a recent prospective case-control study of men in whom prostate cancer was diagnosed, Fradet et al.[138] found that survival was inversely associated with saturated fat intake. As compared to men ingesting less than 10.8% of dietary calories from saturated fat, those ingesting more than 13.2% had three times the risk of dying from prostate cancer (RR = 3.13) and were more likely to develop bone metastasis (RR = 3.4) at a median follow-up of 5.2 years.[138]

Evidence supporting a relationship between prostate cancer and dietary fat also comes from animal studies. Wang et al.[139] injected prostate cancer cells (LNCaP) into mice and placed them on a "typical American" diet containing 40% fat. In 3 weeks, prostate tumor growth was noted. The researchers then divided the animals into subgroups receiving diets containing approximately 40%, 30%, 20%, 10%, and 2% of calories as fat. Progression of prostate cancer ceased or was reversed in some animals placed on 10% to 20% fat diets. This was in contrast to continued tumor growth in groups ingesting higher amounts of fat. PSA levels were also lower in mice on the 2% fat diet as compared to those on the 40% fat diet.[139]

On a molecular level, much remains unknown. Myers and Ghosh[140] recently postulated that the risk seen with high fat intake may be linked to 5-lipoxygenase products of arachidonic acid (a ubiquitous fatty acid found in animal fat) and that inhibition of 5-lipoxygenase could lead to prostate cancer cell death and apoptosis. However, the significance of genetic polymorphisms for 5-lipoxygenase and the role of other fatty acid metabolic pathways in prostate cancer risk remain elusive.

The worldwide difference in prostate cancer incidence may also be associated with dietary intake of soy proteins. In Asian countries such as Japan and the Republic of Korea, where prostate cancer incidence and mortality are just a fraction of that in North America, consumption of soy in the form of tofu, soy milk, tempeh, and miso is noted to be up to 90-fold higher than soy consumption in the United States.[134] In a cross-national study of more than 40 nations, Hebert et al.[134] found soy, on a per-calorie basis, to be the most protective dietary factor. This protective role may be associated with soy's phytoestrogenic components genistein and daidzein. Genistein and daidzein are isoflavonoids with weak estrogenic effect that may have the ability to delay growth of precancerous prostate lesions and prostate tumors.[116,141] Davis et al.[141] showed that genistein inhibits prostate cancer cell growth in culture and induces apoptosis through cell-cycle gene regulation in a dose-dependent manner. Others have demonstrated that genistein is an inhibitor of tyrosine kinase and suggest that genistein may act through inhibition of up-regulated tyrosine kinases in proliferative cancerous states.[131,142,143] Although the association between soy and cancer risk seems convincing, a causal role remains obscure and awaits the rigors of prospective randomized studies. However, given that soy products are generally well tolerated and provide a cost-effective source of isoflavonoids, the scientific community's interest in soy as a chemopreventive agent will likely continue.[120]

To explain the difference in cancer incidence and mortality between nations, researchers have also suggested a chemopreventive role for green tea, a beverage consumed in high quantities in Asia.[117,144] *In vitro* studies by Yang et al.[145] showed that polyphenol extracts from tea inhibited growth of cancerous cell lines and induced cellular apoptosis in a dose-dependent manner. Furthermore, *in vivo* studies by Mohan and Gupta et al.[146,147] found that tea polyphenols inhibited ornithine decarboxylase, a testosterone-induced enzyme that is up-regulated in prostate cancer. Tea polyphenols' inhibition of ornithine decarboxylase in effect attenuates testosterone in the prostatic milieu and may be an important target for chemoprevention.

Tomatoes are rich sources of the carotenoid lycopene. With its potent antioxidant activity, lycopene may protect cellular components from reactive oxygen radical species and lower prostate cancer risk. Epidemiologic data show that lycopene consumption is associated with decreased risk as well as a possible reduction in prostate tumor growth.[148] In a cohort study of approximately 14,000 Adventist men over a 6-year period, consumption of tomato products was associated with lower prostate cancer risk.[149] This finding was substantiated in a prospective cohort study from the Health Professionals Study, where lycopene intake from tomato-based foods was found to be inversely associated with risk.[150] The investigators reported that men ingesting two or more servings of tomato sauce per week had a 36% reduction in cancer risk as compared to counterparts who did not consume tomato sauce. Little is known, however, regarding lycopene's exact mechanism of action or the specific role of different isomers in prostate tissue metabolism.

The role of another antioxidant, vitamin E, as a chemopreventive remains controversial. Epidemiologic and *in vivo* data are often conflicting, despite promising *in vitro* studies.[118,151–154] Part of the difficulty in elucidating vitamin E's effect in chemoprevention is that oral supplements frequently contain different forms of vitamin E than that found naturally in foods. Given the fact that vitamin E exists as potentially eight different compounds, and that isoforms such as γ-tocopherol have been shown to have greater inhibitory effects on prostate cancer cell growth than α-tocopherol, further evaluation of vitamin E is warranted.[154]

Selenium has also been reported to lower prostate cancer risk. In a double-blinded clinical trial designed to determine whether selenium could lower skin cancer recurrences, Clark et al.[155] found that men randomized to receiving selenium had a 63% reduction in prostate cancer incidence as compared to those randomized to receiving placebo. Similar findings were demonstrated in a nested case-control trial of the Health Professionals Follow-Up Study. The investigators found that higher selenium intake, as reflected in nail selenium levels, was significantly protective (odds ratio = 0.35 when comparing the highest and lowest quintile).[156] *In vivo* studies in the human prostate cancer cell lines have also shown that selenium inhibits cancer cell growth at physiologic doses and that its protective effect may be mediated through an androgen-sensitive gene that encodes for a selenium-binding protein.[157,158]

Attention has also focused on vitamin D's antiproliferative and prodifferentiation effect on the prostate.[159,160] Investigators have demonstrated that 1,25-dihydroxyvitamin D_3 [$1,25(OH)_2D_3$], the active metabolite of vitamin D, inhibits cellular proliferation in primary prostate cancer tissue cultures and in prostate cancer cell lines such as PC3, DU145, and LNCaP.[119,161,162] Moreover, epidemiologic evidence shows an inverse relationship between prostate cancer risk and ultraviolet radiation, the primary source of endogenous vitamin D synthesis.[163,164] This observation has led some to suggest that higher rates of prostate cancer in the elderly may be due in part to decreased sun exposure or a decline in the body's ability to synthesize $1,25(OH)_2D_3$ with aging.[160] Similarly, others have proposed that the higher risk in men of African descent may be related to higher skin melanin content, which would decrease endogenous vitamin D production.[114] Taken together, vitamin D and its synthetic analogues may prove to be useful chemopreventive agents for prostate cancer.

Although a relationship between diet and prostate cancer is apparent, whether manipulating the diet will lead to changes in cancer risk is the subject of ongoing clinical trials. In considering the future development of rational chemoprevention trials and test compounds, one must appreciate the interdependence between the practical aspects of clinical trial design and the mechanisms in disease progression.[165,166] A better understanding of the latter may lead to clinical trials that are less restrained by the need for large sample populations and prolonged follow-up. For example, it has been shown that urokinase-mediated cell surface proteolysis and angiogenesis in human prostate cancer cells are important in metastasis and that specific inhibition could decrease the metastatic potential of cancerous cells.[167,168] From this work, one could postulate the design of a chemopreventive agent aimed at preventing metastasis in patients who present with localized disease. As compared to primary chemoprevention, this may be easier to implement clinically as patients are more likely to be motivated and compliant with chronic therapy. Thus, a multidisciplinary approach that reflects our understanding of prostate carcinogenesis and tumor invasion is critical to study design of future chemoprevention trials.

PROSTATE CANCER EARLY DETECTION

Prostate cancer screening or early detection has been accomplished using DRE, measurement of serum PSA (and its various forms), transrectal ultrasonography (TRUS), and combinations of these tests. Although DRE can detect prostate cancer, it detects fewer cancers than does PSA testing and, unfortunately, many cancers detected using DRE are either locally or regionally advanced.[169] Although serum PSA is a better screening test than DRE, DRE should not be abandoned, as it may detect some cancers associated with a normal serum PSA level. Therefore, DRE should be combined with serum PSA testing. TRUS should not be used a first-line screening study as it lacks high specificity, is relatively expensive, and adds little information to that already gained by the use of serum PSA testing and DRE.[170] TRUS is used to guide prostate biopsy in those patients who have an elevated serum PSA level, an abnormal DRE, or both (Fig. 34-4.3).

PSA is a serine protease produced by benign and malignant prostate tissues. Although it is produced in small amounts elsewhere, including breast tissue, endometrium, and in a few malignancies other than prostatic cancer, it should be considered to be organ-specific clinically.[171–175] PSA circulates in the serum as uncomplexed (free or unbound) or complexed (bound) forms.[176–178] Serum PSA is largely complexed by endogenous protease inhibitors, the most common being α_1-antichymotrypsin. Other proteins bind a smaller fraction.

Serum PSA may be elevated transiently in cases of prostatitis and after endoscopic urethral manipulation, prostatic biopsy and, to a more limited extent, ejaculation.[179,180] Routine DRE actually has little effect on serum PSA, but most physicians defer PSA testing after such an examination.[181] The half-life of serum PSA is 2.2 to 3.2 days.[182,183] Therefore, one should wait approximately 4 to 8 weeks after significant prostate manipulation, such as that which occurs with prostatitis or prostate biopsy, before obtaining serum PSA. It should be emphasized that the most common cause for an elevated serum PSA level is BPH, the incidence of which increases with age, as does the incidence of prostate cancer.

Serum PSA concentrations can be decreased by treatment with agents that lower serum testosterone, such as luteinizing hormone–releasing hormone (LHRH) agonists and antagonists, antiandrogens such as flutamide, and the 5α-reductase inhibitor finasteride, which is used for the management of presumed BPH and male-pattern baldness. Finasteride also lowers PSA levels by an average of 50%.[184] Therefore, one can correct for the effect of finasteride on PSA by doubling the PSA level.[185] Use of α-adrenergic antagonists such as terazosin (also used to manage obstructive voiding symptoms) has no appreciable effect on serum PSA levels.[186]

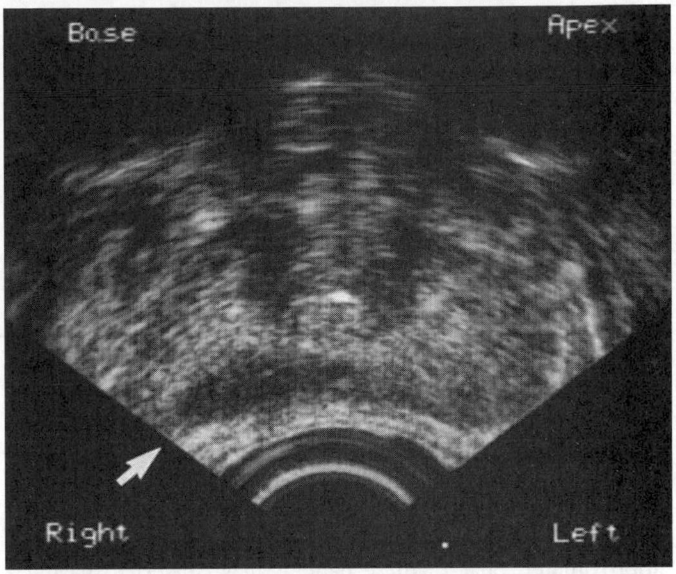

FIGURE 34.4-3. Transrectal ultrasound image showing a characteristic hypoechoic abnormality *(arrow)* consistent with prostate cancer.

USE OF TOTAL SERUM PROSTATE-SPECIFIC ANTIGEN LEVEL AND DIGITAL RECTAL EXAMINATION FOR PROSTATE CANCER EARLY DETECTION

The risk of prostate cancer correlates with serum PSA concentrations and DRE findings. The positive predictive value of a serum PSA level between 4.0 ng/mL and 10 ng/mL is approximately 20% to 30%.[187–191] For levels in excess of 10 ng/mL, the positive predictive value increases to 42% to 71.4%. The use of DRE complements serum PSA testing (Table 34.4-3).

The majority of cancers (>80%) detected by serum PSA are clinically significant as defined by cancer grade and volume.[192] In contrast to the use of DRE alone for early detection of prostate cancer, the majority of PSA-detected cancers are confined *clinically*. However, as many as 40% of cancers detected by the

TABLE 34.4-3. Probability of Prostate Cancer Based on Serum Prostate-Specific Antigen and Digital Rectal Examination

	PSA <4.0 ng/mL		*PSA >4.0 ng/mL*	
Study	–DRE	+DRE	–DRE	+DRE
Cooner et al.[188]	9%	17%	25%	62%
Catalona et al.[189]	—	10%	32%	49%
Hammerer and Huland[370]	4%	21%	12%	72%
Ellis et al.[190]	6%	13%	24%	42%

DRE, digital rectal examination; PSA, prostate-specific antigen.
(Adapted from ref. 171.)

TABLE 34.4-4. Age-Adjusted Prostate-Specific Antigen Reference Ranges

	White[371]		*African American*[372]		*Asian*[373]	
Age Range (y)	Reference Range (ng/mL)	Specificity (%)	Reference Range (ng/mL)	Specificity (%)	Reference Range (ng/mL)	Specificity (%)
40–49	0.0–2.5	95	0.0–2.0	93	0.0–2.0	95
50–59	0.0–3.5	95	0.0–4.0	88	0.0–3.0	95
60–69	0.0–4.5	95	0.0–4.5	81	0.0–4.0	95
70–79	0.0–6.5	95	0.0–5.5	78	0.0–5.0	95

(Adapted from ref. 171.)

use of serum PSA and DRE may have evidence of ECE, usually capsular penetration, if the prostate is removed surgically and examined pathologically.[192]

The frequency of PSA testing remains a matter of some debate. In men with a normal DRE and a PSA level in excess of 2.5 ng/mL, PSA testing should be performed annually, as approximately 50% of these patients may convert to having a PSA level exceeding 4.0 ng/mL.[193,194] The test can be performed biannually in those with a normal DRE and serum PSA level lower than 2.5 ng/mL, as conversion in this group is much less likely. The likelihood of curable prostate cancer, either organ-confined or with ECE associated with low to intermediate cancer grade, is similar in men who have prostate cancer associated with serum PSA levels lower than 4.0 ng/mL and in those with levels of 4.0 to 5.0 ng/mL. Therefore, cure is not likely to be compromised in those with very low serum PSA levels initially who experience a limited rise in the PSA level over time.

Enhancing Prostate-Specific Antigen Test Performance

A number of different strategies have been developed to enhance PSA test performance, by increasing sensitivity in certain populations or specificity in others. These strategies include use of age-specific reference ranges, PSA velocity, PSA density, and the molecular forms of PSA (free or complexed PSA).

PSA density is a measurement that attempts to correct for elevated PSA levels due to BPH. *PSA density* is defined as the total serum PSA level divided by the prostate gland volume (in milliliters) measured by TRUS.[195] As prostate gland volume increases with increasing amounts of BPH, PSA should rise as well. Prostate cancer releases more PSA into the serum than does BPH.[196] The use of PSA density is limited by the need to perform TRUS, variations in the accuracy of TRUS to measure volume, and the fact that PSA levels due to BPH are a product of the ratios of both the stromal and epithelial components of BPH, which vary from patient to patient. Some have suggested that a PSA density cutoff of 0.15 may better discriminate between patients with elevated serum PSA levels due to BPH and those with elevated levels due to cancer.[197] Catalona et al.[198] showed that as many as 50% of prostate cancers may be missed if one uses this PSA density cutoff to determine the need for prostate biopsy. Still others have failed to show any utility for the use of PSA density in men with a normal DRE and PSA levels between 4.0 and 10.0 ng/mL.[199] As BPH tends to occur in the transitional zone of the prostate and not in the central or peripheral zones, attempts to improve prostate cancer detection using transitional zone PSA density have been developed.[200,201] However, like PSA density, these calculations are subject to error, require TRUS, and do not seem to be superior to the use of PSA testing alone in most patients. In addition, the failure to identify prostate cancer in those with larger prostate glands may simply be a product of biopsy sampling errors rather than true absence of the disease.

Age-specific PSA reference ranges are an attempt to compensate for the fact that the standard reference range of 0.0 to 4.0 ng/mL does not reflect age-related volume changes in the prostate due to BPH. A single cutoff may, therefore, be inappropriate for all ages. Many investigators have proposed age-related reference ranges to improve test sensitivity in younger men (who have less BPH and, therefore, would be expected to have lower levels of PSA) and to improve test specificity in older men (who are more likely to have BPH and higher PSA values that accompany it).[202] Race may also have an impact on PSA levels, an issue that has been addressed by several authors (Table 34.4-4). Using age-specific reference ranges, cancer detection rates will increase 8% to 18% in men younger than 60 years and will decrease 4% to 22% in older men. Use of age-specific reference ranges decreases the overall biopsy rate in men undergoing screening. The biopsy rate has been shown to decrease approximately 21% in older men undergoing screening if age-specific reference ranges are used. However, the overall cancer detection rate will also decrease, as fewer elderly men, the group most likely to have prostate cancer, will undergo prostate biopsy. In one series, the overall cancer detection rate fell from 5.7% using the standard PSA cutoff point of 4.0 ng/mL to 3.8% using age-specific reference ranges. Of the T1c or nonpalpable cancers missed in the older patient population, the vast majority have favorable pathologic features suggesting that they may be of low biologic potential in this age group and that failure to detect them may have little impact on patient mortality or morbidity. Use of age-specific reference ranges remains controversial: Some investigators have shown no benefit to their use as compared to use of the standard cutoff point of 4.0 ng/mL. Others have also argued cogently the likelihood that organ-confined cancers are similar in men with serum PSA values between 2.5 and 6.0 ng/mL, suggesting that any lead time gained by use of age-specific reference ranges will not likely translate into improved outcomes and that the increased costs—monetary, physical, and psychological—associated with the increased biopsy rates in men younger than 60 years may not be justified.

PSA velocity refers to the rate of changes in serum PSA over time. PSA velocity is calculated using the following equation: 1/2 (PSA2 − PSA1/time 1) + (PSA3 − PSA2/time 2), where *PSA1* is the first, *PSA2* the second, and *PSA3* the third PSA measurement. Time represents the interval (in years) between PSA measurements. At least three PSA measurements obtained over 24 months or at least 12 to 18 months apart are required for maximal accuracy. In the initial study, significant differences in PSA velocity were noted in patients found to have cancer and BPH many years before cancer diagnosis. Carter et al.[203,204] found that a PSA velocity exceeding 0.75 ng/mL was highly predictive of prostate cancer using one assay (sensitivity 72% and specificity 95%). The use of PSA velocity is limited by the fact that multiple measurements using the same assay over a relatively long period are necessary for accuracy. In addition, there is substantial biologic and laboratory variability in serum PSA testing, and some suggest that only increases in serum PSA greater than 25% are likely to represent changes due to prostatic disease (BPH or cancer).

Perhaps the greatest enhancement of PSA testing has been based on the knowledge that PSA exists in the serum in both free (or unbound) and complexed forms (bound to serum proteins). Stenman et al.[176] made the observation that the free form of serum PSA exists in a higher fraction in men without prostate cancer than in those with the disease. Others observed that the specificity of PSA testing for the detection of prostate cancer could be enhanced by calculating the free-to-total PSA ratio as compared to using total PSA alone.[205] Partin et al.[206] conducted a multiinstitutional trial evaluating the performance of both total and free-to-total PSA for the detection of prostate cancer in men with serum PSA levels between 4.0 and 10.0 ng/mL using the Hybritech assay (Hybritech, Inc., San Diego, CA). All men had a normal DRE and underwent systematic TRUS-guided prostate biopsy. Of 773 men, 379 (49%) were ultimately found to have prostate cancer. As expected, the total PSA was higher and free fraction was lower in those with prostate cancer as compared to those without the disease. Using a free PSA cutoff of 20% to provide 95% sensitivity, these researchers could achieve a specificity of 20%, eliminating 20% of unnecessary biopsies. For patients who had a normal DRE and total PSA concentration between 4.0 and 10.0 ng/mL, the probability of prostate cancer was 56%, 20%, and 8% for those with free PSA fractions of 0% to 10%, 15% to 20%, and more than 25%, respectively. Catalona et al.[206] also demonstrated that the use of the percentage of free PSA in men with total serum PSA concentrations between 4.0 and 10 ng/mL could eliminate 29% of unnecessary biopsies, if a cutoff of 20% free PSA was used as an indicator for prostate biopsy. Others have performed similar studies using the same or different assays and patient populations (i.e., ranges of total PSA).[205,207–213] In these studies, the sensitivity and specificity for cancer detection varied from 71% to 100% and 24% to 95%, respectively, using cutoff points ranging from 14% to 28%.

As 13% to 20% of men with serum PSA concentrations between 2.6 and 4.0 ng/mL (upper limit of normal) will be found to have prostate cancer within 5 years, some have examined the usefulness of percentage of free PSA for the early detection of prostate cancer in these men.[171,176,214] Catalona et al.[208] used percentage of free PSA to screen 914 men aged 50 years or older who had normal DREs and total PSA concentrations between 2.6 and 4.0 ng/mL. Using a cutoff point of 27% free PSA, 90% of cancers were detected and 18% of unnecessary biopsies were eliminated. The positive predictive value of percentage of free PSA at this cutoff point was 24%, and 81% of 52 men who underwent radical prostatectomy were found to have organ-confined cancers. Of these cancers, 83% were considered to be clinically significant based on cancer volume, stage, and grade. Others have shown similar findings using a different PSA cutoff point.[215]

The percentage of free PSA may also be of value in predicting cancer aggressiveness. Carter et al.[216] measured both total and percentage of free PSA serially in men from whom serum had been stored before the diagnosis of prostate cancer. Stored sera from men with aggressive cancers as defined by stage (≥T3, nodal or bone metastases), grade (≥7), or positive margins at the time of radical prostatectomy were compared to sera from men with less aggressive cancers (none of the previously mentioned features). Although total PSA levels were not different between both groups measured serially before the diagnosis, a statistically significant difference between the two groups with respect to percentage of free PSA was noted. All eight patients with aggressive cancers from whom serum was available for testing 10 years before diagnosis had free PSA fractions of 14% or less.

Clinicians should be aware of several issues when determining whether to use percentage of free PSA and in interpreting results of the assay. Age, prostate volume, and method of serum storage before processing may influence PSA ratios. Samples should be processed within 3 hours or stored at −70°C if processing is delayed; otherwise, the free PSA fraction may be degraded.[217] Lower free PSA cutoff points may be possible in smaller gland volumes (i.e., <40 cm^3) while still maintaining an acceptable detection sensitivity of 90%.[207] Several analytical issues must be understood. Assays performed by different methods may yield different results.[191,218,219] The percentage of free PSA cutoff point advised by manufacturers of these assays varies. Therefore, clinicians must be well acquainted with the methods used for free PSA testing before interpreting the results. Finally, it must be emphasized that use of percentage free PSA improves specificity of detection; some cancers will be missed. Both physicians and patients must be aware of this, as some will find any decrement in sensitivity unacceptable. Percentage of free PSA testing may be used best when determining the need for a second prostate biopsy in patients with a normal DRE, a total serum PSA between 4.0 and 10 ng/mL, and a previously negative biopsy.

Future Refinements

Similar to use of percentage of free PSA, several investigators have assessed the measurement of complexed PSA (PSA bound to α_1-antichymotrypsin) for the detection of prostate cancer. Brawer et al.[220] measured total, complexed, and free PSA in 75 men with prostate cancer and in 225 who had benign findings on prostate biopsy. At 95% sensitivity, the specificities of total, free, and complexed PSA were 21.8%, 15.4%, and 26.5%, respectively. Sokoll et al.[221] reported similar findings and improved specificity for complexed PSA as compared to total PSA in men with total serum PSA concentrations between 4.0 and 10.0 ng/mL.

The ProstAsure Index (Horus Global HealthNet, Hilton Head Island, SC) examines the relationships between several variables, such as PSA, age, and prostatic acid phosphatase, using an artificial neural network to predict the risk of prostate cancer. Babaian et al.[222] compared the ProstAsure Index with percentage of free PSA for prostate cancer detection in 54 men with prostate cancer, 77 with BPH, and 94 with no evidence of either. A comparison of the receiver operating characteristics curves for both tests demonstrated that the area under the curve for the ProstAsure Index was higher than that for percentage of free PSA (0.95 vs. 0.86, respectively), suggesting a small but significant advantage for the index.

Other serum proteins have been identified that may, in the future, play a role in prostate cancer detection and evaluation. Prostate-specific membrane antigen (PSMA) is a 750–amino acid type 2 transmembrane glycoprotein distinct from PSA. Serum levels of PSMA are increased in patients with prostate cancer. Human kallikrein-2 is a serum protease that bears considerable homology to PSA. Neither PSMA nor human kallikrein-2 currently is being used routinely for prostate cancer early detection, but refinements in development of serum assays, as well as novel imaging and treatment techniques targeting these and yet-to-be discovered proteins, may have a significant impact on prostate cancer early detection, staging, and treatment.

PROSTATE BIOPSY AND ITS IMPACT ON RISK ASSESSMENT

Prostate biopsy is indicated in men with an elevated serum PSA level, an abnormal DRE, or a combination of the two. Prostate biopsy is best performed under TRUS guidance using a spring-loaded biopsy device coupled to the transrectal probe.[223,224] Although prostate biopsy can be done using a transperineal approach, the transrectal approach facilitates more accurate needle placement and tissue sampling. Rather than just sampling an area abnormal on the basis of DRE or TRUS imaging, systematic biopsy strategies have been developed that improve cancer detection and risk assessment. DRE and TRUS each lack the sensitivity and specificity to guide performance of lesion-directed biopsy only. Traditionally, six (sextant) biopsies have been taken in most patients along a parasagittal line between the lateral edge and the midline of the prostate at the apex, midgland, and base bilaterally (Fig. 34.4-4).[225] Recently, several investigators have assessed the impact of increasing the number of biopsies as well as sampling specific portions or zones of the prostate.[225–227] Investigators have shown that more laterally directed biopsies of the peripheral zone will increase detection rates by 14% to 20% over the more traditional sextant technique. Chang et al.[225] analyzed a biopsy scheme that involved tissue from a minimum of eight sites, including bilateral apex, midlobar midgland, parasagittal midgland, and lateral base (see Fig. 34.4-4). They found that the parasagittal biopsies at the base added very little unique information to this scheme.

As up to 30% of lesions may originate in the transitional zone, many investigators have examined the utility of specific transitional zone biopsies.[228–231] Most have found that routine transitional zone biopsies add little unique information to that gained from routine peripheral zone biopsy schemes. Therefore, transitional zone biopsy should be considered in those with a high suspicion of prostate cancer based on serum PSA level and who have undergone previous peripheral zone biopsy without cancer detection. Patients should be advised that a negative prostate biopsy does not completely exclude cancer, as 13% to 31% of patients with an initially negative biopsy will be found to have cancer on subsequent biopsy.[232,233]

Although the primary goal of prostate biopsy is cancer detection, the information gained from the results, if positive,

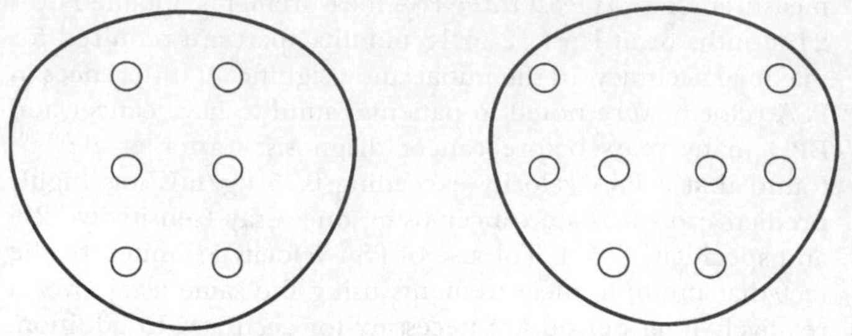

FIGURE 34.4-4. Prostate biopsy schemes. **A:** Traditional sextant (six-biopsy) technique. **B:** More contemporary technique, which samples the peripheral zone more laterally and improves cancer detection rates. (From ref. 225, with permission.)

can be of considerable value in initial risk assessment. The number of cores with cancer as well as the cancer grade determined by biopsy correlate with the risk of ECE and cancer progression. As biopsy samples only a portion of the prostate, accurate grading may be hampered by sampling errors. Grade as measured by biopsy will correlate exactly with that determined by analysis of the entire prostate after radical prostatectomy 31% to 59% of the time.[234,235] Most often, needle biopsy underestimates cancer grade. Grading errors appear to be more limited with the use of contemporary biopsy schemes, which have increased (>6) the number of cores taken.[236]

Prostate cancer volume correlates with both the risk of extracapsular disease and outcome after treatment. Although cancer volume currently is not well assessed by imaging, analysis of the number of biopsy cores involved with cancer as well as the extent of cancer within each core appears to be of value in this regard. Patients with multiple positive biopsies are at an increased risk of both ECE and recurrence after initial therapy. One series reported on 257 consecutive radical prostatectomy patients and demonstrated that the number of positive sextant biopsies and the Gleason score correlated with ECE (P<.0001 and P = .0004, respectively) in a comparison of patients with and without ECE.[237] With respect to serologic recurrence, patients with fewer than three positive biopsies and a Gleason score of less than 7 were at a low risk for recurrence irrespective of preoperative PSA levels (14% risk with a mean follow-up of 2 years).[237] Other investigators have substantiated these findings, noting that patients in whom more than 50% of biopsy cores are involved with cancer are at an increased risk of both ECE and disease recurrence after radical prostatectomy.[238–240] Knowledge of the number of cores involved may give important information not provided by analysis of the PSA level, Gleason grade, and local T stage alone.[241]

Although TRUS-guided prostate biopsy usually is very well tolerated by patients, approximately 24% of those undergoing the procedure will find it very painful. Hematospermia and hematuria are common, occurring in approximately 40% to 50% of patients.[242–244] High fever is rare, occurring in 2.9% to 4.2% of patients. Antibiotic prophylaxis is commonly given, although the necessity for it has been questioned by some.[242] Recent use of aspirin or nonsteroidal antiinflammatory agents is not a contraindication for this procedure.[244]

TO SCREEN OR NOT TO SCREEN?

The case for prostate cancer screening is supported by the following facts: The disease is burdensome; PSA testing improves

TABLE 34.4-5. Average Life Expectancy and Life Expectancy Correlated with Patient's Perception of Health Status

Age (y)	*Average Life Expectancy (y)*	*Good–Excellent Range (y)*	*Fair–Poor Range (y)*
65	15	17–20	11–13
70	12	13–17	8–11
75	10	10–14	6–8
80	7	8–11	3–6

(From ref. 374, with permission.)

detection of clinically important tumors without significantly increasing the detection of unimportant tumors; most PSA-detected tumors are curable using current techniques; and there is no cure for metastatic disease. In addition, several investigators have shown a reduction in cause-specific mortality with screening.[245–247] In a community-based, prospective, randomized trial of men between the ages of 45 and 80 years, Labrie et al.[245] showed that patients randomized to PSA screening had a cause-specific mortality equal to one-third that of unscreened men. However, this study must be interpreted with caution, as fewer than 20% of men in this study were randomized to screening. In an independent, population-based, case-control study that looked at screening with DRE, Jacobsen et al.[246] showed an association between decreased mortality and screening. However, the causal relationship between screening and decreased mortality remains to be proven. In the Prostate, Lung, Colon, Ovarian Trial supported by the National Cancer Institute, men are randomized to screening (with DRE and PSA testing) and to no screening, with cancer-specific mortality as the end point. However, the fact that therapy is not standardized and that screening will occur over only a limited period may make interpretation of results difficult. The efficacy of treatment also is currently being examined in Scandinavia, where two randomized trials compare watchful waiting with radiation or radical prostatectomy. A similar trial, Prostatectomy Versus Observation for Clinically Localized Carcinoma of the Prostate (PIVOT), is accruing patients in the United States. Patients must be informed of the risks and benefits of screening before it is carried out. It appears that many men who undergo screening in certain health care settings have no knowledge of having the test performed, suggesting that more discussion of this test with patients must occur.[248] If screening and eventual treatment are to be offered to asymptomatic patients, they should be offered to those whose age and health status are such that they may benefit from early detection of a disease that may have a protracted natural history (Table 34.4-5). An algorithm for early detection is outlined in Figure 34.4-5.

INITIAL CANCER STAGING AND RISK ASSESSMENT

Historically, initial risk assessment was based on clinical staging—that is, the assessment of anatomic extent of the disease on the basis of physical examination and imaging. Although clinical stage (TNM) correlates with outcome, in a large percentage of patients who are believed to have organ-confined disease, evidence of disease beyond the prostate is identified at the time of radical prostatectomy. Alternatively, some patients with high-risk pathologic features may not experience disease recurrence. Therefore, many clinicians have focused their efforts on better risk assessment schemes that predict the likelihood of disease recurrence if patients are treated and the likelihood of clinical progression if patients undergo initial surveillance. This more modern concept of risk assessment is a product of the knowledge that disease may be better characterized by analyzing many criteria (e.g., serum PSA level, Gleason grade, cancer volume) in combination with clinical stage, as compared to the use of staging alone.

An accurate assessment of risk before definitive treatment is attempted would allow for a more realistic assessment of the likelihood of cure with various treatment options and, therefore, better treatment selection. In addition, such assessment would allow for more accurate prediction of who may be candidates for neoadjuvant or adjuvant treatment or novel clinical trials owing to the presence of high-risk cancer features.

IMAGING

Imaging plays an important role in staging. Both cross-sectional imaging of the pelvis and imaging of the bones (with radionuclide bone scanning) often are performed. However, imaging can be costly, and patients at low risk of advanced disease can be spared the cost and morbidity of cross-sectional imaging and radionuclide bone scanning. With the advent of widespread screening for prostate cancer, considerable stage migration has occurred, and the incidence of metastatic and regionally advanced prostate cancer has decreased. Several investigators have proposed guidelines for prostate cancer imaging that limit costs without compromising significantly the accuracy of staging. However, a recent analysis of the use of cross-sectional imaging [computed tomography (CT) or magnetic resonance imaging (MRI)] and bone scanning in a large cohort of patients cared for by urologists suggests that bone scans, CT, and MRI are overused, certainly in low-risk patients (i.e., PSA <10 ng/mL, stage <T2c, grade <7).[249] In this latter group, 66% of patients were undergoing bone scans, and 24% either CT or MRI.

Radionuclide bone scanning has replaced the use of plain films for the detection of prostate cancer metastases. Although sensitive, bone scans have a low specificity. False-positive scans can occur due to trauma, degenerative disease, or Paget's disease. Lee and Oesterling et al.[250,251] have conducted investigations to assess the ability of serum PSA level to predict bone scan findings (Fig. 34.4-6). In a cancer population representative of newly diagnosed patients in the United States, serum PSA level was the best predictor of bone scan results. Of 852 patients with newly detected prostate cancer, 66% had a serum PSA concentration of less than 10 ng/mL. The likelihood of a positive bone scan due to metastases was 0.6% and 2.6% for those with serum PSA concentrations between 10.1 and 15 ng/mL and 15.1 and 20 ng/mL, respectively. Use of tumor grade, local tumor stage, or a combination of these variables did not enhance the predictive power of PSA testing. Many others have confirmed these results.[252,253] On the basis of these results, one can omit the bone scan in patients with newly diagnosed, untreated prostate cancer who are asymptomatic and have serum PSA concentrations of less than 20 ng/mL and certainly in those with serum PSA concentrations of less than 15 ng/mL.

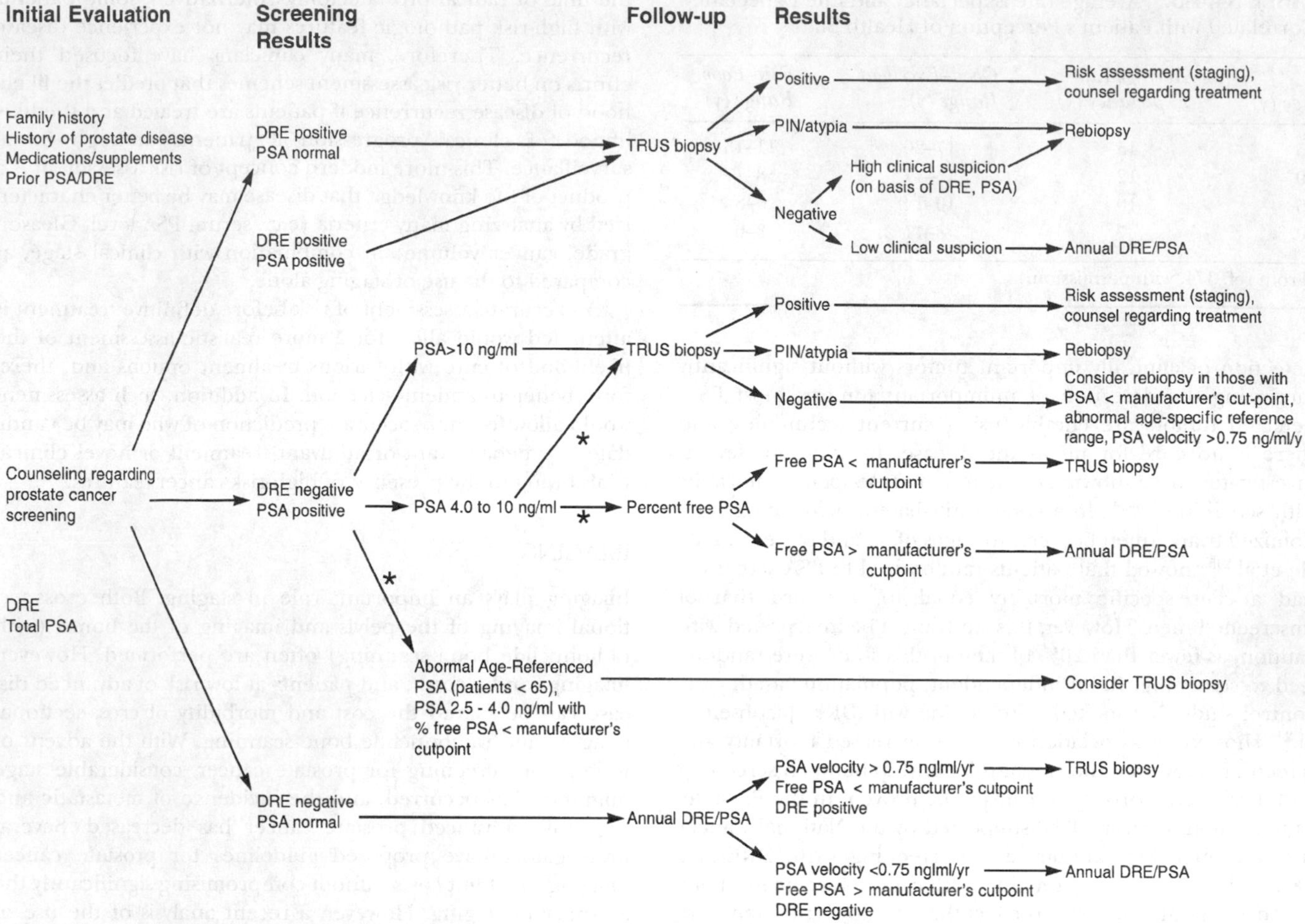

FIGURE 34.4-5. Algorithm for the early detection of prostate cancer. *Whether one uses total prostate-specific antigen (PSA) or its variations (i.e., percentage free or age-referenced prostate-specific antigen testing) for the initial screening for the disease is a matter of debate (see text). DRE, digital rectal examination; PIN, prostatic intraepithelial neoplasia; TRUS, transrectal ultrasonography.

Given that there is some risk of bone metastases in this population, it is reasonable to perform a bone scan in those patients with either very high-grade or very high-stage disease.

Cross-sectional imaging of the pelvis with CT or MRI in patients with prostate cancer generally is performed to exclude lymph node metastases in patients who are believed to be candidates for definitive local therapy (Fig. 34.4-7). However, the incidence of lymph node metastases is currently low (<5%), and imaging is costly and its sensitivity limited. One review of the literature encompassing 15 series and 1354 patients with an incidence of lymph node metastases of 22% revealed a sensitivity of CT and MRI of approximately 36% and a specificity of 97%.[254] The authors of this review suggested that only those patients with a very high risk of lymph node metastases (i.e., 45%) would benefit from cross-sectional imaging. Such patients would include those with a normal bone scan, Gleason score greater than 6, a palpable abnormality on DRE (i.e., T2 to T4 disease), and a serum PSA level of greater than 25 ng/mL.[255]

Radiolabeled monoclonal antibodies directed at PSMA have been used to stage newly diagnosed patients and identify sites of cancer recurrence after definitive therapy. Prostascint (Cytogen Corporation, Princeton, NJ) uses a murine monoclonal antibody labeled with indium 111 for the detection of lymph node and other soft tissue metastases.[256,257] Imaging is performed 72 to 120 hours after administration of the agent. The sensitivity, specificity, and positive predictive value of the test in one patient population with a 37% incidence of nodal metastases was 75%, 86%, and 79%, respectively. In a more recent study of 160 patients imaged before pelvic lymph node dissection, the sensitivity, specificity, and positive and negative predictive values for immunoscintigraphy were 62%, 72%, 62%, and 72%, respectively.[258] The authors found the test, when considered in conjunction with certain combinations of PSA level and Gleason score, was effective in predicting the risk of lymph node metastases. The test has not gained wide popularity owing to difficulties with accurate interpretation, its cost, and the fact that similar information about risk may be gained by use of the serum PSA level, cancer grade, and cancer stage.

Whereas metastatic and regionally advanced disease are relatively uncommon at presentation, ECE and seminal vesicle invasion are not uncommon, occurring in approximately 20% to 40% and 8% of patients at presentation, respectively. Such patients are at an increased risk of recurrence with various forms of local therapy, and pretreatment knowledge of ECE

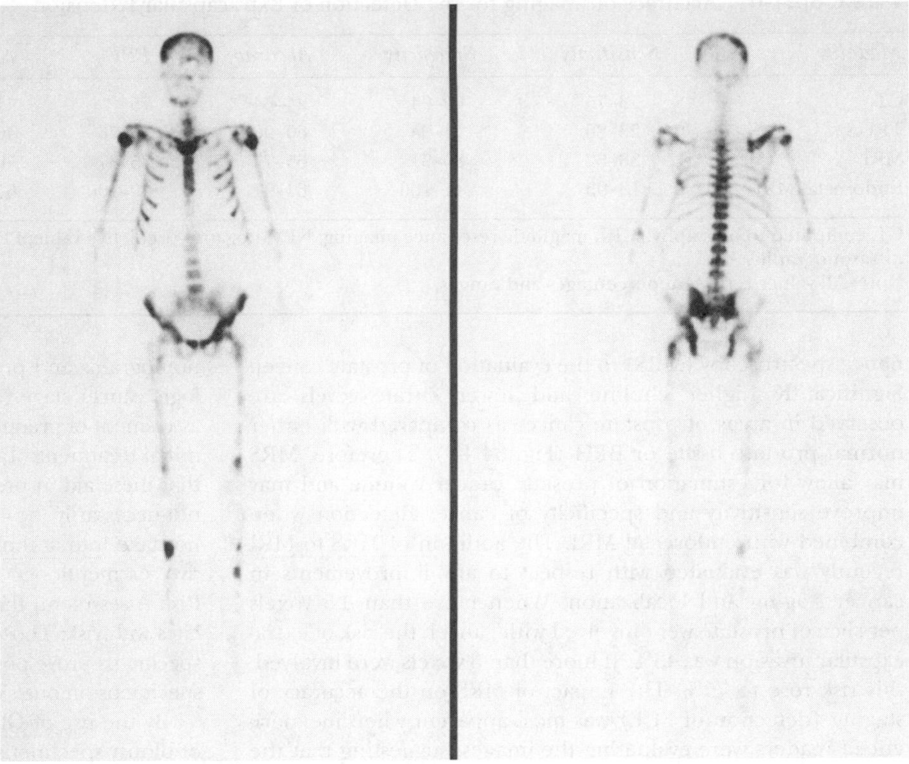

FIGURE 34.4-6. Radionuclide bone scan showing increased uptake consistent with prostate cancer metastases.

would allow for more effective local therapy to be delivered (e.g., wide surgical excision, wider field, higher dose or combination radiation therapy). Whereas CT is a less reliable and efficient test for assessment of ECE or seminal vesicle invasion, as compared to other imaging modalities, both MRI using an endorectal probe and TRUS are used commonly to assess the integrity of the prostatic capsule and seminal vesicles. The performance of CT, MRI (body coil alone and endorectal coil), and TRUS in this regard is reviewed in Tables 34.4-6 and 34.4-7. Given the wide range of test performance noted, other parameters of risk such as cancer grade, serum PSA level, and the number of positive biopsy samples must be taken into account when interpreting the results of either endorectal MRI or TRUS. Whereas TRUS is performed at the time of biopsy, endorectal MRI is, for the most part, used for staging only after a diagnosis has been made. Endorectal MRI may be of some value in staging intermediate-risk patients but provide little additional information in both low- and high-risk patients.

The routine use of endorectal imaging is limited due to problems with interobserver variability and variable diagnostic accuracy. The development of endorectal surface coils has allowed the application of three-dimensional magnetic reso-

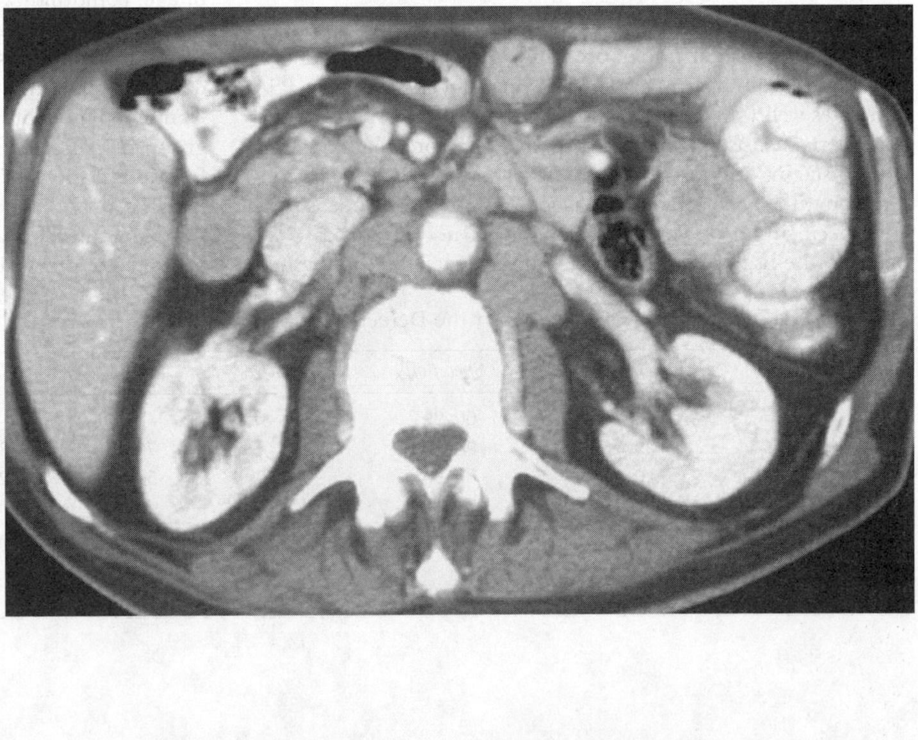

FIGURE 34.4-7. A computed tomography scan showing the presence of retroperitoneal adenopathy due to metastatic prostate cancer.

TABLE 34.4-6. Accuracy of Imaging for the Detection of Extracapsular Extension

Modality	*Sensitivity*	*Specificity*	*Accuracy*	*PPV*	*NPV*	*Reference*
CT	3–75	60–94	24–64[375]	75	41	375–378
TRUS	23–86	71–94	60–90	50–76	46–69	375,378–380
MRI	38–62	80–91	65–77	75–87	50–69	375,381–383
Endorectal MRI	13–95	47–100	64–91	40–100	67–90	260,270,379,380,383–388

CT, computed tomography; MRI, magnetic resonance imaging; NPV, negative predictive value; PPV, positive predictive value; TRUS, transrectal ultrasonography.
Note: All values represent percentages and ranges.

nance spectroscopy (MRS) to the evaluation of prostate cancer. Significantly higher choline and lower citrate levels are observed in areas of prostate cancer as compared with either normal prostate tissue or BPH (Fig. 34.4-8). Therefore, MRS may allow for estimation of prostate cancer volume and may improve sensitivity and specificity of cancer detection when combined with endorectal MRI. The addition of MRS to MRI recently was evaluated with respect to any improvements in cancer staging and localization. When more than 4.5 voxels per slice of prostate were involved with cancer, the risk of extracapsular invasion was 43%. If more than 6 voxels were involved, this risk rose to 75%. The impact of MRS on the accuracy of staging (detection of ECE) was most apparent when inexperienced readers were evaluating the images, suggesting that the use of such technology may be most helpful in improving the accuracy of radiologists with less experience in magnetic resonance interpretation.[259,260] With regard to cancer localization in patients with biopsy-proven prostate cancer, MRS in conjunction with MRI allows for improved ability to localize cancer to a sextant.[261] When either MRI or MRS was positive for cancer, a sensitivity of 91% was achieved. When both were positive at the same site, a specificity of 92% was achieved. Nonetheless, more experience with this technique is necessary before it can be used routinely to guide and deliver treatment.

PRETREATMENT SERUM PROSTATE-SPECIFIC ANTIGEN LEVEL, TUMOR STAGE, CANCER GRADE, AND VOLUME

Pretreatment serum PSA level is used extensively in both pretreatment risk stratification and in predicting the outcome after definitive local treatment.[262–264] The serum concentration of PSA correlates well with cancer volume and stage. However, considerable overlap exists, making use of serum PSA alone inaccurate for clinical staging in most patients. Use of serum PSA level in conjunction with cancer grade and stage adds considerable sensitivity and specificity to the prediction of lymph node status as compared to the use of PSA level alone. Investigators have published nomograms and probability curves that aid in predicting pathologic cancer stage.[265–268] Use of such nomograms allows a better assessment of preoperative risk and more appropriate selection of initial treatment (Table 34.4-8). It is important to note, however, that these aid in predicting the pathologic extent of disease and not necessarily the cure rates with treatment. In addition, they do not take into account other cancer features that may be predictive. As mentioned earlier in Prostate Biopsy and Its Impact on Risk Assessment, the number of positive prostate biopsies correlates with risk: Those patients in whom more than 50% of biopsy specimens prove positive or in whom two to three of three biopsy specimens on one side are positive are more likely to have ECE.

By the use of Gleason grade, local tumor stage, percentage of biopsy specimens involved with cancer, and serum PSA level, pretreatment risk may be assigned. Table 34.4-9 is a summary of the findings from multiple analyses and can serve as a broad-based guide for pretreatment risk stratification. Future refinements in imaging and the use of molecular markers may further improve risk assessment.[269–271]

THE IMPACT OF RISK ASSESSMENT ON TREATMENT SELECTION

The information presented suggests that risk assessment is possible and that it provides both patients and clinicians with important information. Low-risk patients are very good candidates for definitive local therapy using standard techniques. On the basis of age, comorbidity, and the long natural history of this disease in some cases, certain patients may be candidates for surveillance alone. High-risk patients are unlikely to be cured with standard therapy and are ideal candidates for clinical trials. Combined-modality therapy may be especially important in this group of patients.[272] Intermediate-risk patients are candidates for modifications of standard therapy, given a significant risk of recurrence and the emerging knowledge that wide surgical excision and adjuvant radiation therapy may be useful after radical prostatectomy and that dose escalation, improved targeting, and

TABLE 34.4-7. Accuracy of Imaging for the Detection of Seminal Vesicle Invasion

Modality	*Sensitivity*	*Specificity*	*Accuracy*	*PPV*	*NPV*	*Study*
CT	6–36	60–99	69–81	—	—	376–378
TRUS	29–75	98–100	77	75	98	378–380
MRI	20–83	86–96	71–94	50	72–73	381–383
Endorectal MRI	23–100	83–100	77–92	40–100	80–96	270,379,380,383–388

CT, computed tomography; MRI, magnetic resonance imaging; NPV, negative predictive value; PPV, positive predictive value; TRUS, transrectal ultrasonography.
Note: All values represent percentages and ranges.

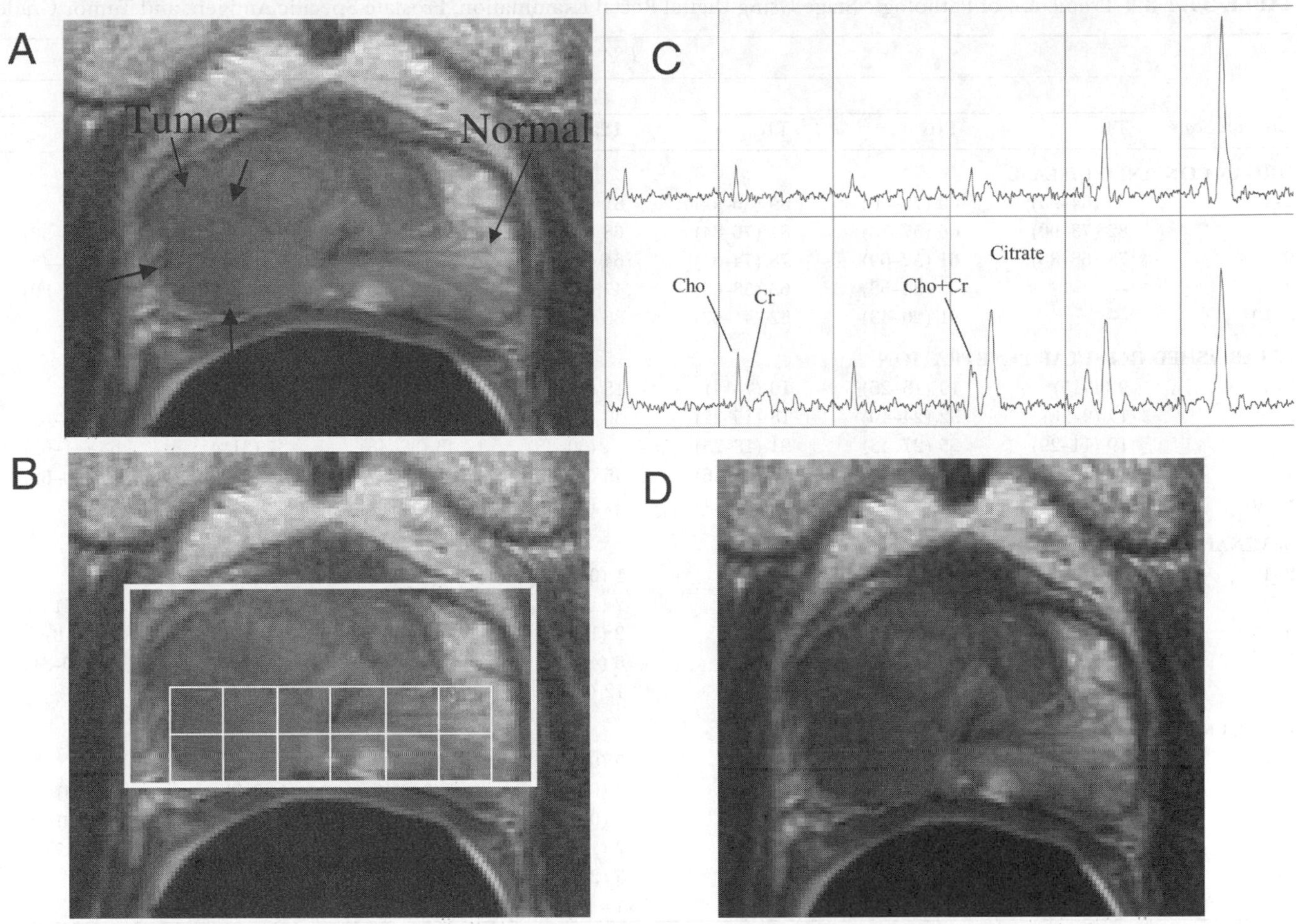

FIGURE 34.4-8. **A:** Representative reception-profile corrected T2-weighted fast spin-echo axial image taken from a volume data set demonstrating a large tumor in the right midgland: low T2-weighted signal intensity (*arrow*). **B:** T2-weighted fast spin-echo axial image with overlying point resolved spectroscopy (PRESS) selected volume (*bold white box*) and phase-encoded grid (*fine white line*) taken from a three-dimensional array of spectra. **C:** Corresponding 0.24-mL proton spectra with the major prostatic metabolites (choline-, creatine-, and citrate-labeled). Spectra in regions of cancer (left side of image) demonstrate elevated choline and reduced citrate relative to regions of healthy peripheral zone tissue. The prostate metabolite levels that are observed in different regions of zonal anatomy, benign prostatic hypertrophy, and cancer are described in detail in the text. **D:** Images can also be created from prostatic metabolite levels and overlaid on the corresponding anatomic images. The red area is where (choline + creatine) citrate ratios were greater than 3 standard deviations of healthy peripheral zone values. (See Color Fig. 34.4-8 in the CD-ROM and on the Web at www.LWWoncology.com.)

combined-modality radiation therapy may have value over standard radiation therapy techniques in this population.[273–277]

TREATMENT SELECTION FOR NONMETASTATIC (T1–T3N0M0) DISEASE

There is no consensus as to what constitutes the best form of treatment for any stage of prostatic disease. Treatment is indicated in those who are symptomatic and those who are at high risk of dying of prostate cancer or developing symptoms of the disease. Given that most patients in whom the disease is currently being detected fall into either the low- or intermediate-risk groups, immediate and aggressive treatment may not be necessary in some patients. Such patients must be informed of the potential risks and benefits of all forms of treatment as well as surveillance, which is an option for some patients. Treatment decisions should be based on cancer stage and grade as well as patient age and health. Both patient and physician bias may play a strong role in treatment selection, inasmuch as precise guidelines for treatment are not available for the majority of patients. Given the protracted and, in some cases, indolent nature of the disease, disease progression may be avoided using a variety of treatment methods. Indeed, the morbidity of different treatment regimens may guide treatment selection in some patients.

Both patients and physicians must interpret the results (morbidity and cancer control rates) of various forms of treatment with caution. Often, the morbidity of treatment is reported using physicians' estimates. However, physicians generally underestimate the impact of the disease in almost all health-related quality-of-life domains.[278] Given the protracted nature of prostate cancer, only a limited number of patients may die of their disease. Therefore, outcome often is assessed using end points other than cause-specific survival, the most common being PSA levels. After radical prostatectomy, the PSA level should fall to undetectable, usually within 6 weeks of surgery. A

TABLE 34.4-8. Prediction of Pathologic Stage Using Digital Rectal Examination, Prostate-Specific Antigen, and Tumor Grade

	PSA = 0–4 ng/mL						
	Clinical Stage						
Gleason Score	T1a	T1b	T1c	T2a	T2b	T2c	T3a
ORGAN-CONFINED DISEASE							
2–4	90 (84–95)	80 (72–86)	89 (86–92)	81 (75–86)	72 (65–79)	77 (69–83)	—
5	82 (73–90)	66 (57–73)	81 (76–84)	68 (63–72)	57 (50–62)	62 (55–69)	40 (26–53)
6	78 (68–88)	61 (52–69)	78 (74–81)	64 (59–68)	52 (46–57)	57 (51–64)	35 (22–48)
7	—	43 (34–53)	63 (58–68)	47 (41–52)	34 (29–39)	38 (32–45)	19 (11–29)
8–10	—	31 (20–43)	52 (41–62)	36 (27–45)	24 (17–32)	27 (18–36)	—
ESTABLISHED CAPSULAR PENETRATION							
2–4	9 (4–15)	19 (13–26)	10 (7–14)	18 (13–23)	25 (19–32)	21 (14–28)	—
5	17 (9–26)	32 (24–40)	18 (15–22)	30 (26–35)	40 (34–46)	34 (27–40)	51 (38–65)
6	19 (11–29)	35 (27–43)	21 (18–25)	34 (30–38)	43 (38–48)	37 (31–43)	53 (41–65)
7	—	44 (35–54)	31 (26–36)	45 (40–50)	51 (46–57)	45 (38–52)	52 (40–63)
8–10	—	43 (32–56)	34 (27–44)	47 (38–56)	48 (40–57)	42 (35–52)	—
SEMINAL VESICLE INVOLVEMENT							
2–4	0 (0–2)	1 (0–3)	1 (0–1)	1 (0–2)	2 (1–5)	2 (1–5)	—
5	1 (0–3)	2 (0–4)	1 (1–2)	2 (1–3)	3 (2–4)	3 (2–6)	7 (3–4)
6	1 (0–3)	2 (0–4)	1 (1–2)	2 (1–3)	3 (2–4)	4 (2–5)	7 (4–13)
7	—	6 (1–13)	4 (2–7)	6 (4–9)	10 (6–14)	12 (7–17)	19 (10–31)
8–10	—	11 (2–23)	9 (5–16)	12 (7–19)	17 (11–25)	21 (12–31)	—
LYMPH NODE INVOLVEMENT							
2–4	0 (0–1)	0 (0–1)	0 (0–0)	0 (0–0)	0 (0–1)	0 (0–1)	—
5	0 (0–2)	1 (0–2)	0 (0–0)	0 (0–1)	1 (0–2)	1 (0–2)	2 (0–4)
6	1 (0–7)	2 (1–5)	0 (0–1)	1 (0–1)	2 (1–3)	2 (1–4)	5 (2–9)
7	—	6 (2–13)	1 (1–3)	2 (1–4)	5 (2–8)	5 (2–9)	9 (4–17)
8–10	—	14 (5–27)	4 (2–7)	5 (2–9)	10 (5–17)	10 (4–18)	—
	PSA = 10.1–20 ng/mL						
ORGAN-CONFINED DISEASE							
2–4	76 (65–68)	58 (46–69)	75 (68–82)	60 (52–70)	48 (39–58)	53 (42–64)	—
5	61 (47–78)	40 (31–50)	60 (54–65)	43 (38–49)	32 (26–37)	36 (29–43)	18 (10–27)
6	—	33 (25–42)	55 (51–59)	38 (34–43)	26 (23–31)	31 (25–37)	14 (8–22)
7	33 (19–57)	17 (11–24)	35 (31–40)	22 (18–26)	13 (11–16)	15 (11–19)	6 (3–10)
8–10	—	9 (5–16)	23 (16–32)	14 (9–19)	7 (5–11)	8 (5–12)	3 (1–5)
ESTABLISHED CAPSULAR PENETRATION							
2–4	20 (10–32)	36 (26–46)	22 (16–29)	35 (26–43)	43 (34–53)	37 (27–47)	—
5	33 (18–47)	50 (39–59)	35 (30–40)	50 (45–56)	57 (51–63)	51 (43–57)	59 (47–69)
6	—	49 (38–59)	38 (34–42)	52 (48–57)	57 (51–62)	50 (44–57)	54 (44–64)
7	38 (18–61)	46 (34–60)	45 (40–50)	55 (50–60)	51 (45–57)	45 (39–52)	40 (30–50)
8–10	—	33 (21–51)	40 (33–49)	46 (38–55)	38 (30–47)	33 (24–42)	26 (17–37)
SEMINAL VESICLE INVOLVEMENT							
2–4	2 (0–7)	4 (1–10)	2 (1–5)	4 (1–8)	7 (12–14)	8 (2–16)	—
5	3 (0–9)	5 (1–10)	3 (2–5)	5 (3–8)	8 (5–11)	9 (6–15)	15 (8–25)
6	—	4 (1–9)	4 (3–5)	5 (3–7)	7 (5–10)	9 (6–13)	14 (8–21)
7	8 (0–28)	11 (3–22)	12 (8–16)	14 (10–19)	18 (13–24)	22 (16–29)	28 (18–39)
8–10	—	15 (4–32)	20 (13–28)	22 (15–31)	25 (18–34)	30 (21–40)	34 (21–47)
LYMPH NODE INVOLVEMENT							
2–4	0 (0–7)	2 (0–8)	0 (0–2)	1 (0–2)	1 (0–5)	1 (0–6)	—
5	3 (0–14)	5 (2–11)	1 (0–2)	2 (1–3)	4 (1–7)	4 (1–7)	7 (3–15)
6	—	13 (6–24)	3 (2–5)	4 (3–6)	10 (7–13)	10 (6–14)	18 (10–27)
7	18 (0–57)	24 (10–41)	8 (5–11)	9 (6–13)	17 (12–23)	18 (12–25)	26 (16–38)
8–10	—	40 (19–60)	16 (10–24)	17 (11–25)	29 (21–38)	29 (19–40)	37 (24–52)

PSA, prostate-specific antigen.
Note: Numbers represent percentage predictive probability (95% confidence interval).
(From ref. 265, with permission.)

PSA = 4.1–10 ng/mL						
Clinical Stage						
T1a	T1b	T1c	T2a	T2b	T2c	T3a
ORGAN-CONFINED DISEASE						
84 (75–92)	70 (60–79)	83 (78–88)	71 (64–78)	61 (52–69)	66 (57–74)	43 (27–58)
72 (60–85)	53 (44–63)	71 (67–75)	55 (51–60)	43 (38–49)	49 (42–55)	27 (17–39)
67 (55–82)	47 (38–57)	67 (64–70)	51 (47–54)	38 (34–43)	43 (38–49)	23 (14–34)
49 (34–68)	29 (21–38)	49 (45–54)	33 (29–38)	22 (18–26)	25 (20–30)	11 (6–17)
35 (18–62)	18 (11–28)	37 (28–46)	23 (16–31)	14 (9–19)	15 (10–22)	6 (3–10)
Established capsular penetration						
14 (7–23)	27 (18–37)	15 (11–20)	26 (19–33)	35 (26–43)	29 (21–37)	44 (30–59)
25 (14–36)	42 (32–51)	27 (23–30)	41 (36–46)	50 (45–55)	43 (37–50)	57 (46–68)
27 (15–39)	44 (35–53)	30 (27–33)	44 (41–48)	52 (48–56)	46 (40–51)	57 (47–67)
36 (20–51)	48 (38–60)	40 (35–44)	52 (48–57)	54 (49–59)	48 (42–54)	48 (37–58)
34 (17–58)	42 (28–57)	40 (33–49)	49 (42–57)	46 (39–53)	40 (31–48)	34 (24–46)
SEMINAL VESICLE INVOLVEMENT						
1 (0–4)	2 (0–6)	1 (0–3)	2 (1–5)	4 (1–9)	5 (1–10)	10 (3–23)
2 (0–5)	3 (1–7)	2 (1–3)	3 (2–5)	5 (3–8)	6 (4–10)	12 (6–20)
2 (0–6)	3 (1–6)	2 (2–3)	3 (2–4)	5 (4–7)	6 (4–9)	11 (6–18)
6 (0–19)	9 (2–18)	8 (5–11)	10 (8–13)	15 (11–19)	18 (13–24)	26 (17–36)
10 (0–34)	15 (4–29)	15 (10–22)	19 (13–26)	24 (17–31)	28 (20–37)	35 (23–48)
Lymph node involvement						
0 (0–2)	1 (0–3)	0 (0–1)	0 (0–1)	1 (0–2)	1 (0–2)	1 (0–5)
1 (0–5)	2 (1–5)	0 (0–1)	1 (0–1)	2 (1–3)	2 (1–3)	3 (1–7)
3 (0–15)	5 (2–11)	1 (1–2)	2 (1–3)	4 (3–6)	4 (3–6)	9 (5–15)
8 (0–32)	12 (5–23)	3 (2–5)	4 (3–6)	9 (6–12)	9 (6–13)	15 (8–23)
18 (0–55)	23 (10–43)	8 (4–12)	9 (5–13)	16 (11–24)	17 (10–26)	24 (13–38)
PSA >20 ng/mL						
ORGAN-CONFINED DISEASE						
—	38 (26–52)	58 (46–68)	41 (31–52)	29 (20–40)	—	—
—	23 (15–32)	40 (32–49)	26 (19–33)	17 (12–22)	19 (14–26)	8 (4–14)
—	17 (11–25)	35 (27–42)	22 (16–27)	13 (10–17)	15 (11–20)	6 (3–10)
—	—	18 (13–23)	10 (7–14)	5 (4–8)	6 (4–9)	2 (1–4)
—	3 (2–7)	10 (6–16)	5 (3–9)	3 (2–4)	3 (2–5)	1 (0–2)
ESTABLISHED CAPSULAR PENETRATION						
—	47 (33–61)	34 (24–44)	48 (36–58)	52 (39–65)	—	—
—	57 (44–68)	49 (40–56)	60 (52–68)	61 (53–69)	55 (46–64)	54 (40–67)
—	51 (37–64)	49 (43–56)	60 (53–66)	57 (50–64)	51 (43–59)	46 (34–58)
—	—	46 (39–54)	51 (44–58)	43 (35–50)	37 (29–45)	29 (19–40)
—	24 (13–42)	34 (27–45)	37 (28–48)	28 (20–37)	23 (16–31)	17 (11–26)
SEMINAL VESICLE INVOLVEMENT						
—	9 (1–22)	7 (2–15)	10 (3–20)	14 (4–29)	—	—
—	10 (2–21)	9 (5–14)	11 (6–17)	15 (9–23)	19 (11–28)	26 (14–41)
—	8 (2–17)	8 (6–12)	10 (7–15)	13 (9–19)	17 (11–24)	21 (13–33)
—	—	22 (15–28)	24 (17–32)	27 (20–34)	32 (24–42)	36 (25–49)
—	20 (6–43)	31 (21–42)	33 (22–45)	33 (24–45)	38 (26–51)	40 (25–55)
LYMPH NODE INVOLVEMENT						
—	4 (0–17)	1 (0–4)	1 (0–5)	3 (0–11)	—	—
—	10 (3–21)	3 (1–6)	3 (1–7)	7 (3–13)	7 (3–13)	11 (4–22)
—	23 (10–40)	7 (4–11)	8 (5–13)	16 (11–23)	17 (11–25)	26 (16–38)
—	—	14 (9–21)	14 (9–22)	25 (18–33)	25 (16–34)	32 (20–45)
—	51 (25–72)	24 (15–36)	24 (15–35)	36 (25–48)	35 (23–48)	42 (27–58)

TABLE 34.4-9. Pretreatment Risk Assessment

Risk Group	*Criteria*	*Recurrence after Local Therapy (Ranges)*	*Risk; Lower*	*Risk; Higher*	*Need for Routine Imaging*
Low	PSA <10 ng/mL; Gleason score ≤6 (no grade 4–5); T1, T2a	6–20%	<50%; positive biopsies; PSA <6 ng/mL; Gleason score 2–4	>50%; positive biopsies	None
Intermediate	PSA 10–20 ng/mL; Gleason score 7; T2b, T3a	34–60%	<50%; positive biopsies; PSA <15 ng/mL; Gleason score 3/4	>50%; positive biopsies; Gleason score 4/3	Bone scan for PSA >15 ng/mL
High	PSA >20 ng/mL; Gleason score 8–10; T3b	50–100%			Bone scan, CT, MRI of pelvis

CT, computed tomography; MRI, magnetic resonance imaging; PSA, prostate-specific antigen.
(Data compiled from refs. 237–241, 255, 262, 265, 266, 273, 274, 322, 354, 359, 389–401.)

persistently detectable PSA level predicts clinical recurrence, although disease may not return for many years and may not lead to death.[279] After cryotherapy and radiation therapy, PSA continues to be produced in most patients. What constitutes an acceptable PSA level after either form of treatment is a matter of some debate. Whereas some argue that low (i.e., <0.5 ng/mL) nadir levels should be reached, the American Society for Therapeutic Radiology and Oncology (ASTRO) defines biochemical recurrence after radiation therapy as three consecutive rises in serum PSA level above nadir.[280,281] Failure cannot occur until nadir is reached. This method of defining outcome is very sensitive to the length of follow-up and the frequency of PSA testing.

NATURAL HISTORY AND SURVEILLANCE ALONE

Certain prostate cancers may grow slowly. In addition, many patients with this disease are elderly and may have concomitant illnesses. Therefore, watchful waiting or surveillance alone may be an appropriate form of management for selected patients with prostate cancer. Contemporary series documenting the true natural history of untreated prostate cancer are limited. Many series are composed of only carefully selected patients, many of whom may have received some form of treatment, often androgen deprivation, during follow-up.

Several investigators have reported the likelihood of local and distant tumor progression in patients who were untreated or who were treated with noncurative intent (i.e., androgen deprivation) (Table 34.4-10). The risk of local progression in these series ranges from 8% to 84%, while the risk of progression to metastatic disease ranges from 6% to 74%. The results should be interpreted with caution, as most patients were older (i.e., >70 years old) and had low-grade or low-stage disease (or both). Furthermore, follow-up in these studies ranged from 4 to 14 years after diagnosis, and such differences likely account for the wide

TABLE 34.4-10. Estimates of Local and Metastatic Tumor Progression in Prostate Cancer Patients Who Remain Untreated and in Those Who Are Treated with Noncurative Intent

Study	*Year*	*No. of Patients*	*Mean Follow-Up (y)*	*Local Tumor Progression*	*Metastatic Tumor Progression*
Egawa et al.[282]	1993	107	6.2	8% of patients	23% of patients
George[284]	1988	120	7	84% of patients	11% of patients
Warner and Whitmore[286]	1994	75	11.2–13.5	77.3% of patients; median time to progression, 78 mo	Median time to progression, 186 mo
Byar and Corle[296]	1981	50	6.8–7.7	N/A	6% of patients
Adolfsson et al.[289] (clinical T3)	1999	50	7.75	66% of patients	22% at 5 y, 34% at 10 y
Adolfsson et al.[287] (clinically localized)	1997	122	9.1	N/A	18% at 10 y, 52% at 15 y
Adolfsson and Carstensen[285] (age <70 y)	1991	61	8.0	49% at 5 y, 72% at 10 y	8% at 5 y, 23% at 10 y
Rana et al.[283]	1994	199	4.2	26% of patients	46% of patients
Johansson et al.[288]	1997	223	14	33% of untreated patients with localized disease	13% of untreated patients with localized disease
Chodak et al.[297]	1994	828	6.6	N/A	19% of grade 1, 42% of grade 2, 74% of grade 3 at 10 y

N/A, data not available.

TABLE 34.4-11. Estimates of Disease-Specific Survival in Prostate Cancer Patients Who Remain Untreated and in Those Who Are Treated with Noncurative Intent

Study	*Year*	*No. of Patients*	*Follow-Up (y)*	*Disease-Specific Survival*
George[284]	1988	120	7.0	80% at 5 y, 75% at 7 y after diagnosis
Byar and Corle[296]	1981	50	6.8–7.7	60%–84% at 5 y (overall survival)
Johansson et al.[288]	1997	223	14	86% at 10 y, 81% at 15 y after diagnosis
Chodak et al.[297]	1994	828	6.6	87% well- or moderately differentiated, 34% poorly differentiated at 10 y after diagnosis
Rana et al.[283]	1994	199	4.2	70% at 5 y, 50% at 10 y after diagnosis
Warner and Whitmore[286]	1994	75	11.2–13.5	Median survival, 156 mo after diagnosis
Egawa et al.[282]	1993	107	6.2	78% at 5 y, 71% at 10 y after diagnosis
Adolfsson et al.[287] (clinically localized)	1997	122	9.1	90% at 10 y, 62% at 15 y after diagnosis
Adolfsson and Carstensen[285] (age <70 y)	1991	61	8.0	98% at 5 y, 92% at 10 y after diagnosis
Adolfsson et al.[289] (clinical T3)	1999	50	7.75	90% at 5 y, 74% at 10 y, 70% at 12 y after diagnosis

range of local and distant progression reported. Therefore, the results may underestimate the risk of disease progression in the general population of patients with prostate cancer, most notably in those who present at a younger age (i.e., <65 years). The definition of local progression in the majority of these series was based on changes in DRE, which is an imprecise measure. Two studies by Egawa et al.[282] and Rana et al.[283] have defined local progression by the development of bladder outlet obstructive symptoms necessitating surgical intervention. These were the only studies in which distant progression exceeded local progression. Finally, it must be emphasized that the use and timing of androgen deprivation therapy varied between studies.[282–289]

The risk of death due to prostate cancer in these series varies. Prostate cancer caused or contributed to death in 34% to 62% of the patients who died.[290–295] In a study of 514 prostate cancer patients, all of whom died between 1988 and 1991 and received immediate or deferred androgen deprivation therapy only, Aus et al.[291] found that prostate cancer caused or contributed to death in 62% of the study population. When analyzing only those patients with clinically localized disease at diagnosis (M0), 50% still died as a result of prostate cancer. Gronberg et al.[293] examined 6514 similar patients, in all of whom prostate cancer was diagnosed in Northern Sweden between 1971 and 1987. Follow-up in this series ranged from 7 to 23 years after initial diagnosis. Fifty-five percent of the patients who died during this time died as a result of prostate cancer. In a series of 451 prostate cancer patients from the Connecticut Tumor Registry, Albertsen et al.[290] reported that prostate cancer was the underlying cause of death in 34% of those who died after a mean follow-up of 15.5 years.

Brasso et al.[295] found that prostate cancer caused a significant excess mortality in untreated patients, with the number of actual deaths being approximately 1.6-fold greater than the expected number of deaths in the general population. Similarly, Rana et al.[283] reported that actuarial survival was 17% less at 5 years and 15% less at 10 years after diagnosis for 199 prostate cancer patients who were managed conservatively, as compared to age-matched controls. Others have shown that patients with prostate cancer may lose a significant number of years of life when their disease is managed conservatively.[290,294] Stattin et al.[294] reported a life expectancy of 6.3 years in 186 prostate cancer patients who were managed with delayed androgen deprivation after transurethral prostatectomy, as compared to a 10.2-year life expectancy for age-matched controls. Finally, several investigators have reported disease-specific survival for prostate cancer patients who were untreated or treated with noncurative intent. Disease-specific survival ranged from 60% to 98% at 5 years, 34% to 92% at 10 years, and 62% to 81% at 15 years after diagnosis (Table 34.4-11).[282–289,296,297]

The risk of prostate cancer progression is intimately related to stage and grade of the disease at the time of diagnosis.[283,285,287–289,291,294,295,298] Patients with metastatic disease at the time of diagnosis fare significantly worse than do patients with clinically localized disease at presentation. Brasso et al.[295] reported that the median survival was 3.7 years for patients with clinically localized prostate cancer, 1.8 years for patients with regionally advanced disease, and only 1.1 years for patients with metastatic disease at diagnosis. In the subset of patients surviving for at least 10 years after diagnosis, prostate cancer was the underlying cause of death in 61% of patients with clinically localized disease and in 76% of patients with advanced disease at diagnosis. Johansson et al.[288] reported outcomes for 642 patients, most of whom were treated with immediate or delayed androgen deprivation. While the 15-year corrected survival was 81% for patients with clinically organ-confined disease (stage T0 to T2) and 57% for patients with clinical stage T3 or T4 disease at diagnosis, the 15-year corrected survival was only 6% for patients with metastases at diagnosis. In a study of 514 prostate cancer patients treated with immediate or deferred androgen deprivation, Aus et al.[291] reported that the median survival of patients with localized disease at diagnosis was 82 months, as compared to only 26 months for patients with metastases at diagnosis. In those with clinically localized disease, T stage correlates with outcome. The risk of local and distant cancer progression and, ultimately, death rises with T stage. The risk of metastatic progression at 10 to 15 years after diagnosis is approximately 25% to 34% for those with T3 disease, whereas it is 13% to 20% for those with stage T1 and T2 disease.[285,287,288] Similarly, 10- to 15-year overall and disease-specific survival is better for those with T1 and T2 disease (62% to 90%), as compared to that associated with T3 and T4 disease (57% to 70%).[288,289,298] It should be noted that the risk of progression from stage T1 or T2 disease to T3 disease is approximately 70% at 10 years in those managed conservatively.[285] Aus et al.[291] found that 10% of patients with clinical stage T1a disease, 47% with clinical stage T1b disease, 52% with clinical stage T2a disease, 53% with clinical stage T2b to T3 disease, and 70% with clinical stage T4 disease ultimately died of prostate cancer.[291]

TABLE 34.4-12. Outcome of Conservative Management of Prostate Cancer According to Histologic Tumor Grade

Study	*No. of Patients*	*Follow-Up (y)*	*Outcome*	*Well-Differentiated (%)*	*Moderately Differentiated (%)*	*Poorly Differentiated (%)*
Johansson et al.[288]	642	14	Death from prostate cancer	16	38	68
Albertsen et al.[290]	451	15.5	Death from prostate cancer at 15 y	9	28	51
Chodak et al.[297]	828	6.6	Disease-specific survival at 10 y	87 (well- and moderately differentiated)	N/A	34
Gronberg et al.[293]	6514	7–23	No. of prostate cancer deaths/total no. of deaths	40	54	72
Albertsen et al.[299]	767	10–20	Probability of death from prostate cancer	4–7	6–11 (Gleason score 5); 10–30 (Gleason score 6)	42–70 (Gleason score 7); 60–87 (Gleason score 8)
Egawa et al.[282]	107	6.2	Disease-specific survival at 10 y	89	87	29
Aus et al.[291]	514	All patients followed until death	Risk of prostate cancer–related death	43	48	60

N/A, data not available.

Tumor grade may be the most important factor predicting disease progression and survival in prostate cancer patients managed conservatively. In a review of 828 prostate cancer patients obtained from six nonrandomized studies of men treated with observation and delayed androgen deprivation, Chodak et al.[297] reported that poorly differentiated disease was the single most important predictor of disease-specific survival. The likelihood of remaining metastasis-free 10 years after diagnosis for patients with well-, moderately, and poorly differentiated tumors was 81%, 58%, and 26%, respectively. Disease-specific survival 10 years after diagnosis was 87% for patients with well- or moderately differentiated disease and only 34% for patients with poorly differentiated disease.[297] Similar results with respect to disease-specific survival and prostate cancer–related death have been reported in a number of other studies (Table 34.4-12).[282,290,291,299] Moreover, poorly differentiated disease remains a significant predictor of prostate cancer–related death when adjusting for other factors such as tumor stage and patient age.[282,283,294,297] In these studies, the relative risk of prostate cancer–related death ranges from 2.6 to 3.6 for patients with moderately differentiated disease and from 6.1 to 12.9 for patients with poorly differentiated disease as compared to patients with well-differentiated prostate cancers.

In one of the best-performed studies on prostate cancer natural history done to date, Albertsen et al.[290,299] examined the impact of tumor grade on long-term survival among prostate cancer patients who were treated with either observation or immediate or delayed androgen deprivation. In their initial study, these authors determined that tumor grade correlated with death due to prostate cancer. Nine percent of patients with well-differentiated, 28% of patients with moderately differentiated, and 51% of patients with poorly differentiated disease died as a result of their prostate cancer within 15 years of diagnosis.[290] These authors also compared the survival of prostate cancer patients treated conservatively with the expected survival of the general population. Age-adjusted survival for men with well-differentiated, Gleason score 2 to 4 tumors was not significantly different from that of the general population. In contrast, the maximum expected loss-of-life expectancy was 4 to 5 years for men with Gleason score 5 to 7 tumors and 6 to 8 years for men with Gleason score 8 to 10 tumors as compared to the general population.[290] In a subsequent study, these authors developed a competing risk analysis to estimate the probability of dying from prostate cancer in 767 men, aged 55 to 74 years, all of whom remained untreated or received immediate or delayed androgen deprivation only.[299] Tumor grade had the most important impact on the risk of prostate cancer–related death for these patients: 4% to 7% of men with Gleason score 2 to 4 disease, 6% to 11% of patients with Gleason score 5 disease, 18% to 30% of patients with Gleason score 6 disease, 42% to 70% of patients with Gleason score 7 disease, and 60% to 87% of patients with Gleason score 8 to 10 disease died of prostate cancer within 15 years of diagnosis.[299] Others have reported similar findings (see Table 34.4-12).

Watchful waiting or surveillance alone for prostate cancer is an option for all patients with the disease. However, progression is likely in many, and the risk correlates with cancer stage and grade. Patients best suited for this approach may be those who are older and have low-grade or low-stage disease and in those with significant comorbidity. In such patients, the morbidity of treatment may outweigh the risks of significant disease progression. Patients being followed up with surveillance only need to be advised that end points for intervention for those on watchful waiting regimens have not been defined.

RADICAL PROSTATECTOMY

Radical prostatectomy can be performed through a lower abdominal incision (radical retropubic prostatectomy) or through a perineal incision (radical perineal prostatectomy). With the former technique, lymphadenectomy can be performed simultaneously. With radical perineal prostatectomy, lymphadenectomy can be performed through a separate incision, laparoscopically, or deleted in those at very low risk of lymph node metastases. Recently, a laparoscopic approach to radical prostatectomy has been developed.[300,301] Although early reports suggest that this technique is feasible and is associated with limited morbidity and acceptable positive margin and biochemical control rates, long-term follow-up in suitable patient populations is not yet available.

Contemporary series of patients with localized prostate cancers suggest that few patients harbor lymphatic disease (4% to 9%), and the risk of lymph node metastases can be quantitated as described previously in Imaging. Whereas high-risk patients benefit from lymphadenectomy, low-risk patients may forgo lymphadenectomy and be treated with definitive local therapy, whether irradiation or radical prostatectomy.[302,303]

Lymphadenectomy should be considered if the Gleason score is 5 to 6 and the PSA level is at least 20 ng/mL or if the Gleason score is 7 or higher and the PSA level is at least 15 ng/mL. Patients with clinical stage C (T3) disease should also be considered as candidates for the procedure.

Radical retropubic prostatectomy is performed through a lower midline incision. The rectus abdominis muscles are separated in the midline, and the retropubic space is entered. A fixed retractor is placed. Lymphadenectomy may be performed selectively as described. Lymph node dissection has been modified over the last several years to include lymph node tissue in areas most likely to harbor disease. The limits of dissection, therefore, most often include the obturator nerve posteriorly, the common iliac artery superiorly, the circumflex iliac vein inferiorly, and the internal aspect of the external iliac vein laterally.

Exposure of the prostate when performing a radical retropubic prostatectomy is undertaken by first incising the endopelvic fascia from the area of the puboprostatic ligaments along the lateral edge of the prostate to its base (Fig. 34.4-9). Fibers of the levator ani are separated from the apex of the prostate. The fascia and overlying dorsal vein complex generally are gathered and suture-ligated to facilitate exposure and prevent bleeding from the complex once it is cut to allow access to the urethra (Fig. 34.4-10). The puboprostatic ligaments, which provide anterior support of the urethra, are left intact over the urethra, but any attachments to the prostate are incised. Preservation of the puboprostatic ligaments facilitates earlier and more complete return of urinary continence as compared to previous techniques, which incised these ligaments over the urethra. Care is taken during the apical dissection of the prostate simultaneously to preserve the urethra's distal continence mechanism and to excise all prostate tissue. The urethral incision should be carried posteriorly beyond the urethra to include Denonvilliers' fascia, thereby ensuring complete cancer excision.

Penile erection is a neurovascular phenomenon, and the nerves and arterial blood supply (neurovascular bundles) crucial to potency run posterolaterally along either side of the prostate (Fig. 34.4-11). These bundles may be spared during surgery in an effort to preserve potency. However, ECE, when it does occur, may occur in the region of the neurovascular bundles. These bundles should be preserved cautiously in those at high risk of ECE. In addition, return of potency after a nerve-sparing radical prostatectomy is not only a function of technique but also of patient age and preoperative function. Older patients and those with poor preoperative potency may not benefit from a nerve-sparing approach. The neurovascular bundles can be located

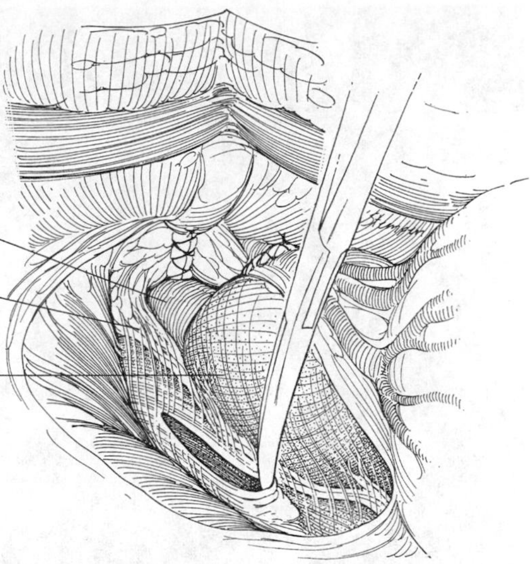

FIGURE 34.4-9. Radical prostatectomy. Incision is made in the lateral prostatic fascia to allow for nerve preservation or excision, depending on clinical stage and grade of disease.

using anatomic landmarks. During nerve-sparing radical prostatectomy, the lateral prostatic fascia is incised. The neurovascular bundles run deep to this fascia at approximately the 5 and 7-o'clock positions along the posterolateral surface of the prostate. Small vascular branches to the prostate may be taken using small clips or sutures. The neurovascular bundles are at the most risk for damage at the time of urethral dissection and transection, ligation of the lateral pedicles, and dissection of the seminal vesicles. However, a nerve stimulation device may facilitate identification and preservation.[304,305] Electrical stimulation may result in smooth muscle relaxation of penile tissue and expan-

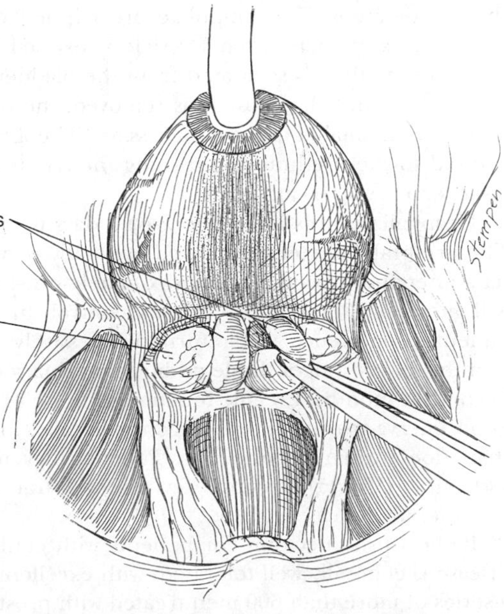

FIGURE 34.4-10. Radical prostatectomy, showing exposure of the seminal vesicles and ligation of the ampullae.

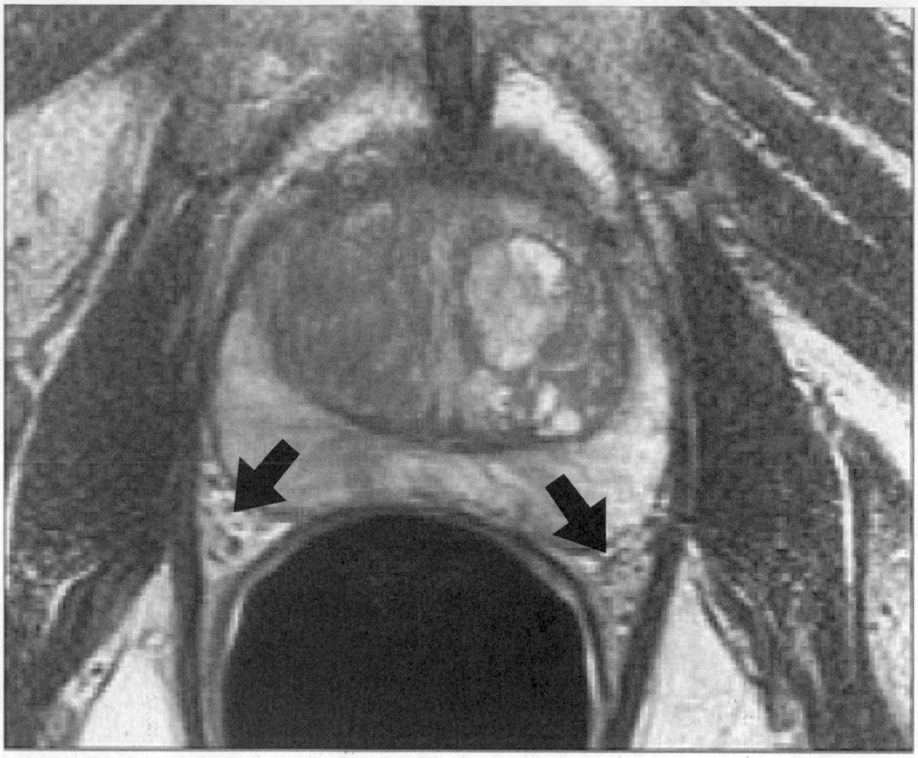

FIGURE 34.4-11. Typical endorectal magnetic resonance image of the prostate demonstrating the relationship of the neurovascular bundles (*arrows*) to the prostate.

sion of corporal sinusoids, resulting in increased penile blood flow, girth, and length. Either intracavernous pressure or penile circumference monitoring can note such changes. Early experience using a commercially available intraoperative, nerve-stimulating device and continuous monitoring of penile circumference during stimulation suggests that use of such a device may allow for better preservation of erectile function.

The lateral pedicles, branches of the prostatic and rectal arteries, are located alongside the prostate. Dissection proceeds superiorly, exposing the seminal vesicles and ampullae of the vas deferens. The ampullae are clipped or tied before being cut, and each seminal vesicle is excised in its entirety. The prostate then is separated from the bladder neck circumferentially. Once the prostate is removed, the bladder neck is closed to a smaller size, if necessary. The bladder neck is sutured to the urethral stump using interrupted suture material over a urethral catheter.

Hospitalization is limited to 2 or 3 days in most situations. The urethral catheter is removed generally between 5 and 14 days after the procedure. Approximately one-half of patients will gain almost immediate urinary control. In the remaining patients, continence will return progressively within 3 to 6 months, rarely longer. Little additional urinary control occurs beyond 12 months. Erectile function in those who have undergone a nerve-sparing approach generally takes longer to return than does urinary continence. Patients may require use of sildenafil (Viagra), vacuum devices, or intracavernous injection therapy, at least initially.

Radical prostatectomy for patients with clinically localized disease is generally well tolerated, with excellent outcomes. In a series of more than 600 men treated with prostatectomy, Trapasso et al.[306] reported a 10-year crude survival rate of 86% and a cause-specific survival of 94%. In an independent analysis of 3170 men treated at a different institution, Zincke et al.[307] reported similar 10-year crude and cause-specific survival rates of 75% and 90%, respectively. In addition, Zincke's group found that crude survival rates at 10 and 15 years after surgery were similar to those of age-matched men from the general population.[307] This finding suggests that carefully selected patients with clinically localized prostate cancer that is treated with prostatectomy can expect to live as long as cohorts without prostate cancer in their community.

However, clinical disease staging is far from perfect, as up to 50% of patients believed to have organ-confined prostate cancer at the time of surgery are later found to have disease beyond the prostate.[262,265,307–309] In addition, cancer recurrences are not uncommon in intermediate- to high-risk patients.[59] Given the protracted nature of this disease and the fact that residual and recurrent disease may respond to salvage therapy such as radiation or hormonal ablation, postoperative follow-up with sensitive serum PSA assays has become increasingly important.[262,310–313] Today, most clinical investigators report patient outcomes in terms of freedom from biochemical failure as well as clinical disease-free survival, in addition to crude and cause-specific survival. *Biochemical failure* is defined as either the persistence of a detectable PSA level postoperatively or the elevation of postoperative PSA to a detectable from a previously undetectable postoperative level. Total serum PSA has a half-life of 2 to 3 days, and its clearance follows first-order elimination kinetics; thus, the duration between surgery and PSA nadir generally takes several weeks and varies as a function of the patient's preoperative PSA level.[314] Postoperative follow-up regimens reflect PSA elimination kinetics and usually consist of symptom assessment and measurement of serum PSA every 3 months for the first year, biannually for the second year and third year, and annually thereafter. Clinical disease-free survival refers to freedom from

TABLE 34.4-13. Comparison of Actuarial Survival Outcomes for Patients Treated with Radical Prostatectomy

Institution	*No. of Patients*	*5-Y (%)*	*10-Y (%)*	*Outcome*	*Follow-Up (y)*
Washington University[318]	925	78	61	PSA <0.6 ng/mL	2.3 (mean)
Duke[321]	1319	65–70	—	PSA <0.5 ng/mL	4 (median)
Baylor[320]	500	77	74	PSA <0.4 ng/mL	2.7 (median)
UCLA[306]	601	69	47	PSA <0.4 ng/mL	2.8 (median)
		86	78	Clinically free of disease	
Mayo Clinic[307]	3170	70	52	PSA <0.2 ng/mL	5.0 (mean)
		85	72	Clinically free of disease	
Cleveland Clinic[262]	423	59	—	PSA <0.2 ng/mL	4.3 (median)
		84	—	Clinically free of disease	
Johns Hopkins[322]	1623	80	68	PSA <0.2 ng/mL	5.0 (mean)
UCSF	543	73	—	PSA <0.2 ng/mL	2.4 (mean)

PSA, prostate-specific antigen; UCLA, University of California at Los Angeles; UCSF, University of California at San Francisco.

detectable local or metastatic disease as assessed by the physician using physical examination, DRE, needle biopsy, radioisotope studies, and other traditional imaging modalities. Of note, studies from the early PSA era frequently used higher PSA cutoffs (e.g., 0.6 ng/mL). However, as the sensitivity of PSA assays improved over the last decade, most clinical investigators now use much lower cutoff points.

In the majority of cases, the first sign of disease recurrence or persistence is biochemical failure.[262,279,315,316] In two contemporary prostatectomy series from the Cleveland Clinic and Johns Hopkins Hospital totaling more than 2000 patients, not one patient showed signs of clinical disease in the absence of PSA failure.[262,279] Indeed, with the current patient follow-up regimen, nearly all recurrent clinical and metastatic disease is preceded by a rising PSA level, and only a few sporadic cases have been reported in the absence of detectable serum PSA.[317] After biochemical (PSA) failure, up to 68% of men will progress to detectable clinical disease at a median follow-up of 19 months. With adjuvant therapy such as irradiation or androgen deprivation at the time of PSA failure, the rate of progression to clinical disease is reportedly lower, at 21%.[262] Metastatic disease after PSA failure occurs in 34% of patients without adjuvant or salvage therapy, and investigators have reported a median actuarial time to metastases of 8 years from the time of PSA failure.[279] For those who develop metastatic disease, the median actuarial time to death was 5 years from the time of metastasis.

Several academic institutions have reported their experience in treating patients with clinically localized disease. The overall 5- and 10-year actuarial PSA progression-free rates range from 59% to 83% and 47% to 74%, respectively (Table 34.4-13).[262,306,307,318–322] The variability in outcomes likely reflects differences in patient selection, surgical technique, and definition of biochemical failure, as those with higher preoperative serum PSA levels, Gleason scores, disease stage, and positive surgical margin status tend to fare worse than counterparts with lower values or negative margins.[262,322,323] Reflecting the natural history of disease progression, clinical disease-free rates are higher, at 84% to 86% (5 years) and 72% to 78% (10 years).

The risk of disease progression and adverse outcomes varies directly with increasing pathologic disease stage, preoperative PSA level, and prostatectomy Gleason scores.[59,262,308,322,324] Whereas PSA relapse-free survival is approximately 80% to 84% for those with T2 disease, it falls to 57% to 67% for those with T3 disease. If one looks at all T stages, those patients who present with serum PSA levels of 10 ng/mL or less have PSA relapse-free survival rates of 80% to 95%, as compared to those with initial serum PSA levels of 10.1 to 20 ng/mL (48% to 75%) and those with levels in excess of 20 ng/mL (31% to 55%). Cancers with Gleason scores of 6 or less are associated with PSA relapse-free survival rates of 75% to 92%, as compared to PSA relapse-free survival rates of approximately 62% to 67% and 38% to 52% for Gleason 7 and 8 to 10 cancers, respectively. PSA relapse-free survival correlates with the risk assessment scheme outlined in Table 34.4-9. At the University of California at San Francisco (UCSF), 92%, 75%, and 44% of low-, intermediate-, and high-risk patients, respectively, managed by radical prostatectomy were free of relapse at 5 years. DNA aneuploidy, seminal vesicle invasion, and positive surgical margin status have also been reported to influence survival outcomes negatively.[59,273,323]

Complications

With increasing experience, the mortality and morbidity associated with radical prostatectomy has declined dramatically. Perioperative mortality in academic centers is exceedingly rare, at approximately 0.2%.[307,325] Intraoperative rectal injury and the need for a colostomy has decreased from 1% and 0.2%, respectively, for the period prior to 1988 to 0.6% and 0.06% for the period after. Similarly, complications such as myocardial infarction (0.1% to 0.4%), deep venous thrombosis (1.1%), pulmonary embolism (0.75%), blood transfusions (<5%), anastomotic stricture (4%), inguinal hernia (1%), and incisional hernia (0.6%) are becoming less common. In the series by Catalona et al.,[325] the incidence of stricture decreased with surgical experience from 6.0% for the first 1000 patients treated to 1.1% in the last 870 patients. As surgical experience continues to grow and techniques are refined, complication rates are likely to decrease further.

A more frequent surgical complication that can significantly influence patients' quality of life is incontinence, both urinary and fecal. Urinary continence is normally maintained by the bladder neck, prostatic smooth muscle, and external striated sphincter.[8] After surgery, the immediate postoperative incontinence rate may be as high as 80%, though more contemporary series report a much lower rate of immediate incontinence.[326,327] Fortunately, the majority of patients (86% to 92%) recover urinary continence within the first postoperative year with observation.[326,327] Some investigators have recommended pelvic floor exercises in the early postoperative period to enhance and expedite recovery of continence; however, the long-term benefits remain unclear.[328,329]

Depending on the patient's age, definition of incontinence, method of assessment, and surgical technique, incontinence rates at 1 year vary from 3% to 36%.[307,325,327,330–333] Across three institutions that included nearly 3000 patients, approximately 90% will be continent at 1 year, when continence is defined as no regular use of pads or no leakage with moderate exercise.[325–327] In a multivariate analysis of risk factors for urinary incontinence, Eastham et al.[327] reported that decreasing age, preservation of both neurovascular bundles, an absence of an anastomotic stricture, and use of a modified surgical technique about the striated urinary sphincter were independently associated with superior urinary outcomes. Continence appears to be equally well preserved with both the retropubic and perineal approaches.[327,334] Severe and persistent incontinence, defined as leakage with normal activity or the need for three or more pads per day, occurs in 1% to 6% of patients, and the use of an artificial sphincter, collagen injection therapy, or surgical sling procedure should be considered in such patients.[307,327,335–338]

A rare complication of surgery is fecal incontinence. Defined as the involuntary loss of liquid or solid stool, fecal incontinence may be caused by direct injury to the internal and external sphincters during perineal prostatectomy or by prolonged retraction of these segments during the procedure leading to neurologic compromise. However, the exact mechanism of injury remains elusive. In a validated patient survey, Bishoff et al.[327] initially evaluated 227 patients treated at two institutions and reported new-onset fecal incontinence rates of 5% and 18% for patients treated with the retropubic and perineal surgical approach, respectively. Although fecal incontinence was most often very limited, patients treated with perineal prostatectomy fared worse in terms of incontinence frequency and volume of leakage. Given the negative impact on patients' quality of life and that patients with fecal incontinence may not report their problem to health care providers, physicians must take a proactive role in assessing this complication.

Maintenance of sexual function has been a major concern for patients and physicians alike. With the advent of the nerve-sparing approach to radical retropubic prostatectomy, more than two-thirds of preoperatively potent patients treated by an experienced surgical team can anticipate return of potency without sacrificing cancer control.[279,325,339,340] Such rates are not reported by all investigators.[341,342] Return of potency after radical prostatectomy depends on many factors, including preoperative potency status, cancer stage, patient age, and whether one or both neurovascular bundles are spared. In clinical studies, *potency* usually is defined as the ability to sustain an erection sufficient for penetration and intercourse. Catalona et al.[325] reported recovery of potency in 68% and 47% of preoperatively potent men treated with bilateral or unilateral nerve-sparing surgery, respectively. Furthermore, younger patients reported superior outcomes. With a follow-up period of at least 18 months, 90% of men between the ages of 40 and 49 years were potent, as compared to 80%, 60%, and 47% of counterparts in their 50s, 60s, and 70s, respectively. Although not statistically significant, the authors reported a trend for better potency outcomes in men with lower preoperative PSA levels and lower disease stage. All studies suggest that the patients most likely to benefit from nerve-sparing surgery are those who are young, potent, and sexually active and have focal disease. It also appears that return of spontaneous erections after nerve-sparing surgery may be improved with early use of either sildenafil or intracavernous injection therapy.[343,344]

In summary, radical prostatectomy is a safe operation for properly selected patients and offers excellent cancer control. Cause-specific survival at 10 years is greater than 90%, and 70% of patients will be free of any signs of disease at 5 years. Major complications are rare, and the complication rate decreases with the surgeon's experience. With current refinements in technique, significant urinary incontinence is rare, and preservation of potency is possible in selected patients. Patients most likely to benefit from this approach are those who have long life expectancies and have either organ-confined disease or limited ECE, which can be excised completely.

Recurrence after Radical Prostatectomy and Role of Neoadjuvant and Adjuvant Therapy

Given the cancer recurrence and secondary treatment rates after radical prostatectomy, some investigators have tested the hypothesis that these rates could be reduced by neoadjuvant androgen deprivation.[345] Such therapy could decrease the likelihood of positive surgical margins, leading to a decrease in local recurrence rates. Every randomized trial performed to date has shown that neoadjuvant androgen deprivation significantly decreases the rate of positive surgical margins.[346–348] The rates of positive surgical margins were decreased by approximately 40% to 60% with neoadjuvant androgen deprivation. Unfortunately, this has not translated into any improvement in clinical or biochemical control rates. In a contemporary trial reported by Klotz and other members of the Canadian Urologic Oncology Group,[349] 213 patients with localized prostate cancer were randomized to radical prostatectomy alone (n = 101) or 12 weeks of cyproterone acetate followed by surgery (n = 112). The probability of biochemical progression at 36 months was similar for the groups treated by surgery alone or cyproterone acetate followed by surgery: 30.1% versus 40.2% ($P = .3233$), respectively. This and similar trials are ongoing. Failure to demonstrate a small, but significant, benefit to neoadjuvant therapy may be due to insufficient follow-up, short duration of androgen deprivation, insufficient power of some trials to demonstrate a benefit, or inclusion in the trials of large numbers of either very low-risk or high-risk patients. Most trials used 3 months of androgen deprivation preoperatively. Some suggest that extending the length of time of neoadjuvant androgen deprivation before surgery may translate into improved outcomes, as further decreases in prostate and cancer volume and serum PSA levels occur after 3 months.[350,351] It is clear, however, that neoadjuvant androgen deprivation cannot substitute for careful preoperative risk assessment and meticulous surgical technique.

For those who have undergone radical prostatectomy, several models have been proposed to identify patients at very high risk for relapse. Partin et al.[352] developed a model from a cohort of patients from one center and validated it on a second cohort of patients from the same center. Additional independent validation was performed.[353] In this model, 80% of failures occur within 4 years of radical prostatectomy, with a median time to failure of 14 to 16 months. The model was defined as: $R_w = (0.061 \times PSA_{ST}) + (0.54 \times \text{postoperative Gleason sum}) + (1.87 \times \text{specimen confined})$. Variables were defined as follows: $PSA_{ST} = 10/(1 + e^{6.8704 - 0.9815 \times PSA})$; *specimen confined* was defined as 1 if there was capsular penetration with positive surgical margins or positive seminal vesicles and was otherwise defined as 0. Patients were considered to be at high risk for serologic relapse, as demonstrated by an R_w exceeding 5.75. From a practical standpoint, an R_w will exceed 5.75 if (1) the cancer is confined to the surgical specimen, PSA level is at least 7.3, and Gleason score is 10; (2) there is ECE with positive margins or seminal vesicle invasion, PSA level is at least 5.4, and the Gleason score is 7; or (3) there is ECE with positive margins or seminal vesicle invasion and the Gleason score exceeds 8.

A second model for patients with pathologically capsule-confined prostate cancer has been proposed by D'Amico et al.[354] The model was defined as: V_{ca} = cancer-specific PSA/PSA leak into serum per cubic centimeter of cancer. Variables were defined as follows: *cancer-specific PSA* = PSA (preoperative) – [0.2 × 0.33 × TRUS prostate volume]. PSA leak is a constant, as a function of Gleason sum. V_{ca} will exceed 4.0 cc in patients with pathologically capsule-confined prostate cancer if (1) Gleason score is 6 and PSA level exceeds 18, (2) Gleason score is 7 and PSA level exceeds 14, or (3) Gleason score is 8, 9, or 10. Recently, Kattan et al.[355] developed a preoperative nomogram for disease recurrence after radical prostatectomy. The nomogram is used by locating a patient's position on a number of predictor variable scales. Each scale has corresponding prognostic points. The point total for all variables is summed, and this sum corresponds to the 5-year PSA progression-free survival likelihood.

From the preceding information, one can broadly identify patients who would be at high risk of relapse for whom adjuvant therapy after radical prostatectomy may be of most benefit. High-risk patients would be those having the following clinical and pathologic findings: (1) positive seminal vesicles, (2) Gleason score 6 and PSA level greater than 18, (3) Gleason score 7 and PSA level greater than 14, (4) Gleason score 8, 9, or 10 and any PSA level, and (5) those with positive surgical margins. Low-risk patients include those with a low pretreatment PSA level (i.e., <10 ng/mL), stage T1c or T2a disease, Gleason grades 1 through 3 disease, and clear surgical margins.

Optimal treatment for patients with adverse disease characteristics, as well as the timing of such treatment, remains controversial. Standard second treatment options after radical prostatectomy include radiation therapy with or without androgen deprivation or androgen deprivation alone. Adjuvant treatment, if given, can be tailored to the risk of relapse as well as to the pattern of suspected relapse (local vs. distant). Distant relapse may be more likely in those with high-grade disease, lymph node metastasis, and very high pretreatment PSA levels, as well as in those patients whose serum PSA level fails to fall to undetectable levels immediately after surgery. Patients at high risk of distant relapse are ideal candidates for experimental adjuvant systemic therapy, whereas those at risk of local relapse are candidates for radiation delivered to the prostatic bed.

The impact of positive surgical margins on outcome is a matter of controversy. Despite careful case selection before radical prostatectomy, between 14% and 41% of patients have tumor extending to the surgical margin on final pathologic analysis, with 33% to 62% of these patients failing radical prostatectomy based on the presence of a detectable serum PSA level.[356–359]

TABLE 34.4-14. Likelihood of Maintaining an Undetectable Serum Prostate-Specific Antigen in Patients with a Positive Surgical Margin

Author	*Undetectable PSA (%)*	*Actuarial Follow-Up*
Paulson[357]	42	5 y
Epstein[367]	57.6	5 y
Ohori[356]	64	5 y
D'Amico[359, a]	50	2 y
Lowe[368]	70	45 mo[b]
UCSF	52	3 y

PSA, prostate-specific antigen; UCSF, University of California at San Francisco.
[a]Patients with a tumor Gleason score greater than 7 or seminal vesicle invasion were excluded from the estimate.
[b]Median follow-up.

Radiation therapy may be given after surgery (adjuvant radiation), on the basis of adverse disease characteristics such as positive surgical margins, or after a documented disease recurrence (therapeutic radiation), on the basis of either biopsy-proven recurrence or biochemical failure alone. Proponents of adjuvant radiation argue that treatment is more effective when the local tumor burden is minimal and that series to date show that patients who undergo adjuvant radiation have been shown to achieve and maintain an undetectable serum PSA level in 77% to 94% of such cases.[360–363] However, despite improved local tumor control, no survival advantage has been demonstrated with adjuvant radiation. Studies have shown that between 42% and 70% of patients with positive surgical margins will maintain undetectable serum PSA levels without adjuvant therapy (Table 34.4-14).[364–368] Pathologic factors such as the location, extent, and number of positive margins may have an impact on the likelihood of disease recurrence in this setting.[368]

To date, no published studies have compared immediate versus delayed treatment in a prospective randomized fashion. Although the Southwest Oncology Group has instituted a randomized trial examining this question, the results of this study are not yet available. A decision to give adjuvant radiation is based on (1) the likelihood of cancer recurrence with adjuvant radiation, (2) the likelihood of cancer recurrence with surveillance alone, (3) the efficacy of radiation when given for biochemical recurrence (efficacy of therapeutic radiation), and (4) the morbidity of radiation. Grossfeld et al.[369] at UCSF created and tested a decision analysis model to help determine the preferred management of a positive surgical margin after radical prostatectomy. The model suggested that immediate radiation may be the preferred course of management for patients with a positive surgical margin and a high likelihood of recurrent local (rather than distant) disease. Such patients included those with low- to intermediate-grade disease (Gleason score <8), multiple positive margins, and no evidence of seminal vesicle invasion. For patients with no evidence of seminal vesicle invasion and all tumor grades, the model gave an equal value to surveillance and immediate adjuvant radiation. Surveillance was still recommended for patients with a preoperative PSA level of less than 15 ng/mL and for those with a single positive margin. However, the authors stressed that their model, which was based on literature-

and institution-based estimates of the efficacy of adjuvant and delayed radiation, may be useful to physicians and patients who can apply individualized probability estimates and utility values for determining their preferred course of management postoperatively. Further research is needed to confirm these results and to determine whether adjuvant radiation therapy is appropriate for patients with other adverse disease characteristics such as established ECE.

RADIATION THERAPY

Curative Potential of Radiation Therapy

Radiation therapy was introduced as a curative modality for localized prostate cancer in the 1950s, largely due to the work of Malcolm Bagshaw[409,410] of Stanford University. Using emerging techniques of megavoltage radiation therapy, it became possible to deliver tumoricidal dose levels to prostate tumors without excessive damage to the skin and the normal tissues surrounding the prostate.[409,410] This approach continues to represent the basic tenet of curative radiation therapy in prostate cancer, although systems of treatment planning and delivery have since advanced to improve precision and decrease toxicity. The ability of radiation to cure localized prostate cancer has thus improved consistently over the past three decades.[410–415]

Failure of radiation therapy to control localized prostate cancer results most frequently from resistance of tumor clonogens to the dose levels used and from failure to cover the entire target volume with the prescribed tumor dose. Before CT became available for treatment planning, tumor target volumes were assumed from planar radiographic images and frequently were inaccurate.[416] To compensate for target volume uncertainties, treatment volumes were classically increased to include a wide safety margin, thus including substantial portions of bladder and rectum in the high-dose region. Because of the high sensitivity of pelvic organs to radiation, the ability to deliver prostate doses exceeding 70 Gy with conventional megavoltage techniques was seriously compromised.[417–419] Whereas clinical data have indicated a need for higher doses to achieve maximal local tumor control,[420] conventional radiation therapy techniques have, in many cases, fallen short of the levels required to eradicate the tumor.[421] Further, while CT-assisted treatment planning has significantly improved the anatomic definitions of the tumor target,[422,423] wide safety margins have remained a common practice to compensate for uncertainties in patient positioning and organ motion. Finally, because computers available for treatment planning were, until recently, slow and limited in performance, calculations of dose distributions were restricted to a limited number of planes within the target volume, and the dose to the rest of the tumor was assumed based on reasonable, albeit imprecise, projections. Hence, the problem of geographic misses and tumor underdosage have continued to contribute to a high frequency of local tumor failure.

Advances in computer technology have enabled the implementation of three-dimensional conformal radiation therapy (3D-CRT) as an approach to overcome some of these problems.[415,421] Three-dimensional treatment planning is based on the ability to define each pixel anatomically within the entire 3D space of irradiated tissues and to calculate precisely the dose delivered at each point. It uses advanced imaging technology for tumor and normal organ segmentation, new algorithms for dose calculations, and computer-aided optimization to generate treatment plans that conform the prescribed dose to the tumor while maximally excluding the adjacent normal organs. The ability to exclude the normal tissues from the volume receiving high-dose irradiation has permitted significant increases in tumor dose without a concomitant increase in normal tissue toxicity.[415] The improved precision also decreased the risks of anatomic tumor misses and underdosage, further improving the potential for local tumor cure. Indeed, a recent outcome assessment involving the use of postirradiation biopsies provided conclusive evidence for the effects of 3D-CRT and dose escalation on the local cure of prostate cancer, thus defining new standards for curative radiation therapy in this disease.[415]

Effect of Dose on Local Tumor Control

Several studies have addressed the relationship between radiation dose and local control in prostate cancer.[415,424–429] The biologic effects of radiation on tumor and normal tissues result in dose-response patterns that translate into sigmoid-shaped curves when plotted graphically.[430,431] Because human tumors consist of heterogeneous clonogen populations with regard to radiation sensitivity,[432] it was suggested that tumor control curves would be relatively shallow, representing population averages for clones of different radiosensitivities.[433,434] The available clinical data mostly confirm this hypothesis, reporting tumor control curves with $\gamma 50$ values of approximately 2.[435–441] The validity of this model to prostate cancer was confirmed recently at the Memorial Sloan-Kettering Cancer Center (MSKCC) in a postirradiation biopsy study of 150 patients who did not receive neoadjuvant androgen deprivation therapy.[415,442] The diagnostic accuracy of posttreatment biopsies depends, among other factors, on the time interval from completion of treatment to biopsy.[443–446] For example, Scardino and Wheeler[443] reported that 32% of patients with a positive biopsy at 12 months after radiation therapy had a negative pathologic specimen at 24 months. As recommended by the ASTRO consensus statement,[447] biopsies were performed in the MSKCC study at 2.5 years or longer after 3D-CRT. The tumor dose was increased gradually in consecutive groups of patients, from 64.8 Gy to 81.0 Gy by increments of 5.4 Gy. Figure 34.4-12 shows that the rate of negative biopsies increased linearly from 48% in patients receiving 64.8 Gy to 94% after 81 Gy. The calculated $\gamma 50$ value for this set of data is 2.22. There was a concomitant increase in PSA relapse-free survival in patients receiving the high-dose range, providing further evidence for a significant effect of dose escalation on the cure of human prostate cancer.

Serum Prostate-Specific Antigen as a Surrogate for Defining Tumor Control after Radiation Therapy

After pelvic irradiation, serum PSA level generally declines over 1 to 2 years, but usually it is not reduced to undetectable levels, as 70% of patients receiving radiation therapy for rectal and other nonprostatic tumors have PSA levels of less than 1.0 ng/mL for extended periods after irradiation.[448] On the basis of these data, it was suggested that cure of localized prostate cancer with radiation would be associated with maintained PSA

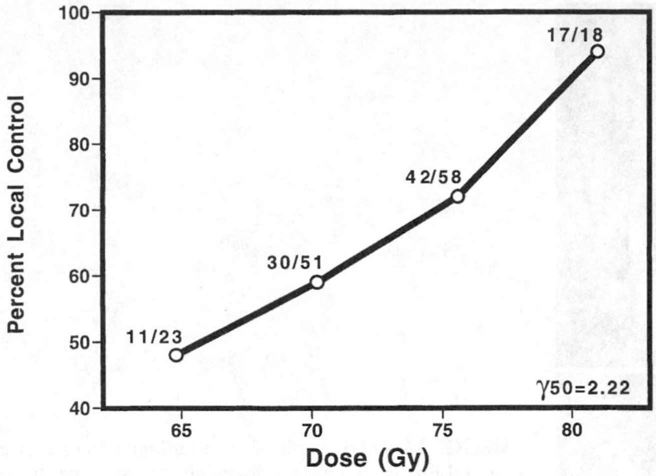

FIGURE 34.4-12. Tumor control curve, showing effect of radiation dose on the rate of negative prostate biopsies.

profiles of less than 1.0 ng/mL.[449,450] It also was suggested that an increased serum PSA level from such postirradiation nadir values can serve as an indicator of disease relapse. Reviewing the emerging data in the field, the ASTRO consensus statement[451] has established a definition for PSA relapse as three consecutive rising PSA values from an established nadir value. The date of failure was defined as the midpoint between the last postirradiation nadir value and the first of the three consecutive increases. This guideline did not stipulate a specific nadir value that is associated with a complete response. However, multiple studies employing multivariate analyses have indicated that a PSA nadir of less than 1 ng/mL represents an independent variable in predicting long-term PSA relapse-free survival.[450,452,453] For example, Kavadi et al.[450] reported that the 5-year PSA relapse-free survival for patients who achieved nadir levels of less than 1.0 ng/mL was 17%, as compared to 70% for patients with posttreatment nadir levels exceeding 1.0 ng/mL. In this study, nadir levels of 50.5 ng/mL did not provide for improved prediction of outcome. The Eastern Virginia Medical School,[453] however, reported 5-year PSA relapse-free survival of 91% and 72% in patients with postirradiation nadir levels of less than 0.5 ng/mL and 0.5 to 1.0 ng/mL, respectively ($P = .06$).

Shipley et al.[454] defined the long-term pattern of PSA response in an outcome study of a multiinstitutional pooled cohort of 1765 patients with T1 to T2 prostate cancer, treated with advanced external-beam techniques to doses ranging from 63 to 79 Gy (median dose, 69.4 Gy). Nadir posttreatment PSA values of ≤1.0 ng/mL were recorded in 80% of the patients, and only 12.8% had values in excess of 2.0 ng/mL. The overall 5-year PSA relapse-free survival was 65.8%, and of the 448 patients followed for more than 5 years, only 5% relapsed from the fifth to the eighth year. Though this study provided evidence that the majority of PSA relapses occur within the first 5 years after radiation therapy, it did not provide evidence that PSA relapse connotes anatomic relapse and that a nonrising profile correlates with lack of tumor relapse. The MSKCC posttherapy biopsy study[415,442] did, however, address this issue. Of patients undergoing biopsy at more than 2.5 years after treatment, 50 of 51 (98%) with a posttreatment PSA nadir of not more than 1.0 ng/mL and a nonrising PSA profile had negative biopsies, as compared with only 21 of 42 (50%) of those with a similar nadir but with a rising PSA profile ($P < .001$). Of patients with a PSA nadir of more than 1.0 ng/mL, 7 of 10 (70%) of those with a nonrising PSA profile and 21 of 47 (45%) with a rising PSA profile had negative biopsy specimens ($P = .2$). Taken together, these data strongly suggest that in early-stage patients in whom PSA levels of not more than 1.0 ng/mL are nadir, a maintained PSA relapse-free profile serves to indicate a 95% likelihood of permanent tumor control after radiation therapy.

Definition of Target Volume

Carcinoma of the prostate is frequently multifocal, involving more than one lobe of the gland.[455] Therefore, the clinical target volume (CTV) for irradiation consists of the total prostatic gland, including the seminal vesicles, as visualized on CT. Capsular involvement with or without periprostatic invasion has been demonstrated in 15% to 66% of radical prostatectomy specimens from patients with stage TI or T2 disease.[456–458] Hence, the prostatic capsule and the immediate periprostatic tissues are incorporated in the CTV. The planning target volume (PTV) encompasses the CTV and an additional 1.0-cm margin of tissue to compensate for patient setup uncertainties and organ motion.[459,460]

The inclusion of pelvic lymph nodes in the CTV has been an issue of continued controversy. Lymph node metastases are common in prostate cancer, and their frequency correlates with stage, tumor volume, and histologic grade.[461–463] The major lymph node–bearing areas that drain the prostate include the external iliac, hypogastric, presacral, and internal pudendal nodes. These chains of nodes can be encompassed by treatment fields that involve a major portion of the pelvis.[464] Several old retrospective studies have suggested that pelvic irradiation in addition to limited prostatic fields improves disease-free survival and results in fewer pelvic failures in T2 or T3 patients.[465–467] Most studies were conducted in the pre-PSA era and without staging laparotomies, leaving open questions regarding the extent of lymph node involvement and their response to therapy. However, Seaward et al.[467] described treatment results in 201 patients considered to be at high risk for lymph node involvement based on combined pretreatment profiles of PSA levels and Gleason scores. The risk of positive nodes (N+ ≥15%) was calculated using the equation [$N+ = 2/3(PSA) + (GS - 6) \times 10$], as suggested by Roach et al.[468] Freedom from PSA failure was significantly improved in 117 patients who received whole pelvis irradiation, as compared to 84 patients whose treatment was limited to the prostate only (median PSA relapse-free survival of 34.3 months vs. 21.0 months; $P = .0001$). Prospective randomized studies in patients undergoing staging laparotomy, carried out by the Stanford group,[469,470] suggested that prophylactic lymph node irradiation may be of benefit only in patients with T1 and T2 disease. However, multiple other studies failed to demonstrate a benefit of prophylactic whole pelvis irradiation.[471–476] The Radiation Therapy Oncology Group study (RTOG 77-06), which randomized 449 patients with T1b or T2N0M0 tumors to receive either prostatic or prostatic plus whole pelvis irradiation after bipedal lymphography or staging laparotomy,[475,476] reported no significant differences in local control and survival (median follow-up of 12 years). The actuarial rates of local relapse at 12 years were 27% for prostate irradia-

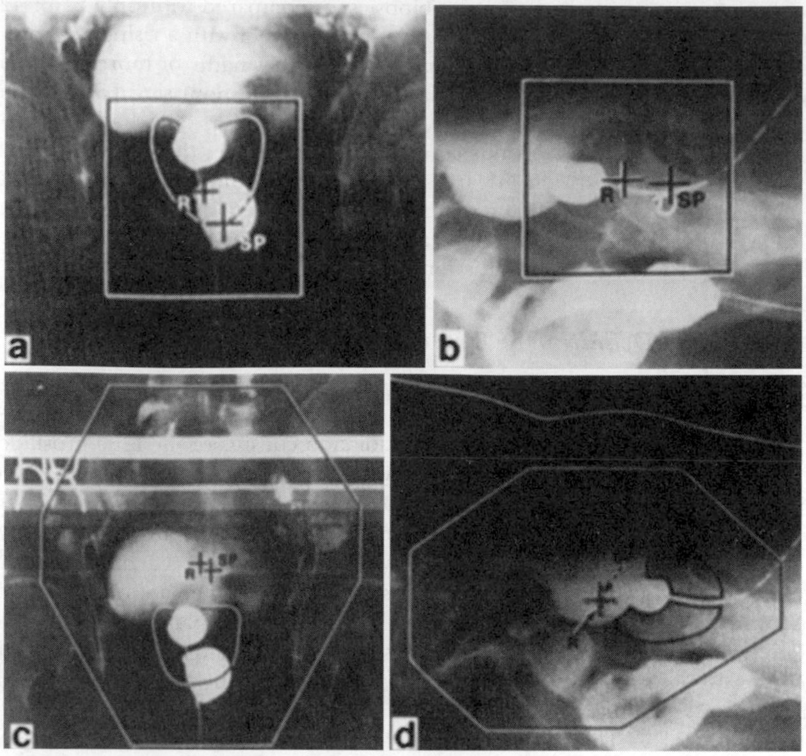

FIGURE 34.4-13. Simulation radiographs of a case planned for treatment with four-field conventional technique. **A:** Anteroposterior localization film of the prostate planning target volume (PTV) and the planned rectangular treatment field. Contrast material (Hypaque) has been placed in the urinary bladder and the rectum, and the balloons of the Foley catheters placed in the bladder and rectum. The setup point (SP) is marked on the patient's skin. The center point for the treatment field is designated (R). **B:** Lateral localization of the prostate PTV and the prostatic field **(C)** and **(D)**. Pelvic fields designed in this patient to treat the pelvic lymph nodes electively. (From ref. 464, with permission.)

tion alone and 22% for prostate plus pelvic irradiation ($P = .2$), and the actuarial survival rates were 43% and 38%, respectively ($P = .4$). Based on these observations, it is generally accepted that elective pelvic irradiation is unlikely to affect the outcome of treatment, and pelvic lymph nodes generally are not included in the CTV for treatment planning.

Simulation and Treatment Planning

CONVENTIONAL (TWO-DIMENSIONAL) EXTERNAL-BEAM RADIATION THERAPY. Treatment is most frequently planned in the supine position at 100 cm source-axis distance, and immobilization devices are increasingly used to reduce patient motion during treatment. Localization skin marks are placed on the patient that correspond to a standardized treatment isocenter, a midline point near the center of the prostate located 1 cm inferior and 6 cm posterior to the upper border of the symphysis pubis. Simulation radiographs are obtained in the treatment position from the level of L5-S1 to 1.0 cm caudal to the ischial tuberosities. The target volume and the surrounding normal organs are drawn on orthogonal planar radiographs produced on conventional simulators or on digitally reconstructed radiographs generated from CT images obtained by CT simulators. To assist in defining the PTV, it is customary to use urinary bladder and rectal catheters and contrast media. A No. 16 Foley catheter is introduced into the bladder, and the balloon is inflated with 5 mL of 90% Hypaque solution. The balloon is pressed against the bladder trigone with light pressure, and the catheter is taped to the thigh. In addition, 30 mL of low-density Hypaque (30%) is introduced into the bladder. A second Foley catheter is placed in the rectum and the balloon is inflated with air and pressed against the internal sphincter of the rectum to indicate the location of the anus. Low-density Hypaque (30%) is also placed in the rectum to outline the rectal wall.

The superior border of the prostatic field usually is located approximately 2 cm above the Foley balloon and includes nearly 30% of the bladder detected by the contrast media (Fig. 34.4-13*A,B*). The inferior border is located short of the internal anal sphincter. The anterior margin is at the posterior cortex of the pubic bone, and the posterior border extends 6 to 10 mm posterior to the anterior rectal wall, sparing the posterior rectal wall. The right and left lateral margins are usually marked at 3.5 to 4.0 cm from the isocenter (see Fig. 34.4-13*A,B*). When there is an indication to treat the pelvic nodes, the inferior border usually is extended to the ischial tuberosities and the superior border to the top surface of L5 (see Fig. 34.4-13*C,D*). The lateral borders are placed approximately 1 cm lateral to the widest diameter of the pelvic inlet, but the superior and inferior corners are trimmed to protect as much bone marrow as possible. The anterior border of the lateral field extends to the anterior aspect of the pubic symphysis, while the posterior margin is established at the midlumen of the rectum inferiorly and at the midsacral bone superiorly (see Fig. 34.4-13*C,D*). The patient receives tattoo marks at the anterior and two lateral triangulation points in a single transverse plane, corresponding to the isocenter of the treatment field.

Treatment plans typically consist of an isocentric four-field box, designed to include the prostate, seminal vesicles, and periprostatic tissues. The cross sections of the beams may be shaped with Cerrobend blocks to protect, surrounding normal tissues, as the situation permits. The daily PTV dose is 1.8 to 2.0 Gy, delivered five times per week with all fields treated at each session, to a total dose of 65 to 70 Gy in 7 to 8 weeks. When the pelvic nodes are treated, radiation is planned first to the entire pelvic field to a dose of 45 to 50 Gy in 5 weeks. The prostate

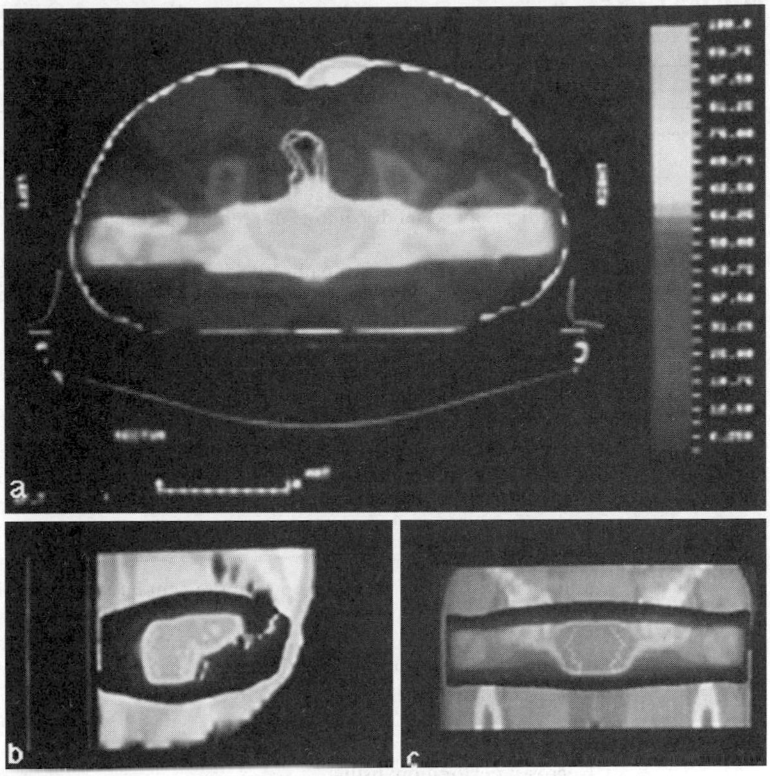

FIGURE 34.4-14. Color wash displays of the dose distribution of a six-field coplanar prostate three-dimensional conformal radiation therapy plan with 15-MV x-rays. The planned treatment consists of one pair of lateral and two pairs of oblique fields. The dose distribution is shown on **(A)** axial, **(B)** sagittal, and **(C)** coronal computed tomography reconstructions of the prostate and surrounding normal tissue at the mid-plan of planning target volume (PTV). The boundaries of the PTV are shown in yellow dots. The red region represents the prescription isodose distribution, and the yellow region corresponds to approximately 70% to 80%, green to 45% to 70%, and blue to 45% or less of the prescription dose. (See Color Fig. 34.4-14 in the CD-ROM and on the Web at www.LWWoncology.com.)

PTV then is boosted to a dose of 20 Gy, raising the dose to the primary prostatic tumor to a total of 65 to 70 Gy. To improve the tolerance of treatment, a "sandwich" technique has been proposed in which the delivery to the large pelvic field is split and the small boost field is delivered in between.[477] This technique permits a rest period and a partial recovery of the bowel and bladder from the toxic effects of the initial pelvic field irradiation.

THREE-DIMENSIONAL CONFORMAL RADIATION THERAPY. Although 3D treatment-planning systems vary in detail, all are based on common principles. The simulation consists of a combination of conventional and CT-assisted procedures. Conventional simulators can be used to determine the positioning of the patient, to define a provisional isocenter, and to produce reference localization skin marks. CT images are used to segment the prostate and normal organs and to generate high-resolution 3D reconstructions. The CT data are also used in calculations of dose distribution, as modern dose calculation formalisms are based on electron density ratios of the anatomic structures included in the treatment fields.[421] Several algorithms are in use for 3D dose calculations, but the more advanced methods, such as the pencil-beam convolution algorithm with pixel-by-pixel inhomogeneity corrections,[421] are required for maximal accuracy.

Treatment is planned in the supine or prone position[478] within individually fabricated immobilization casts to ensure reproducible positioning during repeated treatment sessions.[479] Because prostatic displacement during a course of radiation therapy was shown to be affected by rectal and bladder volumes,[480] some studies have recommended that the simulation and each treatment session be carried out with the patient's bladder and rectum emptied, to reduce daily variations in prostate location and geometry. The tumor target and the critical normal structures are segmented on every CT slice where they appear. The PTV extends from 1.0 cm caudal to the apex of the prostate to 1.0 cm cephalad to the superior tips of the seminal vesicles and encompasses the prostate with a 1.0-cm margin, except posteriorly at the interface with the rectum, where some investigators have suggested the use of a 0.6-cm margin to reduce the risk of rectal toxicity.[479] The target volume and the normal organs then are reconstructed by the computer in 3D and are displayed with the beam's-eye view technique.[481] The most commonly used beam arrangement consists of six coplanar fields (two lateral opposed fields and two pair of oblique fields) shaped to conform the PTV.[482] Dose calculations then are performed and the adequacy of target coverage by the prescription dose is evaluated on displays of isodose or color-wash distributions (Fig. 34.4-14) and by dose-volume histograms.[483] The target dose is either prescribed to the median International Commission on Radiation Units and Measurement ($ICRU_{50}$) reference point[484] or to the maximum isodose surface distribution that completely encompasses the PTV.[482] Some investigators have suggested that the rectal wall dose be restricted to no more than 30% of the prescription dose, the bladder wall dose to 50%, and the bowel dose (when bowel happens to be included in the PTV) to 65%, to decrease the risk of toxicity.[485] When radiation cannot be administered without exceeding these limits, a 3-month course of neoadjuvant androgen deprivation has been suggested to decrease the target volume. Significant reductions in PTV and, consequently, in normal tissue volumes carried to the prescription dose have been observed in nearly 90% of patients treated with this approach.[485] Beam apertures are automatically shaped by the treatment planning computer, applying continuously varying apertures with a margin of 0.5 cm around the outline of the tumor target, to account for beam penumbra. Cerrobend blocks or multileaf collimators then are used to

TABLE 34.4-15. Radiation Therapy Oncology Group–European Organization for Research and Treatment of Cancer Scoring Scheme for Acute and Late Rectal and Bladder Morbidity

Grade	*Rectal*	*Bladder*
Acute disease		
0	No toxicity	No toxicity
1	Increased frequency or change in quality of bowel habits not requiring medication; rectal discomfort not requiring analgesics	Frequency of urination or nocturia less frequent than every hour; dysuria, urgency, bladder spasm requiring local anesthetic
2	Diarrhea requiring parasympatholytic drugs [e.g., diphenoxylate (Lomotil)]; mucous discharge not necessitating sanitary pads; rectal or abdominal pain requiring analgesics	Frequency of urination or nocturia less frequent than every hour; dysuria, urgency, bladder spasm requiring local anesthetic
3	Diarrhea requiring parenteral support; severe mucous or bloody discharge necessitating sanitary pads; abdominal distended bowel loops	Frequency with urgency and nocturia hourly or more frequently; dysuria, pelvic pain, or bladder spasm requiring regular, frequent narcotic; gross hematuria with or without clot passage
4	Acute or subacute obstruction, fistula, or perforation; gastrointestinal bleeding requiring transfusion; abdominal pain or tenesmus requiring tube decompression or bowel diversion	Hematuria requiring transfusion; acute bladder obstruction not secondary to clot passage, ulceration, or necrosis
Chronic disease		
0	No toxicity	No toxicity
1	Mild diarrhea; mild cramping; bowel movement 5 times daily; slight rectal discharge or bleeding	Slight epithelial atrophy; minor telangiectasia; microscopic hematuria
2	Moderate diarrhea and colic; bowel movement >5 times daily; excessive rectal mucus or intermittent bleeding	Moderate frequency; generalized telangiectasia; intermittent microscopic hematuria
3	Obstruction or bleeding requiring surgery	Severe frequency and dysuria; severe generalized telangiectasia (often with petechiae); frequent hematuria; reduction in bladder capacity (<150 mL)
4	Necrosis; perforation; fistula	Necrosis; constructed bladder (capacity <100 mL); severe hemorrhagic cystitis

shape the planned treatment fields. To assure that treatment is delivered as planned, automated on-line electronic portal imaging has also become available recently. In the future, portal imaging may also provide on-line automated corrections of patient setup errors during the treatment session through computer-driven feedback mechanisms.

INTENSITY-MODULATED RADIATION THERAPY. For details of simulation and treatment planning using intensity-modulated radiation therapy (IMRT), see Chapter 29.4.

Tolerance of Treatment and Late Complications

Doses of 70 Gy or less, when delivered with conventional (two-dimensional) external-beam irradiation, are fairly well tolerated. However, grade 2 [RTOG/European Organization for Research and Treatment of Cancer (EORTC) scoring scheme; Table 34.4-15] or higher acute rectal morbidity or urinary symptoms requiring medication (or both) occur in approximately 60% of patients.[486] Symptoms typically appear during the third week of treatment and resolve within days to weeks after its completion. Acute intestinal symptoms, especially those associated with whole pelvis irradiation, are most commonly relieved with diet manipulations. Otherwise, medications such as diphenoxylate hydrochloride (Lomotil) are appropriate to relieve symptoms. Internal and external hemorrhoids may become inflamed during a course of therapy. These symptoms often are best treated with sitz baths and cortisone suppositories. Acute urinary symptoms are treated with phenazopyridine hydrochloride (Pyridium), nonsteroidal antiinflammatory agents, or α-adrenergic blockers such as terazosin. Zelefsky et al.[487] recently reported that α-adrenergic blockers were significantly more effective than nonsteroidal antiinflammatory agents, resulting in significant resolution of urinary symptoms in 66% and moderate improvement in 22%; in only 12% was minimal relief to no improvement observed. In contrast, among patients treated with ibuprofen, only 16% experienced significant symptom relief, 28% exhibited moderate improvement, and 56% demonstrated minimal to no response.

Late complications develop within 3 to 6 months after completion of radiation therapy. Zelefsky et al.[415] reported that the median time to onset of grade 2 or worse late rectal toxicity was 12 months, with a range of 3 to 39 months. Similarly, Teshima et al.[488] from the Fox Chase Cancer Center reported median times to occurrence of grade 2 and 3 rectal toxicities at 13 and 18 months, respectively. The incidence of late complications in patients receiving conventional radiation therapy doses of 70 Gy is low. An analysis of 1020 patients treated in two large RTOG trials demonstrated an incidence of chronic urinary sequelae (i.e., cystitis, hematuria, urethral stricture, or bladder contracture) requiring hospitalization in 7.3% of cases, but the incidence of urinary complications requiring major surgical interventions was only 0.5%.[489] More than one-half of chronic urinary complications were urethral strictures, occurring mostly in patients who had undergone a previous transurethral radical prostatectomy. The incidence of chronic intestinal sequelae (chronic diarrhea, proctitis, rectal or anal stricture, rectal bleeding, or ulcer) requiring hospitalization for diagnosis and minor intervention was 3.3%, with only 0.6% of patients experiencing bowel obstruction or perforation. Fatal complications were extremely uncommon (0.2%).

The risk of late complications increases when radiation doses exceed 70 Gy. Leibel et al.[490] reported 6.9% grade 3 to 4 complications in 174 prostate cancer patients treated with doses exceeding 70 Gy, as compared with 3.5% after treatment with less than 70 Gy. Sandler et al.[491] reported that the actuarial incidence of grade 3 to 4 rectal toxicity for patients who received doses in excess of 68 Gy was 9% at 3 years, as compared to 2% for those who received lower doses. Schultheiss et al.[492] reported late toxicity in 712 patients treated with conventional or conformal radiation techniques. The risk of late toxicity strongly correlated with the central axis dose. The 5-year incidence of grade 2 or 3 late rectal toxicity was 27%, 35%, 43% for central axis doses of 71 to 74 Gy, 74 to 77 Gy, and 77 Gy or more, respectively ($P<.001$).

Rectal complications have also been correlated with the volume of anterior rectal wall receiving a given dose (the so-called volume effect). Benk et al.,[493] from the Massachusetts General Hospital, reported dose-volume patterns and their relationship with rectal bleeding in patients treated with 50.4 Gy whole pelvis photon-beam radiation therapy followed by 25.2 cobalt-gray equivalents (CGE) delivered via a 160-MeV perineal proton beam boost. A logistic regression analysis revealed ten dose-volume combinations that were more likely associated with late rectal bleeding, ranging from 60 CGE delivered to 70% of the anterior rectal wall to 75 CGE involving 30% of the rectal wall. When portions of the anterior rectal wall were exposed to 75 CGE, the actuarial incidence of bleeding at 40 months was 61% when 40% or more of the wall received this dose, as compared with 19% when less than 40% of the wall was exposed ($P = .0036$). Lee et al.[494] reported that among patients receiving PTV doses of less than 76 Gy, the use of a rectal block significantly reduced the incidence of grade 2 to 3 rectal toxicity, from 22% without a block to 7% with a block ($P = .003$). These data indicated the need to spare the rectal wall maximally when protocols of high-dose therapy are implemented, to improve the local outcome in prostate cancer.

3D-CRT has been developed, in part, to address this issue. The ability of the 3D approach to reduce rectal and bladder toxicities has been demonstrated in several studies. The Fox Chase Cancer Center[495] reported acute grade 2 gastrointestinal or genitourinary morbidity with 3D-CRT in 84 of 247 patients (34%), as compared with 93 of 162 patients (57%) treated with conventional radiation therapy techniques ($P<.001$). Dearnaley et al.[496] randomized patients to receive a dose of 64 Gy with conformal or conventional techniques. The late grade 2 rectal toxicity was 5% for 3D-CRT patients, as compared with 15% for the conventional plan ($P = .01$). Leibel et al.[442] have recently updated the MSKCC series of 1100 patients treated with 3D-CRT. In consecutive groups of patients, the tumor dose was gradually increased from 64.8 Gy to 86.4 Gy by increments of 5.4 Gy. The rate of grade 3 rectal bleeding requiring one or more transfusions or one or more laser cauterization procedures was 1%, and the rate of grade 3 urethral stricture was 1%. All strictures occurred in patients who previously underwent transurethral prostate resec-

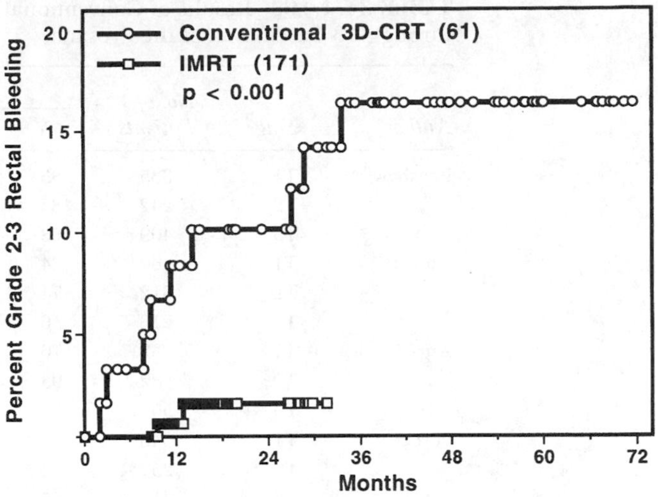

FIGURE 34.4-15. Radiation toxicity. Actuarial risk of grade 2–3 rectal bleeding in 232 patients treated with conventional three-dimensional conformal radiation therapy (3D-CRT) or intensity-modulated radiation therapy (IMRT).

tions. The 5-year actuarial risk of grade 2 rectal bleeding for patients receiving 64.8 to 70.2 Gy was 6%, as compared to 17% for those treated with 75.6 to 81 Gy ($P<.001$).

The rising rate of grade 2 rectal bleeding with increasing 3D-CRT dose[442] indicated that dose escalation would require improved 3D-CRT techniques to decrease the volume of exposed rectal wall and decrease the risk of rectal toxicity. IMRT provides this option. A recent study from MSKCC compared 20 patients in whom concomitant 3D-CRT and IMRT were planned.[497] Only 9% ± 3% of the rectal wall would have received 75 Gy with the IMRT plan, as compared with 14% ± 3% with a routine six-field 3D-CRT plan ($P<.01$). There was also a significant improvement of the percentage PTV receiving the prescription dose (81 Gy) with IMRT. These data indicated that IMRT significantly improves the conformality of the radiation treatment in prostate cancer. To validate the expected decrease in toxicity, the incidence of rectal bleeding was recorded in 61 patients treated to 81 Gy with routine six-field 3D-CRT and was compared with the rates in 171 patients treated to the same dose with IMRT. Figure 34.4-15 shows that the 2-year actuarial risk of grade 2 to 3 rectal bleeding was 2% for IMRT and 10% for conventional 3D-CRT ($P<.001$). Only one patient in each treatment group developed grade 3 rectal bleeding.

Sexual function is preserved in 73% to 82% within the first 12 to 15 months after irradiation,[498,499] but erectile potency diminishes with advancing time, with only 30% to 61% of patients maintaining their potency at 5 years or longer after irradiation.[500] The etiology of erectile dysfunction after radiation therapy appears to be related to vascular disruption caused by treatment as opposed to radiation damage to the nerve bundles.[501] Doppler blood flow studies of the corporal vasculature in patients with erectile dysfunction after radiation therapy suggested that arteriogenic rather than cavernosal or neurogenic dysfunction underlie this toxicity.[501] Patients who develop impotence after radiation therapy can be effectively treated with intracavernosal prostaglandin injection therapy.[502] Preliminary observations with sildenafil in these patients dem-

TABLE 34.4-16. Results of Conventional External-Beam Radiation Therapy in Stage T1 through T3 Carcinoma of the Prostate

			Survival (%)			*Local Relapse-Free Survival (%)*		
Author	*Stage*	*No. of Patients*	5-Y	10-Y	15-Y	5-Y	10-Y	15-Y
Bagshaw[498]	T1	335	85	65	40	90	85	90
	T2	242	83	55	35	80	70	65
	T3	409	68	38	20	76	63	40
Hanks[505]	T1	60	84	54	51	96	96	83
	T2	312	74	43	22	83	71	65
	T3	216	56	32	23	70	65	60
Zagars[507b]	T1	32	76	68	—	100	100	—
	T2	82	93	70	—	97	88	—
	T3	551	72	47	27	88	81	75
Perez[507a]	T1	48	85	70	—	90	80	—
	T2	252	82	65	—	85	76	—
	T3	412	65	42	—	72	60	—

onstrated a 74% response rate.[503] Improved responses to the medication were noted among patients with normal erectile function prior to radiation therapy, as compared to those with declining pretreatment function.[503]

Results of Treatment

Before the PSA era, the outcome of radiation therapy was assessed by DRE, radiography, and isotope scans. Although outcome assessment by this method is somewhat imprecise, especially with regards to local control, it nonetheless appeared that the long-term results of radiation therapy in TI and T2 disease were similar to those observed with radical prostatectomy.[411,412,455–458,477] Using a hazard function over successive 5-year intervals, Coleman et al.[504] reported that with the exception of very small tumors, there was a similar constant risk of relapse for surgery and radiation therapy throughout a follow-up period of 20 years. Stage for stage, the survival outcome was similar for the surgical and radiation series. Hanks[411,505] reported a 14% 10-year cause-specific mortality in 104 lymphadenectomy-staged patients with stages T1b to T2N0 disease treated in the RTOG trial 77-06. Eighty-seven percent of the patients were clinically free of local recurrences, 79% were free of distant metastases, and 67% were free of any failure. The survival rate was nearly identical to the expected survival in a life table for an age-matched control population throughout the 10 years of observation (63% observed vs. 59% expected at 10 years).[411,505] It has been frequently stated that although the results of radiation and radical surgery are comparable up to 10 years, at longer follow-up periods there may be a selective, rapid decrement in survival and disease-free survival for irradiated patients. Table 34.4-16 summarizes published long-term results with conventional external-beam irradiation, indicating outcome data for irradiated patients at 15 years that are similar to published data for radical prostatectomy.[412,505–507a,b]

With the introduction of PSA level as a surrogate for defining tumor control after definitive therapy, it became evident that more failures can be documented after definitive therapy than had previously been appreciated. For example, Zietman et al.[508] reported clinical relapse-free survival of 65% at 10 years in 504 T1 or T2 patients, as compared with freedom from PSA relapse in only 40% of patients. Other studies have confirmed that PSA relapse precedes evidence of anatomic relapse, frequently by more than 2 years.[509,510] The study by Zietman et al.[508] also reported that of the 60% of patients who exhibited a PSA relapse, local progression by 10 years was found in only 13%. These data suggest that most of the rise in PSA level originates from distant metastases. However, Zagars et al.[511] reported that in 80% of PSA relapsing patients, the rise in PSA was associated with a local failure only. The latter study also reported that the rate of PSA relapse in stage T1 or T2a patients was 26% at 5 years, suggesting that radiation therapy cure may occur substantially less frequently than had previously been assumed.

This issue was addressed further by Kupelian et al.,[512] who reviewed 298 stage T1 or T2 patients treated with radical prostatectomy and 253 treated with radiation therapy. The 5-year PSA relapse-free survival rates for radiation versus surgery were 43% and 57%, respectively. Multivariate analysis of time to failure showed that pretreatment PSA level and biopsy Gleason scores were independent predictors of PSA relapse. Based on these parameters, a low risk (pretreatment PSA of ≤10.0 ng/mL and Gleason score ≤6) and high risk (PSA >10.0 ng/mL or Gleason score ≥7) were defined. For low-risk patients, the 5-year PSA relapse-free survival rates for radiation versus surgery were 81% and 80%, while for the high-risk group the rates were 26% versus 37%, respectively. Zagars[510] reported 94% 6-year PSA relapse-free survival in T1 or T2 patients with a PSA level of 4 ng/mL or less and a Gleason score of 2 to 6, 70% for patients with a PSA level of 4 ng/mL or less and a Gleason score of 7 to 10, or a PSA level of 4 to 10 ng/mL and a Gleason score of 2 to 7, and 60% for patients with a PSA level exceeding 4 and a Gleason score of 8 or more.

Shipley et al.[454] further defined the prognostic subgroups for PSA outcome in T1 and T2 patients treated with radiation therapy. This study entailed a multiinstitutional pooled cohort of 1765 patients treated with advanced external-beam techniques to doses ranging from 63 to 79 Gy (median dose, 69.4 Gy). The overall 5-year PSA relapse-free survival was 65.8%. Recursive partitioning analysis of initial PSA, palpation stage, and Gleason score yielded four prognostic groups. Patients with a PSA level of less than 9.2 ng/mL had a 5-year PSA relapse-free survival rate of 81%, whereas for patients with PSA levels between 9.2 and 19.7

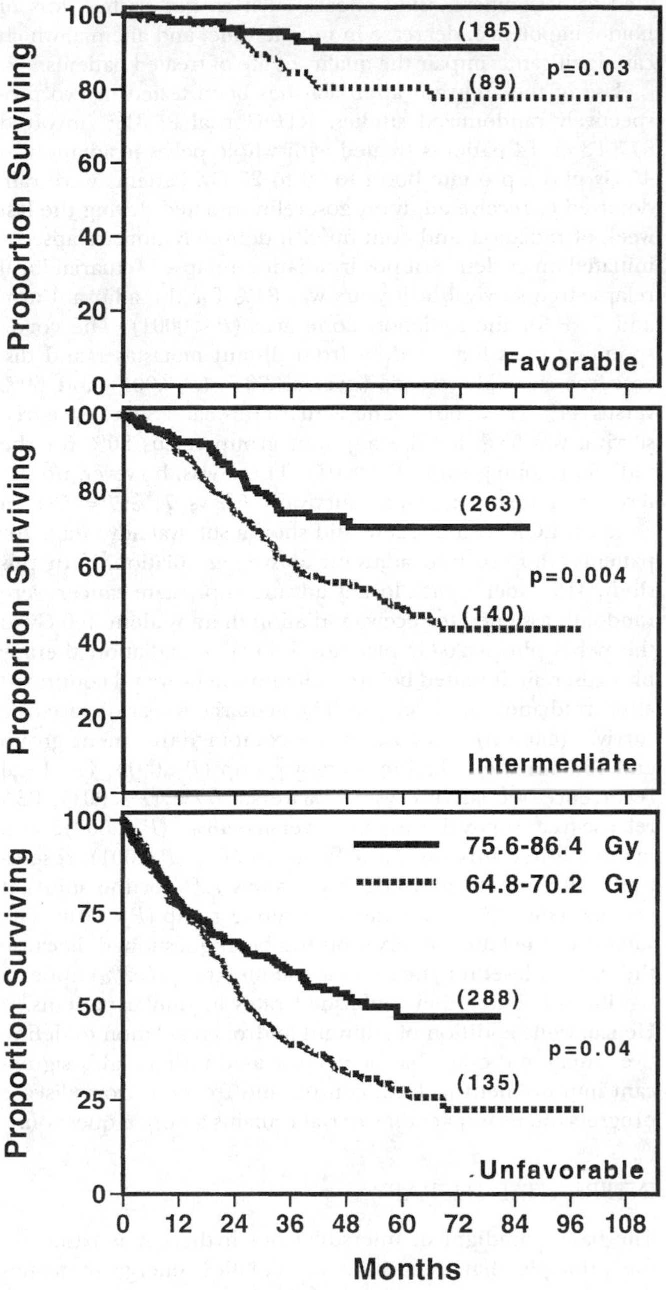

FIGURE 34.4-16. Risk of treatment failure after three-dimensional conformal radiation therapy. (Data from refs. 415, 442.)

ng/mL, it was 69%; for those whose PSA level was at least 19.7 ng/mL and who had a Gleason score of 2 to 6, it was 47%, and for patients with a PSA level of 19.7 ng/mL or more and a Gleason score of 7 to 10, the rate was 29%.

The validity of patient stratification by pretreatment variables as an approach to predict the outcome of treatment has been confirmed by multiple groups and has become standard in the field. Using proportional hazard regression analysis, most studies have identified pretreatment PSA, palpation stage, the Gleason score, and the dose as independent variables that affect long-term outcome. Different combinations of these prognostic variables have been suggested to generate risk groups for PSA relapse. Figure 34.4-16 shows the outcome data generated from the MSKCC 3D-CRT dose escalation database.[415,442] The tumor dose was gradually increased by increments of 5.4 Gy from 64.8 Gy to 86.4 Gy. A dose of 64.8 Gy was given to 96 patients, 70.2 Gy to 268 patients, 75.6 Gy to 446 patients, 81.0 Gy to 250 patients, and 86.4 Gy to 40 patients. The 5-year actuarial PSA relapse-free survival for patients with favorable prognostic indicators (stage T1 or T2, pretreatment PSA level ≤10.0 ng/mL, and Gleason score ≤6) receiving 64.8 to 70.2 Gy was reported as 80%, compared to 91% for those receiving at least 75.6 Gy ($P = .03$). The corresponding rates for patients with intermediate prognosis (one of the prognostic indicators having a higher value) were 47% versus 70% ($P = .004$) and, for the group with unfavorable prognosis (two or more of the prognostic indicators having higher values), were 27% versus 47% ($P = .04$). Androgen deprivation did not improve PSA relapse-free survival in any of the risk groups. This study defines the critical role of dose in affecting the long-term cure of prostate cancer with radiation. Combined with the results of posttreatment biopsies obtained in patients followed for 2.5 years (see Fig. 34.4-12), these data suggest that at least 81 Gy may be required for a maximal probability of cure. The data also demonstrate that a significant proportion of patients with unfavorable prognostic indicators may still have disease that is confined to the prostate and therefore is potentially curable with radiation alone.

Investigators from the Fox Chase Cancer Center[513] have reported a direct relationship between radiation dose and 5-year PSA relapse-free survival in patients treated to doses ranging from 66 to 79 Gy. The study matched by stage and grade 357 patients treated with at least 74 Gy 3D-CRT and 357 patients treated with less than 74 Gy with either conventional or conformal techniques. The 5-year PSA relapse-free survival rates were 71% and 56% for the high- and low-dose groups, respectively ($P = .003$). There was also a dose effect on 5-year freedom from distant metastases (97% vs. 88%; $P = .0004$), cause-specific survival (99% vs. 94%; $P = .007$), and overall survival (88% vs. 79%; $P = .01$). Roach et al.[514] reported an advantage for using higher doses of 3D-CRT in patients with poorly differentiated histologies. Among 50 patients with pretreatment PSA levels of less than 20 ng/mL, the PSA relapse-free survival at 3 years was 83% for patients treated with more than 71 Gy and 0% for those treated to lower doses ($P = .03$).

Zagars et al.[515] also observed a dose effect on the outcome in a retrospective analysis of 94 patients with localized prostate cancer treated with high-dose 3D-CRT (74 to 78 Gy) and 844 patients treated with conventional-dose irradiation (60 to 70 Gy). For analysis, patients were divided into three groups reflecting low (<67 Gy), intermediate (67 to 77 Gy), and high (>77 Gy) treatment dose. The 3-year PSA relapse-free survival rates were 61%, 74%, and 96%, for the low-, intermediate-, and high-dose groups, respectively ($P < .01$). When patients were stratified by the pretreatment PSA level, clinical stage (T1 or T2 vs. T3 or T4), or Gleason score (≤6 vs. 7 to 10), statistically improved PSA outcome was observed in all subgroups except for those with pretreatment PSA levels of less than 4.0 ng/mL. To further prove the impact of dose on the outcome, these investigators randomized 304 patients to receive either 70 Gy using a four-field conventional technique or the same treatment plus a six-field conformal boost to a total dose of 78 Gy.[516] The overall 4-year PSA relapse-free survival was 72% for the 70-Gy patients and 77% for the 78-Gy patients ($P = .21$). A significant difference was nonetheless observed in patients with a pretreatment PSA level exceeding 10 ng/mL (47% for the 70-

Gy and 68% for the 78-Gy patients; $P<.01$), with the most striking effect observed in T1 and T2 patients in this subgroup (55% for the 70-Gy and 93% for the 78-Gy patients; $P = .003$). The difference in the PSA outcome for patients with a pretreatment PSA level of less than 10 ng/mL was not significant. Further follow-up will be required to assess the impact of dose on the latter group of patients.

ANDROGEN ABLATION PLUS RADIATION THERAPY

The discovery that both normal and tumor prostate cells are sensitive to androgen ablation has led to its use as either neoadjuvant or adjuvant treatment in combination with radiation therapy. The rationale for this neoadjuvant approach is to debulk large prostate glands prior to irradiation and possibly to sensitize the tumor to the lethal effect of radiation, whereas adjuvant therapy is designed to eradicate residual disease, remaining either locally or at remote sites, after radiation therapy. Several groups have demonstrated the effectiveness of neoadjuvant androgen deprivation in decreasing the size of the prostate prior to radiation therapy, thus improving the ability to deliver maximal radiation doses without exceeding normal tissue tolerance.[517–519] For example, Zelefsky et al.[519] demonstrated that 3 months of leuprolide acetate and flutamide (Eulexin) reduced the prostate PTV by a mean of 25% (range, 3% to 52%). Further, two posttreatment biopsy series demonstrated improved local control when neoadjuvant androgen ablation was used, suggesting either an additive effect or a sensitizing effect induced by androgen deprivation. Zelefsky et al.[415] reported a 10% incidence of positive biopsies (3 of 31) in patients pretreated for 3 months with androgen deprivation, as compared with 46% (48 of 105) in those patients who received radiation therapy alone ($P<.001$). The relative distribution of the prognostic risk groups and the prescribed dose did not differ significantly between the two groups. Laverdiere et al.[520] reported preliminary results of a randomized trial of stage T2 and T3 prostate cancer patients who underwent biopsy at 24 months after radiation therapy. Patients treated for 3 months with neoadjuvant androgen deprivation followed by 64 Gy of radiation therapy had a 28% incidence of tumor-positive biopsy specimens, as compared to a 65% incidence in those patients receiving radiation alone. However, androgen deprivation given for 3 months before and 6 months after 64-Gy radiation therapy was associated with only a 5% rate of positive biopsies, consistent with an additive rather than a radiation-sensitizing effect.

The clinical value of the neoadjuvant approach was tested in RTOG trial 86-10.[521] Patients with large T2, T3, and T4 prostate tumors were randomized to either receive 2 months of leuprolide and Eulexin before and during radiation therapy or radiation without androgen ablation. The cumulative incidence of local progression at 5 years was 46% for patients undergoing androgen ablation and 71% for patients receiving radiation alone ($P<.001$). Progression-free survival rates, including the ability to maintain normal PSA levels, were 36% and 15%, respectively ($P<.001$). There was, however, no difference in survival. The use of neoadjuvant androgen ablation in patients with locally confined disease (stage T1 to T2a) and a good prognosis currently is being tested by RTOG trial 94-08. Patients are stratified by pretreatment PSA level and Gleason score. It should be emphasized, however, that the use of androgen ablation is associated with significant side effects, such as hot flashes, loss of libido, impotence, decrease in muscle tone, and anemia, which can significantly impair the quality of life of treated patients.

Use of the adjuvant approach has been tested in two prospectively randomized studies. RTOG trial 85-31[522] involved 977 T3 or T4 patients treated with whole pelvis irradiation to 45 Gy plus a prostate boost to 20 to 25 Gy. Patients were randomized to receive adjuvant goserelin initiated during the last week of radiation and continued indefinitely until relapse or initiated on evidence of postirradiation relapse. Actuarial local relapse-free survival at 5 years was 84% for the adjuvant arm and 71% for the radiation-alone arm ($P<.0001$). The corresponding rates for freedom from distant metastases and disease-free survival were 83% versus 70% ($P<.001$) and 60% versus 44% ($P<.0001$). The actuarial 5-year PSA relapse-free survival was 53% for the adjuvant group versus 20% for the radiation-alone group ($P<.0001$). There was, however, no difference in the overall 5-year survival (75% vs. 71%; $P = .52$). In contrast, EORTC trial 22863 did show a survival advantage for patients who received adjuvant androgen ablation.[523] In this study, 415 patients with locally advanced prostate cancer were randomly assigned to receive radiation therapy alone (50 Gy to the pelvis plus a 20-Gy prostatic boost) or radiation therapy plus goserelin initiated before radiation therapy and continued after irradiation until relapse. The actuarial 5-year disease-free survival (clinical) was 85% in the combined-treatment group and 48% for the radiation therapy group ($P<.001$). The local recurrence-free survival was 97% versus 77% ($P<.001$), PSA relapse-free survival was 81% versus 43% ($P<.001$), and metastasis-free survival was 98% versus 56% ($P<.001$), respectively. The overall survival at 5 years was 79% for the adjuvant group versus 62% for the radiation alone group ($P = .001$). The validity of the latter observation has been questioned, because the survival level for the radiation-alone group (62%) appears significantly lower than published rates in similar patients.[524] Hence, while addition of adjuvant androgen ablation to definitive radiation therapy has been associated with a highly significant improvement in local control and freedom from disease progression, its impact on survival remains an open question.

INTERSTITIAL THERAPY

The basic paradigm of interstitial brachytherapy is based on the principle that deposition of radiation energy in tissues decreases exponentially as a square function of the distance from the radiation source. Thus, while tumor tissue infiltrated with radioactive sources would receive maximal doses of radiation, there will be a rapid falloff of the dose in surrounding normal tissues. Over the years, a range of isotopes (e.g., ^{226}Ra, ^{198}Au, ^{125}I, ^{192}Ir, ^{103}Pd) have been tested, and the techniques have evolved from free-hand implantation to ultrasonography- and CT-guided template systems.[525–529] Retropubic implantation of the prostate with ^{125}I sources was the technique of choice until a decade ago.[525,527,529] Long-term follow-up, however, indicated that local failure was significantly increased within nearly all stages as compared with external-beam–treated patients.[529–531] The causes for local failure in these patients are not fully known, but difficulties in achieving a geometrically acceptable distribution of seeds and a homogeneous dose distribution within the prostate have been regarded as major factors affecting this outcome.

More recently, new approaches of percutaneous transperineal implantation have been developed. These systems use sophisticated diagnostic localization procedures for source placement and new methods of dosimetry and computer-aided optimization of treatment planning that improve the ability to produce homogeneous dose distribution within the target volume.[526,527,532,533] The most popular approach has been the TRUS-guided implantation of ^{125}I or ^{103}Pd sources with or without supplemental external-beam irradiation.[527,532,533] Treatment planning is based on CT or TRUS, with images obtained at 5-mm intervals. Isodose distributions are provided at each 5-mm increment throughout the treatment volume to determine the precise localization of seed placement and the source strength required to achieve a dose of 160 Gy with ^{125}I or ^{115}Gy with ^{103}Pd. Implantation is performed while the patient lies in a dorsal lithotomy position and is under spinal anesthesia. A needle guidance template is attached to an ultrasound apparatus and is placed against the perineum. Needles containing the radioactive sources are inserted through the template under TRUS guidance with supplemental fluoroscopy. Compliance of source placement with the pretreatment plan is determined by direct visualization on biplanar ultrasonography. After implantation, 5-mm-thick CT images of the prostate are obtained, and isodose contours are calculated to evaluate the dose that will actually be delivered to the prostate and the surrounding normal tissues. Wallner et al.[526,534] has recently described a method for 3D CT-based pretreatment planning and an implantation technique using individualized template devices that permit more precise source placement within the target volume.

The technologic improvements in transperineal ultrasound-based or CT-planned permanent seed implantation have enhanced the ability of this modality to target high radiation doses to the prostate more precisely than in the past. Concomitantly, treatment results have improved significantly, especially in patients with favorable-risk disease. Three- to 5-year PSA relapse-free survival rates have ranged between 76% and 96%.[535–538] A recent study by Blasko et al.[535] reported the results in 138 T1c to T2 patients with Gleason scores of 6 or less. PSA decreased gradually to levels of less than 1.0 ng/mL over the first 4 years after implantation in 97%, and the actuarial PSA relapse-free survival at 5 years was 93%. Priestly and Beyer[536] reported a rate of 94% PSA relapse-free survival at 5 years for T1 patients, 70% for T2a and T2b patients, and 34% for T1c patients. In contrast, Storey et al.[537] failed to demonstrate effects of stage and Gleason score on the PSA outcome in 206 patients. Freedom from PSA failure correlated, however, with pretreatment PSA levels. Actuarial 5-year freedom from failure was 76% in patients with a pretreatment PSA level of not more than 10 ng/mL, 51% for patients with values of in excess of 10 ng/mL, and 84% for patients with a PSA level of less than 4 ng/mL. Stock et al.[538] demonstrated a dose response for ^{125}I prostate implants. Using TG43 guidelines, dose-volume histograms were calculated. The dose delivered to the gland was defined as the *D90* (dose delivered to 90% of prostate tissue as defined by CT). Patients receiving a D90 dose of less than 140 Gy had a 4-year relapse-free survival of 68%, as compared with 92% for those receiving a D90 dose of at least 140 Gy (P = .02). Two-year posttreatment biopsies were negative in 70% (33 of 47) of patients with a D90 of less than 140 Gy, as compared with a rate of 83% (24 of 29) in patients with a D90 of at least 140 Gy (P = .2).

In the absence of a randomized trial comparing 3D-CRT and permanent interstitial implantation for early-stage prostatic cancer, it has become a challenge to select the most appropriate treatment for a given patient. Zelefsky et al.[539] recently addressed this issue. Their study compared patients with favorable-risk prostate cancer treated with either 3D-CRT (n = 137) or transperineal ^{125}I implantations (n = 145). The 3D-CRT dose range was 64.8 to 81.0 Gy, and the implant dose range was 110 to 257 Gy (median, 150 Gy). The 5-year PSA relapse-free survival rates for the 3D-CRT and the implant groups were 88% and 82%, respectively (P = .09). Protracted grade 2 urinary symptoms persisting for 12 to 70 months were observed in 45 (31%) of the implant patients. In contrast, the 5-year actuarial likelihood of late grade 2 urinary toxicity for the 3D-CRT group was only 8%. The 5-year actuarial likelihood of developing a urethral stricture (grade 3 urinary toxicity) for the 3D-CRT and implant groups was 2% and 12%, respectively (P <.0002). The 5-year actuarial probabilities of rectal toxicity were not significantly different. The 5-year likelihood of posttreatment erectile dysfunction among patients who were potent prior to treatment was 43% for the 3D-CRT and 53% for the implant group (P = .52). These data demonstrated that 3D-CRT and transperineal ^{125}I implantation are each associated with an excellent PSA outcome, but issues of quality of life associated with treatment toxicities may serve as guidelines for therapy selection in the individual patient.

CRYOTHERAPY

Loening et al.,[540] at the University of Iowa, first popularized cryosurgical ablation of prostate cancer in 1969. In their technique, the posterior surface of the prostate, seminal vesicles, and bladder base were exposed through a perineal incision. A cryoprobe then was inserted first into the perivesical fascia and later into the ampullae, seminal vesicles, and entire prostate. The technique was monitored by visual and tactile inspection only. Such therapy resulted in coagulative necrosis of epithelial elements and replacement with fibrous stroma. Outcomes (survival and recurrence) were related to stage and grade. Approximately 41% of patients eventually had evidence of persistent or recurrent disease. At that time, the technique compared favorably with other treatment modalities with respect to survival. However, morbidity was significant and included urethral sloughing of tissue, urethrorectal or urethrocutaneous fistula development, bladder neck obstruction, and urinary incontinence. Porter et al.[541] updated the outcomes of 51 men who underwent cryosurgery alone using this early technique for the management of prostate cancer between 1973 to 1977. Cancer recurrence was documented in 78.4% of the men, and 47.1% died of prostate cancer. Local recurrence was documented in at least 67% of those undergoing the procedure. Kaplan-Meier analyses demonstrated median progression-free and overall survival times of 34 and 75 months, respectively.

Despite this early experience, there has been a resurgence of interest in cryosurgery as a less invasive form of treatment for localized prostate cancer. This interest stems from technical innovations including improved percutaneous techniques, expertise in TRUS, improved cryotechnology, and a better understanding of cryobiology.

Freezing of the prostate is carried out using a multiprobe cryosurgical device.[542] The two parameters that correlate with the likelihood of cell destruction are the cooling rate during freezing and the lowest temperature achieved.[543] Damage may occur due to chemical injury or intracellular ice formation. Cellular destruction occurs as a result of freezing of the extracellular compartment and withdrawal of water from the cells occurring at –15°C, intracellular ice formation occurring at –20° to –40°C, thawing (which results in recrystallization), and tissue thrombosis.[544] Cell death requires temperatures lower than –20°C. However, temperatures as low as –40°C may be necessary to ensure complete freezing of the intracellular compartment. This fact has important clinical implications to the urologist performing cryosurgery, as the hyperechoic edge of the ice ball visualized is 0° to –2°C, and temperatures as low as –20° to –40°C are inside this edge. Therefore, one must extend the ice ball well beyond the edge of the prostate to ensure adequate tissue ablation. Rapid freezing allows for minimal loss of intracellular water and, therefore, the maximal chance of intracellular ice formation. Passive warming, which occurs slowly (over 15 to 20 minutes) after the cryoprobes are allowed to thaw, results in formation of larger ice crystals, a process called *recrystallization*, and this process further destroys tissues. After one episode of freezing, the cells are very vulnerable to additional cycles, and a second freezing cycle will allow for destruction of surviving cells. The destructive process may be facilitated by thrombosis of small vessels and the resulting tissue anoxia.

The ice balls generated by current methods are elliptic in shape, with the maximal radius at the tip. The radius is directly proportional to the rate of flow of liquid nitrogen. At high flow rates, the gradient from the outer edge—which, as mentioned, is at 0°C—to the zone at 20°C is narrow, approximately 2 mm. At low flow rates, this gradient is widened. The ice ball is approximately 4 cm long. Therefore, it is frequently necessary to pull the cryoprobes back toward the apex of the prostate after the initial freezing at the base, to ensure complete destruction of the gland.

Patients, after induction of regional or general anesthesia, are placed in the lithotomy position. A urethral warming device is placed to preserve the urethra and avoid sloughing of tissue postoperatively. This device circulates heated water. An ultrasound transducer is inserted into the rectum, and volume measurements are made of the prostate and cancer or cancers. Using a needle guide, an 18-gauge, hollow-core needle is inserted into the prostate under TRUS guidance. Once in position, a 0.038 J-tipped guidewire is advanced through the needle to the proximal extent of the prostatic capsule. Cannulas and dilators are passed over the wires to facilitate placement of five or more cryoprobes. Generally, two probes are placed anteromedially, two posterolaterally, and one posteriorly. Liquid nitrogen is circulated through these needles, and the resulting freezing zones, or ice balls, can be monitored by ultrasonography. The anterior probes are activated first and allowed to extend posteriorly and laterally. Once these have reached the desired position, thawing is begun, and the posterior probes are activated. Most often, two freeze-thaw cycles are performed, certainly in the area of cancer. In addition, if the ice ball does not adequately extend to the apex of the prostate, the cryoprobes are pulled backward into the apex, and additional freezing is carried out. In areas of ECE, greater propagation of the freeze zone is permitted laterally. If necessary, an additional probe may be placed in any area of gross ECE.

Androgen deprivation before cryosurgery should be considered in patients with large glands or extensive local disease, as such therapy serves to shrink the prostate and cancer, allows for even distribution of the cryoprobes, eliminates steep temperature gradients between the probes, reduces bulky extracapsular disease, and may allow for widening of the periprostatic space and better protection of surrounding structures.

Patients who undergo cryosurgery alone rarely require hospitalization, and the procedure usually is performed on a "come and go" basis. A urethral catheter is left in place for 3 weeks, as such a period of urethral catheterization appears to be associated with a lower likelihood of postoperative tissue sloughing and urinary retention as compared to use of a suprapubic tube alone or shorter periods of urethral catheterization. Patients are followed with serial PSA measurements and assessment of symptom scores. TRUS-guided biopsies of the prostate should be considered in most patients at 6 to 12 months after the procedure, certainly in those who fail to reach PSA nadirs of less than 0.4 ng/mL or in those whose serum PSA falls to a low level initially but rises later.

The efficacy of various forms of treatment for prostate cancer can be assessed by analyzing several end points. Commonly, patients who have been treated with cryotherapy have undergone repeat prostatic biopsy 6 to 12 months after the procedure. The positive biopsy rate after cryoablation ranged between 7.7% and 25%. These results must be analyzed cautiously as not all patients treated underwent biopsy, some patients received neoadjuvant androgen deprivation (which could have affected biopsy data), and false-negative biopsy results are not uncommon, certainly in those with limited disease before treatment. Not surprisingly, there is a relationship between clinical stage and the likelihood of a positive posttreatment biopsy after cryotherapy. The likelihood of a positive biopsy is approximately 9% for those with clinical stage T1 or T2 disease and at least 21% for those with T3 disease.[545,546] Interestingly, benign epithelium, often very focal, has been seen in up to 71% of patients after cryotherapy. The significance of benign epithelium is unknown, and such findings may represent areas of the prostate not frozen to low temperatures, perhaps, in the area of the urethral warmer.

It must be recognized that certain areas of the prostate or seminal vesicles are more likely to be sites of treatment failure. It appears that recurrence is more common in cancers located at the apex (9.5%) and seminal vesicles (43.8%), in contrast to those located in the midgland (4.1%) and base (0%).[547] Similarly, Bahn et al.[548] noted that the apex and, to some extent, the seminal vesicles were more likely to harbor residual disease as compared to the rest of the prostate.

Serum PSA level after definitive treatment such as radical prostatectomy or radiation therapy has been shown to be an important determinant of eventual outcome. What constitutes an acceptable PSA level after cryotherapy has not been well evaluated. Radiation or cryotherapy does not result in complete destruction of all prostate tissue. Detectable levels of PSA may be due to either malignant or benign epithelial elements. Therefore, a low but stable PSA after cryotherapy may not be associated with disease progression. A similar situation has been noted for patients who undergo radiation therapy. This issue was addressed recently at UCSF by Shinohara et al.,[549] who correlated the rates of biochemical and biopsy failure with the PSA nadir after cryosurgical treatment of prostate cancer in 132 patients who underwent 145 cryosurgical ablation procedures. Follow-up included PSA testing at 3, 6, and 12 months and every 6 months thereafter. Biopsies were performed at 6 months, and biochemical failure was defined as a PSA nadir of at least 0.5 ng/mL or subsequent PSA elevation of at least 0.2 ng/mL. Biochemical and biopsy failures were correlated with PSA nadir values after cryosurgery (<0.1 ng/mL, 0.1 to 0.4 ng/mL, 0.5 to 1.5 ng/mL, and >1.5 ng/mL). Biochemical failure (subsequent rise in PSA of 0.2 ng/mL or more) was lowest in those who achieved PSA nadirs of less than 0.1 ng/mL (21%) but was common in those with higher nadir values. Biopsy failure was lowest in those with nadirs of less than 0.1 ng/mL (1.5%) and in those with nadirs of not more than 0.4 ng/mL (10%). In contrast, 55% of the patients with nadir values of 0.5 ng/mL or more had biopsy failure. Both biochemical and biopsy failure tended to occur within the first 12 months after treatment (i.e., 96% and 88% of the biochemical and biopsy failures, respectively). Based on this single study, a PSA nadir of not more than 0.4 ng/mL should be achieved after cryotherapy. Higher values are associated with a significant risk of continued PSA elevation and a high likelihood of residual disease detected on prostatic biopsy.

Greene et al.[550] similarly showed that a serum PSA level in excess of 0.5 ng/mL was highly predictive of biopsy and biochemical failure after cryotherapy. Long[551] recently analyzed a very well-characterized series of 145 patients. The crude rates of maintaining either a negative biopsy or a serum PSA level of less than 0.3 ng/mL at 6 and 24 months after the procedure were 87% and 73%, respectively. However, the overall actuarial rate at 42 months of maintaining a serum PSA level of less than 0.3 ng/mL was 59%.

Koppie et al.[552] recently reported intermediate-terms results of cryotherapy in 176 patients who underwent 207 cryosurgical procedures for clinically localized (stages T1 through T4) prostate cancer using a multiprobe cryosurgical device. The patient population was composed of men who generally had intermediate- or high-risk disease (T3 or T4 disease in 61%). Actuarial biochemical recurrence-free survival rates at 1 year and 3 years after treatment for those patients undergoing primary cryosurgery (excluding repeat procedures and patients who failed previous radiation or radical prostatectomy) were 62% and 49%, respectively. PSA nadir ($P = .001$) and pretreatment serum PSA level ($P = .008$) were significantly associated with outcome after cryosurgery. Outcome correlated with pretreatment risk status. Actuarial biochemical recurrence-free survival 1 year and 3 years after cryosurgery was 82% and 69% for low-risk patients and 58% and 45% for intermediate- to high-risk patients, respectively ($P = .048$). Neoadjuvant androgen deprivation was not shown to improve outcome significantly after cryosurgery. Prostate biopsy was performed after 167 procedures and proved to be positive in 64 (38%) such cases.

Impotence is the most common complication of cryotherapy, occurring in more than 80% of the men who are potent before cryotherapy and who undergo complete (bilateral) treatment of the prostate. Impotence is a product of damage to the neurovascular bundles during the freezing process. Clearly, some patients who are impotent just after the procedure will regain erectile function with time. However, this number appears to be limited, and most men who become impotent after the procedure require long-term treatment for this condition.

Sloughing of tissue occurs in approximately 3% to 10% of patients. The likelihood of either urinary retention due to necrotic tissue obstruction or stricture formation is related to the type of urethral warmer used. Sloughing of urethral tissue, urinary retention, incontinence, and stricture disease are much less common in those patients treated with effective, commercially available urethral warming devices.[553] In addition, leaving the urethral catheter in place for a prolonged period rather than relying on suprapubic urinary drainage will further decrease the likelihood of this complication. Sosa et al.,[553] in a multicenter review, reported the following incidence of early complications: urinary retention for longer than 1 month, 6.8%; pain, 9.4%; infections, 13.4%; and fistula formation, 1.4%. Complications are much more common in those who undergo cryoablation for management of local disease recurrence after radiation therapy. In this patient population, urinary incontinence is common, occurring in 42% of patients, and is usually moderate to severe in nature.[554] Resolution of incontinence will occur in approximately one-half of these patients within 1 year of treatment. Therefore, early and aggressive treatment of incontinence should be delayed until it is ascertained that resolution will not occur.

Options for treatment of incontinence, should it persist, are limited. Collagen injection should be delayed 12 to 15 months after the procedure to allow for healing. Although complete resolution of incontinence is unlikely, significant improvement may be noted in some patients after collagen injection. The use of an artificial sphincter is an option, but additional endoscopic procedures may be necessary, and revision is likely in some patients.

MANAGEMENT OF LOCAL FAILURE AFTER SURGERY, RADIATION THERAPY, AND CRYOTHERAPY

A significant number of men who undergo standard local treatment for prostate cancer will experience biochemical recurrence, which may herald the development of clinical recurrence in some. A recent analysis of patients enrolled in a disease registry of prostate cancer patients demonstrated that 22% of patients who received initial treatment with radical prostatectomy, radiation therapy, or cryotherapy required a second form of prostate cancer treatment within 3 years of initial therapy.[555] Similar results have been reported by others.[556]

Serial PSA measurements provide the most reliable method of detecting recurrence, as tumor progression rarely occurs in the absence of PSA elevation. Distinguishing between local recurrence and distant failure is crucial to subsequent treatment decisions. Physical examination of the prostate or surgical bed by DRE is neither sensitive nor specific for the detection of local recurrence after any form of local therapy. PSA kinetics, in conjunction with pretreatment pathologic stage and grade, may provide the best means of identifying the location of tumor recurrence. Patients with low-grade or low-stage disease and PSA levels of less than 10 ng/mL at the time of initial therapy are most at risk for local recurrence, whereas those with seminal vesicle invasion, high-grade cancers (Gleason score >7), positive lymph nodes, or initial serum PSA levels exceeding 20 ng/mL are more likely to experience failure distantly. A PSA velocity of less than 0.75 ng/mL/y was observed in 94% of patients with local recurrence after radical prostatectomy.[557] Conversely, more than 50% of men with metastatic disease had a PSA velocity greater than 0.75 ng/mL/y. Clearly, a PSA doubling time of less than 6 months suggests distant disease.[306]

Patients with detectable or increasing PSA levels after either surgery or radiation therapy, respectively, may be candidates for local imaging complemented by TRUS-guided biopsy. After

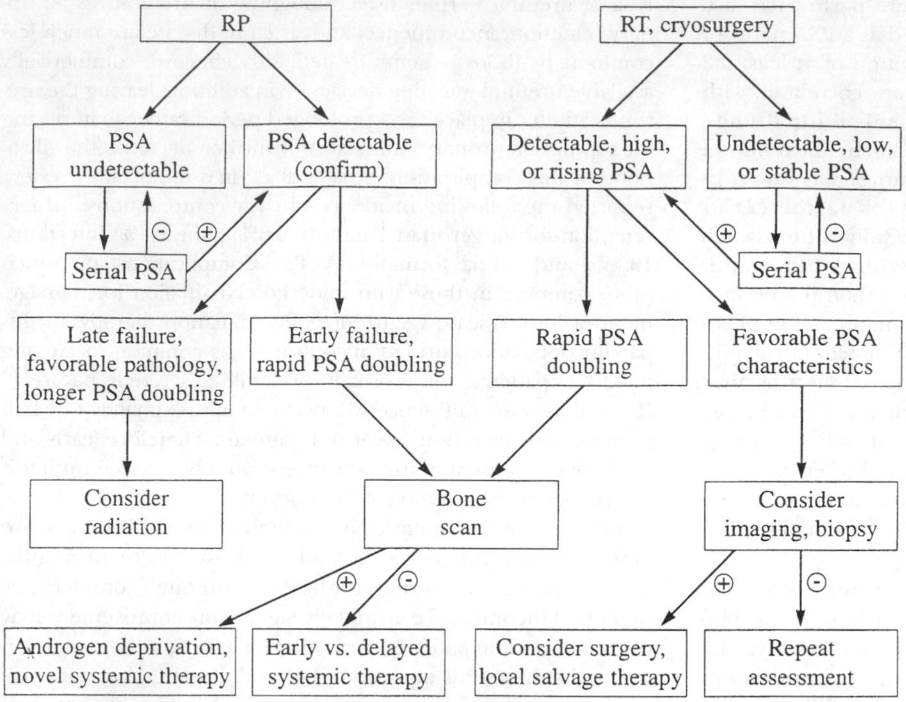

FIGURE 34.4-17. Algorithm for evaluation of those with biochemical failure after radical prostatectomy (RP), radiation therapy (RT), or cryotherapy for presumed localized prostate cancer. PSA, prostate-specific antigen.

surgery, anastomotic biopsy may be positive for local recurrence in 40% to 50% of patients with detectable levels of PSA.[558] However, anastomotic biopsy generally is not necessary after radical prostatectomy, as treatment decisions can be made on the basis of PSA kinetics alone. Indications for TRUS-guided biopsy after either radiation or other forms of focal therapy such as cryotherapy are not clear. Most would agree that such biopsies should be considered in those patients treated with radiation therapy or cryotherapy who show serial elevations in serum PSA level after reaching a PSA nadir. Nadir levels of PSA usually are reached within 8 to 18 months after external-beam irradiation, longer with brachytherapy, and within 3 months after cryotherapy. Both endorectal MRI complemented by spectroscopy and monoclonal antibody imaging may complement the use of PSA kinetics to define the site of recurrence after local therapy.[559] However, CT, MRI, and bone scans rarely are required in the early evaluation of asymptomatic patients with biochemical failure after radical prostatectomy, radiation therapy, and cryoablation (Fig. 34.4-17). In the absence of symptoms, the probability of a positive bone scan due to metastatic disease is less than 5% until the serum PSA level exceeds 40 ng/mL.[560,561] Radioimmunoscintigraphy using an antibody to PSMA has been used to identify the site of recurrence in those patients who experience biochemical failure after radical prostatectomy. The sensitivity and specificity for the detection of recurrence is highly variable, ranging between 44% and 90% and 36% and 86%, respectively.[562] In most patients, this procedure may add little prognostic information over that gained by analysis of posttreatment PSA kinetics and pretreatment cancer grade, stage, and serum PSA level.

Treatment options after radical prostatectomy include surveillance alone, systemic therapy, or radiation to the prostatic bed. In general, 30% to 65% of men who undergo therapeutic, or salvage, radiation therapy after radical prostatectomy will develop and maintain undetectable PSA levels (Table 34.4-17). Schild et al.[563] reported an overall 50% disease-free survival at 3 years; however, 78% of those patients with a pre–radiation therapy PSA level of less than 1.0 ng/mL were disease-free, whereas only 18% of men with a PSA level greater than 1.0 ng/mL remained disease-free. Others have reported similar findings, suggesting that therapeutic radiation after surgery should be applied early. Patients most likely to benefit from salvage radiation after prostatectomy include

TABLE 34.4-17. Probability of an Undetectable Prostate-Specific Antigen Level after Therapeutic Radiation for a Detectable Prostate-Specific Antigen Level after Prostatectomy

Author	*No. of Patients*	*Undetectable PSA (%) Durable Response*	*Follow-Up after RT*
Hudson and Catalona[402]	21	29	12.6 mo (mean)
Schild et al.[403]	46	50	5 y (actuarial)
Wu et al.[404]	53	23	2 y (actuarial)
McCarthy et al.[360]	37	54	27.5–36.0 mo (median)
Morris et al.[405]	48	47	3 y (actuarial)
Forman et al.[406,a]	47	73[c]	36 mo (median)
Cadeddu et al.[407,b,c]	30	37	At least 2 y
vander Kooy et al.[408,a]	30	56	8 y (actuarial)
Coetzee et al.[361,b]	45	51	33 mo (mean)
UCSF	47	41	3 y (actuarial)

PSA, prostate-specific antigen; RT, radiation therapy; UCSF, University of California at San Francisco.
[a]Biochemical failure defined by PSA increase after nadir.
[b]Includes only patients with positive margins.
[c]Does not include patients with seminal vesicle invasion or lymph node involvement by tumor.

those with low- to moderate-grade tumors with an undetectable postoperative PSA that rises after more than 1 year. The exact timing of radiation therapy has yet to be determined, although a pre-radiation therapy PSA cutoff of 2.0 ng/mL currently appears reasonable. Such therapy is usually well tolerated, although transient changes in bowel and bladder function may occur. In a study of 294 men who underwent radiation therapy after surgery, no significant long-term impact of postoperative radiation was seen on either urinary continence or erectile dysfunction.[564,565] Although both brachytherapy and cryotherapy have been used to manage local recurrences after radical prostatectomy, the experience with these modalities is very limited.

Androgen deprivation is the most common form of secondary treatment (88%) after radiation therapy.[566] Such therapy generally is considered palliative rather than curative.

Curative forms of secondary treatment should be considered in properly selected patients. Salvage radical prostatectomy is one option. Cause-specific survival after this procedure ranges from 70% to 90% and 30% to 50% at 8 to 10 years, respectively. In a series from Tefilli et al.,[564] all patients with organ-confined disease were disease-free at 34 months. Amling et al.[569] reported a 10-year disease-free survival of 43% in 108 patients, similar to the results from Rogers et al.[567] and Moul et al.[568] DNA ploidy, preoperative serum PSA level, and Gleason score were significant predictors of outcome postoperatively. Those patients most likely to benefit from salvage surgery include those with favorable disease characteristics before radiation therapy and those with PSA kinetics after radiation therapy consistent with local rather than distant recurrence. Complications of salvage prostatectomy are more common than after primary prostatectomy. Urinary incontinence is seen in 20% to 60% of patients, bladder neck contracture occurs in approximately 20%, and impotence is virtually universal. Rectal injury occurs in fewer than 10% of patients and rarely necessitates fecal diversion. Contemporary series report better outcomes due to improved patient selection, earlier identification of failure, and improved surgical technique.

The largest series of patients treated with cryoablation for local recurrence after primary radiation therapy was reported by Greene and Pisters et al.[550,570] from the M. D. Anderson Cancer Center. Negative sextant biopsies were noted in 77% of patients 6 months after cryoablation. However, only 45 of 150 patients (30%) had a persistently undetectable PSA level with a mean follow-up of 13.5 months. Incontinence was common, and up to 50% of such patients may require transurethral resection for urinary retention and obstructive voiding symptoms. Impotence occurred in at least 80% of men. An effective urethra warming device was determined to be essential to minimize tissue sloughing. Complications such as urethrorectal fistula, abscess formation, and urethral stricture were rare. Additional radiation is an option also.

Grado et al.[571] followed 49 patients treated with brachytherapy after biopsy-proven primary radiation therapy failure. Actuarial biochemical-free survival was 34% at 5 years and was associated with a post-salvage PSA nadir of less than 0.5 ng/mL. Local disease control was 98%; only a single patient demonstrated local, clinical failure. These results are encouraging, especially given the treatment population. The median age was 73.3 years, and 71% had locally advanced disease at initial presentation. Ninety percent of the cancers were moderately to poorly differentiated on prebrachytherapy biopsies. Complications were similar to those seen in patients undergoing primary brachytherapy.

For those patients whose cancers recur after cryotherapy, the choice of secondary treatment is not well defined. Repeat freezing has been reported, as has salvage prostatectomy. In the subset of patients at UCSF who underwent multiple cryotherapy procedures, 67% had no cancer on subsequent biopsies but only 33% achieved long-term, favorable PSA values.[552] Radical prostatectomy is an option, but morbidity may be significant. Radiation treatment can be used after cryoablation and, unlike cryotherapy after radiation, salvage radiation therapy after cryotherapy appears to be associated with minimal morbidity.

New forms of salvage therapy are being developed and refined. Both high-intensity focused ultrasonography and radiofrequency interstitial ablation are being studied and appear to have promise in local control of prostate cancer.[572,573] These methods induce coagulative necrosis of tissue. In preliminary studies, primary high-intensity focused ultrasonography achieved short-term, local control in 60% to 80% of patients. Radiofrequency ablation was able to produce predictable lesions in prostates prior to radical prostatectomy. The long-term efficacy and morbidity of these new forms of focal therapy require further study.

Finally, many patients in whom local therapy fails, as evidenced by rising PSA levels, may not develop clinical evidence of disease.[279] Therefore, observation alone is an option in low-risk, asymptomatic patients in whom primary therapy fails. In such patients, the morbidity and cost of secondary therapy must be carefully considered and compared to the risk of clinical progression of disease.

TREATMENT SELECTION FOR ADVANCED DISEASE: METASTATIC AND LOCAL REGIONAL DISEASE

The spectrum of advanced prostate cancer has changed considerably over the last 10 years since the introduction and widespread use of PSA screening. Prostate cancer is diagnosed in fewer patients at a time when their disease is overtly metastatic. Most cancers are detected earlier, frequently at an asymptomatic stage. Nonetheless, a large number of patients still die of prostate cancer despite earlier detection, which reflects the existence of occult metastatic disease.[1] A redefinition of advanced disease in the current era would seem appropriate, given these changes. Advanced disease might include patients who, at time of diagnosis, have poor-risk features but no overt metastases. One might include two other subsets of patients as having advanced disease: patients who demonstrate cancer progression after either local therapy or androgen ablative therapy, as evidenced solely by a rise in the serum PSA level. With improvements in our understanding of risk stratification, the traditional stage-based therapy may become obsolete, replaced by multifactor stratification schemes and biologically based therapies. However, until the paradigm has changed, we must discuss treatment based on stage or modality.

ANDROGEN DEPRIVATION

Overview

Androgen deprivation remains the mainstay of therapy for patients with advanced prostate cancer. Because androgen may play a role as both a survival factor and a growth factor for prostatic carcinoma cells, interference with the androgen-signaling pathway will generate clinically meaningful remissions in the majority of patients. These remissions are manifest by a reduction in symptoms related to disease, if they exist, and a reduction in the serum PSA level. A decline in serum PSA level reflects, in part, a decrease in the cellular production of PSA, as the PSA gene promoter is, in part, androgen-regulated[574]; thus, withdrawal of androgen will reduce the production of PSA protein. In addition, the reduction in serum PSA level may reflect the consequence of metabolic changes in the cell or a reduction in the prostate cancer cell mass, presumably through induction of cell death pathways. It is likely that the remission sustained by the vast majority of patients reflects a composite of all of these phenomena, although conceivably one or another mechanism may dominate in any one individual.

The majority of circulating androgen is produced by the testicles in the form of testosterone, and the remainder is produced by the adrenal glands, which synthesize the so-called adrenal androgens. These adrenal androgens may contribute up to 40% of the androgen detected within the prostate.[575] Androgen deprivation is achieved through surgical (orchiectomy) or chemical (gonadotropin-releasing hormone analogues) castration. Estrogens and progestational agents, which are less frequently used, will also reduce androgen levels through nuclear receptor–mediated activity. Antiandrogens (androgen receptor antagonists) or agents that interfere with the adrenal production of androgens, such as ketoconazole or aminoglutethimide, also are used.

Most of the data that currently exists regarding the comparative efficacy of androgen ablative strategies and the overall management of patients with advanced disease have been acquired through studies involving patients with radiographic evidence of metastatic disease (M+). How applicable the results of these studies are to patients with earlier stages of advanced prostate cancer is uncertain. Nonetheless, in the M+ population, response durations to androgen deprivation average 12 to 18 months.[576] Even in this far-advanced group of patients, heterogeneity exists, as evidenced by the fact that a minority of patients will demonstrate no biochemical or clinical disease progression 5 years after initiating therapy. An increase in serum PSA level remains the earliest indicator of relapse, although a small subset of patients (<5%) will experience relapse even in the absence of serum PSA progression. Optimal therapy for patients with earlier disease (i.e., locally advanced patients or those who experience relapse after local therapy) remains undefined. Significant side effects exist as a result of treatment with androgen deprivation therapy, and the cost of therapy can be significant as well. Thus, the choice and timing of treatment depends on several factors, including the stage of disease, whether symptoms are present, the rate of disease progression, patient preference, and a full knowledge of the toxicity profiles of the drugs used.

Timing of Androgen Deprivation Therapy

Although it is assumed that androgen deprivation therapy is life-prolonging, this has never been formally proven. Nonetheless, it is likely that androgen deprivation therapy delays the onset of radiographic progression or symptoms in an otherwise asymptomatic man, presumably by reducing the overall tumor cell mass. Whether the earlier initiation of androgen deprivation therapy increases survival duration has long been debated. In theory, it seems reasonable that the earlier the initiation of androgen deprivation therapy, the better the outcome. This would follow from the assumption that, as tumors evolve and acquire more genetic change, the proportion of hormone-refractory cells in the tumor increases.

Three studies now offer evidence that supports the earlier initiation of androgen deprivation therapy. In a study conducted by Bolla et al.,[577] 415 men with locally advanced or high-grade prostate cancer were randomized to receive either external-beam radiation therapy alone or external-beam radiation therapy plus 3 years of androgen deprivation therapy. Cyproterone acetate (a steroidal antiandrogen) and goserelin administration were begun at the time of radiation. The cyproterone acetate was continued for a duration of 1 month, whereas the goserelin was continued for 3 years. Patients were followed for a median duration of 3 years. The actuarial 5-year survival for the radiation-alone group was 62% [95% confidence interval (CI), 52% to 72%] and for the radiation-plus-goserelin group was 79% (95% CI, 72% to 86%) (P = .001). The survival benefit observed in the combination-therapy arm suggested a benefit to the earlier institution of androgen deprivation therapy. This study has been criticized for the relatively brief duration of follow-up (median, 3 years) at the time of publication and for the long duration of androgen deprivation therapy.[578]

Another study, conducted by the British Medical Research Council (MRC),[579] enrolled and randomized 938 men with locally advanced or metastatic prostate cancer to receive either early androgen deprivation therapy (orchiectomy or LHRH analogue) or delayed androgen deprivation therapy. In this study, disease progression (defined as a conversion from M0 to M+ or, alternatively, local progression requiring treatment) occurred more frequently and earlier in the delayed treatment arm (P <.001). In addition, deaths attributable to prostate cancer occurred more frequently in the delayed-therapy arm (257 vs. 203; P = .001). This study has been criticized because of the potential bias created by differing follow-up schedules between arms, resulting in some of the men never actually receiving androgen deprivation therapy in the delayed androgen deprivation therapy arm.[578]

The third study that supports earlier intervention is a study by Messing et al.,[580] in which 98 men who had undergone a radical prostatectomy and were found to have pathologically documented metastatic disease to lymph nodes were randomized to receive either early androgen deprivation therapy (LHRH analogue or orchiectomy plus an antiandrogen) or deferred therapy. A dramatic and statistically significant difference in survival duration in favor of the early androgen deprivation therapy arm was found. After a median of 7.1 years, 7 of 47 men in the immediate therapy arm, as compared to 18 of 51 men in the delayed therapy arm, had died (P = .02). Three men died of prostate cancer in the immediate therapy arm, as compared to 16 men in the delayed therapy arm (P <.01). At the time of the last follow-up, 36 men in the immediate treatment arm versus 9 in the delayed treatment arm were alive without evidence of detectable serum PSA or clinical evidence of disease (P <.001).

Although these three studies suggest that early androgen deprivation therapy may confer a survival advantage over delayed therapy, these studies do not define the optimal timing of androgen deprivation therapy for patients in the modern era. Little justification can be made for withholding androgen deprivation therapy when radiographic evidence of metastatic disease is present. However, for patients earlier in their disease course (i.e., patients who have undergone definitive local therapy but who are at high risk of relapse or patients with rising serum PSA levels after local therapy), the appropriate timing of treatment remains to be defined. Given the heterogeneity in the biologic behavior of tumors in the patient population with rising serum PSA levels after local therapy, several factors should be considered during decision making regarding timing. These factors include those that predict the rapidity of onset of clinical symptoms such as PSA velocity, tumor grade, and the time since local therapy was implemented.[581] In addition, patient factors that potentially affect quality of life should be taken into account. These include patient anxiety, on the one hand, and the short-term and long-term impact of androgen deprivation, on the other.

Prognostic Factors

Most of the studies that have analyzed predictive and prognostic factors of response and survival in patients undergoing androgen deprivation therapy have done so in patients with radiographic evidence of metastatic disease (M+). In such studies, factors that reflect more extensive disease are associated with a poorer prognosis.[582–587] Two such factors are performance status and the presence or absence of symptoms. More quantifiable parameters include the number of bone metastases, the presence of appendicular bone disease in addition to axial bone disease, and higher serum alkaline phosphatase levels. Serum PSA levels are not consistently a predictor of response duration or survival. This apparent paradox may reflect the high variability in PSA production between tumors at the cellular level. In addition, the fact that less well differentiated tumors produce less PSA may mute a direct relationship.[588] As a posttreatment dynamic factor, some studies indicate that normalization of serum PSA level may be associated with a better outcome.[583,589,590] However, Eisenberger et al.[591] found in a randomized study of more than 1300 men with metastatic prostate cancer in which orchiectomy was compared to orchiectomy plus flutamide that, although the serum PSA level normalized (PSA <4) more frequently in men receiving the combination treatment, no difference in survival between the two arms was seen. Patients with visceral metastases[582,583] and patients with lower serum testosterone levels[587] prior to treatment appear to have a poorer outcome. To date, no molecular markers that predict response and response duration to androgen deprivation therapy have been identified.

Monotherapy

ORCHIECTOMY. Surgical castration (orchiectomy) remains the standard for patients who will require permanent androgen deprivation therapy. It has the advantages of convenience and cost (as compared to other modalities) and abrogates compliance issues. In addition, clinical response is rapid after the procedure is performed. In patients with symptomatic metastatic disease, significant improvement in symptoms can be achieved within 24 to 48 hours after orchiectomy. Many patients will choose alternative treatments because of the psychological impact of surgical castration or the desire to be treated with androgen deprivation in an intermittent fashion.

LUTEINIZING HORMONE–RELEASING HORMONE ANALOGUES. Peptide analogues of LHRH, which possess partial agonistic or antagonistic affects, have been used extensively in the treatment of prostate cancer. The commercially approved agents goserelin and leuprolide are partial agonists. These agents will initially cause a transient increase in luteinizing hormone (LH) and follicle-stimulating hormone production, followed by a decline. Consequently, serum testosterone levels decrease within weeks of initial administration. In patients with radiographic evidence of metastases, there is concern that this "flare" in serum LH and testosterone levels within the first couple of weeks after therapy is initiated may worsen existing disease.[592,593] Thus, these agents are commonly used in conjunction with an antiandrogen such as flutamide, nilutamide, or bicalutamide, which blocks ligand binding to the androgen receptor. In one trial, flutamide was shown to abrogate the clinical effects of the serum LH and testosterone flare.[594]

The LHRH analogues are as effective as other modalities in the treatment of patients with advanced prostate cancer. Randomized studies have demonstrated the equal efficacy of LHRH analogues to orchiectomy[595] and to diethylstilbestrol (DES).[596] Depot formulations have been developed that permit monthly or, alternatively, every-3- and -4-month administration. Depot formulations allowing yearly dosing will soon become available. Pure LHRH antagonists have been developed and are currently in clinical trials. Their niche may be in the treatment of patients with symptomatic metastatic disease who are initiating androgen ablative therapy. Because an LH flare should not occur with these agents, their use may obviate the need for concomitant use of an antiandrogen.

ESTROGENS. Estrogens such as DES inhibit LHRH production by the hypothalamus and LH production by the pituitary and, thus, reduce serum levels of testosterone. Whether the entire salutary effect of estrogens is a result of their ability to lower testosterone, which is well established, or a result of other independent mechanisms remains unknown. The presence of estrogen receptors in prostate epithelium suggests that there may be a direct effect.[597] Estrogen therapy was the first exogenous therapy for prostate cancer. In the first Veterans Administration Cooperative Urological Research Group study (VACURG I), patients were randomized to one of four arms: DES, 5 mg alone; orchiectomy alone; DES, 5 mg, plus orchiectomy; or DES, 5 mg, plus placebo.[598] Although the overall survival of patients randomized to DES was the same as for those randomized to orchiectomy, the cancer-specific mortality was lower in the DES-treated group. In this study, the possible therapeutic benefit of DES, 5 mg/d, was offset by an increase in cardiovascular mortality. In VACURG II, patients were randomized to different doses of DES (0.2 mg, 1 mg, and 5 mg) or placebo.[598] The survival of men treated with 1 mg and 5 mg was equivalent, but there was greater toxicity with 5 mg. In another study, men were randomized to leuprolide, 1 mg/d, or to DES, 3 mg/d. Equal efficacy was seen, although the cardiovascular complication rate was higher with DES, 3 mg/d, as compared to leuprolide. Although DES, 1 mg/d, appears to be effective in patients with advanced disease, a significant proportion of men do not achieve castration levels of serum testosterone.[599] In practice, estrogens are used infrequently because of their side effects and their lack of availability, although there is a resurgence of interest in agents that target the estrogen receptor.

ANTIANDROGENS. The antiandrogens are competitive inhibitors of testosterone at the androgen receptor. Two classes of antiandrogens are in clinical use, the first of which is the steroidal antiandrogens, which include cyproterone acetate (Androcur) and megestrol acetate (Megace). The second group is nonsteroidal antiandrogens, which include flutamide (Eulexin), bicalutamide (Casodex), and nilutamide (Anandron). The steroidal antiandrogens have broader activity than their nonsteroidal counterparts. In addition to their effect on the androgen receptor, they possess progestational and glucocorticoid activity. The steroidal antiandrogens suppress testosterone through their feedback effects at the pituitary and hypothalamus. As monotherapy, neither cyproterone acetate nor megestrol acetate is capable of suppressing serum androgen levels completely or indefinitely and, as a result, these agents rarely are used as monotherapy.

In contrast, nonsteroidal antiandrogens act principally through the androgen receptor. Through theses agents' stimulation of the hypothalamus, serum testosterone levels may increase or remain unchanged as compared to pretherapy levels. The nonsteroidal antiandrogens have been used in three clinical settings: first, as part of combined androgen blockade (in conjunction with surgical or chemical castration); second, as salvage monotherapy in patients who were previously treated with androgen deprivation therapy; and third, as initial therapy without surgical or chemical castration. When used in this last setting, they have the potential advantage of allowing potency to be maintained as serum levels of testosterone are maintained. Small clinical trials[600] have been conducted that demonstrated both their efficacy (as determined by their ability to lower serum PSA levels) as sole agents and in conjunction with 5α-reductase inhibitors[601] (which inhibit conversion of testosterone to the more potent form, DHT) and their ability to preserve potency in a proportion of men. However, in two randomized studies, nonsteroidal antiandrogens were found not to be as effective as castration. In one study of 92 patients with M+ prostate cancer, flutamide (250 mg t.i.d.) was compared to DES (1 mg t.i.d.).[602] A significant difference in survival was observed in favor of DES. Median survivals were 43.2 and 28.5 months, respectively ($P = .04$). In another study, orchiectomy was compared to 50 mg/d of bicalutamide.[603] In this study, survival duration was superior with orchiectomy. It should be noted that, in retrospect, this dose of bicalutamide was suboptimal. Another study in which patients were randomized to goserelin plus flutamide or to bicalutamide, 150 mg/d, was conducted.[604] Progression-free and overall survival were equivalent in both arms. In two other studies that were combined for publication, bicalutamide, 150 mg/d, was equivalent to orchiectomy or goserelin for M0 patients but proved inferior for M+ patients.[605] Antiandrogens should therefore not be used as monotherapy in patients with M+ disease. Their use as monotherapy in patients with earlier disease may be equivalent to castration; however, longer follow-up is needed.

COMPARISON OF MONOTHERAPEUTIC AGENTS. Numerous trials have compared the efficacy of the various monotherapeutic agents. The most comprehensive analysis of these studies was performed by the Technology Evaluation Center, an evidence-based practice center for the Agency of Health Care Policy and Research.[606] The conclusions, based on a metaanalysis of ten trials that included 1908 patients, were that no difference in survival existed between patients treated with LHRH agonists or patients treated with orchiectomy or DES and no difference in survival existed between patients treated with the different LHRH agonists.

Combined Androgen Blockade

The role of adrenal androgens in supporting prostate cancer cell growth is uncertain. The adrenal androgens are relatively weak as compared to testosterone. The concept of combined androgen blockade (CAB) was developed by Labrie et al.[607] in an effort to try to suppress testicular androgen production and block adrenal androgens to afford a better androgen deprivation strategy. In the mid-1980s, Labrie et al.[607] demonstrated dramatic responses of patients with metastatic prostate cancer to a combination of chemical or surgical castration and an antiandrogen. In 1989, Crawford et al.[608] published the results of a National Cancer Institute–sponsored intergroup trial (INT-0036) in which 603 men with M+ prostate cancer were randomized to either leuprolide, 1 mg/d SC, or to leuprolide plus flutamide, 250 mg PO t.i.d. CAB resulted in a significant improvement to disease progression over time and a significant difference in median survival in favor of CAB (median survival, 28.3 months vs. 35.6 months; $P = .035$), as compared to leuprolide alone.

Two other studies demonstrated an improvement in survival associated with CAB. In the EORTC trial, 326 men were randomized to either goserelin, 3.6 mg SC for 4 weeks plus flutamide 250 mg PO t.i.d., or orchiectomy.[609] An improvement in median survival was again observed with CAB (34.4 months vs. 27.1 months; $P = .02$). In the other study, 457 men were randomized to orchiectomy or to orchiectomy plus nilutamide.[610] An improvement in survival was again observed (37.1 months vs. 29.8 months; $P = .04$) in favor of CAB.

Most randomized studies to date, however, have not shown an advantage of CAB, although some of these studies have been criticized for being too small, having inadequate follow-up, or for using steroidal antiandrogens. The largest study to date (INT-105) was a study of 1387 men with M+ prostate cancer in which orchiectomy was compared to orchiectomy plus flutamide.[591] Interestingly, although there was a difference in the frequency with which patients achieved a serum PSA level of less than 4.0 ng/mL [74% (95% CI, 69.4 to 78.2) vs. 61.5% (95% CI, 56.4 to 66.4); $P < .001$], there was no difference in overall survival between the two groups.

A metaanalysis was performed by the Prostate Cancer Trialists' Collaborative Group,[611] which sought to reconcile all the studies of CAB. Overall, no benefit was observed for CAB. Criticisms of this particular metaanalysis included the validity of combining studies in which steroidal and nonsteroidal antiandrogens were used and the inclusion of trials that used LHRH analogues but did not use short-term antiandrogen therapy to block the flare. In a second metaanalysis, which excluded studies published only as abstracts, those that did not present data on survival, and those that used short-term antiandrogens, a benefit was seen for CAB (RR, 0.78; 95% CI, 0.67 to 0.90).[612] In a third metaanalysis, no benefits were seen at 2 years, although a modest benefit was observed at 5 years (hazard ratio, 0.861; 95% CI, 0.78 to 0.95).[613] In summary, if a benefit exists for CAB in patients with M+ disease, it is extremely modest.

One caveat in drawing conclusions from these studies is that the majority of patients who were randomized were patients with M+ disease. Far fewer M0 patients were included. Thus, while it is reasonable to conclude that the benefits of CAB in patients with M+ prostate cancer is minimal, at best, for patients with earlier disease, it is less clear. In current practice, antiandrogens should be used at least for a short duration (1 to 2 months) when an LHRH analogue is used in patients with M+ disease. In M+ patients, antiandrogens are of uncertain value when an orchiectomy is performed. However, for patients with earlier forms of disease, given the paucity of relevant data, CAB is a reasonable option. Furthermore, it is important to note that the binding affinity of the currently used antiandrogens for the androgen receptor is relatively low. As more potent or more specific antiandrogens are developed, these issues may need to be readdressed.

PERIPHERAL ANDROGEN BLOCKADE. The efficacy of antiandrogens as monotherapy may be less than that of chemical or surgical castration. Nonetheless, this therapy has the potential appeal of sparing sexual function and reducing other treatment-related side effects, including hot flashes. The strategy of combining an antiandrogen with a 5α-reductase inhibitor (which reduces the conversion of testosterone to DHT) has also been explored. In one study, the addition of a 5α-reductase inhibitor (finasteride) added further antiandrogenic effect to that which already was achieved by an antiandrogen alone, as measured by a further reduction in serum PSA level after the achievement of a nadir with flutamide.[601] Other studies have demonstrated PSA responses and the maintenance of potency in men treated with the combination.[600,614] In one randomized phase II study, there was no difference in the percentage of decrease in serum PSA level when finasteride plus flutamide was compared to goserelin plus flutamide or to goserelin plus finasteride.[615] This approach, although appealing, should still be regarded as experimental. Larger studies have not yet been completed, nor have phase III randomized studies yet been performed that compare this strategy to standard therapies, with survival as an end point.

INTERMITTENT HORMONAL THERAPY. The scientific basis for intermittent hormonal therapy is that hormonally dependent clones of prostate cancer cells may potentially prevent the growth of hormonally independent cells through the elaboration of growth inhibitory factors. Alternatively, the reintroduction of androgen after androgen withdrawal may result in the generation of differentiated tumor cells.[616] It might be advantageous, therefore, to allow the reintroduction of androgen after androgen withdrawal to delay the emergence of an androgen-independent phenotype. This has been substantiated in some tumor models (Shionogi and LNCaP)[617,618] but not others (Dunning).[619] Practically speaking, this treatment involves continuing androgen ablation until adequate testosterone suppression is achieved and then maintaining suppression for some time. This is followed by the discontinuance of therapy and then readministration of therapy at an arbitrary point determined by serum PSA progression. A number of pilot studies testing the feasibility of this approach have been performed.[616,620,621] In general, these studies have suggested that the quality of life of patients treated with this approach may be better and that patients can be maintained off of androgen deprivation therapy for significant periods. Although this approach has wide appeal, it still should be regarded as investigational. A large, randomized intergroup study is now under way comparing continuous hormonal therapy to intermittent hormonal therapy.

Side Effects of Therapy

Although there is a growing appreciation of the breadth and significance of side effects of androgen ablation, comprehensive prospective studies are lacking and, therefore, the frequency of side effects is difficult to quantify. The most frequently described side effects of testosterone suppression are loss of libido, decreased sexual performance, and hot flashes.[613] It appears that the majority of patients are so affected. More subtle, nonquantifiable effects include fatigue and mood changes.[613] The fatigue that results is probably multifactorial. Decreases in serum testosterone level result in a reduction of muscle and red cell mass. In addition, psychological effects, which result in fatigue, may be operable. Other observable side effects are decreased body hair, peripheral edema, and gynecomastia.[613] Peripheral edema appears to be more common with LHRH analogues, whereas gynecomastia is more frequent and more severely associated with estrogens, with antiandrogen monotherapy, or with combined antiandrogen and 5α-reductase inhibitor use. The observed incidence of cardiovascular events, including thromboembolic events, is relatively low with all agents and may well be the anticipated rate in the generally elderly population having an underlying malignancy.[613] The exception to this is estrogens, which reproducibly are associated with higher rates of thromboembolic and cardiovascular events,[613] although this effect may depend on dose and route of administration. Although the incidence of osteopenia and vitamin D deficiency in middle-aged and elderly men has been underappreciated, androgen ablative therapy is likely associated with further bone loss,[622–624] which may result in the greater potential for osteoporotic fractures. Whether bisphosphonates or other agents will prevent these side effects or whether selective androgen receptor modulators will decrease the degree of bone loss is under investigation.

Recurrent Disease after Primary Androgen Ablative Therapy

After androgen ablation, the serum PSA level almost always decreases and achieves a nadir value. This nadir is maintained for a variable period, reflecting (presumably) the inherent composition of the tumor with regard to sensitivity to androgen ablation and the growth kinetics of the remaining androgen-independent cell population. The earliest manifestation of relapse, in most circumstances, is a rise in serum PSA level. Although some patients will manifest a clinical relapse without a rise in their serum PSA level, this is unusual and may be more frequently associated with prostate cancers that exhibit neuroendocrine differentiation. It is important to note that although the serum PSA level in general correlates with tumor cell mass in all stages of disease, this relationship is altered after androgen deprivation therapy. Serum PSA levels generally are lower per tumor cell volume as compared to pretherapy levels. The velocity of serum PSA increase at the time of relapse after androgen therapy may or may not parallel the serum PSA velocity prior to androgen deprivation therapy, presumably reflecting the kinetics of the tumor in these two different stages. In general, however, the serum PSA increase that is seen after androgen ablative therapy predates the onset of radiographic and clinical evidence of disease progression by months, if not years. The PSA velocity in this setting is predictive of survival.

The mechanism by which prostate cancer cells grow independent of androgen is uncertain. Whether this represents clonal evolution of cells acquiring an androgen-independent phenotype through mutations or epigenetic phenomena or through the growth of a preexistent cell type, such as a stem cell, the growth of which was always androgen-independent is uncertain. Nonetheless, the designations assigned to this stage of disease, including *androgen-independent, androgen-refractory, hormone-independent,* and *hormone-refractory,* have been used often and interchangeably. Until better genetic stratification of tumors in this stage of disease occurs, there is little value in separating out by name these different categories.

SECONDARY HORMONAL THERAPY

Prostate cancer epithelial cells maintain their ability to grow in response to the administration of androgens even after primary androgen deprivation therapy stops working. Two trials in which androgen was readministered to patients demonstrated more rapid disease progression.[625,626] Two studies have compared the outcomes of patients in a retrospective fashion if primary androgen deprivation was maintained. In one study, discontinuance of androgen deprivation after failure was an independent predictor of survival,[627] while it failed to be a factor in another study.[628] It is current practice to maintain androgen deprivation (castrate levels of testosterone) even after primary androgen withdrawal stops working. Tumor progression after primary androgen ablation is poorly understood mechanistically and is likely multifactorial. A small subset of patients who experience relapse actually have noncastrate levels of testosterone. Therefore, it is reasonable to check serum testosterone levels at this point and to recommend surgical castration if castrate levels have not been achieved. It had not been until the advent and use of PSA testing that there was some appreciation of the utility of secondary hormonal manipulations after primary androgen deprivation therapy had failed. The implication of serum PSA decline with secondary therapy has not been studied but, in general, for the sake of consistency, a 50% decline in serum PSA level in this setting has been considered a benchmark for response.

Antiandrogen Withdrawal Responses

One of the most interesting observations made in the last decade was the recognition that the withdrawal of antiandrogen therapy (while maintaining testosterone suppression) may be associated with biochemical (PSA) and, in some cases, symptomatic and objective responses.[629] Such responses were described initially in the context of withdrawal of flutamide[630–632] but have since been described on withdrawal of bicalutamide[633,634] and nilutamide.[635,636] Withdrawal responses occur in approximately 25% of patients (range, 15% to 50%). The likelihood of response may correlate with the duration of exposure to the antiandrogen. Other factors such as the type of initial therapy used, whether the antiandrogen was used as part of CAB or was added at the time of disease progression, and other clinical variables have not proven to be predictive of an antiandrogen withdrawal response. Antiandrogen responses generally are observed within a few weeks after withdrawal of the antiandrogen. Responses that occur after withdrawal of bicalutamide may occur later (i.e., up to 8 weeks), perhaps because of this agent's longer serum half-life.[633] The typical duration of antiandrogen withdrawal response is 3 to 4 months, although withdrawal responses may last several years. The mechanism of antiandrogen withdrawal has not yet been defined; however, it is likely that at least one mechanism is the emergence of prostate cancer cells with mutated androgen receptors that respond to an antiandrogen as an agonist rather than an antagonist.[637–641] In fact, when studies have been performed looking for mutated androgen receptors, they are almost exclusively detected in the context of treatment with CAB. Because of the potential benefit of discontinuance of the antiandrogen and the fact that this maneuver is nontoxic and usually is required for enrollment into most clinical trials, it is very reasonable to initiate antiandrogen withdrawal as the first approach for patients whose disease is progressing while they are being treated with antiandrogen therapy. Whether subsequent reintroduction of the same antiandrogen is useful has not been studied.

As mentioned, secondary hormonal maneuvers will elicit responses in patients whose tumors are progressing while they are on primary androgen ablative therapy. The mechanism of these responses probably is multifactorial and likely includes (1) a further reduction in testosterone in those patients who have not achieved a complete reduction of testosterone, (2) blockade of the effect of residual serum androgens through binding of the androgen receptor, (3) reduction in adrenal androgen production, and (4) binding of agents to other nuclear receptors, such as the estrogen receptor, in the prostate cancer cell.

Antiandrogens

Although the nonsteroidal antiandrogens bind the androgen receptor, it is interesting that non–cross-resistance exists between these agents. Scher et al.[642] treated 51 patients who had tumor progression after primary androgen ablative therapy with bicalutamide (200 mg/d). Twelve (24%) patients responded. More frequent responses (in 10 of 26 patients, or 38%) were seen in patients previously treated with flutamide. In another study, Joyce et al.[643] treated 31 patients with bicalutamide, 150 mg/d. Seven patients responded, six of whom had received prior flutamide. Interestingly, the two most impressive responses were those patients who had experienced a flutamide withdrawal response. Responses to nilutamide after flutamide have also been noted.[644] However, no reports of flutamide activity after bicalutamide treatment have been published.

Adrenal Androgen Inhibitors

The rationale behind using adrenal androgen inhibitors is that approximately 5% to 10% of circulating androgen is derived from the adrenal gland and that a higher proportion of androgen within prostate cancer cells may be of adrenal origin. The two most commonly used agents in this setting are aminoglutethimide and ketoconazole, both of which have frequently been used in conjunction with corticosteroids. Therefore, it is difficult to ascertain the true activity of aminoglutethimide and ketoconazole as single agents, as corticosteroids have activity in this disease. Ketoconazole, which inhibits cytochrome P-450 and suppresses both testicular and adrenal androgen production, has significant activity. In one study of men treated with ketoconazole (1200 mg/d) plus hydrocortisone, 30 of 48 patients experienced a decline in serum PSA of greater than 50%.[645] The median duration of response was 3.5 months. Ketoconazole is active at lower doses (i.e., 200 mg t.i.d.) and less toxic, though the comparative efficacy of low versus higher doses has not been studied. The need to combine ketoconazole with a corticosteroid particularly at the lower dose is uncertain. Because ketoconazole requires an acidic stomach pH for optimal absorption, patients are instructed not to take antacids, H_2 blockers, or proton pump inhibitors. The drug should be ingested between meals. Ketoconazole causes nausea and vomiting in 15% of patients, which necessitates discontinuance in some cases. In addition, liver function test abnormalities are seen and, therefore, liver function should be monitored.

Glucocorticoids

Glucocorticoids also have significant activity in prostate cancer. Kelly et al.[646] treated 30 men with hormone-refractory prostate cancer with hydrocortisone, 40 mg/d, and observed a response rate of 20%. Tannock et al.[647] compared prednisone, 10 mg/d, to prednisone plus mitoxantrone. Twenty-two percent of patients treated with glucocorticoids alone responded. This was also seen in a CALGB study comparing hydrocortisone, 40 mg/d, to hydrocortisone plus mitoxantrone.[648] Twenty-two percent of patients responded (PSA decline) to hydrocortisone alone. In another study, 16% of 230 patients receiving hydrocortisone responded, as assessed by declines in serum PSA level.[649]

Megestrol acetate has very modest activity in prostate cancer. Dawson et al.[650] found that, in a randomized study of 160 mg versus 640 mg of megestrol acetate, 12% of patients responded (PSA decline). Because megestrol acetate, which is more commonly used to treat anorexia or hot flashes, may cause a clinical flare in disease, patients in whom this agent is used should be monitored closely.

Estrogens

DES has activity as secondary therapy in patients with hormone-refractory prostate cancer. In one study, 9 of 21 (43%) patients responded by PSA criteria.[651] Interestingly, PC-SPES, a nutritional supplement consisting of eight different herbs, clearly has activity in prostate cancer. DiPaola et al.[652] demonstrated that this concoction had estrogenic activity *in vitro* and serum PSA–lowering activity in men with prostate cancer. It was associated with estrogen-like side effects, including gynecomastia. Interestingly, however, Kameda et al.[653] treated with PC-SPES 34 patients with androgen-independent prostate cancer; all patients had rising serum PSA levels after androgen deprivation and had undergone antiandrogen withdrawal. Fifty-three percent of the patients had a greater than 50% decline in PSA level. Whether the activity of PC-SPES in patients with hormone-refractory prostate cancer is strictly through its estrogenic properties or is modulated by other mechanisms remains to be determined.

MEASURING RESPONSE

One of the most difficult issues in assessing the potential benefits of different forms of therapy in hormone-refractory prostate cancer is the difficulty in measuring response. Few patients have measurable disease, as most patients have osteoblastic bone metastases in which changes are difficult to quantify. Many studies have suggested that a decline in serum PSA level is of biologic importance and clinical significance. Myers et al.[654] demonstrated that a decline in PSA of 50% or greater was associated with prolonged survival in patients treated with suramin. Similarly, an analysis of 110 patients treated at MSKCC with a variety of agents demonstrated that a 50% or greater decline in PSA level was associated with a 21-month median survival, as compared to an 8-month median survival in those without such declines.[655] In the CALGB study comparing hydrocortisone to hydrocortisone plus mitoxantrone, patients who achieved a greater than 50% decline in PSA level survived longer than those who did not.[648] A 75% decrease in PSA level was not associated with better survival than was a 50% decline. In this study, minor (<50%) declines in PSA level were not associated with altered survival.

These studies formed the foundation for the consensus report of the PSA working group in assessing clinical trials in hormone-refractory prostate cancer.[656] The benchmark was set at a minimum 50% decline in PSA level. Although this is a useful benchmark, it is important to note that some potentially effective agents may not decrease PSA. It also is important to note that some agents have direct effects on PSA production such that it may be difficult to assess their activity through serum PSA changes alone.

PROGNOSTIC FACTORS

The main utility of prognostic factors in patients with advanced cancers is that they help to stratify patients into groups entering into clinical trials. In addition, use of prognostic factors may give some insight into predictive factors for response. Although many studies have addressed this issue, few have been useful. In a recent review,[657] nine studies contained sufficient numbers of patients to perform multivariate analysis.[658–665] The most reproducibly important factors that emerged were performance status and hemoglobin level. Other factors of importance appeared to be serum levels of lactate dehydrogenase, alkaline phosphatase, and acid phosphatase.

CHEMOTHERAPY

The traditional view of cytotoxic chemotherapy for prostate cancer is that it had little or no impact on the natural history of the disease. In 1985, Eisenberger et al.[666] reviewed 17 randomized clinical trials that involved 1464 patients. The complete and partial response rate in these trials was 4.5%. In a review of 26 chemotherapy trials performed between 1987 and 1991, the overall response rate was 8.7%.[667] Over the last 5 to 10 years, however, increasing evidence of clinical efficacy of chemotherapy in prostate cancer has emerged. Nonetheless, no trial to date has demonstrated a survival benefit for patients treated with chemotherapy for prostate cancer. The perception of increased efficacy of chemotherapy is the result of several factors. Increased use of the serum PSA level in monitoring activity in clinical trials has suggested that some of the older drugs that previously were believed to be inactive are, in fact, active in this disease. Patients are being placed on clinical trials at an earlier stage because of the recognition that elevations in serum PSA level precede clinical relapse. Furthermore, newer drug combinations have been developed that have greater activity and, finally, better supportive measures, including antiemetics and growth factor support, have allowed clinicians to treat a relatively elderly population in a safer fashion.

Two recently published phase III trials demonstrated the utility of mitoxantrone plus a corticosteroid in hormone-refractory prostate cancer. The first study compared prednisone (10 mg/d) to prednisone (10 mg/d) plus mitoxantrone (12 mg IV every 3 weeks).[647] One hundred and sixty-one patients with hormone-refractory prostate cancer and pain requiring analgesics were entered into the trial. The primary end point in this trial was a significant impact on pain as measured by a drop of 2 points on a 6-point pain scale. Twenty-three (29%) of 80 patients who received mitoxantrone plus prednisone, as compared to 10 (12%) of 81 patients who received prednisone alone, achieved this palliative response ($P = .01$). In addition, the duration of the palliation was longer for those patients who received mitoxantrone plus prednisone (median duration, 43 weeks vs. 18 weeks; $P < .0001$). In another study, hydrocortisone given as a split dose of 30 mg in the morning and 10 mg in the evening was compared to hydrocortisone plus mitoxantrone, 14 mg/m^2 given every 3 weeks.[648] Two hundred and forty-two patients with metastatic hormone-refractory prostate cancer were randomized in this trial. The primary end point for this study was an improvement in survival with mitoxantrone plus hydrocortisone as compared to hydrocortisone alone. No difference in survival was observed (12.6 months vs. 12.3 months). More patients responded (as measured by a greater than 50% decline in PSA level) with mitoxantrone plus hydrocortisone than with hydrocortisone alone (38% vs. 22%; $P = .008$). Pain responses were more frequent in the combination arm. These two studies led to U.S. Food and Drug Administration approval of mitoxantrone for the treatment of hormone-refractory prostate cancer.

Estramustine-Based Chemotherapy

Estramustine is a conjugate of estrogen mustard and estradiol. Originally synthesized to permit the selective delivery of an alkylating agent into an estrogen receptor–positive cancer cell, more recent studies have shown that estramustine possesses little alkylating activity and may work by inhibiting mitosis through binding microtubular proteins in the nuclear matrix. Estramustine preferentially enters cells that possess the estramustine-binding protein, a protein in high concentration in prostatic epithelial cells. As a single agent, estramustine has modest activity. Its activity is related in part to its estrogenic properties but, in addition, perhaps to its microtubular inhibitory properties. Eighteen phase II trials involving 634 patients with hormone-refractory disease demonstrated an objective response rate to estramustine of 19%.[668]

When it was realized that estramustine had microtubular inhibitory properties, *in vitro* studies were performed that demonstrated synergy of this drug with other agents involved in microtubular assembly. Three trials were conducted involving estramustine and vinblastine.[669–671] The doses chosen in these studies generally were estramustine, 10 mg/kg/d, along with weekly vinblastine, 4 mg/m^2. Of 92 patients entered into these three phase II studies, PSA responses were observed in 44 of 88 patients (50%), and objective responses were seen in 6 of 25 patients (24%) with measurable disease. The value of adding estramustine to vinblastine was questioned in a randomized study in which 201 patients with hormone-refractory prostate cancer were randomized to either vinblastine alone, 4 mg/m^2/wk, or vinblastine plus estramustine, 600 mg/m^2/d.[672] Although there was a difference in median survival between the two groups—11.9 months for the combination versus 9.2 months for vinblastine alone—this did not reach statistical significance ($P = .08$). Patients who were treated with the combination had a longer progression-free survival (3.7 months vs. 2.2 months; $P < .001$). PSA responses were more frequent in the combination arm (25.2% vs. 3.2%; $P < .0001$). Interestingly, more frequent gastrointestinal toxicity but less frequent granulocytopenia was seen in the estramustine arm. This study supported the concept that estramustine added activity to vinblastine.

Other estramustine combinations have been investigated. The combination of estramustine and etoposide also showed *in vitro* synergy. Four trials have been conducted with this combination, enrolling a total of 205 patients.[664,673–675] PSA responses were seen in 106 of 190 patients (56%), and measurable responses were noted in 40 of 82 patients (49%). Estramustine has been combined with vinorelbine in three trials.[676–678] One of seven patients with measurable disease responded, and 21 of 47 patients (45%) had a PSA response. Another strategy has been to combine estramustine with the taxanes. Interestingly, one small study of 23 patients with hormone-refractory prostate cancer examined the activity of taxol given as a 24-hour constant infusion at a dose of 135 to 170 mg/m^2.[679] In that study, one patient had a partial response, but no patient had a decline in serum PSA level of greater than 50%. In the one published study in which estramustine was combined with paclitaxel, 4 of 9 patients (44%) had a measurable response, and 17 of 32 (53%) had a PSA response.[680] In a parallel strategy, docetaxel was combined with estramustine. Picus and Schultz[681] demonstrated that docetaxel, when given alone, was active in prostate cancer. In this study, 16 of 35 patients (46%) responded to docetaxel (75 mg/m^2) given every 3 weeks. Petrylak et al.[682] treated 34 patients with estramustine, 280 mg t.i.d., plus docetaxel, 40 to 80 mg/m^2 every 21 days. Twenty of 34 patients (59%) had more than a 50% decline in PSA level. Kreis et al.[683] observed that 14 of 17 patients (82%) treated with estramustine, 14 mg/kg, and docetaxel, 40 to 80 mg/m^2, responded. The dose-limiting toxicity was grade IV leukopenia and grade III fatigue and diarrhea. CALGB completed a phase II study of estramustine and docetaxel in 40 patients with hormone-refractory prostate cancer.[684] Eleven of nineteen men (58%) who were evaluable for response had a PSA response. Because of the significant activity seen with estramustine plus docetaxel, a comparative study is now under way comparing docetaxel plus estramustine to mitoxantrone plus prednisone.

Three-drug regimens have emerged, including estramustine, etoposide, and paclitaxel. In a study of 40 patients, 10 of 22 patients (45%) with measurable disease responded, and 26 of 40 patients (65%) had a PSA response.[663] In another study, estramustine, etoposide, and vinorelbine were used.[685] Two of three patients with measurable disease responded, and 14 of 25 patients (56%) had a PSA response. Kelly et al.[686] treated 56 patients with a combination of carboplatin (AUC 6), taxol (60 to 100 mg/m^2/wk), and estramustine (10 mg/m^2 in three divided doses). A 50% PSA decline was seen in 63% of patients (95% CI, 50% to 76%). Unfortunately, the incidence of deep venous thrombosis reported in this study was 25%.

Clearly, these three-drug combinations are active. Some questions still remain about estramustine-based regimens. First and foremost, are they active enough to prolong survival? Second, what is the contribution of estramustine to these combinations and what is the optimal dosing of estramustine? What are the optimal doses and schedules of the taxanes, and what are the comparative values of three-drug versus two-drug combinations? Finally, what are the details of their activity in early disease?

Other Agents

A number of other drugs are active in patients with hormone-refractory prostate cancer, including cyclophosphamide. Raghaven et al.[687] treated 30 patients with hormone-refractory prostate cancer with oral cyclophosphamide at a dose 100 mg/m^2 for 14 days. Eighteen (60%) had significant improvement in symptoms, whereas 6 (20%) had objective responses.

Doxorubicin has been used in the context of hormone-refractory prostate cancer as well. No study has looked at a single-agent doxorubicin regimen in the post-PSA era. However, this drug has been combined with other agents. A popular regimen was the combination of 5-fluorouracil, doxorubicin, and mitomycin C. In one trial, 48% of 62 patients (i.e., 30 patients) responded.[688] However, in two larger, multicenter studies, response rates were much lower.[689,690] Another combination that has been tried is doxorubicin and cyclophosphamide. In one study, 5 of 15 patients (33%) with measurable disease had a response, and 46% of patients enrolled had a greater than 50% decline in PSA levels.[691]

A regimen popularized at the M. D. Anderson Cancer Center has been a combination of doxorubicin and ketoconazole. In one study, 39 patients were treated with weekly doxorubicin (20 mg/m^2) and daily ketoconazole (1200 mg/d).[692] A PSA decline of greater than 50% was seen in 21 of 38 patients (55%). Seven of twelve patients had a measurable partial response. This regimen has been used as an alternating regimen with estramustine and vinblastine. In one study at the M. D. Anderson Cancer Center of 46 patients with hormone-refractory prostate cancer, 31 patients (67%) had a greater than 50% decline in PSA level, and 12 of 16 patients (75%) had a measurable response.[693]

PALLIATION

Bisphosphonates

Prostate cancer has a strong propensity to spread to bone. Osteoblastic metastases are seen most commonly, principally in the axial structures (pelvis, vertebral bodies) but also in the appendicular structures (long bones, ribs, etc.). This propensity has been a subject of research for many years. One explanation was that tumor cells gained access to vertebral and pelvic bones by retrograde flow through Batson's plexus of paravertebral veins. Other explanations include a similarity between the growth factor requirements that support prostate cancer cell growth and osteoblast growth. Some such factors include osteopontin, osteonectin, insulin-like growth factor (IGF), fibroblast growth factor, transforming growth factor-β, and endothelin-1 (ET-1).[694] Although prostate cancer is primarily an osteoblastic disease, as evidenced by the preponderance of sclerotic bone lesions, it is not uncommon to see mixed blastic and lytic disease. The extent of bone turnover of metastatic bone sites, as measured by a variety of parameters, is high. Bone resorption is mediated through various factors via osteoclastic activity. The value of bisphosphonates in reducing biochemical and clinical parameters of prostate cancer–mediated bone disease is uncertain. Several large, multiinstitutional, randomized trials have now been completed that should clarify these issues. Bisphosphonates have also been used in the context of preventing osteoporosis in patients undergoing androgen deprivation therapy. The value in this setting also remains uncertain, although randomized studies should answer this question.

Radiopharmaceuticals

Radiopharmaceuticals in use are of two general types. The first type are bone-seeking radioisotopes. Strontium 89 is the only approved agent of this type. In a randomized study, strontium 89 was shown to be superior to placebo with respect to bone pain palliation.[695] Pain relief usually occurs within a few weeks after treatment, although 15% of patients will experience a flare in pain within the first 2 weeks. Strontium 89 requires redosing every 3 months. It is generally well tolerated, although progressive bone marrow suppression may occur with repeat dosing. The mechanism of its activity is uncertain, but it is rare to see pain relief coupled with a decline in serum PSA level.

Two trials have been completed that test the value of adding strontium 89 at the time of radiation therapy for symptomatic bone pain relief. In one study, 305 patients with symptomatic bone pain were randomized, after receiving radiation therapy, to receive strontium 89 or hemibody radiation.[696] Twelve weeks after treatment, there was no difference in the degree of improvement in bone pain. However, fewer patients developed new painful areas when strontium 89 was used (47% vs. 65%; $P<.01$). In another trial, patients who had undergone palliative radiation therapy to a bone lesion were randomized to either strontium 89 therapy or no further therapy.[697] There was no difference in overall survival. However, analgesic consumption was reduced when strontium 89 was used. Fewer patients had new painful lesions, and the interval before additional radiation therapy was needed was longer for those receiving strontium 89.

The second general type of radiopharmaceutical in clinical use is a radioisotope coupled to a bisphosphonate. For these agents, homing to bone is based on the ability of bisphosphonate to adhere to the surface of bone. The currently approved agent in this class is samarium 153 ETDMP (ethylenediaminetetramethylene phosphonate) which, in addition to emitting short-range β-particles, is a γ-particle emitter as well. Because of this, imaging is possible.

FUTURE THERAPIES: NOVEL TARGETS

GROWTH FACTOR AND GROWTH FACTOR RECEPTORS AS TARGETS

Some of the most promising targets for cancer therapy are growth factors and growth factor (tyrosine kinase) receptors. Some of the relevant pathways include such growth factor and receptor pathways as epidermal growth factor (EGF), transforming growth factor-β, IGF-1 and IGF-2, and platelet-derived growth factor (PDGF). For several reasons, these growth factors and their tyrosine kinase receptors can be viewed as potential targets in prostate cancer. First, epidemiologic studies suggest that growth factor levels may be involved in either the development or progression of prostate cancer (e.g., IGF-1).[698] Second, some of these growth factors or receptors are dysregulated in different stages of prostate cancer.[699,700] Third, therapeutics such as small molecules and antibodies have been developed against these targets. Finally, there is evidence that targeting these pathways will be effective in cancer therapy. Specifically, an inhibitor of the Abl tyrosine kinase used for the treatment of chronic myelogenous leukemia has been shown to be effective. Furthermore, Herceptin, an antibody directed against Her-2/neu, is an effective therapeutic agent when coupled with chemotherapy in the treatment of breast cancer.[701]

A number of growth factors and receptors are potential targets in prostate cancer, as altered expression of growth factor or receptor can be demonstrated particularly in the context of hormone-refractory prostate cancer. Her-2/neu overexpression can be demonstrated in prostate cancers.[702–704] Overexpression of Her-2/neu may be a mechanism of androgen-independent growth, perhaps through activation of the androgen receptor pathway.[705] Clinical trials involving Herceptin alone and coupled with chemotherapeutic agents currently are under way. The EGF family of receptors is present in normal and malignant prostate epithelium.[706] EGF receptors, when activated by EGF or TGF-α, can stimulate prostate epithelial cell growth. Mechanistically, this may occur through activation of the androgen receptor pathway, suppression of p27, or activation of mitogen-activated protein (MAP) kinase. The EGF pathway is potentially a good target for prostate cancer. Antibodies directed against the receptor (C225), as well as small-molecule inhibitors, have been developed and are in clinical trials.

PDGF has been shown to regulate prostate epithelial stromal interactions in a paracrine fashion.[707] The receptor may be overexpressed in metastatic, hormone-refractory disease.[708] Small-molecule inhibitors have been developed, but clinical trials have not yet been reported.

Nerve growth factor (NGF) is highly concentrated in the prostate.[709] NGF and a related family of peptides, the neurotrophins, influence proliferation, differentiation, and survival of epithelial cells through activation of trk receptors. Trk receptors are expressed in most malignant prostate epithelial tumors.[710] Trk receptor antagonists have been developed and are in clinical trials.

IGF-1 levels may be related to prostate cancer development and progression. *In vitro*, IGF-1 is mitogenic to prostate cancer cell lines.[711] Although the development of specific IGF-1 receptor inhibitors is in progress, none are in clinical testing. Somatostatin analogues have been used because of their ability to lower serum IGF-1 levels. Thus far, no activity has been noted.

ET-1, a potent vasoconstrictor and mitogen for malignant epithelial cells, is overexpressed in the prostatic epithelium.[712] Receptors for ET-1 are expressed in the stroma (ET-B) and epithelium (ET-A). ET-1 plasma levels are higher in patients with advanced disease as compared to those with localized disease or normal controls.[713] An ET-A receptor antagonist, ABT-627, has recently undergone clinical testing and has shown promising results with respect to pain control and disease stabilization.

SIGNAL TRANSDUCTION PATHWAYS

The downstream target pathways of the cell surface growth factor receptors are the MAP kinase, phosphoinositide 3 (PI3) kinase, and phospholipase C pathways. The MAP kinase cascade involves a series of serine threonine and tyrosine kinases that are activated by cell surface signals. EGF, NGF, PDGF, and Her-2/neu all activate MAP kinases and, thus, this pathway may be a relevant target. Currently, inhibitors of MAP kinase are being developed.

The PI3-kinase pathway also is activated by cell surface receptors and may turn out to be a highly relevant pathway in prostate cancer. PTEN, a dual-specificity phosphatase, has been demonstrated to have tumor suppressor activity.[714] In the case of prostate cancer, PTEN is frequently mutated.[715] In addition, PTEN expression appears to correlate with tumor aggressiveness.[716] PTEN normally dephosphorylates lipid substrates of PI3-kinase, including Akt. It appears that Akt is up-regulated in PTEN-mutated cells. Akt, in turn, has the capability of activating several pathways that control proliferation and cell survival. Components of this pathway are, therefore, potentially critical targets in the treatment of prostate cancer. Inhibitors of PI3-kinase and Akt are in development, though they are not yet in clinical trials.

DIFFERENTIATION THERAPY

Differentiation therapy refers to a form of treatment that causes cancer cells to differentiate into a less malignant phenotype or to undergo programmed cell death. This has been demonstrated to be an effective modality for the treatment of promyelocytic leukemia. Several agents are currently in clinical trials in prostate cancer, including phenylacetate and phenylbutyrate and several nuclear receptor agonists, including vitamin D analogues, retinoic acid analogues, and peroxisome proliferator–activated receptor gamma (PPARγ) analogues.

Phenylacetate and phenylbutyrate cause growth arrest and differentiation of prostate cancer cells in culture.[717] These agents have a range of effects including histone acetylation, inhibition of isoprenylation, glutamine depletion, alterations in lipid metabolism, and DNA methylation. Both agents have shown activity in early clinical trials in prostate cancer patients.

The retinoids are compounds that bind to two classes of nuclear receptors, the retinoic acid receptors and the retinoid X receptors. The retinoids cause differentiation of epithelial cells. *In vitro*, the activity of different retinoids is variable, ranging from growth inhibition to growth stimulation. Thus far, clinical trials with retinoids in prostate have been disappointing. The drug liarazole, which has a range of activities including inhibition of retinoid acid metabolism, has shown activity in prostate cancer.[718] In one phase III study comparing liarazole to cyproterone acetate, 20% of patients with hormone-refractory prostate cancer responded to liarazole.[719]

Interest in vitamin D and its analogues is based on epidemiologic data linking low levels of vitamin D and vitamin D receptor polymorphisms to prostate cancer risk,[720,721] as well as *in vitro* data demonstrating a growth-inhibitory effect of these compounds. Noncalcemic vitamin D analogues are now in clinical trials.

PPARγ, a receptor involved in fat cell differentiation, is also present in epithelial cells.[722] Agonists of PPARγ have a growth-inhibitory effect on prostatic cancer cells *in vitro*.[723] Promising results have been achieved with troglitazone in very early studies.

ANTIMETASTATIC THERAPY

The process of metastasis is complex and involves multiple steps. A fundamental step in this process is degradation of the extracellular matrix, which involves enzymes known as *matrix metalloproteinase*. One agent, Marimastat, a selective but non-specific matrix metalloprotease inhibitor, has been tested in patients with prostate cancer.[724] The drug is well tolerated and now is the subject of a prospective, randomized, controlled trial.

IMMUNOTHERAPY

Several immunotherapeutic approaches are currently being investigated in patients with prostate cancer. One such regimen is a coupled antibody approach, in which antibodies are directed against tumor-specific antigens coupled to a toxin or radioisotope. Currently in clinical trials is an antibody directed against PSMA coupled to an α-particle emitter. Another approach is vaccination with antigens enriched on tumor cells, such as specific complex carbohydrate moieties. Still another approach involves mucin 1 (MUC1), an epithelial mucin glycoprotein vaccination with an adjuvant. Incorporating the PSA gene into a herpesvirus vector is another immunotherapeutic modality. A novel approach employs dendritic cells (antigen-presenting cells) loaded with a specific tumor antigen such as PSA, PSMA, or acid phosphatase. The loaded dendritic cells are infused into the patient in an effort to stimulate an immune response. Several clinical trials of this nature are in progress.

One can also augment the production of specific cytokines that stimulate the immune system. One popular approach has been the use of granulocyte-megakaryocyte colony-stimulating factor administered exogenously or delivered in autologous or allogeneic prostate cancer cells. Clinical trials incorporating these different approaches are currently being conducted.

ANGIOGENIC APPROACHES

Angiogenesis is a complex, multistep process that is fundamental to tumor growth and metastasis. This process appears to be important in the growth and progression of localized prostate cancer, as evidenced by a correlation between microvessel density and prognosis in this disease. Whether angiogenesis is important in the establishment of bone metastasis in prostate cancer is uncertain. One of the important mediators of angiogenesis is vascular endothelial growth factor (VEGF). A number of strategies have been developed and directed at VEGF, including VEGF antibodies and small-molecule inhibitors of the VEGF receptors (Flk and KDR). These agents are in clinical trials currently.

A number of additional agents with *in vitro* antiangiogenic properties have been developed (TNP-470, endostatin, etc.) and also are in clinical trials.

REFERENCES

1. Cancer statistics, 1999. *CA Cancer J Clin* 1999;49:8.
2. Brooks JD, Chao WM, Kerr J. Male pelvic anatomy reconstructed from the visible human data set. *J Urol* 1998;159:868.
3. Di Lollo S, Menchi I, Brizzi E, et al. The morphology of the prostatic capsule with particular regard to the posterosuperior region: an anatomical and clinical problem. *Surg Radiol Anat* 1997;19:143.
4. Sattar AA, Noel JC, Vanderhaeghen JJ, Schulman CC, Wespes E. Prostate capsule: computerized morphometric analysis of its components. *Urology* 1995;46:178.
5. Steiner MS. The puboprostatic ligament and the male urethral suspensory mechanism: an anatomic study. *Urology* 1994;44:530.
6. Oelrich TM. The urethral sphincter muscle in the male. *Am J Anat* 1980;158:229.
7. Light JK, Rapoll E, Wheeler TM. The striated urethral sphincter: muscle fibre types and distribution in the prostatic capsule. *Br J Urol* 1997;79:539.
8. Burnett AL, Mostwin JL. In situ anatomical study of the male urethral sphincteric complex: relevance to continence preservation following major pelvic surgery. *J Urol* 1998;160:1301.
9. Myers RP, Goellner JR, Cahill DR. Prostate shape, external striated urethral sphincter and radical prostatectomy: the apical dissection. *J Urol* 1987;138:543.
10. Myers RP. Male urethral sphincteric anatomy and radical prostatectomy. *Urol Clin North Am* 1991;18:211.
11. Myers RP. Anatomical variation of the superficial preprostatic veins with respect to radical retropubic prostatectomy. *J Urol* 1991;145:992.
12. Elbadawi A, Mathews R, Light JK, Wheeler TM. Immunohistochemical and ultrastructural study of rhabdosphincter component of the prostatic capsule. *J Urol* 1997;158:1819.
13. Hollabaugh RS Jr, Dmochowski RR, Steiner MS. Neuroanatomy of the male rhabdosphincter. *Urology* 1997;49:426.
14. Shafik A, Doss S. Surgical anatomy of the somatic terminal innervation to the anal and urethral sphincters: role in anal and urethral surgery. *J Urol* 1999;161:85.
15. Strasser H, Klima G, Poisel S, Horninger W, Bartsch G. Anatomy and innervation of the rhabdosphincter of the male urethra. *Prostate* 1996;28:24.
16. Vaalasti A, Hervonen A. Autonomic innervation of the human prostate. *Invest Urol* 1980;17:293.
17. Zvara P, Carrier S, Kour NW, Tanagho EA. The detailed neuroanatomy of the human striated urethral sphincter. *Br J Urol* 1994;74:182.
18. McNeal JE. The prostate and prostatic urethra: a morphologic synthesis. *J Urol* 1972;107:1008.
19. Cotran RS, Kumar V, Robbins SL. *Robbins pathologic basis of disease,* 5th ed. Philadelphia: WB Saunders, 1994:1023.
20. Mostofi FK, Davis CJ Jr, Sesterhenn IA. Pathology of carcinoma of the prostate. *Cancer* 1992;70:235.
21. Wojno KJ, Epstein JI. The utility of basal cell-specific anti-cytokeratin antibody (34 beta E12) in the diagnosis of prostate cancer. A review of 228 cases. *Am J Surg Pathol* 1995;19:251.
22. McNeal JE. Origin and development of carcinoma in the prostate. *Cancer* 1969;23:24.
23. Gleason DF, Mellinger GT. Prediction of prognosis for prostatic adenocarcinoma by combined histological grading and clinical staging. *J Urol* 1974;111:58.
24. Gleason DF. Histologic grading of prostate cancer: a perspective. *Hum Pathol* 1992;23:273.
25. McNeal JE, Reese JH, Redwine EA, Freiha FS, Stamey TA. Cribriform adenocarcinoma of the prostate. *Cancer* 1986;58:1714.
26. McNeal JE, Alroy J, Villers A, et al. Mucinous differentiation in prostatic adenocarcinoma. *Hum Pathol* 1991;22:979.
27. Bostwick DG, Kindrachuk RW, Rouse RV. Prostatic adenocarcinoma with endometrioid features. Clinical, pathologic, and ultrastructural findings. *Am J Surg Pathol* 1985;9:595.
28. Ro JY, Ayala AG, Wishnow KI, Ordonez NG. Prostatic duct adenocarcinoma with endometrioid features: immunohistochemical and electron microscopic study. *Semin Diagn Pathol* 1988;5:301.
29. Ro JY, Grignon DJ, Ayala AG, et al. Mucinous adenocarcinoma of the prostate: histochemical and immunohistochemical studies. *Hum Pathol* 1990;21:593.
30. Torbenson M, Dhir R, Nangia A, Becich MJ, Kapadia SB. Prostatic carcinoma with signet ring cells: a clinicopathologic and immunohistochemical analysis of 12 cases, with review of the literature. *Mod Pathol* 1998;11:552.
31. Saito S, Iwaki H. Mucin-producing carcinoma of the prostate: review of 88 cases. *Urology* 1999;54:141.
32. Tannenbaum M. *Urologic pathology: the prostate.* Philadelphia: Lea & Febiger, 1977:419.
33. Grignon DJ, Ro JY, Ordonez NG, Ayala AG, Cleary KR. Basal cell hyperplasia, adenoid basal cell tumor, and adenoid cystic carcinoma of the prostate gland: an immunohistochemical study. *Hum Pathol* 1988;19:1425.
34. Young RH, Frierson HF Jr, Mills SE, et al. Adenoid cystic-like tumor of the prostate gland. A report of two cases and review of the literature on "adenoid cystic carcinoma" of the prostate. *Am J Clin Pathol* 1988;89:49.
35. Mott LJ. Squamous cell carcinoma of the prostate: report of 2 cases and review of the literature. *J Urol* 1979;121:833.
36. Little NA, Wiener JS, Walther PJ, Paulson DF, Anderson EE. Squamous cell carcinoma of the prostate: 2 cases of a rare malignancy and review of the literature. *J Urol* 1993;149:137.
37. Okamoto T, Ogiu K, Sato M, et al. Primary squamous cell carcinoma of the prostate: a case report. *Hinyokika Kiyo* 1996;42:67.
38. Corder MP, Cicmil GA. Effective treatment of metastatic squamous cell carcinoma of the prostate with Adriamycin. *J Urol* 1976;115:222.
39. Sarma DP, Weilbaecher TG, Moon TD. Squamous cell carcinoma of prostate. *Urology* 1991;37:260.
40. Reese JH, Freiha FS, Gelb AB, Lum BL, Torti FM. Transitional cell carcinoma of the prostate in patients undergoing radical cystoprostatectomy. *J Urol* 1992;147:92.
41. Alexander SJ, Lee SS, Bekhrad A. Transitional cell carcinoma of the prostate: response to treatment with cisplatinum and cyclophosphamide. *J Urol* 1984;131:975.
42. Matzkin H, Braf Z. Paraneoplastic syndromes associated with prostatic carcinoma. *J Urol* 1987;138:1129.
43. Tetu B, Ro JY, Ayala AG, et al. Small cell carcinoma of prostate associated with myasthenic (Eaton-Lambert) syndrome. *Urology* 1989;33:148.
44. Efros MD, Fischer J, Mallouh C, Choudhury M, Georgsson S. Unusual primary prostatic malignancies. *Urology* 1992;39:407.
45. Bostwick DG. Pathology of the prostate. In: *Contemporary issues in surgical pathology,* vol 15. New York: Churchill Livingstone, 1990:250.
46. Schild HH, Schweden FJ, Lang EK. *Computed tomography in urology.* Stuttgart: Thieme Medical Publishers, 1992:381.
47. Agrons GA, Wagner BJ, Lonergan GJ, Dickey GE, Kaufman MS. From the archives of the AFIP. Genitourinary rhabdomyosarcoma in children: radiologic-pathologic correlation. *Radiographics* 1997;17:919.
48. Limon J, Dal Cin P, Sandberg AA. Cytogenetic findings in a primary leiomyosarcoma of the prostate. *Cancer Genet Cytogenet* 1986;22:159.
49. Claikens B, Oyen R, Goethuys H, Boogaerts M, Baert AL. Non-Hodgkin's lymphoma of the prostate in a young male. *Eur Radiol* 1997;7:238.
50. Narayan P. Neoplasms of the prostate gland. In: Tanagho EA, McAninch JW, eds. *Smith's general urology,* 14th ed. Norwalk, CT: Appleton & Lange, 1995:392.
51. Epstein JI. Nonpalpable preneoplastic lesions of the prostate. In: Raghavan D, Scher HI, Leibel SA, Lang P, eds. *Principles and practice of genitourinary oncology.* Philadelphia: Lippincott-Raven Publishers, 1997:387.

52. Qian J, Wollan P, Bostwick DG. The extent and multicentricity of high-grade prostatic intraepithelial neoplasia in clinically localized prostatic adenocarcinoma. *Hum Pathol* 1997;28:143.
53. de la Torre M, Haggman M, Brandstedt S, Busch C. Prostatic intraepithelial neoplasia and invasive carcinoma in total prostatectomy specimens: distribution, volumes and DNA ploidy. *Br J Urol* 1993;72:207.
54. Erbersdobler A, Gurses N, Henke RP. Numerical chromosomal changes in high-grade prostatic intraepithelial neoplasia (PIN) and concomitant invasive carcinoma. *Pathol Res Pract* 1996;192:418.
55. Bostwick DG, Leske DA, Qian J, Sinha AA. Prostatic intraepithelial neoplasia and well differentiated adenocarcinoma maintain an intact basement membrane. *Pathol Res Pract* 1995;191:850.
56. Park S, Shinohara K, Grossfeld GD, Presti JCJ, Carroll PR. Prostate cancer on repeat biopsy in men with an initial biopsy of atypical adenomatous hyperplasia or high grade prostatic intraepithelial neoplasia. *J Urol* 1999;161:1243.
57. Wilcox G, Soh S, Chakraborty S, Scardino PT, Wheeler TM. Patterns of high-grade prostatic intraepithelial neoplasia associated with clinically aggressive prostate cancer. *Hum Pathol* 1998;29:1119.
58. Di Silverio F, D'Eramo G, Buscarini M, et al. DNA ploidy, Gleason score, pathological stage and serum PSA levels as predictors of disease-free survival in C-D1 prostatic cancer patients submitted to radical retropubic prostatectomy. *Eur Urol* 1996;30:316.
59. Lerner SE, Blute ML, Bergstralh EJ, et al. Analysis of risk factors for progression in patients with pathologically confined prostate cancers after radical retropubic prostatectomy. *J Urol* 1996;156:137.
60. Hawkins CA, Bergstralh EJ, Lieber MM, Zincke H. Influence of DNA ploidy and adjuvant treatment on progression and survival in patients with pathologic stage T3 (PT3) prostate cancer after radical retropubic prostatectomy. *Urology* 1995;46:356.
61. Cheville JC, Lloyd RV, Sebo TJ, et al. Expression of p27kip1 in prostatic adenocarcinoma. *Mod Pathol* 1998;11:324.
62. Miller GJ. Pathology of palpable prostate cancer. In: Raghavan D, Scher HI, Leibel SA, Lang P, eds. *Principles and practice of genitourinary oncology*. Philadelphia: Lippincott-Raven Publishers, 1997: 395.
63. Franks LM. Latent carcinoma of the prostate. *J Pathol Bacteriol* 1954;68:603.
64. Stamey TA, Freiha FS, McNeal JE, et al. Localized prostate cancer. Relationship of tumor volume to clinical significance for treatment of prostate cancer. *Cancer* 1993;71:933.
65. Jacobsen SJ, Katusic SK, Bergstralh EJ, et al. Incidence of prostate cancer diagnosis in the eras before and after serum prostate-specific antigen testing. *JAMA* 1995;274:1445.
66. Gann PH. Interpreting recent trends in prostate cancer incidence and mortality [editorial]. *Epidemiology* 1997;8:117.
67. Smith DS, Catalona WJ. The nature of prostate cancer detected through prostate specific antigen based screening. *J Urol* 1994;152:1732.
68. Catalona WJ, Smith DS, Ratliff TL, Basler JW. Detection of organ-confined prostate cancer is increased through prostate-specific antigen-based screening. *JAMA* 1993;270:948.
69. Parkin DM, Pisani P, Ferlay J. Global cancer statistics. *CA Cancer J Clin* 1999;49:33.
70. Breslow N, Chan CW, Dhom G, et al. Latent carcinoma of prostate of autopsy in seven areas. *Int J Cancer* 1977;20:680.
71. Holund B. Latent prostatic cancer in a consecutive autopsy series. *Scand J Urol Nephrol* 1980;14:29.
72. Guileyardo JM, Johnson WD, Welsh RA, Akazaki K, Correa P. Prevalence of latent prostate carcinoma in two U.S. populations. *J Natl Cancer Inst* 1980;65:311.
73. Billis A. Latent carcinoma and atypical lesions of prostate. An autopsy study. *Urology* 1986;28:324.
74. Sakr WA, Haas GP, Cassin BF, Pontes JE, Crissman JD. The frequency of carcinoma and intraepithelial neoplasia of the prostate in young male patients. *J Urol* 1993;150:379.
75. Shiraishi T, Watanabe M, Matsuura H, et al. The frequency of latent prostatic carcinoma in young males: the Japanese experience. *In Vivo* 1994;8:445.
76. Chang CK, Yu HJ, Chan KW, Lai MK. Secular trend and age-period-cohort analysis of prostate cancer mortality in Taiwan. *J Urol* 1997;158:1845.
77. Powell IJ, Schwartz K, Hussain M. Removal of the financial barrier to health care: Does it impact on prostate cancer at presentation and survival? A comparative study between black and white men in a Veterans Affairs system. *Urology* 1995;46:825.
78. Ndubuisi SC, Kofie VY, Andoh JY, Schwartz EM. Black-white differences in the stage at presentation of prostate cancer in the District of Columbia. *Urology* 1995;46:71.
79. Burks DA, Littleton RH. The epidemiology of prostate cancer in black men. *Henry Ford Hosp Med J* 1992;40:89.
80. Whittemore AS, Kolonel LN, Wu AH, et al. Prostate cancer in relation to diet, physical activity, and body size in blacks, whites, and Asians in the United States and Canada. *J Natl Cancer Inst* 1995;87:652.
81. Krongrad A, Lai H, Lamm SH, Lai S. Mortality in prostate cancer. *J Urol* 1996;156:1084.
82. Haas GP, Sakr WA. Epidemiology of prostate cancer. *CA Cancer J Clin* 1997;47:273.
83. Conlisk EA, Lengerich EJ, Demark-Wahnefried W, Schildkraut JM, Aldrich TE. Prostate cancer: demographic and behavioral correlates of stage at diagnosis among blacks and whites in North Carolina. *Urology* 1999;53:1194.
84. Pienta K, Demers R, Hoff M, et al. Effect of age and race on the survival of men with prostate cancer in the metropolitan Detroit tricounty area, 1973 to 1987. *Urology* 1995;45:93.
85. Polednak AP. Cancer mortality in a higher-income black population in New York State. Comparison with rates in the United States as a whole. *Cancer* 1990;66:1654.
86. Osegbe DN. Prostate cancer in Nigerians: facts and nonfacts. *J Urol* 1997;157:1340.
87. Glover FE Jr, Coffey DS, Douglas LL, et al. The epidemiology of prostate cancer in Jamaica. *J Urol* 1998;159:1984.
88. Ross R, Bernstein L, Judd H, et al. Serum testosterone levels in healthy young black and white men. *J Natl Cancer Inst* 1986;76:45.
89. Coetzee GA, Ross RK. Re: prostate cancer and the androgen receptor [letter]. *J Natl Cancer Inst* 1994;86:872.
90. Giovannucci E, Stampfer MJ, Krithivas K, et al. The CAG repeat within the androgen receptor gene and its relationship to prostate cancer. *Proc Natl Acad Sci U S A* 1997;94:3320.
91. Ross RK, Pike MC, Coetzee GA, et al. Androgen metabolism and prostate cancer: establishing a model of genetic susceptibility. *Cancer Res* 1998;58:4497.
92. Shimizu H, Ross RK, Bernstein L, et al. Cancers of the prostate and breast among Japanese and white immigrants in Los Angeles County. *Br J Cancer* 1991;63:963.
93. Hirayama T. Epidemiology of prostate cancer with special reference to the role of diet. *Natl Cancer Inst Monogr* 1979;(53):149.
94. Kakehi Y. Epidemiology and clinical features of prostate cancer in Japan. *Nippon Rinsho* 1998;56:1969.
95. Keetch DW, Rice JP, Suarez BK, Catalona WJ. Familial aspects of prostate cancer: a case control study. *J Urol* 1995;154:2100.
96. Bratt O, Kristoffersson U, Lundgren R, Olsson H. Familial and hereditary prostate cancer in southern Sweden. A population-based case-control study. *Eur J Cancer* 1999;35:272.
97. Schuurman AG, Zeegers MP, Goldbohm RA, van den Brandt PA. A case-cohort study on prostate cancer risk in relation to family history of prostate cancer. *Epidemiology* 1999;10:192.
98. Gibbs M, Stanford JL, McIndoe RA, et al. Evidence for a rare prostate cancer–susceptibility locus at chromosome 1p36. *Am J Hum Genet* 1999;64:776.
99. Cooney KA. Hereditary prostate cancer in African-American families. *Semin Urol Oncol* 1998;16:202.
100. Norrish AE, McRae CU, Cohen RJ, Jackson RT. A population-based study of clinical and pathological prognostic characteristics of men with familial and sporadic prostate cancer. *BJU Int* 1999;84:311.
101. Zhu K, McKnight B, Stergachis A, Daling JR, Levine RS. Comparison of self-report data and medical records data: results from a case-control study on prostate cancer. *Int J Epidemiol* 1999;28:409.
102. Taylor KL, DiPlacido J, Redd WH, et al. Demographics, family histories, and psychological characteristics of prostate carcinoma screening participants. *Cancer* 1999;85:1305.
103. Giovannucci E, Ascherio A, Rimm EB, et al. A prospective cohort study of vasectomy and prostate cancer in US men. *JAMA* 1993;269:873.
104. Giovannucci E, Tosteson TD, Speizer FE, et al. A retrospective cohort study of vasectomy and prostate cancer in US men. *JAMA* 1993;269:878.
105. Hsing AW, Wang RT, Gu FL, et al. Vasectomy and prostate cancer risk in China. *Cancer Epidemiol Biomarkers Prev* 1994;3:285.
106. Platz EA, Yeole BB, Cho E, et al. Vasectomy and prostate cancer: a case-control study in India. *Int J Epidemiol* 1997;26:933.
107. Zhu K, Stanford JL, Daling JR, et al. Vasectomy and prostate cancer: a case-control study in a health maintenance organization. *Am J Epidemiol* 1996;144:717.
108. Bernal-Delgado E, Latour-Perez J, Pradas-Arnal F, Gomez-Lopez LI. The association between vasectomy and prostate cancer: a systematic review of the literature. *Fertil Steril* 1998;70:191.
109. John EM, Whittemore AS, Wu AH, et al. Vasectomy and prostate cancer: results from a multiethnic case-control study. *J Natl Cancer Inst* 1995;87:662.
110. Lesko SM, Louik C, Vezina R, Rosenberg L, Shapiro S. Vasectomy and prostate cancer. *J Urol* 1999;161:1848.
111. Szarka CE, Grana G, Engstrom PF. Chemoprevention of cancer. *Curr Probl Cancer* 1994;18:6.
112. Lippman SM, Benner SE, Hong WK. Cancer chemoprevention. *J Clin Oncol* 1994;12:851.
113. Kelloff GJ, Lieberman R, Steele VE, et al. Chemoprevention of prostate cancer: concepts and strategies. *Eur Urol* 1999;35:342.
114. Ekman P. Genetic and environmental factors in prostate cancer genesis: identifying high-risk cohorts. *Eur Urol* 1999;35:362.
115. Feigl P, Blumenstein B, Thompson I, et al. Design of the Prostate Cancer Prevention Trial (PCPT). *Control Clin Trials* 1995;16:150.
116. Moyad MA. Soy, disease prevention, and prostate cancer. *Semin Urol Oncol* 1999;17:97.
117. Gupta S, Ahmad N, Mukhtar H. Prostate cancer chemoprevention by green tea. *Semin Urol Oncol* 1999;17:70.
118. McCormick DL, Rao KV. Chemoprevention of hormone-dependent prostate cancer in the Wistar-Unilever rat. *Eur Urol* 1999;35:464.
119. Skowronski RJ, Peehl DM, Feldman D. Actions of vitamin D_3, analogs on human prostate cancer cell lines: comparison with 1,25-dihydroxyvitamin D_3. *Endocrinology* 1995;136:20.
120. Barnes S, Peterson TG, Coward L. Rationale for the use of genistein-containing soy matrices in chemoprevention trials for breast and prostate cancer. *J Cell Biochem Suppl* 1995;22:181.
121. Gormley GJ. Chemoprevention strategies for prostate cancer: the role of 5 alpha-reductase inhibitors. *J Cell Biochem Suppl* 1992;16H:113.
122. Thompson IM Jr, Coltman CA Jr, Crowley J. Chemoprevention of prostate cancer: the Prostate Cancer Prevention Trial. *Prostate* 1997;33:217.
123. Coltman CA Jr, Thompson IM Jr, Feigl P. Prostate Cancer Prevention Trial (PCPT) update. *Eur Urol* 1999;35:544.
124. Bologna M, Muzi P, Biordi L, Festuccia C, Vicentini C. Finasteride dose-dependently reduces the proliferation rate of the LnCap human prostatic cancer cell line in vitro. *Urology* 1995;45:282.
125. Klocker H, Culig Z, Eder IE, et al. Mechanism of androgen receptor activation and possible implications for chemoprevention trials. *Eur Urol* 1999;35:413.
126. Mooradian AD, Morley JE, Korenman SG. Biological actions of androgens. *Endocr Rev* 1987;8:1.
127. Lu S, Tsai SY, Tsai MJ. Regulation of androgen-dependent prostatic cancer cell growth: androgen regulation of CDK2, CDK4, and CKI p16 genes. *Cancer Res* 1997;57:4511.
128. Sudduth SL, Koronkowski MJ. Finasteride: the first 5 alpha-reductase inhibitor. *Pharmacotherapy* 1993;13:309.
129. Ross RK, Bernstein L, Lobo RA, et al. 5-Alpha-reductase activity and risk of prostate cancer among Japanese and US white and black males. *Lancet* 1992;339:887.
130. Presti JC Jr, Fair WR, Andriole G, et al. Multicenter, randomized, double-blind, placebo controlled study to investigate the effect of finasteride (MK-906) on stage D prostate cancer. *J Urol* 1992;148:1201.

131. Denis L, Morton MS, Griffiths K. Diet and its preventive role in prostatic disease. *Eur Urol* 1999;35:377.
132. Clinton SK, Giovannucci E. Diet, nutrition, and prostate cancer. *Annu Rev Nutr* 1998;18:413.
133. Yip I, Heber D, Aronson W. Nutrition and prostate cancer. *Urol Clin North Am* 1999;26:403.
134. Hebert JR, Hurley TG, Olendzki BC, et al. Nutritional and socioeconomic factors in relation to prostate cancer mortality: a cross-national study. *J Natl Cancer Inst* 1998;90:1637.
135. Gann PH, Hennekens CH, Sacks FM, et al. Prospective study of plasma fatty acids and risk of prostate cancer. *J Natl Cancer Inst* 1994;86:281.
136. Giovannucci E, Rimm EB, Colditz GA, et al. A prospective study of dietary fat and risk of prostate cancer. *J Natl Cancer Inst* 1993;85:1571.
137. Hankin JH, Zhao LP, Wilkens LR, Kolonel LN. Attributable risk of breast, prostate, and lung cancer in Hawaii due to saturated fat. *Cancer Causes Control* 1992;3:17.
138. Fradet Y, Meyer F, Bairati I, Shadmani R, Moore L. Dietary fat and prostate cancer progression and survival. *Eur Urol* 1999;35:388.
139. Wang Y, Corr JG, Thaler HT, et al. Decreased growth of established human prostate LNCaP tumors in nude mice fed a low-fat diet. *J Natl Cancer Inst* 1995;87:1456.
140. Myers CE, Ghosh J. Lipoxygenase inhibition in prostate cancer. *Eur Urol* 1999;35:395.
141. Davis JN, Singh B, Bhuiyan M, Sarkar FH. Genistein-induced upregulation of p21WAF1, downregulation of cyclin B, and induction of apoptosis in prostate cancer cells. *Nutr Cancer* 1998;32:123.
142. Akiyama T, Ishida J, Nakagawa S, et al. Genistein, a specific inhibitor of tyrosine-specific protein kinases. *J Biol Chem* 1987;262:5592.
143. Griffiths K, Morton MS, Denis L. Certain aspects of molecular endocrinology that relate to the influence of dietary factors on the pathogenesis of prostate cancer. *Eur Urol* 1999;35:443.
144. Katiyar SK, Mukhtar H. Tea consumption and cancer. *World Rev Nutr Diet* 1996;79:154.
145. Yang GY, Liao J, Kim K, Yurkow EJ, Yang CS. Inhibition of growth and induction of apoptosis in human cancer cell lines by tea polyphenols. *Carcinogenesis* 1998;19:611.
146. Mohan RR, Challa A, Gupta S, et al. Overexpression of ornithine decarboxylase in prostate cancer and prostatic fluid in humans. *Clin Cancer Res* 1999;5:143.
147. Gupta S, Ahmad N, Mohan RR, Husain MM, Mukhtar H. Prostate cancer chemoprevention by green tea: in vitro and in vivo inhibition of testosterone-mediated induction of ornithine decarboxylase. *Cancer Res* 1999;59:2115.
148. Gann PH, Ma J, Giovannucci E, et al. Lower prostate cancer risk in men with elevated plasma lycopene levels: results of a prospective analysis. *Cancer Res* 1999;59:1225.
149. Mills PK, Beeson WL, Phillips RL, Fraser GE. Cohort study of diet, lifestyle, and prostate cancer in Adventist men. *Cancer* 1989;64:598.
150. Giovannucci E, Ascherio A, Rimm EB, et al. Intake of carotenoids and retinol in relation to risk of prostate cancer. *J Natl Cancer Inst* 1995;87:1767.
151. Chan JM, Stampfer MJ, Giovannucci EL. What causes prostate cancer? A brief summary of the epidemiology. *Semin Cancer Biol* 1998;8:263.
152. Kamat AM, Lamm DL. Chemoprevention of urological cancer. *J Urol* 1999;161:1748.
153. Hsing AW, Comstock GW, Abbey H, Polk BF. Serologic precursors of cancer. Retinol, carotenoids, and tocopherol and risk of prostate cancer. *J Natl Cancer Inst* 1990;82:941.
154. Moyad MA, Brumfield SK, Pienta KJ. Vitamin E, alpha- and gamma-tocopherol, and prostate cancer. *Semin Urol Oncol* 1999;17:85.
155. Clark LC, Dalkin B, Krongrad A, et al. Decreased incidence of prostate cancer with selenium supplementation: results of a double-blind cancer prevention trial. *Br J Urol* 1998;81:730.
156. Yoshizawa K, Willett WC, Morris SJ, et al. Study of prediagnostic selenium level in toenails and the risk of advanced prostate cancer. *J Natl Cancer Inst* 1998;90:1219.
157. Yang M, Sytkowski AJ. Differential expression and androgen regulation of the human selenium-binding protein gene hSP56 in prostate cancer cells. *Cancer Res* 1998;58:3150.
158. Webber MM, Perez-Ripoll EA, James GT. Inhibitory effects of selenium on the growth of DU-145 human prostate carcinoma cells in vitro. *Biochem Biophys Res Commun* 1985;130:603.
159. Konety BR, Johnson CS, Trump DL, Getzenberg RH. Vitamin D in the prevention and treatment of prostate cancer. *Semin Urol Oncol* 1999;17:77.
160. Peehl DM. Vitamin D and prostate cancer risk. *Eur Urol* 1999;35:392.
161. Feldman D, Skowronski RJ, Peehl DM. Vitamin D and prostate cancer. *Adv Exp Med Biol* 1995;375:53.
162. Peehl DM, Skowronski RJ, Leung GK, et al. Antiproliferative effects of 1,25-dihydroxyvitamin D3 on primary cultures of human prostatic cells. *Cancer Res* 1994;54:805.
163. Schwartz GG, Hulka BS. Is vitamin D deficiency a risk factor for prostate cancer? (Hypothesis). *Anticancer Res* 1990;10:1307.
164. Hanchette CL, Schwartz GG. Geographic patterns of prostate cancer mortality. Evidence for a protective effect of ultraviolet radiation. *Cancer* 1992;70:2861.
165. Sylvester R, Collette L. Statistical considerations of chemoprevention clinical trials in prostate cancer. *Eur Urol* 1999;35:519.
166. van der Meijden AP. Practical aspects of clinical trials on chemoprevention of prostate cancer. *Eur Urol* 1999;35:515.
167. Crowley CW, Cohen RL, Lucas BK, et al. Prevention of metastasis by inhibition of the urokinase receptor. *Proc Natl Acad Sci U S A* 1993;90:5021.
168. Evans CP, Elfman F, Parangi S, et al. Inhibition of prostate cancer neovascularization and growth by urokinase-plasminogen activator receptor blockade. *Cancer Res* 1997;57:3594.
169. Thompson IM, Ernst JJ, Gangai MP, Spence CR. Adenocarcinoma of the prostate: results of routine urological screening. *J Urol* 1984;132:690.
170. Coley CM, Barry MJ, Fleming C, et al. Should Medicare provide reimbursement for prostate-specific antigen testing for early detection of prostate cancer? II: Early detection strategies. *Urology* 1995;46:125.
171. Polascik TJ, Oesterling JE, Partin AW. Prostate specific antigen: a decade of discovery—what we have learned and where we are going. *J Urol* 1999;162:293.
172. Yu H, Diamandis EP, Sutherland DJ. Immunoreactive prostate-specific antigen levels in female and male breast tumors and its association with steroid hormone receptors and patient age. *Clin Biochem* 1994;27:75.
173. Yu H, Diamandis EP. Prostate-specific antigen in milk of lactating women. *Clin Chem* 1995;41:54.
174. Yu H, Diamandis EP. Measurement of serum prostate specific antigen levels in women and in prostatectomized men with an ultrasensitive immunoassay technique. *J Urol* 1995;153:1004.
175. Levesque M, Hu H, D'Costa M, Diamandis EP. Prostate-specific antigen expression by various tumors. *J Clin Lab Anal* 1995;9:123.
176. Stenman UH, Leinonen J, Alfthan H, et al. A complex between prostate-specific antigen and alpha 1-antichymotrypsin is the major form of prostate-specific antigen in serum of patients with prostatic cancer: assay of the complex improves clinical sensitivity for cancer. *Cancer Res* 1991;51:222.
177. Lilja H, Christensson A, Dahlen U, et al. Prostate-specific antigen in serum occurs predominantly in complex with alpha 1-antichymotrypsin. *Clin Chem* 1991;37:1618.
178. McCormack RT, Rittenhouse HG, Finlay JA, et al. Molecular forms of prostate-specific antigen and the human kallikrein gene family: a new era. *Urology* 1995;45:729.
179. Nadler RB, Humphrey PA, Smith DS, Catalona WJ, Ratliff TL. Effect of inflammation and benign prostatic hyperplasia on elevated serum prostate specific antigen levels. *J Urol* 1995;154:407.
180. Tchetgen MB, Song JT, Strawderman M, Jacobsen SJ, Oesterling JE. Ejaculation increases the serum prostate-specific antigen concentration. *Urology* 1996;47:511.
181. Chybowski FM, Bergstralh EJ, Oesterling JE. The effect of digital rectal examination on the serum prostate specific antigen concentration: results of a randomized study. *J Urol* 1992;148:83.
182. Oesterling JE, Chan DW, Epstein JI, et al. Prostate specific antigen in the preoperative and postoperative evaluation of localized prostatic cancer treated with radical prostatectomy. *J Urol* 1988;139:766.
183. Stamey TA, Yang N, Hay AR, et al. Prostate-specific antigen as a serum marker for adenocarcinoma of the prostate. *N Engl J Med* 1987;317:909.
184. Guess HA, Heyse JF, Gormley GJ. The effect of finasteride on prostate-specific antigen in men with benign prostatic hyperplasia. *Prostate* 1993;22:31.
185. Gormley GJ, Ng J, Cook T, et al. Effect of finasteride on prostate-specific antigen density. *Urology* 1994;43:53.
186. Roehrborn CG, Oesterling JE, Olson PJ, Padley RJ. Serial prostate-specific antigen measurements in men with clinically benign prostatic hyperplasia during a 12-month placebo-controlled study with terazosin. HYCAT Investigator Group. Hytrin Community Assessment Trial. *Urology* 1997;50:556.
187. Woolf SH. Screening for prostate cancer with prostate-specific antigen. An examination of the evidence. *N Engl J Med* 1995;333:1401.
188. Cooner WH, Mosley BR, Rutherford CL Jr, et al. Prostate cancer detection in a clinical urological practice by ultrasonography, digital rectal examination and prostate specific antigen. *J Urol* 1990;143:1146.
189. Catalona WJ, Richie JP, Ahmann FR, et al. Comparison of digital rectal examination and serum prostate specific antigen in the early detection of prostate cancer: results of a multicenter clinical trial of 6,630 men. *J Urol* 1994;151:1283.
190. Ellis WJ, Chetner MP, Preston SD, Brawer MK. Diagnosis of prostatic carcinoma: the yield of serum prostate specific antigen, digital rectal examination and transrectal ultrasonography. *J Urol* 1994;152:1520.
191. Brawer M. Prostate-specific antigen. *CA Cancer J Clin* 1999;49:264.
192. Epstein JI, Walsh PC, Carmichael M, Brendler CB. Pathologic and clinical findings to predict tumor extent of nonpalpable (stage T1c) prostate cancer. *JAMA* 1994;271:368.
193. Carter HB, Epstein JI, Chan DW, Fozard JL, Pearson JD. Recommended prostate-specific antigen testing intervals for the detection of curable prostate cancer. *JAMA* 1997;277:1456.
194. Smith DS, Catalona WJ, Herschman JD. Longitudinal screening for prostate cancer with prostate-specific antigen. *JAMA* 1996;276:1309.
195. Benson MC, Whang IS, Pantuck A, et al. Prostate specific antigen density: a means of distinguishing benign prostatic hypertrophy and prostate cancer. *J Urol* 1992;147:815.
196. Stamey TA, Kabalin JN, McNeal JE, et al. Prostate specific antigen in the diagnosis and treatment of adenocarcinoma of the prostate: II. Radical prostatectomy treated patients. *J Urol* 1989;141:1076.
197. Seaman E, Whang M, Olsson CA, et al. PSA density (PSAD). Role in patient evaluation and management. *Urol Clin North Am* 1993;20:653.
198. Catalona WJ, Richie JP, deKernion JB, et al. Comparison of prostate specific antigen concentration versus prostate specific antigen density in the early detection of prostate cancer: receiver operating characteristic curves. *J Urol* 1994;152:2031.
199. Brawer MK, Aramburu EA, Chen GL, Preston SD, Ellis WJ. The inability of prostate specific antigen index to enhance the predictive value of prostate specific antigen in the diagnosis of prostatic carcinoma. *J Urol* 1993;150:369.
200. Kalish J, Cooner WH, Graham SD Jr. Serum PSA adjusted for volume of transition zone (PSAT) is more accurate than PSA adjusted for total gland volume (PSAD) in detecting adenocarcinoma of the prostate. *Urology* 1994;43:601.
201. Zlotta A, Djavan B, Marberger M, Schulman C. Prostate specific antigen density of the transition zone: a new effective parameter for prostate cancer prediction. *J Urol* 1997;157:1315.
202. Oesterling JE, Cooner WH, Jacobsen SJ, Guess HA, Lieber MM. Influence of patient age on the serum PSA concentration. An important clinical observation. *Urol Clin North Am* 1993;20:671.
203. Carter HB, Pearson JD, Waclawiw Z, et al. Prostate-specific antigen variability in men without prostate cancer: effect of sampling interval on prostate-specific antigen velocity. *Urology* 1995;45:591.
204. Carter HB, Pearson JD. Prostate-specific antigen velocity and repeated measures of prostate-specific antigen. *Urol Clin North Am* 1997;24:333.
205. Christensson A, Bjork T, Nilsson O, et al. Serum prostate specific antigen complexed to alpha 1-antichymotrypsin as an indicator of prostate cancer. *J Urol* 1993;150:100.
206. Catalona WJ, Smith DS, Wolfert RL, et al. Evaluation of percentage of free serum prostate-specific antigen to improve specificity of prostate cancer screening. *JAMA* 1995;274:1214.

207. Partin AW, Catalona WJ, Southwick PC, et al. Analysis of percent free prostate-specific antigen (PSA) for prostate cancer detection: influence of total PSA, prostate volume, and age. *Urology* 1996;48:55.
208. Catalona WJ, Smith DS, Ornstein DK. Prostate cancer detection in men with serum PSA concentrations of 2.6 to 4.0 ng/mL and benign prostate examination. Enhancement of specificity with free PSA measurements. *JAMA* 1997;277:1452.
209. Chen YT, Luderer AA, Thiel RP, et al. Using proportions of free to total prostate-specific antigen, age, and total prostate-specific antigen to predict the probability of prostate cancer. *Urology* 1996;47:518.
210. Luderer AA, Chen YT, Soriano TF, et al. Measurement of the proportion of free to total prostate-specific antigen improves diagnostic performance of prostate-specific antigen in the diagnostic gray zone of total prostate-specific antigen. *Urology* 1995;46:187.
211. Bangma CH, Rietbergen JB, Kranse R, et al. The free-to-total prostate specific antigen ratio improves the specificity of prostate specific antigen in screening for prostate cancer in the general population. *J Urol* 1997;157:2191.
212. Elgamal AA, Cornillie FJ, Van Poppel HP, et al. Free-to-total prostate specific antigen ratio as a single test for detection of significant stage T1c prostate cancer. *J Urol* 1996;156: 1042.
213. Prestigiacomo AF, Lilja H, Pettersson K, Wolfert RL, Stamey TA. A comparison of the free fraction of serum prostate specific antigen in men with benign and cancerous prostates: the best case scenario. *J Urol* 1996;156:350.
214. Gann PH, Hennekens CH, Stampfer MJ. A prospective evaluation of plasma prostate-specific antigen for detection of prostatic cancer. *JAMA* 1995;273:289.
215. Vashi AR, Wojno KJ, Henricks W, et al. Determination of the "reflex range" and appropriate cutpoints for percent free prostate-specific antigen in 413 men referred for prostatic evaluation using the AxSYM system. *Urology* 1997;49:19.
216. Carter HB, Partin AW, Luderer AA, et al. Percentage of free prostate-specific antigen in sera predicts aggressiveness of prostate cancer a decade before diagnosis. *Urology* 1997;49:379.
217. Woodrum D, French C, Shamel LB. Stability of free prostate-specific antigen in serum samples under a variety of sample collection and sample storage conditions. *Urology* 1996;48:33.
218. Brawer M, Daum P, Petteway J, Werner M. Assay variability in serum prostate specific antigen determination. *Prostate* 1995;26:1.
219. Nixon R, Meyer G, Blase A, et al. Comparison of 3 investigational assays for the free form of prostate specific antigen. *J Urol* 1998;160:420.
220. Brawer M, Meyer G, Letran J. Measurement of complexed PSA improves specificity for early detection of prostate cancer. *Urology* 1998;52:372.
221. Sokoll L, Bruzek D, Cox J, et al. Is complexed PSA alone clinically useful? *J Urol* 1998;159:234.
222. Babaian RJ, Fritsche HA, Zhang Z, et al. Evaluation of prostAsure index in the detection of prostate cancer: a preliminary report. *Urology* 1998;51:132.
223. Hodge KK, McNeal JE, Terris MK, Stamey TA. Random systematic versus directed ultrasound guided transrectal core biopsies of the prostate. *J Urol* 1989;142:71.
224. Hodge KK, McNeal JE, Stamey TA. Ultrasound guided transrectal core biopsies of the palpably abnormal prostate. *J Urol* 1989;142:66.
225. Chang JJ, Shinohara K, Bhargava V, Presti JC Jr. Prospective evaluation of lateral biopsies of the peripheral zone for prostate cancer detection. *J Urol* 1998;160:2111.
226. Eskew LA, Bare RL, McCullough DL. Systematic 5 region prostate biopsy is superior to sextant method for diagnosing carcinoma of the prostate. *J Urol* 1997;157:199.
227. Norberg M, Egevad L, Holmberg L, et al. The sextant protocol for ultrasound-guided core biopsies of the prostate underestimates the presence of cancer. *Urology* 1997;50:562.
228. Terris MK, Pham TQ, Issa MM, Kabalin JN. Routine transition zone and seminal vesicle biopsies in all patients undergoing transrectal ultrasound guided prostate biopsies are not indicated. *J Urol* 1997;157:204.
229. Chang JJ, Shinohara K, Hovcy RM, Montgomery C, Presti JC Jr. Prospective evaluation of systematic sextant transition zone biopsies in large prostates for cancer detection. *Urology* 1998;52:89.
230. Bazinet M, Karakiewicz PI, Aprikian AG, et al. Value of systematic transition zone biopsies in the early detection of prostate cancer. *J Urol* 1996;155:605.
231. Fleshner NE, Fair WR. Indications for transition zone biopsy in the detection of prostatic carcinoma. *J Urol* 1997;157:556.
232. Durkan GC, Greene DR. Elevated serum prostate specific antigen levels in conjunction with an initial prostatic biopsy negative for carcinoma: who should undergo a repeat biopsy? *BJU Int* 1999;83:34.
233. Fogarty KT, Arger PH, Shibutani Y, et al. Follow-up of benign hypoechoic peripheral zone lesions of the prostate gland: US characteristics and cancer prevalence. *Radiology* 1994;191:69.
234. Babaian RJ, Grunow WA. Reliability of Gleason grading system in comparing prostate biopsies with total prostatectomy specimens. *Urology* 1985;25:564.
235. Bostwick DG. Gleason grading of prostatic needle biopsies. Correlation with grade in 316 matched prostatectomies. *Am J Surg Pathol* 1994;18:796.
236. Thickman D, Speers WC, Philpott PJ, Shapiro H. Effect of the number of core biopsies of the prostate on predicting Gleason score of prostate cancer. *J Urol* 1996;156:110.
237. Huland H, Hammerer P, Henke RP, Huland E. Preoperative prediction of tumor heterogeneity and recurrence after radical prostatectomy for localized prostatic carcinoma with digital rectal, examination prostate specific antigen and the results of 6 systematic biopsies. *J Urol* 1996;155:1344.
238. D'Amico AV, Whittington R, Malkowicz SB, et al. Combined modality staging of prostate carcinoma and its utility in predicting pathologic stage and postoperative prostate specific antigen failure. *Urology* 1997;49:23.
239. Borirakchanyavat S, Bhargava V, Shinohara K, et al. Systematic sextant biopsies in the prediction of extracapsular extension at radical prostatectomy. *Urology* 1997;50:373.
240. Presti JC Jr, Shinohara K, Bacchetti P, Tigrani V, Bhargava V. Positive fraction of systematic biopsies predicts risk of relapse after radical prostatectomy. *Urology* 1998;52:1079.
241. Wills ML, Sauvageot J, Partin AW, Gurganus R, Epstein JI. Ability of sextant biopsies to predict radical prostatectomy stage. *Urology* 1998;51:759.
242. Enlund AL, Varenhorst E. Morbidity of ultrasound-guided transrectal core biopsy of the prostate without prophylactic antibiotic therapy. A prospective study in 415 cases. *Br J Urol* 1997;79:777.
243. Rietbergen JB, Kruger AE, Kranse R, Schroder FH. Complications of transrectal ultrasound-guided systematic sextant biopsies of the prostate: evaluation of complication rates and risk factors within a population-based screening program. *Urology* 1997;49:875.
244. Rodriguez LV, Terris MK. Risks and complications of transrectal ultrasound guided prostate needle biopsy: a prospective study and review of the literature. *J Urol* 1998;160:2115.
245. Labrie F, Candas B, Dupont A, et al. Screening decreases prostate cancer death: first analysis of the 1988 Quebec prospective randomized controlled trial. *Prostate* 1999;38:83.
246. Jacobsen SJ, Bergstralh EJ, Katusic SK, et al. Screening digital rectal examination and prostate cancer mortality: a population-based case-control study. *Urology* 1998;52:173.
247. Roberts RO, Bergstralh EJ, Katusic SK, Lieber MM, Jacobsen SJ. Decline in prostate cancer mortality from 1980 to 1997, and an update on incidence trends in Olmsted County, Minnesota. *J Urol* 1999;161:529.
248. Federman D, Goyal S, Kamina A, Peduzzi P, Concato J. Informed consent for PSA screening: Does it happen? *Effect Clin Pract* 1999;2:152.
249. Kindrick AV, Grossfeld GD, Stier DM, et al. Use of imaging tests for staging newly diagnosed prostate cancer: trends from the CaPSURE database. *J Urol* 1998;160:2102.
250. Lee CT, Oesterling JE. Using prostate-specific antigen to eliminate the staging radionuclide bone scan. *Urol Clin North Am* 1997;24:389.
251. Oesterling JE, Martin SK, Bergstralh EJ, Lowe FC. The use of prostate-specific antigen in staging patients with newly diagnosed prostate cancer. *JAMA* 1993;269:57.
252. Levran Z, Gonzalez JA, Diokno AC, Jafri SZ, Steinert BW. Are pelvic computed tomography, bone scan and pelvic lymphadenectomy necessary in the staging of prostatic cancer? *Br J Urol* 1995;75:778.
253. Gleave ME, Coupland D, Drachenberg D, et al. Ability of serum prostate-specific antigen levels to predict normal bone scans in patients with newly diagnosed prostate cancer. *Urology* 1996;47:708.
254. Wolf JS Jr, Cher M, Dall'era M, et al. The use and accuracy of cross-sectional imaging and fine needle aspiration cytology for detection of pelvic lymph node metastases before radical prostatectomy. *J Urol* 1995;153:993.
255. Rees MA, Resnick MI, Oesterling JE. Use of prostate-specific antigen, Gleason score, and digital rectal examination in staging patients with newly diagnosed prostate cancer. *Urol Clin North Am* 1997;24:379.
256. Kahn D, Williams RD, Seldin DW, et al. Radioimmunoscintigraphy with ^{111}Indium labeled CYT-356 for the detection of occult prostate cancer recurrence. *J Urol* 1994; 152:1490.
257. Hinkle GH, Burgers JK, Neal CE, et al. Multicenter radioimmunoscintigraphic evaluation of patients with prostate carcinoma using indium-111 capromab pendetide. *Cancer* 1998;83:739.
258. Manyak MJ, Hinkle GH, Olsen JO, et al. Immunoscintigraphy with indium-111-capromab pendetide: evaluation before definitive therapy in patients with prostate cancer. *Urology* 1999;54:1058.
259. Tsuda K, Yu KK, Coakley FV, et al. Detection of extracapsular extension of prostate cancer: role of fat suppression endorectal MRI. *J Comput Assist Tomogr* 1999;23:74.
260. Yu KK, Scheidler J, Hricak H, et al. Prostate cancer: prediction of extracapsular extension with endorectal MR imaging and three-dimensional proton MR spectroscopic imaging. *Radiology* 1999;213:481.
261. Scheidler J, Hricak H, Vigneron DB, et al. Prostate cancer: localization with three-dimensional proton MR spectroscopic imaging—clinicopathologic study. *Radiology* 1999;213:473.
262. Kupelian PA, Katcher J, Levin HS, Klein EA. Stage T1-2 prostate cancer: a multivariate analysis of factors affecting biochemical and clinical failures after radical prostatectomy. *Int J Radiat Oncol Biol Phys* 1997;37:1043.
263. Narayan P, Gajendran V, Taylor SP, et al. The role of transrectal ultrasound-guided biopsy-based staging, preoperative serum prostate-specific antigen, and biopsy Gleason score in prediction of final pathologic diagnosis in prostate cancer. *Urology* 1995;46:205.
264. Oesterling JE. Prostate specific antigen: a critical assessment of the most useful tumor marker for adenocarcinoma of the prostate. *J Urol* 1991;145:907.
265. Partin AW, Kattan MW, Subong EN, et al. Combination of prostate-specific antigen, clinical stage, and Gleason score to predict pathological stage of localized prostate cancer. A multi-institutional update. *JAMA* 1997;277:1445.
266. Kleer E, Larson-Keller JJ, Zincke H, Oesterling JE. Ability of preoperative serum prostate-specific antigen value to predict pathologic stage and DNA ploidy. Influence of clinical stage and tumor grade. *Urology* 1993;41:207.
267. Kleer E, Oesterling JE. PSA and staging of localized prostate cancer. *Urol Clin North Am* 1993;20:695.
268. Kattan MW, Eastham JA, Stapleton AM, Wheeler TM, Scardino PT. A preoperative nomogram for disease recurrence following radical prostatectomy for prostate cancer. *J Natl Cancer Inst* 1998;90:766.
269. Yu KK, Hricak H, Grossfeld GD, Carroll PR. Prediction of patient outcome after radical prostatectomy by imaging: choice of outcome measure. *Acad Radiol* 1998;5[Suppl 2]:S347.
270. D'Amico AV, Schnall M, Whittington R, et al. Endorectal coil magnetic resonance imaging identifies locally advanced prostate cancer in select patients with clinically localized disease. *Urology* 1998;51:449.
271. D'Amico AV, Chang E, Garnick M, et al. Assessment of prostate cancer volume using endorectal coil magnetic resonance imaging: a new predictor of tumor response to neoadjuvant androgen suppression therapy. *Urology* 1998;51:287.
272. Bolla M, Gonzalez D, Warde P, et al. Improved survival in patients with locally advanced prostate cancer treated with radiotherapy and goserelin. *N Engl J Med* 1997;337:295.
273. Epstein JI, Pound CR, Partin AW, Walsh PC. Disease progression following radical prostatectomy in men with Gleason score 7 tumor. *J Urol* 1998;160:97.
274. Epstein JI. The role of perineural invasion and other biopsy characteristics as prognostic markers for localized prostate cancer. *Semin Urol Oncol* 1998;16:124.

275. Hanks GE, Hanlon AL, Schultheiss TE, et al. Dose escalation with 3D conformal treatment: five year outcomes, treatment optimization, and future directions. *Int J Radiat Oncol Biol Phys* 1998;41:501.
276. Hanks GE. Strategies for improving the outcome of patients with poor prognosis prostate cancers. *Acta Oncol* 1998;37:5.
277. Hanks GE, Hanlon AL, Pinover WH, Horwitz EM, Schultheiss TE. Survival advantage for prostate cancer patients treated with high-dose three-dimensional conformal radiotherapy. *Cancer J Sci Am* 1999;5:152.
278. Litwin MS, Lubeck DP, Henning JM, Carroll PR. Differences in urologist and patient assessments of health related quality of life in men with prostate cancer: results of the CaPSURE database. *J Urol* 1998;159:1988.
279. Pound CR, Partin AW, Eisenberger MA, et al. Natural history of progression after PSA elevation following radical prostatectomy. *JAMA* 1999;281:1591.
280. Critz FA, Levinson AK, Williams WH, Holladay DA, Holladay CT. The PSA nadir that indicates potential cure after radiotherapy for prostate cancer. *Urology* 1997;49:322.
281. Panel A. Consensus statement: guidelines for PSA following radiation therapy. *Int J Radiat Oncol Biol Phys* 1997;37:1035.
282. Egawa S, Go M, Kuwao S, et al. Long-term impact of conservative management on localized prostate cancer. A twenty-year experience in Japan. *Urology* 1993;42:520.
283. Rana A, Chisholm GD, Khan M, Rashwan HM, Elton RA. Conservative management with symptomatic treatment and delayed hormonal manipulation is justified in men with locally advanced carcinoma of the prostate. *Br J Urol* 1994;74:637.
284. George NJ. Natural history of localised prostatic cancer managed by conservative therapy alone. *Lancet* 1988;1:494.
285. Adolfsson J, Carstensen J. Natural course of clinically localized prostate adenocarcinoma in men less than 70 years old. *J Urol* 1991;146:96.
286. Warner J, Whitmore WF Jr. Expectant management of clinically localized prostatic cancer. *J Urol* 1994;152:1761.
287. Adolfsson J, Steineck G, Hedlund PO. Deferred treatment of clinically localized low-grade prostate cancer: actual 10-year and projected 15-year follow-up of the Karolinska series. *Urology* 1997;50:722.
288. Johansson JK, Holmberg L, Johansson S, Bergstrom R, Adami HO. Fifteen-year survival in prostate cancer: a prospective population-based study in Sweden. *JAMA* 1997;277:467.
289. Adolfsson J, Steineck G, Hedlund PO. Deferred treatment of locally advanced nonmetastatic prostate cancer: a long-term followup. *J Urol* 1999;161:505.
290. Albertsen PC, Fryback DG, Storer BE, Kolon TF, Fine J. Long-term survival among men with conservatively treated localized prostate cancer. *JAMA* 1995;274:626.
291. Aus G, Hugosson J, Norlen L. Long-term survival and mortality in prostate cancer treated with noncurative intent. *J Urol* 1995;154:460.
292. Hugosson J, Aus G, Bergdahl C, Bergdahl S. Prostate cancer mortality in patients surviving more than 10 years after diagnosis. *J Urol* 1995;154:2115.
293. Gronberg H, Damber L, Jonson H, Damber JE. Prostate cancer mortality in northern Sweden, with special reference to tumor grade and patient age. *Urology* 1997;49:374.
294. Stattin P, Bergh A, Karlberg L, Tavelin B, Damber JE. Long-term outcome of conservative therapy in men presenting with voiding symptoms and prostate cancer. *Eur Urol* 1997;32:404.
295. Brasso K, Friis S, Juel K, Jorgensen T, Iversen P. Mortality of patients with clinically localized prostate cancer treated with observation for 10 years or longer: a population based registry study. *J Urol* 1999;161:524.
296. Byar DP, Corle DK. VACURG randomized trial of radical prostatectomy for stages I and II prostate cancer. *Urology* 1981;17[Suppl]:7.
297. Chodak GW, Thisted RA, Gerber GS, et al. Results of conservative management of clinically localized prostate cancer. *N Engl J Med* 1994;330:242.
298. Adolfsson J. Deferred treatment of low grade stage T3 prostate cancer without distant metastases. *J Urol* 1993;149:326.
299. Albertsen PC, Hanley JA, Gleason DF, Barry MJ. Competing risk analysis of men aged 55 to 74 years at diagnosis managed conservatively for clinically localized prostate cancer. *JAMA* 1998;280:975.
300. Guillonneau B, Vallancien G. Laparoscopic radical prostatectomy: the Montsouris experience. *J Urol* 2000;163:418.
301. Guillonneau B, Vallancien G. Laparoscopic radical prostatectomy: the Montsouris technique. *J Urol* 2000;163:1643.
302. Bishoff JT, Reyes A, Thompson IM, et al. Pelvic lymphadenectomy can be omitted in selected patients with carcinoma of the prostate: development of a system of patient selection. *Urology* 1995;45:270.
303. Narayan P, Fournier G, Gajendran V, et al. Utility of preoperative serum prostate-specific antigen concentration and biopsy Gleason score in predicting risk of pelvic lymph node metastases in prostate cancer. *Urology* 1994;44:519.
304. Klotz L, Herschorn S. Early experience with intraoperative cavernous nerve stimulation with penile tumescence monitoring to improve nerve sparing during radical prostatectomy. *Urology* 1998;52:537.
305. Klotz L. Advances in nerve sparing for radical prostatectomy. *Urology* 1999;54:956.
306. Trapasso JG, deKernion JB, Smith RB, Dorey F. The incidence and significance of detectable levels of serum prostate specific antigen after radical prostatectomy. *J Urol* 1994; 152:1821.
307. Zincke H, Oesterling JE, Blute ML, et al. Long-term (15 years) results after radical prostatectomy for clinically localized (stage T2c or lower) prostate cancer. *J Urol* 1994;152:1850.
308. Blute ML, Bostwick DG, Seay TM, et al. Pathologic classification of prostate carcinoma: the impact of margin status. *Cancer* 1998;82:902.
309. Badalament RA, Miller MC, Peller PA, et al. An algorithm for predicting nonorgan confined prostate cancer using the results obtained from sextant core biopsies with prostate specific antigen level. *J Urol* 1996;156:1375.
310. Medini E, Medini I, Reddy PK, Levitt SH. Delayed/salvage radiation therapy in patients with elevated prostate specific antigen levels after radical prostatectomy. A long term follow-up. *Cancer* 1996;78:1254.
311. Eulau SM, Tate DJ, Stamey TA, Bagshaw MA, Hancock SL. Effect of combined transient androgen deprivation and irradiation following radical prostatectomy for prostatic cancer. *Int J Radiat Oncol Biol Phys* 1998;41:735.
312. Do T, Parker RG, Do C, et al. Salvage radiotherapy for biochemical and clinical failures following radical prostatectomy. *Cancer J Sci Am* 1998;4:324.
313. Ditonno P, Battaglia M, Selvaggi FP. Adjuvant hormone therapy after radical prostatectomy: indications and results. *Tumori* 1997;83:567.
314. Sokoll LJ, Chan DW. Prostate-specific antigen. Its discovery and biochemical characteristics. *Urol Clin North Am* 1997;24:253.
315. Lange P, Ercole CJ, Lightner D, et al. The value of serum prostate specific antigen determinations before and after radical prostatectomy. *J Urol* 1989;141:873.
316. Stein A, deKernion JB, Smith RB, Dorey F, Patel H. Prostate specific antigen levels after radical prostatectomy in patients with organ confined and locally extensive prostate cancer. *J Urol* 1992;147:942.
317. Safa AA, Reese DM, Carter DM, et al. Undetectable serum prostate-specific antigen associated with metastatic prostate cancer: a case report and review of the literature. *Am J Clin Oncol* 1998;21:323.
318. Catalona WJ, Smith DS. 5-year tumor recurrence rates after anatomical radical retropubic prostatectomy for prostate cancer. *J Urol* 1994;152:1837.
319. Partin AW, Pound CR, Clemens JQ, Epstein JI, Walsh PC. Serum PSA after anatomic radical prostatectomy. The Johns Hopkins experience after 10 years. *Urol Clin North Am* 1993;20:713.
320. Ohori M, Abbas F, Wheeler TM, et al. Pathological features and prognostic significance of prostate cancer in the apical section determined by whole mount histology. *J Urol* 1999;161:500.
321. Iselin CE, Box JW, Vollmer RT, et al. Surgical control of clinically localized prostate carcinoma is equivalent in African-American and white males. *Cancer* 1998;83:2353.
322. Pound CR, Partin AW, Epstein JI, Walsh PC. Prostate-specific antigen after anatomic radical retropubic prostatectomy. Patterns of recurrence and cancer control. *Urol Clin North Am* 1997;24:395.
323. Epstein JI, Partin AW, Sauvageot J, Walsh PC. Prediction of progression following radical prostatectomy. A multivariate analysis of 721 men with long-term follow-up. *Am J Surg Pathol* 1996;20:286.
324. Patel A, Dorey F, Franklin J, deKernion JB. Recurrence patterns after radical retropubic prostatectomy: clinical usefulness of prostate specific antigen doubling times and log slope prostate specific antigen. *J Urol* 1997;158:1441.
325. Catalona WJ, Carvalhal GF, Mager DE, Smith DS. Potency, continence and complication rates in 1,870 consecutive radical retropubic prostatectomies. *J Urol* 1999;162:433.
326. Goluboff ET, Saidi JA, Mazer S, et al. Urinary continence after radical prostatectomy: the Columbia experience. *J Urol* 1998;159:1276.
327. Bishoff JT, Motley G, Optenberg SA, et al. Incidence of fecal and urinary incontinence following radical perineal and retropubic prostatectomy in a national population. *J Urol* 1998;160:454.
328. Mathewson-Chapman M. Pelvic muscle exercise/biofeedback for urinary incontinence after prostatectomy: an education program. *J Cancer Educ* 1997;12:218.
329. Chang PL, Tsai LH, Huang ST, et al. The early effect of pelvic floor muscle exercise after transurethral prostatectomy. *J Urol* 1998;160:402.
330. Kerr LA, Zincke H. Radical retropubic prostatectomy for prostate cancer in the elderly and the young: complications and prognosis. *Eur Urol* 1994;25:305.
331. Heathcote PS, Mactaggart PN, Boston RJ, et al. Health-related quality of life in Australian men remaining disease-free after radical prostatectomy. *Med J Aust* 1998;168:483.
332. Ojdeby G, Claezon A, Brekkan E, Haggman M, Norlen BJ. Urinary incontinence and sexual impotence after radical prostatectomy. *Scand J Urol Nephrol* 1996;30:473.
333. Dore B, Gremmo E, Ingrand P, et al. Simplified vesico-urethral anastomosis after radical retropubic prostatectomy for cancer. A preliminary comparative study. *J Urol* 1995;101:113.
334. Gray M, Petroni GR, Theodorescu D. Urinary function after radical prostatectomy: a comparison of the retropubic and perineal approaches. *Urology* 1999;53:881.
335. Haab F, Trockman BA, Zimmern PE, Leach GE. Quality of life and continence assessment of the artificial urinary sphincter in men with minimum 3.5 years of followup. *J Urol* 1997;158:435.
336. Huland H. The risks outweigh the benefits of radical prostatectomy in localised prostate cancer: the argument against. *Eur Urol* 1996;29:31.
337. Smith DN, Appell RA, Rackley RR, Winters JC. Collagen injection therapy for post-prostatectomy incontinence. *J Urol* 1998;160:364.
338. Schaeffer AJ, Clemens JQ, Ferrari M, Stamey TA. The male bulbourethral sling procedure for post-radical prostatectomy incontinence. *J Urol* 1998;159:1510.
339. Walsh PC, Donker PJ. Impotence following radical prostatectomy: insight into etiology and prevention. *J Urol* 1982;128:492.
340. Walsh PC, Partin AW, Epstein JI. Cancer control and quality of life following anatomical radical retropubic prostatectomy: results at 10 years. *J Urol* 1994;152:1831.
341. Talcott JA, Rieker P, Propert KJ, et al. Patient-reported impotence and incontinence after nerve-sparing radical prostatectomy. *J Natl Cancer Inst* 1997;89:1117.
342. Litwin MS, Hays RD, Fink A, et al. Quality-of-life outcomes in men treated for localized prostate cancer. *JAMA* 1995;273:129.
343. Zippe CD, Kedia AW, Kedia K, Nelson DR, Agarwal A. Treatment of erectile dysfunction after radical prostatectomy with sildenafil citrate (Viagra). *Urology* 1998;52:963.
344. Lowentritt BH, Scardino PT, Miles BJ, et al. Sildenafil citrate after radical retropubic prostatectomy. *J Urol* 1999;162:1614.
345. Gleave ME, Sato N, Goldenberg SL, et al. Neoadjuvant androgen withdrawal therapy decreases local recurrence rates following tumor excision in the Shionogi tumor model. *J Urol* 1997;157:1727.
346. Fair WR, Cookson MS, Stroumbakis N, et al. The indications, rationale, and results of neoadjuvant androgen deprivation in the treatment of prostatic cancer: Memorial Sloan-Kettering Cancer Center results. *Urology* 1997;49:46.

347. Soloway MS, Sharifi R, Wajsman Z, et al. Randomized prospective study comparing radical prostatectomy alone versus radical prostatectomy preceded by androgen blockade in clinical stage B2 (T2bNxM0) prostate cancer. The Lupron Depot Neoadjuvant Prostate Cancer Study Group. *J Urol* 1995;154:424.
348. Goldenberg SL, Klotz LH, Srigley J, et al. Randomized, prospective, controlled study comparing radical prostatectomy alone and neoadjuvant androgen withdrawal in the treatment of localized prostate cancer. Canadian Urologic Oncology Group. *J Urol* 1996;156:873.
349. Klotz LH, Goldenberg SL, Jewett M, et al. CUOG randomized trial of neoadjuvant androgen ablation before radical prostatectomy: 36-month post-treatment PSA results. Canadian Urologic Oncology Group. *Urology* 1999;53:757.
350. Gleave ME, Goldenberg SL, Jones EC, et al. Optimal duration of neoadjuvant androgen withdrawal therapy before radical prostatectomy in clinically confined prostate cancer. *Semin Urol Oncol* 1996;14:39.
351. Gleave ME, Goldenberg SL, Jones EC, Bruchovsky N, Sullivan LD. Biochemical and pathological effects of 8 months of neoadjuvant androgen withdrawal therapy before radical prostatectomy in patients with clinically confined prostate cancer. *J Urol* 1996;155:213.
352. Partin AW, Piantadosi S, Sanda MG, et al. Selection of men at high risk for disease recurrence for experimental adjuvant therapy following radical prostatectomy. *Urology* 1995;45:831.
353. Bauer JJ, Connelly RR, Seterhenn IA, et al. Biostatistical modeling using traditional preoperative and pathological prognostic variables in the selection of men at high risk for disease recurrence after radical prostatectomy for prostate cancer. *J Urol* 1998;159:929.
354. D'Amico A, Whittington R, Schultz D, et al. Outcome based staging for clincally localized adenocarcinoma of the prostate. *J Urol* 1997;158:1422.
355. Kattan MW, Wheeler TM, Scardino PT. Postoperative nomogram for disease recurrence after radical prostatectomy for prostate cancer. *J Clin Oncol* 1999;17:1499.
356. Ohori M, Wheeler TM, Kattan MW, Goto Y, Scardino PT. Prognostic significance of positive surgical margins in radical prostatectomy specimens. *J Urol* 1995;154:1818.
357. Paulson DF. Impact of radical prostatectomy in the management of clinically localized disease. *J Urol* 1994;152:1826.
358. Watson RB, Civantos F, Soloway MS. Positive surgical margins with radical prostatectomy: detailed pathological analysis and prognosis. *Urology* 1996;48:80.
359. D'Amico AV, Whittington R, Malkowicz SB, et al. A multivariate analysis of clinical and pathological factors that predict for prostate specific antigen failure after radical prostatectomy for prostate cancer. *J Urol* 1995;154:131.
360. McCarthy JF, Catalona WJ, Hudson MA. Effect of radiation therapy on detectable serum prostate specific antigen levels following radical prostatectomy: early versus delayed treatment. *J Urol* 1994;151:1575.
361. Coetzee LJ, Hars V, Paulson DF. Postoperative prostate-specific antigen as a prognostic indicator in patients with margin-positive prostate cancer, undergoing adjuvant radiotherapy after radical prostatectomy. *Urology* 1996;47:232.
362. Petrovich Z, Lieskovsky G, Freeman J, et al. Surgery with adjuvant irradiation in patients with pathologic stage C adenocarcinoma of the prostate. *Cancer* 1995;76:1621.
363. Zietman AL, Coen JJ, Shipley WU, Althausen AF. Adjuvant irradiation after radical prostatectomy for adenocarcinoma of prostate: analysis of freedom from PSA failure. *Urology* 1993;42:292.
364. Syndikus I, Pickles T, Kostashuk E, Sullivan LD. Postoperative radiotherapy for stage pT3 carcinoma of the prostate: improved local control. *J Urol* 1996;155:1983.
365. Freeman JA, Lieskovsky G, Cook DW, et al. Radical retropubic prostatectomy and postoperative adjuvant radiation for pathological stage C (PcN0) prostate cancer from 1976 to 1989: intermediate findings. *J Urol* 1993;149:1029.
366. Gibbons RP, Cole BS, Richardson RG, et al. Adjuvant radiotherapy following radical prostatectomy: results and complications. *J Urol* 1986;135:65.
367. Epstein JI. Incidence and significance of positive margins in radical prostatectomy specimens. *Urol Clin North Am* 1996;23:651.
368. Lowe BA, Lieberman SF. Disease recurrence and progression in untreated pathologic stage T3 prostate cancer: selecting the patient for adjuvant therapy. *J Urol* 1997;158:1452.
369. Grossfeld GD, Tigrani VS, Nudell D, et al. Management of a positive surgical margin after radical prostatectomy: decision analysis. *J Urol* 2000 (*in press*).
370. Hammerer P, Huland H. Systematic sextant biopsies in 651 patients referred for prostate evaluation. *J Urol* 1994;151:99.
371. Oesterling JE, Jacobsen SJ, Chute CG, et al. Serum prostate-specific antigen in a community-based population of healthy men. Establishment of age-specific reference ranges. *JAMA* 1993;270:860.
372. Morgan TO, Jacobsen SJ, McCarthy WF, et al. Age-specific reference ranges for prostate-specific antigen in black men. *N Engl J Med* 1996;335:304.
373. Oesterling JE, Kumamoto Y, Tsukamoto T, et al. Serum prostate-specific antigen in a community-based population of healthy Japanese men: lower values than for similarly aged white men. *Br J Urol* 1995;75:347.
374. Welch HG, Albertsen PC, Nease RF, Bubolz TA, Wasson JH. Estimating treatment benefits for the elderly: the effect of competing risks. *Ann Intern Med* 1996;124:577.
375. Ebert T, Schmitz-Drager BJ, Burrig KF, et al. Accuracy of imaging modalities in staging the local extent of prostate cancer. *Urol Clin North Am* 1991;18:453.
376. Engeler CE, Wasserman NF, Zhang G. Preoperative assessment of prostatic carcinoma by computerized tomography. Weaknesses and new perspectives. *Urology* 1992;40:346.
377. Platt JF, Bree RL, Schwab RE. The accuracy of CT in the staging of carcinoma of the prostate. *AJR Am J Roentgenol* 1987;149:315.
378. Salo JO, Kivisaari L, Rannikko S, Lehtonen T. Computerized tomography and transrectal ultrasound in the assessment of local extension of prostatic cancer before radical retropubic prostatectomy. *J Urol* 1987;137:435.
379. Bates TS, Gillatt DA, Cavanagh PM, Speakman M. A comparison of endorectal magnetic resonance imaging and transrectal ultrasonography in the local staging of prostate cancer with histopathological correlation. *Br J Urol* 1997;79:927.
380. Presti JC Jr, Hricak H, Narayan PA, et al. Local staging of prostatic carcinoma: comparison of transrectal sonography and endorectal MR imaging. *AJR Am J Roentgenol* 1996;166:103.
381. Deasy NP, Conry BG, Lewis JL, et al. Local staging of prostate cancer with 0.2 T body coil MRI. *Clin Radiol* 1997;52:933.
382. Tuzel E, Sevinc M, Obuz F, Sade M, Kirkali Z. Is magnetic resonance imaging necessary in the staging of prostate cancer? *Urol Int* 1998;61:227.
383. Rorvik J, Halvorsen OJ, Albrektsen G, et al. MRI with an endorectal coil for staging of clinically localised prostate cancer prior to radical prostatectomy. *Eur Radiol* 1999;9:29.
384. Ikonen S, Karkkainen P, Kivisaari L, et al. Magnetic resonance imaging of clinically localized prostatic cancer. *J Urol* 1998;159:915.
385. Bates TS, Cavanagh PM, Speakman M, Gillatt DA. Endorectal MRI using a 0.5 T mid-field system in the staging of localized prostate cancer. *Clin Radiol* 1996;51:550.
386. Perrotti M, Kaufman RP Jr, Jennings TA, et al. Endo-rectal coil magnetic resonance imaging in clinically localized prostate cancer: Is it accurate? *J Urol* 1996;156:106.
387. Bartolozzi C, Menchi I, Lencioni R, et al. Local staging of prostate carcinoma with endorectal coil MRI: correlation with whole-mount radical prostatectomy specimens. *Eur Radiol* 1996;6:339.
388. Sheu MH, Wang JH, Chen KK, Chiang H, Teng MH. Prostate cancer: local staging with endorectal magnetic resonance imaging. *Chung Hua I Hsueh Tsa Chih (Taipei)* 1998; 61:243.
389. Anderson PR, Hanlon AL, Patchefsky A, Al-Saleem T, Hanks GE. Perineural invasion and Gleason 7-10 tumors predict increased failure in prostate cancer patients with pretreatment PSA <10 ng/ml treated with conformal external beam radiation therapy. *Int J Radiat Oncol Biol Phys* 1998;41:1087.
390. Bluestein DL, Bostwick DG, Bergstralh EJ, Oesterling JE. Eliminating the need for bilateral pelvic lymphadenectomy in select patients with prostate cancer. *J Urol* 1994;151:1315.
391. D'Amico AV, Whittington R, Malkowicz SB, et al. A multivariable analysis of clinical factors predicting for pathological features associated with local failure after radical prostatectomy for prostate cancer. *Int J Radiat Oncol Biol Phys* 1994;30:293.
392. D'Amico AV, Whittington R, Malkowicz SB, et al. Role of percent positive biopsies and endorectal coil MRI in predicting prognosis in intermediate-risk prostate cancer patients. *Cancer J Sci Am* 1996;2:343.
393. Gerber G, Thisted R, Chodak G, et al. Results of radical prostatectomy in men with locally advanced prostate cancer: multi-insititutional pooled analysis. *Eur Urol* 1997;32:385.
394. Green GA, Hanlon AL, Al-Saleem T, Hanks GE. A Gleason score of 7 predicts a worse outcome for prostate carcinoma patients treated with radiotherapy. *Cancer* 1998;83:971.
395. Hanks GE, Lee WR, Schultheiss TE. Clinical and biochemical evidence of control of prostate cancer at 5 years after external beam radiation. *J Urol* 1995;154:456.
396. Kuban DA, el-Mahdi AM, Schellhammer PF. Prostate-specific antigen for pretreatment prediction and posttreatment evaluation of outcome after definitive irradiation for prostate cancer. *Int J Radiat Oncol Biol Phys* 1995;32:307.
397. Roach M 3rd, Lu J, Pilepich MV, et al. Long-term survival after radiotherapy alone: radiation therapy oncology group prostate cancer trials. *J Urol* 1999;161:864.
398. Schellhammer PF, el-Mahdi AM, Kuban DA, Wright GL Jr. Prostate-specific antigen after radiation therapy. Prognosis by pretreatment level and post-treatment nadir. *Urol Clin North Am* 1997;24:407.
399. Zagars GK, Pollack A, Kavadi VS, von Eschenbach AC. Prostate-specific antigen and radiation therapy for clinically localized prostate cancer. *Int J Radiat Oncol Biol Phys* 1995;32:293.
400. Zagars GK, Ayala AG, von Eschenbach AC, Pollack A. The prognostic importance of Gleason grade in prostatic adenocarcinoma: a long-term follow-up study of 648 patients treated with radiation therapy. *Int J Radiat Oncol Biol Phys* 1995;31:237.
401. Zincke H, Bergstralh EJ, Blute ML, et al. Radical prostatectomy for clinically localized prostate cancer: long-term results of 1,143 patients from a single institution. *J Clin Oncol* 1994;12:2254.
402. Hudson MA, Catalona WJ. Effect of adjuvant radiation therapy on prostate specific antigen following radical prostatectomy. *J Urol* 1990;143:1174.
403. Schild SE, Buskirk SJ, Wong WW, et al. The use of radiotherapy for patients with isolated elevation of serum prostate specific antigen following radical prostatectomy. *J Urol* 1996;156:1725.
404. Wu JJ, King SC, Montana GS, McKinstry CA, Anscher MS. The efficacy of postprostatectomy radiotherapy in patients with an isolated elevation of serum prostate-specific antigen. *Int J Radiat Oncol Biol Phys* 1995;32:317.
405. Morris MM, Dallow KC, Zietman AL, et al. Adjuvant and salvage irradiation following radical prostatectomy for prostate cancer. *Int J Radiat Oncol Biol Phys* 1997;38:731.
406. Forman JD, Meetze K, Pontes E, et al. Therapeutic irradiation for patients with an elevated post-prostatectomy prostate specific antigen level. *J Urol* 1997;158:1436.
407. Cadeddu JA, Partin AW, DeWeese TL, Walsh PC. Long-term results of radiation therapy for prostate cancer recurrence following radical prostatectomy. *J Urol* 1998;159:173.
408. vander Kooy MJ, Pisansky TM, Cha SS, Blute ML. Irradiation for locally recurrent carcinoma of the prostate following radical prostatectomy. *Urology* 1997;49:65.
409. Bagshaw MA, Kaplan HS, Sagerman RH. Linear accelerator supervoltage therapy: VII. Carcinoma of the prostate. *Radiology* 1965;85:121.
410. Ray GR, Cassady JR, Bagshaw MA. Definitive radiation therapy of carcinoma of the prostate: a report of 15 years experience. *Radiology* 1973;106:407.
411. Hanks GE, Asbell S, Krall JM, et al. Outcome for lymph node dissection negative T1-b, T2 (A2,B) prostate cancer treated with external beam radiation therapy in RTOG 77-06. *Int J Radiat Oncol Biol Phys* 1991;21:1099.
412. Perez CA, Hanks GE, Leibel SA, et al. Localized carcinoma of the prostate (stages T1B, T1C, T2, and T3). Review of management with external beam radiation therapy. *Cancer* 1993;72:3156.
413. Horwitz EM, Hanlon AL, Hanks GE. Update on the treatment of prostate cancer with external beam irradiation. *Prostate* 1998;37:195.

414. Shipley WU, Thames HD, Sandler HM, et al. Radiation therapy for clinically localized prostate cancer. A multi-institutional pooled analysis. *JAMA* 1999;281:1598.
415. Zelefsky MJ, Leibel SA, Gaudin PB, et al. Dose escalation with three-dimensional conformal radiation therapy affects the outcome in prostate cancer. *Int J Radiat Oncol Biol Phys* 1988;41:491.
416. Ten Haken RK, Perez-Tamayo C, Tesser RJ, et al. Boost treatment of the prostate using shaped fixed fields. *Int J Radiat Oncol Biol Phys* 1989;16:193.
417. Lawton CA, Won M, Pilepich MV, et al. Long-term treatment sequelae following external beam irradiation for adenocarcinoma of the prostate: analysis of RTOG studies 7506 and 7706. *Int J Radiat Oncol Biol Phys* 1991;21:935.
418. Leibel SA, Hanks GE, Kramer S. Patterns of care outcomes studies: results of the national practice in adenocarcinoma of the prostate. *Int J Radiat Oncol Biol Phys* 1984;10:401.
419. Smit WGJM, Helle PA, Van Putte WLJ, et al. Late radiation damage in prostate cancer patients treated by high dose external radiotherapy in relation to rectal dose. *Int J Radiat Oncol Biol Phys* 1990;18:23.
420. Hanks GE, Martz KL, Diamond JJ. The effect of dose on local control of prostate cancer. *Int J Radiat Oncol Biol Phys* 1988;15:1299.
421. Fuks Z, Leibel SA, Kutcher GJ, Mohan R, Ling CC. Three dimensional conformal treatment: a new frontier in radiation therapy. In: DeVita VT Jr, Hellman S, Rosenberg SA, eds. *Important advances in oncology.* Philadelphia: JB Lippincott Co, 1991:151.
422. Munzenrider JE, Pilepich M, Rene-Ferrero JB, Tchakarova I, Carter BL. Use of body scanner in radiotherapy treatment planning. *Cancer* 1979;40:170.
423. Goitein M. The utility of computed tomography in radiation therapy: an estimate of outcome. *Int J Radiat Oncol Biol Phys* 1979;5:1799.
424. Zelefsky MJ, Leibel SA, Kutcher GJ, et al. The feasibility of dose escalation with three-dimensional conformal radiotherapy in patients with prostatic carcinoma. *Cancer J Sci Am* 1995;1:42.
425. Forman JD, Duclos M, Shamsa F, Porter AT, Orton C. Hyperfractionated conformal radiotherapy in locally advanced prostate cancer: results of a dose escalation study. *Int J Radiat Oncol Biol Phys* 1996;34:655.
426. Roach M 3rd, Meehan S, Kroll S, et al. Radiotherapy for high grade clinically localized adenocarcinoma of the prostate. *J Urol* 1996;156:1719.
427. Pollack A, Zagars GK. External beam radiotherapy dose response of prostate cancer. *Int J Radiat Oncol Biol Phys* 1997;39:1011.
428. Hanks GE, Hanlon AL, Pinover WH, Horwitz EM, Schultheiss TE. Survival advantage for prostate cancer patients treated with high-dose three-dimensional conformal radiotherapy. *Cancer J Sci Am* 1999;5:152.
429. Hanks GE, Hanlon AL, Schultheiss TE, et al. Dose escalation with 3D conformal treatment: five year outcomes, treatment optimization, and future directions. *Int J Radiat Oncol Biol Phys* 1998;41:501.
430. Porter EH. The statistical dose-cure relationships for irradiated tumors. *Br J Radiol* 1980;53:336.
431. Hendry JH, Moore JV. Is the steepness of dose-incidence curves for tumour control or complications due to variation before or as a result of irradiation? *Br J Radiol* 1984;57:1045.
432. Roberts SA, Hendry JH. A realistic closed-form radiobiological model of clinical tumor-control data incorporating intertumor heterogeneity. *Int J Radiat Oncol Biol Phys* 1998;41:689.
433. Zagars GK, Schultheiss TE, Peters LP. Inter-tumor heterogeneity and radiation dose control curves. *Radiother Oncol* 1987;8:353.
434. Thames HD, Schultheiss TE, Hendry JH, et al. Can modest escalations of dose be detected as increased tumor control? *Int J Radiat Oncol Biol Phys* 1994;22:241.
435. Moore JV, Hendry JH, Hunter RD. Dose-incidence curves for tumour control and normal tissue injury, in relation to the response of clonogenic cells. *Radiother Oncol* 1983;1:143.
436. Thames HD Jr, Peters LJ, Spanos WS Jr, Fletcher GF. Dose response of squamous cell carcinomas of the upper respiratory and digestive tracts. *Br J Cancer* 1980;41[Suppl 4]:35.
437. Metz CE, Tokars RP, Kronman HB, Griem ML. Maximum likelihood estimation of dose-response parameters for therapeutic operating characteristic (TOC) analysis of carcinoma of the nasopharynx. *Int J Radiat Oncol Biol Phys* 1982;8:1185.
438. Harwood AR, Beale FA, Cummings BJ, et al. Supraglottic laryngeal carcinoma: an analysis of dose-time-volume factors in 410 patients. *Int J Radiat Oncol Biol Phys* 1983;9:311.
439. Peters LJ, Fletcher GH. Causes of failure of radiotherapy in head and neck cancer. *Radiother Oncol* 1983;1:53.
440. Williams MV, Denekamp J, Fowler JF. Dose-response relationships for human tumors: implications for clinical trials of dose modifying agents. *Int J Radiat Oncol Biol Phys* 1984;10:1703.
441. Fowler JF. Potential for increasing the differential response between tumors and normal tissues: can proliferation rate be used? *Int J Radiat Oncol Biol Phys* 1986;12:641.
442. Leibel SA, Fuks Z, Zelefsky MJ, et al. The treatment of localized prostate cancer with three-dimensional conformal and intensity modulated radiation therapy at the Memorial Sloan-Kettering Cancer Center. In: Purdy J, Grant W III, Palta J, Butler B, Perez C, eds. *3D conformal radiation therapy and intensity modulated radiation therapy in the next millennium.* Madison, WI: Advanced Medical Publishing (*in press*).
443. Scardino PT, Wheeler TM. Local control of prostate cancer with radiotherapy: frequency and prognostic significance of positive results of post-irradiation biopsy. *Natl Cancer Inst Monogr* 1988;7:95.
444. Kuban DA, El-Mahdi AM. Local control after radiation for prostatic carcinoma: significance and assessment. *Semin Radiat Oncol* 1993;3:221.
445. Crook JM, Bahadur YA, Robertson SJ, Perry GA, Esche BA. Valuation of radiation effect, tumor differentiation, and prostate specific antigen staining in sequential prostate biopsies after external beam radiotherapy for patients with prostate carcinoma. *Cancer* 1997;79:81.
446. Laverdiere J, Gomez JL, Cusan L, et al. Beneficial effect of combination hormonal therapy administered prior and following external beam radiation therapy in localized prostate cancer. *Int J Radiat Oncol Biol Phys* 1997; 37:247.
447. Consensus Statements on Radiation Therapy of Prostate Cancer. Guidelines for prostate re-biopsy after radiation and for radiation therapy with rising prostate-specific antigen levels after radical prostatectomy. *J Clin Oncol* 1999;17:1155.
448. Willett CG, Zietman AL, Shipley WU, Coen JJ. The effect of pelvic radiation therapy on serum levels of prostate specific antigen. *J Urol* 1994;151:1579.
449. Zietman AL, Coen JJ, Shipley WU, Willett CG, Efird JT. Radical radiation therapy in the management of prostatic adenocarcinoma: the initial prostate specific antigen value as a predictor of treatment outcome. *J Urol* 1994;151:640.
450. Zelefsky MJ, Leibel SA, Wallner KE, Whitmore WF Jr, Fuks Z. The significance of normal serum PSA in the follow-up after definitive radiation therapy for prostatic cancer. *J Clin Oncol* 1995; 13:459.
451. Consensus Statement: Guidelines for PSA following radiation therapy. American Society for Therapeutic Radiology and Oncology Consensus Panel. *Int J Radiat Oncol Biol Phys* 1997;37:1035.
452. Kavadi VS, Zagars GK, Pollack A. Serum prostate-specific antigen after radiation therapy for clinically localized prostate cancer: prognostic implications. *Int J Radiat Oncol Biol Phys* 1994;30:279.
453. Schellhammer PF, el-Mahdi AM, Wright GL Jr, Kolm P, Ragle R. Prostate-specific antigen to determine progression-free survival after radiation therapy for localized carcinoma of prostate. *Urology* 1993;42:1320.
454. Shipley WU, Thames HD, Sandler HM, et al. Radiation therapy for clinically localized prostate cancer: a multi-institutional pooled analysis. *JAMA* 1999;281:1598.
455. Byar DP, Mostofi FK. Carcinoma of the prostate: prognostic evaluation of certain pathologic features in 208 radical prostatectomies examined by the step-section technique. *Cancer* 1972;30:5.
456. Stamey TA, Villers AA, McNeal JE, Link PC, Freiha FS. Positive surgical margins at radical prostatectomy: importance of the apical dissection. *J Urol* 1990;143:1166.
457. Catalona WJ, Bigg SW. Nerve-sparing radical prostatectomy: evaluation of results after 250 patients. *J Urol* 1990;143:538.
458. Walsh PC. Radical prostatectomy, preservation of sexual function, cancer control: the controversy. *Urol Clin North Am* 1987;14:663.
459. ICRU Report 50. *Prescribing, recording, and reporting photon beam therapy.* Bethesda: International Commission on Radiation Units and Measurements, 1993.
460. Kutcher GJ, Mageras GS, Leibel SA. Control, correction. and modeling of setup errors and organ motion. *Semin Radiat Oncol* 1995;5:134.
461. Barzell W, Beam MA, Hilaris BS, Whitmore WF. Prostatic adenocarcinoma: relationship of grade and local extent to the pattern of metastases. *J Urol* 1977;118:278.
462. Fowler JE, Whitmore WE. The incidence and extent of pelvic lymph node metastases in apparently localized prostatic cancer. *Cancer* 1981;47:2941.
463. Donahue RE, Mani JH, Whitesel JA, et al. Pelvic lymph node dissection: guide to patient management in clinically locally confined adenocarcinoma of the prostate. *Urology* 1982;20:559.
464. Bagshaw MA. A technique for external beam radiotherapy of carcinoma of the prostate. In: Levitt SH, Tapley NV, eds. *Technological basis of radiotherapy: practical clinical applications.* Philadelphia: Lea & Febiger, 1984:244.
465. McGowan DG. The value of extended field radiation therapy in carcinoma of the prostate. *Int J Radiat Oncol Biol Phys* 1981;7:1333.
466. Ploysongsang SS, Aron BS, Shehata WM. Radiation therapy in prostate cancer: Whole pelvis with prostate boost or small field to prostate? *Urology* 1992;40:18.
467. Seaward SA, Weinberg V, Lewis P, et al. Improved freedom from PSA failure with whole pelvic irradiation for high-risk prostate cancer. *Int J Radiat Oncol Biol Phys* 1998;42:1055.
468. Roach M 3rd, Marquez C, Yuo HS, et al. Predicting the risk of lymph node involvement using the pre-treatment prostate specific antigen and Gleason score in men with clinically localized prostate cancer. *Int J Radiat Oncol Biol Phys* 1994;28(1):33.
469. Bagshaw MA. Radiotherapetic treatment of prostatic carcinoma with pelvic node involvement. *Urol Clin North Am* 1984;2:297.
470. Spaas PG, Bagshaw MA, Cox RS. The volume of extended field irradiation in surgically staged carcinoma of the prostate. *Int J Radiat Oncol Biol Phys* 1988;15:Sl.
471. Zagars GK, von Eschenbach AC, Johnson DE, Oswald MJ. Stage C adenocarcinoma of the prostate: an analysis of 551 patients treated with external beam radiation. *Cancer* 1987; 60:1489.
472. Rosen E, Cassady JR, Connolly J, Chaffey JT. Radiotherapy for prostate carcinoma: the JCRT experience (1968–1978) II. Factors related to tumor control and complications. *Int J Radiat Oncol Biol Phys* 1985;11:725.
473. Aristizabal SA, Steinbronn D, Heusinkveld RS. External beam radiotherapy in cancer of the prostate: the University of Arizona experience. *Radiother Oncol* 1984;1:309.
474. Perez AA, Pilepich MV, Zivnuska F. Tumor control in definitive irradiation of localized carcinoma of the prostate. *Int J Radiat Oncol Biol Phys* 1986;12:523.
475. Asbell SO, Krall JM, Pilepich MV, et al. Elective pelvic irradiation in stage A2, B carcinoma of the prostate: analysis of RTOG 77-06. *Int J Radiat Oncol Biol Phys* 1988;15:1307.
476. Asbell SO, Caplan RJ, Perez CA, et al. Impact of surgical staging on evaluating the radiotherapeutic outcome in RTOG #77-06. A phase III study for T1b-T2N0M0 prostatic carcinoma. *Int J Radiat Oncol Biol Phys* 1995;32:S1.
477. Bagshaw MA, Kaplan ID, Cox RC. Radiation therapy for localized disease. *Cancer* 1993;71:939.
478. Zelefsky MJ, Happersett L, Leibel SA, et al. The effect of treatment positioning on normal tissue dose in patients with prostate cancer treated with three-dimensional conformal radiotherapy. *Int J Radiat Oncol Biol Phys* 1997;37:13.
479. Leibel SA, Kutcher GJ, Mohan R, et al. Three-dimensional conformal radiation therapy at the Memorial Sloan-Kettering Cancer Center. *Semin Radiat Oncol* 1992; 2:274.
480. Zelefsky MJ, Crean D, Mageras GS, et al. Quantification and predictors of prostate position variability in 50 patients evaluated with multiple CT scans during conformal radiotherapy. *Radiother Oncol* 1999;50:225.

481. Goitein M, Abrams M, Rowell D, Pollari H, Wiles J. Multi-dimensional treatment planning: II. Beam's eye-view, back projection, and projection through CT sections. *Int J Radiat Oncol Biol Phys* 1983;9:789.
482. Leibel SA, Zelefsky MJ, Kutcher GJ, et al. Three-dimensional conformal radiation therapy in localized carcinoma of the prostate: interim report of a phase I dose-escalation study. *J Urol* 1994;152:1792.
483. Drzymala RE, Mohan R, Brewster L, et al. Dose-volume histograms. *Int J Radiat Oncol Biol Phys* 1991;21:71.
484. ICRU Report 50. *Prescribing, recording, and reporting photon beam therapy.* Bethesda: International Commission on Radiation Units and Measurements, 1993.
485. Zelefsky MJ, Lebiel SA, Burman CM, et al. Neoadjuvant hormonal therapy improves the therapeutic ration in patients with bulky prostatic cancer treated with three-dimensional conformal radiation therapy. *Int J Radiat Oncol Biol Phys* 1994;29:755.
486. Soffen EM, Hanks GE, Hunt MA, Epstein BE. Conformal static field radiation therapy treatment of early prostate cancer versus non-conformal techniques: a reduction in acute morbidity. *Int J Radiat Oncol Biol Phys* 1992;24:485.
487. Zelefsky MJ, Ginor RX, Fuks Z, Leibel SA. Efficacy of selective alpha1 blocker therapy in the treatment of acute urinary symptoms during radiotherapy for localized prostate cancer. *Int J Radiat Oncol Biol Phys* 1999;45:567.
488. Teshima T, Hanks GE, Hanlon AL, Peter RS, Schultheiss TE. Rectal bleeding after conformal 3D treatment of prostate cancer: time to occurrence, response to treatment and duration of morbidity. *Int J Radiat Oncol Biol Phys* 1997;39:77.
489. Lawton CA, Wong M, Pilepich MV, et al. Long-term treatment sequelae following external beam irradiation for adenocarcinoma of the prostate: analysis of RTOG studies 7506 and 7706. *Int J Radiat Oncol Biol Phys* 1991;21:935.
490. Leibel SA, Hanks GE, Kramer S. Patterns of care outcomes studies: results of the national practice in adenocarcinoma of the prostate. *Int J Radiat Oncol Biol Phys* 1984;10:401.
491. Sandler HM, McLaughlin PW, Ten Haken RK, et al. Three dimensional conformal radiotherapy for the treatment of prostate cancer: low risk of chronic rectal morbidity observed in a large series of patients. *Int J Radiat Oncol Biol Phys* 1995;33:797.
492. Schultheiss TE, Lee WR, Hunt MA, et al. Late GI and GU complications in the treatment of prostate cancer. *Int J Radiat Oncol Biol Phys* 1997;37:3.
493. Benk VA, Adams JA, Shipley WU, et al. Late rectal bleeding following combined x-ray and proton high dose irradiation for stages T3-T4 prostate cancer. *Int J Radiat Oncol Biol Phys* 1993;26:551.
494. Lee WR, Hanks GE, Hanlon AL, Schultheiss TE, Hunt MA. Lateral rectal shielding reduces late rectal morbidity following high dose three-dimensional conformal radiation therapy for clinically localized prostate cancer: further evidence for a significant dose effect. *Int J Radiat Oncol Biol Phys* 1996;35:251.
495. Hanks GE, Schultheiss TE, Hunt MA, Epstein B. Factors influencing incidence of acute grade 2 morbidity in conformal and standard radiation treatment of prostate cancer. *Int J Radiat Oncol Biol Phys* 1995;31:25.
496. Dearnaley DP, Khoo VS, Norman AR, et al. Comparison of radiation side-effects of conformal and conventional radiotherapy in prostate cancer: a randomised trial. *Lancet* 1999;353:267.
497. Zelefsky MJ, Fuks Z, Happersett L, et al. Clinical experience with intensity modulated radiation therapy (IMRT) in prostate cancer. *Radiother Oncol* 1999 (*in press*).
498. Bagshaw MA, Cox RS, Ray GR. Status of radiation treatment of prostate cancer at Stanford University. *Natl Cancer Inst Monogr* 1988;7:4760.
499. Banker FL. The preservation of potency after external beam irradiation for prostate cancer. *Int J Radiat Oncol Biol Phys* 1991;15:219.
500. Shipley WU, Zietman AL, Hanks GE, et al. Treatment related sequelae following external beam radiation for prostate cancer: a review with an update in patients with stages TI and T2 tumor. *J Urol* 1994;152:1799.
501. Zelefsky MJ, Eid JF. Elucidating the etiology of erectile dysfunction after definitive therapy for prostatic cancer. *Int J Radiat Oncol Biol Phys* 1998;40:129.
502. Pierce LJ, Whittington R, Hanno PM, et al. Pharmacologic erection with intracavernosal injection for men with sexual dysfunction following irradiation: a preliminary report. *Int J Radiat Oncol Biol Phys* 1991;21:1311.
503. Zelefsky MJ, McKee AB, Lee H, Leibel SA. Efficacy of oral sildenafil in patients with erectile dysfunction after radiotherapy for carcinoma of the prostate. *Urology* 1999;53:775.
504. Coleman CN, Beard CJ, Kantoff PW, Gelman R. Rate of relapse following treatment for localized prostate cancer: a critical analysis of retrospective reports. *Int J Radiat Oncol Biol Phys* 1994;28:303.
505. Hanks GE, Krall JM, Hanlon AL, et al. Patterns of care and RTOG studies in prostate cancer: long-term survival, hazard rate observations, and possibilities of cure. *Int J Radiat Oncol Biol Phys* 1994;28:39.
506. Zietman AL, Shipley WU. Randomized trials in loco-regionally confined prostate cancer: past, present and future. *Semin Radiat Oncol* 1993;3:210.
507a. Perez CA, Lee HK, Georgiou A, et al. Technical and tumor-related factors affecting outcome of definitive irradiation for localized carcinoma of the prostate. *Int J Radiat Oncol Biol Phys* 1993;26:581.
507b. Zagars GK, von Eschenbach AC, Johnson DE, Oswald MJ. The role of radiation therapy in stages A2 and B adenocarcinoma of the prostate. *Int J Radiat Oncol Biol Phys* 1988;14:701.
508. Zietman AL, Shipley WU, Willett GC. Residual disease after radical surgery or radiation therapy for prostate cancer. Clinical significance and therapeutic implications. *Cancer* 1993;71:959.
509. Pollack A, Zagars GK, Kavadi VS. Prostate-specific antigen doubling time and disease relapse after radiotherapy for prostate cancer. *Cancer* 1994;74:670.
510. Zagars GK. Prostate-specific antigen as an outcome variable for TI and T2 prostate cancer treated by radiation therapy. *J Urol* 1994;152:1786.
511. Zagars GK, Pollack A, von Eschenbach AC. Prostate cancer and radiation therapy—the message conveyed by serum prostate-specific antigen. *Int J Radiat Oncol Biol Phys* 1995;33:23.
512. Kupelian P, Katcher J, Levin H, et al. Eternal beam radiotherapy versus radical prostatectomy for clinical stage T1-2 prostate cancer: therapeutic implications of stratification by pretreatment PSA levels and biopsy Gleason scores. *Cancer J Sci Am* 1997;3:78.
513. Hanks GE, Hanlon AL, Pinover WH, Horwitz EM, Schultheiss TE. Survival advantage for prostate cancer patients treated with high-dose three-dimensional conformal radiotherapy. *Cancer J Sci Am* 1999;5:152.
514. Roach M 3rd, Meehan S, Kroll S, et al. Radiotherapy for high grade clinically localized adenocarcinoma of the prostate. *J Urol* 1996;156:1719.
515. Zagars GK, Pollack A, von Eschenbach AC. Prognostic factors for clinically localized prostate carcinoma: analysis of 938 patients irradiated in the prostate specific antigen era. *Cancer* 1997;79:1370.
516. Pollack A, Zagars GK, Smith LG, Antolak JA, Rosen II. Preliminary results of a randomized dose escalation study comparing 70 Gy to 78 Gy for the treatment of prostate cancer. *Int J Radiat Oncol Biol Phys* 1999;45:146.
517. Green N, Bodner H, Broth E, et al. Improved control of bulky prostate carcinoma with sequential estrogen and radiation therapy. *Int J Radiat Oncol Biol Phys* 1984;10:971.
518. Sandler HM, Perez-Tamayo C, Ten Haken RK, Lichter AS. Dose escalation for stage C (T3) prostate cancer: minimal rectal toxicity observed using conformal therapy. *Radiother Oncol* 1992;23:53.
519. Zelefsky MJ, Lebiel SA, Burman CM, et al. Neoadjuvant hormonal therapy improves the therapeutic ration in patients with bulky prostatic cancer treated with three-dimensional conformal radiation therapy. *Int J Radiat Oncol Biol Phys* 1994;29:755.
520. Laverdiere J, Gomez JL, Cusan L, et al. Beneficial effect of combination hormonal therapy administered prior and following external beam radiation therapy, in localized prostate cancer. *Int J Radiat Oncol Biol Phys* 1997;37:247.
521. Pilepich MV, Krall JM, al-Sarraf M, et al. Androgen deprivation with radiation therapy compared with radiation therapy alone for locally advanced prostatic carcinoma: a randomized comparative trial of the Radiation Therapy Oncology Group. *Urology* 1995;45:616.
522. Pilepich MV, Caplan R, Byhardt RW, et al. Phase III trial of androgen suppression using goserelin in unfavorable prognosis carcinoma of the prostate treated with definitive radiotherapy: report of Radiation Therapy Oncology Group Protocol 85-31. *J Clin Oncol* 1997;15:1013.
523. Bolla M, Gonzalez D, Warde P, et al. Improved survival in patients with locally advanced prostate cancer treated with radiotherapy and goserelin. *N Engl J Med* 1997;337:295.
524. Pollack A, Zagars GK. Androgen ablation in addition to radiation therapy for prostate cancer: Is there true benefit? *Semin Radiat Oncol* 1998;8(2):95.
525. Whitmore WF Jr, Hilaris B, Grabstald H. Retropubic implantation of iodine 125 in the treatment of prostatic cancer. *J Urol* 1972;108:918.
526. Wallner K, Chiu-tsao ST, Roy J, et al. An improved method for computerized tomography–planned transperineal 125 iodine prostate implants. *J Urol* 1991;146:90.
527. Blasko JC, Ragde H, Grimm PD. Transperineal ultrasound-guided implantation of the prostate: morbidity and complications. *Scand J Urol Nephrol Suppl* 1991;137:113.
528. Seyed NAM, Puthawala A, Austin P, et al. Temporary iridium 192 implant in the management of carcinoma of the prostate. *Cancer* 1992;69:2515.
529. Kuban DA, EL-Mahdi AM, Schellhammer PF. I-125 interstitial implantation for prostate cancer. What have we learned in 10 years? *Cancer* 1989;69:2515.
530. Fuks Z, Leibel SA, Wallner KE, et al. The effect of local control on metastatic dissemination in carcinoma of the prostate: long-term results in patients treated with ^{125}I implantation. *Int J Radiat Oncol Biol Phys* 1991;21:537.
531. Kuban DA, EL-Mahdi AM. Local control after radiation for prostatic carcinoma: significance and assessment. *Semin Radiat Oncol* 1993;3:221.
532. Blasko J, Grimm PD, Ragde H. Brachytherapy and organ preservation in the management of carcinoma of the prostate. *Semin Radiat Oncol* 1993;3:240.
533. Anderson LL. Plan optimization and dose evaluation in brachytherapy. *Semin Radiat Oncol* 1993;3:290.
534. Wallner K, Roy J, Harrison L. Dosimetry guidelines to minimize urethral and rectal morbidity following transperineal I-125 prostate brachytherapy. *Int J Radiat Oncol Biol Phys* 1995;32:465.
535. Blasko JC, Wallner K, Grimm PD, Ragde H. Prostate specific antigen based disease control following ultrasound guided 125 iodine implantation for stage T1/T2 prostatic carcinoma. *J Urol* 1995;154:1096.
536. Priestly JB Jr, Beyer DC. Guided brachytherapy for treatment of confined prostate cancer. *Urology* 1992;40:27.
537. Storey MR, Landgren RC, Cottone JL, et al. Transperineal 125 iodine implantation for treatment of clinically localized prostate cancer: 5-year tumor control and morbidity. *Int J Radiat Oncol Biol Phys* 1999;43:565.
538. Stock RG, Stone NN, Tabert A, Iannuzzi C, DeWyngaert JK. A dose-response study for I-125 prostate implants. *Int J Radiat Oncol Biol Phys* 1998;41:101.
539. Zelefsky MJ, Wallner KE, Ling CC, et al. Comparison of the 5-year outcome and morbidity of three-dimensional conformal radiotherapy versus transperineal permanent iodine-125 implantation for early-stage prostatic cancer. *J Clin Oncol* 1999;17:517.
540. Loening S, Bonney W, Fallon B, et al. Cryotherapy. *Prostate* 1984;5:199.
541. Porter M, Ahaghotu C, Loening S, See W. Disease-free and overall survival after cryosurgical monotherapy for clinical stages B and C carcinoma of the prostate: a 20-year followup. *J Urol* 1997;158:1466.
542. Chang Z, Finkelstein J, Ma H, et al. Development of a high performance multiprobe cryosurgical device. *Biomed Instrum Technol* 1994;28:383.
543. Mazur P. Cryobiology: the freezing of biological systems. *Science* 1970;168:939.
544. Zippe C. Cryosurgical ablation for prostate cancer. *Semin Urol* 1995;13:148.
545. Connolly J, Shinohara K, Presti J, Carroll P. Should cryosurgery be considered a therapeutic option in localized prostate cancer? *Urol Clin North Am* 1996;23:623.
546. Connolly J, Shinohara K, Carroll P. Cryosurgery for locally advanced prostate cancer. *Semin Urol Oncol* 1997;15:244.
547. Shinohara K, Rhee B, Presti J, Carroll P. Cryosurgical ablation of the prostate: patterns of cancer recurrence. *J Urol* 1997;158:2206.

548. Bahn D, Lee F, Solomon H, et al. Prostate cancer: US-guided percutaneous cryoablation. *Radiology* 1995;194:551.
549. Shinohara K, Rhee B, Presti J, Carroll P. Cryosurgical ablation of prostate cancer: patterns of cancer recurrence. *J Urol* 1997;158:2206.
550. Greene G, Pisters L, Scott S, Eschenbach AV. Predictive value of prostate specific antigen nadir following salvage cryotherapy. *J Urol* 1997;157:419A.
551. Long J. Preliminary outcomes following cryosurgical ablation of the prostate in patients with clinically localized prostate carcinoma. *J Urol* 1998;159:477.
552. Koppie TM, Shinohara K, Grossfeld GD, Presti JC Jr, Carroll PR. The efficacy of cryosurgical ablation of prostate cancer: the University of California, San Francisco experience. *J Urol* 1999;162:427.
553. Sosa R, Martin T, Lynn K. Cryosurgical treatment of prostate cancer: a multicenter review of complications. *J Urol* 1996;155:401A.
554. Cespedes R, Pisters L, Eschenbach AV, McGuire E. Long-term followup of incontinence and obstruction after salvage cryosurgical ablation of the prostate: results in 143 patients. *J Urol* 1997;157:237.
555. Grossfeld GD, Stier DM, Flanders SC, et al. Use of second treatment following definitive local therapy for prostate cancer: data from the caPSURE database. *J Urol* 1998;160:1398.
556. Lu-Yao GL, Potosky AL, Albertsen PC, et al. Follow-up prostate cancer treatments after radical prostatectomy: a population-based study. *J Natl Cancer Inst* 1996;88:166.
557. Partin AW, Pearson JD, Landis PK, et al. Evaluation of serum prostate-specific antigen velocity after radical prostatectomy to distinguish local recurrence from distant metastases. *Urology* 1994;43:649.
558. Connolly JA, Shinohara K, Presti JC Jr, Carroll PR. Local recurrence after radical prostatectomy: characteristics in size, location, and relationship to prostate-specific antigen and surgical margins. *Urology* 1996;47:225.
559. Silverman JM, Krebs TL. MR imaging evaluation with a transrectal surface coil of local recurrence of prostatic cancer in men who have undergone radical prostatectomy. *AJR Am J Roentgenol* 1997;168:379.
560. Freitas JE, Gilvydas R, Ferry JD, Gonzalez JA. The clinical utility of prostate-specific antigen and bone scintigraphy in prostate cancer follow-up. *J Nucl Med* 1991;32:1387.
561. Cher ML, Bianco FJ Jr, Lam JS, et al. Limited role of radionuclide bone scintigraphy in patients with prostate specific antigen elevations after radical prostatectomy. *J Urol* 1998;160:1387.
562. Elgamal AA, Troychak MJ, Murphy GP. ProstaScint scan may enhance identification of prostate cancer recurrences after prostatectomy, radiation, or hormone therapy: analysis of 136 scans of 100 patients. *Prostate* 1998;37:261.
563. Schild SE, Buskirk SJ, Wong WW, et al. The use of radiotherapy for patients with isolated elevation of serum prostate specific antigen following radical prostatectomy. *J Urol* 1996;156:1725.
564. Tefilli MV, Gheiler EL, Tiguert R, et al. Quality of life in patients undergoing salvage procedures for locally recurrent prostate cancer. *J Surg Oncol* 1998;69:156.
565. Formenti SC, Lieskovsky G, Simoneau AR, et al. Impact of moderate dose of postoperative radiation on urinary continence and potency in patients with prostate cancer treated with nerve sparing prostatectomy. *J Urol* 1996;155:616.
566. Grossfeld G, Steir D, Flanders S, et al. Use of second treatment following definitive local therapy for prostate cancer: data from the CaPSURE database. *J Urol* 1998;160:1398.
567. Rogers E, Ohori M, Kassabian VS, Wheeler TM, Scardino PT. Salvage radical prostatectomy: outcome measured by serum prostate specific antigen levels . *J Urol* 1995;153: 104.
568. Moul JW, Paulson DF. The role of radical surgery in the management of radiation recurrent and large volume prostate cancer. *Cancer* 1991;68:1265.
569. Amling CL, Lerner SE, Martin SK, et al. Deoxyribonucleic acid ploidy and serum prostate specific antigen predict outcome following salvage prostatectomy for radiation refractory prostate cancer. *J Urol* 1999;161:857.
570. Pisters LL, Perrotte P, Scott SM, Greene GF, von Eschenbach AC. Patient selection for salvage cryotherapy for locally recurrent prostate cancer after radiation therapy. *J Clin Oncol* 1999;17:2514.
571. Grado GL, Collins JM, Kriegshauser JS, et al. Salvage brachytherapy for localized prostate cancer after radiotherapy failure. *Urology* 1999;53:2.
572. Gelet A, Chapelon JY, Bouvier R, Pangaud C, Lasne Y. Local control of prostate cancer by transrectal high intensity focused ultrasound therapy: preliminary results. *J Urol* 1999;161:156.
573. Zlotta AR, Djavan B, Matos C, et al. Percutaneous transperineal radiofrequency ablation of prostate tumour: safety, feasibility and pathological effects on human prostate cancer. *Br J Urol* 1998;81:265.
574. Spitzweg C, Zhang S, Bergert ER, et al. Prostate-specific antigen (PSA) promoter-driven androgen-inducible expression of sodium iodide symporter in prostate cancer cell lines. *Cancer Res* 1999;59(9):2136.
575. Geller J, Albert JD, Nochstein DA, et al. Comparison of prostatic cancer tissue dehydrotestosterone levels at the time of relapse following orchiectomy or estrogen therapy. *J Urol* 1984;132:693.
576. Crawford ED, Eisenberger MA, McLeod DG, et al. A controlled trial of leuprolide with and without flutamide in prostatic carcinoma. *N Engl J Med* 1989;321:419.
577. Bolla M, Gonzalez D, Warde P, et al. Improved survival in patients with locally advanced prostate cancer treated with radiotherapy and goserelin. *N Engl J Med* 1997;337(5):295.
578. Raghavan D. Prostate cancer management under scrutiny: one man's meta-analysis is another man's poisson. *J Clin Oncol* 199917(11):3371.
579. Immediate versus differed treatment for advanced prostatic cancer: initial results of the Medical Research Council trial. Medical Research Council Prostate Cancer Working Party Investigators Group. *Br J Urol* 1997;79:235.
580. Messing EM, Manola J, Sarosdy M, et al. Immediate hormonal therapy compared with observation after radical prostatectomy and pelvic lymphadenectomy in men with node-positive prostate cancer. *N Engl J Med* 1999;341(24):1781.
581. Pound CR, Partin AW, Eisenberger MA, et al. Natural history or progression after PSA elevation following radical prostatectomy. *JAMA* 1999;281(17):1591.
582. Crawford ED, Eisenberger MA, McLeod DG, et al. A controlled trial of leuprolide with and without flutamide in prostatic carcinoma. *N Engl J Med* 1989;321:419.
583. Eisenberger MA, Crawford ED, Wolf M, et al. Prognostic factors in stage D2 prostate cancer: important implications for future trials. Results of a Cooperative Intergroup Study (INT 0036). *Semin Oncol* 1994;21:613.
584. Soloway MS, Hardeman SW, Hickey D, et al. Stratification of patients with metastatic prostate cancer based on extent of disease on initial bone scan. *Cancer* 1988;61:195.
585. Mulders PFA, Dijkman GA, Fernandez del Morel P, et al. Analysis of prognostic factors in disseminated prostatic cancer: an update. *Cancer* 1990;65:2758.
586. De Voogt HJ, Suciu S, Sylvester R, et al. Multivariate analysis of prognostic factors in patients with advanced prostatic cancer: results from 2 European Organization for Research on Treatment of Cancer trials. *J Urol* 1989;141:883.
587. Chodak GW, Vogelzang NJ, Caplan RJ, et al. Independent prognostic factors in patients with metastatic (stage D2) prostate cancer: the Zoladex Study Group. *JAMA* 1991; 265:618.
588. Partin AW, Carter HB, Chan DW, et al. Prostate specific antigen in the staging of localized prostate cancer: influence of tumor differentiation, tumor volume and benign hyperplasia. *J Urol* 1990;143:747.
589. Miller JI, Ahmann FR, Drach GW, et al. Clinical usefulness of serum prostate specific antigen after hormonal therapy of metastatic prostate cancer. *J Urol* 1992;147:956.
590. Matzkin H, Eber P, Todd B, et al. Prognostic significance of changes in prostate-specific markers after endocrine treatment of stage D2 prostatic cancer. *Cancer* 1992;70: 2302.
591. Eisenberger MA, Blumenstein BA, Crawford ED, et al. Bilateral orchiectomy with or without flutamide for metastatic prostate cancer. *N Engl J Med* 1998;339(15):1036.
592. Waxman J, Man A, Hendry WF, et al. Importance of early tumor exacerbation in patients treated with long-acting analogues of gonadotrophin releasing hormone for advanced prostatic cancer. *Br Med J* 1985;291:1387.
593. Thompson IM, Zeidman EJ, Rodriguez FR. Sudden death due to disease flare with luteinizing hormone-releasing hormone agonist therapy for carcinoma of the prostate. *J Urol* 1990;144:1479.
594. Labrie F, Dupont A, Belanger A, Lachance R. Flutamide eliminates the risk of disease flare in prostatic cancer patients treated with a luteinizing hormone-releasing hormone agonist. *J Urol* 1987;138(4):804.
595. Soloway MS, Chodak G, Vogelzang NJ, et al. Zoladex versus orchiectomy in treatment of advanced prostate cancer: a randomized trial. *Urology* 1991;37:46.
596. The Leuprolide Study Group. Leuprolide versus diethylstilbestrol for metastatic prostate cancer. *N Engl J Med* 1984;311:1281.
597. Bonkhoff H, Fixemer T, Hunsicker I, Remberger K. Estrogen receptor expression in prostate cancer and premalignant prostatic lesions. *Am J Pathol* 1999;155(2):641.
598. Byar DP. The Veterans Administration Cooperative Urological Research Group's studies of cancer of the prostate. *Cancer* 1973;32:1126.
599. Shearer RJ, Hendry WF, Sommerville IF, et al. Plasma testosterone: an accurate monitor of hormone treatment of prostatic cancer. *Br J Urol* 1973;45:668.
600. Fleshner NE, Fair WR. Anti-androgenic effects of combination finasteride plus flutamide in patients with prostatic carcinoma. *Br J Urol* 1996;78(6):907.
601. Brufsky A, Fontaine-Rothe P, Berlane K, et al. Finasteride and flutamide as potency-sparing androgen-ablative therapy for advanced adenocarcinoma of the prostate. *Urology* 1997;49(6):913.
602. Chang A, Yeap B, Davis T, et al. Double-blind, randomized study of primary hormonal treatment of stage D2 prostate carcinoma: flutamide versus diethylstilbestrol. *J Clin Oncol* 1996;14(8):2250.
603. Iversen P, Tveter K, Varenhorst E. Randomized study of Casodex 50 MG monotherapy vs. orchiectomy in the treatment of metastatic prostate cancer. The Scandinavian Casodex Cooperative Group. *Scand J Urol Nephrol* 1996;30(2):93.
604. Boccardo F, Rubagotti A, Barichello M, et al. Bicalutamide monotherapy versus flutamide plus goserelin in prostate cancer patients: results of an Italian Prostate Cancer Project study. *J Clin Oncol* 1999;7:2027.
605. Tyrrell CJ, Kaisary AV, Iversen P, et al. A randomised comparison of "Casodex" (bicalutamide) 150 mg monotherapy versus castration in the treatment of metastatic and locally advanced prostate cancer. *Eur Urol* 1998;33(5):447.
606. Agency for Health Care Policy and Research. Relative effectiveness and cost-effectiveness of methods of androgen suppression in the treatment of advanced prostatic cancer. *Evidence Report/Technology Assessment*, no. 4:51, 1999.
607. Labrie F, Dupont A, Belanger A, et al. Combination therapy with flutamide and castration (LHRH agonist or orchiectomy) in advanced prostate cancer: a marked improvement in response and survival. *J Steroid Biochem* 1985;23:833.
608. Crawford ED, Eisenberger MA, Mcleod DG, et al. A controlled trial of leuprolide with or without flutamide in prostatic carcinoma. *N Engl J Med* 1989;321:419.
609. Denis LJ, Keuppens F, Smith PH, et al. Maximal androgen blockade: final analysis of EORTC phase III trial 30853. EORTC genitourinary tract cancer cooperative group and the EORTC data center. *Eur Urol* 1998;33(2):144.
610. Janknegt RA, Abbou CC, Baroletti R, et al. Orchiectomy and nilutamide or placebo as treatment of metastatic prostatic cancer in a multinational double-blind randomized trial. *J Urol* 1993;149:77.
611. Prostate Cancer Trialists' Collaborative Group. Maximum androgen blockade in advanced prostate cancer: an overview of 22 randomized trials with 3283 deaths in 5710 patients. *Lancet* 1995;346(8970):265.
612. Caubet JF, Tosteson TD, Dong EW, et al. Maximum androgen blockade in advanced prostate cancer: a meta-analysis of published randomized controlled trials using nonsteroidal antiandrogens. *Urology* 1997;49(1):71.

613. Agency for Health Care Policy and Research. Relative effectiveness and cost-effectiveness of methods of androgen suppression in the treatment of advanced prostatic cancer. *Evidence Report/Technology Assessment,* no. 4:73.
614. Sandhu SS, Matveev VB, Kaisary AV. Finasteride plus flutamide for prostatic carcinoma. *Br J Urol* 1997;80(2):360.
615. Kirby R, Robertson C, Turkes A, et al. Finasteride in association with either flutamide or goserelin as combination hormonal therapy in patients with stage M1 carcinoma of the prostate gland. International Prostate Health council (IPHC) Trial Study Group. *Prostate* 1999;402(2);105.
616. Kirby R, Robertson C, Turkes A, et al. Finasteride in association with either flutamide or goserelin as combination hormonal therapy in patients with stage M1 carcinoma of the prostate gland. International Prostate Health Council (IPHC) Trial Study Group. *Prostate* 1999;402(2):105.
617. Klotz LH, Herr HW, Morse MJ, Whitmore WF Jr. Intermittent endocrine therapy for advanced prostate cancer. *Cancer* 1986;58(11):2546.
618. Sato N, Gleave ME, Bruchovsky N, et al. Intermittent androgen suppression delays progression to androgen-independent regulation of prostate-specific antigen gene in the LNCaP prostate tumor model. *J Steroid Biochem Mol Biol* 1996;58(2):139.
619. Trachtenberg J. Experimental treatment of prostatic cancer by intermittent hormonal therapy. *J Urol* 1987;137(4):785.
620. Oliver RT, Williams G, Paris AM, Blandy JP. Intermittent androgen deprivation after PSA-complete response as a strategy to reduce induction of hormone-resistant prostate cancer. *Urology* 1997;49(1):79.
621. Goldenberg SL, Bruchovsky N, Gleave ME, Sullivan LD, Akakura K. Intermittent androgen suppression in the treatment of prostate cancer: a preliminary report. *Urology* 1995;45(5):839.
622. Wei JT, Gross M, Jaffe CA, et al. Androgen deprivation therapy for prostate cancer results in significant loss of bone density. *Urology* 1999;54(4):607.
623. Townsend MF, Sanders WH, Northway RO, Graham SD Jr. Bone fractures associated with luteinizing hormone-releasing hormone agonists used in the treatment of prostate carcinoma. *Cancer* 1997;79(3):545.
624. Daniell HW, Dunn SR, Ferguson DW, et al. Progressive osteoporosis during androgen deprivation therapy for prostate cancer. *J Urol* 2000;163(1):181.
625. Fowler JE, Whitmore WF. The response of metastatic adenocarcinoma of the prostate to exogenous testosterone. *J Urol* 1981;126:372.
626. Manni A, Bartholomew M, Caplan R, et al. Androgen priming and chemotherapy in advanced prostate cancer: evaluation of determinants of clinical outcome. *J Clin Oncol* 1988;6:1456.
627. Taylor CD, Elson P, Trump DL. Importance of continued testicular suppression in hormone refractory prostate cancer. *J Clin Oncol* 1993;11:2167.
628. Hussain M, Wolf M, Marshall E, et al. Effects of continued androgen-deprived therapy and other prognostic factors on response and survival in phase II chemotherapy trials for hormone-refractory prostate cancer: a Southwest Oncology Group Report. *J Clin Oncol* 1994;12:1868.
629. Scher HI, Zhang Z-F, Cohen L, et al. Hormonally relapsed prostatic cancer: lessons from the flutamide withdrawal syndrome. *Adv Urol* 1995;8:61.
630. Small EJ, Srinivas S. The antiandrogen withdrawal syndrome: experience in a large cohort of unselected patients with advanced prostate cancer. *Cancer* 1995;76:1428.
631. Figg WD, Sartor O, Cooper MR, et al. Prostate specific antigen decline following the discontinuation of flutamide in patients with stage D2 prostate cancer. *Am J Med* 1995;98:412.
632. Herrada J, Dieringer P, Logothetis CJ. Characterization of patients with androgen-independent prostatic carcinoma whose serum prostate specific antigen decreased following flutamide withdrawal. *J Urol* 1996;155:620.
633. Schellhammer P, Venner P, Haas G, et al. Prostate specific antigen decrease after withdrawal of antiandrogen therapy with bicalutamide or flutamide in patients receiving combined androgen blockade. *J Urol* 1997;157:1731.
634. Nieh PT. Withdrawal phenomenon with the antiandrogen Casodex. *J Urol* 1995;153:1070.
635. Gomella LG, Ismail M, Nathan FE. Antiandrogen withdrawal syndrome with nilutamide. *J Urol* 1997;157:1366.
636. Huan SD, Gerridzen RG, Yau JC, et al. Antiandrogen withdrawal syndrome with nilutamide. *Urology* 1997;49:632.
637. Gaddipati JP, McLeod DG, Heidenberg HB, et al. Frequent detection of codon 877 mutation in the androgen receptor gene in advanced prostate cancers. *Cancer Res* 1994;54:2861.
638. Taplin ME, Bubley GJ, Shuster TD, et al. Mutation of the androgen-receptor gene in metastatic androgen-independent prostate cancer. *N Engl J Med* 1995;332:1393.
639. Tilley WD, Buchanan G, Hickey TE, et al. Mutations in the androgen receptor gene are associated with progression of human prostate cancer to androgen independence. *Clin Cancer Res* 1996;2:277.
640. Figg WD, McCall NA, Reed E, et al. The *in vitro* response of four antisteroid receptor agents on the hormone responsive prostate cancer cell line LNCaP. *Oncol Rep* 1995;2:295.
641. Wilding G, Chen M, Gelman EP. Aberrant response *in vitro* of hormone-responsive prostate cancer cells to antiandrogens. *Prostate* 1989;14:103.
642. Scher HI, Liebertz C, Kelly WK, et al. Bicalutamide for advanced prostate cancer: the natural versus treated history of disease. *J Clin Oncol* 1997;15:2928.
643. Joyce R, Fenton MA, Rode P, et al. High dose bicalutamide for androgen independent prostate cancer: effect of prior hormonal therapy. *J Urol* 1997;159:149.
644. Eastham JA, Sartor O. Nilutamide response after flutamide failure in postorchiectomy progressive prostate cancer. *J Urol* 1998;159:990.
645. Small EJ, Baron AD, Fippin L, et al. Ketoconazole retains activity in advanced prostate cancer patients with progression despite flutamide withdrawal. *J Urol* 1997;4:1204.
646. Kelly WK, Curley T, Leibertz C, et al. Prospective evaluation of hydrocortisone and suramin in patients with androgen-independent prostate cancer. *J Clin Oncol* 1995;13:2208.
647. Tannock I, Osoba D, Stockler M, et al. Chemotherapy with mitoxantrone plus prednisone alone for symptomatic hormone-resistant prostate cancer: a Canadian randomized study with palliative end points. *J Clin Oncol* 1996;14:1756.
648. Kantoff P, Halabi S, Conaway M, et al. Hydrocortisone with or without mitoxantrone in men with hormone-refractory prostate cancer: results of the CALGB 9182 study. *J Clin Oncol* 1999;17:2506.
649. Small EJ, Marshall ME, Reyno L, Meyers F, Natale R. Superiority of suramin + hydrocortisone (S + H) over placebo + hydrocortisone (P + H): results of a multi-center double-blind phase III study in patients with hormone refractory prostate cancer (HRPC). *Am Soc Clin Oncol* 1998;17:308a.
650. Dawson NA, Small EJ, Conaway M, et al. Megestrol acetate (MA) in men with hormone-refractory prostate cancer (HRPC): prostate specific antigen (PSA) response and anti-androgen withdrawal (AAWD). Cancer and Leukemia Group B (CALGB) 9181 [abstract]. *Proc Am Soc Clin Oncol* 1996;15:241.
651. Smith DC, Redman BG, Flaherty LE, et al. A phase II trial of oral diethylstilbestrol as a second-line hormonal agent in advanced prostate cancer. *Urology* 1998;52(2):257.
652. DiPaola RS, Zhang H, Lambert GH, et al. Clinical and biologic activity of an estrogenic herbal combination (PC-SPES) in prostate cancer. *N Engl J Med* 1998;339(12):785.
653. Kameda H, Small EJ, Reese DM, et al. A phase II study of PC-SPES, an herbal compound for the treatment of advanced prostate cancer. *Proc Am Soc Clin Oncol* 1999;18:320a(abst 1230).
654. Myers C, Cooper M, Stein C, et al. Suramin: a novel growth factor antagonist with activity in hormone-refractory metastatic prostate cancer. *J Clin Oncol* 1992;10:881.
655. Kelly WK, Scher HI, Mazumdar M, et al. Prostate specific antigen as a measure of disease outcome in hormone-refractory prostatic cancer. *J Clin Oncol* 1993;11:607.
656. Bubley GJ, Carducci M, Dahut W, et al. Eligibility and response guidelines for phase II clinical trials in androgen-independent prostate cancer: recommendations from the prostate-specific antigen working group. *J Clin Oncol* 1999;11:3461.
657. George DJ, Kantoff PW. Prognostic indicators in hormone refractory prostate cancer. *Urol Clin North Am* 1999;26(2):303.
658. Dewys WD, Begg CB, Brodovsky H, et al. A comparative clinical trial of Adriamycin and 5-Flu-orouracil in advanced prostatic cancer: prognostic factors and response. *Prostate* 1983;4:1.
659. Emrich LJ, Priore RL, Murphy GP, et al. Prognostic factors in patients with advanced prostate cancer. *Cancer Res* 1985;45:5173.
660. Fossa SD, Paus E, Lindegaard M, et al. Prostate-specific antigen and other prognostic factors in patients with hormone-resistant prostate cancer undergoing experimental treatment. *Br J Urol* 1992;69:175.
661. Petrylak DP, Scher HI, Li Z, et al. Prognostic factors for survival of patients with bidimensionally measureable metastatic hormone-refractory prostate cancer treated with single-agent chemotherapy. *Cancer* 1992;70:2870.
662. Langlotz C, Schnall M, Pollack H. Staging of prostate cancer: accuracy of MRI imaging. *Radiology* 1995;194:645.
663. Sridhara R, Eisenberger MA, Sinibaldi VJ, et al. Evaluation of prostate-specific antigen as a surrogate marker for response of hormone-refractory prostate cancer to suramin therapy. *J Clin Oncol* 1995;13:2944.
664. Pienta KJ, Redman B, Hussain M, et al. Phase II evaluation or oral estramustine and oral etoposide in hormone-refractory adenocarcinoma of the prostate. *J Clin Oncol* 1994;12:2005.
665. Smith DC, Dunn RL, Strawderman MS, et al. Change in serum prostate-specific antigen as a marker for response to cytotoxic therapy for hormone-refractory prostate cancer. *J Clin Oncol* 1998;16:1835.
666. Eisenberger MA, Simon R, O'Dwyer PJ, et al. A re-evaluation of nonhormonal cytotoxic chemotherapy in treatment of prostatic carcinoma. *J Clin Oncol* 1985;3:827.
667. Yagoda A, Petrylak D. Cytotoxic chemotherapy for advanced hormone-resistant prostate cancer. *Cancer* 1993;71[Suppl 3]:1098.
668. Benson R, Hartley-Asp B. Mechanisms of action and clinical uses of estramustine. *Cancer Invest* 1990;8(3–4):375.
669. Amato RJ, Ellerhorst J, Bui C, et al. Estramustine and vinblastine for patients with progressive androgen-independent adenocarcinoma of the prostate. *Urol Oncol* 1995;1:168.
670. Seidman AD, Scher HI, Petrylak D, et al. Estramustine and vinblastine: use of prostate specific antigen as a clinical trial end point for hormone refractory prostatic cancer. *J Urol* 1992;147:931.
671. Hudes GR, Greenberg R, Krigel RL, et al. Phase II study of estramustine and vinblastine, two microtubule inhibitors, in hormone-refractory prostate cancer. *J Clin Oncol* 1992;10:1754.
672. Hudes G, Einhorn L, Ross E, et al. Vinblastine versus vinblastine plus oral estramustine phosphate for patients with hormone-refractory prostate cancer: a Hoosier Oncology Group and Fox Chase Network phase III trial. *J Clin Oncol* 1999;17(10):3160.
673. Pienta KJ, Redman BG, Bandekar R, et al. A phase II trial of oral estramustine and oral etoposide in hormone refractory prostate cancer. *Urology* 1997;50:401.
674. Dimopoulos MA, Panopoulos C, Bamia C, et al. Oral estramustine and oral etoposide for hormone refractory prostate cancer. *Urology* 1997;50:754.
675. Cruciani G. Phase II oral estramustine and oral etoposide in hormone refractory adenocarcinoma of the prostate: Instituto Oncologico Romagnolo, Gruppo Onco-Urologico. *Proc Am Soc Clin Oncol* 1998;17:329a.
676. Reese D, Burris H, Belledgrun A, et al. A phase I/II study of navelbine (vinorelbine) and estramustine in the treatment of hormone refractory prostate cancer (HRPC). *Proc Am Soc Clin Oncol* 1996;15:A673[abst].
677. Natale RB, Zarefsky S. Phase I/II trial of estramustine with Taxotere (T) or Vinorelbine (V) in patients (pts) with metastatic hormone refractory prostate cancer. *Proc Am Soc Clin Oncol* 1998;17:338a.
678. Carles J, Domenech M, Gelabert-Mas A, et al. Phase II study of estramustine and vinorelbine in hormone refractory prostate carcinoma patients. *Acta Oncol* 1998;37:187.
679. Roth BJ, Yeap BY, Wilding G, et al. Taxol in advanced, hormone-refractory carcinoma of the prostate: a phase II trial of the Eastern Cooperative Oncology Group. *Cancer* 1993;72:2457.

680. Hudes GR, Nathan F, Khater C, et al. Phase II trial of 96-hour paclitaxel plus oral estramustine phosphate in metastatic hormone refractory prostate cancer. *J Clin Oncol* 1997;15:3156.
681. Picus J, Schultz M. Docetaxel (Taxotere) as monotherapy in the treatment of hormone-refractory prostate cancer: preliminary results. *Semin Oncol* 1999;26[Suppl 17]:14.
682. Petrylak DP, Macarthur RB, O'Connor J, et al. Phase I trial of docetaxel with estramustine in androgen-independent prostate cancer. *J Clin Oncol* 1999;17:958.
683. Kreis W, Budman DR, Fetten J, et al. Phase I trial of the combination of daily estramustine phosphate and intermittent docetaxel in patients with metastatic hormone refractory prostate carcinoma. *Ann Oncol* 1999;10:33.
684. Savarese D, Taplin ME, Halabi S, et al. A phase II study of docetaxel (Taxotere), estramustine, and low-dose hydrocortisone in men with hormone-refractory prostate cancer: preliminary results of cancer and leukemia group B Trial 9780. *Semin Oncol* 1999;26[Suppl 17]:39.
685. Colleoni M, Graiff C, Vicario G, et al. Phase II study of estramustine, oral etoposide, and vinorelbine in hormone refractory prostate cancer. *Am J Clin Oncol* 1997;20:383.
686. Kelly WK, Curley T, Slovin S, et al. Paclitaxel, estramustine phosphate and carboplatin (TEC) in patients with advanced prostate cancer (submitted).
687. Raghaven D, Cox K, Pearson BS, et al. Oral cyclophosphamide for the management of hormone refractory prostate cancer. *Br J Urol* 1993;72:625.
688. Logothetis CJ, Samuels ML, von Eschenbach AC, et al. Doxorubicin, mitomycin-C, and 5-fluorouracil (DMF) in the treatment of metastatic hormonal refractory adenocarcinoma of the prostate, with a note on the staging of metastatic prostate cancer. *J Clin Oncol* 1983;1:368.
689. Blumenstein B, Crawford ED, Saiers JH, et al. Doxorubicin, mitomycin C and 5-fluorouracil in the treatment of hormone refractory adenocarcinoma of the prostate: a Southwest Oncology Group study. *J Urol* 1993;150:411.
690. Laurie JA, Hahn RG, Therneau TM, et al. Chemotherapy for hormonally refractory advanced prostate carcinoma: a comparison of combined versus sequential treatment with mitomycin C, doxorubicin, and 5-fluorouracil. *Cancer* 1992;69:1440.
691. Small EJ, Srinivas S, Egan B, et al. Doxorubicin and dose-escalated cyclophosphamide with granulocyte colony-stimulating factor for the treatment for hormone-resistant prostate cancer. *J Clin Oncol* 1996;14:1617.
692. Sella A. Kilbourn R, Amato R, et al. Phase II study of ketoconazole combined with weekly doxorubicin in patients with androgen-independent prostate cancer. *J Clin Oncol* 1994;12:683.
693. Ellerhorst JS, Tu S-M, Amato RJ, et al. Phase II trial of alternating weekly chemohormonal therapy for patients with androgen-independent prostate cancer. *Clin Cancer Res* 1997;3:2371.
694. Eisenberger MA, Reyno LM, Jodrell DI, et al. Suramin: an active drug for prostate cancer. Interim observations in a phase I trial. *J Natl Cancer Inst* 1993;85:611.
695. Reyno LM, Egorin MJ, Eisenberger MA, et al. Development and validation of a pharmacokinetically based fixed dosing scheme for suramin. *J Clin Oncol* 1995;13:2187.
696. Bolger JJ, Dearnaley DP, Kirk D, et al. Strontium-89 (Metastron) versus external beam radiotherapy in patients with painful bone metastases secondary to prostatic cancer: preliminary report of a multicenter trial. *Semin Oncol* 1993;20:32.
697. Porter AT, McEwan AJB, Powe JE, et al. Results of a randomized phase III trial to evaluate the efficacy of strontium-89 adjuvant to local field external beam irradiation in the management of endocrine resistant prostate cancer. *Int J Radiat Oncol Biol Phys* 1993;25:805.
698. Chan JM, Stampfer MJ, Giovannucci E, et al. Plasma insulin–like growth factor-I and prostate cancer risk: a prospective study. *Science* 1998;279(5350):563.
699. Ware JL. Growth factor network disruption in prostate cancer progression. *Cancer Metastasis Rev* 1998;17:443.
700. Foster BA, Kaplan PJ, Greenberg NM. Peptide growth factors and prostate cancer: new models, new opportunities. *Cancer Metastasis Rev* 1998;17:317.
701. Pegram MD Lipton A, Hayes DF, et al. Phase II study of receptor-enhanced chemosensitivity using recombinant humanized anti-p185HER/neu monoclonal antibody plus cisplatin in patients with HER-2/neu-overexpressing metastatic breast cancer refractory to chemotherapy treatment. *J Clin Oncol* 1998;16:2659.
702. Ross JS, Sheehan C, Hayner-Buchan AM, et al. HER-2/neu gene amplification status in prostate cancer by fluorescence in situ hybridization. *Hum Pathol* 1997;28:827.
703. Kallakury BV, Sheehan CE, Ambros RA, et al. Correlation of p34cdc2 cyclin-dependent kinase overexpression, CD44s downregulation, and HER-2/neu oncogene amplification with recurrence in prostatic adenocarcinomas. *J Clin Oncol* 1998;16: 1302.
704. Mark HF, Feldman D, Das S, et al. Fluorescence in situ hybridization study of HER-2/neu oncogene amplification in prostate cancer. *Exp Mol Pathol* 1999;66:170.
705. Craft N, Shostak Y, Carey M, et al. A mechanism for hormone-independent prostate cancer through modulation of androgen signaling by the Her-2/neu tyrosine kinase. *Nat Med* 1999;5:280.
706. Maddy SQ, Chisholm GD, Hawkins RA, et al. Localization of epidermal growth factor receptors in the human prostate by biochemical and immunocytochemical methods. *J Endocrinol* 1987;113:147.
707. Peehl DM, Sellers RG. Basic FGF, EGF, and PDGF modify TGFβ-induction of smooth muscle cell phenotype in human prostatic stromal cells. *Prostate* 1998;35:125.
708. Fudge K, Wang CY, Stearns ME. Immunohistochemistry analysis of platelet-derived growth factor A and B chains and platelet-derived growth factor alpha and beta receptor expression in benign prostatic hyperplasias and Gleason-graded human prostate adenocarcinomas. *Mod Pathol* 1994;7(5):549.
709. Harper GP, Barde YA, Burnstock YA, et al. Guinea pig prostate is a rich source of nerve growth factor. *Nature* 1979;350:678.
710. Pflug BR, Dionne C, Kaplan DR, et al. Expression of a trk high affinity nerve growth factor receptor in human prostate. *Endocrinology* 1995;136:262.
711. Iwamura M, Sluss PM, Casamento JB, et al. Insulin-like growth factor I: action and receptor characterization in human prostate cancer cell lines. *Prostate* 1993;22(3):243.
712. Casey ML, Byrd W, MacDonald PC. Massive amounts of immunoreactive endothelin in human seminal fluid. *J Clin Endocrinol Metab* 1992;74:223.
713. Kobayashi S, Tang R, Wang B, et al. Localization of endothelin receptors in the human prostate. *J Urol* 1994;151(3):763.
714. Myers MP, Pass I, Batty IH, et al. The lipid phosphatase activity of PTEN is critical for its tumor suppressor function. *Proc Natl Acad Sci U S A* 1998;95:13513.
715. Wu X, Senechal K, Neshat MS, Whang YE, Sawyers CL. The PTEN/MMAC1 tumor suppressor phosphatase functions as a negative regulator of the phosphoinositide 3-kinase/Akt pathway. *Proc Natl Acad Sci U S A* 1998;95(26):15587.
716. Ali IU, Division of Cancer Prevention, National Cancer Institute. Mutational spectra of PTEN/MMAC1 gene: a tumor suppressor with lipid phosphatase activity. *J Natl Cancer Inst* 1999,91(22).1922.
717. Samid D, Shack S, Myers CE. Selective growth arrest and phenotype reversion of prostate cancer cells in vitro by nontoxic pharmacological concentrations of phenylacetate. *J Clin Invest* 1993;91(5):2288.
718. Dijkman GA, Gernandez del Moral P, Bruynseels J, et al. Liarozole (R75251) in hormone-resistant prostate cancer patients. *Prostate* 1997;33:26.
719. Debruyne FMJ, Murray R, Fradet Y, et al. Liarozole—a novel treatment approach for advanced prostate cancer: results of a large randomized trial versus cyproterone acetate. *Urology* 1998;52:72.
720. Corder EH, Guess HA, Hulka BS, et al. Vitamin D and prostate cancer: a prediagnostic study with stored sera. *Cancer Epidemiol Biomarkers Prev* 1993;2(5):467.
721. Ingles SA, Ross RK, Yu MC, et al. Association of prostate cancer risk with genetic polymorphisms in vitamin D receptor and androgen receptor. *J Natl Cancer Inst* 1997;89(2): 166.
722. Tontonoz P, Hu E, Spiegelman BM. Stimulation of adipogenesis in fibroblasts by PPARγ2, a lipid-activated transcription factor. *Cell* 1994;79:1147.
723. Kubota T, Koshizuka K, Williamson EA, et al. Ligand for Peroxisome Proliferator-activated receptor γ (Troglitazone) has potent anti-tumor effect against human prostate cancer both in vitro and in vivo. *Cancer Res* 1998;58:3344.
724. Steward WP. Marimastat (BB2516): current status of development. *Cancer Chemother Pharmacol* 1999;43:S56.

HARRY W. HERR
GUIDO DALBAGNI
DEAN F. BAJORIN
WILLIAM U. SHIPLEY

SECTION 5

Cancer of the Urethra and Penis

Primary cancer of the urethra and penis is uncommon. The rarity of tumors involving the penis and urethra has contributed to the lack of a standardized approach in the management of patients with these neoplasms.

Squamous cell carcinoma is the most common cancer in the penis and urethra. The patterns of spread, treatment approaches, and prognosis are related to the extent of disease and the region of the urethra or penis involved by the tumor. Carcinoma of the penis often remains localized for prolonged periods. When metastasis occurs, it follows a stepwise pattern; first, to the inguinal (groin) lymph nodes and, second, to the pelvic lymph nodes. Distant dissemination occurs later. A favorable natural history permits cure of most localized penile cancers and of many with inguinal metastases. Urethral carcinoma in both males and females tends to invade locally and metastasize to regional lymph nodes early in its evolution. Most of these tumors are far advanced locally when diagnosed. This feature accounts for the relative poor prognosis of urethral cancer despite aggressive management.[1]

CARCINOMA OF THE MALE URETHRA

Carcinoma of the male urethra is extremely rare. Approximately 600 cases have been reported. Urethral carcinoma has been reported in boys as young as 13 years of age and in men in their 90s, although most patients are older than 50 years of age. Significant etiologic factors have not been identified, but chronic inflammation appears to play a role in the initiation of disease, because many patients have prior sexually transmitted disease, urethritis, or urethral stricture. The incidence of urethral stricture in men with carcinoma of the urethra ranges from 24% to 76%. The most frequent site of stricture and malignancy is the bulbomembranous urethra. No racial predisposition has been noted.

SYMPTOMS

The lesion is often insidious at onset with symptoms attributed to benign urethral disease with stricture rather than to malignancy. Men often present with a palpable urethral mass or obstructive symptoms. On occasion, pain associated with urethral fistula or periurethral abscess may herald the presence of a male urethral cancer. Urethral stricture or bleeding in a man without a history of trauma or venereal disease should suggest the possibility of urethral carcinoma. Because of the nonspecific nature of the symptoms, diagnosis is often delayed.[2] The most common presenting symptoms are listed in Table 34.5-1. Most reflect local involvements by the lesion.

TABLE 34.5-1. Cancer of the Urethra and Penis

Symptoms[a]	*Number of Patients (%)*
Palpable urethral mass	34 (72)
Obstructive symptoms (with or without retention)	32 (65)
Pain	12 (26)
Urethral fistula or periurethral abscess	10 (21)
Hematuria	10 (21)
Palpable inguinal mass	9 (19)

[a]Presenting symptoms of 47 patients.
(From Fair WR, Yang CR. Urethral carcinoma in males. In: Resnick M, Kursch E, eds. *Current therapy in surgery.* Toronto: BC Decker, 1987, with permission.)

PATHOLOGY

Tumors of the male urethra can be categorized according to histology of the cells lining the anatomic region of origin (Fig. 34.5-1). The epithelium of the prostatic urethra gives rise to transitional cell carcinoma that is histologically and clinically distinct from adenocarcinoma commonly associated with the prostatic glands, but that is identical to the bladder urothelium. Tumors originating in the area of the trigone or bladder neck with direct extension into the prostatic urethra may be mistakenly diagnosed as primary urethral carcinoma unless careful examination and biopsy excludes the vesical neck as the site of origin. Male urethral carcinoma occurs in the bulbomembranous urethra in 60%, penile urethra in 30%, and prostatic urethra in 10%. Histologically, 80% of male urethral cancers are squamous cell carcinoma, 15% are transitional cell carcinoma, and approximately 5% are adenocarcinoma and undifferentiated tumors.[1]

Male urethral carcinoma spreads by direct extension to adjacent structures and usually involves the vascular spaces of the corpus spongiosum and the periurethral tissues. Carcinoma of the bulbomembranous urethra extends to the urogenital diaphragm, prostate, perineum, and scrotal skin. Hematogenous spread is uncommon except in advanced disease. Metastasis occurs by lymphatic embolization to regional lymph nodes. The lymphatics from the anterior urethra drain into the superficial and deep inguinal lymph nodes and occasionally to the external iliac lymph nodes. The lymphatics from the posterior urethra drain into the external iliac, obturator, and hypogastric nodes. Tumors of the anterior urethra usually metastasize to the inguinal nodes, and tumors of the posterior urethra most commonly spread to the pelvic nodes, although exceptions occur. Palpable inguinal lymph nodes occur in approximately 20% of cases and almost always represent metastatic disease.[3]

EVALUATION AND STAGING

The diagnosis is made by transurethral biopsy. The extent of local involvement is determined by careful inspection and palpation of the external genitalia and perineum at the time of cystourethroscopy and by bimanual examination with the patient under anesthesia. Needle biopsy is occasionally helpful in determining local extent of neoplasm. Cytologic studies of voided urine may be helpful for diagnosing some patients. Computed tomography (CT) or magnetic resonance imaging (MRI) may

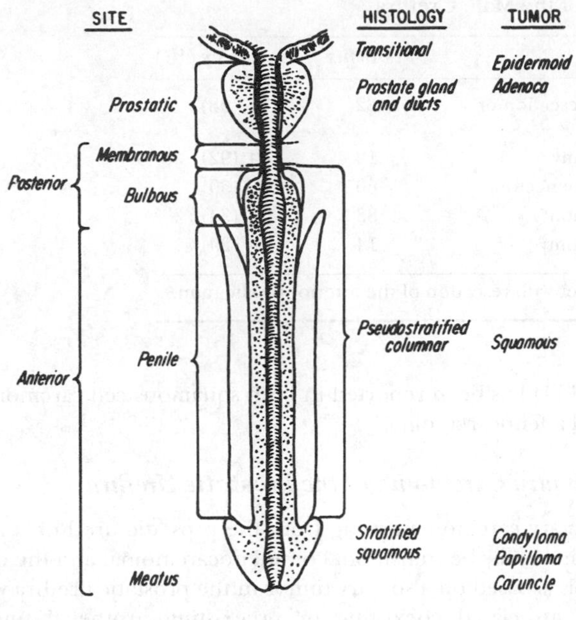

FIGURE 34.5-1. Anatomy and pathology of male urethral carcinoma.

help to evaluate the pelvic and paraaortic nodes. Local soft tissue and bone extension are best evaluated by an MRI scan.

The tumor, node, and metastasis (TNM) staging system is commonly used to assess carcinoma of the urethra[4] (Table 34.5-2). The TNM staging classification is based on depth of invasion of the primary tumor, the presence or absence of regional lymph node involvement, and distant metastasis.

TREATMENT

Surgical excision is the primary therapy for carcinoma of the male urethra. The extent of surgery depends on the location and stage of the tumor. In general, anterior urethral carcinoma is more amenable to surgical control and has a better prognosis than posterior urethral carcinoma. Although some instances of tumor control by irradiation have been reported, in general, radiation has been reserved for patients with early-stage lesions of the anterior urethra who refuse surgery. Radiation therapy has the advantage of preserving the penis but may result in urethral stricture and chronic edema and does not prevent new tumor occurrences in the retained urethra. Combination chemotherapy has achieved encouraging results in patients with metastatic urothelial cancer and is now being integrated more frequently with irradiation and definitive surgery in patients with locally advanced urethral carcinomas.[5]

SURGERY

Table 34.5-3 shows 5-year survival rates in cancer of the male urethra according to stage, site, and surgical treatment.[6–10]

Carcinoma of the Distal Urethra

Carcinoma of the penile urethra may be treated by transurethral resection (TUR), local excision, partial amputation, or radical amputation with or without emasculation. For a superficial papillary or an *in situ* tumor, TUR and fulguration is sufficient. For a tumor infiltrating the corpus and localized to the distal half of the penis, a partial amputation with a 2-cm margin proximal to the visible or palpable tumor is the accepted treatment. If the infiltrating tumor is located in the proximal penile urethra or involves the entire urethra, radical amputation is necessary. This procedure may involve emasculation if the scrotal skin or genitalia are involved. Ilioinguinal groin node dissection is indicated only if the inguinal nodes are palpable. There is no evidence of benefit from prophylactic groin dissection. Carcinoma involving the distal or penile urethra generally enjoys a more favorable prognosis than cancers involving the entire or more proximal regions of the urethra.

TABLE 34.5-2. Tumor (T), Node (N), Metastasis (M) Classification of Carcinoma of the Urethra

PRIMARY TUMOR (MALE AND FEMALE)	
TX	Primary tumor cannot be assessed
T0	No evidence of primary tumor
Ta	Noninvasive papillary, polypoid, or verrucous carcinoma
Tis	Carcinoma *in situ*
T1	Tumor invades subepithelial connective tissue
T2	Tumor invades the corpus spongiosum or the prostate, or the periurethral muscle
T3	Tumor invades the corpus cavernosum or beyond the prostatic capsule, or the anterior vagina or bladder neck
T4	Tumor invades other adjacent organs
REGIONAL LYMPH NODES	
NN	Regional lymph nodes cannot be assessed
N0	No regional lymph node metastasis
N1	Metastasis in a single lymph node, 2 cm or less in greatest dimension
N2	Metastasis in a single lymph node, more than 2 cm but not more than 5 cm in greatest dimension; or multiple lymph nodes, none more than 5 cm in greatest dimension
N3	Metastasis in a lymph node more than 5 cm in greatest dimension
DISTANT METASTASIS	
MX	Presence of distant metastasis cannot be assessed
M0	No distant metastasis
M1	Distant metastasis

(From ref. 4, with permission.)

Carcinoma of the Bulbomembranous Urethra

Transurethral or segmental resection may be adequate for treatment of early superficial tumors involving the bulbomembranous urethra, but such cases are rare. Most patients present with an infiltrating bulky tumor with invasion of surrounding structures. Approximately one-third of these patients are locally understaged and later prove to have pelvic or groin metastasis. The overall survival of patients in this group is poor despite a distinctly radical surgical approach, but radical excision offers the best opportunity for long-term disease control and the lowest incidence of local recurrence. Postoperative morbidity is high. Despite the dismal prognosis, experience suggests that when local control of the tumor can be achieved, overall long-term results are favorable. Such tumors tend to be locally extensive and are apt to recur

TABLE 34.5-3. Five-Year Survival Rate in Cancer of the Male Urethra

Stage	*Site*	*Treatment*	*Patients*	*Survivors (%)*
Superficial	Anterior or posterior	Transurethral resection or fulguration	82	81 (98)
Invasive	Fossa navicularis	Partial penectomy	12	11 (92)
	Penile	Partial or total penectomy	66	33 (50)
	Bulbomembranous	Extended excision[a]	83	28 (34)
	Prostatic	Cystoprostatectomy	14	4 (29)

[a]*En bloc* excision of the penis, scrotum, prostate, and bladder with resection of the inferior public rami.

locally with inadequate local treatment. Metastasis appears to be a late event, which has led to aggressive combined therapy approaches in patients with bulky posterior urethral carcinoma.

Treatment Results for Carcinoma of the Bulbomembranous and Anterior Urethra

Surgery alone gives suboptimal results in the management of male urethral carcinoma. In the Dinney et al. series,[11] two of five patients with tumors of the anterior urethra and none of the four patients with tumors of the bulbomembranous urethra were alive after being treated by surgery alone. In the Dalbagni et al. series,[12] 7 of 18 patients (38%) with tumors of the anterior urethra are disease-free, and 4 of 28 patients (14%) with tumors of the bulbar urethra are disease-free.

Radiation therapy alone was ineffective, as summarized by Zeidman et al.[13] Patients who receive radiation therapy followed by salvage surgery seem to fare worse than if surgery was performed in integrated fashion. A combination of preoperative irradiation (20 to 60 cGy) followed by surgical excision of the inferior pubic rami with partial symphysiectomy, anterior perineum, urogenital diaphragm, and genitalia, *en bloc* with the pelvic organs and lymph nodes, may improve local control and survival.[10] Results suggest that approximately one-third of patients undergoing such extended excision of locally advanced neoplasms can be salvaged.

The integration of chemotherapy used as systemic therapy, and radiosensitization followed by surgery, can be successful in both the bulbomembranous and prostatic urethra. Anecdotal reports document successful treatment using M-VAC [methotrexate, vinblastine, Adriamycin (doxorubicin), and cisplatin] for transitional cell tumors and 5-fluorouracil (FU) plus either mitomycin-C or cisplatin for squamous cell carcinoma.[5,14–19] Three reports substantiate the use of mitomycin-C plus FU chemotherapy integrated with radiation therapy and surgery for squamous cell carcinoma. Baskin and Turzan[16] reported the first case of penile-preserving surgery for carcinoma of the male urethra with combined FU plus mitomycin-C and radiotherapy followed by distal urethrectomy. Licht et al.[17] reported one complete response among two patients treated with similar chemotherapy and radiation for a squamous cell carcinoma of the urethra with lymph node metastasis. Oberfield[18] reported genital preservation in two patients with an invasive squamous cell carcinoma of the bulbar urethra with this chemotherapy regimen plus radiation. In the series by Gheiler et al.,[19] four patients with high-stage tumors were treated with neoadjuvant chemotherapy and radiation before surgery, two of whom were rendered disease-free. Success using cisplatin and FU has been reported in both squamous cell carcinoma[14] and adenocarcinoma.[20]

Primary Carcinoma of the Prostatic Urethra

Primary carcinoma arising from the prostatic urethra is rare. Tumors may be transitional or adenocarcinoma, and the diagnosis is based on a solitary tumor in the prostatic urethra without associated coexisting or preexisting urothelial tumors within the bladder and the bladder neck. There are no characteristic symptoms of this lesion. Patients generally present with hematuria or obstructive urinary symptoms. Prostatic induration on rectal examination represents advanced disease. The serum prostate-specific antigen and acid phosphatase values are normal. Diagnosis depends on transurethral biopsy of the prostate.

Superficial lesions of the prostatic urethra are managed successfully by transurethral resection in the majority of patients. However, such tumors are uncommon. In most instances, the tumor involves the bulk of the prostate with variable extension to the bulbomembranous urethra or to the bladder neck and trigone. In this situation, cystoprostatectomy and urethrectomy is the treatment of choice. In limited experience, the overall 5-year survival rate of patients treated with radical surgery, with or without preoperative irradiation, is poor. Combined modality therapy offers a prospect for improved results. For example, a total of 11 patients with advanced tumors of the prostate, prostatic urethra, or bulbomembranous urethra received neoadjuvant chemotherapy (i.e., M-VAC). Of ten evaluable patients, four (40%) were downstaged to complete clinical remission, including three of five with transitional cell tumors of the prostate and prostatic urethra.[5] In selected responding patients, conservative transurethral resection or prostatectomy rather than pelvic exenteration can be entertained. Most patients, however, are best treated with a combination of aggressive surgery, irradiation, and chemotherapy, although the optimal strategy using these modalities is not established.[14,15]

RADIATION THERAPY

Radiation therapy alone and postoperative radiation are rarely implemented in the management of men with urethral carcinoma. The most common approach has been external-beam radiotherapy, using various techniques to deliver 50 to 60 cGy in 5 to 9 weeks. The long-term results of radiotherapy have been mixed, with the best results reported for patients with distal lesions, for whom the outcome is similar to that reported with surgery.[21]

CARCINOMA OF THE FEMALE URETHRA

Carcinoma of the urethra is unusual among genitourinary tract neoplasms in that it occurs more often in women than in men. Tumors present most commonly in postmenopausal and older women, with 75% of patients older than 50 years of age. The disease is more prevalent among whites than other races.

ETIOLOGY

The cause of urethral carcinoma in women has not been established with certainty, although a causal relationship is reported with chronic irritation, urinary tract infection, and malignancy. Proliferative lesions, such as caruncles, papillomas, adenomas, and polyps, have been associated with subsequent malignancy. Leukoplakia of the urethra is considered a premalignant lesion and is treated with wide local excision.

SYMPTOMS

Most patients present with urinary frequency, hesitancy, obstruction, and a palpable urethral mass. Tumors may present as a papillary growth within the urethra and may later become a soft fungating mass that bleeds easily. Ulcerative lesions may produce a foul-smelling discharge. The lesion may be detected first as a submucosal mass in the anterior wall of the vagina. Spread from the primary lesion is by local extension and infiltration with subsequent involvement of the bladder neck, vagina, or vulva. It may be difficult on initial physical examination to differentiate malignant tumors of the urethra from those of the vulva or vagina.

Lymphatics of the anterior urethra and labia drain to the superficial and then deep inguinal nodes, whereas the posterior urethra drains to the external iliac, hypogastric, and obturator lymph nodes. These boundaries are not distinct, and anatomic crossovers are possible. Clinically palpable inguinal nodes are found in one-third of patients, but histologic confirmation of malignancy is made in more than 90% of this group.[22,23] Pelvic node involvement occurs in 20%, and an additional 15% of patients develop metastatic nodal disease during follow-up. Metastasis outside the pelvis at the time of initial presentation is uncommon.

PATHOLOGY

Stratified squamous epithelium lines the distal two-thirds of the female urethra, and transitional epithelium lines the proximal one-third (Fig. 34.5-2). The submucosa of the urethra contains numerous periurethral glands. Tumor histology is a reflection of the site, with squamous cell carcinoma being the predominant tumor type and usually presenting in the proximal two-thirds of the urethra. In general, carcinomas of the anterior urethra are low grade and less extensive. Carcinomas of the proximal or entire urethra are of higher grade and locally advanced. Squamous cell carcinoma accounts for approximately 60%; transitional cell carcinoma, 20%; adenocarcinoma, 10%; undifferentiated tumors and sarcomas, 5%; and melanoma, 2%. Histologic characteristics do not appear to significantly affect the prognosis, and different histologic types are often treated in a similar fashion.

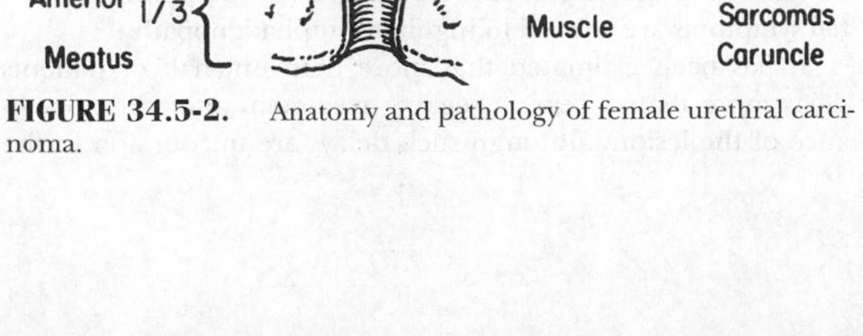

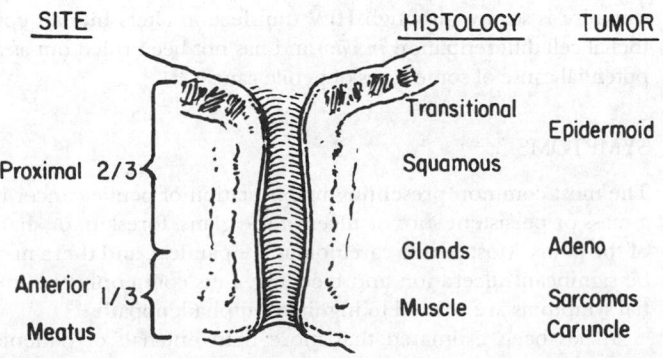

FIGURE 34.5-2. Anatomy and pathology of female urethral carcinoma.

TABLE 34.5-4. Five-Year Survival Rate in Female Urethral Cancer

Stage	*Treatment*	*Patients*	*Survivors (%)*
Early	Radiotherapy	140	94 (67)
	Surgery	24	20 (83)
	Radiotherapy plus surgery	5	4 (80)
Advanced	Radiotherapy	157	34 (34)
	Radiotherapy plus surgery	39	21 (54)

(Adapted from refs. 8 and 24, with permission.)

EVALUATION AND STAGING

A pelvic examination under anesthesia combined with urethroscopy, cytoscopy, and biopsies is performed. Cytologic evaluation of the urine may be of value. Radiographic evaluation consists of a chest x-ray and CT scan of the abdomen and pelvis. A barium enema and bone scan should be obtained in symptomatic patients.

There has been no universally accepted staging system for female urethral carcinoma. The TNM staging system has been adapted to female urethral cancer (see Table 34.5-2), but the practical fact is that staging, treatment, and prognosis are simplified by dividing tumors into anterior and low-stage versus posterior or entire urethra and advanced stage.

TREATMENT

The most significant prognostic factor for local control and survival is the anatomic location and extent of the tumor. Treatment is based primarily on the tumor stage at the time of presentation. Table 34.5-4[8,24] shows 5-year survival rates in female urethral cancer of both early and advanced stage after treatment.

Most urethral cancers in women are locally advanced when detected and involve the proximal one-third or entire urethra. Such lesions clearly do worse than localized, low-grade, anterior urethral lesions. Poor prognosis attributed to urethral cancers in women is because of the advanced stage (high tumor volume), adjacent organ involvement, inability to obtain a clear surgical margin (because of soft tissue infiltration), nodal disease, morbidity of extensive treatment, and inadequate systemic therapy for metastatic tumor. Single-modality therapy often fails for advanced cases and is successful only in selected cases.

SURGERY

Local excision is often sufficient in selected patients with carcinoma of the distal urethra. For example, meatal tumors, if diagnosed early, are associated with an excellent 5-year survival rate. Such tumors are superficial and well localized. The incidence of lymph node metastasis with distal urethral carcinoma is low. Local excision controls the primary tumor, and urinary continence is maintained.

For tumors involving the proximal urethra or extending beyond the urethra into the adjacent structures, more aggressive treatment is required. When surgery is considered, extensive resection is necessary, including total urethrectomy, cystectomy with pelvic lymph node dissection, and removal of most (if not all) of the vagina. Extended excision to include resection of adjacent pubic symphysis and urogenital diaphragm similar to that for proximal male urethral cancer has resulted in local control of a few cases of far advanced urethral carcinoma. Even extensive surgery, however, often fails because of soft tissue infiltration by the tumor beyond the confines of the bladder neck, urethra, and vagina. Local recurrence after surgery alone is common. Anterior exenteration alone led to 10% to 17% 5-year survival and a local recurrence rate of 67%.[25] Garden et al.[26] reported 41% and 31% 5- and 10-year actuarial survival rates, respectively, with a 5-year local control rate of 64% with radiation therapy. Dalbagni et al.[27] reported an overall 5-year survival rate of 32%—that is, the rates were 78% for low-stage and 22% for high-stage tumors, 54% for tumors of the anterior urethra, and 25% and 18% for tumors of the posterior and whole urethra, respectively. No difference was found in survival between women treated with radiation or surgery.[27]

In cases of palpable inguinal nodes, inguinal lymphadenectomy has been advocated. Inguinal lymph node dissection is usually not performed in the absence of palpable disease in the groin.[28,29]

RADIATION THERAPY

Irradiation alone, as with surgical excision, may control small lesions in the distal urethra. Radiation of these small lesions can be accomplished with brachytherapy without additional external-beam irradiation.[30] Interstitial or intracavitary irradiation delivering a 50 to 65 Gy tumor dose has been demonstrated to be sufficient to control small distal urethral lesions.

Tumors of the proximal urethra, bladder neck invasion, or involvement of the entire urethra require combined external irradiation and brachytherapy. External irradiation is delivered to the primary tumor site and regional lymph node. The groin should receive prophylactic irradiation to 50 Gy if there is no palpable adenopathy. In the presence of palpable inguinal lymph nodes, bolus is added to the groin and the total dose is increased from 60 to 65 Gy. The pelvis is treated to 50 Gy by the combined whole pelvis and split field technique. The pelvic side wall can be boosted to 60 Gy in the presence of lymphadenopathy as detected by CT scan. The primary tumor site is boosted with brachytherapy (one or two implants using iridium 192) to bring the total tumor dose from 70 to 80 Gy, depending on tumor size. Complications from irradiation include bowel obstruction, fistula formation, urethral stricture, and incontinence. Radiation therapy alone controls only approximately one-third of cases of advanced disease, and severe complications occur in 15% to 40% of patients.[31–34]

COMBINED MODALITY THERAPY

Although the number of cases of advanced female urethral carcinoma is small, it is obvious that either extensive surgery alone or high-dose irradiation alone produces an unacceptably high morbidity rate and low tumor control rate. This fact has led to combined treatment strategies with chemotherapy, radiation therapy, and surgery in women with advanced urethral cancer. M-VAC chemotherapy and irradiation followed by surgery have been used in patients with transitional cell carcinoma, and those with squamous cell carcinoma have received combined mitomycin-C and 5-fluorouracil and irradiation followed by surgery.[3,35–37] Long-term results from combined modality therapy are unavailable.

CANCER OF THE PENIS

Carcinoma of the penis represents 2% of urogenital cancers. Although rare in North America, tumors of the penis account for 10% to 12% of all malignancies in males among populations in which circumcision is not a common practice.[38]

Penile cancer is the most common genitourinary cancer in Paraguay, representing 45% to 76% of all genitourinary malignancies.[39] In Uganda, where circumcision is usually not performed, penile cancer is the most commonly diagnosed cancer in males.[40] Although malignant penile lesions have been found in young men, most patients are older than 50 years.

ETIOLOGY

Most penile cancers occur in uncircumcised men, suggesting an irritative effect of smegma combined with poor hygiene. Carcinoma is rare among men who were circumcised in the neonatal period, but circumcision performed at puberty or in adulthood does not have the same protective potential as circumcision at birth.[41,42] Although the annual age-adjusted incidence of carcinoma of the penis for males in the United States is only 1 per 100,000, the lifetime risk of penile cancer developing in uncircumcised males may be as high as 1 in 600.[42] Smegma, the product of bacterial action on desquamated epithelial cells is carcinogenic in animal systems, although the specific component responsible for malignant degeneration in human males has not been identified.

Conflicting reports support and deny the association of penile carcinoma with cervical carcinoma in sexual partners or with herpetic infection. No compelling data support the assertion that penile cancer is a sexually transmitted disease.[43] No persistent etiologic relation has been documented between carcinoma of the penis and the venereal diseases of syphilis, granuloma inguinale, or chancroid. Evidence that human papillomavirus (HPV) may be causative is scanty, although HPV transfection alters human epithelial cell differentiation *in vitro* and has not been ruled out as a potential cause of some cases of penile cancer.[44]

SYMPTOMS

The most common presenting manifestation of penile cancer is a mass or persistent sore or ulcer of the glans, foreskin, or shaft of the penis. Most penile carcinomas are painless, and there may be significant ulceration and bleeding. Less commonly, the initial symptoms are related to inguinal lymphadenopathy.[45]

It has been estimated that more than one-half of patients delay more than 1 year in seeking treatment after the appearance of the lesion, although such delays are uncommon in the

TABLE 34.5-5. Premalignant Lesions of the Penis

Lesion	*Characteristic*	*Treatment*
Leukoplakia	White plaque	Local excision
Erythroplasia of Queyrat	Raised, red, velvet lesion; cellular disorientation with multiple mitoses; identical to carcinoma *in situ* of skin; 10% to 20% may develop areas of squamous cell carcinoma; may be painful	Local excision; topical 5-fluorouracil; radiation therapy
Bowen's disease	Red plaque	Local excision
Balanitis xerotica obliterans	Scaly, atrophic with fissure or ulceration; meatus often involved	Local excision; topical steroids (?)
Buschke-Lowenstein tumor	Large verrucous lesion, histologically benign; may undergo malignant degeneration	Local excision with negative margins; topical therapy doubtful; radiation therapy has limited effectiveness

United States. Any delay in the recognition, diagnosis, and therapy of penile carcinoma significantly worsens its prognosis.[45]

PATHOLOGY

Penile carcinoma is most often squamous cell in origin, although malignant melanoma, basal cell carcinoma, Bowen's disease (carcinoma *in situ*), mesenchymal tumors (including Kaposi's sarcoma), metastatic lesions, and leukemic or lymphomatosis infiltrates may involve the penis. Several premalignant lesions have been identified (Table 34.5-5).

STAGING

The initial diagnosis is made by incisional or excisional biopsy. Physical examination determines the extent of local invasion and the status of the inguinal lymph nodes that are essential to proper staging. A CT or MRI scan to evaluate the pelvic and abdominal lymph nodes may also be helpful. The TNM classification (Table 34.5-6) is used to determine the stage of the primary tumor and to quantify nodal metastasis. Nodal status is the most significant prognostic variable predicting survival.[46] The incidence of groin metastasis (palpable or not) increases with T category of the primary lesion. Nodal disease occurs in 20% of T1 tumors and in 47% to 66% of T2–4 penile cancers.[47]

TREATMENT

Treatment depends on the local extent of the primary neoplasm and the status of the regional lymph nodes. Wide excision or partial penectomy with or without inguinal lymph node dissection is the most commonly accepted treatment for small and well localized tumors.[48,49] Radiotherapy may be effective for some patients with noninvasive small lesions and may avoid the functional sacrifice associated with penectomy.[50] Radiation may be associated with necrosis or urethral stenosis, resulting in a nonfunctioning penis. Several investigations have demonstrated that local relapses after radiotherapy can be salvaged by a partial or total amputation of the penis without apparently affecting the prognosis, although this approach remains controversial.[51]

Paramount to treatment planning is a consideration of the lymphatic drainage of the penis (Fig. 34.5-3). The skin of the penis and the lymphatics of the prepuce drain primarily into the superficial inguinal nodes. Bilateral drainage occurs as a result of the freely anastomosing system and crossover at the base of the penis. The glans is drained by the superficial inguinal nodes, but along with those of the corpora, the lymphatics of the glans penis empty into the deep inguinal and iliac nodes. The superficial nodes are located in the deep portion of Camper's fascia above the deep fascia of the thigh, the fascia lata. The superficial lymphatics drain into the deep inguinal lymphatics surrounding the femoral vessels and then to the external iliac, common iliac, and paraaortic lymphatic channels. Tumor invasion of the corpora cavernosa or the posterior urethra may lead to deep pelvic lymphatic metastasis to internal iliac and obturator nodes.

SURGERY

Surgery aims to control the primary neoplasm and is involved in the evaluation and therapy of nodal disease. Bilateral pelvic and inguinal node dissection is indicated, where possible, for any positive groin metastasis detected at the time of or within 6 months of treatment of the penile tumor. This is because lymphatic crossover at the base of the penis accounts for at least 60% contralateral groin metastasis, even in the face of unilateral palpable inguinal nodes.[50,52] Delayed (6 months or more) appearance of unilateral groin metastasis requires only ipsilateral ilioinguinal node dissection.

Treatment of Primary Lesion

Surgical therapy involves removal of the lesion with adequate margins to minimize the risk of local recurrence. Small tumors that are limited to the prepuce are treated by circumcision alone. Lesions that on physical examination involve only the skin may be controlled by wide excisional biopsy. Partial or total

TABLE 34.5-6. Tumor (T), Node (N), Metastasis (M) Classification of Penile Cancer

Stage	*Description*
Ta	Noninvasive verrucous cancer
T1	Tumor less than 2 cm, superficial or exophytic
T2	Tumor greater than 2 cm but less than 3 cm, or tumor invades subepithelial connective tissue
T3	Tumor greater than 5 cm, or tumor invades corpus spongiosum or cavernosum, or urethra
T4	Tumor invades other adjacent structures
N0	No regional lymph node metastasis
N1	Movable, unilateral inguinal lymph node involvement
N2	Movable, bilateral inguinal lymph node involvement
N3	Fixed inguinal lymph node or pelvic node involvement
M0	No evidence of distant metastasis
M1	Evidence of distant metastasis

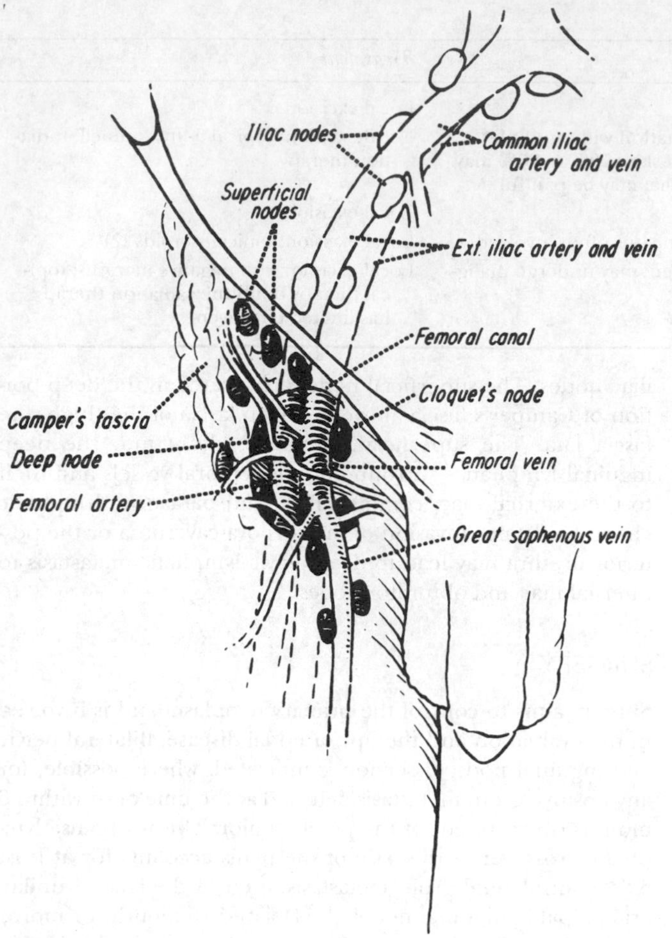

FIGURE 34.5-3. Lymphatic drainage of the penis.

penectomy is indicated for lesions that because of their size, invasiveness, or location on the shaft are not amenable to more conservative treatment. Partial penectomy includes a 2-cm margin of normal shaft proximal to the primary tumor. For extensive lesions approaching the base of the penis, total penectomy is accomplished with excision of both corpora and creation of a perineal urethrostomy. Local recurrence after a properly planned and executed partial or total penectomy is rare.[52–54]

Management of Regional Lymph Nodes

Several factors determine the role of regional lymphadenectomy in patients with penile cancer. First, 50% of patients with squamous cell penile cancer have palpable inguinal lymph nodes at diagnosis. In one-half of these cases, inguinal adenopathy represents benign inflammatory changes associated with ulcerated or infected penile lesions. Clinical assessment of the lymph nodes should be delayed until after a 4- to 6-week course of antibiotic therapy. Persistent adenopathy after 6 weeks warrants biopsy and therapy. Second, approximately 20% of patients with no palpable adenopathy have occult lymphatic metastases. Third, lymph node dissection can be curative for the majority of patients with isolated tumor-bearing inguinal nodes.

Overall, 50% of patients with positive inguinal nodes can be rendered disease-free by surgical resection.[53] The volume of lymph node disease and its location appear to be important predictors of success. In one study of 119 patients, unilateral inguinal node involvement had a median 5-year survival rate of 56%, compared with 9% of patients with bilateral inguinal node metastases, extranodal disease, or iliac node involvement.[54,55] Cure is unlikely by surgical means if the pelvic lymph nodes are involved.

The primary controversy in the surgical management of penile cancer concerns the role of lymph node dissection if there is no clinically identifiable inguinal disease. The overall incidence of false-negative nodes in T1 and T2 disease is approximately 20%, but late nodal extension to the groin after adequate excision of the primary occurs in only 5% to 11% of patients. Routine lymph node dissection is therefore difficult to justify for low-stage primary disease. In patients with advanced (T3, T4) invasive primary tumors, the likelihood of nodal metastases increases, and in some series, two-thirds of patients with clinically negative nodes have histologically confirmed metastasis on lymph node dissection.[56] The significant morbidity that may accompany groin dissection and the lack of controlled prospective studies to document the benefit of early "prophylactic" versus late "therapeutic" groin dissection has led many surgeons and centers to delay lymphadenectomy until clinical evidence of lymph node involvement exists.

Ekstrom and Edsmyr[52] identified a 50% disease control rate among patients who had node dissection delayed until adenopathy was evident. Frew and colleagues[57] could identify no cancer deaths among patients in whom lymph node excision was deferred until clinical node disease was found. Beggs and Spratt[58] reported no significant adverse effect on survival in patients with delayed groin dissection. However, others have reported a significant decrease in 5-year survival rates in patients with therapeutic rather than prophylactic groin dissection and have suggested that delayed surgery is inappropriate.[59] One study showed that 62% of patients survived 5 years if the lymph node dissection was done concomitantly with the primary therapy of the penile lesion, as opposed to an 8% survival rate among those who underwent lymphadenectomy when it became obvious that the nodes were pathologically involved.[47] Most patients who benefited from groin dissection had locally advanced penile cancers. The current recommendation is that, among patients with low-stage (T1, T2) penile cancer and palpably negative groins, expectant management is reasonable in that delayed inguinal lymph node dissection for clinically positive nodes does not seem to compromise long-term survival when compared with patients who never develop inguinal lymphadenopathy.[60] However, for locally advanced (T3, T4) tumors, a "prophylactic" bilateral lymph node dissection may result in improved survival among patients with clinically undetected inguinal metastasis.[56]

Cabanas[61] described a technique of "sentinel node" biopsy followed by formal node dissection if metastatic disease is found. In Cabanas' series, inguinal-femoral-iliac node involvement was not demonstrated without a positive sentinel node biopsy. However, Perinetti and colleagues[62] have reported patients with negative sentinel node biopsies who later developed unresectable bilateral groin disease. A modified or extended sentinel lymph node dissection also has been advocated to cure those patients with limited inguinal disease and to reduce the morbidity of a formal radical ilioinguinal lymphadenectomy. However, Pettaway[63] reported that, among 14 patients who underwent a negative modified superficial inguinal dissection, 5 relapsed with incurable groin metastasis from 3 to 21 months later. Thus, radical ilioinguinal lymphadenectomy is the procedure of choice if groin dissection is indicated.

The operation is performed essentially as described by Whitmore and Vagaiwala.[64] Bilateral pelvic lymph node dissection is performed. The dissection limits are defined by the genitofemoral nerve laterally, the bladder medially, the bifurcation of the common iliac artery superiorly, and the fascia covering the obturator internus and levator ani muscles inferiorly. Cloquet's node is removed from the femoral canal.

The inguinal incision is planned to provide adequate margins surrounding lymph nodes containing obvious tumor and simultaneously to remove the area of skin at greatest risk of devitalization and necrosis. An elliptical incision is made over the inguinal ligament from the anterosuperior iliac spine to the pubic tubercle. The borders of the ellipse parallel the inguinal ligament and extend 4 to 6 cm in vertical diameter at the widest point. Because penile cancers appear to involve the inguinal lymph nodes by tumor embolization rather than through permeation of lymphatic channels, wide thin skin flaps and a thorough dissection, skeletonizing the femoral vessels as is required for malignant melanoma, are not required. The nodes in the superficial and deep inguinal areas are completely removed from the inguinal ligament to the apex of the femoral triangle in the groin (Fig. 34.5-4). With this technique, the incidence of postoperative wound necrosis is markedly reduced.

Radiation Therapy

The main advantage for radiation therapy in penile tumors is that it provides an option of functional preservation of the penis. However, for radiation to represent an alternative to surgery, it must yield comparable local control rates with minimal toxic effects. Several series report initial rates of local control in 80% to 90% of patients treated with radiotherapy, but 10% to 20% eventually relapse and require surgical salvage.[65–67] Furthermore, inadequate control of the primary tumor risks interval metastasis and a reduced cure rate.

Radiation techniques have included interstitial implantation of radium needles, ^{192}Ir sources, or external-beam radiotherapy. The use of brachytherapy has been limited to small tumors. Results from a series of 50 patients implanted with ^{192}Ir wires showed that the tumor was controlled in 95% of the patients with noninfiltrating tumors of 4 cm or less, with the penis conserved in 80% without major impairments of function.[68] When external-beam radiotherapy is used, treatment is usually delivered with a custom-made plastic or wax mold to ensure a uniform dose distribution and to overcome the skin-sparing effects of supervoltage beams. Circumcision is usually recommended before radiotherapy to minimize radiation morbidity associated with cellulitis of the prepuce and the adjacent structures. The whole shaft of the penis is treated to 40 Gy in 20 fractions in 4 weeks, and the primary lesion is boosted to a total dose of 60 Gy. Superficial small lesions can be treated with localized fields using superficial x-rays or electron beams carried to a similar dose.

External-beam radiotherapy of low-stage tumors usually produces 70% to 80% local success rates. Local failures appear in 20% of patients, but some can be salvaged with surgery. If prophylactic or therapeutic lymph node dissection cannot be performed, external-beam radiotherapy to the inguinal and pelvic lymph nodes carried to 50 Gy may provide palliation for some patients.[69,70]

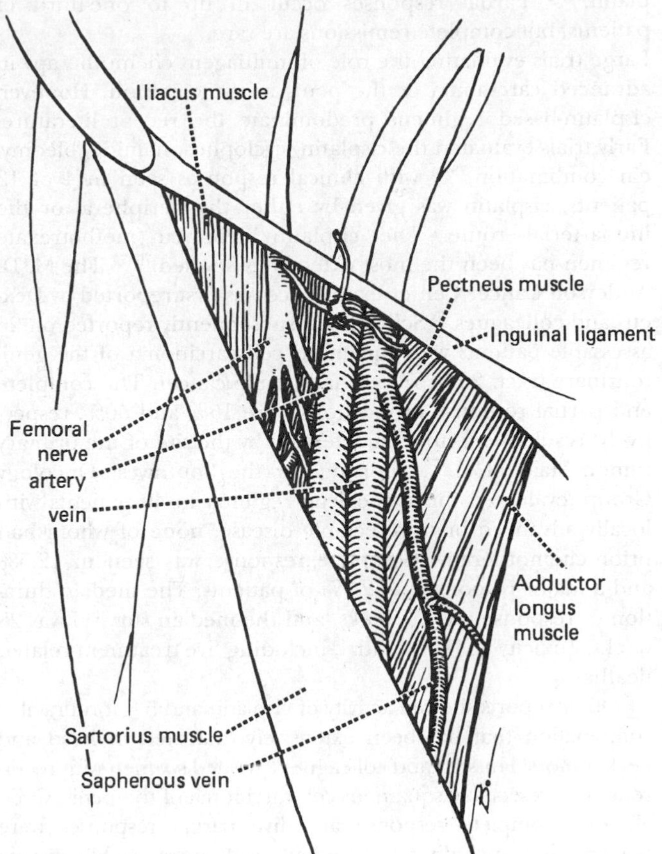

FIGURE 34.5-4. Anatomic limits of groin dissection.

The Royal Marsden Hospital has recently updated their experience with treating 101 patients with radiation for carcinomia of the penis. This group reported an 30% local recurrence rate in patients treated with at least 60Gy of external-beam radiation therapy. However, local control was eventually achieved in 71 of 74 patients with stage I disease, which included retreatment with salvage surgery in 17 patients who had local recurrence following radiation. Unfortunately, very little quality of life information has been published following treatment of penile cancer. However, a recent study from the Norwegian Radium Hospital reports clear results of sexual performance using a formal prospective analysis. This study found that the overall sexual function was preserved or only slightly diminished in 10 of the 12 irradiated patients. However, the analysis also showed that the overall sexual function was normal in only one of five men following wide local excision and in only two of nine men after partial penectomy.

CHEMOTHERAPY

Chemotherapy for urethral and penile carcinoma varies with the histology of the lesion. For patients with pure transitional tumors, cisplatin-combination regimens have shown efficacy. The results with chemotherapy for squamous cell tumors of the penis vary according to the extent of disease, with higher rates of response for locoregional (inguinal) than metastatic (pelvic and beyond) disease. Antitumor activity has been demonstrated with single-agent bleomycin, methotrexate, and cis-

platin.[71,72] Partial responses occur in up to one-third of patients, but complete remissions are rare.
Large trials evaluating the role of multiagent chemotherapy in advanced carcinoma of the penis are uncommon. However, cisplatin-based regimens predominate the recent literature. Early trials evaluated the cisplatin/cyclophosphamide/bleomycin combination,[73,74] with clinical responses seen in 4 of 13 patients; cisplatin was given by either the peripheral or the intraarterial route. The cisplatin/bleomycin/methotrexate regimen has been the most extensively studied.[75–77] The M. D. Anderson Cancer Center experience was first reported by Dexeus and colleagues.[75] Sella et al.[76] subsequently reported on 26 assessable patients with squamous cell carcinoma of the genitourinary tract, 20 of whom had penile cancer. The complete and partial response proportions were 15% and 50%, respectively; results were not characterized by the site of the primary tumor. Haas et al.[77] reporting for the Southwest Oncology Group, evaluated this three-drug regimen in 40 patients with locally advanced or unresectable disease, none of whom had prior chemotherapy. Complete response was seen in 12.5% and a major response in 32.5% of patients. The median duration of response was 16 weeks, and the median survival was 28 weeks. Toxicity was substantial, including five treatment-related deaths.

Other reports showed activity of cisplatin and 5-fluorouracil, a combination that has been extensively evaluated in head and neck tumors. Hussein and colleagues[78] treated six men with recurrent or unresectable squamous cell carcinoma of the penis. Overall, one complete response and five partial responses were documented, including two patients with unresectable disease who were rendered disease-free by surgery. Fisher and coworkers[79] treated five patients with biopsy-proven unresectable disease and reported major responses in four patients, including two men who were pathologically free of disease at surgery. Shammas et al.[80] treated eight patients, two of whom responded.

Most regimens studied in penile cancer use older agents. More recent studies have identified new, active agents in squamous cell carcinoma of the cervix and head and neck, including ifosfamide, paclitaxel, docetaxel, gemcitabine, and vinorelbine (Navelbine). Single and multiagent regimens that include these new drugs are active in squamous cell carcinoma of other origins; they have not been pursued as yet in penile cancer. In summary, chemotherapy is sufficiently active in penile cancer to consider its inclusion in multimodality therapy for patients with bulky or fixed inguinal metastases.

REFERENCES

1. Grabstalt H. Tumors of the urethra in men and women. *Cancer* 1973;32:1236.
2. Mandeler JT, Pool TL. Primary carcinoma of the male urethra. *J Urol* 1966;96:67.
3. Hopkins SG, Nag SK, Soloway MS. Primary carcinoma of male urethra. *Urology* 1984;23:128.
4. Beahrs O, Henson D, Hutter R, Kennedy BJ. *Manual for staging of cancer*, 4th ed. Philadelphia: JB Lippincott Co, 1992:209.
5. Scher HI, Yagoda A, Herr HW, et al. Neoadjuvant M-VAC chemotherapy for extravesical urinary tract tumors. *J Urol* 1988;139:470.
6. Ray B, Canto AK, Whitmore WF. Experience with primary carcinoma of the male urethra. *J Urol* 1977;177:591.
7. Zeidman EJ, Desmond P, Thompson IM. Surgical treatment of carcinoma of the male urethra. *Urol Clin North Am* 1992;19:359.
8. Grigsby PW. Carcinoma of the urethra in women. *Int J Rad Onc Biol Phys* 1998;41:535.
9. Stewart PAH, Anderson CK, Williams RE, et al. Urethral tumors. *Br J Urol* 1978;50:583.
10. Klein FA, Whitmore WF, Herr HW, et al. Inferior pubic rami resection with *en bloc* radical excision of invasive proximal urethral carcinoma. *Cancer* 1983;51:1238.
11. Dinney CPN, Johnson DE, Swanson DA, et al. Therapy and prognosis for male anterior urethral carcinoma: an update. *Urology* 1994;43:506.
12. Dalbagni G, Zhang ZE, Lacombe L, Herr H. Male urethral carcinoma: analysis of treatment outcome. *Urology* 1999;53:1126.
13. Zeidman EJ, Desmond P, Thompson IM. Surgical treatment of carcinoma of the urethra. *Urol Clin North Am* 1992;19:359.
14. Hussein AM, Benedetto P, Sridhar A. Chemotherapy with cisplatin and 5-fluorouracil for penile and urethra squamous cell carcinomas. *Cancer* 1990;65:433.
15. Johnson DW, Kessler JF, Ferrigni RG, et al. Low-dose combined chemotherapy/radiotherapy for management of locally advanced urethral squamous cell carcinoma. *J Urol* 1989;141:615.
16. Baskin LS, Turzan C. Carcinoma of the male urethra: management of locally advanced disease with combined chemotherapy, radiotherapy and penile-preserving surgery. *Urology* 1992;39:21.
17. Licht MR, Klein EA, Bukowski R, et al. Combination radiation and chemotherapy for the treatment of squamous cell carcinoma of the male and female urethra. *J Urol* 1995;153:1616.
18. Oberfeld RA, Zinman LN, Leibenhaut M, et al. Management of invasive squamous cell carcinoma of the bulbomembranous male urethra with co-ordinated chemo-radiotherapy and genital preservation. *Br J Urol* 1996;78:573.
19. Gheiler EL, Tefeli MV, Tiguert R, et al. Management of primary urethral cancer. *Urology* 1998;52:487.
20. Tefilli MV, Gheiler EL, Shekarriz B, et al. Primary adenocarcinoma of the urethra with metastasis to the glans penis: successful treatment with chemotherapy and radiation therapy. *Urology* 1998;52:517.
21. Heysek RV, Parsons JR, Drylie DM, et al. Carcinoma of the male urethra. *J Urol* 1985;134:753.
22. Grabstalt H, Hilaris B, Henschike U, et al. Cancer of the female urethra. *JAMA* 1966;197:835.
23. Desai S, Libertino JA, Zinman L. Primary carcinoma of the female urethra. *J Urol* 1973;110:693.
24. Narayan P, Conety B. Surgical treatment of female urethral carcinoma. *Urol Clin North Am* 1992;19:373.
25. Terry PJ, Cookson MS, Sarosdy MF. Carcinoma of the urethra and scrotum. In: Raghavan D, Scher HI, Leibel SA, Lange P, eds. *Principles and practice of genitourinary oncology*. Philadelphia: Lippincott–Raven Publishers, 1997:347.
26. Garden AS, Zagars GK, Declos L. Primary carcinoma of the female urethra: results of radiation therapy. *Cancer* 1993;71:3102.
27. Dalbagni G, Zhang ZF, Lacombe L, Herr HW. Female urethral carcinoma. Analysis of treatment outcome and a plea for a standardized management strategy. *Br J Urol* 1998;82:835.
28. Bracken RB, Johnson DE, Miller LS, et al. Primary carcinoma of the female urethra. *J Urol* 1976;116:188.
29. Hopkins SC, Vider M, Nag SK, et al. Carcinoma of the female urethra: reassessment of the modes of therapy. *J Urol* 1983;129:958.
30. Mayer R, Fowler JE, Clayton M. Localized urethral cancer in women. *Cancer* 1987;60:1548.
31. Grigsby PW, Corn BW. Localized urethral tumors in women: indications for conservative versus exenterative therapies. *J Urol* 1992;147:1516.
32. Sailer SL, Shipley WU, Wang CC. Carcinoma of the female urethra: a review of results with radiation therapy. *J Urol* 1988;140:1.
33. Taggart CG, Castro JR, Rutledge FN. Carcinoma of the female urethra. *AJR Am J Roengenol* 1972;114:145.
34. Prempree T, Amoremarn R, Patanaphan V. Radiation therapy in primary carcinoma of the female urethra. *Cancer* 1984;54:729.
35. Johnson DW, Kessler JF, Ferrigni RC, et al. Low dose combined chemotherapy/radiotherapy in the management of locally advanced urethral squamous cell carcinoma. *J Urol* 1989;141:615.
36. Calra J, Cortes E, Chen S, et al. Effective multimodality treatment for advanced epidermoid carcinoma of the female genital tract. *J Clin Oncol* 1985;3:917.
37. Tran LN, Krieg RM, Szabo RJ. Combination chemotherapy and radiotherapy for a locally advanced squamous cell carcinoma of the urethra: a case report. *J Urol* 1995;153:422.
38. Hanash K, Furlow W, Utz D, et al. Carcinoma of the penis: a clinicopathologic study. *J Urol* 1970;140:291.
39. Riveros M, Lebrone RF. Geographical pathology of cancer of the penis. *Cancer* 1963;16:798.
40. Dodge OG, Owor R, Templeton AC. Tumors of the male genitalia: recent results. *Cancer Res* 1973;41:132.
41. Jackson SM. The treatment of carcinoma of the penis. *Br J Surg* 1966;53:33.
42. Koenen M, McCurdy S. Circumcision and the risk of cancer of the penis: a life-able analysis. *Am J Dis Child* 1980;134:484.
43. Hellberg D, Valentin J, Eklun D, et al. Penile cancer: is there an epidemiological role for smoking and sexual behavior? *BMJ* 1987;295:1306.
44. Moriyama N, Hagasey Y, Ukei T, et al. *In situ* hybridization study of human papilloma virus from penile cancer. *Jpn J Urol* 1990;81:1706.
45. Hardner GJ, Bhanalaph T, Murphy GP, et al. Carcinoma of the penis: analysis of therapy in 100 consecutive cases. *J Urol* 1972;108:428.
46. Horenblas S, Van Tinteren H. Squamous cell carcinoma of the penis: prognostic factors of survival; analysis of tumor, nodes and metastasis classification system. *J Urol* 1994;151:1239.
47. Ornellas AA, Seixas AL, Marota A, et al. Surgical treatment of invasive squamous cell carcinoma of the penis: retrospective analysis of 350 cases. *J Urol* 1994;151:1244.
48. Skinner DJ, Ledbetter WR, Kelley SP. The surgical management of squamous cell carcinoma of the penis. *J Urol* 1972;107:273.
49. Persky L, DeKernion JD. Carcinoma of the penis. *CA Cancer J Clin* 1986;36:258.
50. Fraley EE, Zhang G, Lange PH. Cancer of the penis: prognosis and treatment plans. *Cancer* 1985;55:1618.

51. Sagerman RH, Yu WS, Chun CT, et al. External beam irradiation of carcinoma of the penis. *Radiology* 1984;152:183.
52. Ekstrom T, Edsmyr F. Cancer of the penis: a clinical study of 292 cases. *Acta Chir Scand* 1958;155:25.
53. Johnson DE, Lo RK. Management of regional lymph nodes in penile carcinoma: five year results following therapeutic groin dissection. *Urology* 1984;24:308.
54. Horenblas S, Van Tinteren H, Delemarre JFM, et al. Squamous cell carcinoma of the penis: treatment of the primary tumor. *J Urol* 1992;147:1533.
55. Srinivas V, Morse MJ, Herr HW, et al. Penile cancer: relation of extent of nodal metastasis to survival. *J Urol* 1987;137:880.
56. Horenblas S, Van Tinteren H, Delemare JFM, et al. Squamous cell carcinoma of the penis: treatment of the regional nodes. *J Urol* 1993;149:492.
57. Frew ID, Jeffries JD, Swinney J. Carcinoma of the penis. *Br J Urol* 1967;39:398.
58. Beggs JH, Spratt JS. Epidermoid carcinoma of the penis. *J Urol* 1964;91:166.
59. McDougal WS, Kirchner FK, Edwards RH, et al. Treatment of carcinoma of the penis: the case of primary lymphadenectomy. *J Urol* 1986;136:38.
60. Theodorescu D, Fair WR, Herr HW, et al. Pure expectant management of patients with T1-4 N0M0 penile cancer. *J Urol* 1995;153:247A.
61. Cabanas RM. An approach for the treatment of penile carcinoma. *Cancer* 1977;39:456.
62. Perinetti EP, Crane DD, Catalona WJ. Unreliability of sentinel lymph node biopsy for staging penile carcinoma. *J Urol* 1980;124:734.
63. Pettaway CA, Pisters LL, Dinney CN, et al. Sentinel lymph node dissection for penile carcinoma. *J Urol* 1995;154:1999.
64. Whitmore WF, Vagaiwala MR. A technique of ilioinguinal lymph-node dissection of carcinoma of the penis. *Surg Gynecol Obstet* 1984;159:573.
65. Grabstalt H, Kelley CD. Radiation therapy of penile cancer: six to ten years follow-up. *Urology* 1980;15:575.
66. Haile K, Delcos L. The place of radiation therapy in the treatment of carcinoma of the distal end of the penis. *Cancer* 1987;45:1980.
67. Salverria JC, Hope-Stone HF, Paris AMI, et al. Conservative treatment of carcinoma of the penis. *Br J Urol* 1979;51:32.
68. Mazeron JJ, Langlois D, Lobo PA, et al. Interstitial radiation therapy for carcinoma of the penis using iridium 192 wires. *J Radiat Oncol Biol Phys* 1984;10:1891.
69. Gerbaulet A, Labin P. Radiation therapy of cancer of the penis: indications, advantages and pitfalls. *Urol Clin North Am* 1992;19:325.
70. Jones WG, Fossa SD, Hammers H, et al. Penis cancer: a review by the joint radiotherapy committee of the European Organization for Research and Treatment of Cancer (EORTC) genitourinary and radiotherapy groups. *J Surg Oncol* 1989;40:227.
70a. Farin R, Norman AR, Steele CG, et al. Treatment results and prognostic factors in 101 men treated with squamous carcinoma of the penis. *Int J Rad Onc Biol Phys* 1997;38:713.
70b. Opjordsmoen S, Waehre H, Aass N, et al. Sexuality in patients treated for penile cancer: patients' experience and doctors' judgement. *Eur J Urol* 1994;73:554.
71. Ahmed T, Sklaroff R, Yagoda A. Sequential trials of methotrexate, cisplatin and bleomycin for penile cancer. *Cancer* 1984;132:465.
72. Gagliano R, Blumenstein BA, Crawford ED, et al. Cisplatin in the treatment of advanced epidermoid carcinoma of the penis: a Southwest Oncology Group study. *J Urol* 1989;141:66.
73. Dexeus FH, Logothetics CJ, Sipahi H. Chemotherapy for advanced squamous carcinoma of the male external genital track and urethra. In: Johnson DE, Logothetics CJ, Von Eschenbach AC, eds. Systemic therapy for genitourinary cancers. Chicago: Year Book Medical Publishers, 1989:255.
74. Eisenberger MA. Chemotherapy for carcinomas of the penis and urethra. *Urol Clin North Am* 1992;19:333.
75. Dexeus FH, Fitz K, Avishay S, et al. Chemotherapy (CHEMO) for advanced squamous cell carcinoma (SC) of the male genital tract: the MD Anderson experience. *J Urol* 1990;143:352A.
76. Sella A, Robinson E, Carrasco CH, et al. Phase II study of methotrexate, cisplatin, and bleomycin combination chemotherapy (CHT) system. *Proc Am Soc Clin Oncol* 1994;13:252.
77. Haas GP, Blumenstein BA, Gagliano RG, et al. Cisplatin, methotrexate and bleomycin for the treatment of carcinoma of the penis: a Southwest Oncology Group study. *J Urol* 1999;161:1823.
78. Hussein AM, Benedetto P, Sridkar KS. Chemotherapy with cisplatin and 5-fluorouracil for penile and urethral squamous cell carcinomas. *Cancer* 1990;65:433.
79. Fisher HAG, Baroda JH, Horton J, et al. Neoadjuvant therapy with cisplatin and 5-fluorouracil for stage III squamous cell carcinoma of the penis. *J Urol* 1990;143:352A.
80. Shammas FV, Ous S, Fossa SD. Cisplatin and 5-fluorouracil in advanced cancer of the penis. *J Urol* 1992;147:630.

George J. Bosl
Dean F. Bajorin
Joel Sheinfeld
Robert J. Motzer
R. S. K. Chaganti

CHAPTER 35

Cancer of the Testis

Cancers of the testis make up a morphologically and clinically diverse group of neoplasms (Table 35-1). The overwhelming majority are primary in the testis, and most of these are germ cell tumors (GCTs). The management of each neoplasm is dependent on the histology and influenced by the anatomy of the testis and its lymphatic and vascular drainage. GCT is a highly curable disease requiring proper management at all stages.

BACKGROUND: INCIDENCE

GCTs are the most common solid tumor in men between the ages of 20 and 35 years. There are three modal peaks: infancy, ages 25 to 40, and approximately age 60. A solid testicular mass in a man aged 50 or greater is usually a lymphoma. The incidence of GCTs appears to be increasing. An estimated 7000 new cases (6900 testis) and 300 deaths caused by germ cell tumors of all primary sites will be reported in the United States in 2000.[1] The incidence of testis cancer varies significantly according to geographic area. The reported incidence is highest in Scandinavia, Switzerland, Germany, and New Zealand; intermediate in the United States and Great Britain; and lowest in Africa and Asia. The rising risk of testicular GCT incidence is associated with a birth cohort effect in both the United States and Europe.[2,3]

EPIDEMIOLOGY

GCTs are seen principally in young whites, and rarely in African Americans. The published ratio between white and African American patients is approximately 4:1 to 5:1, although it was closer to a 40:1 ratio in the U.S. military.[4] In African Americans, GCT behaves similarly to that of the general population.[5] Familial clustering has been observed, particularly among siblings.[6]

The cause of GCT is unknown. Random genetic events occurring during the early stages of meiosis seem to be responsible for the malignant transformation of germ cells (see Biology, later in this chapter). A few congenital developmental defects predispose to the disease.

CRYPTORCHIDISM

The risk of GCT occurring in the cryptorchid testis is several times the risk in normally descended testes. Between 5% and 20% of patients with a history of cryptorchidism develop a tumor in the *normally* descended testis.[7] An abdominal cryptorchid testis is more likely to develop GCT than an inguinal cryptorchid testis.[7] The protective effect of orchiopexy is difficult to quantify, but most data suggest a reduced likelihood of GCT if orchiopexy is performed before puberty. If the testis is inguinal, hormonally functioning, and easily examined, surveillance is recommended. If the testis is not amenable to orchiopexy or cannot be adequately examined, orchiectomy is recommended.

DIETHYLSTILBESTROL

Exogenous administration of estrogens to pregnant mice causes testicular maldescent and dysgenesis in offspring. Cryptorchidism and dysgenesis have also been reported in the male children of women exposed to diethylstilbestrol or oral contraceptives. Despite anecdotes associating diethylstilbestrol exposure with the development of GCT, epidemiologic studies have failed to identify such an association.[8]

KLINEFELTER'S SYNDROME

Klinefelter's syndrome is characterized by testicular atrophy, absence of spermatogenesis, a eunuchoid habitus, and gyneco-

TABLE 35-1. Histologic Classification of Testicular Neoplasms

A. Germ cell tumors (demonstrating one or more of the following components)
  1. Seminoma
    a. Classic (typical) seminoma
    b. Anaplastic seminoma
    c. Spermatocytic seminoma
  2. Embryonal carcinoma
  3. Teratoma
    a. Mature
    b. Immature
    c. Mature or immature teratoma with malignant transformation
  4. Choriocarcinoma
  5. Yolk sac tumor (endodermal sinus tumor; embryonal adenocarcinoma of the prepubertal testis)
B. Sex cord–stromal (gonadal stromal) tumors
  1. Leydig cell tumor
  2. Sertoli cell tumor
  3. Granulosa cell tumor (adult and juvenile types)
C. Both germ cell and gonadal stromal elements
  1. Gonadoblastoma
D. Adnexal and paratesticular tumors
  1. Mesothelioma
  2. Soft tissue origin (e.g., sarcomas)
  3. Adnexal (e.g., adenocarcinoma) of the rete testis
E. Miscellaneous neoplasms
  1. Carcinoid
  2. Lymphoma
  3. Cysts
F. Metastatic neoplasms

mastia. It is diagnosed by a 47,XXY karyotype. Klinefelter's syndrome patients have an increased incidence of mediastinal GCT.

OTHERS

A history of trauma is frequently noted by patients with testicular cancer; however, no evidence supports a direct causal relationship. Rather, the trauma usually prompts examination. Viral orchitis, usually secondary to mumps, may result in testicular atrophy. However, epidemiologic studies have failed to identify viral infection as a cause. More recently, testicular cancer has been reported in men infected with the human immunodeficiency virus. However, too few data support a higher incidence in individuals infected with human immunodeficiency virus, and the results of treatment are similar.[9,10] Reports implicating vasectomy as a cause of GCT have not been confirmed in cohort analysis.[11]

INITIAL PRESENTATION AND MANAGEMENT

SYMPTOMS AND SIGNS

The pathognomonic presentation of a primary testicular tumor is a painless testicular mass that may range in size from a few millimeters to several centimeters. However, the painless testicular mass occurs in only a minority of patients. The majority present with more diffuse testicular pain, swelling, hardness, or some combination of these findings. Since infectious epididymitis or orchitis, or a combination of the two, is more common, a trial of antibiotic therapy is often required in questionable cases. Acute testicular pain, simulating testicular torsion, occurs less frequently and may represent intratumoral hemorrhage. If the testicular discomfort does not abate or findings do not revert to normal within 2 to 4 weeks, a testicular ultrasound is indicated. On ultrasound, the typical testicular tumor is intratesticular and may produce one or more discrete hypoechoic masses. A pattern of multiple, diffuse calcifications in the testis has been associated with GCT.[12] Higher stage at presentation has been associated with delay in diagnosis,[13] and the experience of the treatment unit with the management of GCT appears to influence survival.[14–16]

DIAGNOSIS

A radical inguinal orchiectomy, using an inguinal incision with early high ligation of the spermatic cord at the deep inguinal ring, minimizes local tumor recurrence and aberrant lymphatic spread and is the only acceptable therapeutic and diagnostic procedure. The vasal and vascular components are doubly clamped and divided separately; their respective stumps are pushed into the retroperitoneal space to facilitate removal of the gonadal vessels at the time of retroperitoneal lymph node dissection (RPLND). The testicle and spermatic cord are removed *en bloc*, avoiding any spillage, and meticulous hemostasis is achieved. A transscrotal orchiectomy is contraindicated, because it permits the development of alternate lymphatic drainage pathways to the inguinal and pelvic lymph nodes and leaves intact the spermatic cord from the external to the internal ring. In the rare situation in which the diagnosis of a testicular tumor is in question, then an inguinal incision is required for an open biopsy. The testis can then be examined *in situ* in a sterile field and an appropriate biopsy taken with minimal risk of scrotal or inguinal contamination. Regardless of the preoperative diagnosis, all potential, primary testicular malignancies should be managed through an inguinal approach.

Extragonadal GCTs account for fewer than 10% of GCT. The mediastinum and retroperitoneum are the most common primary sites. Pineal tumors, occurring most frequently in children, are usually GCT. Because of their unique access to the meninges, the metastatic pattern of pineal GCT includes intradural sites along the neuraxis and is infrequently systemic. The management of pineal GCT is discussed in Chapter 43. In extremely rare circumstances, primary GCTs have been found in unusual sites such as the sacrum, thyroid, paranasal sinuses, and soft tissues of the head and neck.[17,18] In patients with extragonadal presentations of GCT, a testicular ultrasound is required. The management of extragonadal and testicular GCT is the same, and primary site is an independent factor in staging and risk classification.

HISTOLOGY

GCT is classified into two major subgroups: seminoma and nonseminoma. Three classifications are summarized in Table 35-2. The Mostofi adaptation of the Dixon/Moore classification[19] was largely adopted by the World Health Organization and is the classification most commonly used in North America and Europe.[20]

TABLE 35-2. Comparison of Three Classifications of Germ Cell Tumors

Dixon and Moore[19]	*World Health Organization*[20]	*British Tumor Panel*[21]
Seminoma	Seminoma Typical (classical) Anaplastic	Seminoma
Embryonal carcinoma	Embryonal carcinoma	Malignant teratoma, undifferentiated
Teratoma	Teratoma Mature Immature With malignant differentiation	Malignant teratoma, differentiated
Choriocarcinoma	Choriocarcinoma	Malignant teratoma, trophoblastic
Yolk sac tumor (endodermal sinus tumor)	Yolk sac tumor	Yolk sac tumor
Teratocarcinoma Teratoma + embryonal carcinoma ± other elements	Mixed germ cell tumors (specify components)	Malignant teratoma, intermediate

The British Tumor Panel's modification of the classification developed by Pugh is widely used in Great Britain and Australia.[21]

CARCINOMA *IN SITU*

Carcinoma *in situ* (CIS)[22] (intratubular germ cell neoplasia) precedes invasive testicular GCT in virtually all cases of typical and anaplastic seminoma and all nonseminomatous histologies in the adult. CIS is frequently present in retroperitoneal presentations and is rarely, if ever, present in mediastinal presentations.[23] It has not been described in spermatocytic seminoma and rarely in tumors arising in prepubertal patients.[24,25] Cytologically, CIS preceding seminoma and nonseminoma is identical. The median time for progression of CIS to invasive disease is 5 years.[26,27] In the general population, the incidence of CIS is low,[28] whereas in men with impaired fertility, the incidence is approximately 0.5%.[29,30] The incidence of CIS is 2% to 5% in both cryptorchid testes and the contralateral testis in patients with a documented prior testicular GCT.[31,32]

SEMINOMA

Seminoma accounts for approximately 50% of all GCT and most frequently appears in the fourth decade of life. The typical or classic form consists of sheets of large cells with abundant cytoplasm and round, hyperchromatic nuclei with prominent nucleoli. A lymphocytic infiltrate, granulomatous reaction with giant cells, or both, are frequently present. Trophoblastic giant cells capable of producing human chorionic gonadotropin (HCG) are present in 15% to 20% of tumors. The presence of syncytiotrophoblastic giant cells in an otherwise pure seminoma does *not* influence prognosis or treatment. *Anaplastic* seminoma is an older term used when three or more mitotic figures are seen per high-power field, and it has no clinical or prognostic importance. Stage for stage, anaplastic seminoma is similar in response and prognosis to classical seminoma.[33]

An *atypical* form of seminoma has been described with unusual immunohistochemical features. Although the cells cytologically resemble classical seminoma, lymphocytic infiltrate and granulomatous reaction are absent, necrosis is more common, and the nuclear to cytoplasmic ratio is higher. These tumors must be distinguished morphologically from solid variants of embryonal carcinoma and yolk sac tumor. Atypical seminoma frequently shows cytoplasmic expression of low-molecular-weight keratin or the type 1 precursor to the blood group antigens, whereas typical seminoma stains negative.[34] Electron microscopic studies have shown that the individual tumor cells acquire cytoplasmic cytokeratin intermediate filaments, suggesting epithelial differentiation. There has been no specific association of atypical seminoma with an adverse prognosis, and its management is currently the same as any other seminoma.

Spermatocytic seminoma is a rare histologic variant seen almost exclusively in men above the age of 45. The relationship of spermatocytic seminoma to other GCTs is not clear, since it is not associated with CIS or bilaterality, does not express placental alkaline phosphatase (PLAP) (see Immunohistochemical Markers, later in this chapter), and has not been shown to have the same genetic abnormalities as other GCTs. Metastatic potential is minimal.

NONSEMINOMATOUS GERM CELL TUMORS

Nonseminomatous histology makes up approximately 50% of all GCTs and most frequently presents in the third decade of life. Most tumors are mixed, consisting of two or more cell types. Seminoma may be a component, but the definition of a pure seminoma *excludes* the presence of any nonseminomatous cell type. The presence of any nonseminomatous cell type (other than syncytiotrophoblasts) imparts the prognosis and management principles of a nonseminomatous tumor.

Embryonal Carcinoma

Embryonal carcinoma is the most undifferentiated somatic cell type. Individual cells are epithelioid in appearance and may be arranged in glandular or tubular nests and cords or as solid sheets of cells. Tumor necrosis and hemorrhage are frequently observed.

Choriocarcinoma

Choriocarcinoma, by definition, consists of both cytotrophoblasts and syncytiotrophoblasts. If cytotrophoblasts are not present, then the diagnosis of choriocarcinoma cannot be made. Pure choriocarcinoma is an extremely rare presentation usually associated with widespread hematogenous metastases and high levels of HCG. Hemorrhage into the primary tumor is frequent and is an occasional severe complication when it spontaneously occurs at a metastatic site.[35] Elements of choriocarcinoma are frequently found in mixed tumors but appear to have no prognostic importance.[36] Syncytiotrophoblastic giant cells can be seen as a component of any GCT (including pure seminoma). They impart no prognostic value by themselves.

Yolk Sac Tumor

Yolk sac tumor (endodermal sinus tumor) is often confused with a glandular form of embryonal carcinoma. This tumor mimics the yolk sac of the embryo and produces α-fetoprotein (AFP). The cells may have a papillary, glandular, microcystic, or solid appearance and may be associated with Schiller-Duval bodies, which are perivascular arrangements of epithelial cells with an intervening extracellular space. Rarely, *embryoid bodies* resembling the early embryo can be seen. Yolk sac histology is infrequently the only histologic subtype in adult GCT except in the mediastinum where pure yolk sac tumors account for a minority of primary tumors.

Teratoma

Teratoma is composed of somatic cell types from two or more germ layers (ectoderm, mesoderm, or endoderm) and is derived from a totipotential, malignant precursor cell (embryonal carcinoma or yolk sac tumor). *Mature teratoma* consists of adult-type differentiated elements such as cartilage, glandular epithelium, nerve tissue, or other differentiated cell types. *Immature teratoma* generally refers to a tumor with partial somatic differentiation, similar to that seen in a fetus. Both mature and immature teratomas are histologically benign. *Teratoma with malignant transformation* refers to a form of teratoma in which one of its components, either immature or mature, develops aggressive growth and histologically resembles another malignancy. These usually take the form of sarcomas (most frequently embryonal rhabdomyosarcoma), and, less frequently, carcinomas (e.g., enteric-type adenocarcinoma), neuroectodermal tumors, or combinations of these.[37] Acute nonlymphocytic leukemias have arisen in the context of mediastinal nonseminomatous GCT, but not from other primary sites.[38] In a review of 41 cases of pure mature or immature teratoma of the testis, 26 (63%) displayed retroperitoneal or systemic metastases, with or without increased levels of serum tumor markers.[39] Therefore, a primary testicular tumor in a postpubertal boy or man that displays only histologically mature or immature teratoma must be considered to be a fully malignant GCT, and management should proceed as if malignant components are present.

BIOLOGY

Adult human male GCTs make up a unique system for the study of the mechanism of transformation of a totipotential germ cell in lineage differentiation. The pluripotentiality of the tumor cells manifests as histologic differentiation into germ cell–like undifferentiated (seminoma), primitive zygotic (embryonal carcinoma), embryonal-like somatically differentiated (teratoma), and extraembryonically differentiated (choriocarcinoma and yolk sac tumor) phenotypes. Until fairly recently, the molecular mechanisms of germ cell transformation, GCT differentiation, or GCT chemotherapy sensitivity and resistance were poorly understood. More recent studies of GCTs have suggested that (1) overexpression of cyclin D2 is an early, possibly oncogenic, event in germ cell tumorigenesis; (2) differentiation in GCTs may be governed by several possibly interacting pathways such as loss of regulators of germ cell totipotentiality and of embryonic development, and genomic imprinting; and (3) chemotherapy sensitivity and resistance may be rooted in part in a p53-dependent apoptotic pathway.

Mechanism of Germ Cell Transformation

Genetic analysis of male GCTs has yielded important data relevant to the mechanism of germ cell transformation.[40] Virtually 100% of tumors show increased copy number of 12p, as one or more copies of i(12p) or as tandem duplications of 12p, *in situ* or transposed elsewhere in the genome (Fig. 35-1).[40] This chromosomal marker has been observed as early as CIS, suggesting that it is among the earliest, if not the earliest, genetic change associated with the origin of these tumors.[40] A candidate gene, *CCND2*, mapped to 12p13, has been identified as the possible driver gene on 12p whose deregulated expression may lead to GCT development.[41] It is abundantly expressed in CIS as well as in many lineages of GCTs.[41] Cyclin D2 is one of the D-type cyclins that, along with the cyclin-dependent kinases cdk4, cdk6, or both, regulates the phosphorylation of pRB and controls the G_1/S cell-cycle checkpoint.[42] Disruption of this checkpoint through amplification or overexpression of D-type cyclins is known to be one of the important pathways in human tumor development.[42]

The precursor of all GCTs is considered to be CIS; however, the stage of germ cell development at which transformation occurs is not known. Two models of origin of CIS cells have been proposed. One model proposed by Skakkebaek and colleagues[43,44] suggested that fetal gonocytes that have escaped normal development into spermatogonia may undergo abnormal cell division mediated by a kit receptor/stem cell factor (kit ligand) paracrine loop, leading to uncontrolled proliferation of gonocytes. Such gonocytes have been postulated to be susceptible to subsequent invasive growth through the mediation of postnatal and pubertal gonadotrophin stimulation. This hypothesis is based on a consideration of immunophenotypic markers expressed by gonocytes and CIS cells, types of abnormal germ cells seen in developmental disorders that predispose to GCTs, and epidemiology of GCT incidence.[43] A second model proposed by Chaganti and colleagues takes into account four established genetic properties of GCTs, namely, increased 12p copy number, expression of cyclin D2 in CIS, consistent near triploid-tetraploid chromosome numbers, and abundant expression of wild-type p53.[45] According to this model, aberrant chromatid exchange events during meiotic crossing over may lead to increased 12p copy number and overexpression of cyclin D2. In a cell containing unrepaired DNA breaks (recombination-associated), overexpressing cyclin D2 may block a p53-dependent apoptotic response and lead to reinitiation of cell-cycle and genomic instability.[45] A role for cyclin D2 in the development of GCTs has also been suggested by Sicinski et al.[46] through studies of mice homozygously inactivated (mutant) for the *CCND2* gene, and expression of *CCND2* mRNA in ovarian granulosa cell tumors and testicular GCT cell lines. In germ cells that have reentered cell cycle following cyclin D2 activation, downstream events such as loss of tumor suppressor genes (TSGs) brought about by genomic instability may lead to neoplastic progression. Extensive molecular genetic analysis has identified genomic, functional (expression), or both kinds of loss of several known TSGs such as *RB1*, *DCC*, and *NME*, and genomic loss at several previously recognized as well as novel chromosomal sites.[40,47]

Embryonal-Like Differentiation in Germ Cell Tumors

Male GCTs display, albeit in a spatially and temporally abnormal manner, patterns of differentiation that mimic stages normally undergone by the developing zygote. Among GCTs, seminoma can be viewed as transformed germ cells that have retained the inhibitory mechanism for zygotic-like differentiation, a feature of germ cells before fertilization. The *in vivo*

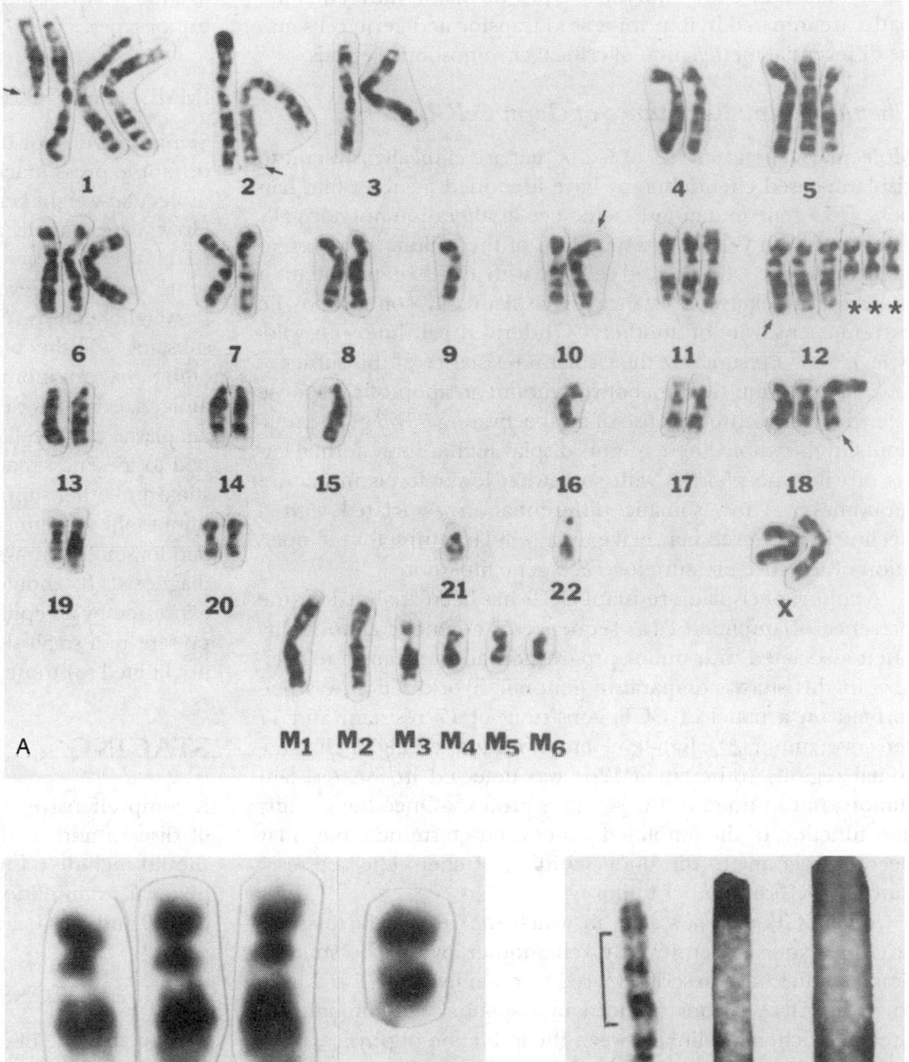

FIGURE 35-1. **A:** Karyotype of a male germ cell tumor cell line with hyperdiploid chromosome number containing three copies (***) of i(12p) chromosomes. Arrows indicate abnormal chromosomes. M1 through M6 are unidentified marker chromosomes. **B:** Abnormalities of 12p in male germ cell tumor showing three normal chromosomes 12 and an i(12p). **C:** Tandem duplication of 12p in i(12p) negative tumor. Abnormally banded marker chromosome (left) revealed chromosome 12 material by chromosome 12 painting probe (middle) and 12p painting probe identified the region of amplification to be 12p (right).

expression patterns of kit receptor and stem cell factor in GCTs are consistent with such a view. Thus, the kit receptor, which normally is expressed by spermatogonia and primary spermatocytes,[48] is expressed mainly by CIS and seminoma.[49] On the other hand, nonseminoma appear to down-regulate kit and up-regulate stem cell factor, consistent with their loss of germ cell phenotype and acquisition of somatic fates.[49] The key developmental difference between seminoma and nonseminoma appears to be the loss of ability to retain germ cell–like totipotentiality by the former.

A great deal of effort has been directed toward understanding the mechanistic basis of decisions that determine the nature and regulation of proliferation and differentiation signals in the developing zygote.[50,51] In this context, GCTs and derived embryonal carcinoma cell lines provide a unique opportunity to study embryonal versus extraembryonal pathways of differentiation, as well as development of somatic lineage. Analysis of genome-wide allelic loss in GCTs showed an overall higher loss in the highly differentiated teratomas compared with the less differentiated embryonal carcinomas.[52] These studies identified chromosomal sites that may harbor effector genes such as transcription factors whose loss may prompt either induction of differentiation or lineage decision.

The ability of GCTs to undergo an embryonal-like developmental program without the contribution of a maternal complement has obvious implications to genomic imprinting. Parental imprints are erased in normal germ cells before meiosis, and new imprinting patterns are laid down during gametogenesis and again during embryogenesis.[53,54] Therefore, the target cell for transformation proposed in our model, the meiotic spermatocyte, would be imprint-erased, which is consistent with observations of biallelic expression in GCTs of *IGF2* and *H19* genes which normally show monoallelic expression in postfertilization somatic tissues.[55,56] A possible mechanism by which embryonal and extraembryonal types of major differentiation paths are initiated in imprint-erased transformed germ cells may be differential methylation of critical chromosomal regions.

Chemotherapy Resistance of Germ Cell Tumors

Molecular genetic studies of GCTs that are clinically resistant to cisplatin-based chemotherapy have identified a subset that harbors *TP53* gene mutations,[57] a molecular alteration not normally associated with GCTs.[58,59] Evaluation of the cellular response to cisplatin in one GCT-derived cell line with a *TP53* gene mutation indicated a relative resistance to cisplatin, in contrast to the extreme sensitivity of another GCT-derived cell line with wild-type *TP53*.[57] Presumably, the cisplatin resistance of this subset of GCTs is rooted in their inability to mount an apoptotic response after drug exposure because of an inactivating *TP53* gene mutation. On the whole, these tumors display higher than normal levels of wild-type p53,[60,61] with somewhat lower levels in mature teratomas.[62] Thus, somatic differentiation associated with a decline in p53 levels may make up a cellular setting for the operation of selective pressure for *TP53* gene mutation.

A cohort of cisplatin-resistant GCTs has been analyzed for the presence of amplified DNA sequences,[63] a genetic abnormality often associated with tumor progression and resistance to therapy. In this study, comparative genomic hybridization was performed on a panel of GCTs consisting of 17 resistant and 17 sensitive tumors.[63] High-level amplification of eight chromosomal regions (other than 12p) was detected in five resistant tumors, but in none of the sensitive group.[63] Once the identity and function of the amplified genes are determined, they may become relevant to the understanding of chemotherapy resistance of GCTs and other tumor types.

Male GCTs offer a system in which the cellular factors portending exquisite sensitivity to chemotherapy can be studied. Some studies have described a reduced ability of GCT cell lines to repair DNA lesions induced by cisplatin.[64,65] Although the precise biochemical link between the induction of physical damage in DNA and the cellular response to it is unclear, in general, cells treated with DNA-damaging agents respond either by induction of a delay in the cell cycle at the G_1 to S phase boundary, or by the induction of apoptosis, both of which are thought to be mediated by p53.[66] It has also been suggested that the rapid apoptotic response of GCTs on exposure to chemotherapeutic agents may be caused by a high ratio of the proapoptotic bax protein to the antiapoptotic bcl-2 protein, favoring apoptosis.[67] This has been substantiated in a limited number of GCT cell lines and needs to be further investigated at the *in vivo* level.[67] However, other *in vitro* studies have suggested that bcl-x_L, a bcl-2-related antiapoptotic protein, may act as the regulator of DNA damage-induced cell death in GCTs, rather than bcl-2.[68] In these studies, exogenous overexpression of bcl-2 in a GCT cell line resulted in sensitization of the cell line to DNA damage-induced cell death. Associated with this sensitization was a decreased endogenous expression of bcl-x_L with little or no change in the level of bax expression. A much attenuated apoptotic response to cisplatin has been observed in somatically differentiated GCT cell lines, reflecting the relative resistance of teratoma elements of GCT specimens.[69] The elucidation of the molecular mechanisms whereby the unique apoptotic response to chemotherapeutic agents is achieved in GCTs will contribute to the understanding of how such a response is achieved, as well as show how resistance may be circumvented in GCTs and other tumor types.

IMMUNOHISTOCHEMICAL MARKERS

Seminoma do not display differentiation *in vitro* or *in vivo* and do not express markers of somatic differentiation such as low-molecular-weight keratins, vimentin, or blood group antigens.[34,70] However, essentially all seminoma express PLAP and kit receptor CD117.[49,71,72] Embryonal carcinoma and yolk sac tumor do display some somatic differentiation. Surface expression of low-molecular-weight keratins (e.g., AE-1, CAM 5.2) and the type 1 precursor substance of the blood group antigens is invariable.[34,70] Most embryonal carcinoma, but not seminoma, also express the CD30 antigen, originally described as a marker of Hodgkin's disease and anaplastic large cell lymphoma.[73–75] Vimentin expression is limited to mesenchymal components of mature teratoma and interstitial and other support cells. In tumors of uncertain histogenesis, immunohistochemical studies that include PLAP, kit receptor, and low-molecular-weight keratins may be useful in establishing a diagnosis. It should be remembered that cytokeratins are expressed by all epithelial tumors, and PLAP immunoreactivity is present in a small subset of epithelial neoplasms, especially (but not limited to) those of Müllerian origin.

STAGING

A comprehensive evaluation is necessary to define the extent of disease and to determine the appropriate treatment, and should include pathologic examination of the primary tumor, physical examination, determination of serum concentrations of AFP and HCG, and radiographic studies.

ANATOMIC CONSIDERATIONS

The initial route of metastasis is lymphatic drainage to retroperitoneal lymph nodes (Fig. 35-2). From the testes, several lymphatic vessels emerge from the mediastinum testis and accompany the gonadal vessels in the spermatic cord. Where the spermatic vessels cross ventral to the ureter, some of these lymphatics diverge medially and drain into the retroperitoneal lymph node chain, whereas others follow the spermatic vessels to their origin. Lymph nodes located lateral or anterior to the inferior vena cava are called paracaval or precaval nodes, respectively. Interaortocaval nodes are those nodes between the inferior vena cava and the aorta. Nodes anterior or lateral to the aorta are preaortic or paraaortic nodes, respectively. The primary *landing zone* for a right testicular tumor lies in the interaortocaval nodes immediately below the renal vessels, and the ipsilateral distribution includes the paracaval, preaortic, and right common iliac. The primary landing zone for a left testicular tumor lies in the true paraaortic nodes just below the left renal vessels, and the ipsilateral distribution for the left testis includes the paraaortic, preaortic, and left common iliac nodes. Metastatic nodal disease in more caudal areas such as the common iliac, external iliac, or inguinal lymph nodes is usually secondary to large volume of disease with retrograde spread. If the patient has undergone a herniorrhaphy, vasectomy, or other transscrotal procedure unrelated to the tumor, additional attention should be paid to pelvic and inguinal lymph nodes.

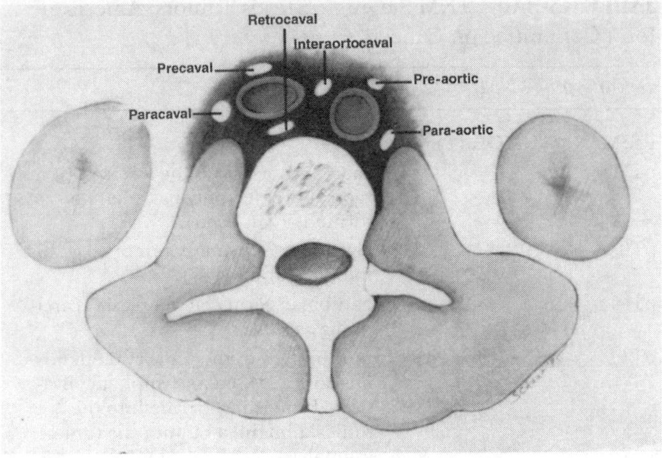

FIGURE 35-2. Retroperitoneal lymph nodes.

Contralateral retroperitoneal metastasis is represented by involvement of nodes usually associated with a tumor from the opposite side. For example, paraaortic lymphadenopathy in the presence of a right-sided primary tumor is considered contralateral. Contralateral spread is more common with right-sided tumors, rare with left-sided primaries, and usually in the setting of large-volume disease.

Retroperitoneal lymphatics continue cephalad and empty into the cisterna chyle via the right and left lumbar trunks. Lymphatic involvement above the retroperitoneal nodes results in involvement of the retrocrural nodes. Supradiaphragmatic spread occurs via the thoracic duct, leading to posterior mediastinal and left supraclavicular lymph node involvement. The anterior mediastinum is not part of this usual nodal hierarchy.

TUMOR IMAGING

Plain chest radiography and computed tomography (CT) are the most important radiologic investigations in determining extent of disease and treatment. The role of magnetic resonance imaging (MRI) is limited.

Computed Tomography

CT is the most effective radiographic technique for identifying metastatic involvement both above and below the diaphragm. Well-circumscribed pulmonary lesions less than 5 mm may be detected, and although these may represent metastases, many lesions in this size range represent benign processes, and their clinical importance depends on clinical stage. In seminoma, such lesions are usually benign.

CT scan of the abdomen is the best technique for identifying retroperitoneal lymphadenopathy and has replaced intravenous pyelography and lymphangiography. The abdominal CT scan is normal in 70% of newly diagnosed seminoma and at least one-third of newly diagnosed nonseminoma. Because GCTs may grow rapidly, treatment decisions should be made within 4 weeks of the last abdominal CT scan. Lymph nodes in the primary landing zones measuring 10 to 20 mm are involved by GCT approximately 70% of the time and those measuring 4 to 10 mm are involved 50% of the time.[76–79] The duodenum and proximal jejunum must be adequately opacified by oral contrast. In evaluation of the postchemotherapy mass, the CT scan is unable to distinguish between residual malignant tumor, teratoma, and necrosis or fibrosis; a *normal* postchemotherapy CT scan does not preclude the presence of disease.

Magnetic Resonance Imaging

Like CT scanning, MRI can identify enlarged lymph nodes. Although MRI occasionally provides valuable preoperative information regarding vascular anatomy and the patency of the great vessels in patients with bulky retroperitoneal disease following chemotherapy, it adds little in the management of most patients with GCT. Both MRI and CT are equally unable to detect viable GCT after chemotherapy.

Lymphangiography

Historically, lymphangiography was used to determine the extent of retroperitoneal involvement in both seminoma and nonseminoma. In most patients, CT scanning has replaced it. The role of lymphangiography is limited to patients with stage I seminoma. In patients with seminoma, lymphangiography may reduce normal tissue irradiation by permitting more precise ports and identifying where a *boost* of radiation may be needed for abnormal nodes seen on lymphangiography but not evident on CT scan.

Positron Emission Tomography

Studies have compared positron emission tomography (PET) with CT for the evaluation of patients with newly diagnosed disease or residual disease after chemotherapy. Although early studies suggest that PET may be more sensitive than CT, disease less than 0.5 cm was not detected.[80] In patients with residual disease, PET has not been consistently able to identify residual viable malignant GCT and does not detect teratoma.[81–83] Therefore, insufficient data exist to recommend PET as part of staging or in the evaluation of residual disease after chemotherapy.

SERUM TUMOR MARKERS

α-Fetoprotein

AFP is a 70,000 molecular-weight glycoprotein produced in the liver, gastrointestinal tract, and fetal yolk sac, and its secretion in GCT is restricted to nonseminomatous histology, usually embryonal cell carcinoma or endodermal sinus tumor. AFP is detected by radioimmunoassay and reported in nanograms per milliliter. The normal adult concentration is usually less than 15 ng/mL. The serum half-life is 5 to 7 days. In patients with pure seminoma, elevated serum concentrations of AFP reflect an undetected nonseminomatous element. An increased serum AFP concentration is present in 10% to 20% of clinical stage I, 20% to 40% of low-burden clinical stage II, and 40% to 60% of high-burden disease. Because of stage migration, the frequency and degree of increased AFP concentrations in patients with advanced tumors has declined.[84]

Human Chorionic Gonadotropin

HCG is a glycoprotein composed of two subunits and is produced by syncytiotrophoblasts. The α subunit is identical to that of luteinizing hormone, follicle-stimulating hormone, and thyroid-stimulating hormone. The β subunits of HCG, luteinizing hormone, follicle-stimulating hormone, and thyroid-stimulating hormone are homologous but have distinct amino acid sequences.[85] Elevated serum concentrations can be found in patients with pure seminoma as well as those with nonseminomatous GCT. Most vendors have adopted the World Health Organization Third International Standard (code number 75/537) resulting in some uniformity in the radioimmunoassays to detect the HCG β subunit. The serum half-life is 18 to 36 hours.

Approximately 10% to 20% of clinical stage I, 20% to 30% of low-volume clinical stage II, and 40% of patients with advanced nonseminomatous GCT present with elevated serum concentrations of HCG; the frequency and degree to which the HCG is elevated has decreased over time.[84] Approximately 15% to 25% of patients with advanced pure seminoma have increased serum concentrations of HCG.[86] False elevations of HCG secondary to either cross-reactivity of the antibody with luteinizing hormone, treatment-induced hypogonadism, or pituitary production of HCG have been reported.[87–89]

Lactate Dehydrogenase

The serum level of lactate dehydrogenase (LDH) has independent prognostic significance in patients with advanced GCT and should be determined in all patients. Increases in the serum concentration are a reflection of tumor burden, growth rate, and cellular proliferation. LDH comprises multiple isoenzymes, but, in practice, the combined LDH value for all isoenzymes is used for clinical decision making. Comparison of one laboratory with another is possible by using ratios of the detected level to the upper limit of normal for the individual assay.[90] Increased serum LDH concentrations are observed in approximately 60% of nonseminomatous GCT patients with advanced disease and in 80% of patients with advanced seminoma.[86,91]

STAGING CLASSIFICATIONS

Revised tumor, nodes, and metastases (TNM) and stage groupings of the American Joint Committee on Cancer and the Union Internationale Centre le Cancre were adopted in 1997 (Table 35-3).[92] For the first time, an *S* category for the serum concentrations of AFP, HCG, and LDH was incorporated because of its independent prognostic significance. Broadly, stage I disease is confined to the testis, stage II disease is restricted to the retroperitoneum, and stage III disease represents involvement of supradiaphragmatic or other nodal sites, or visceral disease. Levels of AFP, HCG, and LDH determine overall stage.

Factors Affecting Staging of the Primary Tumor (T Stage)

The T stage of the primary lesion (not size), histology, and serum tumor marker concentrations predict the likelihood of retroperitoneal disease. For nonseminomatous GCT, the presence of either lymphatic or vascular invasion or both has been associated with a higher likelihood of retroperitoneal metastases (approximately 50%) and is now included in the definition of T2 invasion through the tunica albuginea into tunica vaginalis (also T2), spermatic cord (T3), or scrotum (T4) is an additional adverse feature.

TABLE 35-3A. TNM Staging of Testis Tumors: American Joint Committee on Cancer[92]

Definition of TNM	
PRIMARY TUMOR (T)	
pTX	Primary tumor cannot be assessed (if no radical orchiectomy has been performed, TX is used).
pT0	No evidence of primary tumor (e.g., histologic scar in testis).
pTis	Intratubular germ cell neoplasia (carcinoma *in situ*).
pT1	Tumor limited to the testis and epididymis and no vascular/lymphatic invasion. Tumor may invade into the tunica albuginea but not the tunica vaginalis.
pT2	Tumor limited to the testis and epididymis with vascular/lymphatic invasion or tumor extending through the tunica albuginea with involvement of tunica vaginalis.
pT3	Tumor invades the spermatic cord with or without vascular/lymphatic invasion.
pT4	Tumor invades the scrotum with or without vascular/lymphatic invasion.
REGIONAL LYMPH NODES (N)	
Clinical	
NX	Regional lymph nodes cannot be assessed.
N0	No regional lymph node metastasis.
N1	Lymph node mass 2 cm or less in greatest dimension; or multiple lymph nodes, none more than 2 cm in greatest dimension.
N2	Lymph node mass more than 2 cm but not more than 5 cm in greatest dimension; or multiple lymph nodes, any one mass greater than 2 cm but not more than 5 cm in greatest dimension.
N3	Lymph node mass more than 5 cm in greatest dimension.
Pathologic	
pN0	No evidence of tumor in lymph nodes.
pN1	Lymph node mass 2 cm or less in greatest dimension and less than or equal to five nodes positive, none greater than 2 cm in greatest dimension.
pN2	Lymph node mass more than 2 cm but not more than 5 cm in greatest dimension; more than five nodes positive, none greater than 5 cm; evidence of extranodal extension of tumor.
pN3	Lymph node mass more than 5 cm in greatest dimension.
DISTANT METASTASES (M)	
M0	No evidence of distant metastases.
M1	Nonregional nodal or pulmonary metastases.
M2	Nonpulmonary visceral metastases.

TABLE 35-3B. TNM Staging of Testis Tumors: American Joint Committee on Cancer[92]

	Lactate Dehydrogenase	Human Chorionic Gonadotropin (mIu/mL)	α-Fetoprotein (ng/mL)	
SERUM TUMOR MARKERS (S)				
S1	<1.5 × N[a]	<5000	<1000	
S2	1.5–10.0 × N	5000–50,000	1000–10,000	
S3	>10 × N	>50,000	>10,000	
STAGE GROUPING				
	T	N	M	S
Stage I				
IA	T1	N0	M0	S0
IB	T2	N0	M0	S0
	T3	N0	M0	S0
	T4	N0	M0	S0
IS	T_{ANY}	N0	M0	S_{ANY}
Stage II				
IIA	T_{ANY}	N1	M0	S0
	T_{ANY}	N1	M0	S1
IIB	T_{ANY}	N2	M0	S0
	T_{ANY}	N2	M0	S1
IIC	T_{ANY}	N3	M0	S0
	T_{ANY}	N3	M0	S1
Stage III				
IIIA	T_{ANY}	N_{ANY}	M1	S0
IIIB	T_{ANY}	N_{ANY}	M0	S2
IIIC	T_{ANY}	N_{ANY}	M1	S3

[a]N indicates the upper limit of normal for the lactate dehydrogenase assay.

Reproducible prognostic factors predicting retroperitoneal disease in seminoma have not been identified. A Princess Margaret Hospital study of seminoma patients treated with radiation therapy identified anaplastic histology, invasion of the tunica, and invasion of the epididymis as prognostic for relapse.[93] However, other studies have failed to confirm these findings.[94,95] Similarly, the presence of increased serum concentrations of HCG are not consistently associated with a poor prognosis.[86,96,97]

Factors Affecting Staging of Regional (Retroperitoneal) Nodes (N Stage)

Metastatic disease to retroperitoneal lymph nodes is considered to be stage II disease. The classification of retroperitoneal lymph node involvement is based either on pathologic evaluation after RPLND or clinical evidence of retroperitoneal lymph node involvement (see Table 35-3).

PATHOLOGIC STAGING. The number and size of retroperitoneal lymph nodes found at RPLND have prognostic importance.[98–102] Most retrospective studies report a less than or equal to 35% incidence of recurrent disease when fewer than six nodes are involved with tumor, *and* the largest node is less than 2 cm, *and* no extranodal tumor extension is evident. More extensive tumor involvement is generally associated with a recurrence rate of greater than or equal to 50%. Once lymph node involvement is demonstrated, the histology of the primary tumor, and the presence or absence of vascular invasion in the primary tumor do not appear to add prognostic value.

CLINICAL STAGING. The transverse diameter of the largest lymph node has been used to subcategorize stage II disease (see Table 35-3). For seminoma, the size of retroperitoneal adenopathy usually dictates the treatment modality. Relapse proportions after definitive radiation therapy for seminoma increase progressively from approximately 15% for nodes less than 5 cm to approximately 40% to 60% for nodes greater than 5 cm.[93,103] In nonseminoma, treatment decisions are based on retroperitoneal lymph node size, location of the adenopathy, and the presence and degree of increase in serum tumor marker concentrations.

Prognostic Factors in Advanced Disease

Because 70% to 80% of patients with advanced GCT are cured with modern cisplatin-based chemotherapy, it has become necessary to stratify patients according to the likelihood of cure. Although survival is the best reflection of cure, complete response is often used as a surrogate for cure, since few patients relapse after being rendered free of disease. Histology, metastatic site, primary site, and serum tumor marker concentrations are independent prognostic variables and have been shown to predict the likelihood of cure. Patients who are more likely to be cured (good-risk or good-prognosis subgroup) constitute the majority of GCT patients with advanced disease and should be treated with regimens that have maximum efficacy with minimal toxicity. In contrast, patients who are unlikely to be cured (poor risk or poor prognosis) constitute the minority of patients. For them, more effective therapy is needed; toxicity is an important but secondary issue.

Between 1980 and 1997, several classification algorithms were used to assign good- and poor-risk status based on the extent of disease, specific sites of disease, pretreatment serum tumor marker concentrations, or all these factors. The Memorial Sloan-Kettering Cancer Center (MSKCC)[104] and Indiana University[105] allocation criteria were the most frequently used criteria in the United States and Medical Research Council and European Organization for the Research and Treatment of Cancer (EORTC)[106] criteria in Europe (Table 35-4). A comparison of these four risk criteria in advanced nonseminomatous GCT demonstrated marked differences and revealed that the allocation to either good- or poor-risk categories was in agreement in only 56% of patients.[107] Substantial numbers of patients assigned good-risk status by stringent criteria were classified as poor risk by those that were less stringent. The proportion cured in the poor-risk group increases with less stringent algorithms.[107]

The International Germ Cell Cancer Collaborative Group (IGCCCG), representing GCT clinical trialists from Europe, North America, and Australia, analyzed data from over 5000 patients treated with platinum-based chemotherapy in order to develop a common classification system. The IGCCCG found

TABLE 35-4. Comparison of Four Poor-Risk Classification Algorithms

	Memorial Sloan-Kettering[104]	*Indiana University*[105]	*European Organization for the Research and Treatment of Cancer*[106]	*International*[108]
Primary site	Yes	No	No	Mediastinum
α-Fetoprotein	No	No	>1000 IU/μL	>10,000 ng/mL
Human chorionic gonadotropin	Continuous	No	>10,000 IU/μL	>50,000 mIu/mL
Lactate dehydrogenase	Continuous	No	No	>10 × normal[a]
Metastatic sites	No	Bone, liver, brain	Bone, liver	Bone, liver, brain

[a] Normal defined as the upper limit of normal for the specific assay.

that the independent prognostic factors for progression-free survival for patients with nonseminomatous GCT included pretreatment levels of LDH, HCG, and AFP; site of the primary tumor (i.e., mediastinal vs. testis or retroperitoneal); and the presence of nonpulmonary visceral metastases (such as bone, brain, or liver metastases).[108] Nonpulmonary visceral metastasis was the only significant prognostic factor in seminoma patients. Investigators agreed on three strata of good-, intermediate-, and poor-prognosis patients with nonseminomatous GCT; no poor-risk stratum could be defined in seminoma (Table 35-5). The marker cutoff values were incorporated into the revised TNM classification.[92] Hence, the IGCCCG grouping should be used in future clinical trials and in treatment decision making for patients requiring initial chemotherapy for advanced disease.

MANAGEMENT OF CLINICAL STAGE I DISEASE

SEMINOMA

Radiation Therapy

Radiation therapy remains the treatment of choice for patients with clinical stage I seminoma. The ipsilateral hemiscrotum does not require therapy unless gross tumor spillage has taken place. A randomized trial shows that a simple paraaortic portal excluding the ipsilateral iliac and pelvic nodes is as effective as the dog-leg portal in overall survival. Although more pelvic relapses may be seen, the toxicity appears less (Fig. 35-3*A*).[109] This more restricted portal may be considered a standard of care. Conventional fractionation for clinical stage I disease is 150 to 180 cGy/d for five sessions per week using high-energy linear accelerator beams to a total dose of 2500 to 3000 cGy. Elective, prophylactic radiation therapy to the mediastinum is contraindicated.[110] The contralateral testis should be shielded during treatment. Proper shielding results in an exposure less than 1% of the total dose. For left-sided primary testicular tumors, the left renal hilum must be encompassed. Treatment of pelvic lymph nodes is sometimes required for T4 primary tumors or for scrotal violations with tumor spillage. An involved spermatic cord margin at the internal ring may also require field extension. The relapse rate within the irradiated portal after adequate radiation therapy is negligible. The systemic relapse rate, usually presenting as a supraclavicular mass, averages 4% to 5% (Table 35-6), and the death rate is under 2%.[95,109–114]

Observation

Although the dose of radiation therapy is low and the cure rate exceptionally high, long-term sequelae include the potential for an increased incidence of gastrointestinal neoplasms (see Treatment Sequelae, later in this chapter).[115,116] As a consequence, surveillance has been studied as the only management after orchiectomy, to be followed by chemotherapy at relapse (Table 35-7).[93,117] The relapse rate is approximately 15%, but the median time to relapse is approximately 12 months, longer than that observed for nonseminomatous GCT. Moreover, relapses have occurred at intervals more than 5 years from diagnosis.[93] In addition, over 5 years of follow-up, surveillance is also approximately 30% less expensive.[118] Therefore, in the United States, observation for clinical stage I seminoma is not considered routine.

TABLE 35-5. Germ Cell Tumor Risk Classification: International Consensus[108]

	Seminoma	*Nonseminoma*
Good risk	Any HCG Any LDH Nonpulmonary visceral metastases absent Any primary site	AFP <1000 ng/mL HCG <5000 mIu/mL LDH <1.5 × upper limit of normal Nonpulmonary visceral metastases absent Gonadal or retroperitoneal primary tumor
Intermediate risk	Nonpulmonary visceral metastases present Any HCG Any LDH Any primary site	AFP 1000–10,000 ng/mL HCG 5000–50,000 mIu/mL LDH 1.5–10.0 times upper limit of normal Nonpulmonary visceral metastases absent Gonadal or retroperitoneal primary site
Poor risk	—	Mediastinal primary site Nonpulmonary visceral metastases present (e.g., bone, liver, brain) AFP ≥10,000 ng/mL HCG ≥ 50,000 mIu/mL LDH ≥10 × upper limit of normal

AFP, α-fetoprotein; HCG, human chorionic gonadotropin; LDH, lactate dehydrogenase.

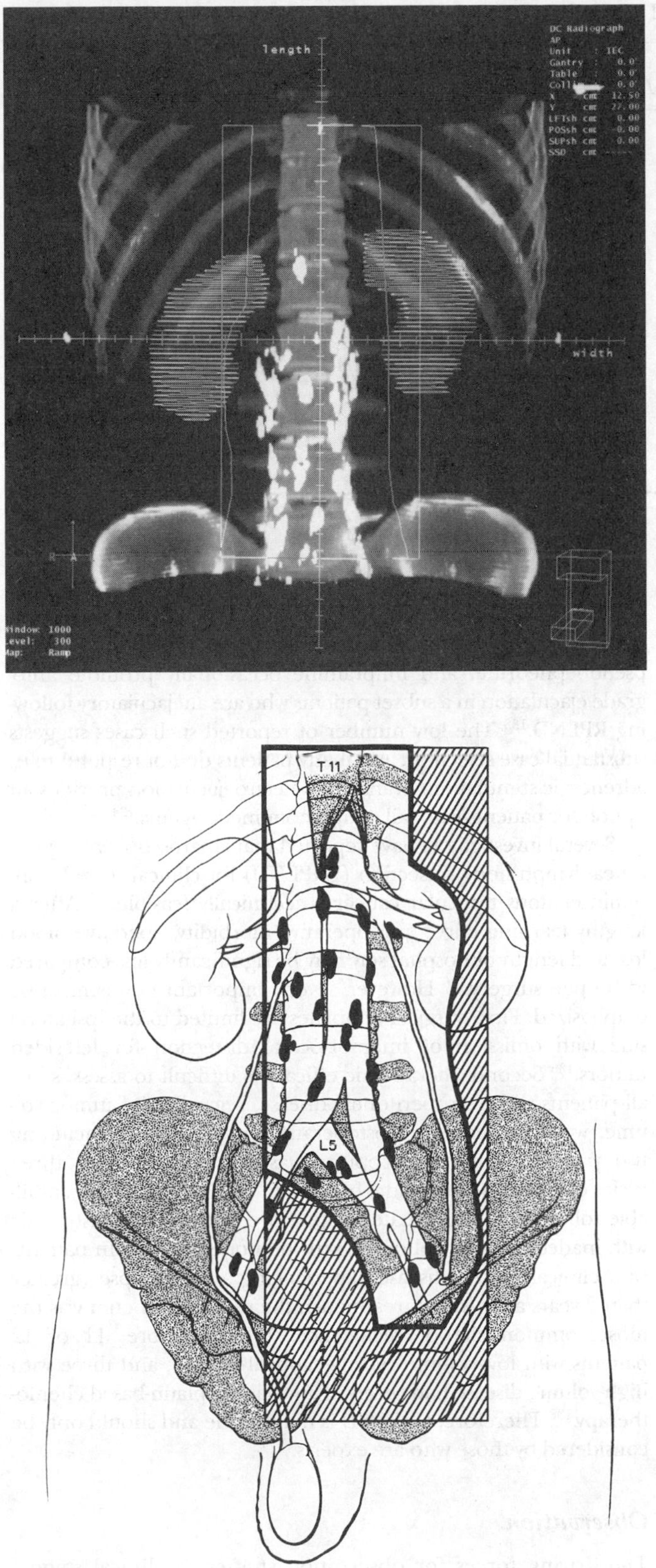

A

B

FIGURE 35-3. **A:** Paraaortic portal for clinical stage I seminoma. **B:** Contoured anterior and posterior radiation treatment fields for men with clinical stage IIA or IIB left testicular cancer. The diagonally shaded area is an individually made, 8-cm-thick Cerrobend block.

TABLE 35-6. Treatment of Seminoma with Radiation Therapy: Outcome and Relapse Patterns

			Relapse Sites(%)	
Stage	*Patients*	*Relapse (%)*	Med/ SCLN	Other ± Med/SCLN
Stage I[95,109–114]	1854	81(4)	33 (41)	48 (59)
Stage IIA/B or nonpalpable[110,112,113,148]	206	14 (7)	3 (21)	11 (79)
Stage IIC or palpable[110,112,148,157]	90	43 (48)	12 (28)	31 (72)

SCLN, supraclavicular lymph node.

NONSEMINOMATOUS GERM CELL TUMORS

Nonseminomatous GCT is thought to be radioresistant, although one randomized trial reported no retroperitoneal relapse after radiation therapy.[119] However, radiation therapy plays no role in its initial management, since chemotherapy for subsequent relapse might be compromised and the systemic relapse rate is higher than for seminoma.[119] If a patient has clinical stage I disease at the conclusion of initial staging, the choice of management options depends on specific histologic features and the status of serum tumor marker concentrations.

Retroperitoneal Lymph Node Dissection

Because of predictable lymphatic metastatic spread, the conventional approach to patients with clinical stage I nonseminomatous GCT has been the modified, bilateral RPLND (Fig. 35-4*A*). Adequate exposure for RPLND can be achieved through either a thoracoabdominal or transabdominal approach. The standard bilateral infrahilar RPLND template, which remains the standard against which therapeutic alternatives are judged, includes the precaval, paracaval, interaortocaval, preaortic, paraaortic, and common iliac lymph nodes bilaterally.

Despite refinement of radiologic imaging, 15% to 40% of patients are clinically understaged. Retroperitoneal metastases are found in approximately 30% of patients judged preoperatively to be clinical stage I. Retroperitoneal relapse occurs in approximately 20% to 25% of patients on clinical stage I surveillance protocols.[120–123]

Infield recurrence is rare after a properly performed RPLND, which is a curative procedure, and surgical mortality is less than 1%. Major complications are unusual but can include pancreatitis, renal vascular or ureteral injuries, chylous ascites, aortic wall necrosis, bowel obstruction, pulmonary emboli, hemorrhage, and wound dehiscence. Minor complications include lymphocele, atelectasis, wound infection, and prolonged ileus.[124,125]

In the past, most patients undergoing bilateral RPLND experienced retrograde ejaculation and subsequent infertility. An improved understanding of the neuroanatomy of seminal emission and ejaculation, the pattern of retroperitoneal metastasis for right- and left-sided tumors, and surgical mapping studies[126,127] led to modification of infrahilar surgical boundaries and techniques.

NEUROANATOMY. Antegrade ejaculation requires coordination of three separate events: (1) closure of the bladder neck,

TABLE 35-7. Observation in the Management of Clinical Stage I Germ Cell Tumors

	Reference	*Patients*	*Relapses (%)*	*Median Disease-Free Interval (mo; Range)*	*Died of Disease (%)*	*Median Follow-Up*
Seminoma	93	113	15 (13)	11 (6–64)	0 (0)	33 mo
	117	202	31 (15)	12 (0.3–9.0 y)	1 (0.5)	5.3 y; 84.1% actuarial 5-y progression-free rate
Subtotal	—	315	46 (15)	—	1 (0.3)	—
Nonseminomatous germ cell tumors	121	154	42 (27)	4 (2–24)	2 (1.3)	7 y
	122	373	100 (27)	<7	4 (1)	5 y; >3% actuarial 5-y progression-free rate
	123	85	25 (29)	7 (2–68)	3 (3)	>10 y
	140	170	48 (28)	6.9 (2.4–20.8)	1 (<1)	6.3 y
	141	105	27 (6)	5	3	6.8 y
Subtotal	—	810	222 (27)	—	12 (1.5)	—

(2) seminal emission, and (3) ejaculation. The sympathetic fibers that mediate seminal emission emanate primarily from the T-12 to L-3 thoracolumbar spinal cord. In the midretroperitoneum, after leaving the sympathetic trunk, the fibers converge toward midline and form the hypogastric plexus near the aortic bifurcation. From the hypogastric plexus, sympathetic fibers travel via pelvic nerves to innervate the vas deferens, seminal vesicles, prostate, and bladder neck. Ejaculation is mediated by combined autonomic and somatic innervation originating at the sacral and lumbar spinal cord levels. Sympathetic stimulation tightens the bladder neck, while pudendal somatic innervation from S-2 to S-4 causes relaxation of the external urethral sphincter and rhythmic contraction of bulbourethral and perineal muscles. Preservation of ejaculatory capacity requires preservation of paravertebral sympathetic ganglia and their fibers, which converge at the superior hypogastric plexus around the aortic bifurcation. Sympathetic chains and postganglionic sympathetic fibers can be prospectively identified, meticulously dissected, and preserved.

NERVE-SPARING RETROPERITONEAL LYMPH NODE DISSECTION. Nerve-sparing RPLND may be of two types: nerve-dissecting or nerve-avoiding. Despite pathologic stage II disease in patients selected for this procedure, recurrences in the retroperitoneum are rare.[128–130] Modified, nerve-avoiding RPLND templates were designed to avoid the hypogastric plexus and contralateral sympathetic fibers responsible for ejaculation in clinical stage I or IIA disease (Figs. 35-4*B* and *C*). These template dissections do not attempt to identify specific nerve fibers. Rather, their design minimizes trauma to the hypogastric plexus by limiting the contralateral dissection to the level above the takeoff of inferior mesenteric artery. This method avoids transsection of the contralateral nerves and results in preservation of ejaculation rates in approximately 50% to 80% of patients.[128,131,132] These rates are higher for a right-sided, nerve-avoiding template dissection compared with modified, left-sided dissection.

Preservation of ejaculation appears to be more successful when nerves are prospectively identified and spared, compared with modified template dissection, although duration of operation is usually longer for the former. With nerve dissection, approximately 95% of patients are left with normal ejaculatory status postoperatively. Regardless of technique, retrograde ejaculation is a potential risk with any RPLND; therefore, preoperative sperm banking is recommended. α-Adrenergic drugs such as ephedrine, pseudoephedrine, and imipramine occasionally promote antegrade ejaculation in a subset patients who are anejaculatory following RPLND.[133] The low number of reported such cases suggests substantial case selection, and many patients do not respond to α-adrenergic stimulation. Transrectal electroejaculation provides an option for patients who fail sympathomimetic agents.[134]

Several investigators have reported that laparoscopic retroperitoneal lymph node dissection (LRPLND) for clinical stage I nonseminomatous testicular cancer is technically feasible.[135] After a lengthy learning curve, postoperative morbidity, operative blood loss and length of hospital stay may be significantly less compared with open surgery.[136] However, several important points must be emphasized. First, surgical templates are limited to the ipsilateral side with omission of interaortocaval dissection for left-sided tumors.[136] Second, therapeutic efficacy is difficult to assess, since all patients with retroperitoneal disease, regardless of tumor volume, were treated with postoperative chemotherapy, including two patients with microscopic metastases who received three cycles of cisplatin, etoposide, bleomycin (BEP).[136,137] Finally, available follow-up is short. Late relapses are potentially catastrophic with inadequate control of the retroperitoneum.[138,139] In patients with clinical stage I disease experiencing a late relapse (greater than 2 years after initial treatment), the retroperitoneum was the most common site of recurrence.[138] Furthermore, 11 of 12 patients with low-volume retroperitoneal disease, and three with high-volume disease had received adjuvant cisplatin-based chemotherapy.[138] Therefore, LRPLND is not routine and should only be considered by those who are experts.

Observation

The driving forces for observation studies in clinical stage I patients were the infertility resulting from RPLND (due to retrograde ejaculation), the frequent absence of therapeutic benefit (i.e., orchiectomy was a curative procedure or systemic disease occurred in the absence of retroperitoneal disease), and the ability of cisplatin-based chemotherapy to cure systemic disease. Approximately 25% of patients with T1N0M0 disease and normal serum tumor markers relapse during sur-

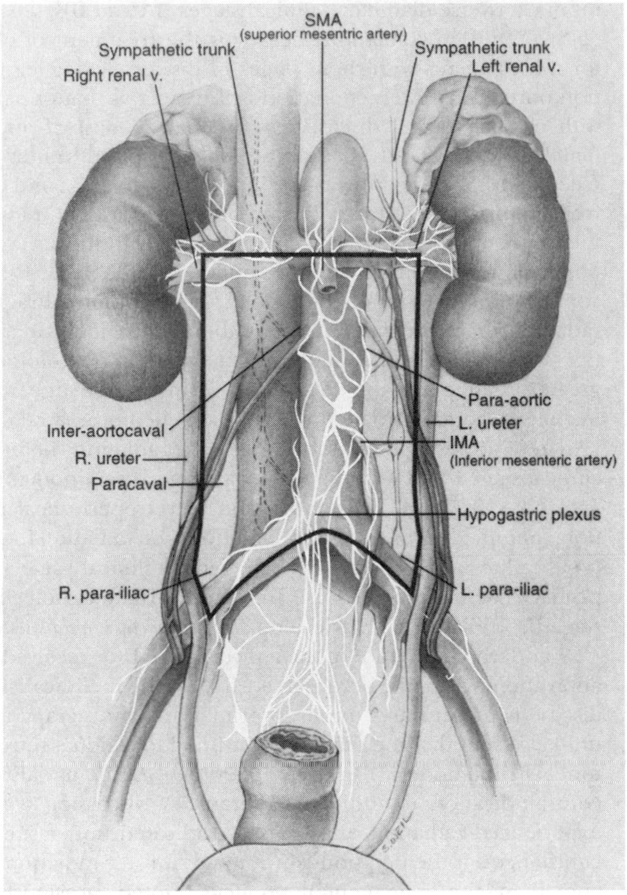

A

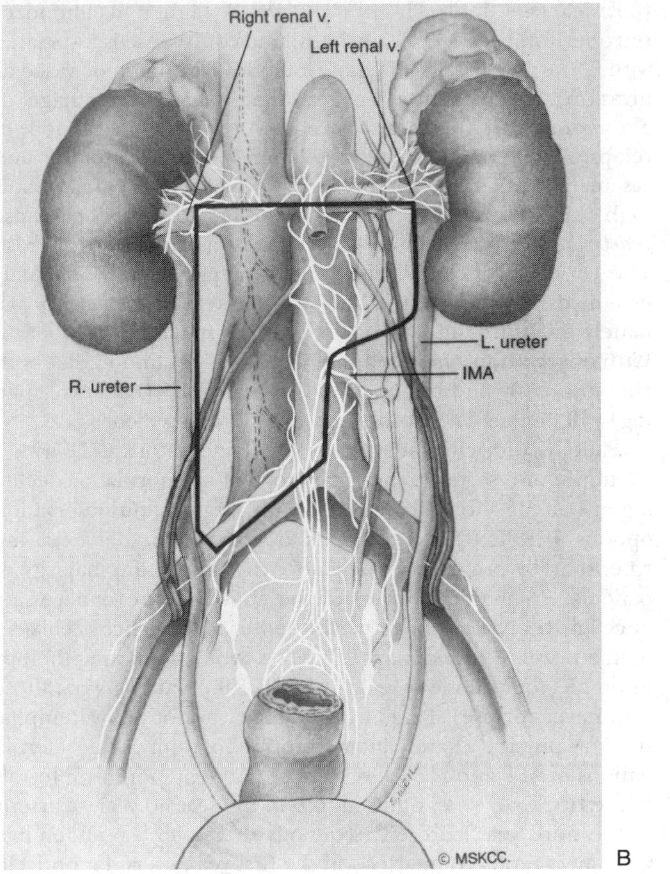

B

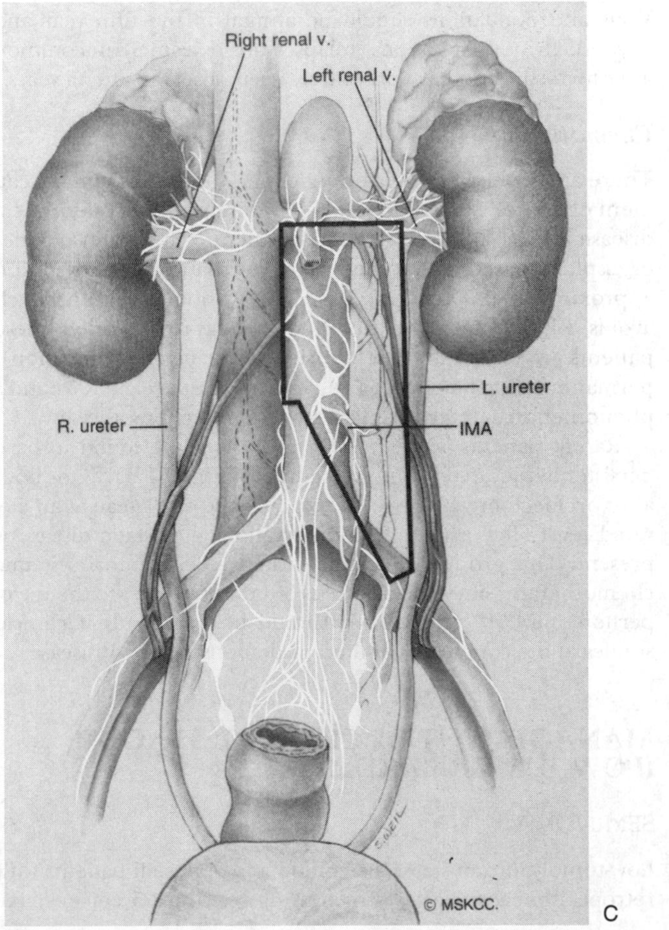

C

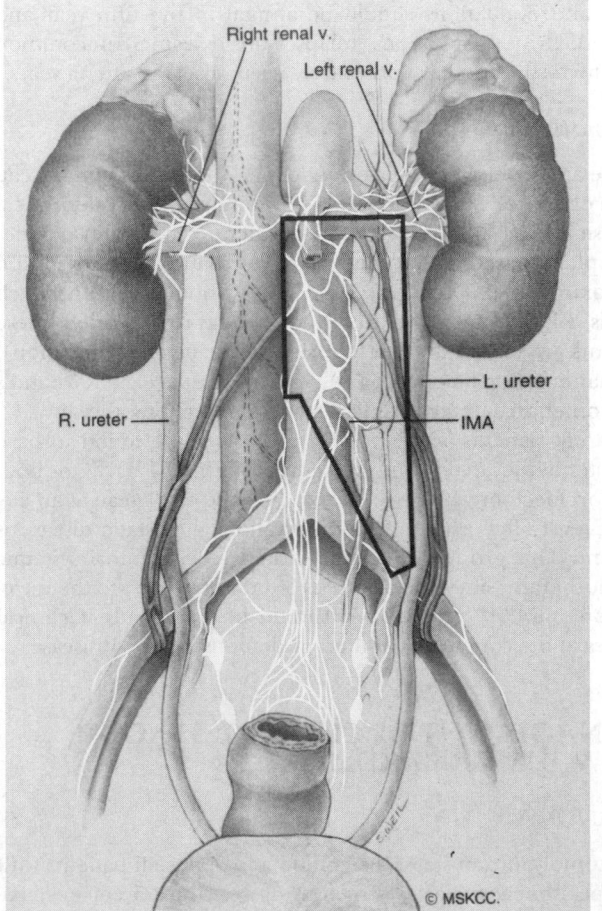

FIGURE 35-4. **A:** Standard modified bilateral retroperitoneal lymph node dissection. **B:** Modified nerve-avoiding template for right testicular tumors. **C:** Modified nerve-avoiding template for left testicular tumors. L., left; R., right; v., vein.

veillance (see Table 35-7).[121–123,140,141] A higher likelihood of retroperitoneal, systemic, or both kinds of relapse is associated with T2 to T4 tumors (T2 now includes lymphatic or vascular invasion). Some studies suggest that a high percentage of embryonal carcinoma also predicts a higher likelihood of relapse.[141,142] However, the correlation between lymphatic and vascular invasion and the presence of embryonal carcinoma is high, and general agreement on histologic criteria for relapse *independent* of vascular or lymphatic invasion does not exist. The retroperitoneum is the site of relapse in approximately two-thirds of patients, the lungs or markers alone in approximately one-third, and other visceral sites much less frequently. With observation, there is a slightly higher likelihood that both chemotherapy and modified bilateral RPLND (*not* nerve-sparing) will be needed in order to achieve the same cure rate.

Patients with clinical stage I nonseminomatous GCT with a T1 tumor and serum tumor markers that are normal or declining at half-life should be offered both surgical and observation options. If RPLND is chosen, it should be of the nerve-sparing type, thereby preserving ejaculatory capacity in the majority of patients. Frequent CT scans of the abdomen are unnecessary once an RPLND has been performed. If surveillance is chosen, then a possibly unnecessary RPLND is avoided, limiting therapy to orchiectomy alone in at least 70% of the patients (i.e., those who never relapse). Patient compliance cannot be overemphasized. A physical examination, chest radiography, and determinations of AFP and HCG levels are required at monthly intervals in the first year, every other month in the second year, quarterly in the third year, and less frequently thereafter. An abdominal CT scan is required quarterly in the first year, every 4 months in the second year, and every 6 months beginning in the third year. Visits and evaluations should be annual in the fifth year and beyond. In both situations, relapses are extremely uncommon after two years and have only rarely been observed after 5 years.

Chemotherapy

There are limited data regarding chemotherapy as initial treatment of clinical stage I disease when the risk of retroperitoneal disease is high. In three reports of patients receiving two cycles of cisplatin-based chemotherapy, fewer than 5% relapsed and approximately 1% died of GCT.[143–145] Although this approach avoids RPLND and the duration of therapy is brief, these patients are exposed to the transient (e.g., myelosuppression), permanent (e.g., neuropathy), and delayed (e.g., Raynaud's phenomenon, acute leukemia) toxicities of chemotherapy.

Rarely, patients with *clinical stage I disease* are found to have persistently elevated serum concentrations of AFP, HCG, or both after orchiectomy. If these markers increase or plateau at an elevated level after a period of observation, metastatic disease is present. This group of patients should receive initial systemic chemotherapy, since the disease is often not limited to the retroperitoneum.[146,147] An RPLND should be done only if clinical studies at the conclusion of therapy demonstrate new disease.

MANAGEMENT OF CLINICAL STAGE II (LOW TUMOR BURDEN)

SEMINOMA

Low-tumor-burden stage II seminoma includes all patients with retroperitoneal metastases measuring less than 5 cm in maximum transverse diameter (clinical stages IIA and IIB; see Table 35-6).[110,112,113,148] Radiation therapy is the treatment of choice for most patients with these stages of disease. A dog-leg radiation portal is used. Fractionation is the same as that of patients with clinical stage I disease, except that a boost of approximately 500 to 750 rads is administered to involved lymph nodes (see Fig. 35-3*B*). Relapses occur in from 5% to 15%, and death from seminoma is rare. Prophylactic mediastinal radiation therapy is not indicated, since relapses solely in the anterior or posterior mediastinum are infrequent (see Table 35-6). The combination of supradiaphragmatic and infradiaphragmatic radiation therapy results in chemotherapy intolerance, a high rate of treatment-related mortality due to chemotherapy, and a greater than expected death rate from disease due to the inability to administer adequate doses of chemotherapy.[149]

There are exceptions to the need for radiation therapy for clinical stage I and nonbulky clinical stage II seminoma. (1) A *horseshoe kidney* is a contraindication to retroperitoneal radiation therapy due to the high likelihood of radiation-induced renal failure. Observation is preferred in clinical stage I, and primary chemotherapy is the treatment of choice for clinical stage II. (2) Patients who develop a *second metachronous testicular GCT* and who have undergone a prior RPLND or received radiation therapy should be observed frequently if clinical stage I disease is present and undergo primary chemotherapy in the unlikely event that the disease is confined to residual retroperitoneal lymph nodes. (3) *Inflammatory bowel disease* may also be a contraindication to radiation therapy. A discussion with an experienced radiation oncologist is indicated under such circumstances. If the decision is not to administer radiation therapy, then the management policies noted previously for patients with a *horseshoe kidney* should be followed.

NONSEMINOMATOUS GERM CELL TUMORS

Low-tumor-burden clinical stage II nonseminomatous GCT encompasses disease ipsilateral to the primary tumor, at or below the renal hilum, not associated with tumor-related back pain, and limited to the primary landing zone. The presence of suprahilar or retrocrural lymphadenopathy, bilateral retroperitoneal nodal metastases, back pain, or contralateral lymph nodes (even if the ipsilateral lymph nodes do not appear to be involved) generally implies unresectable disease (e.g., tumor-associated back pain) or a higher likelihood of metastatic disease (suprahilar and retrocrural adenopathy), and initial chemotherapy is preferred. Ipsilateral solitary lymph nodes less than 3 cm are best handled by RPLND. Lymph nodes between 3 to 5 cm, even if solitary, may be associated with more extensive disease than can be detected on abdominal CT scan.

Retroperitoneal Lymph Node Dissection

The standard approach to patients with clinical stage IIA and some IIB tumors has been RPLND. The priority is to perform a definitive therapeutic operation, following which there is a minimum likelihood of infield recurrence. Margins of resection should not be compromised in an attempt to maintain ejaculatory function. Nerve-sparing dissection may be possible, depending on the location and volume of disease.

An important exception to this approach may be patients with clinical stage IIA or IIB and elevated serum tumor markers. Investigators at MSKCC reported that elevated serum tumor markers

TABLE 35-8. Pathologic Stage II Nonseminomatous Germ Cell Tumors: Surveillance for Minimal Nodal Involvement at Retroperitoneal Lymph Node Dissection

Reference	*Tumor Bulk*	*Patients*	*Relapse (%)*
98	Microscopic involvement only	6	2 (33)
101	<6 nodes; no node >2 cm; no extranodal extension	39	3 (8)
102	<6 nodes; no node >2 cm; no extranodal extension	47	21 (44)
152[a]	Solitary node <2 cm; <6 nodes; no node >2 cm; no extranodal extension	49	1 (2)
153	<6 nodes; no node >2 cm; no extranodal extension	50	11 (22)
Total		191	38 (20)

[a]Included patients treated with dactinomycin with and without additional agents, but did not include cisplatin.

pre-RPLND were the most significant predictor for (1) relapse in patients with low-volume (pN1) retroperitoneal disease who did not receive adjuvant chemotherapy, and (2) for persistent nonseminomatous GCT (usually persistent marker elevation) despite complete resection of high-volume (pN2, pN3) retroperitoneal disease.[150] Elevated serum tumor markers usually reflect systemic disease, and these patients should be considered for primary cisplatin-based chemotherapy. However, for patients with apparent low-volume disease and normal markers, RPLND is often therapeutic and cost effective.[151]

Adjuvant Chemotherapy

Surveillance is a treatment choice for compliant patients with fewer than six involved nodes and none greater than 2 cm (Table 35-8).[98,101,102,152,153] Surveillance requires close monitoring, and chemotherapy is reserved for patients who relapse. Patient compliance, psychological factors, age, or other issues may make adjuvant chemotherapy the preferred choice in rare patients. Three or four cycles of cisplatin-based therapy are required at relapse according to disease status at that time.

Adjuvant chemotherapy remains a strong consideration in patients when greater than or equal to six nodes are involved, any node is greater than 2 cm, or there is extranodal extension. In the late 1970s, treatment programs based on cisplatin, vinblastine, and bleomycin were given as adjuvant therapy following RPLND, and nearly 100% of patients survived relapse free.[98,154] Considerable treatment-related morbidity was associated with these regimens, prompting efforts to reduce toxicity. Two cycles of cisplatin-based chemotherapy are nearly always effective in preventing relapse (Table 35-9).[99,102,154–156] A randomized trial showed that observation with standard treatment at relapse and two cycles of adjuvant chemotherapy had equivalent survival.[102] Etoposide has replaced vinblastine in adjuvant regimens. A more recent study showed that etoposide plus cisplatin alone is adequate, and that bleomycin is unnecessary as part of adjuvant therapy.[156]

IDENTIFICATION OF RELAPSE

Careful periodic follow-up after locoregional therapy is required after radiation therapy for clinical stage I, IIA, and IIB seminoma during observation for clinical stage I nonseminomatous GCT, and after RPLND without adjuvant chemotherapy. After radiation therapy, a chest radiograph, determination of serum concentrations of AFP and HCG, and a physical examination should be performed every 6 weeks to 3 months in the first year, every 3 to 4 months in the second year, and less frequently thereafter. An abdominal CT scan should be done at the conclusion of radiation therapy. Following RPLND, a chest radiograph, determinations of serum concentrations of AFP and HCG, and a physical examination are required every 1 to 2 months in the first year, every 2 to 3 months in the second, and less frequently in the third year and beyond, with annual visits to detect late relapse and second primary tumors after the fifth year. Provided that follow-up has been adequate, virtually all of these patients relapse with low-volume disease and are cured with chemotherapy.

MANAGEMENT OF STAGE II AND STAGE III DISEASE (HIGH TUMOR BURDEN)

High-burden disease includes all patients with extensive or bulky retroperitoneal, supradiaphragmatic nodal or visceral metastases,

TABLE 35-9. Cisplatin-Containing Adjuvant Chemotherapy Trials

Reference	*Stage*[a]	*Regimen*	*Cycles*	*Patients (%N2,N3)*	*Patients Alive and Relapse Free (%)*	*Median Follow-Up*
99	N2B,3	VAB-3	2	29 (100)	100	24
102	N1–3	PVB or VAB-4	2	97 (45)	99[b]	>48
154	N1–3	PVB	2	114 (NS)	95	42
		PVB	4	111 (NS)	99	44
155	N2B,3	VAB-6	2	42 (100)	98	24
156	N2B,3	EP	2	50 (100)	100	35

EP, etoposide + cisplatin; NS, not stated; PVB, cisplatin + vinblastine + bleomycin; VAB-3, VAB-4, VAB-6, contain cisplatin + vinblastine + bleomycin + actinomycin D + cyclophosphamide.

[a]See section Pathologic Staging in text for these older style groupings.

[b]Five patients who relapsed on adjuvant therapy arm never received adjuvant chemotherapy.

TABLE 35-10. Commonly Used Chemotherapy Regimens for Metastatic Germ Cell Tumors

A. Previously untreated, good risk
1. Etoposide, 100 mg/m^2 IV daily × 5 days
   Cisplatin, 20 mg/m^2 IV daily × 5 days
   Four cycles administered at 21-day intervals
2. Etoposide, 100 mg/m^2 IV daily × 5 days
   Cisplatin, 20 mg/m^2 IV daily × 5 days
   Bleomycin, 30 U IV weekly on days 2, 9, and 16
   Three cycles administered at 21-day intervals

B. Previously untreated, poor risk
   Etoposide, 100 mg/m^2 IV daily × 5 days
   Cisplatin, 20 mg/m^2 IV daily × 5 days
   Bleomycin, 30 U IV weekly on days 2, 9, and 16
   Four cycles administered at 21-day intervals

C. Previously treated, first-line salvage therapy
   Ifosfamide, 1.2 g/m^2 IV daily × 5 days
   Mesna, 400 mg/m^2 IV every 8 hours × 5 days
   Cisplatin, 20 mg/m^2 IV daily × 5 days
   plus either
   Vinblastine, 0.11 mg/kg IV days 1 and 2
   or
   Etoposide, 75 mg/m^2 IV daily × 5 days

including patients with stage IIC seminoma. This last group has a high relapse rate with radiation therapy alone (see Table 35-6).[110,111,148,157] Cisplatin-based chemotherapy cures 70% to 80% of those patients. Early clinical trials developed effective regimens such as cisplatin, vinblastine, and bleomycin[158] and cisplatin, vinblastine, bleomycin, dactinomycin, and cyclophosphamide,[91] eliminated maintenance therapy,[159] and replaced vinblastine with etoposide.[158] Adjunctive surgery was shown to be essential to achieving a disease-free state. Although the majority of patients was cured, significant adverse events were observed, including treatment mortality, myelosuppression, pulmonary fibrosis, Raynaud's phenomenon, coronary artery disease, nephrotoxicity, and intestinal ileus.[158,160,161] Good- and poor-risk allocation algorithms were developed and clinical trials performed to address issues represented by different risks of treatment failure. The commonly used standard treatment regimens are summarized in Table 35-10.

GOOD-PROGNOSIS GERM CELL TUMOR

Good-risk patients are those with a high likelihood of cure. All good-risk allocation criteria identify patients with a high probability of complete response. Response proportions range from 88% to 95% with favorable survival distributions.[107] Since the advent of good-risk stratification, trials have focused on eliminating bleomycin from treatment regimens, reducing the number of cycles of therapy, and substituting carboplatin for cisplatin (Table 35-11).[162–168]

A randomized trial performed by Indiana University examined the duration of therapy[162] in 184 patients who received either four cycles of BEP administered over 12 weeks or three cycles administered over 9 weeks. Bleomycin was discontinued for any clinically evident pulmonary toxicity. A disease-free status was achieved by 98% of patients receiving three cycles, and 92% survived, compared with a 97% disease-free status and 92% survival among patients treated with four cycles.

Three randomized clinical trials have evaluated the elimination of bleomycin from regimens containing etoposide and cisplatin. Etoposide and cisplatin (EP) for four cycles was compared with a five-drug, bleomycin-containing regimen (cisplatin, vinblastine, bleomycin, dactinomycin, and cyclophosphamide) in 164 evaluable patients and was found to be therapeutically equivalent.[163] A subsequent analysis evaluated late relapse in patients receiving EP, and none were observed with a median follow-up of 5 years.[169] A randomized trial of cisplatin and etoposide with (BEP) and without bleomycin (EP) was

TABLE 35-11. Randomized Trials in Good-Prognosis Germ Cell Tumors

Reference	*Good-Risk Criteria*	*Regimens (Cycles)*	*Complete Response (%)*	*Durable Response (%)*	*Conclusion*
162	Indiana	BEP(4)	97	92	Regimens equivalent
		BEP(3)	98	92	
163	MSKCC	VAB-6(3)	96	85	Regimens equivalent
		EP(4)	93	82	
164	EORTC	BEP(4)	95	91	BEP superior; survival same
		EP(4)	87	83	
165	Indiana	BEP(3)	94	86[a]	EP(3) inferior
		EP(3)	88	69	
166	MSKCC	EC(4)	90	87	EC inferior
		EP(4)	88	76	
167	MRC/EORTC	CEB(4)	87	77[b]	CEB inferior
		BEP(4)	94	91	
168	GETUG	BEP(3)	92	—	Regimens equivalent
		EP(4)	91	—	

B, bleomycin; C, carboplatin; E, etoposide; EORTC, European Organization for the Research and Treatment of Cancer; GETUG, Genito-Urinary Group of the French Federation of Cancer Centers; MRC, Medical Research Council; MSKCC, Memorial Sloan-Kettering Cancer Center; NS, not stated; P, cisplatin; VAB-6, cisplatin + vinblastine + dactinomycin + bleomycin + cyclophosphamide.
[a]Failure-free survival.
[b]Response defined as failure-free, 1-year survival.

performed by the EORTC in 395 patients. The dose of etoposide in this study was 360 mg/m² per cycle, with the dose modifications for thrombocytopenia in contrast to 500 mg/m² per cycle without dose attenuations in American trials. The bleomycin arm was more toxic, including Raynaud's phenomenon in 8% of patients and two patients who died of pulmonary toxicity. Complete response was lower in EP patients (87% vs. 95%, P = .0075), but no differences were observed in relapses, time to progression, or survival with over 7 years of follow-up.[164] It can be concluded from this study that bleomycin cannot be deleted from good-risk therapy when European doses of etoposide are used.

A French trial directly compared three cycles of BEP to four cycles of EP in 250 patients. This trial used standard doses of bleomycin (30 U/week days 1, 8, and 15 of each cycle) and an etoposide dose of 100 mg/m² on days 1 through 5 (total 500 mg/m²/cycle) in both arms of the trial.[168] The criteria for good risk were those developed by the Institute Gustave Roussy; 97% of patients were good-risk by the IGCCCG criteria. With a median follow-up of 24 months, the survival was similar in both arms [97% for BEP (three cycles) vs. 96% for EP (four cycles)]. Finally, three cycles of BEP were compared with three cycles of EP in 166 patients.[165] The number of patients with persistent or progressive carcinoma, relapse or viable cancer at postchemotherapy surgery was the end point. An interim analysis revealed an increased number of adverse events in the two-drug arm, resulting in early termination of the study.

Two randomized trials have evaluated the substitution of carboplatin for cisplatin. In a multiinstitutional trial of 265 patients, four cycles of carboplatin plus etoposide were compared with four cycles of EP.[166] Although the proportions of complete response did not differ significantly, patients receiving carboplatin plus etoposide had an inferior event-free (incomplete response or relapse) (P = .02) and relapse-free (P = .005) survival, and significantly worse myelosuppression requiring platelet transfusions and hospitalization for granulocytopenic fever. In subset analysis, carboplatin plus etoposide was inferior to EP in both seminoma and nonseminoma patients. The Medical Research Council and EORTC conducted a confirmatory, randomized trial comparing carboplatin, etoposide, and bleomycin with BEP in 598 patients. Bleomycin was administered at 30 U once every 3 weeks. Complete response was greater in patients allocated to BEP (94% vs. 87%, P= .009). Survival was inferior in carboplatin, etoposide, and bleomycin (P = .003), with BEP patients experiencing a 3-year survival of 97% compared with 90% for carboplatin, etoposide, and bleomycin patients. Conventional dose carboplatin therapy is inferior to cisplatin therapy in GCT patients.

Although good-risk studies differ in eligibility criteria, an efficacy threshold has been reached. Cisplatin-based therapy (greater than or equal to 100 mg/m²/cycle) is required; there is no role for carboplatin-based therapy. Four cycles of EP and three cycles of BEP using a 500 mg/m² cumulative dose of etoposide per course are therapeutically equivalent in randomized comparison.[168]

POOR- (AND INTERMEDIATE-) RISK GERM CELL TUMOR

Between 20% and 30% of patients with advanced GCT fail to achieve durable, complete response to first-line, cisplatin-containing chemotherapy. In general, clinical trials for the poor-risk subgroup attempt to improve efficacy by evaluating regimens that have been effective in salvage therapy, substituting a new agent for an existing one or incorporating a dose-intensive regimen. Numerous studies have evaluated the importance of increased serum tumor marker concentrations, number of metastatic sites, size of specific tumor site, site of metastasis (e.g., liver), site of primary tumor (extragonadal or gonadal), and histology[104,105] in an attempt to identify poor-risk patients. Unlike good-risk criteria, the choice of poor-risk selection algorithm is critical. If the criteria are insufficiently stringent, then a proportion of good-risk patients will be treated and unnecessarily exposed to the enhanced toxicity of intensive therapy. In addition, the response proportion will be inflated, making therapy appear more effective than is warranted. The lack of uniform predictive criteria was addressed by the IGCCCG criteria.[108] Durable complete responses occur in 75% and 40% of intermediate- and poor-risk patients, respectively. Because the optimal chemotherapy regimen has not been determined, clinical trials designed to cure an increased proportion of patients remain a priority, and such patients should be treated on clinical trials.

Conventional Dose Therapy

The results of randomized studies conducted in poor-risk patients are shown in Table 35-12.[106,158,170–173] A randomized trial comparing BEP to cisplatin, vinblastine, and bleomycin showed that etoposide-containing therapy was superior to vinblastine-based therapy in the subset of poor-risk patients (Indiana *advanced* disease class).[158] One randomized trial suggested that a regimen with cisplatin, 200 mg/m², etoposide, vinblastine, and bleomycin was superior to cisplatin, 100 mg/m², vinblastine, and bleomycin.[170] A subsequent randomized trial showed that BEP, 200 mg/m², had equal efficacy but greater toxicity than standard BEP[171]; the apparently improved efficacy of cisplatin, 200 mg/m², etoposide, vinblastine, and bleomycin was attributable to etoposide. The role of ifosfamide was tested in a randomized trial; there was no therapeutic benefit of ifosfamide, cisplatin, and etoposide over BEP, and toxicity with ifosfamide, cisplatin, and etoposide was more severe.[174] These results paralleled the absence of survival benefits among consecutive phase II trials of conventional dose, cisplatin-based therapy conducted at MSKCC.[91,175] Therefore, in poor-risk patients, four cycles of BEP remain the standard regimen with which investigational regimens should be compared. Likewise, in intermediate-risk patients by IGCCCG criteria, four cycles of BEP is considered standard therapy.

High-Dose Therapy

The success of high-dose, carboplatin-containing chemotherapy in the treatment of patients with refractory disease led to its incorporation into initial therapy. Stringent selection criteria and rapid hematopoietic reconstitution are required to minimize treatment-related morbidity and mortality.

Two pilot studies clarify high-dose therapy requirements in this setting. In these studies conducted at MSKCC, 58 poor-risk patients were first identified based on clinical presentation, and further selected to receive high-dose therapy based on the clearance of AFP, HCG, or both from serum during standard induction therapy. If the half-life was prolonged, treatment was changed to two-drug, high-dose therapy (etoposide plus carbo-

TABLE 35-12. Results of Randomized Trials in Patients with Poor-Risk Germ Cell Tumors

Reference	*Criteria*	*Treatment*	*No. of Patients*	*% Complete Response*	*% Durable*	*Benefit Over Standard Arm*
106	EORTC	PEB	102	74	NS	
		PEB/PVB	102	75	NS	No
158	Indiana	PVB	37	38	NS	
		PEB	35	63	NS	Yes[a]
170	Indiana	PEB	77	73	61	
		P(200)EB	76	68	63	No
171	NCI	PVB	18	67	50	
		P(200)BVE	34	88	73	Yes
172	Indiana	PEB	141	60	57	
		VIP	145	63	56	No
173	EORTC/MRC	BEP/EP	185	57	55	No
		BOP/VIP-B	186	54	53	

B, bleomycin; E, etoposide; EORTC, European Organization for the Research and Treatment of Cancer; I, ifosfamide; MRC, Medical Research Council; NCI, National Cancer Institute; NS, not stated; O, vincristine; P, cisplatin, 100 mg/m^2; P(200), cisplatin, 200 mg/m^2; SWOG, Southwest Oncology Group; V, vinblastine.
[a]Subset analysis only. No difference in the clinical trial as a whole.

platin).[176,177] Hematopoietic reconstitution was rapid, only one treatment-related death was observed, and an improved survival trend was observed when this approach was compared with historic poor-risk experience with conventional dose, cisplatin-combination therapy.[176,177]

One randomized trial of dose-intensified therapy failed to show a therapeutic benefit.[178] Greater treatment-related morbidity and mortality and lower survival were observed in the high-dose therapy arm. However, the trial was flawed because of a lower dose intensity of cisplatin and a lower total dose of cisplatin in the *high-dose* arm. Since cisplatin, 200 mg/m^2, is not superior to cisplatin 100 mg/m^2,[171] the choice of cisplatin over carboplatin did not permit an adequate dose escalation to overcome resistance.

An ongoing national randomized trial is comparing four cycles of BEP to two cycles of BEP followed by two cycles of three-drug, high-dose therapy in poor- and intermediate-risk patients, and patients should participate if possible.

MANAGEMENT OF RESIDUAL DISEASE

Adjunctive surgical resection of residual disease after chemotherapy is an integral part of the comprehensive management of all patients with advanced GCT.[179,180] In general, surgical exploration is indicated when serum tumor marker concentrations have normalized and residual radiographic abnormalities are present. Increased serum concentrations of AFP and HCG after chemotherapy are often characterized by unresectable, viable GCT, and *salvage chemotherapy* is usually recommended for these patients.[179] Necrotic debris and fibrosis, teratoma, and viable carcinoma can be found at any resected site. Since the relapse rate of patients with necrosis and fibrosis or mature or immature teratoma is 5% to 10% following complete resection of residual disease at all sites, no further therapy is required.[181–184] If viable GCT is present at any site but all disease is completely resected, 30% to 50% of patients relapse following two additional cycles of therapy. Survival is poor among those who do not receive additional chemotherapy.[183,185]

Retroperitoneum

NONSEMINOMATOUS GERM CELL TUMORS. In the retroperitoneum, necrosis and fibrotic debris make up 45% to 50% of pathologic findings, teratoma another 35%, and viable GCT the remaining 15% to 20% (Table 35-13).[181,183,184,186–189] A bilateral RPLND is required, and retrograde ejaculation is the principal long-term consequence.

There is general agreement over the need to resect all sites of measurable residual disease. Since nearly 50% of resected residual retroperitoneal tumors have only necrosis and fibrosis, many studies have attempted to predict their presence. Among 80 patients with sequential CT scans before and after chemotherapy at Indiana University, neither viable GCT nor teratoma was found among 15 patients if no teratoma was present in the primary tumor and the retroperitoneal tumor volume (not diameter) by CT scan had decreased by less than or equal to 90%.[183] Conversely, teratoma in the primary tumor predicts the presence of teratoma or viable GCT in the postchemotherapy resection despite reduction in the original tumor mass.[181,183,184]

Other data suggest that RPLND may be needed regardless of postchemotherapy size. The definition of a normal CT scan has not been consistent. Lymph node diameters of less than or equal

TABLE 35-13. Pathologic Findings in the Retroperitoneum after Chemotherapy in Patients with Advanced Germ Cell Tumors

Reference	*No. of Patients*	*Necrosis*	*Teratoma*	*Carcinoma*
181	122	57	48	17
183	80	35	33	12
184	78	51	22	5
186	73	25	32	16
189	556	250	236	70
Total	909	418 (46%)	371 (41%)	120 (13%)

to 10 mm,[190] less than or equal to 15 mm,[191] and less than or equal to 20 mm[192] have been reported to represent normal CT scans after chemotherapy. Fossa et al. reported that 12 of 37 (30%) patients with normal postchemotherapy serum tumor marker concentrations and CT scan (all nodes less than or equal to 10 mm) had teratoma, and one patient had viable GCT.[191] Toner et al. reported that 8 of 39 (21%) patients with residual masses less than 1.5 cm had viable residual malignancy or teratoma.[181] CT criteria alone are not sufficiently reliable to distinguish viable tumor or teratoma from necrosis. PET scanning has been studied as a technique to detect necrosis and fibrosis, but teratoma was not reliably predicted.[81,82]

The decision to recommend postchemotherapy surgery depends on the frequency of viable carcinoma, the biologic potential of teratoma, and the morbidity of RPLND. If viable carcinoma is present, it is partially drug-resistant and will progress. The cure rate of relapsed disease to ifosfamide-based therapy is approximately 25%.[193–195] If viable disease is completely resected and two additional cycles of cisplatin-based therapy are administered, the cure rate is 50% to 70%.[181,185] Teratoma may be found in metastatic sites despite its absence in the primary tumor. Toner et al. reported that among 75 patients without teratoma in the primary tumor who underwent resection of a residual mass, 25 (33%) had teratoma at a metastatic site.[181] Mature teratoma may grow rapidly (*growing teratoma syndrome*),[196,197] become unresectable, or cause vascular or ureteral obstruction.[198] Malignant transformation of teratoma (i.e., the development of non–germ cell malignant elements such as sarcoma or carcinoma) is present in a minority of resected retroperitoneal teratoma.[37,199] These are clonal in origin with the original GCT and do not represent second primary cancers.[200–202] Surgery is the only therapy (except for leukemia) for this subset of tumors that would otherwise recur and fail to respond to additional chemotherapy. Late local recurrence (defined as greater than 2 years after therapy) of both teratoma and viable GCT is more common when teratoma is present at a metastatic site,[139,203,204] underscoring the need for initial complete surgical resection. Late recurrences of malignant GCT are often chemotherapy resistant, and chance of survival is poor.[203–207]

The complication rate of RPLND following chemotherapy is higher than that of primary RPLND.[124,208] Large-volume residual disease, postchemotherapy desmoplastic reaction, prior exposure to bleomycin, and more extensive retroperitoneal dissection increase the technical demands of the procedure. Careful monitoring of intraoperative and postoperative oxygen concentration (particularly in patients who have received bleomycin), meticulous fluid management with strict replacement criteria, and an emphasis on colloid rather than crystalloid have reduced pulmonary toxicity and nearly eliminated perioperative death from acute respiratory distress syndrome.[179]

Ejaculatory dysfunction and sterility are common sequelae of the standard, modified bilateral RPLND, particularly after primary chemotherapy.[124] Nerve-avoiding RPLND templates are not acceptable alternatives for residual disease after chemotherapy, since there is a higher risk of disease in sites outside the limits of the nerve-avoiding template in patients with a prior high-volume disease.[209] However, in selected patients without severe postchemotherapy desmoplastic changes, it is occasionally technically possible to identify individual sympathetic nerves. Wahle et al. reported that among 296 patients who underwent postchemotherapy RPLND, a select subset of 40 (13.5%) patients underwent nerve-dissecting RPLND after chemotherapy.[210] The majority of these 40 patients had relatively low-volume unilateral adenopathy before induction chemotherapy. With a minimum of 1-year follow-up, 34 of 38 (89%) patients reported normal ejaculation; nine patients reported ten pregnancies. There were no infield recurrences.[210] The best oncologic approach in patients requiring postchemotherapy RPLND remains a bilateral dissection with a nerve-sparing approach limited to a minority of patients.

In summary, all residual retroperitoneal disease should be resected. The need for postchemotherapy RPLND is controversial when the postchemotherapy CT scan, usually of the retroperitoneum, is interpreted as normal. Multivariate analyses show that approximately 20% of patients predicted to have necrosis (fibrosis) have either teratoma or viable GCT.[181,211] No single criterion or combination of criteria predict a negative pathology with sufficient accuracy to eliminate the risk of residual teratoma or viable GCT and obviate postchemotherapy RPLND. The risks of residual teratoma must be weighed against the growth and metastatic potential of viable GCT and the morbidity of the procedure.

SEMINOMA. The approach to the patient with pure seminoma and a postchemotherapy residual mass is controversial. Two important features distinguish seminoma from nonseminomatous tumors. First, teratoma in the residual mass is rare. Second, a complete RPLND following chemotherapy is often not technically feasible, secondary to the severe desmoplastic reaction and obliteration of tissue planes.[212] Consequently, perioperative morbidity has been reported to be higher for seminoma than for nonseminomatous GCT.[213,214]

A number of studies evaluated this issue in seminoma patients.[149, 212–217] Loehrer et al. reported that among 62 patients, 13 underwent attempted surgical excision of residual disease and three (23%) had residual malignancy.[149] The size of residual mass was not considered predictive. Fossa et al. reported 39 patients, 15 of whom received prior radiation therapy.[214] Twelve patients underwent exploration for residual disease; three (25%) had viable seminoma. One postoperative death due to pulmonary toxicity was observed. In a cohort of 45 patients, the size of residual mass was highly correlated with the site of the initial tumor but was not associated with the risk of recurrence.[212] These data support the notion that the majority of patients with persistent radiographic abnormalities do not have residual malignant disease.

The experience at MSKCC differed. Bilateral RPLND was not usually possible or attempted; surgery was often limited to resection of the residual mass or multiple biopsies of the residual radiographic abnormality. In an initial cohort of 104 patients, 8 of 30 (27% of patients with a residual mass greater than 3 cm) relapsed or had residual seminoma.[217] No postoperative deaths occurred. Conversely, among 74 tumors measuring less than 3 cm in diameter, no viable tumor was identified, and only two patients (3%) relapsed at the site of residual disease. Neither of these had undergone operation. Fewer tumors greater than 3 cm were present among patients treated after 1987 compared with those treated before 1987. Those investigators concluded that resection or biopsy of the residual masses greater than or equal to 3 cm was preferable to observation. If viable seminoma was documented, additional therapy was required.[217]

In summary, residual masses less than 3 cm should be observed. Controversy exists regarding the minority of patients with a residual mass measuring greater than or equal to 3 cm. Radiation therapy to the area of residual disease is feasible, but

TABLE 35-14. Ifosfamide-Based Salvage Regimens for Relapsed and Refractory Germ Cell Tumors

Reference	*Regimen*	*No. of Prior Regimens*	*Evaluable*	*Complete Response (%)*	*Durable Complete Response (%)*
193	VIP	1	30	10 (33)	1 (3)
194	VeIP	1	124	56 (45)	29 (23)
195	VIP or VeIP	1 and ≥2	62	21 (34)	15 (24)
226	VIP or VeIP	≥2	56	20 (36)	15 (27)
227	VIP	1 and ≥2	19	9 (47)	NS
228	VIP	1	32	22 (69)	16 (50)

VeIP, vinblastine, ifosfamide, and cisplatin; VIP, etoposide, ifosfamide, and cisplatin.

approximately 75% of patients would receive it unnecessarily and it did not appear to reduce the likelihood of recurrence.[212] Careful observation is an alternative, but relapse with subsequent ifosfamide-based salvage chemotherapy has a low cure rate (see Prognostic Factors: Salvage Chemotherapy, later in this chapter). Surgical resection that can identify residual disease and direct immediate therapy has low morbidity given modern techniques and perioperative care.[217] All factors (e.g., size, site, patient age) must be considered in making this therapeutic decision.

Lung and Mediastinal Resections

Resection of residual disease at sites other than the retroperitoneum is less controversial. There is a higher likelihood of teratoma, viable cancer at nonretroperitoneal sites, or both, with the highest likelihood seen in the mediastinum, probably because residual disease in the mediastinum is usually associated with a mediastinal primary tumor.[181] Size of the pretreatment and the postchemotherapy pulmonary nodule does not correlate with final histology. Different histologies may also be present in each lung. Therefore, residual intrathoracic disease should always be resected.[218,219]

Other Procedures

A small percentage of patients requires operation at multiple sites, usually the retroperitoneum and lung and (less frequently) the neck.[220] Histology at different sites is not predictable based on histology at one site. When the histologic specimen from the retroperitoneum is compared with that from a second site, the histologies are dissimilar in approximately 35% of cases.[182,218,219] When the lung and retroperitoneum are simultaneously involved, multiple, separate procedures may be required, but simultaneous bilateral thoracic and retroperitoneal resections are possible.[221] If a primary testis tumor is present and an orchiectomy is not performed *before* chemotherapy, then it should be performed *after* chemotherapy, as that testis may harbor viable residual disease.[222,223] Studies confirm that all sites of residual disease should generally be resected regardless of histologic findings at the initial procedure.

MANAGEMENT OF RELAPSE AFTER CHEMOTHERAPY

Twenty percent to 30% of patients with advanced GCT relapse or fail to achieve a complete response to conventional cisplatin-based chemotherapy. Effective (and curative) second- and third-line salvage offer further treatment options.

CONVENTIONAL DOSE SALVAGE THERAPY

After the single-agent activity of ifosfamide was identified,[224,225] it was combined with cisplatin and etoposide or cisplatin and vinblastine in patients whose disease was resistant to two prior regimens (Table 35-14).[193–195,226–228] In this heavily pretreated group, between 25% and 35% of patients achieved a complete response, and 15% to 27% remained in durable complete remission.[226,229] Nephrotoxicity and severe neutropenia were extremely common. Results suggesting an improved complete response rate when paclitaxel is substituted for vinblastine await completion of ongoing phase II studies.[230]

HIGH-DOSE THERAPY

The chemosensitivity of GCT, the dose-response phenomena for individual drugs, the rare occurrence of bone marrow metastasis, and a young patient population permit consideration of high-dose therapy. More recent studies have included carboplatin and etoposide with or without an oxazaphosphorine (cyclophosphamide or ifosfamide) and show that a proportion of patients can be cured. In three relatively large series conducted in patients with refractory, progressive GCT, 15% to 21% of patients remained alive and disease-free with long-term follow-up (Table 35-15).[231–234] While these series demonstrate the curative potential of high-dose therapy, the majority of patients with cisplatin-refractory GCT die of disease, and new drugs and strategies are still needed. Studies incorporating paclitaxel are ongoing.

The major toxicities of dose-intensive therapy are hematologic and infectious, with most studies reporting a 10% to 12% treatment-related death rate.[235] Hematopoietic growth factor support decreases the duration of neutropenia and hospitalization.[236] Peripheral blood-derived stem cells have largely replaced the use of autologous bone marrow, and a randomized trial showed that peripheral blood-derived stem cells result not only in rapid neutrophil reconstitution but also faster platelet engraftment.[237]

PROGNOSTIC FACTORS: SALVAGE CHEMOTHERAPY

Despite an occasional cure, the majority of patients receiving salvage chemotherapy fail to achieve a durable complete response and are subsequently considered for high-dose chemotherapy. Prognostic factors can be used to predict which

TABLE 35-15. High-Dose Carboplatin-Containing Chemotherapy in Patients with Refractory, Progressive Germ Cell Tumor

Institution	*Indiana*[231]	*Vienna*[232]	*MSKCC*[233]	*Germany*[234]
Patients	40	42	58	68
Agents	Carboplatin, etoposide ± ifosfamide	Carboplatin, etoposide, cyclophosphamide	Carboplatin, etoposide, cyclophosphamide	Carboplatin, etoposide, ifosfamide
Percent complete response	30	26	40	51
Percent alive, disease-free	15	21	21	37
Median follow-up of survivors (mo)	>24	25	28	NS

patients are most likely to benefit from conventional dose salvage therapy. Patients with a testis primary site *and* a prior complete response have a better prognosis, and conventional dose cisplatin salvage therapy (vinblastine, ifosfamide, and cisplatin) is reasonable in these patients.[238] Patients with an incomplete response to initial therapy or a relapsing extragonadal nonseminomatous GCT have a less than 10% 3-year survival response to conventional dose, cisplatin-containing salvage therapy.[238] In these circumstances, a dose-intensive program, a novel treatment strategy, or a new agent should be considered. The contribution of serum tumor marker concentrations to prognosis in this group of patients has not been established.

Prognostic factors can also be used to identify patients most likely to benefit from salvage high-dose, stem cell–supported, carboplatin containing chemotherapy. Patients with primary mediastinal GCT refractory to initial and salvage chemotherapy, patients with *absolute refractory* disease (rising markers or radiographic evidence of progressive disease within 4 weeks of cisplatin therapy), and patients with high HCG levels rarely achieve a complete response.[233,239] These patients should be considered for phase II studies. All other patients are candidates for a high-dose approach.

NEW AGENTS

A number of single-agent trials have been conducted against refractory GCT.[240–245] Of note, ifosfamide, paclitaxel, and oral etoposide and gemcitabine have demonstrated antitumor activity.[239,245–247] Because paclitaxel is synergistic with cisplatin and oxazaphosphorines *in vitro*, it is being studied in dose-intensive therapy with peripheral blood-derived, stem cell support, and in conventional dose therapy with ifosfamide plus cisplatin. Oral etoposide plays a palliative role in refractory GCT.

ROLE OF SURGERY

Histologic findings of resected masses following second-line or salvage chemotherapy differ from those observed following primary therapy. Viable tumor occurs in approximately 50% of specimens, teratoma in 40%, and necrosis in only 10%.[185] Additional standard-dose chemotherapy adds no benefit to patients with viable nonseminomatous GCT in the resected specimen after *salvage* chemotherapy, as opposed to clear benefit with two additional cycles following complete resection of nonseminomatous GCT after primary chemotherapy.

In general, surgery should be avoided in patients in whom serum tumor marker concentrations remain elevated. While this general rule holds true, surgery has curative potential in a highly select group of patients with increased marker levels, even after salvage chemotherapy. In a study at Indiana University, 38 of 48 (79%) such patients were rendered grossly free of disease, 29 (60%) normalized markers, and ten (21%) had no evidence of disease with a median follow-up of 46 months.[248] Eastham et al. observed that 6 of 16 (31%) patients undergoing resection of residual disease in the face of elevated serum tumor markers were cured.[249] Five of these six patients had retroperitoneal disease only. Finally, Wood et al. examined 15 patients refractory to cisplatin-based therapy who underwent surgical resection of a solitary site of residual disease despite elevated markers at MSKCC.[250] Seven patients (47%) remained free of disease. These are all highly selected patients. At MSKCC, only 4% of patients with refractory disease were surgical candidates when markers were elevated after salvage chemotherapy. Only a small subset of patients with chemotherapy-resistant disease can be cured with surgery. Patients with a solitary retroperitoneal mass and increased AFP seemed to be the best candidates. Technically difficult, this surgery should be performed at a tertiary center.

TREATMENT SEQUELAE

CHEMOTHERAPY

Acute and subacute chemotherapy toxicity frequently occurs but is generally controllable. Control of nausea and vomiting is extremely important in order to maintain adequate hydration. Concurrent administration of a 5-HT_3 antagonist with dexamethasone is superior to a 5-HT_3 antagonist alone.[251] Since cisplatin induces delayed emesis, administration of oral metoclopramide and a benzodiazepine plus dexamethasone for 2 to 4 days after therapy is sometimes necessary. While these antiemetic regimens now permit the administration of 5-day, low-dose, cisplatin-based programs in the office or other outpatient settings, an occasional patient develops severe nausea and vomiting and should be hospitalized in order to protect renal function.

Nephrotoxicity from cisplatin occurs to some extent in all patients and is cumulative. Due to the effect of cisplatin on proximal tubules, progressive reduction in glomerular filtration and cumulative hypomagnesemia may result, associated with an increase in serum creatinine from pretreatment baseline,[252,253] particularly after ifosfamide-based salvage chemotherapy.[229] Nephrotoxicity may be severe in patients receiving high-dose chemotherapy in the salvage setting but does not appear to influence response rate or hematologic recovery.[254] Reports of an increased frequency of diastolic hypertension and cardiac events have appeared,[255] and longer follow-up is needed to establish this association with greater certainty. There are also reports of increased mean cholesterol levels, increased low-density and decreased high-density lipoprotein levels, and increased weight years after chemotherapy for GCT.[256,257]

Myelosuppression frequently occurs.[158,163,166,193,195] Anemia occurs in virtually all patients, but infrequently results in the need for red blood cell transfusions in those previously untreated. Grade 4 thrombocytopenia (platelet count less than 50,000) is distinctly uncommon with primary cisplatin-based therapy, but frequent during salvage chemotherapy. Neutropenic fever occurs in approximately 10% to 15% of patients receiving EP, is more common with the addition of bleomycin, and occurs in more than 50% of patients receiving salvage chemotherapy. Hematopoietic growth factors are recommended prophylactically following neutropenic fever but do not improve survival when given.[258] Severe anemia, neutropenia and neutropenic fever, and thrombocytopenia often accompany ifosfamide-based salvage therapy; hematopoietic growth factor support should be used prophylactically from the beginning of salvage therapy.

Peripheral neuropathy occurs in a majority of patients receiving vinblastine.[259,260] Replacing vinblastine with etoposide decreased the frequency of neuropathy, although cisplatin still causes symptomatic neuropathy in a minority of patients. Auditory toxicity from cisplatin is often associated with reduced high-tone hearing and, less frequently, tinnitus, but patients rarely require hearing aids.

Pulmonary toxicity from bleomycin is rare but can be fatal. In one randomized trial, it resulted in approximately one-half of the treatment-induced deaths.[158] In good-risk patients, a reduction in the number of bleomycin doses from 12 to 9 resulted in no bleomycin-related, treatment-related deaths.[162] Pulmonary function tests (vital capacity and diffusion capacity of carbon monoxide) have been used to dictate changes in bleomycin administration.[91,163] However, the diffusion capacity of carbon monoxide may not predict clinically significant bleomycin-induced lung damage.[261]

Vascular toxicity, most prominently as Raynaud's phenomenon, occurs in a minority (less than 10%) of patients receiving bleomycin administered by weekly bolus. It occurs in the absence of cisplatin (albeit less frequently).[158,160,260] The substitution of etoposide for vinblastine did not reduce the incidence of Raynaud's phenomenon.[158] Erectile dysfunction may be associated with Raynaud's phenomenon as a sign of microvascular angiopathy.[262] Other vascular events include pulmonary emboli,[91] angina and myocardial infarction.[161,260] Coronary artery disease resulting from mediastinal radiation therapy is well recognized and emphasizes the need to avoid mediastinal radiation therapy in the management of patients with seminoma.

Infertility is an important consideration. A minority of patients is infertile at diagnosis. Reduced spermatogenesis and higher follicle-stimulating hormone levels compared with healthy men are frequent in newly diagnosed patients.[263] A similar impairment of testicular function occurs in men with CIS (intratubular germ cell neoplasia).[264] However, paternity in patients on surveillance for clinical stage I disease did not seem to be reduced.[265] A standard, modified bilateral RPLND causes retrograde ejaculation in nearly all patients. Nerve-dissecting and nerve-avoiding RPLND reduce, but do not eliminate, that risk. Chemotherapy may affect the germinal epithelium directly, and Leydig cell insufficiency is frequent.[266,267] After chemotherapy, persistent oligospermia and abnormal forms and motility have been reported,[268] but conception may occur despite oligospermia.

Second malignancies are rare. Metachronous GCT appearing in the contralateral testis occurs in approximately 2% to 3% of all patients.[269] After the second orchiectomy, replacement testosterone is required to maintain normal serum testosterone levels, secondary sexual characteristics, and sexual function. Etoposide causes secondary leukemia characterized by translocations involving chromosome 11q in fewer than 0.5% of patients receiving a total dose less than 2000 mg/m^2 [270,271] and as many as 6% of patients receiving total etoposide doses of greater than 3000 mg/m^2.[272] However, reports showed acute leukemia in 0.8% to 1.3% of patients receiving median cumulative etoposide doses greater than 2400 mg/m^2.[273] The latent period is short, averaging 2 to 4 years.

The incidence of gastrointestinal malignancies increased after radiation therapy or radiation therapy plus chemotherapy.[115,116] The relative risk increases with time and is greatest after 10 years.[115] Stomach cancer is the most prevalent gastrointestinal tumor. An excess of soft tissue sarcoma has also been observed.[115,274] The latent interval is long, and radiation therapy was implicated in the majority.[116,274] These second malignancies do not outweigh the enormous benefits of treatment intervention. Along with the risk of recurrence, these second primary neoplasms emphasize the need for long-term follow-up of treated patients.

Sarcoidosis appears more frequently in GCT patients.[275] Strictly speaking, it is not a sequela of therapy. It occurs both before and after GCT diagnosis. Paratracheal adenopathy or pulmonary nodules without retroperitoneal adenopathy or elevated serum tumor marker levels, particularly in patients with seminoma, suggest the possible presence of sarcoidosis and should lead to biopsy.

MIDLINE TUMORS OF UNCERTAIN HISTOGENESIS

A subset of patients with poorly differentiated carcinoma of unknown histogenesis and uncertain primary site achieve complete response and long-term survival following treatment with cisplatin-combination therapy.[276,277] In a series of 220 patients, 26% of patients achieved a complete response; the 10-year actuarial survival was 16%.[277] Because of cisplatin sensitivity, predominant midline tumor distribution, and occurrence in relatively young patients, the presence of unrecognized extragonadal GCT was suggested despite the absence of increased serum concentration of AFP, HCG, or both in most cases.[276,277] Since i(12p) is a specific chromosomal marker characterizing GCT,[200] genetic analysis was undertaken. i(12p) and chromosome 12 aneuploidy were identified by conventional or molecular cytogenetic analysis or Southern blot analysis for 12p copy number, permitting a diagnosis of GCT in approximately 30% of such tumors.[278] A significantly greater complete plus partial response proportion to cisplatin-based therapy and longer survival were associated with the presence of a GCT genetic marker.[278] Genetic analyses also identified other tumors such as primitive neuroectodermal tumors, lymphoma, desmoplastic small cell tumor, melanoma, and clear cell sarcoma, indicating that this group of midline tumors has a heterogeneous histogenesis. Therefore, genetic analysis using conventional and molecular techniques has both diagnostic and prognostic value.

OTHER TESTICULAR TUMORS

LEYDIG CELL TUMORS

Leydig cell (interstitial cell) tumors account for approximately 2% of testicular tumors.[279,280] Approximately 75% appear in adults who present with a palpable mass or testicular swelling indistinguishable from GCT. A minority has gynecomastia or decreased libido. The remaining 25% of cases present in children, sometimes with signs of sexual pseudoprecocity such as pubic hair, voice change, or enlarged genitalia.[279] A testicular mass associated with virilization in a prepubertal patient is a Leydig cell tumor until proven otherwise. There is no association between Leydig cell tumors and cryptorchidism. These tumors consist of tightly packed polygonal cells with eosinophilic granular cytoplasm and round nuclei with prominent nucleoli. Characteristic intracytoplasmic inclusion bodies (Rinke crystals) are seen in approximately 25% to 40% of cases.[280] A radical inguinal orchiectomy is required, and clinical staging includes a chest radiography, CT scan of the abdomen and pelvis, and studies for urinary and serum steroids.

Most Leydig cell tumors are benign. Malignant potential is difficult to predict. Vascular invasion, cellular atypia, tumor necrosis, infiltrative margins, increased mitotic rate, tumor size less than 5 cm and older age at presentation have been reported to be predictive of malignant potential.[280–282] Metastases are the only reliable criteria of malignancy. The most frequent sites of metastatic spread are the regional lymph nodes followed by lung, liver, and bone. RPLND is reasonable in selected cases with adverse features.[282] Metastatic Leydig cell tumors are radioresistant and chemoresistant. For metastatic disease, particularly that which secretes steroids, ortho-para-DDD, a potent inhibitor of steroidogenesis, has produced responses, but cure is not possible.[283]

SERTOLI CELL TUMORS

Sertoli cell tumors (SCT) account for fewer than 1% of primary testicular neoplasms. They are subclassified into classic, large cell calcifying (LCCSCT), and sclerosing.[284,285] SCT present as a painless, enlarging mass requiring a radical inguinal orchiectomy. LCCSCT are noted for multifocality, familial tendency, and bilaterality. An association has been reported between LCCSCT, pituitary adenoma, adrenocortical hyperplasia, cardiac myxoma, and pigmented skin and mucosal lesions.[286] Precocious puberty is commonly noted in boys with LCCSCT, whereas feminization occurs in approximately 25% of classical SCT but is rare in LCCSCT.[284] A testicular mass associated with feminization in a prepubertal patient is a classic SCT until proven otherwise.

Most SCT are benign and require RPLND only if accompanied by retroperitoneal adenopathy. Metastases are the only reliable indicator of malignancy, occurring in fewer than 10% of cases.[279] The most common sites for metastatic spread are retroperitoneal lymph nodes, mediastinal nodes, lungs, liver, and bone. Sclerosing SCT and LCCSCT have minimal metastatic potential. Radiation therapy and chemotherapy are ineffective.

GRANULOSA CELL TUMORS

Granulosa cell tumors histologically resemble adult-type granulosa cell tumors of the ovary. Gynecomastia and increased estrogen secretion are common. These tumors are extremely rare; their metastatic potential appears limited. Radical orchiectomy is required.

Juvenile granulosa cell tumors are the most common gonadal stromal neoplasms in early childhood, and the morphology may be confused with a yolk sac tumor. These patients usually present with maldescended testes, ambiguous genitalia, and an abnormal karyotype.

GONADOBLASTOMA

Gonadoblastoma are composed of sex cord elements admixed with germ cells. Often bilateral, they occur in men with chromosome abnormalities and those with dysgenetic gonads. Metastases from the GCT element may occur.

MESOTHELIOMA

Mesothelioma of the tunica vaginalis may invade the testis and frequently extend to the internal ring. Surgical intervention requires radical orchiectomy and complete excision of the spermatic cord and hemiscrotum. Retroperitoneal or inguinal metastases may occur if the testis is invaded or if vascular invasion is present. Aggressive surgery is the only useful therapy.

SARCOMAS

Primary sarcomas may arise from the peritesticular and spermatic cord soft tissue elements and should be managed like other sarcomas (see Chapter 39). Radical orchiectomy is required. Subsequent adjuvant radiation therapy is occasionally required, depending on size and tumor grade.[287]

ADENOCARCINOMA OF THE RETE TESTIS

This highly malignant neoplasm arises from the collecting system of the testis.[2,279] Located posteriorly, it often invades adjacent structures such as the cord and epididymis. Over one-half of patients present with metastatic disease. Survival rates are poor, with 30% to 50% dying within 1 year. These tumors generally do not respond to either radiation therapy or chemotherapy.[279] Following radical orchiectomy, RPLND may be curative in some patients with minimal retroperitoneal involvement.

EPIDERMOID CYST

Epidermoid cysts of the testis usually present between the second and fourth decades.[288] They are usually asymptomatic and discovered incidentally. These tumors are round, firm, and sharply demarcated on gross examination. Microscopically, the cyst is lined with stratified squamous epithelium. The adjacent testicular parenchyma is benign, and no CIS is present. The histogenesis of these tumors is uncertain. The clinical behavior of these tumors is uniformly benign; consequently, patients require no further therapy following resection. Testicular ultrasound may be diagnostic, in which case enucleation of the mass is sufficient treatment. Nevertheless, thorough histologic sampling must be performed to rule out a mature teratoma.

LYMPHOMA

Lymphoma is the most common secondary tumor of the testicle and the most frequent testicular neoplasm in men older than age 50.[279,280] Approximately 40% of patients report systemic symptoms such as fatigue, weight loss, and fever. Painless testicular enlargement is common, whereas bilateral involvement occurs in approximately one-third of patients.[289] Radical orchiectomy establishes the diagnosis and cures a small subset of patients. However, most cases are associated with systemic disease. Central nervous system as well as bone marrow diseases are common. Survival is generally poor. Management of lymphoma is discussed in Chapter 45.

Metastatic Carcinoma

Metastatic carcinoma to the testicle is rare and usually associated with diffuse systemic disease.[279] Bilateral involvement is noted in 15% of cases. The most common primary sites include prostate, lung, melanoma, and kidney. Treatment may include radical orchiectomy with further therapy dictated by the primary tumor.

REFERENCES

1. Greenlee RT, Murray T, Bolden S, Wingo PA. Cancer statistics 2000. *CA: Cancer J Clin* 2000;50:7.
2. McKiernan JM, Goluboff E, Liberson G, Golden R, Fisch H. Rising risk of testicular cancer by birth cohort in the United States from 1973 to 1995. *J Urol* 1999;162:361.
3. Bergstrom R, Adami H-O, Mohner M, et al. Increase in testicular cancer incidence in six European countries: a birth cohort phenomenon. *J Natl Cancer Inst* 1996;88:727.
4. Daniels JL, Stutzman R, McLeod D. A comparison of testicular tumors in black and white patients. *J Urol* 1981;125:341.
5. Moul J, Schanne F, Thompson I, et al. Testicular cancer in blacks. A multicenter experience. *Cancer* 1994;73:388.
6. Forman D, Olier R, Brett A, et al. Familial testicular cancer: a report of the UK family register, estimation of risk and an HLA Class 1 sib-pair analysis. *Br J Cancer* 1992;65:255.
7. Batata M, Chu F, Hilaris B, Whitmore W, Golbey R. Testicular cancer in cryptorchids. *Cancer* 1982;49:1023.
8. Schottenfeld D, Warshauer M, Sherlock S, et al. The epidemiology of testicular cancer in young adults. *Am J Epidemiol* 1980;112:232.
9. Timmerman J, Northfelt D, Small E. Malignant germ cell tumors in men infected with the human immunodeficiency virus: natural history and results of therapy. *J Clin Oncol* 1995;13:1291.
10. Bernardi D, Salvioni R, Vaccher E, et al. Testicular germ cell tumors and human immunodeficiency virus infection: a report of 26 cases. *J Clin Oncol* 1995;13:2705.
11. Moller H, Knudsen L, Lynge E. Risk of testicular cancer after vasectomy: cohort study of over 73,000 men. *Br J Med* 1994;309:295.
12. Renshaw AA. Testicular calcifications: incidence, histology and proposed pathological criteria for testicular microlithiasis. *J Urol* 1998;160:1625.
13. Bosl GJ, Vogelzang NJ, Goldman A, et al. Impact of delay in diagnosis on clinical stage of testicular cancer. *Lancet* 1981;2:970.
14. Feuer E, Frey C, Brawley O, et al. After a treatment breakthrough: a comparison of trial and population-based data for advanced testicular cancer. *J Clin Oncol* 1994;12:368.
15. Collette L, Sylvester RJ, Stenning SP, et al. Impact of the treating institution on survival of patients with "poor-prognosis" metastatic nonseminoma. *J Natl Cancer Inst* 1999;91:839.
16. Feuer EJ, Sheinfeld J, Bosl GJ. Does size matter? Association between number of patients treated and patient outcome in metastatic testicular cancer. *J Natl Cancer Inst* 1999;91:816.
17. Dehner L, Mills A, Talerman A, et al. Germ cell neoplasms of head and neck soft tissues: a pathologic spectrum of teratomatous and endodermal sinus tumors. *Hum Pathol* 1990;21:309.
18. Heffner D, Hyams V. Teratocarcinosarcoma (malignant teratoma?) of the nasal cavity and paranasal sinuses: a clinicopathologic study of 20 cases. *Cancer* 1984;53:2140.
19. Dixon FJ, Moore RA. *Atlas of tumor pathology.* Washington, DC: Armed Forces Institute of Pathology, 1952:32.
20. Mostofi FK, Sesterhenn IA. Revised International Classification of Testicular Tumors. In: Jones WG, Harnden P, Appleyard I, eds. *Germ cell tumors III.* Oxford: Pergamon, 1994:153.
21. Pugh RCB. *Pathology of the testis.* Oxford: Blackwell, 1976.
22. Jacobsen G, Henriksen OB, von der Maase H. Carcinoma in situ of testicular tissue adjacent to malignant germ-cell tumors: a study of 105 cases. *Cancer* 1981:2660.
23. Daugaard G, von der Masse H, Olsen J, Rorth M, Skakkebaek NE. Carcinoma-in-situ testis in patients with assumed extragonadal germ-cell tumors. *Lancet* 1987;2:528.
24. Muller J, Skakkebaek NE, Parkins MC. The spermatocytic seminoma: views on pathogenesis. *Int J Androl* 1987;10:1047.
25. Manivel JC, Simonton S, Wold LE, Dehner L. Absence of intratubular germ cell neoplasia in testicular yolk sac tumors in children. An histochemical and immunohistochemical study. *Arch Pathol Lab Med* 1988;112:641.
26. Skakkebaek ME, Berthelsen JG, Muller J. Carcinoma in situ of the undescended testis. *Urol Clin North Am* 1982;8:377.
27. von der Maase H, Rorth M, Walbom-Jorgensen S, et al. Carcinoma in situ of contralateral testis in patients with testicular germ cell cancer: study of 27 cases in 500 patients. *BMJ (Clin Res)* 1986;293:293.
28. Giwercman A, Muller J, Skakkebaek NE. Prevalence of carcinoma in situ and other histopathological abnormalities in testes from 399 men who suffered sudden unexpected death. *J Urol* 1991;145:77.
29. Pryor JP, Cameron KM, Chilton CP, et al. Carcinoma in situ in testicular biopsies from men presenting with infertility. *Br J Urol* 1983;55:780.
30. Skakkebaek NE. Carcinoma in situ of the testis: frequency and relationship to invasive germ cell tumors in infertile men. *Histopathology* 1978;2:157.
31. Berthelsen JG, Skakkebaek NE, von der Maase H, Sorensen B. Screening for carcinoma in situ of the contralateral testis in patients with germinal testicular cancer. *BMJ* 1982;285:1683.
32. Giwercman A, Grindsted J, Hansen B, et al. Testicular cancer risk in boys with maldescended testis: a cohort study. *J Urol* 1987;138:1214.
33. Cockburn A, Vugrin D, Batata M, Hajdu S, Whitmore W. Poorly differentiated (anaplastic) seminoma of the testis. *Cancer* 1984;53:1991.
34. Motzer RJ, Reuter VE, Cordon Cardo C, Bosl GJ. Blood group-related antigens in human germ cell tumors. *Cancer Res* 1988;48:5342.
35. Motzer RJ, Bosl GJ. Hemorrhage: a complication of metastatic testicular choriocarcinoma. *Urology* 1987;30:119.
36. Bosl GJ, Geller N, Cirrincione C, et al. Interrelationships of histopathology and other clinical variables in patients with germ cell tumors of the testis. *Cancer* 1983;51:2121.
37. Motzer RJ, Amsterdam A, Prieto V, et al. Teratoma with malignant transformation: diverse malignant histologies arising in men with germ cell tumors. *J Urol* 1998;159:133.
38. Nichols C, Roth B, Heerema NA, et al. Hematologic neoplasia associated with primary mediastinal germ cell tumors. *N Engl J Med* 1990;322:1425.
39. Leibovitch I, Foster R, Ulbright T, Donohue J. Adult primary pure teratoma of the testis. The Indiana Experience. *Cancer* 1995;75:2244.
40. Chaganti RSK, Murty VVVS, Bosl GJ. Molecular genetics of male germ cell tumors. In: Vogelzang NJ, Shipley WU, Scardino PT, Coffey DS, eds. *Comprehensive textbook of genitourinary oncology.* Baltimore: Williams & Wilkins, 1996:932.
41. Houldsworth J, Reuter V, Bosl G, Chaganti R. Aberrant expression of cyclin D2 is an early event in male germ cell tumorigenesis. *Cell Growth Differ* 1997;8:293.
42. Weinberg RA. The retinoblastoma protein and cell cycle control. *Cell* 1995;81:323.
43. Skakkebaek NE, Rajpert-de Meyts E, Jorgensen N, et al. Germ cell cancer and disorders of spermatogenesis: an environmental connection? *APMIS* 1998;106:3.
44. Skakkebaek NE, Berthelsen JG, Giwercman A, Muller J. Carcinoma in situ of the testis: possible origin from gonocytes and precursors of all types of germ cell tumors except spermatocytoma. *Int J Androl* 1987;10:19.
45. Chaganti RSK, Houldsworth J. The cytogenetic theory of the pathogenesis of human adult male germ cell tumors. *APMIS* 1998;106:80.
46. Sicinski P, Donaher JL, Geneg Y, et al. Cyclin D2 is an FSH-responsive gene involved in gonadal cell proliferation and oncogenesis. *Nature* 1996;384:470.
47. Murty VVVS, Chaganti RSK. A genetic perspective of male germ cell tumors. *Semin Oncol* 1998;25:133.
48. Loveland KL, Schlatt S. Stem cell factor and c-kit in the mammalian testis: lessons originating from Mother Nature's gene knockouts. *J Endocrinol* 1997;153:337.
49. Rajpert-de Meyts E, Skakkeback NE. Expression of the c-kit protein product in carcinoma in situ and invasive testicular germ cell tumors. *Int J Androl* 1994;17:85.
50. Conlon I, Raff M. Size control in animal development. *Cell* 1999;96:235.
51. Edlund T, Jessell TM. Progression from extrinsic to intrinsic signaling in cell fate specification: a view from the nervous system. *Cell* 1999;96:211.
52. Murty VVVS, Bosl GJ, Houldsworth J, et al. Allelic loss and somatic differentiation in human male germ cell tumors. *Oncogene* 1994;9:2245.
53. Barlow D. Imprinting: a gamete's point of view. *Trends Genet* 1993;9:285.
54. Lyon MF. Epigenetic inheritance in mammals. *Trends Genet* 1993;9:123.
55. Van Grup RJHLM, Oosterhuis JW, Kalscheuer V, Marimas ECM, Looijenga LHJ. Biallelic expression of the H19 and IGF2 genes in human testicular germ cell tumors. *J Natl Cancer Inst* 1994;86:1070.
56. Looijenga LHJ, Verkerk AJMH, Dekker MC, et al. Genomic imprinting in testicular germ cell tumours. *APMIS* 1998;106:187.
57. Houldsworth J, Xiao H, Murty VV, et al. Human male germ cell tumor resistance to cisplatin is linked to TP53 gene mutation. *Oncogene* 1998;16:2345.
58. Heimdal K, Lothe LA, Lystad S, et al. No germline TP53 mutations detected in familial and bilateral testicular cancer. *Genes Chromosomes Cancer* 1993;6:92.
59. Peng H-Q, Hogg D, Malkin D, et al. Mutations of the p53 gene do not occur in testis cancer. *Cancer Res* 1993;53:3574.
60. Bartkova J, Bartek J, Lukas J, et al. p53 Protein alterations in human testicular cancer including pre-invasive intratubular germ-cell neoplasia. *Int J Cancer* 1991;49:196.
61. Schenkman NS, Sesterhenn IA, Washington L, et al. Increased p53 protein does not correlate to p53 gene mutations in microdissected testicular germ cell tumors. *J Urol* 1995;154:617.
62. Heidenreich A, Schenkman NS, Sesterhenn IA, et al. Immunohistochemical and mutational analysis of the p53 tumor suppressor gene and the bcl-2 oncogene in primary testicular germ cell tumours. *APMIS* 1998;106:90.
63. Rao PH, Houldsworth J, Palanisamy N, et al. Chromosomal amplification is associated with cisplatin resistance of human male germ cell tumors. *Cancer Res* 1998;58:4260.
64. Koberle B, Grimaldi KA, Sunters A, et al. DNA repair capacity and cisplatin sensitivity of human testis tumour cells. *Int J Cancer* 1997;70:551.
65. Koberle B, Masters JRW, Hartley JA, Wood RD. Defective repair of cisplatin-induced DNA damage caused by reduced XPA protein in testicular germ cell tumours. *Curr Biol* 1999;9:273.

66. Levine AJ. p53, the cellular gatekeeper for growth and division. *Cell* 1997;88:323.
67. Chresta C, Masters J, Hickman J. Hypersensitivity of human testicular tumours to etoposide-induced apoptosis is associated with functional p53 and a high Bax-Bcl-2 ratio. *Cancer* 1996;56:1834.
68. Arriola EL, Rodriguez-Lopez AM, Hickman JA, Chresta CM. Bcl-2 overexpression results in reciprocal downregulation of Bcl-X(L) and sensitizes human testicular germ cell tumours to chemotherapy-induced apoptosis. *Oncogene* 1999;18:1457.
69. Timmer-Bosscha H, de Vries EG, Meijer C, Oosterhuis JW, Muldcer NH. Differential effects of all-trans retinoic acid, docsahexaenoic acid, and hexadecylphosphocholiine on cisplatin-induced cytotoxicity and apoptosis in a cisplatin sensitive and resistant human embryonal carcinoma cell line. *Cancer Chemother Pharmacol* 1998;41:469.
70. Battifora H, Sheibani K, Tubbs R, Kopinski M, Sun T-T. Antikeratin antibodies in tumor diagnosis. *Cancer* 1984;54:843.
71. Manivel J, Jessurun J, Wick M, Dehner L. Placental alkaline phosphatase immunoreactivity in testicular germ-cell neoplasms. *Am J Surg Pathol* 1987;11:21.
72. Izquierdo M, VanDer Valk P, Van Ark-Otte J, et al. Differential expression of the c-kit proto-oncogene in germ cell tumours. *J Pathol* 1995;177:253.
73. Ferreiro JA. Ber-H2 expression in testicular germ cell tumors. *Hum Pathol* 1994;25:522.
74. Hittmair A, Rogatsch H, Hobisch A, Mikuz G, Feichtinger H. CD30 expression in seminoma. *Hum Pathol* 1996;27:1166.
75. Suster S, Huxzar M, Bubis JJ, Geiger B. Fibrosarcoma of the urinary bladder: study of a case showing extensive chondroid differentiation. *Arch Surg* 1987;111:767.
76. Lien H, Stenwig A, Ous S, Fossa S. Influence of different criteria for abnormal lymph node size on reliability of computed tomography in patients with nonseminomatous testicular cancer. *Acta Radiol Diagn* 1986;27:199.
77. Fernandez E, Moul J, Foley J, Colon E, McLeod D. Retroperitoneal imaging with third and fourth generation computed axial tomography in clinical stage I nonseminomatous germ cell tumors. *Urology* 1994;44:548.
78. Leibovitch I, Foster R, Kopecky K, Donohue J. Improved accuracy of computerized tomography based clinical staging in low stage nonseminomatous germ cell cancer using size criteria of retroperitoneal lymph nodes. *J Urol* 1995;154:1759.
79. Hilton S, Herr H, Teitcher J, Begg C, Castellino R. CT detection of retroperitoneal lymph node metastases in patients with clinical stage I testicular nonseminomatous germ cell cancer: assessment of size and distribution criteria. *AJR* 1997;169:521.
80. Albers P, Bender H, Yilmaz H, et al. Positron emission tomography in the clinical staging of patients with stage I and II testicular germ cell tumors. *Urology* 1999;53:808.
81. Stephens AW, Gonin R, Hutchins GD, Einhorn L. Positron emission tomography evaluation of residual radiographic abnormalities in postchemotherapy germ cell tumor patients. *J Clin Oncol* 1996;14:1637.
82. Cremerius U, Effert PJ, Adam G, et al. FDG PET for detection and therapy control of metastatic germ cell tumor. *J Nucl Med* 1998;39:815.
83. Ganjoo KN, Chan RJ, Sharma M, Einhorn LH. PET scans in the evaluation of post-chemotherapy (PC) residual masses in patients with seminoma. *J Clin Oncol* 1999;17:3457.
84. Bosl GJ, Geller NL, Chan EY. Stage migration and the increasing proportion of complete responders in patients with advanced germ cell tumors. *Cancer Res* 1988;48:3524.
85. Vaitukaitis JL. Human chorionic gonadotropin as a tumor marker. *Ann Clin Lab Sci* 1974;4:276.
86. Mencel PJ, Motzer RJ, Mazumdar M, et al. Advanced seminoma: treatment results, survival, and prognostic factors in 142 patients. *J Clin Oncol* 1994;12:120.
87. Catalona WJ, Vaitukaitis JL, Fair WR. Falsely positive specific human chorionic gonadotropin assays in patients with testicular tumors: conversion to negative with testosterone administration. *J Urol* 1979;122:126.
88. Odell WD, Griffin J. Pulsatile secretion of human chorionic gonadotropin in normal adults. *N Engl J Med* 1987;317:1688.
89. Fowler JE, Platoff GE, Kubrock CA, Stutzman RE. Commercial radioimmunoassay for beta subunit of human chorionic gonadotropin: falsely positive determinations due to elevated serum luteinizing hormone. *Cancer* 1982;49:136.
90. Bajorin D, Mazumdar M, Meyers M, et al. Metastatic germ cell tumors: modeling for response to chemotherapy. *J Clin Oncol* 1998;16:707.
91. Bosl GJ, Gluckman R, Geller N, et al. VAB-6: An effective chemotherapy regimen for patients with germ-cell tumors. *J Clin Oncol* 1986;4:1493.
92. Fleming I, et al., ed. *AJCC Cancer Staging Handbook.* Philadelphia: Lippincott–Raven, 1998.
93. Warde P, Gospodarowicz MK, Panzarella T, et al. Stage I testicular seminoma: results of adjuvant irradiation and surveillance. *J Clin Oncol* 1995;13:2255.
94. Vaeth M, Schultz HP, von der Maase H, et al. Prognostic factors in testicular germ cell tumors. *Acta Radiol Oncol* 1984;23:271.
95. Zagars GK, Babian RJ. Stage I testicular seminoma: rationale for postorchidectomy radiation therapy. *Int J Radiat Oncol Biol Phys* 1987;13:155.
96. Butcher DN, Gregory WM, Gunter PA, et al. The biological and clinical significance of HCG-containing cells in seminoma. *Br J Cancer* 1985;51:473.
97. Peckham MJ. Surveillance following orchiectomy for clinical stage I testicular germ-cell malignancy. *Prog Clin Biol Res* 1985;203:523.
98. Vogelzang NJ, Fraley EE, Lange PH, et al. Stage II nonseminomatous testicular cancer: a 10-year experience. *J Clin Oncol* 1983;1:171.
99. Vugrin D, Whitmore W, Cvitkovic E, et al. Adjuvant chemotherapy with VAB-3 of stage II-B testicular cancer. *Cancer* 1981;48:233.
100. Ozols RF, Ihde DC, Linehan WM, Young RC. Management of high risk patients with advanced testis cancer: National Cancer Institute approach. *Semin Oncol* 1988;15:335.
101. Richie JP, Kantoff PW. Is adjuvant chemotherapy necessary for patients with stage B1 testicular cancer? *J Clin Oncol* 1991;9:1393.
102. Williams SD, Stablein DM, Einhorn LH, et al. Immediate adjuvant chemotherapy versus observation with treatment at relapse in pathological stage II testicular cancer. *N Engl J Med* 1987;317:1433.
103. Zagars G, Babaian J. The role of radiation in stage II testicular seminoma. *Int J Radiat Oncol Biol Phys* 1987;13:163.
104. Bosl GJ, Geller N, Cirrincione C, et al. Multivariate analysis of prognostic variables in patients with metastatic testicular cancer. *Cancer Res* 1983;43:3403.
105. Birch R, Williams S, Cone A, et al. Prognostic factors for favorable outcome in disseminated germ cell tumors. *J Clin Oncol* 1986;4:400.
106. de Wit R, Stoter G, Sleijfer DT, et al. Four cycles of BEP versus an alternating regimen of PVB and BEP in patients with poor-prognosis metastatic testicular non-seminoma; a randomised study of the EORTC Genitourinary Tract Cancer Cooperative Group. *Br J Cancer* 1995;71:1311.
107. Bajorin D, Katz A, Chan E, et al. Comparison of criteria for assigning germ cell tumor patients to "good risk" and "poor risk" studies. *J Clin Oncol* 1988;6:786.
108. IGCCCG. International Germ Cell Consensus classification: a prognostic factor-based staging system for metastatic germ cell cancers. *J Clin Oncol* 1997;15:594.
109. Fossa SD, Horwich A, Russell JM, et al. Optimal planning target volume for stage I testicular seminoma: a Medical Research Council randomized trial. *J Clin Oncol* 1999;17:1146.
110. Thomas G, Rider W, Dembo A, et al. Seminoma of the testis: results of treatment and patterns of failure after radiation therapy. *Int J Radiat Oncol Biol Phys* 1982;8:165.
111. Hamilton C, Horwich A, Easton D, Peckham M. Radiotherapy for stage I seminoma testis: results of treatment and complications. *Radiother Oncol* 1986;6:115.
112. Willan B, McGowan D. Seminoma of the testis: a 22-year experience with radiation therapy. *Int J Radiat Oncol Biol Phys* 1985;11:1769.
113. Hanks G, Herring D, Kramer S. Patterns of care outcome studies: results of the national practice in seminoma of the testis. *Int J Radiat Oncol Biol Phys* 1981;7:1413.
114. Fossa S, Aass N, Kaalhus O. Radiotherapy for testicular seminoma stage I: treatment results and long-term post-irradiation morbidity in 365 patients. *Int J Radiat Oncol Biol Phys* 1989;16:383.
115. van Leeuwen F, Stiggelbout A, van den Belt-Dusebout A, et al. Second cancer risk following testicular cancer: a followup study of 1,909 patients. *J Clin Oncol* 1993;11:415.
116. Wanderas EH, Fossa SD, Tretli S. Risk of subsequent non-germ cell cancer after treatment of germ cell cancer in 2006 Norwegian male patients. *Eur J Cancer* 1997;33:253.
117. Horwich A. Surveillance for stage I seminoma of the testis. In: Horwich A, ed. *Testicular cancer: investigation and management.* London: Chapman and Hall, 1991:109.
118. Sharda NN, Kinsella TJ, Ritter MA. Adjuvant radiation versus observation: a cost analysis of alternate management schemes in early-stage testicular seminoma. *J Clin Oncol* 1996; 14:2933.
119. Rorth M, Jacobsen GK, von der Maase H, et al. Surveillance alone versus radiotherapy after orchiectomy for clinical stage I nonseminomatous testicular cancer. Danish Testicular Cancer Study Group. *J Clin Oncol* 1991;9:1543.
120. Sharir S, Jewett MAS, Sturgeon JFG, et al. Progression detection of stage I nonseminomatous testis cancer on surveillance: implications for the followup protocol. *J Urol* 1999;161:472.
121. Gels M, Hoekstra H, Sleijfer D, et al. Detection of recurrence in patients with clinical stage I nonseminomatous testicular germ cell tumors and consequences for further followup: a single-center 10-year experience. *J Clin Oncol* 1995;13:1188.
122. Read G, Stenning S, Cullen M, et al. Medical Research Council prospective study of surveillance for stage I testicular teratoma. *J Clin Oncol* 1992;10:1762.
123. Nicolai N, Pizzocaro G. A surveillance study of clinical stage I nonseminomatous germ cell tumors of the testis: 10-year followup. *J Urol* 1995;154:1045.
124. Baniel J, Foster R, Rowland R, Donohue J. Complications of primary retroperitoneal lymph node dissection. *J Urol* 1994;152:424.
125. Birhle R, Donohue J, Foster R. Complications of retroperitoneal lymph node dissection. *Urol Clin North Am* 1988;15:237.
126. Donohue J, Zachary J, Maynard B. Distribution of nodal metastases in nonseminomatous testis cancer. *J Urol* 1982;128:315.
127. Ray B, Hadju S, Whitmore WFJ. Distribution of retroperitoneal lymph node metastases in testicular germinal tumors. *Cancer* 1974;33:340.
128. Donohue JP, Thornhill JA, Foster RS, Rowland RG, Bihrle R. Retroperitoneal lymphadenectomy for clinical stage A testis cancer (1965 to 1989): modifications of technique and impact on ejaculation. *J Urol* 1993;149:237.
129. Jewett MAS. Nerve sparing technique for retroperitoneal lymphadenectomy in testis cancer. *Urol Clin North Am* 1990;17:449.
130. Donohue JP, Foster RS. Retroperitoneal lymphadenectomy in staging and treatment. The development of nerve-sparing techniques. *Urol Clin North Am* 1998;25:461.
131. Richie J. Clinical stage I testicular cancer: the role of modified retroperitoneal lymphadenectomy. *J Urol* 1990;144:1160.
132. Fossa S, Klepp O, Ous S, et al. Unilateral retroperitoneal lymph node dissection in patients with nonseminomatous testicular tumor in clinical stage I. *Eur Urol* 1984;10:17.
133. Nijman J, Jager S, Boer P, et al. The treatment of ejaculation disorders after retroperitoneal lymph node dissection. *Cancer* 1982;50:2967.
134. Ohl D. Electroejaculation. *Urol Clin North Am* 1993;20:181.
135. Rassweiler JJ, Seemann O, Henkel TO, et al. Laparoscopic retroperitoneal lymph node dissection for nonseminomatous germ cell tumor: indication and limitation. *J Urol* 1996;156:1108.
136. Janetschek G, Hobisch A, Holtl L, et al. Retroperitoneal lymphadenectomy for clinical stage I nonseminomatous testicular tumor: laparoscopy versus open surgery and impact of learning curve. *J Urol* 1996;156:89.
137. Bianchi G, Beltrami P, Giusti G, et al. Unilateral laparoscopic retroperitoneal lymph node dissection for clinical stage I nonseminomatous germ cell testicular neoplasm. *Eur Urol* 1998;33:190.
138. Baniel J, Foster RS, Einhorn L, Donohue J. Late relapse of clinical stage I testicular cancer. *J Urol* 1995;154:1370.
139. Cespedes RD, Peretsman SJ. Retroperitoneal recurrences after retroperitoneal lymph node dissection for low-stage nonseminomatous germ cell tumors. *Urology* 1999;54:548.

140. Dunphy C, Ayala A, Swanson D, Ro J, Logothetis C. Clinical stage I nonseminomatous and mixed germ cell tumors of the testis. *Cancer* 1988;62:1202.
141. Sogani PC, Perrotti M, Herr HW, et al. Clinical stage I testis cancer: long-term outcome of patients on surveillance. *J Urol* 1998;159:855.
142. Heidenreich A, Sesterhenn IA, Mostofi FK, Moul JW. Prognostic risk factors that identify patients with clinical stage I nonseminomatous germ cell tumors at low risk and high risk for metastasis. *Cancer* 1998;83:1002.
143. Pont J, Holtl W, Kosak D, et al. Risk-adapted treatment choice in stage I nonseminomatous testicular germ cell cancer by regarding vascular invasion in the primary tumor: a prospective trial. *J Clin Oncol* 1990;8:16.
144. Oliver RTD, Raja M, Ong J, Gallagher C. Pilot study to evaluate impact of a policy of adjuvant chemotherapy for high risk stage I malignant teratoma on overall relapse rate of stage I cancer patients. *J Urol* 1992;148:1453.
145. Cullen M, Stenning S, Parkinson M, et al. Short course adjuvant chemotherapy in high risk stage I nonseminomatous germ cell tumours of the testis (NSGCTT): an MRC(UK) study report. *Proc ASCO* 1995;14:244(abst).
146. Davis B, Herr H, Fair W, Bosl GJ. The management of patients with nonseminomatous germ cell tumors of the testis with serologic disease only after orchiectomy. *J Urol* 1994;152:111.
147. Saxman S, Nichols C, Foster R, et al. The management of patients with clinical stage I nonseminomatous testicular tumors and persistently elevated serologic markers. *J Urol* 1996;155:587.
148. Gregory C, Peckham M. Results of radiotherapy for stage II testicular seminoma. *Radiother Oncol* 1986;6:285.
149. Loehrer PJ, Birch R, Williams SD, Greco A, Einhorn LH. Chemotherapy of metastatic seminoma: the Southeastern Cancer Study Group experience. *J Clin Oncol* 1987;5:1212.
150. Sheinfeld J, Rabbani F, Mohsein H, et al. Elevated serum tumor markers (STM) prior to 1o RPLND predicts clinical outcome and requirements for systemic chemotherapy in patients with pN1, N2 and N3 nonseminomatous germ cell tumor (NSGCT). *Proc ASCO* 1999;18:308a.
151. Baniel J, Roth B, Foster R, Donohue J. Cost and risk benefit in the management of clinical stage II nonseminomatous testicular tumors. *Cancer* 1995;75:2897.
152. Harlapp J, Weissbach L, Bussar-Maatz R. Adjuvant chemotherapy in nonseminomatous testicular tumor stage II. *Int J Androl* 1987;10:277.
153. Rabbani F, Sheinfeld J, Mohseni H, et al. Prognostic factors for relapse in patients with low volume (pN1) nonseminomatous germ cell tumor (NSGCT) following primary retroperitoneal lymphadenectomy (RPLND). *J Urol* 1999;161:157.
154. Weissbach L, Hartlapp JH. Adjuvant chemotherapy of metastatic stage II nonseminomatous testis tumor. *J Urol* 1991;146:1295.
155. Vugrin D, Whitmore WF, Herr HW, Sogani P, Golbey RB. VAB-6 combination chemotherapy in resected stage II-B testis cancer. *Cancer* 1983;51:5.
156. Motzer RJ, Sheinfeld J, Mazumdar M, et al. Etoposide and cisplatin adjuvant therapy for patients with pathologic stage II germ cell tumors. *J Clin Oncol* 1995;13:2700.
157. Warde P, Gospodarowicz M, Panzarella T, et al. Management of stage II seminoma. *J Clin Oncol* 1998;16:290.
158. Williams SD, Birch R, Einhorn LH, et al. Treatment of disseminated germ-cell tumors with cisplatin, bleomycin, and either vinblastine or etoposide. *N Engl J Med* 1987;316:1435.
159. Einhorn LH, Williams SD, Troner M, Birch R, Greco FA. The role of maintenance therapy in disseminated testicular cancer. *N Engl J Med* 1981;305:727.
160. Vogelzang NJ, Bosl GJ, Johnson K, Kennedy BJ. Raynaud's phenomenon: a common toxicity after combination chemotherapy for testicular cancer. *Ann Intern Med* 1981;95:288.
161. Vogelzang NJ, Frenning DH, Kennedy BJ. Coronary artery disease after treatment with bleomycin and vinblastine. *Cancer Treat Rep* 1980;64:1159.
162. Einhorn LH, Williams SD, Loehrer PJ, et al. Evaluation of optimal duration of chemotherapy in favorable-prognosis disseminated germ cell tumors: a Southeastern Cancer Study Group protocol. *J Clin Oncol* 1989;7:387.
163. Bosl GJ, Geller NL, Bajorin D, et al. A randomized trial of etoposide + cisplatin versus vinblastine + bleomycin + cisplatin + cyclophosphamide + dactinomycin in patients with good-prognosis germ cell tumors. *J Clin Oncol* 1988;6:1231.
164. de Wit R, Stoter G, Kaye SB, et al. Importance of bleomycin in combination chemotherapy for good-prognosis testicular nonseminoma: a randomized study of the European Organization for Research and Treatment of Cancer Genitourinary Tract Cooperative Group. *J Clin Oncol* 1997;15:1837.
165. Loehrer PJ, Johnson DH, Elson P, Einhorn LH, Trump D. Importance of bleomycin in favorable-prognosis disseminated germ cell tumors: an Eastern Cooperative Oncology Group Trial. *J Clin Oncol* 1995;13:470.
166. Bajorin DF, Sarosdy MF, Pfister DG, et al. Randomized trial of etoposide and cisplatin versus etoposide and carboplatin in patients with good-risk germ cell tumors: a multi-institutional study. *J Clin Oncol* 1993;11:598.
167. Horwich A, Sleijfer D, Fossa S, et al. Randomized trial of bleomycin, etoposide, and cisplatin compared with bleomycin, etoposide, and carboplatin in good-prognosis metastatic nonseminomatous germ cell cancer: a multi-institutional medical research council/European Organization for Research and Treatment of Cancer trial. *J Clin Oncol* 1997;15:1844.
168. Culine S, Kerbrat P, Bouzy J, et al. Are 3 cycles of bleomycin, etoposide and cisplatin (3BEP) or 4 cycles of etoposide and cisplatin (4EP) equivalent regimens for patients (pts) with good-risk metastatic non seminomatous germ cell tumors (NSGCT)? Preliminary results of a randomized trial. *Proc ASCO* 1999;18:309.
169. Bajorin DF, Geller NL, Weisen SF, Bosl GJ. Two-drug therapy in patients with metastatic germ cell tumors. *Cancer* 1991;67:28.
170. Nichols CR, Williams SD, Loehrer PJ, et al. Randomized study of cisplatin dose intensity in poor-risk germ cell tumors: a Southeastern Cancer Study Group and Southwest Oncology Group protocol. *J Clin Oncol* 1991;9:1163.
171. Ozols RF, Ihde DC, Linehan WM, et al. A randomized trial of standard chemotherapy vs a high-dose chemotherapy regimen in the treatment of poor prognosis nonseminomatous germ-cell tumors. *J Clin Oncol* 1988;6:1031.
172. Nichols CR, Loehrer PJ, Einhorn LH, Propert K, Vogelzang NJ. Phase III study of cisplatin, etoposide and bleomycin (PVP16B) or etoposide, ifosfamide and cisplatin (VIP) in advanced stage germ cell tumors; an intergroup trial. *Proc ASCO* 1995;1995.
173. Kaye S, Mead G, Fossa S, et al. Intensive induction-sequential chemotherapy with BOP/VIP-B compared with treatment with BEP/EP for poor-prognosis metastatic nonseminomatous germ cell tumor: a randomized Medical Research Council/European Organization for Research and Treatment of Cancer study. *J Clin Oncol* 1998;16:692.
174. Nichols CR, Catalano P, Crawford ED, et al. Randomized comparison of cisplatin and etoposide and either bleomycin or ifosfamide in treatment of advanced disseminated germ cell tumors; an Eastern Cooperative Oncology Group, Southwest Oncology Group, and Cancer and Leukemia Group B study. *J Clin Oncol* 1998;16:1287.
175. Bosl G, Geller N, Vogelzang N, et al. Alternating cycles of etoposide plus cisplatin and VAB-6 in the treatment of poor-risk patients with germ cell tumors. *J Clin Oncol* 1987;5:436.
176. Motzer RJ, Mazumdar M, Gulati SC, et al. Phase II trial of high-dose carboplatin and etoposide with autologous bone marrow transplantation in first-line therapy for patients with poor-risk germ cell tumors. *J Natl Cancer Inst* 1993;85:1828.
177. Motzer RJ, Mazumdar M, Bajorin DF, et al. High-dose carboplatin, etoposide, and cyclophosphamide with autologous bone marrow transplantation in first-line therapy for patients with poor-risk germ cell tumors. *J Clin Oncol* 1997;15:2546.
178. Chevreau C, Droz J, Pico J, et al. Early intensified chemotherapy with autologous bone marrow transplantation in first line treatment of poor risk non-seminomatous germ cell tumours. *Eur Urol* 1993;23:213.
179. Sheinfeld J, Bajorin D. Management of the postchemotherapy residual mass. *Urol Clin North Am* 1993;20:133.
180. Einhorn LH, Williams SD, Mandelbaum I, Donohue JP. Surgical resection in disseminated testicular cancer following chemotherapeutic cytoreduction. *Cancer* 1981;48:904.
181. Toner GC, Panicek D, Heelan R, et al. Adjunctive surgery after chemotherapy for nonseminomatous germ cell tumors: recommendations for patient selection. *J Clin Oncol* 1990;8:1683.
182. Donohue JP, Rowland RG. The role of surgery in advanced testicular cancer. *Cancer* 1984;54:2716.
183. Donohue J, Rowland R, Kopecky K, et al. Correlation of computerized tomographic changes and histological findings in 80 patients having radical retroperitoneal lymph node dissection after chemotherapy for testis tumor. *J Urol* 1987;137:1176.
184. Fossa SD, Qvist H, Stenwig AE, et al. Is postchemotherapy retroperitoneal surgery necessary in patients with nonseminomatous testicular cancer and minimal residual tumor masses? *J Clin Oncol* 1992;10:569.
185. Fox EP, Weathers T, Williams S, et al. Outcome analysis for patients with persistent germ cell nonteratomatous germ cell tumor in post-chemotherapy retroperitoneal lymph node dissections. *J Clin Oncol* 1993;11:1294.
186. Tait D, Peckham MJ, Hendry WF, et al. Post-chemotherapy surgery in advanced non-seminomatous germ cell testicular tumors: the significance of histology with particular reference to differentiated (mature) teratoma. *Br J Cancer* 1984;50:601.
187. Gelderman WA, Schraffordt Koops H, Sleijfer DT, et al. Results of adjuvant surgery in patients with stage III and IV nonseminomatous testicular tumors after cisplatin-vinblastine- bleomycin chemotherapy. *J Surg Oncol* 1988;38:227.
188. Harding MJ, Brown IL, MacPherson SG, Turner MA, Kaye SB. Excision of residual masses after platinum based chemotherapy for non-seminomatous germ cell tumours. *Eur J Cancer Clin Oncol* 1989;25:1689.
189. Steyerberg EW, Keizer HJ, Fossa SD, et al. Resection of residual retroperitoneal masses in testicular cancer: evaluation and improvement of selection criteria. The ReHiT study group. Re-analysis of histology in testicular cancer. *Br J Cancer* 1996;74:1492.
190. Fossa SD, Aass N, Ous S, et al. Histology of tumor residuals following chemotherapy in patients with advanced nonseminomatous testicular cancer. *J Urol* 1989;142:1239.
191. Fossa SD, Ous S, Lien HH, et al. Post-chemotherapy lymph node histology in radiologically normal patients with metastatic nonseminomatous testicular cancer. *Urology* 1989;141:557.
192. Mead G, Stenning S, Parkinson M. The second Medical Research Council study of prognostic factors in nonseminomatous germ cell tumors. *J Clin Oncol* 1991;10:85.
193. Harstrick A, Schmoll HJ, Wilke H, et al. Cisplatin, etoposide, and ifosfamide salvage therapy for refractory or relapsing germ cell carcinoma. *J Clin Oncol* 1991;9:1549.
194. Loehrer P, Gonin R, Nichols C, et al. Vinblastine plus ifosfamide plus cisplatin as initial salvage therapy in recurrent germ cell tumor. *J Clin Oncol* 1998;15:2500.
195. Motzer RJ, Bajorin DF, Vlamis V, Weisen S, Bosl GJ. Ifosfamide-based chemotherapy for patients with resistant germ cell tumors: the Memorial Sloan-Kettering Cancer Center Experience. *Semin Oncol* 1992;19:8.
196. Panicek DM, Toner GC, Heelan RT, Bosl GJ. Nonseminomatous germ cell tumors: enlarging masses despite chemotherapy. *Radiology* 1990;175:499.
197. Lorigan JG, Eftekhari F, David CL, et al. The growing teratoma syndrome: an unusual manifestation of treated nonseminomatous germ cell tumors of the testis. *AJR Am J Roentgenol* 1988;151:325.
198. Morgentaler A, Garnick MB, Richie JP. Metastatic testicular teratoma invading the inferior vena cava. *J Urol* 1988;140:149.
199. Little J, Foster R, Ulbright T, Donohue J. Unusual neoplasms detected in testis cancer patients undergoing postchemotherapy retroperitoneal lymphadenectomy. *J Urol* 1994;152:1144.
200. Bosl GJ, Ilson DH, Rodriguez E, et al. Clinical relevance of the i(12p) marker chromosome in germ cell tumors. *J Natl Cancer Inst* 1994;86:349.
201. Chaganti RSK, Ladanyi M, Samaniego F, et al. Leukemic differentiation of a mediastinal germ cell tumor. *Genes Chromosomes Cancer* 1989;1:83.
202. Rodriguez E, Reuter VE, Mies C, et al. Abnormalities of 2q: a common genetic link between rhabdomyosarcoma and hepatoblastoma? *Genes Chromosomes Cancer* 1991;3:122.
203. Loehrer PJ, Hui S, Clark S, et al. Teratoma following cisplatin-based combination chemotherapy for nonseminomatous germ cell tumors: a clinicopathological correlation. *J Urol* 1986;135:1183.

204. Sonneveld DJA, Sleijfer DT, Koops HS, et al. Mature teratoma identified after postchemotherapy surgery in patients with dissected nonseminomatous testicular germ cell tumors. *Cancer* 1998;82:1343.
205. Bajorin DF, Herr HW, Motzer RJ, Bosl GJ. Current perspectives on the role of adjunctive surgery in combined modality treatment of patients with germ cell tumors. *Semin Oncol* 1992;19:148.
206. Borge N, Fossa SD, Ous S, et al. Late recurrence of testicular cancer. *J Clin Oncol* 1988;6:1248.
207. Roth BJ, Greist A, Kubilis PS, Williams SD, Einhorn LH. Cisplatin-based combination chemotherapy for disseminated germ cell tumors: long-term follow-up. *J Clin Oncol* 1988;6:1239.
208. Skinner DG, Melamud A, Lieskovsky G. Complications of thoracoabdominal retroperitoneal lymph node dissection. *J Urol* 1982;127:1107.
209. Wood DPJ, Herr H, Heller G, Bosl G. Distribution of retroperitoneal metastases after chemotherapy in patients with nonseminomatous germ cell tumors of the testis. *J Urol* 1992;148:1812.
210. Wahle G, Foster R, Bihrle R, et al. Nerve sparing retroperitoneal lymphadenectomy after primary chemotherapy for metastatic testicular carcinoma. *J Urol* 1994;152:428.
211. Streyerberg E, Keizer H, Fossa S, et al. Prediction of residual retroperitoneal mass histology after chemotherapy for metastatic nonseminomatous germ cell tumor: multivariate analysis of individual patient data from six study groups. *J Clin Oncol* 1995;13:1177.
212. Horwich A, Paluchowska B, Norman A, et al. Residual mass following chemotherapy of seminoma. *Ann Oncol* 1997;8:37.
213. Ellison MF, Mostofi FK, Flanigan RC. Treatment of the residual retroperitoneal mass after chemotherapy for advanced seminoma. *J Urol* 1988;140:618.
214. Fossa SD, Borge L, Gass N, et al. The treatment of advanced metastatic seminoma: experience in 55 cases. *J Clin Oncol* 1987;5:1071.
215. Friedman EL, Garnick MB, Stomper PC, et al. Therapeutic guidelines and results in advanced seminoma. *J Clin Oncol* 1985;3:1325.
216. Peckham MJ, Horwich A, Hendry WF. Advanced seminoma: treatment with cis-platinum-based combination chemotherapy or carboplatin (JM8). *Br J Cancer* 1985;52:7.
217. Puc H, Heelan R, Mazumdar M, et al. Management of residual mass in advanced seminoma: results and recommendations from the Memorial Sloan-Kettering Cancer Center. *J Clin Oncol* 1996;14:454.
218. Tiffany P, Morse MJ, Bosl G, et al. Sequential excision of residual thoracic and retroperitoneal masses after chemotherapy for stage III germ cell tumors. *Cancer* 1986;57:978.
219. Gels ME, Hoekstra HJ, Sleijfer DT, et al. Thoracotomy for postchemotherapy resection of pulmonary residual tumor mass in patients with nonseminomatous testicular germ cell tumors: aggressive surgical resection is justified. *Chest* 1997;112:967.
220. See WA, Laurenzo JF, Dreicer R, Hoffman HT. Incidence and management of testicular carcinoma metastatic to the neck. *J Urol* 1996;155:590.
221. Brenner PC, Herr HW, Morse MJ, et al. Simultaneous retroperitoneal, thoracic, and cervical resection of postchemotherapy residual masses in patients with metastatic nonseminomatous germ cell tumors of the testis [see comments]. *J Clin Oncol* 1996;14:1765.
222. Leibovitch I, Little JSJ, Foster RS, et al. Delayed orchiectomy after chemotherapy for metastatic nonseminomatous germ cell tumors. *J Urol* 1996;155:952.
223. Simmonds P, Mead G, Lee A, et al. Orchiectomy after chemotherapy in patients with metastatic testicular cancer. *Cancer* 1995;75:1018.
224. Wheeler BM, Loehrer PJ, Williams SD, Einhorn LH. Ifosfamide in refractory male germ cell tumors. *J Clin Oncol* 1986;4:28.
225. Scheulen ME, Niederle N, Bremer K, et al. Efficacy of ifosfamide in refractory malignant disease and uroprotection by mesna: results of a phase II study with 151 patients. *Cancer Treat Rep* 1983;10:93.
226. Loehrer PJ, Lauer R, Roth BJ, et al. Salvage therapy in recurrent germ cell cancer: ifosfamide and cisplatin plus either vinblastine or etoposide. *Ann Intern Med* 1988;109:540.
227. Ghosn M, Droz JP, Theodore C, et al. Salvage chemotherapy in refractory germ cell tumors with etoposide (VP-16) plus ifosfamide plus high-dose cisplatin. *Cancer* 1988;62:24.
228. Pizzocaro G, Salvoni R, Piva L. High activity, moderate toxicity modified cisplatin, etoposide, ifosfamide (PEI) salvage therapy for germ-cell testicular tumors (GCTT). *Proc ASCO* 1990;9:131.
229. Motzer RJ, Cooper K, Geller NL, et al. The role of ifosfamide plus cisplatin-based chemotherapy as salvage therapy for patients with refractory germ cell tumors. *Cancer* 1990;66:2476.
230. Motzer R, Green G, McCaffrey J, et al. Paclitaxel (T), ifosfamide (I), and cisplatin (P) as first-line salvage therapy for relapsed germ cell tumor (GCT) patients with favorable prognostic features. *Proc ASCO* 1998;17:322A.
231. Broun ER, Nichols CR, Kneebone P, et al. Long-term outcome of patients with relapsed and refractory germ cell tumors treated with high-dose chemotherapy and autologous bone marrow rescue. *Ann Intern Med* 1992;117:124.
232. Linkesch W, Greinix HT, Hocker P, Krainer M, Wagner A. Longterm follow up of phase I/II trial of ultra-high carboplatin, VP16, cyclophosphamide with ABMT in refractory or relapsed NSGCT. *Proc ASCO* 1993;12:232(abst).
233. Motzer R, Mazumdar M, Bosl G, et al. High-dose carboplatin, etoposide, and cyclophosphamide for patients with refractory germ cell tumors: treatment results and prognostic factors for survival and toxicity. *J Clin Oncol* 1996;14:1098.
234. Siegert W, Beyer J, Strohscheer I, et al. High-dose treatment with carboplatin, etoposide, and ifosfamide followed by autologous stem-cell transplantation in relapsed or refractory germ cell cancer: a phase I/II study. *J Clin Oncol* 1994;12:1223.
235. Motzer RJ, Gulati SC, Crown JP, et al. High-dose chemotherapy and autologous bone marrow rescue for patients with refractory germ cell tumors: early intervention is better tolerated. *Cancer* 1992;69:550.
236. Motzer RJ, Gulati SC, Tong WP, et al. Phase I trial with pharmacokinetic analyses of high-dose carboplatin, etoposide, and cyclophosphamide with autologous bone marrow transplantation in patients with refractory germ cell tumors. *Cancer Res* 1993;53:3730.
237. Beyer J, Schwella N, Zingsem J, et al. Hematopoietic rescue after high-dose chemotherapy using autologous peripheral-blood progenitor cells or bone marrow: a randomized comparison. *J Clin Oncol* 1995;13:1328.
238. Motzer RJ, Geller NL, Tan CC, et al. Salvage chemotherapy for patients with germ cell tumors. The Memorial Sloan-Kettering Cancer Center experience (1979–1989). *Cancer* 1991;67:1305.
239. Beyer J, Kramar A, Mandanas R, et al. High-dose chemotherapy as salvage treatment in germ cell tumors: a multivariate analysis of prognostic variables. *J Clin Oncol* 1996;14:2638.
240. Murphy BA, Motzer RJ, Bosl G. Phase II study of iproplatin (CHIP) in patients with cisplatin-refractory germ cell tumors; the need for alternative strategies in the investigation of new agents in GCT. *Invest New Drugs* 1992;10:327.
241. Motzer RJ, Dmitrovsky E, Miller WH, et al. Suramin for germ cell tumors: in vitro growth inhibition and results of a phase II trial. *Cancer* 1993;72:3313.
242. Moasser M, Motzer R, Khoo K-S, et al. all-trans Retinoic acid for treating germ cell tumors. *Cancer* 1995;16:680.
243. Puc H, Bajorin D, Bosl GJ, Amsterdam A, Motzer R. Phase II trial of topotecan in patients with cisplatin-refractory germ cell tumors. *Invest New Drugs* 1995;13:163.
244. Motzer RJ, Bajorin DF, Schwartz LH, et al. Phase II trial of paclitaxel shows antitumor activity in patients with previously treated germ cell tumors. *J Clin Oncol* 1994;12:2277.
245. Motzer RJ, Mazumdar M, Sheinfeld J, et al. Sequential dose-intensive paclitaxel, ifosfamide, carboplatin, and etoposide salvage therapy for germ cell tumor patients. *J Clin Oncol* 2000;18:1173.
246. Einhorn L, Stender M, Williams S. Phase II trial of gemcitabine in refractory germ cell tumors. *J Clin Oncol* 1999;17:509.
247. Bokemeyer C, Gerl A, Schöffski P, et al. Gemcitabine in patients with relapsed or cisplatin-refractory testicular cancer. *J Clin Oncol* 1999;17:512.
248. Murphy B, Breeden E, Donohue J, et al. Surgical salvage of chemorefractory germ cell tumors. *J Clin Oncol* 1993;11:324.
249. Eastman J, Wilson T, Russell C, Ahlering T, Skinner D. Surgical resection in patients with nonseminomatous germ cell tumor who fail to normalize serum tumor markers after chemotherapy. *Urology* 1994;43:3275.
250. Wood DP, Herr HW, Motzer RJ, et al. Surgical resection of solitary metastases after chemotherapy in patients with non-seminomatous germ cell tumors and elevated serum tumor markers. *Cancer* 1992;70:2354.
251. Research TIGfA. Dexamethasone, granisetron, or both for the prevention of nausea and vomiting during chemotherapy for cancer. *N Engl J Med* 1995;332:2.
252. Vogelzang NJ, Torkenson JL, Kennedy BJ. Hypomagnesemia, renal dysfunction, and Raynaud's phenomenon in patients treated with cisplatin, vinblastine, and bleomycin. *Cancer* 1985;56:2765.
253. Bosl GJ, Leitner S, Atlas S, et al. Increased plasma renin and aldosterone in patients treated with cisplatin-based chemotherapy for metastatic germ cell tumors. *J Clin Oncol* 1986;4:1684.
254. Beyer J, Rick O, Weinknecht S, et al. Nephrotoxicity after high-dose carboplatin, etoposide and ifosfamide in germ-cell tumors: incidence and implications for hematologic recovery and clinical outcome. *Bone Marrow Transplant* 1997;20:813.
255. Hansen S, Groth S, Daugaard G, Rossing N, Rorth M. Long-term effects on renal function and blood pressure of treatment with cisplatin, vinblastine, and bleomycin in patients with germ cell cancer. *J Clin Oncol* 1988;6:1728.
256. Gietema J, Sleijfer D, Willemse P, et al. Long-term follow-up of cardiovascular risk factors in patients given chemotherapy for disseminated nonseminomatous testicular cancer. *Ann Intern Med* 1992;116:709.
257. Raghavan D, Cox K, Childs A, Grygiel J, Sullivan D. Hypercholesterolemia after chemotherapy for testis cancer. *J Clin Oncol* 1992;10:1386.
258. Fossa S, Kaye S, Mead G, et al. Filgrastim during combination chemotherapy of patients with poor-prognosis metastatic germ cell malignancy. *J Clin Oncol* 1998;16:716.
259. Hansen SW, Helweg-Larsen S, Trojaborg W. Long-term neurotoxicity in patients treated with cisplatin, vinblastine, and bleomycin for metastatic germ cell cancer. *J Clin Oncol* 1989;7:1457.
260. Meinardi MT, Gietema JA, Van Der Graff WTA, et al. Cardiovasular morbidity in long-term survivors of metastatic testicular cancer. *J Clin Oncol* 2000;18:1725.
261. McKeage M, Evans B, Atkinson C, et al. Carbon monoxide diffusing capacity is a poor predictor of clinically significant bleomycin lung. *J Clin Oncol* 1990;8:779.
262. van Basten J, Hoekstra H, van Driel M, et al. Sexual dysfunction in nonseminoma testicular cancer patients is related to chemotherapy-induced angiopathy. *J Clin Oncol* 1997;15:2442.
263. Petersen PM, Skakkebaek NE, Vistisen K, Rorth M, Giwercman A. Semen quality and reproductive hormones before orchiectomy in men with testicular cancer. *J Clin Oncol* 1999;17:941.
264. Petersen PM, Giwercman A, Hansen SW, et al. Impaired testicular function in patients with carcinoma-in-situ of the testis. *J Clin Oncol* 1999;17:173.
265. Herr H, Bar-Chama N, O'Sullivan M, Sogani P. Paternity in men with stage I testis tumors on surveillance. *J Clin Oncol* 1998;16:733.
266. Howell SJ, Radford JA, Ryder WDJ, Shalet SM. Testicular function after cytotoxic chemotherapy: evidence of Leydig cell insufficiency. *J Clin Oncol* 1999;17:1493.
267. Brennemann W, Stoffel-Wagner B, Helmers A, et al. Gonadal function of patients treated with cisplatin based chemotherapy for germ cell cancer. *J Urol* 1997;158:844.
268. Stephenson W, Poirier S, Rubin L, Einhorn L. Evaluation of reproductive capacity in germ cell tumor patients following treatment with cisplatin, etoposide, and bleomycin. *J Clin Oncol* 1995;13:2278.
269. Wanderas EH, Fossa SD, Tretli S. Risk of a second germ cell cancer after treatment of a primary germ cell cancer in 2201 Norwegian male patients. *Eur J Cancer* 1997;33:244.
270. Bajorin DF, Motzer RJ, Rodriquez E, Murphy B, Bosl GJ. Acute nonlymphocytic leukemia in germ cell tumor patients treated with etoposide-containing chemotherapy. *J Natl Cancer Inst* 1993;85:60.
271. Nichols CR, Breeden ES, Loehrer PJ. Secondary leukemia associated with a conventional dose of etoposide: review of serial germ cell tumor protocols. *J Natl Cancer Inst* 1993;85:36.

272. Pedersen-Bjergaard J, Hansen ST, Larsen SO, et al. Increased risk of myelodysplasia and leukemia after etoposide, cisplatin, and bleomycin for germ-cell tumors. *Lancet* 1991;338:359.
273. Kollmannsberger C, Beyer J, Droz JP, et al. Secondary leukemia following high cumulative doses of etoposide in patients treated for advanced germ cell tumors. *J Clin Oncol* 1998;16:3386.
274. Jacobsen G, Mellemgaard A, Engelholm S, Moller H. Increased incidence of sarcoma in patients treated for testicular seminoma. *Eur J Cancer* 1993;29A:664.
275. Toner GC, Bosl GJ. Sarcoidosis, "sarcoid-like lymphadenopathy," and testicular germ cell tumors. *Am J Med* 1990;89:651.
276. Hainsworth JD, Greco FA. Poorly differentiated carcinoma and poorly differentiated adenocarcinoma of unknown primary site. *Semin Oncol* 1993;20:279.
277. Hainsworth JD, Johnson DH, Greco FA. Cisplatin-based combination chemotherapy in the treatment of poorly differentiated carcinoma and poorly differentiated adenocarcinoma of unknown primary site: results of a 12-year experience. *J Clin Oncol* 1992;10:912.
278. Motzer R, Rodriguez E, Reuter V, et al. Molecular and cytogenetic studies in the diagnosis of patients with poorly differentiated carcinomas of unknown primary site. *J Clin Oncol* 1995;13:274.
279. Thrasher J, Frazier H. Non-germ cell testicular tumors. *Probl Urol* 1994;8:167.
280. Mostofi F, Price EJ. Tumors of the male genital system. In: Hartmann W, Cowan W, eds. *Atlas of tumor pathology.* Washington: Armed Forces Institute of Pathology, 1973:85.
281. Grem J, Robins H, Wilson K, et al. Metastatic Leydig cell tumor of the testis: report of three cases and review of the literature. *Cancer* 1986;58:2116.
282. Kim I, Young R, Scully R. Leydig cell tumors of the testis: a clinicopathological analysis of 40 cases and review of the literature. *Am J Surg Pathol* 1985;9:177.
283. Schwarzman MI, Russo P, Bosl GJ, Whitmore WF. Hormone-secreting metastatic interstitial cell tumor of the testis. *J Urol* 1989;141:620.
284. Anderson G. Sclerosing Sertoli cell tumor of the testis: a distinct histological subtype. *J Urol* 1995;154:1756.
285. Proppe K, Scully R. Large-cell calcifying Sertoli cell tumor of the testis. *Am J Clin Pathol* 1980;74:607.
286. Carney J, Gordon H, Carpenter P, Shenoy B, Go V. The complex myxomas, spotty pigmentation, and endocrine overactivity. *Medicine* 1985;64:270.
287. Russo P, Brady MS, Conlon K, et al. Adult urologic sarcoma. *J Urol* 1992;147:1032.
288. Gilbaugh J, Kelalis P, Dockerty M. Epidermoid cysts of the testes. *J Urol* 1967;97:876.
289. Sussman E, Hajdu S, Kieberman P, et al. Malignant lymphoma of the testis: a clinicopathologic study of 37 cases. *J Urol* 1977;118:1004.

CHAPTER **36**

Gynecologic Cancers

SECTION **1** SETSUKO KUKI CHAMBERS

Molecular Biology of Gynecologic Cancers

ENDOMETRIAL CANCER

Although endometrial cancer, the most common gynecologic cancer, carries the best prognosis, it is important to differentiate between the classic endometrioid tumors, which tend to be estrogen-dependent and well differentiated, from other less common high-risk uterine malignancies, such as uterine papillary serous carcinomas (UPSC), clear cell carcinomas, mixed Müllerian tumors, or sarcomas, which appear to have a different biology.

MICROSATELLITE INSTABILITY

The replication error (RER+) phenotype is characteristic of cancers arising in hereditary nonpolyposis colorectal cancer (HNPCC) kindreds (a familial cancer syndrome with a high incidence of colon, endometrial, and gastric cancers, and a lower incidence of ovarian and pancreatic cancers), and also is found in approximately 20% to 25% of sporadic endometrial cancers. Microsatellite instability appears to occur at the same frequency in the acknowledged precursor of endometrial cancer, complex atypical hyperplasia, as it does in the sporadic endometrial cancer cases.[1] The RER+ phenotype per se does not appear to correlate with clinicopathologic features of the tumors or clinical outcome; thus, the hereditary form of endometrial cancer alone does not appear to portend a worse prognosis than the sporadic form. Mutation of the transforming growth factor-β (TGF-β) type II receptor gene is common in RER+ colon and gastric cancers but uncommon in RER+ endometrial cancers, even those arising in HNPCC kindreds.[2] This suggests that the genesis of RER+ tumors, even within the same familial cancer syndrome, is not the same. Although inactivation of both alleles of either hMSH2 and hMLH1 (DNA mismatch repair genes) appears to underlie microsatellite instability in tumors of HNPCC kindreds, similar to the findings in sporadic colon cancers, sporadic endometrial cancers have not been associated with mutations of any of the known human mismatch repair genes.[3] Instead, hypermethylation of the hMLH1 promoter region (which is linked to attenuation of MLH1 expression in sporadic RER+ colorectal carcinomas) was observed in 71% of sporadic RER+ endometrial cancer cases.[3] In contrast, 25% of uterine sarcomas, an entity not recognized to be part of a familial cancer syndrome, exhibit microsatellite instability that may be related to a mutation in the hMSH2 gene.[4] Microsatellite instability does not appear to be a feature of the UPSC or clear cell carcinomas.[5]

LOSS OF HETEROZYGOSITY STUDIES AND TUMOR SUPPRESSOR GENES

Unlike most other cancers studied to date, regions of sustained allelic loss in most chromosomes characterize endometrial cancer. Regions of chromosomal abnormality commonly found in this disease are listed in Table 36.1-1. Chromosome 17p is frequently involved, which contains the p53 gene known to confer a poor prognosis in endometrial cancers when mutated, and which plays an important role in the transition to carcinoma from atypical

TABLE 36.1-1. Common Regions of Chromosomal Abnormalities

Endometrial cancer	1, 3p, 8q, 10p, 10q, 13q, 17p, 18q
Epithelial ovarian cancer	1p, 1q, 3q, 4q, 5q, 6p, 6q, 7q, 8q, 9p, 10q, 11p, 13q, 17p, 17q, 18q, 19p, 20p, 20q, 22q, Xp, Xq
Cervical cancer	3p, 3q, 6p, 11q, 18q

hyperplasia. Other frequently involved regions include 3p, 10q, and 18q. The PTEN tumor suppressor gene is contained on chromosome 10q; mutations of this gene occur in complex atypical hyperplasia, as well as in one-third of endometrial cancers,[1] but it is not a common feature of UPSC.[6] Unexpectedly, in endometrial cancers, this finding mutation of PTEN tumor suppressor gene is associated with lack of overexpression of p53, as well as with early stage and improved clinical outcome.[6] Chromosome 18q contains the DCC gene, a putative tumor suppressor gene frequently mutated in colon cancers. Chromosome 18 was found to be capable of suppressing tumorigenicity of endometrial cancer cells in nude mice by the procedure of microcell fusion, with DCC expression elevated in most of the suppressed hybrids.[7]

ONCOGENES

K-ras activating point mutations in codons 12 and 13 have been implicated in the development of atypical endometrial hyperplasias and endometrioid carcinomas in Asian women, as well as in colon cancers. Studies of endometrial cancers arising in women in the United States, however, show the prevalence of such mutations to be significantly lower.[8] Notable was the almost complete absence of K-ras mutations in UPSC when compared to the usual endometrioid tumors.[8] In contrast, mutation-dependent and -independent inactivation of p53 is observed in the large majority of UPSC cases.[9]

Overexpression of HER-2/*neu* has been associated with advanced-stage, deep myometrial invasion, and poor survival in endometrial cancers in several studies. Gene amplification did not underlie all cases of HER-2/*neu* overexpression, although both gene amplification and overexpression were each associated with poor outcome.[10] When multivariate analysis was used to determine whether HER-2/*neu* was an independent prognostic factor in endometrial cancers when taking into account other molecular features such as DNA ploidy, epidermal growth factor receptor (EGFR), or p53 status, HER-2/*neu* did not achieve significance.[11] Both c-myc gene amplification and c-fms[12] overexpression also have been associated with advanced-stage and high-grade endometrial cancers.

HORMONE-RELATED MOLECULAR ABNORMALITIES

Estrogen acts as a tumor promoter for the classic endometrioid cancers, with the well- and moderately differentiated tumors containing significant levels of estrogen or progesterone receptors or both. Aromatase cytochrome P-450 is part of the complex responsible for conversion of C19 steroids to estrogen; its increased expression in endometrial cancers but not in normal endometria suggest a role in promotion of neoplastic proliferation.[13] Two different functional isoforms of both the estrogen and progesterone receptors have been described that may account for some of the tissue-specific differences in the effects of hormones and their antagonists on the breast as compared with the endometrium.

Tamoxifen, an estrogen receptor antagonist/agonist, has been associated with an increased risk of development of endometrial cancers. Although studies using murine models have been generally reassuring in regards to the safety of the selective estrogen receptor modulator, raloxifene, on the endometrium, clinical studies to date have been plagued by short follow-up. The molecular mechanisms for the antiestrogenic actions of raloxifene relate to a specific molecular perturbation at aspartate 351 of the ligand-binding domain of the estrogen receptor, on its binding to raloxifene.[14]

MOLECULES INVOLVED IN ADHESION AND INVASION

Integrin (cell adhesion molecules) expression inversely correlates with grade in endometrial cancers, with the loss of the β_1 integrin associated with lymph node metastases.[15] Variant forms of CD44 (a molecule important for cell adhesion and migration) are less frequently expressed in endometrial cancers than in normal endometria, and its absence was significantly associated with an increased propensity for lymph–vascular space invasion.[16] These data suggest that CD44 may play an important role in the function of the normal endometria, where it is strongly expressed near the basement membrane, and its loss may be related to invasion and metastasis.

OVARIAN CANCER

Most of the breakthroughs in understanding the molecular basis for ovarian cancer have been in the area of hereditary epithelial ovarian cancer syndromes, which affect 5% to 10% of ovarian cancer patients. Much work is still needed to understand the biology underlying sporadic ovarian cancers, which invariably present as advanced-stage disease and have a poor long-term outcome.

CLONALITY

In the search for the precursors of invasive epithelial ovarian cancer, molecular studies have been performed on normal ovaries; on benign, borderline, and invasive cancers; and on cancers with adjacent benign-appearing cysts. Such studies have been greatly aided by the ability to culture normal, immortalized, and transformed ovarian surface epithelial cells, as well as transformed cells originating from benign ovarian neoplasms. Evidence for a unifocal origin for these cancers appears to predominate, with bilateral ovarian cancers and metastases sharing common molecular features. Studies of microsatellite instability (which occurs in 17% of cases but appears not to be related to family history[17]) and studies of X chromosome inactivation support the clonal origin of these cancers. This is contrasted to the multifocal origin proposed for a proportion (25%) of the papillary serous carcinomas of the peritoneum; these tumors of multifocal origin are associated with germline BRCA1 (breast cancer gene) mutations.[18] Interestingly, loss of heterozygosity studies, and K-ras and p53 mutation analyses, do not demonstrate shared findings between borderline or benign neoplasms and invasive cancers, suggesting that these entities are not the precursors of invasive epithelial ovarian cancers. For instance, frequent loss of heterozygosity of a portion of Xq on the inactive X chromosome was seen in borderline tumors, but not in low-grade invasive ovarian cancers.[19] Notably, p53 mutations, which are absent in solitary borderline and benign neoplasms, are present along with allelic loss of chromosome 11p in benign-appearing cysts adjacent to the invasive cancers.[20] Similarly, common genetic alterations (such as loss of heterozygosity involving the same allele) were observed in endometrioid and clear cell ovarian carcinomas and adjacent endometriosis.[21]

BRCA1 AND BRCA2 GENES

Unlike most epithelia, division of normal ovarian surface epithelial cells gives rise to two daughter cells with equal growth potential.[22] This provides a mechanism for the involvement of tumor suppressor genes in the development of ovarian cancer, in that repeated division of these cells can unmask such recessive mutations. In addition to being a tumor suppressor gene, BRCA1 may function as a transcription factor, as well as conferring protection against DNA damage. The latter mechanism also has been proposed as a function of BRCA2. Mutations of BRCA1 (unlike BRCA2) can account for the large majority of the familial cases of breast-ovarian cancer syndrome and site-specific ovarian cancers.[23] Among breast-ovarian cancer families, there is significant evidence for heterogeneity of risk among BRCA1-mutation carriers. Assuming two BRCA1 alleles exist, one allele would confer a lifetime breast cancer risk of 62% and an ovarian cancer risk of 11%, whereas the other allele confers a 39% breast cancer risk and a 42% ovarian cancer risk by age 60 years, with the first allele representing 71% of the mutations.[24] BRCA1 mutations specifically localized to the 5' region may increase the risk for ovarian cancer in these patients.[25] BRCA2 mutations confer susceptibility to ovarian cancer with a significantly lower penetrance than for BRCA1. Compared to population-control cases, familial ovarian cancer in general, including disease associated with BRCA1 or BRCA2 mutations, are more frequently associated with advanced stage and, hence, a poorer clinical outcome.[26] Stage for stage, however, BRCA1 mutations do not appear to result in a survival difference. Serous tumors appear to be a hallmark of BRCA1 mutation–associated ovarian cancers, and germline BRCA1 mutations have been reported to occur in papillary serous carcinomas of the peritoneum with a frequency comparable to that in epithelial ovarian cancers.[27] However, no morphologic changes can differentiate normal ovaries removed prophylactically from carriers of a BRCA1 or BRCA2 mutation from ovaries removed from noncarriers; thus, identification of a premalignant lesion remains elusive.[28]

In sporadic ovarian cancer, which represents 95% of ovarian cancer cases, few mutations of BRCA1 or BRCA2 were detected, whereas frequent allelic losses that included the BRCA1 region of chromosome 17q were demonstrated (see Table 36.1-1 for regions of chromosomal abnormality commonly associated with ovarian cancer).[29] These and other data suggest the involvement of additional tumor suppressor genes in the etiology of most of the sporadic ovarian cancers, including one or two that possibly are localized distal to the BRCA1 gene. An intriguing finding is the fact that, present in the germline of patients with sporadic ovarian cancer, is a Taq1 restriction fragment length polymorphism in an intron within the sequences encoding the hormone-binding domain of the progesterone receptor gene.[30] This finding may be associated with coding region mutations of the gene and may contribute to tumorigenesis.

OTHER TUMOR SUPPRESSOR GENES

Functional wild-type p53 has been shown to be required for sensitivity to a variety of chemotherapeutic drugs and radiation, playing a crucial role in the execution of the common end pathway of apoptosis. p53 mutation of one allele predisposes the cell to the loss of wild-type p53 function, which has been shown in ovarian cancer cells to lead to the development of platinum resistance *in vitro*.[31] In ovarian cancers, p53 mutations, which are seen in 50% of advanced cases,[32] are associated with high grade and poor survival, but not with clinical chemoresistance. p53 mutations appear to arise before the onset of ovarian cancer metastasis, but are not present in the germline of patients with familial ovarian cancer phenotypes.[33] p53 has been explored as a target for gene therapy in ovarian cancer by several groups. Similarly, other proapoptotic genes, such as the BAX gene, have been the focus of gene therapy efforts at ovarian selective tumor expression.[34]

Other putative tumor suppressor genes in ovarian cancer include GPC3 (whose promoter is hypermethylated leading to gene silencing), Noey2 (ARH1, an imprinted tumor suppressor gene), OVCA1, and DOC-2, among others. The widespread loss of heterozygosity found in invasive ovarian cancers indicates that there may be several other tumor suppressor genes inactivated during tumorigenesis. The search for such genes (and likewise oncogenes) in ovarian cancer has been greatly facilitated by the advent of technologies such as complementary DNA microarray,[35] comparative genomic hybridization, differential display, and serial analysis of gene expression.

ONCOGENES AND GROWTH FACTORS

Cytokines which may act via autocrine or paracrine routes on ovarian cancer cells include EGF, TGF-β, tumor necrosis factor, interleukin-6 (IL-6), lysophosphatidic acid (LPA), heregulin, vascular endothelial growth factor (VEGF), and the macrophage colony-stimulating factor (CSF-1). Ovarian cancer cells have been shown to contain receptors for these cytokines and thus are capable of responding by phenotypic change, including growth stimulation or inhibition depending on the stimuli. Coexpression of CSF-1 and the protooncogene c-fms (which encodes for the CSF-1 receptor) in ovarian cancer metastases portends a poor outcome.[36] Other oncogenes activated in ovarian cancer include K-ras (mutated in 40% of mucinous tumors), HER-2/*neu* (which does not appear to be related to poor prognosis in ovarian cancer, unlike breast cancer), c-myc, PIK3CA [the catalytic subunit of phosphatidylinositol 3-kinase(PI3-kinase)], and AKT-2 (which is activated by several mitogenic growth factors and serves as a downstream effector of PI3-kinase). Of interest, BRCA1- or BRCA2-linked ovarian cancers do not appear to develop through mutations of K-ras or amplification of HER-2/*neu*, c-myc, or AKT-2.[37] Both tyrosine kinase growth factor receptors and protein tyrosine phosphatases (PTP) may also play an important role: overexpression of PTP1B in ovarian cancers has been correlated with the expression of the tyrosine kinase receptors EGFR, HER-2/*neu*, and c-fms.[38]

DRUG RESISTANCE

The phenomenon of platinum resistance remains the most germane for ovarian cancer patients, although with the inclusion of paclitaxel in first-line therapy, acquired classic multidrug resistance (mdr) is also a relevant mechanism. The first relationship between genomic aberrations in ovarian cancer (gains at specific loci on chromosomes 1q and 13q) and platinum resistance has been described.[39]

Augmented DNA repair at several levels appears to contribute significantly to platinum resistance. In ovarian cancers, elevated levels of ERCC-1 and XPAC, rate-limiting DNA repair genes, are found in clinically platinum-resistant tumors. However, because overexpression of ERCC-1 *in vitro* leads to increased platinum sensitivity, the relative role of the different DNA repair genes in this process remains unclear. Elevated intracellular levels of glutathione, which lead to increased intracellular detoxification of platinum, generally correlate with *in vitro* platinum resistance and have been reported to confer poor survival.[40] In platinum-resistant ovarian cancer cells, an elevated level of γ-glutamylcysteine synthetase, an enzyme that contributes to biosynthesis of glutathione, is associated with increased c-jun expression.[41] On the other hand, glutathione S-transferase (GST) levels do not consistently correlate with platinum resistance *in vitro* or *in vivo.* In ovarian cancer, two GST null genotypes have been found to be associated with lack of responsiveness to platinum or other alkylating agents and with poor survival, which is thought to be due to the contribution of the GST null phenotype to loss of p53 function.[42]

Other interactions between cytokines or oncogenes and modulation of platinum activity have been reported in ovarian cancer. IL-6 has been shown to block apoptosis induced by platinum in ovarian cancer cells.[43] The addition of antibody to HER-2/*neu* enhances chemosensitization of platinum in ovarian cancer cells.[44] Similarly, antisense down-regulation of c-raf or c-myc has been used to sensitize activity of platinum in several tumors. Anti-fas antibody-mediated apoptosis is enhanced by low-dose platinum in resistant ovarian cancers.[45]

On the other hand, overexpression of BAX is associated with chemosensitivity to platinum and paclitaxel, as well as to an improved disease-free survival rate in ovarian cancer.[46] p53 mutations result in the loss of ability of p53 to transactivate BAX in platinum-resistant ovarian cancer cells.[47] IL-1α, through inhibition of DNA repair, also sensitizes the activity of platinum in ovarian cancer cells[48]; and tumor necrosis factor, an apoptosis inducer, can ameliorate platinum resistance in ovarian cancer cells. Transfection of the cytokeratin 18 gene, which encodes an intermediate filament protein into platinum-resistant ovarian cancer cells, leads to a marked increase in platinum sensitivity.[49]

The prevalence of MDR-1 overexpression in ovarian cancer appears to depend on the sensitivity of the methodology used. There is agreement, however, that acquired mdr is clinically relevant for these patients. Mutated p53 can contribute to classic mdr because it can transcriptionally activate the MDR-1 promoter, a phenomenon that is repressed by wild-type p53. Proteins associated with the mdr phenotype and expressed in MDR-1–negative cancers are MRP (MDR-associated protein involved in glutathione conjugate transport) and LRP (lung resistance protein). LRP appears to correlate with clinical chemoresistance (remarkably, both to agents associated with classic mdr, as well as to the class of platinum/alkylating agents) among ovarian cancer patients.[50]

Aside from mdr, the other major mechanism of paclitaxel resistance involves stimulation of expression of the β-tubulin genes in the resistant ovarian cancers.[51] Antisense down-regulation of β-tubulin sensitizes these cells to paclitaxel.

MOLECULES INVOLVED IN ADHESION, MOTILITY, INVASION, ANGIOGENESIS, AND METASTASIS

The cell adhesion molecules CD44 and E-cadherin both are expressed when ovarian cancer cells are attached to peritoneal mesothelium, but such expression is lost when the cells are found in ascites fluid.[52] The β_1 integrin is also found to be an important mediator of ovarian cancer cell adhesion to peritoneal cells.[53] Urokinase-type plasminogen activator is the primary plasminogen activator found in ovarian cancer tissues and, along with the matrix metalloproteinases (in particular, MMP-2 and -9), are important to the biology of invasion and metastasis of ovarian cancer. Inhibitors of urokinase[54] have been shown to block invasive capacity of ovarian cancer cells, whereas a synthetic matrix metalloproteinase inhibitor decreases tumor burden (an effect that is even more pronounced in the presence of platinum[55]) in mice bearing human ovarian cancer xenografts. Urokinase has been shown to be inducible by CSF-1, a cytokine important to *in vivo* metastasis in ovarian cancer,[56] with CSF-1–induced invasion being mediated by urokinase activity,[54] and CSF-1–induced motility being mediated by PAI-1 activity. Urokinase-stimulated invasion is also induced by LPA, which also enhances drug resistance.[57] VEGF, a critical mediator of tumor angiogenesis, is expressed in abundant amounts in ascites and in the malignant ovary.[58] It is notable that molecules important to these related biologic phenotypes, such as E-cadherin and nm23 (associated with absence of lymph node metastasis), also may have putative tumor suppressor function, based on loss of heterozygosity studies or sequence analysis.

CERVICAL AND VULVAR CANCER

The study of the role of viruses in the carcinogenesis of lower genital tract malignancies (thought to be a field effect) has focused on cervical cancer, the third most common gynecologic cancer in the United States. Extension of those studies to vulvar cancer have led to support for two separate etiologies of vulvar cancer: one related to human papillomavirus (HPV), with epidemiologic risk factors similar to that for cervical cancer, and the other not appearing to be HPV-related.

HUMAN PAPILLOMAVIRUS

That HPV is a critical factor for cervical carcinogenesis and that the HPV E6 and E7 genes are oncogenic is clearly established. Infection of human keratinocytes by the oncogenic HPV subtypes leads to abnormalities in differentiation and growth; however, only after long-term culture of immortalized cells does an occasional clone become tumorigenic in nude mice, suggesting that HPV infection alone is not sufficient for cervical carcinogenesis. This theory is supported by data from transgenic mice studies, in which E6/E7 genes can give rise to hyperplastic and neoplastic lesions of epithelial cell types after a latent period;

however, epidermoid cervical cancers have not been noted. Cervical cancers of mesenchymal origin were noted to arise after a long latent period in some of the female progeny of transgenic mice into whom HPV-18 LCR/E6/E7 was introduced.[59] Although the majority of invasive cancers contain integrated forms of HPV, usually at fragile sites, which result in cis activation of protooncogenes such as c-myc, and the large majority of dysplasias contain episomal forms of HPV, this is not always the case. In invasive cancers, HPV-18 is always found to be integrated in the host genome, whereas HPV-16 can be found in an episomal location one-third of the time. When DNA integration occurs, it does so by preferentially disrupting the E2 open reading frame (thus the negative effect of the E2 protein on E6/E7 transcriptional activity) or in such a way that transcriptional initiation from host sequences give rise to overexpression of E6/E7. High-level transcription of E6/E7 is seen in cervical intraepithelial neoplasia grade 3 (CIN 3) and invasive cancers when compared to CIN 1 and CIN 2. On immortalization of normal cells, E7 appears to be responsible for chromosomal instability and aneuploidy, whereas E6 may have a promoting effect by inhibition of DNA repair through interfering with wild-type p53 function. When inoculated in nude mice, those clones that are not tumorigenic display low-level E6/E7 transcription, whereas those which are tumorigenic continue to express high levels of E6/E7.

HUMAN PAPILLOMAVIRUS E6/E7 GENES

On binding with the retinoblastoma (Rb) protein, E7, a potent viral oncoprotein that cooperates with activated ras in transforming assays, frees key cell-cycle proteins from Rb-imposed negative transcriptional regulation. Whereas for the high-risk HPV subtypes 16/18, E7/Rb binding is five- to tenfold more efficient than for HPV 6/11, mutations that affect E7 binding to Rb do not interfere with the capacity to confer immortalization. Similarly, mutations that interfere with E7's transforming properties do not appear to affect Rb binding; thus, the picture is complex.

Likewise, the mechanism for E6 promotion of oncogenesis is not clear. E6 promotes ubiquitin binding to p53, which tags such cells for degradation; thus, on DNA damage, the normal cellular response of induction of wild-type p53 is not seen in HPV-infected cells. Experimental evidence suggests that a p53 polymorphism with arginine at codon 72 is more susceptible to E6-induced degradation *in vivo* than with proline at that site.[60] However, the observation that individuals homozygous for the arginine-encoding allele may be more susceptible to HPV-associated squamous cell cancers than heterozygotes[60] has not been confirmed by larger studies.[61] The suggestion has been made that, instead, this p53 polymorphism may predispose to the development of cervical adenocarcinomas in Asians.[62] Although E6 binds to p53 protein in HPV 16/18 subtypes (not in HPV 6/11), no such correlation is seen *in vivo* between low p53 expression and E6 overexpression. Furthermore, there is evidence that endogenous p53 protein in HPV-infected cancer cells is competent to activate a downstream target gene, despite coexpression of the viral E6 protein.[63]

The development of HPV vaccines has been an intense focus of investigation. Prophylactic HPV vaccine strategies have used noninfective, non–viral DNA-containing, antigenic papilloma virus–like particles. Development of therapeutic HPV vaccines has been somewhat more problematic in that sustained cellular immunity against oncogenic E6 or E7 proteins has been difficult to achieve. New approaches include the use of autologous dendritic cells pulsed with HPV-specific tumor antigens, such as E7, to stimulate tumor-specific cytotoxic T lymphocytes (CTLs).[64] Dendritic cells are thought to be effective stimulators not only to produce and maintain primary CTLs, but also to stimulate established CTL lines.

MOLECULAR COFACTORS IMPORTANT TO CERVICAL CARCINOGENESIS

Because HPV infection is not sufficient for cervical carcinogenesis, attention has focused on molecular cofactors important to this process, such as co-infection by herpes simplex virus 2, and the presence of activated Ha-ras; the latter results in rearrangements and amplifications of the HPV-16 sequence. Many positive and negative transcriptional regulators of E6/E7 transcription have been identified. The presence of the glucocorticoid response element 5' of the HPV genome probably underlies the clinical progression of HPV infection seen in pregnancy. Although retinoic acid represses HPV transcription in normal and malignant cells, its induction of retinoic acid receptor beta is restricted to normal cells. Both the retinoic acid receptor beta gene and a locus on chromosome 11q23 may have tumor-suppressive properties in squamous cell cancers. Loss of heterozygosity studies demonstrate allelic loss of many chromosomes, including 11q, but most frequently involving 3p, 6p, and 18q (see Table 36.1-1).[65]

The immune response is likely to be key in determining malignant transformation of HPV-infected cervical epithelium. The consequences of human immunodeficiency virus (HIV) infection include a dramatic increase in the risk for cervical dysplasia and invasive cancer, the degree of which correlates with the level of immunosuppression. Loss of expression of HLA class I alleles, along with interference with the transporter associated with antigen presentation in cervical cancers, is common; such changes may influence specific immunogenic presentation by tumors.[66] In addition, the finding of certain HLA class II haplotypes in the cancer (when compared to cervical DNA from controls), which may influence the immune response to specific HPV-encoded epitopes, may contribute to the development of cervical neoplasia.[67] In fact, the HLA DQB1 locus shows evidence for allelic association with invasive cervical cancer in HPV-positive patients.[68] This genotype thus appears to increase the risk for development of cervical cancer in these patients. Similar findings are seen when HLA class II haplotypes in CIN were compared to controls; the HLA DQB1 haplotype was significantly more highly associated with CIN.[69]

In general, more than 90% of squamous cell cervical cancers contain HPV DNA, and only rarely are p53 mutations seen. Nuclear c-myb expression is correlated with the presence of HPV; c-myb can transactivate the HPV-16 promoter,[70] as it can transactivate HIV-1 and c-myc. In most studies, HPV status was not a strong independent prognosticator of outcome in cervical cancer patients[71]; however, there appears to be a trend for HPV-negative tumors to do worse. Among HPV-negative cancers, p53 mutations appear to be more common, although HPV-negative cancers that do not contain p53 mutations exist. The latter also do not contain MDM2 gene (capable of binding to p53) amplifications.[72] Among HPV-negative tumors, c-myc overexpression has been associated with an increased risk of metastasis in early-stage disease.

MOLECULAR ABNORMALITIES IN CERVICAL ADENOCARCINOMAS

The presence of both HPV-16 and -18 has been demonstrated in cervical adenocarcinomas, with HPV-18 predominating in cervical adenocarcinoma cell lines. p53 mutations in this disease are associated with advanced-stage and high-grade cases, whereas those tumors containing HPV DNA tend to be of an early stage and low grade. Overexpression of HER-2/*neu* is seen in 25% of cervical adenocarcinomas, which is strongly associated with advanced stage. Reduced expression of nm23 and overexpression of HER-2/*neu* may relate to poor prognosis in these tumors.[73] Molecular findings in cervical adenocarcinomas appear to differ from those seen in adenocarcinomas arising in the endometrium, which do not contain HPV DNA. The frequency of K-ras mutations and the pattern of p53 mutations differ between the two groups[74]; K-ras mutations appear to be an infrequent event in cervical cancers in most studies, which is in contrast to endometrial adenocarcinomas.

NON–HUMAN PAPILLOMAVIRUS-RELATED MOLECULAR ABNORMALITIES IN CERVICAL CANCERS

Expression of cell-cycle genes, such as bcl-1 and bcl-2, have been studied in cervical cancer. Bcl-1 (cyclin D1) is capable of binding to the Rb protein and is overexpressed or amplified in the majority of cervical and vulvar cancer cell lines[75]; its level of expression is elevated by activated c-fms. Overexpression of bcl-2, which protects against apoptosis and differentiation, was not found to relate to HPV status but was more likely to be seen in CIN 3 rather than low-grade dysplasias. Thus, its expression may be an early event important to malignant transformation.[76] *In vitro*, increased bcl-2 expression is noted in cervical cancer cell lines which contain an inactive p53.[77] *In vivo*, overexpression of bcl-2 is strongly correlated with radioresistance,[78] and on multivariate analysis, poor outcome.[79] Overexpression of EGFR also is found to be an independent predictor for poor prognosis in cervical cancer.[80]

Proteinases capable of degrading extracellular matrix may underlie the propensity of cervical cancer to invade adjacent tissues. Both the expression[81] and activity of metalloproteinases have been described in cervical cancers, with more activity seen in this disease than in ovarian or endometrial cancers.[82] Expression of MMP-2 is correlated with that of TIMP-2 in cervical cancer cells, and their coexpression is associated with advanced stage and poor survival.[83] The opposite finding is seen for expression of TIMP-1, a specific inhibitor of the matrix metalloproteinases. In fact, the ratio of matrix metalloproteinases to TIMP-1 is increased in those cervical cancers and their surrounding stroma that have a poor prognosis.[81] Furthermore, morphologic and immunohistochemical markers of angiogenesis correlate with poor outcome in cervical cancer.[84] Many cervical cancers secrete significant levels of VEGF, the adenocarcinomas in particular.[85]

MOLECULAR ABNORMALITIES IN VULVAR CANCERS

Molecular studies support two etiologies of vulvar cancer: (1) vulvar intraepithelial neoplasia grade 3 associated with basaloid and warty carcinomas, the majority of which appear to be associated with the presence of HPV and epidemiologic risk factors similar to that seen for cervical cancer, such as smoking and herpes simplex virus 2 infection; and (2) keratinizing squamous cell carcinomas, which contain little HPV DNA.[86] Thus, HPV is detected less often in vulvar cancers (approximately one-half of the cases contain HPV-16 or -18) than in cervical cancers, with those being HPV-positive having a better prognosis.[87] Similar to cervical cancers, there is higher prevalence of p53 mutations in HPV-negative vulvar cancers when compared to HPV-positive tumors,[88] and p53 overexpression in vulvar cancers appears to relate to poor overall survival.[89] Vulvar squamous cell carcinomas exhibit a broad range of allelic losses, irrespective of HPV status.[90] Furthermore, the divergent patterns of loss of heterozygosity observed suggest that only some, but not most, genetic alterations in adjacent vulvar epithelium or vulvar intraepithelial neoplasia are related to the invasive cancers.[91]

REFERENCES

1. Yoshinaga K, Sasano H, Furukawa T, et al. The PTEN, BAX, and IGFRII genes are mutated in endometrial atypical hyperplasia. *Jpn J Cancer Res* 1998;89:985.
2. Myeroff LL, Parsons R, Kim SJ, et al. A transforming growth factor β receptor type II gene mutation common in colon and gastric but rare in endometrial cancers with microsatellite instability. *Cancer Res* 1995;55:5545.
3. Gurin CC, Federici MG, Kang L, Boyd J. Causes and consequences of microsatellite instability in endometrial carcinoma. *Cancer Res* 1999;59:462.
4. Risinger JI, Umar A, Boyer JC, et al. Microsatellite instability in gynecological sarcomas and in hMSH2 mutant uterine sarcoma cell lines defective in mismatch repair activity. *Cancer Res* 1995;55:5664.
5. Berchuck A, Maxwell GL, Risinger JI, et al. Mutation of the PTEN and beta-catenin genes and microsatellite instability are characteristic of endometrioid endometrial cancers. *Int J Gynecol Cancer* 1999;9[suppl 1]:78.
6. Risinger JI, Hayes K, Maxwell GL, et al. PTEN mutation in endometrial cancers is associated with favorable clinical and pathologic characteristics. *Clin Cancer Res* 1998;4:3005.
7. Yamada H, Sasaki M, Honda T, et al. Suppression of endometrial carcinoma cell tumorigenicity by human chromosome 18. *Genes Chromosomes Cancer* 1995;13:18.
8. Caduff RF, Johnston CM, Frank TS. Mutations of the Ki-ras oncogene in carcinoma of the endometrium. *Am J Pathol* 1995;146:182.
9. Kovalev S, Marchenko ND, Gugliotta BG, et al. Loss of p53 function in uterine papillary serous carcinoma. *Human Pathol* 1998;29:613.
10. Saffari B, Jones LA, El-Naggar A, et al. Amplification and overexpression of HER-2/neu (c-erbB2) in endometrial cancers: correlation with overall survival. *Cancer Res* 1995;55:5693.
11. Lukes AS, Kohler MF, Pieper CF, et al. Multivariate analysis of DNA ploidy, p53, and HER-2/neu as prognostic factors in endometrial cancer. *Cancer* 1994;73:2380.
12. Kacinski BM, Carter D, Mittal K, et al. High level expression of fms proto-oncogene mRNA is observed in clinically aggressive human endometrial adenocarcinomas. *Int J Radiat Oncol Biol Phys* 1988;15:823.
13. Bulun SE, Economos K, Miller D, Simpson ER. CYP19 (aromatase cytochrome P450) gene expression in human malignant endometrial tumors. *J Clin Endocrinol Metab* 1994:79:1831.
14. Levenson AS, Jordan VC. The key to the antiestrogenic mechanism of raloxifene is amino acid 351 (aspartate) in the estrogen receptor. *Cancer Res* 1998;58:1872.
15. Lessey BA, Albelda S, Buck CA, et al. Distribution of integrin cell adhesion molecules in endometrial cancer. *Am J Pathol* 1995;146:717.
16. Fujita N, Yaegashi N, Ide Y, et al. Expression of CD44 in normal human versus tumor endometrial tissues: possible implication of reduced expression of CD44 in lymph-vascular space involvement of cancer cells. *Cancer Res* 1994;54:3922.
17. King BL, Carcangiu ML, Carter D, et al. Microsatellite instability in ovarian neoplasms. *Br J Cancer* 1995;72:376.
18. Schorge JO, Muto MG, Welch WR, et al. Molecular evidence for multifocal papillary serous carcinoma of the peritoneum in patients with germline BRCA1 mutations. *J Natl Cancer Inst* 1998;90:797.
19. Cheng PC, Gosewehr JA, Kim TM, et al. Potential role of the inactivated X chromosome in ovarian epithelial tumor development. *J Natl Cancer Inst* 1996;88:510.
20. Zheng J, Benedict WF, Xu HJ, et al. Genetic disparity between morphologically benign cyst contiguous to ovarian carcinomas and solitary cystadenomas. *J Natl Cancer Inst* 1995;87:1146.
21. Jiang X, Morland SJ, Hitchcock A, Thomans EJ, Campbell IG. Allelotyping of endometriosis with adjacent ovarian carcinoma reveals evidence of a common lineage. *Cancer Res* 1998;58:1707.
22. Godwin AK, Testa JR, Hamilton TC. The biology of ovarian cancer development. *Cancer* 1993;71:530.
23. Gayther SA, Russell P, Harrington P, et al. The contribution of germline BRCA1 and BRCA2 mutations to familial ovarian cancer: no evidence for other ovarian cancer-susceptibility genes. *Am J Hum Genet* 1999;65:1021.
24. Easton DF, Ford D, Bishop DT, and the Breast Cancer Linkage Consortium. Breast and ovarian cancer incidence in BRCA1-mutation carriers. *Am J Hum Genet* 1995;56:265.

25. Shattuck-Eidens D, McClure M, Simard J, et al. A collaborative survey of 80 mutations in the BRCA1 breast and ovarian cancer susceptibility gene: implications for presymptomatic testing and screening. *JAMA* 1995;273:535.
26. Pharoah PDP, Easton DF, Stockton DL, et al. Survival in familial, BRCA1-associated, and BRCA2-associated epithelial ovarian cancer. *Cancer Res* 1999;59:868.
27. Bandera CA, Muto MG, Schorge JO, et al. BRCA1 gene mutations in women with papillary serous carcinoma of the peritoneum. *Obstet Gynecol* 1998;92:596.
28. Stratton JF, Buckley CH, Lowe D, Ponder BA. Comparison of prophylactic oophorectomy specimens from carriers and noncarriers of a BRCA1 or BRCA2 gene mutation. *J Natl Cancer Inst* 1999;91:626.
29. Takahashi H, Behbakht K, McGovern PE, et al. Mutation analysis of the BRCA1 gene in ovarian cancers. *Cancer Res* 1995;55:2998.
30. McKenna NJ, Kieback DG, Carney DN, et al. A germline Taq1 restriction fragment length polymorphism in the progesterone receptor gene in ovarian carcinoma. *Br J Cancer* 1995; 71:451.
31. Brown R, Clugston C, Burns P, et al. Increased accumulation of p53 protein in cisplatin-resistant ovarian cell lines. *Int J Cancer* 1993;55:678.
32. Berchuk A, Kohler MF, Marks JR, et al. The p53 tumor suppressor gene frequently is altered in gynecologic cancers. *Am J Obstet Gynecol* 1994;170:246.
33. Buller RE, Skilling JS, Kaliszewski S, Neimann T, Anderson B. Absence of significant germ line p53 mutations in ovarian cancer patients. *Gynecol Oncol* 1995;58:368.
34. Tai YT, Strobel T, Kufe D, Cannistra SA. *In vivo* cytotoxicity of ovarian cancer cells through tumor-selective expression of the BAX gene. *Cancer Res* 1999;59:2121.
35. Wang K, Gan L, Jeffery E, et al. Monitoring gene expression profile changes in ovarian carcinomas using cDNA microarray. *Gene* 1999;229:101.
36. Rhei E, Bogomolniy F, Federici MG, et al. Molecular genetic characterization of BRCA1- and BRCA2-linked hereditary ovarian cancers. *Cancer Res* 1998;58:3193.
37. Chambers SK, Kacinski BM, Ivins CM, Carcangiu ML. Overexpression of epithelial CSF-1 and CSF-1 receptor: a poor prognostic factor in epithelial ovarian cancer; contrasted with a positive effect of stromal CSF-1. *Clin Cancer Res* 1997;3:999.
38. Weiner JR, Hurteau JA, Kerns BJM, et al. Overexpression of the tyrosine phosphatase PTP1B is associated with human ovarian carcinomas. *Am J Obstet Gynecol* 1994;170:1177.
39. Kudoh K, Takano M, Koshikawa T, et al. Gains of 1q21-q22 and 13q12-q14 are potential indicators for resistance to cisplatin-based chemotherapy in ovarian cancer patients. *Clin Cancer Res* 1999;5:2526.
40. Tanner B, Hengstler JG, Dietrich B, et al. Glutathione, glutathione S-transferase A and aldehyde dehydrogenase content in relationship to drug resistance in ovarian cancer. *Gynecol Oncol* 1997;65:54.
41. Yao KS, Godwin AK, Johnson SW, et al. Evidence for altered regulation of γ-glutamylcysteine synthetase gene expression among cisplatin-sensitive and cisplatin-resistant human ovarian cancer cell lines. *Cancer Res* 1995:55:4367.
42. Howells REJ, Redman CWE, Dhar KK, et al. Association of glutathione S-transferase GSTM1 and GSTT1 null genotypes with clinical outcome in epithelial ovarian cancer. *Clin Cancer Res* 1998;4:2439.
43. Ishioka S, van Haaften-Day C, Sagae S, Kudo R, Hacker NF. Interleukin-6 (IL-6) does not change the expression of Bcl-2 protein in the prevention of cisplatin-induced apoptosis in ovarian cancer cell lines. *J Obstet Gynaecol Res* 1999;25:23.
44. Langton-Webster BC, Xuan JA, Brink JR, Salomon DS. Development of resistance to cisplatin is associated with decreased expression of the gp185$^{c\text{-}erbB\text{-}2}$ protein and alterations in growth properties and responses to therapy in an ovarian tumor cell line. *Cell Growth Differ* 1994;5:1367.
45. Uslu R, Jewett A, Bonavida B. Sensitization of human ovarian tumor cells by subtoxic CDDP to anti-fas antibody-mediated cytotoxicity and apoptosis. *Gynecol Oncol* 1996;62:282.
46. Tai YT, Lee S, Niloff E, Weisman C, Strobel T, Cannistra SA. Bax protein expression and clinical outcome in epithelial ovarian cancer. *J Clin Oncol* 1998;16:2583.
47. Perego P, Giarola M, Righetti SC, et al. Association between cisplatin resistance and mutation of p53 gene and reduced bax expression in ovarian carcinoma cell systems. *Cancer Res* 1996;56:556.
48. Benchekroun MN, Parker R, Dabholkar M, Reed E, Sinha BK. Effects of interleukin-1 alpha on DNA repair in human ovarian carcinoma (NIH:OVCAR-3) cells: implications in the mechanism of sensitization of cis-diamminedichloroplatinum(II). *Mol Pharmacol* 1995;47:1255.
49. Parekh HK, Simpkins H. The differential expression of cytokeratin 18 in cisplatin-sensitive and -resistant human ovarian adenocarcinoma cells and its association with drug sensitivity. *Cancer Res* 1995;55:5203.
50. Izquierdo MA, Scheffer GL, Flens MJ, et al. Major vault protein LRP-related multidrug resistance. *Eur J Cancer* 1996;32A:979.
51. Kavallaris M, Kuo DYS, Burkhart CA, et al. Taxol-resistant epithelial ovarian tumors are associated with altered expression of specific beta-tubulin isotypes. *J Clin Invest* 1997;100:1282.
52. Cannistra SA, Kansas GS, Niloff J, et al. Binding of ovarian cancer cells to peritoneal mesothelium *in vitro* is partly mediated by CD44H. *Cancer Res* 1993;53:3830.
53. Lessan K, Aguiar DJ, Oegema T, Siebenson L, Skubitz AP. CD44 and beta 1 integrin mediate ovarian carcinoma cell adhesion to peritoneal mesothelial cells. *Am J Pathol* 1999;154:1525.
54. Chambers SK, Wang Y, Gertz RE, Kacinski BM. Macrophage colony stimulating factor mediates invasion of ovarian cancer cells through urokinase. *Cancer Res* 1995;55:1578.
55. Giavazzi R, Garofalo A, Ferri C, et al. Batimastat, a synthetic inhibitor of matrix metalloproteinases, potentiates the antitumor activity of cisplatin in ovarian carcinoma xenografts. *Clin Cancer Res* 1998;4:985.
56. Folk NL, Azodi M, Ivins CM, et al. Enhanced ovarian cancer metastasis by the macrophage colony stimulating factor (CSF-1). 2000 (*submitted*).
57. Xu Y, Gaudette DC, Boynton JD, et al. Characterization of an ovarian cancer activating factor in ascites from ovarian cancer patients. *Clin Cancer Res* 1995;1:1223.
58. Sowter HM, Corps AN, Evans AL, et al. Expression and localization of the vascular endothelial growth factor family in ovarian epithelial tumors. *Lab Invest* 1997;77:607.
59. Comerford SA, Maika SD, Laimins LA, et al. E6 and E7 expression from the HPV 18 LCR: development of genital hyperplasia and neoplasia in transgenic mice. *Oncogene* 1995;10:587.
60. Storey A, Thomas M, Kalita A, et al. Role of a p53 polymorphism in the development of human papillomavirus-associated cancer. *Nature* 1998;393:229.
61. Sonoda Y, Saigo PE, Boyd J. p53 and genetic susceptibility to cervical cancer. *J Natl Cancer Inst* 1999;9:557.
62. Yang YC, Chang CL, Chen ML. Effect of p53 polymorphism on susceptibility of cervical cancer in Taiwan. *Int J Gynecol Cancer* 1999;9:104(abst).
63. Butz K, Whitaker N, Denk C, et al. Induction of the p53-target gene GADD45 in HPV-positive cancer cells. *Oncogene* 1999;18:2381.
64. Santin AD, Hermonat PL, Ravaggi A, et al. Induction of human papillomavirus-specific CD4(+) and CD8(+) lymphocytes by E7-pulsed autologous dendritic cells in patients with human papillomavirus type 16- and 18-positive cervical cancer. *J Virol* 1999;73:5402.
65. Mullokandov MR, Kholodilov NG, Atkin NB, et al. Genomic alterations in cervical carcinoma: losses of chromosome heterozygosity and human papilloma virus tumor status. *Cancer Res* 1996;56:197.
66. Keating PJ, Cromme FV, Duggan-Keen M, et al. Frequency of down-regulation of individual HLA-A and -B alleles in cervical carcinomas in relation to TAP-1 expression. *Br J Cancer* 1995:72:405.
67. Apple RJ, Erlich HA, Klitz W, et al. HLA DR-DQ associations with cervical carcinoma show papillomavirus-type specificity. *Nat Genet* 1994;6:157.
68. Neuman RJ, Huettner PC, Lina LI, et al. Association between DQB1 and cervical cancer in patients with human papillomavirus and family controls. *Obstet Gynecol* 2000;95:134.
69. Odunsi K, Terry G, Ho L, Cuzick J, Ganesan TS. Susceptibility to human papillomavirus-associated cervical intra-epithelial neoplasia is determined by specific HLA DR-DQ alleles. *Int J Cancer* 1996;67:595.
70. Nurnberg W, Artuc M, Nawrath M, et al. Human c-myb is expressed in cervical carcinomas and transactivate the HPV-16 promoter. *Cancer Res* 1995;55:4432.
71. Ikenberg H, Sauerbrei W, Schottmuller U, Spitz C, Pfleiderer A. Human papillomavirus DNA in cervical carcinoma—correlation with clinical data and influence on prognosis. *Int J Cancer* 1994;59:322.
72. Miwa K, Miyamoto S, Kato H, et al. The role of p53 inactivation in human cervical cell carcinoma development. *Oncogene* 1995;10:219.
73. Mandal M, Konishi I, Koshiyama M, et al. Altered expression of nm23-H1 and c-erbB-2 proteins have prognostic significance in adenocarcinoma but not in squamous cell carcinoma of the uterine cervix. *Cancer* 1995;75:2523.
74. Jiko K, Tsuda H, Sato S, Hirohashi S. Pathogenic significance of p53 and c-Ki-ras gene mutations and human papillomavirus DNA integration in adenocarcinoma of the uterine cervix and uterine isthmus. *Int J Cancer* 1994;59:601.
75. Kurzrock R, Ku S, Talpaz M. Abnormalities in the PRAD1 (CYCLIN D1/BCL-1) oncogene are frequent in cervical and vulvar squamous cell carcinoma cell lines. *Cancer* 1995;75:584.
76. Saegusa M, Takano Y, Hashimura M, Shoji Y, Okayasu I. The possible role of bcl-2 expression in the progression of tumors of the uterine cervix. *Cancer* 1995;76:2297.
77. Liang XH, Mungal S, Ayscue A, et al. Bcl-2 protooncogene expression in cervical carcinoma cell lines containing inactive p53. *J Cell Biochem* 1995;57:509.
78. Pillai MR, Jayaprakash PG, Nair MK. Bcl-2 immunoreactivity but not p53 accumulation associated with tumour response to radiotherapy in cervical carcinoma. *J Cancer Res Clin Oncol* 1999;125:55.
79. Tjalma W, DeCuyper E, Weyler J, et al. Expression of bcl-2 in invasive and *in situ* carcinoma of the uterine cervix. *Am J Obstet Gynecol* 1998;178:113.
80. Kersemaekers AM, Fleuren GJ, Kenter GG, et al. Oncogene alterations in carcinomas of the uterine cervix: overexpression of the epidermal growth factor receptor is associated with poor prognosis. *Clin Cancer Res* 1999;5:577.
81. Nuovo GJ, MacConnell PB, Simsir A, Valea F, French DL. Correlation of the *in situ* detection of polymerase chain reaction–amplified metalloproteinase complementary DNAs and their inhibitors with prognosis in cervical carcinoma. *Cancer Res* 1995;55:267.
82. Tamakoshi K, Kikawa F, Nawa A, et al. Characterization of extracellular matrix–degrading proteinase and its inhibitor in gynecologic cancer tissues with clinically different metastatic form. *Cancer* 1995;76:2565.
83. Davidson B, Goldberg I, Kopolovic J, et al. MMP-2 and TIMP-2 expression correlates with poor prognosis in cervical carcinoma—a clinicopathologic study using immunohistochemistry and mRNA *in situ* hybridization. *Gynecol Oncol* 1999;73:372.
84. Tjalma W, Van Marck E, Weyler J, et al. Quantification and prognostic relevance of angiogenic parameters in invasive cervical cancer. *Br J Cancer* 1998;78:170.
85. Santin AD, Hermonat PL, Ravaggi A, et al. Secretion of vascular endothelial growth factor in adenocarcinoma and squamous carcinoma of the uterine cervix. *Obstet Gynecol* 1999;94:78.
86. Trimble CL, Hildesheim A, Brinton LA, Shah KV, Kurman RJ. Heterogeneous etiology of squamous carcinoma of the vulva. *Obstet Gynecol* 1996;87:59.
87. Ansink AC, Krul MRL, DeWeger RA, et al. Human papillomavirus, lichen sclerosus, and squamous cell carcinoma of the vulva: detection and prognostic significance. *Gynecol Oncol* 1994;52:180.
88. Lee YY, Wilczynski SP, Chumakov A, Chih D, Koeffler HP. Carcinoma of the vulva: HPV and p53 mutations. *Oncogene* 1994;9:1655.
89. Kohlberger P, Kainz C, Breitenecker G, et al. Prognostic significance of immunohistochemically detected p53 expression in vulvar carcinoma. *Cancer* 1995;76:1786.
90. Pinto AP, Lin MC, Mutter GL, et al. Allelic loss in human papillomavirus–positive and –negative vulvar squamous cell carcinomas. *Am J Pathol* 1999;154:1009.
91. Lin MC, Mutter GL, Trivijsilp P, et al. Patterns of allelic loss (LOH) in vulvar squamous carcinomas and adjacent noninvasive epithelia. *Am J Pathol* 1998;152:1313.

PATRICIA J. EIFEL
JONATHAN S. BEREK
JAMES T. THIGPEN

SECTION **2**

Cancer of the Cervix, Vagina, and Vulva

CARCINOMA OF THE CERVIX

EPIDEMIOLOGY

The American Cancer Society estimated that 12,800 new cases of invasive cervical cancer would be diagnosed in the United States in 1999.[1] During the same year, 4800 patients were expected to die of cervical cancer; this represents approximately 1.8% of all cancer deaths in women and 18% of deaths from gynecologic cancers. However, for women aged 20 to 39 years, cervical cancer remains the second leading cause of cancer deaths after breast cancer.[1] In the United States, age-adjusted death rates from cervical cancer have declined steadily since statistics on the disease were first collected in the 1930s. Although this improvement is primarily because of the adoption of routine screening programs including pelvic examinations and cervical cytologic evaluation, the death rates from cervical cancer had begun to decrease before the implementation of Papanicolaou (Pap) screening, suggesting that other unknown factors may have played some role.[2,3]

Squamous cell carcinoma of the cervix and its intraepithelial precursor follow a pattern typical of sexually transmitted disease. The risk of cervical cancer is increased in prostitutes and in women who have first coitus at a young age, have multiple sexual partners, have sexually transmitted diseases, or bear children at a young age. Promiscuous sexual behavior in male partners is also a risk factor.[4,5] Other factors that may be associated with cervical cancer include cigarette smoking, immunodeficiency, vitamin A or C deficiency, and oral contraceptive use.[6] In the United States, the incidence of cervical cancer is greatest in American Indian, African American, Vietnamese, and Hispanic women.[7–9]

International incidences of cervical cancer tend to reflect differences in cultural attitudes toward sexual promiscuity and the penetration of mass screening programs. Some of the lowest incidences are in the United States, China, North Africa, and the Middle East, where estimated crude rates of cervical cancer are less than 10 per 100,000.[10] However, cervical cancer continues to be the leading cause of cancer deaths for women in many developing countries. Incidences are particularly high in Latin America, Southern and Eastern Africa, India, and Polynesia.[10,11] In the United States, Hispanic women have approximately twice the incidence and Vietnamese women approximately five times the incidence of white women.[12] The incidence is also higher in African Americans than in whites, although this difference has been steadily decreasing, particularly for women less than 50 years old.

A number of studies suggest that the incidence of cervical adenocarcinoma has been increasing, particularly among women in their 20s and 30s.[13–15] Several investigators have reported a correlation between cervical adenocarcinoma and prolonged oral contraceptive use.[16,17] However, the likelihood of a causative relationship is less certain because of the many potential confounding risk factors.[18]

Molecular and epidemiologic studies have demonstrated a strong relationship between human papillomavirus (HPV), cervical intraepithelial neoplasia (CIN), and invasive carcinomas of the cervix.[19,20] HPV DNA has been identified in more than 95% of cervical carcinomas[21]; HPV DNA transcripts and protein products have also been identified in invasive cervical carcinomas.[22–24] In high-grade CIN and invasive carcinoma, papillomavirus DNA is typically integrated into the human genome rather than remaining in an intact viral capsid.[25] It has been theorized that integration of HPV DNA in the human genome, possibly at the E2 site, causes persistent transcription of the E6 and E7 genes. Functional inactivation of p53 by E6 protein or of Rb by E7 protein disrupts normal cell-cycle control mechanisms.[26–28] As the sensitivity and specificity of tests for HPV DNA have improved, it has become increasingly apparent that most of the covariables that have historically been associated with an increased risk of cervical cancer (e.g., age at first coitus, number of partners, socioeconomic status, and so forth) are surrogates for HPV infection.[29,30] Investigators have suggested a number of cofactors that may contribute to disease progression. However, in more recent epidemiologic studies, cigarette smoking was the only consistent independent contributor to the risk of cervical cancer development after controlling for HPV infection.[30] Taken together, the molecular and epidemiologic data provide compelling evidence that HPV infection plays a central causative role in the development of cervical neoplasia.[29–31]

More than 100 HPV subtypes have been identified, and many of these have now been isolated, sequenced, and cloned.[32,33] Approximately 25 subtypes are tropic to the genital tract mucosa. Types 6 and 11 usually cause benign genital warts (condyloma acuminata) but are occasionally associated with invasive cervical lesions. Types 16, 18, 31, 35, and 39 are commonly associated with high-grade CIN and invasive cervical cancer (Table 36.2-1).[34] HPV 18 has been associated with poorly differentiated carcinomas, an increased incidence of lymph node involvement, a poor response to treatment, and a high rate of disease recurrence, whereas HPV 16 has been associated with large cell keratinizing tumors and a lower recurrence rate.[35–37] Although the overall prevalence of HPV DNA is similar between countries, significant variation has been found in the prevalence of some less common HPV types; for example, HPV 45 is most common in western Africa, whereas HPV 39 and HPV 59 are rarely found outside Central and South America.[21] The strong correlation between high-risk HPV subtypes and carcinoma has led to the suggestion that HPV detection and typing be incorporated into mass screening programs[38,39] and has encouraged efforts to develop a prophylactic HPV vaccine.[40]

In 1993 the Centers for Disease Control and Prevention added cervical cancer to the list of acquired immunodeficiency syndrome–defining neoplasms.[41] However, the impact of acquired immunodeficiency syndrome and human immunodeficiency virus (HIV) on the incidence and virulence of cervical cancer remains uncertain.[42–46] Although several studies suggest that the incidence of CIN is higher in HIV-positive women than in the general population,[47,48] overlap in risk factors for the two diseases may influence these results. Although Serraino et al.[46] reported a possible increase in the risk of invasive cervical cancer in European HIV-positive women, several studies in Africa[42] and a large epidemiologic study in the United States[44] have failed to

TABLE 36.2-1. Relationship between Human Papillomavirus Type and Cervical Pathology

	Cervical Diagnosis				
Viral Type	Normal Mild Atypia	Low-Grade Squamous Invasive Lesion	High-Grade Squamous Invasive Lesion	Cancer	*Total*
HPV negative	1671 (91.0%)	115 (30.5%)	33 (12.6%)	16 (10.5%)	1835 (69.8%)
HPV 6, 11, 42, 43, 44, two unclassified types	80 (4.4%)	111 (29.4%)	26 (10.0%)	8 (5.2%)	225 (8.6%)
HPV 16, 18, 31, 33, 35, 45, 51, 52, 56, 58	85 (4.6%)	151 (40.1%)	202 (77.4%)	129 (84.3%)	567 (21.6%)
Total	1836 (100%)	377 (100%)	261 (100%)	153 (100%)	2627 (100%)

HPV, human papillomavirus.
(Modified from Loricez AL, Reid R, Jenson AB, et al. Human papillomavirus infection of the cervix: relative risk associations of 15 common anogenital types. *Obstet Gynecol* 1992;79:328.)

reveal any significant linkage. However, changes in cell-mediated immunity may play a role in the development of cervical cancer,[48–50] and some investigators[43,51,52] have suggested that cervical cancer is a more aggressive disease in immunosuppressed patients. For these reasons, regular surveillance with Pap smears, pelvic examination, and colposcopy (when indicated) should be part of the routine care of HIV-positive women.

NATURAL HISTORY AND PATTERN OF SPREAD

Most cervical carcinomas arise at the junction between the primarily columnar epithelium of the endocervix and the squamous epithelium of the ectocervix. This junction is a site of continuous metaplastic change; this change is most active *in utero*, at puberty, and during a first pregnancy and declines after menopause. The greatest risk of neoplastic transformation coincides with periods of greatest metaplastic activity. Virally induced atypical squamous metaplasia developing in this region can progress to higher grade squamous intraepithelial lesions.

The mean age of women with CIN is approximately 15 years younger than that of women with invasive cancer, suggesting a slow progression of CIN to invasive carcinoma.[53,54] In a 13-year observational study of women with CIN 3, Miller[55] found that disease progressed in only 14%, whereas it remained the same in 61% and disappeared in the remainder. Syrjanen et al.[56] reported spontaneous regression in 38% of high-grade HPV-associated squamous intraepithelial lesions. However, in a large prospective study, Richart and Barron[57] reported mean times to development of carcinoma *in situ* of 58, 38, and 12 months for patients with mild, moderate, or severe dysplasia, respectively, and predicted that 66% of all dysplasias would progress to carcinoma *in situ* within 10 years.

Once tumor has broken through the basement membrane, it may penetrate the cervical stroma directly or through vascular channels. Invasive tumors may develop as exophytic growths protruding from the cervix into the vagina or as endocervical lesions that can cause massive expansion of the cervix despite a relatively normal-appearing cervical portio. From the cervix, tumor may extend superiorly to the lower uterine segment, inferiorly to the vagina, or into the paracervical spaces by way of the broad or uterosacral ligaments. Tumor may become fixed to the pelvic wall by direct extension or by coalescence of central tumor with regional adenopathy. Tumor may also extend anteriorly to involve the bladder or posteriorly to the rectum, although rectal mucosal involvement is a rare finding at initial presentation.

The cervix has a rich supply of lymphatics organized in three anastomosing plexuses that drain the mucosal, muscularis, and serosal layers.[58] The lymphatics of the cervix also anastomose extensively with those of the lower uterine segment, possibly explaining the high frequency of uterine extension from endocervical primary tumors. The most important lymphatic collecting trunks exit laterally from the uterine isthmus in three groups (Fig. 36.2-1).[58,59] The upper branches, which originate in the anterior and lateral cervix, follow the uterine artery, are sometimes interrupted by a node as they cross the ureter, and terminate in the uppermost hypogastric nodes. The middle branches drain to deeper hypogastric (obturator) nodes. The lowest branches follow a posterior course to the inferior and superior gluteal, common iliac, presacral, and subaortic nodes. Additional posterior lymphatic channels arising from the posterior cervical wall may drain to superior rectal nodes or may continue upward in the retrorectal space to the subaortic nodes overlying the sacral promontory. Anterior collecting trunks pass between the cervix and bladder along the superior vesical artery and terminate in the internal iliac nodes.

Table 36.2-2 summarizes the reported incidences of pelvic and paraaortic node involvement for patients who underwent lymphadenectomy as part of primary surgical treatment or before radiotherapy for cervical carcinomas.[60–83] The incidences reported for patients who underwent radical hysterectomy vary widely, probably reflecting differences in the criteria used by surgeons to select patients for radical surgery rather than for primary radiation treatment. Many series excluded patients with extrapelvic disease. Variations in the completeness of lymphadenectomies and histologic processing may also lead to underestimates of the true incidence of regional spread from carcinomas of the cervix.[60,84]

Cervical cancer usually follows a relatively orderly pattern of metastatic progression initially to primary echelon nodes in the pelvis, then to paraaortic nodes and distant sites. Even patients with locoregionally advanced disease rarely have detectable hematogenous metastases at initial diagnosis of their cervical cancer. The most frequent sites of distant recurrence are lung, extrapelvic nodes, liver, and bone.[85,86] Although early studies suggested that the lumbar spine was a relatively frequent site of skeletal metastases, more recent studies using abdominal imaging demonstrate that most patients with isolated lumbar spine

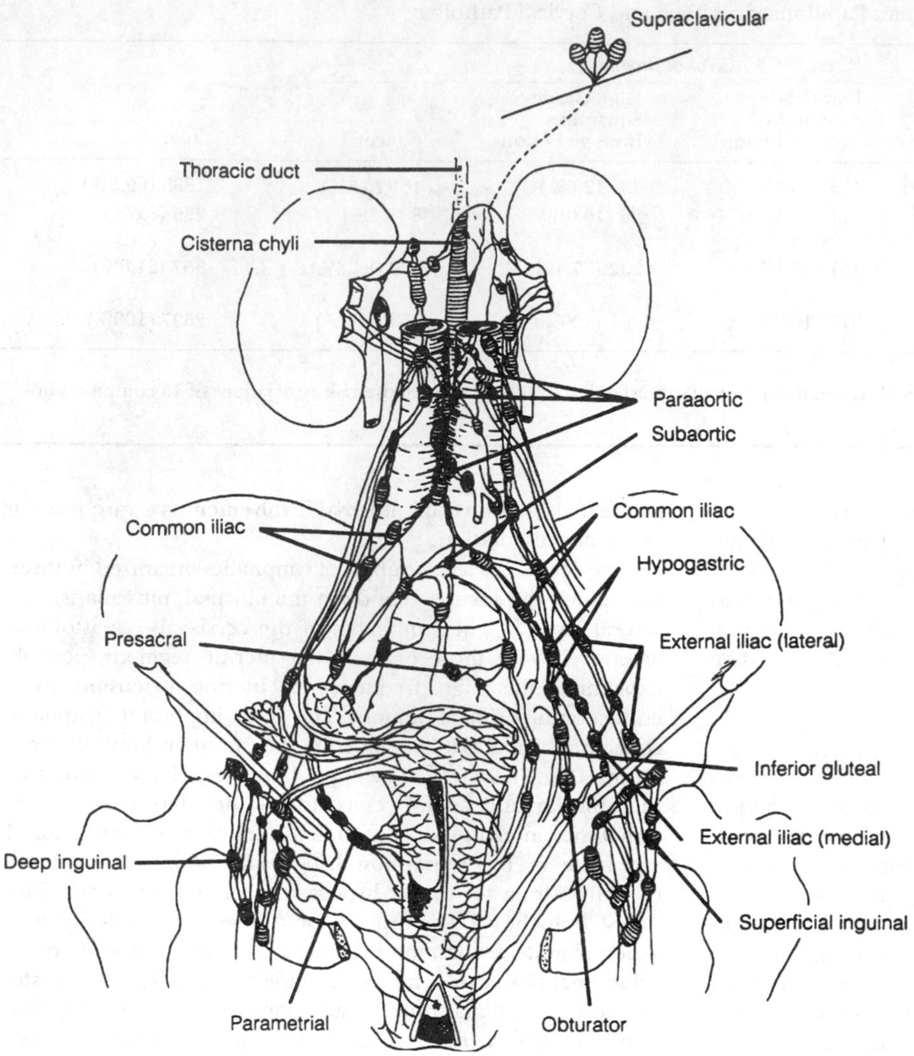

FIGURE 36.2-1. The lymphatic system of the female genital organs. [Reprinted from ref. 481, with permission; adapted from Meigs JV (ed). *Surgical treatment of cancer of the cervix.* New York: Grune & Stratton, 1954:90.]

involvement actually have direct extension of disease from paraaortic nodes.[87]

PATHOLOGY

Cervical Intraepithelial Neoplasia

Several systems have been developed for classifying cervical cytologic findings (Table 36.2-3). Although criteria for the diagnosis of CIN vary somewhat between pathologists, the important characteristics of this lesion are cellular immaturity, cellular disorganization, nuclear abnormalities, and increased mitotic activity. The degree of neoplasia is determined on the basis of the extent of the mitotic activity, immature cell proliferation, and nuclear atypia. If mitoses and immature cells are present only in the lower third of the epithelium, the lesion is usually designated CIN 1. Lesions involving the middle or upper third are diagnosed as CIN 2 or CIN 3, respectively.

The term *cervical intraepithelial neoplasia,* as proposed by Richart,[88] refers only to a lesion that may progress to invasive carcinoma. Although CIN 1 to 2 is sometimes referred to as mild to moderate dysplasia, *CIN* is now preferred over *dysplasia.* Because the word *dysplasia* means "abnormal maturation," proliferating metaplasia without mitotic activity has sometimes been erroneously called dysplasia.

The Bethesda system of classification, designed to further standardize reporting of cervical cytologic findings, was developed after a National Cancer Institute consensus conference in 1988 and was refined in 1991.[89] This system, which separates condylomata and CIN 1, classified as low-grade squamous intraepithelial lesions, from high-grade squamous intraepithelial lesions, is meant to replace the Papanicolaou system and is now widely used in the United States. The Bethesda system introduced the term *atypical squamous cells of undetermined significance.* This uncertain diagnosis is now the most common abnormal Pap test result.[90] In United States laboratories, 1.6% to 9.0% of Pap smears are reported as having atypical squamous cells of undetermined significance.[91] Although most reflect a benign process, approximately 5% to 10% are associated with underlying high-grade squamous intraepithelial lesions, and one-third or more of high-grade squamous intraepithelial lesions are heralded by a finding of atypical squamous cells of undetermined significance on a Pap smear.[92]

Adenocarcinoma In Situ

The diagnosis of adenocarcinoma *in situ* (AIS) is made when normal endocervical gland cells are replaced by tall, irregular columnar cells with stratified, hyperchromatic nuclei and increased mitotic activity, but the normal branching pattern of the endocer-

TABLE 36.2-2. Rates of Lymph Node Metastasis in Patients with Carcinoma of the Cervix

		FIGO Stage											
		IB			IIA			IIB			III		
	Primary Treatment	No. of Patients	Pelvic Nodes	PA Nodes	No. of Patients	Pelvic Nodes	PA Nodes	No. of Patients	Pelvic Nodes	PA Nodes	No. of Patients	Pelvic Nodes	PA Nodes
Girardi and Haas[60]	RH	163	31%		8	0%		249	45%				
Averette et al.[61]	RH	866	14%	5%	95	21%	8%						
Kamura et al.[62]	RH	211	12%		48	17%		86	34%				
Alvarez et al.[63]	RH	401	12%	1%									
Ayhan et al.[64]	RH	207	21%	6%	38	37%	(0/6)	25	40%	(4/8)			
Delgado et al.[65]	RH	645	16%										
Lee et al.[66]	RH	596	13%		250	27%		108	35%				
Fuller et al.[67]	RH	285	15%		133	22%							
Barber et al.[68]	RH/EX	273	14%					283[a]	28%		67	42%	
Burghardt et al.[69]	RH	122	31%		8	25%		195	44%				
Creasman et al.[70]	RH	258	14%		10	10%							
Boyce et al.[71]	RH	138	14%										
Piver and Chung[72]	RH		27%										
Boronow et al.[73]	RH	73	26%										
Sudarsanam et al.[74]	RH/RT	155		7%	21		14%	22		18%	19		19%
Stehman et al.[75]	RT							321	18%		188	23%[b]	
LaPolla et al.[76]	RT	8	75%	50%	8	38%	0%	39	33%	15%	38	55%	37%
Berman et al.[77]	RT	158		5%	25		12%	240		17%	180		25%
Ballon et al.[78]	RT	22	27%	23%	16	38%	19%	32	16%	19%	24	38%	17%
Lagasse et al.[79]	RT	143		6%	22		18%	58		33%	64		30%
Buchsbaum[80]	RT	16		25%	4		0%	15		7%	104		33%
Wharton et al.[81]	RT	21	38%	0%				67[a]	35%	18%	42	29%[b]	33%
Nelson et al.[82]	RT				16		13%	47		15%	39		38%
Guthrie et al.[83]	RT										37		35%

EX, exenteration; FIGO, International Federation of Gynecology and Obstetrics; PA, paraaortic; RH, radical hysterectomy; RT, radiation therapy.
[a]Stages IIA and IIB combined.
[b]Patients with positive paraaortics excluded.

vical glands is maintained and there is no obvious stromal invasion. Approximately 20% to 50% of women with cervical AIS also have squamous CIN, and AIS is often an incidental finding in patients operated on for squamous carcinoma.[93,94] Because AIS is frequently multifocal, cone biopsy margins are unreliable.[93,95]

Microinvasive Carcinoma

Because the definition of microinvasive carcinoma is based on the maximum depth and linear extent of involvement, this diagnosis can only be made after examination of a specimen that includes the entire neoplastic lesion and cervical transformation zone. This requires a cervical cone biopsy.

The earliest invasion appears as a protrusion of cells from the stromoepithelial junction; these cells are better differentiated than the adjacent noninvasive cells and have abundant pink-staining cytoplasm, hyperchromatic nuclei, and small- to medium-sized nucleoli.[96] As the tumor progresses, invasion occurs at multiple sites, and its depth and linear extent become measurable. The depth of invasion should be measured with a micrometer from the base of the epithelium to the deepest point of invasion. Lesions that have invaded less than 3 mm [International Federation of Gynecology and Obstetrics (FIGO) stage IA1] rarely metastasize; 5% to 10% of tumors that invade 3 to 5 mm (FIGO stage IA2) have positive pelvic lymph nodes.[97–99]

Although investigators occasionally label small adenocarcinomas as *microinvasive,* the term probably should not be used for these tumors. Because invasive adenocarcinomas may originate either from the mucosal surface or from the periphery of underlying glands, no reliable method has been found for measuring the depth of invasion of these tumors. For this reason adenocarcinomas are generally classified as either AIS or invasive carcinoma (FIGO stage IB).

Invasive Squamous Cell Carcinoma

Between 80% and 90% of cervical carcinomas are squamous. A number of systems have been used to grade and classify squa-

TABLE 36.2-3. Comparison of Cytology Classification Systems

Bethesda System	*Dysplasia/CIN System*		*Papanicolaou System*
Within normal limits	Normal		Class I
Infection (specify organism)	Inflammatory atypia (organism)		Class II
Reactive and reparative changes			
Squamous cell abnormalities			
Atypical squamous cells of undetermined significance	Squamous atypia		Class IIR
Low-grade squamous intraepithelial lesion	Human papillomavirus atypia		Class IIR
	Mild dysplasia	CIN 1	Class III
High-grade squamous intraepithelial lesion	Moderate dysplasia	CIN 2	Class III
	Severe dysplasia	CIN 3	
	Carcinoma *in situ*	CIN 3	Class IV
Invasive squamous carcinoma	Invasive squamous carcinoma		Class V

CIN, cervical intraepithelial neoplasia.

mous carcinomas, but none have consistently been demonstrated to predict prognosis. One of the most commonly used systems categorizes squamous neoplasms as large cell keratinizing, large cell nonkeratinizing, or small cell carcinoma.[100] Small cell squamous carcinomas have small- to medium-sized nuclei, open chromatin, small or large nucleoli, and abundant cytoplasm. Most authorities believe that patients with small cell squamous carcinoma have a poorer prognosis than those with large cell neoplasms with or without keratin. However, small cell squamous carcinoma should not be confused with anaplastic small cell carcinoma. The latter resembles oat cell carcinoma of the lung because it contains small tumor cells that have scanty cytoplasm, small round to oval nuclei, small or absent nucleoli, finely granular chromatin, and high mitotic activity.[101] Approximately 30% to 50% of anaplastic small cell carcinomas display neuroendocrine features. Small cell anaplastic carcinomas behave more aggressively than poorly differentiated small cell squamous carcinomas; most investigators report survival rates of less than 50% even for patients with early stage I disease.[102–104]

Adenocarcinoma

Invasive adenocarcinoma may be pure or mixed with squamous cell carcinoma (adenosquamous carcinoma). A wide variety of cell types, growth patterns, and degrees of differentiation have been observed. Approximately 80% of cervical adenocarcinomas are made up predominantly of cells whose differentiated features resemble endocervical glandular epithelium with intracytoplasmic mucin production. The remaining tumors are populated by endometrioid cells, clear cells, intestinal cells, or a mixture of more than one cell type. By histologic examination alone, some of these tumors are indistinguishable from those arising elsewhere in the endometrium or ovary.

Minimal-deviation adenocarcinoma (adenoma malignum) is a rare, extremely well differentiated adenocarcinoma that is sometimes associated with Peutz-Jeghers syndrome.[105,106] Because the branching glandular pattern strongly resembles normal endocervical glands, minimal-deviation adenocarcinoma may not be recognized as malignant in small biopsy specimens. Earlier studies reported a dismal outcome for women with this tumor, but more recently, patients have been reported to have a favorable prognosis if the disease is detected early.[107,108]

Young and Scully[109] have described a villoglandular papillary subtype of adenocarcinoma that primarily affects young women, appears to metastasize infrequently, and has a favorable prognosis. Glucksmann and Cherry[110] were the first to describe glassy cell carcinoma, a form of poorly differentiated adenosquamous carcinoma with cells that have abundant eosinophilic, granular, ground-glass cytoplasm; large round to oval nuclei; and prominent nucleoli. Other rare variants of adenosquamous carcinoma include adenoid basal carcinoma and adenoid cystic carcinoma.[111] Adenoid basal carcinoma is a well-differentiated tumor that histologically resembles basal cell carcinoma of the skin and tends to have a favorable prognosis. Adenoid cystic carcinomas consist of basaloid cells in a cribriform or cylindromatous pattern and tend to have aggressive behavior with frequent metastases, although the natural history of these tumors may be long. Whether the prognoses of these rare subtypes are different from those of other adenocarcinomas of similar grade is uncertain.

A variety of neoplasms may infiltrate the cervix from adjacent sites presenting differential diagnostic problems. In particular, it may be difficult or impossible to determine the origin of adenocarcinomas involving the endocervix and uterine isthmus. Although endometrioid histology suggests endometrial origin and mucinous tumors in young patients are most often of endocervical origin, both histologic types can arise in either site.[112] Metastatic tumors from the colon, breast, or other sites may involve the cervix secondarily. Malignant mixed Müllerian tumors, adenosarcomas, and leiomyosarcomas arise occasionally in the cervix but more often involve it secondarily. Primary lymphomas and melanomas of the cervix are extremely rare.

CLINICAL MANIFESTATIONS

Preinvasive disease is usually detected during routine cervical cytologic screening. Early invasive disease may not be associated with any symptoms and is also detected during screening examinations. The earliest symptom of invasive cervical cancer is usually abnormal vaginal bleeding, often following coitus or vaginal douching. This may be associated with a clear or foul-smelling vaginal discharge. Pelvic pain may result from locoregionally invasive disease or from coexistent pelvic inflammatory disease. Flank pain may be a symptom of hydronephrosis, often complicated by pyelonephritis. The triad of sciatic pain, leg edema, and hydronephrosis is almost always associated with extensive pelvic wall involvement by tumor. Patients with advanced tumors may have hematuria or incontinence from a vesicovaginal fistula caused by direct extension of tumor to the bladder. External compression of the rectum by a massive primary tumor may cause constipation, but the rectal mucosa is rarely involved at initial diagnosis.

DIAGNOSIS, CLINICAL EVALUATION, AND STAGING

Diagnosis

The long preinvasive stage of cervical cancer, the relatively high prevalence of the disease in unscreened populations, and the sensitivity of cytologic screening make cervical carcinoma an ideal target for cancer screening. In the United States, screening with cervical cytologic examination and pelvic examination has led to more than a 70% decrease in the mortality from cervical cancer since 1940.[1,113] Only nations with comprehensive screening programs have experienced substantial decreases in cervical cancer death rates during this period.

Authorities disagree about the optimal frequency of cervical cancer screening. In a 1988 consensus statement, the American Cancer Society and other medical groups recommended annual Pap smears beginning at age 18 years or with the onset of sexual activity and added that, after three or more consecutive normal annual examinations, the cytologic evaluation could be performed less frequently at the discretion of the physician.[114,115] For patients who have had repeated negative test results, the marginal gain from screening more often than every 3 years decreases sharply.[116–118] The United States Preventative Services Task Force has recommended that screening be discontinued after age 65 years if results have been consistently normal, and the Canadian Task Force suggests that the screening interval be extended to 5 years after age 35 if previous studies have been normal.[115] Although these groups have suggested tailoring the frequency of Pap smears to patient risk, practical definitions of low and high risk remain controversial. As a result, most clinicians continue to recommend that their patients be screened more frequently than recommended by the national guidelines.[115] The rate of false-negative findings on the Pap test is approximately 10% to 15% in women with invasive cancer.[53,54,114] The sensitivity of the test may be improved by ensuring adequate sampling of the squamocolumnar junction and the endocervical canal; smears without endocervical or metaplastic cells are inadequate and must be repeated. Because AIS originates near or above the transformation zone, it may be missed with conventional cervical smears. Detection of high endocervical lesions may be improved when specimens are obtained with a cytobrush. Also, because hemorrhage, necrosis, and intense inflammation may obscure the results, the Pap smear is a poor way to diagnose gross lesions; these should always be biopsied.

Patients with abnormal findings on cytologic examination who do not have a gross cervical lesion must be evaluated by colposcopy and directed biopsies. Following application of a 3% acetic acid solution, the cervix is examined under 10- to 15-fold magnification with a bright, filtered light that enhances the acetowhitening and vascular patterns characteristic of dysplasia or carcinoma. The skilled colposcopist can accurately distinguish between low- and high-grade dysplasia,[119–121] but microinvasive disease cannot consistently be distinguished from intraepithelial lesions on colposcopy.[122,123]

If no abnormalities are found on colposcopic examination or if the entire squamocolumnar junction cannot be visualized in a patient with an atypical Pap smear result, endocervical curettage should be performed. Some authorities advocate the routine addition of endocervical curettage to colposcopic examination to minimize the risk of missing occult cancer within the endocervical canal.[122–124] However, it is probably reasonable to omit this step in previously untreated women if the entire squamocolumnar junction is visible with a complete ring of unaltered columnar epithelium in the lower canal.

Cervical cone biopsy is used to diagnose occult endocervical lesions and is an essential step in the diagnosis and management of microinvasive carcinoma of the cervix. The geometry of the cone is individualized and tailored to the geometry of the cervix, the location of the squamocolumnar junction, and the site and size of the lesion. Cervical cone biopsy yields an accurate diagnosis and decreases the incidence of inappropriate therapy when (1) the squamocolumnar junction is poorly visualized on colposcopy and a high-grade lesion is suspected, (2) a high grade dysplastic epithelium extends into the endocervical canal, (3) the cytologic findings suggest a high-grade dysplasia or carcinoma *in situ*, (4) a microinvasive carcinoma is found on directed biopsy, (5) the endocervical curettage specimens show high-grade CIN, or (6) the cytologic findings are suspicious for AIS.[55,114,125]

Clinical Evaluation of Patients with Invasive Carcinoma

All patients with invasive cervical cancer should be evaluated with a detailed history and physical examination, with particular attention paid to inspection and palpation of the pelvic organs with bimanual and rectovaginal examinations. Standard laboratory studies should include a complete blood cell count and renal function and liver function tests. All patients should have chest radiography to rule out lung metastases and an intravenous pyelogram [or computed tomography (CT)] to determine the kidney's location and to rule out ureteral obstruction by tumor. Cystoscopy and either a proctoscopy or a barium enema study should be done in patients with bulky tumors.

Many clinicians obtain CT or magnetic resonance imaging (MRI) scans to evaluate regional nodes, but the accuracy of these studies is compromised by their failure to detect small metastases and because patients with bulky necrotic tumors often have enlarged reactive lymph nodes.[126,127] In a large Gynecologic Oncology Group (GOG) study that compared the results of radiographic studies with subsequent histologic findings, Heller et al.[126] found that 79% of the cases with paraaortic lymph node involvement were detected by lymphangiography, whereas only 34% were detected by CT. Unfortunately, lymphangiography is no longer available in many centers. More recent studies suggest that positron emission tomography may be a sensitive noninvasive method of evaluating the regional nodes of patients with cervical cancers.[128] MRI can provide use-

TABLE 36.2-4. International Federation of Gynecology and Obstetrics Staging of Carcinoma of the Cervix (1994)

Stage 0	Carcinoma *in situ*, intraepithelial carcinoma; *Cases of stage 0 should not be included in any therapeutic statistics for invasive carcinoma.*
Stage I	The carcinoma is strictly confined to the cervix (*extension to the corpus should be disregarded.*)
Stage IA	Invasive cancer identified only microscopically. All gross lesions, even with superficial invasion, are stage IB cancers. Invasion is limited to measured stromal invasion with a maximum depth of 5 mm and no wider than 7 mm. (*The depth of invasion should not be more than 5 mm taken from the base of the epithelium, either surface or glandular, from which it originates. Vascular space involvement, either venous or lymphatic, should not alter the staging.*)
Stage IA1	Measured invasion of stroma no greater than 3 mm in depth and no wider than 7 mm.
Stage IA2	Measured invasion of stroma greater than 3 mm and no greater than 5 mm in depth and no wider than 7 mm.
Stage IB	Clinical lesions confined to the cervix or preclinical lesions greater than IA.
Stage IB1	Clinical lesions no greater than 4 cm in size.
Stage IB2	Clinical lesions greater than 4 cm in size.
Stage II	The carcinoma extends beyond the cervix, but has not extended onto the pelvic wall; the carcinoma involves the vagina, but not as far as the lower third.
Stage IIA	No obvious parametrial involvement.
Stage IIB	Obvious parametrial involvement. The carcinoma has extended onto the pelvic wall; on rectal examination there is no cancer-free space between the tumor and the pelvic wall; the tumor involves the lower third of the vagina; all cases with a hydronephrosis or nonfunctioning kidney should be included, unless they are known to be due to another cause.
Stage III	No extension onto the pelvic wall, but involvement of the lower third of the vagina.
Stage IIIA	Extension onto the pelvic wall or hydronephrosis or nonfunctioning kidney.
Stage IIIB	The carcinoma has extended beyond the true pelvis or has clinically involved the mucosa of the bladder or rectum.
Stage IV	The carcinoma has extended beyond the true pelvis or has clinically involved the mucosa of the bladder or rectum.
Stage IVA	Spread of the growth to adjacent organs.
Stage IVB	Spread to distant organs.

(From ref. 135, with permission.)

ful information about the distribution and depth of invasion of tumors in the cervix[129–131] but tends to yield less accurate assessments of the parametrium.[132,133]

Clinical Staging

FIGO has defined the most widely accepted staging system for carcinomas of the cervix.[134,135] The latest (1994) update of this system is summarized in Table 36.2-4. Since the earliest versions of the cervical cancer staging system[136] there have been numerous changes, particularly in the definition of stage I disease.[137] Preinvasive disease was not placed in a separate category until 1950, and the stage IA category for "cases with early stromal invasion" was first described in 1962. Cases of early stromal invasion and occult invasion were redistributed between stages IA1, IA2, and IB_{occult} several times until 1985, when FIGO eliminated stage IB_{occult} and provided the first specific definitions of microinvasive disease (stages IA1 and IA2). In 1994 these definitions were changed again, and, for the first time, stage IB tumors were subdivided according to tumor diameter (see Table 36.2-4). Although these changes have gradually improved the discriminatory value of the staging system, the many fluctuations in the definitions of stages IA and IB have complicated our ability to compare the outcomes of patients whose tumors were staged and treated during different periods.[137] In addition, many gynecologic oncologists in the United States use the Society of Gynecologic Oncologists' definition of a microinvasive carcinoma (i.e., tumor that "invades the stroma in one or more places to a depth of 3 mm or less below the base of the epithelium and in which lymphatic or vascular involvement is not demonstrated"), a definition that still differs from the current FIGO classification.[138]

FIGO stage is based on careful clinical examination and the results of specific radiologic studies and procedures. These should be performed and the stage should be assigned before any definitive therapy is administered. The clinical stage should never be changed on the basis of subsequent findings. When it is doubtful to which stage a particular case should be allotted, the case should be assigned to the earlier stage. According to FIGO,[134] "a growth fixed to the pelvic wall by a short and indurated, but not nodular, parametrium should be allotted to stage IIb." A case should be classified as stage III "only if the parametrium is nodular to the pelvic wall or if the growth itself extends to the pelvic wall." In its rules for clinical staging, FIGO states that palpation, inspection, colposcopy, endocervical curettage, hysteroscopy, cystoscopy, proctoscopy, intravenous urography, and radiographic examination of the lungs and skeleton may be used for clinical staging. Suspected bladder or rectal involvement should be confirmed by biopsy. Findings of bullous edema or malignant cells in cytologic washings from the urinary bladder are not sufficient to diagnose bladder involvement. FIGO specifically states that findings on examinations such as lymphangiography, laparoscopy, CT scan, and MRI are of value for planning therapy but, because these are not yet generally available and the interpretation of results is variable, should not be the basis for changing the clinical stage. Examination under anesthesia is desirable but not required. The rules and notes outlined in the FIGO staging system are integral parts of the clinical staging system and should be strictly observed to minimize inconsistencies in staging between institutions.

Although most clinicians use the FIGO classification system, a number of European groups use a staging system that divides stage IIB tumors according to the extent of parametrial involvement and divides stage III tumors according to whether there is unilateral or bilateral pelvic wall fixation. Until the mid 1980s most reports from The University of Texas M. D. Anderson Cancer Center used a similar staging system that also categorized patients with bulky endocervical tumors in a special category.[137] Although surgically treated patients are sometimes classified according to a tumor, node, metastases (TNM) pathologic staging system, this practice has not been widely accepted because it cannot be applied to patients who are treated with primary radiotherapy.[139]

Surgical Evaluation of Regional Spread

In the 1970s, studies of diagnostic preradiation lymph node dissection used a transperitoneal approach that led to unacceptable morbidity and mortality from radiation-related bowel complications, particularly after treatment with high radiation doses and extended fields.[81,140] More recently, extraperitoneal dissection, which induces fewer bowel adhesions, has been recommended. With this approach, postradiation bowel complications occur in fewer than 5% of patients.[141] A number of groups are currently investigating the use of laparoscopic lymph node dissection to evaluate patients with cervical cancer.[142,143] This approach reduces the length of postoperative hospitalization. However, the rate of late complications from radiotherapy following laparoscopic lymphadenectomy has not yet been determined.

Although the indications for surgical staging are controversial, advocates argue that the procedure identifies patients with microscopic paraaortic or common iliac node involvement who can benefit from extended-field irradiation. Some investigators have also suggested, on the basis of first principles and encouraging results with regard to control of pelvic disease, that debulking of large pelvic nodes before radiotherapy may improve outcome.[144,145] Because patients with radiographically positive pelvic nodes are at greatest risk for occult metastasis to paraaortic nodes, these patients may have the greatest chance of benefiting from surgical staging.

Some authors have advocated pretreatment blind biopsy of the scalene node in patients with positive paraaortic nodes and in patients with a central recurrence who are being considered for pelvic exenteration. The reported incidence of supraclavicular metastasis varies widely (5% to 20% or more) for patients with positive paraaortic lymph nodes.[146,147]

Prognostic Factors

Although rates of survival and control of pelvic disease in cervical cancer patients are correlated with FIGO stage, prognosis is also influenced by a number of tumor characteristics that are not included in the staging system. Clinical tumor diameter is strongly correlated with prognosis for patients treated with radiation (Fig. 36.2-2)[148,149] or surgery.[63,65,150,151] For this reason, FIGO modified the stage I category so that these tumors are subdivided according to clinical tumor diameter (i.e., less than or equal to 4 or greater than 4 cm).[135] For patients with more advanced disease, other estimates of tumor bulk, such as the presence of medial versus lateral parametrial involvement in FIGO stage IIB tumors or of unilateral versus bilateral parametrial or pelvic wall involvement, have also been correlated with outcome.[152–154] The predictive value of the staging system itself may, in part, reflect an association between the stage categories and the primary tumor volume. Operative findings often do not agree with clinical estimates of parametrial or pelvic wall involvement,[69,155,156] and some authors have found that the predictive power of stage diminishes or is lost when comparisons are corrected for differences in clinical tumor diameter.[75,157]

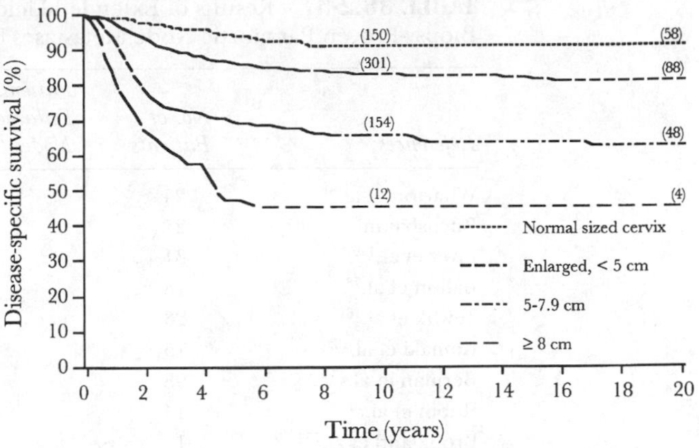

FIGURE 36.2-2. Relationship between tumor diameter and the disease-specific survival rates of 1526 patients with stage IB squamous cell carcinomas of the cervix treated with radiotherapy at M. D. Anderson Cancer Center. Numbers in parentheses represent the number of patients at risk at 10 or 20 years. (Reprinted from ref. 148, with permission.)

Lymph node metastasis is also an important predictor of prognosis. For patients treated with radical hysterectomy for stage IB disease, survival rates are usually reported as 85% to 95% for patients with negative nodes and 45% to 55% for those with lymph node metastases.[61,63,158] Inoue and Morita[159] reported that survival was correlated with the size of the largest node, and several authors have reported correlations between the number of involved pelvic lymph nodes and survival.[62,150,158,160] Survival rates for patients with positive paraaortic nodes treated with extended-field radiotherapy vary between 10% and 50% depending on the extent of pelvic disease and paraaortic lymph node involvement (Table 36.2-5).[77,78,80,81,140,161–168]

For patients treated with radical hysterectomy, other histologic parameters that have been associated with a poor prognosis are lymph-vascular space invasion (LVSI) (Table 36.2-6),[62,150,151,158,169–173] deep stromal invasion (greater than or equal to 10 mm or greater than 70% invasion),[62,63,67,71,150,151,158] and parametrial extension.[62,71,155,174] Roman and colleagues[175] reported a correlation between the quantity of LVSI (percent of histopathologic sections containing LVSI) and the incidence of lymph node metastases. A strong inflammatory response in the cervical stroma tends to predict a good outcome.[176] Uterine body involvement is associated with an increased rate of distant metastases in patients treated with radiation or surgery.[177–180]

Several investigators have reported similar survival rates for patients with squamous carcinomas and those with adenocarcinomas.[84,181–185] However, other investigators have drawn the opposite conclusion, noting unusually high pelvic relapse rates in patients treated surgically for adenocarcinomas and poorer survival rates among patients treated with surgery or irradiation for cervical adenocarcinomas.[186–191] In a multivariate analysis of 1767 patients treated with radiation for FIGO stage IB disease, Eifel and colleagues[188] reported a highly significant independent correlation between histologic features and survival. Using Cox regression analysis, the relative risk of death from cancer for 106 patients with adenocarcinomas 4 cm or more in diameter was determined to be 1.9 times that for patients with squamous

TABLE 36.2-5. Results of Extended-Field Radiation Therapy to the Paraaortic Nodes for Biopsy-Proven Paraaortic Node Metastases from Carcinoma of the Cervix

References	*No. of Patients*	*Patients with Grossly Enlarged Paraaortic Nodes (%)*	*Patients with FIGO Stage III or IVA Tumors (%)*	*5-Y Survival Rate (%)*
Wharton et al.[81]	24	—	58	13
Buchsbaum[80]	21	—	—	21
Piver et al.[140]	31	71	65	10
Ballon et al.[78]	18	—	22	23
Tewfik et al.[161]	23	65[b]	74	22
Komaki et al.[162]	15	—	7	40
Berman et al.[77]	98	76	45	25[a]
Rubin et al.[163]	14	—	0	50
Brookland et al.[164]	15	—	20	40[a]
Nori et al.[165]	27	81	—	29
Podczaski et al.[166]	33	76	30	31
Cunningham et al.[167]	24	35	0	48
Kim et al.[168]	43	—	21	24

FIGO, International Federation of Gynecology and Obstetrics.
[a]Three-year survival.
[b]Clinically enlarged nodes.

tumors (P <.01) (Fig. 36.2-3). Pelvic disease control rates were similar for patients with squamous carcinomas and those with adenocarcinomas, but there was a significantly higher incidence of distant metastases in patients with adenocarcinomas. Although the prognostic significance of histologic grade has been disputed for squamous carcinomas, there is a clear correlation between the degree of differentiation and the clinical behavior of adenocarcinomas.[189,192–195]

Several studies have demonstrated a relationship between hemoglobin level and prognosis in patients with locally advanced cervical cancer.[196–198] The strongest evidence that anemia plays a causative role in pelvic recurrence comes from a small 1978 randomized study conducted at the Princess Margaret Hospital.[196] All patients were maintained at a hemoglobin level of at least 10 gm%, but those in the treatment arm were maintained, through the use of transfusions, at hemoglobin levels of at least 12.5 gm%. The locoregional recurrence rate was significantly higher for the 25 anemic patients in the control arm than it was for the patients who received transfusions. Unfortunately, the results of this small study have never been confirmed, and subsequent studies aimed at overcoming the theoretical radiobiologic consequences of intratumoral hypoxia (hypoxic cell sensitizers, hyperbaric oxygen breathing, neutron therapy) have not been successful.[199–205] Several investigators have correlated low intratumoral oxygen tension levels with a high rate of lymph node metastases and poor survival.[206–208]

TABLE 36.2-6. Relationship between Lymph-Vascular Space Invasion, Pelvic Node Involvement, and Recurrence Rate in Patients Treated with Radical Hysterectomy

	Positive Lymph Nodes (%)		*Recurrence Rate (%)*	
References	LVSI	No LVSI	LVSI	No LVSI
Chung et al.[171]	63	13	50	6
Fuller et al.[172]	40	14		
Nahhas et al.[173]	22	8	20	12
Boyce et al.[169]	32	6	36	4
Burke et al.[170]			38	9
Delgado et al.[158]			23	11
Kamura et al.[62]			18	9
Sevin et al.[151]			38	15
Kristensen et al.[150]			29	9

LVSI, lymph-vascular space invasion.

The serum concentration of squamous cell carcinoma antigen appears to correlate with the stage and size of squamous carcinomas and the presence of lymph node metastases.[209–212] However, investigators disagree about the independent predictive value of this test. Other clinical and biologic features that have been investigated for their predictive power, with variable results, include patient age,[158,213–216] peritoneal cytology,[217,218] platelet count,[219,220] tumor vascularity,[221,222] DNA ploidy or S phase,[223,224] and HPV subtype.[35,225,226] In two studies of patients with histologically negative lymph nodes, investigators have reported higher rates of disease recurrence when a polymerase chain reaction assay of the lymph nodes was strongly positive for HPV DNA.[227,228]

TREATMENT

A number of factors may influence the choice of local treatment, including tumor size, stage, histologic features, evidence of lymph node involvement, risk factors for complications of surgery or radiation, and patient preference. However, as a rule, intraepithelial lesions are treated with superficial ablative techniques; microinvasive cancers invading less than 3 mm (stage IA1) are managed with conservative surgery (excisional conization or extrafascial hysterectomy); early invasive cancers

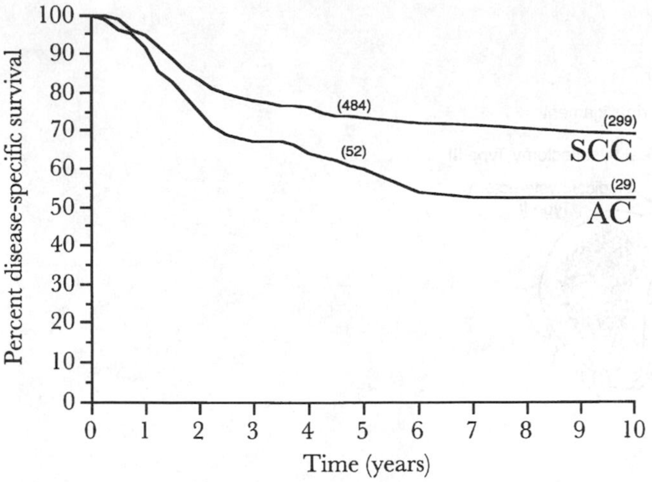

FIGURE 36.2-3. Relationship between histologic type and the disease-specific survival rates of 903 patients treated at M. D. Anderson Cancer Center for stage IB carcinomas of the cervix measuring 4 cm or greater in diameter. Numbers in parentheses represent the number of patients at risk at 10 or 20 years. AC, adenocarcinoma; SCC, squamous cell carcinoma. (Reprinted from ref. 188, with permission.)

(stages IA2 and IB1 and some small stage IIA tumors) are managed with radical surgery or radiotherapy; and locally advanced cancers (stages IB2 through IVA) are managed with radiotherapy. Selected patients with centrally recurrent disease after maximum radiotherapy may be treated with radical exenterative surgery; pelvic recurrence after hysterectomy is treated with irradiation. The results of randomized trials[229–233] have led to the addition of concurrent cisplatin-containing chemotherapy to radiotherapy for patients whose cancers have a high risk of local-regional recurrence.

Preinvasive Disease (Stage 0)

Patients with noninvasive squamous lesions can be treated with superficial ablative therapy (cryosurgery or laser therapy) or with loop excision if (1) the entire transformation zone has been visualized colposcopically, (2) directed biopsies are consistent with Pap smear results, (3) endocervical curettage findings are negative, and (4) there is no suspicion of occult invasion on cytologic or colposcopic examination. If patients do not meet these criteria, a conization should be performed.

With cryotherapy, abnormal tissue is frozen with a supercooled metal probe until an ice ball forms that extends 5 mm beyond the lesion. Because cryonecrosis tends to be patchy and may be inadequate after a single freeze, the tissue should be frozen a second time after it has visibly thawed.[234,235] Another common and equally effective technique ablates tissue with a carbon dioxide laser beam. After laser ablation there is less distortion and more rapid healing of the cervix, but the procedure requires more training and more expensive equipment than does cryosurgery.

Many practitioners now consider loop diathermy excision to be the preferred treatment for noninvasive squamous lesions. With this technique, a charged electrode is used to excise the entire transformation zone and distal canal. Although control rates are similar to those achieved with cryotherapy or laser ablation,[236] loop diathermy is easily learned, is less expensive than laser excision, and preserves the excised lesion and transformation zone for histologic evaluation.[237–240] However, some authorities think that low-grade lesions may be overtreated with this method.[241] Because loop excision may inadequately treat disease within the cervical canal and complicate further treatment, this technique should not be considered an alternative to formal excisional conization when microinvasive or invasive cancer is suspected or for patients with AIS.

Cryotherapy, laser excision, and loop excision are all outpatient office procedures that preserve fertility. Although recurrence rates are low (10% to 15%) and progression to invasion rare (less than 2% in most series), life long surveillance of these patients must be maintained. The risk of recurrence may be somewhat increased in women with HPV type 16 or 18.[236] Treatment with vaginal or type I abdominal hysterectomy currently is reserved for women who have other gynecologic conditions that justify the procedure; invasive cancer still must be excluded before surgery to rule out the need for a more extensive operative procedure.

Microinvasive Carcinoma (Stage IA)

The standard treatment for patients with stage IA1 disease is total (type I) or vaginal hysterectomy. Because the risk of pelvic lymph node metastases from these minimally invasive tumors is less than 1%, pelvic lymph node dissection is not usually recommended.[71,123,242]

Selected patients with tumors that meet the Society of Gynecologic Oncologists' definition of microinvasion (FIGO stage IA1 disease without LVSI) and who wish to maintain fertility may be adequately treated with a therapeutic cervical conization if the margins of the cone are negative. In 1991, Burghardt et al.[243] reported one recurrence (which was fatal) in 93 women followed for more than 5 years after therapeutic conization for minimal (less than 1 mm) microinvasion. Morris et al.[244] reported no invasive recurrences in 14 patients followed for a mean of 26 months after conization for tumors invading 0.5 to 2.8 mm. However, patients who have this conservative treatment must be followed closely with periodic cytologic evaluation, colposcopy, and endocervical curettage.

Diagnostic or therapeutic conization for microinvasive disease is usually performed with a cold knife or carbon dioxide laser on a patient under general or spinal anesthesia. Because an accurate assessment of the maximum depth of invasion is critical, the entire specimen must be sectioned and carefully handled to maintain its original orientation for microscopic assessment. Complications occur in 2% to 12% of patients, are related to the depth of the cone, and include hemorrhage, sepsis, infertility, stenosis, and cervical incompetence.[245] The width and depth of the cone should be tailored to produce the least amount of injury while providing clear surgical margins.

For patients whose tumors invade 3 to 5 mm into the stroma (FIGO stage IA2), the risk of nodal metastases is approximately 5%.[65,99] Therefore, a bilateral pelvic lymphadenectomy should be performed in conjunction with a modified radical (type II) hysterectomy. Modified radical hysterectomy is a less extensive procedure than a classic radical hysterectomy (Fig. 36.2-4). The cervix, upper vagina, and paracervical tissues are removed after careful dissection of the ureters to the point of their entry to the bladder. The medial half of the cardinal ligaments and

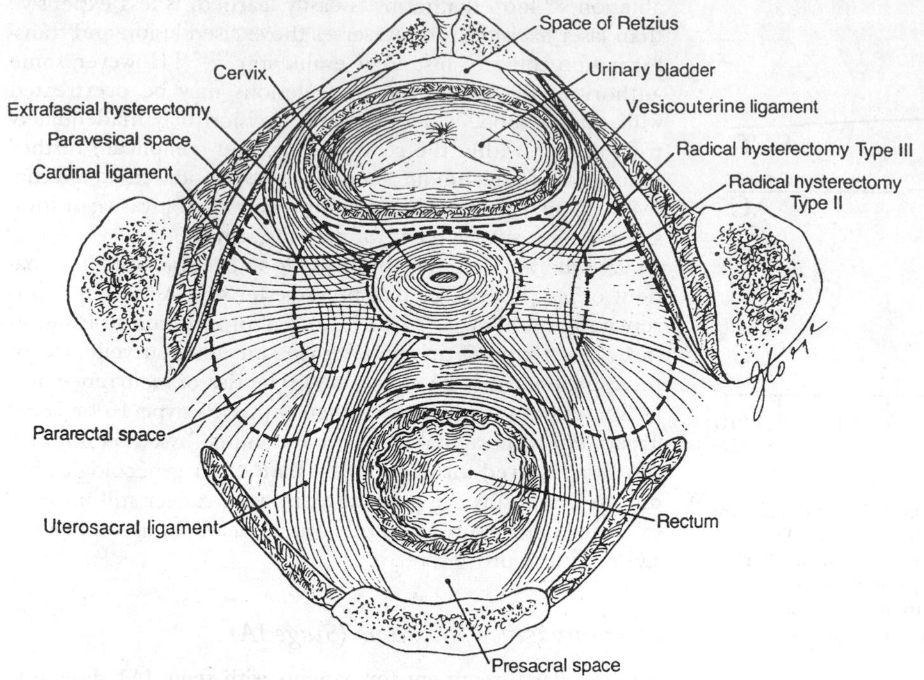

FIGURE 36.2-4. The pelvic ligaments and spaces. Dotted lines indicate the tissues removed with a type II or type III hysterectomy. (Reprinted from ref. 541, with permission.)

the uterosacral ligaments are also removed. With this treatment, significant urinary tract complications are rare and cure rates exceed 95%.[246–248]

Although surgical treatment is standard for *in situ* and microinvasive cancer, patients with severe medical problems or other contraindications to surgical treatment can be successfully treated with radiotherapy. Grigsby and Perez[249] reported a 10-year progression-free survival rate of 100% in 21 patients with carcinoma *in situ* and in 34 patients with microinvasive carcinoma treated with radiation alone. Hamberger et al.[250] reported that all patients with stage IA disease and 89 (96%) of 93 patients with small stage IB disease (less than one cervical quadrant involved) were disease free 5 years after treatment with intracavitary irradiation alone.

Stages IB and IIA

Early stage IB cervical carcinomas can be treated effectively with combined external-beam irradiation and brachytherapy or with radical hysterectomy and bilateral pelvic lymphadenectomy. The goal of both treatments is to destroy malignant cells in the cervix, paracervical tissues, and regional lymph nodes. Studies indicate that selected subgroups of patients who require radiotherapy also benefit from concurrent chemotherapy.[229–231]

Overall survival rates for patients with stage IB cervical cancer treated with surgery or radiation usually range between 80% and 90%, suggesting that the two treatments are equally effective (Table 36.2-7).[63,66,67,72,148,149,251–262] However, biases introduced by patient selection, variations in the definition of stage IA disease, and variable indications for postoperative radiotherapy or adjuvant hysterectomy confound comparisons about the efficacy of radiotherapy versus surgery. Because young women with small, clinically node-negative tumors tend to be favored candidates for surgery and because tumor diameter and nodal status are inconsistently described in published series, it is difficult to compare the results reported for patients treated with the two modalities.

In 1997, Landoni and colleagues reported results from the only prospective trial comparing radical surgery with radiotherapy alone.[263] In their study, patients with stage IB or IIA disease were randomly assigned to receive treatment with type III radical hysterectomy or a combination of external-beam and low dose-rate intracavitary radiotherapy. In the surgical arm, findings of parametrial involvement, positive margins, deep stromal invasion, or positive nodes led to the use of postoperative pelvic irradiation in 62 (54%) of 114 patients with tumors 4 cm or smaller in diameter and in 46 (84%) of 55 patients with tumors measuring less than 4 cm. Patients in the radiotherapy arm received a relatively low total dose of radiation to the cervix, with a median dose to point A of 76 Gy. With a median follow-up of 87 months, the 5-year actuarial disease-free survival rates for patients treated in the surgery and radiotherapy groups were 80% and 82%, respectively, for patients with tumors that were 4 cm or smaller and 63% and 57%, respectively, for patients with larger tumors. The authors reported a significantly higher rate of complications in the patients treated with initial surgery, and they attributed this finding to the frequent use of combined modality treatment in this group.

For patients with stage IB1 squamous carcinomas, the choice of treatment is based primarily on patient preference, anesthetic and surgical risks, physician preference, and an understanding of the nature and incidence of complications with radiotherapy and hysterectomy (described in detail here). For patients with similar tumors, the overall rate of major complications is similar with surgery and radiotherapy, although urinary tract complications tend to be more frequent after surgical treatment and bowel complications are more common after radiotherapy. Surgical treatment tends to be preferred for young women with small tumors because it permits preservation of ovarian function and may cause less vaginal shortening.

TABLE 36.2-7. Five-Year Survival Rates for Patients with International Federation of Gynecology and Obstetrics Stage IB Carcinoma of the Cervix

		Radiation Therapy		Radical Hysterectomy	
References	*Year*	Patients	5-Y Survival Rate	Patients	5-Y Survival Rate
Liu and Meigs[254]	1955			116	74%
Piver and Chung[72]	1975			157	80%
Hoskins et al.[255]	1976			194	87%
Boyce et al.[251]	1981	33	63%	103	81%
Volterrani et al.[256]	1983	127	91%	123	89%
Inoue et al.[257]	1984	59	80%	362	91%
Fuller et al.[67]	1989			285	86%
Kenter et al.[258]	1989			178	87%
Lee et al.[66]	1989			237	86%
Alvarez et al.[63]	1991			401	85%
Hopkins et al.[259]	1991			213	89%
Burghardt et al.[260]	1992			443	83%
Montana et al.[261]	1987	197	83%		
Horiot et al.[253]	1988	218	89%		
Coia et al.[262]	1990	168	74%		
Lowrey et al.[252]	1992	130	81%		
Perez et al.[149]	1992	394	85%		
Eifel et al.[148]	1994	1494	81%		
Barillot et al.[152]	1997		83.5%		
Landoni et al.[263]	1997	167[a]	74%	170[a]	74%

[a]Thirteen percent of patients had International Federation of Gynecology and Obstetrics stage IIA disease.

Radiotherapy is often selected for older, postmenopausal women to avoid the morbidity of a major surgical procedure.

Some surgeons have also advocated the use of radical hysterectomy as initial treatment for patients with stage IB2 tumors.[264–266] However, patients who have tumors measuring more than 4 cm in diameter usually have deep stromal invasion and are at high risk for lymph node involvement and parametrial extension. Because patients with these risk factors have an increased rate of pelvic disease recurrence, surgical treatment is usually followed by postoperative irradiation, which means that the patient is exposed to the risks of both treatments. Consequently, many gynecologic and radiation oncologists believe that patients with bulky (stage IB2) carcinomas are better treated with radical radiotherapy.

Two prospective randomized trials[229,230] indicate that patients who are treated with radiation for bulky central disease benefit from concurrent administration of cisplatin-containing chemotherapy. A third study suggests that patients who require postoperative radiation because of findings of lymph node metastasis or involved surgical margins also benefit from concurrent chemoradiation.[231] These studies are discussed in more detail in the following sections.

RADICAL HYSTERECTOMY. The standard surgical treatment for stage IB and stage IIA cervical carcinomas is radical (type III) hysterectomy and bilateral pelvic lymph node dissection. This procedure involves *en bloc* removal of the uterus, cervix, and paracervical, parametrial, and paravaginal tissues to the pelvic side walls bilaterally, with removal of as much of the uterosacral ligaments as possible (see Fig. 36.2-4). The uterine vessels are ligated at their origin, and the proximal third of the vagina and paracolpium are resected. For women younger than 40 to 45 years, the ovaries usually are not removed. If intraoperative findings suggest a need for postoperative pelvic irradiation, the ovaries may be transposed out of the pelvis.

Intraoperative and immediate postoperative complications of radical hysterectomy include blood loss (average 0.8 L), ureterovaginal fistula (1% to 2%), vesicovaginal fistula (less than 1%), pulmonary embolus (1% to 2%), small bowel obstruction (1% to 2%), and postoperative fever secondary to deep vein thrombosis, pulmonary infection, pelvic cellulitis, urinary tract infection, or wound infection (25% to 50%).[267] Subacute complications include lymphocyst formation and lower extremity edema, the risk of which is related to the extent of the node dissection. Lymphocysts may obstruct a ureter, but hydronephrosis usually improves with drainage of the lymphocyst.[268] The risk of complications may be increased in patients who receive preoperative or postoperative irradiation.

Although most patients have transient decreased bladder sensation after radical hysterectomy, with appropriate management severe long-term bladder complications are infrequent. However, chronic bladder hypotonia or atony occurs in approximately 3% to 5% of patients, despite careful postoperative bladder drainage.[269,270] Bladder atony probably results from damage to the bladder's innervation and may be related to the extent of the parametrial and paravaginal dissection.[271,272] Radical hysterectomy may be complicated by stress incontinence, but reported incidences vary widely and may be influenced by the addition of postoperative radiotherapy.[273,274] Patients may also experience constipation and, rarely, chronic obstipation after radical hysterectomy.

RADIOTHERAPY AFTER RADICAL HYSTERECTOMY. The role of postoperative irradiation in patients with cervical carcinoma is still being defined. Most investigators have reported that postoperative irradiation decreases the risk of pelvic recurrence in patients whose tumors have high-risk features (lymph node metastasis, deep stromal invasion, insecure operative margins, or parametrial involvement).[275–280] However, because the patients who received postoperative radiotherapy in these studies were selected for the high-risk features of their tumors, it is difficult to determine the impact of adjuvant irradiation on survival.

The GOG[281] reported results of a prospective trial testing the benefit of adjuvant pelvic irradiation in patients who have an intermediate risk of recurrence after radical hysterectomy for stage IB carcinoma. Patients were eligible if they had at least two of the following risk factors: greater than one-third stromal invasion, lymphatic space involvement, or clinical diameter of at least 4 cm. Patients with metastases to the pelvic lymph nodes were excluded. After radical hysterectomy, 277 patients were randomly assigned to receive 46.0 to 50.6 Gy of adjuvant radiotherapy to the pelvis or no further treatment. Overall, there was a 47% reduction in the risk of recurrence with adjuvant radiotherapy ($P = .008$). In this preliminary analysis, follow-up was too immature for a significance level to be assigned to the overall survival comparison, but there were 18 deaths (13%) in the radiotherapy arm versus 30 (21%) in the radical hysterectomy only arm (relative mortality, 0.64).[281]

Although pelvic irradiation also reduces the risk of recurrence for patients with pelvic lymph node metastases or parametrial involvement, the risk of pelvic and distant recurrence remains high for these women.[278,282] Some authors have hypothesized that the dose of radiation that can be given safely after surgery may be inadequate to control microscopic disease in a surgically disturbed, hypovascular site.[283] If this were true, it would be an argument for primary radiotherapeutic management of tumors with known high-risk features. Preliminary results of a prospective study conducted by the Southwest Oncology Group suggest that administration of cisplatin-containing chemotherapy concurrent with adjuvant pelvic irradiation may improve the rate of control of pelvic disease and the rate of survival for patients with lymph node metastases, parametrial involvement, or involved surgical margins.[231]

The overall risk of major complications (particularly small bowel obstruction) is probably increased in patients who receive postoperative pelvic irradiation, but inconsistencies in the methods of analysis and the relatively small number of patients in most series make studies of this subject difficult to interpret.[263,265,280,284–288] Bandy et al.[289] reported that patients who were irradiated after hysterectomy had more long-term problems with bladder contraction and instability than those treated with surgery alone.

RADICAL RADIOTHERAPY. Radiotherapy also achieves excellent survival and pelvic disease control rates in patients with stage IB cervical cancers. Eifel et al.[148] reported a 5-year disease-specific survival rate of 90% for 701 patients treated with radiation alone for stage IB1 squamous tumors less than 4 cm in diameter. The central and pelvic tumor control rates were 99% and 98%, respectively. Disease-specific survival rates were 86% and 67% for patients with tumors measuring 4.0 to 4.9 cm or 5 cm or more in diameter, respectively. Pelvic tumor control was achieved in 82% of patients with tumors of 5 cm or more in diameter. Perez et al.[149] and Lowrey et al.[252] reported similar excellent disease control rates for patients with stage IB tumors treated with radiotherapy. Survival rates for patients with FIGO stage IIA disease treated with irradiation range between 70% and 85% and are also strongly correlated with tumor size.[149,152,252] For patients with bulky tumors, studies suggest that results may be improved further with concurrent administration of chemotherapy.[229,230]

As with radical surgery, the goal of radiation treatment is to sterilize disease in the cervix, paracervical tissues, and regional lymph nodes in the pelvis. Patients are usually treated with a combination of external-beam irradiation to the pelvis and brachytherapy. Clinicians balance external and intracavitary treatment in different ways for these patients, weighting one or the other component more heavily. However, brachytherapy is a critical element in the curative radiation treatment of all carcinomas of the cervix. Even relatively small tumors that involve multiple quadrants of the cervix are usually treated with total doses of 80 to 85 Gy to point A. The dose may be reduced by 5% to 10% for small superficial tumors. Although patients with small tumors may be treated with somewhat smaller fields than patients with more advanced locoregional disease, care must still be taken to cover adequately the obturator, external iliac, low common iliac, and presacral nodes. Radiation technique is discussed in more detail in the next section.

IRRADIATION FOLLOWED BY HYSTERECTOMY. In a 1969 report from M. D. Anderson Cancer Center, Durrance and colleagues[290] reported a lower pelvic recurrence rate for patients with bulky endocervical tumors (greater than or equal to 6 cm) treated with external-beam and intracavitary irradiation followed by extrafascial hysterectomy than for those treated with radiation alone. Many groups subsequently adopted combined treatment as a standard approach to bulky stage IB or IIA disease. However, in a 1992 update of the M. D. Anderson experience, Thoms and colleagues[157] suggested that the differences observed in earlier reports may have resulted from a tendency to select patients with massive tumors (greater than or equal to 8 cm) or clinically positive nodes for treatment with radiation alone. When these patients were excluded, pelvic disease control rates were similar with the two approaches.

In 1991, Mendenhall et al.[291] reported no difference in pelvic disease control or survival rates for patients treated before or after the University of Florida adopted a policy (in the mid-1970s) of using combined treatment for patients with bulky (greater than or equal to 6 cm) tumors. In a study of 1526 patients with stage IB squamous carcinomas, Eifel and colleagues[148] reported central tumor recurrence rates of less than 10% for tumors as large as 7.0 to 7.9 cm treated with radiation alone, suggesting that the margin for possible improvement with adjuvant hysterectomy is small. Perez and Kao[292] also found that central recurrences were rare if adequate doses of irradiation (greater than 80 Gy to point A) were delivered. Addition of concurrent chemotherapy should further reduce the margin for improvement with adjuvant hysterectomy.[230]

There is, therefore, no clear evidence that adjuvant hysterectomy improves the outcome of patients with a bulky stage IB or IIA tumor, although many clinicians continue to recommend combined treatment.[293] When combined treatment is planned, the dose of intracavitary irradiation is usually reduced by 15% to

TABLE 36.2-8. Response Rates to Neoadjuvant Chemotherapy in Patients with Previously Untreated Locally Advanced Cervical Cancer

Author	*Year*	*No. of Patients*	*Drugs*	*Response Rate*[a]	*Complete Response Rate*
NEOADJUVANT CHEMOTHERAPY FOLLOWED BY RADIATION THERAPY					
Symonds et al.[369]	1987	30	BOP	57%	0
Kirsten et al.[370]	1987	47	PVB	66%	11%
Lara et al.[371]	1990	24	IP	63%	—
Tobias et al.[372]	1990	32	BIP	69%	6%
Chauvergne et al.[373]	1990	75	MtxCVP	43%	1%
Sardi et al.[374]	1990	151	PVB	79%	21%
Park et al.[375]	1991	113	PF[b]	87%	27%
Souhami et al.[376]	1991	39	BOMP	62%	26%
Tattersall et al.[377]	1992	26	PVB	54%	—
Kumar et al.[378]	1994	94	BIP	72%	5%
Tattersall et al.[379]	1995	129	EpP	63%	6%
Sundfør et al.[380]	1996	43	PF	72%	5%
Leborgne et al.[381]	1997	130	BOP	59%	10%
NEOADJUVANT CHEMOTHERAPY FOLLOWED BY RADICAL HYSTERECTOMY					
Fontanelli et al.[384]	1992	27	PB	78%	11%
Dottino et al.[383]	1991	28	BOMP	100%	36%
Kim et al.[382]	1989	35	PVB	89%	46%
Lai et al.[385]	1997	59	BOP	81%	19%
Sardi et al.[299]	1997	102	BOP	88%	
Benedetti-Panici et al.[297]	1991	75	PBMtx	83%	15%

B, bleomycin; C, chlorambucil; Ep, epirubicin; F, 5-fluorouracil; I, ifosfamide; M, mitomycin C; Mtx, methotrexate; O, vincristine; P, cisplatin; V, vinblastine.
[a]Partial plus complete responses.
[b]Nine patients with adenocarcinomas received platinum, cyclophosphamide (Cytoxan), and doxorubicin (Adriamycin).

25%. A type I, extrafascial hysterectomy is usually performed, in which the cervix, adjacent tissues, and a small cuff of the upper vagina in a plane outside the pubocervical fascia are removed. This procedure involves minimal disturbance of the bladder and ureters. Intrafascial hysterectomy is not used for cervical cancer because it does not remove all cervical tissue,[294] and radical hysterectomy is avoided after high-dose irradiation because of an increased risk of urinary tract complications.[295]

In 1991, the GOG completed a prospective randomized trial of irradiation with or without extrafascial hysterectomy in patients with stage IB tumors of 4 cm or more in diameter. Preliminary analysis demonstrated no significant improvement in the survival rate of patients who had an adjuvant hysterectomy.[296]

CHEMOTHERAPY FOLLOWED BY RADICAL SURGERY. During the 1990s, a number of investigators reported the results of treating patients with bulky stage IB or stage II cervical carcinomas with a combination of neoadjuvant chemotherapy followed by radical surgery.[297–299] Neoadjuvant chemotherapy has usually included cisplatin and bleomycin plus one or two other drugs (Table 36.2-8). The results of uncontrolled studies cannot be easily compared with the results with more traditional treatments because the series are small and often have short follow-up and the criteria for patient selection are not always clear. Some or all of the patients in each of these series received postoperative pelvic irradiation, but detailed descriptions of this additional treatment are not always given. Only one prospective randomized trial has compared radical hysterectomy followed by postoperative radiotherapy with chemotherapy followed by surgery and irradiation.[299] In this study, Sardi et al. observed similar outcomes with the two treatments for patients who had tumors smaller than 60 cm^3 (measured ultrasonographically), but they reported a significantly better projected 4-year disease-free survival with neoadjuvant chemotherapy for patients who had larger tumors. However, most patients had been followed for less than 3 years at the time of the report. Ultimately, the cost and morbidity of this triple-modality treatment may only be justified if it proves to be more effective than treatment with radiation or chemoradiation alone. However, studies comparing these approaches have not yet been reported.

Stages IIB, III, and IVA

Radiotherapy is the primary local treatment for most patients with locoregionally advanced cervical carcinoma. The success of treatment depends on a careful balance between external-beam radiotherapy and brachytherapy, optimizing the dose to tumor and normal tissues and the overall duration of treatment. Five-year survival rates of 65% to 75%, 35% to 50%, and 15% to 20% are reported for patients treated with radiotherapy alone for stage IIB, IIIB, and IV tumors, respectively.[134,149,152,154,214,252] In a French Cooperative Group study of

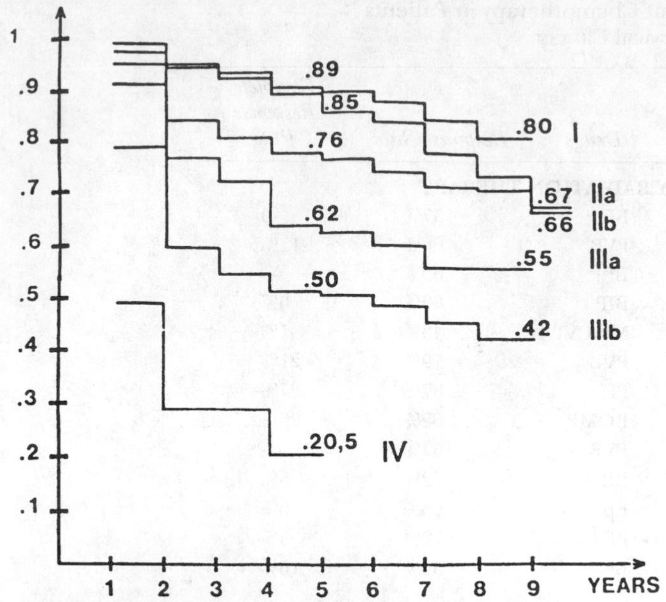

FIGURE 36.2-5. Relationship between International Federation of Gynecology and Obstetrics stage and the actuarial survival rates of 1383 patients with invasive carcinoma of the cervix treated with radiotherapy. (Reprinted from ref. 253, with permission.)

1875 patients treated with radiotherapy according to Fletcher guidelines, Barillot et al.[152] reported 5-year survival rates of 70%, 45%, and 10% for patients with stage IIB, IIIB, and IVA tumors, respectively (Fig. 36.2-5). With appropriate radiotherapy, even patients with massive locoregional disease have a significant chance for cure.

external-beam irradiation is used to deliver a homogeneous dose to the primary cervical tumor and to potential sites of regional spread. An initial course of external irradiation may also improve the efficacy of subsequent intracavitary treatment by shrinking bulky endocervical tumor (bringing it within the range of the high-dose portion of the brachytherapy dose distribution) and by shrinking exophytic tumor that might prevent satisfactory placement of vaginal applicators. For this reason, patients with locally advanced disease usually begin with a course of external-beam treatment. Subsequent brachytherapy exploits the inverse square law to deliver a high dose to the cervix and paracervical tissues while minimizing the dose to adjacent normal tissues.

Although many clinicians delay intracavitary treatment until pelvic irradiation has caused some initial tumor regression, breaks between external-beam and intracavitary therapy should be discouraged, and every effort should be made to complete the entire treatment in less than 7 to 8 weeks. The favorable results documented in reports from large single-institution studies have been based on policies that dictate relatively short overall treatment durations (less than 8 weeks),[300] and several studies in patients with locally advanced cervical cancer have suggested that longer treatment courses are associated with decreased pelvic disease control and survival rates.[301–305]

EXTERNAL-BEAM TECHNIQUE. High-energy photons (15 to 18 MV) are usually preferred for pelvic treatment because they spare superficial tissues that are unlikely to be involved with tumor. At these energies, the pelvis can be treated either with four fields (anterior, posterior, and lateral fields) or with anterior and posterior fields alone (Fig. 36.2-6). When high-energy beams are not available, four fields are usually used because less-penetrating 4- to 6-MV photons often deliver an unacceptably high dose to superficial tissues when only two fields are treated. However, lateral fields must be designed with great care because clinicians' estimates of the location of potential sites of disease on a lateral radiographic view may be inaccurate. In particular, *standard* anterior and posterior borders that have been described in the past may shield regions at risk for microscopic regional disease in the presacral and external iliac nodes and in the presacral and cardinal ligaments; care must also be taken not to underestimate the posterior extent of central cervical disease in patients with bulky tumors.[306–308]

The caudad extent of disease can be determined by placing radiopaque seeds in the cervix or at the lowest extent of vaginal disease. Information gained from radiologic studies can also improve estimates of disease extent. Lymphangiograms are helpful in tailoring blocks, particularly at the anterior border of lateral fields. MRI and CT scans can improve clinicians' understanding of uterine position and thus help clinicians design anterior and posterior field borders. In fact, some investigators have argued that these studies should be obtained routinely for patients with bulky disease to avoid errors in lateral field design.[309] However,

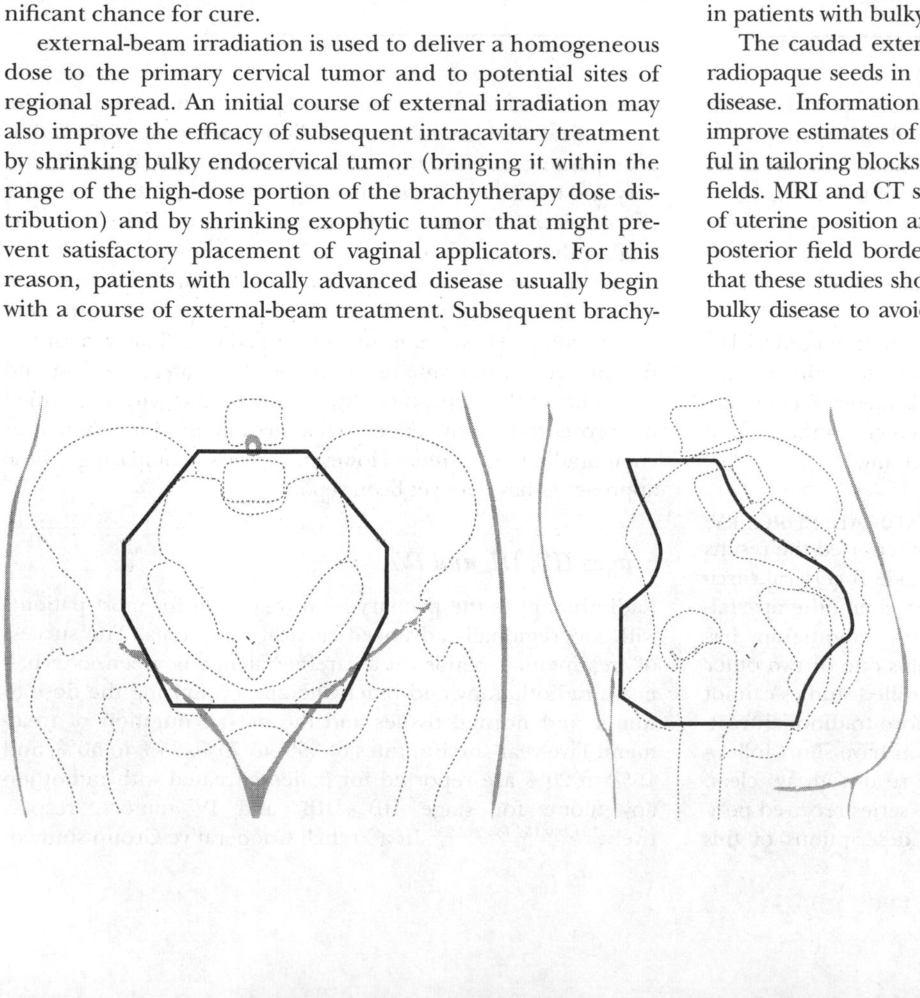

FIGURE 36.2-6. Typical fields used to treat the pelvis with a four-field technique. When lateral fields are used to treat cervical cancers, particular care must be taken to adequately encompass the primary tumor and potential sites of regional spread in the radiation fields.

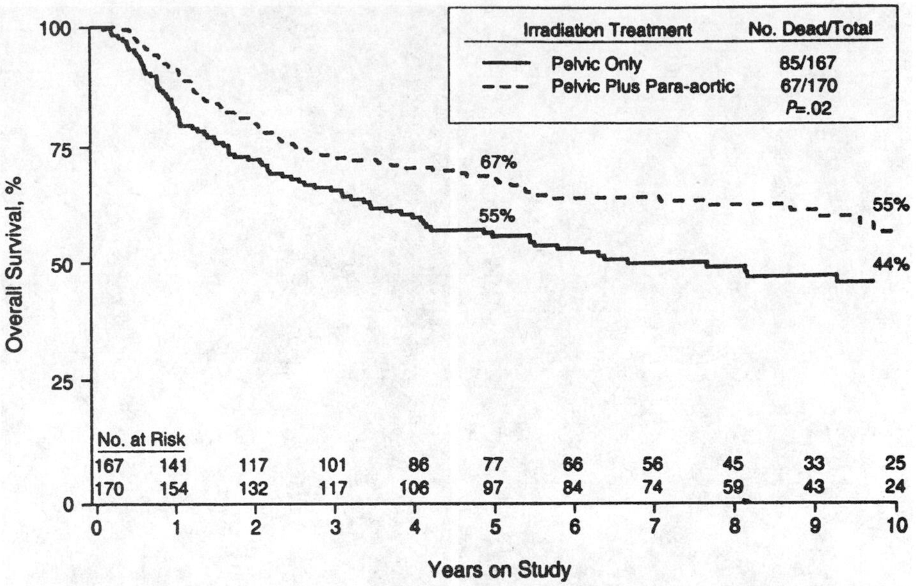

FIGURE 36.2-7. Overall survival rates for patients with stage IB, IIA, or IIB carcinoma of the cervix treated with irradiation to the pelvis alone or to the pelvic and paraaortic nodes on Radiation Therapy Oncology Group study 79-20. (Reprinted from ref. 312, with permission.)

when all these factors are considered, differences in the volume treated with a four-field or a high-energy two-field technique may be small. For this reason, some clinicians prefer to use the simpler technique for patients with bulky tumors.

Tumor response should be evaluated with periodic pelvic examinations to determine the best time to deliver brachytherapy. Some practitioners prefer to maximize the brachytherapy component of treatment and begin as soon as the tumor has responded enough to permit a good placement (with very bulky tumors this may still require greater than or equal to 40 Gy). Subsequent pelvic irradiation is delivered with a central block. A somewhat higher total paracentral dose can be delivered with this approach, but greater reliance is placed on the complex match between the brachytherapy dose distribution and the border of the central shield. This may result in overdoses to medial structures such as the ureters[310] or underdosage of posterior uterosacral disease.[311] For these reasons, other clinicians prefer to give an initial dose of 40 to 45 Gy to the whole pelvis, believing that the ability to deliver a homogeneous distribution to the entire region at risk for microscopic disease and the additional tumor shrinkage achieved before brachytherapy outweighs other considerations. However, external-beam doses of more than 40 to 50 Gy to the central pelvis tend to compromise the dose deliverable to paracentral tissues and increase the risk of late complications.[154]

ROLE OF PARAAORTIC IRRADIATION. The role of extended field irradiation in the treatment of cervix cancer is still being defined. Numerous small series of patients with documented paraaortic node involvement demonstrate that some enjoy long-term survival (see Table 36.2-5).[77,80,140,161–164,166,167] Patients with microscopic involvement have a better survival than do those with gross lymphadenopathy, but even 10% to 15% of patients with gross lymphadenopathy appear to be curable with aggressive management. Survival is also strongly correlated with the bulk of central disease. A 1991 study by Cunningham et al.[167] reported a 48% 5-year survival rate in patients who had paraaortic node involvement discovered at exploration for radical hysterectomy that was then aborted. This experience with patients who had small, radiocontrollable primary disease demonstrates that patients with paraaortic node metastases can often be cured if their primary disease can be sterilized. This indicates that patients may have extensive regional spread without distant metastases and provides an argument for surgical staging in high-risk patients.

Two randomized prospective trials have addressed the role of prophylactic paraaortic irradiation in patients without known paraaortic node involvement. In a study conducted by the Radiation Therapy Oncology Group, 367 patients with primary stage IIB or stage IB or IIA tumors more than 4 cm in diameter were randomly assigned to receive either standard pelvic radiotherapy or extended-field radiotherapy before brachytherapy.[312] No consistent method was used to evaluate the paraaortic nodes. For the 337 evaluable patients, absolute survival was significantly better for those treated with extended fields than for those treated with standard pelvic radiotherapy (67% vs. 55% at 5 years; $P = .02$) (Fig. 36.2-7). There was no significant difference in disease-free survival ($P = .56$).

A second trial, from the European Organization for Research and Treatment of Cancer, involved a similar randomization between pelvic irradiation and extended fields but had very different eligibility criteria.[313] This study included patients with bulky stage IIB (involving distal vagina or lateral parametrium) and III disease and patients with stage I disease or less bulky stage IIB disease who had positive pelvic nodes on lymphangiography or at surgery. The 4-year disease-free survival rates for patients treated with pelvic or extended fields were not significantly different (49.8% and 53.3%, respectively). However, the rate of paraaortic node recurrence was significantly higher in the pelvic field group, and for patients in whom local control was achieved, the rate of distant metastases was 2.8 times greater if treatment was with pelvic irradiation only ($P < .01$).

Both studies revealed an increased rate of enteric complications in patients treated with extended fields. In the Radiation Therapy Oncology Group study,[312] most small bowel obstructions occurred in patients who had undergone pretreatment transperitoneal staging. The European Organization for Research and

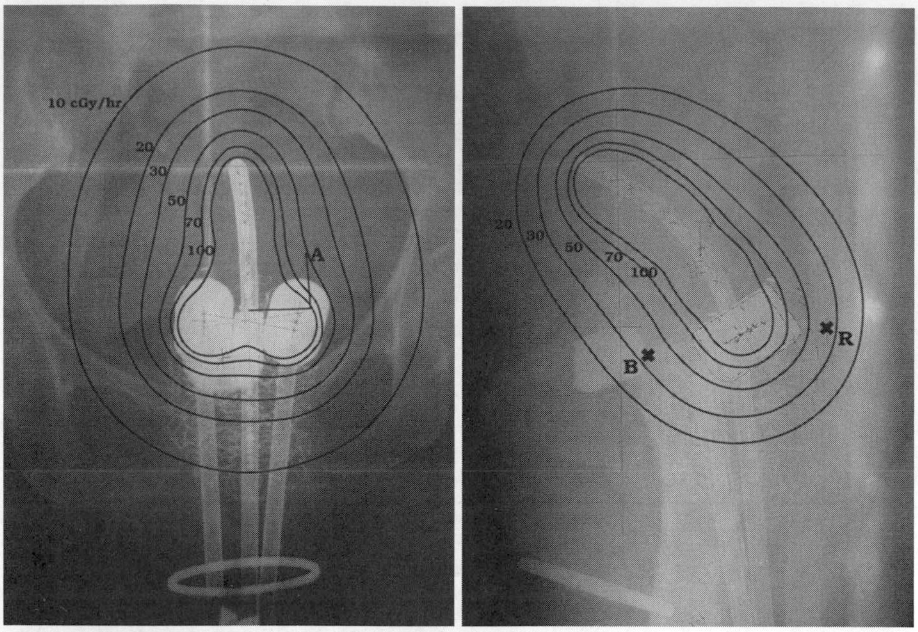

FIGURE 36.2-8. Posteroanterior and lateral views of a Fletcher-Suit-Delclos applicator system in a patient with invasive carcinoma of the cervix. Units on the isodose contours are cGy/h. A, point A; B, bladder reference point; R, rectal reference point.

Treatment of Cancer[313] did not mention a relationship between surgical staging and enteric complications.

Taken together, these data clearly indicate that some paraaortic metastases are not detected by radiographic studies and that patients with occult disease can be cured if the paraaortic nodes are included in radiation fields. However, the addition of concurrent chemotherapy to the regimen of many patients with locally advanced disease increases the importance of careful selection of patients for large field irradiation because of the greater acute toxicity when chemotherapy is combined with extended-field radiotherapy.[314–316]

BRACHYTHERAPY TECHNIQUE. Fletcher described three conditions that should be met for successful cervical brachytherapy: (1) the geometry of the radioactive sources must prevent underdosed regions on and around the cervix, (2) an adequate dose must be delivered to the paracervical areas, and (3) mucosal tolerance must be respected.[317] Although some clinicians have proposed a number of variations on the low-rate intracavitary brachytherapy techniques practiced at M. D. Anderson, Fletcher's conditions continue to dictate the character, intensity, and timing of brachytherapy for cervical cancer.

Brachytherapy is usually delivered using afterloading applicators that are placed in the uterine cavity and vagina. A number of different intracavitary systems have been used; in the United States, variations of the Fletcher-Suit-Delclos low dose-rate system are still used most commonly.[293,317–320] The intrauterine tandem and vaginal applicators are carefully positioned, usually with the patient under anesthesia, to provide an optimal relationship between the system and adjacent tumor and normal tissues. Vaginal packing is used to hold the tandem and colpostats in place and to maximize the distance between the sources and the bladder and rectum. Radiographs should be obtained at the time of insertion to verify accurate placement, and the system should be repositioned if positioning can be improved. Encapsulated radioactive sources are inserted in the applicators after the patient has returned to her hospital bed, reducing exposure to personnel during applicator placement. Remote afterloading devices that further reduce personnel exposure are often used in departments that treat many patients with gynecologic disease. Although ^{226}Ra was used to treat most patients before the 1980s, it has gradually been replaced by ^{137}Cs, which produces a similar dose distribution and avoids the radiation protection problems caused by the radon gas by-product of radium decay.

Brachytherapy Dose. Ideal placement of the uterine tandem and vaginal ovoids produces a pear-shaped distribution, delivering a high dose to the cervix and paracervical tissues and a reduced dose to the rectum and bladder (Fig. 36.2-8).

Treatment dose has been specified in a number of ways, making it difficult to compare experiences. Paracentral doses are most frequently expressed at a single point, usually designated *point A.* This reference point has been calculated in a number of different ways, but it is usually placed 2 cm lateral and 2 cm superior to the external cervical os, in the central plane of the intracavitary system (see Fig. 36.2-8). Point A lies approximately at the crossing of the ureter and the uterine artery, but it bears no consistent relationship to the tumor or target volume. Point A was originally developed as part of the Manchester treatment system (a modification of the earlier Paris system). It was meant to be used in the context of a detailed set of rules governing the placement and loading of the intracavitary system. Today this context is often lost.

Other measures have been used to describe the intensity of intracavitary treatment. *Mg-hrs* or *mgRaEq-hrs* are proportional to the dose of radiation at relatively distant points from the system and therefore give a sense of the dose to the whole pelvis. In 1985 the International Commission on Radiation Units and Measurements recommended use of total reference air Kerma, expressed in mGy at 1 m, as an alternative to mg-hrs that allows for the use of various radionuclides.[321] The International Commission on Radiation Units and Measurements also defined reference points for estimating the dose to the bladder and rectum. These points have been widely, although not universally, accepted. Although normal tissue reference points provide useful information about the dose to a portion of normal tissue, several studies have demonstrated that they consistently underestimate the maximum dose to those tissues.[322–324]

Whatever system of dose specification is used, emphasis should always be placed on optimizing the relationship between the intracavitary applicators and the cervical tumor and other pelvic tissues. Source strengths and positions should be carefully chosen to provide optimal tumor coverage without exceeding normal tissue tolerance. However, optimized source placement can rarely correct for a poorly positioned applicator.

A detailed description of the characteristics of an ideal intracavitary system and of the considerations that influence source strength and position are beyond the scope of this chapter but can be found elsewhere.[320,321,325] However, an effort should always be made to deliver at least 85 Gy (with low dose-rate brachytherapy) to point A for patients with bulky central disease. If the intracavitary placement has been optimized, this can usually be accomplished without exceeding a dose of 75 Gy to the bladder reference point or 70 Gy to the rectal reference point, doses that are usually associated with an acceptably low risk of major complications.[326,327] The dose to the surface of the lateral wall of the apical vagina should not usually exceed 130 to 140 Gy.[325] Suboptimal placements occasionally force compromises in the dose to tumor or normal tissues. To choose a treatment that optimizes the therapeutic ratio in these circumstances requires experience and a detailed understanding of factors that influence tumor control and normal tissue complications.

A total dose (external-beam and intracavitary) of 50 to 55 Gy appears to be sufficient to sterilize microscopic disease in the pelvic nodes in most patients. It is customary to boost the dose to a total of 60 to 65 Gy in lymph nodes known to contain gross disease and in heavily involved parametria.

Brachytherapy Dose Rate. Traditionally, cervical brachytherapy has been performed with sources that yield a dose rate at point A of approximately 40 to 50 cGy/h. These low dose rates permit repair of sublethal cellular injury, preferentially spare normal tissues, and optimize the therapeutic ratio. In an effort to reduce the 3 to 4 days of hospitalization needed to deliver an appropriate dose of low dose-rate irradiation, some investigators have explored the use of *intermediate* dose-rate brachytherapy (80 to 100 cGy/h). However, in a randomized trial, Haie-Meder et al.[328] reported a significant increase in complications when the dose rate was doubled from 40 to 80 cGy/h, indicating that the total dose must be reduced and the therapeutic ratio of treatment may be compromised with higher dose rates. On the basis of laboratory studies, Amdur and Bedford have suggested that differences in the magnitude of the dose-rate effect between tumor and normal tissues may in part reflect differences in the half-times for repair of sublethal radiation damage.[329]

During the past two decades, computer technology has made it possible to deliver brachytherapy at very high dose rates (greater than 100 cGy/min) using a high-activity ^{60}Co or ^{192}Ir source and remote afterloading. High dose-rate intracavitary therapy is now being used for radical treatment of cervical cancer by a number of groups, including several in Japan, Canada, and Europe, and more recently by some groups in the United States.[330–338] Clinicians have found this approach attractive because it does not require that patients be hospitalized and may be more convenient for the patient and the physician. However, unless it is heavily fractionated, high dose-rate brachytherapy loses the radiobiologic advantage of low dose-rate treatment, potentially narrowing the therapeutic window for complication-free cure.[339,340] Advocates of high dose-rate treatment disagree about the number of fractions and total dose that should be delivered. Published experiences suggest that survival rates are roughly similar to those achieved with traditional low dose-rate treatment, but these experiences are difficult to compare because of the same potential problems of selection bias that confound other nonrandomized comparisons.[336,339] Many of the retrospective reviews provide incomplete descriptions of tumor and treatment details.[336] Two purported randomized trials[335,337] also have been criticized for methodologic flaws. The use of high dose-rate brachytherapy for cervical cancer continues to be a source of controversy.

INTERSTITIAL BRACHYTHERAPY. Several groups have advocated the use of interstitial brachytherapy to treat patients whose anatomy or tumor distribution make it difficult to obtain an ideal intracavitary placement. Interstitial implants are usually placed transperineally, guided by a Lucite template that encourages parallel placement of hollow needles that penetrate the cervix and paracervical spaces; needles are usually loaded with ^{192}Ir. Advocates of the procedure describe the relatively homogeneous dose distribution achieved with this method, the ease of inserting implants in patients whose uteri are difficult to probe, and the ability to place sources directly into the parametrium. Early reports were enthusiastic, describing these theoretical advantages and high initial local control rates, but these early reports rarely included sufficient numbers of patients or had long enough follow-up to provide long-term survival rates.[341–345]

In two of the larger early series, Syed and colleagues reported an encouraging projected 5-year survival rate of 53% for 26 patients with stage IIIB disease,[345] and Martinez and colleagues reported an 83% local control rate in 37 patients with stage IIB and IIIB disease.[344] However, survival results from two more recent reports have been disappointing. In a 1995 review of the combined experiences of Stanford and the Joint Center for Radiation Therapy, the 3-year disease-free survival rates for patients with stage IIB and IIIB disease were only 36% and 18%, respectively. Local control rates were 22% and 44%, respectively, and for patients with local control, the rate of complications requiring surgical intervention was high.[346] A 1997 report of the Irvine experience also described disappointing survival rates of 21% and 29%, respectively, for stage IIB and IIIB, again with a high rate of major complications.

Several groups have been exploring the use of transrectal ultrasound, MRI, or laparoscopic guidance,[347–349] interstitial hyperthermia,[350] and high dose-rate interstitial therapy[351] to improve local control and complication rates. However, outside of an investigational setting, interstitial treatment of primary cervical cancers should probably be limited to patients who cannot accommodate intrauterine brachytherapy and patients with distal vaginal disease that requires a boost with interstitial brachytherapy.

COMPLICATIONS OF RADICAL RADIOTHERAPY. During radiotherapy of the pelvis, most patients have mild fatigue and mild to moderate diarrhea that usually is controllable with antidiarrheal medications; some patients have mild bladder irritation. When extended fields are treated, patients may have nausea, gastric irritation, and mild depression of peripheral blood counts. Acute symptoms may be increased in patients receiving concurrent chemotherapy. Unless the ovaries have been transposed, all premenopausal patients who receive pelvic radiotherapy experience ovarian failure by the completion of treatment.

Perioperative complications of intracavitary therapy include uterine perforation, fever, and the usual risks of anesthesia. Thromboembolisms are rare.[352,353] In a review of 4043 patients who had 7662 intracavitary applications for cervical cancer, Jhingran and Eifel[354] reported 11 patients (0.3%) with thromboembolisms, four of which were fatal. All four fatal pulmonary embolisms were in patients with advanced pelvic wall disease.

Estimates of the risk of late complications of radical radiotherapy vary according to the grading system, duration of follow-up, method of calculation, treatment method, and prevalence of risk factors in the study population. However, most reports quote an overall risk of major complications (requiring transfusion, hospitalization, or surgical intervention) of 5% to 15%. In a report from the Patterns of Care Study, Lanciano et al.[355] reported an actuarial risk of 8% at 3 years. In a study of 1784 patients with stage IB disease, Eifel et al.[356] reported an overall actuarial risk of major complications of 7.7% at 5 years. Although the actuarial risk was greatest during the first 3 years of follow-up, there was a continuing risk to surviving patients of approximately 0.3% per year, resulting in an overall actuarial risk of 14% at 20 years. In a 1999 review of 1456 patients treated with radiation alone, Perez et al.[326] reported a crude incidence of severe complications (requiring surgical intervention or more than 4 weeks of hospitalization) of 5% for patients with stage IB cervical cancer and 9% to 10% for patients with more advanced disease.

During the first 3 years after treatment, rectal complications are most common and include bleeding, stricture, ulceration, and fistula. In the study by Eifel and colleagues,[356] the risk of major rectosigmoid complications was 2.3% at 5 years. Major gastrointestinal complications were rare 3 years or more after treatment, but a constant low risk of urinary tract complications persisted for many years (Fig. 36.2-9). The actuarial risk of developing a fistula of any type was 1.7% at 5 years.

Small bowel obstruction is an infrequent complication of standard radiotherapy for patients without special risk factors. The risk is increased dramatically in patients who have undergone transperitoneal lymph node dissection.[141,355,356] However, there appears to be little added risk if the operation is performed with a retroperitoneal approach.[141] Other factors that can increase the risk of small bowel complications in patients treated for cervical cancer include pelvic inflammatory disease, thin body habitus, and the use of high doses or large volumes of external-beam irradiation, particularly with low-energy treatment beams and large daily fraction sizes.[154,355-358]

Most patients treated with radical radiotherapy have some agglutination and telangiectasia of the apical vagina. More significant vaginal shortening can occur, particularly in elderly, postmenopausal women and those with extensive tumors treated with a high dose of irradiation.[356,359] Vaginal function can be optimized with appropriate estrogen support and vaginal dilatation.

CONCURRENT CHEMORADIATION. Reports of five prospective randomized trials[229–233] have provided compelling evidence that the addition of concurrent cisplatin-containing chemotherapy to standard radiotherapy improves the pelvic disease control and survival rates in selected patients with local, regionally advanced cervical cancer. Although these studies differed in their inclusion criteria, treatment specifics, and control treatments, each demonstrated reduction in the relative risk of recurrence of 30% to 50% with cisplatin-containing chemoradiation (Table 36.2-9).

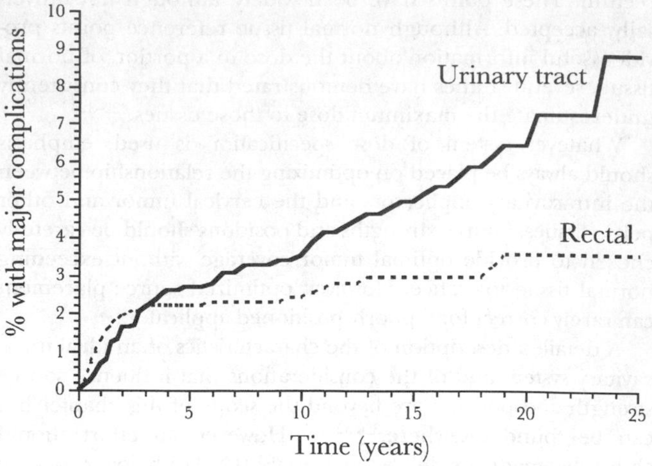

FIGURE 36.2-9. Rates of major rectal and urinary tract complications in 1784 patients with stage IB carcinomas of the cervix treated with radiotherapy. Complication rates were calculated actuarially, and patients who died without experiencing a major complication were censored at the time of death. (Reprinted from ref. 356, with permission.)

Individual investigators and multiinstitutional groups have been exploring combinations of chemotherapy and radiation in patients with cervical cancer for more than 25 years. However, until relatively recently, studies had failed to demonstrate a clear benefit. An early GOG study compared radiation alone with radiation and concurrent hydroxyurea.[360] This study appeared to show some benefit from the combination, but it was criticized because many patients were treated without brachytherapy or with very low doses of radiation and because 93 (49%) of the 190 patients randomized were excluded from the analysis as ineligible or unevaluable. Nevertheless, the GOG continued to include hydroxyurea in the control arm of subsequent studies. The first of these[361] compared hydroxyurea (80 mg/kg given twice per week during external-beam irradiation) with misonidazole, a nitroimidazole hypoxic cell sensitizer that has since been demonstrated to be of no benefit in several trials that compared misonidazole with a placebo.[202,204] Final analysis of this study[361] showed a marginal advantage in progression-free survival (P = .05) and survival (P = .07) for patients treated with hydroxyurea.

Two subsequent GOG studies[232,233] randomly assigned patients with stage IIB to IVA disease to receive either hydroxyurea or cisplatin-containing chemotherapy during external-beam irradiation. All three of the cisplatin-containing arms had local control and survival rates superior to those for the control (hydroxyurea and radiation) arms. In a third study,[229] patients with stage IB tumors measuring at least 4 cm in diameter were randomly assigned to receive radiation alone or radiation plus weekly cisplatin before extrafascial hysterectomy. Patients who received cisplatin were more likely to have a com-

TABLE 36.2-9. Prospective Randomized Trials That Investigate the Role of Concurrent Radiotherapy and Cisplatin-Containing Chemotherapy for Patients with Loco-Regionally Advanced Cervical Cancer

Authors	*Eligibility*	*Chemotherapy in Investigational Arm*	*Chemotherapy in Control Arm*	*Relative Risk of Recurrence (90% Confidence Interval)*	*P*
Rose et al.[232]	FIGO IIB–IVA, PA nodes negative (dissection)	Cisplatin, 40 mg/m^2 (weeks 1–6)	Hydroxyurea, 3 g/m^2 (twice weekly, weeks 1–6)	0.57 (0.42–0.78)	<.001
		Cisplatin, 50 mg/m^2 (days 1 and 29) 5-Fluorouracil, 4 g/m^2 (96-hour infusion, days 1, 29) Hydroxyurea, 2 g/m^2 (twice weekly, weeks 1–6)	Hydroxyurea, 3 g/m^2 (twice weekly, weeks 1–6)	0.55 (0.40–0.75)	<.001
Morris et al.[230]	FIGO IB–IIA (≥5 cm), IIB–IVA, or pelvic lymph nodes positive PA nodes negative (dissection or lymphangiogram)	Cisplatin, 75 mg/m^2 (days 1 and 22, and with second brachytherapy) 5-Fluorouracil, 4 g/m^2 (96-hour infusion days 1, 22, and with second brachytherapy)	None[a]	0.48 (0.35–0.66)	<.001
Keys et al.[229]	FIGO IB (≥4 cm) PA nodes negative (computed tomography or lymphangiogram)	Cisplatin, 40 mg/m^2 (weeks 1–6)[b]	None[b]	0.51 (0.34–0.75)	.001
Whitney et al.[233]	FIGO IIB–IVA, PA nodes negative (dissection)	Cisplatin, 50 mg/m^2 (days 1 and 29) 5-Fluorouracil, 4 g/m^2 (96-hour infusion days 1, 29)	Hydroxyurea, 80 mg/kg (twice weekly during external beam RT)	0.79 (0.62–0.99)	.03
Peters et al.[231]	FIGO I–IIA after radical hysterectomy with findings of: 1) Pelvic lymph node metastases 2) Positive margins 3) Parametrial involvement PA nodes negative	Cisplatin, 70 mg/m^2 (days 1 and 29) 5-Fluorouracil, 4 g/m^2 (96-hour infusion days 1, 29)	None	0.50 (0.29–0.84)	.01

FIGO, International Federation of Gynecology and Obstetrics; PA, paraaortic; RT, radiotherapy.
[a]Patients in control arm had prophylactic paraaortic irradiation.
[b]All patients had extrafascial hysterectomy after radiotherapy.

plete histologic response and were more likely to be disease free at the time of preliminary analysis. A fourth study, cosponsored by the Southwest Oncology Group and the GOG,[231] included patients who were treated with radical hysterectomy and were found to have pelvic lymph node metastases, positive margins, or parametrial involvement. Patients were randomly assigned to receive postoperative pelvic irradiation alone or combined with cisplatin and 5-fluorouracil (5-FU). In a preliminary analysis, patients who received chemotherapy in this study also had a better disease-free survival rate.

During this time, the Radiation Therapy Oncology Group[230] also conducted a trial in which radiotherapy alone (including prophylactic paraaortic irradiation) was compared with pelvic irradiation plus concurrent cisplatin and 5-FU. This is the only study in which chemotherapy was administered during both the brachytherapy and external-beam components of treatment. The results of this trial were released early when highly significant differences were detected in the rates of local control, distant metastasis, overall survival, and disease-free survival favoring the treatment arm that included chemotherapy. Although acute toxic effects of treatment were greater with chemotherapy, the dose and duration of radiation were similar in the two arms, and in an early analysis, there was no significant difference in the incidence of late treatment-related complications.

This work clearly demonstrates that the addition of concurrent cisplatin-containing chemotherapy benefited patients with locally advanced cervical cancer who were treated with radiation in these studies. However, all of the studies explicitly excluded patients with evidence of paraaortic lymph node metastases, poor performance status, or impaired renal function. In the future, clinicians will be challenged to determine how these favorable results can be generalized to patients with cervical cancer who may not have been included in the prospective trials because of severe medical or social problems and to the developing nations where invasive cervical cancer is epidemic.

These studies raise other interesting questions that will undoubtedly be the subjects of future studies. Of four different cisplatin-containing regimens, only two were compared directly.

TABLE 36.2-10. Results of Prospective Randomized Trials That Compared Neoadjuvant Chemotherapy Followed by Radiation Therapy with Radiation Therapy Alone in Patients with Locally Advanced Cervical Cancer

					Survival Rate			
Author	*Year*	*Patients*	*Stages*	*Drugs*	Chemotherapy + Radiation Therapy (%)	Radiation Therapy Alone (%)	*P*	*End Point*
Kumar et al.[378]	1994	184	IIB–IVA	BIP	38	43	0.5	OS at 32 mo
Tattersall et al.[377]	1992	71	IIB–IVA	PVB	44[a]	40[a]	NS	OS at 48 mo
Chauvergne et al.[373]	1990	107	IIIB	MtxCVP	47[a]	50[a]	NS	OS at 48 mo
Tattersall et al.[379]	1995	260	IIB–IVA	EpP	50[a]	69[a]	0.02	OS at 36 mo
Sundfør et al.[380]	1996	94	IIIB–IVA	PF	34[a]	37[a]	0.9	OS at 48 mo
Leborgne et al.[381]	1997	96	IB2–IVA	BOP	38	45	0.4	Disease-free survival at 60 mo
Souhami et al.[376]	1991	107	IIIB	BOMP	23	39	0.02	OS at 60 mo

B, bleomycin; C, chlorambucil; Ep, epirubicin; F, 5-fluorouracil; I, ifosphamide; M, mitomycin C; Mtx, methotrexate; O, vincristine; OS, overall survival; P, cisplatinum; V, vinblastine.
[a]Percentages were estimated from survival curves.

It is unclear from the results which regimen achieves the most favorable therapeutic ratio and whether the inclusion of 5-FU in several of the studies contributed importantly to the results. However, smaller studies have suggested that 5-FU is an effective radiation sensitizer in cervical cancers,[362,363] and the GOG is currently comparing radiation plus continuous-infusion 5-FU with radiation and cisplatin in patients with locally advanced disease. Other drugs that are being studied for their radiosensitizing effects in patients with advanced disease are paclitaxel,[364] carboplatin,[365] and mitomycin C.[366,367] Extended-field irradiation (including the aortic nodes) has proven effective in the treatment of patients with known or suspected aortic node metastasis,[312] but the role of extended-field irradiation needs to be clarified in the context of these new results. Combinations of extended-field irradiation and chemotherapy appear to be feasible, but the acute toxicity is considerable, and late toxicity may be greater than with extended-field radiation alone.[314,316,368]

NEOADJUVANT CHEMOTHERAPY. A number of investigators have explored the use of neoadjuvant chemotherapy for locally advanced cervical carcinoma, trying to exploit the encouraging response rates that have been reported for multiple-agent, cisplatin-containing regimens in previously untreated patients (see Table 36.2-8).[297,299,369–385] To test this approach, a number of prospective randomized trials were conducted comparing radiation alone with neoadjuvant chemotherapy followed by radiation (Table 36.2-10).[373,376–381] Unfortunately, of the seven trials that have been published, five[373,377,378,380,381] demonstrated no benefit from neoadjuvant therapy and two[376,379] demonstrated a significantly better survival rate with radiation alone. In one small trial from South America,[376] patients treated with bleomycin, vincristine, methotrexate, and cisplatin followed by radiation had a significantly poorer survival rate than did those treated with radiation alone. In addition, patients who failed to complete radiotherapy (and were excluded from the analysis) were more frequent in the neoadjuvant chemotherapy arm. Bleomycin toxicity (responsible for four of the deaths) contributed to the poor survival rate of patients treated with neoadjuvant chemotherapy in this study. Tattersall and colleagues[379] compared neoadjuvant chemotherapy (cisplatin and epirubicin) followed by radiotherapy with radiotherapy alone. This study was discontinued when an interim analysis revealed a significantly poorer outcome for patients who received neoadjuvant chemotherapy ($P = .02$).

In another interesting study, published by Chauvergne and colleagues,[373] patients who had a complete or partial response to chemotherapy followed by radiotherapy had a significantly better outcome than did those who had a poorer response to neoadjuvant chemotherapy. However, there were no significant differences in the overall response rates, disease-free survival rates, or median survival between patients treated with neoadjuvant chemotherapy and those treated with radiation alone.

In summary, despite the high rate of response of locally advanced cervical cancers to initial chemotherapy, none of the randomized studies reported to date has demonstrated an improvement in outcome when neoadjuvant chemotherapy was added to radical radiotherapy. In many ways this recapitulates the experience with treatment of locally advanced head and neck cancers, in which it has been hypothesized that the failure of neoadjuvant chemotherapy to influence outcome may reflect cross-resistance of tumor cells to drugs and radiation or accelerated repopulation of tumor clones induced by neoadjuvant chemotherapy.[386–388]

More recently, a number of investigators have begun to explore combinations of neoadjuvant chemotherapy with radical surgery in patients with bulky central disease.[297,299,383–385,389] Only one randomized trial addressing this approach has been published,[299] although a number of other studies have been completed or are in progress. In their study, Sardi and colleagues[299] randomly assigned 205 patients to receive radical hysterectomy with or without neoadjuvant chemotherapy. All patients received postoperative pelvic irradiation. The authors reported a higher rate of resectability (100% vs. 85%) and a better survival rate (81% vs. 66%) for patients treated with neoadjuvant chemotherapy. There have not yet been any comparisons between this approach and radiotherapy alone or combined with chemotherapy.

TABLE 36.2-11. Cytotoxic Drugs Active Against Squamous Cell Carcinoma of the Cervix (Response Rate ≥15%)

Drug	*Response Rate*[a] *(%)*
Cyclophosphamide[393,394]	38/251 (15%)
Chlorambucil[393,411]	11/44 (25%)
Dibromodulcitol[396,397]	23/102 (23%)
Galactitol[398]	7/36 (19%)
Ifosfamide[400–403,405,430]	47/189 (25%)
Melphalan[393]	4/20 (20%)
Carboplatin[406]	27/175 (15%)
Cisplatin[408–412]	190/185 (23%)
Doxorubicin[413–419]	45/266 (17%)
Porfiromycin[420]	17/78 (22%)
Baker's Antifol[421]	5/32 (16%)
5-Fluorouracil[419,421,422]	29/142 (20%)
Methotrexate[413,419]	17/96 (18%)
Vincristine[420]	10/55 (18%)
Vindesine[420]	5/21 (24%)
Vinorelbine[426]	6/33 (18%)
Irenotecan[423–425]	28/142 (20%)
Hexamethylmelamine[420]	12/64 (19%)
Razoxane[427]	5/28 (18%)
Topotecan[691]	8/43 (19%)
Paclitaxel[428,429]	17/84 (20%)

[a]Combined complete and partial response rate.

INTRAARTERIAL CHEMOTHERAPY. Intraarterial infusion of chemotherapeutic agents delivered in the neoadjuvant setting, concurrent with radiotherapy, or as salvage treatment for recurrent disease has generated interest for some years because of the distinct arterial supply to the central pelvis.[362,390–392] A number of drugs have been used in small pilot studies, but 5-FU and cisplatin have been the most popular in this setting. Unfortunately, this technique is difficult and invasive, the toxicity reported in some series has been substantial, and the results have been variable in several small series of patients. However, occasional optimistic reports have maintained some interest in this approach, particularly for concurrent intraarterial chemotherapy and irradiation.

Stage IVB

Patients who present with disseminated disease almost always have incurable disease. The care of these patients must emphasize palliation of symptoms with appropriate pain medications and localized radiotherapy. Tumors may respond to chemotherapy, but responses are usually short.

SINGLE-AGENT CHEMOTHERAPY. Many drugs have been studied for their activity in patients with recurrent or metastatic carcinoma of the cervix. Approximately 20 have yielded response rates (partial and complete) of at least 15% and may be of therapeutic value (Table 36.2-11).[363,393–429]

Several of the platinum compounds have been evaluated in greater detail. Cisplatin has been studied in a variety of doses and schedules.[409,411,412] These studies have demonstrated activity of the drug at a dose of 50 mg/m^2 given intravenously at a rate of 1 mg/min every 3 weeks. Although there appears to be a small but statistically significant increase in the response rate with a doubling of the dose to 100 mg/m^2, this has not resulted in a detectable improvement in the rates of progression-free or overall survival. More prolonged infusion of the same dose over 24 hours yields a similar response rate with less nausea and vomiting, although the development of more effective antiemetic agents reduces the clinical importance of this observation. The response rates with other platinum compounds (i.e., carboplatin and iproplatin) are lower than those observed with cisplatin, which remains the platinum compound of choice for patients with cervical carcinomas.

Ifosfamide has been studied as a single agent in patients with recurrent cervical cancer in at least five phase II trials.[399,402,403,405,430] Response rates ranged between 33% and 50% in three studies that were conducted in patients who had received no previous chemotherapy.[399,403,405,430] However, the response rates were much lower in two phase II trials that included patients who had received prior systemic chemotherapy, with only three partial responses (8%) in 36 patients.[399,402]

COMBINATION CHEMOTHERAPY. Most reports of combination chemotherapy for carcinoma of the cervix have described small, uncontrolled phase II trials of drug combinations that have included at least some agents with known activity. Although response rates have varied widely, data from these phase II studies provide no firm evidence that any of the studied combinations are superior to single-agent therapy for patients with disseminated or recurrent cervical cancer.[431] However, combinations based on ifosfamide and cisplatin and those based on 5-FU and cisplatin have attracted significant interest and deserve further discussion.

Several small phase II studies have evaluated treatment with combinations of ifosfamide and either cisplatin or carboplatin in patients who had not received prior radiotherapy. Response rates for these combinations ranged between 50% and 62% (Table 36.2-12).[404,432–434] A number of investigators have combined bleomycin with ifosfamide and a platinum compound. Three studies that included patients who had not had prior radiotherapy reported response rates of 65% to 100%.[435–437] Reports of treatment with these drugs in previously irradiated patients have yielded mixed but generally lower response rates of between 13% and 72%.[434–438]

Combinations of cisplatin and continuous infusion 5-FU,[439–441] cisplatin and paclitaxel,[442] or cisplatin and vinorelbine[443] also produce high response rates in previously untreated patients. Again, response rates decrease significantly if patients have had previous irradiation.[440,444]

In 1996, the GOG[445] reported results of a large prospective randomized trial comparing cisplatin alone with cisplatin plus ifosfamide and cisplatin plus mitolactol in patients with advanced or recurrent cervical cancers. The addition of ifosfamide to cisplatin improved the response rate (33% vs. 19%, $P = .02$) and progression-free survival rate (4.6 vs. 3.2 months, $P < .05$), but was associated with significantly greater toxicity (leukopenia, peripheral neuropathy, renal toxicity, and encephalopathy) and did not significantly improve the overall median survival. The addition of mitolactol did not improve the response rate or survival duration. Other phase III randomized trials that are ongoing or have been completed recently will evaluate the benefit of adding bleomycin to cisplatin and

TABLE 36.2-12. Platinum-Containing Chemotherapy Combinations Used to Treat Cervical Carcinomas: Contrast between Results in Patients Treated before or after Pelvic Irradiation

Combination	*Responses (%)*
NO PRIOR RADIOTHERAPY	
Cisplatin (20 mg/m^2, d 1–5), ifosfamide[a] (1.5 g/m^2, d 1–5)[432]	15/24 (62%)
Cisplatin (20 mg/m^2, d l–5), ifosfamide (2.5 g/m^2, d l–5)[404]	15/30 (50%)
Carboplatin (300 mg/m^2, d l), ifosfamide (5 g/m^2, d l)[433]	19/32 (59%)
Cisplatin (50 mg/m^2, d l), ifosfamide (5 g/m^2, d l), bleomycin (30 mg, d l)[435]	17/26 (65%)
Cisplatin (50 mg/m^2, d l), ifosfamide (1 g/m^2, d l–5), bleomycin (15 mg, d l)[436]	9/9 (100%)
Carboplatin (200 mg/m^2, d l), ifosfamide (2 g/m^2, d l–3), bleomycin (30 U, d l)[437]	16/18 (89%)
Cisplatin (100 mg/m^2, d l), 5-fluorouracil (1 g/m^2/24 h, d l–5)[440]	20/29 (69%)
Cisplatin (75 mg/m^2, d l), paclitaxel (175 mg/m^2, d l)[442]	—
PRIOR RADIOTHERAPY	
Cisplatin (50 mg/m^2, d l), ifosfamide (5 g/m^2, d l), bleomycin (30 mg, d l)[434]	3/24 (13%)
Cisplatin (50 mg/m^2, d l), ifosfamide (1.2 g/m^2, d l), bleomycin (30 mg, d l)[438]	4/14 (29%)
Cisplatin (50 mg/m^2, d l), ifosfamide (5 g/m^2, d l), bleomycin (30 mg, d l)[435]	26/36 (72%)
Cisplatin (50 mg/m^2, d l), ifosfamide (1 g/m^2, d l–5), bleomycin (15 mg, d l)[436]	5/12 (42%)
Carboplatin (200 mg/m^2, d l), ifosfamide (2 g/m^2, d l–3), bleomycin (30 mg, d l)[437]	5/17 (29%)
Cisplatin (100 mg/m^2, d l), 5-fluorouracil (1 g/m^2/24 h, d l–5)[440]	3/16 (29%)
Cisplatin (100 mg/m^2, d l), 5-fluorouracil (1 g/m^2/24 h, d l–4)[b 441]	14/52 (27%)
Cisplatin (50 mg/m^2, d l), 5-fluorouracil (1 g/m^2/24 h, d l–5)[439]	12/55 (22%)
Cisplatin (75 mg/m^2, d l), paclitaxel (175 mg/m^2, d l)[442]	(57%)

[a]Ifosfamide given with mesna in all combinations.
[b]Allopurinol also given with this regimen.

ifosfamide and will test the addition of paclitaxel or topotecan to cisplatin.

PALLIATIVE RADIOTHERAPY. Localized radiotherapy can provide effective pain relief for symptomatic metastases in bone, brain, lymph nodes, or other sites. A rapid course of pelvic radiotherapy can also provide excellent relief of pain and bleeding for patients who present with incurable disseminated disease.[446–448]

Special Problems

TREATMENT OF LOCALLY RECURRENT CARCINOMA OF THE CERVIX.

After Radical Surgery. Patients should be evaluated for possible recurrent disease if a new mass develops; if, in irradiated patients, the cervix remains bulky or nodular or cervical cytologic findings are abnormal 3 months or more after irradiation; or if symptoms of leg edema, pain, or bleeding develop after initial treatment. The diagnosis must be confirmed with a tissue biopsy, and the extent of disease should be evaluated with appropriate radiographic studies, cystoscopy, proctoscopy, and serum chemistry studies before treatment is administered.

The treatment of choice for patients who have an isolated pelvic recurrence after initial treatment with radical hysterectomy alone is aggressive radiotherapy. Treatment for patients with an isolated central recurrence is similar to that for patients with a primary carcinoma of the vagina. Most patients are treated with external-beam radiotherapy with or without brachytherapy. Implants may need to be inserted under laparoscopic or laparotomy guidance. Pelvic wall recurrences are often treated with external-beam irradiation alone, although intraoperative therapy may contribute to local control in selected patients.[449–451] Reported survival rates usually range between 20% and 40% for patients treated with radical radiotherapy.[452–455] Patients with central recurrence usually have a better prognosis than those with pelvic wall recurrence. Ijaz and colleagues[452] reported a survival rate of 69% 5 years after radical radiotherapy for 16 patients who had isolated vaginal recurrences that did not involve the pelvic wall. Only 18% of patients who had recurrences that were fixed to the pelvic wall or that involved pelvic lymph nodes survived 5 years. Several authors have reported significantly lower salvage rates for patients with locally recurrent adenocarcinoma.[452,456] Thomas and colleagues[457] reported encouraging results in a group of patients treated with radiation and concurrent chemotherapy, but further studies will be needed to determine whether this approach is superior to radiotherapy alone.

After Definitive Irradiation. In some cases, patients who have an isolated central recurrence after radiotherapy can be cured with surgical treatment. Because the extent of disease may be difficult to evaluate and the risk of serious urinary tract complications from pelvic surgery is high after high-dose radiotherapy, surgical salvage treatment usually requires a total pelvic exenteration. Less extensive operations, such as radical hysterectomy or anterior exenteration, are reserved for selected patients with small tumors confined to the cervix or lesions that do not encroach on the rectum, respectively.[458–460]

Tumor involvement of the pelvic sidewall is a contraindication to exenteration but may be difficult to assess if there is extensive radiation fibrosis. The triad of unilateral leg edema, sciatic pain, and ureteral obstruction almost always indicates unresectable disease on the sidewall. Although advanced age is usually considered a contraindication to pelvic exenteration, Matthews and colleagues[461] reported a 5-year survival rate of 46% and an operative mortality of 11% for selected patients who underwent exenteration at the age of 65 years or older compared with a 5-year survival rate of 45% and an operative mortality of 8.5% for younger patients. In all cases, preparation for total pelvic exenteration must involve careful counseling of the patient and family regarding the extent of surgery and postoperative expectations.

The operation begins with a thorough inspection of the abdomen for evidence of intraperitoneal spread or disease in the pelvic sidewall or paraaortic lymph nodes. Despite careful preoperative evaluation, approximately 30% of operations are aborted intraoperatively.[462] Frozen section biopsies are done of suspicious areas. If the biopsy findings are negative, the surgeon proceeds to remove the bladder, rectum, vagina, uterus, ovaries, fallopian tubes, and all other supporting tissues in the true pelvis. A urinary conduit, a transverse or sigmoid colostomy, and a neovagina are created.

Postoperative recuperation may take as long as 3 months. The surgical mortality is less than 10%, with most postoperative complications and deaths related to sepsis, pulmonary thromboembolism, and intestinal complications such as small bowel obstruction and fistula formation.[463,464] Gastrointestinal complications may be reduced by using unirradiated segments of bowel and by closing pelvic floor defects with omentum, rectosigmoid colon, or myocutaneous flaps.[267] Advances in low colorectal anastomosis and techniques for creating continent urinary reservoirs have improved the quality of life for selected patients.[465–467]

The 5-year survival rates for patients who undergo anterior or total pelvic exenteration are 33% to 60% and 20% to 46%, respectively.[459,465,468–470] Several groups are exploring the role of intraoperative irradiation to treat patients with recurrent disease that involves the pelvic wall.[449–451] However, patients with bulky central disease, positive lymph nodes, or 1 year or less between initial treatment and exenteration have a poor prognosis.[469]

TREATMENT AFTER SIMPLE HYSTERECTOMY WITH UNSUSPECTED INVASIVE CANCER. Every patient who undergoes a planned hysterectomy should be carefully screened to rule out invasive cervical cancer before the procedure.[471] However, whenever an unexpected diagnosis of invasive cancer is made in a hysterectomy specimen, the patient should be immediately referred for additional treatment because pelvic radiotherapy produces excellent pelvic disease control rates and survival rates for most patients in this setting.[472–475]

Patients may be classified according to the extent of disease at the time of referral for posthysterectomy treatment into the following groups: (1) microinvasive cancer, (2) tumor confined to the cervix with negative surgical margins, (3) positive surgical margins but no gross residual tumor, (4) gross residual tumor by clinical examination documented by biopsy, and (5) patients referred for treatment more than 6 months after hysterectomy (usually for recurrent disease).[472] In a report of the results of radiotherapy in 123 patients, Roman et al.[475] reported survival rates of 79% and 59% for patients in groups 2 and 3, respectively. In contrast, the survival rate for 30 patients with gross disease (groups 4 and 5) was 41% ($P = .0001$).

Patients with less than 3 mm of invasion without lymph-vascular invasion usually require no treatment after simple hysterectomy. Patients with more extensive involvement who have negative margins require 45 to 50 Gy of pelvic radiotherapy to treat the pelvic nodes and paracolpal tissues. Most clinicians follow this with vaginal intracavitary therapy, delivering an additional vaginal surface dose of 30 to 50 Gy. Patients with positive margins may benefit from a somewhat higher dose of external-beam irradiation through reduced fields designed to include the region at highest risk (e.g., parametria, posterior bladder wall). Patients in groups 3 and 4 reported in the series by Roman and colleagues[475] were usually treated with 65 Gy of external-beam therapy with or without intracavitary therapy. The role of interstitial therapy in this setting is not well documented.

CARCINOMA OF THE CERVICAL STUMP

Although supracervical hysterectomy was once a popular treatment for benign uterine conditions, enthusiasm for the procedure has declined since the 1950s and it is rarely performed today. As a result, carcinomas of the cervical stump are less common than they once were and are usually seen in elderly women. Tumors are usually subclassified as coincidental tumors (diagnosed within 2 years of supracervical hysterectomy) or true cervical stump carcinomas (diagnosed less than 2 years after hysterectomy). Tumors classified as coincidental were probably present at the time of supracervical hysterectomy and are said to have a relatively poor prognosis, although the number of cases in most series is small.

The natural history, staging, and workup of cervical stump carcinomas are the same as for carcinomas of the intact uterus. If possible, the cervix should be probed at the beginning of treatment to determine the length of the uterine canal. MRI may be an important aid to treatment planning in these patients.

Patients with stage IA1 disease may be treated with simple trachelectomy, and selected stage IA2 or small stage IB tumors may be treated with radical trachelectomy and pelvic lymph node dissection. However, most patients are treated with irradiation alone using a combination of external-beam therapy and brachytherapy.

The altered geometry and short uterine canal in these patients complicate treatment planning. However, in most cases the endocervical canal is 2 cm or longer and, after a course of external-beam irradiation, patients can be adequately treated with intracavitary therapy. The endocervical canal is usually loaded with 20 to 30 mgRaEq of cesium, depending on the length of the endocervical canal, and vaginal ovoids are loaded according to their diameter and position. Remote afterloading systems provide somewhat greater flexibility in source loading. If the endocervical canal cannot accommodate any sources, a boost dose may be delivered to the tumor with interstitial therapy, transvaginal irradiation, or reduced fields of external-beam irradiation. However, brachytherapy should be used whenever possible. Barillot et al.[476] reported a survival rate of 81.5% for patients treated with combined brachytherapy and external-beam irradiation versus 38.5% for those treated with external-beam irradiation alone. Several authors have advocated interstitial therapy, using techniques described for apical vaginal carcinomas, for patients with bulkier lesions. Vaginal ovoids alone rarely deliver an adequate dose to the cervix.

Most investigators have reported survival rates similar to those for patients with carcinomas of the intact cervix. In a series of 263 patients, Miller and colleagues[477] reported survival rates of 91%, 77%, and 40% for patients with stage I, II, and III tumors, respectively. Similar survival rates have been reported in other large series.[476,478,479] Miller and colleagues[477] reported a somewhat higher complication rate for cervical stump carcinomas than for carcinomas of the intact cervix, but others have not observed this difference.[476,479]

CARCINOMA OF THE CERVIX DURING PREGNANCY

Estimates of the incidence of invasive cervical cancer during pregnancy range from 0.02% to 0.9%.[480,481] Estimates of the incidence of pregnancy in patients with invasive cervical cancer usually range between 0.5% and 5.0%. Hacker and colleagues[480] reported an incidence of cervical carcinoma *in situ* of 0.013% in pregnant women.

Diagnosis is often delayed because bleeding is erroneously attributed to pregnancy-related complications. All pregnant patients should have a careful pelvic examination and Pap smear at their first antenatal visit. Any suspicious lesion should be biopsied. If the Pap smear result is positive for malignant cells and the diagnosis of invasive cancer cannot be made with colposcopy and biopsy, a diagnostic conization may be necessary. Because conization subjects the mother and fetus to complications, it should be performed only in the second trimester and only in patients with inadequate colposcopy and strong cytologic evidence of invasive cancer. Conization in the first trimester of pregnancy is associated with an abortion rate of up to 33%.[480,482] Conservative conization under colposcopic guidance may reduce the risk.[483]

It appears to be safe to delay definitive treatment of patients with carcinoma *in situ* or stage IA disease until the fetus has matured.[480,481,484] Patients with less than 3 mm of invasion and no LVSI may be followed to term and delivered vaginally. A vaginal hysterectomy may be performed 6 weeks after childbirth if further childbearing is not desired. Patients with 3 to 5 mm of invasion and those with LVSI may also be followed to term. The infant may be delivered by a cesarean section, which is followed immediately by modified radical hysterectomy and pelvic lymph node dissection.[485]

Patients with more than 5 mm of invasion should be treated as having frankly invasive carcinoma of the cervix. Treatment depends on the stage of gestation and the wishes of the patient. Modern neonatal care affords a 75% survival rate for infants delivered at 28 weeks of gestational age and 90% for those delivered at 32 weeks. Fetal pulmonary maturity can be determined by amniocentesis, and prompt treatment can be instituted when pulmonary maturity is documented. It is probably wise to avoid delays in therapy of more than 4 weeks whenever possible although this guideline is controversial.[481,482,486] For most women with stage IB1 tumors, the recommended treatment is classic cesarean section followed by radical hysterectomy with pelvic lymph node dissection. There should be a thorough discussion of the risks and options with both parents before any treatment is undertaken.

Patients with stage II to IV tumors and some patients with bulky stage IB cervical cancers should be treated with radiotherapy. If the fetus is viable, it is delivered by classic cesarean section and radiotherapy is begun postoperatively. If the pregnancy is in the first trimester, external-beam irradiation can be started with the expectation that spontaneous abortion will occur before the delivery of 40 Gy. In the second trimester, a delay of therapy may be entertained to improve the chances of fetal survival. If the patient wishes to delay therapy, it is important to ensure fetal pulmonary maturity before delivery is undertaken.

Compared with other cervical cancer patients, those with cervical cancer during pregnancy have slightly better overall survival because an increased proportion have stage I disease. The diagnosis of cancer in the postpartum period tends to be associated with a more advanced clinical stage and a corresponding decrease in survival. However, studies differ in their conclusions about whether pregnancy has an independent influence on the prognosis of patients with cervical cancer.[481,487,488] Patients who are diagnosed with invasive cervical cancer shortly after a vaginal delivery appear to be at risk for recurrence in the site of their episiotomy. At least 13 cases demonstrating this unusual pattern of failure have been reported.[489–491]

CARCINOMA OF THE VAGINA

Carcinomas of the vagina are rare, accounting for only approximately 2% to 3% of gynecologic malignancies.[492,493] According to FIGO, cases should be classified as vaginal carcinomas only when "the primary site of the growth is in the vagina."[494] A tumor that is limited to the urethra should be classified as a primary urethral cancer, and a tumor that has extended from the vulva to involve the vagina should be classified as a primary vulvar cancer. Also, according to FIGO, any tumor that has extended to the cervical portio and has reached the area of the external os should be classified as a cervical carcinoma. For this reason, in patients with an intact uterus, it is probable that many tumors that originated in the apical vagina are actually classified as cervical cancers. This may explain why a large percentage (30% to 50%) of patients diagnosed with vaginal carcinoma have had a prior hysterectomy (preventing classification of their tumors as primary cervical cancers).[495–498]

More commonly, the vagina is a site of metastasis or direct extension from tumors originating in other genital sites, such as the cervix or endometrium, or from extragenital sites, including the rectum and bladder.

EPIDEMIOLOGY

Vaginal intraepithelial neoplasia (VAIN) often accompanies CIN and is thought to have a similar etiology.[499] VAIN lesions are more often seen in the upper third of the vagina and may be either extensions from adjacent areas of CIN or separate lesions.[500] Kalogirou and associates[501] found 41 cases of VAIN in 993 patients followed with cytologic examination and colposcopy after hysterectomy for CIN. Most VAIN lesions were in the upper vagina, particularly in the vault angles of the suture line.

Because the vagina does not have a transformation zone of immature epithelial cells susceptible to HPV infection, HPV-induced vaginal lesions are thought to arise in areas of squamous metaplasia that develop during healing of mucosal abrasions caused by coitus, tampon use, or other trauma.[499] Invasive vaginal carcinoma has also been associated with chronic irritant vaginitis, particularly that caused by chronic use of a vaginal pessary.[502] Schraub et al.[503] reported that 80% of vaginal cancers arising in patients who used pessaries were in the posterior fornix or posterior wall of the vagina. Investigators have also reported an association between vaginal carcinoma and infection with HPV similar to that found for invasive cervical cancer.[502,504] Ikenberg and colleagues[504] found HPV DNA in 10 of 18 patients with invasive vaginal cancer.

Pride and colleagues[505] suggested that pelvic irradiation might be a predisposing factor in some cases. However, viral and other risk factors independent of the mode of treatment undoubtedly place some of these patients at risk for multiple primary tumors. In a review of 301 patients with vaginal cancer, Chyle and associates[495] found that 56 had a prior history of carcinoma *in situ* of the cervix, 22 had a history of invasive cervical cancer, and two had prior *in situ* carcinomas of the vagina.

Primary invasive carcinoma of the vagina is predominantly a disease of elderly women, with 70% to 80% of cases presenting in women older than 60 years.[494] However, FIGO data[494] suggest that the age of peak incidence may have decreased since the early 1960s, when the highest incidence was among women in their 80s. Except for clear cell carcinomas, which are associated with maternal diethylstilbestrol (DES) exposure, invasive vaginal carcinomas are extremely rare in women younger than 40 years.[494,506]

In 1971, Herbst and colleagues[507] first reported a highly significant association between clear cell carcinomas of the vagina and maternal ingestion of DES during pregnancy. This led to the establishment of a registry to gather information about cases of clear cell carcinoma in the United States. The peak number of DES-associated cases occurred in 1975, when 33 were reported to the registry.[508] The peak risk period for exposed women in the United States is between the ages of 15 and 22 years; the youngest patient reported was 7 years old. The oldest patient reported so far was 42 years old at diagnosis, but the risk to women older than 40 years is still unknown because women in the first exposed cohort are just reaching their fifth decade. Because only approximately 1 of every 1000 women exposed to DES *in utero* develops clear cell carcinoma,[509] investigators have tried to define other risk factors for development of the disease. The risk of clear cell carcinoma has been associated with initiation of DES early during pregnancy, a maternal history of early miscarriage, and premature birth.[508,510] Sharp and Cole[510] found a correlation between adolescent obesity in exposed girls and the development of vaginal clear cell carcinoma. Infection with HPV may be a cofactor in some cases.[511] Among 14 cases of clear cell carcinoma studies by Waggoner and colleagues,[511] three contained HPV 31 DNA; ten of the remaining HPV-negative tumors had p53 protein detected by immunohistochemistry, suggesting a mutation of *p53*.

Although the risk of clear cell carcinoma of the vagina is small in DES-exposed women, 45% of these patients have areas of vaginal adenosis, and 25% have structural abnormalities of the uterus, cervix, or vagina. Fortunately, awareness of the risks of *in utero* DES exposure has led to a dramatic reduction in the use of high doses of estrogen to prevent miscarriage, and the number of young women who need to be followed for this problem is declining. There is as yet no evidence that DES-exposed women are at risk for malignancies other than clear cell carcinoma.[512]

NATURAL HISTORY AND PATTERN OF SPREAD

Approximately 50% of vaginal cancers arise in the upper third of the vagina.[495,498,506,513] Although Plentl and Friedman[513] reported that tumors arise more commonly on the posterior wall, more recent reviews have reported a more even distribution of lesions arising on the anterior, posterior, and lateral walls.[495,498] Tumors may exhibit an exophytic or ulcerative, infiltrating pattern of growth.

Tumors may invade directly to involve adjacent structures such as the urethra, bladder, and rectum. Despite the proximity of these structures, fewer than 10% of vaginal cancers are found to be stage IVA at presentation.[494,498,506,514] However, extensive infiltration of the suburethra or rectovaginal septum is common and frequently influences treatment planning. Vaginal cancers may also spread laterally to the paravaginal space and pelvic wall. Although tumors arising in the vagina undoubtedly can spread superiorly to involve the cervix and uterus, this usually leads to their classification as cervical cancers, according to FIGO convention.

The vagina is supplied with a fine anastomosing network of lymphatics in the mucosa and submucosa. Despite the continuity of lymphatic vessels within the vagina, Plentl and Friedman[515] found a regular pattern of regional drainage from specific regions of the vagina. The lymphatics of the vaginal vault communicate with those of the lower cervix, draining laterally to the obturator and hypogastric nodes. The lymphatics of the posterior wall anastomose with those of the anterior rectal wall, draining to the superior and inferior gluteal nodes. The lymphatics of the lower third of the vagina communicate with those of the vulva and drain either to the pelvic nodes or with the vulvar lymphatics to the inguinofemoral lymph nodes. Plentl and Friedman summarized their description of the lymphatic drainage of the vagina with the comment that, except for the lateral external iliac group, all lymph nodes of the pelvis may at one time or other serve as primary sites of regional drainage for vaginal lymph.[515]

Few data are available concerning the incidence of spread of vaginal cancer to the pelvic lymph nodes. In a review of early reports, Plentl and Friedman[515] quoted an overall incidence of positive nodes of 21%. More recent studies suggest that the incidence of positive pelvic nodes in patients with stage II disease is at least 25% to 30%, emphasizing the importance of regional treatment for these patients.[516,517] Inguinal node metastases generally occur only in patients whose tumors involve the lower third of the vagina.[495,514]

The most frequent site of hematogenous metastasis is the lung. Less frequently, vaginal cancers may metastasize to liver, bone, or other sites.[494,495]

PATHOLOGY

Eighty percent to 90% of primary vaginal malignancies are squamous cell carcinomas.[492,494] Grossly, these tumors may be nodular, ulcerative, or exophytic plaques of any size. Histologically, they are similar to squamous tumors from other sites. Approximately one-third of these tumors are keratinizing, and more than one-half are nonkeratinizing, moderately differentiated lesions.

Verrucous carcinoma is an uncommon variant of squamous cell carcinoma that presents as a warty, fungating mass.[518] Histologically, verrucous carcinoma is composed of large papillary fronds covered by dense keratin. Its deep margin creates a pushing border of well-oriented rete ridges. This tumor rarely metastasizes but can extensively infiltrate into surrounding tissues, including the rectum and coccyx. Wide surgical excision is the treatment of choice in this situation.

TABLE 36.2-13. International Federation of Gynecology and Obstetrics Clinical Staging of Carcinoma of the Vagina

Stage 0	Carcinoma *in situ*, intraepithelial carcinoma.
Stage I	The carcinoma is limited to the vaginal wall.
Stage II	The carcinoma has involved the subvaginal tissues but has not extended onto the pelvic wall.
Stage III	The carcinoma has extended onto the pelvic wall.
Stage IV	The carcinoma has extended beyond the true pelvis or has clinically involved the mucosa of the bladder or rectum. Bullous edema as such does not permit a case to be allotted to stage IV.
Stage IVA	Spread of the growth to adjacent organs, direct extension beyond the true pelvis, or both.
Stage IVB	Spread to distant organs.

Approximately 5% to 10% of primary vaginal neoplasms are adenocarcinomas, although the incidence may vary with the proportion of women in the population who were exposed to DES *in utero*.[492,494,507] Clear cell carcinomas of the vagina are usually polypoid but may have tubulocystic or solid patterns. Adenocarcinomas not associated with DES exposure occur primarily in postmenopausal women. The differential diagnosis of adenocarcinoma occurring in the vagina is often difficult, as it must be distinguished from metastatic tumors originating in other sites.[519] Histologic patterns include clear cell, mucinous, adenosquamous, papillary, and undifferentiated. It has been hypothesized that these tumors may arise in foci of adenosis, from mesonephric rests, or from foci of endometriosis in the vagina.[520,521]

Primary small cell carcinomas of the vagina are rare; fewer than 20 cases have been reported in the literature.[522–524] They are histologically indistinguishable from neuroendocrine small cell carcinomas of the lung or cervix and like these tumors may coexist with squamous or adenocarcinoma elements.

Primary vaginal melanomas represent approximately 3% of primary vaginal cancers and fewer than 20% of genital melanomas.[492,494] Primary vaginal melanomas are thought to arise from melanocytes in areas of melanosis or atypical melanocytic hyperplasia.[525] They usually originate in the lower third of the vagina and occur at a mean age of 55 years, with an age range of 22 to 83 years. They tend to have a poorer prognosis than vulvar melanomas, with 5-year survival rates of 15% to 20% after treatment with surgery, radiation, or both.[526,527]

Approximately 3% of vaginal cancers are sarcomas; approximately two-thirds of these are leiomyosarcomas, but endometrial stromal sarcomas, malignant mixed Müllerian tumors, and other types have been reported.[528] Embryonal rhabdomyosarcoma (sarcoma botryoides) is a highly malignant sarcoma that occurs in children up to 6 years of age. This tumor usually forms soft nodules that fill and protrude from the vagina. The prognosis for children with this tumor has improved with the use of multimodality therapy including surgery, chemotherapy, and radiation.[529]

DIAGNOSIS, CLINICAL EVALUATION, AND STAGING

Most patients with VAIN and approximately 10% to 20% of patients with invasive disease are asymptomatic at presentation; in these cases carcinoma is usually diagnosed during investigation of an abnormal Pap smear result. Colposcopic evaluation in the case of abnormal cytologic findings should always include a detailed examination of the entire vagina and cervix, even when there is an obvious cervical lesion, because patients can present with multiple areas of abnormality. Women who have persistent positive Pap smear results after treatment of CIN should be examined carefully for VAIN.

Approximately 50% to 60% of patients with invasive cancer present with abnormal vaginal bleeding, frequently after coitus or vaginal douching. Patients may also present with complaints of vaginal discharge, a palpable mass, dyspareunia, or pain in the perineum or pelvis.[506,530–532]

According to FIGO, the rules for clinical staging of patients with carcinoma of the vagina are the same as those for clinical staging of patients with cervical cancer.[494] The workup should include careful examination of the cervix and vagina and bimanual examination. All patients should have chest roentgenography, complete blood count, and biochemical profile. Cystoscopy and ureteroscopy are strongly recommended for patients with large tumors or tumors involving the anterior vaginal wall. Proctoscopy is indicated for lesions involving the posterior vaginal wall. A barium enema or skeletal films may also be needed in selected cases. The kidneys should be localized and the rare case of hydronephrosis ruled out with either classical intravenous pyelography or a pyelography obtained with a CT scan. However, it should again be emphasized that the FIGO rules for clinical staging prohibit the use of other information obtained from CT, MRI, lymphangiography, or surgical staging to change clinical stage even though these studies may aid in the determination of disease extent.

The FIGO categories for staging of vaginal cancers are listed in Table 36.2-13.[494] Because this is a clinical staging system, the classification of lesions as stage I or II is probably subjective. In general, thin (less than 0.5 cm), relatively exophytic tumors tend to be classified as stage I, and thicker, infiltrating tumors and those with obvious paravaginal nodularity tend to be classified as stage II. Perez and colleagues[511] use a modification of the FIGO system that distinguishes tumors that infiltrate the parametrium (stage IIB) from those with paravaginal submucosal extension only (stage IIA). They reported a 5-year survival rate of 55% for patients whose tumors were classified as stage IIA versus 35% for those whose tumors were classified as stage IIB.[514]

FIGO does not specify how tumors should be classified when the inguinal nodes are clinically positive. The stage descriptions state that tumors that have spread beyond the true pelvis should be classified as stage IVB, but many clinicians ignore inguinal node status in assigning stage and thus gener-

TABLE 36.2-14. Carcinoma of the Vagina: Survival Rates According to Clinical Stage

	Stage I		*Stage II*		*Stage III*		*Stage IV*		
	Patients	Survival (%)	Patients	Survival (%)	Patients	Survival (%)	Patients	Survival (%)	*Calculation Method*
Pride et al.[505]	9	66	22	49	4	25	8	0	5-y, crude, uncorrected
Nori et al.[536]	14	71	6	66	3	33	13	0	5-y, disease-free
Rubin et al.[537]	12	75	29	48	13	54	12	0	5-y, crude, corrected
Macnaught et al.[535]	14	68	22	34	18	29	7	14	5-y, actuarial
Perez et al.[514]	59	80	64 (IIA)	55	20	38	15	0	10-y, actuarial, disease-free
			34 (IIB)	35					
Spiritos et al.[532]	18	94	5	80	10	50	5	0	5-y, actuarial, disease-free
Davis et al.[517]	44	82	45	53					5-y, actuarial, uncorrected
Eddy et al.[534]	25	73	39	39	15	38	12	25	5-y, actuarial, corrected
Kucera et al.[530]	73	77	110	45	174	31	77	14	5-y, crude, uncorrected
Lee et al.[546]	17	94	6 (IIA)	80	10	80	6	67	5-y, actuarial, cause specific
			10 (IIB)	39					
Kirkbride et al.[506]	40	77	38	78	42	60	19	41	5-y, actuarial, cause specific
Chyle et al.[495]	59	55	104	51	55	37	16	40	10-y, actuarial, uncorrected
		76		69		47		27	10-y, freedom from relapse
Stock et al.[498]	23	67	58	53	9	0	10	15	5-y, actuarial, disease-free

ate confusion in the literature on this subject. The American Joint Committee on Cancer[533] has suggested a TNM staging system that classifies patients with unilateral inguinal metastases as N1 (stage III) and those with bilateral nodes as N2 (stage IVA), but this system is rarely used. Patients with inguinal metastases are sometimes cured with locoregional treatment; Kucera and Vavra[530] report uncorrected 5-year survival rates of 29% for patients with clinically suspicious inguinal nodes and 44% for patients with clinically negative groins.

PROGNOSTIC FACTORS

The rates of local control, distant metastasis, and survival in vaginal carcinoma are all correlated strongly with tumor stage (Table 36.2-14).[495,506,514,530,532,534–537] Tumor size also appears to be an important predictor of outcome. Chyle and colleagues[495] reported a higher rate of local and distant failure for tumors larger than 5 cm in diameter; Kirkbride and associates[506] reported a significantly better survival rate for patients with tumors smaller than 4 cm in diameter; and Stock and colleagues[498] reported better survival when disease was limited to one-third of the vaginal canal.

Most investigators have been unable to find a correlation between tumor site and outcome.[495,506,514,530,532,534,535] However, Chyle and colleagues[495] reported higher rates of local recurrence and overall relapse in patients with posterior wall lesions, and Kucera and Vavra[530] reported a better survival rate for patients whose tumors involved the upper third of the vagina. Tumors that involve the entire vagina tend to have a poorer prognosis, probably reflecting the larger size of these lesions.[495,530] Exophytic tumors may have a better prognosis than those with infiltrating or necrotic lesions.[514] Investigators disagree about the influence of histologic grade and type on outcome. Several investigators have reported a correlation between increasing grade of squamous carcinomas and recurrence,[495,538,539] whereas others have found no correlation.[497,505,540] Chyle and coinvestigators[495] reported significantly poorer survival and local control rates for patients with adenocarcinoma, but other investigators[506,517,540] found no difference in outcome for patients with squamous carcinomas or adenocarcinomas.

TREATMENT

Stage 0

Patients with only HPV infection or VAIN 1 do not require treatment. These lesions often regress spontaneously, are frequently multifocal, and recur quickly after attempts at ablative therapy. VAIN 2 is usually treated by laser ablation. However, VAIN 3 is more likely to harbor an invasive lesion. Hoffman and colleagues[499] reported finding occult invasion in upper vaginectomy specimens from 9 (28%) of 32 patients who had surgery for VAIN 3. It has been recommended that VAIN 3 lesions located in dimples of the vaginal cuff of older patients be locally excised before definitive treatment to rule out occult invasion.[541]

VAIN 3 lesions that have been adequately sampled to rule out invasion can be treated with laser ablation. Cryosurgery should not be used in the vagina because the depth of injury cannot be controlled and inadvertent injury to the bladder or rectum may occur. Superficial fulguration with electrosurgical ball cautery may be used under colposcopic control, with the epithelial tissue wiped away as it is ablated to allow observation of the depth of destruction. Local excision is an excellent method of treatment for small upper vaginal lesions. Rarely, total vaginectomy is required for extensive VAIN 3 lesions. The vagina should then be reconstructed with a split-thickness skin graft. However, this aggressive treatment should not be used for VAIN 2.

Although progression of stage 0 lesions to invasive disease is uncommon, the risk is sufficient to warrant close follow-up of patients treated for VAIN. In a review of 136 cases of carcinoma *in situ* of the vagina, Benedet and Saunders[542] found only four cases (3%) that progressed to invasive cancer with up to 30 years of follow-up. Cheng and colleagues[543] reported four cases of invasive cancer that developed in 35 patients who were followed after wide local excision for VAIN.

VAIN can also be treated effectively with intracavitary radiotherapy,[495,506,514] but this treatment is usually reserved for patients with multifocal, multiply recurrent disease or high operative risk. Treatment is usually delivered using ^{137}Cs loaded in a plastic vaginal cylinder 3 to 4 cm in diameter. Chyle et al.[495] reported a 17% recurrence rate at 10 years in 37 patients treated with a vaginal surface dose of 70 to 80 Gy. Perez et al.[514] reported only one recurrence (5%) in 20 patients treated with a vaginal surface dose of 60 to 70 Gy. The single vaginal recurrence was distal to the region treated with brachytherapy, and the authors emphasize the importance of treating the entire vagina to avoid marginal recurrences. More recently, some authors have reported results using fractionated high-dose-rate intracavitary therapy to treat VAIN. MacCloud and colleagues[544] reported control of VAIN 3 in 11 of 14 patients followed for 36 to 115 months after treatment; in these patients, the vaginal surface was treated with a total dose of 34 to 45 Gy in four to ten fractions. One patient had progression to invasive disease. The authors observed no severe complications with this treatment. However, Ogino and colleagues[545] reported adhesive vaginitis and rectal bleeding in two patients treated to the entire vagina with a less conservative fractionation schedule.

Stage I

Radiotherapy is often the treatment of choice for stage I disease because if surgery is used, total vaginectomy or even exenteration may be needed to obtain satisfactory resection margins. However, surgery has a definite role in selected cases.[498] Early tumors that involve the upper posterior vagina can be removed with a radical hysterectomy and partial vaginectomy (if the uterus is *in situ*) or with a radical upper vaginectomy (if the patient has had a prior hysterectomy) and bilateral pelvic lymphadenectomy. Some surgeons advocate broader indications for surgical treatment of stage I disease.[498,517] Stock and associates[498] reported a 5-year disease-free survival rate of 56% for 15 patients with stage I disease treated with surgery alone (local excision, partial vaginectomy, or radical vaginectomy). One patient in whom disease recurred had successful salvage treatment with irradiation, and two patients who received postoperative irradiation were cured of their disease. Among six patients in the series of Stock et al. who[498] were treated with definitive irradiation, the disease-free survival rate was 80%; one patient in whom disease recurred had successful salvage treatment with pelvic exenteration. For patients with a prior history of pelvic irradiation, radical surgery (usually pelvic exenteration) is indicated and is often curative.

Disease-specific survival rates for patients with stage I disease treated with definitive irradiation range from 75% to 95%.[495,514,530,532,546] Selected patients with small, superficial tumors may be treated with brachytherapy alone. Perez et al.[514] achieved pelvic tumor control in 22 (88%) of 25 selected patients with stage I disease treated with brachytherapy alone. They recommended a dose of 60 to 70 Gy calculated 5 mm beyond the plane of the implant or vaginal mucosa (vaginal surface dose of 80 to 120 Gy). Thicker stage I tumors should be treated with a combination of external-beam irradiation and brachytherapy with an aim to deliver 40 to 50 Gy to the pelvic nodes and 70 to 75 Gy to the tumor.

Stage II

Because investigators rarely define their criteria for distinguishing stage I from stage II disease or for selecting patients for various treatments, different institutional experiences cannot be easily compared. Reported disease-specific survival rates range from 50% to 80%. Data suggest that most patients with stage II disease require treatment with a combination of external-beam irradiation and brachytherapy. Perez and colleagues[514] achieved pelvic tumor control in only 4 (36%) of 11 selected patients with stage II tumors treated with brachytherapy alone, compared with 54 (67%) of 81 patients treated with a combination of external-beam irradiation and brachytherapy. Chyle et al.[495] reported a local recurrence rate (in the vagina) of 11% in 18 patients treated with brachytherapy (usually interstitial implant) alone, but did not report the rate of pelvic wall relapse in this patient subset.

Brachytherapy should be tailored to the volume and distribution of the tumor and its response to external-beam irradiation. For tumors that flatten to less than 5 mm in thickness, the dose to the vagina may be boosted using intracavitary sources in a vaginal cylinder. Because the thickness of apical vaginal tumors may be difficult to assess in patients who have had a hysterectomy, an examination under anesthesia is often needed to determine whether intracavitary therapy will cover the tumor adequately. Transvaginal ultrasound or MRI may also be helpful in treatment planning. When the uterus is intact, tumors high in the posterior fornix can often be treated with a tandem and ovoids. Larger tumors usually require a boost with interstitial therapy or additional external-beam irradiation. Most authors emphasize the importance of brachytherapy in the treatment of vaginal cancer.[514,532,546] However, brachytherapy must be designed to treat the entire vaginal tumor. Chyle and colleagues[495] argue that tumors that cannot adequately be covered with brachytherapy can often be cured with external-beam irradiation alone using carefully designed shrinking fields. They reported three (11%) vaginal recurrences in 28 patients with stage II disease treated with external-beam irradiation alone, compared with 12 (21%) recurrences in 58 patients treated with combined external-beam irradiation and brachytherapy.

Selected patients with stage II disease may be cured with radical surgery.[498] However, total radical vaginectomy or pelvic exenteration is often required to remove the tumor, and results with radical surgery do not appear better than those achieved with radiotherapy alone. Primary radical surgery is usually indicated for patients who have previously had pelvic radiotherapy.

Stages III and IVA

Most authors report disease-specific survival rates of between 30% and 50% for patients with stage III disease and between 15% and 30% for patients with stage IVA disease.[495,506,514,530] Stage III and IVA tumors are usually bulky, highly infiltrative lesions involving most or all of the vagina as well as the pelvic wall, bladder, or rectum. The extent of these tumors and the proximity of critical normal tissue structures make their management a formidable technical challenge. Pelvic recurrence rates are high in most series; the risk of distant metastasis is also relatively high, although distant relapse is often accompanied by locoregional recurrence.

All patients require treatment with external-beam irradiation. Most authors advocate the use of brachytherapy whenever possible. However, Chyle and colleagues[495] reported a fairly high rate of freedom from relapse (47% at 10 years) in a series of patients with stage III disease in which the majority of patients (40 of 55) were treated with external-beam irradiation alone. Brachytherapy is undoubtedly an important part of disease management in some patients. However, in some cases interstitial therapy does not provide adequate coverage of tumors that are large and intimately associated with critical structures. In these cases, it may be appropriate to place greater emphasis on external-beam treatment.

For selected patients with stage IVA disease who are in otherwise good medical condition, a pelvic exenteration with vaginal reconstruction using a gracilis myocutaneous flap or rectus abdominis myocutaneous flap may be the treatment of choice, particularly if a rectovaginal or vesicovaginal fistula is present.[465,516,547]

RADIOTHERAPY TECHNIQUE. external-beam fields must include the primary lesion and the regional lymph nodes. Fields should be individualized according to the primary site. Radiopaque markers placed at the distal edge of the tumor help to define the lower border, which often includes a portion of the introitus. Treating the patient in an open (frog-leg) position can often reduce the severity of vulvar cutaneous reactions.

When tumors involve the lower third of the vagina, pelvic fields should be enlarged to include at least the medial inguinal lymph nodes. When four fields are used to treat the pelvis, care must be taken to cover all the draining lymph nodes. Lateral fields should adequately cover posterior perirectal nodes, particularly when the primary lesion involves the posterior vaginal wall.

Intracavitary brachytherapy is of little value in the treatment of locally advanced vaginal cancers because the dose falls off rapidly from the surface of a vaginal cylinder. In general, the dose at a 5-mm depth is only 50% to 65% of the dose at the vaginal surface. Interstitial brachytherapy can provide better coverage of thick vaginal tumors. Vaginal implants can be inserted free-hand, a technique that requires experience but permits

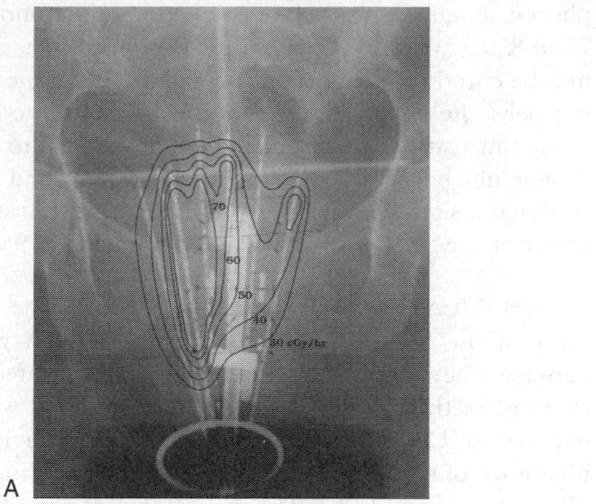

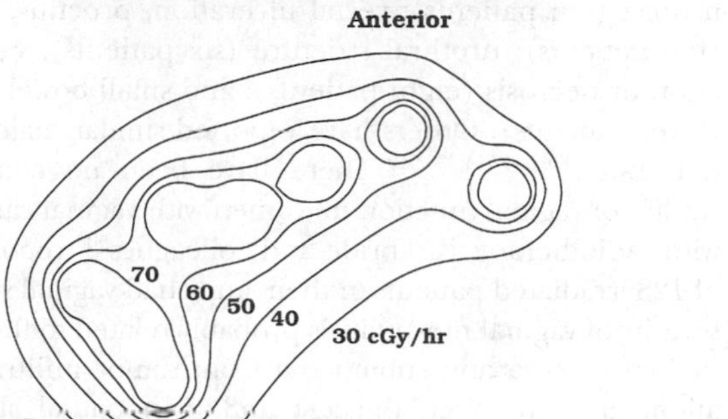

FIGURE 36.2-10. Interstitial implant of a squamous carcinoma involving the anterior and right lateral wall of the vagina. Needles were placed transperineally, while the position of the needles was monitored by fingers in the vagina and rectum. A plastic cylinder in the vagina displaced uninvolved tissues away from the needles, which were loaded with iridium 192 sources. Needles were placed and sources were selected to deliver a somewhat higher dose to the thickest portion of the tumor on the right lateral wall of the vagina. Isodose contours represent the dose rates (in cGy/h) delivered to tissues in a coronal plane at the approximate center of the implant **(A)** and in a transverse plane through the center of the implant **(B)**.

excellent control of the position of sources with respect to the vaginal surface and rectal mucosa, which can be palpated as the needles are positioned (Fig. 36.2-10). Vaginal implants may also be positioned using a perineal template. This technique provides a more homogeneous dose distribution because it facilitates parallel positioning of sources, but the template interferes somewhat with the brachytherapist's ability to monitor the placement of needles with respect to the rectal and vaginal mucosa. When tumors involve the vaginal apex in patients who have had a hysterectomy, laparoscopic or laparotomy guidance may be needed to ensure accurate needle placement.

Several authors have reported a correlation between higher doses of radiation and lower rates of pelvic recurrence.[514,532,540] Chyle and associates[495] did not report a significant correlation between tumor dose and outcome. However, dose-response analyses can be misleading because the total dose of radiation prescribed for a vaginal tumor is often influenced by its size, extent, and initial response to irradiation, all of which determine the feasibility of delivering high-dose brachytherapy. When good brachytherapy coverage of the tumor can be accomplished, an effort should be made to treat the tumor to a dose of 75 to 85 Gy. When brachytherapy is not possible, some patients may be cured with external-beam irradiation alone using shrinking pelvic fields to deliver a tumor dose of 60 to 66 Gy. Treatment can usually be completed in less than 6 to 7 weeks and should not be protracted unnecessarily. Lee and colleagues[546] reported a significantly lower pelvic recurrence rate in patients whose entire treatment course was completed in 9 weeks or less.

COMPLICATIONS OF RADIOTHERAPY. The close proximity of the bladder and rectum makes them vulnerable to damage when invasive vaginal cancers are treated with radiotherapy. In their review of 301 patients treated with definitive irradiation, Chyle and colleagues[495] reported a 19% actuarial incidence of serious complications at 20 years (the crude complication rate was 13%). The most frequent complications were fistulae (ten patients); rectal ulceration, proctitis, or stricture (ten patients); urethral stricture (six patients); vaginal ulceration or necrosis (eight patients); and small bowel obstruction (seven patients). Others have reported similar major complication rates.[496,506,514,530,540] There have been no comprehensive studies of vaginal function in women with vaginal cancer treated with radiotherapy. Kirkbride and colleagues[506] reported that 45 of 128 irradiated patients in their study had vaginal stenosis. The severity of vaginal morbidity is probably related to the damage to vaginal mucosa and submucosa from tumor infiltration, ulceration, and infection; the age and menopausal status of the patient; and the radiation dose and the amount of vaginal tissue treated to high doses.

Vaginal Clear Cell Carcinoma

The treatment of vaginal clear cell carcinoma is similar to that of squamous cell carcinoma. However, most women with vaginal clear cell carcinoma are young, so an effort should be made to preserve vaginal and ovarian function whenever possible. Conventional treatments for stage I and II disease include radical hysterectomy, vaginectomy, and lymphadenectomy with formation of a neovagina using a split-thickness skin graft, and radical radiotherapy. Senekjian and colleagues[548] reported on the use of local therapy alone in 43 patients with stage I disease who were reported to the Registry for Research on Hormonal Transplacental Carcinogenesis. Patients treated with local excision alone had a recurrence rate of more than 40% at 10 years. However, 17 patients who were treated with local irradiation (brachytherapy or transvaginal orthovoltage cone irradiation) with or without local excision had a 10-year recurrence rate of less than 10%. Of 41 assessable patients treated with local therapy in Senekjian and colleagues'[548] report, eight had had 15 pregnancies and 12 live births. Retroperitoneal lymphadenectomy may be indicated when local treatment is considered for stage I lesions, which are reported to have an overall rate of pelvic lymph node metastases of 17%.[549] When larger or more advanced lesions are treated with whole pelvic irradiation, ovarian transposition should be considered before radiotherapy.

The overall actuarial 10-year survival rate for patients treated for vaginal clear cell carcinoma is 79%. The survival rates for patients with stage I and II tumors are 90% and 80%, respectively.[548,550,551] Most recurrences occur within 3 years of initial therapy. However, recurrences have been reported to occur as many as 10 to 20 years after treatment.[552,553] Approximately one-third of relapses are first detected at distant sites, most commonly the lungs or extrapelvic lymph nodes.

ROLE OF CHEMOTHERAPY. Because primary vaginal carcinomas are rare, few reports have specifically addressed the role of chemotherapy in the treatment of this disease. Chemotherapeutic management is usually based on extrapolations from experience with the treatment of carcinomas of the cervix. For this reason, patients who have metastatic or recurrent vaginal carcinoma that is no longer amenable to locoregional treatment are sometimes treated with cisplatin-based chemotherapy even though the efficacy of this treatment is not well documented in the literature. Thigpen and colleagues[554] reported one complete and no partial responses in 16 patients with vaginal cancers treated with cisplatin 50 mg/m^2 every 3 weeks. In another GOG study, no responses were observed in 16 patients treated with etoposide for advanced vaginal cancers.[555] Reports of the use of neoadjuvant chemotherapy or concurrent chemoradiation are anecdotal.[556–558] However, vaginal carcinoma resembles cervical carcinoma in its location, pattern of spread, histologic appearance, relationship to HPV infection, and response to radiotherapy. It may therefore be reasonable to extrapolate from randomized trials demonstrating a benefit from concurrent chemoradiation in patients with locally advanced cervical cancer[229,230,232,559] to justify a similar approach in selected patients with high-risk invasive vaginal cancers.

CARCINOMA OF THE VULVA

EPIDEMIOLOGY

Invasive vulvar carcinoma is a rare disease that accounts for approximately 4% of gynecologic cancers.[1,560] In the United States, invasive vulvar cancer occurs with an average annual age-adjusted incidence rate of 1.2 cases per 100,000 woman-years.[561] The median age of patients diagnosed with invasive vulvar cancer is approximately 65 to 70 years; the incidence peaks in women older than 75 years at approximately 20 per 100,000.[560–562] In contrast, vulvar intraepithelial neoplasia (VIN) tends to occur in younger women; the median age of women diagnosed with VIN is 45 to 50 years. Although investigators have not demonstrated an overall increase in the incidence of invasive vulvar cancer, studies in the United States and Europe suggest that the incidence of VIN has more than doubled since the early 1970s.[561,563,564] This increase has been particularly marked in women younger than 55 years.[561,563] The relatively stable incidence of invasive cancer despite a steady increase in patients diagnosed with VIN could suggest that the etiologic factors for the two conditions are different, that diagnostic procedures have improved, or that effective treatment of VIN has prevented a significant increase in the incidence of invasive disease.

Evidence that HPV may play a role in the pathogenesis of cervical cancer has led investigators to look for HPV infection in patients with vulvar neoplasms. Eighty percent to 90% of VIN lesions contain HPV 16 or other HPV types. However, although more than 90% of invasive cervical cancers are associated with HPV, only 30% to 50% of invasive vulvar carcinomas are associated with evidence of HPV infection.[565–569]

Epidemiologic, histopathologic, and viral data suggest that patients with invasive squamous cell carcinomas of the vulva

TABLE 36.2-15. Relationship between Depth of Stromal Invasion and Inguinal Lymph Node Metastases in Patients with Squamous Cell Carcinomas of the Vulva

	Patients with Positive Lymph Nodes/Total No. of Patients				
Depth of Invasion (mm)	≤1.0	1.1–2.0	2.1–3.0	3.1–5.0	>5
Binder et al.[582]	0/7	0/23	3/14	6/25	15/31
Ross and Erhmann[585]	0/17	1/9	1/13	4/15	0/1
Hoffman et al.[584]	0/24	0/19	2/17	8/15	7/13
Hacker et al.[654]	0/34	2/19	2/17	1/7	3/7
Andreasson and Nyboe[579]	0/8	1/13	3/12	5/32	19/57
Total	0/90	4/83 (5%)	11/73 (15%)	24/94 (26%)	44/109 (40%)

can be divided into at least two groups whose tumors may have different etiologies: one that is associated with HPV infection and one that is not.[561,566,568,570,571] HPV-positive tumors tend to occur in younger women (35 to 55 years), are often associated with VIN, are frequently multifocal, and tend to form less keratin than do HPV-negative tumors. Patients with HPV-positive tumors are also more likely to have CIN and to have the risk factors typically associated with cervical cancers (multiple sexual partners, early age at first intercourse, low socioeconomic status, and cigarette smoking).[571–573] In contrast, HPV-negative tumors usually occur in older women (55 to 85 years), are often associated with vulvar inflammation or lichen sclerosis (but rarely with VIN), are generally unifocal, and are usually well differentiated with exuberant keratin formation.[566–569] Although a number of investigators have reported this distinct grouping of patients with vulvar cancer, others have found greater overlap.[570,574,575]

Several investigators have reported a high incidence of p53 mutations in HPV-negative tumors.[576–578] Lee and colleagues[576] found missense mutations of p53 in four (44%) of nine HPV-negative tumors but in only one (8%) of 12 HPV-positive tumors. They postulated that alteration in p53 activity, either through point mutations or through E6-mediated loss of p53 function in HPV-infected cells, could be important in the development of vulvar neoplasms.

NATURAL HISTORY AND PATTERN OF SPREAD

The female external genitalia include the mons pubis, labia majora, labia minora, clitoris, vestibular bulb, vestibular glands (including Bartholin's glands), and vestibule of the vagina. Together, these structures form the vulva. The region between the posterior commissure of the labia and the anus is termed the *gynecologic perineum*. Approximately 70% of vulvar squamous carcinomas involve the labia majora or minora, most frequently the labia majora.[579–581] Approximately 15% to 20% involve the clitoris, and a similar proportion involve or arise in the perineum. In approximately 10% of cases, the lesion is too extensive to permit determination of the original site, and in approximately 5% of cases, the lesion is multifocal. Vulvar tumors may extend locally to invade adjacent structures, including the vagina, urethra, and anus; advanced vulvar tumors may invade adjacent pelvic bones.

A rich network of anastomosing lymphatics that frequently crosses the midline drains the vulva. Even minimally invasive vulvar tumors may spread to regional lymph nodes (Table 36.2-15).[579,582–585] In most cases, initial regional metastasis is to the superficial inguinal lymph nodes that are located between Camper's fascia and the fascia lata; tumors may then metastasize secondarily to the deep femoral lymph nodes located along the femoral vessels and then to the pelvic lymph nodes (Fig. 36.2-11).[580,586] However, metastases have been reported to the deep femoral lymph nodes without involvement of the superficial inguinal lymph nodes, especially from carcinomas of the clitoris and Bartholin's glands.[580,586–588] Theoretically, tumors involving the clitoris can also spread directly to the obturator nodes through lymphatics that follow the dorsal vein of the clitoris, although evidence of this route is rarely seen in practice. Despite the extensive anastomosis of lymphatics in the region, metastasis of vulvar carcinoma to contralateral lymph nodes is uncommon in patients with well-lateralized T1 lesions.[541]

The lungs are the most common sites of hematogenous metastasis.

PATHOLOGY

As classified by the International Society for the Study of Vulvar Disease, nonneoplastic epithelial disorders of the vulva (previously termed *vulvar dystrophies*) include lichen sclerosis, squamous hyperplasia, and other dermatoses.[589] Approximately 10% of these lesions have cellular atypia and are termed VIN. Histologically, VIN is characterized by disruption of the normal epithelial architecture, varying degrees of cytoplasmic and nuclear maturation, and giant cells with abnormal nuclei.[570,590] VIN lesions are assigned a grade from one to three according to their degree of maturation. Invasive cancers have been associated with two types of VIN.[570] The most common VINs contain nuclear atypia throughout the epithelial layers and are frequently associated with HPV. These lesions are sometimes subdivided into warty and basaloid types, which have greater and lesser degrees of differentiation, respectively.[570] In the second subset of VINs, atypia is largely confined to the basal layers of the epithelium. These lesions tend to occur in older women and are not usually associated with HPV but are commonly adjacent to areas of lichen sclerosis or hyperplasia. Buscema and Woodruff[591] estimated that approximately 4% of patients treated for VIN develop a subsequent invasive cancer.

Paget's disease of the vulva, a rare intraepithelial lesion located in the epidermis and skin adnexa, accounts for 1% to 5% of vulvar neoplasms. Histologically, vulvar Paget's disease is characterized by large, pale, mucopolysaccharide-rich cells that are positive for periodic acid–Schiff. Electron microscopic

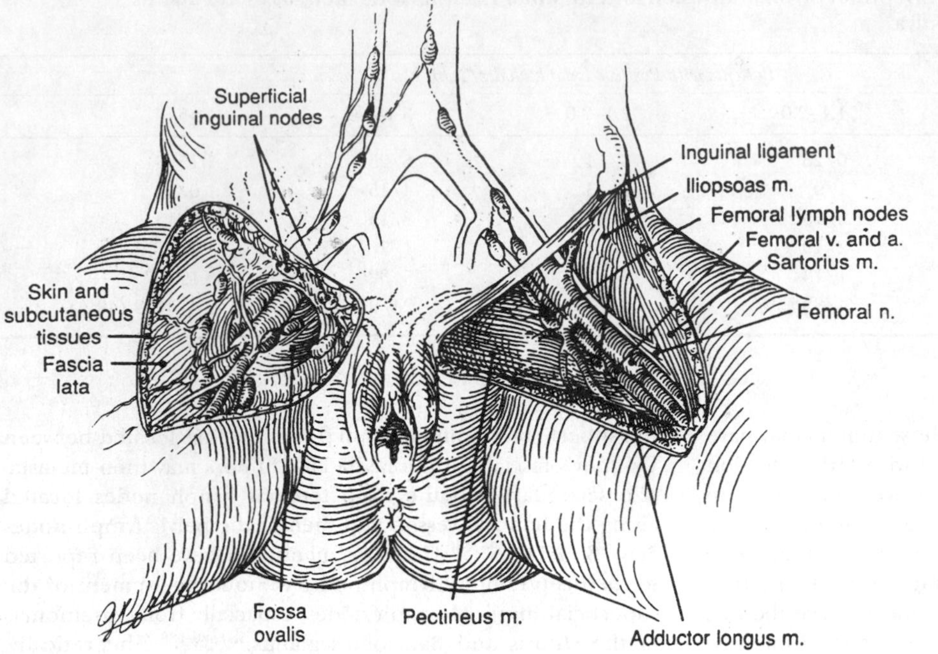

FIGURE 36.2-11. Inguinal-femoral lymph nodes. (From Hacker NF. Vulvar cancer. In: Hacker NF, Moore JG, eds. *Essentials of obstetrics and gynecology.* Philadelphia: WB Saunders, 1992:618,with permission.)

studies have suggested that Paget's cells derive from apocrine cells in the stratum germinativum of the epidermis.[592] Paget's disease usually occurs in postmenopausal women, who often present with symptoms of vulvar pruritus and discomfort.[593] Grossly, Paget's lesions appear eczematoid or, when extensive, may be raised and velvety with persistent weeping.[594] Approximately 5% to 10% of newly diagnosed Paget's lesions are associated with underlying adenocarcinoma arising locally in a vulvar vestibular gland or skin appendage or from a distant site such as the breast or rectum.[593] It has been suggested that Paget's disease with underlying adenocarcinoma represents a different process than other types of intraepithelial Paget's disease because the other types rarely progress to invasive adenocarcinoma.[595]

The term *microinvasive carcinoma of the vulva* should be used with caution. The methods and criteria used to define microinvasive carcinoma of the cervix cannot be applied to carcinoma of the vulva. Stromal invasion by vulvar carcinomas is not measured in a uniform manner, and strict criteria for the diagnosis of microinvasive vulvar cancer have not been defined. VIN is not routinely seen adjacent to invasive vulvar cancer, and the transition from normal tissue to invasive cancer can be abrupt. Elongated rete pegs may extend 6 mm or more from the basement membrane and are sometimes misconstrued as invasive cancer. The International Society of Gynecologic Pathologists recommends that the depth of stromal invasion be measured vertically from the most superficial basement membrane to the deepest tumor. Tumor thickness is defined as the distance between the granular layer of epidermis and the deepest tumor. Lymph node metastases from tumors less than 1 mm in depth or thickness are extremely rare (see Table 36.2-15).[579,582–584] For this reason, FIGO now includes a stage IA subcategory in its staging system for tumors that invade less than 1 mm (Table 36.2-16).[560] However, the risk of inguinal lymph node metastasis rises steeply as the depth of invasion exceeds 1 mm.

More than 90% of invasive vulvar cancers are squamous cell carcinomas. Atypical keratinization is the hallmark of invasive vulvar cancer. Most squamous carcinomas are well differentiated, but mitoses may be noted.[596] Approximately 5% of vulvar cancers are anaplastic carcinomas that may consist of large immature cells, spindle sarcomatoid cells, or small cells. Vulvar carcinomas consisting of small cells may resemble small cell anaplastic carcinomas of the lung or Merkel's cell tumors and have demonstrated an aggressive biologic behavior in the few reported cases.[597–599] Verrucous carcinoma is a rare, very well-differentiated form of vulvar carcinoma that usually presents in the fifth or sixth decade of life as a large, locally invasive lesion.[598] On microscopic examination, the tumor has a papillary, exophytic appearance; tumor cells retain a normal appearance of maturation and demonstrate minimal atypia. Even with extensive local invasion, lymph node metastasis from verrucous carcinoma is rare.

The diagnosis of Bartholin's gland carcinoma is based on clinical findings of a tumor arising in the anatomic location of Bartholin's glands and on the histologic appearance. Biopsy of a tumor arising from a Bartholin's gland usually reveals adenocarcinoma, but squamous cell carcinomas, transitional cell carcinomas (arising from the duct and histologically indistinguishable from transitional cell carcinoma of the bladder), and adenoid cystic carcinomas have also been reported.[588]

Rare cases of primary mammary adenocarcinoma of the vulva have been reported, presumably arising in aberrant mammary tissue occurring along the embryonic milk line.[600] Other rare carcinomas that may occur in the vulva include basal cell carcinomas[601] and sebaceous carcinomas.[602]

Malignant melanomas of the vulva account for approximately 2% to 4% of primary vulvar malignancies and 1% to 3% of melanomas arising in women.[603,604] Vulvar melanoma occurs most frequently in women older than 60 years of age, but 10% to 20% of vulvar melanomas occur in women younger than 40 years.[604] Approximately 50% of vulvar melanomas involve the labium

TABLE 36.2-16. International Federation of Gynecology and Obstetrics Staging of Carcinoma of the Vulva (1994)

Stage I	Lesions 2 cm or less in size confined to the vulva or perineum (T1).[a] No nodal metastases (N0).
Stage IA	Lesions 2 cm or less in size confined to the vulva or perineum and with stromal invasion no greater than 1.0 mm.[b] No nodal metastases.
Stage IB	Lesions 2 cm or less in size confined to the vulva or perineum and with stromal invasion greater than 1.0 mm.[b] No nodal metastases.
Stage II	Tumor confined to the vulva, perineum, or both, or more than 2 cm in the greatest dimension (T2). No nodal metastasis (N0).
Stage III	Tumor of any size with adjacent spread to the lower urethra, vagina, or both, or the anus (T3), and/or unilateral regional node metastasis (N1).
Stage IVA	Tumor invades any of the following: upper urethra, bladder mucosa, rectal mucosa, pelvic bone (T4), and/or bilateral regional node metastasis (N2).
Stage IVB	Any distant metastasis, including pelvic lymph nodes (M1).

[a]Equivalent tumor, node, metastasis (TNM) groupings according to the TNM Committee of the International Union Against Cancer are indicated in parentheses.[540]
[b]The depth of invasion is defined as the measurement of the tumor from the epithelial-stromal junction of the adjacent most superficial dermal papilla to the deepest point of invasion.
(Reprinted from ref. 105, with permission.)

majus, but tumors may also arise on the labium minus, clitoris, or perineum.[604–606] In a large Swedish series, 57% of vulvar melanomas were of the mucosal lentiginous type, 22% were nodular, and 16% were superficial spreading or lentiginous.[606] Most investigators have reported a correlation between depth of invasion or Breslow thickness and outcome.[605,607,608] However, because the vulvar epithelium sometimes lacks a well-developed papillary dermis, which makes it difficult to assign Clark's levels of invasion, Chung and colleagues proposed a modification of the Clark system that is often used to categorize patients with vulvar melanoma.[609,610] Other factors that have been associated with a poorer prognosis are ulceration, clinical amelanosis, and older age.[607] Diagnosis is made by biopsy of any suspicious pigmented or nonpigmented lesion, particularly if it is nodular or indurated or has a perilesional halo.

Vulvar sarcomas constitute 1% to 2% of vulvar malignancies and include leiomyosarcomas, rhabdomyosarcomas, angiosarcomas, neurofibrosarcomas, and epithelioid sarcomas. The prognosis appears to depend on three main determinants: lesion size, tumor contour, and mitotic activity. Lesions greater than 5 cm in diameter with infiltrating margins, extensive necrosis, and more than five mitotic figures per ten high-power fields are the most likely to recur after surgical resection.[611,612]

DIAGNOSIS, CLINICAL EVALUATION, AND STAGING

Patients with VIN may complain of vulvar pruritus, irritation, or a mass, but up to 50% of these patients are asymptomatic at the time of diagnosis.[613,614] Patients with invasive vulvar cancer usually complain of a vulvar mass and chronic vulvar pruritus. Advanced lesions may bleed and are often exquisitely tender.

Because VIN can have many manifestations, any new vulvar lesion should be biopsied. Once the diagnosis of VIN has been established, the entire vulva, cervix, and vagina should be carefully examined because patients often have multifocal or multicentric involvement.[613–615] Colposcopic examination may help to define the extent of disease.

Diagnosis of invasive vulvar lesions requires a wedge biopsy of the lesion with surrounding skin and with underlying dermis and connective tissue so the pathologist can adequately evaluate the depth of stromal invasion. This procedure can usually be performed in the physician's office under local anesthesia. Excisional biopsy is preferred for lesions smaller than 1 cm in diameter.

Patients with invasive disease require additional evaluation for regional and metastatic disease. All patients with invasive disease require a careful physical examination including a detailed pelvic examination, chest radiography, and biochemical profile. Cystoscopy and proctoscopy should be performed in patients with advanced lesions or with tumors that are near the urethra or anus, respectively. Patients who complain of bone pain or who have tumor fixed to pelvic bones should have appropriate skeletal radiography. CT or MRI scans can be obtained to evaluate deep inguinal and pelvic lymph nodes for possible regional metastasis.

In 1983, FIGO adopted a clinical TNM staging system for vulvar cancer. This system was based on a clinical assessment of the primary tumor and regional lymph nodes. However, several studies have demonstrated poor correlation between clinical assessment of the inguinal lymph nodes and pathologic findings.[251,616,617] In a study of 588 patients with tumors that invaded 5 mm or deeper, Homesley and colleagues[616] reported that although 93% of patients with fixed or ulcerated nodes had metastatic tumor, 24% of those with clinically negative nodes had inguinal lymph node metastases and 24% of patients with suspicious but mobile nodes had negative findings at lymphadenectomy. In 1988 the FIGO staging system was modified to incorporate the more accurate information gained from surgical assessment of regional lymph nodes. The staging system was revised again in 1994 to create a separate stage IA for minimally invasive lesions (see Table 36.2-16).[560]

PROGNOSTIC FACTORS

The risk of regional metastases of vulvar carcinoma and the prognosis for cure after treatment are correlated with a number of clinical and pathologic features. Clinical tumor diameter is strongly predictive of outcome and has been incorporated in

TABLE 36.2-17. Relative Survival by Tumor Diameter and Surgical Groin Node Status

	No. of Positive Groin Nodes									
	None		One		Two Unilateral		≥3 or Bilateral		Total	
Tumor Diameter (cm)	No.	Survival (%)	No.	Survival (%)	No.	Survival (%)	No.	Survival (%)	No.	Survival (%)
≤2	154	97.9	18	94.4	9	88.9	9	38.1	190	94.4
2.1–8.0	214	86.9	61	76.6	18	70.5	72	28.9	365	73.3
>8	13	65.8	3	66.7	3	50.0	3	0.0	22	55.7
Total	381	90.9	82	79.7	30	74.0	84	29.0	577[a]	90.9

[a]Three patients had an undetermined number of positive nodes and eight had unknown lesion diameter.
(Adapted from ref. 619.)

the FIGO staging system (Table 36.2-17; see Table 36.2-16). Other factors that have consistently been correlated with outcome include depth of invasion, tumor thickness, and the presence or absence of LVSI.[251,616,618–620] These features tend to be correlated with one another, and all are predictive of lymph node metastasis. More than 75% of patients with LVSI have positive inguinal nodes.[582,616,621] Studies of the relationship between tumor grade and outcome have drawn varying conclusions, possibly reflecting the inconsistent criteria used to grade vulvar tumors.[259,582,616,617,621,622] Other factors that tend to be associated with prognosis include the amount of keratin, the mitotic rate, and the tumor growth pattern.[582,618,623,624] Aneuploid tumors appear to have a poorer prognosis than diploid tumors, but ploidy tends to be correlated with other prognostic factors and may not be an independent predictor of outcome.[625,626] Several authors have reported that tumors containing HPV DNA have a poorer prognosis than HPV-negative tumors.[565,569] Some investigators have reported a worse prognosis for patients aged 70 years or older, whereas others have found no correlation between prognosis and age.[579,616,622,623]

Prognosis is strongly correlated with the presence and number of inguinal node metastases (see Table 36.2-17). In a study of 586 patients treated in two GOG trials, Homesley and colleagues[619] reported 5-year survival rates of 91% for patients with negative inguinal lymph nodes and 75%, 36%, and 24%, respectively, for patients with one or two, three or four, or five or six positive nodes. None of the 16 patients with seven or more nodes involved with tumor survived. Patients with bilateral node involvement had a survival rate of 25%, compared with 71% for those with unilateral node involvement. The authors did not state whether patients with bilateral nodal disease had a poorer prognosis than did patients with a similar number of unilateral metastases. Homesley and colleagues[627] reported that patients with pelvic node metastases had a particularly poor survival rate: Among patients treated with surgery alone, 3-year survival rates were 23% for patients with pelvic node metastases versus 73% for patients with only inguinal node involvement. For this reason, FIGO has categorized tumors that have spread to the pelvic nodes as stage IV. However, it should be remembered that most of these series include patients who did not receive postoperative irradiation. It is not possible from available data to define the prognosis of patients who received multidisciplinary treatment for vulvar cancer metastatic to pelvic lymph nodes.

In 1995, van der Velden and colleagues[628] published a detailed study of nodal prognostic factors in 71 patients with inguinal node metastases from vulvar carcinomas. Patients with extranodal spread or more than two positive nodes received adjuvant radiotherapy to an unspecified dose. The most powerful predictor of outcome in their study was extranodal tumor extension: 28 (63%) of 44 patients with extranodal tumor died of disease versus three (14%) of 22 without this finding. In Cox regression analysis, none of the other factors studied (tumor size, number of nodes, FIGO stage, nodal size, degree of nodal replacement, laterality) added to the predictive power of extranodal extension. Origoni and colleagues reported similar findings in a series of 53 patients with positive nodes.[629]

Studying the relationship between surgical margins and tumor recurrence, Heaps and colleagues[618] reported no local failures in 91 patients whose closest tumor margin (deep or at the skin surface) was 8 mm or more in the fixed specimen. Ten (43%) of 23 patients with margins of 4.8 mm or less experienced a local recurrence, as did 8 (62%) of 13 patients with margins between 4.8 mm and 8.0 mm.

TREATMENT

The traditional operative approach to invasive carcinoma of the vulva, radical *en bloc* resection of the vulva and inguinofemoral nodes, was developed at the beginning of the twentieth century, was popularized during subsequent decades, and remained the standard of care until the early 1980s.[630–632] Radiotherapy was thought to have little role in the treatment of vulvar cancer. Although this surgical approach achieved 5-year survival rates of 60% to 70%, the surgery caused significant physical and psychological complications, and patients with multiple positive nodes continued to have a poor prognosis. In 1981, Hacker and colleagues[633] demonstrated that a less morbid surgical approach, operating through separate vulvar and groin incisions, achieved cure rates similar to those achieved with the traditional radical vulvectomy. Since then, there has been a continuing trend toward less radical surgery for early-stage disease. In addition, prospective and retrospective studies have established the role of radiotherapy in the curative management of locoregionally advanced disease.

Preinvasive Disease (Vulvar Intraepithelial Neoplasia)

After invasive carcinoma has been excluded by a sufficient number of excisional biopsies, the treatment of VIN should be as conservative as possible. Focal lesions can be simply excised. Multiple lesions can be excised separately or, if confluent, with a larger single excision. This approach is generally well tolerated and provides material for histologic assessment. When there is more extensive VIN, the lesions can be vaporized with a CO_2 laser. This method may provide an alternative to more extensive operations but does not yield a specimen for histologic inspection.

Extensive, diffuse VIN may require a wider excision, particularly if the lesion involves the perianal skin. These lesions are sometimes treated with a partial vulvectomy of the superficial skin (called *skinning vulvectomy*). Whenever possible, the vulvar skin should be sutured primarily, but a split-thickness skin graft is sometimes needed to close the defect.

VIN often recurs at or near the margins of resection, even when the histopathologic analysis demonstrates that the initial lesions were completely resected. Presumably this phenomenon reflects the multifocal nature of the condition.[615] In fact, VIN can recur within the donor skin from split-thickness grafts.[541]

T1 and T2

Invasive vulvar tumors can usually be treated effectively without the complications of *en bloc* radical vulvectomy and inguinal node dissection. Today, most gynecologic oncologists advocate an individualized approach to early invasive vulvar carcinomas.[583,634–638] Overall 5-year disease-specific survival rates for stage I (T1N0M0) and stage II (T2N0M0) disease are approximately 98% and 85%, respectively.[619]

Most T1 and selected T2 lesions can be controlled locally with a radical wide local excision. A wide and deep excision of the lesion is performed, with the incision extended down to the inferior fascia of the urogenital diaphragm. An effort should be made to remove the lesion with a 2-cm margin of normal tissue in all directions unless this would require sacrifice of the anus or urethra. The surgical defect is closed in two layers. Small T1 lesions that invade 1 mm or less can be managed with local resection alone because the risk of regional spread is small (see Table 36.2-15). Patients with more invasive tumors must also have surgical or radiation treatment of the inguinal nodes as discussed here.

Larger T2 tumors may require radical vulvectomy to obtain acceptable tumor clearance with negative margins. *En bloc* resection of the vulva and inguinal nodes was once believed to be necessary to prevent recurrences in the soft tissue intervening between the vulva and regional nodes; however, most surgeons now perform the operation through separate vulvar and groin incisions. Although recurrences have been reported in this *tissue bridge*, these appear to be rare, and the risk of complications is significantly decreased when separate incisions are used.[633,637–640]

Wound seroma is the most common acute complication of radical vulvectomy and inguinal node dissection, occurring in approximately 15% of cases.[583,635] Other acute complications include urinary tract infection, wound cellulitis, temporary anterior thigh anesthesia from femoral nerve injury, thrombophlebitis, and, rarely, pulmonary embolus.[583,627,635,637,639] The most common chronic complication is leg edema, but this risk has decreased from approximately 30% to 15% with the use of separate groin incisions.[638] Other chronic complications including genital prolapse, urinary stress incontinence, temporary weakness of the quadriceps muscle, and introital stenosis. Rare late complications include pubic osteomyelitis, femoral hernia, and rectoperineal fistula. These risks are less when separate incisions are used and are further reduced when radical local excision of the primary lesion is done instead of radical vulvectomy.[635,638,641,642]

T3 and T4

Primary tumors that involve the anus, rectum, rectovaginal septum, or proximal urethra pose a difficult problem because adequate surgical clearance can be obtained only by combining a pelvic exenteration with radical vulvectomy and bilateral groin node dissection. Although some patients may be cured with this ultraradical surgery, the risks of acute and long-term complications of the procedure are substantial.[643–645] For this reason, a number of investigators have explored the use of combined surgery and irradiation to spare critical structures in patients with locally advanced disease.

In some cases, patients with T3 tumors that minimally involve the external urethra or anus can undergo initial vulvectomy without sacrifice of major organ function if close margins are accepted near critical structures. Postoperative radiotherapy can then be delivered to prevent local recurrence.[646–648] Although local recurrences are frequently successfully controlled with additional surgery, Faul and colleagues[649] reported an overall 5-year survival rate of only 40% after the first local recurrence and emphasized the importance of achieving local control. These authors reported a significant reduction in the local failure rate (from 58% to 16%) when tumors that were within 8 mm of the operative margins were irradiated after surgery.[649] In such cases, the vulva may be treated with opposed anterior and posterior photon fields (if the inguinal regions also require treatment) or with an appositional perineal electron beam.[648,650] The vulva should receive a total dose of 50 to 65 Gy depending on the proximity of disease to the surgical margin.

In the early 1980s, several investigators[651–655] reported results of preoperative radiotherapy in small series of patients with locally advanced disease. These reports indicated that modest doses of radiation (45 to 55 Gy) produced dramatic tumor responses in some patients with T3 and T4 disease, permitting organ-sparing surgery without sacrifice of tumor control. Hacker and colleagues[654] reported that four of eight patients with T3 to T4 tumors treated preoperatively with 44 to 54 Gy had no residual tumor in the vulvectomy specimen and that seven of these eight had local control of their disease. More recently, investigators have emphasized the use of concurrent chemoradiation in this setting.

Chemotherapy in Locoregionally Advanced Disease

To reduce the need for morbid ultraradical surgery and to improve locoregional control rates, a number of investigators have explored combinations of chemotherapy with radiation and surgery in patients with locally advanced vulvar carcinoma.[556,656–668] Most studies have used combinations of cisplatin, 5-FU, and mitomycin C, extrapolating from the high response rates observed with use of this treatment for locally advanced carcinomas of the cervix and head and neck and from studies that have demonstrated the efficacy of these drugs as radiosensitizers in the treatment of carcinomas of the anus. Treatment schedules usually include a 4- to 5-day infusion of 5-FU combined with one of the other two drugs, with this course repeated every 3 to 4 weeks (Table 36.2-18). Studies have usu-

TABLE 36.2-18. Concurrent Chemoradiotherapy in the Management of Locally Advanced or Recurrent Carcinoma of the Vulva

Investigator	*No. of Patients*	*Chemotherapy*	*Radiation Therapy Dose (Gy)*	*No. with Recurrent or Persistent Local Disease after Radiation Therapy ± Surgery*	*Follow-up (mo)*
Moore et al.[656]	73	5-FU + CDDP	47.6	15 (21%)	22–72
Cunningham et al.[657]	14	5-FU + CDDP	45–50	4 (29%)	7–81
Landoni et al.[658]	58	5-FU + Mito	54	13 (22%)	4–48
Lupi et al.[659]	31	5-FU + Mito	54	7 (23%)	22–73
Wahlen et al.[660]	19	5-FU + Mito	45–50	1 (5%)	3–70
Eifel et al.[661]	12	5-FU + CDDP	40–50	5 (42%)	17–30
Koh et al.[662]	20	5-FU ± CDDP or Mito	30–54	9 (45%)	1–75
Russell et al.[663]	25	5-FU ± CDDP	47–72	6 (24%)	4–52
Scheistroen et al.[664]	42	Bleomycin	45	39 (93%)	7–60
Berek et al.[665]	12	5-FU + CDDP	44–54	0	7–60
Thomas et al.[666]	24	5-FU ± Mito	44–60	10 (42%)	5–43
Evans et al.[556]	4	5-FU + Mito	25–70	2 (50%)	20–29
Levin et al.[667]	6	5-FU + Mito	18–60	0	1–25
Iverson et al.[668]	15	Bleomycin	15–40	11 (83%)[a]	4

CDDP, cisplatinum; 5-FU, 5-fluorouracil; Mito, mitomycin C.
[a]Most patients had unresectable, stage IV lesions.

ally included small numbers of patients with advanced local or regional disease. However, most investigators have observed impressive responses that often appear to be better than would be expected with radiation alone. Randomized trials have not been done and may be difficult to perform because of the small number of patients with locally advanced vulvar cancer. However, trials that demonstrated improved local control and survival when concurrent cisplatin-containing chemotherapy was added to radiation treatment of cervical cancers[229,230,232] and improved colostomy-free survival when mitomycin C and 5-FU were added to radiation treatment of anal cancer[669] suggest that this approach may be also be useful treatment of women with vulvar cancer.

Only one study has investigated the role of neoadjuvant chemotherapy in the treatment of locally advanced vulvar cancer. Benedetti-Panici and colleagues[670] treated 21 patients with stage IVA vulvar cancers with two to three cycles of cisplatin, bleomycin, and methotrexate followed by radical surgery. Two (10%) of 21 patients had partial responses of their vulvar tumors, and 14 (67%) had partial responses of regional nodes. Ninety percent of the tumors were considered operable, but the 3-year survival rate was only 24%.

Caution is warranted in designing aggressive treatment protocols for patients with vulvar cancers, who typically are elderly and often have concurrent medical problems. Serious pulmonary toxicity has been observed in a number of patients treated on studies that included bleomycin.[664,668,671] In the largest published series of patients treated with mitomycin C and 5-FU, hematologic tolerance was acceptable, but the administered dose of mitomycin C was somewhat lower than that generally used in the treatment of anal cancers.[666]

Treatment of Regional Disease

Effective regional treatment is the single most important factor in the curative management of early vulvar cancer. Although patients with vulvar recurrences can often have their disease successfully controlled with additional local treatment, patients who suffer inguinal recurrences are rarely curable.

All patients with primary tumors that invade more than 1 mm must have their inguinal nodes treated. Traditional management includes a bilateral radical inguinal lymph node dissection. Today, this is usually performed through separate groin incisions. An ellipse of skin is removed 1 cm below and parallel to the groin crease.[633] The incision is extended down to the fascia lata and 2 cm above the inguinal ligament to remove the inguinal nodes. The saphenous vein is tied off, the fascia lata is split, and the femoral nodes are dissected. A suction drain is placed, and the wound closed in two layers.

At one time, pelvic node resection was also performed in all patients with invasive vulvar cancer. When subsequent studies demonstrated that pelvic node metastases were found only in patients with clinically suspicious or multiple positive inguinal nodes, use of the procedure was limited to patients determined intraoperatively to have positive inguinal nodes.[672–674]

Then, in 1986, Homesley and colleagues[627] published results of a randomized, prospective study that compared pelvic node resection with inguinal and pelvic irradiation in patients with inguinal node metastases from carcinoma of the vulva. All patients were initially treated with radical vulvectomy and inguinal lymphadenectomy. Patient randomization was done intraoperatively after frozen section evaluation of the inguinal nodes. This trial was closed prematurely, after 114 eligible patients had been entered, when interim analysis revealed a survival advantage for the radiation treatment arm ($P = .03$). The difference was most marked for patients with clinically positive or multiple histologically positive groin nodes (Fig. 36.2-12). For patients with two or more positive nodes, the 2-year survival rates were 63% and 37% for the radiotherapy and pelvic node resection groups, respectively. Analysis of failure patterns reveals that the largest difference between treatment groups was in the number of inguinal failures (Fig. 36.2-13). With the publication of

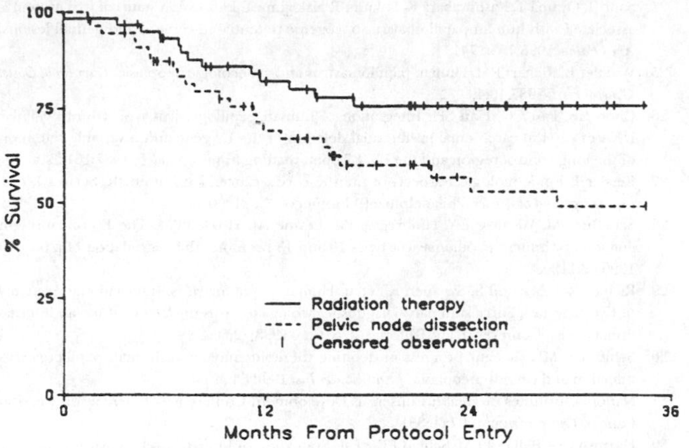

FIGURE 36.2-12. Survival rates of 114 patients with invasive squamous cell carcinoma of the vulva who were entered on a Gynecologic Oncology Group protocol in which patients with positive groin nodes after radical vulvectomy and bilateral inguinal lymphadenectomies were randomly assigned to receive pelvic lymph node dissection or postoperative irradiation to the pelvis and inguinal nodes ($P = .004$). (From ref. 627, with permission.)

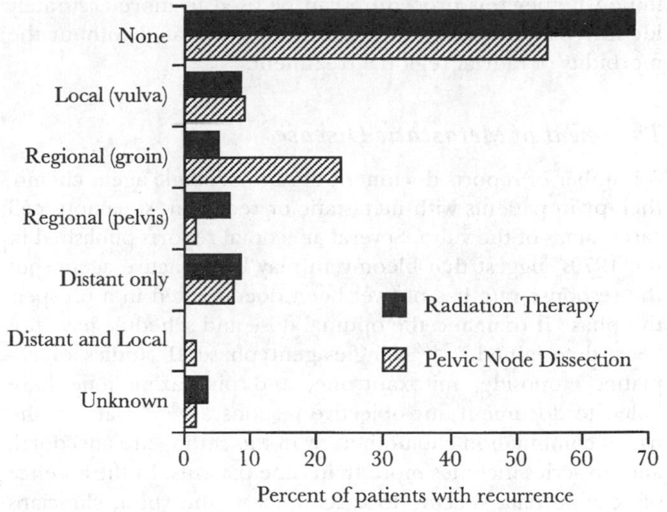

FIGURE 36.2-13. Sites of recurrence in 114 patients with invasive squamous cell carcinoma of the vulva who were entered on a Gynecologic Oncology Group protocol in which patients with positive groin nodes after radical vulvectomy and bilateral inguinal lymphadenectomies were randomly assigned to receive pelvic lymph node dissection or postoperative irradiation to the pelvis and inguinal nodes. (From ref. 627, with permission.)

this study, most practitioners abandoned routine pelvic node dissection, and postoperative radiotherapy became standard for most patients with inguinal node metastases.

Most of the serious acute and subacute complications of radical vulvectomy are related to the lymph node dissection, although these risks have decreased somewhat with the use of separate groin incisions.[674–677] Complications include wound disruption or infection in 50% to 75% of cases, chronic lymphedema in 20% to 50%, and a perioperative mortality of 2% to 5%. Patients who undergo vulvectomy without inguinal node dissection have significantly shorter hospital stays and fewer complications.[674,675,677]

Although radical inguinal lymphadenectomy has historically been considered the treatment of choice for regional management of invasive vulvar carcinoma, several retrospective studies have suggested that regional radiotherapy may be an effective and less morbid way of preventing recurrence in patients with clinically negative groins. In a review of 91 patients who had elective treatment of the inguinal nodes for cancers with primary drainage to the inguinal nodes, Henderson and colleagues[678] observed only two recurrences after treatment with 45 to 50 Gy over 5 weeks, and both of these occurred outside the treatment fields. In a retrospective review of 42 patients with invasive vulvar carcinomas, Petereit and colleagues[675] found no difference in the groin recurrence rate for patients with clinically negative inguinal nodes treated with radical lymphadenectomy or radiotherapy, even though the irradiated patients in their series had more advanced primary tumors. The complications of treatment, including lymphedema, wound separation, and infection, and the length of hospitalization were greater for patients who had had lymphadenectomy. Leiserowitz and colleagues[679] reported no groin recurrences in 23 patients with locally advanced, clinically N0 vulvar cancers after prophylactic treatment of the groins with concurrent chemoradiation.

In 1992 the GOG reported the results of a trial that randomly assigned patients with clinically negative inguinal nodes to receive inguinal node irradiation or radical lymphadenectomy (followed by inguinopelvic irradiation in patients with positive nodes) after resection of the primary tumor.[677] The study was closed after entry of only 58 patients, when an interim analysis demonstrated a significantly higher rate of inguinal recurrence and death in the irradiated group. The authors concluded that lymphadenectomy was the superior treatment, although the morbidity rate of lymphadenectomy was greater than that of groin irradiation. However, the radiotherapy techniques used in this study have since been criticized. CT scans were not consistently obtained to verify the position and size of inguinal nodes. Patients were treated with anterior appositional fields, the dose was prescribed at a depth of 3 cm, and the use of electrons (usually 12 meV) was emphasized. This method of treatment can lead to significant underdosage of the inguinofemoral nodes, which frequently extend to a depth of more than 5 to 8 cm.[680,681] Because of these criticisms, the study's results and the role of radiation in the primary management of clinically negative inguinal nodes remains controversial.

Some surgeons have tried to reduce surgical complications by reducing the extent of lymph node dissections. Burke and colleagues[641] reported four (5%) groin recurrences in 74 patients with T1 to T2 tumors treated with wide local excision and superficial inguinal lymphadenectomy (unilateral or bilateral depending on the location of the tumor). In a prospective study of patients with favorable primary lesions (T1, less than or equal to 5 mm thick, no LVSI), the GOG[682] reported nine (7%) inguinal recurrences in 121 patients who had negative findings on ipsilateral superficial inguinal lymphadenectomy. A number of investigators have explored the use of intraoperative lymphatic mapping to identify a *sentinel* node that would predict the presence or absence of regional metastases.[683–686] Preliminary studies suggest that a sentinel node can be identified in most patients. Further study will be needed to determine whether this procedure can be used to more accurately identify patients who can be successfully treated without the morbidity of radical regional treatment.

Treatment of Metastatic Disease

A number of reports document the use of single-agent chemotherapy in patients with metastatic or recurrent squamous cell carcinomas of the vulva. Several anecdotal reports published in the 1970s suggest that bleomycin may be an active agent, but the response rate has not yet been documented in a prospective phase II trial, and the optimal dose and schedule have not been determined.[687–689] Single-agent phase II studies of cisplatin, etoposide, mitoxantrone, and piperazinedione have failed to document any objective responses.[555,690] Data on the use of combination chemotherapy in this setting are anecdotal, and no series includes more than nine patients. In the absence of reliable data specific to carcinoma of the vulva, clinicians often use combinations that have had some activity in the treatment of cervical cancer. However, there are as yet few data to indicate that chemotherapy can provide effective palliation for patients with metastatic or recurrent vulvar carcinoma that is not amenable to locoregional treatments.

REFERENCES

1. Landis SH, Murray T, Bolden S, et al. Cancer statistics, 1999. *CA Cancer J Clin* 1999;49:8.
2. Brinton LA, Tashima KT, Lehman HF, et al. Epidemiology of cervical cancer by cell type. *Cancer Res* 1987;47:1706.
3. Wingo PA, Tong T, Bolden S. Cancer statistics, 1995. *CA Cancer J Clin* 1995;45:8.
4. Bosch FX, Castellsague X, Munoz N, et al. Male sexual behavior and human papillomavirus DNA: key risk factors for cervical cancer in Spain. *J Natl Cancer Inst* 1996;88:1060.
5. Skegg DCG, Corwin PA, Paul C. Importance of the male factor in cancer of the cervix. *Lancet* 1982;2:581.
6. Meanwell CA. The epidemiology and etiology of cervical cancer. In: Blackledge GRP, Jordan JA, Shingleton HM, eds. *Textbook of gynecologic oncology.* Philadelphia: WB Saunders, 1991:250.
7. American Cancer Society. *Cancer facts and figures—1997.* Atlanta, GA: American Cancer Society, 1997.
8. Baquet CR, Horm JW, Gibbs T, et al. Socioeconomic factors and cancer incidence among blacks and whites. *J Natl Cancer Inst* 1991;83:551.
9. Freeman HP. Cancer in the socioeconomically disadvantaged. *CA Cancer J Clin* 1989;39:266.
10. Parkin DM, Pisani P, Ferlay J. Estimates of the worldwide incidence of 25 major cancers in 1990. *Int J Cancer* 1999; 80:827.
11. Whelan SL, Parkin DM, Masuyer E. *Patterns of cancer in five continents.* Lyons: International Agency for Research on Cancer, 1990.
12. Herrero R. Epidemiology of cervical cancer. *J Natl Cancer Inst Monogr* 1996;21:1.
13. Parazzini F, LaVecchia C. Epidemiology of adenocarcinoma of the cervix. *Gynecol Oncol* 1990;39:40.
14. Vizcaino AP, Moreno V, Bosch FX, Munoz N, Barros-Dios XM, Parkin DM. International trends in the incidence of cervical cancer. I. Adenocarcinoma and adenosquamous cell carcinomas. *Int J Cancer* 1998;75:536.
15. Zheng T, Holford TR, Ma Z, et al. The continuing increase in adenocarcinoma of the uterine cervix: a birth cohort phenomenon. *Int J Epidemiol* 1996;25:252.
16. Thomas DB, Ray RM. Oral contraceptives and invasive adenocarcinomas and adenosquamous carcinomas of the uterine cervix. The World Health Organization Collaborative Study of Neoplasia and Steroid Contraceptives. *Am J Epidemiol* 1996;144:281.
17. Ursin G, Peters RK, Henderson BE, et al. Oral contraceptive use and adenocarcinoma of cervix. *Lancet* 1994;344:1390.
18. Stubblefield PG. Oral contraceptives and neoplasia. *J Reprod Med* 1984;29:524.
19. Bergeron C, Barrasso R, Beaudenon S, et al. Human papillomaviruses associated with cervical intraepithelial neoplasia. Great diversity and distinct distribution in low- and high-grade lesions. *Am J Surg Pathol* 1992;16:641.
20. Durst M, Gissman L, Ikenberg H, Hausen H. A papillomavirus DNA from a cervical carcinoma and its prevalence in cancer biopsy specimens from different geographic regions. *Proc Natl Acad Sci U S A* 1983;80:3812.
21. Bosch FX, Manos MM, Munoz N, et al. Prevalence of human papillomavirus in cervical cancer: a worldwide perspective. International Biological Study on Cervical Cancer (IBSCC) Study Group [see comments]. *J Natl Cancer Inst* 1995;87:796.
22. Arends MJ, Buckley CH, Wells M. Aetiology, pathogenesis, and pathology of cervical neoplasia. *J Clin Pathol* 1998;51:96.
23. Pillai MR, Halabi S, McKalip A, et al. The presence of human papillomavirus-16/-18 E6, p53, and Bcl-2 protein in cervicovaginal smears from patients with invasive cervical cancer. *Cancer Epidemiol Biomarkers Prev* 1996;5:329.
24. Sano T, Oyama T, Kashiwabara K, Fukuda T, Nakajima T. Expression status of p16 protein is associated with human papillomavirus oncogenic potential in cervical and genital lesions. *Am J Pathol* 1998;153:1741.
25. Winkler B, Richart RM. Human papillomavirus and gynecologic neoplasia. *Curr Probl Obstet Gynecol Fertil* 1987;10:49.
26. Choo KB, Pan CC, Han SH. Integration of human papillomavirus type 16 into cellular DNA of cervical carcinoma: preferential deletion of the E2 gene and invariable retention of the long control region and the E6/E7 open reading frames. *Virology* 1987;161:259.
27. Kessler I. Epidemiological aspects of uterine cervix cancer. In: Lurain JR, Sciarra J, eds. *Gynecology and obstetrics.* Philadelphia: JB Lippincott Co, 1990:1.
28. Scheffner M, Werness BA, Huibregtse JM, Levine AJ, Howley PM. The E6 oncoprotein encoded by human papillomavirus types 16 and 18 promotes the degradation of p 53. *Cell* 1990;63:1129.
29. Richart RM, Masood S, Syrjanen KJ, et al. Human papillomavirus. International Academy of Cytology Task Force summary. Diagnostic cytology towards the 21st century: an international expert Conference and Tutorial. *Acta Cytol* 1998;42:50.
30. Schiffman MH. Recent progress in defining the epidemiology of human papillomavirus infection and cervical neoplasia. *J Natl Cancer Inst* 1992;84:394.
31. National Institutes of Health Consensus Development Conference Statement on Cervical Cancer. *Gynecol Oncol* 1997;66:351.
32. Harnish DG, Belland LM, Scheid EE, et al. Evaluation of human papillomavirus-consensus primers for HPV detection by the polymerase chain reaction. *Mol Cell Probes* 1999;13:9.
33. Bernard HU, Chan SY, Manos MM, et al. Identification and assessment of known and novel human papillomaviruses by polymerase chain reaction amplification, restriction fragment length polymorphisms, nucleotide sequence, and phylogenetic algorithms. *J Infect Dis* 1994;170:1077.
34. Joste NE, Rushing L, Granados R, et al. Bethesda classification of cervicovaginal smears: reproducibility and viral correlates. *Hum Pathol* 1996;27:581.
35. Burger RA, Monk BJ, Kurosaki T, et al. Human papillomavirus type 18: association with poor prognosis in early stage cervical cancer [see comments]. *J Natl Cancer Inst* 1996;88:1361.
36. Tseng CJ, Tseng LH, Lai CH, et al. Identification of human papillomavirus types 16 and 18 deoxyribonucleic acid sequences in bulky cervical cancer after chemotherapy. *Am J Obstet Gynecol* 1997;176:865.
37. Walker J, Bloss JD, Liao SV, et al. Human papillomavirus genotype as a prognostic indicator in carcinoma of the uterine cervix. *Obstet Gynecol* 1989;74:781.
38. Fait G, Daniel Y, Kupferminc MJ, et al. Does typing of human papillomavirus assist in the triage of women with repeated low-grade, cervical cytologic abnormalities? [see comments]. *Gynecol Oncol* 1998;70:319.
39. Meijer CJ, Helmerhorst TJ, Rozendaal L, et al. HPV typing and testing in gynaecological pathology: has the time come? [comment]. *Histopathology* 1998;33:83.
40. Sherman ME, Schiffman MH, Strickler H, et al. Prospects for a prophylactic HPV vaccine: rationale and future implications for cervical cancer screening. *Diagn Cytopathol* 1998;18:5.
41. Buehler JW, Ward JW. A new definition for AIDS surveillance. *Ann Intern Med* 1993;118:390.
42. Beral V, Newton R. Overview of the epidemiology of immunodeficiency-associated cancers. *J Natl Cancer Inst Monogr* 1998;23:1.
43. Franceschi S, Dal Maso L, Arniani S, et al. Risk of cancer other than Kaposi's sarcoma and non-Hodgkin's lymphoma in persons with AIDS in Italy. Cancer and AIDS Registry Linkage Study. *Br J Cancer* 1998;78:966.
44. Goedert JJ, Cote TR, Virgo P, et al. Spectrum of AIDS-associated malignant disorders. *Lancet* 1998;351:1833.
45. Rabkin CS, Biggar RJ, Baptiste MS, et al. Cancer incidence trends in women at high risk of human immunodeficiency virus (HIV) infection. *Int J Cancer* 1993;55:208.
46. Serraino D, Carrieri P, Pradier C, et al. Risk of invasive cervical cancer among women with, or at risk for, HIV infection. *Int J Cancer* 1999;82:334.
47. Maiman M, Fruchter RG, Guy L, et al. Human immunodeficiency virus infection and invasive cervical carcinoma. *Cancer* 1993;71:402.
48. Schafer A, Friedmann W, Mielke M, et al. The increased frequency of cervical dysplasia-neoplasia in women infected with the human immunodeficiency virus is related to the degree of immunosuppression. *Am J Obstet Gynecol* 1991;164:593.
49. Buehler JW, Hanson DL, Chu SY. The reporting of HIV/AIDS deaths in women. *Am J Public Health* 1992;82:1500.
50. Castello G, Esposito E, Stellato G, et al. Immunological abnormalities in patients with cervical carcinoma. *Gynecol Oncol* 1986;25:61.
51. Schwartz LB, Carcangiu ML, Bradham L, et al. Rapidly progressive squamous cell carcinoma of the cervix coexisting with human immunodeficiency virus infection: clinical opinion. *Gynecol Oncol* 1991;41:255.
52. Serur E, Fruchter RG, Maiman M, et al. Age, substance abuse, and survival of patients with cervical carcinoma. *Cancer* 1995;75:2530.
53. Kivlahan C, Ingram E. Papanicolaou smears without endocervical cells. Are they inadequate? *Acta Cytol* 1986;30:258.
54. Walton RJ. Editorial: the task force on cervical cancer screening programs. *Can Med Assoc J* 1976;114:981.
55. Miller AB. Control of carcinoma of the cervix by exfoliative cytology screening. In: Coppleson M, ed. *Gynecologic oncology. Fundamental principles and clinical practice.* Edinburgh: Churchill Livingstone, 1981:381.
56. Syrjanen KV, Kataja V, Vyliskoski M, et al. Natural history of cervical human papillomavirus lesions does not substantiate the biological relevance of the Bethesda system. *Obstet Gynecol* 1992;79:675.
57. Richart RM, Barron BA. A follow-up study of patients with cervical dysplasia. *Am J Obstet Gynecol* 1969;105:386.
58. Plentl AA, Friedman EA. Lymphatics of the cervix uteri. In: *Lymphatic system of female genitalia.* Philadelphia: WB Saunders, 1971:75.
59. Netter FH. *The CIBA collection of medical illustrations.* Vol. 2. Reproductive system. Summit, NJ: CIBA Pharmaceutical, 1988.

60. Girardi F, Haas J. The importance of the histologic processing of pelvic lymph nodes in the treatment of cervical cancer. *Int J Gynecol Cancer* 1993;3:12.
61. Averette HE, Nguyen HN, Donato DM, et al. Radical hysterectomy for invasive cervical cancer. A 25-year prospective experience with the Miami technique. *Cancer* 1993;71:1422.
62. Kamura T, Tsukamoto N, Tsuruchi N, et al. Multivariate analysis of the histopathologic prognostic factors of cervical cancer in patients undergoing radical hysterectomy. *Cancer* 1992;69:181.
63. Alvarez RD, Potter ME, Soong SJ, et al. Rationale for using pathologic tumor dimensions and nodal status to subclassify surgically treated stage IB cervical cancer patients. *Gynecol Oncol* 1991;43:108.
64. Ayhan A, Tuncer ZS. Radical hysterectomy with lymphadenectomy for treatment of early stage cervical cancer: clinical experience of 278 cases. *J Surg Oncol* 1991;47:175.
65. Delgado G, Bundy BN, Fowler WC, et al. A prospective surgical pathological study of stage I squamous carcinoma of the cervix: a Gynecologic Oncology Group study. *Gynecol Oncol* 1989;36:314.
66. Lee Y-N, Wang KL, Lin M-H, et al. Radical hysterectomy with pelvic lymph node dissection for treatment of cervical cancer: a clinical review of 954 cases. *Gynecol Oncol* 1989;32:135.
67. Fuller AF, Elliott N, Kosloff C, et al. Determinants of increased risk for recurrence in patients undergoing radical hysterectomy for stage IB and IIA carcinoma of the cervix. *Gynecol Oncol* 1989;33:34.
68. Barber H. Cervical cancer: pelvic and para-aortic lymph node sampling and its consequences. *Baillieres Clin Obstet Gynaecol* 1988;2:769.
69. Burghardt E, Pickel H, Haas J, et al. Prognostic factors and operative treatment of stages IB to IIB cervical cancer. *Am J Obstet Gynecol* 1987;156:988.
70. Creasman WT, Soper JT, Clarke-Pearson D. Radical hysterectomy as therapy for early carcinoma of the cervix. *Am J Obstet Gynecol* 1986;155:964.
71. Boyce J, Fruchter R, Nicastri A, et al. Prognostic factors in stage I carcinoma of the cervix. *Gynecol Oncol* 1981;12:154.
72. Piver MS, Chung WS. Prognostic significance of cervical lesion size and pelvic node metastases in cervical carcinoma. *Obstet Gynecol* 1975;46:507.
73. Boronow RC. Stage I cervix cancer and pelvic node metastasis. *Am J Obstet Gynecol* 1977; 127:135.
74. Sudarsanam A, Charyulu K, Belinson J, et al. Influence of exploratory celiotomy on the management of carcinoma of the cervix. A preliminary report. *Cancer* 1978;41:1049.
75. Stehman FB, Bundy BN, Disaia PJ, et al. Carcinoma of the cervix treated with radiation therapy. I. A multivariate analysis of prognostic variables in the Gynecologic Oncology Group. *Cancer* 1991;67:2776.
76. LaPolla JP, Schlaerth JB, Gaddis O, et al. The influence of surgical staging on the evaluation and treatment of patients with cervical carcinoma. *Gynecol Oncol* 1986;24:194.
77. Berman ML, Keys H, Creasman W, et al. Survival and patterns of recurrence in cervical cancer metastatic to periaortic lymph nodes (a Gynecologic Oncology Group study). *Gynecol Oncol* 1984;19:8.
78. Ballon SC, Berman ML, Lagasse LD, et al. Survival after extraperitoneal pelvic and paraaortic lymphadenectomy and radiation therapy in cervical carcinoma. *Obstet Gynecol* 1981;57:90.
79. Lagasse LD, Creasman WT, Singleton HM, et al. Results and complications of operative staging in cervical cancer: experiences of the Gynecologic Oncology Group. *Gynecol Oncol* 1980;9:90.
80. Buchsbaum H. Extrapelvic lymph node metastases in cervical carcinoma. *Am J Obstet Gynecol* 1979;133:814.
81. Wharton JT, Jones HWI, Day T, et al. Preirradiation celiotomy and extended-field irradiation for invasive carcinoma of the cervix. *Obstet Gynecol* 1977;49:333.
82. Nelson JH, Boyce J, Macasaet M, et al. Incidence, significance, and follow-up of para-aortic lymph node metastases in late invasive carcinoma of the cervix. *Am J Obstet Gynecol* 1977;128:336.
83. Guthrie RT, Buchsbaum HJ, White AJ, et al. Para-aortic lymph node irradiation in carcinoma of the uterine cervix. *Cancer* 1974;34:166.
84. Kjorstad KE, Kjolvenstvedt A, Strickert T. The value of complete lymphadenectomy in radical treatment of cancer of the cervix, stage IB. *Cancer* 1984;54:2215.
85. Fagundes H, Perez CA, Grigsby PW, et al. Distant metastases after irradiation alone in carcinoma of the uterine cervix. *Int J Radiat Oncol Biol Phys* 1992;24:197.
86. Van Nagell JR, Rayburn W, Donaldson ES, et al. Therapeutic implications of patterns of recurrence in cancer of the uterine cervix. *Cancer* 1979;44:2354.
87. Kim RY, Weppelmann B, Salter MM, et al. Skeletal metastases from cancer of the uterine cervix: frequency, patterns, and radiotherapeutic significance. *Int J Radiat Oncol Biol Phys* 1987;13:705.
88. Richart RM. *Cervical intraepithelial neoplasia. Pathology annual.* Vol 8. East Norwalk, CT: Appleton-Century-Crofts, 1973:301.
89. Kurman RJ, Solomon D. *The Bethesda system for reporting cervical/vaginal cytologic diagnoses: definitions, criteria, and explanatory notes for terminology and specimen adequacy.* New York: Springer-Verlag, 1994.
90. Manos MM, Kinney WK, Hurley LB, et al. Identifying women with cervical neoplasia: using human papillomavirus DNA testing for equivocal Papanicolaou results [see comments]. *JAMA* 1999;281:1605.
91. Davey DD, Naryshkin S, Nielsen ML, et al. Atypical squamous cells of undetermined significance: interlaboratory comparison and quality assurance monitors. *Diagn Cytopathol* 1994;11:390.
92. Kinney WK, Manos MM, Hurley LB, et al. Where's the high-grade cervical neoplasia? The importance of minimally abnormal Papanicolaou diagnoses. *Obstet Gynecol* 1998;91:973.
93. Azodi M, Chambers SK, Rutherford TJ, et al. Adenocarcinoma in situ of the cervix: management and outcome. *Gynecol Oncol* 1999;73:348.
94. Jaworski RD, Pacey NF, Greenberg ML, et al. The histologic diagnosis of adeno-carcinoma in situ and related lesions of the cervix uteri: adeno-carcinoma in situ. *Cancer* 1988;61:1171.
95. Wolf JK, Levenback C, Malpica A, et al. Adenocarcinoma in situ of the cervix: significance of cone biopsy margins. *Obstet Gynecol* 1996;88:82.
96. Fu YS, Berek JS. Minimal cervical cancer: definition and histology. *Rec Res Cancer Res* 1988; 106:47.
97. Creasman WT, Zaino RJ, Major FJ, et al. Early invasive carcinoma of the cervix (3 to 5 mm invasion): risk factors and prognosis. A Gynecologic Oncology Group study. *Am J Obstet Gynecol* 1998;178:62.
98. Fu YS, Reagan J. *Pathology of the uterine cervix, vagina, and vulva.* Philadelphia: WB Saunders, 1989.
99. Maiman MA, Fruchter RG, DiMaio TM, et al. Superficially invasive squamous cell carcinoma of the cervix. *Obstet Gynecol* 1988;72:399.
100. Robert ME, Fu YS. Squamous cell carcinoma of the uterine cervix: a review with emphasis on prognostic factors and unusual variants. *Semin Diagn Pathol* 1990;7:173.
101. Albores-Saavedra J, Gersell D, Gilks CB, et al. Terminology of endocrine tumors of the uterine cervix: results of a workshop sponsored by the College of American Pathologists and the National Cancer Institute. *Arch Pathol Lab Med* 1997;121:34.
102. Abeler VM, Holm R, Nesland JM, et al. Small cell carcinoma of the cervix. A clinicopathologic study of 26 patients. *Cancer* 1994;73:672.
103. Morris M, Gershenson DM, Eifel PJ, et al. Treatment of small cell carcinoma of the cervix with cisplatin, doxorubicin, and etoposide. *Gynecol Oncol* 1992;47:62.
104. Sevin BU, Method MW, Nadji M, et al. Efficacy of radical hysterectomy as treatment for patients with small cell carcinoma of the cervix. *Cancer* 1996;77:1489.
105. Gilks CB, Young R, Aguirre P, et al. Adenoma malignum (minimal deviation adenocarcinoma) of the uterine cervix. A clinicopathological and immunohistological analysis of 26 cases. *Am J Surg Pathol* 1989;13:717.
106. Kaku T, Enjoji M. Extremely well-differentiated adenocarcinoma ("adenoma malignum"). *Int J Gynecol Pathol* 1983;2:28.
107. Hirai Y, Takeshima N, Haga A, et al. A clinicocytopathologic study of adenoma malignum of the uterine cervix. *Gynecol Oncol* 1998;70:219.
108. Kaminski PF, Norris HJ. Minimal deviation carcinoma ("adeonoma malignum") of the cervix. *Int J Gynecol Pathol* 1983;2:141.
109. Young RH, Scully RE. Villoglandular papillary adenocarcinoma of the uterine cervix. A clinicopathologic analysis of 13 cases. *Cancer* 1989;63:1773.
110. Glucksmann A, Cherry CP. Incidence, histology, and response to radiation of mixed carcinomas (adenoacanthomas) of the uterine cervix. *Am J Surg Pathol* 1956;12:134.
111. Ferry JA, Scully RE. "Adenoid cystic" carcinoma and adenoid basal cell carcinoma of the uterine cervix: a study of 28 cases. *Am J Surg Pathol* 1988;12:134.
112. Ross JC, Eifel PJ, Cox RS, et al. Primary mucinous adenocarcinoma of the endometrium. A clinicopathologic and histochemical study. *Am J Surg Pathol* 1983;7:715.
113. Koss LG, Stewart FW, Foote FW, et al. Some histological aspects of behavior of epidermoid carcinoma in situ and related lesions of the uterine cervix. *Cancer* 1963;16:1160.
114. American College of Obstetrics and Gynecology. *Technical Bulletin.* Washington, DC: ACOG, 1987.
115. Dewer MA, Hall K, Perchalski J. Cervical cancer screening. Past success and future challenge. *Prim Care* 1992;19:589.
116. Boyce JG, Fruchter RG. Lengthening the interval between Pap smears. *Contemp Obstet Gynecol* 1992;37a:82.
117. Eddy GL. Screening for cervical cancer. *Ann Intern Med* 1990;113:214.
118. Fahs MC, Mandelblatt J, Schechter C, et al. Cost effectiveness of cervical cancer screening for the elderly. *Ann Intern Med* 1992;117:520.
119. Reid R, Herschman BR, Crum CP, et al. Genital warts and cervical cancer. V. The tissue basis of colposcopic change. *Am J Obstet Gynecol* 1984;149:293.
120. Reid R, Stanhope CR, Herschman BR, et al. Genital warts and cervical cancer. IV. A colposcopic index for differentiating subclinical papillomaviral infection from cervical intraepithelial neoplasia. *Am J Obstet Gynecol* 1984;149:815.
121. Reid R, Scalzi P. Genital warts and cervical cancer. VII. An improved colposcopic index for differentiating benign papillomaviral infections from high-grade cervical intraepithelial neoplasia. *Am J Obstet Gynecol* 1985;153:611.
122. Benedet JL, Anderson GH, Boyes DA. Colposcopic accuracy in the diagnosis of microinvasive and occult invasive carcinoma of the cervix. *Obstet Gynecol* 1985;65:557.
123. Kolstad P. Follow-up study of 232 patients with stage Ia1 and 411 patients with stage Ia2 squamous cell carcinoma of the cervix (microinvasive carcinoma). *Gynecol Oncol* 1989;33:265.
124. Townsend DE, Richart RM. Diagnostic errors in colposcopy. *Gynecol Oncol* 1981;12:259.
125. Van Nagell JR, Greenwell N, Powell DF, et al. Microinvasive carcinoma of the cervix. *Am J Obstet Gynecol* 1983;145:981.
126. Heller PB, Malfetano JH, Bundy BN, et al. Clinical-pathologic study of stage IIB, III, and IVA carcinoma of the cervix: extended diagnostic evaluation for paraaortic node metastasis—a Gynecologic Oncology Group study. *Gynecol Oncol* 1990;38:425.
127. Roy C, Le Bras Y, Mangold L, et al. Small pelvic lymph node metastases: evaluation with MR imaging. *Clin Radiol* 1997;52:437.
128. Rose PG, Adler LP, Rodriguez M, et al. Positron emission tomography for evaluating paraaortic nodal metastasis in locally advanced cervical cancer before surgical staging: a surgicopathologic study. *J Clin Oncol* 1999;17:41.
129. Hawnaur JM, Johnson RJ, Buckley CH, et al. Staging, volume estimation and assessment of nodal status in carcinoma of the cervix: comparison of magnetic resonance imaging with surgical findings. *Clin Radiol* 1994;49:443.
130. Martin AJ, Poon CS, Thomas GM, et al. MR evaluation of cervical cancer in hysterectomy specimens: correlation of quantitative T2 measurement and histology. *J Magn Reson Imaging* 1994;4:779.
131. Toita T, Kakinohana Y, Shinzato S, et al. Tumor diameter/volume and pelvic node status assessed by magnetic resonance imaging (MRI) for uterine cervical cancer treated with irradiation. *Int J Radiat Oncol Biol Phys* 1999;43:777.
132. Lien HH, Blomlie V, Iversen T, et al. Clinical stage I carcinoma of the cervix. Value of MR imaging in determining invasion into the parametrium. *Acta Radiol* 1993;34:130.
133. Shiraiwa M, Joja I, Asakawa T, et al. Cervical carcinoma: efficacy of thin-section oblique axial T2-weighted images for evaluating parametrial invasion. *Abdom Imaging* 1999;24:514.

134. Benedet J, Odicino F, Maisonneuve P, et al. Carcinoma of the cervix uteri. *J Epidemiol Biostat* 1998;3:5.
135. International Federation of Gynecology and Obstetrics. Staging announcement. FIGO staging of gynecologic cancers; cervical and vulva. *Int J Gynecol Cancer* 1995;5:319.
136. League of Nations Health Organization. *Inquiry into the results of radiotherapy in cancer of the uterus.* Atlas illustrating the division of cancer of the uterine cervix into four stages according to the anatomo-clinical extent of the growth. Stockholm: Norstedt & Söner, 1938.
137. Eifel PJ. Problems with the clinical staging of carcinoma of the cervix. *Semin Radiat Oncol* 1994;4:1.
138. Seski JC, Murray RA, Morley G. Microinvasive squamous carcinoma of the cervix. Definition, histologic analysis, late results of treatment. *Obstet Gynecol* 1977;50:410.
139. American Joint Committee on Cancer. Cervix uteri. In: Beahrs O, Henson D, Hutter R, et al., eds. *Manual for staging of cancer.* Philadelphia: JB Lippincott Co, 1988:151.
140. Piver MS, Barlow JJ, Krishnamsetty R. Five-year survival (with no evidence of disease) in patients with biopsy-confirmed aortic node metastases from cervical carcinoma. *Am J Obstet Gynecol* 1981;139:575.
141. Weiser EB, Bundy BN, Hoskins WJ, et al. Extraperitoneal versus transperitoneal selective paraaortic lymphadenectomy in the pretreatment surgical staging of advanced cervical carcinoma (a Gynecologic Oncology Group study). *Gynecol Oncol* 1989;33:283.
142. Chi DS, Curtin JP. Gynecologic cancer and laparoscopy. *Obstet Gynecol Clin North Am* 1999;26:201.
143. Possover M, Krause N, Plaul K, et al. Laparoscopic para-aortic and pelvic lymphadenectomy: experience with 150 patients and review of the literature. *Gynecol Oncol* 1998;71:19.
144. Cosin JA, Fowler JM, Chen MD, et al. Pretreatment surgical staging of patients with cervical carcinoma: the case for lymph node debulking. *Cancer* 1998;82:2241.
145. Hacker NF, Wain GV, Nicklin JL. Resection of bulky positive lymph nodes in patients with cervical carcinoma. *Int J Gynecol Cancer* 1995;5:250.
146. Manetta A, Podczaski ES, Larson JE, et al. Scalene lymph node biopsy in the preoperative evaluation of patients with recurrent cervical cancer. *Gynecol Oncol* 1989;33:332.
147. Vasilev SA, Schlaerth JB. Scalene lymph node sampling in cervical carcinoma: a reappraisal. *Gynecol Oncol* 1990;37:120.
148. Eifel PJ, Morris M, Wharton JT, et al. The influence of tumor size and morphology on the outcome of patients with FIGO stage IB squamous cell carcinoma of the uterine cervix. *Int J Radiat Oncol Biol Phys* 1994;29:9.
149. Perez CA, Grigsby PW, Nene SM, et al. Effect of tumor size on the prognosis of carcinoma of the uterine cervix treated with irradiation alone. *Cancer* 1992;69:2796.
150. Kristensen GB, Abeler VM, Risberg B, et al. Tumor size, depth of invasion, and grading of the invasive tumor front are the main prognostic factors in early squamous cell cervical carcinoma. *Gynecol Oncol* 1999;74:245.
151. Sevin BU, Lu Y, Bloch DA, et al. Surgically defined prognostic parameters in patients with early cervical carcinoma. A multivariate survival tree analysis. *Cancer* 1996;78:1438.
152. Barillot I, Horiot JC, Pigneux J, et al. Carcinoma of the intact uterine cervix treated with radiotherapy alone: a French cooperative study: update and multivariate analysis of prognostics factors. *Int J Radiat Oncol Biol Phys* 1997;38:969.
153. Lanciano RM, Won M, Hanks GE. A reappraisal of the International Federation of Gynecology and Obstetrics staging system for cervical cancer. *Cancer* 1992;69:482.
154. Logsdon MD, Eifel PJ. FIGO stage IIIB squamous cell carcinoma of the uterine cervix: an analysis of prognostic factors emphasizing the balance between external-beam and intracavitary radiation therapy. *Int J Radiat Oncol Biol Phys* 1999;43:763.
155. Inoue T, Okumura M. Prognostic significance of parametrial extension in patients with cervical carcinoma stages IB, IIA, and IIB. A study of 628 cases treated by radical hysterectomy and lymphadenectomy with or without postoperative irradiation. *Cancer* 1984; 54:1714.
156. Schmitz H. The classification of uterine carcinoma for the study of the efficacy of radiation therapy. *AJR Am J Roentgenol* 1920;7:383.
157. Thoms WW, Eifel PJ, Smith TL, et al. Bulky endocervical carcinomas: a 23-year experience. *Int J Radiat Oncol Biol Phys* 1992;23:491.
158. Delgado G, Bundy B, Zaino R, et al. Prospective surgical-pathological study of disease-free interval in patients with stage IB squamous cell carcinoma of the cervix: a Gynecologic Oncology Group study. *Gynecol Oncol* 1990;38:352.
159. Inoue T, Chihara T, Morita K. The prognostic significance of the size of the largest nodes in metastatic carcinoma from the uterine cervix. *Gynecol Oncol* 1984;19:187.
160. Inoue T, Morita K. The prognostic significance of number of positive nodes in cervical carcinoma stages IB, IIA, and IIB. *Cancer* 1990;65:1923.
161. Tewfik HH, Buchsbaum HJ, Latourette HB, et al. Para-aortic lymph node irradiation in carcinoma of the cervix after exploratory laparotomy and biopsy-proven positive aortic nodes. *Int J Radiat Oncol Biol Phys* 1982;8:13.
162. Komaki R, Mattingly RF, Hoffman RG, et al. Irradiation of para-aortic lymph node metastases from carcinoma of the cervix or endometrium: preliminary results. *Radiology* 1983;147:245.
163. Rubin SC, Brookland R, Mikuta JJ, et al. Para-aortic nodal metastases in early cervical carcinoma: long-term survival following extended-field radiotherapy. *Gynecol Oncol* 1984;18:213.
164. Brookland RK, Rubin S, Danoff BF. Extended-field irradiation in the treatment of patients with cervical carcinoma involving biopsy proven para-aortic nodes. *Int J Radiat Oncol Biol Phys* 1984;10:1875.
165. Nori D, Valentine E, Hilaris BS. The role of paraaortic node irradiation in the treatment of cancer of the cervix. *Int J Radiat Oncol Biol Phys* 1985;11:1469.
166. Podczaski E, Stryker JA, Kaminski P, et al. Extended-field radiation therapy for carcinoma of the cervix. *Cancer* 1990;66:251.
167. Cunningham M, Dunton C, Corn B, et al. Extended-field radiation therapy in early-stage cervical carcinoma: survival and complications. *Gynecol Oncol* 1991;43:51.
168. Kim PY, Monk BJ, Chabra S, et al. Cervical cancer with paraaortic metastases: significance of residual paraaortic disease after surgical staging. *Gynecol Oncol* 1998;69:243.
169. Boyce JG, Fruchter RG, Nicastri AD, et al. Vascular invasion in stage I carcinoma of the cervix. *Cancer* 1984;53:1175.
170. Burke TW, Hoskins WJ, Heller PB, et al. Prognostic factors associated with radical hysterectomy failure. *Gynecol Oncol* 1987;26:153.
171. Chung CK, Nahhas WA, Stryker JA, et al. Analysis of factors contributing to treatment failures in stages IB and IIA carcinoma of the cervix. *Am J Obstet Gynecol* 1980;138:550.
172. Fuller AF, Elliott N, Kosloff C, et al. Lymph node metastases from carcinoma of the cervix, stages IB and IIA: implications for prognosis and treatment. *Gynecol Oncol* 1982;13:165.
173. Nahhas WA, Sharkey FE, Whitney CW, et al. The prognostic significance of vascular channel involvement and deep stromal penetration in early cervical carcinoma. *Am J Clin Oncol* 1983;6:239.
174. Zreik TG, Chambers JT, Chambers SK. Parametrial involvement, regardless of nodal status: a poor prognostic factor for cervical cancer. *Obstet Gynecol* 1996;87:741.
175. Roman T, Souhami L, Freeman C, et al. High dose rate afterloading intracavitary therapy in carcinoma of the cervix. *Int J Radiat Oncol Biol Phys* 1991;20:921.
176. Kainz C, Gitsch G, Tempfer C, et al. Vascular space invasion and inflammatory stromal reaction as prognostic factors in patients with surgically treated cervical cancer stage IB to IIB. *Anticancer Res* 1994;14:2145.
177. Grimard L, Genest P, Girard A, et al. Prognostic significance of endometrial extension in carcinoma of the cervix. *Gynecol Oncol* 1986;31:301.
178. Mitani Y, Yukinari S, Jimi S, Iwasaki H. Carcinomatous infiltration into the uterine body in carcinoma of the uterine cervix. *Am J Obstet Gynecol* 1964;89:984.
179. Noguchi H, Shiozawa I, Kitahara T, et al. Uterine body invasion of carcinoma of the uterine cervix as seen from surgical specimens. *Gynecol Oncol* 1988;30:173.
180. Perez CA, Camel HM, Askin F, et al. Endometrial extension of carcinoma of the uterine cervix: a prognostic factor that may modify staging. *Cancer* 1981;48:170.
181. Grigsby PW, Perez CA, Kuske RR, et al. Adenocarcinoma of the uterine cervix: lack of evidence for a poor prognosis. *Radiother Oncol* 1988;12:289.
182. Kilgore LC, Soong SJ, Gore H, et al. Analysis of prognostic features in adenocarcinoma of the cervix. *Gynecol Oncol* 1988;31:137.
183. Miller BE, Flax SD, Arheart K, et al. The presentation of adenocarcinoma of the uterine cervix. *Cancer* 1993;72:1281.
184. Shingleton HM, Gore H, Bradley DH, et al. Adenocarcinoma of the cervix. I. Clinical evaluation and pathologic features. *Obstet Gynecol* 1981;139:799.
185. Waldenström A-C, Hrovath G. Survival of patients with adenocarcinoma of the uterine cervix in western Sweden. *Int J Gynecol Cancer* 1999;9:18.
186. Chen RJ, Lin YH, Chen CA, et al. Influence of histologic type and age on survival rates for invasive cervical carcinoma in Taiwan. *Gynecol Oncol* 1999;73:184.
187. Eide TJ. Cancer of the uterine cervix in Norway by histologic type, 1970–1984. *J Natl Cancer Inst* 1987;79:199.
188. Eifel PJ, Burke TW, Morris M, et al. Adenocarcinoma as an independent risk factor for disease recurrence in patients with stage IB cervical carcinoma. *Gynecol Oncol* 1995;59:38.
189. Hopkins M, Morley GW. A comparison of adenocarcinoma and squamous cell carcinoma of the cervix. *Obstet Gynecol* 1991;77:912.
190. Kleine W, Rau K, Schwoeorer D, et al. Prognosis of adenocarcinoma of the cervix uteri: a comparative study. *Gynecol Oncol* 1989;35:145.
191. Lai C-H, Hsueh S, Hong J-H, et al. Are adenocarcinomas and adenosquamous carcinomas different from squamous carcinomas in stage IB and II cervical cancer patients undergoing primary radical surgery? *Int J Gynecol Cancer* 1999;9:28.
192. Eifel PJ, Burke TW, Delclos L, et al. Early stage I adenocarcinoma of the uterine cervix: treatment results in patients with tumors <4 cm in diameter. *Gynecol Oncol* 1991;41:199.
193. Berek JS, Hacker NS, Fu YS, et al. Adenocarcinoma of the uterine cervix: histologic variables associated with lymph node metastasis and survival. *Obstet Gynecol* 1985;65:46.
194. Matthews CM, Burke TW, Tornos C, et al. Stage I cervical adenocarcinoma: prognostic evaluation of surgically treated patients. *Gynecol Oncol* 1993;49:19.
195. Raju K, Kjorstad KE, Abeler V. Prognostic factors in the treatment of stage IB adenocarcinoma of the cervix. *Int J Gynaecol Obstet* 1991;1:69.
196. Bush R. The significance of anemia in clinical radiation therapy. *Int J Radiat Oncol Biol Phys* 1986;12:2047.
197. Girinski T, Pejovic-Lenfant M, Bourhis J, et al. Prognostic value of hemoglobin concentrations and blood transfusions in advanced carcinoma of the cervix treated by radiation therapy: results of a retrospective study of 386 patients. *Int J Radiat Oncol Biol Phys* 1989;16:37.
198. Kapp DS, Fischer D, Gutierrez E, et al. Pretreatment prognostic factors in carcinoma of the uterine cervix: a multivariable analysis of the effect of age, stage, histology and blood counts on survival. *Int J Radiat Oncol Biol Phys* 1983;9:445.
199. Brady LW, Plenk HP, Hanley JA, et al. Hyperbaric oxygen therapy for carcinoma of the cervix stages IIB, IIIA, IIIB and IVA: results of a randomized study by the Radiation Therapy Oncology Group. *Int J Radiat Oncol Biol Phys* 1981;7:990.
200. Dische S, Anderson PJ, Sealy R, et al. Carcinoma of the cervix—anaemia, radiotherapy and hyperbaric oxygen. *Br J Radiol* 1983;56:251.
201. Dische S, Chassagne D, Hope-Stone HF, et al. A trial of Ro 03-8799 (pimonidazole) in carcinoma of the uterine cervix: an interim report from the Medical Research Council Working Party on Advanced Carcinoma of the Cervix. *Radiother Oncol* 1993;26:93.
202. Grigsby PW, Winter K, Wasserman TH, et al. Irradiation with or without misonidazole for patients with stages IIIB and IVA carcinoma of the cervix: final results of RTOG 80-05. Radiation Therapy Oncology Group. *Int J Radiat Oncol Biol Phys* 1999;44:513.
203. Maor MH, Gillespie BW, Peters LJ, et al. Neutron therapy in cervical cancer: results of a phase III RTOG study. *Int J Radiat Oncol Biol Phys* 1988;14:885.
204. Overgaard J, Bentzen SM, Kolstad P, et al. Misonidazole combined with radiotherapy in the treatment of carcinoma of the uterine cervix. *Int J Radiat Oncol Biol Phys* 1989;16:1069.
205. Sundfør K, Trope C, Suo Z, et al. Normobaric oxygen treatment during radiotherapy for carcinoma of the uterine cervix. Results from a prospective controlled randomized trial. *Radiother Oncol* 1999;50:157.

206. Fyles AW, Milosevic M, Wong R, et al. Oxygenation predicts radiation response and survival in patients with cervix cancer [published erratum appears in *Radiother Oncol* 1999;50:371]. *Radiother Oncol* 1998;48:149.
207. Höckel M, Vorndran B, Schlenger K, et al. Tumor oxygenation: a new predictive parameter in locally advanced cancer of the uterine cervix. *Gynecol Oncol* 1993;51:141.
208. Sundfør K, Lyng H, Rofstad EK. Tumour hypoxia and vascular density as predictors of metastasis in squamous cell carcinoma of the uterine cervix. *Br J Cancer* 1998;78:822.
209. Bolger BS, Dabbas M, Lopes A, et al. Prognostic value of preoperative squamous cell carcinoma antigen level in patients surgically treated for cervical carcinoma. *Gynecol Oncol* 1997;65:309.
210. Duk JM, Groenier KH, de Bruijn HWA, et al. Pretreatment serum squamous cell carcinoma antigen: a newly identified prognostic factor in early-stage cervical carcinoma. *J Clin Oncol* 1996;14:111.
211. Hong JH, Tsai CS, Chang JT, et al. The prognostic significance of pre- and posttreatment SCC levels in patients with squamous cell carcinoma of the cervix treated by radiotherapy. *Int J Radiat Oncol Biol Phys* 1998;41:823.
212. Massuger LF, Koper NP, Thomas CM, et al. Improvement of clinical staging in cervical cancer with serum squamous cell carcinoma antigen and CA 125 determinations. *Gynecol Oncol* 1997;64:473.
213. Alvarez RD, Soong SJ, Kinney WK, et al. Identification of prognostic factors and risk groups in patients found to have nodal metastasis at the time of radical hysterectomy for early-stage squamous carcinoma of the cervix. *Gynecol Oncol* 1989;35:130.
214. Lanciano RM, Won M, Coia L, et al. Pretreatment and treatment factors associated with improved outcome in squamous cell carcinoma of the uterine cervix: a final report of the 1973 and 1978 Patterns of Care Studies. *Int J Radiat Oncol Biol Phys* 1991;20:667.
215. Rutledge FN, Mitchell MR, Munsell M, et al. Youth as a prognostic factor in carcinoma of the cervix: a matched analysis. *Gynecol Oncol* 1992;44:123.
216. Spanos WJ, King A, Keeney E, et al. Age as a prognostic factor in carcinoma of the cervix. *Gynecol Oncol* 1989;35:66.
217. Estape R, Angioli R, Wagman F, et al. Significance of intraperitoneal cytology in patients undergoing radical hysterectomy. *Gynecol Oncol* 1998;68:169.
218. Kashimura M, Sugihara K, Toki N, et al. The significance of peritoneal cytology in uterine cervix and endometrial cancer. *Gynecol Oncol* 1997;67:285.
219. Hernandez E, Heller PB, Whitney C, et al. Thrombocytosis in surgically treated stage IB squamous cell cervical carcinoma (a Gynecologic Oncology Group study). *Gynecol Oncol* 1994;55;328.
220. Lopes A, Daras V, Cross PA, et al. Thrombocytosis as a prognostic factor in women with cervical cancer. *Cancer* 1994;74:90.
221. Höckel M, Schlenger K, Mitze M, et al. Tumor vascularity—a novel prognostic factor in advanced cancer of the uterine cervix. *Proc Soc Gynecol Oncol* 1995:48.
222. Wiggins DL, Granai CO, Steinhoff MM, et al. Tumor angiogenesis as a prognostic factor in cervical carcinoma. *Gynecol Oncol* 1995;56:353.
223. Gasinska A, Urbanski K, Jakubowicz J, et al. Tumour cell kinetics as a prognostic factor in squamous cell carcinoma of the cervix treated with radiotherapy. *Radiother Oncol* 1999;50:77.
224. Kristensen GB, Kaern J, Abeler VM, et al. No prognostic impact of flow-cytometric measured DNA ploidy and S-phase fraction in cancer of the uterine cervix: a prospective study of 465 patients. *Gynecol Oncol* 1995;57:79.
225. Lombard I, Vincent-Salomon A, Validire P, et al. Human papillomavirus genotype as a major determinant of the course of cervical cancer. *J Clin Oncol* 1998;16:2613.
226. Duggan MA, McGregor SE, Benoit JL, et al. The human papillomavirus status of invasive cervical adenocarcinoma: a clinicopathological and outcome analysis. *Hum Pathol* 1995;26:319.
227. Ikenberg H, Wiegering I, Pfisterer J, et al. Human papillomavirus DNA in tumor-free regional lymph nodes: a potential prognostic marker in cervical cancer. *Cancer J Sci Am* 1996;2:28.
228. Kobayashi Y, Yoshinouchi M, Tianqi G, et al. Presence of human papilloma virus DNA in pelvic lymph nodes can predict unexpected recurrence of cervical cancer in patients with histologically negative lymph nodes. *Clin Cancer Res* 1998;4:979.
229. Keys HM, Bundy BN, Stehman FB, et al. Cisplatin, radiation, and adjuvant hysterectomy for bulky stage IB cervical carcinoma. *N Engl J Med* 1999;340:1154.
230. Morris M, Eifel PJ, Lu J, et al. Pelvic radiation with concurrent chemotherapy compared with pelvic and paraaortic radiation for high-risk cervical cancer. *N Engl J Med* 1999;340:1137.
231. Peters WAI, Liu PY, Barrett R, et al. Concurrent chemotherapy and pelvic radiation therapy compared with pelvic radiation therapy alone as adjuvant therapy after radical surgery in high-risk early-stage cancer of the cervix. *J Clin Oncol* 2000;18:1606.
232. Rose PG, Bundy BN, Watkins J, et al. Concurrent cisplatin-based chemotherapy and radiotherapy for locally advanced cervical cancer. *N Engl J Med* 1999;340:1144.
233. Whitney CW, Sause W, Bundy BN, et al. A randomized comparison of fluorouracil plus cisplatin versus hydroxyurea as an adjunct to radiation therapy in stages IIB-IVA carcinoma of the cervix with negative para-aortic lymph nodes: a Gynecologic Oncology Group and Southwest Oncology Group study. *J Clin Oncol* 1999;17:1339.
234. Creasman WT, Hinshaw WM, Clarke-Pearson DL. Cryosurgery in the management of cervical intraepithelial neoplasia. *Obstet Gynecol* 1984;63:145.
235. Schantz A, Thormann L. Cryosurgery for dysplasia of the uterine ectocervix. A randomized study of the efficacy of the single- and double-freeze technique. *Acta Obstet Gynecol Scand* 1984;1984:417.
236. Mitchell MF, Tortolero-Luna G, Cook E, et al. A randomized clinical trial of cryotherapy, laser vaporization, and loop electrosurgical excision for treatment of squamous intraepithelial lesions of the cervix. *Obstet Gynecol* 1998;92:737.
237. Gunasekera PC, Phipps JM, Lewis BV. Large loop excision of the transformation zone (LLETZ) compared to carbon dioxide laser in the treatment of CIN: a superior mode of treatment. *Br J Obstet Gynecol* 1990;97:995.
238. Murdoch JB, Grimshaw RN, Monaghan JM. Loop diathermy excision of the abnormal cervical transformation zone. *Int J Gynecol Cancer* 1991;1:105.
239. Burger MPM, Hollema H. The reliability of the histologic diagnosis in colposcopically directed biopsy. A plea for LETZ. *Int J Gynecol Cancer* 1993;3:385.
240. Wright TC, Richart RM, Ferenczy A, et al. Comparisons of specimens removed by CO_2 laser conization and loop electrosurgical excision procedure. *Obstet Gynecol* 1992;79:147.
241. Alvarez RD, Helm CW, Edwards R, et al. Prospective randomized trial of LLETZ versus laser ablation in patients with cervical intraepithelial neoplasia. *Gynecol Oncol* 1994; 52:175.
242. Simon NL, Gore H, Shingleton HM, et al. A study of superficially invasive carcinoma of the cervix. *Obstet Gynecol* 1986;68:19.
243. Burghardt E, Girardi F, Lahousen M, et al. Microinvasive carcinoma of the uterine cervix (International Federation of Gynecology and Obstetrics stage IA). *Cancer* 1991;67:1037.
244. Morris M, Mitchell MF, Silva EG, et al. Cervical conization as definitive therapy for early invasive squamous carcinoma of the cervix. *Gynecol Oncol* 1993;51:193.
245. Luesley DM, McCrum A, Terry PB, et al. Complications of cone biopsy related to the dimensions of the cone and the influence of prior colposcopic assessment. *Br J Obstet Gynecol* 1985;92:158.
246. Magrina JF, Goodrich MA, Weaver AL, et al. Modified radical hysterectomy: morbidity and mortality. *Gynecol Oncol* 1995;59:277.
247. Sevin BU, Nadji M, Avarette HE, et al. Microinvasive carcinoma of the cervix. *Cancer* 1992;70:2121.
248. Copeland LJ, Silva EG, Gershenson DM, et al. Superficially invasive squamous cell carcinoma of the cervix. *Gynecol Oncol* 1992;45:307.
249. Grigsby PW, Perez CA. Radiotherapy alone for medically inoperable carcinoma of the cervix: stage IA and carcinoma in situ. *Int J Radiat Oncol Biol Phys* 1991;21:375.
250. Hamberger AD, Fletcher GH, Wharton JT. Results of treatment of early stage I carcinoma of the uterine cervix with intracavitary radium alone. *Cancer* 1978;41:980.
251. Boyce J, Fruchter RG, Kasambilides E, et al. Prognostic factors in carcinoma of the vulva. *Gynecol Oncol* 1985;20:364.
252. Lowrey GC, Mendenhall WM, Million RR. Stage IB or IIA-B carcinoma of the intact uterine cervix treated with irradiation: a multivariate analysis. *Int J Radiat Oncol Biol Phys* 1992;24:205.
253. Horiot JC, Pigneux J, Pourquier H, et al. Radiotherapy alone in carcinoma of the intact uterine cervix according to G. H. Fletcher guidelines: a French cooperative study of 1383 cases. *Int J Radiat Oncol Biol Phys* 1988;14:605.
254. Liu W, Meigs JV. Radical hysterectomy and pelvic lymphadenectomy. A review of 473 cases including 244 for primary invasive carcinoma of the cervix. *Am J Obstet Gynecol* 1955;69:1.
255. Hoskins WJ, Ford J, Lutz M, et al. Radical hysterectomy and pelvic lymphadenectomy for the management of early invasive cancer of the cervix. *Gynecol Oncol* 1976;4:278.
256. Volterrani F, Feltre L, Sigurta D, et al. Radiotherapy *versus* surgery in the treatment of cervix stage Ib cancer. *Int J Radiat Oncol Biol Phys* 1983;9:1781.
257. Inoue T. Prognostic significance of the depth of invasion relating to nodal metastases, parametrial extension, and cell types. A study of 628 cases with stage IB, IIA, and IIB cervical cancer. *Cancer* 1984;54:3035.
258. Kenter GG, Ansink AC, Heintz APM, et al. Carcinoma of the uterine cervix stage I and IIA: results of surgical treatment: complications, recurrence, and survival. *Eur J Surg Oncol* 1989;15:55.
259. Hopkins MP, Reid GC, Vettrano I, et al. Squamous cell carcinoma of the vulva: prognostic factors influencing survival. *Gynecol Oncol* 1991;43:113.
260. Burghardt E, Hofmann HMH, Ebner F, et al. Results of surgical treatment of 1028 cervical cancers studied with volumetry. *Cancer* 1992;70:648.
261. Montana GS, Fowler WC, Varia MA, et al. Analysis of results of radiation therapy for stage IB carcinoma of the cervix. *Cancer* 1987;60:2195.
262. Coia L, Won M, Lanciano R, et al. The Patterns of Care Outcome Study for cancer of the uterine cervix. Results of the second national practice survey. *Cancer* 1990;66:2451.
263. Landoni F, Maneo A, Colombo A, et al. Randomised study of radical surgery versus radiotherapy for stage Ib-IIa cervical cancer. *Lancet* 1997;350:535.
264. Alvarez RD, Gelder MS, Gore H, et al. Radical hysterectomy in the treatment of patients with bulky early stage carcinoma of the cervix uteri. *Surg Gynecol Obstet* 1993;176:539.
265. Bloss JD, Berman ML, Mukhererjee J, et al. Bulky stage IB cervical carcinoma managed by primary radical hysterectomy followed by tailored radiotherapy. *Gynecol Oncol* 1992;47:21.
266. Rettenmaier MA, Casanova DM, Micha JP, et al. Radical hysterectomy and tailored postoperative radiation therapy in the management of bulky stage IB cervical cancer. *Cancer* 1989;63:2220.
267. Orr JW, Shingleton HM, Hatch KD, et al. Correlation of perioperative morbidity and conization-radical hysterectomy interval. *Obstet Gynecol* 1982;59:726.
268. Hatch KD, Parham G, Shingleton H, et al. Ureteral strictures and fistulae following radical hysterectomy. *Gynecol Oncol* 1984;19:17.
269. Green T. Ureteral suspension for prevention of ureteral complications following radical Wertheim hysterectomy. *Obstet Gynecol* 1966;28:1.
270. Mann WJ, Orr JW, Shingleton HM, et al. Perioperative influences on infectious morbidity in radical hysterectomy. *Gynecol Oncol* 1981;11:207.
271. Forney JP. The effect of radical hysterectomy on bladder physiology. *Am J Obstet Gynecol* 1980;138:374.
272. Sasaki H, Yoshida T, Noda K, et al. Urethral pressure profiles following radical hysterectomy. *Obstet Gynecol* 1982;59:101.
273. Ralph G, Tamussino K, Lichtenegger W. Urological complications after radical hysterectomy with or without radiotherapy for cervical cancer. *Arch Gynecol Obstet* 1990;248:61.
274. Farquharson DI, Shingleton HM, Soong SJ, et al. The adverse effects of cervical cancer treatment on bladder function. *Gynecol Oncol* 1987;27:15.
275. Gonzales DG, Ketting BW, Van Bunningen B, et al. Carcinoma of the uterine cervix stage IB and IIA: results of postoperative irradiation in patients with microscopic infiltration in the parametrium and/or lymph node metastases. *Int J Radiat Oncol Biol Phys* 1989;16:389.
276. Hogan WM, Littman P, Griner L, et al. Results of radiation therapy given after radical hysterectomy. *Cancer* 1982;49:1278.

277. Kinney WK, Alvarez RD, Reid GC, et al. Value of adjuvant whole-pelvis irradiation after Wertheim hysterectomy for early-stage squamous carcinoma of the cervix with pelvic nodal metastasis: a matched-control study. *Gynecol Oncol* 1989;34:258.
278. Morrow CP. Is pelvic radiation beneficial in the postoperative management of stage Ib squamous cell carcinoma of the cervix with pelvic node metastases treated by radical hysterectomy and pelvic lymphadenectomy? *Gynecol Oncol* 1980;10:105.
279. Remy JC, Di Maio T, Fruchter RG, et al. Adjunctive radiation after radical hysterectomy in stage IB squamous cell carcinoma of the cervix. *Gynecol Oncol* 1990;38:161.
280. Soisson AP, Soper JT, Clarke-Pearson DL, et al. Adjuvant radiotherapy following radical hysterectomy for patients with stage IB and IIA cervical cancer. *Gynecol Oncol* 1990;37:390.
281. Sedlis A, Bundy BN, Rotman MZ, et al. A randomized trial of pelvic radiation therapy versus no further therapy in selected patients with stage IB carcinoma of the cervix after radical hysterectomy and pelvic lymphadenectomy: a Gynecologic Oncology Group Study. *Gynecol Oncol* 1999;73:177.
282. Chatani M, Nose T, Masaki N, et al. Adjuvant radiotherapy after radical hysterectomy of cervical cancer. Prognostic factors and complications. *Strahlenther Onkol* 1998;174:504.
283. Russell AH, Tong DY, Figge DC, et al. Adjuvant postoperative pelvic radiation for carcinoma of the uterine cervix: pattern of cancer recurrence in patients undergoing elective radiation following radical hysterectomy and pelvic lymphadenectomy. *Int J Radiat Oncol Biol Phys* 1984;10:211.
284. Barter JF, Soong SJ, Shingleton HM, et al. Complications of combined radical hysterectomy—postoperative radiation therapy in women with early stage cervical cancer. *Gynecol Oncol* 1989;32:292.
285. Fiorca JV, Roberts WS, Greenberg H, et al. Morbidity and survival patterns in patients after radical hysterectomy and postoperative adjuvant pelvic radiotherapy. *Gynecol Oncol* 1990; 36:343.
286. Montz FJ, Holschneider CH, Solh S, et al. Small bowel obstruction following radical hysterectomy: risk factors, incidence and operative findings. *Gynecol Oncol* 1994;53:114.
287. Snijders-Keilholz A, Hellebrekers BW, Zwinderman AH, et al. Adjuvant radiotherapy following radical hysterectomy for patients with early-stage cervical carcinoma (1984–1996). *Radiother Oncol* 1999;51:161.
288. Thomas GM, Dembo AJ. Is there a role for adjuvant pelvic radiotherapy after radical hysterectomy in early stage cervical cancer? *Int J Gynecol Cancer* 1991;1:1.
289. Bandy LC, Clarke-Pearson DL, Soper JT, et al. Long-term effects on bladder function following radical hysterectomy with and without postoperative radiation. *Gynecol Oncol* 1987;26:160.
290. Durrance FY, Fletcher GH, Rutledge FN. Analysis of central recurrent disease in stages I and II squamous cell carcinomas of the cervix on intact uterus. *AJR Am J Roentgenol* 1969;106:831.
291. Mendenhall WM, McCarty PJ, Morgan LS, et al. Stage IB-IIA-B carcinoma of the intact uterine cervix greater than or equal to 6 cm in diameter: is adjuvant extrafascial hysterectomy beneficial? *Int J Radiat Oncol Biol Phys* 1991;21:899.
292. Perez CA, Kao MS. Radiation therapy alone or combined with surgery in the treatment of barrel-shaped carcinoma of the uterine cervix (stages IB, IIA, IIB). *Int J Radiat Oncol Biol Phys* 1985;11:1903.
293. Eifel PJ, Moughan J, Owen JB, et al. Patterns of radiotherapy practice for patients with squamous carcinoma of the uterine cervix. A Patterns of Care Study. *Int J Radiat Oncol Biol Phys* 1999;43:351.
294. Piver MS, Rutledge F, Smith JP. Five classes of extended hysterectomy for women with cervical cancer. *Obstet Gynecol* 1974;44:265.
295. Rotman M, John MJ, Moon SH, et al. Limitations of adjunctive surgery in carcinoma of the cervix. *Int J Radiat Oncol Biol Phys* 1979;5:327.
296. Keys H, Bundy B, Stehman F, et al. Adjuvant hysterectomy after radiation therapy reduces detection of local recurrence in "bulky" stage IB cervical cancer without improving survival: results of a prospective randomized GOG trial. *Cancer J Sci Am* 1997;3:117.
297. Benedetti Panici P, Scambia G, Greggi S, et al. Neoadjuvant chemotherapy and radical surgery in locally advanced cervical carcinoma. Prognostic factors for response and survival. *Cancer* 1991;67:372.
298. Eddy GL. Neoadjuvant chemotherapy before surgery in cervical cancer. *J Natl Cancer Inst Monogr* 1996;21:93.
299. Sardi JE, Giaroli A, Sananes C, et al. Long-term follow-up of the first randomized trial using neoadjuvant chemotherapy in stage Ib squamous carcinoma of the cervix: the final results. *Gynecol Oncol* 1997;67:61.
300. Eifel P, Thames H. Has the influence of treatment duration on local control of carcinoma of the cervix been defined? *Int J Radiat Oncol Biol Phys* 1995;32:1527.
301. Fyles AW, Pintilie M, Kirkbride P, et al. Prognostic factors in patients with cervix cancer treated by radiation therapy: results of a multiple regression analysis. *Radiother Oncol* 1995;35:107.
302. Girinski T, Rey A, Roche B, et al. Overall treatment time in advanced cervical carcinomas: a critical parameter in treatment outcome. *Int J Radiat Oncol Biol Phys* 1993;27:1051.
303. Lanciano RM, Pajak TF, Martz K, et al. The influence of treatment time on outcome for squamous cell cancer of the uterine cervix treated with radiation: a Patterns-of-Care Study. *Int J Radiat Oncol Biol Phys* 1993;25:391.
304. Perez CA, Grigsby PW, Castro-Vita H, et al. Carcinoma of the uterine cervix. I. Impact of prolongation of overall treatment time and timing of brachytherapy on outcome of radiation therapy. *Int J Radiat Oncol Biol Phys* 1995;32:1275.
305. Petereit DG, Sarkaria JN, Chappell R, et al. The adverse effect of treatment prolongation in cervical carcinoma. *Int J Radiat Oncol Biol Phys* 1995;32:1301.
306. Greer BE, Koh WJ, Figge DC, et al. Gynecologic radiotherapy fields defined by intraoperative measurements. *Gynecol Oncol* 1990;38:421.
307. Kim RY, McGinnis LS, Spencer SA, et al. Conventional four-field pelvic radiotherapy technique without CT treatment planning in cancer of the cervix: potential geographic miss. *Radiother Oncol* 1994;30:140.
308. Thomas L, Chacon B, Kind M, et al. Magnetic resonance imaging in the treatment planning of radiation therapy in carcinoma of the cervix treated with the four-field pelvic technique. *Int J Radiat Oncol Biol Phys* 1997;37:827.
309. Russell AH. Contemporary radiation treatment planning for patients with cancer of the uterine cervix. *Semin Oncol* 1994;21:30.
310. McIntyre JF, Eifel PJ, Levenback C, et al. Ureteral stricture as a late complication of radiotherapy for stage IB carcinoma of the uterine cervix. *Cancer* 1995;75:836.
311. Chao C, Williamson JF, Grigsby PW, et al. Uterosacral space involvement in locally advanced carcinoma of the uterine cervix. *Int J Radiat Oncol Biol Phys* 1998;40:397.
312. Rotman M, Pajak M, Choi K, et al. Prophylactic extended-field irradiation of para-aortic lymph nodes in stages IIB and bulky IB and IIA cervical carcinomas. Ten-year treatment results of RTOG 79-20. *JAMA* 1995;274:387.
313. Haie C, Pejovie MH, Gerbaulet A, et al. Is prophylactic para-aortic irradiation worthwhile in the treatment of advanced cervical carcinoma? Results of a controlled clinical trial of the EORTC radiotherapy group. *Radiother Oncol* 1988;11:101.
314. Grigsby PW, Lu JD, Mutch DG, et al. Twice-daily fractionation of external irradiation with brachytherapy and chemotherapy in carcinoma of the cervix with positive para-aortic lymph nodes: phase II study of the Radiation Therapy Oncology Group 92-10. *Int J Radiat Oncol Biol Phys* 1998;41:817.
315. Malfetano JH, Keys H. Aggressive multimodality treatment for cervical cancer with paraaortic lymph node metastases. *Gynecol Oncol* 1991;42:44.
316. Varia MA, Bundy BN, Deppe G, et al. Cervical carcinoma metastatic to para-aortic nodes: extended-field radiation therapy with concomitant 5-fluorouracil and cisplatin chemotherapy: a Gynecologic Oncology Group study. *Int J Radiat Oncol Biol Phys* 1998; 42:1015.
317. Fletcher GH. Female pelvis. In: Fletcher GH, ed. *Textbook of radiotherapy.* Philadelphia: Lea & Febiger, 1980.
318. Delclos L, Fletcher GH, Sampiere V, et al. Can the Fletcher gamma ray colpostat system be extrapolated to other systems? *Cancer* 1978;41:970.
319. Delclos L, Fletcher GH, Moore EB, et al. Minicolpostats, dome cylinders, other additions and improvements of the Fletcher-Suit afterloadable system: indications and limitations of their use. *Int J Radiat Oncol Biol Phys* 1980;6:1195.
320. Delclos L. Gynecologic cancers: pelvic examination and treatment planning. In: Levitt S, Tapley N, eds. *Technological basis of radiation therapy: practical clinical applications.* Philadelphia: Lea & Febiger, 1984:193.
321. International Commission on Radiation Units and Measurements. *Dose and volume specification for reporting intracavitary therapy in gynecology.* Vol. 38. Bethesda, MD: International Commission on Radiation Units and Measurements, 1985:1.
322. Kapp KS, Stuecklschweiger GF, Kapp DS, et al. Dosimetry of intracavitary placements for uterine and cervical carcinoma: results of orthogonal film, TLD, and CT-assisted techniques. *Radiother Oncol* 1992;24:137.
323. Ling CC, Schell MC, Working KR, et al. CT-assisted assessment of bladder and rectum dose in gynecological implants. *Int J Radiat Oncol Biol Phys* 1987;13:1577.
324. Schoeppel SL, LaVigne ML, Martel MK, et al. Three-dimensional treatment planning of intracavitary gynecologic implants: analysis of ten cases and implications for dose specification. *Int J Radiat Oncol Biol Phys* 1994;28:277.
325. Eifel PJ, Morris M, Delclos L, et al. Radiation therapy for cervical carcinoma. In: Dilts PVJ, Sciarra JJ, eds. *Gynecology and obstetrics.* Philadelphia: JB Lippincott Co, 1993:1.
326. Perez CA, Grigsby PW, Lockett MA, et al. Radiation therapy morbidity in carcinoma of the uterine cervix: dosimetric and clinical correlation. *Int J Radiat Oncol Biol Phys* 1999;44:855.
327. Roeske JC, Mundt AJ, Halpern H, et al. Late rectal sequelae following definitive radiation therapy for carcinoma of the uterine cervix: a dosimetric analysis. *Int J Radiat Oncol Biol Phys* 1997;37:351.
328. Haie-Meder C, Kramar A, Lambin P, et al. Analysis of complications in a prospective randomized trial comparing two brachytherapy low dose rates in cervical carcinoma. *Int J Radiat Oncol Biol Phys* 1994;29:1195.
329. Amdur RJ, Bedford JS. Dose-rate effects between 0.3 and 30 Gy/h in a normal and a malignant human cell line [see comments]. *Int J Radiat Oncol Biol Phys* 1994;30:83.
330. Akine Y, Arimoto H, Ogino T, et al. High-dose-rate intracavitary irradiation in the treatment of carcinoma of the uterine cervix: early experience with 84 patients. *Int J Radiat Oncol Biol Phys* 1988;14:893.
331. Ito H, Kumagaya H, Shigematsu N, et al. High dose rate intracavitary brachytherapy for recurrent cervical cancer of the vaginal stump following hysterectomy. *Int J Radiat Oncol Biol Phys* 1991;20:927.
332. Kapp KS, Stuecklschweiger GF, Kapp DS, et al. Prognostic factors in patients with carcinoma of the uterine cervix treated with external-beam irradiation and IR-192 high-dose-rate brachytherapy. *Int J Radiat Oncol Biol Phys* 1998;42:531.
333. Newman H, James K, Smith C. Treatment of cancer of the cervix with a high-dose-rate afterloading machine (the Cathetron). *Int J Radiat Oncol Biol Phys* 1983;9:931.
334. Orton CG, Seyedsadr M, Somnay A. Comparison of high and low dose rate remote afterloading for cervix cancer and the importance of fractionation. *Int J Radiat Oncol Biol Phys* 1991;21:1425.
335. Patel FD, Sharma SC, Neigi PS, et al. Low dose rate vs. high dose rate brachytherapy in the treatment of carcinoma of the uterine cervix: a clinical trial. *Int J Radiat Oncol Biol Phys* 1993;28:335.
336. Petereit DG, Pearcey R. Literature analysis of high dose rate brachytherapy fractionation schedules in the treatment of cervical cancer: is there an optimal fractionation schedule? *Int J Radiat Oncol Biol Phys* 1999;43:359.
337. Shigematsu Y, Nishiyama K, Masaki N, et al. Treatment of carcinoma of the uterine cervix by remotely controlled afterloading intracavitary radiotherapy with high-dose rate: a comparative study with a low-dose rate system. *Int J Radiat Oncol Biol Phys* 1983;9:351.
338. Stitt JA, Fowler JF, Thomadsen BR, et al. High dose rate intracavitary brachytherapy for carcinoma of the cervix: the Madison system: I. Clinical and radiobiological considerations. *Int J Radiat Oncol Biol Phys* 1992;24:383.

339. Eifel PJ. High dose-rate brachytherapy for carcinoma of the cervix: high tech or high risk? *Int J Radiat Oncol Biol Phys* 1992;24:383.

340. Scalliet P, Gerbaulet A, Dubray B. HDR versus LDR gynecological brachytherapy revisited. *Radiother Oncol* 1993;28:118.

341. Aristizabal SA, Woolfitt B, Valencia A, et al. Interstitial parametrial implants in carcinoma of the cervix stage II-B. *Int J Radiat Oncol Biol Phys* 1987;13:445.

342. Fontanesi J, Dylewski G, Photopulos G, et al. Impact of dose on local control and development of complications in patients with advanced gynecological malignancies treated by interstitial template boost technique. *Endocuriether Hyperther Oncol* 1993;9:115.

343. Gaddis O, Morrow CP, Klement V, et al. Treatment of cervical carcinoma employing a template for transperineal interstitial Ir^{192} brachytherapy. *Int J Radiat Oncol Biol Phys* 1983; 9:819.

344. Martinez A, Edmundson GK, Cox RS, et al. Combination of external-beam irradiation and multiple-site perineal applicator (MUPIT) for treatment of locally advanced or recurrent prostatic, anorectal, and gynecologic malignancies. *Int J Radiat Oncol Biol Phys* 1985;11:391.

345. Syed AMN, Puthwala AA, Neblett D, et al. Transperineal interstitial-intracavitary "Syed-Neblett" applicator in the treatment of carcinoma of the uterine cervix. *Endocuriether Hyperther Oncol* 1986;2:1.

346. Hughes-Davies L, Silver B, Kapp D. Parametrial interstitial brachytherapy for advanced or recurrent pelvic malignancy: the Harvard/Stanford experience. *Gynecol Oncol* 1995;58:24.

347. Stock RG, Chan K, Terk M, et al. A new technique for performing Syed-Neblett template interstitial implants for gynecologic malignancies using transrectal-ultrasound guidance. *Int J Radiat Oncol Biol Phys* 1997;37:819.

348. Recio FO, Piver MS, Hempling RE, et al. Laparoscopic-assisted application of interstitial brachytherapy for locally advanced cervical carcinoma: results of a pilot study. *Int J Radiat Oncol Biol Phys* 1998;40:411.

349. Erickson B, Gillin MT. Interstitial implantation of gynecologic malignancies. *J Surg Oncol* 1997;66:285.

350. Gupta AK, Vicini FA, Frazier AJ, et al. Iridium-192 transperineal interstitial brachytherapy for locally advanced or recurrent gynecological malignancies. *Int J Radiat Oncol Biol Phys* 1999;43:1055.

351. Demanes DJ, Rodriguez RR, Bendre DD, et al. High dose rate transperineal interstitial brachytherapy for cervical cancer: high pelvic control and low complication rates. *Int J Radiat Oncol Biol Phys* 1999;45:105.

352. Corn BW, Shaktman BD, Lanciano RM, et al. Intra- and perioperative complications associated with tandem and colpostat application for cervix cancer. *Int J Radiat Oncol Biol Phys* 1997;64:224.

353. Dusenbery KE, Carson LF, Potish RA. Perioperative morbidity and mortality of gynecologic brachytherapy. *Cancer* 1991;67:2786.

354. Jhingran A, Eifel PJ. Perioperative and postoperative complications of intracavitary radiation for FIGO stage I-III carcinoma of the cervix. *Int J Radiat Oncol Biol Phys* 1998;42:151.

355. Lanciano RM, Martz D, Montana GS, et al. Influence of age, prior abdominal surgery, fraction size, and dose on complications after radiation therapy for squamous cell cancer of the uterine cervix. A Patterns of Care Study. *Cancer* 1992;69:2124.

356. Eifel PJ, Levenback C, Wharton JT, et al. Time course and incidence of late complications in patients treated with radiation therapy for FIGO stage IB carcinoma of the uterine cervix. *Int J Radiat Oncol Biol Phys* 1995;32:1289.

357. Potish RA. Importance of predisposing factors in the development of enteric damage. *Am J Clin Oncol* 1982;5:189.

358. Van Nagell JR, Parker JC, Maruyama Y, et al. The effect of pelvic inflammatory disease on enteric complications following radiation therapy for cervical cancer. *Am J Obstet Gynecol* 1977;128:767.

359. Bruner DW, Lanciano R, Keegan M, et al. Vaginal stenosis and sexual function following intracavitary radiation for the treatment of cervical and endometrial carcinoma. *Int J Radiat Oncol Biol Phys* 1993;27:825.

360. Hreshchyshyn MM, Aron BS, Boronow RC, et al. Hydroxyurea or placebo combined with radiation to treat stages IIIB and IV cervical cancer confined to the pelvis. *Int J Radiat Oncol Biol Phys* 1979;5:317.

361. Stehman FB, Bundy BN, Thomas G, et al. Hydroxyurea versus misonidazole with radiation in cervical carcinoma: long-term follow-up of a Gynecologic Oncology Group trial. *J Clin Oncol* 1993;11:1523.

362. Chaney AW, Eifel PJ, Logsdon MD, et al. Mature results of a pilot study of pelvic radiotherapy with concurrent continuous infusion intra-arterial 5-FU for stage IIIB-IVA squamous cell carcinoma of the cervix. *Int J Radiat Oncol Biol Phys* 1999;45:113.

363. Thomas G, Dembo A, Ackerman I, et al. A randomized trial of standard versus partially hyperfractionated radiation with or without concurrent 5-fluorouracil in locally advanced cervical cancer. *Gynecol Oncol* 1998;69:137.

364. Chen MD, Paley PJ, Potish RA, et al. Phase I trial of taxol as a radiation sensitizer with cisplatin in advanced cervical cancer. *Gynecol Oncol* 1997;67:131.

365. Muderspach LI, Curtin JP, Roman LD, et al. Carboplatin as a radiation sensitizer in locally advanced cervical cancer: a pilot study. *Gynecol Oncol* 1997;65:336.

366. Rakovitch E, Fyles AW, Pintilie M, et al. Role of mitomycin C in the development of late bowel toxicity following chemoradiation for locally advanced carcinoma of the cervix. *Int J Radiat Oncol Biol Phys* 1997;38:979.

367. Christie DR, Bull CA, Gebski V, et al. Concurrent 5-fluorouracil, mitomycin C and irradiation in locally advanced cervix cancer. *Radiother Oncol* 1995;37:181.

368. Malfetano JH, Keys H, Cunningham MJ, et al. Extended-field radiation and cisplatin for stage IIB and IIIB cervical carcinoma. *Gynecol Oncol* 1997;67:203.

369. Symonds RP, Habeshaw T, Watson ER, et al. Combination chemotherapy prior to radical radiotherapy for stage III and IV carcinoma of the cervix. *Clin Radiol* 1987;38:273.

370. Kirsten F, Atkinson K, Coppleson J, et al. Combination chemotherapy followed by surgery or radiotherapy in patients with locally advanced cervical cancer. *Br J Obstet Gynecol* 1987;94:583.

371. Lara PC, Garcia-Puche JL, Pedraza V. Cisplatin-ifosphamide as neoadjuvant chemotherapy in stage IIIB cervicaluterine squamous-cell carcinoma. *Cancer Chemother Pharmacol* 1990;26(Suppl):36.

372. Tobias J, Buxton EJ, Blackledge G, et al. Neoadjuvant bleomycin, ifosfamide and cisplatin in cervical cancer. *Cancer Chemother Pharmacol* 1990;26(Suppl):59.

373. Chauvergne J, Rohart J, Héron JF, et al. Essai randomisé de chimiothérapie initiale dans 151 carcinomes du col utérin localement étendus (T2b-N1, T3b, MO). *Bull Cancer* 1990; 77:1007.

374. Sardi J, Sananes C, Giarole A, et al. Neoadjuvant chemotherapy in locally advanced carcinoma of the cervix uteri. *Gynecol Oncol* 1990;38:486.

375. Park TK, Choi DH, Kim SN, et al. Role of induction chemotherapy in invasive cervical cancer. *Gynecol Oncol* 1991;41:107.

376. Souhami L, Gil R, Allan S, et al. A randomized trial of chemotherapy followed by pelvic radiation therapy in stage IIIB carcinoma of the cervix. *Int J Radiat Oncol Biol Phys* 1991;9:970.

377. Tattersall MHN, Ramirez C, Coppleson M. A randomized trial comparing platinum-based chemotherapy followed by radiotherapy vs. radiotherapy alone in patients with locally advanced cervical cancer. *Int J Gynecol Cancer* 1992;2:244.

378. Kumar L, Kaushal R, Nandy M, et al. Chemotherapy followed by radiotherapy versus radiotherapy alone in locally advanced cervical cancer: a randomized study. *Gynecol Oncol* 1994;54:307.

379. Tattersall MHN, Larvidhaya V, Vootiprux V, et al. Randomized trial of epirubicin and cisplatin chemotherapy followed by pelvic radiation in locally advanced cervical cancer. *Am J Clin Oncol* 1995;13:444.

380. Sundfør K, Trope CG, Hogberg T, et al. Radiotherapy and neoadjuvant chemotherapy for cervical carcinoma. A randomized multicenter study of sequential cisplatin and 5-fluorouracil and radiotherapy in advanced cervical carcinoma stage 3B and 4A. *Cancer* 1996;77:2371.

381. Leborgne F, Leborgne JH, Doldán R, et al. Induction chemotherapy and radiotherapy of advanced cancer of the cervix: a pilot study and phase III randomized trial. *Int J Radiat Oncol Biol Phys* 1997;37:343.

382. Kim DS, Moon H, Kim KT, et al. Two-year survival: preoperative adjuvant chemotherapy in the treatment of cervical cancer stages Ib and II with bulky tumor. *Gynecol Oncol* 1989;33:225.

383. Dottino PR, Plaxe S, Beddoe A, et al. Induction chemotherapy followed by radical surgery in cervical cancer. *Gynecol Oncol* 1991;40:7.

384. Fontanelli R, Spatti G, Raspagliesi F, et al. A preoperative single course of high-dose cisplatin and bleomycin with glutathione protection in bulky stage IB/II carcinoma of the cervix. *Ann Oncol* 1992;3:117.

385. Lai CH, Hsueh S, Chang TC, et al. Prognostic factors in patients with bulky stage IB or IIA cervical carcinoma undergoing neoadjuvant chemotherapy and radical hysterectomy. *Gynecol Oncol* 1997;64:456.

386. Potish RA, Twiggs LB. On the lack of demonstrated clinical benefit of neoadjuvant cisplatinum therapy for cervical cancer. *Int J Radiat Oncol Biol Phys* 1993;27:975.

387. Tannock IF, Browman G. Lack of evidence for a role of chemotherapy in the routine management of locally advanced head and neck cancer. *J Clin Oncol* 1986;4:1121.

388. Withers HR, Taylor JMG, Maciejewski B. The hazard of accelerated tumor clonogen repopulation during radiotherapy. *Acta Oncol* 1988;27:131.

389. Kim D, Moon H, Hwang Y, et al. Preoperative adjuvant chemotherapy in the treatment of cervical cancer stage IB, IIA, and IIB with bulky tumor. *Gynecol Oncol* 1988;29:321.

390. Morris M, Eifel PJ, Burke TW, et al. Treatment of locally advanced cervical cancer with concurrent radiation and intra-arterial chemotherapy. *Gynecol Oncol* 1995;57:72.

391. Rettenmaier MA, Moran MF, Ramsinghani NF, et al. Treatment of advanced and recurrent squamous carcinoma of the uterine cervix with constant intraarterial infusion of cisplatin. *Cancer* 1988;61:1301.

392. Roberts WS, Lapolla JP, Greenberg H, et al. Continuous intra-arterial cisplatin combined with radiotherapy in locally advanced squamous carcinoma of the cervix: a Gynecologic Oncology Group pilot study. *Int J Gynecol Cancer* 1995;5:335.

393. Muscato M, Perry M, Yarbro J. Chemotherapy of cervical carcinoma. *Semin Oncol* 1982; 9:373.

394. Omura G, Velez G, Birch R. Phase II randomized study of doxorubicin, vincristine, and 5-FU. *Cancer Treat Rep* 1981;65:901.

395. Thigpen T, Vance R, Balducci, et al. Chemotherapy in the management of advanced or recurrent cervical and endometrial carcinoma. *Cancer* 1981;48:658.

396. Lira-Puerto V, Piccart M, Wiemik P, et al. A comparison of U.S. and Mexican experience with single drug therapy in advanced cervical cancer (NCI-PAHO and ECOG study). *Proc ASCO* 1985;4:117.

397. Stehman FB, Blessing JA, McGehee R, et al. A phase II evaluation of mitolactol in patients with advanced squamous cell carcinoma of the cervix: a Gynecologic Oncology Group study. *J Clin Oncol* 1989;7:1892.

398. Stehman FB, Blom J, Blessing JA, et al. Phase II trial of galactitol 1,2:5,6-dianhydro (NSC 132313) in the treatment of advanced gynecologic malignancies: a Gynecologic Oncology Group study. *Gynecol Oncol* 1983;15:381.

399. Sutton GP, Blessing JA, Adcock L, et al. Phase II study of ifosfamide and mesna in patients with previously treated carcinoma of the cervix: a Gynecologic Oncology Group study. *Invest New Drugs* 1989;7:341.

400. Sutton GP, Blessing JA, Photopoulos G, et al. Phase II experience with ifosphamide/mesna in gynecologic malignancies: preliminary report of Gynecologic Oncology Group studies. *Semin Oncol* 1989;15:381.

401. Thigpen T, Lambuth B, Vance R. Ifosfamide in the management of gynecologic cancers. *Semin Oncol* 1990;17:11.

402. Perez C, Kurman R, Stehman F, et al. Uterine cervix. In: Hoskins W, Perez C, Young R, eds. *Principles and practice of gynecologic oncology.* Philadelphia: JB Lippincott Co, 1992:591.

403. Meanwell C, Mould J, Blackledge G, et al. Phase II study of ifosfamide in cervical cancer. *Cancer Treat Rep* 1986;70:727.

404. Cervellino JC, Araujo CE, Sanchez O, et al. Cisplatin and ifosfamide in patients with advanced squamous cell carcinoma of the uterine cervix. *Acta Oncol* 1995;34:257.

405. Hannigan EV, Dinh TV, Doherty MG. Ifosfamide with mesna in squamous carcinoma of the cervix: phase II results in patients with advanced or recurrent disease. *Gynecol Oncol* 1991;43:123.
406. McGuire WP, Arseneau J, Blessing JA, et al. A randomized comparative trial of carboplatin and iproplatin in advanced squamous carcinoma of the uterine cervix: Gynecologic Oncology Group study. *J Clin Oncol* 1989;7:1462.
407. Baker L. Cis-platin in treatment of cervical and endometrial cancer patients. In: Prestayko J, Crooke S, Carter S, eds. *Cisplatin: current status and new developments.* New York: Academic Press, 1980:403.
408. Baker L, Boutselis J, Alberts D, et al. Combination chemotherapy for patients with disseminated carcinoma of the uterine cervix. *Proc ASCO* 1985;4:120.
409. Bonomi P, Blessing J, Stehman F, et al. Randomized trial of three cisplatin dose schedules in squamous-cell carcinoma of the cervix: a Gynecologic Oncology Group study. *J Clin Oncol* 1985;3:1079.
410. Cohen C, Castro-Marin A, Deppe G, et al. Chemotherapy of advanced or recurrent cervical cancer with platinum II—a preliminary report. *Proc ASCO* 1978;19:401.
411. Thigpen T, Shingleton H, Homesley H, et al. Cis-platinum in treatment of advanced or recurrent squamous cell carcinoma of the cervix. *Cancer* 1981;48:899.
412. Thigpen JT, Blessing JA, DiSaia PJ, et al. A randomized comparison of a rapid versus prolonged (24 hr) infusion of cisplatin in therapy of squamous cell carcinoma of the uterine cervix: a Gynecologic Oncology Group study. *Gynecol Oncol* 1989;32:198.
413. Cavins J, Geisler H. Treatment of advanced, unresectable, cervical carcinoma already subjected to complete irradiation therapy. *Gynecol Oncol* 1978;6:256.
414. Freeman R, Herson J, Wharton T, et al. Single agent chemotherapy for recurrent carcinoma of the cervix. *Cancer Clin Trials* 1980;3:345.
415. Greenberg B, Kardinal C, Pajek T, et al. Adriamycin versus adriamycin and bleomycin in advanced epidermoid carcinoma of the cervix. *Cancer Treat Rep* 1977;61:1383.
416. Malkasian G, Decker D, Green S, et al. Treatment of recurrent and metastatic carcinoma of the cervix: comparison of doxorubicin with a combination of vincristine and 5-fluorouracil. *Gynecol Oncol* 1981;11:235.
417. Piver M, Barlow J, Xynos F. Adriamycin alone or in combination in 100 patients with carcinoma of the cervix or vagina. *Am J Obstet Gynecol* 1978;131:311.
418. Wallace H, Hreshchyshyn M, Wilbanks G, et al. Comparison of the therapeutic effect of adriamycin alone versus adriamycin plus vincristine versus adriamycin plus cyclophosphamide in the treatment of advanced carcinoma of the cervix. *Cancer Treat Rep* 1978;62:1435.
419. Wasserman T, Carter S. The integration of chemotherapy into combined modality treatment of solid tumors: VIII. Cervical cancer. *Cancer Treat Rep* 1977;4:25.
420. Thigpen JT. Single agent chemotherapy in carcinoma of the cervix. In: Surwit E, Alberts D, eds. *Cervix cancer.* Boston: Martinus Nijhoff, 1987:119.
421. Arseneau JC, Bundy B, Dolan T, et al. Phase II study of Baker's antifol in advanced squamous cell carcinoma of the cervix. *Am J Clin Oncol* 1982;5:61.
422. Malkasian G, Decker D, Jorgensen E. Chemotherapy of carcinoma of the cervix. *Gynecol Oncol* 1976;5:109.
423. Look KY, Blessing JA, Levenback C, et al. A phase II trial of CPT-11 in recurrent squamous carcinoma of the cervix: a gynecologic oncology group study. *Gynecol Oncol* 1998;70:334.
424. Takeuchi S, Dobashi K, Fujimoto S, et al. A late phase II study of CPT-11 on uterine cervical cancer and ovarian cancer. Research Groups of CPT-11 in Gynecologic Cancers. *Gan To Kagaku Ryoho* 1991;18:1681.
425. Verschraegen CF, Levy T, Kudelka AP, et al. Phase II study of irinotecan in prior chemotherapy-treated squamous cell carcinoma of the cervix. *J Clin Oncol* 1997;15:625.
426. Morris M, Brader KR, Levenback C, et al. Phase II study of vinorelbine in advanced and recurrent squamous cell carcinoma of the cervix. *J Clin Oncol* 1998;16:1094.
427. Conroy JF, Lewis GCJ, Blessing JA, et al. ICRF-159 in patients with advanced squamous cell carcinoma of the uterine cervix. *Am J Clin Oncol* 1984;7:131.
428. Kudelka AP, Winn R, Edwards CL, et al. Activity of paclitaxel in advanced or recurrent squamous cell cancer of the cervix. *Clin Cancer Res* 1996;2:1285.
429. McGuire WP, Blessing JA, Moore D, et al. Paclitaxel has moderate activity in squamous cervix cancer. A Gynecologic Oncology Group study. *J Clin Oncol* 1996;14:792.
430. Cervellino J, Araujo C, Pirisi C, et al. Ifosfamide and mesna at high doses for the treatment of cancer of the cervix: a GETLAC study. *Cancer Chemother Pharmacol* 1990;26:S1.
431. Thigpen T, Vance R, Khansur T. Carcinoma of the uterine cervix: current status and future directions. *Semin Oncol* 1994;21(Suppl 2):543.
432. Chiara S, Consoli R, Falcone A, et al. Cisplatin and 5-fluorouracil in advanced and recurrent cervical cancer. *Tumori* 1988;74:471.
433. Kuhnle H, Meerpohl HG, Eiermann W, et al. Phase II study of carboplatin/ifosfamide in untreated advanced cervical cancer. *Cancer Chemother Pharmacol* 1990;26:S33.
434. Ramm K, Vergote I, Kaem J, et al. Bleomycin-ifosfamide-cisplatinum (BIP) in pelvic recurrence of previously irradiated cervical carcinoma: a second look. *Gynecol Oncol* 1992;46:203.
435. Buxton EJ, Meanwell CA, Hilton C, et al. Combination bleomycin, ifosfamide, and cisplatin chemotherapy in cervical cancer. *J Natl Cancer Inst* 1989;81:359.
436. Kumar L, Bhargava V. Chemotherapy in recurrent and advanced cervical cancer. *Gynecol Oncol* 1991;40:107.
437. Murad AM, Triginelli SA, Ribalta JCL. Phase II trial of bleomycin, ifosfamide, and carboplatin in metastatic cervical cancer. *J Clin Oncol* 1994;12:55.
438. Tay SK, Lai FM, Soh LT, et al. Combined chemotherapy using cisplatin ifosfamide and bleomycin (PIB) in the treatment of advanced and recurrent cervical carcinoma. *Aust N Z J Obstet Gynaecol* 1993;32:263.
439. Bonomi P, Blessing J, Ball H, et al. A phase II evaluation of cisplatin and 5-fluorouracil in patients with advanced squamous cell carcinoma of the cervix: a Gynecologic Oncology Group study. *Gynecol Oncol* 1989;37:354.
440. Kaern J, Trope C, Kjorstad KE, et al. A phase II study of 5-fluorouracil/cisplatin in recurrent cervical cancer. *Tidsskr Nor Laegeforen* 1990;110:2759.
441. Weiss G, Green S, Hannigan E, et al. A phase II trial of cisplatin and 5-fluorouracil with allopurinol for recurrent or metastatic carcinoma of the uterine cervix: a Southwest Oncology Group trial. *Gynecol Oncol* 1990;37:354.
442. Papadimitriou CA, Sarris K, Moulopoulos LA, et al. Phase II trial of paclitaxel and cisplatin in metastatic and recurrent carcinoma of the uterine cervix. *J Clin Oncol* 1999;17:761.
443. Pignata S, Silvestro G, Ferrari E, et al. Phase II study of cisplatin and vinorelbine as first-line chemotherapy in patients with carcinoma of the uterine cervix. *J Clin Oncol* 1999;17:756.
444. Brader KR, Morris M, Levenback C, et al. Chemotherapy for cervical carcinoma: factors determining response and implications for clinical trial design. *J Clin Oncol* 1998;16:1879.
445. Omura GA, Blessing J, Vaccarello L, et al. A randomized trial of cisplatin versus cisplatin + mitolactol versus cisplatin + ifosfamide in advanced squamous cell carcinoma of the cervix by the Gynecologic Oncology Group. *Gynecol Oncol* 1996;60:120.
446. Boulware RJ, Caderao JB, Delclos L, et al. Whole pelvis megavoltage irradiation with single doses of 1000 rad to palliate advanced gynecologic cancers. *Int J Radiat Oncol Biol Phys* 1979;5:333.
447. Spanos WJ, Wasserman T, Meoz R, et al. Palliation of advanced pelvic malignant disease with large fraction pelvic radiation and misonidazole: final report of RTOG phase I/II study. *Int J Radiat Oncol Biol Phys* 1987;13:1479.
448. Spanos WJ, Perez CA, Marcus S, et al. Effect of rest interval on tumor and normal tissue response—a report of phase III study of accelerated split course palliative radiation for advanced pelvic malignancies (RTOG-8502). *Int J Radiat Oncol Biol Phys* 1993;25:399.
449. Höckel M, Baussmann E, Mitze M, et al. Are pelvic side-wall recurrences of cervical cancer biologically different from central relapses? *Cancer* 1994;74:648.
450. Mahé MA, Gérard JP, Dubois JB, et al. Intraoperative radiation therapy in recurrent carcinoma of the uterine cervix: report of the French Intraoperative Group on 70 patients. *Int J Radiat Oncol Biol Phys* 1996;34:21.
451. Stelzer KJ, Koh WJ, Greer BE, et al. The use of intraoperative radiation therapy in radical salvage for recurrent cervical cancer: outcome and morbidity. *Am J Obstet Gynecol* 1995;172:1881.
452. Ijaz T, Eifel PJ, Burke T, et al. Radiation therapy of pelvic recurrence after radical hysterectomy for cervical carcinoma. *Gynecol Oncol* 1998;70:241.
453. Jobsen JJ, Leer JWH, Cleton FJ, et al. Treatment of locoregional recurrence of carcinoma of the cervix by radiotherapy after primary surgery. *Gynecol Oncol* 1989;33:368.
454. Potter ME, Alvarez RD, Gay FL, et al. Optimal therapy for pelvic recurrence after radical hysterectomy for early-stage cervical cancer. *Gynecol Oncol* 1990;37:74.
455. Larson DM, Copeland LJ, Stringer CA, et al. Recurrent cervical carcinoma after radical hysterectomy. *Gynecol Oncol* 1988;30:381.
456. Wang CJ, Lai CH, Huang HJ, et al. Recurrent cervical carcinoma after primary radical surgery. *Am J Obstet Gynecol* 1999;181.
457. Thomas GM, Dembo AJ, Black B, et al. Concurrent radiation and chemotherapy for carcinoma of the cervix recurrent after radical surgery. *Gynecol Oncol* 1987;27:254.
458. Coleman RL, Burke TW, Morris M, et al. Intra-operative radiographs to confirm the adequacy of lymph node resection in patients with suspicious lymphangiograms. *Gynecol Oncol* 1994;51:362.
459. Hatch KD, Shingleton H, Soong S, et al. Anterior pelvic exenteration. *Gynecol Oncol* 1988; 31:205.
460. Rutledge S, Carey MS, Prichard H, et al. Conservative surgery for recurrent or persistent carcinoma of the cervix following irradiation: is exenteration always necessary? *Gynecol Oncol* 1994;52:353.
461. Matthews CM, Morris M, Burke TW, et al. Pelvic exenteration in the elderly patient. *Obstet Gynecol* 1992;79:773.
462. Miller B, Morris M, Rutledge F, et al. Aborted exenterative procedures in recurrent cervical cancer. *Gynecol Oncol* 1993;50:94.
463. Orr JWJ, Shingleton HM, Hatch KD, et al. Gastrointestinal complications associated with pelvic exenteration. *Am J Obstet Gynecol* 1983;145:325.
464. Roberts WS, Cavanaugh D, Bryson SC, et al. Major morbidity after pelvic exenteration: a seven-year experience. *Obstet Gynecol* 1987;69:617.
465. Berek JS, Hacker NF, Lagasse LD. Rectosigmoid colectomy and reanastamosis to facilitate resection of primary and recurrent gynecologic cancer. *Obstet Gynecol* 1984;64:715.
466. Rowland RG, Mitchell ME, Bihrle R. Alternative techniques for a continent urinary reservoir. *Urol Clin North Am* 1987;14:797.
467. Penalver MA, Barreau G, Sevin BU, et al. Surgery for the treatment of locally recurrent disease. *J Natl Cancer Inst Monogr* 1996;21:117.
468. Rutledge RN, Smith JP, Wharton JT, et al. Pelvic exenteration: an analysis of 296 patients. *Am J Obstet Gynecol* 1977;129:881.
469. Shingleton HM, Soong SJ, Gelder MS, et al. Clinical and histopathologic factors predicting recurrence and survival after pelvic exenteration for cancer of the cervix. *Obstet Gynecol* 1989;73:1027.
470. Stanhope CR, Webb MJ, Podratz KC. Pelvic exenteration for recurrent cervical cancer. *Clin Obstet Gynecol* 1990;33:897.
471. Roman L, Morris M, Eifel P, et al. Reasons for inappropriate simple hysterectomy in the presence of invasive cancer of the cervix. *Obstet Gynecol* 1992;79:485.
472. Andras EJ, Fletcher G, Rutledge F. Radiotherapy of carcinoma of the cervix following simple hysterectomy. *Am J Obstet Gynecol* 1973;115:647.
473. Heller PB, Barnhill DR, Mayer AR, et al. Cervical carcinoma found incidentally in a uterus removed for benign disease. *Obstet Gynecol* 1986;67:187.
474. Hopkins MP, Peters WA, Anderson W, et al. Invasive cervical cancer treated initially by standard hysterectomy. *Gynecol Oncol* 1990;36:7.
475. Roman LD, Morris M, Mitchell MF, et al. Prognostic factors for patients undergoing simple hysterectomy in the presence of invasive cancer of the cervix. *Gynecol Oncol* 1993;50:179.
476. Barillot I, Horiot JC, Cuisenier J, et al. Carcinoma of the cervical stump: a review of 213 cases. *Eur J Cancer* 1993;29A:1231.
477. Miller BE, Copeland LJ, Hamberger AD, et al. Carcinoma of the cervical stump. *Gynecol Oncol* 1984;18:100.
478. Igobeli P, Kapp DS, Lawrence R, et al. Carcinoma of the cervical stump: comparison of

radiation therapy factors, survival, and patterns of failure with carcinoma of the intact uterus. *Int J Radiat Oncol Biol Phys* 1983;9:153.
479. Kovalic JJ, Perez CA, Grigsby PW, et al. The effect of volume of disease in patients with carcinoma of the uterine cervix. *Int J Radiat Oncol Biol Phys* 1991;21:905.
480. Hacker NF, Berek JS, Lagasse LD, et al. Carcinoma of the cervix associated with pregnancy. *Obstet Gynecol* 1982;59:735.
481. Shingleton HM, Orr JW. *Cancer of the cervix.* Philadelphia: JB Lippincott Co, 1995:344.
482. Averette HE, Nasser N, Yakow SL, et al. Cervical conization in pregnancy. Analysis of 180 operations. *Am J Obstet Gynecol* 1970;106:543.
483. Tseng CJ, Horng SG, Soong YK, et al. Conservative conization for microinvasive carcinoma of the cervix. *Am J Obstet Gynecol* 1997;176:1009.
484. Woodrow N, Permezel M, Butterfield L, et al. Abnormal cervical cytology in pregnancy: experience of 811 cases. *Aust N Z J Obstet Gynaecol* 1998;38:161.
485. Seago DP, Roberts WE, Johnson VK, et al. Planned cesarean hysterectomy: a preferred alternative to separate operations. *Am J Obstet Gynecol* 1999;180:1385.
486. Duggan B, Muderspach LI, Roman L, et al. Cervical cancer in pregnancy: reporting on planned delay in therapy. *Obstet Gynecol* 1993;82:598.
487. Hopkins MP, Morley GW. The prognosis and management of cervical cancer associated with pregnancy. *Obstet Gynecol* 1992;80:9.
488. Zemlickis D, Lishner M, Degendorfer P, et al. Maternal and fetal outcome after invasive cervical cancer in pregnancy. *J Clin Oncol* 1991;9:1956.
489. Cliby WA, Dodson MK, Podratz KC. Cervical cancer complicated by pregnancy: episiotomy site recurrences following vaginal delivery. *Obstet Gynecol* 1994;84:179.
490. Copeland LJ, Saul PB, Sniege N. Cervical adenocarcinoma: tumor implantation in the episiotomy sites of two patients. *Gynecol Oncol* 1987;28:230.
491. Van den Broek NR, Lopes AD, Ansink A, et al. "Microinvasive" adenocarcinoma of the cervix implanting in an episiotomy scar. *Gynecol Oncol* 1995;59:297.
492. Creasman WT, Phillips JL, Menck HR. The National Cancer Data Base report on cancer of the vagina. *Cancer* 1998;83:1033.
493. Parker SL, Tong T, Bolden S, et al. Cancer statistics, 1997. *CA Cancer J Clin* 1997;47:5.
494. Shepherd J, Sideri M, Benedet J, et al. Carcinoma of the vagina. *J Epidemiol Biostat* 1998;3:103.
495. Chyle V, Zagars GK, Wheeler JA, et al. Definitive radiotherapy for carcinoma of the vagina: outcome and prognostic factors. *Int J Radiat Oncol Biol Phys* 1996:891.
496. Eddy GL, Jenrette JMI, Creasman WT. Effect of radiotherapeutic technique on local control in primary vaginal carcinoma. *Int J Gynecol Cancer* 1993;3:399.
497. Gallup DG, Talledo OE, Shah KJ, Hayes C. Invasive squamous cell carcinoma of the vagina: a 14-year study. *Obstet Gynecol* 1987;69:782.
498. Stock RG, Chen ASJ, Seski J. A 30-year experience in the management of primary carcinoma of the vagina: analysis of prognostic factors and treatment modalities. *Gynecol Oncol* 1995;56:45.
499. Hoffman MS, De Cesare LS, Roberts WS, et al. Upper vaginectomy for *in situ* and occult, superficially invasive carcinoma of the vagina. *Am J Obstet Gynecol* 1992;166:30.
500. Lenehan PM, Meffe F, Lickrish GM. Vaginal intraepithelial neoplasia: biological aspects and management. *Obstet Gynecol* 1986;68:333.
501. Kalogirou D, Antoniou G, Karakitsos P, et al. Vaginal intraepithelial neoplasia (VAIN) following hysterectomy in patients treated for carcinoma in situ of the cervix. *Eur J Gynaecol Oncol* 1997;18:188.
502. Merino MJ. Vaginal cancer: the role of infectious and environmental factors. *Am J Obstet Gynecol* 1991;165:1255.
503. Schraub S, Sun XS, Maingon P, et al. Cervical and vaginal cancer associated with pessary use. *Cancer* 1992;69:2505.
504. Ikenberg H, Runge M, Göppinger A, et al. Human papillomavirus DNA in invasive carcinoma of the vagina. *Obstet Gynecol* 1990;76:432.
505. Pride GL, Schultz AE, Chuprevich TW, et al. Primary invasive squamous carcinoma of the vagina. *Obstet Gynecol* 1979;53:218.
506. Kirkbride P, Fyles A, Rawlings GA, et al. Carcinoma of the vagina—experience at the Princess Margaret Hospital (1974–1989). *Gynecol Oncol* 1995;56:435.
507. Herbst AL, Ulfelder H, Poskanzer DC. Adenocarcinoma of the vagina: an association of maternal stilboestrol therapy with tumour appearing in young women. *N Engl J Med* 1971;284:878.
508. Herbst AL, Anderson SA, Hubby MM, et al. Risk factors for the development of diethylstilbestrol associated clear cell adenocarcinoma: a case-control study. *Am J Obstet Gynecol* 1986;154:814.
509. Melnick S, Cole P, Anderson D, et al. Rates and risks of diethylstilbestrol-related clear-cell adenocarcinoma of the vagina and cervix. An update. *N Engl J Med* 1987;316:514.
510. Sharp GB, Cole P. Identification of risk factors for diethylstilbestrol-associated clear cell adenocarcinoma of the vagina: similarities to endometrial cancer. *Am J Epidemiol* 1991;134:1316.
511. Waggoner SE, Anderson SM, Van Eyck S, et al. Human papillomavirus detection and p53 expression in clear-cell adenocarcinoma of the vagina and cervix. *Obstet Gynecol* 1994;84:404.
512. Hatch EE, Palmer JR, Titus-Ernstoff L, et al. Cancer risk in women exposed to diethylstilbestrol in utero. *JAMA* 1998;280:630.
513. Plentl AA, Friedman EA. Clinical significance of the vaginal lymphatics. In: *Lymphatic system of female genitalia.* Philadelphia: WB Saunders, 1971:57.
514. Perez CA, Grigsby PW, Garipagaoglu M, et al. Factors affecting long-term outcome of irradiation in carcinoma of the vagina. *Int J Radiat Oncol Biol Phys* 1999;44:37.
515. Plentl AA, Friedman EA. Lymphatics of the vagina. In: *Lymphatic system of female genitalia.* Philadelphia: WB Saunders, 1971:51.
516. Al-Kurdi M, Monagnan JM. Thirty-two years experience in management of primary tumors of the vagina. *Br J Obstet Gynecol* 1981;88:1145.
517. Davis KP, Stanhope CR, Garton GR, et al. Invasive vaginal carcinoma: analysis of early-stage disease. *Gynecol Oncol* 1991;42:131.
518. Isaacs JH. Verrucous carcinoma of the female genital tract. *Gynecol Oncol* 1976;4:259.
519. Matias-Guiu X, Lerma E, Prat J. Clear cell tumors of the female genital tract. *Semin Diagn Pathol* 1997;14:233.
520. Addison WA, Hammond CB, Parker RT. The occurrence of adenocarcinoma in endometriosis of the rectovaginal septum during progestational therapy. *Gynecol Oncol* 1979;8:193.
521. Yaghesezian H, Palazzo JP, Finkel GC, et al. Primary vaginal adenocarcinoma of the intestinal type associated with adenosis. *Gynecol Oncol* 1992;45:62.
522. Joseph RE, Enghardt MH, Doering DL, et al. Small cell neuroendocrine carcinoma of the vagina. *Cancer* 1992;70:784.
523. Miliauskas JR, Leong AS. Small cell (neuroendocrine) carcinoma of the vagina. *Histopathology* 1992;21:371.
524. Prasad CJ, Ray JA, Kessler S. Primary small cell carcinoma of the vagina arising in a background of atypical adenosis. *Cancer* 1992;70:2484.
525. Lee RB, Buttoni L, Dhru K, et al. Malignant melanoma of the vagina: a case report of progression from preexisting melanosis. *Gynecol Oncol* 1984;19:238.
526. Buchanan DJ, Schlaerth J, Kurosaki T. Primary vaginal melanoma: thirteen-year disease-free survival after wide local excision and review of recent literature. *Am J Obstet Gynecol* 1998;178:1177.
527. Ragnarsson-Olding B, Johansson H, Rutqvist LE, et al. Malignant melanoma of the vagina. *Cancer* 1993;71:1893.
528. Peters WA, Kumar NB, Andersen WA, et al. Primary sarcoma of the adult vagina: a clinicopathologic study. *Obstet Gynecol* 1985;65:699.
529. Andrassy RJ, Wiener ES, Raney RB, et al. Progress in the surgical management of vaginal rhabdomyosarcoma: a 25-year review from the Intergroup Rhabdomyosarcoma Study Group. *J Pediatr Surg* 1999;34:731.
530. Kucera H, Vavra N. Radiation management of primary carcinoma of the vagina: clinical and histopathological variables associated with survival. *Gynecol Oncol* 1991;40:12.
531. Manetta A, Pinto J, Larson J, et al. Primary invasive carcinoma of the vagina. *Obstet Gynecol* 1988;72:77.
532. Spiritos N, Doshi B, Kapp D, et al. Radiation therapy for primary squamous cell carcinoma of the vagina: Stanford University experience. *Gynecol Oncol* 1989;35:20.
533. American Joint Committee on Cancer. Vagina. In: Beahrs O, Henson D, Hutter R, et al., eds. *Manual for staging of cancer.* Philadelphia: JB Lippincott Co, 1988:169.
534. Eddy GL, Marks RD, Miller MC, et al. Primary invasive vaginal carcinoma. *Am J Obstet Gynecol* 1991;165:292.
535. Macnaught R, Symonds R, Hole D, et al. Improved control of primary vaginal tumours by combined external-beam and interstitial radiotherapy. *Clin Radiol* 1986;37:29.
536. Nori D, Hilaris B, Stanimir G, et al. Radiation therapy of primary vaginal carcinoma. *Int J Radiat Oncol Biol Phys* 1983;9:1471.
537. Rubin SC, Young J, Mikuta JJ. Squamous carcinoma of the vagina: treatment, complications, and long-term follow-up. *Gynecol Oncol* 1985;20:346.
538. Vavra N, Seifert M, Kucera H, et al. Die Strahlentherapie des primären Vaginalkarzinoms und der Einfluß histologischer und klinischer Faktoren auf die Prognose. *Strahlenther Onkol* 1991;167:1.
539. Marcus R, Million R, Daly J. Carcinoma of the vagina. *Cancer* 1978;42:2507.
540. Peters W, Kumar N, Morley G. Carcinoma of the vagina. Factors influencing outcome. *Cancer* 1985;55:892.
541. Berek JS, Hacker NF. *Practical gynecologic oncology.* Baltimore: Williams & Wilkins, 1994.
542. Benedet JL, Saunders BH. Carcinoma in situ of the vagina. *Am J Obstet Gynecol* 1984;148:695.
543. Cheng D, Ng TY, Ngan HY, et al. Wide local excision (WLE) for vaginal intraepithelial neoplasia (VAIN). *Acta Obstet Gynecol Scand* 1999;78:648.
544. MacLeod C, Fowler A, Dalrymple C, et al. High-dose-rate brachytherapy in the management of high-grade intraepithelial neoplasia of the vagina. *Gynecol Oncol* 1997;65:74.
545. Ogino I, Kitamura T, Okajima H, et al. High-dose-rate intracavitary brachytherapy in the management of cervical and vaginal intraepithelial neoplasia [see comments]. *Int J Radiat Oncol Biol Phys* 1998;40:881.
546. Lee WR, Marcus RB, Sombeck MD, et al. Radiotherapy alone for carcinoma of the vagina. the importance of overall treatment time. *Int J Radiat Oncol Biol Phys* 1994;29:983.
547. Benson C, Soisson AP, Carlson J, et al. Neovaginal reconstruction with a rectus abdominis myocutaneous flap. *Obstet Gynecol* 1993;81:871.
548. Senekjian E, Frey K, Anderson D, et al. Local therapy in stage I clear cell adenocarcinoma of the vagina. *Cancer* 1987;60:1319.
549. Scully RE, Welch WR. Pathology of the female genital tract after prenatal exposure to diethylstilbestrol. In: Herbst AL, Bern HA, eds. *Developmental effects of diethylstibestrol (DES) in pregnancy.* New York: Thieme-Stratton, 1981:26.
550. Senekjian E, Frey K, Stone C, et al. An evaluation of stage II vaginal clear cell adenocarcinoma according to substages. *Gynecol Oncol* 1988;31:56.
551. Wharton J, Fletcher G, Delclos L. Invasive tumors of the vagina: clinical features and management. In: Coppleson M, ed. *Gynecologic oncology: fundamental principles and clinical practice.* Vol. 1. New York: Churchill Livingstone, 1981:345.
552. Fishman DA, Williams S, Small W Jr, et al. Late recurrences of vaginal clear cell adenocarcinoma. *Gynecol Oncol* 1996;62:128.
553. Jones WB, Tan LK, Lewis JL. Late recurrence of clear cell adenocarcinoma of the vagina and cervix: a report of three cases. *Gynecol Oncol* 1993;51:266.
554. Thigpen T, Blessing J, Homesley HD, et al. Phase II trial of cisplatin in advanced or recurrent cancer of the vagina: a Gynecologic Oncology Group study. *Gynecol Oncol* 1986;23:101.
555. Slayton R, Blessing J, Beecham J, et al. Phase II trial of etoposide in the management of advanced or recurrent squamous cell carcinoma of the vulva and carcinoma of the vagina. *Cancer Treat Rep* 1987;71:869.
556. Evans LS, Kersh CR, Constable WC, et al. Concomitant 5-fluorouracil, mitomycin-C, and radiotherapy for advanced gynecologic malignancies. *Int J Radiat Oncol Biol Phys* 1988;15:901.
557. Umesaki N, Kawamura N, Tsujimura A, et al. Stage II vaginal cancer responding to chemotherapy with irinotecan and cisplatin: a case report. *Oncol Rep* 1999;6:123.
558. Yordan E, Deppe G, Malviya V, et al. Chemotherapy of vulvar and vaginal malignancies. In: Deppe G, ed. *Chemotherapy of gynecologic cancer.* New York: Wiley-Liss, 1990:107.

559. Eifel PJ. Concurrent chemotherapy and radiation: a major advance for women with cervical cancer [editorial; comment]. *J Clin Oncol* 1999;17:1334.
560. Shepherd J, Sideri M, Benedet J, et al. Carcinoma of the vulva. *J Epidemiol Biostat* 1998;3:111.
561. Sturgeon SR, Brinton LA, Devesa SS, et al. *In situ* and invasive vulvar cancer incidence trends (1973–1987). *Am J Obstet Gynecol* 1992;166:1482.
562. Mabuchi K, Bross DS, Kessler II. Epidemiology of cancer of the vulva. A case-control study. *Cancer* 1985;55:1843.
563. Iversen T, Tretli S. Intraepithelial and invasive squamous cell neoplasia of the vulva: trends in incidence, recurrence, and survival rate in Norway. *Obstet Gynecol* 1998;91:969.
564. Jones RW, Baranyai J, Stables S. Trends in squamous cell carcinoma of the vulva: the influence of vulvar intraepithelial neoplasia. *Obstet Gynecol* 1997;90:448.
565. Ansink AC, Krul MR, De Weger RA, et al. Human papillomavirus, lichen sclerosus, and squamous cell carcinoma of the vulva: detection and prognostic significance. *Gynecol Oncol* 1994;52:180.
566. Bloss JD, Liao SY, Wilczynski SP, et al. Clinical and histologic features of vulvar carcinomas analyzed for human papillomavirus status: evidence that squamous cell carcinoma of the vulva has more than one etiology. *Hum Pathol* 1991;22:711.
567. Crum CP. Carcinoma of the vulva: epidemiology and pathogenesis. *Obstet Gynecol* 1992; 79:448.
568. Hørding U, Junge J, Daugaard S, et al. Vulvar squamous cell carcinoma and papillomaviruses: indications for two different etiologies. *Gynecol Oncol* 1994;52:241.
569. Monk BJ, Burger RA, Lin F, et al. Prognostic significance of human papillomavirus (HPV) DNA in primary invasive vulvar cancer. *Obstet Gynecol* 1995;85:709.
570. Crum CP, McLachlin CM, Tate JE, et al. Pathobiology of vulvar squamous neoplasia. *Curr Opin Obstet Gynecol* 1997;9:63.
571. Trimble CL, Hildesheim A, Brinton LA, et al. Heterogeneous etiology of squamous carcinoma of the vulva. *Obstet Gynecol* 1996;87:59.
572. Hording U, Daugaard S, Junge J, et al. Human papillomaviruses and multifocal genital neoplasia. *Int J Gynecol Pathol* 1996;15:230.
573. Mitchell MF, Prasay CJ, Silva EG, et al. Second genital primary squamous neoplasms in vulvar carcinoma: viral and histopathologic correlates. *Obstet Gynecol* 1993;81:13.
574. Park JS, Jones RW, McLean MR, et al. Possible etiologic heterogeneity of vulvar intraepithelial neoplasia. A correlation of pathologic characteristics with human papillomavirus detection by in situ hybridization and polymerase chain reaction. *Cancer* 1991;67:1599.
575. Haefner HK, Tate JE, McLachlin CM, et al. Vulvar intraepithelial neoplasia: age, morphological phenotype, papillomavirus DNA, and coexisting invasive carcinoma. *Hum Pathol* 1995;26:147.
576. Lee YY, Wilczanski SP, Chumakov A, et al. Carcinoma of the vulva: HPV and p53 mutations. *Oncogene* 1994;9:1655.
577. Pilotti S, D'Amato L, Della Torre G, et al. Papillomavirus, p53 alteration, and primary carcinoma of the vulva. *Diagn Mol Pathol* 1995;4:239.
578. Sliutz G, Schmidt W, Tempfer C, et al. Detection of p53 point mutations in primary human vulvar cancer by PCR and temperature gradient gel electrophoresis. *Gynecol Oncol* 1997;64:93.
579. Andreasson B, Nyboe J. Predictive factors with reference to low-risk of metastases in squamous cell carcinoma in the vulvar region. *Gynecol Oncol* 1985;21:196.
580. Plentl AA, Friedman EA. Clinical significance of the vulvar lymphatics. In: *Lymphatic system of female genitalia.* Philadelphia: WB Saunders, 1971:27.
581. Shimm DS, Fuller AF, Orlow EL, et al. Prognostic variables in the treatment of squamous cell carcinoma of the vulva. *Gynecol Oncol* 1986;24:343.
582. Binder SW, Huang I, Fu YS, et al. Risk factors for the development of lymph node metastasis in vulvar squamous carcinoma. *Gynecol Oncol* 1990;37:9.
583. Hacker NF, Berek JS, Lagasse LD, et al. Individualization of treatment for stage I squamous cell vulvar carcinoma. *Obstet Gynecol* 1984;63:155.
584. Hoffman JS, Kumar NB, Morley GW. Microinvasive squamous carcinoma of the vulva: search for a definition. *Obstet Gynecol* 1983;61:615.
585. Ross MJ, Ehrmann RL. Histologic prognosticators in stage I squamous cell carcinoma of the vulva. *Obstet Gynecol* 1987;70:774.
586. DiSaia PJ, Creasman WT, Rich WM. An alternative approach to early cancer of the vulva. *Am J Obstet Gynecol* 1979;133:825.
587. Chu J, Tamimi HK, Figge DC. Femoral node metastases with negative superficial inguinal nodes in early vulvar cancer. *Am J Obstet Gynecol* 1983;61:408.
588. Leuchter RL, Hacker NF, Voet RL, et al. Primary carcinoma of the Bartholin gland: a report of 14 cases and review of the literature. *Obstet Gynecol* 1982;60:361.
589. Ridley CM, Frankman O, Jones IS, et al. New nomenclature for vulvar disease: report of the Committee on Terminology of the International Society for the Study of Vulvar Disease. *J Reprod Med* 1990;35:483.
590. Wilkinson EJ. The 1989 presidential address. International Society for the Study of Vulvar Disease. *J Reprod Med* 1990;35:981.
591. Buscema J, Woodruff JD. Progressive histobiologic alterations in the development of vulvar cancer. *Am J Obstet Gynecol* 1980;138:146.
592. Koss LG, Brockunier AJ. Ultrastructural aspects of Paget's disease of the vulva. *Arch Pathol* 1969;87:592.
593. Fanning J, Lambert HC, Hale TM, et al. Paget's disease of the vulva: prevalence of associated vulvar adenocarcinoma, invasive Paget's disease, and recurrence after surgical excision. *Am J Obstet Gynecol* 1999;180:24.
594. Lee RA, Dahlin DC. Paget's disease of the vulva with extension into the urethra, bladder and ureters: a case report. *Am J Obstet Gynecol* 1981;140:834.
595. Hart WR, Millman JB. Progression of intraepithelial Paget's disease of the vulva to invasive carcinoma. *Cancer* 1977;40:2333.
596. Buscema J, Stern JL, Woodruff JD. Early invasive carcinoma of the vulva. *Am J Obstet Gynecol* 1981;140:563.
597. Gil-Moreno A, Garcia-Jimenez A, Gonzalez-Bosquet J, et al. Merkel cell carcinoma of the vulva. *Gynecol Oncol* 1997;64:526.
598. Japese H, van Dinh T, Woodruff JD. Verrucous carcinoma of the vulva: study of 24 cases. *Obstet Gynecol* 1982;60:462.
599. Loret de Mola JR, Hudock PA, Steinetz C, et al. Merkel cell carcinoma of the vulva. *Gynecol Oncol* 1993;51:272.
600. Irvin WP, Cathro HP, Grosh WW, et al. Primary breast carcinoma of the vulva: a case report and literature review. *Gynecol Oncol* 1999;73:155.
601. Feakins RM, Lowe DG. Basal cell carcinoma of the vulva: a clinicopathologic study of 45 cases. *Int J Gynecol Pathol* 1997;16:319.
602. Carlson JW, McGlennen RC, Gomez R, et al. Sebaceous carcinoma of the vulva: a case report and review of the literature. *Gynecol Oncol* 1996;60:489.
603. Raber G, Mempel V, Jackisch C, et al. Malignant melanoma of the vulva. Report of 89 patients. *Cancer* 1996;78:2353.
604. Weinstock MA. Malignant melanoma of the vulva and vagina in the United States: patterns of incidence and population-based estimates of survival. *Am J Obstet Gynecol* 1994;171:1225.
605. Phillips GL, Bundy BN, Okagaki T, et al. Malignant melanoma of the vulva treated by radical hemivulvectomy. A prospective study of the Gynecologic Oncology Group. *Cancer* 1994;73:2626.
606. Ragnarsson-Olding BK, Kanter-Lewensohn LR, Lagerlof B, et al. Malignant melanoma of the vulva in a nationwide, 25-year study of 219 Swedish females: clinical observations and histopathologic features. *Cancer* 1999;86:1273.
607. Ragnarsson-Olding BK, Nilsson BR, Kanter-Lewensohn LR, et al. Malignant melanoma of the vulva in a nationwide, 25-year study of 219 Swedish females: predictors of survival. *Cancer* 1999;86:1285.
608. Trimble EL, Lewis JL, Williams LL, et al. Management of vulvar melanoma. *Gynecol Oncol* 1992;45:254.
609. Chung AF, Woodruff JM, Lewis JLJ. Malignant melanoma of the vulva: a report of 44 cases. *Obstet Gynecol* 1975;45:638.
610. Tasseron EWK, van der Esch EP, Hart AAM, et al. A clinicopathological study of 30 melanomas of the vulva. *Gynecol Oncol* 1992;46:170.
611. Curtin JP, Saigo P, Slucher B, et al. Soft-tissue sarcoma of the vagina and vulva: a clinicopathologic study. *Obstet Gynecol* 1995;86:269.
612. Nirenberg A, Östör AG, Slavin J, et al. Primary vulvar sarcomas. *Int J Gynecol Pathol* 1995;14:55.
613. Bernstein SG, Kovac BR, Townsend DE, et al. Vulvar carcinoma *in situ*. *Obstet Gynecol* 1983; 61:304.
614. Friedrich EG, Wilkenson EJ, Fu YS. Carcinoma *in situ* of the vulva: a continuing challenge. *Am J Obstet Gynecol* 1980;136:830.
615. Kuppers V, Stiller M, Somville T, et al. Risk factors for recurrent VIN. Role of multifocality and grade of disease. *J Reprod Med* 1997;42:140.
616. Homesley HD, Bundy BN, Sedlis A, et al. Prognostic factors for groin node metastasis in squamous cell carcinoma of the vulva (a Gynecologic Oncology Group study). *Gynecol Oncol* 1993;49:279.
617. Sedlis A, Homesley H, Bundy BN, et al. Positive groin lymph nodes in superficial squamous cell vulvar cancer. A Gynecologic Oncology Group study. *Am J Obstet Gynecol* 1987;156:1159.
618. Heaps JM, Fu YS, Montz FJ, et al. Surgical-pathologic variables predictive of local recurrence in squamous cell carcinoma of the vulva. *Gynecol Oncol* 1990;38:309.
619. Homesley HD, Bundy BN, Sedlis A, et al. Assessment of current International Federation of Gynecology and Obstetrics staging of vulvar carcinoma relative to prognostic factors for survival (a Gynecologic Oncology Group study). *Am J Obstet Gynecol* 1991;164:997.
620. Husseinzadeh N, Wesseler T, Schellhas H, et al. Significance of lymphoplasmocytic infiltration around tumor cell in the prediction of regional lymph node metastases in patients with invasive squamous cell carcinoma of the vulva: a clinico-pathologic study. *Gynecol Oncol* 1989;34:200.
621. Husseinzadeh N, Wesseler T, Schneider D, et al. Prognostic factors and the significance of cytologic grading in invasive squamous cell carcinoma of the vulva: a clinicopathologic study. *Gynecol Oncol* 1990;36:192.
622. Kürzl R, Messerer D. Prognostic factors in squamous cell carcinoma of the vulva: a multivariate analysis. *Gynecol Oncol* 1989;32:143.
623. Pinto AP, Signorello LB, Crum CP, et al. Squamous cell carcinoma of the vulva in Brazil: prognostic importance of host and viral variables. *Gynecol Oncol* 1999;74:61.
624. Smyczek-Gargya B, Volz B, Geppert M, et al. A multivariate analysis of clinical and morphological prognostic factors in squamous cell carcinoma of the vulva. *Gynecol Obstet Invest* 1997;43:261.
625. Kaern J, Iversen T, Tropé EO, et al. Flow cytometric DNA measurements in squamous cell carcinoma of the vulva: an important prognostic method. *Int J Gynecol Cancer* 1992;2:169.
626. Mariani L, Conti L, Atlante G, et al. Vulvar squamous carcinoma: prognostic role of DNA content. *Gynecol Oncol* 1998;71:159.
627. Homesley HD, Bundy BN, Sedlis A, et al. Radiation therapy versus pelvic node resection for carcinoma of the vulva with positive groin nodes. *Obstet Gynecol* 1986;68:733.
628. van der Velden J, Lindert ACM, Lammes FB, et al. Extracapsular growth of lymph node metastases in squamous cell carcinoma of the vulva. The impact on recurrence and survival. *Cancer* 1995;75:2885.
629. Origoni M, Sideri M, Garsia S, et al. Prognostic value of pathological patterns of lymph node positivity in squamous cell carcinoma of the vulva stage III and IVA FIGO. *Gynecol Oncol* 1992;45:313.
630. Bassett A. Traitement chirurgical operatoire de l'epithelioma primitif du clitoris. *Rev Chir* 1912;46:546.
631. Taussig FJ. Cancer of the vulva: an analysis of 155 cases. *Am J Obstet Gynecol* 1940;40:764.
632. Way S. Carcinoma of the vulva. *Am J Obstet Gynecol* 1960;79:692.
633. Hacker NF, Leuchter RS, Berek JS, et al. Radical vulvectomy and bilateral inguinal lymphadenectomy through separate groin incisions. *Obstet Gynecol* 1981;58:574.
634. Burke TW, Stringer CA, Gershenson DM, et al. Radical wide excision and selective inguinal node dissection for squamous cell carcinoma of the vulva. *Gynecol Oncol* 1990;38:328.
635. Farias-Eisner R, Cirisano FD, Grouse D, et al. Conservative and individualized surgery for early squamous carcinoma of the vulva: the treatment of choice for stage I and II (T_{1-2} N_{0-1} M_0) disease. *Gynecol Oncol* 1994;53:55.
636. Iverson T, Abeler V, Aalders J. Individualized treatment of stage I carcinoma of the vulva. *Obstet Gynecol* 1981;57:85.

637. Lin JY, DuBeshter V, Angel C, et al. Morbidity and recurrence with modifications of radical vulvectomy and groin dissection. *Gynecol Oncol* 1992;47:80.
638. Magrina JF, Gonzalez-Bosquet J, Weaver AL, et al. Primary squamous cell cancer of the vulva: radical versus modified radical vulvar surgery. *Gynecol Oncol* 1998;71:116.
639. Grimshaw RN, Murdoch JB, Monaghan JM. Radical vulvectomy and bilateral inguinal-femoral lymphadenectomy through separate incisions—experience with 100 cases. *Int J Gynecol Cancer* 1993;3:18.
640. Schulz MJ, Penalver M. Recurrent vulvar carcinoma in the intervening tissue bridge in early invasive stage I disease treated by radical vulvectomy and bilateral groin dissection through separate incisions. *Gynecol Oncol* 1989;35:383.
641. Burke TW, Levenback C, Coleman RL, et al. Surgical therapy of T1 and T2 vulvar carcinoma: further experience with radical wide excision and selective inguinal lymphadenectomy. *Gynecol Oncol* 1995;57:215.
642. Thuesen B, Andreasson B, Bock JE. Sexual function and somatopsychic reactions after local excision of vulvar intra-epithelial neoplasia. *Acta Obstet Gynecol Scand* 1992;71:126.
643. Grimshaw RN, Ghazal Aswad S, Monaghan JM. The role of ano-vulvectomy in locally advanced carcinoma of the vulva. *Int J Gynecol Cancer* 1991;1:15.
644. Hoffman MS, Cavanagh D, Roberts WS, et al. Ultraradical surgery for advanced carcinoma of the vulva: an update. *Int J Gynecol Cancer* 1993;3:369.
645. Hopkins MP, Morley GW. Pelvic exenteration for the treatment of vulvar cancer. *Cancer* 1992;70:2835.
646. Alberti W, Katsilieris I, Schulz U, et al. Indikationen und Ergebnisse der postoperativen Radiotherapie des Vulvakarzinoms. *Stralentherapie und Onkologie* 1986;162:488.
647. Pao WM, Perez CA, Kuske RR, et al. Radiation therapy and conservation surgery for primary and recurrent carcinoma of the vulva: report of 40 patients and a review of the literature. *Int J Radiat Oncol Biol Phys* 1988;14:1123.
648. Perez CA, Grigsby PW, Chao C, et al. Irradiation in carcinoma of the vulva: factors affecting outcome. *Int J Radiat Oncol Biol Phys* 1998;42:335.
649. Faul CM, Mirmow D, Huang Q, et al. Adjuvant radiation for vulvar carcinoma: improved local control. *Int J Radiat Oncol Biol Phys* 1997;38:381.
650. Perez CA, Grigsby PW, Galakatos A, et al. Radiation therapy in management of carcinoma of the vulva with emphasis on conservation therapy. *Cancer* 1993;71:3707.
651. Acosta AA, Given FT, Frazier AB, et al. Preoperative radiation therapy in the management of squamous cell carcinoma of the vulva: preliminary report. *Am J Obstet Gynecol* 1978;132:198.
652. Boronow RC. Combined therapy as an alternative to exenteration for locally advanced vulvo-vaginal cancer: rationale and results. *Cancer* 1982;49:1085.
653. Fairey RN, MacKay PA, Benedet JL, et al. Radiation treatment of carcinoma of the vulva, 1950–1980. *Am J Obstet Gynecol* 1985;151:591.
654. Hacker NF, Berek JS, Juillard GJF, et al. Preoperative radiation therapy for locally advanced vulvar cancer. *Cancer* 1984;54:2056.
655. Jafari K, Magalotti M. Radiation therapy in carcinoma of the vulva. *Cancer* 1981;47:686.
656. Moore DH, Thomas GM, Montana GS, et al. Preoperative chemoradiation for advanced vulvar cancer: a phase II study of the Gynecologic Oncology Group. *Int J Radiat Oncol Biol Phys* 1998;42:79.
657. Cunningham MJ, Goyer RP, Gibbons SK, et al. Primary radiation, cisplatin, and 5-fluorouracil for advanced squamous carcinoma of the vulva. *Gynecol Oncol* 1997;66:258.
658. Landoni F, Maneo A, Zanetta G, et al. Concurrent preoperative chemotherapy with 5-fluorouracil and mitomycin C and radiotherapy (FUMIR) followed by limited surgery in locally advanced and recurrent vulvar carcinoma. *Gynecol Oncol* 1996;61:321.
659. Lupi G, Raspagliesi F, Zucali R, et al. Combined preoperative chemoradiotherapy followed by radical surgery in locally advanced vulvar carcinoma. A pilot study. *Cancer* 1996;77:1472.
660. Wahlen SA, Slater JD, Wagner RJ, et al. Concurrent radiation therapy and chemotherapy in the treatment of primary squamous cell carcinoma of the vulva. *Cancer* 1995;75:2289.
661. Eifel PJ, Morris M, Burke TW, et al. Preoperative continuous infusion cisplatinum and 5-fluoruouracil with radiation for locally advanced or recurrent carcinoma of the vulva. *Gynecol Oncol* 1995;59:51.
662. Koh WJ, Wallace HJ, Greer BE, et al. Combined radiotherapy and chemotherapy in the management of local-regionally advanced vulvar cancer. *Int J Radiat Oncol Biol Phys* 1993;26:809.
663. Russell AH, Mesic JB, Scudder SA, et al. Synchronous radiation and cytotoxic chemotherapy for locally advanced or recurrent squamous cancer of the vulva. *Gynecol Oncol* 1992;47:14.
664. Scheistroen M, Trope C. Combined bleomycin and irradiation in preoperative treatment of advanced squamous cell carcinoma of the vulva. *Acta Oncol* 1992;32:657.
665. Berek JS, Heaps JM, Fu YS, et al. Concurrent cisplatin and 5-fluorouracil chemotherapy and radiation therapy for advanced-stage squamous carcinoma of the vulva. *Gynecol Oncol* 1991;42:197.
666. Thomas G, Dembo A, DePetrillo A, et al. Concurrent radiation and chemotherapy in vulvar carcinoma. *Gynecol Oncol* 1989;34:263.
667. Levin W, Goldberg G, Altaras M, et al. The use of concomitant chemotherapy and radiotherapy prior to surgery in advanced stage carcinoma of the vulva. *Gynecol Oncol* 1986;25:20.
668. Iversen T. Irradiation and bleomycin in the treatment of inoperable vulval carcinoma. *Acta Obstet Gynecol Scand* 1982;61:195.
669. Cummings B. Anal canal carcinomas. In: Meyer JL, Vaeth JM, eds. *Frontiers in radiation oncology.* Vol. 26. Basel: Karger, 1992:131.
670. Benedetti-Panici P, Greggi S, Scambia G, et al. Cisplatin, bleomycin, and methotrexate preoperative chemotherapy in locally advanced vulvar carcinoma. *Gynecol Oncol* 1993;50:49.
671. Mäkinen J, Salmi T, Grönroos M. Individually modified treatment of invasive squamous cell vulvar cancer: 10-year experience. *Ann Chir Gynaecol* 1987;76(Suppl):68.
672. Figge DC, Gaudenz R. Invasive carcinoma of the vulva. *Am J Obstet Gynecol* 1974;119:382.
673. Hacker NF, Berek JS, Lagasse LD, et al. Management of regional lymph nodes and their prognostic influence in vulvar cancer. *Obstet Gynecol* 1983;61:408.
674. Morley GW. Infiltrative carcinoma of the vulva: results of surgical treatment. *Am J Obstet Gynecol* 1976;124:874.
675. Petereit DG, Mehta MP, Buchler DA, et al. A retrospective review of nodal treatment for vulvar cancer. *Am J Clin Oncol* 1993;16:38.
676. Podratz KC, Symmonds RE, Taylor WF. Carcinoma of the vulva: analysis of treatment failures. *Am J Obstet Gynecol* 1982;143:340.
677. Stehman FB, Bundy BN, Thomas G, et al. Groin dissection versus groin radiation in carcinoma of the vulva: a Gynecologic Oncology Group study. *Int J Radiat Oncol Biol Phys* 1992; 24:39.
678. Henderson RH, Parsons JT, Morgan L, et al. Elective ilioinguinal lymph node irradiation. *Int J Radiat Oncol Biol Phys* 1984;10:811.
679. Leiserowitz GS, Russell AH, Kinney WK, et al. Prophylactic chemoradiation of inguinofemoral lymph nodes in patients with locally extensive vulvar cancer. *Gynecol Oncol* 1997;66:509.
680. Eifel PJ. Vulvar carcinoma: radiotherapy or surgery for the lymphatics? *Front Radiat Ther Oncol* 1994;28:218.
681. Koh WJ, Chiu M, Stelzer KJ, et al. Femoral vessel depth and the implications for groin node radiation. *Int J Radiat Oncol Biol Phys* 1993;27:969.
682. Stehman FB, Bundy BN, Dvoretsky PM, et al. Early stage I carcinoma of the vulva treated with ipsilateral superficial inguinal lymphadenectomy and modified radical hemivulvectomy: a prospective study of the Gynecologic Oncology Group. *Obstet Gynecol* 1992;79:490.
683. Ansink AC, Sie-Go DM, van der Velden J, et al. Identification of sentinel lymph nodes in vulvar carcinoma patients with the aid of a patent blue V injection: a multicenter study. *Cancer* 1999;86:652.
684. Bowles J, Terada KY, Coel MN, et al. Preoperative lymphoscintigraphy in the evaluation of squamous cell cancer of the vulva. *Clin Nucl Med* 1999;24:235.
685. Levenback C, Burke TW, Morris M, et al. Potential applications of intraoperative lymphatic mapping in vulvar cancer. *Gynecol Oncol* 1995;59:216.
686. Terada KY, Coel MN, Ko P, et al. Combined use of intraoperative lymphatic mapping and lymphoscintigraphy in the management of squamous cell cancer of the vulva. *Gynecol Oncol* 1998;70:65.
687. Deppe G, Cohen C, Bruckner H. Chemotherapy of squamous cell carcinoma of the vulva: a review. *Gynecol Oncol* 1979;7:345.
688. Sirisabya N. Clinical trials of bleomycin on female genital cancer: a preliminary report. *J Med Assoc Thai* 1974;56:101.
689. Yahia C, Fuller AF, Cloud LP. Successful long-term palliation of stage IV vulvar carcinoma with operation and bleomycin sulfate. *Am J Obstet Gynecol* 1978;130:360.
690. Thigpen JT, Blessing JA, Homesley H, et al. Phase II trials of cisplatin and piperazinedione in advanced or recurrent squamous cell carcinoma of the vulva: a Gynecologic Oncology Group study. *Gynecol Oncol* 1986;23:358.

THOMAS W. BURKE
PATRICIA J. EIFEL
FRANCO M. MUGGIA

SECTION 3

Cancers of the Uterine Body

ENDOMETRIAL CARCINOMA

CLINICAL OVERVIEW

Tumors of the uterine fundus comprise the most common group of gynecologic malignancies. Annual incidence figures for the United States have remained stable at approximately 36,000 cases during the 1990s. Deaths from disease occur in 6000 women per year.[1] The large proportion of survivors with these cancers reflects a disease course characterized by early onset of symptoms and well-established diagnostic guidelines. Nevertheless, women with high-risk or advanced disease have a poor prognosis and account for the most uterine cancer deaths.[2]

A general classification of uterine fundal cancers is provided in Table 36.3-1. Approximately 90% of tumors arise within the epithelium of the uterine lining and are categorized as endometrial carcinomas. Within this group, 90% of cancers are typical endometrial adenocarcinomas.[3] The typical endometrial carcinomas are further subdivided into three architectural grades based on the percentage of solid tumor growth: Grade 1 cancers have identifiable endometrial glands

TABLE 36.3-1. Classification of Uterine Fundal Cancer

Tumor Type	*Approximate Frequency (%)*
Epithelial tumors (endometrioid, papillary endometrioid, papillary serous, clear cell, mucinous)	90
Mesenchymal tumors (endometrial stromal sarcoma, leiomyosarcoma, other nonspecific sarcomas)	5
Mixed tumors (malignant mixed Müllerian, adenosarcoma)	3
Secondary tumors (metastasis, direct local extension: cervix, ovary, colon)	2

and are well differentiated (Fig. 36.3-1), whereas grade 3 tumors demonstrate a solid growth pattern and are poorly differentiated.[4] Rare cell types, including papillary serous carcinoma, clear cell carcinoma, papillary endometrioid carcinoma, and mucinous carcinoma, account for the remaining 10% of cases. Adenosquamous carcinomas are now classified as typical endometrial adenocarcinomas with squamous differentiation. In general, all of these uncommon cell types are associated with a later age of onset, greater risk for extrauterine metastases, and poorer prognosis when compared with typical grade 1 adenocarcinomas.[5–14]

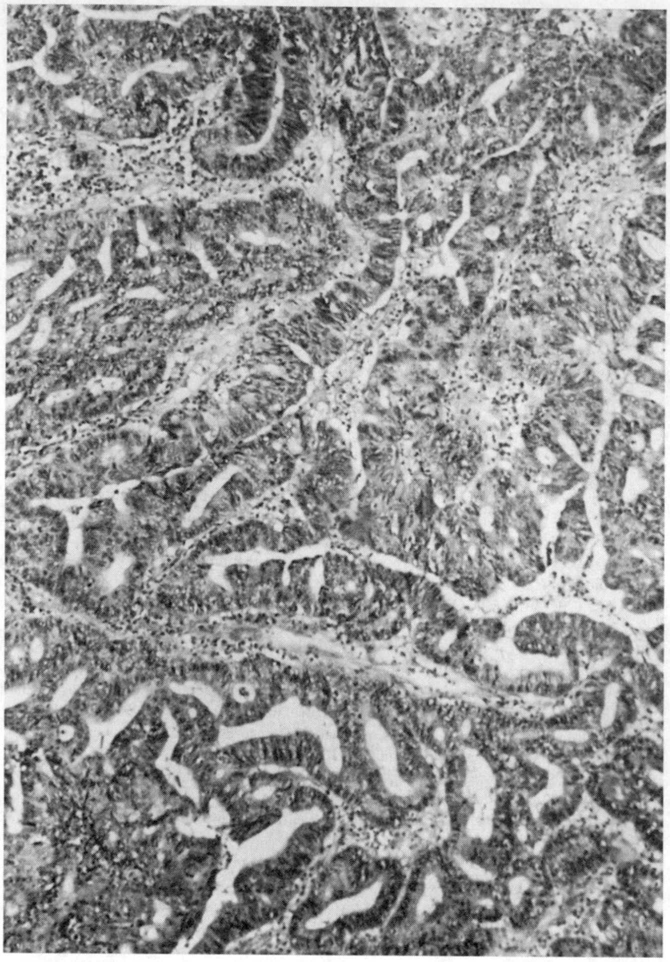

FIGURE 36.3-1. Adenocarcinomas of the endometrium are graded on the basis of their architectural pattern. A complex, branching, glandular pattern without solid areas, as seen in this photomicrograph, is characteristic of grade 1 cancers.

EPIDEMIOLOGY

The normal endometrium is a hormonally responsive tissue. Estrogenic stimulation produces cellular growth and glandular proliferation, which is cyclically balanced by the maturational effects of progesterone.[15] Abnormal proliferation and neoplastic transformation of the endometrium has been associated with chronic unopposed exposure to estrogenic stimulation. It is currently believed that estrogen-associated endometrial cancers progress through a premalignant stage described as *atypical adenomatous hyperplasia.* This phase is characterized by increases in gland number and complexity as well as cytologic atypia. Although serial observations of women with adenomatous hyperplasia are scarce, it is estimated that at least one-third of such cases progress to carcinoma.[16]

The best-recognized risk factors for the development of endometrial carcinoma can be related to chronic estrogen exposure. These include oral intake of exogenous estrogen (without progestins), estrogen-secreting tumors, low parity, extended periods of anovulation, early menarche, and late menopause.[17–25] Pregnancy represents a 9-month period of relatively intense progesterone stimulation by the placenta. Consequently, women with multiple pregnancies have a lower risk of endometrial lesions on the basis of this protective hormonal effect. Both menarche and menopause are commonly associated with absent or irregular ovulation, so women who experience early onset or late cessation of ovarian function are more likely to have additional estrogenic exposure.[26] Morbidly obese women also have a greater risk of endometrial cancer, presumably because their adipocytes are able to convert androstenedione of adrenal origin to estrone, a weak circulating estrogen.

Epidemiologic studies have consistently identified women with diabetes mellitus and hypertension as having an increased risk of endometrial carcinoma. This risk remains independent of other known factors in multivariate analyses. It has not been possible to connect these relatively common medical conditions to the "estrogenic hypothesis" of endometrial carcinogenesis. Epidemiologic risk factors for endometrial cancer are listed in Table 36.3-2.

There is extensive current interest in the potential connection between long-term tamoxifen use as adjuvant therapy for women with breast cancer and the development of endometrial cancers. Although primarily an estrogen antagonist, tamoxifen also has some agonist properties. The diagnosis of endometrial cancer among a few women taking tamoxifen on the National Surgical Adjuvant Breast and Bowel Project trial has raised concerns about the safety of such therapy.[27] Some pathology reviews of tamoxifen-associated endometrial tumors have identified a preponderance of poor-prognosis tumors, whereas others have noted a majority of low-risk lesions.[28–33] A confounding variable is the known increased risk of endometrial tumors in women with breast cancer.[34] This issue is complex and evolving. On the basis of current information, it seems reasonable to conclude that (1) if an association between tamoxifen and endometrial carcinoma exists, the over-

TABLE 36.3-2. Epidemiologic Risk Factors for Endometrial Carcinoma

Factors	*Relative Risk*
CHRONIC ESTROGENIC STIMULATION	
Estrogen replacement (no progestin)	2–12
Early menarche/late menopause	1.6–4.0
Nulliparity	2–3
Anovulation	ND
Estrogen-producing tumors	ND
DEMOGRAPHIC CHARACTERISTICS	
Increasing age	4–8
Caucasian race	2
High socioeconomic status	1.3
European/North American country	2–3
Family history of endometrial cancer	2
ASSOCIATED MEDICAL ILLNESS	
Diabetes mellitus	3
Gallbladder disease	3.7
Obesity	2–4
Hypertension	1.5
Prior pelvic radiotherapy	8

ND, no data.
Table compiled from multiple sources.

all risk is small compared with the risk of recurrent breast cancer, and (2) women receiving long-term tamoxifen therapy should be monitored carefully for uterine abnormalities. Ultrasonic assessment of the contour and thickness of the endometrium is frequently used to monitor such patients, but its value is unproven. Certainly, any woman with abnormal vaginal bleeding should be evaluated promptly by biopsy. Exposure to adjuvant tamoxifen therapy should be limited to 5 years. The development of new selective estrogen receptor modulators that do not have stimulatory effects on the endometrium should eliminate all such risk for women who may benefit from antiestrogen therapy.

NATURAL HISTORY AND ROUTES OF SPREAD

Endometrial carcinoma is a disease of postmenopausal women. The average age at diagnosis is usually about 60 years. Women with high-risk tumors, such as grade 3 adenocarcinoma, papillary serous carcinoma, and clear cell carcinoma, tend to be slightly older. All endometrial lesions originate in the glandular component of the uterine lining. Their initial growth forms a polypoid mass within the uterine cavity (Fig. 36.3-2). This tumor mass is friable and often contains areas of superficial necrosis. Consequently, postmenopausal bleeding is the hallmark symptom for more than 90% of patients. Because most women and their physicians recognize that this as an ominous finding, prompt diagnosis is common.

With further growth, the primary tumor may extend to involve a greater proportion of the endometrial surface and ultimately extend to the lower uterine segment and cervix. Invasion into the myometrium occurs simultaneously. The

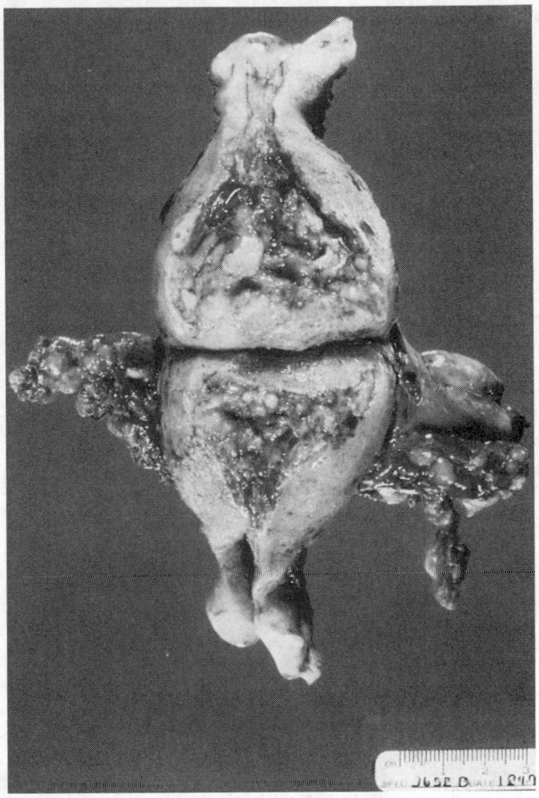

FIGURE 36.3-2. Endometrial cancers develop as polypoid lesions that gradually expand to fill the uterine cavity. This well-differentiated tumor involves both the anterior and posterior uterine walls throughout the entire fundus. Scattered areas of superficial necrosis give rise to the hallmark symptom of postmenopausal bleeding.

uterus has a rich and complex lymphatic network. Channels draining the superior portion of the fundus parallel the ovarian vessels and empty into the paraaortic lymph nodes in the upper abdomen. Lymphatics from the middle and lower portions of the uterus travel through the broad ligaments to the pelvic nodes. A few small lymphatic vessels course through the round ligaments to the superficial inguinal nodes. As a result of this extensive network, nodal metastases can occur at any level and in any combination.[35]

Tumors that penetrate the uterine serosa may directly invade adjacent tissues, such as the bladder, colon, or adnexae, or they may exfoliate into the abdominal cavity to form implant metastases. Small tumor fragments may also gain access to the peritoneal cavity by traversing the fallopian tubes. However, the clinical importance of this potential mechanism of spread is uncertain. Hematogenous dissemination is observed but uncommon. Sites of distant spread include lung, liver, bone, and brain.

DIAGNOSIS AND PRETHERAPY EVALUATION

A diagnosis of endometrial carcinoma should be considered in postmenopausal women with any vaginal bleeding, perimenopausal women with heavy or prolonged bleeding, and premenopausal women with abnormal bleeding patterns who are obese or oligo-ovulatory. Although a formal dilatation and curettage has been the standard technique for diagnosis, outpatient endometrial biopsy has replaced it in most situations.[36–38] A correctly performed endometrial biopsy includes an ade-

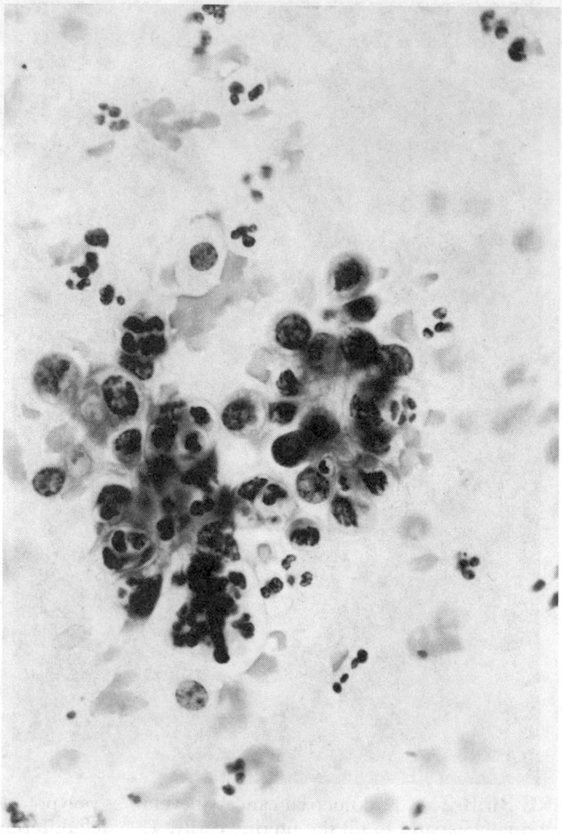

FIGURE 36.3-3. This photomicrograph shows two small tissue fragments demonstrating the typical features of adenocarcinoma. Although not universally seen, such findings are sometimes identified on routine cervical cytology specimens and lead to the diagnosis of endometrial cancer in an asymptomatic woman.

quate amount of tissue obtained from multiple passes through the uterus, and it has a diagnostic accuracy equivalent to that of surgical curettage under anesthesia. Operative sampling may be necessary in unusual patients, such as those with cervical stenosis, inadequate outpatient biopsy, or inability to tolerate an outpatient examination and procedure. Asymptomatic women with endometrial cancer occasionally have abnormal glandular components detected by routine cervical cytology (Fig. 36.3-3). Because the Papanicolaou (Pap) smear is designed to sample the cervical epithelium, this method of diagnosis is uncommon. Fewer than 50% of women with known endometrial cancer have an abnormal Pap smear.[39,40]

Endometrial carcinoma is a surgically treated and staged tumor. Consequently, the focus of the pretreatment evaluation is on the detection of unresectable disease and a determination of operative risk. For patients with disease that is clinically limited to the uterus by physical examination, a straightforward evaluation that includes laboratory studies, a chest radiograph, and an electrocardiogram is adequate. A serum CA-125 assay should be considered in women with high-risk histologic types because it may be predictive of occult extrauterine disease and may be useful as a tumor marker.[41–43] More sophisticated imaging studies such as ultrasound, computed tomography, intravenous pyelography, and magnetic resonance imaging rarely provide information that is not determined after surgical exploration. These studies should be reserved for patients with advanced disease or prohibitive surgical risks. Many women with endometrial cancer are elderly and have associated medical conditions, particularly obesity, diabetes, and hypertension. The pretreatment medical evaluation should be individualized based on findings obtained from the medical history and general physical examination.

RISK FACTORS

Histopathologic risk factors have been extensively evaluated since the late 1970s.[44–49] For convenience, these can be grouped into uterine and extrauterine categories. Major prognostic factors associated with the uterine component of the tumor are grade or cell type, depth of myometrial invasion, and tumor extension to the cervix. Less important are extent of uterine cavity involvement,[50] lymph–vascular space invasion,[51] and tumor vascularity. Obviously, women whose tumors have spread beyond the uterus have a poorer prognosis. The major extrauterine risk factors are adnexal metastases, pelvic or paraaortic lymph node spread, positive peritoneal cytology, peritoneal implant metastases, and distant organ metastases.

A detailed analysis of nearly 1000 patients has been presented by the Gynecologic Oncology Group (GOG).[49] The relative risks for the various histologic factors evaluated in that study are summarized in Table 36.3-5. The risk for developing recurrent disease was greatest in women whose tumors had metastasized to pelvic or paraaortic lymph nodes, demonstrated gross intraperitoneal spread, or contained unequivocal lymph–vascular space invasion. Not surprisingly, an exceptionally high incidence of recurrence was noted in cases with two or more risk factors. Based on the findings of this and other surgical staging trials, the International Federation of Gynecology and Obstetrics (FIGO) adopted a surgical staging system for uterine fundal cancers in 1988.[4]

In addition to the more classic histologic risk factors, several studies have examined archival specimens to evaluate a number of potential molecular markers. Data suggesting a prognostic role for DNA ploidy, S-phase fraction, oncogenes, tumor suppressor genes, AgNOR, and nuclear morphometric features should be considered preliminary.[52–59] Further prospective study in larger numbers of fresh tissue specimens may lead to a refinement of risk assessment. This would be particularly useful if it permitted the identification of the small percentage of otherwise low-risk patients who are destined to develop recurrent disease. Data reported by Lim and colleagues[60] suggest that this approach is possible using ploidy and p53 overexpression as markers.

Some women have a genetic predisposition for endometrial cancer. Endometrial tumors are a component of some of the cancer family syndromes identified and evaluated by Lynch and colleagues.[61,62] Within these unique families, the risk of developing endometrial cancer may approach 50%. However, cancer syndromes account for relatively few cases of endometrial carcinoma overall. Endometrial cancer is also more common in women with a previous cancer of the breast, colon, or ovary. Dual neoplasms may occur simultaneously or metachronously. The time interval between the diagnosis of the two neoplasms may be as long as 10 years.[34]

TABLE 36.3-3. Clinical Staging of Uterine Fundal Tumors[a]

Stage	*Description*
I	The tumor is limited to the uterine fundus.
IA	The uterine cavity measures 8 cm or less.
IB	The length of the uterine cavity is greater than 8 cm.
II	The tumor extends to the uterine cervix.
III	The tumor has spread to the adjacent pelvic structures.
IV	There is bulky pelvic disease or distant spread.
IVA	Tumor invades the mucosa of the bladder or rectosigmoid.
IVB	Distant metastases are present.

[a]International Federation of Gynecology and Obstetrics, 1971.

TABLE 36.3-4. Surgical Staging of Uterine Fundal Tumors[a]

Stage	*Description*
I	The tumor is confined to the uterine fundus.
IA	The tumor is limited to the endometrium.
IB	The tumor invades less than one-half of the myometrial thickness.
IC	The tumor invades more than one-half of the myometrial thickness.
II	The tumor extends to the cervix.
IIA	Cervical extension is limited to the endocervical glands.
IIB	The tumor invades the cervical stroma.
III	There is regional tumor spread.
IIIA	The tumor invades the uterine serosa or adnexa, or there is positive peritoneal cytology.
IIIB	Vaginal metastases are present.
IIIC	The tumor has spread to pelvic or paraaortic lymph nodes.
IV	There is bulky pelvic disease or distant spread.
IVA	Tumor invades the mucosa of the bladder or rectosigmoid.
IVB	Distant metastases are present.

[a]International Federation of Gynecology and Obstetrics, 1988.

STAGING

Before 1988, uterine fundal cancers were staged clinically. The clinical staging system stratified patients with early disease on the basis of a fractional biopsy specimen from both the endocervix and the endometrium as well as the depth of the uterine cavity and physical examination (Table 36.3-3). These techniques for assessment of disease volume and spread were found to be erroneous in as many as one-third of cases when compared with histopathologic findings at the time of laparotomy.[63,64] In addition, women with small-volume disease in retroperitoneal nodes or the peritoneal cavity were rarely identified during clinical staging. The clinical system was abandoned because the accumulating data from surgical staging reports was more accurate and allowed stratification of similar risk groups for adjuvant and adjunctive therapy trials. Consequently, the surgical staging system approved at the 1988 FIGO meeting is currently used for most patients with uterine fundal cancers (Table 36.3-4). Risk factors incorporated into this system include depth of myometrial invasion, tumor extension to the cervix, tumor spread to adnexal organs, peritoneal cytology, retroperitoneal lymph node metastases, and spread to abdominal or distant sites. The clinical staging criteria have been retained for patients who do not undergo surgical exploration as a part of their initial treatment. Patients in this group are those with obviously advanced cancers who would not benefit from tumor resection by hysterectomy and those with medical conditions that preclude an operative procedure.

TREATMENT OF PRIMARY DISEASE

Surgical Resection and Operative Staging

Resection of the primary tumor by total abdominal hysterectomy and bilateral salpingo-oophorectomy is the mainstay of therapy for uterine cancers.[65] Because endometrial cancer originates in the fundus, adequate surgical margins can usually be achieved by simple extrafascial hysterectomy. Salpingo-oophorectomy is recommended because the ovary is a relatively common site of occult metastasis and because most women are already postmenopausal and no longer have hormonal function from the organ. Removal of the uterus is curative treatment for most stage I cases. The more extensive radical hysterectomy has been recommended for selected patients with gross tumor involvement of the cervix.[66,67] However, combined therapy, using both external-beam pelvic irradiation and extrafascial hysterectomy, is more frequently used in such cases.[68–72] The increased expansion of endoscopic surgery has permitted its application in endometrial cancer. The staging portion of the operation is performed endoscopically followed by a transvaginal hysterectomy. Among surgical teams skilled in these techniques, the results appear to be equivalent to those obtained by open laparotomy.[73] Some evidence also suggests that aggressive cytoreduction may improve survival in women with extrauterine disease.[74]

The surgical staging system for uterine fundal tumors identifies certain histopathologic prognostic features for stage and substage assignment but does not define a specific surgical approach required to accomplish staging. The additional operative procedures associated with surgical staging produce a small, but definite, increase in operative risk. Most reported complications are related to organ injury during biopsy or hemorrhage from vascular injury during node sampling.[75–77] Patients who have extensive intraperitoneal staging procedures also have a greater risk of bowel injury if they receive postoperative external irradiation.[78]

Who should undergo surgical staging? Some advocate an extended staging procedure for all women with endometrial cancer. Our approach has been to limit surgical staging to patients at risk for occult disease spread. We routinely perform staging procedures in women with grade 2 or 3 adenocarcinomas and those with variant histologic tumor types. This group typically represents approximately one-third of cases. For patients with grade 1 adenocarcinoma, we estimate the depth of myometrial invasion intraoperatively by making a visual estimate[79] and evaluating a frozen section (Fig. 36.3-4). Extended staging procedures are only performed when significant myometrial invasion (more than 50%) is identified. Using this stratified approach to surgical staging minimizes surgical

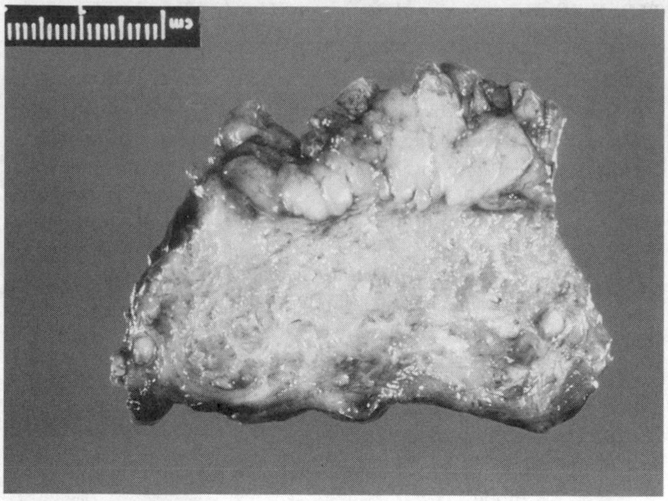

FIGURE 36.3-4. The depth of myometrial invasion can be estimated by visually examining a cut section of the uterine wall taken at the level of the tumor. A clear line distinguishes polypoid tumor growth from myometrium in this surgical specimen. The accuracy of intraoperative visual estimates can be enhanced by using frozen section analysis in selected cases.

risk for patients with low-risk tumors while maximizing the chance for detecting occult extrauterine disease in those patients at risk (Fig. 36.3-5).

An equally important question is what procedures constitute an adequate staging effort. After the collection of cytology specimens and completion of the hysterectomy, the staging assessment is focused on two general areas—the peritoneal cavity and the retroperitoneal lymph nodes. Many gynecologic oncologists have adopted a staging approach similar to that used for women with epithelial ovarian carcinoma. Evaluation of the peritoneal cavity begins with a careful visual and palpatory inspection. Abnormal areas from peritoneal or serosal surfaces are biopsied. In the absence of obvious disease spread, random biopsies from multiple peritoneal sites are obtained. Cytology or histology samples, or both, are also taken from the diaphragm. A portion of the omentum is removed. When we examined our peritoneal staging procedures in a group of at-risk women, we found that occult peritoneal spread is relatively uncommon.[80] Although directed biopsy of palpably suspicious areas often detected metastatic disease, random biopsies were rarely positive. Peritoneal cytology and omental biopsy, coupled with directed biopsy from abnormal sites, provided accurate and reliable information regarding intraperitoneal disease.

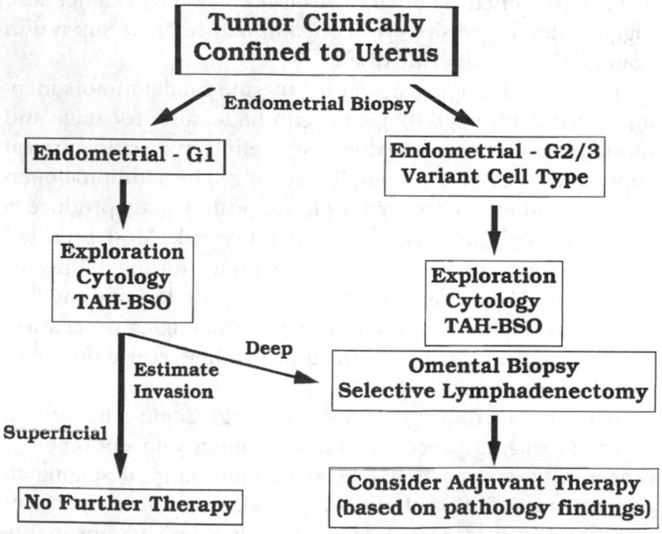

FIGURE 36.3-5. Schematic representation of a staging algorithm. Patients with grade 1 (G1) typical endometrial adenocarcinoma have an exploratory laparotomy with peritoneal cytology, total abdominal hysterectomy (TAH), and bilateral salpingo-oophorectomy (BSO). The depth of myometrial invasion and extension to the cervix are evaluated intraoperatively. Those with low-risk features have no further therapy, whereas those with high-risk features undergo an extended staging operation. All patients with grade 2 or 3 (G2/3) endometrial tumors and those with variant histologic types (papillary serous, papillary endometrioid, clear cell) undergo an extended staging procedure.

The lymphatic drainage of the uterine fundus is complex. Cancers may access either the pelvic or paraaortic nodes, and occasionally the inguinal nodes, on either side. Consequently, detecting retroperitoneal lymph node spread is a potentially difficult problem. Various techniques for lymph node evaluation have been proposed, including palpation with biopsy of abnormal nodes, single lymph node biopsy, selective lymphadenectomy, and full node dissection.[81–83] We believe that a systematic and selective approach to lymphadenectomy reliably detects occult metastases and accurately portrays the true lymph node status.[84] More limited approaches are clearly less accurate. Kilgore and colleagues' suggestion that complete lymphadenectomy may carry a therapeutic advantage deserves further investigation.[85]

The primary goal of surgical staging is to provide an accurate assessment of disease spread at the time therapy is initiated. For patients with tumors confined to the uterus, those in the low-risk subgroup (grade 1 tumor with superficial myometrial invasion) are adequately treated by hysterectomy alone. Fortunately, such cases account for most women with endometrial cancer. Women with tumors demonstrating high-risk features have an incidence of recurrent disease of 25% to 40% and are excellent candidates for adjuvant therapy trials. Patients with more advanced disease warrant additional postoperative adjunct treatment.

Radiotherapy

HISTORICAL PERSPECTIVE. Within a few years of Marie Curie's discovery in 1895, radium was used to treat uterine cancers. Early reports of pathologic complete responses to radiation, encouraging survival rates with combined treatment, and the reduction of postoperative vaginal recurrences fueled enthusiasm for combined treatment.[86,87] By the 1950s, preoperative irradiation followed by hysterectomy had become standard treatment for early-stage endometrial cancer in the United States and other countries, although a few clinicians argued the advantages of selective postoperative irradiation.[88,89] The development of megavoltage radiotherapy in the 1950s reduced the risk of pelvic irradiation and increased the use of this modality to prevent pelvic recurrences. In more recent years, clinicians increasingly have come to appreciate the value of operative findings as a guide to the selection of adjuvant treatment. Because preoperative irradiation has never been proven to be more effective than tailored postoperative radiation therapy, its use has declined in favor of treatment with initial surgery.[65,90,91] Moreover, although radiation therapy has been clearly demonstrated to reduce the rate of pelvic

TABLE 36.3-5. Frequency of Recurrence in Patients with Positive Risk Factors

	Frequency of Recurrence[a]			
Positive Risk Factor	Radiation Therapy	No Radiation Therapy	Total (%)	*Comment*
Specific factor				
Pelvic node	4/16 (1P)	1/2 (1P)	5/18 (27.7)	
Aortic node	0/2	2/3	2/5 (40.0)	
Adnexa	1/5	0/2	1/7 (14.3)	
Gross disease	1/2	0/2	1/4 (25.0)	
Cytology	5/18 (1P)	1/14	6/32 (18.8)	2/4 with implants only
CSI	8/30	1/4	9/34 (26.5)	0/2 with implants only
Isthmus/cervix	8/65 (2P, 3V)	7/29 (4P, 1V)	15/94 (16.0)	0/8 with implants only
Total[b]				
One factor	27/138 (19.6%)	12/56 (21.4%)	39/194 (20.1)	2/140 with implants only
Two factors	25/58 (4P, 1V)	6/14 (1P, 1V)	31/72 (20.1)	0/2 with implants only
Three or more factors	24/42 (5P, 1V)	13/18 (5P, 2V)	38/60 (63.3)	

CSI, capillary-like space involvement; P, pelvic recurrence; V, vaginal recurrence.
[a]Number of cases with recurrence/total number in group.
[b]Twenty-eight patients with one positive factor did not have sufficient follow-up. Eighteen patients with two or more positive factors did not have sufficient follow-up.
(From ref. 49, with permission.)

disease recurrence after hysterectomy, the influence of adjuvant irradiation on the survival rate of patients with endometrial carcinoma has never been clearly determined. As a result, investigators continue to disagree about the role that adjuvant radiotherapy should play in the management of uterine carcinomas.

Several factors have made it difficult to study the value of adjuvant treatment. Because most newly diagnosed endometrial carcinomas are clinically confined to the uterus, with cure rates of 80% to 90% after treatment with hysterectomy alone, the margin for improvement is small. To detect any advantage from adjuvant treatment, studies must have many patients or must be confined to subgroups that are at high risk for recurrence. The influences of physicians' biases on the selection of patients for adjuvant treatment have limited the value of retrospective studies. Retrospective experiences are also difficult to compare because of changes that have been made in the classification systems for staging and grading neoplasms and the relatively recent recognition of special high-risk histologic subtypes. For these reasons, the selection of treatment is based primarily on clinicians' understandings of the risk factors for recurrence and the natural history of the disease, impressions gained from inconclusive studies, and physician or patient preference.

PREOPERATIVE IRRADIATION. The primary goal of preoperative intracavitary irradiation is to prevent vaginal recurrences. Bedwinek et al.[92] observed an inverse correlation between the dose of intracavitary treatment and the incidence of distant metastases in their patients, but other investigators have not confirmed this result. Intrauterine applicators are usually loaded with 35 to 40 mgRaEq of cesium and left in place for approximately 72 hours for a total exposure of 3500 to 4000 mgRaEq-hr. Vaginal applicators are loaded to deliver 60 to 70 Gy to the surface of the apical vagina over the same period. Inserting additional sources in the form of Heyman or Simon capsules may increase the dose to the fundus. After this dose of radiation, hysterectomy can be safely performed within 2 to 3 days.[93,94] Immediate hysterectomy is usually preferred because important prognostic information about the depth of tumor infiltration is retained. Although the popularity of preoperative irradiation has declined, some groups still support its use for patients with grade 2 or 3 tumors. Preoperative irradiation is not indicated for patients with grade 1 tumors that are clinically confined to the uterus, because low-grade carcinomas are usually superficial and have a very low risk of recurrence after treatment with hysterectomy alone.

The theoretical arguments for preoperative irradiation are strongest for patients with uterine cancers that grossly involve the cervix, because preoperative intracavitary techniques deliver a greater dose to the paracervical tissues than is possible with postoperative vaginal irradiation. Combined preoperative external-beam and intracavitary irradiation may be indicated for patients with nonserous tumors that extensively infiltrate the cervix. However, when external-beam irradiation is given preoperatively, hysterectomy should be delayed 4 to 6 weeks.

Because radiation therapy has been used to treat high-risk endometrial carcinoma for many years, few unselected series of patients treated with surgery alone have been reported. In early series, overall vaginal recurrence rates were as high as 15% to 25%[87,95] However, changes in the staging of disease and methods of reporting results make it difficult to relate these results to current experience. A few authors have reported much lower vaginal recurrence rates after surgery alone and have suggested that the wide range of reported local recurrence rates may, in part, reflect variations in surgical technique that influence the risk of tumor cell implantation.[96,97]

Most data suggest that irradiation reduces the incidence of vaginal recurrence from 10% to 15% to less than 5% for patients with high-risk disease. In a compilation of series published between 1967 and 1973, Jones[87] reported an overall incidence of vaginal recurrences of 4.6% in patients treated with preoperative radium compared with 10.6% in patients treated with surgery alone. Subsequent series reported vaginal relapse rates of 0% to 5% for patients with clinical stage I disease treated with preoperative intracavitary irradiation (Table 36.3-5).[93,94,97–103] However,

TABLE 36.3-6. Rates of Vaginal Recurrence for Patients Treated with Hysterectomy for Endometrial Carcinoma

Reference	*Preoperative ICRT (%)*	*Postoperative EBRT ± ICRT (%)*	*Postoperative ICRT Only (%)*	*Surgery Alone (%)*
Jones[a] [87] (1975)	1378 (4.6)	—	16 (5.2)	770 (10.3)
Ohlsen et al.[93] (1977)	0/99	—	—	—
Underwood et al.[94] (1977)	0/182	—	—	—
Bean et al.[98] (1978)	0/130	1/41 (2.4)[b]	0/2	1/107 (0.9)[c]
Piver et al.[99] (1979)	4/87 (4.6)	—	0/49	4/53 (7.5)
Reddy et al.[100] (1979)	2/66 (3)	0/17	—	7/94 (7.4)
Eifel et al.[97] (1983)	1/63 (1.6)	0/15	—	3/178 (1.7)
Torrisi et al.[106] (1989)	—	2/46 (4.3)[b]	—	—
Kucera et al.[107] (1990)	—	3/229 (1.3)[b]	1/376 (0.2)[c]	—
Sause et al.[102] (1990)	2/112 (1.7)	3/117 (2.5)	—	—
Calais et al.[101] (1990)	7/121 (5.8)	—	3/63 (4.8)	—
Piver and Hempling[108] (1990)	—	0/41[b]	0/92[c]	—
Sorbe and Smeds[135] (1990)	—	—	3/404 (0.7)	—
Randall et al.[118] (1990)	—	10/154 (6.5)[b]	—	—
Grigsby et al.[103] (1991)	14/685 (2)	3/152 (2)	—	—
Stryker et al.[109] (1991)	—	2/86 (2.3)[b]	—	—
Bliss and Cowie[117] (1992)	—	4/91 (4.4)[b]	—	0/31[c]
Elliott et al.[136] (1994)	—	—	8/358 (2.2)	29/453 (6.4)
Carey et al.[111] (1995)	—	5/129 (4)[b]	—	6/227 (2.6)[c]
Noyes et al.[141] (1995)	—	—	0/63[c]	—
Poulsen et al.[273] (1996)	—	—	—	17/641 (3)[c]
MacLeod et al.[140] (1998)	—	—	2/143[c] (1.4)	—

EBRT, external-beam radiotherapy; ICRT, intracavitary radiotherapy.
[a]Compiled from ten series published between 1967 and 1973.
[b]Includes only patients described as high risk.
[c]Includes only patients described as low risk.

these results cannot be compared with the recurrence rates of patients not treated with radiation because, in nearly all studies, patients who had a higher risk of recurrence were selected to receive combined treatment (Table 36.3-6).

POSTOPERATIVE REGIONAL IRRADIATION. For many years, the only prospective randomized study that had evaluated the benefit of postoperative pelvic irradiation was one conducted at the Norwegian Radium Hospital and published in 1980.[104] Patients with clinical stage I adenocarcinomas underwent total abdominal hysterectomy and bilateral salpingo-oophorectomy. Those proven to have metastases at laparotomy were excluded from the study, but no consistent surgical evaluation was performed. The remaining 540 patients received 60 Gy with brachytherapy to the surface of the apical vagina and were then randomized either to receive 40 Gy of pelvic radiotherapy or no further treatment.

Although patients who received pelvic irradiation in this study had a lower rate of pelvic recurrences, there was no significant improvement in overall disease-specific survival. The data suggested that the survival rate of patients with deeply invasive grade 3[104] tumors may be improved with radiotherapy, but the number of patients in this subset was small, and the result was not statistically significant. The authors suggested that regional irradiation may have failed to improve the survival rate because patients whose pelvic disease was controlled recurred instead at distant sites. However, local control appeared to be most improved for patients with tumors that deeply invaded the myometrium, whereas the higher rate of distant metastases was seen primarily in irradiated patients with superficial or no muscle invasion. However, although the Norwegian study is one of the largest published series of patients with endometrial cancer, few patients with high-risk disease and relatively few disease-related deaths were reported. As a result, the study was unable to demonstrate or rule out moderate differences in survival rates between patient subgroups.

Several studies that document 80% to 90% survival rates for patients with high-risk disease treated with postoperative radiotherapy provide indirect evidence of the efficacy of regional irradiation.[49,105–111] Carey and colleagues[111] reported an 81% 5-year relapse-free survival rate for 157 patients with clinical stage I disease and high-risk features (deep myometrial invasion, grade 3, adenosquamous histology, or cervical involvement) who were prospectively treated with a standardized treatment protocol. The local recurrence rate was 29% in 28 patients who refused recommended pelvic radiotherapy compared with 4% in those who received the treatment as per protocol ($P = .03$). Overall recurrence rates (29% vs. 16%) were not significantly different. In another prospective phase II trial, Piver and Hempling[108] reported a 5-year survival rate of 88% in 41 patients who received postoperative pelvic radiotherapy for deeply invasive or grade 3 tumors that were surgically staged with a finding of negative paraaortic nodes. Only one patient had disease recurrence within the radiation treatment field. Kucera et al.[107] reported a survival rate of 88% for 229 patients who had infiltration of the outer one-third of the myometrium or grade 2 or 3 tumors that involved the middle third. This survival rate was not significantly different from that of 376 patients who had more favorable tumors treated with hysterectomy and vaginal irradiation alone (91%). The GOG reported a 70% projected 5-year survival rate in 63 patients who had metastases to the pelvic nodes without paraaortic node involvement.[49] Of these studies, only one (that by Carey and colleagues[111]) excluded patients with papillary serous neoplasms from the analysis. Because the tendency of serous tumors to recur intraperitoneally is not adequately addressed with local treatment, their inclusion in studies of adjuvant pelvic irradiation tends to obscure its possible benefit to patients with high-risk endometrioid tumors.

The GOG completed a randomized trial comparing surgery with surgery plus pelvic radiation therapy in 448 women with intermediate risk endometrial adenocarcinoma.[112] The dose of pelvic radiation was 50.4 Gy, and brachytherapy was not used in either arm. All patients underwent complete surgical staging and only those with FIGO stage IB, IC, or occult stage II disease were eligible. With a median follow-up of 56 months, the estimated 2-year progression-free interval was 96% for patients who received adjuvant radiation therapy versus 88% for those treated only with surgery (P = .004). Disease recurred in the pelvis in three patients treated with adjuvant radiation and in 17 patients treated with surgery alone. Overall survival rates for patients treated with or without adjuvant radiation were 96% and 89%, respectively, at 36 months; this difference was not statistically significant (P = .09). This study clearly confirms the ability of postoperative irradiation to reduce local recurrence, although some of this reduction may have been achievable with brachytherapy alone. Opponents of adjuvant irradiation argue that survival was not improved by adjuvant treatment. However, follow-up of this study is still incomplete, and the inclusion of patients with very favorable (e.g., stage IB, grade 1) tumors may dilute a survival benefit to remaining patients (if it exists).

These studies suggest that pelvic radiotherapy is indicated for patients with endometrioid or mucinous tumors that are confined to the pelvis and have features that predict a high risk of recurrence in the pelvis. The potential benefit of treatment should be carefully balanced against the risk of complications, particularly for patients with a history of pelvic infection, multiple abdominal surgical procedures, or severe diabetes mellitus. Patients whose tumors invade the myometrium by more than 50% or involve the cervical stroma, lymph–vascular spaces, or pelvic lymph nodes are at highest risk for pelvic recurrence and are usually treated with external-beam radiation to the true pelvis. Other risk factors may be used to select treatment for tumors with intermediate risk factors (e.g., grade 2 tumors invading to the middle third of the myometrium). Schink et al.[113] reported that tumors measuring less than 2 cm in diameter rarely involved pelvic nodes, whereas those involving the entire uterine cavity had a high risk of pelvic nodal involvement and disease recurrence even when the outer half of the myometrium was not invaded. Patients with intermediate risk factors in the uterus who have had extensive nodal dissections without demonstration of nodal involvement are less likely to benefit from regional irradiation, particularly in view of the possible increased risk of late complications in patients who have had staging lymphadenectomies.[114–116]

Pelvic radiotherapy is usually delivered using a four-field technique or anteroposterior opposed fields with 15 to 20 MV photons to a total dose of 40 to 50 Gy. Serious complications are observed in 2% to 5% of patients who receive this treatment, but complications may be greater for patients who have had a staging lymphadenectomy.[114–116] Corn and colleagues[116] also reported a correlation between external-beam irradiation and the risk of complications. Some clinicians give additional intracavitary irradiation to the vaginal cuff after pelvic radiotherapy, although investigators disagree about the benefit of this treatment. Bliss and Cowie[117] reported a lower vaginal recurrence rate (10% vs. 0%) in patients who had intracavitary irradiation added to external-beam irradiation, but gastrointestinal toxicity was also increased. In contrast, Randall et al.[118] reported no difference in local control or complication rates when the vaginal cuff received an intracavitary radiation boost. Several authors[117,119,120] have reported increased complication rates when an intracavitary boost was added to 45 to 50 Gy of external-beam radiotherapy to the pelvis; however, these groups tended to give relatively high doses (more than 50 Gy) or rapid dose rates (more than 70 cGy/hr) to the vaginal surface.

TABLE 36.3-7. Survival Rate of Patients Treated with Extended-Field Irradiation for Endometrial Carcinoma Metastatic to Paraaortic Lymph Nodes

Reference	*Number of Patients*	*5-Y Survival Rate (%)*
Komaki et al.[121]	7	60
Potish[129]	15	40
Feuer and Calanog[122]	18	50
Morrow et al.[49]	48	37
Rose et al.[125]	17	53
Corn et al.[124]	50	46
Hicks et al.[126]	11	27
Blythe et al.[127]	13	54
Onda et al.[128]	20	75[a]

[a]Patients also received three cycles of cisplatin-containing chemotherapy before radiation therapy.

EXTENDED-FIELD IRRADIATION. Extended-field irradiation appears to be effective treatment for patients with nonserous endometrial cancer metastatic to paraaortic nodes. Between 30% and 50% of patients survive 5 years with this treatment (Table 36.3-7).[49,121–128] Survival rates are not clearly different for patients with gross or microscopic nodal involvement.[125,129] In their review of 50 patients, Corn et al.[124] reported a lower rate of recurrence in paraaortic lymph nodes in patients who had had a lymph node dissection in addition to extended-field irradiation. However, multivariate analysis suggested that the risk of recurrence was not significantly decreased by combined treatment. In another study, Onda and colleagues[128] reported a 5-year survival rate of 75% for 20 patients treated with lymphadenectomy followed by cisplatin-containing chemotherapy and extended-field irradiation. Further study is needed to determine whether this excellent survival rate is reproducible.

WHOLE ABDOMINAL IRRADIATION. The poor prognosis of uterine papillary serous carcinomas and their tendency to spread and recur intraabdominally have led radiation oncologists to explore the value of treatment with whole abdominal irradiation. The 68% abdominal recurrence rate reported by Greven et al.[130] in patients with pathologic stage III papillary serous or clear cell carcinomas after treatment with pelvic or extended-field radiotherapy demonstrate why smaller radiation fields are usually inadequate for this disease. Although whole abdominal radiotherapy is accepted by many clinicians as a standard treatment for papillary serous carcinoma, there are as yet only anecdotal reports supporting its efficacy.[123,131,132] Potish[123] reported long-term survival in five (57%) of nine patients who had intraperitoneal spread from uterine papillary serous carcinoma at diagnosis, and Malipeddi et al.[131] reported survival durations of 102 to 133 months in five of ten patients treated with whole abdominal irradiation. Three of the patients who survived more than 5 years had been diagnosed with pathologic stage IIIA disease. Treatment techniques are similar to those used to treat patients with primary ovarian carcinomas.

Some authors have advocated the use of whole abdominal irradiation for patients with tumors of other histologic subtypes.[133] The number of patients treated in these series is insufficient to determine whether the treatment is better than locoregional irradiation or even whether it is beneficial. Most studies suggest that intraabdominal dissemination is an uncommon pattern of spread in patients with nonserous histologic subtypes, even when malignant cells are seen in peritoneal washings taken at the time of hysterectomy. Although some have advocated whole abdominal irradiation to treat patients with positive peritoneal cytology, there is little evidence that this finding predicts a pattern of intraabdominal recurrence in patients with the more common endometrioid subtypes of endometrial carcinoma. Thus, treatment directed specifically at the positive cytology may not be warranted.[134]

The GOG is comparing whole abdominal radiation therapy with chemotherapy (cisplatin and doxorubicin) for patients with FIGO (1988) stage III and IV disease (less than 2 cm residual).[133] This study will be of particular interest for its comparison of the two treatments in patients with papillary serous tumors, although it will also include patients with nonserous stage III tumors for whom the risk of intraabdominal dissemination is probably small.

POSTOPERATIVE VAGINAL IRRADIATION. Some patients with minimally invasive grade 2 or noninvasive grade 3 tumors have a significant risk of vaginal recurrence despite a relatively low risk of pelvic node metastases. Implantation of tumor cells in the vaginal cuff incision may be an important mechanism of recurrence in these cases.

Postoperative intracavitary irradiation appears to be a very effective method of preventing vaginal cuff recurrences. Calais et al.[101] reported no differences between the survival and vaginal recurrence rates of patients treated with preoperative or postoperative intracavitary radiation. Reported rates for central recurrence range from 0% to 5% for patients treated with postoperative intracavitary irradiation alone, with the variation partly reflecting the different selection criteria used by various groups.[87,98,99,101,107,108,111,135,136]

A variety of different types of intracavitary applicators have been used to treat the vaginal cuff. Radioactive sources are usually placed in vaginal ovoids or in a plastic dome-shaped vaginal cylinder. The arrangement of sources and shape of the cylinder are designed to deliver a homogeneous dose to the apical vaginal surface. Additional sources may be used to treat the midvagina if desired. Because the dose of radiation decreases rapidly to approximately 50% to 60% of the surface dose at a depth of 0.5 cm beneath the vaginal mucosa, the dose to adjacent normal tissues is substantially less than the vaginal surface dose.

In the past, radiation was usually administered at low dose rates. Typically, the apical one-third to one-half of the vaginal surface was treated to a total dose of 60 to 70 Gy (30 to 40 Gy at 0.5 cm depth) at a dose rate of 90 to 100 cGy/hr (50 to 60 cGy/hr at 0.5 cm depth). With this treatment, most investigators report a risk of major complications of approximately 1% to 2%.[98,103,104,108,119] The complication rates tend to be higher with higher total doses and when more than one-half of the vaginal length is treated, although this has not been studied rigorously.

Today, fractionated high dose-rate intracavitary irradiation is increasingly being used as an alternative to low dose-rate irradiation to treat the vaginal cuff. This approach is more convenient for the patient and the physician and less costly than inpatient low dose-rate irradiation.[137] The use of high dose-rate brachytherapy has been less controversial in this setting than in the treatment of primary cervical cancer because only a modest dose of radiation is needed to prevent tumor recurrence in the vagina and because placement of the vaginal cylinder requires little manipulation and no sedation.

There is no clear consensus about the ideal dose or fractionation schedule for high dose-rate vaginal brachytherapy. Sorbe and Smeds[135] compared four fractionation schemes—4 × 9.0 Gy, 5 × 6.0 Gy, 6 × 5.0 Gy, and 6 × 4.5 Gy, prescribed at a tissue depth of 1.0 cm—in 404 patients who received intracavitary irradiation alone (without external-beam irradiation) after hysterectomy. The rates of acute and late complications were strongly correlated with fraction size. Eighty-eight percent of patients treated with 4 × 9.0 Gy had significant late rectal complications. Because the authors prescribed treatment at 1.0-cm depth, the total dose and dose per fraction at the mucosal surface were much higher than the specified dose.

Most authors have recommended more conservative fractionation schemes. Treatment is usually prescribed at the surface or 5 mm beneath the mucosa. When the dose is prescribed at 5 mm beneath the mucosa, it should be remembered that the rectal mucosa will receive a total dose (and dose per fraction) that is similar to the prescribed dose. In some reports, investigators have recommended a number of fractionation schemes including, for example, 6 × 6 Gy,[138] 3 × 7 Gy,[139] 4 × 8.5 Gy,[140] and 2 × 16.2 Gy,[141] with doses specified at the vaginal surface. All have reported vaginal recurrence rates of less than 1.5% for patients with relatively favorable tumors.

RADIOTHERAPY ALONE. Although hysterectomy is the primary treatment of most endometrial carcinomas, radiotherapy alone is also an effective treatment that is sometimes indicated for patients who are medically inoperable or who have unresectable disease. Most authors report disease-specific survival rates of 75% to 85% and local recurrence rates of 10% to 20% for patients with clinical stage I to II disease treated with radiation alone. Prognosis is usually correlated with clinical stage and histologic grade.[142–148] Kupelian et al.[146] found that the survival rate of patients with papillary serous tumors was significantly poorer than that for patients with other histologic types of endometrial cancer. However, the disease-specific survival rate of 43% was not obviously different from that commonly reported for treatment of this tumor with hysterectomy alone.

Some authors recommend treatment with a combination of external-beam and intracavitary irradiation.[144,147,148] However, very good local control and survival rates also have been reported after treatment with brachytherapy alone.[145,146] Patients who have low-grade tumors that do not expand the uterus are probably effectively treated with intracavitary irradiation alone. Patients with large uterine cavities, cervical involvement, or grade 3 tumors may benefit from a course of external-beam irradiation before intracavitary treatment.

Brachytherapy must cover the uterine fundus adequately when treatment will not include a hysterectomy. A single uterine tandem with increased activity in the highest source may be sufficient for patients who have a very small uterine cavity. A number of applicator systems, such as the Heyman capsule or Simon afterloading systems, have been devised to improve the dose to the fundus in patients with larger uterine cavities. Both of these afterloading systems are used to pack the uterine cavity with radium or cesium sources to expand the dose distribution to the fundus. In some cases, two tandems can be placed in the right and left cornua of the uterus and loaded to achieve the desired distribution. Magnetic resonance imaging may be helpful in planning treatment.

Several groups have reported results of treatment with high dose-rate intracavitary radiation for patients with inoperable endometrial cancer.[149–151] In the largest of these series, Knocke and colleagues[150] reported results for 280 patients, most of whom had clinical stage I to II disease. Treatment appeared to be well tolerated, but the local recurrence rates were somewhat higher than those reported from earlier series. In particular, local control rates for patients with clinical stage IB and II tumors were only approximately 60%. This rate may possibly reflect a suboptimal distribution to the uterine fundus from the single-channel tandem applicator used in their treatments. Nguyen and Petereit[151] reported good uterine disease control rates (88%) but a high rate of perioperative morbidity and two perioperative deaths in 36 patients treated with high dose-rate brachytherapy for clinical stage I disease. Although this approach may offer advantages over low dose-rate brachytherapy for selected patients who are deemed medically inoperable, sedation may still be required to optimize applicator insertion. Deep venous thrombosis, a possible complication of prolonged bed rest during low dose-rate applications, can also be encouraged by prolonged lithotomy positioning for high dose-rate procedures.[151,152] Whatever method of brachytherapy is used, these patients should only be treated by experienced brachytherapists in a well-controlled environment with adequate monitoring and emergency medical support.

Systemic Adjuvants

HORMONES

Historical Background. The original observations by Kelley and Baker[153] documenting the responsiveness of metastatic endometrial adenocarcinoma to progestogens encouraged the organization of the Endometrial Surgical Adjuvant Study Group in 1965, the forerunner of the GOG. This group's initial trial failed to demonstrate an effect of medroxyprogesterone acetate (MPA) on recurrences after surgical treatment of stage I endometrial cancer.[154] Nevertheless, it stimulated the interest of gynecologic oncologists in collaborative clinical trials and led directly to a grant application in support of GOG activities that began in May 1971. More recent studies have focused on the role of adjuvant progestogens on higher risk populations with stage I or clinically occult stage II cancer.

Adjuvant Hormonal Studies. Progestogens have been widely used to treat metastatic endometrial cancer. Although no adjuvant effect of MPA was shown in the initial randomized study, optimistic results were obtained using adjunctive progestogens in women with stage I endometrial cancer compared retrospectively with patients treated only with local modalities.[155,156] Subsequent randomized studies, however, again failed to demonstrate survival differences.[157–159] Accordingly, some have argued for performing clinical trials on a better-selected population—for example, those with a greater chance of recurrence or with features that might render them more responsive to progestogens. However, such selection criteria produce the paradox that higher-risk tumors are less likely to be hormone responsive. Subset analyses have documented an unfavorable relative survival in "receptor-poor" versus "receptor-rich" stage I endometrial cancer treated with MPA. Studies have been initiated in Germany comparing higher doses of MPA (1000 mg orally daily) with tamoxifen and with observation in patients with stage I cancer and with nonrandomized use of MPA in women with stage II disease. However, because no fully published results from such newer adjuvant therapy trials have appeared, adjuvant hormonal therapy can only be recommended in the context of clinical trials. Similarly, nonrandomized experience with progestogens given as induction therapy before, or in lieu of, surgery in patients with preinvasive or minimally invasive disease, or in patients who are poor surgical risks, attests to their biologic activity but does not represent an established indication.[160]

In addition to the use of adjuvant progestogens alone, a large Italian study of women with FIGO stage I cancers randomized patients with invasion beyond one-third of the myometrium to either external radiation or external irradiation plus MPA. No differences were seen among arms.[158]

CYTOTOXIC CHEMOTHERAPY. Cytotoxic chemotherapy has been considered as an adjuvant treatment in certain circumstances when the risk of distant recurrence exceeds 20%. These circumstances include (1) any stage II tumor, (2) clear cell or papillary serous histology, (3) absence of hormone receptors, (4) preoperative finding of elevated CA-125, and (5) selected stage I disease with deep myometrial invasion. A study from the M. D. Anderson Cancer Center in patients with some of these adverse prognostic factors reported a favorable experience after adjuvant cisplatin, doxorubicin, and cyclophosphamide therapy.[161,162] Confirmation from randomized studies is lacking, however.

Because the only randomized study of adjuvant chemotherapy yielded negative results (GOG 34, a study comparing adjuvant doxorubicin to no further therapy after surgery and radiation for stage I and occult stage II high-risk endometrial cancer),[49] the GOG has subsequently launched studies to evaluate other adjunct modalities. In July 1995, GOG 99, which randomized all cell types (except papillary serous and clear cell) of surgical stage I or occult stage II endometrial cancers to either no additional treatment or pelvic radiotherapy, was closed to accrual. In a simultaneous trial, GOG 94 treated all papillary serous and clear cell tumors, regardless of stage, with whole abdominal radiation. Patients with other cell types and optimally debulked clinical stage III or IV were also eligible for this study.

New clinical trials have been proposed to compare combination chemotherapy (doxorubicin and cisplatin) and pelvic radiation in women with stage IB, IC, IIA, and IIB endometrial cancers. It is hoped that better patient selection, higher dose intensity, use of a more active drug regimen, and avoidance of the toxicities seen in GOG 34 from doxorubicin after pelvic radiation will allow systemic therapy to demonstrate a benefit, even though this combination regimen does not enhance survival in patients with advanced disease.[163] A resurgence of interest in consolidation therapy with simultaneous irradiation and chemotherapy is likely as paclitaxel and cisplatin are more tolerable in such situations than doxorubicin. In addition, drug combinations have been proposed before local irradiation in high-risk patients (those with papillary serous/clear cell histology, pathologic stage III and IVA disease, and earlier stages beyond IA if they have at least any two of the following unfavorable risk factors: grade 3 disease, more than one-third myometrial invasion, cervical stromal invasion, and vascular space involvement).

TREATMENT OF RECURRENT DISEASE

Treatment Failure

Treatment failure in low-risk patients is exceedingly rare. In our series investigating surveillance strategies, we had only one failure in this group.[164] Tumor recurrence is most common in women with advanced-stage disease or those with high-risk features in their primary tumor. Late recurrence is uncommon, and virtually all failures are clinically evident within 3 years of original diagnosis.[164–166]

One-half of patients whose tumors recur are symptomatic. A targeted examination and diagnostic evaluation should readily lead to the correct diagnosis. The remaining group with treatment failure have their recurrence detected during routine surveillance. Although the Pap smear and chest radiograph may detect an asymptomatic recurrence, this clinical scenario is rare. Most recurrences are detected by physical examination. Serum CA-125 levels may be useful in monitoring patients for the development of recurrent disease, especially those who have papillary serous carcinomas or intraperitoneal disease.[42,167] Follow-up intervals of 6 to 12 months coupled with prompt evaluation of symptomatic patients seems to be an appropriate approach to surveillance. Routine use of diagnostic studies beyond cytology and the selective use of CA-125 is probably not cost effective.

The patterns of recurrence depend on initial disease distribution. Patients with advanced primary disease tend to have abdominal or systemic failure. Approximately one-third of recurrences seen in women whose primary tumors were confined to the uterus are limited to the pelvis; the remaining two-thirds have some component of distant failure.[3] It is important to identify those cases with isolated pelvic recurrence because some can be salvaged by radiotherapy or ultraradical surgery.[168,169] Conversely, treatment of systemic recurrence is largely palliative.

Systemic Agents

HORMONE THERAPY

Overview of Clinical Studies. Progestogens have been used in the management of recurrent endometrial cancer after the original report by Kelly and Baker in 1961[153] used the parenterally administered hydroxyprogesterone caproate.[153,170–172] Beneficial results from these trials were mostly confined to a subset of patients with well-differentiated tumor, metastases to the lung, and a long disease-free interval between diagnosis of the primary tumor and the development of metastases. Subsequent trials, using MPA or megestrol acetate, explored the use of high-dose progestogen therapy on better-selected patients through the study of hormone receptor content of tumors and limiting therapy to receptor-positive cases, paralleling breast cancer strategies.[172,173] Overall, fewer than 30% of patients (even with the best selection) show objective responses, and the survival of patients with metastatic disease is disappointingly short, except for a rare, extremely hormone-responsive patient. Earlier series reporting very long median survival rates reflect carefully selected patients or loose criteria of response.[153,170]

No dose-response effect for progestogens has been proven.[174] Although some responders have very long survival rates, the median duration of response in most studies does not exceed 10 months. The results of treatment with tamoxifen are generally inferior to those obtained with progestogens.[175] It remains to be seen whether tamoxifen in sequential combination with progestogens (to modulate receptors) will have an advantage over progestogen therapy alone.

Other hormonal manipulations are increasingly under study. These include not only combinations of tamoxifen and MPA, but also other selective estrogen receptor modulators such as raloxifene, luteinizing hormone–releasing hormone (LHRH) agonists and antagonists, aromatase inhibitors, and miscellaneous other drugs (Table 36.3-8).[176–180] It is likely that the same subset of patients responds to these hormonally directed therapies, and no obvious advantage of one agent over another has emerged to date. Moreover, results from small studies may be discordant, reflecting the importance of patient selection in maximizing the probability of response.

Biologic and Pharmacologic Considerations. The presence of estrogen and progesterone receptors in tumors has been shown to correlate with well-differentiated cancers and with response to progestogens.[181–184] Sequentially alternating tamoxifen and MPA or megestrol acetate regimens are based on the concept of up-regulation of progesterone receptors by the antiestrogen.[179] Other laboratory studies indicate the presence of specific binding sites for LHRH and for androgen receptors.[185] Supplementing clinical observations with molecular correlates of response may bring out some differences that are currently not apparent and also possibly lead to crossover hormonal therapies, a concept that has been useful in breast cancer treatment. The rational selection of specific hormonal manipulations from laboratory findings may become more feasible with the wider applicability of molecular immunohistochemical probes.

CYTOTOXIC CHEMOTHERAPY

Overview of Clinical Trials. Most women with recurrent or stage IV endometrial cancers, except for those with well-differentiated and receptor-positive metastases, must be assessed for treatment with cytotoxic chemotherapy. Doxorubicin and its analogue epirubicin have shown reproducible antitumor activity in phase II and III trials.[186,187] These phase III studies have indicated that the addition of cyclophosphamide to doxorubicin improves neither response nor survival rates and suggest that the incorporation of progestogens does not improve results[187–189]

TABLE 36.3-8. Selected Series of Hormonally Based Therapy in Women with Advanced Endometrial Cancer

Reference	*Drug (Class)*	*Patients*	*Response Rate (%)*	*End Points/Comments/Median Survival*
Reifenstein[170]	HPC (progestogen)	314	30	20 mo
Lentz et al.[173]	MA (progestogen)	54	24	Median PFS 2.5 mo, survival 7.6 mo
Thigpen et al.[174]	MPA 200 (progestogen)	145	25	Median PFS 3.2 mo, survival 11.1 mo
	MPA 1000 (progestogen)	144	15	Median PFS 2.5 mo, survival 7 mo
Thigpen et al.[175]	Tamoxifen (antiestrogen)	68	10	Median PFS 1.9 mo, survival 8.8 mo
Jeyarajah et al.[176]	Leuprolide (Gn RH analogue)	32	28	5 mo
Covens et al.[177]	Leuprolide (Gn RH analogue)	25	0	6 mo
Rose et al.[178]	Anastrazole	23	9	6 mo
Blessing[179]	Danazol	—	—	Ongoing GOG study
Blessing[179]	Tamoxifen + MPA	60	—	Final analysis pending
Mandeli[180]	Letrozole (aromatase inhibitor)	—	—	Ongoing study of New York GOG

Gn RH, gonadotropin-releasing hormone; GOG, Gynecologic Oncology Group; HPC, hydroxyprogesterone caproate; MA, megestrol acetate; MPA, medroxyprogesterone acetate; PFS, progression-free survival.

(Table 36.3-9). A number of other drugs studied by the GOG and others also have shown little efficacy but often have been used in combinations. On the other hand, cisplatin and carboplatin both show consistent antitumor activity,[187,191–197] and a phase III study combining cisplatin with doxorubicin showed superior progression-free survival over doxorubicin alone.[190] However, the overall median survival rate for patients receiving doxorubicin plus cisplatin was not improved. Other agents with single-agent activity include paclitaxel,[198,199] ifosfamide,[200] and oral etoposide.[201,202] Paclitaxel (250 mg/m^2) given on a 24-hour infusion schedule and requiring cytokine support with filgrastim showed remarkable activity,[198] with four complete responses and six partial responses among 28 patients. A 24-hour infusion of 150 mg/m^2 is being tested in phase III studies in combination with doxorubicin. Shorter infusions of paclitaxel have activity with less myelosuppression[199] and are often used in combination with carboplatin[203] or in three-drug combinations.[204] Regimens of platinums and taxanes also have activity against papillary serous cancers[205] and are, therefore, replacing doxorubicin-containing regimens in this condition.[167] On the other hand, the addition of intraperitoneal cisplatin to doxorubicin plus cyclophosphamide did not have an encouraging outcome.[206] In ongoing pilot studies with radiation, platinums and particularly cisplatin are favored.[207]

Carboplatin is the preferred drug when added to paclitaxel because of its lower incidence of severe neurotoxicity relative to cisplatin.

Biologic and Pharmacologic Considerations. Laboratory and clinical studies should better define the role of systemic chemotherapy in relation to various known biologic factors in an analogous way to how pathologic features and hormone receptors have assisted

TABLE 36.3-9. Cytotoxic Drug Trials Showing Activity in Women with Endometrial Carcinoma

Series	*Drug(s), Doses (mg/m^2)*	*n*	*CR + PR (%)*	*End Points*
Horton et al.[188]	DOX, 40	56	4 + 11 (27)	Median survival 27 wk
	CAF, 250/30/300	58		Median survival 27 wk
Cohen et al.,[189] GOG 28 (1984)	MEL + FU, 7/525 × 4 d	77	12 + 17 (38)	Not reported
	CAF, 250/30/300	78		Not reported
Thigpen et al.,[187] GOG 48 (1994)	DOX, 60	132	7 + 22 (22)	PFS 3.2 mo, survival 6.9 mo
	AC, 60/500	144	18 + 25 (30)	PFS 3.9 mo, survival 7.3 mo
Thigpen et al.,[190] GOG 107 (1993)	DOX, 60	137	12 + 25 (27)	PFS 3.4 mo
	AP, 60/60	155	24 + 29 (46)	PFS 5.4 mo
GOG 139	AP, 60/60	175	—	Final analysis pending
	AP Circadian, 60/60	177	—	
GOG 163	AP, 60/50	160	—	Final analysis pending
	AT, 50/150	168	—	
GOG 177	AP, 60/50	—	—	Still accruing
	TAP, 160/45/50	—	—	

AC, doxorubicin + cyclophosphamide; AP, doxorubicin + cisplatin; AT, doxorubicin + paclitaxel; CAF, cyclophosphamide + doxorubicin + 5-fluorouracil; CR, complete response; DOX, doxorubicin; FU, 5-fluorouracil; GOG, Gynecologic Oncology Group; MEL, melphalan; PFS, progression-free survival; PR, partial response; TAP, paclitaxel (Taxol) + doxorubicin + cisplatin.

in refining hormonal therapies. Endometrial cancers commonly express P-glycoprotein (Pgp). Studying the mechanisms of drug resistance mediated by multidrug resistance gene 1(MDR1)-mediated Pgp may assist in identifying doxorubicin- and paclitaxel-resistant tumors.[208] Moreover, mutations in p53 occur somewhat concordantly with the expression of Pgp and may help to define a more resistant subpopulation. A relationship between progesterone and the expression of Pgp also has been postulated[209]; prior progestogen therapy might lead to changes in Pgp expression. The epidermal growth factor receptor and HER-2/neu are also likely to be important in determining chemosensitivity and outcome, as well as therapeutic targets.[210,211] Studies are beginning to focus on special subtypes, such as papillary serous and clear cell carcinomas, that not only have a propensity to metastasize early but may also have altered drug sensitivities. Several investigators have known that p53 mutations are more frequent in these cell types and are indicative of poor prognosis. Microsatellite instability, persistence of bcl-2191, and high proliferation indices may also be of prognostic significance.

Radiotherapy

Vaginal recurrences of endometrial carcinomas can often be successfully treated with radiation therapy if there is no evidence of extrapelvic disease. For patients whose initial treatment was hysterectomy alone, vaginal recurrence is usually treated with a combination of external-beam irradiation and intracavitary or interstitial brachytherapy, depending on the extent and distribution of disease. Technical considerations are similar to those for primary vaginal carcinoma.

With this treatment, reported 5-year survival rates for patients who have isolated recurrences in the vaginal apex are usually 40% to 60%.[212–218] Outcome is correlated with the recurrent tumor's grade, size, and extent and the time to recurrence.[212,214–216] Sears et al.[216] reported 5-year survival rates of 74% and 30% for patients with tumors measuring 2 cm or less, or more than 2 cm, respectively, which suggests that early detection and treatment may be important. These authors also reported significantly better survival rates for patients who had a portion of their treatment given with brachytherapy. Distal vaginal recurrences are less common but may also be cured with irradiation if there is no other evidence of recurrent cancer.[212,213,216,219,220] If possible, the inguinal nodes should be treated when the distal vagina is involved.

The prognosis is much poorer for patients who have recurrent tumor on the pelvic wall.[213,214,216] However, there are anecdotal reports of prolonged disease-free survival after locoregional treatment.[213,216] Recurrence isolated to inguinal nodes should be treated aggressively because cures have been reported after treatment with irradiation.[221]

Surgery

Surgery plays a limited role in the management of recurrent endometrial cancer. Although cytoreduction is probably valuable for women with advanced primary cancers, secondary cytoreduction after failure of primary therapy has no real role because of the lack of effective regional or systemic therapy. Two legitimate indications for surgical management are attempted curative resection of central pelvic recurrence by exenteration and palliative treatment in selected clinical situations.

Historically, ultraradical resection of recurrent endometrial cancer has not been recommended because of the perception that systemic spread was too common. However, reviews that have examined carefully evaluated patients have identified a subset of women whose recurrence is limited to the pelvis.[222] Cure rates of 40% to 50% have been obtained after resection by pelvic exenteration. These values are comparable to those reported for the treatment of central recurrence in patients with cervix cancer.[223,224] Consequently, patients who have recurrent disease that is clinically limited to the central pelvis and have not been successful with radiotherapy should be considered candidates for curative resection. A diligent search for subclinical metastatic disease should be carried out before exploration and at the time of operation.

Palliative surgery is largely limited to patients with intraabdominal recurrences causing bowel obstruction or pain. Candidates for palliative operations must have realistic expectations as to the goals of surgery, and the planned procedure should have a reasonable chance of achieving the desired goal. The patient's life expectancy and clinical status should be adequate for the proposed procedure and the anticipated recovery. The operation performed should be the minimum procedure with the lowest risk capable of correcting the problem. Heroic operations attempted in patients with no chance for long-term survival are pointless.

OUTCOME AND SURVIVAL

Long-term survival of patients with endometrial cancer is clearly related to their surgical stage and substage. Representative 5-year survival rates by stage are 90% for stage I, 60% for stage II, 40% for stage III, and 5% for stage IV. Because the vast majority of patients have stage I disease and because there is a wide variation in survival based on risk profile within this stage, most research into postoperative adjuvant therapy is aimed at subsets of stage I patients. It is anticipated that the routine use of surgical staging will result in a more homogeneous subgrouping of similar risk patients and allow a more reliable prediction of survival potential. Selected patients with advanced disease that can be encompassed by surgical resection with or without adjunctive irradiation can be cured. However, few patients meet such criteria. Although patients with disseminated disease frequently respond to cytotoxic therapy, such responses tend to be short and provide a limited improvement in progression-free survival. As was suggested earlier, posttreatment surveillance for recurrence should be used to identify candidates for clinical trials of new agents or therapeutic approaches.

UTERINE SARCOMAS

TUMOR TYPES

Tumors with a malignant mesenchymal component account for approximately 10% of uterine fundal neoplasms. Pure uterine sarcomas of the homologous type arise from native elements, as is seen in endometrial stromal sarcoma, leiomyosarcoma, and sarcomas of nonspecific supporting tissues (fibrous tissue, vessels, lymphatics). Heterologous sarcomas may contain elements with nonnative differentiation, such as skeletal muscle, bone, and cartilage.[225] The malignant mixed Müllerian tumor (MMT) is a mixture of carcinoma and sarcoma. Although any combination is possible, serous carcinoma admixed with endometrial stromal sarcoma is the most common histologic type. The adenosarcoma is a rare mixed tumor in which a benign epithelial component is mixed with a sarcomatous element.

CLINICAL PRESENTATION

Uterine sarcomas exhibit the typical gross features of similar tumors at other sites—firm, fleshy growth with areas of hemorrhage and necrosis. The initial growth phase of most sarcomas is within the fundal portion of the uterus. If the tumor involves the endometrial cavity, postmenopausal or abnormal vaginal bleeding is common. Tumors that have a polypoid growth configuration may prolapse through the cervix to present as an upper vaginal mass. This presentation is most often seen with MMTs.

Extensive local growth is another common clinical presentation. Once the tumor has penetrated the uterine serosa, it can rapidly attach to adjacent pelvic structures or loops of bowel positioned in the pelvis (Fig. 36.3-6). This locally advanced pelvic tumor presentation is typical of leiomyosarcoma. Patients with locally advanced cancers have symptoms related to an expanding pelvic mass (fullness, pressure, pain, urinary frequency) or to entrapment and destruction of adjacent organs (hematuria, tenesmus, rectal bleeding, bowel obstruction, fistula).

As is seen for epithelial tumors of the uterus, distant spread from uterine sarcomas may occur by a variety of mechanisms. Intraabdominal and retroperitoneal nodal metastases are frequently associated with the MMT.[226] This is not surprising because the epithelial component is usually papillary serous carcinoma and predominates within metastatic sites. Consequently, patients with advanced MMT follow a clinical pattern similar to that of women with epithelial ovarian cancer. All uterine sarcomas have a propensity for hematogenous dissemination. Pulmonary metastases are most frequently observed. Other sites include liver, bone, and brain. Women with distant spread at the time of diagnosis have symptoms and examination findings based on the location of their disease.

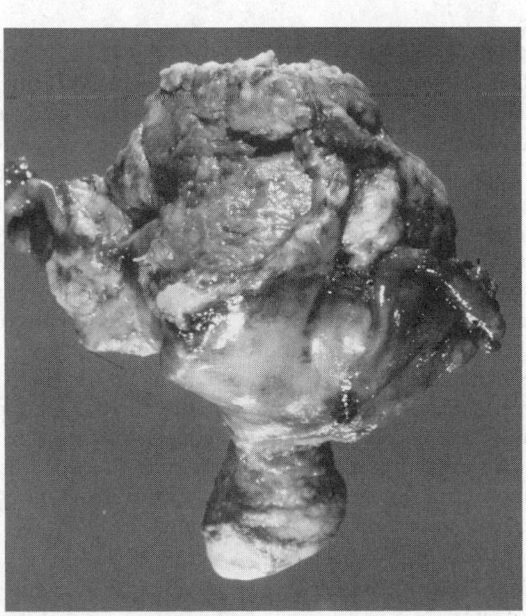

FIGURE 36.3-6. Uterine sarcomas tend to present as large, fleshy central pelvic tumors. This leiomyosarcoma has replaced most of the uterine fundus and penetrated the serosa to engulf the adnexa and directly contact intraperitoneal structures.

EVALUATION

Uterine sarcoma should be suspected in any postmenopausal women with an enlarging central pelvic mass. If the tumor projects into the uterine cavity or has partially prolapsed through the cervix, an endometrial or direct biopsy should provide a tissue diagnosis. Evaluation by an experienced pathologist is critical because uterine sarcomas are rare and the biopsy material is often fragmented or necrotic. Tumors originating within the uterine wall require exploratory laparotomy and hysterectomy to establish a diagnosis. Because primary therapy usually includes hysterectomy, the preoperative evaluation should focus on a search for disease at common metastatic sites and assessment of operative risk.

When the diagnosis of sarcoma is known or suspected, the pretreatment evaluation should include a careful history and physical examination, chest radiograph, and laboratory studies. The CA-125 level may be elevated in some cases, particularly in MMT tumors with peritoneal spread. Other markers have not been consistently useful. Computed tomography of the abdomen and pelvis may be helpful in identifying occult extrauterine disease. Cystoscopy, proctosigmoidoscopy, and barium enema should be performed in patients with advanced pelvic disease. Brain, bone, or liver imaging should be considered in patients with abnormal physical or laboratory findings.

TREATMENT

Surgery

Patients in whom the diagnosis of uterine sarcoma is not anticipated often undergo hysterectomy for a presumed diagnosis of uterine leiomyoma or "central" pelvic mass. Although most of these cases are not surgically staged, many are apparently stage I tumors. When the diagnosis of sarcoma is established and hysterectomy is technically feasible, surgical resection of the primary tumor should be attempted. Such surgery may be curative for tumors confined to the uterus. Because of the overall poor prognosis associated with uterine sarcomas, we proceed with extended surgical staging similar to that used for patients with endometrial adenocarcinoma when disease is clinically limited to the uterus. Although a survival benefit to surgical staging has not been demonstrated, knowledge of the true extent of disease is helpful in selecting therapy options.

In more extensive disease cases, resection or debulking of the central tumor can provide important palliation of bleeding and pain. Tumor reduction may enhance the ability of postoperative adjunctive therapy to extend survival, but this concept is not as well established as in epithelial ovarian tumors. The aggressiveness of the surgical approach must include a balance between the desire to remove as much tumor as possible and the risks of additional operative procedures. Patients with widespread or bulky unresectable disease should not be subjected to high-risk operations under the guise of cytoreduction.

Occasionally, surgical intervention is indicated in women with advanced or recurrent disease, but such situations are clinically uncommon. Some women have obtained long-term survival and apparent cure after resection of an isolated pulmonary metastasis.[167,227,228] Exploration to palliate bowel obstruction or

TABLE 36.3-10. Selected Cytotoxic Drug Trials in Uterine Leiomyosarcomas

Reference	*Drug(s) (mg/m²)*	*Evaluable Patients*	*CR + PR (%)*	*End Points/Comments*
Omura et al.[246]	DOX, 60	28	0 + 7 (25)	Not reported by subset
	DOX + DTIC, 250 × 5 d	20	6 (30)	Not reported by subset
Muss et al.[247]	DOX, 60	38	3 (8)	Not separated by arm, cell type
	DOX + CTX, 60 + 500			
Sutton et al.[248]	IFX, 1.5 × 5 d	35	0 + 6 (17)	Response duration 3.8 mo, survival 6 mo
Sutton et al.[200]	DOX + IFX, 50 + 5 g	33	1 + 9 (30)	Response duration 4.1 mo, survival 9.6 mo
Thigpen et al.[252]	CDDP,[a] 50	33	0 + 1 (3)	Response duration 3.4 mo, survival 7.8 mo
Thigpen et al.[251]	CDDP,[b] 50	19	0 + 1 (5)	
Slayton et al.[253]	VP-16, 100 × 3 d (1,3,5)	28	1 + 2 (11)	
Thigpen et al.[254]	VP-16, 100 × 3 d (1–3)	28	0	PFS 2.1 mo, survival 9.2+ mo
Rose et al.[274]	VP-16, 150 oral × 21 d	29	0 + 2 (6.9)	AML, 1 patient
Currie et al.[256]	HED, 2g, 100 × 3 d, 700	38	2 + 5 (18)	Response duration 12 mo, survival 15 mo
Sutton et al.[255]	Taxol, 175	33	3 + 0 (10)	
Miller et al.[275]	Topotecan, 1.5 × 5 d	36	1 + 3 (11)	Response duration 3.3 mo
Blessing[179]	Taxol,[b] 175	—	—	Ongoing GOG study
Blessing[179]	Gemcitabine,[b] 1000	—	—	Ongoing GOG study

AM, acute myelogenous leukemia; CDDP, cisplatin; CR, complete response; CTX, cyclophosphamide; DOX, doxorubicin (Adriamycin); DTIC, dimethyl triazenoimidazole carboxamide; GOG, Gynecologic Oncology Group; HED, hydroxyurea + etoposide + dacarbazine; IFX, ifosfamide; PFS, progression-free survival; PR, partial response; VP-16, etoposide.
[a]Subset of uterine sarcoma series.
[b]Previously treated.

fistula is appropriate in selected refractory disease patients who have a good performance status and reasonable projected survival time. Potentially morbid palliative operations in women with terminal disease should be avoided whenever possible.

Radiotherapy

MIXED MÜLLERIAN TUMOR. The role of radiation therapy in the management of carcinosarcoma is controversial. Patients are frequently treated with postoperative pelvic radiotherapy, but irradiation has never been proven to influence survival. Retrospective comparisons of treatments are invariably biased by physicians' tendencies to select treatment on the basis of known prognostic indicators. No randomized study has directly compared patients with similar prognostic features who were treated with or without radiotherapy.

Most retrospective reviews of patients with carcinosarcoma have demonstrated a lower rate of pelvic tumor recurrence in patients who received postoperative pelvic irradiation.[229–239] In most cases, this has not resulted in a demonstrable improvement in the survival rate. However, few studies have evaluated risk factors that could have influenced treatment selection. Potential bias and the small number of patients in most studies have made it impossible to determine the efficacy of treatment.

The GOG retrospectively evaluated its experience in two studies.[233,240] Hornback et al.[233] reviewed the influence of pelvic radiotherapy in a study originally designed to evaluate the role of doxorubicin. In this study, radiotherapy was given at the discretion of the investigator. In 109 patients with stage I or II disease (95 of whom had carcinosarcoma), the pelvis was the first site of recurrence in five of 49 patients (10%) who had radiation therapy versus 14 of 60 patients (23%) treated with surgery alone. However, irradiated patients had a higher rate of distant metastasis, and no significant difference in the 2-year survival rate was reported. In a more recent review of another GOG study, the pelvis was reported to be the first site of recurrence in 17% and 24% of patients with carcinosarcoma treated with or without postoperative irradiation, respectively. The overall relapse rates were not significantly different. As with other reviews, because the tumor stage, grade, and depth of invasion and rates of lymph node involvement were not compared for patients receiving different treatments, the efficacy of radiotherapy cannot be determined from these studies.

LEIOMYOSARCOMA AND ENDOMETRIAL STROMAL SARCOMA. Few studies have separately reported control rates for patients treated with radiotherapy for leiomyosarcoma, and the numbers of patients are too small to evaluate efficacy.[233,236,240] Patients with close surgical margins may benefit from postoperative irradiation. Because lymph node metastasis from leiomyosarcoma is uncommon, treatment of the operative bed (usually the lower pelvis) may be sufficient in most cases.

Several authors reporting small series of patients with endometrial stromal tumors have commented on the role of radiotherapy, either suggesting that it is effective[241–243] or ineffective.[244] Berchuck et al.[242] reported dramatic responses in two of three patients who had measurable tumor. One patient remained free of disease for more than 10 years after treatment. However, reports of radiotherapy for these tumors are little more than anecdotal, and further study is needed to define the role of radiotherapy adequately.

Chemotherapy and Hormonal Therapy

Differences in the management of metastatic uterine leiomyosarcomas and MMTs with respect to systemic chemotherapy have been established, and separate trials are conducted for these two entities (Tables 36.3-10 and 36.3-11). Endometrial

TABLE 36.3-11. Selected Cytotoxic Drug Trials in Uterine Mixed Mesodermal Tumors

Reference	*Drug(s) (mg/m²)*	*n*	*CR + PR (%)*	*End Points/Comments*
Omura et al.[246]	DOX, 60	41	4 (10)	Not reported by subset
	DOX + DTIC, 250 × 5 d	31	—	Not reported by subset
Muss et al.[247]	DOX	51	3 + 2 (10)	Not separated by arm, cell type
	DOX + CTX, 60 + 500	—	—	—
Sutton et al.[257]	IFX	28	5 + 4 (31)	Not reported
Sutton et al.[258]	IFX, 1.5 × 5	102	37 (36)	PFS 4.0 mo, survival 7.6 mo
	CDDP + IFX, 20 × 5, 1.5 × 5	92	50 (54)	PFS 6.0 mo, survival 9.4 mo
Slayton et al.[a253]	VP-16, 100 (d 1, 3, 5)	31	0 + 2	Response duration 2 mo, survival 6 mo
Currie et al.[276]	HED, 2g, 100 × 3 d, 700	32	2 + 3 (16)	Response duration 6.3 mo
Thigpen et al.[a277]	CDDP, 50	63	5 + 7 (19)	Response duration 9.3 mo, survival 7.0 mo
Thigpen et al.[b254]	CDDP, 50	28	5 (18)	
Blessing[179]	Taxol, 175	—	—	Ongoing GOG study

CDDP, cisplatin; CR, complete response; CTX, cyclophosphamide; DOX, doxorubicin (Adriamycin); DTIC, dimethyl triazenoimidazole carboxamide; GOG, Gynecologic Oncology Group; HED, hydroxyurea + etoposide + dacarbazine; IFX, ifosfamide; PFS, progression-free survival; PR, partial response; VP-16, etoposide.
[a]Subset of uterine sarcoma series.
[b]Previously treated.

stromal sarcomas are less common and usually not included in clinical trials. Because antitumor activity of chemotherapy regimens has been documented in advanced stages, several trials are ongoing or planned in earlier stages of disease. Evidence to support the use of chemotherapy as an adjuvant to surgery is not yet forthcoming. One randomized study of the addition of doxorubicin after surgery in stage I and II uterine sarcomas yielded no advantage for the adjuvant chemotherapy group.[245]

In mixed mesodermal tumors of stage I, II, and III, a GOG trial begun in 1993 is comparing whole abdominal radiation to chemotherapy with cisplatin and ifosfamide.[179] These trials require several years to complete, a difficulty compounded by the evolving nature of the adjuvant treatments that are applied.

LEIOMYOSARCOMA. Doxorubicin was shown to be an effective drug against leiomyosarcomas arising in the uterus.[246] Drug combinations were claimed to improve results in both childhood and adult sarcomas of extrauterine origin, but the addition of dacarbazine to doxorubicin did not improve the survival of patients with metastatic uterine sarcomas beyond that obtained with doxorubicin alone.[246] Response rates were, however, significantly better in the doxorubicin plus dacarbazine arm. A subsequent randomized study also performed by the GOG failed to show that the addition of cyclophosphamide in modest doses was advantageous over doxorubicin by itself.[247] The alkylating agent ifosfamide has modest activity[248] but does not add substantially to the therapeutic efficacy of doxorubicin.[249,250] Other drugs, such as cisplatin,[251,252] etoposide,[253,254] and paclitaxel,[179,255] also have been evaluated and have modest to minimal activity. A combination of hydroxyurea, etoposide, and dacarbazine had antitumor activity without major toxicities.[256]

MIXED MÜLLERIAN TUMOR. Ifosfamide[257] and cisplatin[254] have greater antitumor activity against uterine MMT than does doxorubicin. Accordingly, the two drugs in combination have been explored in all stages and also compared with ifosfamide alone[258] in advanced, persistent, or recurrent disease. The results indicate an advantage for the combination in terms of responses and progression-free survival, but nearly equivalent median survival at a cost of increasing toxicity. The combination is being administered to completely resected stage I and II MMTs of the uterus (GOG 117), but the assessment will require a comparison to historical controls. Taxanes, such as paclitaxel, have been evaluated,[179] and this agent has already formed part of an active combination with the pegylated liposomal doxorubicin, Doxil.[259] Experience with a number of other platinum-based combinations has been reported in very small series. These should be regarded as leads for future trials rather than a reliable indicator of activity.[260]

ENDOMETRIAL STROMAL SARCOMA. The systemic treatment of endometrial stromal sarcoma is guided by reports from individual institutions[242,244,261,262] and case reports.[263,264] The tumor's relative rarity does not support the conduct of clinical trials. Because of the presence of hormonal receptors in low-grade (fewer than ten mitoses per high-power field) tumors, hormonal therapy has been advocated.[261,265] However, high-grade tumors are treated with chemotherapy.[263,265] Investigation of biologic and pharmacologic issues may point the way for hypothesis-driven drug trials.

BIOLOGIC AND PHARMACOLOGIC CONSIDERATIONS. The growth of benign leiomyomas is under both estrogenic and progestogenic control.[266,267] Accordingly, the study of receptors and hormone-action inhibitors for antitumor activity may be relevant to the management of malignant smooth muscle tumors.[268] Receptors also have been studied in endometrial stromal sarcomas[269,270] and justify exploration of inhibition or depletion of hormonal mediators in the management of these tumors. Overexpression in MDR2 and mutations in p53 have been noted in some uterine sarcomas, but not in leiomyomas.[271] For the development of cytotoxic therapy, the role of MDR1-mediated Pgp expression in determining resistance to doxorubicin has been investigated in a cell line from a leiomyosarcoma of the uterus and its doxorubicin-resistant derivative.[271] Drugs that are substrates for Pgp may restore sensitivity to doxorubicin in this resistant variant. Trials of such resistance-reversing agents, including the cyclosporin analogue PSC-833, may lead to a reassessment of the potential for drugs such as doxorubicin, taxanes, and vinca alkaloids in the treatment of these traditionally refractory tumors.[272]

OUTCOME AND SURVIVAL

Stage is the most significant predictor of outcome for women with uterine sarcomas. Patients whose tumors are confined to the uterus have a survival rate of 60% to 70% after surgical resection. Major sites of failure include the pelvis, upper abdomen, and lung. Few well-conducted prospective adjuvant therapy trials have been accomplished, so a precise role for either adjuvant irradiation or chemotherapy remains undefined. As has been noted for endometrial carcinoma, adjuvant pelvic irradiation may reduce the rate of pelvic failure without improving survival if more patients succumb to distant failure. Pelvic irradiation and local tumor control may be an important issue in tumors with extension to the cervix. However, so few patients are placed in this category that meaningful treatment data are not available.

Very few patients with tumor spread outside of the uterus can be curatively treated. Some women with small-volume regional disease have obtained long-term survival after external-beam irradiation. However, most patients with advanced or recurrent disease ultimately experience disease progression and die. These women are excellent candidates for new therapeutic trials.

REFERENCES

1. Landis SH, Murray T, Bolden S, et al. Cancer statistics, 1999. *CA Cancer J Clin* 1999;49:8.
2. Boronow RC. Endometrial cancer: not a benign disease. *Obstet Gynecol* 1976;47:630.
3. Burke TW, Heller PB, Woodward JE, et al. Treatment failure in endometrial carcinoma. *Obstet Gynecol* 1990;75:96.
4. Creasman WT. New gynecologic cancer staging. *Obstet Gynecol* 1990;75:287.
5. Ng ABP, Reagan JW, Storasli JP, et al. Mixed adenosquamous carcinoma of the endometrium. *Am J Clin Pathol* 1973;59:765.
6. Silverberg SG, De Giorgi LS. Clear cell carcinoma of the endometrium: clinical, pathologic, and ultrasonic findings. *Cancer* 1973;31:1127.
7. Kurman RJ, Scully RE. Clear cell carcinoma of the endometrium: an analysis of 21 cases. *Cancer* 1976;37:872.
8. Salazar OM, DePapp EW, Bonfiglio TA, et al. Adenosquamous carcinoma of the endometrium: an entity with an inherent poor prognosis? *Cancer* 1977;40:119.
9. Alberhasky RC, Connelly PJ, Christopherson WM. Carcinoma of the endometrium. IV. Mixed adenosquamous carcinoma: a clinical-pathological study of 68 cases with long-term follow-up. *Am J Clin Pathol* 1982;77:655.
10. Christopherson WM, Alberhasky RC, Connelly PJ. Carcinoma of the endometrium. I. A clinicopathologic study of clear-cell carcinoma and secretory carcinoma. *Cancer* 1982;49:1511.
11. Hendrickson M, Ross J, Eifel P, et al. Uterine papillary serous carcinoma: a highly malignant form of endometrial adenocarcinoma. *Am J Surg Pathol* 1982;6:93.
12. Jeffrey JF, Krepart GV, Lotocki RJ. Papillary serous adenocarcinoma of the endometrium. *Obstet Gynecol* 1986;67:670.
13. Chambers JT, Merino M, Kohorn EI, et al. Uterine serous papillary carcinoma. *Obstet Gynecol* 1987;69:109.
14. Sutton GP, Brill L, Michael H, et al. Malignant papillary lesions of the endometrium. *Gynecol Oncol* 1987;27:294.
15. Ehrlich CA, Young PCM, Cleary RE. Cytoplasmic progesterone and estradiol receptors in normal, hyperplastic, and carcinomatous endometrial: therapeutic implications. *Am J Obstet Gynecol* 1981;141:539.
16. Kurman RJ, Kaminski PF, Norris HJ. The behavior of endometrial hyperplasia: a long-term study of "untreated" hyperplasia in 170 patients. *Cancer* 1985;56:403.
17. Wynder EL, Escher GC, Mantel N. An epidemiological investigation of cancer of the endometrium. *Cancer* 1966;19:489.
18. MacMahon B. Risk factors for endometrial cancer. *Gynecol Oncol* 1974;2:122.
19. Smith DC, Prentice R, Thompson DJ, et al. Association of exogenous estrogen and endometrial carcinoma. *N Engl J Med* 1975;293:1164.
20. Ziel HK, Finkle WD. Increased risk of endometrial carcinoma among users of conjugated estrogens. *N Engl J Med* 1975;297:1167.
21. Gray LA, Christopherson WM, Hoover RN. Estrogens and endometrial cancer. *Obstet Gynecol* 1977;49:385.
22. Antunes CMF, Stolley PD, Rosenshein NB. Endometrial cancer and estrogen use: report of a large case-control study. *N Engl J Med* 1979;300:9.
23. Davies JL, Rosenshein NB, Antunes CMF. A review of the risk factors for endometrial carcinoma. *Obstet Gynecol Surv* 1981;36:107.
24. Ernster VL, Bush TL, Huggins GR, et al. Benefits and risks of menopausal estrogen and/or progestin hormone use. *Prev Med* 1988;17:201.
25. Parazzina F, La Vecchia C, Bocciolone L, et al. Review: the epidemiology of endometrial cancer. *Gynecol Oncol* 1991;41:1.
26. McPherson CP, Sellers TA, Potter JD, et al. Reproductive factors and endometrial cancer. The Iowa Women's Health Study. *Am J Epidemiol* 1996;143:1195.
27. Fisher B, Constantino JP, Redmond CK, et al. Endometrial cancer in tamoxifen-treated breast cancer patients: findings from the National Surgical Adjuvant Breast and Bowel Project (NSABP) B-14. *J Natl Cancer Inst* 1994;86:527.
28. Killackey MA, Hakes TB, Pierce VK. Endometrial adenocarcinoma in breast cancer patients receiving antiestrogens. *Cancer Treat Rep* 1985;69:237.
29. Malfetano JH. Tamoxifen-associated endometrial carcinoma in postmenopausal breast cancer patients. *Gynecol Oncol* 1990;39:82.
30. DeMuylder X, Neven P, DeSomer M. Endometrial lesions in patients undergoing tamoxifen therapy. *Int J Gynecol Obstet* 1991;36:127.
31. Gal D, Kopel S, Bashevkim M, et al. Oncogenic potential of tamoxifen on endometrial of postmenopausal women with breast cancer: a preliminary report. *Gynecol Oncol* 1992;42:120.
32. Barakat RR, Wong G, Curtin JP, et al. Tamoxifen use in breast cancer patients who subsequently develop corpus cancer is not associated with a higher incidence of adverse histologic features. *Gynecol Oncol* 1994;95:164.
33. Silva EG, Tornos CS, Mitchell MF. Malignant neoplasms of the uterine corpus in patients treated for breast carcinoma: the effects of tamoxifen. *Int J Gynecol Pathol* 1994;13:248.
34. Mitchell MF, Reddoch J, Atkinson EN, et al. Patients with both breast and endometrial hyperplasia or cancer. *Gynecol Oncol* 1993;49:143(abst).
35. Burke TW, Levenback C, Tornos C, et al. Intraabdominal lymphatic mapping to direct selective pelvic and paraaortic lymphadenectomy in women with high-risk endometrial cancer: results of a pilot study. *Gynecol Oncol* 1996;62:169.
36. Greenwood SM, Wright DJ. Evaluation of the office endometrial biopsy in the detection of endometrial carcinoma and atypical hyperplasia. *Cancer* 1979;43:1474.
37. Koss LG, Schreiber K, Moussouris H, et al. Endometrial carcinoma and its precursors: detection and screening. *Clin Obstet Gynecol* 1982;25:44.
38. Grimes DA. Diagnostic office curettage–heresy no longer. *Contemp Obstet Gynecol* 1986;28:96.
39. Eddy GL, Strumpf KB, Wojtowycz MA, et al. Biopsy findings in five hundred thirty-one patients with atypical glandular cells of uncertain significance as defined by the Bethesda system. *Am J Obstet Gynecol* 1997;177:1188.
40. Eddy GL, Wojtowycz MA, Piraino PS, Mazur MT. Papanicolaou smears by the Bethesda system in endometrial malignancy: utility and prognostic importance. *Obstet Gynecol* 1997;90:999.
41. Patsner B, Mann WJ, Cohen H, et al. Predictive value of preoperative serum CA 125 levels in clinically localized and advanced endometrial carcinoma. *Am J Obstet Gynecol* 1988;158:399.
42. Rose PG, Sommers RM, Reale FR, et al. Serial CA-125 measurements for evaluation of recurrence in patients with endometrial carcinoma. *Obstet Gynecol* 1994;84:12.
43. Sood AK, Buller RE, Burger RA, et al. Value of preoperative CA 125 level in the management of uterine cancer and prediction of clinical outcome. *Obstet Gynecol* 1997;90:441.
44. Connelly PJ, Alberhasky RC, Christopherson WM. Carcinoma of the endometrium. III. Analysis of 865 cases of adenocarcinoma and adenoacanthoma. *Obstet Gynecol* 1982;59:569.
45. Hendrickson M, Ross J, Eifel P, et al. Adenocarcinoma of the endometrium: analysis of 265 cases with carcinoma limited to the uterine corpus. *Gynecol Oncol* 1982;13:373.
46. Christopherson WM, Connelly PJ, Alberhasky RC. Carcinoma of the endometrium. V. An analysis of prognosticators in patients with favorable subtypes and stage I disease. *Cancer* 1983;51:1705.
47. Boronow RC, Morrow CP, Creasman WT, et al. Surgical staging in endometrial cancer: clinical-pathologic findings of a prospective study. *Obstet Gynecol* 1984;63:823.
48. DiSaia PJ, Creasman WT, Boronow RC, et al. Risk factors and recurrence patterns in stage I endometrial cancer. *Am J Obstet Gynecol* 1985;151:1009.
49. Morrow C, Bundy B, Kurman R, et al. Relationship between surgical-pathological risk factors and outcome in clinical stage I and II carcinoma of the endometrium: a Gynecologic Oncology Group study. *Gynecol Oncol* 1991;40:55.
50. Schink JC, Lurain JR, Wallemark CB, et al. Tumor size in endometrial cancer: a prognostic factor for lymph node metastasis. *Obstet Gynecol* 1987;70:216.
51. Hanson MB, van Nagell JR Jr, Powell DE, et al. The prognostic significance of lymph-vascular space invasion in stage I endometrial cancer. *Cancer* 1985;55:1753.
52. Wilkinson N, Buckley CH, Chawner L, et al. Nucleolar organizer regions in normal, hyperplastic, and neoplastic endometrial. *Int J Gynecol Pathol* 1990;9:55.
53. Enomoto T, Inoue M, Perantoni AO, et al. K-ras activation in premalignant and malignant epithelial lesions of the human uterus. *Cancer Res* 1991;51:5308.
54. Hetzel DJ, Wilson TO, Kenney GL, et al. HER-2/neu expression: a major prognostic factor in endometrial cancer. *Gynecol Oncol* 1992;47:179.
55. Lukes AS, Kohler MF, Pieper CF, et al. Multivariable analysis of DNA ploidy, p53, and HER-2/neu as prognostic factors in endometrial cancer. *Cancer* 1994;73:2380.
56. Miller B, Morris M, Silva E. Nucleolar organizer regions: a potential prognostic factor in adenocarcinoma of the endometrium. *Gynecol Oncol* 1994;54:137.
57. Trere D, Melchiorri C, Chieco P, et al. Interphase AgNOR quantity and DNA content in endometrial adenocarcinoma. *Gynecol Oncol* 1994;53:202.

58. Pisani AL, Barbuto DA, Chen D, et al. HER-2/neu, p53, and DNA analyses as prognosticators for survival in endometrial carcinoma. *Obstet Gynecol* 1995;85:729.
59. Heffner HM, Freedman AN, Asirwatham JE, Lele SB. Prognostic significance of p53, PCNA, and c-erbB-2 in endometrial adenocarcinoma. *Eur J Gynaecol Oncol* 1999;20:8.
60. Lim P, Aquino-Parsons CF, Wong F, et al. Low-risk endometrial carcinoma: assessment of a treatment policy based on tumor ploidy and identification of additional prognostic indicators. *Gynecol Oncol* 1999;73:191.
61. Lynch HT, Krush AJ, Larsen AL, et al. Endometrial carcinoma: multiple primary malignancies, constitutional factors and heredity. *Am J Med Sci* 1966;252:381.
62. Lynch HT, Krush AJ, Thomas RJ, et al. Cancer family syndrome. In: Lynch EHT. *Cancer genetics.* Springfield, IL: Charles C. Thomas Publisher, 1976:355.
63. Cowles TA, Magrina JF, Masterson BJ, et al. Comparison of clinical and surgical staging in patients with endometrial carcinoma. *Obstet Gynecol* 1985;66:413.
64. Creasman WT, DeGeest K, DiSaia PJ, et al. Significance of true surgical pathologic staging: a Gynecologic Oncology Group study. *Am J Obstet Gynecol* 1999;181:31.
65. Society of Gynecologic Oncologists. Practice guidelines: uterine corpus-endometrial cancer. *Oncology* 1998;12:122.
66. Park RC, Patow WE, Petty WM, Zimmerman EA. Treatment of adenocarcinoma of the endometrium. *Gynecol Oncol* 1974; 2:60.
67. Rutledge F. The role of radical hysterectomy in adenocarcinoma of the endometrium. *Gynecol Oncol* 1974;2:331.
68. Hernandez W, Nolan JF, Morrow CP, et al. Stage II endometrial carcinoma: two modalities of treatment. *Am J Obstet Gynecol* 1978;131:171.
69. Kinsella TJ, Bloomer WD, Lavin PT, et al. Stage II endometrial carcinoma: 10-year follow-up of combined radiation and surgical treatment. *Gynecol Oncol* 1980;10:290.
70. Onsrud M, Aalders J, Abeler V, et al. Endometrial carcinoma with cervical involvement (stage II): prognostic factors and value of combined radiological-surgical treatment. *Gynecol Oncol* 1982;13:76.
71. Eltabbakh GH, Moore AD. Survival of women with surgical stage II endometrial cancer. *Gynecol Oncol* 1999;74:80.
72. Feltmate CM, Duska LR, Chang YC, et al. Predictors of recurrence in surgical stage II endometrial adenocarcinoma. *Gynecol Oncol* 1999;73:407.
73. Childers JN, Brzechffa PR, Hatch KD, et al. Laparoscopic assisted surgical staging (LASS) of endometrial carcinoma. *Gynecol Oncol* 1993;51:33.
74. Chi DS, Welshinger M, Venkatraman ES, Barakat RR. The role of surgical cytoreduction in stage IV endometrial carcinoma. *Gynecol Oncol* 1997;67:56.
75. Moore DH, Fowler WC Jr, Walton LA, et al. Morbidity of lymph node sampling in cancers of the uterine corpus and cervix. *Obstet Gynecol* 1989;74:180.
76. Clarke-Pearson D, Cliby W, Soper J, et al. Morbidity and mortality of selective lymphadenectomy in early stage endometrial cancer. *Gynecol Oncol* 1991;40:168(abst).
77. Orr JW, Holloway RW, Orr P, et al. Surgical staging of uterine cancer: an analysis of perioperative morbidity. *Gynecol Oncol* 1991;42:209.
78. Weiser EB, Bundy BN, Hoskins WJ, et al. Extraperitoneal versus transperitoneal selective paraaortic lymphadenectomy in the pretreatment surgical staging of advanced cervical carcinoma (a Gynecologic Oncology Group study). *Gynecol Oncol* 1989;33:283.
79. Doering DL, Barnhill DR, Weiser EB, et al. Intraoperative evaluation of depth of myometrial invasion in stage I endometrial adenocarcinoma. *Obstet Gynecol* 1989;74:930.
80. Marino BD, Burke TW, Tornos C, et al. Staging laparotomy for endometrial carcinoma: assessment of peritoneal spread. *Gynecol Oncol* 1995;56:34.
81. Larson DM, Johnson K, Olson KA. Pelvic and para-aortic lymphadenectomy for surgical staging of endometrial cancer: morbidity and mortality. *Obstet Gynecol* 1992;79:998.
82. Girardi F, Petru E, Heydarfadai M, et al. Pelvic lymphadenectomy in surgical treatment of endometrial cancer. *Gynecol Oncol* 1993;49:177.
83. Kim YB, Niloff JM. Endometrial carcinoma: analysis of recurrence in patients treated with a strategy minimizing lymph node sampling and radiation therapy. *Obstet Gynecol* 1993;82:175.
84. Chuang L, Burke TW, Tornos C, et al. Staging laparotomy for endometrial carcinoma: assessment of retroperitoneal lymph nodes. *Gynecol Oncol* 1995;58:189.
85. Kilgore L, Partridge E, Alvarez R, et al. Adenocarcinoma of the endometrium: survival comparisons of patients with and without pelvic node biopsies. *Gynecol Oncol* 1995;56:29.
86. Heyman J. The so-called Stockholm method and the results of treatment of uterine cancer at the Radiumhemmet. *Acta Radiol* 1935;22:129.
87. Jones HW. Treatment of adenocarcinoma of the endometrium. *Obstet Gynecol Surv* 1975;30:147.
88. Javert C, Douglas R. Treatment of endometrial adenocarcinoma. *AJR Am J Roentgenol* 1956;75:580.
89. Keller D, Kempson FL, Levine G, et al. Management of the patient with early endometrial carcinoma. *Cancer* 1974;33:1108.
90. Partridge EE, Shingleton HM, Menck HR. The National Cancer Data Base report on endometrial cancer. *J Surg Oncol* 1996;61:111.
91. Maggino T, Romagnolo C, Landoni F, et al. An analysis of approaches to the management of endometrial cancer in North America: a CTF study. *Gynecol Oncol* 1998;68:274.
92. Bedwinek J, Galakatos A, Camel M, et al. Stage I, grade III adenocarcinoma of the endometrium treated with surgery and irradiation. Sites of failure and correlation of failure rate with irradiation technique. *Cancer* 1984;54:40.
93. Ohlsen JD, Johnson GH, Stewart JR, et al. Combined therapy for endometrial carcinoma: preoperative intracavitary irradiation followed promptly by hysterectomy. *Cancer* 1977;39:659.
94. Underwood PB, Lutz MH, Kreutner A, et al. Carcinoma of the endometrium: radiation followed immediately by operation. *Am J Obstet Gynecol* 1977;128:86.
95. Rutledge FN, Tan SK, Fletcher GH. Vaginal metastases from adenocarcinoma of the corpus uteri. *Am J Obstet Gynecol* 1958;75:167.
96. Lewis GC, Mortel R, Slack NH. Adenocarcinoma of the body of the uterus. *J Obstet Gynecol Br Comm* 1977;77:342.
97. Eifel PJ, Ross J, Hendrickson M, et al. Adenocarcinoma of the endometrium. Analysis of 256 cases with disease limited to the uterine corpus: treatment options. *Cancer* 1983;52:1026.
98. Bean HA, Bryant AJS, Carmichael JA, et al. Carcinoma of the endometrium in Saskatchewan: 1966 to 1971. *Gynecol Oncol* 1978;6:503.
99. Piver MS, Yazigi R, Blumenson L, et al. A prospective trial comparing hysterectomy, hysterectomy plus vaginal radium, and uterine radium plus hysterectomy in stage I endometrial carcinoma. *Obstet Gynecol* 1979;54:85.
100. Reddy S, Lee MS, Hendrickson FR. Pattern of recurrences in endometrial carcinoma and their management. *Radiology* 1979;133:737.
101. Calais G, Vitu L, Descamps P, et al. Preoperative or postoperative brachytherapy for patients with endometrial carcinoma stage I and II. *Int J Radiat Oncol Biol Phys* 1990;19:523.
102. Sause WT, Fuller DB, Smith WG, et al. Analysis of preoperative intracavitary cesium application vs postoperative external beam radiation in stage I endometrial carcinoma. *Int J Radiat Oncol Biol Phys* 1990;18:1013.
103. Grigsby PW, Perez CA, Kuten A, et al. Clinical stage I endometrial cancer: results of adjuvant irradiation and patterns of failure. *Int J Radiat Oncol Biol Phys* 1991;21:379.
104. Aalders J, Abeler V, Kolstad P, et al. Postoperative external irradiation and prognostic parameters in stage I endometrial carcinoma. *Obstet Gynecol* 1980;56:419.
105. Marchetti DL, Piver MS, Tsukada Y, et al. Prevention of vaginal recurrence of stage I endometrial adenocarcinoma with postoperative vaginal radiation. *Obstet Gynecol* 1986;67:399.
106. Torrisi JR, Barnes WA, Popescu G, et al. Postoperative adjuvant external-beam radiotherapy in surgical stage I endometrial carcinoma. *Cancer* 1989;64:1414.
107. Kucera H, Vavra N, Weghaupt K. Benefit of external irradiation in pathologic stage I endometrial carcinoma: a prospective clinical trial of 605 patients who received postoperation and additional pelvic irradiation in the presence of unfavorable prognostic factors. *Gynecol Oncol* 1990;38:99.
108. Piver MS, Hempling RE. A prospective trial of postoperative vaginal radium/cesium for grade 1-2 less than 50% myometrial invasion and pelvic radiation therapy for grade 3 or deep myometrial invasion in surgical stage I endometrial adenocarcinoma. *Cancer* 1990;66:1133.
109. Stryker JA, Podczaski E, Kaminski P, et al. Adjuvant external beam therapy for pathologic stage I and occult stage II endometrial carcinoma. *Cancer* 1991;67:2872.
110. Podczaski E, Kaminski P, Gurski K, et al. Detection and patterns of treatment failure in 300 consecutive cases of "early" endometrial cancer after primary surgery. *Gynecol Oncol* 1992;47:323.
111. Carey MS, O'Connell GJ, Johanson CR, et al. Good outcome associated with a standardized treatment protocol using selective postoperative radiation in patients with clinical stage I adenocarcinoma of the endometrium. *Gynecol Oncol* 1995;57:138.
112. Roberts JA, Brunetto VI, Keys HM, et al. A phase III randomized study of surgery vs surgery plus adjunctive radiation therapy in intermediate-risk endometrial adenocarcinoma (GOG No. 99). *Gynecol Oncol* 1998;68:135(abst).
113. Schink JC, Rademaker AW, Miller DS, et al. Tumor size in endometrial cancer. *Cancer* 1991;67:2791.
114. Lewandowski G, Torrisi J, Potkul RK, et al. Hysterectomy with extended surgical staging and radiotherapy versus hysterectomy alone and radiotherapy in stage I endometrial cancer: a comparison of complication rates. *Gynecol Oncol* 1990;36:401.
115. Greven KM, Lanciano RM, Herbert SH, et al. Analysis of complications in patients with endometrial carcinoma receiving adjuvant irradiation. *Int J Radiat Oncol Biol Phys* 1991;21:919.
116. Corn BW, Lanciano RM, Greven KM, et al. Impact of improved irradiation technique, age and lymph node sampling on the severe complication rate of surgically staged endometrial cancer patients: a multivariate analysis. *J Clin Oncol* 1994;12:510.
117. Bliss P, Cowie VJ. Endometrial carcinoma: does the addition of intracavitary vault caesium to external beam therapy postoperatively result in improved control or increased morbidity? *Clin Oncol* 1992;4:373.
118. Randall ME, Wilder J, Greven K, et al. Role of intracavitary cuff boost after adjuvant external irradiation in early endometrial carcinoma. *Int J Radiat Oncol Biol Phys* 1990;19:49.
119. Murrell DS, Orton CG. Survival and complications in stage I carcinoma of corpus uteri receiving post-operative irradiation. *Radiother Oncol* 1988;12:281.
120. Jereczek-Fossa B, Jassem J, Nowak R, et al. A. Late complications after postoperative radiotherapy in endometrial cancer: analysis of 317 consecutive cases with application of linear-quadratic model. *Int J Radiat Oncol Biol Phys* 1998;41:329.
121. Komaki R, Mattingly RF, Hoffman RG, et al. Irradiation of para-aortic lymph node metastases from carcinoma of the cervix or endometrium: preliminary results. *Radiology* 1983;147:245.
122. Feuer G, Calanog A. Endometrial carcinoma. Treatment of positive paraaortic nodes. *Gynecol Oncol* 1987;27:104.
123. Potish RA. Abdominal radiotherapy for cancer of the uterine cervix and endometrium. *Int J Radiat Oncol Biol Phys* 1989;16:1453.
124. Corn B, Lanciano R, Greven K, et al. Endometrial cancer with para-aortic adenopathy: patterns of failure and opportunities for cure. *Int J Radiat Oncol Biol Phys* 1992;24:223.
125. Rose P, Cha S, Tak W, et al. Radiation therapy for surgically proven para-aortic node metastasis in endometrial carcinoma. *Int J Radiat Oncol Biol Phys* 1992;24:229.
126. Hicks ML, Piver MS, Puretz JL, et al. Survival in patients with paraaortic lymph node metastases from endometrial adenocarcinoma clinically limited to the uterus. *Int J Radiat Oncol Biol Phys* 1993;26:607.
127. Blythe JG, Edwards E, Heimbecker P. Paraaortic lymph node biopsy: a twenty-year study. *Am J Obstet Gynecol* 1997;176:1157.
128. Onda T, Yoshikawa H, Mizutani K, et al. Treatment of node-positive endometrial cancer with complete node dissection, chemotherapy and radiation therapy. *Br J Cancer* 1997; 75:7836.

129. Potish R. Radiation therapy of periaortic node metastases in cancer of the uterine cervix and endometrium. *Radiology* 1987;165:567.
130. Greven KM, Lanciano RM, Corn B, et al. Pathologic stage III endometrial carcinoma. Prognostic factors and patterns of recurrence. *Cancer* 1993;71:3697.
131. Malipeddi P, Kapp DS, Teng NN. Long-term survival with adjuvant whole abdominopelvic irradiation for uterine papillary serous carcinoma. *Cancer* 1993;71:3076.
132. Grice J, Ek M, Greer B, et al. Uterine papillary serous carcinoma: evaluation of long-term survival in surgically staged patients. *Gynecol Oncol* 1998;69:69.
133. Randall ME, Spirtos NM, Dvoretsky P. Whole abdominal radiotherapy versus combination chemotherapy with doxorubicin and cisplatin in advanced endometrial carcinoma (phase III): Gynecologic Oncology Group study no. 122. *Monogr Natl Cancer Inst* 1995;19:13.
134. Kadar N, Homesley H, Malfetano J. Positive peritoneal cytology is an adverse factor in endometrial carcinoma only if there is other evidence of extrauterine disease. *Gynecol Oncol* 1991;46:145.
135. Sorbe BG, Smeds AC. Postoperative vaginal irradiation with high dose rate afterloading technique in endometrial carcinoma stage I. *Int J Radiat Oncol Biol Phys* 1990;18:305.
136. Elliott P, Green D, Coates A, et al. The efficacy of postoperative vaginal irradiation in preventing vaginal recurrence in endometrial cancer. *Int J Gynecol Cancer* 1994;4:84.
137. Pinilla J. Cost minimization analysis of high-dose-rate versus low-dose-rate brachytherapy in endometrial cancer. Gynecology Tumor Group. *Int J Radiat Oncol Biol Phys* 1998;42:87.
138. Thomas H, Pickerine GL, Dunn P, et al. Treating the vaginal vault in carcinoma of the endometrium using the Buchler afterloading system. *Br J Radiol* 1991;64:1044.
139. Weiss E, Hirnle P, Arnold-Bofinger H, et al. Adjuvant vaginal high-dose-rate afterloading alone in endometrial carcinoma: patterns of relapse and side effects following low-dose therapy. *Gynecol Oncol* 1998;71:72.
140. MacLeod C, Fowler A, Duval P, et al. High-dose-rate brachytherapy alone post-hysterectomy for endometrial cancer. *Int J Radiat Oncol Biol Phys* 1998;42:1033.
141. Noyes WR, Bastin K, Edwards SA, et al. Postoperative vaginal cuff irradiation using high dose rate remote afterloading: a phase II clinical protocol. *Int J Radiat Oncol Biol Phys* 1995;32:1439.
142. Landgren RC, Fletcher GH, Delclos L, Wharton JT. Irradiation of endometrial cancer in patients with medical contraindication to surgery or with unresectable lesions. *AJR Am J Roentgenol* 1976;126:148.
143. Jones D, Stout R. Results of intracavitary radium treatment for adenocarcinoma of the body of the uterus. *Clin Radiol* 1986;37:169.
144. Grigsby P, Kuske R, Perez C, et al. Medically inoperable stage I adenocarcinoma of the endometrium treated with radiotherapy alone. *Int J Radiat Oncol Biol Phys* 1987;13:483.
145. Lehoczky O, Bosze P, Ungar L, et al. Stage I endometrial carcinoma: treatment of nonoperable patients with intracavitary radiation therapy alone. *Gynecol Oncol* 1991;43:211.
146. Kupelian PA, Eifel PJ, Tornos C, et al. Treatment of endometrial carcinoma with radiation therapy alone. *Int J Radiat Oncol Biol Phys* 1993;27:817.
147. Rose PG, Baker S, Kern M, et al. Primary radiation therapy for endometrial carcinoma: a case controlled study. *Int J Radiat Oncol Biol Phys* 1993;27:585.
148. Rouanet P, Dubois JB, Gely S, et al. Exclusive radiation therapy in endometrial carcinoma. *Int J Radiat Oncol Biol Phys* 1993;26:223.
149. Nguyen C, Souhami L, Roman TN, et al. High-dose-rate brachytherapy as the primary treatment of medically inoperable stage I-II endometrial carcinoma. *Gynecol Oncol* 1995;59:370.
150. Knocke TH, Kucera H, Weidinger B, et al. Primary treatment of endometrial carcinoma with high-dose-rate brachytherapy: results of 12 years of experience with 280 patients. *Int J Radiat Oncol Biol Phys* 1997;37:359.
151. Nguyen TV, Petereit DG. High-dose-rate brachytherapy for medically inoperable stage I endometrial cancer. *Gynecol Oncol* 1998;71:196.
152. Petereit DG, Sarkaria JN, Chappell RJ. Perioperative morbidity and mortality of high-dose-rate gynecologic brachytherapy. *Int J Radiat Oncol Biol Phys* 1998;42:1025.
153. Kelley RM, Baker W. Progestational agents in the treatment of carcinoma of the endometrium. *N Engl J Med* 1961;264:216.
154. Lewis GC, Slack NH, Mortel R, et al. Adjuvant progestogen therapy in primary definitive treatment of endometrial cancer. *Gynecol Oncol* 1974;2:368.
155. Bonte J. Hormonothérapie adjuvante par medroxyprogestérone dans le traitement de l'adénocarcinome endométrial au stade I. *Med et Hyg* 1977;35:4193.
156. Kauppila A, Grönroos M, Neiminen U. Adjuvant progestin therapy in endometrial carcinoma. *Prog Cancer Res Ther* 1983;25:219.
157. Kauppila A. Progestin therapy of endometrial breast and ovarian carcinoma. *Acta Obstet Gynecol Scand* 1984;63:441.
158. DePalo G, Merson M, Del Vecchio M, et al. A controlled clinical study of adjuvant medroxyprogesterone acetate (MPA) therapy in pathologic stage I endometrial carcinoma with myometrial invasion. *Proc Ann Meet Am Soc Clin Oncol* 1985;4:121(abst).
159. Macdonald RR, Thorogood J, Mason MK. A randomized trial of progestogens in the primary treatment of endometrial carcinoma. *Br J Obstet Gynaecol* 1988;95:166.
160. Piver MS. Progesterone therapy for malignant peritoneal cytology surgical stage I endometrial adenocarcinoma. *Semin Oncol* 1988;15:50.
161. Stringer CA, Gershenson DM, Burke TW, et al. Adjuvant chemotherapy with cisplatin, doxorubicin, and cyclophosphamide (PAC) for early-stage high-risk endometrial cancer: a preliminary analysis. *Gynecol Oncol* 1990;38:305.
162. Burke TW, Gershenson DM, Morris M, et al. Postoperative adjuvant cisplatin, doxorubicin, and cyclophosphamide (PAC) chemotherapy in women with high-risk endometrial carcinoma. *Gynecol Oncol* 1994;55:47.
163. Morrow CP, Bundy BN, Homesley HD. Doxorubicin as an adjuvant following surgery and radiation therapy in patients with high-risk endometrial carcinoma, stage I, and occult stage II: a Gynecologic Oncology Group study. *Gynecol Oncol* 1990;36:166.
164. Reddoch JM, Burke TW, Morris M, et al. Surveillance for recurrent endometrial carcinoma: development of a follow-up scheme. *Gynecol Oncol* 1995;59:221.
165. Shumsky AG, Stuart GCE, Brasher P, et al. An evaluation of routine follow-up of patients treated for endometrial carcinoma. *Gynecol Oncol* 1994;55:229.
166. Salvesen HB, Akslen LA, Iversen T, Iversen OE. Recurrence of endometrial carcinoma and the value of routine follow up. *Br J Obstet Gynaecol* 1997;104:1302.
167. Levenback C, Burke TW, Silva E, et al. Uterine papillary serous carcinoma (UPSC) treated with cisplatin, doxorubicin, and cyclophosphamide (PAC). *Gynecol Oncol* 1992;46:317.
168. Brown JM, Dockerty MB, Symmonds RE, et al. Vaginal recurrence of endometrial carcinoma. *Am J Obstet Gynecol* 1968;100:544.
169. Phillips GL, Prem KA, Adcock LL, et al. Vaginal recurrence of adenocarcinoma of the endometrium. *Gynecol Oncol* 1982;13:232.
170. Reifenstein EC. Hydroxyprogesterone caproate therapy in advanced endometrial cancer. *Cancer* 1971;27:485.
171. Piver MS, Barlow JJ, Lurain JR, et al. Medroxyprogesterone acetate (Depo-Provera) vs hydroxyprogesterone caproate (Delalutin) in women with metastatic endometrial adenocarcinoma. *Cancer* 1980;45:268.
172. Podratz KC, O'Brien PC, Malkasian GD, et al. Effects of progestational agents in treatment of endometrial carcinoma. *Obstet Gynecol* 1985;66:106.
173. Lentz SS, Brady MF, Major FJ, et al. High dose megestrol acetate in advanced or recurrent endometrial cancer: a Gynecologic Oncology Group study. *J Clin Oncol* 1996;14:357.
174. Thigpen JT, Brady M, Alvarez RD, et al. Oral medroxy-progesterone acetate in the treatment of advanced or recurrent endometrial carcinoma: a dose-response study by the Gynecologic Oncology Group. *J Clin Oncol* 1999;17:1736.
175. Thigpen JT, Brady MF, Homesley HD, et al. Tamoxifen in the treatment of advanced or recurrent endometrial carcinoma: a Gynecologic Oncology Group study. *J Clin Oncol* (*submitted*).
176. Jeyarajah AR, Gallagher CJ, Blake PR, et al. Long-term follow-up of gonadotrophin-releasing hormone analog treatment for recurrent endometrial cancer. *Gynecol Oncol* 1996;63:47.
177. Covens A, Thomas G, Shaw P, et al. A phase II study of leuprolide in advanced/recurrent endometrial cancer. *Gynecol Oncol* 1997;64:126.
178. Rose PG, Van Le L, Bell J, Walker JL, Lee JB. A phase II study of anastrazole in advanced or persistent endometrial carcinoma: a Gynecologic Oncology Group study. *Gynecol Oncol.* (*submitted*).
179. Blessing J. Gynecologic Oncology Group Statistical Office, Buffalo, NY. Unpublished data.
180. Mandeli J. New York Gynecologic Oncology Group, Mt. Sinai Hospital, New York. Unpublished data.
181. Rendina GM, Donadio C, Fabri M, et al. Tamoxifen and medroxyprogesterone therapy for advanced endometrial carcinoma. *Eur J Obstet Gynecol Reprod Biol* 1984;17:285.
182. Creasman WT, Soper JT, McCarty KS Jr, et al. Influence of cytoplasmic steroid receptor content on prognosis of early stage endometrial carcinoma. *Am J Obstet Gynecol* 1985;151:922.
183. Liao BS, Twiggs LB, Leung BS, et al. Cytoplasmic estrogen and progesterone receptors as prognostic parameters in primary endometrial carcinoma. *Obstet Gynecol* 1986;67:463.
184. Ehrlich CE, Young PCM, Stehman FB, et al. Steroid receptors and clinical outcome in patients with adenocarcinoma of the endometrium. *Am J Obstet Gynecol* 1988;158:796.
185. Chatzaki E, Bax CM, Eidne KA, et al. The expression of gonadotropin-releasing hormone and its receptor in endometrial cancer, and its relevance as an autocrine growth factor. *Cancer Res* 1996;56:2059.
186. Calero F, Rodriguez-Escudero F, Jimeno J, et al. Clinical evaluation of epirubicin in endometrial adenocarcinoma and uterine cervix carcinoma. *Proc Am Soc Clin Oncol* 1989;8:156.
187. Thigpen JT, Blessing JA, DiSaia PJ, et al. A randomized comparison of doxorubicin alone versus doxorubicin plus cyclophosphamide in the management of advanced or recurrent endometrial carcinoma: a Gynecologic Oncology Group study. *J Clin Oncol* 1994;12:1408.
188. Horton J, Elson P, Gordon P, Hahn R, Creech R. Combination chemotherapy for advanced endometrial cancer. An evaluation of three regimens. *Cancer* 1982;49:2441.
189. Cohen CJ, Bruckner HW, Deppe G, et al. Multidrug treatment of advanced and recurrent endometrial carcinoma: a Gynecologic Oncology Group study. *Obstet Gynecol* 1984;63:719.
190. Thigpen T, Blessing J, Homesley H, et al. Phase III trial of doxorubicin ± cisplatin in advanced or recurrent endometrial carcinoma: a Gynecologic Oncology Group (GOG) study. *Proc Am Soc Clin Oncol* 1993;12:(abst 830):261.
191. Tropé C, Grundsell H, Johnsson JE, et al. A phase II study of cisplatinum for recurrent corpus cancer. *Eur J Cancer* 1980;16:1025.
192. Seski JC, Edwards CL, Herson J, et al. Cisplatin chemotherapy for disseminated endometrial cancer. *Obstet Gynecol* 1982;59:225.
193. Thigpen JT, Blessing JA, Lagasse LD, et al. Phase II trial of cisplatin as second-line chemotherapy in patients with advanced or recurrent endometrial carcinoma: a Gynecologic Oncology Group study. *Am J Clin Oncol* 1984;7:253.
194. Long HJ, Pfeifle DM, Wieand HS, et al. Phase II evaluation of carboplatin in advanced endometrial carcinoma. *J Natl Cancer Inst* 1988;80:276.
195. Thigpen JT, Blessing JA, Homesley J, et al. Phase II trial of cisplatin as first-line chemotherapy in patients with advanced and recurrent endometrial carcinoma: a Gynecologic Oncology Group study. *Gynecol Oncol* 1989;33:68.
196. Green JB, Green S, Alberts DS, et al. Carboplatin therapy in advanced endometrial cancer. *Obstet Gynecol* 1990;75:696.
197. Burke TW, Munkarah A, Kavanagh JJ. Treatment of advanced or recurrent endometrial carcinoma with single-agent carboplatin. *Gynecol Oncol* 1993;51:397.
198. Ball HG, Blessing JA, Lentz SS, et al. A phase II trial of Taxol in advanced and recurrent adenocarcinoma of the endometrium: a Gynecologic Oncology Group study. *Gynecol Oncol* 1996;62:278.
199. Lincoln S, Blessing JA, Lee RB, et al. Evaluation of paclitaxel (Taxol) in the treatment of recurrent or persistent endometrial carcinoma: a Gynecologic Oncology Group study. *Gynecol Oncol* (*submitted*).
200. Sutton GP, Blessing JA, DeMars LR, et al. A phase II Gynecologic Oncology Group trial of ifosfamide and mesna in advanced or recurrent adenocarcinoma of the endometrium. *Gynecol Oncol* 1996;63:25.
201. Rose PG, Blessing JA, Lewandowski GS, et al. A phase II trial of prolonged oral etoposide

(VP-16) as second-line therapy for advanced and recurrent endometrial carcinoma: a Gynecologic Oncology Group study. *Gynecol Oncol* 1996;63:101.

202. Poplin EA. Phase II trial of oral etoposide in recurrent or refractory endometrial adenocarcinoma: a Southwest Oncology Group study. *Gynecol Oncol* 1999;74:432.
203. Price FV, Edwards RP, Kelley JL, Kunschner AJ, Hart LA. A trial of outpatient paclitaxel and carboplatin for advanced, recurrent, and histologic high-risk endometrial carcinoma: preliminary report. *Semin Oncol* 1997;24[Suppl 15]:78.
204. Lissoni A, Gabriele A, Gorga G, et al. Cisplatin-, epirubicin- and paclitaxel-containing chemotherapy in uterine adenocarcinoma. *Ann Oncol* 1997;8:969.
205. Le TD, Yamada SD, Rutgers JL, et al. Complete response of a stage IV uterine papillary serous carcinoma to neoadjuvant chemotherapy with Taxol and carboplatin. *Gynecol Oncol* 1999;73:461.
206. Chambers JT, Chambers SK, Kohorn EI, et al. Uterine papillary serous carcinoma treated with intraperitoneal cisplatin and intravenous doxorubicin and cyclophosphamide. *Gynecol Oncol* 1996;60:438.
207. Reisinger SA, Asbury R, Liao SY, et al. A phase I study of weekly cisplatin and whole abdominal radiation for the treatment of stage III and IV endometrial carcinoma: a Gynecologic Oncology Group pilot study. *Gynecol Oncol* 1996;63:299.
208. Pastan I, Gottesman M. Multiple-drug resistance in human cancer. *N Engl J Med* 1987;316:1388.
209. Yang CP, DePinho SG, Greenberger LM, et al. Progesterone interacts with P-glycoprotein in multidrug-resistant cells and in the endometrium of gravid uterus. *J Biol Chem* 1989;264:782.
210. Berchuck A, Soisson AP, Olt GJ, et al. Epidermal growth factor receptor expression in normal and malignant endometrium. *Am J Obstet Gynecol* 1989;161:1247.
211. Esteller M, Garcia A, Martinez i Palones JM, Cabero A, Reventos J. Detection of c-erbB-2/neu and fibroblast growth factor-3/INT-2 but not epidermal growth factor receptor gene amplification in endometrial cancer by differential polymerase chain reaction. *Cancer* 1995;75:2139.
212. Curran WJ, Whittington R, Peters AJ, et al. Vaginal recurrences of endometrial carcinoma: the prognostic value of staging by a primary vaginal carcinoma system. *Int J Radiat Oncol Biol Phys* 1988;15:803.
213. Poulsen MG, Roberts SJ. The salvage of recurrent endometrial carcinoma in the vagina and pelvis. *Int J Radiat Oncol Biol Phys* 1988;15:809.
214. Kuten A, Grigsby PW, Perez CA, et al. Results of radiotherapy in recurrent endometrial carcinoma: a retrospective analysis of 51 patients. *Int J Radiat Oncol Biol Phys* 1989;17:29.
215. Morgan JD, Reddy S, Sarin P, et al. Isolated vaginal recurrences of endometrial carcinoma. *Radiology* 1993;189:609.
216. Sears JD, Greven KM, Hoen HM, et al. Prognostic factors and treatment outcome for patients with locally recurrent endometrial cancer. *Cancer* 1994;74:1303.
217. Ackerman I, Malone S, Thomas G, et al. Endometrial carcinoma—relative effectiveness of adjuvant irradiation vs therapy reserved for relapse [see comments]. *Gynecol Oncol* 1996;60:177.
218. Charra C, Roy P, Coquard R, et al. Outcome of treatment of upper third vaginal recurrences of cervical and endometrial carcinomas with interstitial brachytherapy. *Int J Radiat Oncol Biol Phys* 1998;40:421.
219. Aalders JG, Abeler V, Kolstad P. Recurrent adenocarcinoma of the endometrium: a clinical and histopathological study of 379 patients. *Gynecol Oncol* 1984;17:85.
220. Greven KM. Interstitial radiation for recurrent cervix or endometrial cancer in the suburethral region. *Int J Radiat Oncol Biol Phys* 1998;41:831.
221. Foote RL, Schray MF, Wilson TO, Malkasian GD Jr. Isolated peripheral lymph node recurrence of endometrial carcinoma. *Cancer* 1988;61:2561.
222. Morris M, Alvarez RD, Kinney WK, et al. Treatment of recurrent adenocarcinoma of the endometrium with pelvic exenteration. *Gynecol Oncol* 1996;60:288.
223. Barber HRK, Brunschwig A. Treatment and results of recurrent cancer of corpus uteri in patients receiving anterior and total pelvic exenteration, 1947–1963. *Cancer* 1968;22:949.
224. Rutledge FN. Pelvic exenteration: an update of the University of Texas M. D. Anderson Hospital experience and review of the literature. In: Rutledge FN, Gershenson DM, eds. *Gynecologic cancer: diagnosis and treatment strategies*, vol 7. Austin, TX: University of Texas Press, 1987.
225. Ober WB. Uterine sarcomas: histogenesis and taxonomy. *Ann N Y Acad Sci* 1959;75:568.
226. Spanos WJ Jr, Peters LJ, Oswald MJ. Patterns of recurrence in malignant mixed müllerian tumor of the uterus. *Cancer* 1986;57:155.
227. McCormack PM, Martin M. The changing role of surgery for pulmonary metastases. *Ann Thorac Surg* 1979;28:139.
228. Mountain CF, McMurtrey MJ, Hermes KE. Surgery for pulmonary metastasis: a 20-year experience. *Ann Thorac Surg* 1984;38:323.
229. Salazar OM, Dunne ME. The role of radiation therapy in the management of uterine sarcomas. *Int J Radiat Oncol Biol Phys* 1980;6:899.
230. Sorbe B. Radiotherapy and/or chemotherapy as adjuvant treatment of uterine sarcomas. *Gynecol Oncol* 1985;20:281.
231. Wheelock JB, Krebs HB, Schneider V, et al. Uterine sarcoma: analysis of prognostic variables in 71 cases. *Am J Obstet Gynecol* 1985;151:1016.
232. George M, Pejovic MH, Kramar A. Uterine sarcomas: prognostic factors and treatment modalities—study on 209 patients. *Gynecol Oncol* 1986;24:58.
233. Hornback NB, Omura G, Major FJ. Observations on the use of adjuvant radiation therapy in patients with stage I and II uterine sarcoma. *Int J Radiat Oncol Biol Phys* 1986;12:2127.
234. Echt G, Jepson J, Steel J, et al. Treatment of uterine sarcomas. *Cancer* 1990;66:35.
235. Larson B, Silfverswärd C, Nilsson B, et al. Endometrial stromal sarcoma of the uterus. A clinical and histopathological study. The Radiumhemmet series 1936–1981. *Eur J Obstet Gynecol Reprod Biol* 1990;35:239.
236. Moskovic E, Macsweeney E, Law M, et al. Survival, patterns of spread and prognostic factors in uterine sarcoma: a study of 76 patients. *Br J Radiol* 1993;66:1009.
237. Gerszten K, Faul C, Kounelis S, et al. The impact of adjuvant radiotherapy on carcinosarcoma of the uterus. *Gynecol Oncol* 1998;68:8.
238. Chauveinc L, Deniaud E, Plancher C, et al. Uterine sarcomas: the Curie Institut experience. Prognosis factors and adjuvant treatments. *Gynecol Oncol* 1999;72:232.
239. Ferrer F, Sabater S, Farrus B, et al. Impact of radiotherapy on local control and survival in uterine sarcomas: a retrospective study from the Grup Oncologic Catala-Occita. *Int J Radiat Oncol Biol Phys* 1999;44:47.
240. Major FJ, Blessing JA, Silverberg SG, et al. Prognostic factors in early-stage uterine sarcoma. *Cancer* 1993;71:1702.
241. Rose PG, Boutselis JG, Sachs L. Adjuvant therapy for stage I uterine sarcoma. *Am J Obstet Gynecol* 1987;156:660.
242. Berchuck A, Rubin SC, Hoskins WJ, et al. Treatment of endometrial stromal tumors. *Gynecol Oncol* 1990;36:60.
243. Larson B, Silfverswärd C, Nilsson B, et al. Mixed Müllerian tumours of the uterus—prognostic factors: a clinical and histopathologic study of 147 cases. *Radiother Oncol* 1990;17:123.
244. DeFusco PA, Gaffey TA, Malkasian GD, et al. Endometrial stromal sarcoma: review of Mayo Clinic experience, 1945–1980. *Gynecol Oncol* 1989;35:8.
245. Omura GA, Blessing JA, Major FJ, et al. A randomized clinical trial of adjuvant Adriamycin in uterine sarcoma: a GOG study. *J Clin Oncol* 1985;3:1240.
246. Omura GA, Major FJ, Blessing JA, et al. A randomized study of Adriamycin with and without dimethyl triazenoimidazole carboxamide in advanced uterine sarcomas. *Cancer* 1983;52:626.
247. Muss HB, Bundy B, DiSaia PJ, et al. Treatment of recurrent or advanced uterine sarcoma. A randomized trial of doxorubicin versus doxorubicin and cyclophosphamide (a phase III trial of the Gynecologic Oncology Group). *Cancer* 1985;55:1648.
248. Sutton GP, Blessing JA, Barrett RJ, et al. Phase II trial of ifosfamide and mesna in leiomyosarcoma of the uterus: a Gynecologic Oncology Group study. *Am J Obstet Gynecol* 1992;166:556.
249. Hawkins RE, Wiltshaw E, Mansi JL. Ifosfamide with and without Adriamycin in advanced uterine leiomyosarcoma. *Cancer Chemother Pharmacol* 1990;26:S26.
250. Sutton G, Blessing JA, Malfetano HH. Ifosfamide, doxorubicin and mesna in the treatment of metastatic uterine leiomyosarcomas. *Gynecol Oncol* 1996;62:226.
251. Thigpen JT, Blessing JA, Wilbanks GD. Cisplatin as second-line chemotherapy in the treatment of advanced or recurrent leiomyosarcoma of the uterus. A phase II trial of the Gynecologic Oncology Group. *Am J Clin Oncol* 1986;9:18.
252. Thigpen JT, Blessing JA, Beecham J, et al. Phase II trial of cisplatin as first-line chemotherapy in patients with advanced or recurrent uterine sarcomas: a Gynecologic Oncology Group study. *J Clin Oncol* 1991;9:162.
253. Slayton RE, Blessing JA, Angel C, et al. Phase II trial of etoposide in the management of advanced and recurrent leiomyosarcoma of the uterus: a Gynecologic Oncology Group study. *Cancer Treat Rep* 1987;71:1303.
254. Thigpen T, Blessing JA, Yordan E, et al. Phase II trial of etoposide in leiomyosarcoma of the uterus: a Gynecologic Oncology Group study. *Gynecol Oncol* 1996;63:120.
255. Sutton G, Blessing JA, Ball H. Phase II trial of paclitaxel in leiomyosarcoma of the uterus: a Gynecologic Oncology Group study. *Gynecol Oncol* 1999;74:346.
256. Currie JL, Blessing JL, Muss HB, et al. Combination chemotherapy with hydroxyurea, dacarbazine (DTIC), and etoposide in treatment of uterine leiomyosarcoma: a Gynecologic Oncology Group study. *Gynecol Oncol* 1996;61:27.
257. Sutton GP, Blessing JA, Rosenshein N, et al. Phase II trial of ifosfamide and mesna in mixed mesodermal tumors of the uterus (a Gynecologic Oncology Group study). *Am J Obstet Gynecol* 1989;161:309.
258. Sutton GP, Brunetto V, Kilgore L, et al. A phase III trial of ifosfamide alone or in combination with cisplatin in the treatment of advanced, persistent, or recurrent carcinosarcoma of the uterus: a Gynecologic Oncology Group study. *Gynecol Oncol* 1998;68:137(abst).
259. Hornreich G, Muggia FM, Wadler S, et al. Phase II combination Doxil-paclitaxel (PacliDox) in uterine carcinomas and sarcomas—an active regimen. A NYGOG study. *Gynecol Oncol* 2000;76:265(abstr).
260. Thigpen JT. Cisplatin in gynecologic carcinosarcoma (correspondence). *J Clin Oncol* 1992;10:1365.
261. Gadducci A, Sartori E, Landoni F, et al. Endometrial stromal sarcoma: analysis of treatment failures and survival. *Gynecol Oncol* 1996;63:247.
262. Nordal RR, Kristensen GB, Kaern J, et al. The prognostic significance of surgery, tumor size, malignancy grade, menopausal status, and DNA ploidy in endometrial stromal sarcoma. *Gynecol Oncol* 1996;62:254.
263. Yamawaki T, Shimizu Y, Hasumi K. Treatment of stage IV "high-grade" endometrial stromal sarcoma with ifosfamide, Adriamycin, and cisplatin [Case Report]. *Gynecol Oncol* 1997;64:265.
264. Irvin W, Pelkey T, Rice L, et al. Endometrial stromal sarcoma of the vulva arising in extraovarian endometriosis: a case report and literature review. *Gynecol Oncol* 1998;71:313.
265. Scribner DR Jr, Walker JL. Low-grade endometrial stromal sarcoma preoperative treatment with Depo-Lupron and Megace. *Gynecol Oncol* 1998;71:458.
266. Sutton GP, Stehman FB, Michael H, et al. Estrogen and progesterone receptors in uterine sarcomas. *Obstet Gynecol* 1986;68:709.
267. Hitti IF, Glasber SS, McKenzie C, et al. Uterine leiomyosarcoma with massive necrosis diagnosed during gonadotropin releasing hormone analog therapy for presumed uterine fibroid. *Fertil Steril* 1991;56:778.
268. Madsen WE, Das Gupta TK, Walker MJ. The influence of glucocorticoids on the growth of a human leiomyosarcoma cell line, SK-LMS-1. *Int J Cancer* 1989;44:1034.
269. Katz L, Merino M, Sakamoto H, et al. Endometrial stromal sarcoma: a clinicopathologic study of 11 cases with determination of estrogen and progestin receptor levels in three tumors. *Gynecol Oncol* 1987;26:87.
270. Tosi P, Sforza V, Sanpietro R. Estrogen receptor content, immunohistochemically determined by monoclonal antibodies in endometrial stromal sarcoma. *Obstet Gynecol* 1989;73:75.
271. Hall KL, Teneriello MG, Taylor RR, et al. Analysis of Ki-ras, p53, and MDM2 genes in uterine leiomyomas and leiomyosarcomas. *Gynecol Oncol* 1997;65:330.

272. Gosland MP, Lum BL, Sikic BI. Reversal by cefoperazone of resistance to etoposide, doxorubicin, and vinblastine in multidrug resistant human sarcoma cells. *Cancer Res* 1989;49:6905.
273. Poulsen HK, Jacobsen M, Bertelsen K, et al. Adjuvant radiation therapy is not necessary in the management of endometrial carcinoma stage I, low-risk cases. *Int J Gynecol Cancer* 1996;6:38.
274. Rose PG, Blessing JA, Soper JT, et al. Prolonged oral etoposide in recurrent or advanced leiomyosarcoma of the uterus: a Gynecologic Oncology Group study. *Gynecol Oncol* 1998;70:267.
275. Miller DA, Blessing JA, Kilgure LJ, et al. A phase II trial of topotecan in patients with advanced, persistent or recurrent uterine leiomyosarcomas: a Gynecologic Oncology Group study. *Am J Clin Oncol* (*in press*).
276. Currie JL, Blessing JA, McGehee R, Soper JT, Berman M. Phase II trial of hydroxyurea, dacarbazine (DTIC), and etoposide (VP-16) in mixed mesodermal tumors of the uterus: a Gynecologic Oncology Group study. *Gynecol Oncol* 1996;61:94.
277. Thigpen JT, Blessing JA, Orr JW, et al. Phase II trial of cisplatin in the treatment of patients with advanced or recurrent mixed mesodermal sarcomas of the uterus: a Gynecologic Oncology Group study. *Cancer Treat Rep* 1986;70:271.

FRANCO M. MUGGIA
PATRICIA J. EIFEL
THOMAS W. BURKE

SECTION 4

Gestational Trophoblastic Diseases

Gestational trophoblastic disease encompasses a spectrum of interrelated conditions spanning proliferative changes resulting from an abnormal fertilization to highly malignant lesions such as choriocarcinoma. Four distinct clinicopathologic entities have been described: molar pregnancy (including complete and partial hydatidiform moles), invasive mole (chorioadenoma destruens), placental-site trophoblastic tumors, and choriocarcinoma. Although these constitute fewer than 1% of gynecologic malignancies, they are highly important to recognize because of their life-threatening potential and their high curability if treated early and by experienced centers.

EPIDEMIOLOGY

Gestational trophoblastic disease most commonly follows molar pregnancy but may also occur after normal or ectopic pregnancies and spontaneous or therapeutic abortions. Its incidence varies widely among various populations, with figures as high as 1 in 120 pregnancies in some areas of Asia and South America, compared to 1 in 1200 in the United States.[1] The risk is fivefold greater in women older than 40 years[2] and is also increased in those younger than 20 years.[2] Prior molar pregnancies, lower socioeconomic status, and blood group A women married to group O men are at higher risk.[1–3] Parity, ethnicity, nutritional factors, and cigarette smoking have been examined as risk factors, but no clear association has been found. However, oral contraceptives and the number of sexual partners before the index pregnancy appear to double the risk of gestational trophoblastic tumors.[4]

PATHOLOGY AND BIOLOGY

Hydatidiform moles (complete and partial) are characterized by clusters of hydropic villi, and trophoblastic hyperplasia with atypia. Partial moles show a variable amount of focal trophoblastic hyperplasia and have identifiable fetal or embryonic tissues. Invasive moles (chorioadenoma destruens) have findings similar to complete moles but display a greater tendency to invade surrounding tissues. The rare placental-site trophoblastic tumors[5]—initially named *trophoblastic pseudotumors*—are derived from intermediate trophoblast cells [which secrete placental lactogen in greater amounts than human chorionic gonadotropin (HCG)], and they present clinically as nodules in the endometrium and myometrium after removal of a mole. Microscopically, these tumors show no chorionic villi and are characterized by a proliferation of cells with oval nuclei and abundant eosinophilic cytoplasm. They usually arise after nonmolar abortion or a term pregnancy, but occasionally after hydatidiform mole and, in one case, after a metastatic gestational trophoblastic neoplasia.[6] Choriocarcinomas consist of invasive and anaplastic trophoblastic tissue made up of cytotrophoblastic and syncytiotrophoblastic elements, obligatory secretion of HCG, and rich vascularity. Commonly accompanying the trophoblastic neoplasia are one or more theca lutein ovarian cysts that are a result of HCG stimulation. Rarely, the malignancy can coexist with an intact pregnancy.[7] Treatment has evolved based on prognostic-factor risk classification and staging and not on pathologic features.

Cytogenetics has provided clues as to the origin of hydatidiform moles: Most complete moles have a 46XX karyotype, with the minority being 46XY. All X chromosomes are from paternal origin. These are believed to arise from fertilization of an empty ovum by a haploid sperm that then undergoes duplication. Maternal mitochondrial DNA has been identified.[8] On the other hand, partial moles contain both maternal and parental chromosomes, are triploid, and their sex chromosomes are typically XXY. Presumably, as a result of fertilization of a normal ovum by two sperms, if the extra haploid set is of parental origin, a partial mole arises. If the extra haploid set is of maternal origin, then a trisomic fetus develops.[9,10]

The molecular biology of trophoblastic malignant transformation has been explored; insulin-like growth factor from parental chromosomes, and growth factors released through immunologic mechanisms have been studied.[11,12] Overexpression of the epidermal growth factor receptor has been described.[13] The epidermal growth factor is capable of modulating the expression of placental lactogen in a rat choriocarcinoma line.[14] Mutations in p53 have not been found.[15]

CLINICAL DIAGNOSIS AND HUMAN CHORIONIC GONADOTROPIN

A molar pregnancy is suspected with first-trimester bleeding, a uterus larger than expected for gestational age, and absence of fetal heart sounds and fetal parts in association with a markedly elevated HCG level. Iron-deficiency anemia is common at diagnosis because of recurrent bleeding. Other signs include hyperemesis, the passage of "prune juice–like" clots and even actual grape-like villi, toxemia during the first or second trimester, presence of ovarian enlargement with theca lutein

TABLE 36.4-1. Prognostic Scoring System for Gestational Trophoblastic Disease

	Score			
Factor	0	1	2	4
Age	—	<39 y	—	>39 y
Antecedent pregnancy	Mole	Abortion	Term	—
Interval from pregnancy (months)	<4	4–6	7–12	>12
Serum human chorionic gonadotropin	$<10^3$ IU/L	10^3–10^4 IU/L	10^4–10^5 IU/L	$>10^5$ IU/L
ABO groups	—	O or A	B or AB	—
Largest tumor	<3 cm	3–5 cm	>5 cm	—
Metastatic sites	Lung	Spleen, kidney	Gastrointestinal tract, liver	Brain
Number of metastases	—	1–3	4–8	>8
Prior chemotherapy	—	—	One drug	Two or more drugs

(Reprinted from ref. 24, with permission.)

cysts, and hyperthyroidism. Invasive moles may cause rupture of the uterus. Rupture of an ovarian cyst and metastatic disease may rarely be the presentation of an otherwise unrecognized or silent gestational trophoblastic disease. In fewer than 1% of molar pregnancies, a normal fetal (twin) pregnancy may coexist. Radiologic procedures, particularly ultrasonography, are used to suggest the diagnosis. HCG determinations are of central importance in the diagnosis, treatment, follow-up, and likely pathogenesis of gestational trophoblastic disease.

HCG consists of α and β chains, and its primary function is the maintenance of the corpus luteum during pregnancy. The α chain is cross-reactive with luteinizing hormone and with thyrotropin (previously thyroid-stimulating hormone). The β-2 subunit (β-HCG) is unique to HCG and has been used for the radioimmunoassay of HCG in the presence of luteinizing hormone.[16] Normally, HCG peaks at 10 to 12 weeks of gestation, and actual levels and serial changes in β-HCG are essential to diagnose and track the outcome of trophoblastic disease. After evacuation of a molar pregnancy, β-HCG titers usually disappear in 8 to 10 weeks.[17] Persistence may indicate local and, less often, metastatic disease: From the New England Trophoblastic Disease Center experience, 15% of women with a complete mole and 5.5% of women with partial moles developed nonmetastatic trophoblastic disease.[18] A β-HCG level of 100,000 mIU/mL or more, a uterine size greater than expected from gestational age, and the presence of theca lutein ovarian cysts larger than 6 cm in diameter identify women at high risk for persistent gestational trophoblastic disease after evacuation of a complete mole. For these women, the risk of subsequent nonmetastatic manifestations is 31%, and 8.8% develop metastases, contrasting with 3.5% and 0.6%, respectively, for women without these risk factors. Such a risk may be reduced by chemoprophylaxis with short courses of methotrexate and dactinomycin.[19] Although such use of preventive chemotherapy is controversial, serial β-HCG measurements are essential in both high- and low-risk groups. Weekly HCG measurements until three nondetectable determinations, followed by monthly tests for 6 months, are advised. In addition, effective contraception during the entire period of follow-up is essential to avoid confusing the clinical picture.

Other tumor marker measurements may assist in the management of gestational trophoblastic disease: The placental-site trophoblastic tumor produces low levels of HCG but may be identified by measurement of placental lactogen.[20] The serum CA-125 has been found useful as a predictor of persistence of molar disease.[21] Finally, the ratio of serum to cerebrospinal fluid β-HCG has been used to identify brain metastases if such a ratio is less than 60:1.[22]

CHORIOCARCINOMA

CLINICAL FEATURES AND STAGING

Metastatic disease occurs in 4% of patients after local management of hydatidiform moles and very rarely after term pregnancies (1 in 40,000) or abortions. Rapid growth and a high propensity for hemorrhage make this tumor a medical emergency. Metastases are found in lung (80%), vagina (30%), pelvis (20%), brain (10%), and liver (10%). Other rare sites are the spleen, kidneys, and gastrointestinal tract.[18] The lungs are often involved with multiple lesions, and at times this involvement is massive at presentation, leading to respiratory insufficiency.[23] On the other hand, early detection in the asymptomatic state may take place through computed tomography in cases with persistent moles. The central nervous system is seldom involved in the absence of pulmonary metastases.

Anatomic staging of choriocarcinoma (I, confined to corpus; II, metastases to pelvis and vagina; III, pulmonary metastases with or without uterine, pelvic, or vaginal involvement; and IV, other metastases, such as brain, liver, kidneys, or gastrointestinal tract) is seldom used. Therapeutic planning relies on the scoring system based on prognostic factors that was developed at the Charing Cross Hospital by Bagshawe[24] and later adopted by other groups, including the World Health Organization (Table 36.4-1). The importance of this scoring system lies in the identification of a high-risk choriocarcinoma that requires more intensive use of drug combinations to achieve cures and prevent emergence of resistance.

The total score for a patient is obtained by adding the individual scores for each prognostic factor, with a score of 4 being considered low risk, a score of 5 to 7 as intermediate risk, and a score of greater than 7 as high risk.

TREATMENT

Chemotherapy is highly effective for all forms of gestational trophoblastic disease. The curative effects of methotrexate in a

TABLE 36.4-2. Drug Regimens for Gestational Trophoblastic Disease

LOW RISK (SINGLE AGENTS)

Methotrexate[a]: 30–50 mg/m^2 IM weekly; 0.4 mg/kg IM or IV daily × 5 d (repeat in 2 wk); or 1 mg/kg IM or IV on days 1, 3, 5, and 7 (repeat in 2 wk) plus folinic acid (leucovorin), 0.1 mg/kg or IV on days 2, 4, 6, and 8

Dactinomycin: 1.25 mg/m^2 IV (repeat in 2 wk), or 10 μg/kg (up to 0.5 mg) IV daily × 5 d (repeat in 2 wk)

INTERMEDIATE OR HIGH RISK (DRUG COMBINATIONS)

EMA-CO consists of alternating cycles of EMA (days 1 and 2) and CO (day 8)

Day 1 EMA: *etoposide*, 100 mg/m^2 IV; and *dactinomycin*, 0.5 mg IV; and *methotrexate*, 100 mg IV push followed by 200 mg/m^2 12-h IV

Day 2 EMA: *etoposide*, 100 mg/m^2 IV; *dactinomycin*, 0.5 mg IV; and *folinic acid*, 15 mg IV or PO every 12 h × 4, 24 h after start of methotrexate

Day 8 CO: *vincristine*, 1 mg/m^2 IV; and *cyclophosphamide*, 600 mg/m^2 IV

SALVAGE REGIMENS

PEBA: cisplatin, etoposide, bleomycin, doxorubicin[32]

VIP: etoposide, ifosfamide, and cisplatin (doses as per germ cell regimen)

Single agents: taxanes, platinum and vinca analog, topoisomerase I inhibitors, ifosfamide, gemcitabine[33]

[a]Requires normal renal and bone marrow function and no stomatitis.

disease that had previously resulted in the death of 60% of patients with disease confined to the uterus and 90% of patients with metastatic disease heralded the era of modern chemotherapy.[25] The current challenges are to provide the proper follow-up after evacuation of hydatidiform moles, to balance drug administration with surgical interventions when more invasive trophoblastic disease is present, and finally to tailor the type of chemotherapy to the risk group of gestational trophoblastic disease that has been identified. The scoring system in Table 36.4-1 assists in reaching decisions, but the expertise of a multidisciplinary team cannot be overemphasized. In particular, hysterectomy and single-agent chemotherapy must be considered in stage I disease depending on the patient's desire for future fertility. In this circumstance, chemotherapy reduces dissemination during surgery and treats any occult metastases not previously detected.

The therapeutic regimens for low-risk disease based on the scoring that has been developed have sought to maximize efficacy while minimizing toxicity. As shown in Table 36.4-2, these regimens have consisted of methotrexate by itself or with leucovorin rescue or dactinomycin. Monitoring with β-HCG to document a prompt 1 log or greater reduction in the titer in 18 days, along with continued monthly monitoring of negative values for 1 year, is standard practice. In small series, most patients failing to achieve a satisfactory response to methotrexate were adequately treated with dactinomycin[26] or etoposide.[27] Myeloid leukemia and secondary cancers are a concern with etoposide,[28] which is not encouraging for its use in low-risk patients. Therefore, current Gynecologic Oncology Group studies for low-risk disease are comparing methotrexate with dactinomycin and also assessing dactinomycin in patients not responding to methotrexate.

In intermediate- and high-risk patients, combination chemotherapy is the treatment of choice, and the serum EMA-CO (etoposide, dactinomycin, and folinic acid; vincristine and cyclophosphamide) combination (see Table 36.4-2) is most commonly used. This combination was introduced after recognition of the activity of etoposide, even after failure of other drug regimens, including those for low risk plus cyclophosphamide, vincristine, doxorubicin, hydroxyurea, and 5-fluorouracil.[24] The Gynecologic Oncology Group has used a combination of methotrexate, dactinomycin, and chlorambucil (MAC) with excellent results in intermediate risk patients.[29] Familiarity with one regimen ensures greater safety and proper application.

Results with EMA-CO are excellent in intermediate risk and most high-risk disease patients.[24] However, approximately 20% of patients, predominantly high-risk or intermediate risk who are methotrexate resistant,[30] do not show a complete response. Some of these patients may be salvaged, or could be treated when methotrexate resistance is identified, with regimens containing cisplatin. Deaths from choriocarcinoma usually result either from very late presentations leading to complications such as respiratory failure or central nervous system hemorrhage, or from the development of drug resistance if the tumor burden is excessive at the outset or if treatment has not been sufficiently aggressive. In any event, as for germ cell tumors and other gynecologic cancer, resistance to cisplatin determines an unfavorable outcome. Experimental strategies to overcome such resistance include dose intensification, analog development, and use of new drugs such as taxanes and topoisomerase I inhibitors, although experience is limited.[29] In addition, radiation and surgical resection of metastases may play a role. Specifically, radiation given concomitantly with chemotherapy has been advocated from the outset in patients who have brain metastases to decrease the risk of hemorrhage. A dose of 3000 cGy given over 10 fractions has been found satisfactory.[31]

REFERENCES

1. Buckley JD. The epidemiology of molar pregnancy and choriocarcinoma. *Clin Obstet Gynecol* 1984;27:153.
2. Bagshawe KD, Dent J, Webb J. Hydatidiform mole in England and Wales. 1973–1983. *Lancet* 1986;2:673.
3. Bagshawe KD, Rawlings G, Pike MC, et al. The ABO group in trophoblastic neoplasia. *Lancet* 1971;1:553.
4. Palmer JR, Driscoll SG, Rosenberg L, et al. Oral contraceptive use and risk of gestational trophoblastic tumors. *J Natl Cancer Inst* 1999;91:635.
5. Kurman RJ, Main CS, Chen HC. Intermediate trophoblast: a distinctive form of trophoblast with specific morphological, biochemical, and functional features. *Placenta* 1984;5:349.
6. Steigrad SJ, Cheung AP, Osborn RA. Choriocarcinoma co-existent with an intact pregnancy: case report and review of the literature. *J Obstet Gynaecol Res* 1999;25:197.
7. Schneider D, Halperin R, Segal M, Bukovsky I. Placental-site trophoblastic tumor following metastatic gestational trophoblastic neoplasia. *Gynecol Oncol* 1996;63:267.
8. Wallace DC, Surti U, Adams CW, et al. Complete moles have paternal chromosomes but maternal mitochondrial DNA. *Hum Genet* 1982;61:145.
9. Lawler S, Fisher RA, Dent J. A prospective genetic study of complete and partial hydatidiform moles. *Am J Obstet Gynecol* 1991;164:1270.
10. McFadden DE, Kalousek DK. Two different phenotypes of fetuses with chromosomal triploidy: correlation with parental origin of the extra haploid set. *Am J Med Genet* 1991;38:535.
11. Cross JC, Werb Z, Fisher SJ. Implantation and the placenta: key pieces of the development puzzle. *Science* 1994;266:1508.
12. Roberts DJ, Mutter GL. Advances in the molecular biology of gestational trophoblastic disease. *J Reprod Med* 1994;39:201.
13. Steller MA, Mok SC, Yeh J. Effects of cytokines on epidermal growth factor receptor expression by malignant trophoblast cells *in vitro*. *J Reprod Med* 1994;39:208.
14. Sun Y, Robertson MC, Duckworth ML. The effects of epidermal growth factor/transforming growth factor alpha on the expression of placental lactogen I and II mRNAs in a rat choriocarcinoma cell line. *Endocrinol J* 1998;45:297.
15. Cheung AN, Srivastava G, Chung LP, et al. Expression of the p53 gene in trophoblastic cells in hydatidiform moles and normal human placentas. *J Reprod Med* 1994;39:223.

16. Vaitukaitis JL, Braunstein GID, Ross GT. A radioimmunoassay which specifically measures human chorionic gonadotropin in the presence of human luteinizing hormone. *Am J Obstet Gynecol* 1976;38:453.
17. Goldstein DP. Endocrine assay in chorionic tumors. *Clin Obstet Gynecol* 1978;18:41.
18. Berkowitz RS, Bernstein MR, Laborde O, et al. Subsequent pregnancy experience with gestational trophoblastic disease. New England Trophoblastic Disease Center, 1965–1992. *J Reprod Med* 1994;39:228.
19. Berkowitz RS, Goldstein DP, Bernstein MR. Ten years' experience with methotrexate and folinic acid as primary therapy for gestational trophoblastic disease. *Gynecol Oncol* 1986;23:111.
20. Driscoll SG. Placental site chorioma: the neoplasm of the implantation site trophoblast. *J Reprod Med* 1984;29:821.
21. Koonings PP, Schlaerth JB. CA125: a marker for persistent gestational trophoblastic disease? *Gynecol Oncol* 1993;49:240.
22. Athanassiou A, Begent RHL, Newlands ES, et al. Central nervous system metastases of choriocarcinoma: twenty-three years' experience at Charing Cross Hospital. *Cancer* 1983;52:1728.
23. Kelly MP, Rustin GJS, Ivory C, et al. Respiratory failure due to choriocarcinoma: a study of 103 dyspneic patients. *Gynecol Oncol* 1988;29:199.
24. Bagshawe KD. Treatment of high-risk choriocarcinoma. *J Reprod Med* 1984;29:813.
25. Li MC, Hertz R, Spence DB. Effect of methotrexate therapy upon choriocarcinoma and chorioadenoma. *Proc Soc Exp Biol Med* 1956;93:361.
26. Hoffman MS, Fiorica JV, Gleeson NC, et al. A single institution experience with weekly intramuscular methotrexate for nonmetastatic gestational trophoblastic disease. *Gynecol Oncol* 1996;60:292.
27. Mangili G, Garavaglia E, Frigerio L, et al. Management of low-risk gestational trophoblastic tumors with etoposide (VP16) in patients resistant to methotrexate. *Gynecol Oncol* 1996;61:218.
28. Soto-Wright V, Goldstein DP, Bernstein MR, Berkowitz RS. The management of gestational trophoblastic tumors with etoposide, methotrexate, and actinomycin D. *Gynecol Oncol* 1997;64:156.
29. Curry SL, Blessing JA, DiSaia PJ, et al. A prospective randomized comparison of methotrexate, dactinomycin and chlorambucil versus methotrexate, dactinomycin, cyclophosphamide doxorubicin, melphalan, hydroxyurea and vincristine in "poor prognosis" metastatic gestational trophoblastic disease: a Gynecologic Oncology Group study. *Obstet Gynecol* 1989;73:357.
30. Kim SJ, Bae SN, Kim JH, et al. Risk factors for the prediction of treatment failure in gestational trophoblastic tumors treated with EMA/CO regimen. *Gynecol Oncol* 1998;71:247.
31. Yordan EL Jr, Schlaerth JB, Gaddis O, et al. Radiation therapy in the management of gestational choriocarcinoma metastatic to the central nervous system. *Obstet Gynecol* 1987;69:627.
32. Li-Pai C, Shu-No C, Jian-Xuan F, et al. PEBA regimen (cisplatin, etoposide, bleomycin, and Adriamycin) in the treatment of drug-resistant choriocarcinoma. *Gynecol Oncol* 1995;56:231.
33. Sutton GP, Soper JT, Blessing JA, et al. Ifosfamide alone and in combination in the treatment of refractory malignant gestational trophoblastic disease. *Am J Obstet Gynecol* 1992;167:489.

ROBERT F. OZOLS
PETER E. SCHWARTZ
PATRICIA J. EIFEL

SECTION **5**

Ovarian Cancer, Fallopian Tube Carcinoma, and Peritoneal Carcinoma

OVARIAN CANCER

On the basis of distinct clinical and pathologic features, ovarian carcinomas can be separated into three major entities: epithelial carcinomas, germ cell tumors, and stromal carcinomas. The vast majority of ovarian carcinomas are epithelial in origin, accounting for more than 90% of the estimated 25,200 new cases of ovarian cancer diagnosed in 1999 in the United States.[1] Fallopian tube carcinomas and extraovarian peritoneal carcinomas are much less common, but because of marked similarities to ovarian epithelial carcinomas in their biology and clinical presentation, these tumors also are considered in this chapter. Approximately 14,500 women died in the United States of ovarian cancer in 1999, making this tumor the leading cause of death from a gynecologic cancer.[1] Overall, ovarian cancer accounts for 4% of all cancer diagnoses and 5% of all cancer deaths. The lifetime risk of further development of ovarian cancer is approximately 1.5%, and 1 woman in 100 will die of the disease.[2]

The vast majority of epithelial ovarian carcinomas are diagnosed in postmenopausal women, and the median age at diagnosis is 63 years. The age-specific incidence increases from 15 to 16 per 100,000 in the 40 to 44 age group to a peak rate of 57 per 100,000 in the 70 to 74 age group.[3] Since the late 1970s, there has been little change in incidence or mortality rates.[4] However, a statistically significant increase in 5-year survival rates has been seen—36% in 1970 versus 50% in 1994.[1] This improvement in survival is likely the result of more effective platinum-based chemotherapy and improvements in surgery and supportive care. African American women in the United States have a lower incidence (10.3 per 100,000 women) compared with white women,[5] and the stage-specific 5-year survival rates for white and African American women are similar: localized disease, 96% versus 91%; regional, 80% versus 78%; and advanced disease, 28% versus 24%, respectively.[1]

The biology and carcinogenesis of ovarian cancer is detailed elsewhere in this text (see Chapter 36.1). Hormonal, environmental, and genetic factors all have been identified as playing an important role in the development of ovarian cancer.

A family history is the single most important risk factor for the development of ovarian cancer. However, the vast majority of ovarian cancers are sporadic in nature. Fewer than 10% of cases can be defined as hereditary ovarian cancer (at least two first-degree relatives with ovarian cancer) in which predisposition for the disease follows a classic pattern of autosomal dominant transmission with a variable degree of penetrance. Two distinct clinical syndromes associated with hereditary ovarian cancer have been identified in which there is a germline inheritance of a mutant gene that is transmitted in an autosomal dominant manner and leads to increased susceptibility to ovarian cancer. The hereditary breast-ovarian cancer syndrome (HBOC) is the most common of these and accounts for 85% to 90% of all hereditary ovarian cancer cases currently identified.[5] The majority of these tumors are associated with mutations of the BRCA1 locus, in which more than 100 mutations have been thus far identified. A second breast-ovarian cancer susceptibility gene, BRCA2, has been localized to chromosome 13q12.[6] BRCA2 shares structural and functional similarities with BRCA1 and also appears to be involved in cell progression and cell differentiation.

Initial family pedigree studies revealed multiple cases of ovarian cancer without any increase in breast cancer, and this finding led to the possibility of a site-specific form of ovarian cancer.[7] However, linkage studies have failed to identify additional loci other than BRCA1, which suggests site-specific manifestation is not a distinct hereditary syndrome but rather represents a variant of HBOC in which early-onset breast cancer is infrequent.[5] It also has been demonstrated that hereditary ovarian cancer is a component of the hereditary nonpolyposis colorectal cancer syndrome (HNPCC).[8] HNPCC is an autosomal dominant genetic syndrome that is also known as *Lynch syndrome II*.[9]

Ovarian cancer associated with germline mutations of BRCA1 appears to present with distinct clinical and pathologic features compared with sporadic ovarian cancer.[10] The vast majority of BRCA1-associated cancers are serous adenocarcinomas, with an average age at diagnosis of 48 years. BRCA1-associated cancer may have a more favorable course than sporadic ovarian cancer. In a study by Rubin et al.[10] they reported a median survival of 77 months in 43 patients with advanced BRCA1-associated disease compared with 29 months for matched controls. These results have been confirmed in some, but not all, retrospective studies. A large prospective study is currently in progress by the Gynecologic Oncology Group (GOG) to compare the clinical course of sporadic ovarian cancer with that associated with BRCA1 and BRCA2 mutations.

Close surveillance and screening with transvaginal sonography is frequently used in women at high risk for hereditary ovarian cancer, although there is no evidence yet that such an approach decreases mortality.[11] The National Institutes of Health Consensus Development Panel has recommended that prophylactic oophorectomy be strongly considered in women with hereditary ovarian cancer at age 35 years or after childbearing is completed. However, an increased risk remains for peritoneal carcinomatosis in women with hereditary ovarian cancer, which persists after prophylactic oophorectomy. Oral contraceptives, however, may reduce the risk of ovarian cancer in women with mutations in the BRCA1 or BRCA2 gene. Narod et al.[12] demonstrated that use of oral contraceptives for 6 or more years is associated with a 60% reduction in risk in a study of 207 women with hereditary ovarian cancer with 161 of their sisters as controls. These data strongly suggest that oral contraceptive use should be considered in the prevention of cancer in women with BRCA1 or BRCA2 mutations. In addition, it is essential that patient education and counseling by trained geneticists be part of any risk-assessment program.

PATHOGENESIS

The common epithelial tumors account for 60% of all ovarian neoplasms and for 80% to 90% of ovarian malignancies. The remaining tumors arise from germ or stromal cells. The epithelial tumors arise from the surface epithelium, or serosa, of the ovary. During embryogenesis, the lining of the celomic cavity consists of mesothelial cells of mesodermal origin, and the gonadal ridge is covered by serosal epithelium. Müllerian ducts, which give rise to the fallopian tubes, uterus, and vagina, are the result of invagination of the mesothelial lining. When the epithelium becomes malignant, it can express a variety of Müllerian-type differentiations. Serous carcinomas can resemble the fallopian tube, mucinous tumors the endocervix, endometrioid carcinomas the endometrium, and clear cell tumors can resemble endometrial glands occurring in pregnancy. It is thought that germ cell tumors originate in a primitive streak and can migrate to the gonads. The mesenchyma gives rise to the ovarian stroma, and stromal tumors arise from this cell type.

The most common form of dissemination of epithelial tumors throughout the peritoneal cavity is by exfoliation of malignant cells through the surface of the ovarian capsule. The circulation of the peritoneal fluid to the undersurface of the right hemidiaphragm facilitates the widespread dissemination of malignant tumor cells. All intraperitoneal surfaces are at risk. In addition, the omentum is a frequent site of tumor growth. Tumor spread also occurs via the lymphatics from the ovary. A primary source of drainage follows the ovarian blood supply in the infundibulopelvic ligament to lymph nodes around the aorta and vena cava to the level of the renal vessels. There is also lymphatic drainage through the broad ligament and parametrial channels; consequently, pelvic sidewall lymphatics, including the external iliac, obturator, and hypergastric chains, are also frequent sites of lymphatic metastases from ovarian primary tumors. More rarely, spread may occur along the course of the round ligament, resulting in involvement of inguinal lymph nodes. Spread to lymph node is common, and approximately 10% of patients with ovarian cancer that appears to be localized to the ovaries have metastases to paraaortic lymph nodes. Retroperitoneal lymph node involvement is found in the majority of cases of advanced ovarian cancer when the disease has spread throughout the peritoneal cavity.

The dissemination of ovarian cancer can be clinically occult. As is described later in the section Staging, surgical staging requires meticulous histologic examination of visually normal tissues throughout the peritoneal cavity because microscopic disease frequently is detected in the undersurfaces of the diaphragm and other peritoneal sites. Hematogenous metastases to extraabdominal sites can occur but is uncommon. There can be direct extension of the tumor from the ovary to involve the peritoneal surfaces of the bladder, rectosigmoid, and pelvic peritoneum.

HISTOLOGIC CLASSIFICATION OF EPITHELIAL TUMORS

Table 36.5-1 details the classification of common epithelial tumors that has been developed by the World Health Organization and the International Federation of Gynecology and Obstetrics.[13] The nomenclature for these tumors reflects the cell type, location of the tumor, and degree of malignancy, ranging from benign epithelial tumors to tumors of low malignant potential to invasive carcinomas. Tumors of low malignant potential ("borderline malignancy") have an excellent prognosis compared with invasive carcinomas, and their clinical behavior and management is described later in the section Borderline Tumors. Tumors of low malignant potential are characterized by epithelial papillae with atypical cell clusters, cellular stratification, nuclear atypia, and increased mitotic activity. The differentiation between these tumors and carcinomas is primarily made on the architectural basis of invasion. Frankly malignant tumors are characterized by an infiltrative destructive growth pattern, with malignant cells growing in a disorganized pattern and dissection into stromal planes.

The invasive epithelial carcinomas are characterized by histologic type and grade (the degree of cellular differentiation). The histologic type has limited prognostic significance independent of clinical stage. Histologic grade is an important independent prognostic factor in patients with early-stage epithelial tumors. Grading systems have been based on cytologic detail or a pattern grading classification based on the degree to which a tumor forms papillary structures or glands versus solid tumor. The relative prognostic value of histologic subtype and grade compared with other surgical and biologic factors is discussed in the section Prognostic Factors.

DIAGNOSIS AND SYMPTOMS

Epithelial cancers of the ovary have been described as a silent killer because the overwhelming majority of patients present with disease that has spread outside of the ovary and indeed outside of the pelvis at the time of initial presentation. Approx-

TABLE 36.5-1. World Health Organization Classification of Malignant Ovarian Tumors

COMMON EPITHELIAL TUMORS
Malignant serous tumor
Adenocarcinoma, papillary adenocarcinoma, papillary cystadenocarcinoma
Surface papillary carcinoma
Malignant adenofibroma, cystadenofibroma
Malignant mucinous tumor
Adenocarcinoma, cystadenocarcinoma
Malignant adenofibroma, cystadenofibroma
Malignant endometrioid tumor
Carcinoma
Adenocarcinoma
Adenoacanthoma
Malignant adenofibroma, cystadenofibroma
Endometrioid stromal sarcoma
Mesodermal (Müllerian) mixed tumor: homologous and heterologous
Clear cell (mesonephroid) tumor, malignant
Carcinoma and adenocarcinoma
Brenner tumor, malignant
Mixed epithelial tumor, malignant
Undifferentiated carcinoma
Unclassified
SEX CORD–STROMAL TUMORS
Granulosa-stromal cell tumor
Granulosa cell tumor
Tumor in the thecoma-fibroma group
Fibroma
Unclassified
Androblastoma: Sertoli-Leydig cell tumor
Well differentiated
Tubular androblastoma, Sertoli cell tumor (tubular adenoma of Pick)
Tubular androblastoma with lipid storage, Sertoli cell tumor with lipid storage
Sertoli-Leydig cell tumor (tubular adenoma with Leydig cells)
Leydig cell tumor, hilus cell tumor
Of intermediate differentiation
Poorly differentiated (sarcomatoid)
With heterologous elements
Gynandroblastoma
Unclassified
Germ cell tumor
Dysgerminoma
Endodermal sinus tumor
Embryonal carcinoma
Polyembryoma
LIPID (LIPOID) CELL TUMORS
Choriocarcinoma
Teratoma
Immature
Mature dermoid cyst with malignant transformation
Monodermal and highly specialized
Struma ovarii
Carcinoid
Struma ovarii and carcinoid
Others
Mixed forms
GONADOBLASTOMA
Pure
Mixed with dysgerminoma or other form of germ cell tumor

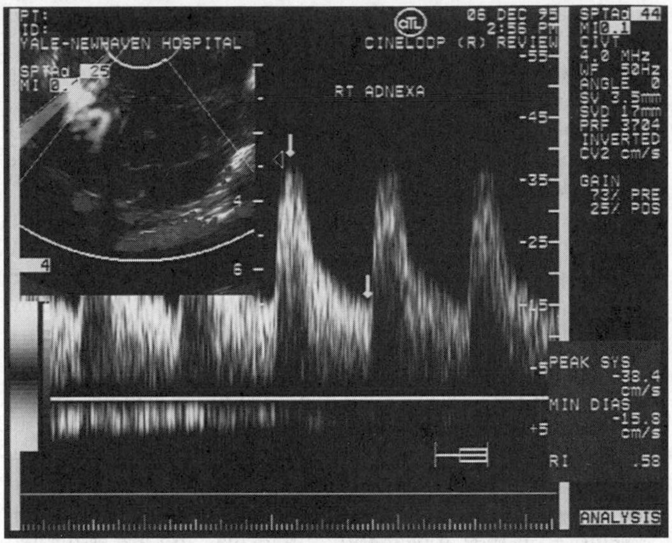

FIGURE 36.5-1. Endovaginal ultrasound with color Doppler flow studies demonstrating an epithelial ovarian cancer. (Courtesy of Dr. Kenneth J. W. Taylor.) (See Color Fig. 36.5-1 in the CD-ROM and on the Web at www.LWWoncology.com.)

imately 70% of patients with epithelial cancers of the ovary present with stage III or IV disease, whereas 70% of patients with germ cell ovarian malignancies present with stage I disease.[11] Unlike epithelial cancers, ovarian germ cell malignancies tend to stretch and twist the infundibulopelvic ligament, causing severe pain while the disease is still confined to the ovary. Functioning ovarian tumors of the sex cord–stromal type may present with symptoms suggestive of excessive endogenous estrogen or androgen production. Granulosa cell tumors occurring in premenarchal women present with precocious puberty. Women in the reproductive years with granulosa cell tumors present with amenorrhea, and postmenopausal women may present with postmenopausal bleeding. Sertoli-Leydig cell tumors may present with symptoms of virilization.

Abdominal discomfort and bloating are the most common symptoms experienced by women with epithelial ovarian cancers, followed by vaginal bleeding, gastrointestinal symptoms, and urinary tract symptoms. Patients presenting with nonspecific lower abdominal discomfort and bloating require a prompt and careful pelvic examination. Not performing routine rectovaginal pelvic examinations may result in women with relatively early-stage ovarian cancer having a delay in diagnosis. Papanicolaou smear screening is inadequate for identifying ovarian cancer, although 1% to 2% of women seen at the Yale–New Haven Medical Center with ovarian cancer have an abnormality on their Papanicolaou smear suggesting the presence of an adenocarcinoma not of cervical origin.

Barber and Graber[15] have recommended that a palpable ovary in a postmenopausal woman is an indication for surgery. This report in 1971 predated the modern era of ultrasound technology. The identification of an adnexal mass on routine pelvic examination is now an indication for diagnostic ultrasound evaluation. Advances in endovaginal ultrasound and color Doppler flow techniques have resulted in identifying characteristics of pelvic masses that either make them highly suggestive to be benign or highly suggestive for malignancy (Fig. 36.5-1). Morphology indices have been developed to indicate the likelihood of pelvic masses being malignant. Kurjak et al.[16] has reported that particular color Doppler flow patterns and resistive indices

are characteristic of malignant pelvic masses. Taylor and Schwartz[17] have presented data suggesting that resistive indices and pulsatility indices are not always effective in distinguishing benign masses from pelvic masses. As a general rule, an adnexal mass suspicious for malignancy by ultrasound morphology criteria is probably the best technique available short of biopsying the mass to identify which masses are most likely malignant.

The most common complaints associated with ovarian malignancies in the pediatric population are pain, abdominal swelling, and pelvic mass. Ovarian masses in premenarchal women require prompt evaluation and an exploratory laparotomy, because functional cysts do not occur in this group. Most premenarchal women with adnexal masses have benign disease.

Small ovarian cysts are often identified with use of ultrasound examinations of postmenopausal ovaries. Approximately 8% to 9% of postmenopausal women who do not have clinically palpable ovaries are found by ultrasound examination to have ovarian cysts between 1.5 to 3.0 cm in size.[18] These cysts do not need to be removed if they appear to be unilocular and are associated with a normal level of CA-125 and normal color Doppler flow studies. Postmenopausal women with complex pelvic masses, simple cysts in association with elevated serum CA-125 levels, or simple cysts in association with abnormal color Doppler flow studies should undergo prompt surgery.

Enlarged ovaries in reproductive-age women are relatively common and frequently are due to either functioning ovarian cysts, such as endometriomas and corpus luteum cysts, or to benign ovarian cysts. Women found to have such cysts are evaluated with serum CA-125 levels. CA-125 levels are often elevated in such patients and can be misleading if one uses the standard cutoff of 35 U/mL to distinguish benign cysts from malignancy in menstruating women. Studies suggest that a CA-125 cutoff from 65 to 200 U/mL is necessary to distinguish benign cysts from malignant cysts in premenopausal women.[19]

Cysts that appear by ultrasound criteria to be functional in nature may be followed through several menstrual cycles. Often they disappear over this short observation interval. Functional cysts may also disappear when oral contraceptives are used. Neoplastic cysts do not disappear under the influence of oral contraceptives. Rising values of serial CA-125 assays obtained during the observation period are an indication that a malignancy may be present. In turn, CA-125 values that are stable or declining generally reflect the presence of a functional cyst. CA-125 assays should always be obtained when a woman is not actively menstruating, because menses have been associated with marked elevation of serum CA-125.

Computed tomographic (CT) scans are useful in preoperatively evaluating the extent of disease when a pelvic mass is present. CT scans are most useful when combined with oral and intravenous contrast. They allow assessment of retroperitoneal lymph nodes in the paraaortic area and the identification of intraperitoneal and mesenteric implants.

Diagnostic laparoscopy is now being used for evaluation of unexplained pelvic pain and small adnexal masses. The difficulty with the laparoscopic approach to the evaluation of pelvic masses is rupturing a malignant tumor. In general, if a stage IA ovarian tumor can be removed intact, there is little evidence that additional therapy has a major impact on survival. Survival in this situation is extremely good. However, once an ovarian malignancy has been ruptured, patients are treated with either radiation therapy or cytotoxic chemotherapy.[20] Both treatment modalities carry with them physical as well as psychological trauma. Although there is no solid evidence that rupture of an early-stage ovarian malignancy decreases survival, avoidance of rupture of an ovarian neoplasm should be the routine method of approaching ovarian masses suspicious for malignancy.

Another technique for the diagnosis of ovarian cancer is peritoneal cytology. Aspiration of obvious ascites for cytologic assessment is routinely performed to identify malignant cells. If no ascites is present, saline may be instilled percutaneously or through the vaginal apex to flush the abdominal cavity and pelvis. The fluid is then withdrawn and sent for cytologic assessment. This diagnostic technique is quite uncomfortable for the patient and has been associated with poor patient acceptance and high false-positive results. Culdocentesis is not routinely used in the United States for the evaluation of a woman with possible ovarian cancer.

Serum CA-125 is the gold standard for tumor markers in the evaluation of pelvic masses, particularly epithelial ovarian cancers. Serum α-fetoprotein (AFP) and human chorionic gonadotropin (HCG) have been helpful in recognizing preoperatively the presence of an endodermal sinus tumor, embryonal carcinoma, choriocarcinoma, or mixed germ cell tumor.[14] However, most young women with these diseases are not recognized preoperatively to have a malignancy. Levels of AFP and HCG are best applied in serially monitoring the effectiveness of therapy. Failure to identify preoperatively elevations of these markers does not preclude one from using them postoperatively in determining efficacy and duration of treatment for these diseases.[14]

In summary, a woman suspected of having ovarian cancer requires a preoperative workup that should include a CT scan to evaluate the extent of disease in both the pelvis and the upper abdomen and to rule out occult alternative primary sites for the origin of the disease, such as the pancreas. A serum CA-125 measurement is useful because 80% of women with advanced ovarian cancer have elevations of CA-125. The marker may be used as a secondary support for ovarian cancer being present preoperatively, and it may be used postoperatively to confirm the effectiveness of therapy. Radiologic studies of the upper intestinal tract as well as the lower tract are not routinely recommended unless the patient is having symptoms related to the intestinal tract. A barium enema or Hypaque enema can be very helpful in determining whether there is compromise of the sigmoid colon lumen in women with obstructive symptoms.

Patients with a preoperative evaluation consistent with the diagnosis of ovarian cancer would do best if referred to a gynecologic oncologist. Survival data suggests that those patients operated on by gynecologic oncologists for early-stage and late-stage disease do better in terms of progression-free and overall survival, at least in part because of more aggressive cytoreductive surgery performed by gynecologic oncologists and more appropriate surgical staging of the patient before initiating treatment.

STAGING

Ovarian cancer is a surgically staged disease. Thus, it is important for physicians to be thoroughly familiar with the International Federation of Gynecologists and Obstetricians (FIGO) staging system for primary carcinomas of the ovary[21] (Table 36.5-2). As described earlier in the section Pathogenesis, ovarian cancer spreads by direct extension to neighboring organs by exfoliating cells into the peritoneal cavity that can implant

TABLE 36.5-2. International Federation of Gynecologists and Obstetricians Stage Grouping for Primary Carcinoma of the Ovary (1998)

Stage	*Description*
I	Growth limited to the ovaries.
IA	Growth limited to one ovary; no ascites. No tumor on the external surface; capsule intact.
IB	Growth limited to both ovaries; no ascites. No tumor on the external surface; capsule intact.
IC[a]	Tumor either stage IA or IB but with tumor on the surface of one or both ovaries, or with capsule ruptured, or with ascites present containing malignant cells, or with positive peritoneal washings.
II	Growth involving one or both ovaries with pelvic extension.
IIA	Extension and/or metastases to the uterus and/or tubes.
IIB	Growth involving one or both ovaries with pelvic extension.
IIC[a]	Tumor either stage IIA or IIB but with tumor on the surface of one or both ovaries, or with capsule(s) ruptured, or with ascites present containing malignant cells, or with positive peritoneal washings.
III	Tumor involving one or both ovaries with peritoneal implants outside the pelvis and/or positive retroperitoneal or inguinal nodes. Superficial liver metastases equals stage III. Tumor is limited to the true pelvis but with histologically verified malignant extension to small bowel or omentum.
IIIA	Tumor grossly limited to the true pelvis with negative nodes but with histologically confirmed microscopic seeding of abdominal peritoneal surfaces.
IIIB	Tumor of one or both ovaries with histologically confirmed implants of abdominal peritoneal surfaces, none exceeding 2 cm in diameter. Nodes negative.
IIIC	Abdominal implants greater than 2 cm in diameter and/or positive retroperitoneal or inguinal nodes.
IV	Growth involving one or both ovaries with distant metastasis. If pleural effusion is present, cytologic test results must be positive to allot a case to stage IV. Parenchymal liver metastasis equals stage IV.

[a] To evaluate the impact on prognosis of the different criteria for allotting cases to stage IC or IIC, it is of value to know if rupture of the capsule was spontaneous or caused by the surgeon, and if the source of malignant cells detected was peritoneal washings or ascites.

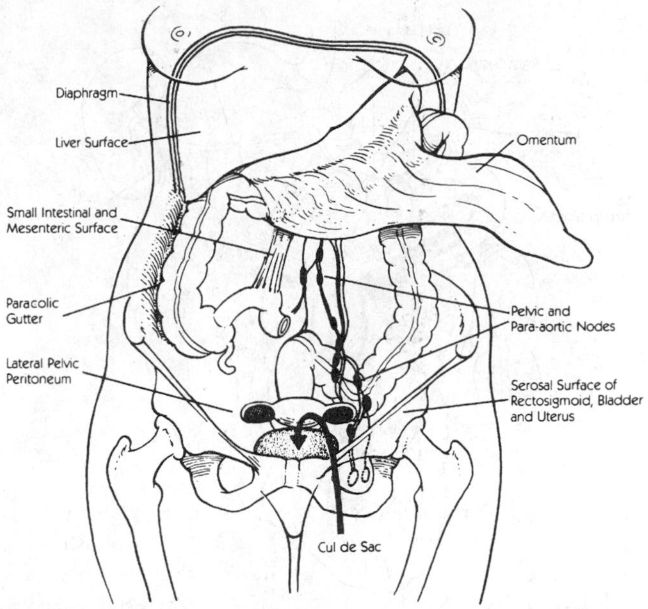

FIGURE 36.5-2. Ovarian cancer spread pattern. (From Young RC, Perez CA, Hoskins WV. Cancer of the ovary. In: DeVita VT Jr, Hellman S, Rosenberg SA, eds. *Cancer: principles and practice of oncology*, 4th ed. Philadelphia: JB Lippincott Co, 1993:1226, with permission.)

on parietal and visceral peritoneum throughout the peritoneal cavity. It also disseminates by lymphatic spread, particularly to the pelvic sidewall lymph nodes (external iliac and obturator chains) and along the gonadal vessels to the upper common iliac and paraaortic lymph node chains (Fig. 36.5-2). Surgical staging procedures must evaluate sites to which ovarian cancer is likely to spread.

Complete surgical staging is a necessity to properly evaluate the patient and to determine whether additional therapy should be recommended. Proper surgical staging requires that a vertical incision be used that extends from the pelvis into the upper abdomen. Subumbilical incisions do not allow the surgeon to perform complete surgical staging. On entering the peritoneal cavity, any fluid present should be aspirated and sent for cytologic studies. Peritoneal fluid, even if limited to the pelvis, is more likely to yield malignant cells than are cytologic washings.[22] If no fluid is present, however, one should routinely irrigate the pelvis and paracolic spaces with normal saline. The fluid is then aspirated and sent to the cytology lab for evaluation. Careful inspection of the abdominal cavity should then be performed. Adhesions should be lysed to restore normal anatomy. Samples of the adhesions should be sent for microscopic evaluation.

If intraperitoneal carcinomatosis is not present, it is most appropriate to first resect the ovarian tumor and then to proceed with surgical staging. For women who are operated on for a tumor seemingly limited to one ovary, if preservation of fertility is an issue, the grossly normal opposite ovary should be biopsied or any implants on the ovarian surface should be excised. Preservation of fertility should be considered in any women of reproductive age with either a borderline malignant tumor of the ovary or an invasive epithelial cancer grossly confined to one ovary. A frozen section assessment of any abnormality involving the contralateral ovary helps guide the surgeon in determining whether to remove that ovary. Samples of pelvic peritoneum from the area of the ipsilateral infundibulopelvic and round ligaments, the cul-de-sac of Douglas, and urinary bladder are obtained. Pelvic retroperitoneal lymph nodes are removed in all patients with unilateral tumors. Patients in whom bilateral disease is suspected undergo bilateral pelvic lymph node sampling. Any enlarged pelvic retroperitoneal lymph nodes are removed, regardless of their locations. Lymphadenectomy is an important part of staging ovarian cancers, particularly when the disease is grossly limited to one ovary. In this situation, up to 20% of women have been found to have paraaortic lymph node metastases.[23]

The vertical incision is then extended to assess disease in the upper abdomen. If gross disease is not present in the omentum, an intracolic omentectomy is sufficient for diagnostic purposes. When disease is present in the omentum, the omentum should be excised from the greater curvature of the

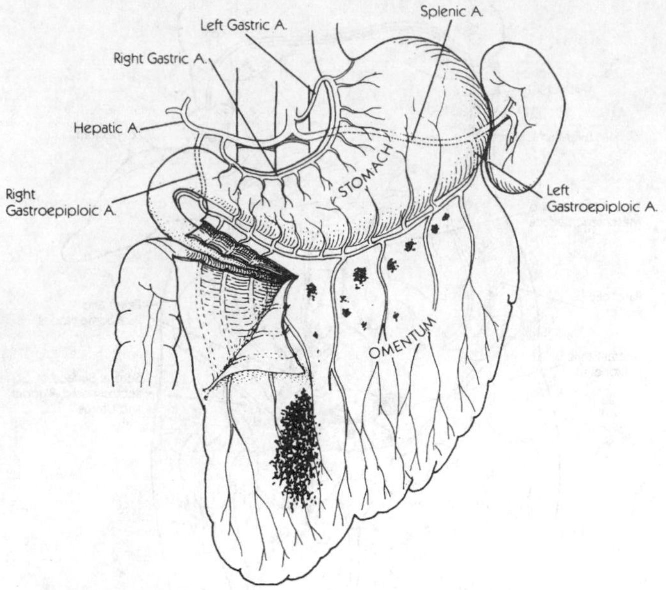

FIGURE 36.5-3. Excising omentum off stomach. A, artery. (From Young RC, Perez CA, Hoskins WV. Cancer of the ovary. In: DeVita VT Jr, Hellman S, Rosenberg SA, eds. *Cancer: principles and practice of oncology*, 4th ed. Philadelphia: JB Lippincott Co, 1993:1226, with permission.)

stomach (Fig. 36.5-3). The upper abdominal evaluation continues with a careful inspection of the right hemidiaphragm, liver serosa, and parenchyma. If no disease is visually present, a 1 cm × 2 cm piece of peritoneum is excised off of the suprahepatic diaphragm, care being given not to remove underlying musculature and create a pneumothorax. The spleen is then carefully inspected, as is the left diaphragm. The paracolic spaces are then evaluated, and large strips of peritoneum (3 cm × 5 cm) are removed from the left and right paracolic spaces if no obvious disease is present. The large bowel is then carefully inspected. The small intestine is evaluated, and any implants present on bowel or its mesentery are removed. The colon, either the ascending or the descending colon, is then mobilized to expose the paraaortic area. If the peritoneal cavity has been freed of bulky tumor such that the maximum residual tumor is less than 1 cm in stage III patients, retroperitoneal lymph nodes are removed by taking the fat pad from the upper half of the common iliac artery up to the level of the renal vessels. However, if bulky residual disease (greater than 1 cm) is left in the upper abdomen, there is no role for paraaortic lymphadenectomy.[24] An international prospective randomized trial is now being conducted to determine the role of systematic pelvic and paraaortic lymphadenectomy for advanced ovarian cancer in women with 1 cm or smaller intraperitoneal residual tumor.[25] In postmenopausal women or women in whom fertility is no longer desired, one should routinely perform a bilateral salpingo-oophorectomy and total abdominal hysterectomy. The hysterectomy is performed because the serosal surface of the uterus is a large peritoneal surface for implantation of malignant cells. In addition, field effects may be present whereby the epithelium of the fallopian tubes or uterus are involved with premalignant or malignant processes. The latter changes cannot be grossly recognized at the time of surgery.

POSTSURGICAL STAGING

Understaging occurs rather frequently at the time of the initial surgery for ovarian malignancies, especially when the preoperative diagnosis is that of a benign process. This leads to use of inappropriate incisions that does not allow complete surgical staging when the diagnosis of a malignancy is recognized intraoperatively. At other times, it is due to a lack of familiarity with commonly accepted surgical staging procedures.

The issue of the inadequately staged early-stage patient with ovarian cancer is a difficult one. The simplest solution for such patients is to subject them to a properly performed staging laparotomy performed by a gynecologic oncologist. However, if this is not possible or practical, an alternative is to obtain a CT scan and a CA-125. If the CT scan and CA-125 are normal and the tumor was one of low malignant potential, no further therapy is recommended at the Yale–New Haven Medical Center. If the tumor is an invasive epithelial malignancy, we would consider giving single-agent chemotherapy, such as carboplatin, to such a patient. However, no prospective randomized series of patients have been reported using this approach. If the CT scan is positive, a surgical procedure to remove gross disease should be performed.

Postoperative reevaluation by laparotomy or laparoscopy has been advocated by some authors.[26] Earlier laparoscopic surgical staging papers revealed that as much as 30% to 40% of patients originally thought to have FIGO stage I or II disease actually had disease in the upper abdomen.[26] Complications as a result of earlier laparoscopic procedures had been relatively limited and included pneumothorax, bleeding requiring transfusions, wound infections, and hypotension.[26] More recently, more thorough laparoscopic techniques have been described that allow for paraaortic lymph node dissections and omentectomies.[27] As the degree of the aggressiveness of laparoscopic surgical procedures advances, the complications become more significant.

SCREENING

Successful screening for ovarian cancer, by definition, would decrease mortality and morbidity from the disease. With currently available tests, routine screening for ovarian cancer cannot be recommended. Successful screening for any malignancy requires detection either at a time when the disease is in its early stages or in a precancerous stage without invasive features. Although the patterns of spread of ovarian cancer have been well defined, the precise natural history is poorly understood. It has not been established that untreated stage I routinely progresses to more advanced stages. Even if an orderly progression from stage I to stage IV takes place, the time frame for such a progression remains to be established. The entire peritoneum is at risk because peritoneal carcinomatosis may develop after an oophorectomy. Furthermore, the syndrome of extraovarian peritoneal carcinomatosis is characterized by widespread intraperitoneal epithelial carcinoma in the presence of histologically normal ovaries. In addition, there is no direct evidence for a premalignant lesion in ovarian cancer. As noted, no experimental data suggest that an ovarian cyst can progress to a borderline tumor that can, in turn, lead to an invasive carcinoma.

The primary reason that screening is not recommended, however, is because the currently available screening techniques (ovarian palpation, transvaginal ultrasound, and serum

CA-125 determinations) are not sufficiently accurate for general screening. These tests have been limited by their sensitivity and specificity. Because a laparotomy is required to diagnose ovarian cancer, the positive predictive value (PPV) for screening is the primary consideration due to the cost, morbidity, and even mortality associated with unnecessary laparotomies for a false-positive screening test.[28] The PPV is defined as the ratio of a true-positive test (laparotomy) to true-positive plus false-positives. Most investigators think that the PPV of a laparotomy should be at least 10%.[29]

Whereas pelvic examinations continue to be routinely recommended for women, ovarian palpation has not been established as a useful screening procedure. Most screening studies have used either serum tumor markers or ultrasonography or both. Although serum CA-125 levels correlate with progression or regression of established disease[29] and are also useful in the preoperative evaluation of a pelvic mass, the test does not have sufficient specificity to be used as a routine screen for ovarian cancer.[28] Besides ovarian cancer, many other conditions can be associated with an elevated CA-125 level, including cirrhosis, peritonitis, pancreatitis, endometriosis, uterine leiomyomata, benign ovarian cysts, and pelvic inflammatory disease.

In a Swedish study,[30] CA-125 levels were measured annually in 550 women older than 40 years. In women with levels greater than 30 U/mL, sequential CA-125 levels were obtained every 3 months, along with pelvic examinations and transabdominal ultrasounds performed every 6 months. In this study, 175 women were found to have elevated CA-125 levels, and six ovarian cancers were detected.

Transvaginal ultrasonography is a more specific alternative to both transabdominal ultrasonography[31] and CA-125 screening. In studies from the University of Kentucky of more than 3000 asymptomatic postmenopausal women, the PPV was less than 10%.[32] In an effort to improve the unacceptably high rate of false-positive results with transvaginal ultrasonography, color Doppler imaging also has been studied in an effort to identify areas of vascularization that are associated with malignancy.[33] However, the addition of color Doppler imaging has not yet been established to improve the overall efficacy of ultrasonographic screening.

Several large screening trials have used a sequential combination of serum CA-125 and ultrasonography. In an English study, 22,000 volunteers without a family history of ovarian cancer underwent screening with serum CA-125 that was followed by abdominal ultrasonography for elevations of greater than 30 U/mL.[34] Women underwent a laparotomy for any detectable ovarian abnormality. In this study, 11 women had ovarian cancer, seven with stage III or IV disease. The PPV was less than 10% for early-stage disease. Table 36.5-3 summarizes the results of uncontrolled trials of ovarian cancer screening in more than 36,000 women.[35] A total of 41 cases of ovarian cancer were identified, but only 12 were in women with stage I disease. In the 29 women who were diagnosed with advanced-stage ovarian cancer, it is unlikely that survival would have been significantly improved by an earlier diagnosis because the disease had already spread throughout the peritoneal cavity. Screening may ultimately be more effective in women with a positive family history of ovarian cancer.[36] At this point, however, no evidence shows that even screening such a high-risk population has an impact on morbidity and mortality.

Several large ovarian cancer screening trials are currently in progress. The National Cancer Institute's Prostate, Lung, Colon, Ovarian Cancer (PLCO) trial compares screening with an annual CA-125 measurement, transvaginal ultrasound, and pelvic examination to usual medical care in 76,000 women aged 60 through 74.[37] The participants in the study will be followed for 10 years. A European multicentric study headquartered at St. Bartholomew's Hospital in London will evaluate 120,000 postmenopausal women randomized to receive no screening or screening with transvaginal ultrasound followed by color flow Doppler examinations in women with abnormal transvaginal ultrasounds. In addition, serial CA-125 levels will be used to determine which participants should go on to the next stage of screening. Studies are also in progress to identify more sensitive tumor markers. Macrophage colony-stimulating factor (M-CSF) has been detected in epithelial ovarian tumors and in 70% of the serum or ascites of patients with diagnosed carcinomas.[38] Serum M-CSF levels, together with CA-125 levels, may be more predictive than CA-125 levels alone. Similarly, OVX-1 is a newly developed antibody that may also complement CA-125.[39] The combination of these two antibodies has been more accurate in predicting the presence of residual disease at second-look surgical procedures. Furthermore, a panel of CA-125, M-CSF, and OVX-1 was shown to identify early-stage ovarian cancer with extremely high sensitivity and moderate specificity in preliminary studies.[40] The levels of these tumor markers and their rate of change over time are being prospectively analyzed to help identify an individual's risk of ovarian cancer. Lysophosphatidic acid, which had previously been shown to be elevated in malignant ascites, may also have utility as a predictive biomarker for ovarian cancer, because an elevated level was found in nine of ten patients with early-stage disease.[41] Additional studies of sensitivity and specificity are in progress.

Inasmuch as screening has not been effective in diagnosing early-stage ovarian cancers, prophylactic oophorectomies have been advocated by some for women in high-risk groups. However, women still are at risk for peritoneal carcinomatosis even after normal ovaries have been removed. A multicenter prospective evaluation of the role of prophylactic oophorectomy in high-risk individuals is in progress. Preliminary results support a protective effect of an oophorectomy, although peritoneal carcinomatosis occurs at a higher rate in this group of women than in the general population.[42] Karlan et al.[43] have reported on the findings of peritoneal serous papillary carcinoma in women at high risk by family history for ovarian cancer. These investigators performed BRCA1 and BRCA2 gene mutation studies on four patients who developed serous carci-

TABLE 36.5-3. Uncontrolled Trials of Ovarian Cancer Screening

Country	*Reference*	*Participants*	*Ovarian Cancers Diagnosed* Stage I	Total
Sweden	30	5550	2	6
United Kingdom	31	5479	5	9
United Kingdom	34	21,959	3	11
United States	32	3220	2	3
Total		**36,208**	**12**	**29**

(From ref. 99, with permission.)

nomas of the peritoneum and found that three of the four had BRCA1 mutations. None of the patients with peritoneal serous papillary carcinomas was recognized before intraabdominal carcinomatosis was evident.[43]

PROGNOSTIC FACTORS

At the conclusion of a comprehensive laparotomy, the clinical findings and the histology are used to select postoperative therapy. In addition, new prognostic factors are being evaluated that may be used to identify groups of patients in whom more specific biologic treatments or more aggressive therapy is indicated.

Clinicopathologic findings determined to be clinically useful include the following:

- FIGO stage
- Histologic subtype
- Histologic grade
- Factors associated with tumor dissemination
- Malignant ascites
- Malignant peritoneal washings
- Tumor excrescences on ovarian surface
- Ruptured capsule
- Dense ovarian adhesions
- Volume of residual disease after cytoreductive surgery

The tumor stage remains the most important prognostic variable. Few trials provide an accurate assessment regarding the long-term survival of patients with early-stage ovarian cancer because earlier studies often included inadequately staged patients. Stage I patients with well- or moderately well–differentiated tumors have a greater than 90% 5-year survival rate.[20] Patients with stage I disease with poor prognostic features are often included in treatment protocols for patients with stage II disease. This group of patients has been termed *early-stage disease with unfavorable characteristics.* However, limited information is available regarding the actual survival impact of some of the factors used to characterize patients as having an unfavorable prognosis. Rupture of the capsule increases the stage to IC. In a Swedish series, however, no adverse effect on survival could be established for early-stage patients in whom the capsule was ruptured during surgery.[44] Furthermore, in contrast to the established adverse effect of malignant ascites, there is limited information regarding the prognostic significance of positive peritoneal cytology. Recently, tumor adherence in the presence of dense adhesions has also been considered an adverse prognostic factor, and such patients should be considered as having stage II disease even in the absence of pathologic confirmation.[45] Tumor size, bilaterality, and cytologically negative ascites have no prognostic significance. The most reliable long-term survival data on accurately staged early-stage ovarian cancer patients is derived from studies of the GOG. In these studies, unfavorable prognosis early-stage ovarian cancer patients have a five-year survival rate of approximately 80%.[20]

Patients with stage III disease have a 5-year survival rate of approximately 15% to 20% that is dependent in large part on the volume of disease present in the upper abdomen. Patients with stage IV disease have less than a 5% 5-year survival.

Volume of residual disease after cytoreductive surgery for patients with advanced ovarian cancer has a significant impact on survival. After the administration of postoperative cisplatin-based combination chemotherapy, 5-year survival rates for patients with optimal stage III disease (defined as no residual nodule greater than 1 cm in diameter) is approximately 35%.[46]

The true prognostic impact of histologic subtype and grade in patients with epithelial ovarian cancer remains to be determined. In patients with early-stage ovarian cancer, grade is an accepted determinant of risk and used to assign postoperative therapy as discussed earlier in the section Management of Early-Stage Disease. Studies have also identified an adverse prognostic effect of clear cell histology in early-stage ovarian cancer.[20,47] In advanced-stage patients, mucinous histology and clear cell histology also have been shown to have an adverse prognostic significance.[47] In a GOG analysis, no negative second-look laparotomies in patients with mucinous or clear cell tumors were performed. Some studies also have demonstrated that histologic grade has an impact on survival in patients with advanced-stage disease.

Serum CA-125 levels frequently reflect the volume of disease and, as such, in multivariate analysis, preoperative levels have not exerted an independent prognostic effect on survival.[48] However, postoperative CA-125 levels were shown to be an independent prognostic variable.[49] Most studies also have demonstrated that serum CA-125 levels after three cycles of chemotherapy are accurate predictors for the probability of a patient achieving a complete remission.[49] However, the CA-125 level after three cycles of chemotherapy cannot be used as a guide for treatment decisions because of the lack of predictive power.

The prognostic significance of age on survival of patients with ovarian cancer has been recognized.[50] Median survival is at least 2 years longer in women younger than age 65 compared with those older than 65.

The prognostic significance of DNA ploidy and S-phase fraction have been examined in ovarian cancer.[51] Investigators in Europe have now included aneuploidy in their selection of high-risk early-stage ovarian cancer patients for adjuvant therapy.[51] Controversy remains, however, as to the nature of the relationship between histologic grade and degree of aneuploidy. In the GOG, aneuploidy has not been included as a criteria for risk in early-stage disease.

A series of new molecular factors have been proposed to have prognostic significance in ovarian cancer (Table 36.5-4).[52–54] These factors include markers of proliferation, drug resistance, serum cytokine levels, growth factor receptors or signal transduction pathways, genes associated with metastases, and oncogene expression. Most of these factors have been identified in retrospective studies without multivariate analysis or confirmation in larger studies. These factors were developed from experimental studies in the biology of ovarian cancer (described in Chapter 36.1). Currently, none of these markers is routinely used to select therapy for patients with ovarian cancer.

MANAGEMENT OF EARLY-STAGE DISEASE

A subset of patients with early-stage ovarian cancer definitely has been shown not to require any additional postoperative therapy after a comprehensive staging laparotomy. Patients with stage IA or IB disease with well- or moderately well–differentiated tumors have a 5-year survival rate of more than 90% without any adjuvant treatment.[20] Patients with favorable prognosis early-stage ovarian cancer (stage IA and IB with grade 1 and 2 tumors) were randomized in an earlier GOG study to receive no treatment or oral intermittent melphalan (0.2 mg/

TABLE 36.5-4. Experimental Prognostic Factors in Ovarian Cancer

Morphometry	
DNA ploidy and S-phase fraction	
Drug resistance markers	
	P glycoprotein immunoreactivity
	Glutathione S-transferase pi
	c-erbB-2
	Multidrug resistance proteins (Lrp)
	Nucleotide excision DNA repair genes ERCC1 and XPAC
	BAX
Oncogene	
	Mutant p53 expression
	AKT-2
Markers of proliferation	
	Ki67
	Proliferating cell nuclear antigen
Markers of tumor spread	
	Metastasis-related genes (nm23-H1)
	Cathepsin D
	Urokinase-type plasminogen activators
	Colony-stimulating factor 1
	CD44 molecules
Cytokine levels and other active proteins	
	Heat-shock protein
	Interleukin-6
	Platelet derived growth factor

kg daily for 5 days) with repeat cycles every 4 to 6 weeks for a total of 12 courses or 18 months of therapy. With a median follow-up of more than 6 years, only six deaths have been reported in 81 patients: four in the observation group and two in patients who received melphalan. Disease-free survival and overall survival is shown in Figure 36.5-4. Patients with favorable prognosis early-stage ovarian cancer can be spared the acute and chronic toxicities of chemotherapy, including myeloproliferative disorders such as leukemia.

The optimum treatment of early-stage ovarian cancer patients with unfavorable prognosis remains an area of controversy. Opinions differ as to not only what modality of treatment should be used (external-beam radiotherapy, intraperitoneal radioisotopes, or chemotherapy) but also with regard to the role of immediate therapy or to delay of treatment until disease progression. Furthermore, as noted, consensus has not been established as to the prognostic significance of some clinicopathologic features, such as positive peritoneal cytologies and a surgically ruptured capsule with contamination of the pelvis with cyst fluid. Clinicopathologic factors currently used by the GOG to define unfavorable prognosis early-stage disease include FIGO stage II and IC, clear cell histology, and grade 3 tumors.

External-Beam Radiotherapy

Although cisplatin- or paclitaxel-containing chemotherapy has become the standard initial treatment for patients with unfavorable prognosis early-stage ovarian cancer in all but a few centers, a number of studies have demonstrated that carefully applied whole abdominal radiotherapy is also a highly effective treatment for some patients.

Early nonrandomized studies suggested that pelvic disease control and survival were improved when patients with early-stage ovarian carcinoma were treated with postoperative pelvic radiation. In particular, patients with stage II disease had consistently better survival rates if the pelvis was treated (Table 36.5-5).[55–62] However, these studies also demonstrated the importance of the coelomic pattern of metastatic spread, which limited the benefit of pelvic irradiation.

On the basis of these findings and encouraging responses of ovarian carcinoma to alkylating agents, investigators at the M. D. Anderson Cancer Center conducted a prospective trial that compared pelvic and whole abdominal irradiation with pelvic irradia-

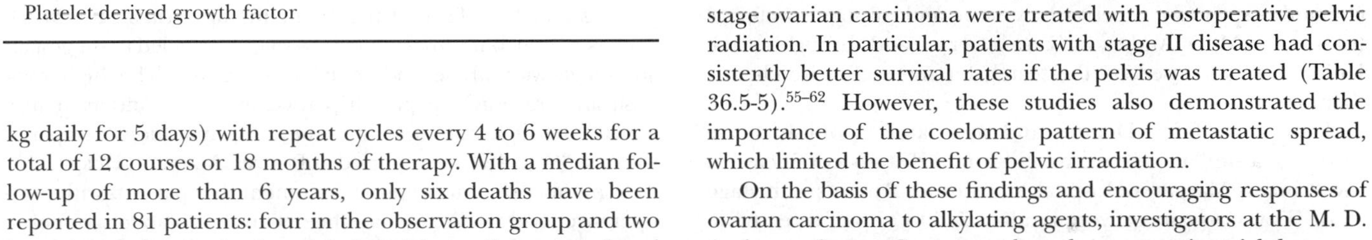

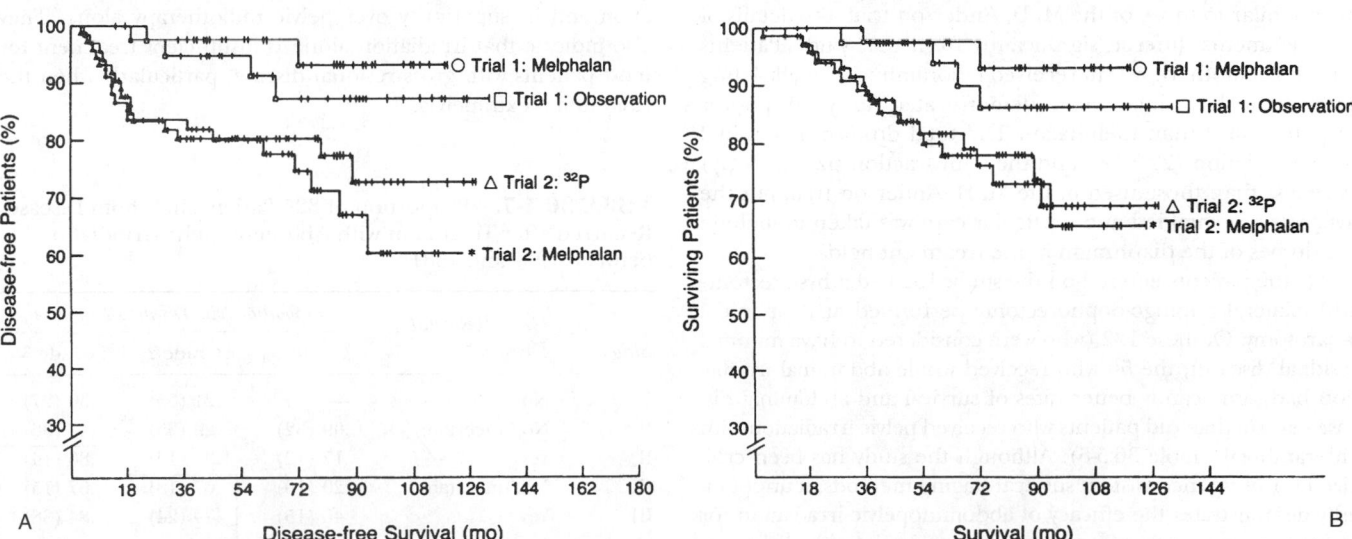

FIGURE 36.5-4. Disease-free (**A**) and overall (**B**) survival of patients with early-stage ovarian cancer. The top two curves represent patients with favorable prognoses randomized to observation or melphalan. The lower two curves represent patients with unfavorable prognoses randomized to either phosphorus 32 or melphalan. (From ref. 20, with permission.)

TABLE 36.5-5. Results of Early Series Comparing Postoperative Pelvic or Lower Abdominal Radiation versus Surgery Alone for Stage II Carcinoma of the Ovary

	Treatment	
Reference	Surgery Alone (%)	Surgery and Radiation (%)
Kent and McKay[59]	9/32 (28)	19/36 (53)
Van Orden[62]	2/8 (25)	8/22 (36)
Ross[61]	1/9 (11)	5/23 (22)
Munnell[60]	0/16	9/29 (31)
Dalley[57]	0/5	7/51 (13)
Barr[55]	9/27 (33)	43/91 (47)
Clark[56]	1/6 (17)	16/51 (31)

(Modified from ref. 58, with permission.)

TABLE 36.5-6. Survival Rates and Relapse Sites for 116 Patients with Stage IB, II, and Asymptomatic III Ovarian Cancer Who Had a Total Hysterectomy and Bilateral Salpingo-Oophorectomy Completed at Initial Operation[a]

	Number of Patients (%)			
		Site of Failure		*4-Y Survival*
Treatment	Total	Pelvis	Abdomen	*Rate*
Pelvic RT[b]	31	8 (27)	8 (27)	50%
Pelvic RT plus chlorambucil	51	10 (20)	13 (25)[c]	55%[d]
Pelvic plus whole abdominal RT	50	11 (22)	0 (0)	81%[d]

RT, radiation therapy.
[a]Princess Margaret Hospital (Toronto) randomized trial.
[b]Stage IB and II only.
[c]$P<.01$.
[d]$P<.02$.
(From ref. 64, with permission.)

tion and single-agent chemotherapy (melphalan).[63] Patients who had stage I to III ovarian carcinomas with less than 2 cm of residual disease after surgery were included. Abdominal treatment was delivered with cobalt (^{60}Co) using the moving strip technique. Each strip was treated with 26 to 28 Gy in 8 to 12 fractions with partial shielding of the liver and kidneys. The authors reported that survival rates were similar for patients treated in the two arms, but the rate of serious bowel complications was higher for patients who received whole abdominal irradiation. It was concluded that chemotherapy was a superior treatment, and subsequent clinical trials at the M. D. Anderson Cancer Center and throughout the United States focused on the search for more effective chemotherapy.

Four years later, Dembo and associates[64] published the results of a similar prospective randomized study conducted at the Princess Margaret Hospital in Toronto. Patients with stage IB or II ovarian cancer were randomized to one of three treatment arms: pelvic irradiation, pelvic plus whole abdominal irradiation, or pelvic irradiation plus single-agent chemotherapy. Patients with "asymptomatic" stage III disease were randomized only between the last two arms. Although the treatment arms were similar to those of the M. D. Anderson trial, the details of the treatments differed significantly from that study. Patients on the chemotherapy arm received chlorambucil, an alkylating agent that has since been demonstrated to yield poorer response rates than melphalan. The total dose of abdominal strip irradiation (22.5 Gy) and the daily fraction size (2.25 Gy) were less than those used in the M. D. Anderson trial, but the liver was not shielded and particular care was taken to include the domes of the diaphragm in the treatment fields.

Of 190 patients entered on the study, 132 had a hysterectomy and bilateral salpingo-oophorectomy performed at their initial laparotomy. Of these 132 (who were considered to have minimal residual disease), the 50 who received whole abdominal irradiation had significantly better rates of survival and abdominal disease control than did patients who received pelvic irradiation with chlorambucil (Table 36.5-6). Although the study has been criticized for using inconsistent surgical staging methods, it undoubtedly demonstrates the efficacy of abdominopelvic irradiation for at least some subsets of patients with minimal residual disease. Subsequent analysis of patients treated at Princess Margaret Hospital demonstrated that patients who had grade 1; stage I or II, grade 2; or stage I or II, grade 3 disease and no gross residual tumor after surgery were most likely to have a prolonged disease-free interval after abdominopelvic irradiation (Table 36.5-7).[65,66]

Differences in the chemotherapy and radiotherapy techniques described above may explain the apparently contradictory results of the two trials. An imbalance in the proportion of stage IA patients may have favored the chemotherapy arm in the M. D. Anderson trial, but subset analysis by stage also failed to suggest an advantage with whole abdominal irradiation.[65] The high total dose and fraction size per strip used at M. D. Anderson may explain the high rate of severe enteric complications compared with the 3% to 4% rate reported at Princess Margaret Hospital.[67]

A number of other reports document that patients with postoperative residual disease have been cured with abdominopelvic irradiation alone; relapse-free survival rates of 40% to 60% at 10 to 15 years have been reported for patients with residual gross disease measuring less than 2 cm (Table 36.5-8).[68–74] Collectively, these studies demonstrate the efficacy of abdominopelvic irradiation and its superiority over pelvic radiotherapy alone. They also indicate that irradiation alone is insufficient treatment for most patients with gross residual disease, particularly when the residuum is extrapelvic.

TABLE 36.5-7. Proportion of 325 Patients in Whom Disease Recurred after Treatment with Abdominopelvic Irradiation between 1971 and 1981

		Proportion with Disease Recurrence		
Stage	*Gross Residual Disease*	Grade 1	Grade 2	Grade 3
I	No	—	.21 (33)	.30 (27)
II	No/uncertain	.09 (32)	.29 (35)	.47 (36)
II	Yes	.17 (12)	.38 (16)	.86 (14)
III	No/uncertain	.20 (10)	.67 (18)	.67 (15)
III	Yes	.40 (15)	.79 (24)	.84 (38)

Numbers in parentheses are the number of patients treated in each group.
(From ref. 67, with permission.)

TABLE 36.5-8. Evidence for Cure of Ovarian Cancer by Abdominopelvic Radiotherapy: Long-Term Outcome in Patients with Stage II and III Disease and Macroscopic Residuum

	Size of Residuum		
Study Center	<2 cm	>2 cm	*End Point*
Princess Margaret Hospital[66]	38 (91)	6 (91)	10-y relapse-free rate
Stanford[73]	50 (42)	14 (54)	15-y failure-free rate
Salt Lake City[69]	62 (12)	0 (10)	10-y relapse-free survival
Walter Reed Hospital[74]	42 (24)	10 (20)	10-y survival rate
Yale[72]	41 (27)	—	~6-y surviving fraction

Numbers in parentheses are the number of patients treated in each group.
(Modified from ref. 68, with permission.)

Randomized data comparing abdominopelvic irradiation with modern cisplatin- or paclitaxel-based chemotherapy have been difficult to obtain. Although retrospective studies do not demonstrate a clear advantage of one treatment over the other for patients with minimal residual disease, physician biases are strong and several multiinstitutional trials addressing this question have been closed prematurely because of inadequate patient accrual. In 1993, Redman and coworkers[75] published the results of a randomized trial comparing abdominopelvic irradiation with single-agent cisplatin in 40 patients with microscopic residual disease, stages IC to III. The 5-year survival rates were 58% and 62% in the two arms, respectively, but the power of the study was weak because of the small number of patients. In 1994, Chiara and colleagues[76] reported results of a second study comparing whole abdominal radiotherapy with cisplatin and cyclophosphamide in 70 patients with high-risk stage I or II disease. This study was compromised by poor accrual and protocol violations; 8 (24%) of the 34 patients assigned to receive radiotherapy were treated with chemotherapy. Projected 5-year survival rates for those treated with radiation (25 patients) or chemotherapy (44 patients) were 53% and 71%, respectively ($P = .16$).

However, these studies still leave us with an incomplete understanding of the role of radiotherapy in initial management of ovarian cancer. Although pelvic irradiation was routinely added to early treatments with single alkylating agents, it generally has been abandoned since platinum-containing regimens became standard. Early studies of pelvic radiation therapy alone and the success of whole abdominal plus pelvic irradiation in selected patients indicate that radiation is an active agent and suggest that pelvic irradiation may be a useful addition to chemotherapy for selected patients who have a high risk of pelvic recurrence. However, no study has ever been done to determine whether pelvic irradiation could improve the control rates achieved with modern chemotherapy.

Whole Abdominal Radiotherapy Technique

The ^{60}Co moving strip technique was developed at the M. D. Anderson Cancer Center in the 1960s to improve the acute tolerance of patients to large whole abdominal fields of radiation. The abdomen was divided into horizontal strips of 2.5 cm each; two to four contiguous strips were treated each day, moving down gradually until the whole abdomen had received the prescribed dose of irradiation. Subsequent studies suggested that large stationary megavoltage fields could be tolerated, and they were technically less difficult to deliver.[58] Dembo and coworkers[77] subsequently reported a randomized comparison of open field whole abdominal irradiation (22 Gy in 22 fractions) with the moving strip technique (22.5 Gy in ten fractions per strip), demonstrating lower complication rates and comparable tumor control with the simpler open field technique.

The high rate of subdiaphragmatic recurrences observed after treatment with early "whole abdominal" fields that did not completely cover the diaphragms illustrate the critical importance of covering the entire peritoneal cavity. More recently, in a review of a prospective multiinstitutional trial, Klaassen and colleagues[78] reported a significantly poorer survival rate for patients whose whole abdominal radiation fields were found to deviate seriously from protocol specifications.

Patients should always be simulated under fluoroscopy, and fields should provide a 1-cm margin on the maximum cephalad excursion of the diaphragmatic domes under quiet respiration. It is often necessary to flash the lateral abdominal wall and to include the entire bony pelvis in whole abdominal fields to avoid excluding peritoneal surfaces. In obese patients with poor abdominal tone, the fields may need to extend laterally beyond the bony pelvis. This is particularly true when the patient is treated in the prone position. The thickness of the abdominal wall should be considered in choosing the energy of the radiation beam. When fields are designed using CT scans of the whole abdomen, coverage of peritoneal surfaces can be assured. The total dose of whole abdominal irradiation varies between 22 and 30 Gy depending on the fractionation scheme, use of concurrent chemotherapy, and patient tolerance. Posterior kidney blocks are placed to limit the renal dose to 15 to 18 Gy, and a portion of the liver may be shielded during part of the treatment, limiting the dose to 22 to 25 Gy. The true pelvis is usually treated to a higher dose of 45 to 50 Gy, either after whole abdominal irradiation or concurrently as a "field within a field" (not to exceed a total daily dose to the pelvis of 180 cGy). Martinez and coworkers[73] have suggested boosting the dose to the paraaortic nodes and medial diaphragms with a T-shaped field in selected patients. Chemotherapy that is given before or after irradiation can influence normal tissue tolerance and should be considered in estimations of organ tolerance.

Intraperitoneal Radioisotopes

The characteristic transcolonic pattern of dissemination of ovarian cancer first led clinicians to treat patients with intraperitoneal isotopes in the 1950s, and this treatment is still used by some practitioners for a selected group of patients with minimal disease. The isotope that is usually used is chromic phosphate (^{32}P). ^{32}P decays with a half-life of 14.3 days, emitting β-particles with a mean energy of 0.69 MeV. Because the average penetration of these particles in soft tissue is less than 1 to 2 mm, treatment with chromic phosphate is inappropriate for patients who have macroscopic residual disease. Because the goal is to distribute the isotope evenly over peritoneal surfaces, patients with intraabdominal adhesions that inhibit the flow of the isotope-containing fluid are poor candidates for this treatment.

Intraabdominal distribution is usually evaluated before treatment by scanning the patient after an intraabdominal injection of technetium 99m sulfur colloid. If a good distribution is confirmed, the patient is treated with 10 to 20 mCi of chromic phosphate diluted in saline and then is positioned to optimize distribution. It is estimated that this dose delivers 20 to 40 Gy of radiation to the peritoneal surface. However, nonuniform distribution can produce variations in the dose of tenfold or more.

A GOG study, published in 1990, randomized 141 patients with poorly differentiated stage IA to B, stage IC, or completely resected stage II disease to receive either melphalan (0.2 mg/kg/d for 5 days, repeated every 4 to 6 weeks for 12 cycles) or intraperitoneal ^{32}P (15 mCi at the time of surgery).[20] The 5-year survival rates of 81% and 78% for patients treated with melphalan or ^{32}P, respectively, were not significantly different. Toxic effects were acceptable for most patients on both arms. However, four (6%) patients treated with ^{32}P required an operation for small bowel obstruction, and two (3%) patients treated with melphalan developed leukemia. The authors concluded that intraabdominal ^{32}P was the preferred treatment for these patients because of its limited toxicity and no known risk for causing leukemia.

Three randomized studies have compared ^{32}P with cisplatin-containing chemotherapy[79–81]; none demonstrated a significant difference in survival between the two treatments. Vergote and colleagues[80] randomized 347 patients who had no gross residual disease after laparotomy to receive intraperitoneal ^{32}P (7 to 10 mCi) or cisplatin (six courses of 50 mg/m^2 each). The estimated 5-year survival rates were 83% and 81%, respectively (P = .6). Although the dose of ^{32}P was relatively low, 12 (9%) of 136 patients who had this treatment experienced small bowel obstructions compared with 2% of patients treated with cisplatin. For this reason, the authors recommended cisplatin as standard treatment.

In a GOG study, Young and colleagues[81] compared intraabdominal ^{32}P with combination chemotherapy (cisplatin and cyclophosphamide) for patients with high-risk early-stage disease. The 5-year survival rates were 76% and 84%, respectively (P = .08). One toxic death was reported in each treatment arm, but these authors also concluded that the greater risk of bowel complications with ^{32}P outweighed the hematologic complications of chemotherapy; on this basis, the authors recommended chemotherapy as the preferred treatment.

The most common complication of ^{32}P administration is transient abdominal pain in 15% to 20% of patients. Chemical or infectious peritonitis is a rare complication that occurs in 2% to 3% of patients. The most serious late complication of treatment is small bowel obstruction, which has been reported in 5% to 10% of patients treated with ^{32}P alone. This risk increases to an unacceptable rate of 20% to 30% when intraperitoneal ^{32}P is combined with external-beam radiotherapy, an approach that is no longer recommended.

These clinical trials, however, did not establish whether any form of adjuvant therapy was, in fact, superior to no immediate treatment for patients with early-stage ovarian cancer with unfavorable prognostic features. The Italian Interregional Cooperative Group of Gynecologic Oncology has conducted a randomized trial with a no-treatment arm in patients with stage I or IB, grade 2 or 3 tumors who are randomized to receive cisplatin (50 mg/m^2 for six cycles) or to observation.[82] With a median observation time of 76 months, overall survival rates between the two treatment arms is similar (88% with cisplatin vs. 82% in the control group), although there is a marked improvement in disease-free survival for patients treated with cisplatin (83% vs. 65%). The absence of a larger difference in overall survival reflects the ability of cisplatin-based chemotherapy to salvage patients at the time of recurrence. Two additional trials, in which there is a no-treatment arm, are also in progress in Europe for early-stage ovarian cancer patients (Table 36.5-9). The Scandinavian randomized trial is similar in design to that of the Italian study. In an English trial, however, the randomization is between observation and treatment with single-agent carboplatin. Unlike the Scandinavian study, the English trial has no requirement for extensive surgical staging.

The current GOG trial for patients with early-stage ovarian cancer with unfavorable prognosis compares three cycles against six cycles of a treatment with paclitaxel and carboplatin (see Table 36.5-9). The details of this combination are discussed later in the section Paclitaxel Combination Therapy.

It is apparent that the optimum postoperative treatment for patients with early-stage ovarian cancer with unfavorable prognostic features remains to be established. Pending the results of the ongoing clinical trials, treatment options include chemotherapy with cisplatin or carboplatin, total abdominal and pelvic irradiation, and paclitaxel-based chemotherapy. In addition, a no-treatment option can be considered, although this choice has been shown to be associated with a decrease in dis-

TABLE 36.5-9. Clinical Trials in Early-Stage Ovarian Cancer

	Randomization	*Results*
GOG trials		
GOG protocol 157	Paclitaxel (175 mg/m^2 in a 3-hr infusion) plus carboplatin (dosed to an AUC of 7.5): three versus six cycles	Closed for accrual; no survival data available
GOG protocol 175	Three cycles of paclitaxel (175 mg/m^2 in a 3-hr infusion) plus carboplatin (AUC = 6) followed by randomization to observation or 24 weekly administrations of paclitaxel (40 mg/m^2)	Open for accrual 1999; no data available
ICON I trial	Carboplatin (AUC = 5) versus observation	Comprehensive staging not mandatory in this trial; no survival data yet available
Scandinavian trial	Carboplatin (AUC = 6) versus observation	Includes aneuploidy as a poor prognostic feature; no survival data available

AUC, area under the curve; GOG, Gynecologic Oncology Group; ICON I, International Collaborative Ovarian Neoplasms trial I.

ease-free survival. Second-look operations after completion of adjuvant therapy are not routinely recommended.

TREATMENT OF ADVANCED-STAGE OVARIAN CANCER

The generally accepted treatment for patients with either stage III or IV (advanced stage) ovarian cancer has been similar—cytoreductive surgery, when feasible, followed by chemotherapy.

Cytoreduction

Aggressive surgery to remove virtually all gross tumor (i.e., cytoreductive surgery or tumor debulking surgery) has become an integral part of initial surgery for management of ovarian cancer. The theoretical benefits of cytoreductive surgery are to remove large necrotic tumors with poor blood supplies and to remove large tumors that are in a slower growth phase, leaving behind tumors that are more sensitive to the effects of chemotherapy. Theoretically, all patients with stage III and IV disease are candidates for cytoreductive surgery. Stage IV patients, based on the presence of parenchymal liver disease, enlarged retrocrural lymph nodes, supraclavicular lymph nodes, mediastinal metastases, and parenchymal lung metastases may not be candidates for optimal cytoreductive surgery. In addition, we have found that women who have disease on CT scan that involves the porta hepatis or is associated with suprarenal lymphadenopathy or omental metastases that extend into the hilum of the spleen frequently have such advanced disease at the time of the cytoreductive surgery that the likelihood of optimal cytoreduction being accomplished is virtually nil. Women with stage IV disease based only on the presence of malignant pleural effusion have been able to undergo optimal cytoreductive surgery. Its impact on their survival has been questioned.[83] Studies have suggested that an optimal surgical cytoreductive effort should be performed in women with stage IV disease, even when parenchymal liver disease is recognized preoperatively.[84,85] If patients can be optimally cytoreduced to less than 1 to 2 cm maximum diameter of residual tumor, their median survival has varied from 25 to 40 months, whereas those women who were suboptimally cytoreduced had median survival rates of 10 to 18 months. Interestingly, the stage IV patients optimally cytoreduced in three of the four series had a superior survival to optimally cytoreduced patients with stage III ovarian cancer treated in prospective randomized trials by the GOG.[46]

Successful surgical management of stage III or IV ovarian cancer requires meticulous attention to surgical techniques to avoid complications and a thorough knowledge of abdominal and pelvic anatomy to allow the successful accomplishment of cytoreductive surgery. In general, it is wisest to start with an incision in the lower abdomen to free the pelvis of cancer, then work up into the upper abdomen to attempt to clear it of cancer, then complete the procedure with paraaortic and pericaval retroperitoneal lymph node sampling or resection if optimal cytoreduction has been accomplished within the peritoneal cavity. The goal of optimal cytoreductive surgery is complete removal of all palpable or visible tumor. A minimal goal of cytoreductive surgery is to reduce the residual tumor to less than 1 cm and preferably less than 0.5 cm in maximum diameter.

On entering the abdominal cavity, normal anatomy is restored by lysing adhesions and freeing organs from adherent tumor. Frequently the pelvis is completely filled with tumor. By identifying the round ligaments and suture ligating and dividing them, the pelvic retroperitoneum can be entered and the external iliac arteries and veins, the hypogastric arteries, and the ureters can be rapidly identified. Accomplishing this allows ligation of the infundibulopelvic ligaments with the ovarian vessels; resection of peritoneum, along with the attached vessels down to the tumor mass; and dissection of the ovarian mass off of, or with, the underlying peritoneum to elevate the mass from the pelvic sidewall. By dividing the utero-ovarian ligaments and fallopian tubes, one can then remove the mass. At times, it may be necessary to resect small bowel or sigmoid colon in continuity with the ovarian mass. An end-to-end or side-to-side anastomosis restores bowel continuity. Less frequently a colostomy is necessary. Once each of the ovaries has been removed, a hysterectomy is performed. At times, ovarian cancers infiltrate into the uterus and it is necessary to take the uterus out *en bloc* with the ovarian tumor. Implants in the cul-de-sac may be resected using retroperitoneal dissection. Sigmoid colon implants usually involve epiploic appendices, which can be resected without performing a sigmoid colon resection. Retroperitoneal lymph nodes are routinely removed from the external iliac artery and vein, hypogastric arteries, and the obturator fossa. An appendectomy is routinely performed.

Having resected the pelvic disease, a complete omentectomy is performed and large masses implanting on peritoneal surfaces, including the diaphragm, are removed. Once the abdomen has been cleared of disease, or the maximum residual disease is less than 1 cm, the fat pad overlying and surrounding the aorta and vena cava is removed, as are lymph nodes involved with metastatic disease in this area. In general, if large residual tumor volume is left within the peritoneal cavity, there is not much benefit in resecting retroperitoneal disease. However, when intraperitoneal disease has been optimally cytoreduced to less than 1-cm maximal residual tumor volume, retroperitoneal lymphadenectomies are appropriate.

Impact of Primary Cytoreductive Surgery

The clinical rationale for cytoreductive surgery has been ascribed to Griffiths,[86] who demonstrated in 1974 that survival was directly effected by the initial degree of cytoreductive surgery for women with advanced-stage ovarian cancer. In a retrospective review, patients with no residual disease had a mean survival of 39 months compared with 29 months for residual disease of less than 0.5 cm, 18 months for residual disease of 0.6 to 1.5 cm, and 11 months for those who were not cytoreduced below 1.5 cm. None of the latter patients survived beyond 26 months. Women who underwent optimal cytoreductive surgery had similar survival rates to women who had minimal-size abdominal metastases at the initial surgery. Subsequent to that report, numerous series have confirmed that aggressive cytoreductive surgery to 2 cm of residual tumor or less significantly enhances survival for patients. Most patients participated in trials in which multidrug chemotherapy was used, usually involving cisplatin-based chemotherapy. A review of nine reports, in which primary cytoreductive surgery resulted in disease of less than 2 cm or greater than 2 cm, demonstrated a mean survival in the optimally cytoreduced group of 29.4 months compared with 13.4 months in the group in whom cytoreductive surgery was suboptimal[86–94] (Table 36.5-10).

TABLE 36.5-10. Effect of Residual Disease at the Conclusion of Primary Cytoreductive Surgery on Survival

Investigators	*Treatment*	*Residual Disease*	*Survival*
Griffiths (1975)[86]	L-PAM	0	39
		0–0.5	29
		0.6–1.5	18
		>1.5	11
Hacker et al. (1983)[87]	Varied	<0.5	40
		0.6–1.5	18
		>1.5	6
Vogl et al. (1983)[88]	CHAP	<2 cm	>40
		>2 cm	16
Pohl et al. (1984)[89]	Varied	<2 cm	45
		>2 cm	16
Delgado et al. (1984)[90]	Varied	<2 cm	45
		>2 cm	16
Redman et al. (1986)[93]	CAP	<3 cm	38
		>3 cm	26
Conte et al. (1986)[94]	CAP, CP	<2 cm	>40
		>2 cm	16
Neijt et al. (1991)[92]	CHAP or CP	<1 cm	40
		>1 cm	21
Piver et al. (1988)[91]	PAC	<2 cm	48
		>2 cm	21
Totals			**Mean 36.7 (optimal)** **Mean 16.6 (suboptimal)**

CAP, cyclophosphamide, Adriamycin, and cisplatin; CHAP, cyclophosphamide, hexamethylmelamine, Adriamycin, and cisplatin; CP, cyclophosphamide and cisplatin; L-PAM, melphalan; PAC, cisplatin, doxorubicin, and cyclophosphamide.
(Modified from Young RC, Perez CA, Hoskins WV. Cancer of the ovary. In: DeVita VT Jr, Hellman S, Rosenberg SA, eds. *Cancer: principles and practice of oncology,* 4th ed. Philadelphia: JB Lippincott Co, 1993:1226, with permission.)

Two metaanalyses gave conflicting views on the survival impact of cytoreductive surgery.[95,96] Hunter et al.[95] reviewed a total of 58 separate studies containing 6962 patients to determine whether maximum cytoreduction surgery benefits the survival of women with advanced ovarian cancer. These authors looked at the median survival times of groups of women with advanced ovarian cancer and used multiple linear regression techniques to analyze the effects on median survival. The variables studied were the proportion of each cohort undergoing maximum cytoreductive surgery, the use of cisplatin chemotherapy, the dose intensity of the chemotherapy, the proportion of each cohort with stage IV disease, and the year of publication of the study. The use of cisplatin chemotherapy resulted in an increased survival time of 53% [95% confidence intervals (CI), 35% to 73%]. For each 0.2 unit increase in dose intensity, the increase in median survival time was 11.1% (95% CI, 6% to 17%, *P* = .001). Stage IV disease had a negative impact on survival. For each 10% increase in the number of stage IV patients in the study, a negative survival increase of 2.6% (95% CI, –0.1% to –5.4%) was found. For each 10% increase in the percentage of women who underwent maximum cytoreductive surgery, the increase in survival was only 4.1% (95% CI, –0.6% to 9.1%, *P* = .089) (Fig. 36.5-5). This study concluded that cytoreductive surgery has only a small effect on the survival of women with advanced ovarian cancer and that the type of treatment used (i.e., cisplatin) was far more important.

Allen et al.[96] performed metaanalyses on 12 reports of women with stage III ovarian cancer in which they could determine that patients either had no residual disease, residual disease less than or equal to 2 cm, or residual disease greater than 2 cm, and on four reports of stage IV ovarian cancer for which similar analyses were possible. The results of these metaanalyses were consistent with survival benefits accruing to patients with no residual disease and residual disease less than or equal to 2 cm after surgery for stage III and IV disease when compared with patients with residual tumor masses greater than 2 cm. These authors, however, indicated that the survival benefit for women with small residual tumor probably reflects more the biology of the tumor and suggests that less-invasive tumors may be more chemotherapy-sensitive than those tumors in which optimum cytoreductive surgery was not possible. To date, no prospective randomized trials have been performed assessing the value of cytoreductive surgery in advanced ovarian cancer.

Three GOG studies give important insight into the impact of cytoreductive surgery in advanced ovarian cancer. The first demonstrated that removing all gross tumor defines true optimal cytoreductive surgery. Women treated with cisplatin-based chemotherapy who had no gross disease left had a progression-free interval of 42 months compared with 20 months for those with residual disease of less than 1 cm.[97] The second study revealed that women who had 1 to 2 cm residual tumor had a significant survival improvement compared with those who had more than 2 cm of residual tumor.[98] This third study refuted early data suggesting that women undergoing optimal cytoreductive surgery have similar survival as those patients initially found at surgery to have low-volume disease.[46] The latter study reported on 348 women with 1 cm or less residual tumor, 200 of whom initially had abdominal disease of 1 cm or less. When implants were present on parietal or visceral peritoneum, even when optimally cytoreduced, survival rates significantly decreased. Indeed, the best survival for stage III patients observed were those whose initial macroscopic tumor was less than 1 cm in the omentum and associated with either no disease or microscopic disease in other abdominal sites (*P* = .0001). Those with the poorest survival had tumors initially greater than 1 cm involving omentum and had gross disease in other abdominal sites (Fig. 36.5-6). This study refutes early data suggesting that women undergoing optimal cytoreductive surgery have the same survival as those patients initially found at surgery to have low-volume disease. The study demonstrates that biologic factors responsible for bulk disease may be as important as technical ability to resect the disease.

Aggressive cytoreductive surgery incurs complications. Chen and Bochner[99] reported on 60 patients who underwent optimal cytoreductive surgery. These patients had a 5% operative morbidity. Blythe and Wahl[100] have looked at quality of life in optimal residual disease (less than 2 cm in diameter) and suboptimal residual disease (more than 2 cm in diameter) and found that 75% of the optimal group were judged to have good or good-to-fair quality of life, but only 18% of the suboptimal group achieved this quality of life. It has been argued that perhaps those women who are able to be optimally cytoreduced have biologically less virulent disease than those patients in

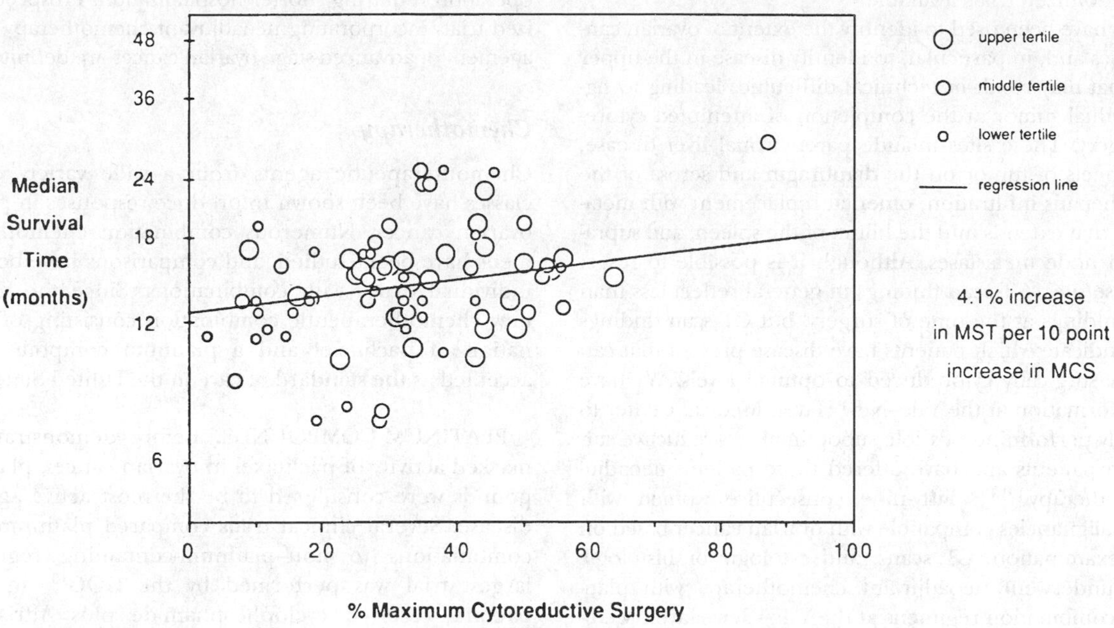

FIGURE 36.5-5. Graph of log median survival time (MST; in months) versus percent maximum cytoreductive surgery (MCS) for 76 cohorts for which dose intensity could be calculated after adjustments for effects of dose intensity, percent stage IV, and platinum chemotherapy. (From ref. 95, with permission.)

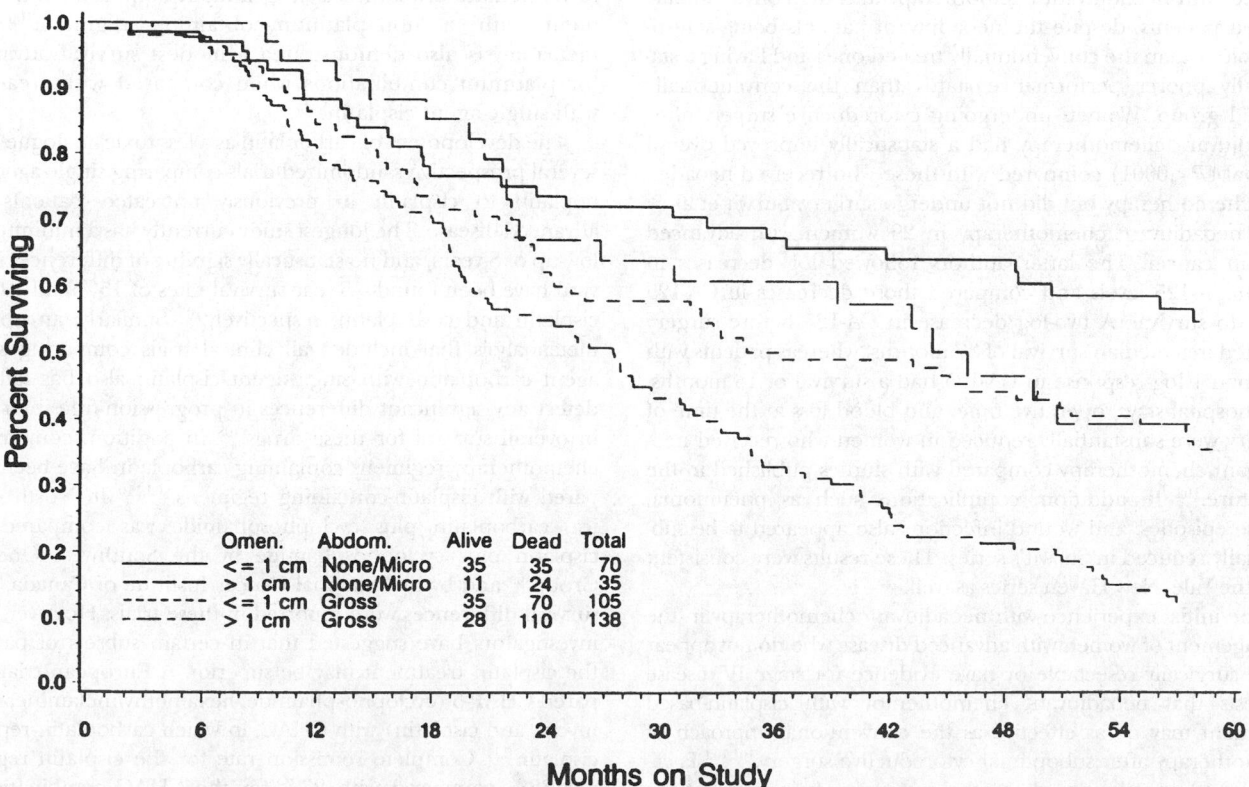

FIGURE 36.5-6. Survival time by initial maximum omental (Omen.) and abdominal (Abdom.) tumor diameter. Micro, microscopic. (From ref. 46, with permission.)

whom optimal cytoreductive surgery cannot be achieved. This question has yet to be answered as there are no data from prospective randomized trials available.

CT scans have been used to identify the extent of ovarian cancer metastases and, in particular, to identify disease in the upper abdomen that may result in technical difficulties leading to significant residual tumor at the completion of attempted cytoreductive surgery. These sites include parenchymal liver disease, confluent sheets of tumor on the diaphragm and serosa of the liver, porta hepatis infiltration, omental replacement with metastatic tumor that extends into the hilum of the spleen, and suprarenal lymph node metastases. Although it is possible to resect some of these sites, CT scan findings in general reflect less than the actual findings at the time of surgery, but CT scan findings frequently indicate which patients have disease present that can be routinely surgically cytoreduced to optimal levels. We have used this information at the Yale–New Haven Medical Center to avoid initially performing possible suboptimal cytoreductive surgery in such patients and have offered those patients neoadjuvant chemotherapy.[101,102] Fifty-nine consecutive women with advanced malignancies compatible with ovarian cancer based on a physical examination, CT scans, and cytologic or histologic specimens underwent neoadjuvant chemotherapy with platinum-based combination regimens at the Yale–New Haven Medical Center.[103] Forty-one subsequently underwent cytoreductive surgery. Their overall progression-free survival rates were compared with those of 206 consecutive women with stage III and IV epithelial ovarian cancers treated with conventional cytoreductive surgery followed by the same platinum-based combination chemotherapy.[103] No statistical difference was observed in the overall survival or in progression-free survival between the group treated with neoadjuvant chemotherapy and the conventionally treated patients, despite the neoadjuvant patients being statistically older than the conventionally treated ones and having a statistically poorer performance status than the conventionally treated group. Women undergoing cytoreductive surgery after neoadjuvant chemotherapy had a statistically improved overall survival ($P < .0001$) compared with those who received neoadjuvant chemotherapy but did not undergo surgery. Surwit et al.[104] used neoadjuvant chemotherapy in 29 women with advanced ovarian cancer. The latter authors followed log decreases in serum CA-125 levels and compared those decreases in CA-125 levels to survival. A two-log decrease in CA-125 before surgery resulted in a median survival of 37 months, whereas patients with less than 1 log response in CA-125 had a survival of 18 months. The hospital stays, operative time, and blood loss at the time of surgery were substantially reduced in women who received neoadjuvant chemotherapy compared with studies published in the literature.[104] In addition, complications such as pneumonia, febrile episodes, and wound infections also appeared to be substantially reduced in Surwit's series. These results were consistent with the Yale–New Haven series as well.

The initial experience with neoadjuvant chemotherapy in the management of women with advanced disease who do not appear to be surgically resectable or have evidence for stage IV disease suggests that neoadjuvant chemotherapy with cisplatin-based treatment may be as effective as the conventional approach of chemotherapy after suboptimal cytoreductive surgery.[101,102] Paclitaxel-based neoadjuvant chemotherapy is now being used at the Yale–New Haven Medical Center. Potential advantages of neoadjuvant chemotherapy appear to be a much more rapid improvement in quality of life, a less expensive treatment program for patients and, when surgery is ultimately performed, an easier operation requiring shorter hospitalization. Prospective randomized trials incorporating neoadjuvant chemotherapy in the management of advanced-stage ovarian cancer are definitely needed.

Chemotherapy

Chemotherapeutic agents from a wide variety of different classes have been shown to produce responses in patients with ovarian cancer. Numerous combination chemotherapy regimens have been studied, and comparisons have been made of individual drugs with combinations. Since the mid-1990s, a new chemotherapeutic combination consisting of the combination of paclitaxel and a platinum compound has been accepted as the standard of care in the United States.

PLATINUM COMPOUNDS. Before demonstration of the marked activity of paclitaxel in ovarian cancer, platinum compounds were considered to be the most active agents in this disease. Several clinical trials compared platinum-containing combinations to non–platinum-containing regimens. The largest trial was performed by the GOG[105] in which 120 patients received cyclophosphamide plus Adriamycin and were compared with 107 patients who were treated with cyclophosphamide, Adriamycin, and cisplatin (CAP). The CAP regimen was deemed superior based on a higher overall response rate (51% vs. 26%), longer progression-free duration (13.1 months vs. 7.7 months), and an improvement in overall survival rate (15.7 months vs. 9.7 months). A metaanalysis of 45 clinical trials in ovarian cancer confirmed the survival benefit of immediate cisplatin-based treatment compared with treatment with a non–platinum-containing regimen.[106] The metaanalysis also demonstrated a modest survival advantage for platinum combinations when compared with treatment with single-agent cisplatin.

The development of carboplatin as a less toxic analogue led to several prospective randomized trials comparing single-agent carboplatin to cisplatin in previously untreated patients with advanced disease. The longest study currently has a minimum follow-up of 8 years, and no statistically significant differences in survival have been found—5-year survival rates of 15% and 19% for cisplatin and carboplatin, respectively.[107] Similarly, an updated metaanalysis that included all clinical trials comparing single-agent carboplatin with single-agent cisplatin also has failed to detect any significant differences in progression-free interval or in overall survival for these drugs.[108] In addition, combination chemotherapy regimens containing carboplatin have been compared with cisplatin-containing regimens.[109,110] In North America, carboplatin plus cyclophosphamide was compared with cisplatin plus cyclophosphamide by the Southwest Oncology Group[109] and by the National Cancer Institute of Canada.[110] No survival differences were reported in these trials. However, some investigators have suggested that in certain subsets of patients, the cisplatin treatment may be superior. A European trial compared CHAP-5 (cyclophosphamide, hexamethylmelamine, Adriamycin, and cisplatin) with CHAC, in which carboplatin replaced cisplatin.[111] Complete remission rate for the cisplatin regimen was 32% compared with 27% for the CHAC combination. A trend toward improvement in the survival rate was seen for patients with less than 1 cm of disease who were randomized to

TABLE 36.5-11. Randomized Trials of Cisplatin Dose Intensity

Country	*References*	*Randomization*	*Number of Patients*	*Result*	*Comment*
Hong Kong	115	Cisplatin, 120 mg/m^2 versus 60 mg/m^2	65	Increased survival for high dose	Nonuniform staging and low statistical power
United States	116	100 mg/m^2 cisplatin plus 1000 mg/m^2 cyclophosphamide × four cycles versus 50 mg/m^2 cisplatin plus 500 mg/m^2 cyclophosphamide × eight cycles	485	No difference in survival	Dose intensity of cisplatin doubled
Italy	117	75 mg/m^2 cisplatin every 3 wk × six cycles versus 50 mg/m^2 weekly × eight cycles	295	No difference in survival	Dose intensity of cisplatin doubled
Italy	118	100 mg/m^2 or 50 mg/m^2 cisplatin plus epidoxorubicin 60 mg/m^2 and cyclophosphamide 600 mg/m^2	145	No difference in response or survival	Three-drug dose-intense combination leading to more toxicity but no survival benefit
Scotland	119,120	100 mg/m^2 cisplatin plus 750 mg/m^2 cyclophosphamide versus 50 mg/m^2 cisplatin plus 750 mg/m^2 cyclophosphamide	165	Improved survival in high-dose arm	Survival difference is decreasing with longer follow-up

the cisplatin regimen. In patients with bulky disease, no survival differences were found.

In these studies, platinum-based regimens were routinely administered for six cycles. Prospective randomized trials have compared five cycles with ten cycles[112] or six with 12,[113] and no statistically significant differences have been reported in survival for patients treated with the greater number of cycles. However, numerous questions remain regarding the role of dose and dose intensity of these agents in the overall treatment of patients with ovarian cancer. Cisplatin dose intensity (expressed as mg/m^2/wk) was studied retrospectively in 33 published trials in ovarian cancer.[114] This retrospective analysis provided evidence for the importance of dose with regard to response and survival. Doses of cisplatin beyond 100 mg/m^2 have been associated with unacceptable toxicity, primarily neurotoxicity. Several prospective clinical trials have compared differences in cisplatin dose intensity (Table 36.5-11). In the GOG trial, 485 patients with bulky stage III or IV disease were randomized to receive either eight cycles of cisplatin (50 mg/m^2) plus cyclophosphamide (500 mg/m^2) every 3 weeks, or four cycles of cisplatin (100 mg/m^2) plus cyclophosphamide (1000 mg/m^2) every 3 weeks.[116] This study demonstrated that a regimen could be administered at double the dose intensity of cisplatin with increased grade 3 and 4 myelotoxicity. However, no significant difference was noted in overall response rate or survival for patients who received the high-dose regimens. Two similar studies from Italy also were not able to demonstrate any improvement for patients who received double-dose intensity of cisplatin.[117,118] In contrast, the study from the West Scotland's Clinical Trial Group compared two different cisplatin plus cyclophosphamide regimens and initially reported an improvement in survival for patients receiving the higher-dose intensity.[214] In this trial, patients with stage IC to IV disease were randomized to treatment with either 50 mg/m^2 (low dose) or 100 mg/m^2 (high dose) cisplatin, with all patients receiving 750 mg of cyclophosphamide. With the longer follow-up, the differences in survival appear to be decreasing.[120] There currently is no evidence that a dose of cisplatin greater than 75 mg/m^2/cycle should be routinely used in combination chemotherapy for patients with advanced ovarian cancer.

In contrast to cisplatin, carboplatin is rapidly excreted in the kidney. The area under the concentration-time curve is dependent on glomerular filtration rate (GFR). Retrospective studies have identified a correlation between response and toxicity and area under the curve (AUC), with a plateau reached for response at an AUC of 6 to 7.[121] Formulas have been developed to individualize dose based on AUC and patients' renal function. In Calvert's formula, the dose (mg) = AUC × [GFR + 25].[122] In these studies, GFR was estimated by ^{51}CrEDTA clearance. Creatinine clearance, however, can be used to approximate GFR and can be measured or estimated with age and serum creatinine. Prospective randomized trials have been performed in which patients with advanced ovarian cancer have been randomized to different AUCs covering a twofold difference in dose intensity. In a study from the Danish Ovarian Cancer Study Group, there was no increased efficacy for patients randomized to receive an AUC of 4 versus 8.[123] All patients in this trial also received cyclophosphamide. In the trial from the United Kingdom,[125] patients received carboplatin dosed to an AUC of 6 or 12. Greater grade 4 toxicity in patients scheduled to receive an AUC of 12 subsequently was found, which led to substantial dose reduction.

Several randomized trials also have explored cisplatin plus cyclophosphamide versus doxorubicin-containing combinations. In the GOG trial,[125] 349 patients with advanced disease were randomized to receive either cisplatin plus cyclophosphamide or a PAC combination (cisplatin, doxorubicin, and cyclophosphamide). No significant differences were reported with regard to complete remission rates (30% vs. 33%), progression-free interval (median, 22.7 months vs. 24.6 months), or overall survival rate (median, 31.2 vs. 38.9 months). In contrast, a large Italian trial has reported a significantly higher, surgically confirmed, complete remission rate (62% vs. 40%) and a 10-month increase in median survival for patients treated with PAC compared with cyclophosphamide and cisplatin (CP).[126] Two separate metaanalyses pooling the data from these clinical trials has identified a survival benefit between 5% and 7% from years 2 to 6 for patients with the doxorubicin regimens.[127,128] Direct comparison of these regimens, however, has

TABLE 36.5-12. Randomized Trials of Paclitaxel plus Platinum in Advanced Ovarian Cancer

Trial and Randomization	*Reference*	*Number of Patients/Stage*	*CCR (%)*	*PFS Median (mo)*	*OS Median (mo)*
GOG 111	133	386; suboptimal stage II and IV			
Cisplatin (75 mg/m^2) plus paclitaxel (135 mg/m^2 in 24 hr)			51	18	38
Cisplatin (75 mg/m^2) plus cyclophosphamide (750 mg/m^2)			31	13	24
OV-10	134	668; stage IIB–IV			
Cisplatin (75 mg/m^2) plus paclitaxel (175 mg/m^2 in 3 hr)			50	16	35
Cisplatin (75 mg/m^2) plus cyclophosphamide (750 mg/m^2)			36	12	25
GOG 132	135	615; suboptimal stage III–IV			
Cisplatin (75 mg/m^2) plus paclitaxel (135 mg/m^2 in 24 hr)			NA	14.1	26.6
Paclitaxel (200 mg/m^2)			NA	11.4	26
Cisplatin (100 mg/m^2)			NA	16.4	30.2
ICON III[a]	136	2075; stage I–IV			
Carboplatin (AUC = 5–6) plus paclitaxel (175 mg/m^2)			NA	NA	NA
Carboplatin (AUC = 5–6)			NA	NA	NA
Cisplatin (50 mg/m^2) plus doxorubicin (50 mg/m^2) plus cyclophosphamide (500 mg/m^2)			NA	NA	NA

AUC, area under the curve; CCR, clinical complete remission; GOG, Gynecologic Oncology Group; ICON III, International Collaborative Ovarian Neoplasms trial III; NA, not available; OS, overall survival; PFS, progression-free survival.
[a]Preliminary results reported no difference between any treatment group. Mature survival results are pending.

been somewhat limited by differences in toxicity and dose intensity. Only the GOG study was performed with regimens that produced comparable hematologic toxicity. Although the metaanalysis suggested that the addition of doxorubicin slightly prolonged survival, a large prospective comparison [International Collaborative Ovarian Neoplasms (ICON) trial II] of single-agent carboplatin (AUC = 5) versus the PAC regimen did not demonstrate any differences in either progression-free survival or overall survival rates.[129]

Before the demonstration of the role of paclitaxel in the initial chemotherapy of patients with advanced ovarian cancer, standard chemotherapy regimens in the United States consisted primarily of either cisplatin (75 mg/m^2) or carboplatin (dosed to an AUC of 6 to 7, or approximately 350 mg/m^2) together with cyclophosphamide (at a dose of 600 to 750 mg/m^2). In contrast, many clinicians in Europe continue to use the PAC regimen or single-agent carboplatin.

PACLITAXEL COMBINATION CHEMOTHERAPY. Taxanes are a new class of cytotoxic agents with a unique mechanism of action. Paclitaxel and docetaxel both have been demonstrated to have activity in platinum-resistant patients.[130,131] The taxanes exert their cytotoxicity primarily by their effect on microtubules. Taxanes bind to microtubules and shift their equilibrium toward microtubular assembly, leading to a cell-cycle arrest in G_2/M. Premedication with steroids, cimetidine, and diphenhydramine has essentially eliminated the hypersensitivity reactions that limited early phase I trials. Of particular importance in the phase II trials, which demonstrate an overall response rate of 30% to 40%, was the observation that paclitaxel was active in patients who had disease progression while receiving cisplatin or had a duration of remission of less than 6 months. In the GOG trial of 43 patients, 27 were defined as platinum-resistant.[130] The overall response rate in this subset of patients was 33%, compared with the overall response rate of 37%. Toxicities of paclitaxel include alopecia, myalgia, and myelosuppression (primarily neutropenia with little effect on platelets). The activity of paclitaxel was confirmed in other phase II trials.[132]

Based on these results, a series of prospective randomized trials have compared platinum and paclitaxel versus regimens without paclitaxel (Table 36.5-12). The GOG study[133] randomized almost 400 patients with suboptimal stage III and IV disease to paclitaxel plus cisplatin or to cyclophosphamide plus cisplatin. The paclitaxel regimen was superior with regard to response rate, complete remission, second-look rate, progression-free survival, and overall survival (Fig. 36.5-7). In this group of patients with poor prognosis and advanced disease, a 14-month improvement in median survival (24 months vs. 38 months) is seen in patients treated with the paclitaxel combination. The results of this study were confirmed by a European/Canadian trial that had a similar randomization.[134] In this trial, however, paclitaxel was administered at 175 mg/m^2 in a 3-hour infusion instead of the 24-hour infusion used in the GOG trial. Furthermore, in the latter trial, in contrast to GOG 111, patients initially randomized to the nonpaclitaxel combination were frequently crossed over at the time of disease pro-

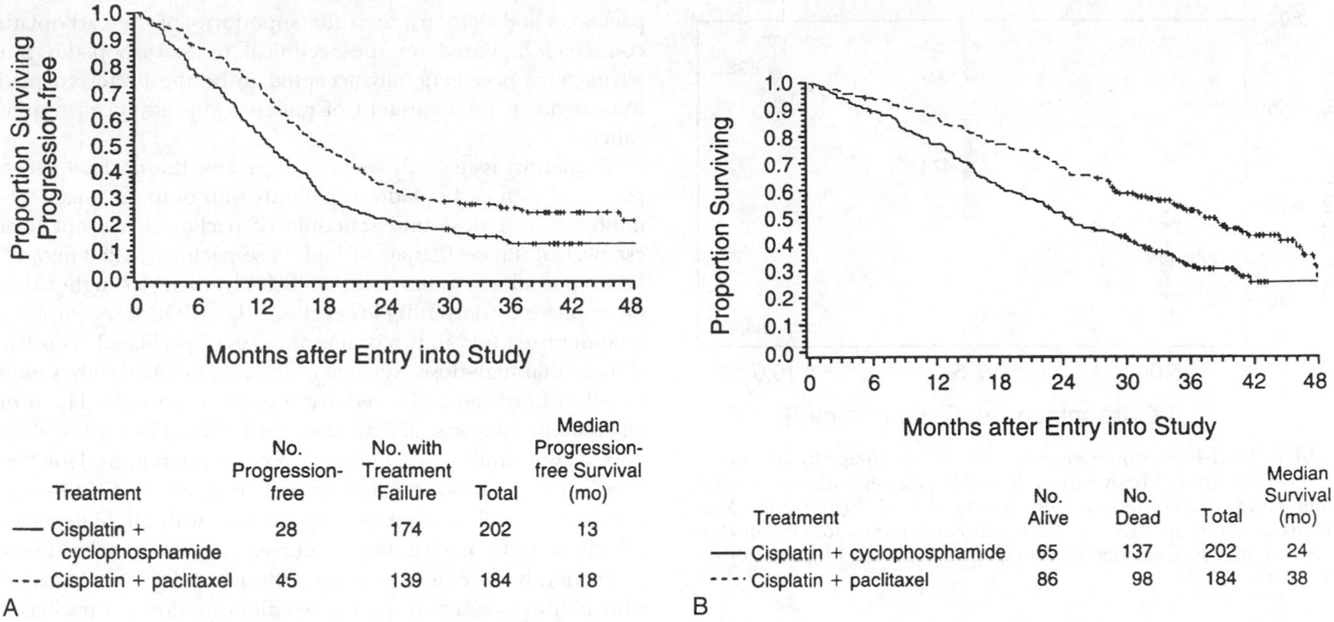

FIGURE 36.5-7. Disease-free **(A)** and overall **(B)** survival of patients with suboptimal stage III and IV ovarian cancer randomized to treatment with cisplatin plus cyclophosphamide (*solid line*) or cisplatin plus paclitaxel (*dotted line*). (From ref. 133, with permission.)

gression if they were initially randomized to cisplatin plus cyclophosphamide. Nevertheless, the results of this trial also showed a 10-month improvement in overall survival for patients treated initially with paclitaxel plus cisplatin.[134] The subsequent trial by the GOG in the same group of patients was a three-arm study in which patients were randomized to receive single-agent cisplatin (100 mg/m^2), single-agent paclitaxel (200 mg/m^2), or the combination of cisplatin plus paclitaxel as described earlier in this section.[135] In this protocol (GOG 132), most patients randomized to single-agent treatment actually received both drugs in sequence, as patients were routinely crossed to the other arm before clinical progression was noted through either persistent disease radiographically or findings of residual disease at second-look laparotomy. Although no difference was found in median survival between any treatment approach and GOG 132, six cycles of combination chemotherapy were judged to be the preferable regimen because of decreased toxicity.

The preliminary results of the European trial (ICON III) comparing carboplatin plus paclitaxel versus single-agent carboplatin or combination chemotherapy versus a PAC regimen also have been reported.[136] Mature survival data and subset analysis are awaited. Although the initial results did not demonstrate any significant difference in survival rate, the current recommendation that initial chemotherapy consist of paclitaxel plus a platinum compound was not altered by the results of this trial.

Although a series of prospective randomized trials and two metaanalyses demonstrated equivalent activity of carboplatin versus cisplatin, concern still remained that carboplatin was the inferior platinum compound in patients with optimal stage III disease. Consequently, three prospective randomized trials have been performed throughout the world comparing cisplatin plus paclitaxel versus carboplatin plus paclitaxel (Table 36.5-13).[137–139] Bookman et al.[140] initially reported that these two drugs could be combined at full therapeutic doses if carboplatin was dosed

TABLE 36.5-13. Randomized Trials of Carboplatin plus Paclitaxel versus Cisplatin plus Paclitaxel

Trial and Randomization	*Reference*	*Number of Patients/Stage*	*PFS (Median)*	*OS (Median)*
GOG 158	137	840; optimal stage III		
Carboplatin (AUC = 7.5) plus paclitaxel (175 mg/m^2 in 3 hr)			22 mo	NA
Cisplatin (75 mg/m^2) plus paclitaxel (135 mg/m^2)			21.7 mo	NA
AGO	138	798; stage IIB–IV		
Carboplatin (AUC = 6) plus paclitaxel (185 mg/m^2 in 3 hr)			69 wk	NA
Cisplatin (75 mg/m^2) plus paclitaxel (185 mg/m^2 in 3 hr)			73 wk	NA
NETHERLANDS-DANISH	139	190; stage IIB–IV		
Carboplatin (AUC = 5) plus paclitaxel (175 mg/m^2 in 3 hr)			ND	NA
Cisplatin (75 mg/m^2) plus paclitaxel (175 mg/m^2 in 3 hr)			ND	NA

AGO, Arbeitsgemeinschaft Gynaekologische Onkologie; AUC, area under the curve; GOG, Gynecologic Oncology Group; NA, not available; ND, no difference reported; OS, overall survival; PFS, progression-free survival.

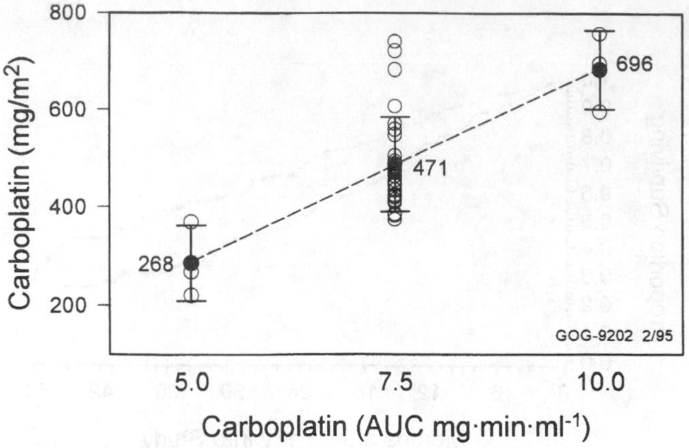

FIGURE 36.5-8. Comparison of carboplatin dosage by area under the curve (AUC) and body surface in ovarian cancer patients receiving combination chemotherapy with paclitaxel and carboplatin. Most patients received an AUC of 7.5, which corresponds to a mean dose (based on body surface area) of 471 mg/m^2. (From ref. 140, with permission.)

according to AUC considerations and if paclitaxel was administered at 175 mg/m^2 in a 3-hour infusion. The selection of a 3-hour paclitaxel infusion was based on a prior European/Canadian trial[132] in which patients with previously treated advanced ovarian cancer were randomized in a two-by-two bifactor design to receive paclitaxel by 24- or 3-hour infusion and one of two different doses of paclitaxel (175 mg/m^2 or 135 mg/m^2). A 3-hour infusion at 175 mg/m^2 was the preferred paclitaxel dose schedule for patients with ovarian cancer because of decreased neutropenia and a trend toward increased efficacy at the higher dose. The GOG pilot study demonstrated the safety and efficacy of paclitaxel (175 mg/m^2) in a 3-hour infusion together with carboplatin (dosed to an AUC of 7.5).[140] The overall response rate to this combination was 75%, with 67% of 24 patients with measurable disease achieving a clinical complete remission. The median dose of carboplatin was 470 mg/m^2 when using the Calvert formula to select an AUC of 7.5 (Fig. 36.5-8). This dose of carboplatin, even when combined with paclitaxel at 175 mg/m^2, was higher than that usually used in combinations when the drug is empirically dosed based on body surface area (300 to 350 mg/m^2).

All three randomized trials comparing cisplatin plus paclitaxel versus carboplatin with paclitaxel have been presented in preliminary form and all have come to the same conclusion. GOG 158[137] was the largest of these trials and was different from the European studies in that only patients with optimal stage III disease were eligible. More than 800 patients were randomized to cisplatin (75 mg/m^2) plus paclitaxel (135 mg/m^2 at 24-hour infusion) versus carboplatin (AUC = 7.5) plus paclitaxel (175 mg/m^2 in a 3-hour infusion). Patients were well balanced for prognostic factors. No difference was found in median times to progression between these two regimens, and the hazard ratio was 0.90 (95% CI, 0.76 to 1.11), which essentially excludes the possibility that carboplatin plus paclitaxel is inferior to cisplatin plus paclitaxel. In addition, increased metabolic and gastrointestinal toxicity was associated with the cisplatin regimen. Survival comparisons between the two treatment arms await further penetration of the data. The Arbeitsgemeinschaft Gynaekologische Onkologie trial[138] incorporated the quality-of-life instrument in its comparison of cisplatin plus paclitaxel versus carboplatin plus paclitaxel and demonstrated the superiority of the carboplatin combination. Based on these clinical trials, carboplatin plus paclitaxel is now generally accepted to be the preferred platinum regimen for treatment of patients with advanced ovarian cancer.

Numerous issues still remain regarding the optimal use of paclitaxel with carboplatin in patients with ovarian cancer. The importance of dose and schedule of paclitaxel has not been established. Phase II trials of high-dose paclitaxel (250 mg/m^2) had reported a response rate of 48%,[141] which was higher than other phase II trials using lower doses. The GOG has completed a randomized trial of two different doses of paclitaxel. This trial showed that high-dose paclitaxel (250 mg/m^2) had only a modest effect in patients with recurrent ovarian cancer.[142] The overall response rate was 36% versus 27.5% for a 175 mg/m^2 dose. Survival was similar—12.5 months versus 11.9 months. However, even with granulocyte colony-stimulating factor (G-CSF) support, substantially greater toxicity was seen with the higher dose schedule. Additional studies are currently in progress in Europe in previously untreated patients with advanced ovarian cancer who are randomized to receive two different doses of paclitaxel, with all patients receiving the same carboplatin dose. No survival data are yet available from these trials. The optimal number of cycles of paclitaxel plus carboplatin to be used as initial therapy for patients also remains to be determined. No evidence suggests that increasing the number of cycles of cisplatin plus cyclophosphamide improves outcome. Prospective randomized trials are, however, in progress in which patients who achieve a clinical complete remission with paclitaxel plus carboplatin are randomized to maintenance paclitaxel therapy for 3 to 12 months. Until the completion of these trials, standard chemotherapy for patients with advanced ovarian cancer consists of six cycles of paclitaxel (175 mg/m^2 in a 3-hour infusion) plus carboplatin dosed to an AUC of 5.0 to 7.5.

Management after Induction Chemotherapy

The majority of previously untreated patients achieve a clinical complete remission after induction chemotherapy. Clinical complete remission is defined as no evidence of disease on physical examination or by radiographic studies, together with a normal CA-125. However, between 50% and 75% of advanced-disease patients ultimately relapse from a clinical remission. Even patients who are surgically confirmed to be in a complete remission (negative second look) still remain at high risk with a relapse rate of 30% to 50% after platinum-based chemotherapy.

SECOND-LOOK SURGERY. Second-look surgery is a carefully planned systematic surgical approach to evaluating patients who have completed a program of chemotherapy and who, by clinical examination and by diagnostic imaging studies, are free of evidence of persistent cancer. The purpose of the second-look operation is to completely explore the abdominal cavity, sample any abnormalities found, and biopsy peritoneal surfaces where microscopic ovarian cancer is likely to be found. If disease is present, additional therapy should be routinely recommended.

Second-look operations were originally introduced by Wangenstein et al.[143] for evaluating patients with colon cancer. It was then applied in a series of studies to ovarian cancer management. The surgery is performed through a vertical incision that allows access to the peritoneal cavity from the pelvis to the diaphragm.

On entering the abdominal cavity, washings of the paracolic and pelvic spaces are performed. Adhesions are lysed and sent for histologic assessment. Sampling then begins in the pelvis with removal of large strips of peritoneum (2 cm × 3 cm) from the pelvic side walls in the areas of the round ligaments and the infundibulopelvic ligaments, from the bladder flap peritoneum, and from the cul-de-sac peritoneum. Epiploic appendices of the sigmoid colon are removed. The retroperitoneal spaces are examined, and any residual lymph node or fatty tissues surrounding the external iliac artery, vein, or hypogastric artery are removed.

Remnants of omentum are then removed, as are large strips (3 cm × 5 cm) of peritoneum in the right and left pericolic spaces. The diaphragm is carefully inspected; any abnormalities are removed. If no abnormalities are present, a strip of peritoneum overlying the inferior surface of the diaphragm also is removed. The bowel is carefully inspected. Any nodules on the bowel surfaces are removed. Any mesenteric implants are removed. The retroperitoneal space is then explored by mobilizing the bowel. The paraaortic and vena cava areas are explored, and nodularities and fat pads are removed. The anterior abdominal wall peritoneum is also sampled. At the completion of the procedure, somewhere between 20 and 40 biopsies of peritoneum and fat pads, including the retroperitoneal lymph node–bearing areas, should have been obtained. The thoroughness of the second-look operation is determined less by the number of samples obtained and more by the size of the sheets of peritoneum that are stripped off. The larger the volume of tissue available for the pathologist to inspect, the greater the chances are that occult disease will be identified.

The most important factors determining whether a second-look operation is negative are cancer stage at the initial operation and the volume of residual disease at that operation.[144,145] Patients with stage I disease have a very high incidence of negative second-look operations, whereas those with advanced disease have a significantly lower incidence of negative second-look surgeries. Patients with no residual disease after primary cytoreductive surgery have a 77% incidence of negative second-look operations. Those with less than 2 cm of residual disease have an approximately 45% incidence of negative second-look surgeries, and those with disease greater than 2 cm have no more than a 25% incidence.[145] The timing of second-look surgery has changed over the years. With the introduction of cisplatin and doxorubicin chemotherapy in the 1970s, prolonged chemotherapy was no longer indicated. As noted, randomized clinical trials did not demonstrate any improvement after six cycles of platinum-based treatment. Second-look operations only are routinely recommended for women participating in clinical trials.

Second-look operations are not without complications. A report by Rubin and Lewis[145] analyzing 682 second-look surgeries suggested that the overall rate of morbidity was approximately 19%. A typical problem associated with this operation is infections in the surgical incision, the urinary tract, and the lungs. Some reports also have indicated the presence of bleeding and the need for blood transfusions. Experience at the Yale–New Haven Medical Center would suggest that incidence of recurrent ovarian cancer after a negative second-look operation was in the 15% to 20% range; however, others have reported recurrence rates as high as 50% within 1 year.

The greatest value of second-look surgery is assessing patients on clinical protocols in which an answer to a question regarding therapeutic efficacy is being asked or for patients who are willing to go on to second-line therapy in a research format when the status of their cancer is important to answer clinical research questions.

Advances in laparoscopic surgery have led to recommendations for laparoscopy as an alternative to laparotomy.[27,146] Laparoscopic surgery can be useful if the patient is found to have disseminated miliary-type cancer and can avoid a laparotomy. However, if the patient has focal disease, it may be missed at second-look laparoscopy because of technical reasons, or it may not be resectable through a laparoscope and a second-look laparotomy must be performed. Gynecologic oncologists skilled with advanced laparoscopic techniques are now providing data suggesting that, in their hands, laparoscopic second-look operations are comparable to laparotomies.

Patients at highest risk for recurrent disease after achieving a complete remission are those who had large-volume disease before initiation of chemotherapy and those with more poorly differentiated tumors.[147] The overall survival rate for patients with recurrent ovarian cancer is poor, and it depends on a multiplicity of factors, the most important being the length of the initial disease-free interval. However, the vast majority of patients with recurrent ovarian cancer ultimately succumb to their disease. Consequently, numerous clinical strategies are being studied in an effort to prevent or delay recurrences in patients who achieve a clinical complete remission.

RADIOTHERAPY AFTER OR COMBINED WITH CHEMOTHERAPY. Numerous small phase I and II studies have used whole abdominal irradiation as salvage treatment for patients with minimal residual disease after chemotherapy. Some authors have reported 3-year progression-free survival rates as high as 25% to 35% and occasional 10- to 15-year disease-free survivors among patients treated with abdominal irradiation after an incomplete response to chemotherapy.[148–151] However, others have reported high complication rates and have been discouraged by the short duration of most remissions, particularly for patients with high-grade disease or macroscopic residual tumor.[152,153] Reported 5-year survival rates for patients treated with abdominal irradiation after a negative second-look laparotomy have been approximately 60% to 70%, but are not clearly different from reported survival rates with platinum-based chemotherapy alone.

Two randomized trials have compared whole abdominal irradiation with additional consolidative chemotherapy for patients with minimal disease after surgical cytoreduction and platinum-containing chemotherapy. Bruzzone and associates[154] randomized patients who had minimal or no residual disease after chemotherapy [doxorubicin, cyclophosphamide (Cytoxan), and cisplatin or carboplatin] to receive whole abdominal irradiation or three more cycles of chemotherapy. The study was closed after accruing only 41 patients because disease progression had been observed in 55% of patients treated with radiation versus 29% of those treated with additional chemotherapy ($P = .08$). The authors recommended treatment with chemotherapy, but the small number of patients and short median follow-up weaken the conclusions of their study. In a second study by Lambert and coworkers,[155] 254 patients with stage IIB to IV disease received five monthly courses of carboplatin and second-look laparotomy. The 117 patients who had residual disease of 2 cm or less after secondary cytoreduction were then randomized to receive either five additional courses of carboplatin or whole abdominal irradiation (24 Gy in 5 weeks). The authors reported no statistical difference in survival or disease-free survival rates between the two treatment arms.

Although a small proportion of patients treated with whole abdominal irradiation for microscopic residual disease after chemotherapy enjoy long disease-free intervals, the control rates appear to be much poorer than those reported for patients treated with initial radiation for a similar volume of residual disease. A number of factors may contribute to these disappointing results. Patients who have not responded completely to chemotherapy may have disease that is inherently more aggressive than that of patients chosen for primary treatment with whole abdominal irradiation. Radiotherapy is often compromised because of poor hematologic tolerance after aggressive chemotherapy, which further decreases the probability of the tumor being sterilized. It also has been suggested that cytoreductive treatments (surgery, irradiation, or chemotherapy) may stimulate the proliferation of clonogenic tumor cells. Consequently, to overcome rapid repopulation, higher doses of radiation may be required to sterilize tumor cells that remain after a course of chemotherapy.

Hoskins and colleagues[156] have reported encouraging results for a regimen that integrated whole abdominal irradiation in the initial treatment of patients with minimal residual disease after cytoreduction. In their study, radiation was given after the first three of six cycles of cisplatin and cyclophosphamide. Comparison with the results of similar patients treated during a later time with six cycles of chemotherapy alone favored the alternating regimen, particularly for patients with stage I disease ($P = .04$).

Clinical trials of other modalities focused on preventing or delaying recurrence after initial chemotherapy are in progress: consolidation with high-dose chemotherapy, whole abdominal irradiation, intraperitoneal ^{32}P, intraperitoneal chemotherapy with cisplatin, intraperitoneal immunotherapy, and additional cycles of systemic chemotherapy and hormonal therapy with agents such as tamoxifen. Randomized trials addressing these modalities have been limited by slow accrual, and currently there is no evidence that consolidation treatment is able to improve survival after six cycles of initial treatment with paclitaxel plus a platinum compound.

TREATMENT OF RECURRENT OVARIAN CANCER

The selection of treatment modalities and drug regimens for patients with recurrent ovarian cancer is based on the initial chemotherapy regimen used and on the nature of the initial response to treatment. Patients with recurrent ovarian cancer can be broadly divided into two subsets with a markedly different prognosis. Patients whose disease recurs with a disease-free interval of less than 6 months have a worse prognosis that approaches that of patients who progress while receiving their initial chemotherapeutic regimen. In contrast, patients who have a disease-free interval of more than 6 months or 1 year have a markedly improved prognosis, primarily because of the increased efficacy of salvage chemotherapy. In patients with a long disease-free interval, secondary cytoreductive surgery can be considered in select subsets of patients.

Secondary Cytoreductive Surgery

Primary cytoreductive surgery has well-documented benefits in the management of women with advanced ovarian cancer. The possibility that secondary cytoreductive surgery (i.e., surgery performed to remove known persistent or recurrent disease after initiating chemotherapy) may be beneficial to patients has been suggested by numerous authors.[144] Berek et al.[157] reported that secondary cytoreductive surgery could be performed on 12 of 32 patients (38%), and their tumors were reduced to less than 1.5 cm of residual disease. The median survival for that group was 20 months, compared with 5 months for the 20 patients whose disease could not be optimally cytoreduced. The patients most likely to undergo optimal cytoreductive surgery were those who previously had optimal primary cytoreduction, less than 1000 mL of ascites, and a tumor size of less than 5 cm at the second operation. The interval from the primary to secondary surgery should be longer than 12 months. Factors that did not have an impact on secondary cytoreductive surgery included patient age, tumor grade, type of chemotherapy, and the presence or absence of bowel obstruction. Subsequently, Segna et al.[158] reported their experience with secondary cytoreductive surgery. They too were able to show that if optimal secondary cytoreductive surgery could be performed, patients lived longer before succumbing to ovarian cancer. Factors that influenced successful efforts in cytoreductive surgery were a time interval of more than 1 year between the original operation and the secondary cytoreductive surgery and having optimal cytoreductive surgery performed at the initial operation. It is the current recommendation at the Yale–New Haven Medical Center that women who would be suitable for secondary cytoreductive surgery at the time of recurrence are those who have had more than a 1-year time interval between the initial operation and the diagnosis of recurrence. These women preferably had optimal cytoreductive surgery performed at the initial operation. However, if a review of the operative report suggests that an aggressive attempt at optimal cytoreductive surgery was not performed, this would make them suitable for secondary cytoreductive surgery.

Neijt et al.[159] compared the survival of women who underwent optimal cytoreductive surgery with the survival of women who were unsuccessfully optimally cytoreduced but in whom, generally after three cycles of cisplatin-based chemotherapy, a secondary cytoreductive surgery was attempted. Those patients who underwent optimal secondary cytoreductive surgery had a statistically improved survival rate compared with those who were unable to undergo optimal secondary cytoreductive surgery. However, those patients who were optimally secondarily cytoreduced did not have a survival rate comparable to those patients who had optimal cytoreduction performed at the initial operation (Fig. 36.5-9).

van der Burg et al.[160] reported on the European Organization for Research and Treatment of Cancers (EORTC) experience with debulking surgery after induction chemotherapy for advanced ovarian cancer. Three hundred nineteen of 425 patients with advanced epithelial ovarian cancer who had more than 1 cm in diameter of residual tumor after primary surgery received three cycles of cyclophosphamide and cisplatin and were randomized to undergo secondary cytoreductive surgery or no surgery. Both groups received additional chemotherapy. The progression-free and overall survival rates were both significantly longer in the group that underwent surgery ($P = .01$) (Fig. 36.5-10). The difference in survival was 6 months. At 2 years after initial diagnosis, 56% of the group that underwent surgery were alive, as opposed to 46% of the group that did

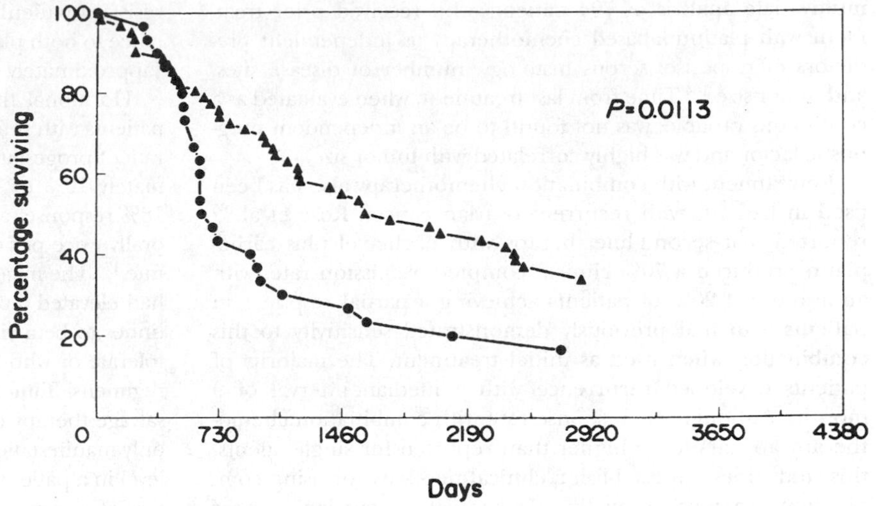

FIGURE 36.5-9. Survival after cytoreductive surgery leading to tumor residuals of 1 cm or smaller at the staging laparotomy (staging) or during chemotherapy (intervention cytoreductive surgery). (From ref. 159, with permission.)

not. In an update, the 5-year survival rate was 23% for the surgery group and 12% for the nonsurgery group.[161] A multivariate analysis determined that debulking surgery was an independent prognostic factor (P = .012) for survival. After adjusting for all other prognostic factors, the risk of dying was reduced by 33% (95% CI, 10% to 50%; P = .008). This study statistically confirmed improved survival with optimal secondary cytoreductive surgery. However, secondary cytoreductive surgery does not make up for inadequate cytoreductive surgery performed at the initial operation.

Palliative surgery may be necessary in women with advanced ovarian cancer. This surgery may involve a colostomy for relief of a large bowel obstruction, lyses of adhesions, and surgical management of small bowel obstruction. Small bowel obstruction is a common complication as ovarian cancer advances and becomes refractory to chemotherapy. In considering surgery to relieve small bowel obstruction, the time from the original diagnosis and treatment of the ovarian cancer to the time of the obstruction is important, as is the adequacy of the initial cytoreductive surgery. Women who present with small bowel obstruction during the initial course of chemotherapy and who have not undergone optimal cytoreductive surgery generally have biologically aggressive tumors for which the role for surgery of the small bowel is minimal. A palliative gastrostomy tube may be most appropriate in this situation. In turn, women who have had prolonged periods during which they were free of disease, usually lasting more than 1 year from the original diagnosis, do benefit from small bowel surgery to relieve obstruction. However, a pseudo–small bowel obstruction pattern can be seen in women with advanced ovarian cancer with intraabdominal carcinomatosis, which occurs when ovarian cancer cells infiltrate the myenteric plexus of the small bowel. Surgery generally plays no role in management of these patients. Medical treatment with metoclopramide, which stimulates motility of the upper gastrointestinal tract without stimulating gastric, biliary, or pancreatic secretions, may at times be helpful. Large bowel obstruction, particularly sigmoid colon obstruction, is relieved by performing colostomies and can allow the patient to have significant prolongation of life and improved quality of life if the disease is confined to the pelvis.

Chemotherapy for Recurrent Disease

Patients with ovarian cancer who had a response to chemotherapy and then relapsed after a disease-free interval of more than 6 months are considered drug sensitive. These patients are routinely retreated with single-agent carboplatin or paclitaxel. The likelihood of achieving a secondary response to either of these agents is based on the length of the disease-free interval.[162] Single-agent carboplatin has a more favorable toxicity profile than cisplatin and remains the preferable platinum compound for treatment of recurrent disease. Some studies have suggested that the weekly administration of paclitaxel may be superior to the use of the traditional 3-week schedule in patients with recurrent ovarian cancer,[163] although prospective randomized trials comparing these two different schedules are currently in progress. In addition to the "platinum-free" interval, the probability of response to second-line chemotherapy is related to additional clinical factors. Eisenhauer et al.[164] identified three factors in a

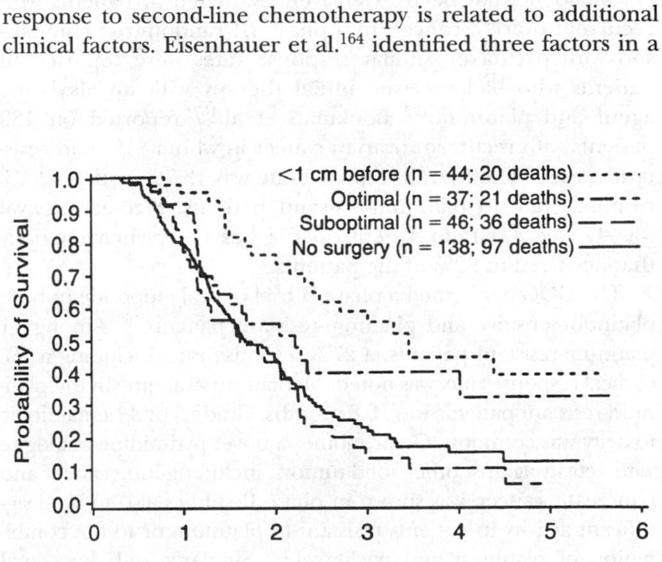

FIGURE 36.5-10. Survival of patients with advanced epithelial ovarian cancer who did not have debulking surgery and patients who had such surgery, according to whether the lesions were less than 1 cm in diameter before cytoreduction, less than 1 cm after cytoreduction (optimal), or more than 1 cm after cytoreduction (suboptimal). (From ref. 160, with permission.)

multivariate analysis of 704 patients who received prior treatment with platinum-based chemotherapy as independent predictors of response: serous histology, number of disease sites, and tumor size.[164] Time from last treatment, when evaluated as a continuous variable, was not found to be an independent prognostic factor and was highly correlated with tumor size.

Retreatment with combination chemotherapy also has been used in patients with recurrent ovarian cancer. Rose et al.[165] reported that second-line therapy with paclitaxel plus carboplatin produced a 70% clinical complete remission rate, with an additional 20% of patients achieving a partial response in patients who had previously demonstrated sensitivity to this combination when used as initial treatment. The majority of patients developed recurrence with a median interval of 9 months. Although the response rate with combination chemotherapy appears to be higher than reported for single agents, this study does not establish a clinical necessity for using combination chemotherapy in drug-sensitive ovarian cancer patients at the time of recurrence. It is possible that the same long-term survival rates could have been achieved by use of these drugs in sequence. For most patients, the appropriate choice of second-line treatment consists of single-agent chemotherapy with combinations reserved primarily for patients who have a prolonged disease-free interval.

For patients who did not respond to platinum- or paclitaxel-based retreatment or who developed resistance to these drugs when used as second-line agents, numerous other agents have been shown to have activity. However, response rates are significantly lower in patients who have platinum- or paclitaxel-resistant ovarian cancer, and these patients should be encouraged to enter experimental clinical trials. Drugs that have been shown to be active in patients with platinum- and paclitaxel-resistant ovarian cancer include topotecan,[166,167] oral etoposide,[168] gemcitabine,[169] liposomal doxorubicin,[170] and vinorelbine.[171]

Topotecan, a second-generation semisynthetic camptothecin analogue, has been extensively evaluated in patients with recurrent ovarian cancer. In a phase III randomized comparison with paclitaxel, similar response rates were reported in patients who had received initial therapy with an alkylating agent and platinum.[172] Bookman et al.[167] reported on 139 patients with recurrent ovarian cancer in whom 81% had resistant disease. The overall response rate was 13.7%, with a 12.4% response rate in platinum-resistant patients. Median survival was 47 weeks. Grade 4 neutropenia was the primary toxicity that occurred in 82% of the patients.

The GOG performed a phase II trial of oral etoposide in both platinum-sensitive and platinum-resistant patients.[168] Among 41 platinum-resistant patients, a 27% response rate, including a 7% clinical response rate, was noted. Median survival time in the platinum-resistant patients was 10.8 months. Grade 3 or 4 hematologic toxicity was common. Gemcitabine, a novel pyrimidine analogue with activity against other solid tumors, including lung cancer and pancreatic cancer, was shown in phase II studies also to have significant activity in patients resistant to platinum or to the combination of platinum and paclitaxel.[169] Similarly, with liposomal doxorubicin, a response rate of 26% was observed in platinum-resistant patients with a median progression-free survival rate of 5.7 months. Grade 3 and 4 nonhematologic skin and mucosal toxicities were common.

In addition to these newer drugs, older agents, such as hexamethylmelamine and ifosfamide, also have activity in platinum-resistant patients, although it appears that in patients with resistance to both platinum and paclitaxel, the response rates are low (approximately 10%).

Hormonal therapy has long been used in the treatment of patients with refractory ovarian cancer.[173,174] The overall response rate of progestational agents and antiestrogens has been approximately 10% to 15%. A large GOG study, however, reported an 18% response rate for tamoxifen administered at a dose of 20 mg orally twice per day, including a 10% clinical complete remission rate.[173] The majority of patients achieving a response in this study had elevated levels of estrogen receptor. Hormonal therapy continues to be a viable therapeutic option for patients who cannot tolerate or who have been unsuccessful with numerous cytotoxic regimens. Tamoxifen also has been recommended as the initial salvage therapy for patients who have a rising CA-125 level as the only manifestation of their disease.[174,175] Although a rising CA-125 level in a patient in a clinical complete remission is highly predictive of a symptomatic recurrence (median time to physical or radiographic evidence of recurrent disease is 4 to 6 months), there is no evidence that immediate treatment with salvage chemotherapy is more effective than reserving such treatment for when other manifestations of recurrent disease appear. A trial is ongoing in the United Kingdom in which patients with elevated markers are randomized to immediate systemic therapy or to treatment at the time of symptomatic progression.

Palliative Radiotherapy

Radiation therapy can play an important role in palliation of patients with incurable ovarian cancer. Symptoms from a growing pelvic mass frequently dominate the final months of life for patients with terminal ovarian cancer, causing pain, bleeding, and rectal narrowing. Palliative pelvic radiotherapy can provide rapid relief and, in some cases, may prevent or delay the need for diverting colostomy.

Palliative treatment courses are designed to be convenient and to achieve rapid symptom relief. At the M. D. Anderson Cancer Center, palliation of pelvic disease has been achieved using two single-fraction treatments of 10 Gy each to the true pelvis delivered 1 month apart.[176] Treatment is delivered using 18 to 25 MeV photons. In a report of 42 patients who had advanced ovarian cancer and were treated with this approach, Adelson and coworkers[176] reported that tumors in 19% of patients partially or completely responded to irradiation after one fraction and 75% responded after two fractions. Toxicity was minimal if treatment was limited to two fractions (20 Gy). However, they reported major hemorrhagic complications in four of eight patients who survived more than 6 months after three fractions. Spanos and colleagues[177] reported a high rate of gastrointestinal complications (49% at 1 year) in patients who were treated with three fractions of 10 Gy each and misonidazole for a variety of advanced pelvic malignancies.

The Radiation Therapy Oncology Group investigated the efficacy of a multiple daily fraction split-course regimen (14.8 Gy delivered at 3.7 Gy per fraction in 2 days) in patients with advanced pelvic malignancies.[178] Treatment was repeated every 2 to 4 weeks for a total dose of up to 44.4 Gy. A complete or partial tumor response was reported in 34% of patients (42% of those completing three courses), and toxic effects were acceptable. The interval between fractions had no significant influence on the response rate.

TABLE 36.5-14. Pharmacokinetic Advantage Associated with Intraperitoneal Administration of Selected Cytotoxic Agents

Agent	*Peak Peritoneal Cavity to Plasma Concentration Ratio*
Doxorubicin	474
Mitoxantrone	620
Cisplatin	20
Carboplatin	18
Mitomycin	71
5-Fluorouracil	298
Methotrexate	92
Paclitaxel	1000

(From ref. 181, with permission.)

Other authors have reported relief of pelvic pain, bleeding, large bowel obstruction, pulmonary compromise, bone pain, and other symptoms of metastatic disease with radiotherapy using a variety of fractionation schemes.[179] Patients with isolated cerebral metastases should be treated with combined surgical resection, postoperative whole brain irradiation, and chemotherapy, if possible.[180] With this treatment, some patients survive for more than 3 years. Survival after treatment with radiation alone is usually less than 6 months.

Intraperitoneal Chemotherapy

Clinical trials evaluating direct intraperitoneal installation of antineoplastic agents were based on the biology of ovarian cancer and on pharmacologic modeling studies.[181] Physiologic and anatomic characteristics of the peritoneal cavity and the chemical properties of antineoplastic drugs suggested that the intraperitoneal administration of anticancer agents in a large volume would lead to a pharmacologic advantage compared with intravenous therapy. A series of phase I studies demonstrated that large-volume intermittent dialysis was feasible via a semipermanent Tenckhoff catheter (Table 36.5-14). These studies demonstrated that, despite a significant number (20% to 30%) of instances in which uniform distribution of drugs containing dialysate could not be achieved because of adhesions, overall intraperitoneal therapy was technically feasible and associated with a marked pharmacologic advantage defined as the ratio of antineoplastic agent in the dialysate compared with blood levels. The development of implantable peritoneal access devices (Port-A-Cath) facilitated patient acceptance and decreased the complication rate. Most recently, paclitaxel has been evaluated via the intraperitoneal route.[181] Intraperitoneal administration led to a marked pharmacologic advantage, and 61% of patients who had microscopic disease before intraperitoneal paclitaxel achieved a response to therapy.

Phase II trials demonstrated that cisplatin had the highest activity when administered via the intraperitoneal route to patients with recurrent ovarian cancer. Intraperitoneal chemotherapy had no advantage in patients with bulky disease. However, in patients with small-volume residual ovarian cancer, responses were observed (40%) in those patients who had prior response to intravenous cisplatin.[182] Because this is the same group of patients who also had the greatest benefit from retreatment with systemic cisplatin,[183] the possibility remained that the primary benefit of intraperitoneal therapy in these trials was due to systemic absorption and delivery to the tumor via the microcirculation.

More recently, intraperitoneal chemotherapy has been compared with intravenous therapy in randomized trials. A large prospective randomized study of intraperitoneal cisplatin (100 mg/m^2) combined with intravenous cyclophosphamide (600 mg/m^2) compared with intravenous cisplatin (100 mg/m^2) and intravenous cyclophosphamide in patients with optimal advanced ovarian cancer was initiated in the late 1980s[184] (Table 36.5-15). Patients eligible for this intergroup study all had residual tumor masses of less than 2 cm at the completion of cytoreductive surgery. The intraperitoneal arm was considered to be superior based on pathologically confirmed complete remission (40% vs. 31%, $P = .10$) and patient survival (median survival, 49 months vs. 41 months) and a decrease in the death-hazard ratio to 0.76 for the patients treated with intraperitoneal therapy. In addition, clinical hearing loss and neutropenia were more frequent and more severe in patients receiving intravenous cisplatin. During the long duration of this study, standard intravenous chemotherapy for ovarian cancer has changed from cisplatin plus cyclophosphamide to carboplatin plus paclitaxel. Consequently, it remains to be determined whether intraperitoneal cisplatin produces a similar advantage when combined with intravenous paclitaxel. A prospective randomized trial comparing intravenous cisplatin and paclitaxel to an experimental arm consisting of two cycles of carboplatin dosed to an AUC of 9 followed by six cycles of intraperitoneal cisplatin and intravenous paclitaxel has been completed.[185] Recurrence-free survival was increased in the experimental arm by 5.1 months, although there is no statisti-

TABLE 36.5-15. Intraperitoneal Cisplatin in Previously Untreated Ovarian Cancer

	Intraperitoneal Cisplatin (100 mg/m^2) plus Cyclophosphamide (600 mg/m^2)	*Intravenous Cisplatin (100 mg/m^2) plus Cyclophosphamide (600 mg/m^2)*
Stage III with less than 2.0 cm residual disease	263 patients	276 patients
Response: negative second look	62/156 (40%)	52/168 (31%)
Median survival	49 mo	41 mo
Intraperitoneal versus intravenous death hazard ratio	.76	—
Toxicity	—	Hearing loss, neutropenia

(From ref. 184, with permission.)

cally significant difference in overall survival. The experimental arm had significantly increased toxicity. Based on these results and the activity of intraperitoneal paclitaxel, the GOG is conducting another randomized trial in which patients with optimal stage III disease are comparing standard intravenous paclitaxel plus cisplatin to an experimental regimen of intravenous paclitaxel on day 1, intraperitoneal cisplatin on day 2, and intraperitoneal paclitaxel on day 8.

A separate phase III trial of intraperitoneal chemotherapy is in progress in Europe. Patients with a surgically confirmed complete remission to standard induction chemotherapy are randomized to receive six cycles of intraperitoneal cisplatin as a consolidation regimen compared with observation. No results are available from this trial.

EXPERIMENTAL THERAPY

High-Dose Chemotherapy with Hematologic Support

Standard-dose chemotherapy produces response rates in more than 70% of patients with advanced ovarian cancer. However, most patients develop disease recurrence, at which point salvage therapy has limited curative potential. Because of the high response rate to standard-dose chemotherapy and because of retrospective studies identifying a relationship between dose intensity and response, numerous clinical studies have evaluated high-dose chemotherapy with hematologic support. However, no established role has yet been determined for high-dose chemotherapy with hematologic support in the routine treatment of patients with advanced ovarian cancer.

The initial trials used autologous bone marrow rescue in heavily treated patients who were treated with single agents followed by transplantation. Subsequently, combinations of high-dose alkylating agents and platinum compounds were evaluated. Shpall et al.[186] summarized the results of phase I and phase II trials in ovarian cancer patients. The overall response rate is approximately 70% to 80%; however, the median duration of response is less than 10 months.

More recently, Stiff et al.[187] reported on the results with high-dose chemotherapy with hematologic support in 100 patients with recurrent or persistent ovarian cancer. They performed a univariate and multivariate analysis to identify factors associated with prolonged survival after high-dose chemotherapy. Cisplatin sensitivity and bulk of disease were identified as the best predictors for progression-free survival. Median progression-free and overall survival rates for 20 patients with platinum-sensitive disease with less than 1 cm of volume were 19 and 30 months, respectively. In the absence of a prospective randomized trial, there is no evidence that this approach produces superior results in patients with platinum-sensitive small-volume disease compared with what could be achieved with traditional second-line chemotherapy.

In this and other studies, it is apparent that the most favorable group of patients in whom additional trials with high-dose chemotherapy are indicated consists of patients who have both chemotherapy-sensitive tumors as well as a low tumor burden. Preclinical and clinical studies also suggest that multiple applications of high-dose chemotherapy may be superior to single courses. The combination of peripheral stem cell transfusions with hematopoietic growth factors has permitted the evaluation of multiple courses of high-dose therapy in patients with ovarian cancer. Investigators at the Memorial Sloan-Kettering Cancer Center[188] performed phase I and II studies of dose escalation of paclitaxel with high-dose cyclophosphamide and peripheral blood stem cell transfusions in chemotherapy-naïve patients with advanced ovarian cancer. Induction therapy consisted of two cycles of cyclophosphamide (3 g/m^2) plus escalating doses of paclitaxel (from 150 to 350 mg/m^2) followed by G-CSF and leukopheresis to harvest peripheral stem cells. Patients then received four courses of rapidly cycled carboplatin and cyclophosphamide (1500 mg/m^2 per course) with hematopoietic rescue. Multiple cycles of high-dose chemotherapy could be safely administered with hematopoietic support. The overall response rate was 100%, with 34% of the patients achieving a surgically confirmed complete response. A similar trial was reported by Schilder et al.[189] in previously untreated patients using a regimen that included high-dose carboplatin, paclitaxel, and topotecan. In high-risk patients with bulky disease, a 67% clinical complete response rate was reported.

Based on these results, the GOG is conducting a pilot study of multiple cycles of high-dose chemotherapy followed by peripheral stem cell transfusion in patients with small-volume disease. If it can be demonstrated that such an approach is feasible in a multicenter study, then a larger prospective randomized comparison against standard doses of chemotherapy in previously untreated patients will be performed. In addition, clinical trials are planned in evaluating the role of multiple cycles of high-dose chemotherapy as a consolidation treatment in patients who achieve an initial response to induction chemotherapy. There is no evidence from clinical trials that high-dose chemotherapy has significant curative potential in patients who have either bulky residual disease or drug-resistant tumors. At present, high-dose chemotherapy with hematologic support should be considered an experimental procedure, and patients should be entered on clinical trials evaluating safety and efficacy.

New Drug Combinations

The standard chemotherapy for ovarian cancer now consists of paclitaxel plus a platinum compound. Although the majority of patients achieve a response to therapy, time to progression is 22 months for patients with optimal stage III disease and 18 months for patients with suboptimal stage III and stage IV disease. As noted earlier in the section Chemotherapy for Recurrent Disease, a series of new agents have been shown to have activity in ovarian cancer, including topotecan, gemcitabine, oral etoposide, and encapsulated doxorubicin. New combinations based on the activity of paclitaxel and platinum are currently being evaluated.

Hansen et al.[190] reported on a phase II trial of gemcitabine in combination with paclitaxel and carboplatin. This combination resulted in a response rate of 100%, with the majority of patients having suboptimal disease. Herben et al.[191] reported that the three-drug combination of paclitaxel, cisplatin, and topotecan also produced a high response rate (60% clinical complete response and 27% partial response) in previously untreated patients, but was associated with significant neutropenia that required large dose reductions in all three agents and G-CSF support. With the large number of active compounds available for recurrent disease, numerous new potential combinations and sequences are under consideration. Currently, preclinical models have not been shown to be predictive in identifying the clinical activity of new combinations. Empirical phase I and phase II trials are in progress and will be followed by prospective randomized comparisons of three-drug combinations and sequential therapy to determine if there is any clinical benefit in the combination of paclitaxel and carboplatin compared with standard treatment.

Reversal of Drug Resistance

The molecular mechanisms associated with drug resistance, the primary factor that limits the curative potential of any salvage therapy in patients with ovarian cancer, are being extensively studied. Resistance to alkylating agents and platinum compounds has been shown to be multifactorial, and specific biochemical resistance pathways include (1) decreases in drug accumulation; (2) increased inactivation in the cytosol via detoxification enzymes, such as glutathione S-transferase, or by direct binding to nonprotein thiols such as glutathione; and (3) increased activity of DNA repair enzymes that remove lethal DNA adducts. For the taxanes, at least two mechanisms of acquired resistance have been identified in cells made resistant by prolonged exposure *in vitro*. In paclitaxel-resistant cells, increased expression of the membrane P glycoprotein efflux pump is seen, which leads to partial cross-resistance to bulky natural products, including vinca alkaloids and anthracyclines. In addition, paclitaxel-resistant cells have structure alterations in α and β tubulin protein subunits, which form an integral part of microtubules.

The inhibitor of γ-glutamylcysteine synthetase, buthionine sulfoximine, has entered phase II trials based on a phase I trial that demonstrated the agent could be safety administered while producing an 80% reduction in growth-stimulating hormone levels in circulating lymphocytes in the majority of drug-resistant patients.[192] Furthermore, growth-stimulating hormone depletion in tumor cells was also documented in this study. In the phase II trial, drug-resistant patients are receiving the combination of buthionine sulfoximine plus melphalan.

Additional clinical trials aimed at reversing drug resistance to platinum compounds are focused on DNA repair pathways. In platinum-resistant tumors, increased expression of nucleotide excision repair enzymes has been demonstrated, in particular XPA and ERCC1.[193] Previous studies had demonstrated that platinum sensitivity could be restored by inhibition of DNA polymerase α with aphidicolin.[194] Clinical evaluation of aphidicolin has been limited by drug availability. Current clinical trials are using inhibitors of ribonucleotide reductase (e.g., gemcitabine and hydroxyurea) in combination with cisplatin.

Combinations of cyclosporin and cisplatin have also been studied in platinum-resistant patients.[195] Cyclosporin and non-nephrotoxic and nonimmunosuppressive analogues, such as PSC 833, have the potential to reverse platinum resistance by down-regulation of oncogenes involved in signal transduction, which are elevated in platinum-resistant tumors.[193] These drugs are also potent inhibitors of the multidrug resistance (MDR)-1 efflux pump, although this pathway is not involved in platinum resistance. A GOG trial[195] reported a 25% response rate in platinum-resistant patients treated with cyclosporin and cisplatin. Larger trials with the less toxic PSC 833 are in progress.

Platinum resistance also has been linked to increased expression of c-erbB-2. Antibodies to c-erbB-2 in combination with cisplatin have shown synergistic cell kill *in vitro*.[196] Clinical evaluation of such a combination is in progress.

Numerous clinical trials have explored the potential to reverse the multidrug resistance phenotype in ovarian cancer. Three distinct patterns of this phenotype have been identified: (1) the classic MDR-1 (P glycoprotein) mechanism associated with natural products, such as the vinca alkaloids and doxorubicin; (2) altered topoisomerase (atypical MDR) phenotype, primarily associated with drugs involving inhibition of topoisomerase II, such as etoposide; and (3) multidrug resistance–associated protein (MRP). The clinical importance of each of these mechanisms of drug resistance in ovarian cancer has not been established. Tumors from doxorubicin-treated patients (approximately 30% to 50%) have higher levels of immunostaining of P glycoprotein than do tumors from untreated patients (approximately 10% to 15%), suggesting that MDR expression is at least associated with resistance to natural products.[197] However, because doxorubicin has not been routinely used as part of induction regimens, clinical trials of MDR inhibition in ovarian cancer have had decreased interest. The identification of the prominent role of paclitaxel in ovarian cancer has led to new interest in modulation of natural product resistance. It is clear, however, that paclitaxel resistance is multifactorial and includes alteration in molecular species and levels of tubulin, which may be more important than MDR.

Clinical studies have identified the association of MRP expression and drug resistance.[198] The frequency of MRP expression in ovarian cancer remains to be determined. One study suggests that an associated drug-resistant protein (Lrp) may have prognostic significance in ovarian cancer.[199]

Immunotherapy and Gene Therapy in Ovarian Cancer

Genetic alterations in oncogene and suppressor gene function and the immunobiology of ovarian cancer are reviewed elsewhere in this text. Abnormalities in suppressor gene function, particularly TP53, are common in ovarian cancer. Cisplatin sensitivity is associated with TP53 function, with loss of function usually resulting in resistance.[193] Loss of TP53 function may inhibit the drug-induced pathways of apoptosis. In experimental models of gene therapy, sensitivity to cisplatin can be restored in resistant cell lines by reintroduction of p53 into tumor cells.[200]

An additional potential gene therapy in ovarian cancer relates to molecular chemotherapy in which a gene product can selectively sensitize tumor cells to an agent not ordinarily toxic. Adenoviral-mediated delivery of herpes simplex virus thymidine kinase has been shown to selectively synthesize human ovarian cancer cells to ganciclovir, and clinical evaluation is planned for this combination.

The immunotherapy of ovarian cancer has evolved from the administration of nonspecific immunostimulants, such as *Corynebacterium parvum* to more specific therapies targeting antigens and surface receptors present on tumor cells. Interleukin-2 (IL-2) has been studied extensively in ovarian cancer patients, either as a single agent administered intraperitoneally or as part of adoptive immunotherapy together with lymphokine activated killer cells. In initial studies with IL-2 and lymphokine activated killer cells, peritoneal toxicity was unacceptable.[201] Subsequent trials with lower doses of IL-2 produced acceptable toxicity, and the preliminary report described apparent durable responses in selected patients with recurrent ovarian cancer treated with intraperitoneal IL-2.[202]

Antibody conjugates (either with antineoplastic drug, biologic toxin, or radioisotopes) also have been evaluated in early trials in ovarian cancer patients. On the basis of prolonged survival observed in a pilot study in patients with small-volume residual disease treated with iodine 131–labeled monoclonal antibody directed against an ovarian cancer phosphatase,[203] a larger confirmatory trial of this conjugate is planned in Europe.

BORDERLINE TUMORS

Epithelial tumors of low malignant potential (borderline malignant potential tumors), are unusual in that they have the capacity to metastasize yet the required treatment seems to be limited to surgery for the overwhelming majority of patients. The different pathologic and biologic natures of these tumors were not recognized by FIGO until 1971 and the World Health Organization in 1973.[204] Borderline malignant potential tumors are distinguished from benign mucinous and serous tumors by the presence of epithelial budding, multilayering of the epithelium, increased mitotic activity, and nuclear atypia. However, they are also associated with absence of stromal invasion. These tumors can be quite large in size, with the serous tumors having mean diameters varying between 7 and 12 cm and bilaterality ranging from 33% to 75%.[205] Mucinous tumors of borderline malignant potential tend to be larger, with a mean diameter of 17 to 20 cm, and can be associated with pseudomyxoma peritonei. One must always be certain to rule out the possibility of a synchronous appendiceal primary tumor when dealing with the latter entity.

Borderline malignant potential tumors represent approximately 4% to 14% of all ovarian malignancies. The mean age of women developing tumors of low malignant potential is 40 years, approximately 20 years earlier than the mean age for women with epithelial cancers of the ovary. Ovarian tumors of low malignant potential have been associated with infertility and ovulation induction.[206]

Ovarian tumors of low malignant potential are staged in the same manner as epithelial cancers (see Table 36.5-1). However, their survival rate, stage for stage, is far superior. Kurman and Trimble[207] reported that the survival for 538 women with tumors of low malignant potential who had stage I disease was 99% with a mean follow-up of 7 years. The survival for 415 women with stage II and III disease was 92% with a mean follow-up of 7 years. The causes of death in this review were radiation-associated complications in three patients, chemotherapy-associated complications in nine, and bowel obstruction in eight. Eight women died from invasive carcinoma, and 18 died of disease without any additional information. Noteworthy was the fact that more patients died of treatment-related complications than died of bowel obstruction from progressive disease.

Management of patients with low malignant potential tumors of the ovary is similar to that of the surgical management of invasive cancer. However, preservation of fertility should be routinely performed in young women. Tazelaar et al.[208] found no evidence of microscopic disease in grossly normal ovaries that were bivalved in 61 patients with stage I low malignant potential tumors of the ovary. Women with advanced disease or who have completed childbearing should undergo total abdominal hysterectomy and bilateral salpingo-oophorectomy with complete cancer staging. If intraabdominal disease is present, aggressive cytoreductive surgery should be performed.

The evidence is scant to suggest that treatment beyond that of the initial surgery has any beneficial role. This is true for stage II and III disease as well as for stage I disease. Appropriate adjuvant therapy has yet to be identified in the management of women with tumors of low malignant potential. Trope et al.[209] studied adjuvant therapy in 253 women with stage I and II ovarian tumors of low malignant potential in four randomized trials at the Norwegian Radium Hospital between 1970 and 1984. Adjuvant treatment consisted of (1) external radiation and intraperitoneal radioactive gold, or external radiation alone; (2) intraperitoneal radioactive gold or phosphorus followed by no further treatment or thiotepa; (3) thiotepa versus no further treatment; and (4) cisplatin versus intraperitoneal phosphorus. No differences in the two arms in any of the four randomized studies could be identified. It was recommended that adjuvant radiation and chemotherapy were not indicated in patients with stage I or II ovarian tumors of low malignant potential. A series of 94 patients reported by Chambers et al.[210] from Yale–New Haven Medical Center did not reveal any significant impact on adjuvant therapy for women with ovarian tumors of low malignant potential. Barnhill et al.[211] reported on 146 women with stage I serous tumors of low malignant potential. No adjuvant therapy was offered, and with a median follow-up of 42.4 months (range 1.6 to 108.0), no patient has developed a recurrence.

Attempts to identify women who might be at increased risk for recurrence based on flow cytometry studies have not demonstrated consistent results.[212,213] Evidence has yet to be presented confirming that routinely treating patients whose tumors are aneuploid provides survival benefit. Surgery should be the main treatment approach for this disease. Chemotherapy should be reserved for progressive disease that does not respond to surgical management.

SEX CORD–STROMAL TUMORS

Ovarian sex cord–stromal tumors represent approximately 5% of all ovarian cancers. In general, they tend to present with stage I disease and frequently are associated with hormonal effects, such as precocious puberty, amenorrhea, postmenopausal bleeding, or virilizing symptoms. Granulosa cell tumors are the most common of the sex cord–stromal tumors and may be associated with endometrial hyperplasia and endometrial carcinoma. One cannot always tell the steroid production of the malignancies based on histologic appearance. For example, granulosa cell tumors have been reported to be associated with virilization. Sertoli-Leydig cell tumors have been associated with endometrial cancer.[214] Pascale et al.[215] have demonstrated that, in virilized women, the findings of increased serum testosterone with normal gonadotropin levels and gonadotropin-releasing hormone agonist suppression of gonadotropins leading to normalization of testosterone levels suggest that various ovarian androgen-secreting tumors are not autonomous but apparently depend on gonadotropin stimulation.

Willemsen et al.[216] reported on 12 patients who developed granulosa cell tumors. All patients in the series underwent ovarian hyperstimulation for the treatment of infertility. All patients received clomiphene citrate and gonadotropins or both. Willemsen et al.[216] postulated that granulosa cell tumors may already be present in the ovaries and are simply waiting for a hormone trigger or that the increased follicle-stimulating hormone concentrations used in ovulation induction are oncogenic to granulosa cells.[216] However, it is also possible that the discovery of granulosa cells during ovarian stimulation is coincidental.

Surgical staging of sex cord–stromal tumors is the same as that for epithelial ovarian cancers (see Table 36.5-1). Surgical management of sex cord–stromal tumors is based on the stage of the tumor as well as the age of the patient. In general, premenarchal women or patients presenting in the reproductive years tend to have stage I disease in most series. A unilateral salpingo-oophorectomy is all that is routinely necessary for the management of this disease. The role for adjuvant therapy in younger women has not been demonstrated. However, in women who have completed childbearing, surgery should be more aggressive, including a bilateral salpingo-oophorectomy and total abdominal hysterectomy along with standard surgical staging. Women older than age 40 at diagnosis are more likely to experience a recurrence of granulosa cell tumors, and it is for that reason that adjuvant therapy is recommended by some[214] in the older age population, although definitive evidence for its efficacy in preventing or delaying recurrences is lacking.

Patients with advanced-stage disease (i.e., stage II to IV) may benefit from additional therapy. Cisplatin-based combination chemotherapy has been the most frequently used treatment. However, few series have been reported, and they involve small numbers of women with granulosa cell tumors. Colombo et al.[217] demonstrated that primary treatment of six women with advanced granulosa cell tumor was effective using cisplatin, vinblastine, and bleomycin (the PVB regimen). However, their experience with the PVB regimen in five patients with recurrent disease was complicated by significant toxicity, leading to two deaths.[217] Pectasides et al.[218] reported on ten patients with advanced or recurrent granulosa cell tumor treated with cisplatin, Adriamycin, and cyclophosphamide (CAP). Five complete and one partial response was obtained. One of the pathologically complete respondents, however, relapsed 48 months after the onset of chemotherapy. Homesley et al.[219] reported a collaborative group experience using bleomycin, etoposide, and cisplatin combination chemotherapy in the treatment of women with sex cord–stromal tumors. Forty-eight of the 57 tumors were granulosa cell tumors. For the series as a whole, 35 patients (61.4%) receiving this combination chemotherapy regimen had complete responses. Eighteen of the 35 underwent second-look surgery. Fourteen of the 18 patients had pathologically negative second-look results, four patients had a partial response, 14 patients had stable disease, and two patients had progression of disease among the 55 patients evaluable for response. Sixteen patients received the chemotherapy after primary surgery, nine of whom had received the chemotherapy because of positive peritoneal cytology and seven for the treatment of gross residual disease. Eleven of 16 primary treatment patients (68.8%) are free of progressive disease, whereas 21 of 41 (51.2%) were free of disease when they were treated only after recurrent disease was noted.

The overall survival in two large series of granulosa cell tumors was 85% and 90%, with one series reporting 100% survival for stage I disease and the other reporting 94% survival for stage I disease at 5 years.

The current recommendations at Yale–New Haven Medical Center for women with early-stage granulosa cell tumors are surgery only for those younger than 40 and surgery followed by etoposide and carboplatin chemotherapy for women older than 40 who have stage I disease. For women older than 40 or for any woman with advanced-stage or recurrent disease, we recommend doxorubicin, cisplatin, and etoposide. Serum inhibin levels may be useful in monitoring for relapse.[220] However, there is at least anecdotal experience that it may be elevated for unexplained reasons. Another tumor marker, Müllerian inhibiting substance (MIS), is usually undetectable in females before puberty.[221] Gustafson et al.[221] reported that elevated MIS levels dramatically declined in two girls with granulosa cell tumors after surgery. MIS may be an effective marker for granulosa cell tumors and Sertoli-Leydig cell tumors. Lane et al.[222] have demonstrated preoperative elevations of MIS in six of eight subjects (75%) with juvenile granulosa cell tumors and seven of nine (78%) with adult granulosa cell tumors. None of 21 women with normal or nondetectable MIS levels developed recurrent granulosa cell tumors, but incompletely resected or recurrent disease was associated with elevated MIS levels in 6 of 15 patients.

Roush et al.[223] performed flow cytometric DNA ploidy and S-phase fraction analysis on 18 women with granulosa cell tumors of the ovary. Eleven of the tumors were diploid and 7 were aneuploid. Only one of ten (10%) with euploid tumors died of disease, whereas four out of five (80%) with aneuploid tumors died of the disease. This observation did not reach statistical correlation. Perhaps in the future flow cytometric studies may be useful in identifying which group of patients might benefit from adjuvant therapy as opposed to observation.

Sertoli-Leydig cell tumors occur much less often than granulosa cell tumors yet are the second most common sex cord–stromal tumor. Their management is the same as that of granulosa cell tumors in terms of staging, surgical management, and adjuvant chemotherapy. Rare forms of sex cord–stromal tumors include sex cord tumors with annular tubules associated with the Peutz-Jeghers syndrome that are usually confined to the ovaries and can be treated with surgery alone. Thecomas rarely are malignant. Malignant thecomas would be treated in the same manner as granulosa cell tumors.

Recurrent sex cord–stromal tumors are treated with surgical resection followed by adjuvant therapy. If the recurrence is isolated and could be encompassed in a radiation field, older literature suggests that radiation therapy may be of value if the malignancy is a granulosa cell tumor. The natural history of granulosa cell tumors is to be slow growing. Although late recurrences occur, it is difficult to know for certain whether it is the resection of the recurrent cancer or resection followed by the radiation therapy that has had an impact on prolonging patient survival. Patients with extensive recurrences should be treated with cisplatin-based combination chemotherapy.

EXTRAOVARIAN PERITONEAL CARCINOMA

The diagnosis and management of women who present with intraperitoneal carcinomatosis can represent a diagnostic and therapeutic problem. In some patients, the primary site is unknown, and peritoneal carcinomatosis can present as part of the syndrome of adenocarcinomas of unknown primary site. Adenocarcinomas of unknown primary site who present with peritoneal carcinomatosis can respond to chemotherapy with platinum-based regimens. In a series of 18 women treated with a platinum-based regimen, median survival was 23 months, and five patients had complete remissions and long-term survival.[224] The histologic classification and nomenclature of peritoneal carcinomatosis has been unclear and has included terms such as *mesothelioma, peritoneal papillary serous carcinoma, extraovarian serous carcinoma,* and *paraovarian cystadenocarcinoma.* Although embryologically the germinal epithelium of the ovary and the mesothelium of the peritoneal cavity are derived from the same celomic epithelium, a subset of peritoneal tumors can be morphologically identified that have a more favorable clinical behavior in response to therapy compared with peritoneal mesotheliomas.[225] It has been proposed that the former disease process be termed *peritoneal adenocarcinoma (serous) of Müllerian type.*[225] The serous type of peritoneal carcinomatosis is the most common. However, other histologic types of peritoneal carcinomatosis resulting from the common ancestry of celomic epithelium are possible, including mucinous, endometrioid, clear cell, and mixed peritoneal adenocarcinoma of Müllerian type. Using the proposed terminology, when an uncommon subtype other than serous is present, it can be encompassed in the description. Malignant mesotheliomas have a different histologic pattern and, in most cases, can be separated from the Müllerian-type peritoneal adenocarcinomas. Peritoneal mesotheliomas are more aggressive tumors, with a survival rate of usually less than 1 year. Furthermore, in women they are relatively less common than peritoneal adenocarcinomas of Müllerian type.

Most patients with extraovarian peritoneal carcinomatosis have signs and symptoms similar to those women who present with advanced-stage ovarian cancer. At surgery, these women frequently have ascites with diffuse peritoneal carcinomatosis. Attempts at cytoreductive surgery usually are made, although no evidence supports survival benefit in those women with peritoneal carcinomatosis who undergo optimum cytoreductive surgery. This may be due to the fact that although no tumor nodule larger than 1.5 cm is left behind, these women have innumerable such nodules throughout the peritoneal cavity and their actual tumor burden after cytoreductive surgery remains substantial. It appears that approximately 50% of patients with peritoneal carcinomatosis can be successfully surgically cytoreduced. Survival for patients with Müllerian peritoneal adenocarcinoma is similar to that reported for advanced ovarian cancer. In a large study from the University of California, Los Angeles, the median survival of patients who received chemotherapy after primary cytoreductive surgery was 28.4 months.[225] Patients who received cisplatin-based chemotherapy had a substantially longer survival rate (57% living longer than 23 months) than patients who were not treated with cisplatin-based regimens. Based on the pattern of metastases and chemosensitivity to platinum-based chemotherapy, it seems prudent that current therapy for this group of patients should include cytoreductive surgery followed by chemotherapy with paclitaxel plus a platinum compound.

GERM CELL TUMORS OF THE OVARY

Germ cell tumors of the ovary are much less common than epithelial ovarian neoplasms. However, because they are highly curable and because they affect primarily young women of childbearing potential, appropriate management by specialists is exceedingly important. Germ cell tumors account for 2% to 3% of all ovarian cancers in Western countries. They almost always occur in younger women, and their peak incidence is in the early 20s. An increased incidence of germ cell tumors is found in Asian and black societies, and these tumors represent as many as 15% of all ovarian cancers in these populations.

PATHOLOGY

Table 36.5-1 provides the World Health Organization classification for germ cell tumors of the ovary. Serum tumor markers for HCG and AFP are useful in the diagnosis and management of these tumors. They are often divided clinically into dysgerminoma and nondysgerminoma germ cell tumors.

DIAGNOSIS

Abdominal pain, pelvic fullness, and urinary symptoms are common in patients with germ cell tumors of the ovary. In a minority of patients (approximately 10%), abdominal pain can be severe, usually the result of hemorrhage, rupture, or torsion of the tumor. Abdominal distention can also be a symptom and often is associated with ascites.

Patients frequently have a palpable adnexal mass that should be ultrasonographically evaluated. Surgical exploration is usually required in masses of 8 cm or larger. Serum levels of HCG and AFP are useful in the diagnosis of some germ cell tumors.

PATTERNS OF METASTASIS

In contrast to epithelial tumors, approximately 60% to 70% of germ cell tumors are stage I at diagnosis.[226] Stage II and IV are relatively uncommon, and stage III accounts for approximately 25% to 30% of tumors. Primary germ cell tumors can be very large and often are greater than 20 mL in size. With the notable exception of dysgerminoma, bilateral ovarian involvement is not common. Multiple peritoneal surfaces are often involved in addition to frequent lymph node involvement. These tumors also appear to have a greater tendency for hematogenous metastases compared with epithelial tumors, and liver and lung involvement can be observed. Ascites is infrequent (approximately 20% of cases).

SURGICAL MANAGEMENT

The importance of initial surgical approach for the treatment of germ cell tumors of the ovary cannot be overemphasized.[226] Most patients can have fertility preserved, and the type of operative procedure is dictated by operative findings. In most cases, the contralateral ovary and the uterus can be preserved. Even in those situations of dysgerminoma in which the incidence of bilaterality is more common, bilateral oophorectomy is not routinely necessary because postoperative chemotherapy is curative and fertility can be preserved. In cases in which the contralateral ovary is grossly abnormal, cystectomy or biopsy can be performed and bilateral salpingo-oophorectomy performed in the case of a dysgenetic gonad.

The principles with regard to surgical staging of germ cell tumors are similar to those described for epithelial tumors. After a large transverse incision, the entire peritoneal cavity

TABLE 36.5-16. Second-Look Laparotomy in Germ Cell Tumors of the Ovary

	Second-Look Results		
Initial Therapy	*Negative*	Mature Teratoma	Immature Teratoma
Complete resection of tumor at initial therapy	38	5	2
Incomplete resection of tumor at initial therapy			
No teratoma in primary tumor (48 patients)	45	—	—
Teratoma in primary tumor (24 patients)	4	16	4

should be carefully inspected. In the absence of ascites, peritoneal washings should be obtained and all fluids should be histologically examined. If disease is grossly confined to the pelvis, random biopsies should be performed analogous to surgical staging of early-stage epithelial ovarian carcinomas. Particular emphasis should be paid to paraaortic and pelvic lymph nodes because these are more commonly involved than in epithelial tumors. Although sampling of suspicious nodes is indicated for staging, no evidence suggests that lymphadenectomy is beneficial. Cytoreductive surgery is recommended as for epithelial tumors of the ovary. However, it must be emphasized that, even in the presence of widespread metastatic disease, because of the efficacy of chemotherapy, the contralateral ovary can frequently be preserved.

There is no role for routine second-look operations in patients with a germ cell tumor who are clinically free of disease after chemotherapy. In particular, if the primary tumor was completely resected and did not contain teratoma, second-look procedures after chemotherapy are of no established benefit[227] (Table 36.5-16). In some patients with a teratomatous tumor, however, a second-look procedure may be beneficial. Such patients may have residual mature teratoma, particularly if the initial resection was incomplete and postchemotherapy removal of benign teratomas is beneficial. Unresected teratomas in males with testicular cancer have been known to progress and lead to significant morbidity unless completely resected. Although experience with germ cell tumors of the ovary is not as extensive, the presumption remains that teratomas can lead to life-threatening complications and should be removed after initial chemotherapy.

MANAGEMENT OF DYSGERMINOMAS

Dysgerminomas are the most common malignant germ cell tumors of the ovary and often have been considered the female equivalent of a seminoma. In contrast to nondysgerminomatous tumors, dysgerminomas are more frequently stage I, involve both ovaries, spread to retroperitoneal lymph nodes, and are markedly sensitive to radiotherapy. Because these tumors are also exquisitely sensitive to cisplatin-based chemotherapy, the role of curative radiation therapy has decreased. Furthermore, current chemotherapy usually does not result in ovarian ablation.

The vast majority of patients with dysgerminoma are diagnosed with early-stage disease. Because preservation of fertility is an important issue for most of these women, all carefully staged patients with stage IA disease can be observed without compromising cure because only 15% to 25% of patients recur and they can be successfully salvaged.[227,228] Until the demonstration that metastatic dysgerminoma could be cured with cisplatin-based chemotherapy, most patients with stage I disease and all patients with higher stages were treated with radiotherapy. Virtually all early-stage patients were cured of their disease. Even in patients with stage III disease treated with radiation therapy, the 5-year survival rate was 80% to 90%, although recurrence-free survival was substantially lower.

The GOG evaluation of platinum-based chemotherapy in dysgerminomas has followed reports on the efficacy of different regimens in testicular cancer.[228] In the early 1980s, ovarian germ cell tumors were treated with the PVB regimen.[229] Subsequently, based on studies in testicular cancer that demonstrated increased efficacy and less toxicity for the bleomycin, etoposide, and cisplatin (BEP) regimen, this regimen has been used in patients with metastatic germ cell tumors, including dysgerminoma (see Table 36.5-16). With a median follow-up of more than 2 years, 17 of 18 patients with advanced-stage dysgerminoma treated with one of these platinum-based regimens are disease free.[228] Based on these results in advanced disease, the current approach within the GOG is to examine the role of carboplatin (400 mg/m^2) and etoposide (120 mg/m^2 on days 1 to 3) in completely resected stage IB to III patients with dysgerminoma.

NONDYSGERMINOMATOUS GERM CELL TUMORS

The vast majority of nondysgerminomatous germ cell tumors of the ovary are treated with surgery followed by combination chemotherapy.

The immature teratomas are the second most common germ cell malignancy, accounting for 10% to 20% of all ovarian tumors seen in women younger than 20 years. The tumors rarely occur in postmenopausal women and most commonly occur between the ages of 10 and 20 years. These tumors contain elements resembling embryologically derived tissues and can occur in combination with other germ cell tumors (mixed germ cells). Occasionally, they are the source of excessive steroids, and patients can present with sexual pseudoprecosity. Tumor markers for AFP and HCG are negative unless a mixed germ cell tumor is present.

The most important prognostic feature, and that which is used to dictate therapy, is the grade of the lesion. In stage IA, grade 1 lesions, 5-year survival rates are greater than 90%, and no evidence suggests that chemotherapy improves outcome. However, this is the only subset of patients with immature teratomas in whom chemotherapy should not be used. Even patients with stage IA, grade 2 and 3 disease have such a high relapse rate that postoperative chemotherapy is indicated.[226–229]

In patients whose tumors are confined to the ovary, unilateral oophorectomy or salpingo-oophorectomy should be performed. As noted, contralateral tumor involvement is rare in germ cell tumors other than dysgerminoma. The most frequent sites of dissemination are the peritoneum and retroperitoneal lymph nodes. Widespread dissemination to lungs, liver, or brain are uncommon. Before the development of effective

TABLE 36.5-17. Bleomycin, Etoposide, and Cisplatin Regimen in Germ Cell Tumors

Cisplatin	20 mg/m^2/d × 5 d
Etoposide (VP-16)	100 mg/m^2/d × 5 d
Bleomycin	20 U/m^2/wk

Cycles are administered every 21 days.

chemotherapy, prognosis for patients with advanced-stage germ cell tumor was poor. The same combination that was found to be curative in disseminated testicular cancer quickly replaced nonplatinum regimens such as vincristine, dactinomycin, and cyclophosphamide. The PVB regimen produced a survival rate of 71% in a heterogeneous group of germ cell patients.[229] The current chemotherapy regimen of choice for patients with nondysgerminomatous germ cell tumors is the BEP regimen (Table 36.5-17). In the GOG trial, 89 of 93 stage I, stage II, and stage III patients with completely resected tumor are disease free after three courses of this regimen.[229]

Although no prospective comparison has been performed between PVB and BEP in patients with advanced-stage germ cell tumor of the ovary, the latter regimen is preferred because of the results of the randomized trial in patients with advanced testicular cancer in which the superiority of BEP was established.[230] In that trial, PVB produced a 70% 4-year survival rate in patients with metastatic, far-advanced testicular tumors, which was inferior to results obtained with BEP. Furthermore, the BEP regimen was less toxic than PVB because of elimination of vinblastine-related neuromuscular toxicities.

Endodermal sinus (yolk sac) tumors are derived from the primitive yolk sac and are the third most frequent germ cell tumor of the ovary. These tumors secrete AFP, which can be used as a marker for response and recurrence. Similar to other germ cell tumors, a unilateral oophorectomy can be performed because the tumors are rarely, if ever, bilateral. Most patients have early-stage disease, but all patients, regardless of stage and extent of initial surgery, are treated with platinum-based chemotherapy.[231] No evidence supports a correlation between extent of initial surgery and survival. Before the development of effective chemotherapy, 2-year survival was only 20%. However, with platinum-based chemotherapy, the complete response rate is approximately 60%.

Embryonal carcinoma and nongestational choriocarcinoma of the ovary are both extremely rare. Embryonal carcinomas can secrete both AFP and HCG, whereas pure choriocarcinomas secrete only HCG. Due to the rarity of these tumors, long-term results with chemotherapy have not been specifically described. However, the recommended treatment approach consists of unilateral oophorectomy or salpingo-oophorectomy followed by combination chemotherapy with the BEP regimen.[231] Similarly, mixed germ cell tumors of the ovary that contain two or more elements should also be treated with surgery followed by combination chemotherapy. Prognosis in mixed germ cell tumors is related to the relative amount of the most aggressive malignant component. The most frequent combination consists of elements of endodermal sinus tumor and dysgerminoma. Mixed germ cell tumors may secrete any combination of markers, depending on the histologic components of the tumor.

FALLOPIAN TUBE CANCER

Primary malignant neoplasms of the fallopian tube are exceedingly rare, and only a few hundred new cases are diagnosed annually in the United States, making it the least common site of origin for a malignant neoplasm of the female genital tract. Most fallopian tube carcinomas present as papillary serous adenocarcinomas. Intraperitoneal dissemination of fallopian tube carcinomas is similar to that observed with epithelial ovarian cancer. However, there appears to be a higher propensity to spread outside the peritoneal cavity. Survival has been shown to be dependent on the depth of invasion of the tumor in the fallopian tube.[232] For intermucosal lesions, 5-year survival is 91%, compared with 53% for tumors with mucosal wall invasion, and less than 25% in those situations in which the tumor has penetrated the tubal serosa. In addition to the depth of invasion, histologic differentiation and lymphatic capillary space involvement also have been shown to be of prognostic significance.[233] In cases of metastatic disease, the distinction between metastatic ovarian carcinoma can be difficult. Criteria frequently used to confirm the diagnosis of a primary fallopian tube carcinoma include tumor in the fallopian tube and rising from the endosalpinx, histologic pattern reproducing the epithelium of the mucosa with a papillary pattern, evidence for transition between benign and malignant tubal epithelium in the wall, and less tumor in the ovaries than in the tubes. In difficult cases, tumors are at times referred to as *tubo-ovarian carcinoma.* A minority of fallopian tube carcinomas are bilateral at the time of diagnosis. In contrast to patients with ovarian cancer, the majority of patients with tubal carcinoma are diagnosed with disease confined to the tubes and pelvic structures.

Patients with fallopian tube carcinomas appear to have a shorter history of symptoms compared with those with epithelial ovarian carcinomas.[233] The most common symptom is postmenopausal vaginal bleeding. Abdominal pain and leukorrhea are also common. Tubal distention produces more intense pain than is usually reported by patients with ovarian cancer, and these symptoms may account for the fact that more patients present with earlier stage carcinoma than patients with epithelial ovarian cancer in whom the absence of specific symptoms may account for more disseminated disease.

The surgical management of patients with fallopian tube carcinoma is identical to those with epithelial ovarian cancer.[233] Survival is improved in that group of patients in whom cytoreductive surgery is successful. Similarly, postoperative chemotherapy for fallopian tube carcinoma is analogous to that for patients with epithelial ovarian cancer. Currently, no data have been reported on the role of paclitaxel in this tumor. However, based on similar responses to cisplatin-based chemotherapy, it appears that the combination of paclitaxel plus a platinum compound should be considered the current chemotherapy regimen of choice for fallopian tube carcinoma.

REFERENCES

1. Landis SH, Murray T, Bolden S, Wingo PA. Cancer statistics. *CA Cancer J Clin* 1999;49:8.
2. Yancik R. Ovarian cancer. Age contrasts in incidence, histology, disease stage at diagnosis, and mortality. *Cancer* 1993;71:517.
3. Yancik R, Ries LG, Yates JW. Ovarian cancer in the elderly: an analysis of surveillance, epidemiology and end results program data. *Am J Obstet Gynecol* 1986;154:639.
4. Ries LAG, Kosary CL, Hankey BF, et al., eds. SEER cancer statistics review: 1973–1994. NIH publication no. 97-2789. Bethesda, MD: National Cancer Institute, 1997.

5. Boyd J. Molecular genetics of hereditary ovarian cancer. *Oncology* 1998;12:399.
6. Wooster R, Neuhausen SL, Mangion J, et al. A strong candidate for the breast and ovarian cancer susceptibility gene BRCA2. *Science* 1994;266:66.
7. Lynch HT, Bewtra C, Lynch JF. Familial ovarian cancer clinical nuances. *Am J Med* 1983;81:1073.
8. Bewtra C, Watson P, Conway T, et al. Hereditary ovarian cancer: a clinicopathologic study. *Int J Gynecol Pathol* 1992;11:180.
9. Lynch HT, Kimberling W, Albano WA, et al. Hereditary nonpolyposis colorectal cancer. (Lynch syndrome I and II). I. Clinical description of resource. *Cancer* 1985;56:934.
10. Rubin SC, Benjamin I, Behbakht K, et al. Clinical and pathological features of ovarian cancer in women with germ-line mutations of BRCA1. *N Engl J Med* 1996;335:1413.
11. Boyd J, Rubin SC. Hereditary ovarian cancer: molecular genetics and clinical implications. *Gynecol Oncol* 1997;64:196.
12. Narod SA, Risch H, Moslehi R, et al. Oral contraceptives and the risk of hereditary ovarian cancer. *N Engl J Med* 1998;339:424.
13. Scully RE. Tumors of the ovary and maldeveloped gonads, fallopian tube, and broad ligament. In: Young RH, Clement PB, eds. *Atlas of tumor pathology*, 3rd series. Washington, DC: Armed Forces Institute of Pathology, 1996:27.
14. Fishman DA, Schwartz PE. Current approaches to diagnosis and treatment of ovarian germ cell malignancies. *Curr Opinion Obstet Gynecol* 1994;6:98.
15. Barber HRK, Graber EA. The PMPO syndrome. *Obstet Gynecol* 1971;38:921.
16. Kurjak A, Shalan H, Kupesic S, et al. An attempt to screen asymptomatic women for ovarian and endometrial cancer with transvaginal color and pulsed Doppler sonography. *J Ultrasound Med* 1994;13:295.
17. Taylor KJW, Schwartz PE. Screening for early ovarian cancer. *Radiology* 1994;192:1.
18. Schwartz PE, Taylor KJW. Ovarian cancer: epidemiological perspectives with developments in early diagnosis. In: Popkin DR, Peddle LJ, eds. *Women's health today. Perspective on current research and clinical practice.* The proceedings of the XIV World Congress of Gynecology and Obstetrics, Montreal, September 1994. New York: Parthenon Publishing Group, 1994:257.
19. Chen D, Schwartz PE, Li X, Yang Z. Evaluation of CA125 levels in differentiating malignant from benign tumors in patients with pelvic masses. *Obstet Gynecol* 1988;72:23.
20. Young RC, Walton LA, Ellenberg SS, et al. Adjuvant therapy in stage I and stage II epithelial ovarian cancer: results of two prospective randomized trials. *N Engl J Med* 1990;322:1021.
21. Pecorelli S, Odicino F, Maisonneuve P, et al. Carcinoma of the ovary. *J Epidemiol Biostat* 1998;3:75.
22. Schwartz PE, Chambers SK, Chambers JT, Tilton K, Foemmer R. CA125 in peritoneal washings and fluid: correlation with plasma CA125 and peritoneal cytology. *Obstet Gynecol* 1989;73:339.
23. Delgado G, Chun B, Caglar H, et al. Para-aortic lymphadenectomy in gynecologic malignancies confined to the pelvis. *Obstet Gynecol* 1978;50:418.
24. Scarabelli C, Gallo A, Zarrelli A, Visentin C, Campagnutta E. Systematic pelvic and para-aortic lymphadenectomy during cytoreductive surgery in advanced ovarian cancer: potential benefit on survival. *Gynecol Oncol* 1995;56:328.
25. Hacker NF. Systematic pelvic and para-aortic lymphadenectomy for advanced ovarian cancer—therapeutic advance or surgical folly? *Gynecol Oncol* 1995;56:325.
26. Ozols RF, Fisher RI, Anderson T, Makuch R, Young RC. Peritoneoscopy in the management of ovarian cancer. *Am J Obstet Gynecol* 1981;140:611.
27. Childers JM, Lang J, Surwit EA, Hatch KD. Laparoscopic surgical staging of ovarian cancer. *Gynecol Oncol* 1995;59:25.
28. Schapira MM, Matchar DB, Young MJ. The effectiveness of ovarian cancer screening. A decision analysis model. *Ann Intern Med* 1993;118:838.
29. Jacobs I. Genetic, biochemical, and multimodal approaches to screening for ovarian cancer. *Gynecol Oncol* 1994;55:S22.
30. Einhorn N, Sjövall K, Knapp RC, et al. Prospective evaluation of serum CA 125 levels for early detection of ovarian cancer. *Obstet Gynecol* 1992;80:14.
31. Campbell S, Bhan V, Royston P, Whitehead MI, Collins WP. Transabdominal ultrasound screening for early ovarian cancer. *BMJ* 1989;299:1363.
32. DePriest PD, van Nagell JR, Gallion HH, et al. Ovarian cancer screening in asymptomatic postmenopausal women. *Gynecol Oncol* 1993;51:205.
33. Karlan BY, Platt LD. The current status of ultrasound and color Doppler imaging in screening for ovarian cancer. *Gynecol Oncol* 1994;55:S28.
34. Jacobs I, Davies AP, Bridges J, et al. Prevalence screening for ovarian cancer in postmenopausal women by CA 125 measurement and ultrasonography. *BMJ* 1993;306:1030.
35. Westhoff C. Current status of screening for ovarian cancer. *Gynecol Oncol* 1994;55:S39.
36. Bourne TH, Campbell S, Reynolds K, et al. The potential role of serum CA 125 in an ultrasound-based screening program for familial ovarian cancer. *Gynecol Oncol* 1994;52:379.
37. Kramer BS, Gohagan J, Prorok PC, Smart C. A National Cancer Institute sponsored screening trial for prostatic, lung, colorectal, and ovarian cancers. *Cancer* 1993;71:589.
38. Ramakrishnan S, Xu FJ, Brandt SJ, et al. Elevated levels of macrophage colony stimulating factor (M-CSF) in serum and ascites from patients with epithelial ovarian cancer. *Proc Soc Gynecol Oncol* 1990:21:40.
39. Xu FJ, Yu YH, Daly L, et al. OVX1 radioimmunoassay complements CA-125 for predicting the presence of residual ovarian carcinomas at second-look surgical surveillance procedures. *J Clin Oncol* 1993;11:1506.
40. Woolas RP, Xu FJ, Jacobs IJ, et al. Elevation of multiple serum markers in patients with stage I ovarian cancer. *J Natl Cancer Inst* 1993;85:1748.
41. Xu Y, Shen Z, Wiper DW, et al. Lysophosphatidic acid as a potential biomarker for ovarian and other gynecologic cancers. *JAMA* 1998;280:719.
42. Struewing JP, Watson P, Easton DF, et al. Effectiveness of prophylactic oophorectomy in inherited breast/ovarian cancer families. *Am J Human Genetics* 1994;55:384,A70(abst).
43. Karlan BY, Baldwin RL, Lopez-Luevanos ES, et al. Peritoneal serous papillary carcinoma, a phenotypic variant of familial ovarian cancer: implications for ovarian cancer screening. *Am J Obstet Gynecol* 1999;180:917.
44. Sjövall K, Nilsson B, Einhorn N. Different types of rupture of the tumor capsule and the impact of survival in early ovarian carcinoma. *Int J Gynecol Cancer* 1994;4:333.
45. Dembo AJ, Davy M, Stenwj AE, et al. Prognostic factors in patients with stage I epithelial ovarian cancer. *Obstet Gynecol* 1990;75:263.
46. Hoskins WJ, Bundy BN, Thigpen JT, Omura GA. The influence of cytoreductive surgery on recurrence-free interval and survival in small volume stage III epithelial ovarian cancer: a Gynecologic Oncology Group study. *Gynecol Oncol* 1992;47:159.
47. Omura GA, Brody MF, Homesley HD, et al. Long-term follow-up and prognostic factor analysis in advanced ovarian carcinomas: the Gynecologic Oncology Group experience. *J Clin Oncol* 1991;9:1138.
48. Makar APH, Kristensen GB, Kaern J, et al. Prognostic value of pre- and postoperative serum CA-125 levels in ovarian cancer: new aspects and multivariate analysis. *Obstet Gynecol* 1992;79:1002.
49. Fayers PM, Rustin G, Wood R, et al. The prognostic value of serum CA-125 in patients with advanced ovarian carcinoma: an analysis of 573 patients by the Medical Research Council Working Party on gynaecological cancer. *Int J Gynecol Cancer* 1993;3:285.
50. Markman M, Lewis JL, Saigo P, et al. Impact of age on survival of patients with ovarian cancer. *Gynecol Oncol* 1993;49:236.
51. Kaern J, Trope CG, Kristensen GB, Tveit KM, Pettersen EO. Evaluation of deoxyribonucleic acid ploidy and S-phase fraction as prognostic parameters in advanced epithelial ovarian carcinoma: a prospective study. *Am J Obstet Gynecol* 1994;170:479.
52. Bookman MA. Factoring outcomes in ovarian cancer [Editorial]. *J Clin Oncol* 1996;14:325.
53. van der Zee AGJ, Hollema HH, deBruijn A, et al. Cell biological markers of drug resistance in ovarian carcinoma. *Gynecol Oncol* 1995;58:165.
54. van der Zee AGJ, Hollema H, Suurmeijer AJH, et al. Value of P-glycoprotein, glutathione S-transferase pi, c-erb B-2, and p53 as prognostic factors in ovarian carcinomas. *J Clin Oncol* 1995;13:70.
55. Barr W, Cowell MAC, Chatfield WR. The management of ovarian carcinoma—a review of 420 cases. *Scott Med J* 1970;15:250.
56. Clark DGC, Hilaris B, Roussis C, Brunschwig A. The role of radiation therapy (including isotopes) in the treatment of carcinoma of the ovary. Results of 614 patients treated at Memorial Hospital, New York, NY. In: Ariel IM, ed. *Progress in clinical cancer*, vol 5. New York: Grune & Stratton, 1973:227.
57. Dalley VM. Radiotherapy in malignant disease of the ovary. *Proc Royal Soc Med* 1969; 62:359.
58. Fuks F. External radiotherapy of ovarian cancer: standard approaches and new frontiers. *Semin Oncol* 1975;2:253.
59. Kent SW, McKay DG. Primary cancer of the ovary. An analysis of 349 cases. *Am J Obstet Gynecol* 1960;80:430.
60. Munnell LW. The changing prognosis and treatment in cancer of the ovary. *Am J Obstet Gynecol* 1968;100:790.
61. Ross WM. Primary carcinoma of the ovary. A review of 150 cases with an appraisal of the fallopian tube as a pathway of spread. *Cancer Med Assoc J* 1966;94:1035.
62. Van Orden DA. Ovarian carcinoma. The problems of staging and grading. *Am J Obstet Gynecol* 1966;94:195.
63. Delclos L, Smith JP. Ovarian cancer with special regard to types of radiotherapy. *Natl Cancer Inst Monogr* 1975;42:129.
64. Dembo A, Bush R, Beale F, et al. Ovarian carcinoma: improved survival following abdominopelvic irradiation in patients with a completed pelvic operation. *Am J Obstet Gynecol* 1979;134:793.
65. Carey MS, Dembo AJ, Simm JE, et al. Testing the validity of a prognostic classification in patients with surgically optimal ovarian carcinoma: a 15-year review. *Int J Gynecol Cancer* 1993;3:24.
66. Dembo A. The sequential multiple modality treatment of ovarian cancer. *Radiother Oncol* 1985;3:187.
67. Dembo AJ. Abdominopelvic radiotherapy in ovarian cancer. *Cancer* 1985;55:2285.
68. Dembo AJ. Epithelial ovarian cancer: the role of radiotherapy. *Int J Radiat Oncol Biol Phys* 1992;22:835.
69. Fuller DB, Sause WT, Plenk HP, Menlove RL. Analysis of postoperative radiation therapy in stage I through III epithelial ovarian carcinoma. *J Clin Oncol* 1987;5:897.
70. Goldberg N, Peschel RE. Postoperative abdominopelvic radiation therapy for ovarian cancer. *Int J Radiat Oncol Biol Phys* 1988;14:425.
71. Leers WH, Kock HCLV. The evaluation of postoperative irradiation in patients with early-stage ovarian cancer. *Gynecol Oncol* 1987;28:41.
72. Lindner H, Willich H, Atzinger A. Primary adjuvant whole abdominal irradiation in ovarian carcinoma. *Int J Radiat Oncol Biol Phys* 1990;19:1203.
73. Martinez A, Schray MF, Howes AE, Bagshaw MA. Postoperative radiation therapy for epithelial ovarian cancer: the curative role based on a 24-year experience. *J Clin Oncol* 1985;3:901.
74. Weiser EB, Burke TW, Heller PB, et al. Determinants of survival of patients with epithelial ovarian carcinoma following whole abdomen irradiation (WAR). *Gynecol Oncol* 1988;30:201.
75. Redman CWE, Mould J, Warwick J, et al. The West Midlands epithelial ovarian cancer adjuvant therapy trial. *Clin Oncol* 1993;5:1.
76. Chiara S, Conte P, Franzone P, et al. High-risk early-stage ovarian cancer. Randomized clinical trial comparing cisplatin plus cyclophosphamide versus whole abdominal radiotherapy. *Am J Clin Oncol* 1994;17:72.
77. Dembo AJ, Bush RS, Beale FA, et al. A randomized clinical trial of moving strip versus open field whole abdominal irradiation in patients with invasive epithelial cancer of ovary. *Int J Radiat Oncol Biol Phys* 1983;9:97.

78. Klaassen D, Shelley W, Starreveld A, et al. Early stage ovarian cancer: a randomized clinical trial comparing whole abdominal radiotherapy, melphalan, and intraperitoneal chromic phosphate: a National Cancer Institute of Canada Clinical Trials Group report. *J Clin Oncol* 1988;6:1254.
79. Bolis G, Colombo N, Pecorelli S, et al. Adjuvant treatment for early epithelial ovarian cancer: results of two randomized clinical trials comparing cisplatin to no further treatment or chromic phosphate (^{32}P). *Am J Clin Oncol* 1995;6:887.
80. Vergote IB, Vergote-De Vos LN, Abeler VM, et al. Randomized trial comparing cisplatin with radioactive phosphorus or whole-abdomen irradiation as adjuvant treatment of ovarian cancer. *Cancer* 1992;69:741.
81. Young RC, Brady MF, Nieberg RM, et al. Randomized clinical trial of adjuvant treatment of women with early (FIGO I–IIA high risk) ovarian cancer—GOG #95. *Proc Am Soc Clin Oncol* 1999;18:357a(abst).
82. Bolis G, Colombo N, Pecorelli S, et al. Adjuvant treatment for early epithelial ovarian cancer: results of two randomised clinical trials comparing cisplatin to no further treatment or chromic phosphate (^{32}P). *Ann Oncol* 1995;6:887.
83. Goodman HM, Harlow BL, Sheets EE, et al. The role of cytoreductive surgery in the management of stage IV epithelial ovarian cancer. *Gynecol Oncol* 1992;46:367.
84. Bristow RE, Montz FJ, La Gasse LD, Leuchter RS, Karlan BY. Survival impact of surgical cytoreduction in stage IV epithelial ovarian cancer. *Gynecol Oncol* 1999;72:278.
85. Curtin JP, Mauk R, Venkatraman ES, Barakat RR, Hoskins WJ. Stage IV ovarian cancer: impact of surgical debulking. *Gynecol Oncol* 1997;64:9.
86. Griffiths CT. Surgical resection of tumor bulk in the primary treatment of ovarian carcinoma. *Natl Cancer Inst Monogr* 1975;42:101.
87. Hacker NF, Berek JS, Lagasse LD, et al. Primary cytoreductive surgery for epithelial ovarian cancer. *Obstet Gynecol* 1983;61:413.
88. Vogl SE, Pagano M, Kaplan BH, et al. Cisplatin based combination chemotherapy for advanced ovarian cancer: high overall response rate with curative potential only in women with small tumor burdens. *Cancer* 1983;51:2024.
89. Pohl R, Dallenback-Hellweg G, Plugge T, et al. Prognostic parameters in patients with advanced malignant ovarian tumors. *Eur J Gynaecol Oncol* 1984;3:160.
90. Delgado G, Oram DH, Petrilli ES. Stage III ovarian cancer: the role of a maximal surgical reduction. *Gynecol Oncol* 1984;19:293.
91. Piver MS, Lele SB, Marchetti DL, et al. The impact of aggressive debulking surgery and cisplatin chemotherapy on progression-free survival in stage III and IV ovarian carcinoma. *J Clin Obstet Gynecol* 1988;6:983.
92. Neijt JP, ten Bokkel Huinink WW, van der Burg ME, et al. Long-term survival in ovarian cancer. *Eur J Cancer* 1991;27:1367.
93. Redman JR, Petrini GR, Saigo PE, et al. Prognostic factors in advanced ovarian carcinoma. *J Clin Oncol* 1986;4:515.
94. Conte PF, Bruzzone M, Hiara S, et al. A randomized trial comparing cisplatin plus cyclophosphamide versus cisplatin, doxorubicin, and cyclophosphamide in advanced ovarian cancer. *J Clin Oncol* 1986;4:965.
95. Hunter RW, Alexander NDE, Soutter WP. Meta-analysis of surgery in advanced ovarian carcinoma: is maximum cytoreductive surgery an independent determinant of prognosis? *Am J Obstet Gynecol* 1992;166:504.
96. Allen DG, Heintz APM, Touw FWMM. A meta-analysis of residual disease and survival in stage III and IV carcinoma of the ovary. *Eur J Gynaecol Oncol* 1995;16:349.
97. Omura GA, Bunda BN, Berek JS, et al. Randomized trial of cyclophosphamide plus cisplatin with or without doxorubicin in ovarian carcinoma: a Gynecologic Oncology Group study. *J Clin Oncol* 1989;7:457.
98. Hoskins WJ, McGuire WP, Brady MF, et al. The effect of diameter of largest residual disease on survival after primary cytoreductive surgery in patients with suboptimal residual epithelial ovarian cancer. *Am J Obstet Gynecol* 1994;170:974.
99. Chen SS, Bochner R. Assessment of morbidity in primary cytoreductive surgery for advanced ovarian cancer. *Gynecol Oncol* 1985;20:190.
100. Blythe JG, Wahl TP. Debulking surgery: does it increase the quality of survival? *Gynecol Oncol* 1982;14:396.
101. Chambers JT, Chambers SK, Voyneck IM, Schwartz PE. Neoadjuvant chemotherapy in stage X ovarian carcinoma. *Gynecol Oncol* 1990;37:327.
102. Schwartz PE, Chambers JT, Makuch R. Neoadjuvant chemotherapy for advanced ovarian cancer. *Gynecol Oncol* 1994;53:33.
103. Schwartz PE, Rutherford TJ, Chambers JT, Kohorn EI, Thiel RP. Neoadjuvant chemotherapy for advanced ovarian cancer: long-term survival. *Gynecol Oncol* 1999;72:93.
104. Surwit E, Childers J, Atlas I, et al. Neoadjuvant chemotherapy for advanced ovarian cancer. *Int J Gynecol Cancer* 1996;6:356.
105. Omura G, Blessing JA, Ehrlich CE, et al. A randomized trial of cyclophosphamide and doxorubicin with or without cisplatin in advanced ovarian carcinoma. *Cancer* 1987;56:1725.
106. Stewart LA, for the Advanced Ovarian Cancer Trialists Group (AOCTG). Chemotherapy in advanced ovarian cancer: an overview of randomized clinical trials. *BMJ* 1991;303:884.
107. Taylor AE, Wiltshaw E, Gore MR, et al. Long-term follow-up of the first randomized study of cisplatin using carboplatin for advanced epithelial ovarian cancer. *J Clin Oncol* 1994;12:2066.
108. Aabo K, Adams M, Adnitt P, et al. Chemotherapy in advanced ovarian cancer: four systematic meta-analyses of individual patient data from 37 randomized trials. *Br J Cancer* 1998;78:1749.
109. Alberts DS, Green S, Hannigan EV, et al. Improved therapeutic index of carboplatin plus cyclophosphamide versus cisplatin plus cyclophosphamide: final report by the Southwest Oncology Group of a phase III randomized trial in stages III and IV ovarian cancer. *J Clin Oncol* 1992;10:706.
110. Swenerton K, Jeffrey J, Stuart G, et al. Cisplatin-cyclophosphamide versus carboplatin-cyclophosphamide in advanced ovarian cancer: a randomized phase III study of the National Cancer Institute of Canada Clinical Trials Group. *J Clin Oncol* 1992;10:718.
111. ten Bokkel Huinink WW, van der Burg MEL, van Oosterom AT, et al. Carboplatin in combination therapy for ovarian cancer. *Cancer Treat Rev* 1988;15:9.
112. Hakes T, Hoskins W, Jones W, et al. Randomized prospective trial of 5 versus 10 cycles of cyclophosphamide, doxorubicin and cisplatin (CAP) in stage III and IV ovarian cancer. *Proc Am Soc Clin Oncol* 1990;9:156.
113. Bertelsen K, Jakobsen A, Stroyer I, et al. A prospective randomized comparison of 6 and 12 cycles of cyclophosphamide, Adriamycin, and cisplatin in advanced epithelial ovarian cancer: a Danish Ovarian Study Group trial (DACOVA). *Gynecol Oncol* 1993;49:30.
114. Levin L, Hryniuk WM. Dose intensity analysis of chemotherapy regimens in ovarian carcinoma. *J Clin Oncol* 1978:5:756.
115. Hong Kong Ovarian Carcinoma Study Group. A randomized study of high dose versus low dose cisplatin combined with cyclophosphamide in the treatment of advanced ovarian cancer. *Chemotherapy* 1989;35:221.
116. McGuire WP, Hoskins WJ, Brady MF, et al. Assessment of dose-intensive therapy in suboptimally debulked ovarian cancer: a Gynecologic Oncology Group study. *J Clin Oncol* 1995;13:1589.
117. Columbo N, Piltelli MR, Parma G, et al. Cisplatin dose intensity in ovarian cancer. *Proc Am Soc Clin Oncol* 1993;12:255.
118. Conte PF, Bruzzone M, Carino F, et al. High dose versus low dose cisplatin in combination with cyclophosphamide and epidoxorubicin in suboptimal ovarian cancer: a randomized study of the Gruppo Oncologico Nord-Ovest. *J Clin Oncol* 1996;14:351.
119. Kaye SB, Lewis CR, Paul J, et al. Randomised study of two doses of cisplatin with cyclophosphamide in epithelial ovarian cancer. *Lancet* 1992;340:329.
120. Kaye SB, Paul J, Cassidy J, et al. Mature results of a randomized trial of two doses of cisplatin for the treatment of ovarian cancer. *J Clin Oncol* 1996;14:2113.
121. Jodrell DI, Egorin MJ, Canetta RM, et al. Relationships between carboplatin exposure and tumor response and toxicity in patients with ovarian cancer. *J Clin Oncol* 1992;10:520.
122. Calvert AH, Newell DR, Gumbrell LA, et al. Carboplatin dosage: prospective evaluation of a simple formula based on renal function. *J Clin Oncol* 1989;7;1748.
123. Jakobsen A, Bertelsen K, Andersen JE, et al. Dose-effect study of carboplatin in ovarian cancer: a Danish Ovarian Cancer Group study. *J Clin Oncol* 1997;15:193.
124. Gore ME, Mainwaring PN, Ahern R, et al. Randomized trial of dose-intensity with single-agent carboplatin in patients with epithelial ovarian cancer. *J Clin Oncol* 1998;16:2426.
125. Omura G, Bundy B, Berek J, et al. Randomized trial of cyclophosphamide plus cisplatin with or without doxorubicin in ovarian carcinoma: a Gynecologic Oncology Group study. *J Clin Oncol* 1989;7:457.
126. Conte PD, Bruzzone M, Chiara S, et al. A randomized trial comparing cisplatin plus cyclophosphamide versus cisplatin, doxorubicin, and cyclophosphamide in advanced ovarian cancer. *J Clin Oncol* 1986;4:965.
127. Omura GA, Buyse M, Marsoni S, et al. CP versus CAP chemotherapy of ovarian carcinoma: a meta-analysis. *J Clin Oncol* 1991;9:1668.
128. A'Hern RP, Gore ME. Impact of doxorubicin on survival in advanced ovarian cancer. *J Clin Oncol* 1995;13:726.
129. The ICON Collaborators. ICON 2: randomized trial of single-agent carboplatin against three-drug combination of CAP (cyclophosphamide, doxorubicin, and cisplatin) in women with ovarian cancer. *Lancet* 1998;352:1571.
130. Thigpen JT, Blessing JA, Ball H, et al. Phase II trial of paclitaxel in patients with progressive ovarian carcinoma after platinum-based chemotherapy: a Gynecologic Oncology Group study. *J Clin Oncol* 1994;12:1748.
131. Piccart MJ, Gore M, ten Bokkel Huinink W, et al. Docetaxel: an active new drug for treatment of advanced epithelial ovarian cancer. *J Natl Cancer Inst* 1995;87:676.
132. Eisenhauer EA, ten Bokkel Huinink WW, Swenerton KD, et al. European-Canadian randomized trial of paclitaxel in relapsed ovarian cancer: high-dose versus low-dose and long versus short infusion. *J Clin Oncol* 1994;12:2654.
133. McGuire WP, Hoskins WJ, Brady MF, et al. Cyclophosphamide and cisplatin compared with paclitaxel and cisplatin in patients with stage III and stage IV ovarian cancer. *N Engl J Med* 1996;334:1.
134. Stuart G, Bertelsen K, Mangioni C, et al. Updated analysis shows a highly significant improved overall survival (OS) for cisplatin-paclitaxel as first line treatment of advanced ovarian cancer: mature results of the EORTC-GCCG, NOCOVA, NCIC CTG and Scottish Intergroup trial. *Proc Am Soc Clin Oncol* 1998;17:361a.
135. Muggia FM, Braly PS, Brady MR, et al. Phase III trial of cisplatin or paclitaxel versus their combination in suboptimal stage III and IVE epithelial ovarian cancer: Gynecologic Oncology Group study #132. *Proc Am Soc Clin Oncol* 1997;16:A1257.
136. Harper P, ICON collaborators. A randomized comparison of paclitaxel (T) and carboplatin (J) versus a control arm of single agent carboplatin (J) or CAP (cyclophosphamide, doxorubicin, and cisplatin): 2075 patients randomized into the 3rd International Collaborative Ovarian Neoplasms study (ICON3). *Proc Am Soc Clin Oncol* 1999;18:356a.
137. Ozols RF, Bundy BN, Clarke-Pearson D, et al. Randomized phase III study of cisplatin (CIS)/paclitaxel (PAC) versus carboplatin (CARBO)/PAC in optimal stage III epithelial ovarian cancer (OC): a Gynecologic Oncology Group trial (GOG 158). *Proc Am Soc Clin Oncol* 1999;18:356a(abst 1373).
138. duBois A, Lueck HJ, Meier W, et al. Cisplatin/paclitaxel vs carboplatin/paclitaxel in ovarian cancer: update of an Arbeitsgemeinschaft Gynaekologische Onkologie (AGO) study group trial. *Proc Am Soc Clin Oncol* 1999;18:356a(abst 1374).
139. Neijt JP, Hansen M, Hansen SW, et al. Randomized phase III study in previously untreated epithelial ovarian cancer FIGO stage IIB, IIC, III, IV comparing paclitaxel-cisplatin and paclitaxel-carboplatin. *Proc Am Soc Clin Oncol* 1997;16:1259.
140. Bookman MA, McGuire WP, Kilpatrick D, et al. Carboplatin and paclitaxel in ovarian carcinoma: a phase I study of the Gynecologic Oncology Group. *J Clin Oncol* 1996;14:1895.
141. Kohn EC, Sarosy G, Bicher A, et al. Dose-intense Taxol: high response rate in patients with platinum-resistant recurrent ovarian cancer. *J Natl Cancer Inst* 1994;86:18.
142. Omura GA, Brady MF, Delmore JE, et al. A randomized trial of paclitaxel (T) at 2 dose

levels and filgrastim (G; G-CSF) at 2 doses in platinum (P) pretreated epithelial ovarian cancer (OVCA): a Gynecologic Oncology Group, SWOG, NCCTG and ECOG study. *Proc Am Soc Clin Oncol* 1996;15:280(abst 755).
143. Wangenstein OH, Lewis FJ, Tongen L. The second look in cancer surgery. *Lancet* 1951;71:303.
144. Schwartz PE, Smith JP. Second look operations in ovarian cancer. *Am J Obstet Gynecol* 1980;138:1124.
145. Rubin SR, Lewis JLJ. Second look surgery in ovarian carcinoma. *Crit Rev Oncol Hemat* 1988;8:75.
146. Berek JS, Griffiths CT, Levinthal JM. Laparoscopy for second-look evaluation in ovarian cancer. *Obstet Gynecol* 1981;58:192.
147. Rubin S, Hoskins W, Saigo P, et al. Prognostic factors for recurrence following negative second-look laparotomy in ovarian cancer patients treated with platinum-based chemotherapy. *Gynecol Oncol* 1991;42:137.
148. Cmelak AJ, Kapp DS. Long-term survival with whole abdominopelvic irradiation in platinum-refractory persistent or recurrent ovarian cancer. *Gynecol Oncol* 1997;65:453.
149. Fein DA, Morgan LS, Marcus RB Jr, et al. Stage III ovarian carcinoma: an analysis of treatment results and complications following hyperfractionated abdominopelvic irradiation for salvage. *Int J Radiat Oncol Biol Phys* 1994;29:169.
150. Morgan L, Chafe W, Mendenhall W, Marcus R. Hyperfractionation of whole-abdomen radiation therapy: salvage treatment of persistent ovarian carcinoma following chemotherapy. *Gynecol Oncol* 1988;31:122.
151. Schray M, Martinez A, Howes A, et al. Advanced epithelial ovarian cancer: salvage whole abdominal irradiation for patients with recurrent or persistent disease after combination chemotherapy. *J Clin Oncol* 1988;6:1433.
152. Fuks Z, Rizel S, Biran S. Chemotherapeutic and surgical induction of pathological complete remission and whole abdominal irradiation for consolidation does not enhance the cure of stage III ovarian carcinoma. *J Clin Oncol* 1988;6:509.
153. Hoskins W, Lichter A, Wittingham R, et al. Whole abdominal and pelvic irradiation in patients with minimal disease at second-look surgical reassessment for ovarian carcinoma. *Gynecol Oncol* 1985;20:271.
154. Bruzzone M, Repetto L, Chiara S, et al. Chemotherapy versus radiotherapy in the management of ovarian cancer patients with pathological complete response or minimal residual disease at second look. *Gynecol Oncol* 1990;38:392.
155. Lambert HE, Rustin GJS, Gregory WM, Nelstrop AE. A randomized trial comparing single-agent carboplatin with carboplatin followed by radiotherapy for advanced ovarian cancer: a North Thames Ovary Group study. *J Clin Oncol* 1993;11:440.
156. Hoskins PJ, Swenerton KD, Wong F, et al. Platinum plus cyclophosphamide plus radiotherapy is superior to platinum alone in "high-risk" epithelial ovarian cancer (residual negative and either stage I or II, grade III, or stage III, any grade). *Int J Gynecol Cancer* 1995;5:134.
157. Berek JS, Hacker NF, Lagasse LD, et al. Survival of patients following secondary cytoreductive surgery in ovarian cancer. *Obstet Gynecol* 1983;61:189.
158. Segna RA, Dottino P, Mandeli P, Konsker K, Cohen CJ. Secondary cytoreduction for ovarian cancer following cisplatin therapy. *J Clin Oncol* 1993;11:434.
159. Neijt J, ten Bokkel Huinink W, van der Burg ME, et al. Randomized trial comparing two combination chemotherapy regimens (CHAP-5 vs CP) in advanced ovarian carcinoma. *J Clin Oncol* 1987;5:1157.
160. van der Burg ME, van Lent M, Buyse M, et al. The effect of debulking surgery after induction chemotherapy on the prognosis in advanced epithelial ovarian cancer. Gynecologic Cancer Cooperative Group of the European Organization for Research and Treatment of Cancer. *N Engl J Med* 1995;332:629.
161. van der Burg MEL, van Lent M, Kobierska A, et al. After 6 years follow-up intervention debulking surgery remains an independent prognostic factor for survival in advanced epithelial ovarian cancer. An EORTC Gynecologic Cancer Cooperative Group study. *Int J Gynecol Cancer* 1997;7[Suppl 2]:28.
162. Ozols RF. Treatment of recurrent ovarian cancer: increasing options—"recurrent" results. *J Clin Oncol* 1997;15:2177.
163. Fennelly D, Aghajanian C, Shapiro F, et al. Phase I pharmacologic study of paclitaxel administered weekly in patients with relapsed ovarian cancer. *J Clin Oncol* 1997;15:187.
164. Eisenhauer EA, Vermorken JB, van Glabbeke M. Predictors of response to subsequent chemotherapy in platinum pretreated ovarian cancer: a multivariate analysis of 704 patients. *Ann Oncol* 1997;8:963.
165. Rose PG, Fusco N, Fluellen L, Rodriguez M. Second-line therapy with paclitaxel and carboplatin for recurrent disease following first-line therapy with paclitaxel and platinum in ovarian or peritoneal carcinoma. *J Clin Oncol* 1998;16:1494.
166. Hoskins P, Eisenhauer E, Beare S, et al. Randomized phase II study of two schedules of topotecan in previously treated patients with ovarian cancer: a National Cancer Institute of Canada Clinical Trials Group study. *J Clin Oncol* 1998;16:2233.
167. Bookman MA, Malmstrom H, Bolis G, et al. Topotecan for the treatment of advanced epithelial ovarian cancer: an open-label phase II study in patients treated after prior chemotherapy that contained cisplatin or carboplatin and paclitaxel. *J Clin Oncol* 1998;16:3345.
168. Rose PG, Blessing JA, Mayer AR, Homesley HD. Prolonged oral etoposide as second-line therapy for platinum-resistant and platinum-sensitive ovarian carcinoma: a Gynecologic Oncology Group study. *J Clin Oncol* 1998;16:405.
169. Lund B, Hansen OP, Theilade K, Hansen M, Neijt JP. Phase II study of gemcitabine (2',2'-difluorodeoxycytidine) in previously treated ovarian cancer patients. *J Natl Cancer Inst* 1994;86:1530.
170. Muggia FM, Hainsworth JD, Jeffers S, et al. Phase II study of liposomal doxorubicin in refractory ovarian cancer: antitumor activity and toxicity modification by liposomal encapsulation. *J Clin Oncol* 1997;15:987.
171. Bajetta E, DiLeo A, Biganzoli L, et al. Phase II study of vinorelbine in patients with pretreated advanced ovarian cancer: activity in platinum-resistant disease. *J Clin Oncol* 1996;14:2546.
172. ten Bokkel Huinink W, Gore M. Carmichael J, et al. Topotecan versus paclitaxel for the treatment of recurrent epithelial ovarian cancer. *J Clin Oncol* 1997;15:2183.
173. Hatch KD, Beecham JB, Blessing JA, Creasman WT. Responsiveness of patients with advanced ovarian carcinoma to Tamoxifen. *Cancer* 1991;68:269.
174. van der Velden J, Gitsch G, Wain GV, Friedlander ML, Hacker NF. Tamoxifen in patients with advanced epithelial ovarian cancer. *Int J Gynecol Cancer* 1995;5:301.
175. Ozols RF. Update of the NCCN ovarian cancer practice guidelines. *Oncology* (Huntingt) 1997;11:95.
176. Adelson MD, Wharton JT, Delclos L, Copeland L, Gershenson D. Palliative radiotherapy for ovarian cancer. *Int J Radiat Oncol Biol Phys* 1987;13:17.
177. Spanos WJ, Wasserman T, Meoz R, et al. Palliation of advanced pelvic malignant disease with large fraction pelvic radiation and misonidazole: final report of RTOG phase I/II study. *Int J Radiat Oncol Biol Phys* 1987;13:1479.
178. Spanos WJ, Perez CA, Marcus S, et al. Effect of rest interval on tumor and normal tissue response—a report of phase III study of accelerated split course palliative radiation for advanced pelvic malignancies (RTOG-8502). *Int J Radiat Oncol Biol Phys* 1993;25:399.
179. Corn BW, Lanciano RM, Boente M, et al. Recurrent ovarian cancer. Effective radiotherapeutic palliation after chemotherapy failure. *Cancer* 1994;74:2979.
180. Rodriguez GC, Soper JT, Berchuck A, et al. Improved palliation of cerebral metastases in epithelial ovarian cancer using a combined modality approach including radiation therapy, chemotherapy, and surgery. *J Clin Oncol* 1992;10:1553.
181. Markman M. Intraperitoneal therapy of ovarian cancer. *Semin Oncol* 1998;25:356.
182. McClay EF, Howell SB. A review: intraperitoneal cisplatin in the management of patients with ovarian cancer. *Gynecol Oncol* 1990;36:1.
183. Markman M, Rothman R, Hakes T, et al. Second-line platinum therapy in patients with ovarian cancer previously treated with cisplatin. *J Clin Oncol* 1991;9:389.
184. Alberts DS, Liu PY, Hannigan EV, et al. Intraperitoneal cisplatin plus intravenous cyclophosphamide versus intravenous cisplatin plus intravenous cyclophosphamide for stage III ovarian cancer. *N Engl J Med* 1996;335:1950.
185. Markman M, Bundy B, Benda J, et al. Randomized phase III study of intravenous (IV) cisplatin (CIS)/paclitaxel (PAC) versus moderately high dose IV carboplatin (CARB) followed by IV PAC and intraperitoneal (IP) CIS in optimal residual ovarian cancer (OC): an intergroup trial (GOG, SWOG, ECOG). *Proc Am Soc Clin Oncol* 1998;17:361a.
186. Shpall E, Slemmer S, Bearman S. High dose chemotherapy with autologous bone marrow support for the treatment of epithelial ovarian cancer. In: Markman M, Hoskins WJ, eds. *Cancer of the ovary.* New York: Raven Press, 1993:327.
187. Stiff PJ, Bayer R, Kerger C, Potkul RK, et al. High-dose chemotherapy with autologous transplantation for persistent/relapsed ovarian cancer: a multivariate analysis of survival for 100 consecutively treated patients. *J Clin Oncol* 1997;15:1309.
188. Aghajanian C, Fennelly D, Shapiro F, et al. Phase II study of "dose-dense" high-dose chemotherapy treatment with peripheral-blood progenitor-cell support as primary treatment for patients with advanced ovarian cancer. *J Clin Oncol* 1998;16:1852.
189. Schilder RJ, Johnson S, Gallo J, et al. Phase I trial of multiple cycles of high-dose chemotherapy supported by autologous peripheral blood stem cells. *J Clin Oncol* 1999;17:2198.
190. Hansen SW, Anderson H, Boman K, et al. Gemcitabine, carboplatin, and paclitaxel (GCP) as first-line treatment of ovarian cancer FIGO stages IIB–IV. *Proc Am Soc Clin Oncol* 1999;18:357a.
191. Herben VMM, Nannan Panday VR, Richel DJ, et al. Phase I and pharmacologic study of the combination of paclitaxel, cisplatin, and topotecan administered intravenously every 21 days as first-line therapy in patients with advanced ovarian cancer. *J Clin Oncol* 1999;17:747.
192. O'Dwyer PJ, Hamilton TC, LaCreta FP, et al. Phase I trial of buthionine sulfoximine in combination with melphalan in patients with cancer. *J Clin Oncol* 1996;14:249.
193. Dabholkar M, Reed E. Cisplatin. *Cancer Chemother Biol Response Modif* 1996;16:88.
194. Masuda H, Ozols RF, Lai GM, et al. Increased DNA repair as a mechanism of acquired resistance to *cis*-diamminedichloroplatinum(II) in human ovarian cancer cells lines. *Cancer Res* 1988;48:5713.
195. Manetta A, Borman M, Boyle J, et al. Cyclosporin enhancement of cisplatin activity in refractory ovarian cancer. *Gynecol Oncol* 1992;45:80.
196. Pietras RJ, Fendly BM, Chazin VR, et al. Antibody to HER-2/neu receptor blocks DNA repair after cisplatin in human breast and ovarian cancer cells. *Oncogene* 1994;9:1829.
197. Bourhis J, Goldstein LJ, Riou G, et al. Expression of a human multidrug resistance gene in ovarian carcinomas. *Cancer Res* 1989;49:5062.
198. Kruh GD, Chan A, Myers K, et al. Expression complementary DNA library transfer establishes mrp as a multidrug resistance gene. *Cancer Res* 1994;54:1649.
199. Izquierdo MA, van der Zee AGJ, Vermorken JB, et al. Drug resistance–associated marker lrp for prediction of response to chemotherapy and prognoses in advanced ovarian carcinoma. *J Natl Cancer Inst* 1994;87:1220.
200. Berchuck A, Bast RC. p53-based gene therapy of ovarian cancer: magic bullet? *Gynecol Oncol* 1995;59:169.
201. Steis RG, Urba WJ, van der Molen LA, et al. Ten-year follow-up of patients receiving cisplatin, doxorubicin, and cyclophosphamide chemotherapy for advanced epithelial ovarian carcinoma. *J Clin Oncol* 1989;7:223.
202. Edwards RP, Lembersky BC, Kunschner AJ. Intraperitoneal interleukin-2 (IL-2) produces durable responses for refractory ovarian cancer. *Proc Am Soc Clin Oncol* 1995;14:333.
203. Epenetos AA, Hooker G, Krausz T, et al. Antibody-guided irradiation of advanced ovarian cancer with intraperitoneally administered radiolabeled monoclonal antibodies. *J Clin Oncol* 1987;5:1980.
204. Serov SF, Scully RE, Sobin LH. *International histologic classification and staging of tumors. 9. Histologic typing of ovarian tumors.* Geneva: World Health Organization, 1973.
205. Trimble EL, Trimble CL. Epithelial ovarian tumors of low malignant potential. In: Markman M, Hoskins WJ, eds. *Cancer of the ovary.* New York: Raven Press, 1993:415.
206. Goldberg GL, Runowicz CD. Ovarian carcinoma of low malignant potential, infertility, and induction of ovulation—is there a link? *Am J Obstet Gynecol* 1992;166:853.

207. Kurman RJ, Trimble CL. The behavior of serous tumors of low malignant potential: are they ever malignant? *Int J Gynecol Pathol* 1993;12:120.
208. Tazelaar HD, Bostwick DG, Ballon SC, Hendrickson MR, Kempson RL. Conservative treatment of borderline ovarian tumors. *Obstet Gynecol* 1985;66:417.
209. Trope C, Kaern J, Vergote IB, Kristensen G, Abeler V. Are borderline tumors of the ovary overtreated both surgically and systemically? A review of four prospective randomized trials including 253 patients with borderline tumors. *Gynecol Oncol* 1985;51:236.
210. Chambers JT, Merino MJ, Kohorn EI, Schwartz PE. Borderline ovarian tumors. *Am J Obstet Gynecol* 1988;159:1088.
211. Barnhill OR, Kurman RJ, Brady MF, et al. Preliminary analysis of the behavior of stage I ovarian serous tumors of low malignant potential: a Gynecologic Oncology Group study. *J Clin Oncol* 1995;13:2752.
212. Friedlander ML, Hedley DW, Swanton C, Russell P. Prediction of long-term survival by flow cytometric analysis of the cellular DNA content in patients with advanced ovarian cancer. *J Clin Oncol* 1988;6:282.
213. Kaern J, Trope C, Kjorstad KE, Abeler V, Pettersen EO. Cellular DNA content as a new prognostic tool in patients with borderline tumors of the ovary. *Gynecol Oncol* 1990;38:452.
214. Schwartz PE, Smith J. Management of ovarian stromal tumors. *Am J Obstet Gynecol* 1976; 125:402.
215. Pascale MM, Pugeat M, Roberts M, et al. Androgen suppressive effects of GnRH agonist in ovarian hyperthecosis and virilizing tumours. *Clin Endocrinol* 1994;41:571.
216. Willemsen W, Kruitwagen R, Bastiaans B, Hanselaar T, Rolland R. Ovarian stimulation and granulosa-cell tumour. *Lancet* 1993;341:986.
217. Colombo N, Sessa C, Landoni F, et al. Cisplatin, vinblastine, and bleomycin combination chemotherapy in metastatic granulosa cell tumor of the ovary. *Obstet Gynecol* 1986; 67:265.
218. Pectasides D, Alevizakos N, Athanassiou AE. Cisplatin-containing regimen in advanced or recurrent granulosa cell tumours of the ovary. *Ann Oncol* 1992;3:316.
219. Homesley HD, Bundy BN, Hurteau JA, Roth LM. Bleomycin, etoposide and cisplatin combination therapy of ovarian granulosa cell tumors and other stromal malignancies: a Gynecologic Oncology Group study. *Gynecol Oncol* 1999;72:131.
220. Healy KL, Burger HG, Mamers P, et al. Elevated serum inhibin concentrations in postmenopausal women with ovarian tumors. *N Engl J Med* 1993;329:1539.
221. Gustafson ML, Lee MM, Asmundson L, MacLaughlin DT, Donahoe PK. Müllerian inhibiting substance in the diagnosis and management of intersex and gonadal abnormalities. *J Pediatr Surg* 1993;28:439.
222. Lane AH, Fuller AF Jr, Kehas J, Donahoe PK, MacLaughlin DT. Diagnostic utility of müllerian inhibiting substance determination in patients with primary and recurrent granulosa cell tumor. *Gynecol Oncol* 1999;73:51.
223. Roush GR, El-Naggar AK, Abdul-Karim FW. Granulosa cell tumor of the ovary: a clinicopathologic flow cytometric DNA analysis. *Gynecol Oncol* 1995;56:430.
224. Strand CM, Grosh WW, Baxter J, et al. Peritoneal carcinomatosis of unknown primary site in women. *Ann Intern Med* 1989;111:213.
225. Fowler JM, Nieberg RK, Schooler TA, Berek JS. Peritoneal adenocarcinoma (serous) of müllerian type: a subgroup of women presenting with peritoneal carcinomatosis. *Int J Gynecol Cancer* 1994;4:43.
226. Williams SD. Current management of ovarian germ cell tumors. *Semin Oncol* 1994;8:53.
227. Williams SD. Ovarian germ cell tumors: an update. *Semin Oncol* 1998;25:407.
228. Williams SD, Blessing JA, Hatch KD, Homesley HD. Chemotherapy of advanced dysgerminoma: trials of the Gynecologic Oncology Group. *J Clin Oncol* 1991;9:1950.
229. Williams SD, Blessing JA, Moore DH, Homesley HD, Adcock L. Cisplatin, vinblastine, and bleomycin in advanced and recurrent ovarian germ-cell tumors. *Ann Intern Med* 1989;111:22.
230. Williams SD, Birch R, Einhorn L, et al. Disseminated germ cell tumors: chemotherapy with cisplatin plus bleomycin plus either vinblastine or etoposide. *N Engl J Med* 1987;316:1435.
231. Williams S, Blessing JA, Liao SY, Ball H, Hanjani P. Adjuvant therapy of ovarian germ cell tumors with cisplatin, etoposide, and bleomycin: a trial of the Gynecologic Oncology Group. *J Clin Oncol* 1994;12:701.
232. Schiller HM, Silverberg SG. Staging and prognosis in primary carcinoma of the fallopian tube. *Cancer* 1971;28:389.
233. Markman M, Zaino R, Busowski J, Barakat R. Carcinoma of the fallopian tube. In: Hoskins WJ, Perez CA, Young RC, eds. *Principles and practice of gynecologic oncology*. Philadelphia: JB Lippincott Co, 1992:783.

CHAPTER 37

Cancer of the Breast

SECTION 1 Molecular Biology of Breast Cancer

ROBERT B. DICKSON
MARC E. LIPPMAN

GENETICS

FAMILIAL DISEASE

The purpose of this chapter is to provide an introduction to the cellular, genetic, biochemical, and molecular bases of breast cancer. Although the roles of steroid hormones have occupied breast cancer researchers since the 1950s, the roles of growth factors did not begin to emerge until the 1980s. The 1980s also saw the discovery of many of the oncogenes and suppressor genes driving progression of the disease and highlighted their connections to growth factor and steroid regulatory pathways. The 1990s witnessed the discovery of genes causing the familial forms of breast cancer. The final decade of the twentieth century also ushered in major advances in our understanding of the cell cycle, DNA repair, and cell death (apoptosis) and their regulation.

Much excitement has been generated over the successes in identifying the inherited defects in somatic genes responsible for hereditary and familial breast cancers (Table 37.1-1). Although hereditary breast cancers occurring in defined syndromes are characterized by a very high penetrance of multiple types of cancer, breast cancer families may also display a lower penetrance and not be so clearly associated with elevated risk for multiple other types of cancer. The incidence of the former category is estimated at 1% of breast cancer cases, whereas the latter make up approximately 5% to 10% of cases.[1] Most researchers in the field of hereditary genetics of breast cancer have focused on genes that conformed to the two-hit hypothesis, which states that a point mutation might be inherited in one allele of a candidate gene at a putative susceptibility locus and that loss of heterozygosity (LOH) or another genetic alteration might occur in the other allele of that locus later in life, leading to cancer.

The first triumph in the identification of genes leading to the multicancer syndromes that include breast cancer was the demonstration that the *TP53* gene (on chromosome 17p13) is responsible for the Li-Fraumeni syndrome of hereditary breast cancers, sarcomas, and other tumor types.[1–3] As is discussed later in the section The Cell Cycle and Cell Death, mutations in this gene had been previously described in the context of progression of sporadic cancers of the breast and other organs. More recently, mutations in the *PTEN* (or *MMAC1*) gene (on chromosome 10q22-23) have been described in Cowden's syndrome of hereditary breast cancers and multicutaneous lesions.[4] This gene also is discussed later in the context of growth factor signal transduction, but it may not be commonly mutated in sporadic breast cancers. Other studies have implicated mutations of the *STK11/LKB1* gene (on chromosome 19) in the Peutz-Jeghers syndrome of hamartomatous polyps, breast cancers, gastrointestinal cancers, and reproductive cancers,[5] and the *MLH1* and *MLH2* genes in the Muir-Torre syndrome of gastrointestinal and genitourinary tumors and breast cancer.[6] Finally, although initially proposed to do so, mutations in the *ataxia telangiectasia* gene do not appear to contribute to the risk of developing breast cancer.[7]

Two important genes that confer risk for the more pervasive, familial forms breast cancer have been identified. Carriers of

TABLE 37.1-1. Major Genetic Defects in Breast Cancer

ESTABLISHED FAMILIAL BREAST GENES (ALL TUMOR SUPPRESSORS)

Gene	*Chromosomal Location*	*Disease*
TP53 (p53)	17p13 (mutated, LOH)	Li-Fraumeni syndrome of multiple hereditary cancers
PTEN	10q23 (mutated, LOH)	Cowden's syndrome of multiple hereditary cancers
BRCA-1	17q21 (mutated, LOH)	Familial female breast and ovarian cancers
BRCA-2	13q14 (mutated, LOH)	Familial female and male breast cancers

ESTABLISHED BREAST CANCER PROGRESSION GENES

Gene	*Chromosomal Location*	*Class*	*Function*
C-ERBB2	17q12	Oncogene (amplified)	Growth factor receptor subunit
C-MYC	8q24	Oncogene (amplified)	Cell-cycle/cell death regulator; protein synthesis
CCND1 (cyclin D1)	11q13	Oncogene (amplified)	Cell-cycle G_1 regulator
CDKN2 (p16)	9p21	Suppressor gene (methylated, LOH)	Cell-cycle G_1 regulator
RB-1	13q14	Suppressor gene (mutated, LOH)	Cell-cycle G_1 and G_1/S regulator
TP53 (p53)	17p13	Suppressor gene (mutated, LOH)	Cell-cycle/cell death/DNA repair regulator
CDH1 (E-cadherin)	16q22-23	Suppressor gene (methylated, LOH)	Cell-cell adhesion protein

LOH, loss of heterozygosity.

these mutant genes may display a wide range of levels of increased risk of cancer, and the genes are quite prevalent in certain populations. King and coworkers[8] first localized *BRCA-1* (for breast cancer and ovarian cancer-1) to chromosome 17q21. The gene was subsequently cloned and found to be novel, containing an amino terminal, a zinc- and DNA-binding "ring finger" motif, a carboxyl terminal BRCT (BRCA carboxy terminal) domain, and a nuclear localization sequence as recognizable motifs.[9] Interestingly, mutations in this gene are particularly prevalent in breast cancer of Ashkenazi Jewish women; however, some of these women belong to families nearly devoid of multiple afflicted members.[1] The detection of *BRCA-1* mutations in women with no familial association of the disease also has been reported in other studies comparing different carrier populations, emphasizing the variable penetrance of inherited risk conferred by this gene. Mutations in the *BRCA-1* gene have been verified in familial breast and ovarian cancer patients, but surprisingly, mutations have not been detected in sporadic breast cancers. Thus, *BRCA-1* does not appear to be a classic tumor suppressor gene of relevance to both tumor onset and progression. However, studies have observed that the *BRCA-1* protein may have an aberrant, cytoplasmic localization in breast cancer cell lines from sporadic tumors, suggesting that a nonclassic mode of functional inactivation could be at work in this tumor type.[10] Other studies have suggested that decreased expression of the BRCA-1 protein also occurs during the progression of sporadic breast cancers.[11] Consistent with these findings are observations that antisense oligonucleotides directed against the *BRCA-1* messenger RNA (mRNA) enhance the proliferation of breast tumor cells and mammary epithelial cells in culture *in vitro*. Correspondingly, other studies have demonstrated that retroviral transfer of the nonmutated *BRCA-1* gene selectively inhibits growth of breast cancer cells *in vitro* and *in vivo* in nude mice.[12]

A separate body of work has identified a separate locus, termed *BRCA-2* (on chromosome 13q13), which is associated with familial cancers of the female and male breast and, to a lesser extent, of the ovaries. This gene also has been cloned; it shares homology with *BRCA-1*[13] and its encoded protein is now thought to function biochemically in a fashion very similar to BRCA-1. However, although *BRCA-2* confers risk of female breast cancer, its effects on risk of ovarian cancer appear smaller than the risk conferred by *BRCA-1*. In addition, mutations of *BRCA-2* confer risk of male breast cancer and (to a more limited extent) several other cancers, such as prostate cancer, pancreatic cancer, non-Hodgkin's lymphoma, basal cell carcinoma, bladder carcinoma, and fallopian tube tumors. Breast cancers of *BRCA* carriers are, overall, of similar prognostic significance when matched for other characteristics to the sporadic cases of breast cancer in noncarriers, although they also show more often a high nuclear grade and p53 mutations.[1]

As already noted, the structure and function of the two BRCA proteins appear to be similar. Each appears to serve as an important regulator of cell-cycle "checkpoint control" mechanisms, involving cell-cycle arrest, cell death (apoptosis), and DNA repair. BRCA-1 appears to directly interact with the p53 protein (leading to induction of a cell-cycle inhibitor, p21), the RNA polymerase holoenzyme, the transcription factor CREB, and two novel proteins termed BAP1 and BARD1. Both BRCA-1 and BRCA-2 are also found in complexes with Rad51, a protein important for the cellular response to DNA damage.[1] In addition, BRCA-1 is phosphorylated by the ATM (ataxia telangiectasia mutated) kinase in response to DNA damage.[14] Thus, the roles of both BRCA proteins are now emerging as central gatekeepers of genomic stability.[1] In studies of mice bearing a conditional knockout of the *BRCA-1* gene, its further functions have emerged: mammary ductal morphogenesis and checkpoint control in the G_2/M phase of the cell cycle.[15,16] Finally, and perhaps most interesting of all, the normal BRCA-1 protein appears to function to suppress the signaling of mammary epithelial cells by the estrogen receptor.[17] This observation may place the BRCA proteins at center stage in control of the sex steroid–regulated pathways, long suspected to induce breast cancer.[18]

CYTOGENETIC STUDIES

Breast cancers, like other forms of malignancy, are thought to progress by accumulation of a series of genetic and resulting phenotypic changes in the pathways regulating cellular proliferation, differentiation, death (apoptosis or necrosis), DNA repair, tissue compartmentalization, and responses to therapy. Although several specific genetic alterations (discussed later in Oncogenes and Suppressor Genes of Breast Cancer Progression) have been identified with high frequency and proven relevance in breast cancer, certainly many more important genetic changes remain to be fully elucidated. Using classic cytogenetic methodologies and studies of LOH, genetic regions identified as frequently rearranged, amplified, deleted, or otherwise altered have been commonly detected on chromosomes 1, 3, 6, 7, 8, 9, 11, 13, 15, 16, 17, 18, and 20. More recently, the powerful techniques of comparative genomic hybridization and chromosome painting followed by spectral karyotyping have allowed implication of additional chromosome regions, including areas of 10, 12, and 22.[19,20] Although they have only begun to be used in this type of study, the techniques of comparative genomic hybridization and spectral karyotyping allow rapid analysis of subtle genomic imbalances and chromosomal rearrangements. Using these techniques, the benign lesions termed *fibroadenomas* are observed to be largely devoid of genetic imbalances (although they do contain some chromosomal defects), whereas aneuploid breast tumors contain far more chromosomal aberrations than diploid breast tumors.[20] Considering genetic changes on a broad scale, it appears that breast cancer (in contrast to certain other common epithelial tumors, such as colon cancer) is primarily characterized by chromosomal instability, as opposed to point mutagenesis. These chromosomal changes may arise from defects in the centrosomes and in the associated spindle apparatus of mammary epithelial cells. However, the exact pathogenesis of these defects remains obscure.[21,22]

ONCOGENES AND SUPPRESSOR GENES OF BREAST CANCER PROGRESSION

The most common genetic abnormalities in the progression both of sporadic and familial breast cancers (as in many other types of solid tumors) appear to be losses of heterozygosity at multiple loci (see Table 37.1-1). As noted earlier, an LOH event uncovers the functional consequences of a mutation in an allele of a tumor suppressor gene by removal of the dominant, normal allele. At the present time, in addition to the *TP53* gene and the two *BRCA* loci noted earlier, LOH on 13q, 9p, and 16q are known to involve specifically the tumor suppressor genes *RB-1* (retinoblastoma-1), *CDKN2* (encoding the p16 protein), and *CDH1* (encoding the E-cadherin protein), respectively. *RB-1* and *CDKN2* regulate the cell cycle, whereas *CDH1* primarily regulates differentiation and tissue compartmentalization. Other suspected tumor suppressor genes involved in the progression of breast cancer have been proposed to reside on 6q, 7q, 11p, 11q, 15q, 17q, 20, and 22. It is notable that two types of DNA alteration can lead to suppressor gene inactivation on one allele, before LOH of the other allele. For example, although point mutation may be more common for *TP53* and *Rb*, gene methylation may be more common for *CDKN2* and *CDH1*.[23] In some cases, genomic areas containing tumor suppressor genes also are susceptible to complete loss or deletion of both alleles. Certain tumor suppressor gene candidates, such as the gene encoding the p27 cell-cycle regulatory protein,[24] exhibit the characteristic of haploid insufficiency, whereby (in contrast to *TP53, BRCA-1, BRCA-2, PTEN, CDKN2,* and *CDH1*) a single normal copy of the gene is not fully suppressive of cancer. For this type of suppressor gene, mutation deletion and LOH are not common.[24]

The second most common type of cytogenetic alteration in breast cancer appears to be gene amplification. The initial step in gene amplification is thought to be the formation of extrachromosomal, self-replicating units termed *double-minute chromosomes.* These genetic elements then later become permanently incorporated into chromosomal regions and are termed *homogeneous-staining regions.* An amplified genetic unit (amplicon) is initially much larger than the actual size of the principal gene of biologic importance to tumorigenesis. Thus, silent or irrelevant genes may be detected coamplified with one or more expressed genes on an amplicon. The principal, best-established amplified and functional genes for tumorigenesis (also called *dominant oncogenes*) detected to date in breast cancer are the growth factor receptor *c-ERBB*$_2$, the nuclear transcription factor *c-MYC,* and the cell-cycle kinase regulator *CCND1.* A significant amount of work remains to be done to identify other potentially important oncogenes in breast cancer. For example, DNA gains are common on 6q, 8p, 8q, 11q, 12q, 13q, and 20q. In each of these cases, however, the specific genes involved in driving the chromosome amplification process are still under active investigation.[20,25]

STEROID AND GROWTH FACTOR PATHWAYS OF CELLULAR REGULATION

STEROID RECEPTORS

The estrogen and progesterone receptors are dimeric, gene-regulatory proteins. Estrogen and progesterone are well-established endocrine steroid regulators that modulate multiple aspects of mammary gland pathology. These two hormones work together to direct mammary epithelial growth, differentiation, and survival.[18,26,27] Although both steroids are commonly thought to be of primary importance for tumors arising in the reproductively competent years between puberty and menopause, local aromatization of adrenal androgens provides additional estrogens in the postmenopausal years. Both estrogen and progesterone act through their nuclear receptors (ER and PR, respectively) to modulate transcription of target genes.[26] Genes encoding the receptors for each class of steroids are members of a single large superfamily of transcription-modulating factors. ERs may exist in either homodimeric or heterodimeric species, composed of α and β receptors. In contrast, the PR is always a heterodimeric protein. Research on each system has defined additional, alternately spliced and mutated receptor forms. The biologic roles of these additional variant receptor subunits is under current investigation. Each steroid receptor dimer is also associated with other proteins, including heat-shock proteins, to allow ligand-binding association with its cognate, palindromic DNA elements. Other studies also have defined coactivational and corepressive proteins (CBP/p300, SRC-1, TIF2, AIB-1, N-CoR, SMRT, NSD1), which also interact with steroid receptors and function to modulate histone acetylation and deacetylation, a critical process thought to allow full access of the DNA to steroid receptors. DNA interaction of steroid receptors occurs through zinc finger structures of the receptors and promotes formation of a stable initiation complex to facilitate the transcription of responsive genes. Of considerable interest is the observation that the cell-cycle regulator cyclin D1 (product of the *CCND1* gene) also interacts with the ER to promote its transcriptional activity.[26,27] Superimposed on this complexity, each receptor is able to adopt multiple conformations, depending on the characteristics of interaction of the steroid (or nonsteroid ligand) with the receptor binding pocket. For example, the estrogen receptor can adopt at least three distinct conformations, depending on the antiestrogen bound.[28] Other studies suggest that the signal transduction pathways induced by growth factors and hormones may directly or indirectly regulate steroid receptor function. For example, cyclic adenosine monophosphate (cAMP), epidermal growth factor (EGF), heregulin (an EGF family member), and insulin-like growth factor (IGF)-1 appear to be able to modulate the activity of the estrogen receptor through phosphorylation; receptor phosphorylation modulates as well the steroid specificity of receptors for transactivation of steroid responsive genes.[26,29,30] The steroids are also well known for their ability to modulate directly the expression of cell-cycle regulatory genes known as *nuclear protooncogenes*, such as *c-MYC*, and the EGF receptor (EGFR)/HER-2 growth factor–receptor pathways.[31,32] The nuclear protooncoproteins and other cell-cycle regulatory proteins, such as cyclin D1, represent points of regulatory convergence of both steroid and growth factor pathways in cells. These findings describe a complex role for growth factors in the expression of progressively more malignant phenotypes and in escape from normal hormonal control.

Because the growth of breast cancer is often regulated by the female sex steroids, determinations of the cellular concentrations of ER and PR in the tumor are currently used to predict which patients have a good prognosis and which may also benefit from antihormonal therapy. Although these assays were originally designed as radioligand techniques, they are more commonly performed today using radioimmunoassay and immunohistochemical technologies. Although extremely useful, it has been repeatedly noted that these assays do not provide perfect prognostic tools for the disease. Although more than 60% of human breast cancers are ER-positive, no more than two-thirds of these ER-positive tumors respond to endocrine therapy.[26,33–36] In addition, 5% to 10% of the patients designated as ER-negative appear initially to respond to endocrine therapy.[26,37] To improve the value of determinations of the ER for tumor prognosis, the presence of the estrogen-regulated PR protein is now routinely performed. In many breast tumor cell lines and in normal ER-containing tissues, such as the endometrium and brain, PR expression also has been shown to be positively regulated by estrogen.[26,38] It is still not known whether ER regulates PR in normal human mammary epitheliums in precisely the same subpopulation of ductal and lobular luminal cells, although this supposition is considered to be likely. It is of interest that the ER and PR appear to be strongly up-regulated in ductal carcinoma *in situ* and in hormone-dependent breast cancer, relative to normal mammary epithelium. Whereas the ER- and PR-positive epithelial cell populations are distinct from the majority of proliferative cells in the normal gland, in cancer these cells grow rapidly. It is of interest that in histologically normal breast tissue adjacent to cancer, the epithelium also displays an aberrant, proliferative response to estrogen.[39,40] As already noted, other studies have made a connection between the ER and the tumor suppressor BRCA-1; expression of the normal form of BRCA-1 suppresses the transactivational activity of the ER.[17]

It is not clear what relationship exists between ER-positive and ER-negative forms of the disease. Several ER-negative breast cancer cell lines do not transcribe the ER mRNA because of an extensive methylation of the 5' promoter of the gene.[41] Treatment of ER-negative breast cancer cells *in vitro* with azacytidine, an inhibitor of gene methylation, resulted in expression of a functional ER.[42] However, the generality of this mechanism to clinical breast cancer is not yet certain. Central questions in breast cancer research focus on mechanisms of desensitization of the disease to antihormonal therapy and design of strategies to maintain antihormonal responses in patients. Studies have suggested that tamoxifen resistance of breast cancer may be associated with cellular hypersensitization to the weakly estrogenic effects of the drug, perhaps due to expression of receptor-associated regulatory proteins, receptor mutation, or selection for variant receptor isoforms.[26,43–45] Several variant receptor isoforms are under investigation with respect to the latter possibility. An exon 5–deleted ER variant lacks the hormone binding domain, displaying constitutively active, hormone-independent, transactivational characteristics. This receptor isoform is elevated in tamoxifen-relapsing breast cancer. Expression of an exon 4–deleted ER variant correlates with low histologic grade and high PR. Expression of other deletions in exons 2 and 4 or 3 to 7 are associated with high grade and high ER content.[26]

Although measurement of PR improves the predictability of hormone dependency of a tumor, this relationship remains imperfect. Retrospective clinical studies have demonstrated that, among ER-positive tumors, only 70% of those that are also PR-positive, and 25% to 30% of PR-negative tumors, respond to hormone therapy. The reasons for these discrepancies are unclear but may include laboratory error, differential metabolism of tamoxifen, the ability of a mutated ER or PR to regulate gene expression in the absence of ligand, the ability of defective or phosphorylated ER or PR to bind ligand but not regulate gene expression, or the ability of either defective or phosphorylated receptors to induce constitutive synthesis of otherwise regulated proteins.[26] Clearly, a challenge for the future is the development of routine, potentially more informative assays of ER and PR functionally. Another major hope is that study of other genetic changes in breast cancer, including those in growth factors, their receptors, and their signaling, will also improve our ability to predict functionality of the steroid receptor pathways relative to therapeutic outcomes.

The ER cannot be clearly classified either as an oncoprotein or tumor suppressor protein. Although it is thought to mediate the onset and progression of the disease, unexpected results were obtained when the ER was expressed endogenously in ER-positive breast cancer lines and compared to its heterotypic expression in formerly ER-negative lines. In striking contrast to its normal function in ER-positive cell lines, ER expressed in ER-negative cell lines functions to suppress cell growth, in spite of its normal action to regulate expression of certain hormonally responsive genes.[46,47] Thus, the multiple differences between ER-positive and ER-negative breast cancer appear to include incompatible growth regulatory mechanisms. We also do not understand the molecular basis for a lack of expression of PR in certain ER-positive breast cancers. A cell hybridization study with an antiestrogen resistant, ER-positive, but PR-negative sublime of MCF-7 has shown that loss of PR expression is a recessive phenotype in this system.[48] Finally, it should be noted that pathways of estrogen metabolism may be modulated in the pathophysiology of the disease. For example, the enzyme aromatase, which is responsible for conversion of adrenal androgens to estrogen in the postmenopausal breast and in other tissues, has been suggested as a potential, oncoprotein-like molecule in breast cancer.[49]

Increased expression and altered isozyme patterns of the family of cellular enzymes termed *protein kinase C* (PKC) also have been implicated during malignant progression of breast cancer.[50] This enzyme family can act to down-modulate ER mRNA, to activate ER function, to independently induce some estrogen-responsive genes with *AP-1* sites in their promoters, and to allow expression of more invasive cellular characteristics.[51] The PKC family contains at least nine cytoplasmic-nuclear enzymes, each of which possesses serine-threonine specificity for phosphate in addition to other cellular proteins[52]; different isotypes serve different cellular functions. The activity of PKC is known to be regulated by hormones and growth factors during normal lactational differentiation and to contribute to the regulation of casein expression.[52] PKC activity has been suggested to be elevated in ER-negative and drug-resistant breast cancer relative to ER-positive breast cancer. Treatment of ER-positive breast cancer with an activator of PKC, such as the phorbol ester 12-O-tetradecanoyl phorbol-13-acetate, leads to rapid down-regulation of ER, destabilization of its mRNA, and phosphorylation of the ER protein, coincident with modulation of its function.[53–56] Phosphorylation of ER and PR (induced by estrogen itself) by growth factor pathways (such as IGF-1), heregulin, cAMP, dopamine agonists, and other hormones may also constitutively activate the steroid receptors.[57–60] Other current studies have suggested that receptors for other steroids (potential cancer prevention agents, retinoids, vitamin D) may modulate ER/PR function by modulating their chromatic interactions.[61,62]

GROWTH FACTOR PATHWAYS IN THE NORMAL AND MALIGNANT GLAND

The natural secretory products of the mammary epithelial cell, colostrum and milk, are abundant sources of growth factors.[63] Growth factors in the normal gland probably serve multiple purposes in the development of the newborn, in mammary growth, and in mammary carcinogenesis. A large body of literature has shown that estrogen, antiestrogens, progestins, and antiprogestins strongly regulate certain growth factors and receptors of the EGF and transforming growth factor-β (TGF-β) families, as well as growth factors, receptors, and secreted binding proteins of the IGF family (Table 37.1-2).[64,65] EGF, apparently the most abundant milk-derived growth factor, is an important regulator both of the proliferation and the differentiation of the mouse mammary gland *in vivo* and of mouse mammary explants *in vitro*.[66,67] It also has been observed that circulating mouse salivary gland–derived EGF may potentiate spontaneous mammary tumor formation in the mouse model and promote the growth of the tumors once they are formed.[66,68] EGF, or other members of this growth factor family, are also required supplements for the clonal anchorage-dependent growth, *in vitro*, of normal human mammary epithelial cells.[69] In contrast, human breast cancer cells in culture are largely independent of this exogenous requirement. However, most breast cancer cell lines retain EGFRs and appear to be stimulated in their growth by their own autocrine or paracrine production of this family of factors.[33,65]

TABLE 37.1-2. Sex Hormone Regulation of Growth Factor Systems in Breast Cancer

EGF FAMILY
Growth factors: EGF, TGF-α, amphiregulin
Receptors: EGFR, c-erbB$_2$
IGF FAMILY
Growth factors: IGF-2
Receptors: IGF-1R, IGF-2R, insulin receptor
Binding proteins: BP-2, BP-3, BP-4, BP-5
TGF-β FAMILY
Growth factors: TGF-β$_1$, TGF-β$_2$, TGF-β$_3$
PDGF FAMILY
Growth factors: PDGF-1, PDGF-2

BP, binding protein; EGF(R), epidermal growth factor (receptor); IGF, insulin-like growth factor; PDGF, platelet-derived growth factor; TGF, transforming growth factor.

Direct modulation of signal transduction pathways of EGF and its family members, as well as their indirect regulation by other unrelated growth factors are proving to be critical during mammary development. The EGF family consists of, at present, four receptors and more than six growth factors in mammals, and an additional half-dozen growth factors encoded only by certain mammalian viruses. TGF-α and amphiregulin, close structural and functional homologs of EGF, can produce qualitatively the same proliferative effects as EGF in mouse mammary explants and in cultured human and mouse mammary epithelial cell lines.[65,67] Each of these factors is also produced in proliferative, early ductal development; amphiregulin is also produced in the lobuloalveolar development of pregnancy.[70] However, the detailed localization patterns and functions of each family member differ.[71,72] For example, an immunohistochemical study in the mouse gland has revealed that expression of TGF-α is highest in the basal epithelial, proliferative end-bud cap cells, whereas expression of EGF is in scattered ductal luminal secretory cells.[73] Hepatocyte growth factor, a non-EGF family factor, also appears to be involved in ductal morphogenesis.[74] The EGF-related neuregulin subfamily of isoforms (including heregulin) is expressed primarily in the mammary stroma and appears to modulate the lobuloalveolar development of pregnancy.[75] TGF-α, a heparin-binding family member termed *amphiregulin*, and their common receptor, the

EGFR, are all detected *in vitro* in proliferating human mammary epithelial cells in culture. TGF-α mRNA levels are relatively low in explanted, primary cultures of resting epithelial organoids[76,77]; the entire system appears tightly coupled to proliferation in the normal gland. TGF-α and amphiregulin are known to act as autocrine autostimulatory growth factors in normal and immortalized human mammary epithelial cells in mass culture; an anti-EGFR antibody or heparin, respectively, reversibly inhibited proliferation.[77–79] Although the majority of work on the biology of the EGF family has focused on regulation of proliferation, it is now clear that many other aspects of mammary biology may be under its control, such as cell differentiation and survival. The complex heterodimerization pattern of the EGFR family may play a role in governing the multiple responses of this system.[80,81]

Since the early work of DeLarco, Todaro, Sporn, and others, overexpression of EGF family members has been thought to contribute to progression of multiple types of cancer. Specifically, in early studies, the level of secretion of TGF-α in breast cancer, fibroblasts, and other cell types was correlated with expression of oncogenes. In breast cancer, a direct correlation among TGF-α production, expression of the *c-ras*^{H} oncogene, and malignant transformation was demonstrated *in vitro*.[82–89] Subsequent work in human breast cancer and in benign proliferative breast disease has also established that TGF-α overexpression is very common.[84,85]

The development of transgenic technology has allowed additional correlation of expression of TGF-α, amphiregulin, and cripto-1 (another EGF family member, but with an unrelated receptor type) with mammary tumors induced by a wide range of oncogenes.[86] This technology also has allowed study of the effect of overexpression of TGF-α under the control of mammary-selective mouse mammary tumor virus (MMTV) or metallothionine promoters in the mammary glands of mice. The multiple conclusions of these studies implicate TGF-α–induced proliferation, TGF-α–blocked differentiation, and TGF-α–suppressed, postlactational glandular regression in mammary hyperplasia and tumorigenesis.[87–92] More recently, transgenic expression of the EGF subfamily known as *neuregulins* also has been shown to lead to mammary tumorigenesis.

Although observations of overexpression of EGF family growth factors have led to significant biologic insights into breast cancer, the greatest clinical impact has come from study of EGF family receptors. Gene amplification and resultant overexpression of EGFR-related c-erbB$_2$ (HER-2/neu) protein is found in approximately 25% of human breast cancer cases[93] (see Table 37.1-1). In addition, expression of the EGFR occurs in 40% of breast tumors, but in the absence of gene amplification. Expression of each protein signifies poor prognosis for the patient.[94] Current studies are addressing the frequency and relevance of expression of the additional, EGFR-related c-erbB$_3$ and c-erbB$_4$ receptors in breast cancer. Transgenic mouse studies also have been successfully used to confirm the oncogenic potential of the c-erbB$_2$ oncoprotein. Interestingly, activational mutations in the extracellular domain of the c-erbB$_2$ oncoprotein were commonly detected in transgenic mouse mammary carcinomas, but this type of mutation has not been described in human breast cancer.[95] Stimulation of cells through the EGFR family may also sensitize cells to other carcinogenic insults. For example, expression of a TGF-α transgene accelerates the progression of carcinogen-initiated mouse mammary tumors.[96] In summary, the etiologic evidence is compelling for EGF family growth factors and their receptors in mammary tumorigenesis after combining data from human pathologic studies and from transgenic mouse models.

In human breast cancer cell lines *in vitro*, autocrine growth dependence of cells on the TGF-α/EGFR system also has been documented in one ER-negative breast cancer cell line—the MDA-MB-468. It is clear in this line that a rare gene amplification of the EGFR sensitizes the cells to autocrine function of TGF-α. This line, thus representative only of a small percentage of breast cancers, expresses more than 10^6 EGFRs (per cell). TGF-α and amphiregulin are also induced by estrogen in hormone-dependent MCF-7 breast cancer cells. Antisense TGF-α complementary DNA, anti–TGF-α antibodies, and anti-erbB$_2$ ribozymes partially block estrogen-induced growth *in vitro*,[97–102] strongly suggesting a hormone-inducible type of autocrine system. The potential clinical relevance of this type of system is significant. Possible autocrine functions of other EGF family members in breast cancer have not yet been fully evaluated, although high expression of neuregulins has been reported in some cell lines *in vitro*. A number of studies have more closely addressed the functions of the neuregulin subfamily in their interactions with the EGFR-related c-erbB$_3$ and c-erbB$_4$ proteins in breast cancer. The neuregulins appear to act *in vitro* with biphasic effects: Low levels are proliferative, whereas higher levels may inhibit epithelial proliferation. The neuregulins also appear to promote differentiation and induce casein synthesis in the developing gland and in breast cancer cells.[75,103,104] To summarize available data, autocrine function of the EGFR ligand system may be most critical in normal gland growth and early stages of breast tumorigenesis, as contrasted with later stages of the disease. Paracrine, tumor-host interactive functions of this family of factors (discussed later in The Process of Malignant Progression) may then begin to dominate its functions as the disease progresses. Strategies using toxic, genetically engineered EGFR ligand bacterial toxin fusion proteins (termed *oncotoxins*) or humanized, anti–c-erbB$_2$ or anti-EGFR antibodies, either alone or coupled with toxins or other therapeutic drugs (*immunotoxins*), could possibly find future therapeutic utility, because a large portion of hormone-independent breast cancers express significant levels of these receptors.[83,93,105,106]

A second growth factor family of potential importance in cancer is the fibroblast growth factor (FGF) family.[107] Members of this family also have been implicated in mammary gland growth and malignant transformation. These growth factors bind to heparin, require a heparin cofactor for proper presentation to and interaction with receptors, and accumulate in the extracellular matrix after their release from cells. Some FGF isoforms do not possess a signal sequence of secretion, but all forms appear to be released by cells by one or more mechanisms. Although FGF-1 and FGF-4 are expressed during the ductal growth phase of the mouse mammary gland in luminal ductal epithelial cells, expression of FGF-2 and FGF-7 are primarily stromal. FGF-1, FGF-2, and FGF-7 have been detected in mammary preneoplasias, tumors, and cell lines, but not in levels significantly higher than normal. FGF-3 (also known in the mouse as *int-2*) is a well-known oncogenic growth factor activated in the mouse mammary gland by MMTV insertional mutagenesis. FGF-4 also has been associated with metastasis of certain mouse mammary tumors.[108]

However, although amplification of the genes encoding FGF-3 and FGF-4 have been observed in human breast cancer, these two genes are seldom expressed at the protein level. This finding appears to be the result of their co-amplification with other more important genes located nearby on the chromosomes (genes encoding c-erbB_2 and cyclin D1, respectively). In the human mammary gland, FGF-1 and FGF-2 have been localized both to myoepithelial and to epithelial cells. Although studies *in vitro* have implicated FGF-2 as an autocrine growth factor in immortalized human mammary epithelial cells,[109] expression of FGF-2 in clinical human breast cancer is correlated with a good prognosis. Although FGF-1 also has been detected in human breast cancer, it is localized primarily to macrophages[110]; its biologic role is not fully known, but it could potentially contribute to inflammation and angiogenesis. FGF receptors (FGFR) 1–4 each have been localized (and the gene encoding FGFR1 occasionally amplified) in human breast cancer.[111–113] Receptor heterodimerization is likely to represent a locus of control for FGFR function. Several of the FGF family members have been shown to promote tumor growth and dissemination of metastasis in xenograft models of human breast cancer, at least partially through effects on the tumor vasculature. However, the complete relevance of these observations to the pathophysiology of human breast cancer is still under investigation.[114]

TGF-β, a family of at least three growth factors distinct from FGF and EGF families, is also present in the normal and malignant mammary epithelium and in human milk.[115,116] Receptors for TGF-βs comprise a family of heterodimeric serine-threonine kinases.[117] TGF-βs are profoundly negative in their proliferative effects on ductal epithelial proliferation in mouse mammary glands *in vivo*[27] and on most other epithelial cell types. Expression of TGF-β family members is suppressed by estrogen and progesterone.[27,65] All three TGF-β isoforms are detected at the mRNA level in the developing mouse mammary epithelium. All isoforms of TGF-β, once produced, are retained in the stromal matrix surrounding the mammary ducts, but TGF-β is absent from the matrix of growing end buds and lateral branches.[118] Glandular production of TGF-β decreases, along with its stromal accumulation around alveoli during midpregnancy and lactation; TGF-β is suppressive of lactation.[119–121] However, TGF-β is again elevated as postlactational glandular regression occurs.[122] The role of TGF-β also has been examined by using a transgenic mouse approach. Targeted expression of TGF-β in the pregnant mammary epithelium with an MMTV promoter leads to inhibition of both alveolar development and lactation.[120] All three TGF-β isoforms have been detected in the human gland, with a similar distribution to that observed in the mouse. Paradoxically, TGF-β production increases with malignant progression in breast cancer. Its accumulation may have significance for development of the characteristic fibrous desmoplastic stroma of breast cancer,[123] tumor angiogenesis, and immune suppression.[124] Thus, although serving a growth-inhibitory role in the normal gland, progression to cancer may be associated with desensitization of this pathway. Overproduction of TGF-β may thus contribute to aberrant tumor-host interactions in breast cancer.[118,125,126] It is of interest, at least in some cell lines *in vitro*, that TGF-β may even stimulate tumor cell invasion.[127] An active area of current investigation involves study of inactivating mutations in the TGF-β receptor. To date, however, loss of TGF-β receptor by mutation or by loss of expression has been observed in colon cancer and retinoblastoma, respectively.[128]

A complex regulatory system is also emerging from studies of the insulin-like growth factors. Whereas the IGF-1 receptor (IGF-1R) is a heterodimeric tyrosine kinase, closely related to the insulin receptor, the IGF-2R is an unrelated binding protein also capable of interacting with TGF-β and with cathepsin D. IGF-2 production, as well as cellular responsiveness to IGFs, is stimulated by estrogen and inhibited by antiestrogens in some hormone-dependent breast cancer cell lines. IGF-2 is thought to be a potential autocrine growth factor in breast cancer; in contrast, IGF-1 is synthesized in the tumor stroma and is considered to have important paracrine growth and survival-stimulatory actions in the disease. Transgenic mouse models have demonstrated that mammary expression of IGF-1 causes ductal hypertrophy and suppression of postlactational involution and that IGF-2 expression can lead to mammary cancer. The cellular responsiveness to IGFs appears to be modulated by estrogens and antiestrogens as a result of regulation of both receptors (type 1 being induced and type 2 repressed); IGF-binding proteins 2, 4, and 5 (each of which are estrogen-induced); IGF-binding protein 3 (which is estrogen inhibited), and the signal transduction docking phosphoprotein insulin receptor substrate 1 (IRS-1) (which is estrogen-induced). The biologic functions of the IGF binding proteins (BP) are not fully understood, although BP-1 appears inhibitory of the actions of IGF-1, even with *in vivo* models. Although BP-3 may contribute to poor prognosis of breast cancer, BP-4 and IGF-1R correlates with good prognosis. IGF-2R is under active investigation as a tumor suppressor gene in cancers of the breast and other tissues. Its gene is subject to frequent LOH and, possibly, mutations in breast cancer.[129–132]

It should be noted that, at present, several dozen other growth factors have been identified in breast cancer, but their consideration is beyond the scope of this chapter; this information is reviewed elsewhere.[133] To summarize some of these data, prolactin[134] and mammary-derived growth factor-1 might be autocrine positive factors in breast cancer, and mammary-derived growth inhibitor and mammostatin may serve negative growth functions.[133] In addition, hepatocyte growth factor/scatter factor is a stromal-derived paracrine-acting stimulator both of epithelial growth and of tumor angiogenesis. Finally, vascular endothelial growth factor, pleiotropin, and platelet-derived growth factor may serve as angiogenic, vascularization-inducing factors in breast cancer.[65,133] Other growth factors under hormonal regulation in breast cancer probably remain undiscovered; future investigations should evaluate this possibility. Many studies have also established that steroid regulation of growth factors is important in the uterus and, possibly, the prostate gland, as well as in the breast.[133]

SIGNAL TRANSDUCTION AND NUCLEAR ONCOGENES

Unifying, mechanistic links between the proliferative actions of growth- and survival-modulatory steroids, growth factors, and integrins in diverse tissues are represented by the multiple classes of nuclear protooncogenes and other transcription factors (see Table 37.1-1).[65,135] These transcription-regulating proteins mediate convergent pathways of regulatory stimuli directly through steroid action, through growth factor–induced mitogen-activated protein (MAP) kinases, through other cytoplasmic tyrosine kinases (Fak, Src) or phospholipase C–PKC, through cytokine-induced JAK-STAT pathways, through TGF-β family–induced SMAD molecules, and through integrin-induced Fak/Src pathways. The MAP kinase pathways are central pathways for the proliferative and survival stimuli exerted through the EGFR, the c-erbB_2 receptor, and the insulin receptor type 1 families. Receptors trigger this pathway through autophosphorylation and subsequent binding to src homology 2/3 (SH2/SH3) or phosphotyrosine-binding (PTB) domains of signal transduction adaptor proteins. After mitogenic growth factor treatment of many types of cells, including normal and malignant breast epithelial cells, and a cascade of protein phosphorylations, c-Myc, AP-1–acting (c-fos, c-Jun, and Jun B), c-Myb, and Ets protooncogenes and ATF, EIK, SRF, and NFKB transcription factors are commonly observed to be induced. The protein products of at least three nuclear protooncogenes, *c-MYC, c-FOS,* and *c-JUN,* are also induced by both estrogen and progesterone in breast cancer. Progestins additionally induce *c-JUNB.*[133,135] Not surprisingly, tamoxifen down-modulates c-MYC expression during treatment-induced regression of patient tumors.[136] c-MYC, c-FOS, and c-JUN induction also have been shown to occur in human mammary epithelial cells *in vitro* and in the rat uterus in response to estrogen treatment *in vivo.*[137–139] Cyclin D1 also appears to be a central nuclear protooncogene-like molecule further downstream of AP-1 and other mitogenic transcriptional controls. Not only does it regulate the G_1 phase of the cell cycle, but similar to the AIB-1 (amplified in breast cancer) protein, it also appears to directly modulate in a positive way the transactivational ability of the estrogen receptor.[140,141]

c-Fos and c-Jun proteins contain specific domains that allow them to form a heterodimeric complex that can interact with the gene promoter consensus sequence termed *AP-1.* In an analogous manner, the c-Myc protein, of central importance to estrogenic stimulation of breast cancer cells, dimerizes with another protein termed *Max* (or *Myn* in the mouse) to modulate genes through a different consensus sequence, termed an *E-box* (and possibly other sequences). The cellular supply of Max that is available for productive dimerization with c-Myc depends on its interaction with its other family members, termed *Mad* and *Mxi1.* The interaction of Max with either of these proteins serves to reduce its availability for interactions with Myc and may exert negative transactivational through E-box sites. Myc-Max dimers are known to induce proliferation, apoptosis, and chromosomal instability, depending on the cellular context and degree of expression. Myc-Max interaction with the TATA binding protein represents one transactivational mechanism to stimulate basal transcription. A second specific transactivational mechanism involves E-box promoter genes such as those encoding the CAD (carbamoyl phosphate synthetase–aspartate transcarbamoylase–dihydro orotase), DHFR (dihydrofolate reductase), and ODC (ornithine decarboxylase) enzymes.[142] However, multiple c-Myc–regulated genes do not appear to possess E-boxes, and E-box–interactive sequences do not appear to be required for c-Myc effects on proliferation and apoptosis.[143]

Several other c-Myc–interactive proteins exist in addition to the TATA binding protein and Max; they include TRRAP, BIN1, DAM, p107, YY1, MIZ1, and TFII-1. Thus, multiple other potential mechanisms may exist for transactivational and transcriptional suppressive effects of c-Myc.[142] Estrogen and progesterone induce c-Myc; the latter appears to primarily modulate the mammary epithelial cell cycle both by inducing the synthesis of cyclin E and the CDC25A phosphatase and by triggering the degradation of p27 (kip1), resulting in an active CDK2. Activation of CDK2 results in inhibitory phosphorylation of Rb and promotes cell-cycle progression though G_1/S. Additional primary effects of c-Myc appear to be induction of cyclin A to activate CDK2 and induction of the E_2F_1 transcription factor to promote cell-cycle progression through S.[142,144,145]

Although much is known about the cellular and molecular biology of c-Myc, it is clearly an understudied oncoprotein in breast cancer. It appears to be central to the disease in two respects. First, antisense oligonucleotides directed against the c-Myc mRNA have been used to block estrogen-induced proliferation in breast cancer cells.[146] Second, amplification of the *c-MYC* gene is now known to be one of the most common genetic alterations in breast cancer; approximately one-fifth of breast cancers contain this genetic change. A putative (but currently unidentified) suppressor gene on chromosome 1p32-pter is proposed to control *c-MYC* amplification in breast cancer.[144,147] Despite its apparent importance, study of *c-MYC* gene expression in breast cancer has been slow because of difficulties in measuring its encoded protein in tumor biopsies. Specifically, the protein has a very short half-life,[148] and there have been a lack of suitable monoclonal antibodies capable of staining paraffin sections. A few studies focusing on gene amplification have shown that *c-MYC* is associated with poor prognosis, high S phase, and postmenopausal disease, although the latter has not been confirmed.[144,147] Based on several investigations in various epithelial malignancies, including those of the ovary and liver, *c-MYC* amplification is thought to cooperate with TGF-α with EGFR overexpression and with downstream signaling pathways. Thus, dual stimulation of the EGFR pathway and c-Myc may serve a general cooperative function in epithelial transformation.[149–151]

The c-Myc protein may, therefore, act in multiple systems to regulate gene expression, promote cell proliferation, inhibit differentiation, modulate cell adhesion, and effect immune recognition. Central to these effects is its role to specifically regulate initiation of DNA replication. Overall, gene regulatory activities of the protein also encompass both activation and suppression of gene expression; modulation of the cell cycle; activation of apoptosis (programmed cell death); and modulation of DNA metabolism, DNA dynamics, energy metabolism, and macromolecular synthesis. It is also known that the c-Myc protooncogene product can immortalize cells. Of current interest, the role of c-Myc to induce apoptosis depends on $p19^{ARF}$-mediated activation of the p53 tumor suppressor gene, at least in fibroblasts. However, this mechanism has not yet been demonstrated in mammary cancer.[142,148] A variety of other malignancy-associated biologic consequences of *c-MYC* amplification also have been described. Very pertinent to the process of malignant progression, some reports have suggested that expression of the *c-MYC* gene may allow amplification of other genes, (e.g., *ODC* and *DHFR*)[142], alter cellular resistance to *cis*-platinum and other DNA strand scission–inducing drugs,[152] and act to suppress differentiation in association with the decrease of collagen gene transcription.[153] The c-Myc protein may also inhibit transcription of the rat *neu* oncogene (*c-ERB2* homologue).[154] However, the importance of this interaction for human breast cancer is not yet known. Nevertheless, *c-MYC* amplification appears not to be closely associated with *c-ERBB2* amplification in primary breast cancer. c-Myc may also relate to the aging and senescence process; increased expression of c-Myc in multiple tissue types with aging may reflect cumulative proliferation-associated disregulation and has been proposed to contribute to aberrant mitogenic responses of the tissue in postmenopausal breast cancer.[155] However, increased expression of the c-Myc partner Mxil is also enhanced during aging and may attenuate the effects of c-Myc.[156]

The *c-MYC* gene and other oncogenes have been introduced into immortalized human or mouse mammary epithelial cells using an amphotrophic retroviral vector. These studies have observed that either c-Myc or the simian virus 40T nuclear oncoproteins (but not v-Ras^H or v-Mos cytoplasmic oncoproteins) allowed the cells to grow in soft agar in response to FGF-1, FGF-2, EGF, or TGF-α.[157] Because mammary fibroblasts produce EGF- and FGF-related growth factors[158] and because their conditioned media could support transforming growth of nuclear oncogene–transfected mammary epithelial cells, these observations have supported a role *in vivo* for stromal-epithelial interactions. Such a synergistic interaction has been observed *in vitro* in TGF-α/c-Myc bitransgenic mice. Co-overexpression of these two gene products allows rapid (10 weeks) onset of highly proliferative mammary tumors, independent of sex hormones in either gender.[150,151] Thus, an amplified *c-MYC* gene may function in breast cancer to allow growth factors or hormones to act to drive aberrant, transformed growth.[145]

THE CELL CYCLE AND CELL DEATH

TUMOR SUPPRESSOR GENES

Seminal studies by Broca in the nineteenth century[159] established that breast cancer can have a familial pattern of onset in 5% to 10% of cases. In addition, it has been observed that families with a very high incidence of the disease sometimes display a high incidence of additional cancer(s), such as ovarian cancer. A hypothesis has been proposed that such families inherit a defective or lost allele encoding a tumor suppressor gene. This hypothesis was based largely on work by Knudson, who suggested that the inactivation of two alleles of a gene was required in the disease known as retinoblastoma,[160] and Harris, who demonstrated that certain chromosomes could suppress malignancy *in vitro* in cell hybrid studies.[161] This concept has led to the discovery of several tumor suppressor genes in breast cancer, some regulating the cell cycle and cell death, and others regulating different aspects of the progression of the disease.

The first tumor suppressor gene shown to confer risk of an inherited breast cancer syndrome was termed *TP53*, and more recently, the *PTEN* gene was implicated in this respect. Also, the two *BRCA* genes (see Table 37.1-1) are responsible for a larger group of patients with an inherited pattern of breast cancer (*BRCA-2*) and breast plus ovarian cancers (*BRCA-1*). It is now widely accepted that *BRCA-1, BRCA-2,* and *PTEN* all function as tumor suppressor genes. However, in contrast to *TP53*, their mutations are uncommon in sporadic breast cancers. Conversely, three other well-established tumor suppressor genes, *CDKN2* (p16), *RB-1*, and *CDH1* (E-cadherin), are commonly altered (mutation, methylation, LOH, and deletion) in sporadic breast cancer but do not appear to be involved in conferring familial risk of the disease (see Table 37.1-1).

During the malignant progression of breast cancer to its fully metastatic state, mutation, inactivation, loss, or down-regulated expression of tumor suppressing genes commonly occurs. Estimated incidences of these processes for the relevant, known suppressor genes are as follows: *TP53*, 30% to 40%; *RB-1*, 15% to 20%; *CDKN2*, 20% to 30%; and *CDH1*, 20% to 30%.[135] Tumor suppressor genes appear to function in four major ways: as antiproliferative or antisurvival factors, as DNA-repair inducers, and as differentiation-promoting agents. BRCA-1 and BRCA-2 serve roles to direct repair of damaged DNA. The ATM protein (described earlier as a suspected tumor suppressor) detects the damage and transmits the signal to the BRCA proteins, while multiple other proteins, such as Rad51 and p53, serve roles downstream of the BRCAs.[162,163] E-cadherin, a suppressor that works through an unrelated pathway, serves to strengthen homotypic interactions of mammary epithelial cells and maintain their differentiated status; in addition, it promotes sequestration of β-catenin (a proliferation-promoting protein that regulates the T-cell factor (TCF) class of transcription factors).[164] p53, by inducing the p21 protein (Waf-1/CIP-1), also inhibits proliferation, whereas the p16 protein also serves to inhibit the cell cycle; both p53 and p16 suppressor proteins ultimately promote phosphorylation and inactivation of Rb to block G_1 and G_1/S transit of the cell cycle.[165,166] Although Rb is thought to be a central tumor suppressor protein in breast cancer, it appears to be understudied at present, particularly with respect to its mutation status. PTEN serves to suppress cell survival and proliferation by dephosphorylating phosphoinositides to prevent their activation of the three AKT signal transduction kinases.[167–169] Beyond the scope of this chapter is the consideration of literally dozens of additional candidate tumor suppressor genes that also function on these cellular pathways (see also the section The Process of Malignant Progression).[135]

Study of the *TP53* gene has provided remarkable insights into multiple areas of cancer biology. *TP53* is a tumor suppressor gene, but when mutated in one of several sensitive regions, its conformation changes, its stability increases, and its regulatory properties are radically altered. Mutation can confer a loss of tumor suppressor activity and gain of tumor promotion function.[170] The nonmutated p53 gene product is an oligomeric DNA binding protein that functions to trigger cellular responses to DNA damage; it has been termed the "guardian of the genome." p53 functions both by protein-protein interactions and by regulation of transcription. The p53 protein appears to function in the context of DNA damage as a G_1/S and G_2/M checkpoint controller to slow cell growth and induce DNA repair; cell death is triggered in a process termed *apoptosis* if damage is too severe for repair. It is of particular importance for the progression of many cancers, including breast cancer, that mutation of p53 is associated with enhanced genetic instability.[171] Certain viral proteins, although they are probably not relevant to breast cancer, are known to inactivate p53 as a critical event in viral carcinogenesis.[170]

It is not yet fully clear what molecular events induce (through protein stabilization) the p53 protein. However, it is well known that UV irradiation and double-strand DNA breaks are strong inducers of p53 stabilization through the DNA-dependent protein kinase and the ATM gene product. ATM is a signal transduction protein with high homology to phosphatidyl–insitol-3 kinase.[172] Of uncertain molecular bases are observations that inhibitors of PKC inhibitors, serine-threonine phosphatases, and cAMP can prevent p53-mediated responses. On a molecular level, p53 induces growth arrest in multiple points of the cell cycle through induction of p21, a multipotent inhibitor of cyclin-dependent kinases (CDKs), which blocks cell-cycle progression (discussed later in Cyclins, Cyclin-Dependent Kinases, and Inhibitors); p21 also blocks a catalytic inhibitor of a DNA replication termed *proliferating cell nuclear antigen* (PCNA). A very important, specific consequence of p21 induction is the inhibition of cyclin E–CDK2-catalyzed phosphorylation of the Rb protein. Hypophosphorylation of Rb allows its function as an additional cell-cycle inhibitor. p53 is also thought to directly modulate transcription of Rb and to directly bind a partner of Rb (termed *p107*) at the protein level.[173] Additionally, p53 induces transcription of genes encoding cyclin G, ERCC (excision repair cross-complementing), and Gadd 45 (growth arrest DNA damage protein), all proteins thought to be involved in DNA repair. A third general process triggered by p53 is apoptotic death. This process is quite distinct from necrotic death in that it requires ATP, the cell condenses the chromation of its nucleus, the nucleus undergoes fragmentation, and the cell maintains an intact plasma membrane until the final stage, at which point terminal cells are consumed by macrophages.[170,173] Negative regulators of p53 are thought to include its phosphorylation by several kinases, its nuclear exclusion by unknown mechanisms, and its complexation with a protein called *MDM-2* (murine double-minute gene-2), itself a p53-inducible protein and an oncogene (at least in some cancers other than breast cancer).[173]

The most extreme result of p53 induction is apoptosis. A protein whose transcription is directly inhibited on this pathway is Bcl-2[174] (Table 37.1-3). Bcl-2 is an apoptosis-preventing protein, commonly expressed in breast cancer in p53-mutated cells.[175] Bcl-2 is localized in the mitochondria, nuclear membrane, and endoplasmic reticulum. It functions, along with a homologue termed *Bclx*$_L$, to suppress the function of Bax, a death-inducing protein; many Bcl family members act to form mitochondrial pores of differential ionic permeability. Several other stimulatory and inhibitory family members exist, including Bclx$_S$, a promoter of apoptotic death. This entire system functions to regulate death by regulating a series of regulatory cysteine proteases within the cell. The apoptotic system is thought to be triggered by hypoxia or by a shift in the redox potential of the cell; Bcl-2 and Bclx$_L$ protect against death (induced by proapoptotic Bax) by modulating mitochondrial permeability and regulating mitochondrial release of cytochrome C.[170,171] In addition, two family members of *p53*, called *p73* and *p63*, are under current study for their p53-like properties.[176,177]

Although quite complex, the balance of life/apoptosis is critically regulated in cancer progression and response to therapy (see Table 37.1-3). Estrogen, progesterone, TGF-α, EGF, and insulin all appear to suppress apoptosis and promote survival of breast cancer model systems. Antiestrogens, antiprogestins, TGF-β, and the overexpressed c-Myc oncoprotein can induce apoptosis unless countered with a survival-promoting, environmental influence. Current research is focused on how these factors regulate the apoptotic pathway(s).[178,179] The system has clear implications for response of breast cancer to radiation, antihormonal and biologic therapies, chemotherapy, and even gene therapy. For example, it has been suggested that estrogen promotes chemotherapy resistance of breast cancer by induction of Bcl-2,[180] that p53 mutation results in resistance to chemotherapy,[181] and that experimental gene therapy with *bclx* can differentially kill tumor cells and sensitize them to chemotherapy but spare bone marrow cells.[182,183] Gene therapy addressing the *p53* gene directly has also been proposed.[170]

TABLE 37.1-3. Cell Death (Apoptosis) Regulatory Factors in Breast Cancer

SURVIVAL FACTORS
Extracellular signals
Estrogen, progesterone
EGF, TGF-α
Insulin, IGF-1, IGF-2
Extracellular matrix
Signal transduction pathways
P13K, AKT, ERK1/2 MAPKs, PDK1, RSKs, CREB
Mitochondrial protectors
Bcl-2, Bcl-X$_L$
Caspase activation protectors
Flip
ADED family
Protectors of effector caspases
IAPs
DEATH FACTORS
Extracellular signals
Chemotherapy, radiation therapy
Antiestrogens, antiprogestins
Cytotoxic cytokines: FasL, TNF, TGF-β
Oxidative stress, hypoxia
Growth factor deprivation
Cell detachment
Signal transduction pathways
p53, JNK, p38 MAPK
Mitochondrial activators
BAD, Bax
Caspase activators
Cytochrome C, APAF1
Fadd
Caspase cascades
Caspase 8, 10; effector caspases 3, 6, 7
Caspase 9; effector caspases 3, 6, 7

ADED, antideath domain; AKT, protein kinase B; APAF1, apoptotic protease activating factor-1; CREB, cyclic adenosine monophosphate–responsive element binding protein; EGF, epidermal growth factor; ERK1/2 MAPKs , extracellular signaling regulated kinases 1/2 mitogen-activated protein kinases; IGF, insulin-like growth factor; IAP, inhibitor of apoptotic proteases; JNK, Jun terminal kinase; PDK1, phosphoinositide-dependant kinase 1; RSK, ribosomal S6 kinase; TGF, transforming growth factor; TNF, tumor necrosis factor.

The *RB-1* gene product also has tumor suppressor functions and is a nuclear protein. When mutated in one of several critical regions, the function of the gene product is inactivated. The Rb protein is also functionally inactivated by phosphorylation; this phosphorylation is catalyzed by one or more cyclin-dependent protein kinases. It is of interest that a large number of cellular growth regulatory proteins, such as members of the c-Myc, CDK, and E$_2$F-1 families, bind the Rb protein or its family members. Rb appears to function to restrict cellular entry into the S phase of the cell cycle (Table 37.1-4). Hypophosphorylated Rb binds E$_2$F-1 and DF-1 family members to restrict access of these transcription factors to the chromatin. The

TABLE 37.1-4. The Cell Cycle

Phase	*Cellular Regulator*	*Cell-Cycle Kinase*	*Cyclin*	*Cell-Cycle Kinase Inhibitors*	*Cell-Cycle Phosphatase*	*Cell-Cycle Kinase Effectors*
G_1	Estrogen, progesterone, growth factors, c-Myc/Max, p53	CDK4, CDK6	D1, D2, D3	p15,[a] p18, p16, p19, p21, p27, p57	CDC25A	Rb/E_2F
G_1/S	c-Myc/Max, extracellular matrix, cell-cell junctions	CDK2	E	p21, p57, p27	CDC25B	Rb/E_2F/DB-1
S	—	CDK2	A	p21, p27, p57	—	—
G_2/M	p53/MDM-2	CDK1	B/A	p21, p27, p57	CDC25C	—

CDC, cell division cycle; CDK, cyclin-dependent kinase; DP, DNA-binding partner of E_2F; MDM-2, murine double-minute gene-2; Rb, retinoblastoma.
[a]The gene encoding this inhibitor also encodes, in an alternate reading frame, *p19*[ARF] an inhibitor of MDM-2, the protein that inhibits the function of p53.

result is a blockade of transcription from genes involved in G_1/S progression and S phase in the cell cycle.[165,184]

CYCLINS, CYCLIN-DEPENDENT KINASES, AND INHIBITORS

Growth factors and inhibitors, as well as oncogenes and tumor suppressors, function to a large extent in the G_1 phase of the cell cycle. The cell cycle (see Table 37.1-4) is directly controlled by an ordered series of CDKs, their positive regulatory subunits (cyclins), and their inhibitors. Early G_1 is driven by the three cyclin D family members bound to CDK4 and CDK6. In the next portion of the cycle, the G_1/S transition is driven by cyclin E–CDK2. The S phase is driven by cyclin A–CDK2, and then the G_2/M transition is driven by cyclin B/A–CDC2 (CDK1).

As important regulators of the epithelial cell cycle in breast cancer, tyrosine kinase receptor-acting growth factors and sex steroids induce both c-Myc and cyclin D1. c-Myc itself appears to suppress D1 in cycling cells, induce cyclin E (and possibly CDC25A), and trigger the proteosome-mediated destruction of the CDKI p27 (kip1) and activation of CDK2. Cyclin D1–CDK4 is inhibited by the CDKI called *p15* (INK4), by the tumor suppressive CDKI p16 (MTS1 or INK4b), and by p18 and p19, more recently defined CDKIs of the same family. Cyclin D–CDK4 and cyclin E–CDK2 are also each inhibited by the CDKI termed *p21* (Waf-1/CIP-1), which is induced by p53; by p27 (kip1); and by p57 (kip2), which may be involved in cellular senescence. It has been shown that synthesis of CDK4 is inhibited by TGF-β; overexpression of CDK4 leads to TGF-β resistance. p27 is also of note because it is induced by growth-inhibitory TGF-β. Rb is phosphorylated and inactivated both by the cyclin D–CDK4 and by the cyclin E–CDK2 kinases. Many the effects of multiple regulators of G_1 and G_1/S are thus integrated by their collective effects on phosphorylation of Rb. c-Myc also disregulates S phase by inducing cyclin (to activate CDK1) and E_2F-1. P53 also functions later in the cycle; its mutation not only abrogates the G_1/S checkpoint, but also a post–M spindle assembly checkpoint.[135,185,186]

As should now be evident, a major body of work has begun to implicate cyclins as likely oncogenes and CDK inhibitors as likely tumor suppressors (see Table 37.1-1). These studies have shown that the genes encoding cyclin D1 and cyclin E are commonly amplified and deregulated, respectively, in breast cancer. The amplification of the cyclin D1 (*CCND1*) gene occurs in approximately 30% of breast cancer cases; its prognostic significance is under current investigation.[187,188] It is of note that the genes for both cyclin D1 and cyclin E can function as mammary cancer–inducing oncogenes when driven by the MMTV promoter in the transgenic mouse.[189] Deletion of the gene-encoding cyclin D1 (*ccnd1*) in a mouse model results in failure of lobuloalveolar development of the mammary gland.[190] More recent studies, initially in cancer cell lines, have also implicated the cyclin inhibitor p16 [MTS-1(multiple tumor suppressor-1)] and p27 (kip-1) as major tumor suppressors; the *CDKN2* gene (encoding p16) is commonly inactivated by gene methylation,[191] whereas the gene encoding p27 is commonly down-regulated. Finally, the *RB-1* gene is commonly mutated, deleted, and down-regulated in breast cancer. The result of all of these common aberrations seems to be similar—defective G_1/S transitions in the mammary epithelial cell cycle.[192]

PROCESS OF MALIGNANT PROGRESSION

Evidence is rapidly accumulating that the development of cancer is a process that not only involves disregulation of proliferative factors and activation of oncogenes but also disregulation of inhibitory factors and loss of suppressor gene function (Fig. 37.1-1). Studies in breast cancer have served to underscore the role of germline deletion or mutation of suppressor genes in the familial forms of the disease, and somatic gene amplifications, mutations, deletions, and rearrangements during malignant progression of the disease. Malignant progression of breast cancer involves a progressive deterioration of the normal mechanisms of cell-cycle progression. DNA repair, apoptotic controls, and tissue compartmentalization break down (through angiogenesis and tumor invasion) until the highly abnormal state of metastatic disease is reached. Early aberrations in proliferation probably only slightly perturb the pathways activated by systemic hormones (estrogen and progesterone) and local growth fac-

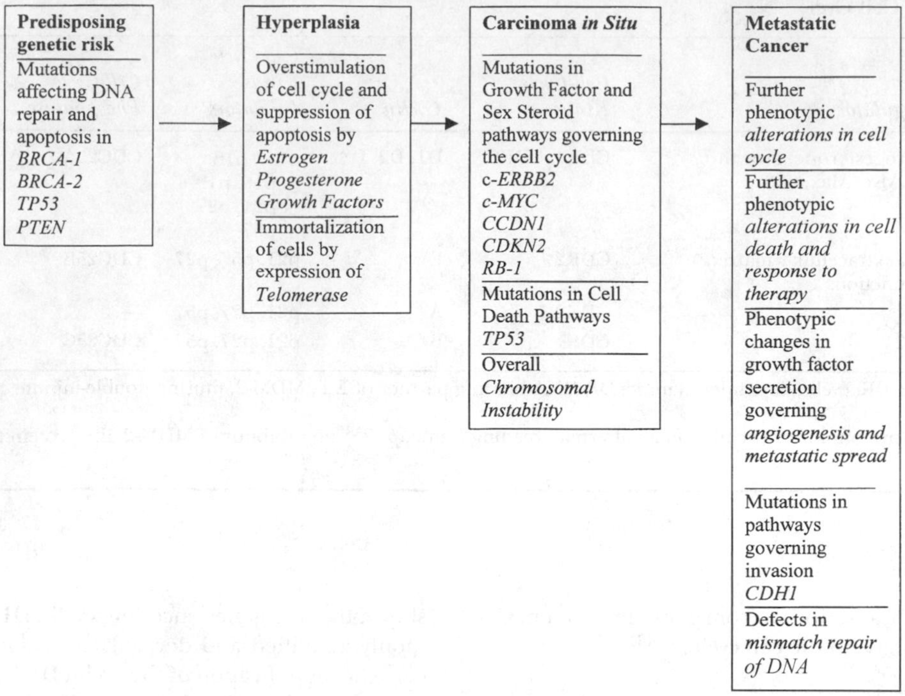

FIGURE 37.1-1. Summary of the genetic and phenotypic alteration of mammary epithelial cells associated with the onset and progression of breast cancer.

tors (such as TGF-α). The actual mechanisms for these early hyperactive proliferative controls to induce benign breast disease or premalignant atypical ductal or lobular carcinoma are not at all clear at the present time. Some studies have shown that genetic damage is minimal in these early lesions, although this area of study is only in its earliest stages.[193]

An interesting, current area of research into mechanisms of onset of breast cancer involves the DNA replication–associated enzyme telomerase. High levels of expression of this enzyme have been shown to lead to cell immortalization, a widely hypothesized early step in human tumorigenesis. One study has implicated the catalytic subunit of this enzyme (hTERT) plus two oncogenes—simian virus 40T (a viral oncogene that inactivates both p53 and Rb) and the mutant form of the signal transduction protein c-RasH—in converting human embryonic kidney cells to cancer.[194] Telomerase overexpression has been detected in the earliest stages of breast cancer; it is known to be induced both by estrogen and by c-Myc. Thus, telomerase disregulation may serve a subtle, early function in breast tumorigenesis—replicative immortality.[195–198]

The next steps in tumorigenesis almost entirely involve spontaneous gene amplification, LOH, and mutations, which arise because of overactive cell cycles or defective cell death that are largely due to abnormal cell-cycle checkpoint controls. Once these types of genetic alterations begin to occur, a cascade of further genetic changes occurs, resulting from overall genomic and chromosomal instability. Familial disease may bypass one or more steps in this cascade. The mechanisms for genetic instability and accumulation of further mutations in other cancers, such as colon cancer, have been proposed to initially depend on overexpression of a mutator gene termed *MSH2*.[199] To date, however, these mechanisms have not been fully evaluated for breast cancer, and mismatch repair defects appear to be associated primarily with later stages of progression and metastasis of breast cancer. In contrast to colon cancer, centrosomal defects appear to predominate in early breast cancer, potentially causing the chromosomal type of instability.[22]

Almost certainly, the most important consequences of these molecular changes initially relate to limited effectiveness of antihormonal therapy, chemotherapy, and radiation therapy. The mechanisms of failure of antihormonal therapy in hormone receptor–positive disease may potentially relate to sensitization of the tumor to very low levels of sex hormones and to the partially estrogenic properties of the clinically utilized hormonal antagonists, such as tamoxifen. Chemotherapy resistance in breast cancer is also not fully understood, but probably involves altered cell death responses and altered metabolism of the drugs.[200,201] Resistance to radiation is also not fully understood, but probably involves defects in the ATM pathway (including BRCA proteins and p53), leading to DNA damage–induced death.[172] Full consideration of mechanisms of resistance to each of these therapeutic modalities is beyond the scope of this chapter; however, the answers probably lie in the events made possible by genetic instability, aberrant proliferation, and defective death mechanisms. During treatment-associated malignant progression, as additional amplifications, LOHs, and mutations occur, the cancer cells with the greatest capacity for growth, invasion, or survival undergo positive selection. Other cells may be more susceptible to necrotic or apoptotic death.[202,203] Some studies have detected genetic changes in histologically normal tissue surrounding breast tumors, consistent with this clonal evolution hypothesis.[204,205]

The oncogenes, suppressor genes, growth factors, and sex hormones discussed in this chapter may also interact in critical patterns during treatment-associated disease progression. For example, certain common patterns of cytogenetic alterations exist in breast tumors, possibly the signature of distinct pathways of progression.[206] Many studies have now used cell lines *in vitro* and in the transgenic mouse in an attempt to sort out the biologic roles of likely tumor etiologic factors and their interactions.[207] From these studies, it appears that certain acquired genetic changes may interact unfavorably with residual growth regulatory pathways operant in the normal tissue. One example already discussed is the unfavorable interaction between cyclin D1 and the estrogen receptor.[140] Several other examples may include the interaction of amplified *c-ERBB2* or *c-MYC* genes in the presence of an autocrine- or paracrine-activated EGFR system.[207,208] *c-ERBB2* amplification in association with downstream overexpression of the signal transduction *c-RASH* gene is also an unfavorable interaction.[208,209] The tyrosine kinase signal transduction pathways (such as c-Ras^H) that govern proliferation, survival, or both, also clearly interact with c-Myc in cellular models *in vitro* and in transgenic mouse models of mammary cancer.[151,207,209–211] Another type of synergistic interaction may result from c-Myc expression in association with overexpression of apoptosis-suppressing Bcl-2. A final example is that of p53. Mutated p53 may interact unfavorably with c-$crbB_2$ by blocking apoptotic pathways.[207,212]

Study of the interactions of growth regulatory pathways with mutations in genes involved in signal transduction cell-cycle and cell-death pathways is thus in its infancy. A major approach for the future understanding of this phenomenon will involve increased use of the transgenic and gene knockout mouse models, with the eventual hope of establishing the biochemical and cellular bases of various patterns of malignant progressions. Future studies aimed at detailed characterization of the interaction of ER, PR, growth factors, protooncogenes, and suppressor genes with various therapeutic approaches in these animal models are thus likely to shed much light on their interactive roles in the onset and progression of breast cancer. At present, however, few studies *in vivo* have focused on combinations of genetic alterations thought to be important in human disease or on the use of transgenic models for studies of treatment-induced resistance and disease progression to metastasis.

The ultimate event that leads to mortality from breast cancer is metastasis. Two separate but apparently interactive cellular processes seem to occur to allow metastasis of the disease: tumor angiogenesis and loss of proper tissue compartmentalization (invasion). It is not yet fully established whether genetic or phenotypic changes underlie these alterations. However, several molecular determinants have been proposed to relate to each process. Loss of cell-cell attachment, altered cell substratum attachment, and altered cytoskeletal organization play a role in regulating cellular invasion. In addition, cell locomotion, proteolysis, and the ability to survive and proliferate at distant sites also must contribute.[213–215] Although acquisition of this group of characteristics is responsible for a cancer to locally invade host tissue, the ability of a tumor to distribute itself to distant sites also requires the development of a tumor vasculature—the complex process of angiogenesis.[216,217] Some studies have shown that metastatic alterations may have at least some genetic basis[218] and that distant metastases are more likely to exhibit dominance of a malignant clone than primary tumors.[219] Because of space limitations, we cannot discuss the processes of angiogenesis and metastasis further here; the reader is directed to the more general chapter covering some of these processes earlier in this volume (Chapter 9).

IMPLICATIONS OF MOLECULAR BIOLOGY FOR TUMOR PREVENTION, EARLY DETECTION, PROGNOSIS, AND RESPONSE TO THERAPY

A major hope in the study of genetic changes in breast cancer is that they lead to development of new prevention and early detection strategies, therapies, and prognostic tools. In the area of prevention, there is much current work to establish more rapid, accurate, and cost-effective assays of *BRCA-1* and *BRCA-2* mutations to better identify women with a familial propensity for breast cancer. In addition, the gene(s) responsible for a significant number of breast cancer families remain to be identified, and the bases (genetic and/or environmental) for the variable penetrance of the *BRCA* genes remain to be determined. Women at high risk will undoubtedly be the population of emphasis for future prevention trials. Although the benefits of prophylactic mastectomy and oophorectomy are now established, tamoxifen is also known to be an effective prevention strategy. A major, current trial is comparing tamoxifen to raloxifene (an antiestrogen thought to produce fewer endometrial cancers and to provide other benefits). However, new pharmacologic or dietary strategies are needed, particularly to prevent ER-negative breast cancer.[220–222]

In the area of early detection, we now know that overproduction of growth factors such as TGF-α and hepatocyte growth factor are very common, but they have not yet been shown to distinguish benign proliferative disease from malignant disease.[223–225] However, exciting results have been reported in the area of chromosomal instability. It is possible that detection of telomerase expression or the ability to detect subtle genetic alterations will provide useful new approaches for marking the onset of cancer. Development of new nipple aspirate methodologies and blood and urinary assays for growth factors, growth factor receptors, autoantibodies to oncoproteins, and tumor DNA are also currently under way.[226–229]

In the area of prognosis and response to therapy, much hope has been vested in development of more accurate and rapid methods for immunohistochemical and fluorescent *in situ* methodologies for characterization of oncogenes, suppressor genes, and related proteins.[230] Serum and plasma assays for growth factors are also of interest, in addition to more classical tumor markers of CA15.3 and CEA (carcinoembryonic antigen) for determining prognosis and response to therapy. Sensitive assays to detect tumor-derived cells and DNA in the blood are also under development. Obviously, detection of ER and PR in tumors has led the way for integration of molecular markers into clinical decisions regarding prognosis and response to therapy. Pure antiestrogens and aromatase inhibitors are now in clinical trials for ER-positive, relapsing tumors. More recently, detection of the c-$erbB_2$ oncoprotein has also proven its value for characterization of poor-prognosis tumors, as well as for those that are likely to have a poor response to adjuvant hormonal therapy and chemotherapy. Although technically more difficult to measure, EGFR is of interest for future study of tumors likely to have a poor prognosis and poor response to hormonal therapy. Because of common expression or overexpression of these two receptors in breast cancer, they are now targets of new experimental therapies that use antibodies to their extracellular domains and couple or gene-fuse these antibodies to toxic moieties.[231–233]

A large group of studies have confirmed that 20% to 30% of breast tumors contain an amplification of the *c-ERBB2* gene and overexpress the encoded receptor protein. *c-ERBB2* is also overexpressed in a very high portion of ductal carcinoma *in situ*.[234,235] Expression of the c-erbB_2 protein is associated with an elevated mitotic rate; it correlates with poor clinical response to certain chemotherapeutic and antihormonal drugs (5-fluorouracil, methotrexate, Cytoxan, and tamoxifen-containing regimens) and insensitivity to tamoxifen *in vitro*.[235,236] c-erbB_2 expression is also associated with poor prognosis in patients who do not receive treatment with chemotherapeutic or antihormonal drugs.[237–241] Although one might postulate that *c-ERBB2* gene amplification directly modulates metastatic capacity based on data with tumor models, its association with poor prognosis would appear to relate to other features of tumor biology still to be fully elucidated.

The c-erbB_2 protein also holds significant interest for breast tumor immunology. Certain antibodies to the extracellular domain of the c-erbB_2 protein seem to sensitize cells to killing by *cis*-platinum, carboplatinum, and doxorubicin *in vivo*. It is thought that the mechanism of this effect is interference with DNA repair mechanisms.[242,243] The shed extracellular domain of c-erbB_2 protein may represent a useful, antigenic blood-borne marker of breast cancer burden,[244] and the c-erbB_2 protein itself may be a new target of immunotherapy of cancer,[243,245,246] as with EGFR.[247] Specifically, a humanized, anti–c-erbB_2 antibody termed *herceptin* is showing promise in clinical trials.[243] More recent results also suggest the possibility of active immunotherapy targeting the c-erbB_2 protein; a lymphoplasmacytic infiltrate in breast cancer was shown to indicate good prognosis for an erbB_2-positive subset of patients. This study noted production of growth-inhibitory antibodies by peripheral lymphocytes from these patients.[243,248]

Although many studies have demonstrated the prognostic significance of c-erbB_2 expression for lymph node–positive patients, the role of the oncoprotein in the malignant process is not clear. For example, many established human breast cancer cell lines overexpressing c-erbB_2 are frequently of poor tumorigenicity in the nude mouse. This fact could theoretically be due to a lack of coexpression of a heterodimeric receptor partner or a ligand, or to coinduction of a suppressive phosphatase.[249] Overexpression of c-erbB_2 in immortalized breast epithelial and breast cancer cell lines has suggested that it is only weakly transforming *in vitro*, and it has not significantly induced or enhanced a tumorigenic phenotype *in vivo* in several studies.[250] However, in the transgenic mouse, c-erbB_2 expression results in long-latency, metastatic breast tumors.[251] Association of the c-erbB_2 protein with, and activation of, the c-Src oncoprotein in this model are thought to be critical in the tumorigenic pathway. Because the c-erbB_2 protein can heterodimerize with other receptor family members, co-overexpression of all family members and cross-dimerization must eventually be taken into account in prognostic and therapeutic studies. Of interest in this respect are studies identifying a constitutively active, variant form of EGFR in human cancers.[252]

As we have emphasized, nuclear protooncogenes are common mechanistic links between the actions of growth-promoting steroids and growth factors in diverse tissues. Although amplification of the c-*MYC* nuclear protooncogene is one of the most common genetic alterations in breast cancer (approximately 20% of breast cancers contain this amplicon), it must be the target of much future investigation because of its central role in a diversity of cellular processes.[147,253–257] Study of *c-MYC* gene expression in breast cancer has been hampered by immunologic and stability difficulties in measuring the protein in tumor biopsies, but new fluorescence *in situ* and polymerase chain reaction methodologies are likely to improve c-Myc studies in human breast cancer. The c-Myc protein has a very short half-life, and only now are high-quality monoclonal antibodies capable of staining paraffin sections becoming available. In spite of these difficulties, several studies have shown that amplification of the *c-MYC* gene is clearly associated with poor prognosis.[147,256,257] In addition, in *in vivo* and *in vitro* models, EGF family growth factors have been shown to dramatically interact with the c-Myc oncogene product in tumorigenesis. These studies provide food for thought in development of future clinical studies, such as those targeting the EGFR or c-erbB_2 together with c-Myc.[258]

There also is significant hope that studies of c-Myc will aid in the prediction of tumor response to therapy. Expression of Myc may also alter cellular resistance to *cis*-platinum and other DNA strand scission–inducing drugs,[259] and it may suppress differentiation in association with decreased collagen gene transcription.[260] c-*MYC* amplification is clearly not associated with c-*ERBB2* amplification in primary breast cancer[261]; rather, it identifies a subset of biologically different, poor-prognosis tumors. These studies also suggest that tumors containing either of these two important amplicons may be of such different biologic significance that the amplicons are mutually incompatible.[262–264]

Another major effort in better understanding breast tumor prognosis and response to therapy surrounds the genes involved in controlling cell death and DNA repair. Specifically, the *TP53* gene, whose protein product has the potential to mediate apoptotic death induced by virtually all forms of adjuvant therapy, is easily measured by immunohistochemical methodology. A major caveat is that pathologists cannot be certain that the accumulation of p53 protein they measure is due to mutation rather than to induction from a proapoptotic stimulus. Much effort will go into improvements in p53 methodology. Data, so far, clearly indicate that *TP53* overexpression confers poor prognosis and likelihood of a poor response to endocrine therapy and chemotherapy,[265,266] but much additional study needs to apply high-throughput mutation analysis to routine assay. *TP53* also is widely discussed as a potential gene for gene therapy trials of cancer. Three regulators downstream of p53 are also promising. First, loss of Rb detected by immunohistochemistry appears to indicate poor prognosis,[267] as does expression of bcl-2 and down-regulation of Bax.[268–271] However, more studies must be carried out on *RB-1* mutation analyses and detection of other Bcl family members. Finally, a new area of study is the identification of poor-prognosis and response-to-therapy genes by use of high throughput complementary DNA chip assay analyses. Such studies have the potential to improve tumor diagnosis and prognosis.[272,273]

Studies of metastasis have suggested that quantification of tumor angiogenesis and deposition of the extracellular matrix protein (termed *tenascin*) may be of value in evaluating this critical transition of the disease. To supplement the traditional lymph node biopsy measurements, promising new drugs are in clinical trial for blockade of angiogenesis.[274] Metastasis itself seems to depend on the elaboration of proteases (such as urokine/plasminogen activator and matrix metalloproteases), the most promising of which for prognostic significance is the cognate inhibitor urokinase PAI-1 (plasminogen activator inhibitor-1). New drugs, such as marimastat, are currently in clinical trials studying blockade of proteases. This will be a very active area of future drug development.[275,276] Finally, the adhesive changes that metastatic cells undergo are of major interest. Loss of expression of E-cadherin (and acquisition of a mesenchymal phenotype marked by the intermediate filament vimentin), loss of $\alpha_2\beta_1$ integrin, overexpression of a 67-kD laminin binding protein, and overexpression of a variant form of the hyaluronic acid receptor (CD44) are all of poor prognosis or correlated with poor tumor grade in early clinical studies.[277–283] Much larger studies are needed to fully evaluate the clinical significance of these metastasis-associated cellular changes.

In summary, although a very large number of genetic and phenotypic alterations have been suggested in breast cancer, only a handful have been fully identified and brought to clinical study. It is quite encouraging that study of each of these genes and phenotypic changes has provided its own unique perspective to the biology of the disease. The challenge for the future, however, is to take advantage of this knowledge to improve detection of familial risk; develop prevention strategies; improve early detection, clinical diagnosis, and prediction of therapeutic outcome; develop therapies; and rapidly apply more novel biologic therapeutics.[284] It is our prediction that future discovery in breast cancer will focus on the molecular bases of processes involved in treatment failure—invasion, angiogenesis, metastasis, and resistance to therapy. Central to these hopes are the development of new technologies for high throughput analyses of pathologic material (such as laser capture microdissection techniques, fluorescence *in situ* hybridization, and other molecular cytogenetic methods), complementary DNA chip array assay methods, SAGE (serial analysis of gene expression), and other cutting-edge RNA and protein analysis techniques. It is essential that new technologies be brought to improve tumor diagnosis and prediction of response to existing therapies. These approaches should also result in discovery of new targets for more biologic-based therapies and prevention strategies for breast cancer. Prospects for clinical translation of basic molecular biologic results appear to be bright.

REFERENCES

1. De Michele A, Weber BL. Inherited genetic factors. In: Harris JR, Lippman ME, Morrow M, Osborne CK, eds. *Diseases of the breast,* 2nd ed. Philadelphia: Lippincott Williams & Wilkins, 2000:221.
2. Malkin D, Li FP, Strong LC, et al. Germ line p53 mutations in a familial syndrome of breast cancer, sarcomas, and other neoplasms. *Science* 1990;250:1233.
3. Srivastava S, Zou ZQ, Pirollo K, Blattner W, Chang EH. Germ line transmission of a mutated p53 gene in a cancer-prone family with Li Fraumeni syndrome. *Nature* 1990;348:747.
4. Liaw D, Marsh DJ, Li J, et al. Germline mutations of the PTEN gene in Cowden disease, an inherited breast and thyroid cancer syndrome. *Nature Genet* 1997;16:64.
5. Hamminki A, Tomlinson I, Markie D. Localization of a susceptibility locus for PJS to 19p using comparative genomic hybridization and targeted linkage analysis. *Nature Genet* 1997;115:87.
6. Anderson DE. An inherited form of large bowel cancer: Muir's syndrome. *Cancer* 1980;45[Suppl 15]:1103.
7. Fitzgerald MG, Bean JM, Hedge SR, et al. Heterozygous ATM mutations do not contribute to early onset of breast cancer. *Nature Genet* 1997;15:307.
8. Hall JM, Lee MK, Newman B, et al. Linkage of early-onset familial breast cancer to chromosome 17q21. *Science* 1990;250:1684.
9. Miki Y, Swensen J, Shattuck-Eidens D, et al. A strong candidate for the breast and ovarian cancer susceptibility gene BRCA-1. *Science* 1994;266:66.
10. Chen Y, Chen C, Riley D, et al. Aberrant subcellular localization of BRCA-1 in breast cancer. *Science* 1995;270:789.
11. Thompson ME, Jensen RA, Obermiller PS, Page DL, Holt JT. Decreased expression of brca1 accelerates growth and is often present during sporadic breast cancer progression. *Nature Genet* 1995;9:444.
12. Holt JT, Thompson ME, Szabo C, et al. Growth retardation and tumour inhibition by BRCA1. *Nature Genet* 1996;12:298.
13. Wooster R, Bignell G, Lancaster J, et al. Identification of the breast cancer susceptibility gene BRCA2. *Nature* 1995;378:789.
14. Cortez D, Wang Y, Qin J, Elledge SJ. Requirement of ATM-dependent phosphorylation of brca1 in the DNA damage response to double-strand breaks. *Science* 1999;286:1162.
15. Xu X, Wagner KU, Larson D, et al. Conditional mutation of BRCA1 in mammary epithelial cells results in blunted ductal morphogenesis and tumour formation. *Nature Genet* 1999;22:37.
16. Xu X, Weaver Z, Linke SP, et al. Centrosome amplification and a defective G_2-M cell cycle checkpoint induce genetic instability in BRCA1 exon 11 isoform-deficients cells. *Mol Cell* 1999;3:389.
17. Fan S, Wang JA, Yuan R, et al. BRCA1 inhibition of estrogen receptor signaling in transfected cells. *Science* 1999;284:1354.
18. Dickson RB, Stancel G. Estrogen-mediated processes in normal and cancer cells. *J Natl Cancer Inst* 2000 (*in press*).
19. Schrock E, du Manoir S, Veldman T, et al. Multicolor spectral karyotyping of human chromosomes. *Science* 1996;273:494.
20. Ried T, Just KE, Holtgreve-Grez H, et al. Comparative genomic hybridization of formalin fixed, paraffin embedded breast tumors reveals different patterns of chromosomal gains and losses in fibroadenomas and diploid and aneuploid carcinomas. *Cancer Res* 1995;55:5415.
21. Nicolson GL. Breast cancer metastasis–associated genes: role in tumour progression to the metastatic state. *Biochem Soc Symp* 1996;63:231.
22. Pihan GA, Purohit A, Wallace J, et al. Centrosome defects and genetic instability in malignant tumors. *Cancer Res* 1998;58:3974.
23. Brenner AJ, Aldaz CM. Chromosome 9p allelic loss and p16/CDKN2 in breast cancer and evidence of p16 inactivation in immortal breast epithelial cells. *Cancer Res* 1995;55:2892.
24. Fero ML, Randel E, Gurley KE, Roberts JM, Kemp CJ. The murine gene p27Kip1 as haplo-insufficient for tumor suppression. *Nature* 1998;396:177.
25. Knuulila S, Borkquist AM, Autio K, et al. DNA copy number amplification in human neoplasms. *Am J Pathol* 1998;152:1107.
26. Elledge RM, Fuqua SAW. Estrogen and progesterone receptors. In: Harris JR, Lippman ME, Morrow M, Osborne CK, eds. *Diseases of the breast,* 2nd ed. Philadelphia: Lippincott Williams & Wilkins, 2000:471.
27. Dickson RB, Russo J. Biochemical control of breast development. In: Harris JR, Lippman ME, Morrow M, Osborne CK, eds. *Diseases of the breast,* 2nd ed. Philadelphia: Lippincott Williams & Wilkins, 2000:15.
28. Spencer TE, Jenster G, Burcin MM, et al. Steroid receptor coactivator-1 is a histone acetyltransferase. *Nature* 1997;389:194.
29. McDonnell DP, Clemm DL, Hermann T. Analysis of the estrogen receptor function *in vitro* reveals three distinct classes of antiestrogen. *Mol Endocrinol* 1995;9:659.
30. Fujimoto N, Katzenellenbogen BS. Alteration in the agonist/antagonist balance of antiestrogens by activation of protein kinase A signaling pathways in breast cancer cells: antiestrogen selectivity and promoter dependence. *Mol Endocrinol* 1994;8:296.
31. Suchard M, Landers JP, Sandhu NP, Spelsberg TC. Steroid hormone regulation of nuclear proto-oncogenes. *Endocrine Rev* 1993;14:659.
32. Dickson RB, Lippman ME. Estrogenic regulation of growth and polypeptide growth factor secretion in human breast carcinoma. *Endocrine Rev* 1987;8:29.
33. Osborne CK, Hamilton B, Titus G, Livingston RB. Epidermal growth factor stimulation of human breast cancer cells in culture. *Cancer Res* 1980;40:2361.
34. Allegra JC, Lippman ME. Estrogen receptor status and the disease-free interval in breast cancer. *Recent Results Cancer Res* 1980;71:20.
35. DeSombre E, Green G, Jensen E. Estrophilin and endocrine responsiveness of breast cancer. In: McGuire W, ed. *Hormones, receptors and breast cancer.* New York: Raven Press, 1978:1.
36. Paridaens R, Sylvester RJ, Ferrazzi E, et al. Clinical significance of the quantitative assessment of estrogen receptors in advanced breast cancer. *Cancer* 1980;46:2889.
37. Edwards DP, Chamness GC, McGuire WL. Estrogen and progesterone receptor proteins in breast cancer. *Biochim Biophys Acta* 1979;560:457.
38. Eckert RL, Katzenellenbogen BS. Human endometrial cells in primary tissue culture: modulation of the progesterone receptor level by natural and synthetic estrogens *in vitro. J Clin Endocrinol Metab* 1981;52:699.
39. Clarke RB, Howell A, Anderson E. Estrogen sensitivity of normal human breast tissue *in vivo* and implanted into athymic nude mice: analysis of the relationship to progesterone receptor expression. *Breast Cancer Res Treat* 1998;45:121.
40. Khan SA, Sachdeva A, Naim S, et al. The normal breast epithelium of women with breast cancer displays an aberrant response to estradiol. *Cancer Epidemiol Biomarkers Prev* 1999;8:867.
41. Ottaviano YL, Issa JP, Parl FF, et al. Methylation of the estrogen receptor gene CpG island marks loss of estrogen receptor expression in human breast cancer cells. *Cancer Res* 1994;54:2552.
42. Ferguson AT, Lapidus RG, Baylin SB, Davidson NE. Demethylation of the estrogen receptor gene in estrogen receptor–negative breast cancer cells can reactivate estrogen receptor gene expression. *Cancer Res* 1995;55:2279.

43. Masamura S, Santer SJ, Heitjan DF, et al. Estrogen deprivation causes estradiol hypersensitivity in human breast cancer cells. *Endocrinology* 1995;136:2918.
44. Catherino WH, Wolf DM, Jordan VC. A naturally occurring estrogen receptor mutation results in increased estrogenicity of a tamoxifen analog. *Mol Endocrinol* 1995;9:1053.
45. Murphy LC, Hilsenbeck SG, Dotzlaw H, et al. Relationship of clone 4 estrogen receptor variant messenger RNA expression to human breast cancer. *Clin Cancer Res* 1995;1:235.
46. Jiang SY, Jordan VC. Growth regulation of estrogen receptor–negative breast cancer cells transfected with complementary DNAs for estrogen receptor. *J Natl Cancer Inst* 1992;84:580.
47. Touitou I, Vignon F, Cavailles V, Rochefort H. Hormonal regulation of cathepsin D following transfection of the estrogen or progesterone receptor into three sex steroid hormone resistant cancer cell lines. *J Steroid Biochem Mol Biol* 1991;40:231.
48. Paik S, Hartmann DP, Dickson RB, Lippman ME. Antiestrogen resistance in ER positive breast cancer cells. *Breast Cancer Res Treat* 1994;31:301.
49. Tekmal RR, Santen RJ. Local estrogen production: is aromatase an oncogene? In: Manni A, ed. *Contemporary endocrinology: endocrinology of breast cancer.* Totowa, NJ: Humana Press, 1999:79.
50. Martinez-Lacaci I, Dickson RB. Dual regulation of mitogenic growth factor pathways in breast cancer by sex steroids and protein kinase C. *J Steroid Biochem Mol Biol* 1996;57.
51. Ways DK, Kukoly CA, de Vente J, et al. MCF-7 breast cancer cells transfected with protein kinase C-alpha exhibit altered expression of other protein kinase C isoforms and display a more aggressive neoplastic phenotype. *J Clin Invest* 1995;95:1906.
52. Dekker LV, Parker PJ. Protein kinase C—a question of specificity. *Trends Biochem Sci* 1994;19:73.
53. Tzukerman M, Zhang XK, Pfahl M. Inhibition of estrogen receptor activity by the tumor promoter 12-O-tetradecanylphorbol-13-acetate: a molecular analysis. *Mol Endocrinol* 1991;5:1983.
54. Saceda M, Knabbe C, Dickson RB, et al. Post-transcriptional destabilization of estrogen receptor mRNA in MCF-7 cells by 12-O-tetradecanoylphorbol-13-acetate. *J Biol Chem* 1991;266:17809.
55. Joel PB, Traish AM, Lannigan DA. Estradiol and phorbol ester cause phosphorylation of serine 118 in the human estrogen receptor. *Mol Endocrinol* 1995;9:1041.
56. Kato S, Endoh H, Masuhiro Y, et al. Activation of the estrogen receptor through phosphorylation by mitogen-activated protein kinase. *Science* 1995;270:1491.
57. Power RF, Conneely OM, O'Malley BW. New insights into activation of the steroid hormone receptor superfamily. *Trends Pharmacol Sci* 1992;13:318.
58. Power RF, Mani SK, Codina J, Conneely OM, O'Malley BW. Dopaminergic and ligand-independent activation of steroid hormone receptors. *Science* 1991;254:1636.
59. Aronica SM, Katzenellenbogen BS. Stimulation of estrogen receptor–mediated transcription and alteration in the phosphorylation state of the rat uterine estrogen receptor by estrogen, cyclic adenosine monophosphate, and insulin-like growth factor-1. *Mol Endocrinol* 1993;7:743.
60. Pietras RJ, Arboleda J, Reese DM, et al. HER-2 tyrosine kinase pathway targets estrogen receptor and promotes hormone-independent growth in human breast cancer cells. *Oncogene* 1995;10:2435.
61. Segars JH, Marks MS, Hirschfeld S, et al. Inhibition of estrogen-responsive gene activation by the retinoid X receptor beta: evidence for multiple inhibitory pathways [published erratum appears in *Mol Cell Biol* 1993;13:3840]. *Mol Cell Biol* 1993;13:2258.
62. Salbert G, Fanjul A, Piedrafita FJ, et al. Retinoic acid receptors and retinoid X receptor-alpha down-regulate the transforming growth factor-beta 1 promoter by antagonizing AP-1 activity. *Mol Endocrinol* 1993;7:1347.
63. Grosvenor CE, Picciano MF, Baumrucker CR. Hormones and growth factors in milk. *Endocr Rev* 1993;14:710.
64. Cullen KJ, Lippman ME. Stromal-epithelial interactions in breast cancer. *Cancer Treat Res* 1992;61:413.
65. Dickson R, Lippman ME. Growth factors in breast cancer. *Endocrine Rev* 1995;16:559.
66. Kurachi H, Okamoto S, Oka T. Evidence for the involvement of the submandibular gland epidermal growth factor in mouse mammary tumorigenesis. *Proc Natl Acad Sci U S A* 1985;82:5940.
67. Vonderhaar BK. Regulation of development of the normal mammary gland by hormones and growth factors. *Cancer Treat Res* 1988;40:251.
68. Oka T, Tsutsumi O, Kurachi H, Okamoto S. The role of epidermal growth factor in normal and neoplastic growth of mouse mammary epithelial cells. *Cancer Treat Res* 1988;40:343.
69. Ram TG, Kokeny KE, Dilts CA, Ethier SP. Mitogenic activity of neu differentiation factor/heregulin mimics that of epidermal growth factor and insulin-like growth factor-I in human mammary epithelial cells. *J Cell Physiol* 1995;163:589.
70. Liscia DS, Merlo G, Ciardiello F, et al. Transforming growth factor-alpha messenger RNA localization in the developing adult rat and human mammary gland by *in situ* hybridization. *Dev Biol* 1990;140:123.
71. Martinez-Lacaci I, Bianco C, DeSantis M, Salomon DS. Epidermal growth factor–related peptides and their cognate receptors in breast cancer. In: Bowcock A, ed. *Breast cancer: molecular genetics, pathogenesis, and therapeutics.* Totowa, NJ: Humana Press, 1999:31.
72. Brandt BH, Roetger A, Dittmar T, et al. c-erbB-2/EGFR as dominant heterodimerization partners determine a motogenic phenotype in human breast cancer cells. *FASEB J* 1999;13:1939.
73. Snedeker SM, Brown CF, Di Augustine RP. Expression and functional properties of transforming growth factor alpha and epidermal growth factor during mouse mammary gland ductal morphogenesis. *Proc Natl Acad Sci U S A* 1991;88:276.
74. Wang Y, Selden AC, Morgan N, Stamp GW, Hodgson HJ. Hepatocyte growth factor/scatter factor expression in human mammary epithelium. *Am J Pathol* 1994;144:675.
75. Yang U, Spitzer E, Meyer D, et al. Sequential requirement of scatter factor/hepatocyte growth factor (SF/HGF) and neu differentiation factor/heregulin (NDF/HRG) in the morphogenesis and differentiation of the mammary gland. *J Cell Biol* 1995;131:215.
76. Valverius EM, Ciardiello F, Heldin NE, et al. Stromal influences on transformation of human mammary epithelial cells overexpressing c-myc and SV40T. *J Cell Physiol* 1990;145:207.
77. Bates SE, Valverius EM, Ennis BW, et al. Expression of the transforming growth factor-alpha/epidermal growth factor receptor pathway in normal human breast epithelial cells. *Endocrinology* 1990;126:596.
78. Li S, Plowman GD, Buckley SD, Shipley GD. Heparin inhibition of autonomous growth implicates amphiregulin as an autocrine growth factor for normal human mammary epithelial cells. *J Cell Physiol* 1992;153:103.
79. Kenney N, Johnson G, Selvam M, et al. Transforming growth factor α (TGFα) and amphiregulin (AR) as autocrine growth factors in nontransformed, immortalized 184A1N4 human mammary epithelial cells. *Mol Cell Differ* 1993;1:163.
80. Earp HS, Dawson TL, Li X, Yu H. Heterodimerization and functional interaction between EGF receptor family members: a new signaling paradigm with implications for breast cancer research. *Breast Cancer Res Treat* 1995;35:115.
81. Pinkas-Kramarski R, Alroy I, Yarden Y. ErbB receptors and EGF-like ligands: cell lineage determination and oncogenesis through combinatorial signaling. *J Mammary Gland Biol Neoplasia* 1997;2:97.
82. Ciardiello F, McGeady ML, Kim N, et al. Transforming growth factor-alpha expression is enhanced in human mammary epithelial cells transformed by an activated c-Ha-ras protooncogene but not by the c-neu protooncogene, and overexpression of the transforming growth factor-alpha complementary DNA leads to transformation. *Cell Growth Differ* 1990;1:407.
83. Dickson R, Lippman M. Control of human breast cancer by estrogen, growth factors, and oncogenes. In: Lippman M, Dickson R, eds. *Breast cancer: cellular and molecular biology.* Boston: Kluwer Academic Publishers, 1988:119.
84. Graus-Porta D, Beerli RR, Daly JM, Hynes NE. ErbB-2, the preferred heterodimerization partner of all ErbB receptors, is a mediator of lateral signaling. *EMBO J* 1997;16:1647.
85. Parham DM, Jankowski J. Transforming growth factor alpha in epithelial proliferative diseases of the breast. *J Clin Pathol* 1992;45:513.
86. Kenney N, Smith G, Maroulakou I, et al. Detection of amphiregulin and Cripto-1 in mammary tumors from transgenic mice. *Mol Carcinog* 1996;15:44.
87. Jhappan C, Stahle C, Harkins RN, et al. TGF alpha overexpression in transgenic mice induces liver neoplasia and abnormal development of the mammary gland and pancreas. *Cell* 1990;61:1137.
88. Coleman S, Daniel CW. Inhibition of mouse mammary ductal morphogenesis and down-regulation of the EGF receptor by epidermal growth factor. *Dev Biol* 1990;137:425.
89. Sandgren EP, Luetteke NC, Palmiter RD, Brinster RL, Lee DC. Overexpression of TGF alpha in transgenic mice: induction of epithelial hyperplasia, pancreatic metaplasia, and carcinoma of the breast. *Cell* 1990;61:1121.
90. Matsui Y, Halter SA, Holt JT, Hogan BL, Coffey RJ. Development of mammary hyperplasia and neoplasia in MMTV-TGF alpha transgenic mice. *Cell* 1990;61:1147.
91. Smith GH, Sharp R, Kordon EC, Jhappan C, Merlino G. Transforming growth factor alpha promotes mammary tumorigenesis through selective survival and growth of secretory epithelial cells. *Am J Pathol* 1995;147:1081.
92. Sandgren EP, Schroeder JA, Qui TH, et al. Inhibition of mammary gland involution is associated with transforming growth factor alpha but not c-myc-induced tumorigenesis in transgenic mice. *Cancer Res* 1995;55:3915.
93. Hynes NE, Stern DF. The biology of ErbB-2/neu/HER-2 and its role in cancer. *Biochim Biophys Acta* 1994;1198:165.
94. Chrysogelos SA, Dickson RB. EGF receptor expression, regulation, and function in breast cancer. *Breast Cancer Res Treat* 1994;29:29.
95. Dankort DL, Muller WJ. Transgenic models of breast cancer metastasis. In: Dickson RB, Lippman ME, eds. *Mammary tumor cell cycle, differentiation, and metastasis.* Boston: Kluwer Academic Publishers, 1996:71.
96. Coffey RJ Jr, Meise KS, Matsui Y, et al. Acceleration of mammary neoplasia in transforming growth factor alpha transgenic mice by 7,12-dimethylbenzanthracene. *Cancer Res* 1994;54:1678.
97. Kenney NJ, Saeki T, Gottardis M, et al. Expression of transforming growth factor alpha antisense mRNA inhibits the estrogen-induced production of TGF alpha and estrogen-induced proliferation of estrogen-responsive human breast cancer cells. *J Cell Physiol* 1993;156:497.
98. Bates SE, McManaway ME, Lippman ME, Dickson RB. Characterization of estrogen responsive transforming activity in human breast cancer cell lines. *Cancer Res* 1986;46:1707.
99. Reddy K, Yee D, Hilsenbeck S, et al. Inhibition of estrogen-induced breast cancer cell proliferation by reduction in autocrine transforming growth factor α expression. *Cell Growth Differ* 1994;5:1215.
100. Qi CF, Liscia DS, Normanno N, et al. Expression of transforming growth factor alpha, amphiregulin and Cripto-1 in human breast carcinomas. *Br J Cancer* 1994;69:903.
101. Martinez-Lacaci I, Saceda M, Plowman GD, et al. Estrogen and phorbol esters regulate amphiregulin expression by two separate mechanisms in human breast cancer cell lines. *Endocrinology* 1995;136:3983.
102. Tang CK, Concepcion SZW, Milan M, et al. Ribozyme-mediated down-regulation of ErbB-4 in estrogen receptor–positive breast cancer cells inhibits proliferation both *in vitro* and *in vivo*. *Cancer Res* 1999;59:5315.
103. Holmes WE, Sliwkowski MX, Akita RW, et al. Identification of heregulin, a specific activator of p185ErbB2. *Science* 1992;256:1205.
104. Wen D, Peles E, Cupples R, et al. Neu differentiation factor: a transmembrane glycoprotein containing an EGF domain and an immunoglobulin homology unit. *Cell* 1992;69:559.
105. Ennis B, Valverius E, Lippman M, et al. Anti EGF receptor antibodies inhibit the autocrine stimulated growth of MDA-MB-468 breast cancer cells. *Mol Endocrinol* 1989;3:1830.

106. Pastan I, Chaudhary V, FitzGerald DJ. Recombinant toxins as novel therapeutic agents. *Annu Rev Biochem* 1992;61:331.
107. Kern FG. The role of fibroblast growth factors in breast cancer pathogenesis and progression. In: Bowcock A, ed. *Breast cancer: molecular genetics, pathogenesis, and therapeutics.* Totowa, NJ: Humana Press, 1999:59.
108. Coleman-Krnacik S, Rosen JM. Differential temporal and spatial gene expression of fibroblast growth factor family members during mouse mammary gland development. *Mol Endocrinol* 1994;8:218.
109. Souttou B, Hamelin R, Crepin M. FGF2 as an autocrine growth factor for immortal human breast epithelial cells. *Cell Growth Differ* 1994;5:615.
110. Kern FG. The role of angiogenesis in the transition to hormone independence and acquisition of the metastatic phenotype. In: Manni A, ed. *Endocrinology of breast cancer.* Totowa, NJ: Humana Press, 1999:169.
111. Adnane J, Gaudray P, Dionne CA, et al. BEK and FLG, two receptors to members of the FGF family, are amplified in subsets of human breast cancers. *Oncogene* 1991;6:659.
112. McLeskey SW, Ding IY, Lippman ME, Kern FG. MDA-MB-134 breast carcinoma cells overexpress fibroblast growth factor (FGF) receptors and are growth-inhibited by FGF ligands. *Cancer Res* 1994;54:523.
113. Theillet C, Adelaide J, Lonason G, et al. FGFR1 and PLAT genes and DNA amplification at 8p12 in breast and ovarian cancers. *Genes Chromosomes Cancer* 1993;7:219.
114. McLeskey SW, Zhang L, Kharbanda S, et al. Fibroblast growth factor–overexpressing models of angiogenesis and metastasis in breast cancer. *Breast Cancer Res Treat* 1996;39:103.
115. McCune BK, Mullin BR, Flanders KC, et al. Localization of transforming growth factor-beta isotypes in lesions of the human breast. *Hum Pathol* 1992;23:13.
116. Koli KM, Arteaga CL. Transforming growth factor-beta and breast cancer. In: Bowcock A, ed. *Breast cancer: molecular genetics, pathogenesis, and therapeutics.* Totowa, NJ: Humana Press, 1999:95.
117. Wrana JL, Attisano L, Wieser R, Ventura F, Massague J. Mechanism of activation of the TGF-beta receptor. *Nature* 1994;370:341.
118. Koli KM, Arteaga CL. Complex role of tumor cell transforming growth factor (TGF)-betas on breast carcinoma progression. *J Mammary Gland Biol Neoplasia* 1996;1:373.
119. Knabbe C, Lippman ME, Wakefield LM, et al. Evidence that transforming growth factor-beta is a hormonally regulated negative growth factor in human breast cancer cells. *Cell* 1987;48:417.
120. Robinson SD, Silberstein GB, Roberts AB, Flanders KC, Daniel CW. Regulated expression and growth inhibitory effects of transforming growth factor-beta isoforms in mouse mammary gland development. *Development* 1991;113:867.
121. Mieth M, Boehmer FD, Ball R, Groner B, Grosse R. Transforming growth factor-beta inhibits lactogenic hormone induction of beta-casein expression in HC11 mouse mammary epithelial cells. *Growth Factors* 1990;4:9.
122. Jhappan C, Geiser AG, Kordon EC, et al. Targeting expression of a transforming growth factor beta 1 transgene to the pregnant mammary gland inhibits alveolar development and lactation. *EMBO J* 1993;12:1835.
123. Schedin PJ, Thackray LB, Malone P, et al. Programmed cell death and mammary neoplasia. In: Dickson RB, Lippman ME, eds. *Mammary tumor cell cycle, differentiation, and metastasis.* Boston: Kluwer Academic Publishers, 1996:3.
124. Stampfer MR, Yaswen P, Alhadeff M, Hosoda J. TGF beta induction of extracellular matrix associated proteins in normal and transformed human mammary epithelial cells in culture is independent of growth effects. *J Cell Physiol* 1993;155:210.
125. Arteaga CL, Hurd SD, Winnier AR, et al. Anti-transforming growth factor (TGF)-beta antibodies inhibit breast cancer cell tumorigenicity and increase mouse spleen natural killer cell activity: implications for a possible role of tumor cell/host TGF-beta interactions in human breast cancer progression. *J Clin Invest* 1993;92:2569.
126. Zugmaier G, Paik S, Wilding G, et al. Transforming growth factor beta 1 induces cachexia and systemic fibrosis without an antitumor effect in nude mice. *Cancer Res* 1991;51:3590.
127. Welch DR, Fabra A, Nakajima M. Transforming growth factor beta stimulates mammary adenocarcinoma cell invasion and metastatic potential. *Proc Natl Acad Sci U S A* 1990;87:7678.
128. Brattain MG, Ko Y, Banerji SS, Wu G, Willson JKV. Defects of TGF-beta receptor signaling in mammary cell tumorigenesis. *J Mammary Gland Biol Neoplasia* 1996;1:365.
129. Richert MM, Wood TL. Expression and regulation of insulin-like growth factors and their binding proteins in the normal breast. In: Manni A, ed. *Contemporary endocrinology: endocrinology of breast cancer.* Totowa, NJ: Humana Press, 1999:39.
130. Cullen KJ, Kaup SS, Rasmussen AA. Interactions between stroma and epithelium in breast cancer: implications for tumor genesis growth and progression. In: Manni A, ed. *Contemporary endocrinology: endocrinology of breast cancer.* Totowa, NJ: Humana Press, 1999:155.
131. Lee AV, Yee D. Role of the IGF system in breast cancer proliferation and progression. In: Manni A, ed. *Contemporary endocrinology: endocrinology of breast cancer.* Totowa, NJ: Humana Press, 1999:187.
132. Oates AJ, Schumaker LM, Jenkins SB, et al. The mannose 6-phosphate/insulin-like growth factor 2 receptor (M6P/IGF2R), a putative breast tumor suppressor gene. *Breast Cancer Res Treat* 1998;47:269.
133. Dickson RB, Lippman ME. Autocrine and paracrine growth factors in the normal and neoplastic breast. In: Harris JR, Lippman ME, Morrow M, Osborne CK, eds. *Diseases of the breast,* 2nd ed. Philadelphia: Lippincott Williams & Wilkins, 2000:303.
134. Vonderhaar BK. Prolactin and its receptors in human breast cancer. In: Manni A, ed. *Contemporary endocrinology: endocrinology of breast cancer.* Totowa, NJ: Humana Press, 1999:261.
135. Dickson RB, Lippman ME. Oncogenes and suppressor genes. In: Harris JR, Lippman ME, Morrow M, Osborne CK, eds. *Diseases of the breast,* 2nd ed. Philadelphia: Lippincott Williams & Wilkins, 2000:281.
136. Le Roy X, Escot C, Brouillet JP, et al. Decrease of c-erbB-2 and c-myc RNA levels in tamoxifen-treated breast cancer. *Oncogene* 1991;6:431.
137. Chiappetta C, Kirkland JL, Loose-Mitchell DS, Murthy L, Stancel GM. Estrogen regulates expression of the jun family of protooncogenes in the uterus. *J Steroid Biochem Mol Biol* 1992;41:113.
138. Murphy LJ. Estrogen induction of insulin-like growth factors and myc proto-oncogene expression in the uterus. *J Steroid Biochem Mol Biol* 1991;40:223.
139. Leygue E, Gol-Winkler R, Gompel A, et al. Estradiol stimulates c-myc proto-oncogene expression in normal human breast epithelial cells in culture. *J Steroid Biochem Mol Biol* 1995;52:299.
140. Neuman E, Ladha MH, Lin N, et al. Cyclin D1 stimulation of estrogen receptor transcriptional activity independent of cdk4. *Mol Cell Biol* 1997:17:5338.
141. Anzick SL, Kononen J, Walker RL, et al. AIB1, a steroid receptor coactivator amplified in breast and ovarian cancer. *Science* 1997;277:965.
142. Dang CV. c-Myc target genes involved in cell growth, apoptosis, and metabolism. *Mol Cell Biol* 1999;19:1.
143. Xiao Q, Claassen G, Shi J, et al. Transactivation-defective c-MycS retains the ability to regulate proliferation and apoptosis. *Genes Dev* 1998;12:3803.
144. Nass SJ, Dickson RB. Defining a role for c-myc in breast tumorigenesis. *Breast Cancer Res Treat* 1997;44:1.
145. Nass SJ, Dickson RB. Epidermal growth factor–dependent cell cycle progression is altered in mammary epithelial cells which overexpress c-myc. *Clin Cancer Res* 1998;4:1813.
146. Watson PH, Pon RT, Shiu RPC. Inhibition of c-myc expression by phosphorothioate antisense oligonucleotide identifies a critical role for c-myc in the growth of human breast cancer. *Cancer Res* 1991;51:3996.
147. Deming SL, Nass SJ, Dickson RB, Trock BJ. C-Myc amplification in breast cancer: a meta analysis of its frequency and association with risk factors. *Proc Annu Meet AACR* 1999;40:1358(abst).
148. Dang CV, Resar LMS, Emison E, et al. Function of the c-myc oncogenic transcription factor. *Exp Cell Res* 1999;253:63.
149. Lee LW, Raymond VW, Tsao MS, et al. Clonal cosegregation of tumorigenicity with overexpression of c-myc and transforming growth factor α genes in chemically transformed rat liver epithelial cells. *Cancer Res* 1991;51:5238.
150. Amundadottir LT, Nass S, Berchem G, Johnson MD, Dickson RB. Cooperation of TGFα and c-myc in mouse mammary tumorigenesis: coordinated stimulation of growth and suppression of apoptosis. *Oncogene* 1996;13:757.
151. Amundadottir LT, Johnson MD, Merlino GT, Smith GH, Dickson RB. Synergistic interaction of transforming growth factor α and c-myc in mouse mammary and salivary gland tumorigenesis. *Cell Growth Differ* 1995;6:737.
152. Sklar MD, Prochownik EV. Modulation of cis-platinum resistance in friend erythroleukemia cells by c-myc. *Cancer Res* 1991;51:2118.
153. Yang BS, Geddes TJ, Pogulis RJ, de Crombrugghe B, Freytag SO. Transcriptional suppression of cellular gene expression by c-myc. *Mol Cell Biol* 1991;11:2291.
154. Suen TC, Hung MC. c-myc reverses neu-induced transformed morphology by transcriptional repression. *Mol Cell Biol* 1991;11:354.
155. Semsei I, Ma S, Cutler RG. Tissue and age specific expression of the myc protooncogene family throughout the lifespan of the C57BL/6J mouse strain. *Oncogene* 1989;4:465.
156. Schreiber-Agus N, Meng Y, Hoang T, et al. Role of Mxi1 in ageing organ systems and the regulation of normal and neoplastic growth. *Nature* 1998;393:483.
157. Valverius EM, Ciardiello F, Heldin NE, et al. Stromal influences on transformation of human mammary epithelial cells overexpressing c-myc and SV40T. *J Cell Physiol* 1990;145:207.
158. Cullen KJ, Lippman ME. Stromal-epithelial interactions in breast cancer. In: Lippman ME, Dickson RB, eds. *Genes, oncogenes and hormones.* Boston: Kluwer Academic Publishers, 1992:413.
159. Broca P. *Traite des Tumeurs.* Paris: Asselin, 1866.
160. Knudson AG Jr. Mutation and cancer: statistical study of retinoblastoma. *Proc Natl Acad Sci U S A* 1971;68:820.
161. Harris H, Miller OJ, Klein G, Worst P, Tachibana T. Suppression of malignancy by cell fusion. *Nature* 1969;223:363.
162. Venkitaraman AR. Breast cancer genes and DNA repair. *Science* 1999;286:1100.
163. Chen CF, Li S, Zhong Z, et al. Association of BRCA1 with the hRad50. *Science* 1999;285:747.
164. Christofori G, Semb H. The role of the cell-adhesion molecule E-cadherin as a tumour-suppressor gene. *Trends Biochem Sci* 1999;24:73.
165. Kaelin WG Jr. Functions of the retinoblastoma protein. *Bioessays* 1999;21:950.
166. Fung YK, T'Ang A. The role of the retinoblastoma gene in breast cancer development. *Cancer Treat Res* 1992;61:59.
167. Ahmad S, Singh N, Glazer RI. Role of AKT1 in 17B-estradiol- and insulin-like growth factor I (IGF-I)-dependent proliferation and prevention of apoptosis in MCF-7 breast carcinoma cells. *Biochem Pharmacol* 1999;58:425.
168. Datta SR, Brunet A, Greenberg ME. Cellular survival: a play in three Akts. *Genes Dev* 1999;13:2905.
169. Weng LP, Smith WM, Dahia PLM, et al. PTEN suppresses breast cancer cell growth by phophatase activity–dependent G1 arrest followed by cell death. *Cancer Res* 1999;59:5808.
170. Elledge RM, Lee W. Life and death of p53. *Bioessays* 1995;17:923.
171. Cullotta E, Koshland D. Molecules of the year: p53 sweeps through cancer research. *Science* 1993;262:1958.
172. Lavin MF, Khanna KK, Beamish H, et al. Relationship of the ataxia-telangiectasia protein ATM to phosphoinositide 3-kinase. *Trends Biochem Sci* 1996;20:382.
173. Cox LS, Lane DP. Tumor suppressors, kinases and clamps: how p53 regulates the cell cycle in response to DNA damage. *Bioessays* 1996;18:501.
174. Hockenbery DM. Bcl-2, a novel regulator of cell death. *Bioessays* 1995;17:631.
175. Silvestrini R, Veneroni S, Daidone MG, et al. The bcl-2 protein: a prognostic indicator strongly related to p53 protein in lymph node–negative breast cancer patients. *J Natl Cancer Inst* 1994;86:499.

176. Reed JC. Dysregulation of apoptosis in cancer. *J Clin Oncol* 1999;17:2941.
177. Agarwal ML, Taylor WR, Chernov MV, Chernova OB, Stark GR. The p53 network. *J Biol Chem* 1998;273:1.
178. Wang T, Phang J. Effects of estrogen on apoptotic pathways in human breast cancer cell line MCF-7. *Cancer Res* 1995;55:2487.
179. Merlo GR, Basolo F, Fiore L, Duboc L, Hynes NE. p53-dependent and p53-independent activation of apoptosis in mammary epithelial cells reveals a survival function of EGF and insulin. *J Cell Biol* 1995;128:1185.
180. Teixeira C, Reid JC, Pratt MA. Estrogen promotes chemotherapeutic drug resistance by a mechanism involving bcl-2 proto-oncogene expression in human breast cancer cells. *Cancer Res* 1995;55:3902.
181. Foekens JA, Buessecker F, Peters HA, et al. Plasminogen activator inhibitor-2: prognostic relevance in 1012 patients with primary breast cancer. *Cancer Res* 1995;55:1423.
182. Clark M, Apel I, Benedict M, et al. A recombinant bcl-x_s adenovirus selectively induces apoptosis in cancer cells but not in normal bone marrow cells. *Proc Natl Acad Sci U S A* 1995;92:11024.
183. Sumantran VN, Ealovega MW, Nunez G, Clarke MF, Wicha MS. Overexpression of Bcl-XS sensitizes MCF-7 cells to chemotherapy-induced apoptosis. *Cancer Res* 1995;55:2507.
184. Chellappan SP, Hiebert S, Mudryj M, Horowitz JM, Nevins JR. The E2F transcription factor is a cellular target for the RB protein. *Cell* 1991;65:1053.
185. Obaya AJ, Mateyak MK, Sedivy JM. Mysterious liaisons: the relationship between c-myc and the cell cycle. *Oncogene* 1999;18:2934.
186. Nijjar T, Wigington D, Garbe JC, et al. p57KIP2 expression and loss of heterozygosity during immortal conversion of cultured human mammary epithelial cells. *Cancer Res* 1999;59:5112.
187. Zukerberg LR, Yang WI, Gadd M, et al. Cyclin D1 (PRAD1) protein expression in breast cancer: approximately one-third of infiltrating mammary carcinomas show overexpression of the cyclin D1 oncogene. *Mod Pathol* 1995;8:560.
188. Keyomarsi K, Conte D Jr, Toyofuku W, Fox MP. Deregulation of cyclin E in breast cancer. *Oncogene* 1995;11:941.
189. Wang TC, Cardiff RD, Zukerberg L, et al. Mammary hyperplasia and carcinoma in MMTV-cyclin D1 transgenic mice. *Nature* 1994;369:669.
190. Sicinski P, Donaher JL, Parker SB, et al. Cyclin D1 provides a link between development and oncogenesis in the retina and breast. *Cell* 1995;82:621.
191. Herman JG, Merlo A, Mao L, et al. Inactivation of the cDK2N2/p16/MTS1 gene is frequently associated with aberrant methylation in all common human cancers. *Cancer Res* 1995;55:4525.
192. Nielsen NH, Loden M, Cajander J, Emdin SO, Landberg G. G1-S transition defects occur in most breast cancers and predict outcome. *Breast Cancer Res Treat* 1999;56:105.
193. Lizard-Nacol S, Lidereau R, Collin F, et al. Benign breast disease: absence of genetic alterations at several loci implicated in breast cancer malignancy. *Cancer Res* 1995;55:4416.
194. Hahn WC, Counter CM, Lundberg AS, et al. Creation of human tumour cells with defined genetic elements. *Nature* 1999;400:464.
195. Zakien VA. Telomeres. Beginning to understand the end. *Science* 1995;270:1601.
196. Hiyama E, Gollahon L, Kataoka T, et al. Telomerase activity in human breast tumors. *J Natl Cancer Inst* 1996;88:116.
197. Greenberg RA, O'Hagan RC, Deng H, et al. Telomerase reverse transcriptase gene is a direct target of c-myc but is not functionally equivalent in cellular transformation. *Oncogene* 1998;18:1219.
198. Kyo S, Takakura M, Kanaya T, et al. Estrogen activates telomerase. *Cancer Res* 1999;59:5917.
199. Fishel R, Lescoe MK, Rao MR, et al. The human mutator gene homolog MSH2 and its association with hereditary nonpolyposis colon cancer. *Cell* 1994;77:167.
200. Dickson RB, Lippman ME. *Drug and hormonal resistance in breast cancer.* New York: Ellis Horwood, 1996:1.
201. Aoyagi H, Dickson RB. Programmed cell death and its resistance in breast cancer chemotherapy. *Pathogenesis* 1999;1:143.
202. Sato T, Akiyama F, Sakamoto G, Kasumi F, Nakamura Y. Accumulation of genetic alterations and progression of primary breast cancer. *Cancer Res* 1991;51:5794.
203. Callahan R, Cropp C, Merlo GR, et al. Genetic and molecular heterogeneity of breast cancer cells. *Clin Chim Acta* 1993;217:63.
204. Deng G, Lu Y, Zolotnikov G, et al. Loss of heterozygosity in normal tissue adjacent to breast carcinomas. *Science* 1996;274:2057.
205. O'Connell P, Pekkel V, Fuqua SAW, et al. Analysis of loss of heterozygosity in 399 premalignant breast lesions at 15 genetic loci. *J Natl Cancer Inst* 1998;90:697.
206. Dickson RB. The molecular basis of breast cancer. In: Kurzrock R, Talpaz M, eds. *Molecular biology in cancer medicine,* 2nd ed. London: Martin Dunitz, 1999:287.
207. Amundadottir LT, Merlin GT, Dickson RB. Transgenic models of breast cancer. *Breast Cancer Res Treat* 1996;39:119.
208. Ciardiello F, Gottardis M, Basolo F, et al. Additive effects of c-erbB-2, c-Ha-ras, and transforming growth factor-alpha genes on *in vitro* transformation of human mammary epithelial cells. *Mol Carcinog* 1992;6:43.
209. Dati C, Muraca R, Tazartes O, et al. C-erbB-2 and ras expression levels in breast cancer are correlated and show a co-operative association with unfavorable clinical outcome. *Int J Cancer* 1991;47:833.
210. Rosfjord EC, Dickson RB. Growth factors, apoptosis, and survival of mammary epithelial cells. *J Mammary Gland Biol Neoplasia* 1999;4:229.
211. Sinn E, Muller W, Pattengale P, et al. Coexpression of MMTV/v-Ha-ras and MMTV/c-myc genes in transgenic mice: synergistic action of oncogenes *in vivo.* *Cell* 1987;49:465.
212. Li B, Rosen J, McMenamin-Balano J, et al. Neu/erbB$_2$ in transgenic cooperates with p53-172H during mammary tumorigenesis in transgenic mice. *Mol Cell Biol* 1997;17:3155.
213. Liotta LA, Steeg PS, Stetler-Stevenson WG. Cancer metastasis and angiogenesis: an imbalance of positive and negative regulation. *Cell* 1991;64:327.
214. Sierra A, Lloveras B, Castellsague X, et al. Bcl-2 expression is associated with lymph node metastasis in human ductal breast carcinoma. *Int J Cancer* 1995;60:54.
215. Rosfjord E, Dickson RB. Cell adhesion and metastasis. In: Bowcock A, ed. *Contemporary approaches to breast cancer.* Totowa, NJ: Humana Press, 1999:285.
216. Ellis LM, Nicolson GL, Fidler IJ. Concepts and mechanisms of breast cancer metastasis. In: Bland KI, Copeland EM, eds. *The breast,* 2nd ed. Philadelphia: WB Saunders, 1998:564.
217. Folkman J. Angiogenesis in breast cancer. In: Bland KI, Copeland EM, eds. *The breast,* 2nd ed. Philadelphia: WB Saunders, 1998:586.
218. Davies BR, Barraclough R, Rudland PS. Induction of metastatic ability in a stably diploid benign rat mammary epithelial cell line by transfection with DNA from human malignant breast carcinoma cell lines. *Cancer Res* 1994;54:2785.
219. Cornetta K, Moore A, Johannessohn M, Sledge GW. Clonal dominance detected in metastases but not primary tumors of retrovirally marked human breast carcinoma injected into nude mice. *Clin Exp Metastasis* 1994;12:3.
220. Lerman C, Peshkin BN. Psychosocial issues in BRCA1/2 testing. In: Bowcock AM, ed. *Breast cancer: molecular genetics, pathogenesis, and therapeutics.* Totowa, NJ: Humana Press, 1998:247.
221. Jordan VC, Costa AF. Chemoprevention. In: Harris JR, Lippman ME, Morrow M, Osborne CK, eds. *Diseases of the breast,* 2nd ed. Philadelphia: Lippincott Williams & Wilkins, 2000:265.
222. Jordan C, Morrow M. Tamoxifen, raloxifene, and the prevention of breast cancer. *Endocr Rev* 1999;20:253.
223. Gregory H, Thomas CE, Willshire IR, et al. Epidermal and transforming growth factor alpha in patients with breast tumours. *Br J Cancer* 1989;59:605.
224. Perroteau I, Salomon D, De Bortoli M, et al. Immunological detection and quantitation of alpha transforming growth factors in human breast carcinoma cells. *Breast Cancer Res Treat* 1986;7:201.
225. Macias A, Perez R, Hagerstrom T, Skoog L. Identification of transforming growth factor alpha in human primary breast carcinomas. *Anticancer Res* 1987;7:1271.
226. Eckert K, Granetzny A, Fischer J, Nexo E, Grosse R. A mr 43,000 epidermal growth factor–related protein purified from the urine of breast cancer patients. *Cancer Res* 1990;50:642.
227. Li Z, Bustos V, Miner J, et al. Propagation of genetically altered tumor cells derived from fine-needle aspirates of primary breast carcinoma. *Cancer Res* 1998;58:5271.
228. Khan SA, Masood S, Miller L, Numann PJ. Random fine needle aspiration of the breast of women at increased breast cancer risk and standard risk controls. *Breast J* 1998;4:420.
229. Salven P, Perhoniemi V, Tykka H, Maenpaa H, Joensuu H. Serum VEGF levels in women with a benign breast tumor or breast cancer. *Breast Cancer Res Treat* 1999;53:161.
230. Hayes DR, Bast RC, Desch CE, et al. Tumor marker utility grading system: a framework to evaluate clinical utility of tumor markers. *J Natl Cancer Inst* 1996;88:1456.
231. Muss HB, Thor AD, Berry DA, et al. C-erbB-2 expression and response to adjuvant therapy in women with node-positive early breast cancer [published erratum appears in *N Engl J Med* 1994;331:211]. *N Engl J Med* 1994;330:1260.
232. Berns EM, Foekens JA, van Staveren IL, et al. Oncogene amplification and prognosis in breast cancer: relationship with systemic treatment. *Gene* 1995;159:11.
233. Fox S, Smith K, Hollyer J. The epidermal growth factor receptor as a prognostic marker: results of 370 patients and a review of 3009 patients. *Breast Cancer Res Treat* 1994;29:41.
234. Gusterson B, Machin L, Gullick W, et al. Immunohistochemical distribution of c-erbB-2 in infiltrating and *in situ* breast cancer. *Int J Cancer* 1988;42:842.
235. Paik S, Hazan R, Fisher ER, et al. Pathologic findings from the national surgical adjuvant breast and bowel project: prognostic significance of erbB-2 protein overexpression in primary breast cancer. *J Clin Oncol* 1990;8:103.
236. Benz C, Sarup J, Scott G, et al. Estrogen-dependent, tamoxifen-resistant tumorigenic growth of MCF-7 cells transfected with Her2/neu. *Breast Cancer Res Treat* 1992;24:85.
237. Thor AD, Berry DA, Budman DR, et al. Erb B_2, p53, and efficacy of adjuvant therapy in lymph node–positive cancer. *J Natl Cancer Inst* 1998;90:1346.
238. Sunderland MC, McGuire WL. Oncogenes as clinical prognostic indicators. *Cancer Treat Res* 1991;53:3.
239. Gusterson B, Gelber R, Bettelheim R, et al. Prognostic importance of c-erbB-2 expression in breast cancer. *J Clin Oncol* 1992;10:1049.
240. Anbazhagan R, Gelber RD, Bettelheim R, Goldhirsch A, Gusterson BA. Association of c-erbB-2 expression and S-phase fraction in the prognosis of node positive breast cancer. *Ann Oncol* 1991;2:47.
241. Toikkanen S, Helin H, Isola J, Joensuu H. Prognostic significance of HER-2 oncoprotein expression in breast cancer: a 30-year follow-up. *J Clin Oncol* 1992;10:1044.
242. Hancock MC, Langton BC, Chan T, et al. A monoclonal antibody against the c-erbB-2 protein enhances the cytotoxicity of cis-diaminedichloroplatinum against human breast and ovarian tumor cell lines. *Cancer Res* 1991;51:4575.
243. Cheever MA, Disis ML. Immunology and immunotherapy. In: Harris JR, Lippman ME, Morrow M, Osborne CK, eds. *Diseases of the breast,* 2nd ed. Philadelphia: Lippincott Williams & Wilkins, 2000:811.
244. Langton BC, Crenshaw MC, Chao LA, et al. An antigen immunologically related to the external domain of gp185 is shed from nude mouse tumors overexpressing the c-erbB-2 (HER-2/neu) oncogene. *Cancer Res* 1991;51:2593.
245. Wels W, Harwerth IM, Mueller M, Groner B, Hynes NE. Selective inhibition of tumor cell growth by a recombinant single-chain antibody-toxin specific for the erbB-2 receptor. *Cancer Res* 1992;52:6310.
246. Carter P, Presta L, Gorman CM, et al. Humanization of an anti-p185HER2 antibody for human cancer therapy. *Proc Natl Acad Sci U S A* 1992;89:4285.
247. Pastan I, Fitz Gerald D. Recombinant toxins for cancer treatment. *Science* 1991;254:1173.
248. Pupa SM, Menard S, Andreola S, Colnaghi MI. Antibody response against the c-erbB-2 oncoprotein in breast carcinoma patients. *Cancer Res* 1993;53:5864.

249. Zhai Y, Beittenmiller H, Wang B, et al. Increased expression of specific tyrosine protein phosphatases in human breast epithelial cells neoplastically transformed by the neu oncogene. *Cancer Res* 1993;53:2272.
250. Pierce JH, Arnstein P, Di Marco E, et al. Oncogenic potential of erbB-2 in human mammary epithelial cells. *Oncogene* 1991;6:1189.
251. Guy CT, Muthuswamy SK, Cardiff RD, Soriano P, Muller WJ. Activation of the c-Src tyrosine kinase is required for the induction of mammary tumors in transgenic mice. *Genes Dev* 1994;8:23.
252. Ekstrand AJ, Sugawa N, James CD, Collins VP. Amplified and rearranged epidermal growth factor genes in human glioblastomas: effects of type II mutation on receptor function. *Biochem Biophys Res Comm* 1991;178:1413.
253. Bonilla M, Ramirez M, Lopez-Cueto J, Gariglio P. *In vivo* amplification and rearrangement of c-myc oncogene in human breast tumors. *J Natl Cancer Inst* 1988;80:665.
254. Cline MJ, Battifora H, Yokota J. Proto-oncogene abnormalities in human breast cancer: correlations with anatomic features and clinical course of disease. *J Clin Oncol* 1987;5:999.
255. Varley JM, Swallow JE, Brammar WJ, Whittaker JL, Walker RA. Alterations to either c-erbB-2(neu) or c-myc proto-oncogenes in breast carcinomas correlate with poor short-term prognosis. *Oncogene* 1987;1:423.
256. Berns EM, Klijn JG, van Putten WL, et al. c-myc amplification is a better prognostic factor than HER2/neu amplification in primary breast cancer. *Cancer Res* 1992;52:1107.
257. Escot C, Theillet C, Lidereau R, et al. Genetic alteration of the c-myc protooncogene (myc) in human primary breast carcinomas. *Proc Natl Acad Sci U S A* 1986;83:4834.
258. Jamerson MH, Johnson MD, Dickson RB. Dual regulation of proliferation and apoptosis: c-myc in bitransgenic murine mammary tumor models. *Oncogene* 2000;19:1065.
259. Sklar MD, Prochownik EV. Modulation of cis-platinum resistance in friend erythroleukemia cells by c-myc. *Cancer Res* 1991;51:2118.
260. Yang BS, Geddes TJ, Pogulis RJ, de Crombrugghe B, Freytag SO. Transcriptional suppression of cellular gene expression by c-myc. *Mol Cell Biol* 1991;11:2291.
261. Gullick WJ, Tuzi NL, Kumas S, et al. c-erbB$_2$ and c-myc genes and their expression in normal tissues and in human breast cancer. In: *Cancer cells 7: molecular diagnostics of human cancer.* New York: Cold Spring Harbor Press, 1989:393.
262. Baselga J, Norton L, Albanell J, Kim YM, Mendelsohn J. Recombinant humanized anti-HER2 antibody (Herceptin) enhances the antitumor activity of paditaxel and doxorubicin against HER-2/neu overexpressing human breast cancer xenografts. *Cancer Res* 1998;58:2825.
263. Pietras RJ, Poen JC, Gailardo D, et al. Monoclonal antibody to HER-2/neu receptor modulates repair of radiation-induced damage and enhances radiosensitivity of human breast cancer cells overexpressing this oncogene. *Cancer Res* 1999;59:1347.
264. Pietras RJ, Regram MD, Fino RS, Moneval DA, Slamon DJ. Remission of human breast cancer xenografts on therapy with humanized monoclonal antibody to HER-2 receptor and DNA reactive drugs. *Oncogene* 1998;17:2235.
265. Fan S, Smith ML, Rivet DJ II, et al. Disruption of p53 function sensitizes breast cancer MCF-7 cells to cisplatin and pentoxifylline. *Cancer Res* 1995;55:1649.
266. Domagala W, Striker G, Szadowska A, et al. p53 protein and vimentin in invasive ductal NOS breast carcinoma—relationship with survival and sites of metastases. *Eur J Cancer* 1994;30A:1527.
267. Pietilainen T, Lipponen P, Aaltomaa S, et al. Expression of retinoblastoma gene protein (RB) in breast cancer as related to established prognostic factors and survival. *Eur J Cancer* 1995;31A:329.
268. Bhargava V, Kell DL, van de Rijn M, Warnke RA. Bcl-2 immunoreactivity in breast carcinoma correlates with hormone receptor positivity. *Am J Pathol* 1994;145:535.
269. Gasparini G, Barbareschi M, Doglioni C, et al. Expression of bcl-2 protein predicts efficacy of adjuvant treatments in operable node-positive breast cancer. *Clin Cancer Res* 1995;2:189.
270. Krajewski S, Blomqvist C, Franssila K, et al. Reduced expression of proapoptotic gene BAX is associated with poor response rates to combination chemotherapy and shorter survival in women with metastatic breast adenocarcinoma. *Cancer Res* 1995;55:4471.
271. Bonetti A, Zaninelli M, Leone R, et al. bcl-2 but not p53 expression is associated with resistance to chemotherapy in advanced breast cancer. *Clin Cancer Res* 1998;4:2331.
272. Nacht M, Ferguson AT, Zhang W, et al. Combining serial analysis of gene expression and array technologies to identify genes differentially expressed in breast cancer. *Cancer Res* 1999;59:5464.
273. Sgroi DC, Teng S, Robinson G, et al. *In vivo* gene expression profile analysis of human breast cancer progression. *Cancer Res* 1999;59:5656.
274. Fox SB, Harris AL. Angiogenesis as a diagnostic and therapeutic target. In: Harris JR, Lippman ME, Morrow M, Osborne CK, eds. *Diseases of the breast,* 2nd ed. Philadelphia: Lippincott Williams & Wilkins, 2000:799.
275. Duffy MJ, Reilly D, McDermott E, et al. Urokinase plasminogen activator as a prognostic marker in different subgroups of patients with breast cancer. *Cancer* 1994;74:2276.
276. Foekens JA, Peters HA, Look MP, et al. The urokinase system of plasminogen activation and prognosis in 2780 breast cancer patients. *Cancer Res* 2000;60:636.
277. Kaufmann M, Heider KH, Sinn HP, et al. CD44 variant exon epitopes in primary breast cancer and length of survival. *Lancet* 1995;345:615.
278. Montero MD, Zavagno G, Meggiolaro F, et al. Vimentin and proliferating cell nuclear antigen (PCNA) expression on node negative breast carcinomas and their correlations with pathologic variables and prognosis. *Breast J* 1995;4:175.
279. Heimann R, Ferguson D, Gray S, Hellman S. Assessment of intratumoral vascularization (angiogenesis) in breast cancer prognosis. *Breast Cancer Res Treat* 1998;52:147.
280. Locopo N, Fanelli M, Gasparini G. Clinical significance of angiogenic factors in breast cancer. *Breast Cancer Res Treat* 1998;52:159.
281. Linderholm B, Tavelin B, Grankvist K, et al. Vascular endothelial growth factor is of high prognostic value in node-negative breast carcinoma. *J Clin Oncol* 1998;16:3121.
282. Bergers G, Javaherian K, Lo KM, Folkman J, Hanahan D. Effects of angiogenesis inhibitors on multistage carcinogenesis in mice. *Science* 1999;284:808.
283. Malonne H, Langer I, Kiss R, Atassi G. Mechanisms of tumor angiogenesis and therapeutic implications: angiogenesis inhibitors. *Clin Exp Metastasis* 1999;17:1.
284. Rosen N, Sepp-Lorenzino L, Lippman ME. Biologic therapy. In: Harris JR, Lippman ME, Morro M, Osborne CK, eds. *Disease of the breast,* 2nd ed. Philadelphia: Lippincott Williams & Wilkins, 2000:825.

ERIC P. WINER
MONICA MORROW
C. KENT OSBORNE
JAY R. HARRIS

SECTION 2

Malignant Tumors of the Breast

Breast cancer has a major impact on the health of women. Approximately 183,000 women are diagnosed with invasive breast cancer each year and nearly 41,000 women die of the disease.[1] In American women, breast cancer is the most frequently diagnosed cancer and the second leading cause of cancer death.[1] In women aged 40 to 55, breast cancer is the leading cause of all mortality. There has been a slight decline in breast cancer mortality overall,[1] which can be attributed both to the success of early detection programs and to advances in treatment, particularly developments in systemic therapy. Data from the Surveillance, Epidemiology, and End Results (SEER) program indicate that white women in the United States have a 13.1% lifetime risk of developing breast cancer, whereas African American women have a 9.6% lifetime incidence.[2] The lifetime risk of dying from breast cancer is 3.4% for both African American and white women in the United States.

For several decades there had been a dramatic increase in the incidence of invasive breast cancer. While the incidence of invasive breast cancer has leveled off,[1] the number of *in situ* cancers, particularly ductal carcinoma *in situ* (DCIS), has been on the rise. SEER data indicate that there was a 130% increase in *in situ* cancers in whites and a 190% increase in African Americans from 1983 to 1996.[2] It is estimated that *in situ* carcinoma was diagnosed in almost 40,000 women in the United States in 1999.[1] The increase in *in situ* cancers, particularly DCIS, is largely a result of the increasing use of screening mammography.

In this chapter, we describe the salient features of breast cancer, stressing practical information of importance to clinicians and findings that are new since the last edition of this text. The increasing incidence of *in situ* cancer and the more complex management issues surrounding DCIS are reflected in an expanded section dealing with these issues. For more details about breast cancer, the interested reader is referred to a related textbook in this series devoted exclusively to diseases of the breast.[3]

RISK FACTORS FOR BREAST CANCER

Multiple factors are associated with an increased risk of developing breast cancer, including increasing age, family history, exposure to female reproductive hormones (both endogenous and exogenous), dietary factors, benign breast disease, and environmental factors. The majority of these factors convey a small to moderate increase in risk for any individual woman. It has been estimated that approximately 50% of women who develop breast cancer have no identifiable risk factor beyond increasing age and female gender.[4] Since breast cancer is such an overwhelmingly female disease, gender is often not even considered among the risk factors. The importance of age is sometimes overlooked as well. Many women, particularly young women, overestimate their risk of developing breast cancer.[5] As can be seen in Table 37.2-1, age plays a major role in breast cancer risk.[2] In women under 30, breast cancer is extremely uncommon. From 1992 to 1996, the incidence of breast cancer in women aged 35 to 39 was 59 per 100,000; however, in women 55 to 59, the incidence was 296 per 100,000.

TABLE 37.2-1. Surveillance, Epidemiology, and End Results Incidence and Mortality Age-Specific Rates by Race from 1992 to 1996[a]

	Incidence Rates		
Age at Diagnosis (y)	All Races	Whites	African Americans
25–29	7.8	7.4	10.3
30–34	24.4	23.4	31.5
35–39	59.0	58.2	62.3
40–44	117.0	117.6	120.3
45–49	195.7	198.2	199.1
50–54	257.5	264.6	241.4
55–59	296.3	304.0	280.2
60–64	347.3	364.2	294.2
65–69	404.4	423.2	341.9
70–74	455.5	473.9	390.7
75–79	483.3	500.7	424.1
80–84	468.1	487.1	372.8
85+	405.0	416.5	353.0
	Mortality		
Age at Death (y)	All Races	Whites	African Americans
25–29	1.1	0.9	2.2
30–34	4.1	3.6	7.8
35–39	10.5	9.6	17.8
40–44	20.2	18.9	32.6
45–49	34.3	32.7	51.9
50–54	50.1	48.3	71.0
55–59	63.0	62.1	80.5
60–64	78.5	78.5	93.1
65–69	95.7	96.7	103.4
70–74	114.7	115.5	127.3
75–79	133.2	134.5	138.7
80–84	157.0	158.1	164.4
85+	200.5	202.6	200.4

[a]Rates are per 100,000.
(Adapted from ref. 2.)

The annual incidence continues to rise, albeit more gradually, as a woman enters her 60s and 70s.

FAMILIAL FACTORS

A family history of breast cancer has long been recognized as a risk factor for the disease. The majority of women diagnosed with breast cancer do not have a family member with the disease, and only 5% to 10% have a true hereditary predisposition to breast cancer.[6] Many women with a positive family history overestimate their risk of developing breast cancer,[7] and women considering genetic testing have been shown to overestimate their chance of having a mutation.[8] Overall, the risk of developing breast cancer is increased 1.5- to 3.0-fold if a woman has a mother or sister with breast cancer.[9,10] Family history, however, is a heterogeneous risk factor with different implications depending on the number of relatives with breast cancer, the exact relationship, the age at diagnosis, and the number of unaffected relatives. For example, there may be minimal elevation in breast cancer risk for a woman whose mother was diagnosed with breast cancer at an advanced age and who has no other family history of the disease. In contrast, a woman who has multiple family members diagnosed with early-onset breast cancer is at a much higher risk of developing the disease.[11] Even in the absence of a known inherited predisposition, women with a family history of breast cancer face some level of increased risk, likely from some combination of shared environmental exposures, unexplained genetic factors, or both. For women with a limited family history, assessment tools such as the Gail model may be helpful in providing a quantitative estimate of breast cancer risk.[12] Of note, the Gail model was used in the National Surgical Adjuvant Breast Project (NSABP) breast cancer prevention study with tamoxifen.

INHERITED PREDISPOSITION TO BREAST CANCER

The identification of the two tumor suppressor genes BRCA1[13] and BRCA2[14] has provided new insights into the understanding of breast cancer genetics. When a woman has a mutation in either of these genes, she faces a markedly increased lifetime risk of developing breast cancer.[15–17] The possibility of a mutation in either BRCA1 or BRCA2 should be considered when breast cancer is diagnosed at a young age (i.e., less than 45 to 55), when multiple relatives are affected, when there is a history of other cancers in the family (particularly ovarian cancer), or any combination of these factors. Although an increased risk of ovarian cancer is seen in families with both BRCA1 and BRCA2 mutations, the presence of ovarian cancer in a family member of a woman with breast cancer is more consistent with a mutation in BRCA1.[15] Both BRCA1 and BRCA2 are inherited in an autosomal dominant manner and can be passed to offspring through either maternal or paternal lineage. A number of models have been developed to help clinicians estimate the chance of identifying a gene mutation.[18,19]

In 1990, chromosome 17q21 was identified as the likely location for a breast cancer susceptibility gene.[20] The BRCA1 gene was ultimately cloned in 1994.[13] Mutations in BRCA1 are associated with a 50% to 85% risk of developing breast cancer during a woman's lifetime, with a particularly striking predisposition to early-onset breast cancer.[21,22] The risk of ovarian cancer is elevated, though not to the same extent as breast cancer. Nevertheless, the presence of both early-onset breast cancer and ovarian cancer in either a single individual or within a family is highly suggestive of a BRCA1 mutation. Men with BRCA1 mutations do not appear to be at increased risk of breast cancer, but are probably at increased risk of prostate cancer and possibly of colon cancer.[23] The BRCA1 gene is large, with 24 coding regions and 1863 amino acids; hundreds of mutations have been described throughout the gene. As a result, screening for a mutation in BRCA1 is costly and time consuming. Polymorphisms in the gene are not uncommon and probably do not convey an elevated cancer risk.

BRCA2 is located on chromosome 13 and is an even larger gene than BRCA1.[14] Women with BRCA2 mutations are thought to be at a similar risk of developing breast cancer as those with BRCA1 mutations.[16,24] There is an increased risk of ovarian cancer in women with BRCA2 mutations, although to a lesser degree than with BRCA1. Men with BRCA2 mutations develop breast cancer with a lifetime incidence that is estimated to be 6%.[25] In addition, there are a variety of other cancers that appear to be associated with BRCA2; however, studies to date remain limited.

In the general population, it is estimated that between 1 in 500 and 1 in 800 individuals carry a BRCA1 mutation. BRCA2 mutations are even less common.[26] In contrast, mutations in either BRCA1 or BRCA2 occur in approximately 1 in 40 individuals of Ashkenazi Jewish background.[22] Within this population, three founder mutations (185delAG and 5382 insC in BRCA1 and 6174delT in BRCA2) appear to have been passed on for generations. Because of the higher gene frequency in individuals of Ashkenazi descent, the chance of finding a mutation in an Ashkenazi Jewish woman with a personal history, family history, or both of breast cancer, ovarian cancer, or both is much higher than in a non-Ashkenazi. Because of the high frequency of the founder mutations in this group of individuals, genetic testing can begin with an assessment for the presence of the three mutations. In Ashkenazi Jewish women diagnosed with breast cancer at age 40 or earlier, it has been estimated that 20% or more have a mutation.[27]

Genetic testing should be preceded by a careful evaluation of an individual's personal cancer history and family history. The implications of genetic testing for both the individual and the extended family are considerable, and these issues should be addressed in genetic counseling session(s) before any testing. A more extensive discussion of this issue is found elsewhere in this text.

There are many unanswered questions about both BRCA1 and BRCA2. Since the genes are large and mutations can be highly variable in location, an important issue is whether all mutations convey the same level of risk. It is unknown to what extent breast cancer risk is modified by other genes, hormonal factors, or environmental exposures. For example, preliminary reports have suggested that early pregnancy is not protective, [28] although oophorectomy appears to lower breast cancer risk.[29] For women with mutations who have not developed breast cancer, a variety of strategies have been considered to lower risk and are described later, in Breast Cancer Prevention.

Women with BRCA1-associated breast cancers are thought to have a high proportion of high-grade, hormone receptor–negative cancers, although it is not clear that their overall outcome is different from that of women with sporadic breast cancer.[30–32] The tumors in women with BRCA2 mutations do not appear to have distinctive features and bear a closer resemblance to sporadic breast cancer.[32] At this time, it is not known whether a woman's genetic status should influence management decisions when breast cancer is diagnosed. Women with mutations have a higher risk of developing contralateral cancers, but their clinical course has otherwise not been shown to be different from other women with breast cancer.[31] For this reason, there are insufficient data to indicate that either local or systemic management of the patient with a mutation should differ from what is the standard of care based on stage, tumor grade, receptor status, and general health status.

Breast cancer is also observed as part of other familial syndromes, including Li-Fraumeni syndrome,[33] Cowden syndrome,[34] Muir syndrome,[35] and ataxia-telangiectasia.[36]

HORMONAL FACTORS

The development of breast cancer in many women appears to be related to female reproductive hormones. Epidemiologic studies have consistently identified a number of breast cancer risk factors, each of which is associated with increased exposure to endogenous estrogens. Early age at menarche, nulliparity or late age at first full-term pregnancy, and late age at menopause increase the risk of developing breast cancer.[12,37] In postmenopausal women, obesity[38] and postmenopausal hormone therapy,[39] both of which are positively correlated with plasma estrogen levels and plasma estradiol levels,[40,41] are associated with increased breast cancer risk. Furthermore, *in utero* exposure to high concentrations of estrogen may also increase breast cancer risk.[42,43]

The age-specific incidence of breast cancer increases steeply with age until menopause. After menopause, although the incidence continues to increase, the rate of increase decreases to approximately one-sixth of that seen in the premenopausal period. This dramatic slowing of the rate of increase in the age-specific incidence curve suggests that ovarian activity plays a major role in the etiology of breast cancer. The relative risk of developing breast cancer for a woman with natural menopause before age 45 is one-half that of a woman whose menopause occurs after age 55.[44] There is substantial evidence that estrogen deprivation via iatrogenic premature menopause can reduce breast cancer risk. Epidemiologic studies have shown that premenopausal women who undergo oophorectomy without hormone replacement have a markedly reduced risk of breast cancer later in life. Oophorectomy before age 50 decreases breast cancer risk, with an increasing magnitude of risk reduction as the age at oophorectomy decreases.[45] In a small study of women undergoing ovarian ablation as part of adjuvant breast cancer treatment, contralateral breast cancer rates were reduced compared with women not undergoing ovarian ablation.[46] Recent data from women with BRCA1 mutations suggest that early oophorectomy has a substantial protective effect on breast cancer risk in this population as well.[29]

Age at menarche and the establishment of regular ovulatory cycles are strongly linked to breast cancer risk.[47,48] Earlier age at menarche is associated with an increased risk of breast cancer[48]; there appears to be a 20% decrease in breast cancer risk for each year that menarche is delayed.[47] Of note, hormone levels through the reproductive years in women who experience early menarche may be higher than in women who undergo a later menarche.[49] Additionally, late onset of menarche results in a delay in the establishment of regular ovulatory cycles, although there is some controversy over whether this delay confers any additional protective effect.[50,51] From these data regarding menarche and menopause, it seems likely that the total duration of exposure to endogenous estrogen is an important factor in breast cancer risk.

The relationship between pregnancy and breast cancer risk appears more complicated. Age at first full-term pregnancy clearly influences breast cancer risk. Based on epidemiologic studies, women whose first full-term pregnancy occurs after age 30 have a two- to fivefold increase in breast cancer risk in comparison with women who have a first full-term pregnancy before approximately age 18.[52,53] Nulliparous women are at greater risk for the development of breast cancer than parous women, with a relative risk of about 1.4.[52] During pregnancy, mammary cells differentiate into mature breast cells prepared for lactation. After this differentiation, these cells have a longer cell cycle, allowing more time for DNA repair in G_1.[54] Breast cancer risk increases transiently after a pregnancy.[55] The increased risk, which lasts approximately 10 years, is then associated with a more durable protective effect.[55,56] The reason for the increased risk has been hypothesized to be the increase in proliferation, growth, and maturation of breast cells preparing for lactation, leading to the development of mutations. Alternatively, risk may increase secondary to the effect of high levels of hormones on subclinical cancers.

Studies of lactation on breast cancer risk have had inconsistent results. Studies have suggested that a long duration of lactation reduces breast cancer risk in premenopausal women.[57,58]

The effect of abortion, whether spontaneous or induced, on breast cancer risk is less clear. Several studies have found that termination of a pregnancy not only negates any protective effect, but, in fact, increases breast cancer risk.[59] More recent studies, including a large population-based cohort comprised of 1.5 million Danish women,[60] show no increase in long-term risk after early termination of a pregnancy.[61,62] These apparently contradictory effects of pregnancy on risk have been explained in a variety of ways. As breast tissue undergoes differentiation as a result of hormonal changes of a full-term pregnancy, these fully differentiated cells may be less likely to undergo malignant transformation. In incomplete pregnancy, the breast is exposed only to the high estrogen levels of early pregnancy. These unopposed high levels theoretically could be responsible for an increased risk in women who do not carry the pregnancy to term and thus do not experience the full mammary differentiation in preparation for lactation. Despite these theoretical arguments, at this time there is no *conclusive* evidence that early termination of a pregnancy has any effect on breast cancer risk.

The effects of exogenous hormones, in the form of hormone replacement therapy and oral contraceptives, on breast cancer risk have been studied extensively. Metaanalyses of the effect of hormone replacement therapy demonstrate small, but statistically significant, increases in risk (relative risks, 1.02 to 1.35) for users.[39,63,64] Risk appears to increase with current use and duration of use. This finding is consistent with studies demonstrating that postmenopausal women with higher concentrations of endogenous estrogen levels have a greater risk of developing breast cancer than women with lower estrogen levels.[40,41] More recent studies have found statistically significant increases in risk in women taking both estrogen and progestin compared with those taking estrogen alone for hormone replacement.[65,66] It is of interest that several more recent studies suggest that breast cancer arising in women on hormone replacement therapy may be histologically more favorable.[67,68] Furthermore, the increased risk of breast cancer appears to be reduced after cessation of hormone replacement therapy and may actually disappear after approximately 5 years.[68]

Overall, there is no convincing evidence of a significantly increased risk of breast cancer in women who have used oral contraceptives.[69,70] Some studies suggest that a slightly increased risk of breast cancer is seen in women who are younger than 35 and who use oral contraceptives, possibly related to duration and/or recency of use.[69,71] Studies of subsets of patients, including those with a family history of breast cancer or a history of benign breast disease, have not produced consistent findings.[72]

LIFESTYLE AND DIETARY FACTORS

A possible relationship between breast cancer and diet has been suggested by the large international variation in breast cancer incidence rates. Studies of immigrant groups suggest that these differences are not due solely to genetic factors.[73,74] Japanese women immigrating to the United States and first-generation American-born Japanese women were found to have an incidence of breast cancer almost equal to that of whites in the same area and considerably higher than that of women in Japan.[74] Because national per capita fat consumption correlates with incidence and mortality from breast cancer, many investigators have sought to determine the relationship between fat intake and breast cancer risk. Kinlen compared breast cancer rates of nuns who ate no or very little meat with single British women who ate regular diets and observed no differences.[75] Breast cancer mortality among Seventh Day Adventists, a group that adheres to a diet low in animal fats, is not significantly lower than expected when compared with the general population.[76] A pooled analysis of seven prospective cohort studies involving 337,819 women demonstrated no difference in breast cancer risk between women in the highest and lowest quintile of fat intake.[77] Furthermore, this study and other more recent studies have also been unable to detect any relation between risk of breast cancer and consumption of specific types of fats.[77–79] Thus, over the range of fat intake seen in western societies, there is no apparent association between breast cancer risk and fat intake in adults. Any effect of fat intake during childhood or adolescence, however, cannot be ruled out based on available data.

Examination of the relationship between energy balance and breast cancer has been more revealing. Data have been consistent for a positive association between birth weight and breast cancer.[13,80] Most case-control and cohort studies of attained height, a variable highly correlated with age at menarche, and risk of breast cancer suggest a positive relationship.[81] Although being overweight during early adult life has been associated with a lower incidence of premenopausal breast cancer,[38,82] weight gain after age 18 is associated with a significantly increased risk in postmenopausal breast cancer.[38,83] The protection conferred by increased weight early in life is thought to be secondary to increased irregularity of menstrual cycles in these women, suggesting their exposure to endogenous estrogens is decreased.[84] The increased risk with weight gain in later adult life has been explained by increased estrogen levels in these women secondary to increased production in adipose tissue.[38]

These findings are also consistent with the possible influence of physical activity on breast cancer risk. A premenopausal woman's level of physical activity, even if moderate, can have an effect on the likelihood of ovulatory cycles and, for this reason, may alter breast cancer risk.[85,86] Furthermore, physical activity influences body fat stores, the principal source of estrogen in postmenopausal women.

Multiple studies suggest a positive association between alcohol intake and breast cancer risk. A large metaanalysis demonstrated a relative risk of 1.1 for one drink per day, 1.2 for two drinks per day, and 1.4 for three drinks per day.[87] Additional data from prospective studies confirm this increase in risk.[88] The effect of alcohol intake, which is associated with increased estrogen levels, appears to be mitigated by high folic acid intake.[89]

Many investigators have examined the effects of specific dietary components on breast cancer risk. Despite the lack of evidence that fiber or individual vitamins and minerals confer any significant protective effect, it appears that a diet high in fruits and vegetables may decrease breast cancer risk.[90,91]

BENIGN BREAST DISEASE

Benign breast lesions are classified as proliferative or nonproliferative. Nonproliferative disease is not associated with an increased risk of breast cancer, whereas proliferative disease without atypia results in a small increase in risk (relative risk, 1.5 to 2.0). Atypical hyperplasia is associated with a greater risk of cancer development (relative risk, 4.0 to 5.0).[92]

Dupont and Page found a marked interaction between atypia and a family history of a first-degree relative with breast cancer.[92] This subgroup of patients had a risk 11-fold that of women with nonproliferative breast disease. The absolute risk of breast cancer development in women with a positive family history and atypical hyperplasia was 20% at 15 years, compared with 8% in women with atypical hyperplasia and a negative family history of breast carcinoma. Proliferative breast disease appears to be more common in women with a significant family history of breast cancer than in controls, further supporting its significance as a risk factor.[94] Of note, however, the majority of breast biopsies done for clinical indications demonstrate nonproliferative disease. In Dupont and Page's study of 10,000 breast biopsies, 69% had nonproliferative changes and only 3.6% demonstrated atypical hyperplasia.[92] No increased risk of breast cancer development has been observed in women with a diagnosis of proliferative disease who have used estrogens after breast biopsies.[93]

ENVIRONMENTAL FACTORS

Exposure to ionizing radiation, either secondary to nuclear explosion or medical diagnostic and therapeutic procedures, increases breast cancer risk. Because of the long latency period for radiation-induced breast cancers, in addition to the increased sensitivity to mutagenic damage in a developing breast, radiation exposure after age 40 produces a minimal increase in risk, while exposure early in life carries the greatest risk. A markedly increased risk of breast cancer development has been reported in women who received mantle irradiation for the treatment of Hodgkin's disease before age 15.[95] Other environmental factors, including exposure to electromagnetic fields and organochlorine pesticides, have been suggested to increase breast cancer risk, but further data are needed before drawing firm conclusions.

MANAGEMENT OF THE HIGH-RISK PATIENT

A woman's risk of developing breast cancer is influenced by a range of factors. There is no formal definition of what constitutes *high risk.* Without question, women who carry mutations in either BRCA1 or 2 or who have a family history consistent with genetically transmitted breast cancer are considered to be at higher risk than those in the general population.[6,22] A second and much less common group of high-risk women consists of those individuals who have received mantle irradiation, usually for treatment of Hodgkin's disease.[95,96] Women with lobular carcinoma *in situ* (LCIS) or atypical hyperplasia on breast biopsy arc also considered high risk. Although a variety of hormonal factors (e.g., early menarche, late age at first full-term pregnancy) affect breast cancer risk on a population basis, these conditions have a relatively small effect on risk for any individual woman.

In approaching women concerned about breast cancer risk, it is important to recognize that many women overestimate their risk of developing breast cancer.[7,97] In one study, respondents overestimated their probability of dying from breast cancer within 10 years by more than 20-fold.[97] A number of studies have demonstrated that overestimation of risk is associated with psychological morbidity and, in some cases, avoidance of proven screening measures.[98,99] Providing women with an accurate assessment of breast cancer risk may have a number of benefits, including allaying anxiety and facilitating treatment decisions[100] (Table 37.2-2).

The first step in determining a woman's risk of developing breast cancer is to take a thorough history, evaluating for the presence of known risk factors. Of these, family history, age, and the presence of a premalignant lesion on previous breast biopsy are probably the most significant. Because of the substantially higher risk of identifying a BRCA1 or BRCA2 mutation in women of Ashkenazi Jewish descent, ethnic background should also be established. It can be helpful to provide women who are concerned about their breast cancer risk with a numeric risk estimate. A number of models for risk assessment are available, of which the Gail model[14,101] and a model developed by Claus and colleagues from the Cancer and Steroid

TABLE 37.2-2. Potential Benefits of Breast Cancer Risk Assessment

Enhanced understanding of actual risk
Improved medical decision-making regarding:
Hormone replacement therapy after menopause
Mammography in women aged 40–49
Tamoxifen therapy to lower breast cancer risk
Prophylactic mastectomy
Possible psychological benefit of accurate risk perception

(Adapted from ref. 100.)

Hormone Study[11] are the most frequently used. The Gail model, which calculates a woman's risk of developing breast cancer based on age at menarche, age at first live birth, number of previous breast biopsies, the presence or absence of atypical hyperplasia, and the number of first-degree female relatives with breast cancer, has been used in the NSABP breast cancer prevention trials. Efforts to validate the Gail model in different settings have produced variable results. In the Nurses' Health Study cohort, the Gail model was found to overestimate breast cancer risk,[102] although, in other settings, it has proven to be more accurate.[103] In the NSABP prevention trial, the Gail model performed extremely well, with a ratio of observed to predicted cancers in study participants of 1.03 (95% confidence interval, 0.88 to 1.22).[104] In general, the Gail model is thought to underestimate risk in women with strong family histories, at least in part because it only incorporates a family history in first-degree relatives. The Claus model, on the other hand, takes into account both first- and second-degree relatives, although it does not include other risk factors. Not surprisingly, the numeric assessments produced by different models may produce discordant estimates.[105] The widespread use of the Gail model as part of the NSABP prevention trials has led to its general acceptance in clinical practice. In communicating model-based estimates to high-risk women, the limitations of these models should be emphasized. Clinicians should also be aware that women who are anxious about their breast cancer risk may continue to overestimate their risk of developing the disease even after receiving individualized counseling.[7]

Although there is extensive literature on breast cancer screening in the general population, there are few data available on which to base screening recommendations in women with inherited susceptibility genes or other factors that markedly increase breast cancer risk. For high-risk women over the age of 40, annual mammography is recommended.[106] The area of greatest controversy is in screening women under the age of 40. An expert panel has recommended that women with an inherited susceptibility gene should perform monthly breast self-examinations, undergo a clinical breast examination once or twice a year, and have annual mammograms beginning between the ages of 25 and 35.[107] The role of more frequent mammograms (i.e., twice annually), digital mammography, or magnetic resonance imaging (MRI) is uncertain. Ongoing studies are addressing these issues.

BREAST CANCER PREVENTION

The identification of risk factors associated with the development of breast cancer has led to an effort to prevent breast cancer in women at increased risk. Numerous strategies have been considered, including risk factor modification, lifestyle alteration, drug therapy, and prophylactic surgery. Only preliminary evidence suggests that behavioral approaches can be used to alter breast cancer risk,[86,108] and, unfortunately, most of the known risk factors for breast cancer are not easily modifiable. Few women would be willing to modify the age at which they have a first pregnancy in an effort to lower breast cancer risk. While early menopause may be associated with lower breast cancer risk, there are adverse psychological and physical consequences of premature menopause. Some investigators have attempted to alter a woman's natural hormonal milieu to lower breast cancer risk, and it is possible that such approaches might have future promise.[109] To date, however, most efforts to lower a woman's risk of developing breast cancer have focused on pharmacologic interventions.

SELECTIVE ESTROGEN RECEPTOR MODULATORS

Adjuvant trials of tamoxifen have demonstrated clear reductions in the development of contralateral breast cancers in women treated with tamoxifen.[110] These data, as well as preclinical evidence supporting a role for tamoxifen in breast cancer prevention,[111,112] led to the development of the NSABP's Breast Cancer Prevention Trial and to various studies in Europe.

The NSABP trial, known as P-1, randomized over 13,000 patients to either tamoxifen for 5 years or to a placebo.[113] To be eligible, women 35 years of age or older had to have at least a 1.66% chance of developing breast cancer over the ensuing 5 years based on the Gail model. Because of the elevated risk associated with age, any woman over the age of 60 was eligible for the trial. Overall, women randomized to 5 years of tamoxifen experienced a 49% decrease in invasive breast cancer, with similar risk reduction seen in women both younger than 50 and older than 50. The benefits of tamoxifen were seen across all patient subgroups (Table 37.2-3) and were highly statistically significant. Despite the high level of statistical significance, the absolute benefit from tamoxifen is of relatively small magnitude, even if one also considers the cases of DCIS prevented by tamoxifen (69 cases in the placebo arm and 35 in women on tamoxifen). To date, the benefit seen with tamox-

TABLE 37.2-3. Incidence of Invasive Breast Cancer in Women Participating in P-1

	Placebo		*Tamoxifen*		
	No. of Cases	Annual Rate per 1000 Women	No. of Cases	Annual Rate per 1000 Women	*Risk Ratio (95% Confidence Interval)*
All women (n = 13,388)	175	6.76	89	3.43	0.51 (0.39–0.66)
Women younger than 50 y (n = 5177)	68	6.70	38	3.77	0.56 (0.37–0.85)
Women 50 to 59 y (n = 4048)	50	6.28	25	3.10	0.49 (0.29–0.81)
Women 60 y or older (n = 3950)	57	7.73	26	3.33	0.45 (0.27–0.74)
Women with history of lobular carcinoma *in situ* (n = 826)	18	12.99	8	5.69	0.44 (0.16–1.06)
Women with history of atypical hyperplasia (n = 1193)	23	10.11	3	1.43	0.14 (0.03–0.47)

(Adapted from ref. 113.)

ifen only applies to the prevention of estrogen receptor (ER)–positive cancers; in P-1, there was no reduction in the risk of ER-negative cancers. While there is reason to believe that the beneficial effects of tamoxifen may extend beyond 5 years,[110] it is unknown to what degree a 5-year course of tamoxifen affects a woman's lifetime risk of developing breast cancer.

The benefits associated with tamoxifen must also be balanced against the potential risks, in terms of both serious toxicities and adverse consequences with respect to quality of life.[113,114] Increases in both endometrial cancer and thromboembolic events were seen in women on tamoxifen, although more commonly in older women (50 and older) than their younger counterparts. Based on these findings, it is thought that tamoxifen may be most beneficial in younger women with an elevated risk of developing breast cancer.[115]

The findings from NSABP P-1 must also be considered in light of two European studies evaluating tamoxifen.[116,117] Both the Royal Marsden Hospital chemoprevention trial and the Italian prevention trial failed to demonstrate a protective effect of tamoxifen. The studies were considerably smaller than P-1 (2494 in the Royal Marsden trial and a total of 5408 in the Italian), and a number of explanations have been offered to explain the negative results. The Royal Marsden trial, for example, may have included a substantial number of women from families with BRCA1 and BRCA2 mutations, and the Italian study results could have been compromised by poor compliance with the study medication. Nevertheless, the European findings provide a sobering counterpoint to the P-1 study. These results, as well as recognition of the limitations of what has been learned from P-1, underscore the need for further research in this area. At present, the need to individualize decision making about tamoxifen in the prevention setting cannot be overemphasized.

Raloxifene, another selective ER modulator, has also been shown to lower the risk of developing invasive breast cancer. In a randomized trial in postmenopausal women with osteoporosis, two doses of raloxifene (60 or 120 mg) were compared with placebo. Treatment with raloxifene not only led to an improvement in bone density and fracture risk, but also appeared to prevent breast cancer.[118,119] Among 5129 women randomized to raloxifene, there were a total of 13 cases of breast cancer, compared with 27 cases among 2576 who were assigned to placebo (relative risk, 0.24; 95% confidence interval, 0.13 to 0.44). Like tamoxifen, raloxifene increased the risk of thromboembolic disease (relative risk, 3.1; 95% confidence interval, 1.5 to 6.2) but did not appear to increase the risk of endometrial cancer. The follow-up of patients on the trial was relatively short (median, 40 months), and women participating in the trial were generally not at increased risk of developing breast cancer (apart from the increased risk associated with increasing age). The NSABP is now conducting a second-generation prevention trial (P-2) in which tamoxifen and raloxifene are being compared directly in postmenopausal women who are at increased risk of developing breast cancer. Until the results of that trial or additional data are available, the routine use of raloxifene to lower a woman's risk of developing breast cancer cannot be recommended.[120,121]

OTHER PHARMACOLOGIC AGENTS TO LOWER BREAST CANCER RISK

Ongoing trials are evaluating a wide range of other agents to lower a woman's risk of developing breast cancer. A randomized Italian study indicated that fenretinide, a differentiating agent in the retinoid family, lowers the risk of contralateral cancers.[122] Unfortunately, symptomatic nyctalopia is a problem for approximately 10% of patients taking this agent.[123] A U.S. Intergroup trial comparing tamoxifen plus placebo versus tamoxifen plus N-(4-hydroxyphenyl) Retinamide was stopped prematurely, making it unlikely that there will be a definitive answer as to whether N-(4-hydroxyphenyl) Retinamide plays a role in a woman's risk of developing breast cancer. Trials involving other differentiating agents, aromatase inhibitors, and vaccines are ongoing, but it is unlikely that there will be any commercially available agent to lower breast cancer risk in the next several years.

PROPHYLACTIC MASTECTOMY

For years it has been assumed that prophylactic mastectomy would lower a woman's risk of developing breast cancer. Since a small amount of breast tissue remains following mastectomy, the level of protection was debated. In a retrospective but rigorously conducted analysis at the Mayo Clinic, Hartmann et al. have demonstrated a 90% reduction in breast cancer risk as a result of prophylactic mastectomy.[124] Most women and their physicians consider prophylactic mastectomy to be an extreme procedure[125]; however, for certain high-risk women, such as those with an inherited genetic predisposition, it is currently an option. Modeling studies have demonstrated that prophylactic mastectomy in women with BRCA1 mutations may result in a modest improvement in survival.[126,127] The decision to proceed with prophylactic surgery should be considered carefully. Unlike many other choices that high-risk women may face, this is one that is irreversible and should not be made without carefully considering all the available options. Women who are considering prophylactic mastectomy with reconstruction should also recognize the potential short- and long-term complications associated with breast reconstruction (see Breast Reconstruction, later in this chapter).

BIOPSY TECHNIQUES FOR SUSPICIOUS BREAST LESIONS

In this section, the various techniques employed to biopsy suspicious palpable and mammographic breast lesions are described. The major techniques used to diagnose palpable breast masses are fine-needle aspiration (FNA), core-cutting needle biopsy, and excisional biopsy. (Incisional biopsy is occasionally used to diagnose large breast masses, but this technique has largely been replaced by the less invasive aspiration or core biopsy.) The advantages and disadvantages of the three techniques are listed in Table 37.2-4. Both FNA and core biopsy are office procedures. Excisional biopsy, with rare exceptions, is an outpatient procedure that can be done using local anesthesia.

The main issue surrounding the use of FNA is the risk of false-negative results. Large series of FNA have demonstrated a sensitivity of 87%, an incidence of insufficient specimens ranging from 4% to 13%, and a false-negative rate of 4.0% to 9.6%.[128–130] Fibrotic tumors, infiltrating lobular, tubular, and cribriform histologies, and physician inexperience have all been found to be sources of false-negative aspirate results.[128,131,132]

TABLE 37.2-4. Biopsy Techniques for Palpable Masses

Technique	*Advantages*	*Disadvantages*
Fine-needle aspiration cytology	Rapid, painless, inexpensive; no incision before selection of local therapy	Will not distinguish *in situ* from invasive cancer; no histologic detail; false-negative results and insufficient specimens occur; requires experienced cytopathologists
Core biopsy	Rapid, painless, inexpensive; no incision; can be read by any pathologist	False-negative results and incomplete characterization of the lesion can occur
Excisional biopsy	Complete histology before treatment decision; avoids false-negative results and insufficient samples; may serve as definitive lumpectomy	Expensive, more painful, and can be evident cosmetically; creates an incision to be incorporated into definitive surgery

False-positive aspirates are extremely uncommon and are reported in fewer than 1% of cases in most large series.[128–132] FNA does not, however, reliably distinguish invasive cancer from DCIS, potentially leading to the overtreatment of gross DCIS.

Core-cutting needle biopsy has many of the advantages of FNA, in addition to which it provides histologic details of the lesion. The accuracy of core biopsy is similar to that reported for FNA, with sensitivities of 79% to 94%.[133,134] Shabot et al.[135] prospectively compared the diagnostic accuracy of FNA and core-cutting needle biopsy in 81 women. The accuracy of FNA was 96%, compared with 79% for the core-cutting needle technique. No false-positive results were observed in any of these reports.[133–135]

Excisional biopsy has been the standard technique used in diagnosing breast masses. This method affords the physician complete evaluation of tumor size and histologic characteristics before selecting definitive local therapy. When an excisional biopsy is performed, an attempt should be made to remove a small margin of grossly normal tissue around the tumor. Kearney and Morrow[136] used such an approach in 239 patients with cancer and obtained negative margins in 95% of cases, thus avoiding the need for a reexcision as part of definitive breast-conserving therapy. Proper specimen handling with inking of the margins facilitates this approach. There is no evidence that a one-step procedure (i.e., biopsy under general anesthesia followed by definitive surgery if positive) is associated with any survival benefit compared with biopsy followed by definitive surgery at a later time.

Until relatively recently, nonpalpable, mammographically detected lesions have been routinely approached by needle-localized excisional biopsy. The most important factor in the success of this approach is how close the localizing needle is placed to the mammographic abnormality. Gallagher et al.[137] reported wire placement to within 2 mm of the target in 96% of cases, allowing excision with a median specimen volume of 6.0 cm, and 96% of the lesions were removed with a single specimen. Specimen radiography is an essential part of the biopsy procedure done for microcalcifications in order to confirm that the calcifications are present in the biopsy specimen. Although nonpalpable masses can frequently be identified grossly at the time of biopsy, specimen radiography is also useful to ensure that the gross lesion corresponds to the mammographic abnormality. Failure to excise the mammographic lesion is reported in fewer than 5% of cases in most modern series.[138–140] When this occurs, persistence of the lesion on mammogram should be confirmed and repeat biopsy undertaken.

Frozen section is generally reliable in the diagnosis of palpable breast masses, but indications for its use in the evaluation of nonpalpable breast lesions are limited. The abnormalities being sought by needle-localization biopsy are usually small and are often histologically borderline and difficult to diagnose on frozen section. Sacchini et al.[141] noted a discordance rate of 12% between the frozen-section diagnosis and the final histologic diagnosis in a study of 403 nonpalpable lesions. Errors in distinguishing atypical hyperplasia from DCIS accounted for most of the discrepancies. Tinnemans et al.[142] had two false-positive results in a series of 297 nonpalpable lesions diagnosed by frozen section, as well as a 3% incidence of false-negative results. Because needle-localization biopsy is rarely undertaken with a plan to proceed to definitive therapy at the same operation, a careful examination of the entire lesion with paraffin sections is generally the more prudent course.

An alternative approach to the diagnosis of nonpalpable abnormalities is the image-guided breast biopsy, using either stereotactic mammography or ultrasound to guide needle placement. The choice of technique is dependent on the visibility of the lesion. In general, ultrasound guidance is more rapid and does not require breast compression, making it better tolerated. Stereotactic guidance is reserved for lesions not visualized on ultrasound.

A review of seven series comparing stereotactic core biopsies with surgical excision demonstrates sensitivities ranging from 71% to 100% for the core-biopsy technique in a selected group of patients.[143] In a series in which core biopsy was performed using automated 14-gauge biopsy devices, sensitivities of 92% to 100% were reported, and insufficient specimens were rare.[144] Extensive experience has been gained with these techniques, and a number of indications for surgical biopsy after core biopsy have been identified. These include lack of concordance between the radiographic finding and the histologic diagnosis, a diagnosis of radial scar, or atypical hyperplasia.[145] Atypical hyperplasia on a core biopsy is associated with DCIS in 30% to 50% of cases,[145–148] while radial scar may be difficult to distinguish from a well-differentiated carcinoma that has elicited a fibrous reaction.

For mammographic abnormalities that are benign, core biopsy is clearly less traumatic and more cost effective than needle localization and excision. For highly suspicious abnormalities (BI-RADS 5), the benefits are less clear. Two studies have demonstrated that, for experienced surgeons, the likelihood of obtaining negative margins with a single operative procedure for excision of nonpalpable abnormalities is the same whether or not a core-biopsy diagnosis of carcinoma is obtained before surgery.[148,149] However, Morrow et al.[148] prospectively evaluated the number of operations needed to complete local therapy in 409 patients with nonpalpable cancer approached initially with core biopsy or needle localization and excision. Core biopsy reduced the number of operations for all types of lesions except when patients were treated by lumpectomy alone. This suggests that for small calcified lesions with a high likelihood of being pure DCIS, surgical excision may remain the diagnostic procedure of choice.

DUCTAL CARCINOMA *IN SITU*

DCIS, also known as *intraductal carcinoma*, is an entity distinct in both its clinical presentation and its biologic potential from LCIS, the other lesion classified as noninvasive carcinoma. The widespread use of screening mammography has resulted in a significant increase in the detection rate of DCIS, and the acceptance of breast-conserving therapy for the treatment of invasive carcinoma has led to changes in the management of women with DCIS. Uncertainty exists as to the proportion of women with mammographically detected DCIS who will develop invasive carcinoma during their lifetimes. This has led to a debate regarding whether all DCIS should be treated as early-stage carcinoma with either mastectomy or lumpectomy and irradiation, or whether some DCIS can be excised and observed.

An abnormal mammographic report of clustered microcalcifications is currently the most common presentation of DCIS. DCIS can also present as a mass or pathologic nipple discharge, or can be identified as an incidental finding in a breast biopsy. In many reports of mammographically directed biopsies, DCIS accounts for one-half or more of the malignancies identified.[140,150]

The widespread use of screening mammography has resulted in a remarkable increase in the incidence (or detection rate) of DCIS.[151] This increase in the incidence of DCIS has been observed in women both younger than and older than 50 years of age, and in both white and African American women. This dramatic increase in the number of DCIS cases has led some authors to suggest that screening results in the detection of biologically indolent DCIS that is unlikely to become clinically significant during a woman's lifetime. The findings that patients with lesions detected by screening have a higher frequency of grade 3 lesions than patients with lesions not detected by screening[152] and that the risk factors for DCIS and invasive carcinoma are similar[153] argue against this point.

DCIS is characterized pathologically by a proliferation of presumably malignant epithelial cells within the mammary ductal-lobular system, without light microscopic evidence of invasion into the surrounding stroma. However, DCIS encompasses a heterogeneous group of pathologic lesions that differ in their growth pattern and cytologic features. At present, there is no universal agreement as to how best to subclassify these lesions. Proposed classification schemes for DCIS have variously emphasized (1) architectural features or growth pattern of the neoplastic cells within the ductal-lobular system, (2) cytologic features of the neoplastic cells, and (3) cellular necrosis, singly and in combinations. The traditional system for classifying DCIS was based primarily on architectural pattern and recognized five major subtypes: comedo, cribriform, micropapillary, papillary, and solid. DCIS is commonly subdivided into the comedo type and the noncomedo type (which encompasses the other variants). This is based on the observations that the comedo type usually appears more malignant cytologically and is more often associated with invasion[154,155] than are the other DCIS types. Classification systems based primarily on architecture have a number of limitations: (1) many DCIS display a mixture of patterns, (2) the correlation between architecture and nuclear grade is not very high, and (3) interobserver reproducibility in the categorization of DCIS lesions by architectural pattern is poor.[156] Several newer systems classify DCIS lesions primarily on the basis of nuclear grade, necrosis, or both, with architectural pattern given secondary or no consideration.[156–160] In 1997, a consensus conference was convened in an attempt to reach agreement on the classification of DCIS.[161] While the panel did not endorse any one system of classification, there was agreement that certain features be routinely documented in pathology reports of DCIS lesions. These include nuclear grade (low, intermediate, or high grade), the presence of necrosis (comedo or punctate), cell polarization, and architectural pattern(s).

A number of biologic markers in DCIS lesions have been evaluated. These studies have generally shown that comedo or high-grade lesions more frequently than noncomedo or low-grade lesions lack estrogen and PR,[162–164] overexpress the HER-2/*neu* (c-erbB-2) oncogene,[162–166] show mutations of the p53 tumor suppressor gene with accumulation of its protein product,[162–167] and demonstrate angiogenesis in the surrounding stroma.[168,169]

Axillary lymph node involvement in patients with mammographically detected DCIS is a rare event. In one series of 189 patients with DCIS, most of whose tumors were detected by mammography alone, none showed metastases on axillary dissection.[170] A National Cancer Data Base review of 10,946 patients with DCIS who had an axillary dissection between 1985 and 1991 demonstrated that only 406 (3.6%) of this group had axillary metastases.[171]

A frequently encountered issue related to DCIS is the identification of small foci of invasive carcinoma, so-called microinvasion. Unfortunately, this term has not been applied in a consistent, standardized manner, and the histologic diagnosis of microinvasion is not straightforward. In the 1997 edition of the *AJCC Cancer Staging Manual*,[172] microinvasion is defined for the first time as "the extension of cancer cells beyond the basement membrane into the adjacent tissues with no focus more than 0.1 cm in greatest dimension" and are staged as T1mic, a subset of T1 breast cancer. The staging manual further states that "when there are multiple foci of microinvasion, the size of only the largest focus is used to classify the micro-invasion" and that the size of the individual foci should not be added together. Given the problems with both the definition and pathologic diagnosis of microinvasion, the clinical significance of this lesion is controversial. The reported incidence of axillary lymph node involvement in patients given the diagnosis of microinvasion ranges from 0% to 20%.[173–179] The management of this condition is discussed in the next section, Treatment Options.

TREATMENT OPTIONS

A variety of local treatments, ranging from excision alone to mastectomy, have been proposed for DCIS. Making comparisons among retrospective reports is difficult because of differences in patient populations, lack of standardization of surgical and radiotherapeutic techniques, and changes in treatment practice over time. Mastectomy is a curative treatment for approximately 98% to 99% of patients with DCIS, whether gross or mammographic.[180–182] Of note, patients with initial biopsies that showed DCIS but who later had invasive carcinoma identified in the mas-

TABLE 37.2-5. Results of Treatment of Ductal Carcinoma *In Situ* by Excision Alone

Investigators	*No. of Patients*	*Follow-Up (mo)*	*Recurrences*	*Percentage Invasive*
Arnesson and Olsen[191]	169	80[a]	25 (15%)	36
Carpenter et al.[192]	28	38[b]	5 (18%)	20
Schwartz[193]	191	55[a]	28 (14%)	18
Silverstein et al.[194]	256	72	38 (15%)	51
Silverstein et al.[194]	93 (margins >1 cm)	?	2 (2%)	—
Hetelekidis et al.[195]	59	96	10 (9%)	40
Fisher et al. (B-17)[190]	391	90	109 (28%)	53

tectomy specimens were excluded from these reports. Recurrences after mastectomy are almost all invasive carcinomas and may present as a chest wall or axillary recurrence or as distant metastases without evidence of local recurrence. Mastectomy is a highly effective treatment for DCIS, but it is a relatively radical approach to a lesion that may not progress to invasive carcinoma during the patient's lifetime. It also seems somewhat paradoxical that a woman with an invasive carcinoma should be able to preserve her breast, whereas the reward for screening and early detection is a mastectomy. The acceptance of breast-conserving therapy for the treatment of invasive carcinoma has led to its use also as a treatment for DCIS.

Treatment of DCIS by mastectomy has not been directly compared with treatment by excision and irradiation, and it is unlikely that such a trial will ever be done. In many cases, the assumption has been made that since these two treatments result in equivalent survival for patients with invasive carcinoma, the same will be true for patients with DCIS. This assumption is flawed, due to the difference in the risk of metastatic disease between patients with invasive carcinoma and those with DCIS. In patients with invasive carcinoma, the risk of metastatic disease is largely present at diagnosis and is not greatly altered by local recurrence in the breast. In patients with DCIS, on the other hand, the risk of metastases at diagnosis is negligible, and an invasive local recurrence carries with it the potential risk of breast cancer mortality. Therefore, the anticipated incidence of invasive recurrence and the results of salvage therapy should determine the suitability of excision and irradiation as a treatment for DCIS. A number of nonrandomized studies are available to address this issue.[183–187] Solin and associates[183,184] reported the results of 268 women with 271 breasts with DCIS treated with excision and irradiation at ten institutions in Europe and the United States. At a median follow-up of 10.3 years, the 15-year actuarial rate of local failure was 19%. It is noteworthy that although the local failure rate in this study was relatively high, the 15-year cause-specific survival was 96%. The methods of mammographic and pathologic evaluation and the extent of surgical resection employed in this study would probably not be considered adequate today (e.g., only 15% underwent reexcision, and margin status was unknown in 120 cases; 46%). In spite of these caveats, this study is noteworthy for the large number of patients and relatively long duration of follow-up, and the low cause-specific mortality is reassuring. An examination of the subset of patients with mammographically detected lesions from this series (n = 110) did not reveal a significantly lower rate of local failure than that seen in the group as a whole,[188] a finding also reported by Hiramatsu et al.[185]

Because one-half of the local failures seen after breast-conserving therapy for intraductal carcinoma are invasive carcinoma, the outcome of salvage treatment of these recurrences is important. In a separate report, Solin and coworkers[189] described 42 cases of local failure in 274 cases of DCIS treated with excision plus irradiation. The median follow-up after salvage treatment was 3.7 years. Nineteen of the recurrences (45%) were DCIS, and 14 of these were detected by mammography alone. All of the women with DCIS recurrences remain free of disease after mastectomy, with a median follow-up of 4.7 years. Five patients with invasive recurrence had developed distant metastases, either simultaneously with the recurrence (one patient) or subsequently (four patients). Chest wall recurrences were seen in three patients who had salvage mastectomy for an invasive recurrence, and all of these women developed distant metastases. Of the entire group of 42 women with recurrence, 36 patients (86%) were alive and free of disease, 4 patients (10%) died of disease, 1 patient is alive with disease, and 1 patient died of other causes. Similarly high rates of salvage have been reported in other studies[190]; however, the ultimate breast cancer mortality resulting from breast-conserving therapy cannot yet be assessed given the available follow-up in these studies.

A number of investigators have also examined the use of excision alone as a treatment[190–195] (Table 37.2-5). Patients treated with this approach are highly selected, usually on the basis of low histologic grade, small lesion size, or both. The percentage of patients with DCIS in the study population meeting these selection criteria is usually not stated, making it unclear how many women with DCIS are candidates for this type of treatment. In general, the results show rates of local recurrence that are higher than that seen with excision combined with irradiation. A 1999 publication by Silverstein et al. suggests that the rate of local recurrence will be low if there is an adequate margin of resection (defined as greater than 10 mm).[194] There are, however, several limitations of the study that are worth noting. First, the group of 93 patients treated by wide excision alone who had margins greater than 10 mm is highly selected. The median size of the lesion was only 9 mm, and only 23% showed comedo necrosis. The patients were cared for by a dedicated team of surgeons, radiologists, and pathologists, and the specimens were routinely handled by total sequential embedding, an ideal technique for assessing margins, but uncommonly used because of its expense. In addition, since these patients were seen more recently in the series compared with the irradiated patients, their follow-up time is shorter, estimated to be approximately 5 years as a median, with many less than 3 years. Therefore, this data set

TABLE 37.2-6. Results of Randomized Clinical Trials Testing the Value of Radiation Therapy after Excision

Trial	*No. of Patients*	*Median Follow-Up (mo)*	*End Point*	*Excision (%)*	*Excision and Radiation Therapy*
National Surgical Adjuvant Breast and Bowel Project B-17[190]	818	90	8-y local recurrence rate	26.8	12.1%; $P<.000005$
			8-y ductal carcinoma *in situ* recurrence rate	13.4	8.2%; $P=.007$
			8-y invasive recurrence rate	13.4	3.9%; $P<.000005$
European Organization for Research and Treatment of Cancer 10853[196]	1010	51	4-y local recurrence rate	16	9%; $P=.005$
			4-y ductal carcinoma *in situ* recurrence rate	8	5%; $P=.06$
			4-y invasive recurrence rate	8	4%; $P=.04$

does not allow the conclusion that the full range of DCIS lesions can be managed by wide excision alone.

To date, there have been two clinical trials with published results in women with DCIS randomized to excision alone or excision plus radiation therapy (RT)[190,196] (Table 37.2-6). Both trials involved patients with DCIS treated with an excision yielding histologically negative surgical margins defined as tumor-filled ducts not touching an inked surface. The NSABP has reported the 8-year results of trial B-17.[190] In this study, 818 women were randomized to excision alone or excision plus 5000 cGy of irradiation to the breast. Eighty percent of the women in the study had tumors detected by mammographic screening. At 90 months of follow up, a persistent reduction was seen with RT. The 8-year incidence of invasive recurrence was significantly reduced from 13.4% to 3.9% by irradiation, and the incidence of recurrent DCIS was also significantly reduced from 13.4% to 8.2%. The European Organization for Research and Treatment of Cancer has reported the 4-year results of trial 10853.[196] In this study, 1010 women were randomized to excision alone or excision plus 5000 cGy of irradiation to the breast. Seventy-one percent of the women in the study had tumors detected by mammographic screening. With a median follow-up of 51 months, a 38% reduction in the annual incidence of ipsilateral breast recurrence was observed in the irradiated group. The 4-year incidence of invasive recurrence was significantly reduced from 8% to 4% by irradiation and the incidence of recurrent DCIS was also reduced from 8% to 5%. The overall survival is the same for the two groups, as is the incidence of distant metastases. Of note, the baseline recurrence rate with excision alone was similar in the two trials, but the reduction with RT was somewhat greater in the NSABP trial (59% reduction) compared with the European Organization for Research and Treatment of Cancer trial (38% reduction). In addition, the local benefit of RT for both DCIS trials is lower than that seen for trials of RT for invasive cancers treated by excision.

The identification of women at high risk of developing invasive carcinoma after breast-conserving therapy for apparently localized DCIS would be extremely helpful. The NSABP has reported the results of two analyses of the pathologic features of 623 of the 824 patients enrolled in protocol B-17.[197,198] In the initial report, moderate or marked comedo necrosis and uncertain or involved margins were associated with an increased risk of local failure. While radiation reduced the risk of failure in all subgroups, the absolute benefit was greatest in those patients at highest risk for recurrence.[197] After 8 years, an analysis of nine histologic features, including margins, histologic type, nuclear grade, tumor size, and comedo necrosis, demonstrated that only comedo necrosis significantly predicted for an increased risk of ipsilateral breast recurrence in multivariate analyses. Breast recurrence was much greater in unirradiated patients with moderate or marked comedo necrosis compared with patients with absent or slight comedo necrosis. The addition of RT eliminated most of the risk associated with this factor, with 13% of those with absent or slight comedo necrosis and 14% with moderate or marked comedo necrosis recurring after RT at 8 years.[198] Margin involvement was of borderline significance, but only a minority of patients had involved margins.

Several studies have suggested that age may influence the risk of local recurrence after breast-conserving therapy. Solin et al.[184] noted a 25% incidence of local failure in patients aged 50 or younger treated with excision and irradiation compared with 2% in patients older than 50, in spite of the fact that nuclear grade, tumor size, and margin status did not differ between groups. The median time to local failure was also shorter in the younger patients (4.9 vs. 8.7 years). Similar findings using a cutoff of 40 years was noted by Van Zee et al. and Fourquet et al.[199,200] Other studies have suggested that a family history of breast cancer may affect the risk of local failure after excision and irradiation.[185,186]

Attempts have been made to incorporate the size of the lesion, its histologic features, and the extent of the surgical excision into a prognostic index that would direct treatment selection. One such index is the Van Nuys Prognostic Index, which assigns equally weighted scores of 1, 2, or 3 for histologic type, width of the surgical margin, and size of the lesion.[201] Lesions with low Van Nuys Prognostic Index scores are said to be suitable for excision alone; those with intermediate scores (5 to 7) require the addition of irradiation; and those with high scores require mastectomy. While such a simplification of the decision-making process is attractive, there are a number of limitations to this index.[202] As noted previously, the latest information from this group now suggests that margin width is the key prognostic factor, with lesion size and histologic type much less important.[194] Until the Van Nuys Prognostic Index is validated, it should not substitute for an individualized assessment of the risks and benefits of the available treatment options for DCIS.

Tamoxifen has been shown to reduce the risk of both invasive and intraductal carcinoma in women at increased risk for breast cancer development[112] and to reduce contralateral breast cancer incidence when used as an adjuvant treatment in women with breast cancer.[203] The initial results of NSABP protocol B-24, in which 1804 patients with DCIS treated by lumpectomy and RT were randomized to tamoxifen (20 mg daily) or placebo for 5 years, have been reported with a mean

TABLE 37.2-7. Results of National Surgical Adjuvant Breast Project Protocol B-24: Addition of Tamoxifen to Lumpectomy and Radiotherapy

	Placebo (n = 902)			*Tamoxifen (n = 902)*				
	No. of Events	Annual Rate per 100 Patients	Cumulative 5-Y Percentage	No. of Events	Annual Rate per 100 Patients	Cumulative 5-Y Percentage	*Relative Risk*	*P Value*
Recurrent invasive breast carcinoma	29	0.77	3.4	16	0.42	2.1	0.53	.04
Recurrent noninvasive breast carcinoma	42	1.12	5.2	37	0.96	4.3	0.85	.46
All first breast cancer events (ipsilateral and contralateral)	104	2.76	13.0	71	1.84	8.8	0.66	.007

(Adapted from ref. 204.)

follow-up of 62 months[204] (Table 37.2-7). Overall, the risk of ipsilateral recurrence of any type (invasive or noninvasive) or of new contralateral breast cancers was reduced from 13.0% to 8.8% at 5 years, a highly significant reduction. These benefits need to be weighed against the potential risks of treatment, which are lowest in patients aged less than 50[201] and those who have had a prior hysterectomy.

The available information on DCIS suggests that, although all patients can be treated with mastectomy, many are candidates for treatment with excision and irradiation, and a smaller group may be appropriately treated with excision alone. When thinking about treatment selection, it is useful to consider (1) the risk for breast cancer recurrence, (2) the risk for an invasive breast cancer, and (3) the risk for dying of breast cancer as well as the patient's perception of the risks and benefits of the treatment options. The available data on breast-conserving treatment (BCT) with irradiation generally show recurrence rates of 10% to 15% at 10 years. Approximately one-half of these recurrences are invasive carcinoma, for a 10-year risk of 5% to 7%. Assuming that the risk of dying of breast cancer is one-third or less the risk of developing an invasive cancer, the risk of breast cancer death with BCT is approximately 2% at 10 years. (If the risk of local recurrence is 5% to 10%, then the breast cancer mortality risk is reduced proportionally.) The risk for death 10 years after a mastectomy for DCIS is 1% to 2%, with nearly all breast cancer mortality seen by that time. In contrast, given the long-term risk of a breast cancer recurrence after BCT, comparisons of breast cancer mortality 30 years after treatment could show greater differences in survival between women having mastectomy and those treated with excision and RT. However, the use of tamoxifen will significantly reduce the risk of invasive recurrence. Whether RT is necessary for all patients with DCIS treated with a breast-sparing approach remains uncertain. Retrospective data indicate that highly selected patients, usually those with small, low-grade (none or slight comedo necrosis) DCIS with widely negative margins, have a low local recurrence rate after excision alone. The effect of tamoxifen on recurrence when RT is not given is uncertain, since this approach has not been directly studied in clinical trials.

While developments in molecular biology may one day allow us to predict more precisely which lesions progress to invasive carcinoma, efforts must now be directed toward minimizing local recurrence in women treated with a breast-conserving approach. The initial step in the evaluation of patients with DCIS is determination of the extent of the lesion. Because most patients with DCIS have nonpalpable mammographic lesions, careful mammographic evaluation before treatment selection is critical. The routine use of magnification views as part of the mammographic evaluation allows the detection of additional calcifications that reduce the discrepancy between the pathologic and the mammographic extent, particularly for well-differentiated DCIS. The goals of surgery are to remove all suspicious microcalcifications and to achieve negative margins of resection. Needle localization should be used to guide the biopsy, and, if the calcifications are extensive, bracketing wires are useful to aid in complete excision. Specimen mammography is essential to confirm the excision of calcifications. In cases in which calcifications are extensive or approach the edge of the surgical specimen (even when the margins are negative), postexcision mammography is useful to confirm the removal of all suspicious calcifications. It is important to recognize that, although DCIS lesions are not clinically detectable, they may be quite large. Morrow et al. found that contraindications to breast preservation were present in 33% of patients with DCIS compared with only 10% of patients with stage I invasive carcinoma.[205] Extensive disease, which could not be encompassed with a cosmetic resection, was the major contraindication to BCT in patients with DCIS.

A detailed pathologic evaluation is also needed and should include orientation and inking of the specimen before sectioning as well as measurement of both specimen and, if present, tumor size. Because accurate measurement of microscopic DCIS is often difficult, reporting the number of blocks in which DCIS is present and the total number of blocks is useful. If DCIS is present on only one slide, then it is useful to note its size. The correlation of microcalcifications with DCIS (i.e., calcifications noted in DCIS, calcifications in adjacent benign breast tissue, or both) and the margin status should be noted. If margins are involved, the extent of involvement should be stated, and when negative, the proximity of the lesion to the margin should be noted.

Clinical trials currently in design or open for accrual in the United States include (1) a randomization following excision to clear margins of 3 mm and tamoxifen to RT or no RT (Radiation Therapy Oncology Group, Intergroup) and (2) trials of wide excision alone (Harvard, Eastern Cooperative Oncology Group).

MICROINVASIVE CARCINOMA

As previously discussed, microinvasive carcinoma has been a poorly defined pathologic entity. Similar to DCIS, it is being diagnosed more frequently because of the increased use of screening mammography.

The limited available data on patients with microinvasive carcinoma suggest that axillary lymph node metastases are infrequent and the prognosis after surgical treatment is excellent.[173–176,178,179,206–208] Because of variability in the definition of microinvasion, results from the literature are applicable to an individual patient only if microinvasion is defined in the same way. Since the incidence of axillary node metastases is low, axillary dissection is not routinely indicated. Survival in patients with microinvasive carcinoma seems to be intermediate between that for DCIS and that for small invasive carcinomas. The use of BCT in these patients should follow the same guidelines for careful mammographic and pathologic evaluation with the requirement for negative margins of resection as for patients with an extensive intraductal component–positive invasive carcinoma.

SUMMARY

DCIS represents a heterogeneous group of lesions of varying malignant potential. Total (simple) mastectomy is associated with a cure rate of 98% to 99% for all types of DCIS. Patients with localized DCIS are candidates for breast-sparing surgery and irradiation. Detailed mammography and careful pathologic evaluation are essential to confirm the localized nature of the lesion and judge the adequacy of resection. The goals of surgery are to remove all suspicious microcalcifications and to achieve negative margins of resection. Excision alone may be an appropriate treatment for selected women with small (less than 1 to 2 cm) low-grade DCIS lesions with clearly negative margins. Axillary dissection is not indicated in DCIS. In women with large high-grade lesions undergoing mastectomy, a low axillary sampling obviates the need for reoperation if invasion is identified. The use of tamoxifen should be considered to reduce the risk of ipsilateral breast tumor recurrence after breast-conserving surgery and to reduce the risk of contralateral breast cancer. A detailed discussion of the risks and benefits of the various options must be undertaken to allow each woman with DCIS to make an informed treatment choice.

LOBULAR CARCINOMA *IN SITU*

LCIS is not detectable on macroscopic examination and is always an incidental microscopic finding in breast tissue removed for another reason.[209] Given this, the incidence of LCIS in the general population is unknown. Reviews of large series of benign breast biopsies done for clinical abnormalities have found that only 0.5% to 3.6% are LCIS.[210–213] LCIS is also an uncommon finding in autopsy studies.[214] In all reports, LCIS is noted to be more common in younger women, with the mean age at diagnosis usually reported to be between 44 and 46 years, with 80% to 90% of cases of LCIS occurring in premenopausal women.[210–213] LCIS is reported to occur approximately ten times more frequently in white women than in African American women in the United States.[215] The frequency with which LCIS is diagnosed is increasing, with one series[216] reporting a 15% increase in the number of cases seen from 1973 to 1988. Although some of this increase is due to greater recognition of LCIS as a pathologic entity, the major factor responsible appears to be the increased number of breast biopsies that are performed as a result of screening mammography. A review[217] of 6287 mammographically generated biopsies showed that LCIS was present in 2.3% of total cases, accounting for 9.8% of mammographically detected lesions classified as malignancies. No specific mammographic findings are associated with LCIS. Several studies have examined the distribution of LCIS in an involved breast and the contralateral breast. Multicentric LCIS is identified in 60% to 80% of mastectomy specimens.[218–220] In addition, LCIS is frequently noted to be bilateral.[211]

In contrast with DCIS, which is heterogeneous in its histologic appearance, the histologic features of LCIS show little variation and are usually easily recognized. LCIS is most often characterized by a solid proliferation of small cells, with small, uniform, round-to-oval nuclei, and variably distinct cell borders. Some cases of LCIS are, however, characterized by larger cells with larger nuclei that show some degree of pleomorphism. LCIS is typically present in the terminal duct-lobular units and distends and distorts the involved spaces. In some instances, LCIS cells involve extralobular ducts. The growth within these ducts may be either solid or pagetoid (i.e., the LCIS cells are insinuated between the duct basement membrane and the native ductal epithelial cells).

LCIS has a low proliferative rate,[221,222] is typically positive for ER,[221–223] and rarely, if ever, shows overexpression of HER-2/*neu*[221,222] or accumulation of the p53 protein.[221,222] In addition, LCIS is characterized by loss of expression of the adhesion molecule E-cadherin.[224] While the diagnosis of LCIS is usually straightforward, there is no sharp dividing line between atypical lobular hyperplasia and LCIS. In some patients, LCIS may involve foci of sclerosing adenosis and produce a pattern that mimics invasive carcinoma. Also, the distinction between LCIS and DCIS is sometimes problematic.[225]

The major issue in the management of LCIS is the risk for invasive carcinoma after a diagnosis of LCIS. Six series[210–213,215,225] with long-term follow-up address the malignant potential of LCIS after biopsy alone (Table 37.2-8). With the exception of one study,[225] the studies show that LCIS is associated with an increased risk for the development of breast carcinoma that is approximately seven to ten times that of the index population. In addition, the five studies with long-term follow-up agree that the risk for subsequent cancer development is equal in both

TABLE 37.2-8. Follow-Up Studies of Lobular Carcinoma *In Situ*

Author	*No.*	*Percentage Invasive Cancer*	*Follow-Up (y)*	*Relative Risk*
Haagensen et al.[211]	287	18.0	16.3	6.9
Rosen et al.[215]	99	34.5[a]	24	9.0
Wheeler et al.[212]	32	12.5	17.5	—
Andersen[213]	47	26.4[b]	15	12.0
Page et al.[210]	44	23.0	18	9.0
Salvadori et al.[227]	80	6.3	5	10.3
Ottesen et al.[228]	69	11.6	5	11.0
Bodian et al.[226]	236	26.0[c]	18	5.4
Fisher et al.[225]	182	3.3	5	—

[a]Percentage calculated for 85 patients with follow-up.
[b]Includes two patients with bilateral cancers counted separately.
[c]Includes ductal carcinoma *in situ* and invasive carcinoma.

breasts. Most carcinomas that develop in women with LCIS are infiltrating ductal, not infiltrating lobular carcinoma.[211,212,227] However, the incidence of infiltrating lobular carcinoma is significantly elevated compared with the 5% to 10% incidence observed among breast cancers in the general population. More recent information about invasive cancer risk associated with a diagnosis of LCIS comes from the NSABP tamoxifen prevention trial.[113] There were 826 women with LCIS in this study, and the average annual rate of invasive carcinoma development among the placebo group was 12.99 per 1000 women. The use of tamoxifen reduced this risk to 5.69, a relative risk of 0.44.

The observations that most women with LCIS do not develop breast cancer, that the risk for breast cancer is bilateral, and that most tumors are infiltrating ductal carcinomas give credence to the hypothesis that LCIS is a risk factor for cancer development. One management option for the woman with LCIS is careful observation, as would be done for any woman known to be at increased risk for breast cancer development due to a positive family history or prior personal history of breast cancer. The use of tamoxifen in women electing observation only is worthy of consideration. An alternative for women unwilling to accept the risk for breast cancer development (approximately 1% per year) associated with a policy of careful observation is bilateral simple mastectomy, usually with immediate reconstruction. Treatment strategies addressing one breast, such as unilateral simple mastectomy with contralateral biopsy, would seem illogical because the risk of LCIS is bilateral regardless of the findings of the contralateral biopsy. The effectiveness of a program of careful follow-up in detecting potentially curable carcinoma in a population of high-risk women is uncertain. A metaanalysis of 389 reported cases of LCIS followed for a mean of 10.9 years reported a breast cancer mortality of 2.8%, although 16.4% of the group developed carcinoma.[229] In contrast, of 391 women treated initially with mastectomy, breast cancer mortality was 0.9%. However, many of these series antedate the use of modern mammography, and uniform clinical follow-up was not used.

Wide surgical excision and histologically negative margins are not needed when careful follow-up is chosen given that LCIS is known to be a multifocal lesion. Similarly, RT has no role in the management of LCIS. When observation is elected, it is recommended that women with LCIS be examined at 4- to 6-month intervals and obtain annual mammograms. Because the increased risk of breast cancer persists indefinitely, observation must last for the patient's lifetime. The choice between careful observation with or without tamoxifen and bilateral prophylactic mastectomy can only be made by the patient who thoroughly understands the risk she assumes. Surgical treatment of LCIS is not an emergency, and detailed discussions of treatment options are important for patients to overcome the confusion often associated with this diagnosis.

STAGING OF BREAST CANCER

Staging refers to the grouping of patients according to the extent of their disease. It is useful in (1) determining the choice of treatment for individual patients, (2) estimating their prognosis, and (3) comparing the results of different treatment programs. Staging can be based on either clinical or pathologic findings. Currently, staging of cancer is determined by the American Joint Committee on Cancer (AJCC), which is jointly sponsored by the American Cancer Society and the American College of Surgeons. The AJCC system is a clinical and pathologic staging system and is based on the TNM system, in which *T* refers to tumor, *N* to nodes, and *M* to metastasis. The current edition, the fifth, published in 1997[172] is given verbatim below. It provides rules for classification, definition of the anatomy, and stage groupings. Of particular note in the 1997 classification are the new changes: (1) the designation of T1mic for invasive cancers with microinvasion measuring 0.1 cm or less in greatest dimension, and (2) the designation of pN1a for nodal micrometastasis (none larger than 0.2 cm).

The many changes in the AJCC system over time and its complexity have limited its use and usefulness. In addition, the current system does not address present-day issues, such as a patient's suitability for BCT or the risk of distant relapse with and without systemic therapy. In practice, most clinicians simply use the tumor size and the histologic findings of axillary dissection, often grouped for convenience into negative, one to three positive nodes, four to nine positive nodes, and ten or more positive nodes.

AMERICAN JOINT COMMITTEE ON CANCER RULES FOR CLASSIFICATION

Clinical Staging

Clinical staging includes physical examination, with careful inspection and palpation of the skin, mammary gland, and lymph nodes (axillary, supraclavicular, and cervical), imaging, and pathologic examination of the breast or other tissues to establish the diagnosis of breast carcinoma. The extent of tissue examined pathologically for clinical staging is less than that required for pathologic staging (see next section, Pathologic Staging). Appropriate operative findings are elements of clinical staging, including the size of the primary tumor and chest wall invasion, and the presence or absence of regional or distant metastasis.

Pathologic Staging

Pathologic staging includes all data used for clinical staging, surgical exploration, and resection as well as pathologic examination of the primary carcinoma, including not less than excision of the primary carcinoma with no macroscopic tumor in any margin of resection by pathologic examination. A case can be classified pT for pathologic stage grouping if there is only microscopic, but not macroscopic, involvement at the margin. If there is tumor in the margin of resection by macroscopic examination, it is coded TX because the extent of the primary tumor cannot be assessed. If there is no clinical evidence of axillary metastasis, resection of at least the low axillary lymph nodes (level 1; i.e., those lymph nodes located lateral to the lateral border of the pectoralis minor muscle) should be performed for pathologic (pN) classification. Such a resection ordinarily includes six or more lymph nodes. Metastatic nodules in the fat adjacent to the mammary carcinoma within the breast, without evidence of residual lymph node metastases are classified as regional lymph node metastases (N). Pathologic stage grouping includes any of the following combinations: pT pN pM, or pT pN cM, or cT cN pM.

ANATOMY

Primary Site

The mammary gland, situated on the anterior chest wall, is composed of glandular tissue within a dense fibroareolar stroma. The glandular tissue consists of approximately 20 lobes, each of which terminates in a separate excretory duct in the nipple.

Regional Lymph Nodes

The breast lymphatics drain by way of three major routes: axillary, transpectoral, and internal mammary. Intramammary lymph nodes are considered with, and coded as, axillary lymph nodes for staging purposes; metastasis to any other lymph node is considered distant (M1), including supraclavicular, cervical, or contralateral internal mammary. The regional lymph nodes are presented here:

1. Axillary (ipsilateral): interpectoral (Rotter's) nodes and lymph nodes along the axillary vein and its tributaries that may be (but are not required to be) divided into the following levels:
   a. Level I (low axilla): lymph nodes lateral to the lateral border of pectoralis minor muscle
   b. Level II (midaxilla): lymph nodes between the medial and lateral borders of the pectoralis minor muscle and the interpectoral (Rotter's) lymph nodes
   c. Level III (apical axilla): lymph nodes medial to the medial margin of the pectoralis minor muscle including those designated as subclavicular, infraclavicular, or apical

   Note: Intramammary lymph nodes are coded as axillary lymph nodes.
2. Internal mammary (ipsilateral): lymph nodes in the intercostal spaces along the edge of the sternum in the endothoracic fascia

Any other lymph node metastasis is coded as a distant metastasis (M1), including supraclavicular, cervical, or contralateral internal mammary lymph nodes.

Metastatic Sites

All distant visceral sites are potential sites of metastasis. The four major sites of involvement are bone, lung, brain, and liver, but this widely metastasizing disease has been found in many other sites.

TUMOR, NODE, METASTASIS CLASSIFICATION

Primary Tumor

The clinical measurement used for classifying the primary tumor (T) is the one judged to be most accurate for that particular case (e.g., physical examination or imaging such as a mammogram). The pathologic tumor size for classification (T) is a measurement of *only the invasive component.* For example, if there is a 4.0-cm intraductal component and a 0.3-cm invasive component, the tumor is classified T1a. The size of the primary tumor is measured for T classification before any tissue is removed for special studies, such as for ERs.

Microinvasion of Breast Carcinoma

Microinvasion is the extension of cancer cells beyond the basement membrane into the adjacent tissues with no focus more than 0.1 cm in greatest dimension. When there are multiple foci of microinvasion, the size of only the largest focus is used to classify the microinvasion. (Do not use the sum of all the individual foci.) The presence of multiple foci of microinvasion should be noted, as it is with multiple larger invasive carcinomas.

Multiple Simultaneous Ipsilateral Primary Carcinomas

The following guidelines are used when classifying multiple simultaneous ipsilateral primary (infiltrating, macroscopically measurable) carcinomas. These criteria do not apply to one macroscopic carcinoma associated with multiple separate microscopic foci: (1) Use the largest primary carcinoma to classify T. (2) Enter into the record that this is a case of multiple simultaneous ipsilateral primary carcinomas. Such cases should be analyzed separately.

Simultaneous Bilateral Breast Carcinomas

Each carcinoma is staged as a separate primary carcinoma in a separate organ.

Inflammatory Carcinoma

Inflammatory carcinoma is a clinicopathologic entity characterized by diffuse brawny induration of the skin of the breast with an erysipeloid edge, usually without an underlying palpable mass. Radiologically there may be a detectable mass and characteristic thickening of the skin over the breast. This clinical presentation is due to tumor embolization of dermal lymphatics. The tumor of inflammatory carcinoma is classified T4d.

Paget's Disease of the Nipple

Paget's disease of the nipple without an associated tumor mass (clinical) or invasive carcinoma (pathologic) is classified Tis. Paget's disease with a demonstrable mass (clinical) or an invasive component (pathologic) is classified according to the size of the tumor mass or invasive component.

Skin of Breast

Dimpling of the skin, nipple retraction, or any other skin change except those described under T4b and T4d may occur in T1, T2, or T3 without changing the classification.

Chest Wall

Chest wall includes ribs, intercostal muscles, and serratus anterior muscle, but not pectoral muscle.

DEFINITION OF TUMOR, NODE, METASTASIS CLASSIFICATION

Definitions for classifying the primary tumor (T) are the same for clinical and for pathologic classification (Table 37.2-9). The telescoping method of classification can be applied. If the measurement is made by physical examination, the examiner will

TABLE 37.2-9. Tumor, Node, and Metastasis Classification of Breast Cancer

PRIMARY TUMOR (T)[a]

TX	Primary tumor cannot be assessed
T0	No evidence of primary tumor
Tis	Carcinoma *in situ*: Intraductal carcinoma, lobular carcinoma *in situ*, or Paget's disease of the nipple with no tumor
T1	Tumor 2 cm or less in greatest dimension
T1mic	Microinvasion 0.1 cm or less in greatest dimension
T1a	Tumor more than 0.1 but not more than 0.5 cm in greatest dimension
T1b	Tumor more than 0.5 cm but not more than 1 cm in greatest dimension
T1c	Tumor more than 1 cm but not more than 2 cm in greatest dimension
T2	Tumor more than 2 cm but not more than 5 cm in greatest dimension
T3	Tumor more than 5 cm in greatest dimension
T4	Tumor of any size with direct extension to (a) chest wall or (b) skin, only as described below:
T4a	Extension to chest wall
T4b	Edema (including peau d'orange) or ulceration of the skin of the breast or satellite skin nodules confined to the same breast
T4c	Both (T4a and T4b)
T4d	Inflammatory carcinoma (see definition of inflammatory carcinoma given previously)

REGIONAL LYMPH NODES (N)

NX	Regional lymph nodes cannot be assessed (e.g., previously removed)
N0	No regional lymph node metastasis
N1	Metastasis to movable ipsilateral axillary lymph node(s)
N2	Metastasis to ipsilateral axillary lymph node(s) fixed to one another or to other structures
N3	Metastasis to ipsilateral internal mammary lymph node(s)

PATHOLOGIC CLASSIFICATION (PN)

pNX	Regional lymph nodes cannot be assessed (e.g., previously removed or not removed for pathologic study)
pN0	No regional lymph node metastasis
pN1	Metastasis to movable ipsilateral axillary lymph node(s)
pN1a	Only micrometastasis (none larger than 0.2 cm)
pN1b	Metastasis to lymph node(s), any larger than 0.2 cm
pN1bi	Metastasis in one to three lymph nodes, any more than 0.2 cm and all less than 2 cm in greatest dimension
pN1bii	Metastasis to four or more lymph nodes, any more than 0.2 cm and all less than 2 cm in greatest dimension
pN1biii	Extension of tumor beyond the capsule of a lymph node metastasis less than 2 cm in greatest dimension
pN1biv	Metastasis to a lymph node 2 cm or more in greatest dimension
pN2	Metastasis to ipsilateral axillary lymph nodes that are fixed to one another or to other structures
pN3	Metastasis to ipsilateral internal mammary lymph node(s)

DISTANT METASTASIS (M)

MX	Distant metastasis cannot be assessed
M0	No distant metastasis
M1	Distant metastasis (includes metastasis to ipsilateral supraclavicular lymph node[s])

STAGE GROUPING

Stage 0	Tis	N0	M0
Stage I	T1[b]	N0	M0
Stage IIA	T0	N1	M0
	T1[b]	N1[c]	M0
	T2	N0	M0
Stage IIB	T2	N1	M0
	T3	N0	M0
Stage IIIA	T0	N2	M0
	T1[b]	N2	M0
	T2	N2	M0
	T3	N1	M0
	T3	N2	M0
Stage IIIB	T4	Any N	M0
	Any T	N3	M0
Stage IV	Any T	Any N	M1

[a]Paget's disease associated with a tumor is classified according to the size of the tumor.
[b]T1 includes T1mic.
[c]The prognosis of patients with N1a is similar to that of patients with pN0.

TABLE 37.2-10. Histopathologic Types and Grades

HISTOPATHOLOGIC TYPES

Carcinoma, not otherwise specified
Ductal
- Intraductal (*in situ*)
- Invasive with predominant intraductal component
- Invasive, not otherwise specified
- Comedo
- Inflammatory
- Medullary with lymphocytic infiltrate
- Mucinous (colloid)
- Papillary
- Scirrhous
- Tubular
- Other

Lobular
- *In situ*
- Invasive with predominant *in situ* component
- Invasive

Nipple
- Paget's disease, not otherwise specified
- Paget's disease with intraductal carcinoma
- Paget's disease with invasive ductal carcinoma

Other
- Undifferentiated carcinoma

HISTOPATHOLOGIC GRADE (G)

GX	Grade cannot be assessed
G1	Well differentiated
G2	Moderately differentiated
G3	Poorly differentiated
G4	Undifferentiated

use the major headings (T1, T2, or T3). If other measurements, such as mammographic or pathologic, are used, the telescoped subsets of T1 can be used.

HISTOPATHOLOGIC TYPE

The histologic types and grades are presented in Table 37.2-10.

LOCAL MANAGEMENT OF INVASIVE BREAST CANCER

This section describes the multidisciplinary approach to the local management of breast cancer by addressing the use of mastectomy, conservative surgery (CS), and RT in a coordinated fashion, as well as by considering the integration of local and systemic treatment.

Modified radical mastectomy is still the most common surgical treatment for patients with invasive breast cancer in the United States.[230,231] The term *modified radical mastectomy* is used to describe a variety of surgical procedures, but all involve complete removal of the breast, the underlying pectoral fascia, and some of the axillary nodes. Whereas the modified radical mastectomy may not seem to differ significantly from the radical mastectomy, it represents a major departure from Halstedian principles of *en bloc* cancer surgery. The switch to modified radical mastectomy occurred when it became recognized that treatment failure after breast cancer surgery usually is caused by the systemic dissemination of cancer cells before surgery, rather than an inadequate operative procedure. In addition, by the 1970s, fewer patients with large tumors with fixation to the pectoral muscle were being seen, making modified radical mastectomy feasible for most women. Two prospective randomized trials demonstrated no difference in survival between patients treated with modified radical and radical mastectomy. These findings were confirmed in two prospective randomized trials.[232,233] Perhaps the most influential of the studies refuting the Halstedian concept was the NSABP B-04 trial.[234] In this trial, clinically node-negative patients were randomized to radical mastectomy, simple mastectomy and nodal irradiation, or simple mastectomy with axillary observation and delayed dissection if positive nodes developed. The failure of this trial to demonstrate a difference in survival between groups was the final proof that the Halstedian concept of breast cancer did not apply to the majority of patients and was a landmark in our understanding of the local therapy of breast cancer. Today, there are few, if any, indications for radical mastectomy.

The strategy behind BCT is to remove the bulk of the tumor surgically and to use moderate doses of radiation to eradicate any residual cancer. The application of this strategy requires an understanding of the extent and distribution of cancer in a breast with an apparently localized tumor. This issue has been clarified as a result of the work of Holland and coauthors.[235,236] In their initial study,[235] mastectomy specimens with unicentric tumors 4 cm or less in size were evaluated using 5-mm sections, radiography of these thin slices, and an average of 20 blocks per specimen for histologic evaluation. Only 39% of specimens showed no evidence of cancer beyond the reference tumor. In 20%, there was additional cancer, but this was confined to within 2 cm of the reference tumor. Forty-one percent of cases had residual cancer more than 2 cm from the reference tumor; of these, two-thirds had pure intraductal carcinoma and one-third had mixed intraductal and invasive carcinoma (Fig. 37.2-1). Local recurrence in the breast

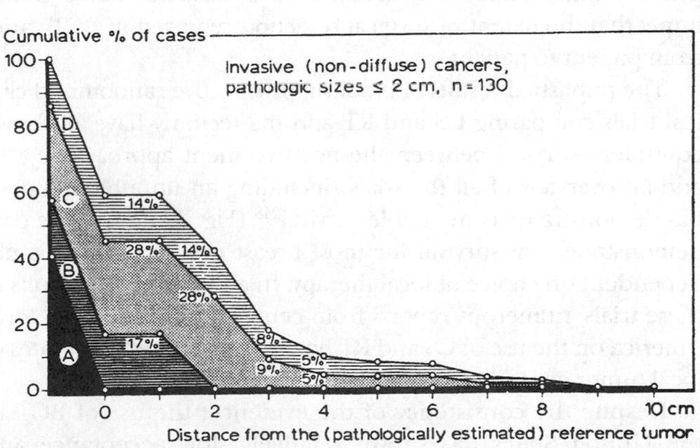

FIGURE 37.2-1. Frequency of additional cancer foci at increasing distance from a clinically unifocal reference tumor. Two hundred sixty-four mastectomy specimens were studied from patients with breast cancers measuring 4 cm or less and judged to be unifocal based on clinical findings. Thirty-nine percent of cases (group A) showed no additional cancer foci beyond the reference tumor. In 20% of cases (group B), additional foci were found but were restricted to within 2 cm of the reference tumor. Forty-one percent of the cases showed cancer foci further than 2 cm from the reference tumor, including 27% in which the additional foci were entirely intraductal (group C) and 14% in which they were invasive and intraductal (group D).

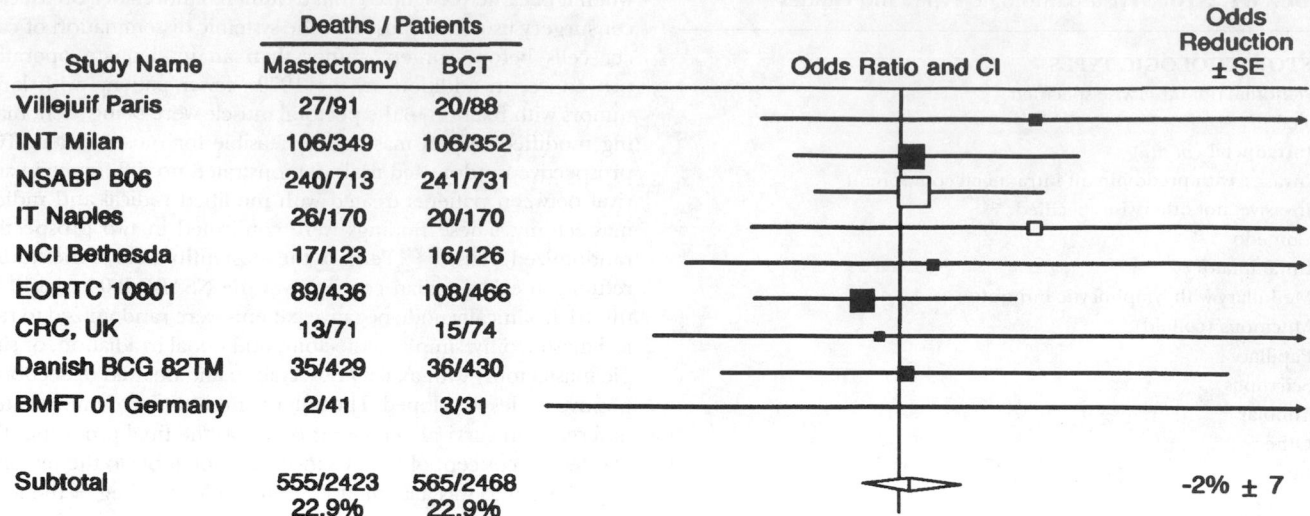

Study Name	Deaths / Patients: Mastectomy	Deaths / Patients: BCT	Odds Reduction ± SE
Villejuif Paris	27/91	20/88	
INT Milan	106/349	106/352	
NSABP B06	240/713	241/731	
IT Naples	26/170	20/170	
NCI Bethesda	17/123	16/126	
EORTC 10801	89/436	108/466	
CRC, UK	13/71	15/74	
Danish BCG 82TM	35/429	36/430	
BMFT 01 Germany	2/41	3/31	
Subtotal	555/2423 22.9%	565/2468 22.9%	-2% ± 7

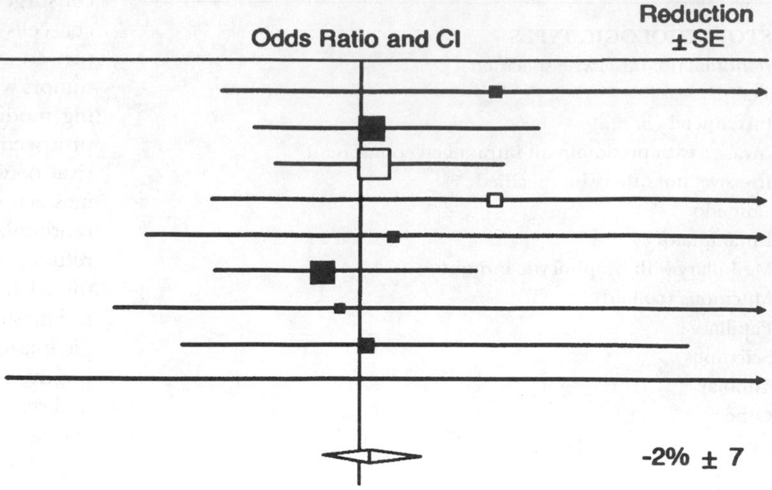

FIGURE 37.2-2. Overview analysis of trials of conservative surgery and radiotherapy versus mastectomy. The squares represent the odds ratio of the annual death rate in the radiotherapy group compared with the control group. The vertical line is an odds ratio of 1, and the 99% confidence interval (CI) is shown by the horizontal line. Squares to the right of the vertical indicate a survival benefit for mastectomy. BCG, Breast Cancer Group; BCT, breast-conserving treatment; BMFT, Bundesminsterium für Forschung und Techologie; CRC, Cancer Research Campaign; EORTC, European Organization for Research and Treatment of Cancer; INT, Instituto Nazionale per lo studio e al Cura dei Tumori; IT, Instituto Tumori; NCI, National Cancer Institute; NSABP, National Surgical Adjuvant Breast Project; SE, standard error. (Reprinted from Anonymous. Effects of radiotherapy and surgery in early breast cancer. An overview of the randomized trials. Early Breast Cancer Trialists Collaborative Group. *N Engl J Med* 1995;333(22):1444, with permission.)

occurs at or near the site of the primary tumor in most cases,[237–240] emphasizing that this multifocal involvement is biologically important. In a subsequent study, the amount of residual intraductal carcinoma was evaluated.[236] Approximately 10% of patients had prominent intraductal carcinoma (defined as a total of six or more low-power fields of intraductal carcinoma) extending more than 2 cm from the reference tumor. These studies indicate that the extent and amount of microscopic cancer in the vicinity of a primary tumor, known as *multifocality*, is variable. These results imply that the extent of surgical resection required in BCT varies from patient to patient.

The published results of modern, prospective randomized clinical trials comparing CS and RT and mastectomy have all shown equivalent survival between the two treatment approaches,[241–247] and an overview of all the trials (including an unpublished one) has demonstrated comparable survival[248] (Fig. 37.2-2). These data demonstrate that survival for most breast cancer patients is not dependent on choice of local therapy. In addition to the results of these trials, numerous reports from centers in Europe and North America on the use of CS and RT have demonstrated high rates of local tumor control with satisfactory cosmetic results.[249–253]

Despite the consistency of the evidence, the use of BCT in the United States has shown relatively slow acceptance and considerable geographic variation.[230,231] Studies indicate that fewer than 50% of women with stage I and II breast carcinoma are treated with BCT.[230,231] The available data indicate that a minority of patients have contraindications to BCT,[254,255] and that these are readily identified with standard clinical tools, such as physical examination and mammography including magnification views.[256] National studies indicate that physicians continue to use inappropriate selection criteria for BCT.[230]

The rates of recurrence in the breast at 7 to 18 years ranged from 7% to 19% in the randomized studies using widely varying surgical and RT techniques.[241–247] In the corresponding patients treated with mastectomy, 4% to 14% of patients developed local recurrence, emphasizing that mastectomy does not guarantee freedom from local recurrence, even in women with clinical stage I and II breast carcinoma. The nonrandomized studies with the longest follow-up describe a persistent risk of recurrence in the breast through 20 years of follow-up.[251–253,257] These results have been contrasted to those seen after mastectomy, in which most local failures occur in the first 3 years following surgery. The annual incidence rate for a recurrence at or near the primary site is constant for years 2 through 7 after treatment, and then decreases to a low level by 10 years after treatment.[253] In contrast, the annual incidence rate for recurrence elsewhere in the breast increases slowly to a rate of approximately 0.7% per year at 8 years and remains stable.[253] Recurrences in the skin of the treated breast are a rare event associated with a poor prognosis.[258] Whole breast irradiation is effective at eradicating multicentric breast carcinoma, but it does not prevent the subsequent development of new cancers.

A number of factors have been identified that influence the risk for local recurrence after BCT. Young age has consistently been observed to be associated with an increased risk of local recurrence after breast-conserving surgery and RT.[259–263] However, young age has similarly been associated with a worse outcome after mastectomy.[264,265] In young women with a family history suggestive of an inherited breast cancer susceptibility, BCT is associated with a higher rate of opposite breast cancer compared with young women without such a family history.[266] This is consistent with the findings of an increased risk of opposite breast cancer in young patients with mutations undergoing mastectomy.[31,267] The rate of local recurrence in young patients with a positive family history is, if anything, lower than in patients with a negative family history. This might be explained by the findings linking BRCA1

TABLE 37.2-11. Recurrence Rates (%) following Conservative Surgery and Radiation Therapy by Margin Status

Author (Institution)	*No. of Patients (Median Follow-Up)*	*End Point*	*Negative (%)*	*Close (%)*	*Positive (%)*
Borger et al.[276] (the Netherlands)	1026 (5.5 y)	5-y actuarial	2	6	16
Dewar et al.[277] (Gustave-Roussy)	757 (9 y)	10-y actuarial	6	—	14
Freedman et al.[278] (Fox Chase)	1262 (6.3 y)	10-y actuarial	7	14	12
Park et al.[279] (Joint Center for Radiation Therapy)	533 (10.6 y)	8-y crude rate	7	7	14[a]/27[b]
Anscher et al.[280] (Duke)	259 (3.7 y)	5-y actuarial	2	—	10
Smitt et al.[281] (Stanford)	303 (6 y)	10-y actuarial	2	16	0[a]/9[b]
Peterson et al.[282] (University of Pennsylvania)	1021 (6.8 y)	8-y actuarial	9	17	11
Wazer et al.[283] (Tufts)	498 (6 y)	10-y actuarial	2	2	15
Pittinger et al.[284] (University of Rochester)	211 (4.5 y)	Crude rate (follow-up, 54 mo)	3	3	—
Cowen et al.[285] (Marseilles)	152 (6 y)	5-y actuarial	—	—	20

[a]Focally positive.
[b]More than focally positive.

and 2 with radiation repair genes,[268,269] or by a greater likelihood of localized (extensive intraductal component–negative) cancers in patients with mutations compared with patients without mutations.[270] However, patients with mutations appear to be at risk for late new primaries in the treated breast.[271] Of note, patients with a mutation do not appear to be at an increased risk for adverse effects from RT.[272,273] Thus, BCT appears to be an acceptable option for patients with a suspected or known mutation, although these patients need to be apprised of the increased risk of a second breast cancer, either in the opposite or, over time, in the treated breast. Many of these patients, particularly those with favorable presentations, elect bilateral mastectomy. A modeling study suggests that bilateral mastectomy may be associated with a modest gain in survival.[127]

An extensive intraductal component has been shown to be an important risk factor for local recurrence when margins of resection are not evaluated.[274] An extensive intraductal component has been found to be a marker for a large residual tumor burden in the involved quadrant of the breast[236,275] such that moderate-dose RT is not able to eradicate it. In such patients, a larger breast resection is commonly required to ensure adequate removal. Results have shown that the microscopic margins of resection are the major selection factor for BCT (Tables 37.2-11 and 37.2-12). Patients with negative margins of excision (typically defined as the absence of either invasive or ductal *in situ* disease directly at an inked surface) have generally been observed to have low rates of local recurrence following treatment with CS and RT.[276–285] In particular, patients with an extensive intraductal component, but with negative inked margins of excision, are not at an increased risk of local recurrence.[279–281,286] The outcome of patients with close margins of excision has been less clear. In part, this reflects variability in the definition of *close margins* and, perhaps, the effect of institutional policies calling for escalated radiation doses based on the proximity of cancer cells to the margin of resection. In the Joint Center for Radiation Therapy (JCRT) experience shown in Table 37.2 12, there was no significant difference in recurrence rates between patients with close margins (less than or equal to 1 mm) compared with patients with margins greater than 1 mm using similar doses.[279] Some studies have suggested a high rate of local recurrence at 10 years in patients with close margins; however, the number of patients in these series and the actual follow-up time is limited.[278,281]

Long-term data on the use of BCT in patients with positive margins are more limited. In most analyses, positive margins have been associated with a high risk of breast cancer recurrence.[276–280,283–285] At the JCRT, patients with positive margins had a considerably higher risk of breast cancer recurrence than patients with negative margins.[279] The 8-year crude rate of breast recurrence was 18% for patients with positive margins. However, patients with focally positive margins (any invasive or *in situ* ductal carcinoma at the margin in three or fewer low-power microscopic fields) had a 14% rate of recurrence compared with a 27% rate in patients with greater than focally positive margins. These data suggest that patients with focally positive margins can be considered for BCT. As discussed in this section, the use of adjuvant systemic therapy results in a large reduction in local recurrence in patients treated with CS

TABLE 37.2-12. Eight-Year Outcome Related to Margins of Resection (Joint Center for Radiation Therapy)

Margin Status	*No. of Patients*	*Percentage Local Resection*	*Percentage with Distant or Regional Failure or Opposite Breast Cancer Resection*	*Percentage Died without Recurrence*	*Percentage with No Evidence of Disease*
Negative	204	7	25	4	63
Close[a]	94	7	28	6	59
Focally positive[b]	122	14	25	7	54
Greater than focally positive	66	27	35	3	35

[a]Any *in situ* or invasive disease within 1 mm of inked surface, but not present at surface.
[b]*In situ* or invasive disease at inked surface, but in three or fewer low-power fields.

and RT. In the JCRT series, among the 45 patients with focally positive margins who received adjuvant systemic therapy, the 8-year local recurrence rate was 8% (95% confidence interval, 1% to 18%).[279] Additional experience is needed to confirm this finding. Patients with more than focally positive margins require more surgery given the significantly higher rate of breast cancer recurrence.

The use of *adjuvant systemic therapy* is an important factor associated with recurrence in the breast when used in conjunction with CS and RT. This is most clearly demonstrated in three randomized clinical trials. In the NSABP B-13 trial, node-negative, ER-negative patients were randomized to chemotherapy or to a no-treatment control group. Among the 235 patients treated with CS and RT, the 8-year rate of recurrence in the ipsilateral breast was 13.4% without chemotherapy and only 2.6% with chemotherapy.[287] Similar results are seen with adjuvant tamoxifen. In NSABP trial B-14, node-negative, ER-positive patients were randomized to tamoxifen or to a placebo. Among the 1062 patients treated with CS and RT, the 10-year rate of recurrence in the ipsilateral breast was 14.7% without tamoxifen and only 4.3% with tamoxifen.[288] A similar result was seen in the Stockholm Breast Cancer Study Group among node-negative patients randomized to tamoxifen or to a placebo.[289] Among the 432 patients treated with CS and RT, the 10-year rate of recurrence in the ipsilateral breast was 12% without tamoxifen and only 3% with tamoxifen.

GUIDELINES FOR PATIENT SELECTION

Based on the extensive information available from prospective and retrospective studies, there is a general consensus on the criteria for patient selection for the use of BCT. It is now established that, in most cases, BCT results in a cosmetically satisfactory breast and that it provides survival rates equivalent to those seen after mastectomy. The American College of Surgeons, the American College of Radiology, the College of American Pathologists, and the Society of Surgical Oncology have jointly provided standards of care for BCT and most recently published their report in 1998.[290] Key portions of this report are summarized here and additional comments are provided in parentheses.

CONTRAINDICATIONS FOR BREAST-CONSERVATION TREATMENT WITH RADIATION THERAPY

Absolute Contraindications

- Women with two or more primary tumors in separate quadrants of the breast or with diffuse malignant-appearing microcalcifications are not considered candidates for breast-conservation treatment.
- A history of previous therapeutic irradiation to the breast region that, combined with the proposed treatment, would result in an excessively high total radiation dose to a significant volume is another absolute contraindication.
- Pregnancy is an absolute contraindication to the use of breast irradiation. However, in many cases, it may be possible to perform breast-conserving surgery in the third trimester and to treat the patient with irradiation after delivery.
- Finally, persistent positive margins after reasonable surgical attempts absolutely contraindicate BCT with radiation. The importance of a single focally positive microscopic margin needs further study and may not be an absolute contraindication (see updated results from the JCRT in Local Management of Invasive Breast Cancer, earlier in this chapter).

Relative Contraindications

- A history of collagen vascular disease is a relative contraindication to BCT because published reports indicate that such patients tolerate irradiation poorly.[291] Most radiation oncologists will not treat patients with scleroderma or active lupus erythematosus, considering either an absolute contraindication. In contrast, rheumatoid arthritis is not a contraindication.[292]
- Patients with multiple gross tumors in the same quadrant and indeterminate calcifications must be carefully assessed for suitability because studies in this area are not definitive.
- Tumor size is not an absolute contraindication to BCT, although few reports have been published about treating patients with tumors larger than 4 to 5 cm. However, a relative contraindication is the presence of a large tumor in a small breast in which an adequate resection would result in significant cosmetic alteration.
- Breast size can be a relative contraindication. Women with large or pendulous breasts can be treated by irradiation if reproducibility of patient setup can be ensured and it is technically possible to obtain adequate dose homogeneity.

NONMITIGATING FACTORS

- The presence of clinical or pathologic involvement in axillary nodes should not prevent the treatment.
- Concern about not being able to detect a recurrence is not a contraindication. The changes associated with recurrence can usually be detected at an early stage by physical examination and mammography.
- The delivery of irradiation to the breast does not result in a meaningful risk of second tumors in the treated area or in the untreated area.
- Tumor location is not a factor in the choice of treatment. Tumors in a superficial subareolar location occasionally may require the resection of the nipple-areolar complex so that negative margins can be achieved, but this does not affect outcome. The patient and her physician need to assess whether such a resection is preferable to mastectomy.
- A family history of breast cancer is not a contraindication to breast conservation. Little is known about the risk of breast recurrence in patients with hereditary breast cancer, but currently this is not a contraindication to BCT. (However, such patients should be apprised of their increased risk of a second breast cancer.)
- A high risk of systemic relapse is not a contraindication for breast conservation, but is a determinant of the need for adjuvant therapy.

CONSERVATIVE SURGERY WITHOUT RADIATION THERAPY

An unresolved question is whether RT is necessary in all patients with invasive breast cancer after CS. Six randomized clinical trials with published results have compared CS alone with CS and RT in

TABLE 37.2-13. Outcome in the Trials Comparing Conservative Surgery with and without Radiation Therapy

		Local Recurrences		*Survival*		
Trial	*Median Follow-Up (mo)*	Conservative Surgery (%)	Conservative Surgery + Radiation Therapy (%)	Conservative Surgery (%)	Conservative Surgery + Radiation Therapy (%)	*Analysis*
National Surgical Adjuvant Breast Project B-06[241]	144	35	10	58	62	12-y actuarial
Swedish[379]	106	24	9	78	78	10-y actuarial
Ontario[294]	91	35	11	76	79	8-y crude
Milan III[242]	52	18[a]	2[a]	No difference		5-y actuarial
Scottish[295]	68	25	6	No difference		5-y actuarial
English[296]	71	35	13	Not available		6-y crude

[a]Estimated from curves.

patients with early-stage breast cancer.[241,242,293–296] These trials vary with regard to patient selection, the details of the surgery and RT, the use of adjuvant systemic therapy, and the length of follow-up. The results of these various trials are shown in Table 37.2-13. These trials all show a large reduction in the rate of local recurrence after RT, with an average crude rate of reduction of approximately 75% (range, 63% to 89%). None of the six trials shows a significant survival benefit for RT; however, in the trials with published data, the survival rate is slightly better for irradiated patients than for nonirradiated patients. A large trial (or perhaps a metaanalysis of multiple smaller trials) is necessary to detect a small, but clinically significant difference in survival, if it in fact exists.

Attempts have been made to identify a subgroup of patients (based on various clinical and histologic features) that has a low risk of local recurrence after CS alone. It was not possible to identify such a subgroup within the Ontario and NSABP randomized trials. Local recurrence rates are generally lower in trials using more extensive surgery than in those using lumpectomy and in older patients than in younger patients. The JCRT attempted to identify such a subgroup in a prospective single-arm trial in which patients with favorable disease were offered the option of CS alone. The criteria for entry onto this protocol were tumor size of 2 cm or less, histologically negative axillary nodes, absence of both lymphatic vessel invasion and an extensive intraductal component in the cancer, and no cancer cells visualized within 1 cm of inked margins.[297] All but one patient had a negative reexcision. This trial was stopped shortly before reaching its accrual goal of 90 patients because of stopping rules ensuring against an excessively high local recurrence rate. The latest analysis includes the results in 81 patients. The median age of patients in this trial was 66 years, and median pathologic size of the cancers was 9 mm. With a median follow-up of 92 months, 19 of the patients have developed a recurrence in the ipsilateral breast, for a crude local recurrence rate of 23%. Based on the results of this prospective study, it was concluded that, even in a highly selected group of breast cancer patients, there is a substantial risk of early local recurrence after treatment with wide excision alone.

The use of adjuvant systemic therapy substantially reduces the rate of local recurrence in patients treated with CS and RT,[287–289] but does not seem to reduce greatly the rate of local recurrence after CS alone. There are no published trials directly comparing CS with and without either chemotherapy or tamoxifen. Information on this is available from indirect comparisons within randomized clinical trials for both adjuvant chemotherapy and tamoxifen. In the NSABP trial B-06, an indirect comparison of the effect of adjuvant chemotherapy can be made. Node-positive patients treated with lumpectomy and adjuvant chemotherapy but without RT had a 12-year rate of recurrence in the breast of 41% compared with only 5% for node-positive patients treated with lumpectomy, RT, and chemotherapy ($P < .001$).[241] In comparison, node-negative patients treated with lumpectomy without RT had a 12-year rate of recurrence in the breast of 32% compared with 12% for node-negative patients treated with lumpectomy with RT. A similar observation, suggesting that systemic therapy further decreases the rate of local recurrence when combined with RT, but not in its absence, is also seen in indirect comparisons within the Milan trials.[242] In the Scottish trial, patients with ER-negative cancers were treated with adjuvant cyclophosphamide, methotrexate, and 5-fluorouracil (CMF) chemotherapy. With a median follow-up of approximately 5.7 years, the crude rate of local regional recurrence was 44% among patients treated with CS, but without RT, compared with only 14% among patients treated with RT.[295]

There is particular interest in avoiding RT in older patients. It is often less convenient for such patients to receive RT, and their local recurrence rate appears lower after CS alone compared with younger patients.[298–300] The results of retrospective studies of CS alone with or without adjuvant tamoxifen have shown variable results.[301–302] The Cancer and Leukemia Group B (CALGB) and other groups in North America have completed a prospective randomized clinical trial testing the value of RT in older breast cancer patients treated by CS and tamoxifen; at this time there are no results from the trial. In NSABP B-21, women with tumors smaller than 1 cm with negative axillary lymph nodes were randomized to tamoxifen alone, breast irradiation alone, or breast irradiation plus tamoxifen. With an average follow-up of 73 months, 24.4% of women in the tamoxifen-only arm had an ipsilateral recurrence, compared to 11.7% of women who received breast irradiation plus tamoxifen. The difference was highly statistically significant. Based on these results, the investigators thought it unlikely that tamoxifen could be substituted for radiation in this patient population.[300a]

In conclusion, the use of breast irradiation after CS is associated with a large reduction in the rate of local recurrence. The available data from the randomized trials do not show a survival benefit; however, none of the available trials has the statistical power to eliminate a small survival difference. A subset at low risk of local recurrence following CS has not been clearly identified, and RT is currently considered standard. The addition of adjuvant systemic therapy to CS alone has not been demonstrated to decrease local recurrence. In elderly patients, particularly those with significant comorbidity, RT is commonly omitted because of the practical difficulties of delivering such therapy in this group of patients.

PREOPERATIVE CHEMOTHERAPY

The successful application of preoperative chemotherapy in locally advanced breast cancer has led to a number of studies in patients with stage I and II breast carcinoma to determine if the use of preoperative chemotherapy would allow breast conservation in patients who would otherwise be treated with mastectomy. Early studies demonstrated a high response rate to preoperative chemotherapy with conversion of patients initially thought to be unsuitable for BCT to be considered reasonable candidates for breast conservation.[303,304] In addition to increasing the number of patients who can undergo BCT, a second goal of preoperative therapy is to improve survival. The available randomized trials suggest that the use of preoperative chemotherapy does reduce the use of mastectomy, but does not improve survival.[305–307] Of note, however, in the NSABP trial B-18,[306] an analysis of breast recurrence rates among patients initially eligible for lumpectomy and those who were eligible only after down-staging by chemotherapy demonstrated a local failure rate of 6.9% in those thought to be candidates for lumpectomy before chemotherapy compared with 14.5% in those who required down-staging ($P = .04$). Similar findings were noted in a trial from France.[308] Further experience is therefore needed to identify down-staged patients who can be effectively managed by BCT. A major practical problem with the use of preoperative chemotherapy to increase rates of BCT is the determination of the extent of residual viable tumor that must be resected. The clinical assessment of response is relatively inaccurate using clinical examination and mammography. Given this, we approach these patients by initially resecting any clinically or mammographically abnormal tissue. If viable tumor is present throughout the specimen, a reexcision is carried out even if the initial margins are negative. If further viable tumor is present in the reexcised specimen, a reevaluation of the patient's suitability for BCT is undertaken. Marking the extent of the tumor before chemotherapy with stereotactically placed clips or skin tattoos is useful for determining the tumor location in patients who have a complete clinical response and may aid in assessing the need for resection of residual abnormalities in patients with a partial response.

The definitive role of neoadjuvant therapy in operable breast cancer remains undefined. There appears to be no rationale, outside of a clinical trial, for its routine use in patients who are suitable candidates for BCT. Initial chemotherapy is appropriate when a large tumor in a small breast would necessitate mastectomy and the patient desires BCT. However, in the study of Morrow et al.,[254] this contraindication to BCT was present in only 6% of 336 patients with stage I and stage II carcinoma. The potential for a higher risk of breast recurrence should be discussed with the patient, and the pathology carefully reviewed before deciding that the patient is a suitable candidate for BCT.

TECHNIQUE AND COMPLICATIONS OF BREAST-CONSERVING SURGERY

The goal of breast-conserving surgery is to minimize the risk of local recurrence while leaving the patient with a cosmetically acceptable breast. The most common form of breast-conserving surgery used in the United States is referred to as *lumpectomy*. The surgical technique of lumpectomy differs from that used for mastectomy in that lumpectomy is not an *en bloc* cancer operation. Quadrantectomy is another type of breast-conserving surgery that is designed to remove an anatomic segment of breast tissue and frequently includes removal of the overlying skin and underlying pectoral fascia. Because excision of a large amount of breast tissue is the major factor responsible for a poor cosmetic outcome after BCT, lumpectomy is considered the appropriate initial surgical approach in the United States. Other surgical factors that influence the cosmetic appearance are the size and placement of the incision, the management of the lumpectomy cavity, and the extent of axillary dissection.

A number of technical aspects of lumpectomy are worth emphasizing. In general, the incision should be placed directly over the area of the tumor. This is true even when a biopsy is performed for a mammographically detected lesion. In the upper part of the breast, incisions should be curvilinear or transverse and follow the natural skin creases (Langer's lines) of the breast. In the lower part of the breast, the choice of a curvilinear or radial incision depends on the contour of the patient's breast, the distance from the skin to the tumor, and the amount of breast tissue to be resected. It is not necessary to remove skin (except for superficial tumors) or to remove needle tracks from core-needle biopsies or FNAs. Preservation of the subcutaneous fat and the avoidance of thin skin flaps is also important in maintaining normal breast contour. Raising flaps is necessary only to allow access to the tumor. Meticulous hemostasis is important because a large hematoma distorts the appearance of the breast and makes reexcision and follow-up evaluation more difficult. The presence of a postbiopsy hematoma, however, is not a contraindication to BCT. It is best to avoid reapproximation of the breast tissue since this can result in distortion of the breast contour, which may not be apparent with the patient supine on the operating table. The best cosmetic results usually are obtained by allowing the lumpectomy cavity to fill in with serum and fibrin. Drainage of the lumpectomy cavity should be avoided. Finally, the incision should be closed with a subcuticular suture to avoid cross-hatching of the skin.

A critical step in lumpectomy is the evaluation of the completeness of excision of the tumor. To allow adequate histologic evaluation, the specimen should be removed as a single piece of tissue and should not be transected unless the pathologist is present. The use of marking sutures to orient the specimen for the pathologist allows reporting of the status of individual margins. Gross inspection of the specimen in the operating room allows identification of positive or close margins, facilitating immediate reexcision. Frozen-section histologic study is sometimes useful to evaluate grossly suspicious areas, but the routine use of frozen sections to evaluate grossly normal margins is of doubtful value. The ideal amount of grossly normal breast tissue around the tumor that should be resected as part of a lumpectomy is uncertain. A resection of 0.5 to 1.0 cm of grossly normal breast tissue results in histologically negative margins in a large percentage of patients.[136] Larger resections may be necessary for invasive ductal carcinomas with an extensive intraductal component[309] and for infiltrating lobular carcinomas.[310]

When axillary dissection is performed as part of breast-conserving surgery, a separate incision should be used, except in patients with tumors high in the tail of the breast. A curvilinear incision at the edge of the hair-bearing axillary skin provides the best cosmetic result. The incision should not extend anterior to the fold of the pectoralis major or posterior to the latissimus dorsi.

The primary indications for a reexcision are positive or unknown histologic margins of resection on the initial excision. Several studies have demonstrated residual carcinoma in approximately one-half of cases when reexcision is performed for positive or unknown margins.[308,311] No consensus exists on the best technique for reexcision. When reexcision is done within 1 to 2 weeks of the biopsy, it is not usually possible to reexcise an entire biopsy cavity as a single specimen without sacrificing large amounts of breast tissue. One author's (M. M.) technique of reexcision in most cases is to reexcise each of the walls of the biopsy cavity separately. If the initial specimen is marked with orienting sutures, reexcision can be limited to the involved margins. Otherwise, thin pieces of tissue are shaved off each wall of the biopsy cavity and sent as separate specimens, with the new margin surface marked for the pathologist. When longer intervals have elapsed between the biopsy and the time of reexcision, contraction of the biopsy cavity may allow excision of the entire cavity as a single specimen without sacrificing excessive amounts of breast tissue. The status of the final margin should be used to determine the patient's suitability for BCT. Kearney and Morrow[136] found that 86 of 90 patients undergoing reexcision for positive or unknown margins were satisfactory candidates for BCT.

There are relatively few complications of breast-conserving surgery. Wound infection is infrequent, although rates of infection may be increased when reexcision is performed. The late occurrence of breast abscess after BCT has been reported.[312] The median time to abscess development was 5 months (range, 1.5 to 8.0 months). The only factor found to correlate with abscess formation was larger size of the lumpectomy specimen. Cellulitis of the breast occurring at a median of 4 months after BCT also has been reported in approximately 3% of cases.[313]

TECHNIQUE AND COMPLICATIONS OF MASTECTOMY

Modified radical mastectomy involves the complete removal of the breast tissue, the underlying fascia of the pectoralis major muscle, and the removal of some of the axillary lymph nodes. Modified radical mastectomy is performed through an elliptical transverse incision, which encompasses the nipple-areola complex and the biopsy scar if an open biopsy has been performed. The nipple-areola complex and the biopsy incision must be removed, but the remainder of the skin of the breast can be preserved in early-stage breast cancer if needed for breast reconstruction. With a skin-sparing procedure, additional exposure to allow complete excision of the breast tissue is achieved by incision rather than excision of the skin. Skin flaps are created in the plane between the subcutaneous fat and the underlying breast tissue. Because of the variability in the amount of subcutaneous fat, no single thickness is appropriate for all skin flaps. To encompass all breast tissue, the dissection should extend superiorly to the inferior border of the clavicle, medially to the lateral border of the sternum, inferiorly to the superior extent of the rectus sheath, and laterally to the latissimus dorsi muscle. The fascia of the pectoralis major muscle can safely be preserved when needed for breast reconstruction. In general, however, excision posterior to the fascia provides a convenient plane for ensuring removal of most of the breast tissue. With the breast attached inferiorly and laterally, axillary dissection is carried out. Closed suction drains are then placed in the apex of the axilla and beneath the inferior skin flap. Skin closure is accomplished with a subcuticular suture. Pressure dressings are not needed with suction drains and may compromise blood supply.

The term *total mastectomy* refers to the removal of the entire breast including the axillary tail of Spence, with preservation of both pectoral muscles and the axillary nodes. The indications for total mastectomy include (1) patients with DCIS who elect mastectomy, (2) patients undergoing prophylactic surgery to prevent the development of breast cancer, (3) patients who develop a recurrence in the breast after BCT that had included an axillary dissection, and, on rare occasion, (4) patients with metastatic disease undergoing mastectomy for local control of the primary tumor.

Mastectomy is an extremely safe operative procedure.[314] For patients with serious comorbid conditions who are at an unacceptably high risk for general anesthesia, mastectomy can be done using a combination of local anesthesia, intercostal blocks, and intravenous sedation. The reported incidence rate of wound infection with mastectomy ranges from 6% to 14%.[315,316] The most common organisms are streptococcus or *Staphylococcus aureus*.[316] Factors that predispose to infection include the use of a two-step procedure (i.e., open biopsy preceding mastectomy) and prolonged suction catheter drainage.[316,317] A single dose of antibiotics (86% cephalosporin) has been shown to reduce the incidence of wound infection by 38%.[318,319] However, because the overall incidence of infection in these patients is so low, the cost effectiveness of routine antibiotic prophylaxis for all patients undergoing mastectomy has not been established. A selective policy of antibiotic administration to high-risk patients (e.g., prior biopsy, anticipation of long operating time) seems to be most appropriate. Necrosis of the skin flaps is a relatively uncommon problem today, but was reported in 8% to 60% of cases, particularly in earlier series of patients undergoing radical mastectomy.[320,321] Factors associated with skin-flap necrosis include denuding the subcutaneous fat from the flaps, closure under tension, infection, and use of a vertical incision and occlusive pressure dressings.[315,316,322] Skin incisions should be planned to allow tension-free closure. Pressure dressings are not necessary when suction drains are used, and suspected cellulitis should be promptly treated with antibiotics. Seroma formation occurs in 100% of patients after mastectomy and should be considered a side effect, rather than a complication, of the procedure. Prolonged lymphatic drainage after mastectomy is primarily related to extensive node involvement followed by obesity and the performance of a two-step procedure.[323] Prolonged seroma formation, in addition to requiring multiple physician visits, may be associated with delayed wound healing and an increased risk of infection.[315,316,320] Seroma formation can be minimized by leaving drains in place until their combined output is less than 40 mL/24 hours. Fluid collections should be managed by aspiration every other day. Some advocated the use of tacking sutures to obliterate the axillary dead space and attach the skin flaps to the pectoral muscle,[321] but this has not been established. Phantom breast syndrome has been long recognized.[324] In one prospective study,[325] phantom pain was reported in 13% of patients at 3 weeks, and nonpainful phantom sensations were present in an additional 15%. Similar incidences were seen at 1 year and at 6 years. The cause of this syndrome is unknown.

ONCOLOGIC CONSIDERATIONS IN IMMEDIATE RECONSTRUCTION

The switch from radical mastectomy to modified radical mastectomy and advances in plastic surgical technique have made immediate breast reconstruction an option for most patients who undergo mastectomy. A number of concerns about immediate reconstruction have been raised and the available information addressing these concerns comes from retrospective studies. The incidence of local failure in patients undergoing breast reconstruction appears to be comparable with patients treated by mastectomy alone.[326–328] Similarly, the ability to detect local recurrence does not appear altered by immediate reconstruction.[329–331] There is, however, a greater risk of problems in patients undergoing immediate reconstruction who require postmastectomy RT, specifically among patients receiving implants.[332,333] This includes patients in whom the implants are placed beneath latissimus dorsi or transverse rectus abdominis myocutaneous (TRAM) flaps. In contrast, patients reconstructed with the TRAM flap without an implant appear to tolerate postoperative RT better.[334,335] Immediate reconstruction does create technical problems in the administration of RT. With immediate reconstruction, it can be more difficult to treat the internal mammary nodes and to boost the chest wall. Communication before mastectomy between the surgeon and the radiation oncologist is useful to make decisions on an individual basis. In summary, immediate breast reconstruction has not been shown to increase the incidence of local failure or impede the detection of local recurrence. In the hands of an experienced reconstructive surgeon, the incidence of complications associated with the procedure is low, and the need for postoperative systemic therapy should not be considered a contraindication to immediate reconstruction. In patients with larger tumors or clinically positive nodes, in whom there is a high likelihood that postoperative chest wall RT will be administered, it may be prudent to avoid implant reconstruction or forego immediate reconstruction altogether.

INDICATIONS FOR POSTOPERATIVE RADIATION THERAPY

Postoperative RT refers to the use of irradiation to the chest wall and draining lymph node regions as an adjuvant treatment after mastectomy. Postoperative RT has been clearly shown to reduce the rate of local regional tumor recurrence (i.e., recurrence on the chest wall or in the axillary, internal mammary, or supraclavicular lymph nodes) by treating residual microscopic disease that has spread beyond the margin of surgical resection. In the absence of postoperative RT, there is a substantial risk of local recurrence after modified radical (or even radical) mastectomy, principally related to the presence and extent of axillary nodal involvement. If axillary nodes are involved, local recurrence is seen in 10% to 30% of patients, whereas if axillary nodes are uninvolved, local recurrence is seen in only approximately 5% of patients.[336,337] Once a local recurrence is clinically manifest, it can be effectively controlled in only approximately one-half of patients.[338–340] Therefore, postoperative RT can benefit high-risk patients simply by preventing local recurrence.

Despite the clear-cut improvement in local control with adjuvant RT,[341] its effect on survival remains controversial. Assessing the survival value of postoperative RT requires evaluation within large, prospective randomized clinical trials. There are six published trials in which patients were randomized after radical, modified radical, or total mastectomy to postoperative RT or no further treatment in the absence of systemic therapy.[342–351] Some of these are among the earliest clinical trials performed in medicine. In many of these trials, RT was given using orthovoltage equipment and in most trials techniques were used that delivered considerable doses to the heart and are now considered outmoded. Despite this, the use of postoperative RT clearly reduced the incidence of local recurrence, but none of these trials demonstrated a clear-cut improvement in the survival rate. In addition, some of these trials showed a late increase in cardiac mortality in patients treated with RT compared with unirradiated patients.[342,343] The most modern of these trials was conducted at the Radiumhemmet in Stockholm between 1971 and 1976.[345,346] In this trial, 644 patients with operable breast cancer were treated with modified radical mastectomy and randomized to postoperative RT or no further treatment. With a median follow-up time of 16 years, node-negative patients had a decreased rate of local recurrence with postoperative RT, but there was no effect on distant metastases or survival. For node-positive patients, the use of postoperative RT was associated with not only a decrease in local recurrence, but also a decrease in distant metastasis ($P=$ .02). An overview of randomized trials of postoperative RT after mastectomy with or without axillary dissection showed no difference in survival when patients treated with RT were compared with those treated without RT over the first 10 years after surgery.[352] After 10 years, however, there was a lower rate of survival associated with the use of RT, but this was not statistically significant. When cause-specific mortality data were examined, there was an excess of cardiac deaths among patients treated with RT, but this was offset by a reduced number of deaths from breast cancer, especially in the more recent trials. An overview reanalysis published in 2000 showed similar results.[353] These studies suggest that if increased cardiovascular mortality associated with adjuvant irradiation can be avoided by the use of appropriate techniques, a benefit in survival will be seen.

There are a number of studies that have examined the rate of local recurrence in patients treated with mastectomy and adjuvant chemotherapy, but without RT.[354–357] In the largest of these, the rate of local recurrence in 2016 node-positive patients entered into Eastern Cooperative Oncology Group adjuvant systemic therapy trials was examined.[356] The 10-year rate of local regional recurrence (with or without simultaneous distant failure) was 12.9% for patients with one to three positive nodes and 28.7% with greater than or equal to four positive nodes. Similar results are observed in the other studies.[354,355,357] These studies, as well as the trials described here, demonstrate a moderate risk of local regional recurrence in node-positive patients treated with mastectomy and adjuvant systemic therapy, particularly when four or more nodes are involved.

A number of studies have examined the issue of adding postoperative RT to adjuvant chemotherapy (Table 37.2-14).[357–367] The two largest of these are from the Danish Breast Cancer Cooperative Group (DBCG). In DBCG trial 82b, 1708 premenopausal patients who had undergone mastectomy for pathologic stage II or III breast cancer were randomly assigned to eight cycles of CMF plus local regional RT or to nine cycles of CMF alone.[357]

TABLE 37.2-14. Randomized Trials Testing the Value of Postoperative Radiation Therapy Used in Conjunction with Adjuvant Systemic Therapy

Trial	*Treatment Arms*	*Patients*	*Years*	*Type Radiation Dose (Gy)/Fractions*	*Follow-Up (y)*	*Survival Rate (%)*
Dana-Farber Cancer Institute/Joint Center for Radiation Therapy[360]	CT	100	1974–1984	Supervoltage	5	72
	CT + RT	106		45/20		66
Southeastern Cancer Study Group[361]	CMF × 6[a]	133	1976–1981	Supervoltage	10	36[b]
	CMF × 12[a]	61		50/5 wk		22[b]
	RT + CMF × 6[a]	137				43[b]
Danish Breast Cancer Group[357]	CMF	856	1982–1989	Supervoltage	10	45
	CMF + RT	852		48–50/22–25		54
Danish Breast Cancer Group[358]	Tam	689	1982–1990	Supervoltage	10	36
	Tam + RT	686		48–50/22–25		45
Mayo Clinic[362]	L-PAM	85	1973–1980	Supervoltage	5	56
	CFP	112		50/24[c]		66
	RT + CFP	115				68
Piedmont Oncology[363]	L-PAM	43	1977–?	Supervoltage	10	47
	L-PAM + RT	33		45–50/30		60
	CMF	44				58
	CMF + RT	39				46
Glasgow[364]	RT	103	1976–1982	Orthovoltage	5	59[d]
	RT + CMF	111		37.8/15		68[d]
	CMF	108				63[d]
British Columbia[359]	CMF	154	1979–1986	Supervoltage	15	46
	CMF + RT	164		37.5/16		54
Helsinki[365]	CAFt	52	1981–1984	?	8	69
	RT	50		45/15		55
	CAFt + RT	47				65
	CAFt + RT + Tam	50				67
M. D. Anderson Cancer Center[366]	FAC[e]	54	1978–1980	?	3	69[f]
	FAC + RT[e]	43		?		64[f]
South Sweden[367] (premenopausal)	RT	147	1978–1985	Supervoltage	8	62 (both RT groups)[g]
	RT + C	148		38/20		
	C	139				45[g]
South Sweden[367] (postmenopausal)	RT	236	1978–1985	Supervoltage	8	36 (both RT groups)[g]
	RT + Tam	239		38/20		
	Tam	244				54[g]

C, cyclophosphamide; CAFt, cyclophosphamide, doxorubicin, ftorafur; CFP, cyclophosphamide, 5-fluorouracil, prednisone; CMF, cyclophosphamide, methotrexate, 5-fluorouracil; CT, chemotherapy with L-PAM (L-phenylalanine mustard) or CMF; FAC, fluorouracil, Adriamycin, cyclophosphamide; RT, radiation therapy; Tam, tamoxifen.
[a] >4 positive nodes.
[b] Percentage estimated from curves.
[c] Treatment was delivered in two 12-d blocks separated by a 4-wk interval.
[d] Disease-related mortality.
[e] All patients were randomized to receive FAC with or without bacille Calmette-Guérin.
[f] Disease-free survival (not survival rate).
[g] Median survival (mo).

With a median follow-up of 114 months, the 10-year rate of local regional recurrence was reduced from 32% to 9% with RT, and overall survival was improved from 45% to 54% with RT (both P values <.01) (Fig. 37.2-3). In DBCG trial 82c, 1375 postmenopausal patients who had undergone mastectomy for pathologic stage II or III breast cancer were randomly assigned to tamoxifen for 1 year plus local regional RT or to tamoxifen alone.[358] With a median follow-up time of 123 months, the 10-year rate of local regional recurrence was reduced from 35% to 8% with RT, and overall survival was improved from 36% to 45% with RT (both P values <.05) (Fig. 37.2-4). In a smaller trial from British Columbia, 318 node-positive premenopausal patients treated with modified radical mastectomy were similarly randomized to adjuvant CMF chemotherapy and postoperative RT or to chemotherapy alone. The results of the British Columbia trial were similar to those of the DBCG trial 82b.[359] Of note, the magnitude of the improvement seen in these trials is similar to that seen with adjuvant systemic therapy (chemotherapy, hormonal therapy, or both) and suggests that all node-positive patients should receive postmastectomy RT. A metaanalysis published in 2000 showed a survival benefit for local regional RT in node-positive women treated with modified radical mastectomy and adjuvant systemic therapy.[368]

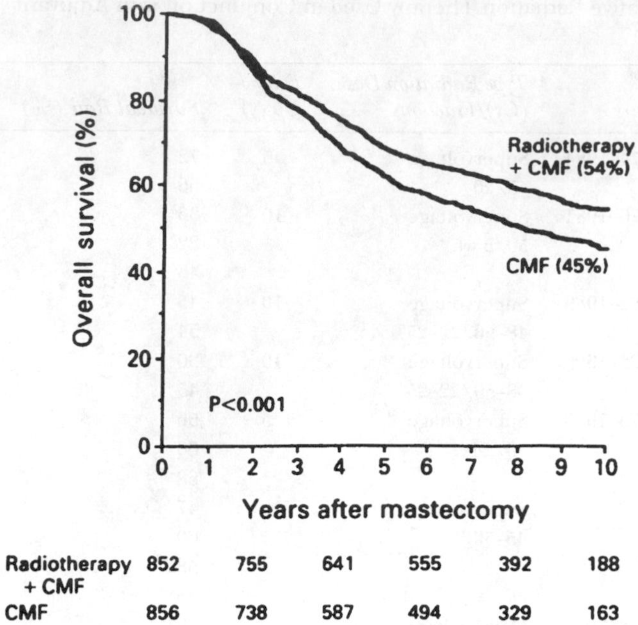

FIGURE 37.2-3. Survival results in the Danish Breast Cancer Cooperative Group trial 82b comparing cyclophosphamide, methotrexate, and 5-fluorouracil (CMF) chemotherapy and radiation therapy with chemotherapy alone in premenopausal patients treated with mastectomy.

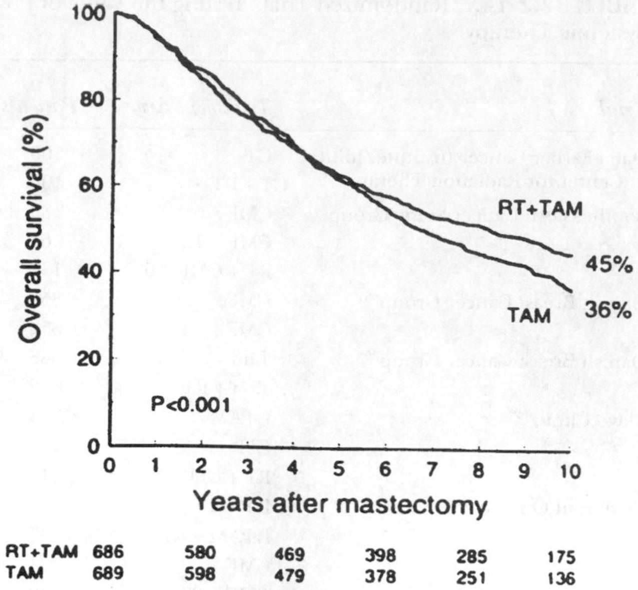

FIGURE 37.2-4. Survival results in the Danish Breast Cancer Cooperative Group trial 82c comparing tamoxifen (TAM) and radiation therapy (RT) with tamoxifen alone in postmenopausal patients treated with mastectomy.

For a number of reasons, however, these trials have not resulted in the universal use of postoperative RT in node-positive patients, particularly those with only one to three positive nodes. One reason is that the worldwide overview of all trials of postoperative RT only shows a small, but not statistically significant survival benefit.[344] A more substantial reason relates to the issue of generalizing from these results due to differing surgical and systemic treatments. The extent of axillary surgery performed in these trials was less than that performed in the United States, and the rates of local regional recurrence, especially axillary recurrences, observed in the Danish trials were greater than observed in U.S. series. In particular, as noted previously, series of patients with one to three positive nodes treated by modified radical mastectomy and adjuvant chemotherapy from the United States show rates of local regional recurrence in the range of 10%,[352–356] compared with approximately 30% in the two Danish trials. Also, systemic therapy in the Danish trials may have been suboptimal by current standards. What seems clear is that these trials address an important principle about the value of establishing local regional control in the presence of systemic therapy. Without detracting from the importance or validity of the principle, it is legitimate to question the clinical implications of these results for practice in the United States. The final reason for the failure of these trials to translate directly into clinical practice is the concern about long-term complications of postoperative RT, especially late cardiac mortality. This is especially relevant in patients receiving chemotherapy with potential cardiac toxicity, such as doxorubicin (Adriamycin). To address the issues raised by the available data on postoperative RT, the American Society of Therapeutic Radiology and Oncology sponsored a symposium on postoperative RT and invited a panel to hear the latest information on this topic and to develop a Consensus Summary Statement. The panel was composed of three radiation oncologists, a medical oncologist, a surgical oncologist, and a consumer activist.

The panel agreed to the statements outlined in the next sections.[369]

Patient Selection

Postoperative RT may be given to improve local control or to improve survival. Patients with four or more positive lymph nodes should receive postoperative RT to improve local control. There may also be a survival benefit in these patients. The data regarding patient selection for survival advantage are less clear, but the most recent evidence suggests that the greatest survival benefit is seen in node-positive patients with low tumor burdens (i.e., fewer positive nodes or smaller tumors). Radiation therapy in these patients for survival benefit is worthy of consideration, pending more definitive data. To establish the survival benefit of postoperative RT in patients with one to three positive nodes, a large randomized clinical trial should be performed. (Such a large Intergroup trial was subsequently approved.)

Technique

Although both recent trials demonstrating a survival benefit with postoperative RT included treatment to the chest wall, axilla, supraclavicular area, and the internal mammary nodes, there is controversy about what sites require treatment. In all patients, the chest wall should be treated. The value of including the internal mammary nodes is uncertain and is currently being studied in a large European randomized controlled trial. In patients with positive axillary nodes, the internal mammary nodes are known to be also involved in approximately 30% of cases. Treatment of this area is, therefore, worthy of serious consideration, provided that it can be done with acceptable morbidity. Following a level I and II axillary dissection, the use of a third field to treat the axillary apex and supraclavicular area is appropriate for selected node-positive patients, particularly those with four or more positive nodes. A posterior axillary radiation field is not routinely indicated after a level I and II axillary dissection. However, if there is concern about the completeness of surgery, the addition of a posterior axillary field may be appropriate. Careful attention must be paid to the morbidity of treatment. In particular, postoperative RT has the potential to cause late cardiac mortality in patients with left-sided cancers. Therefore, the amount of heart (and also lung) in the treatment field must be minimized and documented. Computed tomographic (CT) treatment planning is useful in accomplishing this goal.

COMPLICATIONS OF RADIATION THERAPY

Possible complications of RT include arm edema, brachial plexopathy, decreased arm mobility, soft tissue necrosis, rib fractures, radiation pneumonitis, carcinogenesis (e.g., contralateral breast cancer and sarcoma), and radiation-related heart disease. Information on heart toxicity and carcinogenesis is reviewed here. The data on complications after both postmastectomy RT and RT administered as part of BCT are reviewed.

Injury to the heart is a possible complication after RT. The long-term results from the early trials on postoperative RT using outmoded techniques show an increased risk of cardiac mortality. A more recent population study showed an increased risk of fatal myocardial infarctions for patients receiving left-sided breast RT compared with right-sided breast RT[370]; however, the techniques of RT are not described. A large institution study on patients treated with modern techniques (without adjuvant chemotherapy) did not show an increased risk with long follow-up.[371] In the Stockholm postmastectomy trial discussed previously, late cardiac mortality was seen, but this was clearly related to the amount of heart irradiated.[372] Late cardiac mortality has not been seen in institution-based studies using limited cardiac irradiation with CMF chemotherapy,[373,374] but may possibly occur with RT and high-dose doxorubicin.[375] CT simulation allows for three-dimensional visualization of anatomic structures including the heart and can be useful in selecting techniques to greatly limit the volume of irradiated heart.[376]

One possible complication of RT for breast cancer is the induction of another breast cancer. Breast tissue is known to be sensitive to radiation carcinogenesis. The latency period between exposure and the detection of induced cancers is at least 5 years, and this risk persists for many decades. The risk of carcinogenesis increases with doses up to 10 Gy, then seems to level off and decline so that for doses in the therapeutic range (greater than 45 Gy), the risk seems to be small.[377,378] Because the dose to the opposite breast from a course of RT is in the range of 1 to 3 Gy, tumor induction in the contralateral breast is of greater potential concern than in the ipsilateral breast. Age at exposure to radiation is the other important risk factor for carcinogenesis in human breast tissue.[378–380] The highest risk occurs in female subjects exposed at the youngest age. With increasing age, the risk of carcinogenesis declines. The risk for women older than 40 years of age seems to be negligible, but not zero. A number of studies have addressed the risk of contralateral breast cancer after postoperative RT. Boice and colleagues conducted a case-control study in a cohort of 41,109 patients diagnosed with breast cancer between 1935 and 1982 in Connecticut.[381] Among women who survived for at least 10 years, RT was associated with a small, but marginally significant, elevation in the risk of a contralateral breast cancer (relative risk, 1.33). The increased risk associated with RT was evident among women who were younger than 45 years of age when they were treated (relative risk, 1.59), but not among older women (relative risk, 1.01). In another case-control study from Denmark,[382] the incidence of a second primary breast cancer in the contralateral breast was examined among 56,540 women with a first primary breast cancer diagnosed between 1943 and 1978. In that study, RT was not associated with an increased risk of contralateral breast cancer (relative risk, 1.04). It is possible to estimate the increased absolute risk of contralateral breast cancer given the elevated relative risk for patients aged 45 or younger seen in the study by Boice et al.[381] The risk may actually be lower, as is suggested by the Danish study. For patients aged 45 years or younger, the risk of contralateral breast cancer within 15 years is approximately 11% without RT and increased to approximately 12% to 13% with the addition of RT. The risk of contralateral breast cancer within 30 years is approximately 22% without RT and increases to approximately 25% to 26% with RT. Thus, the risk of contralateral breast cancer in young patients, which is already higher than that for older patients, is likely to be further increased to a small extent by the use of RT.

Sarcomas of soft tissue or bone are a rare, but well-documented complication of RT. In a report from Memorial Sloan-Kettering Cancer Center, a total of 48 patients with a prior history of breast cancer and subsequent treatment-related sarcomas were seen at the institution over a 43-year period.[383] Lymphangiosarcoma of the extremity accounted for 22, or 46%, of the series. Most of these patients had been treated with radical mastectomy and postoperative RT. The other 26 sarcomas occurred within a RT treatment field and were considered radiation related. Twenty-one of these 26 patients were diagnosed with a soft tissue sarcoma and 5 with a bone sarcoma. The median latency interval between the diagnosis of breast cancer and the development of sarcoma was 11 years (range, 4 to 44) and was similar for the two types of sarcomas. The survival of these patients was poor. In a registry study from Sweden, 13,490 patients with breast cancer diagnosed between 1960 and 1980 were followed through 1988.[384] Nineteen sarcomas were reported, whereas 8.7 were expected (relative risk, 2.2; absolute risk, $1.7/10^4$ person-years). Twelve of the sarcomas appeared within the radiation fields. Of particular interest is that a high percentage of sarcomas after treatment with CS and RT are angiosarcomas.[385,386] The typical initial clinical appearance of this sarcoma is as reddish, purplish, or bluish nodules or as skin discoloration. There are often many such areas. These initial findings can be subtle, and diagnosis is commonly not made until more advanced signs are present. Of note, the latency period for this radiation-induced sarcoma is shorter than for other sarcomas, with some occurring before 5 years.

Lung cancer also appears to be increased in patients irradiated for breast cancer. The latency period from RT to diagnosis is approximately 10 years. In a case-referent study reported by Inskip and others[387] using the Connecticut Tumor Registry, there was a small increased risk of lung cancer among 10-year survivors of breast cancer associated with the use of postoperative RT (relative risk, 1.8; 95% confidence interval, 0.8 to 3.8). The relative risk for the period 15 years or more after RT was 2.8

(95% confidence interval, 1.0 to 8.2); however, it can be difficult to distinguish a late metastasis of breast cancer to lung from a new primary lung cancer even with a tissue specimen. This increased relative risk suggests that there would be approximately nine cases of RT-induced lung cancer per year among 10,000 breast cancer patients who survived at least 10 years. Similar findings were noted in a study using the SEER database.[388] Another study from this same group suggested that the effects of smoking and RT are multiplicative,[389] although this relation has not been established with certainty.[390] These studies all examined the risk of lung cancer after local regional irradiation, and the risk may be less after more localized breast irradiation.

Sequencing of Systemic Therapy and Radiation Therapy

Clinicians are now commonly faced with the necessity of combining systemic therapy and RT in patients after CS and after mastectomy. Given (1) the variable agents, duration, and intensity of CT regimens, (2) variations in RT and surgical techniques, and, chiefly, (3) the limited data from randomized clinical trials addressing this question, the optimal sequencing approach is unresolved. The major goal in sequencing is to obtain the highest rate of survival; however, additional important goals are to maintain a low rate of local recurrence and a low rate of complications. The options for combining RT and CT are (1) CT first followed by RT; (2) RT first followed by CT; (3) RT and CT simultaneously; or (4) some number of cycles of CT, then RT, and then more CT (commonly referred to as *sandwich* therapy). In considering this issue, it would be useful to know whether a delay in either CT or RT decreases its effect, what the complication rate is for each sequence option, and whether prior RT affects the ability to give maximal doses of CT. It seems plausible that delays in the initiation of CT will decrease its effectiveness; however, firm data demonstrating this are not available. As previously described, the use of preoperative CT has not clearly improved survival compared with conventionally timed adjuvant chemotherapy.[391] Retrospective reviews of patients treated either with mastectomy or BCT examining the influence of the delay of CT on outcome have demonstrated conflicting results.[392–394] The information available on whether a delay in the initiation of RT to give CT first leads to a increased local recurrence rate is also conflicting.[394–401] The results from two NSABP adjuvant studies in node-positive breast cancer (B-15 and B-16) did not show any effect with delays of 12 weeks.[402]

Prospective randomized clinical trials are required to test formally the effect of sequencing of CT and RT on outcome. The Dana-Farber/Beth Israel/JCRT trial is the only published trial specifically designed to address this issue. In this trial, 244 patients at moderate or high risk for relapse (almost all node-positive) were randomly assigned to receive either (1) RT followed by cyclophosphamide, doxorubicin, methotrexate (with leucovorin), fluorouracil, and prednisone given every 21 days for four cycles or (2) CT followed by RT.[403] With a median follow-up of 58 months, the 5-year crude incidence of first sites of recurrence suggested that local recurrence was greater with delayed RT and distant recurrence was greater with delayed CT. The overall actuarial rate of distant failure was higher in the RT-first arm (37% vs. 25%; $P = .05$), thus favoring the CT-first arm. This trial does not specifically address the question of sequencing in node-negative patients or with longer than 12 weeks of chemotherapy. One can hypothesize that the effect of delay in the initiation of RT is related to the extent of the breast surgery and the final margin status; namely, a delay of 12 to 16 weeks is important only for patients with limited breast surgery and close or positive margins. This hypothesis is suggested by a subset analysis of the JCRT trial; however, this trial was not large enough to allow for such analysis. At this writing, there are two ongoing unpublished trials in France. In the Arcosein trial, approximately 700 patients treated with breast-conserving surgery will be randomized either to (1) mitoxantrone, cyclophosphamide, and fluorouracil given every 3 weeks for six cycles followed by RT, or (2) concurrent CT and RT using the same drugs. In the other trial, patients are randomized either to (1) epirubicin, cyclophosphamide, and fluorouracil followed by RT, or (2) concurrent mitoxantrone, cyclophosphamide, and fluorouracil and RT.

Another important question regarding sequencing is whether RT and CT can be given simultaneously without an increase in complications or a decrease in the cosmetic outcome. The use of simultaneous RT and CT has the advantage of eliminating the necessity for delaying one of the modalities and perhaps providing an additive or synergistic interaction between the RT and CT. It has been reported, however, that the concurrent use of CMF chemotherapy and full-dose RT can result in greater skin reactions compared with patients treated sequentially,[404,405] as well as a decrease in the long-term cosmetic result.[404] It may be possible to combine CMF and RT in other, more tolerable ways. At the University of Pennsylvania, 210 patients were treated with concurrent CF and RT, followed by six cycles of CMF, with excellent results.[406] The JCRT has conducted a prospective pilot study of a modified concurrent CMF and RT regimen using reduced doses of RT designed to lessen treatment side effects by anticipating the known interaction of CMF and RT.[407] One hundred twelve patients with zero to three positive lymph nodes were entered into this prospective study. Patients received six cycles of CMF given every 28 days. On day 14 of cycle 1, patients started tangential field RT, consisting of 39.6 Gy in 22 fractions to the whole breast and a 16-Gy boost to the tumor bed using electrons. The most common acute toxicity observed during or shortly after RT was moist desquamation (seen in 50% of patients). Grade 4 neutropenia was noted in 16 patients during RT, but only one patient required hospitalization. Radiation pneumonitis (grade 2) was noted in only one patient. Fifty-one patients were evaluable for cosmetic scoring by JCRT physicians 2 years (± 6 months) after the end of CT: 47% had excellent, 43% had good, and 10% had fair cosmetic scores. Seventy-nine percent of patients (89 of 112) were evaluable for CT dosages delivered; overall, 93% of patients received at least 85% of all drug doses. Thus, it seems feasible to consider the administration of concurrent treatment with CMF and reduced doses of RT; however, longer term data are required to substantiate this.

Doxorubicin and cyclophosphamide (AC) given every 3 weeks for four cycles are currently used more widely than CMF, given its shorter course and at least equivalent outcome. With the substantial interaction between doxorubicin and RT, it does not seem feasible to combine these modalities concurrently even with reduced doses of RT. When AC is used, the results of the JCRT Upfront-Outback trial provide strong support for the use of AC × 4 followed by RT in all moderate- and high-risk patients. Preliminary results suggest that AC × 4 followed by Taxol × 4 may further improve outcome compared with AC × 4 alone; the optimal timing of RT in this setting is uncertain. Given that the positive results in this trial were obtained using RT after completion of Taxol, it generally seems best to use this approach.[408] Studies are under way testing the feasibility of AC × 4 followed by concurrent Taxol and RT; however, there is a report of early-onset pneumonitis using this approach[503] and another report showing none.[409]

Axillary Treatment

Axillary treatment in the form of a complete dissection was, for many years, standard management in patients with invasive breast cancer. As dictated by the Halstedian concept of breast cancer spread, axillary dissection was considered a critical component of the surgical cure of the disease. The axillary nodes were considered the *filter* before spread of cancer cells to distant sites. Axillary dissection is also known to be useful in assessing prognosis and ensuring local tumor control in the axilla. By the 1970s, there was increasing evidence that axillary dissection had a limited effect on survival. This was most convincingly demonstrated in the NSABP trial B-04. In this trial, patients with clinically negative axillary nodes were randomized to radical mastectomy, total mastectomy with observation of the axillary nodes and a delayed dissection if positive nodes appeared, or total mastectomy with RT to the regional lymphatics.[234] No statistically significant difference in the 10-year survival rate was found among the groups, despite the fact that approximately 40% of the patients undergoing axillary dissection had positive nodes and a similar percentage were presumed to have positive nodes in the observation-only arm. While this study emphasizes that axillary dissection is not of survival benefit for the majority of patients, the number of patients in this trial was insufficient to rule out a small, but clinically important survival benefit.[410] Also of note is that 25% to 30% of the 20-year survivors reported in a series of patients treated with radical mastectomy alone had positive axillary nodes,[411–414] suggesting that, for a small number of patients, axillary dissection may be therapeutic. The therapeutic potential of axillary dissection is also supported by the survival benefits noted in the more recent trials of postmastectomy RT.[415–417]

With the general recognition that axillary dissection was principally a prognostic, rather than therapeutic, procedure, a number of studies were undertaken to determine the extent of axillary surgery needed to determine whether nodes were positive or negative. Many of these studies examined the likelihood of skip metastases (i.e., involvement of nodes in the upper axilla; level III) in the absence of involvement in the lower (level I or II) nodes. Involvement of level III is clearly rare when both levels I and II are negative.[418,419] There is considerable variability in the literature on the risk of skip metastases to level II. Much of this variability may be due to variations in the definition of which nodal tissues constitute levels I and II. These disparate observations have led some authors to conclude that a level I dissection provides accurate staging information,[420] while most have concluded that removal of both levels I and II is required.[421,422] A level I and II dissection is effective at providing local control in the axilla. Among patients treated with a level I and II dissection as part of BCT, axillary recurrence rates of less than 3% have been reported.[423–426] When patients undergo more limited random axillary sampling procedures, the likelihood of local recurrence is related to the number of lymph nodes removed. The 5-year probability of an axillary recurrence is approximately 20% in patients with no lymph nodes examined and approximately 10% when only one to two negative nodes are removed. At least six to ten nodes need to be removed to avoid misclassification and to optimize local control in the axilla.[234,426–429] While a level I and II dissection is generally well tolerated, there are occasionally complications. Major complications, including injury or thrombosis of the axillary vein and injury to the motor nerves of the axilla, are infrequent. Minor complications are more common and include seroma formation, shoulder dysfunction, loss of sensation in the distribution of the intercostobrachial nerve, and edema of the arm and breast.

A number of developments have led to a reexamination of the need for axillary dissection in all patients. Under discussion is the routine use of adjuvant systemic therapy in many patients with node-negative breast cancer, the increasing use of BCT, and the increasing number of patients with small, mammographically detected cancers with a low risk of axillary metastases. One approach to avoiding axillary dissection is to identify cancers with a low risk of nodal metastases. The incidence of axillary nodal involvement is known to be related principally to tumor size. However, axillary node metastases are still seen in 12% to 37% of cancers measuring 1 cm or less,[170,429–435] and in a number of studies, the incidence of metastases does not decrease appreciably even with cancers 0.5 cm or smaller.[429,432,434] The only groups of patients with invasive carcinoma regularly identified as having nodal metastases in fewer than 5% of cases are those with microinvasive tumors, those with grade 1 tumors less than 5 mm,[415] and those with pure tubular carcinomas less than 1 cm.[436,437] However, most patients continue to undergo axillary dissection, even in these favorable groups. A Patterns of Care study examining axillary surgery in 17,151 patients with stage I and II carcinoma undergoing BCT in 1994 found that overall, 93% had an axillary dissection. Even in patients with grade 1 tumors, favorable histologic subtypes, or tumors less than 5 cm, 88% or more underwent axillary dissection.

The new technique of lymphatic mapping and sentinel node biopsy offers the possibility of reliably identifying patients with axillary node involvement with a low-morbidity operation, allowing axillary dissection to be limited to patients with nodal metastases who can benefit from the procedure. The sentinel node is defined as the first node receiving lymphatic drainage from a tumor, and the absence of metastases in the sentinel node reliably predicts the absence of metastases in the remaining axillary nodes. This concept was popularized by Giuliano et al. in malignant melanoma and later adapted to breast cancer.[438] Multiple studies have now confirmed that a sentinel node can be identified in more than 90% of cases, with experience, and predicts the status of the remaining nodes with 90% to 95% accuracy[439–444] (Table 37.2-15).

The sentinel node can be identified using isosulfan blue dye, radiolabeled colloids, or a combination of the two agents. Similar success rates are reported for the techniques, and a randomized trial demonstrated no difference in the rate of sentinel node identification, predictive value of the sentinel node, or learning curve for isosulfan blue dye alone compared with the blue dye plus technetium sulfur colloid.[445] Approximately 20 to 30 cases appear to be necessary to master the sentinel biopsy technique, with individual learning curves varying widely.[444–446]

A number of contraindications to sentinel node biopsy have been identified, including the presence of suspicious axillary

TABLE 37.2-15. Studies of Lymphatic Mapping and Sentinel Node Biopsy

Study	*No. of Patients*	*Technique*	*Sentinel Node Identified (%)*	*Node Positive (%)*	*False-Negative Rate (%)*
Giuliano et al.[439]	107	B	94	42	0
Veronesi et al.[440]	376	R	97	49	6.7
Shons et al.[441]	253	B + R	92	—	0.5
Guenther et al.[442]	145	B	71	30	3.0
Borgstein et al.[443]	130	R	94	43	1.7
Krag et al.[444]	443	R	91	28	11.0

B, blue dye; R, radioactivity.

adenopathy, evidence of locally advanced breast cancer, use of preoperative chemotherapy, multifocal or multicentric tumor, prior axillary surgery, and a pregnant or lactating patient. In addition, virtually no information on accuracy of the procedure for tumors larger than 5 cm is available. Lymphatic mapping and sentinel node biopsy have prompted renewed interest in the role of the internal mammary nodes in breast cancer. A small number of internal mammary node biopsies have been reported in patients whose lymphoscintigraphy results have failed to demonstrate axillary drainage, but the need for internal mammary node biopsy remains to be defined.

Sentinel node biopsy offers the pathologist the opportunity to perform a much more detailed examination of one or two nodes than is possible when evaluating an entire axillary specimen. It has been known for more than 30 years that approximately 20% of lymph nodes in which no tumor is seen after routine processing and light microscopy contain tumor cells that can be identified by serial sectioning or immunohistochemistry.[447–450] Early studies did not find these micrometastases to be prognostically significant, and these techniques were not practical for use on an entire axillary specimen. With the ability to examine only one or two sentinel nodes, there is renewed interest in the possibility of using immunohistochemistry for ultra staging. However, prospective confirmation of the significance of tumor cells detected by immunohistochemistry is lacking. The retrospective studies that indicate prognostic significance show a wide variation in the magnitude of this effect,[451–453] making patient counseling difficult. The results of two prospective clinical trials being carried out by the American College of Surgeons Clinical Oncology Group and the NSABP to address these issues will provide important information regarding the clinical significance of micrometastases.

An additional important unresolved issue is the need for completion axillary dissection when a positive sentinel node is identified. The initial sentinel node studies demonstrated that the sentinel node is the only tumor-containing node in 40% to 60% of cases, and fewer than 20% of patients have more than three involved nodes.[438–445] A positive sentinel node establishes the need for systemic therapy, and, in patients undergoing breast-conserving surgery, radiation of the breast includes a significant portion of the low axilla, helping to maintain local control. However, the possibility that axillary dissection has some therapeutic benefit for patients with involved nodes cannot be excluded, making abandonment of completion axillary dissection unwise. The need for axillary dissection in sentinel node–positive patients is being addressed in a prospective randomized trial by the American College of Surgeons Clinical Oncology Group.

The initial results of lymphatic mapping and sentinel node biopsy are extremely promising. However, data on the long-term outcome of sentinel node biopsy alone in unselected populations and information on the ability of surgeons outside of centers of expertise doing a low volume of breast surgery are needed before it can be determined if sentinel node biopsy will replace axillary dissection as the standard of care for the node-negative or node-positive breast cancer.

LOCAL RECURRENCE

LOCAL RECURRENCE AFTER MASTECTOMY

Local recurrence following mastectomy usually presents as one or more asymptomatic nodules in or under the skin of the chest wall, typically located in or near the scar of the mastectomy.[454] A few patients present with diffuse chest wall involvement, more commonly seen in patients with locally advanced tumors originally. *Carcinoma en cuirasse* is a distinct form of diffuse infiltration of the skin or subcutaneous tissues of the chest wall with woody induration and spread of tumor well beyond the limits of standard surgical or RT boundaries. Approximately 80% of local recurrences appear by 5 years after mastectomy and nearly all occur by 10 years.[264,367,455] However, local recurrences occurring 15 to 50 years after initial surgery have been reported. It is possible that some of these late recurrences may represent new secondary cancer arising in residual breast tissue.[456]

It is unclear how often chest wall recurrences progress to be symptomatic. In some series, only 25% to 30% of patients develop significant morbidity.[367,457] However, in one series of 100 patients with local regional recurrence, 62 had one or more significant symptoms before death.[458] Despite aggressive local treatment, most patients with an isolated local recurrence following mastectomy eventually manifest distant metastases. In a series of patients with local, regional, or both local and regional recurrence treated at the JCRT, the 5- and 10-year actuarial rates of freedom from distant metastases were 30% and 7%, respectively.[459] The corresponding rates of overall survival were 50% and 26%. However, patients surviving without disease 15 or more years after treatment with RT have been described. More recent series appear to include patients with more favorable disease and suggest that favorable subsets of patients with local recurrence can be identified based on factors discussed here.[460–463]

A number of prognostic factors for survival following local recurrence have been identified.[459–465] The interval between mastectomy and local recurrence (called the *disease-free interval*) is the most reliable indicator of the time to subsequent distant failure and overall survival. This likely reflects the intrinsic growth rate of the tumor. For example, at the JCRT, the relapse-free survival at 3 years was 20% for patients treated with aggressive RT who had isolated local recurrences less than 24 months after initial surgery, compared with 36% in patients who had isolated local recurrences at 24 months or longer after surgery.[459] The respective 10-year survival rates were 7% versus 36%, with similar results found in nearly all RT series. Lymph node status at the time of mastectomy and the number of sites and the size of recurrence also appear to influence prognosis. In patients with a long disease-free interval, limited disease capable of being resected, limited initial axillary involvement, or both limited disease and involvement, the prognosis may be favorable.[460–463]

Patients undergoing skin-sparing mastectomy do not appear to be at a greater risk of local recurrence than patients undergoing more conventional mastectomy,[466] but further experience is needed to confirm this.

Patients with local recurrence after mastectomy should have a complete restaging to rule out distant metastases. In particular, a CT scan of the chest and abdomen and a bone scan is recommended since many patients have additional sites of involvement only discovered in this manner.[467] MRI or positron emission tomography scans may provide additional information.[468,469] Limited local excision has been used in some patients, with further local failure occurring in over one-half of patients so treated.[338] For highly selected patients, local control rates in excess of 75% have been reported with wide local excision of skin and subcutaneous tissue or partial or full-thickness chest wall resection, with some patients surviving 5 years or more.[470–472] RT has been the standard form of local treatment for patients with local recurrence after mastectomy. The volume of disease remaining at the time of RT is a critical determinant of the likelihood of achieving long-term local control, and gross excision is recommended if feasible. In patients with initially unresectable disease, the use of initial systemic therapy should be strongly considered. Patients with a recurrence in one portion of the chest wall or draining lymph node areas should receive RT to the entire chest wall. Patients with chest wall recurrence may subsequently have recurrences in the supraclavicular region (and the axillary region if not previously dissected) if only the chest wall is irradiated.[464,465] In general, the higher the dose of RT delivered, the less likely is an in-field failure, and doses in the range of 60 Gy to the site of recurrence are recommended, even following gross excision. However, even with technically optimal RT, further local recurrence is seen in a significant minority of patients. Attempts to improve this have included the addition of hyperthermia; however, this treatment is still limited by technical limitations, complications, and inconclusive support for its use in randomized trials.[473,474] The use of hyperfractionated, accelerated RT has not shown improved results.[475] Photodynamic therapy has shown some utility in previously treated patients,[476] but its role in the primary treatment of local recurrence has not been established.

It is not clear whether using adjuvant systemic therapy in conjunction with local treatment can prolong disease-free or overall survival time. While a number of retrospective studies have suggested a benefit to adjuvant systemic therapy,[464,465,477,478] the only randomized trial addressing this issue is from Switzerland and has only a limited number of patients (n = 167).[479,480] Entry in this trial was restricted to patients with a positive or undetermined ER assay, disease-free interval greater than 1 year, and three or fewer nodules, each 3 cm or smaller in diameter, without fixation. Randomized patients underwent complete gross tumor resection and RT and were randomly allocated to receive either tamoxifen until relapse or to observation. With a median follow-up of 6.3 years, the 5-year relapse-free survival rates were 59% and 36% in the tamoxifen and observation arms, respectively (P = NS). However, this difference had nearly disappeared by 8 to 9 years, and the overall survival rates were the same in both groups. This trial was not large enough to suggest a clinically important advantage for adjuvant systemic therapy.

At present, the available information does not clearly identify which patients benefit from the different available treatments or at what point in the course of the disease treatment should be instituted. Local treatment of patients with no evidence of distant metastases reduces morbidity for many and may increase survival time for some patients and is, therefore, generally recommended. This is particularly true in patients with favorable prognostic factors. In patients with a hormone-receptor–positive cancer, hormonal therapy is often considered in addition to local treatment, given the suggestion of benefit in some studies and the limited toxicities associated with such treatment. While the value of adjuvant chemotherapy in this situation is not established, it appears reasonable to use it for patients who have not been previously treated. In patients with an inoperable recurrence, it is reasonable to use *neoadjuvant* systemic therapy to facilitate definitive local treatment. No information is available regarding the benefits of reapplying chemotherapy in patients who had received initial adjuvant systemic therapy. In patients with concurrent or prior distant metastases, appropriate systemic therapy should be used, with RT reserved for patients with persistent local symptoms.

BREAST RECURRENCE AFTER BREAST-CONSERVING THERAPY

As previously noted, the large majority of recurrences in the treated breast following CS and RT are at or near the site of the primary tumor.[253] The risk of this type of recurrence is relatively constant from years 2 to 7 following treatment and then declines. Recurrences at a distance from the primary tumor are more common at longer follow-up times. Both mammography and physical examination are useful in detecting a recurrence in the breast following CS and RT, with the majority of recurrences evident on mammography with or without findings on physical examination.[481,482] The findings on physical examination associated with a recurrence may be subtle, especially when the primary tumor was of infiltrating lobular histology. Changes in the physical examination that occur more than 2 years following the completion of RT should be viewed as suspicious. Recurrence in the nipple alone, presenting as Paget's disease, can also occur.

There can be substantial overlap in the radiologic appearance between benign and malignant lesions following treatment. Ultrasound is sometimes helpful in distinguishing benign and malignant masses. MRI scans may also be useful, but this is not yet established.[483,484] In patients with suspicious findings, prompt biopsy is recommended. Mammographic or ultrasound-directed core-needle biopsy is an increasingly used approach to confirm the diagnosis.

The large majority of breast recurrences are operable, and the majority of patients are alive 5 years after recurrence.[244,485–489] The results appear to be better than for patients with local recurrence after mastectomy, except possibly for patients with early recurrence for whom prognosis is equally poor after mastectomy and BCT.[490] Factors that influence prognosis in patients with operable disease are not well established. The most important prognostic factor in patients undergoing mastectomy in the JCRT experience was the histology of the recurrence.[485] There was no further evidence of disease among the 24 patients with only noninvasive cancer or predominantly noninvasive disease with only focal areas of invasion. In contrast, 38% of patients (38 of 99) with predominantly infiltrating tumors developed a further recurrence, usually distant. A small minority of patients present with skin involvement following BCT, and these patients have a poor prognosis.[258]

In patients with a breast recurrence, appropriate staging for distant metastases should be performed before definitive therapy. The standard treatment for an isolated breast recurrence is mastectomy. Subsequent chest wall recurrences occur in fewer than 10% of patients treated with mastectomy. Postoperative complications following mastectomy are rare. Wide local excision alone is associated with a substantial risk of further breast failure and uncontrolled local disease.[485,488,491] There is limited experience with reirradiation for patients with a breast recurrence.[492–494] Many patients treated with mastectomy for local recurrence desire breast reconstruction. Immediate reconstruction with a myocutaneous flap is psychologically advantageous and also promotes tissue healing. The risk of complications following reconstruction is slightly greater than in patients who have not had prior RT, and the overall cosmetic results may not be quite as favorable. Previously irradiated patients have tolerated submuscularly placed tissue expanders poorly.

The role of adjuvant systemic therapy following breast recurrence has not been established. In patients with an invasive recurrence, the risk of distant recurrence is substantial, and the use and concerns of adjuvant systemic therapy are similar to those described previously (see Local Recurrence after Mastectomy, earlier in this chapter).

BREAST RECONSTRUCTION

As discussed, breast reconstruction is an important option for a breast cancer patient undergoing mastectomy to consider and should routinely be discussed with the patient before definitive surgery. The only contraindications to breast reconstruction are the presence of significant comorbid conditions that would interfere with the patient's ability to tolerate a longer operative procedure in the case of immediate reconstruction or additional procedures in the case of delayed reconstruction. In patients who may require postoperative chest wall irradiation, implant reconstructions should be avoided since the risk of implant loss is high after RT.[495] However, TRAM flap reconstructions appear to tolerate postoperative RT well.[334] Patient age,[496] need for adjuvant chemotherapy,[330] or poor long-term prognosis are not contraindications to reconstruction.

The simplest technique for breast reconstruction involves the use of available tissue and placement of an implant. This approach is best for women with small or moderate-sized breasts with minimal ptosis and requires adequate skin to cover an implant of a size similar to the contralateral breast. The use of limited skin excision, with operative exposure gained by incision, usually leaves enough skin to cover an implant. Oncologic surgeons now generally agree that the only skin that it is necessary to excise for reasons of cancer control is the nipple-areola complex and the biopsy scar. If insufficient skin is available to achieve symmetry with the contralateral breast or for larger or ptotic breasts, a tissue expander may be employed. This technique involves placement of a prosthesis that is only partially inflated beneath the pectoral muscle. Using a subcutaneous injection port, the prosthesis is gradually filled with saline over a period of weeks to months until the desired breast size and shape are achieved.

Silicone breast implants have been available for over 30 years. In January 1992, the U.S. Food and Drug Administration (FDA) declared that silicone gel–filled implants could not be used until more information was available about their long-term safety. This moratorium, however, did not apply to saline-filled implants, and the FDA later recommended that gel-filled implants be allowed in breast cancer patients pending the results of further study. The major recognized complication of implants is the development of capsular contracture, an excessive scar formation around the implant that may lead to deformity and pain of the breast. Other complications of implants include rupture of the implant and leakage of silicone through the intact implant capsule. The incidence of these complications is uncertain. A major concern regarding the use of silicone implants arose after uncontrolled reports suggested an increased incidence of connective tissue disease in women with implants.[497–499] However, in 1995 the American Society of Rheumatologists concluded that scientific evidence does not support an association between implants and connective tissue disease. A metaanalysis of 13 epidemiologic studies and other publications on this topic identified a relative risk of 0.76 for any connective tissue disease and 0.98 for scleroderma in patients with breast implants.[500] Similar risks were reported by Silverman et al.[501] after a metaanalysis of 4000 cases.

Another technique of reconstruction is the use of myocutaneous flaps to transfer skin, fat, and muscle from distant parts of the body. The most commonly used flaps are the latissimus dorsi and TRAM flaps. The use of a flap for reconstruction requires a more lengthy and involved operative procedure than the implant method, and postoperative recovery is somewhat longer because there are two separate incision sites. The latissimus flap is often used in conjunction with a prosthesis because, in most cases, the flap alone provides insufficient bulk to achieve symmetry. With the latissimus flap, there is only a 1% incidence of complete flap loss.[502] The TRAM flap usually allows an adequate breast mound to be fashioned without the use of a prosthesis, but its blood supply is more tenuous than that of the latissimus flap, with major necrosis reported in 5% of patients and partial necrosis in as many as 31% of patients.[330,503] For some patients, the removal of extra tissue from the lower abdomen is an advantage to this procedure. Abdominal wall herniation is seen in 2% to 5% of patients following this procedure, but this percent is dependent on the skill and experience of the operator. Long-term cigarette smoking (more than 20 pack-years) has an acute and chronic effect on microcirculation and, in many centers, is a contraindication

TABLE 37.2-16. Types of Reconstruction after Mastectomy

Type	*Advantages*	*Disadvantages*
Implant	One-stage procedure; short operative time; minimal prolongation of hospitalization and recovery, and low cost	Capsular contracture; possible rupture or leakage; poor cosmetic outcome in large or ptotic breasts
Tissue expander	Short operative time; low cost; hospitalization and recovery not prolonged	Multiple physician visits; possible rupture or leakage of implant
Latissimus dorsi flap	Reliable flap; autogenous tissue; natural contour	Donor site scar; moderate prolongation of hospitalization and recovery; usually requires an implant
Transverse rectus abdominis flap	Autogenous tissue; natural contour; abdominoplasty	Donor site scar; significant prolongation in hospitalization and recovery; possible flap loss and abdominal wall hernia

to the procedure. If these myocutaneous flaps are not available or suitable for use, it is possible to transfer composite tissues from distant sites and to perform a microvascular anastomosis to nearby vessels.[504] This technique, known as a *free flap*, requires a skilled microsurgeon and prolonged operating time and is only occasionally chosen for primary reconstruction. The potential benefits and complications of the various reconstructive procedures are listed in Table 37.2-16.

Regardless of the technique of reconstruction chosen, the creation of a breast mound is the chief goal in breast reconstruction. Surgery on the contralateral breast, such as reduction or mastopexy, may be required to achieve symmetry. Reconstruction of a nipple-areola complex is another secondary procedure that some patients elect to undergo in order to improve cosmetic appearance. The patient's own nipple should *not* be used for this purpose because recurrent carcinoma due to persistence of breast tissue on the nipple has been reported. Microscopic involvement of the nipple is seen in 30% of mastectomy specimens, but is frequently not apparent at the time of gross pathologic examination. The nipple can be reconstructed using a variety of local flap techniques or by the use of full-thickness skin grafts. Tattooing of the grafts produces a color match to the patient's own areola and allows any site to be used as the donor.[505] Tissue from the contralateral nipple should not be used for nipple reconstruction because of the concern of transferring breast tissue to the reconstruction site.

SPECIAL THERAPEUTIC PROBLEMS

PAGET'S DISEASE OF THE NIPPLE

Paget's disease of the nipple is a rare form of breast cancer that is characterized clinically by eczematoid changes of the nipple. Associated symptoms include itching, erythema, and nipple discharge.[506–508] Paget's disease is diagnosed histologically by the presence of large cells, with pale cytoplasm and prominent nucleoli (known as Paget's cells) involving the epidermis of the nipple. In approximately 45% of women with Paget's disease, a breast mass is detected at presentation, and in most of the remainder, infiltrating or intraductal carcinoma is identified in the mastectomy specimen.[506–509] The average age of women with Paget's disease does not differ from that of women with other forms of breast cancer, but symptoms are frequently present for 6 months or more before diagnosis.[506,509] The relation between the changes observed in the nipple and the underlying breast cancer remains a matter of controversy. One theory suggests that the nipple involvement represents the migration of malignant cells from the underlying breast tumor. The alternate hypothesis suggests that Paget's cells are a separate disease process originating in epidermis.

Paget's disease has traditionally been treated with mastectomy. The rationales for this approach are the need to sacrifice the nipple-areola complex, the fact that the subareolar ducts may be diffusely involved with tumor, and the observation that carcinoma may be found at a considerable distance from the nipple.[506–509] A limited experience with breast-conserving procedures in the management of Paget's disease has been described. Paone and Baker reported five patients who underwent excision of the nipple with a wedge resection of underlying breast tissue, who remained free of disease at 10-year follow-up.[508] Lagios and coworkers reported five patients with no palpable breast mass and negative mammogram results treated by excision of the nipple-areola complex, who remained free of parenchymal recurrence at a mean follow-up of 50 months.[510] One patient, treated with only partial nipple excision, developed recurrent Paget's disease at 12 months, which was resected. In contrast, four of ten patients treated by Dixon et al. with excision alone had local recurrences after a median follow-up of 40 months.[511] Twenty selected patients with Paget's disease without clinical or radiologic evidence of parenchymal breast cancer were treated with RT alone or excision plus RT at the Institut Curie from 1960 to 1984.[512] At a median follow-up of 7.5 years, three patients had recurrent disease in the nipple-areola region and were treated with mastectomy. The 7-year actuarial probability of survival with the breast preserved was 81%. Bulens et al., using similar selection criteria, reported no local or distant failures in a group of 13 patients treated with breast irradiation alone.[513] Osteen collected a total of 79 patients treated by local excision with or without RT, with nine local recurrences.[514]

When considering therapeutic options in Paget's disease, it is helpful to think of the condition as DCIS involving the nipple, usually associated with additional intraductal or invasive carcinoma in the underlying breast parenchyma. The extent of the underlying involvement determines the patient's suitability for BCT. Detailed mammographic evaluation (including magnification views of the subareolar region) and histologic evaluation with margin assessment are essential components of this evaluation. For patients with evidence of diffuse involvement or disease at a distance from the nipple, mastectomy remains the standard therapy. In patients with disease localized to the subareolar area or the nipple-areola complex, BCT can be considered. This treatment requires removal of the entire nipple-areola complex and some of the underlying ductal region. In carefully selected patients, local failure rates with this approach appear to be similar to those reported for other breast carcinomas. The prognosis in Paget's disease is related to the stage of the disease and appears to be similar to that of women with other types of breast carcinoma. If invasive breast cancer is found, adjuvant systemic treatment should follow the same guidelines used for other patients with invasive cancer.

MALE BREAST CANCER

Cancer of the male breast is an uncommon disease, accounting for less than 1% of all cases of breast carcinoma.[515,516] According to SEER data, approximately 1600 cases of male breast cancer and 400 deaths were expected to occur in 1999.[2] In one study, a family history of female breast or ovarian cancer was reported in 30% of men with breast cancer.[517] As described previously (see Inherited Predisposition to Breast Cancer, earlier in this chapter), studies have demonstrated that germline mutations of BRCA2 are associated with an increased risk of male breast cancer, as well as early-onset breast cancer in women. In the absence of a family history, however, a BRCA2 mutation is unlikely to be found in a man with breast cancer. An initial report suggested that BRCA2 might account for approximately 15% of male breast cancer; however, a high percentage of patients in this study had a family history of female breast cancer.[518] The only population-based study using male patients from a cancer registry found a much lower (4%) incidence of BRCA2 mutations.[517] Other factors that increase the risk of male breast cancer include Klinefelter's syndrome, hepatic schistosomiasis, and radiation exposure.[519–521] Except for men with Klinefelter's syndrome, the presence of gynecomastia does not seem to be associated with an increased risk of breast carcinoma; however, microscopic changes of gynecomastia are commonly seen histologically in male breast cancer.[522,523]

Male breast cancer typically presents as a mass beneath the nipple-areola complex.[523,524] Ulceration of the nipple is a frequent sign, although isolated nipple discharge is uncommon. The mean age of men with breast carcinoma is between 60 and 70, slightly higher than that of women with the disease.[525] Infiltrating ductal carcinoma is the most common tumor type, but Paget's disease of the nipple and inflammatory carcinoma have been reported in men.[522,525] LCIS is not seen in the male breast, and infiltrating lobular carcinoma is rare.[522–524] As many as 80% of male breast carcinomas are hormone-receptor positive,[526,527] and an inverse correlation exists between receptor positivity and age, similar to that seen in women.[527]

The standard local treatment for male breast carcinoma is mastectomy. If the tumor is not fixed to the pectoral muscle, a modified radical mastectomy can be performed. If muscle involvement is limited, a portion of this structure can be removed. For patients with extensive involvement of the pectoral muscle, a radical mastectomy may be required.[524] BCT for male breast carcinoma is rarely feasible given the small size of the breast and the subareolar location of the cancer in most men. Patients may, however, occasionally express an interest in this approach to therapy.

The survival rate of men with breast cancer is similar to that of women after controlling for differences in stage.[528,529] As in women, axillary nodal status is the major predictor of outcome.[523,524,530] In a report of 335 cases of male breast cancer, 84% of node-negative patients survived 10 years, compared with 44% of those with one to three positive nodes and 14% with four or more positive nodes, not dissimilar to that seen with female patients.[531] Age at diagnosis and tumor size were also significant in a multivariate analysis of prognostic factors in the study of Hulthorn et al.[530] Borgen and coauthors[524] found that only duration of symptoms and axillary nodal status were significant predictors of outcome.

The benefit of adjuvant systemic therapy in male breast cancer has not been evaluated in randomized clinical trials, although men with metastatic breast cancer are thought to have a similar course and response to treatment as women with the disease.[532] By extrapolation, this experience has guided the approach to adjuvant therapy in men with early-stage disease. The administration of adjuvant tamoxifen to men with stage II and III disease resulted in a 55% 5-year survival, compared with 28% in historic controls receiving no systemic treatment.[533] Two small retrospective studies[534,535] suggest that survival is improved by adjuvant systemic chemotherapy. In the absence of definitive data, guidelines for the use of adjuvant therapy in men should be the same as those employed in women and guided by prognosis and hormone receptor status. Similarly, decisions about the use of radiation should parallel the treatment of female breast cancer. For those men who choose to have CS, radiation is mandatory. Postmastectomy radiation appears to decrease local regional recurrence, but does not have a substantial effect on survival.[536] Two trials that report an overall survival for women undergoing postmastectomy radiation[357,359] suggest that radiation should be considered following mastectomy in men with nodal involvement.

The use of systemic therapy in male patients with metastatic breast cancer should also follow the guidelines set for female patients. Tamoxifen, megestrol acetate (Megace), aromatase inhibitors, and surgical castration are the principal treatments, although antiandrogens and luteinizing hormone-releasing hormone agonists have been reported to be effective.[537] Response rates of 50% to 80% to hormonal therapy are reported, and responses to second-line therapy are commonly seen.[538–540] The traditional method of hormonal manipulation has been orchiectomy. A literature review found a 67% response rate to this treatment, which increased to 80% when only receptor-positive cancers were considered.[538] Tamoxifen has a similar response rate and has become increasingly popular as a first-line hormonal manipulation, but tamoxifen may not be as well tolerated in men as in women.[541] Orchiectomy is now often reserved for patients who have failed multiple other therapies.[539,540,542] Chemotherapy is useful as palliative treatment. In general, the spectrum of activity with chemotherapeutic agents is similar to what has been seen in women with breast cancer, although much of the information is anecdotal.

BREAST CANCER DURING PREGNANCY

Breast cancer is not a common complication of pregnancy; however, when the two occur simultaneously, it presents a complex clinical challenge. Older studies indicated that approximately 7% to 14% of breast cancer occurring in women of childbearing age was complicated by a concurrent pregnancy.[543,544] A review of 416,441 pregnancies found an incidence of 2.2 breast cancers per 10,000 pregnancies.[545] The demographic changes that have led to delays in childbearing have increased the proportion of breast cancer cases that are now associated with pregnancy. It has been suggested that breast cancer may complicate 1 in 1000 pregnancies.[546]

The clinical presentation of breast cancer during pregnancy is typically a palpable mass. The mass or thickening may initially be attributed to the breast changes expected with pregnancy. Nipple discharge, including a thin, sometimes bloody discharge from multiple ducts, may be a normal accompaniment of pregnancy. On the other hand, a persistent, unilateral, bloody discharge during pregnancy requires further investigation.

Mammography is not as useful in pregnant patients as in those who are not pregnant because of the increased density in breast parenchyma associated with pregnancy.[546] Moreover, the increase in breast size during pregnancy also may make detection more difficult. As is the case with nonpregnant patients, an unremarkable mammogram should not lead to a decision to forego biopsy in a patient with a palpable mass. Delays in diagnosis are not uncommon in pregnant women, most likely due to the difficulty of examining the breast of a pregnant woman and the reluctance of many physicians to suspect breast cancer in a relatively young, gravid patient.

Breast cancer during pregnancy has been thought to be a particularly virulent disease, but much of the poor prognosis may be due to advanced disease at the time of diagnosis. Petrek et al. compared 56 pregnant breast cancer patients treated at Memorial Hospital from 1960 to 1980 with 166 nonpregnant women of the same age treated in the same period.[547] Sixty-one percent of the pregnant women and 38% of the nonpregnant women had positive lymph nodes; 31% of the pregnant women had T1 tumors compared with 50% of their counterparts.

After correction for tumor stage and age, most studies indicate that survival in women treated during pregnancy is similar to that seen in nonpregnant women.[547–550] In the series by Petrek et al.,[547] node-negative pregnant patients had a 77% 10-year survival compared with 75% for nonpregnant patients. The corresponding 10-year survival figures for node-positive patients were 25% and 41%, respectively, and were not statistically different. In contrast, a multiinstitutional study of 407 patients aged 20 to 29 at the time of cancer diagnosis found a relative risk of cancer death of 2.83 (95% confidence interval, 1.24 to 6.45) for the 26 patients whose cancer was diagnosed during pregnancy compared with those who had never been pregnant.[551]

After a diagnosis is made, the pregnant patient with breast cancer should meet with a multidisciplinary team, including a medical, surgical, and radiation oncologist, as well as with her obstetrician.[552] In addition, psychosocial support for the patient and her family is critical. An initial evaluation should include an assessment of the extent of the disease, with an emphasis on symptoms suggestive of advanced disease and a thorough physical examination. Mammography can be performed safely throughout the course of pregnancy. Diagnostic studies, such as bone scans and CT scans, should be avoided early in the pregnancy, particularly during the period of organogenesis. These studies are not essential in the initial evaluation of most women with localized breast cancer.

For women in the first or second trimester, the question of pregnancy termination is inevitably raised. While some treatment approaches are feasible during pregnancy, others are contraindicated. Depending on the patient's specific situation, continuing the pregnancy may or may not compromise the usual breast cancer treatment. Even when deviations from the usual treatment are required, it is unclear to what extent such changes or delays affect a woman's odds of remaining free from recurrent breast cancer. The concerns about compromising care must be balanced, by the woman, her family, and her physicians, with the desire to continue the pregnancy. The woman facing these issues must also consider the possibility that if she receives chemotherapy, her ability to conceive another child could be compromised.[553,554] There is no clear evidence that pregnancy termination changes overall survival,[548] but the limitations of all studies that have examined this issue should be recognized. In general, clinicians and patients must understand that the disease outcomes for pregnant women with breast cancer are less well understood than for the general population of women with breast cancer.

In the setting of a pregnancy, options for local therapy need to be considered carefully. Radiation to the breast is contraindicated at all times during pregnancy because of the inability to shield the developing fetus from scatter. If a woman is in her third trimester, the use of CS is reasonable as radiation can be administered after the delivery with only a minimal delay in treatment. For women who are in their first or second trimesters, delaying radiation for 3 to 8 months is of far greater concern as it may increase the risk of local recurrence.[403] However, if a woman is going to receive a course of adjuvant chemotherapy during pregnancy, radiation may not be planned for several months. If the inability to administer radiation during pregnancy leads to a substantially longer time to the initiation of radiation than would usually be the case, serious consideration should be given to proceeding directly to mastectomy. Reconstruction with a TRAM flap is contraindicated because of the effect on the abdominal wall.[555] Other forms of reconstruction are not generally recommended because of the additional anesthesia time required by reconstruction and the difficulty achieving symmetry in a pregnant woman.

The vast majority of young women with breast cancer receive some type of adjuvant systemic therapy as part of their treatment. Such treatment decisions are particularly complex in the pregnant patient. The potential benefits of treatments for the mother must be considered within the context of risks to the fetus. In general, all chemotherapeutic agents should be avoided during the first trimester because of the risk to the fetus. When chemotherapy is administered during the first trimester, there is an increased risk of spontaneous abortion, compromised fetal viability, and major organ malformations.[556,557] Certain agents, such as methotrexate and 5-fluorouracil, appear to be particularly problematic in terms of fetal malformation.[558,559] Cyclophosphamide and other alkylator agents have also been associated with fetal malformation in the first trimester.[558] Exposure of the fetus to chemotherapy after the first trimester does not appear to increase the risk of major fetal malformation.[556] However, there are reports of low birth weight, growth retardation, and fetal demise when exposure occurs after the first trimester.[560] Chemotherapy does cross the placenta, so there is the potential for fetal bone marrow suppression and other organ toxicity. Fetal myocardial necrosis has been reported with the third-trimester administration of an anthracycline,[561] but other fetal abnormalities have not been reported with this agent.[562,563] Many clinicians remain concerned about the potential late cardiac effects of *in utero* anthracycline exposure to the fetus. There are no data concerning the safety of *in utero* taxane exposure.

When adjuvant chemotherapy is administered during pregnancy, many clinicians opt for an anthracycline-based regimen, such as four cycles of doxorubicin and cyclophosphamide. Chemotherapy should not be administered until the second trimester, and even then many physicians try to delay chemotherapy for as many weeks as possible to allow for further fetal development.[556] Adjuvant chemotherapy for women in their third trimesters is often delayed until after delivery, often with the plan of delivering the baby several weeks early.

A regimen of fluorouracil, Adriamycin, and cyclophosphamide chemotherapy has been used by investigators at M. D. Anderson Cancer Center in a total of 24 pregnant women during their second and third trimesters.[552] Birth weights, Apgar scores, and general health of the newborns were reported to be normal. In France, generally favorable short-term outcomes (median follow-up, 42.3 months) have been reported for children exposed to a range of chemotherapy regimens during the second and third trimesters.[564] Adjuvant tamoxifen has not been shown to be safe in women during pregnancy.

In the rare situation that a gravid patient has metastatic disease, treatment decisions are even more difficult and must be tailored to the individual situation. For women with rapidly progressive disease, there may be few options apart from proceeding with systemic therapy, regardless of gestational age.

OCCULT PRIMARY WITH AXILLARY METASTASES

It is relatively uncommon for breast cancer to present as an axillary nodal metastasis without a palpable lesion in the breast. In a study of over 10,000 patients treated for primary breast cancer at Memorial Sloan-Kettering Cancer Center between 1975 and 1988, occult primaries with axillary metastases accounted for 0.35% of the cancers.[565] Similarly, 0.5% of 12,000 breast cancers treated at the National Cancer Institute in Milan were found to be occult primaries with axillary metastases.[566]

Although malignant axillary adenopathy may be secondary to a variety of primary solid tumors, as well as lymphoma, breast cancer is by far the most common diagnosis in a woman presenting with isolated axillary adenopathy. Before undergoing biopsy, a woman should have a complete physical examination and bilateral mammography. Chest radiography should be obtained, particularly in those with a smoking history. Once a diagnosis is established, additional radiologic studies looking for another primary tumor are rarely helpful in the absence of specific symptoms.[565–567] The presence of positive hormone receptors further suggests a diagnosis of breast cancer, although other primary tumors (i.e., lung carcinoma) can also be positive for ER.

Several series suggest that MRI may be able to detect otherwise occult cancers in the breast and may be helpful in planning local therapy.[568] In one small series, MRI identified the primary cancer in 9 of 12 patients presenting with axillary disease.[569] In another series from the University of Pennsylvania, MRI of the breast detected occult cancers in 19 of 22 women with a mean size of 17 mm.[570] A German study using MRI detected occult invasive cancer in 6 of 14 women.[571] Case reports also describe the use of positron emission tomography scanning to identify occult lesions.[572] The absence of a lesion on either mammography or MRI does not rule out the possibility of disease within the breast.

In the past, it was generally recommended that women with axillary disease (in the setting of an occult primary) undergo

TABLE 37.2-17. Results of Mastectomy in 228 Women with Axillary Disease in the Setting of an Occult Primary Tumor

Investigators	*Patients*	*Cancers/ Mastectomies*	*5-Y Survival Rate (%)*
Ashikari et al.[573]	42	22/34 (65%)	79
Baron et al.[565]	35	22/33 (67%)	75
Ellerbroek et al.[567]	42	1/13 (8%)	72
Fitts et al.[578]	13	11/13 (85%)	71
Haagensen[574]	18	13/14 (93%)	57
Kemeny et al.[580]	20	5/11 (45%)	Not stated
Owen et al.[575]	25	15/25 (60%)	50
Patel et al.[576]	29	16/29 (55%)	28
Vezzoni et al.[566]	49	33/44 (75%)	84
Westbrook and Gallagher[577]	18	9/12 (75%)	61
Total		147/228 (64%)	

mastectomy.[573] Table 37.2-17 summarizes the results of mastectomy in 228 patients. Overall, a primary tumor was found in 64% of patients, with the highest rate of detection in some of the older studies in which patients did not routinely undergo mammography. The size of the cancers identified at mastectomy has varied. Contrary to what some might expect, some of the cancers identified are of moderate size. Rosen and Kimmel reported a median tumor size of 1.5 cm (range, 0.1 to 6.6 cm),[579] and Baron et al. noted that 45% of the cancers were multifocal.[565] These findings have important implications for BCT in these women, although it is likely that the use of MRI to detect occult cancers would decrease the proportion of women identified with unsuspected tumors at the time of mastectomy.

There are a number of reports of using BCT in patients with occult primaries.[566,580–583] The obvious objection to this approach is that there may be a relatively large tumor, multifocal disease, or both in the breast that might not be well controlled with radiation. Results with this approach have been mixed. A series of 44 patients treated at the Institut Curie with relatively high-dose whole breast irradiation (median dose, 60 Gy) reported a 9% risk of ipsilateral breast recurrence at 8 years.[581,582] Ellerbroek et al. reported a 17% 5-year actuarial rate of ipsilateral breast recurrence in a group of 16 women treated with breast conservation.[567] There has been no apparent survival difference associated with breast conservation in comparison with mastectomy, but randomized trials in women with occult primaries have not been performed. Furthermore, the series are sufficiently small that it would be misleading to draw anything but the most tentative conclusions regarding the survival equivalence of this approach. Whether or not a mastectomy is performed, some form of axillary surgery should be performed in women presenting with palpable axillary disease because of the limited ability of radiation to control gross axillary disease.

Overall survival for women with occult primary tumors is similar to the survival of patients with comparable axillary involvement in the setting of known primary tumors. Some investigators have suggested that survival may even be slightly better for those with occult primary tumors.[582] Given the fact that tumor size is of prognostic significance even in patients with positive nodes, it is not surprising that those with occult primary tumors (often with minimal disease in the breast) could have a slightly better prognosis than the general population of node-positive patients. Systemic treatment for patients with occult primary tumors and axillary involvement should reflect the current standard of care for patients with node-positive breast cancer.

Phyllodes Tumor

The term *phyllodes tumor* includes a group of lesions of varying malignant potential ranging from completely benign tumors to fully malignant sarcomas. Clinically, phyllodes tumors are smooth, rounded, multinodular lesions that may be indistinguishable from fibroadenomas. Skin ulceration is seen with large tumors, but this is usually due to pressure necrosis rather than invasion of the skin by malignant cells. Histologically, phyllodes tumor, like fibroadenoma, is composed of epithelial elements and a connective tissue stroma.

Phyllodes tumors are classified as benign, borderline, or malignant based on the nature of the tumor margins (pushing or infiltrative) and presence of cellular atypia, mitotic activity, and overgrowth in the stroma.[584] There is disagreement about which of these criteria is most important, although most experts favor stromal overgrowth. The percentage of phyllodes tumors classified as malignant ranges from 23% to 50%.[585,586] Axillary metastases are reported in less than 5% of cases, but are a poor prognostic sign when present. Metastases more commonly follow the pattern seen with sarcomas (with the lung as the most common site) and histologically resemble sarcomas. They occur in 6% to 22% of cases and are considerably more common in the malignant subtype.[584–587] Approximately 20% of phyllodes tumors recur locally if excised with no margin or a margin of a few millimeters of normal breast tissue, regardless of whether they are benign or malignant.[588] A wide excision with a 2-cm margin of normal breast tissue is appropriate therapy for benign and borderline phyllodes tumors unless they are so large that this is not cosmetically feasible. In the past, many authors have advocated mastectomy for the management of malignant phyllodes tumors.[588,589] Since phyllodes tumors are not multicentric, there is no clear-cut biologic rationale for mastectomy, and series have reported the successful treatment of malignant phyllodes tumors with wide excision.[590,591] The use of systemic therapy for malignant phyllodes tumors is based on the guidelines for treating sarcomas.

PROGNOSTIC AND PREDICTIVE FACTORS

Some of the key decisions in the current management of primary breast cancer involve the need for prognostication and the optimal selection of therapy. A *prognostic factor* is defined as a biologic or clinical measurement that is associated with disease-free or overall survival in the absence of adjuvant systemic therapy. A *predictive factor* is any measurement associated with response or lack of response to a particular therapy. Estrogen receptor status has been clearly shown to be a predictive factor for hormonal therapy, in both the adjuvant and metastatic disease settings. Prognostication is especially important in identifying patients whose prognoses are so favorable that adjuvant systemic therapy is unnecessary. Prognostic factors can also be useful in identifying patients whose prognoses with conventional treatment are so poor as to warrant consideration of more aggressive investigational therapies.

It should be stressed that evaluating potential prognostic and predictive factors requires caution. Individual studies often evaluate many factors and report only the statistically significant ones. To be useful, potential factors require validation in a separate large data set in which multivariate analysis allows for the assessment of the potential factor when adjusted for other known factors.[592–594] It has also been recognized that certain prognostic factors may only be important in the first 5 years after primary treatment, but not with long-term follow-up.

The most established prognostic factor is the number of positive axillary lymph nodes based on at least a level I or II axillary dissection and a detailed histologic evaluation. An adequate axillary dissection usually contains at least ten lymph nodes. As the number of involved lymph nodes increases, relapse rates increase, and survival rates decrease.[595] Patients are often grouped as having negative nodes, one to three positive nodes, four to nine positive nodes, or ten or more positive nodes. Given the morbidity of axillary dissection and controversies about its therapeutic value, many patients are now undergoing sentinel node biopsy or no axillary surgery (see Axillary Treatment, earlier in this chapter).

Tumor size, one of the first prognostic variables accurately quantified, is also a valuable prognostic factor. Tumor size refers to the maximal size of the invasive component measured on microscopic sections. Tumor size correlates with the number of histologically involved nodes, but has independent prognostic significance. Tumor size is particularly useful in patients with pathologically negative nodes. Patients with negative nodes and tumor size less than 1 cm have a favorable prognosis.[432,596,597] This appears true even for patients with mammographically detected cancers, except perhaps those showing casting-type calcifications.[598]

Tumor grade is commonly provided on pathology reports, and several investigators have demonstrated that it is an important prognostic factor in individual series. The use of tumor grade, however, has been limited by poor reproducibility.[599,600] The most widely used grading systems for breast cancer are the Scarff-Bloom-Richardson classification and Fisher's nuclear grade, although both systems are frequently used in modified versions.[601,602] Other pathologic factors, such as lymphatic and vascular invasion and the presence of necrosis, have been found to be important prognostic factors in individual series, but are similarly limited by poor reproducibility.

Among clinical factors, young patient age has been reported to be an adverse prognostic factor by some,[260,603] but not all, investigators. In two large studies, breast cancer patients younger than 35 years of age had a worse prognosis than older patients. In both studies, young patients were more likely than older patients to have adverse prognostic factors, but young age remained a significant prognostic factor in multivariate analysis. At the 1998 Sixth International Conference on Adjuvant Therapy of Breast Cancer, young patient age was first recognized as an adverse prognostic factor.[604]

Of the biochemical measurements, the most important is the presence or absence of ER and PR in the tumor. In the past, the receptor status was determined by a dextran-coated charcoal biochemical assay. More recently, nearly all laboratories are using an immunohistochemistry assay (estrogen and progesterone receptor immunohistochemical assay, ERICA and PRICA). ERICA is preferable in that it does not require fresh tissue, allows correlation with histology, and can be performed even on very small lesions. Although hormone receptor status correlates with prognosis, it does so only weakly. Furthermore, several studies have reported that ER is a prognostic factor for 5-year disease-free survival, although the curves tend to merge with longer follow-up.[605,606] This suggests that ER status is a measure of proliferative capacity, rather than metastatic potential. Despite this, hormone receptor determination is of critical importance as a predictive factor for hormonal therapy. In addition, the 1998 Overview on the use of adjuvant chemotherapy [see Adjuvant Drug (Systemic) Therapy, later in this chapter] showed that its effectiveness was somewhat greater in ER-poor cancers than in ER-positive cancers, thus establishing ER as a weak predictive factor for adjuvant chemotherapy.

The identification of micrometastases in bone marrow using antibodies to various epithelial antigens has also been evaluated for its prognostic significance. A metaanalysis of 20 published studies reported in 1998, including 2494 patients using a variety of techniques, concluded that the presence of micrometastases did not contribute independent prognostic information.[607] More recently, a group using a monoclonal antibody to bind an antigen on cytokeratins not present on bone marrow cells showed a strong correlation between the presence of cytokeratin-positive cells in the bone marrow and 4-year survival.[608] This study raised the possibility that standardized procedures for (1) the preparation of bone marrow specimens, (2) the use of antibodies and staining technique, and (3) the criteria for defining positively stained cells may allow for the routine use of this procedure. Additional follow-up and future studies are needed to establish this before its use in routine clinical practice.

Measures of proliferation have been another area for the evaluation of prognostic factors. This includes mitotic index, thymidine labeling index, flow cytometry, and several antibodies to cell-cycle–associated antigens. One of the concerns in the use of these various measures of proliferation is ensuring standardization. The most thoroughly evaluated of these in the United States has been DNA flow cytometry. Flow cytometry can be performed on fresh tissue specimens, frozen biopsy samples, needle aspirates taken directly from the tumor, or paraffin-embedded tissues. The technique produces a measure of DNA content (DNA ploidy) and the distribution of cells in the cell cycle. Of particular interest has been the percent of cells in the S phase. In 1997, a review of the experience with S-phase fraction determined by flow cytometry concluded that standardization and quality control must be improved before it can be routinely used.[609]

Studies are also under way to determine whether S-phase fraction is a predictive factor for the use of chemotherapy. Studies using antibodies to Ki-67 and proliferating cell nuclear antigen have shown encouraging early results but are not established. To date, there have been relatively few studies that have directly compared different measures of proliferation.

There has also been interest in the prognostic value of growth factors and their receptors. Of these growth factors, the greatest interest has been in HER-2/*neu*. The gene is located on chromosome 17q21 and is transcribed into a 4.5-kb mRNA, which is translated into a 185-kD glycoprotein. While multiple studies have demonstrated the negative impact of HER-2/*neu* overexpression on the progress of node-positive patients, the role of HER-2/*neu* in node-negative patients is less clear.[610] There is evidence, however, that HER-2/*neu* may be a useful predictive factor. Several retrospective studies suggest that only patients whose tumors have little or no detectable levels of HER-2/*neu* derive considerable benefit from cyclophosphamide (Cytoxan), methotrexate, and 5-fluorouracil regimens, and, in a study from CALGB, that patients whose tumors have high levels of HER-2/*neu* derive greater benefit from dose-intensive Cytoxan, Adriamycin, and 5-fluorouracil regimens.[611] A study from the NSABP that compared adjuvant treatment with and without Adriamycin demonstrated that patients with HER-2/*neu*–negative tumors had the same outcome with or without Adriamycin, whereas patients with HER-2/*neu*–positive tumors who did not receive Adriamycin had significantly worse prognoses.[612] Similar results were also seen in a trial from the Southwest Oncology Group study.[613] With the growing use of HER-2/*neu* testing, the most reliable method to determine HER-2/*neu* status must be established.[614]

It has also been suggested that HER-2/*neu* status may predict response to endocrine therapy.[615] Among patients treated with adjuvant tamoxifen, those with HER-2/*neu*–positive tumors tend to have shorter disease-free and overall survival times compared with patients with low HER-2/*neu* levels.[616] However, the data supporting an interaction between HER-2/*neu* expression and adjuvant tamoxifen therapy is not conclusive, and patients with ER-positive and HER-2/*neu*–positive cancers should still receive adjuvant hormonal therapy. Ongoing trials are testing the combined use of tamoxifen and trastuzumab (Herceptin) in these patients.

There are a large number of investigations of other potential prognostic and predictive factors; however, it is beyond the scope of this chapter to review each of them. None has been established for routine use in clinical care, including nm23, p53, cathepsin D, and other measures of tumor invasiveness, measures of angiogenesis, and evolving microarray technology.

ADJUVANT DRUG (SYSTEMIC) THERAPY

It is thought that occult metastases (or *micrometastases*) are commonly present when patients first present with operable breast cancer. This view is based on the fact that, even following effective local treatment, many patients develop metastatic involvement over time and improvements in local control have been shown to provide, at best, only a small decrease in distant metastases.[248,617] Given this, improving the long-term outlook for newly diagnosed breast cancer patients with early-stage disease can only be accomplished with improvements in systemic therapy.

Beginning more than three decades ago, many clinical trials were organized to test the value of various drugs as an adjunct or *adjuvant* to local treatment. These trials, described in detail here, have demonstrated significant improvements in survival for treated patients compared with controls. Adjuvant chemotherapy, hormonal therapy, or both are now in widespread use around the world. Since its introduction, there has been a decrease in the death rate from breast cancer, suggesting a beneficial effect on public health. In many populations, it has been difficult to distinguish the life-saving effects of screening mammography from those of adjuvant systemic therapy since these two interventions were introduced at approximately the same time. In one large population-based study from British Columbia in which this issue was studied, the use of adjuvant systemic therapy by itself had a direct beneficial effect on the death rate from breast cancer.[617]

TABLE 37.2-18. Adjuvant Drug Therapy: Percentage Reduction in the Annual Odds of Either Recurrence or Death (from Any Cause)

Patient Age (y)	*Therapy*	*Reduction in Annual Odds of Recurrence (%)*	*Reduction in Annual Odds of Death (%)*
<50	Tamoxifen × 5 y vs. no therapy	45 ± 8	32 ± 10
50–59	Tamoxifen × 5 y vs. no therapy	37 ± 6	11 ± 8
60–69	Tamoxifen × 5 y vs. no therapy	54 ± 5	33 ± 6
<40	Polychemotherapy vs. none	37 ± 7	27 ± 8
40–49	Polychemotherapy vs. none	35 ± 5	27 ± 5
50–59	Polychemotherapy vs. none	22 ± 4	14 ± 4
60–69	Polychemotherapy vs. none	18 ± 4	8 ± 4

(Adapted from refs. 110 and 619.)

Over 100 prospective randomized clinical trials of adjuvant therapy have been conducted. More than 15 years ago, the Early Breast Cancer Trialists' Collaborative Group was formed to organize this vast body of information. This group has provided a composite analysis of all randomized trials of the treatment of primary breast cancer performed worldwide.[618] The major portion of this activity has focused on adjuvant drug therapy; the results of the 1995 Overview are summarized in Table 37.2-18.[110,619] The 1995 Overview (published in 1998) provided important new insights related to the value of tamoxifen in premenopausal women and the utility of chemotherapy in postmenopausal women.

In the Overview, the number of events (either relapse or death) in the treatment and control arms of individual trials are scored to determine an expected-minus-observed value and an odds ratio indicative of the value of the treatment. When a treatment is beneficial in a given trial, the expected-minus-observed value is negative, and the odds ratio is less than 1.0. Similar studies are grouped together, and a combined expected-minus-observed value and overall odds ratio can then be calculated. In combining the results of similar studies, each expected-minus-observed value and odds ratio are weighted by the relative size of each experiment so that a large study with more events counts more. This statistical method provides an estimate of the effectiveness of a certain therapy based on the entirety of all available data from randomized trials (see Table 37.2-18).

In examining the results of the Overview, it is important to distinguish those results that are generated from a direct comparison of randomized arms and those results that are indirect comparisons of treatment results across different studies. For example, an indirect comparison would use data from trials comparing chemotherapy versus no treatment with trials comparing ovarian ablation versus no treatment to compare the relative benefits of chemotherapy versus ovarian ablation. The results of direct comparisons provide solid information for use in making treatment decisions, whereas the results of indirect comparisons should be used in generating hypotheses to be

TABLE 37.2-19. Absolute Reduction in Mortality at 10 Years per 100 Patients Treated

	Proportional Reduction in Annual Mortality (%)		
	.50	.30	.10
Estimated mortality at 10-y with no therapy			
70% (multiple positive nodes)	23 (70 47)	13 (70 57)	4 (70 66)
30% (moderate risk, node-negative)	12 (30 18)	7 (30 23)	2 (30 28)
10% (<1-cm tumor, node-negative)	5 (10 5)	3 (10 7)	1 (10 9)

(Adapted from ref. 110.)

The results of the breast cancer metaanalysis suggest an important principle; namely, that the proportional reduction in the risk of relapse as a result of a treatment is generally constant regardless of the patient's absolute risk of relapse (Table 37.2-19). To illustrate this, assume that a therapy reduces the annual odds of relapse by one-third. If we treat patients who are expected to have recurrences at a rate of 15% per year, only approximately 20% of patients would be free of disease at the end of 10 years without therapy. Reducing the rate of recurrence by one-third with therapy reduces the annual relapse rate to 10%. At this reduced recurrence rate, 35% of patients would be free of disease at 10 years, for an absolute improvement of 15%. If we apply the same therapy to a group of patients expected to develop recurrent disease at 1.5% per year, we would lower the recurrence rate to 1.0% per year with therapy. In turn, the percentage of patients who develop recurrence would decline from 14% to 10% at 10 years. In this situation, the absolute improvement is only 4%. In some situations, such as a woman with a tumor that is less than 1 cm with negative nodes, the absolute benefits might be even smaller.

Clinicians should consider the effect of an adjuvant therapy in terms of both disease-free and overall survival. Ultimately, the goal of adjuvant treatment is to prolong survival. Some clinicians would argue that an improvement in disease-free survival, in and of itself, justifies the use of adjuvant treatment since recurrence is often associated with substantial morbidity. Any improvement in disease-free survival must be considered in the context of the short- and long-term toxicity of adjuvant treatment. In general, improvement in disease-free survival usually translates into survival benefits as well. For this reason, it is reasonable to consider disease-free survival in making treatment decisions, particularly if the studies in question have a sufficiently short follow-up such that an overall survival advantage would not yet emerge.

ADJUVANT TAMOXIFEN

Tamoxifen was initially considered a promising candidate for adjuvant treatment because of its efficacy against advanced disease and relative lack of toxicity. In the Overview analysis, over 37,000 patients were randomized in 55 trials examining the effect of adjuvant tamoxifen at a dose of 20 to 40 mg/d for at least 1 year. The trial has yielded no clear evidence that 40 mg is superior to 20 mg, in addition to which, the higher dose is more expensive and possibly more toxic. As a result, the standard dose of tamoxifen is 20 mg/d.

TABLE 37.2-20. Effects of Tamoxifen for 5 Years According to Estrogen-Receptor Level

Estrogen-Receptor Level	*Reduction in Annual Odds of Recurrence (%)*	Reduction in Annual Odds of Death (%)
Poor (<20 fmol/mg)	6 ± 11	−3 ± 11
Unknown	37 ± 8	21 ± 9
Positive	50 ± 4	28 ± 5
10–99 fmol/mg	43 ± 5	23 ± 6
≥100 fmol/mg	60 ± 6	36 ± 7

(Adapted from ref. 110.)

As shown in Table 37.2-18, the benefits of tamoxifen are substantial and are seen in both premenopausal and postmenopausal women. Tamoxifen, taken for approximately 5 years, reduces the annual odds of disease recurrence by 47% and the annual odds of death by 26%. The degree of benefit is similar in younger and older women. The benefits of tamoxifen administered for 5 years were similar despite the presence or absence of chemotherapy. This finding represented a change from the previous Overview, at least for premenopausal women. Importantly, the benefits seen with tamoxifen were only seen in women with ER-positive tumors. There appeared to be no benefit from adjuvant tamoxifen in ER-poor patients in terms of either recurrence or death (Table 37.2-20).[110]

In terms of duration of tamoxifen therapy, 5 years of treatment is the standard of care (Table 37.2-21).[110] Once women with ER-poor tumors were excluded from the analysis, indirect comparisons indicated that 5 years were superior to 2 years or less. This finding is supported by the results of two individual studies comparing 2 years versus 5 years of tamoxifen.[620,621] It remains uncertain whether more than 5 years of tamoxifen could be superior to 5 years. In both the NSABP B-14 trial and a trial from Scotland, patients randomized to more than 5 years of therapy appeared to have a greater risk of recurrence.[288,622] An Eastern Cooperative Oncology Group trial suggested that the continuation of tamoxifen beyond 5 years may delay relapse in ER-positive patients; however, there was no difference in survival in this study.[623] At present, the available data would support stopping tamoxifen at 5 years. Of note, there are both preclinical and clinical data (withdrawal responses in the metastatic setting) to suggest that tamoxifen may act as a growth agonist after variable periods of exposure.[624] If this is the case, it is not difficult to imagine that the withdrawal of tamoxifen could, in and of itself, be of benefit. Tamoxifen lowers the risk of disease recurrence even after it has been discontinued.[110] Women randomized to 5 years of tamoxifen had a 33% annual reduction in recurrence after 5 years (when they were no longer taking tamoxifen) compared with women who never took tamoxifen. For mortality, the proportional reduction after 5 years was similar to the proportional reduction seen during the first 5 years.

TABLE 37.2-21. Duration of Tamoxifen

Group	*Reduction in Annual Odds of Recurrence (%)*	*Reduction in Annual Odds of Death (%)*
Tamoxifen 1 y		
<50	2 ± 7	−2 ± 8
50–59	28 ± 6	21 ± 6
All	20 ± 3	11 ± 3
Tamoxifen 2 y		
<50	14 ± 5	10 ± 6
50–59	32 ± 4	19 ± 5
All	29 ± 3	17 ± 3
Tamoxifen 5 y		
<50	45 ± 8	32 ± 10
50–59	37 ± 6	11 ± 8
All	47 ± 3	26 ± 4

(Adapted from ref. 110.)

In general, tamoxifen appears to have greater benefit in women with strongly positive ERs.[110] In the trials evaluating 5 years of tamoxifen, the proportional reduction in annual recurrence was 43% for patients who had moderately ER-positive tumors (less than 100 fmol) and 60% for women with strongly ER-positive tumors (greater than 100 fmol). Similar trends were seen for mortality. Despite the predictive value of progesterone receptors (PR) in patients with advanced disease, PR status did not appear to affect the benefits of tamoxifen in patients with ER-positive tumors. There were insufficient numbers of patients with ER-negative, PR-positive tumors in the Overview to draw any definite conclusions about the benefits of tamoxifen in this subgroup. In clinical practice, such patients are usually considered to have hormonally responsive disease, and similar recommendations for adjuvant tamoxifen therapy should be made for ER-negative, PR-positive patients as for those with ER-positive tumors.

As noted previously, the substantial benefits of adjuvant tamoxifen appear to be confined to patients with positive hormone receptor results. This finding represents a change from previous publications of the Overview. A total of 8000 women with ER-poor tumors were randomized to tamoxifen or no tamoxifen. Although the 10% reduction in the annual odds of recurrence is statistically significant, the absolute benefit is of small magnitude. The proportional reduction in terms of mortality is even smaller, and there is no trend for improved outcome with longer duration of treatment. Given these results, women who are shown to have negative hormone receptor status should not be treated with tamoxifen to prevent a systemic recurrence.

With growing interest in the measurement of HER-2/*neu* or c-erbB-2, there has been concern raised about the role of tamoxifen in women with both positive hormone receptors and HER-2/*neu* overexpression. In the metastatic setting, trials have suggested relative resistance to hormonal therapy in patients with HER-2/*neu* overexpression.[625] In the adjuvant setting, a retrospective analysis of the Italian GUN-1 trial suggested that patients with ER-positive, HER-2/*neu* overexpressing tumors had a worse outcome with tamoxifen than those who received no hormonal intervention.[626] A retrospective analysis of a large CALGB trial failed to detect a negative interaction between tamoxifen and HER-2/*neu*.[627] At this time, HER-2/*neu* overexpression does not preclude the use of adjuvant tamoxifen in a patient who is otherwise an appropriate candidate.

In addition to its effect on recurrence and mortality in trials of 5 years of therapy, tamoxifen has also been shown to reduce the incidence of contralateral tumors. There was a 47% reduction in the annual odds of developing a contralateral cancer.

TABLE 37.2-22. Adverse Effects of Tamoxifen

Serious, but Rare	*Less Serious, but More Common*	*Not Proven, but a Concern for Many Patients*
Thromboembolic events	Hot flashes	Depression
Endometrial cancer	Vaginal discharge	Weight gain
Cataracts	Sexual dysfunction	

The reduction in contralateral tumors was independent of the hormone receptor status of the primary tumor. These findings are consistent with the results of individual trials,[288] the NSABP tamoxifen prevention trial,[113] and the results seen with the use of tamoxifen in women with DCIS.[204]

The serious toxicities of tamoxifen and the common side effects are listed in Table 37.2-22. In individual trials, the Overview, and the tamoxifen prevention trial, there has been an unequivocal increase in the incidence of endometrial cancer in women taking tamoxifen. The excess risk over 10 years is estimated to be four cases of endometrial cancer per 1000 women. In NSABP B-14, there was a 0.16% annual risk of developing endometrial cancer on tamoxifen.[113] The breast cancer prevention trial has strongly suggested that endometrial cancer is primarily a problem for women over 50.[113] Thromboembolic complications were also seen more frequently in older women.

Tamoxifen has been reported to have positive effects on bone density in postmenopausal women.[628] In the NSABP prevention study, there was a reduction in osteoporotic fractures with tamoxifen that almost reached statistical significance.[113] The clinical significance of this finding is uncertain, and the effects of tamoxifen on bone have not been compared with the bone effects of agents approved to prevent or treat osteoporosis. In premenopausal women, there has been concern raised about accelerated bone loss.[629] Although tamoxifen does lower cholesterol levels,[630] there was no improvement in cardiac or vascular events with tamoxifen in the Overview.[110] In the NSABP prevention study, there was no difference in the frequency of fatal myocardial infarction, nonfatal myocardial infarction, or angina requiring surgical intervention.[113]

In patients who are receiving chemotherapy, tamoxifen can be administered either following the completion of treatment or concurrently with chemotherapy. While there have been theoretical concerns raised about tamoxifen reducing tumor growth rates and interfering with the effects of chemotherapy,[631] this has not been observed clinically. Clinical studies indicate that thromboembolic complications are increased when the two treatments are administered concurrently.[632] Outside of a clinical trial, either approach is reasonable. A similar concern has been raised about a potential negative interaction of tamoxifen and radiation, but this has not been supported by clinical data. Tamoxifen, which was administered concurrently with radiation, lowered the rate of ipsilateral breast recurrences by 61% in NSABP B-14.[113]

Which patients with invasive breast cancer should receive tamoxifen? It is possible to answer this question with less equivocation than in the past. All women who have positive lymph nodes or tumors greater than 1 cm in the setting of positive hormone receptors should receive adjuvant tamoxifen for a period of 5 years. For women with small tumors (T1a or T1b) and negative lymph nodes, the risk of a systemic recurrence is relatively low, and decisions about tamoxifen need to be considered carefully. For the majority of such women, the benefits of tamoxifen probably outweigh the risks. This is particularly the case for a woman who has undergone CS plus radiation and in whom tamoxifen will not only decrease the risk of a systemic recurrence but will also lower the chance of an ipsilateral recurrence or a new contralateral primary. Since the life-threatening toxicities of tamoxifen (endometrial cancer and thromboembolic disease) are more common in women over 50, these toxicities should be considered when making decisions about tamoxifen in this older group of women who are at low risk of recurrence. The decision to continue tamoxifen needs to be reevaluated in women who experience unpleasant side effects. While tamoxifen is usually well tolerated, some patients have a more difficult time with side effects than others. In summary, it is reasonable to consider the use of tamoxifen and to discuss the pros and cons of treatment in any woman diagnosed with a hormone receptor–positive or unknown breast cancer. Tamoxifen should not be administered to women with negative hormone receptor status unless the main goal of treatment is to prevent a second primary tumor. It should be recognized, however, that for the majority of women with invasive breast cancer, the risk of a systemic recurrence is far higher than the risk of developing a second primary tumor.

HORMONAL INTERVENTIONS OTHER THAN TAMOXIFEN

Although tamoxifen is the mainstay of adjuvant hormonal therapy for patients with breast cancer, questions still remain about the role of ovarian ablation in the management of women with stage I or II disease. If anything, this area has become even more complex in recent years as a result of new findings from clinical trials.

Twelve randomized trials using either surgical or radiation ablation were judged to be of adequate quality to be included in the Overview.[633,634] Of these studies that included 3456 women, seven evaluated ovarian ablation as the sole adjuvant treatment and five looked at ovarian ablation in combination with chemotherapy. Many of the trials were underpowered; some included both premenopausal and postmenopausal women, and only the trials that included chemotherapy had information on ER assays. Despite the fact that most of the individual trials had failed to detect a difference in overall survival, the combined analysis of the 12 studies indicated a highly significant improvement in both recurrence rates and survival for ovarian ablation (Table 37.2-23).[634] Not surprisingly, this benefit was confined to women who were under 50 at the time of randomization. There was no significant benefit seen with ovarian ablation in the 1354 women

TABLE 37.2-23. Metaanalysis of the Effects of Ovarian Ablation

Group	*Reduction in Annual Odds of Recurrence (%)*	*Reduction in Annual Odds of Death (%)*
Ovarian ablation vs. no adjuvant therapy (age <50)	25 ± 7	24 ± 7
Ovarian ablation + chemotherapy vs. chemotherapy	10 ± 9	8 ± 10

(Adapted from ref. 634.)

who were over 50, most of whom would have already experienced menopause. The absolute improvement in survival at 15 years associated with ovarian ablation in the older subgroup was 2.5%, a difference that was not statistically significant. Of interest, the benefits of ovarian ablation appeared to be far less dramatic in women who also received chemotherapy. The explanation for this finding may lie in the fact that at least some of the benefit associated with chemotherapy may be due to treatment-induced menopause that occurs in a substantial proportion of premenopausal women.

A U.S. Intergroup Trial prospectively studied the value of adding a luteinizing hormone–releasing hormone agonist to a course of adjuvant cyclophosphamide, Adriamycin, and 5-fluorouracil in premenopausal, receptor-positive, node-positive patients.[635] Women were randomized to chemotherapy alone, chemotherapy plus 5 years of goserelin, or chemotherapy plus 5 years of goserelin and 5 years of tamoxifen. The addition of goserelin and tamoxifen resulted in an improvement in 5-year relapse-free survival from 67% to 78% ($P < .01$), a difference that is likely attributable to tamoxifen. The addition of goserelin alone resulted in much smaller improvement in relapse-free survival that was not statistically significant. In a subset analysis, there was the suggestion of greater benefit with goserelin in women under the age of 40, who would be less likely to experience chemotherapy-induced menopause.[635]

Several European studies have also addressed the role of ovarian ablation in women with early-stage breast cancer. Investigators in Sweden randomized 732 premenopausal women with positive hormone receptors to nine cycles of intravenous CMF every 3 weeks or ovarian ablation. After a median follow-up of 68 months, there was no difference in either disease-free or overall survival.[636] In another trial, the combination of goserelin for 3 years and tamoxifen for 5 years was compared with six cycles of intravenous CMF (day 1, 8 every 28 days) in 1045 premenopausal women with hormone receptor–positive breast cancer.[637] There was no difference in survival between the two arms, although patients on the hormonal therapy had a statistically significant improvement in relapse-free survival after a median follow-up of 42 months. Finally, in a smaller but more mature trial, there was no difference seen between intravenous CMF (every 3 weeks for six to eight cycles) and ovarian ablation in approximately 300 premenopausal women.[638] In women with higher levels of ER expression, there was the suggestion of a better outcome with ovarian ablation; conversely, women with low ER expression appeared to have a better outcome with chemotherapy.

The results of these studies are of great interest, and indirect comparisons in the Overview suggest that ovarian ablation and chemotherapy are similar in the magnitude of their effects. It remains unclear where ovarian ablation fits into the treatment paradigm for women with early-stage breast cancer. Any conclusions must be tempered by the recognition that the database on ovarian ablation is far less extensive than on either chemotherapy or tamoxifen. While ovarian ablation may be comparable with chemotherapy in selected premenopausal patients, there are insufficient data to suggest that ovarian ablation should be substituted for chemotherapy as a routine practice. The potential negative consequences of ovarian ablation in women with breast cancer have not been fully investigated and could be even greater in some women than a course of chemotherapy. It also remains unclear to what extent ovarian ablation adds to benefits seen with tamoxifen in premenopausal women. For many clinicians, the pressing clinical question is whether ovarian ablation is of additional benefit in the premenopausal woman who has received chemotherapy, is taking tamoxifen, and continues to have menstrual cycles. In the absence of additional data, there are insufficient data to recommend such a treatment approach at this time.

Far more limited data are available about other adjuvant hormonal therapies. While toremifene has been shown to be equivalent to tamoxifen in the metastatic setting,[639] its activity in the adjuvant setting has not been established. There are insufficient data to support the use of any other antiestrogens as adjuvant treatment for early-stage breast cancer, including raloxifene.

In postmenopausal women, ongoing studies are evaluating aromatase inhibitors in place of tamoxifen, in conjunction with tamoxifen, and following 2 to 5 years of tamoxifen. Given the activity of aromatase inhibitors in the metastatic setting, these agents may ultimately play a role in the adjuvant therapy of postmenopausal women.

ADJUVANT CHEMOTHERAPY

The first trials of adjuvant chemotherapy were launched in the 1950s, but it was not until the late 1960s that the first modern trials of combination chemotherapy were initiated. Since the 1970s, randomized trials have addressed many fundamental questions related to adjuvant chemotherapy. Adjuvant chemotherapy initially was administered to women with positive nodes; a series of trials published in the late 1980s extended the use of adjuvant chemotherapy to node-negative women as well.[640–642]

Two early trials had a major effect on the care of women with breast cancer and the design of future studies.[643,644] The NSABP compared the use of melphalan for 2 years versus no adjuvant therapy in 349 women with node-positive disease. At the same time, Bonadonna and colleagues in Milan evaluated 12 months of CMF versus no adjuvant treatment in 386 women. Both studies showed a statistically significant improvement in disease-free survival, with subset analyses strongly suggesting most of the benefit was in women under the age of 50. The studies demonstrated a trend toward improved survival with chemotherapy, although the survival comparisons did not reach statistical significance. CMF quickly became the standard care for node-positive patients, particularly those who were premenopausal at the time of diagnosis. Twenty-year follow-up of the Milan trial has demonstrated a persistent advantage for the premenopausal women who received CMF, with a difference in survival of 47% versus 22%.[645]

Additional randomized trials have been completed since 1980. Many of these trials have been substantially larger than the early studies, thereby increasing the power of the trials to detect small but clinically meaningful differences. These trials have contributed to our understanding of the optimal duration of therapy,[646] the role anthracyclines play,[647,648] and the benefits of treatment in both node-negative[640] and postmenopausal patients.[649,650]

There are many unanswered questions about the optimal use of adjuvant chemotherapy in women with operable breast cancer, however, one can argue that more is known about adjuvant chemotherapy for women with breast cancer than almost any other topic in clinical oncology. At the present time, there

TABLE 37.2-24. Effects of Combination Chemotherapy across Entire Patient Population in Overview Analysis

Regimen	*Total No. of Patients Analyzed*	*Reduction in Annual Odds of Recurrence (%)*	*Reduction in Annual Odds of Death (%)*
All polychemotherapy regimens	18,788	23.5% (± 2.1); $2P<.00001$	15.3% (± 2.4); $2P<.00001$
Cyclophosphamide, methotrexate, and 5-fluorouracil	8150	24% (± 3); $2P<.00001$	14% (± 4); $2P<.00009$
Cyclophosphamide, methotrexate, and 5-fluorouracil + additional cytotoxics	3218	20% (± 5); $2P<.00004$	15% (± 5); $2P<.003$
Other polychemotherapy	7420	25% (± 4); $2P<.00001$	17% (± 4); $2P=.00004$

(Adapted from ref. 619.)

is no woman with invasive breast cancer for whom we can say there is no benefit associated with adjuvant chemotherapy, but for many women the absolute benefit is exceedingly small. In such settings, the potential benefits of treatment need to be carefully balanced against the side effects and potential risks of treatment. Breast cancer is a heterogeneous malignancy with a highly variable natural history. While the extent of disease (or stage of disease) partially reflects the underlying biology of the cancer, a more comprehensive understanding of the molecular biology and genetics of breast cancer is needed. Ultimately, this understanding will allow us to tailor therapies for specific patient subgroups and to target therapies to different tissue types. Until we gain a better understanding of subgroup differences, we are forced to consider the risks and benefits of treatments across broad populations, as best exemplified by the Overview analysis.[619]

It is difficult to overestimate the importance of the Oxford Overview analysis[618,619] in furthering our understanding of the role that adjuvant chemotherapy plays in women with breast cancer. The results of 69 randomized trials involving approximately 30,000 women were included in the third and most recent analysis and publication of the Overview.[619] Although any metaanalysis has limitations, the large number of women included in the analysis allows for comparisons that cannot be made in individual trials.

Table 37.2-24 outlines the benefits of polychemotherapy (combination chemotherapy) in comparison with no chemotherapy in a total of 47 trials involving 17,000 women. In some of these trials, women received additional treatment (i.e., tamoxifen) as well, but all study participants were randomized to receive multiple courses of combination chemotherapy or no chemotherapy. As can be seen, there is a highly significant benefit for combination chemotherapy compared with no chemotherapy. For the population as a whole, polychemotherapy reduced the annual odds of recurrence by approximately 25% and the annual odds of death by approximately 15%. The reduction in recurrence as a result of chemotherapy was greatest during the first 5 years following diagnosis, although there was still a significant, although smaller, proportional reduction in recurrence as a result of chemotherapy even after 5 years. The effect of chemotherapy on survival was seen during the first 5 years and persisted to an equal or greater extent during the next 5 years. The fact that the survival curves continued to separate after 5 years is not surprising; recurrences of breast cancer during the first 5 years after a diagnosis may lead to death from breast cancer during the subsequent 5-year period. This finding underscores the importance of following women with early-stage breast cancer for an extended period of time to obtain a full picture of the effect of a therapy on long-term survival. The effect of adjuvant chemotherapy on women under age 50 is illustrated in Figure 37.2-5.

In the Overview analysis, the proportional reductions in recurrence and mortality are similar in node-negative and node-positive patients.[619] Given the better prognosis of node-negative patients, especially those node-negative patients with small tumors (i.e., less than 1 cm), the absolute benefit of therapy in women with negative lymph nodes is much smaller than in those who have positive nodes. It is estimated from the Overview data that an average node-negative patient under age 50 would have an absolute improvement in survival at 10 years of 7% (an improvement from 71% to 78%). In contrast, the absolute improvement for a node positive patient under age 50 is estimated to be 11% (an improvement from 42% to 53%).[619] Given the mix of trials included in the Overview, the actual benefits of chemotherapy may be somewhat greater in a compliant patient population without significant comorbidity in whom full doses are delivered.[651]

There is a strong relationship in the Overview between age and the magnitude of benefit seen with chemotherapy, with younger women having a proportionally greater reduction in both recurrence and mortality than women aged 50 to 69. The Overview includes data on only approximately 600 women aged 70 or older, thus limiting any conclusions that can be drawn regarding this subgroup. Since over one-third of all women diagnosed with breast cancer in the United States are over the age of 70,[1] it is unfortunate that additional data are not available. The reductions in recurrence and mortality by age are detailed in Table 37.2-25. Although the benefit of chemotherapy is less in older women, the Overview shows a statistically significant advantage for chemotherapy across all age groups (up to age 69).

The age-related findings in the Overview are consistent with observations made in the earlier trials[643,644] (i.e., that the benefit of chemotherapy is greater in younger women than in an older patient population). The more substantial benefit of chemotherapy in younger patients, as well as the established benefits of ovarian ablation in premenopausal women,[634] suggests that adjuvant chemotherapy may be working both through a direct cytotoxic effect on the tumor and an endocrine effect by way of the induction of menopause (which occurs in a substantial number of premenopausal women receiving chemotherapy).[553] It should be noted, however, that not all studies show a consistent relationship between the induction of menopause secondary to chemotherapy and disease outcome.[652,653] It has been difficult to separate the effects of age and menopausal status because of their high degree of correlation. It is of interest, however, that in the Overview, post-

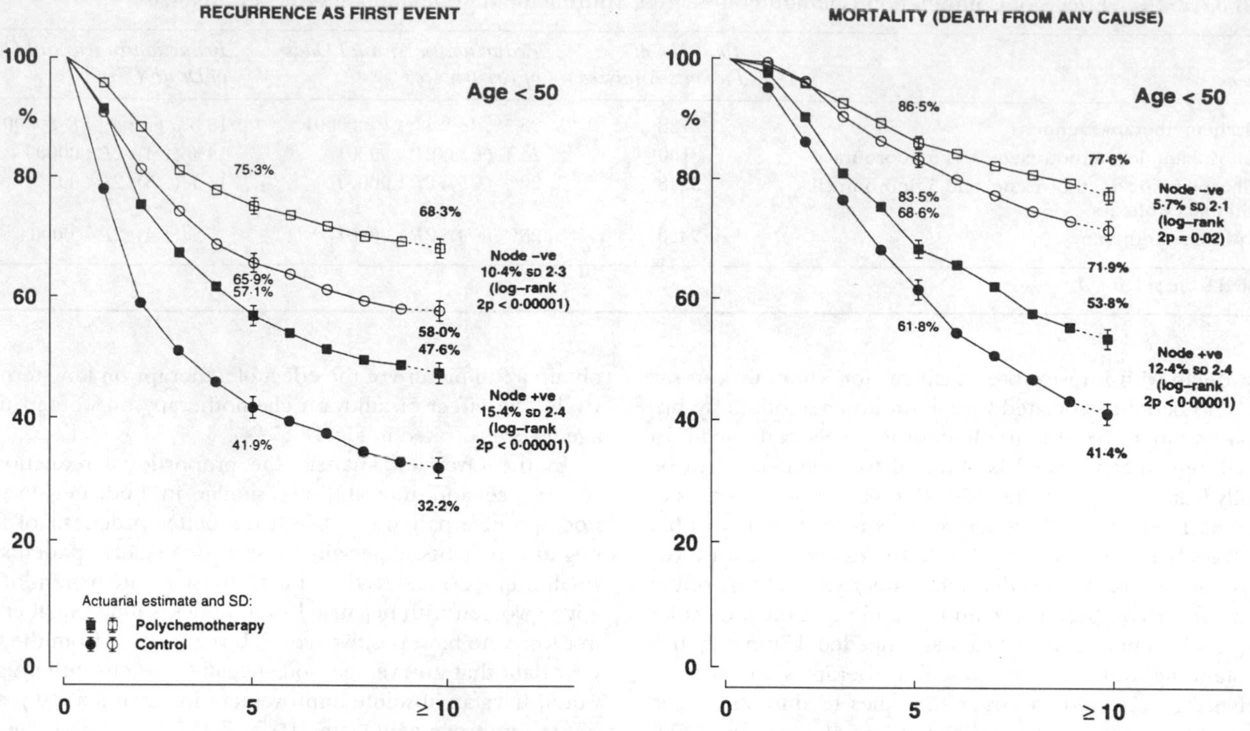

FIGURE 37.2-5. Effect of polychemotherapy on recurrence and mortality in women less than 50 years of age. (From ref. 619, with permission.)

menopausal women under the age of 50 appeared to derive a similar benefit from chemotherapy as did premenopausal women under 50.[619] This finding would suggest that chemotherapy-induced ovarian ablation is not the primary factor leading to improvement in disease-free survival and overall survival with chemotherapy. If chemotherapy is less effective in older women, there are multiple possible explanations for this phenomenon apart from the ovarian ablation hypothesis. Women over the age of 50 may have a different biologic mix of tumors; the fact that there are age-related differences in tumor biology is suggested by the differences in hormone receptor status across age. Older women may also tend to receive lower doses of therapy and are more subject to competing causes of mortality. Finally, it should be noted that several studies[640,642,643] have suggested that the age-related differences in outcome with adjuvant chemotherapy may be less significant than was previously thought.

Other subjects addressed in the 1998 Overview include the influence of hormone receptor status on decisions regarding therapy and the utility of tamoxifen in conjunction with adjuvant chemotherapy.[619] While chemotherapy was beneficial to a highly significant degree in patients with both ER-negative and ER-positive tumors, there was a trend for greater benefit in women with ER-negative tumors. This finding was seen particularly in women aged 50 to 69 in whom the proportional reduction in recurrence was almost twice as great (30% ± 5 vs. 18% ± 4) in patients with ER-negative tumor compared with those who had ER-positive tumors. The administration of tamoxifen (in addition to chemotherapy) did not appear to have a substantial effect on the benefits of chemotherapy. In other words, the proportional risk reductions from chemotherapy were similar whether or not a woman received tamoxifen; however, the number of younger women receiving chemoendocrine therapy in the Overview was small.[619]

TABLE 37.2-25. Effect of Age on Outcome with Adjuvant Chemotherapy

Age (y)	*Reduction in Annual Odds of Recurrence (%)*	*Reduction in Annual Odds of Death (%)*
<40	37 ± 7	27 ± 5
40–49	34 ± 5	27 ± 5
50–59	22 ± 4	14 ± 4
60–69	18 ± 4	8 ± 4

(Adapted from ref. 619.)

The Overview has provided additional findings of clinical significance. Among these findings, shorter duration therapy (3 to 6 months) appears to be as effective as longer therapy. In addition, anthracycline-containing regimens appear to be superior to non–anthracycline-containing regimens. A total of 11 randomized trials involving 5942 patients compared CMF with an anthracycline-containing regimen. Overall, anthracycline-containing therapy resulted in a proportional recurrence reduction of 12% and a proportional mortality reduction of 11%. The mortality reduction, which resulted in an absolute improvement in survival at 5 years of 2.7%, was of borderline statistical significance.[619] Finally, the Overview did not demonstrate a preponderance of deaths from other causes as a result of chemotherapy, including deaths from other neoplasms and deaths from vascular events.[619]

USE OF ANTHRACYCLINES IN THE ADJUVANT SETTING

The use of anthracycline-based therapy merits further comment. The finding from the Overview, suggesting a small incremental benefit with anthracyclines, has been seen in some individual trials as well.[654] A U.S. Intergroup trial involving almost 2700 patients compared six cycles of CMF with six cycles of cyclophosphamide, doxorubicin, and fluorouracil (CAF) in high-risk, node-negative patients.[648] The trial demonstrated a 2% improvement (one-sided $P = .03$) in survival for the Adriamycin-containing arm in both premenopausal and postmenopausal women. A Canadian trial comparing CMF and CEF (cyclophosphamide, epirubicin, fluorouracil) demonstrated an improvement in both disease-free and overall survival for the epirubicin-containing arm.[647] This trial led to the Food and Drug Administration's approval of epirubicin as adjuvant therapy in the United States. To date, epirubicin-containing adjuvant regimens have been much more popular in Europe than in the United States.

NSABP B-15 randomized node-positive patients to CMF or four cycles of AC administered every 3 weeks. Although there was no difference in disease-free survival or overall survival between the two arms, the AC arm has been widely adopted as a standard of care. The shorter duration of the treatment of the regimen and the relative ease of administration has led to the regimen's popularity. Whether or not four cycles of AC (lasting approximately 3 months) is equivalent to one of the longer anthracycline-containing regimens (which have often included fluorouracil) remains uncertain. Of interest, using a nonanthracycline regimen, the International Breast Cancer Study Group demonstrated that three cycles of CMF was inferior to six.[655]

Retrospective analyses from a number of studies suggest that the HER-2/*neu* status of the tumor may influence the relative benefit of anthracycline-containing regimens. Studies have suggested that either more intensive anthracycline-containing regimens[611] or the mere addition of an anthracycline to a non–anthracycline-containing regimen[612,613] may be particularly beneficial in patients whose tumors overexpress HER-2/*neu*. Patients who were HER-2/*neu*–negative in these studies appeared to derive far less benefit from the addition or intensification of an anthracycline.[612,613] Small retrospective studies have also suggested relative resistance of HER-2–positive disease to CMF-type regimens.[656] Given the retrospective nature of all of the analyses described previously, it remains uncertain to what extent the benefit of anthracyclines reported in individual trials and in the Overview is a function of HER-2/*neu* status. The use of an anthracycline-containing regimen has become the standard of care in patients with HER-2/*neu* overexpression (who are receiving chemotherapy) and in most patients with multiple positive lymph nodes. In women with HER-2/*neu*–negative tumors who are at low to moderate risk of recurrence, CMF-type regimens represent a reasonable standard of care. CMF-type regimens are also appropriate for patients who cannot tolerate an anthracycline. There is great interest in investigating the newer nonanthracycline regimens in this population as well.

DOSE INTENSITY AND DOSE DENSITY IN ADJUVANT TREATMENT

Dose intensity in adjuvant therapy has been of major interest since 1980. A retrospective review of the initial Milan CMF study suggested that patients who received a greater proportion of the intended chemotherapy dose had a superior outcome to those who had more extensive dose reductions.[657] This study, as well as trials in the metastatic setting and preclinical models, led to the development of a series of prospective randomized trials that tested the hypothesis that more dose-intensive treatment would improve clinical outcome for patients with node-positive breast cancer.

The Cancer and Leukemia Group B compared three doses and schedules of CAF chemotherapy. Approximately 1550 patients were randomized to either (1) four cycles of low-dose CAF; (2) six cycles of moderate-dose CAF; or (3) four cycles of high-dose CAF. The total doses in the moderate- and high-dose arms were identical, and the low-dose arm received one-half of the total dose of either of the other groups. The high-dose arm used doses of cyclophosphamide and Adriamycin (600 mg/m^2 and 60 mg/m^2, respectively) that are now considered the standard of care.[653,658] A statistically significant improvement in disease-free survival and overall survival at a median follow-up of 9 years in favor of the moderate- or high-dose arms in comparison with the low-dose arm ($P < .0001$ and $P < .004$ for the two comparisons) was seen. The absolute improvement in 5-year survival between the high- and low-dose arms was 7% (79% vs. 72%). These results are consistent with either a dose-response relationship (progressive improvement in outcome with dose escalation) or a threshold effect.[653]

Three additional trials have evaluated dose escalations with either cyclophosphamide, doxorubicin, or both. In an Intergroup trial, four cycles of AC chemotherapy were administered to over 3100 women with node-positive breast cancer. The dose of cyclophosphamide was fixed at 600 mg/m^2, but women were randomized to Adriamycin doses of 60 mg/m^2, 75 mg/m^2, and 90 mg/m^2. Despite increased acute toxicity with higher doses of doxorubicin, there was no evidence of an improvement in either disease-free survival or overall survival.[659] Although the median follow-up from the trial is relatively brief, the results do not support the use of more than 60 mg/m^2 per cycle. In two NSABP trials (B-22 and B-25), the dose of Adriamycin was kept constant at 60 mg/m^2, and women were randomized to receive 600 or 1200 mg/m^2 of cyclophosphamide. Despite the increased dose, there was no improvement in disease-free survival or overall survival.[660] In B-25, the cyclophosphamide dose was escalated from 1200 to as high as 2400 mg/m^2 for four cycles. Toxicity on the higher dose arms appeared to be greater, including an increased number of cases of acute leukemia and myelodysplasia. Although a subset analysis of women with four to nine nodes suggested a slight improvement for the high-dose arm in terms of disease-free survival and overall survival, this was not seen in other nodal subgroups. Dose escalation of cyclophosphamide beyond 600 mg/m^2 as part of combination adjuvant therapy is unlikely to be of substantial benefit and does not appear to be worth the added toxicity. While other studies have used higher than standard doses of cyclophosphamide, at present there is no established role for escalating doses above the 600 mg/m^2 cycle range in clinical practice.[661]

The ultimate test of dose intensity has been the use of very high doses of chemotherapy, usually alkylating agents, in combination with autologous bone marrow or peripheral stem cell support. An initial report from Peters et al. suggested that this approach, when used in women with ten or more positive nodes, improved disease-free survival in comparison with historical controls.[662] A series of randomized trials have been conducted over the past decade comparing high-dose chemotherapy with less intensive treatment programs. Many of these trials have been reported, while others are still accruing or maturing.

TABLE 37.2-26. Results of Adjuvant Trial Comparing High-Dose Chemotherapy with Bone Marrow Support versus Intermediate-Dose Chemotherapy

	Intermediate-Dose Chemotherapy	*High-Dose Therapy with Bone Marrow Support*	*P*
Event-free survival	64%	68%	.7
Overall survival	80%	78%	.1
Relapses	28%	20%	
Toxic deaths	0	29	

(Adapted from ref. 663.)

To date, there is little evidence that the use of high-dose chemotherapy with autologous bone marrow or peripheral stem cell support improves disease outcomes in the adjuvant setting. In the largest of the adjuvant trials, Peters et al. randomized over 800 women with ten or more positive lymph nodes to four cycles of CAF chemotherapy followed by an intermediate-dose consolidation versus the same induction therapy followed by high-dose cisplatin, carmustine, and cyclophosphamide with stem cell support.[663] With a median follow-up of 37 months, there was no significant difference in either event-free or overall survival (Table 37.2-26). Of note, the overall survival in the intermediate-dose group was 70%, far higher than many would have anticipated from the historic controls. While there were fewer relapses in the high-dose arm, this difference was offset by an increase in the number of toxic deaths on the high-dose arm. Additional follow-up is still needed, but other randomized trials have failed to demonstrate a significant benefit for treatment with high-dose chemotherapy administered with bone marrow or stem cell support.[664,665] It is premature to draw definite conclusions, but at this time, high-dose chemotherapy with peripheral stem cell support cannot be recommended as adjuvant therapy outside of controlled clinical trials.

INCORPORATION OF THE TAXANES INTO ADJUVANT THERAPY

Because of the demonstrated activity of the taxanes in the treatment of metastatic breast cancer,[666,667] both paclitaxel and docetaxel have been incorporated into adjuvant chemotherapy trials. While the results of trials with docetaxel are not yet available, four cycles of paclitaxel have been shown to improve disease-free and overall survival in node-positive patients. Henderson et al. randomized women to AC × 4 followed by paclitaxel (175 mg/m^2 every 3 weeks × 4) or no additional treatment. The addition of paclitaxel resulted in a 22% proportional reduction in the risk of recurrence and a 26% proportion reduction in mortality. These data were recently updated at an FDA hearing; at 36 months' follow-up, 73% of patients randomized to AC were alive and disease-free compared with 77% of women who received paclitaxel. The absolute improvement in survival was 3% (84% to 87%).[795] The benefit of paclitaxel was similar in premenopausal and postmenopausal women, but patients with hormone receptor–negative tumors appeared to have a greater reduction in risk than those with positive hormone receptor status [Taxol (paclitaxel) package insert].

Although four cycles of AC followed by four cycles of paclitaxel have become a widely accepted standard program for node-positive breast cancer, there are many questions remaining about this regimen. First, is the improvement in women who received paclitaxel entirely due to paclitaxel itself or is it related to the longer duration of therapy? Second, is the benefit of paclitaxel in hormone receptor–positive patients sufficiently large that it should be a routine component of the adjuvant regimen? This question is particularly relevant in the woman with positive receptors who has a small tumor, generally favorable prognostic factors, and a small number of positive lymph nodes. Finally, how will the use of other paclitaxel schedules (i.e., weekly treatment) and the use of docetaxel compare with the benefit seen in the study described previously? Ongoing trials are addressing these issues.

SELECTION OF ADJUVANT REGIMEN AND DECISION MAKING ABOUT ADJUVANT TREATMENT

There is no single adjuvant regimen that has emerged as the treatment of choice for all women with breast cancer. Although anthracycline-containing regimens have gained tremendous popularity in clinical practice and are, in some cases, superior to CMF,[619,647,648] there remains a role for CMF-type regimens in many women with breast cancer. Table 37.2-27 lists the adjuvant regimens that are acceptable in a nonprotocol setting.

It is impossible to identify a group of women with invasive breast cancer in which there is absolutely no benefit to be gained from adjuvant chemotherapy. In some patient subgroups, the benefits are of extremely small magnitude and should be carefully considered in light of the risks associated with treatment. Women with tumors less than or equal to 0.5 cm (T1a) with negative lymph nodes should not be treated with chemotherapy because of their favorable natural history.[669] Because of the limited toxicities associated with tamoxifen, the reduction in recurrence risk as a result of tamoxifen treatment, and the possibility that chemotherapy may be somewhat less effective in patients with ER-positive tumors,[619] the decision to add chemotherapy to tamoxifen in a woman who is at relatively low risk of recurrence can be particularly difficult. The acute side effects of chemotherapy (e.g., myelosuppression, emesis, mucositis, infection, fatigue) can have a substantial effect on short-term quality of life. In addition, the persistent or late effects of treatment, such as premature menopause, weight gain, and a slightly increased risk of leukemia, must also be considered.[670]

Patient preferences play an important role in decision making about adjuvant therapy. Surveys have demonstrated that some women are willing to accept the side effects of chemotherapy for small improvements in their risk of recurrence or

TABLE 37.2-27. Acceptable Adjuvant Regimens Outside of a Clinical Trial

FAC × 4–6 cycles
AC × 4 cycles
AC × 4 cycles followed by paclitaxel × 4 cycles
CEF × 6 cycles
CMF × 6 months (preferably oral)[650,668]
A × 4 cycles followed by CMF × 8 cycles (rarely used)[669]

AC, doxorubicin and cyclophosphamide; CEF, cyclophosphamide, epirubicin, fluorouracil; CMF, cyclophosphamide, methotrexate, and 5-fluorouracil; FAC, fluorouracil, Adriamycin, and cyclophosphamide.

death from breast cancer.[671,672] In one survey, the median acceptable life extension in exchange for a course of chemotherapy was 3 to 6 months, and over one-half of those surveyed indicated that they would take chemotherapy for a survival benefit of 1% or less.[672] It is unclear to what extent such surveys are representative of the general population, but there are clearly many women who accept the short-term toxicity and inconvenience of chemotherapy in exchange for a small improvement in outcome. In most preference studies, there is considerable variability across patients.[671,672] Ultimately, it is hoped that adjuvant therapy will be better tailored to the tumor, so that women do not need to consider such tradeoffs (i.e., a toxic treatment for a small benefit). Until we succeed in this endeavor, it is incumbent on oncologists to describe the potential advantages and disadvantages of adjuvant treatment to their patients.

PREOPERATIVE CHEMOTHERAPY

For the past two decades, preoperative chemotherapy has been administered to patients with locally advanced breast cancer. More recently, a number of randomized trials have been performed in which preoperative therapy has been administered to women with operable disease.[307,673,674] In general, preoperative therapy has been successful in downstaging tumors, both decreasing the size of the tumor and decreasing the number of axillary lymph nodes involved with tumor. It is extremely rare for tumors to progress during preoperative therapy, and the proportion of women who can undergo CS following preoperative treatment is increased.[306] The response to preoperative therapy is a predictor of disease-free and overall survival.[673] To date, however, there is no evidence that preoperative therapy improves overall survival when compared with postoperative treatment.[306,675] Ongoing studies may be helpful in determining whether the response to preoperative therapy can be used to individualize postsurgical treatment. Until additional data are available, the primary advantage of preoperative therapy is to increase the chance of breast-conserving CS in women who are otherwise borderline candidates for this procedure.

THERAPY OF LOCALLY ADVANCED AND INFLAMMATORY BREAST CANCER

The term *locally advanced breast cancer* encompasses a heterogeneous group of patients including those with neglected, slow-growing tumors as well as those with biologically aggressive disease. Locally advanced breast cancer is a relatively uncommon presentation in the economically developed world, accounting for only 5% of cases in major centers, and no more than 20% in other locations. In most other parts of the world, however, locally advanced breast cancer is more common, accounting for at least one-half of all cases. This difference is thought to be due to variations in public awareness and attitudes, as well as the availability of medical resources, including screening mammography. Biologic differences between populations may also play a role (as discussed later, in Inflammatory Breast Cancer). The relative infrequency of locally advanced breast cancer has limited the speed of clinical progress in this area.

The definition of locally advanced breast cancer is variable. All investigators include patients with inoperable stage IIIB, while some also include patients with operable stage III, stage IV by virtue of positive supraclavicular lymph nodes, or both. Management recommendations and prognosis might vary according to which of these definitions is used. For example, it might not be necessary to recommend preoperative chemotherapy for a patient with IIIA breast cancer that could be removed surgically. A reader of this literature needs to be certain which of the various definitions is used.

ROLE OF SYSTEMIC THERAPY

Historically, the results in treating patients with locally inoperable breast cancer using surgery and RT were uniformly poor. More aggressive local treatment did little to improve survival rates, but did result in increased complications. The results, however, improved greatly with the development of effective chemotherapy.[676–679] This is related in part to the ability of chemotherapy to convert most cases of inoperable primary breast cancer to operable disease. In addition, these patients likely experience the same benefit in decreasing rates of recurrence and death as do patients with stage I and II disease treated with postoperative chemotherapy. Since systemic therapy results in a proportional reduction in the risk of systemic recurrence, the absolute benefit in patients with locally advanced disease may be considerable. In the Overview analysis, the benefit of systemic therapy was equally apparent in adjuvant trials that included stage III patients.

The response rates to preoperative chemotherapy are high, possibly related to the presence of an intact blood supply. The use of preoperative treatment allows (1) the early initiation of systemic therapy in a disease with a high distant failure rate, (2) a reduction in the extent of the operative procedure needed to render the patient grossly free of disease, and (3) the opportunity to observe directly the response to treatment (an *in vivo* chemosensitivity assay). Should the tumor not respond to the initial chemotherapy regimen, substitution with other drugs or the timely initiation of RT may be beneficial. Clinical response is usually determined by physical examination, but can be supplemented by mammography and/or ultrasonography. It is important to note, however, that clinical response does not always correlate with pathologic response.[680] Up to one-third of patients found to be histologically free of disease have residual abnormalities by palpation or imaging after induction chemotherapy. Conversely, approximately one-third of patients thought to be in complete remission on clinical grounds still have residual disease on pathologic examination. Pathologic response is the best indicator of response to treatment, and patients with a complete pathologic response have a favorable prognosis.[681] Newer imaging methods, such as MRI,[682] may improve the ability to judge response.

A wide variety of chemotherapy regimens have been used as preoperative treatment, with most incorporating doxorubicin. These regimens generally produce response rates in at least two-thirds of patients with a complete pathologic remission rate of approximately 10% to 20%. There is no evidence that one doxorubicin-containing regimen is better than another; neoadjuvant treatment is generally given to maximal response. The optimal duration and sequencing of preoperative and postoperative therapy has not been determined.[683] Attempts are under way to determine if there are molecular predictors of response to neoadjuvant therapies.[684–686] Tamoxifen is used in patients with hormone receptor–positive cancers, although it is generally administered following the completion of chemotherapy.

INTEGRATION OF SYSTEMIC AND LOCAL THERAPIES

Following successful neoadjuvant chemotherapy, a variety of options for local treatment have been investigated. These include RT alone, simultaneous RT and chemotherapy, and surgery alone. In many but not all cases, further chemotherapy is employed after local treatment. Surgery following neoadjuvant chemotherapy permits a pathologic assessment of response, the rapid reintroduction of chemotherapy, and the use of lower doses of RT. The most typical approach is to use an anthracycline-containing chemotherapy as induction, followed by modified radical mastectomy, additional chemotherapy, and then consolidative RT. It appears feasible to do an immediate breast reconstruction using a flap in this setting,[687] although it may delay the initiation of adjuvant chemotherapy and make RT technically more difficult. Clinical trials and experience have confirmed that a combined modality approach is an effective way to achieve local control and also to provide a substantial rate of long-term survival.[676]

The high response rates seen with induction chemotherapy have stimulated interest in the use of BCT for selected patients with locally advanced breast cancer. Good results have been reported in some series,[676,688,689] but the experience using this approach is still limited, and data from randomized, prospective trials are not available. Should breast conservation be contemplated, all of the usual considerations apply, including a mammographic evaluation that does not demonstrate diffuse disease. The conservative resection should obtain clear margins with an acceptable cosmetic result. Criteria for determining the extent of surgery in a conservative resection following induction chemotherapy have not been established, and the long-term local control rates remain uncertain.

In general, prognostic factors predictive of good outcome in patients with locally advanced breast cancer are the same as in lower stages of primary breast cancer; namely, smaller tumor size, slower growth rate, better differentiation, and fewer involved axillary lymph nodes. In addition to these classical factors, the response of locally advanced cancers to preoperative chemotherapy is an additional important prognostic factor. As noted, evidence from many series indicates that patients with rapidly responding cancers and those who achieve a complete remission have a better outcome than patients who do not have a good response to chemotherapy. Patients with inflammatory breast cancer appear to have a different clinical course than other patients with locally advanced cancer. An important distinction should be drawn between locally advanced disease by virtue of rapid growth and those that are locally advanced by virtue of neglect of a slowly growing cancer. Patients with these neglected cancers have a more indolent course than similarly staged patients with rapidly growing cancer. This distinction is better discerned by a careful history than by any laboratory study including flow cytometry.

INFLAMMATORY BREAST CANCER

Although frequently grouped with other locally advanced cases, inflammatory breast cancer is a distinct clinical and pathologic entity. It is defined by the presence of diffuse brawny edema of the skin of the breast with an erysipeloid edge, usually without an underlying palpable mass. The clinical presentation is due to tumor embolization of dermal lymphatics. While dermal lymphatic invasion is required for the diagnosis as specified by the current AJCC staging system, patients with the clinical presentation, but without evidence of dermal lymphatic invasion, also have a poor prognosis with local treatment only. It is common for patients with inflammatory breast cancer to give a history of having been treated unsuccessfully with antibiotics before their referral to a breast cancer specialist. Inflammatory breast cancer is uncommon in the United States and in most of Europe, but is seen much more frequently in North Africa. European women living in Morocco have presented with this particularly virulent form of primary breast cancer, suggesting the existence of a specific etiologic agent. The identity of such a putative agent remains elusive. Inflammatory breast cancer has become more common in the United States. Data from SEER show that between 1975 and 1977 and 1990 and 1992, the incidence doubled, increasing among whites from 0.3 to 0.7 cases per 100,000 person-years and among African Americans from 0.6 to 1.1 cases.[690]

Nearly all patients with inflammatory breast cancer are dead within 5 years in the absence of systemic therapy. In addition, the historic results of surgical treatment demonstrate a difficulty in obtaining clear margins and a high local recurrence rate. Preoperative chemotherapy in patients with inflammatory breast cancer produces a response rate in the vicinity of 80%, and most patients can go on to surgical resection with clear margins. As in other patients with locally advanced breast cancer, the most typical approach is to use an anthracycline-containing chemotherapy as induction, followed by surgery, then additional chemotherapy, and then consolidative RT. With the combined modality approach, over 70% of patients achieve local tumor control. This is particularly true in patients whose tumors respond well to initial chemotherapy. In patients with inflammatory breast cancer who successfully complete a combined modality treatment, prognosis is dramatically improved when compared with the prechemotherapy era. Currently, approximately one-half of patients treated with combined modality treatment survive for 5 years and approximately 35% of the patients have been reported to be disease free at 10 years.[676,691] This improvement may reflect the biology of rapidly growing disease and its preferential effect of chemotherapy.

Improving the results in locally advanced breast cancer can be achieved by a number of means. It may be possible to decrease the incidence of locally advanced breast cancer by diminishing any socioeconomic factors that impede early diagnosis. Further improvements in the results of treating patients with locally advanced breast cancer require even better systemic therapy. In this regard, there is great interest in including patients with locally advanced disease in clinical trials of novel systemic therapies. Locally advanced disease affords a special research opportunity (i.e., the ability to obtain primary tumor tissue before and after chemotherapy to correlate with response and other clinical parameters).

FOLLOW-UP AFTER PRIMARY TREATMENT

There are over 2 million breast cancer survivors in the United States. As screening programs identify more patients with earlier stage disease, and as the number of women diagnosed with DCIS continues to rise, there will be even more women living with a personal history of breast cancer. Women with a history of invasive breast cancer are at risk of developing metastatic disease. Most recurrences are detected within 5 to 10 years

TABLE 37.2-28. Goals of Follow-Up Care after Treatment for Early-Stage Breast Cancer

Area of Concern	*Rationale and/or Goal*
Identification of second primary breast cancer or ipsilateral breast recurrence	Women with a personal history of breast cancer are at increased risk of new primary; early detection may improve survival; similar principles apply to ipsilateral recurrence
Identification of metastatic disease	Prompt identification of metastatic disease may prevent women from suffering progressive symptoms of advanced disease (e.g., bone pain) without treatment; rare recurrences, such as limited chest wall disease, may be treated with curative intent
Identification of complications related to breast cancer treatment	Surgery, chemotherapy, hormonal therapy, and radiation can all result in rare, but serious complications
Provide knowledgeable advice about other health issues	Many health issues (e.g., the decision to use hormonal replacement therapy) may be affected by a woman's history of breast cancer; a balanced view of these issues may assist women in making optimal health decisions
Provide psychosocial support	A diagnosis of breast cancer and subsequent treatment is a major event in many patients' lives; recognition of the psychosocial and psychosexual sequelae of breast cancer with institution of treatment, as needed, is part of comprehensive clinical care

after diagnosis, but later recurrences can occur.[692] Women with both invasive and noninvasive breast cancer face a 0.5% to 1.0% annual risk of developing a contralateral cancer,[693] and this risk is even higher in women diagnosed with a first breast cancer at a younger age and those with an inherited predisposition.[694] In addition, women who have been treated for breast cancer are at risk for complications related to their treatment and face a variety of health-related decisions (e.g., pregnancy, hormone replacement therapy, prevention of osteoporosis) that may need to be carefully considered in light of their breast cancer history.[671]

Although extensive testing to identify early presentations of metastatic disease is probably not warranted, there is a strong rationale for having a physician knowledgeable about breast cancer care follow the patient after completion of treatment. While many follow-up visits after breast cancer treatment may seem routine to the physician, the visit provides both the clinician and the patient with the opportunity to address a wide range of issues. Table 37.2-28 outlines the specific goals of follow-up care.

Contrary to what many patients expect,[695] early diagnosis of metastatic disease by performing frequent, extensive, or both kinds of testing has not been shown to improve survival. Two randomized trials have compared simple follow-up regimens consisting of periodic physical examination and routine mammography with more intensive evaluation including radiographic studies (chest radiography, bone scan, liver ultrasound) and laboratory studies (complete blood counts and liver function tests) in women after treatment of early-stage breast cancer.[696,697] More intensive follow-up resulted in a slightly earlier time at which systemic recurrences were detected; however, there was no difference in overall survival. Some physicians have argued that more intensive follow-up schedules might improve quality of life by providing patients with added reassurance, allowing treatment of metastatic disease before a patient develops symptoms, or both. These arguments are not supported by quality-of-life assessments performed as part of one of the large randomized follow-up studies.[696] With the development of ever more accurate methods of detecting low-volume metastatic disease (i.e., spiral CT or positron emission tomographic scanning), there is the potential to detect metastatic disease even earlier than in the randomized trials discussed previously. The routine monitoring of tumor markers may also allow for the detection of metastatic disease at an earlier point in a patient's clinical course.[698] There is little reason to believe that early detection of metastatic disease as a result of monitoring tumor markers would result in an improvement in either survival or quality of life; the routine use of tumor markers in patients who have completed breast cancer therapy is generally not recommended and can be particularly problematic.[699] An elevated marker may be the first sign of an impending recurrence, but a thorough search for metastatic disease may be negative even in the presence of an elevated marker.[700] There is no treatment that has proven to be of benefit to patients with elevated tumor markers who have no evidence of disease, and such situations are almost always anxiety provoking for patients. Early intervention in asymptomatic patients with metastatic breast cancer has not been demonstrated to improve clinical outcome. For this reason, the identification of metastatic disease in an asymptomatic patient could theoretically lead to the initiation of toxic therapy that could have a negative effect on a patient's quality of life and, at the same time, not improve her overall survival.[700]

The American Society of Clinical Oncology has published evidence-based recommendations for follow-up care after a diagnosis of breast cancer.[701] A physical examination and history (emphasizing symptoms that could be due to metastatic disease) are recommended every 3 to 6 months for the first 3 years after diagnosis and every 6 to 12 months for the subsequent 2 years. Even for patients who are 5 or more years postdiagnosis, annual follow-up is recommended. Women should be advised to do breast self-examinations on a monthly basis and to have annual mammography and gynecologic examinations. Routine laboratory testing (including tumor markers) and radiologic studies are not recommended. Patients with signs or symptoms of recurrent disease should be rigorously evaluated. These recommendations have been issued in the context of the presently available therapies for patients with recurrent breast cancer. If treatments become available in the years ahead that can prolong the lives of women diagnosed with asymptomatic, low-volume, metastatic disease, recommendations for follow-up care will need to be altered.

MANAGEMENT OF PATIENTS WITH METASTATIC BREAST CANCER

The management of patients with metastatic breast cancer is a topic familiar to most medical oncologists. Although the major-

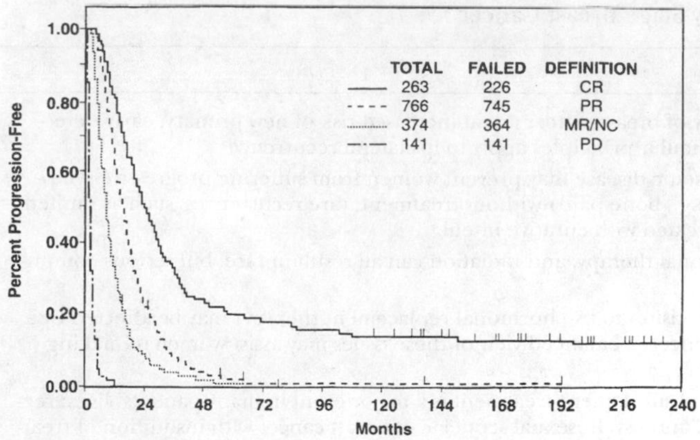

FIGURE 37.2-6. Overall survival curves of 1544 patients (excluding 37 patients with insufficient information to determine response status) with metastatic breast cancer receiving front-line chemotherapy according to response to therapy. Deaths from any cause were included. CR, complete response; MR, minimal response; NC, no change; PD, progressive disease; PR, partial response.

ity of women diagnosed with breast cancer today will never experience a systemic recurrence, approximately 41,000 women in the United States will die of metastatic breast cancer in 2000.[1] The median survival for women with metastatic breast cancer is in the range of 2 to 3 years, but there is great variability. Indeed, there are even a small number of patients with metastatic disease who will receive a course of chemotherapy and remain relapse-free for a decade or longer (Fig. 37.2-6).[702]

The heterogeneity of patients with metastatic breast cancer must be emphasized. Rarely, patients with metastatic breast cancer succumb to their disease within weeks of a diagnosis; others live with the disease for many years. Many patients have metastatic involvement that is confined to bone or soft tissue, while others have predominantly visceral disease. CNS involvement is relatively unusual as a presenting sign or symptom of metastatic disease.[703] It is important, both in the approach to individual patients and in considering clinical trial results, to have an understanding of the variability of metastatic breast cancer. Table 37.2-29 outlines the clinical and laboratory characteristics of patients with metastatic breast cancer who have an indolent versus aggressive clinical course. No single factor explains the heterogeneity that is seen clinically. It is uncertain to what extent the administration of prior adjuvant therapy affects a patient's prognosis in the setting of advanced disease. There are reports of patients responding to chemotherapy in the metastatic setting even after receiving the identical therapy in the adjuvant setting.[704] On the other hand, a patient who develops an early recurrence following treatment with an effective adjuvant regimen (i.e., CA followed by paclitaxel followed by tamoxifen) almost certainly has a relatively poor outlook in the metastatic setting.

GOALS OF THERAPY IN PATIENTS WITH METASTATIC BREAST CANCER

The two primary goals in the treatment of patients with metastatic breast cancer are (1) improvement or maintenance of quality of life and (2) prolongation of survival. The measurement of response rates in either clinical trials or clinical practice is useful only to the extent that response is a surrogate for survival, quality of life, or both. Maintenance of quality of life is achieved by controlling disease-related symptoms, minimizing toxicity from treatment, and limiting the intrusion of the patient's disease and treatment on her life. Historically, it has been difficult to demonstrate that treatment prolongs survival, but there has been an assumption on the part of many medical oncologists that treatment of metastatic breast cancer extends survival. More recently, several trials have demonstrated that more effective therapy has been able to prolong survival in women with metastatic breast cancer. These trials have included studies of hormonal agents, chemotherapeutic agents, and combinations of chemotherapy and Herceptin.[666,667,705,706] While the median prolongation in survival has been a matter of months, these trials have demonstrated an important principle (i.e., more effective treatment of metastatic breast cancer can extend the lives of our patients). In selecting a treatment program, close attention must be paid to the patient's symptoms, the pace of her disease, and her preferences and ability to tolerate the therapy.

EVALUATION OF PATIENTS WITH SUSPECTED METASTATIC BREAST CANCER

All patients who are thought to have metastatic breast cancer should undergo a careful physical examination and a thorough history. Historically, it was considered mandatory to biopsy a first site of metastatic disease to confirm the diagnosis. In the case of patients with chest wall or lymph node involvement, pleural effusions, or other easily assessable disease, obtaining biopsy or cytologic proof of metastatic disease can be accomplished with minimal difficulty. If a more complicated procedure is needed, which could place the patient at greater discomfort or risk, physician judgment must be exercised. In the patient with a history of breast cancer who has unequivocal radiologic evidence of advanced breast cancer, a biopsy can often be deferred. If there is any question as to whether the patient has cancer or any suspicion that the patient may have a second primary (i.e., widespread pure lytic bone lesions and anemia suggestive of multiple myeloma) that would require alternative treatment, a biopsy is essential. In the case of a woman with a history of breast cancer who presents with a solitary pulmonary nodule, a resection of the lesion is usually required since a high percentage of these lesions may be primary lung cancers.[707] A biopsy to establish metastatic disease provides an opportunity to reassess the hormone receptor status of the tumor. While few tumors evolve from ER negative to ER positive, more frequently there can be loss of hormone receptors over time.[624] With the availability of Herceptin, the result of a HER-2/*neu* assay is often important in making treatment decisions, although this can often be assessed from specimens of the primary tumor.

Recommendations for the laboratory and radiographic evaluation of patients with newly diagnosed metastatic breast cancer have been established by the National Cancer Center Network.[120] Routine blood work consisting of complete blood counts and liver function tests are recommended. In addition, chest radiographs and bone scans are recommended. The decision to proceed with other radiographic studies can be based on symptoms, although many physicians obtain a baseline assessment of liver involvement with a CT scan or MRI, particularly if the presence of liver metastases would change treatment. Since intracranial involvement is extremely rare in newly diagnosed

TABLE 37.2-29. Factors That Affect Prognosis in Patients with Metastatic Breast Cancer

Favorable Prognosis (Indolent Clinical Course)	*Unfavorable Prognosis (Aggressive Clinical Course)*
Long disease-free interval (usually considered at least 2 y from initial diagnosis)[a]	Short disease-free interval (usually considered less than 2 y from initial diagnosis)[a]
Hormone receptor positivity	Hormone receptor negativity
Response to prior therapy	Lack of response to prior therapy
Lack of visceral involvement	Presence of visceral involvement, CNS involvement, or both
Limited sites and bulk of disease	Multiple sites of disease and extensive involvement at these sites
HER-2/*neu* negativity	HER-2/*neu* positivity[b]

[a]Although 2 years is often used as an arbitrary cutoff in separating early recurrences from later recurrences, the longer the disease-free interval, the more indolence one can expect in terms of tumor behavior.
[b]It is not clear that HER-2/*neu* positivity remains an adverse prognostic factor with the availability of trastuzumab.

patients in the absence of CNS symptoms, a CT or MRI of the brain is not usually recommended for a woman with a new diagnosis in the absence of symptoms.[700] The use of tumor markers in the management of patients with breast cancer remains controversial.[708] It is reasonable to obtain a carcinoembryonic antigen and CA 27-29 level, looking for an elevation in either of these proteins. If elevated, they can be followed to determine if rising or falling levels correlate with the patient's disease status. Caution should be used in changing a treatment regimen based on tumor makers alone. If tumor makers are negative at the time of diagnosis, they can be checked again when the patient has disease progression, as they are more commonly elevated in patients with more extensive disease.

LOCAL VERSUS SYSTEMIC THERAPY

Patients with a chest wall recurrence, a single site of bone involvement, pleural disease, or other localized sites can often be managed with local therapy alone. In such situations, systemic therapy may be delayed until there is evidence of disease progression. There is a small group of patients with isolated metastatic disease who remain disease-free for an extended period of time after local therapy to the involved site. This situation is best exemplified by the patient who presents with an isolated chest wall recurrence. Although patients with isolated chest wall recurrence should receive definitive local treatment, local therapy is not mandatory in minimally symptomatic patients who present with isolated sites of distant disease (i.e., a single bone lesion). As previously mentioned, isolated pulmonary nodules generally should be resected because these often represent a second primary. There are reports of resection of hepatic metastases,[709] but this approach cannot be recommended as standard practice.

In certain situations, patients treated with local therapy for an isolated recurrence may also be considered for adjuvant systemic therapy. A phase II trial of fluorouracil, Adriamycin, and cyclophosphamide chemotherapy for patients with stage IV but no evidence of disease suggested an improvement in relapse-free survival in comparison with historic controls. It should be noted, however, that the majority of these patients had not received prior adjuvant chemotherapy.[710] A retrospective review of 96 patients with isolated recurrence demonstrated an improvement in disease-free survival and overall survival for those patients who received some form of systemic therapy although the majority received hormonal therapy as opposed to chemotherapy.[711] Other investigators have reported less promising results with the use of chemotherapy in this setting.[464] In such situations, the toxicity of a course of chemotherapy must be balanced against the largely theoretical benefits. The use of chemotherapy in the patient with stage IV but no evidence of disease has its greatest appeal in the patient with a hormone receptor–negative tumor who has never received cytotoxic chemotherapy, but the benefits in this setting remain uncertain. In contrast, it is reasonable to have a lower threshold to prescribe a hormonal therapy in the patient with positive hormone receptors, with the hope that treatment will delay the time to progression. A randomized trial in 167 ER-positive patients with locoregional recurrence demonstrated an improvement in median disease-free survival (26 vs. 82 months) with the addition of tamoxifen to locoregional treatment.[479] This difference was largely related to a reduction in local recurrence; there was no difference in 5-year overall survival. The role of second-line hormonal therapy in women who develop a breast recurrence on tamoxifen is unknown.

In patients with widespread disease, local therapy is often used to provide palliation for specific symptoms. Radiation to bone lesions, CNS disease, or, less commonly, soft tissue disease, can be effective in controlling disease. At times, local therapy is administered in conjunction with systemic therapy, although one must be careful about the potential increase in toxicity that may be seen with the concurrent administration of chemotherapy and radiation. Decisions about the use of local therapy in the patient with advanced disease can be complex. Such decisions should be guided by the patient's symptoms or impending symptoms, the extent to which those symptoms can be relieved by supportive care, and the chance that a change in systemic therapy will provide effective palliation for the local disease.

Administration and Choice of Systemic Therapy

The vast majority of patients with metastatic breast cancer receive some form of systemic therapy. The initial question is whether to consider hormonal therapy or chemotherapy. Because of the limited toxicity with most hormonal therapies, patients who have hormone receptor–positive tumors and a limited to moderate disease burden should generally receive hormonal therapy. Patients with both estrogen and progesterone receptor positivity are more likely to respond to hormonal therapy than are those with ER-positive/PR-negative or ER-negative/PR-positive tumors.[624] A trial of hormonal therapy may be justified even in the presence of negative hormone receptors since a small number of patients with ER-negative/PR-negative tumors respond to a hormonal intervention.[712] The key issues that the

TABLE 37.2-30. Hormonal Therapy for Women with Metastatic Breast Cancer

Premenopausal	*Postmenopausal*
Tamoxifen	Antiestrogens
Ovarian ablation	Tamoxifen
Oophorectomy	Toremifene
Luteinizing hormone–releasing hormone agonist	Aromatase inhibitors
	Anastrozole
Progestins	Letrozole
Androgens	Exemestane
High-dose estrogens	Progestins
	Androgens
	High-dose estrogens

clinician must consider in proceeding with initial hormonal therapy are whether or not the patient is likely to respond to the treatment and whether the patient would be adversely affected if she did not respond to treatment and was started on chemotherapy 2 to 3 months later. Visceral disease, particularly low-volume and asymptomatic disease, is not a contraindication to the use of hormonal therapy; however, the patient with extensive visceral disease is probably better served by chemotherapy. If a patient with a hormone receptor–positive cancer is initially treated with chemotherapy, the clinician should consider returning to hormonal therapy at some point in the future.

Table 37.2-30 lists the commercially available hormonal therapies for premenopausal and postmenopausal women. In general, there is little evidence that one hormonal therapy is substantially more effective than another. As a result, the ease of administration and tolerability usually dictates the choice of treatment.

In premenopausal women who have never received hormonal therapy, tamoxifen is generally the treatment of choice. A small randomized trial has suggested that tamoxifen and ovarian ablation are equivalent in efficacy.[713] In patients who respond to tamoxifen, the duration of response is often in excess of a year and may extend for several years in a minority of patients.[714] Medical or surgical ovarian ablation is usually the second-line hormonal therapy of choice in women who are premenopausal, particularly those who have responded to tamoxifen. European trials have evaluated the use of a combination of ovarian ablation and tamoxifen in patients with metastatic breast cancer. In some studies, there has been a suggestion of an improved overall response rate,[715,716] but it remains unclear if this approach is superior to sequential therapy. Aromatase inhibitors are not active in premenopausal women because of the high levels of circulating estrogen from the ovaries. Aromatase inhibitors can be used in conjunction with ovarian ablation, although there is little published information about this combination. Megestrol acetate remains the usual third-line hormonal therapy. The subgroup of premenopausal women with hormone receptor–positive tumors can, at times, have an extended survival in the metastatic setting. Faulkson et al. have reported a median survival of approximately 5 years in a group of hormone receptor–positive, premenopausal women who were initially treated with chemotherapy plus oophorectomy.[717] If anything, many clinicians may tend to undervalue the benefits of hormonal therapy in premenopausal women with positive hormone receptor status.

In postmenopausal women, tamoxifen remains the usual first-line therapy. In the metastatic setting, toremifene is an acceptable alternative based on the equivalence demonstrated between the two agents in randomized trials.[625] Since many women with metastatic breast cancer have either developed disease progression on tamoxifen or have had a recent course of adjuvant tamoxifen, there are fewer and fewer patients receiving antiestrogens when they present with metastatic disease. The aromatase inhibitors (i.e., anastrozole, letrozole, and exemestane) have all been demonstrated in randomized clinical trials to be equivalent or superior to megestrol acetate.[718,719] Exemestane, a steroidal aromatase inhibitor that irreversibly inhibits aromatase activity, has been shown to have a survival advantage in comparison with Megace.[719] All three agents are generally well tolerated and are not associated with the bothersome weight gain that is seen with Megace.[718] It is unknown, at this time, if one aromatase inhibitor is superior to another. A randomized trial demonstrated the equivalence of anastrozole (Arimidex) and tamoxifen in patients who had had no prior hormonal therapy,[720] making it reasonable to consider these agents as first-line therapy even in patients who have never received tamoxifen. Objective response rates to the aromatase inhibitors have been in the 10% to 20% range, but a substantial number of patients in these trials have had disease stabilization for 6 months or longer.[718,719,721] Megestrol acetate remains a third-line therapy, and patients rarely are treated with either androgens or high-dose estrogen as fourth- and fifth-line therapy.

In both premenopausal and postmenopausal women, occasional responses can be seen with withdrawal of either high-dose estrogen (now rarely used), tamoxifen, or progestins.[722,723] Withdrawal responses are relatively rare and are more commonly seen when a patient has had a prior response to the hormonal manipulation. The possibility of withdrawing tamoxifen (without additional therapy) can be considered in the patient with low-volume, indolent, ER-positive disease who has either been on adjuvant tamoxifen for several years or has had a documented response in the metastatic setting.

Assessing the response of patients to hormonal therapy can be complex. Many patients treated with hormonal therapy have bone-only disease, making response assessment complex. In addition, it can take up to several months to see a response in some patients, whereas others have more rapid disease regressions. A flare phenomenon with worsening bone pain, increasing soft tissue lesions, hypercalcemia, or all three is seen in a small percentage of patients who are started on hormonal therapy.[724,725] Flares have been seen with high-dose estrogen, tamoxifen, progestins, and androgens and occur within the first days to weeks of treatment. A portion of patients who have a flare go on to respond to endocrine therapy. With either hormonal therapy or chemotherapy, there can be a rise in tumor marker levels, alkaline phosphatase, or both early in the course of therapy, with a subsequent decline. Clinicians should not continue hormonal therapy in patients with rapid or unequivocal evidence of disease progression. In the minimally symptomatic patient, it is often prudent to continue therapy for several months if there is an uncertainty concerning the response to treatment. In these situations, it is important to explain to patients that a change in therapy in the near future may be necessary, but that there is little to be lost by continuing the hormonal approach with close monitoring of disease status.

A question that often arises is how many hormonal regimens to administer before moving on to chemotherapy. In a patient who has had a prior response to (or extended disease stabilization with) hormonal therapy, there is a reasonable chance of observing a response with another hormonal approach. There are patients who respond to a second hormonal therapy, even if their disease progressed through a first agent.[721] In making a clinical decision as to whether to consider a second, third, or even fourth hormonal approach, the clinician needs to weigh the therapeutic index of another hormonal agent versus that of chemotherapy. The chance of observing a response with each successive hormonal regimen decreases. However, if the patient continues to have relatively indolent disease and will not be harmed by delaying therapy that may have a higher chance of producing an objective response (i.e., chemotherapy), it is reasonable to try another hormonal therapy, even if the likelihood of obtaining a response is small. For that matter, it is important to reconsider the potential advantages of another trial of hormonal therapy, even in a patient who has received intervening chemotherapy.

Resistance to hormonal therapies ultimately develops in virtually all patients with advanced disease. The mechanisms responsible for resistance to hormonal therapy are not fully understood[726] and are currently being investigated. Identifying new hormonal agents, such as pure antiestrogens, new selective ER modulators, and antiprogestins, is a priority. Ongoing studies are also addressing the potential of using hormonal therapies with other agents, such as differentiating compounds, to enhance disease control.

CYTOTOXIC CHEMOTHERAPY FOR METASTATIC BREAST CANCER

Although hormonal therapy is usually the treatment of choice for patients with hormone receptor–positive cancer, almost all patients eventually develop hormone-refractory disease, and many patients with metastatic breast cancer have negative hormone receptor status. For these patients, chemotherapy is the treatment of choice, with the goal of ongoing symptom control and modest prolongation of survival. The use of chemotherapy for metastatic breast cancer has evolved since 1990. Multiple new agents are now available,[727] many of which have a favorable toxicity profile. Clinical trials have addressed a variety of fundamental issues related to the administration of chemotherapy to patients with metastatic breast cancer, such as the value of single agents versus combination therapy and the appropriate duration of therapy.

Table 37.2-31 lists the agents commercially available for patients with advanced breast cancer. While some of these have official Food and Drug Administration approval for the treatment of breast cancer, others have simply become part of the standard armamentarium as a result of general clinical acceptance. There is no rigid order in which agents or regimens should be administered. CMF and CAF were long considered the standard of care for initial chemotherapy treatment of advanced disease, but the development of the taxanes and a variety of other agents has given physicians and patients far greater flexibility in making treatment decisions. The taxanes and doxorubicin are usually considered the most active agents for the treatment of advanced disease, but the activity of any agent is most dependent on the characteristics of the patient population, particularly the extent of prior therapy. There are few compelling data that one regimen is markedly superior to another or promotes improved long-term survival.[728] The precise order in which treatments are administered is unlikely to affect overall survival. The CALGB has demonstrated that initial treatment with an investigational agent (in patients who did not have visceral crisis) does not compromise either overall survival or response to a subsequent doxorubicin-based regimen.[729] The availability of new agents, such as the taxanes, has improved overall survival,[666,667] but the order in which treatments are delivered (i.e., taxane as first-line vs. second-line therapy) is unlikely to have a major effect on long-term outcome.

TABLE 37.2-31. Active Chemotherapeutic Agents in the Treatment of Metastatic Breast Cancer

Anthracyclines and related agents
Adriamycin[a]
Epirubicin
Mitoxantrone
Liposomal doxorubicin[b]
Alkylating agents
Cyclophosphamide[c]
Melphalan
Thiotepa
Vinca alkaloids
Vinorelbine[b]
Vinblastine
Taxanes
Paclitaxel[a]
Docetaxel[a]
Antimetabolites
5-Fluorouracil[c]
(± Leucovorin)
Capecitabine[b]
Methotrexate[c]
Gemcitabine[b]

[a]Commonly used as first-line therapy.
[b]Commonly used at some point in disease course.
[c]Usually administered with other agents in first-line therapy.

In patients who have received no prior chemotherapy in the metastatic setting, objective response rates of 25% to 55% have been seen in multicenter randomized trials.[667,730–732] Higher response rates are seen in single-institution, phase II trials.[733,734] It is likely that the percentage of patients who derive some palliative benefit from chemotherapy is higher than the reported response rates in multicenter trials. The median duration of response with most first-line chemotherapy regimens is in the range of 6 to 12 months, with a shorter duration of response seen in patients who are treated in the second- and third-line setting.

COMBINATION VERSUS SINGLE-AGENT CHEMOTHERAPY

For several decades, the use of combination chemotherapy was considered the standard of care. More recently, several trials have compared combination therapy with the use of single agents in the treatment of advanced breast cancer.[666,667,730,735] In a large Eastern Cooperative Oncology Group trial, Sledge and colleagues randomized patients to one of three arms: single-agent Adriamycin, single-agent paclitaxel, or a combination of the two. Patients initially randomized to the single-agent arms were crossed over to the alternate agent at the time of progression. Although there was a statistically significant improvement in response rate and time to progression on the combination arm, there was no difference in either survival or quality of life.[730,736] If one considers the secondary responses with the crossover therapy, there is even less reason to view combination therapy as a superior approach. A Finnish trial that randomized patients to combination or single-agent therapy in both the first- and second-line setting also failed to show any appreciable difference in disease outcomes.[735] A major advantage of single-agent therapy is the ability to assess whether a given agent is of benefit to the patient. When a patient responds to combination therapy, it is never clear whether she is benefiting from a single drug in the regimen or from all of the agents. While the administration of combination therapy remains a common practice, it is most appropriate in highly symptomatic patients in whom the higher response rate seen with combination therapy may be worth the added toxicity. Numerous trials have also compared the use of chemotherapy alone versus the combination of chemotherapy and hormonal agents.[737,738] In general, these trials have demonstrated either higher response rates, longer time to progression, or both with the combination treatment, as well as a benefit in terms of survival.

DURATION OF CHEMOTHERAPY

Several trials have examined how long chemotherapy should be continued in patients with stable or responding disease. Muss and colleagues treated 250 patients with initial CAF chemotherapy and randomized almost 150 women with stable or responsive disease to maintenance chemotherapy or observation. Although there was a 6-month prolongation in time to disease progression for women on maintenance therapy, there was no difference in overall survival.[739] Findings from other investigators have been quite similar.[740] Of note, a very brief course of treatment may not only shorten time to progression, but it may also compromise quality of life.[741] Coates and colleagues randomized Australian patients to continuous chemotherapy versus intermittent therapy (three cycles only) with reinstitution of treatment at the time of disease progression.[741] The two groups had an equivalent overall survival, but the intermittent group had a lower response rate, shorter time to progression, and inferior quality of life. Since the maximal response to chemotherapy often occurs after approximately 4 to 6 months of treatment, one interpretation of this trial is that the failure to treat patients until they achieved a maximal response to therapy perhaps compromised quality of life.

The question of how long to continue chemotherapy is frequently raised in discussions with patients. Assuming a patient has had 4 to 6 months of chemotherapy and has stable or responsive disease, there is no evidence that continuing treatment will have an effect on her overall survival. When a patient experiences progression of disease, treatment (at times with the same regimen) can always be resumed. In the patient who was initially symptomatic, has had excellent palliation of her symptoms, and has minimal toxicity with treatment, chemotherapy can be continued with the goal of delaying disease progression.

DOSE AND SCHEDULE OF CHEMOTHERAPY

A large number of trials have addressed questions that relate to either the dose or schedule of chemotherapy. In general, higher response rates have been seen with regimens that are in the standard-dose range than those in which the doses are reduced substantially. Low-dose CMF has been found to be inferior to standard-dose therapy (600 mg/m^2; 40 mg/m^2; 600 mg/m^2).[742] Lower responses rates or more rapid disease progression have been demonstrated with other agents when doses have been reduced below the usually accepted range.[743,744] The clinician must balance the potential benefits and toxicities of different dose levels. To date, there is little convincing evidence to show that escalating doses of chemotherapy to levels that require growth factor support has a substantial effect on disease outcome. In addition, some of these regimens result in a marked increase in toxicity.[745]

Questions exist about the optimal schedule for many cytotoxic agents. By changing the schedule of many agents, there is the suggestion that both efficacy and toxicity can be altered. The NSABP compared 3-hour versus 24-hour paclitaxel administration in patients with locally advanced or metastatic disease.[746] Although a significantly higher response rate was observed with the longer infusion (54% vs. 44%), there was no difference in survival, and the longer infusion was much more inconvenient. Initial reports of weekly taxanes[734,747] have been encouraging, and these dose-dense schedules are being compared with the standard every 3 week regimens in randomized trials of interest. A European trial compared classical CMF (day 1 and 8 with oral cyclophosphamide) with an every 3 week regimen. The classical regimen, which is more dose dense, resulted in a higher response rate and an improvement in overall survival.[748] With the availability of oral fluorouracil agents[749] and liposomally encapsulated agents, such as doxorubicin (Doxil),[750] it is possible to increase the duration of exposure to cytotoxic agents without committing patients to ambulatory infusion pumps or frequent clinic visits.

HIGH-DOSE CHEMOTHERAPY WITH HEMATOPOIETIC SUPPORT

Beginning in the mid-1980s, trials were initiated evaluating the role of high-dose chemotherapy with autologous bone marrow support. These studies were based on preclinical models and the hope that dose escalation would result in prolongation of survival.[751] Multiple phase I and II trials in women with metastatic breast cancer suggested that high-dose chemotherapy resulted in high response rates, generally in excess of 70%. In addition, a small proportion of patients (approximately 10% to 15%) remained free of disease progression for several years following therapy.[752–754] In general, patients with a low disease burden, long disease-free interval, and absence of visceral involvement appeared to have the most favorable outcome after high-dose therapy.[755–757] Based on preliminary trials, thousands of women in the United States underwent treatment with high-dose chemotherapy throughout the late 1980s and 1990s.

More recently, the mature results of a randomized trial comparing high-dose chemotherapy with prolonged conventional chemotherapy have been published. Stadtmauer and colleagues enrolled 553 women with metastatic breast cancer onto a trial designed to determine if high-dose chemotherapy would improve disease outcomes.[758] Of the original cohort, 310 women had a response to initial chemotherapy, and 199 of these women were ultimately randomized to receive either high-dose chemotherapy with stem cell support versus prolonged treatment with CMF. With a median follow-up of 37 months, there was no evidence that high-dose therapy improved either time to progression or overall survival. Subgroup analyses looking at demographic variables, response (complete vs. partial response) to induction treatment, and disease characteristics failed to identify a population of patients that had a better outcome with high-dose therapy than with CMF. In another study, Berry et al. retrospectively compared the outcomes of 560 women registered with the Autologous Bone Marrow Transplant Registry with 657 patients who participated in a series of CALGB trials using conventional dose chemotherapy.[759] All patients included in the analysis were 60 years of age or younger and had chemotherapy-sensitive disease. In a multivariate model, there was no difference in survival between the two groups of patients. The investigators could not identify any patient subgroup who had a better outcome with high-dose therapy. Thus, despite the initial enthusiasm for high-dose chemotherapy for metastatic breast cancer, this approach appears unlikely to have a substantial effect on the natural history of the disease.[760]

TRASTUZUMAB (HERCEPTIN)

The development of Herceptin has been a major advance in the treatment of HER-2/*neu*–positive metastatic breast cancer. As previously noted, approximately 25% to 30% of all breast cancers overexpress HER-2/*neu*, a 185-kD transmembrane glycoprotein receptor. These tumors have a more aggressive natural history, a higher risk of recurrence, a higher frequency of visceral disease at first recurrence, and a lower likelihood of ER positivity. Herceptin, a humanized recombinant anti–HER-2/*neu* antibody, has been evaluated in a series of clinical trials as both a single agent and in combination with chemotherapy.

In a multinational trial, women with HER-2/*neu*–overexpressing metastatic breast cancer were randomized to receive chemotherapy alone or chemotherapy plus Herceptin.[705,761] Patients who had not received an anthracycline in the adjuvant setting were randomized to AC with or without Herceptin. Those patients who had received an adjuvant anthracycline-containing regimen received paclitaxel with or without Herceptin. Chemotherapy was continued in stable or responding patients for a minimum of six cycles. In the absence of disease progression, Herceptin was administered weekly at a dose of 2 mg/kg for 1 year or longer. Table 37.2-32 summarizes the results of the trial.

The benefit of Herceptin was seen both in patients who received AC and in those who received paclitaxel. In addition, the survival benefit was noted despite the fact that approximately two-thirds of the women randomized to chemotherapy alone ultimately received Herceptin on an open-label extension protocol at the time of disease progression. While Herceptin was generally well tolerated, there was a 19% incidence of grade III or IV cardiac dysfunction on the AC plus Herceptin arm; with the combination of Herceptin and paclitaxel, the frequency of serious cardiac toxicity was only 4%.[705]

In a large single-agent trial, Cobleigh and colleagues treated 222 women with refractory metastatic breast cancer (one or two prior chemotherapy regimens).[762] As a single agent, Herceptin was well tolerated. Five percent of the study population developed cardiac dysfunction; however, all these patients had either received prior anthracyclines or had preexisting cardiac disease. The overall response rate in this group of pretreated patients was 15%, with a median duration of response of 9.1 months. In another single-agent trial, Vogel et al. reported a response rate of 25% in 112 women with HER-2/*neu*–overexpressing metastatic breast cancer.[763] Although none of these patients had received chemotherapy in the metastatic setting, over one-half had received prior doxorubicin in the adjuvant setting. Taken together, these two trials clearly demonstrate the activity of Herceptin administered as a single agent.

TABLE 37.2-32. Benefit of Herceptin When Added to Chemotherapy

	Chemotherapy	*Chemotherapy + Herceptin*	*P Value*
Response rate	29%	45%	<.0001
Time to progression	4.5 mo	7.2 mo	<.0001
Median survival	20.3 mo	25.4 mo	= .025

(Adapted from refs. 705 and 761.)

There is compelling evidence to consider the use of Herceptin in the initial management of women with HER-2/*neu*–positive, hormone-refractory metastatic breast cancer; however, there are a multitude of unanswered questions about the use of Herceptin in clinical practice. It is unknown how long Herceptin should be administered, whether it should be continued with second-line chemotherapy after disease progression, or if single-agent therapy (followed by chemotherapy) is better or worse than combination treatment. Many of these questions will be answered through future clinical trials; others will depend on gaining a fuller understanding of the complex mechanism of action of Herceptin and its probable role in sensitizing breast cancer to the effects of chemotherapy. It is unlikely that there is any role for Herceptin in patients whose tumors do not overexpress HER-2/*neu*. Discussions continue regarding the optimal methods to assess HER-2/*neu* overexpression. Additional trials are needed to test combinations of Herceptin with other cytotoxic agents. Promising preliminary reports have appeared using combinations of Herceptin plus vinorelbine,[764] Herceptin plus docetaxel,[765] and Herceptin plus weekly paclitaxel.[766] Finally, the role of Herceptin in both the neoadjuvant and adjuvant setting will be the focus of a number of clinical trials in the years ahead.

QUALITY OF LIFE AND SUPPORTIVE CARE ISSUES

A growing emphasis has been placed on quality-of-life issues in women with metastatic breast cancer. This interest has been reflected by an increasing effort to measure quality of life in clinical trials.[736,741,767,768] Although only a small number of randomized trials in women with metastatic breast cancer have demonstrated differences in quality of life,[741,769] this research has likely led to a greater awareness of quality-of-life issues in clinical practice.

Many of the newer chemotherapy and hormonal agents have fewer side effects, or at least a more manageable side-effect profile than agents that were available a decade ago. In many ways, the emphasis on single-agent therapy can be viewed as a step forward from a quality-of-life standpoint. There is also an ongoing effort to make breast cancer treatment more convenient for patients. Virtually all therapy is administered in the outpatient setting, and there is a growing interest in the development of oral chemotherapeutic agents. Patient surveys have documented a strong preference for oral treatment, but only if the oral therapy can be administered without compromising efficacy.[770,771]

With the heightened interest in quality-of-life issues, there has also been a greater emphasis on supportive care measures. The use of bisphosphonates in women with lytic bone lesions has become a standard of practice.[772] Treatment with bisphosphonates does not improve survival, but does have an important effect on the frequency of bone-related complications such as pain, the need for palliative radiation, and hypercalcemia. There is a growing awareness of fatigue, its relationship with anemia, and the potential benefits of treatment with erythropoietin.[773] Nausea and vomiting, while still a problem with many chemotherapy regimens, are far better controlled with the judicious use of some of the newer antiemetic agents.[774] While the availability of these newer supportive care measures represents a major advance in the care of women with breast cancer, the clinician needs to weigh carefully the advantages and disadvantages of each of these supportive care interventions.

NEW TREATMENT APPROACHES

It is difficult to know which of the therapies currently in development will have a future role in the treatment of women with breast cancer. There is renewed interest in immune-based treatments, including vaccines, monoclonal antibodies, and approaches using dendritic cells. Ongoing trials are evaluating a range of novel therapeutics, including differentiating agents and angiogenesis inhibitors. As our basic understanding of breast cancer grows, it is likely that there will be a whole new generation of targeted molecular therapies, allowing clinicians to increase the efficacy and decrease the toxicity of treatment for women with breast cancer.

REFERENCES

1. Greenlee RT, Murray T, Bolden S, Wingo PA. Cancer statistics, 2000. *CA Cancer J Clin* 2000;50:7.
2. Ries LAG, Kosary CL, Hankey BF, et al., eds. *SEER Cancer Statistics Review, 1973–1996*. Bethesda, MD: National Cancer Institute, 1999.
3. Harris JR, Lippman ME, Morrow M, Osborne CK, eds. *Diseases of the breast*, 2nd ed. Philadelphia: Lippincott Williams & Wilkins, 2000.
4. Madigan M, Ziegler R, Benichon C, et al. Proportion of breast cancer cases in the United States explained by well established risk factors. *J Natl Cancer Inst* 1995;87:1681.
5. Phillips KA, Glendon G, Knight J. Putting the risk of breast cancer in perspective. *N Engl J Med* 1999;340:141.
6. Claus EB, Schildkraut JM, Thompson WE, Risch NJ. The genetic attributable risk of breast and ovarian cancer. *Cancer* 1996;77:2318.
7. Lerman C, Lustbader E, Rimer B, et al. Effects of individualized breast cancer risk counseling: a randomized trial. *J Natl Cancer Inst* 1995;87:286.
8. Bluman LG, Rimer BK, Berry DA, et al. Attitudes, knowledge and risk perceptions of women with breast and/or ovarian cancer considering testing for BRCA1 and BRCA2. *J Clin Oncol* 1999;17:1040.
9. Ottman R, King M, Pike M, et al. Practical guide to estimating risk in familial breast cancer. *Lancet* 1983;2:556.
10. Anderson D. Genetic study of breast cancer: identification of a high risk group. *Cancer* 1974;34:1090.
11. Claus EG, Risch N, Thompson WD. Autosomal dominant inheritance of early-onset breast cancer: implications for risk prediction. *Cancer* 1994;73:643.
12. Gail MH, Brinton LA, Byar DP, et al. Projecting individualized probabilities of developing breast cancer for white females who are being examined annually. *J Natl Cancer Inst* 1989;81:1879.
13. Miki Y, Swensen J, Shattuck-Eidens D, et al. A strong candidate for the breast and ovarian cancer susceptibility gene BRCA1. *Science* 1994;266:66.
14. Wooster R, Neuhausen SL, Mangion J, et al. Localization of a breast cancer susceptibility gene, BRCA2, to chromosome 13q12-13. *Science* 1994;265:2088.
15. Frank TS, Manley SA, Olopade OI, et al. Sequence analysis of BRCA1 and BRCA2: correlation of mutations with family history and ovarian cancer risk. *J Clin Oncol* 1998;16:1969.
16. Easton DF, Steele L, Fields P, et al. Cancer risks in two large breast cancer families linked to BRCA2 on chromosome 13q 12-13. *Am J Hum Genet* 1997;61:120.
17. Easton DF, Ford D, Bishop T, and the Breast Cancer Linkage Consortium. Breast and ovarian cancer incidence in BRCA1-mutation carriers. *Am J Hum Genet* 1995;56:265.
18. Berry DA, Parmigiani G, Sanchez J, et al. Probability of carrying a mutation of breast-ovarian cancer gene BRCA1 based on family history. *J Natl Cancer Inst* 1997;89:227.
19. Couch FJ, DeShano ML, Blackwood MA, et al. BRCA1 mutations in women attending clinics that evaluate the risk of breast cancer. *N Engl J Med* 1997;336:1416.
20. Hall JM, Lee MK, Newman B, et al. Linkage of early-onset familial breast cancer to chromosome 17q21. *Science* 1990;250:1684.
21. Ford D, Easton D, Bishop T, et al. Risks of cancer in BRCA1 mutation carriers. *Lancet* 1994;343:692.
22. Struewing JP, Hartge P, Wacholder S, et al. The risk of cancer associated with specific mutations of BRCA1 and BRCA2 among Ashkenazi Jews. *N Engl J Med* 1997;336:1401.
23. Arason A, Barkardottir RB, Elgisson V. Linkage analysis of chromosome 17q markers and breast-ovarian cancer in Icelandic families, and possible relationship to prostatic cancer. *Am J Hum Genet* 1993;52:711.
24. Phelan CM, Lancaster JM, Tonin P, et al. Mutation analysis of the BRCA2 gene in 49 site-specific breast cancer families. *Nat Genet* 1996;13:120.
25. Wooster R, Bignell G, Lancaster J. Identification of the breast cancer susceptibility gene BRCA2. *Nature* 1995;378:789.
26. Ford D, Easton DF, Peto J. Estimates of the gene frequency of BRCA1 and its contribution to breast and ovarian cancer incidence. *Am J Hum Genet* 1995;57:1457.
27. Fitzgerald MG, MacDonald DJ, Krainer M, et al. Germ-line BRCA1 mutations in Jewish and non-Jewish women with early-onset breast cancer. *N Engl J Med* 1996;334:143.
28. Jernstrom H, Lerman C, Ghadirian P, et al. Pregnancy and risk of early breast cancer in carriers of BRCA1 and BRCA2. *Lancet* 1999;354:1846.
29. Rebbeck TR, Levin AM, Eisen A, et al. Breast cancer risk after bilateral prophylactic oophorectomy in BRCA1 mutation carriers. *J Natl Cancer Inst* 1999;91:1475.
30. Lee JS, Wacholder S, Struewing J, et al. Survival after breast cancer in Ashkenazi Jewish BRCA1 and BRCA2 mutation carriers. *J Natl Cancer Inst* 1999;92:259.
31. Robson M, Gilewski T, Haas B, et al. BRCA-associated breast cancer in young women. *J Clin Oncol* 1998;16:1642.
32. Noguchi S, Kasugai T, Miki Y, et al. Clinicopathologic analysis of BRCA1 or BRCA2 associated hereditary breast carcinoma in Japanese women. *Cancer* 1999;85:2200.
33. Malkin D, Li F, Strong L, et al. Germ line p53 mutations in a familial syndrome of breast cancer, sarcomas, and other neoplasms. *Science* 1990;250:1233.
34. Brownstein M, Wolf M, Bikowski J. Cowden's disease: a cutaneous marker of breast cancer. *Cancer* 1978;41:2393.
35. Hall N, Williams M, Murday V, et al. Muir-Torre syndrome: a variant of the cancer family syndrome. *J Med Genet* 1994;31:627.
36. Swift M, Reitnauer P, Morrell D, et al. Breast and other cancers in families with ataxia-telangiectasia. *N Engl J Med* 1987;316:1289.
37. Rosner B, Colditz G. Nurses' Health Study. Log-incidence model of breast cancer incidence. *J Natl Cancer Inst* 1996;88:359.
38. Huang Z, Hankinson SE, Colditz GA, et al. Dual effects of weight and weight gain on breast cancer risk. *JAMA* 1997;278:1407.
39. Collaborative Group on Hormonal Factors in Breast Cancer. Breast cancer and hormone replacement therapy: collaborative reanalysis of data from 51 epidemiological studies of 52,705 women with breast cancer and 108,411 women without breast cancer. *Lancet* 1997;350:1047.
40. Hankinson SE, Willett WC, Manson JE, et al. Plasma sex steroid hormone levels and risk of breast cancer in postmenopausal women. *J Natl Cancer Inst* 1998;90:1292.
41. Cauley JA, Lucas FL, Kuller LH, et al. Elevated serum estradiol and testosterone concentrations are associated with a high risk for breast cancer. *Ann Intern Med* 1999;130:270.
42. Trichopoulos D. Hypothesis: does breast cancer originate in utero? *Lancet* 1990;335:939.
43. Ekbom A, Hsieh C, Lipworth L, et al. Intrauterine environment and breast cancer risk in women: a population-based study. *J Natl Cancer Inst* 1997;89:71.
44. Trichopoulos D, MacMahon B, Cole P. Menopause and breast cancer risk. *J Natl Cancer Inst* 1972;48:605.
45. Helzlsouer KJ. Epidemiology, prevention, and early detection of breast cancer. *Curr Opin Oncol* 1995;7:489.
46. Nissen-Meyer R. Primary breast cancer: the effect of primary ovarian irradiation. *Ann Oncol* 1991;2:343.
47. MacMahon B, Trichopoulos D, Brown J. Etiology of human breast cancer: a review. *J Natl Cancer Inst* 1973;50:21.
48. Kelsey JL, Gammon MD, John EM. Reproductive factors and breast cancer. *Epidemiol Rev* 1993;15:233.
49. MacMahon B, Trichopoulos D, Brown J. Age at menarche, urine estrogens and breast cancer risk. *Int J Cancer* 1982;30:427.
50. Henderson B, Ross R, Ludd H. Do regular ovulatory cycles increase breast cancer risk? *Cancer* 1985;45:1206.
51. MacMahon B, Trichopoulos D, Brown J. Age at menarche, probability of ovulation and breast cancer risk. *Int J Cancer* 1982;29:12.
52. MacMahon B, Cole P, Lin T. Age at first birth and breast cancer risk. *Bull WHO* 1970;43:209.
53. Trichopoulos D, Hsieh C, MacMahon B. Age at first birth and breast cancer risk. *Int J Cancer* 1983;31:701.
54. Russo J, Tay L, Russo I. Differentiation of the mammary gland and susceptibility to carcinogenesis. *Breast Cancer Res Treat* 1982;2:5.
55. Bruzzi P, Negri E, La Vecchia C. Short term increase in risk of breast cancer after full term pregnancy. *BMJ* 1988;47:757.
56. Rosner B, Colditz G, Willett W. Reproductive risk factors in a prospective study of breast cancer: the Nurses' Health Study. *Am J Epidemiol* 1994;139:819.

57. Newcomb P, Storer B, Longnecker M, et al. Lactation and a reduced risk of premenopausal breast cancer. *N Engl J Med* 1994;330:81.
58. Prevention of cancer in the next millennium: report of the Chemoprevention Working Group of the American Association for Cancer Research. *Cancer Res* 1999;59:4743.
59. Brind J, Chinchilli V, Severs W, Summy-Long J. Induced abortion as an independent risk factor for breast cancer: a comprehensive review and meta-analysis. *J Epidemiol Comm Health* 1996;50:481.
60. Melbye M, Wohlfahrt J, Olsen J. Induced abortion and the risk of breast cancer. *N Engl J Med* 1997;336:81.
61. Adami H, Bergstrom R, Lund E, et al. Absence of association between reproductive variables and the risk of breast cancer in young women in Sweden and Norway. *Br J Cancer* 1990;62:122.
62. Newcomb P, Storer B, Longnecker M, et al. Pregnancy termination in relation to risk of breast cancer. *JAMA* 1996;275:283.
63. Steinberg K, Thacker S, Smith S, et al. A meta-analysis of the effect of estrogen replacement therapy on the risk of breast cancer. *JAMA* 1991;265:1985.
64. Sillero-Arenas M, Delgado-Rodriguez M, Rodigues-Canteras R, et al. Menopausal hormone replacement therapy and breast cancer: a meta-analysis. *Obstet Gynecol* 1992;79:286.
65. Schairer C, Lubin J, Troisi R, et al. Menopausal estrogen and estrogen-progestin replacement therapy and breast cancer risk. *JAMA* 2000;283:485.
66. Ross R, Paganini-Hill A, Wan P, Pike M. Effect of hormone replacement therapy on breast cancer risk: estrogen versus estrogen plus progestin. *J Natl Cancer Inst* 2000;16:328.
67. Salmon R, Ansquer Y, Asselain B, et al. Clinical and biological characteristics of breast cancers in post-menopausal women receiving hormone replacement therapy for menopause. *Oncol Rep* 1999;6:699.
68. Gapstur S, Morrow M, Sellers T. Hormone replacement therapy and risk of breast cancer with a favorable histology: results of the Iowa Women's Health Study. *JAMA* 1999;281:2091.
69. Collaborative Group on Hormonal Factors in Breast Cancer. Breast cancer and hormonal contraceptives: collaborative reanalysis of individual data on 53,297 women with breast cancer and 100,239 women without breast cancer from 54 epidemiological studies. *Lancet* 1996;47:1713.
70. Hankinson S, Colditz G, Manson J, et al. A prospective study of oral contraceptive use and risk of breast cancer (Nurses' Health Study, United States). *Cancer Causes Control* 1997;8:65.
71. Wingo P, Lee N, Ory H, et al. Age specific differences in the relationship between oral contraceptive use and breast cancer. *Obstet Gynecol* 1991;78:161.
72. Collaborative Group on Hormonal Factors in Breast Cancer. Breast cancer and hormonal contraceptives: further results. *Contraception* 1996;54(Suppl):1S.
73. McMichael A, Giles G. Cancer in migrants to Australia: extending descriptive epidemiological data. *Cancer Res* 1988;48:751.
74. Buell P. Changing incidence of breast cancer in Japanese-American women. *J Natl Cancer Inst* 1973;51:1479.
75. Kinlen L. Meat and fat consumption and cancer mortality: a study of strict religious orders in Britain. *Lancet* 1982;1:946.
76. Phillips R, Garfinkel L, Kuzma J. Mortality among California Seventh Day Adventists for selected cancer sites. *J Natl Cancer Inst* 1980;65:1097.
77. Hunter D, Spiegelman D, Adami H, et al. Cohort studies of fat intake and the risk of breast cancer—a pooled analysis. *N Engl J Med* 1996;334:356.
78. Willett W, Stampfer M, Colditz G. Dietary fat and risk of breast cancer. *N Engl J Med* 1987;316:22.
79. Holmes M, Hunter D, Colditz G, et al. Association of dietary intake of fat and fatty acids with risk of breast cancer. *JAMA* 1999;281:914.
80. Michels K, Trichopoulos D, Robins J, et al. Birthweight as a risk factor for breast cancer. *Lancet* 1996;348:1542.
81. Hunter D, Willett W. Diet, body size, and breast cancer. *Epidemiol Rev* 1993;15:110.
82. Rich-Edwards J, Goldman M, Willett W, et al. Adolescent body mass index and ovulatory infertility. *Am J Obstet Gynecol* 1994;171:171.
83. Ziegler R, Hoover R, Nomura A, et al. Relative weight, weight change, height, and breast cancer risk in Asian-American women. *J Natl Cancer Inst* 1996;88:650.
84. Hankinson S, Willett W, Manson J, et al. Alcohol, height, and adiposity in relation to estrogen and prolactin levels in postmenopausal women. *J Natl Cancer Inst* 1994;87:1297.
85. Thune I, Brenn T, Lund E, Gaard M. Physical activity and the risk of breast cancer. *N Engl J Med* 1997;336:1269.
86. Rockhill B, Willett W, Hunter D, et al. A prospective study of recreational physical activity and breast cancer risk. *Arch Intern Med* 1999;159:2290.
87. Longnecker M. Alcoholic beverage consumption in relation to risk of breast cancer: meta-analysis and review. *Cancer Causes Control* 1994;5:73.
88. Gapstur S, Potter J, Sellers T, et al. Increased risk of breast cancer with alcohol consumption in postmenopausal women. *Am J Epidemiol* 1992;136:1221.
89. Zhang S, Hunter D, Hankinson S, et al. A prospective study of folate intake and the risk of breast cancer. *JAMA* 1999;281:1632.
90. Freudenheim J, Marshall J, Vena J, et al. Premenopausal breast cancer risk and intake of vegetables, fruits, and related nutrients. *J Natl Cancer Inst* 1996;88:340.
91. American Institute for Cancer Research WCRF. *Food, nutrition and the prevention of cancer: a global perspective.* Washington, DC: American Institute for Cancer Research, 1997.
92. Dupont W, Page D. Risk factors for breast cancer in women with proliferative breast disease. *N Engl J Med* 1985;312:146.
93. Dupont W, Page D, Parl F, et al. Estrogen replacement therapy in women with a history of proliferative breast disease. *Cancer* 1999;85:1277.
94. Skolnick M, Cannon-Albright L, Goldgar D, et al. Inheritance of proliferative breast disease in breast cancer kindreds. *Science* 1990;250:1715.
95. Gervais-Fagnou DD, Girouard C, Laperriere N, Pintillie M, Goss PE. Breast cancer in women following supradiaphragmatic irradiation for Hodgkin's disease. *Oncology* 1999;57:224.
96. Aisenberg AC, Finkelstein DM, Doppke KP, et al. High risk of breast carcinoma after irradiation of young women with Hodgkin's disease. *Cancer* 1997;79:1203.
97. Black WC, Nease RF Jr, Tosteson AN. Perceptions of breast cancer risk and screening effectiveness in women younger than 50 years of age. *J Natl Cancer Inst* 1995;87:720.
98. Cappelli M, Surh L, Humphreys L, et al. Psychological and social determinants of women's decisions to undergo genetic counseling and testing for breast cancer. *Clin Genet* 1999;55:419.
99. Watson M, Lloyd S, Davidson J, et al. The impact of genetic counseling on risk perception and mental health in women with a family history of breast cancer. *Br J Cancer* 1999;79:868.
100. Armstrong K, Eiszen A, Weber B. Assessing the risk of breast cancer. *N Engl J Med* 2000;342:564.
101. Benichou J, Gail MJ, Mulvihil JJ. Graphs to estimate an individualized risk of breast cancer. *J Clin Oncol* 1996;14:103.
102. Spiegelman D, Colditz GA, Huner D, Hertzmark E. Validation of the Gail et al model for predicting individual breast cancer risk. *J Natl Cancer Inst* 1994;86:600.
103. Bondy M, Lustbader ED, Halabi S, Ross E, Vogel VG. Validation of a breast cancer risk assessment model in women with a positive family history. *J Natl Cancer Inst* 1994;86:620.
104. Costantino JP, Gail MH, Pee D, et al. Validation studies for models projecting the risk of invasive and total breast cancer incidence. *J Natl Cancer Inst* 1999;91:1541.
105. McGuigan KA, Ganz PA, Breant C. Agreement between breast cancer risk estimation methods. *J Natl Cancer Inst* 1996;88:1315.
106. Gail M, Rimer B. Risk-based recommendations for mammographic screening for women in their forties. *J Clin Oncol* 1998;19:3105.
107. Burke W, Daly M, Garber J, et al. Recommendations for follow-up care of individuals with an inherited predisposition to cancer: II. BRCA1 and BRCA2. *JAMA* 1997;277:997.
108. Verloop J, Rookus MA, van der Kooy K, van Leeuwen FE. Physical activity and breast cancer risk in women aged 20-54 years. *J Natl Cancer Inst* 2000;92:128.
109. Spicer DV, Ursin G, Parisky YR. Changes in mammographic densities induced by a hormonal contraceptive designed to reduce breast cancer risk. *J Natl Cancer Inst* 1994;86:408.
110. Early Breast Cancer Trialists' Collaborative Group. Tamoxifen for early breast cancer: an overview of the randomised trials. *Lancet* 1998;352:930.
111. Nayfield SG, Karp JE, Ford LG, Dorr FA, Kramer FS. Potential role of tamoxifen in prevention of breast cancer. *J Natl Cancer Inst* 1991;83:1450.
112. Radmacher MD, Simon R. Estimation of tamoxifen's efficacy for preventing the formation and growth of breast tumors. *J Natl Cancer Inst* 2000;92:48.
113. Fisher B, Costantino JP, Wickerham DL, et al. Tamoxifen for prevention of breast cancer: report of the National Surgical Adjuvant Breast and Bowel Project P-1 study. *J Natl Cancer Inst* 1998;90:1371.
114. Day R, Ganz PA, Costantino JP. Health-related quality of life and tamoxifen in breast cancer prevention: a report from the National Surgical Adjuvant Breast and Bowel Project P-1 Study. *J Clin Oncol* 1999;17:2659
115. Gail MH, Costantino JP, Bryant J, et al. Weighing the risks and benefits of tamoxifen treatment for preventing breast cancer. *J Natl Cancer Inst* 1999;91:1829.
116. Powles T, Eeles R, Ashley S, et al. Interim analysis of the incidence of breast cancer in the Royal Marsden Hospital tamoxifen randomised chemoprevention trial. *Lancet* 1998;352:98.
117. Veronesi U, Maisonneuve P, Costa A, et al. Prevention of breast cancer with tamoxifen: preliminary findings from the Italian randomised trial among hysterectomised women. Italian Tamoxifen Prevention Study. *Lancet* 1998;352:93
118. Ettinger B, Black DM, Mitlak BH, et al. Reduction of vertebral fracture risk in postmenopausal women with osteoporosis treated with raloxifene: results from a 3-year randomized clinical trial. Multiple Outcomes of Raloxifene Evaluation (MORE) Investigators. *JAMA* 1999;282:637.
119. Cummings SR, Eckert S, Krueger KA, et al. The effect of raloxifene on risk of breast cancer in postmenopausal women: results from the MORE randomized trial. *JAMA* 1999;281:2189.
120. NCCN Breast Cancer Risk-Reduction Guidelines. *Oncology* 1999;13:241.
121. Chlebowski RT, Collyar DE, Somerfield MR, Pfister DG. American Society of Clinical Oncology technology assessment on breast cancer risk reduction strategies: tamoxifen and raloxifene. *J Clin Oncol* 1999;17:1939.
122. Veronesi U, De Palo G, Marubini E, et al. Randomized trial of fenretinide to prevent second breast malignancy in women with early breast cancer. *J Natl Cancer Inst* 1999;91:1847.
123. Decensi A, Fontana V, Fioreto M, et al. Long-term effects of fenretinide on retinal function. *Eur J Cancer* 1997;33:80.
124. Hartmann LC, Schaid DJ, Woods JE, et al. Efficacy of bilateral prophylactic mastectomy in women with a family history of breast cancer. *N Engl J Med* 1999;340:77.
125. Eisen A, Weber BL. Prophylactic mastectomy—the price of fear. *N Engl J Med* 1999;340:137.
126. Schrag D, Kuntz KM, Garber JE, Weeks JC. Decision analysis—effects of prophylactic mastectomy and oophorectomy on life expectancy among women with BRCA1 or BRCA2 mutations. *N Engl J Med* 1997;336:1465.
127. Schrag D, Kuntz KM, Garber JE, Weeks JC. Life expectancy gains from cancer prevention strategies for women with breast cancer and BRCA1 or BRCA2 mutations. *JAMA* 2000;283:617.
128. Kline T, Joshi L, Neal H. Fine needle aspiration of the breasts: diagnoses and pitfalls. *Cancer* 1979;44:1458.
129. Bell D, Hajdu S, Urban J, et al. Role of aspiration cytology in the diagnosis and management of mammary lesions in office practice. *Cancer* 1983;51:1182.
130. Hammond S, Keyhi-Rofagha S, O'Toole R. Statistical analysis of fine needle aspiration of the breast: a review of 678 cases plus 4,265 cases from the literature. *Acta Cytol* 1987;31:276.
131. Lamb J, Anderson T. Influence of cancer histology on the success of fine needle aspiration of the breast. *J Clin Pathol* 1989;42:733.
132. Barrow G, Anderson J, Lamb J, et al. Fine needle aspiration of breast cancer: relationship of clinical factors to cytology results in 689 primary malignancies. *Cancer* 1986;58:1493.
133. Fentiman I, Millis R, Hayward J. Value of needle biopsy in outpatient diagnosis of breast cancer. *Arch Surg* 1980;115:652.

134. Minkowitz S, Moskowitz R, Khafif R, et al. Tru-Cut needle biopsy of the breast: an analysis of its specificity and sensitivity. *Cancer* 1986;57:320.
135. Shabot M, Goldberg I, Schick P, et al. Aspiration cytology is superior to Tru-Cut needle biopsy in establishing the diagnosis of clinically suspicious breast masses. *Ann Surg* 1982;196:122.
136. Kearney T, Morrow M. Effect of re-excision on the success of breast conserving surgery. *Ann Surg Oncol* 1995;2:303.
137. Gallagher W, Cardenosa G, Rubens J, et al. Minimal-volume excision of nonpalpable breast lesions. *AJR Am J Roentgenol* 1989;153:957.
138. Meyer J, Eberlein T, Stomper P, et al. Biopsy of occult breast lesions. *JAMA* 1990;263:2341.
139. Thompson W, Bowen J, Dorman B, et al. Mammographic localization and biopsy of nonpalpable breast lesions: a 5-year study. *Arch Surg* 1991;126:730.
140. Alexander H, Candela F, Dershaw D, et al. Needle localized mammographic lesions: results and evolving treatment strategy. *Arch Surg* 1990;125:1441.
141. Sacchini V, Luini A, Agresti R, et al. Nonpalpable breast lesions: analysis of 952 operated cases. *Breast Cancer Res Treat* 1995;32:59.
142. Tinnemans J, Wobbes T, Holland R, et al. Mammographic and histopathologic correlation of nonpalpable lesions of the breast and the reliability of frozen section diagnosis. *Surg Gynecol Obstet* 1987;165:523.
143. Morrow M. When can stereotactic core biopsy replace excisional biopsy? A clinical perspective. *Breast Cancer Res Treat* 1995;36:1.
144. Venta LH. Image-guided biopsy of nonpalpable breast lesions. In: Harris JR, Lippman ME, Morrow M, Osborne CK, eds. *Diseases of the breast.* Philadelphia: Lippincott Williams & Wilkins, 2000.
145. Bassett L, Winchester DP, Caplan RB, et al. Stereotactic core-needle biopsy of the breast: a report of the Joint Task Force of the American College of Radiology, American College of Surgeons, and College of American Pathologists. *CA Cancer J Clin* 1997;47:171.
146. Liberman L, Cohen MA, Dershaw DD, et al. Atypical ductal hyperplasia diagnosed at stereotaxic core biopsy of breast lesions: an indication for surgical biopsy. *AJR Am J Roentgenol* 1995;164:1111.
147. Burbank F. Stereotactic breast biopsy of atypical ductal hyperplasia and ductal carcinoma in situ lesions: improved accuracy with directional, vacuum-assisted biopsy. *Radiology* 1997;202:843.
148. Morrow M, Venta L, Stinson T, et al. Is core biopsy the diagnostic procedure of choice for all mammographic abnormalities? *Proc Am Soc Clin Oncol* 1999;18:79a.
149. Liberman L, LaTrenta LR, Dershaw DD, et al. Impact of core biopsy on the surgical management of impalpable breast cancer. *AJR Am J Roentgenol* 1997;168:495.
150. Morrow M, Schmidt R, Cregger B, Hassett C, Cox S. Preoperative evaluation of abnormal mammographic findings to avoid unnecessary breast biopsy. *Arch Surg* 1994;129:1091.
151. Ernster VL, Barclay J, Kerlikowske K, Grady D, Henderson IC. Incidence and treatment for ductal carcinoma in situ of the breast. *JAMA* 1996;275:913.
152. Pandya S, Mackarem G, Lee AKC, et al. Ductal carcinoma in situ: the impact of screening on clinical presentation and pathologic features. *Breast J* 1998;4:146.
153. Gapstur S, Morrow M, Ellman A, Sellers TA. Risk factors for breast cancer differ by histologic type: results of the Iowa Women's Health Study. *JAMA* 1999;281:2091.
154. Schwartz GF, Patchefsky AS, Finklestein SD, et al. Nonpalpable in situ ductal carcinoma of the breast: predictors of multicentricity and microinvasion and implications for treatment. *Arch Surg* 1989;124:29.
155. Silverstein MJ, Waisman JR, Gamagami P, et al. Intraductal carcinoma of the breast (208 cases): clinical factors influencing treatment choice. *Cancer* 1990;66:102.
156. European Commission Working Group on Breast Screening Pathology. Consistency achieved by 23 European pathologists in categorizing ductal carcinoma in situ of the breast using five classifications. *Hum Pathol* 1998;9:1056.
157. Lagios MD, Margolin FR, Westdahl PR, Rose MR. Mammographically detected duct carcinoma in situ: frequency of local recurrence following tylectomy and prognostic effect of nuclear grade on local recurrence. *Cancer* 1989;63:618.
158. Poller DN, Silverstein MJ, Galea M, et al. Ductal carcinoma in situ of the breast: a proposal for a new simplified histological classification association between cellular proliferation and c-erbB-2 protein expression. *Mod Pathol* 1994;7:257.
159. Silverstein MJ, Poller DN, Waisman JR, et al. Prognostic classification of breast ductal carcinoma in situ. *Lancet* 1995;345:1154.
160. Holland R, Peterse JL, Millis RR, et al. Ductal carcinoma in situ: a proposal for a new classification. *Semin Diagn Pathol* 1994;11:167.
161. The Consensus Conference Committee. Consensus conference of the classification of ductal carcinoma in situ. *Cancer* 1997;80:1798.
162. Bose S, Lesser ML, Norton L, Rosen PP. Immunophenotype of intraductal carcinoma. *Arch Pathol Lab Med* 1996;120:81.
163. Albonico G, Querzoli P, Ferretti, S, Rinaldi R, Nenci I. Biological profile of in situ breast cancer investigated by immunohistochemical technique. *Cancer Detect Prev* 1998;22:313.
164. Rudas M, Neumayer R, Gnant MF, et al. p53 protein expression, cell proliferation, and steroid hormone receptors in ductal and lobular in situ carcinomas of the breast. *Eur J Cancer* 1997;33:39.
165. Mack L, Kerkvliet N, Doig G, O'Malley FP. Relationship of a new histological categorization of ductal carcinoma in situ of the breast with size and the immunohistochemical expression of p53, c-erbB-2, bcl-2 and ki-67. *Hum Pathol* 1997;28:974.
166. Poller DN, Roberts EC, Bell JA, et al. p53 protein expression in mammary ductal carcinoma in situ: relationship to immunohistochemical expression of estrogen receptor c-erbB-2 protein. *Hum Pathol* 1993;24:463.
167. O'Malley FP, Vnencak-Jones CL, Dupont WD. p53 mutations are confined to comedo type ductal carcinoma in situ of the breast: immunohistochemical and sequencing data. *Lab Invest* 1994;71:67.
168. Guidi AJ, Fischer L, Harris JR, Schnitt SJ. Microvessel density and distribution in ductal carcinoma in situ of the breast. *J Natl Cancer Inst* 1994;85:614.
169. Engels K, Fox SB, Whitehouse RM, Gatter KC, Harris AL. Distinct angiogenic patterns are associated with high-grade in situ ductal carcinomas of the breast. *J Pathol* 1997;181:207.
170. Silverstein MJ, Gierson ED, Waisman JR, et al. Axillary lymph node dissection for T1a breast carcinoma: is it indicated? *Cancer* 1994;73:664.
171. Winchester DP, Menck HR, Osteen RT, Kraybill W. Treatment trends for ductal carcinoma in situ of the breast. *Ann Surg Oncol* 1995;2:207.
172. American Joint Committee on Cancer. *AJCC cancer staging manual.* Philadelphia: Lippincott–Raven, 1997:172.
173. Schuh ME, Nemoto T, Penetrante R, Rosner D, Dao TL. Intraductal carcinoma. Analysis of presentation, pathologic findings, and outcome of disease. *Arch Surg* 1986;121:1303.
174. Rosner D, Lane WW, Penetrante R. Ductal carcinoma in situ with microinvasion. A curable entity using surgery alone without need for adjuvant therapy. *Cancer* 1991;67:1498.
175. Wong JH, Kopald KH, Morton DL. The impact of microinvasion on axillary node metastases and survival in patients with intraductal breast cancer. *Arch Surg* 1990;125:1298.
176. Lagios MD. Microinvasion in ductal carcinoma in situ. In: Silverstein MJ, ed. *Carcinoma in situ of the breast.* Baltimore: Williams & Wilkins, 1997:241.
177. Elston CW, Ellis IO, eds. *Diagnostic histopathology of the breast.* Edinburgh: Churchill Livingstone, 1998:242.
178. Silver SA, Tavassoli FA. Mammary ductal carcinoma in situ with microinvasion. *Cancer* 1998;82:2382.
179. Silverstein MJ. Ductal carcinoma in situ with microinvasion. In: Silverstein MJ, ed. *Ductal carcinoma in situ of the breast.* Baltimore: Williams & Wilkins, 1997:557.
180. Silverstein MJ. Van Nuys experience by treatment. In: Silverstein MJ, ed. *Ductal carcinoma in situ of the breast.* Baltimore: Williams & Wilkins, 1997:443.
181. Kinne DW, Petrek JA, Osborne MP, et al. Breast carcinoma in situ. *Arch Surg* 1989; 124:33.
182. Cataliotti L, Distante V, Pacini P. Florence experience. In: Silverstein MJ, ed. *Ductal carcinoma in situ of the breast.* Baltimore: Williams & Wilkins, 1997:449.
183. Solin LJ, Recht A, Fourquet A, et al. Ten-year results of breast-conserving surgery and definitive irradiation for intraductal carcinoma (ductal carcinoma in situ) of the breast. *Cancer* 1991;68:2337.
184. Solin LJ, Kurtz J, Fourquet A, et al. Fifteen year results of breast-conserving surgery and definitive breast irradiation for the treatment of ductal carcinoma in situ of the breast. *J Clin Oncol* 1996;14:754
185. Hiramatsu H, Bornstein BA, Recht A, et al. Local recurrence after conservative surgery and radiation therapy for ductal carcinoma in situ: possible importance of family history. *Cancer J Sci Am* 1995;1:55.
186. McCormick B, Rosen PP, Kinne D, Cox L, Yahalom J. Duct carcinoma in situ of the breast: an analysis of local control after conservation surgery and radiotherapy. *Int J Radiat Oncol Biol Phys* 1991;21:289.
187. Kestin LL, Goldstein NS, Lacerna MD, et al. Factors associated with local recurrence of mammographically detected ductal carcinoma in situ in patients given breast-conserving therapy. *Cancer* 2000;88:596.
188. Solin LJ, McCormick B, Recht A, et al. Mammographically detected clinically occult ductal carcinoma in situ (intraductal carcinoma) treated with breast-conserving surgery and definitive breast irradiation. *Cancer J Sci Am* 1996;2:158.
189. Solin LJ, Fourquet A, McCormick B, et al. Salvage treatment for local recurrence following breast conserving surgery and definitive irradiation for ductal carcinoma in situ (intraductal carcinoma) of the breast. *Int J Radiat Oncol Biol Phys* 1994;30:3.
190. Fisher B, Dignam J, Wolmark N, et al. Lumpectomy and radiation therapy for the treatment of intraductal breast cancer: findings from National Surgical Adjuvant Breast and Bowel Project B-17. *J Clin Oncol* 1998;16:441.
191. Arnesson LG, Olsen K. Linköping experience. In: Silverstein MJ, ed. *Ductal carcinoma in situ of the breast.* Baltimore: Williams & Wilkins, 1997:373.
192. Carpenter R, Boulter PS, Cooke T, et al. Management of screen detected ductal carcinoma of the female breast. *Br J Surg* 1989;76:564
193. Schwartz GF. Treatment of subclinical ductal carcinoma in situ by local excision and surveillance: a personal experience. In: Silverstein MJ, ed. *Ductal carcinoma in situ of the breast.* Baltimore: Williams & Wilkins, 1997:353.
194. Silverstein MJ, Lagios MD, Groshen S, et al. The influence of margin width on local control of ductal carcinoma in situ of the breast. *N Engl J Med* 1999;340:1455.
195. Hetelekidis S, Collins L, Silver B, et al. Predictors of local recurrence following excision alone for ductal carcinoma in situ. *Cancer* 1999;85:427.
196. Julien J-P, Bijker N, Fentiman IS, et al. Radiotherapy in breast conserving treatment for ductal carcinoma in situ: first results of EORTC randomized phase III trial 10853. *Lancet* 2000;355:528.
197. Fisher ER, Costantino J, Fisher B, et al. Pathologic findings from the National Surgical Adjuvant Breast Project (NSABP) Protocol B-17. Intraductal carcinoma (ductal carcinoma in situ). *Cancer* 1995;75:1310.
198. Fisher ER, Dignam J, Tan-Chiu E, et al. Pathologic findings from the National Surgical Adjuvant Breast Project (NSABP) eight-year update Protocol B-17. *Cancer* 1999; 86:429.
199. Van Zee K, Liberman L, Samli B, et al. Long-term follow up of women with ductal carcinoma in situ treated with breast-conserving surgery. *Cancer* 1999;86:1757.
200. Fourquet A, Zafrani B, Campana F, Clough KB. Institut Curie experience. In: Silverstein MJ, ed. *Ductal carcinoma in situ of the breast.* Baltimore: Williams & Wilkins, 1997:391.
201. Silverstein MJ, Lagios MD, Craig PH, et al. A prognostic index for ductal carcinoma in situ of the breast. *Cancer* 1996;77:2267.
202. Schnitt SJ, Harris JR, Smith BL. Developing a prognostic index for ductal carcinoma in situ of the breast. Are we there yet? *Cancer* 1996;77:2189.
203. Mamounas EP, Bryant J, Fisher B, Wickerham DL, Wolmark N. Primary breast cancer (PBC) as a risk factor for subsequent contralateral breast cancer (CBC): NSABP experience from nine randomized adjuvant trials. *Breast Cancer Res Treat* 1998;50:230.
204. Fisher B, Dignam J, Wolmark N, et al. Tamoxifen in treatment of intraductal breast can-

cer: National Surgical Adjuvant Breast and Bowel Project B-24 randomized controlled trial. *Lancet* 1999;353:1993.
205. Morrow M, Bucci C, Rademaker A. Medical contraindications are not the major factor in the underutilization of breast conserving therapy. *J Am Coll Surg* 1998;186:269.
206. Akhtar S, Zablow A, Michaelson RA, Hutter RVP, Leitner SP. Predictors of axillary lymph node metastases in small (one centimeter or less) T1a,b primary breast cancer. *Proc Am Soc Clin Oncol* 1998;17:120a(abst).
207. Penault-Llorca F, Le Bouedec G, Pomel C, et al. Microinvasive carcinoma of the breast: is axillary lymph node dissection indicated? *Lab Invest* 1998;78:25A(abst).
208. Prasad ML, Giri G, Hoda S. Clinicopathologic features of microinvasive (<1mm) carcinoma of the breast. *Lab Invest* 1998;78:25A(abst).
209. Foote FW Jr, Stewart FW. Lobular carcinoma in situ: a rare form of mammary carcinoma. *Am J Pathol* 1941;17:491.
210. Page DL, Kidd TE Jr, Dupont WD, et al. Lobular neoplasia of the breast: higher risk for subsequent invasive cancer predicted by more extensive disease. *Hum Pathol* 1991;22:1232.
211. Haagensen CD, Bodian C, Haagensen DE. *Lobular neoplasia (lobular carcinoma in situ) breast carcinoma: risk and detection.* Philadelphia: WB Saunders, 1981:238.
212. Wheeler JE, Enterline HT, Roseman JM, et al. Lobular carcinoma in situ of the breast: long-term follow-up. *Cancer* 1974;34:554.
213. Andersen JA. Lobular carcinoma in situ of the breast: an approach to rational treatment. *Cancer* 1977;39:2597.
214. Alpers CE, Wellings SR. The prevalence of carcinoma in situ in normal and cancer associated breasts. *Hum Pathol* 1985;16:796.
215. Rosen PP, Kosloff C, Lieberman PH, Adair F, Braun DW Jr. Lobular carcinoma in situ of the breast. Detailed analysis of 99 patients with average follow-up of 24 years. *Am J Surg Pathol* 1978;2:225.
216. Lemanne D, Simon M, Martino S, et al. Breast carcinoma in situ: greater rise in ductal carcinoma in situ vs lobular carcinoma in situ. *Proc Am Soc Clin Oncol* 1991;10:45.
217. Frykberg ER, Bland KI. In situ breast carcinoma. *Adv Surg* 1993;26:29.
218. Lewison EF, Finney GG Jr. Lobular carcinoma in situ of the breast. *Surg Gynecol Obstet* 1968;126:1280.
219. Carter D, Smith RL. Carcinoma in situ of the breast. *Cancer* 1977;40:1189.
220. Lambird PA, Shelley WM. The spatial distribution of lobular in situ mammary carcinoma. Implications for size and site of breast biopsy. *JAMA* 1969;210:689.
221. Albonico G, Querzoli P, Ferretti S, Rinaldi R, Nenci I. Biological profile of in situ breast cancer investigated by immunohistochemical technique. *Cancer Detect Prev* 1998;22:313.
222. Rudas M, Neumayer R, Gnant MF, et al. p53 protein expression, cell proliferation and steroid hormone receptors in ductal and lobular in situ carcinomas of the breast. *Eur J Cancer* 1997;33:39.
223. Bur ME, Zimarowski MJ, Schnitt SJ, Baker S, Lew R. Estrogen receptor immunohistochemistry in carcinoma in situ of the breast. *Cancer* 1992;69:1174.
224. Vos CB, Cleton-Jansen AM, Berx G, et al. E-cadherin inactivation in lobular carcinoma in situ of the breast; an early event in tumorigenesis. *Br J Cancer* 1997;76:1131.
225. Fisher ER, Costantino J, Fisher B, et al. Pathologic findings from the National Surgical Adjuvant Breast Project (NSABP) protocol B-17. Five-year observations concerning lobular carcinoma in situ. *Cancer* 1996;78:1403.
226. Bodian CA, Perzin KH, Lattes R. Lobular neoplasia. Long term risk of breast cancer and relation to other factors. *Cancer* 1996;78:1024.
227. Salvadori B, Bartolic C, Zurrida S, et al. Risk of invasive cancer in women with lobular carcinoma in situ of the breast. *Eur J Cancer* 1991;27:35.
228. Ottesen GL, Graversen HP, Blichert-Toft M, Zedeler K, Andersen JA. Lobular carcinoma in situ of the female breast: short-term results of a prospective nationwide study. *Am J Surg Pathol* 1993;17:14.
229. Bradley SJ, Weaver DW, Bouwman DL. Alternatives in the surgical management of in situ breast cancer: a meta-analysis of outcome. *Am Surg* 1990;58:428.
230. Morrow M, Winchester DP, Chmiel JS, et al. Factors responsible for the under-utilization of breast-conserving therapy. *Proc Am Soc Clin Oncol* 1998;17:98a(abst).
231. Lazovich D, Solomon CC, Thomas DB, et al. Breast conservation therapy in the United States following the 1990 National Institutes of Health Consensus Development Conference on the treatment of patients with early stage breast cancer. *Cancer* 1999;86:628.
232. Turner L, Swindell R, Bell W. Radical versus modified radical mastectomy for breast cancer. *Ann R Coll Surg Engl* 1981;63:239.
233. Maddox W, Carpenter J, Laws H, et al. A randomized prospective trial of radical (Halsted) mastectomy versus modified radical mastectomy in 311 breast cancer patients. *Ann Surg* 1983;198:207.
234. Fisher B, Redmond C, Fisher ER, et al. Ten-year results of a randomized clinical trial comparing radical mastectomy and total mastectomy with or without radiation. *N Engl J Med* 1985;312:674.
235. Holland R, Veling S, Mravunac M, Hendriks JH. Histologic multifocality of T_{is}, T_{1-2} breast carcinomas: implications for clinical trials of breast conserving treatment. *Cancer* 1985;56:979.
236. Holland R, Connolly J, Gelman R, et al. Histologic multifocality of Tis, T1-2 breast carcinomas: implications for clinical trials of breast conserving treatment. *J Clin Oncol* 1990;8:113.
237. Lagios M, Richards V, Rose M, Yee E. Segmental mastectomy without radiotherapy: short-term follow-up. *Cancer* 1983;52:2173.
238. Montgomery A, Greening W, Levene A. Clinical study of recurrence rate and survival time of patients with carcinoma of the breast treated by biopsy excision without any other therapy. *J R Soc Med* 1978;71:339.
239. Targart R. Partial mastectomy for breast cancer. *BMJ* 1978;2:1268.
240. Freeman C, Belliveau N, Kim T, Boivin JF. Limited surgery with or without radiotherapy for early breast carcinoma. *J Can Assoc Radiol* 1981;32:125.
241. Fisher B, Anderson S, Redmond CK, et al. Reanalysis and results after 12 years of follow-up in a randomized clinical trial comparing total mastectomy with lumpectomy with or without irradiation in the treatment of breast cancer. *N Engl J Med* 1995;333:1456.
242. Veronesi U, Salvadori B, Luini A, et al. Breast conservation is a safe method in patients with small cancer of the breast. Long-term results of three randomized trials on 1,973 patients. *Eur J Cancer* 1995;31A:1574.
243. Jacobson JA, Danforth DN, Cowan KH, et al. Ten-year results of a comparison of conservation with mastectomy in the treatment of stage I and II breast cancer. *N Engl J Med* 1995;332:907.
244. van Dongen JA, Bartelink H, Fentiman IS, et al. Factors influencing local relapse and survival and results of salvage treatment after breast conserving therapy in operable breast cancer: EORTC trial 1081, breast conservation compared with mastectomy in TNM stage I and II breast cancer. *Eur J Cancer* 1992;28A:801.
245. Arriagada R, Le MG, Rochard F, Contesso G, for the Institut Gustave-Roussy Breast Cancer Group. Conservative treatment versus mastectomy in early breast cancer: patterns of failure with 15 years of follow-up data. *J Clin Oncol* 1996;14:1558.
246. van Dongen JA, Bartelink H, Fentiman IS, et al. Randomized clinical trial to assess the value of breast-conserving therapy in stage I and II breast cancer: EORTC 10801 trial. *J Natl Cancer Inst* 1992;11:15.
247. Blichert-Toft M, Rose C, Andersen JA, et al. Danish randomized trial comparing breast conservation therapy with mastectomy: six years of life-table analysis. *J Natl Cancer Inst Monogr* 1992;11:19.
248. Early Breast Cancer Trialists' Collaborative Group. Effects of radiotherapy and surgery in early breast cancer: an overview of the randomized trials. *N Engl J Med* 1995;333:1444.
249. Clark RM, Wilkinson RH, Mahoney LJ, Reid JG, MacDonald WD. Breast cancer: a 21-year experience with conservative surgery and radiation. *Int J Radiat Oncol Biol Phys* 1982;8:967.
250. Fowble B, Solin L, Schultz D, Goodman RL. Ten-year results of conservative surgery and irradiation for stage I and II breast cancer. *Int J Radiat Oncol Biol Phys* 1991;21:269.
251. Fourquet A, Campana F, Zafrani B, et al. Prognostic factors of breast recurrence in the conservative management of early breast cancer: a 25-year follow-up. *Int J Radiat Oncol Biol Phys* 1989;17:719.
252. Kurtz J, Amalric R, Brandone H, et al. Local recurrence after breast-conserving surgery and radiotherapy: frequency, time course, and prognosis. *Cancer* 1989;63:1912.
253. Gage I, Recht A, Gelman R, et al. Long-term outcome following breast conserving surgery and radiation therapy. *Int J Radiat Oncol Biol Phys* 1995;33:245.
254. Morrow M, Bucci C, Rademaker A. Medical contraindications are not a major factor in the underutilization of breast conserving therapy. *J Am Coll Surg* 1998;186:269.
255. Foster RS, Farwell ME, Costanza MC. Breast therapy for breast cancer: patterns of care in a geographic region and estimation of potential applicability. *Ann Surg Oncol* 1995;2:275.
256. Morrow M, Schmidt R, Hassett C. Patient selection for breast conservation therapy with magnification mammography. *Surgery* 1995;118:621.
257. Harris J, Recht A, Amalric R, et al. Time course and prognosis of local recurrence following primary radiation therapy for early breast cancer. *J Clin Oncol* 1984;2:37.
258. Gage I, Schnitt S, Recht A, et al. Skin recurrences after breast conserving therapy for early stage breast cancer. *J Clin Oncol* 1998;16:480.
259. Kurtz J, Jacquemier J, Amalric R, et al. Why are local recurrences (LR) after breast-conserving surgery more frequent in younger patients? *J Clin Oncol* 1990;8:591.
260. Nixon AJ, Neuberg D, Hayes EF, et al. Relationship of patient age to pathologic features of the tumor and prognosis for patients with stage I or II breast cancer. *J Clin Oncol* 1994;12:888.
261. de la Rochefordiere A, Mouret-Fourme E, de Ricke Y, et al. Local and distant relapses in relation to age following breast-conserving surgery and irradiation in premenopausal patients with breast cancer. *Int J Radiat Oncol Biol Phys* 1998;42:180(abst).
262. Vrieling C, Collette L, Fourquet A, et al. The higher local recurrence rate after breast conserving therapy in young patients explained by larger tumor size and incomplete excision at first attempt? *Int J Radiat Oncol Biol Phys* 1998;42:125(abst).
263. de la Rochefordiere A, Asselain B, Campana G, et al. Age as a prognostic factor in premenopausal breast carcinoma. *Lancet* 1993;341:1039.
264. Donegan W, Perez-Mesa C, Watson F. A biostatistical study of locally recurrent breast carcinoma. *Surg Gynecol Obstet* 1966;122:529.
265. Matthews R, McNeese M, Montague E, Oswald MJ. Prognostic implications of age in breast cancer patients treated with tumorectomy and irradiation or with mastectomy. *Int J Radiat Oncol Biol Phys* 1988;14:659.
266. Chabner E, Nixon A, Gelman R, et al. Family history and treatment outcome in young women after breast-conserving surgery and radiation therapy for early-stage breast cancer. *J Clin Oncol* 1998;16:2045.
267. Verhoog LC, Brekelmans CTM, Seynaeve C, et al. Survival and tumour characteristics of breast cancer patients with germline mutations of BRCA1. *Lancet* 1998;351:316.
268. Scully R, Chen J, Plug A, et al. Association of BRCA1 with Rad51 in mitotic and meiotic cells. *Cell* 1997;88:265.
269. Sharan SK, Morimatsu M, Albrecht U, et al. Embryonic lethality and radiation hypersensitivity mediated by Rad51 in mice lacking BRCA. *Nature* 1997;386:804.
270. Marcus JN, Watson P, Page DL, et al. Hereditary breast cancer: pathobiology, prognosis, and BRCA1 and BRCA2 gene linkage. *Cancer* 1996;77:697.
271. Smith TE, Harrold EV, Matloff BC, et al. BRCA 1,2 status, family history and ipsilateral breast tumor relapse following conservative surgery and radiation therapy. *Proc Am Soc Clin Oncol* 1999;18:624a(abst).
272. Pierce L, Strawderman M, Narold S, et al. No deleterious effects of radiotherapy in women who are heterozygous for a BRCA-1 or BRCA-2 mutation following breast conserving therapy. *Proc Am Soc Clin Oncol* 1999;18:86a(abst).
273. Gaffney DK, Brohet RM, Lewis CM, et al. Response to radiation therapy and prognosis in breast cancer patients with BRCA1 and BRCA2 mutations. *Radiother Oncol* 1998;47:129.
274. Harris JR. Breast-conserving therapy as a model for creating new knowledge in clinical oncology. *Int J Radiat Oncol Biol Phys* 1996;35:641.
275. Schnitt S, Connolly J, Khettry U, et al. Pathologic findings on reexcision of the primary site in breast cancer patients considered for treatment by primary radiation therapy. *Cancer* 1987;59:675.

276. Borger J, Kemperman H, Hart A, et al. Risk factors in breast-conservation therapy. *J Clin Oncol* 1994;12:653.
277. Dewar JA, Arriagada R, Benhamou S, et al. Local relapse and contralateral tumor rates in patients with breast cancer treated with conservative surgery and radiotherapy (Institute Gustave-Roussy 1970–1982). IGR Breast Cancer Group. *Cancer* 1995;76:2260.
278. Freedman G, Fowble B, Hanlon A, et al. Patients with close or positive margins treated with conservative surgery and radiation have an increased risk of breast recurrence that is delayed by adjuvant systemic therapy. *Int J Radiat Oncol Biol Phys* 1999;44:1005.
279. Park CC, Mitsumori M, Nixon A, et al. Outcome at 8 years after breast conserving surgery and radiation therapy for invasive breast cancer: influence of margin status and systemic therapy on local recurrence. *J Clin Oncol* 2000;18(8)1668.
280. Anscher MS, Jones P, Prosnitz LR, et al. Local failure and margin status in early-stage breast carcinoma treated with conservation surgery and radiation therapy. *Ann Surg* 1993;218:22.
281. Smitt MC, Nowels KW, Zdeblich MJ, et al. The importance of the lumpectomy surgical margin status in long term results of breast conservation. *Cancer* 1995;76:259.
282. Peterson ME, Schultz DJ, Reynolds C, et al. Outcomes in breast cancer patients relative to margin status after treatment with breast-conserving surgery and radiation therapy: the University of Pennsylvania experience. *Int J Radiat Oncol Biol Phys* 2000 *(in press).*
283. Wazer DE, Schmidt-Ullich RK, Ruthazer R, et al. Factors determining outcome for breast-conserving irradiation with margin-directed dose escalation to the tumor bed. *Int J Radiat Oncol Biol Phys* 1998;40:851.
284. Pittinger TP, Maronian NC, Poulter CA, Peacock JL. Importance of margins status in outcome of breast-conserving surgery for carcinoma. *Surgery* 1994;116:605.
285. Cowen D, Largillier R, Bardou V-J, et al. Positive margins after conservative treatments impacts local control and possibly survival in node-negative breast cancer. *Int J Radiat Oncol Biol Phys* 1998;42:126(abst).
286. Fisher ER, Sass R, Fisher B, et al. Pathologic findings from the National Surgical Adjuvant Breast Project (Protocol 6) II: relation of local breast recurrence to multicentricity. *Cancer* 1986;57:1717.
287. Fisher B, Dignam J, Mamounas HP, et al. Sequential methotrexate and fluorouracil for the treatment of node-negative breast cancer patients with estrogen-receptor negative tumors: eight year results from NSAPB B-13 and first report of findings from NSABP B-10 comparing methotrexate and fluorouracil with conventional cyclophosphamide, methotrexate and fluorouracil. *J Clin Oncol* 1996;14:1982.
288. Fisher B, Dignam J, Bryant J, et al. Five versus more than five years of tamoxifen therapy for breast cancer patients with negative lymph nodes and estrogen receptor-positive tumors. *J Natl Cancer Inst* 1996;88:1529.
289. Dalberg K, Johansson H, Johansson U, Rutqvist L, for the Stockholm Breast Cancer Study Group. A randomized trial of long term adjuvant tamoxifen plus postoperative radiation therapy versus radiation therapy for patients with early stage breast carcinoma treated with breast-conserving surgery. *Cancer* 1998;82:2204.
290. American College of Radiology, American College of Surgeons, College of American Pathologists and the Society of Surgical Oncology. Standards for diagnosis and management of invasive breast carcinomas. *CA Cancer J Clin* 1998;48:83.
291. Fleck R, McNeese MD, Ellerbroek NA, Hunter TA, Holmes FA. Consequences of breast irradiation in patients with pre-existing collagen vascular diseases. *Int J Radiat Oncol Biol Phys* 1989;17:829.
292. Morris MM, Powell SN. Irradiation in the setting of collagen vascular disease: acute and late complications. *J Clin Oncol* 1997;15:2728.
293. Liljegren G, Holmberg L, Bergh J, et al. 10-year results after resection with and without postoperative radiotherapy for stage I breast cancer. A randomized trial. *J Natl Cancer Inst* 1999;17:2326.
294. Clark RM, Whelan T, Levine M, et al. Randomized clinical trial of breast irradiation following lumpectomy and axillary dissection for node-negative breast cancer: an update. Ontario Clinical Oncology Group. *J Natl Cancer Inst* 1996;88:1659.
295. Forrest AP, Stewart HJ, Everington D, et al. Randomised controlled trial of conservation therapy for breast cancer: 6-year analysis of the Scottish trial. Scottish Cancer Trials Breast Group. *Lancet* 1996;348:708.
296. Renton SC, Gazet JC, Ford HT, Corbishley C, Sutcliffe R. The importance of the resection margin in conservative surgery for breast cancer. *Eur J Surg Oncol* 1996;22:17.
297. Lim M, Nixon A, Gelman R, et al. A prospective study of conservative surgery alone without radiotherapy in selected patients with stage I breast cancer. *Breast Cancer Res Treat* 1999;57:34(abst).
298. Nemoto T, Patel J, Rosner D, et al. Factors affecting recurrence in lumpectomy without irradiation for breast cancer. *Cancer* 1991;67:2079.
299. Kantorowitz DA, Poulter CA, Sischy B, et al. Treatment of breast cancer among elderly women with segmental mastectomy or segmental mastectomy plus postoperative radiotherapy. *Int J Radiat Oncol Biol Phys* 1995;15:263.
300. Reed MWR, Morrison JM. Wide local excision as the sole primary treatment in elderly patients with carcinoma of the breast. *Br J Surg* 1989;76:898.
300a. Wolmark N, Dignam J, Margolese R, et al. The role of radiotherapy and tamoxifen in the management of node negative invasive breast cancer <1 cm treated with lumpectomy: preliminary results of NSABP protocol B-21. Proc ASCO 2000;19;abst 271.
301. Martelli G, DePalo G, Rossi N, et al. Long-term follow-up of elderly patients with operable breast cancer treated with surgery without axillary dissection plus adjuvant tamoxifen. *Br J Surg* 1995;72:1251.
302. Lee KS, Plowman PN, Gilmore OJA, Gray R. Tamoxifen in breast conservation therapy. *Int J Clin Pharmacol Ther* 1995;33:281.
303. Bonadonna G, Veronesi U, Brambilla C, et al. Primary chemotherapy to avoid mastectomy in tumors with diameters of three centimeters or more. *J Natl Cancer Inst* 1990; 82:1539.
304. Smith IE, Jones AL, O'Brien ME, et al. Primary medical (neoadjuvant) chemotherapy for operable breast cancer. *Eur J Cancer Clin Oncol* 1993;29A:1796.
305. Powles TJ, Hickish TF, Makris A, et al. Randomized trial of chemoendocrine therapy started before or after surgery for treatment of primary breast cancer. *J Clin Oncol* 1995;13:547.
306. Fisher B, Brown A, Mamounas E, et al. Effect of preoperative chemotherapy on local-regional disease in women with operable breast cancer: findings from National Surgical Adjuvant Breast and Bowel Project B-18. *J Clin Oncol* 1997;15:2483.
307. Fisher B, Bryant J, Wolmark N, et al. Effect of preoperative chemotherapy on the outcome of women with operable breast cancer. *J Clin Oncol* 1998;16:2672.
308. Avril A, Faucher A, Bussieres E, et al. Results of 10 years of a randomized trial of neoadjuvant chemotherapy in breast cancers larger than 3 cm. *Chirurgie* 1998;123:247.
309. Vicini F, Eberlein T, Connolly J, et al. The optimal extent of resection for patients with stages I or II breast cancer treated with conservative surgery and radiotherapy. *Ann Surg* 1992;214:200.
310. Clarke D, Martinez A. Identification of patients who are at high risk for locoregional breast cancer recurrence after conservative surgery and radiotherapy: a review article for surgeons, pathologists, and radiation and medical oncologists. *J Clin Oncol* 1992;10:474.
311. Gwin J, Eisenberg B, Hoffman J, et al. Incidence of gross and microscopic carcinoma in specimens from patients with breast cancer after re-excision lumpectomy. *Ann Surg* 1993;218:729.
312. Keidan R, Hoffman J, Weese J, et al. Delayed breast abscesses after lumpectomy and radiation therapy. *Am Surg* 1990;56:440.
313. Rescigno J, McCormick B, Brown A, Myskowski PL. Breast cellulitis after conservative surgery and radiotherapy. *Int J Radiat Oncol Biol Phys* 1994;29:163.
314. Schneiderman M, Axtell L. Deaths among female patients with carcinoma of the breast treated by a surgical procedure only. *Surg Gynecol Obstet* 1979;148:193.
315. Say C, Donegan W. A biostatistical evaluation of complications from mastectomy. *Surg Gynecol Obstet* 1974;138:370.
316. Aitken D, Minton J. Complications associated with mastectomy. *Surg Clin North Am* 1983;63:1331.
317. Beatty J, Robinson G, Zaia J, et al. A prospective analysis of nosocomial wound infection after mastectomy. *Arch Surg* 1983;118:1421.
318. Platt R, Zucker J, Zaleznik D, et al. Perioperative antibiotic prophylaxis and wound infection following breast surgery. *J Antimicrob Chemother* 1993;(Suppl B)31:43.
319. Platt R, Zucker J, Zaleznik D, et al. Prophylaxis against wound infection following herniorrhaphy or breast surgery. *J Infect Dis* 1992;166:556.
320. Budd D, Cochran R, Sturtz O, Fouty WJ Jr. Surgical morbidity after mastectomy operations. *Am J Surg* 1978;135:218.
321. Chilson T, Chan F, Lonser R, Wu TM, Aitken DR. Seroma prevention after modified radical mastectomy. *Am Surg* 1992;58:750.
322. Jolly P, Viar W. Reduction of morbidity after radical mastectomy. *Am Surg* 1981;47:377.
323. Petrek JA, Peters M, Nori S, et al. Axillary lymphadenopathy: a prospective randomized trial of thirteen factors influencing drainage, including early or delayed arm mobilization. *Arch Surg* 1991;125:378.
324. Jamison K, Wellisch DK, Katz RL, Pasnau RO. Phantom breast syndrome. *Arch Surg* 1979;114:93.
325. Kroner K, Knudsen UB, Lundley H, Hvid H. Long-term phantom breast syndrome after mastectomy. *Clin J Pain* 1992;8:346.
326. Johnson C, Van Heerden J, Donohue J, et al. Oncological aspects of immediate breast reconstruction following mastectomy for malignancy. *Arch Surg* 1989;124:819.
327. Petit J, Le M, Mouriesse H, et al. Can breast reconstruction with gel-filled silicone implants increase the risk of death and second primary cancer in patients treated by mastectomy for breast cancer? *Plast Reconstr Surg* 1994;94:115.
328. Kroll S, Ames F, Singletary S, et al. The oncologic risks of skin preservation at mastectomy when combined with immediate reconstruction of the breast. *Surg Gynecol Obstet* 1991;172:17.
329. Noone R, Frazier T, Noone G, et al. Recurrence of breast carcinoma following immediate reconstruction: a 13-year review. *Plast Reconstr Surg* 1994;90:96.
330. Eberlein T, Crespo L, Smith B, et al. Prospective evaluation of immediate reconstruction after mastectomy. *Ann Surg* 1993;218:29.
331. Noone R, Murphy J, Spear S, et al. A six-year experience with immediate reconstruction for mastectomy for cancer. *Plast Reconstr Surg* 1985;76:258.
332. Victor SJ, Brown DM, Horwitz EM, et al. Treatment outcome with radiation therapy after breast augmentation or reconstruction in patients with primary breast carcinoma. *Cancer* 1998;82:1303.
333. Evans GRD, Schusterman MA, Kroll SS, et al. Reconstruction and the radiated breast: is there a role for implants? *Plast Reconstr Surg* 1995;96:1111.
334. Hunt KA, Baldwin BJ, Strom E, et al. Feasibility of postmastectomy radiation therapy after TRAM flap breast reconstruction. *Ann Surg Oncol* 1997;4:377.
335. Williams JK, Carlson GW, Bostwick J 3rd, Bried JT, Mackay G. The effects of radiation treatment after TRAM flap breast reconstruction. *Plast Reconstr Surg* 1997;100:1153.
336. Valagussa P, Bonadonna G, Veronesi U. Patterns of relapse and survival following radical mastectomy: analysis of 716 consecutive patients. *Cancer* 1978;41:1170.
337. Fisher B, Wolmark N, Bauer M, Redmond C, Gebhardt M. The accuracy of clinical nodal staging and of limited axillary dissection as a determinant of histologic nodal status in carcinoma of the breast. *Surg Gynecol Obstet* 1981;152:765.
338. Bedwinek J, Lee J, Fineberg B, Ocwieza M. Prognostic indicators in patients with isolated local–regional recurrence of breast cancer. *Cancer* 1981;47:2232.
339. Aberizk W, Silver B, Henderson IC, Cady B, Harris JR. The use of radiotherapy for treatment of isolated local–regional recurrence of breast cancer after mastectomy. *Cancer* 1986;58:1214.
340. Chen K, Montague E, Oswald M. Results of irradiation in the treatment of loco-regional breast cancer recurrence. *Cancer* 1985;56:1269.
341. Early Breast Cancer Trialists' Collaborative Group. Effects of radiotherapy in early breast cancer. An overview of the randomized trials. *N Engl J Med* 1995;1444:55.
342. Jones JM, Ribeiro GG. Mortality patterns over 34 years of breast cancer patients in a clinical trial of post-operative radiotherapy. *Clin Radiol* 1989;40:204.
343. Host H, Brennhovd IO, Loeb M. Postoperative radiotherapy in breast cancer—long-term results from the Oslo study. *Int J Radiat Oncol Biol Phys* 1986;12:727.

344. Early Breast Cancer Trialists' Group. *Treatment of early breast cancer; world-wide experience, 1985–1990.* Vol. 1. Oxford, UK: Oxford University Press.
345. Rutqvist L, Pettersson D, Johansson H. Adjuvant radiation therapy versus surgery alone in operable breast cancer: long-term follow-up in a randomized clinical trial. *Radiother Oncol* 1993;26:104.
346. Rutqvist LE, Lax I, Fornander T, Johansson H. Cardiovascular mortality in a randomized trial of adjuvant radiation therapy versus surgery alone in primary breast cancer. *Int J Radiat Oncol Biol Phys* 1992;22:887.
347. Fisher B, Slack NH, Cavanaugh PJ, Gardner B, Ravdin IG. Postoperative radiotherapy in the treatment of breast cancer: results of the NSABP clinical trial. *Ann Surg* 1970;172:711.
348. Lythgoe JP, Palmer MK. Manchester regional breast study: 5 and 10 year results. *Br J Surg* 1982;69:693.
349. Haybittle JL, Brinkley D, Houghton J, A'Hern RP, Baum M. Postoperative radiotherapy and late mortality: evidence from the Cancer Research Campaign trial for early breast cancer. *BMJ* 1989;298:1611.
350. Stewart H, Jack W, Forrest A, et al. South-east Scottish trial of local therapy in node negative breast cancer. *Breast* 1994;3:31.
351. Turnbull AR, Turner DT, Chant AD, et al. Treatment of early breast cancer. *Lancet* 1978;2:7.
352. Cuzick J, Stewart H, Rutqvist L, et al. Cause-specific mortality in long-term survivors of breast cancer who participated in trials of radiotherapy. *J Clin Oncol* 1994;12:447.
353. Anonymous. Favourable and unfavourable effects on long-term survival of radiotherapy for early breast cancer: an overview of the randomised trials. Early Breast Cancer Trialists Collaborative Group. *Lancet* 2000;355(9217)1757.
354. Stefanik D, Goldberg R, Byrne P, et al. Local–regional failure in patients treated with adjuvant chemotherapy for breast cancer. *J Clin Oncol* 1985;3:660.
355. Fowble B, Gray R, Gilchrist K, et al. Identification of a subgroup of patients with breast cancer and histologically positive axillary nodes receiving adjuvant chemotherapy who may benefit from postoperative radiotherapy. *J Clin Oncol* 1988;6:1107.
356. Recht A, Gray R, Davidson N, et al. Locoregional failure 10 years after mastectomy and adjuvant chemotherapy with or without tamoxifen without irradiation: experience of the Eastern Cooperative Oncology Group. *J Clin Oncol* 1999;17:1689.
357. Overgaard M, Hansen PS, Overgaard J, et al. Postoperative radiotherapy in high-risk premenopausal women with breast cancer who receive adjuvant chemotherapy. Danish Breast Cancer Cooperative Group 82b Trial. *N Engl J Med* 1997;337:949.
358. Overgaard M, Jensen M-B, Overgaard J, et al. Randomized controlled trial evaluating postoperative radiotherapy in high-risk postmenopausal breast cancer patients given adjuvant tamoxifen: report from the Danish Breast Cancer Cooperative Group DBCG g2c Trial. *Lancet* 1999;353:1641.
359. Ragaz J, Jackson SM, Le N, et al. Adjuvant radiotherapy and chemotherapy in node-positive premenopausal women with breast cancer. *N Engl J Med* 1997;337:956.
360. Griem KL, Henderson IC, Gelman R, et al. The 5-year results of a randomized trial of adjuvant radiation therapy after chemotherapy in breast cancer patients treated with mastectomy. *J Clin Oncol* 1987;5:1546.
361. Velez-Garcia E, Carpenter JT Jr, Moore M, et al. Postsurgical adjuvant chemotherapy with or without radiotherapy in women with breast cancer and positive axillary nodes: a South-Eastern Cancer Study Group (SEG) Trial. *Eur J Cancer* 1992;28A:1833.
362. Martinez A, Ahmann D, O'Fallon J, et al. An interim analysis of the randomized surgical adjuvant trial for patients with unfavorable breast cancer. *Int J Radiat Oncol Biol Phys* 1984;10(Suppl 2):106.
363. Muss H, Cooper R, Brockschmidt J, et al. A randomized trial of adjuvant chemotherapy with and without radiation therapy for stage II breast cancer: 11-year follow-up of Piedmont Oncology Association (protocol no. 74176). *Breast Cancer Res Treat* 1989;14:185.
364. McArdle C, Crawford D, Dykes E, et al. Adjuvant radiotherapy and chemotherapy in breast cancer. *Br J Surg* 1986;73:264.
365. Blomqvist C, Tiusanen K, Elomaa I, et al. The combination of radiotherapy, adjuvant chemotherapy (cyclophosphamide-doxorubicin-ftorafur) and tamoxifen in stage II breast cancer. Long-term follow-up results of a randomised trial. *Br J Cancer* 1992;66:1171.
366. Buzdar AJ, Blumenschein GR, Smith TL, et al. Adjuvant chemotherapy with fluorouracil, doxorubicin, and cyclophosphamide, with or without Bacillus Calmette-Guerin and with or without irradiation in operable breast cancer. A prospective randomized trial. *Cancer* 1984;53:384.
367. Tennvall-Nittby L, Tengrup I, Landberg T. The total incidence of loco-regional recurrence in a randomized trial of breast cancer TNM stage II. The South Sweden Breast Cancer Trial. *Acta Oncol* 1993;32:641.
368. Whelan TJ, Julian J, Wright J, et al. Does locoregional radiation therapy improve survival in breast cancer? A meta-analysis. *J Clin Oncol* 2000;18:1220.
369. Harris JR, Halpin-Murphy P, McNeese M, et al. Consensus statement on postmastectomy therapy. *Int J Radiat Oncol Biol Phys* 1999;44:989.
370. Paszat L, Mackillop WJ, Groome PA, et al. Mortality from myocardial infarction following postlumpectomy radiotherapy for breast cancer: a population-based study in Ontario, Canada. *Int J Radiat Oncol Biol Phys* 1999;43:755.
371. Nixon AJ, Manola J, Gelman R, et al. No long-term increase in cardiac-related mortality after breast-conserving surgery and radiation therapy using modern techniques. *J Clin Oncol* 1998;16:1374.
372. Gyenes G, Rutqvist LE, Liedberg A, Fornander T. Long-term cardiac morbidity and mortality in a randomized trial of pre- and postoperative radiation therapy versus surgery alone in primary breast cancer. *Radiother Oncol* 1998;48:185.
373. Gustavsson A, Bendahl P-O, Cwikiel M, et al. No serious late cardiac effects after adjuvant radiotherapy following mastectomy in premenopausal women with early breast cancer. *Radiother Oncol* 1999;43:745.
374. Hojris I, Overgaard M, Christensen JJ, et al. Morbidity and mortality of ischemic heart disease in 3083 high-risk breast cancer patients given adjuvant systemic treatment with or without postmastectomy irradiation. *Radiother Oncol* 1998;48(Suppl 1):S120(abst).
375. Shapiro CL, Hardenbergh PH, Gelman R, et al. Cardiac effects of adjuvant doxorubicin and radiation therapy in breast cancer patients. *J Clin Oncol* 1998;16:3493.
376. Lu H-M, Cash E, Nixon A, et al. The impact of CT-simulation on the planning of tangential fields for left breast treatment. *Int J Radiat Oncol Biol Phys* 1999;45:159(abst).
377. Goss PE, Sierra S. Current perspectives on radiation-induced breast cancer. *J Clin Oncol* 1998;16:338.
378. Mattsson A, Ruden B-I, Hall P, Wilking N, Rutqvist LE. Radiation-induced breast cancer: long-term follow-up of radiation for benign breast disease. *J Natl Cancer Inst* 1993;85:1679.
379. Committee on the Biological Effects of Ionizing Radiations, Board on Radiation Effects Research Commission on Life Sciences, National Research Council. *Health effects of exposure to low levels of ionizing radiation: BEIR V.* Washington, DC: National Academy, 1990.
380. Tokunaga M, Land C, Tokuoka S, et al. Incidence of female breast cancer among atomic bomb survivors, 1950–1985. *Radiat Res* 1994;138:209.
381. Boice JD Jr, Harvey EB, Blettner M, Stovall M, Flannery JT. Cancer in the contralateral breast after radiotherapy for breast cancer. *N Engl J Med* 1992;326:781.
382. Storm H, Andersson M, Boice J Jr, et al. Adjuvant radiotherapy and risk of contralateral breast cancer. *J Natl Cancer Inst* 1992;84:1245.
383. Brady MS, Garfein CF, Petrek JA, Brennan MF. Post-treatment sarcoma in breast cancer patients. *Ann Surg Oncol* 1994;1:66.
384. Karlsson P, Holmberg E, Johansson K-A, et al. Soft tissue sarcoma after treatment for breast cancer. *Radiother Oncol* 1996;38:25.
385. Strobbe LJ, Peterse HL, van Tinteren H, et al. Angiosarcoma of the breast after conservative therapy for invasive cancer, the incidence and outcome. An unforseen sequela. *Breast Cancer Res Treat* 1998;47:101.
386. Marchal C, Weber B, de Lafontan B, et al. Nine breast angiosarcomas after conservative treatment for breast carcinoma: a survey from French comprehensive cancer centers. *Int J Radiat Oncol Biol Phys* 1999;4:113.
387. Inskip P, Stovall M, Flannery J. Lung cancer risk and radiation dose among women treated for breast cancer. *J Natl Cancer Inst* 1994;86:983.
388. Neugut AI, Robinson E, Lee WC, et al. Lung cancer after radiation therapy for breast cancer. *Cancer* 1993;71:3054.
389. Neugut A, Murray T, Santos J, et al. Increased risk of lung cancer after breast cancer radiation therapy in cigarette smokers. *Cancer* 1994;73:1615.
390. Inskip P, Boice J Jr. Radiotherapy-induced lung cancer among women who smoke [Editorial]. *Cancer* 1994;73:1541.
391. Smith IE, Gregory K. The sequencing of systemic and local therapies in primary breast cancer. *Semin Breast Dis* 1999;2:110.
392. Glucksberg H, Rivkin S, Rasmussen S, et al. Combination chemotherapy (CMFVP) versus L-phenylalanine mustard (L-PAM) for operable breast cancer with positive axillary nodes: a Southwest Oncology Group study. *Cancer* 1982;50:423.
393. Buzdar A, Smith T, Powell KC, et al. Effect of timing of initiation of adjuvant chemotherapy on disease-free survival in breast cancer. *Breast Cancer Res Treat* 1982;2:163.
394. Recht A, Come S, Gelman R, et al. Integration of conservative surgery, radiotherapy, and chemotherapy for the treatment of early-stage node-positive breast cancer: sequencing, timing, and outcome. *J Clin Oncol* 1991;9:1662.
395. Buchholz T, Austin-Seymour M, Moe R, et al. Effect of delay in radiation in the combined modality treatment of breast cancer. *Int J Radiat Oncol Biol Phys* 1993;26:23.
396. Buchholz TA, Hunt KK, Amosson CM, et al. Sequencing of chemotherapy and radiation in lymph node-negative breast cancer. *Cancer J Sci Am* 1999;5:159.
397. Hartsell W, Recine D, Griem K, Murthy AK. Delaying the initiation of intact breast irradiation for patients with lymph node positive breast increases the risk of local recurrence. *Cancer* 1995;76:2497.
398. Buzdar A, Kau S, Smith T, et al. The order of administration of chemotherapy and radiation and its effect on local control of operable breast cancer. *Cancer* 1993;71:3680.
399. McCormick B, Norton L, Yao TJ, Yahalom J, Petrek JA. The impact of the sequence of radiation and chemotherapy on local control after breast-conserving surgery. *Cancer J Sci Am* 1996;2:39.
400. Wallgren A, Bernier J, Gelber RD, et al. Timing of radiotherapy and chemotherapy following breast conserving surgery for patients with node-positive breast cancer. *Int J Radiat Oncol Biol Phys* 1996;35:649.
401. Leonard CE, Wood ME, Zhen B, et al. Does administration of chemotherapy before radiotherapy in breast patients treated with conservative surgery negatively impact local control? *J Clin Oncol* 1995;13:2906.
402. Mamounas EP, Fisher B, Bryant J, et al. Does delaying breast irradiation in order to administer adjuvant chemotherapy increase the rate of ipsilateral breast tumor recurrence (IBTR)? Results from two NSABP adjuvant studies in node-positive breast cancer (B-15 and B-16). *Breast Cancer Res Treat* 1996;41:219(abst).
403. Recht A, Come SE, Henderson IC, et al. The sequencing of chemotherapy and radiation therapy after conservative surgery for patients with early-stage breast cancer. *N Engl J Med* 1996;334:1356.
404. Botnick L, Come S, Rose C, et al. Primary breast irradiation and concomitant adjuvant chemotherapy. In: Harris J, Hellman S, Silen W, eds. *Conservative management of breast cancer.* Philadelphia: JB Lippincott, 1983:321.
405. Meek A, Order S, Abeloff M, et al. Concurrent radiochemotherapy in advanced breast cancer. *Cancer* 1983;51:1001.
406. Markiewicz DA, Fox KR, Schultz DJ, et al. Concurrent chemotherapy and radiation for breast conservation treatment of early-stage breast cancer. *Cancer J Sci Am* 1998;4:185.
407. Dubey AK, Recht A, Come SE, et al. Concurrent CMF and radiation therapy for early stage breast cancer: results of a pilot study. *Int J Radiat Oncol Biol Phys* 1999;45:877.
408. Taghian AG, Assad S, Kuter I, et al. Increased risk of radiation pneumonitis in breast cancer patients treated by concomitant taxol and radiation therapy. *Int J Radiat Oncol Biol Phys* 1999;45:316(abst).

409. Bellon JR, Lindsley KL, Ellis GK, et al. Feasibility of concurrent radiation therapy and paclitaxel or docetaxel chemotherapy in the management of locally advanced breast cancer. *Int J Radiat Oncol Biol Phys* 1999;45:309(abst).
410. Harris J, Osteen R. Patients with early breast cancer benefit from effective axillary treatment. *Breast Cancer Res Treat* 1985;5:17.
411. Adair F, Berg J, Joubert L, et al. Long term follow-up of breast cancer patients: the 30 year report. *Cancer* 1974;33:1145.
412. Brinkley D, Haybittle J. The curability of breast cancer. *Lancet* 1975;2:95.
413. Fentiman I, Cuzick J, Millis R. Which patients are cured of breast cancer? *BMJ* 1984;289:1108.
414. Rosen P, Groshen S, Saigo P, et al. A long-term follow-up study of survival in stage I (T1N0M0) and stage II (T1N1M0) breast carcinoma. *J Clin Oncol* 1989;7:355.
415. Ravdin PM. Can patient and tumor characteristics allow prediction of axillary lymph node status? *Semin Breast Dis* 1998;1:141.
416. Brenin D, Morrow M, Moughan J, et al. Management of axillary lymph nodes in breast cancer: a national pattern of care study of 17,151 patients. *Ann Surg* 1999;230:686.
417. Morton DL, Duan-Ren W, Wong JH, et al. Technical details of intraoperative lymphatic mapping and sentinel node biopsy in the management of primary melanoma. *Arch Surg* 1992;127:392.
418. Rosen P, Martin M, Kinne D, et al. Discontinuous or "skip" metastases in breast carcinoma: analysis of 1228 axillary dissections. *Ann Surg* 1983;197:276.
419. Veronesi U, Rilke F, Luini A, et al. Distribution of axillary node metastases by level of invasion. *Cancer* 1987;59:682.
420. Boova R, Bonanni R, Rosato F. Patterns of axillary nodal involvement in breast cancer. *Ann Surg* 1982;196:642.
421. Danforth D, Findlay P, McDonald H, et al. Complete axillary lymph node dissection for stage I-II carcinoma of the breast. *J Clin Oncol* 1986;4:655.
422. Pigott J, Nichols R, Maddox W, et al. Metastases to the upper levels of the axillary nodes in carcinoma of the breast and its implications for nodal sampling procedures. *Surg Gynecol Obstet* 1984;158:255.
423. Halverson K, Taylor M, Perez C, et al. Regional nodal management and patterns of failure following conservative surgery and radiation therapy for stage I and II breast cancer. *Int J Radiat Oncol Biol Phys* 1993;26:593.
424. Recht A, Pierce S, Abner A, et al. Regional node failure conservative surgery and radiotherapy for early stage breast carcinoma. *J Clin Oncol* 1991;9:988.
425. Siegel B, Mayzel K, Love S. Level I and II axillary dissection in the treatment of early-stage breast cancer. *Arch Surg* 1990;125:1144.
426. Fowble B, Solin L, Schultz D, et al. Frequency sites of relapse, and outcome of regional node failures following surgery and radiation for early breast cancer. *Int J Radiat Oncol Biol Phys* 1989;17:703.
427. Kjaergaard J, Blichert-Toft M, Andersen J, et al. Probability of false negative nodal status in conjunction with partial axillary dissection in breast cancer. *Br J Surg* 1985;72:365.
428. Graversen H, Blichert-Toft M, Andersen J, et al. Breast cancer: risk of axillary recurrence in node-negative patients following partial dissection of the axilla. *Eur J Surg Oncol* 1988;14:407.
429. Axelsson C, Mouridsen H, Zedeler K, et al. Axillary dissection of level I and II lymph nodes is important in breast cancer classification. *Eur J Cancer* 1992;28A:1415.
430. Cady B, Stone M, Wayne J. New therapeutic possibilities in primary invasive breast cancer. *Ann Surg* 1993;183:338.
431. Baker L. Breast Cancer Detection Demonstration Project: five-year summary report. *Cancer* 1982;32:194.
432. Carter C, Allen C, Henson D. Relation of tumor size, lymph node status and survival in 24,740 breast cancer cases. *Cancer* 1989;63:181.
433. Chadha M, Chabon A, Friedmann P, et al. Predictors of axillary lymph node metastases in patients with T1 breast cancer. *Cancer* 1994;73:359.
434. Dewar J, Sarrazin D, Benhamou E, et al. Management of the axilla in patients treated at Institut Gustave-Roussy. *Int J Radiat Oncol Biol Phys* 1987;13:475.
435. Wilson R, Donegan W, Mettlin C, et al. The 1982 national survey of carcinoma of the breast in the United States by the American College of Surgeons. *Surg Gynecol Obstet* 1984;159:309.
436. McDivitt R, Boyce W, Gersell D. Tubular carcinoma of the breast: clinical and pathological observations concerning 135 cases. *Am J Surg Pathol* 1982;6:401.
437. Peters G, Wolff M, Haagensen C. Tubular carcinoma of the breast: clinical-pathologic correlations based on 100 cases. *Ann Surg* 1981;193:138.
438. Giuliano AE, Kirgan DM, Guenther JM, Morton DL. Lymphatic mapping and sentinel lymphadenectomy for breast cancer. *Ann Surg* 1994;220:391.
439. Giuliano AE, Jones RC, Brennan M, Statman R. Sentinel lymphadenectomy in breast cancer. *J Clin Oncol* 1997;15:2345.
440. Veronesi U, Paganelli G, Vitale G, et al. Sentinel lymph node biopsy and axillary dissection for breast cancer: results in a large series. *J Natl Cancer Inst* 1999;91:368.
441. Shons A, Joseph E, Cox CE, et al. Predictors of sentinel lymph node metastases in the lymphatic mapping of breast cancer patients. *Breast Cancer Res Treat* 1997;46:24(abst).
442. Guenther JM, Krishnamoorthy M, Tan LR. Sentinel lymphadenectomy for breast cancer in a community managed care setting. *Cancer J Sci Am* 1997;3:336.
443. Borgstein PJ, Pijpers R, Comans EF, et al. Sentinel lymph node biopsy in breast cancer: guidelines and pitfalls of lymphoscintigraphy and gamma probe detection. *J Am Coll Surg* 1998;186:275.
444. Krag D, Weaver D, Ashikaga T, et al. The sentinel node in breast cancer. A multicenter validation study. *N Engl J Med* 1998;337:941.
445. Morrow M, Rademaker AW, Bethke KP, et al. Learning sentinel node biopsy: results of a prospective randomized trial of two techniques. *Surgery* 1999;126:714.
446. Cox CE, Pendas S, Cox JM, et al. Guidelines for lymphatic mapping of patients with breast cancer. *Ann Surg* 1998;227:645.
447. Pickren JW. Significance of occult metastases. A study of breast cancer. *Cancer* 1961;14:1266.
448. Fisher ER, Swamidoss S, Lee CM, et al. Detection and significance of occult axillary node metastases in patients with invasive breast cancer. *Cancer* 1978;42:2025.
449. Rosen PP, Saigo PE, Braun DW Jr, Beattie EJ Jr, Kinne DW. Occult axillary lymph node metastases from breast cancers with intramammary lymphatic tumor emboli. *Am J Surg Pathol* 1982;6:639.
450. Wilkinson EJ, Hause LL, Hoffman RG, et al. Occult axillary lymph node metastases in invasive carcinoma: characteristics of the primary tumor and significance of the metastases. *Pathol Annu* 1982;17:67.
451. International (Ludwig) Breast Cancer Study Group. Prognostic importance of occult axillary lymph node micrometastases from breast cancers. *Lancet* 1990;335:1565.
452. McGuckin MA, Cummings MC, Walsh MD, et al. Occult axillary node metastases in breast cancer: their detection and prognostic significance. *Br J Cancer* 1996;73:88.
453. Clare SE, Sener SF, Wilkens W, et al. Prognostic significance of occult lymph node metastases in node-negative breast cancer. *Ann Surg Oncol* 1997;4:447.
454. Gilliland MD, Barton RM, Copeland EM. The implications of local recurrence of breast cancer as the first site of therapeutic failure. *Ann Surg* 1983;197:284.
455. Zimmerman K, Montague E, Fletcher G. Frequency, anatomical distribution and management of local recurrences after definitive therapy for breast cancer. *Cancer* 1966;19:67.
456. Mackarem G, Roche CA, Silverman ML, Hughes KS. The development of new, primary non-invasive carcinoma of the breast 29 years after bilateral radical mastectomy. *Breast J* 1998;4:51.
457. Marshall K, Redfern A, Cady B. Local recurrences of carcinoma of the breast. *Surg Gynecol Obstet* 1974;139:406.
458. Bedwinek JM, Fineberg B, Lee J, Ocwieza M. Analysis of failures following local treatment of isolated local-regional recurrence of breast cancer. *Int J Radiat Oncol Biol Phys* 1981;7:581.
459. Aberizk WJ, Silver B, Henderson IC, Cady B, Harris JR. The use of radiotherapy for treatment of isolated locoregional recurrence of breast carcinoma after mastectomy. *Cancer* 1986;58:1214.
460. Ballo MT, Strom EA, Singletary SE, et al. Predicting outcome in patients with locoregionally recurrent breast carcinoma after mastectomy. *Int J Radiat Oncol Biol Phys* 1999;45:310(abst).
461. Hsi RA, Antell A, Schultz DJ, Solin LJ. Radiation therapy for chest wall recurrence of breast cancer after mastectomy in a favorable subgroup of patients. *Int J Radiat Oncol Biol Phys* 1998;42:495.
462. Kamby C, Sengelov L. Pattern of dissemination and survival following isolated locoregional recurrence of breast cancer. A prospective study with more than 10 years of follow up. *Breast Cancer Res Treat* 1997;45:181.
463. Willner J, Kiricuta IC, Kolbl O. Locoregional recurrence of breast cancer following mastectomy: always a fatal event? Results of univariate and multivariate analysis. *Int J Radiat Oncol Biol Phys* 1997;37:853.
464. Halverson KJ, Perez CA, Kuske RR, et al. Locoregional recurrence of breast cancer: a retrospective comparison of irradiation alone versus irradiation and systemic therapy. *Am J Clin Oncol* 1992;15:93.
465. Schwaibold F, Fowble BL, Solin LJ, Schultz DJ, Goodman RL. The results of radiation therapy for isolated local regional recurrence after mastectomy. *Int J Radiat Oncol Biol Phys* 1991;21:299.
466. Newman LA, Kuerer HM, Hunt KK, et al. Presentation, treatment, and outcome of local recurrence after skin-sparing mastectomy and immediate breast reconstruction. *Ann Surg Oncol* 1998;5:620.
467. Cheng JC, Cheng SH, Lin K-J, et al. Diagnostic thoracic-computed tomography in radiotherapy for loco-regional recurrent breast carcinoma. *Int J Radiat Oncol Biol Phys* 1998;41:607.
468. Kramer S, Schulz-Wendtland R, Hagedorn K, Bautz W, Lang N. Magnetic resonance imaging in the diagnosis of local recurrences in breast cancer. *Anticancer Res* 1998;18(3C):2159.
469. Hathaway PB, Mankoff DA, Maravilla KR, et al. Value of combined FDG PET and MR imaging in the evaluation of suspected recurrent local-regional breast cancer: preliminary experience. *Radiology* 1999;210:807.
470. Salvadori B, Rovini D, Squicciarini P, et al. Surgery for local recurrences following deficient radical mastectomy for breast cancer: a selected series of 39 cases. *Eur J Surg Oncol* 1992;18:438.
471. McCormack PM, Bains MS, Burt ME, et al. Local recurrent mammary carcinoma failing multimodality therapy: a solution. *Arch Surg* 1989;124:158.
472. Kroll SS, Schusterman MA, Larson DL, Fender A. Long-term survival after chest-wall reconstruction with musculocutaneous flaps. *Plast Reconstr Surg* 1990;86:697.
473. International Collaborative Hyperthermia Group. Radiotherapy with or without hyperthermia in the treatment of superficial localized breast cancer: results from five randomized controlled trials. *Int J Radiat Oncol Biol Phys* 1996;35:731.
474. Lee HK, Antell AG, Perez CA, et al. Superficial hyperthermia and irradiation for recurrent breast carcinoma of the chest wall: prognostic factors in 196 tumors. *Int J Radiat Oncol Biol Phys* 1998;40:365.
475. Ballo MT, Strom EA, Singletary SE, et al. Local-regional control of recurrent breast carcinoma after mastectomy: does hyperfractionated accelerated radiotherapy improve local control? *Int J Radiat Oncol Biol Phys* 1999;44:105.
476. Mang TS, Allison R, Hewson G, Snider W, Moskowitz R. A phase II/III clinical study of tin ethyl etiopurpurin (Purlytin)-induced photodynamic therapy for the treatment of recurrent cutaneous metastatic breast cancer. *Cancer J Sci Am* 1998;4:378.
477. Mora EM, Buzdar AU, Johnston DA. Aggressive therapy for locoregional recurrence after mastectomy in stage II and III breast cancer patients. *Ann Surg Oncol* 1996;3:162.
478. Juan O, Lluch A, de Paz L, et al. Prognostic factors in patients with isolated recurrences of breast cancer (stage IV-NED). *Breast Cancer Res Treat* 1999;53:105.
479. Borner M, Bacchi M, Goldhirsch A, et al. First isolated locoregional recurrence following mastectomy for breast cancer: results of a phase III multicenter trial comparing systemic treatment with observation after excision and radiation. *J Clin Oncol* 1994;12:2071.

480. Borner MM, Bacchi M, Castiglione M. Possible deleterious effect of tamoxifen in premenopausal women with locoregional recurrence of breast cancer. *Eur J Cancer* 1996;32A:2173.
481. Sadowsky NL, Semine A, Harris JR. Breast imaging: a critical aspect of breast conserving treatment. *Cancer* 1990;65:2113.
482. Dershaw DD. Mammography in patients with breast cancer treated by breast conservation (lumpectomy with or without radiation). *AJR Am J Roentgenol* 1995;164:309.
483. Dao TH, Rahmouni A, Campana F, et al. Tumor recurrence versus fibrosis in the irradiated breast: differentiation with dynamic gadolinium-enhanced MR imaging. *Radiology* 1993;187:751.
484. Mumtaz H, Davidson T, Hall-Craggs MA, et al. Comparison of magnetic resonance imaging and conventional triple assessment in locally recurrent breast cancer. *Br J Surg* 1997;84:1147.
485. Abner AL, Recht A, Eberlein T, et al. Prognosis following salvage mastectomy for recurrence in the breast after conservative surgery and radiation therapy for early-stage breast cancer. *J Clin Oncol* 1993;11:44.
486. Doyle TH, Schultz DJ, Peters CA, Solin LJ. Long term results of local recurrence after breast conservation therapy for invasive breast cancer. *Int J Radiat Oncol Biol Phys* 1999;45:309(abst).
487. Kemperman H, Borger J, Hart A, et al. Prognostic factors for survival after breast conserving therapy for stage I and II breast cancer. The role of local recurrence. *Eur J Cancer* 1995;31A:690.
488. Dalberg K, Mattsson A, Sandelin K, Rutqvist LE. Outcome of treatment for ipsilateral breast tumor recurrence in early-stage breast cancer. *Breast Cancer Res Treat* 1998;49:69.
489. Chaudary MA, Nagadowska M, Smith P, Gregory W, Fentiman IS. Local recurrence after breast conservation treatment: outcome following salvage mastectomy. *Breast* 1998;7:33.
490. van Tienhoven G, Voogd AC, Peterse JL, et al. Prognosis after treatment for locoregional recurrence after mastectomy or breast conserving therapy in two randomised trials (EORTC 10801 and DBCG-82TM). *Eur J Cancer* 1999;35:32.
491. Spitalier J-M, Ayme Y, Brandone H, Amalric R, Kurtz JM. Treatment of mammary recurrences after breast conservation. *Breast Dis* 1991;4:20(abst).
492. Resch A, Mock U, Fellner C, et al. Breast conserving surgery and PDR-brachytherapy for recurrent breast cancer after primary breast conserving treatment including EBT and HDR-brachytherapy—preliminary results. *Eur J Cancer* 1997;33:S159(abst).
493. Mullen EE, Deutsch M, Bloomer WD. Salvage radiotherapy for local failures of lumpectomy and breast irradiation. *Radiother Oncol* 1997;42:25.
494. Deutsch M. Repeat high dose partial breast irradiation after lumpectomy for in-breast tumor recurrences following initial lumpectomy and radiotherapy. *Int J Radiat Oncol Biol Phys* 1998;42:255(abst).
495. Barreau-Pouhaer L, Le M, Rietjens M, et al. Risk factors for failure of immediate breast reconstruction with prosthesis after total mastectomy for breast cancer. *Cancer* 1992;70:1145.
496. August D, Wilkins E, Rea T. Breast reconstruction in older women. *Surgery* 1994;115:663.
497. Weissman M, Vecchione D, Albert L, et al. Connective tissue disease following breast augmentation: a preliminary test of the human adjuvant disease hypothesis. *Plast Reconstr Surg* 1988;82:626.
498. van Nunen S, Gatenby P, Basten A. Post-mammoplasty connective tissue disease. *Arthritis Rheum* 1982;25:694.
499. Kumagai Y, Shiokawa Y, Medsger T, et al. Clinical spectrum of connective tissue disease after cosmetic surgery. *Arthritis Rheum* 1984;27:1.
500. Perkins LL, Clark BD, Klein PJ, Cook RR. A metaanalysis of breast implants and connective tissue disease. *Ann Plast Surg* 1995;35:561.
501. Silverman BS, Brown SL, Bright RA, Kaczmarek TS. A critical assessment of the relationship between silicone breast implants and connective tissue diseases. *Regul Toxicol Pharmacol* 1996;23:74.
502. Schneider W, Hill L, Brown R. Latissimus dorsi myocutaneous flap for breast reconstruction. *Br J Plast Surg* 1981;30:286.
503. Bunkis J, Walton R, Mathes S. Experience with the transverse lower rectus abdominis operation for breast reconstruction. *Plast Reconstr Surg* 1983;72:819.
504. Shaw W. Microvascular free flap breast reconstruction. *Clin Plast Surg* 1984;11:333.
505. Becker H. The use of intradermal tattoo to enhance the final result of nipple areola reconstruction. *Plast Reconstr Surg* 1986;77:673.
506. Nance F, DeLoach D, Welsh R, et al. Paget's disease of the breast. *Ann Surg* 1970;171:684.
507. Ashikari R, Park K, Huvos A. Paget's disease of the breast. *Cancer* 1970;26:680.
508. Paone J, Baker R. Pathogenesis and treatment of Paget's disease of the breast. *Cancer* 1981;48:825.
509. Maier W, Rosemond G, Harasym E. Paget's disease in the female breast. *Surg Gynecol Obstet* 1969;128:1253.
510. Lagios M, Westdahl P, Rose M, Concanon S. Paget's disease of the nipple: alternative management in cases without and with minimal extent of underlying breast carcinoma. *Cancer* 1984;54:545.
511. Dixon R, Galea MH, Ellis IO, Elston CW, Blamey RW. Paget's disease of the nipple. *Br J Surg* 1991;78:722.
512. Fourquet A, Campana F, Viehl P. Paget's disease of the nipple without detectable breast tumor: conservative management with radiation therapy. *Int J Radiat Oncol Biol Phys* 1987;13:1463.
513. Bulens P, Vanuytsel L, Rinders A, et al. Breast conserving treatment of Paget's disease. *Radiother Oncol* 1990;17:305.
514. Osteen R. Paget's disease of the nipple. In: Harris J, Hellman S, Henderson I, Kinne D, eds. *Breast diseases.* Philadelphia: JB Lippincott, 1991:797.
515. Sasco AJ, Lowenfels AB, Pasker-DeJong P. Epidemiology of male breast cancer: a meta-analysis of published case-control studies and discussion of selected aetiological factors. *Int J Cancer* 1993;53:538.
516. Gradishar WJ. Male breast cancer. In: Harris J, Lippman M, Morrow M, Osborne CK, eds. *Diseases of the breast.* Philadelphia: Lippincott Williams & Wilkins, 2000.
517. Friedman LS, Gayther SA, Kurosaki T, et al. Mutation analysis of BRCA1 and BRCA2 in a male breast cancer population. *Am J Hum Genet* 1997;60:313.
518. Couch FJ, Farid LM, DeShano ML, et al. BRCA2 germline mutations in male breast cancer cases and breast cancer families. *Nat Genet* 1996;13:123.
519. Jackson A, Muldal S, Ockey C, et al. Carcinoma of the male breast in association with Klinefelter syndrome. *BMJ* 1965;1:223.
520. El Gazarerli M, Abdul-Aziz A. On biliharziasis and male breast cancer in Egypt: a preliminary report and review of the literature. *Br J Cancer* 1963;17:566.
521. Eldar S, Nash E, Abrahamson J. Radiation carcinogenesis in the male breast. *Eur J Surg Oncol* 1989;15:274.
522. Axelsson J, Andersson A. Male breast cancer. *World J Surg* 1983;7:281.
523. Heller K, Rosen P, Schottenfeld D. Male breast cancer: a clinicopathologic study of 97 cases. *Ann Surg* 1978;188:60.
524. Borgen P, Wong G, Vlamis V, et al. Current management of male breast cancer: a review of 104 cases. *Ann Surg* 1992;215:451.
525. Thomas DB. Breast cancer in men. *Epidemiol Rev* 1993;15:220.
526. Treves N. Inflammatory carcinoma of the breast in the male patient. *Surgery* 1953;34:810.
527. Friedman M, Hoffman P, Dandolos E. Estrogen receptors in male breast cancer: clinical and pathologic correlations. *Cancer* 1981;47:134.
528. Vetto J, Jun SY, Padduch D, Eppich H, Shih R. Stages at presentation, prognostic factors, and outcome of breast cancer in males. *Am J Surg* 1999;177:379.
529. Willsher PC, Leach IH, Ellis IO, et al. A comparison outcome of male breast cancer with female breast cancer. *Am J Surg* 1997;173:185.
530. Hulthorn R, Friberg S, Hulthorn K. Male breast carcinoma. II. A study of the total material reported to the Swedish Cancer Registry 1958–1967 with respect to treatment, prognostic factors, and survival. *Acta Oncol* 1987;26:327.
531. Guincc V, Olsson H, Moller T, et al. The prognosis of breast cancer in males: a report of 335 cases. *Cancer* 1993;71:154.
532. Goss PE, Reid C, Pintilie M, Lim R, Miller N. Male breast carcinoma: a review of 229 patients who presented to the Princess Margaret Hospital during 40 years: 1955–1996. *Cancer* 1999;85:629.
533. Ribeiro G, Swindell R. Adjuvant tamoxifen for male breast cancer. *Br J Cancer* 1992;65:252.
534. Bagley C, Wesley M, Young R, et al. Adjuvant chemotherapy in males with cancer of the breast. *Am J Clin Oncol* 1987;10:55.
535. Patel H, Buzdar A, Hortobagyi G. Role of adjuvant chemotherapy in male breast cancer. *Cancer* 1989;64:1583.
536. Schuchardt U, Seegenschmiedt MH, Mirschner MJ, Renner H, Sauer R. Adjuvant radiotherapy for breast carcinoma in men: a 20-year clinical experience. *Am J Clin Oncol* 1996;19:330.
537. Jaiyesimi I, Buzdar A, Sahin A, et al. Carcinoma of the male breast. *Ann Intern Med* 1992;117:771.
538. Volm M, Gradishar W. How to diagnose and manage male breast cancer. *Contemp Oncol* 1994;4:17.
539. Anelli M, Anelli A, Tran K, et al. Tamoxifen administration is associated with a high rate of treatment-limiting symptoms in male breast cancer patients. *Cancer* 1994;74:74.
540. Bezwoda W, Hesdorffer C, Dansey R. Breast cancer in men: clinical features, hormone receptor status, and response to therapy. *Cancer* 1987;60:1337.
541. Kraybill W, Kaufman R, Kinne D. Treatment of advanced male breast cancer. *Cancer* 1981;47:2185.
542. Lopez M, DiLauro L, Lazzaro B, et al. Hormonal treatment of disseminated male breast cancer. *Oncology* 1985;42:345.
543. Applewhite R, Smith L, Divicenu F. Carcinoma of the breast with pregnancy and lactation. *Ann Surg* 1973;39:101.
544. Treves N, Holleb A. A report of 549 cases of breast cancer in women 35 years of age or younger. *Surg Gynecol Obstet* 1958;107:271.
545. Torres J, Mickal A. Carcinoma of the breast in pregnancy. *Clin Obstet Gynecol* 1975;18:219.
546. Sorosky JI, Scott-Conner CE. Breast disease complicating pregnancy. *Obstet Gynecol Clin North Am* 1998;25:353.
547. Petrek J, Dukoff R, Rogatko A. Prognosis of pregnancy associated breast cancer. *Cancer* 1991;67:869.
548. King R, Welch J, Martin J, et al. Carcinoma of the breast associated with pregnancy. *Surg Gynecol Obstet* 1985;160:228.
549. Deemarksy L, Neishadt E. Breast cancer and pregnancy. *Breast* 1989;7:17.
550. Anderson B, Petrek J, Byrd D, et al. Pregnancy influences breast cancer stage at diagnosis in women 30 years of age and younger. *Ann Surg Oncol* 1996;3:204.
551. Guinee V, Olsson H, Moller T, et al. Effect of pregnancy on prognosis for young women with breast cancer. *Lancet* 1994;343:1587.
552. Berry DL, Theriault RL, Holmes FA, et al. Management of breast cancer during pregnancy using a standardized protocol. *J Clin Oncol* 1999;17:855.
553. Burstein HJ, Winer EP. Reproductive issues. In: Harris JR, Lippman ME, Morrow ME, Osborne CK, eds. *Diseases of the breast.* Philadelphia: Lippincott Williams & Wilkins, 2000:1051.
554. Bines J, Oleske DM, Cobleigh MA. Ovarian function in premenopausal women treated with adjuvant chemotherapy for breast cancer. *J Clin Oncol* 1996;14:1718.
555. Lawrence WT, McDonald HD. Pregnancy after breast reconstruction with a transverse rectus abdominis musculocutaneous flap. *Ann Plast Surg* 1986;16:354.
556. Partridge AH, Garber JE. Long-term outcomes of children exposed to antineoplastic agents in utero. *(in press).*
557. Doll DC, Ringenberg S, Yarbro JW. Antineoplastic agents and pregnancy. *Semin Oncol* 1989;16:337.
558. Weibe VJ, Sipila PEH. Pharmacology of antineoplastic agents in pregnancy. *Crit Rev Oncol Hematol* 1994;16:75.

559. Caligiuri MA, Mayer RJ. Pregnancy and leukemia. *Semin Oncol* 1989;16:388.
560. Zemlickis D, Lishner M, Degendorfer P, et al. Fetal outcome after in utero exposure to cancer chemotherapy. *Arch Intern Med* 1992;152:573.
561. Schaison G, Jacquillat C, Auclerc G, et al. Les fisques foeto-embryonnaines des chimiotherapies. *Bull Cancer* 1979;66:165.
562. Turchi JJ, Villasis C. Anthracyclines in the treatment of malignancy in pregnancy. *Cancer* 1988;61:435.
563. Garber JE. Long-term follow-up of children exposed in utero to antineoplastic agents. *Semin Oncol* 1989;16:437.
564. Giacalone PL, Laffargue F, Benos A. Chemotherapy for breast carcinoma during pregnancy: a French national survey. *Cancer* 1999;86:2266.
565. Baron P, Moore M, Kinne D. Occult primary cancer presenting with axillary metastases. *Arch Surg* 1990;125:210.
566. Vezzoni P, Balestrazi A, Bignami P. Axillary lymph node metastases from occult carcinoma of the breast. *Tumori* 1979;65:87.
567. Ellerbroek N, Holmes F, Singletary E. Treatment of patients with isolated axillary nodal metastases from an occult primary carcinoma consistent with breast origin. *Cancer* 1990;66:1461.
568. Henry-Tillman RS, Harms SE, Westbrook KC, Korourian S, Klimberg VS. Role of breast magnetic resonance imaging in determining breast as a source of unknown metastatic lymphadenopathy. *Am J Surg* 1999;178:496.
569. Morris EA, Schwartz LH, Dershaw DD, et al. MR imaging of the breast in patients with occult primary breast carcinoma. *Radiology* 1997;205:437.
570. Orel SG, Weinstein SP, Schnall MD, et al. Breast MR imaging in patients with axillary node metastases and unknown primary malignancy. *Radiology* 1999;212:543.
571. Schorn C, Fischer U, Luftner-Nagel S, Westerhof JP, Grabbe E. MRI of the breast in patients with metastatic disease of unknown primary. *Eur Radiol* 1999;9:470.
572. Scoggins CR, Vitola JV, Sandler MP, Atkinson JB, Frexes-Steed M. Occult breast cancer presenting as an axillary mass. *Am Surg* 1999;65:1.
573. Ashikari R, Rosen PP, Urban JA, Senoo T. Breast cancer presenting as an axillary mass. *Ann Surg* 1976;183:415.
574. Haagensen C. In: *Diseases of the breast*, 2nd ed. Philadelphia: WB Saunders, 1971:486.
575. Owen H, Dockerty M, Gray H. Occult carcinoma of the breast. *Surg Gynecol Obstet* 1954;98:302.
576. Patel J, Nemoto T, Rozner D, et al. Axillary lymph node metastasis from an occult breast cancer. *Cancer* 1981;47:2923.
577. Westbrook K, Gallagher H. Breast carcinoma presenting as an axillary mass. *Am J Surg* 1963;106:460.
578. Fitts WT, Steiner GC, Enterline HT. Prognosis of occult carcinoma of the breast. *Am J Surg* 1963;106:460.
579. Rosen P, Kimmel M. Occult breast carcinoma presenting with axillary lymph node metastases: a followup study of 48 patients. *Hum Pathol* 1990;21:518.
580. Kemeny M, Rivera D, Terz J, et al. Occult primary adenocarcinoma with axillary metastases. *Am J Surg* 1986;152:43.
581. Campana F, Forquet A, Ashby M. Presentation of axillary lymphadenopathy without detectable breast primary (T0N1B): experience at Institut Curie. *Radiol Oncol* 1989;15:321.
582. Forquet A, de la Rochefordiere A, Campana C. Occult primary cancer with axillary metastases. In: Harris J, Lippman M, Morrow M, Hellman S, eds. *Diseases of the breast*, 2nd ed. Philadelphia: Lippincott–Raven, 2000:703.
583. Whillis D, Brown PW, Rodger A. Adenocarcinoma from an unknown primary presenting in women with an axillary mass. *Clin Oncol* 1990;2:189.
584. Rowell M, Perry R, Hsiu J, et al. Phyllodes tumor. *Am J Surg* 1993;165:376.
585. Treves N. A study of cystosarcoma phyllodes. *Ann NY Acad Sci* 1964;114:922.
586. Salvadori B, Cusumano F, Del Bo R, et al. Surgical treatment of phyllodes tumors of the breast. *Cancer* 1989;63:2532.
587. Oberman H. Cystosarcoma phyllodes: a clinicopathologic study of hypercellular periductal stromal neoplasms of the breast. *Cancer* 1965;18:697.
588. Petrek J. Phyllodes tumors. In: Harris J, Lippman M, Morrow M, Hellman S, eds. *Diseases of the breast*, 1st ed. Philadelphia: Lippincott–Raven, 1996:863.
589. West L, Weiland L, Clagett O. Cystosarcoma phyllodes. *Ann Surg* 1971;173:520.
590. Reinfuss M, Mitus J, Smolak K, et al. Malignant phyllodes tumors of the breast: a clinical and pathological analysis of 55 cases. *Eur J Cancer* 1993;29A:1252.
591. Palmer M, De Risi D, Pelikan A, et al. Treatment options and recurrence potential for cystosarcoma phyllodes. *Surg Gynecol Obstet* 1990;170:193.
592. McGuire WL. Breast cancer prognostic factors: evaluation guidelines. *J Natl Cancer Inst* 1991;83:154.
593. Gasparini G, Pozza F, Harris AL. Evaluating the potential usefulness of new prognostic and predictive indicators in node-negative breast cancer patients. *J Natl Cancer Inst* 1993;85:1206.
594. Hayes DF, Trock B, Harris AL. Assessing the clinical impact of prognostic factors: when is "statistically significant" clinically useful? *Breast Cancer Res Treat* 1998;52:305.
595. Saez RA, McGuire WL, Clark GM. Prognostic factors in breast cancer. *Semin Surg Oncol* 1989;5:102.
596. Rosen PP, Groshen S, Saigo PE, et al. A long-term follow-up study of survival in stage I ($T_1N_0M_0$) and stage II ($T_1N_1M_0$) breast carcinoma. *J Clin Oncol* 1989;7:355.
597. McGuire WL, Clark GM. Prognostic factors and treatment decisions in axillary-node-negative breast cancer. *N Engl J Med* 1992;326:1756.
598. Tabar L, Chen H-H, Duffy SW, et al. A novel method for prediction of long-term outcome of women with T1a, T1b, and 10-14 mm invasive breast cancers: a prospective study. *Lancet* 2000;355:429.
599. Harvey JM, de Klerk NH, Sterrett GF. Histological grading in breast cancer: interobserver agreement, and relation to other prognostic factors including ploidy. *Pathology* 1992;24:63.
600. Dalton LW, Page DL, Dupont WD. Histologic grading of breast carcinoma. A reproducibility study. *Cancer* 1994;73:2765.
601. Fisher ER, Redmond C, Fisher B. Histologic grading of breast cancer. *Pathol Ann* 1980;15:239.
602. le Doussal V, Tubiana-Hulin M, Friedman S, et al. Prognostic value of histologic grade nuclear components of Scarff-Bloom-Richardson (SBR): an improved score modification based on a multivariate analysis of 1262 invasive ductal breast carcinomas. *Cancer* 1989;64:1914.
603. Albain KS, Allred DC, Clark GM. Breast cancer outcome and predictors of outcome: are there age differentials? *J Natl Cancer Inst* Mongr 1994;16:35.
604. Goldhirsch A, Glick JH, Gelber RD, Senn H-J. Meeting highlights: international consensus panel on the treatment of breast cancer. *J Natl Cancer Inst* 1998;90:1601.
605. Adami H-O, Graffman S, Lindgren A, et al. Prognostic implication of estrogen receptor content in breast cancer. *Breast Cancer Res Treat* 1985;5:293.
606. Mason BH, Holdaway IM, Mullins PR, et al. Progesterone and estrogen receptors as prognostic variables in breast cancer. *Cancer Res* 1983;43:2985.
607. Funke I, Schraut W. Meta-analysis of studies on bone marrow micrometastases: an independent prognostic impact remains to be substantiated. *J Clin Oncol* 1998;16:557.
608. Braun S, Pantel K, Muller P, et al. Cytokeratin-positive cells in the bone marrow and survival of patients with stage I, II or II breast cancer. *N Engl J Med* 2000;342:525.
609. Wenger CR, Clark GM. S-phase fraction and breast cancer: a decade of experience. *Breast Cancer Res* 1997;51:255.
610. Ravdin PM, Chamness GC. The c-erbB-2 proto-oncogene as a prognostic and predictive marker in breast cancer: a paradigm for the development of other macromolecular markers—a review. *Gene* 1995;159:19.
611. Thor AD, Berry DA, Budman D, Muss HB, Kute T. erbB-2, p 53, and efficacy of adjuvant therapy in lymph node-positive breast cancer. *J Natl Cancer Inst* 1998;90:1346.
612. Paik S, Bryant J, Park C, et al. erbB-2 and response to doxorubicin in patients with axillary lymph node-positive, hormone receptor-negative breast cancer. *J Natl Cancer Inst* 1998;90:1361.
613. Ravdin PM, Green S, Albain KS, et al. Initial report of the SWOG biological correlative study of c-erbB-2 expression as a predictor of outcome in a trial comparing adjuvant CAF T with tamoxifen (T) alone. *Proc Am Soc Clin Oncol* 1998;17:97a(abst).
614. Clark GM. Should selection of adjuvant chemotherapy for patients with breast cancer be based on erbB-2 status? [editorial]. *J Natl Cancer Inst* 1998;90:1320.
615. De Placido S, Carlomagno C, De Laurentiis M, et al. c-cerbB2 expression predicts tamoxifen efficacy in breast cancer patients. *Breast Cancer Res Treat* 1998;52:55.
616. Sjögren S, Inganäs M, Lindgren A, et al. Prognostic and predictive value of c-erbB-2 overexpression in primary breast cancer, alone and in combination with other prognostic markers. *J Clin Oncol* 1998;16:462.
617. Fisher B, Redmond C, Poisson R, et al. Eight-year results of a randomized clinical trial comparing total mastectomy and lumpectomy with or without irradiation in the treatment of breast cancer. *N Engl J Med* 1989;320:822.
618. Early Breast Cancer Trialists' Collaborative Group. Systemic treatment of early breast cancer by hormonal, systemic or immune therapy: 133 randomized trials involving 31,000 recurrences and 24,000 deaths among 75,000 women. *Lancet* 1992;339:1.
619. Early Breast Cancer Trialists' Collaborative Group. Polychemotherapy for early breast cancer: an overview of the randomised trials. *Lancet* 1998;352:930.
620. Swedish Breast Cancer Cooperative Group. Randomized trial of two versus five years of adjuvant tamoxifen for postmenopausal early stage breast cancer. *J Natl Cancer Inst* 1996;88:1543.
621. Current Trials Working Party of the Cancer Research Campaign Breast Cancer Trials Group. Evaluating tamoxifen duration in women aged fifty years or older with breast cancer. *J Natl Cancer Inst* 1996;88:1834.
622. Stewart HJ, Forrest AP, Everington D, et al. Randomized comparison of 5 years of adjuvant tamoxifen with continuous therapy for operable breast cancer. The Scottish Cancer Trials Breast Group. *Br J Cancer* 1996;74:297.
623. Tormey DC, Gray R, Falkson HC (for the Eastern Cooperative Oncology Group). Postchemotherapy adjuvant tamoxifen therapy beyond five years in patients with lymph node-positive breast cancer. *J Natl Cancer Inst* 1996;88:1828.
624. Osborne CK. Tamoxifen in the treatment of breast cancer. *N Engl J Med* 1999;339:1609.
625. Hayes DF, Van Zyl JA, Hacking A, et al. Randomized comparison of tamoxifen and two separate doses of toremifene in postmenopausal patients with metastatic breast cancer. *J Clin Oncol* 1995;13:2556.
626. Carlomagno C, Perrone F, Gallo C, et al. c-erbB2 overexpression decreases the benefit of adjuvant tamoxifen in early-stage breast cancer without axillary lymph node metastases. *J Clin Oncol* 1996;14:2702.
627. Muss H, et al. Lack of interaction of tamoxifen (T) use and ErbB2/HER-2/neu expression in CALGB 8541: a randomized adjuvant trial of three different doses of cyclophosphamide, doxorubicin and fluorouracil (CAF) in node positive primary breast cancer. *Proc Am Soc Clin Oncol* 1999;18:68a(abst 256).
628. Love RR, Mazess RB, Barden HS, et al. Effects of tamoxifen on bone mineral density in postmenopausal women with breast cancer. *N Engl J Med* 1992;326:852.
629. Powles TJ, Hickish T, Kanis JA, Tidy A, Ashley S. Effect of tamoxifen on bone mineral density measured by dual-energy x-ray absorptiometry in healthy premenopausal and postmenopausal women. *J Clin Oncol* 1996;14:78.
630. Love RR, Wiebe DA, Newcomb PA, et al. Effects of tamoxifen on cardiovascular risk factors in postmenopausal women. *Am Intern Med* 1991;115:860.
631. Osborne CK, Kitten L, Arteaga CL. Antagonism of chemotherapy induced cytotoxicity for human breast cancer by antiestrogens. *J Clin Oncol* 1989;7:710.
632. Pritchard KI, Paterson AH, Paul NA, et al. Increased thromboembolic complications with concurrent tamoxifen and chemotherapy in a randomized trial of adjuvant therapy for women with breast cancer. National Cancer Institute of Canada Clinical Trials Group Breast Cancer Site Group. *J Clin Oncol* 1996;14:2731.
633. Early Breast Cancer Trialists' Collaborative Group. Effects of adjuvant tamoxifen and of cytotoxic therapy on mortality in early breast cancer: an overview of 61 randomised trials among 28,896 women. *N Engl J Med* 1988;319:1681.

634. Early Breast Cancer Trialists' Collaborative Group. Ovarian ablation in early breast cancer: overview of the randomised trials. *Lancet* 1996;348:1189.
635. Davidson N, O'Neil A, Habermann T, et al. Effect of chemohormonal therapy in premenopausal node(+), receptor(+) breast cancer: an Eastern Cooperative Group Phase III Intergroup Trial. *Proc Am Soc Clin Oncol* 1999;18(abst 249).
636. Ejlertsen B, Dombernowsky P, Mouridsen HT, et al. Comparable effect of ovarian ablation and CMF chemotherapy in premenopausal hormone receptor positive breast cancer patients. *Proc Am Soc Clin Oncol* 1999;18(abst 248).
637. Jakesz R, Hausmaninger H, Samonigg H, et al. Comparison of adjuvant therapy with tamoxifen and goserelin vs. CMF in premenopausal stage I and II hormone-responsive breast cancer patients: four-year results of Austrian Breast Cancer Study Group (ABCSG). *Proc Am Soc Clin Oncol* 1999;18(abst 250).
638. Scottish Cancer Trials Breast Group and ICFR Breast Unity, Guy's Hospital. Adjuvant ovarian ablation versus CMF chemotherapy in premenopausal women with pathological stage II breast carcinoma: the Scottish Trial. *Lancet* 1993;341:1293.
639. Hayes DF, Van Zyl JA, Hacking A, et al. Randomized comparison of tamoxifen and two separate doses of toremifene in postmenopausal patients with metastatic breast cancer. *J Clin Oncol* 1995;13:2556.
640. Fisher B, Redmond C, Dimitrov NV, et al. A randomized clinical trial evaluating sequential methotrexate and fluorouracil in the treatment of patients with node-negative breast cancer who have estrogen-receptor-negative tumors. *N Engl J Med* 1989;320:473.
641. Mansour EG, Gray R, Shatila AH, et al. Efficacy of adjuvant chemotherapy in high-risk node-negative breast cancer intergroup study. *N Engl J Med* 1989;320:485.
642. Mansour EG, Gray R, Shatila AH, et al. Survival advantage of adjuvant chemotherapy in high-risk node-negative breast cancer: ten-year analysis—an intergroup study. *J Clin Oncol* 1998;16:3486.
643. Bonadonna G, Brusamolino E, Valagussa P, et al. Combination chemotherapy as an adjuvant treatment in operable breast cancer. *N Engl J Med* 1976;294:405.
644. Fisher B, Carbone P, Economou SG, et al. L-Phenylalanine mustard (L-PAM) in the management of primary breast cancer: a report of early findings. *N Engl J Med* 1975;292:117.
645. Bonadonna G, Valagussa P, Moliterni A, Zambetti M, Brambilla C. Adjuvant cyclophosphamide, methotrexate, and fluorouracil in node-positive breast cancer: the results of 20 years of follow-up. *N Engl J Med* 1995;332:901.
646. Tancini G, Bonadonna G, Valagussa P, et al. Adjuvant CMF in breast cancer: comparative 5-year results of 12 versus 6 cycles. *J Clin Oncol* 1983;1:2.
647. Levine MD, Bramwell VH, Pritchard KI, et al. Randomized trial of intensive cyclophosphamide, epirubicin, and fluorouracil chemotherapy compared with cyclophosphamide, methotrexate, and fluorouracil in premenopausal women with node-positive breast cancer. *J Clin Oncol* 1998;16:2651.
648. Hutchins L, Green S, Ravdin P, et al. CMF versus CAF with and without tamoxifen in high-risk node-negative breast cancer patients and a natural history follow-up study in low-risk node-negative patients: first results of intergroup trial INT 0102. *Proc Am Soc Clin Oncol* 1998;17:1a(abst 2).
649. Fisher B, Redmond C, Legault-Poisson S, et al. Postoperative chemotherapy and tamoxifen compared with tamoxifen alone in the treatment of positive-node breast cancer patients aged 50 years and older with tumors responsive to tamoxifen: results from the National Surgical Adjuvant Breast and Bowel Project B-16. *J Clin Oncol* 1990;8:1005.
650. Fisher B, Dignam J, Wolmark N. Tamoxifen and chemotherapy for lymph node-negative, estrogen receptor-positive breast cancer. *J Natl Cancer Inst* 1997;89:1673.
651. Osborne CK, Ravdin PM. Adjuvant systemic therapy of primary breast cancer. In: Harris JR, Lippman ME, Morrow M, Osborne CK, eds. *Diseases of the breast,* 2nd ed. Philadelphia: Lippincott Williams & Wilkins, 2000:599.
652. Pagani O, O'Neil A, Castiglione M, et al. Prognostic impact of amenorrhoea after adjuvant chemotherapy in premenopausal women with axillary node involvement: results of the International Breast Cancer Study Group Trial VI. *Eur J Cancer* 1998;34:632.
653. Budman DR, Berry D, Cirrincione CT, et al. Dose and dose intensity as determinates of outcome in the adjuvant treatment of breast cancer. *J Natl Cancer Inst* 1998;90:1205.
654. Fisher B, Redmond C, Wickerham DL, et al. Doxorubicin-containing regimens for the treatment of stage II breast cancer: the National Surgical Adjuvant Breast and Bowel Project experience. *J Clin Oncol* 1989;7:572.
655. International Breast Cancer Study Group. Duration and reintroduction of adjuvant chemotherapy for node-positive premenopausal breast cancer patients. *J Clin Oncol* 1996;14:1885.
656. Gusterson BA, Gelber RD, Goldhirsch A, et al. Prognostic importance of c-erbB-2 expression in breast cancer. International (Ludwig) Breast Cancer Study Group. *J Clin Oncol* 1992;10:1049.
657. Bonadonna G, Valagussa P. Dose-response effect of adjuvant chemotherapy in breast cancer. *N Engl J Med* 1981;304:10
658. Wood WC, Budman DR, Korzun AH, et al. Dose and dose intensity of adjuvant chemotherapy for stage II, node-positive breast carcinoma. *N Engl J Med* 1994;330:1253.
659. Henderson IC, Berry D, Demetri G, et al. Improved disease-free and overall survival (OS) from the addition of sequential paclitaxel but not from the escalation of doxorubicin dose level in the adjuvant chemotherapy of patients with node-positive primary breast cancer. *Proc Am Soc Clin Oncol* 1998;17:101a(abst 390A).
660. Fisher B, Anderson S, Wickerham L, et al. Increased intensification and total dose of cyclophosphamide in a doxorubicin-cyclophosphamide regimen for the treatment of primary breast cancer: findings from the National Surgical Adjuvant Breast and Bowel Project B-22. *J Clin Oncol* 1997;15:1858.
661. Fisher B, Anderson S, CeCillis A, et al. Further evaluation of intensified and increased dose of cyclophosphamide for the treatment of primary breast cancer: findings from the National Surgical Adjuvant Breast and Bowel Project B-25. *J Clin Oncol* 1999;17:3374.
662. Peters WP, Ross M, Vredenburgh JJ, et al. High-dose chemotherapy and autologous bone marrow support as consolidation after standard-dose adjuvant therapy for high-risk primary breast cancer. *J Clin Oncol* 1993;11:1132.
663. Peters W, Rosner G, Vredenbergh J, et al. A prospective, randomized comparison of two doses of combination alkylating agents as consolidation after CAF in high-risk primary breast cancer involving ten or more axillary lymph nodes. *Proc Am Soc Clin Oncol* 1999;18:1a(abst 2).
664. Hortobagyi GN, Buzdar AU, Theriault RL, et al. Randomized trial of high-dose chemotherapy and blood cell autografts for high-risk primary breast carcinoma. *J Natl Cancer Inst* 2000;92:225.
665. Rodenhuis S, Richel DJ, van der Wall E, et al. Randomised trial of high-dose chemotherapy and haemopoietic progenitor-cell support in operable breast cancer with extensive axillary lymph-node involvement. *Lancet* 1998;352:515.
666. Nabholtz JM, Senn HJ, Bezwoda WR, et al. Prospective randomized trial of docetaxel versus mitomycin plus vinblastine in patients with metastatic breast cancer progressing despite previous anthracycline-containing chemotherapy. 304 Study Group. *J Clin Oncol* 1999;17:1413.
667. Bishop JF, Dewar J, Toner GC, et al. Initial paclitaxel improves outcome compared with CMFP combination chemotherapy as front-line therapy in untreated metastatic breast cancer. *J Clin Oncol* 1999;17:2355.
668. Goldhirsch A, Coates AS, Colleoni M, Castiglione-Gertsch M, Gelber RD. Adjuvant chemoendocrine therapy in postmenopausal breast cancer: cyclophosphamide, methotrexate, and fluorouracil dose and schedule may make a difference. International Breast Cancer Study Group. *J Clin Oncol* 1998;16:1358.
669. Bonadonna G, Zambetti M, Valagussa P. Sequential or alternating doxorubicin and CMF regimens in breast cancer with more than three positive nodes. *JAMA* 1995;273:542.
670. Burstein HJ, Winer EP. Primary care for survivors of breast cancer. *N Engl J Med* 2000 *(in press).*
671. Lindley C, Vasa S, Sawyer W, Winer E. Quality of life and preferences for treatment following systemic adjuvant therapy for early stage breast cancer. *J Clin Oncol* 1998;16:1380.
672. Ravdin PM, Siminoff IA, Harvey JA. Survey of breast cancer patients concerning their knowledge and expectations of adjuvant therapy. *J Clin Oncol* 1997;15:515.
673. Bonadonna G, Valagussa P, Brambilla C, et al. Primary chemotherapy in operable breast cancer: eight-year experience at the Milan Cancer Institute. *J Clin Oncol* 1998;16:93.
674. Wolff AC, Davidson NE. Primary systemic therapy in operable breast cancer. *J Clin Oncol* 2000;18:1558.
675. Hortobagyi GN. Treatment of breast cancer. *N Engl J Med* 1998;339:974.
676. Hortobagyi GN, Singletary SE, Strom EA. Treatment of locally advanced and inflammatory breast cancer. In: Harris JR, Lippman ME, Morrow M, Osborne CK, eds. *Diseases of the breast,* 2nd ed. Philadelphia: Lippincott Williams & Wilkins, 2000:645.
677. DeLena M, Zucali R, Viganotti G, Valagussa P, Bonadonna G. Combined chemotherapy-radiotherapy approach in locally advanced (T_{3b}-T_4) breast cancer. *Cancer Chemother Pharmacol* 1978;1:53.
678. Valagussa P, Zambetti M, Bignami PD, et al. T3b-T4 breast cancer: factors affecting results in combined modality treatment. *Clin Exp Metastasis* 1983;1:191.
679. Swain SM, Sorace RA, Bagley CS, et al. Neoadjuvant chemotherapy in the combined modality approach of locally advanced nonmetastatic breast cancer. *Cancer Res* 1987;47:3889.
680. Herrada J, Iyer RB, Atkinson EN, et al. Relative value of physical examination, mammography, and breast sonography in evaluating the size of the primary tumor and regional lymph node metastases in women receiving neoadjuvant chemotherapy for locally advanced breast carcinoma. *Clin Cancer Res* 1997;3:1565.
681. Kuerer HM, Newman LA, Smith TL, et al. Clinical course of breast cancer patients with complete pathologic primary tumor and axillary lymph node response to doxorubicin-based neoadjuvant chemotherapy. *J Clin Oncol* 1999;17:460
682. Trecate G, Ceglia E, Stabile F, et al. Locally advanced breast cancer treated with primary chemotherapy: comparison between magnetic resonance imaging and pathologic evaluation of residual disease. *Tumori* 1999;85:220.
683. Zambetti M, Oriana S, Quattrone P, et al. Combined sequential approach in locally advanced breast cancer. *Ann Oncol* 1999;10:305.
684. Mackay HJ, Cameron D, Rahilly M, et al. Reduced MLH1 expression in breast tumors after primary chemotherapy predicts disease-free survival. *J Clin Oncol* 2000;18:87.
685. Willsher PC, Pinder SE, Gee JM, et al. c-erbB2 expression predicts response to preoperative chemotherapy for locally advanced breast cancer. *Anticancer Res* 1998;18:3695.
686. Honkoop AH, van Diest PJ, de Jong JS, et al. Prognostic role of clinical, pathological and biological characteristics in patients with locally advanced breast cancer. *Br J Cancer* 1998;77:621.
687. Newman LA, Kuerer HM, Hunt KK, et al. Feasibility of immediate breast reconstruction for locally advanced breast cancer. *Ann Surg* 1999;230:72.
688. Merajver SD, Weber BL, Cody R, et al. Breast conservation and prolonged chemotherapy for locally advanced breast cancer: the University of Michigan experience. *J Clin Oncol* 1997;15:2873.
689. Clark J, Rosenman J, Cance W, Halle J, Graham M. Extending the indications for breast-conserving treatment to patients with locally advanced breast cancer. *Int J Radiat Oncol Biol Phys* 1998;42:345.
690. Chang S, Parker SL, Pham T, Buzdar AU, Hursting SD. Inflammatory breast carcinoma incidence and survival: the surveillance, epidemiology, and end results program of the National Cancer Institute, 1975–1992. *Cancer* 1998;82:2366.
691. Ueno NT, Buzdar AU, Singletary SE, et al. Combined-modality treatment of inflammatory breast carcinoma: twenty years of experience at M. D. Anderson Cancer Center. *Cancer Chemother Pharmacol* 1997;40:321.
692. Saphner T, Tormey DC, Gray R. Annual hazard rates of recurrence for breast cancer after primary therapy. *J Clin Oncol* 1996;14:2738.
693. Dawson LA, Chow E, Goss PE. Evolving perspectives in contralateral breast cancer. *Eur J Cancer* 1998;34:2000.
694. Bernstein LJ, Thompson WD, Risch N, Holford TR. The genetic epidemiology of second primary breast cancer. *Am J Epidemiol* 1992;136:937.

695. Muss HB, Tell GS, Case LK, Roberson P, Atwell BM. Perceptions of follow-up care in women with breast cancer. *Am J Clin Oncol* 1991;14:55.
696. GIVIO Investigators. Impact of follow-up testing on survival and health-related quality of life in breast cancer patients. *JAMA* 1994;271:1587.
697. Del Turco MR, Palli D, Cariddi A, et al. Intensive diagnostic follow-up after treatment of primary breast cancer. *JAMA* 1994;271:1593.
698. Chan DW, Beveridge RA, Muss H, et al. Use of Truquant BR radioimmunoassay for early detection of breast cancer recurrence in patients with stage II and stage III disease. *J Clin Oncol* 1997;15:2322.
699. American Society of Clinical Oncology. Clinical practice guidelines for the use of tumor markers in breast and colorectal cancer. *J Clin Oncol* 1996;14:2843.
700. Hayes DF. Evaluation of patients after primary therapy. In: Harris JR, Lippman ME, Morrow M, Osborne CK, eds. *Diseases of the breast*, 2nd ed. Philadelphia: Lippincott Williams & Wilkins, 2000:709.
701. American Society of Clinical Oncology. Recommended breast cancer surveillance guidelines. *J Clin Oncol* 1997;15:2149.
702. Greenberg PAC, Hortobagyi GN, Smith TL, et al. Long-term follow-up of patients with complete remission following combination chemotherapy for metastatic breast cancer. *J Clin Oncol* 1996;14:2197.
703. Posner JB. *Neurologic complications of cancer*. Philadelphia: FA Davis, 1995.
704. Valagussa P, Tancini G, Bonadonnna G. Salvage treatment of patients suffering relapse after adjuvant chemotherapy. *Cancer* 1986;58:1411.
705. Norton L, Slamon D, Leyland-Jones, B, et al. Overall survival advantage to simultaneous chemotherapy plus the humanized anti-HER2 monoclonal antibody Herceptin in HER2-overexpressing metastatic breast cancer. *Cancer* 1998;83:1142.
706. Kaufmann M, Bajetta E, Diriz LY, et al. Exemestane is superior to megestrol acetate after tamoxifen failure in postmenopausal women with advanced breast cancer: results of a phase III randomized double-blind trial. *J Clin Oncol* 2000;18:1399.
707. Cahan WG, Castro EB. Significance of a solitary lung shadow in patients with breast cancer. *Ann Surg* 1975;181:137.
708. Hayes DF, Bast RC, Desch CE, et al. Tumor marker utility grading system: a framework to evaluate clinical utility of tumor markers. *J Natl Cancer Inst* 1996;88:1456.
709. Seifert JK, Weigel TF, Gonner V, Boltger TC, Junginer T. Liver resection for breast cancer metastases. *Hepato-Gastroenterology* 1999;46:2935.
710. Blumenchein GR, Pinnameni K, Buzdar A, et al. Combined regional and systemic therapy in breast cancer patients with an isolated metastasis with or without prior chemotherapy. *Adjuvant Ther Cancer* 1984;4:316.
711. Juan O, Lluch A, de Paz L, et al. Prognostic factors in patients with isolated recurrences of breast cancer (stage IV-NED). *Breast Cancer Res Treat* 1999;53:105.
712. Osborne CK, Yochmowitz MG, Knight WA IIII, McGuire W. The value of estrogen and progesterone receptors in the treatment of breast cancer. *Cancer* 1980;46:(Suppl):2884.
713. Ingle JN, Krook JE, Green SJ, et al. Randomized trial of bilateral oophorectomy versus tamoxifen in premenopausal women with metastatic breast cancer. *J Clin Oncol* 1986;4:178.
714. Sunderland MC, Osborne CK. Tamoxifen in premenopausal patients with metastatic breast cancer: a review. *J Clin Oncol* 1991;9:1283.
715. Klijn JGM, Blamey RW, Boccardo F, et al. Combination LHRH-agonist plus tamoxifen treatment is superior to medical castration alone in premenopausal metastatic breast cancer. *Breast Cancer Res Treat* 1998;50:227.
716. Jonat W, Kaufmann M, Blamey RW, et al. A randomized study to compare the effect of the luteinising hormone releasing hormone (LHRH) analogue goserelin with or without tamoxifen in pre- and perimenopausal patients with advanced breast cancer. *Eur J Cancer* 1995;2:137.
717. Faulkson G, Holcroft C, Gelman RS, et al. Ten-year follow-up study of premenopausal women with metastatic breast cancer: an Eastern Cooperative Oncology Group study. *J Clin Oncol* 1995;13:1453.
718. Buzdar A, Jonat W, Howell A, Jones S, Blomqvist C. Anastrozole, a potent and selective aromatase inhibitor, versus megestrol acetate in postmenopausal women with advanced breast cancer: results of overview analysis of two phase III trials. *J Clin Oncol* 1996;14:2000.
719. Kaufmann M, Bajetta E, Yves Dirix L, et al. Exemestane is superior to megestrol acetate after tamoxifen failure in postmenopausal women with advanced breast cancer: results of a phase III randomized double-blind trial. *J Clin Oncol* 2000;18:1399.
720. Nabholtz JM, Bonneterre J, Buzdar AU, et al. Preliminary results of two multi-center trials comparing the efficacy and tolerability of Arimidex (anastrozole) and tamoxifen in postmenopausal women with advanced breast cancer. *Breast Cancer Res Treat* 1999;57:31(abst 27).
721. Dombernowsky P, Smith I, Falkson G, et al. Letrozole, a new oral aromatase inhibitor for advanced breast cancer: double-blind randomized trial showing a dose effect and improved efficacy and tolerability compared with megestrol acetate. *J Clin Oncol* 1998;16:453.
722. Howell A, Dodwell DJ, Anderson H, Redford J. Response after withdrawal of tamoxifen and progestens in advanced breast cancer. *Cancer* 1992;3:611.
723. Belani CP, Pearl P, Whitley NO, Aisner J. Tamoxifen withdrawal response. Report of a case. *Arch Intern Med* 1989;149:449.
724. Clarysse A. Hormone induced tumor flare. *Eur J Cancer Clin Oncol* 1985;21:585.
725. Plotkin D, Lechner JJ, Jung WE, Rosen PJ. Tamoxifen flare in advanced breast cancer. *JAMA* 1978;240:2644.
726. Ellis MJ, Hayes DF, Lippman ME. Treatment of metastatic breast cancer. In: Harris JR, Lippman ME, Morrow M, Osborne CK, eds. *Diseases of the breast*, 2nd ed. Philadelphia: Lippincott Williams & Wilkins 2000:749.
727. Burstein HJ, Bunnell CA, Winer EP. New agents and schedules for advanced breast cancer. *Semin Oncol (in press)*.
728. Fossati R, Confalonieri C, Torri V, et al. Cytotoxic and hormonal treatment for metastatic breast cancer: a systematic review of published randomized trials involving 31,510 women. *J Clin Oncol* 1998;16:3439.
729. Constanza ME, Weiss RB, Henderson IC, et al. Safety and efficacy of using a single agent or a phase II agent before instituting standard combination chemotherapy in previously untreated metastatic breast cancer patients: reports of a randomized study—CALGB 8642. *J Clin Oncol* 1999;17:1397.
730. Sledge GW Jr, Neuberg D, Ingle J, Martino S, Wood W. Phase III trial of doxorubicin vs. paclitaxel vs. doxorubicin + paclitaxel as first-line therapy for metastatic breast cancer: an intergroup trial. *Proc Am Soc Clin Oncol* 1997;16:1a(abst 2).
731. Chan S, Friedrichs K, Noel D. Prospective randomized trial of docetaxel versus doxorubicin in patients with metastatic breast cancer. *J Clin Oncol* 1999;17:2341.
732. Paridaens R, Biganzoli L, Bruning P. Paclitaxel versus doxorubicin as first-line single-agent chemotherapy for metastatic breast cancer: a European organization for research and treatment of cancer randomized study with cross-over. *J Clin Oncol* 2000;18:724.
733. Ravdin PM, Burris HA, Cook G, et al. Phase II trial of docetaxel in advanced anthracycline-resistant or anthracenedione-resistant breast cancer. *J Clin Oncol* 1995;13:2879.
734. Seidman AD, Hudis CA, Albanel J, et al. Dose-dense therapy with weekly 1 hour paclitaxel infusions in the treatment of metastatic breast cancer. *J Clin Oncol* 1998;16:3353.
735. Joensuu H, Holli K, Heikkinen M, et al. Combination chemotherapy versus single-agent therapy as first- and second-line treatment in metastatic breast cancer: a prospective randomized trial. *J Clin Oncol* 1998;16:3720.
736. Neuberg D, Sledge GW Jr, Fettig J, Cella D, Wood W. Changes in quality of life (QOL) during induction therapy in patients enrolled in a randomized trial of Adriamycin, Taxol, and Adriamycin plus Taxol in metastatic breast cancer. *Proc Am Soc Clin Oncol* 1997;16:54a(abst 185).
737. Sledge GW, Hu P, Falkson G. Comparison of chemotherapy with chemohormonal therapy as first-line therapy for metastatic, hormone-sensitive breast cancer: an Eastern Cooperative Oncology Group study. *J Clin Oncol* 2000;18:262.
738. Perry MC, Kardinal CG, Korzun AH, et al. Chemohormonal therapy in advanced carcinoma of the breast: Cancer and Leukemia Group B Protocol 8081. *J Clin Oncol* 1987;5:1534.
739. Muss H, Case LD, Richards F. Interrupted versus continuous chemotherapy in patients with metastatic breast cancer. The Piedmont Oncology Association. *N Engl J Med* 1991;325:1342.
740. Gregory RK, Powles RJ, Chang JC, Ashley S. A randomized trial of six versus twelve courses of chemotherapy in metastatic carcinoma of the breast. *Eur J Cancer* 1997;33:2194.
741. Coates A, Gebski V, Bishop JF, et al. Improving the quality of life during chemotherapy for advanced breast cancer. A comparison of intermittent and continuous treatment strategies. *N Engl J Med* 1987;317:1490.
742. Tannock I, Boyd N, De Boer G, et al. A randomized trial of two dose levels of cyclophosphamide, methotrexate, and fluorouracil chemotherapy for patients with metastatic breast cancer. *J Clin Oncol* 1988;6:1377.
743. Bastolt L, Dalmark M, Gjedde SB, et al. Dose-response relationship of epirubicin in the treatment of postmenopausal patients with metastatic breast cancer: a randomized study of epirubicin at four different dose levels performed by the Danish Breast Cancer Cooperative Group. *J Clin Oncol* 1990;14:1146.
744. Nabholtz JM, Gelmon K, Bontenbal M, et al. Multicenter, randomized comparative study of two doses of paclitaxel in patients with metastatic breast cancer. *J Clin Oncol* 1996;14:1858.
745. Winer E, Berry D, Duggan D, et al. Failure of higher dose paclitaxel to improve outcome in patients with metastatic breast cancer—results from CALGB 9342. *Proc Am Soc Clin Oncol* 1998;17:101a(abst 388).
746. Smith RE, Brown AM, Mamounas EP. Randomized trial of 3-hour versus 24-hour infusion of high-dose paclitaxel in patients with metastatic or locally advanced breast cancer: National Surgical Adjuvant Breast and Bowel Project protocol B-26. *J Clin Oncol* 1999;17:3403.
747. Burstein HJ, Manola J, Younger J, et al. Docetaxel administered on a weekly basis for metastatic breast cancer. *J Clin Oncol* 2000;18:1212.
748. Engelsman E, Klijn JCM, Rubens RD, et al. "Classical" CMF versus a 3-weekly intravenous CMF schedule in postmenopausal patients with advanced breast cancer: an EORTC Breast Cancer Cooperative phase III trial (10808). *Eur J Cancer* 1991;27:966.
749. Blum JL, Jones SE, Buzdar AU, et al. Multicenter phase II study of capecitabine in paclitaxel-refractory metastatic breast cancer. *J Clin Oncol* 1999;17:485.
750. Ranson MR, Carmichael J, O'Byrne K, et al. Treatment of advanced breast cancer with sterically stabilized liposomal doxorubicin: results of a multicenter phase II trial. *J Clin Oncol* 1997;15:3185.
751. Hryniuk W, Bush H. The importance of dose intensity in chemotherapy of metastatic breast cancer. *J Clin Oncol* 1994;2:1281.
752. Peters WP, Shpall EJ, Jones RB, et al. High-dose combination alkylating agents with bone marrow support as initial treatment for metastatic breast cancer. *J Clin Oncol* 1988;6:1368.
753. Kennedy MJ, Beveridge RA, Rowley SD, et al. High-dose chemotherapy with reinfusion of purged autologous bone marrow following dose-intense induction as initial therapy for metastatic breast cancer. *J Natl Cancer Inst* 1991;83:920.
754. Antman K, Ayash L, Elias A, et al. A phase II study of high-dose cyclophosphamide, thiotepa, and carboplatin with autologous marrow support in women with measurable advanced breast cancer responding to standard-dose therapy. *J Clin Oncol* 1992;10:102.
755. Ayash LJ, Wheeler C, Fairclough D, et al. Prognostic factors for prolonged progression-free survival with high dose autologous stem cell support for breast cancer in North America. *J Clin Oncol* 1995;13:2043.
756. Rizzieri DA, Vredenburgh JJ, Jones R. Prognostic and predictive factors for patients with metastatic breast cancer undergoing aggressive induction therapy followed by high-dose chemotherapy with autologous stem-cell support. *J Clin Oncol* 1999;17:3064.
757. Rowlings PA, Williams SF, Antman KH. Factors correlated with progression-free survival after high-dose chemotherapy and hematopoietic stem cell transplantation for metastatic breast cancer. *JAMA* 1999;282:1335.
758. Stadtmauer E, O'Neill A, Goldstein L. Conventional-dose chemotherapy compared with high dose-chemotherapy plus autologous hematopoietic stem-cell transplantation for metastatic breast cancer. *N Engl J Med* 2000;342:1069.
759. Berry DA, Broadwater G, Perry MC, et al. Conventional- vs high-dose therapy for metastatic breast cancer: comparison of Cancer and Leukemia Group B and Blood and Marrow Transplant Registry patients. *Proc Am Soc Clin Oncol* 1999;18:128a(abst 490).

760. Lippman M. Editorial: high-dose chemotherapy plus autologous bone marrow transplantation for metastatic breast cancer. *N Engl J Med* 2000;15:1119.
761. Slamon D, Leyland-Jones B, Shak S, et al. Addition of Herceptin (humanized anti-HER2 antibody) to first line chemotherapy for HER2 overexpressing metastatic breast cancer markedly increases anticancer activity: a randomized multinational controlled phase III trial. *Proc Am Soc Clin Oncol* 1998;17:98a(abst 377).
762. Cobleigh MA, Vogel C, Tripathy D, et al. Multinational study of the efficacy and safety of humanized anti-HER2 monoclonal antibody in women who have HER2 overexpressing metastatic breast cancer that has progressed after chemotherapy for metastatic disease. *J Clin Oncol* 1999;17:2639.
763. Vogel CL, Cobleigh MA, Tripathy D, et al. Efficacy and safety of Herceptin as a single agent in first-line treatment of HER2 overexpressing metastatic breast cancer. *Breast Cancer Res Treat* 1998:50(abst 23).
764. Burstein HJ, Kuter I, Richadson PG, et al. Herceptin and vinorelbine for HER2-positive metastatic breast cancer: a phase II study. *Proc Am Soc Clin Oncol* 2000:19(abst 392).
765. Burris HA 3rd. Docetaxel (Taxotere) in HER-2-positive patients and in combination with trastuzumab (Herceptin). *Semin Oncol* 2000;27(2 Suppl 3):19.
766. Fornier M, Seidman AD, Esteva FJ, et al. Weekly Herceptin + 1 hour Taxol: phase II study in HER2 overexpressing and non-overexpressing metastatic breast cancer. *Proc Am Soc Clin Oncol* 1999;126a(abst 482).
767. Winer EP. Quality-of-life research in patients with breast cancer. *Cancer* 1994;74(Suppl):410.
768. Tao ML, Ganz PA. Techniques in the assessment of quality of life. In: Harris JR, Lippman ME, Morrow ME, Osborne CK, eds. *Diseases of the breast*, 2nd ed. Philadelphia: Lippincott Williams & Wilkins, 2000:1103.
769. Kornblith AB, Hollis DR, Zuckerman E, et al. Effect of megestrol acetate on quality of life in a dose-response trial in women with advanced breast cancer. The Cancer and Leukemia Group B. *J Clin Oncol* 1993;11:2081.
770. Liu G, Franssen E, Fitch MI, Warner E. Patient preferences for oral versus intravenous palliative chemotherapy. *J Clin Oncol* 1997;15:110.
771. DeMario MD, Ratain MJ. Oral chemotherapy: rationale and future directions. *J Clin Oncol* 1999;17:3362.
772. Hortobagyi GN, Theriault RL, Porter L, et al. Efficacy of pamidronate in reducing skeletal complications in patients with breast cancer and lytic bone metastases. Protocol 19 Aredia Breast Cancer Study Group. *N Engl J Med* 1996;335:1785.
773. Demetri GD, Kris M, Wade J, Cella D. Quality-of-life benefit in chemotherapy patients treated with epoietin alfa is independent of disease response or tumor type: results from a prospective community oncology study. Procrit Study Group. *J Clin Oncol* 1998;16:3412.
774. Gralla RJ, Osoba D, Kris MG, et al. Recommendations for the use of antiemetics: evidence-based, clinical practice guidelines. American Society of Clinical Oncology. *J Clin Oncol* 1999;17:2971.

SECTION **3**

JOSEPH J. DISA
JEANNE A. PETREK

Rehabilitation after Treatment for Cancer of the Breast

Breast reconstruction after mastectomy has grown in popularity since the 1970s. The era of diagnosis with less extensive cancers has ushered in less extensive total mastectomies, including "skin sparing" with an incision only around the areola. Presently, the typical patient has many choices, not only regarding the cancer management but also regarding multiple surgical options after mastectomy.

The first consideration after mastectomy is whether to reconstruct the breast. Not performing breast reconstruction is the simplest approach. The patient then faces postmastectomy appearance and the need, in most women, for an external prosthesis to restore appearance and weight balance. Mastectomy forms first began as individually made cotton fluff-filled forms. Then foam rubber forms were manufactured with holes in the back for metal weights to add stability and gravity. Now almost all weighted breast prostheses are made of solid silicone materials. The variably shaped breast forms are also available in several skin colors. It is very rare, but possible, to require custom manufacturing of the form for irregular mastectomy defects.

The external prosthesis is completely concealed in a bra with an adjustable built-in pocket specially constructed to accommodate it. Wearing the weighted prosthesis should help the body maintain its posture and balance and may prevent back and neck strain. With the concern that the prosthesis could become dislodged, even with such a specially fitted bra or swimsuit, adherent forms have now become popular. Using a variety of surgical adhesives, the form adheres to the chest wall or to a backing on the skin of the chest wall, so that the form can be removed every night while the backing can remain for a week or more. In retrospective studies,[1,2] the differences among those opting for breast reconstruction, those wearing external prostheses, and those doing neither were explored.

The American Cancer Society sponsors the program Reach to Recovery (1-800-ACS-2345), which began in 1952, a time in which all volunteers had undergone mastectomy. Today, the survivor-to-patient outreach and support include volunteers who have had breast conservation and postmastectomy reconstruction. At the physician's request, trained volunteers meet with the patient to discuss several aspects of recovery, including physiologic, psychological, and cosmetic rehabilitation. Resources for the patient include breast prostheses information with knowledge of local resources, clothing suggestions, and even an exercise booklet and aids.

DELAYED VERSUS IMMEDIATE RECONSTRUCTION

If breast reconstruction is elected, the next decision is timing, immediate (at the time of the mastectomy) or delayed. The traditional concept of performing the mastectomy, proceeding with adjuvant therapy, and delaying reconstruction until the completion of adjuvant therapy is being supplanted by the increasing use of immediate reconstruction. In a mastectomy without immediate reconstruction, it is difficult to "save" any extra native breast skin because, with the volume of the breast missing, there is excess skin folding and wrinkling. The first large report of immediate reconstruction was in 1982 by Georgiade et al.[3] In their series of 62 patients, the authors concluded that immediate breast reconstruction in selected patients offered the advantages of improved aesthetic results, decreased cost, less morbidity, and no adverse effect on cancer management.

Because the mastectomy and reconstruction are performed under a single anesthetic, the total hospital costs and convalescent time are reduced when compared to mastectomy and delayed reconstruction.[4] Immediate reconstruction reduces physical morbidity by limiting the total number of anesthetics and reducing the need for a symmetry procedure on the opposite breast.[5] Critical landmarks for optimizing breast form and symmetry are the inframammary fold, which is preserved, and the breast skin envelope, which can be preserved and maintained in its native state with immediate reconstruction.

Current methods of reconstruction can be broadly classified into autologous tissue or prosthetic material. Autologous tissue reconstruction uses the patient's own tissue (skin, subcutaneous tissue, and muscle) from another site to reconstruct the missing breast. Prosthetic reconstruction uses a process known as *tissue expansion* to create a "pocket" for the ultimate placement of a breast implant. There are occasional indications for a combination of both autologous tissue and an implant. The selection of the reconstructive technique is based on anatomic patient factors, including the laxity and thickness of the remaining chest wall skin, the condition of the chest wall musculature, the size of the opposite breast, and the availability of suitable autologous tissue donor sites. To identify the appropriate method of reconstruction, the anatomic factors are considered with cancer treatment goals and the patient's expectations, as well as, most important, clinical factors (diabetes, obesity, other chronic illnesses) because operative complexity and postoperative recovery varies.

PROSTHETIC RECONSTRUCTION

Breast reconstruction using prosthetic materials involves the use of tissue expanders and permanent breast implants. Initially, implants were placed directly under the skin in the mastectomy space, but the results were limited by the available skin envelope and capsular contracture.[6,7] The development of tissue expanders allowed for greater control over the size of the skin envelope, thus resulting in the ability to use larger prostheses for symmetry. Current techniques use a complete submuscular placement of the tissue expander, with coverage by pectoralis major, serratus anterior, and occasionally the anterior rectus sheath.[6]

A biodimensional textured surface tissue expander is placed either at the time of mastectomy, which increases the operative time of less than 1 hour, or in a delayed fashion, during a separate later operation. The area is allowed to heal for approximately 10 to 14 days, at which time fluid expansion is commenced. Using an integrated valve within the expander, saline is injected into the expander percutaneously until the appropriate size is reached (Fig. 37.3-1). Adjuvant chemotherapy can be commenced during the expansion process. The exchange to a permanent breast implant takes place after the chemotherapy course. Using a two-stage method of implant reconstruction allows for maximum control of the implant pocket and optimal symmetry with the contralateral breast (Fig. 37.3-2). When indicated, contralateral symmetry procedures such as augmentation mammoplasty, reduction mammoplasty, or mastopexy (breast lift), are accomplished when the tissue expander is exchanged to a permanent implant.

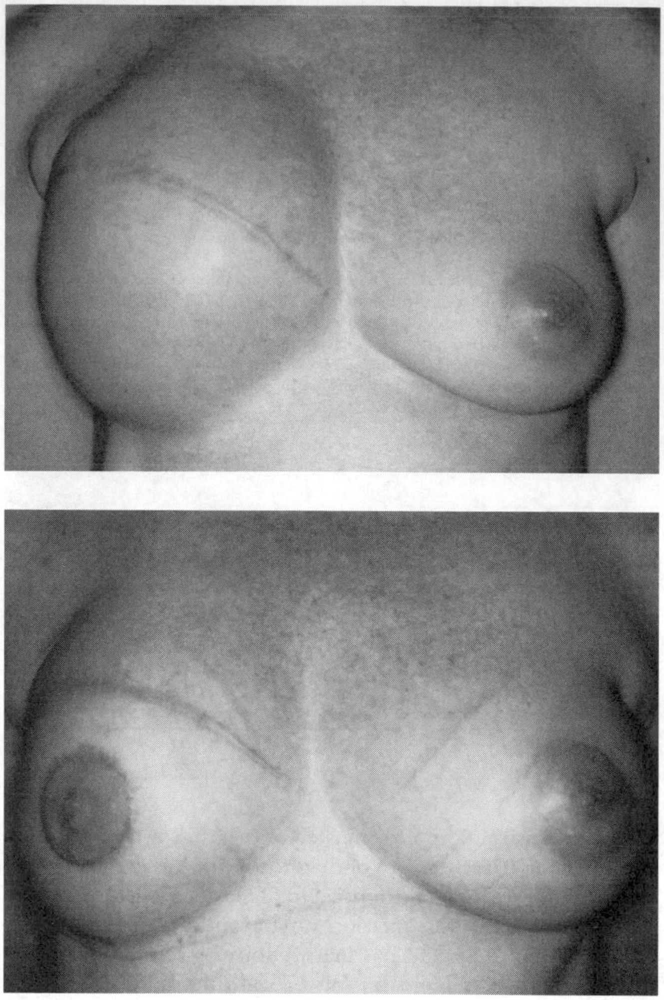

A

B

FIGURE 37.3-2. **A:** After expansion is complete, the pocket is overexpanded relative to the normal breast to maximize ptosis and implant projection. **B:** The same patient subsequent to exchange of the tissue expander to a permanent saline breast implant followed by nipple-areola reconstruction and tattooing.

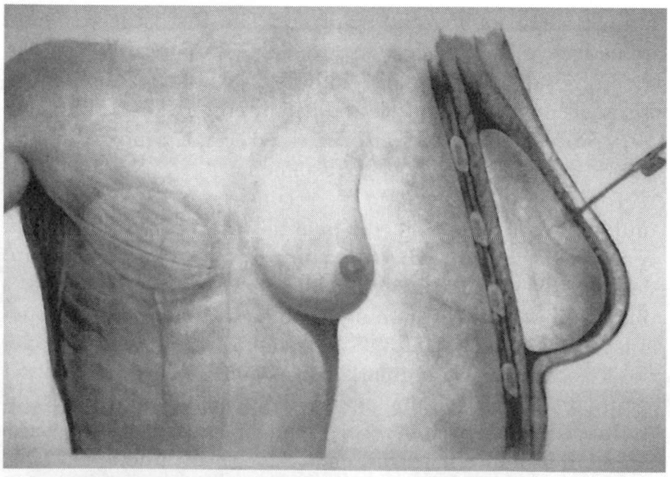

FIGURE 37.3-1. Complete submuscular placement of the tissue expander at the time of mastectomy (*left*). Percutaneous approach to expansion using a complete submuscular integrated valve tissue expander (*right*).

The author (J. J. D.) reported results with 770 consecutive patients undergoing tissue expansion over a 10-year period. In this series, premature removal of the tissue expander secondary to wound-related complications or persistent disease was necessary in only 1.8% of the patients.[8] The advantages of tissue expander implant reconstruction are the simplicity, reliability, and avoidance of donor site morbidity. The disadvantages of this technique relate to the use of prosthetic material and include infection, leakage of the implant, capsular contracture, and differences in texture and symmetry when compared to the contralateral breast, which can lead to multiple surgical procedures on the opposite breast.

Breast implants available for reconstruction vary in size, shape, surface texturing, and fill material. In general, implants

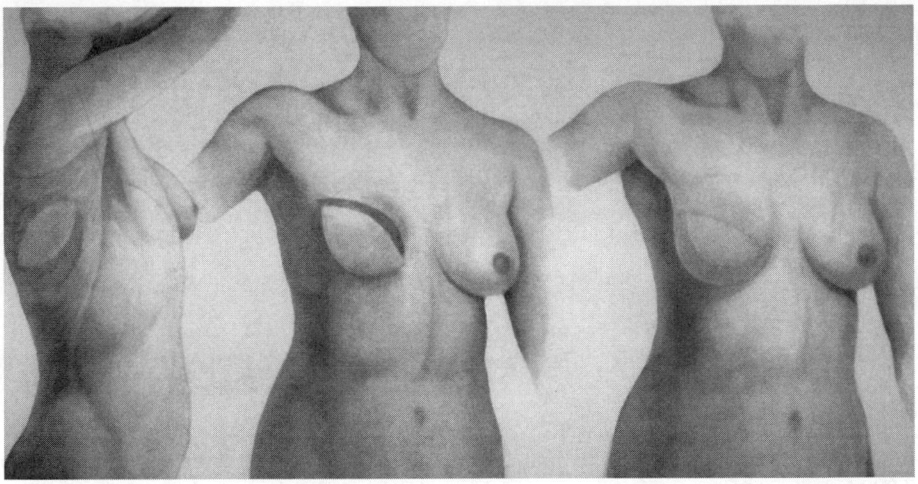

FIGURE 37.3-3. Design of the latissimus flap and skin island (*left*). Transposition of the myocutaneous latissimus dorsi flap into the mastectomy defect (*center*). Latissimus flap breast reconstruction with the placement of a breast implant underneath the latissimus dorsi flap (*right*).

are either round or anatomic in shape, with a smooth or textured surface, and saline or silicone gel–filled. Currently, saline-filled breast implants are available, and use of silicone gel implants requires enrollment in a silicone adjunct study sponsored by the implant manufacturers, U.S. Food and Drug Administration, and the Institution Review Board where the procedure is being performed. Despite the moratorium placed on the general use of silicone gel implants, to date there is no convincing cause and effect between "human adjuvant disease" and the use of silicone gel implants.[9]

AUTOLOGOUS TISSUE RECONSTRUCTION

The most predictable results in breast reconstruction involve the use of autologous tissue. In general, use of the patient's own tissue results in a reconstruction that can closely match the opposite breast in size, shape, and texture. Depending on the volume of the tissue transferred and the volume of the contralateral breast, autologous tissue breast reconstruction sometimes also requires an implant.

Methods of autologous tissue breast reconstruction include local flaps and distant flaps. Local flaps, including the latissimus dorsi myocutaneous flap and the pedicled transverse rectus abdominus myocutaneous (TRAM) flap, rely on transposition of muscle, subcutaneous tissue, and skin into the mastectomy defect based on the attached native blood supply of the muscle. Distant flap breast reconstruction mandates the use of microvascular free tissue transfer. The most common distant tissue donor site is the free TRAM flap. Other donor sites include the inferior gluteal flap, the superior gluteal flap, the deep inferior epigastric artery perforator flap, and the Rubens flap. Reconstruction using these tissues relies on harvesting the flap with its discreet vascular pedicle. The vascular pedicle is then anastomosed using microsurgical technique to appropriate recipient vessels in the mastectomy site, usually the thoracodorsal and internal mammary vessels.

The latissimus dorsi myocutaneous flap with an overlying skin island can be transposed from the back into the mastectomy defect (Fig. 37.3-3). The advantages of the latissimus flap are in its ease of harvest and minimal donor site morbidity, compared to other sites.[10] The chief disadvantage of the latissimus flap is that concomitant use of a breast implant is often necessary due to the limited volume of tissue provided (Fig. 37.3-4). Without a simultaneous implant placement, the latissimus dorsi flap is reserved for small breasts.

The most common method of autologous tissue breast reconstruction is with the TRAM flap[11] because of the texture and the large volume, both of which match the other breast (Fig. 37.3-5). The blood supply to the skin island and lower abdominal fat is derived from perforating vessels through the underlying rectus abdominus muscle. Depending on the

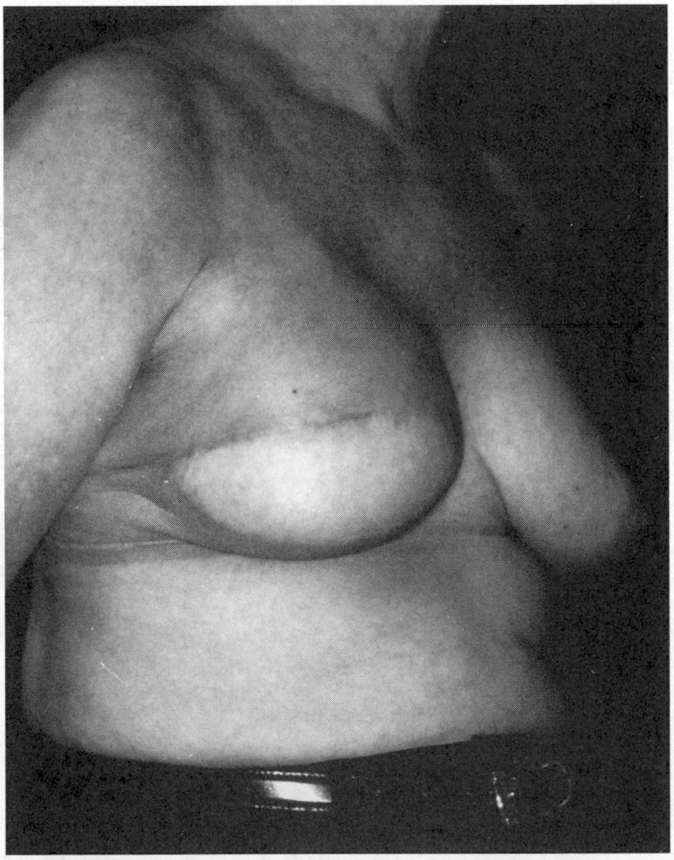

FIGURE 37.3-4. Right breast reconstruction with latissimus dorsi myocutaneous flap and permanent implant. The implant was necessary to achieve symmetry with the opposite breast.

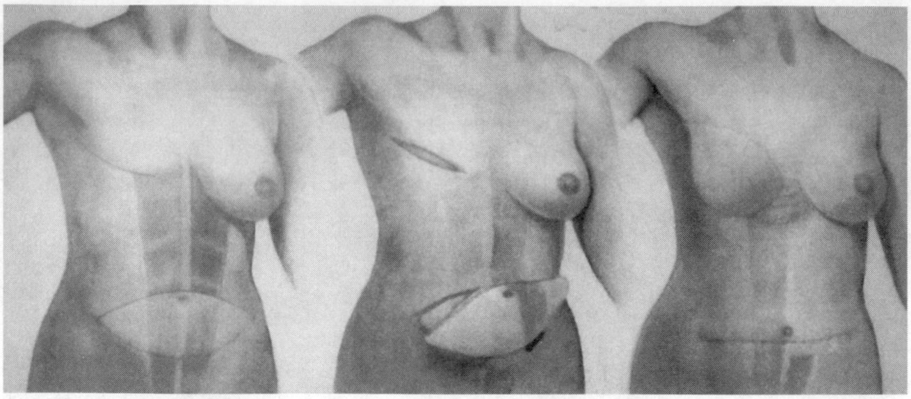

FIGURE 37.3-5. Design of an unipedicled transverse rectus abdominus myocutaneous (TRAM) flap on the lower abdomen (*left*). Elevation of the TRAM flap based on the left rectus abdominus muscle (*center*). Right breast reconstruction with unipedicled TRAM flap after closure of donor site and inset of flap (*right*).

increasing volume necessary to match the other breast, the TRAM flap can be transferred on a single pedicle (usually the contralateral superior epigastric), double pedicle (using both rectus muscles and their associated superior epigastric vessels), or as a free flap (based on the deep inferior epigastric vessels)[12] (Fig. 37.3-6).

The TRAM flap allows the reconstructive surgeon the most versatility and design. Thus, the flap can be sculpted to closely match the contralateral breast in unilateral reconstruction, or itself in bilateral reconstruction (Fig. 37.3-7). The use of a breast implant is rarely indicated with a TRAM flap, because an ample amount of tissue exists in properly selected patients. The lower abdominal donor site scar is easily hidden with conventional clothing. Despite the obvious advantages of the TRAM flap, not everyone is a candidate. Thin patients may not have an adequate amount of tissue at the donor site, whereas obese patients have a much higher risk for local and systemic complications.[13] Total flap loss with the free TRAM flap can occur, but the risk is generally accepted to be less than 2%.[14,15] Use of the rectus abdominus muscle results in 10% loss in abdominal wall strength in unilateral reconstruction and 40% loss when both muscles are harvested.[16] Lower abdominal bulging and hernia formation occurs in fewer than 10% of patients and can be minimized by surgical techniques that maximize preservation of the rectus muscles.[17]

Other methods of autologous tissue reconstruction include the gluteus free flap based on the superior or inferior gluteal vessels, and the Rubens flap based on the deep circumflex iliac artery. These techniques are technically demanding and do not offer the same high-quality tissue available with a TRAM flap.

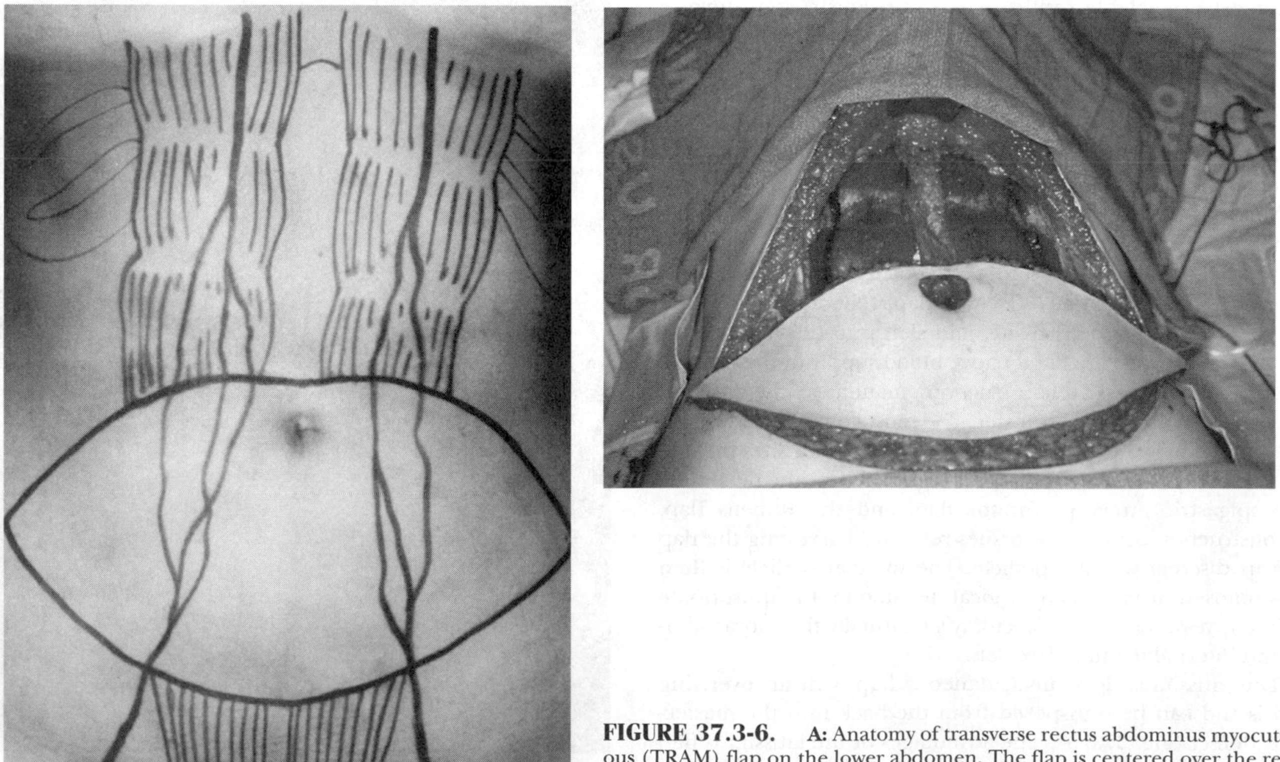

A

B

FIGURE 37.3-6. **A:** Anatomy of transverse rectus abdominus myocutaneous (TRAM) flap on the lower abdomen. The flap is centered over the rectus abdominus muscles and is supplied by the superior epigastric vessels and the deep inferior epigastric vessels. **B:** Intraoperative appearance of a bipedicled TRAM flap after harvest and before transposition into the mastectomy defect.

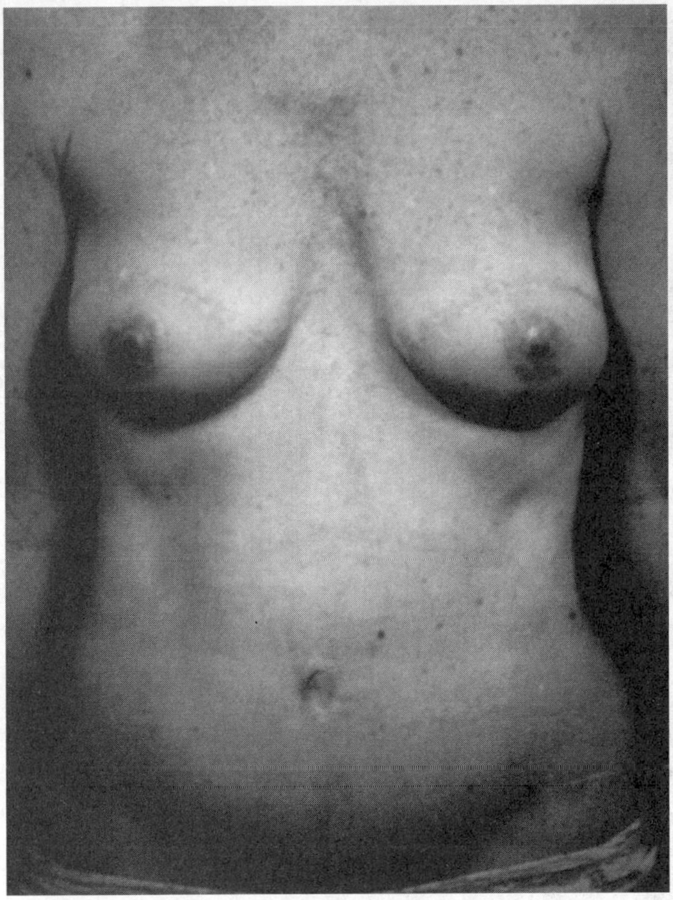

FIGURE 37.3-7. Bilateral breast reconstruction with transverse rectus abdominus myocutaneous flaps and subsequent nipple-areola reconstruction. The use of autologous tissue conveys a natural appearance to the breast reconstruction.

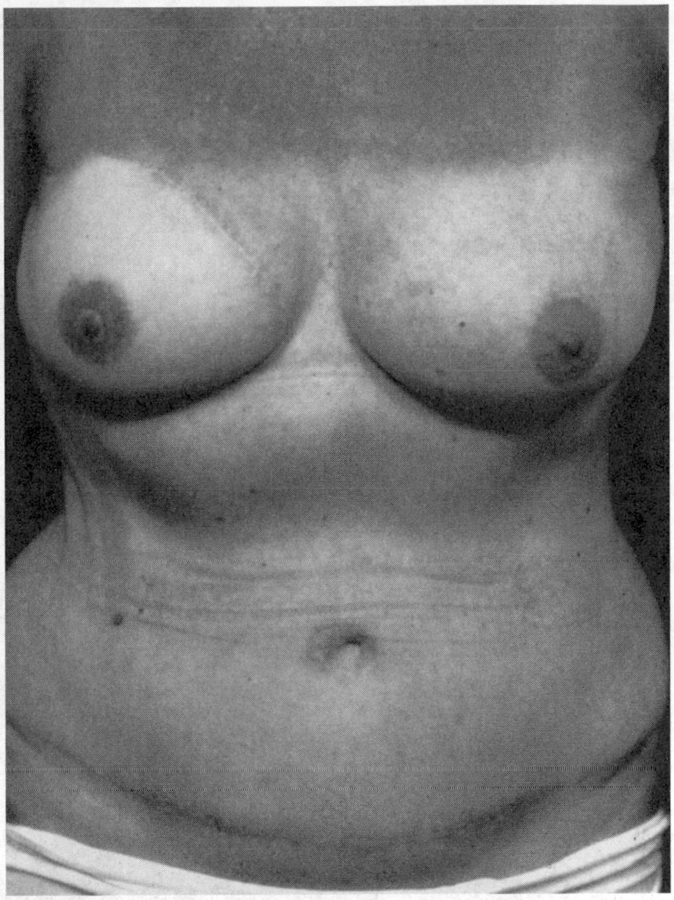

FIGURE 37.3-8. Right breast reconstruction after mastectomy for failed breast-conservation therapy with an unipedicled transverse rectus abdominus myocutaneous (TRAM) flap. The skin island on the TRAM flap has been used to replace the radiated skin from the breast mound.

Therefore, their use is reserved for patients desiring breast reconstruction that are not candidates for more conventional methods.

POSTMASTECTOMY AFTER BREAST IRRADIATION

Breast reconstruction after local failure in the irradiated breast presents a unique challenge for both the oncologic and reconstructive surgeon. The late effects of radiation are characterized clinically by a loss of skin elasticity, fibrosis, and decreased blood supply. The postradiation fibrosis severely limits the ability of the tissue expander to create a satisfactory pocket for the permanent implant. There is an increased incidence of infection, skin necrosis, and expander extrusion when attempting to expand the irradiated skin and muscle chest wall, as well as a high rate of capsular contracture in the final result. The lack of projection of the permanent implant and capsular contracture detracts from the final aesthetic result.[18,19]

Increasing the success of breast reconstruction after prior irradiation involves the use of autologous tissue. Depending on the method, this procedure can be performed with or without a breast implant. The transfer of the ipsilateral latissimus dorsi muscle with a cutaneous skin island into the mastectomy defect delivers a large volume of healthy nonirradiated tissue into the defect. In conjunction with a tissue expander, the flap can be expanded without difficulty, and ultimately a permanent implant can be placed with improved aesthetics and a decreased incidence of complications.[20]

In a series[21,22] of 680 consecutive patients who underwent TRAM flap breast reconstruction, 108 patients had had previous irradiation, and no difference was found in flap survival in the two groups. There was, however, increased incidence of infection and fat necrosis in the radiated group, which detracts from the final aesthetic result. The effects of irradiation on the mastectomy flaps predisposes to ischemia and may increase scar formation.[20]

SKIN-SPARING MASTECTOMY WITH IMMEDIATE RECONSTRUCTION

Although autologous tissue breast reconstruction can create a breast mound that resembles the breast in shape and consistency, one drawback is the color difference between the native breast skin and the flap skin (from the distant site), which conveys a "patch-like" appearance (Fig. 37.3-8). The technique of skin-sparing mastectomy is accomplished through one incision

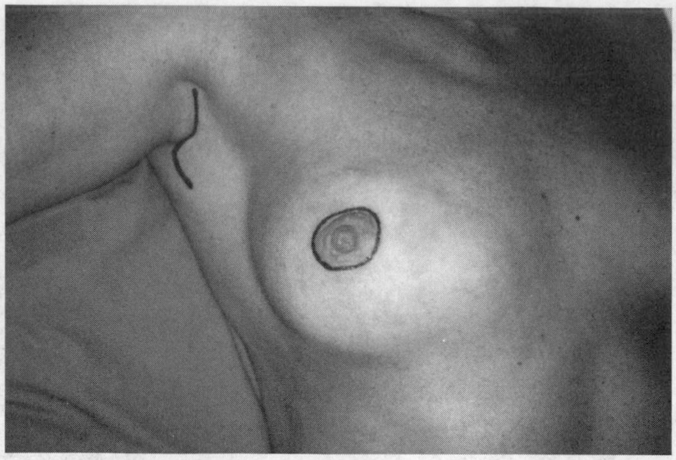

A

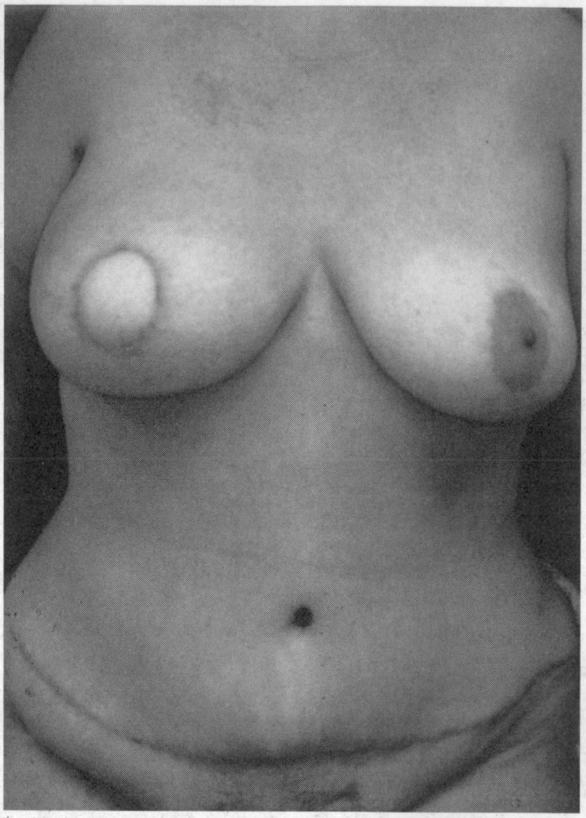

B

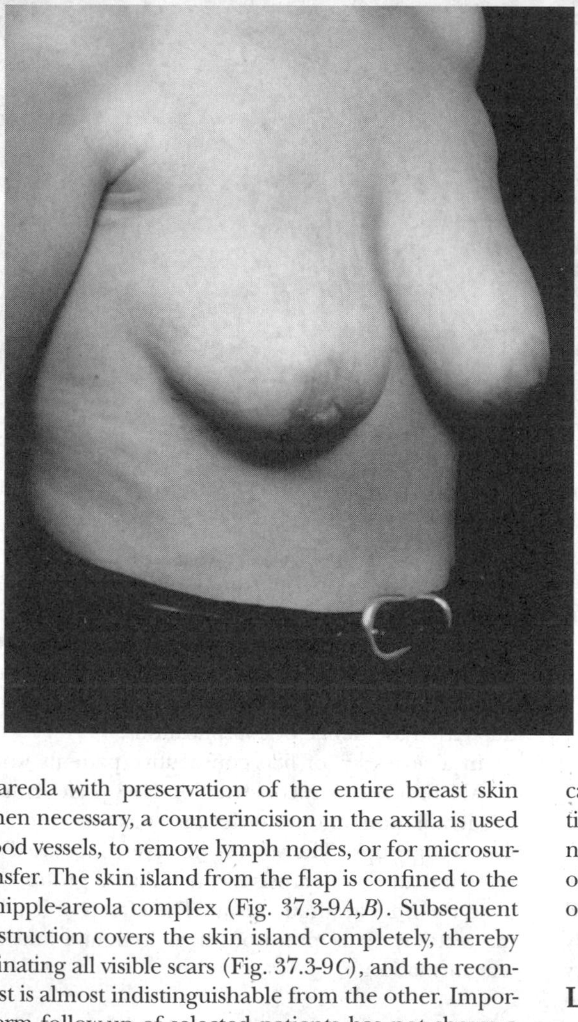

C

FIGURE 37.3-9. **A:** Design of circumareolar incision for complete skin-sparing mastectomy and axillary counterincision for exposure of lymph nodes and blood vessels. **B:** Complete skin-sparing mastectomy with free transverse rectus abdominus myocutaneous (TRAM) flap and reconstruction before nipple-areola reconstruction in another patient. **C:** Right breast reconstruction with a free TRAM flap after complete skin-sparing mastectomy. The patient has undergone right nipple-areola reconstruction and tattooing. Using this complete skin-sparing approach, the periareolar mastectomy incision is barely visible.

around the areola with preservation of the entire breast skin envelope. When necessary, a counterincision in the axilla is used to expose blood vessels, to remove lymph nodes, or for microsurgical flap transfer. The skin island from the flap is confined to the zone of the nipple-areola complex (Fig. 37.3-9*A,B*). Subsequent nipple reconstruction covers the skin island completely, thereby virtually eliminating all visible scars (Fig. 37.3-9*C*), and the reconstructed breast is almost indistinguishable from the other. Importantly, long-term follow-up of selected patients has not shown a difference in local recurrence rates after skin-sparing mastectomy versus traditional mastectomy.[23–25] Technical advances using complete skin-sparing techniques have resulted in reconstructed breasts that are virtually indistinguishable from the native breast in terms of color, texture, and appearance.[23]

Nipple-areola reconstruction can be accomplished simply in the outpatient setting. One method is simply tattooing a nipple and areola onto the breast mound to imitate the color and size of the opposite nipple-areola complex. Alternatively, a local flap can be raised on the breast mound to create the nipple projection, or a skin graft can be placed (Fig. 37.3-10). Although the nipple reconstruction lacks sensation and the erectile function of the natural nipple, it provides an important visual suggestion of normalcy and decreases the stigmata of mastectomy.

LYMPHEDEMA

Aside from recurrence, lymphedema is the most dreaded sequelae of breast cancer treatment. Approximately 15% to 20% of breast cancer patients have developed lymphedema after breast cancer treatment. Therefore, of perhaps 2 million current breast cancer survivors after axillary dissection, approximately 400,000 cope daily with the disfigurement, discomfort, and disability of arm and hand swelling.

Lymphedema is the result of a functional overload of the lymphatic system in which lymph volume exceeds transport capabili-

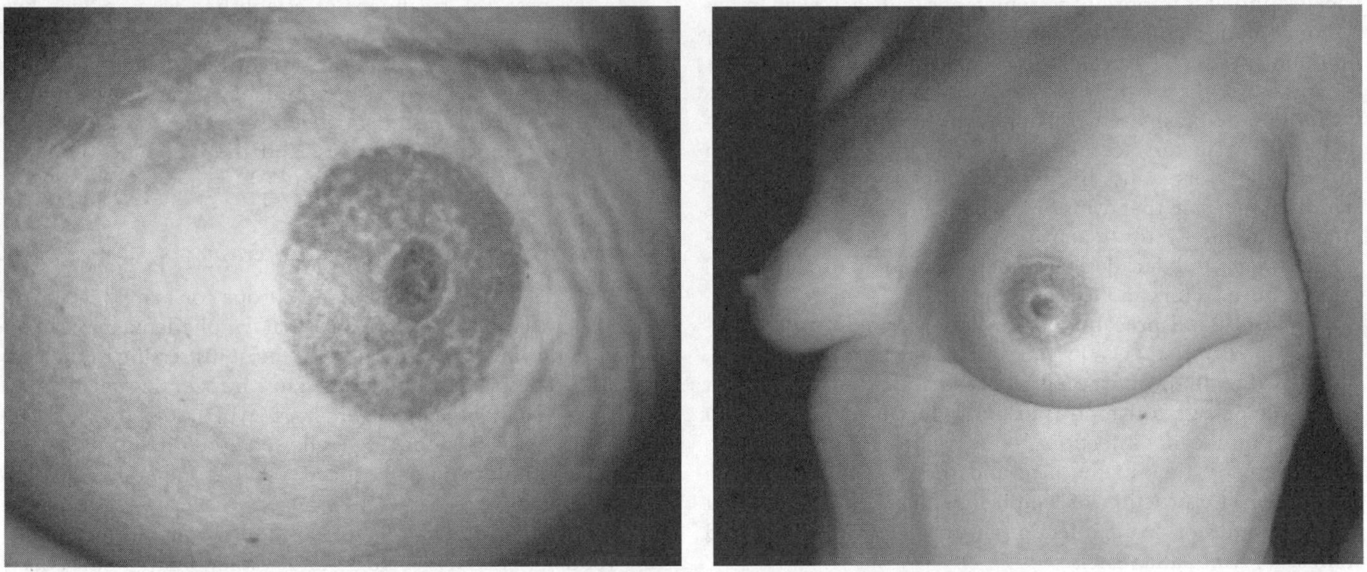

A B

FIGURE 37.3-10. **A:** Nipple-areola reconstruction using a tattooing technique only. **B:** Left breast reconstruction after complete skin-sparing mastectomy with a pedicled transverse rectus abdominus myocutaneous flap, and subsequent nipple-areola reconstruction using a local flap followed by tattooing.

ties. The functioning lymph system removes large molecules that reach the interstitial space by filtration, cellular metabolism, or secretion. The buildup of interstitial macromolecules leads to an increase in oncotic pressure in the tissues, producing more edema, and the blocked lymphatic vessels raise hydrostatic pressure proximally in the system. Persistent swelling and stagnant protein eventually lead to fibrosis and provide an excellent culture medium for repeated bouts of cellulitis and lymphangitis. With dilatation of the lymphatics, the internal valves become incompetent, causing further stasis.

The reported incidence of lymphedema has varied greatly and depends in part on the extent of axillary treatment, the interval between axillary treatment and measurement, methods used to define lymphedema, and the completeness of the patient population follow-up.

All reports on the incidence of lymphedema, including the seven selected ones from a review,[26] are retrospective, and in each of these reports, the denominator (i.e., the number of patients at risk for developing lymphedema in a particular population) is imprecise or unknown. The incidence varied from 6% to 30%, with the lowest incidence of lymphedema having the shortest follow-up.[26]

ETIOLOGIC FACTORS

Almost all previous studies find that the incidence and the degree of lymphedema is correlated to the extent of surgical dissection as more nodes are excised. However, two large studies[27,28] could not demonstrate this relationship, perhaps because rather small differences in extent of axillary dissection were assessed. Regardless of the number of lymph nodes excised, surgeons should attempt to carefully preserve the fatty axillary tissue containing the invisible lymphatic trunks around the vein and to dissect the tissue only inferior to the axillary vein.

In every study that has evaluated this issue, the addition of radiation therapy directed to the dissected axilla was a strong predictor of lymphedema.[26] Of particular importance is that even when the intent is to radiate the breast only (such as after lumpectomy), some radiation dosage may reach the axilla depending on radiotherapy technique and patient anatomy. Specific breast radiotherapy techniques with the goal to avoid the dissected axilla and the pathophysiology of radiation-related lymphedema have been reviewed.[29] For precise radiation technique, it may be helpful for the surgeon to mark axillary dissection by radiopaque clips, and the area can then be seen on the simulation films.

It is biologically intuitive that sentinel lymph node biopsy of one or few nodes should decrease the risk of lymphedema. However, the sentinel node operation is not always so limited, and it is theoretically possible that indeed the sentinel node may be at the level of the axillary vein (and the lymph trunks), thereby theoretically predisposing the patient to lymphedema. The risk of lymphedema has not yet been assessed in the follow-up of patients treated with sentinel lymph node technology. Furthermore, if axillary radiotherapy is added after sentinel node biopsy, there is the risk of lymphedema. In series reporting axillary radiotherapy but no axillary surgery at all, lymphedema incidence ranged from 2% to 5%.[29]

Beyond these two definite factors—extent of surgical dissection and radiation to the axilla—a wide range of possible etiologic factors has not been evaluated systematically. Older age at diagnosis was reported to be a significant factor in one study,[30,31] but was unrelated to lymphedema incidence in another,[32] and curiously was not noted in others. Similar disagreement holds for dominant hand on the operated side,[32,33] obesity,[27,34] surgical technique,[31] and postoperative course.[35,36]

PREVENTION OF LYMPHEDEMA AFTER AXILLARY TREATMENT

Because controlling lymphedema requires daily attention, and because "curing" lymphedema has not been accomplished, emphasis must be placed on prevention. Nevertheless, without evidence-based knowledge of etiologic factors, the list of post-treatment arm precautions is based on intuitive reasoning. As a background, it is important to remember that each woman has a congenitally different anatomy, which also is probably uniquely prone to degenerative conditions, similar to the remainder of the vascular system. This has been studied thus far in a limited fashion with lymphoscintigraphy.[37] The individual patient factors, combined with surgical and radiation treatment factors, must be the main determinants, notwithstanding the fact that lymphedema may occur several years after treatment. Events or activities, such as exercise, in the subsequent years and decades have not been studied to state which are causative factors and to what degree.

Arm and hand precautions are loosely based on two overarching principles: (1) Do not increase lymph production, which is directly proportional to blood flow, and (2) do not increase blockage to lymph transport. Heat (such as that in a sauna), significant infections, and vigorous arm exercise increase blood flow in the arm and thereby increase lymph production. Obstruction of lymph flow may result from tight arm garments or from infections with ensuing fibrosis and stenosis of lymphatic vessels.

The patient is instructed as follows:

1. Avoid puncturing or injuring the skin in any way. Use meticulous skin and nail/cuticle care. Pay immediate attention and use standard first aid care.
2. Avoid vaccinations, injections, blood pressure monitoring, blood drawing, and intravenous administration in that arm.
3. Avoid constricting sleeves or jewelry and wear a padded bra strap (to avoid supraclavicular area compression).
4. Avoid heat, such as with sunburns or tanning, baths, and saunas.
5. Avoid violent exercises and strenuous exertion. Consider vigorous aerobic arm exercise only when compression garments support the arm.

No data govern any of these recommendations. In the only studies that reported on bilateral axillary dissections, there was no higher risk of lymphedema in those women over those who had unilateral axillary dissection.[26,38] This calls into question whether blood drawing, intravenous administration, blood pressure monitoring, and injections are proven to hasten the development of lymphedema. On the other hand, breaking the skin barrier, even during medical procedures, could theoretically predispose to infection, and blood pressure monitoring could cause soft tissue trauma. Data for any of the other arm and hand precautions are also intuitive and not evidence-based.

All patients after axillary dissection are instructed in the arm and hand care precautions, which may, however, be too severe for those at low risk and yet not aggressive enough for those at highest risk. Because lymphedema development may occur even several decades[39] after the axillary treatment, patients are admonished to follow these demanding precautions for the remainder of their lives.

LYMPHEDEMA TREATMENTS

Therapeutic nihilism (i.e., no treatment at all) is deplorable, although common. The fact that the average clinician is ill-prepared to recognize early signs of lymphedema must be remedied because the sooner the treatment is started, the less treatment is required to prevent further progression.

In the past, the treatment of established lymphedema has varied from none at all to a host of aggressive surgical procedures. Between the extremes are various combined conservative treatments, the most important of which are elevation, compression garments, centripetal massage and exercises, pneumatic compression devices, and the complete (or complex) decongestive physiotherapy (CDP) program.

Complete Decongestive Physiotherapy

CDP has been widely available in Europe for many years. The program was founded on the fact that lymphedema exists in an entire body quadrant, although it is most distressing in the arm or hand. The program includes skin care, gentle specific massage known as *manual lymph drainage* (MLD), low stretch multilayer compression bandaging (followed by a fitted compression garment when edema is reduced), and therapeutic exercises with the garment or bandages in place.

The modification and features of the various CDP programs by Vodder,[40] Leduc,[41] Foldi,[42] and Casley-Smith[43] have been reviewed in the 1998 American Cancer Society Workshop on Breast Cancer Treatment–Related Lymphedema. Although the principles followed are the same for each school, the massage techniques vary somewhat in the degree of pressure, motion, and timing of strokes. Additionally, the Leduc technique uses low intermittent pneumatic pressure (<40 mm Hg) pumps, and the Casley-Smith group uses benzopyrone medication.

A typical program is given below. CDP must be performed by skilled, specially trained therapists. During the treatment phase, the patient is given one or two daily 75 to 90 minute treatments over 1 to 4 weeks. In the maintenance phase, which is continued indefinitely, the patient maintains and optimizes the results by applying some of the techniques learned in the treatment phase, such as wearing an elastic sleeve during the day, bandaging (as described below) the affected limb overnight, and exercising for 15 minutes a day while wearing the bandages.

MLD, or manual lymph therapy, is a delicate massage technique that stimulates lymph vessels to contract more frequently and that directs and channels fluid toward adjacent, functioning lymph basins. MLD begins with stimulation of the lymph vessels and nodes in unaffected and opposite basins (neck, contralateral axilla, ipsilateral groin). Edema fluid and obstructed lymphatics are made to drain toward functioning lymph basins across the midline of the body, down toward the groin, over the top of the shoulder, around the back, and so forth. Finally, in segmented order, massage of the involved trunk, then shoulder, upper arm, forearm, wrist, and hand is performed. Multilayer low-stretch bandaging is done immediately after MLD. Bandages are wrapped from the fingertips to the axilla with maximal pressure distally and less pressure proximally. This is done by using many layers of minimally elastic cotton bandages, beneath which layers of foam rubber padding are inserted to ensure uniform pressure distribution or to increase pressure in areas that are particularly fibrotic. The bandaged patient is next guided through exercises involving active range of motion with the muscles and joints functioning within the closed space of the bandaging. Isometric exercise is generally avoided.

After volume reduction has been accomplished, well-fitted custom-made compressive garments (see next section) continue ongoing control of edema. The patient should be re-measured and the garment replaced every 3 months. The prescribed exercises continue in the low-stretch multilayer bandages, which are also worn overnight. The patient and family is trained to continue the maintenance program at home. Follow-up visits to the center usually take place at least at 6-month intervals.

Although this increasingly popular technique appears more successful in reversing lymphedema than other modalities, the availability of patient services and treatment centers that can practice CDP are limited. The patient availability[44] and the professional education for physical therapists[45] has been reviewed. The theory and clinical application of the four schools of manual lymphatic technique are reviewed in the American Cancer Society monograph by their representative faculty.[40-43]

Elevation and Elastic Garments

Although elevation is helpful in reducing swelling through use of gravity, it is impractical. A patient with lymphedema should be fitted with an elastic sleeve from wrist to axilla, if the edema is mild, or after swelling reduction, if the edema is moderate. A separate gauntlet or handpiece allows the patient to wash her hands without removing the sleeve.

The compression classes are as follows:

I. 20 to 30 mm Hg
II. 30 to 40 mm Hg
III. 40 to 50 mm Hg
IV. 50 to 60 mm Hg

For upper extremity lymphedema, a class II or III support is generally required. The person measuring the lymphedematous arm and hand should be specifically trained in fitting such garments and in instructing the patient in proper application. A statistically significant reduction in edema has been reported in women who wore garments for 6 consecutive hours per day.[46] Using these garments during exercise, physical activity, and air travel is recommended.

Pneumatic Pumps

The standard sequential system is a multichamber pump that delivers the compression at the same pressure in each garment section from distal to proximal tissues. The gradient sequential system delivers pressures that differ by approximately 10 mm Hg between each chamber, with the higher pressures delivered to the distal chamber. A minimum of 1 hour each pumping session with the arm elevated is required, and lower pressures for longer periods are more effective than higher pressures for a shorter time. Individualized and tailored pumping programs should be prescribed by a physical therapist, based on measurable efficacy and tolerability, as known by the serial assessment before the patient is placed on a home program.

The various devices have been reported in several controlled studies[47-49] to reduce lymphedema. Although theoretically attractive to use machinery for the pumping action on the arm lymphatics, pumping has not been as clinically effective as would be hoped. It has been hoped that pneumatic compression devices or "pumps" could duplicate the beneficial effects of massage.[50] However, the pumps force protein-rich edema fluid toward the shoulder but not through the axillary blockage. Rationale and controversies about pumps have been reviewed.[50,51]

MEDICATIONS

Diuretics are not effective in high-protein edemas such as lymphedema. Although the diuretics can temporarily mobilize water, the osmotic pressure from the increased protein in the interstitial space causes rapid re-accumulation of edema.

Benzopyrones belong to a group of drugs that include the bioflavonoids and the coumarins. The former occurs widely in nature, especially in fruits and vegetables. Benzopyrones may improve chronic lymphedema by stimulating macrophage activity for increased proteolysis and thereby removal of stagnant, excess protein in the tissue spaces, which results in less oncotic pressure and edema fluid. In 1993, a randomized, double-blind, placebo-controlled, crossover trial of 5,6-benzo-α-pyrone demonstrated its efficacy in an Australian study.[52] Although the effect was mild, it was statistically significant. However, in a similar study design, a larger number of breast cancer patients in an American multicenter study led by the Mayo Clinic were reported. No value was found with the benzopyrone beyond the placebo effect.[53] Furthermore, 6% of these study subjects had serious elevation of liver function tests.

REFERENCES

1. Hart SS, Meyerowitz BE, Apolone G, et al. Quality of life among mastectomy patients using external breast prostheses. *Tumori* 1997;83:581.
2. Reaby LL. Breast restoration decision making: enhancing the process. *Cancer Nurs* 1998;21:196.
3. Georgiade G, Georgiade N, McCarty KS Jr, Seigler HF. Rationale for immediate reconstruction of the breast following modified radical mastectomy. *Ann Plast Surg* 1982;8:20.
4. Khoo A, Kroll SS, Reece GP, et al. A comparison of resource costs of immediate and delayed breast reconstruction. *Plast Reconstr Surg* 1998;101:964.
5. Elliot LF, Hartrampf CR Jr. Breast reconstruction: progress in the past decade. *World J Surg* 1990;14:763.
6. Gruber RP, Kahn RA, Lash H, Maser MR. Breast reconstruction following mastectomy: a comparison of submuscular and subcutaneous techniques. *Plast Reconstr Surg* 1981;67:312.
7. Asplund O. Capsular contracture in silicone gel and saline filled breast implants after reconstruction. *Plast Reconstr Surg* 1984;73:270.
8. Disa JJ, Ad-El DD, Cohen SM, et al. The premature removal of tissue expanders in breast reconstruction. *Plast Reconstr Surg* 1999;104:1662.
9. Gabriel SE, O'Fallon WM, Kurland LT, et al. Risk of connective-tissue diseases and other disorders after breast implantation. *N Engl J Med* 1994;330:1697.
10. Bostwick J III, Scheflan M. The latissimus dorsi musculocutaneous flap: a one stage breast reconstruction. *Clin Plast Surg* 1980;7:71.
11. Hartrampf CR, Scheflan M, Black PW. Breast reconstruction with a transverse abdominal island flap. *Plast Reconstr Surg* 1982;69:216.
12. Grotting JC, Urist MM, Maddox WA, Vasconez LO. Conventional TRAM flap versus free microsurgical TRAM flap for immediate breast reconstruction. *Plast Reconstr Surg* 1989; 83:828.
13. Kroll SS, Netscher DT. Complications of TRAM flap breast reconstruction in obese patients. *Plast Reconstr Surg* 1989;84:886.
14. Hidalgo DA, Disa JJ, Cordeiro PG, Hu Q. A review of 716 consecutive free flaps for oncologic surgical defects: refinement in donor-site selection and technique. *Plast Reconstr Surg* 1998;102:722.
15. Schusterman MA, Kroll SS, Miller MJ, et al. The free transverse rectus abdominus musculocutaneous flap for breast reconstruction: one center's experience with 211 consecutive cases. *Ann Plast Surg* 1994;32:234.
16. Kind GM, Rademaker AW, Mustoe TA. Abdominal-wall recovery following TRAM flap: a functional outcome study. *Plast Reconstr Surg* 1997;99:417.
17. Reece GP, Kroll SS. Abdominal wall complications: prevention and treatment. *Clin Plast Surg* 1998;25:235.
18. Disa JJ, Petrek JA. Surgical management after local failure in the irradiated breast. *Semin Breast Dis* 1999;2:252.
19. Schuster RH, Kuske RR, Young VL, Fineberg B. Breast reconstruction in women treated with radiation therapy for breast cancer: cosmesis, complications, and tumor control. *Plast Reconstr Surg* 1992;90:445.
20. Kroll SS, Schusterman MA, Reece GP, et al. Breast reconstruction with myocutaneous flaps in previously irradiated patients. *Plast Reconstr Surg* 1994;93:460.
21. Williams JK, Bostwick J III, Bried JT, et al. TRAM flap breast reconstruction after radiation treatment. *Ann Surg* 1995;221:756.
22. Williams JK, Carlson GW, Bostwick J III, et al. The effects of radiation treatment after TRAM flap breast reconstruction. *Plast Reconstr Surg* 1997;100:1153.
23. Hidalgo DA, Borgen PJ, Petrek JA, et al. Immediate reconstruction after complete skin-sparing mastectomy with autologous tissue. *J Am Coll Surg* 1998;187:17.
24. Toth BA, Forley BG, Calabria R. Retrospective study of skin-sparing mastectomy in breast reconstruction. *Plast Reconstr Surg* 1999;104:77.

25. Carlson GW, Bostwick J III, Styblo TM, et al. Skin-sparing mastectomy: oncologic and reconstructive considerations. *Ann Surg* 1997;225:570.
26. Petrek JA, Heelan MC. Incidence of breast carcinoma-related lymphedema. *Cancer* 1998;83:2776.
27. Werner RS, McCormick B, Petrek JA, et al. Arm edema in conservatively managed breast cancer: obesity is a major predictive factor. *Ther Radiol* 1991;180:177.
28. Dewar JA, Sarrazin D, Benhamou E, et al. Management of the axilla in conservatively treated breast cancer: 592 patients treated at Institut Gustave-Roussy. *Int J Radiat Oncol Biol Phys* 1987;13:475.
29. Meek AG. Breast radiotherapy and lymphedema. *Cancer* 1998;83:2788.
30. Delouche G, Bachelot F, Premont M, et al. Conservation treatment of early breast cancer: long term results and complications. *Int J Radiat Oncol Biol Phys* 1987;13:29.
31. Pezner RD, Patterson MP, Hill LR, et al. Arm lymphedema in patients treated conservatively for breast cancer: relationship to patient age and axillary node dissection technique. *Int J Radiat Oncol Biol Phys* 1986;12:2079.
32. Kissin MW, Querci della Rovere G, Easton D, et al. Risk of lymphoedema following the treatment of breast cancer. *Br J Surg* 1986;73:580.
33. Ivens D, Hoe AL, Podd CR, et al. Assessment of morbidity from complete axillary dissection. *Br J Cancer* 1992;66:136.
34. Larson D, Weinstein M, Goldberg I, et al. Edema of the arm as a function of the extent of axillary surgery in patients with stage I–II carcinoma of the breast treated with primary radiotherapy. *Int J Radiat Oncol Biol Phys* 1986;12:1575.
35. Tadych K, Donegan WL. Postmastectomy seromas and wound drainage. *Surg Gynecol Obstet* 1987;165:483.
36. West JP, Ellison JB. A study of the causes and prevention of edema of the arm following radical mastectomy. *Surg Gynecol Obstet* 1959;109:359.
37. Bourgeois P, Leduc O, Leduc A. Imaging techniques in the upper management and prevention of posttherapeutic upper limb edemas. *Cancer* 1998;83:2805.
38. Mortimer PS, Bates SO, Brassington HD, et al. The prevalence of arm lymphedema following treatment for breast cancer. *QJM* 1996;89:377.
39. Brennan MJ, Weitz J. Lymphedema 30 years after radical mastectomy. *Am J Phys Med Rehabil* 1992;71:12.
40. Kasseroller RG. The Vodder school: the Vodder method. *Cancer* 1998;83:2840.
41. Leduc O, Leduc A, Bourgeois P, Belgrado JP. The physical treatment of upper limb edema. *Cancer* 1998;83:2835.
42. Foldi E. The treatment of lymphedema. *Cancer* 1998;83:2833.
43. Casley-Smith JR, Boris M, Weindorf S, Lasinski B. Treatment for lymphedema of the arm—the Casley-Smith method: a noninvasive method produces continued reduction. *Cancer* 1998;83:2843.
44. Thiadens SRJ. Current status of education and treatment resources for lymphedema. *Cancer* 1998;83:2864.
45. Augustine E, Corn M, Danoff J. Lymphedema management training for physical therapy students in the United States. *Cancer* 1998;83:2869.
46. Bertelli G, Venturini M, Forno G, et al. An analysis of prognostic factors in response to conservative treatment of postmastectomy lymphedema. *Surg Gynecol Obstet* 1992;175:455.
47. Pappas CJ, O'Donnell TF Jr. Long-term results of compression treatment for lymphedema. *J Vasc Surg* 1992;16:555.
48. Richmond DM, O'Donnell TF Jr, Zelikovski A. Sequential pneumatic compression for lymphedema: a controlled trial. *Arch Surg* 1985;120:1116.
49. Zanolla R, Monzeglio C, Balzarini A, et al. Evaluation of the results of three different methods of postmastectomy lymphedema treatment. *J Surg Oncol* 1984;26:210.
50. Brennan MJ, Miller LT. Overview of treatment options and review of the current role and use of compression garments, intermittent pumps, and exercise in the management of lymphedema. *Cancer* 1998;83:2821.
51. Rinehart-Ayres ME. Conservative approaches to lymphedema treatment. *Cancer* 1998; 83:2828.
52. Casley-Smith JR, Morgan RG, Piller NB. Treatment of lymphedema of the arms and legs with 5,6-benzo-pyrone. *N Engl J Med* 1993;16:1158.
53. Loprinzi CL, Kugler JW, Sloan JA, et al. Lack of effect of coumarin in women with lymphedema after treatment for breast cancer. *N Engl J Med* 1999;340:346.

CHAPTER 38

Cancer of the Endocrine System

SECTION 1

TERRY C. LAIRMORE
SAMUEL A. WELLS, JR.
JEFFREY F. MOLEY

Molecular Biology of Endocrine Tumors

The transformation of a cell from the normal to the malignant phenotype is a result of a stepwise accumulation of genetic defects that render the cell unresponsive to or independent of normal cellular growth signals. Defects in a variety of oncogenes and tumor suppressor genes have been described in endocrine neoplasms. Characterization of these specific molecular defects has yielded insight into the mechanisms of tumorigenesis in these tissues and, in some cases, provided clinically applicable diagnostic or prognostic information. Identification of the germline mutations associated with the multiple endocrine neoplasia types 1 and 2 (MEN 1, MEN 2) syndromes has led to the advent of direct DNA testing for individuals at risk. In patients with a hereditary form of medullary thyroid carcinoma (MTC), early thyroidectomy may be performed on the basis of DNA mutational analysis at a time when the MTC is occult and likely curable. Finally, the molecular defects that occur in tumors arising in the familial endocrine neoplasia syndromes have been found to play an important role in tumorigenesis of sporadic neoplasms arising in the same endocrine tissues.

MULTIPLE ENDOCRINE NEOPLASIA SYNDROMES

MULTIPLE ENDOCRINE NEOPLASIA TYPE 1

Clinical Features

MEN 1 is characterized by the development of parathyroid hyperplasia, neuroendocrine tumors of the pancreas and duodenum, and adenomas of the anterior pituitary gland.[1] In addition, affected patients develop bronchial and thymic carcinoids, benign thyroid and adrenocortical tumors, subcutaneous lipomas, cutaneous angiofibromas,[2] and spinal ependymomas[3] with increased frequency. More than 90% of patients inheriting a *MEN1* gene mutation develop hyperparathyroidism (HPT) by the second or third decade of life. Depending on the method of study, 35% to 75% of mutation carriers develop neuroendocrine tumors of the pancreas and duodenum that are frequently malignant. The neuroendocrine tumors in patients with MEN 1 result in symptoms due to either excess secretion of a specific hormone product or the effects of the tumoral process itself. The malignant duodenopancreatic tumors and intrathoracic tumors account for the majority of the disease-related morbidity and mortality in *MEN1* gene mutation carriers.[4,5]

Genetics

MEN1 TUMOR SUPPRESSOR GENE. In 1988, the *MEN1* predisposition gene was mapped to chromosome 11q13 by a combination of studies of the loss of chromosome sequences in tumor DNA and genetic linkage analysis using markers from chromosome 11.[6] The frequent occurrence of chromosome deletions encompassing the 11q13 interval in tumor DNA supports the hypothesis that the *MEN1* gene is a classic tumor suppressor gene. The normal protein encoded by a tumor suppressor gene is presumed to function as a negative control or "brake" on unregulated cellular growth and proliferation, such that complete elimination of its function by mutation or deletion of both homologous copies would be expected to result in unregulated cell growth. The multifocal involvement characteristically observed in affected endocrine tissues presumably reflects the chance occurrence of multiple "second hits."

The *MEN1* tumor suppressor gene encodes a predicted 610–amino acid protein product termed *menin.*[7] The structure of the *MEN1* gene consists of ten exons, with the first exon being untranslated. The 2.8-kilobase menin messenger RNA (mRNA) transcript is ubiquitously expressed and may be detected in lymphocytes, thymus, pancreas, thyroid, the gonads, and other tissues. Similar to the protein products of most previously described tumor suppressor genes, evidence has been provided that menin is a nuclear protein.[8]

The diverse array of reported *MEN1* mutations includes missense, nonsense, frameshift, and mRNA splicing defects that are distributed throughout the nine coding exons as well as the intervening intronic sequences. The *MEN1* gene mutations in a series of 25 separate kindreds with MEN 1 are depicted graphically in Figure 38.1-1. To date, more than 100 germline *MEN1* mutations have been reported in the literature,[7,9–16] and there are almost as many distinct mutations as there are separate families. Approximately two-thirds of the reported mutations in the *MEN1* gene result in truncation of the C-terminal portion of the menin protein. No specific genotype-phenotype correlations have been established to date.

CELLULAR BIOLOGY OF MENIN PROTEIN PRODUCT. The precise role of menin in the regulation of cell growth has yet to be elucidated. Menin binds to the JunD transcriptional regulation factor and may function to inhibit JunD-activated transcription.[17] The nucleotide sequence of menin is highly conserved, with an overall homology of 97% between the human and murine genes.[18] In the mouse embryo, *MEN1* expression appears as early as gestational day 7 and ultimately is detectable at high levels in diverse tissue, including testis and the central nervous system. These findings support a broad role for the menin protein product in regulating cell growth that is not limited to the tissues affected in MEN 1. Lymphocytes from patients with a heterozygous germline mutation in the *MEN1* gene have been shown to exhibit increased premature centromere division in cell culture when exposed to an alkylating agent.[19] The finding of increased chromosomal instability suggests that the *MEN1* gene product may normally function in part to maintain the integrity of DNA.

MULTIPLE ENDOCRINE NEOPLASIA TYPE 2 SYNDROMES

Clinical Features

The MEN 2 syndromes include MEN 2A, MEN 2B, and familial, non-MEN medullary thyroid carcinoma (FMTC). These syndromes are inherited in an autosomal dominant fashion and are caused by germline mutations in the *RET* protooncogene. The most consistent feature of MEN 2 syndromes is MTC, which is multifocal, bilateral, and usually occurs at a young age (Fig. 38.1-2). There is almost complete penetrance of MTC in these syndromes; almost all persons who inherit the disease allele develop MTC. Other features of the syndromes are variably expressed, with incomplete penetrance. These features are summarized in Table 38.1-1.

MTCs are derived from the thyroid C cells, also called *parafollicular cells,* which migrate from the neural crest. C cells comprise 1% of the total thyroid mass and are dispersed throughout the gland, with the highest concentration in the upper poles (Fig. 38.1-3). The C cells are so named because of their unique ability to secrete the hormone calcitonin. Calcitonin is a specific tumor marker for MTC. It is extremely useful in the screening of individuals predisposed to the hereditary forms of the disease and in the follow-up of patients who have been treated. C cells also are capable of secreting other hormones, including carcinoembryonic antigen.

Patients with MEN 2A develop multifocal, bilateral MTC, associated with C-cell hyperplasia. Approximately 42% of affected patients develop pheochromocytomas, which may also be multifocal and bilateral and usually are associated with adrenal medullary hyperplasia. HPT develops in 25% to 35% of patients and is due to hyperplasia, which may be asymmetric, with one or more glands becoming enlarged.[20] Parathyroid carcinoma has been

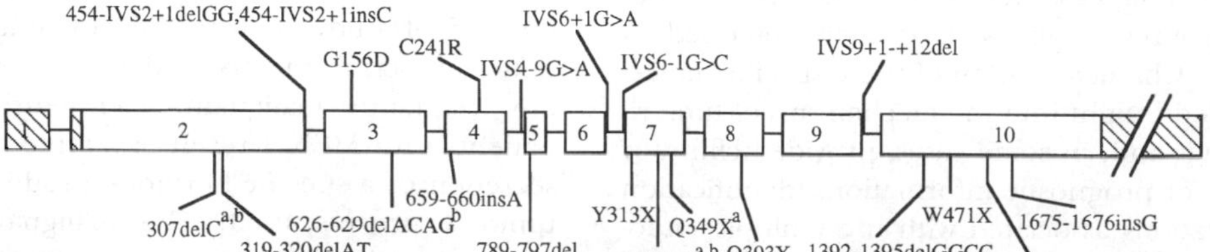

FIGURE 38.1-1. Germline mutations in the *MEN1* gene in a set of 25 independent kindreds. The mutations are distributed throughout the nine coding exons of the gene. Five splicing defects and two missense mutations are depicted above the *MEN1* gene, and seven nonsense and six frameshift mutations are depicted below the *MEN1* gene. The position of the mutation is reported as the codon in which it occurs relative to the open reading frame. The position of the splicing defects are reported as the number of bases 3' or 5' to the nearest exon [(+) indicates 3' direction and (–) indicates 5' direction relative to the exon]. For the deletions, insertions, and splicing defects, uppercase letters refer to exon nucleotides and lowercase letters refer to intron nucleotides. [a]Previously reported mutations; [b]mutations that occur in more than one family. (Reprinted from ref. 16, with permission.)

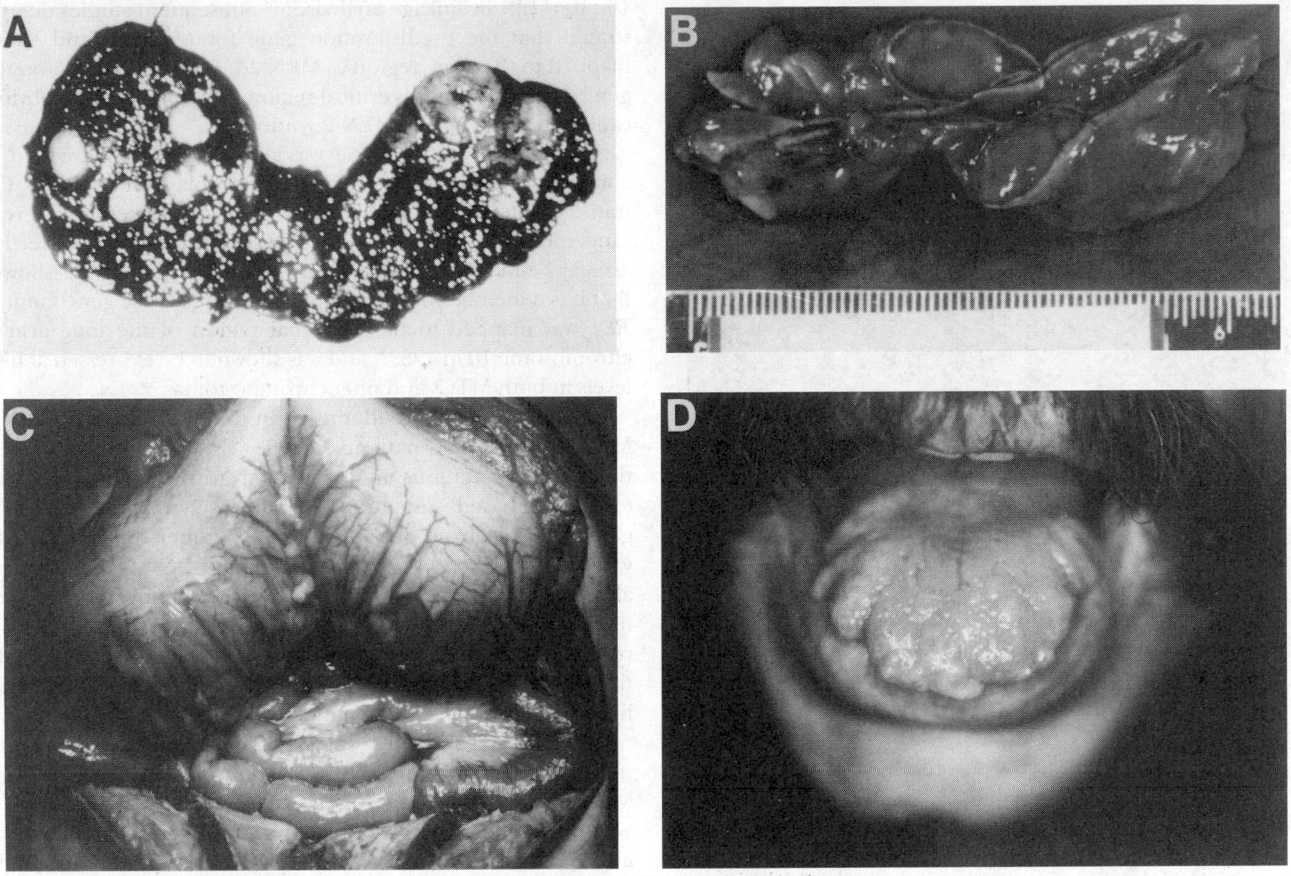

FIGURE 38.1-2. Features of patients with hereditary medullary thyroid carcinoma (MTC). **A:** Bisected thyroid gland from a patient with multiple endocrine neoplasia type 2A (MEN 2A), showing multicentric, bilateral foci of MTC. **B:** Adrenalectomy specimen from patient with multiple endocrine neoplasia type 2B (MEN 2B), demonstrating pheochromocytoma. **C:** Megacolon in patient with MEN 2B. **D:** Midface and tongue of patient with MEN 2B, showing characteristic tongue notching secondary to plexiform neuromas. (**A** courtesy of Dr. S. A. Wells. **B–D** courtesy of Dr. R. Thompson. Reprinted from JF Moley, Medullary thyroid carcinoma. In: Clark O, Duh Q-Y, eds. *Textbook of endocrine surgery*. Philadelphia: WB Saunders, 1997, with permission.)

reported in one patient with MEN 2A.[21] Cutaneous lichen amyloidosis has been described in some patients with MEN 2A.[22] In this entity, macular amyloidosis presents as brownish plaques of multiple tiny papules, usually in the interscapular area. Microscopically, these lesions demonstrate a hyperplastic epidermis, acanthosis, lymphocytic infiltrate, and amyloid goblets. Hirschsprung's disease is infrequently associated with MEN 2A.[23–25] This disease is characterized by the absence of autonomic ganglion cells within the distal colonic parasympathetic plexus, resulting in obstruction and megacolon.

TABLE 38.1-1. Clinical Features of Sporadic MTC, MEN 2A, MEN 2B, and FMTC

Clinical Setting	*Features of MTC*	*Inheritance Pattern*	*Associated Abnormalities*	*Genetic Defect*
Sporadic MTC	Unifocal	None	None	Somatic *RET* mutations in >20% of tumors
MEN 2A	Multifocal, bilateral	Autosomal dominant	Pheochromocytomas, hyperparathyroidism	Germline missense mutations in extracellular cysteine codons of *RET*
MEN 2B	Multifocal, bilateral	Autosomal dominant	Pheochromocytomas, mucosal neuromas, megacolon, skeletal abnormalities	Germline missense mutation in tyrosine kinase domain of *RET*
FMTC	Multifocal, bilateral	Autosomal dominant	None	Germline missense mutations in extracellular or intracellular cysteine codons of *RET*

FMTC, familial, non-MEN medullary thyroid carcinoma; MEN 2A, multiple endocrine neoplasia type 2A; MEN 2B, multiple endocrine neoplasia type 2B; MTC, medullary thyroid carcinoma.
(Adapted from JF Moley, Medullary thyroid carcinoma. In: Clark O, Duh Q-Y, eds. *Textbook of endocrine surgery*. Philadelphia: WB Saunders, 1997, with permission.)

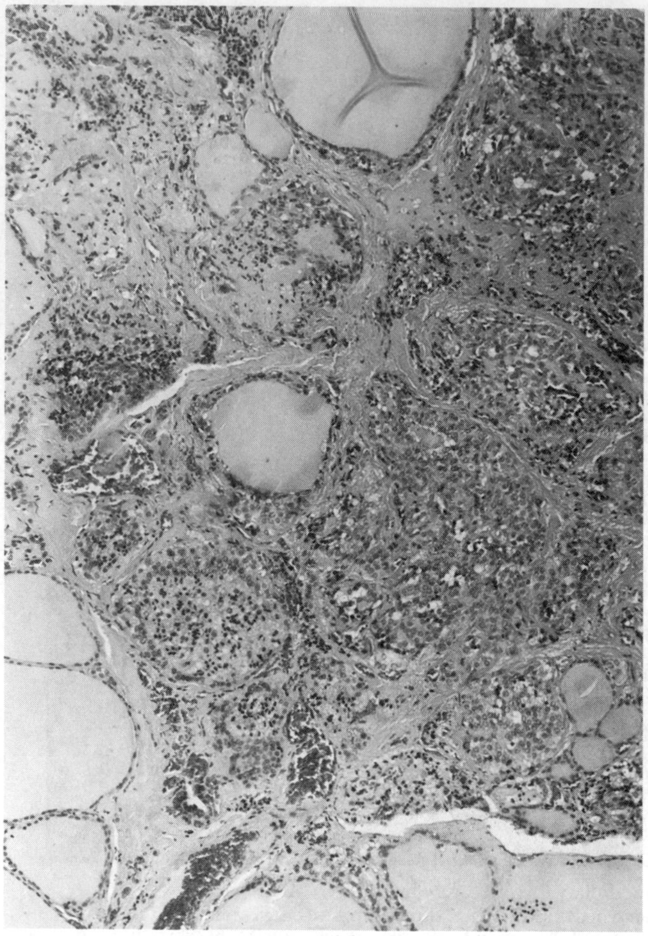

FIGURE 38.1-3. Photomicrograph of medullary thyroid carcinoma showing nests and sheets of small, uniform cells with scant to moderate amounts of amphophilic cytoplasm infiltrating around normal thyroid follicles. (Reprinted from Moley JF, Lairmore TC, Phay JE, Hereditary endocrinopathies. *Curr Probl Surg* 1999;36:653, with permission.)

In MEN 2B, 40% to 50% of patients develop pheochromocytomas, and all individuals develop neural gangliomas, particularly in the mucosa of the digestive tract, conjunctiva, lips, and tongue. MEN 2B patients also have megacolon, skeletal abnormalities, and markedly enlarged peripheral nerves. MEN 2B patients do not develop HPT. MTC develops at a very young age (infancy) and appears to be the most aggressive form of hereditary MTC, although its aggressiveness may be related more to the extremely early age of onset than to the biologic virulence of the tumor. MTC in MEN 2B is rarely curable.

FMTC is characterized by the development of MTC without any other endocrinopathies.[26] MTC in these patients has a later age of onset and follows a more indolent clinical course than MTC in patients with MEN 2A and MEN 2B. Occasional patients with FMTC never manifest clinical evidence of MTC (symptoms or a lump in the neck), though biochemical testing and histologic evaluation of the thyroid usually demonstrates MTC.

Genetics

THE *RET* PROTOONCOGENE. In 1987, the gene for MEN 2A was localized to the pericentromeric region of chromosome 10 (10q11.2) by linkage analysis.[27,28] Subsequent studies demonstrated that the predisposition gene for MEN 2B and FMTC mapped to the same region as MEN 2A.[29,30] The *RET* protooncogene resides within this critical region, which made it an obvious candidate gene for the MEN 2 syndromes.

The *RET* protooncogene was first discovered based on its ability to transform mouse NIH 3T3 fibroblasts in culture.[31] The transforming *RET* sequences first identified represented a rearrangement of *RET* that occurred *in vitro* during the transfection assay.[32] Sequence analysis of the *RET* protooncogene showed that it is a member of the receptor tyrosine kinase gene family.[33] *RET* was mapped to the proximal region of the long arm of chromosome 10 in 1989[34] and was shown to be expressed at high levels in both MTCs and pheochromocytomas.[35]

RET mutations were identified in the constitutional DNA of MEN 2A and FMTC patients in 1993.[36,37] Mulligan et al.[36] identified *RET* mutations in association with MEN 2 using an expression-based mutational analysis system. Analysis of genomic DNA from MEN 2A family members proved that the variants identified in the complementary DNAs (cDNAs) were also in the constitutional DNA of affected family members and not in individuals unaffected by MEN 2A. All mutations resulted in substitution of cysteine residues clustered near the transmembrane domain of *RET*. In all but one, MEN 2A tumor heterozygosity for the mutant and wild-type *RET* allele was retained. Mulligan et al.[36] suggested a dominant or dominant-negative mechanism for *RET* mutation in the development of MTC and pheochromocytomas in MEN 2A.[36]

Donis-Keller et al.[37] used single-strand conformational variant (SSCV) and sequence analysis to identify mutations in *RET* in the constitutional DNA of patients with MEN 2A and FMTC. Both MEN 2A and FMTC were shown to be associated with mutations that result in substitution of cysteine residues in the extracellular portion of *RET* immediately adjacent to the transmembrane domain. Unexpectedly, the same mutations were found to characterize MEN 2A and FMTC kindreds.

Subsequent investigations demonstrated mutations of *RET* in MEN 2B patients.[38,39] In 95% of cases of MEN 2B, the *RET* protooncogene mutation is a missense methionine-to-threonine (ATG to ACG) change at codon 918 in exon 16. This codon is positioned within the tyrosine kinase catalytic core of the intracellular domain. Two families with MEN 2B have been described that have a codon 883 mutation in the tyrosine kinase domain of *RET*.[40]

More than 30 missense mutations have been described in MEN 2A and FMTC kindreds (Table 38.1-2).[41,42] Most of these mutations result in nonconservative changes in cysteine residues, although changes in Glu, Val, Met, Leu, and Tyr have also been described. Several of these mutations have been shown to result in "gain-of-function" in the *RET* protein product, with increased intrinsic tyrosine kinase activity or alterations of substrate recognition (or both) and transforming capability.[43] The *RET* protooncogene encodes a protein with three domains: a cysteine-rich extracellular receptor domain, a hydrophobic transmembrane domain, and an intracellular tyrosine kinase catalytic domain (Fig. 38.1-4). The *RET* gene consists of at least 20 exons[44] and is expressed as five major mRNA species.[45,46] The *RET* gene product is expressed in a limited number of cell types in the normal individual, including the thyroid C cells, the adrenal medulla, and parts of the brain. The gene is important in the embryonic development of the enteric nervous system and the kidneys.[47]

TABLE 38.1-2. *RET* Mutations in Hereditary Medullary Thyroid Carcinoma

	Missense Germline Mutations in the RET Protooncogene	
Syndrome	Exon	Codon
MEN 2A, FMTC	10	609
		611
		618
		620
	11	631[a]
		634
	13	790
		791
FMTC	11	630
	13	768
	14	804
		844[a]
	15	891
MEN 2B	16	918
		883

FMTC, familial, non-MEN medullary thyroid carcinoma; MEN 2A, multiple endocrine neoplasia type 2A; MEN 2B, multiple endocrine neoplasia type 2B.
[a]Clinical features not yet characterized.
(Reprinted from Moley JF, Lairmore TC, Phay JE. Hereditary endocrinopathies. *Curr Probl Surg* 1999;36:653, with permission.)

Glial-derived neurotrophic factor (GDNF) and neurturin are ligands to the receptor domain of the *RET* gene product.[48–54] GDNF is a 32-kD protein dimer that was first purified from glial cell lines and is a potent neurotrophic survival factor for motor neurons. A glycophosphatidylinositol-linked protein called *GDNF receptor-a* (GDNFR-α) is a cofactor in the signaling heterodimeric complex with *RET*. Current evidence suggests that GDNF binds directly to GDNFR-α and indirectly with *RET*. When triggered by ligand, wild-type *RET* dimerizes with another *RET* molecule, and this dimerization is responsible for phosphorylation and activation of the tyrosine kinase domain, with subsequent downstream signal transduction events. *RET* molecules that contain MEN 2A-type mutations are constitutively dimerized and therefore activated. In contrast, the mutation responsible for MEN 2B does not result in constitutive dimerization but changes the substrate specificity of the tyrosine kinase domain, which results in transformation.

OTHER *RET* GENOTYPE-PHENOTYPE CORRELATIONS

Cutaneous Lichen Amyloidosis. Interscapular lesions of cutaneous lichen amyloidosis (CLA) have been described in several families with MEN 2A.[22] The total number of patients described with this entity is fewer than 100. In a 634→Tyr mutation was reported in one family with MEN 2A and CLA, and in two other families, a 634→Arg mutation was described that segregated with both *MEN2A* and CLA.[55]

Hyperparathyroidism. HPT in MEN 2A is caused by parathyroid hyperplasia; the hypercalcemia is mild and often asymptomatic. HPT clusters in some families with MEN 2A. Whether specific *MEN2A* mutations are associated with a higher incidence of HPT remains controversial. Mulligan et al.[56] previously described a strong correlation between C634R mutation and HPT in families with MEN 2A, but other studies have been unable to confirm this relationship definitively.[57–59]

Hirschsprung's Disease. Hirschsprung's disease is characterized by absence of autonomic ganglion cells within the distal colonic parasympathetic plexus, resulting in obstruction and proximal megacolon. Approximately 80% of Hirschsprung's disease cases are sporadic, and the remainder are familial. A subset of familial Hirschsprung's cases have been found to be associated with germline mutations of *RET*.[24,56] Most of these are inactivating and loss-

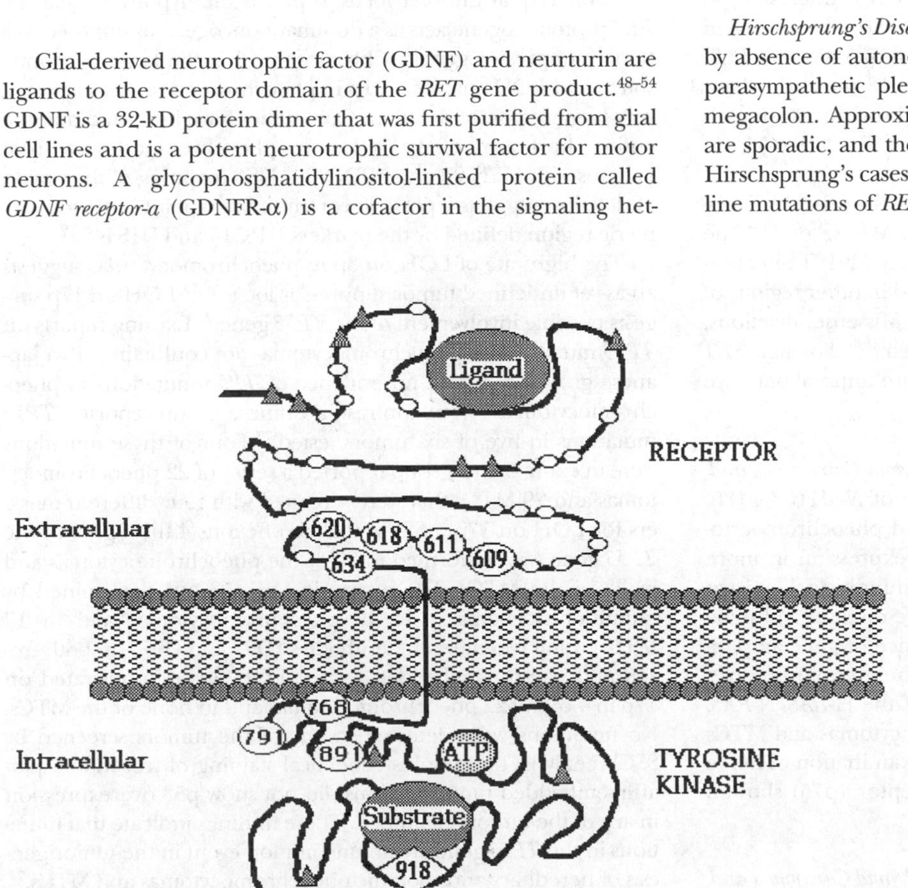

FIGURE 38.1-4. Diagram of *RET* gene product delineating locations of germline mutations found in multiple endocrine neoplasia type 2A and familial, non-MEN medullary thyroid carcinoma (*ovals*), germline mutations in multiple endocrine neoplasia type 2B (*diamond*), and mutations in hereditary Hirschsprung's disease (*triangles*). As mentioned in the text, the *RET* gene product is thought to create a dimer that forms a complex with glial-derived neurotrophic factor receptor-α or neurturin. The *RET* gene product is divided into the intracellular, transmembrane, and extracellular domains. ATP, adenosine triphosphate. (Adapted from Moley JF, Kim S, *Molecular genetics in surgical oncology.* Austin: RG Landes, 1994, with permission.)

TABLE 38.1-3. Loss of Heterozygosity in Pheochromocytomas and Medullary Thyroid Carcinomas

Study	*Chromosomal Arms Tested*	*LOH in Pheos (No. LOH/No. Informative)*	*LOH in MTCs (No. LOH/No. Informative)*
Khosla et al.[178]	1p, 2p, 3p, 5q, 10q, 13q, 16p, 17p, 17q, 22q	1p-13/31, 2p-1/34, 3p-4/24, 10q-1/22, 17p-7/27, 22q-5/18	1p-1/11, 22-1/7
Moley et al.[69]	1p, 1q	1p-12/18 (9/9 from MEN 2A and 2B patients)	1p-3/24
Yang et al.[179]	1p	1p-5/8	
Mathew et al.[180]	1p, 1q, 5, 6, 7, 11, 12	1p-4/6	1p-3/8
Shin et al.[181]	1p, 22q	1p-12/22, 22q-8/20	
Mulligan et al.[70]	1-22, both arms	1p-15/25, 3p-10/18, 3q-9/15, 5q-1/7, 6q-1/7, 8p-1/8, 11p-3/19, 11q-2/23, 13-2/17, 17p-3/20, 17q-1/20, 22-8/20	1p-7/28, 3p-1/19, 3q-2/14, 7p-1/17, 10p-1/18, 10q-1/25, 11p-1/16, 13-2/22, 15-1/9, 21-1/8, 22-4/22
Dou et al.[73]	2-23	3q-13/13 F, 6/8 S, 21q-4/6 F, 2/7 S, 22q-7/13 F, 1/10 S, 11q-2/6 F, 3/7 S	3q-2/7 F, 1/8 S, 22q-4/15 F, 2/8 S
Herfarth et al.[74]	17p	17p-4/22	17p-0/14

F, familial (MEN 2A and 2B); LOH, loss of heterozygosity; MEN 2A, multiple endocrine neoplasia type 2A; MEN 2B, multiple endocrine neoplasia type 2B; MTCs, medullary thyroid carcinomas; Pheos, pheochromocytomas; S, sporadic (MEN 2A and 2B).
Note: If arm tested is not listed in LOH column, LOH was not found.
(Adapted from J Moley, Molecular events in the development and progression of medullary thyroid cancer and pheochromocytoma. In: Nelkin B, ed., *Genetic mechanisms in multiple endocrine neoplasia type 2.* Austin: RG Landes, 1996, with permission.)

of-function (frameshift and nonsense) mutations and are not associated with the MEN 2A phenotype. Several families, however, have been described in which Hirschsprung's disease cosegregates with either *MEN2A* or *FMTC* (missense codon 618 or 620 mutations).[60] Additionally, a few Hirschsprung's disease patients have been described with missense mutations in codon 609 or 620 who have no evidence of MEN 2A or MTC.[23,25,56] It is interesting to note that the Hirschsprung's disease phenotype can be associated with either loss-of-function or gain-of-function mutations of *RET*. All patients with MEN 2B (missense codon 918 mutation) have megacolon and chronic colonic motility disturbances, though they usually do not require surgery for this (see Fig. 38.1-2*C*).[61]

RET Mutations in Sporadic Tumors. Mutations in the *RET* protooncogene have also been found in sporadic MTCs.[37,40,62–64] The most frequent mutation in sporadic MTCs is the M918T mutation found in MEN 2B. Mutations have been found in other regions of the extracellular and intracellular domains. Missense, deletions, and insertion mutations have been described.[41,65] Somatic *RET* mutations in sporadic pheochromocytomas are unusual but have also been described.[41]

Other Dominant Oncogenes in Medullary Thyroid Carcinomas and Pheochromocytomas. Absence of amplification of *N-MYC, C-MYC,* and *ERB-B2* has been reported in MTCs and pheochromocytomas. Roncalli et al.[66] reported that N-myc expression in more than 10% of tumor cells, as detected by immunohistochemistry, was associated with poorer survival, sporadic disease, and male gender. These investigators found no evidence of gene amplification and did not determine the basis for the overexpression.[66] Our group reported absence of mutation of the H-*RAS*, N-*RAS*, and K-*RAS* genes in a series of pheochromocytomas and MTCs analyzed by direct sequencing.[67] Likewise, examination of nerve growth factor and nerve growth factor receptor (p75) showed no abnormality at the DNA or RNA levels.[68]

Other Tumor Suppressor Genes in Medullary Thyroid Carcinoma and Pheochromocytoma. Several studies have evaluated loss of heterozygosity (LOH) at tumor suppressor loci in pheochromocytomas and MTCs; these are summarized in Table 38.1-3. The cumulative data indicate a higher-than-background incidence of LOH in pheochromocytomas on chromosome arms 1p, 3p, 17p, and 22q.[69,70] In MTCs, the report by Mulligan et al.[70] suggests a significant incidence of 1p LOH; however, evaluation of other chromosomal arms yielded no consistent findings. Lack of significant LOH on 10q, at the *RET* locus, supports the hypothesis that the *RET* protooncogene acts as a dominant oncogene as opposed to a tumor suppressor gene.[71] Chromosome 1 is the largest chromosome, and LOH analysis on 1p in pheochromocytomas suggests a very large region of deletion. Our studies have indicated that the entire short arm of 1p is lost in pheochromocytomas from patients with MEN 2A and MEN 2B.[69] Fine mapping of the region of deletion suggests a possible common breakpoint in the centromeric region defined by the markers D1S514 and D1S442.[72]

The high rate of LOH on 3p in pheochromocytomas suggests an as-yet undefined tumor suppressor locus.[70,73] LOH on 17p suggests possible involvement of the *TP53* gene.[74] Existing reports on *TP53* mutations in pheochromocytomas are conflicting. Two Japanese groups reported no evidence of *TP53* mutations in pheochromocytomas.[75,76] In contrast, a Chinese group reported *TP53* mutations in five of six tumors tested.[77] Four of these mutations were in exon 4. Our group reported a series of 22 pheochromocytomas and 29 MTCs that were screened with four different markers for LOH on 17p.[74] SSCV analysis of exons 4 through 9 of the *TP53* gene was performed in 20 of the pheochromocytomas and in 22 of the MTCs. The expression of p53 was determined by immunohistochemistry in 19 pheochromocytomas and in 17 MTCs, using two different antibodies (D01 and D07) on both frozen and paraffin-embedded tissues. LOH was demonstrated on 17p in 4 of the 22 pheochromocytomas and in none of the MTCs. No mutations were detected in any of the tumors screened by SSCV analysis. Immunohistochemical staining of frozen and paraffin-embedded tumor sections did not show p53 overexpression in any of the tumors examined. These findings indicate that mutations in the *TP53* gene are an uncommon event in the tumorigenesis of hereditary and sporadic pheochromocytomas and MTCs.[74]

Pheochromocytomas also occur in neurofibromatosis type 1 (NF1) and von Hippel-Lindau (VHL) disease, both of which are caused by mutations in tumor suppressor genes. *NF1* gene expression was decreased or absent in 7 of 20 pheochromocytomas from patients with MEN 2 and sporadic disease.[78] Because *NF1* is ubiquitously expressed, its lack of expression indicates that *NF1* may play a role in the development or progression of pheochromocytomas from patients who do not have NF1. Because of the extremely large size of the *NF1* gene, mutational analysis has not yet been performed. Mutational analysis of the *VHL* gene in non-VHL pheochromocytomas has not been reported.

There have been no reports of the involvement of DNA repair genes (*MLH1, MSH2*) in development or progression of pheochromocytomas or MTCs, and replication error or repeats have not been a consistent finding in these tumors (J. F. Moley, unpublished data).

Preventive Surgery for MEN 2A *Gene Carriers*

Individuals with MEN 2A and FMTC are virtually certain to develop MTC at some point in their lives (usually before age 30 years). Therefore, at-risk family members who are found to have inherited a *RET* gene mutation are candidates for thyroidectomy, regardless of their stimulated plasma calcitonin levels. In a series from Washington University in St. Louis, Wells et al.[79] reported the performance of preventive surgery in 13 asymptomatic *RET* mutation carriers. One hundred thirty-two individuals from seven different kindreds affected by MEN 2A were screened. Of the 132 individuals, 48 had an established diagnosis of MEN 2A, and 58 were at 50% risk for inheriting the disease but had no clinical evidence of endocrine neoplasia. Twenty-six unaffected spouses of MEN 2A kindred members served as controls. All individuals were evaluated for the presence of *RET* gene mutations. PCR- and sequence-based direct mutation analysis of genomic DNA from the 58 individuals at 50% risk for MEN 2A identified 21 individuals who had inherited a *RET* mutation associated with disease. The other thirty-seven family members had two normal *RET* alleles. All 26 unaffected control individuals had normal *RET* alleles. After meeting with genetic counselors, who informed them of the pattern of disease inheritance and the basis for the genetic tests, total thyroidectomy was offered to all 21 individuals who were found to have inherited a *RET* mutation. The patients ranged in age from 6 to 21 years (mean, 13.2 years). In 12 of the 21 patients (mean age, 12 years; range, 6–21 years), the stimulated plasma calcitonin levels were within normal limits. In the remaining nine patients (mean age, 15.1 years, range, 8–20 years), the stimulated plasma calcitonin levels were elevated.

Of the 12 genetically positive individuals with normal stimulated plasma calcitonin levels, 6 patients (or, in the case of minors, their parents) decided against having an immediate thyroidectomy, for reasons of convenience of timing or because they preferred to wait until calcitonin levels were elevated. Of the nine family members with elevated stimulated plasma calcitonin levels, two wished to delay thyroidectomy for several months for personal reasons. In the remaining 13 individuals (six with normal plasma calcitonin levels and seven with elevated levels), total thyroidectomy, lymph node dissection, and parathyroid autotransplantation were performed. After thyroidectomy and parathyroid autotransplantation, patients were placed on thyroid hormone, calcium, and vitamin D supplementation. Approximately 8 weeks after the operation, the oral calcium and vitamin D were stopped. Two weeks after the oral calcium and vitamin D replacement were stopped, the serum calcium concentration was within the normal range in each patient. Of the seven patients whose preoperative plasma calcitonin levels were elevated, each had microscopic evidence of MTC on histologic examination. Two of the seven had macroscopic disease. Of the six patients with normal preoperative plasma calcitonin levels, macroscopic MTC (n = 1), microscopic MTC (n = 2), or C-cell hyperplasia only (n = 3) was evident. A total of 212 lymph nodes were resected from the central zone of the neck (14.5 per patient), none of which was found, on histologic examination, to contain metastases. In each of the 13 patients, the stimulated plasma calcitonin levels were normal after total thyroidectomy.

Lips et al.,[80] in a series from the Netherlands, identified 14 young members of families affected by MEN 2A who had normal calcitonin testing but who were found to be *MEN2A* gene carriers by DNA testing. Thyroidectomy was performed on 8 of these 14, and foci of MTC were identified in all 8.

In a later report of preventive thyroidectomies in *RET* mutation carriers, Wells et al.[81] at Washington University in St. Louis reported a series of 49 children with MEN 2A and MEN 2B. In this series, 14 children had a prophylactic thyroidectomy based on genetic testing. The average age of the children at the time of surgery was 10.5 years. Postoperative calcitonin levels were all undetectable, and no evidence of recurrent MTC was found during a mean follow-up of 1.3 years. In an interim report of 3-year follow-up of the earliest group of 18 patients, no recurrence of disease was noted.[82]

The finding of carcinoma in the thyroid glands of many of these young patients with normal stimulated calcitonin testing indicates that the operation was therapeutic, not prophylactic.[81,83] There is some urgency, therefore, to applying this genetic test to other at-risk individuals and performing thyroidectomy on those who test positive genetically. The ideal age for performance of thyroidectomy in those patients found to be genetically positive has not been determined unequivocally. It is reasonable to perform surgery in 6-year-old patients with MEN 2A and FMTC. Patients with MEN 2B should undergo thyroidectomy during infancy, because of the aggressiveness and earlier age of onset of MTC in these patients.[61,84] Patient follow-up over the next decades will determine whether there is a significant rate of recurrence after preventive thyroidectomy. At present, it is advisable to follow up these patients with stimulated plasma calcitonin levels every 1 to 2 years. These patients must also continue to be followed for the development of pheochromocytomas and HPT.

MOLECULAR PATHOGENESIS OF SPORADIC THYROID NEOPLASMS

The thyroid follicular cell is highly differentiated, with the ability to concentrate iodide and synthesize thyroglobulin. Thyroid-stimulating hormone (TSH) is the major regulator of differentiated function of follicular cells and also functions as a growth factor for follicular cells via a cyclic adenosine monophosphate–mediated signal transduction pathway. In addition, thyroid cell growth and proliferation are influenced by a variety of growth factors and cytokines, as well as by the amount of iodine in the diet. Presumably, a host of genetic and environmental factors may result in unregulated growth or loss of differentiated func-

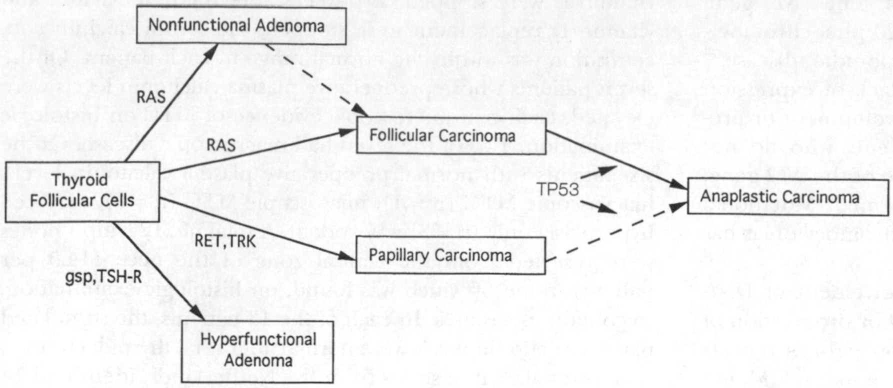

FIGURE 38.1-5. Flow diagram of proven and postulated events in thyroid follicular cell tumorigenesis. Mutations in the *RAS* oncogene are believed to be early events in the genesis of follicular neoplasms. Activation of the *RET* and *TRK* receptor tyrosine kinases is specific to papillary thyroid carcinomas. The association of mutations in the *TP53* tumor suppressor gene with undifferentiated thyroid tumors suggests that mutations in *TP53* are a critical event in the progression of follicular carcinoma to anaplastic carcinoma.

tion and confer a proliferative advantage to certain follicular cells, resulting in nodule formation.[85] Progression of benign adenomatous nodules to differentiated carcinoma is speculative at present, but good evidence exists for the development of anaplastic carcinomas from well-differentiated tumors.[86–88] A schematic model of the proposed events in thyroid follicular cell tumorigenesis is shown in Figure 38.1-5.

EPIDEMIOLOGIC AND GENETIC FACTORS ASSOCIATED WITH THYROID NEOPLASIA

Papillary thyroid carcinoma accounts for 85% of differentiated thyroid carcinomas in iodine-sufficient countries.[89] In areas of iodine deficiency or endemic goiter, an overall increased incidence of thyroid cancer is noted, attributable to a higher proportion of follicular carcinomas and anaplastic thyroid carcinomas (which often arise from preexisting follicular carcinomas).[90–93] The incidence of thyroid neoplasia is also increased in certain hereditary syndromes, including familial adenomatous polyposis coli, Cowden's disease, and MEN 1. Exposure to external radiation in childhood is a strong risk factor for the subsequent development of benign and malignant thyroid nodules.[94–98] Point mutations of K-*RAS* have been detected in 60% of radiation-related thyroid tumors.[99]

FOLLICULAR ADENOMAS

A local proliferative advantage may be provided to a thyroid follicular cell by genetic mutational events, environmental factors, or the local influence of cytokines or growth factors. Clonal expansion of cells with a growth advantage leads to nodule formation.

Mutations in all three members of the *RAS* oncogene family (K-*RAS*, N-*RAS*, and H-*RAS*) have been detected in thyroid neoplasms.[100] *RAS* mutations are detected with equal frequency in benign and malignant thyroid neoplasms[101] and are believed to represent an early event in follicular cell tumorigenesis.[102] *RAS* mutations occur predominantly in follicular thyroid carcinomas, with most of the mutations occurring at codon 61 of H-*RAS* and N-*RAS*.[101,103,104] By contrast, *RAS* mutations are a rare event in papillary thyroid carcinomas. It appears that *RAS* mutations are not sufficient for transformation of the thyroid cell; additional genetic events are required. In cooperation with other oncogenes,[105] transformation of thyroid cells *in vitro* with mutant *RAS* is associated with loss of differentiation, including decreased iodide uptake and expression of thyroid peroxidase.[106]

Mutational events affecting receptors or intermediates along the adenylate cyclase–cyclic adenosine monophosphate signal transduction pathway may contribute to the formation of hyperfunctioning adenomas. A subset of hyperfunctioning adenomas has been shown to harbor somatic mutations in the gene encoding the TSH receptor (*TSHR*) that result in constitutive activation of downstream events.[107] Mutations in the G protein intracellular mediator of adenylate cyclase (G_S) have been detected in 25% of hyperfunctioning thyroid nodules.[108,109] Therefore, a unifying molecular theme in the pathogenesis of hyperfunctioning nodules is inappropriate activation of the TSH signal transduction pathway, which is a result of specific gene mutations altering a key mediator of an otherwise well-balanced cascade.

Finally, deletion of chromosomal sequences from the 11q13 region has been demonstrated in 14% of follicular adenomas,[110] suggesting that inactivation of a tumor suppressor gene in this region may play a role in follicular cell tumorigenesis in a subset of tumors.

PAPILLARY THYROID CARCINOMA

Activation of receptor tyrosine kinases (*RET/PTC*, *NTRK1*, *MET*), whether by chromosomal rearrangement or gene amplification, is associated with the transformation of follicular cells to papillary thyroid carcinoma.[111,112] The *RET* protooncogene was first discovered based on its ability to transform mouse NIH 3T3 fibroblasts in culture.[31] The transforming *RET* sequences first identified represented a rearrangement of *RET* that occurred *in vitro* during the transfection assay.[32] Fusco et al.[113] subsequently demonstrated that DNAs from 25% of papillary carcinomas or their lymph node metastases also were positive in transfection assays. The transforming sequences in papillary carcinomas, originally believed to be a unique oncogene termed *PTC* (for *p*apillary *t*hyroid *c*arcinoma), were shown to represent *in vivo* chromosomal rearrangements that resulted in the juxtaposition of sequences encoding the intracellular tyrosine kinase domain of *RET* with 5' sequences from one of three unrelated genes.[111,113–117] The most frequent form of activated *RET/PTC* results from a paracentric inversion of chromosome 10q,[116] which in turn incites the gene fusion of D10S170 (H4) sequences with the catalytic domain of *RET* (Fig. 38.1-6). The frequency of *RET* rearrangements in papillary carcinomas may be as high as 33%,[113,118] but a lower frequency has been found in other studies,[119,120] perhaps reflecting either racial or environmental factors influencing thyroid tumorigenesis in different geographic regions.

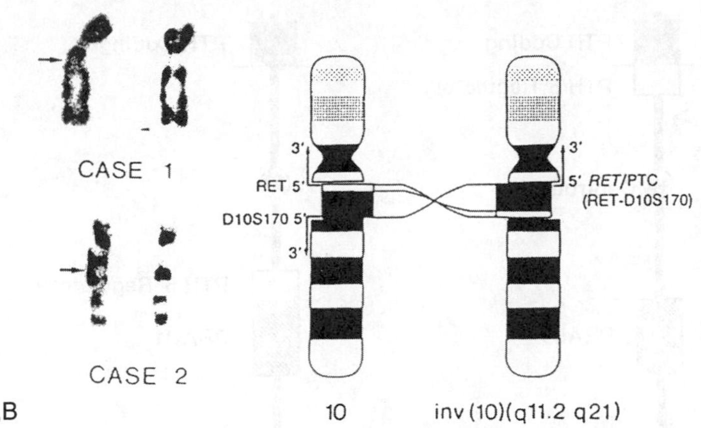

FIGURE 38.1-6. Chromosome 10q inversion in papillary thyroid carcinoma. **A:** Two representative chromosome 10 homologues from tumor cells of patients 1 and 2 showing inv(10)(q11.2q21) (*arrows*). **B:** Schematic view of the paracentric inversion of chromosome 10q generating the transforming sequence *RET/PTC*. (From ref. 116, with permission.)

Activation of *NTRK1* (tropomyosin receptor kinase), which encodes a cell surface receptor for nerve growth factor, has also been detected in some papillary carcinomas.[111] The *NTRK1* oncogene is generated by a chromosomal rearrangement that juxtaposes the tyrosine kinase domain of *NTRK1* and the 5' region of the TPR gene, both mapping to chromosome 1q23-24.[121,122] Finally, the *MET* oncogene, which also encodes a receptor tyrosine kinase, is amplified and overexpressed in 70% of papillary and poorly differentiated carcinomas but in only 25% of follicular carcinomas.[123,124] Activation of *MET* by amplification[124] and the presence of a rearranged, activated form of *RET*[125–127] have been suggested as predictors of aggressive biologic behavior and poor prognosis in papillary carcinomas. However, because of the generally excellent prognosis of these tumors, larger studies will be required to confirm these observations.

Activation of receptor tyrosine kinases by the common mechanism of gene rearrangement that brings the tyrosine kinase domain under the control of inappropriate upstream regulators derived from any of several "activating genes" appears to be specific for the transformation of follicular cells into papillary thyroid carcinoma.

FOLLICULAR THYROID CARCINOMA

Numerous chromosomal deletions have been detected in thyroid neoplasms, suggesting a role for multiple tumor suppressor genes in the initiation or progression of these tumors. Although sporadic follicular thyroid tumors exhibit allelic chromosomal loss of chromosome 11q13 sequences with increased frequency,[110] one study failed to find accompanying mutations in the *MEN1* gene in the remaining normal allele, suggesting that a tumor suppressor gene other than *MEN1* might be involved in tumorigenesis of these neoplasms.[128] In addition to the 11q13 deletions described in follicular adenomas, Herrmann et al.[129] have presented evidence for chromosome 3p deletions specific to follicular carcinomas and proposed that inactivation of a tumor suppressor gene on chromosome 3p is important in the progression from follicular adenoma to carcinoma.

ANAPLASTIC THYROID CARCINOMA

Point mutations in the *TP53* tumor suppressor gene are frequent in anaplastic thyroid carcinomas but not in differentiated thyroid tumors.[130,131] This suggests that the *TP53* mutation is a critical event in the progression of follicular carcinoma to anaplastic carcinoma. Wild-type *TP53* encodes a nuclear phosphoprotein that functions as a transcriptional regulator believed to influence cell-cycle arrest or programmed cell death in response to genetic damage. Disruption of this protective function appears to be relevant to the progression of thyroid neoplasms to an aggressive, undifferentiated phenotype. Codons 273[130,131] and 248[131] are hot spots for *TP53* mutation in anaplastic thyroid carcinoma.

MEDULLARY THYROID CARCINOMA

The molecular genetic alterations associated with sporadic medullary carcinoma of the thyroid were discussed earlier in Other *RET* Genotype-Phenotype Correlations.

GENETIC ABNORMALITIES IN PARATHYROID NEOPLASMS

BENIGN PARATHYROID NEOPLASMS

Neoplasms of the parathyroid glands are almost always benign and occur with increased frequency in postmenopausal women, after neck irradiation, or as a component of several distinct familial syndromes. Benign parathyroid adenomas in patients with primary HPT have a proliferative defect (increase in cellular mass) as well as a defect in regulating parathyroid hormone (PTH) release in response to the extracellular calcium concentration (set-point abnormality).[132] In different parathyroid tumors, at least three specific genetic defects have been uncovered, including activation of an oncogene, inactivation of the *MEN1* tumor suppressor gene, and mutations in the cell surface calcium-sensing receptor.

MUTATIONS IN THE *MEN1* GENE AND ROLE OF OTHER TUMOR SUPPRESSOR GENES

Patients with MEN 1 inherit one mutated copy of the *MEN1* gene in the germline and therefore require only one chance additional somatic event (deletion, point mutation) to result in the loss of the remaining functional copy of the gene within an individual parathyroid cell. Presumably, the relatively likely combined occurrence of these genetic events leads to the asynchronous development of multiglandular parathyroid neoplasms (parathyroid hyperplasia) in affected individuals. LOH for markers in the *MEN1* gene region has been demonstrated not only in MEN 1–related parathyroid tumors but also in approximately 30% of sporadic parathyroid adenomas.[133–136] As previously suspected from studies of chromosome 11q13 LOH in DNA from sporadic parathyroid adenomas, loss of *MEN1* gene function now is known to be responsible for a subset of the parathyroid adenomas in patients with sporadic primary HPT. In this subset, the occurrence of a sporadic parathyroid adenoma presumably requires the chance occurrence of two somatic inactivating events (one involving each homologous copy of the *MEN1* gene).

A study by Heppner et al.[137] identified somatic mutations in one allele of the *MEN1* gene in tumor DNA from 7 of 33 parathyroid adenomas. In each of these tumors, a chromosome

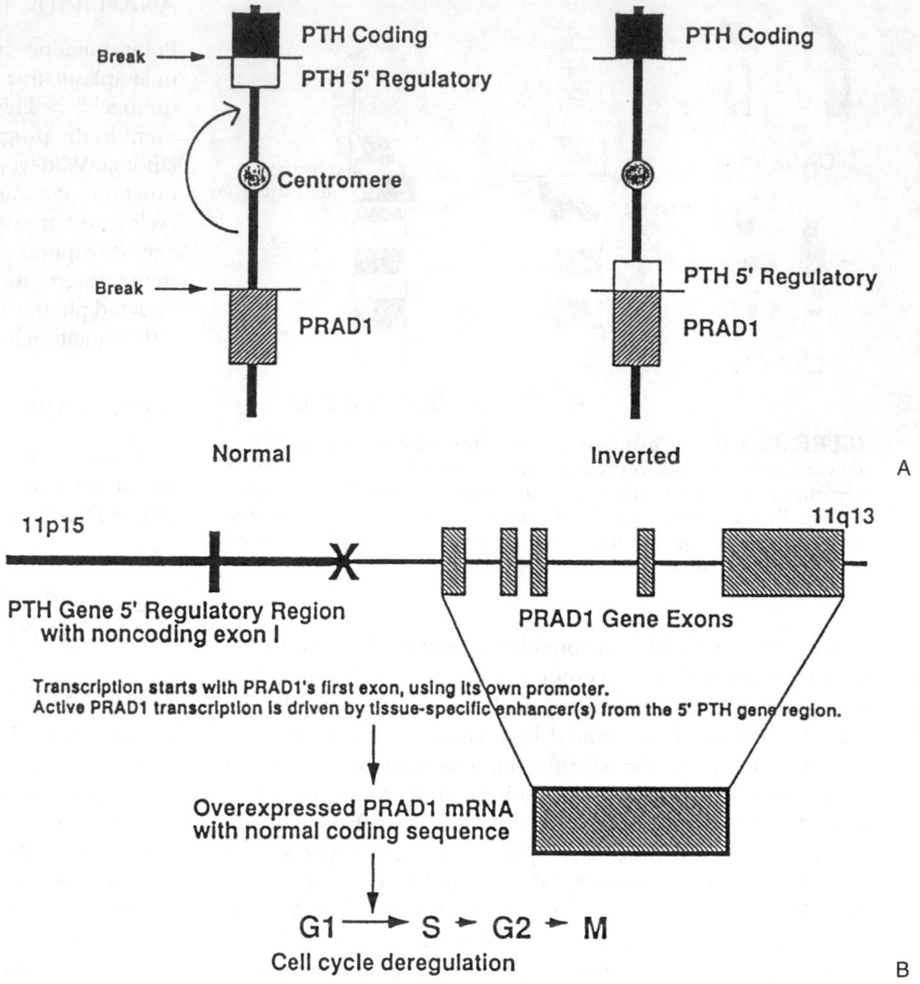

FIGURE 38.1-7. **A:** Schematic diagram illustrating the pericentromeric inversion of chromosome 11 deduced to have caused the observed rearrangement involving the PTH gene and the *PRAD1* gene in a subset of parathyroid adenomas. The tumor's other copy of chromosome 11, which contains an intact PTH gene, is not shown. **B:** Diagram of the directly observed molecular structure of the PTH/*PRAD1* DNA rearrangement in a subset of parathyroid adenomas and its functional consequences. X represents the chromosome breakpoint between the PTH gene regulatory region, plus PTH noncoding exon 1 (*solid light vertical bar*) and part of its first intron, from 11p15 (*left*), and the intact promoter and 5 exons of the PRAD1 gene from 11q13. (Reprinted from ref. 132, with permission.)

deletion was detected that eliminated the remaining wild-type copy of the *MEN1* gene in tumor DNA. Farbeno et al.[138] screened 45 sporadic adenomas from 40 patients with nonfamilial HPT by LOH and SSCV analysis. LOH for chromosome 11q13 was present in 13 (29%) of the tumors and, in six of these cases, somatic mutation was detected in the remaining copy of the *MEN1* gene. These findings suggest that a subset of sporadic parathyroid adenomas is caused by a combination of somatic genetic events within a parathyroid cell that inactivate both copies of the *MEN1* tumor suppressor gene.

ACTIVATION OF THE PRAD1 PROTOONCOGENE BY CHROMOSOMAL GENE REARRANGEMENT

In a small subset of parathyroid adenomas (approximately 5%), a pericentromeric inversion of chromosome 11 has been detected that results in a gene rearrangement involving the PTH gene on 11p15 and the parathyroid adenoma 1 (*PRAD1*) oncogene or cyclin D1 on 11q13.[139,140] As a consequence of the breakpoint and rejoining in 11q13, the PTH transcriptional regulatory sequences and its noncoding exon 1 are placed immediately upstream of the *PRAD1* protooncogene intact promoter and its five exons (Fig. 38.1-7). This rearrangement results in inappropriate or unregulated expression of *PRAD1* in response to the parathyroid tissue–specific transcriptional regulatory elements of the PTH gene. It has been suggested that the subset of patients with the *PRAD1* chromosomal rearrangement tend to have larger tumors and are more often symptomatic than are other patients with this disease.[132]

OTHER GENETIC LOCI IMPLICATED IN FAMILIAL HYPERCALCEMIC SYNDROMES

FAMILIAL BENIGN HYPERCALCEMIA

Familial benign hypercalcemia (hypocalciuric hypercalcemia)[141,142] is a dominantly inherited condition characterized by mild hypercalcemia, low urinary calcium excretion, and the absence of symptoms or the complications of hypercalcemia. The features of familial benign hypercalcemia are important to recognize and distinguish from other hypercalcemic disorders, because surgery fails to result in correction of the calcium level.[143–149]

Pollak et al.[150] demonstrated that mutations in the human calcium-sensing receptor gene are associated with familial benign hypocalcemia as well as neonatal severe HPT (NSHPT). Parathyroid cells from patients with familial benign hypercalcemia are characterized by an abnormally increased set point for extracellular calcium.[151]

The germline mutations that are associated with familial benign hypercalcemia are heterozygous, inactivating mutations in the calcium-sensing receptor gene.[152] The reported mutations include point mutations, nonsense mutations, or insertions that are postulated to result in varying degrees of loss of the receptor's calcium-sensing function.[150,153–156]

NEONATAL SEVERE HYPERPARATHYROIDISM

NSHPT is characterized by severe hypercalcemia, failure to thrive, dehydration, pathologic fractures and rib cage deformities, respiratory distress, and hypotonia in the newborn. The disorder usually requires urgent total parathyroidectomy in the first few weeks of life, although some have achieved a favorable outcome with intensive medical management.[157]

In some cases, NSHPT results from homozygous mutations (mutations on both homologous alleles) that cause loss of function of the calcium-sensing receptor gene.

HEREDITARY HYPERPARATHYROIDISM–JAW TUMOR SYNDROME

The autosomal dominant inheritance of HPT without any associated features and without any apparent association to the MEN syndromes has been described in several families.[158–160] HPT–jaw tumor syndrome (HPT-JT) is recognized as a distinct syndrome characterized by the autosomal dominant inheritance of recurrent parathyroid adenomas, fibroosseous jaw tumors, Wilms' tumor, and parathyroid carcinoma.[161] The onset of hypercalcemia typically occurs in childhood or the second decade of life. The association may not be recognized in many cases because the jaw lesions occur asynchronously in relation to the parathyroid tumors and may occur in some patients without HPT. The parathyroid tumors may be single or multiple but have a tendency toward recurrence after subtotal parathyroidectomy. The parathyroid adenomas in the familial HPT-JT syndrome often are cystic, a finding that occasionally is noted in primary sporadic HPT. The specific gene responsible for the HPT-JT syndrome remains to be identified.[161,162]

PARATHYROID CARCINOMA

Molecular defects with a possible role in progression to the malignant phenotype have also been sought in tumor DNA from parathyroid carcinomas. Although one study failed to detect evidence of mutations in exons 5, 7, and 8 of the *TP53* gene in parathyroid carcinomas,[163] another study reported allelic loss of *TP53* in two of six informative parathyroid carcinomas.[164] None of 20 informative parathyroid adenomas exhibited deletions of *TP53*. Most recently, the retinoblastoma tumor suppressor gene has been shown to be inactivated in most parathyroid carcinomas but not in adenomas.[165]

GENETIC ABNORMALITIES IN ADRENAL NEOPLASMS

SPORADIC PHEOCHROMOCYTOMAS

The molecular genetic alterations associated with sporadic pheochromocytomas were discussed earlier in Genetics under Multiple Endocrine Neoplasia Type 2 Syndromes.

FAMILIAL PHEOCHROMOCYTOMAS ARISING IN PATIENTS WITH VON HIPPEL-LINDAU SYNDROME AND NEUROFIBROMATOSIS TYPE 1

Pheochromocytomas occur in association with the VHL and NF1 syndromes. VHL syndrome is characterized by the development of retinal, cerebellar, and spinal hemangioblastomas, pancreatic and renal cysts, renal carcinomas, pheochromocytomas, neuroendocrine tumors of the pancreas, epididymal cysts, and endolymphatic sac tumors. The original mapping of the *VHL* gene by positional cloning to chromosome 3p was reported in 1993.[166] The *VHL* tumor suppressor gene encodes a protein that regulates the transcription of DNA to mRNA by RNA polymerase II.[167] Clinical heterogeneity exists in patients with the VHL syndrome. In type 1, pheochromocytomas do not occur. Pheochromocytomas are associated with type 2a, but renal cell carcinomas do not occur. Finally, in type 2b, both pheochromocytomas and renal cell carcinomas develop. The preceding classification has been related also to apparent genotype-phenotype correlations associated with mutations in the *VHL* gene.[168]

Mutations in the tumor suppressor gene for NF1 on chromosome 17q were identified in 1990.[169,170] Pheochromocytomas occur in approximately 1% to 2% of patients with NF1. Bilateral tumors occur with increased frequency compared with sporadic cases of pheochromocytomas.

ADRENOCORTICAL ADENOMAS AND CARCINOMAS

Several lines of evidence suggest a role for mutation or loss of the *TP53* tumor suppressor gene in adrenocortical neoplasms. First, LOH for markers from 17p has been consistently demonstrated in adrenocortical carcinomas but not in benign adrenocortical adenomas or hyperplasia.[171] Frequent LOH has also been detected for markers on chromosome 11p and 13q.[171] It is of interest to note that adrenocortical carcinomas occur with increased frequency in patients with the Li-Fraumeni syndrome, who have been shown to harbor germline mutations in *TP53*,[172] and in patients with the Beckwith-Wiedemann syndrome, which is associated with a defect on chromosome 11p15.[173] Sequence analysis has also demonstrated point mutations in the *TP53* gene in adrenocortical carcinomas[174] and in adrenal adenomas in some[77] but not all[174] studies. Point mutations of G protein genes have been detected in a variety of endocrine tumors, including adrenocortical tumors.[108,175] Mutations of the adrenocorticotropic hormone receptor have not been detected in adrenal neoplasms.[176]

In one study of 35 adrenocortical lesions (six hyperplasias, 19 adenomas, ten adrenocortical carcinomas), LOH at 11q13 was detected in 31% of the tumors analyzed.[177] The frequency of LOH for this region was significantly greater in adrenocortical carcinomas (60%) than in benign lesions (11%). However, inactivating mutations of the *MEN1* gene were demonstrated in almost none of the tumors with LOH at 11q13. The authors concluded that the *MEN1* gene appears not to play a significant role in the development of benign or malignant adrenocortical neoplasms.[177]

SUMMARY

A variety of genetic abnormalities in both oncogenes and tumor suppressor genes have been identified in endocrine neoplasms. The study of tumors developing in the inherited endocrine cancer syndromes has provided valuable insight into genetic events that likely play a role in the genesis of sporadic tumors developing in the same endocrine tissues. The advent of direct DNA testing for germline mutations in the *RET* protooncogene that are responsible for the MEN 2 syndromes has made possible early thyroidectomy at a time when hereditary MTC is likely occult and curable. The identification of germline mutations in the *MEN1* gene will allow direct genetic testing and an enhanced understanding of the mechanisms of tumorigenesis of related endocrine tumors.

REFERENCES

1. Marx S, Spiegel AM, Skarulis MC, et al. Multiple endocrine neoplasia type 1: clinical and genetic topics. *Ann Intern Med* 1998;129:484.
2. Darling TN, Skarulis MC, Steinberg SM, et al. Multiple facial angiofibromas and collagenomas in patients with multiple endocrine neoplasia type 1. *Arch Dermatol* 1997;133:853.
3. Kato H, Uchimura I, Morohoshi M, et al. Multiple endocrine neoplasia type 1 associated with spinal ependymoma. *Intern Med* 1996;35:285.
4. Wilkinson S, Teh BT, Davey KR, et al. Cause of death in multiple endocrine neoplasia type 1. *Arch Surg* 1993;128:683.
5. Doherty GM, Olson JA, Frisella MM, et al. Lethality of multiple endocrine neoplasia type 1. *World J Surg* 1997;22:581.
6. Larsson C, Skogseid B, Öberg K, et al. Multiple endocrine neoplasia type 1 gene maps to chromosome 11 and is lost in insulinoma. *Nature* 1988;332:85.
7. Chandrasekharappa SC, Guru SC, Manickamp P, et al. Positional cloning of the gene for multiple endocrine neoplasia-type 1. *Science* 1997;276:404.
8. Guru SC, Goldsmith PK, Burns AL, et al. Menin, the product of the *MEN1* gene, is a nuclear protein. *Proc Natl Acad Sci USA* 1998;95:1630.
9. Lemmens I, Van de Ven WJM, Kas K, et al. Identification of the multiple endocrine neoplasia type 1 (MEN1) gene. *Hum Mol Genet* 1997;6:1177.
10. Agarwal SK, Kester MB, Debelenko LV, et al. Germline mutations in the *MEN1* gene in familial multiple endocrine neoplasia type 1 and related states. *Hum Mol Genet* 1997;6:1169.
11. Mayr B, Apenberg S, Rothamel T, et al. Menin mutations in patients with multiple endocrine neoplasia. *Eur J Endocrinol* 1997;137:684.
12. Shimizu S, Tsukada T, Futami H, et al. Germline mutations of the *MEN1* gene in Japanese kindreds with multiple endocrine neoplasia type 1. *Jpn J Cancer Res* 1997;88:1029.
13. Bassett JHD, Forbes SA, Pannett AAJ, et al. Characterization of mutations in patients with multiple endocrine neoplasia type 1. *Am J Hum Genet* 1998;62:232.
14. Kishi M, Tsukada T, Shimizu SW, et al. A large germline deletion of the *MEN1* gene in a family with multiple endocrine neoplasia type 1. *Jpn J Cancer Res* 1998;89:1.
15. Olufemi SE, Green JS, Manickam P, et al. Common ancestral mutation in the *MEN1* gene is likely responsible for the prolactinoma variant of MEN 1 (MEN1 Burin) in four kindreds from Newfoundland. *Hum Mutat* 1998;11:264.
16. Mutch MG, Dilley WG, Sanjurjo F, et al. Germline mutations in the multiple endocrine neoplasia type 1 gene: evidence for frequent splicing defects. *Hum Mutat* 1999;13:175.
17. Agarwal SK, Guru SC, Heppner C, et al. Menin interacts with the AP1 transcription factor JunD and represses JunD-activated transcription. *Cell* 1999;96:143.
18. Stewart C, Parente F, Piehl F, et al. Characterization of the mouse *Men1* gene and its expression during development. *Oncogene* 1998;17:2485.
19. Sakurai A, Katai M, Itakura Y, et al. Premature centromere division in patients with multiple endocrine neoplasia type 1. *Cancer Genet Cytogenet* 1999;109:138.
20. Howe JR, Norton JA, Wells SA Jr. Prevalence of pheochromocytoma and hyperparathyroidism in multiple endocrine neoplasia type 2A: results of long-term follow-up. *Surgery* 1993;114:1070.
21. Jenkins PJ, Satta MA, Simmgen M, et al. Metastatic parathyroid carcinoma in the MEN 2A syndrome. *Clin Endocrinol* 1997;47:747.
22. Gagel RF, Levy ML, Donovan DT, et al. Multiple endocrine neoplasia type 2A associated with cutaneous lichen amyloidosis. *Ann Intern Med* 1989;111:802.
23. Romeo G, Ronchetto P, Luo Y, et al. Point mutations affecting the tyrosine kinase domain of the *RET* proto-oncogene in Hirschsprung's disease. *Nature* 1994;367:377.
24. Edery P, Lyonnet S, Mulligan LM, et al. Mutations of the *RET* proto-oncogene in Hirschsprung's disease. *Nature* 1994;367:378.
25. Decker RA, Peacock ML. Occurrence of MEN 2A in familial Hirschsprung's disease: a new indication for genetic testing of the RET proto-oncogene. *J Pediatr Surg* 1998;33:207.
26. Farndon JR, Leight GS, Dilley WG, et al. Familial medullary thyroid carcinoma without associated endocrinopathies: a distinct clinical entity. *Br J Surg* 1986;73:278.
27. Mathew CGP, Chin KS, Easton DF, et al. A linked genetic marker for multiple endocrine neoplasia type 2A on chromosome 10. *Nature* 1987;328:527.
28. Simpson NE, Kidd KK, Goodfellow PJ, et al. Assignment of multiple endocrine neoplasia type 2A to chromosome 10 by genetic linkage. *Nature* 1987;328:528.
29. Norum RA, Lafreniere RG, O'Neal LW, et al. Linkage of the multiple endocrine neoplasia type 2B gene (MEN2B) to chromosome 10 markers linked to MEN2A. *Genomics* 1990;8:313.
30. Lairmore TC, Howe JR, Korte JA, et al. Familial medullary thyroid carcinoma and multiple endocrine neoplasia type 2B map to the same region of chromosome 10 as multiple endocrine neoplasia type 2A. *Genomics* 1991;9:181.
31. Takahashi M, Ritz J, Cooper GM. Activation of a novel human transforming gene, *ret*, by DNA rearrangement. *Cell* 1985;42:581.
32. Takahashi M, Cooper GM. *ret* transforming gene encodes a fusion protein homologous to tyrosine kinases. *Mol Cell Biol* 1987;7:1378.
33. Takahashi M, Buma Y, Iwamoto T, et al. Cloning and expression of the *ret* proto-oncogene encoding a tyrosine kinase with two potential transmembrane domains. *Oncogene* 1988;3:571.
34. Ishizaka Y, Itoh F, Tahira T, et al. Human *ret* proto-oncogene mapped to chromosome 10q11.2. *Oncogene* 1989;4:1519.
35. Santoro M, Rosati R, Grieco M, et al. The *ret* proto-oncogene is consistently expressed in human pheochromocytomas and thyroid medullary carcinomas. *Oncogene* 1990;5:1595.
36. Mulligan LM, Kwok JBJ, Healey CS, et al. Germ-line mutations of the *RET* proto-oncogene in multiple endocrine neoplasia type 2A. *Nature* 1993;363:458.
37. Donis-Keller H, Dou S, Chi D, et al. Mutations in the RET proto-oncogene are associated with MEN 2A and FMTC. *Hum Mol Genet* 1993;2:851.
38. Hofstra RMW, Landsvater RM, Ceccherini I, et al. A mutation in the *RET* proto-oncogene associated with multiple endocrine neoplasia type 2B and sporadic medullary thyroid carcinoma. *Nature* 1994;367:375.
39. Carlson KM, Dou S, Chi D, et al. Single missense mutation in the tyrosine kinase catalytic domain of the *RET* protooncogene is associated with multiple endocrine neoplasia type 2B. *Proc Natl Acad Sci USA* 1994;91:1579.
40. Smith DP, Houghton C, Ponder BAJ. Germline mutation of *RET* codon 883 in two cases of *de novo* MEN 2B. *Oncogene* 1997;15:1213.
41. Eng C, Mulligan LM. Mutations of the RET proto-oncogene in the multiple endocrine neoplasia type 2 syndromes, related sporadic tumors, and Hirschprung disease. *Hum Mutat* 1997;9:97.
42. Berndt I, Reuter M, Saller B, et al. A new hot spot for mutations in the ret proto-oncogene causing familial medullary thyroid carcinoma and multiple endocrine neoplasia type 2A. *J Clin Endocrinol Metab* 1998;83:770.
43. Santoro M, Carlomagno F, Romano A, et al. Activation of *RET* as a dominantly transforming gene by germline mutations of MEN2A and MEN2B. *Science* 1995;267:381.
44. Kwok JBJ, Gardner E, Warner JP, et al. Structural analysis of the human *ret* proto-oncogene using exon trapping. *Oncogene* 1993;8:2575.
45. Tahira T, Ishizaka Y, Itoh F, et al. Characterization of *ret* proto-oncogene mRNAs encoding two isoforms of the protein product in a human neuroblastoma cell line. *Oncogene* 1990;5:97.
46. Tahira T, Ishizaka Y, Itoh F, et al. Expression of the *ret* proto-oncogene in human neuroblastoma cell lines and its increase during neuronal differentiation induced by retinoic acid. *Oncogene* 1991;6:2333.
47. Schuchardt A, D'Agati V, Larsson-Blomberg L, et al. Defects in the kidney and enteric nervous system of mice lacking the tyrosine kinase receptor Ret. *Nature* 1994;367:380.
48. Sánchez MP, Silos-Santiago I, Frisén J, et al. Renal agenesis and the absence of enteric neurons in mice lacking GDNF. *Nature* 1996;382:70.
49. Pichel JG, Shen L, Sheng HZ, et al. Defects in enteric innervation and kidney development in mice lacking GDNF. *Nature* 1996;382:73.
50. Moore MW, Klein RD, Farinas I, et al. Renal and neuronal abnormalities in mice lacking GDNF. *Nature* 1996;382:76.
51. Trupp M, Arenas E, Fainzilber M, et al. Functional receptor for GDNF encoded by the c-*ret* proto-oncogene. *Nature* 1996;381:785.
52. Durbec P, Macos-Gutierrez CV, Kilkenny C, et al. GDNF signalling through the Ret receptor tyrosine kinase. *Nature* 1996;381:789.
53. Jing S, Wen D, Yu Y, et al. GDNF-Induced activation of the ret protein tyrosine kinase is mediated by GDNFR-a, a novel receptor for GDNF. *Cell* 1996;85:1113.
54. Treanor JJS, Goodman L, de Sauvage F, et al. Characterization of a multicomponent receptor for GDNF. *Nature* 1996;382:80.
55. Hofstra RM, Sijmons RH, Stelwagen T, et al. Ret mutation screening in familial cutaneous lichen amyloidosis associated with multiple endocrine neoplasia. *J Invest Dermatol* 1996;107:215.
56. Mulligan LM, Eng C, Healey CS, et al. Specific mutations of the *RET* proto-oncogene are related to disease phenotype in MEN 2A and FMTC. *Nat Genet* 1994;6:70.
57. Schuffenecker I, Billaud M, Calender A, et al. Ret proto-oncogene mutations in French MEN 2A and FMTC families. *Hum Mol Genet* 1994;3:1939.
58. Frank-Raue K, Hoppner W, Frilling A, et al. Mutations of the ret proto-oncogene in German multiple endocrine neoplasia families: relation between genotype and phenotype. *J Clin Endocrinol Metab* 1996;81:1780.
59. Schuffenecker I, Virally-Monod M, Brohet R, et al. Risk and penetrance of primary hyperparathyroidism in multiple endocrine neoplasia type 2A families with mutations at codon 634 of the RET proto-oncogene. *J Clin Endocrinol Metab* 1998;83:487.
60. Borst MJ, VanCamp JM, Peacock ML, Decker RA. Mutational analysis of multiple endocrine neoplasia type 2A associated with Hirschsprung's disease. *Surgery* 1995;117:386.
61. O'Riordain DS, O'Brien T, et al. Multiple endocrine neoplasia type 2B: more than an endocrine disorder. *Surgery* 1995;118:936.
62. Eng C, Smith DP, Mulligan LM, et al. A novel point mutation in the tyrosine kinase domain of the *RET* proto-oncogene in sporadic medullary thyroid carcinoma and in a family with FMTC. *Oncogene* 1995;10:509.
63. Bolino A, Schuffenecker I, Luo Y, et al. *RET* mutations in exons 13 and 14 of FMTC patients. *Oncogene* 1995;10:2415.
64. Marsh KJ, Learoyd DL, Andrew SD, et al. Somatic mutations in the RET proto-oncogene in sporadic medullary thyroid carcinoma. *Clin Endocrinol* 1996;44:249.
65. Musholt P, Musholt T, Goodfellow P, et al. "Cold" SSCV for mutation analysis of the RET proto-oncogene. *Surgery* 1997;122:363.
66. Roncalli M, Viale G, Grimelius L, et al. Prognostic value of N-myc immunoreactivity in medullary thyroid carcinoma. *Cancer* 1994;74:134.
67. Moley JF, Brother MB, Wells SA, et al. Low frequency of *ras* gene mutations in neuroblastomas, pheochromocytomas, and medullary thyroid cancers. *Cancer Res* 1991;51:1596.

68. Moley JF, Wallin GK, Brother MB, et al. Oncogene and growth factor expression in MEN 2 and related tumors. *Henry Ford Hosp Med J* 1992;40:284.
69. Moley J, Brother M, Fong C, et al. Consistent association of 1p loss of heterozygosity with pheochromocytomas from patients with multiple endocrine neoplasia type 2 syndromes. *Cancer Res* 1992;52:770.
70. Mulligan LM, Gardner E, Smith BA, et al. Genetic events in tumour initiation and progression in multiple endocrine neoplasia type 2. *Genes Chromosomes Cancer* 1993;6:166.
71. Nelkin BN, Nakamura Y, White RW, et al. Low incidence of loss of chromosome 10 in sporadic and hereditary human medullary thyroid carcinoma. *Cancer Res* 1989;49:4114.
72. Moley JF, Marshall HN. 1p deletions in human pheochromocytomas share a common pericentromeric breakpoint and do not involve imprinting. *Am J Hum Genet* 1994;55:A347.
73. Dou S, Toshima K, Liu L, et al. Identification of chromosomal loci for tumor suppressor loci implicated in progression of pheochromocytoma and medullary thyroid carcinoma. *Am J Hum Genet* 1994;55[Suppl]:A20.
74. Herfarth K, Wick M, Marshall H, et al. Absence of TP53 alterations in pheochromocytomas and medullary thyroid carcinomas. *Genes Chromosomes Cancer* 1997;20:24.
75. Yoshimoto K, Iwahana H, Fukuda A, et al. Role of p53 mutations in endocrine tumorigenesis: mutation detection by polymerase chain reaction–single strand conformation polymorphism. *Cancer Res* 1992;52:5061.
76. Yana I, Nakamura T, Shin E, et al. Inactivation of the p53 gene is not required for tumorigenesis of medullary thyroid carcinoma or pheochromocytoma. *Jpn J Cancer Res* 1992;83:1113.
77. Lin SR, Lee YJ, Tsai JH. Mutations of the p53 gene in human functional adrenal neoplasms. *J Clin Endocrinol Metab* 1994;78:483.
78. Gutmann DH, Geist RT, Rose K, et al. Loss of neurofibromatosis type I (NF1) gene expression in pheochromocytomas from patients without NF1. *Genes Chromosomes Cancer* 1995;13:104.
79. Wells SA Jr, Chi D, Toshima K, et al. Predictive DNA testing and prophylactic thyroidectomy in patients at risk for multiple endocrine neoplasia type 2A. *Ann Surg* 1994;220:237.
80. Lips CJM, Landsvater RM, Höppener JWM, et al. Clinical screening as compared with DNA analysis in families with multiple endocrine neoplasia type 2A. *N Engl J Med* 1994;331:828.
81. Skinner MA, DeBenedetti MK, Moley JF, et al. Medullary thyroid carcinoma in children with multiple endocrine neoplasia types 2A and 2B. *J Pediatr Surg* 1996;31:177.
82. Wells SA Jr, Skinner MA. Prophylactic thyroidectomy, based on direct genetic testing, in patients at risk for the multiple endocrine neoplasia type 2 syndromes. *Exp Clin Endocrinol Diabetes* 1998;106:29.
83. Lairmore TC, Frisella MM, Wells SAJ. Genetic testing and early thyroidectomy for inherited medullary thyroid carcinoma. *Ann Med* 1996;28:401.
84. Norton JA, Froome LC, Farrell RE, et al. Multiple endocrine neoplasia type IIb. *Symp Endocr Surg* 1979;59:109.
85. Farid NR, Shi Y, Zou M. Molecular basis of thyroid cancer. *Endocr Rev* 1994;15:202.
86. Williams ED. The aetiology of thyroid tumors. *Clin Endocrinol Metab* 1979;8:193.
87. Moore JHJ, Bacharach B, Choi HY. Anaplastic transformation of metastatic follicular carcinoma of the thyroid. *J Surg Oncol* 1985;29:216.
88. Venkatesh YS, Ordonez NG, Schultz PN, et al. Anaplastic carcinoma of the thyroid: a clinicopathologic study of 121 cases. *Cancer* 1990;66:321.
89. Hay ID. Papillary thyroid carcinoma. *Endocrinol Metab Clin North Am* 1990;19:545.
90. Wahner HW, Cuello C, Correa P, et al. Thyroid carcinoma in an endemic goiter area, Cali, Colombia. *Am J Med* 1966;40:58.
91. Heitz P, Moser SH, Staub JJ. Thyroid cancer. A study of 573 thyroid tumors and 161 autopsy cases observed over a thirty year period. *Cancer* 1976;37:2329.
92. Williams ED, Doniach I, Bjarnason O, et al. Thyroid cancer in an iodide rich area: a histopathological study. *Cancer* 1977;39:215.
93. Belfiore A, La Rosa GL, La Porta GA, et al. Cancer risk in patients with cold thyroid nodules: relevance of iodine intake, sex, age and multinodularity. *Am J Med* 1992;93:363.
94. Rallison ML, Dobyns BM, Keating FR, et al. Thyroid nodularity in children. *JAMA* 1975;233:1069.
95. McTiernan AM, Weiss NS, Daling JR. Incidence of thyroid cancer in women in relation to previous exposure to radiation therapy and history of thyroid disease. *J Natl Cancer Inst* 1984;73:575.
96. Schneider AB, Shore-Freedman E, Ryo UY, et al. Radiation-induced tumors of the head and neck following childhood irradiation. *Medicine* 1985;64:1.
97. Shore RE, Woodard E, Hildreth N, et al. Thyroid tumors following thymus irradiation. *J Natl Cancer Inst* 1985;74:1177.
98. Hamilton TE, van Belle G, LoGerfo JP. Thyroid neoplasia in Marshall islanders exposed to nuclear fallout. *JAMA* 1987;258:629.
99. Wright PA, Williams ED, Lemoine NR, et al. Radiation-associated and "spontaneous" human thyroid carcinomas show a different pattern of ras oncogene mutation. *Oncogene* 1991;6:471.
100. Suarez HG, du Villard JA, Severino M, et al. Presence of mutations in all three ras genes in human thyroid tumors. *Oncogene* 1990;5:565.
101. Karga H, Lee JK, Vickery ALJ, et al. Ras oncogene mutations in benign and malignant thyroid neoplasms. *J Clin Endocrinol Metab* 1991;73:832.
102. Namba H, Rubin SA, Fagin JA. Point mutations of ras oncogenes are an early event in thyroid tumorigenesis. *Mol Endocrinol* 1990;4:1474.
103. Shi YF, Zou MJ, Schmidt H, et al. High rates of ras codon 61 mutation in thyroid tumors in an iodide-deficient area. *Cancer Res* 1991;51:2690.
104. Lemoine NR, Mayall ES, Wyllie FS, et al. High frequency of *ras* oncogene activation in all stages of human thyroid tumorigenesis. *Oncogene* 1989;4:159.
105. Fusco A, Berlinghieri MT, Di Fiore PP, et al. One- and two-step transformation of rat thyroid epithelial cells by retroviral oncogenes. *Mol Cell Biol* 1987;7:3365.
106. Francis-Lang H, Zannini M, De Felice M, et al. Multiple mechanisms of interference between transformation and differentiation in thyroid cells. *Mol Cell Biol* 1992;12:5793.
107. Parma J, Duprez L, Van Sande J, et al. Somatic mutations of the thyrotropin receptor gene cause hyperfunctioning thyroid adenomas. *Nature* 1993;365:649.
108. Lyons J, Landis CA, Harsh G, et al. Two G protein oncogenes in human endocrine tumors. *Science* 1990;249:635.
109. Suarez HG, du Villard JA, Caillou B, et al. Gsp mutations in human thyroid tumors. *Oncogene* 1991;6:677.
110. Matsuo K, Tang S-H, Fagin JA. Allelotype of human thyroid tumors: loss of chromosome 11q13 sequences in follicular neoplasms. *Mol Endocrinol* 1991;5:1873.
111. Bongarzone I, Pierotti MA, Monzini N, et al. High frequency of activation of tyrosine kinase oncogenes in human papillary thyroid carcinoma. *Oncogene* 1989;4:1457.
112. Santoro M, Carlomagno F, Hay ID, et al. Ret oncogene activation in human thyroid neoplasms is restricted to the papillary cancer subtype. *J Clin Invest* 1992;89:1517.
113. Fusco A, Grieco M, Santoro M, et al. A new oncogene in human thyroid papillary carcinomas and their lymph-nodal metastases. *Nature* 1987;328:170.
114. Grieco M, Santoro M, Berlingieri MT, et al. PTC is a novel rearranged form of the *ret* proto-oncogene and is frequently detected in vivo in human thyroid papillary carcinomas. *Cell* 1990;60:557.
115. Ishizaka Y, Ushijima T, Sugimura T, et al. cDNA cloning and characterization of ret activated in a human papillary carcinoma cell line. *Biochem Biophys Res Commun* 1990;168:402.
116. Pierotti MA, Santoro M, Jenkins RB, et al. Characterization of an inversion on the long arm of chromosome 10 juxtaposing D10S170 and RET and creating the oncogenic sequence RET/PTC. *Proc Natl Acad Sci USA* 1992;89:1616.
117. Sozzi G, Bongarzone I, Miozzo M, et al. A t(10;17) translocation creates the RET/PTC2 chimeric transforming sequence in papillary thyroid carcinoma. *Genes Chromosomes Cancer* 1994;9:244.
118. Bongarzone I, Butti MG, Coronelli S, et al. Frequent activation of ret protooncogene by fusion with a new activating gene in papillary thyroid carcinomas. *Cancer Res* 1994;54:2979.
119. Wajjwalku W, Nakamura S, Hasegawa Y, et al. Low frequency of rearrangements of the *ret* and *trk* proto-oncogenes in Japanese thyroid papillary carcinomas. *Jpn J Cancer Res* 1992;83:671.
120. Zou M, Shi Y, Farid NR. Low rate of *ret* proto-oncogene activation (PTC/retTPC) in papillary thyroid carcinomas from Saudi Arabia. *Cancer* 1994;73:176.
121. Morris CM, Hao QL, Heisterkamp N, et al. Localization of the TRK proto-oncogene to human chromosome bands 1q23-1q24. *Oncogene* 1991;6:1093.
122. Greco A, Pierotti MA, Bongarzone I, et al. TRK-T1 is a novel oncogene formed by the fusion of TPR and TRK genes in human papillary thyroid carcinomas. *Oncogene* 1992;7:237.
123. Di Renzo MF, Narsimhan RP, Olivero M, et al. Expression of the Met/HGF receptor in normal and neoplastic human tissues. *Oncogene* 1991;6:1977.
124. Di Renzo MF, Olivero M, Ferro S, et al. Overexpression of the c-MET/HGF receptor gene in human thyroid carcinomas. *Oncogene* 1992;7:2549.
125. Jhiang SM, Caruso DR, Gilmore E, et al. Detection of the PTC/ret^{TPC} oncogene in human thyroid cancers. *Oncogene* 1992;7:1331.
126. Jhiang SM, Smanik PA, Mazzaferri EL. Development of a single-step duplex RT-PCR detecting different forms of *ret* activation, and identification of the third form of in vivo *ret* activation in human papillary thyroid carcinomas. *Cancer Lett* 1994;78:69.
127. Jhiang SM, Mazzaferri EL. The ret/PTC oncogene in papillary thyroid carcinoma. *J Lab Clin Med* 1994;123:331.
128. Nord B, Larsson C, Wong FK, et al. Sporadic follicular thyroid tumors show loss of a 200-kb region in 11q13 without evidence for mutations in the *MEN1* gene. *Genes Chromosomes Cancer* 1999;26:35.
129. Herrmann MA, Hey ID, Bartelt DHJ, et al. Cytogenetic and molecular genetic studies of follicular and papillary thyroid cancers. *J Clin Invest* 1991;88:1596.
130. Fagin JA, Matsuo K, Karmarkar A, et al. High prevalence of mutations of the p53 gene in poorly differentiated human thyroid carcinomas. *J Clin Invest* 1992;91:179.
131. Ito T, Seyama T, Mizuno T, et al. Unique association of p53 mutations with undifferentiated but not with differentiated carcinomas of the thyroid gland. *Cancer Res* 1992;52:1369.
132. Arnold A. Genetic basis of endocrine disease 5. Molecular genetics of parathyroid gland neoplasia. *J Clin Endocrinol Metab* 1993;77:1108.
133. Thakker RV, Bouloux P, Wooding C, et al. Association of parathyroid tumors in multiple endocrine neoplasia type 1 with loss of alleles on chromosome 11. *N Engl J Med* 1989;321:218.
134. Radford DM, Ashley SW, Wells SA Jr, et al. Loss of heterozygosity of markers on chromosome 11 in tumors from patients with multiple endocrine neoplasia syndrome type 1. *Cancer Res* 1990;50:6529.
135. Byström C, Larsson C, Blomberg C, et al. Localization of the *MEN1* gene to a small region within chromosome 11q13 by deletion mapping in tumors. *Proc Natl Acad Sci U S A* 1990;87:1968.
136. Friedman E, DeMarco L, Gejman PV, et al. Allelic loss from chromosome 11 in parathyroid tumors. *Cancer Res* 1992;52:6804.
137. Heppner C, Kester MB, Agarwal SK, et al. Somatic mutation of the *MEN1* gene in parathyroid tumours. *Nat Genet* 1997;16:375.
138. Farnebo F, Teh BT, Kytola S, et al. Alterations of the MEN1 gene in sporadic parathyroid tumors. *J Clin Endocrinol Metab* 1998;83:2627.
139. Arnold A, Hyung GK, Gaz RD, et al. Molecular cloning and chromosomal mapping of DNA rearranged with the parathyroid hormone gene in a parathyroid adenoma. *J Clin Invest* 1989;83:2034.
140. Motokura T, Bloom T, Kim HG, et al. A novel cyclin encoded by a bcl1-linked candidate oncogene. *Nature* 1991;350:512.
141. Jackson CE, Boonstra CE. The relationship of hereditary hyperparathyroidism to endocrine adenomatosis. *Am J Med* 1967;43:727.
142. Foley TPJ, Harrison HC, Arnaud CD, et al. Familial benign hypercalcemia. *J Pediatr* 1972;81:1060.
143. Heath HI, Purnell DC. Urinary cyclic 3',5'-adenosine monophosphate responses to exogenous and endogenous parathyroid hormone in familial benign hypercalcemia and primary hyperparathyroidism. *J Lab Clin Med* 1980;96:974.

144. Marx SJ, Attie MF, Levine MA, et al. The hypocalciuric or benign variant of familial hypercalcemia: clinical and biochemical features in fifteen kindreds. *Medicine* 1981;60:397.
145. Paterson CR, Gunn A. Familial benign hypercalcaemia. *Lancet* 1981;2:61.
146. Attie MF, Gill JRJ, Stock JL, et al. Urinary calcium excretion in familial hypocalciuric hypercalcemia: persistence of relative hypocalciuria after induction of hypoparathyroidism. *J Clin Invest* 1983;72:667.
147. Law WMJ, Bollman S, Kumar R, et al. Vitamin D metabolism in familial benign hypercalcemia (hypocalciuric hypercalcemia) differs from that in primary hyperparathyroidism. *J Clin Endocrinol Metab* 1983;58:744.
148. Law WM, Heath HI. Familial benign hypercalcemia (hypocalciuric hypercalcemia): clinical and pathogenetic studies in 21 families. *Ann Intern Med* 1985;102:511.
149. Heath HI. Familial benign (hypocalciuric) hypercalcemia, a troublesome mimic of mild primary hyperparathyroidism. *Endocrinol Metab Clin North Am* 1989;18:723.
150. Pollak MR, Brown EM, Chou Y-HW, et al. Mutations in the Ca^{2+}-sensing receptor gene cause familial hypocalciuric hypercalcemia and neonatal severe hyperparathyroidism. *Cell* 1993;75:1297.
151. Khosla S, Ebeling PR, Firek AF, et al. Calcium infusion suggests a "set-point" abnormality of parathyroid gland function in familial benign hypercalcemia and more complex disturbances in primary hyperparathyroidism. *J Clin Endocrinol Metab* 1993;76:715.
152. Brown EM. Mutations in the calcium-sensing receptor and their clinical implications. *Horm Res* 1997;48:199.
153. Aida K, Koishi S, Inoue M, et al. Familial hypocalciuric hypercalcemia associated with mutation in the human Ca^{2+}-sensing receptor gene. *J Clin Endocrinol Metab* 1995;80:2594.
154. Chou Y-H, Pollak M, Brandi M, et al. Mutations in the human Ca^{2+}-sensing receptor gene that cause familial hypocalciuric hypercalcemia. *Am J Hum Genet* 1995;56:1075.
155. Janicic N, Pausova Z, Cole DEC, et al. Insertion of an Alu sequence in the Ca^{2+}-sensing receptor gene in familial hypocalciuric hypercalcemia and neonatal severe hyperparathyroidism. *Am J Hum Genet* 1995;56:880.
156. Pearce S, Trump D, Wooding C, et al. Calcium-sensing receptor mutations in familial benign hypercalcaemia and neonatal severe hyperparathyroidism. *J Clin Invest* 1995;96:2683.
157. Heath HI. Familial hypocalciuric hypercalcemia. In: Bilezikian J, Marcus R, Levine M, eds. *The parathyroids.* New York: Raven Press, 1994:699.
158. Goldsmith RE, Sizemore GW, Chen I-W, et al. Familial hyperparathyroidism; description of a large kindred and a review of the literature. *Ann Intern Med* 1976;84:36.
159. Wassif WS, Moniz CF, Friedman E, et al. Familial isolated hyperparathyroidism: a distinct genetic entity with an increased risk of parathyroid cancer. *J Clin Endocrinol Metab* 1993;77:1485.
160. Jackson CE, Norum RA, Boyd SB, et al. Hereditary hyperparathyroidism and multiple ossifying jaw fibromas: a clinically and genetically distinct syndrome. *Surgery* 1990;108:1006.
161. Szabó J, Heath B, Hill VM, et al. Hereditary hyperparathyroidism–jaw tumor syndrome: the endocrine tumor gene HRPT2 maps to chromosome 1q21-q31. *Am J Hum Genet* 1995;56:944.
162. Teh BT, Farnebo F, Twigg S, et al. Familial isolated hyperparathyroidism maps to the hyperparathyroidism–jaw tumor locus in 1q21-q32 in a subset of families. *J Clin Endocrinol Metab* 1998;83:2114.
163. Hakim JP, Levine MA. Absence of p53 point mutations in parathyroid adenoma and carcinoma. *J Clin Endocrinol Metab* 1994;78:103.
164. Cryns VL, Rubio MP, Thor AD, et al. p53 abnormalities in human parathyroid carcinoma. *J Clin Endocrinol Metab* 1994;78:1320.
165. Cryns VL, Thor A, Xu H-J, et al. Loss of the retinoblastoma tumor-suppressor gene in parathyroid carcinomas. *N Engl J Med* 1994;330:757.
166. Latif F, Tory K, Gnarra J, et al. Identification of the von Hippel-Lindau disease tumor suppressor gene. *Science* 1993;260:1317.
167. Duan DR, Pause A, Burgess WH, et al. Inhibition of transcription elongation by the VHL tumor suppressor protein. *Science* 1995;269:1402.
168. Crossey PA, Richards FM, Foster K, et al. Identification of intragenic mutations in the von Hippel-Lindau disease tumour suppressor gene and correlation with disease phenotype. *Hum Mol Genet* 1994;3:1303.
169. Cawthon RM, Weiss R, Xu G, et al. A major segment of the neurofibromatosis type 1 gene: cDNA sequence, genomic structure, and point mutations. *Cell* 1990;62:193.
170. Wallace MR, Marchuk DA, Andersen LB, et al. Type 1 neurofibromatosis gene: identification of a large transcript disrupted in three NF1 patients. *Science* 1990;249:181.
171. Yano T, Linehan M, Anglard P, et al. Genetic changes in human adrenocortical carcinomas. *J Natl Cancer Inst* 1989;7:518.
172. Srivastava S, Zou Z, Pirollo K, et al. Germ-line transmission of a mutated p53 gene in a cancer-prone family with Li-Fraumeni syndrome. *Nature* 1990;348:747.
173. Ping AJ, Reeve AE, Law DJ, et al. Genetic linkage of Beckwith-Wiedemann syndrome to 11p15. *Am J Hum Genet* 1989;44:720.
174. Reincke M, Karl M, Travis WH, et al. p53 mutations in human adrenocortical neoplasms: immunohistochemical and molecular studies. *J Clin Endocrinol Metab* 1994;78:790.
175. Williamson EA, Johnson SJ, Foster S, et al. G protein gene mutations in patients with multiple endocrinopathies. *J Clin Endocrinol Metab* 1995;80:1702.
176. Latronico AC, Reincke M, Mendonça BB, et al. No evidence for oncogenic mutations in the adrenocorticotropin receptor gene in human adrenocortical neoplasms. *J Clin Endocrinol Metab* 1995;80:875.
177. Gortz B, Roth J, Speel EJM, et al. *MEN1* gene mutation analysis of sporadic adrenocortical lesions. *Int J Cancer* 1999;80:373.
178. Khosla S, Patel VM, Hay ID, et al. Loss of heterozygosity suggests multiple genetic alterations in pheochromocytomas and medullary thyroid carcinomas. *J Clin Invest* 1991;87:1691.
179. Yang K-P, Nguyen CV, Castillo SG, et al. Deletion mapping on the distal third region of chromosome 1p in multiple endocrine neoplasia type IIA. *Anticancer Res* 1990;10:527.
180. Mathew CGP, Smith BA, Thorpe K, et al. Deletions of genes on chromosome 1 in endocrine neoplasia. *Nature* 1987;328:524.
181. Shin E, Fujita S, Takami K, et al. Deletion mapping of chromosome 1p and 22q in pheochromocytoma. *Jpn J Cancer Res* 1993;84:402.

SECTION **2**

DOUGLAS L. FRAKER
MONICA SKARULIS
VIRGINIA LIVOLSI

Thyroid Tumors

Cancers of the endocrine glands or organs are rare, as they will account for only 1.5% of the estimated 1.22 million new cases of non–skin cancer and 0.21% of the estimated 563,100 cancer deaths in the United States in 1999.[1] Thyroid cancer is overwhelmingly the most common type of endocrine malignancy, accounting for the majority of the deaths due to endocrine cancers. It was estimated that in 1999 there would be 18,100 new cases of thyroid cancer (more than 90% of the total new endocrine cancers) and 1400 deaths due to thyroid cancer, which is 60% of the total deaths due to endocrine malignancies (Table 38.2-1).[1] Compared to the number of thyroid cancers, there are approximately 800 cases of endocrine pancreas tumors (not all malignant),[2] 550 adrenal cancers, 130 pituitary gland cancers, and 65 parathyroid gland cancers. The discrepancy between the total number of cases of all endocrine cancers arising in the thyroid (91%) and the total proportion of endocrine cancer deaths (60%) reflects the relatively indolent nature and long-term survival associated with thyroid malignancies.

Within the broad category of thyroid cancers, there are many types, each with a distinctive epidemiology, natural history, treatment, and prognosis. The general categories of thyroid cancer are well-differentiated malignancies, anaplastic cancer, medullary thyroid cancer (MTC), and other unusual cancers, such as lymphoma, sarcoma, and other rare malignancies.[3] The normal thyroid is composed histologically of two main parenchymal cell types. Follicular cells line the colloid follicles, concentrate iodine, and are involved in the production of thyroid hormone. These cells give rise to well-differentiated cancers and, almost certainly, anaplastic thyroid cancer (ATC). The second cell type is the parafollicular or C cell, which produces calcitonin and is the cell of origin for MTC. Stromal and immune cells of the thyroid are responsible for sarcoma and lymphoma, respectively. Of the 18,100 new cases of thyroid cancer each year, approximately 90% of malignant thyroid nodules are well-differentiated cancers, 5% to 9% are MTC, 1% to 2% are anaplastic cancers, 1% to 3% are lymphoma, and fewer than 1% are sarcoma and other rare tumors.[3]

Within the category of well-differentiated thyroid cancers, there are various histologic subtypes. These descriptive subgroupings have evolved since the 1980s with an improved understanding of the biology of these different types. Initial categories included papillary, follicular, and mixed tumor with variable

TABLE 38.2-1. Incidence and Proportion of All Endocrine Cancers and Relative Proportions of Different Primary Thyroid Cancer Subtypes

	Number	*Percentage of Total*
All endocrine cancers[a]		
Thyroid	18,100	91
Endocrine pancreas	800	4
Adrenal	550	2.8
Thymus	425	2.1
Pineal gland	128	0.6
Pituitary gland	77	0.4
Parathyroid	48	0.2
Carotid body, paraganglia	33	0.16
Primary thyroid cancers[b]		
Well-differentiated		87–90
Papillary		75
Follicular		10
Hürthle cell		2–4
Anaplastic		1–2
Medullary thyroid cancer		5–9
Sporadic		6
Familial		3
Lymphoma		1–3
Sarcoma and others		<1

[a]Adapted from ref. 1.
[b]Adapted from ref. 3.

areas of both papillary and follicular histology. Several studies have documented that these mixed tumors with any area of papillary features have the same natural history and prognosis as papillary thyroid cancer without follicular feratures.[3,4] This category of mixed papillary and follicular carcinoma should be grouped with papillary carcinoma; even those that are composed entirely of follicles should be included (diagnosed as the follicular variant of papillary carinoma). The major cytologic feature shared by all members of this group, regardless of the histologic pattern, is the characteristic nucleus. A third category of lesions grouped with differentiated thyroid carcinoma is the Hürthle cell or oncocytic carcinoma. Although there are controversies about whether Hürthle cell neoplasms can behave in a benign fashion, most authors now accept the concept of benign and malignant lesions with this cytology.[5] The clinical behavior of these lesions is somewhat more aggressive than usual follicular carcinomas, and some authors prefer to include these lesions in the intermediate malignancy group. The distribution of well-differentiated thyroid cancer subgroups in some reports shows that 80% to 85% are papillary, with 10% to 15% of cases being follicular and 3% to 5% Hürthle cell carcinomas.[3] These published figures may not reflect adequate pathologic recognition of the follicular variant of papillary carcinoma, and true follicular carcinoma may represent 5% or fewer of well-differentiated thyroid cancers in countries with iodine-sufficient diets.[4] Therefore, as 90% of all thyroid cancers are well-differentiated and 85% to 95% of all well-differentiated tumors are papillary tumors, papillary thyroid cancer accounts for 75% to 80% of all thyroid cancers.

This chapter is organized to present the key clinical aspects of well-differentiated thyroid cancers, anaplastic cancers, MTCs, thyroid lymphoma, and secondary thyroid malignancies. As the vast majority of thyroid cancers present as thyroid nodules, yet only a minority of all thyroid nodules are malignant, a general discussion of the incidence, evaluation, and management of thyroid nodules precedes discussion of specific clinical conditions.

THYROID NODULES

The prevalence of thyroid nodules depends on the population under study; gender, age, and history of exposure to ionizing radiation strongly influence the results of various large studies, as does the method by which the nodules are being detected (physical examination, ultrasonography, or pathology). There is clearly an age-dependent increase in thyroid nodules[6]; in one pathologic study, up to 90% of women older than 70 years and 60% of men older than 80 years had nodular goiter.[7] All studies show that women develop nodules more frequently than men, although reports of the female to male ratio vary from 1.2:1 to 4.3:1.[8] An increased tendency to develop thyroid nodules is demonstrated in groups exposed to ionizing radiation, especially during childhood. In a study at the Michael Reese Hospital, 38.4% of patients who received radiation before age 16 years developed palpable thyroid nodules.[9] In patients with Hodgkin's disease treated with mantle radiation, 3% developed thyroid nodules.[10]

Most thyroid nodules are found in asymptomatic patients either during routine physical examination of the neck or because the patient notices a mass in the neck. By obtaining information from the history and physical examination, one assesses the risk of malignancy in that individual. In general, there is a 5% to 10% chance of malignancy in all thyroid nodules for the total population[11]; however, men and patients at the extremes of age are at higher risk for malignancy. Nodules found in a patient with a history of childhood neck irradiation carry a 33% to 37% chance of malignancy.[12,13] The presence of a solitary nodule is of greater concern than a thyroid with multiple nodules; however, a dominant nodule or a nodule that changes size in the setting of a multinodular goiter should be investigated to exclude carcinoma. Patients with Graves' disease who develop a nodule may have a higher risk of cancer.[14,15] Whether the co-occurrence of Graves' disease affects the aggressiveness of the thyroid carcinoma is a topic of controversy.[16,17] However, the occurrence of carcinoma in autonomously functioning nodules is extremely rare.[8]

Although not specific for malignancy, a history of rapid increase in size, dyspnea, dysphagia, hoarseness, and the development of a Horner's syndrome are worrisome symptoms. Tender nodules are more often associated with thyroiditis and are likely to be benign. A family history of thyroid cancer or pheochromocytoma should suggest MTC in the setting of multiple endocrine neoplasia type 2a (MEN 2A) or MEN 2B.[19] Other inherited disorders to be aware of are Gardner's syndrome[20] and Cowden's disease,[21] both of which are associated with benign and malignant thyroid neoplasms. On examination of the neck, attention to the firmness, mobility, and size of the nodules, their adherence to surrounding structures, and the presence of adenopathy are important clues to the presence of carcinoma. However, these features, with the exception of cervical lymphadenopathy, lack specificity for malignancy.[22]

Thyroid function testing should be performed to identify underlying thyroid pathology and not to differentiate benign from malignant nodules. Subclinical hyperthyroidism, sometimes seen only as a suppressed thyroid-stimulating hormone (TSH), may be secondary to an autonomously functioning nodule. In this case, one determines whether the nodule is functional with a radionuclide scan by iodine uptake. Tests of serum thyroglobulin (Tg) levels are not helpful in distinguishing benign from malignant thyroid nodules.[18] Routine measurement of serum calcitonin may be useful to identify patients with sporadic medullary carcinoma of the thyroid preoperatively[23]; however, the cost-effectiveness of this practice requires further evaluation.[24] The majority of both benign and malignant thyroid nodules are hypofunctional when compared to normally functioning thyroid tissue; thus, the finding of a "cold nodule" on ^{123}I or ^{99}Tc scanning is nonspecific. Radionuclide scans are also helpful in determining the functional status of nodules in patients with multinodular thyroid disease to focus a biopsy on cold nodules.[18] A hyperfunctioning or hot nodule is rarely malignant in an adult.[18]

High-resolution ultrasonography is a useful adjunct to the clinical examination for size assessment of nodules, for the detection of multiple nodules not discerned by palpation, and for assisting in fine-needle aspiration biopsy (FNAB) of nodules.[25,26] Despite advances in technology allowing more sensitive detection of blood flow in thyroid pathology, differences in echogenicity or vascularity cannot distinguish benign from malignant lesions.[27] Ultrasonography identifies whether a lesion is cystic or solid, and the vast majority of cystic lesions are benign. A more cost-effective method to identify a cyst is fine-needle aspiration (FNA) with return of fluid and disappearance of the nodule after aspiration. Cysts larger than 4 cm in size and having a partially solid component and those that recur after three aspirations may warrant biopsy, as these conditions are more likely to be associated with malignancy.[3]

The single most important study in the evaluation of thyroid nodules is the FNAB. The impact this procedure has had on clinical practice is reflected by a reduction of the total number of thyroid surgeries performed, a greater proportion of malignancies removed at surgery, and an overall reduction in the cost of managing patients with nodules.[8] The accuracy of cytologic diagnosis from fine-needle biopsy ranges from 70% to 97%[25] and is highly dependent on the skill of the person performing the biopsy and that of the cytopathologist interpreting it. The results of FNAB are most commonly divided into the following categories: benign or negative (colloid nodule or hyperplastic nodule), indeterminate (all follicular neoplasms, including those with Hürthle cell changes), suspicious or malignant (papillary, anaplastic, medullary, and lymphoma), and insufficient sample. Reviews of this technique provide insight into the results typically obtained at the time of fine-needle biopsy of the nodules: 70% are classified as benign (range, 53% to 90%), 4.0% as malignant (range, 1% to 10%), 10% as suspicious or indeterminate (range, 5% to 23%), and 17% as insufficient sample (range, 15% to 20%).[28]

The malignant potential of follicular neoplasms cannot be determined by cytologic evaluation; thus, the biopsies from all such lesions are generally classified as suspicious or indeterminate, and most come to surgical resection. The cells from follicular adenomas and follicular carcinomas appear identical; only by identifying capsular or vascular invasion can cancer be diagnosed.[18] Specimens with predominantly Hürthle cells must be treated in the same fashion; however, extensive Hürthle cell changes can be seen in Hashimoto's thyroiditis. Malignancy is found in 10% to 20% of follicular nodules that are classified as indeterminate on biopsy.[18,29]

Attempts to develop more discriminating cytologic subclassifications to improve the yield of malignancy found at surgery have not proven highly successful, nor are they easily adopted at other institutions. A new technique to improve the sensitivity of FNA in this situation has been to perform polymerase chain reaction analysis for telomerase, which is an enzyme expressed in virtually all malignant cancers but not expressed in benign or normal tissue.[30] Preliminary studies have demonstrated increased telomerase activity in thyroid cancers, and this may serve as a useful adjunct to improve the sensitivity of this category of suspicious or indeterminate FNAB with more appropriate surgical procedures.[31,32]

Biopsies classified as benign or negative are safely followed up medically with the caveat that false-negative results occur in 1% to 6% of cases.[28] Clinical judgment should dictate the course of action in these cases; if a large, hard nodule is fixed to surrounding tissue and is painful, surgery should be performed despite a negative aspirate. Sampling error occurring during biopsy of large, cystic hemorrhagic nodules or simple misdiagnosis account for many of the false-negative results.[33] False-positive results for malignancy occur in 3% to 6% of all biopsies.[28] The cytologic features of Hashimoto's thyroiditis frequently lead to these false-positive interpretations.[33] With experienced cytopathologists, this false-positive rate should decrease to less than 1%.[34]

Benign thyroid nodules can be followed up carefully by routine physical examination or, more precisely, by ultrasonography and do not generally require repeat biopsy.[18] Thyroxine suppression therapy is widely used; however, randomized controlled studies have indicated that thyroxine therapy is not superior to placebo.[35–37]

Attention to potential side effects of long-term thyroxine therapy has stirred controversy. The creation of a subclinical hyperthyroid state by suppressive doses of thyroxine increases the incidence of osteoporosis.[15] There is evidence that postmenopausal women who are not on estrogen replacement therapy are at higher risk for bone demineralization while on suppressive doses of thyroxine.[38] Patients on long-term suppressive therapy may have cardiac symptoms (tachycardia, arrhythmias),[39] and those at high risk for recurrence of thyroid cancer may receive less aggressive suppression and judicious use of β-adrenergic blockers to prevent atrial arrhythmias.[39]

WELL-DIFFERENTIATED THYROID CARCINOMA

DEMOGRAPHICS AND EPIDEMIOLOGY

The incidence of both papillary and follicular thyroid carcinomas in terms of gender distribution is similar, with approximately a 2.5-fold excess in favor of female individuals as compared to male individuals (Table 38.2-2).[3,40–46] The median age at diagnosis is earlier in women than in men for both papillary and follicular subtypes and tends to be earlier for papillary cancer as compared to follicular cancer in either gender (see Table 38.2-2).[42–46] Specifically, median age at diagnosis in white

TABLE 38.2-2. Age, Gender Distribution, Proportion of Papillary or Follicular and Extent of Disease at Presentation for Several Institutional Series of Well-Differentiated Thyroid Cancer

					Papillary[a]			*Follicular*		
Institution	*Interval*	*No.*	*Mean Age (y)*	*F/M Ratio*	No.	LN at Dx	Distant Met	No.	LN at Dx	Distant Met
UCSF[90]	1942–1970	443	—	—	399	43%	2%	44	11%	2%
Brigham[91]	1948–1982	210	—	—	164	46%	—	46	32%	—
Hartford[35]	1960–1984	223	46.3	3:1	178	—	—	45	—	—
Lahey Clinic[36]	1961–1980	309	—	2.1:1	244	—	1%	65	—	0%
Ohio State[37]	1962–1993	1355	35.7	2.2:1	1077	40%	2%	278	25%	5%
Toronto[38]	1963–1983	1578	45	3:1	1074	27%	6%	504	12%	13%
Mayo Clinic[39,b]	1946–1970	959	45	2.3:1	859	37%	—	100	6%	12%
University of Michigan[40,c]	1962–1982	37	45	2.4:1	0	—	—	37	8%	16%

Distant Met, distant metastases documented at diagnosis; F/M, female-male; LN at Dx, lymph node metastases present at diagnosis; UCSF, University of California, San Francisco.
[a]Series with mixed tumors reported are grouped together as papillary in this table.
[b]Mayo Clinic series reported as two separate studies combined in this table.
[c]University of Michigan series reported as group that had only follicular lesions.

women is between 40 and 41 years, whereas for white men, it is 44 to 45 years for papillary carcinoma.[3] For follicular thyroid carcinoma, the median age at diagnosis is 48 for white women as compared to 53 for white men.[3] Well-differentiated thyroid cancer has a greater incidence in whites than in blacks of both genders.[7] The relative proportion of age-adjusted incidence rates is slightly more than twofold higher for whites. One significant difference in the incidence in terms of race is that the proportion of well-differentiated thyroid carcinomas that are follicular is increased greatly in blacks as compared to whites. It is reported that follicular carcinoma accounts for 15% of all well-differentiated tumors in whites as compared to 34% in blacks.[3]

ETIOLOGY

Radiation exposure to the thyroid gland is the only risk factor known definitively to increase the incidence of well-differentiated thyroid cancer.[47,48] Thyroid exposure to radiation can occur in two ways: from external sources or from ingestion of radioactive material. Data regarding external exposure to the thyroid comes primarily from two sources. One is medically administered external-beam irradiation, and the second is environmental exposure, previously related to nuclear weapons attacks or weapons testing and, more recently, from nuclear power plant accidents. Internal exposure occurs by ingestion of radioisotopes of iodine that concentrate in the thyroid gland from either medical treatment with radioactive iodine or by ingestion of these radioisotopes from the fallout from nuclear weapons explosions or power plant accidents. The relative risks of radiation exposure from these different sources has been well studied, and variables, such as age at exposure, radiation dose, and latent period to developing cancers, have been defined.[48] However, radiation accounts for only a small portion of the total annual cases of well-differentiated thyroid cancer.[49] Other potential factors that may predispose to thyroid neoplasms include diet (particularly content of iodine), effects of steroid hormones, and other occupational exposures.[47,50]

Case-control studies,[51,52] as well as detailed institutional reviews of large populations of patients[9,53] undergoing childhood irradiation, show that there is an inverse relationship between increased risk of thyroid cancer and age of exposure to radiation. Relative risk is also linearly related to exposure dose, at least up to 2000 rads.[9,54] The latent period after exposure is at least 3 to 5 years, and there is no apparent drop-off in the increased risk even after 40 years after the radiation exposure.[54] One of the best analyzed databases regarding childhood radiation for medical purposes comes from Schneider et al.[9,53,54] at the University of Chicago. They have intensively analyzed more than 3000 patients who were irradiated between 1939 and 1962. More than one-third of these patients developed thyroid nodules, and 318 patients were documented to have thyroid cancer.[53] The large populations studied by Schneider et al. showed that increased relative risk of thyroid carcinoma was low and thyroid cancers were rare between 5 and 10 years after radiation exposure.[54] The majority of cases occurred between 20 and 40 years after exposure. However, even after 40 years, the relative risk as compared to a nonirradiated population was still increased.[54] For these reasons, the large cohort of patients who underwent childhood irradiation for benign medical conditions between 1920 and 1960 are now between the ages of 40 and 80, and this population still has an increased risk of developing thyroid carcinoma as compared to nonirradiated patients.

Although the use of radiation for benign conditions has not been practiced since the 1960s, there is increased use of radiation treatments for neoplastic conditions, including infants, children, and young adults.[55] The majority of this patient population is made up of patients with either Hodgkin's or non-Hodgkin's lymphoma but also includes long-term survivors of Wilms' tumor of the kidneys or neuroblastoma in which there is some scatter to the thyroid gland.[10,55] The young age at treatment for neuroblastoma and Wilms' tumor (mean age, 2 and 3 years, respectively) and the relatively high-dose of thyroid exposure (660 rads and 310 rads, respectively) has led to a dramatic increase in relative risk of 350 for neuroblastoma patients and 132 for survivors of Wilms' tumors for the development of thyroid cancer.[51] Relative risks between 16 and 80 have been reported in this patient population of adolescents and young adults treated for lymphoma.[10,55] In the adult patient population treated with therapeutic radiation for malignancies, there is a drop-off in risk reflecting the importance of age at exposure. A large study of more than 150,000 women treated with radiation for cervical cancer had an estimated thyroid exposure of 11 rads, with a relative risk of 2.35, compared to nonirradiated age-matched controls.[56]

A second type of radiation exposure to the thyroid gland is via ingestion of radioisotopes that concentrate in the thyroid. These isotopes come from two sources: medical administration either for diagnostic or therapeutic purposes using radioactive iodine,[57] and environmental exposure to fallout from nuclear weapons or nuclear accidents. The most common exposure is due to ^{131}I administered for diagnostic thyroid scans. A typical nuclear medicine study exposes the thyroid to the equivalent of approximately 50 rads of external-beam radiation exposure.[58] A large study of more than 35,000 diagnostic scans between 1951 and 1969 showed a very minimal increase in the number of thyroid cancers, with 50 actual cases versus 39.4 cases predicted.[58] A second, more significant medical exposure is therapeutic ^{131}I administered for ablation of thyroid tissue, with the equivalent of 6000 to 10,000 mL to treat Graves' disease.[59] Despite this high radiation dose, there is a standardized increased incidence ratio of only 1.32 for thyroid cancer,[59] as the high-dose ^{131}I most likely destroys the thyroid parenchyma.

A more dangerous type of ingestion of radioisotopes of iodine comes from exposure to nuclear fallout.[60,61] Data from fallout exposure comes from nuclear weapon–testing sites at the Marshall Islands[60] and Nevada in the 1950s,[61] as well as the 1986 nuclear power plant explosion at Chernobyl.[62] The positive results in these studies compared to the lack of risk of the medical use of ^{131}I is most likely due to other high-energy short-lived isotopes, such as ^{129}I and ^{132}I to ^{135}I present in fallout that are more damaging but are not present in radioisotope drugs. An early study completed 4.5 years after the event at Chernobyl suggested no increased risk of thyroid nodules.[63] More recent studies show a steady sequential increase in the diagnosis of pediatric thyroid cancer as early as 3 years and increasing from 5 to now 10 years since the incident.[62] This data reflect the importance of age at exposure, as this increased incidence occurs primarily in children.

The natural history and pathology of radiation-associated thyroid cancer has been well documented in the aforementioned epidemiologic studies.[9,50] The vast majority of cases have a papillary histology, and these behave in the same way as nonradiation-associated papillary cancers.[9]

Although the data relating radiation exposure of the thyroid gland and subsequent development of carcinoma are definitive, the majority of patients who developed well-differentiated thyroid carcinoma have absolutely no history of radiation exposure. A study from the Connecticut Tumor Registry shows that 9% of thyroid cancer could be related to radiation exposure, meaning 91% of cases have no identifiable risk factor.[49] Other factors, including dietary influences, sex hormones, environmental exposures, or increased genetic susceptibility, have been studied, with very mixed results and no clear associations. Dietary influences have primarily focused on the level of iodine in the diet.[47,50,64] Iodine-deficient diets or diets that include a large intake of vegetables from the crucifer family (which block iodine uptake) may lead to increased TSH levels and are considered goitrogenic, with a modest increase in follicular cancers.[64] Increased iodine intake due to shellfish occurs in the geographic areas with the highest incidence of predominantly papillary thyroid cancer, such as Iceland, Norway, and Hawaii.[65]

There is no clear familial syndrome or genetic disease associated with the development of well-differentiated thyroid cancer, although one study has suggested a propensity to multifocal well-differentiated thyroid cancer in a small number of families.[66] However, none of the described oncogenes for well-differentiated thyroid cancer (RET, MNG-1, TCO) were found to be involved in evaluation of 56 kindreds.[67,68] This contrasts with MTC, in which a variety of genetic syndromes now are being defined at the molecular level (see later in Treatment of Familial Medullary Thyroid Cancer and Table 38.2-10).[65]

PATHOLOGY

Thyroid malignancies are derived from either follicular cells (papillary, follicular, Hürthle cell, and anaplastic carcinomas) or C cells (medullary carcinoma, described later in Medullary Thyroid Cancer).[69,70] The degree of clinical malignancy varies greatly among the types of carcinoma: It is convenient to consider these tumors as falling into three categories with increasing clinical aggressiveness: well-differentiated (papillary carcinoma, follicular carcinoma), intermediate differentiation (Hürthle cell carcinoma, some variants of papillary carcinoma, insular carcinoma), and undifferentiated (anaplastic carcinoma).

Papillary carcinoma constitutes approximately 80% to 85% of malignant epithelial thyroid tumors in developed countries where sufficient iodine is present in the diet.[3,71] Grossly, papillary carcinomas have a variable appearance from minute subcapsular white scars to large tumors greater than 5 to 6 cm that grossly extend outside the thyroid gland. Cystic change, calcification, and even ossification may be identified.

Microscopically, papillary carcinomas are characterized by the presence of papillae, but some variants contain no papillary areas, are totally follicular in pattern, and are identified as a follicular variant.[72] The term *mixed papillary and follicular carcinoma* is no longer used, because the great majority of papillary carcinomas of the thyroid do contain some follicular areas (Fig. 38.2-1). Biologically, all these tumors, independent of their degree of follicular pattern, show similar clinical characteristics.[69,70,73] The World Health Organization defines papillary thyroid cancer as "a malignant epithelial thyroid neoplasm with a distinctive set of nuclear features. The nuclei of papillary carcinoma are enlarged and ovoid and contain thick nuclear membranes, small nucleoli often pressed against the nuclear membrane, intranuclear grooves, and intranuclear cytoplasmic inclusions."[73,74] Because the nuclei are enlarged, they frequently overlap each other, which is a helpful clue in both the cytologic preparations and histologic slides. Papillary carcinoma has a propensity to invade lymphatic spaces and, therefore, leads to microscopic multifocal lesions in the gland as well as a high incidence of regional lymph node metastases.[73] The latter may be the presenting symptom of a thyroid papillary carcinoma as, in some cases, a primary tumor is very small (less than a few millimeters).

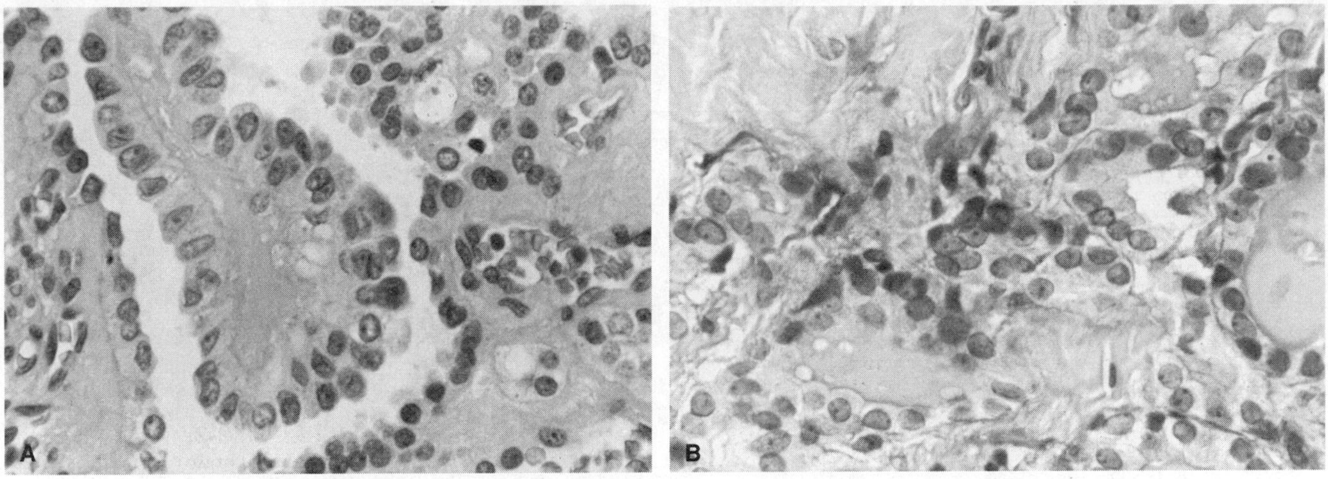

FIGURE 38.2-1. **A:** Classic papillary carcinoma. Note the papilla with its fibrovascular core. The nuclei are enlarged, are elongated rather than round, and have irregular nuclear outlines. (Hematoxylin and eosin, ×250.) **B:** Follicular variant of papillary carcinoma. The tumor cells are arranged in follicles; note the characteristic nuclei throughout the lesion. (Hematoxylin and eosin, ×250.)

Certain variants of papillary carcinoma have been shown to be more aggressive clinically, but these make up a minority of all papillary carcinomas. The more aggressive variants include the so-called tall cell variant, in which the cells are at least twice as long as they are wide[75]; the columnar variant, which shows a curious clear cytoplasm[76]; and the diffuse sclerosis variant, which is found more commonly in young individuals and adolescents.[77] This sclerosis variant permeates the thyroid lymphatics and has a 100% incidence of regional lymph node metastases at the time of diagnosis. All these high-risk variants are associated with significant mortality at 5 years, ranging between 25% and 90%.[75,78]

True follicular thyroid carcinoma is a rare tumor comprising approximately 5% to 10% of thyroid malignancies in nonendemic goiter areas of the world.[3] Before iodine prophylaxis via iodinated salt, follicular carcinoma was much more frequently diagnosed. In addition, the pathologic dictum—that any tumor with a pattern that is 50% or more characteristic of follicular carcinoma should be diagnostically placed in a follicular carcinoma category—has been shown to be incorrect. Indeed, most of the follicular pattern thyroid malignancies represent the follicular variant of papillary carcinoma and share its biological features, natural history, and prognosis.[73] Follicular thyroid carcinoma is unifocal and thickly encapsulated and shows invasion of the capsule or the vessels. Because of the diagnostic confusion, it is difficult to collect statistics about the survival rate or the metastatic potential of true follicular carcinoma.[79] Most studies show that if capsular invasion but not vascular invasion is present, the prognosis is excellent, with 85% to 100% of patients surviving at least 10 years of follow-up.[79,80]

A variant of follicular neoplasms is the Hürthle cell neoplasm. In 1894, Hürthle described a thyroid cell that was later shown to be the parafollicular C cell.[5] For this reason, the designation of cells and their tumors as Hürthle cells is historically incorrect as these lesions are actually derived from thyroid follicular cells.[5] The preferred pathologic term is *oncocytic*. However, because a large body of literature exists on the subject of Hürthle cells and Hürthle cell neoplasms, this nomenclature will be used. The Hürthle cell tumor of the thyroid is one of the most controversial lesions in this organ. Initially, all such lesions, despite the histologic features, were considered to be malignant; hence, it was recommended that they all be treated aggressively.[81] However, many studies have evaluated the clinical pathologic features of thyroid Hürthle cell tumors and have shown that, on average, only 33% show histologic evidence of malignancy or invasive growth and may metastasize.[82,83] Hürthle cell tumors that do not demonstrate invasion microscopically behave as adenomas and may be treated conservatively.

CLINICAL FINDINGS IN WELL-DIFFERENTIATED THYROID CANCER

The typical clinical presentation for a patient with well-differentiated thyroid cancer is development of an asymptomatic thyroid nodule.[8,11] Other symptoms may infrequently precede or occur simultaneously with development of a nodule, including hoarseness, dyspnea, and dysphagia, reflecting local invasion of the recurrent laryngeal nerve, the trachea, and the esophagus, respectively.[84,85] A small subset of patients present with palpable cervical lymphadenopathy without an identifiable mass in the thyroid. Because most patients with well-differentiated thyroid cancer are euthyroid, complaints related to thyroid dysfunction are rare, and thyroid function test results tend to be normal. Certain aspects of the clinical history are relevant to the differential diagnosis, including a prior history of radiation exposure (increased risk of papillary cancer), family history (increased risk of familial MTC), and rapid rate of growth of the thyroid nodule (increased likelihood of ATC or thyroid lymphoma), but may also represent a spontaneous hemorrhage into a benign cyst. A second category of patients diagnosed with thyroid nodules consists of those in whom the nodule is not palpable but is diagnosed by imaging studies obtained for other clinical indications.[86] For example, patients undergoing neck ultrasonography for parathyroid disease or undergoing neck magnetic resonance imaging studies for cervical spine disease may have unappreciated nodular disease within the thyroid.[87]

Any new palpable thyroid nodule or any lesion larger than 1.0 cm identified by neck imaging should be initially assessed by FNAB (described previously in Thyroid Nodules).[88] Nodules

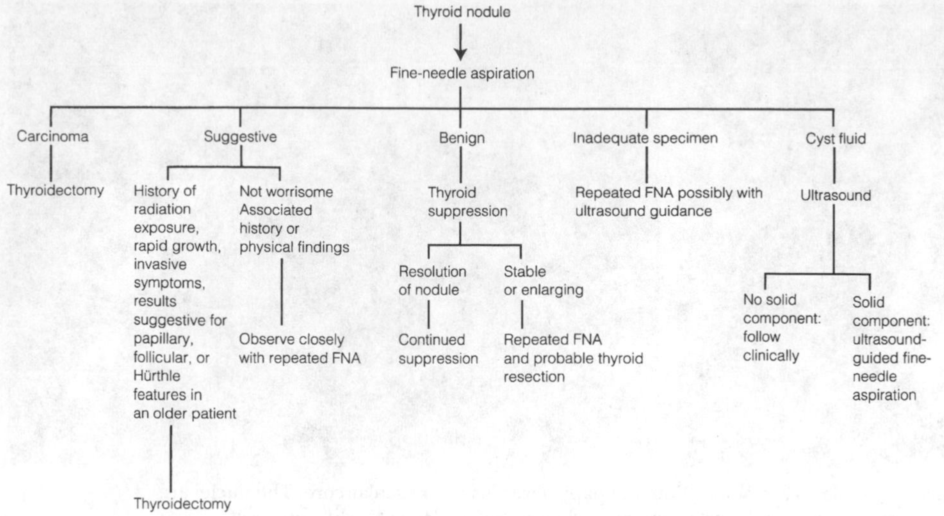

FIGURE 38.2-2. A flow diagram for management of thyroid nodules based on fine-needle aspiration as the initial procedure.

smaller than 1.0 cm may be followed intermittently (6 to 12 months) with ultrasonography and should be subjected to biopsy only when the nodule becomes larger than 1.0 cm.[18] Management decisions in these patients are based on the FNA results modified by certain factors of the clinical history.[8,28] Potential management options include careful observation typically combined with thyroid suppression, alternative or repeat diagnostic studies, or surgical excision. The goal of management of these patients is to avoid missing an enlarging carcinoma that could be morbid to the patients if the disease is not recognized and treated balanced against the goal of avoiding unnecessary surgical procedures for benign pathology.[8,89] An algorithm of management based on FNA as the initial procedure is shown in Figure 38.2-2. Decisions regarding patient management in four of the five categories of possible results from the FNA are relatively straightforward. Patients with malignant lesions detected by FNA should undergo surgical resection. The extent of this resection is controversial and is discussed in detail later in Treatment of Well-Differentiated Thyroid Cancer: Surgery. Patients with a benign FNA result should be followed up intermittently, and nodules that enlarge should be resubmitted to biopsy.[18] The controversial point regarding these patients is the use of thyroid suppression.[35–37] Although common clinical practice is to suppress patients who have benign nodules by FNA using thyroid hormone, objective data that this practice alters the clinical course are lacking. Some investigators argue that patients with a prior history of radiation should have all thyroid lesions surgically resected once they are noted without a biopsy.[3] Although the proportion of these patients with carcinoma is relatively increased, the majority (65%) still do not have malignant lesions.[9]

Patients with an inadequate biopsy should submit to a repeat biopsy, as one-half of the time this provides definitive results.[33] Often, patients with small lesions that are not discrete and are difficult to palpate as well as patients with large lesions with areas of necrosis or hemorrhage have inadequate sampling results. Repeat FNA with ultrasonographic guidance to ensure that the aspiration specimen is taken from a solid component of the lesion may be helpful.[26,86] Nodules in patients in whom a diagnosis cannot be obtained by repeat FNA even with ultrasonographic assistance should be studied with nuclear medicine scans to determine the functional status of the nodule.[27] Functional nodules have a small chance of being malignant, whereas hyperfunctional nodules in adults are unlikely to harbor malignant lesions and require no further study other than close follow-up.[18]

Cystic lesions should be aspirated until all the fluid is removed.[90] After the cyst fluid aspiration, the area is studied with ultrasonography, and any residual solid component is sent for biopsy by FNA using ultrasound guidance. Cysts that have a complex cyst and solid component, are recurrent after three separate aspirations, and are larger than 4 cm may warrant open biopsy, as these conditions are more likely to be associated with malignancies.[3,90] Patients who have a cyst resolve and then recur should undergo repeat cyst aspiration, with biopsy reserved for patients with recurrent lesions despite three prior successful aspirations.

Most investigators recommend surgical resection of lesions classified as indeterminate or suspicious by FNA to establish definitive diagnosis.[91] Analysis of subgroups in this category show the majority of aspirates "suggestive of a follicular neoplasm" and, to a lesser extent, "suspicious for papillary" or "Hürthle cell features."[92] In a large series from the M. D. Anderson Cancer Center, 22% of patients with suspicious FNA eventually were shown to have cancer; of these patients, virtually all biopsies suggested papillary cancer on the initial cytology report, and the majority with follicular or Hürthle features and who were older were the patients who proved to have malignant lesions.[92] Analyses such as these may establish criteria for selective surgical management of patients with suspicious nodules on FNA. Any patients with an indeterminate or suspicious FNA with other risk factors, such as prior radiation exposure or local symptoms, should have nodules surgically resected. For patients with no risk factors and stable nodules, some investigators have advocated using nuclear medicine thyroid scans to determine patient management.[3] A cold mass clearly has a higher risk for being a carcinoma as compared to a warm or hot mass by this nuclear medicine scan, and patients with functional or hyperfunctioning nodules can be followed up clinically.

NATURAL HISTORY AND PROGNOSIS

The natural history and prognosis of well-differentiated thyroid cancer has been intensively studied since the 1980s.[93–99] Clear definition of risk factors associated with poor outcome have allowed more selective and less morbid treatment recommendations. In general, well-differentiated thyroid cancer is one of

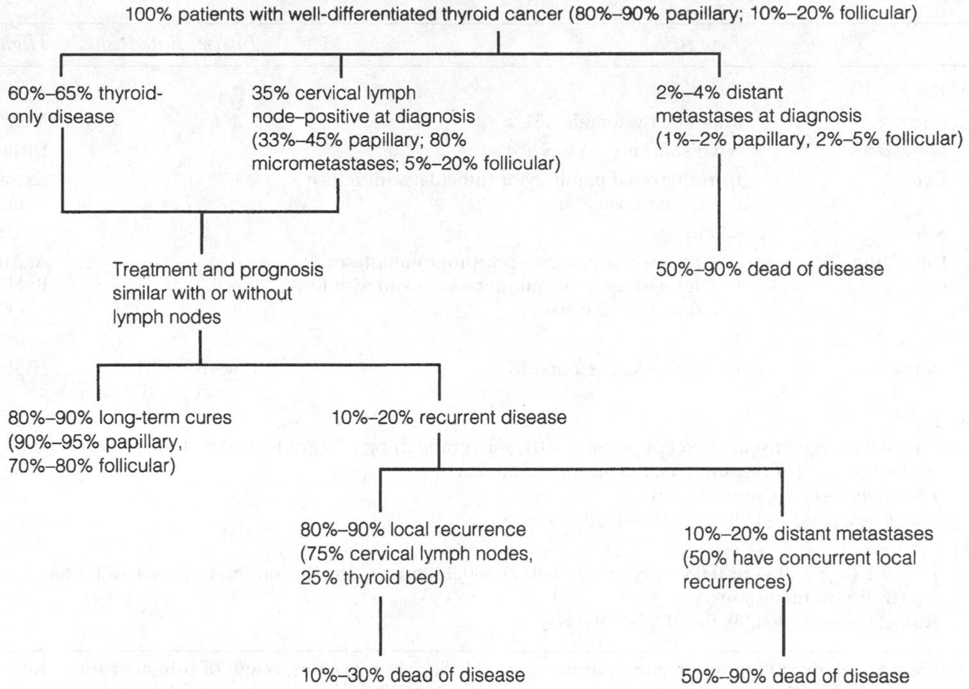

FIGURE 38.2-3. A flow diagram for well-differentiated thyroid cancer showing the extent of disease at the time of diagnosis, the natural history, and the outcome-based specific disease patterns. (Adapted from refs. 5 and 49.)

the most indolent solid neoplasms, with favorable long-term survival.[94,96] However, a small proportion of patients with papillary cancer and a slightly larger proportion of patients with follicular thyroid cancer do die from disease-related causes.[94–98] As opposed to other solid neoplasms, one major difference is that regional lymph node metastases appear to have no strong correlation with overall survival in most,[94–96,99] but not all, series[93,98] but do consistently correlate with local recurrence.

At presentation, approximately two-thirds of patients have disease that is localized to the thyroid. The median size of tumors is between 2.0 and 2.5 cm in most large series.[40–42,100,101] Patients with papillary carcinomas smaller than 1.0 cm are considered to have minimal or occult papillary thyroid cancer (papillary microcarcinoma).[3] In North American studies, the incidence of occult papillary tumors ranges between 0.5% and 14.0%, with a greater proportional incidence in older age groups. Studies from Scandinavia report up to one-third of patients with minimal papillary thyroid cancers.[3] There is clearly a large discrepancy between this incidence of one-fourth to one-third of patients having occult papillary thyroid cancer and the incidence of 40 per 1 million patient population of clinically significant disease. This discrepancy would argue strongly that these minimal lesions have a different biology than the clinically apparent thyroid cancers. For this reason, standard practice is not to investigate or submit to biopsy nodules that are smaller than 1.0 cm, except in the setting of familial MTC.[88] However, a proportion of patients who present with metastases to cervical lymph nodes may have a clinically occult lesion.[102]

Approximately 33% to 61% of patients with papillary thyroid cancer will have involvement of clinically apparent cervical lymph nodes at the time of diagnosis (see Table 38.2-2).[42,43,45,100,101,103] The reported incidence of positive cervical lymph node metastases in follicular thyroid cancers is much lower, ranging between 5% and 20%, with a median of approximately 10%.[42,43,45,57,100,101] However, this is probably an overestimate, as many series of follicular thyroid carcinomas include follicular variants of papillary carcinoma that have the natural history of papillary thyroid cancer and metastasize to lymph nodes with a high incidence. Some argue that the frequency of true lymphatic metastases from follicular thyroid carcinoma to regional lymph nodes may be extremely unusual, being less than 1%,[4] although one report from Memorial Sloan-Kettering Cancer Center (MSKCC) reported a 31% incidence of lymph node metastases in follicular carcinoma.[103] If patients with papillary cancer have lymph nodes studied in great detail, the incidence of micrometastases in lymph nodes increases to 80%.[3] The clinical significance of these micrometastases in some ways parallels the significance of the microscopic foci of intrathyroidal disease, as it is very common but does not progress and change clinical outcome.

Hürthle cell neoplasms generally have the same natural history and survival as follicular tumors[79]; however, the incidence of nodal metastases is greater than that of follicular carcinomas but not as high as papillary cancers.[103] Another difference that may have an impact on outcome is that these lesions do not tend to take up radioactive iodine with the efficiency of papillary tumors.[104]

Only a small minority of patients have metastatic hematogenous disease at the time of diagnosis.[32,36,41,100] In a large series from Mazzaferri and Jhiang,[42] 1% to 2% of papillary thyroid cancer patients and 2% to 5% of follicular thyroid cancer patients had distant metastases outside the neck or mediastinum at the time of diagnosis (Fig. 38.2-3). One series of 1038 patients from the MSKCC reported 44 patients (47%) presenting with metastases at diagnosis, including 2.3% of patients with papillary cancer and 11% with follicular cancer.[105] Having distant metastases at the time of presentation is a strong predictor of very poor outcome. Between 50% and 90% of these patients die secondary to their thyroid malignancy.[42] In the 44 patients in this category in the MSKCC series, there was a 43% long-term survival.[105]

In the overall population with papillary thyroid cancer, there is a 90% to 95% long-term disease-free survival and a

TABLE 38.2-3. Schema for Categorizing Patients with Well-Differentiated Thyroid Cancer by Prognostic Risk Categories

	Low Risk	*Intermediate Risk*	*High Risk*
AMES[107]			
Age	Males <41 y, female <51 y		Male >40 y, female >50 y
Metastases	No distant metastases		Distant metastases
Extent	Intrathyroidal papillary or follicular with minor capsule inversion		Extrathyroidal papillary or follicular with major invasion
Size	<5 cm		>5 cm
Definition	A: Any low-risk age group without metastases B: High-risk age without metastases and with low-risk extent and size		A: Any patient with metastases B: High-risk age with either high-risk extent or size
DAMES[112]			
Definition	Low-risk AMES + euploid	Low-risk AMES + aneuploid	High-risk AMES + aneuploid
AGES[109]			
PS = 0.05 × age in years (except pt <40 y = 0), + 1 (grade 2) or + 3 (grade 3–4), + 1 (if extrathyroidal) or + 3 (if distant metastases), + 0.2 × tumor size (in centimeters, maximum diameter)			
PS range: 0–11.65; median, 2.6			
Risk categories: 0–3.99; 4–4.99; 5–5.99; >6			
MACIS[113]			
PS = 3.1 (age <39 y) or 0.08 × age (if age >40 y), + 0.3 × tumor size (in centimeters), + 1 (if incompletely resected), + 1 (if locally invasive), + 3 (if distant metastases)			
Risk categories: 0–5.99; 6–6.99; 7–7.99; >8			

AGES, *a*ge, tumor *g*rade, tumor *e*xtent, tumor *s*ize; AMES, *a*ge, *m*etastases, *e*xtent of primary cancer, tumor *s*ize; DAMES, AMES system modified by tumor cell *D*NA content measured by flow cytometry; MACIS, *m*etastasis, *a*ge, *c*ompleteness of resection, *i*nvasion, *s*ize; PS, prognostic score.

70% to 80% long-term disease-free survival for patients with follicular cancers. The 20% of patients in this group who develop recurrent disease includes a majority with local cervical recurrences either in lymph nodes or the thyroid bed and a minority of patients with distant metastases to the lung, bone, and liver.[3,42] Once again, patients who do develop distant metastases have a poorer outcome, with 50% to 90% disease-specific deaths, whereas patients with locally recurrent disease in the neck have long-term survivals between 70% and 90% even in the presence of persistent cervical disease.[42]

Overall survival in well-differentiated thyroid carcinoma from various institutional series shows a better 10-year survival for papillary cancer, ranging between 74% and 93% as compared to follicular cancer, with 10-year survivals of 43% to 94%.[106] Although many institutions have reported their data based on these histologic subcategories, a more meaningful system is to categorize patients according to defined risk factors more pertinent to generating prognostic information. Groups at both the Lahey Clinic[41,107,108] and the Mayo Clinic[44,45,109–111] have considerable databases that define prognostic risk factors for well-differentiated thyroid cancer. The two dominant factors in both series are the age at diagnosis and the presence of distant metastases.[107,109] All systems also include some measurement of the size of the lesion and other factors, such as local invasion or grade of the tumor, which have impact on outcome. In general, younger patients do well with well-differentiated thyroid cancer. Cady and Rossi[107] defined low-risk age categories as men younger than 40 and women younger than 50 years. The Mayo Clinic takes age into account using a numerical factor in a formula calculating a prognostic score (PS) that does not discriminate according to gender. Although historical data report follicular cancer as having worse outcome than papillary thyroid cancer, Donohue et al.[100] showed that if one corrects for age and other prognostic variables, the outcome is similar within these two pathologic subcategories.

As stated, patients who have distant metastatic disease either at presentation or with recurrence do much worse.[42,106] Similarly, patients with local invasion or high-grade lesions have a worse prognosis. The risk categorization schema developed by the Lahey Clinic group incorporating these components carries the acronym AMES (*a*ge, *m*etastatic disease, *e*xtrathyroidal extension, *s*ize) (Table 38.2-3).[107] Using this system, low-risk patients can be identified who have a long-term overall survival of 98% and overall disease-free survival of 95% as compared to 54% and 45%,

TABLE 38.2-4. Survival or Disease-Free Survival in Patients with Well-Differentiated Thyroid Cancer Based on Various Prognostic Classification Schemes

Risk Group	*Low (%)*	*Intermediate (%)*	*High (%)*	
AMES[107]				
Overall survival	98		54	
Disease-free survival	95		45	
DAMES[114]				
Disease-free survival	92	45	0	
	Prognostic Score			
AGES[109]	<4	4–5	5–6	>6
20-Y survival	99	80	33	13
	Prognostic Score			
MACIS[113]	<6	6–7	7–8	>8
20-Y survival	99	89	56	24

AMES, *a*ge, *m*etastases, *e*xtent of primary cancer, tumor *s*ize; DAMES, AMES system modified by tumor cell *D*NA content measured by flow cytometry; AGES, *a*ge, tumor *g*rade, tumor *e*xtent, tumor *s*ize; MACIS, *m*etastasis, *a*ge, *c*ompleteness of resection, *i*nvasion, *s*ize.

TABLE 38.2-5. American Joint Committee on Cancer Staging System for Thyroid Cancer

TNM classification				
Tumor (T)				
T0	No evidence of primary tumor			
T1	Tumor <1 cm			
T2	Tumor >1 cm but <4 cm			
T3	Tumor >4 cm limited to thyroid			
T4	Tumor of any size extending beyond thyroid capsule			
Nodal involvement (N)				
Nx	Nodes cannot be assessed			
N0	No nodal metastases			
N1	Regional node metastasis			
N1a	Ipsilateral cervical lymph nodes			
N1b	Bilateral cervical or mediastinal lymph nodes			
Metastases (M)				
Mx	Distant metastases cannot be assessed			
M0	No distant metastases			
M1	Distant metastases			
Staging group				
Papillary-follicular cancer				
Age <45 y	Stage 1	Any T	Any N	M0
Age >45 y	Stage 1	T1	N0	M0
	Stage 2	T2/T3	N0	M0
	Stage 3	T4	N0	M0
		or		
		Any T	N1	M0
	Stage 4	Any T	Any N	M1
Medullary cancer				
	Stage 1	T1	N0	M0
	Stage 2	T2-4	N0	M0
	Stage 3	Any T	N1	M0
	Stage 4	Any T	Any N	M1
Anaplastic				
All cases are stage IV				

(Adapted from ref. 116.)

respectively, for high-risk patients (Table 38.2-4). A group from Canada added an assessment of DNA content by flow cytometry to the AMES categorization and showed that high-risk patients with aneuploid tumors have essentially zero long-term survival in a small number of patients.[112] The initial system developed by the Mayo Clinic group[109] carried the acronym AGES (*a*ge, tumor *g*rade, tumor *e*xtent, tumor *s*ize; see Table 38.2-3). A mathematical formula to develop a PS with different weights on these factors was developed. The scoring system showed that patients with a PS of less than 4 had a 99% 20-year survival, whereas patients with a PS greater than 6 had a 13% 20-year survival, with graded categories in between (see Table 38.2-4).[109] A more recent modification of this system is seen in MACIS (*m*etastasis, *a*ge at diagnosis, tumor extent subdivided into *c*ompleteness of resection and *i*nvasion, and tumor *s*ize).[113] Using this system, the score of less than 6 yields a 20-year survival of 99%, and a score of more than 8 results in a 20-year survival of only 24%. On the basis of these scoring systems that have been verified by other institutions, the aggressiveness of treatment can be balanced against the possible treatment risks and costs. Clearly, if subgroups of patients with 99% 20-year survivals can be prospectively identified, aggressive therapy with potential life-long complications cannot be justified in this subpopulation. Sanders and Cady[114] reexamined the AMES criteria for a group of thyroid cancer patients treated between 1980 and 1990. Survival rate for the low-risk groups was 98% and for the high-risk group was 47%, consistent with data collected over the previous four decades. As has been published by this group before, there was no significant improvement in survival with total thyroidectomy or radioactive iodine therapy (discussed later in Radioiodine Therapy).[155]

The Mayo Clinic group applied the AMES criteria to its long-term database, evaluating 1685 patients treated between 1940 and 1991 in the low-risk category with papillary thyroid cancer.[115] The 30-year rate for disease-specific mortality was 2%; for distant metastases, it was 3% in this patient population. With 20-year follow-up, there was a 4% rate of local recurrence and an 8% rate of nodal recurrence. These two reports verify the criteria established much earlier for prediction of outcome in well-differentiated thyroid cancer.[114,115] The importance of age, extrathyroidal extension, and distant metastases play an important role in the American Joint Committee on Cancer staging of thyroid cancer (Table 38.2-5).[116]

There is no large database that has verified this adaptation of the AMES and MACIS staging system into the TNM (tumor-node-metastasis) classification used by the American Joint Committee on Cancer. However, a very similar staging system was developed by the National Thyroid Cancer Treatment Cooperative Study registry, which initiated collection of data in 1987.[117] A report of more than 1500 patients analyzed by this staging system showed that 5-year disease-specific survivals for papillary thyroid cancer in stage I and II were 100%, 93.8% for stage III, and 78.5% for stage IV (<.0001).[117] The disease-free survival similarly showed a high correlation with stages I through IV papillary carcinoma, having survivals of 94.4%, 92.5%, 82.7%, and 30%, respectively (P<.0001). A comparison of the ability of this prospective registry to predict for patients being disease-free over long-term follow-up produced slightly higher correlation values than the AMES classification but slightly lower than the MACIS and TNM classifications.[117]

TREATMENT OF WELL-DIFFERENTIATED THYROID CANCER

Surgery

The key decisions in the surgical management of thyroid nodules or cancers (or both) is whom to operate on and how extensive a resection to perform. The development of FNAB and the proven accuracy of those results since the mid-1980s has significantly decreased the number of patients who present with thyroid nodules and need to undergo surgical exploration for diagnosis.[8,89] Consequently, FNA has increased the proportion of nodules that are surgically excised and turn out to be cancer. The algorithm outlined in Figure 38.2-2 is a guide for deciding which patients should undergo surgical resection based on an initial assessment by FNAB.

Before the development and widespread use of preoperative FNA of thyroid nodules, surgeons frequently relied on frozen-section test results obtained during the procedure to guide them.[118] The utility of frozen-section diagnosis for thyroid nodules is controversial. The situations in which the frozen section may be useful is for patients who have suspicious FNA results. Specifically, patients with suspicious cytology (e.g., follicular neoplasm or possible follicular variant of papillary carcinoma) or patients with a nondiagnostic FNA on repeated biopsies underwent surgical resection with an unknown diagnosis of malignancy. Most of the lesions in the indeterminate FNA category are follicular neoplasms, the majority of which are benign. As previously described in the section Pathology, capsular and vascular invasion determine malignancy, and the ability to render an accurate interpretation on frozen-section analysis is very limited. A large series from Chen et al.[119] at Johns Hopkins University examined this patient population. They reported that 87% of frozen sections rendered no useful information, whereas 5% gave inaccurate results. Their conclusions were that obtaining frozen sections did more harm than good in addition to the expense incurred. A similar series from Bonner et al.[120] also reported that frozen-section interpretation of lesions diagnosed as follicular or Hürthle cell neoplasms on FNA is fraught with error. The recommended approach in this group of patients is to perform excision of the thyroid lobe harboring the nodule and to wait for the definitive pathologic report. If the lesion turns out to be a follicular carcinoma with characteristics that place a patient at high risk, such as significant capsular invasion or angioinvasion,[18] a completion total or near total thyroidectomy is performed during a second operation to remove the contralateral thyroid lobe.[121,122] In cases suspicious for a follicular variant of papillary carcinoma, the presence of specific nuclear features that define papillary thyroid cancer may be identifiable on frozen-section analysis. For this reason, patients with FNA results that are read as follicular neoplasm with some features of papillary nuclei should undergo lobectomy and intraoperative assessment (frozen section, touch preparation) to attempt identification of a follicular variant of papillary thyroid cancer.

A long-standing controversy among endocrine surgeons has existed regarding the extent of surgical resection for well-differentiated thyroid cancer.[3] This question may never be answered definitively by a clinical trial, as the expense and number of patients needed for trials of this indolent low-risk disease are overwhelming.[123] Acceptable surgical procedures to remove a thyroid neoplasm include a lobectomy, a subtotal thyroidectomy, a near-total thyroidectomy, and a total thyroidectomy. The entire thyroid lobe on the side of the primary cancer is taken out as completely as possible for any of these procedures. The difference comes in the management of the contralateral lobe and how this choice relates to outcome as well as operative morbidity. Arguments typically put forth for either more conservative therapy or more aggressive surgery are listed in Table 38.2-6. In a thyroid lobectomy, the contralateral lobe is not dissected but is simply examined visually and by palpation for abnormalities. A subtotal thyroidectomy leaves a rim of 2 to 4 g of tissue in the upper lateral portion of the contralateral thyroid lobe.[124] By leaving thyroid in this location, two things are accomplished. First,

TABLE 38.2-6. Arguments for and against Conservative or More Radical Surgery for Well-Differentiated Thyroid Cancer

Issue	*Conservative Surgery*	*Radical (Total Thyroidectomy) Surgery*
Prognostic risk factors	Systems to define risk can accurately identify patients who have 20-y survival of 99% and 20-y disease-free survival >95%	Occasional low-risk patient develops recurrence (small lesions may grow aggressively; multifocality in >25% of cases)
Safety of surgery	Risks of permanent hypocalcemia and recurrent laryngeal nerve injury greatly reduced with lobar or subtotal thyroidectomy	Experienced surgeon can perform these procedures with very minimal or no long-term complications
Postoperative iodine	If necessary, ^{131}I ablation of thyroid remnant can be accomplished with no morbidity	Thyroid ablation with ^{131}I is complicated by pain if a gross thyroid remnant exists; decreased efficacy of ^{131}I with residual thyroid
Anaplastic cancer	Local recurrences able to be managed; risk of conversion to anaplasia is <1%	Potential for local recurrence with possible dedifferentiation to a more aggressive tumor

(From refs. 108, 111, with permission.)

TABLE 38.2-7. Long-Term Complications of Total versus Subtotal Thyroidectomy

Study	*Number*	*Hypocalcemia (%)*	*Recurrent Laryngeal Nerve (%)*
Subtotal thyroidectomy			
Hay et al.[109,a]	722	2 (0.3)	13 (1.8)
Brooks et al.[101]	179	0 (0)	1 (0.69)
Flynn et al.[125]	28	0 (0)	0 (0)
Rossi et al.[108]	309	1 (0.3)	1 (0.3)
Total thyroidectomy			
Hay et al.[109,a]	136	44 (32)	2 (1.5)
Brooks et al.[101]	43	3 (7)	3 (7)
Flynn et al.[125]	45	4 (9)	0 (0)
Rossi et al.[108]	0	—	—

[a]Ref. 109 represents an older series between 1946 and 1970, as compared with other reports that are from the last two decades.

the recurrent laryngeal nerve as it enters the larynx at the ligament of Berry is not dissected and consequently does not present a risk for injury. Second, the blood supply to the superior parathyroid gland on that side is less likely to be disrupted by leaving a rim of tissue in this location. A near-total thyroidectomy leaves a much smaller amount of normal tissue (<1 g) immediately adjacent to the ligament of Berry. This maneuver may offer some protection to the recurrent laryngeal nerve, but it offers minimal benefit in terms of preserving the blood supply of the upper parathyroid. A total thyroidectomy implies that every effort is made to excise all thyroid tissue, leaving no gross or macroscopic residual thyroid in either lobe. The difference between a total thyroidectomy and a near-total thyroidectomy usually depends on the particular anatomy of the thyroid in any given patient. There may be a small ledge of thyroid tissue, called the *tubercle of Zuckerkandl*, at the ligament of Berry that may limit safe resection of the entire thyroid.

The real increased risk of performing a total thyroidectomy versus a lesser resection may be in the long-term incidence of hypocalcemia (Table 38.2-7). A study from the Mayo Clinic spanning the years between 1946 and 1970 reported a 32% incidence of permanent hypocalcemia after total thyroidectomy versus only a 0.3% incidence after a subtotal procedure.[109] More recent series report much less permanent morbidity and show variable results comparing the patients undergoing subtotal with those undergoing total thyroidectomy. Virtually all experienced surgeons should be able to perform total thyroidectomies with less than 1% recurrent nerve injuries, with the long-term risk of hypoparathyroidism of 2% to 9%.[125]

The most compelling argument for performing a unilateral lobectomy or a subtotal thyroidectomy are the data that come from the definition of prognostic factors for this disease. These rating scales identified by the acronyms AMES or AGES have been used to evaluate thousands of patients (see later in Natural History and Prognosis).[107,109,113] A low-risk patient defined by the AMES criteria has a 20-year survival of 99% with a 20-year disease-free survival of more than 95%.[106] If prognostic factors can accurately diagnose patients with such excellent outcome, the added benefit of a total thyroidectomy as well as postoperative iodine therapy may not be worth the potential morbidity for the patient. However, careful medical surveillance for cancer in the contralateral lobe as well as recurrence must be maintained. Furthermore, in situations in which a small thyroid remnant is left, the true morbidity of treating this patient with ablative doses of ^{131}I (if indicated) is relatively minimal.[126] In fact, it is typical for patients with a surgical report of a "total thyroidectomy" that there is residual thyroid tissue within the bed of the thyroid identified on the postresection diagnostic scan, as actually a near-total thyroidectomy was performed. This small thyroid remnant is then ablated with postoperative ^{131}I treatments. Radioiodine ablation of an intact lobe of the thyroid lobectomy is associated with considerably more symptoms.[127]

A very large review from the Mayo Clinic of 1685 patients with papillary thyroid cancer treated between 1940 and 1991 has been reported with a long-term follow-up.[115] Based on surgeons' preference, 1468 patients underwent a near-total or total thyroidectomy (87%), while 195 patients (12%) had a unilateral resection. With a 20-year follow-up, the incidence of local recurrence with unilateral resection was 14% and, for bilateral resection, it was 2%.[115] Similarly, the incidence of recurrent cervical lymph node metastases after unilateral resection was 19% as compared to 6% after bilateral resection ($P = .0001$). Despite this very clear difference in recurrence rates, there was no translation of benefit in terms of disease-specific survival or distant metastases. The overall mortality at 30 years for patients with either unilateral resection or bilateral resection was approximately 2%. These results further confirm the excellent predictive outcome of the AMES low-risk criteria with long-term follow-up.[115] The authors concluded that although no survival benefit is gained from bilateral thyroid resection, the significant improvement in local recurrence with a minimal operative morbidity in the hands of experienced surgeons would lead to recommendation of near-total or total thyroidectomy for even this low-risk category of patients. Arguing with the opposing viewpoint, Sanders and Cady also provided a long-term review of their personal series and came to the conclusion that there was no benefit in performing bilateral resection versus unilateral resection for low-risk patients.

For patients in a high-risk category, there is much less disagreement regarding the extent of surgery, although there are still some proponents of less than total or near-total thyroidectomy. An analysis of 303 patients with high-risk papillary thyroid cancer showed an improvement in overall survival (relative risk ratio, 0.37) but not cancer-specific mortality or disease-free survival.[128] In this nonrandomized study, no effect of extent of surgery was seen in patients with follicular thyroid cancer.[128] A report by Wanebo et al.[129] in a smaller number of high-risk patients reported that 10-year disease-specific survival was 82% with total thyroidectomy, 78% with subtotal thyroidectomy, and 89% with unilateral lobectomy. Again, neither of these retrospective reviews was a prospective randomized study and, for reasons discussed later in Radioactive Therapy, in terms of effectiveness of adjuvant postoperative radioiodine treatments and ease of follow-up with serum Tg measurements, the vast majority of investigators would agree that a total or near-total thyroidectomy is indicated for high-risk patients. For patients with extrathyroidal extension, the *en bloc* resection of invaded structures should be performed. If the tumor is on the anterior thyroid, this provides minimal morbidity to the patients, as resection of the overlying strap muscles, such as the sternal thyroid, causes no symptoms postoperatively. For posterior tumors, direct invasion of the trachea and esophagus should be resected with either partial tracheal resection and primary closure or resection of the esophagus muscular layer, again with closure and drainage.[130] This aggressive strategy for extrathyroidal extension at the first operation offers the best chance for local control.

The surgical management of lymph node metastases from well-differentiated thyroid cancer is also somewhat controversial.[131–133] Most experts agree that a procedure somewhere between "berry-picking" of clinically positive nodes and a formal modified radical neck dissection is the ideal treatment. For patients who have bulky and obviously pathologic lymph node metastases, a formal neck dissection is indicated.[134] As noted in Natural History and Prognosis, particularly in lower-risk younger patients, the presence of metastatic disease to lymph nodes does not carry the connotation of worse prognosis of other solid neoplasms. Although lymph node metastases correlate with increased local recurrence, they do not carry a worse prognosis in several series.[94,96,99] The lymph nodes typically involved are the level VI on paratracheal lymph nodes in the cervical compartment and the level III and IV lymph nodes lateral to the internal jugular vein in the midneck or lower neck. During any thyroid resection, these lymph node areas should be palpated. Lymph nodes that are abnormal because they are firm or large should be subjected to biopsy with frozen-section pathologic evaluation. If positive for metastatic cancer, these lymph node areas should be completely dissected.

The technique of sentinel lymph node biopsy that has been used for melanoma and breast cancer has been applied to thyroid cancer using isosulfan blue.[135] Seventeen patients had thyroid mapping, with successful removal of sentinel lymph nodes in 15 (88%) and 2 failures due to retrosternal lymph nodes. Of 12 patients with cancer, 5 had positive lymph nodes (42%: 3 level VI, 2 level IV) for metastases and, in 2 patients, the sentinel node was the only node positive for cancer.[135] Whether this technique has a role in thyroid cancer in which the significance of nodal metastases is less than in breast cancer remains to be seen.

Some investigators have noted a positive correlation with lymph node metastases and outcome[93,95] and have argued for more routine formal dissections on that basis.[136] Tisell et al.,[137] who have widely promoted microdissection of all lymphatic tissue for MTC, reported their results applying the same technique to papillary thyroid cancer. In their series of 195 patients, there was a 70% incidence of lymph node metastases in men and a 4% to 5% incidence of lymph node metastases in women. With long-term follow-up, only three patients (1.6%) of this series died, partially due to locally recurrent thyroid cancer, all living more than 17 years after the initial surgery.[137] A different strategy was used by a group from Germany: For well-differentiated cancer, a modified radical neck dissection was performed routinely only for T4 lesions.[138] For other-stage primary tumors, only if there were positive cervical lymph nodes was a modified radical neck dissection performed at the time of initial surgery. After a mean of 6.5 years of follow-up, 77 patients (31%) underwent reoperation because of regional tumor recurrence. In the subgroup of patients with papillary thyroid cancer, the incidence of regional recurrence for T2 lesions was 45% in those without initial neck dissection versus 3% for those with an initial neck dissection; 77% of patients for T3 lesions without initial lymph node dissection had local recurrence as compared to 36% with initial dissection, and patients with T4 tumors had a 75% recurrence rate without initial node dissection versus 33% with an initial node dissection ($P<.0001$).[138] It is not clear from this study with limited follow-up whether this decreased incidence of regional recurrence has an impact on survival and warrants a modified radical neck dissection for all patients with positive central neck lymph nodes at the time of initial thyroidectomy.

Radioiodine Therapy

The postoperative treatment of patients with well-differentiated thyroid cancer, particularly relating to radioiodine therapy, is controversial. The lack of well-designed, randomized controlled studies and the low probability that any large multicenter treatment studies will ever come to fruition force the clinician to rely on retrospective studies and surveys of practice habits.[139,140]

All patients who have undergone a total or near-total thyroidectomy for a follicular carcinoma or a papillary carcinoma larger than between 1.0 and 1.5 cm should be considered candidates for radioiodine ablation. ^{131}I ablation of residual normal thyroid is important after what is thought to be complete resection of the primary tumor to aid in the detection of metastatic disease and to destroy residual microscopic cancer. Normal thyroid tissue takes up ^{131}I more avidly than does cancer[140] and thus prevents full visualization of the true extent of disease. Furthermore, ^{131}I ablation removes the contribution of normal thyroid tissue serum Tg, an important tumor marker in the follow-up of postoperative patients.[141,142] Most important, many studies have documented that ^{131}I ablation decreases cancer death,[128,143] tumor recurrence,[128,144] and development of distant metastases.[128,145] Despite such data for large patient populations, Cady and Rossi[107] and Sanders and Cady[114] observed that an enhanced survival has not been documented with the use of radioiodine ablation in the Lahey Clinic series, particularly in "low-risk" patients defined by AMES criteria.

The dose of ^{131}I for ablation is not standardized. Some recommend low-dose ablation with less than 30 mCi given on an outpatient basis. This approach should be reserved for low-risk young patients who may benefit from an overall lower radiation exposure and who accept the fact that several low radioiodine doses may be necessary before successful ablation. Several studies demonstrating proper diagnostic scan preparation with sufficiently elevated TSH and adherence to a low-iodine diet describe disparate rates of successful ablations using less than 30 mCi ranging from 27% to 83%.[146,147]

Higher ablative doses ranging from 100 to 150 mCi should be used for older, high-risk patients, particularly those known to have an incomplete resection of the primary tumor, an invasive primary tumor, or metastases. Beierwaltes et al.[148] demonstrated that 87% of their patients were ablated with an initial dose of 100 to less than 200 mCi. No significant differences were noted when doses from 100 to 200 mCi or more were used, leading to a recommendation of an optimal ablative dose of 100 to 149 mCi.[148] The goal of dosimetry is to derive the dose of ^{131}I that will deliver no more than 200 cGy to the blood, with no more than 120 mCi retained at 48 hours or 80 mCi in the presence of pulmonary metastases. This decreases the risk of bone marrow damage and radiation fibrosis in patients with metastatic lung disease. The methods used to perform dosimetry are generally modifications of the protocol developed by

Benua and Leeper[149] and others. One recommended approach is for all patients with metastatic disease treated with repeated therapeutic doses of ^{131}I to undergo dosimetric quantification of the highest, safe dose, using a ceiling of 300 mCi. Other investigators recommend a standard fixed dose that may vary according to the site of uptake.[150] For example, a dose of 150 mCi is given for residual or recurrent thyroid bed carcinoma with or without metastases, up to 200 mCi for bone metastases, and a reduced dose of 75 mCi for diffuse pulmonary metastases to prevent radiation pneumonitis and fibrosis.

Lymph node metastases were found in up to 42% of patients at time of initial therapy in one large study by Mazzaferri and Jhiang.[151] Radioiodine is indicated in these patients to decrease recurrences that may have an impact on long-term survival.[77,152]

Pulmonary metastases are frequently detected exclusively on radioiodine scanning. Sclumberger reported an increase in this observation, noting the rate of negative chest radiograph results in patients with metastatic disease to have increased from 13% to 43%.[141] Earlier detection of pulmonary metastases before development of gross chest film abnormalities is thought to be due to the use of Tg screening and the enhanced sensitivity of ^{131}I scanning. This same group reported on 23 patients who had diffuse pulmonary metastases seen only on radioiodine scanning, of which almost 90% had no further uptake and a decrease in the serum Tg after ^{131}I therapy. Bone metastases may require several modalities for adequate therapy. Surgery may be needed for orthopedic stabilization or palliation of pain. External radiation may be used in combination with radioactive iodine in difficult cases.[154]

Ablation of residual thyroid is typically performed at approximately 6 weeks after near-total or total thyroidectomy. Most, but not all, centers perform a diagnostic scan followed by ablative ^{131}I therapy. To optimize uptake by both residual thyroid and thyroid cancer, patients are rendered hypothyroid with a goal of increasing TSH. To accomplish this, thyroid replacement after thyroidectomy is triiodothyronine, as it has a much shorter half-life than thyroxine, and it is discontinued 2 weeks before treatment. In response to this hypothyroid state, TSH must achieve levels of greater than 25 to 30 µU/mL to obtain optimal uptake of radioiodine. A low-iodine diet is instituted 1 to 2 weeks before scanning to enhance the uptake and retention of radioiodine.[155]

Just as there is lack of consensus regarding ablation and therapeutic doses of ^{131}I, the diagnostic scanning dose is as controversial. The ideal dose achieves high sensitivity in detecting residual thyroid tissue, thyroid cancer, and metastatic foci and reduces the potential for sublethal radiation "stunning" of thyroid tissue that prevents optimal uptake of future ^{131}I therapy. Although it is clear that higher scanning doses improve visualization of thyroid remnants and metastases,[156] even conventional scanning doses of 4 to 5 mCi of ^{131}I were found to diminish therapeutic radioiodine uptake.[157] Park et al.[158] have suggested that diagnostic scanning with ^{123}I may prevent the stunning effect. One strategy is to use a 5-mCi ^{131}I diagnostic dose followed by a whole body scan at 48 hours, with treatment following in most cases in 24 to 96 hours after whole body scanning. A posttherapy whole body scan is obtained after 5 to 7 days to determine the extent of disease.[159] Follow-up diagnostic scanning should be performed at 6- to 12-month intervals, and treatment should continue until there is no further uptake, the serum Tg is in the "athyreotic" range, or complications of ^{131}I therapy arise.

Medical management of malignant lesions includes thyroxine therapy to suppress TSH, which is invaluable in preventing tumor recurrences. The degree to which one suppresses TSH is a point of debate. It is advisable to keep the TSH at or below the normal range (range, 0.5 to 5 µU/mL) in patients who are thought to be without evidence of disease and to maintain a lower TSH (0.1 µU/mL) in patients with residual neck disease, metastases, or recurrent disease. A large review by the National Cancer Treatment Cooperative Registry of 693 patients reported for all papillary thyroid patients that TSH levels did not predict disease progression.[160] In high-risk papillary cancer, patient TSH was a predictor of risk ($P = .03$) but not when radioiodine therapy was included in the analysis ($P = .004$).[160] The degree of thyroid suppression in these cases is dictated by balance of the risk of recurrent thyroid cancer and the overall medical condition of patients, particularly their cardiovascular status.

THYROGLOBULIN MEASUREMENTS. Tg, an important tumor marker in the follow-up of thyroid cancer patients, is the protein that provides a matrix for thyroid hormone synthesis within thyroid follicles and is critical in the storage of thyroid hormone within the thyroid gland.[161] After successful thyroidectomy and ablation of residual normal or cancerous thyroid tissue by radioiodine, the Tg will be in the athyreotic range. Levels above the athyreotic range are indicative of persistent, functioning residual thyroid tissue or carcinoma. If there is detectable serum Tg in the circumstance of suppressive thyroxine therapy, it is a true indicator of persistent or recurrent thyroid carcinoma. However, thyroxine may suppress Tg in patients with metastatic disease; therefore, the test is more sensitive in the setting of thyroid hormone suppressive therapy withdrawal and frank hypothyroidism documented by an elevated TSH.

At the time of thyroid hormone withdrawal for both initial postoperative scans and for subsequent follow-up scans, Tg is measured in conjunction with the diagnostic whole body scan and may be more sensitive than the scan in detecting cancer, as demonstrated by several investigators.[142,162] Pineda et al.[142] treated 17 patients with 150 to 300 mCi ^{131}I who had negative diagnostic whole body scan results but serum Tg measurements above 8 ng/mL (range, 8 to 480 ng/mL) detected at the time of hypothyroidism.[142] Posttherapy scan results were positive in the thyroid bed or at sites of distant metastases in 16 of 17 patients. After repeated therapeutic doses given under similar conditions, 8 of 13 patients had a positive scan result after a second therapeutic dose, and five of five were positive after a third treatment. Lowering of Tg was demonstrated as was a decrease in uptake demonstrated on subsequent posttherapy scans.

Since this initial report,[142] there has been a great deal of debate regarding the optimal management of patients who are whole body iodine scan–negative but Tg-positive. This debate has included discussions of the false-negative rate of Tg, and alternative imaging studies, including positron emission tomography (PET) scans as well as sestamibi, technetium-sestamibi scans, and thallium 201 scans.[140] Without question, there are patients who have negative whole body iodine scan results but have definite recurrent and metastatic well-differentiated thyroid cancer. PET scans have been reported to have sensitivities of identifying the occult disease in 82%[163] and 71%[164] in this patient population. In the series of patients studied at MSKCC, the PET scan result changed clinical management in 19 of 37 patients.[164] In patients with elevated Tg levels, PET

TABLE 38.2-8. Comparison of Whole Body Iodine Scans and Scans Obtained after Injection of Recombinant Human Thyroid-Stimulating Hormone

	T4 Withdrawal Scan	*rhTSH Scan*
Mean TSH level at time of ^{131}I injection	101 ± 77	132 ± 89
Negative scans	68	83
Positive scans	59	44
Uniquely positive scans	18	3
Percentage of ^{113}I uptake (mean ± SEM)	0.4 ± 0.7	03. ± 0.7 (P = .004)
Elevated thyroglobulin[a] (n = 35)	14	13

rhTSH, recombinant human thyroid-stimulating hormone; SEM, standard error of the mean.
[a]Measured at time of radioactive iodine injection.
(Adapted from ref. 171.)

scans had a positive predictive value of 92%; in patients with a low Tg value, PET scans had a negative predictive value of 93%.[164] A study from the University of Southern California reported that 100% of patients imaged by PET with elevated or rising Tg had evidence of disease, although only 17 of these 24 patients had this recurrence confirmed (biopsy or alternative imaging studies).[165] Alternative imaging methods, including sestamibi scans as well as ^{201}Tl scans, could detect thyroid cancer metastases even in patients with false-negative normal Tg level results.[140,166]

The relatively routine use of radioiodine ablation in this patient population who are Tg-positive and whole body scan–negative has been debated in the literature.[140] Most experts agree that a selective approach incorporating prognostic features of the primary tumor (age of patient, extrathyroidal extension) should come into play regarding management of these patients. It should also be understood that a variety of patients with autoantibodies to Tg may have spurious results that are most commonly false-negative results but also have the potential for false-positive test results.[167] The controversy in this area speaks to the need for a randomized trial that may be conducted by one of the North American cooperative groups to answer the question of radioiodine treatment in this patient population. An even more elegant way to detect residual tumor may be use of the polymerase chain reaction technique for application of Tg messenger RNA circulating in peripheral blood.[168] The clinical relevance of this molecular detection method remains to be seen.

ADJUVANTS TO RADIOIODINE THERAPY. The success of radioiodine therapy is dependent on residual thyroid tissue concentrating iodine avidly under the stimulation of elevated TSH. In some circumstances, stimulation by endogenous TSH is impossible, as in the case of hypopituitarism, or is contraindicated, as in patients with central nervous system metastases in whom the hypothyroid state could lead to acute swelling and complications. Lithium can be used to increase the therapeutic effects of ^{131}I by decreasing its turnover and effectively increasing its half-life at oral doses of 400 to 800 mg daily for 7 days.[169] A study from the National Institutes of Health reported an estimated increased radiation exposure to the tumor by taking lithium of 2.29-fold after an ^{131}I treatment dose.[170]

The availability of recombinant human TSH has led to a large study that reported comparing diagnostic whole body iodine scans after standard thyroxine withdrawal compared to scans obtained with recombinant human thyroid-stimulating hormone (rhTSH).[171] In 127 patients with a diagnosis of well-differentiated thyroid cancer in this study, rhTSH, 0.9 mg, was injected once daily intramuscularly for 2 days. The day after the final injection, patients received between 3 and 5 mCi of ^{131}I and were scanned 48 hours later. At least 4 weeks later, patients underwent standard thyroxine withdrawal with an endogenous TSH at least more than 25 U/mL. The results of several parameters of this study are shown in Table 38.2-8.[171] There were 65 patients who had concordant negative scan results (51% of the patient population). In the additional 62 patients (49% of population) who had positive scan results, both scans were positive in 41; only the standard thyroxine withdrawal study result was positive in 18, and only the rhTSH scan result was positive in 3. These results analyzed in a different way demonstrate that the rhTSH scan was equivalent to or better than the standard scan in 86% of the patients but inferior to the standard withdrawal scan in 14% (P<.001).[171] This difference in scan results culminated in an alteration of therapy in 13% of the patients who were then treated with high-dose radioactive iodine based on the standard scan alone. On the other hand, there was a highly significant worsening of symptoms of hypothyroidism (P<.001) and dysphoric mood states (P<.001) after withdrawal of thyroid hormone as compared to rhTSH.[171] The rhTSH was shown to be safe with only some mild nausea side effects. The serum Tg was studied at the point of peak TSH levels before both these scans in 35 patients. It was elevated more than 5 ng/mL in 14 of 35 patients with the standard withdrawal scan and 13 of 35 patients with the rhTSH scan. These results would indicate that in low- to moderate-risk patients, the use of recombinant thyrotropin may be indicated in follow-up annual scans, with near-equivalent efficacy of thyroid withdrawal but none of the morbidity for the patients.

COMPLICATIONS OF RADIOIODINE THERAPY. The most common side effects from radioiodine therapy include sialadenitis, nausea, and temporary bone marrow suppression.[127] Amifostine, (Ethyol) which has been used as a radioprotector of head and neck cancer, significantly reduced sialadenitis from radiation treatment for thyroid cancer.[172] Testicular function and spermatogenesis are transiently impaired but appear to recover with time.[173] In a study comparing fertility rates, birth rates, and prematurity between women treated with ^{131}I and those not treated, there were no significant differences.[174]

One noted that three of six patients who became pregnant within the first year after radioactive treatment had children with significant congenital anomalies.[175]

There is a dose-dependent relationship between ^{131}I therapy and the development of leukemia. The incidence increases when the total cumulative dose is greater than 800 mCi and can be avoided by treating at widely spaced intervals (6 to 12 months) with activity between 100 and 200 mCi.[176] A higher incidence of bladder carcinoma has been seen in patients who have received high cumulative doses of radioiodine.[177] Urine dilution by adequate hydration and frequent voiding can reduce the radiation exposure to the bladder wall.

Chemotherapy and Radiation Therapy

The most effective nonsurgical treatment for well-differentiated thyroid cancer is, without question, ablation with radioiodine.[140,154] Other conventional modes of neoplastic treatment—chemotherapy, and external-beam radiation therapy—demonstrate much poorer results and, consequently, are much less studied. The best single chemotherapeutic agent for this tumor is doxorubicin (Adriamycin) with partial response rates of 30% and up to 45% in some series.[178] Combination therapy with Adriamycin and cisplatin has produced disappointing results that were no better than single-agent trials, and the toxicity was worse.

For surgically unresectable local disease that has not responded to radioiodine, the best treatment may be a combination of hyperfractionated radiation treatments plus Adriamycin. Response rates of more than 80% have been reported using this regimen, although even in this situation, complete responses are rare and limited in duration.[178] Adjuvant radiation therapy for grossly resected well-differentiated thyroid cancer has not generally been thought to be beneficial[179,180] until one recent retrospective study. This study by Farahati et al.,[181] a retrospective review, analyzed patients with T4 primary lesions (evidence of extrathyroidal extension) who underwent radiation (n = 99) compared to those who did not (n = 70).[181] Patients received a uniform treatment course of total thyroidectomy with initial ablative radioactive iodine, with or without 5000 to 6000 rads of external-beam radiation therapy to the neck and mediastinum, followed by a second ablative dose of radioactive iodine. The group that had radiation treatments had recurrent disease in 4% of cases (3 of 75 patients), while the group who did not receive radiation had recurrences in 26% (13 of 50 patients; $P = .0001$).[181] This benefit for radiation extended only to the subgroup of patients with lymph node–positive disease. In patients with papillary thyroid cancer who were lymph node–negative, there were 1 of 47 patients (2%) with recurrence with radiation therapy and 2 of 21 patients (9.5%) without radiation therapy had recurrences, which was not statistically significant ($P = .27$). In patients with T4 lesions and positive lymph nodes who received radiation, there were 2 recurrences in 28 (7.1%) and there were 13 recurrences in 29 patients without radiation therapy (44.8%; $P = .002$). These results would suggest that patients with T4 papillary thyroid cancer, particularly with positive lymph nodes, should undergo external-beam radiation therapy to the neck. This patient population should be studied in a prospective manner to determine the benefit of that additional therapy. This retrospective review showed not only an improvement in local recurrence but an improvement in distant metastases in this subgroup.[181]

ANAPLASTIC THYROID CANCER

ATC is one of the most aggressive and difficult human malignancies to treat and subsequently is one of the most lethal. As opposed to the excellent long-term survival for well-differentiated thyroid carcinoma, ATC in most series has a median survival of 4 to 5 months from the time of diagnosis, with rare long-term survivors.[182–184]

The proportional incidence of ATC compared to the total number of thyroid carcinomas is variable but appears to be declining over time. Historically, ATC was said to constitute 5% to 15% of all thyroid carcinomas in the United States[182] and between 10% to 50% in European series.[3] Current epidemiologic studies indicate that this lethal form of thyroid cancer has decreased to between 1% and 3% of the total number of cases.[183] Institutional reviews over a distinct period support the apparent real decrease in the incidence of ATC. One of the largest single-institution series, from the Mayo Clinic, spans the years 1946 to 1971.[182] During that time, 1161 patients with thyroid cancer had their primary treatment at Mayo Clinic, including 82 cases of ATC or 7.1% of the total. Later single-institution series from Loyola (1966 to 1989)[185] and Roswell Park (1968 to 1992)[183] reported respective incidences of 5% and 2.7%. The decrease over time may be partially related to iodine prophylaxis and an overall decrease in endemic iodine-deficient goiter in North America.

Patients with ATC differ epidemiologically from patients with well-differentiated thyroid neoplasms, with a median age two to three decades older and with a more equal gender distribution (Table 38.2-9).[182–185] Median age at diagnosis ranges between 63 and 74 years. In most series, including the largest one from the Mayo Clinic with 82 patients,[182] there are equal number of male and female patients, but some series show a predilection for women near the ratio that is commonly reported for well-differentiated thyroid cancer.

ATC is commonly related to a prior or a concurrent diagnosis of well-differentiated thyroid cancer or benign nodular thyroid disease. This association of ATC with prior or concurrent well-differentiated thyroid carcinoma suggests two features of the biology of this tumor. First, ATC may arise via the dedifferentiation of prior well-differentiated thyroid cancer, and the aggressive growth pattern of this anaplastic tumor may replace all previous evidence of well-differentiated tumor.[186] Also, the close association between ATC and well-differentiated thyroid cancer suggests that the risk factors are similar.[185]

The natural history, clinical presentation, and outcome of ATC reflect the biology of this tumor as an undifferentiated, rapidly growing neoplasm with invasive characteristics. The patients uniformly present with a palpable mass that is reported to be increasing in size during the period of observation. The median tumor size in patients with ATC from Roswell Park Cancer Institute was 8 to 9 cm, with a range of 3 to 20 cm as compared to the usual size of 2 to 3 cm for well-differentiated thyroid cancer.[183] Invasion to the trachea, larynx, or recurrent laryngeal nerve leads to hoarseness at diagnosis and, in a subset of these patients, an invasion to the esophagus may cause dysphagia.

TABLE 38.2-9. Clinical Series of Anaplastic Thyroid Carcinomas with Demographic Data, Total Percentage of Thyroid Cancer, and Survival

Institution	*Years*	*No.*	*Total Thyroid Cancers*	*Anaplastic Thyroid Cancers (%)*	*Median Age*	*M/F Ratio*	*Median Survival (mo)*	*2-Y Survival (%)*	*5-Y Survival (%)*
Mayo Clinic[182]	1946–1971	82	1161	7.1	65	1:0.7	5	8	3
Loyola University[183]	1966–1989	17	340	5.7	63	1:3.5	12	29	17
Roswell Park[184]	1968–1992	21	771	2.7	65	1:1.1	4.5	14	10
Sweden[185,a]	1984–1992	33			74	1:3.1	4.5	—	—

M/F, male-female.
[a]Series is a collective review from several institutions.

The majority of patients with ATC die from aggressive local regional disease, primarily with upper airway respiratory failure. At the time of diagnosis, 25% to 50% of patients may have synchronous pulmonary metastases.[182–184] However, it is usually the local growth causing obliteration of the airway that causes the patient's demise. For this reason, aggressive local therapy is indicated in all patients who can tolerate it and in whom it is technically possible. As opposed to well-differentiated thyroid cancer, ^{131}I plays no role in the treatment of recurrent or metastatic disease for this tumor. Therefore, total or near-total thyroidectomy is not as important in ATC, except as needed to obtain local control.[182]

Survival after the diagnosis of ATC is very poor. With the median survival in most series being less than 5 months from the time of diagnosis, this is one of the most rapidly lethal tumors known in clinical oncology.[182–184] The majority of patients die due to local recurrence, although distant metastases occur primarily in lung, bone, and liver. External radiation has been used with limited success to treat locally recurrent ATC. One study from London reported 10 of 17 patients with an objective response to accelerated radiation (three complete responses and seven partial responses) but toxicity to the esophagus was considerable.[187] In the mid-1980s, Kim and Leeper[188] reported improved responses with a combination of radiation therapy and relatively low-dose Adriamycin as an apparent synergistic agent, achieving responses in 84% of 19 patients, although still having a median survival of only 12 months. Adriamycin is the single most effective chemotherapeutic for ATC, and it has been shown that Adriamycin plus platinum is more effective than Adriamycin alone. A review from the National Cancer Database reports a 10-year survival of 14% for ATC.[189] Early diagnosis with aggressive surgical therapy supplemented by external-beam radiation therapy and Adriamycin-based chemotherapy is the most appropriate treatment for patients with anaplastic thyroid carcinoma.

MEDULLARY THYROID CANCER

MTC was recognized in the 1950s by Hazard et al.[190] as a distinct clinicopathologic entity. Since this description, sequential pathologic, biochemical, and molecular genetic studies have progressed to render this one of the best characterized solid malignancies of the thyroid.[65,191] In 1959, Hazard described MTC as a solid thyroid neoplasm without follicular histology but with a high degree of lymph node metastases that accounted for 3.5% of thyroid cancers in a review at the Cleveland Clinic.[190] Over the next 10 years, investigators identified and described the parafollicular C cell that produces calcitonin, which lowers serum calcium.[191] In 1966 and 1967, Williams[192,193] suggested that MTC arose from this C-cell population. This hypothesis was confirmed by a number of investigators who documented elevated serum calcitonin from patients with MTC. During the decade of the 1970s, Wells et al[194] extended the measurement of calcitonin by defining a provocative test that rendered this hormonal tumor marker one of the most sensitive and specific in all of oncology. Understanding of the familial associations of MTC with corollary genetic studies reported in the 1980s and early 1990s[191] has defined molecular changes that are important for inherited MTC and may have implications for sporadic MTC as well.[195]

MTC constitutes as few as 3%[4] or as many as 12%[191] of most institutional series of detectible thyroid cancers. As opposed to well-differentiated thyroid cancer, MTC is not associated with radiation exposure, but it does occur in distinct familial syndromes. Sporadic or nonfamilial MTC accounts for 60% to 70% of cases, with three distinct familial syndromes accounting for the remainder.[191] MTC is the most prominent clinical diagnosis in MEN 2a and MEN 2B (Table 38.2-10).[196] In 1986, familial MTC with none of the associated features of MEN 2a or MEN 2B was described.[197] Appreciation of this syndrome has shifted the percentage of incidence of sporadic MTC as a function of the total number of cases of MTC from 80% to 60% and even lower in some series. In addition to the presence or absence of other associated endocrine abnormalities, each of these familial forms of MTC has a unique natural history and prognosis.[191] Furthermore, studies have identified specific genetic changes associated with each type (see Table 38.2-10).[195]

Parafollicular, or C cells, arise embryologically from the neural crest and have characteristics shared with other cells with a similar origin.[171] The C cells are located primarily in the upper and middle thirds of the thyroid lobes, with a particular concentration posteriorly. This feature is important to surgical therapy, as this is the location in which the recurrent laryngeal nerve passes under the ligament of Berry and enters the larynx. Therefore, complete thyroid resection is necessary for this condition, because MTC typically arises in this upper portion of the thyroid gland where the C cells are concentrated.

Grossly, MTC may be circumscribed or infiltrative and is usually yellow. Histologically, this tumor can be described as having a wide variety of patterns, including glandular, solid, spindle-cell, oncocytic, clear cell, papillary pattern, small cell,[198] and giant cell. The nuclei of MTC resemble those of neuroendocrine tumors in other areas of the body. They are usually round and have a stippled "pepper-and-salt" chromatin.[198] Pathologic features associated with a poor prognosis include presence of necrosis ($P = .001$), squamous pattern

TABLE 38.2-10. Characteristics of Sporadic and Various Familial Forms of Medullary Thyroid Cancer

		Familial		
	Sporadic	Non-MEN	MEN 2a	MEN 2B
Age at diagnosis	42–45	43–45	24–27[a]	15–20
Gender (F/M ratio)	1:1	1:1	1:1	1:1
Associated diseases	None	None	Pheochromocytoma, hyperparathyroidism	Pheochromocytoma, marfanoid body habitus, oral and eye mucosal neuromas, gastrointestinal tract ganglioneuromas
Disease extent	Unilateral	Bilateral	Bilateral	Bilateral
Lymph nodes at diagnosis	40–50%	10–20%	14%	38%
Distant metastases at diagnosis	12%	0%	0–3%	20%
Cured of MTC	14–30%	70–80%	56–100%	0%
Dead due to MTC	30%	0%	0–17%	50%
Mutations in RET on chromosome 10	Met 918→Thr (33%) Glu 768→Asp	Mutations in cysteines in extracellular domain near membrane	Mutations in cysteines in extracellular domain near membrane	Met 918→Thr

F/M, female-male; MEN 2a, multiple endocrine neoplasia type 2a; MTC, medullary thyroid carcinoma.
[a]The age at diagnosis at centers performing genetic screening can be at or even before birth. Numbers reported reflect series based on biochemical screening of families at risk.
(Data from refs. 68, 191, 195, 196, 208, 209, and 212.)

($P = .002$), presence of oxyphil cells in the tumor and absence of cells with intermediate cytoplasm ($P = .02$), and less than 50% calcitonin immunoreactivity ($P = .04$).[199]

CLINICAL PRESENTATION AND DIAGNOSIS

The clinical symptoms at the time of presentation vary, dependent on the situation for each patient. Patients with familial MTC who are identified by screening with stimulation tests[191] or with molecular analysis[200] are universally identified before any macroscopic mass or lesion. Sporadic patients typically present with an asymptomatic mass in the thyroid.[191] Patients with bulky disease with extremely high levels of calcitonin may have severe secretory diarrhea as a principal symptom. Before the definition of the molecular change for familial MTC,[200] basal and stimulated serum calcitonin levels were used to screen patients.[191] Sequential calcitonin testing is still important as a tumor marker for following up patients with MTC.

Various nuclear medicine imaging studies have been evaluated in patients with MTC to identify gross and occult metastases. MTC does not concentrate iodine, so ^{131}I thyroid scans are of no utility.[201] Similarly, thallium as well as technetium scans have been used with minimal benefit in this disease. ^{131}I metaiodobenzylguanidine scans have been useful in pheochromocytoma and neuroblastoma and have been studied for MTC but do not identify a large proportion of the lesions.[202] Other studies have used radiolabeled anti–carcinoembryonic antigen antibody[203] or anticalcitonin antibody but with limited success. Several studies have used somatostatin receptor scintigraphy in the setting of MTC.[204,205] Like other amine precursor uptake and decarboxylation (APUD) cells, C cells may express a high level of somatostatin receptors, and pharmacologic developments of radiolabeled agents, based on analogs that bind to somatostatin receptor, have been studied for use in treating MTC. In general, the results are better than any other nuclear medicine agent; however, occult lesions smaller than 1 cm[204] as well as liver lesions still are missed with this technique.

TREATMENT

General Approaches

Chemotherapy and external-beam radiation therapy are ineffective against MTC, rendering surgical resection the only definitive therapy.[206,207] For patients with sporadic MTC who are not identified by biochemical or genetic screening, the appropriate operation in most cases is total thyroidectomy with central node dissection. Total thyroidectomy is indicated in this sporadic setting because a small proportion of lesions may be bilateral and because it may not be clear at the time of operation whether a patient is an index case of familial disease or the disorder is a true sporadic case. Because all familial syndromes have a high propensity for bilateral tumors, total thyroidectomy is indicated except possibly for patients having nonfamilial syndromes and small lesions (<1.0 cm).[208] However, one report of 80 patients with sporadic MTC smaller than 1 cm showed that 11% had clinically involved lymph nodes, 31% had pathologically involved lymph nodes, and 5% had distant metastases.[207] Combined with this thyroid resection, a central lymph node dissection is performed, removing lymphoid tissue from the level of the hyoid bone to the innominate vessels inferiorly and laterally to the jugular vein. Lymph nodes lateral to the jugular vein are sampled and, if there is any evidence of metastatic spread in this area, a formal modified radical neck dissection is performed.[209]

The incidence of positive lymph nodes correlates with the size of the primary lesion at the time of diagnosis. It has been reported that for lesions smaller than 1 cm, there can still be an 11% incidence of positive nodal disease, whereas in patients with tumors larger than 2 cm, 60% will have positive cervical lymph nodes.[208] Combining all cases of MTC, between 15% and 75% have spread to the lymph nodes at the time of diagnosis.[191] For this reason, Duh et al.[208] advocated a formal modified radical neck dissection for any lesion larger than 2 cm on the side in which it is located, with a central node dissection on the contralateral side.

The incidence of distant metastases at the time of diagnosis varies with the clinical setting. Twelve percent of patients with sporadic MTC have distant metastases, whereas 20% of those with MEN 2B have metastatic spread but only 3.3% of patients with MEN 2a.[191,196] Patients with familial non-MEN MTC also have a favorable clinical condition similar to MEN 2a, with 2% of patients presenting with distant metastases.[179] Moley et al.[206] have instituted staging laparoscopy to identify liver metastases in patients undergoing thyroid resection and lymph node dissection. For MTC, liver metastases are often the site of metastatic disease and are often radiologically occult. By performing laparoscopy, the incidence of biochemical cure has increased because patients with unresectable liver disease are eliminated from the therapy pool.

The outcome of treatment of patients with sporadic MTC has improved. An early review published in 1970 reported 5- and 10-year survival rates of 48% and 12%, respectively.[191] More recent studies show a 5-year survival of between 80% and 90% and 10-year survival between 70% and 80% for combined series of familial and sporadic MTC.[208–210] The series from the National Cancer Database confirms this improved survival, with a 75% 10-year survival for MTC.[189] It is interesting to note that the natural history and prognosis for the various subtypes of MTC correlate with described genetic changes. The two groups with the worst outcome (sporadic and MEN 2B) have similar genetic changes in the RET oncogene, as do the two types with favorable outcome (familial non-MEN and MEN 2B).[200]

One controversial area in the surgical management of patients with MTC is the proper approach to patients who have persistently elevated basal or stimulated calcitonin after resection of all gross disease.[205,211–215] In many of these cases, imaging studies with conventional techniques of ultrasonography, computed tomography, or magnetic resonance imaging, plus newer techniques of somatostatin receptor scintigraphy,[204] demonstrate no areas of disease. One strategy to identify the region from which elevated calcitonin is coming is to perform selected venous sampling with systemic pentagastrin or calcium stimulation.[205] The key clinical question is: In these patients, who have occult MTC with no radiographic or clinical evidence by which to localize residual tumor but with persistently abnormal calcitonin levels, is the natural history altered by aggressive attempts to excise the occult disease surgically? Excision attempts generally do not produce normalization of calcitonin levels. The best results come from Tisell, who performs meticulous 12-hour neck dissections, often removing 40 to 60 additional cervical lymph nodes in patients with occult MTC.[214] In a series of 11 patients, he had four that had normalized calcitonin levels, with another four that had dramatic improvement in their calcitonin levels. However, even these improvements in the calcitonin levels do not necessarily translate into improved survival. Thirty-one patients were identified, all of whom had gross disease resected at initial operation at the Mayo Clinic but had documented elevated postoperative calcitonin.[215] With a median follow-up of almost 12 years, only 11 patients developed clinically or radiographically apparent recurrent disease, and these 11 patients were reoperated at that time. None of these patients normalized their calcitonin levels after reoperation. Important is that the overall 5- and 10-year survival rates in this population were 90% and 86%, respectively, with only two patients dying specifically from MTC.[215] Both patients had sporadic MTC with very aggressive invasive primary lesions and died of distant metastases 2 to 2.5 years after diagnosis. Even though there is no alternative therapy to surgical resection for MTC, the data regarding the prognosis of occult MTC plus the lack of success even with very extensive reoperations to normalize calcitonin would argue that the best course of action in this patient population is close follow-up and operation only when clinically apparent disease is present.

For patients with metastatic MTC, surgical resection may still offer the best chance of survival as well as long-term palliation. In 16 patients with metastatic MTC at Johns Hopkins, 21 palliative reoperations were performed. These procedures included neck reoperations in 11 cases but also removal of mediastinal masses and liver metastases as well as other miscellaneous lesions. All patients had clear relief of their index symptoms, typically diarrhea and fatigue, and had a median survival rate of 8.2 years.[216]

The results of MTC treatment with external-beam radiation therapy[217] or chemotherapeutics are disappointing.[218,219] Radiation administered at a dose of more than 5000 rads to a large Y-shaped anterior field without laryngeal shielding necessary to treat these patients causes significant local toxicity. Dysphagia as well as dyspnea can be severe in certain individuals. Furthermore, treatment with this radiation dose has not definitively been shown to decrease local recurrences. One large study from France of 59 patients reported local recurrences within the radiation field in 30% of patients.[217] Chemotherapeutics used in treatment of MTC include Adriamycin, dacarbazine, streptozocin, and 5-fluorouracil.[218] Single-agent response rates are poor, with aggressive Adriamycin regimens producing 20% to 30% objective responses. A study of combination chemotherapy showed that a regimen of 5-fluorouracil, streptozocin, and dacarbazine produces objective responses in only 15%.[218] The poor outcome of treatment of metastatic disease validates the treatment recommendation to diagnose patients with MTC early and treat with initial aggressive surgery.

Due to failure of chemotherapy and radiation therapy to offer significant benefit for patients with MTC, innovative therapeutic strategies for MTC have been developed, such as the use of gene therapy. This technique primarily uses adenovirus to transduce either interleukin-2 or suicide gene, such as herpes simplex virus thymidine kinase.[220,221] Other more directed gene therapies would rely on the expression of calcitonin only from MTC and have use of selective promoter in front of a suicide gene or other targeted transgene.

Treatment of Familial Medullary Thyroid Cancer

An increasing number of patients are identified in one of the three familial settings of MTC that are diagnosed using biochemical or genetic screening.[200] Routine use of provocative biochemical testing to diagnose MTC led to a significant decrease in the age of diagnosis, a significant decrease in the incidence of lymph node metastases, and a significant increase in the number of patients cured biochemically at these earlier operations.[191] This strategy has been extended to an earlier stage with the description of the mutations in the RET oncogene present in the MEN 2a.[200] At Washington University, Wells et al.[200] use a molecular genetic screening technique to identify patients who are carriers of the MEN 2a mutation as infants or young children. Before any abnormality in basal or stimulated calcitonin, these patients undergo a total thyroidectomy, a total parathyroidectomy, and a parathyroid autograft. Pathologic evaluation on these children's thyroid identifies either C-cell hyperplasia or microscopic or macroscopic MTC. In the initial trial, no patients treated with this strategy had evidence of lymph node metastases, and this surgical strategy should be curative.

The genetic test for the mutations in the RET protooncogene have become commercially available, and many individuals are reporting series based on early operation for patients identified by RET mutation. A review has noted that in a total of 209 patients treated in this manner, 3.4% had normal thyroid glands with no evidence of C-cell hyperplasia or MTC.[222] It was also noted that in these patients undergoing prophylactic operations, there was an 8.6% incidence of lymph node metastases. Based on these results, it is thought that a prophylactic central neck dissection should be performed at the time of this prophylactic thyroidectomy, based on genetic testing. Because this oncogene was one of the first to be defined that led to a therapeutic procedure, there has been appropriate attention paid to the psychosocial impact of genetic testing. A study from Lyon, France suggests that patients who are in this situation of being kindreds undergoing genetic testing are frustrated regarding this stressful process.[223]

THYROID LYMPHOMA

Thyroid lymphoma is a relatively rare disease constituting fewer than 1% of all lymphomas and accounting for 2% of extranodal non-Hodgkin's lymphoma (see Chapter 45.3).[224] Almost all these thyroid lymphomas are non-Hodgkin's lymphoma,[225] with the majority (70% to 90%) being intermediate grade and the remainder being high grade.[226] Many are considered mucosa-associated lymphoid tissue lymphomas or *MALTomas* and show plasmacytic differentiation and may be associated with similar lesions in extranodal sites especially in the gastrointestinal tract.[231]

The majority of patients with thyroid lymphoma all have disease on one side of the diaphragm with a proportion confined to the thyroid (stage IE) and the majority with thyroid disease plus cervical or mediastinal lymph nodes (stage IIE).[227] The incidence of this disease may be changing, primarily due to improved recognition and diagnosis of thyroid lymphoma. Henry Ford Hospital in Detroit saw seven cases of thyroid lymphoma in 20 years before 1976 and 30 cases in the 8 years after 1976.[225] One hypothesis to explain the incidence increase is that these patients were previously diagnosed as having anaplastic thyroid carcinoma and, with better understanding and more sophisticated diagnostic tools, such as immunohistochemistry, these patients are being correctly categorized as having thyroid lymphoma.

In most series, there is a strong female predominance, ranging from 3:1 in the large Mayo Clinic series[228] to 6.5:1 from Brown University[227] and up to 8:1 for the Vancouver, British Columbia study.[226] The median age in most series at diagnosis places patients in the seventh decade of life, similar to what is seen for ATC and much older than patients with well-differentiated thyroid cancer.[226–228] Between 10% and 30% of patients report a symptom or combination of symptoms relating to local invasion, including hoarseness, dyspnea with stridor, or dysphagia.[226] Patients with thyroid lymphoma virtually never have hyperthyroidism but frequently have hypothyroidism. These hypothyroid patients have evidence of autoimmune thyroiditis or Hashimoto's thyroiditis, either by biopsy or from the pathologic specimen.[225]

The optimal treatment for thyroid lymphoma has evolved with the success of combination chemotherapy used in the treatment of non-Hodgkin's lymphoma and with the ability to obtain an accurate diagnosis without invasive surgery by large-needle or core needle biopsy. Skarsgard et al.[226] argued that the role of surgery in this disease is simply to obtain adequate tissue for diagnosis and that the primary treatment should be external-beam radiation combined with an Adriamycin-based chemotherapy regimen. Using this strategy at his institution, the 5-year survival was 70%, and the 4-year disease-free survival was also 70%. Others have argued that in the 20% to 30% minority of patients who have no extrathyroidal extension, excellent survival is achieved by surgical excision plus postoperative radiation therapy.[224] Patients with extrathyroidal disease either by direct extension or lymph node involvement should be considered to have systemic disease. Although some endocrine surgeons argue that attempts to clear the trachea to avoid airway obstruction should be performed if at all possible in all patients,[224] others report that the rapid use of radiation therapy (starting the day after the diagnostic biopsy procedure) produces the same beneficial results.[226,227] All would agree that the efficacy in long-term survival using a combination of radiation therapy and chemotherapy render aggressive surgical resection with a sacrifice of recurrent laryngeal nerve or possibly resulting in hypoparathyroidism contraindicated for thyroid lymphoma.

SECONDARY THYROID MALIGNANCY

Involvement of the thyroid gland by malignant metastases from other sites is rare, accounting for fewer than 1% of thyroid malignancies in most clinical series involving surgical resection or FNA biopsies.[229,230] On the other hand, the incidence of thyroid metastases identified on autopsy series is greater and can range between 2% and 26% in autopsy series, probably depending on the thoroughness of the examination by the pathologists.[229] From these autopsy series, the most predominant malignancies metastatic to the thyroid are breast and lung, each accounting for 25% of the total.[229] Melanoma, renal cell carcinoma, and gastrointestinal tract malignancies each account for approximately 10% of these secondary malignancies from autopsy studies. A variety of other miscellaneous diagnoses account for the remainder.

For the more clinically relevant situation in which the thyroid metastasis is detected premortem, the most common primary site is renal cell carcinoma, accounting for 23% of 111 such cases combined from the literature.[229] The next most common sites are breast (16%), lung (15%), melanoma (5%), and colon and larynx (4.5% each). Occasionally, the thyroid metastasis may be the initial presentation of an occult primary from a gastrointestinal source or renal primary. Because FNA biopsy is the diagnostic tool used to evaluate thyroid nodules as the initial step, an awareness of the potential of the secondary metastases is important for interpretation of these biopsy results.

Dependent on the clinical situation, some of these patients may need thyroidectomy for palliation of local symptoms. Thyroid metastases may grow at a rapid rate and can cause airway obstruction. In one large institutional series from Toronto, 8 of 11 patients derived benefit from a thyroidectomy after premortem diagnosis of secondary metastases.[230]

REFERENCES

1. Landis SH, Murray T, Bolden S, Wingo PA. Cancer statistics, 1999. *CA Cancer J Clin* 1999;49:8.
2. Jensen RT, Norton JA. Endocrine tumors of the pancreas. In: Yamada T, Alpers BH, Owyang C, Powell DW, Silverstein FE, eds. *Textbook of gastroenterology*. Philadelphia: JB Lippincott Co, 1995:2131.
3. Jossart GH, Clark OH. Well-differentiated thyroid cancer. *Curr Probl Surg* 1994;31(12):937.
4. LiVolsi VA, Asa SL. The demise of follicular carcinoma of the thyroid gland. *Thyroid* 1994;4(2):233.
5. LiVolsi VA, Bronner MP. Oxyphilic (Ashkenazi-Hürthle cell) tumors of the thyroid: microscopic features predict biologic behavior. *Surg Pathol* 1988;1(2):137.
6. Mariotti S, Franceshi C, Cossarizza A, Pinchera A. The aging thyroid. *Endocrine Rev* 1995;16:686.
7. Denham MJ, Willis EJ. A clinico-pathological survey of thyroid glands in old age. *Gerontology* 1980;26:160.
8. Burch HB. Evaluation and management of the solid thyroid nodule. *Endocrinol Metab Clin North Am* 1995;24:663.
9. Schneider AB. Radiation-induced thyroid tumors. *Endocrinol Metab Clin North Am* 1990;19:495.
10. Hancock SL, Cox RS, McDougall IR. Thyroid diseases after treatment of Hodgkins' disease. *N Engl J Med* 1991;325:599.
11. Mazzaferri EL. Thyroid cancer in thyroid nodules: finding a needle in the haystack. *Am J Med* 1992;93:359.
12. DeGroot LJ, Reilly M, Pinnamenneni K, et al. Retrospective and prospective study of radiation-induced thyroid disease. *Am J Med* 1983;74:852.
13. Schneider AB, Shore-Freedman E, Ryo UY, et al. Radiation-induced tumors of the head and neck following childhood irradiation. *Medicine* 1985;64:1.
14. Farbota LM, Calandra DB, Lawrence AM, et al. Thyroid carcinoma in Graves' disease. *Surgery* 1985;98:1148.
15. Shapiro SJ, Friedman NB, Perzik SL, et al. Incidence of thyroid carcinoma in Graves' disease. *Cancer* 1970;26:1261.
16. Hales IB, McElduff A, Crummer P, et al. Does Graves' disease or thyrotoxicosis affect the prognosis of thyroid cancer? *J Clin Endocrinol Metab* 1992;75:886.
17. Mazzaferri EL. Management of a solitary thyroid nodule. *N Engl J Med* 1993;328:553.
18. Singer PA, Cooper DS, Daniels GH, et al. Treatment guidelines for patients with thyroid nodules and well-differentiated thyroid cancer. *Arch Intern Med* 1996;156(19):2165.
19. Raue F, Frank-Raue K, Grauer A. Multiple endocrine neoplasia type 2: clinical features and screening. *Endocrinol Clin North Am* 1994;23:137.
20. Bell B, Mazzaferri EL. Thyroid cancer in familial polyposis coli: case report and literature review. *Dig Dis Sci* 1993;38:185.
21. Shapiro SD, Lambert WC, Schwartz RA. Cowden's disease. A marker for malignancy. *Int J Dermatol* 1988;27:232.
22. Hammings JF, Goslings BM, Van Steenis GJ, et al. The value of fine needle aspiration biopsy in patients with nodular thyroid disease divided into groups of suspicion of malignant neoplasms on clinical grounds. *Arch Intern Med* 1990;150:113.
23. Pacini F, Fontanelli M, Fugazzola L, et al. Routine measurement of serum calcitonin in nodular thyroid diseases allows the preoperative diagnosis of unsuspected sporadic medullary thyroid carcinoma. *J Clin Endocrinol Metab* 1994;78:826.
24. Dunn JT. When is a nodule a sporadic medullary thyroid carcinoma? [Editorial]. *J Clin Endocrinol Metab* 1994;78:824.
25. Hagag P, Strauss S, Weiss M. Role of ultrasound-guided fine-needle aspiration biopsy in evaluation of nonpalpable thyroid nodules. *Thyroid* 1998;8(11):989.
26. Danese D, Schiacchitano S, Farsetti A, Andreoli M, Pontecorvi A. Diagnostic accuracy of conventional versus sonography-guided fine-needle aspiration biopsy of thyroid nodules. *Thyroid* 1998;8(1):15.
27. Shimamoto K, Endo T, Ishigaki T, et al. Thyroid nodules: evaluation with color Doppler ultrasonography. *J Ultrasound Med* 1993;12:673.
28. Caruso D, Mazzaferri EL. Fine needle aspiration biopsy in the management of thyroid nodules. *Endocrinologist* 1991;1:194.
29. Gharib H, Goellner JR, Zinsmeister AR, et al. Fine-needle aspiration biopsy of the thyroid. *Ann Intern Med* 1984;101:25.
30. Cheng AJ, Lin JD, Chang T, Wang TC. Telomerase activity in benign and malignant human thyroid tissues. *Br J Cancer* 1998;77(12):2177.
31. Saji M, Westra WH, Chen H, et al. Telomerase activity in the differential diagnosis of papillary carcinoma of the thyroid. *Surgery* 1997;122(6):1137.
32. Umbricht CB, Saji M, Westra WH, et al. Telomerase activity: a marker to distinguish follicular thyroid adenoma from carcinoma. *Cancer Res* 1997;57(11):2144.
33. Hall TL, Layfield LJ, Phillippe A, Rosenthal DL. Sources of diagnostic error in fine needle aspiration of the thyroid. *Cancer* 1989;63:718.
34. Carson HJ, Castelli MJ, Gattuso P. Incidences of neoplasia and Hashimoto's thyroiditis: a fine needle aspiration study. *Diagn Cytopathol* 1996;14:38.
35. Gharib H, James EH, Charboneau JW, et al. Suppressive therapy with levothyroxine for solitary thyroid nodules: a double-blind controlled clinical study. *N Engl J Med* 1987;317:70.
36. Cheung PSY, Lee JMH, Boey JH. Thyroxine suppression of benign thyroid nodules: a prospective randomized study. *World J Surg* 1989;13:818.
37. Reverter JL, Lucas A, Salinas I, et al. Suppressive therapy with levothyroxine for solitary thyroid nodules. *Clin Endocrinol (Oxf)* 1992;36:25.
38. Ross DS. Subclinical hyperthyroidism: possible danger of overzealous thyroxine replacement therapy. *Mayo Clin Proc* 1988;63:1223.
39. Biondi B, Fazio S, Carella C, et al. Cardiac effects of long-term thyrotropin-suppressive therapy with levothyroxine. *J Clin Endocrinol Metab* 1993;77:334.
40. Fritts LL, Crombie HD, Allen LW, Deckers PJ. Surgical treatment options for well-differentiated thyroid cancer: more is not necessarily better. *Contemp Surg* 1993;42:197.
41. Cady B, Rossi R, Silverman M, Wool M. Further evidence of the validity of risk group definition in differentiated thyroid carcinoma. *Surgery* 1985;98(6):1171.
42. Mazzaferri EL, Jhiang SM. Long-term impact of initial surgical and medical therapy on papillary and follicular thyroid cancer. *Am J Med* 1994;97:418.
43. Simpson WJ, McKinney SE, Carruthers JS, et al. Papillary and follicular thyroid cancer: prognostic factors in 1,578 patients. *Am J Med* 1987;83:479.
44. Brennan MD, Bergstralh EJ, van Heerden JA, McConahey WM. Follicular thyroid cancer treated at the Mayo Clinic, 1946 through 1970: initial manifestations, pathologic findings, therapy, and outcome. *Mayo Clin Proc* 1991;66:11.
45. McConahey WM, Hay ID, Woolner LB, van Heerden JA, Taylor WF. Papillary thyroid cancer treated at the Mayo Clinic, 1946 through 1970: initial manifestations, pathologic findings, therapy and outcome. *Mayo Clin Proc* 1986;61:978.
46. Harness JK, Thompson NW, McLeod MK, Eckhauser FE, Lloyd RV. Follicular carcinoma of the thyroid gland: trends and treatment. *Surgery* 1984;96(6):971.
47. Francheschi S, Boyle P, Maisonneuve P, et al. The epidemiology of thyroid carcinoma. *Crit Rev Oncogen* 1993;4:25.
48. Shore RE. Issues and epidemiological evidence regarding radiation-induced thyroid cancer. *Radiat Res* 1992;131:98.
49. Ron E, Kleinerman RA, Boice JD Jr, et al. A population-based case-control study of thyroid cancer. *J Natl Cancer Inst* 1987;79:1.
50. Binter G, Lax S, Eber O. The impact of geographical, clinical, dietary and radiation-induced features in epidemiology of thyroid cancer. *Eur J Cancer* 1993;29A:1547.
51. Shore RE, Woodard E, Hildreth N, et al. Thyroid tumors following thymus irradiation. *J Natl Cancer Inst* 1985;74:1177.
52. Ron E, Modan B, Preston D, et al. Thyroid neoplasia following low-dose radiation in childhood. *Radiat Res* 1989;120:516.
53. Schneider AB, Recant W, Pincky SM, et al. Radiation-induced thyroid carcinoma. Clinical course and results of therapy in 296 patients. *Ann Intern Med* 1986;105:405.
54. Schneider AB, Ron E, Lubin J, Stovall M, Gierlowski TC. Dose-response relationships for radiation-induced thyroid cancer and thyroid nodules: evidence for the prolonged effects of radiation on the thyroid. *J Clin Endocrinol Metab* 1993;77:362.
55. Tucker MA, Jones PHM, Boice JD Jr, et al. Therapeutic radiation at a young age is linked to secondary thyroid cancer. *Cancer Res* 1991;51:2885.
56. Boice JD Jr, Engholm G, Lkeinerman RA, et al. Radiation dose and second cancer risk in patients treated for cancer of the cervix. *Radiat Res* 1988;116:3.
57. Hallquist A, Hardell L, Degerman A, Wingren G, Boquist L. Medical diagnostic and therapeutic ionizing radiation and the risk for thyroid cancer: a case control study. *Eur J Cancer Prev* 1994;3:259.
58. Holm LE, Wiklund KE, Lundell GE, et al. Thyroid cancer after diagnostic doses of iodine-131: a retrospective cohort study. *J Natl Cancer Inst* 1988;80:1132.
59. Holm LE, Hall P, Wiklund K, et al. Cancer risk after iodine-131 therapy for hyperthyroidism. *J Natl Cancer Inst* 1991;83:1072.
60. Hamilton TE, van Belle G, LoGerfo JP. Thyroid neoplasia in Marshall islanders exposed to nuclear fallout. *JAMA* 1987;258:629.
61. Kerber RA, Till JE, Simon SL, et al. A cohort study of thyroid disease in relation to fallout from nuclear weapons testing. *JAMA* 1993;270:2076.
62. Nikiforov Y, Gnepp DR. Pediatric thyroid cancer after the Chernobyl disaster. *Cancer* 1994;74:748.
63. Mettler FA Jr, Williamson MR, Royal HD, et al. Thyroid nodules in the population living around Chernobyl. *JAMA* 1992;268:616.
64. Franceschi S, Levi F, Negri E, Fassina A, LaVecchia C. Diet and thyroid cancer: a pooled analysis of four European case-control studies. *Int J Cancer* 1991;48:395.
65. Glattre E, Haldorsen T, Berg JP, Stensvold I, Solvoll K. Norwegian case-control study testing the hypothesis that seafood increases the risk of thyroid cancer. *Cancer Causes Control* 1993;4:11.
66. Grossman RF, Tu SH, Duh QY, et al. Familial nonmedullary thyroid cancer. *Arch Surg* 1995;130:892.
67. Lesueur F, Stark M, Tocco T, et al. Genetic heterogeneity in familial nonmedullary thyroid carcinoma: exclusion of linkage to RET, MNG1, and TCO in 56 families. NMTC Consortium. *J Clin Endocrinol Metab* 1999;84(6):2157.
68. Goodfellow PJ, Wells SA. RET gene and its implications for cancer. *J Natl Cancer Inst* 1995;87(20):1515.
69. Rosai J, Carcangiu ML, DeLellis RA. Tumors of the thyroid gland. In: *Atlas of tumor pathology*, 3rd series, fascicle 5. Washington DC: Armed Forces Institute of Pathology, 1993.
70. LiVolsi VA. *Surgical pathology of the thyroid*. Philadelphia: WB Saunders, 1990.
71. Hay ID. Papillary thyroid carcinoma. *Endocrinol Metab Clin North Am* 1990;19:545.
72. Hay ID. Papillary thyroid carcinoma. *Endocrinol Metab Clin North Am* 1990;19:545.
73. Tielens ET, Sherman SI, Hruban RH, Ladenson PQ. Follicular variant of papillary thyroid carcinoma: a clinicopathologic study. *Cancer* 1994;73(2):425.
74. Chan JK, Saw D. The grooved nucleus. A useful diagnostic criterion of papillary carcinoma of the thyroid. *Am J Surg Pathol* 1986;10:672.
75. Johnson TL, Lloyd RV, Thompson NW, Beierwaltes WH, Sisson JC. Prognostic implications of the tall cell variant of papillary thyroid carcinoma. *Am J Surg Pathol* 1988;12(1):22.

76. Gaertner EM, Davidson M, Wenig B. The columnar cell variant of thyroid papillary carcinoma. *Am J Surg Pathol* 1995;19:940.
77. Carcangiu ML, Bianchi S. Diffuse sclerosing variant of papillary thyroid carcinoma: clinicopathologic study of 15 cases. *Am J Surg Pathol* 1989;13:1041.
78. Ruter A, Nishiyama R, Lennquist S. Tall-cell variant of papillary thyroid cancer: disregarded entity? *World J Surg* 1997;21(1):15.
79. Cooper DS, Schneyer CR. Follicular and Hürthle cell carcinoma of the thyroid. *Endocrinol Metab Clin North Am* 1990;19(3):577.
80. van Heerden JA, Hay ID, Goellner RJ, et al. Follicular thyroid carcinoma with capsular invasion alone: a nonthreatening malignancy. *Surgery* 1992;112:1130.
81. Gundry SR, Burney RE, Thompson NW, Lloyd R. Total thyroidectomy for Hürthle cell neoplasm of the thyroid. *Arch Surg* 1983;118:529.
82. Gosain AK, Clark OH. Hürthle cell neoplasms: malignant potential. *Arch Surg* 1984;119:515.
83. Grant SC, Barr D, Goeliner JR, Hay ID. Benign Hürthle cell tumors of the thyroid: a diagnosis to be trusted? *World J Surg* 1988;12:488.
84. Friedman M. Surgical management of thyroid carcinoma with laryngotracheal invasion. *Otolaryngol Clin North Am* 1990;23(3):495.
85. Ballantyne A. Resections of the upper aerodigestive tract for locally invasive thyroid cancer. *Am J Surg* 1994;168:636.
86. Cochand-Priollet B, Guillausseau PJ, Chagnon S, et al. The diagnostic value of fine-needle aspiration biopsy under ultrasonography in nonfunctional thyroid nodules: a prospective study comparing cytologic and histologic findings. *Am J Med* 1994;97:152.
87. Stark DD, Clark OH, Gooding GAW, Moss AA. High resolution ultrasound and computerized tomography of thyroid lesions in patients with hyperparathyroidism. *Surgery* 1983;94:863.
88. Mazzaferri EL. NCCN thyroid carcinoma practice guidelines. *Oncology* 1999;13:391.
89. Hamburger JI. Diagnosis of thyroid nodules by fine needle biopsy: use and abuse. *J Clin Endocrinol Metab* 1994;70(2):335.
90. Clark OH, Okerlund MD, Cavalieri RR, Greenspan FS. Diagnosis and treatment of thyroid, parathyroid, and thyroglossal duct cysts. *J Clin Endocrinol Metab* 1979;48:983.
91. Block MA, Dailey GE, Robb JA. Thyroid nodules indeterminate by needle biopsy. *Am J Surg* 1983;146:72.
92. Tyler DS, Winchester DJ, Caraway NP, Hickey RC, Evans DB. Indeterminate fine-needle aspiration biopsy of the thyroid: identification of subgroups at high risk for invasive carcinoma. *Surgery* 1994;116:1054.
93. Schelfhout LJDM, Creutzberg CL, Hamming JF, et al. Multivariate analysis of survival in differentiated thyroid cancer: the prognostic significance of the age factor. *Eur J Cancer Clin Oncol* 1988;24(2):331.
94. Joensuu H, Klemi PJ, Paul R, Tuominen J. Survival and prognostic factors in thyroid carcinoma. *Acta Radiol Oncol* 1986;25:243.
95. Torres J, Volpato RD, Power EG, et al. Thyroid cancer. *Cancer* 1985;56:2298.
96. Harness JK, McLeod MK, Thompson NW, Noble WC, Burney RE. Deaths due to differentiated thyroid cancer: a 46-year perspective. *World J Surg* 1988;12:623.
97. Staunton MD. Thyroid cancer: a multivariate analysis on influence of treatment on long-term survival. *Eur J Surg Oncol* 1994;20:613.
98. Akslen LA, Haldorsen T, Thoresen SO, Glattre E. Survival and causes of death in thyroid cancer: a population-based study of 2479 cases from Norway. *Cancer Res* 1991;51:1234.
99. Cunningham MP, Duda RB, Recant W, et al. Survival discriminants for differentiated thyroid cancer. *Am J Surg* 1990;160:344.
100. Donohue JH, Goldfien SD, Miller TR, Abele JS, Clark OH. Do the prognoses of papillary and follicular thyroid carcinomas differ? *Am J Surg* 1984;148:166.
101. Brooks JR, Starnes HF, Brooks DC, Pelkey JN. Surgical therapy for thyroid carcinoma: a review of 1249 solitary thyroid nodules. *Surgery* 1988;104:940.
102. Allo MD, Christianson W, Koivunen D. Not all "occult" papillary carcinomas are "minimal." *Surgery* 1988;104:971.
103. Shaha AR, Shah JP, Loree TR. Patterns of nodal and distant metastasis based on histologic varieties in differentiated carcinoma of the thyroid. *Am J Surg* 1996;172(6):692.
104. Caplan RH, Abellera RM, Kisken WA. Hürthle cell neoplasms of the thyroid gland: reassessment of functional capacity. *Thyroid* 1994;4(3):243.
105. Shaha AR, Shah JP, Loree TR. Differentiated thyroid cancer presenting initially with distant metastasis. *Am J Surg* 1997;174(5):474.
106. Rossi RL, Cady B, Silverman ML, et al. Surgically incurable well-differentiated thyroid carcinoma. *Arch Surg* 1988;123:569.
107. Cady B, Rossi R. An expanded view of risk-group definition in differentiated thyroid carcinoma. *Surgery* 1988;104:947.
108. Rossi RL, Cady B, Silverman ML, Wool MS, Horner TA. Current results of conservative surgery for differentiated thyroid carcinoma. *World J Surg* 1986;10:612.
109. Hay ID, Grant CS, Taylor WF, McConahey WM. Ipsilateral lobectomy versus bilateral lobar resection in papillary thyroid carcinoma: a retrospective analysis of surgical outcome using a novel prognostic scoring system. *Surgery* 1987;102(6):1087.
110. Zimmerman D, Hay ID, Gough IR, et al. Papillary thyroid carcinoma in children and adults: Long-term follow-up of 1039 patients conservatively treated at one institution during three decades. *Surgery* 1988;104:1157.
111. Grant CS, Hay ID, Gough IR, et al. Local recurrence in papillary thyroid carcinoma: Is extent of surgical resection important? *Surgery* 1988;104:954.
112. Pasieka JL, Zedenius J, Auer G, et al. Addition of nuclear DNA content to the AMES risk-group classification for papillary thyroid cancer. *Surgery* 1992;112:1154.
113. Hay I, Bergstralh E, Goellner J, Ebersold J, Grant C. Predicting outcome in papillary thyroid carcinoma: development of a reliable prognostic scoring system in a cohort of 1779 patients surgically treated at one institution during 1940 through 1989. *Surgery* 1993;114:1050.
114. Sanders LE, Cady B. Differentiated thyroid cancer: re-examination of risk groups and outcome of treatment. *Arch Surg* 1998;133(4):419.
115. Hav ID, Grant CS, Bergstralh EJ, et al. Unilateral total lobectomy: is it sufficient treatment for patients with AMES low-risk papillary thyroid carcinoma? *Surgery* 1998;124(6):958.
116. American Joint Committee on Cancer. Thyroid gland. In: Fleming ID, Cooper JS, Henson DE, et al., eds. *AJCC cancer staging manual,* 5th ed. Philadelphia: Lippincott-Raven, 1997:63.
117. Sherman SI, Brierley JD, Sperling M, et al. Prospective multicenter study of thyroid carcinoma treatment. *Cancer* 1998;83(5):1012.
118. Hamburger JI, Hamburger SW. Declining role of frozen section in surgical planning for thyroid nodules. *Surgery* 1985;98(2):307.
119. Chen H, Nicol TL, Udelsman R. Follicular lesions of the thyroid. *Ann Surg* 1995;222(1):101.
120. Bonner MP, Hamilton RH, LiVolsi VA. Utility of frozen section analysis in follicular lesions of the thyroid. *Endocr Pathol* 1994;5:154.
121. DeGroot LJ, Kaplan EL. Second opinion for "completion" of thyroidectomy in treatment of differentiated thyroid cancer. *Surgery* 1991;110:936.
122. DeJong SA, Demeter JG, Lawrence AM, Paloyan E. Necessity and safety of completion thyroidectomy for differentiated thyroid carcinoma. *Surgery* 1992;112:734.
123. Udelsman R, Lakatos E, Ladenson P. Optimal surgery for papillary thyroid carcinoma. *World J Surg* 1996;20(1):88.
124. Friedman M, Pacella BL Jr. Total versus subtotal thyroidectomy. *Otolaryngol Clin North Am* 1990;23(3):413.
125. Flynn MB, Lyons KJ, Tarter JW, Ragsdale TL. Local complications after surgical resection for thyroid carcinoma. *Am J Surg* 1994;168:404.
126. Logue JP, Tsang RW, Brierley JD, Simpson WJ. Radioiodine ablation of residual tissue in thyroid cancer: relationship between administered activity, neck uptake and outcome. *Br J Radiol* 1994;67:1127.
127. DiRusso G, Kern KA. Comparative analysis of complications from I-131 radioablation for well-differentiated thyroid cancer. *Surgery* 1994;116:1024.
128. Taylor T, Specker B, Robbins J, et al. Outcome after treatment of high-risk papillary and non-Hürthle cell follicular thyorid carcinoma. *Ann Intern Med* 1998;129(8):622.
129. Wanebo H, Coburn M, Teates D, Cole B. Total thyroidectomy does not enhance disease control or survival even in high risk patients with differentiated thyroid cancer. *Ann Surg* 1998;227(6):912.
130. Talpos GB. Tracheal and laryngeal resections for differentiated thyroid cancer. *Am Surg* 1999;65(8):754.
131. McGregor GI, Luoma A, Jackson SM. Lymph node metastases from well-differentiated thyroid cancer. *Am J Surg* 1998;149:608.
132. King WWK, Li AKC. What is the optimal treatment of nodal metastases in differentiated thyroid cancer? *Aust N Z J Surg* 1994:64:815.
133. Moley JF, Wells SA. Compartment-mediated dissection for papillary thyroid cancer. *Langenbecks Arch Surg* 1999;384(1):9.
134. Sako K, Marchetta FC, Razack MS, Shedd DP. Modified radical neck dissection for metastatic carcinoma of the thyroid. *Am J Surg* 1985;150:498.
135. Kelemen PR, Van Herle AJ, Giuliano AE. Sentinel lymphadenectomy in thyroid malignant neoplasms. *Arch Surg* 1998;133(3):288.
136. Ozaki O, Ito K, Kobayashi K, Suzuki A, Manabe Y. Modified neck dissection for patients with nonadvanced, differentiated carcinoma of the thyroid. *World J Surg* 1988;12:825.
137. Tissel LE, Nilsson B, Molne J, et al. Improved survival of patients with papillary thyroid cancer after surgical microdissection. *World J Surg* 1996;20(7):848.
138. Simon D, Goretzki PE, Witte J, Roher HD. Incidence of regional recurrence guiding radicality in differentiated thyroid carcinoma. *World J Surg* 1996;20(7):860.
139. Solomon BL, Wartofsky L, Burman KD. Current trends in the management of well differentiated papillary thyroid carcinoma. *J Clin Endocrinol Metab* 1996;81:333.
140. Wartofsky L, Sherman SI, Gopal J, Schlumberger M, Hay ID. The use of radioactive iodine in patients with papillary and follicular thyroid cancer. *J Clin Endocrinol Metab* 1998;83(12):4195.
141. Schlumberger M. Can iodine-131 whole body scan be replaced by thyroglobulin measurement in the postsurgical follow up of differentiated thyroid carcinoma? *J Nucl Med* 1992;33:172.
142. Pineda JD, Lee T, Ain K, Reynolds JC, Robbins J. Iodine-131 therapy for thyroid cancer patients with elevated thyroglobulin and negative diagnostic scan. *J Clin Endocrinol Metab* 1995;80:1488.
143. Krishnamurthy GT, Blahd WH. Radioiodine I-131 therapy in the management of thyroid cancer. A prospective study. *Cancer* 1977;40:195.
144. Samaan NA, Maheshwari YK, Nader S, et al. Impact of therapy for differentiated carcinoma of the thyroid: an analysis of 706 cases. *J Clin Endocrinol Metab* 1983;56:1131.
145. Massin JP, Savoie JC, Garnier H, et al. Pulmonary metastases in differentiated thyroid carcinoma. Study of 58 cases with implication for the primary tumor treatment. *Cancer* 1984;53:982.
146. DeGroot LJ, Reilly M. Comparison of 30- and 50-mCi doses of iodine-131 for thyroid ablation. *Ann Intern Med* 1982;96:51.
147. McCowan KD, Adler RA, Ghaed N, et al. Low-dose radioiodide thyroid ablation in postsurgical patients with thyroid cancer. *Am J Med* 1976;61:52.
148. Beierwaltes WH, Rabbani R, Dmowchowski C, et al. An analysis of "ablation of thyroid remnants" with 131-I in 511 patients from 1947–1984: experience at University of Michigan. *J Nucl Med* 1984;25:1287.
149. Bonua RS, Leeper RD. A method and rationale for treatment thyroid carcinoma with the largest, safe dose of 131-I. In: Medeiros-Neto G, Gaitan E, eds. *Frontiers in thyroidology.* New York: Plenum Medical, 1986:1317.
150. Mazzaferri EL. Carcinoma of follicular epithelium: radioiodine and other treatment and outcomes. In: Braverman LE, Utiger RD, eds. *Werner and Ingbar's the thyroid: a fundamental and clinical text,* 6th ed. Philadelphia: JB Lippincott Co, 1991:1138.
151. Mazzaferri EL, Jhiang SM. Long-term impact of initial surgical and medical therapy on papillary and follicular thyroid cancer. *Am J Med* 1994;97:418.
152. Mazzaferri EL, Young RL, Oertel JE, et al. Papillary thyroid carcinoma: the impact of therapy in 576 patients. *Medicine* 1977;56:171.

153. Harwood J, Diarck OI, Dunphy JE. Significance of lymph node metastasis in differentiated thyroid cancer. *Cancer* 1979;43:810.
154. Sweeney DC, Johnson GS. Radioiodine therapy for thyroid cancer. *Endocrinol Metab Clin North Am* 1995;24:803.
155. Lakshmanan M, Schaffer A, Robbins J, et al. A simplified low iodine diet in 131-I scanning and therapy for thyroid cancer. *Clin Nucl Med* 1988;13:966.
156. Ramanna L, Waxman A, Brachman MB, et al. Treatment rationale in thyroid carcinoma: effect of scan dose. *Clin Nucl Med* 1985;10:687.
157. Jeevanram RK, Shah DH, Sharma M, et al. Influence of initial large dose on subsequent uptake of therapeutic radioiodine in thyroid cancer patients. *Nucl Med Biol* 1986;13:277.
158. Park HM, Perkins OW, Edmondson JW, et al. Influence of diagnostic radioiodines in the uptake of ablative doses of iodine-131. *Thyroid* 1994;4:49.
159. Sherman SI, Tielens ET, Sostre S, et al. Clinical utility of post-treatment radioiodine scans in the management of patients with thyroid carcinoma. *J Clin Endocrinol Metab* 1994;78:629.
160. Cooper DS, Specker B, Ho M, et al. Thyrotropin suppression and disease progression in patients with differentiated thyroid cancer: results from the National Thyroid Cancer Treatment Cooperative Registry. *Thyroid* 1998;8(9):737.
161. Dunn JT. Thyroglobulin: chemistry and biosynthesis. In: Braverman LE, Utiger RD, eds. *Werner and Ingbar's the thyroid: a fundamental and clinical text*, 6th ed. Philadelphia: JB Lippincott Co, 1991:98.
162. Pacini F, Lippi F, Formica N, et al. Therapeutic doses of iodine-131 reveal undiagnosed metastases in thyroid cancer patients with detectable serum thyroglobulin. *J Nucl Med* 1987;28:1888.
163. Dietlein M, Scheidhauer K, Voth E, Theissen P, Schicha H. Fluorine-18 fluorodeoxyglucose positron emission tomography and iodine-131 whole body scintigraphy in the follow-up of differentiated thyroid cancer. *Eur J Nucl Med* 1997;24(11):1342.
164. Wang W, Macapinlac H, Larson SM, et al. [18F]-2-fluoro-2-deoxy-D-glucose positron emission tomography localizes residual thyroid cancer in patients with negative diagnostic ^{131}I whole body scans and elevated serum thyroglobulin levels. *J Clin Endocrinol Metab* 1999;84(7):2291.
165. Conti PS, Durski JM, Bacqai F, Grafton ST, Singer PA. Imaging of locally recurrent and metastatic thyroid cancer with positron emission tomography. *Thyroid* 1999;9(8):797.
166. Seabold JE, Gurll N, Schurrer ME, Aktay R, Kirchner PT. Comparison of 99m Tc-methoxyisobutyl isonitrile and 201T1 scintigraphy for detection of residual thyroid cancer after 131I ablative therapy. *J Nucl Med* 1999;40(9):1434.
167. Spencer CA, Takeuchi M, Kazaroxyan M, et al. Serum thyroglobulin autoantibodies: prevalence, influence on serum thyroglobulin measurement, and prognostic significance in patients with differentiated thyroid carcinoma. *J Clin Endocrinol Metab* 1998;83:1121.
168. Ringel MD, Ladenson PW, Levine MA. Molecular diagnosis of residual and recurrent thyroid cancer by amplification of thyroglobulin mRNA in peripheral blood. *J Clin Endocrinol Metab* 1998;83:4435.
169. Pons F, Carpio I, Estorch M, et al. Lithium as an adjuvant of iodine-131 when treating patients with well-differentiated thyroid carcinoma. *Clin Nucl Med* 1987;8:644.
170. Koong SS, Reynolds JC, Movius EG, et al. Lithium as a potential adjuvant to ^{131}I therapy of metastatic, well differentiated thyroid carcinoma. *J Clin Endocrinol Metab* 1999;84(3):912.
171. Ladenson PW, Braverman LE, Mazzaferri EL, et al. Comparison of administration of recombinant human thyrotropin with withdrawal of thyroid hormone for radioactive iodine scanning in patients with thyroid carcinoma. *N Engl J Med* 1997;337(13):888.
172. Bohuslavizki KH, Brenner W, Klutmann S, et al. Radioprotection of salivary glands by amifostine in high-dose radioiodine therapy. *J Nucl Med* 1998;39(7):1237.
173. Pacini F, Gasperi M, Fugazzda L, et al. Testicular function in patients with differentiated thyroid carcinoma treated with radioiodine. *J Nucl Med* 1994;35:1418.
174. Dottorini ME, Lomuscio G, Mazzuchelli I, et al. Assessment of female fertility and carcinogenesis after 131-I therapy for differentiated thyroid carcinoma. *J Nucl Med* 1995;36:21.
175. Ayala C, Navarro E, Rodriguez JR, et al. Conception after iodine-131 therapy for differentiated thyroid cancer. *Thyroid* 1998;8(11):1009.
176. Van Nostrun D, Neutze J, Atkins F. Side effects of "rational dose" iodine-131 therapy for metastatic well-differentiated thyroid carcinoma. *J Nucl Med* 1986;27:1519.
177. Edmonds CJ, Smith T. The long-term hazards of the treatment of thyroid cancer with radioiodine. *Br J Radiol* 1986;59:45.
178. Ekman ET, Lundell G, Tennvall J, Wallin G. Chemotherapy and multimodality treatment in thyroid carcinoma. *Otolaryngol Clin North Am* 1990;23(3):523.
179. Tubiana M, Haddad E, Schlumberger M, et al. External radiotherapy in thyroid cancers. *Cancer* 1985;55:2062.
180. O'Connell MEA, A'Hern RP, Harmer CL. Results of external beam radiotherapy in differentiated thyroid carcinoma: a retrospective study from the Royal Marsden Hospital. *Eur J Cancer* 1994;30A:733.
181. Farahati J, Reiners C, Stuschke M, et al. Differentiated thyroid cancer. Impact of adjuvant external radiotherapy in patients with perithyroidal tumor infiltration (stage pT4). *Cancer* 1996;77(1):172.
182. Nel CJ, van Heerden JA, Goellner JR, et al. Anaplastic carcinoma of the thyroid: a clinicopathologic study of 82 cases. *Mayo Clin Proc* 1985;60:51.
183. Tan RK, Finley RK, Driscoll D, et al. Anaplastic carcinoma of the thyroid: a 24-year experience. *Head Neck* 1995;17:41.
184. Tennvall J, Lundell G, Hallquist A, et al., Swedish Anaplastic Thyroid Cancer Group. Combined doxorubicin, hyperfractionated radiotherapy, and surgery in anaplastic thyroid carcinoma. *Cancer* 1994;74:1348.
185. Demeter JG, DeJong SA, Lawrence AM, Paloyan E. Anaplastic thyroid carcinoma: risk factors and outcome. *Surgery* 1991;110:956.
186. Harada T, Ito K, Shimaoka K, Hosoda Y, Yakumaru K. Fatal thyroid carcinoma. Anaplastic transformation of adenocarcinoma. *Cancer* 1977;39:2588.
187. Mitchell G, Huddart R, Harmer C. Phase II evaluation of high dose accelerated radiotherapy for anaplastic thyroid carcinoma. *Radiother Oncol* 1999;50(1):33.
188. Kim JH, Leeper RD. Treatment of anaplastic giant and spindle cell carcinoma of the thyroid gland with combination Adriamycin and radiation therapy: a new approach. *Cancer* 1983;52:954.
189. Hundahl SA, Fleming ID, Fremgen AM, Menck HR. A National Cancer Database report on 53,856 cases of thyroid carcinoma treated in the U.S., 1985–1995. *Cancer* 1998;83(12):2638.
190. Hazard JB, Hawk WA, Crile G. Medullary (solid) carcinoma of the thyroid—a clinicopathologic entity. *J Clin Endocrinol Metab* 1959;19:152.
191. Brunt LM, Wells SA Jr. Advances in the diagnosis and treatment of medullary carcinoma. *Endocr Surg* 1987;67(2):263.
192. Williams ED. Histogenesis of medullary carcinoma of the thyroid. *J Clin Pathol* 1966;19:114.
193. Williams ED. Medullary carcinoma of the thyroid gland. *J Clin Pathol* 1967;20:395.
194. Wells SA Jr, Baylin SB, Linehan WM, et al. Provocative agents and the diagnosis of medullary carcinoma of the thyroid gland. *Ann Surg* 1978;188:139.
195. Komminoth P. The RET proto-oncogene in medullary and papillary thyroid carcinoma. Molecular features, pathophysiology and clinical implications. *Virchows Arch* 1997;431(1):1.
196. O'Riordain DS, O'Brien T, Weaver AL, et al. Medullary thyroid carcinoma in multiple endocrine neoplasia types 2A and 2B. *Surgery* 1994;116:1017.
197. Farndon JR, Leight GS, Dilley WG, et al. Familial medullary thyroid carcinoma without associated enodcrinopathies: a distinct clinical entity. *Br J Surg* 1986;73:278.
198. Albores-Saavedra J, LiVolsi VA, Williams ED. Medullary carcinoma. *Semin Diagn Pathol* 1985;2:102.
199. Franc B, Rosenberg-Bourgin M, Caillou B, et al. Medullary thyroid carcinoma: search for histological predictors of survival (109 proband cases analysis). *Hum Pathol* 1998;29(10):1078.
200. Wells SA Jr, Chi DD, Toshima K, et al. Predictive DNA testing and prophylactic thyroidectomy in patients at risk for multiple endocrine neoplasia type 2A. *Ann Surg* 1994;220:237.
201. Sone T, Fukunaga M, Otsuka N, et al. Metastatic medullary thyroid cancer: localization with iodine-131 Metaiodobenzylguanidine. *J Nucl Med* 1985;26:604.
202. Thomas CC, Cowan RJ, Albertson DA, Cooper MR. Detection of medullary carcinoma of the thyroid with I-131 MIBG. *Clin Nucl Med* 1994;19(12):1066.
203. Edington HD, Watson CG, Levine G, et al. Radioimmunoimaging of metastatic medullary carcinoma of the thyroid gland using an indium-11-labeled monoclonal antibody to CEA. *Surgery* 1988;104:1004.
204. Frank-Raue K, Bihl H, Dorrt U, et al. Somatostatin receptor imaging in persistent medullary thyroid carcinoma. *Clin Endocrinol* 1995;42:31.
205. Krausz Y, Rosier A, Guttmann H, et al. Somatostatin receptor scintigraphy for early detection of regional and distant metastases of medullary carcinoma of the thyroid. *Clin Nucl Med* 1999;24(4):256.
206. Moley JF, Debenedetti MK, Dilley WG, Tisell LE, Wells SA. Surgical management of patients with persistent or recurrent medullary thyroid cancer. *J Intern Med* 1998;243(6):521.
207. Evans DB, Fleming JB, Lee JE, Cote G, Gagel RE. The surgical treatment of medullary thyroid carcinoma. *Semin Surg Oncol* 1999;16(1):50.
208. Duh QY, Sancho JJ, Greenspan FS, et al. Medullary thyroid carcinoma. The need for early diagnosis and total thyroidectomy. *Arch Surg* 1989;124:1206.
209. Pelizzo MR, Bernante P, Piotto A, et al. The extent of surgery for thyroid medullary cancer. *Tumori* 1994;80:427.
210. Modigliani E, Cohen R, Campos JM, et al. Prognostic factors for survival and for biochemical cure in medullary thyroid carcinoma: results in 899 patients. The GETC Study Group. *Clin Endocrinol* 1998;48(3):265.
211. Chi DD, Moley JF. Medullary thyroid carcinoma: genetic advances, treatment recommendations, and the approach to the patient with persistent hypercalcitoninemia. *Surg Oncol Clin North Am* 1998;7(4):681.
212. McHenry CR, Oppenheim DS, Murphy T, et al. Familial nonmultiple endocrine neoplasia medullary thyroid carcinoma: an evolving clinical entity. *Surgery* 1992;112:729.
213. Block MA, Jackson CE, Tashjian AH Jr. Management of occult medullary thyroid carcinoma. *Arch Surg* 1978;113:368.
214. Tisell LE, Hansson G, Jansson S, Salander H. Reoperation in the treatment of asymptomatic metastasizing medullary thyroid carcinoma. *Surgery* 1986;99(1):60.
215. van Heerden JA, Grant CS, Gharib H, Hay ID, Ilstrup DM. Long-term course of patients with persistent hypercalcitoninemia after apparent curative primary surgery for medullary thyroid carcinoma. *Ann Surg* 1990;212(4):395.
216. Chen H, Roberts JR, Ball DW, et al. Effective long-term palliation of symptomatic, incurable metastatic medullary thyroid cancer by operative resection. *Ann Surg* 1998;227(6):887.
217. Nguyen TD, Chassard JL, Lagarde P, et al. Results of postoperative radiation therapy in medullary carcinoma of the thyroid: a retrospective study by the French Federation of Cancer Institutes—the Radiotherapy Cooperative Group. *Radiother Oncol* 1992;23:1.
218. Schlumberger M, Abdelmoumene N, Delisle NJ, Couette JE, Groupe d'Etude des Tumeurs a Calcitonine (GETC). Treatment of advanced medullary thyroid cancer with an alternating combination of 5 FU-streptozocin and f FU-dacarbazine. *Br J Cancer* 1995;71:363.
219. Orlandi F, Caraci P, Berruti A, et al. Chemotherapy with dacarbazine and 5-fluorouracil in advanced medullary thyroid cancer. *Ann Oncol* 1994;5:763.
220. Zhang R, Straus FH, DeGroot LJ. Effective genetic therapy of established medullary thyroid carcinomas with murine interleukin-2: dissemination and cytotoxicity studies in a rat tumor model. *Endocrinology* 1999;140(5):2152.
221. Soler MN, Milhaud G, Lekmine F, et al. Treatment of medullary thyroid carcinoma by combined expression of suicide and interleukin-2 genes. *Cancer Immunol Immunother* 1999;48(2–3):91.
222. Kebebew E, Tresler PA, Siperstein AE, Duh QY, Clark OH. Normal thyroid pathology in patients undergoing thyroidectomy for finding a RET gene germline mutation: a report of three cases and review of the literature. *Thyroid* 1999;9(2):127.

223. Freyer G, Dazord A, Schlumberger M, et al. Psychosocial impact of genetic testing in familial medullary-thyroid carcinoma: a multicentric pilot evaluation. *Ann Oncol* 1999;10(1):87.
224. Friedberg MH, Coburn MC, Monchik JM. Role of surgery in stage IE non-Hodgkin's lymphoma of the thyroid. *Surgery* 1994;116:1061.
225. Hamburger JI, Miller JM, Kini SR. Lymphoma of the thyroid. *Ann Intern Med* 1983;99:685.
226. Skarsgard ED, Connors JM, Robins RE. A current analysis of primary lymphoma of the thyroid. *Arch Surg* 1991;126:1199.
227. Rosen IB, Sutcliffe SB, Gospodarowicz MK, Chua T, Simpson WJ. The role of surgery in the management of thyroid lymphoma. *Surgery* 1988;104:1095.
228. Devine RM, Edis AJ, Banks PM. Primary lymphoma of the thyroid: a review of the Mayo Clinic experience through 1978. *World J Surg* 1981;5:33.
229. Haugen BRE, Nawaz S, Cohn A, et al. Secondary malignancy of the thyroid gland: a case report and review of the literature. *Thyroid* 1994;4(3):297.
230. Rosen IB, Walfish PG, Bain J, Bedard YC. Secondary malignancy of the thyroid gland and its management. *Ann Surg* Oncol 1995;2(3):252.
231. Kossev P, LiVolsi VA. Lymphoid lesions of the thyroid: review in light of the Revised European-American Lymphoma Classification and upcoming World Health Organization Classification. *Thyroid* 1999;9:1273.

***SECTION* 3**

DOUGLAS L. FRAKER

Parathyroid Tumors

Parathyroid neoplasia is a common endocrine problem, whereas parathyroid carcinoma is exceptionally rare.[1] Parathyroid carcinomas, as opposed to other endocrine tumors that become less hormonally active when malignant, are hyperfunctional and characterized by severe elevations of serum calcium with associated renal and bone symptoms.[2] The clinical course is variable, but typically follows a pattern of local recurrence in the neck with late distant metastases to lung, bone, and liver.

The initial report of a parathyroid carcinoma was made by de Quervain in 1909.[3] He described a patient with a large locally invasive neck mass that was parathyroid on histologic evaluation. The tumor was definitely malignant as the patient developed lung metastases after removal of the neck mass, but no signs or symptoms of hypercalcemia were described. The initial description of severe hypercalcemia associated with parathyroid cancer was made three decades later by Armstrong.[4] The rarity of parathyroid carcinoma limits reports to primarily small institutional series with occasional reviews of all experience reported in the medical literature. Even institutions such as the Massachusetts General Hospital[5] or the Mayo Clinic[3] with extensive clinical interest in this disease have only one to two dozen cases in clinical reviews spanning four to five decades. A detailed review by Obara and Fujimoto[2] identified 270 cases of parathyroid carcinoma in the English literature between 1933 and 1991. An article from the National Cancer Database in the United States identified 286 cases of parathyroid cancer reported between 1985 and 1995.[6] This single report more than doubles the number of cases in the literature for this rare disease. The epidemiology, pathology, clinical course, treatment, and prognosis of this rare malignancy is described in relation to the much more common diagnoses of parathyroid adenoma and hyperplasia.

PRIMARY HYPERPARATHYROIDISM

The vast majority of parathyroid cancers are functional with excess production of parathyroid hormone (PTH) which results in the clinical syndrome of primary hyperparathyroidism (HPT). The pathology of HPT can be grouped into three general categories: a single parathyroid adenoma (83% to 85% of cases), multiglandular hyperplasia (15%), and parathyroid cancer (0.5% to 3.0%).[7] The proportion of HPT patients who truly have parathyroid cancer is likely to be well under the 2% of cases more recently quoted.[2] The epidemiologic and pathologic characteristics of these three general categories of HPT are shown in Table 38.3-1.

PATHOLOGY

Schantz and Castleman defined the pathologic criteria used to distinguish parathyroid carcinoma from benign parathyroid adenoma in a classic article in 1973.[8] Thick fibrous bands, pleomorphic cells in a trabecular pattern, and a high incidence of mitotic figures are the chief distinguishing features[8,9] (Fig. 38.3-1 and see Table 38.3-1). Invasion of the glandular capsule and vascular invasion are also found with parathyroid carcinoma. However, as with other endocrine neoplasms, the diagnosis of parathyroid carcinoma strictly is difficult on histologic evaluation using the criteria outlined previously.[10] There is a spectrum of these changes present in benign adenomas, atypical adenomas, and true carcinomas.[11] Even histologic evidence of capsular or vascular invasion is not pathognomonic for parathyroid cancer as spontaneous hemorrhage in large benign parathyroid adenomas may result in a similar histologic appearance.[12]

In addition to the histologic criteria, both the clinical course and the gross pathology observed at operation help to define a lesion as parathyroid cancer.[12] The typical clinical presentation is discussed in greater detail here, but parathyroid carcinoma tends to have a higher serum calcium level, more marked symptoms of HPT, and larger lesions that may be palpable in the neck. The operating surgeon finds a large lesion that is more firm than typical adenomas.[10] The color of parathyroid carcinoma is frequently gray-brown versus the red-brown of benign lesions, reflecting the increased fibrous stroma within these tumors.[10] Most important, parathyroid carcinoma may locally invade into adjacent structures such as the ipsilateral thyroid gland or overlying strap muscles of the neck. This gross pathologic feature is infrequently seen with benign lesions.[8–10]

In the past decade, several groups have used flow cytometry to analyze DNA content in parathyroid carcinomas compared with adenomas. In three series, a consistent proportion between 31% and 56% of parathyroid carcinomas were documented to be aneuploid.[13–15] The DNA content of parathyroid adenomas is not as consistent, with one group reporting no aneuploidy in 32 patients[13] and other groups reporting propor-

TABLE 38.3-1. Comparison of the Various Causes of Primary Hyperparathyroidism

Cause	*Frequency*	*Etiologic Factors*	*Gender*	*Pathology*		
				Age (y)	*Gross*	*Microscopic*
Adenoma	83–85%	Radiation exposure	F>M 2–3:1	55–61	Single enlarged soft red-brown gland	Nests of parathyroid chief cells; decreased cytoplasmic fat; possible rim at normal tissue
Hyperplasia	15%	Familial in multiple endocrine neoplasia 1 and 2	M=F	25–40	Asymmetric enlargement with red-brown color of 4+ glands	Similar to adenomas; minimal intercellular fat
Carcinoma	<1%	Familial? Radiation exposure?	M=F	45–50	Single large firm white/gray mass frequently invading thyroid or strap muscle	Trabecular arrangement of tumor cells divided by fibrous bands; mitotic figures present; possible capsular, vascular or adjacent structure invasion

tions in the range of one-third aneuploid similar to parathyroid carcinoma.[2] A second piece of information that these studies report is that aneuploidy is a prognostic indicator for parathyroid carcinoma. August reported that four out of five patients with aneuploid parathyroid carcinoma died of disease with the fifth alive with extensive recurrence, while four of four patients with diploid parathyroid carcinoma were cured with no evidence of recurrence after parathyroid surgery.[15]

EPIDEMIOLOGY

The incidence of parathyroid cancer is most commonly reported in the context of primary HPT. Most endocrine surgeons report 0.5% to 4.0% of all HPT as being parathyroid carcinoma (Table 38.3-2). Because the estimate of the annual incidence of primary HPT is reported to be 1 per 2000,[1] then if 1% of HPT is parathyroid cancer, the incidence of this malignancy would be approximately 0.5 per 100,000 persons. This incidence is clearly an overestimation as it would place the annual number of parathyroid cancers in the United States more than 1000 new cases, which greatly exceeds the actual number. Several tertiary institutions have reported their total experience with parathyroid carcinoma over several decades in the setting of more than 1000 cases of primary HPT. The Mayo Clinic,[3] the Cleveland Clinic,[16] and the University of Michigan[17] reported an overall proportion of parathyroid cancer in HPT of 0.6%, 0.47%, and 0.37% (see Table 38.3-2). However, even these numbers may be overestimates as these tertiary institutions are more likely to be referred these patients with this rare diagnosis. A review from a tertiary referral center in Padua, Italy, reported 5.2% of all patients operated on for HPT between 1980 and 1996 were parathyroid cancers.[18] This unusually high proportion does not appear to be an overestimation due to inaccurate pathology as 13 of 16 had metastases and two had multiple local recurrences. Thompson at the University of Michigan reported an incidence of two parathyroid carcinomas in 1450 initial parathyroid operations for HPT over the past two decades at the University of Michigan for a percentage of 0.14%.[17] The National Cancer Database reported 286 cases of parathyroid cancer in a 10-year period. This group believed that it captured 60% to 80% of all cancers in the United States during that time interval. If that estimate is correct, then there are only 36 to 48 cases of parathyroid cancer annually in the United States. With an incidence of 0.015 per 100,000 population, parathyroid cancer is one of the most rare of all human cancers. Because of this low incidence, there is no American Joint Committee on Cancer Staging system for parathyroid cancer.[6]

The gender distribution is equal or has a slight female preponderance in most series and differs from benign parathyroid adenomas, which have a higher female predominance[2,6,7,9] (see Table 38.3-2). The age at diagnosis can vary between 19 and 81 and the median age in most series is between 45 and 51 years. The large National Cancer Database series had essentially an equivalent gender distribution (51% male and 49% female subjects) and a mean and median age of 54.5 and 55.1 years, respectively. There was also no disproportional incidence by race in this report with 76.2% non-Hispanic white, 12.2% black, 7.3% Hispanic, and 4.2% others.[6] There are no documented etiologic causes for this malignancy, although there is a familial association in a few series. Parathyroid cancer has been reported and documented in members of multiple endocrine neoplasia 1 kindreds.[19] In this autosomal dominant disease, the predominant endocrine abnormality is multiglandular benign hyperplasia of the parathyroids. Familial non–multiple endocrine neoplasia 1 associated parathyroid cancer has been reported in siblings[20] and in one report, several relatives across two generations had parathyroid carcinoma.[21] This study also reported other relatives with primary HPT who had atypical adenomas, implying a connection between this benign pathologic entity and true parathyroid carcinoma. External radiation exposure has been correlated with parathyroid neoplasms, but virtually all reports describe an association between radiation and the more common parathyroid adenoma, although there are isolated case reports of patients with parathyroid carcinoma who had a history of radiation treatments in the distant past.[22] Patients with renal failure typically experience secondary HPT with nonclonal hyperplasia of all parathyroid glands, but 13 cases of parathyroid cancer have been reported in the literature in this clinical setting.[23]

CLINICAL PRESENTATION

Because virtually all parathyroid carcinomas are functional, meaning they produce high and unregulated levels of PTH, the signs and symptoms of this disease relate primarily to the consequences of this hormone excess. Specifically, various manifestations of renal disease associated with hypercalcemia and hypercalciuria such as renal stones, renal colic, nephrocalcinosis,

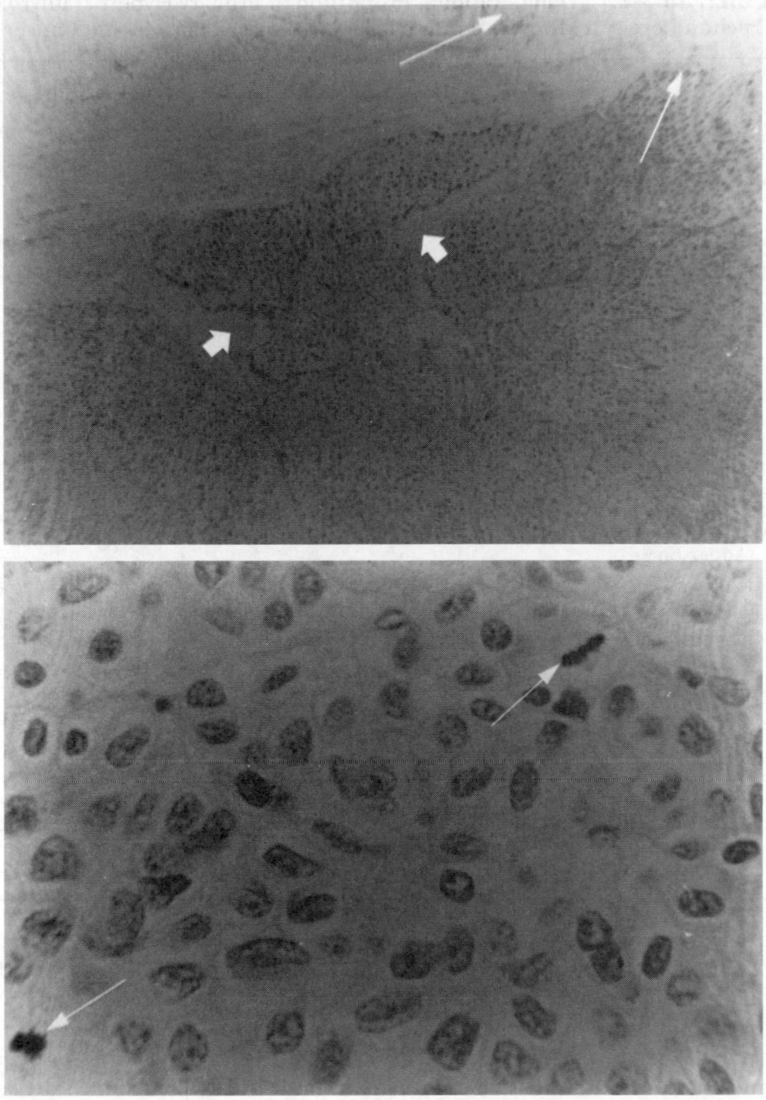

FIGURE 38.3-1. Pathologic characteristics that are used to define a lesion as a parathyroid carcinoma are shown in these two panels. **A:** A low-power view demonstrates dense fibrous bands with the cells arranged in a trabecular pattern (*arrowheads*) and evidence of capsular invasion (*arrows*). **B:** A high-power view documents a high number of mitotic figures (*arrows*) in one single field of view.

renal insufficiency, or all of these manifestations occur in up to 90% of cases[24,25] (Table 38.3-3). Also, the prevalence of bone disease related to calcium absorption with osteoporosis and bone pain is much greater in parathyroid carcinoma than in patients with parathyroid adenoma,[26,27] with up to 70% of patients manifesting the symptoms. In nonmalignant parathyroid disease, it is unusual to have both renal and bone symptomatology documented at the time of diagnosis.[28] However, these symptoms are present simultaneously at diagnosis in up to 50% of patients with parathyroid carcinoma (see Table 38.3-3).

These amplified symptoms reflect the increased magnitude of the biochemical disturbances seen with parathyroid carcinoma. The level of total serum calcium is significantly elevated in virtually all series of parathyroid carcinoma, with the mean values between 15 and 16 mg/dL compared with 11 to 12 mg/dL seen with parathyroid adenomas[2,25] (see Table 38.3-3). Similarly, the PTH level in parathyroid carcinoma is consistently higher than for benign parathyroid disease, with more than 70% of patients having a greater than fivefold increase over the upper limits of normal for PTH.[2,29] Because of the high degree of hypercalcemia, it is unusual for patients to be asymptomatic at presentation with parathyroid carcinoma compared with patients with benign causes of HPT who are asymptomatic in more than 50% of cases in some series.[26,27] Up to 14% of patients with parathyroid carcinoma may present with hypercalcemic crisis manifested by a depressed level of consciousness, dehydration, and extreme hypercalcemia.[5] The size of the typical parathyroid carcinoma is much larger than benign lesions. The median maximal diameter in most series is between 3.0 and 3.5 cm compared with approximately 1.5 cm for benign adenomas[8,9] (see Table 38.3-2). This large mass translates into a significant number of patients who present with a palpable neck mass ranging between 22% and 50% of cases.[9,24,25] Again, it is extremely unusual for patients with benign lesions to have palpable abnormalities in the neck, and this is a clinical sign that strongly suggests parathyroid carcinoma. In 10% of cases, patients with parathyroid carcinoma present with symptoms of hoarseness caused by compression or invasion of recurrent laryngeal nerve and vocal cord paresis.[2]

NATURAL HISTORY

The best information regarding the natural history of parathyroid carcinoma comes from a detailed review of 163 cases

TABLE 38.3-2. Demographics, Proportion of Primary Hyperparathyroidism That Is Parathyroid Cancer, Tumor Size, and Calcium Levels in More Recent Institutional Series of Parathyroid Cancer

Institution	*Years*	*Total Cases* No. of Cases	Total Primary Hyperparathyroidism	*Percentage of Cancer*	*M:F*	*Age Mean/ Range*	*Tumor Size (cm)*	*Serum Weight (g)*	*Ca (mg/dL)*
Mayo Clinic[3]	1928–77	12	2013	0.6	4:8	51, 29–72	—	6.8	14.5
Cleveland Clinic[16]	1938–88	6	1200	0.47	4:3	47, 20–61	—	—	15.3
Lahey Clinic[30]	1942–84	9	301	3.0	3:6	48, 19–64	3.5	—	14.0
Massachusetts General Hospital[5]	1948–83	28	1200	2.3	14:14	45, 28–72	3.0	6.7	13.7
Memorial Sloan-Kettering Cancer Center[28]	1955–91	14	—	—	7:7	48, 27–81	3.3	12.0	14.8
Rochester[49]	1958–90	11	197	5.6	1:10	54, —	—	—	15.2
Emory[38]	1960–82	3	360	0.8	2:1	57, 43–69	2.9	—	16.1
M. D. Anderson[29]	1968–82	14	—	—	7:7	—, 27–61	—	—	16.8
Michigan (total)[17]	1973–90	5	1650	0.37	2:3	46, 35–61	—	—	17.5
Michigan (initial)[17,a]	1973–90	2	1450	0.14					
National Cancer Database[6]	1985–95	286	—	—	1:1	54, 14–88	3/3	—	—
Brazil[36]	1970–95	10	—	—	2:1	51, 27–74	—	—	14.3
Italy[18]	1980–96	16	290	5.2	2:1	60, 30–78	2.9	—	13.5

Ca, calcium.
[a]University of Michigan data reported as total experience and subgroup who underwent initial operation at this institution.

reported between 1981 and 1989[2] (summarized in Table 38.3-4). At initial presentation, few patients with parathyroid carcinoma have metastases either to regional lymph nodes (less than 5%) or distant sites (less than 2%). In the National Cancer Database series of 286 patients, only 16 (5.6%) had lymph node metastases noted at the time of initial surgery.[6] This report did not comment on the incidence of distant metastases and has a relatively short follow-up interval. A higher proportion of parathyroid carcinomas are locally invasive into the thyroid gland, overlying strap muscles, recurrent laryngeal nerve, trachea, or esophagus. Some patients are not identified preoperatively or

TABLE 38.3-3. Comparison of the Incidence of Signs and Symptoms at Presentation in Patients with Parathyroid Carcinoma versus Parathyroid Adenoma

	Adenoma	*Carcinoma (Median Percentage, Range)*
Renal	18%	60% (27–90%)
Skeletal	13–20%	55% (19–64%)
Renal and skeletal	<5%	32% (0–50%)
Peptic ulcer disease	3–13%	18% (0–22%)
Palpable neck mass	<2%	38% (22–48%)
Parathyroid crisis	<2%	14% (0–27%)
Asymptomatic	38–61%	3% (0–27%)
Serum calcium (mg/dL)	11–12	14–16

(Data from refs. 1–3, 5, 8, 9, 24–27, 43, 48, and 50.)

intraoperatively as having parathyroid carcinoma and undergo parathyroid procedures as if to treat parathyroid adenoma. Only after review of the pathology following this resection, or when these patients have either local recurrences or metastases is a correct diagnosis of parathyroid carcinoma made. The incidence of not recognizing parathyroid carcinomas at initial operation ranges between 11% from the Lahey Clinic series (one in nine),[30] to 36% in the M. D. Anderson series (5 of 14),[29] and up to 86% in the Cleveland Clinic series (six of seven).[16]

After surgical treatment, 40% to 60% of patients have recurrent disease at some point typically in the range of 2 to 5 years after the initial resection.[29,31] Since parathyroid carcinomas are functional, serial measurements of calcium or PTH serve as ideal tumor markers for this malignancy. In patients followed closely, hypercalcemia precedes physical evidence of recurrent disease in most cases. The most common location of recurrence is regionally either in the tissues of the neck or in cervical lymph nodes, accounting for two-thirds of the recurrent cases.[2] Often the local recurrences in the neck are difficult to identify as they may be small, multifocal, and involve the scar from the previous procedure. Use of ultrasound, sestamibi-thallium scanning,[32,33] and more recently positron emission tomographic scanning,[34] may aid in this difficult diagnosis. Distant metastases occur in 25% of patients, primarily in the lungs but also in the bone and liver[2,35] (see Table 38.3-4). More recently published series have reported a higher incidence of recurrence than prior studies. In nine patients from Brazil with parathyroid cancer with long-term follow-up, five had local or nodal neck recurrence (55%), three had lung metastases

TABLE 38.3-4. Clinicopathologic Features, Natural History, and Outcome in Patients with Parathyroid Carcinoma

At initial presentation[a]	
Local invasion	23%
Thyroid	15%
Recurrent laryngeal nerve	3.7%
Other (muscle, trachea, esophagus)	4.9%
Lymph node metastases	4.3%
Distant metastases	1.8%
Recurrence after initial resection[a]	
Local recurrence	36%
Lymph node recurrence	17%
Cervical	14%
Mediastinal	6.1%
Distant metastases	25%
Lung	15%
Bone	6%
Liver	4%
Outcome after surgical treatment[b]	
Alive	66%
No evidence of disease	42%
Mean follow-up	4.6 y
Alive with disease	24%
Mean follow-up	7 y
Dead	34%
Caused by parathyroid carcinoma	30%
Caused by unrelated causes	4%

[a]Based on 163 patients.[2]
[b]Based on 108 patients.[2]

(33%), and one had bone metastasis (11%).[36] In a study of 16 patients from Italy, 13 had distant metastases (nine lung alone, four lung plus bone) and 2 others had local neck recurrences.[8] The reasons for this high incidence of recurrence between 94% and 100% may be due to more accurate pathologic diagnosis excluding patients with atypical adenomas.

Patients who experience parathyroid carcinoma typically die of metabolic consequences and not directly from malignant growth.[35] For this reason, surgical treatment to debulk parathyroid carcinoma, if possible, is indicated as medical management of the hypercalcemia of parathyroid carcinoma is difficult (see Treatment, later in this chapter). The median survival after recurrent parathyroid cancer ranges between 3 and 5 years, with isolated case reports of patients surviving several decades with intermittent surgical debulking.[31]

DIFFERENTIAL DIAGNOSIS

Other non-HPT causes of hypercalcemia can be ruled out primarily by the biochemical studies of serum PTH simultaneous with total and ionized serum calcium. Secondary HPT in the setting of renal failure is clinically obvious by the concomitant renal disease. There are isolated reports of development of parathyroid carcinoma in this clinical setting as well, however.[37] Once the diagnosis of primary HPT is established, the histopathologic diagnosis of parathyroid carcinoma may be difficult as discussed previously.[10,12] Supporting evidence of malignancy comes from markedly elevated calcium levels (greater than 14.0 mg/dL) and larger gland sizes (greater than 3.0 cm). In most reported institutional series, it is likely that parathyroid carcinoma is overdiagnosed.[17,38] In one such study, a careful review of the pathology in the context of the clinical course identified more than one-half of the patients with previously diagnosed parathyroid carcinomas as more appropriately considered as benign or atypical adenomas.[38] This difficulty in correctly identifying parathyroid carcinoma is also reflected by the wide variation in clinical outcome between different series. Some series report long-term disease-free survival at rates greater than 75%. One explanation for series in which outcomes are much better than the norm is that they include in their analysis patients with atypical parathyroid adenomas that were not truly malignant.[17] Other investigators take an opposite approach and include only cases in their institutional reviews that recur locally or manifest distant metastases.[28] This approach may underestimate the true incidence of cases of parathyroid carcinoma because there is a subgroup with this disease that may be cured with an aggressive initial resection.

Local recurrence of parathyroid neoplasms after initial resection does not necessarily establish the diagnosis of parathyroid carcinoma. Two patterns of benign lesions that recur locally have been described. First, patients with a single parathyroid adenoma may have partial or incomplete resection of a gland such that there is an isolated regrowth after the initial procedure in the exact position where the first abnormal gland was removed.[39] The recurrent gland grows in an area of fibrosis and scar, and may well give the gross appearance of an invasive carcinoma, but detailed pathologic analysis of the initial or recurrent specimen shows no evidence of carcinoma in terms of mitotic figures, cellular appearance, or fibrous bands. A second category of nonmalignant recurrent disease is a condition called parathyromatosis.[37,40] Parathyromatosis is a diffuse seeding of the cervical tissue with parathyroid cells that implant and grow. This occurs when lesions that are being excised have the capsule ruptured and are spilled or when lesions are partially removed with a raw surface of the adenoma exposed to the field of dissection. This condition is much more difficult to treat than isolated local recurrence and is tantamount to a nonmetastasizing locally recurrent carcinoma, and this condition has been described with lesions that have absolutely no pathologic or clinical manifestations of parathyroid carcinoma.

TREATMENT

The only effective treatment of parathyroid cancer is surgical resection. The most important component to achieve a favorable outcome is recognition by the operating surgeon that a lesion is likely to be a parathyroid cancer, which allows performance of the appropriate *en bloc* resection of the tumor with all potential areas of invasion at the initial operation (Fig. 38.3-2).[30,31] Patients with extremely high serum calcium levels (greater than 13.5 mg/dL) should lead the physician to suspect parathyroid cancer preoperatively. Other clinical features that suggest parathyroid cancer are a palpable mass and hoarseness. Intraoperatively, if a large lesion is identified, particularly if it is firm or scirrhous, then the operating surgeon should assume the lesion is parathyroid cancer and do an *en bloc* resection. The practice of minimally invasive parathyroidectomy, which is appropriate in the vast majority of patients with HPT, should be altered in these clinical situations.[41] Parathyroid cancer typically invades the ipsilateral thyroid lobe, and resection of the tumor

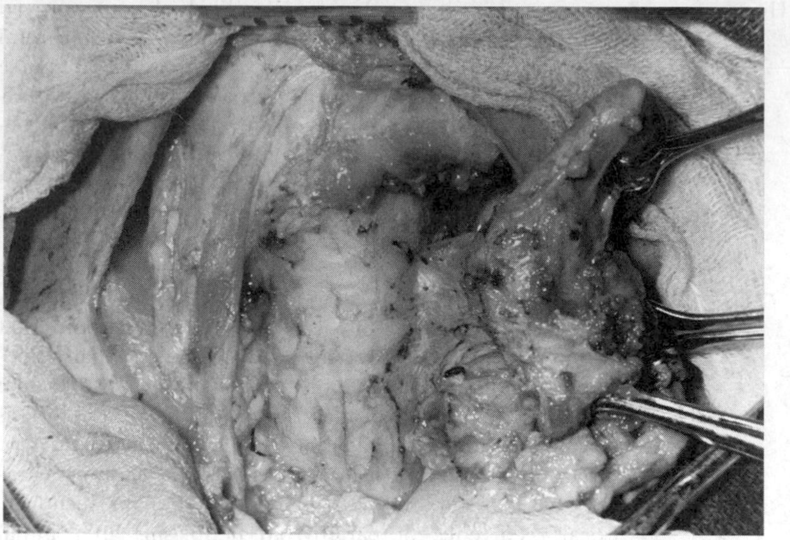

FIGURE 38.3-2. *En bloc* resection of an isolated recurrence of a parathyroid carcinoma as shown after a partial dissection. The parathyroid cancer is resected together with overlying strap muscles and the left lobe of the thyroid gland. This *en bloc* specimen is being retracted laterally in the clamps. The midline structure is the trachea that is completely cleared of surrounding tissues. This patient is alive and well with no evidence of recurrent disease or recurrent hypercalcemia 3 years after this resection for an isolated local recurrence.

with one or both thyroid lobes is frequently required to perform an adequate operation.[30] In most series, long-term results in terms of local recurrence are significantly improved when an *en bloc* excision including thyroid is done as opposed to cases in which only the parathyroid cancer is removed.[30,31] The recognition and diagnosis of parathyroid cancer preoperatively correlates strongly with a favorable outcome. In a small series of seven patients from the Cleveland Clinic, six had parathyroid carcinomas that were not appreciated until after the procedure.[16] All of these patients had recurrences, whereas the one case that was known to be a parathyroid cancer preoperatively underwent an *en bloc* resection with long-term disease-free survival. The recurrent laryngeal nerve may be intimately involved or invaded by the parathyroid cancer. In these situations, patients frequently have preoperative hoarseness due to the tumor invasion of the nerve.[2] Because the nerve is at risk for loss of function due to the malignant process itself, it is appropriate to resect the recurrent laryngeal nerve if necessary to perform an *en bloc* excision during the initial procedure for parathyroid cancer. The increased potential for long-term local control achieved by this approach outweighs the complication of postoperative vocal cord paralysis, which can be improved with techniques such as Teflon injection into the paralyzed cord. Assessment of cervical lymph nodes, particularly level 6 paratracheal nodes and levels 3 and 4 internal jugular nodes, should be performed with node dissection only for enlarged or firm lesions.

For most cases of recurrent parathyroid carcinoma confined to the neck, the most appropriate treatment is aggressive reresection. However, as opposed to the initial procedure in which the success rate is up to 40% to 60%, it is unusual to obtain long-term cures in patients who have to undergo reresection.[5] In a large series from the Mayo Clinic, no patients who underwent reresection were cured.[3] However, there are selective patients described in the literature who have disease-free intervals greater than 10 years after two or three local resections in the neck.[11,17] The benefit of sacrificing the recurrent laryngeal nerve is greatly decreased in patients undergoing reresection for recurrent parathyroid cancer as most recurrences are multifocal. If a recurrent nodule involves the recurrent laryngeal nerve, there are most likely other areas of parathyroid cancer that are adherent to the trachea, esophagus, and great vessels of the neck. Since it is impossible to remove all of these vital structures, one is unlikely to obtain a cure by taking the nerve. However, in certain circumstances in which there is an isolated local recurrence that is involving the nerve, it again should be sacrificed with an *en bloc* resection as those patients' conditions, in rare instances, may be salvaged by an aggressive surgical procedure (see Fig. 38.3-2).

Nonsurgical forms of therapy for parathyroid carcinoma have generally poor results such that surgical treatment of distant metastases is appropriate in certain situations. Pulmonary metastases as well as bone metastases should be resected, if possible, primarily to debulk tumor to decrease the magnitude of the hypercalcemia.[42,43] However, occasionally long-term salvage is achieved in this group of patients with aggressive surgical treatment.

Radiation therapy, in general, does not result in meaningful antitumor responses.[44] Isolated case reports of long-term control exist, and radiation therapy should be used in patients with unresectable recurrent cervical disease.[11] Various chemotherapeutic agents alone or in combination have been used for treatment of parathyroid carcinoma with limited success.[44] Dacarbazine alone or in combination with 5-fluorouracil and cyclophosphamide have been reported to result in objective responses, including one complete response in a patient with pulmonary metastases.[44,45] Other combination therapies have resulted in rare responses. Part of the problem with the medical treatment of parathyroid carcinoma is that the rarity of this disease does not allow systematic evaluation of various combination therapies.

The second aspect of medical management for metastatic parathyroid carcinoma relates to the treatment of the hypercalcemia.[40] Acute therapy of patients with hypercalcemic crises or high serum calcium levels is similar to that used for other causes of symptomatic hypercalcemia. Volume loading with loop diuretics causing a forced diuresis is the initial therapy. For patients with parathyroid carcinoma, the ultimate management of the hypercalcemia is directed at the tumor to decrease the level of PTH, if possible, by surgical treatment. In situations in which surgical resections are no longer possible, the treatment of hypercalcemia is difficult, and this metabolic abnormality is the primary cause of death for the majority of these patients.[26,27,31] The most effective

TABLE 38.3-5. Five- and 10-Year Survival after Surgical Excision of Parathyroid Cancer

Institution	*Time Interval*	*No.*	*5-Y Survival (%)*	*10-Y Survival (%)*
Mayo Clinic[22]	1920–91	43	69	55
National Cancer Institute [42,a]	1933–68	46	50	13
Cleveland Clinic[15]	1938–88	7	85	57
Massachusetts General Hospital, total[5,b]	1948–83	25	80	78
Massachusetts General Hospital, recurrent[5,b]	1948–83	9	44	22
Memorial Sloan-Kettering Cancer Center[25]	1955–91	14	55	55
Columbia[21,a]	1968–81	62	50	35
M. D. Anderson[26]	1968–82	14	36	18
Karolinska, Stockholm[31,a]	1968–90	40	50	35
National Cancer Database[6]	1985–95	286	55.5	49.1
Italy[18]	1980–96	10	20	20
Total		251	57	39

[a]Series that are collective reviews from several institutions.
[b]Massachusetts General Hospital reported survival rates separately for all patients and for the subgroup that had recurrent disease.

agents in this setting are the bisphosphonates that inhibit osteoclast bone resorption.[44,46] Two agents available in the United States are etidronate and pamidronate. Other agents used in other settings of hypercalcemia such as plicamycin (formerly mithramycin) and calcitonin have limited benefit.[44] Gallium nitrate has also been used as an inhibitor of bone reabsorption, but is limited by nephrotoxicity.[17,47] All agents used to date in the setting of high tumor burden from parathyroid carcinoma have a limitation that the patients become refractory after initial treatment. Newer generations of more potent bisphosphonates may hold some promise for symptomatic management of this group of patients.[44]

OUTCOME

The ability to achieve long-term survival in patients with parathyroid carcinoma ranges between 18% and 78% in various series.[2,5,24,25,48] The 5- and 10-year overall survival rates for patients with resected parathyroid carcinoma are shown in Table 38.3-5. A summary of 251 patients analyzed shows a 5-year survival of 57% and a 10-year survival of 39%. The National Cancer Database reported a 5-year survival at 55.5% and a 10-year survival of 49.1% in 286 patients treated.[6] These two large series accounted for the majority of cases of parathyroid cancer in the literature and provides an accurate assessment of outcome. The majority of patients who have recurrences after initial surgery ultimately succumb to this disease because there is a much lower rate of salvage after second or third procedures. For patients with local recurrences or distant metastases, only between 0% and 15% have long-term cures after secondary resections as there is no meaningful nonsurgical therapy.

REFERENCES

1. Heath H 3rd, Hodgson SF, Kennedy MA. Primary hyperparathyroidism: incidence, morbidity, and potential economic impact in a community. *N Engl J Med* 1980;302:189.
2. Obara T, Fujimoto Y. Diagnosis and treatment of patietns with parathyroid carcinoma: an update and review. *World J Surg* 1991;15:738.
3. van Heerden JA, Weiland LH, ReMine WH, et al. Cancer of the parathyroid glands. *Arch Surg* 1979;114:475.
4. Armstrong HG. Primary carcinoma of the parathyroid gland with report of a case. *Bull Acad Med* 1938;11:105.
5. Wang C, Gaz RD. Natural history of parathyroid carcinoma: diagnosis, treatment and results. *Am J Surg* 1985;149:522.
6. Hundahl SA, Fleming ID, Fremgen AM, et al. Two hundred eighty-six cases of parathyroid carcinoma treated in the U.S. between 1985–1995. A National Cancer Database Report. *Cancer* 1999;86:538.
7. Rossi RL, ReMine SG, Clerkin EP. Hyperparathyroidism. *Surg Clin North Am* 1985;65:187.
8. Schantz A, Castleman B. Parathyroid carcinoma: a study of 70 cases. *Cancer* 1973;31:600.
9. Fujimoto Y, Obara T. How to recognize and treat parathyroid carcinoma. *Surg Clin North Am* 1987;56:343.
10. Smith JF, Coombs RRH. Histologic diagnosis of carcinoma of the parathyroid gland. *J Clin Pathol* 1984;37:1370.
11. Levin KE, Galante M, Clark OH. Parathyroid carcinoma versus parathyroid adenoma in patients with profound hypercalcemia. *Surgery* 1987;101:649.
12. LiVolsi VA, Hamilton R. Intraoperative assessment of parathyroid gland pathology: a common view from the surgeon and the pathologist. *Am J Clin Pathol* 1994;102:365.
13. Levin KE, Chew KL, Ljung BM, et al. Deoxyribonucleic acid cytometry helps identify parathyroid carcinomas. *J Clin Endocrinol Metab* 1988;67:779.
14. Obara T, Fujimoto Y, Hirayama A, et al. Flow cytometric DNA analysis of parathyroid tumors with special reference to its diagnostic and prognostic value in parathyroid carcinoma. *Cancer* 1990;65:1789.
15. August DA, Flynn SD, Jones MA, et al. Parathyroid carcinoma: the relationship of nuclear DNA content to clinical outcome. *Surgery* 1993;113:290.
16. Hakaim AG, Esselstyn CB Jr. Parathyroid carcinoma: 50-year experience at The Cleveland Clinic Foundation. *Cleve Clin J Med* 1993;60:331.
17. Sandelin K, Thompson NW, Bondeson L. Metastatic parathyroid carcinoma: dilemmas in management. *Surgery* 1991;110:978.
18. Favia G, Lumachi F, Polistina F, et al. Parathyroid carcinoma: sixteen new cases and suggestions for correct management. *World J Surg* 1998,22:1225.
19. Mallette LE, Bilezikian JP, Ketcham AS, et al. Parathyroid carcinoma in familial hyperparathyroidism. *Am J Med* 1974;57:642.
20. Wassif WS, Moniz CF, Friedman E, et al. Familial isolated hyperparathyroidism: a distinct genetic entity with an increased risk of parathyroid cancer. *J Clin Endocrin Metabol* 1993;77:1485.
21. Streeten EA, Weinstein LS, Norton JA, et al. Studies in a kindred with parathyroid carcinoma. *J Clin Endocrinol Metabol* 1992;75:362.
22. Takeichi N, Dohi K, Ito H, et al. Parathyroid tumors in atomic bomb survivors in Hiroshima: a review. *J Radiat Res Suppl* 1991;189.
23. Takami H, et al. Parathyroid carcinoma in a patient receiving long-term hemodialysis. *Surgery* 1999;125:239.
24. Shane E, Bilezikian JP. Parathyroid carcinoma: a review of 62 patients. *Endocr Rev* 1982;3:218.
25. Wynne AG, van Heerden J, Carney JA, et al. Parathyroid carcinoma: clinical and pathologic features in 43 patients. *Medicine* 1992;71:197.
26. Lafferty FW. Primary hyperparathyroidism. *Arch Intern Med* 1981;141:1761.
27. Nikkila MT, Saaristo JJ, Koivula TA. Clinical and biochemical features in primary hyperparathyroidism. *Surgery* 1989;105:148.
28. Vetto JT, Brennan MF, Woodruf J, et al. Parathyroid carcinoma: diagnosis and clinical history. *Surgery* 1993;114:882.
29. Anderson BJ, Samaan NA, Vassilopoulou-Sellin R, et al. Parathyroid carcinoma: features and difficulties in diagnosis and management. *Surgery* 1983;94:906.
30. Cohn K, Silverman M, Corrado J, et al. Parathyroid carcinoma: the Lahey Clinic experience. *Surgery* 1985;98:1095.
31. Sandelin K, Auer G, Bondeson L, et al. Prognostic factors in parathyroid cancer: a review of 95 cases. *World J Surg* 1992;16:724.

32. Lu G, Shih WJ, Ziu JY. Technetium-99m MIBI uptake in recurrent parathyroid carcinoma and brown tumors. *J Nucl Med* 1995;36:811.
33. Al-Sobhi S, Ashari LH, Ingemansson S. Detection of metastatic parathyroid carcinoma with Tc-99m sestamibi imaging. *Clin Nucl Med* 1999;24:21.
34. Neumann D, Esselstyn CB, Siciliano D, et al. Preoperative imaging of parathyroid carcinoma by positron emission tomography. *Ann Otol Rhinol Laryngol* 1994;103:741.
35. Sandelin K, Tullgren O, Farnebo LO. Clinical course of metastatic parathyroid cancer. *World J Surg* 1994;18:594.
36. Cordeiro AC, Montenegro FLM, Klucsar MAV, et al. Parathyroid carcinoma. *Am J Surg* 1998;175:52.
37. Rosen IB, Young JEM, Archibald SD, et al. Parathyroid cancer: clinical variations and relationship to autotransplantation. *CJS* 1994;37:465.
38. McKeown PP, McGarity WC, Sewell CW. Carcinoma of the parathyroid gland: Is it overdiagnosed? *Am J Surg* 1984;147:292.
39. Fraker DL, Travis WD, Merendino JJ, et al. Locally recurrent parathyroid neoplasms as a cause for recurrent and persistent primary hyperparathyroidism. *Ann Surg* 1991;213:58.
40. Rattner DW, Marrone GC, Kasdon E, et al. Recurrent hyperparathyroidism due to implantation of parathyroid tissue. *Am J Surg* 1985;149:745.
41. Norman J, Denham D. Minimally invasive radioguided parathyroidectomy in the reoperative neck. *Surgery* 1998;124:1088.
42. Flye MW, Brennan MF. Surgical resection of metastatic parathyroid carcinoma. *Ann Surg* 1981;193:425.
43. Obara T, Okamoto T, Ito Y, et al. Surgical and medical management of patients with pulmonary metastasis from parathyroid carcinoma. *Surgery* 1993;114:1040.
44. Shane E. Parathyroid carcinoma. *Curr Ther Endocrinol Metab* 1994;5:522.
45. Calandra DB, Cheijfec G, Foy BK, et al. Parathyroid carcinoma: biochemical and pathologic response to DTIC. *Surgery* 1984;96:1132.
46. Newrick PG, Braatvedt GD, Webb AJ, et al. Prolonged remission of hypercalcaemia due to parathyroid carcinoma with pamidronate. *Postgrad Med J* 1994;70:231.
47. Warrell RP, Issacs M, Alcock NW, et al. Gallium nitrate for treatment of refractory hypercalcemia from parathyroid carcinoma. *Ann Intern Med* 1987;107:683.
48. Holmes EC, Morton DL, Ketcham AS. Parathyroid carcinoma: a collective review. *Ann Surg* 1968;169:631.
49. Shortell CK, Andrus CH, Phillips CE, et al. Carcinoma of the parathyroid gland: a 30-year experience. *Surgery* 1991;110:704.
50. Wise SR, Quigley M, Saxe AW, et al. Hyperparathyroidism and cellular mechanisms of gastric acid secretion. *Surgery* 1990;108:1058.

SECTION **4**

JEFFREY A. NORTON
HOP N. LE

Adrenal Tumors

PATHOLOGY OF THE ADRENAL CORTEX

HYPERPLASIA

The term *hyperplasia* is defined as an increased number of cells.[1] It is a pathologic change associated with increased function or compensatory change. When a pituitary adrenocorticotropic hormone (ACTH)–secreting tumor produces hypercortisolism (Cushing's disease), the most common form of endogenous hypercortisolism, the adrenal gland is approximately twice normal size. The weight of each hyperplastic adrenal is between 6 and 12 g (normal adrenal weighs between 3 and 6 g). Microscopically there is a widened inner zone of the compact zona reticularis and a sharply demarcated outer zone of clear cells. Adrenal glands in ectopic ACTH syndrome are larger in size, weighing between 12 and 30 g. Macronodular adrenal hyperplasia (3-cm adrenocortical nodules weighing between 30 and 100 g) usually is a secondary response of the adrenal to ACTH, but may occur with primary adrenal pathology. Primary pigmented micronodular adrenal hyperplasia (1- to 5-mm nodules with pigmented appearance and normal glandular weight) is more likely to be autonomous and to occur in children[2] and can occur in a familial pattern.[2]

ADRENAL CORTICAL ADENOMA

Adrenal adenoma is a benign neoplasm of adrenal cortical cells that may possess functional autonomy.[1] In general, an adenoma does not exceed 5 cm in diameter nor 100 g in weight. Some cellular pleomorphism and tumor necrosis may be present, but is rare. It is not possible to describe the exact functional type of neoplasm based solely on histology, although there are consistent differences. Adenomas produce syndromes of hypercortisolism and hyperaldosteronism and seldom produce adrenogenital syndromes. Tumors larger than 6 cm that produce adrenogenital syndromes are usually carcinoma. Pleomorphism, tumor necrosis, and mitotic activity are more common in malignant tumors. The prognosis of adrenal cortical adenoma producing Cushing's syndrome is excellent, and surgical resection invariably produces cure. The prognosis of adrenal cortical adenomas producing hyperaldosteronism may not be as favorable. Resection is followed by a favorable response in blood pressure and serum level of potassium; however, 30% of patients develop recurrent hypertension. Adenomas that produce the adrenogenital syndrome have the least favorable outcome, because many of these tumors are really carcinomas.[3]

ADRENAL CORTICAL CARCINOMA

Adrenal cortical carcinoma is a malignant neoplasm of adrenal cortical cells demonstrating partial or complete histologic and functional differentiation. Adrenal cortical carcinomas are rare and compose between 0.05% and 0.20% of all cancers. This incidence translates to a rate of only 2 per million in the world population. Women develop functional adrenal cortical carcinomas more commonly than men. However, men develop nonfunctioning malignant adrenal tumors more often than women. There is a bimodal occurrence by age, with a peak incidence less than 5 years and a second peak in the fourth and fifth decade. Adrenal cortical carcinoma has been described as part of a complex hereditary syndrome, including sarcoma, breast, and lung cancer.[4] Studies suggest that loss of heterozygosity on the short arm of chromosome 11 (11p) may be important in the pathogenesis of adrenocortical cancer.[5] Germline P53 mutations do not appear to be involved.[6] In a study from a region in Brazil with a tenfold higher incidence of adrenocortical cancer, eight of nine tumors had an increase in genetic material in the chromosomal region 9q34, suggesting that these changes may also be important.[7] In addition, deficiency of 21-hydroxylase (P-450c21), an essential enzyme for zona glomerulosa and fasciculata function, has also been implicated. Prevalence of heterozygous germline mutations in the P-450c21 gene has been noted to be increased in patients with adrenocortical tumors.[8] The myriad of genetic changes seen in different studies of these tumors may explain the association of adrenocortical cancer with complex hereditary syndromes.

TABLE 38.4-1. Diagnosis of Malignancy in Adrenal Cortical Neoplasm

Reliability	*Clinical Criteria*	*Pathologic and Genetic Criteria*
Diagnostic of malignancy	Weight loss, feminization, nodal or distant metastases	Tumor weight >100 g, tumor necrosis, fibrous bands, vascular invasion, number of mitoses per high-power field
Consistent with malignancy	Virilism, Cushing's virilism, no hormone production	Nuclear pleomorphism, aneuploidy
Suggestive of malignancy	Elevated urinary 17-ketosteroids	Capsular invasion, inhibin,[a] 21-hydroxylase deficiency[a]
Unreliable	Hypercortisolism, hyperaldosteronism	Tumor giant cells, cytoplasmic size variation, ratio between compact and clear cells

[a]Updated information (see text).

Adrenal cortical carcinomas are greater than 6 cm in size and weigh between 100 and 5000 g. Areas of necrosis and hemorrhage are common. Invasion and metastases also occur. Microscopically, the appearance is variable. Cells with big nuclei, hyperchromatism, and enlarged nucleoli are all consistent with malignancy.[1] Nuclear pleomorphism is more common in tumors larger than 500 g. Vascular invasion and many mitoses are diagnostic of malignancy. Broad desmoplastic bands are associated with metastatic potential of tumors. The diagnosis of malignancy in cortical tumors that weigh between 50 and 100 g is less certain. Furthermore, the distinction between adrenal and renal carcinoma may also be difficult. Immunostaining for vimentin, epithelial membrane antigen, cytokeratin, and blood group antigens may be used to distinguish the two diagnoses. Adrenal tumors stain positive for vimentin, whereas renal carcinoma is negative for vimentin but positive for the others.[9] Although the difference in natural history between benign and malignant adrenal cortical neoplasms is clear, it is not always possible to histologically separate one from the other. The only reliable, single criterion is the presence of nodal or distant metastases. The data used to differentiate benign from malignant adrenocortical neoplasms include whether and what type of hormone is produced, amount of tumor necrosis, fibrosis, inhibin, 21-hydroxylase deficiency, vascular invasion, mitoses, and tumor weight (Table 38.4-1). The detection of mitotic activity and venous invasion suggest a malignant tumor.[10] Aneuploidy is also associated with cancer.[11] Quantitative nuclear analysis demonstrates that nuclei from adrenal cancers are larger than adenomas, and DNA density is diploid in adenomas and aneuploid in carcinomas.[12] A final criterion is based on the observation that cells from carcinomas produce abnormal amounts of androgens and 11-deoxysteroids.[13] However, this is merely suggestive of malignancy, because only 10% of malignant tumors produce masculinization whereas the rest secrete cortisol, aldosterone, or nothing (see Table 38.4-1).

CLINICAL PRESENTATIONS OF ADRENAL CORTICAL NEOPLASMS

CUSHING'S SYNDROME (HYPERCORTISOLISM)

Signs

Cushing's syndrome, or hypercortisolism, is the result of excessive secretion of ACTH by a pituitary tumor, cortisol by an adrenal tumor, or ACTH by an ectopic source. Determining the cause of the hypercortisolism involves performing multiple tests in a logical sequence (Fig. 38.4-1). Treatment should aim to cure the hypercortisolism and eliminate any tumor that threatens the patient's health, while minimizing the chance of endocrine deficiency or long-term dependence on medications.[14] The signs and symptoms of hypercortisolism are ubiquitous and diverse; nearly every organ in the body is affected.[15] However, there is no single symptom or sign that is common to every patient. Although hypercortisolism is the most common presentation for adrenal cortical neoplasms, Cushing's syndrome is rare, with an estimated incidence of only 10 per million population.[16] Cushing's syndrome can also rarely occur in children.[16] The most common cause of hypercortisolism is iatrogenic administration of steroids to treat other diseases. The most common cause of endogenous hypercortisolism is a pituitary tumor that makes ACTH, or Cushing's disease. Hypercortisolism is not usually associated with multiple endocrine neoplasia type 1 (MEN 1), although it can be present in this familial syndrome. It has been reported to be present in 5% of patients with sporadic Zollinger-Ellison syndrome (ZES) and 19% of patients with ZES and MEN 1.[17]

Progressive weight gain is the most universal symptom of patients with hypercortisolism. Obesity is usually truncal, and patients have thin extremities due to muscle wasting. Increased fat in the dorsal neck region combined with kyphosis secondary to osteoporosis gives the appearance of a "buffalo hump." Serial photographs show a rounding of the face. Increased blood pressure is mild and caused by excess mineralocorticoid secretion. Striae are reliable clinical signs of Cushing's syndrome. Hirsutism consists of excessive fine hair on face, upper back, and arms. Virilization, including clitoromegaly, deep voice, and balding, suggest adrenocortical carcinoma. Glucose intolerance with hyperglycemia is common, and patients may present with diabetes mellitus. Weakness secondary to muscle atrophy is a common complaint and is especially common in ectopic ACTH syndrome with hypokalemia. Menstrual irregularity or amenorrhea is common in women, whereas men with Cushing's syndrome have loss of libido or impotency. In children, the most common presenting sign is obesity and an arrest of normal growth with short stature. Dilatation of blood vessels and thinning of the subcutaneous tissue give the face a ruddy appearance. Mental changes vary from mild depression to severe psychosis and appear to correlate directly with serum levels of cortisol and ACTH. Hypokalemia worsens the weakness associated with Cushing's syndrome and suggests the diagnosis of adrenocortical carcinoma or ectopic ACTH syndrome. Immunosuppression results in unusual infections, including cryptococcosis, aspergillosis, nocardiosis, *Pneumocystis carinii*,

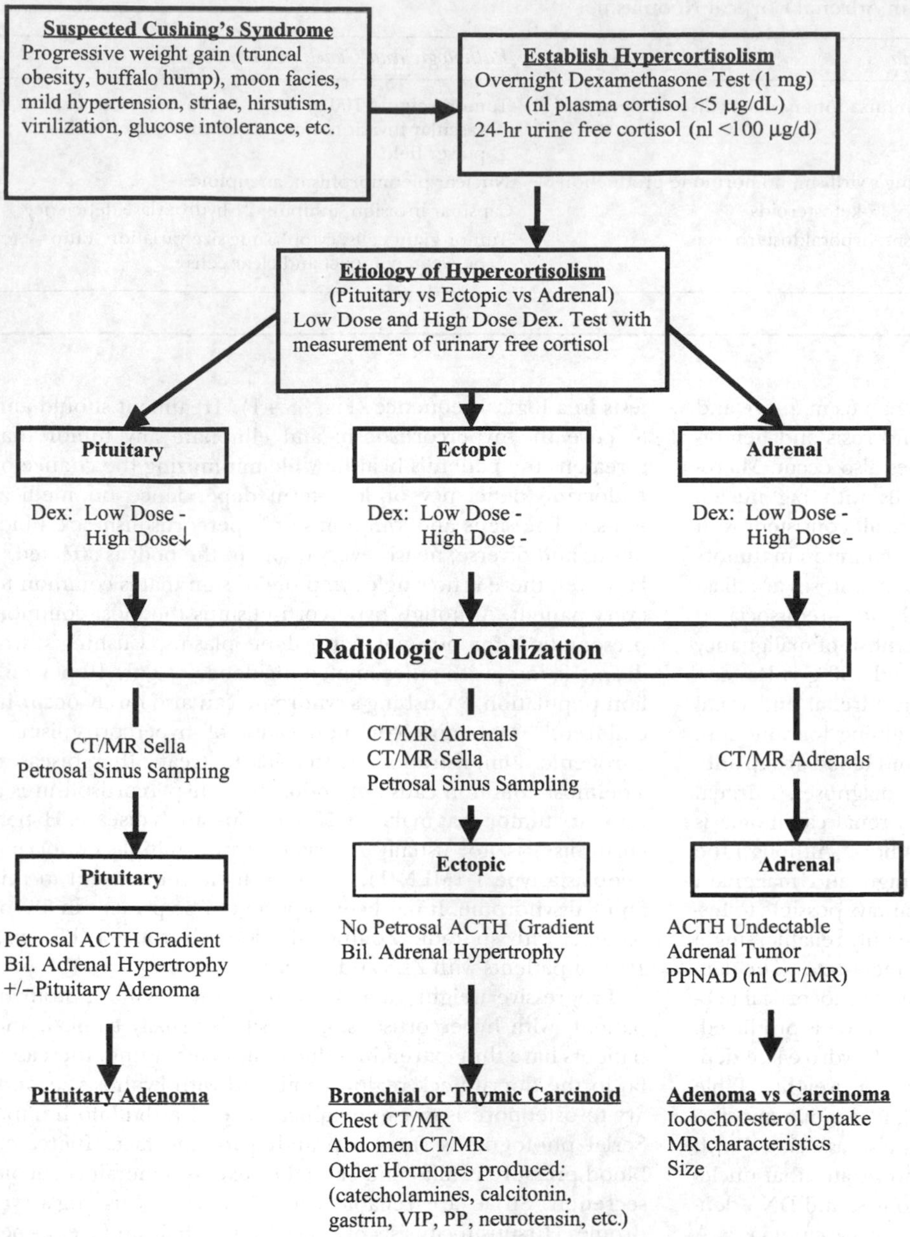

FIGURE 38.4-1. Flow diagram for evaluation of a patient with suspected hypercortisolism. ACTH, adrenocorticotropic hormone; Bil., bilateral; cal, calcitonin; CT, computed tomography; Dex, dexamethasone; MR, magnetic resonance imaging; nl, normal; PP, pancreatic polypeptide; PPNAD, primary pigmented nodular adrenocortical disease; VIP, vasoactive intestinal polypeptide.

and necrotizing fasciitis.[18–21] The early diagnosis of Cushing's syndrome depends primarily on a knowledge of the many different signs and symptoms of the disorder and a high clinical index of suspicion.[22]

Workup and Diagnosis

The initial step in the workup of a patient with presumptive hypercortisolism is to establish biochemically whether hypercortisolism is, in fact, present. The second step is to determine whether the hypercortisolism is "pituitary dependent" or "pituitary independent," and the final step is to determine the exact etiology (see Fig. 38.4-1). Current laboratory testing allows the correct diagnosis in nearly every case.[14,15]

ESTABLISHING HYPERCORTISOLISM. Urinary excretion of unmetabolized ("free") cortisol is directly proportional to the amount of free cortisol in the plasma. As the cortisol-binding globulin becomes saturated (plasma cortisol levels of 20 μg/dL), small increases in cortisol secretion produce exponential increases in urinary free cortisol. This amplification effect makes 24-hour urinary free cortisol the single best measurement to discriminate normal from hypercortisolemic states. The overnight single-dose dexamethasone test (see Fig. 38.4-1) works because of lack of normal feedback (Fig. 38.4-2) that occurs in all forms of hypercortisolism. Normal subjects given 1 mg of dexamethasone orally at 11:00 p.m. have plasma cortisol levels of less than 5 μg/dL at 8:00 a.m. the next day. Patients with endogenous hypercortisolism do not suppress and have cortisol levels greater than 5 μg/dL. The major disadvantage of this test is a 3% incidence of false-negatives (patients with Cushing's syndrome whose levels suppress). This test may also have false-positives (3%), including depression, alcoholism, stress, and primary cortisol resistance. A normal single-

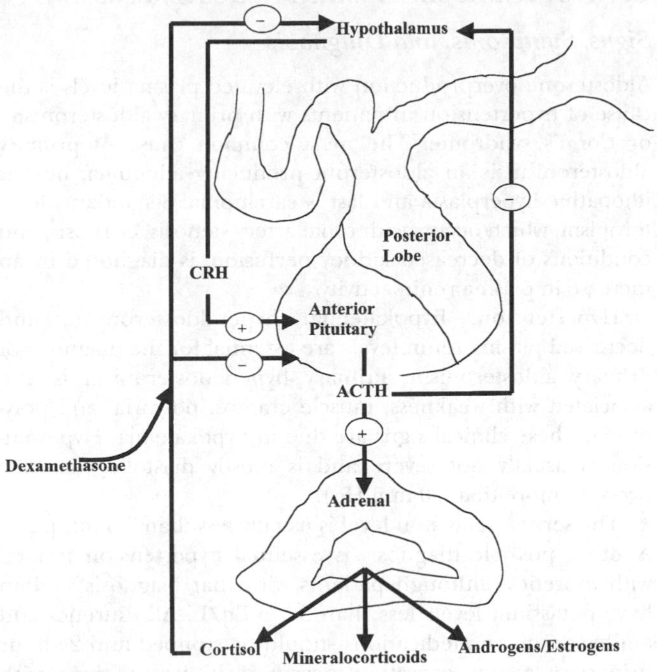

FIGURE 38.4-2. Model of cortisol secretion indicates the mechanism of dexamethasone suppression and corticotropin-releasing hormone (CRH) stimulation of normal cortisol secretion. ACTH, adrenocorticotropic hormone.

dose dexamethasone test and urinary free cortisol (less than 100 μg/d in most laboratories) virtually exclude the diagnosis of hypercortisolism.

ETIOLOGY OF HYPERCORTISOLISM. Patients with pituitary tumor (Cushing's disease) respond to 1 μg/kg corticotropin-releasing hormone (CRH) by increasing plasma ACTH and cortisol levels, whereas patients with depression or other stress diseases have a blunted ACTH response to CRH[23] (see Figs. 38.4-1 and 38.4-2). The CRH test also distinguishes pituitary tumor from ectopic secretion of ACTH. Twenty-nine of 33 patients with Cushing's disease had increased plasma ACTH and cortisol levels after a CRH test, whereas none of 8 with ectopic ACTH responded.[24] Patients with Cushing's syndrome have abnormalities in the diurnal rhythm of plasma levels of cortisol and ACTH. Serial samples over days are necessary because patients with Cushing's disease can have episodic secretion of cortisol. Nevertheless, a low midnight cortisol level (less than 2 μg/dL) excludes the diagnosis of endogenous hypercortisolism. Determination of plasma ACTH levels may also be helpful. Patients with primary adrenal tumors or hyperplasia have undetectable or low plasma ACTH levels, those with pituitary-dependent hypercortisolism have intermediate levels, and those with ectopic ACTH-producing tumors have very high levels; approximately 60% of these patients have ACTH levels greater than 300 pg/mL. Radioimmunoassays for ACTH in plasma have been difficult to perform reliably and interpret because of platelet-associated proteases that degrade ACTH. Samples must be collected using recommended procedures, including prechilled tubes on ice. Urinary 17-ketosteroids can help the differential diagnosis of hypercortisolism. Low levels (less than 10 mg/d) suggest an adrenal adenoma, and very high levels (more than 60 mg/d) occur more commonly in patients with adrenal cancer and ectopic ACTH. Hypokalemia is seen in most patients with ectopic ACTH (16 of 16 in one series) and in only 10% of patients with Cushing's disease.[25]

The standard dexamethasone suppression test is the most useful test in establishing the cause of hypercortisolism (see Figs. 38.4-1 and 38.4-2). The expected results are that urinary free cortisol levels will be markedly suppressed when normal subjects receive a low dose (2 mg) of dexamethasone, but levels do not suppress in patients with Cushing's syndrome. High-dose dexamethasone (8 mg/d) suppresses urinary levels of free cortisol to less than 50% of baseline levels in patients with pituitary-dependent hypercortisolism (Cushing's disease), but it does not suppress levels in patients with primary adrenal causes of hypercortisolism or ectopic ACTH syndrome. This single test makes the diagnosis of Cushing's syndrome and determines the cause of hypercortisolism with an accuracy rate of approximately 95%.

The metyrapone test, which is a stimulation test in patients with pituitary Cushing's disease, can be complementary to the dexamethasone suppression test, and combining both tests results in greater accuracy than with either test alone.[26]

RADIOLOGIC EVALUATION OF HYPERCORTISOLISM. Computed tomography (CT) scans of the sella detect a tumor in only 0% to 15% of patients with pituitary-dependent Cushing's disease, and detect minor abnormalities in 23% to 60%. Most ACTH-secreting tumors are microadenomas (less than 5 mm). Pituitary magnetic resonance imaging (MRI) studies, even with gadolinium, have similar resolution. In patients with pituitary-dependent hypercortisolism, CT and MR may be normal, but bilateral petrosal sinus sampling for ACTH concentrations detects the side with a tumor in most cases.[27] Data indicate that this study is the single best method to differentiate a pituitary from an ectopic ACTH-producing tumor. The study requires bilateral sampling of the inferior petrosal sinus and peripheral veins for plasma ACTH levels before and after CRH. A petrosal sinus to peripheral plasma ACTH level of greater than 3 after CRH administration correctly identifies patients with Cushing's disease (sensitivity, 100%) with few false-positive results (specificity, 100%). Furthermore, petrosal sinus sampling provides correct localization of the ACTH-producing microadenoma in most patients.[27] It is the study of choice both to diagnose and localize pituitary tumors in patients with Cushing's disease.

Adrenal CT can detect normal adrenal glands in most patients. CT can reliably distinguish cortical hyperplasia from tumor.[28] CT has great sensitivity (more than 95%); however, it lacks specificity. In a patient with Cushing's syndrome, early detection of an adrenal neoplasm by CT simplifies the workup. CT can be used to image the primary tumor plus local and distant metastases in patients with cancer. In these cases, the primary tumor is usually greater than 6 cm.[29] Approximately 15% of patients with Cushing's syndrome have a primary adrenal neoplasm as the source of the hypercortisolism. Unilateral adrenal tumors require the detection of a normal adrenal gland on the contralateral side. Adrenal hyperplasia may also be detected if both glands appear enlarged. MRI may be able to add specificity to the sensitivity of CT. MRI may be able to distinguish adrenal adenoma from carcinoma and pheochromocytoma by the appearance on the T2-weighted image. Adenomas appear darker than the liver on the T2 MRI. Carcinomas, whether primary adrenocortical or metastatic, appear as bright as or slightly brighter than the liver on T2 image. Pheochromocytomas appear much brighter (three times) than the liver on T2 MRI.[29]

Radioisotope imaging of adrenals using labeled iodocholesterol, such as ^{131}I-6-β-iodomethylnorcholesteral, can be used to distinguish adenoma from hyperplasia.[30] It can help differentiate a benign cortical neoplasm (adenoma), which usually takes up iodocholesterol (images), from a malignant cortical neoplasm (carcinoma), which usually does not.[31,32] This is not absolute, however, because adrenal cortical carcinomas may take up iodocholesterol and be "hot" on scan.[33] Iodocholesterol scan can be helpful in micronodular hyperplasia in which bilateral uptake confirms the diagnosis. It can image ectopic rests of adrenal tissue. The disadvantages of radioiodocholesterol scans are exposure to radiation, limited isotope availability, and poor imaging of malignant adrenal neoplasms.

INTERPRETATION OF WORKUP FOR CUSHING'S SYNDROME. Once the biochemical tests confirm endogenous hypercortisolism, the remainder of the workup can pinpoint its cause. If it is caused by an adrenal cortical neoplasm, the workup will produce the following results: (1) imaging of the tumor on CT and MRI, (2) low plasma ACTH levels with elevated serum cortisol levels, and (3) no suppression of urinary free cortisol level with high-dose dexamethasone. If criterion number 1 is absent but numbers 2 and 3 are present, primary pigmented nodular adrenocortical disease should be ruled out by iodocholesterol scan (see Fig. 38.4-1). If criteria numbers 1 and 3 are present but ACTH levels are consistently elevated, urinary catecholamines, vanillylmendelic acid (VMA), and metanephrines should be measured because the patient may have an ACTH-producing pheochromocytoma.[34]

In ectopic ACTH syndrome, one finds (1) enlargement of both adrenals on CT, (2) elevated plasma ACTH levels, (3) no suppression with high-dose dexamethasone, and (4) no evidence of pituitary ACTH secretion on petrosal sinus sampling.[35] Bronchial carcinoid tumors are the most common site of ectopic ACTH secretion and are potentially curable. Lobectomy is required, because a significant proportion has nodal metastases. Some bronchial ACTH-producing carcinoid tumors may suppress with dexamethasone, but the false suppression of ectopic ACTH-producing tumors is rare.[35] Malignant tumors, such as Ewing's sarcoma, have been rarely determined to secrete a CRH-like factor that causes Cushing's syndrome.[36] Studies from the Netherlands suggest that OctreoScan (somatostatin receptor scintigraphy) may be useful to image the source of ectopic ACTH. It correctly identifies 80% of ACTH-secreting carcinoid tumors (either bronchial or thymic carcinoids).[37]

In Cushing's disease (pituitary adenoma), one expects to find (1) bilateral hyperplasia of the adrenal glands, (2) normal or mildly elevated plasma ACTH levels, (3) no suppression with low-dose dexamethasone and suppression with high-dose dexamethasone, and (4) localization with petrosal sinus sampling. Occasionally (less than 5% of instances) results may be confused with ectopic ACTH syndrome. This is not common,[38] however, and most studies show that petrosal sinus sampling eliminates the ambiguity.

CONN'S SYNDROME (PRIMARY ALDOSTERONISM)

Signs, Symptoms, and Diagnosis

Aldosterone overproduction with elevated plasma levels is the cause of hypertension in patients with primary aldosteronism, or Conn's syndrome. The most common cause of primary aldosteronism is an aldosterone-producing adenoma; next is idiopathic hyperplasia and last is carcinoma. Secondary aldosteronism, which occurs with renal artery stenosis, cirrhosis, and conditions of decreased kidney perfusion, is diagnosed by an increase in plasma renin activity.

Hypertension, hypokalemia, hyperaldosteronism, and decreased plasma renin levels are essential for the diagnosis of primary aldosteronism. Primary hyperaldosteronism is also associated with weakness, muscle cramps, polyuria, and polydipsia. These clinical signs are due to hypokalemia. Hypertension is usually not severe and is mostly diastolic (diastolic pressure more than 90 mm Hg).

The serum potassium level is usually less than 3.5 mEq/L.[39] Another possible diagnosis is essential hypertension treated with diuretics, although patients with that diagnosis seldom have potassium levels less than 3.5 mEq/L. All diuretics and antihypertensive medications should be stopped and 24-hour urinary potassium excretion measured. In most patients with primary aldosteronism, 24-hour urinary excretion of potassium is greater than 30 mEq. Patients with primary hyperaldosteronism have elevated plasma levels of aldosterone and low levels of renin activity. Measurement of messenger RNA (mRNA) in the kidney and adrenal gland of patients with aldosteronoma also has demonstrated decreased levels of renin mRNA.[40] The plasma aldosterone-renin ratio is usually greater than 30. Final evidence for the diagnosis of primary hyperaldosteronism relies on the inability to lower plasma aldosterone levels and raise plasma renin activity after captopril.[41] The patient takes 25 mg of captopril orally in the morning. Two hours later, plasma levels of aldosterone and renin activity are measured. In normal subjects and patients with essential hypertension, captopril decreases plasma aldosterone levels and increases plasma renin activity. In patients with primary aldosteronism, plasma levels of aldosterone and renin activity do not change. A post-captopril plasma aldosterone level greater than 15 ng/dL and an aldosterone-renin ratio greater than 50 are diagnostic of primary aldosteronism (Table 38.4-2).

TABLE 38.4-2. Diagnosis of Primary Aldosteronism

Measurement	*Result*
Blood pressure	Hypertension
Serum potassium levels	Hypokalemia (serum K^+ <3.5 mEq/L)
Urinary potassium levels	Elevated urinary K^+ excretion (>25–30 mEq/d)
Plasma aldosterone and plasma renin activity	Ratio >30 (elevated aldosterone and low renin)
Urinary aldosterone	Elevated
Captopril suppression test (25 mg orally)	After captopril, aldosterone >15 ng/mL Aldosterone-renin ratio >50
Salt loading (9 g NaCl orally per day for 1–2 wk)	Renin suppression

TABLE 38.4-3. Etiology of Primary Aldosteronism: Idiopathic Adrenal Hyperplasia (IAH) versus Neoplasm

Measurement	*IAH*	*Neoplasm*
Aldosterone response to upright posture	Increase (>20 ng/dL)	No response or decrease (<20 ng/dL)
Serum 18-hydroxycorticosterone	<90 ng/dL	>100 ng/dL
High-resolution computed tomography scan	Normal adrenal glands	Tumor (tumors <7–10 mm may be missed)
Iodocholesterol scan	Symmetric uptake bilaterally	Uptake of tracer by benign adenoma (malignant tumors may not take up tracer)
Spironolactone	Fair response	Good response
Adrenal vein sampling	Aldosterone levels elevated from both adrenal veins and greater than simultaneous peripheral sample	Aldosterone levels elevated on side with tumor; contralateral side equal to simultaneous peripheral samples

Adenoma versus Hyperplasia

Once the diagnosis of primary aldosteronism is established, the next important consideration is the etiology—whether the patient has idiopathic adrenal hyperplasia (IAH) or a tumor that produces aldosterone (Table 38.4-3). The exact cause is critical because drug treatment is indicated for IAH, and surgery is indicated for a neoplasm. Measurement of plasma aldosterone concentrations with respect to postural changes is a relatively quick biochemical test to differentiate between the two. A decrease or no change in the serum level of aldosterone measured at 8:00 a.m. and noon in the upright position after overnight recumbence is consistent with an adenoma. The accuracy of this test is between 75% and 100%.

CT can image approximately 75% to 90% of aldosteronomas.[42] CT may miss small tumors. The contralateral adrenal cortex in a patient with an aldosteronoma appears thin on CT. Iodocholesterol scans with ^{131}I-β-iodomethyl-19-norcholesterol can image 88% of aldosteronomas. The advantage of these nuclear studies over CT is the provision of functional information about the neoplasm. In patients with IAH, the scan shows symmetrical uptake in both adrenal glands; and in patients with adrenal carcinoma causing hyperaldosteronism, the study may show no uptake by the tumor, whereas in adenomas tumor uptake is usually evident.

The single study of choice to determine if hyperaldosteronism is caused by a tumor or hyperplasia is sampling of the adrenal veins for aldosterone.[42] The procedure is performed by simultaneous selective catheterization of both adrenal veins and a peripheral vein. Serum levels of aldosterone and cortisol are measured at each site before and after ACTH. Aldosteronomas make aldosterone in response to ACTH. A unilateral elevation of aldosterone level or of the aldosterone-cortisol ratio indicates the presence of an aldosterone-secreting adenoma. Bilateral levels of aldosterone that are similar and greater than peripheral levels are consistent with IAH. Adrenal venous sampling for aldosterone (96%) is more sensitive than CT (75%) and adrenal venography (78%) in prospective comparisons.[42] If CT is nondiagnostic, venous sampling is the study of choice to distinguish a tumor from hyperplasia.

Treatment

The management of primary aldosteronism depends on the diagnosis. Idiopathic adrenal hyperplasia is best managed medically with spironolactone or amiloride in conjunction with other antihypertensive drugs. Another drug with potential for managing the hypokalemia and hypertension associated with primary aldosteronism (both IAH and adenoma) is the calcium channel blocker nifedipine. Because aldosteronomas are usually small benign adenomas, it is now preferable to use a laparoscopic approach for unilateral adrenalectomy in patients with aldosteronoma. The laparoscopic approach is associated with less pain and morbidity.[43,44]

Results for resection of an aldosteronoma have not been entirely satisfactory. A high percentage of patients initially become normotensive and normokalemic postoperatively (approximately 95% dependent on accurate diagnosis). However, 20% to 30% of patients develop recurrent hypertension within 2 to 3 years. This has caused some physicians to advise against surgery and recommend long-term medical management. This therapy has been demonstrated to effectively control blood pressure and serum level of potassium in patients with aldosteronoma for periods of up to 5 years.[45] Aldosterone-producing adrenocortical carcinomas are rare (2% of all carcinomas).[46] Treatment is similar to other patients with adrenal carcinoma and is discussed later (see the section Treatment of Adrenal Cortical Neoplasms).

INCIDENTAL ADRENAL MASS

High-resolution CT scans have resulted in a new diagnostic problem: an incidental adrenal mass detected by CT. Unexpected adrenal masses are seen in 0.6% of abdominal CT scans. The majority of these are benign adrenal cortical adenomas, which occur in 9% of autopsies.[47] However, one report indicates that an asymptomatic 3-cm adrenal mass that was followed subsequently was found to be metastatic adrenocortical carcinoma.[48] Of 311 incidentally discovered adrenal tumors, adrenocortical carcinoma was diagnosed in 21 cases (7%).[49]

The suggested evaluation of an incidental adrenal mass (incidentaloma) is given in Figure 38.4-3. Two questions arise. Is the tumor functional? Is it cancer?

The first step in evaluation of an incidentally discovered adrenal mass is a careful history and physical examination, including blood pressure.[50] The clinician should examine for evidence of weight change, weakness or hypokalemia, Cushing's syndrome, hypertension, virilization, feminization, change in menstruation, and evidence of occult malignancy (stool guaiac, pap smear, anemia). Laboratory evaluation should consist of a 24-hour urine collection for free cortisol, VMA, metanephrines, and catecholamines. Twenty-four-hour urinary levels of free cortisol are indicated to rule out Cushing's syndrome. Patients with incidentalomas and no stigmata of Cushing's syndrome have

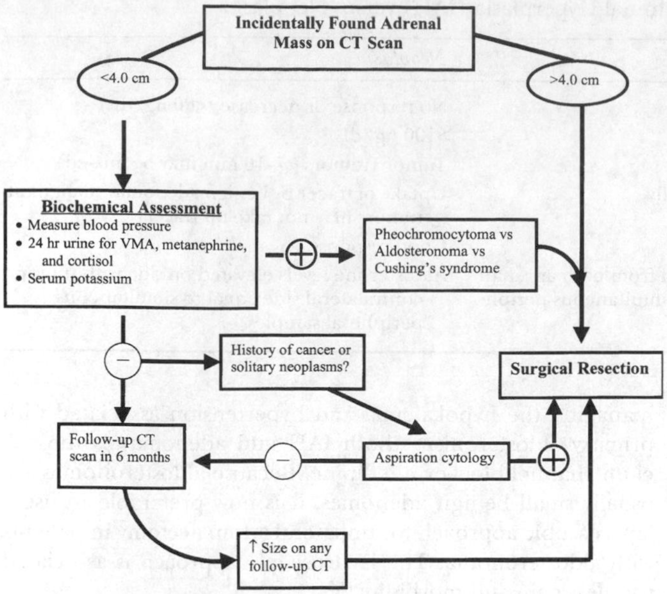

FIGURE 38.4-3. Flow diagram for management of incidentaloma. +, yes; –, no; CT, computed tomography; VMA, vanillylmendelic acid.

been identified who have occult hypercortisolism. These individuals are fairly uncommon but can be identified by measuring a 24-hour urine sample for free cortisol or a low-dose dexamethasone suppression test.[51] If urinary levels of catecholamines or catecholamine metabolites are elevated, the diagnosis is pheochromocytoma (see the section regarding management in Pheochromocytoma, later). In addition, the serum potassium concentration is used to exclude an aldosteronoma. Plasma levels of aldosterone and renin activity should be measured in any patient with hypertension and hypokalemia. Hormonal screening for an excess of androgens or estrogens is limited to patients with clinical signs suggestive of these disorders.[50]

The size of an adrenal mass on CT is an important determinant of a potentially malignant tumor. Adrenal cortical carcinomas are generally greater than 6 cm in diameter, and benign lesions are less than 6 cm. Nevertheless, a smaller lesion should not be totally ignored. Early diagnosis may lead to discovery of a small adrenal cortical carcinoma, which may lead to better prognosis and survival. Patients with primary adrenal cancers less than 5 cm in size have a better prognosis than those with larger tumors. Most recently, because of decreased morbidity with laparoscopic excision, some have advocated surgery for incidentalomas of 4 cm in size, especially in younger patients.[52] CT can accurately image normal glands, hyperplastic adrenal glands, and neoplasms, but it can only distinguish benign from malignant neoplasms by criteria such as size, direct invasion, or distant metastases.[53]

Fine-needle aspiration for cytology of an adrenal mass has limited ability to differentiate benign from malignant primary adrenal lesions. Fine-needle aspiration may be catastrophic in a patient with an unsuspected pheochromocytoma,[53] so urinary catecholamines are indicated to exclude a pheochromocytoma before needle biopsy. In patients with suspected metastatic disease to the adrenal or lymphoma, needle aspiration may be helpful.[47] In patients with known primary cancers, fine-needle aspiration can reliably diagnose adrenal metastasis.[90] Because it cannot distinguish between benign and malignant primary adrenal tumors, fine-needle aspiration cytology is not routinely recommended.

The suggested approach to an asymptomatic adrenal mass is outlined in Figure 38.4-3. Biochemical assessment should be performed to exclude hormonal function of the tumor. The size of the tumor is assessed. Size greater than 4 cm is an indication for surgical resection, especially in a younger patient. The incidence of cancer in solid adrenal masses equal to 6 cm is estimated to be between 35% and 98%.[50] Laparoscopic excision of tumors smaller than 6 cm in size is recommended because of less pain and morbidity. Laparoscopic excision of large adrenal tumors (greater than 6 cm) is not recommended because a high proportion of these tumors are malignant.[54] However, some suggest that size is not a contraindication to the laparoscopic approach.[55] We prefer the open anterior approach to malignant adrenal tumors because of fewer long-term wound complications and higher likelihood of complete tumor excision.[56] If the tumor is hormonally functional, adrenalectomy is indicated and is usually performed laparoscopically. If the patient has a history of cancer, fine-needle aspiration can be considered to exclude adrenal metastases. If the mass is smaller than 4 cm and nonfunctional, a repeat follow-up CT examination in 3 to 6 months is indicated to again determine size. If size increases, surgical excision is necessary.[50] If there is no change at 6 months, it is most likely an adenoma, and subsequent CT scans are unnecessary. It is hoped that the evaluation provides early surgical intervention for functional or malignant adrenal masses and exclusion of nonfunctional benign adrenal adenomas.

SEX HORMONE EXCESS

Adrenocortical carcinoma may present with excessive sex hormone secretion. Virilization or feminization may be combined with hypercortisolism, or the tumor may produce only estrogen or testosterone. In children, the clinical signs of increased androgen production include increased growth, premature development of pubic and facial hair, acne, genital enlargement, increased muscle mass, and deep voice. In women, the clinical signs of excess androgen production include hirsutism, acne, amenorrhea, infertility, increased muscle mass, deep voice, and temporal balding. In children, the clinical signs of increased estrogen production include gynecomastia in boys and precocious breast enlargement and vaginal bleeding in girls. In adult men, hyperestrogenism presents with gynecomastia, decreased sexual drive, impotence, and infertility. In adult women, hyperestrogenism presents primarily with irregular menses in premenopausal women and dysfunctional uterine bleeding or vaginal bleeding in postmenopausal women. The workup requires 24-hour urinary 17-ketosteroids, 17-hydroxysteroids, urinary free cortisol and, depending on virilization or feminization, serum determination of testosterone or estrogen.

Virilization secondary to an adrenal neoplasm may accompany Cushing's syndrome, and if it does occur, it usually indicates adrenal cortical carcinoma. Virilization in the absence of Cushing's syndrome may also occur due to adrenal cortical adenoma[57] or carcinoma.[58] Of course, there are many other disorders that cause virilization in women and children; however, in working up a patient with virilization, an imaging study of both adrenals, either CT or MRI, is indicated to rule out an adrenal neoplasm.

TREATMENT OF ADRENAL CORTICAL NEOPLASMS

ADRENAL CORTICAL ADENOMA

The definitive treatment of benign adrenal adenoma is surgical resection of the adrenal gland with the adenoma. Laparoscopic adrenalectomy is rapidly becoming the procedure of choice to remove benign adrenal tumors.[43,52] It is clearly indicated for smaller tumors (less than 6 cm) because it is associated with less pain and shorter convalescence.[59,60] In patients who are undergoing resection of an adrenal tumor that causes Cushing's syndrome, steroid replacement during and after surgery is necessary. Mineralocorticoid replacement is not required. Postoperative glucocorticoid replacement is indicated until complete recovery of the hypothalamic-pituitary-adrenal axis (see Fig. 38.4-2). Glucocorticoid replacement may be necessary for as long as 2 years.[61] Surgical resection of an adenoma is curative.[61] Larger lesions weighing between 50 and 100 g that appear benign histologically (no mitoses and no vascular invasion) need careful long-term follow-up to exclude carcinoma.

ADRENAL CORTICAL CARCINOMA

The mainstay of treatment of adrenal cortical carcinoma is complete resection of all gross tumor. If the carcinoma is intimately associated with the kidney, liver, or diaphragm on the right or pancreas on the left, it may be necessary to remove part or all of the contiguous structures at the time of definitive surgery. It is important to consider that the best time for curative resection is the initial time. The surgeon needs adequate imaging of the extent of disease, which can be achieved by CT, MRI, or both. CT or MRI should include the chest to rule out metastatic disease above the diaphragm. If the right adrenal is involved and the inferior vena cava is compressed, either an inferior vena cava contrast study or caval ultrasound is useful to assess tumor extension into the cava. If resection of one kidney is indicated, either an intravenous pyelogram or an intravenous contrast CT is necessary to be certain the contralateral kidney is functioning. A complete bowel preparation is used in case the tumor invades the bowel. Even though patients with hypercortisolism have impaired healing, adrenal tumor resection can be performed with acceptable morbidity and an operative mortality of 3%.[62]

Adrenal cortical carcinoma can occur in adults and children. It occurs in children younger than 6 years, with a higher incidence in girls than boys. The median age in children with adrenal cancer is 4 years. Virilization is the most common presenting feature (93%). Some children may also present with precocious puberty or Cushing's syndrome.[63,64] Some children with adrenal cancer can be cured by complete surgical resection. Approximately 65% of children with adrenocortical cancer can be cured by complete surgical resection of tumor.[63] In a multivariate analysis of predictors of outcome, only primary tumor size greater than 200 cm^3 independently identified a poor-prognosis group of children who may require more aggressive adjuvant therapy after surgery.[63] One study of children with adrenocortical cancer demonstrated that virilization was the most common presenting symptom, followed by Cushing's syndrome.[65] The overall 5-year survival rate was 49%, and when all tumor was removed, it was 70%.[65]

The second peak age of occurrence of adrenal cancer is between 40 and 50 years, and approximately 70% of these patients present with hormonal syndromes.[46] The surgical staging of adrenal carcinoma is as follows:

I	Tumor less than 5 cm without local invasion, nodal, or distant metastases
II	Same as stage I except tumor more than 5 cm
III	Tumor with local invasion or positive lymph nodes
IV	Tumor with local invasion and positive lymph nodes or distant metastases (Table 38.4-4)

Most patients (70%) present with stage III or IV disease.[46,66]

The definitive initial treatment for all stage disease, including locally aggressive stage III disease, is *en bloc* resection, which may include the adjacent kidney. This procedure may require a combined thoracoabdominal approach. Surgical resection of localized disease can be curative.[46,66] Some recommend adjuvant mitotane therapy after surgical resection to improve survival.[67] Doses between 1.5 and 2.0 g/d are well tolerated and may prolong survival.[68] However, others do not recommend mitotane therapy because it has not been proven to prolong survival.[69] In an analysis of 105 adult patients with adrenal cancer, only 80 were able to undergo surgery for possible cure, and the median disease-free interval postoperatively was 12 months.[69] The overall 5-year survival rate was 22%.[69] In most series, the 5-year survival rate is between 20% and 35%.[70] In a series from Italy, the 5-year survival rate after surgical resection in 129 cases was 35%.[71] In another series from Goteborg, Sweden, complete surgical resection was routinely combined with 1 year of mitotane therapy. Eighteen patients were treated, and the 5-year survival rate was 58% based on the Kaplan-Maier method.[72] Age over 40 years and the presence of metastases at the time of diagnosis correlated with a poor prognosis.[69] If complete resection of tumor cannot be achieved, tumor debulking should be attempted to decrease the amount of cortisol-secreting tissue and to minimize complications due to tumor mass. Patients who undergo definitive resection should undergo monitoring of steroid hormone levels postoperatively.

TABLE 38.4-4. Staging Criteria for Adrenal Cortical Carcinoma

Stage	*Criteria*
Tumor	
T1	Tumor ≤5 cm, invasion absent
T2	Tumor >5 cm, invasion absent
T3	Tumor outside adrenal in fat
T4	Tumor invading adjacent organs
Lymph nodes	
N0	No positive lymph nodes
N1	Positive lymph nodes
Metastases	
M0	No distant metastases
M1	Distant metastases
Stage grouping	
I	T1, N0, M0
II	T2, N0, M0
III	T1–2, N1, M0; T3, N0, M0
IV	Any T, any N, M1; T3, T4, N1

Accurate measurement of urinary levels requires switching the glucocorticoid replacement therapy from hydrocortisone to dexamethasone. CT and MRI are also used to detect local recurrences and pulmonary metastases. If a recurrence is detected, it can be removed surgically. Prolonged remissions have been reported after resection of hepatic, pulmonary, and cerebral metastases from adrenal cortical carcinoma.[73–75] Patients with recurrent adrenal cortical carcinoma who can be surgically resected have improved survival over those who cannot. In 52 cases of recurrent disease, the 5-year survival rate of reoperated cases was 50% versus 8% for nonoperated cases.[76] When complete resection of tumor metastases is not possible, near total resection may still be helpful in some hormonally productive, slow growing adrenal cortical cancers.[76] Palliation of bony metastases may be achieved by radiation therapy.[46] Abdominal radiation therapy may be useful in 65% of patients with local recurrences not amenable to resection, and the treatment has even relieved bowel obstruction. However, it does not appear to improve the duration of survival.[46]

CHEMOTHERAPY

Once the patient has recurrent or metastatic adrenal cortical carcinoma, chemotherapy with o,p-DDD (mitotane) usually is started.[77] Therapy is initiated at a dose of 2 to 6 g daily in two or three divided doses and increased until adverse reactions occur. Adverse reactions include gastrointestinal toxicity (anorexia, nausea, vomiting, and diarrhea), neuromuscular toxicity (depression, dizziness, tremors, headache, confusion, and weakness), and skin rash. Seventy-nine percent of treated patients develop some gastrointestinal toxicity, 50% develop neuromuscular toxicity, and 15% develop a skin rash.[77] Mitotane is associated with prolongation of the bleeding time and abnormal platelet aggregation.[78] A decrease in urinary 17-hydroxysteroids and 17-ketosteroids occurs in 67% of patients treated due to a direct effect on steroid metabolism, and a partial response occurs in approximately 35% of patients treated with mitotane. It is important to measure blood levels of o,p-DDD and achieve serum levels higher than 14 µg/mL. In one study, patients who had blood levels of less than 10 µg/mL had no demonstrable therapeutic effects, whereas seven of eight patients who had levels greater than 14 µg/mL had objective responses and subsequently lived significantly longer.[79] Unfortunately, the difference between efficacy and toxicity is small, and levels greater than 20 µg/mL are associated with symptoms of neuromuscular toxicity.[79]

Tumor responses usually occur in the first 6 weeks after the initiation of mitotane treatment. Although most patients who demonstrate an objective response to o,p-DDD subsequently relapse, there have been a few long-term survivors with metastatic adrenocortical carcinoma treated with mitotane. Mitotane may be an unpleasant drug, and when clinical toxicity is present, the dose must be adjusted to minimize side effects. Because patients with adrenocortical carcinoma are rare, there have been no controlled studies to establish that mitotane can significantly alter the natural course of adrenocortical carcinoma. Some suggest that adjuvant o,p-DDD improves survival after initial surgery for adrenocortical carcinoma,[67] although most experts do not recommend it as an adjuvant drug after total resection of primary adrenocortical cancer.[69,80] In a report of 59 patients with adrenal cancer who received mitotane therapy at a dose between 7 and 10 g/day, 37 patients were evaluable for tumor response.[69] Of the 37 patients, only 8 (22%) had a documented partial response.[69] Mitotane has been reported to have a 20% response rate.[81] Most experts do not recommend mitotane for the management of patients with adrenocortical cancer.[76,82–84] However, others argue that the dose of drug is critical and that the dose of mitotane must be pushed to toxicity to see reasonable response rates.[85,86] When one achieves a measurable serum mitotane level greater than 14 µg/mL, mitotane appears to have a more favorable impact on survival. Lower serum levels have no impact at all.[86] At best, the response rate with mitotane alone is 60%, and few complete responses have been reported.[87] Mitotane has clear benefit to help control hypercortisolism. In one retrospective review, two inoperable patients were treated preoperatively with mitotane and streptozotocin, and each had a 50% reduction in primary tumor size. One patient also had complete regression of pulmonary metastases. Tumor was resected in both patients, and both were treated with more chemotherapy postoperatively. Both patients have remained completely free of disease for 9 and 5 years postoperatively.[88] Chemotherapy has been combined with mitotane treatment. Eighteen patients with advanced adrenal cortical carcinoma were treated with etoposide (VP16), 100 mg/m^2/day, and cisplatin, 100 mg/m^2, every 4 weeks plus mitotane. A complete response was seen in three cases and a partial response in three cases, for an overall response rate of 33%.[89] Because of the *in vitro* finding that mitotane is able to reverse multidrug resistance, it has also combined with etoposide, doxorubicin, and cisplatin in a (n = 28) Italian multicenter trial of patients with advanced metastatic adrenal cortical carcinoma. A complete response was achieved in two patients and partial responses in 13, for an overall response rate of 54%.[90] Patients treated with mitotane plus chemotherapy have prolonged survival over patients treated with chemotherapy alone.[91]

Chemotherapy regimens besides o,p-DDD have been ineffective against adrenal cortical carcinoma. Partial responses have been reported with regimens based on doxorubicin[84] and alkylating agents. Promising regimens include cisplatin and etoposide. In three studies including these drugs in patients with metastatic adrenal cortical carcinoma who failed mitotane, there were seven responses in eight patients, including one complete response,[92] although the complete responder had a duration of only 1 year. Another active regimen includes 5-fluorouracil, doxorubicin, and cisplatin, which has produced 3 responders in 13 patients treated.[93] One patient had a complete response that lasted for 42 months.[93] Patients who have not responded to mitotane have been effectively treated with a combination of cisplatin and etoposide.[94]

Suramin is known to inhibit the binding of growth factors, including epidermal growth factor, platelet-derived growth factor, and transforming growth factor-β, to tumor receptors and may reduce tumor growth by antagonizing these factors.[95] It has been used as a phase 1 agent in 21 patients with metastatic adrenal cortical cancer who have failed other therapy, and 3 partial responses (14%) were seen with no complete responses.[95,96] Suramin has toxicity related to blood coagulation, and some patients have had thrombocytopenia and hemorrhage (C. A. Stein, R. LaRocca, C. E. Myers, personal communication, 1991). In another study of nine patients with metastatic adrenal cortical carcinoma treated with suramin, cumulative doses between 8 and 30 g were administered over 1 to 15 months. One-third had a partial response, and the remainder had progression or stabilization. Toxicity included

TABLE 38.4-5. Chemotherapy Agents Used to Treat Adrenocortical Carcinoma

Investigations	*Drug*	*Dose*	*Frequency*	*Patients*	*Efficacy*
Gutierrez and Crooke, 1980[77]	Mitotane	1–12 g/d	b.i.d. or t.i.d.	37	22–33% PR
Luton et al., 1990[69]					
Van Slooten et al., 1984[79]					
Venkatesh et al., 1989[83]		7–10 g/d	b.i.d.	72	29% PR
Haak et al., 1994[86]		High dose (serum levels >14 μg/mL)			60% PR, few CR
Kornely and Schlaghecke, 1994[87]		High dose plus streptozotocin		2	CR with surgery plus chemotherapy
Decker et al., 1991[84]		6 g/d		36	22% PR
Stein et al., 1989[95]	Suramin	1.0–1.5 mg/m²	qwk	21	3 PR
Arit et al., 1994[97]		8–30 g		9	3 PR
LaRocca et al., 1990[96]					
Stein et al., 1989[95]	Doxorubicin	60 mg/m	q3wk	16	19% PR
Schlumberger et al., 1991[93]	5-Fluorouracil + Doxorubicin + Cisplatin	500 mg/m² days 1, 2, 3 60 mg/m² day 2 120 mg/m² day 2	q4wk	13	1 CR, 2 PR
Berruti et al., 1992[92]	Etoposide + Doxorubicin + Cisplatin	Not given		3	1 CR 2 PR
Avico et al., 1992[102]	Oncovin Cisplatin Epipodophyllotoxin Cytoxin	Not given		1	1 CR
Berruti et al., 1998[166]	Mitotane + Etoposide + Doxorubicin + Cisplatin	2–4 g/d 100 mg/m² days 5–7 20 mg/m² days 1 and 8 40 mg/m² days 1 and 9	q4wk	28	2 CR 13 PR
Zidan et al., 1996[167]	Mitotane + Cisplatin	Not given		1	1 CR

CR, complete remission; PR, partial remission.

polyneuropathy, coagulopathy, and thrombocytopenia.[97] Suramin has had limited efficacy and serious toxicity.[97] Suramin does not appear to be an effective agent in adrenal cancer.

In vitro studies in a soft agar system suggest that the new midazole tetrazirione compound 8-carbamoyl-3-methylimidazo(5,1-d)-1,2,3,5 tetrazin-4(3H)-1 (temozolomide) is very active against adrenal cortical carcinoma.[98] Paclitaxel also has been shown to be effective against the adrenocortical carcinoma cell line, human NCI-H295, in *in vitro* studies.[99] Taxol also has been effective in *in vitro* studies against a steroid-secreting malignant adrenal cortical carcinoma cell line.[100]

Gossypol has been shown in experimental studies of adrenal cancer to inhibit tumor growth and prolong survival of mice.[101] However, in phase 1 human studies with metastatic adrenal cancer, it had a partial response rate of 20%. One 5-year-old child with metastatic adrenal cancer had a near complete response to oncovin, cisplatin, epipodophyllotoxin, and cytoxan.[102] Steroid hormone receptors have been detected *in vitro* in adrenal cortical carcinomas, indicating dependence on progesterone and glucocorticoid. However, *in vivo* studies of therapy related to manipulation of receptors have not been done. The available chemotherapy agents and results are summarized in Table 38.4-5. Mitotane is a first-line chemotherapy drug, and combination regimens including cisplatin and other drugs are the preferred second-line choices. Adrenal cortical carcinoma is rare and malignant. Most patients present with stage III and IV tumors (see Table 38.4-4). Metastatic sites of adrenal cancer are lymph nodes (68%), lung (71%), liver (42%), and bone (26%).[103] Surgical cure may only be feasible in stage I or stage II tumors (tumors confined to the adrenal gland).

In patients with invasion of contiguous structures at presentation, median survival is 2.3 years.[46] Patients who present with stage I disease have a 50% 5-year survival rate compared with patients who present with either stage II or III disease, who have a 10% 5-year survival rate.[82] In patients with tumors confined to the adrenal gland, the mean duration of survival is 5 years.[46] For all patients, the 5-year survival rate is between 10% and 35%, indicating that most patients present with locally advanced or distant disease.[69,104,105] Most clinicians still recommend aggressive surgical resection of locally recurrent or metastatic cancer in these patients, but one study demonstrates that, even with this aggressive intervention, the 5-year survival rate is only approximately 10% to 20%.[75] These data indicate the poor prognosis of all patients with adrenal cortical carcinoma and support the use of adjuvant systemic chemotherapy or radiotherapy for resectable lesions (stages I to III). Based on the current evidence, however, adjuvant chemotherapy or radiation therapy is not recommended because effective regimens have not yet been documented.

Future challenges for better treatment of adrenal cortical carcinoma include earlier diagnosis and better adjuvants than o,p-DDD. Earlier diagnosis can be facilitated by an index of suspicion of hormonal excess during history and physical examinations. Changes in body appearance and menstrual history are important clues to earlier diagnosis. The use of MRI to differentiate benign from malignant incidentalomas of the adrenal may help clinicians find early resectable adrenal cortical cancers. Drugs such as cisplatin and etoposide or mitotane combined with chemotherapy[106] may be useful in the management of these difficult patients.

ECTOPIC ADRENOCORTICOTROPIC HORMONE SYNDROME

The first report of a patient who exhibited features of Cushing's syndrome had an oat cell carcinoma of the bronchus secreting a peptide now called *corticotrophin*, or ACTH. Similar patients who had adrenal hyperplasia without pituitary tumors were reported over the next 30 years, but it was Christy[107] and Liddle[108] who established the presence of ACTH-like material in tumors other than pituitary tumors, in the blood, and in subnormal quantities in the pituitary itself.[107,108] The name *ectopic ACTH syndrome* was introduced in 1962.[108]

The diagnosis of ectopic ACTH syndrome is based on the metabolic evaluation of the patient who presents with hypercortisolism. An early clue to the diagnosis is the presence of Cushing's syndrome and severe hypokalemia (potassium level under 3.3 mEq/L). The diagnosis is based primarily on high plasma ACTH and cortisol levels, which do not change with high-dose dexamethasone or administration of CRH, and results of petrosal sinus sampling that demonstrate low levels of ACTH draining the pituitary gland that do not change with CRH. Once the diagnosis is established, the primary therapeutic goal is to find and eradicate the neoplasm that is secreting ACTH. When this is accomplished by surgery, chemotherapy, or radiation therapy, long-term cures can be achieved. The main clinical problems have been finding the source of ectopic ACTH in some patients and treating the aggressive underlying tumor in others. The causative tumors, in approximate order of frequency, are as follows:

1. Oat cell or small cell lung cancer
2. Carcinoid tumor of the bronchus
3. Epithelial carcinoma of the thymus or thymic carcinoids
4. Pancreatic islet cell tumor
5. Medullary carcinoma of the thyroid gland
6. Pheochromocytoma
7. Gut carcinoids
8. Ovarian adenocarcinoma
9. Pancreatic cystadenoma
10. Adenocarcinoma of unknown site

Other than small cell carcinoma of the lung, the most common cause of ectopic ACTH syndrome is either bronchial or thymic carcinoid tumors. The recommended radiographic procedures to localize ACTH-producing tumors include chest and abdominal CT, chest and abdominal MRI, urinary catecholamines to screen for pheochromocytoma, plasma levels of calcitonin to rule out medullary thyroid carcinoma, and inferior petrosal sinus sampling with CRH in patients in whom the differential diagnosis of Cushing's disease (pituitary) is unclear. Any suspicious finding in the chest or abdomen can be unequivocally confirmed by fine-needle aspiration and radioimmunoassay for ACTH in the aspirate.

The goal of therapy for patients with ectopic ACTH production is to find and treat (usually resect, unless it is oat cell carcinoma) the neoplasm that is the source of ACTH. Cancer resection is indicated for patients with bronchial carcinoid tumors (lobectomy with lymph nodes) because 50% will have positive lymph node metastases. Despite this clear malignant potential, approximately 75% of patients are cured by surgical resection.[109] The proper therapy for ACTH-producing neoplasms depends on the diagnosis (exact tumor that produces ACTH) and extent of disease.

Any of these tumors may be malignant and may metastasize. Therefore, in some patients with ectopic ACTH production, the primary disease cannot be eradicated and therapy must be directed toward correcting the life-threatening metabolic and hormonal abnormalities. Hypokalemia and excess mineralocorticoid activity may be managed with potassium supplementation and spironolactone. Hypercortisolism may be managed with metyrapone, aminoglutethimide, or mitotane. Bilateral adrenalectomy is recommended for patients who have ectopic ACTH secondary to tumors that cannot be localized despite diligent radiographic efforts and for patients who have stable, but unresectable, metastatic disease whose hypercortisolism cannot be managed medically.

PHEOCHROMOCYTOMA

Pheochromocytomas are rare tumors that rise from chromaffin cells in the adrenal medulla and elsewhere. Pheochromocytomas secrete catecholamines and cause intermittent, episodic, or sustained hypertension. Pheochromocytomas can present with either lactic acidosis or unexplained fever. In autopsy series, only 0.005% to 0.1% of persons have unsuspected pheochromocytomas.[1] When urinary catecholamines are measured in hypertensive patients, pheochromocytoma is present in only 0.1% of patients. Although these tumors are rare, it is important to diagnose and localize pheochromocytomas. Sustained hypertension caused by a pheochromocytoma is curable with tumor resection. Sudden death is associated with pheochromocytoma. Pheochromocytomas may be malignant. Earlier diagnosis and therapy may lessen the probability of death from malignancy and improve the prognosis. Incidence of malignancy in pheochromocytomas is as low as 5% and as high as 46% in different series.[110] Extraadrenal tumors may be more commonly cancerous. Pheochromocytomas may be associated with endocrine and nonendocrine inherited disorders. Bilateral adrenal medullary pheochromocytomas are components of MEN 2a and MEN 2B. Some recommend unilateral adrenalectomy in some MEN 2a patients as long as careful follow-up of the contralateral adrenal gland with urinary catecholamines is maintained.[111] Familial pheochromocytoma also has been described. Affected individuals have bilateral adrenal pheochromocytomas and no other manifestation of MEN syndromes. In other families, extraadrenal pheochromocytomas have been reported, sometimes in the same location (bladder, etc.) in affected individuals. Pheochromocytomas occur in approximately 25% of patients with von Hippel-Lindau (VHL) disease[112] and in fewer than 1% of patients with neurofibromatosis and von Recklinghausen's disease.[113]

Pheochromocytomas produce catecholamines, which result in clinical symptoms of anxiety attacks, episodic hypertension, or sustained hypertension. Severe, symptomatic paroxysmal hypertension with symptoms that are not related to stress or emotional distress are the most common presenting complaint of patients with pheochromocytoma.[114] However, pheochromocytomas may also produce other hormones, including ACTH; therefore, patients may have concomitant Cushing's syndrome. Pheochromocytomas may produce many other peptide hormones, including somatostatin, calcitonin, oxytocin, and vasopressin.

ONCOGENE

Pheochromocytomas originate from the neural crest and may develop by arrest at various points during normal differentiation. The *ras* oncogene does not appear to be involved in the tumoral process of pheochromocytoma, because one study failed to detect any abnormality of *ras* gene sequence in ten pheochromocytomas.[115] Loss of heterozygosity at specific loci may help localize tumor suppressor genes involved in the formation of various familial and sporadic pheochromocytomas. Of 41 tumors tested, significant allelic losses were found on chromosome 1p (42%), 3p (16%), 17p (24%), and 22q (31%). Furthermore, there appeared to be a correlation between loss of heterozygosity on chromosome 1p with urinary excretion of metanephrine and loss of heterozygosity on chromosomes 1p, 3p, and 17p with tumor volume.[116] Because pheochromocytomas are part of the VHL syndrome, investigators have studies the role of the tumor suppressor gene *CUL2*, whose product interacts with the VHL tumor suppressor in the pathophysiology of sporadic pheochromocytomas. It does not appear to have a significant effect, because only 1 of 26 tumors had a mutation.[117]

PATHOLOGY

Pheochromocytomas arise from chromaffin cells. Chromaffin cells are widespread and associated with sympathetic ganglia during fetal life. After birth, most chromaffin cells degenerate, and the majority remain in the adrenal medulla. This may explain why approximately 90% of pheochromocytomas are in the adrenal medulla. Extraadrenal pheochromocytomas may arise anywhere, including the carotid body, intracardiac, along the aorta (both thoracic and abdominal), and within the urinary bladder. The most common extraadrenal location is the organ of Zuckerkandl, which is near the origin of the inferior mesenteric artery to the left of the aortic bifurcation. Extraadrenal pheochromocytomas may more often be malignant. Bilateral adrenal pheochromocytomas occur in familial syndromes, including MEN 2a and MEN 2B.[118]

Data from series of patients with sporadic pheochromocytomas indicate that the right adrenal gland more commonly harbors a tumor than the left gland.[119] Pheochromocytomas resected from hypertensive patients usually measure between 3 and 5 cm in diameter and weigh approximately 100 g.[120] These tumors appear tan to gray in color and have a soft smooth consistency. Larger tumors may be cystic or have necrotic areas and often have calcification. Microscopically, pheochromocytomas resemble the cell of origin. Tumors are usually arranged in cords or alveolar patterns.[1] Tumors may be composed of cords of cells lining vascular structures that have an angiomatous appearance. Tumors are generally clearly separated from the adrenal cortex by a thin band of fibrous tissue. Extension of the pheochromocytoma into the cortex or vascular invasion may occur in benign neoplasms.[1]

TABLE 38.4-6. Differentiation of Benign versus Malignant Pheochromocytomas

Characteristic	*Benign*	*Malignant*
Metastases	–	+
Weight (g)	<200	>500
Occurrence (%)	50–90	10–50
Vascular invasion	+	+
Capsular invasion	+	+
Mitoses	±	++++
Nuclear pleomorphism	+	–
Ploidy	Diploid	Hyperdiploid, triploid
Necrosis	±	++
Tumors with neuropeptide Y gene expression	+	–
Proportion of patients with elevated serum levels of neuron-specific enolase (%)	–	+

+, extent present; –, extent absent.

The pathologic distinction between benign and malignant pheochromocytomas is not clear, and pathologists have relied on the reported benign natural history of most pheochromocytomas. However, some reports indicate that more pheochromocytomas than expected are malignant. In one large series, the tumor recurrence rate was 10% and most recurrences occurred within 5 years.[119] In another series, the recurrence rate was 23%,[121] and in another it was 46%.[122] Certainly these results partly reflect the referral pattern of tertiary institutions, but they may also reflect a true higher malignancy rate than originally suggested. Malignant tumors tend to be larger and weigh more, although this is not an absolute criterion[1] (Table 38.4-6). Staining for the nuclear proliferation marker MIB-1 is positive in 50% of malignant pheochromocytomas and negative in benign tumors. It is preliminary data, but it may be a useful marker for malignancy.[123] The only absolute criterion for malignancy is the presence of secondary tumors in sites where chromaffin cells are not usually present and visceral metastases. Benign pheochromocytomas may demonstrate marked nuclear pleomorphism, whereas paradoxically, malignant ones demonstrate less.[1] Malignant pheochromocytomas usually have many more mitoses than benign tumors, but capsular and vascular invasion occurs with equal frequency in both.[1] Nuclear DNA ploidy may be a predictive indicator of malignant potential.[124] Flow cytometry has been used to define a subgroup of patients with pheochromocytoma who have malignant tumor. Tumor whose DNA ploidy studies demonstrated tetraploidy or polyploidy and aneuploidy had a significantly higher chance of a malignant course than most tumors, which were normally diploid. It has been observed that neuropeptide Y gene expression by tumors may be used to distinguish benign from malignant pheochromocytomas. Neuropeptide Y mRNA was expressed in 9 of 9 benign tumors and only 4 of 11 malignant tumors, suggesting that expression of this gene is seen more often in benign pheochromocytomas.[125] Others have attempted to differentiate patients with benign and malignant pheochromocytomas by serum levels of neuron-specific enolase and neuropeptide Y, but observed differences were not significant.[126] Finally, studies indicate that size of tumor (weight) correlated best with malignant potential, as did amount of necrosis[127] (see Table 38.4-6).

CLINICAL MANIFESTATIONS AND DIAGNOSIS

Patients with pheochromocytomas can present with a range of symptoms, from mild labile hypertension to sudden death secondary to a hypertensive crisis, myocardial infarction, or cerebral vascular accident. The classic patient describes "spells" of paroxysmal headaches, pallor, palpitations, hypertension, and diaphoresis. In 50% of patients, the hypertension is intermittent, whereas in the others it is sustained. In 90% of children with pheochromocytomas, the hypertension is sustained. Patients may have signs of chronic hypovolemia, such as orthostatic hypotension or lactic acidosis secondary to excess α-catecholaminergic stimulation and vasoconstriction. Most patients have mild weight loss, but obesity does not rule out pheochromocytoma. Diabetes mellitus may be induced.

The diagnosis of pheochromocytoma is based on measuring catecholamines and metabolites in the urine (Fig. 38.4-4). If a pheochromocytoma is suspected clinically or a patient has a history of familial pheochromocytoma, MEN 2a, or MEN 2B, the best study is a 24-hour urine test for catecholamines, metanephrine, and VMA. In a report describing the testing of 64 patients, 30 of whom had pheochromocytomas, 24-hour urine collections for VMA, dopamine, epinephrine, and norepinephrine were analyzed. The 24-hour urinary levels of VMA and norepinephrine had the greatest sensitivity (97%), whereas the levels of VMA had the best specificity (91%).[128] Another study also reports that urinary measurement of catecholamine, VMA, and metanephrine levels were the most sensitive screening test.[129] Methods are now available to measure plasma catecholamines using a radioenzymatic assay. This can provide a more direct measurement of catecholamine excess, but there have been conflicting reports comparing the value of urinary or plasma catecholamines in the diagnosis of pheochromocytoma. As the plasma studies become more reliable, they may be a more sensitive and specific method than the urinary assay. However, it depends on the laboratory and the method, because studies still report that urinary measurements are more sensitive than plasma.[130]

The clonidine suppression test has become the test of choice to determine whether a patient with borderline urinary or plasma catecholamine level has a pheochromocytoma.[131] It is the study of choice to diagnose pheochromocytomas in patients with plasma catecholamine concentrations between 500 and 2000 pg/mL.[132] In normal subjects and patients with idiopathic hypertension, clonidine suppresses plasma levels of epinephrine and norepinephrine. In patients with pheochromocytoma, clonidine does not suppress levels. Only two incorrect diagnoses have been reported using the clonidine suppression test: one false-positive and one false-negative.[133] An overnight method of this test has also been reported based on the measurement of urinary levels of norepinephrine and epinephrine.[131]

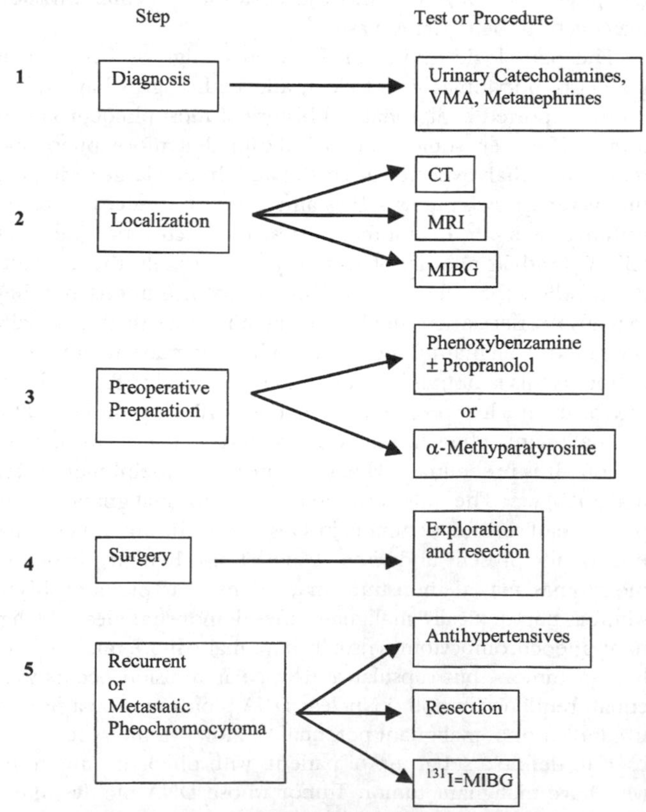

FIGURE 38.4-4. Flow diagram for diagnosis, localization, preoperative preparation, treatment, and follow-up of a patient with a pheochromocytoma. CT, computed tomography; MIBG, metaiodobenzylguanidine; MRI, magnetic resonance imaging; VMA, vanillylmendelic acid.

LOCALIZATION STUDIES

CT and MRI are the two radiologic (nonnuclear medicine) procedures of choice to localize pheochromocytomas (see Fig. 38.4-4). Both are noninvasive and sensitive, being able to detect tumors approximately 1 cm in diameter. MRI may be more specific because of the increased signal intensity on the T2-weighted image. CT has some advantages over MRI. CT scanners currently have greater resolution and greater availability. In a Mayo Clinic study of 52 patients with pheochromocytoma, CT detected 51 of 52 tumors, including 9 of 10 bilateral tumors.[134] In another study, unenhanced high-resolution CT detected pheochromocytomas in six of six patients who had tumors found at surgery, including two extraadrenal retroperitoneal tumors.[135] MRI also has remarkable resolution. In seven patients with pheochromocytomas demonstrated on CT, MRI imaged all primary lesions as well as metastases to the chest, retroperitoneum, and liver. Because it has no radiation exposure, it can be used to image a pheochromocytoma during pregnancy. In one analysis, CT imaged 16 of 19 pheochromocytomas (84%), whereas MRI imaged 12 of 15 (75%) for comparable sensitivity.[136] In addition, MRI successfully imaged an intrapericardial pheochromocytoma and distinguished it from the cardiac chambers and surrounding great vessels, which could not be determined by CT.

Another important technique for the localization of pheochromocytomas is nuclear scanning after the administration of labeled metaiodobenzylguanidine (MIBG) (see Fig. 38.4-4). The compound is similar to norepinephrine and is taken up and concentrated in adrenergic tissue. ^{131}I-MIBG has been studied in 400 patients to localize suspected pheochromocytoma.[137] The sensitivity of MIBG scanning was 78% in sporadic pheochromocytoma, 91% in malignant pheochromocytoma, and 94% in familial pheochromocytoma. The overall sensitivity was 87%. The specificity was nearly 100% in all categories and overall. ^{131}I-MIBG at another institution demonstrated a sensitivity of 77% and a specificity of 96%,[138] and two other institutions had similar findings.[139,140] More recent data confirm previous studies and demonstrate that labeled MIBG is a useful diagnostic and imaging study for the detection and localization of pheochromocytoma.[128] In three studies from three different institutions, it had a sensitivity of 86% and correctly diagnosed and imaged tumor in 71 of 83 patients.[128,136] It appears that MIBG scanning is safe, noninvasive, and efficacious for the localization of pheochromocytomas, including those that arise in nonadrenal sites, and malignant disease. Metastatic bone involvement by pheochromocytoma can be imaged by ^{131}I-MIBG, but standard bone scintigraphy may be more sensitive. In summary, MIBG scanning images catecholamine-producing tumors with a high specificity and sensitivity. Whereas CT and MRI reflect changes in morphology, scintigraphic imaging relies on tissue function.[140] False-positive results with MIBG scintigraphy are rare (but tumors such as medullary thyroid carcinoma and neuroblastoma can image), which accounts for the high specificity (98% to 100%) of the study. False-negative results can occur and have an incidence of approximately 13% to 20%,[128,136] which lowers sensitivity. It appears that these false-negatives may be more common with multiple tumors and metastatic disease in the same patient.

MANAGEMENT

Preoperative Preparation

Once the diagnosis is established and the tumor localized, preoperative preparation includes α-adrenergic blockade. Patients are started on phenoxybenzamine, 10 mg orally two or three times daily (see Fig. 38.4-4). If tachycardia develops (heart rate more than 100 beats/min), β-adrenergic blocking agents (propranolol) are added before surgery. Propranolol should never be started before α blockade because unopposed vasoconstriction may worsen hypertension. Phenoxybenzamine increases the total blood and plasma volume in patients with pheochromocytoma. In addition, lactic acidosis may be present in patients with pheochromocytoma related to the effect of catecholamines on peripheral circulation. The measurement and correction of arterial blood pH should be performed in all patients before the induction of anesthesia and surgery.

α-Methyltyrosine is a competitive inhibitor of tyrosine hydroxylase, the rate-limiting step in catecholamine biosynthesis. Treatment with α-methyltyrosine (metyrosine) reduces catecholamine production by 50% to 80% in patients with pheochromocytoma. The usual dose is 250 mg four times daily, which may be increased to a maximum dose of 3 to 4 g/day.[141] It has been used preoperatively to prepare some patients with pheochromocytoma and unusual cardiac complications for surgery, and it may be used to treat hypertensive crisis in patients with pheochromocytoma.[140,142] Studies suggest that it is most effective when combined with phenoxybenzamine.[143] Others have successfully used the calcium-antagonist nifedipine with phenoxybenzamine or nicardipine alone (60 to 120 mg every 24 hours) to control labile hypertensive episodes in patients with pheochromocytoma.[144] Either of these newer drug strategies appear to work as well as or better than the more traditional strategy of phenoxybenzamine.

Intraoperative Management

If the patient is elderly or has had cardiac complications, he or she should be transferred to the intensive care unit the day before surgery and a Swan-Ganz catheter should be inserted. This allows correction of hemodynamic imbalances and optimization of cardiac performance. The morning of operation, an arterial catheter and peripheral intravenous catheters should be inserted. Arterial blood gas should be measured to rule out acidosis. During surgery, especially during manipulation of the tumor, marked increases in blood pressure may occur; hypertensive episodes should be controlled with either α-adrenergic blocking agents like regitine or agents that directly relax arterial and venous smooth muscle like sodium nitroprusside. Nitroprusside is the preferred drug because of its rapid onset and short duration. It is administered via a continuous intravenous infusion with a pump, and the blood pressure is continuously titrated to acceptable levels. The use of preoperative preparation with oral α-adrenergic blocking agents and intraoperative adjustment and regulation of blood pressure with nitroprusside has greatly facilitated the surgical resection of pheochromocytoma and has reduced operative morbidity and mortality.

The operation is performed using a transabdominal incision, either a bilateral subcostal or a long midline incision. Preoperative localization studies, such as CT, MRI, and ^{131}I-MIBG, guide the exploration, but the entire abdomen should be carefully visualized and palpated. Others argue that localization procedures are so sensitive and specific that more direct approaches may be preferred.[145] Small intraadrenal pheochromocytomas have been removed using laparoscopic techniques. Laparoscopic procedures appear to decrease pain and shorten the time to recovery. Most pheochromocytomas are well localized. However, in instances of malignant pheochromocytomas or multiple pheochromocytomas in known or unsuspected MEN syndromes, some tumors may be missed. Extraadrenal pheochromocytomas may be difficult to find. The most common locations of intraabdominal extraadrenal pheochromocytoma are in the hilar region of the kidneys and in the chromaffin tissue along the aorta from the celiac axis to the aortic bifurcation. The organ of Zuckerkandl at the aortic bifurcation is the most common extraadrenal location. Pheochromocytomas have been described within the urinary bladder. Multiple locations, metastatic potential, and multiple tumors all support the necessity for a complete exploration of the entire abdominal cavity. The "rule of ten" may be of value in the management of pheochromocytomas: Ten percent are malignant, 10% are extraadrenal, and 10% are bilateral. In patients with MEN 2, some suggest that nearly 100% either have or will develop bilateral benign adrenal medullary pheochromocytomas,[146] whereas others suggest that the incidence of bilaterality, although high, may be significantly less (70%).[147]

MALIGNANT PHEOCHROMOCYTOMAS

Malignant pheochromocytomas are thought not to occur in MEN syndromes and to be present in approximately 10% of patients with pheochromocytoma. Two reports indicate that substantially more than 10% of sporadic pheochromocytoma may be malignant.[121,122] In one study, 25 of 69 (36%) patients had malignant pheochromocytomas diagnosed by recurrent or metastatic disease[121]; in another study using the same criteria, 81 of 176 (46%) patients with pheochromocytomas had malignant disease.[122] In the later study, original histologic review by blinded pathologists did not discriminate malignant versus benign neoplasms with accuracy. Pathologic analysis was not helpful in predicting which tumors were malignant.[122] Patients who developed metastases did not develop them until 0.2 to 28.7 years after their initial surgery. Incidence of detection for the first 9 years was 5% per year. Males were more likely to develop metastatic pheochromocytoma. Imaging with ^{131}I-MIBG was usually able to detect recurrent or metastatic pheochromocytoma. Some recommend yearly ^{131}I-MIBG scans to detect recurrent disease in all patients after resection of pheochromocytoma.[122] New studies indicate that octreotide scintigraphy may also be useful to image malignant metastatic pheochromocytoma.[148] If the tumor is imaged by somatostatin receptor scintigraphy, octreotide therapy may have potent antitumor effects.[149] Others recommend lifetime follow-up with measurement of blood pressure and urinary levels of catecholamines.[121] The detection of recurrent or metastatic pheochromocytoma should be based on the same methods as detection of primary or initial pheochromocytoma. These methods include urinary and serum catecholamine measurement, the clonidine suppression test, CT scanning, MRI, and ^{131}I-MIBG scanning. Careful follow-up requires some, but not necessarily all, of these studies on a yearly basis (see Fig. 38.4-4). It appears that with careful follow-up the incidence of malignant pheochromocytoma may be greater than 10% and may approach 30% to 50%.

The basic principles in the treatment of malignant pheochromocytoma have been to surgically resect recurrences or metastases whenever possible and to treat hypertensive symptoms by catecholamine blockade.[150] Even in pediatric patients, surgical resection of metastatic and recurrent pheochromocytoma has been shown to prolong survival.[151] Painful bony metastases, which may be diagnosed by either ^{131}I-MIBG scans or standard bone nuclide scans, respond well to radiotherapy. Soft tissue masses or bony masses generally respond well to radiation therapy if doses of 40 Gy or more can be administered.[124] Localized or solitary soft tissue masses, even when metastatic to the liver or lung, may be successfully resected surgically. Standard chemotherapy regimens including doxorubicin plus streptozotocin and carmustine plus doxorubicin have not had efficacy in the treatment of malignant pheochromocytomas.

Survival data of patients with malignant pheochromocytoma are difficult to obtain because of the rarity and indolence of the tumor. In a large series from the Mayo clinic, the 5-year survival rate was 36%.[150] Others report a 5-year survival rate of 60% in 15 patients with malignant pheochromocytoma.[152] In this study, patients were treated primarily by aggressive surgery and medical blood pressure control.[152] In a final series, patients who succumbed from malignant pheochromocytoma did so within 3 years of the appearance of metastases.[153]

The early success with streptozotocin in the treatment of neuroendocrine tumors of the gastrointestinal tract suggested that it might also be useful in the treatment of malignant pheochromocytomas. Streptozotocin has had mixed responses in patients with malignant pheochromocytoma. Initial work with streptozotocin was disappointing and suggested no role for it in the treatment of malignant pheochromocytoma.[153] However, Feldman[154] treated one patient with a good response and suggested that the dosage schedule might be important in obtaining a beneficial result. He provided additional 3-year follow-up on that patient and noted that the patient maintained an 85% reduction in urinary homovanillic acid levels and a 73% reduction in urinary VMA levels with normal renal function despite 66 g of streptozotocin.[155] Other investigators have tried this regimen and noted no response and deterioration of renal function. It may be that some patients with malignant pheochromocytoma respond to streptozotocin chemotherapy, but many do not, and it does not appear to play a major role in the treatment of patients with these rare tumors.

Because of the high sensitivity (85%) and specificity (100%) of ^{131}I-MIBG to image pheochromocytomas, its use in higher doses to treat recurrent or metastatic pheochromocytomas has been implemented. Current imaging modalities of pheochromocytoma permit relatively accurate dosimetry to the tumor on the basis of the diagnostic dose of ^{131}I-MIBG administered. If uptake by primary or metastases is high, it is possible to deliver very high radiation doses by increasing the administered activity. Specific activity of ^{131}I-MIBG of 200 mCi in 5 mg has now been achieved. With the remarkable ability of MIBG to image tumors, one would expect its ability to treat metastatic or recurrent tumors to be equally effective; however, the results have not been very dramatic. Treatment response in patients with pheochromocytomas can be measured by catecholamine secretion and standard tumor size measurements. Blood pressure control of a few patients with malignant pheochromocytoma has been facilitated by ^{131}I-MIBG therapy.[156] One trial reports the use of ^{131}I-MIBG therapy in 15 patients with malignant pheochromocytoma. Patients were treated with ^{131}I-MIBG (specific activity 740 MBq/mg) every 3 months. The typical patients received three doses. The absorbed cumulative tumor dose was 12 to 155 Gy. A beneficial response to treatment was observed in nine patients (60%), four never responded, and others had a slight response. No complete responses were observed. Five patients had measurable partial responses to treatment, and seven had clear hormonal responses. Toxicity included pancytopenia in one patient that resolved after discontinuation of therapy.[156] In another study of 12 patients treated with ^{131}I-MIBG, 5 (42%) reduced catecholamine levels and 2 decreased tumor size (17%).[157] Vetter and colleagues[158] reported two patients with malignant pheochromocytomas treated with ^{131}I-MIBG who had minor reduction in tumor size but no change in catecholamine secretion. There were no reported complete responses until more recently.[156–158] Targeted radiotherapy with ^{131}I-MIBG is effective in 58% of malignant pheochromocytomas with objective responses.[159] One report documented a 4-year biochemical and imageable complete response with ^{131}I-MIBG treatment in one patient.[160] Another report documents significant partial responses in three patients treated with ^{131}I-MIBG.[156]

Neuroblastomas are aggressive tumors of neural crest origin that occur in children and have no association with hypertension. All patients with neuroblastoma have high plasma levels of dopa. Patients with benign pheochromocytomas have elevated plasma levels of norepinephrine or epinephrine, and

TABLE 38.4-7. Treatment of Metastatic Malignant Pheochromocytoma

Investigations	*Compound*	*Patients*	*Patients with Change in Catecholamine Secretion*	*Result of Imaging and Urine Levels of Catecholamine*
Feldman et al., 1984[157]	^{131}I-MIBG	3	No change	Questionable decrease
Krempf et al., 1991[156]	^{131}I-MIBG	15	7 partial decreases (47%) 4 normal	5 decreases (33%)
Nakabeppu and Nakajo, 1994[160]	^{131}I-MIBG	1	1 normal	1 CR
Feldman 1983[154]	High-dose streptozotocin	1	Marked decrease	Marked decrease
Averbuch et al., 1988[161]	Cyclophosphamide + Vincristine + Dacarbazine	14	2 normal 6 partial decreases (57%)	1 CR 6 PR (50%)
Noshiro et al., 1996[168]	Cyclophosphamide + Vincristine + Dacarbazine	2	1 decrease 1 no change	1 marked decrease
Sisson et al., 1999[165]	^{131}I-MIBG + Cyclophosphamide + Dacarbazine + Vincristine	6	3 decreases	2 PR
Arai et al., 1998[169]	α-Methylparatyrosine + Cyclophosphamide + Dacarbazine + Vincristine	1	1 partial decrease	No change
Tada et al., 1998[164]	α-Methylparatyrosine + Cyclophosphamide + Dacarbazine + Vincristine	3	2 decreases	No change

CR, complete remission; ^{131}I-MIBG, iodine 131–labeled metaiodobenzylguanidine; PR, partial remission.

none have elevated plasma levels of dopa. Sixty percent of patients with malignant pheochromocytomas have elevated plasma levels of dopa, in contrast to benign pheochromocytoma. The similarity between malignant pheochromocytoma and neuroblastoma is further supported by the astonishing responsiveness of malignant pheochromocytomas to therapy that is effective in treating neuroblastomas.[161] Combination of cyclophosphamide, vincristine, and dacarbazine has an 80% response rate for metastatic neuroblastoma[162] and has been used in patients with metastatic pheochromocytoma. The chemotherapy regimen consists of cyclophosphamide, 750 mg/m^2 intravenously, on day 1, vincristine, 1.4 mg/m^2 intravenously, on day 1, and dacarbazine, 600 mg/m^2 intravenously, on days 1 and 2, repeated every 21 days. Doses of cyclophosphamide and dacarbazine have been increased or decreased on the basis of neurotoxicity. This regimen has now been reported in 14 patients with metastatic pheochromocytoma.[161] The ability to respond to the chemotherapy regimen correlated with plasma norepinephrine level before therapy. One patient had a complete response (both biochemical and imageable) that lasted for 9 months. One other patient also had a biochemical complete response, and a total of eight (57%) patients had clear decreases in 24-hour levels of urinary catecholamines. Seven patients (50%) also had at least a 50% decrease in the measurable size of tumor. Biochemical response (urinary catecholamines) correlated well with response evaluated on imaging studies. The median duration of response was greater than 18 months. All responding patients have had dramatic improvement in hypertension control and performance status. The regimen has been well tolerated, and toxicity has been mild.[161] Hypertensive crises after cytotoxic drug therapy in patients with pheochromocytoma have been reported,[162] but this potentially life-threatening complication is not a problem with adequate α-adrenergic blockade. Single cases have been reported to have complete responses with cyclophosphamide, vincristine, and dacarbazine (CVD).[163] Three additional patients have been treated with CVD, resulting in partial responses.[164]

Patients with malignant pheochromocytomas have been treated with both chemotherapy and radioactive MIBG in a study protocol. Six patients with metastatic pheochromocytoma were treated with three doses of ^{131}I-MIBG followed by a year of chemotherapy with CVD given in 21-day cycles. Three patients had significant partial responses to ^{131}I-MIBG, and two patients had further partial responses to chemotherapy. The combination therapy produced additive antitumor effects.[165] Two additional patients with metastatic pheochromocytomas also have been treated with CVD with partial responses.[166] Table 38.4-7 lists possible treatment regimens for metastatic pheochromocytoma.

REFERENCES

1. Page DL, DeLellis RA, Hough AJ. Tumors of the adrenal. In: *Atlas of tumor pathology*. Washington: Armed Forces Institute of Pathology, 1986.
2. Travis WD, Tsokos M, Doppman JL, et al. Primary pigmented nodular adrenocortical disease. *Am J Surg Pathol* 1989;13:921.
3. Hough AJ, Hollifield JW, Page DL, Hartmann WH. Diagnostic factors in adrenal cortical tumors. *Am J Clin Pathol* 1979;72:390.
4. Lynch HT, Katz DA, Bogard PJ, Lynch JF. The sarcoma, breast cancer, lung cancer, and adrenocortical carcinoma syndrome revisited. *Am J Dis Child* 1985;139:134.

5. Henry I, Grandjovans S, Couillin P, et al. Tumor-specific loss of 11 p 15.5 alleles in del 11 p 13 Wilms tumor and in familial adrenocortical carcinoma. *Proc Natl Acad Sci U S A* 1989;86:3247.
6. James LA, Kelsey AM, Birch JM, Varley JM. Highly consistent genetic alterations in childhood adrenocortical tumors detected by comparative genomic hybridization. *Br J Cancer* 1999;81:300.
7. Figueiredo BC, Stratakis CA, Sandrini R, et al. Comparative genomic hybridization analysis of adrenocortical tumors of childhood. *J Clin Endocrinol Metab* 1999;84:1116.
8. Beuschlein F, Schulze T, Mora P, et al. Steroid 21-hydroxylase mutations and 21-hydroxylase messenger ribonucleic acid expression in human adrenocortical tumors. *J Clin Endocrinol Metab* 1998;83:2585.
9. Wick MR, Cherwitz DL, McGlennen RC, Dehner LP. Adrenocortical carcinoma: an immunohistochemical comparison with renal cell carcinoma. *Am J Pathol* 1986;122:343.
10. Weiss LM, Medeiros LJ, Vickery AL. Pathologic features of prognostic significance in adrenocortical carcinoma. *Am J Surg Pathol* 1989;13:202.
11. Hosaka Y, Rainwater LM, Grant CS, et al. Adrenocortical carcinoma: nuclear deoxyribonucleic acid ploidy studied by flow cytometry. *Surgery* 1987;102:1027.
12. Scarpelli M, Montironi R, Mazzucchelli R, Thompson D, Bartels PH. Distinguishing cortical adrenal gland adenomas from carcinomas by their quantitative nuclear features. *Anal Quant Cytol Histol* 1999;21:31.
13. O'Hare MJ, Monaghan P, Neville AM. The pathology of adrenocortical neoplasia: a correlated structural and functional approach to the diagnosis of malignant disease. *Hum Pathol* 1979;10:137.
14. Orth DN. Cushing's syndrome. *N Engl J Med* 1995;332:791.
15. Perry RR, Nieman LK, Cutler GB, et al. Primary adrenal causes of Cushing's syndrome: diagnosis and surgical management. *Ann Surg* 1989;210:59.
16. Magiakou MA, Mastorakos G, Oldfield EH, et al. Cushing's syndrome in children and adolescents: presentation, diagnosis and therapy. *N Engl J Med* 1994;331:629.
17. Maton PN, Gardner JD, Jensen RT. Cushing's syndrome in patients with the Zollinger-Ellison syndrome. *N Engl J Med* 1986;315:1.
18. Kramer M, Corrado ML, Bacci V, et al. Pulmonary cryptococcosis and Cushing's syndrome. *Arch Intern Med* 1983;143:2179.
19. Fulkerson WJ, Newman JH. Endogenous Cushing's syndrome complicated by *Pneumocystis carinii* pneumonia. *Am Rev Respir Dis* 1984;129:188.
20. Graham BS, Tucker WS Jr. Opportunistic infections in endogenous Cushing's syndrome. *Ann Intern Med* 1984;101:334.
21. Cunningham DS, Cutler GB Jr. Spontaneous vulvar necrotizing fasciitis in Cushing's syndrome. *South Med J* 1994;87:837.
22. Corenblum B, Kwan T, Gee S, Wong NC. Bedside assessment of skin-fold thickness. A useful measurement for distinguishing Cushing's disease from other causes of hirsutism and oligomenorrhea. *Arch Int Med* 1994;154:777
23. Chrousos GP, Schuermeyer TH, Doppman J, et al. Clinical applications of corticotropin-releasing factor. *Ann Intern Med* 1985;102:344.
24. Nieman LK, Chrousos GP, Oldfield EH, et al. The ovine corticotropin-releasing hormone stimulation test and the dexamethasone suppression test in the differential diagnosis of Cushing's syndrome. *Ann Intern Med* 1986;105:862.
25. Howlett TA, Drury PL, Perry L, et al. Diagnosis and management of ACTH-dependent Cushing's syndrome: comparison of the features in ectopic and pituitary ACTH production. *Clin Endocrinol* 1986;24:699.
26. Avgerinos PC, Yanovski JA, Oldfield EH, Nieman LK, Cutler GB Jr. The metyrapone and dexamethasone suppression tests for the differential diagnosis of the adrenocorticotropin-dependent Cushing syndrome: a comparison. *Ann Int Med* 1994;121:318.
27. Oldfield EH, Doppman JL, Nieman LK, et al. Petrosal sinus sampling with and without corticotropin-releasing hormone for the differential diagnosis of Cushing's syndrome. *N Engl J Med* 1991;325:897.
28. Doppman JL, Nieman LK, Travis WD, et al. CT or MR imaging of massive macronodular adrenocortical disease: a rare cause of autonomous primary adrenal hypercortisolism. *J Comput Assist Tomogr* 1991;15:773.
29. Dunnick NR. Adrenal carcinoma. *Radiol Clin North Am* 1994;32:99.
30. Bierwaltes WH, Sisson JC, Shapiro JC, Shapiro B. Diagnosis of adrenal tumors with radionuclide imaging. *Spec Top Endocrinol Metab* 1984;6:1.
31. Schteingart DE, Seabold JE, Gross MD, Swanson DP. Iodocholesterol adrenal tissue uptake and imaging in adrenal neoplasms. *J Clin Endocrinol Metab* 1981;52:1156.
32. Fig LM, Gross MD, Shapiro B, et al. Adrenal localization in the adrenocorticotropic hormone–independent Cushing syndrome. *Ann Intern Med* 1988;109:547.
33. Pasieka JL, McLeod MK, Thompson NW, Gross MD, Schteingart DE. Adrenal scintigraphy of well-differentiated (functioning) adrenocortical carcinomas: potential surgical pitfalls. *Surgery* 1992;112:884.
34. Spark RF, Connolly PB, Gluckin DS, et al. ACTH secretion from a functioning pheochromocytoma. *N Engl J Med* 1979;301:416.
35. Limper AH, Carpenter PC, Scherthauer B, Staats BA. The Cushing syndrome induced by bronchial carcinoid tumors. *Ann Intern Med* 1992;117:209.
36. Preeyasombat C, Sirikulchayanonta V, Mahachokelertwattana P, Sriphraprodang A, Boonpucknairig S. Cushing's syndrome caused by Ewing's sarcoma secreting corticotropin releasing factor-like peptide. *Am J Dis Child* 1992;146:1103.
37. de Herden WW, Krenning EP, Malchoff CD. Somatostatin receptor scintigraphy: its value in tumor localization in patients with Cushing's syndrome caused by ectopic corticotropin or corticotropin-releasing hormone secretion. *Am J Med* 1994;96:305.
38. Boggan JE, Tyrrell JB, Wilson CB. Transsphenoidal microsurgical management of Cushing's disease: report of 100 cases. *J Neurosurg* 1983;59:195.
39. Weinberger MH, Grim CE, Hollifield JW, et al. Primary aldosteronism: diagnosis, localization and treatment. *Ann Intern Med* 1979;90:386.
40. Shionoiri H, Hirawa N, Ueda S. Renin gene expression in the adrenal and kidney of patients with primary aldosteronism. *J Clin Endocrinol Metab* 1992;74:103.
41. Lyons DG, Kern DC, Brown RD, et al. Single dose captopril as a diagnostic test for primary aldosteronism. *J Clin Endocrinol Metab* 1983;57:892.
42. Geisinger MA, Zelch M, Bravo E, et al. Primary hyperaldosteronism: comparison of CT, adrenal venography, and venous sampling. *AJR Am J Roentgenol* 1983;141:299.
43. Go H, Takeda M, Imai T, et al. Laparoscopic adrenalectomy for Cushing's syndrome: comparison with primary aldosteronism. *Surgery* 1995;117:11.
44. Querin S, Pomp A. Early experience with laparoscopic approach for adrenalectomy. *Surgery* 1993;114:1120.
45. Ghose RP, Hall PM, Bravo EL. Medical management of aldosterone producing adenomas. *Ann Intern Med* 1999;131:105.
46. Cohn K, Gottesman L, Brennan M. Adrenocortical carcinoma. *Surgery* 1986;100:1170.
47. Candel AG, Gattuso P, Reyes CV, Prinz RA, Castelli MJ. Fine needle aspiration biopsy of adrenal masses in patients with extra-adrenal malignancy. *Surgery* 1993;114:1132.
48. Hofle G, Gasser RW, Lhotta K, et al. Adrenocortical carcinoma evolving after diagnosis of preclinical Cushing's syndrome in an adrenal incidentaloma. A case report. *Horm Res* 1998;50:237.
49. Kasperlik-Zaluska AA, Migdalska BM, Makowska AM. Incidentally found adrenocortical carcinoma. A study of 21 patients. *Eur J Cancer* 1998;34:1721.
50. Ross NS, Aron DC. Hormonal evaluation of the patient with an incidentally discovered adrenal mass. *N Engl J Med* 1990;323:1401.
51. Reincke M, Nieke J, Krestin GP, et al. Preclinical Cushing's syndrome in adrenal "incidentalomas": comparison with adrenal Cushing's syndrome. *J Clin Endocrinol Metab* 1992;75:826.
52. Michel LA, deCanniere L, Hamoir E, et al. Asymptomatic adrenal tumours: criteria for endoscopic removal. *Eur J Surg* 1999;165:767.
53. McCorkell SJ, Miles NL. Fine-needle aspiration of catecholamine-producing adrenal masses: a possibly fatal mistake. *AJR Am J Roentgenol* 1985;145:113.
54. Kolomecki K, Pomorski L, Kuzdak K, Narebski J, Wichman R. The surgical treatment of incidentaloma. *Neoplasma* 1999;46:124.
55. Henry JF, Defechereux T, Gramatica L, Raffaelli M. Should laparoscopic approach be proposed for large and/or potentially malignant adrenal tumors? *Langenbecks Arch Surg* 1999;38:366.
56. Buell JF, Alexander HR, Norton JA, Yu KC, Fraker DL. Bilateral adrenalectomy for Cushing's syndrome: anterior versus posterior approach. *Ann Surg* 1997;225:63.
57. Gabrilove JL, Seman AT, Sabet R, Mitty HA, Nicolis GL. Virilizing adrenal adenoma with studies on the steroid content of the adrenal venous effluent and a review of the literature. *Endocr Rev* 1981;2:462.
58. Gabrilove JL, Frieberg EK, Nicolis GL. Peripheral blood steroid levels in Cushing's syndrome due to adrenocortical carcinoma or adenoma. *Urology* 1983;22:576.
59. Wells SA, Merke DP, Cutler GB Jr, Norton JA, Lacroix A. The role of laparoscopic surgery in adrenal disease. *J Clin Endocrinol Metab* 1998:831:3041.
60. Linos DA, Stylopoulos N, Boukis M, et al. Anterio, posterio, laparoscopic approach for management of adrenal tumors. *Am J Surg* 1997;173:120.
61. Doherty GM, Nieman LK, Cutler GB Jr, Chrousos GP, Norton JA. Time to recovery of the hypothalamic-pituitary-adrenal axis after curative resection of adrenal tumors in patients with Cushing's syndrome. *Surgery* 1990;108:1085.
62. van Heerden JA, Young WF Jr, Grant CS, Carpenter PC. Adrenal surgery for hypercortisolism-surgical aspects. *Surgery* 1995;117:466.
63. Ribeiro RC, Sandrini Neto R, Schell MJ, et al. Adrenocortical carcinoma in children: a study of 40 cases. *J Clin Oncol* 1990;8:67.
64. Chudler RM, Kay R. Adrenocortical carcinoma in children. *Urol Clin North Am* 1989;16:469.
65. Teinturier C, Pauchard MS, Brugieres L, et al. Clinical and prognostic aspects of adrenocortical neoplasms in childhood. *Med Pediatr Oncol* 1999;32:106.
66. Henley DJ, van Heerden JA, Grant CS, Carney JA, Carpenter PC. Adrenal cortical carcinoma: a continuing challenge. *Surgery* 1983;94:226.
67. Kasperlik-Zaluska AA, Migdalska BM, Zgliczynski S, Makowska AM. Adrenal carcinoma: a clinical study and treatment results of 52 patients. *Cancer* 1995;75:2587.
68. Dickstein G, Shechner C, Arad E, Best LA, Nativ O. Is there a role for low doses of mitotane as adjuvant therapy in ACC? *J Clin Endocrinol Metab* 1998;83:3100.
69. Luton JP, Cerdas S, Billaud L, et al. Clinical features of adrenocortical carcinoma: prognostic factors and the effect of mitotane therapy. *N Engl J Med* 1990;322:1195.
70. Demure MJ, Somberg LB. Functioning and nonfunctioning adrenocortical carcinoma: clinical presentation and therapeutic strategies. *Surg Clin North Am* 1998:7:791.
71. Crucitti F, Bellantone B, Ferrante A, Boscherini M, Crucitti P. Italian registry for ACC. *Surgery* 1996;119:161.
72. Khorram-Manesh A, Ahlman H, Jansson S, et al. Adrenocortical carcinoma: surgery and mitotane for treatment and steroid profiles for follow-up. *World J Surg* 1998;22:605.
73. Appelqvist P, Kostiainen S. Multiple thoracotomy combined with chemotherapy in metastatic adrenal cortical carcinoma: a case report and review of the literature. *J Surg Oncol* 1983;24:1.
74. Potter DA, Strott CA, Javadpour N, Roth JA. Prolonged survival following six pulmonary resections for metastatic adrenal cortical carcinoma: a case report. *J Surg Oncol* 1984;25:273.
75. Jensen JC, Pass HI, Sindelar WF, Norton JA. Recurrent or metastatic disease in select patients with adrenocortical carcinoma. *Arch Surg* 1991;126:457.
76. Ballantone R, Ferrante A, Boscherini M, et al. Role of reoperation in recurrence of ACC: results from 188 cases collected in the Italian National Registry for ACC. *Surgery* 1997; 122:1212.
77. Gutierrez ML, Crooke ST. Mitotane (o,p-DDD). *Cancer Treat Rev* 1980;7:49.
78. Ajani JA, Levin B, Wallace S. Systemic and regional therapy of advanced islet cell tumors. *Gastroenterol Clin North Am* 1989;18:923.
79. Van Slooten H, Moolenaar AJ, Van Seters AP, Smeek D. The treatment of adrenocortical carcinoma with o,p-DDD: prognostic implications of serum levels monitoring. *Eur J Clin Oncol* 1984;20:47.

80. Vassilopoulou-Sellin R, Guinee VF, Klein MJ. Impact of adjuvant mitotane on the clinical course of patients with adrenal cancer. *Cancer* 1993;71:3119.
81. Decker RA, Elson P, Hogan TF. ECOG mitotane and Adriamycin in patients with ACC. *Surgery* 1991;110:1006.
82. Bodie B, Novick AC, Pontes JE, et al. The Cleveland Clinic experience with adrenal cortical carcinoma. *J Urol* 1989;141:257.
83. Venkatesh S, Hickey RC, Sellin RV, Fernandez JF, Samoan NA. Adrenal cortical carcinoma. *Cancer* 1989;64:765.
84. Decker RA, Elson P, Hogan TF, et al. Eastern Cooperative Oncology Group study 1989: mitotane and Adriamycin in patients with advanced adrenocortical carcinoma. *Surgery* 1991;110:1006.
85. Haak HR, Van Seters AP, Moolenaar AJ. Mitotane therapy of adrenocortical carcinoma. *N Engl J Med* 1990;322:758.
86. Haak HR, Hermans J, van de Velde CS, et al. Optimal treatment of adrenocortical carcinoma with mitotane: results in a consecutive series of 96 patients. *Br J Cancer* 1994;69:947.
87. Kornely E, Schlaghecke R. Complete remission of metastasized adrenocortical carcinoma under o,p-DDD. *Exp Clin Endocrinol* 1994;102:50.
88. Grondal S, Cedermark B, Eriksson B, et al. Adrenocortical carcinoma. A retrospective study of a rare tumor with a poor prognosis. *Eur J Surg Oncol* 1990;16:500.
89. Bonacci R, Gigliotti A, Baudin E, et al. Cytotoxic therapy with etoposide and cisplatin in advanced adrenocortical carcinoma. *Br J Cancer* 1998;78,546.
90. Berruti A, Terzolo M, Pia A, Angeli A, Dogliotti L. Mitotane associated with etoposide, doxorubicin and cisplatin in treatment of advance ACC. *Cancer* 1998;10:2194.
91. Barzon L, Fallo F, Sonino N, Daniele O, Boscaro M. ACC: experience in 45 patients. *Oncology* 1997;54:490.
92. Berruti A, Terzolo M, Paccotti P. Favorable response of metastatic ACC to etoposide, Adriamycin and cisplatin. *Tumori* 1992;78:345.
93. Schlumberger M, Brugieres L, Gicquel C, et al. 5-Fluorouracil, doxorubicin, and cisplatin as treatment for adrenal cortical carcinoma. *Cancer* 1991;67:2997.
94. Zidan J, Shpendler M, Robinson E. Treatment of metastatic ACC with etoposide and cisplatin after failure with mitotane. *Am J Clin Oncol* 1996;19:229.
95. Stein CA, LaRocca RV, Thomas R, McAtee N, Myers CE. Suramin: an anticancer drug with a unique mechanism of action. *J Clin Oncol* 1989;7:499.
96. LaRocca RV, Stein CA, Danesi R, et al. Suramin in adrenal cancer: modulation of steroid hormone production, cytotoxicity *in vitro* and clinical antitumor effect. *J Clin Endocrinol Metab* 1990;71:497.
97. Arit W, Reincke M, Siekmann L, Winkelmann W, Allolio B. Suramin in adrenocortical cancer: limited efficacy and serious toxicity. *Clin Endocrinol* 1994;41:299.
98. Raymond E, Izbicka E, Soda H, et al. Activity of temozolomide against human tumor colony-forming units. *Clin Cancer Res* 1997;10:1769.
99. Fallo F, Pilon C, Barzon L, et al. Paclitaxel is an effective antiproliferative agent on the human NCI-H295 adrenocortical carcinoma cell line. *Chemotherapy* 1998;44:129.
100. Fallo F, Pilon C, Barzon L, et al. Effects of Taxol on the human NCI-H295 adrenocortical carcinoma cell line. *Endocr Res* 1996;22:709.
101. Wu YW, Chek CL, Knazck RA. An *in vitro* study of antitumor effects of gossypol in human SW-13 adrenocortical carcinoma. *Cancer Res* 1989;49:3754.
102. Avico M, Bossi G, Livieri C. Partial response after intensive chemotherapy in a child. *Med Pediatr Oncol* 1992;20:246.
103. Didolkar MS, Bescher RA, Elias EG, Moore RH. Natural history of adrenal cortical carcinoma: a clinicopathologic study of 42 patients. *Cancer* 1981;47:2153.
104. Icard P, Chapuis Y, Andreassian B, Bernard A, Proye C. Adrenocortical carcinoma in surgically treated patients: a retrospective study on 156 cases by the French Association of Endocrine Surgery. *Surgery* 1992;112:972.
105. Pommier R, Brenna MF. An 11 year experience with adrenocortical cancer. *Surgery* 1992;112:1963.
106. Bates SE, Shieh CY, Mickley LA, et al. Mitotane enhances cytotoxicity of chemotherapy in cell lines expressing a multidrug resistance gene (mdr-1/P-glycoprotein) which is also expressed by adrenocortical carcinomas. *J Clin Endocrinol Metab* 1991;73:18.
107. Christy NP. Adrenocorticotrophic activity in plasma of patients with Cushing's syndrome associated with pulmonary neoplasms. *Lancet* 1961;1:85.
108. Liddle GW, Island D, Meador CK. Normal and abnormal regulation of corticotropin secretion in man. *Recent Prog Horm Res* 1962;18:125.
109. Pass HI, Doppman JL, Nieman L, et al. Management of the ectopic ACTH syndrome due to thoracic carcinoids. *Ann Thorac Surg* 1990;50:52.
110. Proye C, Vix M, Goropoulos A, Kulo P, Leconte-Houcke M. High incidence of malignant pheochromocytomas. *J Endocrinol Invest* 1992;15:651.
111. Lairmore TC, Ball W, Baylin SB, Wells AS Jr. Management of pheochromocytomas in patients with multiple endocrine neoplasia type 2 syndromes. *Ann Surg* 1993;217:595.
112. Loughlin KR, Gittes RF. Urological management of patients with von Hippel-Lindau's disease. *J Urol* 1986;136:789.
113. Nakagawara A. Malignant pheochromocytoma with ganglioneuroblastomatous elements in a patient with von Recklinghausen's disease. *Cancer* 1985;55:2794.
114. Mann SJ. Severe paroxysmal hypertension (pseudopheochromocytoma): understanding the cause and treatment. *Arch Intern Med* 1999;159:670.
115. Moley JF, Brother MB, Wells SA, et al. Low frequency of *ras* gene mutations in neuroblastomas, pheochromocytomas and medullary thyroid cancers. *Cancer Res* 1991;51:1596.
116. Khosia S, Patel VM, Hay ID, et al. Loss of heterozygosity suggests multiple genetic alterations in pheochromocytomas and medullary thyroid carcinomas. *J Clin Invest* 1991; 87:1691.
117. Duerr EM, Gimm O, Neuberg DS, et al. Differences in allelic distribution of two polymorphisms in the VHL-associated gene *CUL2* in pheochromocytoma patients without somatic *CUL2* mutations. *J Clin Endocrinol Metab* 1999;84:3207.
118. Lips KJM, Van der Sluys Veer J, Struyvenberg A, et al. Bilateral occurrence of pheochromocytoma in patients with multiple endocrine neoplasia syndrome type 2a (Sipple's syndrome). *Am J Med* 1981;70:1051.
119. Remine WH, Chong GC, van Heerden JA, Sheps SG, Harison EG. Current management of pheochromocytoma. *Ann Surg* 1974;179:740.
120. Sutton MGS, Sheps SG, Lie JT. Prevalence of clinically unsuspected pheochromocytoma. Review of a 50 year autopsy series. *Mayo Clin Proc* 1981;56:354.
121. Scott HW, Halter SA. Oncologic aspects of pheochromocytoma: the importance of follow-up. *Surgery* 1984;96:1061.
122. Beierwaltes WH, Sisson JC, Shapiro B, et al. Malignant potential of pheochromocytoma. *Proc American Association of Cancer Research* 1986;27:617.
123. Brown HM, Komorowski RA, Wilson SD, Demeure MJ, Zhu YR. Predicting metastasis of pheochromocytomas using DNA flow cytometry and immunohistochemical markers of cell proliferation: a positive correlation between MIB-1 staining and malignant tumor behavior. *Cancer* 1999;86:1583.
124. Sheps SG, Jiang NS, Klec GG, van Heerden JA. Recent developments in the diagnosis and management of pheochromocytoma. *Mayo Clin Proc* 1990;65:88.
125. Helman LJ, Cohen PS, Averbuch SD, et al. Neuropeptide Y expression distinguishes malignant from benign pheochromocytoma. *J Clin Oncol* 1989;7:1720.
126. Grouzmann E, Gicquel C, Pluin PF, et al. Neuropeptide Y and neuron specific enolase levels in benign and malignant pheochromocytomas. *Cancer* 1990;66:1833.
127. Medeiros LJ, Wolf BC, Balogh K, Federman M. Adrenal pheochromocytoma. A clinicopathologic review of 60 cases. *Hum Pathol* 1985;16:580.
128. Hanson MW, Feldman JM, Beam CA, Leight GS, Coleman E. Iodine 131–labelled metaiodobenzylguanidine scintigraphy and biochemical analyses in suspected pheochromocytoma. *Arch Intern Med* 1991;151:1397.
129. Samaan NA, Hickey RC, Shutts PE. Diagnosis, localization and management of pheochromocytoma. *Cancer* 1988;62:2451.
130. Duncan MW, Compton P, Lazarus L, Smythe GA. Measurement of norepinephrine and 3,4-dihydroxyphenylglycol in urine and plasma for the diagnosis of pheochromocytoma. *N Engl J Med* 1988;319:136.
131. MacDougall IC, Isles CG, Stewart H, et al. Overnight clonidine suppression test in the diagnosis and exclusion of pheochromocytoma. *Am J Med* 1988;84:993.
132. Bravo EL, Tarazi RC, Fouad FM, Vidt DG, Gifford RW. Clonidine suppression test: a useful aid in the diagnosis of pheochromocytoma. *N Engl J Med* 1981;305:623.
133. Taylor HC, Mayes D, Anton AH. Clonidine suppression test for pheochromocytoma: examples of misleading results. *J Clin Endocrinol Metab* 1986;63:238.
134. Welch TJ, Sheedy PF, van Heerden JA, et al. Pheochromocytoma: value of computed tomography. *Radiology* 1983;148:501.
135. Radin DR, Ralls PW, Boswell WD, et al. Pheochromocytoma: detection by unenhanced CT. *AJR Am J Roentgenol* 1986;146:741.
136. Velchik MG, Alavi A, Kressel HY, Engelman K. Localization of pheochromocytoma: MIBG, CT and MRI correlation. *J Nucl Med* 1989;30:328.
137. Shapiro B, Copp JE, Sisson JC, et al. Iodine-131 metaiodobenzylguanidine for the locating of suspected pheochromocytoma: experience in 400 cases. *J Nucl Med* 1985; 26:576.
138. Swenson SJ, Brown MJ, Sheps SG, et al. Use of ^{131}I-MIBG scintigraphy in the evaluation of suspected pheochromocytoma. *Mayo Clin Proc* 1985;60:299.
139. Koizumi M, Endo K, Sakahara H, et al. Computed tomography and ^{131}I-MIBG scintigraphy in the diagnosis of pheochromocytoma. *Acta Radiologica Diag* 1986;27:305.
140. Fischer M, Galanski M, Winterberg B, Vetter H. Localization procedures in pheochromocytoma and neuroblastoma. *Cardiology* 1985;72:143.
141. Perry RR, Keiser HR, Norton JA, et al. Surgical management of pheochromocytoma with the use of metyrosine. *Ann Surg* 1990;212:621.
142. Imperato-McGinley J, Gautier T, Ehlers K, et al. Reversibility of catecholamine-induced dilated cardiomyopathy in a child with a pheochromocytoma. *N Engl J Med* 1987;316:793.
143. Steinsapir J, Carr AA, Prisant LM, Bransome ED Jr. Metyrosine and pheochromocytoma. *Arch Intern Med* 1997;157:901.
144. Proye C, Thevenin D, Cecat P, et al. Exclusive use of calcium channel blockers in preoperative and intraoperative control of pheochromocytomas: hemodynamics and free catecholamine assays in ten consecutive patients. *Surgery* 1989;106:1149.
145. Irvin GL, Fishman LM, Sher JA, Yeung LK, Irane H. Pheochromocytoma lateral vs anterior operative approach. *Ann Surg* 1989;209:774.
146. Carneyl JA, Sizemore GW, Sheps SG. Adrenal medullary disease in multiple endocrine neoplasia, type 2. *Am J Clin Pathol* 1976;66:279.
147. Cance WG, Wells SAJ. Multiple endocrine neoplasia type IIa. *Curr Probl Surg* 1985;22:1.
148. Kopf D, Bockisch A, Steinert H, et al. Octreotide scintigraphy and catecholamine response to an octreotide challenge in malignant pheochromocytoma. *Clin Endocrinol* 1997;46:39.
149. Tenenbaum F, Schlumberger M, Lumbroso J, Parmentier C. Beneficial effects of octreotide in a patient with metastatic paraganglioma. *Eur J Cancer* 1996;32:737.
150. van Heerden JA, Sheps SG, Hamberger B, et al. Pheochromocytoma: current status and changing trends. *Surgery* 1982;91:367.
151. Ein SH, Weitzman S, Thornes P, Seagram CG, Filler RM. Pediatric malignant pheochromocytoma. *J Pediatric Surg* 1994;29:1197.
152. Guo JZ, Gong LS, Chen SX, Luo BY, Xu MY. Malignant pheochromocytoma: diagnosis and treatment in fifteen cases. *J Hypertens* 1989;7:261.
153. Scott WH, Reynolds V, Green N, et al. Clinical experience with malignant pheochromocytoma. *Surg Gynecol Obstet* 1982;154:801.
154. Feldman JM. Treatment of metastatic pheochromocytoma with streptozotocin. *Arch Intern Med* 1983;143:1799.
155. Feldman JM. [In reply to a letter to the editor by Gross DJ, Schlank E, Ipp E.] *Arch Intern Med* 1985;145:368.

156. Kreempf M, Lumbroso J, Mornex R, et al. Use of m-[131I]iodobenzylguanidine in the treatment of malignant pheochromocytoma. *J Clin Endocrinol Metab* 1991;72:455.
157. Feldman JM, Frankel N, Coleman RE. Platelet uptake of the pheochromocytoma-scanning agent ^{131}I-meta-iodobenzylguanidine. *Metabolism* 1984;33:397.
158. Vetter H, Fischer M, Muller-Rensing R, Vetter W, Winterberg B. [^{131}I]-meta-iodobenzylguanidine in treatment of malignant pheochromocytomas. *Lancet* 1983;2:107.
159. Troncone L, Rufini V. ^{131}I-MIBG therapy of neural crest tumors [review]. *Anticancer Res* 1997;17:1823.
160. Nakabeppu Y, Nakajo M. Radionuclide therapy of malignant pheochromocytoma with ^{131}I-MIBG. *Ann Nucl Med* 1994;8:259.
161. Averbuch SD, Steakley CS, Young RC, et al. Malignant pheochromocytoma: effective treatment with a combination of cyclophosphamide, vincristine and dacarbazine. *Ann Intern Med* 1988;109:267.
162. Finklestein JZ, Klemperer MR, Evans A, et al. Multiagent chemotherapy for children with metastatic neuroblastoma: a report from children's cancer study group. *Med Pediatr Oncol* 1979;6:179.
163. Tato A, Orte L, Diz P, Quereda C, Ortuno J. Malignant pheochromocytoma, still a therapeutic challenge. *Am J Hypertens* 1997;10:479.
164. Tada K, Okuda Y, Yamashita K. Three cases of malignant pheochromocytomas treated with cyclophosphamide, vincristine and dacarbazine combination chemotherapy and alpha-methyl-p-tyrosine to control hypercatecholaminemia. *Horm Res* 1998;49:295.
165. Sisson JC, Shapiro B, Shulkin BL, et al. Treatment of malignant pheochromocytomas with ^{131}I-MIBG (metaiodobenzylguanidine) and chemotherapy. *Am J Clin Oncol* 1999; 22:364.
166. Berruti A, Terrzolo M, Pia A, Angeli A, Dogliotti L. Mitotane associated with etoposide, doxorubicin, and cisplatin in the treatment of advanced adrenocortical carcinoma. Italian Group for the Study of Adrenal Cancer. *Cancer* 1998;83:2194.
167. Zidan J, Shpendler M, Robinson E. Treatment of metastatic adrenal cortical carcinoma with etoposide (VP-16) and cisplatin after failure with o,p'DDD. Clinical case reports. *Am J Clin Oncol* 1996;19:229.
168. Noshiro T, Honma H, Shimizu K, et al. Two cases of malignant pheochromocytoma treated with cyclophosphamide, vincristine and dacarbazine in a combined chemotherapy. *Endocr J* 1996;43:279.
169. Arai A, Naruse M, Naruse K, et al. Cardiac malignant pheochromocytoma with bone metastases. *Intern Med* 1998;37:940.

SECTION 5

H. RICHARD ALEXANDER
ROBERT T. JENSEN

Pancreatic Endocrine Tumors

INTRODUCTION

Pancreatic endocrine (or neuroendocrine) tumors (PETs) are uncommon neoplasms that share a number of features.[1,2] Histologically, they are classified as apudomas and share cytochemical features with melanoma, pheochromocytoma, carcinoid tumors, and medullary thyroid carcinoma.[2] All amine precursor uptake and decarboxylation (APUD) neoplasms have the capacity to synthesize and secrete polypeptide products that have specific endocrine hormone activity. Except for insulinoma, each is malignant in most (more than 60%), if not all, cases (Table 38.5-1). Each type is a vascular tumor sharing with the other types a similar radiographic appearance and metastatic patterns of spread (primarily to regional lymph nodes and liver).

PETs are considered *functional* if they are associated with a clinical syndrome due to ectopic hormone release or *nonfunctional* if not associated with clinical symptoms. In the latter category are pancreatic polypeptide (PP) tumors (PPomas), as the hormone causes no specific symptoms.[1,3] In addition, some PETS are associated with no known hormone elevation and histologically are indistinguishable from functional tumors.[1]

In general, PETs are uncommon. Functional PETs are reported to have a prevalence of 10 per million population.[4] The prevalence in unselected autopsy studies is 0.5% to 1.5%, with fewer than 1 of 1000 being functional.[1,5] The incidence of clinically significant PETs is 3.6 to 4 per million population per year; nonfunctional PETs or PPomas are reported to account for 15% to 30% of all PETs.[3,6] Gastrinomas or PPomas are the most common malignant PETs, whereas insulinoma is the most common benign PET. Gastrinomas usually are clinically recognized because of the Zollinger-Ellison syndrome (ZES) and have been studied extensively.[7–9] This chapter presents information in a format that reflects the many similarities of PETs, though detailed discussions of each tumor type are provided for those tumors associated with unique issues.

PATHOGENESIS, PATHOLOGIC FEATURES, AND TUMOR BIOLOGY

GENERALLY MALIGNANT NEOPLASMS

In 1955, Zollinger and Ellison described two patients with severe peptic ulcer disease treatable only by total gastrectomy because of extreme hypersecretion of gastric acid associated with a non-β islet cell tumor of the pancreas.[10] Analysis of tumor extracts via enzymatic degradation and amino acid analysis demonstrated that the secretagogue in the tumor was identical to human antral gastrin[11,12]; hence, these tumors are called *gastrinomas.* Studies estimate that the ZES occurs in one-half to three patients per million population per year and varies from half as common to 1.2 times as common as insulinomas.[13]

Almost all the early clinical manifestations are due to gastric acid hypersecretion secondary to hypergastrinemia.[14] Effective control of the gastric hypersecretion either medically or surgically abolishes all clinical manifestations such as peptic ulcer disease or diarrhea.[14,15] Along with basal gastric acid hypersecretion, hypergastrinemia causes trophic changes in the gastric mucosa,[16] with the result that patients with ZES have increased numbers of parietal cells and an increased maximum acid secretory capacity.[14,16] Many patients with ZES have diarrhea and, in some patients, it is the sole presenting manifestation. The diarrhea is a result of acid hypersecretion causing direct injury to the small intestinal mucosa, inactivation of pancreatic lipase, and precipitation of bile acids. ZES patients with diarrhea become asymptomatic when the gastric acid hypersecretion is controlled, even though the hypergastrinemia remains unchanged.[14]

Gastrin in both normal subjects and patients with ZES has been found in a number of different molecular sizes. In gastrinoma, gastrin 17 (G_{17}) is the major gastrin component, composing 74% to 80% of the total immunoreactivity, with "big gastrin" or gastrin 34 (G_{34}), making up most of the remainder.[17] In contrast, in sera from normal subjects and patients without gastrinoma, G_{34} contributes more than 60% of the total gastrin immunoreactivity.[14] In addition to G_{17} and G_{34}, smaller and larger forms of gastrin have been described in sera and gastrinomas from patients with ZES.[2,8,9,18,19] Also, a large-molecular-weight progastrin has been described in plasma and tumors of patients with gastrinomas.[20,21] High amounts of progastrin have been found in patients with gastrinoma metastatic to liver.[20] The relative amount of G_{17}, the amount of NH_2-terminal fragments, and the ratio of the amount of G_{17} amino-terminal immunoreac-

TABLE 38.5-1. Enteropancreatic Endocrine Tumors

Tumor Name	*Syndrome Name*	*Hormone*	*Percentage Malignant*	*Location*
PPoma	PPoma	Pancreatic polypeptide	>60	Pancreas
Nonfunctioning	Nonfunctioning pancreatic endocrine tumor	None	>60	Pancreas
Symptoms due to released hormones				
Gastrinomas	Zollinger-Ellison syndrome	Gastrin	60–90	Pancreas (30–60%)
				Duodenum (30–43%)
				Other (10–20%)
Insulinoma	Insulinoma	Insulin	10–15	Pancreas (>99%)
VIPoma	Pancreatic cholera	Vasoactive intestinal peptide	80	Pancreas (90%)
	Verner-Morrison syndrome			Adrenal gland (10%)
	WDHA			
Glucagonoma	Glucagonoma	Glucagon	60	Pancreas (>99%)
Somatostatinoma	Somatostatinoma	Somatostatin	71	Pancreas (56%)
				Upper small intestine (44%)
GRFoma	GRFoma	Growth hormone–releasing peptide	30	Pancreas (33%)
				Lung (53%)
				Small intestine (10%)
				Other (7%)
ACTHoma	Ectopic Cushing's syndrome	ACTH	>95 (pancreatic)	Pancreas (4–16%)

ACTH, adrenocorticotropic hormone; GRF, growth hormone–releasing factor; WDHA, watery diarrhea, hypokalemia, and achlorhydria.

tivity to the amount of G_{17} carboxy-terminal immunoreactivity have been shown to be predictive of the extent of the gastrinoma by some investigators[22] but not others.[20]

In recent studies, the proportion of gastrinomas found at surgery in the duodenum and in lymph nodes near the pancreatic head has increased to greater than 50%,[23–26] such that 65% to 90% of all gastrinomas found at surgery occur in the pancreatic head and duodenal area (Table 38.5-2).[23,25] Gastrinomas have also been reported to occur occasionally in other sites such as the liver, stomach, jejunum, mesentery, common bile duct, heart, and spleen (Fig. 38.5-1).[14,28] In women, ovarian gastrinomas can occur and are functionally indistinguishable from other gastrinomas.[14,27–29]

At present, the cell of origin of gastrinomas and other PETs remains obscure. Recent studies have provided evidence that duodenal gastrinoma, which usually contains many well-differentiated gastrin-containing (G) cells (in contrast to pancreatic gastrinoma), originates from gastrin cells in the duodenal crypts and Brunner's glands.[30,31] Because pancreatic gastrinomas are pleomorphic with heterogeneous cell types, it has been proposed that they originate from a multipotential, endocrine-programmed stem cell that undergoes somewhat inappropriate and incomplete differentiation toward the G cell.[30,31] As G cells are not normally present in the adult pancreas, pancreatic gastrinomas are generally considered ectopic, whereas gastrinomas in areas that normally contain G cells (duodenum, stomach, jejunum) are considered entopic.[14,32]

TABLE 38.5-2. Sites of Apparent Primary Gastrinoma

Location	*Frequency (%)*
Duodenal	40–50
Pancreatic	30–40
Lymph node	10–15
Ectopic (nonpancreaticoduodenal or nodal)	≤5
Liver	
Common bile duct	
Cardiac	
Mesentery	
Spleen	
Ovary	

In early studies in which patients presented late in the course of their disease, gastrinomas were found at surgery in most patients with ZES (81% to 94%).[33] In subsequent studies of patients undergoing potentially curative surgery, no gastrinomas were found in as many as 50% of patients.[34] Recent studies have shown that almost all the missed gastrinomas were in the duodenum.[25] Now that exploration of the duodenum is being performed routinely, gastrinomas are found in more than 90% of patients.[35]

In early studies, 60% to more than 90% of patients with ZES had a malignant gastrinoma,[32,33,36,37] whereas in recent studies only one-half of patients have a malignant gastrinoma at the time of diagnosis. Metastases usually are to peripancreatic lymph nodes and to the liver.[14] Bone metastases have been reported in approximately 30% of patients with metastatic gastrinoma in the liver.[38–40] The diagnosis of malignancy is complicated by the fact that no histologic criteria predict malignancy, which can be established only by the presence of metastases.[2,14] Even metastatic disease can be difficult to establish, because a number of cases of extrapancreatic gastrinoma localized in lymph nodes have been described with no evidence of primary

A, B

C, D

E, F

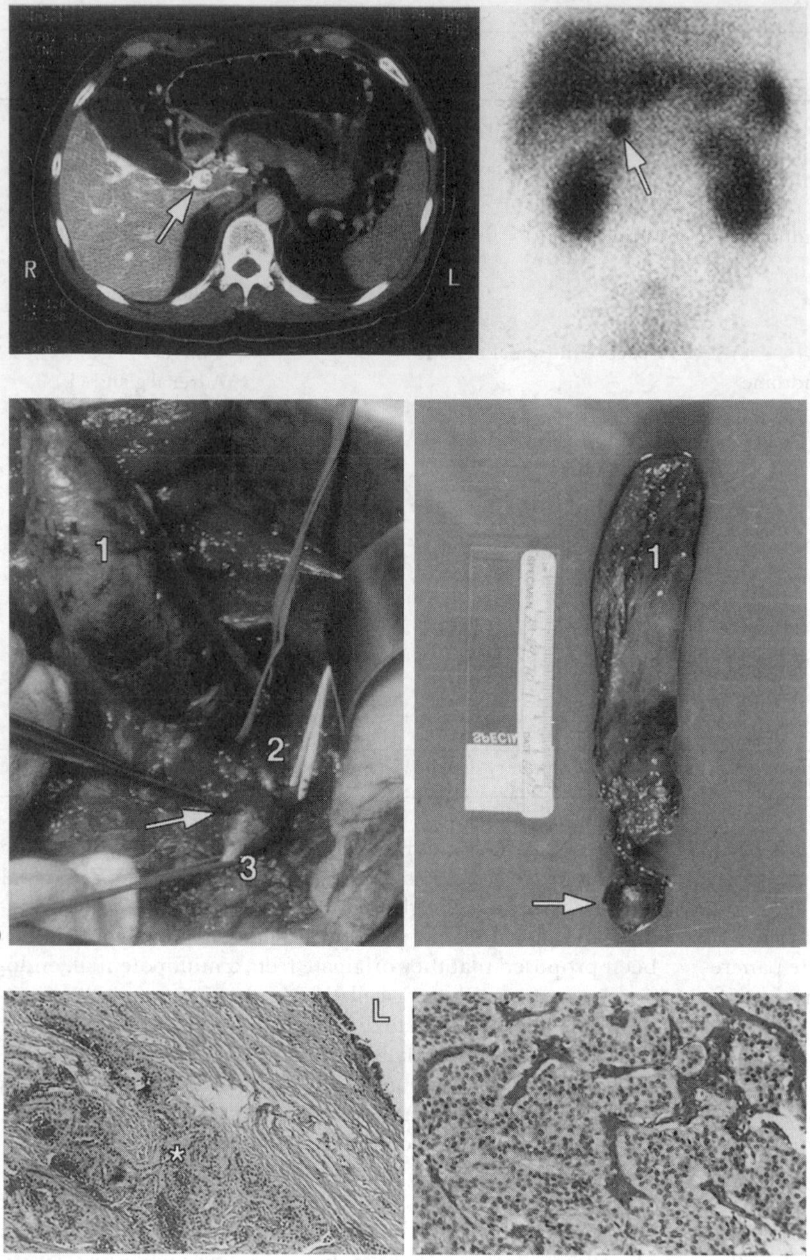

FIGURE 38.5-1. Patient with a primary gastrinoma of the common bile duct, illustrating several important features of the disease. Computed tomography scan after selective angiography **(A)** shows a 1.5-cm enhancing nodule (*arrow*) at neck of gallbladder just above the head of the pancreas, which is also seen on somatostatin receptor scintigraphy **(B)**. **C:** At surgical exploration, a discrete mass is seen within the wall of the common bile duct (*arrow* shows primary tumor; 1, gallbladder; 2, cystic duct; 3, common bile duct). The primary tumor after resection **(D)** was a primary intracholedochal gastrinoma **(E)**, and the adjacent lumen of the bile duct (L) is lined by normal epithelium. The tumor showed typical aggregation of neuroendocrine cells and dense vasculature characteristic of neuroendocrine tumors **(F)**. Immunoperoxidase stained positive for chromogranin, synaptophysin, and gastrin. (From ref. 29.)

tumor. Some of these cases have apparently been cured by excision of lymph nodes, which suggests that the gastrinoma was not metastatic but rather originated in the lymph node.[41]

Numerous studies have attempted to identify predictors of malignancy in gastrinomas as well as other PETs. Clinically, tumor size has been shown to be an important predictor of liver metastases but not lymph node metastases.[26] Liver metastases occurred in 4% of gastrinomas less than 1 cm in diameter, in 28% of tumors measuring 1.1 to 2.9 cm, and in 61% of tumors larger than 3 cm.[26] In several prospective studies, duodenal gastrinomas have been found to be malignant with metastatic spread in 48% to 75% of cases.[25,26,42] In one large study involving 90 patients with ZES with pancreatic or duodenal gastrinomas, an equal percentage had lymph node metastases (48% and 47%, respectively), showing that, as regards lymph node metastases, the malignant potential of ectopic and entopic gastrinomas does not differ.[26] However, in this same study, 5% of patients with duodenal gastrinomas had liver metastases, which was significantly less (P<.00001) than the 52% incidence in patients with pancreatic gastrinomas. Because most duodenal gastrinomas are small (80% <1 cm) and most pancreatic gastrinomas are large (70% ≥3 cm), it remains unclear whether tumor size and location are independent predictors.

Recent studies have attempted to use assessments of nuclear DNA to differentiate benign from malignant gastrinomas and other PETs.[2,43] DNA ploidy analysis in some studies did not predict prognosis.[2] However, in a study of 59 patients with gastrinomas, 54% were diploid, 15% near-diploid, 0% pure tetraploid, and 25% nontetraploid aneuploid, while another 5% exhibited multiple stem line aneuploidy.[44] All patients with multiple stem line aneuploidy had widespread metastases, and the results of the DNA analysis correlated with disease extent.[44] Silver staining of nuclear organizer regions, expression of the proliferating nuclear antigen, and expression of the cell cycle–associated antigen Ki-67, have all been reported to be potentially useful in differentiating benign from malignant PETs.[43] Chromosomal abnormalities have recently been reported in PETs in five of nine patients, but such alterations were not associated with more aggressive tumor behavior.[45] The protooncogene HER-2/*neu* recently was reported to be overexpressed in gastrinomas from 11 patients, with no mutations in the *ras* gene and a mutation in the p53 gene in only 1 of 11 patients.[46] No correlation with malignancy and HER-2/*neu* was found, but a previous study by the same investigators on carcinoid tumors of the gastrointestinal tract found a trend toward increased HER-2/*neu* copy number and aggressiveness.[47] Similarly, no abnormal expression of p53 protein was found in PETs in another study.[43]

One study showed allelic loss on chromosome 11q13 in gastric carcinoids from patients with multiple endocrine neoplasia type 1 (MEN 1) and ZES, suggesting that the pathogenesis of these tumors is similar to that of the pancreatic and parathyroid tumors that develop in MEN 1 patients.[48,49] Using positional cloning, the gene for MEN 1 has been located on chromosome 11q13,[50] and approximately 30% of gastrinomas occurring in the sporadic setting have mutations in the gene.[51]

Approximately 20% of patients with ZES have a familial form and demonstrate evidence of MEN 1 (Wermer's syndrome). MEN 1 is an autosomal dominant trait characterized by hyperplasia or tumors of multiple endocrine organs, hyperparathyroidism being the most common abnormality.[52] Islet cell tumors of the pancreas are the second most common abnormality, occurring in 82% of MEN 1 patients, with 57% having ZES and 25% insulinomas.[52–54] Pituitary and adrenal adenomas are less common. Patients with MEN 1 with ZES differ from sporadic cases in that they frequently present at a younger age; their tumors are almost always multiple and frequently small and, in some studies, patients with MEN 1 have an increased survival rate as compared with sporadic cases.[7,26,54]

Immunocytochemical studies of tumors from patients with ZES have demonstrated gastrin in 90% to 100% in some studies and in 56% to 78% in others.[14] This difference may be due to differences in tissue fixation or type of gastrin antibody used or to a low content of gastrin in small tumors. Recent studies have demonstrated that more than 50% of tumors also demonstrated other peptides, including PP in 17% to 50%, insulin in 20% to 33%, glucagon in 0% to 33%, somatostatin in 0% to 33%, and adrenocorticotropic hormone–like immunoreactivity in 0% to 30%.[14,54] In one report that reviewed seven different immunocytochemical studies involving tumors from 75 patients with ZES, gastrin was found in 80%, insulin in 30%, human PP (HPP) in 35%, glucagon in 29%, and somatostatin in 21%.[55] Therefore, it has become increasingly difficult, if not impossible, to determine which of the hormones found in a tumor by immunocytochemistry are clinically important in a given patient.[14] The endocrine nature of the tumor is not always apparent and, at present, to obtain a precise classification, a combination of clinical and biochemical data and immunocytochemical studies for peptides as well as for chromogranins, neuron-specific enolase, and synaptophysin frequently are necessary.[56,57]

Plasma elevations of peptides other than gastrin frequently occur in ZES.[14] A prospective study in 45 consecutive cases of ZES demonstrated increased concentrations in plasma of another peptide besides gastrin in 62%.[55] Motilin was the peptide most often present at abnormally high levels (29%), and neurotensin and gastrin-releasing peptide were elevated in 20% and 10%, respectively. HPP was elevated in plasma in 27% of patients, which compares with plasma HPP elevations of 10% to 60% described previously.[58,59] Some investigators have proposed that plasma HPP elevations might be a useful marker for identifying patients with metastatic liver disease,[60] but other researchers do not agree.[61] Despite frequent reports of finding insulin, glucagon, or somatostatin by immunocytochemical study, as well as occasional ZES patients with a concomitant insulinoma[62] or glucagonoma, no patient had increased amounts of these peptides in plasma in the aforementioned prospective study of 45 patients.[55] The presence or absence of abnormal plasma levels of a particular peptide or the extent of elevation did not correlate with location of tumor, extent of tumor, or the presence or absence of a particular symptom.[63] Adrenocorticotropic hormone (ACTH) production in PETs, particularly in ZES patients, is associated with a very aggressive tumor phenotype.[40,64]

Elevated concentrations of human chorionic gonadotropin (HCG) subunits (α or β chains) in sera or in the tumor by immunocytochemistry occur in some patients with gastrinoma and may be predictive of malignancy.[57] In a study of 30 patients with ZES, 57% of patients with malignant and 45% with benign disease had elevated concentrations of α-HCG in plasma.[65] Seven patients had elevated levels of β-HCG in plasma, with four having malignant disease. This study demonstrates that elevated plasma concentrations of α- or β-HCG are not useful in predicting malignancy.

Chromogranin A is a 48-kD protein that is co-stored and co-released with peptide hormones from gastrointestinal tract endocrine cells and tumors[57] and is not produced by nonendocrine cells. Immunocytochemical staining for chromogranin A has shown its presence in gastrinomas, carcinoids, antral G cells, and fundic enterochromaffin-like (ECL) cells of the stomach.[57,66] Elevated levels in the plasma are reported to be one of the best markers for PETs, although chromogranin levels also are elevated in carcinoid and other neuroendocrine tumors.[57] In a recent study of 72 patients with PETs or carcinoid tumors, 99% had elevated plasma chromogranin A levels, 88% chromogranin B levels, and 6% chromogranin C levels.[67] In another study, plasma chromogranin A levels were measured in 112 patients with ZES, and the value correlated significantly with fasting serum gastrin (FSG) levels.[68] However, there was no correlation between the plasma level of chromogranin A and the amount of tumor, presence or absence of metastatic disease, or presence or absence of MEN 1.[68]

Histologic studies have demonstrated the general similarity of PETs and carcinoid tumors.[1,2] Different histologic classifications have been proposed based on growth patterns, including a glandular pattern, solid nests of cells (solid pattern), a trabecular or ribbon-like structure (gyriform pattern), and unclassified pattern.[1,2,14] Similar patterns have been demonstrated in tumors from patients with other endocrine tumors, and the type of histologic pattern does not correlate with the type of hormone produced, clinical symptoms, or malignancy. Ultrastructural classifications have all been proposed on the basis of the type of granules seen, but this also does not correlate with malignancy or clinical features.[2,14]

GENERALLY BENIGN NEOPLASMS: INSULINOMA

Insulinomas were first recognized by Whipple,[69] who described 30 patients with hypoglycemia and pancreatic adenomas. Whipple's triad consists of the characteristic symptoms of hypoglycemia associated with blood glucose levels of less than 50 mg/dL and immediate relief after ingestion of glucose and have, for many years, remained the major criteria for the diagnosis of insulinoma.[69] Insulinomas usually occur in patients between the ages of 20 and 75 years. The average age at presentation is between 44 and 46 years, and there is a preponderance of women in most series (60%).[1,70,71]

Insulinomas are the opposite of gastrinomas, in that whereas 60% to 90% of gastrinomas are malignant, only 5% to 11% of insulinomas are malignant.[1,70–73] Most insulinomas are found to be solitary benign pancreatic nodules, often encapsulated, with only 2% to 10% of patients having multiple tumors.[1,70,71] In a patient with multiple insulinomas, MEN 1 should be suspected.[52] Insulinomas are uniformly distributed throughout the entire pancreas and are usually less than 1.5 cm in maximum diameter.[72,73]

CLINICAL PRESENTATION AND DIAGNOSIS

Resection is the only curative modality for patients with PETs, and the success of operation is contingent on establishing the correct diagnosis, determining whether a patient may belong to a MEN kindred, performing appropriate radiographic imaging studies to assess the location of the primary tumor and the extent of regional or distant metastatic spread, and ensuring adequate medical management of the functional sequelae of excess hormone production preoperatively.

GASTRINOMA

Gastrinomas are slightly more common in men (60%) than in women (40%). The mean age at diagnosis is 45 to 50 years, and approximately 20% of patients have MEN 1. The most common presentation in patients with ZES is abdominal pain in 26% to 58%, which usually cannot be differentiated from pain caused by other common acid peptic disorders.[8,9,74] However, in some studies, a significant proportion of individuals (14% to 25%) have no peptic ulcer or abdominal pain at the time of diagnosis.[74] Diarrhea is the initial symptom in 37% to 73% of patients and, in 15% to 18%, it is the only symptom. In one study involving 122 patients with ZES, esophageal symptoms, endoscopic abnormalities, or both were present in 61% of patients.[75] In early studies, up to 93% of patients had a peptic ulcer and, in 36%, the ulcers were multiple or in unusual locations.[8,9] Although the decreased severity of peptic ulcer disease at diagnosis suggests that in patients with ZES diagnoses are being made earlier, in almost all series a delay of 3 to 6 years still exists between the onset of symptoms and diagnosis.[76] Intestinal perforation, especially of the jejunum, is a presenting event in up to 7% of patients with ZES.[77]

The diagnosis should be suspected on the basis of the clinical presentation and established in almost all patients by demonstrating elevated basal gastric acid secretion [basal acid output (BAO)] and fasting hypergastrinemia.[7] Between 38% and 68% of patients have a solitary peptic ulcer, and 14% to 25% have no peptic ulcer. ZES should be suspected in the clinical setting of peptic ulcer with diarrhea, familial peptic ulcer, peptic ulcer in unusual locations, and recurrent or resistant peptic ulcer. ZES should be particularly suspected in patients with peptic ulcers that persist or recur despite treatment for *Helicobacter pylori* infection or with H_2-receptor antagonists, in patients with severe esophagitis, and in patients with duodenal ulcers without *H pylori* infection.[74] *H pylori* is present in 90% to 98% of patients with idiopathic duodenal ulcer disease, and 90% heal with *H pylori* eradication; in ZES, fewer than 50% of patients have *H pylori* infection. In all patients who have peptic ulcer disease severe enough to require gastric surgery, at least one preoperative FSG level should be obtained.

To make the diagnosis of ZES, it is necessary to demonstrate an FSG elevated above 200 pg/mL and an elevated BAO.[8,74,78] The FSG concentration usually is obtained first, and only rarely do normal values occur in patients with ZES.[79,80] Although nearly 32% of patients with ZES have an FSG of at least 1000 pg/mL, in the remaining two-thirds the FSG is elevated but not to the level of 1000 pg/mL.[81] Two general types of disorders other than ZES are also known to cause elevation in FSG: those associated with gastric acid hypersecretion and those associated with hypochlorhydria or achlorhydria, including chronic gastritis, gastric cancer, and pernicious anemia and in postvagotomy patients.[8,9] One of the most common causes of FSG elevation is drug-induced hypergastrinemia due to inhibition of acid secretion with H^+K^+-ATPase inhibitors (omeprazole, lansoprazole).[8] Similarly, *H pylori* infection can, on occasion, cause elevations of FSG in the range seen in ZES.[82] No absolute level of elevation in FSG distinguishes patients with disorders of acid hypersecretion versus hyposecretion; they can be distinguished only by direct assessment of acid output. If facilities are not available to measure the BAO, then a simple determination of the pH of the gastric contents (while the patient is not taking antisecretory medications) should be performed. A pH of 2.5 or higher virtually excludes the diagnosis of ZES.[78]

The most commonly used secretory criteria for diagnosing ZES are a BAO of at least 15 mEq/h in patients who have not undergone previous acid-reducing operations and at least 5 mEq/h in patients who have had previous acid-reducing operations.[8,74] The mean BAO in various series ranged from 34 to 53 mEq/h for patients with a history of previous acid-reducing surgery.[14] A BAO of at least 15 mEq/h will include up to 99% of patients with ZES and exclude 90% of patients with routine duodenal ulcers. In patients who have undergone previous acid-reducing surgery, the mean BAO exceeds 5 mEq/h in most studies but, in 6% to 45% of ZES patients, is less than 5 mEq/h.[78] Patients with ZES also have an elevated maximum acid output (MAO) and an elevated BAO/MAO ratio that often exceeds 0.6.[74,83] However, diagnostic criteria based on the MAO or BAO/MAO ratio offer no advantage over an elevated BAO alone.[8,9]

If a patient has an FSG of at least 1000 pg/mL and a gastric pH of less than 2.5, then the diagnosis of ZES generally is established.[1,74] The only other disorder that can mimic ZES in this capacity is retained gastric antrum syndrome, an uncommon condition that occurs in patients who have undergone a Billroth II gastroenterostomy with a portion of antrum left attached to the excluded proximal duodenal stump. This diagnosis can be excluded in patients after gastric surgery by the secretin stimulation test and by gastric ^{99m}Tc pertechnetate scanning. In patients with only moderately elevated FSG levels and a gastric pH of less than 2.5, ZES must be differentiated from retained gastric antrum syndrome, *H pylori* infection, chronic gastric outlet obstruction, antral G-cell hyperplasia, massive small bowel resection and, rarely, chronic renal failure. These conditions are best distinguished from ZES by the use of various gastrin-provocative tests, including the secretin test,[84,85] calcium infusion test,[53,85] and meal test.[86] The sensitivity of the secretin stimulation test is superior to the calcium and meal-provocative tests and is the one most commonly used.[87] Gastrin levels after secretin increased by 110 pg/mL in 93%, by more than 200 pg/mL in 87%,[81] and by more than 50% in 85%[87] of patients with ZES. Because of its ease, lack of side effects, high sensitivity, and very low occurrence of false-positive outcomes, the secretin test is the diagnostic provocative test of choice; a rise in gastrin of 200 ng/mL is diagnostic. The calcium infusion test should be reserved for the rare patient in whom ZES is strongly suspected but the secretin test is negative.[81]

Antral G-cell hyperplasia is reported to mimic ZES clinically, with elevated FSG and BAO.[88] This syndrome frequently occurs in patients after vagotomy, is due to increased numbers of antral G cells, is curable by antrectomy, may be associated with *H pylori* infections, and is differentiated from ZES by a negative secretin test and an exaggerated (at least 100% increase) postmeal serum gastrin level. Antral G-cell hyperfunction is similar to antral G-cell hyperplasia except that there are normal numbers of G cells and the syndrome is frequently familial, with autosomal dominant inheritance, and is associated with hyperpepsinogenemia I.[89] This syndrome was reported to be distinguishable from ZES by its association with a negative secretin test and an exaggerated increase in postprandial serum gastrin.[81,89] In patients with ZES, only 30% had a greater than 100% increase and 10% had a greater than 150% increase in the postprandial serum gastrin level.[86] Therefore, the meal test actually is frequently positive in patients with ZES and does not reliably differentiate ZES from antral syndromes.

Chronic gastric outlet obstruction can be difficult to distinguish from ZES because the obstruction can be caused by ZES or it can mimic ZES and be secondary to other causes of duodenal obstruction.[90] ZES can be differentiated from the other causes of obstruction by a secretin test and prolonged gastric suction.[91] Massive small bowel resection can cause a transient hypergastrinemia and elevation of BAO and can be distinguished from ZES by history and the secretin test. Chronic renal failure and *H pylori* infections can cause hypergastrinemia, which is usually associated with acid hyposecretion, although occasionally it may be associated with acid hypersecretion[82,92] and can be differentiated from ZES by the secretin test.

INSULINOMA

The clinical symptoms of insulinoma are due to hypoglycemia in almost all instances.[4,70,71] Most symptoms are neuroglycopenic in nature and include visual disturbances (59%), confusion (51%), altered consciousness (38%), and weakness (32%). Seizures occur but are uncommon (23%).[4,70,71] Symptoms also can occur due to excess catecholamine release (adrenergic symptoms), such as sweating (43%) and tremulousness (23%).[71] In one study, 49% of patients had both neuroglycopenic and adrenergic symptoms, 38% had neuroglycopenic symptoms only, and 12% had adrenergic symptoms only.[4] Symptoms are characteristically associated with fasting, a delayed meal, or exercise.

TABLE 38.5-3. Common Diagnostic Criteria for Insulinoma

Symptoms of hypoglycemia (headache, lightheadedness, confusion, drowsiness, seizures)
Symptoms of catecholamine excess (tremors, palpitations)
Hypoglycemia during a monitored fast (<50 mg/dL)
Increased serum insulin (>5–10 μU/mL)
Increased proinsulin (≥25%)
Negative sulfonylurea screen
Relief of symptoms after eating

The diagnosis of insulinoma can be established only by documenting symptomatic hypoglycemia with inappropriately elevated serum insulin levels during a monitored fast (Table 38.5-3).[4] Hypoglycemia usually is defined as a blood glucose level of less than 50 mg/dL in the fasting state. In healthy individuals, the blood glucose value usually does not decrease to less than 70 mg/dL after an overnight fast. In more than 97% of individuals, a supervised fast of 48 hours or less will be sufficient to diagnose insulinoma by the development of clinical symptoms and a plasma glucose level of less than 50 mg/dL.[4] In addition, patients with the diagnosis will usually have serum insulin levels greater than 5 μU/mL, and 97% will have levels greater than 10 μU/mL. An insulin-glucose ratio greater than 0.3 is typical.[93] In some normal obese subjects, because of hyperinsulinemia due to insulin resistance, the fasting plasma insulin-glucose ratio may be elevated and may mimic the pattern in insulinoma.[70,71] In these patients, the fasting glucose is normal and, with prolonged fasting, the blood glucose level does not decrease to less than 55 mg/dL.

A number of other conditions can cause fasting hypoglycemia with increased plasma insulin levels, including causes of organic hyperinsulinism due to pancreatic islet cell disease aside from insulinoma, factitious use of excessive insulin or hypoglycemia agents, or autoantibodies against the insulin receptor.[1,4,70,94,95] To differentiate insulinoma from these other conditions, additional tests are useful, including plasma determination of proinsulin, C-peptide level, antibodies to insulin, and plasma sulfonylurea levels. Because endogenous insulin is synthesized as a precursor, proinsulin, quantification of the higher-molecular-weight component, called the *proinsulin-like component*, is useful. In patients with surreptitious use of insulin or oral hypoglycemia agents, the proinsulin level is either normal or decreased.[95] The measurement of C peptide has proven useful in differentiating organic hypersecretion of insulin from patients surreptitiously using insulin because commercial insulin preparations contain no C peptide. In insulinoma, the characteristic finding is either an elevated or normal plasma C-peptide concentration, whereas in patients surreptitiously using insulin, the plasma insulin level is high and the C-peptide level low.[70,71,95]

NONFUNCTIONING PANCREATIC ENDOCRINE TUMORS

Nonfunctioning PETs and PPomas present in the fourth and fifth decade of life.[4,32,96] PPomas release the hormone pancreatic polypeptide, which has no known functional sequelae.[1]

Originally it was thought that nonfunctioning PETs did not release any hormone products, but these lesions have since been shown to secrete chromogranins, α-HCG or β-HCG subunits, or other peptides that do not cause symptoms.[57] Increasingly, what in the past were believed to be nonfunctioning PETs now are appreciated to have elevated plasma PP levels. In one study, one-half to three-fourths of PETs not associated with any clinical syndrome and classified as nonfunctioning were found to be PPomas. Elevated plasma PP is specific for endocrine pancreatic tumors; of 53 patients with adenocarcinoma of the pancreas, none had elevated plasma PP levels.[97] Currently, no data are available to suggest that nonfunctioning PETs without elevated PP and PPomas differ in biologic behavior or presentation.[1] Immunohistochemically nonfunctioning PETs and PPomas can stain positively for numerous other gastrointestinal peptides. In one series of 30 nonfunctioning tumors, 50% displayed insulin-like immunoreactivity, 30% glucagon, 43% PP, and 13% somatostatin, and only 13% stained for no peptide.[98] With these tumors, symptoms arise largely from mechanical or mass effects of the neoplasm, and therefore the tumors are diagnosed late, when they are quite large and locally invasive.

They are usually solitary tumors except in patients with MEN 1, in whom multiple adenomas are seen.[2,3] The tumors are distributed throughout the pancreas at a pancreatic head-body-tail ratio of 7:1:1.5.[4] The malignancy rate varies from 64% to 92%.[97]

Chromogranin A and B levels are elevated in almost all patients with nonfunctioning PETs.[67] Elevated plasma levels of PP do not establish the diagnosis of a PPoma even when a pancreatic mass is present. Plasma PP levels are reported to be elevated in 22% to 71% of patients with functional PETs in various studies,[1,99] as well as in nonpancreatic carcinoid tumors. Furthermore, elevated plasma levels of PP can occur in other situations such as old age; after bowel resection; with alcohol abuse; during certain infections; in chronic noninfective inflammatory disorders, acute diarrhea, chronic renal failure, diabetes, chronic relapsing pancreatitis, and hypoglycemia; or after eating.[99,100] To increase the specificity of an elevated plasma level for a PPoma, an atropine suppression test may be used. In one study of 48 patients with elevated plasma PP levels, atropine (1 mg intramuscularly) did not suppress PP levels in any of the 18 patients with PETs but did suppress the level by 50% in all patients without tumors.[59]

Patients present with abdominal pain in 36% and jaundice in 28% of cases; in 16% of patients, the tumors are found incidentally at surgery and, in the remaining patients, a variety of symptoms due to the tumor mass are present.[1,101] The average delay from onset of symptoms until diagnosis varied from 5 months to 2 to 7 years.[97]

OTHER RARE PANCREATIC ENDOCRINE TUMORS

The VIPoma syndrome, also commonly called the *Verner-Morrison syndrome,* was first described by Verner and Morrison in 1958.[102] Because of the resemblance of the diarrheal fluid to that seen in patients with cholera, the terms *pancreatic cholera* and *endocrine cholera*[103] and the abbreviation *WDHA*[32] (watery diarrhea, hypokalemia, and achlorhydria) have also been used for this condition. The tumors occur in a bimodal distribution. The mean age for adults at diagnosis is 50 years, with a range of 32 to 81 years. There is a female predominance. In children, the mean age at diagnosis is 2 to 4 years, with a range of 10 months to 9 years.[104]

In adults, more than 80% of VIPomas are located in the pancreas,[1,4] with rare cases caused by intestinal carcinoids or pheochromocytomas that produce vasoactive intestinal peptide (VIP).[105] VIPomas are usually large solitary tumors.[1,106] In one series, only 2% of tumors were multiple, with 50% to 75% reported to be in the pancreatic tail.[105] One- to two-thirds of patients with VIPomas have metastases at the time of diagnosis or surgery.[103] Characteristically in children younger than 10 years, and rarely in adults (5% of cases), VIPoma syndrome is due to a ganglioneuroma or ganglioneuroblastoma. These extrapancreatic tumors are less often malignant (10%) than are pancreatic VIPomas.[105]

Using immunocytochemical studies, 34% to 38% of VIPomas also stain for HPP, 19% for glucagon, 10% for somatostatin, 5% for insulin, and 0% for gastrin.[98,107] VIPomas also elaborate the peptide histidine methionine (PHM-27), a 27–amino acid peptide that shares with VIP a common precursor peptide, pre-pro-VIP/PHM-27.[1,2,103] The presence of immunoreactive VIP is strongly suggestive for VIPoma, as this peptide rarely is found in other pancreatic endocrine tumors (10 of 104 pancreatic endocrine tumors in one study).[107]

Plasma levels of VIP are consistently elevated in patients with the VIPoma syndrome and appear to be responsible for the functional syndrome (Table 38.5-4).[1,103,105] A continuous infusion of VIP for 10 hours in normal human subjects to achieve plasma levels similar to those seen in patients with the VIPoma syndrome produced watery diarrhea in 6 to 7 hours.[108] The principal features of VIPoma syndrome are the presence of severe secretory diarrhea associated with hypokalemia and dehydration.[1,103–105] The diarrhea is copious, all patients with VIPoma producing more than 3 L/d.[103,105] A volume of less than 700 mL/d has been proposed to rule out the diagnosis of VIPoma.[109] Cramping pain or colic is reported in 35% to 63% of patients.[103,105] Gross steatorrhea usually is not present; in one study, none of 52 patients with VIPomas had 24-hour fecal fat greater than 15 g/d[105] and, in another study, 84% of the patients did not have steatorrhea.[103] Weight loss is almost universally present.[105] Erythematous flushing of the head or trunk area is characteristic and reported in 23% of patients. The clinical laboratory studies invariably demonstrate hypokalemia (83% to 100%) and, to a lesser degree, hypercalcemia (41%), hypochlorhydria (70%), and mild hyperglycemia (18%).[1,103–105] Hypokalemia is often severe, potassium levels being less than 2.5 mmol/L at some time in 93% of patients.[105]

The diagnosis of VIPoma requires the documentation of an elevated plasma concentration of VIP and the presence of a

TABLE 38.5-4. Symptoms Commonly Associated with Rare Pancreatic Endocrine Tumors

VIPoma	*Glucagonoma*	*Somatostatinoma*
Diarrhea	Weight loss	Gallbladder disease
Dehydration	Migratory necrolytic erythema	Diabetes mellitus
Weight loss		Weight loss
Crampy pain	Glucose intolerance	Diarrhea
Hypokalemia	Hypoaminoacidemia	Steatorrhea
	Thromboembolic disease	Hypochlorhydria

large volume of secretory diarrhea.[1,103,110] A large number of possible causes for the diarrhea can be excluded by fasting the patient because, in patients with VIPomas, the diarrhea persists during fasting.[1,103,109] The diarrheal fluid should be characteristic of a secretory diarrhea,[109] wherein the stool electrolytes can account for all of the stool water osmolality [(sodium + potassium) × 2 = measured osmolality].[109] Other diseases can produce a chronic, large-volume secretory diarrhea and can be confused with VIPoma, one such syndrome being the *pseudo-VIPoma syndrome.*[109] Other causes of such diarrhea include ZES and chronic laxative abuse.[111] In addition, some cases of secretory diarrhea are of unknown origin.[111,112]

The range for normal fasting plasma VIP levels in most laboratories is 0 to 170 pg/mL.[104,105] In one series of patients with VIPomas, the mean value was 965 pg/mL, and the lowest value was 225 pg/mL.[104] In contrast, in another large study, the mean value in patients with VIPomas was 675 pg/mL, the highest value seen in a normal patient being 53 pg/mL and the lowest value seen in a VIPoma patient being 160 pg/mL.[105]

In 1942, the association of a pancreatic tumor with a skin rash was first described.[113] Then, in 1966, McGavran et al.[114] reported a patient with an elevated fasting glucagon level, dermatitis, diabetes, and a pancreatic endocrine tumor. Later, in 1973, Wilkinson[115] described the rash associated with this endocrine tumor as necrolytic migratory erythema. Mallinson et al.[116] specifically established the association of a cutaneous rash with glucagon-producing tumors of the pancreas when they reported nine cases in 1974.

Most glucagonomas are large at the time of diagnosis, the average size being between 5 and 10 cm. Glucagonomas have a predilection for arising in the pancreatic tail in 50% to 80% of patients.[117] In one study, 22% of these tumors were in the head, 14% in the body, and 51% in the pancreatic tail.[118] Most glucagonomas are malignant, and the most common site of metastatic spread is the liver. Less commonly, there is spread to lymph nodes, bone, and mesentery. In most cases, glucagonomas are within the pancreas; however, a glucagonoma associated with the typical clinical syndrome was found in the proximal duodenum.[117] Glucagonomas usually occur as a single tumor, although in 10% of patients in one series, multiple tumors or diffuse involvement by a single mass was found.[117]

Glucagonomas usually occur in middle to late age, with only 16% of cases occurring in individuals younger than 40 years and most occurring at 50 to 70 years of age.[117] The typical dermatitis occurs in 64% to 90% of patients, diabetes mellitus or glucose intolerance in 83% to 90%, weight loss in 56% to 90%, diarrhea in 14% to 15%, abdominal pain in 12%, and thromboembolic disease with venous thrombosis in 24% and with pulmonary emboli in 11%; occasionally, psychiatric disturbances also are seen (see Table 38.5-4).[1,117–119] Laboratory abnormalities include anemia in 44% to 85% of patients, hypoaminoacidemia in 26% to 100%, hypocholesterolemia in 80%, and renal glycosuria.[1,118]

The pathophysiology of the glucagonoma syndrome is related to the known actions of glucagon. Glucagon stimulates glycogenolysis, gluconeogenesis, ketogenesis, lipolysis, and insulin secretion, as well as affecting gastrointestinal tract secretion, inhibiting pancreatic and gastric secretion, inhibiting intestinal motility, and increasing heart rate and contractility. Hyperglycemia in glucagonoma results from the increased hepatic glycogenolysis and glyconeogenesis. Weight loss has been attributed to the known catabolic effects of glucagon.[119] It has not been clearly established that the skin rash is due to the hyperglucagonemia *per se*, because in numerous patients given large doses of glucagon over extended periods of time, the skin rash did not develop.[1,119] Possibly, the glucagon-induced hypoaminoacidemia that develops in 80% to 95% of patients may be involved, because correction of the hypoaminoacidemia has been shown to correct the dermatitis without changing plasma glucagon concentrations in some patients.[1,119,120] The similarity of the lesions to those seen in patients with zinc deficiencies has resulted in trials of zinc therapy in some patients, with observed benefit[119]; however, plasma zinc levels are normal in most cases.

Glucagon is one of the most frequently recognized peptides in immunocytochemical studies of PETs, though in many cases it is not associated with any syndrome. In one series of 1366 autopsy cases, a frequency of 0.8% adenomas was reported, and all contained glucagon-producing cells.[98,119] The morphology of most glucagon-producing tumors demonstrates no general features that distinguish them from other PETs.[1,98,117,119]

The presence of cutaneous lesions often precedes the diagnosis of the syndrome for long periods, with a mean of 6 to 8 years and a maximum of 18 years. Typically, the rash starts as an erythematous patch, usually at periorofacial or intertriginous areas such as the groin, buttocks, thighs, or perineum, and then spreads laterally. The lesions later become raised, with superficial, central blistering. The top of the bullae frequently detach or rupture, leaving eroded areas that crust. The lesions tend to heal in the center, while the edges continue to spread with a crusting well-defined edge. Healing is associated with the development of hyperpigmentation. This entire sequence characteristically takes 1 to 2 weeks, so that while some new lesions are developing, others are healing; therefore, a mixed pattern of erythema, bullous formation with epidermal separation, crusting, and hyperpigmentation together with normal skin can occur. The histopathology can be as varied as the clinical presentation.[117] Glossitis or angular stomatitis is reported to occur in 34% to 68% of patients.

Once the diagnosis is suspected, it can be confirmed by establishing the presence of a marked elevation in plasma glucagon concentration. In most laboratories, the upper limit of normal for fasting glucagon concentration is 150 to 200 pg/mL. In one large review of glucagonomas, only two patients had a plasma glucagon level of 200 to 500 pg/mL, four patients had a level between 500 and 1000 pg/mL, and 52 patients had a level in excess of 1000 pg/mL.[118] These results are in agreement with another study,[117] in which the mean plasma glucagon concentration in 73 cases of glucagonoma was 2110 ± 334 pg/mL, with a range of 550 to 6600 pg/mL and no result of less than 500 pg/mL. Hyperglucagonemia (generally <500 pg/mL) is reported to occur in chronic renal insufficiency, diabetic ketoacidosis, prolonged starvation, acute pancreatitis, acromegaly, hypercortisolism, septicemia, severe burns, severe stress (trauma, exercise), familial hyperglucagonemia, and hepatic insufficiency.[117,119]

Somatostatinomas release somatostatin, a hormone that inhibits numerous endocrine and exocrine functions. Release of almost all gastrointestinal tract hormones, including insulin, glucagon, gastrin, secretin, cholecystokinin, and motilin, is inhibited by somatostatin. In addition to the inhibition of endocrine secretions, somatostatin has direct effects on a number of target organs, including inhibition of gastric acid secretion, increased intestinal motility, and reduced intestinal absorption of fat. In 1977, the first two cases of somatostatinoma were described by Ganda et al.[121] and Larsson et al.[122] Somatostatinomas are the least common PET, fewer than 50 cases having been described.[123] Patients characteristically have diabetes mellitus, gallbladder disease, diarrhea, weight loss, steatorrhea, and hypochlorhydria (see Table 38.5-4).[1,97,103,124,125]

Somatostatinomas occur in the pancreas in 56% to 75% of cases, and the remainder occur in the upper small intestine.[97,125] The tumors have a predilection for the pancreatic head and occur there two to three times as often as in the body or tail.[97,125] In 90% of patients, the tumors are solitary[125] and range from 1.5 to 10.0 cm in diameter. Tumors demonstrate evidence of metastatic spread at diagnosis or operation in 70% to 92% of patients.[97,125] Metastases usually occur in the liver (75% of patients with metastases) but also in the regional lymph nodes (31%) and, less frequently, in bone.[97,125]

Electron-microscopical studies show that the secretory granules are typical of those in D cells in 89% of the tumors examined.[97,125] Immunocytochemical analysis shows somatostatin-like immunoreactive material in tumors that, in addition, contained insulin (33%), calcitonin (27%), and gastrin (13%).

The mean age of patients is affected with somatostatinomas is 50 years.[97,125] For patients with intestinal somatostatinomas, 43% were women, as compared with 66% with pancreatic tumors.[125] Diabetes mellitus was present in 95% of patients with pancreatic tumors and in 21% of those with intestinal tumors.[97] Gallbladder disease was seen in 94% of pancreatic and 36% of intestinal tumor patients, and weight loss was noted in 90% of pancreatic and 44% of intestinal cases.[97] Steatorrhea and hypochlorhydria occurred in 83% to 86% of pancreatic tumor cases but in only 12% to 17% of intestinal tumor cases.[1,97] Symptoms attributable to excess somatostatin release are seen in no more than 45% of patients in some studies.[123]

GRFomas are the most recently described PET syndrome and feature excessive release of growth hormone–releasing factor (GRF).[126–128] In reviews of GRFomas, 29% to 30% originated in the pancreas, 53% in the lung, and 10% in small intestinal tumors, and there was a rare case in the adrenal gland.[129,130]

Multiple pancreatic tumors have been reported in 30% of patients with GRFomas in one series.[129] Approximately 40% of all GRFomas occur in patients with ZES and, in another 40%, Cushing's syndrome was present.[1,129] Tumors generally are large (>6 cm), varying from 1 to 25 cm in diameter.[129] In one series, tumor size, GRF levels, and the presence of metastases were not related.[129]

On light-microscopical studies, typical features of a PET are seen, the lesion being composed of trabecular or solid nests and sheets of uniform tumor cells.[123,129] In electron-microscopical studies, tumor cells containing 100- to 250-nm secretory granules are seen.[129,131–133] Immunochemical studies demonstrated GRF-immunoreactive material in all tumors examined, with 10% to 80% of cells possessing GRF.[123,129,130] GRF-immunoreactive materials were seen in 31% of all PETs in one study[134] but in 0% to 100% in other pathological studies,[126,127,129,135] although very few of these patients had acromegaly. The known actions of GRF as a stimulant of growth hormone release account for the clinical presentation with acromegaly.[126,127,129,135]

Patients are between 15 and 63 years old, the average age being 38.[123,129,130] Patients with intestinal GRFomas tend to be younger, with two of three patients in one study being younger than 20 years.[129] A female preponderance (73%) is seen for all GRFomas. Acromegalic features are indistinguishable from those of patients with classical acromegaly and include enlargement of hands and feet, facial changes, skin changes, headache, and peripheral nerve entrapment.[123,129,130,135] The diagnosis should be suspected in any patient with acromegaly who does not have a pituitary adenoma imaged by magnetic resonance modalities or with an abdominal mass[123] and is confirmed by measuring plasma GRF levels.

IMAGING AND LOCALIZATION OF PANCREATIC ENDOCRINE TUMORS

Relatively precise localization of the gastrinoma has become an increasingly important factor in evaluating patients with ZES.[83,136] With the increased ability to control gastric acid hypersecretion with antisecretory drugs, emergency total gastrectomy rarely is necessary now, allowing the clinician time to determine the location and extent of the gastrinoma. The ability for long-term control of gastric acid hypersecretion has made tumor growth and possible metastatic spread an increasingly important determinant of long-term survival.[14,15,26,37] Preoperative imaging studies can identify patients with metastatic disease to the liver or other sites so that unnecessary surgery can be prevented. Gastrinomas frequently are multiple and extrapancreatic, and accurate imaging assists in determining the nature of the operative procedure. Imaging studies identify resectable metastatic disease to the liver in up to 15% of patients.[137] For insulinoma, the extent of preoperative imaging necessary to ensure an operative cure has not been clearly defined.[138–141] It is generally agreed that some preoperative localization is essential, primarily because insulinomas are frequently small (90% <2 cm in diameter) and, to a lesser extent, because metastatic spread should be identified to prevent unnecessary surgery. However, the question of the extent of localization studies that should be performed in occult insulinomas has not yet been resolved.[142–144]

A number of different techniques, including abdominal ultrasonography, computed tomography (CT) scanning, magnetic resonance imaging (MRI), selective abdominal angiography, selective venous sampling for gastrin from portal venous tributaries (PVS), intraarterial secretin with hepatic venous gastrin sampling (IAS), somatostatin receptor scintigraphy (SRS), endoscopic ultrasonography (EUS) preoperatively, intraoperative ultrasonography (IOUS), and intraoperative endoscopy (IOE) with transillumination of the duodenum at surgery have all been reported as helpful in localizing gastrinomas.

Ultrasonography has a low sensitivity for localizing both primary and metastatic tumors, but, in a prospective study,[145] it was recommended that this imaging modality continue to be used because it has high specificity, is noninvasive and, on occasion, localizes gastrinomas not found by other modalities.[145] The CT scan detects nearly 50% of all primary and metastatic liver disease; however, its ability to detect primary tumors has been shown to be directly related to tumor size,[136] detecting 0% of tumors less than 1 cm in diameter, 30% of those between 1 and 3 cm, and 95% of tumors more than 3 cm in diameter. Frequently, small primary tumors, which are being increasingly found in the duodenum (<1 cm), usually are missed by CT.[23,25,136,146] Furthermore, CT scan is less sensitive for detecting extrahepatic, extrapancreatic gastrinomas than pancreatic gastrinomas. In a large, prospective study, selective angiography was found to detect 68% of primary tumors and 86% of hepatic metastases.[147] The ability to detect tumors was location-dependent: Of gastrinomas in the pancreatic head, 90% were found, as were 80% in the body, 45% in the tail, and 34% in the duodenum; 50% of extrapancreatic, extrahepatic, and extraduodenal tumors also were found.[147] In a comparative study, angiography detected 20% more hepatic metastases than did CT scanning (68%), and the combination detected 96% of all liver metastases.[38]

Improvements in the sensitivity of MRI have increased its usefulness in localizing gastrinomas and other PETs. A prospective study from the years 1986 to 1987 reported that MRI was less sensitive than either CT scanning or angiography,[148] but a recent study using current, improved MRI technology was more sensitive than either angiography or CT scanning for metastatic disease.[149] However, MRI remains less sensitive than angiography for primary tumor.[149] For insulinomas, ultrasonography localizes 33%, MRI 46%, CT scanning 35%, dynamic CT scanning 66%, selective arteriography 63%, and all imaging studies combined 80%.[1,70,71,143,144]

Pancreatic endocrine tumors frequently have a high density of somatostatin receptors, and scanning after injection of the radiolabeled long-acting somatostatin analog octreotide localizes pancreatic endocrine tumors.[150–154] This technique is one of the most sensitive methods for localizing primary gastrinomas[38,39,152,153,155–159]: 60% of primary gastrinomas and more than 90% of metastases to liver.[38] The sensitivity of SRS in identifying gastrinoma in patients prior to operation increases with tumor size: Only 30% of tumors less than 1.1 cm and 64% of those 1.1 to 2.0 cm are detected, as compared to 96% of tumors larger than 2 cm.[146] SRS appears to be the procedure of choice to screen ZES patients for the presence of bone metastases. In a study of 115 patients with ZES, 8 (7%) were determined to have bone metastases.[160] Bone scan was positive in 52 patients, resulting in a very low specificity. SRS and MRI were positive in 6 and 7 patients, respectively. Because it is noninvasive and highly sensitive and has the ability to image the entire body for metastatic foci, SRS is recommended as the initial procedure of choice in cases of gastrinoma and for all PETs except insulinomas (Fig. 38.5-2).[39] SRS is reported to localize 53% of insulinomas but, because such lesions frequently have low densities of somatostatin receptors, this number may be higher than what can be routinely achieved.[151]

EUS is being used increasingly to localize PETs.[152,161–163] It is reported to localize 75% of primary gastrinomas[152,161–163] and to be particularly useful for intrapancreatic tumors. Whether EUS can image small duodenal gastrinomas is unclear.[164] However, EUS is an invasive procedure, and the additional information obtained over SRS or current MRI techniques is unproven. Recently, EUS was reported to have a high sensitivity, localizing 80% of insulinomas, even though 15% were no more than 1 cm in diameter.[162]

PVS has been reported to be useful for functional localization of gastrinomas.[136] However, in a prospective study, a combination of PVS and standard CT and MRI imaging yielded results only marginally better than imaging alone in identifying gastrinomas.[165] In this study, neither the magnitude of the gastrin gradient nor its presence or absence correlated with whether a gastrinoma would be found at surgery. A gradient greater than 50% is reported to occur in 68% of all patients with ZES. PVS requires expertise, is time-consuming, and is associated with some morbidity, primarily abdominal pain at the catheter insertion site.[165,166] These drawbacks, combined with limited availability and the fact that 70% to 80% of gastrinomas are near the duodenum–pancreatic head, had led most[165] (but not all[167]) investigators to conclude that PVS has limited usefulness in ZES. This experience is in marked contrast to the use of PVS for insulinomas, where it has proven to be extremely valuable in localizing lesions throughout the pancreas.[141,142]

Most gastrinomas (91%) demonstrate a paradoxical release of gastrin with intravenous injection of secretin.[81] This characteristic has been used to localize gastrinomas selectively by

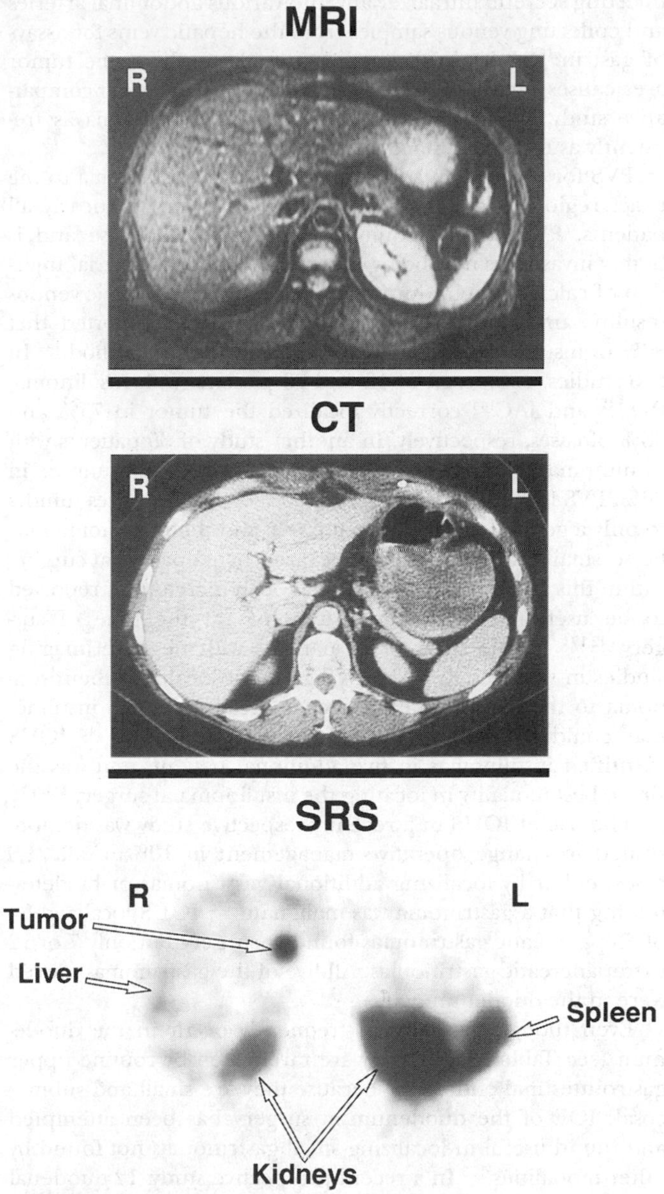

FIGURE 38.5-2. Example of somatostatin receptor scintigraphy sensitivity in detecting gastrinoma. A patient with biochemically confirmed Zollinger-Ellison syndrome underwent initial imaging studies. The magnetic resonance image (MRI) and computed tomography (CT) scan did not show any lesion. However, somatostatin receptor scintigraphy (SRS) showed a positive signal in the right upper quadrant, which was confirmed to be a 1.4-cm gastrinoma resected from the anterior lateral wall of the second part of the duodenum at surgical exploration. (From ref. 39.)

injecting secretin intraarterially into various abdominal arteries and collecting venous samples from the hepatic veins for assays of gastrin.[168] Injection into the arterial supply of the tumor area causes a marked increase in gastrin.[168] In a recent comparative study, IAS was found to localize the gastrinoma as frequently as the much more technically difficult PVS.[169]

PVS for insulin can accurately localize an insulinoma to the exact region of the pancreas (head, body, tail) in nearly all patients. PVS, which requires considerable expertise and is highly invasive, is now being replaced by the intraarterial injection of calcium (IAC) during angiography, with hepatic venous insulin sampling. A recent preoperative study reported that 80% of insulinomas could be localized using this method.[144] In two studies, composed of 12 and 23 patients with insulinoma, PVS[142] and IAC[144] correctly localized the tumor in 75% and 88% of cases, respectively. In another study of 35 patients with insulinoma in whom radiologic studies imaged the tumors in 46%, PVS localized the tumor in 100%.[170] PVS localizes tumors to only a general area of the pancreas, and the insulinoma may be so small that it cannot be localized by palpation at surgery within this area. However, IOUS has been increasingly reported to be useful in localizing insulinomas at the time of surgery.[142,171] In one study of 12 patients with negative imaging studies in whom 75% had a PVS gradient localizing the insulinoma to the appropriate pancreatic area, at surgery insulinomas could be localized by palpation in only 41%.[142] IOUS identified insulinomas in five additional patients and was the single best modality in locating the insulinoma at surgery.[142]

The use of IOUS in a recent prospective study was demonstrated to change operative management in 10% of all ZES cases, either by localizing additional gastrinomas or by determining that a gastrinoma was malignant.[172] IOUS localized 22 of 23 pancreatic gastrinomas found at surgery but only 7 of 12 extrapancreatic gastrinomas. All five of the gastrinomas missed were in the duodenum.[172]

Even though gastrinomas frequently occur in the duodenum (see Table 38.5-2), they are rarely seen by routine upper gastrointestinal endoscopy because they are small and submucosal. IOE of the duodenum at surgery has been attempted and found useful in localizing small gastrinomas not found by other modalities.[173] In a recent prospective study, 12 duodenal gastrinomas were found at surgery in 10 patients.[173] IOE detected 10 of the 12 (83% sensitivity), which was significantly greater than either standard preoperative imaging, which detected 3 (25% sensitivity) or IOUS and palpation, which detected 5 (42% sensitivity). IOE with transillumination detects 20% more duodenal tumors than does palpation,[174] and duodenotomy detects an additional 15%. Endoscopic transillumination also is often helpful in establishing the placement of the duodenotomy incision.[174]

TREATMENT OF RESECTABLE DISEASE

GASTRINOMA

In ZES patients, gastric acid hypersecretion must be controlled because most patients will not be cured after surgical exploration.[76,175] If acid hypersecretion is controlled, patients have an excellent quality of life; however, long-term prognosis is being increasingly determined by the malignant nature of the gastrinoma.[26] As many as 90% of gastrinomas may be malignant; therefore, it is important to consider surgical therapy directed at the primary and metastatic disease, if feasible (Fig. 38.5-3).

Management of Gastric Acid Hypersecretion

Years ago, patients with ZES required total gastrectomy to control gastric acid hypersecretion. Before effective medical management, the operation was commonly done as an emergency procedure and carried a mortality rate of 15%.[33] Operative results were unsatisfactory for patients who had less than a total gastrectomy, with most patients developing recurrent ulcer disease, often with lethal complications, within days of surgery.[33] With the development of increasingly effective medical therapy, the mortality for patients with ZES undergoing total gastrectomy has decreased. Though an early study claimed that total gastrectomy could lead to regression of the gastrinoma in some patients,[176] subsequent studies have failed to substantiate this claim.[37,176,177] There is no evidence that either medical therapy of gastric hypersecretion or total gastrectomy affects the growth rate of the gastrinoma.[14]

Numerous studies have demonstrated that gastric acid hypersecretion can now be controlled medically over the long term in every patient who will reliably take oral medication—the H^+K^+-ATPase inhibitor omeprazole or lansoprazole.[76,175,178,179] The availability of these agents and their long duration of action have greatly simplified management because they can be taken once or twice per day. Therefore, most authorities recommend that total gastrectomy be reserved for patients who are unreliable, do not have access to routine medical follow-up, or cannot or will not take oral medication.[14,76] In all other patients, medical therapy is the treatment of choice. Although parietal cell vagotomy in patients with ZES in whom no tumor was found at surgery decreased the BAO by 66%, most patients still needed some antisecretory drug.[34] At present, routine performance of parietal cell vagotomy is not recommended.[174]

In patients with ZES and the MEN 1 syndrome, medical control of gastric hypersecretion can be greatly facilitated by correction of the hyperparathyroidism that is almost invariably present by the time ZES develops.[52] Correction of hyperparathyroidism may reduce the FSG concentration, increase the responsiveness to a given dose of antisecretory medication, or decrease the BAO.[180] Therefore, in patients with ZES and MEN 1 with hyperparathyroidism, parathyroidectomy should be performed before any contemplated surgical procedure to control acid hypersecretion.

The results of medical treatment of gastric acid hypersecretion have been reviewed extensively.[3,14,76,175] H_2-receptor antagonists (cimetidine, ranitidine, famotidine) alone or in combination with anticholinergic agents (propantheline, isopropamide) and, more recently, the substituted benzimidazole (omeprazole), which functions as an H^+K^+-ATPase inhibitor, have been used successfully in the long-term treatment of gastric hypersecretion in ZES. The number of patients in whom medical therapy fails varies greatly in different series[14,175]: For cimetidine, the reported failure rate varies from 0% to 65%,[14,175,181] for ranitidine from 0% to 40%,[14,175,182] and for omeprazole and lansoprazole from 0% to 7.5%.[14,76,175,178,179] The failure rate for famotidine has been reported as 0% in several series.[14,175,183] In general, studies have shown that relief of symptoms does not adequately reflect the effectiveness of anti-

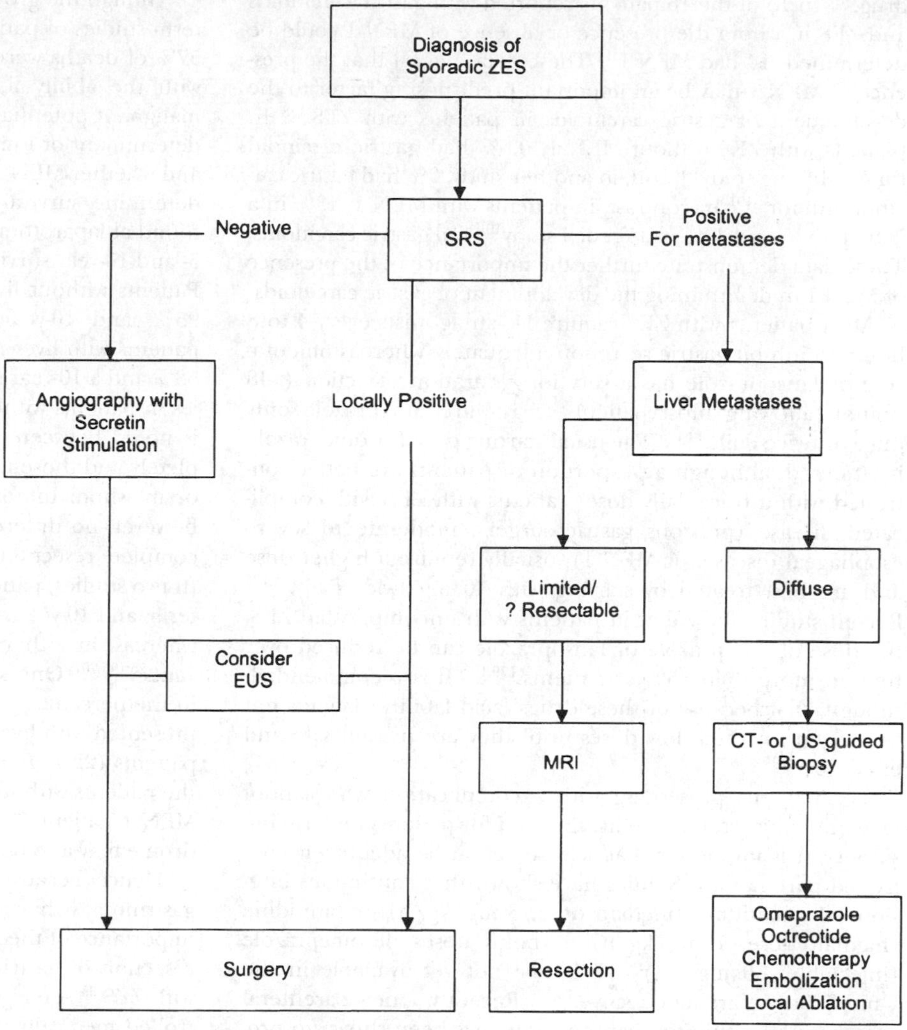

FIGURE 38.5-3. Flow diagram showing a proposed workup for patients with newly diagnosed sporadic Zollinger-Ellison syndrome (ZES). After biochemical confirmation of disease, an initial screening study with somatostatin receptor scintigraphy (SRS) should be performed. Patients who have results positive for metastases should undergo additional imaging studies. If disease is confined to the liver, then resection or other therapies, as shown, should be considered. For patients who have a locally positive result, endoscopic ultrasonography (EUS) should be considered, after which patients undergo exploration with curative intent. If somatostatin receptor scintigraphy is negative, then angiography with selective secretin stimulation should be performed. CT, computed tomography; MRI, magnetic resonance imaging; US, ultrasonography.

secretory therapy. Most studies have demonstrated that in order to assess the adequacy of antisecretory therapy, gastric acid secretion must be measured while the patient is taking medication.[14]

The amount of antisecretory medication varies widely from patient to patient; thus, the optimal dose of medication must be determined for each patient initially and must periodically be reevaluated.[14,175] Recent studies have shown that if enough antisecretory drug is used to decrease gastric acid secretion to less than 10 mEq/h for the hour prior to the next dose of medications in patients with no history of gastric surgery and to less than 5 mEq/h in patients with a history of acid-reducing procedures or severe esophageal disease, peptic ulcers will heal and complications of peptic ulcer disease will be prevented.[14,76,175] To reduce acid output to these levels before the next dose of medication, patients frequently require more than twice the usual dose of H_2-receptor antagonist or three times the usual dose of omeprazole recommended for idiopathic peptic ulcer disease.[14,76,175] In recent studies, the median doses were 3.6 g/d for cimetidine (range, 1.2 to 12.6 g/d), 1.2 g/d for ranitidine (range, 0.45 to 6.0 g/d), 0.25 g/d for famotidine (range, 0.05 to 0.8 g/d), 20 to 80 mg/d for omeprazole (range, 20 to 360 mg/d), and 30 to 120 mg/d for lansoprazole.[14,76,175] The long-term use of these doses of H_2 antagonists and omeprazole has proven to be both effective and safe.[14,175] Except for antiandrogen side effects (impotence, gynecomastia, and breast tenderness) with high-dose cimetidine in up to 60% of male patients, long-term treatment with cimetidine in women or with ranitidine, famotidine, or omeprazole in patients of either gender has been shown to be safe.[14,175] Omeprazole has been associated with the development of hepatitis that resolved after discontinuation of the drug.[184]

The long-term use of omeprazole has caused concern about toxicity, because female rats given long-term omeprazole (or other potent inhibitors of gastric acid secretion) have developed proliferation of gastric ECL cells and, in some cases, carcinoid tumors of the stomach.[16,185] Results from a number of studies have led most[185] (but not all[186]) investigators to conclude that the ECL hyperplasia and gastric carcinoid tumor formation in these animal models were most likely secondary to drug-induced achlorhydria and the resultant hypergastrinemia and not secondary directly to a toxic action of the antisecretory drug. Hyperplasia of gastric endocrine cells occurs in patients with ZES. Quantitative studies indicate that gastric ECL cells are increased approximately twofold, independent of administration of antisecretory agents.[14,187–189] In two studies in which omeprazole treatment was prolonged for up to 4 years, there was no statistical increase in gastric ECL cells owing to use of this drug.[187] In 15 of the 16 patients reported with gastric carcinoids and ZES in whom the presence or absence of MEN 1 could be determined, 14 had MEN 1.[14] These data suggest that the presence of MEN 1 may be an important predisposing factor to the development of gastric carcinoids in patients with ZES.[188] In patients with ZES without MEN 1, 0.6% had gastric carcinoid tumors in one study[190] and, in another study, 0% had gastric carcinoid tumors.[191] In contrast, in patients with MEN 1, 13% in a U.S. study[190] and 30% in a French study[191] had gastric carcinoids. These data demonstrate further the importance of the presence of MEN 1 in determining the development of gastric carcinoids.

Most patients with ZES require H_2 antagonists every 4 to 8 hours to inhibit gastric secretion adequately, whereas omeprazole or lansoprazole has a very long duration of action (>48 hours), allowing most patients to require omeprazole only once or twice daily.[14,175] The usual starting dose for omeprazole is 60 mg/d, although a proportion of patients are better controlled with a twice-daily dose. Patients with ZES with complicated disease (previous gastric surgery, moderate to severe esophageal disease, or MEN 1), usually require a higher dose and are best treated by starting with 40 mg twice daily.[14,175] Recent studies show that in patients with uncomplicated ZES, the dose of omeprazole or lansoprazole can be reduced over time in more than 85% of patients.[179,192] It is recommended, though, that because of these drugs' acid lability, patients not be started on these low doses until they are proven safe and effective.[179,192]

For patients presenting with a complication who cannot take oral antisecretory medication and for patients undergoing surgery, it is important that acid secretion be adequately controlled parenterally. Studies have shown that continuous infusions of cimetidine (median dose, 3 mg/kg/h) or ranitidine (median dose, 1 mg/kg/h) or bolus doses of omeprazole (injectable, 60 mg every 12 hours; not yet available in the United States) are all effective.[14,175] Recently, a new parenteral proton pump inhibitor, pantoprazole, has been shown to produce a dose-dependent decrease in acid output in volunteers stimulated with pentagastrin.[193] These drugs should be continued until oral antisecretory agents can be restarted.

Surgery to Cure Gastrinoma

In a number of studies, the 5-year survival rate for all patients with ZES was 62% to 87%, and the 10-year survival was 47% to 77%.[26,194–199] A recent comprehensive report from the National Institutes of Health cited long-term outcome in 151 consecutive ZES patients who underwent operation with curative intent[35]: Among patients with sporadic gastrinoma, 34% were biochemically and radiographically free of disease at 10 years, as compared to no patients with MEN 1 and ZES. The overall 10-year survival was 94% (Fig. 38.5-4). In another study from the same institution, a multivariate analysis of factors associated with long-term (>5-year) cure was performed.[200] Age, gender, duration of symptoms or disease, and severity of disease (as reflected by the level of BAO, FSG, or secretin stimulation test) did not predict outcome. Only a diagnosis of MEN 1 was inversely correlated with cure. In addition, the status of preoperative imaging studies (either positive or negative), tumor size, and number of tumors resected did not correlate with cure. However, a normal postoperative FSG and secretin stimulation test did independently and significantly predict cure.

Though the growth of gastrinoma is generally slow, in long-term studies of patients originally treated by total gastrectomy, 57% of deaths were due to tumor progression.[33,37] Therefore, with the ability to control gastric acid hypersecretion, the malignant potential of the tumor is an increasingly important determinant of long-term prognosis. The extent of the tumor and whether MEN 1 is present or absent have been reported to determine survival rates.[194,195,201] In patients with no tumor found at laparotomy or in whom tumor is completely resected, 5- and 10-year survival rates are 90% to 100%, respectively.[25,194] Patients without liver metastases had a 5-year survival rate of 95%, and 10-year survival rates were 90%.[26] In contrast, patients with liver metastases had a 5-year survival rate of only 53% and a 10-year survival of 30% (Fig. 38.5-5).[26] In most studies in patients without liver metastases, a difference in survival is noted between patients whose tumors were resected completely and those in whom tumors were resected and recurred or in whom tumors were incompletely resected. There was, however, no difference in survival rate between patients with complete resection and those with no tumor found at surgery. In two studies, patients with MEN 1 are reported to have a better 5- and 10-year survival rate than patients without MEN 1,[194] whereas in other studies, the difference was not significant.[26,195,201] One study demonstrated a significant difference in the percentage of patients with ZES with MEN 1 (6%) who presented with liver metastases, as compared with non–MEN 1 patients (22%, $P = .03$), with no difference in survival rate for the patients without liver metastases between MEN 1 and non–MEN 1 patients.[26] The presence of concurrent Cushing's syndrome may also be associated with a poor prognosis.[202]

Hence, because of the excellent prognosis for patients with gastrinomas that are resected and the evidence of increased importance of the malignancy in determining survival, surgical resection of gastrinoma should be considered in all patients with ZES.[35] After gastric acid hypersecretion is adequately controlled medically, it must be determined whether the patient has sporadic ZES (ZES without MEN 1) or whether ZES is present with MEN 1.[14] The role of surgery is controversial in patients with MEN 1.[203–205]

A recent study has addressed the question of whether surgical resection of the tumor alters its natural history.[206] In this study, only 3% of patients with ZES undergoing tumor resection developed liver metastases during follow-up, whereas significantly more patients treated medically developed liver metastases (26%, $P < .003$) (Fig. 38.5-6). Two deaths occurred owing to metastatic disease in the nonoperated group, as compared with no disease-specific deaths in the surgical group ($P = .085$). Although this was not a randomized study, the two groups did not differ in clinical or laboratory characteristics or time of follow-up (15.4 ± 1.5 years [no surgery] vs. 14.0 ± 0.8 years [surgery] from onset). This study strongly suggests that surgery alters the natural history of ZES and therefore should be recommended in patients without MEN 1. Additional studies reported after 1986 also indicate a higher cure rate, averaging approximately 40%, for patients with ZES who undergo operation; however, there was wide variation, from 17% to 100%.[23,25,195,207–211]

In most recent series, the improvement in outcome after surgical exploration and resection with curative intent is due to a number of factors. First, because gastric acid hypersecretion can be managed in all patients with antisecretory agents, surgical

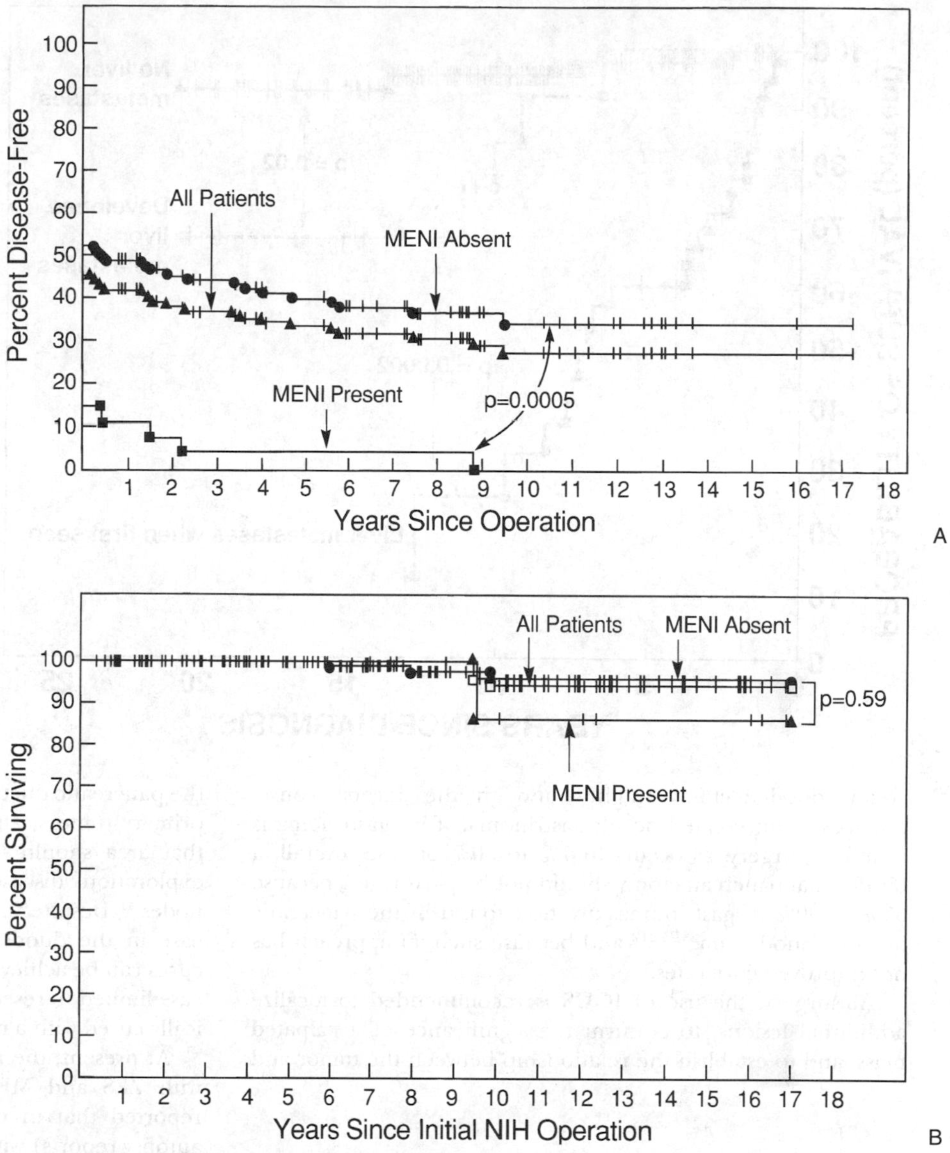

FIGURE 38.5-4. Disease-free (**A**) and disease-specific (**B**) survival in patients with the Zollinger-Ellison syndrome (ZES). **A:** Kaplan-Meier plot of disease-free survival after surgical exploration to resect and potentially cure gastrinoma. Twenty-eight patients with ZES and multiple endocrine neoplasia type 1 underwent 32 surgical explorations, and 123 patients with sporadic ZES underwent 144 surgical explorations. Data are presented based on number of operative procedures rather than number of patients. Results show the percentage of the total number of surgical patients in each group who are disease-free at the indicated time. **B:** Kaplan-Meier plot of survival specific for ZES. Four deaths occurred, secondary to progressive metastatic disease in three cases and a paradoxical cerebral embolus postoperatively through a patent foremen ovale valley in one case. MEN1, multiple endocrine neoplasia type 1; NIH, National Institutes of Health. (From ref. 35.)

exploration can be done electively and safely.[14,25,35,212] Second, patients can be effectively screened to eliminate occult metastatic unresectable disease, thereby improving patient selection for potentially curative surgery.[38,39,152] Furthermore, the knowledge that small duodenal primary tumors are more frequent than previously was appreciated has resulted in increased detection and resection of these lesions than in earlier studies.[35,42,79] In a 10-year prospective analysis of surgical outcome in patients with ZES, the overall percentage of patients free of disease at 5 years was 30%,[25] consistent with the updated outcome from the same institution.[35] In addition, ectopic gastrinoma can occur in a variety of other locations, including small bowel mesentery, common bile duct, and ovary.[29]

At laparotomy, the entire pancreas as well as the duodenum should be dissected and exposed.[23,25,171,213] IOUS and transillumination of the duodenum should be performed.[23,25] Duodenotomy in the anterior wall of the second part of the duodenum also should be performed.[23,25,171,213] Palpation alone can identify 65% of duodenal gastrinomas, endoscopic transillumination an additional 20% of tumors, and duodenotomy an additional 15% of tumors not localized by any other modality.[174] For duodenal tumors, 71% are in the first part of the duodenum, 21% in the second part, and 8% in the third part.[42] Using this approach to carefully evaluate the duodenum, gastrinomas have been found in all patients undergoing operation,[35] 71% of such lesions being duodenal.[76] At laparotomy, if a gastrinoma is found as a solitary lesion in the liver, it should be removed, provided the resection can be performed safely. If gastrinoma is found in the pancreatic head, it should be enucleated.[23,211] If extensive gastrinoma not amenable to eradication is found in the pancreatic head area, performing a pancreaticoduodenectomy (Whipple's operation) for potential cure is controversial.[214,215] A Whipple procedure cured 11 of 12 patients with tumors localized by imaging studies and PVS to the peripancreatic head area.[211] However, no studies have demonstrated an increased survival rate overall in patients with ZES after pancreaticoduodenectomy. Because of the possible morbidity and mortality associated with this operation and the excellent long-term prognosis of these patients, it has not yet been established whether the adverse consequences of a pan-

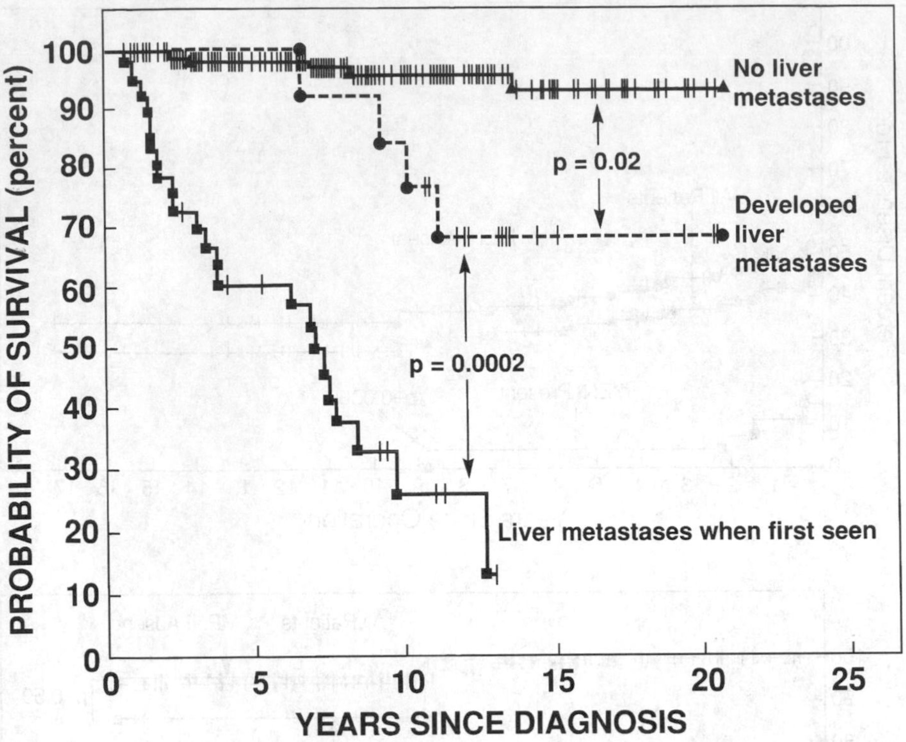

FIGURE 38.5-5. Survival based on the presence or absence of liver metastases in patients with the Zollinger-Ellison syndrome (ZES). Survival rates were evaluated using death due to ZES-related causes. Six of 158 patients with no liver metastases died; 17 patients developed liver metastases during the follow-up period, of whom 4 died; and 23 of 37 patients who presented with liver metastases on initial evaluation have died. (Data from ref. 40.)

creaticoduodenectomy might outweigh the adverse consequences of unresected occult gastrinoma. If no gastrinoma is found at surgery, as occurs in 7% to 30% of cases overall, a blind distal pancreatectomy should not be performed, because 65% to 90% of gastrinomas are now found in the pancreatic head or duodenum[23,25,212] and because such an approach has not improved cure rates.

At surgery, the use of IOUS is recommended to localize additional lesions, to confirm the significance of a palpated mass, and to establish the relationship between the tumor and the pancreatic duct.[172,216–219] For either pancreatic or duodenal primary tumors, any abnormal or suspicious lymph nodes in that area should be excised. In some patients undergoing exploration, disease may be limited to one or more lymph nodes.[41] Despite the inability to identify a primary site of disease in the duodenum or pancreas, long-term biochemical cures can be achieved. In one study of 13 patients who had disease limited to resected lymph nodes, 43% remained biochemically cured with a median follow-up of 5.3 years.[41]

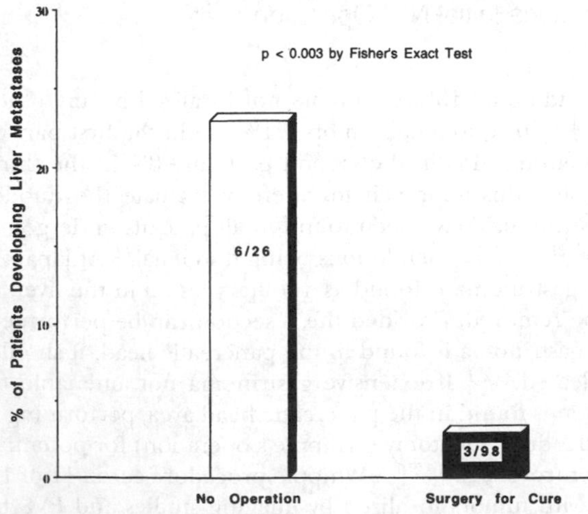

FIGURE 38.5-6. Incidence of liver metastases that developed in patients with the Zollinger-Ellison syndrome, some of whom had undergone surgery with curative intent while others were merely observed. Of 98 patients who underwent operation, 3 developed liver metastases at a mean follow-up of 6 years (range, 0.7 to 16.8 years), as compared to 6 of 26 patients who did not undergo operation, with a mean follow-up of 8.7 years (range, 1.5 to 19.0 years). (From ref. 206.)

At present, the role of surgery in the treatment of patients with ZES and MEN 1 is unclear.[53,54,205,212] A recent study reported that in eight patients (six surgical cases and two autopsy reports) with ZES and MEN 1, gastrinomas were found in the duodenum in all.[220] In all six patients whose tumors were surgically resected, the gastrin values were normal postoperatively, and this study raised the possibility that these patients could be cured. However, a number of limitations exist for this study; for example, cure cannot be established without a secretin provocative test, which was not reported in this study. A recent prospective study involving ten consecutive patients with ZES and MEN 1 demonstrated that no patients could be cured by simple tumor enucleation even after duodenotomy.[221] Cure was not possible short of pancreaticoduodenectomy, because 30% of patients had more than 20 duodenal tumors and 86% of patients had positive lymph nodes. This study also demonstrated that 20% of patients with MEN 1 and ZES had pancreatic gastrinomas.[221] Another recent study reported three patients with MEN 1 and ZES who were cured by a Whipple procedure.[211] In 77 patients with MEN 1 and ZES, the only independent factor associated with the development of liver metastases was a pancreatic primary tumor measuring greater than 3 cm.[222] Operation with curative intent in 118 patients did not influence survival. Currently, because of the excellent prognosis of these patients, the ability to control acid secretion medically, the presence of other pancreatic tumors, and the morbidity of this procedure, it is not routinely recommended. Our recommendation is to operate on patients with MEN 1 and ZES when a tumor of at least 2.5 cm is seen on imaging studies.[8,9,203] This policy is based on the recent observation that metastases to the liver correlated with tumor size.[26] If the tumor is in the pancreatic head, it is enucleated if possible, and, if in the pancreatic tail, it is resected and a duodenal exploration is performed.

Because most patients with sporadic ZES undergoing operation and resection will have persistent or recurrent disease, the role of reoperation in these patients warrants consideration. In a series of 17 patients who had previously undergone an operation with curative intent, reoperations were performed on the basis of biochemically documented recurrent disease and one or more positive imaging studies.[18,223] In those undergoing reoperation, it was possible to identify and resect disease in 17 of 18 cases, with biochemical cures in all, although median follow-up was short (34 months). Of note, the site of recurrent disease identified at reoperation was related to the initial operative findings. For example, in those in whom lymph node disease was resected initially, most patients had lesions identified in the duodenum at reoperation. In contrast, in those who had a primary duodenal or pancreatic lesion initially resected, recurrence was commonly identified in regional lymph nodes. Because of the increased potential risk of complications associated with reoperation in this setting, reoperation should be considered carefully.

INSULINOMA

Medical Therapy for Hypoglycemia of Insulinoma

The simplest form of nonsurgical treatment for insulinoma is dietary management.[1,70–72] Many insulinoma patients begin ingesting frequent small meals to alleviate symptoms prior to seeking medical evaluation, and a significant percentage report weight gain in the year prior to diagnosis. Slowly absorbed oral nutrients such as cornstarch, bread, potatoes, and rice are recommended.[1,224]

A number of drugs have been reported to control the hyperinsulinemia, with octreotide and diazoxide being the most effective.[1,70–72] Diazoxide, a benzthiazide analog, directly inhibits insulin release from β cells through stimulation of α-adrenergic receptors and also has an extrapancreatic hyperglycemic effect, possibly by inhibiting cyclic adenosine monophosphate phosphodiesterase, which enhances glycogenolysis.[1,70–72] The major side effects of diazoxide are sodium retention, gastrointestinal symptoms such as nausea and, occasionally, hirsutism. Edema can result from the sodium retention, and the addition of a diuretic such as trichlormethiazide, a benzothiadiazine derivative, can correct the edema as well as augment the hyperglycemic effect.[1,70–72] Diazoxide should be initiated, with 150 to 200 mg given in two to three divided doses per day and, if not effective, increased to a maximum of 600 to 800 mg/d.[1,70,71] The calcium channel inhibitor verapamil has been used, either alone or in combination with other drugs, to help control hypoglycemia in a small number of patients,[1] as has propranolol.[72,225] Phenytoin (Dilantin) inhibits the release of insulin from β cells and has been used successfully to treat a small number of patients with refractory hypoglycemia.[72,226] Maintenance doses of 300 to 600 mg/d are used, but it is reported that in only one-third or fewer patients is the hyperglycemic effect of phenytoin of any clinical significance.[72] Glucocorticoids (prednisone, 1 mg/kg) and glucagon, either alone or with diazoxide, have also been used in a few patients.[72]

Octreotide controls symptoms and hypoglycemia in 40% to 60% of patients.[1,70,71,227,228] This drug is generally well tolerated and usually is initiated at doses of 50 μg subcutaneously two or three times daily, which can be increased to 1500 μg/d.[228] The main side effects are gastrointestinal, such as bloating and abdominal cramping, and include long-term side effects such as malabsorption and cholelithiasis.[1,70,71,228] Besides improving symptoms, octreotide decreases plasma insulin levels in 65% of patients.[228] However, most patients were treated for less than 1 week preoperatively, so the long-term efficacy is not known in a significant number of patients. Octreotide also decreases plasma glucagon levels and growth hormone secretion; hence, it may worsen the hypoglycemia in some patients.[70]

Surgical Therapy

All insulinomas without evidence of metastases should be surgically removed, regardless of the severity of symptoms. Of all insulinomas, 80% to 90% are benign isolated lesions that are cured by complete surgical removal.[1,70–72,94,138–140] The extent of preoperative imaging necessary for successful outcome of resection of presumed benign solitary pancreatic insulinoma is controversial.[138–140] Because insulinomas are exclusively located within the pancreatic parenchyma, thorough exploration and intraoperative evaluation with inspection, palpation, and IOUS can result in successful resection in the vast majority of patients undergoing operation. IOUS has been advocated as an important adjunct in operation for insulinoma, not only in identifying lesions at the time of surgery but as an aid in enucleating the lesion by identifying the relationship between the tumor in the pancreatic parenchyma and the adjacent pancreatic duct. This is particularly important in the case of lesions located in the head of the pancreas, where a resection other than enucleation would require pancreaticoduodenectomy. Selective arterial stimulation of the splanchnic vessels supplying the pancreas using the secretagogue calcium can produce a subsequent rise in insulin levels obtained from catheters positioned at the orifice of the hepatic veins.[144] The sensitivity of this test is almost 90% and allows one to direct attention to a particular region of the pancreas at the time of operation. Blind distal pancreatectomy has been used in the past in an attempt to cure insulinoma in patients in whom no lesion could be identified, based on the appreciation that insulinomas can be distributed anywhere in the pancreatic parenchyma and resection of a large portion of normal pancreatic tissue should therefore have a reasonable cure rate for occult disease. However, given the current status of available localization studies, this practice should be largely unnecessary. With careful inspection and the use of IOUS, the number of people with occult lesions that cannot be identified at the time of operation should be fewer than 5%.[138,141] In this setting, our recommendation would be to proceed with distal pancreatectomy only in the face of a position insulin step-up in the hepatic veins after selective intraarterial stimulation with calcium demonstrates a *bona fide* step-up in the splenic artery as compared to the gastroduodenal or hepatic arteries.

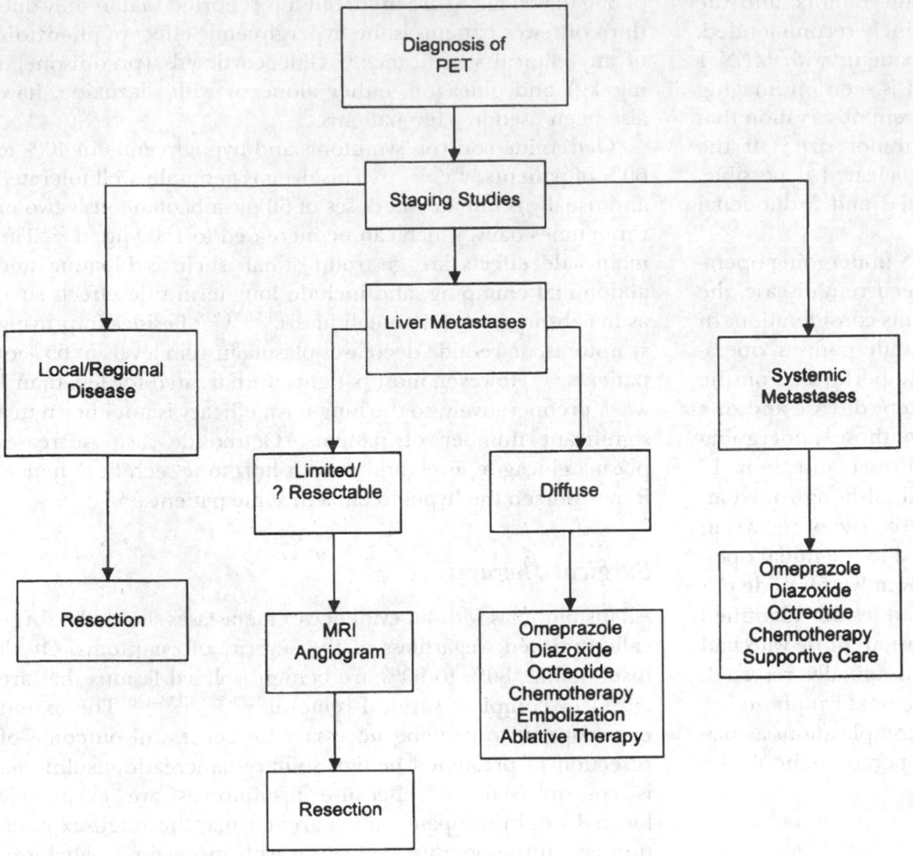

FIGURE 38.5-7. Flow diagram illustrating the general approach and management strategy for patients with pancreatic endocrine tumors (PET). Once the diagnosis has been established, initial staging studies are performed to determine the absence or presence of metastatic disease. A variety of palliative options are available to control the functional sequelae of hormone excess for increasing tumor burden. For those patients who have isolated liver metastases, resection should be performed when possible. Other regional therapies that may cause durable palliation of symptoms or disease control in the liver should be attempted. For those patients who have local regional disease, resection should be considered. MRI, magnetic resonance imaging.

The liver must always be explored for evidence of metastatic disease, and the entire abdomen must be explored to rule out rare extrapancreatic tumors that primarily secrete insulinoma-related growth factors (IGFs). IGF-secreting tumors that cause hypoglycemia usually are of mesodermal origin and have considerable tumor bulk by the time hypoglycemia symptoms occur.[71] The entire pancreas must be explored for other tumors, since multifocal tumors occur in up to 10% of all cases.[1,70,71] Isolated lesions of the tail may be enucleated or removed *en bloc* by distal pancreatectomy. Body and head lesions require enucleation with careful dissection to avoid damage to the main pancreatic duct and its attendant morbidity. Even in cases of documented metastatic disease, refractory debilitating symptoms may be an indication for debulking the pancreatic lesions, as metastases are not always secretory. Removal of peripancreatic lymph nodes may be curative for malignant insulinoma if no liver metastases are present.[93,224]

The documentation of metastatic disease, either at the time of surgery or by imaging studies, is the only accurate means of diagnosing malignant insulinoma. Unlike all other PETs, malignant insulinomas are uncommon, occurring in only 5% to 11% of all cases of insulinoma. Malignant primary insulinomas usually are not occult and have a mean size of 6 cm, which is more than three times as large as benign insulinomas.[1,70–72,229] The median disease-free survival after curative resection of malignant insulinomas was 5 years in one series.[229] The recurrence rate was 63%, the median interval to recurrence was 2.8 years, and the median survival with recurrent tumor was 19 months. Palliative re-resection was associated with a median survival of 4 years, whereas median survival after biopsy was only 11 months.[229] Surgical resection of primary and metastatic insulinomas is desirable when possible.[229] Malignant insulinomas, like other PETs, may respond to chemotherapy and treatment with octreotide.[1,71,228] The use of these agents for all malignant PETs is described later in Treatment of Metastatic Disease.

OTHER PANCREATIC ENDOCRINE TUMORS

The remainder of the PETs are relatively infrequent and include VIP-producing tumors (VIPomas), glucagonomas, ACTHomas, somatostatinomas, and GRF pancreatic tumors (GRFomas). Each of these PETs is usually malignant.

The treatment is surgical, if possible, even in the more than 60% of cases in which metastases are present at the time of diagnosis (Fig. 38.5-7).[3] Of 25 cases of nonfunctional PETS in one series, a Whipple procedure was performed in 20% of patients, partial or total pancreatectomy in 25%, and tumor excision in 10%.[101] The survival rates were 60% at 3 years and 44% at 5 years in this series.[101] The cure rate of these tumors at present is low because of their late recognition.

The first treatment objective in patients with VIPomas, even before considering the diagnosis, is the replenishment of fluid and electrolyte losses to correct the profound hypokalemia, dehydration, and acidosis that usually are present. The patients may require 5 L/d or more of fluid and more than 350 mEq/d of potassium.[104] In the past, numerous drugs have been reported to control, to varying degrees, the diarrheal output in small numbers of VIPoma patients; among these agents are prednisone (60 to 100 mg/d), clonidine, indomethacin, phenothiazines, lithium carbonate, propranolol, metoclopramide, loperamide, lidamidine, angiotensin II, and norepinephrine.[1,103,104]

Octreotide, a long-acting somatostatin analog, can control the diarrhea in both the short and long term in 87% of patients with VIPoma, and it is now the agent of choice.[1,103,227,228] In recent reviews of treatment of 20 and 25 patients with VIPomas with octreotide, the drug completely abolished diarrhea in 10% of patients in the first study and in 65% in the other and improved the diarrhea in 90% in the first study and in 95% in the other.[1,227,228] In some patients, responses have been reported to be short-lived, or a patient may respond initially to a low dose (50 to 100 μg three times daily) but subsequently may require a larger dose to control the diarrhea and may even become refractory to doses up to 1200 μg/d.[228] In nonresponsive patients or in patients whose symptoms recur, the administration of glucocorticoids concomitantly with octreotide has proven effective in a small number of cases.[228] With octreotide treatment, plasma VIP concentrations decreased in 80% to 88% of patients.[226,228]

After imaging studies have been conducted to localize the primary VIPoma and determine the extent of the tumor, surgical excision for cure should be considered in all patients without metastatic disease. In one series, surgical resection of a pancreatic VIPoma relieved all symptoms in 17 patients (33%),[105] and 30% were cured in another series.[230] Surgical removal with complete control of all symptoms was possible in 78% of all patients with VIP-producing ganglioneuroblastomas.[105]

For patients with glucagonomas, medical therapy with octreotide improves dermatitis in 54% to 90% of patients, with complete disappearance of this symptom in up to 30%.[1,227,228] In one study, diarrhea improved in four of six patients and resolved in two of six patients. Diabetes mellitus was not improved with octreotide treatment.[228] The diabetes mellitus was severe enough to require oral hypoglycemia agents in 42% of patients and insulin in 27%. Plasma glucagon levels decreased in 80% to 90% of patients but only decreased to the normal range in 10% to 20% of patients on octreotide treatment.[1,227,228]

In 50% to 80% of patients, metastases are already present at the time of diagnosis.[1,117–119] Surgical resection has been successful in a number of patients with resectable disease,[1,118,119] but the exact percentage of cases that can be cured is not known. In one large review involving 92 cases of glucagonoma, only 16 of the malignant cases were treated by surgical resection alone. Seven cases exhibited normal plasma glucagon levels after resection and, in the five cases that had no evidence of metastatic spread, plasma glucagon levels postoperatively were normal in two. Even if a patient eventually develops a recurrence, an extended disease-free interval may be attained that is beneficial.[119] A number of studies have reported a benefit to patients even if surgical debulking only can be accomplished.[117–119] In patients with widely metastatic disease in whom surgical debulking is not possible, various chemotherapeutic agents are used and are discussed later in Treatment of Metastatic Disease.

Most somatostatinomas are found at the time of laparotomy for cholecystectomy or during gastrointestinal imaging studies for various nonspecific complaints such as abdominal pain or diarrhea.[97,125] The symptoms produced by somatostatinomas are less pronounced and less specific than those seen with other PETs and probably do not reach a detectable level until patients develop high somatostatin blood levels late in the course of the disease. Though the plasma levels of somatostatin usually are elevated in pancreatic somatostatinomas, in duodenal or small-intestinal tumors these levels may fail to be conclusive.[123,231]

Duodenal somatostatinomas are increasingly associated with von Recklinghausen's disease.[231] In a recent review, 27 duodenal somatostatinomas with or without von Recklinghausen's disease were compared with pancreatic somatostatinomas without von Recklinghausen's disease.[231] The cases of somatostatinomas with von Recklinghausen's disease were similar to the sporadic duodenal cases in that they rarely were associated with the somatostatinoma syndrome, additional hormone production was infrequent, and they were less frequently malignant (30% vs. 71%).

The number of patients undergoing successful complete resection ranges from 60% to 80%.[83,96] In one series, 65% of patients were reported to have undergone successful resection, but the percentage actually cured was not stated.[232] In a number of patients, a combination of surgical resection and cytotoxic therapy was used,[97,125,233] and 60% of the patients were alive 6 months to 5 years after diagnosis. Because of the malignant nature of these tumors, if imaging studies demonstrate a possible resectable tumor, results suggest that patients with somatostatinomas will benefit from surgical resection.

In patients without metastatic disease, surgical resection of a GRFoma should be carried out. Surgical resection results in resolution of the GRFoma syndrome,[126,129,234] but the long-term cure rate is unknown. Before surgery and in those patients with nonresectable lesions, various agents may reduce plasma growth hormone levels. Even though dopamine agonists such as bromocriptine are successful and widely used in patients with classic acromegaly,[135] rarely is it possible to normalize plasma growth hormone levels in patients with GRFomas.[123,128] Octreotide is now the agent of choice.[1,123,135] In all cases thus far described, octreotide significantly suppressed or normalized growth hormone and IGF-1 levels[135,228,235–237] and, in some cases, this was associated with pituitary shrinkage.[235,237] In 75% of cases, octreotide decreased plasma GRF levels by more than 50%.[123]

In a few studies in patients with PETs secreting the peptide neurotensin, a neurotensinoma syndrome has been proposed.[1,3,55,97] Clinical features of patients with possible neurotensinomas include hypokalemia, weight loss, diabetes mellitus, cyanosis, hypotension, and flushing in a patient with a PET.[97] In a review of six cases, one-half of the patients were cured by resection of the pancreatic endocrine tumor, and the remaining one-half improved with chemotherapy.[97] Elevated plasma neurotensin levels have been measured in patients with VIPomas, and their symptoms did not differ from those with normal levels; a similar result was found in patients with gastrinomas.[55]

Patients with PETs and Cushing's syndrome (ACTHoma) have been reported.[64,202] In recent studies, 4% to 16% of Cushing's syndrome cases attributable to an ectopic ACTH syndrome originated from a pancreatic tumor. Cushing's syndrome is reported in 19% of patients with the ZES syndrome and MEN 1. In these patients, the disease was of pituitary origin and was mild. Cushing's syndrome also occurs in sporadic cases of ZES and, in one prospective study, it was found in 5% of all cases.[1,202] In these patients, the Cushing's syndrome was severe due to the ectopic ACTH production and occurred with metastatic pancreatic endocrine tumors, which responded poorly to chemotherapy; hence, the disease was associated with a poor prognosis.[202] The occurrence of Cushing's syndrome as the only manifestation of a PET occurs in 37% to 60% of cases and may precede any other hormonal syndrome.

Hypercalcemia resulting from a PET secreting a parathyroid hormone–related protein or to an unknown hypercalcemia substance that mimics the action of parathyroid hormone and causes hyperparathyroidism has been reported.[238–240] The tumor is generally large and metastatic to the liver by the time of diagnosis,[238,240] although in one recent case, radical resection of a pancreatic tail tumor with subsequent treatment with chemotherapy resulted in a total remission for 5 years.[239]

TREATMENT OF METASTATIC DISEASE

The treatment of all metastatic PETs is considered as a unit because, in most respects, cytotoxic protocols and surgical approaches are the same. The long-term natural history of most functional PETs (malignant insulinomas, VIPomas, glucagonomas, GRFomas, somatostatinomas) is not known because, until recently, effective treatment for the functional syndrome did not exist and therefore patients often died of complications of the hormonal excess rather than from the tumor *per se*.[1,40] In a study including 212 patients with ZES who had well-controlled gastric acid hypersecretion, 31% had died at a mean follow-up of almost 14 years.[40] One-half of these deaths were due to tumor progression, particularly in bone and liver, and to ectopic ACTH production. In a recent large study involving 185 patients with ZES in which no patient died from acid-related problems, the 10-year survival rate was not significantly different among patients in whom no tumor was found (only 8%), patients in whom tumor was completely resected, and patients in whom tumor was resected without biochemical cure (84%, 96%, and 93%, respectively).[26] However, in patients with unresectable disease, the 10-year survival rate was only 30%. This study demonstrates that the development of metastatic liver disease is the primary determinant of survival.[26] Currently, no data are available to suggest that survival for patients with other PETs will differ from that for patients with ZES and, in fact, limited data from PPomas, of which most were metastatic, reported mean survival of 4.3 years[3] and a 5-year survival rate of 44%,[101] which is similar to patients with metastatic gastrinomas. Most authorities would agree that treatment directed to metastatic unresectable liver disease is indicated. However, at present, there is no agreement about when therapy should be started or the efficacy of various therapeutic options, because of the small numbers of patients treated with various protocols. Chemotherapy either alone or combined with cytoreductive surgery, hepatic arterial embolization alone or with chemotherapy, hormonal therapy with the long-acting somatostatin analog octreotide, interferon, or hepatic transplantation have all been reported to be useful in small numbers of cases.[241,242]

CHEMOTHERAPY

Almost all studies that include significant numbers of patients and investigate the effects of chemotherapeutic agents on PETs include all types of PETs, often combined with carcinoids. Whether these results can be extrapolated to each histologic type is unclear at present. Three studies have demonstrated no difference in response rates of various PETs to streptozotocin (STZ)[243–245]; however, only small numbers of patients with different type of PETs were included. Other studies have shown a variable response of gastrinomas, glucagonomas, and VIPomas to chemotherapeutic agents such as dacarbazine (DTIC) or STZ, suggesting that differences may exist. Finally, other studies suggest that functioning tumors respond better than nonfunctioning tumors[243,246,247] and, among functioning tumors, insulin and VIP-secreting PETs may be more sensitive to STZ-based therapies.[246,247] Therefore, it should not be considered established that each tumor responds equally to chemotherapy.

Except for STZ[243,244,248,249] or chlorozotocin,[245,250] single-agent chemotherapy with various other agents (doxorubicin,[251] etoposide,[252] carboplatin,[253] DTIC,[254] and tubercidin[255]) has had limited efficacy (Table 38.5-5). STZ, a glycosamine nitrosourea compound originally derived from a *Streptomyces* species, has been in clinical use since 1967.[256,257] In preclinical studies, it was found to have cytotoxic effects on pancreatic islet cells[258] and has generally been used, usually in combination with other agents, for the treatment of metastatic PETs.[13,218,243,245,249,259–265] The current first-line regimen is the combination of STZ and doxorubicin.[245] This recommendation is based on a prospective study that demonstrated that STZ and doxorubicin were superior to STZ and 5-fluorouracil (5-FU) or chlorozotocin alone (response rates of 69%, 45%, and 30%, respectively).[245] Median durations of response were 18 months for the doxorubicin combination, 14 months for the 5-FU combination, and 17 months for the chlorozotocin group. Survival for patients treated with the doxorubicin combination was significantly longer. In a previous prospective study, STZ alone in 42 patients produced a response rate of 36%, with 12% showing a complete response, whereas STZ plus 5-FU had demonstrated a response rate of 63%, with 33% of patients having a complete response.[243]

STZ combined with 5-FU or 5-FU plus doxorubicin causes an objective response in up to 80% of patients with metastatic gastrinoma. For all PETs, the combination of STZ plus 5-FU gave a response rate of 63%, which was significantly better than the 40% response rate with STZ alone.[243] However, in a prospective study of ten patients with progressive metastatic gastrinoma to the liver, chemotherapy with STZ, 5-FU, and doxorubicin resulted in only a 40% objective response rate, no complete remissions, and no statistical difference in survival in responders versus nonresponders.[218] In another study of a similar group of 22 patients, only 5% of patients demonstrated an objective decrease in tumor size.[263] Therefore, the precise role and efficacy of chemotherapy in patients with metastatic gastrinoma has not been established.

Also, when chemotherapy should be initiated in a given patient with metastatic disease has not been clearly determined.[218] Recently, it has become apparent that the time course of tumor progression in patients with metastatic untreated gastrinoma is highly variable.[266] Of 19 patients evaluated, 26% showed no tumor growth over a mean follow-up of 29 months, 32% had marginal progression (<50% increase in tumor volume), and 42% had rapid growth in less than 1 year. Some patients have been followed up for 20 years with stable metastatic disease,[37] although most die within 5 years, with the mean survival being 3 to 5 years.[14,15,137,267] Of the two research groups with considerable experience with metastatic gastrinoma, one group proposed that patients be treated with chemotherapy when they become symptomatic.[243] However, if gastric acid hypersecretion is controlled adequately, symptoms due to the tumor arise only very late in the course of the disease. Another group proposed that, after the initial evaluation, patients be

TABLE 38.5-5. Drug Therapy for Pancreatic Endocrine Tumors and Gastrinomas

Agent	*Patients*	*Objective Response*	*Reference*
ALL PANCREATIC ENDOCRINE TUMORS			
STZ	31	17 (54%)	249
	52	26 (50%)	271
	17	7 (41%)	248
	16	10 (62%)	244
	42	14 (36%)	243
Etoposide	6	0 (0%)	252
Dox	20	4 (20%)	251
Carboplatin	9	0 (0%)	253
CZT	13	7 (53%)	250
	33	10 (33%)	245
DTIC	11	1 (9%)	255
Tubercidin	6	2 (33%)	255
Etoposide and cisplatin	14	2 (14%)	271
CZT + 5-FU	44	14 (32%)	270
STZ + 5-FU	40	25 (63%)	243
	22	1 (5%)	265
	30	19 (68%)	269
	33	15 (45%)	245
STZ + Dox	5	1 (20%)	260
	36	25 (69%)	245
STZ or STZ + 5-FU	45	19 (42%)	262
STZ + 5-FU + Dox	10	4 (40%)	218
5-FU + Dox + cisplatin	5	1 (20%)	
Octreotide	46	8 (17%)	227
	66	8 (11%)	228
	42	0 (0%)	279
	13	0 (0%)	280
Interferon	11	0 (0%)	288
	322	39 (12%)	272
Interferon-α + 5-FU	7	1 (14%)	289
GASTRINOMAS ONLY			
STZ	24	12 (50%)	243
CZT	4	4 (25%)	245
STZ + 5-FU	3	1 (33%)	243
	10	8 (80%)	7
	22	1 (5%)	263
	11	5 (45%)	245
STZ + Dox	1	7 (64%)	245
STZ or 5-FU	28	12 (42%)	262
STZ	17	7 (42%)	262
STZ + 5-FU + Dox	10	4 (40%)	218
Octreotide	9	1 (11%)	285
	16	3 (19%)	227
	22	3 (14%)	228
	6	0 (0%)	280
Interferon	4	2 (50%)	287
	11	0 (0%)	288

CZT, chlorozotocin; Dox, doxorubicin; DTIC, dacarbazine; 5-FU, 5-fluorouracil; STZ, streptozotocin.

reassessed in 3 to 6 months and those patients with evidence of increasing size of hepatic metastases be treated with chemotherapy.[218] No studies have recommended chemotherapy for patients with metastases only to regional lymph nodes.

STZ causes nausea and vomiting in almost all patients, dose-related renal dysfunction (including proteinuria) in 20% to 70%, decrease in creatinine clearance in 20% to 70%, abnormalities in hepatic function in 29%, and leukopenia and thrombocytopenia in 6% to 9%.[218,268,269] In one study, nine patients suffered from chronic renal failure, and seven required dialysis; thus, use of STZ must be carefully monitored.[245] The nausea and vomiting can now be controlled in almost all patients using 5-HT^3 antagonists such as ondansetron, so that the renal dysfunction is the major dose-limiting toxic effect. Chlorozotocin is structurally closely related to STZ,[268,270] but it causes less nausea and vomiting than does STZ. Patient response to chlorozotocin alone[245,250] or in combination with 5-FU[270] is, in general, similar to that to STZ (see Table 38.5-5).

Etoposide, dactinomycin, and cisplatin alone have been used in a few cases but are generally not effective.[248] The combination of etoposide and cisplatin was evaluated in 14 patients with metastatic PETs, and the results were compared with those in metastatic carcinoid tumors (13 patients) or anaplastic neuroendocrine tumors (18 patients: 6 pancreas; 8 stomach or intestine; 1 lung; 3 unknown).[271] This study was performed because recent work has demonstrated that these two agents are effective in small cell lung cancer, which has neuroendocrine features histologically similar to those seen in PETs. Sixty-seven percent of the anaplastic neuroendocrine tumors, 14% of the PETs, and 0% of the metastatic carcinoid tumors demonstrated partial to complete regression.[271]

Other etoposide combinations including doxorubicin, cisplatin, and 5-FU have been tried in a small number of patients with limited success (i.e., response rate of 20%).[272] Glucagonomas are reported to respond frequently to dacarbazine,[1,118,273–276] including some cases of complete remission, whereas in other PETs, the response rate is low.

HORMONAL THERAPY WITH SOMATOSTATIN ANALOGS

Hormonal therapy with the long-acting somatostatin analog octreotide is effective in controlling the symptoms due to a number of different PETs or carcinoid-like tumors, including VIPomas, glucagonomas, GRFomas, insulinomas, gastrinomas, and carcinoids.[277–282] In animal studies, somatostatin analogs can inhibit tumor growth[283] and the growth of transplantable insulinomas and chondrosarcomas.[284] More than 90% of all PETs except insulinomas possess somatostatin receptors,[1,151,154,277] which may mediate the action of somatostatin on these tumors. Hormonal treatment with octreotide is reported to cause a decrease in tumor size in 8 of 66 patients with PETs in one review.[228] A decrease in hepatic metastases in 3 of 22 patients has been noted in different reports of gastrinoma treated with octreotide.[228] However, another study of nine patients with metastatic gastrinoma treated with octreotide for 1 to 11 months reported no benefit.[285] In subsequent studies, octreotide infrequently caused a decrease in PET tumor size,[279,280,282] but stabilization of disease was more commonly seen in 25% to 50% of patients, and increased survival was not demonstrated in these studies.[278–280,282,286] These results must be extended to a larger, multicenter study, but they suggest that octreotide may have a cytostatic effect and, by decreasing the tumor growth rate, may increase survival.

INTERFERON-α

Interferon-α has been reported to be effective at controlling symptoms in patients with PETs.[270,272,279,287] In a review of numerous series involving 322 patients with various neuroendocrine tumors, 43% of the patients showed a biochemical response (>50% decrease in hormone levels) and 12% showed a decrease in tumor size with interferon-α treatment either alone or in combination with other agents.[272] Of 57 patients with PETs, 47% had a biochemical response and 12% experienced decreased tumor size. The mean duration of the response was 20 months (range, 2 to 96 months). Disease stabilization was seen in 25%. There was no difference in the response rate between patients with or without previous chemotherapy.[272]

In another study of 11 patients with metastatic gastrinoma to the liver that was increasing in size, interferon-α (5 million U/d) failed to decrease tumor size in any patients but slowed tumor growth in 3 patients.[288]

These results suggest that the effect of interferon-α on PETs is similar to that of octreotide in that it has minimal tumoricidal activity, with PETs rarely regressing with treatment. However, interferon-α may stabilize the disease in a significant percentage of patients and possibly extend survival, although with PETs this has not yet been proven. Interferon has been used with 5-FU,[289] octreotide,[272] and 5-FU plus STZ,[272] though in such small numbers of patients that clear assessment of any advantages of these combinations is not possible.

HEPATIC ARTERY EMBOLIZATION

Hepatic artery embolization with or without postocclusion chemotherapy has been used successfully in small numbers of patients with metastatic PETs to the liver.[110,247,290–293] It is reported in some studies that 68% to 100% of patients demonstrated symptomatic improvement with this therapy.[290,292,294] In one study involving 111 patients, hepatic arterial occlusion was combined with chemotherapy in 64% of the patients, using doxorubicin plus dacarbazine or STZ plus 5-FU.[247] Objective remissions were observed in 60% of the patients treated with embolization alone and in 80% of patients treated with added chemotherapy.[247] With embolization alone, the median duration of the remission was 4 months and, with chemoembolization, it was 18 months. Chemoembolization using doxorubicin in iodized oil combined with either gelatin powder or sponge particles has recently been reported in two studies to improve symptoms in 68% to 100% of patients and to decrease tumor size or hormonal markers in 57% to 100% of patients.[292,294] Side effects include abdominal pain, nausea, vomiting, and fever usually lasting 3 to 10 days,[290] with severe complications (including hepatic failure, infection, acute renal failure, and death) occurring in 10% to 15%.[290,295] Until recently, it often was difficult to establish the true extent of the metastatic disease and, therefore, to decide which patients might be most helped by this procedure. With the availability of SRS, it should now be possible to accomplish this in most cases. In a patient with a symptomatic PET and diffusely metastatic disease to the liver but minimal or no bone metastases, in whom hormone symptoms cannot be controlled by octreotide, chemotherapy, or other medical treatment, hepatic artery embolization should be considered.

SURGICAL TREATMENT

Systemic removal of all resectable tumor has been recommended in general for PETs[110,296–300] and, if possible, for VIPomas,[103,301] glucagonomas,[118,119] GRFomas,[123] and somatostatinomas.[302] The data of Zollinger et al.[15] suggest that removal of all resectable tumor, termed *debulking* or *cytoreductive surgery*, prolongs life expectancy. No studies to date have evaluated debulking surgery in a controlled, prospective manner. It is important to differentiate between the possible benefit of such surgery in patients with gastrinomas or nonfunctional tumors and the potential benefit in patients with functional PETs for whom poor medical therapy for the hormonal excess state might ensue. In the former group, the procedure must extend life or relieve tumor symptoms to be worthwhile, whereas in the latter group, improved ability to control the hormonal excess state in situations without effective medical therapy may be a major benefit.

A number of studies have provided data dealing with this approach.[296,297,299,300] One study involved 17 patients with potentially resectable metastatic PETs,[296] and the second evaluated 74 patients with metastatic neuroendocrine tumors (50 carcinoid, 23 islet cell, and 1 atypical tumor).[297] In the first study, in 80% of cases, the tumor was completely excised at surgery, and the survival rate was 79% at 5 years, with a mean follow-up of 3 years.[296] In this study, patients with extensive metastatic disease had a 5-year survival rate of 28%, equal to that in inoperable patients, whereas patients with limited resection had significantly prolonged survivals ($P = .02$). In the second study, 36 hepatic lobectomies or extended hepatectomies and 38 nonanatomic liver resections were performed. Perioperative mortality was 2.7%, morbidity 24%, and 4-year survival 73%; 90% of patients experienced symptomatic improvement postoperatively.[297] Norton et al.[137] reported the successful resection of all metastatic disease in 5 of 20 patients with ZES with extensive disease, 2 of whom have maintained normal gastrin levels postoperatively. A series of 38 patients with PETs confined to liver who underwent resection was compared to 23 patients with comparable tumor burden but technically unresectable disease.[299] Survival was significantly longer in those who underwent resection, although other factors may also have influenced outcome. The conclusion of each of these studies was that resection of metastatic disease to liver should be considered in selected patients with neuroendocrine tumors.[110,296,297,299] It is important to remember that this may be possible in only a small proportion (9% in one study[303] and 5% in another[296]) of all patients with metastatic PETs in the liver. Furthermore, at present, whether such an approach actually increases survival is not clear (see Figs. 38.5-3, 38.5-7). This approach may be required in patients with symptomatic tumors in whom octreotide or the use of chemotherapy alone is not reducing plasma hormone levels sufficiently, so that symptoms remain poorly controlled.[1]

LIVER TRANSPLANTATION

Liver transplantation has been attempted in small numbers of patients with metastatic PETs.[304–308] Each of the reported series involves small numbers of cases. All these studies recommend that liver transplantation be considered in selected cases, especially patients without extrahepatic disease. In the largest series of 31 patients who underwent liver transplantation for neuroendocrine tumors, 15 were for carcinoid and 16 were for PETs.[309] Survival rates were significantly higher for the carcinoid patients (69% alive at 5 years) than for the PET patients (8% alive at 4 years). It appears from this small number of cases that long-term cure is uncommon, with recurrence to liver being most common. Whether liver transplantation is more effective in PET cases than in other metastatic tumors and whether it appreciably prolongs survival remains undetermined.

REFERENCES

1. Jensen RT, Norton JA. Management of metastatic pancreatic endocrine tumors. In: Feldman M, Scharschmidt BF, Sleisenger MH, eds. *Gastrointestinal and liver disease.* Philadelphia: WB Saunders, 1998:871.
2. Kloppel G, Schroder S, Heitz PU. Histopathology and immunopathology of pancreatic endocrine tumors. In: Mignon M, Jensen RT, eds. *Endocrine tumors of the pancreas: recent advances in research and management.* Basel: S Karger, 1995:120.
3. Eriksson B, Oberg K. PPomas and nonfunctioning endocrine pancreatic tumors: clinical presentation, diagnosis, and advances in management. In: Mignon M, Jensen RT, eds. *Endocrine tumors of the pancreas: recent advances in research and management.* Basel: S Karger, 1995:208.
4. Metz DC. Diagnosis and treatment of pancreatic neuroendocrine tumors. *Semin Gastrointest Dis* 1995;6:67.
5. Weil C. Gastroenteropancreatic endocrine tumors. *Klin Wochenschr* 1985;63:433.
6. Dent RB, van Heerden JA, Weiland LH. Nonfunctioning islet cell tumors. *Ann Surg* 1981;193:185.
7. Mignon M, Jais P, Cadiot G, Yedder DB, Vatier J. Clinical features and advances in biological diagnostic criteria for Zollinger-Ellison syndrome. In: Mignon M, Jensen RT, eds. *Endocrine tumors of the pancreas: recent advances in research and management.* Basel: S Karger, 1995:223.
8. Jensen RT. Gastrin-producing tumors. In: Arnold A, ed. *Endocrine neoplasms.* Amsterdam: Kluwer Academic Publishers, 1997:293.
9. Jensen RT. Gastrinoma. *Bailliere's Clin Gastroenterol* 1996;10:603.
10. Zollinger RM, Ellison EH. Primary peptic ulceration of the jejunum associated with islet cell tumors of the pancreas. *Ann Surg* 1955;142:709.
11. Gregory RA, Grossman MI, Tracy HJ, Bentley PH. Nature of the gastric secretagogue in Zollinger-Ellison tumors. *Lancet* 1967;2:543.
12. Gregory RA, Tracy JH, Agarwal KL. Amino acid constitution of two gastrins isolated from Zollinger-Ellison tumor tissue. *Gut* 1969;10:603.
13. Eriksson B, Oberg K, Skogseid B. Neuroendocrine pancreatic tumors. *Acta Oncol* 1989;28:373.
14. Jensen RT, Gardner JD. Gastrinoma. In: Go VLW, DiMagno EP, Gardner JD, et al., eds. *The pancreas: biology, pathobiology, and disease.* New York: Raven Press, 1993:931.
15. Zollinger RM, Ellison EC, Fabri PJ, et al. Primary peptic ulceration of the jejunum associated with islet cell tumors: twenty-five year appraisal. *Ann Surg* 1980;192:422.
16. Willems G. Trophic action of gastrin on specific target cells in the gut. In: Mignon M, Jensen RT, eds. *Endocrine tumors of the pancreas: recent advances in research and management.* Basel: S Karger, 1995:30.
17. Dockray GJ, Walsh JH, Passaro E Jr. Relative abundance of big and little gastrins in the tumors and blood of patients with Zollinger-Ellison syndrome. *Gut* 1975;16:353.
18. Dockray GJ, Walsh JH. Amino terminal gastrin fragment in serum of Zollinger- Ellison syndrome patients. *Gastroenterology* 1975;68:222.
19. Hilsted L, Bardram LC. Terminally glycine extended gastrins in serum and tumors from patients with Zollinger-Ellison syndrome. *Can J Physiol Pharmacol* 1986;64:136.
20. Bardram L. Progastrin in serum from Zollinger-Ellison patients: an indicator of malignancy? *Gastroenterology* 1990;98:1420.
21. Pauwels S, Desmond H, Dimaline R, Dockray GJ. Identification of progastrin in gastrinoma antrum and duodenum by a novel radioimmunoassay. *J Clin Invest* 1986;77:376.
22. Kothary PC, Fabri PJ, Gower W, et al. Evaluation of NH_2-terminus gastrins in gastrinoma syndrome. *J Endocrinol Metab* 1986;62:970.
23. Norton JA, Doppman JL, Collen MJ, et al. Prospective study of gastrinoma localization and resection in patients with Zollinger-Ellison syndrome. *Ann Surg* 1986;204:468.
24. Wolfe MM, Alexander RW, McGuigan JE. Extrapancreatic extraintestinal gastrinoma: effective treatment by surgery. *N Engl J Med* 1982;306:1533.
25. Norton JA, Doppman JL, Jensen RT. Curative resection in Zollinger-Ellison syndrome: results of a 10-year prospective study. *Ann Surg* 1992;215:8.
26. Weber HC, Venzon DJ, Fishbein VA, et al. Determinants of metastatic rate and survival in patients with Zollinger-Ellison syndrome (ZES): a prospective long-term study. *Gastroenterology* 1995;108:1637.
27. Maton PN, Macken SM, Norton JA, et al. Ovarian carcinoma as a cause of Zollinger-Ellison syndrome. *Gastroenterology* 1989;97:464.
28. Primrose JN, Maloney M, Wells M, Bulgin O, Johnston D. Gastrin-producing ovarian mucinous cystadenomas: a cause of Zollinger-Ellison syndrome. *Surgery* 1988;104:830.
29. Wu PC, Alexander HR, Bartlett DL, et al. A prospective analysis of the frequency, location, and curability of ectopic (nonpancreaticoduodenal nonnodal) gastrinoma. *Surgery* 1997;122:1176.
30. Solcia E, Capella C, Buffa R, et al. Endocrine cells of the gastrointestinal tract and related tumors. *Pathol Annu* 1979;9:163.
31. Solcia E, Capella C, Buffa R, Frigerio G, Fiocca R. Pathology of the Zollinger-Ellison syndrome. In: Fenoglio CM, Wolff M, eds. *Progress in surgical pathology.* 1980;1:119.
32. Friesen SR. Tumors of the endocrine pancreas. *N Engl J Med* 1982;306:580.
33. Fox PS, Hofmann JW, Wilson SD, DeCosse JJ. Surgical management of the Zollinger-Ellison syndrome. *Surg Clin North Am* 1974;54:394.
34. Richardson CT, Peters MN, Feldman M. Treatment of Zollinger-Ellison syndrome with exploratory laparotomy, proximal gastric vagotomy, and H_2-receptor antagonists. *Gastroenterology* 1985;89:357.
35. Norton JA, Fraker DL, Alexander HR, et al. Surgery to cure the Zollinger-Ellison syndrome. *N Engl J Med* 1999;341:635.
36. Ellison EC, Wilson SD. The Zollinger-Ellison syndrome: re-appraisal and evaluation of 260 registered cases. *Ann Surg* 1964;160:512.
37. Zollinger RM, Martin EW, Carey LC. Observations on the post-operative tumor growth of certain islet cell tumors. *Ann Surg* 19761;84:525.
38. Gibril F, Reynolds JC, Doppman JL, et al. Somatostatin receptor scintigraphy: its sensitivity compared with that of other imaging methods in detecting primary and metastatic gastrinomas. A prospective study. *Ann Intern Med* 1996;125:26.
39. Termanini B, Gibril F, Reynbolds JC, et al. Value of somatostatin receptor scintigraphy: a prospective study in gastrinoma of its effect on clinical management. *Gastroenterology* 1997;112:335.
40. Yu F, Venzon DJ, Serrano J, et al. Prospective study of the clinical course, prognostic factors, causes of death, and survival in patients with long-standing Zollinger-Ellison syndrome. *J Clin Oncol* 1999;17:615.
41. Arnold WS, Fraker DL, Alexander HR, et al. Apparent lymph node primary gastrinoma. *Surgery* 1994;116:1123.
42. Thom AK, Norton JA, Axiotis CA, Jensen RT. Location, incidence, and malignant potential of duodenal gastrinomas. *Surgery* 1991;110:1086.
43. Bordi C, Viale G. Analysis of cell proliferation and tumor antigens of prognostic significance in pancreatic endocrine tumors. In: Mignon M, Jensen RT, eds. *Endocrine tumors of the pancreas: recent advances in research and management.* Basel: S Karger, 1995:45.
44. Metz DC, Kuchnio M, Fraker DL, et al. Flow cytometry and Zollinger-Ellison syndrome: relationship to clinical course. *Gastroenterology* 1993;105:799.
45. Long PP, Hruban RH, Lo R, et al. Chromosome analysis of nine endocrine neoplasms of the pancreas. *Cancer Genet Cytogenet* 1994;77:55.
46. Evers BM, Rady PL, Sandoval K, et al. Gastrinomas demonstrate amplification of the HER-2/*neu* proto-oncogene. *Ann Surg* 1994;219:596.
47. Evers BM, Rady PL, Tyring SK, et al. Amplification of the HER-2/*neu* protooncogene in human endocrine tumors. *Surgery* 1992;112:211.
48. Cadiot G, Laurent-Puig P, Thuille B, et al. Is the multiple endocrine neoplasia type 1 gene a suppressor for fundic argyrophil tumors in the Zollinger-Ellison syndrome? *Gastroenterology* 1993;105:579.
49. Debelenko LV, Zhuang Z, Emmert-Buck MR, et al. Allelic deletions on chromosome 11a13 in multiple endocrine neoplasia type 1–associated and sporadic gastrinomas and pancreatic endocrine tumors. *Cancer Res* 1997;57:2238.
50. Chandrasekharappa SC, Guru SC, Manickam P, et al. Positional cloning of the gene for multiple endocrine neoplasia–type 1. *Science* 1997;276:404.
51. Goebel SU, Heppner C, Burns AL, et al. Genotype/phenotype correlation of multiple endocrine neoplasia type 1 gene mutations in sporadic gastrinomas. *J Clin Endocrinol Metab* 2000;85:116.
52. Eberle F, Grun R. Multiple endocrine neoplasia type I. *Adv Intern Med Pediatr* 1981;5:76.
53. Mignon M, Cadiot G, Rigaud D, et al. Management of islet cell tumors in patients with multiple endocrine neoplasia type 1. In: Mignon M, Jensen RT, eds. *Endocrine tumors of the pancreas: recent advances in research and management.* Basel: S Karger, 1995:342.
54. Metz DC, Jensen RT, Bale AE, et al. Multiple endocrine neoplasia type 1: clinical features and management. In: Bilezekian JP, Levine MA, Marcus R, eds. *The parathyroids.* New York: Raven Press, 1994:591.
55. Chiang H, O'Dorisio TM, Huang SC, et al. Multiple hormone elevations in patients with Zollinger-Ellison syndrome: prospective study of clinical significance and of development of a second symptomatic pancreatic endocrine tumor syndrome. *Gastroenterology* 1990;99:1565.
56. Mukai K, Greider MH, Grotting JC, Rosai J. Retrospective study of 77 pancreatic endocrine tumors using the immunoperoxidase method. *Am J Surg Pathol* 1982;6:387.
57. Eriksson B. Tumor markers for pancreatic endocrine tumors, including chromogranins HCG-alpha and HCG-beta. In: Mignon M, Jensen RT, eds. *Endocrine tumors of the pancreas: recent advances in research and management.* Basel: S Karger, 1995:121.
58. Bloom SR, Adrian TE, Bryant MG, Polak JM. Pancreatic polypeptide: a marker for Zollinger-Ellison syndrome. *Lancet* 1978;1:1155.
59. Adrian TE, Uttenthal LD, Williams SJ, Bloom SR. Secretion of pancreatic polypeptide in patients with pancreatic endocrine tumors. *N Engl J Med* 1986;315:287.
60. Taylor IL, Rotter J, Walsh JH, Passaro E Jr. Is pancreatic polypeptide a marker for Zollinger-Ellison syndrome? *Lancet* 1978;1:845.
61. Langstein HN, Norton JA, Chiang HCV, et al. The utility of circulating levels of human pancreatic polypeptide as a marker of islet cell tumors. *Surgery* 1990;108:1109.
62. Sheppard BC, Norton JA, Doppman JL, et al. Management of islet cell tumors in patients with multiple endocrine neoplasia; a prospective study. *Surgery* 1989;106:1108.
63. Mathew CGP, Easton DF, Nakamura Y, et al. Presymptomatic screening for multiple endocrine neoplasia type 2A with linked DNA markers. *Lancet* 1991;337:7.
64. Amikura K, Alexander HR, Norton JA, et al. Role of surgery in management of adrenocorticotropic hormone–producing islet cell tumors of the pancreas. *Surgery* 1995;118:1125.
65. Bardram L, Agner T, Hagen C. Levels of alpha subunits of gonadotropin can be increased in Zollinger-Ellison syndrome both in patients with malignant tumors and apparently benign disease. *Acta Endocrinol* 1988;118:135.
66. Wiedenmann B, Waldherr R, Buhr H, et al. Identification of gastroenteropancreatic neu-

roendocrine cells in normal and neoplastic human tissue with antibodies against synaptophysin, chromogranin A, secretogranin I (chromogranin B), and secretogranin II. *Gastroenterology* 1988;95:1364.

67. Stridsberg M, Oberg K, Li Q, Engstrom U, Lundqvist G. Measurements of chromogranin A, chromogranin B (secretogranin I), chromogranin C (secretogranin II), and pancreastatin in plasma and urine from patients with carcinoid tumours and endocrine pancreatic tumours. *J Endocrinol* 1995;144:49.
68. Goebel SU, Serrano J, Yu F, et al. Prospective study of the value of serum chromogranin A or serum gastrin levels in the assessment of the presence, extent, or growth of gastrinomas. *Cancer* 1999;85:1470.
69. Whipple AO. The surgical therapy of hyperinsulinism. *J Int Chir* 1938;3:237.
70. Creutzfeldt W. Insulinomas: clinical presentation, diagnosis, and advances in management. In: Mignon M, Jensen RT, eds. *Endocrine tumors of the pancreas: recent advances in research and management.* Basel: S Karger, 1995:148.
71. Comi RJ, Gorden P, Doppman JL. Insulinoma. In: Go VLW, ed. *The pancreas: biology, pathobiology, and disease.* New York: Raven Press, 1993:979.
72. Fajans SS, Vinik AI. Insulin-producing islet cell tumors. *Endocrinol Metab Clin North Am* 1989;18:45.
73. Stefanini P, Carboni M, Patrassi N, Basoli A. Beta-islet cell tumor of the pancreas: results of a study on 1067 cases. *Surgery* 1974;75:597.
74. Hirschowitz BI. Zollinger-Ellison syndrome: pathogenesis, diagnosis, and management. *Am J Gastroenterol* 1997;92:44S.
75. Miller LS, Vinayek R, Frucht H, et al. Reflux esophagitis in patients with Zollinger-Ellison syndrome. *Gastroenterology* 1990;98:341.
76. Jensen RT, Fraker DL. Zollinger-Ellison syndrome: advances in treatment of the gastric hypersecretion and the gastrinoma. *JAMA* 1994;271:1.
77. Waxsman I, Gardner JD, Jensen RT, Maton PN. Peptic ulcer perforation as the presentation of Zollinger-Ellison syndrome. *Dig Dis Sci* 1991;36:19.
78. Maton PN. Zollinger-Ellison syndrome: recognition and management of acid hypersecretion. *Drugs* 1996;52:33.
79. Zimmer T, Stolzel U, Bader M, et al. Brief report: a duodenal gastrinoma in a patient with diarrhea and normal serum gastrin concentrations. *N Engl J Med* 1995;333:634.
80. Jais P, Mignon M. Normal serum gastrin concentration in gastrinoma. *Lancet* 1995;346:1421.
81. Frucht H, Howard JM, Slaff JF. Secretin and calcium provocative tests in patients with Zollinger-Ellison syndrome: a prospective study. *Ann Intern Med* 1989;111:713.
82. Metz DC, Weber HC, Orbuch M, et al. *Helicobacter pylori* infection: a reversible cause of hypergastrinemia and hyperchlorhydria which can mimic Zollinger-Ellison syndrome. *Dig Dis Sci* 1995;40:153.
83. Alexander HR Jr, Jensen RT, Doppman JL. Pancreatic endocrine tumors. In: Torosian M, ed. *Integrated cancer management: surgery, medical oncology, and radiation oncology.* New York: Marcel Dekker, 1999:241.
84. Deveney CW, Deveney KS, Jaffe BM, Janes RS, Way LW. Use of calcium and secretin in the diagnosis of gastrinoma (Zollinger-Ellison syndrome). *Ann Intern Med* 1979;87:680.
85. Isenberg JI, Walsh JH, Passaro E Jr, Moore EW, Grossman MI. Unusual effect of secretin on serum gastrin, serum calcium, and gastric acid secretion in a patient with suspected Zollinger-Ellison syndrome. *Gastroenterology* 1972;62:626.
86. Frucht H, Howard JM, Stark HA, et al. Prospective study of meal provocative gastrin testing in patients with Zollinger-Ellison syndrome. *Am J Med* 1989;87:528.
87. Lamers CBH, van Tongeren JHM. Comparative study of the value of calcium secretin and meal stimulated increase in serum gastrin in the diagnosis of the Zollinger-Ellison syndrome. *Gut* 1979;18:128.
88. Friesen SR, Tomita T. Pseudo-Zollinger-Ellison syndrome. Hypergastrinemia, hyperchlorhydria without tumor. *Ann Surg* 1981;194:481.
89. Taylor IL, Calam JK, Roth JI, et al. Family studies of hypergastrinemic, hyperpepsinogenemic I duodenal ulcer. *Ann Intern Med* 1981;95:421.
90. Hangen D, Maltz GS, Anderson CM. Marked hypergastrinemia in gastric outlet obstruction. *J Clin Gastroenterol* 1989;11:442.
91. Fuerle G, Ketterer H, Becker HD, Creutzfeldt W. Circadian serum gastrin concentrations in control persons and in patients with ulcer disease. *Scand J Gastroenterol* 1972;7:177.
92. Nakanishi T, Shinomura Y, Kanayama S, Matsuzawa Y. Eradication of *Helicobacter pylori* normalizes serum gastrin concentration and antral gastrin cell number in a patient with primary gastrin cell hyperplasia. *Am J Gastroenterol* 1993;88:440.
93. Comi RJ, Gorden P, Doppman HL, Norton JA. Insulinoma. In: Go VLW, Gardner JD, Brooks FP, et al., eds. *The exocrine pancreas: biology, pathology, and diseases.* New York: Raven Press, 1986:745.
94. Moller DE, Flier JS. Insulin resistance—mechanisms, syndromes, and implications. *N Engl J Med* 1991;325:938.
95. Grunberger G, Weiner JL, Silverman R, et al. Factitious hypoglycemia due to surreptitious administration of insulin: diagnosis, treatment, and long-term follow-up. *Ann Intern Med* 1988;108:252.
96. Thompson GB, van Heerden JA, Grant CS, Carney JA, Ilstrup DM. Islet cell carcinomas of the pancreas: a twenty-year experience. *Surgery* 1988;104:1011.
97. Vinik AI, Strodel WE, Eckhauser FE, et al. Somatostatinomas, PPomas, neurotensinomas. *Semin Oncol* 1987;14:263.
98. Heitz PU, Kasper M, Polak JM, Kloppel G. Pancreatic endocrine tumors. *Hum Pathol* 1982;13:263.
99. Vinik AI, Moattari AR. Treatment of endocrine tumors. *Endocrinol Clin North Am* 1989;18:483.
100. Peracchi M, Tagliabue R, Quatrini M, Reschini E. Plasma pancreatic polypeptide response to secretin. *Eur J Endocrinol* 1999;141:47.
101. Kent RB, van Heerden JA, Weiland LH. Nonfunctioning islet cell tumors. *Ann Surg* 1981;193:185.
102. Verner JV, Morrison AB. Islet cell tumor and a syndrome of refractory watery diarrhea and hypokalemia. *Am J Med* 1958;29:529.
103. Matuchansky C, Rambaud JC. VIPomas and endocrine cholera: clinical presentation, diagnosis, and advances in management. In: Mignon M, Jensen RT, eds. *Endocrine tumors of the pancreas: recent advances in research and management.* Basel: S Karger, 1995:166.
104. Mekhjian HS, O'Dorisio TM. VIPoma syndrome. *Semin Oncol* 1987;14:282.
105. Long RG, Bryant MG, Mitchell SJ, et al. Clinicopathological study of pancreatic and ganglioneuroblastoma tumors secreting vasoactive intestinal polypeptide (VIPomas). *Br Med J* 1981;282:1767.
106. Koppel G, Heitz PU. Pancreatic endocrine tumors. *Pathol Res Pract* 1988;183:155.
107. Capella C, Polak JM, Butta R, et al. Morphologic patterns and diagnostic criteria of VIP-producing endocrine tumors. A histologic, histochemical, ultrastructural, and biochemical study of 32 cases. *Cancer* 1983;52:1860.
108. Kane MG, O'Dorisio TM, Krejs GJ. Production of secretory diarrhea by intravenous infusion of vasoactive intestinal peptide. *N Engl J Med* 1983;309:1482.
109. Krejs GJ. VIPomas syndrome. *Am J Med* 1987;82:37.
110. Nagorney DM, Que FG. Cytoreductive hepatic surgery for metastatic gastrointestinal neuroendocrine tumors. In: Mignon M, Jensen RT, eds. *Endocrine tumors of the pancreas: recent advances in research and management.* Basel: S Karger, 1995:416.
111. Morris AI, Turnberg LA. Surreptitious laxative abuse. *Gastroenterology* 1979;77:780.
112. Read NW, Read MG, Krejs GJ, et al. A report of five patients with large volume secretory diarrhea but no evidence of endocrine tumor or laxative abuse. *Dig Dis Sci* 1982;27:193.
113. Becker SW, Kahn D, Rothman S. Cutaneous manifestations of internal malignant tumors. *Arch Dermatol Syph* 1942;45:1069.
114. McGavran MH, Unger RH, Recant L, et al. A glucagon-secreting alpha-cell carcinoma of the pancreas. *N Engl J Med* 1966;274:1408.
115. Wilkinson DS. Necrolytic migratory erythema with carcinoma of the pancreas. *Trans St John's Hosp Dermatol Soc* 1973;59:244.
116. Mallinson CN, Bloom SR, Warin AP, et al. A glucagonoma syndrome. *Lancet* 1974;2:1.
117. Stacpoole PW. The glucagonoma syndrome: clinical features, diagnosis, and treatment. *Endocr Rev* 1981;2:347.
118. Guillausseas PJ, Guillausseau-Scholer C. Glucagonomas: clinical presentation, diagnosis, and advances in management. In: Mignon M, Jensen RT, eds. *Endocrine tumors of the pancreas: recent advances in research and management.* Basel: S Karger, 1995:183.
119. Holst JJ. Glucagon-producing tumors. In: Cohen S, Soloway D, eds. *Hormone producing tumors of the gastrointestinal tract.* New York: Churchill Livingstone, 1985:57.
120. Abravia C, De Bartolo M, Katzen R, Lawrence AM. Disappearance of glucagonoma rash after surgical resection but not during dietary normalization of serum amino acids. *Am J Clin Nutr* 1984;39:351.
121. Ganda PO, Weir GC, Soeldner JS, et al. Somatostatinoma: a somatostatin-containing tumor of the endocrine pancreas. *N Engl J Med* 1977;296:963.
122. Larsson LI, Hirsch MA, Holst J, et al. Pancreatic somatostatinoma clinical features and physiologic implications. *Lancet* 1977;1:666.
123. Sassolas G, Chayvialle JA. GRFomas, somatostatinomas: clinical presentation, diagnosis, and advances in management. In: Mignon M, Jensen RT, eds. *Endocrine tumors of the pancreas: recent advances in research and management.* Basel: S Karger, 1995:194.
124. Lrejs GJ, Orci L, Conlon M, et al. Somatostatinoma syndrome (biochemical, morphological, and clinical features). *N Engl J Med* 1979;301:285.
125. Boden G, Shimoyama R. Somatostatinoma. In: Cohen S, Soloway RD, eds. *Hormone-producing tumors of the gastrointestinal tract.* New York: Churchill Livingstone, 1985:85.
126. Rivier J, Spress J, Thorner M, Vale W. Characterization of a growth-hormone releasing factor from a human pancreatic islet cell tumor. *Nature* 1982;300:276.
127. Thorner MO, Perryman RL, Cronin MJ, et al. Somatotroph hyperplasia. *J Clin Invest* 1982;70:965.
128. Guillemin R, Brazeau P, Bohlen P, et al. Growth hormone–releasing factor from a human pancreatic tumor that caused acromegaly. *Science* 1982;27:774.
129. Sano T, Asa SL, Kovacs K. Growth hormone releasing–producing tumors: clinical, biochemical, and morphological manifestations. *Endocr Rev* 1988;9:357.
130. Losa M, Schopohl J, von Werder K. Ectopic secretion of growth hormone–releasing hormone in man. *J Endocrinol Invest* 1993;16:69.
131. Berger C, Trouillas J, Bloch B, et al. Multihormonal carcinoid tumors of the pancreas: secreting growth hormone–releasing factor as a cause of acromegaly. *Cancer* 1984;54:2097.
132. Moller DE, Moses AC, Jones K, Thorner MO, Vance ML. Octreotide suppresses both growth hormone (GH) and GH-releasing hormone (GHRH) in acromegaly due to ectopic GHRH secretion. *J Clin Endocrinol Metab* 1989;68:499.
133. von Werder K, Losa M, Stalla FK, et al. Long-term treatment of a metastasizing GRFoma with a somatostatin analogue (SMS 201-995) in a girl with gigantism. *Scand J Gastroenterol* 1986;21:238.
134. Christofides ND, Stephanou A, Suzuki H, Yianigou Y, Bloom SR. Distribution of immunoreactive growth hormone–releasing hormone in the human brain and intestine and its production by tumors. *J Clin Endocrinol Metab* 1984;59:747.
135. Barkan AL. Acromegaly: diagnosis and therapy. *Endocrinol Metab Clin North Am* 1989;18:277.
136. Orbuch M, Doppman JL, Strader DB, et al. Imaging for pancreatic endocrine tumor localization: recent advances. In: Mignon M, Jensen RT, eds. *Endocrine tumors of the pancreas: recent advances in research and management.* Basel: S Karger, 1995:268.
137. Norton JA, Sugarbaker PH, Doppman JL, et al. Aggressive resection of metastatic disease in select patients with malignant gastrinoma. *Ann Surg* 1986;203:352.
138. van Heerden JA, Grant CS, Czako PF, Service FJ, Charboneau JW. Occult functioning insulinomas: which localizing studies are indicated? *Surgery* 1992;112:1010.
139. Hashimoto LA, Walsh RM. Preoperative localization of insulinomas is not necessary. *J Am Coll Surg* 1999;189:368.
140. Pasieka JL, McLeod MK, Thompson NW, Burney RE. Surgical approach to insulinomas. Assessing the need for preoperative localization. *Arch Surg* 1992;127:442.
141. Brown CK, Bartlett DL, Doppman JL, et al. Intraarterial calcium stimulation and intraoperative ultrasonography in the localization and resection of insulinomas. *Surgery* 1997;122:1189.

142. Norton JA, Shawker TH, Doppman JL, et al. Localization and surgical treatment of occult insulinomas. *Ann Surg* 1990;212:615.
143. Axelrod L. Insulinoma: cost-effective care in patients with a rare disease. *Ann Intern Med* 1995;123:311.
144. Doppman JL, Chang R, Fraker DL, et al. Localization of insulinomas to regions of the pancreas by intra-arterial stimulation with calcium. *Ann Intern Med* 1995;123:269.
145. London JB, Shawker TH, Doppman HL, et al. Prospective assessment of abdominal ultrasound in patients with Zollinger-Ellison syndrome. *Radiology* 1991;178:763.
146. Alexander HR, Fraker DL, Norton JA, et al. Prospective study of somatostatin receptor scintigraphy and its effect on operative outcome in patients with Zollinger-Ellison syndrome. *Ann Surg* 1998;228:228.
147. Maton PN, Miller DL, Doppman HL, et al. Role of selective angiography in the management of Zollinger-Ellison syndrome. *Gastroenterology* 1987;92:913.
148. Frucht H, Doppman JL, Norton JA, et al. MR imaging of gastrinomas: comparison with computed tomography, angiography, and ultrasound. *Radiology* 1989;171:713.
149. Pisegna JR, Doppman JL, Norton JA, Metz DC, Jensen RT. Prospective comparative study of ability of MR imaging and other imaging modalities to localize tumors in patients with Zollinger-Ellison syndrome. *Dig Dis Sci* 1993;38:1318.
150. Lamberts SWJ, Bakker WH, Reubi JC, Krenning EP. Somatostatin receptor imaging in the localization of endocrine tumors. *N Engl J Med* 1990;323:1246.
151. Krenning EP, Kwekkeboom DJ, Oei HY, et al. Somatostatin-receptor scintigraphy in gastroenteropancreatic tumors. *Ann N Y Acad Sci* 1994;733:416.
152. de Kerviler E, Cadiot G, Lebtahi R, et al. Somatostatin receptor scintigraphy in forty-eight patients with the Zollinger-Ellison syndrome. *J Nucl Med* 1994;21:1191.
153. Gibril F, Reynolds JC, Doppman JL, et al. Does the use of octreoscanning alter management in patients with Zollinger-Ellison syndrome? A prospective study. *Gastroenterology* 1995;108:A356(abst).
154. Kwekkeboom DJ, Krenning EP, Oei HY, van Eyck CHJ, Lamberts SWJ. Use of radiolabelled somatostatin to localize islet cell tumors. In: Mignon M, Jensen RT, eds. *Endocrine tumors of the pancreas: recent advances in research and management.* Basel: S Karger, 1995:298.
155. Lebtahi R, Cadiot G, Sarda L, et al. Clinical impact of somatostatin receptor scintigraphy in the management of patients with neuroendocrine gastroenteropancreatic tumors. *J Nucl Med* 1997;38:853.
156. Cadiot G, Bonnaud G, Lebtahi R, et al. Usefulness of somatostatin receptor scintigraphy in the management of patients with Zollinger-Ellison syndrome. *Gut* 1997;41:107.
157. Cadiot G, Lebtahi R, Sarda L, et al. Preoperative detection of duodenal gastrinomas and peripancreatic lymph nodes by somatostatin receptor scintigraphy. *Gastroenterology* 1996;111:845.
158. Reuter E, Semler P, Baer U, Sigismund R. Detection of a small gastrinoma by combined radiologic and scintigraphic techniques. *Clin Nucl Med* 1997;22:714.
159. van Eijck CJH, Lamberts SWJ, Lemaire LCJM, et al. The use of somatostatin receptor scintigraphy in the differential diagnosis of pancreatic duct cancers and islet cell tumors. *Ann Surg* 1996;224:119.
160. Gibril F, Doppman JL, Reynolds JC, et al. Bone metastases in patients with gastrinomas: a prospective study of bone scanning, somatostatin receptor scanning, and magnetic resonance imaging and their detection, frequency, location, and effect of their detection on management. *J Clin Oncol* 1998;16:1040.
161. Ruszniewski P, Amouyal P, Amouyal G, et al. Endocrine tumors of the pancreatic area: localization by endoscopic ultrasonography. In: Mignon M, Jensen RT, eds. *Endocrine tumors of the pancreas: recent advances in research and management.* Basel: S Karger, 1995:258.
162. Rosch T, Lightdale CJ, Botet JF, et al. Localization of pancreatic endocrine tumors by endoscopic ultrasonography. *N Engl J Med* 1992;326:1721.
163. Thompson NW, Czako PF, Fritts LL, et al. Role of endoscopic ultrasonography in the localization of insulinomas and gastrinomas. *Surgery* 1994;116:1131.
164. Doppman JL. Pancreatic endocrine tumors—the search goes on [Editorial]. *N Engl J Med* 1992;326:1770.
165. Cherner JA, Doppman HL, Norton JA, et al. Selective venous sampling for gastrin to localize gastrinomas. *Ann Intern Med* 1986;105:841.
166. Miller DL, Doppman JL, Metz DC, et al. Zollinger-Ellison syndrome: technique, results, and complications of portal venous sampling. *Radiology* 1992;182:235.
167. Vinik A, Moattari R, Cho K, Thompson N. Transhepatic portal venous catheterization for localization for sporadic and MEN gastrinomas. *Surgery* 1990;107:246.
168. Strader DB, Doppman JL, Orbuch M, et al. Functional localization of pancreatic endocrine tumors. In: Mignon M, Jensen RT, eds. *Frontiers of gastrointestinal research.* Basel: S Karger, 1995:282.
169. Doppman JL, Miller DL, Chang R, et al. Gastrinomas: localization by means of selective intraarterial injection of secretin. *Radiology* 1990;174:25.
170. Vinik AI, Delbridge L, Moattari R, Cho K, Thompson N. Transhepatic portal vein catheterization for localization of insulinomas: a ten-year experience. *Surgery* 1991;109:1.
171. Norton JA. Surgical treatment of islet cell tumors with special emphasis on operative ultrasound. In: Mignon M, Jensen RT, eds. *Endocrine tumors of the pancreas: recent advances in research and management.* Basel: S Karger, 1995:309.
172. Norton JA, Cromack DT, Shawker TH, et al. Intraoperative ultrasonographic localization of islet cell tumors. *Ann Surg* 1988;207:160.
173. Frucht H, Norton JA, London JF, et al. Detection of duodenal gastrinomas by operative endoscopic transillumination a prospective study. *Gastroenterology* 1990;99:1622.
174. Sugg SL, Norton JA, Fraker DL, et al. A prospective study of intraoperative methods to diagnose and resect duodenal gastrinomas. *Ann Surg* 1993;218:2.
175. Metz DC, Jensen RT. Advances in gastric antisecretory therapy in Zollinger-Ellison syndrome. In: Mignon M, Jensen RT, eds. *Endocrine tumors of the pancreas: recent advances in research and management.* Basel: S Karger, 1995:240.
176. Friesen SR. Effect of total gastrectomy on the Zollinger-Ellison tumor: observation by second-look operations. *Surgery* 1967;62:609.
177. Fox PS, Hofmann JW, DeCosse JJ, Wilson SD. The influence of total gastrectomy on survival in malignant Zollinger-Ellison tumors. *Ann Surg* 1974;180:558.
178. Metz DC, Strader DB, Orbuch M, et al. Use of omeprazole in Zollinger-Ellison: a prospective nine-year study of efficacy and safety. *Aliment Pharmacol Ther* 1993;7:597.
179. Jensen RT, Metz DC, Koviack PD, Feigenbaum KM. Prospective study of the long-term efficacy and safety of lansoprazole in patients with Zollinger-Ellison syndrome. *Aliment Pharmacol Ther* 1993;7:41.
180. Norton JA, Cornelius MJ, Doppman JL, et al. Effect of parathyroidectomy in patients with hyperparathyroidism and Zollinger-Ellison syndrome and multiple endocrine neoplasia type 1: a prospective study. *Surgery* 1987;102:958.
181. McCarthy DM, Olinger EJ, May RJ, Long VW, Gardner JD. H_2-histamine receptor blocking agents in the Zollinger-Ellison syndrome. *Ann Intern Med* 1977;87:668.
182. Jensen RT, Doppman JL, Gardner JD. Gastrinoma. In: Go VLW, Brooks FA, DiMagno EP, et al., eds. *The exocrine pancreas: biology, pathobiology, and disease.* New York: Raven Press, 1986:727.
183. Howard JM, Chremos AN, Collen MJ, et al. Famotidine, a new potent, long-acting histamine H_2-receptor antagonist: comparison with cimetidine and ranitidine in the treatment of Zollinger-Ellison syndrome. *Gastroenterology* 1985;88:1026.
184. Koury SI, Stone CK, La Charité DD. Omeprazole and the development of acute hepatitis. *Eur J Emerg Med* 1998;5:467.
185. Ekman L, Hansson E, Havu N, et al. Toxicological studies on omeprazole. *Scand J Gastroenterol* 1985;20:53.
186. Penston J, Wormsley KG. Achlorhydria-hypergastrinaemia: carcinoids—a flawed hypothesis. *Gut* 1987;28:488.
187. Maton PN, Lack EE, Collen MJ, et al. The effect of Zollinger-Ellison syndrome and omeprazole therapy on gastric endocrine cells. *Gastroenterology* 1990;99:943.
188. Solcia E, Capella C, Fiocca R, Cornaggia M, Bosi F. The gastroenteropancreatic endocrine system and related tumors. *Gastroenterol Clin North Am* 1989;18:671.
189. D'Adda T, Corletto V, Pilato FD, et al. Quantitative ultrastructure of endocrine cells of oxyntic mucosa in Zollinger-Ellison syndrome. *Gastroenterology* 1990;99:17.
190. Jensen RT. Gastrinoma as a model for prolonged hypergastrinemia in man. In: Walsh JH, ed. *Gastrin.* New York: Raven Press, 1993:373.
191. Lehy T, Cadiot G, Mignon M, Ruszniewski P, Bonfils S. Influence of multiple endocrine neoplasia type 1 on gastric endocrine cells in patients with the Zollinger-Ellison syndrome. *Gut* 1992;33:1275.
192. Metz DC, Pisegna JR, Fishbeyn VA, et al. Currently used doses of omeprazole in Zollinger-Ellison syndrome are too high. *Gastroenterology* 1992;103:1498.
193. Pisegna JR, Martin P, McKeand W, et al. Inhibition of pentagastrin-induced gastric acid secretion by intravenous pantoprazole: a dose-response study. *Am J Gastroenterol* 1999;94:2874.
194. Zollinger RM, Ellison EC, O'Dorision T, Sparks J. Thirty years' experience with gastrinoma. *World J Surg* 1984;8:427.
195. Ellison EC, Carey LC, Sparks J, et al. Early surgical treatment of gastrinoma. *Am J Med* 1987;82:17.
196. Kisker O, Bastian D, Bartsch D, Nies C, Rothmund M. Localization, malignant potential, and surgical management of gastrinomas. *World J Surg* 1998;22:651.
197. Farley DR, van Heerden JA, Grant CS, Miller LJ, Ilstrup DM. The Zollinger- Ellison syndrome: a collective surgical experience. *Ann Surg* 1992;216:561.
198. Soga J, Yakuwa Y. The gastrinoma/Zollinger-Ellison syndrome: statistical evaluation of a Japanese series of 359 cases. *J Hepatobil Pancreat Surg* 1998;5:77.
199. Stadil F, Bardram L, Gustafsen J, Efsen F. Surgical treatment of the Zollinger-Ellison syndrome. *World J Surg* 1993;17:463.
200. Alexander HR, Bartlett DL, Venzon DJ, et al. Analysis of factors associated with long-term (five or more years) cure in patients undergoing operation for Zollinger-Ellison syndrome. *Surgery* 1998;124:1160.
201. Podevin P, Ruszniewski P, Mignon M, et al. Management of multiple endocrine neoplasia type I (MEN I) in Zollinger-Ellison syndrome. *Gastroenterology* 1990,98:A230.
202. Maton PN, Gardner JD, Jensen RT. The incidence and etiology of Cushing's syndrome in patients with Zollinger-Ellison syndrome. *N Engl J Med* 1986;315:1.
203. Jensen RT. Management of the Zollinger-Ellison syndrome in patients with multiple endocrine neoplasia type 1. *J Intern Med* 1998;243:477.
204. Thompson NW. The surgical management of hyperparathyroidism and endocrine disease of the pancreas in the multiple endocrine neoplasia type 1 patient. *J Intern Med* 1995;238:269.
205. Mignon M, Cadiot G. Diagnostic and therapeutic criteria in patients with Zollinger-Ellison syndrome and multiple endocrine neoplasia type 1. *J Intern Med* 1998;243:489.
206. Fraker DL, Norton JA, Alexander HR, Venzon DJ, Jensen RT. Surgery in Zollinger-Ellison syndrome alters the natural history of gastrinoma. *Ann Surg* 1994;220:320.
207. Vogel SB, Wolfe MM, McGuigan JE. Localization and resection of gastrinomas in Zollinger-Ellison syndrome. *Ann Surg* 1987;205:550.
208. Delcore R Jr, Cheung LY, Friesen SR. Outcome of lymph node involvement in patients with Zollinger-Ellison syndrome. *Ann Surg* 1988;208:291.
209. Delcore R, Hermeck AS, Friesen SR. Selective surgical management of correctable hypergastrinemia. *Surgery* 1989;106:1094.
210. Howard TJ, Zinner MJ, Stabile BE, Passaro E Jr. Gastrinoma excision for cure. *Ann Surg* 1990;211:9.
211. Stadil F. Treatment of gastrinomas with pancreatoduodenectomy. In: Mignon M, Jensen RT, eds. *Endocrine tumors of the pancreas: recent advances in research and management.* Basel: S Karger, 1995:333.
212. Norton JA, Jensen RT. Unresolved surgical issues in the management of patients with Zollinger-Ellison syndrome. *World J Surg* 1991;15:151.
213. Fraker DL, Alexander HR. The surgical approach to endocrine tumors of the pancreas. *Semin Gastrointest Dis* 1995;6:102.
214. Udelsman R, Yeo CJ, Hruban RH, et al. Pancreaticoduodenectomy for selected pancreatic endocrine tumors. *Surg Gynecol Obstet* 1993;177:269.

215. Delcore R, Friesen SR. Role of pancreatoduodenectomy in the management of primary duodenal wall gastrinomas in patients with Zollinger-Ellison syndrome. *Surgery* 1992;112:1016.
216. Charboneau WJ, James EM, van Heerden JA, et al. Intraoperative real-time ultrasonographic localization of pancreatic insulinomas. *J Ultrasound Med* 1983;2:251.
217. Cromack DT, Norton JA, Sigel B, et al. The use of high-resolution intraoperative ultrasound to localize gastrinomas: an initial report of a prospective study. *World J Surg* 1987;11:648.
218. von Schrenck T, Howard JM, Doppman JL, et al. Prospective study of chemotherapy in patients with metastatic gastrinoma. *Gastroenterology* 1988;94:1326.
219. Zeiger MA, Shawker TH, Norton JA. Use of intraoperative ultrasonography to localize islet cell tumors. *World J Surg* 1993;17:448.
220. Pipeleers-Marichal M, Somers G, Willems G, et al. Gastrinomas in the duodenums of patients with multiple endocrine neoplasia type 1 and the Zollinger-Ellison syndrome. *N Engl J Med* 1990;322:723.
221. MacFarlane MP, Fraker DL, Alexander HR, Norton JA, Jensen RT. A prospective study of surgical resection of duodenal and pancreatic gastrinomas. *Surgery* 1995;118:973.
222. Cadiot G, Vuagnat A, Doukhan I, et al. Prognostic factors in patients with Zollinger-Ellison syndrome and multiple endocrine neoplasia type 1. *Gastroenterology* 1999;116:286.
223. Jaskowiak NT, Fraker DL, Alexander HR, et al. Is reoperation for gastrinoma excision indicated in Zollinger-Ellison syndrome? *Surgery* 1996;120:1055.
224. Boden G. Insulinoma and glucagonoma. *Semin Oncol* 1987;14:253.
225. Blum I, Doron M, Laron Z, et al. Prevention of hypoglycemia attacks by propranolol in a patient suffering from insulinoma. *Diabetes* 1975;24:535.
226. Hofeldt FD, Dippe SE, Levin SR, et al. Effects of diphenylhydantoin upon glucose-induced insulin secretion in three patients with insulinoma. *Diabetes* 1974;23:192.
227. Maton PN, Gardner JD, Jensen RT. The use of the long acting somatostatin analogue 201-995 in patients with pancreatic endocrine tumors. *Dig Dis Sci* 1989;34:29.
228. Maton PN. The use of the long-acting somatostatin analogue octreotide in patients with islet cell tumors. *Gastroenterol Clin North Am* 1989;18:897.
229. Danforth DN, Gorden P, Brennan MF. Metastatic insulin secreting carcinoma of the pancreas: clinical course and the role of surgery. *Surgery* 1984;96:1027.
230. Verner JV, Morrison AB. Endocrine pancreatic islet disease with diarrhea: report of a case due to diffuse hyperplasia of nonbeta islet tissue with a review of 54 additional cases. *Arch Intern Med* 1974;133:492.
231. Mao C, Shah A, Hanson DJ, Howard JM. Von Recklinghausen's disease associated with duodenal somatostatinoma: contrast of duodenal versus pancreatic somatostatinomas. *J Surg Oncol* 1995;59:67.
232. Konomi K, Chijiiwa K, Katsuta T, Yamaguchi K. Pancreatic somatostatinoma: a case report and review of the literature. *J Surg Oncol* 1990;43:259.
233. Soldati TK, Delnoce G, Garino M, et al. Pancreatic somatostatinoma. *Pan Minerva Med* 1990;32:141.
234. Sano T, Yamasaki R, Saito H, et al. Growth hormone–releasing hormone (GHRH) secreting pancreatic tumor in a patient with multiple endocrine neoplasia type 1. *Surg Pathol* 1987;11:810.
235. Barkan AL, Shenker Y, Grekin RJ, et al. Acromegaly from ectopic GHRH secretion by a malignant carcinoid tumor: successful treatment with long-acting somatostatin analogue SMS. *Cancer* 1986;61:221.
236. Melmed S, Ziel FH, Braustein GD, et al. Medical management of acromegaly due to ectopic production of GHRH by a carcinoid tumor. *J Clin Endocrinol Met* 1988;67:395.
237. Wilson DM, Hoffman AR. Reduction of pituitary size by the somatostatin analogue SMS 201-995 in a patient with an islet cell tumour secreting growth hormone releasing factor. *Acta Endocrinol* 1986;113:23.
238. Arps H, Dietel M, Schulz A, Janzarik H, Kloppel G. Pancreatic endocrine carcinoma with ectopic PTH-production and paraneoplastic hypercalcaemia. *Virchows Arch* 1986;408:497.
239. Bresler L, Boissel P, Conroy T, Grosdidier J. Pancreatic islet cell carcinoma with hypercalcemia: complete remission 5 years after surgical excision and chemotherapy. *Am J Gastroenterol* 1991;86:635.
240. Mao C, Carter P, Schaefer P, et al. Malignant islet cell tumor associated with hypercalcemia. *Surgery* 1995;117:37.
241. Miller CA, Ellison EC. Therapeutic alternatives in metastatic neuroendocrine tumors. *Surg Oncol Clin N Am* 1998;7:863.
242.. Gibril F, Doppman JL, Jensen RT. Recent advances in the treatment of metastatic pancreatic endocrine tumors. *Semin Gastrointest Dis* 1995;6:114.
243. Moertel CG, Hanley JA, Johnson LA. Streptozotocin alone compared with streptozotocin plus fluorouracil in the treatment of advanced islet-cell carcinoma. *N Engl J Med* 1980;303:1189.
244. Buchanan KD, O'Hare MMT, Russel CJF, Kennedy TL, Hadden DR. Factors involved in the responsiveness of gastrointestinal apudomas to streptozotocin. *Dig Dis Sci* 1986;31:511S.
245. Moertel CG, Lefkopoulo M, Lipsitz S, et al. Streptozotocin-doxorubicin, streptozotocin-fluorouracil, or chlorozotocin in the treatment of advanced islet cell carcinoma. *N Engl J Med* 1992;326:519.
246. Eriksson B, Arnberg H, Lindgren PG, et al. Neuroendocrine pancreatic tumours: clinical presentation, biochemical and histopathological findings in 84 patients. *J Intern Med* 1990;228:103.
247. Moertel CG, Johnson CM, McKusick MA, et al. The management of patients with advanced carcinoid tumors and islet cell carcinomas. *Ann Intern Med* 1994;120:302.
248. Kvols LK, Buck M. Chemotherapy of the metastatic carcinoid and islet cell tumors: a review. *Am J Med* 1987;82:77.
249. Eriksson B, Oberg K. An update of the medical treatment of malignant endocrine pancreatic tumors. *Acta Oncol* 1993;32:203.
250. Bukowski RM, McCracken JD, Balcerzek SP, et al. Phase II study of chlorozotocin in islet cell carcinoma. *Cancer Chemother Pharmacol* 1983;11:48.
251. Moertel CG, Lavin PT, Hahn RG. Phase II trial of doxorubicin for advanced islet cell carcinoma. *Cancer Treat Rep* 1982;66:1567.
252. Kelsen DP, Buckner J, Einzig A, et al. Phase II trial of cisplatin and etoposide in adenocarcinomas of the upper gastrointestinal trac. *Cancer Treat Rep* 1987;71:329.
253. Saltz L, Lauwers G, Wiseberg J, Kelsen D. A phase II trial of carboplatin in patients with advanced APUD tumors. *Cancer* 1993;72:619.
254. Ohshio G, Hosotani R, Imamura M, et al. Gastrinoma with multiple liver metastases: effectiveness of dacarbazine (DTIC) therapy. *J Hepatobil Pancreat Surg* 1998;5:339.
255. Moertel CG. An odyssey in the land of small tumors. *J Clin Oncol* 1987;5:1502.
256. Herr RR, Jahnke HK, Argoudelis AD. The structure of streptozotocin. *J Am Chem Soc* 1967;98:4808.
257. Weiss RB. Streptozotocin: a review of its pharmacology, efficacy, and toxicity. *Cancer Treat Rep* 1982;66:427.
258. Rakieten N, Rakieten ML, Nadkani MV. Studies of the diabetogenic action of streptozotocin (NSC-37917). *Cancer Chemother Rep* 1969;29:91.
259. Hofman JW, Fox PS, Wilson SD. Duodenal wall tumors and the Zollinger-Ellison syndrome. *Arch Surg* 1973;107:334.
260. Kelsen DG, Cheng E, Kemeny N, Magill GB, Yagoda A. Streptozotocin and Adriamycin in the treatment of APUD tumors (carcinoid islet cell and medullary thyroid). *Proc Am Assoc Cancer Res* 1982;23:433.
261. Frame J, Kelsen D, Kemeney N, et al. A phase II trial of streptozotocin and Adriamycin in advanced APUD tumors. *Am J Clin Oncol* 1988;11:490.
262. Bonfils S, Ruszniewski P, Haffar S, Laucournet H. Chemotherapy of hepatic metastases (HM) in Zollinger-Ellison syndrome (ZES). Report of a multicenter analysis. *Dig Dis Sci* 1986;31:51.
263. Ruszniewski PH, Rougier P, Andre-David F, et al. Prospective multicentric study: chemotherapy with streptozotocin (STZ) and 5-fluorouracil (5FU) for liver metastases (LM) in Zollinger-Ellison syndrome (ZES). *Gastroenterology* 1989;96:A431.
264. Arnold R, Frank M. Systemic chemotherapy for endocrine tumors of the pancreas: recent advances. In: Mignon M, Jensen RT, eds. *Endocrine tumors of the pancreas: recent advances in research and management.* Basel: S Karger, 1995:431.
265. Ruszniewski P, Hochlaf S, Rougier P, Mignon M. Chimiotherapie intraveineuse par streptozotocine et 5 fluoro-uracile des metastases hepatiques du syndrome de Zollinger-Ellison. *Gastroenterol Clin Biol* 1991;15:393.
266. Sutliff VE, Doppman JL, Gibril F, et al. Growth of newly diagnosed, untreated metastatic gastrinomas and predictors of growth patterns. *J Clin Oncol* 1997;15:2420.
267. Bonfils S, Landor SH, Mignon M, et al. Results of surgical management in 92 consecutive patients with Zollinger-Ellison syndrome. *Ann Surg* 1981;194:692.
268. Ajani JA, Levin B, Wallace S. Systemic and regional therapy of advanced islet cell tumors. *Gastroenterol Clin North Am* 1989;18:923.
269. Oberg K. The use of chemotherapy in the management of neuroendocrine tumors. *Endocrinol Metab Clin North Am* 1993;22:941.
270. Bukowski RM, Tangen C, Lee R, et al. Phase II trial of chlorozotocin and fluorouracil in islet cell carcinoma: a Southwest Oncology Group. *J Clin Oncol* 1992;10:1914.
271. Moertel CG, Kvols LK, O'Connell MJ, Rubin J. Treatment of neuroendocrine carcinomas with combined etoposide and cisplatin. *Cancer* 1991;68:22.
272. Eriksson B, Oberg K. Interferon therapy of malignant endocrine pancreatic tumors. In: Mignon M, Jensen RT, eds. *Endocrine tumors of the pancreas: recent advances in research and management.* Basel: S Karger, 1995:451.
273. Kvols LK, Buck M. Chemotherapy of endocrine malignancies: a review. *Semin Oncol* 1987;14:343.
274. Marynick SP, Fagadau WR, Duncan LA. Malignant glucagonoma syndrome. Response to chemotherapy. *Ann Intern Med* 1980;93:453.
275. Awrich AE, Peetz M, Fletcher WS. Dimethyltriazenomidazole carboxamide therapy of islet cell carcinomas of the pancreas. *J Surg Oncol* 1981;17:321.
276. Kurose T, Seino Y, Ishida LT, et al. Successful treatment of metastatic glucagonoma with dacarbazine. *Lancet* 1984;1:621.
277. Scarpignato C. Somatostatin analogues in the management of endocrine tumors of the pancreas. In: Mignon M, Jensen RT, eds. *Endocrine tumors of the pancreas: recent advances in research and management.* Basel: S Karger, 1995:385.
278. Angeletti S, Corleto VD, Schillaci O, et al. Single dose of octreotide stabilizes metastatic gastro-entero-pancreatic endocrine tumours. *Ital J Gastroenterol Hepatol* 1999;31:23.
279. Arnold R, Frank M, Kajdan U. Management of gastroenteropancreatic endocrine tumors: the place of somatostatin analogues. *Digestion* 1994;55:107.
280. Arnold R, Neuhaus C, Benning R, et al. Somatostatin analog sandostatin and inhibition of tumor growth in patients with metastatic endocrine gastroenteropancreatic tumors. *World J Surg* 1993;17:511.
281. Vinik AI, Tsai ST, Moattari AR, et al. Somatostatin analogue (SMS-201-995) in the management of gastroentero-pancreatic tumors and diarrhea syndromes. *Am J Med* 1986;81:23.
282. Saltz L, Trochanowski B, Buckley M, et al. Octreotide as an antineoplastic agent in the treatment of functional and nonfunctional neuroendocrine tumors. *Cancer* 1993;72:244.
283. Redding TW, Schally AV. Inhibition of growth of pancreatic carcinomas in animal models by analogs of hypothalamic hormones. *Proc Natl Acad Sci USA* 1984;84:248.
284. Reubi JC. Somatostatin analogue inhibits chondrosarcoma and insulinoma tumor growth. *Acta Endocrinol* 1985;109:108.
285. Kvols LK, Buck M, Moertel CG, et al. Treatment of metastatic islet cell tumors with a somatostatin analogue. *Ann Intern Med* 1987;107:162.
286. Arnold R, Trautmann ME, Creutzfeldt W, et al. Somatostatin analogue octreotide and inhibition of tumour growth in metastatic endocrine gastroenteropancreatic tumours. *Gut* 1996;38:430.
287. Erickson B, Oberg K, Alm G, et al. Treatment of malignant endocrine pancreatic tumors with human leukocyte interferon. *Lancet* 1986;2:1307.
288. Pisegna JR, Slimak GG, Doppman JL, et al. An evaluation of human recombinant alpha interferon in patients with metastatic gastrinoma. *Gastroenterology* 1993;105:1179.
289. Saltz L, Kemeny N, Schwartz G, Kelsen D. A phase II trial of alpha-interferon and 5-fluorouracil in patients with advanced carcinoid and islet cell tumors. *Cancer* 1994;74:958.

290. Valette PJ, Souquet JC. Pancreatic islet cell tumors metastatic to the liver: treatment by hepatic artery chemo-embolization. *Horm Res* 1989;32:77.
291. Arcenas AG, Ajani JA, Carrasco CH, Levin B, Wallace S. Vascular occlusive therapy of pancreatic endocrine tumors metastatic to the liver. In: Mignon M, Jensen RT, eds. *Endocrine tumors of the pancreas: recent advances in research and management.* Basel: S Karger, 1995:439.
292. Perry LJ, Stuart K, Stokes KR, Clouse ME. Hepatic arterial chemoembolization for metastatic neuroendocrine tumors. *Surgery* 1994;116:1111.
293. Venook AP. Embolization and chemoembolization therapy for neuroendocrine tumors. *Curr Opin Oncol* 1999;11:38.
294. Stokes KR, Stuart K, Clouse ME. Hepatic arterial chemoembolization for metastatic endocrine tumors. *J Vasc Intervent Radiol* 1993;4:341.
295. Carrasco CH, Chuang VP, Wallace S. Apudoma metastatic to the liver: treatment by hepatic artery embolization. *Radiology* 1983;149:79.
296. Carty SE, Jensen RT, Norton JA. Prospective study of aggressive resection of metastatic pancreatic endocrine tumors. *Surgery* 1992;112:1024.
297. Que FG, Nagorney DM, Batts KP, Linz LJ, Kvols LK. Hepatic resection for metastatic neuroendocrine carcinomas. *Am J Surg* 1995;169:36.
298. Harrison LE, Brennan MF, Newman E, et al. Hepatic resection for noncolorectal nonneuroendocrine metastases: a fifteen-year experience with ninety-six patients. *Surgery* 1997;121:625.
299. Chen H, Hardacre JM, Uzra A, Cameron JL, Choti MA. Isolated liver metastases from neuroendocrine tumors: Does resection prolong survival? *J Am Coll Surg* 1998;187:88.
300. Frilling A, Rogiers X, Malagó M, et al. Treatment of liver metastases in patients with neuroendocrine tumors. *Langenbecks Arch Surg* 1998;383:62.
301. O'Dorisio TM, Mekhjian H, Gaginella TS. Medical therapy of VIPomas. *Endocrinol Metab Clin North Am* 1989;18:545.
302. McFadden D, Jaffe BN. Surgical approaches to endocrine-producing tumors of the gastrointestinal tract. In: Cohen S, Soloway RD, eds. *Hormone producing tumors of the gastrointestinal tract.* New York: Churchill Livingstone, 1985:139.
303. McEntee GP, Nagorney DM, Kvols LK, et al. Cytoreductive hepatic surgery for neuroendocrine tumors. *Surgery* 1990;108:1091.
304. Dousset B, Houssin D, Soubrane O, et al. Metastatic endocrine tumors: Is there a place for liver transplantation? *Liver Transplant Surg* 1995;1:111.
305. Curtiss SI, Mor E, Schwartz ME, et al. A rational approach to the use of hepatic transplantation in the treatment of metastatic neuroendocrine tumors. *J Am Coll Surg* 1995;180:184.
306. Routley D, Ramage JK, McPeake J, Tan KC, Williams R. Orthotopic liver transplantation in the treatment of metastatic neuroendocrine tumors of the liver. *Liver Transplant Surg* 1995;1:118.
307. Azoulay D, Bismuth H. Role of liver surgery and transplantation in patients with hepatic metastases from pancreatic endocrine tumors In: Mignon M, Jensen RT, eds. *Endocrine tumors of the pancreas: recent advances in research and management.* Basel: S Karger, 1995:461.
308. Le Treut YP, Delpero JR, Dousset B, et al. Results of liver transplantation in the treatment of metastatic neuroendocrine tumors. *Ann Surg* 1997;225:355.
309. Görög D, Toth A, Weltner J. Prognosis of untreated liver metastasis from rectal cancer. *Acta Chir Hung* 1997;36:106.

SECTION **6**

ROBERT T. JENSEN
GERARD M. DOHERTY

Carcinoid Tumors and the Carcinoid Syndrome

PATHOLOGY AND TUMOR HISTOLOGY

Neuroendocrine tumors (NETs) are derived from the diffuse neuroendocrine system, which is made up of peptide- and amine-producing cells with different hormonal profiles depending on their site of origin.[1] Carcinoids are classified as NETs and share cytochemical features with melanomas, pheochromocytomas, medullary carcinoma of the thyroid, and pancreatic endocrine tumors (PETs).[1–5] Carcinoids are composed of monotonous sheets of small round cells with uniform nuclei and cytoplasm.[4] Mitotic figures are rare.[1,2,4] Oberndorfer[6] introduced the term *carcinoid* in 1907 to describe tumors that behaved more indolently than adenocarcinomas.[6] Pathologists cannot differentiate benign from malignant carcinoids based on histology, nor histologically can they differentiate PETs from carcinoids.[3] Malignancy can only be determined if invasion or distant metastases are found. Ultrastructurally, carcinoids possess electron-dense neurosecretory granules, and they contain small clear vesicles that correspond to the synaptic vesicles of neurons.[1,4,7] Carcinoids synthesize bioactive amines and peptides, including neuron-specific enolase; 5-hydroxytryptamine; 5-hydroxytryptophan; synaptophysin; chromogranin A and C; and other peptides, such as insulin, growth hormone, neurotensin, adrenocorticotropic hormone (ACTH), melanocyte-stimulating hormone-β, gastrin, pancreatic polypeptide, calcitonin, substance P, other various tachykinins (e.g., neuropeptide K), growth hormone–releasing hormone, bombesin, and various growth factors such as transforming growth factor-β (TGF-β), platelet-derived growth factor, and basic fibroblast growth factor.[1,3,8]

Most carcinoids are tentatively identified on routine histology.[4,8] However, these tumors are characterized by their histologic staining patterns due to their shared secreted products and certain cytoplasmic proteins.[1,4] Historically, one of the most important was their staining with silver.[1,3,4] Characteristically, carcinoids either take up and reduce silver (argentaffin reaction) or take it up but do not reduce it (argyrophilic).[2,3] Currently, the identification of chromogranin, synaptophysin, or neuron-specific enolase (NSE) is generally used.[1,3,8] The chromogranins (A, B, C) are acidic polypeptides that are the major component of the secretory granules of many neuroendocrine cells.[8,9] Generally, chromogranin A immunoreactivity is more specific than the argyrophil reaction because the latter also identifies other intracellular proteins such as melanin.[8] NSE, the gamma-gamma dimer of the glycolytic enzyme enolase, occurs in the cytoplasm of most neuroendocrine cells and is positive in most carcinoids as well as other APUD (amine precursor uptake and decarboxylation) tumors.[1,8] The advantage of NSE as a marker is that its reactivity is unrelated to secretory granule content. However, NSE can be occasionally misleading because some tumors not considered neuroendocrine, such as fibroadenomas of breast carcinoma and certain lymphomas, may contain a considerable amount of NSE activity.[1] Synaptophysin is a calcium-binding vesicle membrane glycoprotein that is expressed independently of other neuroendocrine proteins.[1]

In addition to the general histologic NET markers, specific markers for carcinoids may identify the tumor as a carcinoid.[1] Serotonin can be identified by various methods, including the use of the argentaffin reaction of Masson or using antibodies to serotonin.[8,10] In general, the argentaffin reaction of Masson is usually positive, and the serotonin antibody localization is frequently weak or negative in midgut carcinoids, whereas in foregut and hindgut carcinoids, serotonin immunoreactivity is detected more often than is the argentaffin reaction.[8,10]

Williams and Sanders[11] proposed classifying carcinoids according to their site of origin because carcinoids with similar sites of origin frequently share functional manifestations, histochemistry, and secretory products (Table 38.6-1). Foregut carcinoids generally have a low serotonin [5-hydroxytryptamine (5-HT)] content, are argentaffin-negative but argyrophilic, occasionally secrete 5-

TABLE 38.6-1. Classification of Carcinoid Tumors

	Origin		
Histochemistry and Products	Foregut[a]	Midgut[b]	Hindgut[c]
Histochemistry			
Silver staining	Argentaffin-negative, argyrophilic or negative	Argentaffin-positive	Argentaffin-negative (75%) or occasional argyrophilic (55%)
Neuron-specific enolase	Positive	Positive	Positive
Chromogranin A	Positive	Positive	Positive (42%)
Cytoplasmic granules (electron microscope)	Round, variable density, 180 nm	Pleomorphic, uniform density, 230 nm	Round, variable density, approximately 190 nm
Products			
Tumor	Low 5-HT content, multihormonal[d]	High 5-HT content, multihormonal[d]	Rarely 5-HT, multihormonal[d]
Blood	5-HTP, histamine, multihormonal,[d] occasionally secrete ACTH	5-HT, multihormonal,[d] rarely secrete ACTH	Rarely release 5-HTP or ACTH
Urine	5-HTP, 5-HT, 5-HIAA, histamine, and others	5-HT, 5-HIAA	Negative
Carcinoid syndrome	Occurs but may be atypical	Occurs frequently (with metastases)	Rarely occurs
Metastasize to bone	Common	Rarely	Common

ACTH, adrenocorticotropic hormone; 5-HIAA, 5-hydroxyindolacetic acid; 5-HT, 5-hydroxytryptamine; 5-HTP, 5-hydroxytryptophan.
[a]Respiratory tract, pancreas, stomach, proximal duodenum.
[b]Jejunum, ileum, appendix, Meckel's diverticulum, ascending colon.
[c]Includes transverse and descending colon, rectum.
[d]Multihormonal includes tachykinins (substance P, substance K, neuropeptide K), neurotensin, peptide YY, enkephalin, insulin, glucagon, gastrin, glicentin, vasoactive intestinal peptide, somatostatin, pancreatic polypeptide, ACTH, or a subunit of human chorionic gonadotropin.

hydroxytryptophan (5-HTP) or ACTH, can be associated with an atypical carcinoid syndrome, are often multihormonal, and may metastasize to bone. Although many foregut carcinoids synthesize peptides, clinical syndromes are rarely produced and elevated plasma hormone levels are generally not detected. Midgut carcinoids are argentaffin-positive, have a high serotonin content, have smaller numbers of endocrine cells than foregut tumors, most frequently cause the classic carcinoid syndrome when they metastasize, release serotonin and tachykinins (substance P, neuropeptide K, substance K), rarely secrete 5-HTP or ACTH, and uncommonly metastasize to bone.[12] Hindgut carcinoid tumors are argentaffin-negative, often argyrophilic, rarely contain serotonin, rarely cause carcinoid syndrome, contain numerous gastrointestinal (GI) hormones, rarely secrete 5-HTP or ACTH, and may metastasize to bone.[12]

Carcinoids within the same site of origin, such as lung, thymus, and pancreas, can differ significantly in characteristics and behavior. Therefore, it has been proposed that the term *carcinoid* be replaced by the designation *neuroendocrine tumor*, and a new classification system has been drawn up.[1,4] In this proposed classification, tumors are divided according to tissue of origin and subdivided by growth behavior. It is proposed that this new classification system better reflects the biology of these tumors and provides better guidelines for tumors with similar behaviors in different tissues.

Carcinoids can be ubiquitous, but most take origin in four sites: bronchus, appendix, rectum, and jejunoileum.[13,14] In the past, carcinoids were most frequently reported in the appendix (approximately 40%); however, more recently the bronchus and lung are the most common site (32%) (Table 38.6-2). The distribution reported from analyses of two large National Cancer Institute databases from 1950 to 1971 and from 1973 to 1991 are contrasted in Table 38.6-2. A number of trends are apparent from comparison of the data from these two periods. The percentages of gastric carcinoids almost doubled, whereas the percentage of appendiceal carcinoids decreased more than fourfold from 38% to 7.6%. Small intestinal carcinoids remained a large group comprising approximately 20% of all carcinoids. Overall, GI carcinoids remain the most frequent, comprising 74% of all carcinoids in the 1973 to 1991 Surveillance, Epidemiology, and End Results (SEER) data,[14] with the respiratory tract being a distant second with 25%.[14]

The exact clinical incidence of carcinoids varies in different studies. An incidence of 7.1 per million for males is reported,[15] with 8.7 per million reported for females[15] in England and Scotland, and 13 cases per million population reported in Ireland. Carcinoids thus occur 11 times more frequently than insulinomas and 26 times more frequently than gastrinomas.[16] In other series, the incidence of clinically significant tumors was 7 per million population per year in Scandinavia, which was two times more frequent than all PETs, seven times more than gastrinomas, and eight times more than insulinomas.[3,17,18] The clinical presentation of carcinoids far underestimates their occurrence, because many are asymptomatic. This fact is demonstrated by SEER data, which report an annual incidence rate of 2.8 per million population for small intestinal carcinoids,[19] whereas in an autopsy study at the Mayo Clinic, 6500 cases per million were reported.[20] In another study, the annual incidence of malignant carcinoids at autopsy was 21 per million population per year,[21] whereas in a Swedish study calculated on autopsy and surgical results, the incidence was 84 cases per million population.[21] The distribution of carcinoid tumors found in various surgical or clinical series differs markedly from that found at autopsy.[22] As many as 76% of all carcinoids are found in the jejunoileum at autopsy, whereas they make up approximately one-fourth of cases in clinical and surgical series.

TABLE 38.6-2. Carcinoid Tumor Location, Frequency of Metastases, and Association with Carcinoid Syndrome

	Location (% of Total)		*Incidence of Metastases (%)*		*Incidence of Carcinoid Syndrome (%)*
	Godwin 1975 (1950–1971) (n = 4349)	Modlin 1997 (1973–1991) (n = 5468)	Godwin 1975 (1950–1971)	Modlin 1997 (1973–1991)	Godwin 1975 (1950–1971)
Foregut					
Esophagus	<1	<1	—	67	—
Stomach	2	3.8	22	31	9.5
Duodenum	2.6	2.1	20	—	3.4
Pancreas	<1	<1	20	76	20
Gallbladder	<1	<1	33	56	5
Bile duct	<1	<1	—	—	—
Ampulla	<1	<1	14	—	—
Larynx	<1	<1	50	0	—
Bronchus, lung	11.5	32.5	20	27	13
Midgut					
Jejunum	1.3	2.3	35	70 (jejunum and ileum)	9
Ileum	23	17.6	35		9
Meckel's diverticulum	1	0.4	18	—	13
Appendix	38	7.6	2	35	<1
Colon	4.3	6.3	60	71	5
Liver	<1	<1	—	29	—
Ovary	<1	<1	6	32	50
Testis	<1	<1	—	—	50
Cervix	<1	<1	24	67	3
Hindgut					
Rectum	13	10	3	14	—

(Data from refs. 13 and 14.)

Approximately 1 in every 200 to 300 appendectomies result in discovery of a carcinoid.[20] Most occur in the tip of the appendix. The majority (i.e., 90%) are less than 1 cm in diameter and are without metastases.[20,23,24] In the SEER data of 1570 appendiceal carcinoids,[25] 62% were localized, 27% had regional lesions, and 8% had distant metastatic disease. Approximately 50% of the carcinoids between 1 and 2 cm in size metastasize to lymph nodes.[26]

Small intestinal carcinoids may be multiple; 70% to 87% are present within the ileum and 40% to 70% within 2 feet of the ileocecal valve.[20,27,28] Forty percent are less than 1 cm in diameter, 32% are 1 to 2 cm, and 29% are more than 2 cm.[28] In an analysis of 12 series, 47% (range, 0% to 100%) were associated with metastases,[28] whereas 35% to 70% were associated with metastases in the National Cancer Institute studies[13,14] (see Table 38.6-2). With the carcinoid, a marked fibrotic reaction can occur that can distort the gut or mesentery and can present clinically with small bowel obstruction or venous mesenteric infarction. Distant metastases occur to the liver (36% to 60%),[27,28] to bone (3%)[28] and, occasionally, to lung (4%).[28] Approximately 20% to 30% of patients with ileal carcinoid have one or more additional ileal primary carcinoids.[27,29] The incidence of metastases from small intestinal carcinoids is dependent on tumor size.[27,29] If the tumor is smaller than 1 cm, metastases occur in fewer than 15% to 25%.[20,27,28] If the tumor is between 1 and 2 cm in size, metastases occur in 58% to 80%.[20,27,28] If the tumor is larger than 2 cm, metastases occur in more than 70%.[20,27,28] In contrast to jejunoileal carcinoids, duodenal carcinoids are often discovered by endoscopy.[30] In two series[13,30] (see Table 38.6-2), 20% to 21% of duodenal carcinoids had metastases. Invasion into the muscularis propria, tumor size, and mitotic activity all correlated with metastatic spread, with invasion being the strongest predictor. No duodenal carcinoid smaller than 1 cm metastasized, whereas 33% of the tumors larger than 2 cm and 35% of tumors invading the muscularis mucosa metastasized.[30]

In approximately 1 in every 2500 proctoscopies, a small nodule is seen that is diagnosed as a carcinoid.[20] Nearly all rectal carcinoids occur submucosally on the anterior or lateral walls between 4 and 13 cm above the dentate line.[20,31] Sixty-six percent to 80% are less than 1 cm in diameter and rarely metastasize (5%).[31] Tumors 1 to 2 cm can metastasize (5% to 30%),[31–33] and tumors larger than 2 cm, which are uncommon, metastasize in more than 70%.[20,26,31,32] Colorectal carcinoids are almost entirely limited to the sigmoid colon and rectum, with the vast majority in the rectum. Metastases occurs in approximately 10% to 22%,[31] and in most cases, the tumor is larger than 2 cm in diameter and has invaded the muscularis propria. Invasiveness correlates with the presence of increased mitoses or atypical histology.[33] Colonic carcinoids uncommonly occur in the remainder of the colon, with almost 60% occurring in the cecum or ileocecal area. These tumors tend to be large (90% are larger than 2 cm; 50% are 5 cm or larger)[34] and are associated with metastases (61%).

Bronchial carcinoids resemble intestinal carcinoids and are not related to smoking.[7] Poor prognostic pathologic features include increased mitotic count, nuclear pleomorphism, vascular invasion, undifferentiated growth pattern, and lymphatic invasion.[3] The bronchus is the site of a primary carcinoid in approximately 2% of cases.[35] The classification of bronchial carcinoids has been a subject of debate.[36] Lung NETs have been classified into four categories: the typical carcinoid [also called *bronchial carcinoid* and *Kulchitsky cell carcinoma-I* (KCC-I)], atypical carcinoid (also called *well-differentiated neuroendocrine carcinoma* and *KCC-II*), intermediate small cell neuroendocrine carcinomas, and small cell neuroendocrine carcinomas (also called *KCC-III*).[36–38] Another proposed classification[4] includes these tumors under three general categories of lung NETs: benign or low-grade malignant (typical carcinoid); low-grade malignant (atypical carcinoid); and high-grade malignant (poorly differentiated carcinoma of the large cell or small cell type). The different categories of lung NETs have different prognosis, varying from excellent for typical carcinoids to poor for small cell neuroendocrine carcinomas.[36–39]

Gastric carcinoids account for three of every 1000 gastric neoplasms. Three subtypes of gastric carcinoids are proposed to occur,[40] and they originate from gastric enterochromaffin-like (ECL) cells.[40] Two subtypes are associated with hypergastrinemic states, either chronic atrophic gastritis (80%) (type I) or Zollinger-Ellison syndrome (6%) (type II), which is almost always as part of multiple endocrine neoplasia type 1 (MEN 1).[40,41] Gastric carcinoids types I and II generally pursue a benign course, with 9% to 30% developing metastases. They are usually multiple and small, with infiltration restricted to the mucosa and submucosa.[40] The third type of gastric carcinoids (type III) (sporadic ECL tumors) occur without hypergastrinemia, and they pursue a more aggressive course, with 54% to 66% developing metastases.[40,41] They are often large, single tumors; 50% have atypical histology, and some patients develop carcinoid syndrome.[3,40]

Carcinoids can be classified on their histologic growth patterns as insular, trabecular, glandular, undifferentiated, or mixed.[3,8,42] The midgut carcinoids frequently possess the most typical morphology,[8] with insular-like formation of regular tumor cells surrounded by fibrotic stroma. Most foregut carcinoids show a more mixed growth pattern, with a solid, ribbon-like, trabecular, or acinar pattern. Hindgut carcinoids are frequently solid or trabecular.[8,42] It has been demonstrated that the histologic types have prognostic significance.[42–44] In one classification of decreasing order of median survival time in years, the growth pattern ranked as follows[42]: mixed insular plus glandular (4.4 years), insular (2.9 years), trabecular (2.5 years), mixed insular plus trabecular (2.3 years), glandular (0.9 years), and undifferentiated (0.5 years). In other studies, carcinoids are divided histologically into typical (well-differentiated neuroendocrine tumors) and atypical (nuclear atypia, necrosis, increased mitotic activity),[4] and categorization has been shown to have prognostic significance.[4,33,44]

MOLECULAR PATHOGENESIS

Little is known about the induction of malignant growth or the factors promoting the growth of carcinoids.[3,45–48] For some gastric carcinoids, studies show that gastrin is an important growth factor.[3,40] An increased occurrence of gastric carcinoids occurs in disease states (pernicious anemia, atrophic gastritis, Zollinger-Ellison syndrome) that result in hypergastrinemia.[3,40] The hyperplastic effect of hypergastrinemia is restricted to gastric ECL cells.[49,50] It has been proposed that, with prolonged hypergastrinemia, ECL hyperplasia (simple, linear, micronodular, adenomatoid), dysplasia, and carcinoid formation are increased.[49,50] In pernicious anemia and atrophic gastritis, up to 4% to 11% of patients develop gastric carcinoids.[49,51] Patients with Zollinger-Ellison syndrome also develop gastric carcinoids, although they are much more frequent in the subgroup with MEN 1.[52,53] In patients with Zollinger-Ellison syndrome with MEN 1 with gastric carcinoids, allelic loss occurs at the MEN 1 locus on chromosome 11q13, and thus fundic gastric carcinoids are now included in the spectrum of MEN 1 tumors. Studies suggest that other important growth factors in some carcinoid tumors are TGF-α[50] and TGF-β,[54,55] insulin-like growth factor-1 (IGF-1),[47,50,55] trefoid peptides (TFF1, TFF2, TFF3),[50] platelet-derived growth factor,[47,54] vascular endothelial growth factor,[56] acidic and basic fibroblast growth factor,[47,54,55] and epidermal growth factor.[54,55]

Limited studies have been performed on carcinoids examining the possible role of mutations of protooncogenes and alterations of tumor-suppressor genes in their pathogenesis.[45,47,48] Mutations in common oncogenes, such as K-*ras*, are uncommon in GI carcinoids.[45,48] Overamplification of HER2/NEU, c-myc, and c-jun have been described in some cell lines derived from GI endocrine tumors and some carcinoids.[48,57] In bronchial carcinoids, a high expression of c-fos, c-jun, and c-met occurs early, and a high expression of c-myc and L-myc occurs late. Alterations in the common tumor suppressor gene p53[3,48,58,59] are also uncommon in carcinoids,[3,45,48,58,59] as are alterations in the retinoblastoma gene in typical carcinoids, although they may occur in atypical carcinoids.[24,45,60,61] MEN 1 has been shown to be due to defects in a 10-exon gene on chromosome 11q13 that encodes for a 610–amino acid nuclear protein, MENIN.[62,63] Loss of heterozygosity at this locus has been reported in 26% to 78% of carcinoids,[64–66] and mutations in the MENIN gene were reported to be 18% in one study.[64] Microsatellite instability is rare in carcinoids[67]; however, by comparative genomic hybridization, both frequent gains (of chromosome 5, 14, 17q, 7) and losses (especially of chromosome 9p) are reported.[68]

CLINICAL FEATURES

GENERAL CHARACTERISTICS

The age of onset ranges from 10 to 93 years, with a mean onset of 36 years of age for tumors of the cervix, 63 years for tumors of the small intestine and respiratory tract, and 66 years for tumors of the rectum.[14,22]

CARCINOID TUMORS WITHOUT SYSTEMIC FEATURES

The presentation of carcinoids that do not cause carcinoid syndrome is diverse and related to the site of origin of the tumor as well as the malignant spread of the tumor. In the appendix (see Table 38.6-2), carcinoids are usually found incidentally during surgery for suspected appendicitis.[23] Small intestinal carcinoids in the jejunoileum are the most common location for carcinoids of clinical significance.[20,22,29] Most small intestinal carcinoids found in autopsy studies do not cause symptoms, but these tumors can cause fibrosis of the mesentery, which results in kinking of the bowel, intestinal obstruction, and gut infarction or intussusception. The most common presenting symptoms due to the small intestinal carcinoids *per se* are periodic abdominal pain (51%),[20,22,28,29] intestinal obstruction with ileus and invagination (31%),[28] an abdominal tumor (17%),[28] or GI bleeding (11%).[28] Because of the vagueness of the symptoms, the diagnosis is frequently delayed, with a median time of onset from symptoms to

TABLE 38.6-3. Clinical Characteristics in Patients with Malignant Carcinoid Syndrome

	At Presentation		*During Course of Disease*			
	Davis 1973	Norheim 1987	Thorson 1958	Feldman 1987	Norheim 1987	Soga 1999
No. of Patients	91	91	79	111	91	748
SYMPTOM OR SIGN						
Diarrhea	73%	32%	68%	73%	84%	67%
Flushing	65%	23%	74%	63%	75%	78%
Pain	—	10%	—	—	—	34%
Asthma and wheezing	8%	4%	18%	3%	15%	10%
Pellagra	2%	—	5%	—	—	—
None	12%	—	—	22%	—	—
Carcinoid heart disease present	11%	—	41%	14%	33%	33%
DEMOGRAPHICS						
Male	59%	46%	61%	—	46%	52%
Age						
Mean	57 y	59 y	52 y	—	—	54.5 y
Range	25–79 y	ND	18–80 y	—	—	9–91 y
TUMOR LOCATION						
Foregut	5%	9%	2%	—	9%	33%
Midgut	78%	87%	75%	—	87%	60%
Hindgut	5%	1%	8%	—	1%	1%
Unknown	11%	2%	15%	—	2%	6%

ND, no data.
(Data from refs. 12, 17, 39, 80, and 83.)

diagnosis of approximately 2 years[20,29] and a range up to 20 years. Duodenal and gastric carcinoids are usually found incidentally during endoscopy.[22,30,51] Rectal carcinoids are frequently found incidentally during endoscopy but can be symptomatic.[31,69] The most common symptoms include melena and bleeding (39%), constipation (17%), and diarrhea (12%).[31] Bronchial carcinoids are frequently discovered on chest radiograph. In one large series,[36] 31% of patients were asymptomatic, and the carcinoid was incidentally discovered. The most common symptoms are pneumonia, hemoptysis, and cough.[36] Thymic carcinoids present as anterior mediastinal masses, usually on chest radiograph. Ovarian and testicular carcinoids may present as masses detected by physical examination or ultrasound. Most carcinoids present as an isolated disease, but associations exist between foregut carcinoids and MEN 1,[40,52,53,70] gastric carcinoids and diseases causing hypergastrinemia[40,52,70] ampullary somatostatin-rich carcinoids and von Recklinghausen's disease,[45,71,72] an intestinal carcinoid with myotonic dystrophy,[73] a gastric carcinoid in a patient with primary biliary cirrhosis,[74] and duodenal carcinoid tumors causing Zollinger-Ellison syndrome.[75] Metastatic carcinoids in the liver, presenting as hepatomegaly, may be the initial presentation in a patient who is fully active and productive with minimal symptoms and normal or near-normal liver function tests.[20]

CARCINOID TUMORS WITH SYSTEMIC FEATURES

The most common systemic syndrome caused by carcinoids is the malignant carcinoid syndrome. As already mentioned, carcinoids may contain and secrete a number of biologically active substances. Immunocytochemical or radioimmunoassay studies show that carcinoids can contain ACTH, gastrin, somatostatin, insulin, motilin, growth hormone, gastrin-releasing peptide, serotonin, calcitonin, neurotensin, melanocyte-stimulating hormone-β, tachykinins (substance P, substance K, neuropeptide K), glucagon, pancreatic polypeptide (PP), vasoactive intestinal peptide (VIP), and prostaglandins.[3,27,28,31,44,76,77] These substances may not be released in sufficient amounts to cause symptoms. In various studies of patients with carcinoids, elevated serum concentrations of PP occur in 43%,[17,76] motilin in 14%,[76] and subunits of human chorionic gonadotropin (HCG) in 12%;[17] a slightly elevated level of gastrin was reported in 15%,[17] and none were reported with an elevated VIP[76] or plasma gastrin-releasing peptide level.[76] Even though these GI peptides were present in the serum, it is not apparent that any of these peptides contributed to any clinical symptoms.

Foregut carcinoids are more likely to produce various GI peptides than midgut carcinoids.[78] Ectopic ACTH production with Cushing's syndrome is increasingly seen with foregut carcinoids,[22,78,79] and in some studies, these tumors were the most common cause of the ectopic ACTH syndrome, accounting for 64% of all patients.[79] Acromegaly due to release of growth hormone–releasing factors can occur with a number of carcinoids.[71] The somatostatinoma syndrome due to somatostatin release can occur with duodenal carcinoids.[71,72]

CARCINOID SYNDROME

CLINICAL FEATURES

Flushing attacks occur in 23% to 65% of carcinoid syndrome patients initially and in 63% to 78% at some time during the disease course (Table 38.6-3). The typical flush is the sudden appearance of a deep red erythema of the upper part of the body, primarily the face and neck. Flushes are often associated with an unpleasant feeling of warmth, occasionally with lacrimation, itching, palpitations, facial or conjunctival edema, and diarrhea. Flushes may be spontaneous or precipitated by stress; alcohol; certain foods, such as cheese; exercise; or pharmacologically by injections of agents such as catecholamines, calcium, or pentagastrin.[22,80–82] Flushes may be brief, lasting 2 to 5 minutes, especially initially, or may be prolonged for hours, especially later in the course. They are usually seen with carcinoids of midgut origin but can also occur in some patients with foregut tumors.[22] With bronchial carcinoids, the flushes can be frequently prolonged, lasting for hours to days, reddish in color, associated with salivation, lacrimation, diaphoresis, facial swelling, palpitations, deep furrowing of the forehead, diarrhea, and hypotension.[22,81] The flushing with bronchial carcinoids has a greater tendency to cause diffuse body involvement, and after repeated flushing of this type, patients may develop a constant red or cyanotic coloration.[20] The flush associated with gastric carcinoids is also reddish in color but patchy in distribution over the neck and face. It is frequently provoked by food intake or pentagastrin, with erythema associated with blotches and wheals with central clearing, frequently occurring around the root of the neck and on the arms, and the lesions are frequently associated with pruritus.[20,22,81]

Diarrhea is commonly present in 32% to 73% of patients initially and in 67% to 84% at some time during the disease course (see Table 38.6-3). Diarrhea usually occurs with flushing (85% of cases), but it may occur alone (15% of cases).[3,22,83] The diarrhea is described as watery and, less commonly, as frothy or the pale bulky stool of steatorrhea, with the stool number ranging from 2 to 30 per day, and 60% of patients have output of less than 1 L/d.[22,80,81,84] Steatorrhea is present in 67% and in 46% is more than 15 g/d.[84] Abdominal pain may be present with the diarrhea or independently, and the frequency varies from 10% to 34% (see Table 38.6-3).

Cardiac manifestations occur in 11% to 66% of patients[85–87] (see Table 38.6-3). The cardiac disease is due to fibrosis involving the endocardium, primarily of the right side of the heart, although left side lesions can also occur.[3,81,85,86,88] The fibrous deposits are diffuse and are found most commonly on the ventricular aspect of the tricuspid valve and the associated chordae and less commonly on the pulmonary valve cusps. These fibrous deposits tend to cause constriction of both the tricuspid and pulmonic valves. At the pulmonic valve, stenosis is usually predominant, whereas at the tricuspid valve, the constriction results in the valve being fixed open, and tricuspid regurgitation is usually predominant.[81,85,88] In two series, 80% of the patients with cardiac lesions had evidence of heart failure.[39,80] Lesions on the left side occur in 30% of autopsy studies, are less extensive, and most frequently occur on the mitral valve.[3]

Other clinical manifestations of carcinoid syndrome are wheezing or asthma-like symptoms in 8% to 25% of patients and pellagra-like skin lesions with hyperkeratosis and pigmentation in 2% to 5% of cases (see Table 38.6-3). Rarely reported are rheumatoid arthritis,[39] arthralgias,[39] changes in mental state or confusion, and ophthalmic changes during flushing leading to vessel occlusion.[3,39] A variety of noncardiac problems secondary to increased fibrous tissue have been reported, including retroperitoneal fibrosis leading to ureteral obstruction, or Peyronie's disease of the penis; intraabdominal fibrosis; and occlusion of mesenteric arteries or veins.[22,81] Sexual dysfunction is a common complaint of men with carcinoid syndrome.[22] This may relate to the vascular effect of serotonin on pelvic blood vessels.[22]

PATHOBIOLOGY

Carcinoid syndrome developed in 8% of 8876 patients with carcinoids,[12] with an incidence of 1.7% to 18.4% in six different series.[12,80] Carcinoid syndrome occurs only when sufficient concentrations of the hormonal products released by the tumor reach the systemic circulation. Its occurrence and severity are directly related to tumor size in an area that drains into the systemic circulation.[20] In 91% of cases, this only occurs after distant metastases (especially to the liver) develop.[12,80,81] Rarely, however, primary GI tumors with nodal metastases with extensive invasion retroperitoneally or drainage into the ovarian veins; pancreatic carcinoids with retroperitoneal lymph nodes; or carcinoids, such as those in the lung or ovary, with direct access to the systemic circulation can produce the carcinoid syndrome without hepatic metastases.[12,80,89,90] Rarely, medullary thyroid carcinoma, a duodenal adenoma, or small cell lung cancer also have been reported to cause carcinoid syndrome.[81,91] All carcinoids do not have the same propensity to metastasize and to produce the carcinoid syndrome (see Table 38.6-2). Because midgut tumors are the most common and frequently metastasize, midgut tumors account for 60% to 87% of the carcinoid syndrome, foregut tumors for 2% to 33%, hindgut for 1% to 8%, and an unknown primary location for 2% to 15% (see Table 38.6-3).

Symptoms of carcinoid syndrome were originally attributed to secretion of 5-HT (serotonin) by the tumor.[92] In one study[22] of 380 patients with carcinoid tumors, 56% had evidence of serotonin overproduction; 18% of 500 patients in a second study[80] and 88% of 103 patients with carcinoid tumors in a third study[17] had elevated urinary 5-hydroxyindolacetic acid (5-HIAA), the major metabolite of serotonin (Fig. 38.6-1). When 44 consecutive cases were studied before any resection, 84% of the patients had serotonin overproduction.[22] In various studies, 12% to 26% of patients with evidence of serotonin overproduction did not have symptoms of carcinoid syndrome. In one study[93] of 44 consecutive patients with carcinoids, platelet and urinary serotonin, 5-HIAA, and seven catecholamine metabolites were measured. Platelet serotonin was elevated in 96%, 43%, and 0% of patients with midgut, foregut, and hindgut carcinoids, respectively. Urinary dopamine and catecholamine metabolites were elevated in 38% and 33% of midgut, 20% and 20% of foregut, and 7% and 14% of hindgut carcinoids, respectively. In a large review[12] of 748 cases of carcinoid syndrome, 92% had increased serotonin activity.

Patients may develop either a typical or atypical type of carcinoid syndrome (see Fig. 38.6-1). In patients with the typical carcinoid syndrome, the conversion of tryptophan to 5-HTP is the rate-limiting step. Once formed, the 5-HTP is rapidly converted to 5-HT in the tumor by dopa decarboxylase, either stored in the neurosecretory tumor granules or released into vascular compartments, and most is taken up and stored in the granules of platelets. A small amount remains in the plasma. The majority in the circulation is converted by monamine oxidase and aldehyde dehydrogenase to 5-HIAA, which appears in large amounts in the urine.[3,83] Characteristically, patients with carcinoid syndrome have expansion of the serotonin pool size, increase in blood and

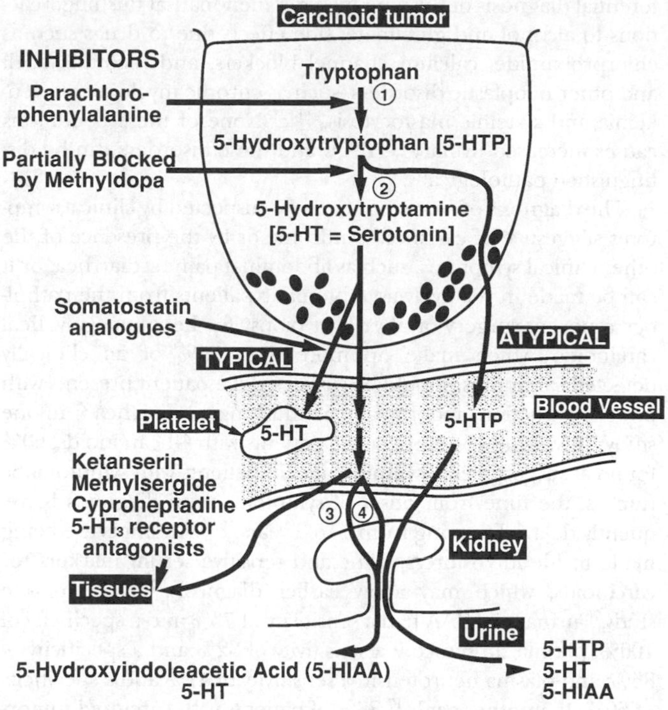

FIGURE 38.6-1. Synthesis, secretion, and metabolism of serotonin [5-hydroxytryptamine (5-HT)] and 5-hydroxytryptophan in patients with typical and atypical carcinoid syndrome, and site of drug action. (1) Tryptophan hydroxylase. (2) Aromatic 1-amino acid decarboxylase (dopa decarboxylase). (3) Monoamine oxidase. (4) Aldehyde dehydrogenase. Arrows indicate the sites of action of therapeutic agents used in the treatment of carcinoid syndrome. Somatostatin analogues include octreotide and lanreotide. Serotonin receptor subtype 3 antagonists ($5\text{-}HT_3$) include ondansetron, tropisetron, and alosetron.

platelet concentrations of serotonin, and elevations of 5-HIAA in the urine.[3,93,94] This is the typical pattern in argentaffin- and argyrophil-positive tumors such as midgut carcinoids, which characteristically secrete large amounts of serotonin and which make up to 60% to 87% of all cases of carcinoid syndrome (see Table 38.6-3). Some carcinoids cause an atypical carcinoid syndrome[22,95] and are thought to be deficient in the enzyme dopa decarboxylase; thus, they cannot convert 5-HTP to 5-HT (serotonin), and 5-HTP is secreted into the bloodstream (see Fig. 38.6-1). Plasma serotonin levels are normal in these patients, but urinary levels are usually elevated because some of the 5-HTP is decarboxylated in the kidney and excreted as serotonin (5-HT). Patients with this type of carcinoid tumor may have a marked increase in urinary 5-HT and 5-HTP levels but normal or only slightly elevated 5-HIAA levels.[22,83] Foregut carcinoids are more likely to excrete high levels of 5-HT and 5-HTP in the urine and give the atypical carcinoid syndrome.[22]

The exact cause of flushing in carcinoid syndrome remains unclear.[94,96] Flushing is not thought to be due to serotonin overproduction, because serotonin antagonists generally have no effect on the flushing.[94,97–101] Using a specific radioenzymatic assay during spontaneous flushing in patients with midgut carcinoids, increased plasma serotonin and norepinephrine levels were found with higher levels in the external jugular than the antecubital veins.[94] This result suggests a possible role for these bioamines in the pathogenesis of flushing with midgut carcinoids. The exact etiology of the flushing in patients with carcinoid syndrome may differ depending on the different tumor types. In patients with gastric carcinoids, the red, patchy, pruritic flush is thought to be caused by histamine,[82] because this type of flushing can be prevented by the use of H_1- and H_2-receptor antagonists.[3,82] In addition to serotonin, other candidates for mediators of flushing include the tachykinins (substance P, neuropeptide K), various GI peptides, and prostaglandins.[83,98,99] However, other studies generally have concluded that prostaglandins are unlikely to be major mediators of the flushing or diarrhea.[83,102]

Studies demonstrate that numerous tachykinins are stored in carcinoids and are released during flushing.[17,76,99,103–106] In some studies, changes in plasma substance P or neuropeptide K levels did not correlate with the occurrence of flushing, leading the authors to conclude that circulating tachykinins have only a minor role, if any, in causing the flushing.[83,98,107] One study[99] demonstrated that all eight patients with midgut carcinoids had elevated plasma substance P levels; however, 88% of patients with PETs and 71% of patients with idiopathic flushing also had elevated levels. In one study,[99] octreotide relieved pentagastrin-induced flushing in all patients without necessarily altering the substance P response. Furthermore, pentagastrin caused flushing in some patients without rises in plasma substance P, suggesting that mediators other than substance P must be important in inducing the flushing.[99] Even though various GI peptides have been proposed to be involved in the flush, no changes in plasma levels of VIP, GIP, neurotensin, PP, motilin, insulin, glucagon, or enteroglucagon have been detected with provocation of the flush.[108]

Patients with carcinoid syndrome have been shown to have increased colonic motility with a shortened transit time and, possibly, a secretory or absorptive alteration.[84,96,109,110] Serotonin is thought to be predominantly responsible for the diarrhea in some patients by its effects on gut motility and intestinal electrolyte and fluid secretion.[83,84] Serotonin receptor antagonists (especially $5\text{-}HT_3$-receptor antagonists such as ondansetron[101]) relieve the diarrhea.[97,98,100,101] In one study,[100] diarrhea was improved by ondansetron in six of six patients with carcinoid syndrome (100%) and nausea in three of four patients (75%), whereas flushing was improved in none of five patients (0%). This finding suggests that $5\text{-}HT_3$ receptors are mediating the diarrhea and nausea. This conclusion is further supported by the demonstration that alosetron, another $5\text{-}HT_3$-receptor antagonist, decreased proximal colonic emptying in patients with carcinoid syndrome.[111] One study[110] provides evidence that prostaglandin E_2 and tachykinins may also be important mediators of carcinoid diarrhea. Patients with carcinoid syndrome had decreased absorption of sodium, potassium, chloride, and water in the jejunum and increased intraluminal nonsubstance P tachykinin and prostaglandin E_2 concentrations compared with normal controls.[96] In combination with histamine, serotonin may be responsible for producing asthma[112] and may be involved in the fibrotic reactions causing heart disease, Peyronie's disease, and ureteral obstruction.[81,98] The pathogenetic link between the carcinoid and heart disease remains a subject of controversy.[22] No relationship between the severity of the heart disease and other common manifestations, such as flushing, diarrhea, or duration of disease, has been established.[22,113] It was reported[85,113] that patients with heart disease have higher urinary 5-HIAA excretion and higher plasma levels of neurokinin A[113] and substance P[113,113] than those without heart disease. A study[114] examining cardiac tissue specimens obtained at operation demonstrated, using immunocytochemistry, increased amounts of TGF-β1 and TGF-β3 but not TGF-β2. It was proposed[114] that TGF-βs may play an important role in proliferation in carcinoid heart disease.

DIAGNOSIS

Diagnosis of carcinoid syndrome relies on the measurement of urinary or plasma serotonin or its metabolites (5-HIAA) in the urine, with the measurement of 5-HIAA in a 24-hour urine sample the most commonly used test (see Fig. 38.6-1). False-positives may occur if the patient is eating serotonin-rich foods, such as bananas, plantains, pineapple, kiwi fruit, walnuts, hickory nuts, pecans, and avocados, which falsely elevate urinary levels.[115,116] Medications, including cough medicine containing guaifenesin, acetaminophen, salicylates, and L-dopa, should also be avoided because they may affect urinary 5-HIAA levels.[116,117] If one properly controls dietary and medicinal intake, the normal range for urinary 5-HIAA excretion is between 2 and 8 mg per 24 hours,[22] although other researchers suggest that using a level of 15 mg/d may reduce false-positive results.[116] Many patients with serotonin-secreting carcinoids have urinary 5-HIAA excretion in the range of 8 to 30 mg per 24 hours.[118] The measurement of urinary 5-HIAA levels is the current method of choice to diagnose carcinoid syndrome.[118] In one study,[83] 5-HIAA determinations alone had a 73% sensitivity and a 100% specificity for carcinoid syndrome.[83]

Most physicians rely totally on the measurement of urinary 5-HIAA for diagnosis. However, urinary and platelet measurement of serotonin itself may give additional information; thus, it has been recommended that these should also be measured.[22,83,93] In two studies,[119] platelet serotonin levels not only were more sensitive than urinary 5-HIAA and urinary serotonin levels, they were not affected by the patient's diet, as are the 5-HIAA levels. In one comparative study of 44 consecutive carcinoid patients, the platelet serotonin levels,[93] urine 5-HIAA, and urinary serotonin levels were measured. In 14 foregut carcinoids, the sensitivities were 50%, 29%, and 55%, respectively; for 25 midgut carcinoids, the sensitivities were 100%, 92%, and 82%, respectively; and for hindgut carcinoids, the sensitivities were 20%, 0%, and 60%, respectively. The data demonstrate the increased sensitivity of measuring platelet serotonin levels. Elevations of 5-HIAA can occur in malabsorption states and a number of other conditions.[81,116] It is important to remember that foregut carcinoids tend to produce an atypical carcinoid syndrome with increased plasma 5-HTP but not serotonin, because they lack the appropriate decarboxylase (see Fig. 38.6-1), with the result that urinary 5-HIAA may not be markedly increased.[22] In such patients with a normal or minimally elevated 5-HIAA and for whom there is a strong suspicion of carcinoid syndrome, they should be screened for other urinary metabolites of tryptophan,[118] and platelet serotonin levels should be measured. However, this screening is usually not necessary because some of the 5-HTP is decarboxylated in the intestine and other tissues, and many of these patients have elevated urinary 5-HT or 5-HIAA levels.[118]

Diagnostic difficulties may arise in patients who flush for reasons other than carcinoid syndrome,[22,120] in patients with carcinoid syndrome in whom flushing is not apparent, in patients with certain carcinoids (especially foregut tumors in whom 5-HIAA may be normal or minimally elevated),[118] or in the rare patient without metastatic disease who presents with flushing.[89] The differential diagnosis of flushing includes menopausal flushing; reactions to alcohol and glutamate; side effects due to drugs such as chlorpropamide, calcium channel blockers, and nicotinic acid; and other neoplastic disorders, such as chronic myelogenous leukemia and systemic mastocytosis.[120,121] None of these conditions causes increased urinary 5-HIAA, and these disorders can be distinguished pathologically.

The diagnosis of a carcinoid may be suspected by clinical symptoms suggestive of carcinoid syndrome or by the presence of the other clinical symptoms, such as abdominal pain or diarrhea, or it can be made in relatively asymptomatic patients from the pathology report at surgery or after liver biopsy for hepatomegaly. Ileal carcinoids, which make up more than 25% of all clinically detected carcinoids, should be suspected if a patient presents with bowel obstruction, abdominal pain, flushing, or diarrhea.[22] In one study[26] involving 154 consecutive patients with GI carcinoids, 60% found at surgery were asymptomatic. In patients with symptomatic tumors, the time from onset of symptoms until diagnosis is frequently delayed, varying from 1 to 2 years.[17,20] Attempts are being made to identify more specific and sensitive serum markers for carcinoids, which may allow earlier diagnosis.[17,22,76,83] In one study,[76] urinary 5-HIAA had a sensitivity of 73% and a specificity of 100%; plasma substance P a sensitivity of 32% and a specificity of 85%; and plasma neurotensin a sensitivity of 41% and a specificity of 60%. In another study,[17] 88% of patients with carcinoid tumors (93% with hepatic metastases) had an elevated 5-HIAA; 66% an elevated plasma neuropeptide K; and 43% an elevated plasma PP concentration. A number of studies[122–124] demonstrate that serum chromogranin A levels are elevated in 56% to 100% of patients with carcinoids, and the level correlates with tumor bulk. Serum chromogranin A elevations are not specific for carcinoids because increased levels occur with high frequency in patients with PETs[9,122,123,125] and certain other NETs.[123,125] The α (α-HCG) or β (β-HCG) subunits of HCG are detected frequently by immunocytochemistry in carcinoids, and elevated plasma levels of HCG are reported in 28% of carcinoids[126] and 13% of patients with carcinoid syndrome.[127] NSE also is used as a plasma marker of carcinoid tumors,[126] but it is less sensitive than chromogranin A, being positive in only 17% to 47% of patients.[122,123]

LOCALIZATION

A number of techniques, including GI endoscopy, barium radiographs, chest radiographs, imaging studies [ultrasound, computed tomographic (CT) scan, magnetic resonance imaging, angiography], endoscopic ultrasound, selective venous sampling for various hormones, positron emission tomography scanning, and various forms of radionuclide scanning [radiolabeled somatostatin receptor scintigraphy (SRS), iodinated metaiodobenzylguanidine (MIBG)], all have been used to determine the location of the primary tumor as well as tumor extent.[3,22,128–131]

Bronchial carcinoids are usually detected by chest radiography, CT or, occasionally, by bronchoscopy.[22,36,38] They appear frequently (37%) as opacities with sharp or often notched margins.[132] They are slow growing and often induce airway compression with resultant atelectasis. Enlarged hilar lymph nodes from metastasis are rare.[132] Rectal, duodenal, colonic, and gastric carcinoids are almost always detected by GI endoscopy, with barium radiographs being generally negative.[26,69] When positive, barium radiographs show dilated loops of small bowel or extrinsic filling defects but rarely detect a mucosal lesion,[26] whereas ileal, cecal, and right colon tumors are often diagnosed on radiographic studies.[133]

The main problem is localizing small bowel carcinoids, which may be very small and frequently missed by barium studies, and small carcinoids in other GI tissues.[3] Some of these tumors can be localized by angiography, SRS, or CT,[3] but many are not seen with these modalities. Liver metastases usually are detected by CT or, more recently, SRS. Angiography is more sensitive than CT for detecting liver metastases.[3,22] At present, CT and SRS are the primary diagnostic modality for tumor staging. CT frequently misses the primary tumor, especially if it is small (less than 1.5 cm).[134] However, CT is generally helpful in evaluating the presence of liver metastases and retroperitoneal lymphadenopathy.[3,134]

Carcinoids possess high-affinity receptors for somatostatin in 88% to 100% of cases.[55,128,135] The somatostatin receptors are present in both the primary tumor and metastases. Five subtypes (numbered sst_1 to sst_5) of somatostatin receptors have been described.[135] Octreotide binds with high affinity to sst_2 and with a lower affinity to sst_3 and sst_5 and has a very low affinity for sst_1 and sst_4.[135] Studies show almost all carcinoids (90% to 100%) possess sst_2; 50% to 60% sst_5; 10% to 100% sst_3; 70% to 100% sst_1; and 20% to 100% sst_4.[55] [^{111}In-DTPA-DPhe] octreotide has been approved for localizing carcinoids using radionuclide scanning.[135] SRS images tumor in 73% to 89% of patients with carcinoids.[128,134,135] In one comparative study of 40 patients,[129] SRS localized tumors in 78% and CT in 82%. SRS detected primary tumors in two patients missed on CT, and in 16% of cases it detected lesions not previously seen.[129] Numerous other studies[134,135] have demonstrated that SRS has greater sensitivity for localizing carcinoids, especially the extent of metastatic spread, than conventional imaging studies (Fig. 38.6-2). More recent studies demonstrate that it has a higher specificity than bone scanning and equal or greater sensitivity.[136,137] In general, SRS has excellent specificity, but it is important to remember that high densities of somatostatin receptors exist on a number of other normal and abnormal cells that can lead to increased uptake and a false-positive response.[138] These include granulomas (e.g., sarcoid, tuberculosis), activated lymphocytes (wound infections, lymphomas), thyroid diseases (goiter, thyroiditis), PETs, and other endocrine tumors. In one study,[138] 12% of SRS localizations were false-positives; however, by considering the clinical context the number of false-positives was reduced to less than 4%. Because of its sensitivity and ability to image all body areas, SRS should be the initial imaging procedure to localize and establish the extent of carcinoids.

Bone metastases are increasingly being recognized in patients with metastatic carcinoid and other PETs.[3,136] In one study[137] of 30 patients with carcinoid tumors, bone metastases were found in four (13%) using SRS and bone scanning. In general, technetium 99m bone scanning and SRS have been found to be more sensitive than conventional radiographs for detecting bone metastases.[3,22,139]

Positron emission tomography scanning with 5-hydroxytryptophan [^{11}C-labeled 5-HTP] has been compared with CT in 16 patients with carcinoids.[131] Positron emission tomography was more sensitive in ten of the patients than CT and was equally sensitive to CT in the others.[131] During treatment, a close correlation ($r = 0.91$) was found between changes in the positron emission tomography scan transport rate constant and changes in urinary 5-HIAA, suggesting that positron emission tomography scanning may be useful for monitoring the results of therapy.[131]

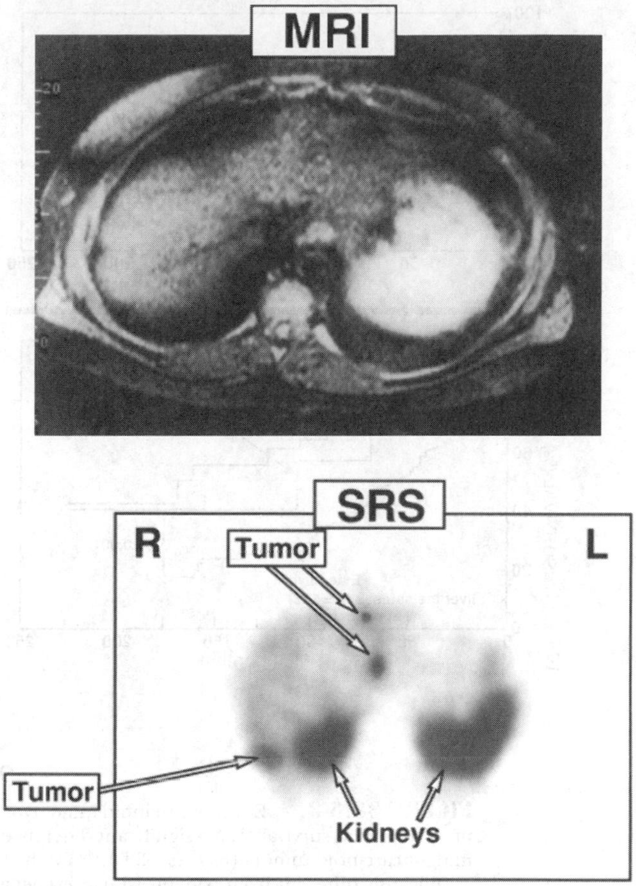

FIGURE 38.6-2. Comparison of the ability of magnetic resonance imaging (MRI) and somatostatin receptor scintigraphy (SRS) to localize hepatic metastases in a patient with carcinoid syndrome and metastatic gastric carcinoid to the liver. MRI was negative for tumor, whereas SRS demonstrated liver metastases (labeled *tumor*) in the left and right hepatic lobes. The imaging results in this patient demonstrate the greater sensitivity of SRS for localizing hepatic metastases from a carcinoid tumor over conventional imaging studies.

PROGNOSIS

Clinically, carcinoid syndrome is generally a manifestation of advanced disease.[3,12,20,80] Two in every three patients with carcinoid syndrome have physical signs of cancer, such as an abdominal mass or hepatomegaly.[20] A clear positive correlation exists between tumor mass and urinary 5-HIAA levels[20,43,80]; therefore, the laboratory test measuring 5-HIAA levels is a good marker for extent of disease.

Carcinoids from different locations not only differ in the percentage that are malignant and the percentage that develop carcinoid syndrome (see Table 38.6-2), but also in their aggressiveness. The percentage of carcinoids in different locations having localized disease, regional metastases, or distant metastases varies widely. The highest percentage of nonlocalized disease is with pancreatic (91%), colonic (77%), and small intestinal carcinoids (75%), whereas the highest percentage with localized disease is the larynx (100%), followed by the ovary, appendix, and rectum (62% to 95%). Overall metastases are present at the time of diagnosis in 45% of patients in the SEER group data.[14] In one study,[140] no difference was found in the overall 5-year survival rate of patients with foregut (60%) or midgut carcinoids (63%) (Fig. 38.6-3A).

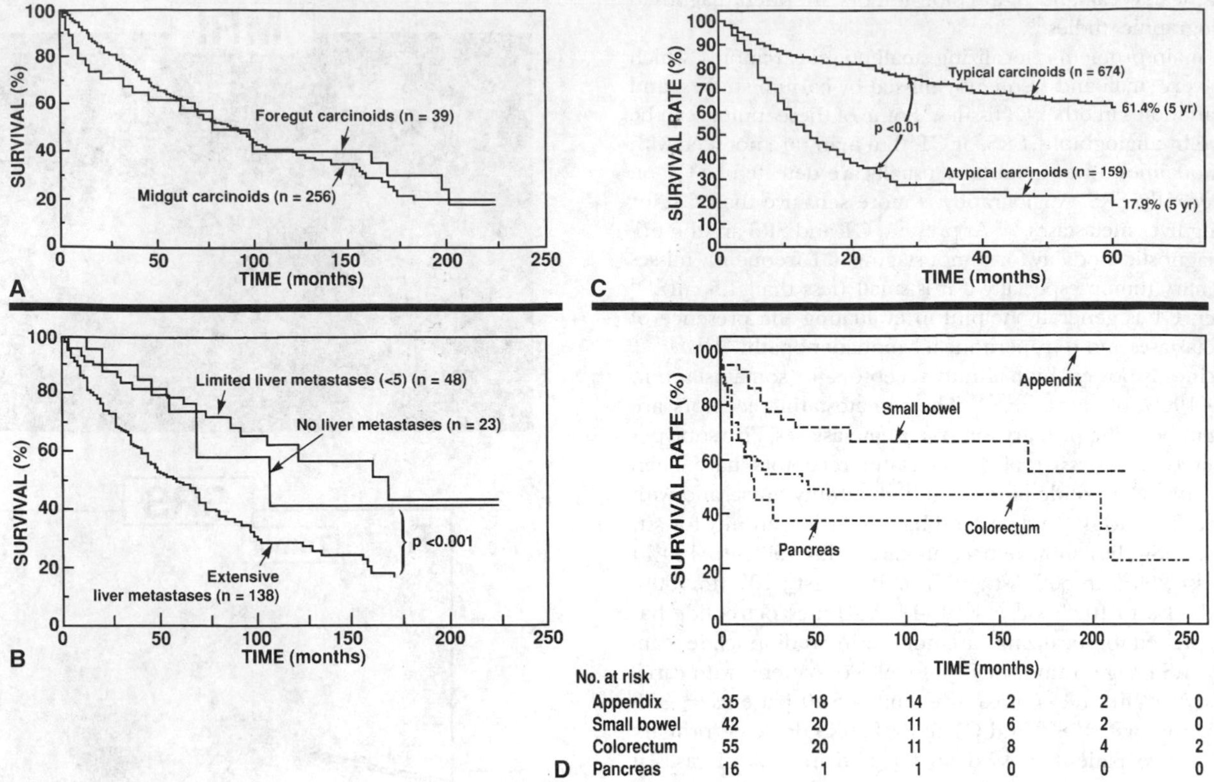

FIGURE 38.6-3. Effect of carcinoid tumor type, extent of metastases, histologic pattern, or localization of primary tumor on survival. **A:** No significant difference was noted in 5-year survival rates for patients with foregut or midgut carcinoid tumors (60% vs. 63%).[140] **B:** The 5-year survival rate of patients with no liver metastases was not significantly different from patients with a few hepatic metastases (fewer than 5) (73% vs. 79%), but was significantly (P<.001) greater than those patients with extensive hepatic metastases (more than 5) (47%).[140] **C:** Effect of the histologic pattern of the carcinoid tumor in 833 patients, with the 5-year survival rates for both patterns, is shown.[44] **D:** The number of patients at risk at different times are shown. Patients with an appendiceal primary tumor had a significantly (P<.01) better prognosis than those with pancreatic or colorectal carcinoids.

Survival rates with different carcinoids depend on both the site and the extent of tumor[13,14,141] (Tables 38.6-4 and 38.6-5; see Fig. 38.6-3*D*). For all 8305 patients in the SEER data[14] with local disease only, the 5-year survival rate was 80%, varying from 0% for liver and 65% for small intestine and ileum to 94% for appendix. In patients with regional involvement, the 5-year survival rate was 51% overall, varying from 0% for the pancreas and gallbladder to 85% for the appendix. For patients with distant metastases, the

TABLE 38.6-4. Five-Year Survival Rates of Carcinoid Tumors by Site and Stage

	Localized (%)	*Regional (%)*	*Distant (%)*	*Unstaged (%)*	*All Stages (%)*
Carcinoid site					
Stomach	64	40	10	66	49
Small intestine	65	66	36	53	55
Colon (except appendix)	71	44	20	68	42
Appendix	94	85	34	78	86
Rectum	81	47	18	75	72
Liver	0	N/A	0	N/A	22
Gallbladder	83	0	N/A	N/A	41
Pancreas	N/A	0	26	57	34
Retroperitoneum	N/A	N/A	N/A	N/A	50
Other and ill-defined digestive tract	N/A	3	25	N/A	11
Trachea/bronchi/lung	85	70	14	65	77
Ovary	95	N/A	13	N/A	66
All sites (mean ± SEM)	80 ± 4	51 ± 10	22 ± 3	66 ± 3	50 ± 6

SEM, standard error of the mean.
(From ref. 14, with permission.)

TABLE 38.6-5. Prognostic Factors in Carcinoid Tumors

UNIVARIATE ANALYSIS
Age (P = .001) [<50–97%; ≥50–63%]
Gender (P<.01) [5-y survival: female (66%) > male (47%)]
Primary tumor site (P<.01) (survival rate: appendix > small bowel > colorectal > pancreas)
Depth of invasion (P<.001)
Presence of lymph node metastases (P<.001) [5-y survival: no (94%) vs. yes (43%)]
Tumor size (P<.005) [5-y survival: 1 cm (100%) > 1.1–2.0 cm (82%) > 2.1+ cm(39%)]
Presence of liver metastases (P<.001) [5-y survival: no (88%) vs. yes (25%)]
Extent of hepatic metastases (P<.001) [extensive, 47% vs. limited (<5), 79%]
Mode of discovery (P<.001) (incidentally > symptomatic)
Operative intent (P<.001) [5-y survival: cure (91%) vs. palliative (25%)]
Presence of a second malignancy
Histologic features (typical or atypical)
Flow cytometry features (i.e., aneuploidy)
Mitotic counts (P<.001) (<10 per ten high-power fields vs. >10 per ten high-power fields)
Ki-67 index (P<.05)
Proliferative cell nuclear antigen expression
Presence of carcinoid syndrome
Laboratory results [extent of increase of serum chromogranin A (P <.01), urinary 5-HIAA (P<.01), plasma neuropeptide K (P<.05)]
MULTIVARIATE ANALYSIS
Death due to all causes
Gender (RR, 2.78; 95% CI, 1.2–6.5)
Death due to the disease
Presence of metastases (RR, 3.87; 95% CI, 1.0–14.5)

CI, confidence interval; 5-HIAA, 5-hydroxyindolacetic acid; Ki-67, proliferative associated nuclear antigen recognized by monoclonal antibody Ki-67; RR, relative risk.
All results are from ref. 142 except age (refs. 3, 44, 144), extent of hepatic metastases (ref. 140), histologic features (refs. 3, 44), flow cytometry features (refs. 3, 156, 158, 159), mitotic counts (ref. 146), Ki-67 index (ref. 147), proliferative cell nuclear antigen expression (ref. 290), presence of carcinoid syndrome (refs. 3, 161), and laboratory results (refs. 140, 161).

overall 5-year survival rate was 22%, varying from 0% for the liver to 36% for the small intestine. In different studies for the common carcinoids, the 5-year survival rate was the highest for carcinoids of the appendix (86% to 100%),[13,20,25,142,143] followed by lung (77% to 87%),[13,14] rectum (62% to 72%),[13,14,26,31,143] small intestine (42% to 73%),[3,13,14,20,27–29,142,143] and colon and stomach (42% to 75%).[13,14,34,142,143]

One of the main determinants of survival is the presence of liver metastases (see Tables 38.6-4 and 38.6-5 and Fig. 38.6-3).[3,14,28,31,141,143] In a multivariant analysis of 188 cases of patients with carcinoids,[142] the one factor independently predictive of death was the presence of metastases. Additional prognostic factors are summarized in Table 38.6-5. The extent of hepatic metastases is also an important prognostic factor (see Fig. 38.6-3*B*; Table 38.6-5). In one study,[140] the survival rate was similar in patients with limited hepatic metastases (fewer than five) or no metastases, and it was significantly greater (P <.001) than for patients with extensive metastases. Female gender is associated with a better prognosis,[142,143] as is younger age.[140,143–145] The level of tissue invasion is an important predictor of the probability of developing liver metastases.[28,31,142] The likelihood of finding regional invasion, metastatic disease, and decreasing survival rates is directly proportional to the size of the primary tumor.[3,20,27,32,33,142] With carcinoids of less than 1 cm in diameter, fewer than 15% to 30% in the small bowel have metastatic disease; in the rectum, fewer than 0% to 20%; and in the appendix, fewer than 0% to 2%.[17,20,23,31,32] In contrast, for those tumors more than 2 cm in diameter, 33% to 95% in the small bowel have metastases; in the rectum, more than 70% have metastatic disease; and in the appendix, 33% have metastatic disease.[20,27–29,31,32] For all patients with carcinoids the 5-year survival rate varies from 11% to 86% in different studies[13,14,17] (see Table 38.6-4).

The histologic features as well as the stage of the carcinoid have been shown to correlate with disease-specific survival and the risk of metastases[26,28,30,33,34,44,142] (see Table 38.6-5 and Fig. 38.6-3*C*). In one study,[142] for patients with bowel tumors invading only the submucosa (T1), the 5-year survival rate was 100%; with tumors invading the muscularis propria (T2), it was 81%; with tumors invading to the subserosa (T3), it was 70%; and with tumors involving the visceral peritoneum or directly invading other structures (T4), it was 52%. These results are consistent with numerous studies that have demonstrated that, for carcinoids, the probability of developing liver metastases is closely related to the level of tissue invasion.[3,27,28,31,32,34,44] With bronchial carcinoids,[38] the most important variables affecting prognosis are increasing age, tumor diameter larger than 3 cm, T stage, N stage, lymph node involvement, and number of lymph nodes involved. For all pulmonary NETs, which include typical and atypical carcinoids, and for large cell and small cell neuroendocrine carcinomas,[146] the histologic features, number of mitoses, degree of necrosis, vascular invasion, and extent of nuclear pleomorphism all had a significant effect on survival.[146] Histologic features such as necrosis, increased mitotic count, nuclear pleomorphism, vascular or lymphatic invasion, and undifferentiated growth pattern are used to classify carcinoids histologically as typical or atypical,[4,38] and this variable can have a marked effect on survival (see Fig. 38.6-3*C* and Table 38.6-5).[27,33,34,38,44,146] Measures of proliferation, such as Ki-67 activity or proliferative cell nuclear antigen expression, correlate with tumor aggressiveness or survival in some studies,[147–149] but not in others.[150] Flow cytometry has been used to attempt to define the malignant potential for both GI and bronchial carcinoids.[38,149,151–156] In two studies[3,151] of GI carcinoids, the presence of metastases or decreased survival correlated with the presence of aneuploidy,[152,153] whereas in other studies,[149,154,157] no correlation was found. In bronchial carcinoids, aneuploidy was reported to occur in 50% to 79%,[3] and in some studies,[156,158,159] but not others,[157,160] the flow cytometric result was predictive of the presence of metastases or decreased survival. In one study,[158] aneuploidy was seen significantly more frequently in atypical (74% of cases) than in typical (18%) bronchial carcinoids.

In various studies in the before-octreotide era,[17,80] the median survival of patients with carcinoid syndrome from the time of onset of symptoms varied from 3.5 to 8.5 years, and the presence of carcinoid syndrome was associated with decreased survival. The mean survival after recognition of abnormal excretion of 5-HIAA was 23 months,[80] and the 5-

year survival rates after onset of symptoms in two studies were 30% and 67%.[17,80] In a number of studies,[140,161] the level of 5-HIAA excretion has been correlated with survival (see Table 38.6-5). In one study, patients excreting 10 to 49 mg/d had a median survival of 29 months; those with 50 to 149 mg/d had a survival rate of 24 months, and those with more than 150 mg/d had a mean survival rate of 13 months.[80] Octreotide treatment has been proposed to extend survival. Studies show the level of plasma chromogranin A elevation is predictive of survival,[140] as is the plasma level of the tachykinin neuropeptide K.[140,161] In one study,[140] patients with a plasma chromogranin A level of less than 5000 μg/L had significantly (P <.001) longer survival than those with higher values (56 months vs. 33 months, respectively). A number of studies[28,31] have provided evidence that patients with carcinoids are at increased risk of developing a synchronous adenocarcinoma (7% to 10%), with the most common site being the large intestine. The development of a second malignancy is associated with a worse prognosis.[144]

The most immediate life-threatening complication of carcinoid syndrome, the carcinoid crisis, is observed more frequently in patients who have intense symptoms from foregut carcinoids or who have greatly elevated urinary 5-HIAA levels (more than 200 mg per 24 hours).[162] The carcinoid crisis may occur spontaneously, or it may be associated with stress, anesthesia, chemotherapy, or even biopsy of hepatic metastases.[3,20,135,163,164] Patients usually develop flushing, diarrhea, and abdominal pain. Mentation is altered, ranging from light-headedness to coma. Cardiac abnormalities also occur, including tachycardia, hypertension, or profound hypotension.[3] The carcinoid crisis may be successfully treated, but in some patients it may also be a terminal event.[20,162] In one study[165] of 21 patients with abdominal carcinoids, of whom 90% had an elevated urinary 5-HIAA level, 80% had evidence of cardiovascular instability during surgery, primarily hypotension. In five cases pretreated with octreotide, the changes in blood pressure were less and responded easily to additional octreotide.[165] Other investigators also have described the value of octreotide in the treatment and prevention of carcinoid crises.[3,135,163–166]

TREATMENT

Many patients with hepatic metastases from carcinoid tumors remain active and well except for occasional episodes of flushing or diarrhea. Treatment of these patients includes avoiding stress and conditions or substances that precipitate flushing, and dietary supplementation with nicotinamide (Fig. 38.6-4). Heart failure may require diuretics; wheezing may require oral bronchodilators such as salbutamol, a bronchodilator that interacts with β-adrenergic receptors and does not induce flushing, or aminophylline; and mild diarrhea may respond to antidiarrheal agents such as loperamide or diphenoxylate. If patients still have carcinoid syndrome symptoms, serotonin receptor antagonists or somatostatin analogues are the drugs of choice, although a number of other drugs also have been shown to be effective in small numbers of patients[3,77] (see Figs. 38.6-1 and 38.6-4).

These various agents act in a variety of ways, including by inhibiting the synthesis of serotonin (parachlorophenylalanine, α-methyldopa), by functioning as serotonin receptor antagonists and blocking the action of 5-HT on target tissues, or by inhibiting the release of various vasoactive substances (octreotide, interferon-α) (see Figs. 38.6-1 and 38.6-4). Parachlorophenylalanine, which blocks the hydroxylase enzyme that converts tryptophan to 5-HTP, relieves diarrhea and improves flushing in some patients and reduces urinary 5-HIAA.[162,167] However, its side effects include hypersensitivity reactions and psychiatric disturbances, making it intolerable for long-term clinical use.[162,167] α-Methyldopa blocks the conversion of 5-HTP to serotonin; however, its effect is partial. It occasionally relieves flushing, which may be secondary to inhibiting catecholamine-stimulated release of vasoactive substances, and has little effect on GI symptoms.[78,81] Phenoxybenzamine, an α-adrenergic antagonist, as well as phenothiazines, possibly acting as α-adrenergic receptor antago-

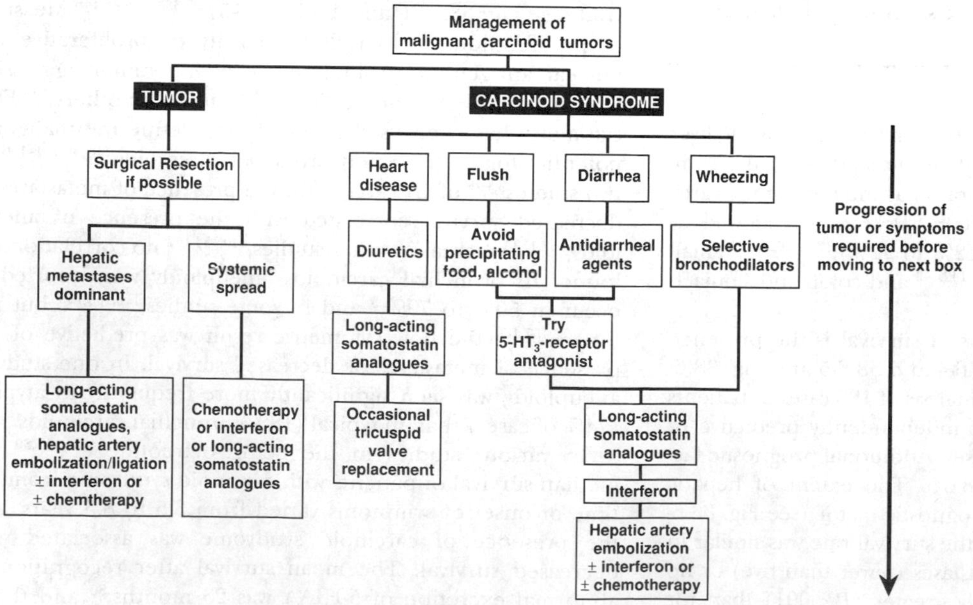

FIGURE 38.6-4. Algorithm for the treatment of malignant carcinoid tumors. *Somatostatin analogues* refers to the use of octreotide, lanreotide, or their long-acting depot formulations (long-acting–release octreotide or sustained-release lanreotide). 5-HT$_3$, 5-hydroxytryptamine subtype 3.

nists, may block flushing provoked by alcohol or other agents, although patients frequently become refractory.[78,81,97] Fourteen subclasses of serotonin (5-HT) receptors have been described.[168] The 5-HT_1 and 5-HT_2 receptor antagonists methylsergide,[93,97,169] cyproheptadine,[169,170] and ketanserin[169,171,172] frequently decrease the GI symptoms but usually do not decrease the flushing. In one study,[20] cyproheptadine used at a dose of 3 to 8 mg three times per day reduced diarrhea in 50% of patients, with minimal, if any, effect on flushing or excretion of 5-HIAA. Cyproheptadine also is reported to have antitumor activity.[3,173] The use of methysergide is limited because it can cause or enhance retroperitoneal fibrosis. In various studies,[166,171,172,174] ketanserin diminished frequency and severity of flushing in 6% to 100% and diarrhea in 30% to 100% of patients. 5-HT_3-receptor antagonists (ondansetron, tropisetron, alosetron) usually control diarrhea and nausea and, occasionally, flushing.[93,100,101,111,169] A combination of histamine H_1- and H_2-receptor antagonists are effective in carcinoid syndrome that is caused by gastric carcinoids.[82] Prednisone in doses of 20 mg/d gives occasional relief in some cases with severe flushing; however, it is ineffective in controlling the GI symptoms.[78,81] Tamoxifen was reported to cause symptomatic improvement in two patients with carcinoid syndrome[3]; however, in a study involving 16 patients with malignant carcinoids, no improvement or sustained reduction in 5-HIAA occurred with tamoxifen administration.[175]

Native somatostatin reduces symptoms in patients with carcinoid syndrome.[176] However, its use is limited by its short half-life (2.5 to 3.0 minutes). With the availability of synthetic, long-acting somatostatin analogues, octreotide (half-life, 90 minutes),[177] and lanreotide, treatment can be given subcutaneously every 6 to 12 hours.[178] These drugs are now the drugs of choice to control the symptoms of patients with carcinoid syndrome.[110,135,164,179–190] These somatostatin analogues are effective at relieving symptoms and decreasing hormone levels when self-administered every 6 to 12 hours subcutaneously in patients with carcinoid syndrome.[20,110,135,164,179–189,189–191] Octreotide[192] decreases 5-HT and neuropeptide K release and synthesis from midgut carcinoids by a direct action on tumor cells. In an analysis of 62 published studies,[164] octreotide controlled symptoms in more than 80% of patients. When doses in excess of 375 µg/day were used, diarrhea improved in more than 80%.[135,164,179] If more than 400 µg/d of octreotide were used, flushing was controlled in more than 80%.[135,164,179] At least 70% of patients had a higher than 50% decrease in 5-HIAA.[164,179] It was recommended[164] that, in patients with carcinoid syndrome with mild to moderate symptoms, treatment should be initiated with 100 µg subcutaneously every 8 hours. Individual responses vary and some patients require higher doses, with doses increased as high as 3000 µg/d.[164] Forty percent of patients escaped from control after a median time of 4 months, with the remaining patients having sustained control for up to 2.5 years; all responded for more than 1 year, and one-third responded for more than 2 years.[20]

Results similar to octreotide have been described with lanreotide.[181,183,185] In patients with life-threatening features of carcinoid syndrome or the carcinoid crises, somatostatin analogues are effective at both treating these as well as preventing their possible development during known precipitating events, such as surgery, anesthesia, chemotherapy, or stress.[135,163,165,193] It has been recommended[179] that patients with carcinoids scheduled for surgery should be given 150 to 250 µg of octreotide subcutaneously every 6 to 8 hours beginning 24 to 48 hours before anesthesia. In patients receiving chemotherapy, 250 to 300 µg subcutaneously 1 to 2 hours before chemotherapy is recommended.[179]

Sustained-release preparations of somatostatin have been developed that facilitate treatment. These include monthly octreotide-LAR (long-acting release) or biweekly lanreotide-SR (sustained release) formulations.[84,181,182,194] With octreotide-LAR (30 mg/month) a plasma level of 1 ng/mL or more is maintained for 25 days, whereas this requires three to six injections per day of the non–sustained-release form.[84,195] Similar to the nondepot forms, the sustained-release preparations are highly effective at controlling symptoms of carcinoid syndrome.[181–183,194]

Short-term side effects of somatostatin analogues have been minimal, occurring in 40% to 50% of patients.[3,135,181,196] Pain at the injection site and effects related to the GI tract (discomfort in 59% and nausea/diarrhea in 15%) are most common. Most are short-lived and therapy is not interrupted.[135] Important long-term side effects include gallstone formation, steatorrhea, and deterioration in glucose tolerance.[3,135,181,197,198] In various studies,[135] the incidence of gallstones in patients treated long term with octreotide has varied from 5% to 80%, and in a review[135,199] of 13 studies involving 213 acromegalic patients, 29% developed gallstones.[135,199] In a study[197] of 45 patients with metastatic carcinoid or PETs treated long term with octreotide, the overall incidence of gallstones, biliary sludge, or both was 52%, with 7% having symptomatic disease requiring surgical treatment.

Interferon-α is effective in carcinoid syndrome, either alone[200–204] or combined with hepatic artery embolization.[203,205] In more than 300 patients with carcinoids and carcinoid syndrome treated with interferon,[204] the overall biochemical response rate was 42%. In 111 patients[201,204] from one center given interferon-α (1.5 to 7.0 mU three to seven times per week), 42% had a biochemical response (a more than 50% decrease in tumor marker) with a median duration of 32 months. In 70% of patients, an improvement in flushing or diarrhea was seen. In another study,[206] high doses of interferon-α were used (24 mU/m^2/d); 39% of patients had a decrease in 5-HIAA secretion, flushing improved in 65%, and diarrhea improved in 33%. However, these responses were transient, lasting a median of only 7 weeks. Interferon-α has been combined with hepatic embolization[205] in seven patients and compared with interferon given alone in 12 patients (5 mU/d) for the treatment of carcinoid syndrome. Evaluation after 1 year of treatment showed that, with interferon alone, 50% of patients had decreased urinary levels of 5-HIAA, and when combined with embolization, 71% of patients had a decrease. With interferon alone,[205] 58% had decreased flushing and 67% had decreased diarrhea, whereas with the addition of embolization, 86% had decreased flushing and 43% had decreased diarrhea.

Patients with carcinoid syndrome who have no response to octreotide or interferon-α alone have been treated with a combination of both agents.[184,204] In one study[204] involving 24 patients, all demonstrating increased urinary 5-HIAA levels and 19 having classic carcinoid syndrome, complete biochemical remission occurred in 18% and partial biochemical remission occurred in 59%. For a patient with severe carcinoid syndrome not responsive to other measures, hepatic artery embolization or ligation either alone or combined with interferon or chemotherapy may be effective[20,203,205,207–213] (see Fig. 38.6-4). In two studies[214,215] involving 32 patients with metastatic liver disease with carcinoid syndrome, embolization or ligation resulted in at least a 50% decrease in urinary 5-HIAA levels in 63% of patients. In the largest study,[215] 100% of patients had disappearance of diarrhea and flushing immediately after the procedure, and at 1 year postprocedure, 61% were free of symptoms. Chemoembolization,[20,207,208,210–212] which is embolization with Gelfoam and simultaneous chemotherapy (doxorubicin, mitomycin C, cisplatin, 5-fluorouracil) or interferon,[213] was reported to result in symptomatic improvement in a significant number of patients with carcinoid syndrome. In one large study[212] involving 42 patients with carcinoid tumors, 83% had a decrease in 5-HIAA with chemoembolization followed by treatment with doxorubicin plus dacarbazine [(dimethyltriazeno)imidazole carboxamide; DTIC] and streptozotocin plus 5-fluorouracil, and the mean decrease was 87%. Among patients responding, 98% had improvement in flushing and 88% had improvement in diarrhea.[212] In another study[207] of 15 patients who were unsuccessfully treated with chemotherapy and somatostatin analogue, hepatic artery chemoembolization with 5-fluorouracil, adriamycin, cisplatin, and mitomycin C controlled diarrhea in 75%, flushing in 58%, and pain in 75%. Hepatic artery occlusion or embolization can have significant side effects, with nausea, vomiting, liver pain, and fever.[208,209,212] Major complications occurred in 12% to 17% of patients,[208,212] including hepatorenal syndrome, sepsis, gallbladder perforation or necrosis, upper GI bleeding, and abscess formation. In two studies,[209,216] 5% to 7% of patients died of a complication of hepatic artery occlusion. In the literature, the mortality rate is reported as less than 3%, pain occurs in 100%, and pyrexia and leukocytosis are reported in 50%, as well as occasional acute gangrenous cholecystitis from obstruction of the cystic artery, hepatic abscess, paralytic ileus, and renal failure.[214]

The approach to treatment of carcinoid syndrome at present is summarized in Figure 38.6-4. After symptomatic treatment, patients should avoid precipitating food and alcohol and use oral antidiarrheal agents for mild diarrhea and oral selective bronchodilators for wheezing. Serotonin receptor antagonists, particularly the new 5-HT_3 antagonists (ondansetron, tropisetron), may be effective, particularly for diarrhea and nausea. Octreotide or lanreotide are the drugs of choice, self-administered by the patient. If tachyphylaxis develops, the dose can be increased. If symptoms recur, are severe, and do not respond to an increased octreotide dose, other serotonin receptor antagonists, such as cyproheptadine or ketanserin, should be considered. If this strategy is ineffective, then interferon alone or subsequently combined with somatostatin analogues should be considered (see Fig. 38.6-4).

TREATMENT OF THE CARCINOID TUMOR

Resection of local or regional nodal metastatic disease can result in cure in some patients.[217–219] Because in the case of most carcinoids the possibility of metastatic disease is directly related to primary size, the extent of surgical resection for possible cure should be determined accordingly. In the case of appendiceal tumors smaller than 1 cm without gross metastases, which pertains to the majority,[20,25,217,219] a simple appendectomy is sufficient.[20,217,219] Of 103 such patients treated with a simple appendectomy, of whom 103 were followed for 5 years and 83 for 10 to 35 years, no patient developed a local recurrence or metastatic disease.[20,23] With rectal carcinoids smaller than 1 cm, local resection usually is adequate and results in cure.[3,20,32,69,220,221] The depth of invasion is also an important prognostic factor[32] and should also be assessed in all tumors.[32] If no invasion of the muscularis propria is present for rectal carcinoids smaller than 2 cm, local resection is adequate.[32] With small intestinal carcinoids smaller than 1 cm, complete agreement about treatment has not been reached. In most series, 15% to 20% of tumors smaller than 1 cm have metastases. In another series, however, 69% of tumors smaller than 0.5 cm were associated with metastases,[222] and in another series,[28] 32% of tumors 0.6 to 1.0 cm in size had metastases, leading one group[222] to conclude that, with midgut carcinoids, malignancy is independent of size. This has led some to recommend a wide *en bloc* resection of the adjacent lymph node–bearing mesentery for all small intestinal carcinoids.[26] If the carcinoid is 2 cm or larger, which is uncommon in the case of carcinoids of the rectum or appendix and occurs in 40% of small bowel carcinoids,[20] a full-scale cancer operation should be done.[20] In the case of carcinoids of the appendix that are 2 cm or larger, a right hemicolectomy is the operation of choice.[20,23,26,217,219] In a tumor larger than 2 cm in the rectum or a smaller tumor with invasion through the muscularis propria, an abdominoperineal resection or a low anterior resection with primary anastomosis is recommended by some[3,26,32,223] but not by others.[33] In two studies[33,221] in patients with rectal carcinoids larger than 2 cm, all patients died from or developed metastatic disease to the liver despite abdominoperineal or low anterior resection, and the authors concluded that radical surgery is inappropriate if anorectal carcinoids can be removed by local excision. In the case of a small intestinal carcinoid of 2 cm or more, a wide resection is recommended with *en bloc* resection of the adjacent lymph node–bearing mesentery.[26] For carcinoids of the appendix 1 to 2 cm in size, simple appendectomy is recommended by some,[20,23,217] whereas others favor more aggressive surgery, such as a partial cecectomy or formal right hemicolectomy for those lesions located at the base of the appendix to ensure clear margins[26] or in patients with invasion of the mesoappendix or vascular invasion.[217] For carcinoids of the rectum 1 to 2 cm in size, it is estimated that 11% to 47% have metastases,[31–33] and thus it is recommended by some that these tumors be locally resected with a wide, local, full-thickness excision[221] and that those tumors found to invade the muscularis propria undergo abdominoperineal or low anterior resection.[20,26,217,223] In another study,[33] however, 47% of these patients had metastases and 50% without metastatic disease developed metastases on follow-up, leading the authors to conclude that extensive surgery is not routinely warranted in these patients. With gastric carcinoids, treatment is generally stratified by whether hypergastrinemia is present (type I or II) or not (type III).[40,224–228] Most recommend that, in patients with type I or II with small lesions of less than 1 cm, the carcinoids should be removed endoscopically.[226,228,229] In patients with type I or II gastric carcinoids, if the tumor is larger than 2 cm or if there is local invasion, some recommend total gastrectomy,[26,230] whereas others recommend it be removed surgically with resection, with antrectomy performed for type 1 (pernicious anemia) lesions.[40,228] For type I or II lesions of 1 to 2 cm, no general agreement has been reached on treatment; some recommend that these lesions should be treated surgically,[224] whereas others recommend endoscopic treatment.[228]

In type III gastric carcinoids not associated with hypergastrinemia, which tend to be larger and more aggressive, if they are larger than 2 cm, excision and regional lymph node clearance is recommended.[224–226,228] Some recommend a similar approach for any carcinoid larger than 1 cm, whereas others recommend it be reserved for tumors in this size range showing histologic invasion. Most tumors smaller than 1 cm are treated endoscopically.[224–226]

Resection of isolated hepatic metastases may also be beneficial or curative in select patients.[162,217–219,231,232] In one study,[232] 22% of patients had unilobar disease and could have all tumor resected, whereas in other studies, fewer than 10% of patients were surgical candidates because of more disseminated disease.[231,233] In the 20% with all metastatic disease resected,[232] 5-HIAA levels were normal and 10-year survival was 100%. The role of cytoreductive or debulking surgery in patients in whom all tumor cannot be removed is unclear. No prospective randomized trials have addressed this question. A number of retrospective analyses suggest that such an approach should be considered in selected cases.[20,162,217–219,231,232,234–236] A number of studies[218,219,222,231,236,237] recommend debulking mesenteric metastases and removal of compromised intestinal segments, even in the presence of liver metastases. In one study[222] of 138 patients with midgut carcinoids of whom 51 patients were subjected to surgery with the principal aim of removing the primary tumor and debulking mesenteric metastases, the authors concluded that this surgery provided considerable symptomatic relief. A similar study[237] of 75 patients with advanced abdominal carcinoids, all of whom underwent exploratory laparotomy [33% had debulking procedures (excluding liver)], demonstrated a significantly longer survival in those patients who underwent debulking procedures (excluding liver), whether or not liver metastases were present.

The role of cytoreductive hepatic resection or of cryotherapy for patients with multiple hepatic metastases from carcinoids is also unclear.[218,231,235,236,238] In a review of 47 cases of patients with metastatic carcinoids who underwent partial hepatectomy, the mortality rate was 4.3% and the mean survival rate was 6.2 years.[231] In 60% of the patients, the symptoms of carcinoid syndrome resolved after resection. The authors of this review concluded that resection of hepatic metastases may relieve clinical endocrinopathies and that the symptomatic response may last several months.[231] It was recommended that if more than 90% of the imaged tumor could be safely removed, resection should be considered. In a study[238] of 13 patients with metastatic NETs to the liver (including seven patients with carcinoids), complete ablation of all visible tumor was achieved at surgery by cryotherapy in all but one patient. With a mean follow-up of 13.5 months, 92% of the patients were alive and only 17% of the patients with complete ablation had recurrent tumor.[238]

In one study,[239] radiation therapy was used in 44 patients with symptomatic metastatic unresectable carcinoid tumors. Survival was not prolonged; however, substantial palliation was achieved in most cases, with an overall response rate of 80%, including 76% (16 of 21) for abdominal tumors, 92% (12 of 13) for spinal metastases, 63% (five of eight) for brain metastases, and 89% (eight of nine) for bone metastases. Of eight patients with intracranial lesions,[239] none demonstrated progression during follow-up (median dose, 3300 cGy). At present, radiotherapy is primarily used for symptomatic bone metastases, especially to the spine.

Because MIBG is frequently taken up by carcinoids and concentrated, the possibility of using radiolabeled MIBG therapeutically has been evaluated in a small number of patients.[3,240–243] Iodine 125 MIBG or iodine 131 MIBG has been reported to decrease 5-HIAA urine concentrations and control symptomatic metastases in a small number of cases.

CHEMOTHERAPY

No general agreement on has been reached about when, or even if, chemotherapy should be started in patients with malignant carcinoids. One group with considerable experience[20] suggests that only patients with significant symptoms or disability from malignant disease or syndromes or who have a poor prognosis should undergo chemotherapy. Chemotherapy for metastatic carcinoids has, in general, been disappointing[3,244,245] (Table 38.6-6). Single-agent therapy with doxorubicin,[162,246] 5-fluorouracil,[162] DTIC,[166,247–249] actinomycin D,[247] cisplatin,[250] alkylating agents,[78] etoposide,[251] streptozotocin,[78] and carboplatin,[252] has provided low tumor response rates of 0% to 30%. In general, the duration of responses is short, usually less than 1 year. Combination chemotherapy for metastatic carcinoid has not been shown to have any clear advantage compared with single-agent chemotherapy. Two-dose combinations have been used of streptozotocin and 5-fluorouracil[43,166,201,246,253,254]; streptozotocin and cyclophosphamide[43]; streptozotocin and doxorubicin[253]; etoposide and cisplatin[255]; DTIC and 5-fluorouracil[256]; and lomustine and 5-fluorouracil[257] with low response rates of 0% to 40% and no apparent significant improvement over the use of single agents alone. Three-drug combinations with 5-fluorouracil, doxorubicin, and cisplatin[258]; DTIC, 5-fluorouracil, and epirubicin[259,260]; and streptozotocin, cyclophosphamide, and 5-fluorouracil[261]; or four-drug combinations of streptozotocin, doxorubicin, cyclophosphamide, and 5-fluorouracil[261] also gave low response rates of 10% to 31% and showed no additional therapeutic advantage over a single agent. Remissions were short-lived, with an average duration of 4 to 7 months.[20,162,166,244] It can be concluded that no combination therapy has clearly had a beneficial effect in the treatment of malignant carcinoids. Given the indolent nature of the tumor, poor efficacy, and undisputed toxicity of chemotherapy and the availability of excellent symptomatic therapy (octreotide and interferon), chemotherapy usually is reserved for advanced tumors with evidence of progression late in the disease course. Selective hepatic artery infusion of 5-fluorouracil had a similar response rate as that reported for systemic 5-fluorouracil.[78]

BIOTHERAPY

Analogues such as octreotide or lanreotide, in addition to controlling symptoms and reducing secretion of 5-HIAA or various peptides, also have been assessed for their antitumor effects[181,183,185,189,191,201,262–265] (see Table 38.6-6). In general, these analogues have a poor tumoricidal effect, decreasing tumor size in only 0% to 17% of patients. However, both somatostatin analogues (lanreotide, octreotide) have a tumoristatic effect, stabilizing the growth of metastatic disease and, in some studies, prolonging survival.[135,181,185,265] The mean survival in the 66 patients treated with octreotide in the Mayo Clinic studies[191,264] was 3 years, which was significantly longer than the 9 to 12 months in the 92 patients treated with chemotherapy in the Eastern Coop-

TABLE 38.6-6. Antitumor Drug Therapy of Carcinoids

Agent	*No. of Patients*	*Patients with Objective Response*[a]	*Reference*
SINGLE AGENT			
Dox	81	17 (21%)	246
	33	7 (21%)	162
5-FU	19	5 (26%)	162
DTIC	18	3 (17%)	166
	7	2 (29%)	248
	56	9 (16%)	249
Actinomycin D	17	1 (6%)	247
Cisplatin	15	1 (7%)	250
Alkylating agents	39	9 (23%)	78
ETOP	17	0 (0%)	251
STZ	23	7 (30%)	78
Carboplatin	20	0 (0%)	252
Interferon			
Human leukocyte	36	4 (11%)	200
	13	2 (15%)	202
	7	1 (14%)	269
Interferon-α	16	4 (25%)	273
	20	4 (20%)	206
	10	1 (10%)	202
	10	0 (0%)	262
	111	16 (14%)	201
	18	2 (11%)	272
	22	4 (18%)	271
	34	4 (12%)	270
	9	2 (22%)	275
Octreotide	25	4 (16%)	191
	23	2 (9%)	189, 201
	10	0 (0%)	263
	23	4 (17%)	264
	20	0 (0%)	265
	55	1 (2%)	266
Lanreotide	13	1 (8%)	185
	39	0 (0%)	181
Lanreotide-SR	10	0 (0%)	183
Hepatic artery occlusion or embolization	27	10 (37%)	215
	4	3 (75%)	214
	23	16 (70%)	212
	29	11 (38%)	209
	40	17 (42%)	232
COMBINATION			
STZ + 5-FU	43	3 (7%)	201, 254
	42	14 (33%)	43, 166
	80	18 (22%)	246
	10	4 (40%)	253
STZ + CTX	47	12 (26%)	43
STZ + Dox	10	4 (40%)	253
Interferon-α + octreotide	24	0 (0%)	278
	9	0 (0%)	184
Interferon-α + 5-FU	14	1 (7%)	279
Interferon-α + -γ	10	0 (0%)	280
DTIC + 5-FU	9	1 (11%)	256
CCNU + 5-FU	18	3 (17%)	257
ETOP + cisplatin	13	0 (0%)	255
5-FU + Dox + cisplatin	20	2 (10%)	258
DTIC + 5-FU + epirubicin	20	2 (10%)	259
	9	1 (11%)	260
STZ + CTX + 5-FU	9	2 (22%)	261
STZ + Dox + CTX + 5-FU	56	17 (30%)	261
STZ + Dox + interferon-α	11	0 (0%)	274
Hepatic artery embolization + Dox	18	6 (33%)	282
	13	13 (100%)	283
	23	8 (35%)	284
	15	12 (80%)	285
Hepatic artery embolization + 5-FU	10	6 (60%)	210
Hepatic artery occlusion + interferon α2β	17	9 (53%)	213
Hepatic artery embolization + cisplatin	17	13 (77%)	211
Hepatic artery embolization + Dox + cisplatin	16	8 (50%)	208
Hepatic artery occlusion + DTIC + Dox and 5-FU + STZ	42	28 (67%)	212
Hepatic artery embolization + Dox + cisplatin + mitomycin C	15	10 (67%)	207

CCNU, lomustine; CTX, cyclophosphamide; Dox, doxorubicin; DTIC, dacarbazine; ETOP, etoposide; 5-FU, 5-fluorouracil; SR, sustained release; STZ, streptozotocin.

[a]Objective response is defined as a decrease in tumor size using the criteria of the author. Changes in tumor markers or functional improvement were not included as an objective response.

erative Oncology Group studies. Similarly, in a phase II study[265,266] examining the effect of octreotide, 150 to 250 mg three times per day, on survival and tumor growth in 20 patients with metastatic carcinoids, 50% of patients had a CT-documented stabilization of metastatic disease that was maintained a minimum of 2 months (median, 5 months). The median survival was not reached at 29 months. Similar results were reported in prospective studies with octreotide or lanreotide in Germany,[267] in Sweden,[185] and in two studies in Italy[183,268] in which 45%, 70%, 80%, and 100% of the patients did not demonstrate tumor progression during treatment, respectively. No prospective study has proven that this tumor stabilization results in increased survival.

Studies[200–202,206,262,266,269–275] show that human leukocyte interferon or interferon-α causes a decrease in tumor size in a small number (0% to 20%) of patients with metastatic tumors (see Table 38.6-6). However, similar to octreotide, interferon appears to have a tumoristatic effect, stopping further tumor growth and stabilizing the extent of metastatic disease, which may lead to prolonged survival.[201,204,276] In a large prospective study[201] of interferon-α in 111 patients with metastatic disease, 16 patients (14%) demonstrated a greater than 50% reduction in tumor size, whereas 66% demonstrated a stabilization of disease and 19% progressed. In this study, the survival of patients treated with interferon was prolonged compared with the survival of those treated with streptozotocin and 5-fluorouracil. Interferon treatment (3 million to 9 million units three times per week) was associated with tolerable but significant side effects, including flu-like symptoms in 89%, fatigue in 70%, weight loss in 57%, reduction of blood counts in 31% (anemia in 31%, leukopenia in 3%, thrombocytopenia in 14%), increased serum levels of triglycerides in 32%, and increased liver enzymes in 31%.[201] Clinical thyroid disease developed in 76% of patients with thyroid antibodies.[3] In 22 patients,[277] it was found that the induction of the enzyme 2R,5R-oligoadenylate synthetase with interferon treatment correlated with the development of a clinical response; however, it is unknown if this response is predictive of changes in tumor size with interferon treatment. The optimal dose for long-term treatment seems to be 5 to 10 mU three to five times per week; subsequently, however, it is important to titrate the dose individually for each patient.[204] It is recommended that the leukocyte count be used as an indication of the antiproliferative effect of interferon-α, with the goal of reducing the leukocytes to less than 3×10^9 per liter.[204]

Because of their separate tumoristatic effects and ability to control symptoms, the combination of octreotide and interferon-α were assessed in small numbers of patients with malignant carcinoid syndrome, either alone or in combination with other agents (see Table 38.6-6). With octreotide and interferon,[184,266,278] interferon-α plus 5-fluorouracil,[279] interferon-α and -β,[280] and streptozotocin with doxorubicin and interferon-α,[274] only low rates (0% to 10%) of decrease in tumor size occurred, which was similar to interferon-α alone. Although some of these combinations, such as octreotide and interferon-α, were more effective than either agent alone at controlling symptoms of the carcinoid syndrome or decreasing 5-HIAA excretion,[204] no clearly increased tumoricidal effect was apparent. In one study[184] involving 21 patients with metastatic NETs (including nine with carcinoids) who were unresponsive to monotherapy with octreotide, an interferon-α plus octreotide combination caused inhibition of tumor growth in 67%. In one patient (6%), a decrease in tumor was noted, whereas in the other 61%, the response was a stabilization of tumor size without further growth over a median period of 12 months (range, 3 to 52 months).[184]

Studies[281] demonstrate that somatostatin analogues (lanreotide, octreotide), but not interferon, can induce apoptosis in carcinoid. In contrast, treatment with interferon-α[276] induced increased expression of bcl-2 in the carcinoids, whereas treatment with somatostatin analogues did not. It was proposed that this induced bcl-2 expression may contribute to keeping the malignant carcinoid cells at G_0 and therefore be one of the mechanisms of the antiproliferative effects of interferon.[276]

EMBOLIZATION AND CHEMOEMBOLIZATION

Surgical hepatic artery ligation or embolization via interventional radiology has been reported to reduce hepatic tumor bulk alone[20,209,212,214,215,232]; combined with interferon[213]; or as chemoembolization combined with chemotherapy with DTIC, cisplatin, doxorubicin, 5-fluorouracil, or streptozotocin[208,210–213,282–285] (see Table 38.6-6). In one study[209] of 29 patients with metastatic carcinoids, 38% had a decrease in tumor size after embolization; 38% had a greater than 50% decrease in hormone levels and 52% had either. Overall growth stabilization[209] was achieved in 38% for a median duration of 7 months. In two other studies involving 31 patients,[214,215] 19 patients had temporary liver dearterialization and 12 were treated with chemoembolization. After temporary liver dearterialization, 41% had a decrease in metastatic hepatic tumor size, whereas with embolization 50% showed a decrease, and in almost all cases the reduction was present for more than 12 months. Hepatic artery occlusion with chemotherapy or chemoembolization may be more effective than embolization or hepatic artery occlusion alone.[212] In one large study,[212] the percentage of patients who had tumor regression after hepatic artery ligation alone was similar to that for patients receiving chemoembolization (treatment with DTIC and doxorubicin alternating with streptozotocin and 5-fluorouracil) (67% vs. 69%, respectively) (see Table 38.6-6). However, the duration of the response was decreased (4 months vs. 18 months for the combination).

In nine recent studies involving chemoembolization (embolization combined with doxorubicin in ethiodized oil or with 5-fluorouracil, DTIC, doxorubicin, cisplatin, mitomycin C, or streptozotocin),[3,207,208,210,211,282–285] a decrease in tumor size was seen in 33% to 100% of the patients (see Table 38.6-6). The average decrease in size in one study was 84%.[283] In one study,[283] 47% of patients survived 2 years (median survival, 17 months), and in another study the median survival time was 15 months.[208] Interferon has been compared with and without hepatic artery embolization in 42 patients with metastatic carcinoid tumors.[213] Seventeen patients were embolized and received interferon for 1 year, and the remaining 25 patients received only interferon. At 1 year, 82% with embolization had stable disease or decrease in metastases, whereas 64% of those treated with interferon had stable decrease.[213] Also at 1 year, all patients responding to interferon and those with stable disease were randomized to no interferon or continued interferon (3 mU 3 days per week). One year later, all patients receiving interferon had stable disease as compared with only 40% of those taking no interferon. Survival was significantly longer in patients remaining on interferon. Embolization combined with interferon caused a significantly higher rate of tumor shrinkage than embolization alone in this study but did not prolong survival.[213]

LIVER TRANSPLANTATION

In contrast to other metastatic tumors to the liver in which liver transplantation has generally given poor results and has been largely abandoned, interest in liver transplantation is increasing for patients with metastatic carcinoids and PETs.[71,286–289] In a review of 103 patients[287] with malignant NETs who underwent liver transplantation (43 carcinoids, 48 PETs), the 2-year and 5-year survival rates were 60% and 47%, respectively. However, recurrence-free survival was less than 24%.[287] Univariate analysis defined favorable prognostic factors as age younger than 50 years, primary tumor in lung or bowel, and pretransplantation somatostatin therapy. Multivariate analysis identified the adverse prognostic factors as begin age older than 50 years and transplantation combined with upper abdominal exenteration or Whipple's resection ($P<.01$). It was concluded[287] that liver transplantation may be justified, particularly in young patients with only hepatic disease.

REFERENCES

1. Kloppel G, Heitz PU. Classification of normal and neoplastic neuroendocrine cells. *Ann N Y Acad Sci* 1994;733:18.
2. Langley K. The neuroendocrine concept today. *Ann N Y Acad Sci* 1994;733:1.
3. Jensen RT, Norton JA. Carcinoid tumors and the carcinoid syndrome. In: DeVita VT Jr, Hellman S, Rosenberg SA, eds. *Cancer: principles and practice of oncology, 5th ed.* Philadelphia: Lippincott–Raven, 1997:1704.
4. Capella C, Heitz PU, Hofler H, Solcia E, Kloppel G. Revised classification of neuroendocrine tumours of the lung, pancreas and gut. *Virchows Arch* 1995;425:547.
5. Kulke MH, Mayer RJ. Carcinoid tumors. *N Engl J Med* 1999;340:858.
6. Oberndorfer S. Karzinoide tumoren des dunndarms. *Frankf Z Pathol* 1907;1:426.
7. Caplin ME, Buscombe JR, Hilson AJ, et al. Carcinoid tumour. *Lancet* 1998;352:799.
8. Wilander E. Diagnostic pathology of gastrointestinal and pancreatic neuroendocrine tumours. *Acta Oncol* 1989;28:363.
9. Eriksson B. Tumor markers for pancreatic endocrine tumors, including chromogranins, HCG-alpha and HCG-beta. In: Mignon M, Jensen RT, eds. *Endocrine tumors of the pancreas: recent advances in research and management.* Frontiers of Gastrointestinal Research Series. Basel: S Karger, 1995:121.
10. Wilander E, Lundqvist M, el-Salhy M. Serotonin in fore-gut carcinoids. A survey of 60 cases with regard to silver stains, formalin-induced fluorescence and serotonin immunocytochemistry. *J Pathol* 1985;145:251.
11. Williams ED, Sandler M. The classification of carcinoid tumours. *Lancet* 1963;1:238.
12. Soga J, Yakuwa Y, Osaka M. Carcinoid syndrome: a statistical evaluation of 748 reported cases. *J Exp Clin Cancer Res* 1999;18:133.
13. Godwin JD II. Carcinoid tumors. An analysis of 2,837 cases. *Cancer* 1975;36:560.
14. Modlin IM, Sandor A. An analysis of 8305 cases of carcinoid tumors. *Cancer* 1997;79:813.
15. Newton JN, Swerdlow AJ, dos Santos Silva IM, et al. The epidemiology of carcinoid tumours in England and Scotland. *Br J Cancer* 1994;70:939.
16. Watson RG, Johnston CF, O'Hare MM, et al. The frequency of gastrointestinal endocrine tumours in a well-defined population—Northern Ireland 1970–1985. *QJM* 1989;72:647.
17. Norheim I, Oberg K, Theodorsson-Norheim E, et al. Malignant carcinoid tumors. An analysis of 103 patients with regard to tumor localization, hormone production, and survival. *Ann Surg* 1987;206:115.
18. Eriksson B, Oberg K, Skogseid B. Neuroendocrine pancreatic endocrine tumors. Clinical findings in a prospective study of 84 patients. *Acta Oncologia* 1989;28:373.
19. Weiss NS, Yang CP. Incidence of histologic types of cancer of the small intestine. *J Natl Cancer Inst* 1987;78:653.
20. Moertel CG. Karnofsky memorial lecture. An odyssey in the land of small tumors. *J Clin Oncol* 1987;5:1502.
21. Berge T, Linell F. Carcinoid tumours. Frequency in a defined population during a 12-year period. *Acta Pathol Microbiol Scand* 1976;84:322.
22. Feldman JM. Carcinoid tumors and the carcinoid syndrome. *Curr Probl Surg* 1989;26:835.
23. Moertel CG, Dockerty MB, Judd ES. Carcinoid tumors of the vermiform appendix. *Cancer* 1968;21:270.
24. Pearce SH, Trump D, Wooding C, et al. Loss of heterozygosity studies at the retinoblastoma and breast cancer susceptibility (BRCA2) loci in pituitary, parathyroid, pancreatic and carcinoid tumours. *Clin Endocrinol* 1996;45:195.
25. Sandor A, Modlin IM. A retrospective analysis of 1570 appendiceal carcinoids. *Am J Gastroenterol* 1998;93:422.
26. Thompson GB, Van Heerden JA, Martin JK Jr, et al. Carcinoid tumors of the gastrointestinal tract: presentation, management, and prognosis. *Surgery* 1985;98:1054.
27. Burke AP, Thomas RM, Elsayed AM, Sobin LH. Carcinoids of the jejunum and ileum. *Cancer* 1997;79:1086.
28. Soga J. Carcinoids of the small intestine: a statistical evaluation of 1102 cases collected from the literature. *J Exp Clin Cancer Res* 1997;16:353.
29. Moertel CG, Sauer WG, Dockerty MB, Baggenstoss AH. Life history of the carcinoid tumor of the small intestine. *Cancer* 1961;14:901.
30. Burke AP, Sobin LH, Federspiel BH, Shekitka KM, Helwig EB. Carcinoid tumors of the duodenum. A clinicopathologic study of 99 cases. *Arch Pathol Lab Med* 1990;114:700.
31. Soga J. Carcinoids of the rectum: an evaluation of 1271 reported cases. *Surg Today* 1997;27:112.
32. Naunheim KS, Zeitels J, Kaplan EL, et al. Rectal carcinoid tumors—treatment and prognosis. *Surgery* 1983;94:670.
33. Koura AN, Giacco GG, Curley SA, et al. Carcinoid tumors of the rectum. *Cancer* 1997;79:1294.
34. Soga J. Carcinoids of the colon and ileocecal region: a statistical evaluation of 363 cases collected from the literature. *J Exp Clin Cancer Res* 1998;17:139.
35. Hasleton PS, Gomm S, Blair V, Thatcher N. Pulmonary carcinoid tumours: a clinico-pathological study of 35 cases. *Br J Cancer* 1986;54:963.
36. Dusmet M, McKneally MF. Bronchial and thymic carcinoid tumors: a review. *Digestion* 1994;55:70.
37. Bonato M, Cerati M, Pagani A, et al. Differential diagnostic patterns of lung neuroendocrine tumours. *Virchows Arch A Pathol Anat Histopathol* 1992;420:201.
38. Hasleton PS. Histopathology and prognostic factors in bronchial carcinoid tumours. *Thorax* 1994;49:S56.
39. Thorson AH. Studies on carcinoid disease. *Acta Med Scand* 1958;334[Suppl]:1.
40. Rindi G, Bordi C, Rappel S, et al. Gastric carcinoids and neuroendocrine carcinomas: pathogenesis, pathology, and behavior. *World J Surg* 1996;20:168.
41. Granberg D, Wilander E, Stridsberg M, et al. Clinical symptoms, hormone profiles, treatment, and prognosis in patients with gastric carcinoids. *Gut* 1998;43:223.
42. Johnson LA, Lavin PT, Moertel CG, et al. Carcinoids: the prognostic effect of primary site histologic type variations. *J Surg Oncol* 1986;33:81.
43. Moertel CG, Hanley JA. Combination chemotherapy trials in metastatic carcinoid tumor and the malignant carcinoid syndrome. *Cancer Clin Trials* 1979;2:327.
44. Soga J. Statistical evaluation of 2001 carcinoid cases with metastases, collected from literature: a comparative study between ordinary carcinoids and atypical varieties. *J Exp Clin Cancer Res* 1998;17:3.
45. Weber HC, Jensen RT. Pancreatic endocrine tumors and carcinoid tumors: recent insights from genetic and molecular biologic studies. In: Dervenis CG, ed. *Advances in pancreatic disease. Molecular biology, diagnosis and treatment.* Stuttgart, Germany: Georg Thieme Verlag, 1996:55.
46. Oberg K. Biology, diagnosis, and treatment of neuroendocrine tumors of the gastrointestinal tract. *Curr Opin Oncol* 1994;6:441.
47. Rindi G, Capella C, Solcia E. Pathobiology and classification of gut endocrine tumors. In: Mignon M, Colombel JF, eds. *Recent advances in the pathophysiology and management of inflammatory bowel diseases and digestive endocrine tumors.* Paris: John Libbey Eurotext, 1999:177.
48. Calender A. New insights in genetics of digestive neuroendocrine tumors. In: Mignon M, Colombel JF, eds. *Recent advances in the pathophysiology and management of inflammatory bowel diseases and digestive endocrine tumors.* Paris: John Libbey Eurotext, 1999:155.
49. Helander HF, Bordi C. Morphology of gastric mucosa during prolonged hypergastrinemia. In: Mignon M, Jensen RT, eds. *Endocrine tumors of the pancreas: Recent advances in research and management.* Frontiers in Gastrointestinal Research Series. Basel, Switzerland: S Karger, 1995:372.
50. Modlin IM, Tang LH. Cell and tumour biology of the gastric enterochromaffin-like cell. *Ital J Gastroenterol Hepatol* 1999;31:S117.
51. Kokkola A, Sjoblom SM, Haapiainen R, et al. The risk of gastric carcinoma and carcinoid tumours in patients with pernicious anaemia. *Scand J Gastroenterol* 1998;33:88.
52. Jensen RT. Gastrinoma as a model for prolonged hypergastrinemia in man. In: Walsh JH, ed. *Gastrin.* New York: Raven Press, 1993:373.
53. Lehy T, Cadiot G, Mignon M, Ruszniewski P, Bonfils S. Influence of multiple endocrine neoplasia type 1 on gastric endocrine cells in patients with the Zollinger-Ellison syndrome. *Gut* 1992;33:1275.
54. Oberg K. Expression of growth factors and their receptors in neuroendocrine gut and pancreatic tumors, and prognostic factors for survival. *Ann N Y Acad Sci* 1994;733:46.
55. Wulbrand U, Wied M, Zofel P, et al. Growth factor receptor expression in human gastro-enteropancreatic neuroendocrine tumours. *Eur J Clin Invest* 1998;28:1038.
56. Terris B, Scoazeck JY, Rubbia L, et al. Expression of vascular endothelial growth factor in digestive neuroendocrine tumours. *Histopathology* 1998;32:133.
57. Evers BM, Rady PL, Tyring SK, et al. Amplification of the HER-2/*neu* protooncogene in human endocrine tumors. *Surgery* 1992;112:211.
58. Gibril F, Reynolds JC, Doppman JL, et al. Somatostatin receptor scintigraphy: its sensitivity compared with that of other imaging methods in detecting primary and metastatic gastrinomas: a prospective study. *Ann Intern Med* 1996;125:26.
59. O'Dowd G, Gosney JR. Absence of overexpression of p53 protein by intestinal carcinoid tumours. *J Pathol* 1995;175:403.
60. Barbareschi M, Girlando S, Mauri FA, et al. Tumour suppressor gene products, proliferation, and differentiation markers in lung neuroendocrine neoplasms. *J Pathol* 1992;166:343.
61. Cagle PT, el-Naggar AK, Xu HJ, Hu SX, Benedict WF. Differential retinoblastoma protein expression in neuroendocrine tumors of the lung. *Am J Pathol* 1997;150:393.
62. Guru SC, Goldsmith PK, Burns AL, et al. Menin, the product of the MEN1 gene, is a nuclear protein. *Proc Natl Acad Sci U S A* 1998;95:1630.
63. Chandrasekharappa SC, Guru SC, Manickam P, et al. Positional cloning of the gene for multiple endocrine neoplasia-type 1. *Science* 1997;276:404.
64. Gortz B, Roth J, Krahenmann A, et al. Mutations and allelic deletions of the MEN1 gene are associated with a subset of sporadic endocrine pancreatic and neuroendocrine tumors and not restricted to foregut neoplasms. *Am J Pathol* 1999;154:429.
65. Jakobovitz O, Nass D, DeMarco L, et al. Carcinoid tumors frequently display genetic abnormalities involving chromosome 11. *J Clin Endocrinol Metab* 1996;81:3164.
66. D'Adda T, Keller G, Bordi C, Hofler H. Loss of heterozygosity in 11q13-14 regions in gastric neuroendocrine tumors not associated with multiple endocrine neoplasia type 1 syndrome. *Lab Invest* 1999;79:671.
67. Ghimenti C, Lonobile A, Campani D, Bevilacqua G, Caligo MA. Microsatellite instability and allelic losses in neuroendocrine tumors of the gastro-entero-pancreatic system. *Int J Oncol* 1999;15:361.
68. Terris B, Meddeb M, Marchio A, et al. Comparative genomic hybridization analysis of sporadic neuroendocrine tumors of the digestive system. *Genes Chromosomes Cancer* 1998;22:50.
69. Jetmore AB, Ray NE, Gathright JB Jr, et al. Rectal carcinoids: the most frequent carcinoid tumor. *Dis Colon Rectum* 1992;35:717.
70. Metz DC, Jensen RT, Bale AE, et al. Multiple endocrine neoplasia type 1: clinical features and management. In: Bilezekian JP, Levine MA, Marcus R, eds. *The parathyroids.* New York: Raven Press, 1994:591.
71. Jensen RT, Norton JA. Endocrine neoplasms of the pancreas. In: Yamada T, Alpers DH, Owyang C, Powell DW, Silverstein FE, eds. *Textbook of gastroenterology.* Philadelphia: JB Lippincott, 1998:2193.
72. Mao C, Shah A, Hanson DJ, Howard JM. Von Recklinghausen's disease associated with duodenal somatostatinoma: contrast of duodenal versus pancreatic somatostatinomas. *J Surg Oncol* 1995;59:67.
73. Reimund JM, Duclos B, Chamouard P, et al. Intestinal carcinoid tumor and myotonic dystrophy. A new association. *Dig Dis Sci* 1992;37:1922.

74. Mork H, Jakob F, Al-Taie O, Gassel AM, Scheurlen M. Primary biliary cirrhosis and gastric carcinoid: a rare association? *J Clin Gastroenterol* 1997;24:270.
75. Jensen RT, Gardner JD. Gastrinoma. In: Go VLW, DiMagno EP, Gardner JD, et al., eds. *The pancreas: biology, pathobiology and disease.* New York: Raven Press, 1993:931.
76. Feldman JM, O'Dorisio TM. Role of neuropeptides and serotonin in the diagnosis of carcinoid tumors. *Am J Med* 1986;81:41.
77. Norton JA, Levin B, Jensen RT. Cancer of the endocrine system. In: DeVita VT Jr, Hellman S, Rosenberg SA, eds. *Cancer: principles and practice of oncology.* Philadelphia: JB Lippincott, 1993:1333.
78. Bouchier IAD. *Carcinoid tumours and the carcinoid syndrome.* London: Bailliere Tindall, 1984.
79. Becker M, Aron DC. Ectopic ACTH syndrome and CRH-mediated Cushing's syndrome. *Endocrinol Metab Clin North Am* 1994;23:585.
80. Davis Z, Moertel CG, McIlrath DC. The malignant carcinoid syndrome. *Surg Gynecol Obstet* 1973;137:637.
81. Grahame-Smith DG. The carcinoid syndrome. *Am J Cardiol* 1968;21:376.
82. Roberts LJ II, Marney SR Jr, Oates JA. Blockade of the flush associated with metastatic gastric carcinoid by combined histamine H_1 and H_2 receptor antagonists. *N Engl J Med* 1979;300:236.
83. Feldman JM. Carcinoid tumors and syndrome. *Semin Oncol* 1987;14:237.
84. Jensen RT. Overview of chronic diarrhea caused by functional neuroendocrine neoplasms. *Semin Gastrointest Dis* 1999;10:156.
85. Jacobsen MB, Nitter-Hauge S, Bryde PE, Hanssen LE. Cardiac manifestations in mid-gut carcinoid disease. *Eur Heart J* 1995;16:263.
86. Anderson AS, Krauss D, Lang R. Cardiovascular complications of malignant carcinoid disease. *Am Heart J* 1997;134:693.
87. Lundin L, Landelius J. Echocardiography for carcinoid heart disease. *Ann N Y Acad Sci* 1994;733:437.
88. Roberts WC, Sjoerdsma A. The cardiac disease associated with the carcinoid syndrome (carcinoid heart disease). *Am J Med* 1964;36:5.
89. Feldman JM, Jones RS. Carcinoid syndrome from gastrointestinal carcinoids without liver metastasis. *Ann Surg* 1982;196:33.
90. Ricci C, Patrassi N, Massa R, Mineo C, Benedetti-Valentini FJ. Carcinoid syndrome in bronchial adenoma. *Am J Surg* 1973;126:671.
91. Betchen SA, Cirigliano M, Furth EE, et al. Tubulovillous adenoma of the duodenum. A new etiology for flushing and urinary 5-HIAA elevation. *Dig Dis Sci* 1998;43:1474.
92. Pernow B, Waldenstrom J. Paroxysmal flushing and other symptoms caused by 5-hydroxytryptamine and histamine in patients with malignant tumours [Preliminary communication]. *Lancet* 1954;2:951.
93. Kema IP, deVries GE, Sloof MJH, Biesma B, Muskiet FAJ. Serotonin, catecholamines, histamine, and their metabolites in urine, platelets, and tumor tissue of patients with carcinoid tumors. *Clin Chem* 1994;40:86.
94. Matuchansky C, Luanay JM. Serotonin, catecholamines, and spontaneous midgut carcinoid flush: plasma studies from flushing and nonflushing sites. *Gastroenterology* 1995;108:743.
95. Feldman JM. Serotonin metabolism in patients with carcinoid tumors: incidence of 5-hydroxytryptophan-secreting tumors. *Gastroenterology* 1978;75:1109.
96. Makridis C, Theodorsson E, Akerstrom G, Oberg K, Knutson L. Increased intestinal nonsubstance P tachykinin concentrations in malignant midgut carcinoid disease. *J Gastroenterol Hepatol* 1999;14:500.
97. Grahame-Smith DG. *The carcinoid syndrome.* London: William Heinemann Medical Books, 1972.
98. Creutzfeldt W, Stockmann F. Carcinoids and carcinoid syndrome. *Am J Med* 1987;82:4.
99. Vinik AI, Gonin J, England BG, et al. Plasma substance-P in neuroendocrine tumors and idiopathic flushing: the value of pentagastrin stimulation tests and the effects of somatostatin analog. *J Clin Endocrinol Metab* 1990;70:1702.
100. Wymenga AN, de Vries EG, Leijsma MK, Kema IP, Kleibeuker JH. Effects of ondansetron on gastrointestinal symptoms in carcinoid syndrome. *Eur J Cancer* 1998;34:1293.
101. Wilde MI, Markham A. Ondansetron: a review of its pharmacology and preliminary clinical findings in novel applications. *Drugs* 1996;52:773.
102. Metz SA, McRae JR, Robertson RP. Prostaglandins as mediators of paraneoplastic syndromes: review and up-date. *Metabolism* 1981;30:299.
103. Theodorsson-Norheim E, Norheim I, Oberg K, et al. Neuropeptide K: a major tachykinin in plasma and tumor tissues from carcinoid patients. *Biochem Biophys Res Commun* 1985;131:77.
104. Emson PC, Gilbert RF, Martensson H, Nobin A. Elevated concentrations of substance P and 5-HT in plasma in patients with carcinoid tumors. *Cancer* 1984;54:715.
105. Norheim I, Theodorsson-Norheim E, Brodin E, Oberg K. Tachykinins in carcinoid tumors: their use as a tumor marker and possible role in the carcinoid flush. *J Clin Endocrinol Metab* 1986;63:605.
106. Schaffalitzky de Muckadell OB, Aggestrup S, Stentoft P. Flushing and plasma substance P concentration during infusion of synthetic substance P in normal man. *Scand J Gastroenterol* 1986;21:498.
107. Oates JA. The carcinoid syndrome [Editorial]. *N Engl J Med* 1986;315:702.
108. Lucas KJ, Feldman JM. Flushing in the carcinoid syndrome and plasma kallikrein. *Cancer* 1986;58:2290.
109. von der Ohe MR, Camilleri M, Kvols LK, Thomforde GM. Motor dysfunction of the small bowel and colon in patients with the carcinoid syndrome and diarrhea. *N Engl J Med* 1993;329:1073.
110. Saslow SB, O'Brien MD, Camilleri M, et al. Octreotide inhibition of flushing and colonic motor dysfunction in carcinoid syndrome. *Am J Gastroenterol* 1997;92:2250.
111. Saslow SB, Scolapio JS, Camilleri M, et al. Medium term effects of a new $5HT_3$ antagonist, alosetron, in patients with carcinoid diarrhoea. *Gut* 1998;42:628.
112. Herxheimer H. Further observations on the influence of 5-hydroxytryptamine on bronchial function. *J Physiol* 1953;122:49.
113. Lundin L, Norheim I, Landelius J, Oberg K, Theodorsson-Norheim E. Carcinoid heart disease: relationship of circulating vasoactive substances to ultrasound-detectable cardiac abnormalities. *Circulation* 1988;77:264.
114. Waltenberger J, Lundin L, Oberg K, et al. Involvement of transforming growth factor-β in the formation of fibrotic lesions in carcinoid heart disease. *Am J Pathol* 1993;142:71.
115. Feldman JM, Lee EM. Serotonin content of foods: effect on urinary excretion of 5-hydroxyindoleacetic acid. *Am J Clin Nutr* 1985;42:639.
116. Nuttall KL, Pingree SS. The incidence of elevations in urine 5-hydroxyindoleacetic acid. *Ann Clin Lab Sci* 1998;28:167.
117. Feldman JM, Butler SS, Chapman BA. Interference with measurement of 3-methoxy-4-hydroxymadelic acid and 5-hydroxyindoleacetic acid by reducing metabolites. *Clin Chem* 1974;20:607.
118. Feldman JM. Urinary serotonin in the diagnosis of carcinoid tumors. *Clin Chem* 1986;32:840.
119. DeVrie EGE, Kema IP, Slooff MJH, et al. Recent developments in diagnosis and treatment of metastatic carcinoid tumours. *J Gastroenterol* 1993;28:87.
120. Wilkin JK. Flushing reactions: consequences and mechanisms. *Ann Intern Med* 1981; 95:468.
121. Jensen RT. Gastrointestinal abnormalities and involvement in systemic mastocytosis. *Hematol Oncol Clin North Am* 2000;14:579.
122. Baudin E, Gigliotti A, Ducreux M, et al. Neuron-specific enolase and chromogranin A as markers of neuroendocrine tumours. *Br J Cancer* 1998;78:1102.
123. Nobels FR, Kwekkeboom DJ, Coopmans W, et al. Chromogranin A as serum marker for neuroendocrine neoplasia: comparison with neuron-specific enolase and the alpha-subunit of glycoprotein hormones. *J Clin Endocrinol Metab* 1997;82:2622.
124. Stridsberg M, Oberg K, Li Q, Engstrom U, Lundqvist G. Measurements of chromogranin A, chromogranin B (secretogranin I), chromogranin C (secretogranin II) and pancreastatin in plasma and urine from patients with carcinoid tumours and endocrine pancreatic tumours. *J Endocrinol* 1995;144:49.
125. Goebel SU, Serrano J, Yu F, et al. Prospective study of the value of serum chromogranin A or serum gastrin levels in assessment of the presence, extent, or growth of gastrinomas. *Cancer* 1999;85:1470.
126. Oberg K, Wide L. hCG and hCG subunits as tumour markers in patients with endocrine pancreatic tumours and carcinomas. *Acta Endocrinol (Copenh)* 1981;98:256.
127. Grossmann M, Trautmann ME, Poertl S, et al. Alpha-subunit and human chorionic gonadotropin-β immunoreactivity in patients with malignant endocrine gastroenteropancreatic tumours. *Eur J Clin Invest* 1994;24:131.
128. Krenning EP, Kwekkeboom DJ, Oei HY, et al. Somatostatin-receptor scintigraphy in gastroenteropancreatic tumors. *Ann N Y Acad Sci* 1994;733:416.
129. Westlin JE, Janson ET, Arnberg H, et al. Somatostatin receptor scintigraphy of carcinoid tumours using the [^{111}In-DTPA-D-Phe^{1}]-octreotide. *Acta Oncol* 1993;32:783.
130. Gibril F, Doppman JD, Jensen RT. Comparative analysis of tumor localization techniques for neuroendocrine tumors. *Yale J Biol Med* 1997;70:481.
131. Orlefors H, Sundin A, Ahlstrom H, et al. Positron emission tomography with 5-hydroxytryptophan in neuroendocrine tumors. *J Clin Oncol* 1998;16:2534.
132. Nessi R, Basso Ricci P, Basso Ricci S, et al. Bronchial carcinoid tumors: radiologic observations in 49 cases. *J Thorac Imaging* 1991;6:47.
133. Jeffree MA, Barter SJ, Hemingway AP, Nolan DJ. Primary carcinoid tumours of the ileum: the radiological appearances. *Clin Radiol* 1984;35:451.
134. Schillaci O, Scopinaro F, Danieli R, et al. Single photon emission computerized tomography increases the sensitivity of indium-111-pentetreotide scintigraphy in detecting abdominal carcinoids. *Anticancer Res* 1997;17(3B):1753.
135. Jensen RT. Peptide therapy. Recent advances in the use of somatostatin and other peptide receptor agonists and antagonists. In: Lewis JH, Dubois A, eds. *Current clinical topics in gastrointestinal pharmacology.* Malden, MA: Blackwell Science, 1997:144.
136. Gibril F, Doppman JL, Reynolds JC, et al. Bone metastases in patients with gastrinomas: a prospective study of bone scanning, somatostatin receptor scanning, and MRI in their detection, their frequency, location and effect of their detection on management. *J Clin Oncol* 1998;16:1040.
137. Lebtahi R, Cadiot G, Delahaye N, et al. Detection of bone metastases in patients with endocrine gastroenteropancreatic tumors: bone scintigraphy compared with somatostatin receptor scintigraphy. *J Nucl Med* 1999;40:1602.
138. Gibril F, Reynolds JC, Chen CC, et al. Specificity of somatostatin receptor scintigraphy: a prospective study and the effects of false positive localizations on management in patients with gastrinomas. *J Nucl Med* 1999;40:539.
139. Kisker O, Weinel RJ, Geks J, et al. Value of somatostatin receptor scintigraphy for preoperative localization of carcinoids. *World J Surg* 1996;20:162.
140. Janson ET, Holmberg L, Stridsberg M, et al. Carcinoid tumors: analysis of prognostic factors and survival in 301 patients from a referral center. *Ann Oncol* 1997;8:685.
141. Jensen RT. Natural history of digestive endocrine tumors. In: Mignon M, Colombel JF, eds. *Recent advances in pathophysiology and management of inflammatory bowel diseases and digestive endocrine tumors.* Paris: John Libbey Eurotext, 1999:192.
142. McDermott EWM, Guduric B, Brennan MF. Prognostic variables in patients with gastrointestinal carcinoid tumours. *Br J Surg* 1994;81:1007.
143. Shebani KO, Souba WW, Finkelstein DM, et al. Prognosis and survival in patients with gastrointestinal tract carcinoid tumors. *Ann Surg* 1999;229:815.
144. Greenberg RS, Baumgarten DA, Clark WS, Isacson P, McKeen K. Prognostic factors for gastrointestinal and bronchopulmonary carcinoid tumors. *Cancer* 1987;60:2476.
145. Makridis C, Ekbom A, Bring J, et al. Survival and daily physical activity in patients treated for advanced midgut carcinoid tumors. *Surgery* 1997;122:1075.
146. Travis WD, Rush W, Flieder DB, et al. Survival analysis of 200 pulmonary neuroendocrine tumors with clarification of criteria for atypical carcinoid and its separation from typical carcinoid. *Am J Surg Pathol* 1998;22:934.
147. Bordi C, Viale G. Analysis of cell proliferation and tumor antigens of prognostic significance in pancreatic endocrine tumors. In: Mignon M, Jensen RT, eds. *Endocrine tumors of*

the pancreas: recent advances in research and management. Frontiers of Gastrointestinal Research Series. Basel, Switzerland: S Karger, 1995:45.
148. Chaudhry A, Oberg K, Wilander E. A study of biological behavior based on the expression of a proliferating antigen in neuroendocrine tumors of the digestive system. *Tumour Biol* 1992;13:27.
149. von Herbay A, Sieg B, Schurmann G, et al. Proliferative activity of neuroendocrine tumours of the gastroenteropancreatic endocrine system: DNA flow cytometric and immunohistological investigations. *Gut* 1991;32:949.
150. Tomita T. p53 and proliferating cell nuclear antigen in endocrine tumors of pancreas and intestinal carcinoids. *Pathology* 1997;29:147.
151. Santinelli A, Ranaldi R, Baccarini M, Mannello B, Bearzi I. Ploidy, proliferative activity, p53 and bcl-2 expression in bronchopulmonary carcinoids: relationship with prognosis. *Pathol Res Pract* 1999;195:467.
152. Tsushima K, Nagorney DM, Weiland LH, Lieber MM. The relationship of flow cytometric DNA analysis and clinicopathology in small-intestinal carcinoids. *Surgery* 1989;105:366.
153. Tsioulias G, Muto T, Kubota Y, et al. DNA ploidy pattern in rectal carcinoid tumors. *Dis Colon Rectum* 1991;34:31.
154. Kujari H, Joensuu H, Klemi P, Asola R, Nordman E. A flow cytometric analysis of 23 carcinoid tumors. *Cancer* 1988;61:2517.
155. Wilander E, Bjelkenkrantz K, Risberg B. Nuclear DNA recordings in gastric carcinoids. A cytofluorometric study on single tumour cells. *Pathol Res Pract* 1987;182:331.
156. Jones DJ, Hasleton PS, Moore M. DNA ploidy in bronchopulmonary carcinoid tumours. *Thorax* 1988;43:195.
157. Fitzgerald SD, Meagher AP, Moniz-Pereira P, et al. Carcinoid tumor of the rectum. DNA ploidy is not a prognostic factor. *Dis Colon Rectum* 1996;39:643.
158. el-Naggar AK, Ballance W, Karim FW, et al. Typical and atypical bronchopulmonary carcinoids. A clinicopathologic and flow cytometric study. *Am J Clin Pathol* 1991;95:828.
159. Thunnissen FB, Van Eijk J, Baak JP, et al. Bronchopulmonary carcinoids and regional lymph node metastases. A quantitative pathologic investigation. *Am J Pathol* 1988;132:119.
160. Travis WD, Linnoila RI, Tsokos MG, et al. Neuroendocrine tumors of the lung with proposed criteria for large-cell neuroendocrine carcinoma. An ultrastructural, immunohistochemical, and flow cytometric study of 35 cases. *Am J Surg Pathol* 1991;15:529.
161. Janson EMT, Oberg KE. Carcinoid tumours. *Clin Gastroenterol* 1996;10:589.
162. Moertel CG. Treatment of the carcinoid tumor and the malignant carcinoid syndrome. *J Clin Oncol* 1983;1:727.
163. Vaughan DJ, Brunner MD. Anesthesia for patients with carcinoid syndrome. *Int Anesthesiol Clin* 1997;35:129.
164. Harris AG, Redfern JS. Octreotide treatment of carcinoid syndrome: analysis of published dose-titration data. *Aliment Pharmacol Ther* 1995;9:387.
165. Veall GRQ, Peacock JE, Bax NDS, Reilly CS. Review of the anaesthetic management of 21 patients undergoing laparotomy for carcinoid syndrome. *Br J Anaesth* 1994;72:335.
166. Kvols LK. Therapy of the malignant carcinoid syndrome. *Endocrinol Metab Clin North Am* 1989;18:557.
167. Sjoerdsma A, Lovenberg W, Engelman K, et al. Serotonin now: clinical implications of inhibiting its synthesis with para-chlorophenylalanine. *Ann Intern Med* 1970;73:607.
168. Alexander SPH, Peters JA. *1997 receptor and ion channel nomenclature supplement,* 8th ed. Cambridge: Elsevier Trends Journals, 1997.
169. Gregor M. Therapeutic principles in the management of metastasising carcinoid tumors: drugs for symptomatic treatment. *Digestion* 1994;55[Suppl 3]:60.
170. Berry EM, Maunder C, Wilson M. Carcinoid myopathy and treatment with cyproheptadine (Periactin). *Gut* 1974;15:34.
171. Robertson JI. Carcinoid syndrome and serotonin: therapeutic effects of ketanserin. *Cardiovasc Drugs Ther* 1990;1:53.
172. Gustafsen J, Lendorf A, Raskov H, Boesby S. Ketanserin versus placebo in carcinoid syndrome. A clinical controlled trial. *Scand J Gastroenterol* 1986;21:816.
173. Moertel CG, Kvols LK, Rubin J. A study of cyproheptadine in the treatment of metastatic carcinoid tumor and the malignant carcinoid syndrome. *Cancer* 1991;67:33.
174. Sullivan PA, O'Donovan M. Ketanserin, a 5-HT antagonist, in symptomatic treatment of carcinoid syndrome. *Ir J Med Sci* 1986;155:436.
175. Moertel CG, Engstrom PF, Schutt AJ. Tamoxifen therapy for metastatic carcinoid tumor: a negative study. *Ann Intern Med* 1984;100:531.
176. Frolich JC, Bloomgarden ZT, Oates JA, McGuigan JE, Rabinowitz D. The carcinoid flush. Provocation by pentagastrin and inhibition by somatostatin. *N Engl J Med* 1978;299:1055.
177. Pless J, Bauer W, Briner U, et al. Chemistry and pharmacology of SMS 201-995, a long-acting octapeptide analogue of somatostatin. *Scand J Gastroenterol Suppl* 1986;119:54.
178. Kutz K, Nuesch E, Rosenthaler J. Pharmacokinetics of SMS 201-995 in healthy subjects. *Scand J Gastroenterol Suppl* 1986;119:65.
179. Harris AG, O'Dorisio TM, Woltering EA, et al. Consensus statement: octreotide dose titration in secretory diarrhea. Diarrhea management consensus development panel. *Dig Dis Sci* 1995;40:1464.
180. Oberg K. Advances in chemotherapy and biotherapy of endocrine tumors. *Curr Opin Oncol* 1998;10:58.
181. Ruszniewski P, Ducreux M, Chayvialle JA, et al. Treatment of the carcinoid syndrome with the long-acting somatostatin analogue lanreotide: a prospective study in 39 patients. *Gut* 1996;39:279.
182. Rubin J, Ajani J, Schirmer W, et al. Octreotide acetate long-acting formulation versus open-label subcutaneous octreotide acetate in malignant carcinoid syndrome. *J Clin Oncol* 1999;17:600.
183. Tomassetti P, Migliori M, Gullo L. Slow-release lanreotide treatment in endocrine gastrointestinal tumors. *Am J Gastroenterol* 1998;93:1468.
184. Frank M, Klose KJ, Wied M, et al. Combination therapy with octreotide and α-interferon: effect on tumor growth in metastatic endocrine gastroenteropancreatic tumors. *Am J Gastroenterol* 1999;94:1381.
185. Eriksson B, Renstrup J, Imam H, Oberg K. High-dose treatment with lanreotide of patients with advanced neuroendocrine gastrointestinal tumors: clinical and biological effects. *Ann Oncol* 1997;8:1041.
186. Schonfeld WH, Elkin EP, Woltering EA, et al. The cost-effectiveness of octreotide acetate in the treatment of carcinoid syndrome and VIPoma. *Int J Tech Assess Health Care* 1996;14:514.
187. Bajetta E, Carnaghi C, Ferrari L, et al. The role of somatostatin analogues in the treatment of gastro-enteropancreatic endocrine tumours. *Digestion* 1996;57:72.
188. Stewart PM, Stewart SE, Clark PMS, Sheppard MC. Clinical and biochemical response following withdrawal of a long-acting, depot injection form of octreotide (Sandostatin-LAR). *Clin Endocrinol* 1999;50:295.
189. Oberg K, Norheim I, Theodorsson E. Treatment of malignant midgut carcinoid tumours with a long-acting somatostatin analogue octreotide. *Acta Oncol* 1991;30:503.
190. Arnold R, Frank M. Gastrointestinal endocrine tumours: medical management. *Clin Gastroenterol* 1996;10:737.
191. Kvols LK, Moertel CG, O'Connell MJ, et al. Treatment of the malignant carcinoid syndrome: evaluation of a long-acting somatostatin analogue. *N Engl J Med* 1986;315:663.
192. Wangberg B, Nilsson O, Theodorsson E, Dahlstrom A, Ahlman H. The effect of a somatostatin analogue on the release of hormones from human midgut carcinoid tumour cells. *Br J Cancer* 1991;64:23.
193. Ahlman H, Ahlund L, Dahlstrom A, et al. SMS 201-995 and provocation tests in preparation of patients with carcinoids for surgery or hepatic arterial embolization. *Anesth Analg* 1988;67:1142.
194. Gillis JC, Noble S, Goa KL. Octreotide long-acting release (LAR). A review of its pharmacological properties and therapeutic use in the management of acromegaly. *Drugs* 1997;53:681.
195. Lancranjan I, Bruns C, Grass P, et al. Sandostatin LAR: pharmacodynamics, efficacy, and tolerability in acromegalic patients. *Metabolism* 1995;44[Suppl 1]:18.
196. Dunne MJ, Elton R, Fletcher T, Hofker P, Shui I. Therapeutic considerations in Sandostatin in the treatment of GEP endocrine tumors. In: O'Dorisio TM, ed. *Sandostatin and gastroenteropancreatic endocrine tumors.* Berlin: Springer-Verlag, 1989:93.
197. Trendle MC, Moertel CG, Kvols LK. Incidence and morbidity of cholelithiasis in patients receiving chronic octreotide for metastatic carcinoid and malignant islet cell tumors. *Cancer* 1997;79:830.
198. Avila NA, Shawker TH, Roach P, et al. Sonography of gallbladder abnormalities in acromegaly patients following octreotide and ursodiol therapy: incidence and time course. *J Clin Ultrasound* 1998;26:289.
199. Newman CB, Melmed S, Snyder PJ, et al. Safety and efficacy of long-term octreotide therapy of acromegaly: results of a multicenter trial in 103 patients—a clinical research center study. *J Clin Endocrinol Metab* 1995;80:2768.
200. Oberg K, Norheim I, Lind E, et al. Treatment of malignant carcinoid tumors with human leukocyte interferon: long-term results. *Cancer Treat Rep* 1986;70:1297.
201. Oberg K, Eriksson B. The role of interferons in the management of carcinoid tumors. *Acta Oncol* 1991;30:519.
202. Nobin A, Lindblom A, Mansson B, Sundberg M. Interferon treatment in patients with malignant carcinoids. *Acta Oncol* 1989;28:445.
203. Hanssen LE, Schrumpf E, Jacobsen MB, et al. Extended experience with recombinant alpha-2b interferon with or without hepatic artery embolization in the treatment of midgut carcinoid tumors. *Acta Oncol* 1991;30:523.
204. Oberg K, Eriksson B, Janson ET. The clinical use of interferons in the management of neuroendocrine gastroenteropancreatic tumors. *Ann N Y Acad Sci* 1994;733:471.
205. Hanssen LE, Schrumpf E, Kolbenstvedt AN, Tausjo J, Dolva LO. Treatment of malignant metastatic midgut carcinoid tumors with recombinant human α2b interferon with or without prior hepatic artery embolization. *Scand J Gastroenterol* 1989;24:787.
206. Moertel CS, Rubin J, Kvols LK. Therapy of metastatic carcinoid tumor and the malignant carcinoid syndrome with recombinant leukocyte A interferon. *J Clin Oncol* 1989;7:865.
207. Drougas JG, Anthony LB, Blair TK, et al. Hepatic artery chemoembolization for management of patients with advanced metastatic carcinoid tumors. *Am J Surg* 1998;175:408.
208. Kim YH, Ajani JA, Carrasco CH, et al. Selective hepatic arterial chemoembolization for liver metastases in patients with carcinoid tumor or islet cell carcinoma. *Cancer Invest* 1999;17:474.
209. Eriksson BK, Larsson EG, Skogseid BM, et al. Liver embolizations of patients with malignant neuroendocrine gastrointestinal tumors. *Cancer* 1998;83:2293.
210. Diaco DS, Hajarizadeh H, Mueller CR, et al. Treatment of metastatic carcinoid tumors using multimodality therapy of octreotide acetate, intra-arterial chemotherapy, and hepatic arterial chemoembolization. *Am J Surg* 1995;169:523.
211. Diamandidou E, Ajani JA, Yang DJ, et al. Two-phase study of hepatic artery vascular occlusion with microencapsulated cisplatin in patients with liver metastases from neuroendocrine tumors. *AJR Am J Roentgenol* 1998;170:339.
212. Moertel CG, Johnson CM, McKusick MA, et al. The management of patients with advanced carcinoid tumors and islet cell carcinomas. *Ann Intern Med* 1994;120:302.
213. Jacobsen MB, Hanssen LE, Kolmannskog F, et al. Interferon-α2β, with or without prior hepatic artery embolization: clinical response and survival in mid-gut carcinoid patients. *Scand J Gastroenterol* 1995;30:789.
214. Marlink RG, Lokich JJ, Robins JR, Clouse ME. Hepatic arterial embolization for metastatic hormone-secreting tumors. Technique, effectiveness, and complications. *Cancer* 1990;65:2227.
215. Nobin A, Mansson B, Lunderquist A. Evaluation of temporary liver dearterialization and embolization in patients with metastatic carcinoid tumour. *Acta Oncol* 1989;28:419.
216. Moertel CG, May GR, Martin JK. Sequential hepatic artery occlusion and chemotherapy for metastatic islet carcinoid tumor and islet cell carcinoma. *Proc Am Soc Clin Oncol* 1985;4:80.
217. Loftus JP, Van Heerden JA. Surgical management of gastrointestinal carcinoid tumors. *Adv Surg* 1995;28:317.
218. Norton JA. Surgical management of carcinoid tumors: role of debulking and surgery for patients with advanced disease. *Digestion* 1994;55[Suppl 3]:98.

219. Rothmund M, Kisker O. Surgical treatment of carcinoid tumors of the small bowel, appendix, colon and rectum. *Digestion* 1994;55[Suppl 3]:86.
220. Andaker L, Lamke LO, Smeds S. Follow-up of 102 patients operated on for gastrointestinal carcinoid. *Acta Chir Scand* 1985;151:469.
221. Sauven P, Ridge JA, Quan SH, Sigurdson ER. Anorectal carcinoid tumors. Is progressive surgery warranted? *Ann Surg* 1990;211:67.
222. Makridis C, Oberg K, Juhlin C, et al. Surgical treatment of midgut carcinoid tumors. *World J Surg* 1990;14:377.
223. Mani S, Modlin IM, Ballantyne G, Ahlman H, West B. Collective reviews: carcinoids of the rectum. *J Am Coll Phys* 1994;179:231.
224. Ahlman H, Kolby L, Lundell L, et al. Clinical management of gastric carcinoid tumors. *Digestion* 1994;55:77.
225. Gilligan CJ, Phil M, Lawton GP, et al. Gastric carcinoid tumors: the biology and therapy of an enigmatic and controversial lesion. *Am J Gastroenterol* 1995;90:338.
226. Akerstrom G. Management of carcinoid tumors of the stomach, duodenum, and pancreas. *World J Surg* 1996;20:173.
227. Bordi C, Falchetti A, Azzoni C, et al. Aggressive forms of gastric neuroendocrine tumors in multiple endocrine neoplasia type I. *Am J Surg Pathol* 1997;21:1075.
228. Ahlman H. Surgical treatment of carcinoid tumours of the stomach and small intestine. *Ital J Gastroenterol Hepatol* 1999;31:S198.
229. Stuart RC. Primary gastric carcinoids. *Br J Surg* 1991;78:1013.
230. Shi W, Buchanan KD, Johnston CF, et al. The octreotide suppression test and [^{111}In-DTPA-D-Phe^{1}]-octreotide scintigraphy in neuroendocrine tumours correlate with responsiveness to somatostatin analogue treatment. *Clin Endocrinol* 1998;48:303.
231. Nagorney DM, Que FG. Cytoreductive hepatic surgery for metastatic gastrointestinal neuroendocrine tumors. In: Mignon M, Jensen RT, eds. *Endocrine tumors of the pancreas: recent advances in research and management.* Frontiers of Gastrointestinal Research Series. Basel, Switzerland: S Karger, 1995:416.
232. Wangberg B, Westberg G, Tylen U, et al. Survival of patients with disseminated midgut carcinoid tumors after aggressive tumor reduction. *World J Surg* 1996;20:892.
233. Galland RB, Blumgart LH. Carcinoid syndrome. Surgical management. *Br J Hosp Med* 1986;35:166,168.
234. Thompson NW. Surgical treatment of the endocrine pancreas and Zollinger-Ellison syndrome in the MEN 1 syndrome. *Henry Ford Hosp Med J* 1992;40:195.
235. Que FG, Nagorney DM, Batts KP, Linz LJ, Kvols LK. Hepatic resection for metastatic neuroendocrine carcinomas. *Am J Surg* 1995;169:36.
236. Ahlman H, Westberg G, Wangberg B, et al. Treatment of liver metastases of carcinoid tumors. *World J Surg* 1996;20:196.
237. Soreide O, Berstad T, Bakka A, et al. Surgical treatment as a principle in patients with advanced abdominal carcinoid tumors. *Surgery* 1992;111:48.
238. Seifert JK, Cozzi PJ, Morris DL. Cryotherapy for neuroendocrine liver metastases. *Semin Surg Oncol* 1998;14:175.
239. Schupak KD, Wallner KE. The role of radiation therapy in the treatment of locally unresectable or metastatic carcinoid tumors. *Int J Radiat Oncol Biol Phys* 1991;20:489.
240. Kimmig BN. Radiotherapy for gastroenteropancreatic neuroendocrine tumors. *Ann N Y Acad Sci* 1994;733:488.
241. Britton KE, Ur E, Hawkins L, Grossman AB, Besser GM. Treatment of malignant phaeochromocytoma, paraganglioma and carcinoid tumours with ^{131}I-metaiodobenzylguanidine. *Nucl Med Commun* 1993;14:856.
242. Bauer R, van de Flierdt E, Stettmeier H, Langhammer HR, Pabst HW. I-131 MIBG therapy of carcinoid tumor of intestinal origin. *Eur J Nucl Med* 1988;14:234.
243. Hoefnagel CA, den Hartog Jager FC, Taal BG, Abeling NG, Engelsman EE. The role of I-131- MIBG in the diagnosis and therapy of carcinoids. *Eur J Nucl Med* 1987;13:187.
244. Oberg K. The use of chemotherapy in the management of neuroendocrine tumors. *Endocrinol Metab Clin North Am* 1993;22:941.
245. Rougier P, Ducreux M. Systemic chemotherapy of advanced digestive neuroendocrine tumours. *Ital J Gastroenterol Hepatol* 1999;31:S202.
246. Engstrom PF, Lavin PT, Moertel CG, Folsch E, Douglass HO Jr. Streptozocin plus fluorouracil versus doxorubicin therapy for metastatic carcinoid tumor. *J Clin Oncol* 1984;2:1255.
247. van Hazel GA, Rubin J, Moertel CG. Treatment of metastatic carcinoid tumor with dactinomycin or dacarbazine. *Cancer Treat Rep* 1983;67:583.
248. Ritzel U, Leonhardt U, Stockmann F, Ramadori G. Treatment of metastasized midgut carcinoids with decarbazine. *Am J Gastroenterol* 1995;90:627.
249. Bukowski RM, Tangen CM, Peterson RF, et al. Phase II trial of dimethyltriazenoimidazole carboxamide in patients with metastatic carcinoid. *Cancer* 1994;73:1505.
250. Moertel CG, Rubin J, O'Connell MJ. Phase II study of cisplatin therapy in patients with metastatic carcinoid tumor and the malignant carcinoid syndrome. *Cancer Treat Rep* 1986;70:1459.
251. Kelsen D, Fiore J, Heelan R, Cheng E, Magill G. Phase II trial of etoposide in APUD tumors. *Cancer Treat Rep* 1987;71:305.
252. Saltz L, Lauwers G, Wiseberg J, Kelsen D. A phase II trial of carboplatin in patients with advanced APUD tumors. *Cancer* 1993;72:619.
253. Kelsen DG, Cheng E, Kemeny N, Magill GB, Yagoda A. Streptozotocin and Adriamycin in the treatment of APUD tumors (carcinoid, islet cell and medullary thyroid). *Proc Am Assoc Cancer Res* 1982;23:433.
254. Oberg K, Norheim I, Lundqvist G, Wide L. Cytotoxic treatment in patients with malignant carcinoid tumors. Response to streptozocin—alone or in combination with 5-FU. *Acta Oncol* 1987;26:429.
255. Moertel CG, Kvols LK, O'Connell MJ, Rubin J. Treatment of neuroendocrine carcinomas with combined etoposide and cisplatin. Evidence of major therapeutic activity in the anaplastic variants of these neoplasms. *Cancer* 1991;68:227.
256. Ollivier S, Fonck M, Becouarn Y, Brunet R. Dacarbazine, fluorouracil, and leucovorin in patients with advanced neuroendocrine tumors. *Am J Clin Oncol* 1998;21:237.
257. Kaltsas G, Papamichael D, Plowman PN, et al. 5-Fluorouracil (5-FU) and lomustine (CCNU) combination for the treatment of advanced neuroendocrine tumours (NET). *J Clin Oncol* 1998;17:245a.
258. Rougier P, Oliveira J, Ducreux M, et al. Metastatic carcinoid and islet cell tumours of the pancreas: a phase II trial of the efficacy of combination chemotherapy with 5-fluorouracil, doxorubicin and cisplatin. *Eur J Cancer* 1991;27:1380.
259. Di Bartolomeo M, Bajetta E, Bochicchio AM, et al. A phase II trial of dacarbazine, fluorouracil and epirubicin in patients with neuroendocrine tumours. A study by the Italian Trials in Medical Oncology (ITMO) Group. *Ann Oncol* 1995;6:77.
260. Bajetta E, Rimassa L, Carnaghi C, et al. 5-Fluorouracil, dacarbazine, and epirubicin in the treatment of patients with neuroendocrine tumors. *Cancer* 1998;83:372.
261. Bukowski RM, Johnson KG, Peterson RF, et al. A phase II trial of combination chemotherapy in patients with metastatic carcinoid tumors. *Cancer* 1987;60:2891.
262. Creutzfeldt W, Bartsch HH, Jacubaschke U, Stockmann F. Treatment of gastrointestinal endocrine tumor with interferon-α and octreotide. *Acta Oncologia* 1991;30:529.
263. Vinik A, Moattari AR. Use of somatostatin analog in management of carcinoid syndrome. *Dig Dis Sci* 1989;34:14S.
264. Kvols L, Moertel C, Schutt A, Rubin J. Treatment of the malignant carcinoid syndrome (MCS) with a long acting somatostatin analogue (SMS 201-995): preliminary evidence that more is not better. *Proc ASCO* 1987;6:370.
265. Saltz L, Trochanowski B, Buckley M, et al. Octreotide as an antineoplastic agent in the treatment of functional and nonfunctional neuroendocrine tumors. *Cancer* 1993;72:244.
266. Janson ET, Oberg K. Long-term management of the carcinoid syndrome. Treatment with octreotide alone and in combination with alpha-interferon. *Acta Oncol* 1993;32:225.
267. Arnold R, Neuhaus C, Benning R, et al. Somatostatin analog Sandostatin and inhibition of tumor growth in patients with metastatic endocrine gastroenteropancreatic tumors. *World J Surg* 1993;17:511.
268. Angeletti S, Corleto VD, Schillaci O, et al. Single dose of octreotide stabilize metastatic gastro-entero-pancreatic endocrine tumours. *Ital J Gastroenterol Hepatol* 1999;31:23.
269. Valimaki M, Jarvinen H, Salmela P, et al. Is the treatment of metastatic carcinoid tumor with interferon not as successful as suggested? *Cancer* 1991;67:547.
270. Bajetta E, Zilembo N, di Bartolomeo M, et al. Treatment of metastatic carcinoids and other neuroendocrine tumors with recombinant interferon-alpha-2a. *Cancer* 1993;72:3099.
271. di Bartolomeo MD, Bajetta E, Zilembo N, et al. Treatment of carcinoid syndrome with recombinant interferon alpha-2a. *Acta Oncologia* 1993;32:235.
272. Biesma B, Willemse PHB, Mulder NH, et al. Recombinant interferon alpha-2b in patients with metastatic APUDomas: effect on tumours and tumour markers. *Br J Cancer* 1992;66:850.
273. Schober C, Schmoll E, Schmoll HJ, et al. Antitumour effect and symptomatic control with interferon α_{2b} in patients with endocrine active tumours. *Eur J Cancer* 1992;28A:1664.
274. Janson ET, Ronnblom L, Ahlstrom H, et al. Treatment with alpha-interferon versus alpha-interferon in combination with streptozocin and doxorubicin in patients with malignant carcinoid tumors: a randomized trial. *Ann Oncol* 1992;3:635.
275. Doberauer C, Niederle N, Kloke O, Kurschel E, Schmidt CG. [Treatment of metastasized carcinoid tumor of the ileum and cecum with recombinant alpha-2b interferon]. *Onkologie* 1987;10:340.
276. Imam H, Gobl A, Eriksson B, Oberg K. Interferon-alpha induces bcl-2 proto-oncogene in patients with neuroendocrine gut tumor responding to its antitumor action. *Anticancer Res* 1997;17:4659.
277. Grander D, Oberg K, Lundqvist ML, et al. Interferon-induced enhancement of 2',5'-oligoadenylate synthetase in mid-gut carcinoid tumours. *Lancet* 1990;336:337.
278. Tiensuu-Janson EM, Ahlstrom H, Andersson T, Oberg KE. Octreotide and interferon alfa: a new combination for the treatment of malignant carcinoid tumours. *Eur J Cancer* 1992;28A:1647.
279. Saltz L, Kemeny N, Schwartz G, Kelsen D. A phase II trial of alpha-interferon and 5-fluorouracil in patients with advanced carcinoid and islet cell tumors. *Cancer* 1994;74:958.
280. Janson ET, Kauppinen HL, Oberg K. Combined alpha- and gamma-interferon therapy for malignant midgut carcinoid tumors. *Acta Oncologia* 1993;32:231.
281. Imam H, Eriksson B, Lukinius A, et al. Induction of apoptosis in neuroendocrine tumors of the digestive system during treatment with somatostatin analogs. *Acta Oncol* 1997;36:607.
282. Ruszniewski P, Rougier P, Roche A, et al. Hepatic arterial chemoembolization in patients with liver metastases of endocrine tumors. A prospective phase II study in 24 patients. *Cancer* 1993;71:2624.
283. Stokes KR, Stuart K, Clouse ME. Hepatic arterial chemoembolization for metastatic endocrine tumors. *J Vasc Intervent Radiol* 1993;4:341.
284. Therasse E, Breittmayer F, Roche A, et al. Transcatheter chemoembolization of progressive carcinoid liver metastasis. *Radiology* 1993;189:541.
285. Perry LJ, Stuart K, Stokes KR, Clouse ME. Hepatic arterial chemoembolization for metastatic neuroendocrine tumors. *Surgery* 1994;116:1111.
286. Le Treut YP, Delpero JR, Dousset B, et al. Results of liver transplantation in the treatment of metastatic neuroendocrine tumors. A 31-case French multicentric report. *Ann Surg* 1997;225:355.
287. Lehnert T. Liver transplantation for metastatic neuroendocrine carcinoma. *Transplantation* 1998;66:1307.
288. Anthuber M, Jauch KW, Briegel J, Groh J, Schildberg FW. Results of liver transplantation for gastroenteropancreatic tumor metastases. *World J Surg* 1996;20:73.
289. Dousset B, Saint-Marc O, Pitre J, et al. Metastatic endocrine tumors: medical treatment, surgical resection, or liver transplantation. *World J Surg* 1996;20:908.
290. Wang DG, Johnston CF, Buchanan KD. Oncogene expression in gastroenteropancreatic neuroendocrine tumors: implications for pathogenesis. *Cancer* 1997;80:668.

SECTION 7

GERARD M. DOHERTY
ROBERT T. JENSEN

Multiple Endocrine Neoplasias

The multiple endocrine neoplasia (MEN) syndromes are a group of syndromes characterized by tumors of endocrine organs (Table 38.7-1). MEN 1 affects the parathyroid glands, endocrine pancreas, and pituitary gland, among other organs, whereas MEN 2 affects the thyroid gland, parathyroid glands, and adrenal glands. A great deal has been learned over the last 10 years about the genetics and genotype-phenotype relationships characteristic of these syndromes. Syndromes that were earlier thought to be completely separate [MEN 2B and familial medullary thyroid cancer, (FMTC)] are now known to be closely related to MEN 2A.

MULTIPLE ENDOCRINE NEOPLASIA TYPE 1

Wermer first described the familial occurrence of tumors involving the pituitary gland, parathyroid glands, and pancreatic islets.[1] The syndrome was initially called *Wermer's syndrome,* subsequently called *multiple endocrine adenomatosis type 1,* and now *MEN 1.* It is now clear that the parathyroid disease is always hyperplasia and that the pancreatic endocrine tumors may be malignant.

MEN 1 is inherited as an autosomal dominant trait.[2] Chromosomal linkage studies localized the genetic defect to the long arm of chromosome 11 (q-13 locus).[3] The gene has subsequently been identified and codes a protein called *menin.*[4] This follows the two-hit theory of neoplasia of Knudson[5] in which an inherited mutation in one chromosome is unmasked by a somatic deletion or mutation in the other normal chromosome, thereby removing the suppressor effect of the normal gene. These results are in contrast to patients without MEN 1 who develop pancreatic endocrine tumors, in whom the pancreatic neoplasms develop homozygous inactivation of the MEN 1 gene in 27% to 39% of cases.[6–8]

Studies concerning the etiology of primary hyperparathyroidism in patients with MEN 1 suggest that there is a circulating factor in the plasma that stimulates bovine parathyroid cells to proliferate.[9,10] Subsequently, analysis[10–13] of plasma mitogenic activity in MEN 1 patients demonstrated that basic fibroblast growth factor or a closely related factor was present, and circulating antibodies to it have been identified.[11] However, other studies have demonstrated that there is a monoclonal abnormality in the hyperplastic parathyroid glands of patients with MEN 1, suggesting that the hyperplastic process in these glands may not be totally dependent on a circulating factor but rather through inactivation of the MEN 1 gene in a precursor cell.[14]

CLINICAL PRESENTATION

The peak incidence of symptoms in women with MEN 1 is during the third decade of life, whereas the peak incidence in men is during the fourth decade. In individuals from kindreds, its presence can usually be detected with screening by the age of 18.[15] More than one-half of patients with MEN 1 have adenomas of more than one organ, and approximately 20% have three affected endocrine glands. The frequency of glandular involvement, in descending order, is parathyroid, pancreas, pituitary, adrenal cortex, and thyroid. Both the adrenal cortex and the thyroid typically have benign, nonfunctioning adenomas. Other clinically important tumors these patients develop include gastric carcinoids,[16] bronchial carcinoids (primarily women),[17] and carcinoid tumors of the thymus (primarily men).[18] The frequency of clinical signs and symptoms, in descending order, is hypercalcemia, nephrolithiasis, peptic ulcer disease, hypoglycemia, headache, visual field loss, hypopituitarism, acromegaly, galactorrhea-amenorrhea, and rarely Cushing's syndrome.[19–21] Patients with MEN 1 have a decreased

TABLE 38.7-1. Multiple Endocrine Neoplasia Syndromes and Familial Medullary Thyroid Cancer

Characteristics	*MEN 1*	*MEN 2A*	*MEN 2B*	*Familial Medullary Thyroid Carcinoma*
Chromosome	11q12-13	Pericentromeric 10	Pericentromeric 10	Pericentromeric 10
Genetic defect	*MEN1* mutation	RET mutation	RET mutation	RET mutation
MTC	No	Bilateral	Bilateral	Bilateral
Pheochromocytoma	No	70% bilateral	70% bilateral	No
Parathyroid disease	Hyperplasia	Hyperplasia	No	No
Phenotype	No	No	Bony abnormalities, mucosal neuromas, marfanoid habitus, bumpy lips	No
Mode of inheritance	Autosomal dominant	Autosomal dominant	Autosomal dominant	Autosomal dominant
Course of MTC	No MTC	Variable, frequently indolent	More virulent	Most indolent
Pancreatic endocrine tumors	Yes: pancreatic peptide, 80–100%; gastrinoma, 50%; insulinoma, 20%; growth hormone–releasing factor, vasoactive intestinal peptide (uncommon)	No	No	No

MEN, multiple endocrine neoplasia; MTC, medullary thyroid carcinoma.

life expectancy, with a 50% probability of death by age 50. One-half of the deaths are due to a malignant tumoral process or a sequela of the disease.[22,23]

PARATHYROID GLAND INVOLVEMENT

Primary hyperparathyroidism is the most common abnormality in patients with MEN 1, occurring in 88% to 97% of affected patients.[19,24–26] The diagnosis is dependent on the detection of elevated serum levels of calcium and parathyroid hormone. Primary hyperparathyroidism is usually the initially recognized clinical manifestation of patients with MEN 1, although in prospectively screened patients, other manifestations may be biochemically detected earlier.[15,27] Occasional patients have clinical manifestations of Zollinger-Ellison syndrome (ZES) before primary hyperparathyroidism.[28] Further, pituitary adenomas or hyperinsulinism may be identified before hypercalcemia.[29] The pathology associated with primary hyperparathyroidism is always hyperplasia or multiple gland disease, although some glands may appear grossly normal.[25,26] Basic fibroblast growth factor has been expressed in the hyperplastic parathyroid glands of patients with MEN 1.[30] The surgical management requires removal of three and a half or four parathyroid glands to control the hypercalcemia. If four glands are removed, immediate autograft of some of the parathyroid tissue into the musculature of the nondominant forearm is recommended.[31] The results of surgery have not been ideal. The incidence of recurrent or persistent hyperparathyroidism is 16% to 54%, and the incidence of hypoparathyroidism is between 10% and 25%.[32,33] Primary hyperparathyroidism has been shown to adversely affect the medical management of the gastric acid hypersecretion in MEN 1 patients with ZES. Many clinicians recommend initial parathyroid surgery to control hypercalcemia because it facilitates the management of the gastric acid hypersecretion.[34]

PANCREATIC ENDOCRINE TUMORS

Malignant pancreatic endocrine tumors are the most common MEN 1–related cause of death in MEN 1 kindreds (Table 38.7-2).[23] Pathologic examination of the duodenum and pancreas in patients with MEN 1 demonstrates multiple neuroendocrine tumors.[35–37] Tumors producing pancreatic peptide are the most common pancreatic endocrine tumor in MEN 1 patients, occurring in 80% to 100%.[38] These tumors cause symptoms only due to the tumor mass itself and thus often present when tumor growth is advanced. Many patients develop functional pancreatic endocrine tumors, sometimes coincident with pancreatic peptide–producing tumors, of whom most have gastrinoma, approximately 20% insulinoma, 3% glucagonoma, and 1% vasoactive intestinal peptide (VIPoma)[19,25] (see Table 38.7-1).

A number of studies have suggested that most gastrinomas in patients with ZES and MEN 1 are in the duodenum[37,39] and not in the pancreas. The ideal treatment of the ZES is surgical excision of the gastrinoma; however, in patients with MEN 1, excision of gastrinoma rarely results in normal serum gastrin levels.[40–42] Because of the low probability of cure and the suggestion that the gastrinoma is less malignant in MEN 1, some have recommended that patients with MEN 1 do not undergo surgery.[43,44] However, familial gastrinoma may still have a malignant course.[23,45] Others recommend surgery if a localized gastrinoma is identified by a gastrin gradient on portal venous sampling or secretin angiogram,[45] if the serum pancreatic peptide concentration is elevated,[46] or if a tumor mass is identified by imaging studies.[45,47] Somatostatin receptor scintigraphy can be used to rule out distant metastases and to evaluate for other primary sites (Fig. 38.7-1).[48] At present, the best approach is still unclear.

To date, no studies have demonstrated that surgical resection of gastrinomas in MEN 1 is beneficial. One study suggests that surgical resection of primary gastrinomas in patients with and without MEN 1 decreases the probability of the development of liver metastases,[49] which is the most important negative predictor of survival. Further, when followed for long periods of time, patients with gastrinoma and MEN 1 develop liver metastases at a rate similar to patients with sporadic disease.[50] Therefore, we currently recommend that all patients with ZES and MEN 1 have extensive localization studies including somatostatin receptor scintigraphy. Only patients with unequivocally positive imaging studies and no metastases

TABLE 38.7-2. Multiple Endocrine Neoplasia Type 1–Related Causes of Death in the Washington University Series

Cause	*No. of Patients*	*Age (y), Median (range)*
Malignant islet cell tumor	12	46 (27–89)
Ulcer disease	6	56 (41–72)
Malignant carcinoid tumor	6	53 (42–63)
Hypercalcemia/uremia	3	42 (30–45)
Total	27/59[a] (46%)	

[a]Of 59 patients with multiple endocrine neoplasia type 1 who died, 27 died of causes related to multiple endocrine neoplasia type 1. (From ref. 23, with permission.)

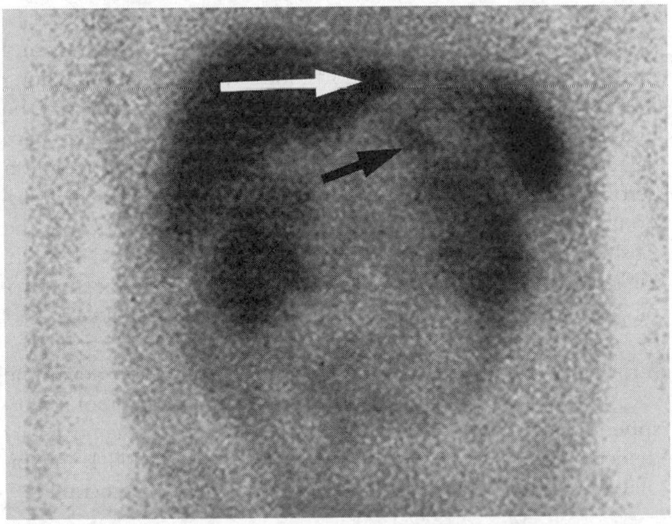

FIGURE 38.7-1. Somatostatin receptor scintigraphy can be helpful to identify sites of distant metastasis or otherwise undetected second primary tumors in the lungs or mediastinum. In this patient with a malignant nonfunctional neuroendocrine tumor in the body of the pancreas (*black arrow*), the scintigram revealed a solitary metastasis in the left lateral segment of the liver (*white arrow*) that was not demonstrated on computed tomographic scan or magnetic resonance imaging.

should undergo surgical exploration with intraoperative ultrasound. Tumors larger than 1 cm identified in the pancreatic head are enucleated, the duodenum is carefully explored by duodenotomy, and solitary or multiple tumors identified are resected; large tumors in the pancreatic body or tail are removed by distal pancreatectomy and splenectomy.[51] Some studies suggest that nearly 50% of large tumors treated in this manner may have lymph node metastases.[47] Other studies have shown that the primary tumor size is not necessarily correlated with the presence of lymph node metastases in particular.[52] Resection of liver metastases from patients with MEN 1 may also be beneficial.[53] Using this approach, while cure of ZES is unusual, resection should reduce the risk of subsequent metastatic disease.[49] No data conclusively demonstrate that this approach increases survival.

MEN 1 is present in 20% of all patients with ZES and 4% of patients with insulinoma.[38,54,55] The exact percentage of patients with VIPoma, glucagonoma, or somatostatinoma with MEN 1 is not known, but is estimated to be low (less than 5%)[38] (see Table 38.7-1). The surgical management of insulinoma and VIPoma in MEN 1 patients has had more frequent biochemical cures than resection for gastrinoma.[56] Medical management of the watery diarrhea in VIPoma is effective using either short-acting or depot somatostatin analogues. Hypoglycemia management in insulinoma is not reliable. Diazoxide and octreotide are available and may be useful for short-term treatment. In patients with MEN 1, insulinoma and VIPoma are frequently solitary large tumors. Resection may result in cure.[45,47,57–59] Some recommend the use of endoscopic ultrasound to identify the insulinoma in patients with MEN 1.[60] Portal venous sampling for insulin or calcium angiography may also be useful.[45,47,61]

PITUITARY TUMORS

Pituitary tumors occur in 54% to 80% of patients with MEN 1.[19,21,25] Symptoms may be due to local encroachment including headache and visual field defects. In a review of series, the most common tumor was a prolactinoma (41% to 76%), followed by growth hormone–secreting tumor, nonfunctional tumor, and rarely adrenocorticotropic hormone– or thyroid-stimulating hormone–secreting tumors.[62] Men with prolactinoma may be unable to achieve a penile erection, whereas women may have galactorrhea. Growth hormone–secreting tumors (25%) result in acromegaly.[21] In one study 20% of patients with MEN 1 and gastrinoma had Cushing's syndrome.[63] In all cases in this series, the Cushing's syndrome was of pituitary origin and was mild. Cushing's syndrome may also result from release of adrenocorticotropic hormone–like material from a pancreatic islet cell tumor[38,63,64] or a foregut carcinoid tumor (ectopic adrenocorticotropic hormone). Prolactinomas are generally treated by dopamine receptor agonists (bromocriptine, pergolide, cabergoline). Transsphenoidal pituitary surgery may be indicated to control any detectable pituitary mass lesion in patients with MEN 1. Incompletely resected patients may also be treated with bromocriptine.

ADRENAL AND THYROID TUMORS AND LIPOMAS

Adrenal abnormalities may occur in 27% to 36% of patients with MEN 1.[19,25,65] The most common abnormality is a benign, nonfunctional cortical adenoma, although adrenal cortical carcinomas and hyperplasia may also occur.[19,25,66] Adrenal cortical hyperfunction may rarely be found secondary to an adrenal tumor. Adrenal cortical neoplasms are usually nonfunctional in patients with MEN 1. Thyroid adenomas also occur in approximately 5% to 30% of patients with MEN 1 and have little clinical significance.[25] Lipomas are seen with greater frequency in patients with MEN 1, as are cutaneous angiofibromas and collagenomas.[67]

CARCINOID TUMORS

Gastric carcinoid tumors develop in 7% to 30% of patients with MEN 1 with ZES.[16,62] They arise from gastric enterochromaffin-like cells and thus are also call *ECLomas*. Approximately 18% have metastases, they are usually multiple, and they generally pursue an indolent course.

Thymic carcinoids occur in 0% to 8% of patients with MEN 1, are almost exclusively in men, are usually asymptomatic, and are not associated with Cushing's or carcinoid syndrome.[18] They pursue an aggressive course with distant metastases and are an increasing cause of death in older men with MEN 1.

Bronchial carcinoid tumors occur in 0% to 8% of patients with MEN 1. Eighty percent are in women and 74% are benign; however, they are an occasional cause of death.[17]

FAMILIAL MEDULLARY THYROID CARCINOMA AND MULTIPLE ENDOCRINE NEOPLASIA TYPES 2A AND 2B

HISTORY AND PATHOLOGY

In 1959, Hazard and coworkers[68] first described medullary thyroid carcinoma (MTC) and its striking histologic characteristics of cellular argentaffin staining and amyloid production. MTC is associated with three distinct familial syndromes: MEN 2A, MEN 2B, and familial non-MEN MTC, a disease characterized by hereditary MTC without associated endocrinopathies (see Table 38.7-1).[69]

In 1961, Sipple reported the unusually high incidence of bilateral pheochromocytomas in patients with thyroid malignancy.[70] These patients were later found to have MTC, and the familial disease was inherited as a mendelian autosomal dominant trait with high gene penetrance[71,72] (see Table 38.7-1). Subsequently, primary hyperparathyroidism was also noted to be part of the syndrome.[73] In 1968, this syndrome of medullary carcinoma of the thyroid gland, pheochromocytomas, and hyperparathyroidism was termed *MEN 2*; now it is called *MEN 2A*. In 1966 Williams and Pollock called attention to the finding that some patients had multiple mucosal neuromas, with or without marfanoid habitus, puffy lips, prominent jaw, pes cavus, and medullated corneal nerves with MTC and pheochromocytomas.[74] For this group of patients the terms *MEN 2B* and *MEN 3* were subsequently suggested.[75] Patients with MEN 2B do not have parathyroid disease. The gene defect in patients with MEN 2A, MEN 2B, and familial MTC is a germline mutation in the RET protooncogene.[76,77]

MTC is a malignant neuroendocrine tumor of the parafollicular thyroid cells or the calcitonin-secreting cells (C cells). Histologically, the MTC in patients with familial MTC, MEN 2A, and MEN 2B appears identical to the MTC occurring sporadically. However, in the familial form of MTC there is bilateral, multifocal involvement, and the cancer usually occupies a position in the superior lateral part of the thyroid lobe at the junction of the upper and middle third. In the sporadic setting, the MTC is usually unilateral. MTC is most malignant in MEN 2B, malignant in MEN 2A, and least virulent in FMTC (see Table 38.7-1). MTC accounts for 5% to 12% of all thyroid cancers, and only 10% of all MTC is familial.[78] In MEN 2A, approximately 42% to 60% of patients develop pheochromocytoma.[79]

The pheochromocytomas in patients with MEN 2A or MEN 2B usually present in the second or third decade of life and are often bilateral.[78,80–82] The size of the tumor or tumors in patients with MEN 2A is usually less than 2 to 3 cm, while it is usually larger in patients with MEN 2B. Even in MEN 2A patients with apparent unilateral pheochromocytomas, the contralateral adrenal gland almost always demonstrates medullary hyperplasia on pathologic analysis.[81] Patients with medullary hyperplasia rarely have symptoms of pheochromocytoma. ^{131}I-metaiodobenzyl guanidine scans in patients with MEN 2A may be useful to predict the presence of a clinically significant pheochromocytoma and can be obtained preoperatively. Pheochromocytomas in patients with MEN 2A or MEN 2B are seldom malignant and are usually within the adrenal gland. Histologically, these tumors are indistinguishable from those occurring sporadically in a nonfamilial setting.

The parathyroid lesions in MEN 2A consist of generalized hyperplasia[26] and should be managed like the parathyroid disease in MEN 1[31,83,84] (see Table 38.7-1). Approximately 35% of patients with MEN 2A develop primary hyperparathyroidism.[82] The primary hyperparathyroidism in MEN 2A is usually less clinically significant and causes fewer symptoms than the primary hyperparathyroidism in MEN 1.[82]

CLINICAL PRESENTATION

Any of the neoplasms that make up the syndromes of MEN 2A or MEN 2B may be the presenting problem; however, MTC is a hallmark feature that occurs in nearly 100% of affected individuals. Of 164 patients with MEN 2A, each had MTC, 35 (21%) had pheochromocytomas, and 28 (17%) had primary hyperparathyroidism.[78] In another study of patients with MEN 2A, each had MTC, 40% had pheochromocytomas, and 60% had parathyroid hyperplasia.[85] In patients with MEN 2B, all have MTC and approximately 60% develop pheochromocytomas.[86]

In patients with MEN 2B the MTC presents at an early age and appears more aggressive, since few patients live beyond 30 years of age.[87] In some kindreds, the MTC in MEN 2B may be less malignant and individuals may live longer.[88] The characteristic appearance of MEN 2B patients is often the first sign of disease (see Fig. 38.7-1) and may suggest the diagnosis before other clinical abnormalities. However, with investigation by measuring calcitonin, the MTC is always present at the time of clinical recognition (see Table 38.7-1).

Patients may initially seek medical advice because of episodic spells with headache, dizziness, or symptoms of irritability and nervousness. It is unusual for patients with MEN 2A to present with symptoms related to parathyroid disease.[69]

PREOPERATIVE EVALUATION AND SCREENING

When a suspicion of FMTC, MEN 2A, or MEN 2B exists, precise diagnosis depends on detection of missense mutations in the RET protooncogene in peripheral leukocytes. Several studies in individuals from families with MEN 2A have been able to predict the inheritance of MEN 2A by detection of missense mutations in RET.[89–93] Screening of new patients or family members for mutations in RET involves polymerase chain reaction amplification and DNA sequence analysis for detection of known point mutations in exons 10 and 11 (codons 609, 611, 618, 620, and 634) for MEN 2A and FMTC and exon 16 (codon 918) for MEN 2B. If a RET mutation is detected, each individual (100%) develops MTC. Further, if a RET mutation is absent, the individual does not need any additional testing. Virtually all patients with MTC have either elevated basal or stimulated plasma levels of calcitonin (CT). Patients who present with clinically apparent disease usually have basal plasma CT levels exceeding 1 ng/mL.[94] Generally, there is a direct correlation between the tumor mass of MTC and plasma calcitonin levels.[95]

Minimal plasma elevations of plasma CT are indicative of MTC in patients who have no other clinical evidence of the neoplasm.[95] Some patients with normal basal plasma CT levels have an increase to abnormal levels following calcium infusion (15 mg/kg over 4 hours) or pentagastrin injection (0.5-mg/kg bolus). Short bolus calcium injection (2 mg of calcium gluconate per kilogram over 1 minute) also provokes elevated plasma CT levels in MTC patients. The peak plasma CT levels in patients with MTC are highest with the combination test of calcium and pentagastrin injection.[96]

The presence of inherited MTC can be currently diagnosed in individuals from kindreds before detectable elevations in plasma calcitonin levels. Surgery performed based solely on detection of RET mutations always demonstrates MTC or C-cell hyperplasia.[92,97,98] It is necessary in patients with MEN 2A or MEN 2B to exclude a pheochromocytoma before undertaking surgery for MTC. Pheochromocytomas can be excluded by measuring normal urinary levels of epinephrine, norepinephrine, vanillylmandelic acid, and metanephrines. If an elevated level is detected, pheochromocytoma localization studies should be done. Abdominal computed tomography and magnetic resonance imaging are frequently helpful in localizing the pheochromocytoma, but additional more sensitive studies may be needed.[99,100] Metaiodobenzylguanidine is concentrated into pheochromocytoma cells and provides a means to functionally localize these tumors using scintigraphy.[100] The sensitivity of this method varies from 79% to 91%, with a specificity of 94% to 99%.[100]

SURGICAL MANAGEMENT

The ability to diagnose MTC in patients at risk for FMTC allows the physician to diagnose and treat this malignancy in an early preclinical stage. Should one diagnose MTC in a patient from a MEN 2A kindred, it is absolutely essential that the remainder of the family members at risk be screened. It is in this situation that RET testing has the greatest utility. Patients diagnosed by genetic testing have surgically curable C-cell hyperplasia or carcinoma confined to the thyroid gland.[92]

MEN 2A or MEN 2B patients with pheochromocytoma merit evaluation of both adrenal glands. Pheochromocytomas in MEN 2 syndromes have not been extraadrenal, nor have they been malignant.[80] Before surgical exploration, all patients need effective α-adrenergic receptor blockade.[86,100] Phenoxybenzamine should be administered 1 to 2 weeks before surgery, starting with a dose of 10 mg twice daily and increased to a usual dose of 10 to 20 mg three times daily.[100] The end point is normotension with mild to moderate asymptomatic postural hypotension (15 mm Hg) accompanied by symptoms of a blockade including nasal stuffiness. β-Adrenergic blockade is usually not required[101] except in patients with persistent sinus tachycardia.[86,100] The β blocker should never be administered before the institution of α-adrenergic blockage, because this may result in unopposed α agonism with hypertensive crisis.[100]

At operation, if a solitary pheochromocytoma is present, it should be resected. Some advocate only resecting abnormal adrenal glands confirmed by palpation,[102] while others recommend routinely resecting both adrenal glands.[81] Some patients have had unilateral adrenalectomy and remained asymptomatic with normal urinary catecholamines for a mean follow-up of 8 to 12 years.[80,102] We use preoperative radioiodinated metaiodobenzyl guanidine scan or magnetic resonance scan to determine unilateral versus bilateral adrenal involvement in these patients. With imaging studies to localize the adrenal tumor, laparoscopic methods are now used to remove it.[103] Patients with MEN 2A undergoing unilateral adrenalectomy should be followed carefully at 6-month or yearly intervals, since a second adrenal tumor may be diagnosed biochemically before it is clinically apparent.

The surgical management of familial MTC is total thyroidectomy with a central lymph node dissection. It is essential that a total thyroidectomy be performed, because the MTC is always bilateral.

POSTOPERATIVE FOLLOW-UP

In patients with MEN 2A and MEN 2B, MTC is the disease that is most frequently lethal. The MTC in patients with MEN 2B seems to be more virulent than in patients with MEN 2A[87] (see Table 38.7-1), although a group of children with MTC in the setting of MEN 2B have been reported, some of whom appear to be cured of MTC. Survival of patients with MEN 2A is dependent on the extent of MTC at initial surgical resection.[94] Data suggest that the survival rate of patients with MTC in the presence of MEN 2A is excellent.[104]

With the widespread availability of reliable radioimmunoassays for CT, an individual patient can be easily followed postoperatively. Detection of an elevated basal plasma CT level or the finding of an abnormal response to calcium and pentagastrin indicates recurrent or persistent disease. In patients with metastatic MTC, it is unclear what is the best strategy. Radioactive iodine ablation, thyroid suppression, and radiation therapy have not been helpful. MTC is relatively insensitive to chemotherapy. Because of the indolent nature of the tumor, most have chosen not to aggressively treat metastatic disease.

The 10-year survival of MTC is approximately 80% to 90%. Aggressive surgical resection has been used to locally control recurrent MTC, and one-third of individuals can be rendered biochemically disease free.[105] However, it must be remembered that in patients with MEN 2A, the MTC may be well tolerated. The average life expectancy of patients with MTC and MEN 2A is over 50 years.[106] The current best therapy for familial MTC is early diagnosis and complete resection of intrathyroidal disease at initial surgery. Ablation of extrathyroidal disease when detected as persistent or recurrent elevations of plasma CT levels following total thyroidectomy requires the development of effective systemic adjuvant treatment.

REFERENCES

1. Wermer P. Endocrine adenomatosis: peptic ulcer in a large kindred. *Am J Med* 1963;35:205.
2. Oberg K, Skogseid B, Ericksson N. Multiple endocrine neoplasia type I. *Acta Oncol* 1989;28:383.
3. Larsson C, Skogseid B, Öberg K, Nakamura Y, Nordenskjöld M. Multiple endocrine neoplasia type 1 gene maps to chromosome 11 and is lost in insulinoma. *Nature* 1988;332:85.
4. Chandrasekharappa SC, Guru SC, Manickam P, et al. Positional cloning of the gene for multiple endocrine neoplasia-type 1. *Science* 1997;276:404.
5. Knudson AG. Mutation and cancer: statistical study of retinoblastoma. *Proc Natl Acad Sci U S A* 1971;68:820.
6. Toliat MR, Berger W, Ropers HH, Neuhaus P, Wiedenmann B. Mutations in the MEN1 gene in sporadic neuroendocrine tumours of gastroenteropancreatic system. *Lancet* 1997;350:1223.
7. Zhuang Z, Vortmeyer AO, Pack S, et al. Somatic mutations of the MEN1 tumor suppressor gene in sporadic gastrinomas and insulinomas. *Cancer Res* 1997;57:4682.
8. Goebel SU, Heppner C, Burns AL, et al. Genotype/phenotype correlation of multiple endocrine neoplasia type 1 gene mutations in sporadic gastrinomas. *J Clin Endocrinol Metab* 2000;85:113.
9. Brandi ML, Aurbach GD, Fitzpatrick LA, et al. Parathyroid mitogenic activity in plasma from patients with familial multiple endocrine neoplasia type I. *N Engl J Med* 1986;314:1287.
10. Brandi ML. Multiple endocrine neoplasia type I: general features and new insights into etiology. *J Endocrinol Invest* 1991;14:61.
11. Zimmering MB, Brandi ML, de Grange DA, et al. Circulating fibroblast growth factor-like substance in familial multiple endocrine neoplasia-type I. *J Clin Endocrinol Metab* 1990;70:149.
12. Zimering MB, Riley DJ, Tjaller-Varia S. Circulating fibroblast growth factor like antibodies in two patients with multiple endocrine neoplasia type 1 and prolactinoma. *J Clin Endocrinol Metab* 1994;79:1546.
13. Zimering MB, Katsumata N, Soto Y. Increased basic fibroblast growth factor in plasma from multiple endocrine neoplasia type 1: relation to pituitary tumor. *J Clin Endocrinol Metab* 1993;76:1182.
14. Thakker RV, Bouloux P, Wooding C, et al. Association of parathyroid tumors in multiple endocrine neoplasia type I with loss of alleles on chromosome 11. *N Engl J Med* 1989;218:224.
15. Skogseid B, Eriksson B, Lundquist G, et al. Multiple endocrine neoplasia type 1: a 10-year prospective screening study in four kindreds. *J Clin Endocrinol Metab* 1991;73:281.
16. Rindi G, Bordi C, Rappel S, et al. Gastric carcinoids and neuroendocrine carcinomas: pathogenesis, pathology and behavior. *World J Surg* 1996;20:168.
17. Duh Q-Y, Hybarger CP, Geist R, et al. Carcinoid associated with multiple endocrine neoplasia syndromes. *Am J Surg* 1987;154:142.
18. Teh BT, Zedenius J, Kytola S, et al. Thymic carcinoids in multiple endocrine neoplasia type 1. *Ann Surg* 1998;228:99.
19. Ballard HS, Frame B, Hartsock RT. Familial multiple endocrine adenoma—peptic ulcer complex. *Medicine* 1964;43:481.
20. Loeb JN. Polyglandular disorders. In: Wyngaarden JB, Smith LH, eds. *Cecil textbook of medicine.* Philadelphia: W.B. Sanders, 1982:1304.
21. Bone HG. Diagnosis of multiglandular endocrine neoplasias. *Clin Chem* 1990;36:711.
22. Wilkinson S, Teh BT, Davey KR, et al. Cause of death in multiple endocrine neoplasia type 1. *Arch Surg* 1993;128:683.
23. Doherty GM, Olson JA, Frisella MM, et al. Lethality of multiple endocrine neoplasia type 1. *World J Surg* 1998;22:581.
24. Radford DM, Ashley SW, Wells SA Jr, Gerhard DS. Loss of heterozygosity of markers on chromosome 11 in tumors with patients with multiple endocrine neoplasia syndrome I. *Cancer Res* 1991;50:1154.
25. Eberle F, Grun R. Multiple endocrine neoplasia type I. *Adv Int Med Pediatr* 1981;5:76.
26. Leight GS, Hensley MI. Management of familial hyperparathyroidism. *Prog Surg* 1987;184:106.
27. Skogseid B, Oberg K. Experience with multiple endocrine neoplasia type 1 screening. *J Intern Med* 1995;238:255.
28. Benya RV, Metz DC, Venzon DJ, et al. Zollinger-Ellison syndrome can be initial endocrine manifestation in patients with multiple endocrine neoplasia type 1. *Am J Med* 1994;97:436.
29. Shepherd JJ. The natural history of multiple endocrine neoplasia type 1. *Arch Surg* 1991;126:935.
30. Mutsuyama I. Expression of basic fibroblast growth factor in hyperplastic parathyroid glands from patients with multiple endocrine neoplasia type 1. *World J Surg* 1994;18:921.
31. Wells SA Jr, Farndon JR, Dale JK, et al. Long-term evaluation of patients with primary parathyroid hyperplasia managed by total parathyroidectomy and heterotopic autotransplantation. *Ann Surg* 1980;192:451.
32. Hellman P, Skogseid B, Oberg K, et al. Primary and reoperative parathyroid operations in hyperparathyroidism of multiple endocrine neoplasia type 1. *Surgery* 1998;124:993.
33. Rizzoli R, Green J III, Marx SJ. Primary hyperparathyroidism in familial multiple endocrine neoplasia type I: long-term follow-up of serum calcium levels after parathyroidectomy. *Am J Med* 1985;78:467.
34. Norton JA, Cornelius MJ, Doppman JL, et al. Effect of parathyroidectomy in patients with hyperparathyroidism, Zollinger-Ellison syndrome, and multiple endocrine neoplasia type 1: a prospective study. *Surgery* 1987;102:958.
35. Thompson NW, Lloyd RV, Nishiyama RH, et al. MEN I pancreas: a histological and immunohistochemical study. *World J Surg* 1984;8:561.
36. Kloppel G, Willemar S, Stamm B, et al. Pancreatic lesions and hormonal profile in pancreatic tumors in multiple endocrine neoplasia type I. *Cancer* 1986;57:1820.
37. Pipeleers-Marichal M, Somers G, Willems G, et al. Gastrinomas in the duodenums of patients with multiple endocrine neoplasic type 1 and the Zollinger-Ellison syndrome. *N Engl J Med* 1990;322:723.
38. Jensen RT, Norton JA. Endocrine tumors of the pancreas in gastrointestinal disease. In: Sleisenger MH, Fordtran JS, eds. *Gastrointestinal disease,* 1993:1695.
39. Norton JA, Jensen RT. Unresolved surgical issues in the management of patients with Zollinger-Ellison syndrome. *World J Surg* 1991;15:151.

40. Jensen RT, Gardner JD. Zollinger-Ellison syndrome: clinical presentation, pathology, diagnosis and treatment. In: Dannenberg A, Zakim D, eds. *Peptic ulcer and other acid-related diseases.* New York: Academic Research Association, 1991:117.
41. Jensen RT, Gardner JD, Raufman JP. Zollinger-Ellison syndrome. NIH combined clinical staff conference. *Ann Intern Med* 1983;98:59.
42. Norton JA. Invited commentary. *World J Surg* 1984;8:572.
43. Fox PS, Hofmann JW, Wilson SD, DeCosse JJ. Surgical management of the Zollinger-Ellison syndrome. *Surg Clin North Am* 1974;54:395.
44. Malagelada JR, Edis AJ, Adson MA, van Heerden JA, Go VLW. Medical and surgical options in the management of patients with gastrinoma. *Gastroenterology* 1983;84:1524.
45. Thompson NW. Surgical considerations in the MEA I syndrome. In: Johnston IDA, Thompson NW, eds. *Endocrine surgery. Butterworths International Medical Reviews.* London: Butterworths, 1983:144.
46. Mutch MG, Frisella MM, DeBenedetti MK, et al. Pancreatic polypeptide is a useful plasma marker for radiographically evident pancreatic islet cell tumors in patients with multiple endocrine neoplasia type 1. *Surgery* 1997;122:1012.
47. Sheppard BC, Norton JA, Doppman JL, et al. Management of islet cell tumors in patients with multiple endocrine neoplasia: a prospective study. *Surgery* 1989;106:1108.
48. Yim JH, Siegel BA, DeBenedetti MK, et al. Prospective study of the utility of somatastatin receptor scintigraphy in the evaluation of patients with multiple endocrine neoplasia type I. *Surgery* 1998;124:1037.
49. Fraker DL, Norton JA, Alexander HR, Venzon DJ, Jensen RT. Surgery in Zollinger-Ellison syndrome alters the natural history of gastrinoma. *Ann Surg* 1994;220:320.
50. Weber HC, Venzon DJ, Lin JT. Determinants of metastatic rate and survival in patients with Zollinger-Ellison syndrome: a prospective long-term study. *Gastroenterology* 1995;108:1637.
51. Lairmore TC, Chen VY, DeBenedetti MK, et al. Duodenopancreatic resections in patients with multiple endocrine neoplasia type 1 (MEN 1). *Ann Surg* 2000;231:909.
52. Lowney JK, Frisella MM, Lairmore TC, Doherty GM. Islet cell tumor metastasis in multiple endocrine neoplasia type I: correlation with primary tumor size. *Surgery* 1998;124:1043.
53. Cherner JA, Sawyers JL. Benefit of resection of metastatic gastrinoma in multiple endocrine neoplasia type I. *Gastroenterology* 1992;102:1049.
54. Jensen RT, Maton PN. Zollinger-Ellison syndrome. In: Gustavsson S, Kumar D, Graham DY, eds. *The stomach.* London: Churchill Livingstone, 1991:341.
55. Norton JA, Fraker DL, Alexander HR, et al. Surgery to cure the Zollinger-Ellison syndrome. *N Engl J Med* 1999;341:635.
56. Jensen RT, Norton JA. Pancreatic endocrine tumors. In: Yamada T, Alpers DH, Owyang C, Powell DW, Silvenstein FE, eds. *Textbook of gastroenterology.* Philadelphia: Lippincott, 1991:1912.
57. Thompson NW, Lloyd RV, Nishiyama RH, et al. MEN-1 pancreas: a histological and immunohistochemical study. *World J Surg* 1984;8:561.
58. Rasbach DA, van Heerden JA, Telandar RL, et al. Surgical management of hyperinsulinism in the multiple endocrine neoplasia, type I syndrome. *Arch Surg* 1985;120:584.
59. O'Riordain DS, O'Brien T, van Heerden JA. Surgical management of insulinoma associated with MEN-1. *World J Surg* 1994;18:488.
60. Thompson NW, Czako PF, Fritts LL. Role of endoscopic ultrasonography in the localization of insulinomas and gastrinomas. *Surgery* 1994;116:1131.
61. Cohen MS, Picus D, Lairmore TC, et al. Prospective study of provocative angiograms to localize functional islet cell tumors of the pancreas. *Surgery* 1997;122:1091.
62. Metz DC, Jensen RT, Bale AE, et al. Multiple endocrine neoplasia type 1: clinical features and management. In: Bilezekian JP, Levine MA, Marcus R, eds. *The parathyroids.* New York: Raven Press, 1994:591.
63. Maton PN, Gardner JD, Jensen RT. The incidence and etiology of Cushing's syndrome in patients with Zollinger-Ellison syndrome. *N Engl J Med* 1986;315:1.
64. Lamers CB, Stadil F, Tongren, JMV. Prevalence of endocrine abnormalities in patients with the Zollinger-Ellison syndrome and their families. *Am J Med* 1981;64:687.
65. Skogseid B, Rastad J, Gobl A, et al. Adrenal lesion in multiple endocrine neoplasia type 1. *Surgery* 1995;118:1077.
66. Skogseid B, Larsson C, Lindgren PG. Clinical and genetic features of adrenocortical lesions in MEN-1. *J Clin Endocrinol Metab* 1992;75:76.
67. Marx S, Spiegel AM, Skarulis MC, et al. Multiple endocrine neoplasia type 1: clinical and genetic topics. *Ann Intern Med* 1998;129:484.
68. Hazard JB, Hawk WH, Creile GJ. Medullary (solid) carcinoma of the thyroid-clinicopathologic entity. *J Clin Endocrinol Metab* 1959;19:704.
69. Norton JA, Wells SA Jr. Medullary thyroid carcinoma and multiple endocrine neoplasia type-II syndromes. *Surg Endocrinol* 1990;5:359.
70. Sipple JH. The association of pheochromocytoma with carcinoma of the thyroid gland. *Am J Med* 1961;31:163.
71. Williams ED. A review of 17 cases of carcinoma of the thyroid and pheochromocytoma. *J Clin Pathol* 1965;18:288.
72. Schimke RN, Hartmann WH. Familial amyloid-producing medullary thyroid carcinoma and pheochromocytoma. A distinct genetic entity. *Ann Intern Med* 1965;63:1027.
73. Manning PC, Molnar GD, Black BM, Priestly JT, Wollner LB. Pheochromocytoma, hyperparathyroidism and thyroid carcinoma occurring coincidentally. *N Engl J Med* 1963;268:68.
74. Williams ED, Pollock DJ. Multiple mucosal neuromata with endocrine tumors: a syndrome alluded to von Rechlinghausen's disease. *J Pathol Bacteriol* 1989;91:71.
75. Chong GC, Beahrs OH, Sizemore GW, Woolner LH. Medullary carcinoma of the thyroid gland. *Cancer* 1975;35:695.
76. Mulligan LM, Kwok JBJ, Healey CS, et al. Germ-line mutation of the RET proto-oncogene in multiple endocrine neoplasia type 2A. *Nature* 1993;363:458.
77. Donis-Keller H, Dou S, Chi D, et al. Mutations in the RET proto-oncogene are associated with MEN 2A and FMTC. *Hum Mol Genet* 1993;2:851.
78. Grun R, Eberle F. Multiple endocrine neoplasia, type II (MEN II). *Ergeb Inn Med Kinderheildk* 1981;46:151.
79. Howe JR, Norton JA, Wells SA Jr. Prevalence of pheochromocytomas and hyperparathyroidism in MEN2A: results of a long-term follow-up. *Surgery* 1993;114:1070.
80. Lairmore TC, Ball DW, Baylin SB, Wells J, Samuel A. Management of pheochromocytomas in patients with multiple endocrine neoplasia type 2 syndromes. *Ann Surg* 1993;217:595.
81. Carney JA, Sizemore GW, Sheps SG. Adrenal medullary disease in multiple endocrine neoplasia, type 2. *Am J Clin Pathol* 1976;66:279.
82. O'Riordain DS, O'Brien T, Grant CS, et al. Surgical management of primary hyperparathyroidism in multiple endocrine neoplasia types 1 and 2. *Surgery* 1993;114:1031.
83. Kraimps J, Duh Q-Y, Demeure M, Clark O. Hyperparathyroidism in multiple endocrine neoplasia syndrome. *Surgery* 1992;112:1080.
84. Herfarth K, Bartsch D, Doherty GM, Wells S, Lairmore T. Surgical management of hyperparathyroidism in patients with multiple endocrine neoplasia type 2A. *Surgery* 1996;120:966.
85. Keiser HR, Beaven MA, Doppman J, et al. Sipple's syndrome: medullary thyroid carcinoma, pheochromocytoma and parathyroid disease. *Ann Intern Med* 1973;78:561.
86. Wells SA Jr. Multiple endocrine neoplasia type II: recent results. *Cancer Res* 1990;18:71.
87. Norton JA, Fromme LC, Farrell RE, Wells SA Jr. Multiple endocrine neoplasia type 2b: the most aggressive form of medullary thyroid carcinoma. *Surg Clin North Am* 1979;59:109.
88. Vasen HF, vanderFeltz M, Raue F. The natural course of MENIIb-18 cases. *Arch Intern Med* 1992;152:1250.
89. Ledger GA, Khosla S, Lindor NM, Thibodeau SM, Gharib H. Genetic testing in the diagnosis and management of multiple endocrine neoplasia type II. *Ann Intern Med* 1995;122:118.
90. Frilling A, Roher HD, Ponder BA. Presymptomatic screening for medullary thyroid carcionoma in patients with multiple endocrine neoplasia type 2A. *World J Surg* 1994;18:577.
91. Lips CJ, Landsvater RM, Hoppener JW. Clinical screening as compared with DNA analysis in families with multiple endocrine neoplasia type 2A. *N Engl J Med* 1994;331:828.
92. Wells SA Jr, Chi DD, Toshima K, et al. Predictive DNA testing and prophylactive thyroidectomy in patients at risk for multiple endocrine neoplasia type 2A. *Ann Surg* 1994;220:237.
93. Tsai MS, Ledger GA, Khosla S, Gharib H, Thibodeau SM. Identification of multiple endocrine neoplasia type 2 gene carriers using linkage analysis and analysis of the RET protooncogene. *J Clin Endocrinol Metab* 1994;78:1261.
94. Wells SA Jr, Baylin SG, Leight GS, et al. The importance of early diagnosis in patients with hereditary medullary thyroid carcinoma. *Ann Surg* 1982;195:505.
95. Wells SA Jr, Baylin SB, Gann DW, et al. Medullary thyroid carcinoma: relationship of method of diagnosis to pathological staging. *Ann Surg* 1978;188:377.
96. Melvin KEW, Miller HH, Tashjian AH Jr. Early diagnosis of medullary carcinoma of the thyroid by means of calcitonin assay. *N Engl J Med* 1971;285:1115.
97. Dralle H, Gimm O, Simon D, et al. Prophylactic thyroidectomy in 75 children and adolescents with hereditary medullary thyroid carcinoma: German and Austrian experience. *World J Surg* 1998;22:744.
98. Learoyd D, Marsh D, Richardson A, et al. Genetic testing for familial cancer: consequences of RET proto-oncogene mutation analysis in multiple endocrine neoplasia, type 2. *Arch Surg* 1997;132:1022.
99. Valk TW, Frager MW, Gross MD, et al. Spectrum of pheochromocytoma in multiple endocrine neoplasia: a scintigraphic portrayal using 131-I-metaiodobenzylguanidine. *Ann Intern Med* 1981;94:762.
100. Shapiro B, Fig LM. Management of pheochromocytomas. *Endocrinol Metab Clin North Am* 1989;18:443.
101. Hull CJ. Pheochromocytoma: diagnosis, preoperative preparation and anesthetic management. *Br J Anaesth* 1986;58:1453.
102. Farndon JR, Fagraeus L, Wells SA Jr. Recent developments in the management of phaechromocytoma. In: Johnston IDA, Thompson NW, eds. *Endocrine surgery.* London: Butterworths, 1983:189.
103. Brunt LM, Doherty GM, Norton JA, et al. Laparoscopic adrenalectomy compared to open adrenalectomy for benign adrenal neoplasms. *J Am Coll Surg* 1996;183:1.
104. Wells SA Jr, Baylin SG, Johnsrude IS, et al. Thyroid venous catheterization in the early diagnosis of familial medullary thyroid carcinoma. *Ann Surg* 1982;196:505.
105. Moley JF, Dilley WG, DeBenedetti MK. Improved results of cervical reoperation for medullary thyroid carcinoma. *Ann Surg* 1997;225:734.
106. Jackson CE, Talpos GB, Kanbouris A, et al. The clinical course after definitive operation for medullary thyroid carcinoma. *Surgery* 1983;94:995.

CHAPTER 39

Sarcomas of the Soft Tissue and Bone

SECTION 1

MURRAY F. BRENNAN
KALED M. ALEKTIAR
ROBERT G. MAKI

Soft Tissue Sarcoma

INCIDENCE

In the United States the incidence of soft tissue sarcoma is approximately 7800 new cases per year. A little more than 50% of these new patients go on to die of the disease.[1] The relatively small number of cases seen and the great diversity in histopathologic presentation, anatomic site, and biologic behavior have made a comprehensive understanding of these disease entities extremely difficult. They are, however, ideal prototypes to demonstrate the important role of multidisciplinary management. It is clear that soft tissue sarcoma, diagnosed at an early stage, is eminently curable. When diagnosed at the time of extensive local or metastatic disease, soft tissue sarcoma is rarely curable.

Analysis of population based data from Connecticut[2] suggests an increase in incidence in both men and women, greater for women.

ETIOLOGY AND GENETICS

Most soft tissue sarcomas have no clearly defined etiology, although multiple associated or predisposing factors have been identified (Table 39.1-1). Data suggest that genetic mutations in pluripotent mesenchymal stem cells give rise to malignant clones that differentiate along pathways that resemble normal histogenesis. Alterations in the RB-1 and p53 genes are detected in a substantial proportion of sarcomas.[3,4] The importance of these cell regulatory genes in the pathogenesis of sarcoma is highlighted by the high incidence of germline mutations in patients with hereditary retinoblastoma, and by identification of germline mutations in p53 in the Li-Fraumeni syndrome.[5,6] A genetic predisposition to soft tissue sarcoma has also been associated with neurofibromatosis,[7,8] and familial adenomatous polyposis.[9]

The most common tumors in patients with neurofibromatosis are in the central nervous system. In a 42-year follow-up study, 47% of all malignancies were nervous system tumors.[10] This review confirms the high incidence of malignant tumors in patients with neurofibromatosis: approximately 46% of all patients with this disease develop either a malignant tumor or a benign central nervous system tumor.[10] This prevalence is slightly higher in those with a family history of neurofibromatosis than in those with sporadic cases, but is common in both. Relatives of such patients, whether with a family history or not, are also at risk of developing malignant tumors. The development of pheochromocytoma also is a complication of neurofibromatosis.[11] Approxi

TABLE 39.1-1. Genetic Predisposition to Soft Tissue Sarcoma

	Sarcoma	*Gene*	*Chromosome*	*Reference*
Neurofibromatosis type I (von Recklinghausen's disease)	Malignant peripheral nerve sheath tumor	NF-1	17q11.2	414
Retinoblastoma	Soft tissue, osteogenic	Rb-1	13q14	415,416
Li-Fraumeni syndrome	Soft tissue, osteogenic	TP53	17p13	6,417
Gardner's syndrome	Fibrosarcoma, desmoid tumor	APC	5q21	418,419
Werner's syndrome (adult progeria)	Soft tissue	WRN	8p12	420
Gorlin's syndrome (nevoid basal cell carcinoma syndrome)	Fibrosarcoma, rhabdomyosarcoma	PTC	9q22.3	2
Carney's triad	Gastrointestinal stromal tumor	Unknown	Unknown	421,422
Tuberous sclerosis (Bourneville disease)	Rhabdomyoma, rhabdomyosarcoma	TSC1 TSC2	9q34 16p13.3	423–425

mately 5% of patients with neurofibromatosis develop malignant peripheral nerve sheath tumors (MPNSTs).[10]

Genetic predisposition to malignancy is well established in the form of an autosomal dominant gene in 8% to 9% of children with soft tissue sarcomas.[12] Survivors of retinoblastoma with the associated Rb gene abnormality often develop tumors later in life with a high incidence of sarcomas; the best documented is osteosarcoma.[13] A follow-up study of members of Li-Fraumeni families with childhood rhabdomyosarcoma found additional cancers including carcinoma of the breast, soft tissue sarcomas, lung cancer, skin cancer, leukemia, pancreatic cancer, and brain tumors.[14]

It is important to emphasize that in patients who have retinoblastoma, the increased risk of a second primary is enhanced by radiotherapy,[15] which is dose dependent.

Familial adenomatous polyposis, a subset of which is Gardner's syndrome, is commonly associated with the development of intraabdominal desmoids.[16] These tumors behave as low-grade fibrosarcomas, although constant debate exists as to the histopathologic classification and distinction between the desmoid tumor and aggressive fibromatosis (see below, in Pathologic Classification). However, their natural history of slow growth with accompanying invasion of contiguous structures increases the risk of subsequent mortality when managed inappropriately.

The development of soft tissue and bone sarcoma as a result of exposure to radiation has been known since 1922.[17] Although uncommon, these sarcomas usually have a poor prognosis. In a review of 160 patients,[18] the antecedent diseases for which the radiation was given were predominantly breast and cervical cancer and lymphoma (Fig. 39.1-1). External radiation therapy was given to 99% of the patients, 14% of whom received additional treatment with temporary or permanent radioisotope implantation. One patient inadvertently ingested radium. The subsequent tumor that developed was most commonly an osteogenic sarcoma, followed by soft tissue tumors, particularly malignant fibrous histiocytoma (MFH) and angiosarcoma or lymphangiosarcoma (see Fig. 39.1-1). No significant difference in survival was found between patients with bone tumors and those with soft tissue sarcomas. Survival was not affected by site, latency period, and the amount of radiation received initially, nor were there any differences for patients receiving chemotherapy for their sarcomas. The three factors in the Cox multivariate analysis that had a significant unfavorable association were presentation with metastatic disease (P = .017), incomplete or no operative resection (P = .004), and tumor size of at least 5 cm (P= .007). Tumor grade was not significant in any analyses, but only 6% of the patients had low-grade tumors.[18]

Given the increased use of radiation therapy as a primary treatment modality for breast cancer, concern has been expressed that an increased incidence of sarcoma might be expected. In one study[19] all 122,991 women with breast cancer in Sweden from 1958 to 1992 were followed, and 116 soft tissue sarcomas were found. There were 40 angiosarcomas and 76 other sarcomas. As expected, angiosarcoma correlated with lymphedema [relative risk = 9.5 (3.2 to 28.0)] but not radiation therapy. For other sarcomas, there was a dose-response relationship with exposure to radiation therapy.

Lymphedema has long been established as a factor in the development of lymphangiosarcoma. The most well-recognized association is with the postmastectomy, postirradiated lymphedematous arm, described by Stewart and Treves.[20] This is not a radiation-induced sarcoma because the lymphangiosar-

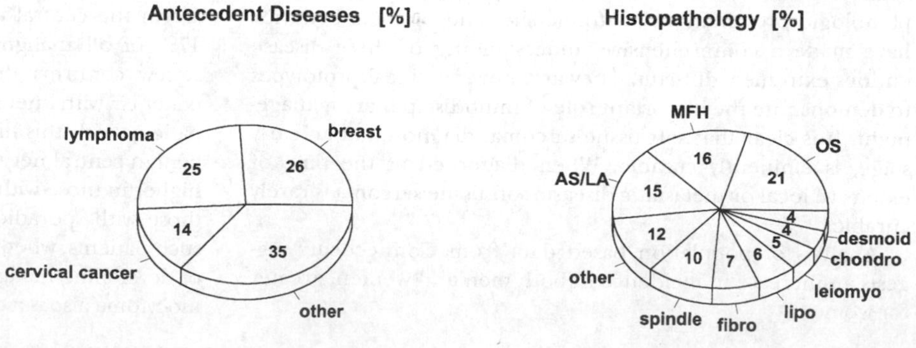

FIGURE 39.1-1. Radiation-associated soft tissue sarcoma: antecedent disease for which radiation was given and histopathology of sarcomas that developed in 160 patients at Memorial Sloan-Kettering Cancer Center. AS, angiosarcoma; LA, lymphangiosarcoma; MFH, malignant fibrous histiocytoma; OS, osteogenic sarcoma. (From ref. 18, with permission.)

coma develops in sites both inside and outside of the irradiated field, in the edematous extremity. Similar advanced sarcomas have been seen following filarial infection and chronic lymphedema. Lymphangiosarcoma can arise in filarial lymphedema and remain localized for relatively long periods of time.[21]

The issue of trauma as a possible predisposing factor is more controversial. Often a minor episode of injury is the factor that draws attention to the presence of a mass, implying a causative association that is not real. Abdominal desmoid tumors commonly follow parturition.[22] However, they can occur in the extremity and may be associated with antecedent vigorous physical activity. They may be multifocal.[23]

Chemical agents have been implicated in the etiology of soft tissue sarcoma. Through the years there have been conflicting reports about the relationship between occupational exposure to phenoxyacetic acids found in some herbicides and chlorophenols (found in some wood preservatives) (Table 39.1-2).[20,24–30] Other authors have pointed to the inherent problems in occupational epidemiology in relationship to the source material for soft tissue sarcoma, among them, (1) possible recall bias in self-reported exposure data; (2) soft tissue sarcomas not consistently classified in the International Classification of Diseases, which is organ based; (3) variation in the operational definition of soft tissue sarcomas; and (4) because of their rarity, difficulty recruiting sufficient patients for a case-control study, and cohorts would have to be extremely large to identify an increase in risk.[31,32] Nevertheless, some studies have suggested a link between phenoxy herbicide exposure in forestry workers, farmers, and railroad workers and subsequent development of sarcoma,[33] whereas other studies from the United States, New Zealand, and Finland have not confirmed this relationship.[26,30,34]

Interestingly, it has been suggested[35] that such exposure may be tissue type specific (i.e., MFH and leiomyosarcoma having a herbicide association, but none being found for liposarcoma).

An increased incidence of soft tissue sarcomas was seen in a cohort of 1520 industrial workers exposed for more than 1 year to 2,3,7,8-tetrachlorodibenzo-p-dioxin,[36] but other studies did not substantiate these findings.[37,38]

The issue of dioxin as a risk factor remains controversial. A population-based case-control study assessed the risk of soft tissue sarcomas in Vietnam veterans, including those potentially exposed to Agent Orange, which contains dioxin, and found no increased risk among any subset of veterans compared with control groups.[39] Another study found no increased risk for Vietnam veterans compared with men who had never been in Vietnam.[40] The risk for subgroups of veterans who were more likely to be exposed to Agent Orange, compared with their unexposed counterparts in Vietnam, was not statistically significant.

Several chemical carcinogens have an established role in the development of hepatic angiosarcomas: thorotrast, vinyl chloride, and arsenic (including Fowler's 1% arsenic solution.[34,41–43] A review of pesticides and cancer[44] has again linked the phenoxy herbicides to soft tissue sarcoma and lymphoma, but again questions the causal relationship of these agents.

Chemotherapy for pediatric malignancies has been associated with the subsequent development of osteogenic sarcomas[45]; a relationship with the development of soft tissue sarcomas has not been demonstrated.

CYTOGENETIC ABNORMALITIES

It is important to emphasize that extensive cytogenetic abnormalities occur in soft tissue sarcoma (Table 39.1-3). These are usually associated with high-grade tumors, but are not consistent between tumors. For example, an analysis of 36 tumors,[46] pleomorphic soft tissue sarcomas were examined. Multiple complex karyotypes were identified and at least 24 recurrent abnormalities (defined by their presence in at least five cases) were detected. However, none of the selected rearrangements was specific for any one of a particular subgroup. It seems unlikely at the present time, therefore, that cytogenetic analysis can help differentiate the pleomorphic sarcomas. Conversely, specific changes have been identified in selected sarcomas. The best examples are the classical translocation in Ewing's sarcoma (primitive neuroectodermal tumor), t(11;22)(q24;q11.2-12), and the translocation seen in synovial sarcoma t(X;18)(p11.2;q11.2). In these situations, these genetic abnormalities can be used as a diagnostic tool.

Multiple other studies of genetic abnormalities have been published. Abnormalities of INK4A (coding for p16 and p19ARF on 9p21) and INK4B have been correlated with poor survival.[47] These chromosomal alterations occur in 15% of patients with high-grade sarcomas. In myxoid liposarcoma, the presence of the TLS-CHOP fusion protein has now been firmly established[48] and is considered a definitive diagnostic tool for these tumors.

DISTRIBUTION

Soft tissue sarcomas can occur in any site throughout the body. Almost 50% of all soft tissue sarcomas appear in the extremities (Fig. 39.1-2), with two-thirds of extremity lesions occurring in

TABLE 39.1-2. Case-Control Studies of Relationship between Exposure to Phenoxy Herbicides and Incidence of Soft Tissue Sarcoma

Location	*Author*	*Year*	*No.*	*Relative Risk*	*95% Confidence Interval*
North Sweden	Hardell and Sandstrom[24]	1979	46	5.3	2.4–11.5
South Sweden	Eriksson et al.[25]	1981	99	6.8	2.6–17.3
New Zealand	Smith et al.[26]	1984	82	1.6	0.7–3.3
England and Wales	Balarajan and Acheson[27]	1984	1961	1.15	0.83–1.59
New York State: Vietnam service	Greenwald et al.[28]	1984	281	0.7	0.17–2.92
Veterans' Administration patients: Vietnam service	Kang et al.[29]	1986	234	0.83	0.63–1.09
Kansas	Hoar et al.[30]	1986	133	1	0.7–1.6

(Adapted from Brennan MF. Management of extremity soft tissue sarcoma. *Am J Surg* 1989;158:71.)

TABLE 39.1-3. Chromosomal Changes in Soft Tissue Sarcoma

Tumor Histology	*Chromosomal Alteration*	*Involved Gene(s)*	*Frequency*	*Reference*
Ewing's sarcoma family[a]	t(11;22) (q24;q12)	EWS-FLI1	85%	426,427
	t(21;22) (q22;q12)	EWS-ERG	5–10%	428
	t(7;22) (p22;q12)	EVT1-EWS	Rare	429
	t(17;22) (q12;q12)	EIAF-EWS	Rare	430
	t(1;16) (q11-25;q11-24)	Unknown	Approximately 10%	431,432
	Trisomy 8	Not applicable	Approximately 50%	432,433
	Trisomy 12	Not applicable	Approximately 30%	433
Myxoid/round cell liposarcoma	t(12;16) (q13;p11)	TLS (FUS)-CHOP	>75%	434,435
	t(12;22) (q13;q12)	EWS-CHOP	Uncommon	436
Low-grade liposarcoma	Giant chromosomes, ring chromosomes	? gene(s) on chromosome 17	60%	437,438
Alveolar rhabdomyosarcoma	t(2;13) (q35;q14)	PAX3-FKHR	Approximately 70%	439
	t(1;13) (p36;q14)	PAX7-FKHR	Approximately 15%	73,439
Malignant melanoma of soft tissues (clear cell sarcoma)	t(12;22) (q13;q12)	EWS-ATF1	>75%	440,441
Desmoplastic small round cell tumor	t(11;22) (p13;q12)	EWS-WT1	>90%	77,165,442,443
Synovial sarcoma	t(X;18) (p11;q11)	SYT-SSX1, SYT-SSX2	>90%	77,165,375,444–446
Extraskeletal myxoid chondrosarcoma	t(9;22) (q22;q12)	EWS-CHN (TEC)	>75%	447,448
Dermatofibrosarcoma protuberans	t(17;22) (q22;q13), ring chromosomes	COL1A1-PDGFB	>50%; ring chromosomes >75%	449,450
Congenital fibrosarcoma	t(12;15) (p13;q25)	ETV6 (TEL)-NTRK3 (TRKC)	Unknown	451
Malignant rhabdoid tumor	del 22(q11.2)	hSNF5/INI1	Approximately 50%[b]	452,453
Uterine leiomyosarcoma (and leiomyoma)	t(12;14) (q14-15;q23-24)	Unknown	Uncommon	454
Embryonal rhabdomyosarcoma	Trisomy 2, trisomy 8	Unknown	Rare	455,456
Epithelioid sarcoma	Loss of heterozygosity (22q); t(8;22) (q22;q11)	?NF2, ?EWS	Rare	457,458
Malignant fibrous histiocytoma	Complex karyotype	Unknown	Common	46

[a]Ewing's sarcoma family includes classical Ewing's sarcoma, peripheral neuroectodermal tumor, Askin's tumor, and peripheral neuroepithelioma.
[b]Mutations seen in other cases, giving greater than 80% with disruption of the hSNF5 gene.

the lower limb, and 30% intraabdominally divided equally between visceral and retroperitoneal lesions.

PATHOLOGIC CLASSIFICATION

Soft tissue tumors generally are categorized according to the normal tissues they mimic.[49,50] Many soft tissue neoplasms have been described, reflecting the diversity of soft tissues in the body (Table 39.1-4).[50] Although most soft tissues arise from

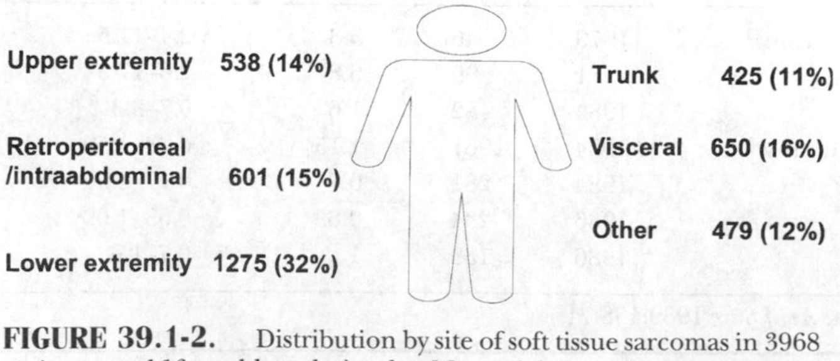

FIGURE 39.1-2. Distribution by site of soft tissue sarcomas in 3968 patients aged 16 or older admitted to Memorial Sloan-Kettering Cancer Center between July 1982 and July 1999.

embryonic mesoderm, tumors of the peripheral nervous system (ectoderm), and some tumors of uncertain histogenesis are included as soft tissue neoplasms.

Soft tissue tumors may be benign or malignant, and a variety of borderline lesions are also recognized. The ratio of benign to malignant tumors is certainly more than 100:1. The soft tissue sarcomas are the malignant tumors that arise in soft tissues. The precise pathogenesis of the vast majority of the sarcomas is uncertain. Unlike carcinomas, sarcomas do not demonstrate *in situ* changes, nor does it appear that sarcomas originate from benign soft tissue tumors. An exception would appear to be the development of MPNST in patients with neurofibromatosis.

Although each of the sarcomas has distinguishing histologic characteristics, the different types of sarcoma have many common clinical and pathologic features. Sarcomas are characterized by local invasiveness. The pattern of metastasis of most sarcomas is hematogenous. Lymph node metastases are uncommon, with the exception of selected cell types usually associated with childhood sarcoma (Table 39.1-5).[51–53] Grossly, most sarcomas are similar, with a pale tan fish flesh appearance (although liposarcomas may be soft and yellow). The clinical behavior of most types of sarcoma also is similar, determined more by anatomic location, grade, and size, than by specific histologic pattern.[54]

TABLE 39.1-4. Histologic Classification of Soft Tissue Sarcoma

FIBROUS TUMORS

A. Benign tumors
  1. Nodular fasciitis (including intravascular and cranial types)
  2. Proliferative fasciitis and myositis
  3. Atypical decubital fibroplasia (ischemic fasciitis)
  4. Fibroma (dermal, tendon sheath, nuchal)
  5. Keloid
  6. Elastofibroma
  7. Calcifying aponeurotic fibroma
  8. Fibrous hamartoma of infancy
  9. Fibromatosis coli
  10. Infantile digital fibromatosis
  11. Myofibromatosis (solitary, multicentric)
  12. Hyaline fibromatosis
  13. Calcifying fibrous pseudotumor

B. Fibromatoses
  1. Superficial fibromatoses
    a. Palmar and plantar (Dupuytren's contracture fibromatoses)
    b. Penile (Peyronie's fibromatosis)
    c. Knuckle pads
  2. Deep fibromatoses
    a. Abdominal fibromatosis (abdominal desmoid)
    b. Extraabdominal fibromatosis (extraabdominal desmoid)
    c. Intraabdominal fibromatosis (intraabdominal desmoid)
    d. Mesenteric fibromatosis (including Gardner's syndrome)
    e. Infantile (desmoid-type) fibromatosis

C. Malignant tumors
  1. Fibrosarcoma
    a. Adult fibrosarcoma
    b. Congenital or infantile fibrosarcoma
    c. Inflammatory fibrosarcoma (inflammatory myofibroblastic tumor)

FIBROHISTIOCYTIC TUMORS

A. Benign tumors
  1. Fibrous histiocytoma
    a. Cutaneous fibrous histiocytoma (dermatofibroma)
    b. Deep fibrous histiocytoma
  2. Juvenile xanthogranuloma
  3. Reticulohistiocytoma
  4. Xanthoma

B. Intermediate tumors
  1. Atypical fibroxanthoma
  2. Dermatofibrosarcoma protuberans (including pigmented form, Bednar's tumor)
  3. Giant cell fibroblastoma
  4. Plexiform fibrohistiocytic tumor
  5. Angiomatoid fibrous histiocytoma

C. Malignant tumors
  1. Malignant fibrous histiocytoma
    a. Storiform-pleomorphic fibrous histiocytoma
    b. Myxoid fibrous histiocytoma
    c. Giant cell fibrous histiocytoma (malignant giant cell tumor of soft parts)
    d. Xanthomatous (inflammatory type) fibrous histiocytoma

LIPOMATOUS TUMORS

A. Benign tumors
  1. Lipoma
    a. Cutaneous lipoma
    b. Deep lipoma
      (i) Intramuscular lipoma
      (ii) Tendon sheath lipoma
      (iii) Lumbosacral lipoma
      (iv) Intraneural and perineural fibrolipoma
    c. Multiple lipomas
  2. Angiolipoma
  3. Spindle cell or pleomorphic lipoma
  4. Myolipoma
  5. Angiomyolipoma
  6. Myelolipoma
  7. Chondroid lipoma
  8. Hibernoma
  9. Lipoblastoma or lipoblastomatosis
  10. Lipomatosis
    a. Diffuse lipomatosis
    b. Cervical symmetric lipomatosis (Madelung's disease)
  11. Atypical lipoma

B. Malignant tumors
  1. Liposarcoma
    a. Well-differentiated liposarcoma
      (i) Lipoma-like liposarcoma
      (ii) Sclerosing liposarcoma
      (iii) Inflammatory liposarcoma
    b. Myxoid liposarcoma
    c. Round cell (poorly differentiated myxoid) liposarcoma
    d. Pleomorphic liposarcoma
    e. Dedifferentiated liposarcoma

SMOOTH MUSCLE TUMORS

A. Benign tumors
  1. Leiomyoma (cutaneous, deep, and pleomorphic)
  2. Angiomyoma (vascular leiomyoma)
  3. Epithelioid leiomyoma
  4. Intravenous leiomyomatosis
  5. Leiomyomatosis peritonealis disseminata

B. Malignant tumors
  1. Leiomyosarcoma
  2. Epithelioid leiomyosarcoma

SKELETAL MUSCLE TUMORS

A. Benign tumors
  1. Adult rhabdomyoma
  2. Genital rhabdomyoma
  3. Fetal rhabdomyoma
  4. Intermediate (cellular) rhabdomyoma

B. Malignant tumors
  1. Rhabdomyosarcoma
    a. Embryonal rhabdomyosarcoma
    b. Botryoid rhabdomyosarcoma
    c. Spindle cell rhabdomyosarcoma
    d. Alveolar rhabdomyosarcoma
    e. Pleomorphic rhabdomyosarcoma
  2. Rhabdomyosarcoma with ganglionic differentiation (ectomesenchymoma)

TUMORS OF BLOOD AND LYMPH VESSELS

A. Benign tumors
  1. Papillary endothelial hyperplasia

(continued)

TABLE 39.1-4. *(Continued)*

2. Hemangioma
   a. Capillary (including juvenile) hemangioma
   b. Cavernous hemangioma
   c. Venous hemangioma
   d. Epithelioid hemangioma (angiolymphoid hyperplasia, histiocytoid hemangioma)
   e. Granulation type hemangioma (pyogenic granuloma)
   f. Tufted hemangioma
3. Deep hemangioma (intramuscular, synovial, perineural)
4. Lymphangioma
5. Lymphangiomyoma and lymphangiomyomatosis
6. Angiomatosis
7. Lymphangiomatosis

B. Intermediate tumors
1. Hemangioendothelioma
   a. Epithelioid hemangioendothelioma
   b. Endovascular papillary angioendothelioma (Dabska's tumor)
   c. Spindle cell hemangioendothelioma

C. Malignant tumors
1. Angiosarcoma and lymphangiosarcoma
2. Kaposi's sarcoma
3. Follicular dendritic cell sarcoma

PERIVASCULAR TUMORS

A. Benign tumors
1. Glomus tumor
2. Glomangiomyoma
3. Hemangiopericytoma

B. Malignant tumors
1. Malignant glomus tumor
2. Malignant hemangiopericytoma

SYNOVIAL TUMORS

A. Benign tumors
1. Tenosynovial giant cell tumor
   a. Localized tenosynovial giant cell tumor
   b. Diffuse tenosynovial giant cell tumor (extraarticular pigmented villonodular synovitis, florid tenosynovitis)

B. Malignant tumors
1. Synovial sarcoma
   a. Biphasic (fibrous and epithelial) synovial sarcoma
   b. Monophasic (fibrous or epithelial) synovial sarcoma
2. Malignant giant cell tumor of tendon sheath

MESOTHELIAL TUMORS

A. Benign tumors
1. Solitary fibrous tumor of pleura and peritoneum (localized fibrous mesothelioma)
2. Multicystic mesothelioma
3. Adenomatoid tumor
4. Well-differentiated papillary mesothelioma

B. Malignant tumors
1. Malignant solitary fibrous tumor of pleura and peritoneum
2. Diffuse mesothelioma
   a. Epithelial diffuse mesothelioma
   b. Fibrous (spindled, sarcomatoid) diffuse mesothelioma
   c. Biphasic diffuse mesothelioma

NEURAL TUMORS

A. Benign tumors
1. Traumatic neuroma
2. Morton's neuroma
3. Multiple mucosal neuromas
4. Neuromuscular hamartoma (benign Triton tumor)
5. Nerve sheath ganglion
6. Schwannoma (neurilemoma)
   a. Cellular schwannoma
   b. Plexiform schwannoma
   c. Degenerated (ancient) schwannoma
   d. Schwannomatosis
7. Neurothekeoma (nerve sheath myxoma)
8. Neurofibroma
   a. Diffuse neurofibroma
   b. Plexiform neurofibroma
   c. Pacinian neurofibroma
   d. Epithelioid neurofibroma
9. Granula cell tumor
10. Melanocytic schwannoma
11. Ectopic meningioma
12. Ectopic ependymoma
13. Ganglioneuroma
14. Pigmented neuroectodermal tumor of infancy (retinal anlage tumor, melanotic progonoma)

B. Malignant tumors
1. MPNST (malignant schwannoma, neurofibrosarcoma)
   a. Malignant Triton tumor (MPNST with rhabdomyosarcoma)
   b. Glandular MPNST (malignant glandular schwannoma)
   c. Epithelioid MPNST (malignant epithelioid schwannoma)
2. Malignant granular cell tumor
3. Clear cell sarcoma (malignant melanoma of soft parts)
4. Malignant melanocytic schwannoma
5. Gastrointestinal autonomous nerve tumor (plexosarcoma)
6. Primitive neuroectodermal tumor
   a. Neuroblastoma
   b. Ganglioneuroblastoma
   c. Neuroepithelioma (peripheral neuroectodermal tumor)
   d. Extraskeletal Ewing's sarcoma

PARAGANGLIONIC TUMORS

A. Benign tumors
1. Paraganglioma

B. Malignant tumors
1. Malignant paraganglioma

EXTRASKELETAL CARTILAGINOUS AND OSSEOUS TUMORS

A. Benign tumors
1. Panniculitis ossificans and myositis ossificans
2. Fibroosseous pseudotumor of the digits
3. Fibrodysplasia (myositis) ossificans progressiva
4. Extraskeletal chondroma or osteochondroma
5. Extraskeletal osteoma

B. Malignant tumors
1. Extraskeletal chondrosarcoma
   a. Well-differentiated chondrosarcoma
   b. Myxoid chondrosarcoma
   c. Mesenchymal chondrosarcoma
2. Extraskeletal osteosarcoma

PLURIPOTENTIAL MESENCHYMAL TUMORS

A. Benign tumors
1. Mesenchymoma

(continued)

TABLE 39.1-4. *(Continued)*

B. Malignant tumors	5. Amyloid tumor
1. Malignant mesenchymoma	6. Parachordoma
MISCELLANEOUS TUMORS	7. Ossifying and nonossifying fibromyxoid tumors
A. Benign tumors	8. Palisaded myofibroblastoma of lymph node
1. Congenital granular cell tumor	B. Malignant tumors
2. Tumoral calcinosis	1. Alveolar soft part sarcoma
3. Myxoma	2. Epithelioid sarcoma
a. Cutaneous myxoma	3. Malignant extrarenal rhabdoid tumor
b. Intramuscular myxoma	4. Desmoplastic small cell tumor
c. Juxtaarticular myxoma	**UNCLASSIFIED TUMORS**
4. Angiomyxoma	

MPNST, malignant peripheral nerve sheath tumor.

GRADING OF SARCOMA

After establishing the diagnosis of sarcoma, the most critical piece of information the pathologist can provide to the clinician is histologic grade. The pathologic features that define grade include cellularity, differentiation, pleomorphism, necrosis, and number of mitoses. Unfortunately, the criteria for grading are neither specific nor standardized. Furthermore, several grading scales are used: a four-grade system (Broders),[55] a three-grade system (low, intermediate, high) as recognized by the American Joint Commission on Cancer (AJCC),[56] and a binary system (high vs. low) as used at Memorial Hospital.[50] Even when there is agreement about the number of grades to be used, expert pathologists disagree about specific criteria for defining grade.[57–60]

The possible clinical implications are obvious. In adjuvant chemotherapy trials high grade was defined differently at different centers, making comparison of results between trials, and combining results of multiple trials, extremely hazardous. For example, tumors of 240 patients who participated in the Scandinavian Sarcoma Group adjuvant trial for high-grade extremity sarcoma were reviewed by a panel of reference pathologists. A four-grade system was used in this trial; only patients with grade III or IV sarcomas were eligible. On review, 5% of the patients were considered ineligible because their tumors actually were low grade.[61,62] Furthermore, although it did not influence eligibility, there was considerable discordance between the original pathologists and the reference pathologists with regard to whether a lesion was grade III or IV. Although the adjuvant regimen did not affect survival (see below, in Adjuvant Chemotherapy), a difference in survival was noted between patients with tumors of these two grades as assigned by the reference pathologists.

Many pathologists consider mitotic activity and degree of necrosis to be the most important pathologic features.[63] To define a practical grading system, the European Organization for Research on the Treatment of Cancer (EORTC) studied the histologic features of tumors from 282 patients who partici-

TABLE 39.1-5. Soft Tissue Sarcomas: Histologic Type and Lymph Node Metastasis

	Weingrad[52,a]		*Mazeron*[53,b]		*Fong*[51,c]	
Histopathology	No. of Nodal Metastases/ All Sarcoma Patients	Percentage of All Lesions	No. of Nodal Metastases/All Sarcoma Patients	Percentage of All Lesions	No. of Nodal Metastases/ All Sarcoma Patients	Percentage of All Lesions
Fibrosarcoma	55/1083	5.1	54/215	25.1	0/162	0
Malignant fibrous histiocytoma	1/30	3.3	84/823	10.2	8/316	2.5
Embryonal rhabdomyosarcoma	108/888	12.2	201/1354	14.8	12/88	13.6
Leiomyosarcoma	10/94	10.6	21/524	4	9/328	2.7
Neurofibrosarcoma, malignant peripheral nerve tumor	0/60	0	3/476	0.6	2/96	2.1
Vascular	—	—	43/376	11.4	—	—
Angiosarcoma	—	—	—	—	5/37	13.5
Lymphangiosarcoma	—	—	—	—	1/4	25.0
Osteosarcoma	20/327	6.1	—	—	0/11	0
Synovial sarcoma	91/535	17	117/851	13.7	2/145	1.4
Liposarcoma	15/288	5.2	16/504	3.2	3/403	0.7
Alveolar soft part sarcoma	6/62	9.7	3/24	12.5	0/13	0
Other	14/148	9.5	25/110	22.7	15/222	6.4
Epithelioid	—	—	14/70	—	2/12	16.7
Total	320/3515	9.1	567/5257	10.8	46/1772	2.6

[a]From a summary of 47 studies.
[b]From a summary of 122 studies.
[c]Database includes only extraskeletal osteosarcomas and chondrosarcomas.

pated in their adjuvant chemotherapy trial, and correlated the pathologic findings with outcome.[64] In multivariate analysis, only mitotic count (less than 3, 3 to 20, and greater than 20 mitoses per 10 consecutive high power fields), the presence or absence of necrosis, and tumor size predicted survival.

Mutation of p53, nuclear overexpression of p53, and a high Ki-67 proliferation index are associated with high grade and poor survival.[65] As yet, however, these biologic markers have not been shown to be independent indicators of prognosis and cannot be used to grade sarcomas.

Several tumors that are considered sarcomas have no recognizable normal tissue counterpart (e.g., alveolar soft part tumor, Ewing's sarcoma, epithelioid sarcoma). These tumors often have unique clinical features and usually are not graded. However, note that Ewing sarcomas are considered high-grade, undifferentiated sarcomas.

DIFFERENTIAL DIAGNOSIS

In addition to sarcoma, the differential diagnosis of a soft tissue mass includes a variety of benign lesions, as well as primary or metastatic carcinoma, melanoma, and lymphoma. Accurate diagnosis requires an adequate and representative biopsy of the tumor, and the tissue must be well fixed and well stained. Antibodies for immunohistochemical staining are available commercially, and this technique is readily applicable to paraffin-embedded tissues. The most useful immunohistochemical markers are the intermediate filaments (e.g., vimentin, keratin, desmin, leukocyte common antigen, S-100). In addition, the pathologist should be prepared to process tissue from selected cases for electron microscopy, cytogenetic studies, or molecular analysis. This implies that certain diagnoses are considered by the clinician, that the diagnostic biopsy is obtained appropriately, and that the clinician and pathologist communicate before the biopsy is performed to ensure that the necessary steps are taken in handling the tissue.

Cytogenetic analyses reveal clonal chromosome alterations in the majority of sarcomas.[66] Consistent chromosomal abnormalities have been identified in several soft tissue tumors,[61,62,67–84] but cytogenetic analysis is labor intensive and requires short-term culture of the sarcoma cells. Fusion genes resulting from chromosomal rearrangements may be detected by reverse transcriptase polymerase chain reaction. This technique has been quite effective in diagnosing and distinguishing among the small cell sarcomas. Table 39.1-3 describes some of the genetic changes identified in soft tissue sarcoma. Fluorescent *in situ* hybridization using probes to locate specific chromosomal abnormalities may become clinically useful, but is unavailable for routine diagnostic use at this time. Supernumerary ring chromosomes, seen in mesenchymal neoplasms of low or borderline malignancy, such as dermatofibrosarcoma protuberans, may be identified with this technique.

As might be expected from a group of rare, diverse, but related tumors, there may be considerable disagreement among pathologists regarding the specific histologic diagnosis in individual cases. When pathologic material from 424 patients who entered into Eastern Cooperative Oncology Group (ECOG) sarcoma trials was reviewed by a panel of expert pathologists, 10% of cases were rejected as not being sarcoma, and for 14% of the remaining cases there was disagreement with respect to the histologic subtype.[85] Similarly, in the Southeastern Cancer Group experience with 216 patients, 6% were determined not to have sarcoma, and in 27% the type of sarcoma was deemed incorrect by the reviewers.[86] In the Scandinavian Sarcoma Group experience, the specific histologic diagnosis was disputed in 20%.[61]

Overall, the three most common histopathologic subtypes are MFH, liposarcoma, and leiomyosarcoma. Some types of sarcoma occur with greater frequency in certain age groups or in specific locations, forming clinicopathologic syndromes that permit standardized treatment strategies. The distribution of common histologic types among different age groups is demonstrated in Figure 39.1-3. The most common extremity sarcomas are liposarcoma, MFH, tendosynovial sarcoma, and fibrosarcoma, although a variety of other histologic types are seen. Most retroperitoneal sarcomas are liposarcomas or leiomyosarcomas. The distribution of histologic type by site is shown in Figure 39.1-4.[87]

The most frequently encountered chest wall sarcomas are desmoids, liposarcomas, and myogenic sarcomas.[88]

Virtually all gastrointestinal sarcomas were previously classified as leiomyosarcomas or leiomyoblastomas.[89] It is now recognized that many gastrointestinal sarcomas do not express markers of myogenic differentiation and are better classified as gastrointestinal stromal tumors, or, if they exhibit neural differentiation, gastrointestinal autonomic nerve tumors (GANT).[90] The pattern of recurrence is intraabdominal, including liver metastasis.[89]

Overall, leiomyosarcoma is the most common type of genitourinary sarcoma in the adult[91] and arises in the bladder, kidney, or prostate, usually in older individuals. Rhabdomyosarcoma arising in paratesticular tissues is a disease of young men. Three major types of uterine sarcoma are recognized: (1) leiomyosarcomas, tumors of the myometrium; (2) mesodermal mixed tumors (malignant mixed Müllerian tumors), composed of elements of carcinoma and sarcoma; and (3) endometrial stromal sarcoma, the least common, which arises from endometrial stroma and usually has an aggressive behavior.

Approximately 10% to 15% of all sarcomas occur in children. The majority of pediatric patients have small cell sarcomas, including embryonal rhabdomyosarcoma and the Ewing's sarcoma and primitive neuroectodermal tumor spectrum (see Chapter 44.2).

CLINICOPATHOLOGIC FEATURES OF SPECIFIC TYPES OF BENIGN AND MALIGNANT SOFT TISSUE TUMORS

TUMORS OF FIBROUS ORIGIN

There are a variety of benign tumors and tumor-like lesions of fibrous tissue that must be distinguished from true fibrosarcoma. These lesions may also be confused with reactive or reparative processes. A variety of names have been used to designate identical or overlapping entities. In addition, there are a variety of fibrous proliferations of infancy and childhood that resemble lesions in the adult, but are associated with a better prognosis. Features of lesions that may be mistaken for sarcoma are summarized in the following sections.

Nodular Fasciitis

Nodular fasciitis, also called *pseudosarcomatous fasciitis,* is a benign lesion usually seen in adults aged 20 to 40, although it has been

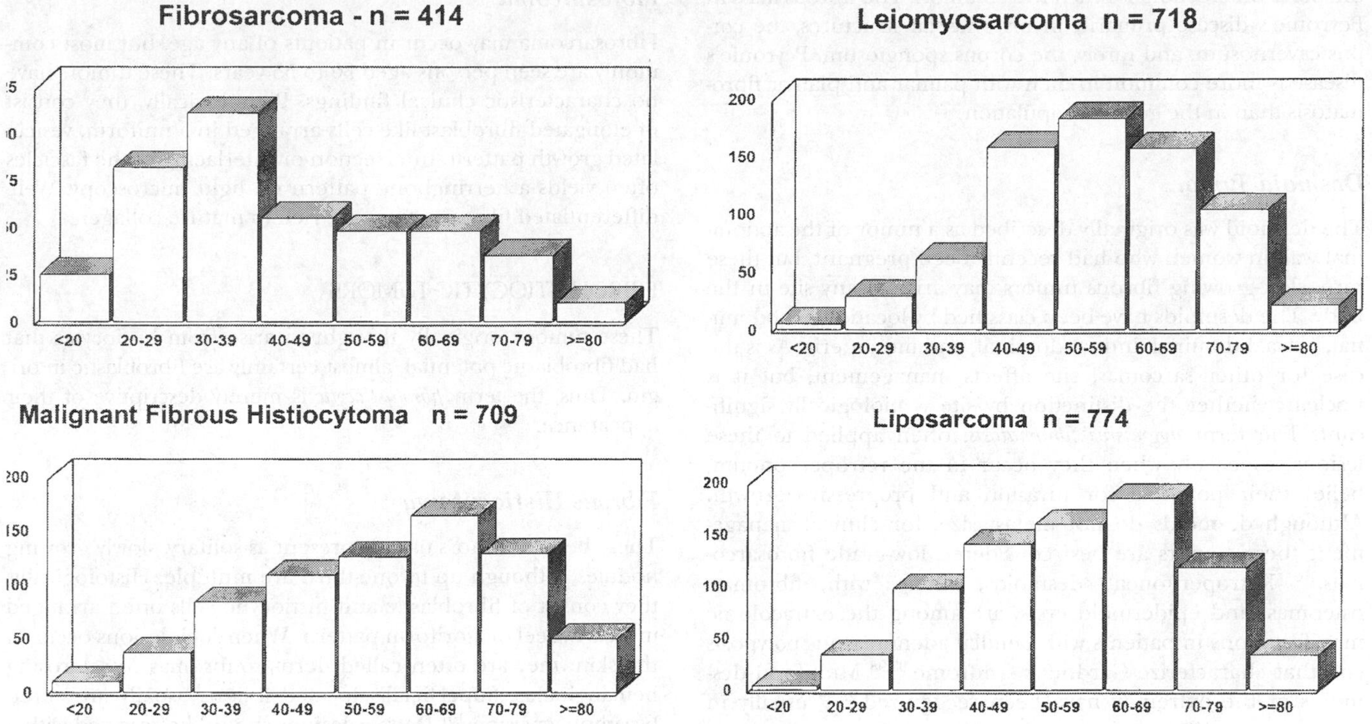

FIGURE 39.1-3. Age distribution of common histologic types of soft tissue sarcomas.

reported in both older and younger patients.[92,93] The typical lesion grows rapidly over several weeks reaching a size of 1 to 2 cm. Growth is usually self-limited, and lesions rarely are larger than 5 cm. Tenderness or soreness is a common complaint. The upper extremity is the most common site, especially the volar aspect of the forearm. Nodular fasciitis generally arises in the subcutaneous fascia or the superficial portions of the deep fascia. Histologically, the lesions are nodular, nonencapsulated masses, consisting of plump, immature fibroblasts arranged in short, irregular bundles or fascicles. Because of their cellularity, rapid growth, and high mitotic activity these lesions may be mistaken for fibrosarcoma. Recurrence is uncommon after simple excision.

Fibroma

Fibroma is a general term that has been applied to a group of poorly defined benign lesions that arise in the skin or soft tissues. Most are effectively treated by simple excision. Fibroma of tendon sheath is a slowly growing dense fibrous nodule that is attached to the tendon sheath, found most frequently in the hands or feet.[94] Recurrence may occur after local excision.

Elastofibroma

Elastofibroma is a rare, slow-growing benign tumor that characteristically arises between the lower portion of the scapula and the chest wall of older individuals.[95,96] These lesions, which typically occur in workers who have done repetitive manual tasks for years, are thought to be reactive. Elastofibromas grow as ill-defined masses, often measuring 5 to 10 cm in diameter. They may occur bilaterally and rarely have a familial association. Histologically, these lesions consist of swollen eosinophilic collagen and elastic fibers, and stain intensely for elastins. Complete excision is curative.

Superficial Fibromatoses

Superficial fibromatoses arise from the fascia or aponeurosis and generally are small and slow growing. Palmar fibromatosis is associated with flexion contractures (Dupuytren's contracture), and is by far the most common form, afflicting as many as one in five persons aged 65 and older. This condition is more common in men than in women and tends to be familial. Although benign, these lesions have a tendency to recur after simple excision. Plantar fibromatosis (Ledderhose's disease) tends to occur in a somewhat younger age group, but may occur with greater frequency in patients with palmar fibromatosis. Penile fibromatosis (Peyronie's disease), which causes pain and curvature of

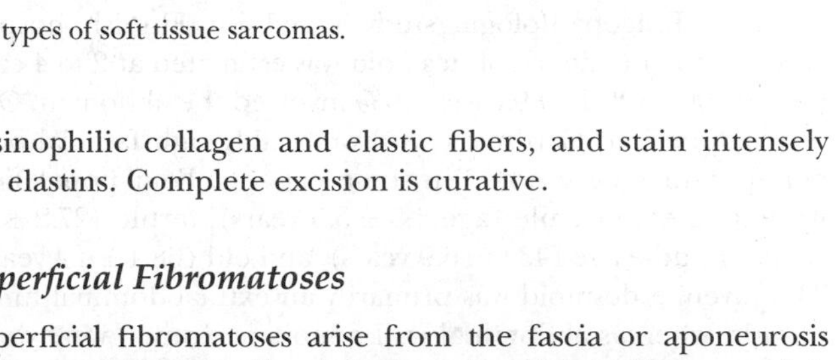

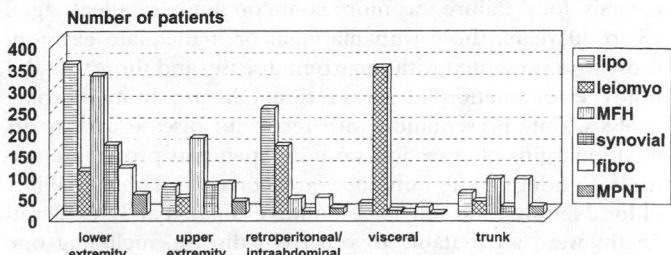

FIGURE 39.1-4. Predominant histology by site of soft tissue sarcomas in 3968 patients aged 16 or older admitted to Memorial Sloan-Kettering Cancer Center between July 1982 and July 1999. MFH, malignant fibrous histiocytoma; MPNT, malignant peripheral nerve tumor.

the penis on erection, is much less common. The fibrous mass in Peyronie's disease primarily involves fascial structures, the corpus cavernosum, and rarely, the corpus spongiosum. Peyronie's disease is more common in men with palmar and plantar fibromatosis than in the general population.

Desmoid Tumor

The desmoid was originally described as a tumor of the abdominal wall in women who had recently been pregnant, but these rare, slow-growing fibrous tumors may arise at any site in the body. The desmoids have been classified by location as abdominal, extraabdominal, intraabdominal, and mesenteric. As is the case for other sarcomas, site affects management, but it is unclear whether the distinction by site is biologically significant. The term *aggressive fibromatosis,* often applied to these lesions, especially when they occur in the retroperitoneum, belies their potential for invasion and progressive growth. Although desmoids do not metastasize, for clinical management these tumors are best considered low-grade fibrosarcomas.[16] Retroperitoneal desmoids, along with fibromas, osteomas, and epidermoid cysts, are among the extracolonic manifestations in patients with familial adenomatous polyposis coli that characterize Gardner's syndrome.[97,98] Multifocal desmoids of the extremity have been recognized,[23,99] usually in young women.

In a clinicopathologic study based on Finnish hospital records, the incidence of desmoid was estimated at 2 to 4 cases per 100,000. Of the 89 cases, 49% involved the abdomen. Only one patient had Gardner's syndrome, although familial bone abnormalities were noted in some patients. Four populations were defined: juvenile (age 4.5 ± 3.5 years), fertile (27.2 ± 4.4 years), middle age (43.9 ± 6.9 years), and old (68.1 ± 4.4 years). The juvenile desmoid was primarily an extraabdominal tumor of girls, whereas abdominal wall tumors of women were dominant in the fertile age group. Among middle-aged patients, abdominal wall tumors predominated, but the proportion of men and women was equal. In the oldest age group, both abdominal and extraabdominal tumors occurred without a gender difference. These investigators reported that the growth rate in premenopausal women was statistically greater than the rate of growth observed in male patients.[100]

Among 131 patients with desmoid tumors treated at Memorial Hospital, of whom 39% presented with recurrent disease, the female to male ratio was 1:6. Approximately one-half of these tumors arose in the extremity; 15% were retroperitoneal, 12% arose in the abdominal wall, and 10% were chest wall tumors. Four patients had Gardner's syndrome. In univariate analysis, local failure was more common among patients aged 18 to 30 years, those with marginal or inadequate excision, those who presented with recurrent disease, and those who did not receive radiation for gross residual disease. In multivariate analysis, only presentation with recurrent disease and inadequate margins of resection were independent prognostic features. Gender had no influence on recurrence. The probability of local failure following excision was estimated at 37%. Eleven deaths were attributable to recurrent disease, including one patient who developed pulmonary metastases; none of the 11 patients had an extremity primary.[16] Management of patients with desmoid tumors is discussed later in this chapter in the section Desmoids (Aggressive Fibromatoses).

Fibrosarcoma

Fibrosarcoma may occur in patients of any age, but most commonly are seen persons aged 30 to 55 years. These tumors have no characteristic clinical findings. Pathologically, they consist of elongated fibroblast-like cells arranged in a uniform, vesiculated growth pattern. Intersection or interlacing of the fascicles often yields a herringbone pattern on light microscopy. Well-differentiated fibrosarcomas are rich in mature collagen.

FIBROHISTIOCYTIC TUMORS

These tumors, originally thought to arise from histiocytes that had fibroblastic potential, almost certainly are fibroblastic in origin. Thus, the term *fibrohistiocytic* is merely descriptive of their appearance.

Fibrous Histiocytoma

These benign tumors usually present as solitary, slowly growing nodules, although up to one-third are multiple. Histologically, they consist of fibroblastic and histiocytic cells often arranged in a cartwheel or storiform pattern. When such lesions occur in the skin, they are often called dermatofibromas or sclerosing hemangiomas. Superficially located lesions usually are cured by simple excision.[101] Deeper lesions should be resected with a wider margin of normal tissue to prevent local recurrence.[102]

Xanthoma

Xanthoma refers to a collection of lipid-laden histiocytes and is seen in diseases associated with hyperlipidemia. These lesions generally occur in cutaneous or subcutaneous locations, but may involve deep soft tissues. Presumably, xanthomas are reactive lesions.

Dermatofibrosarcoma Protuberans

Dermatofibrosarcoma protuberans[103,104] is probably best considered a low-grade sarcoma. This lesion may occur anywhere in the body, but more than 40% occur on the trunk, 20% in the head and neck, and 40% on the extremities. This lesion typically presents in early or midadult life, beginning as a nodular cutaneous mass. The pattern of growth is usually slow and persistent, and as the lesion enlarges over many years, it becomes protuberant. Large lesions often are associated with satellite nodules. Dermatofibrosarcoma protuberans is histologically similar to benign fibrous histiocytoma, but grows in a more infiltrative pattern, spreading along connective tissue septa in deep areas. The central portion of the tumor consists of a uniform population of plump fibroblasts arranged in a distinct ordered pattern. Unlike fibrous histiocytoma, dermatofibrosarcoma protuberans stains positive for CD34, suggesting a neural origin.[105] More than 75% of these tumors have a ring chromosome, probably of chromosome 17 origin, superimposed on a normal karyotype[106] (see Table 39.1-3).

Up to 50% recur after simple excision.[104,107] Occasionally, areas of increased pleomorphism and mitotic activity occur, especially in recurrent lesions. Metastases occur rarely to lung or to lymph nodes.[107] Because of their locally aggressive nature, these lesions may ultimately lead to amputation or even death because of extensive invasion. A variant with melanin pigmentation (Bednar's tumor) also is recognized.[108]

Malignant Fibrous Histiocytoma

The term MFH was first introduced in 1963 to describe a group of malignant soft tissue tumors with a fibrohistiocytic appearance.[109] Since then, this entity has become the most commonly diagnosed extremity sarcoma. A number of subtypes have been described, including myxoid, giant cell, inflammatory, angiomatoid, and pleomorphic types. With advances in pathologic techniques, it has been claimed that a specific line of differentiation can be identified in the overwhelming majority of patients with pleomorphic MFH.[110] Nonetheless, this designation has been useful clinically.

MFH characteristically is a tumor of later adult life with a peak incidence in the seventh decade, although it may occur in younger adults. MFH usually presents as a painless mass; the most common site is the lower extremity, followed by the upper extremity and the retroperitoneum.[111,112]

TUMORS OF ADIPOSE TISSUE

Lipomas

Lipomas are the most common of all benign neoplasm and may arise in any location where fat is normally present. Lipomas may be deep seated in the mediastinum or retroperitoneum where they may attain massive size. Multiple lipomas are occasionally seen in a familial pattern. *Lipomatosis* is a term applied to a poorly circumscribed overgrowth of mature adipose tissue that grows in an infiltrating pattern.

Well-differentiated lipomas are composed of fat cells, but are demarcated from surrounding fat by a thin fibrous capsule. These tumors usually are found within subcutaneous fat, but may occur anywhere in the body. In spindle cell lipoma, mature fat is replaced by collagen-forming spindle cells; this lesion typically arises in the posterior neck and shoulder in men between the ages of 45 and 65. Pleomorphic lipoma is a closely related lesion. Local excision of lipoma and these variants is generally curative. The term *atypical lipoma* is used by some to describe these benign lesions; others use atypical lipoma to describe a well-differentiated liposarcoma that arises in a subcutaneous or intramuscular location.[113,114]

Angiolipomas present as subcutaneous nodules, usually in young adults. The most common site is the upper extremity. Angiolipomas rarely reach more than 2 cm, but they often are painful, especially during their initial growth period. Microscopically, these tumors consist of adipocytes with interspersed vascular structures. Myxoid and fibroblastic angiolipomas are recognized.

Angiomyolipoma

The term *angiomyolipoma* is used for a nonmetastasizing renal tumor that is composed of fat, smooth muscle, and blood vessels. Angiomyolipoma is more common in women than in men and is seen in association with tuberous sclerosis. Although angiomyolipoma is usually well demarcated from normal kidney, it may extend into the surrounding retroperitoneum. Angiomyolipomas may be solitary or multicentric and may produce abdominal pain or hematuria. Wide excision is curative. Angiomyolipomas of the liver have also been described.[115]

Hibernoma

Hibernoma is a rare, slowly growing benign neoplasm that resembles the glandular, brown fat that is found in hibernating animals. The literature consists primarily of case reports, and in most of these the tumor arises within the thorax.[116] Lesions of the trunk, retroperitoneum, or extremities also are reported. Excision is generally curative.

Lipoblastoma and Lipoblastomatosis

Lipoblastoma and lipoblastomatosis are peculiar variants of lipoma that occur almost exclusively in infancy and early childhood.[117] They differ from lipoma by their cellular immaturity and their close resemblance to the myxoid form of liposarcoma.

Liposarcoma

Liposarcoma is primarily a tumor of adults with a peak incidence between age 50 and 65. Next to MFH, it is the most commonly diagnosed soft tissue sarcoma in adults. Liposarcoma may occur anywhere in the body, although the most common sites are the thigh and the retroperitoneum. As with other adult sarcomas, there are no characteristic clinical findings. Several types of liposarcoma are recognized and have different clinical outcomes.[118] Well-differentiated liposarcoma is a nonmetastasizing lesion. It is often difficult to distinguish well-differentiated liposarcoma from atypical lipoma, and the distinction may be irrelevant to the clinician. Sclerosing liposarcoma, also a low-grade lesion, typically occurs in the retroperitoneum.

Myxoid liposarcoma accounts for 40% to 50% of all liposarcomas. The tumor consists of proliferating lipoblasts within a delicate capillary network and has a myxoid matrix. The amount and distribution of the mucoid material may vary widely. Although previously considered a low-grade lesion, it is now clear that a myxoid matrix can be seen in many high-grade liposarcomas. As with other sarcomas, pathologic nomenclature can vary widely between pathologists. Myxoid liposarcoma typically has a t(12;16)(q13-14;p11) translocation.[69] Round cell (or lipoblastic) liposarcoma is characterized by excessive proliferation of small rounded cells. Round cell liposarcoma has the same translocation seen in myxoid liposarcoma,[72] suggesting that these liposarcomas are variants of the same pathogenetic process. Fibroblastic liposarcoma is composed of slender, fibroblast-like cells, and, like round cell liposarcoma, is of higher grade than myxoid liposarcoma. Pleomorphic liposarcoma, as the name implies, is a highly malignant lesion. Mitotic activity is high, and hemorrhage or necrosis is common.

It is not unusual for large liposarcomas to consist of multiple nodules, some of which contain only low-grade elements and others containing intermediate- or high-grade elements. The term *dedifferentiated liposarcoma*[119] has been used to refer to lesions that appear to begin as low-grade lesions, but progress to higher grade tumors and show evidence of nonlipogenic differentiation.[120] This lesion is seen most frequently in the retroperitoneum.

TUMORS OF SMOOTH MUSCLE

Leiomyoma

Benign smooth muscle tumors are quite common in the uterus and in the gastrointestinal tract. Rare cutaneous leiomyomas arise from the piloerector muscles of the skin. Some occur on a familial basis. These lesions are often multiple and may be quite painful.[121,122] Typically, these cutaneous leiomyomas develop in adolescence or early adult life as small discreet papules that eventually form nodules. The extensor surfaces of the extremities are most often affected, and the nodules may follow a dermatomal distribution. Although these tumors are histologically benign, recurrences after surgical incision are seen frequently, and often the lesions are so numerous that surgical incision is not possible. Leiomyoma may also occur deep within the extremities, abdominal cavity, or retroperitoneum.

Angiomyoma is a solitary form of leiomyoma. This lesion tends to occur on the extremity in people between the fourth and sixth decades of life. Women are more commonly afflicted than men.

Intravenous leiomyomatosis is a rare condition in which nodules of benign smooth muscle tissue grow within the veins of the myometrium and may extend into the uterine and hypogastric veins.[123] Rarely, these tumors extend up the inferior vena cava into the heart.[124] Diffuse peritoneal leiomyomatosis is also recognized, often occurring in association with pregnancy.[125] Leiomyomas in children have been associated with human immunodeficiency virus infection.

Leiomyosarcoma

Leiomyosarcoma may arise in any location, but more than half are located in retroperitoneal or intraabdominal sites. These masses often reach quite large proportions, but present insidiously with nonspecific symptoms. In addition, most visceral sarcomas are leiomyosarcoma. Cutaneous leiomyosarcomas usually appear as small solitary extremity nodules.[126] Deep extremity leiomyosarcoma most frequently arises in the thigh and may arise in association with medium or large veins.[127] Although rare, leiomyosarcoma may arise in large vascular structures and present with symptoms of obstruction to the normal flow of blood. The most common arterial site is the pulmonary artery; patients present with symptoms of decreased pulmonary outflow. Leiomyosarcoma of the inferior vena cava, which may present with the Budd-Chiari syndrome, is also described.

The typical cell of the leiomyosarcoma is elongated and has an abundant cytoplasm. Multinucleated giant cells are common. Epithelioid changes, in which the cells become rounded, with concomitant clear cell changes in the neoplasm, may occur in otherwise typical leiomyosarcomas. When the tumor is predominantly or exclusively epithelioid, the term *leiomyoblastoma* has been used. The term *leiomyoblastoma*, however, fails to convey any information with regard to clinical behavior.

Localization of muscle antigens by means of immunohistochemistry proves the diagnosis of leiomyosarcoma. Desmin and smooth muscle actin are the most common immunohistochemical stains. Grading of leiomyosarcoma, however, can be quite difficult, although mitotic activity appears to be the best indicator of prognosis.

TUMORS OF SKELETAL MUSCLE

Benign tumors of striated muscle are rare. Several types of rhabdomyosarcoma are recognized. Embryonal rhabdomyosarcoma is a small cell tumor that usually arises in the orbit or genitourinary tract in children. The botryoid type of embryonal rhabdomyosarcoma, which frequently originates in mucosa-lined visceral organs such as the vagina and the urinary bladder, generally grows as a polypoid tumor. These tumors may disseminate widely, but are responsive to chemotherapy and radiation. Embryonal rhabdomyosarcomas occasionally arise in adults. Although regression of tumor in response to pediatric chemotherapy regimens usually occurs, age is an important prognostic factor for survival, with worse outcomes in older patients.[128] Extremity rhabdomyosarcoma in adolescents and young adults often has an alveolar histology. Alveolar rhabdomyosarcoma is composed of ill-defined aggregates of poorly differentiated round or oval cells that frequently show central loss of cellular cohesion and formation of irregular *alveolar* spaces. These tumors appear to have a worse prognosis than embryonal rhabdomyosarcoma in younger children, but not in adults. A specific translocation, t(2,13)(q37;q14) involving the PAX3 gene on chromosome 2 and the FKHR gene on chromosome 13, is seen in the majority of alveolar rhabdomyosarcomas.[72] In other patients, the translocated chromosome 2 locus is different.[73] Many pediatric studies include all types of rhabdomyosarcoma seen in the pediatric population.

In adults, pleomorphic rhabdomyosarcoma is the most common form of rhabdomyosarcoma. This high-grade lesion is not clinically distinguishable from other high-grade adult sarcomas.

VASCULAR TUMORS

Hemangioma

Hemangiomas are among the most common soft tissue tumors. Most hemangiomas are present at birth and regress spontaneously. Rapid growth with impingement on vital structures may occur, however, and treatment with intralesional injection of interferon has been life-saving.[129] Pulmonary hemangiomatosis, a rare disorder of diffuse microvascular proliferation in the lung, has been treated effectively with systemic interferon. Cavernous hemangioma refers to a benign lesion consisting of large dilated blood vessels with a flattened endothelium.

Lymphangioleiomyomatosis

Pulmonary lymphangioleiomyomatosis is a disease of women of childbearing age. Patients present with cough, hemoptysis, and dyspnea. Grossly, the lungs demonstrate multiple small cystic lesions. On microscopic examination, there is proliferation of normal smooth muscle around the airways and the blood and lymphatic vessels. Tamoxifen does not appear to be useful, but responses to progestational agents have been seen.[130]

Epithelioid Hemangioendothelioma

As its name implies, epithelioid hemangioendothelioma is a vascular tumor that has an epithelial appearance.[131] It has several forms. These lesions may appear as a solitary, slightly painful mass in either superficial or deep soft tissue. Metastases to lung, regional lymph nodes, liver, and bone are reported. Another pattern is that of a diffuse bronchoalveolar infiltrate or multiple small pulmonary nodules. This entity has also been called *IBVAT* (intravascular, bronchiolar, and alveolar tumor of the lung).[132] Patients may present with cough and hemoptysis. Epithelioid hemangioendothelioma can also arise in the liver, often presenting as an incidental finding, or as part of a workup for mild elevation of liver enzymes or vague abdominal pain. Multiple liver nodules are the rule. Although these lesions can metastasize, they usually run an indolent course. Liver transplantation has been performed, even in patients with metastatic disease.[133]

Kaposi's Sarcoma

Classic Kaposi's sarcoma is an unusual vascular sarcoma that occurs in the skin of the lower extremities of elderly men of Mediterranean or Jewish extraction.[134] The disease is usually indolent, although it can spread to the lungs and the gastrointestinal tract. Cutaneous lesions can be palliated with radiation therapy when necessary. Another form of Kaposi's sarcoma occurs in Bantu men in Africa; it may also occur in African children in whom it runs a more aggressive course. Kaposi's sarcoma has arisen in renal allograft recipients who are receiving immunosuppressant therapy.[135] Epidemic Kaposi's sarcoma is a complication of human immunodeficiency virus infection (see Chapter 50.1).

Angiosarcoma

Angiosarcomas may arise in either blood or lymphatic vessels. Cutaneous lymphangiosarcoma may develop in chronically lymphedematous extremities.[136] The classic presentation is the Stewart-Treves syndrome, lymphangiosarcoma in the chronically lymphedematous arms of women who have been treated for breast cancer with radical mastectomy, and, often, axillary irradiation.[20] Hemangiosarcomas are usually located in the skin or superficial soft tissue. Multicentric angiosarcomas occur on the scalp and face of elderly men, where unrelenting progression can cause severe ulceration and infection.[137] Angiosarcoma of the breast is usually an aggressive lesion that recurs locally and may metastasize, primarily to lung; histologic grade has been of prognostic value.[138] Angiosarcomas are known to occur in sites of prior irradiation without chronic lymphedema, in particular the pelvis of women who have received radiation therapy for gynecologic cancers.[139] Soft tissue angiosarcoma, often with epithelioid features, may arise on the extremities or within the abdomen.[140]

PERIVASCULAR TUMORS

Glomus Tumor

Glomus tumors mimic the modified smooth muscle cells of the glomus body, a special form of arteriovenous anastomosis that is located in the skin and participates in thermal regulation. The glomus tumor generally presents as small, blue-red nodule in subcutaneous tissue or in the subungual region of the finger.[141] These tumors are often associated with paroxysmal pain irradiating away from the tumor. Complete excision is the appropriate management.

Hemangiopericytoma

The cells of these tumors resemble pericytes, cells that normally are arranged along capillaries and venules. These rare tumors usually arise in adults, although an infantile hemangiopericytoma is recognized. The adult form is most common in the lower extremity, but also occurs in the pelvis or retroperitoneum or other sites. The tumors tend to be well circumscribed and consist of tightly packed cells around thin-walled vascular channels of varying calibers. The cells of hemangiopericytoma stain immunohistochemically with factor XIIIa and HLA-DR antigen, but not with factor VIII-related antigen.[142] Many hemangiopericytomas have an indolent behavior, although some behave like other high-grade sarcomas.[143]

TUMORS OF SYNOVIAL TISSUE

Nodular Tenosynovitis

A variety of benign tumors and tumor-like lesions arise from the synovium. Nodular tenosynovitis (tenosynovial giant cell tumor) is a giant cell tumor that may occur at any age but is most commonly seen between the ages of 30 to 50. These tumors are somewhat more common in women. They occur with greatest frequency in the hand, but are also seen in the ankles and knees, among other sites. These slow-growing tumors grow as circumscribed lobulated masses and are usually diagnosed when they are less than 5 cm in diameter. Because of their location, excision is often done with close margins and local recurrence is seen in 10% to 20% of patients. A diffuse form occurs in and around joints, most commonly around the knee or ankle. In contrast to most giant cell tumors, this neoplasm grows in expansive sheets without a mature capsule. Malignant giant cell tumors of the tendon sheath are also recognized.

Synovial Sarcoma

Synovial sarcoma usually occurs in young adults.[144] The most common site is around the knee. As opposed to most other soft tissue sarcomas, these lesions occasionally are painful. This tumor is composed of two morphologically distinct types of cells that form a characteristic biphasic pattern. The biphasic synovial sarcoma includes epithelial cells with a surrounding spindle or fibrous component. Calcification, with or without ossification, is seen in up to 30% of tumors. The spindle cells stain positive for keratin and epithelial membrane antigen. Vimentin is demonstrable in spindle cells but absent in epithelial cells. S-100 may be positive as well. Monophasic synovial sarcoma of both fibrous and epithelial types are recognized, although monophasic epithelial synovial sarcoma is extremely rare. Synovial sarcomas contain a characteristic chromosomal translocation, t(X;18)(p11.2;q11.2); a hybrid transcript has been identified.[68]

TUMORS OF THE PERIPHERAL NERVES

Neurofibroma

Solitary neurofibromas are small, slow-growing cutaneous or subcutaneous nodules that usually arise during the third decade of life. By definition, these lesions are not associated with neurofibromatosis. Neurofibromatosis type 1 (NF1, peripheral neurofibromatosis, von Recklinghausen's disease) is one of the most common genetic disorders, affecting approximately 1 in 3000 live births.[145] An autosomal dominant mutation at the 17q11.2 locus has been identified.[146] The clinical features of NF1 include café au lait spots, Lisch nodules (pigmented hamartomas) of the iris, and neurofibromas of several types. Cutaneous neurofibromas, soft, fleshy growths, arise in the skin in all patients with NF1. These lesions may range in size from a few millimeters to 50 to 60 cm. Although some patients have only a few such lesions, others may have hundreds. Subcutaneous neurofibromas are firm and nodular and may be painful. Plexiform neurofibromas are large lesions that affect large segments of a nerve, thickening and distorting the nerve into a tortuous mass. They may cause severe dysesthetic pain.

Benign Schwannoma

Also called *neurilemoma,* this benign lesion occurs most commonly in people aged 20 to 50 years. Common sites include the head and neck and the flexor surfaces of the extremities. It grows slowly and is usually smaller than 5 cm when the diagnosis is made. This encapsulated nerve sheath tumor is distinguished from neurofibroma in that schwannoma consists of two components: a highly ordered cellular region (Antoni A area), and a loose, myxoid component (Antoni B area).

Cellular Schwannoma

This tumor is more cellular than classical schwannoma. It usually presents in patients during the seventh decade of life as a painless paravertebral mass.[147] Complete excision is curative in most patients.

Granular Cell Tumor

The granular cell tumor (also called granular cell myoblastoma) is a rare tumor that probably is of neural origin. This tumor usually presents in adults as a small, poorly circumscribed subcutaneous nodule, although there are patients who have multiple lesions. This entity has a distinct histologic appearance and stains positive for S-100. Granular cell tumor usually runs a benign course, but metastases have been reported.

Malignant Peripheral Nerve Sheath Tumors

MPNSTs have also been called malignant schwannoma, neurofibrosarcoma, or neurogenic sarcoma. The majority of MPNSTs are high grade and characteristically stain for the S-100 protein. The lower extremity and the retroperitoneum are the most common sites, but MPNSTs may arise anywhere in the body.[148] These tumors originate from the nerve sheath, rather than from the nerve itself. Although higher estimates appear in the literature, approximately 5% of patients with NF1 develop MPNSTs,[10,11] usually arising from a plexiform neurofibroma. The majority of patients with MPNST do not have neurofibromatosis, however. After accounting for size and grade, the prognosis of patients with MPSNT in the setting of NF1 is not different from that of other patients. The malignant peripheral nerve tumor that develops in the patient with neurofibromatosis historically has been considered to have a poor prognosis compared with other extremity malignant sarcomas. However, when other factors of known risk for outcome such as grade and size are accounted for, malignant peripheral nerve tumors arising both sporadically and in the presence of neurofibromatosis tend to have a similar outcome to other poor prognosis peripheral sarcomas.[149] MPNSTs tend to present with a greater preponderance of large size and high grade than other soft tissue sarcomas, hence their reputation for aggressivity. The Triton tumor is a malignant peripheral nerve tumor with rhabdomyosarcomatous elements.[149]

Because of evolving concepts and nomenclature, the literature is confusing with regard to MPNST and primitive neuroectodermal tumor. The latter, a small cell tumor of children and young adults, is a variant of Ewing's sarcoma.

Gastrointestinal Autonomic Nerve Tumor

GANT, also called plexosarcoma, presumably arises from the enteric plexus of the gastrointestinal tract. Clinically and microscopically, GANT resembles gastrointestinal leiomyosarcoma, but immunostaining is negative for markers of myogenic differentiation. Neurofilaments are seen by electron microscopy.[90] GANT is usually considered a subset of gastrointestinal stromal tumors (GISTs) and characteristically demonstrates expression of the oncogene c-kit (CD117).

EXTRASKELETAL CARTILAGINOUS AND OSSEOUS TUMORS

Myositis Ossificans

This benign lesion is a self-limiting process that usually is associated with trauma. Despite its name, myositis ossificans is not necessarily confined to the muscle nor is inflammation a prominent feature. The condition usually presents in athletic young adults as a tender, soft tissue mass. Over a period of weeks, the mass usually becomes firm or rock hard. Radiographs show calcification several weeks after the lesion appears. Histologically, the mass consists of fibroblastic tissue, often with prominent mitotic activity. Nonetheless, this process is benign and may be managed conservatively. Obviously, it is important to distinguish between myositis ossificans and sarcoma, especially extraosseous osteogenic sarcoma.

Extraskeletal Chondrosarcoma

Myxoid chondrosarcoma (also called chordoid sarcoma) occurs most commonly in patients over the age of 35. More than two-thirds occur in the extremity.[150] This tumor usually grows slowly, but late recurrence and metastasis is common. A nonrandom reciprocal translocation has been shown in these tumors.[83,84]

Extraosseous Osteogenic Sarcoma

Extraosseous osteogenic sarcoma are rare, high-grade sarcomas defined by their production of malignant osteoid and bone.[151,152] By definition, they are not attached to the skeleton. Unlike typical osteogenic sarcoma of bone, these tumors rarely occur in patients under the age of 20, and most patients are over 50 years of age.[153,154] These high-grade tumors present like other soft tissue sarcomas. Most arise in the extremities, although osteosarcoma of other sites, including breast, retroperitoneum, urinary bladder, or other visceral organs have been reported. There is considerable heterogeneity in the histologic appearance. Spindle cell varieties may resemble MFH, MPNST, or fibrosarcoma, whereas others have a more epithelioid appearance. Giant cells are a common feature. Some lesions that may contain bone or cartilage are hard to distinguish from MFH, but bone in MFH is well differentiated. Nonetheless, extraosseous osteogenic sarcoma resembles MFH in terms of age, sites of distribution, and clinical behavior.

TUMORS OF UNCERTAIN HISTOGENESIS

Myxoma

Intramuscular myxoma is a rare tumor that occurs in adults, usually in the large muscles of the extremities. Myxomas consist of abundant mucoid material but few cells. Although these lesions often measure 5 to 10 cm, their clinical behavior is generally benign.[155] Multiple intramuscular myxomas occur in association with fibrous dysplasia.

Aggressive angiomyxoma[156] is a tumor that usually occurs in women, although male patients have been reported. The lesion generally presents as a mass in the perineal or pelvic area. Local recurrence can result in considerable morbidity given the location of these tumors, but distant metastases do not occur.

Mesenchymoma

Malignant mesenchymoma is defined as a malignant tumor showing at least two types of malignant mesenchymal differentiation in addition to a poorly differentiated fibrosarcomatous element.[157] These rare tumors are generally thought to behave clinically in accordance with the predominant component, although one report suggests that their behavior is not as aggressive as might be expected.[158]

Alveolar Soft Part Tumor

This rare tumor occurs most frequently in patients between 15 and 35 years of age. Women outnumber men, especially in patients less than 20 years of age.[159] Prognosis is better in those patients who present at a younger age. These tumors often present in the lower extremities as slow-growing painless masses. Grossly, alveolar soft part tumors are poorly circumscribed. They typically grow in an organoid or nest-like arrangement. The alveolar spaces actually are necrotic areas. Considerable controversy regarding histogenesis persists. Neural derivation has been suggested, but other data suggest a myogenic origin.[160] Lung, brain, and bone are the most common sites of metastasis. Although this tumor tends to grow slowly, the ultimate prognosis is quite poor. Patients may remain asymptomatic over years, however, even with metastatic disease.

Epithelioid Sarcoma

Epithelioid sarcoma is another tumor of adolescents and young adults. This tumor usually presents as a small, firm nodule in the subcutaneous tissue of the distal extremities.[161,162] Multiple recurrences, which grow along tendons and fascial planes, are a characteristic feature. Unlike most other sarcomas, lymph node metastases are common, and the tumor may appear in the extremity in transit to the regional nodes.[51,161] Lung is the most common site of distant metastasis.

Clear Cell Sarcoma (Malignant Melanoma of Soft Parts)

This tumor, also called clear cell sarcoma of tendons and aponeuroses, presents as a soft tissue mass. Because of the presence of intracellular melanin and the tendency for regional nodal metastasis, it has been suggested that this entity is better considered a melanoma than a soft tissue sarcoma. Despite these clinical features, clear cell sarcoma has a distinct chromosomal translocation, t(12;22)(q13;q13). Size is the most important prognostic factor. Treatment of the primary is similar to that of other sarcomas. There are few reported responses to chemotherapy.

Desmoplastic Small Cell Tumor

This newly appreciated entity is a tumor of adolescents and young adults.[163] It usually presents in the abdomen, often with diffuse peritoneal implants. Because of its multifocal nature, complete resection is usually impossible. Chemotherapy regimens used in the treatment of Ewing's sarcoma have induced responses in patients with this disease, but are rarely curative. A specific translocation between chromosomes 11 and 22 that is different from the translocation of Ewing's sarcoma has been identified.[164,165]

Follicular Dendritic Cell Sarcoma

This unusual lesion is thought to arise from lymphatic tissue[166] and commonly occur in the neck, but has been described in other sites.[167]

CLINICAL PRESENTATION

The presence of soft tissue sarcoma almost invariably is suggested by the development of a mass. This mass is usually large, often painless, and may be associated by the patient with an episode of injury. The majority present at a size greater than 5 cm. The size distribution for 3541 cases admitted to Memorial Sloan-Kettering Cancer Center (MSKCC) is illustrated in Figure 39.1-5. The focus of the clinical evaluation is to determine the likelihood of a benign or malignant soft tissue tumor, the involvement of muscular or neurovascular structures, and the ease with which biopsy or subsequent excision can be obtained.

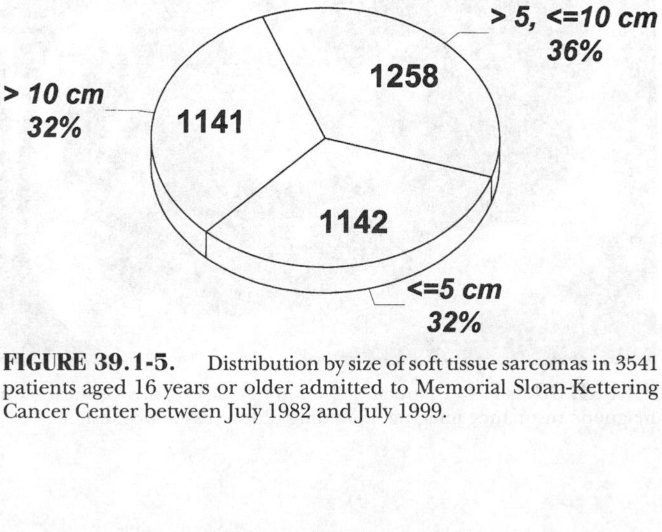

FIGURE 39.1-5. Distribution by size of soft tissue sarcomas in 3541 patients aged 16 years or older admitted to Memorial Sloan-Kettering Cancer Center between July 1982 and July 1999.

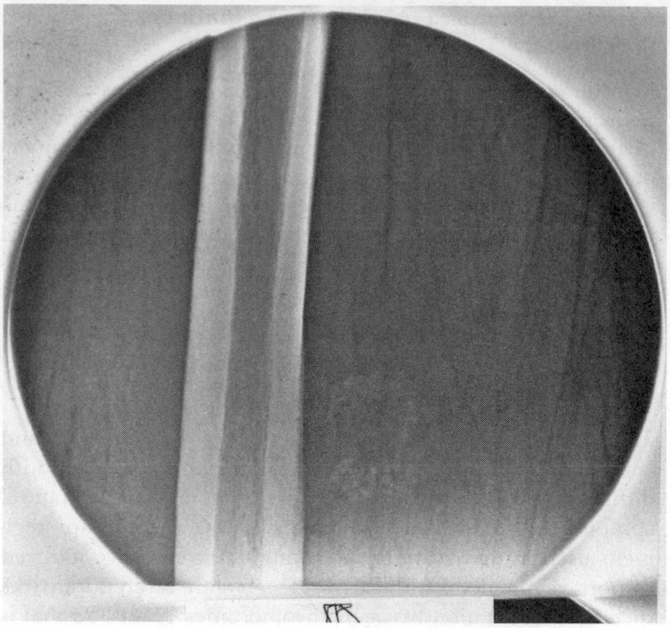

FIGURE 39.1-6. Myositis ossificans suggested by calcification on a plain film.

Size becomes an important feature (see Prognostic Factors for Outcome, later in this chapter) and definitive diagnosis is dependent on biopsy and histologic confirmation.

DIFFERENTIAL DIAGNOSIS

The major concern, when confronted with a soft tissue mass, is whether or not the lesion is benign or malignant. In most patients with small lesions, or even on occasion large lesions, the differentiation is from the most common soft tissue tumor, lipoma. This may be simple but becomes more difficult as the more aggressive and underappreciated inherently benign lesions are considered. Particularly difficult is myositis ossificans. The patient often has an antecedent history of trauma,

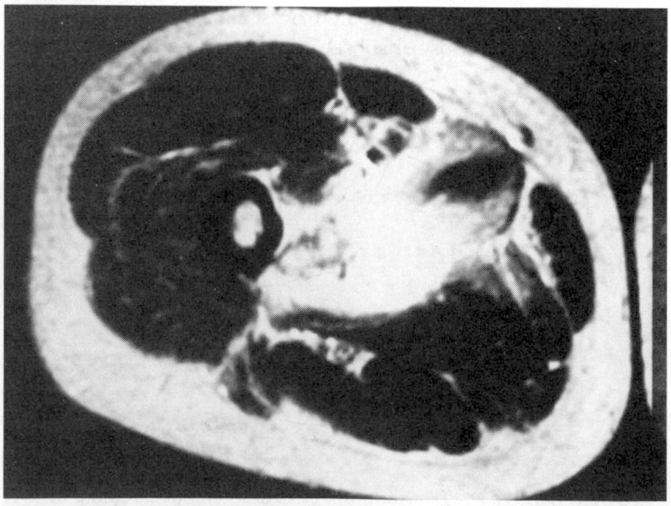

FIGURE 39.1-7. Characteristic findings of myositis ossificans on magnetic resonance imaging, including diffuse tissue expansion.

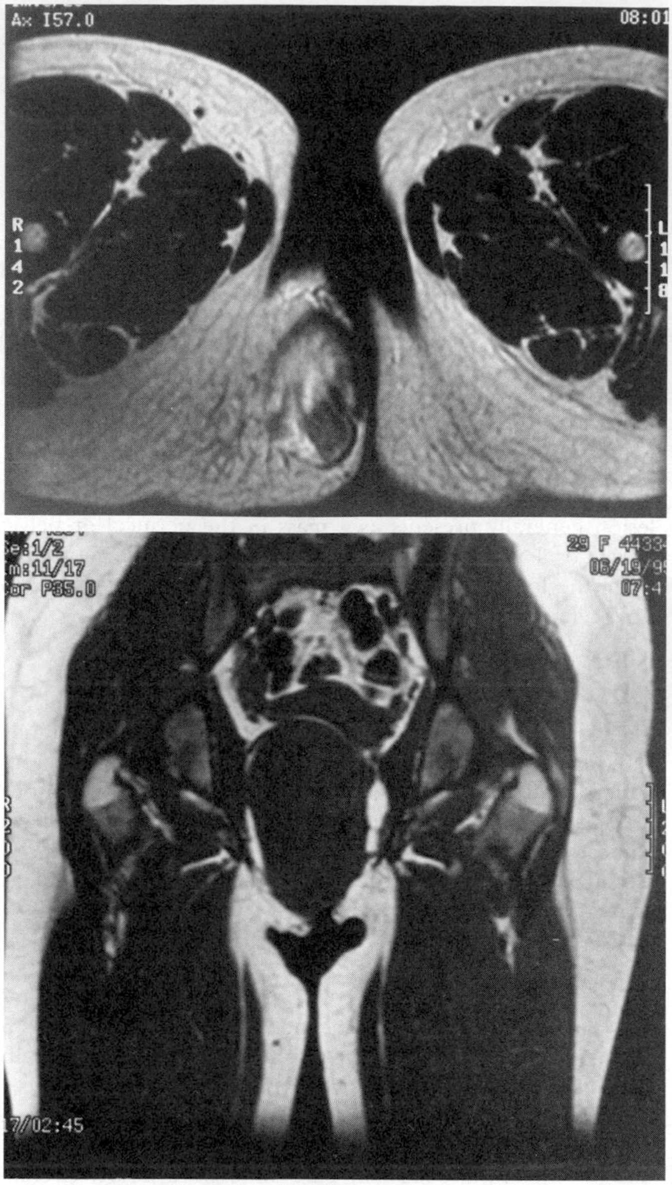

A

B

FIGURE 39.1-8. Other similarly difficult lesions are angiomyxoma, here seen growing as a mass in the perineum **(A)** and pelvis **(B)** in a young woman.

and often presents with a large, firm to hard lesion that, on plain film, may have a telltale sign of intrinsic calcification. This does not preclude a malignant lesion. Tru-Cut (Travenol Laboratories, Deerfield, IL) needle biopsy or open biopsy is often accompanied by aggressive hemorrhage, suggesting a vascular neoplasm. In most cases, diagnosis can be made fairly accurately by either plain film (Fig. 39.1-6) or magnetic resonance imaging (MRI) (Fig. 39.1-7). Certainly, the diagnosis should be suspected when there is a significant history of trauma, the lesion is particularly hard, and there is inherent calcification.

Other difficult lesions are the angiomyolipoma and the rare angiomyxoma (Figs. 39.1-8*A* and *B*), which can also be vascular lesions, and the atypical schwannoma, which can be quite large and often is invasive (Fig. 39.1-9). They can often be quite destructive, causing ureteric obstruction and bone invasion. The management is as difficult as for any sarcoma. Conversely, unless

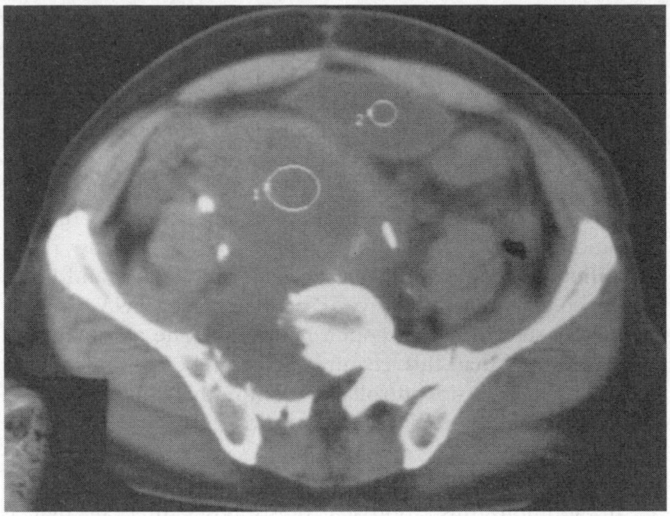

FIGURE 39.1-9. Atypical schwannoma can be quite large and often invasive, as shown here in a man with a 20-year history of having undergone multiple resections for large invasive lesions.

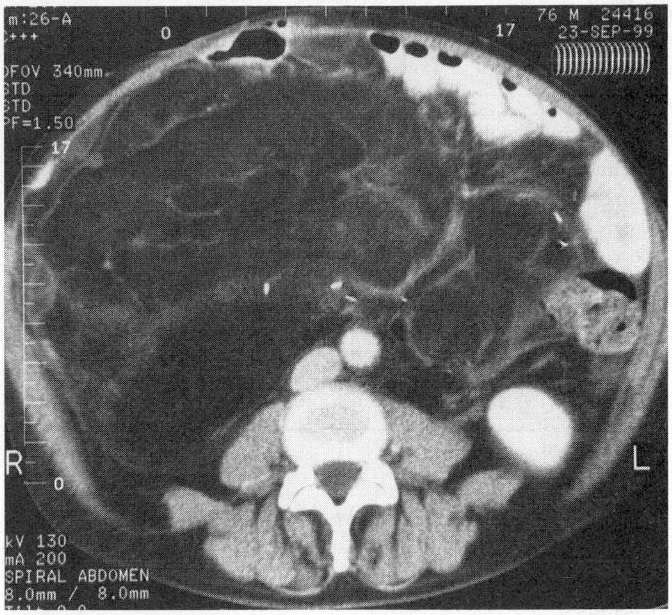

FIGURE 39.1-10. Computed tomography of a massive intraabdominal liposarcoma.

absolutely imperative, multiple radical operations in inherently indolent lesions should be avoided.

IMAGING STUDIES

Imaging studies for soft tissue sarcoma vary, depending to some extent on the site. They involve evaluation both of the primary lesion and the potential site of metastasis. Evaluation of the primary lesion in the extremity, and head and neck, predominantly is either by computed tomography (CT) scan, or magnetic resonance imaging (MRI), which provides some increased definition. In the hands of a knowledgeable radiologist, MRI can provide information over and above that provided by CT.[168] Nevertheless, a Radiology Diagnostic Oncology Group study comparing these modalities has shown no benefit of MRI over CT.[169] What is clear in this era of cost containment is that multiple modalities, all focusing on the same entity, are not required.

An important issue for the primary clinician is identification of the relationship of the sarcoma to neurovascular structures. Angiography is rarely of value. For the primary intraabdominal lesion we prefer CT scan (Fig. 39.1-10), which can identify both primary and potential metastasis, although in lesions known to involve the intestinal tract, MRI may add information.

Positron Emission Tomographic Scan

While positron emission tomographic (PET) scan has been used as an investigational agent for several years, it has yet to gain universal acceptance. It does appear in some studies that grade can be distinguished by this modality. At present, it would appear that the role of PET is primarily in the identification of unsuspected sites of metastasis in patients with recurrent high-grade tumors.

SITES OF METASTATIC DISEASE

As important as imaging studies of the primary lesion is evaluation of possible sites of metastasis. This knowledge is essential. An analysis of patients at MSKCC reveals the common sites of metastasis that can guide investigation (Fig. 39.1-11). Metastatic disease from soft tissue sarcoma is also site-specific. For patients with extremity lesions, most metastases (70%) go primarily to the lung.[170] For patients with retroperitoneal or visceral lesions, a much more common site for metastases would be the liver parenchyma, with lung only a secondary site. Nevertheless, no site is immune from soft tissue sarcoma metastasis, and other unique patterns can be identified (e.g., the unusual presentation of intraabdominal metastasis following an extremity liposarcoma).[171]

Clearly, for small, superficial extremity lesions, either high or low grade, evaluation for sites of metastasis is less important and simple chest roentgenogram suffices. Conversely, with large high-grade lesions, where the risk of metastatic disease is significant, more extensive evaluation is required. For extremity lesions, the primary modality is a chest roentgenogram followed by a CT scan of the chest. For retroperitoneal, visceral, and intraabdominal lesions, then the site of metastasis that is

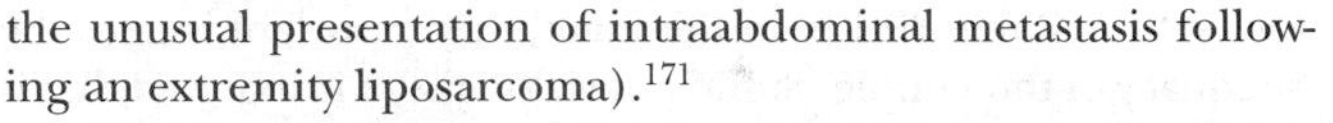

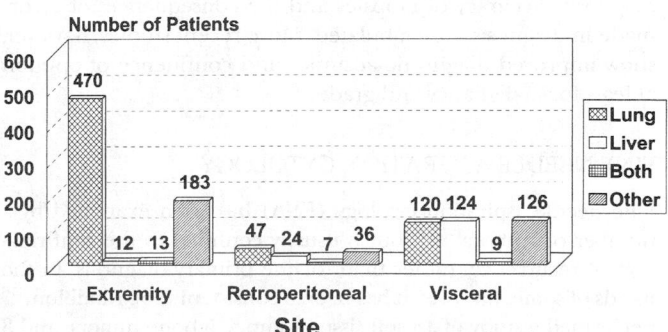

FIGURE 39.1-11. Common sites of metastasis that can guide investigation (from 1171 patients admitted to Memorial Sloan-Kettering Cancer Center between July 1982 and July 1999). The primary site of metastasis for extremity lesions is the lung.

TABLE 39.1-6. Accuracy of Tru-Cut Biopsy[a]

	Tru-Cut	*Incisional*	*Frozen Section*
Number	60	45	36
Adequate tissue (%)	93	100	94
Correct malignancy (%)	95	100	88
Correct grade (%)	88	96	62[b]
Correct histology (%)	75	84	47[b]

[a]Memorial Sloan-Kettering Cancer Center, 1990 through 1995.
[b]Significance by Fisher exact test, $P<.05$, versus Tru-Cut.
(Reprinted from Heslin MJ, Lewis JJ, Woodruff JM, Brennan MF. Core needle biopsy for diagnosis of extremity soft tissue sarcoma. *Ann Surg Oncol* 1997;4:425, with permission.)

most common (i.e., the liver) is evaluated with the modality that is used for evaluation of the primary lesion.

BIOPSY

The primary thrust of biopsy is to obtain adequate tissue for definitive histopathologic confirmation, to evaluate grade, and to identify prognostic factors that would alter the approach to definitive treatment. In the main, for lesions that are less than 5 cm, particularly those that are superficial, excisional biopsy is the preferred approach.

VALUE OF TRU-CUT BIOPSY

Several studies have examined this issue,[172,173] and a summary of the accuracy of Tru-Cut, incisional and frozen section biopsies is included in Table 39.1-6. In the main, the important issue is the adequacy of the sample. Sufficient viable tissue is required that is both representative of the lesion and available for all histopathologic evaluation, immunohistochemistry, and where necessary, electron microscopy. As molecular markers become a factor in prognosis, meticulous attention to the adequacy of biopsy, tissue preservation, and evaluation is paramount. Histopathologic interpretation varies from center to center and may be a major variable in decision making. As with other relatively rare lesions, it is essential that review of the histopathology be made by an experienced group. In a paper from a major center,[174] members of the Musculoskeletal Tumor Society were surveyed and the diagnostic accuracy of biopsies and the consequences of errors made in diagnosis were tabulated. More recent studies, however, show improved diagnostic accuracy and confluence of opinion at least for malignancy and grade.[175]

FINE NEEDLE ASPIRATION CYTOLOGY

Fine needle aspiration cytology (FNA) has been examined by a number of authors[175,176] but is usually confined to the confirmation of recurrence, rather than for the primary diagnosis. In the hands of some, however, it has been a consistent tool. Kindblom[176] performed a study of 18 soft tissue tumors, 5 bone tumors, and 3 metastatic carcinomas thought to be primary soft tissue tumors to examine the relative advantages of a technique using both light and electron microscopy rather than conventional light microscopic aspiration cytology. In their hands FNA was a valuable adjunct used in this manner, but is rarely employed in most centers, other than to identify expected recurrent lesions.

Some authors have argued that biopsy itself is not justified if FNA is available. Rydholm[177] has suggested that no open biopsy is ever really indicated, the argument against its use suggesting the possibility of risking local tumor spread. The author is concerned that antecedent open biopsy increases both the magnitude of the subsequent operation and the need for adjuvant radiation therapy. The author argues that without biopsy, radiation therapy is not needed in the majority of cases and limits the need for more extensive resections. Using FNA, the surgeon proceeds directly to open operation. The author points out, however, that this requires referral before antecedent biopsy, a relatively uncontrollable event in the United States. In addition, other authors suggest that this results in ten patients with benign lesions referred for every sarcoma patient,[178] certainly an untenable situation under our present system.

In addition, this approach presupposes that all that is required is a malignant sarcoma diagnosis and the type or grade of sarcoma does not determine therapy. At MSKCC for extremity lesions we use brachytherapy (BRT) for high-grade lesions and external-beam radiation therapy for low-grade lesions, particularly of large size, that would preclude such an approach. The authors themselves conclude the difficulty if patients should be candidates for pretreatment neoadjuvant therapy to improve survival. However, they argue that immunohistochemistry, electron microscopy, DNA cytology, and chromosomal analysis, all of which can be performed on FNA, ensure the appropriateness of this approach.[179] We still favor adequate tissue from Tru-Cut, excisional, or incisional biopsy to begin such a procedure.

FROZEN SECTION

In some institutions, frozen section is relied on as the diagnostic tool of choice. For many institutions, however, this is unavailable. Our results for frozen section are described in Table 39.1-6. For diagnosis of malignancy, frozen section is accurate but for histopathologic subtypes and grade it is inferior to permanent sections of either Tru-Cut or incisional biopsy.

STAGING

There have been significant changes in the staging of soft tissue sarcoma. The original 1992 staging system was based on a review published in 1977.[180] That staging system has since been considerably modified. The major difference was the inclusion in the original staging system of a subcategory grade [i.e., patients with small (less than 5 cm) lesions that were high grade, were considered as stage IIIA]. Several reviews, however, have suggested that such lesions (small, high grade) have a much more favorable prognosis than outlined in the original 1977 proposal. Reports from two separate institutions[181,182] suggest that survival of these patients is certainly better than 80% and in many patients, 90%. Consequently, size, which had been historically considered a subcategory of grade, was redefined. Clearly, however, size is a continuous variable and the decision to divide tumors into less than 5 cm or greater than 5 cm is clearly arbitrary.[183] An analysis of greater than 1000 patients with localized extremity sarcoma seen at MSKCC between 1982 and 1997 has been published.[184] The new staging system, however, now includes both size and depth. Our analysis of the present modified 1997 staging system makes it more clear

TABLE 39.1-7. Primary Extremity Soft Tissue Sarcoma: Distant Metastases by Stage, Memorial Sloan-Kettering Cancer Center, July 1, 1982 through December 31, 1997 (n = 1059)

	Total (No.)	*Yes (%)*
Old staging system (1992)		
1A	140	2 (1)
1B	221	13 (6)
3A	272	47 (17)
3B	426	144 (34)
New staging system (1997)		
1A	140	2 (1)
1B	30	3 (10)
2A	191	10 (5)
2B	272	47 (17)
2C	23	4 (17)
3A	208	57 (27)
3B	195	83 (43)

(From ref. 183, with permission.)

that stages IB (low-grade, large superficial tumors) are uncommon as are stage IIC (high-grade, large, superficial tumors). They are in such a minority that the ability to use them meaningfully in a staging system must be questioned (Table 39.1-7). In addition, this would suggest that depth, although significant in multiple, overall analyses, is of less value when incorporated with other prognostic factors such as size. In addition, it is clear that size itself is a continuous variable as mentioned previously, and for the high-risk tumors (i.e., the large, less than 5-cm, deep tumors), they can be meaningfully divided into tumors of greater than 5 cm or greater than 10 cm. Using this approach then, distant metastasis-free survival can be quite clearly distinguished into four discriminating groups (Tables 39.1-8 *A*, *B*, and *C* and Fig. 39.1-12).

Stage IV disease from lymph node metastasis, which as previously alluded to, is rare in the majority of adult soft tissue sarcomas, is equivalent to any other metastasis. For example, if one takes patients with lymph node metastasis only or lymph nodes plus other metastasis and contrasts those to other systemic metastasis, then the disease-specific survival is essentially the same (Fig. 39.1-13). Finally, it is important to emphasize that prognostic factors can vary with time. For early recurrence, it would appear that grade is predominant, whereas for late recurrence, size assumes a progressively more important role.[54,185]

Whether or not age should be a determinant in a staging system is as yet unclear. Certainly, when age is examined as an outcome for overall survival, the older patient has a shorter survival

TABLE 39.1-8A. Newer Approaches to Staging System of Soft Tissue Sarcoma: Stage Groupings

Stage	*Grade*	*Tumor*	*Nodes*	*Metastasis*
I	G1–2	T1A–1B or 2A	N0	M0
II	G1–2	T2B	N0	M0
	G3–4	T1A–1B or 2A	N0	M0
III	G3–4	T2B	N0	M0
IV	Any G	Any T	N1	M0
	Any G	Any T	N0	M1

(From ref. 229, with permission.)

TABLE 39.1-8B. Local Recurrence, Disease-Free Survival and Overall Survival in Patients with Modified Staging

Stage		*Freedom from Local Recurrence*	*Disease-Free Survival*	*Overall Survival*
1	Low grade <5 cm Low grade >5 cm superficial	79.09%	77.91%	98.79%
2	Low grade >5 cm deep High grade <5 cm High grade >5 cm superficial	75.16%	63.63%	81.80%
3	High grade >5 cm deep	74.46%[a]	36.27%[b]	51.65%[b]

[a]P = .5.
[b]P = .0001.

than the younger patient. This has usually been arbitrarily divided into less than 50 or greater than 50 years, with a patient over 50 having a worse prognosis. Conversely, a distinction into three groups can show some separation, which we thought were, in the main, disease-dependent rather than age-dependent (Fig. 39.1-14). It certainly seems clear that patients under the age of 16 (i.e., the pediatric age group) have a far different prognosis and a far different response to treatment with sarcoma than do the adults, and this should not be included in the current adults' staging system. An analysis of the most common histopathologic type in children, rhabdomyosarcoma, suggested that the soft tissue sarcomas in children behave in a somewhat different manner than those in adults. It does appear that the early stage of disease and the late stage of disease are similar in both children and adults, but the intermediate stage lesions have a better prognosis in children, which does not appear solely due to their ability to tolerate extent of treatment.[128] Site is also a clear determinant of outcome. Patients with retroperitoneal and visceral sarcomas certainly do worse than patients with extremity lesions (Fig. 39.1-15).

Conversely, there are factors that affect our ability to treat specific sites such as difficulty of radical resections for head and neck tumors and the limitations of radiation therapy in intraabdominal sites.

It does appear that site is a significant factor in survival. However, it is difficult to separate site from adequacy of treatment. It is clear that patients with retroperitoneal sarcoma can and do die of local recurrence, an uncommon event in extremity lesions. The intraabdominal visceral leiomyosarcomas still maintain a high metastatic rate as the primary cause of death.

Bone invasion by soft tissue sarcoma with neurovascular invasion has historically been considered a bad prognostic feature. However, as bone invasion is relatively uncommon in soft tissue

TABLE 39.1-8C. Statistical Test on Three Stages

Study	*Log-Rank Test*	*Wilcoxon Test*
Local recurrence	P = .5	P = .25
Disease-free survival	P = .0001	P = .0001
Overall survival	P = .0001	P = .0001

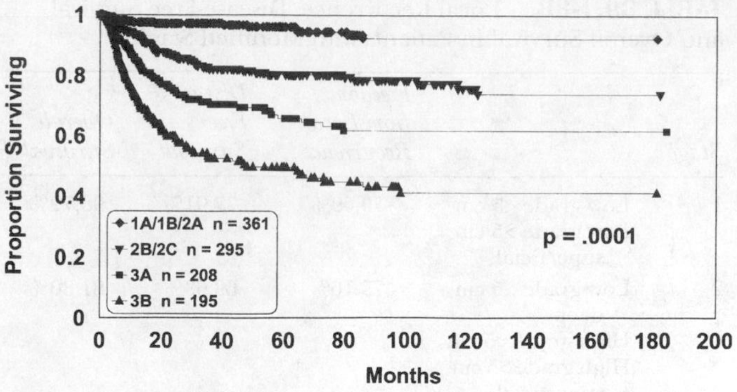

FIGURE 39.1-12. Distant metastasis-free survival for patients with primary extremity soft tissue sarcoma (n = 1059 patients admitted to Memorial Sloan-Kettering Cancer Center between July 1982 and January 1998) by stages, incorporating 1A/1B/2A versus 2B/2C versus 3A versus 3B. Significance describes the overall difference between the curves. (From ref. 183, with permission.)

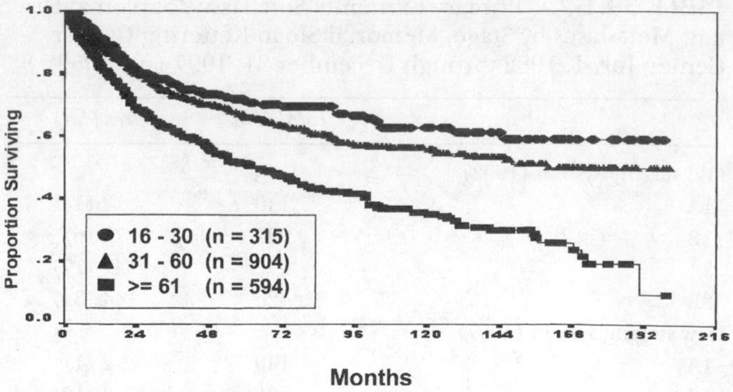

FIGURE 39.1-14. Overall survival for extremity soft tissue sarcoma by age group in 1813 patients aged 16 years or older admitted to Memorial Sloan-Kettering Cancer Center between July 1982 and July 1999 (P <.001). Significance describes the overall difference between the curves.

sarcoma, it has not been uniformly included in any staging system, but should certainly be considered as a poor prognostic factor.

As of the present time, the innumerable molecular markers that have been included and defined for soft tissue sarcoma, some with prognostic implications, have not been included in staging systems, but one that we would expect to become an increasingly important variable.

MANAGEMENT OF EXTREMITY AND SUPERFICIAL TRUNCAL SOFT TISSUE SARCOMA

SURGICAL TREATMENT

A suggested algorithm is shown in Figure 39.1-16. Where appropriate, alternative approaches are discussed in the text (e.g., for patients with lesions less than 5 cm and positive microscopic margins not able to be reresected without major morbidity, radiation therapy can be selectively used). The mainstay of treatment for all soft tissue sarcomas of the extremity and trunk is surgical excision. The issues of debate concern how extensive that surgical excision should be and whether it should be preceded or followed by adjuvant therapy.

Wide *en bloc* resection is used most often. Historical attempts to resect all muscle bundles from origin to exertion have now been supplanted by an encompassing resection, aiming to obtain 2 cm of all uninvolved tissue in all directions. This is often unrealistic, however, because the limiting factor is usually neurovascular juxtaposition or, occasionally, bony juxtaposition. Because most soft tissue sarcomas tend not to invade bone directly, only rarely does bone need to be resected. Soft tissue sarcomas only uncommonly involve the skin, so major skin resection should be limited. In situations of primary or recurrent tumors where skin is involved, or the tumor is so extensive that skin is involved, then consideration of free flap or rotational flap closure becomes important, particularly in those patients who are candidates for subsequent adjuvant radiation therapy.

EXTENT OF SURGICAL RESECTION

The most extensive resection is clearly amputation. This should be only rarely indicated in soft tissue sarcoma at the present time because limb-sparing operations are possible in at least 95% of patients. Experience over the last 25 years at MSKCC indicates that the 50% amputation rate in the late 1960s is now less than 5% (Fig. 39.1-17). Amputation should be

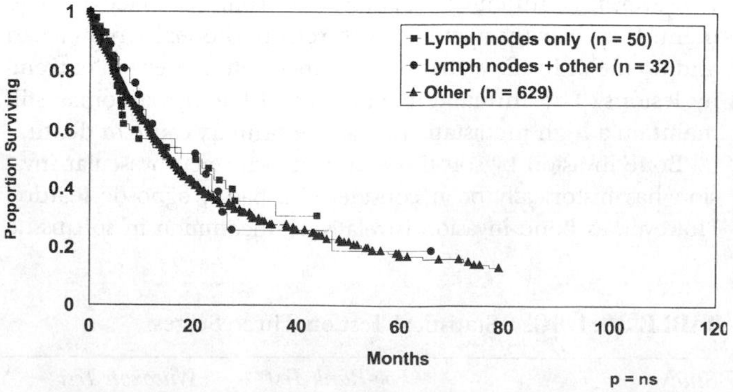

FIGURE 39.1-13. Disease-specific survival for patients with soft tissue sarcoma with metastases (n = 711 patients admitted to Memorial Sloan-Kettering Cancer Center between July 1982 and July 1997); lymph node metastases alone versus lymph node metastases with other metastases versus all other metastases. (From ref. 183, with permission.)

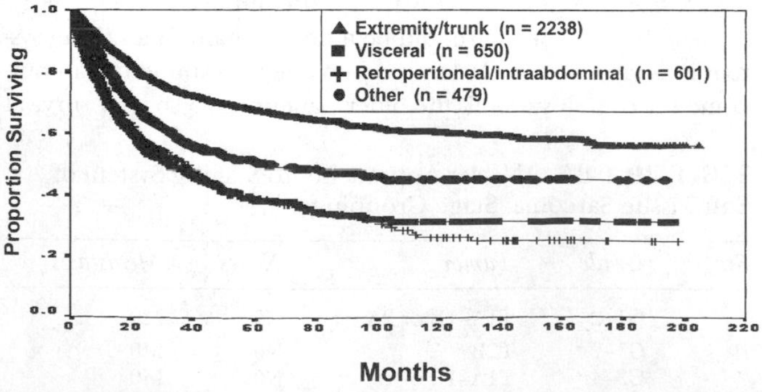

FIGURE 39.1-15. Disease-specific survival by site of soft tissue sarcoma in 3968 patients aged 16 years or older admitted to Memorial Sloan-Kettering Cancer Center between July 1982 and July 1999 (P <.001). Patients with retroperitoneal or visceral sarcomas did worse than patients with extremity lesions. Significance describes the overall difference between the curves.

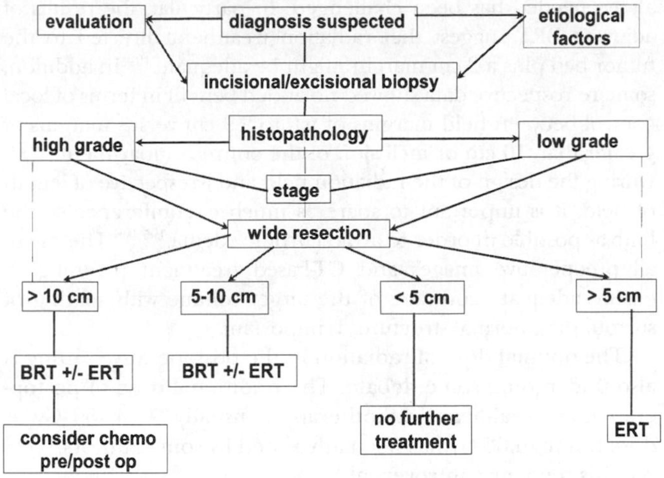

FIGURE 39.1-16. Management algorithm for extremity and superficial truncal soft tissue sarcoma. BRT, brachytherapy; ERT, external-beam radiation therapy.

reserved, in the main, for tumors not able to be resected by any other means, without evidence of metastatic disease and the propensity for good long-term functional rehabilitation. Often these are patients with large, low-grade tumors with considerable cosmetic and functional deformity, who can be rendered free of symptoms by a major amputation.

Major amputation has been contrasted to limb-sparing surgery combined with adjuvant radiation.[186] Local recurrence can occur after the limb-sparing operation, and follow-up data on this study confirm that this is almost invariably salvaged, but there is no effect on long-term survival.[187] The issue of amputation versus limb-sparing surgery for extremity lesions has been addressed by a prospective randomized trial at the National Cancer Institute (NCI). In patients entered into this trial, follow-up is now available for more than 10 years. Although local recurrence is greater in those undergoing limb-sparing operation plus irradiation compared with amputation (Fig. 39.1-18), survival overall is not different (Fig. 39.1-19).

SIZE

Because size is a prognostic factor for outcome both in terms of local recurrence and subsequent metastatic disease, the approach

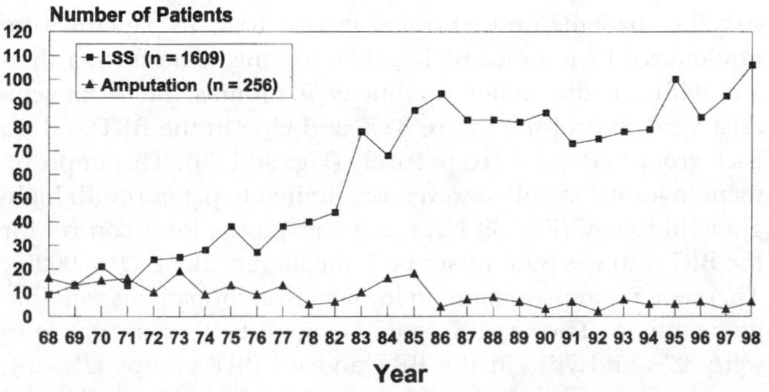

FIGURE 39.1-17. Limb-sparing surgery (LSS) versus amputation for all patients, primary and recurrent. Trends in management over time based on the experience at Memorial Sloan-Kettering Cancer Center from 1968 to 1998.

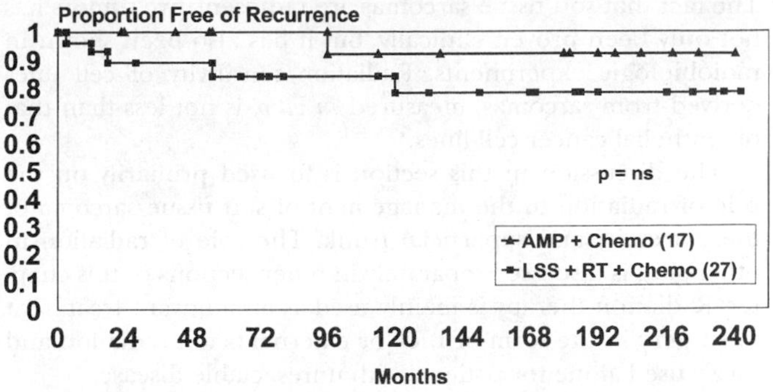

FIGURE 39.1-18. Soft tissue sarcoma, local recurrence according to treatment. Limb-sparing surgery (LSS) plus irradiation (RT) compared with amputation (AMP) at the National Cancer Institute. (Courtesy of J. C. Yang and S. A. Rosenberg.)

these lesions can be varied. In patients with small lesions less than 5 cm, complete surgical excision is usually sufficient, adjuvant therapy being reserved for only those with recurrent lesions. Given the high risk of recurrence and of systemic disease for lesions larger than 10 cm that are high grade, these patients are candidates for investigational approaches, especially neoadjuvant chemotherapy (see below, in Adjuvant Chemotherapy). All patients with lesions larger than 5 cm should be considered for adjuvant radiation therapy as a proven method of limiting local recurrence.[181]

RADIATION THERAPY

Before discussing the role of radiation therapy in the management of soft tissue sarcoma, it is important to differentiate between radiosensitivity and radioresponsiveness. *Radiosensitivity* refers to the inherent response of cancer cells to radiation, and *radioresponsiveness* refers to how quickly a tumor regresses after radiation. These two parameters do not always correlate.

Unfortunately, the slow rate of regression of soft tissue sarcomas even after high doses of radiation, an example of poorly radioresponsive tumors, is often mistaken for radioresistance. This in turn has lead to an extensive debate about the effectiveness of radiation therapy in soft tissue sarcomas. This debate was not settled until the recent past, even though the use of x-rays for the treatment of sarcoma was first proposed in 1902.[188]

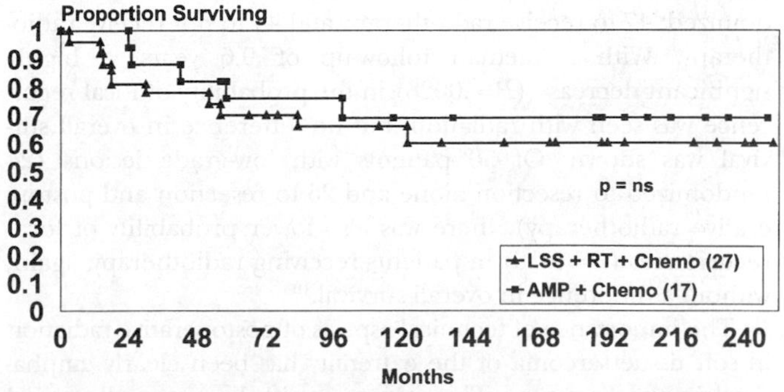

FIGURE 39.1-19. Soft tissue sarcoma, disease-free survival according to treatment. Limb-sparing surgery (LSS) plus irradiation (RT) compared with amputation (AMP) at the National Cancer Institute. (Courtesy of J. C. Yang and S. A. Rosenberg.)

The fact that soft tissue sarcomas are radiosensitive tumors has not only been proven clinically, but it has also been shown in radiobiologic experiments. Radiation sensitivity of cell lines derived from sarcomas, measured *in vitro*, is not less than that of epithelial cancer cell lines.[189–191]

The discussion in this section is focused primarily on the role of radiation in the management of soft tissue sarcoma of the extremity and superficial trunk. The role of radiation in other sites is discussed separately in other sections of this chapter. Radiation therapy is mainly used as an adjuvant treatment to surgery in the form of BRT or external-beam radiation and rarely used alone for patients with unresectable disease.

ADJUVANT RADIATION

The effectiveness of adjuvant radiation has been clearly shown not only through retrospective data but also through three prospective randomized trials that have compared surgery alone with surgery and radiation.[187,192,193] Therefore, the question that we should be asking is not whether radiation is useful, but rather which form of radiation is the most effective in terms of tumor control and function preservation.

POSTOPERATIVE EXTERNAL-BEAM RADIOTHERAPY

The use of postoperative external-beam radiotherapy in soft tissue sarcoma of the extremities has served as an early model for function preserving approach in oncology.

Historically, amputation was considered the standard surgical treatment for soft tissue sarcoma of the extremity, but data that evaluated more conservative surgery followed by postoperative external-beam radiotherapy emerged as a reasonable alternative.[194,195] These encouraging results lead the NCI to perform a randomized prospective trial that compared amputation with wide local excision and postoperative radiation in patients with high-grade soft tissue sarcoma of the extremity. Twenty-seven patients were randomized to conservative surgery and radiotherapy, and 16 received amputation (2:1 randomization). There were four local recurrences in the limb-sparing group and none in the amputation group ($P = .06$). However, there were no differences in disease-free survival rates (71% and 78% at 5 years; $P = .75$) or overall survival rates (83% and 88% at 5 years; $P = .99$) between the limb-sparing group and the amputation treatment groups.[187] In a subsequent trial, investigators at the NCI wanted to determine if adjuvant radiation was needed after wide local excision. Ninety-one patients with high-grade lesions were randomized; 47 to receive radiotherapy and 44 to not receive radiotherapy. With a median follow-up of 9.6 years, a highly significant decrease ($P = .0028$) in the probability of local recurrence was seen with radiation, but no difference in overall survival was shown. Of 50 patients with low-grade lesions (24 randomized to resection alone and 26 to resection and postoperative radiotherapy), there was also lower probability of local recurrences ($P = .016$) in patients receiving radiotherapy, again, without a difference in overall survival.[193]

The importance of technical aspects of postoperative radiation in soft tissue sarcoma of the extremity has been clearly emphasized in the literature. The volume at risk has generally varied from including the whole compartment from origin to insertion, to giving a generous margin around the tumor bed, scar, and drainage sites.[196–198] However, whether such generous margins are always needed has been challenged. In particular, the results of adjuvant BRT suggest that radiation treatment directed to the tumor bed plus a 2-cm margin might be adequate.[199] In addition, some retrospective data showed no added benefit in terms of local control between field margins of 5.0 to 9.9 cm versus margins of greater than 10 cm or inclusion of the entire compartment.[200,201] During the design of the radiation field and irrespective of length of field, it is important to spare as much circumference of the limb as possible in order to avoid chronic edema.[195,196] The use of all preoperative images and CT-based treatment planning to ensure adequate coverage of the target volume with sparing of surrounding normal structures is important.

The optimal dose of radiation in the postoperative setting is also undergoing some debate. The traditional dose of postoperative external-beam radiotherapy is usually 60 to 66 Gy. A dose less than 63 Gy has been advocated by some authors,[200,201] but this remains controversial.

In summary, the effect of postoperative external-beam radiation on local control for soft tissue sarcoma of the extremity, whether it is high or low grade, has been shown in two prospective randomized trials. Most authors recommend that the tumor bed, including scar and drainage site plus at least 5 to 7 cm margins be included in the initial field of treatment. Then, one or two further reductions in the treatment volume should be done to allow maximum sparing of normal tissues. The total dose is usually 60 to 70 Gy depending on tumor grade, size, margin status, and location.

ADJUVANT BRACHYTHERAPY

Although most of the initial experience with adjuvant radiation has revolved around external-beam radiation, BRT is becoming an attractive alternative. With BRT, patients usually leave the hospital having completed all their treatment in approximately 2 weeks compared with a 6- to 7-week course of external-beam radiation. The evaluation of the tumor bed at the time of the operation by both the surgeon and the radiation oncologist can far exceed any imaging modality in its accuracy, and the rapid dose fall off with BRT spares more normal tissue than external radiation. In addition, Janjan et al. reported savings of $1000 per patient treated with BRT as compared with external irradiation.[202]

The initial experience with adjuvant BRT at MSKCC was reported by Hilaris et al. in 1982[203] and based on these encouraging results a prospective randomized trial was initiated at that time. The aim of this trial was to determine whether adjuvant BRT was needed after complete gross resection. One hundred sixty-four patients were enrolled in that trial; 78 patients were randomized to adjuvant BRT and 86 patients to no further therapy. With a median follow-up time of 76 months, the 5-year actuarial local control rates were 82% and 69% in the BRT and no BRT groups ($P = .04$), respectively (Fig. 39.1-20). This improvement in local control, however, was limited to patients with high-grade histology (Fig. 39.1-21). For this group, local control for the BRT arm was 89% versus 66% for surgery alone ($P = .0025$). There was no improvement in local control for patients with low-grade tumors. The 5-year freedom from distant recurrence rates were 83% and 76% in the BRT and no BRT groups ($P = .6$), respectively. Analysis by histologic grade did not demonstrate an effect of BRT on the development of distant metastasis or survival.[192] Even though adjuvant BRT did not show an improvement in local control in patients with low-grade tumors, the local

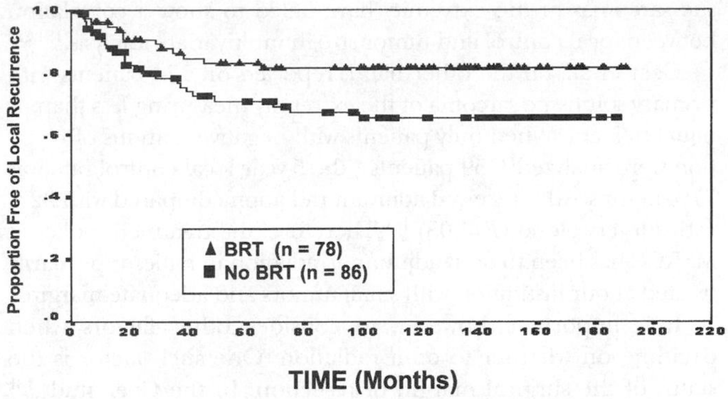

FIGURE 39.1-20. Results of a prospective randomized trial at Memorial Sloan-Kettering Cancer Center of adjuvant brachytherapy (BRT) in patients undergoing limb-sparing surgery (n = 3968 patients admitted to Memorial Sloan-Kettering Cancer Center between July 1982 and July 1992, follow-up to July 1999; *P* = .4). Patients who received adjuvant BRT had a statistically significant improvement in local control. (Updated from ref. 192, with permission.)

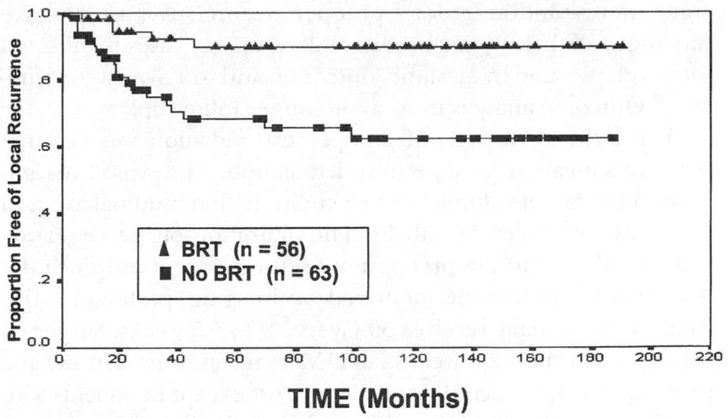

FIGURE 39.1-21. Results of a prospective randomized trial at Memorial Sloan-Kettering Cancer Center of adjuvant brachytherapy (BRT) in patients undergoing limb-sparing surgery (n = 119, from July 1982 to July 1992, follow-up to July 1999; *P* = .002). This local control advantage was limited to patients with high-grade lesions. (Updated from ref. 192, with permission.)

recurrence rates were 22% (no BRT) and 27% (BRT), indicating the need for adjuvant external radiation in those patients.[204]

Other institutions have also reported encouraging results in their experience with BRT in soft tissue sarcoma.[205,206] In most of those cases, BRT was used as a boost in combination with external beam irradiation, but whether this combination is needed in all patients is unclear. Alekhteyar et al. reported on 105 patients with primary or locally recurrent high-grade soft tissue sarcomas who were treated with wide local excision and BRT (87 patients) or BRT and external-beam irradiation (18 patients). With a median follow-up of 22 months, there was no statistically significant difference in the 2-year actuarial local control rates between the two groups; 86% in the BRT group compared with 90% in BRT plus external-beam irradiation group (*P* = .32).[207] At MSKCC, external-beam irradiation is added to BRT only when the geometry of the implant is suboptimal or there is a positive surgical margin.

One of the most attractive aspects of BRT is the ability to deliver further radiation in previously irradiated patients who may otherwise need amputation in order to obtain good local control. Nori et al. and Pearlstone et al. reported a local control rate of 82.5% (33 of 40) and 65% (17 of 26), respectively, when using conservative surgery and reirradiation with BRT.[208,209] Catton et al., on the other hand, reported a local control of only 36% (4 of 11) for patients treated with conservative surgery and no further irradiation.[210]

The technical aspects of BRT are different from external-beam radiotherapy. At the time of the operation, the radiation oncologist and the surgeon jointly evaluate the tumor bed, and the radiation target area is determined by adding 2 cm margin longitudinally and 1.0 to 1.5 cm circumferentially. The radiation oncologist then implants this target area with an array of after-loading catheters, placed percutaneously and spaced 1 cm apart. The loading of the catheters takes place no sooner than the fifth postoperative day to allow enough time for wound healing.[211] Unlike with postoperative irradiation, no attempts are usually made to treat large margins or to include the scar and the drainage site. In patients treated with BRT alone, the dose is usually 45 Gy given over 4 to 6 days, and when given as boost the dose is usually 15 to 20 Gy plus 45 to 50 Gy with external-beam irradiation. The most common isotope used is the low-dose-rate iridium 192; however, high activity iodine 125 is occasionally used in young patients or to protect the gonads. More recently, high-dose-rate iridium 192 has been advocated by some authors to take advantage of its radiation safety aspects as well as its dose-optimization capabilities.[212] Further follow-up, however, is still needed to determine its long-term morbidity and overall efficacy.

PREOPERATIVE EXTERNAL-BEAM RADIOTHERAPY

Of the three types of adjuvant radiation, preoperative external-beam irradiation is the only modality that has not been tested against surgery in a randomized trial. There is, however, a great deal of interest and enthusiasm for this approach. Some of the potential advantages of preoperative external-beam radiation therapy include decreased intraoperative seeding of tumor cells, a smaller radiation target volume compared with postoperative irradiation, and tumor shrinkage that might facilitate later surgery. Suit et al. evaluated the relationship between tumor size and the sequencing of radiation and showed that preoperative radiation was superior to postoperative radiation in terms of local control for patients with tumors greater than 15 cm.[213] However, others have shown no difference.[214] Pollack et al. from M. D. Anderson Cancer Center compared the sequencing effect, not only according to size, but also according to presentation. For patients who presented to their institution with gross disease, the 10-year local control rate was 88% for preoperative radiation compared with 67% with postoperative radiation (*P* = .01). In contrast, for those presenting after an excision elsewhere, the 10-year local control was better with postoperative radiation (88% versus 73%, *P* = .07). It is important to note, however, that on multivariate analysis for predictors of local control for the entire population, the type of radiation was not a determinant of local control.[215] It is evident from this discussion that there are no conclusive data on which adjuvant radiation produces the best results in terms of local control; indeed the results are similar. Therefore, the only way to adequately answer this question would be through a randomized prospective trial. Such a trial was just concluded at the Princess Margaret Hospital in Toronto, Canada, where patients with extremity soft tissue sarcoma were randomized to preoperative versus postoperative radiation. With 1.9 years median follow-up, six cases manifested local relapse and metastatic outcome and survival were similar.[216] Outcome analysis must await longer follow-up.

The technical aspects of preoperative radiation for the large part are similar to postoperative irradiation. The typical margin around the target volume is 5 to 7 cm in the longitudinal axis and 1.5 to 2.0 cm circumferentially. The definition of the target volume is different in the preoperative setting since it only includes the gross tumor volume identified on imaging, preferably MRI. This volume usually receives 50 Gy in 5.0 to 5.5 weeks. Surgery is usually performed 2.5 weeks later. Most institutions that use the preoperative approach do not add a boost except in patients with positive margins, where an additional 15 Gy is given.[198]

SPECIAL CONSIDERATIONS

POSITIVE MARGINS OF RESECTION

Positive microscopic margin was found to be an independent adverse prognostic factor for local relapse in 1041 patients with localized soft tissue sarcoma of the extremity (P = .0001).[184] Although adjuvant radiation has been shown to improve local control in soft tissue sarcoma of the extremity, its effect on patients with positive microscopic margin has not been clearly defined. Data from the Princess Margaret Hospital and Massachusetts General Hospital on patients treated with adjuvant radiation have shown a 10% to 16% increase in the 5-year local recurrence rates in patients with positive margins compared with those with negative margins despite the use of adjuvant irradiation.[217,218] In our trial of adjuvant BRT a total of 29 patients with positive margins were randomized: 15 to the BRT arm and 14 to the no BRT arm.[192] Five local failures were noted in each group (P= .99). These findings then beg the following question, when compared with surgery alone; does adjuvant irradiation improve local control in patients with positive margins of resection? Alektiar et al. evaluated 110 patients with primary high-grade soft tissue sarcoma of the extremity who were treated at MSKCC with surgery alone (19 patients) or with surgery and radiation (91 patients). The 5-year actuarial local control for the whole group was 71%. In the group that received adjuvant radiation the 5-year local control rate was 75% compared with 56% in those treated with surgery alone (P = .01). Adjuvant radiation also retained its significance as an independent prognostic factor for local control when multivariate analysis was performed (P = .01).[219] Whether any radiation modality is better than another in those patients is debatable possibly due to the paucity of data. Alekhteyar et al.[207] demonstrated a trend toward improvement in local control if BRT was supplemented with external-beam radiotherapy in patients with positive margins (90% vs. 59%, P= .08). However, others showed no difference in local control between external-beam irradiation and BRT boost.[218]

SMALL SOFT TISSUE SARCOMAS

Despite the fact that two randomized trials that compared surgery alone with adjuvant radiation have shown an improvement in local control in all patients, there is still considerable debate in the literature on whether all patients need adjuvant irradiation. Two large-scale studies that have looked at prognostic factors in soft tissue sarcomas of the extremity have failed to show a correlation between local control and tumor size in multivariate analysis.[184,220]

Geer et al., on the other hand, reported on 174 patients with primary soft tissue sarcoma of the extremity measuring less than or equal to 5 cm. When only patients with negative margins of resection were analyzed (159 patients), the 5-year local control rate was 77% in those who received adjuvant radiation compared with 92% with surgery alone (P= .08).[181] Therefore, the treatment policy at MSKCC has been to omit adjuvant irradiation in patients primarily treated at our institution with small tumors and adequate margins.

It is important, however, to consider other factors when deciding on whether to omit radiation. One such factor is the status of the surgical margin of resection. In the Geer study,[181] the effect of adjuvant radiation was only analyzed in the subset of patients with negative margins. In fact, patients with positive margins in that study had a 5-year local control rate of only 56% versus 88% in those with negative margins (P= .01). Similar finding were reported by Fleming et al. from M. D. Anderson Cancer Center.[182] Therefore, it is also our policy to treat patients with positive margins even if the tumors were less than or equal to 5 cm. The other factor that should be considered is whether the patient has had a prior unplanned excision. Noria et al. found a significantly higher rate of local recurrence in patients who were treated after unplanned excision on the outside compared with patients who receive their treatment at their institution (22% vs. 7%, P= .03).[221] It is important to remember that the previously mentioned scenario is common in the community settings when small soft tissue lesions are excised under the presumption that they are benign. Therefore, its is our policy to attempt a reexcision if at all feasible, otherwise patients are strongly considered for postoperative irradiation.

SOFT TISSUE SARCOMAS OF THE HANDS AND FEET

Soft tissue sarcomas of the distal extremity deserve special consideration since they pose a formidable challenge to the treating oncologist. For a start, a true wide local excision is the exception rather than the rule in these sites due to the lack of muscular bulk and the proximity to neurovascular structures and bone. In addition, the overall prognosis has been shown to be inferior to other sites in the extremity. Brien et al. showed that even in patients with hand tumors that are less than or equal to 5 cm, the survival rate was significantly lower than other extremity sites (P= .0008).[222]

In the past, the use of adjuvant irradiation was fraught with debate about the functional outcome in regions that have traditionally been considered poorly tolerant of radiation. However, more recently data to the contrary have been demonstrated. Talbert et al. treated 78 patients with nonmetastatic soft tissue sarcoma of the distal extremity with conservative surgery and radiation therapy. The 10-year local control rate was 74% and the salvage rate was 80% in patients who failed locally using this approach. The rate of amputation from complications was 8%.[223] Bray et al. also reported on 25 patients with soft tissue sarcoma of the hand and forearm. Twenty received adjuvant radiation and with a mean follow-up of 37 months, the local control rate was 88%. In addition, 88% of those who survived and did not require amputation were able to return to occupational and activities of daily living with minimal or no functional limitation.[224]

Therefore, conservative surgery and adjuvant radiation should be considered as an acceptable treatment modality for distal soft tissue sarcomas. Special attention, however, needs to be paid to radiation treatment technique in order to minimize complications and preserve function.

DEFINITIVE RADIATION

Surgery remains the main treatment for patients with sarcoma of the extremity, and every effort should be made to attempt resection. However, in some patients with unresectable disease definitive radiation could be considered due to medical reasons or to achieve some palliation. Since sarcoma may be radiocurable in terms of cell killing but not radioresponsive in terms of shrinkage of the mass, this can be perplexing, as such masses could give the false impression that little has been accomplished, whereas in reality the mass is mainly made up of sterilized tumor cells and debris. Tepper and Suit reported on 51 patients treated with definitive photon beam irradiation to a total dose of 64 to 66 Gy. The 5-year local control and survival rate were 33% and 25%, respectively. Local control was better for tumors less than 5 cm (87.5%) than in tumors 5 to 10 cm (53%) or greater than 10 cm (30%).[225] Slater et al. showed similar findings in 57 patients treated with definitive photon irradiation to 44 to 88 Gy. The 5-year local control was 28%.[226]

More recently, hyperfractionated photon radiation was combined with intravenous iododeoxyuridine as a radiosensitizer. Goffman et al. reported on 36 patients treated in this fashion, and with a median follow-up of 4 years the local control rate was 60%.[227]

Other investigators have looked at using neutron radiotherapy either alone or in combination with photon beam radiation. Schwarz et al. reviewed the European experience with such an approach and reported a local control rate of 50%, but the rate of severe complications ranged from 6.6% when neutron therapy was used as a boost to 50% when used alone.[228]

ADJUVANT CHEMOTHERAPY

Surgery remains the mainstay of therapy for soft tissue sarcoma in the control of local disease. As discussed previously, radiation therapy also plays a role in the local control of soft tissue sarcomas. Nonetheless, as many as one-half of all patients with adequate local control of disease develop distant metastasis, usually to the lungs (extremity sarcomas) or liver (abdominal primary).[229] As has been demonstrated in other cancers such as breast and colorectal cancer and osteosarcoma, it was hoped that adjuvant chemotherapy would help decrease the frequency of distant metastases, thus increasing overall survival. At least 15 studies of adjuvant therapy for soft tissue sarcoma have been performed. Since anthracyclines are the most active agents in sarcoma therapy in the metastatic setting, they have been used in nearly all of the adjuvant trials, alone or in combination. Most of these studies are small, and therefore lack the statistical power to detect small changes in overall survival. Accordingly, metaanalyses have been performed on the randomized trials for adjuvant chemotherapy in soft tissue sarcoma. In the following section the data from the individual studies and metaanalyses are examined (Table 39.1-9). Single-agent chemotherapy trials are considered first, followed by studies with combination chemotherapy.

RANDOMIZED ADJUVANT STUDIES OF DOXORUBICIN ALONE

One of the earliest studies to accrue patients in a randomized trial of adjuvant chemotherapy was performed by the Gynecologic Oncology Group for patients with uterine sarcomas.[230] Two hundred twenty-five patients with stage I or II uterine sarcomas of any histopathologic subtype were treated surgically for local control. Radiation was added at the discretion of the physician for local control, then patients were randomized to doxorubicin, 60 mg/m^2 every 3 weeks for eight cycles, or to observation alone. Of 156 evaluable patients, disease-free survival was not different between the two groups, nor was there a statistically significant difference in overall survival (73.7 months in the treated arm versus 55.0 months in the control arm). The addition of radiation therapy did not affect survival, although there was a lower rate of vaginal relapse in the group treated with radiation.

Between 1978 and 1982, the Dana-Farber Cancer Institute, Brigham and Women's Hospital, and Massachusetts General Hospital enrolled AJCC stage IIB to IVA patients in a study in which local therapy consisted of radical surgery, or wide *en bloc* excision followed by radiation.[231] Forty-two patients were randomized to receive five doses of doxorubicin, 90 mg /m^2, every 3 weeks, versus observation. The timing of chemotherapy varied between Dana-Farber Cancer Institute/Brigham and Women's Hospital and Massachusetts General Hospital, with former patients receiving both radiation and chemotherapy postoperatively, and the latter patients receiving radiation and two of the five cycles of chemotherapy before surgery. There was no significant difference in local control, relapse-free survival, or overall survival in this study, although there was a trend (not statistically significant) toward better overall survival of patients with extremity sarcomas who received chemotherapy compared with the patients who did not receive chemotherapy.

Similarly, the ECOG enrolled 47 AJCC stage IIB to IVA patients in a study in which local therapy consisted of radical surgery or wide *en bloc* excision followed by radiation.[232] Patients with local recurrence were permitted on the study as well. Thereafter, patients received doxorubicin, 70 mg/m^2 every 3 weeks for seven cycles. Thirty-two were eligible for analysis. There was no difference in local control, relapse-free survival, or overall survival in the treatment and control arms.

The Intergroup Sarcoma Study Group also examined AJCC stage IIB to IVA patients treated with surgery for local control. Seventy-eight eligible patients were randomized to observation or to doxorubicin at 35 mg/m^2 given as daily bolus doses on two consecutive days.[233,234] Six cycles of doxorubicin were given at 3-week intervals in the chemotherapy arm. There was no significant difference in local recurrence, disease-free survival, or overall survival in the chemotherapy arm compared with the control arm. A trend was noted toward improved disease-free survival for extremity lesions that was of borderline statistical significance ($P = .06$). However, pooling the data from the Boston, ECOG, and Intergroup studies demonstrated no survival benefit for adjuvant doxorubicin.[234]

The Scandinavian Sarcoma Group performed the largest study of doxorubicin as an adjuvant to local therapy for soft tissue sarcomas.[62] Two hundred forty patients were treated with surgery with the option of adjuvant radiation for local control. Patients were then randomized to receive either doxorubicin, 60 mg/m^2, every 4 weeks for nine cycles, or to no chemother-

TABLE 39.1-9. Adjuvant Studies in Soft Tissue Sarcoma

Study	*Regimen*	*Doxorubicin Dose (mg/m²)*	*No. of Patients Evaluable*	*Extremity Patients*	*Median Follow-Up (y)*[a]	*Reported Disease-Free Survival Control (%)*	*Reported Disease-Free Survival Treated (%)*	*Reported Overall Survival Control (%)*	*Reported Overall Survival Treated (%)*	*Reference*
National Cancer Institute extremity	CAM	50–70	65	65	7.1	54[b]	75[b]	60	83	240–242
National Cancer Institute head and neck/trunk/breast	CAM	50–70	31	0	3.0	49	77	58	68	244
National Cancer Institute retroperitoneal	CAM	50–70	15	0	2.4	84	50	100	47	245
Gynecologic Oncology Group	Dox	60	156	0	n/a	47	59	52	60	230
MDA	VACAR	60	47	43	>10	35[b]	55[b]	57	65	246,247
Mayo Clinic	VCAct/VAD	50	61	48	5.4	65	83	70	90	248
European Organization for Research and Treatment of Cancer	CyVADIC	50	317	216	6.7	43[b]	56[b]	55	63	249
Intergroup	Dox	70–90	78	50	1.7	55	73	70	91	233,234
European Cooperative Oncology Group	Dox	70	30	18	>4.9	55	66	52	65	232
Boston	Dox	90	42	25	>3.8	62	67	72	71	231,459
Scandinavian Sarcoma Group	Dox	60	181	155	3.3	n/a	n/a	n/a	n/a	62
Rizzoli	Dox	75	77	77	n/a	45[b,c]	73[b,c]	70[b,c]	91[b,c]	235,236
University of California Los Angeles	Dox	90	119	119	2.3	54[c]	58[c]	80[c]	85[c]	238
Bergonié	CyVADIC	50	59	36	4.4	32[b]	81[b]	54[b]	87[b]	250
RPMI	Dox	60–75	19	0	5.0	46	75	36	63	239
Italian Sarcoma Group	I/Epi	Epi at 120 mg/m²	104	n/a	3.0	37[b]	51[b]	55[b]	72[b]	251
1997 metaanalysis	Any	Various	1568	904	9.4	44[b]	52[b]	53	57	261

CAM, cyclophosphamide, doxorubicin, methotrexate; CyVADIC, cyclophosphamide, vincristine, doxorubicin, dacarbazine; Dox, doxorubicin; I/Epi, ifosfamide, epirubicin; MDA, M. D. Anderson Cancer Center; n/a, not available; RPMI, Roswell Park Memorial Institute; VACAR, vincristine, doxorubicin, cyclophosphamide, actinomycin D; VCAct/VAD, vincristine, cyclophosphamide, actinomycin D alternating with vincristine, doxorubicin, dacarbazine.
[a]Disease-free survival and overall survival are not necessarily indicated at the median follow-up time.
[b]Survival difference reached significance.
[c]Some patients on control arm received chemotherapy.

apy. Chemotherapy was started within 6 weeks of surgery when radiation was not used for local control, or within 10 weeks when radiation was used. One hundred eighty-one patients were evaluable; at a median follow-up of 40 months, there was no difference in local control, disease-free survival, or overall survival for the evaluable patients. Survival data was also assessed for the entire 240 patient cohort; again, there was no difference in disease-free survival or overall survival.

The Istituto Ortopedico Rizzoli examined a heterogeneous group of 77 patients with high-grade extremity sarcomas.[235] For local control some patients had radical surgery alone, surgery and preoperative radiation, or radiation and chemotherapy before surgical resection (the conservative surgery group). Thereafter patients were randomized to receive or not receive doxorubicin, 25 mg/m² given daily as boluses on 3 consecutive days in a 21-day cycle, for a total of six cycles. Relapse-free survival was improved in the chemotherapy arm (79% vs. 45%) at a median 28 months follow-up. In updated data from this study,[236] disease-free and overall survival were improved in the patients receiving chemotherapy. However, in a more recent update,[237] disease-free and overall survival benefit were not seen in the group treated with conservative surgery and chemotherapy versus conservative surgery alone. These data are difficult to analyze owing to the complex randomization scheme of the study as well as contamination of the control arm with patients receiving at least some chemotherapy (those receiving conservative surgery).

Investigators at the University of California, Los Angeles (UCLA) School of Medicine examined patients with high-grade extremity sarcoma, treating 119 patients with intraarterial doxorubicin for 3 days before radiation of the anatomic region and wide excision of the tumor.[238] Thereafter patients were randomized to observation alone versus five cycles of doxorubicin, 45 mg/m^2 daily as a bolus on 2 consecutive days, once a month. At a median follow-up time of 28 months, there was no improvement in either disease-free or overall survival in the chemotherapy arm. There was a statistically insignificant improvement in local control rates in the chemotherapy arm (3 of 21 patients vs. 9 of 27 patients in the control arm relapsed). The use of intraarterial preoperative doxorubicin in the control arm complicates comparison with the other doxorubicin adjuvant studies.

At Roswell Park Memorial Institute, 19 patients with stage I uterine sarcoma were randomized to surgery alone versus surgery plus adjuvant doxorubicin, 60 to 75 mg/m^2 every 4 weeks for six cycles.[239] No statistically significant difference in survival was noted. Six of the patients randomized to the chemotherapy arm refused randomization and were assessed as part of the control group, instead of using an intention-to-treat analysis.

RANDOMIZED ADJUVANT STUDIES OF COMBINATION CHEMOTHERAPY

In 1983 the NCI published the first in a series of publications on adjuvant chemotherapy for soft tissue sarcoma of different anatomic sites. A pilot study examined 26 patients with extremity sarcoma grades II and III, treated for local control with amputation or limb-sparing surgery with radiation.[240] These patients were treated postoperatively with escalating doses of cyclophosphamide (500 to 700 mg/m^2) and doxorubicin (50 to 70 mg/m^2) every 28 days, with a maximum cumulative dose of 550 mg/m^2 of doxorubicin. This combination was followed by six cycles of intermediate dose methotrexate (50 to 250 mg/kg with dose escalation). Patients were randomized to receive chemotherapy with or without C. parvum adjuvant immunotherapy, and were compared with historic controls. There was no effect of the immunologic adjuvant, but the overall survival at 5 years was 73%, better than the 45% seen in the historic controls.

These initial data led to examination of adjuvant chemotherapy alone in a second cohort of patients with extremity sarcomas. Sixty-five patients underwent similar local control as described previously, then were randomized to observation or to the same cyclophosphamide, doxorubicin, and methotrexate regimen of the pilot study.[240,241] Initial data indicated that disease-free survival and overall survival were improved in the chemotherapy arm. With longer follow-up (median, 7.1 years), 5-year disease-free survival was still improved (75% vs. 54% in the control arm), but the difference in overall survival (83% vs. 60% in the control arm) was not statistically significant.[242] Local control was improved in the chemotherapy arm. In long-term follow-up there has been non–tumor-related mortality; there continues to be no survival advantage in either treatment arm (J. Yang, S. Rosenberg, unpublished results).

Fourteen of the 101 patients treated with the NCI regimen developed clinical congestive heart failure. Other patients had radioventriculograms performed confirming a subclinical decrease in cardiac ejection fraction at rest or with exercise. In all, there was an overall event rate of 46% clinical or subclinical cardiomyopathy in the 75 evaluated patients.[243] The high rate of cardiomyopathy led to a third trial examining the same cyclophosphamide, doxorubicin, and methotrexate combination versus a regimen without methotrexate and a doxorubicin ceiling cumulative dose of 350 mg/m^2.[242] No difference in 5-year overall survival was observed (69% for low dose, 75% for high dose), nor was there a difference in 5-year disease-free survival. There was no clinical congestive heart failure documented in the low-dose arm, and the decrease in cardiac ejection fraction by nuclear medicine study was less pronounced than with the high-dose arm.

The NCI has also examined adjuvant chemotherapy for other sites in two other trials, using the same cyclophosphamide, doxorubicin, and methotrexate combination regimen.[244,245] In one study, some of the 37 patients with retroperitoneal sarcoma (15 of whom were prospectively randomized) were given adjuvant chemotherapy.[245] Patients given chemotherapy had a trend to poorer overall survival compared with the control group (P = .06). Analysis of this study is difficult because of the small number of patients and lack of prospective randomization for all patients. A separate NCI study using the same chemotherapy regimen examined 31 patients with soft tissue sarcoma of the head and neck, breast, and trunk.[244] All patients had resection and postoperative radiation, then were randomized to receive chemotherapy or no further therapy. Six patients received C. parvum adjuvant immunotherapy. A trend toward improved disease-free survival was seen in the chemotherapy patients, but there was no statistically significant difference in overall survival.

The M. D. Anderson Cancer Center started one of the earliest adjuvant trials for soft tissue sarcoma.[246,247] Because of their high local relapse rate, patients with head and neck or abdominal sarcomas all received surgery, radiation, and chemotherapy in this study. Forty-three eligible patients with trunk and extremity sarcomas were treated with local therapy (surgery and radiation) with or without chemotherapy. The chemotherapy regimen consisted of vincristine, oral cyclophosphamide, and doxorubicin every 4 weeks. After seven cycles of doxorubicin-based therapy, actinomycin D was substituted for doxorubicin in a maintenance phase to complete 2 years of chemotherapy. The initial results demonstrated poorer disease-free survival in the chemotherapy arm (76% vs. 83% for the control arm, P value not significant) and double the rate of metastasis in the chemotherapy arm (but P >.3), and the study was stopped. However, the original study stratified patients by histology, not by tumor grade. In a reanalysis of this data of the patients with truncal or extremity sarcomas, disease-free survival was improved in the chemotherapy arm (55% vs. 35% at 10 years, P = .05), although there was no difference in overall survival in the two groups.[247]

Another early study of combination chemotherapy was reported by the Mayo Clinic.[248] Sixty-one patients with sarcomas of the trunk or extremities were treated with surgery alone for local control, then randomized to no further therapy or to chemotherapy. The chemotherapy alternated between cycles of vincristine, actinomycin D, and cyclophosphamide and cycles of vincristine, doxorubicin, and dacarbazine, given at 6-week intervals for eight courses. Thirteen patients (randomly selected from either group) were given bacilles Calmette-Guérin methanol extraction residue as nonspecific immunotherapy, but this was discontinued owing to ulceration at the injection site. There was no benefit in overall survival in the chemotherapy arm, and there was a high local recurrence rate, likely due to the omission of radiation in the local control phase of therapy. The chemotherapy regimen used in this study had low dose intensity by today's standards.

The largest single study of adjuvant combination chemotherapy in soft tissue sarcoma was performed by the EORTC.[249] Four hundred sixty-eight patients (excluding only very low grade sarcomas) were treated with surgery for their primary sarcoma, and with adjuvant radiation used for margins less than 1 cm. Patients were randomized to receive or not receive combination chemotherapy with cyclophosphamide, vincristine, doxorubicin, and dacarbazine (CyVADIC; Table 39.1-10), given every 28 days for eight cycles. Disease-free survival and local control were both better in the chemotherapy arm, but overall survival was not significantly different between the two arms. Improvement in local recurrence rates was limited to patients with head, neck, and trunk sarcomas and was not observed for patients with extremity sarcomas. Some criticism has been raised as to the long accrual time of the study (11 years), inability of nearly half of patients to complete all eight cycles of chemotherapy, and the relatively large number of patients ineligible for analysis, which most commonly was due to inappropriate radiation therapy.

A smaller study from the Fondation Bergonié also examined the CyVADIC regimen as adjuvant therapy.[250] Following local therapy with surgery and radiation, 59 eligible patients with AJCC stage IIB to IVA tumors were randomized to receive no chemotherapy or CyVADIC chemotherapy, in doses similar to the EORTC study. In comparison with the EORTC trial, patients were treated with chemotherapy sooner after surgery, and on 21-day cycles, as opposed to 28-day cycles in the EORTC study. More patients with extremity sarcomas were in the chemotherapy group, and the histology of the treated groups was different (e.g., more MFH and no undifferentiated sarcoma in the chemotherapy arm). In contrast to the EORTC trial, local control, distant metastasis-free survival ($P = .003$), and overall survival ($P = .002$) were better in the chemotherapy arm than the control arm. However, in comparison with the EORTC study, the chemotherapy arm fared better (5-year survival 85% vs. 68% for the EORTC study), and the control group performed more poorly (5-year survival under 37%, compared with 63% in the EORTC trial).

The Italian Sarcoma Study Group reported in abstract form the only trial to date to examine an anthracycline plus ifosfamide as adjuvant therapy for extremity sarcoma.[251] After surgery with or without local radiation, 104 patients were randomized to receive no chemotherapy or to receive ifosfamide (1.8 g/m^2 on 5 consecutive days) with epirubicin (60 mg/m^2 on 2 consecutive days), with filgrastim support. Interim analysis in 1996 led to early conclusion of the trial. At a median follow-up of 36 months, overall survival in the chemotherapy arm was 72% compared with 55% for the control arm ($P = .002$). This investigation is promising for its use of the two most active agents against sarcoma in an appropriate cohort of patients. Review of the final

TABLE 39.1-10. Combination Chemotherapy for Sarcoma: A Comparison of Formulations

Regimen	*Dose*	*Comments*
Doxorubicin	60–90 mg/m^2	Bolus or IVCI over 3–4 d q3w
Ifosfamide		
Standard dosing	5 g/m^2	24 hour IVCI with mesna q3–4w
High dose	2–3 g/m^2/d	Bolus or IVCI with mesna for 4 d q3–4w
AD		
Doxorubicin	60 mg/m^2	Bolus, or IVCI over 3–4 d q3w
Dacarbazine	750–1000 mg/m^2	
MAID		
Doxorubicin	60 mg/m^2	Bolus, or divided over 3 d by bolus or IVCI q3–4w
Ifosfamide with mesna	2.0–2.5 g/m^2	Bolus, or IVCI × 3 d q3–4w with mesna
Dacarbazine	900–1000 mg/m^2	Bolus or over 3 d IVCI q3-4w
AI or AIM		
Doxorubicin	50–75 mg/m^2	Bolus, or divided over 2–3 d by bolus or IVCI q3–4w
Ifosfamide (with mesna)	5.0–7.5 g/m^2	Daily over 3 d or IVCI q3–4w with mesna
MAP		
Mitomycin C	8 mg/m^2	Boluses, q3w
Doxorubicin	40 mg/m^2	
Cisplatin	60 g/m^2	
CyVADIC		
Cyclophosphamide	500 mg/m^2	
Vincristine	1 mg/m^2 days 1,5; max 1.5 mg/dose	
Doxorubicin	50 mg/m^2	Bolus q3w
Dacarbazine	250 mg/m^2/d × 5	

IVCI, intravenous continuous infusion.

data will be necessary to assess patient selection and follow-up before conclusions can be drawn concerning this data.

CONCLUSIONS FROM INDIVIDUAL ADJUVANT CHEMOTHERAPY STUDIES

Clearly, the small size of these trials makes interpretation on an individual basis difficult, since such studies have no statistical power to detect small (e.g., 10% to 20%) changes in overall survival. In many of the studies, a significant proportion of patients was ineligible for analysis, raising the question of selection bias. A second example of selection bias arises from the fact that patients who are enrolled on clinical trials are healthier overall than nonrandomized patients, and survive longer, as demonstrated in the Mayo study.[248] Historic controls are inadequate for comparison as there continue to be advances in diagnosis, specific therapy, and supportive care that could affect outcome.[240]

Beyond general problems with randomized studies, staging and dose intensity also affect our ability to draw conclusions about individual studies. A number of patients with low-grade or small tumors are included in the trials described previously. Patients with high-grade sarcomas do well as long as the primary disease is small (less than 5 cm). The improved outcome with small, high-grade tumors has been incorporated into the most recent staging system for sarcoma.[252] Future studies must focus on patients with large tumors at high risk of relapse. Furthermore, dose intensity of doxorubicin is low to moderate in many studies of adjuvant chemotherapy to date, and largely did not have growth factors such as filgrastim available. It is reasonably clear that doxorubicin and ifosfamide show dose-dependent responses,[253–258] and with better supportive care more intensive therapy may lead to improved survival. It is hoped that the first studies evaluating the use of adjuvant chemotherapy using an anthracycline combined with ifosfamide with growth factors[251] will give further direction to future studies in the adjuvant therapy of sarcomas.

METAANALYSES OF RANDOMIZED TRIALS OF ADJUVANT CHEMOTHERAPY FOR SARCOMA

Given the lack of statistical power of the existing randomized trials, it was hoped that combining the data from individual studies of adjuvant chemotherapy for sarcoma would reveal improvement in overall survival that could not be detected in smaller studies. For example, to detect a 10% difference between control group and treatment group with a power of 0.90 would require approximately 1000 patients to be enrolled in a randomized study.

Antman and colleagues[234] pooled the data for three randomized studies (ECOG, Dana-Farber Cancer Institute/Massachusetts General Hospital, and the Intergroup studies). The 168 eligible patients examined in this study make up a smaller group than the EORTC adjuvant trial, but were followed for up to 11 years in some cases. Patients with extremity lesions fared better than those with other sites of disease ($P = .02$), but there was no difference in overall survival in those receiving chemotherapy versus control patients.

Zalupski et al.[259] examined overall and disease-free survival in patients with extremity sarcoma obtained from ten of the adjuvant studies mentioned previously. Data was extracted from the text and tables of each study. The combined data indicated a 10% absolute improvement in overall survival (from 71% to 81%, $P = .0005$) and 15% improvement in disease-free survival (53% vs. 68%, $P < .00001$). Criticism of this metaanalysis includes the fact that potentially inappropriate patients were included (e.g., those from the Rizzoli and UCLA studies who received preoperative chemotherapy). In addition, some of the data were relatively immature as well, such as the EORTC and Bergonié studies.

Tierney and colleagues assessed 15 published studies 2 years later and converted the survival data into the odds of recurrence based on the latest available publication from each trial.[260] Standardization was performed to account for different lengths of follow-up. In all, 1546 patients were included in the study, which showed improved survival at 2 years and at 5 years in the 13 and 11 studies eligible for analysis at each time point, respectively. In contrast to the previous metaanalysis from Zalupski et al.,[259] the Rizzoli data were included in this study, but not the data from UCLA.

The most rigorous metaanalysis was published in 1997.[261] In this study, 23 potential studies were considered, and 14 ultimately included; only 31 potential patients were omitted due to unavailability of data, giving a cohort of 1568 patients to examine. Patient accrual had to be complete by the end of 1992, which excluded one trial. Histology for each patient was recorded, but pathology review was not centralized. Median follow-up was 9.4 years. Analyses were stratified by trial, and hazard ratios were calculated for each trial and combined, allowing for an assessment of the risk of death or recurrence in comparison with control patients. Disease-free survival at 10 years was found to be improved from 45% to 55% and was statistically significant ($P = .0001$). Local disease-free survival at 10 years also favored the chemotherapy arm, improving from 75% to 81% ($P = .016$). However, overall survival, while improving at 10 years from 50% to 54%, was not statistically significant ($P = .12$). The largest difference in overall survival was found in subgroup analysis of the 886 patients with extremity sarcomas, in which absolute overall survival was shown to increase 7% in the group receiving chemotherapy ($P = .029$).

CONCLUSIONS: ADJUVANT CHEMOTHERAPY FOR SOFT TISSUE SARCOMAS

The data from the metaanalyses described previously must be examined with caution. Although the most recent metaanalysis is a useful tool, it still combines studies with different designs, diverse criteria for enrollment, variations in pathologic assessment such as grading, different chemotherapeutic regimens, and different end points. In particular, only one-fourth of the specimens from the 1997 metaanalysis underwent review of tumor grade; approximately 60% were reviewed for histologic subtype. Of 15 published adjuvant studies, only two, the Rizzoli and Bergonié studies, show improved overall survival in the chemotherapy arm. Only one small study included in the 1997 metaanalysis used ifosfamide, another active agent in sarcoma.

If there is a benefit for the adjuvant use of chemotherapy, it appears modest, based on the previously mentioned data. Given no statistically significant benefit in a population of patients typically healthier than patients not enrolled on protocols, the data do not support the routine use of adjuvant chemotherapy for soft tissue sarcoma outside of the setting of a clinical trial. However, moderate to large extremity lesions represent one situation in which adjuvant chemotherapy may be considered on a case-by-case basis. The subset analysis of extremity data from the 1997 metaanalysis indicates this is one situation in which adjuvant chemotherapy can be considered. However, subset analyses are used to generate hypotheses and do not necessarily give definitive results. Publication of the more recent Italian study of epirubicin and ifosfamide as adjuvant therapy for extremity sarcomas may clarify this situation further. With clear definition of a population at high risk for metastatic disease, identification of relatively sensitive histologic subtypes of sarcoma, and use of combinations of active agents, it is hoped that future studies will delineate which clinical situations merit use of adjuvant chemotherapy.

PREOPERATIVE CHEMOTHERAPY

Preoperative chemotherapy has been successful in the management of predominantly pediatric sarcomas such as Ewing's sarcoma and osteosarcoma. With this success, the concept was extended to use in adult soft tissue sarcomas. Preoperative neoadjuvant chemotherapy can make subsequent surgery easier and potentially treats micrometastatic disease earlier before acquisition of resistance. Treating with chemotherapy before surgery also leaves primary vasculature intact for drug delivery. In addition, preoperative chemotherapy can guide postoperative treatment based on pathologic review of the tissue after chemotherapy. In experimental models, preoperative chemotherapy eliminates a postoperative surge in growth of metastases noted after resection of primary tumors.[262,263]

There is relatively little evidence concerning the use of neoadjuvant chemotherapy in the treatment of soft tissue sarcomas. Rouesse et al. retrospectively examined a group of 34 patients with locally advanced sarcomas for whom only amputation or mutilating surgery was feasible.[264] Patients received doxorubicin-based chemotherapy for two to seven cycles before resection. Postoperative radiation was offered to some patients. Partial or complete responses were noted in over one-third of patients; not surprisingly, those patients who had a complete response by any means had a better overall survival than those who did not respond completely. Local recurrence was common in the responding group, as well.

A retrospective trial of 46 patients from M. D. Anderson Cancer Center examined preoperative chemotherapy using cyclophosphamide, doxorubicin, and dacarbazine.[265] Forty percent of patients demonstrated complete, partial, or minor responses to chemotherapy and had better rates of survival than the patients who did not have an objective clinical response to chemotherapy.

A prospective trial was performed at MSKCC in which 29 patients with large, high-grade, primary or recurrent metastases were given two cycles of combination chemotherapy before definitive therapy with surgery and radiation.[266] Clinical and radiologic studies were performed before chemotherapy, and the specimen was assessed for response after surgical resection. Only 1 of 29 patients demonstrated a clinical partial response, although liquefaction, cystic necrosis, and hemorrhage into the tumor were noted regularly in the resected specimen, with three tumors showing greater than 90% necrosis. Most patients did not elect to receive postoperative chemotherapy after surgery, and survival results from this study did not differ significantly from studies of adjuvant doxorubicin or of no chemotherapy.

Assessing the response to preoperative chemotherapy in primary soft tissue sarcomas is difficult. Some softening or liquefaction can be noted clinically without significant change in tumor size, but in the trial from MSKCC neither CT nor MRI provided information that predicted long-term outcome. It appears that there are significantly fewer cases of complete response compared with preoperative adjuvant chemotherapy for sarcoma of bone (osteosarcoma or Ewing's sarcoma), and it is difficult to objectively evaluate responses grossly or microscopically after chemotherapy. Other imaging modalities may demonstrate changes consistent with chemotherapy effect (MRI spectroscopy, PET, gallium scan, thallium scan),[267–271] but these modalities remain investigational.

In sum, preoperative chemotherapy is given to some patients with potentially sensitive sarcoma subtypes such as synovial sarcoma or other high-grade lesions. It is clear from the present AJCC staging system that larger, deep, high-grade lesions have a high risk of metastasis.[252] Thus, it is conceivable that local control could improve with adjuvant chemotherapy, without significantly changing overall survival. Nonetheless, preoperative chemotherapy may be considered during an attempt to maintain function of an extremity, with the possibility that more aggressive surgery could be performed later if needed. Selected patients have had responses that allow for a more conservative resection, avoid an amputation, or both.

INTRAARTERIAL CHEMOTHERAPY

There have been many studies examining the role of intraarterial chemotherapy, with doxorubicin, cisplatinum, or both; in some situations other drugs have been used as well. This infusional approach is to be differentiated from local limb perfusion, discussed later in the section Hyperthermia and Limb Perfusion. Intraarterial chemotherapy has the potential benefit of providing higher doses of chemotherapy to the limb in a first-pass effect. However, pharmacokinetic data have not shown an advantage over intravenous chemotherapy.[272]

Intraarterial chemotherapy has been used in conjunction with radiation as well. Mention has already been made of the UCLA adjuvant study in which patients received 3 days of intraarterial doxorubicin before administration of 35 Gy of external-beam radiation over 10 days, or 17.5 Gy administered over 5 days.[273] Patients were then randomized to receive postoperative doxorubicin intravenously or no further chemotherapy. No difference in survival or local control was noted in this study. Thereafter, a randomized trial by the same group examined preoperative intravenous versus intraarterial chemotherapy before radiation (28 Gy given over 8 days) followed by wide excision. There was no difference in local recurrence or survival between the 45 patients receiving intraarterial doxorubicin and the 54 patients receiving intravenous doxorubicin.[274]

A number of studies have examined intraarterial chemotherapy before radiation and surgery,[275,276] doxorubicin alone,[273,277] or in combination with other drugs such as cisplatin,[275,278,279] single agent intraarterial cisplatin,[280] or intraarterial doxorubicin in combination with intravenous doxorubicin or other agents.[281] Doxorubicin with simultaneous radiation has also been examined.[282,283] In these studies, some patients have been able to avoid amputation. Infusional chemotherapy has its attendant complications as well, including arterial thromboembolism, infection, gangrene, and problems with wound healing, itself requiring amputation. Pathologic fractures have been reported in patients receiving chemotherapy and relatively large doses of radiation. One study[283] reported ten major complications in 13 patients treated intraarterial chemotherapy with simultaneous radiation, emphasizing the investigational nature of this approach. Although there are situations in which such therapy should be considered, intraarterial chemotherapy at present has a limited role in the treatment of extremity sarcomas.

HYPERTHERMIA AND LIMB PERFUSION

In contrast to systemic intraarterial chemotherapy infusion, perfusion of limbs requires isolation of the arterial and venous system of the limb by means of a tourniquet and obtaining access to arteries and veins supplying the limb. The arterial and venous supply of the limb is connected to an extracorporeal circulation system to isolate the limb from the rest of the body. Recirculation of the blood from the limb is performed by a heart-lung machine to reoxygenate the blood. Care is taken after isolation of the limb to ensure no leakage of the circuit into the systemic circulation; technetium-labeled albumin is injected into the circuit and a probe is used over the heart to ensure isolation of the bypass circuit. Since mild hyperthermia may make chemotherapy more effective in some clinical settings (as mentioned in this section), the blood of the circuit is often warmed to 39° to 40°C.

A number of chemotherapeutic agents have been used for limb perfusion, such as melphalan, nitrogen mustard, actinomycin D, and doxorubicin. The most effective agents to date have been melphalan when given with tumor necrosis factor (TNF). The greatest experience with this technique comes from Eggermont et al.[284,285] Two hundred forty-six patients with primary or recurrent sarcomas that would otherwise require amputation or marked loss of function were treated with one and occasionally two isolated limb perfusion sessions. After isolation of the extremity, melphalan (10 to 13 mg/L limb volume) was perfused into the limb with a dose of TNF ten times the lethal dose for humans, under mild hyperthermic conditions. In early studies interferon-α was included in the regimen, but was later dropped, as it did not appear to improve results over melphalan and TNF alone. Both components of the regimen appeared important; the omission of TNF led to a decrease in tissue dose of melphalan, probably from its effects on the tumor vasculature. Surgery to remove residual tumor was performed 2 to 4 months after limb perfusion. With a median follow-up of 3 years, 71% of patients had successful limb salvage.

It is difficult to compare this approach with standard chemotherapy, given the heterogeneity of patients between the two types of studies. In aggregate, the response rate does appear higher in the perfusion studies than in the infusion studies. However, isolated limb perfusion requires substantial expertise and specialized dedicated equipment. Complications of this technique include shock (from systemic leak of TNF); infection; chronic damage to skin, muscles, and nerve; persistent edema; and arterial or venous thrombosis. Experience has led to a decrease in the incidence and severity of complications. Isolated limb perfusion does appear to hold promise for at least a subset of patients who would otherwise require amputation for local control and has been approved for such patients in Europe. Studies are underway to examine the utility of regional limb infusion, which would not require bypass machines, as a simplified means of treating otherwise unresectable extremity sarcomas.

Hyperthermia has been used in other ways to enhance the effects of chemotherapy in patients with locally advanced disease. Whole body hyperthermia using extracorporeal heating of blood has been combined with ifosfamide and carboplatin intravenous chemotherapy, and responses have been seen in patients with otherwise refractory small cell sarcomas.[286] Regional hyperthermia provided through an external magnetic field (phased array) has been examined in combination with ifosfamide and etoposide.[287] Similarly, hyperthermia achieved with an external electromagnetic field has been combined with ifosfamide, etoposide, and doxorubicin.[288] In both studies, partial and complete responses in patients with locally advanced sarcoma have been observed. The hyperthermia used in these protocols is more aggressive than that used with limb perfusion; higher temperatures have led to a higher rate of local complications. Isolated limb perfusion has not been compared directly with simultaneous hyperthermia and chemotherapy. In sum, isolated limb perfusion and hyperthermia-enhanced chemotherapy represent novel ways of attempting to preserve function of limbs in what otherwise would be situations in which amputation would be necessary. In the United States, such procedures remain investigational at present.

SPECIAL FEATURES OF THE MANAGEMENT OF SARCOMAS OF NONEXTREMITY SITES

MANAGEMENT OF VISCERAL/RETROPERITONEAL SARCOMA

Clinical Presentation

Most patients present with an asymptomatic abdominal mass (Fig. 39.1-22). On occasion pain is present and, less commonly, gastrointestinal bleeding, incomplete obstruction, or neurologic symptoms relating to retroperitoneal invasion or pressure on neurovascular structures are present. Weight loss is uncommon and incidental diagnosis is often the norm. In one report,[289] neurologic symptoms related primarily to an expanding retroperitoneal mass were identified in 27% of patients.

On physical examination, a large abdominal mass is often present. Important issues of differential diagnosis, particularly

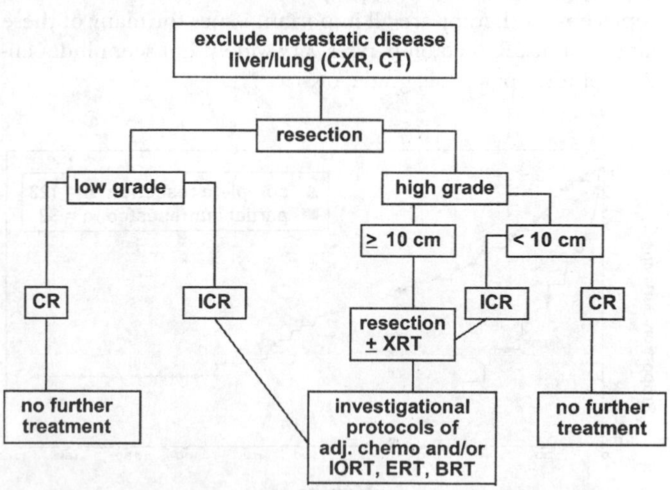

FIGURE 39.1-22. Algorithm for the management of retroperitoneal or visceral sarcoma. BRT, brachytherapy; CR, complete resection; CT, computed tomography; CXR, chest radiography; ERT, external-beam radiation therapy; ICR, incomplete resection; IORT, intraoperative radiation therapy; x-ray therapy.

in the young, are the presence of a germ cell tumor or a primary retroperitoneal tumor arising from the adrenal. Most of such lesions, however, are tumors of mesenchymal origin, either benign or malignant.

USE OF IMAGING STUDIES. In the main, CT remains the primary modality for evaluation of retroperitoneal and visceral sarcomas. Because the most likely site of visceral metastasis is the liver, a CT scan of the abdomen and pelvis usually encompasses description not only of the primary lesion, but also of the most likely source of metastasis. For retroperitoneal lesions, the incidence of metastatic disease to the liver is possible but still low.

Of the histopathologic types, leiomyosarcoma and liposarcoma predominate (see Fig. 39.1-4), whereas other types seen in the extremity, such as MFH, are very uncommon. Most retroperitoneal tumors are high-grade lesions because of the predominance of leiomyosarcoma in the visceral lesions. The retroperitoneal liposarcoma is often predominantly low grade and overall the more common tumor. Nevertheless, with increasing frequency we note the mixed cellularity and grade of some retroperitoneal sarcomas.

Primary surgical resection is the dominant therapeutic modality. Preoperative bowel preparation is important, not because of tumor invasion, but often because of the technical difficulty of resection without encompassing the intestine. Because many tumors involve the retroperitoneum, evaluation of renal function, particularly the establishment of contralateral adequate renal function, is important, to allow nephrectomy where appropriate.

Although resection of adjacent organs is common[289] proof that a more extensive resection of adjacent organs has an effect on long-term survival seems limited. It is clear that complete surgical resection is the primary factor in outcome (Fig. 39.1-23). Once complete resection is accounted for, the predominant factor in outcome is the grade of the lesion.

TECHNICAL ISSUES. The major issue in resection of such lesions is adequate exposure. Thoracoabdominal incisions, rectus-dividing incisions, incisions extending through the inguinal ligament into the thigh, the availability of venovenous bypass, adequate and appropriate anesthetic, and blood replacement therapy are all important issues for many of these large lesions. Resectability rates vary widely, but seem independent of histologic type, grade, or size.[289]

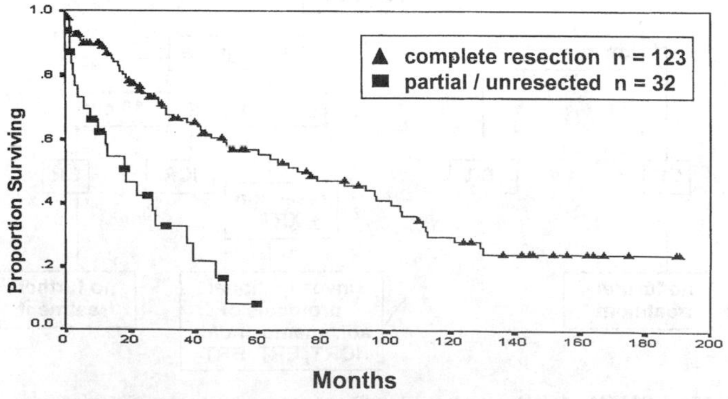

FIGURE 39.1-23. Survival following resection of primary retroperitoneal sarcoma according to resection status in 155 patients aged 16 years or older admitted to Memorial Sloan-Kettering Cancer Center between July 1982 and July 1999 ($P<.001$).

These factors should not preclude attempts at reresection. Complete resection is usually possible in 60% to 70% of patients presenting with a second or subsequent recurrence. In our reviews,[289,290] although nephrectomy was commonly performed (in 46% of cases), the kidney itself was rarely involved. In the report by Jaques and coworkers[289] only 2 of 30 nephrec tomies showed true parenchymal invasion. Nevertheless, the encompassment of the kidney and the involvement of the hilar renal vasculature all make the resection of the kidney on occasions technically necessary.

The overriding principle is not to be reticent about resection of adjacent organs should they be involved by tumor. Conversely, one should not resect uninvolved organs if they are not the limiting factor in the margins. For example, the resection of a kidney, when the vena cava is the closest margin, makes little oncologic sense. Overall, the use of debulking for recurrent lesions is rarely of significant value in terms of long-term survival. More extended resections do not seem to improve local recurrence or survival. It is often difficult to decide how much can be palliated by incomplete removal of tumor. The concept, however, should be that unless palliation can be achieved, operation should be reserved for those patients for whom complete resection is at least possible, if not probable. The basis for unresectability is usually the presence of peritoneal implants or extensive vascular involvement.

Retroperitoneal sarcomas remain a major clinical challenge. Most of these tumors are large, making it difficult to obtain adequate margins of resection. Compounding the problem, the presence of normal organ such as small bowel, large bowel, kidney, and liver make delivery of therapeutic doses of radiation therapy either difficult or impossible.

Jaques and coworkers[289] reported the experience at MSKCC from 1982 to 1987. One-half of the patients presented with liposarcoma, whereas 29% had leiomyosarcoma. Sixty-five percent of primary sarcomas underwent a complete resection, whereas approximately one-half the patients with recurrent retroperitoneal sarcomas could have a complete resection. Despite complete resection, local recurrence developed in approximately 40% to 50% of cases. There is a clear need for adjuvant local therapy. Importantly, local recurrence is a problem for both high-grade and low-grade lesions: The local recurrence rate is similar, but the time to recurrence differs significantly. The median time for recurrence was 15 months for high-grade and 42 months for low-grade sarcomas. Fifty-three percent of patients required adjacent organ resection, and 40% of patients required more than one adjacent organ resection, in order to accomplish complete removal of disease.

Adjuvant external-beam irradiation is limited because of the low tolerance of surrounding normal organs. However, there are data to suggest some improvement in local control with moderate doses of external-beam irradiation.[291,292] Tepper and associates[293] reviewed a cohort of 23 patients with retroperitoneal sarcomas treated with surgery and radiation therapy. For patients who underwent a complete resection, local control was 71%. Radiation dose appeared to influence tumor control, with only 30% of patients locally controlled at doses less than 5000 cGy and 83% of patients controlled with doses greater than 6000 cGy. Obviously, the total dose of radiation that is possible varies with the size and location of that lesion.

With the need to deliver higher doses of radiation to the tumor and lower doses to surrounding tissue, there has been an interest in using intraoperative radiation therapy (IORT).[294,295] Petersen et al. from the Mayo Clinic reported on 87 patients who were treated with IORT that was supplemented by external-beam radiation in 80/87. With a median follow-up of 3 years, the 5-year local control and survival rates were 58% and 50%, respectively.[296] Sindelar and coworkers[297] reported a prospective, randomized clinical trial utilizing intraoperative radiation therapy at the NCI. Thirty-five patients with surgically resected sarcomas of the retroperitoneum were randomized to receive IORT (20 Gy) followed by low-dose external-beam irradiation (35 to 40 Gy) versus external-beam radiation therapy alone (50 to 55 Gy). The study revealed a significant improvement in local control for those who received IORT. There was no effect on survival. Patients who received IORT also received misonidazole, and they had a higher incidence of peripheral neuropathy than those who received external-beam radiation alone. On the other hand, those who received higher dose external-beam radiation alone, without IORT, had a higher incidence of radiation enteritis.

To build on the NCI data, we have begun to examine IORT at MSKCC. Instead of using electron beam IORT, we have used a technique that involves high-dose-rate remote afterloading. All patients had a maximal tumor resection. At the time of surgery, a dose of 12 to 15 Gy was delivered with IORT. Postoperative external irradiation of 45 Gy was added. No misonidazole was given. The concept is that this dose of IORT without misonidazole should result in a significantly lower incidence of neuropathy than the experience of the NCI, and this dose of external-beam irradiation should result in lower risk of radiation enteritis. Alektiar et al. reported on 32 patients treated with such an approach.[298] With a median follow-up of 33 months, the 5-year actuarial local control and overall survival rates were 62% and 45%, receptively. The rate of peripheral neuropathy was 6% and the rate of gastrointestinal toxicity was 19%.

MANAGEMENT OF HEAD AND NECK SARCOMA

Soft tissue sarcomas of the head and neck in adults are rare. They represent approximately 1% of all head and neck malignancies and 10% of all soft tissue sarcomas. Most of these tumors present as a painless subcutaneous or submucosal mass. Any histologic type of soft tissue sarcoma could originate in the head and neck area, but there is preponderance of angiosarcoma in this site. Multimodality approach is the cornerstone for most soft tissue sarcomas of the head and neck. Surgery is the main treatment for these tumors, and every attempt should be made to obtain at least gross total resection, otherwise the results are usually poor. However, unlike extremity sarcomas, head and neck sarcomas are not amenable to wide local excision with generous margin of normal tissue due to anatomic constraints. Therefore, the use of adjuvant radiation is more liberal in this site because local recurrence could be the cause of death in a substantial proportion of patients.

Eeles et al. reported on 103 patients with soft tissue sarcoma of the head and neck area treated by surgery with or without radiation. The 5-year survival rate was 50% and the local control rate was 47%. The only independent prognostic factor for survival was surgery other than biopsy ($P = .003$). For local control the combined use of surgery and radiation as opposed to single modality was also an independent prognostic factor ($P = .002$). In addition, local tumor was the cause of death in 63% of cases.[299] Willers et al. reported on 46 patients with soft tissue sarcoma excluding angiosarcoma who were treated by radiation with or without surgery. The 5-year survival and local control rates were 74% and 69%, respectively. On multivariate analysis survival correlated with low grade, recurrent presentation, and lack of direct extension ($P = .001$, .01, .03, respectively). For local control the only independent prognostic factor was the T stage ($P = .05$). There was also a 15-fold increased risk of dying for patients whose tumor had recurred locoregionally, compared with controlled sarcomas ($P = .004$).[300]

Le et al. reported on 65 patients treated by surgery with or without radiation and found the 5-year survival and local control rates to be 56% and 66%, respectively. On multivariate analysis the independent predictors of improved survival were age less than 55 ($P = .009$), low grade ($P = .0002$), extent of resection ($P = .008$), and negative margin ($P = .0009$). For local control smaller tumor size ($P = .004$) and grade 1 to 2 ($P = .01$) were independent predictors.[301]

Angiosarcoma of the head and neck deserve special consideration due to their poor prognosis compared with other sarcomas in that region.[300,302] Some of the difficulties in managing this disease have to do with its notorious propensity to infiltrate throughout the dermis beyond what is clinically apparent, making wide local excision with negative margins difficult to achieve. In addition, they display a higher incidence of regional lymph node metastasis than other sarcomas with a reported rate of 10% to 15%.[303]

Morrison et al. reported on 14 patients with angiosarcoma of the head and neck treated by radiation with or without surgery. The 5-year overall and distant metastasis-free survival rates were 29% and 37%, respectively. The 5-year above clavicle local control rates were 24% for definitive radiation compared with 40% with adjuvant radiation ($P = .03$).[304] Similar findings were reported by Willers et al. on 11 patients with 5-year overall, distant metastasis-free, and local recurrence-free survival rates of 31%, 42%, and 24%, respectively.[300]

MANAGEMENT OF BREAST SARCOMA

Primary soft tissue sarcomas of the breast are rare, representing approximately 1% of all breast malignancies. They usually present as a painless mass with no distinctive findings on mammography. The main treatment is surgery and the extent of resection is debatable, but most authors believe that wide excision with generous negative margin is adequate.[305] North et al. reported on 25 patients treated by surgery with or without radiation. The 5-year overall survival rate was 61%, which did not vary significantly between those treated with wide excision compared with those who underwent mastectomy ($P = .9$). Five patients received adjuvant radiation and none of them developed local recurrence.[306]

Gutman et al. showed similar findings in 60 cases of breast sarcoma treated by surgery with or without radiation.[307] Johnstone et al. reported on 10 patients treated with mastectomy and adjuvant radiation. The 5-year survival rate was 66% with no local or regional failures.[308]

SERIOUS COMPLICATIONS OF PRIMARY TREATMENT

WOUND COMPLICATIONS

It is well established that radiation and chemotherapy inhibit wound healing. Early studies defined the effects of doxorubicin and x-ray treatment on wound healing in animal models.[309] The authors demonstrated that the timing and the combination of multiple antineoplastic agents were critical to inhibiting wound healing. They suggested that radiation or antineoplastic drugs delivered more than 7 days on either side of the wound were accompanied by minimal inhibition of wound healing. Conversely, the application of radiation or chemotherapy just before, or in close juxtaposition to, the time of wounding, resulted in significant impairment of wound healing as demonstrated by wound-breaking strength. This appeared to be due to inhibition of newly synthesized collagen as determined by hydroxyproline assays.

A comprehensive review of the effect of chemotherapeutic agents on wound healing[310] emphasized the importance of the agents used and the timing of delivery.

In our studies of adjuvant BRT and wound complications, we also demonstrated that when particular attention is paid to the timing of delivery of radiation via afterloading catheters to beyond the fifth postoperative day, the major wound complication rate approaches that with surgery alone.[211]

More recently, wound complications (wound infection or the need for further operative intervention) were analyzed in the randomized BRT trial at MSKCC.[310a] The overall rate was 24% in the BRT arm compared with 14% in the control arm ($P = .13$). However, the rate of reoperation was higher in the BRT group, 10% versus 0% ($P = .006$). The other covariable that contributed to wound reoperation was the width of the excised skin. If the width was greater than 4 cm the rate was 10%, but if the width was less than or equal to 4 cm the rate was 1% ($P = .02$). These types of complications are not unique to BRT but have been shown with external-beam irradiation as well.[311–313] In a randomized trial from Princess Margaret Hospital comparing preoperative and postoperative irradiation, wound complication was a primary end point of the study. Wound complications were defined as secondary wound surgery, hospital admission for wound care, and deep packing or prolonged dressings within 120 days following tumor resection. The investigators found that preoperative radiation had a significantly higher rate of wound complications (35% vs. 17%, $P = .01$).[314]

In situations in which wound complications may be anticipated because of the magnitude of the wound, extent of the resection, prior radiation, and so forth, serious consideration should be given to bringing fresh vascularized tissue in the form of either transpositional or free grafts into the area to cover the defect before the placement or delivery of radiation therapy. With this approach, postoperative morbidity can be markedly diminished.

OTHER COMPLICATIONS

The effect of adjuvant radiation and chemotherapy on the development of bony fracture has been reported in the literature but the data are scant. Stinson et al. reported on 145 patients with soft tissue sarcoma who underwent limb-sparing surgery and postoperative radiation with or without chemotherapy and found a 6% fracture rate.[315] For patients treated with adjuvant BRT in the MSKCC randomized trial, the rate of fracture was 4% compared with 0% in the control arm. This difference, however, was not statistically significant ($P = .2$).[310a] Brant et al. reported a 7.6% rate of pathologic fracture in patients treated with preoperative radiation.[316]

Lin et al. evaluated 205 patients with soft tissue sarcomas of the thigh to determine the contributing factors to pathologic fracture of the femur in patients treated with adjuvant radiation. The 5-year actuarial risk was 8.6%, which on univariate analysis correlated with periosteal stripping ($P = .0001$), location in the anterior compartment ($P = .008$), female sex ($P = .01$), the use of chemotherapy ($P = .02$), age greater than or equal to 50 ($P = .03$), and the use of external-beam radiation instead of BRT ($P = .04$). On multivariate analysis only periosteal stripping retained significance ($P = .01$).[317]

The other type of complication encountered with adjuvant radiation is peripheral nerve damage. In the control arm of the MSKCC randomized trial the rate was 7% compared with 9% in the BRT arm ($P = .8$).[310a] LePechoux et al. reported a rate of 1.6% of peripheral nerve damage in 62 patients treated with postoperative radiation.[318] Brant et al. reported a 3.4% rate for patients treated with preoperative radiation.[316]

PROGNOSTIC FACTORS FOR OUTCOME

As more sophisticated approaches to the analysis of outcome become more widely employed, it becomes clear that the variables being investigated provide different information. Prognostic factors for local recurrence, metastasis, disease-specific survival, and overall survival may all be fine gradations of differing factors, all of which provide considerably different information.

An analysis of long-term follow-up for over 1000 patients with localized soft tissue sarcoma of the extremity has been provided from our group.[184] From prospective data collected from 1041 patients over the age of 16, we have determined the clinical pathologic factors that influence local recurrence, distant recurrence, and disease-specific and overall survival. The 5-year survival rate was 76%, with a median follow-up of 4 years. Factors that increased the risk of local recurrence were age greater than 50 years, recurrent disease at the time of presentation, positive histologic primary margins, histologic subtypes of fibrosarcoma (including desmoid), and malignant peripheral nerve tumors (Table 39.1-11).

Factors that increased distant recurrence rates were tumor size greater than 5 cm, high histologic grade, deep location, recurrent disease at the time of presentation, and histologic subtype leiomyosarcoma. Histology of liposarcoma was favorable for decreased distant recurrence rate when compared with other histologies.

For disease-specific mortality, large tumor size, high histologic grade, deep location, recurrent disease at presentation, positive histologic margins at the time of resection of the primary, lower extremity site, and the histologic types of leiomyosarcoma and malignant peripheral nerve tumor were all factors.

Postmetastasis survival for most patients is independent of factors involved in the primary presentation, although large tumor size has been associated. The determination of recurrence rates and survival rates can depend on which factor is

TABLE 39.1-11. Relative Risk Influence on Recurrence of Localized Extremity Soft Tissue Sarcoma[a]

	Local Recurrence (P)	*Distant Recurrence (P)*	*Disease-Free Survival (P)*
Age	1.6 (.001)	—	—
Recurrent presentation	2.0 (.001)	1.5 (.02)	1.5 (.033)
Fibrosarcoma	2.5 (.006)	—	—
Malignant peripheral nerve tumor	1.8 (.001)	—	1.9 (.008)
Size >5 cm	—	1.9 (.0001)	2.1 (.0001)
Margin positive	1.8 (.0001)		1.7 (.011)
Depth	—	2.5 (.0007)	2.8 (.0002)
High grade	—	4.3 (.0001)	4.0 (.0001)
Leiomyosarcoma	—	1.7 (.024)	1.9 (.012)

[a]Multivariate number = 1041.
(From ref. 184, with permission.)

examined. For example, high-grade lesions have a much greater cumulative hazard rate of developing a distant metastasis in the first 30 months. Low-grade lesions, however, have a continued slow but inexorable progression to a continuing long-term rate of metastasis. This raises the interesting biologic question of whether lack of recognition of the metastatic potential of low-grade sarcomas is caused by inherent sampling error in low-grade lesions, where small foci of potentially metastatic cells are not appreciated. Alternatively, all soft tissue sarcomas may be inherently imbued with metastatic potential. One thing is clear: 5-year survival does not guarantee cure. An analysis of patients who were disease-free 5 years after the diagnosis and treatment of extremity lesions showed 9% would go on to have a further recurrence in the next 5 years (Fig. 39.1-24).[185]

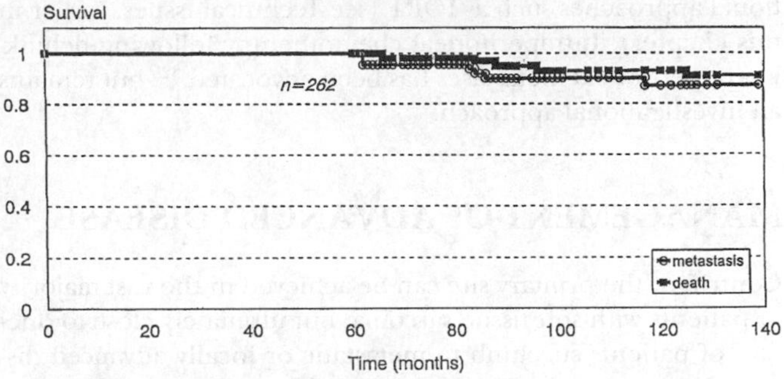

FIGURE 39.1-24. Survival in patients with extremity soft tissue sarcoma who were metastasis-free at 5 years. (From ref. 527, with permission.)

QUALITY OF LIFE AND FUNCTIONAL OUTCOME

Quality of life assessment has gained so much importance in recent years that many randomized trials in the field of oncology are evaluating that issue either as the primary end point or secondary to outcome. This issue is obviously of great significance in patients with soft tissue sarcoma of the extremity who are being treated with conservative surgery and adjuvant therapy in order to preserve function and potentially improve the overall quality of life.

However, in order to determine the effect of adjuvant therapy it is important to look at other potential contributing factors as well. One such factor is the extent of surgical resection. Sugarbaker et al. found no evidence of improved quality of life in patients treated with conservative surgery and adjuvant radiation compared with amputation,[319] but more recently Davis et al. showed a significantly higher levels of handicap in amputated patients compared with those treated with conservative surgery.[320] In patients treated with conservative surgery, the effect of the extent of surgery on functional outcome is not clearly defined. Robinson et al. reported on 54 patients who were disease-free 2 or more years after limb-conserving treatment for soft tissue sarcoma of the leg or pelvic girdle.[324] The extent of surgery was not an independent prognostic factor for limb function, although univariate analysis suggested an association with range of movement ($P<.025$).[81] On the other hand, Bell et al. showed that neural sacrifice performed at the time of wide local excision was associated with poorer outcome on univariate ($P = .002$) and multivariate analysis ($P = .019$).[321] Conventional chemotherapy has not been shown to affect the functional outcome of patients with extremity sarcomas.

The effect of adjuvant radiation and some of its parameters on functional outcome have been studied more extensively. Yang et al. reported that adjuvant postoperative external-beam radiation compared with surgery alone resulted in significantly worse limb strength and edema and range of motion, but these deficits were often transient and had few measurable effects on activities of daily life or global quality of life.[193] Schupak et al. reported on a group of patients who underwent rigorous psychofunctional testing and were part of the BRT randomized trial at MSKCC. There were no significant differences in the functional outcome between the BRT group and the no BRT group. The psychofunctional scores, however, revealed a higher level of anxiety, depression, and appreciation of illness in patients who received adjuvant BRT.[322] Karasek et al. evaluated 41 patients who were treated with surgery and radiation and showed that 83% of them had good or excellent functional outcome. But there was a correlation between volume irradiated to greater than or equal to 55 Gy and poorer functional score, strength, fibrosis, and skin changes.[323] Robinson et al. also found that doses in excess of 60 Gy resulted in increased fibrosis and a worse functional outcome.[324]

TREATMENT OF LOCAL RECURRENCE

The treatment of locally recurrent soft tissue sarcoma in almost any site that is amenable to low morbidity surgical resection is reresection. Local recurrence, however, remains a significant factor in long-term morbidity and mortality. In cases in which surgical resection can be achieved, then adjuvant radiation therapy should be considered in the vast majority of patients with recurrent disease. In patients undergoing systemic recurrence, again surgical resection should be considered.

Analyses of patients undergoing local resection of intraabdominal lesions have been extensively reviewed.[289,290] It is clear that when complete gross resection can be achieved, operation for local recurrence should be attempted along with investigational approaches such as IORT (see Technical Issues, earlier in this chapter). Intraperitoneal chemotherapy following debulking of peritoneal metastases has been advocated,[325] but remains an investigational approach.

MANAGEMENT OF ADVANCED DISEASE

Control of the primary site can be achieved in the vast majority of patients with soft tissue sarcoma, but ultimately close to one-half of patients succumb to metastatic or locally advanced disease. Unfortunately, the most active chemotherapeutic options are of limited value and are associated with serious and potentially life-threatening toxicity. Median survival from the time metastases are recognized is 8 to 12 months, although 20% to 25% of patients with metastatic sarcoma are alive 2 years after diagnosis. Patients with metastatic sarcoma often feel well at the time that a radiograph or CT reveals metastases and may remain free of symptoms for months, or even years. Thus, alleviation of symptoms is not an immediate concern in many patients, although progressive sarcoma is inevitable. Surgical resection can provide selected patients with prolonged periods of freedom from disease, and radiation therapy provides palliation for individual patients who have localized symptomatic metastases. Optimal treatment of patients with unresectable or metastatic soft tissue sarcoma requires an appreciation for the natural history of the disease, close attention to the individual patient, and an understanding of the benefits and limitations of the therapeutic options.

RESECTION OF METASTATIC DISEASE

Approximately 20% of patients with a soft tissue sarcoma of an extremity or the trunk develop pulmonary metastases, and in the majority, the lung remains the only clinically evident site of metastasis. In retrospective series, 20% to 30% of patients who undergo metastasectomy are alive 5 years later.[326–331]

Of 716 patients with primary extremity sarcoma who were treated at Memorial over a period of 6 years, pulmonary-only metastases occurred in 19%, or 135. Of these 135 patients, 58% underwent thoracotomy and 83% of those had a complete resection of their tumor. In the 65 patients who had a complete resection of their tumor, 69% recurred with pulmonary metastases as their only site of disease. Median survival from complete resection was 19 months, and 3-year survival was only 23% of those resected and 11% of those presenting with lung metastasis only. Patients who did not undergo thoracotomy all died within 3 years.[170] Chemotherapy had no obvious effect on survival in either the resected or unresected patients. Incomplete resection was no better than no operation (Fig. 39.1-25). At M. D. Anderson, in contrast to the experience with primary sarcoma, response to chemotherapy administered before pulmonary resection did not predict for improved outcome.[332] Again, there is a glaring need for effective approaches to reducing systemic recurrence in patients rendered free of disease by surgical resection.

In patients who have pulmonary only metastatic disease that is not amenable to resection, an innovative approach under study is isolated lung perfusion.[333] This technique or direct lung infusion can be used to administer chemotherapeutic drugs or biologic agents in a way that results in a high concentration of the agent in the lung, with no systemic exposure.

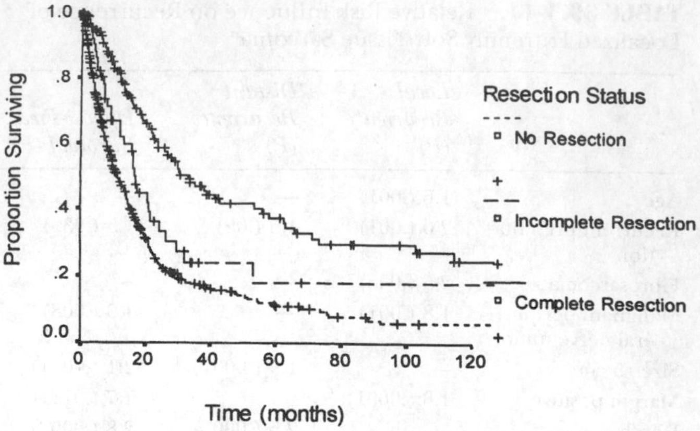

FIGURE 39.1-25. Pulmonary resection of soft tissue sarcoma metastases from the extremity. Comparison of no resection, versus incomplete resection versus complete gross resection of all known metastases. (From ref. 528, with permission.)

SYSTEMIC THERAPY FOR ADVANCED DISEASE

The activity of individual commercially available chemotherapeutic agents in patients with soft tissue sarcoma is summarized in Table 39.1-12. Doxorubicin has been the mainstay of chemotherapy for advanced sarcoma. Whereas early studies suggested overall response rates of 30%,[254,334] in more recent trials the response rate was closer to 20%.[335,336] Subset analysis of patients with soft tissue sarcoma from a large randomized phase II trial of different doses of doxorubicin demonstrated a dose-response relationship in patients with sarcoma.[254] These data have been confirmed in other trials of single-agent doxorubicin and trials with doxorubicin-containing combination therapy.[255–258] Some studies have begun to examine liposomal forms of doxorubicin, which may have fewer side effects than doxorubicin itself; response rates have been low, however.

Ifosfamide has approximately the same efficacy as doxorubicin. In the past, ifosfamide dosing was limited by severe urothelial toxicity (hemorrhagic cystitis). The uroprotective agent mesna has markedly changed the ability to give both ifosfamide and cyclophosphamide, and ifosfamide doses as large as 14 to 18 g/m^2 over several days are given in some studies. There has been a debate as to the relative efficacy of cyclophosphamide versus ifosfamide, in particular whether ifosfamide is truly a different drug or whether differences in dosing of the two drugs accounts for the difference in response. The best study addressing this question came from the EORTC, which performed a randomized phase II trial examining the response rates of ifosfamide, 5 g/m^2, to cyclophosphamide, 1.5 g/m^2. There was greater myelosuppression with cyclophosphamide, but response rates were 7.5% for cyclophosphamide and 18% with ifosfamide; although suggestive, this difference did not achieve statistical significance. Additionally, there is some evidence to suggest a dose-response relationship for ifosfamide.[253] This is also borne out by the large number of phase II trials examining high-dose ifosfamide in metastatic soft tissue sarcoma (see Table 39.1-12); responses to higher doses of ifosfamide are occasionally seen in patients failing lower doses of alkylating agents. The similar response rates of ifosfamide and doxorubicin, even in doxorubicin-resistant patients, suggested a lack of cross-resistance in combination che-

TABLE 39.1-12. Selected Studies of Single-Agent Chemotherapy for Advanced Disease[a]

Regimen	*Dose and Schedule*	*Notes*[b]	*No. of Patients Evaluable*	*No. of Patients Responding*	*Response Rate (%)*	*Reference*
Antibiotics						
Doxorubicin	70 mg/m² q3w	A	148	26	17	Borden[461]
	75 mg/m² q3w	A	83	21	25	Mouridsen[462]
	80 mg/m² q3w	A	90	18	20	Edmonson[336]
Liposomal doxorubicin	75–105 mg/m² q2w		23	3	13	Casper[463]
PEGylated liposomal doxorubicin	55 mg/m² q4w	B	35	2	6	Skubitz[464]
Epirubicin	75 mg/ m² q3w		84	15	18	Mouridsen[462]
Epirubicin ± dexrazoxane	160 mg/m² q3w epirubicin ± 1000 mg/m² dexrazoxane		34	8	24	Lopez[465]
Mitomycin C	12 mg/m² q3w		34	0	0	van Osterom[354]
Bleomycin			32	0	0	Amato[466]
Actinomycin D			30	5	17	Golbey[467]
Alkylating agents						
Cyclophosphamide	1.5g/m² q3w	A	67	8	12	Bramwell[468]
Hexamethylmelamine	—		40	3	7	Borden[469]
Ifosfamide	5 g/m² × 24 h IVCI	A	68	12	18	Bramwell[468]
	2 g/m² × 4 d IVB		95	17	18	Antman[337]
	2 g/m² × 7 d IVB	B	72	21	29	Patel[470]
	1.0 g/m² × 14–21 d IVCI		33	8	24	Frustaci[369]
Cisplatin	50 mg/m²	C	96	13	13	Thigpen[390]
	75 mg/m²		42	3	7	Samson[471]
	200 mg/m²		40	6	15	Budd[472]
Carboplatin	320–400 mg/m²		50	6	12	Goldstein[473]
Antimetabolites						
Gemcitabine	1000 mg/m² qwk × 3–7		19	2	11	Patel[474]
Methotrexate	Various		41	15	36	Subramanian[475]
	≥5g/m² q2w with vincristine		14	2	14	Vaughn[476]
5-Fluorouracil	—		8	1	12	Gold[477]
Microtubule toxins						
Docetaxel	100 mg/m² q3w		29	5	17	Van oesel[478]
Paclitaxel	250 mg/m² q3w		48	6	12	Balcerzak[479]
Vinblastine	1.5 mg/m²/d × 5		15	0	0	Yap[480]
Vinorelbine	30 mg/m² q1w × 8		36	4	11	Fidias[342]
Topoisomerase inhibitors						
Etoposide	100 mg/m²/d × 3d q3w	D	28	0	0	Thigpen[481]
	50 mg/m² PO qd × 21d q4w	D	29	2	7	Rose[482]
Topotecan	1.5 mg/m² qd × 5, q3w		29	3	10	Bramwell[483]
Other agents						
Dacarbazine	Various		53	9	17	Gottlieb[339]
	1200 mg/m²		44	8	18	Buesa[340]
Gallium nitrate	700 mg/m²		24	0	0	Saiki[484]
Mitoxantrone	—		53	0	0	Presant[485]
	—		61	—	2	Bull[486]

IVB, intravenous bolus; IVCI, intravenous continuous infusion.
[a]Only the largest series or unique studies of individual drugs are considered here.
[b]A, one arm of a randomized study; B, includes soft tissue and bone sarcomas; C, uterine leiomyosarcoma and mixed mesodermal sarcoma; D, uterine leiomyosarcoma only.

motherapy. It should be noted that synovial sarcoma appears relatively responsive to ifosfamide.[337,338]

The third drug with modest activity in sarcoma is dacarbazine. Its activity was recognized over 20 years ago,[339] and later confirmed.[340] Dacarbazine has frequently been used in combination chemotherapy with doxorubicin (see Combination Chemotherapy for Advanced Soft Tissue Sarcoma, later in this chapter). Dacarbazine is given in a variety of schedules, from intravenous continuous infusion as part of the mesna, doxorubicin, ifosfamide, and dacarbazine (MAID) protocol[341] (see

TABLE 39.1-13. Selected Studies of Investigational Agents in Sarcoma Therapy[a]

Investigational Agent	*No. of Patients*	*Response Rate (%)*	*Reference*
Antibiotics			
Aclacinomycin	33	3	Earhart[487]
Amsacrine	31	3	Yap[488]
Azotomycin	14	29	Weiss[489]
Carminomycin	48	27	Perevodchikova[490]
Echinomycin	34	0	Taylor[491]
Esorubicin	12	0	Giaccone[492]
Mitozolamide	25	0	Somers[493]
Menogaril	21	5	Buckner[494]
Methoxymorpholin-odoxorubicin	17	12	Taub[495]
PALA + dipyridamole	19	5	Casper[496]
Piritrexim	22	9	Schiesel[497]
Pyrazofurin	21	0	Cormier[498]
Raltitrexed	21	0	Blay[499]
Triazinate	29	0	Thigpen[500]
Trimetrexate	50	12	Eisenhauer[501]
Alkylating agents			
Chlorozotocin	37	3	Amato[466]
CI-980	18	0	Patel[502]
Cystemustine	28	4	Cure[503]
Dibromodulcitol	33	0	Borden[504]
Dianhydrogalactitol	28	0	Thigpen[505]
Trofosfamide	12	3	Blomqvist[506]
Miscellaneous agents			
Amonafide	26[b]	1	Asbury[507]
Bruceantin	34	0	Amato[466]
Diaziquone	40	0	Chan[508]
Diglycoaldehyde	20	0	Vosika[509]
Doxorubicin + VX-710	11	9	Bramwell[510]
Elliptinium	19	0	Somers[511]
Homoharringtonine	16	0	Ajani[512]
ICRF-159	29	3	Borden[504]
MGBG	38	3	Amato[466]
Merbarone	33	3	Kraut[513]
Maytansine	40	0	Borden[504]
TGU	19	0	Rouesse[514]
Vindesine	46	6	Sordillo[515]

MGBG, methylglyoxal bisguanylhydrazone (mitoguazone); PALA, N-phosphonacetyl-L-aspartate; TGU, 1,2,4-triglycidyl urasol.
[a]For editorial reasons, only the largest studies are shown, if there is more than one study for a given investigational drug.
[b]Uterine leiomyosarcoma only.

Table 39.1-10), to one large bolus. The major side effect of dacarbazine is nausea and vomiting, which is abrogated to some extent by dividing the dose over 2 to 4 days. In general, nausea and vomiting from dacarbazine have been substantially reduced with the use of serotonin antagonist antiemetics.

As for other single agents, cisplatin and carboplatin have given occasional responses in phase II trials. However, in contrast to pediatric sarcomas such as Ewing's sarcoma and rhabdomyosarcoma, other agents such as single-agent vincristine, etoposide, and actinomycin D appear to be inactive. The taxanes also show little activity; however, there are data that vinorelbine[342] and gemcitabine[343,344] have modest activity in at least some subtypes of soft tissue sarcoma.

The response rates of other largely investigational agents in soft tissue sarcomas are shown in Table 39.1-13. Few of these drugs have demonstrated meaningful activity in soft tissue sarcoma.

Used in some of the earliest studies in sarcoma adjuvant chemotherapy, immunotherapy for sarcoma treatment is seeing renewed interest, without significant success to date. Cytokines alone appear to be ineffective in sarcoma (Table 39.1-14), as does nonspecific immunotherapy with bacterial cell wall components. A study underway at the NCI is examining vaccination of patients with peptides representing the fusion proteins observed in specific subtypes of sarcoma. Lymphocyte activated killer cell and other T-cell immunotherapy with cytokines was investigated in a small number of patients at the NCI without any observed responses. Dendritic cell vaccines as well as other forms of tumor-specific immunotherapy are undergoing investigation and may be of relevance to patients with soft tissue sarcoma.

Angiogenesis inhibition has emerged as a potential new therapy for solid tumors of all types, including sarcoma. To date, weak angiogenesis inhibitors such as the interferons have shown no efficacy in sarcoma (see Table 39.1-14). Stronger angiogenesis inhibitors such as TNP-470 (AGM-1470), or vascular endothelial growth factor (VEGF)-pathway inhibitor SU5416 have been examined in phase I trials,[345] but there have been only a handful of sarcoma patients treated with these more potent antiangiogenic agents.

Newer biologic agents are beginning to be assessed, based on the biology of specific sarcoma subsets, in particular liposarcoma. The antidiabetic drug troglitazone binds to the receptor PPAR-γ (peroxisome proliferator-activated receptor-γ). This receptor is present on the cell surface of some liposarcomas. When PPAR-γ binds a ligand, it can induce differentiation of the liposarcoma toward an adipocyte, with abundant fat droplet accumulation and decreased S-phase fraction. This laboratory finding led to an

TABLE 39.1-14. Biologic Agents in Sarcoma Therapy

Biologic Agent	*No. of Patients*	*Response Rate*	*Reference*
Interferon-α	16	0	Schuff-Werner[516]
Interferon-α_{2b}	64	5	Borden[517]
Interferon-α_{2b} with tamoxifen	7	0	Jazieh[518]
Interferon-β	20	5	Harris[519]
Interferon-β_{ser}	23	0	Borden[517]
Interleukin-2	6	—	Rosenberg[520]
	12	1	Gravis[521]
Liposomal muramyl tripeptide phosphatidylethanolamine	19	0	Verweij[522]
Tumor necrosis factor	16	0	Rinehart[523]
Troglitazone	3	—	Demetri[346]
SU5416	4	—	Rosen[345]

ongoing trial of troglitazone in patients with advanced liposarcoma.[346] A subset of patients with liposarcoma demonstrates similar lipid accumulation *in vivo* to that noted *in vitro*. To date, there are no data on relapse-free or overall survival of these patients.

COMBINATION CHEMOTHERAPY FOR ADVANCED SOFT TISSUE SARCOMA

A variety of combinations of chemotherapy have been developed and examined in phase II trials. The typical backbone of a combination regimen is doxorubicin (or its analogue epirubicin) with an alkylating agent, with or without other agents (see Table 39.1-10). One of the earliest combinations used was doxorubicin and dacarbazine, which has been well studied by the Southwest Oncology Group. Although initial responses noted a 41% major response rate,[347] subsequent study of either a bolus or continuous infusion of the same regimen yielded a 17% response rate.[348]

CyVADIC has been widely used for sarcoma therapy in the United States and Europe. Although single arm studies showed response rates as high as 71%,[256,257,349] a randomized trial showed no significant difference in overall survival between CyVADIC and doxorubicin as a single agent.[335] The two drug combinations of doxorubicin and ifosfamide[335] or epirubicin and ifosfamide[350–352] have consistently given response rates above 25%. Current studies are investigating higher doses of ifosfamide with fixed doxorubicin dose and growth factor support.

MAID was proven effective in metastatic soft tissue sarcoma in a large phase II trial from the Dana-Farber Cancer Institute.[341] This randomized trial took place before the routine use of growth factors for aggressive chemotherapeutic regimens and examined doxorubicin and dacarbazine versus MAID. The study showed an increased response rate in the MAID arm (32% vs. 17%, $P<.002$).[353] Underscoring the increased toxicity of aggressive chemotherapy regimens, there were eight toxic deaths on the study, seven in the 170 patients treated with the 7.5 g/m^2 total dose of ifosfamide per cycle. This dose was decreased to 6 g/m^2 during the course of the study. All treatment deaths occurred in patients older than 50 years of age. In a univariate analysis, there was a survival advantage for the two-drug arm (13 months vs. 12 months for MAID); however, this difference was not significant in a multivariate analysis. As noted in the later section on Dose Intensity, with the introduction of growth factors, the dose intensity of this regimen has become better tolerated.

The response rates of metastatic sarcoma to cisplatin are low, and response rate to mitomycin C is zero in one small study.[354] However, the combination of the two drugs with doxorubicin (called MAP) yielded a 43% response rate in a study from the Mayo Clinic. The activity of the MAP regimen has been confirmed in an independent ECOG trial.[336,355]

A recent metaanalysis of all of the data from seven large EORTC provided a useful resource to assess response rates to combination chemotherapy in a multiinstitutional setting.[356] The 2185 patients with follow-up in this study were subjected to a univariate and multivariate analysis of survival based on a number of factors, including age, sex, performance status before chemotherapy, presence and site of metastatic disease, histologic subtype, histologic grade, and disease-free interval (time since initial diagnosis of sarcoma). The overall median survival time was 51 weeks. The predictors of overall survival included good performance status, lack of liver involvement, low histopathologic grade, long disease-free interval, and young age ($P<.005$ for all these factors in a multivariate analysis). Although absence of liver involvement, young age, and high histopathologic grade also predicted for response to chemotherapy, so did liposarcoma histology ($P<.01$ for all these factors in a multivariate analysis); leiomyosarcoma histology did not qualify as a factor for response to chemotherapy independent of liver metastasis. Although not stratified by site, these data provide some of the best evidence that response rate does not necessarily correlate with overall survival.

Is combination chemotherapy better than single-agent doxorubicin for overall survival? Again, the concept arises of response rates differing from rates of overall survival. There have been several phase III trials examining the issue of combination chemotherapy versus single agents for patients with metastatic disease (Table 39.1-15); two such trials examined this question in uterine sarcoma. There were improved response rates in several of the trials with combination chemotherapy, but there was no survival advantage over single-agent doxorubicin. Complete responses were rare during these studies and were not durable. These data argue that single agents are as effective as combination chemotherapy for patients with metastatic disease, in terms of overall survival. However, some patients may be eligible for palliative resection of metastatic disease. In these situations in which such aggressive therapy is contemplated, combination chemotherapy, which gives better response rates than single agents, can be considered.

DOSE INTENSITY

It is a central tenet of oncology that response to chemotherapy is a function of dose and dose intensity.[357] A dose-response effect for doxorubicin and ifosfamide has been suggested in a variety of studies.[253,358] However, toxicity limits the amount of chemotherapy that can be given in any one cycle, as illustrated by the phase III trial of the MAID combination chemotherapy noted previously.[353] It is argued that if dose could be increased, better responses might be seen. Better supportive care can help increase dose intensity as outlined in this section.

The use of hematopoietic growth factors has allowed for the study of higher doses of chemotherapy in sarcoma. Some of the aggressive regimens for therapy of metastatic sarcoma satisfy the American Society of Clinical Oncology guidelines for use of growth factors given their high rate of febrile neutropenia.[359] Granulocyte-macrophage colony-stimulating factor (sargramostim), the first granulocyte growth factor used, decreased the myelosuppression seen with CyADIC[360] and MAID[361] chemotherapy, and allowed for increased dose intensity of high-dose ifosfamide.[362] Granulocyte-macrophage colony-stimulating factor allowed for escalation of the dose of doxorubicin when given in combination with 5 g/m^2 of ifosfamide, with improvement in response rate.[363,364] Granulocyte-macrophage colony-stimulating factor has also been shown to allow increased dose intensity of the MAP combination of chemotherapy, allowing addition of ifosfamide.[365]

Similarly, granulocyte colony-stimulating factor (filgrastim) has been widely used to increase dose intensity and decrease myelotoxicity of aggressive chemotherapeutic regimens such as MAID[366] or dose-escalated doxorubicin and ifosfamide.[367] However, with escalated doses (25% increase) in the MAID regimen, there appears to be no significant increased response rate despite use of growth factors.[368] There may be other ways to

TABLE 39.1-15. Selected Randomized Trials in Advanced Disease

Group	Regimen	No. of Patients	Response Rate (Complete Response Rate)	Median Survival (mo)	Reference
GOG[a]	A	80	16% (6%)	7.7	Omura[388]
	AD	66	24% (10%)	7.3	
GOG[a]	A	50	19% (4%)	11.6	Muss[389]
	ACy	54	19% (8%)	10.9	
COG	A	41	17% (2%)	8.5	Cruz[524]
	ActL	25	4%	8.1	
	ActLV	26	0	11.5	
	ActLCyclo	26	0	5.1	
ECOG	A	54	30% (7%)	8.6	Schoenfeld[255]
	CyAV	56	21% (5%)	7.9	
	CyActV	58	12% (2%)	9.5	
ECOG	A	94	18% (5%)	8.0	Borden[460]
	A	88	17% (3%)	8.4	
	ADIC	92	30% (6%)	8.0	
ECOG	A	148	17% (4%)	9.4	Borden[461]
	AVd	143	18% (6%)	9.0	
ECOG	A	90	20% (2%)	< 9	Edmonson[336]
	AI	88	34% (3%)	11	
	MAP	84	32% (7%)	9	
EORTC	A	240	23% (4%)	12.0	Santoro[335]
	AI	231	28% (5%)	12.6	
	CyVADIC	134	28% (8%)	11.7	
CALGB/SWOG	AD	170	17% (2%)	13.3	Antman[353]
	AID	170	32% (2%)	11.9	
EORTC	A	112	14% (2%)	10.4	Nielsen[525]
	Epi	111	15% (3%)	10.8	
	Epi	111	14% (3%)	10.4	
EORTC metaanalysis	Any anthracycline-based regimen	2185	26% (n/a)	11.8	Van Glabbeke[356]

A, doxorubicin; Act, Actinomycin D; CALGB, Cancer and Leukemia and Group B; COG, Central Oncology Group; Cy, cyclophosphamide; Cyclo, cycloleucine; DIC, dacarbazine; Epi, epirubicin; GOG, Gynecologic Oncology Group; I, ifosfamide; L, L-PAM (L-phenylalanine mustard); M, mitomycin C; n/a, not available; P, cisplatin; SWOG, Southwest Oncology Group; V, vincristine; VD, vindesine.
[a]Uterine sarcoma only; response rates are only for subset of patients with measurable disease.

achieve dose intensity. A study of low-dose, long-term (approximately 2-week) ifosfamide showed responses in patients who failed other forms of chemotherapy for their sarcomas.[369] As was seen with previous studies, it may well be that responsiveness to a particular regimen may not translate into increased survival.

Unfortunately, the cardiac toxicity of doxorubicin and nephrotoxicity and central nervous system toxicity of ifosfamide prevent much greater dose escalation than performed in some studies today. The next logical step is to proceed to high-dose therapy with stem cell support, which is currently under study with pediatric sarcomas.[370,371] Such studies show long-term disease-free survival for a handful of patients with Ewing's sarcoma, osteosarcoma, or rhabdomyosarcoma. Even in these relatively chemotherapy-sensitive sarcomas, the majority of patients have relapsed rapidly. Given that complete responses (and therefore chemotherapy sensitivity) are rare in the metastatic setting of adult soft tissue sarcoma, it is not surprising that the few patients with soft tissue sarcoma who undergo high-dose therapy with stem cell rescue relapse quickly. High-dose therapy with stem cell rescue should not be considered for patients with metastatic sarcoma outside the setting of a clinical trial.[372,373] With poor results from high-dose therapy, the pursuit of agents with better activity against soft tissue sarcoma will remain a primary focus for therapy of relapsed disease.

RESPONSE BY HISTOLOGIC SUBTYPE AND SITE

A major focus in critical reading of the literature concerning responses of soft tissue sarcoma to chemotherapy is the variety of patient sarcoma histology. Pediatric sarcomas are known for their relative sensitivity to chemotherapy (Ewing's sarcoma, osteosarcoma, and rhabdomyosarcoma). As for adult sarcomas, synovial sarcomas and fibrosarcomas are generally sensitive to chemotherapy. GISTs, alveolar sarcoma of soft parts, and low- to intermediate-grade chondrosarcomas are notorious for their resistance to chemotherapy. An imbalance in the subtypes of sarcomas in various groups of patients can markedly affect overall outcome for the study in question.

Site of disease is another important factor in determination of outcome for patients with soft tissue sarcoma. For example, patients with large low-grade liposarcoma of the extremity show lower relapse rates than patients with low-grade liposarcomas of the retroperitoneum; the latter are more difficult to control locally. Similarly, formerly called leimyosarcomas of the gastrointestinal tract, both true leiomyosarcomas and gastrointestinal stomal tumors (GISTs), are less responsive to chemotherapy than leiomyosarcoma of other sites (see Leiomyosarcoma, later in this chapter). Anatomy of metastatic disease can also affect overall response rates. For example, metastases to liver are less likely to respond to chemotherapy than metastases to another site[356]; however, this may represent the tendency of GISTs to metastasize to the liver. Variations in the site of disease or metastasis pattern may at least in part account for the different responses noted in randomized trials of chemotherapy for soft tissue sarcoma.

It is clear that specific subtypes of soft tissue sarcomas demonstrate unique biologic behavior. As diagnosis and classification of sarcomas improve, these unique features may become more evident. Examples of specific sites or subtypes of sarcoma and their characteristics are presented here.

LEIOMYOSARCOMA

Leiomyosarcomas are one of the most common forms of soft tissue sarcoma. They are also relatively uniform in histologic appearance, and thus there is greater concordance of pathologists in the diagnosis of leiomyosarcoma than other forms of soft tissue sarcoma. Given their relative frequency and the consistency of diagnosis of leiomyosarcoma, it is useful to examine the sensitivity of this subset of sarcomas to standard chemotherapy.

The response rate of leiomyosarcoma in subset analysis of randomized trials is shown in Table 39.1-16. Subset analyses cannot substitute for primary trials of chemotherapy, but still can be useful in generating hypotheses for further studies. Doxorubicin appears to be active in leiomyosarcomas, but ifosfamide appears to add little to the response rate of this subset of tumors. In one small study of uterine leiomyosarcomas, a modest response to ifosfamide was observed.[374] Ifosfamide, in contrast, appears to be effective in other subtypes of sarcoma.

The primary site of leiomyosarcoma can have an equally important effect on survival. The difference in response rates for different sites of leiomyosarcoma is highlighted in the trials from ECOG and Southwest Oncology Group.[336,353] Although only 20% to 25% of uterine leiomyosarcomas responded to chemotherapy, uterine leiomyosarcoma was approximately twice as responsive to chemotherapy compared with leiomyosarcomas arising from the gastrointestinal tract (GISTs). These data are at odds with the cumulative EORTC metaanalysis of therapy for metastatic sarcomas[356]; however, in the EORTC study, leiomyosarcomas were not stratified with respect to site; poorly responding gastrointestinal stromal tumors were grouped together with better responding leiomyosarcomas of other sites. Given the poor response of gastrointestinal stromal tumors to any chemotherapy, patients with recurrent unresectable disease carrying this diagnosis should be considered candidates for phase I or phase II studies, even before routine chemotherapy with doxorubicin or ifosfamide. Attention to improved histopathologic diagnosis will play a part in the design of future studies of chemotherapy in the adjuvant or metastatic setting.

SYNOVIAL SARCOMA

Synovial sarcoma demonstrates two histologies, a monophasic form and a biphasic form. Specific translocations in this subset of sarcoma between the SSX and SYT genes on chromosomes X and 18 may be prognostic factors for this subtype of sarcoma. Patients with biphasic histology demonstrated SYT-SSX1 gene fusions. These patients fared more poorly than patients with SYT-SSX2 positive tumors that were associated with the monophasic phenotype[375]; such molecular phenotyping represents an attractive method of predicting outcome to therapy and need for more or less intensive therapy.

Patients with synovial sarcoma tend to be younger than patients with other subtypes of soft tissue sarcoma. Patients with synovial sarcoma are therefore likely to have a better per-

TABLE 39.1-16. Response of Leiomyosarcoma to Various Chemotherapy Regimens

Study	*Regimen*	*Total Patients*	*No. of LMSA Patients (% of Study Population)*	*Response Rate (% for All)*	*Response Rate (% for LMSA)*	*Response Rate (% for Non-LMSA)*
Dana-Farber Cancer Institute[337]	I	99	27 (27%)	18	7	22
Gynecologic Oncology Group[374]	I	35[a]	35[a] (100%)	17	17	n/a
Indiana University[526]	AI	42	18 (43%)	36	17	50
Southwest Oncology Group[348]	AD bolus	118	53 (45%)	17	15	19
	AD IVCI	118	52 (44%)	17	—	—
Cancer and Leukemia Group B/ Southwest Oncology Group[353]	AD	170	59 (35%)	17	16	19
	ADI	170	58 (34%)	32	22	37
Eastern Cooperative Oncology Group[336]	A	90	42 (47%)	20	10	30
	AI	88	37 (42%)	34	14	50
	MAP	84	37 (44%)	32	19	45
European Organization for Research and Treatment of Cancer[356]	Any anthracycline-based regimen	2185	492 (26%)	26	22	30

A, doxorubicin; D, dacarbazine; I, ifosfamide; IVCI, intravenous continuous infusion; LMSA, leiomyosarcoma; n/a, not applicable; M, mitomycin C; P, cisplatin.
[a]Uterine leiomyosarcoma only.

formance status than patients with other subtypes of sarcoma, a positive predictor for response to chemotherapy in the EORTC database.[356] The higher response rates in such patients may therefore be in part due to patient selection factors, not just histologic diagnosis.

In patients with advanced synovial sarcoma, ifosfamide (at a high dose of 14 to 18 g/m^2) appears to be an active agent with a 100% response rate in one study of 13 patients.[338] The EORTC metaanalysis of 2185 sarcoma patients included 115 synovial sarcomas evaluable for response to chemotherapy[356]; the response rate was 31%, not significantly different than the overall response rate of 26%. The conflict between these results may be due to dose intensity, as well as the use of an inappropriate group for comparison; the EORTC data examined the response of metastatic sarcoma to anthracyclines and only a portion of patients received ifosfamide (at a maximum dose of 5 g/m^2, a low dose by today's standards).

PEDIATRIC SARCOMAS IN ADULT POPULATIONS

A number of pediatric sarcomas occur in the adults, including Ewing's sarcoma (in soft tissue or bone), rhabdomyosarcoma (usually embryonal), and osteosarcoma. These diseases differ from typical adult sarcomas in that they are considered systemic diseases despite their initial presentation. Ewing's sarcoma and rhabdomyosarcoma are typically much more sensitive to chemotherapy than adult soft tissue sarcomas.[376] In osteosarcoma, long-term survival has been achieved in pediatric patients with the use of adjuvant chemotherapy. Unfortunately, adults with osteosarcoma are generally more resistant to chemotherapy than children. Adjuvant (or neoadjuvant) chemotherapy is the standard of care for adults with a diagnosis of rhabdomyosarcoma or Ewing's sarcoma. In addition, adults with a typical osteosarcoma of bone should receive neoadjuvant or adjuvant chemotherapy in addition to therapy for local control of their tumor. However, in extraskeletal osteosarcoma, the use of chemotherapy as an adjuvant to surgical control of the primary disease remains controversial, largely due to the low response rates to chemotherapy seen in patients with metastatic soft tissue osteosarcoma.[153,377]

Typical regimens for small cell pediatric sarcomas, specifically rhabdomyosarcoma and Ewing's sarcoma, include the combination of vincristine, doxorubicin, and cyclophosphamide (occasionally with actinomycin D), and the combination of ifosfamide and etoposide.[376,378,379] The MAID regimen also shows activity in pediatric sarcomas.[380] There is debate as to whether adults do worse than pediatric patients with the same stage of disease. Adults are less likely than children to tolerate the aggressive regimens of chemotherapy used in these diseases. In addition, adults may present with advanced stage disease relative to children or adolescents. One retrospective study showed older patients with rhabdomyosarcoma tolerated chemotherapy as well as the pediatric population, but fared worse overall[381]; tumor size, site, and response to chemotherapy predicted outcome in another series.[382] In Ewing's sarcoma, the role of age in predicting outcome is controversial.[383,384] A high percentage of patients with pediatric sarcomas are enrolled on protocols examining new therapy in the setting of randomized trials. Adults with diagnosis of sarcoma usually seen in pediatric populations should be included on pediatric protocols whenever feasible to help determine appropriate care for patients with these rare diagnoses.

UTERINE SARCOMAS

Uterine sarcomas are rare, accounting for 3% to 7% of all uterine malignancies. The uterus is a unique site in that at least three different sarcomatous entities may arise from this organ, including leiomyosarcoma, endometrial stromal sarcoma, and carcinosarcoma (also known as malignant mixed Müllerian tumor). The most common histopathologic type is Müllerian tumor.

For localized disease surgery is the main treatment. Whether adjuvant radiation is needed remains a controversial topic. Most studies showed some improvement in local control but not survival.[385,386] More recently, however, Ferrer et al. reviewed the experience of the Grup Oncologic Catala-Occita and found that the addition of radiation to surgery improved local control as well as survival in 103 patients with stage I to IVa.[387] It is hoped that the ongoing EORTC-55874 randomized trial will determine the exact effect of adjuvant radiation in this malignancy.

The Gynecologic Oncology Group performed a prospective randomized trial comparing adjuvant chemotherapy with no further therapy in patients with stage I to II uterine sarcoma. No significant improvement was noted in progression-free interval or overall survival.[230]

In advanced disease, the Gynecologic Oncology Group also compared doxorubicin alone with doxorubicin and dacarbazine in a randomized trial.[388] Response rates and overall survival did not differ between the two arms; the response rate to doxorubicin of 28 women with leiomyosarcoma was 25%. Thereafter, doxorubicin was compared with doxorubicin plus cyclophosphamide; response rates in both arms were 19%, with a 13% response rate to doxorubicin for patients with leiomyosarcoma.[389] Uterine sarcoma overall showed a 22% to 25% response rate to chemotherapy as noted previously.[336,348]

A number of phase II studies have examined responses to various agents for various subtypes of uterine sarcoma. Patients with carcinosarcoma (one form of mixed Müllerian tumor) have been treated with cisplatin,[390,391] or with doxorubicin[391]; there were no responses in the small cohort of patients given doxorubicin.[391] When patients develop metastatic disease from carcinosarcoma, it is usually of the carcinomatous elements, indicating this is the more important characteristic of the tumor to treat. This may explain the responses of this sarcoma to therapy effective for epithelial tumors. Leiomyosarcoma is responsive to doxorubicin as noted previously, less sensitive to ifosfamide (see Leiomyosarcoma, earlier in this chapter), and also relatively unresponsive to cisplatin.[390]

Endometrial stromal sarcomas express estrogen and progesterone receptors,[392] and anecdotal responses to progestins have been noted.[393] However, it is clear that frequency of positive estrogen or progesterone receptor staining is substantially greater than the response rate to hormonal therapy such as tamoxifen. In a prospective trial of tamoxifen in uterine sarcomas, only one patient (with a mixed Müllerian tumor) responded, out of a total 29 patients treated (19 with leiomyosarcoma).[394]

DESMOIDS (AGGRESSIVE FIBROMATOSES)

Desmoid tumors belong to a family of myofibroblastic fibromatoses that are unusual in their bland histology and slow progression. Surgery remains the treatment of choice for these lesions, which cannot truly be called sarcomas because of their lack of metastatic potential.

The role of adjuvant radiation for completely resected primary desmoid tumor is controversial. Most authors agree that for patients with negative resection margins, postoperative radiation is not recommended.[395,396] However, for patients with positive microscopic margins the role of adjuvant radiation is more debatable. Spear et al. from Massachusetts General Hospital reported a local control rate of 61% for patients with primary tumors with positive microscopic margins treated with surgery alone.[395] Others, however, have reported lower local control rates.[397] The conclusion from these studies is that failure does not invariably occur if residual microscopic tumor from a primary lesion is left *in situ* as long as local progression would not cause significant morbidity. When adjuvant radiation is indicated for some primary lesion or in most recurrent tumors, the usual dose is approximately 50 Gy.

In advanced cases desmoids can still cause significant morbidity in proximal extremity lesions and can be fatal if they arise in the retroperitoneum, since such sites are difficult to resect completely.

Although the use of adjuvant radiation is becoming more restricted, the role of definitive radiation is emerging as a reasonable alternative to radical surgery. Ballo et al. reported a 5-year local control rate of 69% for patients treated with radiation for gross disease.[396] Others have shown similar findings.[395,398] The recommended dose for definitive radiation is usually 56 Gy in 2 Gy per fraction to 60 Gy given at 1.8 Gy per fraction.

Desmoids classically arise in pregnancy as an abdominal mass independent of the uterus. Desmoids have been examined for hormone receptors and have binding sites for estrogens and antiestrogens in some cases.[399,400] There are anecdotes of responses to hormonal manipulation such as tamoxifen,[401–403] testolactone,[404] toremifene,[405] goserelin,[406] and progestins.[406,407] There are well-documented responses of desmoids to sulindac[404] and other nonsteroidal antiinflammatory drugs, and reports of responses to vitamin K, vitamin C, and warfarin.[404,408] Responses can take months and continue for years.

Responses have been reported to single-agent doxorubicin chemotherapy[409] as well as to combination chemotherapy at either standard or relatively low doses.[410–412] As noted previously, responses can be slow, and therapy should not be abandoned for stable disease.

In summary, for easily resectable disease, surgery alone would appear to be the optimal approach especially in patients with negative microscopic margin. In advanced cases, a trial of nonsteroidal antiinflammatory drugs or hormonal therapy can be considered in most patients. A period of close observation is also reasonable, because some patients demonstrate regression without any therapy. However, if a patient is symptomatic and not a candidate for surgery, consideration should be given to radiation or chemotherapy to increase the chance of a response.

RECOMMENDATIONS FOR PATIENTS WITH ADVANCED DISEASE

Low-grade tumors grow slowly and may be less responsive to chemotherapy than higher grade lesions. Accordingly, an asymptomatic patient with stable or only slowly progressive disease can be observed only. Resection of metastatic disease, in particular lung metastases, provides some patients with long-term survival and can be considered if the lungs are the only site of remaining disease.[413]

Randomized studies have shown that combination chemotherapy can provide a better probability of a response than single-agent doxorubicin. However, overall survival for any combination chemotherapy has not been proven superior to doxorubicin alone as a single agent. When a clinical response is needed, e.g., before potential surgery for metastases, combinations of agents such as doxorubicin and ifosfamide should be considered, especially for patients with good performance status. For patients with poor performance status, single-agent doxorubicin remains the standard of care, since no other therapy or combination of treatments has proven superior to it for overall survival. Single-agent ifosfamide or dacarbazine can be used as a second-line agent. Dacarbazine demonstrates modest activity in soft tissue sarcoma, and with doxorubicin is a well-studied and well-tolerated combination in metastatic disease. Patients with advanced disease are candidates for phase I and phase II studies of new therapy for sarcoma, since we have but few tools with which to treat such patients presently.

FUTURE DIRECTIONS

Metastatic sarcoma, whether at time of disease presentation, or after local control of primary disease, remains an extremely difficult problem. The search for effective chemotherapeutic and biologic agents will be the focus of continuing research for patients with advanced disease. In the near future, results should be forthcoming of the study of the differentiation agent troglitazone for patients with metastatic or recurrent liposarcoma. Even more potent agonists of the PPAR-γ receptor such as rosiglitazone and pioglitazone will be examined in the metastatic and adjuvant setting for patients with liposarcoma. The study of angiogenesis inhibition is just beginning. The examination of antagonists of the VEGF and other pathways of angiogenesis, may show promise in this class of tumors, using agents such as SU5416, angiostatin, and endostatin. In terms of novel chemotherapeutic agents, ecteinascidin 743 has demonstrated some promise in phase I studies and may provide the first new effective antisarcoma agent since ifosfamide.

In the longer term, it is hoped that new biologic agents for sarcoma therapy can be found that are as potent as TNF in murine models of sarcoma. TNF, interleukin-2, and cytokines appear to be toxic and largely inactive as sarcoma therapy when given systemically. Nonetheless, other biologic interventions may show promise, such as immunotherapy with targeted production of cytokines, or interference with cell-signaling pathways. Characteristic fusion proteins of sarcomas (or peptides thereof) will be tested in the near future for their effectiveness in the appropriate subtypes of sarcomas, such as many pediatric sarcomas. Vaccines incorporating dendritic cells appear to be effective immunogens in preclinical studies. Preparations of heat shock proteins or of immunogenic glycolipids found in sarcoma cell membranes may also provide interesting agents for therapy. Potent agents inhibiting cellular signaling pathways through ras, tyrosine kinases, and other regulators of cell division are just now entering clinical trials. The first tentative steps into the realm of gene therapy for cancer are just now being taken. It is hoped that the continued strides made in understanding molecular and cell biology, such as the mechanisms of sarcoma induction by fusion proteins encoded by specific chromosomal translocations seen in sarcomas, will lead to new therapies that will affect the therapy of this diverse family of tumors.

REFERENCES

1. Landis S, Murray T, Bolden S, Wingo P. Cancer statistics. *CA Cancer J Clin* 1999;9:8.
2. Zahm S, Fraumeni J Jr. The epidemiology of soft tissue sarcoma. *Semin Oncol* 1997;24:504.
3. Latres E, Drobnjak M, Pollack D, et al. Chromosome 17 abnormalities and TP53 mutations in adult soft tissue sarcomas. *Am J Pathol* 1994;145:345.
4. Cance W, Brennan M, Dudas M, et al. Altered expression of the retinoblastoma gene product in human sarcomas. *N Engl J Med* 1990;323:1457.
5. Malkin D. *The Li-Fraumeni syndrome.* Vol. 7. Philadelphia: Lippincott, 1995.
6. Li F, Fraumeni J Jr. Soft tissue sarcomas, breast cancer and other neoplasms. A familial syndrome? *Ann Intern Med* 1969;71:747.
7. D'Agostino A, Soule E, Miller R. Sarcomas of the peripheral nerves and somatic soft tissues associated with multiple neurofibromatosis (von Recklinghausen's disease). *Cancer* 1963;16:1015.
8. Heard G. Malignant disease in von Recklinghausen's neurofibromatosis. *Proc R Soc Med* 1963;56:502.
9. Fraumeni J Jr, Vogel C, Easton J. Sarcomas and multiple polyposis in a kindred. A genetic variety of hereditary polyposis? *Arch Intern Med* 1968;121:57.
10. Sorensen S, Mulvihill J, Nielsen A. Long-term follow-up of von Recklinghausen neurofibromatosis. *N Engl J Med* 1986;314:1010.
11. Riccardi V. Von Recklinghausen neurofibromatosis. *N Engl J Med* 1981;305:1617.
12. Williams W, Strong L. Genetic epidemiology of soft tissue sarcomas in children. In: Muller W, ed. *First International Research Conference. Familial cancer.* Basel, Switzerland: Karger, 1985:151.
13. Draper G, Sanders B, Kingston J. Second primary neoplasms in patients with retinoblastoma. *Br J Cancer* 1986;53:661.
14. Li F, Fraumeni J. Prospective study of a family cancer syndrome. *JAMA* 1982;247:2692.
15. Wong F, Boice J Jr, Abramson D, et al. Cancer incidence after retinoblastoma. Radiation dose and sarcoma risk. *JAMA* 1997;278:1261.
16. Posner M, Shiu M, Newsome J, et al. The desmoid tumor: not a benign disease. *Arch Surg* 1989;124:191.
17. Beck A. Zur frage des Rontgensarkoms, zugleich ein Beitrag zur pathogenese des Sarkoms. *Muench Med Wochenschr* 1922;69:623.
18. Brady M, Gaynor J, Brennan M. Radiation-associated sarcoma of bone and soft tissue. *Arch Surg* 1992;127:1379.
19. Karlsson P, Holmberg E, Samuelsson A, et al. Soft tissue sarcoma after treatment for breast cancer —a Swedish population-based study. *Eur J Cancer* 1998;34:2068.
20. Stewart F, Treves N. Lymphangiosarcoma in post-mastectomy lymphedema. *Cancer* 1943;1:64.
21. Muller R, Hajdu S, Brennan M. Lymphangiosarcoma associated with chronic filarial lymphedema. *Cancer* 1987;59:179.
22. Pack G, Ehrlich H. Neoplasms of the anterior abdominal wall with special consideration of desmoid tumors: experience with 391 cases and collective review of literature. *Int Abst Surg* 1944;79:177.
23. Fong Y, Rosen P, Brennan M. Multifocal desmoids. *Surgery* 1993;114:902.
24. Hardell L, Sandstrom A. A case-control study: Soft tissue sarcoma and exposure to chemical substances: a case referent study. *Br J Cancer* 1979;39:711.
25. Eriksson M, Hardell L, Ber N, et al. Soft tissue sarcomas and exposure to chemical substances: a case referent study. *Br J Ind Med* 1981;38:27.
26. Smith A, Pearce N, Fisher D, et al. Soft tissue sarcoma and exposure to phenoxyherbicides and chlorophenols in New Zealand. *J Natl Cancer Inst* 1984;73:1111.
27. Balarajan R, Acheson E. Soft tissue sarcomas in agriculture and forestry workers. *J Epidemiol Commun Health* 1984;38:113.
28. Greenwald P, Kovasznay B, Collins D, Therriault G. Sarcomas of soft tissue after Vietnam service. *J Natl Cancer Inst* 1984;73:1107.
29. Kang H, Weatherbee L, Breslin P, et al. Soft tissue sarcoma and military service in Vietnam: a case comparison group analysis of hospital patients. *J Occup Med* 1986;28:1215.
30. Hoar S, Blair A, Holmes F, et al. Agricultural herbicide use and risk of lymphoma and soft tissue sarcoma. *JAMA* 1986;256:1141.
31. Kelly S, Guidotti T. Phenoxyacetic acid herbicides and chlorophenols and the etiology of lymphoma and soft tissue neoplasms. *Public Health Rev* 1989/90;17:1.
32. Lynge E, Storn H, Jensen O. The evaluation of trends in soft tissue sarcoma according to diagnostic criteria and consumption of phenoxy herbicides. *Cancer* 1987;60:1896.
33. Hoppin J, Tolbert P, Herrick R, et al. Occupational chlorophenal exposure and soft tissue sarcoma risk among men aged 30–60 years. *Am J Epidemiol* 1998;148:693.
34. Riihimake V, Asp S, Hernberg S. Mortality of 2,4-dichlorophenoxyacetic acid and 2,4,5-trichlorophenoxyacetic acid herbicide applicators in Finland: first report of an ongoing prospective cohort study. *Scand J Work Environ Health* 1982;8:37.
35. Hoppin J, Tolbert P, Flanders W, et al. Occupational risk factors for sarcoma subtypes. *Epidemiology* 1999;10:300.
36. Fingerhut M, Halperin W, Marlow D, et al. Cancer mortality in workers exposed to 2,3,7,8-tetrachlorodibenzo-p-dioxin. *N Engl J Med* 1991;324:212.
37. Wiklund K, Holm L. Soft tissue sarcoma risk in Swedish agricultural and forestry workers. *J Natl Cancer Inst* 1986;76:229.
38. Wiklund K, Dich J, Holm L. Soft tissue sarcoma risk in Swedish licensed pesticide applicators. *J Occup Med* 1988;30:801.
39. Brann E. The association of selected cancers with service in the US military in Vietnam: II. Soft tissue and other sarcomas. *Arch Intern Med* 1990;150:2485.
40. Kang H, Enziger F, Breslin P, et al. Soft tissue sarcoma and military service in Vietnam: a case-control study. *J Natl Cancer Inst* 1987;79:693.
41. DaSilva H, Abbatt J, DaMotta L. Malignancy and other effects following the administration of thorotrast. *Lancet* 1965;2:201.
42. Creech J, Makk L. Liver disease among polyvinyl chloride production workers. *Ann NY Acad Sci* 1973;246:88.
43. Lander J, Stanley R, Summer H. Angiosarcoma of the liver associated with Fowler's solution. *Gastroenterology* 1975;68:1562.
44. Dick J, Zahm S, Hanberg A, Adami H. Pesticides and cancer. *Cancer Causes Control* 1997;8:420.
45. Tucker M, D'Angio G, Bioce J Jr, et al. Bone sarcomas linked to radiotherapy and chemotherapy in children. *N Engl J Med* 1987;317:588.
46. Mertens F, Fletcher C, Dal Cin P, et al. Cytogenetic analysis of 46 pleomorphic soft tissue sarcomas and correlation with morphologic and clinical features: a report of the CHAMP Study Group. Chromosomes and morphology. *Genes Chromosomes Cancer* 1998;22:16.
47. Orlow I, Drobnjak M, Zhang Z, et al. Alteration of INK4A and INK4B genes in adult soft tissue sarcomas: effect on survival. *J Natl Cancer Inst* 1999;91:73.
48. Sreekantaiah C, Karakousis C, Leong S, Sandberg A. Cytogenetic findings in liposarcoma correlate with histopathologic subtypes. *Cancer* 1992;69:2484.
49. Enzinger F, Weiss S. *Soft tissue tumors.* 3rd ed. St. Louis: Year Book Medical, 1995.
50. Hajdu S. *Pathology of soft tissue tumors.* Philadelphia: Lea & Febiger, 1979.
51. Fong Y, Coit D, Woodruff J, Brennan M. Lymph node metastasis from soft tissue sarcoma in adults: analysis of data from a prospective database of 1772 sarcoma patients. *Ann Surg* 1993;218:72.
52. Weingrad D, Rosenberg S. Early lymphatic spread of osteogenic and soft tissue sarcomas. *Surgery* 1978;84:231.
53. Mazeron J, Suit H. Lymph nodes as sites of metastases from sarcomas of soft tissue. *Cancer* 1987;60:1800.
54. Gaynor J, Tan C, Casper E, et al. Refinement of clinicopathological staging for localized soft tissue sarcoma of the extremity: a study of 423 adults. *J Clin Oncol* 1992;10:1317.
55. Broders A, Hargrave R, Meyerding H. Pathological features of soft tissue fibrosarcoma with special reference to the grading of its malignancy. *Surg Gynecol Obstet* 1939;69:267.
56. Beahrs O, Henson D, Hutter R, Kennedy B. *Manual for staging cancer.* 4th ed. Philadelphia: Lippincott, 1992.
57. Costa J, Wesley R, Glatstein E. The grading of soft tissue sarcoma. Results of a clinicohistopathologic correlation in a series of 163 cases. *Cancer* 1984;53:530.
58. Trojani M, Contesso G, Coindre J. Soft tissue sarcoma of adults. Study of pathological prognostic variables and definition of a histopathological grading system. *Int J Cancer* 1984;33:37.
59. Myhre-Jensen O, Kaae S, Madsen E. Histopathological grading of soft tissue sarcomas: relation to survival in 261 surgically treated patients. *Acta Pathol Microbiol Immunol Scand* 1983;91A:145.
60. Markhede G, Angervall L, Stener B. A multivariate analysis of the prognosis after surgical treatment of malignant soft tissue tumors. *Cancer* 1982;49:1721.
61. Alvegard T, Berg N. Histopathology peer review of high-grade soft tissue sarcoma: the Scandinavian Sarcoma Group experience. *J Clin Oncol* 1989;7:1845.
62. Alvegard TA, Sigurdsson H, Mouridsen H, et al. Adjuvant chemotherapy with doxorubicin in high-grade soft tissue sarcoma: a randomized trial of the Scandinavian Sarcoma Group. *J Clin Oncol* 1989;7:1504.
63. Enzinger F. *Recent developments in the classification of soft tissue sarcomas.* Chicago: Year Book Medical, 1977.
64. van Unnik J, Coindre J, Contesso G. Grading of soft tissue sarcomas: experience of the EORTC soft tissue and bone sarcoma group. *Dev Oncol* 1988;55:7.
65. Drobnjak M, Latres E, Pollack D, et al. Prognostic implications of p53 nuclear overexpression and high proliferation index of Ki-67 in adult soft tissue sarcomas. *J Natl Cancer Inst* 1994;86:549.
66. Fletcher J, Kozakewich H, Hoffer F, et al. Diagnostic relevance of clonal chromosome aberrations in malignant soft tissue tumors. *N Engl J Med* 1991;324:436.
67. Limon J, Mrozek K, Mandahl N, et al. Cytogenics of synovial sarcoma: presentation of 10 new cases and review of the literature. *Genes Chromosomes Cancer* 1991;3:338.
68. Clark J, Rocques P, Crew A, et al. Identification of novel genes, SYT and SSX, involved in the t(X;18)(p11.2;q11.2) translocation found in human synovial sarcoma. *Nature Genet* 1994;7:502.
69. Turc-Carel C, Limon J, Dal Cin P, et al. Cytogenetic studies of adipose tissue tumors. II. recurrent reciprocal translocation t(12;16)(q13;p11) in myxoid liposarcomas. *Cancer Genet* Cytogenet 1986;23:291.
70. Crozat A, Aman P, Mandahl N, Ron D. Fusion of CHOP to a novel RNA-binding protein in human myxoid liposarcoma. *Nature* 1993;363:640.
71. Knight J, Renwick P, Cin P, et al. Translocation t(12;16)(q13;p11) in myxoid liposarcoma and round cell liposarcoma: molecular and cytogenetic analysis. *Cancer Res* 1995;55:24.
72. Wang-Wuu S, Soukup S, Ballard E, et al. Chromosomal analysis of sixteen human rhabdomyosarcomas. *Cancer Res* 1988;48:983.
73. Davis R, D'Cruz C, Lovell M, et al. Fusion of PAX7 to FKHR by the variant t(1;13)(p36;q14) translocation in alveolar rhabdomyosarcoma. *Cancer Res* 1994;54:2869.
74. Delattre O, Zucman J, Melot T, et al. The Ewing family of tumors—a subgroup of small round cell tumors defined by specific chimeric transcripts. *N Engl J Med* 1994;331:294.
75. Sorensen P, Lessnick S, Lopez-Terrada D, et al. A second Ewing's sarcoma translocation t(21;22), fuses the EWS gene to another ETS-family transcription factor, ERG. *Nature Genet* 1994;6:146.
76. Giovanni M, Beigel J, Serra M, et al. EWS-erg and EWS-Fli 1 fusion transcripts in Ewing's sarcoma and primitive neuroectodermal tumors with variant translocations. *J Clin Invest* 1994;94:489.

77. Ladanyi M, Gerald W. Fusion of the EWS and WT1 genes in the desmoplastic small round cell tumor. *Cancer Res* 1994;54:2837.
78. Bridge J, Borek D, Neff J, Huntrakoon M. Chromosomal abnormalities in clear cell sarcoma. Implications for histogenesis. *Am J Clin Pathol* 1990;93:26.
79. Fletcher J. Translocation (12;22)(q13-14;q12) is a non-random aberration in soft tissue clear-cell sarcoma. *Genes Chromosomes Cancer* 1992;5:184.
80. Reeves B, Fletcher C, Gusterson B. Translocation t(12;22)(q13;q13) is a nonrandom rearrangement in clear cell sarcoma. *Cancer Genet Cytogenet* 1992;64:101.
81. Rodriguez E, Sreekantaiah C, Reuter V, et al. t(12;22)(q13;q13) and trisomy 8 are nonrandom aberrations in clear cell sarcoma. *Cancer Genet Cytogenet* 1992;64:107.
82. Stenman G, Kindblom L, Angervall L. Reciprocal translocation t(12:22)(q13;q13) in clear cell sarcoma of tendons and aponeuroses. *Genes Chromosomes Cancer* 1992;4:122.
83. Orndal C, Carlen B, Akerman M, et al. Chromosomal abnormality t(9;22)(q22;q12) in an extraskeletal myxoid chondrosarcoma characterized by fine needle aspiration cytology, electron microscopy, immunohistochemistry, and DNA flow cytometry. *Cytopathology* 1991;2:261.
84. Turc-Carel C, Dal Cin P, Rao U. Recurrent breakpoints at 9q31 and 22q12.2 in extraskeletal myxoid chondrosarcoma. *Cancer Genet Cytogenet* 1988;30:145.
85. Shiraki M, Enterline H, Brooks J, et al. Pathologic analysis of advanced adult soft tissue sarcomas, bone sarcomas, and mesothelioma. *Cancer* 1989;64:484.
86. Presant C, Russell W, Alexander R, Fu Y. Soft tissue and bone sarcoma histopathology peer review: the frequency of disagreement in diagnosis and the need for second pathology opinions. The Southeastern Cancer Study Group experience. *J Clin Oncol* 1986; 4:1658.
87. Vezeridis M, Moore R, Karakousis C. Metastic patterns in soft tissue sarcomas. *Arch Surg* 1983;118:915.
88. Gordon M, Hajdu S, Bains M, Burt M. Soft tissue sarcomas of the chest wall. Results of surgical resection. *J Thorac Cardiovasc Surg* 1991;101:843.
89. Conlon K, Casper E, Brennan M. Primary gastrointestinal sarcomas: analysis of prognostic variables. *Ann Surg Oncol* 1995;2:26.
90. Lauwers G, Erlandson R, Casper E, et al. Gastrointestinal autonomic nerve tumors. A clinicopathological, immunohistochemical, and ultrstructural study of 12 cases. *Am J Surg Pathol* 1993;17:887.
91. Russo P, Brady M, Conlon K, et al. Adult urological sarcoma. *J Urol* 1992;147:1032.
92. Bernstein K, Lattes R. Nodular (pseudosarcomatous) fasciitis, a nonrecurrent lesion: clinicopathologic study of 134 cases. *Cancer* 1982;49:1668.
93. Hutter R, Stewart F, Foote F. Fasciitis: a report of 70 cases with follow-up proving the benignity of the lesion. *Cancer* 1962;15:992.
94. Chung E, Enzinger F. Fibroma of tendon sheath. *Cancer* 1979;44:1945.
95. Stemmermann G, Stout A. Elastofibroma dorsi. *Am J Clin Pathol* 1962;38:499.
96. Brown R, Clearkin K, Nakachi K, Burdick C. Elastofibroma dorsi. *N Engl J Med* 1966;275:154.
97. Gardner E, Richards R. Multiple cutaneous and subcutaneous lesions occuring simultaneously with hereditary polyposis and osteomatosis. *Am J Hum Genet* 1953;5:139.
98. Gardner E. Follow up study of a family group exhibiting dominant inheritance for a syndrome including intestinal polyps, osteomas, fibromas, and epidermal cysts. *Am J Hum Genet* 1962;14:376.
99. Antal I, Szendroi M, Kovacs G, et al. Multicentric extraabdominal desmoid tumour: a case report. *J Cancer Res Clin Oncol* 1994;120:490.
100. Reitamo J, Scheinin T, Hayry P. The desmoid syndrome. New aspects in the cause, pathogenesis and treatment of the desmoid tumour. *Am J Surg* 1986;151:230.
101. Franquemont D, Cooper P, Shmookler B, Wick M. Benign fibrous histiocytoma of the skin with potential for local recurrence: a tumor to be distinguished from dermatofibroma. *Mod Pathol* 1990;3:158.
102. Fletcher C. Benign fibrous histiocytoma of subcutaneous and deep soft tissue: a clinicopathologic analysis of 21 cases. *Am J Surg Pathol* 1990;14:801.
103. Burkhardt B, Soule E, Winkelman R, Ivins J. Dermatofibrosarcoma protruberans: study of 56 cases. *Am J Surg* 1966;111:638.
104. Taylor H, Helwig E. Dermatofibrosarcoma protruberans: a study of 115 cases. *Cancer* 1962;15:717.
105. Weiss S, Nickoloff B. CD34 is expressed by a distinctive cell population in peripheral nerve, nerve sheath tumors, and related lesions. *Am J Surg Pathol* 1993;17:1039.
106. Bridge J, Neff J, Sandberg A. Cytogenetic analysis of dermatofibrosarcoma protruberans. *Cancer Genet Cytogenet* 1990;49:199.
107. McPeak C, Druz T, Nicastri A. Dermatofibrosarcoma protruberans: an analysis of 86 cases—five with metastasis. *Am Surg* 1967;166(Suppl 2):803.
108. Bednar B. Storiform neurofibromas of the skin, pigmented and non-pigmented. *Cancer* 1957;10:368.
109. Ozzello L, Stout A, Murray M. Cultural characteristics of malignant histiocytomas and fibrous zanthomas. *Cancer* 1963;16:331.
110. Fletcher C. Pleomorphic malignant fibrous histiocytoma: fact or fiction? *Am J Surg Pathol* 1992;16:213.
111. Pezzi C, Rawlings M, Esgro J, et al. Prognostic factors in 227 patients with malignant fibrous histiocytoma. *Cancer* 1992;69:2098.
112. Rooser B, Willen H, Gustafson P, et al. Malignant fibrous histiocytoma of soft tissue. *Cancer* 1991;67:499.
113. Evans H, Soule E, Winkelman R. Atypical lipoma, atypical intramuscular lipoma, and well differentiated retroperitoneal liposarcoma. *Cancer* 1979;43:574.
114. Azumi N, Curtis J, Kempson R, Hendrickson M. Atypical and malignant neoplasms showing lipomatous differentiation: a study of 111 cases. *Am J Surg Pathol* 1987;11:161.
115. Nonomura A, Mizukami Y, Kadoya M. Angiomyolipoma of the liver: a collective review. *J Gastroenterol* 1994;29:95.
116. Ahn C, Harvey J. Mediastinal hibernoma, a rare tumor. *Ann Thorac Surg* 1990;50:828.
117. Mentzel T, Calonje E, Fletcher C. Lipoblastoma and lipoblastomatosis: a clinicopathological study of 14 cases. *Histopathology* 1993;23:527.
118. Chang H, Hajdu S, Collin C, Brennan M. The prognostic value of histologic subtypes in primary extremity liposarcoma. *Cancer* 1989;64:1514.
119. McCormick D, Mentzel T, Beham A, Fletcher C. Dedifferentiated liposarcoma. Clinicopatholiogic analysis of 32 cases suggesting a better prognostic subgroup among pleomorphic sarcomas. *Am J Surg Pathol* 1994;18:1213.
120. Tallini G, Erlandson R, Brennan M, Woodruff J. Divergent myosarcomatous differentiation in retroperitoneal liposarcoma. *Am J Surg Pathol* 1993;17:546.
121. Fisher W, Helwig E. Leiomyomas of the skin. *Arch Dermatol* 1963;88:510.
122. Fox S. Leiomyomatosis cutis. *N Engl J Med* 1960;263:1248.
123. Norris H, Parmley T. Mesenchymal tumors of the uterus. V. Intravenous leiomyomatosis: a clinical and pathologic study of 14 cases. *Cancer* 1975;36:2164.
124. Suginami H, Kaura R, Ochi H, Matsuura S. Intravenous leiomyomatosis with cardiac extension. *Obstet Gynecol* 1990;76:527.
125. Tavassoli F, Norris H. Peritoneal leiomyomatosis (leiomyomatosis peritonealis disseminata). *Int J Gynecol Pathol* 1982;1:59.
126. Stout A, Hill W. Leiomyosarcoma of the superficial soft tissues. *Cancer* 1958;11:844.
127. Gustafson P, Willen H, Baldetorp B, et al. Soft tissue leiomyosarcoma. *Cancer* 1992;70:114.
128. LaQuaglia M, Heller G, Ghavimi F, et al. The effect of age at diagnosis on outcome in rhabdomyosarcoma. *Cancer* 1994;73:109.
129. White C. Treatment of hemangiomatosis with recombinant interferon alfa [Review]. *Semin Hematology* 1990;27:15.
130. Taylor J, Ryu J, Colby T, Raffin T. Lymphangioleiomyomatosis. Clinical course in 32 patients. *N Engl J Med* 1990;323:1254.
131. Weiss S, Ishak K, Dail D, et al. Epithelioid hemangioendothelioma and related lesions. *Semin Diagn Pathol* 1986;3:259.
132. Dail D, Liebow A, Gmelich J, et al. Intravascular, bronchiolar, and alveolar tumor of the lung (IBVAT). *Cancer* 1983;51:452.
133. Kelleher M, Iwatsuki S, Sheahan D. Epithelioid hemangioendothelioma of liver. Clinicopathological correlation of 10 cases treated hby orthotopic liver transplantation. *Am J Surg Pathol* 1989;13:999.
134. Reynolds W, Winkelman R, Soule E. Kaposi's sarcoma: a clinicopathologic study with particular reference to its relationship to the reticuloendothelial system. *Medicine (Baltimore)* 1965;44:419.
135. Stribling J, Wertzner S, Smith G. Kaposi's sarcoma in renal allograft recipients. *Cancer* 1978;42:442.
136. Woodard A, Ivins J, Soule E. Lymphangiosarcoma arising in chronic lymphedematous extremities. *Cancer* 1972;30:562.
137. Holden C, Spittle M, Jones E. Angiosarcoma of the face and scalp, prognosis and treatment. *Cancer* 1987;59:1046.
138. Rosen P, Kimmel M, Ernsberger D. Mammary angiosarcoma: the prognostic significance of tumor differentiation. *Cancer* 1988;62:2145.
139. Nanus D, Kelsen D, Clark D. Radiation-induced angiosarcoma. *Cancer* 1987;60:777.
140. Fletcher C, Beham A, Bekir S, et al. Epithelioid angiosarcoma of deep soft tissue: a distinctive tumor readily mistaken for an epithelial neoplasm. *Am J Surg Pathol* 1991;15:915.
141. Shugart R, Soule E, Johnson E. Glomus tumor. *Surg Gynecol Obstet* 1963;117:334.
142. Nemes Z. Differentiation markers in hemangiopericytoma. *Cancer* 1992;69:133.
143. Enzinger F, Smith B. Hemangiopericytoma. An analysis of 106 cases. *Hum Pathol* 1976;7:61.
144. Brodsky J, Burt M, Hajdu S, et al. Tendosynovial sarcoma. Clinicopathologic features, treatment and prognosis. *Cancer* 1992;70:484.
145. Riccardi V. *Neurofibromatosis: phenotype, natural history and pathogenesis.* 2nd ed. Baltimore: Johns Hopkins University Press, 1992.
146. Wallace M, Marchuk D, Andersen L, et al. Type I neurofibromatosis gene: identification of a large transcript disrupted in three NF1 patients. *Science* 1990;249:181.
147. White W, Shiu M, Rosenblum M, et al. Cellular schwannoma. *Cancer* 1990;66:1266.
148. Woodruff J, Chernick N, Smith M, et al. Peripheral nerve tumors with rhabdomyosarcomatous differentiation (malignent "Triton" tumors). *Cancer* 1973;32:426.
149. Vauthey J, Woodruff J, Brennan M. Extremity malignant peripheral nerve sheath tumors (neurogenic sarcomas): a 10-year experience. *Ann Surg Oncol* 1995;2:126.
150. Enzinger F, Shiraki M. Extraskeletal myxoid chondrosarcoma: an analysis of 34 cases. *Hum Pathol* 1972;3:421.
151. Sordillo P, Hajdu S, Magill G, Golbey R. Extraosseous osteogenic sarcoma. *Cancer* 1983;51:727.
152. Chung E, Enzinger F. Extraskeletal osteosarcoma. *Cancer* 1987;60:1132.
153. Bane B, Evans H, Ro J, et al. Extraskeletal osteosarcoma. A clinicopathologic review of 26 cases. *Cancer* 1990;76:2762.
154. Lee J, Fetsch J, Wasdhal D, et al. A review of 40 patients with estraskeletal osteosarcoma. *Cancer* 1995;76:2253.
155. Enzinger F. Intramuscular myxoma. *Am J Clin Pathol* 1965;43:104.
156. Steeper T, Rosai J. Aggressive angiomyxoma of the female pelvis and perineum. Report of nine cases of a distinctive type of gynecologic soft tissue neoplasm. *Am J Clin Pathol* 1983;7:463.
157. Stout A, Lattes R. *Malignant mesenchymoma. Tumors of soft tissue.* Armed Forces Institute of Pathology Atlas of Tumor Pathology, 1967:172.
158. Newman P, Fletcher C. Malignant mesenchymoma. Clinicopathologic analysis of a series with evidence of low-grade behaviour. *Am J Surg Pathol* 1991;15:607.
159. Lieberman P, Brennan M, Kimmel M, et al. Alveolar soft-part sarcoma. A clinico-pathologic study of half a century. *Cancer* 1989;63:1.
160. Tallini G, Parham D, Dias P, et al. Myogenic regulatory protein expression in adult soft tissue sarcomas. A sensitive and specific marker of skeletal muscle differentiation. *Am J Pathol* 1994;144:693.
161. Prat J, Woodruff J, Marcove R. Epithelioid sarcoma. *Cancer* 1978;41:1472.
162. Chase D, Enzinger F. Epithelioid sarcoma. *Am J Surg Pathol* 1985;9:241.

163. Gerald W, Miller H, Battifora H, et al. Intraabdominal desmoplastic small round-cell tumor: report of 19 cases of a distinctive type of high-grade polyphenotypic malignancy affecting young individuals. *Am J Surg Pathol* 1991;15:499.
164. Rodriguez E, Sreekantaiah C, Gerald W, et al. A recurring translocation, t(11;22(p13;q11.2), characterizes intraabdominal desmoplastic small round-cell tumors. *Cancer Genet Cytogenet* 1993;69:17.
165. Sawyer J, Tryka A, Lewis J. A novel reciprocal chromosome translocation t(11;22) (p13;q12) in an intraabdominal desmoplastic small round-cell tumor. *Am J Surg Pathol* 1992;16(4):411.
166. Fonesca R, Yamakawa M, Nakamura S, et al. Follicular dendritic cell sarcoma and interdigitating reticulum cell sarcoma: a review. *Am J Hematol* 1998;59:161.
167. Schwarz R, Chugo P, Arber D. Extranodal follicular dendritic cell tumor of the abdominal wall. *J Clin Oncol* 1999;17:2290.
168. Demas B, Heelan R, Lane J, et al. Soft tissue sarcomas of the extremities: prospective comparison of MRI and CT in determination of anatomic extent of disease. *Am J Radiol* 1988;150:615.
169. Panicek D, Gatsonis C, Rosenthal D, et al. CT and MR imaging in local staging of primary malignant musculoskeletal neoplasms; report of the Radiology Diagnostic Oncology Group. *Radiology* 1997;202:237.
170. Gadd M, Casper E, Woodruff J, et al. Development and treatment of pulmonary metastases in adult patients with extremity soft tissue sarcoma. *Ann Surg* 1993;218:705.
171. Cheng E, Dempsey S, Springfield S, Mankin H. Frequent incidence of extrapulmonary sites of initial metastases in patients with liposarcoma. *Cancer* 1995;75:1120.
172. Ball A, Fisher C, Pittam M, et al. Diagnosis of soft tissue tumors by tru-cut biopsy. *Br J Surg* 1990;77:756.
173. Kissin M, Fisher C, Carter R, et al. Value of tru-cut biopsy in the diagnosis of soft tissue tumours. *Br J Surg* 1986;73:742.
174. Mankin H, Lange T, Spanier S. The hazards of biopsy in patients with malignant primary bone and soft tissue tumors. *J Bone Joint Surg* 1982;64:1121.
175. Kissin M, Fisher C, Webb A, Westbury G. Value of fine needle aspiration cytology in the diagnosis of soft tissue tumours: a preliminary study on the excised specimen. *Br J Surg* 1987;74:479.
176. Kindblom L. Light and electron microscopic examination of embedded fine-needle aspiration biopsy specimens in the preoperative diagnosis of soft tissue and bone tumors. *Cancer* 1983;51:2264.
177. Rydhom A. Soft tissue lesions in adults: biopsy—yes or no? *Ann Oncol* 1992;3(Suppl 2):S57.
178. Rooser B, Rydhom A, Alvegard T. Centralization of soft tissue sarcoma. Status in Sweden, 1982. *Acta Orthop Scand* 1987;58:641.
179. Akerman M, Killander D, Rydholm A, Rooser B. Aspiration of musculoskeletal tumors for cytodiagnosis and DNA analysis. *Acta Orthop Scand* 1987;58:525.
180. Russell W, Cohen J, Enzinger F, et al. A clinical and pathological staging system for soft tissue sarcoma. *Cancer* 1977;40:1562.
181. Geer R, Woodruff J, Casper E, Brennan M. Management of small soft tissue sarcoma of the extremity in adults. *Arch Surg* 1992;127:1285.
182. Fleming J, Berman R, Cheng S, et al. Long-term outcome of patients with American Joint Committee on Cancer stage IIB extremity soft tissue sarcomas. *J Clin Oncol* 1999;17:2772.
183. Brennan MF. Staging of soft tissue sarcomas. *Ann Surg Oncol* 1999;6:8.
184. Pisters P, Leung D, Woodruff J, et al. Analysis of prognostic factors in 1,041 patients with localized soft tissue sarcomas of the extremities. *J Clin Oncol* 1996;14:1679.
185. Lewis J, Leung D, Casper E, et al. Multifactorial analysis of long-term follow-up (more than 5 years) of primary extremity sarcoma. *Arch Surg* 1999;134:190.
186. Rosenberg S, Kent H, Costa J, et al. Prospective randomized evaluation of the role of limb-sparing surgery, radiation therapy, and adjuvant chemoimmunotherapy in the treatment of soft tissue sarcoma. *Surgery* 1978;84:62.
187. Rosenberg S, Tepper J, Galtstein E, et al. The treatment of soft tissue sarcoma of the extremities: prospective randomized evaluations of (1) limb-sparing surgery plus radiation therapy compared with amputation and (2) the role of adjuvant chemotherapy. *Ann Surg* 1982;196:305.
188. Pusey W. Cases of sarcoma and of Hodgkin's disease treated by exposure to X-rays: a preliminary report. *JAMA* 1902;38:166.
189. Weichselbaum R, Beckett M, Vijayakumar S, et al. Radiobiological characterization of head and neck and sarcoma cells derived from patient prior to radiotherapy. *Int J Radiat Oncol Biol Phys* 1990;19:313.
190. Kelland L, Bingle L, Edwards S, Steel G. High intrinsic radiosensitivity of a newly established and characterised human embryonal rhabdomyosarcoma cell line. *Br J Cancer* 1989;59:160.
191. Ruka W, Taghian A, Gioioso D, et al. Comparison between the in vitro intrinsic radiation sensitivity of human soft tissue sarcoma and breast cancer cell lines. *J Surg Oncol* 1996;61:290.
192. Pisters P, Harrison L, Leung D, et al. Long term results of a prospective randomized trial of adjuvant brachytherapy in soft tissue sarcoma. *J Clin Oncol* 1996;14:859.
193. Yang J, Chang A, Baker A, et al. Randomized prospective study of the benefit of adjuvant radiation therapy in the treatment of soft tissue sarcomas of the extremity. *J Clin Oncol* 1998;16:197.
194. Lindberg R, Martin R, Romsdahl M. Surgery and postoperative radiotherapy in the treatment of soft tissue sarcomas in adults. *Am J Roentgenol Radium Ther Nucl Med* 1975;123:123.
195. Suit H, Russell W, Martin R. Sarcoma of soft tissue: clinical and histopathologic parameters and response to treatment. *Cancer* 1975;35:1478
196. Suit H, Russell W, Martin R. Management of patients with sarcoma of soft tissue in an extremity. *Cancer* 1973;31:1237.
197. Lindberg R, Martin R, Romsdahl M, Barkley H. Conservative surgery and postoperative radiotherapy in 300 adults with soft tissue sarcomas. *Cancer* 1981;47:2391.
198. Suit H, Sprio I. Role of radiation in the management of adult patients with sarcoma of soft tissue. *Semin Surg Oncol* 1994;10:347.
199. Harrison L, Franzese F, Gaynor J, Brennan M. Long-term results of a prospective randomized trial of adjuvant brachytherapy in the management of completely resected soft tissue sarcomas of the extremity and superficial trunt. *Int J Radiat Oncol Biol Phys* 1993;27:259.
200. Mundt A, Awan A, Sibley G, et al. Conservative surgery and adjuvant radiation therapy in the management of adult soft tissue sarcoma of the extremities: clinical and radiobiological results. *Int J Radiat Oncol Biol Phys* 1995;32:977.
201. Pao W, Pilepich M. Postoperative radiotherapy in the treatment of extremity soft tissue sarcomas. *Int J Radiat Oncol Biol Phys* 1990;19:907.
202. Janjan N, Yasko A, Reece G, et al. Comparision of charges related to radiotherapy for soft tissue sarcomas treated with preoperative external beam radiation versus interstitial implantation. *Ann Surg Oncol* 1994;1:415.
203. Hilaris B, Shiu M, Nori D. Limb-sparing therapy for locally advanced soft tissue sarcomas. *Endocur Hypertherm Oncol* 1985;1:17.
204. Pisters P, Harrison L, Woodruff J, et al. A prospective randomized trial of adjuvant brachytherapy in the management of low-grade soft tissue sarcomas of the extremity and superficial trunk. *J Clin Oncol* 1994;12:1150.
205. Schray M, Gunderson L, Sim F, et al. Soft tissue sarcoma: integration of brachytherapy, resection, and external irradiation. *Cancer* 1990;66:451.
206. Thomas L, Delannes M, Stockle E, et al. Intraoperative interstitial iridium brachytherapy in the management of soft tissue sarcomas: preliminary results of a feasibility phase II study. *Radiother Oncol* 1994;33:99.
207. Alekhteyar K, Leung D, Brennan M, Harrison L. The effect of combined external beam radiotherapy and brachytherapy on local control and wound complications in patients with high-grade soft tissue sarcomas of the extremity with positive microscopic margin. *Int J Radiat Oncol Biol Phys* 1996;36:321.
208. Nori D, Shupak K, Shiu M, Brennan M. Role of brachytherapy in recurrent extremity sarcoma in patients treated with prior surgery and irradiation. *Int J Radiat Oncol Biol Phys* 1991;20:1229.
209. Pearlstone D, Janjan N, Feig B, et al. Re-resection with brachytherapy for locally recurrent soft tissue sarcoma arising in a previously radiated field. *Cancer J Sci Am* 1999;5:26.
210. Catton C, Davis A, Bell R, et al. Soft tissue sarcoma of the extremity. Limb salvage after failure of combined conservative therapy. *Radiother Oncol* 1996;41:209.
211. Ormsby M, Hilaris B, Nori D, Brennan M. Wound complicatons of adjuvant radiation therapy in patients with soft tissue sarcomas. *Ann Surg* 1989;210:93.
212. Alekhteyar K, Porter A, Herskovic A, et al. Preliminary results of hyperfracitonated high dose rate brachytherapy in soft tissue sarcomas. *Endocurietherapy/Hyperthermia Oncology* 1994;10:179.
213. Suit H, Mankin H, Wood W, et al. Treatment of the patient with stage M_0 soft tissue sarcoma. *J Clin Oncol* 1988;6:854.
214. Cheng E, Dusenbery K, Winters M, Thompson R. Soft tissue sarcomas: preoperative versus postoperative radiotherapy. *J Surg Oncol* 1996;61:90.
215. Pollack A, Zagars G, Goswitz M, et al. Preoperative vs. postoperative radiotherapy in the treatment of soft tissue sarcomas: a matter of presentation. *Int J Radiat Oncol Biol Phys* 1998;42:563.
216. O'Sullivan B, Davis A, Group CS, et al. Effect on radiotherapy field sizes in a recently completed Canadian Sarcoma Group and NCI Canada Clinical Trials Group randomized trial comparing pre-operative and post-operative radiotherapy in extremity soft tissue sarcoma. *Int J Radiat Oncol Biol Phys* (abstract) 1999;45:238.
217. LeVay J, O'Sullivan B, Catton C, et al. Outcome and prognostic factors in soft tissue sarcoma in the adult. *Int J Radiat Oncol Biol Phys* 1993;27:1091.
218. Sadoski C, Suit H, Rosenberg A, et al. Preoperative radiation, surgical margins, and local control of extremity sarcomas of soft tissues. *J Surg Oncol* 1993;52:223.
219. Alektiar K, Velasco J, Zelefsky M, et al. Adjuvant radiotherapy for margin positive high-grade soft tissue sarcoma of the extremity. *Int J Radiat Oncol Biol Phys* (*in press*).
220. Coindre J, Terrier P, Bui N, et al. Prognostic factors in adult patients with locally controlled soft tissue sarcoma: a study of 546 patients from the French Federation of Cancer Centers Sarcoma Group. *J Clin Oncol* 1996;14:869.
221. Noria S, Davis A, Kandel R, et al. Residual disease following unplanned excision of a soft tissue sarcoma of an extremity. *J Bone Joint Surg Am* 1996;78:650.
222. Brien E, Terek R, Geer R, et al. Treatment of soft tissue sarcomas of the hand. *J Bone Joint Surg Am* 1995;77:564.
223. Talbert M, Zagars G, Sherman N, Romsdahl M. Conservative surgery and radiation therapy for soft tissue sarcoma of the wrist, hand, ankle, and foot. *Cancer* 1990;66:2482.
224. Bray P, Bell R, Bowen C, et al. Limb salvage surgery and adjuvant radiotherapy for soft tissue sarcomas of the forearm and hand. *J Hand Surg* 1997;22A:495.
225. Tepper J, Suit H. Radiation therapy alone for sarcoma of soft tissue. *Cancer* 1985;56:475.
226. Slater J, McNeese M, Peters L. Radiation therapy for unresectable soft tissue sarcomas. *Int J Radiat Oncol Biol Phys* 1986;12:1729.
227. Goffman T, Tochner Z, Glatstein E. Primary treatment of large and massive adult sarcomas with Iododeoxyuridine and aggressive hyperfractionated irradiation. *Cancer* 1991;67:572.
228. Schwarz R, Krull A, Lessel A, et al. European results of neutron therapy in soft tissue sarcomas. *Recent Results Cancer Res* 1998;150:100.
229. American Joint Committee on Cancer. Soft tissue sarcoma. In: Fleming ID, Cooper JS, Henson DE, et al., eds. *AJCC cancer staging handbook.* 5th ed. Philadelphia: Lippincott–Raven, 1998:139.
230. Omura GA, Blessing JA, Major F, et al. A randomized clinical trial of adjuvant adriamycin in uterine sarcomas: a Gynecologic Oncology Group study. *J Clin Oncol* 1985;3:1240.
231. Antman K, Suit H, Amato D, et al. Preliminary results of a randomized trial of adjuvant doxorubicin for sarcomas: lack of apparent difference between treatment groups. *J Clin Oncol* 1984;2:601.
232. Lerner HJ, Amato DA, Savlov ED, et al. Eastern Cooperative Oncology Group: a comparison of adjuvant doxorubicin and observation for patients with localized soft tissue sarcoma. *J Clin Oncol* 1987;5:613.
233. Baker LH. Adjuvant treatment for soft tissue sarcomas. In: Ryan JR, Baker LH, eds. *Recent concepts in sarcoma treatment.* Dordrecht, The Netherlands: Kluwer, 1988:130.

234. Antman K, Ryan L, Borden E, et al. Pooled results from three randomized adjuvant studies of doxorubicin versus observation in soft tissue sarcomas: 10 year results and review of the literature. In: Salmon SE, ed. *Adjuvant therapy of cancer*, VI. Philadelphia: WB Saunders, 1990:529.
235. Gherlinzoni F, Bacci G, Picci P, et al. A randomized trial for the treatment of high-grade soft tissue sarcomas of the extremities: preliminary observations. *J Clin Oncol* 1986;4:552.
236. Picci P, Bacci G, Gherlinzoni F, et al. Results of a randomized trial for the treatment of localized soft tissue tumors (STS) of the extremities in adult patients. In: Ryan JR, Baker LH, eds. *Recent concepts in sarcoma treatment.* Dordrecht, The Netherlands: Kluwer, 1988:144.
237. Gherlinzoni F, Picci P, Bacci G, Cazzola A. Late results of a randomized trial for the treatment of soft tissue sarcomas (STS) of the extremities in adult patients. *Proc Am Soc Clin Oncol* 1993;12:A1633.
238. Eilber FR, Giuliano AE, Huth JF, Morton DL. Postoperative adjuvant chemotherapy (adriamycin) in high grade extremity soft tissue sarcoma: a randomized prospective trial. In: Salmon SE, ed. *Adjuvant therapy of cancer*, V. Orlando: Grune & Stratton, 1987:719.
239. Piver MS, Lele SB, Marchetti DL, Emrich LJ. Effect of adjuvant chemotherapy on time to recurrence and survival of stage I uterine sarcomas. *J Surg Oncol* 1988;38:233.
240. Rosenberg SA, Tepper J, Glatstein E, et al. Prospective randomized evaluation of adjuvant chemotherapy in adults with soft tissue sarcomas of the extremities. *Cancer* 1983;52:424.
241. Rosenberg SA, Chang AE, Glatstein E. Adjuvant chemotherapy for treatment of extremity soft tissue sarcomas: review of the National Cancer Institute experience. *Cancer Treat Symp* 1985;3:83.
242. Chang AE, Kinsella T, Glatstein E, et al. Adjuvant chemotherapy for patients with high-grade soft tissue sarcomas of the extremity. *J Clin Oncol* 1988;6:1491.
243. Dresdale A, Bonow RO, Wesley R, et al. Prospective evaluation of doxorubicin-induced cardiomyopathy resulting from postsurgical adjuvant treatment of patients with soft tissue sarcomas. *Cancer* 1983;52:51.
244. Glenn J, Kinsella T, Glatstein E, et al. A randomized, prospective trial of adjuvant chemotherapy in adults with soft tissue sarcomas of the head and neck, breast, and trunk. *Cancer* 1985;55:1206.
245. Glenn J, Sindelar WF, Kinsella T, et al. Results of multimodality therapy of resectable soft tissue sarcomas of the retroperitoneum. *Surgery* 1985;97:316.
246. Lindberg RD, Murphy WK, Benjamin RS, et al. Adjuvant chemotherapy in the treatment of primary soft tissue sarcomas: a preliminary report. In: Institute MAAT, ed. *Management of primary bone and soft tissue tumors.* Chicago: Year Book Medical, 1977:343.
247. Benjamin RS, Terjanian TO, Fenoglio CJ, et al. The importance of combination chemotherapy for adjuvant treatment of high-risk patients with soft tissue sarcomas of the extremities. In: Salmon SE, ed. *Adjuvant therapy of cancer*, V. Orlando: Grune & Stratton, 1987:735.
248. Edmonson JH, Fleming TR, Ivins JC, et al. Randomized study of systemic chemotherapy following complete excision of nonosseous sarcomas. *J Clin Oncol* 1984;2:1390.
249. Bramwell V, Rouesse J, Steward W, et al. Adjuvant CyVADIC chemotherapy for adult soft tissue sarcoma—reduced local recurrence but no improvement in survival: a study of the European Organization for Research and Treatment of Cancer Soft Tissue and Bone Sarcoma Group. *J Clin Oncol* 1994;12:1137.
250. Ravaud A, Bui NB, Coindre J-M, et al. Adjuvant chemotherapy with CyVADIC in high risk soft tissue sarcoma: a randomized prospective trial. In Salmon SE, ed. Adjuvant therapy of cancer, VI. Philadelphia: WB Saunders, 1990:556.
251. Frustaci S, Gherlinzoni F, De Paoli A, et al. Maintenance of efficacy of adjuvant chemotherapy (CT) in soft tissue sarcoma (STS) of the extremities. Update of a randomized trial. *Proc Am Soc Clin Oncol* 1999;18:A2108(abst).
252. Fleming ID, Cooper JS, Henson DE, et al. *AJCC cancer staging manual*, 5th ed. Philadelphia: Lippincott–Raven, 1997:131.
253. Benjamin RS, Legha SS, Patel SR, Nicaise C. Single-agent ifosfamide studies in sarcomas of soft tissue and bone: the M.D. Anderson experience. *Cancer Chemother Pharmacol* 1993;31(Suppl 2):S174.
254. O'Bryan RM, Luce JK, Talley RW, et al. Phase II evaluation of adriamycin in human neoplasia. *Cancer* 1973;32:1.
255. Schoenfeld DA, Rosenbaum C, Horton J, et al. A comparison of adriamycin versus vincristine and adriamycin, and cyclophosphamide versus vincristine, actinomycin-D, and cyclophosphamide for advanced sarcoma. *Cancer* 1982;50:2757.
256. Bodey GP, Rodriguez V, Murphy WK, et al. Protected environment —prophylactic antibiotic program for malignant sarcomas: randomized trial during remission induction chemotherapy. *Cancer* 1981;47:2422.
257. Pinedo HM, Bramwell VH, Mouridsen HT, et al. CyVADIC in advanced soft tissue sarcoma: a randomized study comparing two schedules. A study of the EORTC Soft Tissue and Bone Sarcoma Group. *Cancer* 1984;53:1825.
258. Steward WP, Verweij J, Somers R, et al. Granulocyte-macrophage colony-stimulating factor allows safe escalation of dose-intensity of chemotherapy in metastatic adult soft tissue sarcomas: a study of the European Organization for Research and Treatment of Cancer Soft Tissue and Bone Sarcoma Group. *J Clin Oncol* 1993;11:15.
259. Zalupski MM, Ryan JR, Hussein ME, Baker LH. Defining the role of adjuvant chemotherapy for patients with soft tissue sarcoma of the extremities. In Salmon SE, ed. *Adjuvant chemotherapy of cancer*, VII. Philadelphia: Lippincott, 1993:385.
260. Tierney JF, Mosseri V, Stewart LA, et al. Adjuvant chemotherapy for soft tissue sarcoma: review and meta-analysis of the published results of randomised clinical trials. *Br J Cancer* 1995;72:469.
261. Sarcoma Meta-analysis Collaboration. Adjuvant chemotherapy for localised resectable soft tissue sarcoma of adults: meta-analysis of individual data. *Lancet* 1997;350:1647.
262. Fisher B, Gunduz N, Saffer EA. Influence of the interval between primary tumor removal and chemotherapy on kinetics and growth of metastases. *Cancer Res* 1983;43:1488.
263. Simpson-Herren L, Sanford AH, Holmquist JP. Effects of surgery on the cell kinetics of residual tumor. *Cancer Treat Rep* 1976;60:1749.
264. Rouesse JG, Friedman S, Sevin DM, et al. Preoperative induction chemotherapy in the treatment of locally advanced soft tissue sarcomas. *Cancer* 1987;60:296.
265. Pezzi CM, Pollock RE, Evans HL, et al. Preoperative chemotherapy for soft tissue sarcomas of the extremities. *Ann Surg* 1990;211:476.
266. Casper ES, Gaynor JJ, Harrison LB, et al. Preoperative and postoperative adjuvant combination chemotherapy for adults with high grade soft tissue sarcoma. *Cancer* 1994;73:1644.
267. Southee AE, Kaplan WD, Jochelson MS, et al. Gallium imaging in metastatic and recurrent soft tissue sarcoma. *J Nucl Med* 1992;33:1594.
268. Menendez LR, Fideler BM, Mirra J. Thallium-201 scanning for the evaluation of osteosarcoma and soft- tissue sarcoma. A study of the evaluation and predictability of the histological response to chemotherapy. *J Bone Joint Surg Am* 1993;75:526.
269. Koutcher JA, Ballon D, Graham M, et al. 31P NMR spectra of extremity sarcomas: diversity of metabolic profiles and changes in response to chemotherapy. *Magn Reson Med* 1990;16:19.
270. Kern KA, Brunetti A, Norton JA, et al. Metabolic imaging of human extremity musculoskeletal tumors by PET. *J Nucl Med* 1988;29:181.
271. Nieweg OE, Pruim J, Hoekstra HJ, et al. Positron emission tomography with fluorine-18-fluorodeoxyglucose for the evaluation of therapeutic isolated regional limb perfusion in a patient with soft tissue sarcoma. *J Nucl Med* 1994;35:90.
272. Didolkar MS, Kanter PM, Baffi RR, et al. Comparison of regional versus systemic chemotherapy with adriamycin. *Ann Surg* 1978;187:332.
273. Eilber FR, Giuliano AE, Huth JF, Morton DL. A randomized prospective trial using postoperative adjuvant chemotherapy (adriamycin) in high-grade extremity soft tissue sarcoma. *Am J Clin Oncol* 1988;11:39.
274. Eilber F, Giuliano A, Huth J, Mirra J. Neoadjuvant chemotherapy, radiation, and limited surgery for high grade soft tissue sarcoma of the extremity. In: Ryan JR, Baker LH, eds. *Recent concepts in sarcoma treatment.* Dordrecht, The Netherlands: Kluwer, 1988:115.
275. Soulen MC, Weissmann JR, Sullivan KL, et al. Intraarterial chemotherapy with limb-sparing resection of large soft- tissue sarcomas of the extremities. *J Vasc Interv Radiol* 1992;3:659.
276. Wanebo HJ, Temple WJ, Popp MB, et al. Preoperative regional therapy for extremity sarcoma. A tricenter update. *Cancer* 1995;75:2299.
277. Hoekstra HJ, Schraffordt Koops H, Molenaar WM, et al. A combination of intraarterial chemotherapy, preoperative and postoperative radiotherapy, and surgery as limb-saving treatment of primarily unresectable high-grade soft tissue sarcomas of the extremities. *Cancer* 1989;63:59.
278. Rahoty P, Konya A. Results of preoperative neoadjuvant chemotherapy and surgery in the management of patients with soft tissue sarcoma. *Eur J Surg Oncol* 1993;19:641.
279. Chawla SP, Rosen G, Eilber F, et al. Cisplatin and adriamycin as neoadjuvant and adjuvant chemotherapy in the management of soft tissue sarcoma. In Salmon SE, ed. *Adjuvant therapy of cancer*, VI. Philadelphia: WB Saunders, 1990:567.
280. Kempf RA, Irwin LE, Menendez L, et al. Limb salvage surgery for bone and soft tissue sarcoma. A phase II pathologic study of preoperative intraarterial cisplatin. *Cancer* 1991;68:738.
281. Azzarelli A, Quagliuolo V, Casali P, et al. Preoperative doxorubicin plus ifosfamide in primary soft tissue sarcomas of the extremities. *Cancer Chemother Pharmacol* 1993;31(Suppl 2):S210.
282. Levine EA, Trippon M, Das Gupta TK. Preoperative multimodality treatment for soft tissue sarcomas. *Cancer* 1993;71:3685.
283. Mason M, Robinson M, Harmer C, Westbury G. Intra-arterial adriamycin, conventionally fractionated radiotherapy and conservative surgery for soft tissue sarcomas. *Clin Oncol (R Coll Radiol)* 1992;4:32.
284. Eggermont AM, Schraffordt Koops H, Lienard D, et al. Isolated limb perfusion with high-dose tumor necrosis factor-alpha in combination with interferon-gamma and melphalan for nonresectable extremity soft tissue sarcomas: a multicenter trial. *J Clin Oncol* 1996;14:2653.
285. Eggermont AMM, Schraffordt Koops H, Klausner JM, et al. Limb salvage by isolated limb perfusion (ILP) with TNF and melphalan in patients with locally advanced soft tissue sarcomas: outcome of 270 ILPs in 246 patients. *Proc Am Soc Clin Oncol* 1999;18:A2067(abst).
286. Wiedemann GJ, d'Oleire F, Knop E, et al. Ifosfamide and carboplatin combined with 41.8 degrees C whole-body hyperthermia in patients with refractory sarcoma and malignant teratoma. *Cancer Res* 1994;54:5346.
287. Issels RD, Prenninger SW, Nagele A, et al. Ifosfamide plus etoposide combined with regional hyperthermia in patients with locally advanced sarcomas: a phase II study. *J Clin Oncol* 1990;8:1818.
288. Issels RD, Bosse D, Abdel-Rahman S, et al. Preoperative systemic etoposide/ifosfamide/doxorubicin chemotherapy combined with regional hyperthermia in high-risk sarcoma: a pilot study. *Cancer Chemother Pharmacol* 1993;31(Suppl 2):S233.
289. Jaques D, Coit D, Hajdu S, Brennan M. Management of primary and recurrent soft tissue sarcoma of the retroperitoneum. *Ann Surg* 1990;212:51.
290. Bevilacqua R, Rogatko A, Hajdu S, Brennan M. Prognostic factors in primary retroperitoneal soft tissue sarcoma. *Arch Surg* 1991;126:328.
291. Catton C, O'Sullivan B, Kotwall C. Outcome and prognosis in retroperitoneal soft tissue sarcoma. *Int J Radiat Oncol Biol Phys* 1994;29:1005.
292. Fein D, Corn B, Lanciano R. Management of retroperitoneal sarcomas: does dose escalation impact on locoregional control? *Int J Radiat Oncol Biol Phys* 1995;31:129.
293. Tepper JE, Suit HD, Wood WC, et al. Radiation therapy of retroperitoneal soft tissue sarcomas. *Int J Radiat Oncol Biol Phys* 1984;10:825.
294. Willet C, Suit H, Tepper J. Intraoperative electron beam radiation therapy for retroperitoneal soft tissue sarcomas. *Cancer* 1991;68:278.
295. Gunderson L, Najorney D, McIlrath D. External beam and intraoperative electron irradiation for locally advanced soft tissue sarcomas. *Int J Radiat Oncol Biol Phys* 1993;25:647.
296. Petersen I, Haddock M, Donohue J. Use of intraoperative electron beam radiation therapy in the management of soft tissue sarcomas. *Int J Radiat Biol Phys (in press).*
297. Sindelar W, Kinsella T, Chen P. Intraoperative radiotherapy in retroperitoneal sarcomas. *Arch Surg* 1993;128:402.
298. Alektiar K, Hu K, Anderson L, et al. High dose rate intraoperative radiation therapy (HDR-IORT) for retroperitoneal sarcomas. *Int J Radiat Biol Phys* 2000;47:157.

299. Eeles R, Fisher C, A'Hern R, et al. Head and neck sarcomas: prognostic factors and implications for treatment. *Br J Cancer* 1993;68:201.
300. Willers H, Hug E, Spiro I, et al. Adult soft tissue sarcomas of the head and neck treated by radiation and surgery or radiation alone: patterns of failure and prognostic factors. *Int J Radiat Oncol Biol Phys* 1995;33:585.
301. Le Q, Fu K, Kroll S, et al. Prognostic factors in adult soft tissue sarcomas of the head and neck. *Int J Radiat Oncol Biol Phys* 1997;37:975.
302. Lydiatt W, Shaha A, Shah J. Angiosarcoma of the head and neck. *Am J Surg* 1994;168:451.
303. Tran L, Mark R, Meier R, et al. Sarcomas of the head and neck. Prognostic factors and treatment strategies. *Cancer* 1992;70:169.
304. Morrison W, Byers R, Garden A, et al. Cutaneous angiosarcoma of the head and neck: a therapeutic dilemma. *Cancer* 1995;76:319.
305. Moore M, Kinne D. Breast sarcoma. *Surg Clin North Am* 1996;76:383.
306. North J, McPhee M, Arredondo M, Edge S. Sarcoma of the breast: implications of the extent of local therapy. *Am Surg* 1998;64:1059.
307. Gutman H, Pollock R, Ross M, et al. Sarcoma of the breast: implications for extent of therapy. The MD Anderson experience. *Surgery* 1994;116:505.
308. Johnstone P, Pierce L, Merino M, et al. Primary soft tissue sarcomas of the breast: local-regional control with post-operative radiotherapy. *Int J Radiat Oncol Biol Phys* 1993;27:671.
309. Devereux D, Kent H, Brennan M. Time dependent effects of Adriamycin and x-ray therapy on wound healing in the rat. *Cancer* 1980;45:2805.
310. Shamberger R, Devereux D, Brennan M. The effect of chemotherapeutic agents on wound healing. In: Murphy G, ed. *International advances in surgical oncology*. New York: Alan R. Liss, 1981:15.
310a. Alektiar K, Zelefsky M, Brennan M. Morbidity and long term results of adjuvant brachytherapy in soft tissue sarcoma: a prospective randomized trial. *Int J Radiat Oncol Biol Phys* 2000;47:1237.
311. Bell R, Mahoney J, O'Sullivan B, et al. Wound healing complications in soft tissue sarcoma management: comparision of three treatment protocols. *J Surg Oncol* 1991;46:190.
312. Bujko K, Suit H, Springfield D, Convery K. Wound healing after preoperative radiation for sarcoma of soft tissues. *Surg Gynecol Obstet* 1993;176:124.
313. Peat B, Bell R, Davis A, et al. Wound-healing complications after soft tissue sarcoma surgery. *Plast Reconstr Surg* 1994;93:980.
314. O'Sullivan B, Davis A, Bell R, et al. Phase III randomized trial of pre-operative versus post-operative radiotherapy in the curative management of extremity soft tissue sarcoma. A Canadian Sarcoma Group and NCI Canada Clinical Trials Group study. *Proc ASCO* 1999;18:535a.
315. Stinson S, DeLaney T, Greenberg J, et al. Acute and long-term effects on limb function of combined modality limb sparing therapy for extremity soft tissue sarcoma. *Int J Radiat Oncol Biol Phys* 1991;21:1493.
316. Brant T, Parsons J, Marcus R Jr, et al. Preoperative irradiation for soft tissue sarcomas of the trunk and extremities in adults. *Int J Radiat Oncol Biol Phys* 1990;19:899.
317. Lin P, Schupak K, Boland P, et al. Pathologic femoral fracture after periosteal excision and radiation for the treatment of soft tissue sarcoma. *Cancer* 1998;82:2356.
318. LePechoux C, LeDeley M, Delaloge S, et al. Postoperative radiotherapy in the management of adult soft tissue sarcoma of the extremities: results with two different total dose, fractionation, and overall treatment time schedules. *Int J Radiat Oncol Biol Phys* 1999;44:879.
319. Sugarbaker P, Barofsky I, Rosenberg S, Gianola F. Quality of life assessment of patients in extremity sarcoma clinical trials. *Surgery* 1982;91:17.
320. Davis A, Devlin M, Griffin A, et al. Functional outcome in amputation versus limb sparing of patients with lower extremity sarcoma: a matched case-control study. *Arch Phys Med Rehabil* 1999;80:615.
321. Bell R, O'Sullivan B, Davis A, et al. Functional outcome in patients treated with surgery and irradiation for soft tissue tumours. *J Surg Oncol* 1991;48:224.
322. Schupak K, Lane J, Weilepp A, et al. The psychofunctional handicap associated with the use of brachytherapy in the treatment of lower extremity high grade soft tissue sarcomas. Proceedings of the 35th Annual ASTRO Meeting. *Int J Radiat Oncol Biol Phys* 1993;27:293.
323. Karasek K, Constine L, Rosier R. Sarcoma therapy: functional outcome and relationship to treatment parameters. *Int J Radiat Oncol Biol Phys* 1992;24:651.
324. Robinson M, Spruce L, Eeles R, et al. Limb function following conservation treatment of adult soft tissue sarcoma. *Eur J Cancer* 1991;27:1567.
325. Sugerbaker P. Intraperitoneal chemotherapy for treatment and prevention of peritoneal carcinomatosis and sarcomatosis. *Dis Colon Rect* 1994;37:S115.
326. Creagan E, Fleming T, Edmonston J, Pairolero P. Pulmonary resection for metastatic nonosteogenic sarcoma. *Cancer* 1979;44:1908.
327. Putnam J, Roth J, Wesley M, et al. Analysis of prognostic factors in patients undergoing resection of pulmonary metastases from soft tissue sarcomas. *J Thorac Cardiovasc Surg* 1984;87:260.
328. Roth J, Putnam J, Wesley M, Rosenberg S. Differing determinants of prognosis following resection of pulmonary metastases from osteogenic and soft tissue sarcoma patients. *Cancer* 1985;55:1361.
329. Casson A, Putnam J, Natarajan G, et al. Five-year survival after pulmonary metastasectomy for adult soft tissue sarcoma. *Cancer* 1992;69:662.
330. Jablons D, Steinberg S, Roth J, et al. Metastasectomy for soft tissue sarcoma. Further evidence for efficacy and prognostic indicators. *J Thorac Cardiovasc Surg* 1989;97:695.
331. Verazin G, Warneke J, Driscoll D, et al. Resection of lung meastases from soft tissue sarcomas. A multivariate analysis. *Arch Surg* 1992;127:1407.
332. Lanza L, Putnam J Jr, Benajmin R, Roth J. Response to chemotherapy does not predict survival after resection of sarcomatous pulmonary meastases. *Ann Thorac Surg* 1991;51:219.
333. Weksler B, Lenert J, Ng B, Burt M. Isolated single lung perfusion with doxorubicin is effective in eradicating soft tissue sarcoma lung metastases in a rat model. *J Thorac Cardiovasc Surg* 1994;107:50.
334. Benjamin RS, Wiernik PH, Bachur NR. Adriamycin chemotherapy—efficacy, safety, and pharmacologic basis of an intermittent single high-dosage schedule. *Cancer* 1974;33:19.
335. Santoro A, Tursz T, Mouridsen H, et al. Doxorubicin versus CyVADIC versus doxorubicin plus ifosfamide in first- line treatment of advanced soft tissue sarcomas: a randomized study of the European Organization for Research and Treatment of Cancer Soft Tissue and Bone Sarcoma Group. *J Clin Oncol* 1995;13:1537.
336. Edmonson JH, Ryan LM, Blum RH, et al. Randomized comparison of doxorubicin alone versus ifosfamide plus doxorubicin or mitomycin, doxorubicin, and cisplatin against advanced soft tissue sarcomas. *J Clin Oncol* 1993;11:1269.
337. Antman KH, Ryan L, Elias A, et al. Response to ifosfamide and mesna: 124 previously treated patients with metastatic or unresectable sarcoma. *J Clin Oncol* 1989;7:126.
338. Rosen G, Forscher C, Lowenbraun S, et al. Synovial sarcoma. Uniform response of metastases to high dose ifosfamide. *Cancer* 1994;73:2506.
339. Gottlieb JA, Benjamin RS, Baker LH, et al. Role of DTIC (NSC-45388) in the chemotherapy of sarcomas. *Cancer Treat Rep* 1976;60:199.
340. Buesa JM, Mouridsen HT, van Oosterom AT, et al. High-dose DTIC in advanced soft tissue sarcomas in the adult. A phase II study of the E.O.R.T.C. Soft Tissue and Bone Sarcoma Group. *Ann Oncol* 1991;2:307.
341. Elias A, Ryan L, Sulkes A, et al. Response to mesna, doxorubicin, ifosfamide, and dacarbazine in 108 patients with metastatic or unresectable sarcoma and no prior chemotherapy. *J Clin Oncol* 1989;7:1208.
342. Fidias P, Demetri GD, Harmon DC. Navelbine shows activity in previously treated sarcoma patients: phase II results from MGH/Dana-Farber/Partners CancerCare Study. *Proc Am Soc Clin Oncol* 1998;17:A1977(abst).
343. Amodio A, Carpano S, Manfredi C, et al. Gemcitabine in advanced stage soft tissue sarcoma: a phase II study. *Clin Ter* 1999;150:17.
344. Merimsky O, Meller I, Kollender Y, et al. Gemcitabine in patients with sarcoma of soft tissue or bone resistant to standard chemotherapy. *Proc Am Soc Clin Oncol* 1999;18:A2098(abst).
345. Rosen L, Mulay M, Mayers A, et al. Phase I dose-escalating trial of SU5416, a novel angiogenesis inhibitor in patients with advanced malignancies. *Proc Am Soc Clin Oncol* 1999; 18:A618(abst).
346. Demetri GD, Fletcher CD, Mueller E, et al. Induction of solid tumor differentiation by the peroxisome proliferator- activated receptor-gamma ligand troglitazone in patients with liposarcoma. *Proc Natl Acad Sci U S A* 1999;96:3951.
347. Gottlieb JA, Baker LH, Quagliana JM, et al. Chemotherapy of sarcomas with a combination of adriamycin and dimethyl triazeno imidazole carboxamide. *Cancer* 1972;30:1632.
348. Zalupski M, Metch B, Balcerzak S, et al. Phase III comparison of doxorubicin and dacarbazine given by bolus versus infusion in patients with soft tissue sarcomas: a Southwest Oncology Group study. *J Natl Cancer Inst* 1991;83:926.
349. Pfeffer MR, Sulkes A, Biran S. Treatment of advanced soft tissue sarcomas with a modified CyVADIC protocol. *Oncology* 1984;41:308.
350. Frustaci S, Foladore S, Buonadonna A, et al. Epirubicin and ifosfamide in advanced soft tissue sarcomas. *Ann Oncol* 1993;4:669.
351. Toma S, Palumbo R, Canavese G, et al. Ifosfamide plus epirubicin at escalating doses in the treatment of locally advanced and/or metastatic sarcomas. *Cancer Chemother Pharmacol* 1993;31(Suppl 2):S222.
352. Toma S, Coialbu T, Biassoni L, et al. Epidoxorubicin plus ifosfamide in advanced and/or metastatic soft- tissue sarcomas. *Cancer Chemother Pharmacol* 1990;26:453.
353. Antman K, Crowley J, Balcerzak SP, et al. An intergroup phase III randomized study of doxorubicin and dacarbazine with or without ifosfamide and mesna in advanced soft tissue and bone sarcomas. *J Clin Oncol* 1993;11:1276.
354. van Oosterom AT, Santoro A, Bramwell V, et al. Mitomycin C (MCC) in advanced soft tissue sarcoma: a phase II study of the EORTC Soft Tissue and Bone Sarcoma Group. *Eur J Cancer* Clin Oncol 1985;21:459.
355. Edmonson JH, Long HJ, Richardson RL, et al. Phase II study of a combination of mitomycin, doxorubicin and cisplatin in advanced sarcomas. *Cancer Chemother Pharmacol* 1985;15:181.
356. Van Glabbeke M, van Oosterom AT, Oosterhuis JW, et al. Prognostic factors for the outcome of chemotherapy in advanced soft tissue sarcomas: an analysis of 2,185 patients treated with anthracycline containing first-line regimens—an European Organization for Research and Treatment of Cancer Soft Tissue and Bone Sarcoma Study Group. *J Clin Oncol* 1999;17:150.
357. Frei E III, Elias A, Wheeler C, et al. The relationship between high-dose treatment and combination chemotherapy: the concept of summation dose intensity. *Clin Cancer Res* 1998;4:2027.
358. O'Bryan RM, Baker LH, Gottlieb JE, et al. Dose response evaluation of adriamycin in human neoplasia. *Cancer* 1977;39:1940.
359. Ozer H. American Society of Clinical Oncology guidelines for the use of hematopoietic colony-stimulating factors. *Curr Opin Hematol* 1996;3:3.
360. Vadhan-Raj S, Broxmeyer HE, Hittelman WN, et al. Abrogating chemotherapy-induced myelosuppression by recombinant granulocyte-macrophage colony-stimulating factor in patients with sarcoma: protection at the progenitor cell level. *J Clin Oncol* 1992;10:1266.
361. Antman KS, Griffin JD, Elias A, et al. Effect of recombinant human granulocyte-macrophage colony-stimulating factor on chemotherapy-induced myelosuppression. *N Engl J Med* 1988;319:593.
362. Christman KL, Casper ES, Schwartz GK. High-intensity scheduling of ifosfamide in adult patients with soft tissue sarcoma. *Proc Am Soc Clin Oncol* 1993;12:A1642(abst).
363. Schutte J, Mouridsen HT, Steward W, et al. Ifosfamide plus doxorubicin in previously untreated patients with advanced soft tissue sarcoma. *Cancer Chemother Pharmacol* 1993;31(Suppl 2):S204.
364. Steward WP, Verweij J, Somers R, et al. Doxorubicin plus ifosfamide with rhGM-CSF in the treatment of advanced adult soft tissue sarcomas: preliminary results of a phase II study from the EORTC Soft tissue and Bone Sarcoma Group. *J Cancer Res Clin Oncol* 1991;117(Suppl 4):S193.
365. Edmonson JH, Petersen IA, Shives TC, et al. Chemotherapy, irradiation, and surgery for function-preserving curative therapy of primary extremity soft tissue sarcomas: intital treatment with I-MAP + GM-CSF–preliminary report. *Sarcoma* 1999;3:60(abst).
366. Bui BN, Chevallier B, Chevreau C, et al. Efficacy of lenograstim on hematologic tolerance to MAID chemotherapy in patients with advanced soft tissue sarcoma and consequences on treatment dose-intensity. *J Clin Oncol* 1995;13:2629.

367. Bitran JD, Samuels BL, Marsik S, et al. A phase I study of ifosfamide and doxorubicin with recombinant human granulocyte colony-stimulating factor in stage IV breast cancer. *Clin Cancer Res* 1995;1:185.
368. Bui NB, Demaille MC, Chevreau C, et al. qMAID VS MAID + 25% with G-CSF in adults with advanced soft tissue sarcoma (STS). First results of a randomized study of the FNCLCC sarcoma group. *Proc Am Soc Clin Oncol* 1998;17:A1991.
369. Frustaci S, Comandone A, Bearz A, et al. Efficacy and tolerability of an ifosfamide continuous infusion (IFO-C.I.) in soft tissue sarcoma (STS) patients (pts). *Proc Am Soc Clin Oncol* 1998;17:A1993(abst).
370. Walterhouse DO, Hoover ML, Marymont MA, Kletzel M. High-dose chemotherapy followed by peripheral blood stem cell rescue for metastatic rhabdomyosarcoma: the experience at Chicago Children's Memorial Hospital. *Med Pediatr Oncol* 1999;32:88.
371. Lucidarme N, Valteau-Couanet D, Oberlin O, et al. Phase II study of high-dose thiotepa and hematopoietic stem cell transplantation in children with solid tumors. *Bone Marrow Transplant* 1998;22:535.
372. Elias AD. High-dose therapy for adult soft tissue sarcoma: dose response and survival. *Semin Oncol* 1998;25(Suppl 4):19.
373. Seynaeve C, Verweij J. High-dose chemotherapy in adult sarcomas: no standard yet. *Semin Oncol* 1999;26:119.
374. Sutton GP, Blessing JA, Barrett RJ, McGehee R. Phase II trial of ifosfamide and mesna in leiomyosarcoma of the uterus: a Gynecologic Oncology Group study. *Am J Obstet Gynecol* 1992;166:556.
375. Kawai A, Woodruff J, Healey JH, et al. SYT-SSX gene fusion as a determinant of morphology and prognosis in synovial sarcoma [see comments]. *N Engl J Med* 1998;338:153.
376. Grier HE. The Ewing family of tumors. Ewing's sarcoma and primitive neuroectodermal tumors. *Pediatr Clin North Am* 1997;44:991.
377. Patel S, Hays C, Papdopoulos N. Pilot study of high-dose ifosfamide (HDI) + G-CSF in patients (pts) with bone and soft tissue sarcomas (STS). *Proc ASCO* 1995;14:516(abst).
378. Craft A, Cotterill S, Malcolm A, et al. Ifosfamide-containing chemotherapy in Ewing's sarcoma: The Second United Kingdom Children's Cancer Study Group and the Medical Research Council Ewing's Tumor Study. *J Clin Oncol* 1998;16:3628.
379. Kushner B, Meyers P, Gerald W, et al. Very high-dose short-term chemotherapy for poor-risk peripheral primitive neuroectodermal tumors, including Ewing's sarcoma, in children and young adults. *J Clin Oncol* 1995;13:2796.
380. Antman K, Crowley J, Balcerzak SP, et al. A Southwest Oncology Group and Cancer and Leukemia Group B phase II study of doxorubicin, dacarbazine, ifosfamide, and mesna in adults with advanced osteosarcoma, Ewing's sarcoma, and rhabdomyosarcoma. *Cancer* 1998;82:1288.
381. La Quaglia MP, Heller G, Ghavimi F, et al. The effect of age at diagnosis on outcome in rhabdomyosarcoma. *Cancer* 1994;73:109.
382. Singer S, Rubin B, Fletcher CDM, et al. Rhabdomyosarcoma (RMS) in adults: size, location, and response to chemotherapy predicts survival. *Proc Am Soc Clin Oncol* 1999;18:A2106(abst).
383. Baldini EH, Demetri GD, Fletcher CD, et al. Adults with Ewing's sarcoma/primitive neuroectodermal tumor: adverse effect of older age and primary extraosseous disease on outcome. *Ann Surg* 1999;230:79.
384. Ahrens S, Hoffmann C, Jabar S, et al. Evaluation of prognostic factors in a tumor volume-adapted treatment strategy for localized Ewing sarcoma of bone: the CESS 86 experience. Cooperative Ewing Sarcoma Study. *Med Pediatr Oncol* 1999;32:186.
385. Hornback N, Omura G, Major F. Observations on the use of adjuvant radiation therapy in patients with stage I and II uterine sarcoma. *Int J Radiat Oncol Biol Phys* 1986; 12:2127.
386. Chi D, Mychalczak B, Saigo P, et al. The role of whole-pelvic irradiation in the treatment of early-stage uterine carcinosarcoma. *Gynecol Oncol* 1997;65:493.
387. Ferrer F, Sabater S, Farrus B, et al. Impact of radiotherapy on local control and survival in uterine sarcomas: a retrospective study from the Group Oncologic Catala-Occita. *Int J Radiat Oncol Biol Phys* 1999;44:47.
388. Omura GA, Major FJ, Blessing JA, et al. A randomized study of adriamycin with and without dimethyl triazenoimidazole carboxamide in advanced uterine sarcomas. *Cancer* 1983;52:626.
389. Muss HB, Bundy B, DiSaia PJ, et al. Treatment of recurrent or advanced uterine sarcoma. A randomized trial of doxorubicin versus doxorubicin and cyclophosphamide (a phase III trial of the Gynecologic Oncology Group). *Cancer* 1985;55:1648.
390. Thigpen JT, Blessing JA, Beecham J, et al. Phase II trial of cisplatin as first-line chemotherapy in patients with advanced or recurrent uterine sarcomas: a Gynecologic Oncology Group study. *J Clin Oncol* 1991;9:1962.
391. Gershenson DM, Kavanagh JJ, Copeland LJ, et al. Cisplatin therapy for disseminated mixed mesodermal sarcoma of the uterus. *J Clin Oncol* 1987;5:618.
392. Lantta M, Kahanpaa K, Karkkainen J, et al. Estradiol and progesterone receptors in two cases of endometrial stromal sarcoma. *Gynecol Oncol* 1984;18:233.
393. Keen CE, Philip G. Progestogen-induced regression in low-grade endometrial stromal sarcoma. Case report and literature review. *Br J Obstet Gynaecol* 1989;96:1435.
394. Wade K, Quinn MA, Hammond I, et al. Uterine sarcoma: steroid receptors and response to hormonal therapy. *Gynecol Oncol* 1990;39:364.
395. Spear M, Jennings L, Mankin H, et al. Individualizing management of aggressive fibromatoses. *Int J Radiat Oncol Biol Phys* 1998;40:637.
396. Ballo M, Zagars G, Pollack A. Radiation therapy in the management of desmoid tumors. *Int J Radiat Oncol Biol Phys* 1998;42:1007.
397. Goy B, Lee S, Eilber F, et al. The role of adjuvant radiotherapy in the treatment of resectable desmoid tumors. *Int J Radiat Oncol Biol Phys* 1997;39:659.
398. Kamath S, Parsons J, Marcus R Jr, et al. Radiotherapy for local control of aggressive fibromatosis. *Int J Radiat Oncol Biol Phys* 1996;36:325.
399. Reitamo JJ, Scheinin TM, Hayry P. The desmoid syndrome. New aspects in the cause, pathogenesis and treatment of the desmoid tumor. *Am J Surg* 1986;151:230.
400. Lim CL, Walker MJ, Mehta RR, Das Gupta TK. Estrogen and antiestrogen binding sites in desmoid tumors. *Eur J Cancer Clin Oncol* 1986;22:583.
401. Waddell WR, Gerner RE, Reich MP. Nonsteroid antiinflammatory drugs and tamoxifen for desmoid tumors and carcinoma of the stomach. *J Surg Oncol* 1983;22:197.
402. Kinzbrunner B, Ritter S, Domingo J, Rosenthal CJ. Remission of rapidly growing desmoid tumors after tamoxifen therapy. *Cancer* 1983;52:2201.
403. Sportiello DJ, Hoogerland DL. A recurrent pelvic desmoid tumor successfully treated with tamoxifen. *Cancer* 1991;67:1443.
404. Waddell WR, Kirsch WM. Testolactone, sulindac, warfarin, and vitamin K1 for unresectable desmoid tumors. *Am J Surg* 1991;161:416.
405. Brooks MD, Ebbs SR, Colletta AA, Baum M. Desmoid tumours treated with triphenylethylenes. *Eur J Cancer* 1992:28a;1014.
406. Wilcken N, Tattersall MH. Endocrine therapy for desmoid tumors. *Cancer* 1991;68:1384.
407. Lanari A. Effect of progesterone on desmoid tumors (aggressive fibromatosis). *N Engl J Med* 1983;309:1523.
408. Klein WA, Miller HH, Anderson M, DeCosse JJ. The use of indomethacin, sulindac, and tamoxifen for the treatment of desmoid tumors associated with familial polyposis. *Cancer* 1987;60:2863.
409. Seiter K, Kemeny N. Successful treatment of a desmoid tumor with doxorubicin. *Cancer* 1993;71:2242.
410. Patel SR, Evans HL, Benjamin RS. Combination chemotherapy in adult desmoid tumors. *Cancer* 1993;72:3244.
411. Weiss AJ, Lackman RD. Low-dose chemotherapy of desmoid tumors. *Cancer* 1989;64:1192.
412. Weiss AJ, Horowitz S, Lackman RD. Therapy of desmoid tumors and fibromatosis using vinorelbine. *Am J Clin Oncol* 1999;22:193.
413. Gadd MA, Casper ES, Woodruff JM, et al. Development and treatment of pulmonary metastases in adult patients with extremity soft tissue sarcoma. *Ann Surg* 1993;218:705.
414. Jhanwar S, Chen Q, Li F, et al. Cytogenetic analysis of soft tissue sarcomas. Recurrent chromosome abnormalities in malignant peripheral nerve sheath tumors (MPNST). *Cytogenet* 1994;78:138.
415. Hovig E, Lothe R, Farrants G, et al. Chromosome 13 alterations in osteosarcoma cell lines derived from a patient with previous retinoblastoma. *Cancer Genet Cytogenet* 1991; 57:31.
416. Scholz R, Kabisch H, Delling G, Winkler K. Homozygous deletion within the retinoblastoma gene in a native osteosarcoma specimen of a patient cured of a retinoblastoma of both eyes. *Pediatr Hematol Oncol* 1990;7:265.
417. Malkin D, Li F, Strong L, et al. Germ line p53 mutations in a familial syndrome of breast cancer, sarcomas, and other neoplasms. *Science* 1990;250:1233.
418. Okamoto M, Sato C, Kohno Y, et al. Molecular nature of chromosome 5q loss in colorectal tumors and desmoids from patients with familial adenomatous ployposis. *Hum Genet* 1990;85:595.
419. Foulkes W. A tale of four syndromes: familial adenomatous polyposis, Gardner syndrome, attenuated APC and Turcot syndrome. *QJM* 1995;88:853.
420. Goto M, Miller R, Ishikawa Y, Sugano H. Excess of rare cancers in Werner syndrome (adult progeria). *Cancer Epidemiol Biomarkers Prev* 1996;5:239.
421. Carney J. Gastric stromal sarcoma, pulmonary chondroma, and extra-adrenal paraganglioma (Carney triad): natural history, adrenocortical component, and possible familial occurrence. *Mayo Clin Proc* 1999;74:543.
422. Carney J, Sheps S, Go V, Gordon H. The triad of gastric leiomyosarcoma, functioning extra-adrenal paraganglioma and pulmonary chondroma. *N Engl J Med* 1977;296:1517.
423. van Slegtenhorst M, de Hoogt R, Hermans C, et al. Identification of the tuberous sclerosis gene TSC1 on chromosome 9q34. *Science* 1997;277:805.
424. Povey S, Burley M, Attwood J, et al. Two loci for tuberous sclerosis: one on 9q34 and one on 16p13. *Ann Hum Genet* 1994;58:107.
425. Sallee D, Spector M, van Heeckeren D, Patel C. Primary pediatric cardiac tumors: a 17 year experience. *Cardiol Young* 1999;9:155.
426. [No authors listed.] Chromosomal translocations in Ewing's sarcoma. *N Engl J Med* 1983;309:496.
427. Zoubek A, Dockhorn-Dworniczak B, Delattre O, et al. Does expression of different EWS chimeric transcripts define clinically distinct risk groups of Ewing tumor patients? *J Clin Oncol* 1996;14:1245.
428. Kaneko Y, Kobayashi H, Handa M, et al. EWS-ERG fusion transcript produced by chromosomal insertion in a Ewing sarcoma. *Genes Chromosomes Cancer* 1997;18:228.
429. Jeon I, David J, Braun B, et al. A variant Ewing's sarcoma translocation (7;22) fuses the EWS gene to the ETS gene ETV1. *Oncogene* 1995;10:1229.
430. Kaneko Y, Yoshida K, Handa M, et al. Fusion of an ETS-family gene, EIAF, to EWS by t(17;22)(q12;q12) chromosome translocation in an undifferentiated sarcoma of infancy. *Genes Chromosomes Cancer* 1996;15:115.
431. Mugneret F, Lizard S, Aurias A, Turn-Carel C. Chromosomes in Ewing's sarcoma. II. Nonrandom adiditional changes, trisomy 8 and der(16)t(1;16). *Cancer Genet Cytogenet* 1988; 32:239.
432. Douglass E, Rowe S, Valentine M, et al. A second nonrandom translocation, der(16)t(1;16)(q21;q13), in Ewing sarcoma and peripheral neuroectodermal tumor. *Cytogenet Cell Genet* 1990;53:87.
433. Maurici D, Perez-Atayde A, Grier H, et al. Frequency and implications of chromosome 8 and 12 gains in Ewing sarcoma. *Cancer Genet Cytogenet* 1998;100:106.
434. Panagopoulos I, Mandahl N, Ron D, et al. Characterization of the CHOP breakpoints and fusiontranscripts in myxoid liposarcomas with the 12;16 translocation. *Cancer Res* 1994;54:6500.
435. Aoki T, Hisaoka M, Kouho H, et al. Interphase cytogenetic analysis of myxoid soft tissue tumors by fluorescence in situ hybridization and DNA flow cytometry using paraffin-embedded tissue. *Cancer* 1997;79:284.
436. Panagopoulos I, Hoglund M, Mertens F, et al. Fusion of the EWS and CHOP genes in myxoid liposarcoma. *Oncogene* 1996;12:489.

437. Heim S, Mandahl N, Dristoffersson U, et al. Marker ring chromosome—a new cytogenetic abnormality characterizing lipogenic tumors? *Cancer Genet Cytogenet* 1987;24:319.
438. Rosai J, Akerman M, Dal Cin P, et al. Combined morphologic and karyotypic study of 59 atypical lipomatous tumors. Evaluation of their relationship and differential diagnosis with other adipose tissue tumors (a report of the CHAMP Study Group). *Am J Surg Pathol* 1996;20:1182.
439. Kelly K, Womer R, Sorensen P, et al. Common and variant gene fusions predict distinct clinicalphenotypes in rhabdomyosarcoma. *J Clin Oncol* 1997;15:1831.
440. Fletcher J. Translocation (12;22)(q13-14;q12) is a nonrandom aberration in soft tissue clear-cell sarcoma [letter]. *Genes Chromosomes Cancer* 1992;5:184.
441. Peulve P, Michot C, Vannier J, et al. Clear cell sarcoma with t(12;22)(q13-14;q12). *Genes Chromosomes Cancer* 1991;3:400.
442. Rauscher Fd, Benjamin L, Fredericks W, Morris J. Novel oncogenic mutations in the WT1 Wilms' tumor suppressor gene: a t(11;22) fuses the Ewing's sarcoma gene, EWS1, to WT1 in desmoplastic small round cell tumor. *Cold Spring Harb Symp Quant Biol* 1994;59:137.
443. Gerald W, Ladanyi M, de Alava E, et al. Clinical, pathologic, and molecular spectrum of tumors associated with t(11;22)(p13;q12): desmoplastic small round-cell tumor and its variants. *J Clin Oncol* 1998;16:3028.
444. Turc-Carel C, Dal Cin P, Limon J, et al. Translocation X;18 in synovial sarcoma. *Cancer Genet Cytogenet* 1986;23:93.
445. Clark J, Rocques P, Crew A, et al. Identification of novel genes, SYT anbd SSX, involved in the t(X;18)(p11.2;q11.2) translocation found in human synovial sarcoma. *Nat Genet* 1994;7:502.
446. Shipley J, Clark J, Crew A, et al. The (X;18)(p11.2;q11.2) translocation found in human synovial sarcomas involves two distinct loci on the X chromosome. *Oncogene* 1994;9:1447.
447. Sciot R, Dal Cin P, Fletcher C, et al. t(9;22)(q22-31;q11-12) is a consistent marker of extraskeletal myxoid chondrosarcoma: evaluation of three cases. *Mod Pathol* 1995;8:765.
448. Brody R, Ueda T, Hamelin A, et al. Molecular analysis of the fusion of EWS to an orphan nuclear receptor gene in extraskeletal myxoid chondrosarcoma. *Am J Pathol* 1997;150:1049.
449. Pedeutour F, Simon M, Minoletti F, et al. Transolocation, t(17;22)(q22;q13), in dermatofibrosarcoma protuberans: a new tumor-associated chromosome rearrangement. *Cytogenet Cell Genet* 1996;72:171.
450. Simon M, Pedeutour F, Sirvent N, et al. Deregulation of the platelet-derived growth factor B-chain gene via fusion with collagen gene COL1A1 in dermatofibrosarcoma protuberans and giant-cell fibroblastoma. *Nat Genet* 1997;15:95.
451. Knezevich S, McFadden D, Tao W, et al. A novel ETV2-NTRK3 gene fusion in congenital fibrosarcoma. *Nat Genet* 1998;18:184.
452. Versteege I, Sevenet N, Lange J, et al. Truncating mutations of hSNF5/INI1 in aggressive paediatric cancer. *Nature* 1998;394:203.
453. Rousseau-Merck M, Versteege I, Legrand I, et al. hSNF5/INI1 inactivation is mainly associated with homozygous deletions and mitotic recombinations in rhabdoid tumors. *Cancer Res* 1999;59:3152.
454. Nibert M, Heim S. Uterine leiomyoma cytogenetics. *Genes Chromosomes Cancer* 1990;2:3.
455. Rodriguez E, Reuter V, Mies C, et al. Abnormalities of 2q: a common genetic link between rhabdomyosarcoma and hepatoblastoma? *Genes Chromosomes Cancer* 1991;3:122.
456. Dietrich C, Jacobsen B, Starklint H, Heim S. Clonal karyotypic evolution in an embryonal rhabdomyosarcoma with trsiomy 8 as the primary chromosomal abnormality. *Genes Chromosomes Cancer* 1993;7:240.
457. Quezado M, Middleton L, Bryant B, et al. Allelic loss on chromosome 22q in epithelioid sarcomas. *Hum Pathol* 1998;29:604.
458. Cordoba J, Parham D, Meyer W, Douglass E. A new cytogenetic finding in an epithelioid sarcoma, t(8;22)(q22;q11). *Cancer Genet Cytogenet* 1994;72:151.
459. Wilson RE, Wood WC, Lerner HL, et al. Doxorubicin chemotherapy in the treatment of soft tissue sarcoma. Combined results of two randomized trials. *Arch Surg* 1986;121:1354.
460. Borden EC, Amato DA, Rosenbaum C, et al. Randomized comparison of three adriamycin regimens for metastatic soft tissue sarcomas. *J Clin Oncol* 1987;5:840.
461. Borden EC, Amato DA, Edmonson JH, et al. Randomized comparison of doxorubicin and vindesine to doxorubicin for patients with metastatic soft tissue sarcomas. *Cancer* 1990;66:862.
462. Mouridsen HT, Bastholt L, Somers R, et al. Adriamycin versus epirubicin in advanced soft tissue sarcomas. A randomized phase II/phase III study of the EORTC Soft Tissue and Bone Sarcoma Group. *Eur J Cancer Clin Oncol* 1987;23:1477.
463. Casper ES, Schwartz GK, Sugarman A, et al. Phase I trial of dose-intense liposome-encapsulated doxorubicin in patients with advanced sarcoma. *J Clin Oncol* 1997;15:2111.
464. Skubitz KM. A phase II trial of pegylated liposomal doxorubicin (DOXIL) demonstrates activity in refractory sarcoma, mesothelioma, and head and neck cancer. *Proc Am Soc Clin Oncol* 1999;18:A2090(abst).
465. Lopez M, Vici P, Di Lauro K, et al. Randomized prospective clinical trial of high-dose epirubicin and dexrazoxane in patients with advanced breast cancer and soft tissue sarcomas. *J Clin Oncol* 1998;16:86.
466. Amato DA, Borden EC, Shiraki M, et al. Evaluation of bleomycin, chlorozotocin, MGBG, and bruceantin in patients with advanced soft tissue sarcoma, bone sarcoma, or mesothelioma. *Invest New Drugs* 1985;3:397.
467. Golbey R, Li MC, Kaufman RF. Actinomycin in the treatment of soft part sarcomas (abst). *James Ewing Society Scientific Program*, 1968.
468. Bramwell VH, Mouridsen HT, Santoro A, et al. Cyclophosphamide versus ifosfamide: a randomized phase II trial in adult soft tissue sarcomas. The European Organization for Research and Treatment of Cancer [EORTC], Soft Tissue and Bone Sarcoma Group. *Cancer Chemother Pharmacol* 1993;31(Suppl 2):S180.
469. Borden EC, Larson P, Ansfield FJ, et al. Hexamethylmelamine treatment of sarcomas and lymphomas. *Med Pediatr Oncol* 1977;3:401.
470. Patel SR, Vadhan-Raj S, Papadopolous N, et al. High-dose ifosfamide in bone and soft tissue sarcomas: results of phase II and pilot studies—dose-response and schedule dependence. *J Clin Oncol* 1997;15:2378.
471. Samson MK, Baker LH, Benjamin RS, et al. Cis-dichlorodiammineplatinum(II) in advanced soft tissue and bony sarcomas: a Southwest Oncology Group Study. *Cancer Treat Rep* 1979;63:2027.
472. Budd GT, Metch B, Balcerzak SP, et al. High-dose cisplatin for metastatic soft tissue sarcoma. *Cancer* 1990;65:866.
473. Goldstein D, Cheuvart B, Trump DL, et al. Phase II trial of carboplatin in soft tissue sarcoma. *Am J Clin Oncol* 1990;13:420.
474. Patel SR, Jenkins J, Papadopoulos NE, et al. Preliminary results of a two-arm phase 2 trial of gemcitabine in patients with gastroinstestinal leiomyosarcomas and other soft tissue sarcomas (STS). *Sarcoma* 1999;3:56(abst).
475. Subramanian S, Wiltshaw E. Chemotherapy of sarcoma. A comparison of three regimens. *Lancet* 1978;1:683.
476. Vaughn CB, McKelvey E, Balcerzak SP, et al. High-dose methotrexate with leucovorin rescue plus vincristine in advanced sarcoma: a Southwest Oncology Group study. *Cancer Treat Rep* 1984;68:409.
477. Gold G, Hall T, Shnider B, et al. A clinical study of 5-fluorouracil. *Cancer* 1959;19:935.
478. van Hoesel QG, Verweij J, Catimel G, et al. Phase II study with docetaxel (Taxotere) in advanced soft tissue sarcomas of the adult. EORTC Soft Tissue and Bone Sarcoma Group. *Ann Oncol* 1994;5:539.
479. Balcerzak SP, Benedetti J, Weiss GR, Natale RB. A phase II trial of paclitaxel in patients with advanced soft tissue sarcomas. A Southwest Oncology Group study. *Cancer* 1995;76:2248.
480. Yap BS, Benjamin RS, Plager C, et al. A randomized study of continuous infusion vindesine versus vinblastine in adults with refractory metastatic sarcomas. *Am J Clin Oncol* 1983;6:235.
481. Thigpen T, Blessing JA, Yordan E, et al. Phase II trial of etoposide in leiomyosarcoma of the uterus: a Gynecologic Oncology Group study. *Gynecol Oncol* 1996;63:120.
482. Rose PG, Blessing JA, Soper JT, Barter JF. Prolonged oral etoposide in recurrent or advanced leiomyosarcoma of the uterus: a gynecologic oncology group study. *Gynecol Oncol* 1998;70:267.
483. Bramwell VH, Eisenhauer EA, Blackstein M, et al. Phase II study of topotecan (NSC 609 699) in patients with recurrent or metastatic soft tissue sarcoma. *Ann Oncol* 1995;6:847.
484. Saiki J, Stephens R, Fabian C, et al. Phase II evaluation of gallium nitrate (NSC-15200) in soft tissue and bone sarcomas. *Proc Am Assoc Cancer Res* 1981;22:525(abst).
485. Presant CA, Gams R, Bartolucci AA. Treatment of metastatic sarcomas with mitoxantrone. *Cancer Treat Rep* 1984;68:813.
486. Bull FE, Von Hoff DD, Balcerzak SP, et al. Phase II trial of mitoxantrone in advanced sarcoma: a Southwest Oncology Group study. *Cancer Treat Rep* 1985;69:321.
487. Earhart RH, Amato DJ, Chang AY, et al. Phase II trial of 6-diazo-5-oxo-L-norleucine versus aclacinomycin-A in advanced sarcomas and mesotheliomas. *Invest New Drugs* 1990;8:113.
488. Yap BS, Plager C, Benjamin RS, et al. Phase II evaluation of AMSA in adult sarcomas. *Cancer Treat Rep* 1981;65:341.
489. Weiss AJ, Ramirez G, Grage T, et al. Phase II study of azotomycin (NSC-56654). *Cancer Chemother Rep* 1968;52:611.
490. Perevodchikova NI, Lichinitser MR, Gorbunova VA. Phase I clinical study of carminomycin: its activity against soft tissue sarcomas. *Cancer Treat Rep* 1977;61:1705.
491. Taylor SA, Metch B, Balcerzak SP, Hanson KH. Phase II trial of echinomycin in advanced soft tissue sarcomas. A Southwest Oncology Group study. *Invest New Drugs* 1990;8:381.
492. Giaccone G, Donadio M, Calciati A. Phase II study of esorubicin in the treatment of patients with advanced sarcoma. *Oncology* 1989;46:285.
493. Somers R, Santoro A, Verweij J, et al. Phase II study of mitozolomide in advanced soft tissue sarcoma of adults: the EORTC Soft Tissue and Bone Sarcoma Group. *Eur J Cancer* 1992;28A:855.
494. Buckner JC, Edmonson JH, Ingle JN, Schaid DJ. Evaluation of menogaril in patients with metastatic sarcomas and no prior chemotherapy exposure. *Am J Clin Oncol* 1989;12:384.
495. Taub RN, Paciucci AP, Behrens B, et al. Phase II study of methoxymorpholinodoxorubicin in advanced sarcomas [PNU/S2243 (FCE23762)]. *Proc Am Soc Clin Oncol* 1997;16:A1831.
496. Casper ES, Baselga J, Smart TB, et al. A phase II trial of PALA + dipyridamole in patients with advanced soft- tissue sarcoma. *Cancer Chemother Pharmacol* 1991;28:51.
497. Schiesel JD, Carabasi M, Magill G, et al. Oral piritrexim—a phase II study in patients with advanced soft tissue sarcoma. *Invest New Drugs* 1992;10:97.
498. Cormier WJ, Hahn RG, Edmonson JH, Eagan RT. Phase II study in advanced sarcoma: randomized trial of pyrazofurin versus combination cyclophosphamide, doxorubicin, and cis- dichlorodiammineplatinum(II) (CAP). *Cancer Treat Rep* 1980;64:655.
499. Blay J-Y, Judson I, Rodenhuis S, et al. A phase II study of raltitrexed ("Tomudex") as second or third line treatment for patients (pts) with advanced soft tissue sarcomas (ASTS) refractory to doxorubicin-containing regimens. *Sarcoma* 1999;3:56.
500. Thigpen JT, O'Bryan RM, Benjamin RS, Coltman CA Jr. Phase II trial of Baker's antifol in metastatic sarcoma. *Cancer Treat Rep* 1977;61:1485.
501. Eisenhauer EA, Wierzbicki R, Knowling M, et al. Phase II trials of trimetrexate in advanced adult soft tissue sarcoma. Studies of the Canadian Sarcoma Group and the National Cancer Institute of Canada Clinical Trials Group. *Ann Oncol* 1991;2:689.
502. Patel SR, Burgess MA, Papadopolous NE, et al. Phase II study of CI-980 (NSC 635370) in patients with previously treated advanced soft tissue sarcomas. *Invest New Drugs* 1998;16:87.
503. Cure H, Krakowski I, Adenis A, et al. Results of a phase II trial with second-line cystemustine at 60 mg/m^2 in advanced soft tissue sarcoma: a trial of the EORTC Early Clinical Studies Group. *Eur J Cancer* 1998;34:422.
504. Borden EC, Ash A, Enterline HT, et al. Phase II evaluation of dibromodulcitol, ICRF-159, and maytansine for sarcomas. *Am J Clin Oncol* 1982;5:417.
505. Thigpen JT, Samson MK. Phase II trial of dianhydrogalactitol in advanced soft tissue and bony sarcomas: a Southwest Oncology Group study. *Cancer Treat Rep* 1979;63:553.
506. Blomqvist C, Wiklund T, Pajunen M, et al. Oral trofosfamide: an active drug in the treatment of soft tissue sarcoma. *Cancer Chemother Pharmacol* 1995;36:263.
507. Asbury R, Blessing JA, Buller R, et al. Amonafide in patients with leiomyosarcoma of the uterus: a phase II Gynecologic Oncology Group study. *Am J Clin Oncol* 1998;21:145.
508. Chan C, Bartolucci A, Brenner D, et al. Phase II trial of diaziquone in anthracycline-resistant adult soft tissue and bone sarcoma patients: a Southeastern Cancer Study Group Trial. *Cancer Treat Rep* 1986;70:427.

509. Vosika GJ, Briscoe K, Carey RW, et al. Phase II study of diglycoaldehyde in malignant melanomas and soft tissue sarcomas. *Cancer Treat Rep* 1981;65:823.
510. Bramwell V, Morris D, Ernst S, et al. Phase I/II study with the MDR inhibitor INCELTM (biricodar, VX-710)+doxorubicin in anthracycline resistant advanced soft tissue sarcoma (STS). *Proc Am Soc Clin Oncol* 1999;18:A2094(abst).
511. Somers R, Rouesse J, van Oosterom A, Thomas D. Phase II study of elliptinium in metastatic soft tissue sarcoma. *Eur J Cancer Clin Oncol* 1985;21:591.
512. Ajani JA, Dimery I, Chawla SP, et al. Phase II studies of homoharringtonine in patients with advanced malignant melanoma; sarcoma; and head and neck, breast, and colorectal carcinomas. *Cancer Treat Rep* 1986;70:375.
513. Kraut EH, Bendetti J, Balcerzak SP, Doroshow JH. Phase II trial of merbarone in soft tissue sarcoma. A Southwest Oncology Group study. *Invest New Drugs* 1992;10:347.
514. Rouesse JG, van Oosterom AT, Capellaere P, et al. Phase II study of 1,2,4-triglycidyl urasol (TGU) in advanced soft tissue sarcoma. A trial of the EORTC Soft Tissue and Bone Sarcoma Cooperative Group. *Eur J Cancer Clin Oncol* 1987;23:1413.
515. Sordillo PP, Magill GB, Gralla RJ. Phase II evaluation of vindesine sulfate in patients with advanced sarcomas. *Cancer Treat Rep* 1981;65:515.
516. Schuff-Werner P, Bartsch H, Schremi W, Nagel GA. Treatment of soft tissue sarcoma with recombinant alpha-interferon. *Antiviral Res* 1984;3:93(abst).
517. Borden EC, Kim K, Ryan L, et al. Phase II trials of interferons-alpha and -beta in advanced sarcomas. *J Interferon Res* 1992;12:455.
518. Jazieh AR, McIntyre W, Husain M, et al. Phase I clinical trial of tamoxifen and interferon alpha in the treatment of solid tumors. *Proc Am Soc Clin Oncol* 1999; 18: A829(abst).
519. Harris J, Das Gupta T, Vogelzang N, et al. Treatment of soft tissue sarcoma with fibroblast interferon (beta- interferon): an American Cancer Society/Illinois Cancer Council study. *Cancer Treat Rep* 1986;70:293.
520. Rosenberg SA, Lotze MT, Muul LM, et al. A progress report on the treatment of 157 patients with advanced cancer using lymphokine-activated killer cells and interleukin-2 or high-dose interleukin-2 alone. *N Engl J Med* 1987;316:889.
521. Gravis G, Viens P, Delva R, et al. rIL-2 in metastatic soft tissue sarcomas refractory to chemotherapy: response and enhancement of further chemosensitivity. *Anticancer Res* 1998;18:3699.
522. Verweij J, Judson I, Steward W, et al. Phase II study of liposomal muramyl tripeptide phosphatidylethanolamine (MTP/PE) in advanced soft tissue sarcomas of the adult. An EORTC Soft Tissue and Bone Sarcoma Group study. *Eur J Cancer* 1994;6:842.
523. Rinehart J, Balcerzak SP, Hersh E. Phase II trial of tumor necrosis factor in human sarcomas: a Southwest Oncology Group study. *Proc Am Soc Clin Oncol* 1990;9:1229(abst).
524. Cruz AB Jr, Thames EA Jr, Aust JB, et al. Combination chemotherapy for soft tissue sarcomas: a phase III study. *J Surg Oncol* 1979;11:313.
525. Nielsen OS, Dombernowsky P, Mouridsen H, et al. High-dose epirubicin is not an alternative to standard-dose doxorubicin in the treatment of advanced soft tissue sarcomas. A study of the EORTC soft tissue and bone sarcoma group. *Br J Cancer* 1998;78:1634.
526. Loehrer PJ Sr, Sledge GW Jr, Nicaise C, et al. Ifosfamide plus doxorubicin in metastatic adult sarcomas: a multi-institutional phase II trial. *J Clin Oncol* 1989;7:1655.
527. Brennan MF. The surgeon as a leader in cancer care: lessons learned from the study of soft tissue sarcoma. *J Am Coll Surg* 1996;182:520.
528. Billingsley K, Burt M, Jara E, et al. Pulmonary metastases from soft tissue sarcoma: analysis of patterns of disease and postmetastasis survival. *Ann Surg* 1999;229:602.

SECTION **2**

MARTIN M. MALAWER
MICHAEL P. LINK
SARAH S. DONALDSON

Sarcomas of Bone

Malignant tumors arising from the skeletal system are rare, representing only 0.2% of all new cancers. Approximately 2600 new cases occur in the United States each year.[1] Osteosarcoma and Ewing's sarcoma, the two most common bone tumors, occur mainly during childhood and adolescence.[2–4] Other mesenchymal (spindle cell) neoplasms that characteristically arise after skeletal maturity—fibrosarcoma, chondrosarcoma, and malignant fibrous histiocytoma (MFH)—are less common.[5–18] The vast majority of experience reported in the management of bone neoplasms has been obtained in patients with osteosarcoma. As a result, the surgical, chemotherapeutic, and radiotherapeutic principles developed for treatment of osteosarcomas form the basis of the management strategy for most of the spindle cell neoplasms.

Since the late 1970s, an explosion of clinical knowledge and experience in the management of bone neoplasms has been seen.[18–29] The development of centers of specific interest in these tumors has played an important role in the advancement of biologic understanding and surgical management of these lesions and the development of multimodality treatment regimens.[24–28] A surgical staging system that permits standardized preoperative evaluation, analysis, and end-result reporting has been developed.[29]

Amputation has been the standard method of treatment for most bone sarcomas, but the 1990s was witness to the development of limb-sparing surgery for most malignant bone tumors.[30–40] Advances in orthopedics, bioengineering, radiographic imaging, radiotherapy, and chemotherapy have contributed to safer, more reliable surgical procedures.[41–81] Computed tomography (CT), developed during the early 1980s, and, more recently, magnetic resonance imaging (MRI), permit extremely accurate evaluation of the local anatomy and enhance the possibility of safe resection.[82–89] Today, limb-sparing surgery is considered safe and routine for approximately 90% of patients with extremity osteosarcomas. An evaluation system has been developed to determine a patient's functional status.[29] This system, for the first time, permits evaluation and comparison of the various limb-sparing procedures and types of surgical reconstructions.

Paralleling these advances has been the demonstrated effectiveness of adjuvant chemotherapy in dramatically increasing overall survival; specifically, the bleak 15% to 20% survival rate associated with surgery alone before the 1970s rose to 55% to 80% with various adjuvant treatment regimens by the 1980s.[50–53,90–92] Multiple-drug regimens are now considered essential treatment. The timing, mode of delivery, and different combinations of these agents are being investigated at many centers. Preoperative chemotherapy regimens (termed *neoadjuvant* or *induction chemotherapy*) and postoperative regimens are being evaluated to determine their effect on the tumor and their impact on the choice of operative procedure and on overall survival.[93–100]

This chapter focuses only on malignant spindle cell tumors. Ewing's sarcoma is presented in detail in Chapter 39.1. Benign tumors are described briefly, and their significance for the oncologist is described.[2,3] Emphasis is placed on natural history, surgical staging, tumor imaging, criteria of patient selection for amputation versus limb-sparing surgery, and technique of limb-sparing procedures. The development, role, timing, and mode of delivery of adjuvant chemotherapy and its relationship to stage of disease are discussed. The role of radiotherapy in specific clinical situations is presented.

CLASSIFICATION AND TYPES OF BONE TUMORS

Bone consists of cartilaginous, osteoid, and fibrous tissue and bone marrow elements. Each tissue can give rise to benign or malignant spindle cell tumors.[2–4] Bone tumors are classified on the basis of cell type and recognized products of proliferating cells. The classification system, described by Lichtenstein[3,56] and modified by Dahlin,[2] is presented in Table 39.2-1. Jaffe[4]

TABLE 39.2-1. General Classification of Bone Tumors

Histologic Type[a]	*Benign*	*Malignant*
Hematopoietic (41.4%)	—	Myeloma
	—	Reticulum cell sarcoma
Chondrogenic (20.9%)	Osteochondroma	Primary chondrosarcoma
	Chondroma	Secondary chondrosarcoma
	Chondroblastoma	Dedifferentiated chondrosarcoma
	Chondromyxoid fibroma	Mesenchymal chondrosarcoma
Osteogenic (19.3%)	Osteoid osteoma	Osteosarcoma
	Benign osteoblastoma	Parosteal osteogenic sarcoma
Unknown origin (9.8%)	Giant cell tumor	Ewing's tumor
		Malignant giant cell tumor
		Adamantinoma
	(Fibrous) histiocytoma	(Fibrous) histiocytoma
Fibrogenic (3.8%)	Fibroma	Fibrosarcoma
	Desmoplastic fibroma	—
Notochordal (3.1%)	—	Chordoma
Vascular (1.6%)	Hemangioma	Hemangioendothelioma
	—	Hemangiopericytoma
Lipogenic (<0.5%)	Lipoma	—
Neurogenic (<0.5%)	Neurilemmoma	—

[a]Distribution based on Mayo Clinic experience.
(Adapted from ref. 2, with permission.)

recommends that each tumor be considered a separate clinicopathologic entity. Radiographic, histologic, and clinical data are necessary to form an accurate diagnosis and to determine the degree of activity and malignancy of each lesion.

Cartilage tumors are lesions in which cartilage is produced. They are the most common bone tumors. Osteochondroma is the most common benign cartilage tumor; some 1% to 2% of solitary osteochondromas become malignant.[57–58] Enchondroma is a benign cartilage tumor that occurs centrally; in adults, malignant transformation may occur. Chondrosarcoma, the most common malignant cartilage tumor, is either intramedullary or peripheral. Ten percent are secondary, arising from an underlying benign lesion.[2] Most chondrosarcomas are low grade, although 10% dedifferentiate into high-grade spindle cell sarcomas or, rarely, a mesenchymal chondrosarcoma.[2,57]

Osteoid tumors are lesions in which the stroma produce osteoid. The benign forms are osteoid osteoma and osteoblastoma. Osteoid osteomas are never malignant. Osteoblastomas rarely metastasize; when they do, it is only after multiple local recurrences.[59] Osteosarcomas are the most common primary malignant tumors of the bone. Histologically, they are composed of malignant spindle cells and osteoblasts that produce osteoid or immature bone. Several variants are now recognized.[60] Parosteal, periosteal, and low-grade intraosseous osteosarcoma are histologically and radiographically distinct from the "classic" central medullary osteosarcomas and have a more favorable prognosis.[61,63]

Fibrous tumors of bone are rare. Desmoplastic fibroma is a locally aggressive, nonmetastasizing tumor, analogous to fibromatosis of soft tissue.[5,6] Fibrosarcoma of bone appears histologically as its soft tissue counterpart. Multiple sections must be obtained to demonstrate the lack of osteoid production. If osteoid is present, the lesion is classified as an osteosarcoma. MFH, a rare lesion and the counterpart of soft tissue MFH, has been described in bone.[7–9] The pathophysiologic behavior of bone and soft tissue MFH is similar, consisting of a storiform pattern with a histiocytic component. Giant cell tumors of unknown origin were originally called benign but are now considered low-grade sarcomas. They have high rates of local recurrence and malignant transformation.[64,65]

Tumors presumably arising from bone marrow elements are the round cell sarcomas. The two most common are Ewing's sarcoma and the rarer non-Hodgkin's lymphoma.

RADIOGRAPHIC EVALUATION AND DIAGNOSIS

Radiographic evaluation combined with the clinical history and histologic examination is necessary for accurate diagnosis. Bone scans, angiography, CT, and MRI are generally not helpful in determining a diagnosis but are important in delineating the extent of local involvement. A systematic approach to the radiographic evaluation of skeletal lesions has been described by Madewell and colleagues,[66] who studied and correlated several hundred radiographic and pathologic specimens. They considered the radiograph as the gross specimen from which a detailed histologic interpretation could be made and biologic activity accurately diagnosed. According to their system, a bone tumor is evaluated by five radiographic parameters:

1. Anatomic site. Specific anatomic sites of the bone give rise to specific groups of lesions. Johnson[67] explained this by a "field" theory, which hypothesizes that the most active cells of a certain area of bone give rise to tumors that are characteristic of that area. In general, spindle cell sarcomas are metaphyseal, whereas round cell sarcomas tend to be diaphyseal.

2. Borders. The border reflects the growth rate and the response of the adjacent normal bone to the tumor. Most tumors have a characteristic border. Benign lesions (e.g., nonossifying fibromas and unicameral bone cysts) have well-defined borders and a narrow transition area that is often associated with a reactive sclerosis. Aggressive or benign tumors [e.g., chondroblastoma and giant cell tumors (GCTs)] tend to have faint borders and wide zones of transition with very little sclerosis, reflecting a faster-growing lesion. Poorly delineated or absent margins indicate an aggressive or malignant lesion.
3. Bone destruction. Bone destruction is the hallmark of a bone tumor. Three patterns of bone destruction are described[68]: geographic, moth-eaten, and permeative. In general, these patterns are found in the tubular bone rather than in the flat bone and represent a combination of cortical and cancellous destruction. These patterns reflect a progressively increasing growth rate of the underlying tumor.
4. Matrix formation. Calcification of the matrix, or new bone formation, may produce an area of increased density within the lesion. Calcification typically appears as flocculent or stippled rings or clusters. The appearance of the new bone varies from dense sclerosis that obliterates all evidence of normal trabeculae, to small, irregular, circumscribed masses described as "wool" or "clouds." Calcification and ossification may appear in the same lesion. Neither type of matrix formation per se is diagnostic of malignancy.
5. Periosteal reaction. Periosteal reaction is indicative of malignancy but not pathognomonic of a particular tumor. A combination of periosteal changes is often noted. In malignant tumors, periosteal reaction is noncontinuous and thin, with multiple laminations. A parallel or a perpendicular pattern may be present.

The radiographic parameters of benign and malignant tumors are quite different. Benign tumors have round, smooth, well-circumscribed borders. No cortical destruction and, generally, no periosteal reaction are found. Malignant lesions have irregular, poorly defined margins. Evidence of bone destruction and a wide area of transition with periosteal reaction are noted. Soft tissue extension is common.

NATURAL HISTORY

Tumors arising in bone have characteristic patterns of behavior and growth that distinguish them from other malignant lesions.[69,89] These patterns form the basis of a staging system and current treatment strategies. These principles and their relationship to management, as formulated by Enneking and colleagues,[69,89] are described here.

BIOLOGY AND GROWTH

Spindle cell sarcomas form a solid lesion that grows centrifugally. The periphery is the least mature part of this lesion. In contradistinction to a true capsule, which surrounds a benign lesion and is composed of compressed normal cells, a malignant tumor is generally enclosed by a pseudocapsule and consists of compressed tumor cells and a fibrovascular zone of reactive tissue with an inflammatory component that interdigitates with the normal tissue adjacent to and beyond the lesion. The thickness of the reactive zone varies with the degree of malignancy and histiogenic type. The histologic hallmark of sarcomas is their potential to break through the pseudocapsule to form satellite lesions of tumor cells. This characteristic distinguishes a nonmalignant mesenchymal tumor from a malignant one.

High-grade sarcomas have a poorly defined reactive zone that may be invaded and destroyed by the tumor. In addition, tumor nodules in tissue may appear to be normal and not continuous with the main tumor. These are termed *skip metastases.* Although low-grade sarcomas regularly demonstrate tumor interdigitation into the reactive zone, they rarely form tumor nodules beyond this area.

The three mechanisms of growth and extension of bone tumors are: (1) compression of normal tissue, (2) resorption of bone by reactive osteoclasts, and (3) direct destruction of normal tissue. Benign tumors grow and expand by the first two mechanisms, whereas direct tissue destruction is characteristic of malignant bone tumors. Sarcomas respect anatomic borders and remain within one compartment. Local anatomy influences tumor growth by setting the natural barriers to extension. In general, bone sarcomas take the path of least resistance. Most benign bone tumors are unicompartmental; they remain confined and may expand the bone in which they arose. Malignant bone tumors are bicompartmental; they destroy the overlying cortex and go directly into the adjacent soft tissue. The determination of anatomic compartment involvement has become more important with the advent of limb-preservation surgery.

On the basis of biologic considerations and natural history, Enneking and colleagues[69,101] classified bone tumors into five categories, each of which shares certain clinical characteristics and radiographic patterns and requires similar surgical procedures.

1. Benign/latent: lesions whose natural history is to grow slowly during normal growth of the individual and then to stop, with a tendency to heal spontaneously. They never become malignant and, if treated by simple curettage, heal rapidly. Surgery is not indicated unless they become symptomatic.
2. Benign/active: lesions whose natural history is one of progressive growth. Simple curettage leaves a reactive rim with some tumor. Curettage is associated with a high recurrence rate. Wide excision through normal bone results in local control in approximately 95% of all cases.
3. Benign/aggressive: lesions that are locally aggressive but do not metastasize. The tumor extends through the capsule into the reactive zone. Local control can be obtained only by removing the lesion with a margin of normal bone beyond the reactive zone.
4. Malignant/low grade: lesions that have a low potential to metastasize. Histologically, a pseudocapsule rather than a true capsule is found. Tumor nodules exist within the reactive zone but rarely beyond. Local control can be accomplished only by removal of all tumor and reactive tissue with a margin of normal bone. These lesions can be treated successfully by surgery alone.

5. Malignant/high grade: lesions whose natural history is to grow rapidly and metastasize early. Tumor nodules are often found within and beyond the reactive zone and at some distance in the normal tissue. Surgery is necessary for local control, and systemic therapy is warranted to prevent metastasis.

METASTASIS

Bone tumors, unlike carcinomas, disseminate almost exclusively through the blood; bones lack a lymphatic system. Early lymphatic spread to regional nodes has only rarely been reported.[18,102] Lymphatic involvement, which has been noted in 10% of cases at autopsy, is a poor prognostic sign.[70] McKenna and associates[71] noted that 6 of 194 patients (3%) with osteosarcoma who underwent amputation demonstrated lymph node involvement. None of these patients survived 5 years. Hematogenous spread is manifested by pulmonary involvement in its early stage and secondarily by bone involvement.[71–76] Bone metastasis is occasionally the first sign of dissemination. With the use of adjuvant chemotherapy, the skeletal system has become a more common site of initial relapse.[46,103,104]

SKIP METASTASIS

A skip metastasis, as previously defined, is a tumor nodule that is located within the same bone as the main tumor but not in continuity with it. Transarticular skip metastases are located in the joint adjacent to the main tumor.[77] Skip metastases are most often seen with high-grade sarcomas. A skip lesion develops by the embolization of tumor cells within the marrow sinusoids; in effect, they are local micrometastases that have not passed through the circulation. Transarticular skips are believed to occur via the periarticular venous anastomosis. The clinical incidence of skip metastases is less than 1%.[78] These lesions are a prognosticator of poor survival.[77,78]

LOCAL RECURRENCE

Local recurrence of a benign or malignant lesion is due to inadequate removal. The aggressiveness of the tumor determines which surgical procedure is required for local control. Ninety-five percent of all local recurrences, regardless of histology, develop within 24 months of attempted removal.[69,79,80]

TABLE 39.2-2. Surgical Staging of Bone Sarcomas

Stage	*Grade*	*Site*
IA	Low (G1)	Intracompartmental (T1)
IB	Low (G1)	Extracompartmental (T2)
IIA	High (G2)	Intracompartmental (T1)
IIB	High (G2)	Extracompartmental (T2)
III	Any G Regional or distant metastasis (M1)	Any (T)

G, grade; G1, any low-grade tumor; G2, any high-grade tumor; M, regional or distal metastases; M0, no metastases; M1, any metastases; T, site; T1, intracompartmental location of tumor; T2, extracompartmental location of tumor.
(From ref. 19, with permission.)

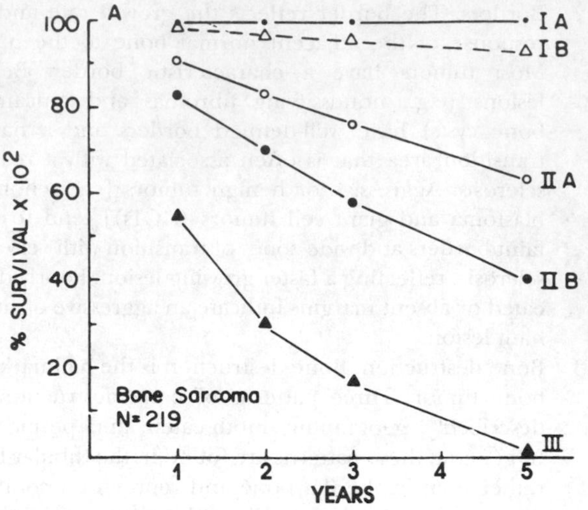

FIGURE 39.2-1. Survival rates over a 5-year period of patients with bone sarcoma according to stage of disease. (From ref. 19, with permission.)

Local recurrence of a high-grade sarcoma decreases overall survival prospects substantially. Local recurrence in patients who have undergone therapy is associated with an even poorer prognosis (Fig. 39.2-1).[75]

STAGING BONE TUMORS

MUSCULOSKELETAL TUMOR SOCIETY CLASSIFICATION

In 1980, the Musculoskeletal Tumor Society (MSTS) adopted a surgical staging system for bone sarcomas (Table 39.2-2).[100] The system is based on the fact that mesenchymal sarcomas of bone behave similarly, regardless of histiogenic type. The surgical staging system, as described by Enneking and colleagues,[101] is based on the GTM classification: grade (G), location (T), and lymph node involvement and metastases (M).

G represents the histologic grade of a lesion and other clinical data. Grade is further divided into two categories: G1 is low grade, and G2 is high grade.

T represents the site of the lesion, which may be intracompartmental (T1) or extracompartmental (T2). Compartment is defined as "an anatomic structure or space bounded by natural barriers or tumor extension." The significance of T1 lesions is easier to define clinically, surgically, and radiographically than that of T2 lesions, and the chance is better for adequate removal of the former without amputation. In general, low-grade bone sarcomas are intracompartmental (T1), whereas high-grade ones are extracompartmental (T2).

Lymphatic spread is a sign of widespread dissemination. Regional lymphatic involvement is equated with distal metastases (M1). Absence of any metastasis is designated as M0.

The surgical staging system developed by Enneking and colleagues[101] for surgical planning and assessment of bone sarcomas is summarized thus:

Stage IA (G1,T1,M0): low-grade intracompartmental lesion, without metastasis

Stage IB (G1,T2,M0): low-grade extracompartmental lesion, without metastasis
Stage IIA (G2,T1,M0): high-grade intracompartmental lesion, without metastasis
Stage IIB (G2,T2,M0): high-grade extracompartmental lesion, without metastasis
Stage IIIA (G1 or G2,T1,M1): intracompartmental lesion, any grade, with metastasis
Stage IIIB (G1 or G2,T2,M1): extracompartmental lesion, any grade, with metastasis

AMERICAN JOINT COMMITTEE ON CANCER BONE TUMOR CLASSIFICATION

In 1983, the American Joint Committee on Cancer Bone Tumor Classification (AJCC) recommended a staging system for the malignant tumors of bone. This system has undergone minimal changes and remains unchanged in the fifth edition of the *AJCC Cancer Staging Manual.* This system is based on two indications: TNM designation [extent of the tumor (T), nodal status (N), and distant metastases (M)] and grade (G). This system is similar to the MSTS classification; however, the AJCC uses four stages instead of three. The four stages are designated *I* to *IV* and may be further modified with *A* or *B.* Stages I and II are defined by the histologic grade (grade I and II) and modified by tumor extent (i.e., cortical involvement, designated E1 to E6) (Table 39.2-3). T(I) indicates that the tumor is confined within the cortex (similar to the MSTS classification A), and T(II) indicates that the tumor extends beyond the cortex (similar to the MSTS classification B). In the AJCC, stage III has remained undefined and stage IV is defined as the presence of metastases. Stage IV tumors are modified by A, which is equivalent to III M1 in the MSTS system (i.e., indicates a nodal metastasis), and B, which is equivalent to III M1 in the MSTS system (i.e., indicates distant metastases).[105]

TABLE 39.2-3. Definitions of Anatomic Extent for Stage IIB Tumors

Maximal Extent	*Definition*
E1	Tumor touches but does not elevate or penetrate the periosteum.
E2	Tumor elevates but does not penetrate the periosteum.
E3	Tumor penetrates into but not through the periosteum.
E4	Minimal extraperiosteal extension, not into a defined structure or space, seen as a nodule of tumor of 1 cm or smaller in fat just outside the periosteum, where muscle does not insert onto bone; the nodule often lies next to a small artery and may represent a small venous embolus that has destroyed the wall of the vein.
E5	Tumor invades any one of the following: tendon, ligament, periarticular structures (tumor is covered by synovial tissue), joint (tumor is intraarticular), muscle, bone, or space (e.g., the popliteal fossa or axilla).
E6	Tumor invades two structures or more.

(From Spanier SS, Schuster JJ, Vander Griend RA. The effect of local extent of the tumor on prognosis in osteosarcoma. *J Bone Joint Surg Am* 1990;72:643, with permission.)

PREOPERATIVE EVALUATION

If the plain radiographs suggest an aggressive or malignant tumor, staging studies should be performed before biopsy. All radiographic studies are influenced by surgical manipulation of the lesion, making interpretation more difficult.[40,69] More important, the biopsy site may be in a location that is not optimal for subsequent *en bloc* removal or radiotherapy.[24,110,111] Bone scintigraphy, MRI, CT, angiography, or a combination of these is required to delineate local tumor extent, vascular displacement, and compartmental localization.[43–47,69,79,83–89]

BONE SCANS

Bone scintigraphy helps determine polyostotic involvement, metastatic disease, and intraosseous extension of tumor.[43,44,46] Malignant bone tumors, although solitary, may in rare cases present with skeletal metastasis.[47] Skip metastases are rarely detected by bone scan, because they are small and localized to the fatty marrow and do not excite cortical response.[77,78]

Appreciation of the intraosseous extension of a bone tumor is important in surgical planning. Removal of bone 3 to 4 cm beyond the area of scintigraphic abnormality has been accepted as a safe margin for limb-sparing procedures after induction chemotherapy.[33]

COMPUTED TOMOGRAPHY

CT allows accurate determination of intra- and extraosseous extension of skeletal neoplasms.[41–45] It accurately depicts the transverse relationship of a tumor. By varying window settings, one can study cortical bone, intramedullary space, adjacent muscles, and extraosseous soft tissue extension. CT should include the entire bone and the adjacent joint. Infusion of intravenous contrast material permits identification of the adjacent large vascular structures. CT evaluation must be individualized. To obtain the maximum benefits from image reconstruction, the surgeon should discuss with the radiologist what information is desired. Three-dimensional reconstruction may be useful. Today, CT and MRI are considered complementary studies for bone sarcomas. Both studies are recommended for most patients.

MAGNETIC RESONANCE IMAGING AND STAGING

MRI has several advantages in the diagnoses of bone sarcomas.[82–89] It has better contrast discrimination than any other modality; furthermore, imaging can be performed in any plane. MRI is ideal for imaging the medullary marrow and thus for detection of tumor as well as the extraosseous component. It has proved especially helpful in several heretofore difficult clinical situations, such as detecting small lesions, evaluating a positive bone scan when the corresponding plain radiograph is negative, determining the extent of infiltrative tumors, and detecting skip metastases.[87–89]

Dynamic MRI is currently being evaluated as a more accurate method of determining intraosseous extension of tumor than conventional MRI. Iwasawa et al.[106] performed a microscopic evaluation of six macrospecimens after tumor resection and chemotherapy. They concluded that the calculation of the slope value of dynamic MRI discriminated regions of microscopic invasion from tumor-free marrow in patients with osteosarcoma after chemotherapy. The slope value of dynamic MRI was greater in the region of microscopic invasion than in the tumor-free marrow and less than in the area showing macroscopic tumor invasion. This technique may provide more accurate determination of intraosseous bony extent than traditional MRI.

ANGIOGRAPHY

The technique of arteriography for bone lesions differs from that used for arterial disease. At least two views (biplane) are necessary to determine the relation of the major vessels to the tumor.[107] Because experience with limb-sparing procedures has increased, it has become essential to determine individual vascular patterns before resection. This is especially crucial for tumors of the proximal tibia, where vascular anomalies are common.[108] Angiography is the most reliable means of determining vascular anatomy and displacement, whereas MRI and CT better demonstrate extraosseous extension. Presently, magnetic resonance angiography is being evaluated in the treatment of bone sarcomas.

THALLIUM SCANS

Thallium 201 scintigraphy has been shown to accumulate in musculoskeletal neoplasms[109,110]; however, it cannot distinguish benign from malignant tumors. Thallium scintigraphy is helpful in following the response to neoadjuvant treatment and detecting local recurrence when MRI cannot be used.[109–112]

CHOOSING A METHOD OF RADIOGRAPHIC EVALUATION

All of the above studies are required in the preoperative evaluation of a bone sarcoma. Each study has unique benefits. Bloem et al.[113] performed a prospective study comparing results of CT, MRI, scintigraphy, and angiography with 56 resected specimens to determine the appropriate choice of procedures. MRI, the single best study, was most accurate for determining intraosseous extent of tumor; scintigraphy and CT were often misleading. Angiography was performed only if the primary tumor was in the vicinity of the major vascular structures. They also reported that CT and MRI were equally accurate in evaluating cortical changes. MRI was superior to CT for detecting muscle involvement in the knee, pelvis, and shoulder.

MRI and CT (transverse data), combined with bone scans and angiography, allow the physician to develop a three-dimensional construct of the local tumor area before surgery and thereby formulate a detailed surgical approach.

BIOPSY TECHNIQUE AND TIMING

The biopsy of a suspected bone tumor must be performed with great care and skill.[114,115] This principle cannot be overemphasized. The consequences of a poorly executed biopsy are often the deciding factor in the choice between a limb-salvage procedure and amputation. Murray and coworkers[114a] from the M. D. Anderson Cancer Center judged that only 19% of patients referred to that institution for treatment of primary bone sarcomas had properly placed biopsies. All of these patients had open (incisional) biopsies, whereas 92% of such procedures performed at the M. D. Anderson Cancer Center over the same period were needle biopsies. Similarly, Mankin et al.[115] compared the results of biopsies performed at the referring institution with those performed at the treatment center. In this study, which involved 329 patients, a major error in diagnosis occurred in 60% of patients from referring hospitals. Importantly, 18.2% of the referred patients had to have less than optimal treatment owing to problems related to the biopsy, and for 8.5% of the total, the prognosis and outcome were thought to have been adversely affected by the biopsy. It is recommended that the biopsy be performed by the surgeon who will make the ultimate decision about the operative procedure. This entails referring some patients who are strongly suspected of having primary bone malignancies to a regional cancer center for biopsy.

Trephine or core biopsy is recommended and often obtains an adequate specimen for diagnosis.[116–118] Multiple samples can be obtained from the same puncture site by slightly changing the angle of approach. Radiographs should be obtained to document the position of the trocar. Core biopsy is preferred if a limb-sparing option exists, because it entails less local contamination than does open biopsy. Core biopsy is especially helpful in difficult areas, such as the spine, pelvis, and hips. If a core biopsy proves to be inadequate, a small incisional biopsy is performed.

Every precaution should be taken to avoid contamination when performing an open biopsy. A tourniquet is used if feasible. If a soft tissue component is present, there is no need to biopsy the underlying bone. To decrease subsequent hemorrhage, polymethylmethacrylate (PMMA) is used to plug a cortical window. Gelfoam is used for hemostasis in the soft tissue. The overlying pseudocapsule is carefully closed to ensure maximum hemostasis. If it is necessary to biopsy the underlying bone, it is essential to use a small, rounded cortical window, especially if the tumor requires primary radiotherapy. Large segments will not reossify, and they often fracture and require late amputations. Regardless of the technique used, tumor cells contaminate all tissue planes and compartments transversed. All biopsy sites must therefore be removed *en bloc* when the tumor is resected or irradiated.

RESTAGING AFTER PREOPERATIVE CHEMOTHERAPY

With the advent of preoperative chemotherapy for osteosarcoma, a need has developed for serial evaluation of the clinical and radiographic response of the tumor before surgery. The staging and preoperative clinical studies previously described are used to evaluate tumor response. These studies have been summarized.[119–125] Complete restaging studies should be obtained after the completion of induction chemotherapy. MRI, CT, thallium scans, and angiography should be evaluated before making a final surgical decision.

CLINICAL EVALUATION

Pain often decreases after induction chemotherapy. Alkaline phosphatase (AP) levels likewise decrease. The tumor shrinks, especially if significant matrix is not present. Conversely, increase of pain, elevated AP values, and increasing tumor size are signs of tumor progression.

PLAIN RADIOGRAPHY

There is a good correlation between radiographic response and the amount of necrosis.[121,124] Smith and colleagues[124] described the radiographic responses seen on serial radiographs: increased ossification of tumor osteoid, marked thickening and new bone formation of the periosteum and tumor border (giving the tumor a more "benign" appearance), and decreased soft tissue mass. The healing ossification is usually solid, homogeneous, and regular and is easily differentiated from tumor osteoid.[121] Less significant changes take place within the intramedullary component, which may include both increased sclerosis and lysis, presumably caused by necrosis and hemorrhage.

ANGIOGRAPHY

After chemotherapy, vascularity decreases markedly.[120,121] Chuang et al.[121] evaluated 53 patients and reported that those with a complete angiographic response had more than 90% necrosis; among those with a partial response, necrosis ranged from 40% to 78%. They concluded that angiographic evaluation was as reliable as pathologic evaluation and that the angiographic features were the best clinical criteria for the evaluation of tumor response.

Carrasco and coworkers[122] from the M. D. Anderson Cancer Center reported on their extensive experience with intraarterial chemotherapy for osteosarcoma (81 patients) and evaluated the angiographic appearance and changes after two and four cycles of preoperative chemotherapy. They developed a simple radiographic system for angiographic changes. They evaluated the midarterial (tumor vascularity) and parenchymal (capillary) phases. They described three types of responses:

1. Angiographic response: complete disappearance of tumor vascularity and stain.
2. Total disappearance of tumor vascularity, with slight persistence of tumor stain (capillary phase).
3. No response: persistence of tumor vascularity and capillary stain.

They reported that 40% of the histologic responders (more than 90% tumor necrosis) and 91% of nonresponders were identified after two cycles. The number of courses was no different between the responders and nonresponders. They concluded that the disappearance of tumor vascularity after two courses of chemotherapy was highly suggestive of a good histologic response and was unlikely to occur in the histologic nonresponders.

COMPUTED TOMOGRAPHY

The most consistent finding in patients who respond to therapy is a decrease in soft tissue mass and the development of a rimlike calcification similar to that seen on plain radiographs.[119] Changes in marrow are not helpful in evaluating response.

BONE SCINTIGRAPHY

Bone scan changes are difficult to evaluate. A decrease in activity generally indicates a favorable response; however, reparative bone formation, signaled by increased activity, may be misleading. Dynamic (quantitative) bone scans, which are based on tumor blood flow and regional plasma clearance by bone and soft tissue, may allow more valid evaluations.[125] Regions that show a greater than 20% decrease in technetium 99m methylene diphosphonate plasma clearance are reported to be associated with necrotic tumor. To quantify bone scans, a tumor to nontumor ratio is obtained after bone scintigraphy. This ratio is then determined preoperatively and after induction chemotherapy on serial scans. A decrease in this ratio is an indication of a good response to chemotherapy.

MAGNETIC RESONANCE IMAGING

Monitoring of neoadjuvant chemotherapy by MRI has become the focus of many studies.[126–128] Holscher and colleagues[126] evaluated 57 patients at the University Hospital of Leiden. T1- and T2-weighted images were obtained in longitudinal, coronal or sagittal, and axial planes. Factors evaluated were margins, homogeneity, hematoma, fibrosis, calcification liquefaction, edema, joint effusion, and fracture. The authors concluded that increased tumor volume or increased or unchanged peritumoral edema and inflammation indicated a poor response. Subjective criteria, such as improved tumor demarcation or an increase in size of area of low signal intensity (presumably necrotic tumor), were independent of tumor response. They concluded that subjective criteria could not predict the good responders.

Conventional MRI is not specific enough to distinguish viable tumor from chemotherapy-related inflammation. On routine T2-weighted images, the signals for tumor, hemorrhage, necrosis, and edema are similar. Tumor cannot be differentiated from inflammation on T1-weighted gadolinium-enhanced images.

THALLIUM SCINTIGRAPHY

Several studies have demonstrated that serial thallium 201 scintigraphy is an accurate way to follow the response of osteosarcoma during the course of neoadjuvant treatment and to predict tumor responses.[109–112] Rosen and associates[110] used this technique to evaluate tumor necrosis after preoperative chemotherapy in 27 patients. They concluded that serial thallium scans can accurately predict a good histologic response and good prognosis. Furthermore, thallium scintigraphy can identify poor responders within the first 2 weeks after the initiation of treatment. They described a simple classification of response: type I, no response; type II, discernible lesion still present; type III, no detectable lesion. All patients with a type III classification and 67% of those with a type II classification were rated as good responders (types II and III constituted a total of nine patients).[110]

POSITRON EMISSION TOMOGRAPHY

Positron emission tomographic scans are nuclear medicine scintigraphy techniques that use 2[^{18}F]-fluoro-2-deoxy-D-glucose as the radiopharmaceutical. This technique is under investigation. It is hoped that it will be able to dynamically evaluate the tumor and the percentage of tumor necrosis after chemotherapy.[129]

SURGICAL MANAGEMENT OF SKELETAL TUMORS

Surgical removal, including curettage, resection, and amputation, is the traditional method of managing skeletal neoplasms. Limb-sparing techniques were developed during the early 1970s.[20–22,29–40] Marcove and associates[130–132] have described cryosurgery for some bony tumors. Enneking and colleagues[101] have formulated means of classifying surgical procedures based on the surgical plane of dissection in relationship to the tumor (Table 39.2-4) and the method of accomplishing the removal (Table 39.2-5). The scheme summarized below affords meaningful comparisons of various operative procedures and gives surgeons a common language.[69,79,101]

Intralesional: An intralesional procedure passes through the pseudocapsule of the neoplasm directly into the lesion. Macroscopic tumor remains, and the entire operative field is potentially contaminated. Curettage is an intralesional procedure.

Marginal: A marginal procedure is one in which the entire lesion is removed in a single piece. The plane of dissection passes through the pseudocapsule or reactive zone around the lesion. When performed for a sarcoma, it leaves macroscopic disease.

Wide (intracompartmental): A wide excision, commonly termed *en bloc resection*, includes the entire tumor, the reactive zone, and a cuff of normal tissue. The entire structure of origin of the tumor is not removed. In patients with high-grade sarcomas, this procedure may leave skip nodules.

Radical (extracompartmental): A radical procedure involves removal of the entire tumor and the structure of origin of the lesion. The plane of dissection is beyond the limiting fascial or bony borders.

It is important to note that any of these procedures may be accomplished either by a local (i.e., limb-sparing) procedure *or* by amputation. Thus, amputation may entail a marginal, wide, or radical excision, depending on the plane through which it passes. Amputation does not necessarily remove all cancer, but it can achieve a specific margin. The local anatomy determines how such a margin can be obtained. Therefore, the aim of preoperative staging is to assess local tumor extent and important local anatomy to enable the surgeon to decide how to achieve a desired margin (i.e., to evaluate the feasibility of one surgical procedure over another). This system allows meaningful comparisons of surgical procedures, end-result reporting, and analysis of combined data. In general, benign bone tumors may be treated adequately by an intralesional procedure (curettage) or a marginal excision. Malignant tumors require either a wide (intracompartmental) or radical (extracompartmental) removal, by an amputation or an *en bloc* procedure. Today, wide excision combined with adjuvant chemotherapy is the treatment for most high-grade bone sarcomas. Radical resections are rare.

TABLE 39.2-4. Classification of Surgical Procedures for Bone Tumors

Margin[a]	*Local*	*Amputation*
Intralesional	Curettage or debulking	Debulking amputation
Marginal	Marginal excision	Marginal amputation
Wide	Wide local excision	Wide through bone, amputation
Radical	Radical local resection	Radical disarticulation

[a]Tumors are classified by the type of margin achieved and whether they are obtained by a local or ablative procedure.
(From ref. 19, with permission.)

TABLE 39.2-5. Surgical Procedure, Plane of Dissection, and Residual Disease for Musculoskeletal Tumors

Type	*Plane of Dissection*	*Result*
Intralesional	Piecemeal debulking or curettage	Leaves macroscopic disease
Marginal	Shell out *en bloc* through pseudocapsule or reactive zone	May leave either satellite or skip lesions
Wide	Intracompartmental *en bloc* with cuff of normal tissue	May leave skip lesions
Radical	Extracompartmental *en bloc*, entire compartment	No residual

(From ref. 19, with permission.)

PRINCIPLES AND TECHNIQUES OF LIMB-SPARING SURGERY

Limb-salvage surgery is a safe operation for selected cases (Fig. 39.2-2).[23–27,133–135] This technique may be used for all spindle cell sarcomas, regardless of histogenesis. Approximately 90% of osteosarcomas can be treated successfully with this technique.[24,26,29,33,40,101] Successful management of localized osteosarcomas and other sarcomas requires careful coordination and timing of staging studies, biopsy, surgery, and preoperative and postoperative chemotherapy or radiation therapy.

PHASES OF OPERATION

Successful limb-sparing procedures consist of three surgical phases[134]:

1. Resection of tumor: Tumor resection follows strictly the principles of oncologic surgery. Avoiding local recurrence is the criterion of success and the main determinant of how much bone and soft tissue are to be removed.
2. Skeletal reconstruction: The average skeletal defect following adequate bone tumor resection measures 15 to 20 cm. Techniques of reconstruction vary and are independent of the resection, although the degree of resection may favor one technique over another.
3. Soft tissue and muscle transfers: Muscle transfers are performed to cover and close the resection site and to restore motor power. Adequate skin and muscle coverage is mandatory. Distal tissue transfers are not used because of the possibility of contamination.

GUIDELINES FOR LIMB-SPARING RESECTION

The surgical guidelines and technique of limb-sparing surgery used by the senior author (MM) are as follows[134]:

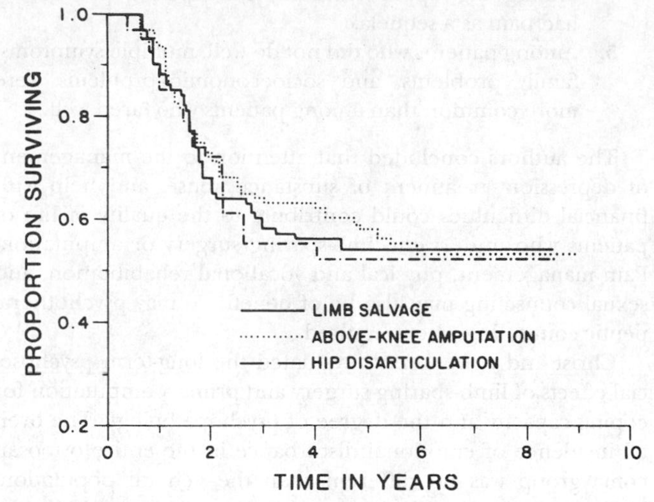

FIGURE 39.2-2. Patient survival after three different types of surgical procedures for osteosarcoma of the distal femur.

1. No major neurovascular tumor involvement
2. Wide resection of the affected bone, with a normal muscle cuff in all directions
3. *En bloc* removal of all previous biopsy sites and potentially contaminated tissue
4. Resection of bone 3 to 4 cm beyond abnormal uptake, as determined by CT or MRI and bone scan
5. Resection of the adjacent joint and capsule
6. Adequate motor reconstruction, accomplished by regional muscle transfers
7. Adequate soft tissue coverage

TYPES OF SKELETAL RECONSTRUCTION

Large skeletal defects are reconstructed after tumor resection by several different modalities. Osteoarticular defects are most often reconstructed by segmental, custom prostheses that are fixed to the remaining intramedullary bone by PMMA (Fig. 39.2-3). The newer knee prostheses allow some rotation as well as flexion and extension, this mobility decreases the forces on the bone-cement interface and thus reduces the risk of loosening.

There has been increasing interest in applying a porous coating to the prosthesis in the hope of obtaining long-term, perhaps even permanent, fixation.[38,136–138] In addition, titanium, a new alloy with superior metallurgical properties, has been introduced. Modular endoprosthetic replacement systems that can be assembled in the operating room are now available and avoid the problem of long delays for custom manufacturing.[38,136] Alternative methods of segmental replacement include large autografts or allografts, used to obtain an arthrodesis, or osteoarticular allografts that may replace the affected joint.[34,136,138,139] Composite allograft (i.e., allograft placed over a prosthesis) has been used. In general, allografts have been used successfully for low-grade sarcomas and for GCTs of bone that do not require chemotherapy or radiotherapy.

Today, most surgeons prefer endoprosthetic replacements. The modular replacement systems can replace the most commonly affected bones: the proximal femur, proximal humerus, distal femur, and proximal tibia.

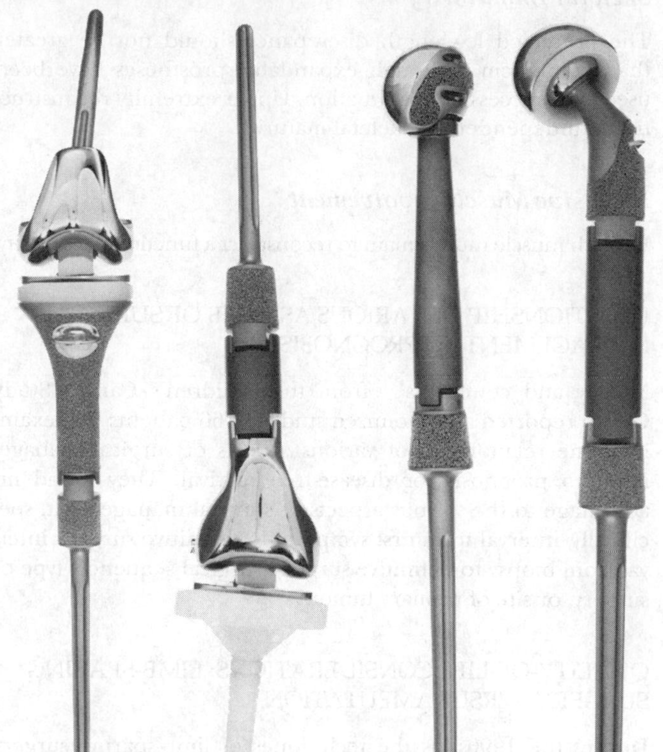

FIGURE 39.2-3. Prostheses used in selected patients for skeletal reconstruction: distal femoral prosthesis **(A)**, proximal tibial prosthesis **(B)**, proximal humeral prosthesis **(C)**, proximal femoral prosthesis **(D)**.

CONTRAINDICATIONS TO LIMB-SPARING SURGERY

Major Neurovascular Involvement

Although vascular grafts may be used, the adjacent nerves are usually at risk, making successful resection less likely. In addition, the magnitude of resection in combination with vascular reconstruction is often prohibitive.

Pathologic Fractures

A fracture through a bone affected by a tumor spreads tumor cells via the hematoma beyond accurately determined limits. The risk of local recurrence increases under such circumstances. If a pathologic fracture heals after neoadjuvant chemotherapy, a limb-salvage procedure may be performed successfully.[140]

Inappropriate Biopsy Sites

An inappropriate or poorly planned biopsy jeopardizes local tumor control by contaminating normal tissue planes and compartments.

Infection

The risk of infection after implantation of a metallic device or an allograft in an infected area is prohibitive. Sepsis jeopardizes the effectiveness of adjuvant chemotherapy.

Skeletal Immaturity

The predicted leg-length discrepancy should not be greater than 6 to 8 cm, although expandable prostheses have been used with success in this situation. Upper extremity reconstruction is independent of skeletal maturity.

Extensive Muscle Involvement

Enough muscle must remain to reconstruct a functional extremity.

RELATIONSHIP OF VARIOUS ASPECTS OF SURGICAL MANAGEMENT TO PROGNOSIS

Makley and coworkers[141] from the Children's Cancer Study Group reported a randomized study of 166 patients that examined the relationship of various aspects of surgical management to prognosis for disease-free survival. They found no advantage to the various aspects of surgical management, specifically, interval from first symptom to definitive surgery, interval from biopsy to definitive surgery, surgical sequence, type of surgery, or site of primary tumor.

QUALITY-OF-LIFE CONSIDERATIONS: LIMB-SPARING SURGERY VERSUS AMPUTATION

During the 1990s, as the techniques of limb-sparing surgery were being developed, it had been assumed that such surgery was superior to amputation. Nonetheless, when complications occurred, many surgeons thought that an amputation might have been preferable. Despite the extensive literature on the various chemotherapy regimens, surgical techniques, and limb-sparing surgery, few studies have focused on the patients' evaluation of their overall quality of life.[142–144] Two studies that have been published are described here.

Greenberg[143] from Massachusetts General Hospital and the Children's Hospital/Dana Farber Cancer Center evaluated 62 osteosarcoma survivors at a mean of 12 years from diagnosis. Of 89 survivors contacted, 62 patients (42 women and 20 men) agreed to be interviewed. These patients responded to a comprehensive battery of psychological questions. In general, most survivors were in good mental and physical health. The results are summarized as follows:

1. The reported rates of psychopathology among amputees and those undergoing limb-sparing surgery did not differ significantly.
2. Fertility was not a problem. Twenty-three normal progeny were born after chemotherapy to eight women and the wives of five men. Only two women were considered infertile; both had undergone radiation therapy associated with other childhood cancers.
3. All responders who had undergone limb-sparing surgery believed the effort to save their limb was worthwhile. Twenty patients rated the effort of limb-salvage very worthwhile, (mean 4.5 out of 5). Those whom the attempt at limb-salvage failed rated the effort as 4.0 (not significantly different than the successful group). Those patients who were less satisfied with surgery had secondary amputations.
4. Pain was usually minimal, but when present, was associated only with lower extremity amputation. The pain pattern suggested deafferentation syndromes. No patients undergoing upper extremity limb-sparing procedures had pain as a sequela.
5. Among patients who did not do well, multiple symptoms, family problems, and socioeconomic problems were more common than among patients who fared well.

The authors concluded that attention to the management of depression, treatment of substance abuse, and help with financial difficulties could contribute to the quality of life of patients who underwent limb-sparing surgery or amputation. Pain management, physical and vocational rehabilitation, and sexual counseling may also be of benefit, as may psychotherapeutic counseling when required.

Christ and coworkers[144] evaluated the long-term psychosocial effects of limb-sparing surgery and primary amputation for coping capacity and the degree of psychopathology. The overall incidence of emotional disturbance in the entire osteosarcoma group was no different than the general population. Unlike patients in other studies, those in the group with initial amputations had substantial difficulty maintaining an optimal functioning level. Their difficulty was even greater than that of limb-salvage patients with a compromised outcome, including those with late amputation. Specifically:

1. An amputee was significantly less likely to have married than a limb-spared patient.
2. Coping mechanisms of those with primary amputations were less effective than those patients in the limb-salvage group. This deficit was still evident several years after surgery.
3. Patients who had limb-salvage without later complications were very pleased with their outcome.
4. Good work experience was an important compensation for physical loss.
5. Male dependency needs were often underestimated. Some men were left to manage their own adaptation tasks, whereas for females the opposite was true. Female patients tended to become excessively dependent.
6. Patients reported no difficulty in enjoying sexual activity. The first postsurgical sexual experience was described as no more traumatic than the first experience that required showing the leg (e.g., swimming).

Despite good social support scores, the amputees had higher psychopathology scores than patients who had undergone limb-sparing procedures. The authors concluded that patients undergoing primary amputation need more intensive support than those whose limbs are spared. They recommend an overall approach similar to that for posttraumatic stress disorder.

AMPUTATIONS

An amputation provides definitive surgical treatment in patients in whom a limb-sparing resection is not a prudent option. A significant number of patients still require amputation, despite the advent of limb-sparing surgery. In contrast to amputations performed for noncancer causes, those for cancer tend to be at a more proximal anatomic level, to occur in younger people (reflecting the incidence of bone sarcomas[145]), and to be technically more difficult.[145] The resultant psychological and cosmetic losses are also more substantial. The amputation experience of the National Cancer Institute since the 1960s has been reviewed; 89% of these procedures were done for sarcomas.[145] Fifty-five percent of the lower extremity amputations were either hip disarticulations or hemipelvectomies. One-half of the upper extremity amputations were interscapulothoracic (forequarter) resections. Osteosarcoma accounted for one-third of all amputations. Large lesions around the pelvis or proximal femur still generally require an amputation, whereas most sarcomas of the shoulder girdle and knee can now be resected. Amputation techniques are well described in the literature.

CRYOSURGERY

Cryosurgery is the use of liquid nitrogen (temperature, –196°C) after curettage of a tumor cavity to kill the remaining tumor cells.[130–132] Necrosis has been shown to occur between –20° and –40°C.[145] In general, a double freeze-thaw cycle is required. The aim of this technique is to enhance local tumor control after a careful curettage and thus avoid resection of the involved bone. Cryosurgery was initially developed by Marcove and colleagues[130,132] at Memorial Hospital for treatment of metastatic bone tumors. They have applied this technique to the treatment of aggressive benign tumors, specifically GCTs, and more recently to low-grade sarcomas as well as chordomas. The local recurrence rate after cryosurgery for these aggressive benign tumors has decreased from more than 30% to 40% to between 5% and 10%.[130–132] This technique is not used for high-grade sarcomas.

CHEMOTHERAPY FOR BONE SARCOMAS

Before the advent of effective adjuvant chemotherapy, the outlook for patients with osteosarcoma was dismal. The overwhelming majority of patients who presented without evidence of metastases and were treated only with surgery ultimately developed metastases and died.[72,146–149] A review of the literature published in 1972 summarized experience with 1337 patients in 11 studies conducted between 1946 and 1971.[149] Approximately one-half of these patients developed metastatic disease—virtually always in the lung—within 6 months after surgery of the primary tumor, and more than 80% developed recurrent disease. Fewer than 20% of the patients survived 5 years. The inescapable conclusion from these studies is that 80% of patients presenting without overt metastases had microscopic subclinical metastases at the time of diagnosis. Thus, the expectation that fewer than 20% of patients would survive beyond 5 years appeared to be reasonable; this expectation served as the background for trials of adjuvant chemotherapy conducted in the 1970s and 1980s. By the late 1970s, the prognosis for patients with osteosarcoma was improving, largely due to the beneficial effects of adjuvant chemotherapy. However, investigators from the Mayo Clinic and elsewhere challenged the apparent contribution of adjuvant chemotherapy, reporting that the patients' prognoses, with or without adjuvant therapy, had apparently improved over time.[150–156]

Two randomized, controlled trials were conducted in the mid-1980s by investigators of the Multi-Institutional Osteosarcoma Study and from the University of California, Los Angeles to resolve the controversy over the role of adjuvant chemotherapy in osteosarcoma. Both studies included a control group treated only with surgery of the primary tumor and no postsurgical adjuvant chemotherapy. Preliminary and mature results of these studies[157–160] confirm the favorable impact of adjuvant chemotherapy in the treatment of osteosarcoma. Furthermore, life tables of event-free survival for patients in the control groups of these studies recapitulated the historical experience *before* 1970. Results of these trials confirm that the natural history of osteosarcoma has not changed since the 1970s; fewer than 20% of patients treated only with surgery of the primary tumor can be expected to survive relapse-free. The bleak historical experience that served as the background for many uncontrolled adjuvant trials in the 1970s appears to be equally valid as a control for studies in the 1980s, 1990s, and beyond. Microscopic, subclinical metastatic disease can be presumed to exist in virtually all patients at the time of diagnosis. Although the more favorable results from the Mayo Clinic for patients treated without adjuvant chemotherapy remain unexplained, it is apparent from the Multi-Institutional Osteosarcoma Study and University of California, Los Angeles studies that adjuvant chemotherapy has a significant favorable influence on outcome and should, therefore, be recommended for all patients with osteosarcoma.

ADJUVANT CHEMOTHERAPY

The rationale for adjuvant chemotherapy of osteosarcoma is derived from experimental evidence that microscopic metastatic disease can be eradicated if the treatment is initiated when the total body burden of metastatic tumor is sufficiently low.[161–163] The strategy of adjuvant chemotherapy after surgical removal of the primary tumor has been applied successfully in the management of other childhood tumors. However, osteosarcoma is a relatively drug-resistant neoplasm, and results of studies of the activity of single agents and drugs in combination against macroscopic osteosarcoma have been disappointing. Few drugs have produced responses in more than 15% of patients, and most responses are partial. Notable exceptions are the responses observed in trials of doxyrubicin,[164] cisplatin,[165–168] high-dose methotrexate (HDMTX) with leucovorin rescue[169–171] and, more recently, ifosfamide.[172] Logic dictates that the application of agents with only modest activity against macroscopic osteosarcoma should not influence the natural history of this disease. Experimental evidence, however, suggests that eradication of microscopic metastases is possible, even with drugs that are marginally effective or even ineffective against gross macroscopic tumors.[161–163,173]

The hopeless prognosis for patients with osteosarcoma led to the enthusiastic application of the available agents, singly or in combination, as adjuvant therapy for patients with nonmetastatic osteosarcoma. An apparent improvement in outcome compared with the historical experience without chemotherapy was demonstrated in a number of these trials. Results of some of the important adjuvant chemotherapy trials of the 1970s and early 1980s are summarized in Table 39.2-6. Concerns have been raised that adjuvant chemotherapy for osteosarcoma may delay, but not prevent, relapse. However, the results of many of the adjuvant studies reported in Table 39.2-6,

TABLE 39.2-6. Reported Results of Representative Trials of Adjuvant Therapy for Osteosarcoma

Adjuvant Regimen	*Investigators*	*Number of Patients*	*% Relapse-Free*	*References*
HDMTX, VCR (Study I)	DFCI	12	42	280,388
HDMTX, VCR ± BCG[a]	NCI	39	38	389
DOX	CALGB	88	39	49,53
DOX ± HDMTX[a]	CALGB	62	50	390
DOX + VCR + HDMTX (Study II)	DFCI	22	59	280
DOX + VCR + HDMTX (weekly) (Study III)	DFCI	46	60	96,280
DOX + VCR + (HDMTX vs. IDMTX)[a]	CCG	166	38	391–393
COMPADRI I (CTX, VCR, DOX, PAM)	SWOG	43	49	392,393
COMPADRI II (CTX, VCR, DOX, PAM, HDMTX)	SWOG	53	35	392,393
COMPADRI III (CTX, VCR, DOX, PAM, HDMTX)	SWOG	84	38	393
DOX + HDMTX + CTX (OSTEO 72)	St. Jude	26	50	395
DOX + HDMTX + CTX (OSTEO 77)	St. Jude	50	56	395
DOX + CDDP	Roswell Park	22	61	97,396
HDMTX + VCR vs. no adjuvant therapy[b]	Mayo Clinic	38	40 (chemotherapy) 44 (no chemotherapy)	156
BCD + HDMTX + DOX + CDDP vs. no adjuvant therapy[c]	MIOS	36 randomized 165 nonrandomized	63 (chemotherapy) 12 (no chemotherapy)	157–159
BCD + HDMTX + VCR + DOX (+ intraarterial DOX + XRT) vs. no adjuvant therapy[c]	UCLA	59	55 (chemotherapy) 20 (no chemotherapy)	92
Whole lung irradiation vs. no adjuvant treatment[d]	EORTC	86	43 (with treatment) 28 (no treatment)	155,394
Whole lung irradiation (+ dactinomycin) vs. no adjuvant treatment[a]	Mayo Clinic	53	40	154
HDMTX + VCR + DOX + CTX (T4 + T5 pooled)	MSKCC	52 (<21 y)	48	50,54,98

BCD, bleomycin, cyclophosphamide, and dactinomycin; BCG, Calmette-Guérin bacillus; CALGB, Cancer and Acute Leukemia Group B; CCG, Children's Cancer Group; CDDP, cisplatin; CTX, Cytoxan (cyclophosphamide); DFCI, Dana-Farber Cancer Institute; DOX, doxorubicin; EORTC, European Organization for Research and Treatment of Cancer; HDMTX, high-dose methotrexate (5 g/m^2 or more) + leucovorin rescue; IDMTX, intermediate-dose methotrexate (750 mg/m^2) + leucovorin rescue; MIOS, Multi-Institutional Osteosarcoma Study; MSKCC, Memorial Sloan-Kettering Cancer Center; NCI, National Cancer Institute; OSTEO, osteosarcoma protocol; PAM, phenylalanine mustard; SWOG, Southwest Oncology Group; UCLA, University of California, Los Angeles; VCR, vincristine; XRT, radiation therapy.

[a]Randomized study; no significant difference in relapse-free survival for patients on each treatment arm of study.

[b]Randomized study; no significant difference in relapse-free survival for patients receiving and not receiving adjuvant HDMTX (see text).

[c]Randomized study; difference in results of treatments highly significant (P>.01) (see text).

[d]Randomized study; difference in results of treatments significant at 6% level.

and more recent trials that include presurgical chemotherapy (Table 39.2-7), some with follow-up beyond 10 years, suggest that life tables of event-free survival have stable plateaus beyond 4 years and that relapses after 3 years are infrequent. The majority of patients surviving 3 years without evidence of recurrence are probably cured.

Examination of the results of chemotherapy trials (see Tables 39.2-6 and 39.2-7) reveals a trend in the direction of improved outcomes for patients treated on more recent, more intensive chemotherapy regimens. Considering that so few drugs have demonstrable activity against macroscopic osteosarcoma, the results reported in adjuvant trials are remarkable. Approximately 60% to 70% of patients with osteosarcoma treated with modern intensive adjuvant chemotherapy regimens survive without recurrence. The development of adjuvant regimens has been largely empirical, and newer, more intensive regimens have resulted in further improvements in outcome. The majority of regimens currently in use incorporate doxorubicin, cisplatin, and HDMTX. The effectiveness of HDMTX in the adjuvant treatment of osteosarcoma has not been universally accepted;[174] reported response rates against macroscopic disease have varied widely, ranging from no response to 80%.[169–171,174,175]

Furthermore, a randomized study conducted by the Children's Cancer Group (CCG)[176] comparing HDMTX and intermediate-dose methotrexate in combination with doxorubicin adjuvant therapy did not show any benefit for patients receiving HDMTX. The overall outcome was not better than that achieved in studies using doxorubicin alone. In contrast, a more recent study from the Instituto Orthopedico Rizzoli[177] demonstrated superior responses in the primary tumor as well as a superior outcome for patients receiving HDMTX as compared with intermediate-dose methotrexate in the context of a multiagent chemotherapy regimen. A trial conducted by the European Osteosarcoma Intergroup compared the combination of doxorubicin and cisplatin alone, or doxorubicin and cisplatin alternating with HDMTX as pre- and postsurgical chemotherapy for patients with osteosarcoma.[178] The disease-free survival for patients receiving the two-drug regimen (without HDMTX) was significantly superior to that of patients treated with all three drugs. However, the intensity of administration of HDMTX was compromised by the design of the study, and the overall outcome of patients in this report is inferior to that observed in other studies.

The role of HDMTX in chemotherapy of osteosarcoma requires further investigation. The effectiveness of this drug

TABLE 39.2-7. Reported Results of Representative Trials Incorporating Presurgical Chemotherapy for Osteosarcoma

Regimen	*Investigators*	*Number of Patients*	*% Relapse-Free*	*References*
HDMTX + VCR + DOX + BCD (T-7 regimen)	MSKCC	54 (younger than 21 y)	74	50,98,199
HDMTX + VCR + DOX + BCD ± CDDP (depending on response) (T-10 regimen)	MSKCC	79 (younger than 21 y)	76	51,98,199
DOX + HDMTX + (BCD or CDDP) ± interferon (COSS 80)[a]	GPO	116	68	99,190
HDMTX + DOX + CDDP	Mount Sinai	25	77	397
HDMTX + VCR + DOX + BCD ± CDDP (depending on response) (CCG-782)	CCG	231	56	192
HDMTX + DOX + CDDP + IFOS (COSS 82)	GPO	125	58	100
DOX + CDDP ± HDMTX[b]	EOIS	231	63 (– HDMTX) 48 (+ HDMTX)	178
IA CDDP + (HDMTX vs. IDMTX) + DOX ± BCD (depending on response)[c]	Instituto Ortopedico Rizzoli	127	51 (overall) 58 (HDMTX) 42 (IDMTX)	177
HDMTX + DOX + IA CDDP ± etoposide, IFOS (postoperative therapy determined based on response to preoperative therapy)	Instituto Ortopedico Rizzoli	164	63	398
(IA CDDP vs. HDMTX) + DOX (postoperative therapy determined based on response to preoperative therapy) (TIOS I)	M. D. Anderson Cancer Center	43	60	193
IA CDDP + DOX ± CTX (depending on response) (TIOS III)	M. D. Anderson Cancer Center	24	—	—
HDMTX + DOX + IFOS ± CDDP	CCG (selected investigators)	95	82	—
HDMTX + DOX + CDDP BCD (POG 8651)[a]	POG	100	70 (presurgical chemotherapy) 73 (immediate surgery)	—
HDMTX + VCR + DOX + BCD + CDDP vs. DOX + CDDP	EOI	391	44	186
HDMTX + BCD + DOX + CDDP (T-12 regimen)	MSKCC	61	76	204
HDMTX + DOX + CDDP ± IFOS ± MTP-PE[d]	CCG and POG	679	67	—

BCD, bleomycin, cyclophosphamide, and dactinomycin; CCG, Children's Cancer Group; CDDP, cisplatin; COSS, Germany-Austria-Swiss Cooperative Osteosarcoma Study; CTX, cyclophosphamide; DOX, doxorubicin; EOI, European Osteosarcoma Intergroup; EOIS, First European Osteosarcoma Intergroup Study; GPO, German Society for Pediatric Oncology; HDMTX, high-dose methotrexate (12 g/m^2 or more) + leucovorin rescue; IA, intraarterial administration; IDMTX, intermediate-dose methotrexate (750 mg/m^2) + leucovorin rescue; IFOS, ifosfamide; MTP-PE, muramyltripeptide phosphatidylethanolamine; MSKCC, Memorial Sloan-Kettering Cancer Center; POG, Pediatric Oncology Group; TIOS, Treatment and Investigation Osteosarcoma Study; VCR, vincristine.

[a]Randomized study; no significant difference in relapse-free survival for patients on each treatment arm of study.

[b]Randomized study; favors treatment without HDMTX (some patients treated only adjuvantly).

[c]Randomized study; difference in results of treatment significant at 7% level.

[d]Randomized study; analysis of results by randomized treatment not yet available.

may be dose-dependent,[179] because dose escalation has produced responses in patients found previously to be unresponsive to treatment.[180] A steep dose-response relationship may also pertain to Adriamycin.[49,163,181] The BCD combination (bleomycin, cyclophosphamide, and dactinomycin) also is used in some regimens,[182] although its effectiveness has been disputed[183] and few modern regimens incorporate it. Carboplatin is an attractive agent to use in place of cisplatin because of possible reduced renal and ototoxicity. However, this analogue may be considerably less active against osteosarcoma than cisplatin,[184] and it cannot yet be recommended.

The optimal chemotherapy regimen for treatment of osteosarcoma continues to be the subject of investigation and heated debate. Although most investigators use intensive, multiagent regimens, the superiority of such regimens as compared to simpler, shorter, less intensive multiagent regimens has been questioned. A large, randomized study conducted by the European Osteosarcoma Intergroup[185] compared the efficacy of six cycles of doxorubicin and cisplatin with the more complicated, more toxic multiagent T-10 regimen pioneered at the Memorial Sloan-Kettering Cancer Center (Fig. 39.2-4). No differences in progression-free (47% at 3 years and 44% at 5 years) and overall survival (65% at 3 years and 55% at 5 years) were detected between the treatment groups, although these results are unsatisfactory when compared with the outcomes achieved on other studies conducted in North America and Europe. Thus, whether any regimen is superior to six cycles of doxorubicin and cisplatin remains an open question.

Further improvements in outcomes for patients with osteosarcoma will likely result from the development of new active agents. The activity of ifosfamide against macroscopic disease has been demonstrated, and this drug has been incor-

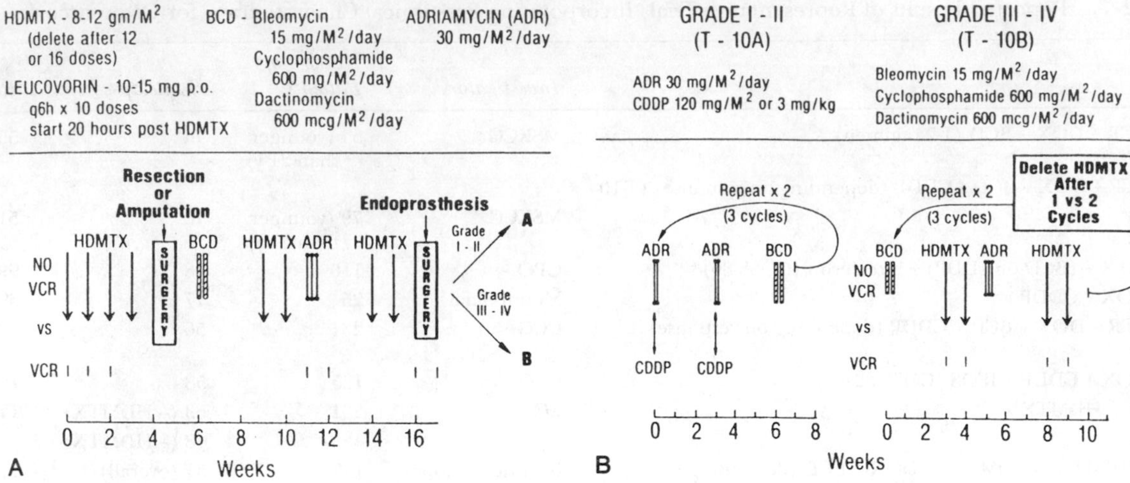

FIGURE 39.2-4. The T-10 regimen from Memorial Sloan-Kettering Cancer Center. **A:** All patients receive the initial 16-week regimen. The presurgical chemotherapy regimen features four weekly courses of high-dose methotrexate (HDMTX) and leucovorin rescue followed by resection or amputation. Patients undergoing endoprosthetic replacement receive 16 weeks of presurgical chemotherapy. **B:** Postoperative chemotherapy is determined by the histologic grade of response of the primary tumor to presurgical chemotherapy. Patients who achieve an unfavorable response in the primary tumor (grades I and II) receive a T-10A regimen postoperatively, featuring doxorubicin, cisplatin (CDDP), and the BCD combination. Patients achieving a favorable response (grades III and IV) receive the T-10B regimen postoperatively and continue to receive HDMTX with doxorubicin and the BCD combination. VCR, vincristine. (From ref. 98, with permission.)

porated into newer regimens under study with promising results.[186,187] The role of ifosfamide in the presurgical and adjuvant settings was addressed specifically in a randomized trial conducted by the American Pediatric Cooperative Oncology Groups. Overall, the projected event-free survival at 3 years is 66% (P. Meyers, personal communication, 1999), but the data are immature, and results pertaining to the contribution of ifosfamide have not yet been analyzed.

PRESURGICAL CHEMOTHERAPY

Presurgical chemotherapy has been used with increasing frequency in the management of osteosarcoma. This strategy evolved concurrently with limb-sparing procedures. Initial attempts at limb salvage at the Memorial Sloan-Kettering Cancer Center in 1973 involved the fabrication of customized endoprostheses for select patients undergoing *en bloc* resection. While the prosthesis was being made (a process requiring up to 3 months), chemotherapy was administered to prevent tumor progression.[54] Retrospectively, it appeared that patients treated with presurgical chemotherapy fared better than did patients treated during the same period with immediate surgery and postoperative adjuvant therapy.[50]

In studies from the Memorial Sloan-Kettering Cancer Center, responsiveness of the primary tumor to preoperative chemotherapy, assessed by histologic evaluation, was found to be a powerful prognostic factor; unfavorable responders were likely to develop distant metastases despite continued use of chemotherapy with the same agents after surgery.[188] The prognostic significance of tumor response to preoperative chemotherapy has been confirmed in multiple studies,[177,189–193] and tumor responsiveness has emerged as one of the most powerful prognostic factors in patients with nonmetastatic extremity osteosarcoma.[194]

Although the initial impetus for presurgical chemotherapy was limb salvage, several theoretical advantages of presurgical chemotherapy apply to all patients with osteosarcoma[50] (Table 39.2-8). Because chemotherapy is administered very soon after biopsy and diagnosis, treatment of the micrometastases known to be present in the majority of patients can be instituted early. This offers a substantial advantage over the traditional adjuvant approach, in which the administration of systemic chemotherapy is delayed by 1 month or more for surgery and wound healing. Earlier administration of systemic treatment may reduce the emergence of drug-resistant cells in the micrometastases.[195,196] For the surgeon, presurgical chemotherapy offers some advantages, because it allows time for fabrication of prostheses and may effect a reduction of bulky tumors, thereby increasing the feasibility of limb-salvage surgery in selected patients.

ASSESSMENT OF TUMOR RESPONSE

Assessment of the response of primary tumors has been based on clinical and radiographic data (see Restaging after Preoperative Chemotherapy, earlier in this chapter); however, the histologic appearance of the resected tumor specimen after presurgical chemotherapy has emerged as the standard for measuring response.[98,188,192,197,198] Several systems for grading the effect of preoperative chemotherapy have been proposed, all of which are based on the degree of cellularity and necrosis in the resected specimen. Grading systems are necessarily imprecise and subject to sampling errors; however, with scrupulous attention to adequate sectioning from many sites of the surgical specimen, the degree of response can be reliably and reproducibly assessed. The grading system designed at Memorial Sloan-Kettering Cancer Center by Huvos and colleagues[98,188] has been used

TABLE 39.2-8. Considerations for Presurgical and Postsurgical Chemotherapy

Timing of Chemotherapy	*Advantages*	*Disadvantages*
Preoperative	Early institution of systemic therapy against micrometastases	High tumor burden (not optimal for first-order kinetics)
	Reduced chance of spontaneous emergence of drug-resistant clones in micrometastases	Increased probability in the selection of drug-resistant cells in primary tumor, which may metastasize
	Reduction in tumor size, increasing the change of limb salvage	Delay in definitive control of bulk disease; increased chance for systemic dissemination
	Provides time for fabrication of customized endoprosthesis	—
	Less chance of viable tumor being spread at the time of surgery	Psychological trauma of retaining tumor
	Individual response to chemotherapy allows selection of different risk groups	Risk of local tumor progression with loss of a limb-sparing option
Postsurgical	Radical removal of bulk tumor decreases tumor burden and increases growth rate of residual disease, making S phase–specific agents more active and optimizing conditions for first-order kinetics	Delay of systemic therapy for micrometastases
	—	No preoperative *in vivo* assay of cytotoxic response
	Decreased probability of selecting a drug-resistant clone in the primary tumor	Possible spread of viable tumor by surgical manipulation

widely (Table 39.2-9). Grade III and IV responses, indicating extensive to complete response in the primary tumor, are considered favorable. Grade I and II responses, indicating minimal destruction of the tumor, are unfavorable. In studies using the Huvos grading system, patients with favorable response (grade III or IV) fare extremely well, whereas those with an unfavorable histologic response to preoperative chemotherapy (grade I or II) are likely to develop distant metastases. Thus, patients at high risk for recurrent disease can apparently be identified early in treatment on the basis of poor response to presurgical chemotherapy. The Huvos grading system has served as a model for other systems for grading tumor response.

Although the predictive value of tumor response to presurgical chemotherapy is now indisputable, a number of problems have surfaced in the application of such response grading to patient management. Different criteria for the definition of favorable and unfavorable response are used in different grading systems, making comparisons among studies difficult. The grading system formerly used by the German Society of Pediatric Oncology (GPO) identifies six categories of response.[197] In the Germany-Austria-Swiss Coooperative Osteosarcoma Study (COSS 80) study conducted by the GPO, favorable response was defined as more than 50% tumor destruction after presurgical chemotherapy; however, in more recent GPO studies,

TABLE 39.2-9. Histologic Grading of the Effect of Preoperative Chemotherapy on Primary Osteosarcoma

Grade	*Effect*
I	Little or no effect identified
II	Area of acellular tumor osteoid, necrotic, or fibrotic material attributable to the effect of chemotherapy, with other areas of histologically viable tumor
III	Predominant areas of acellular tumor osteoid, necrotic, or fibrotic material attributable to the effect of chemotherapy with only scattered foci of histologically viable tumor cells identified
IV	No histologic evidence of viable tumor identified within the entire specimen

(From ref. 98, with permission.)

90% destruction is required. The grading system favored by investigators at the M. D. Anderson Cancer Center divides response into three categories: (1) no effect or doubtful effect with less than 40% tumor destruction; (2) partial effect with 40% to 60% tumor destruction; and (3) definite effect, in which more than 60% of the tumor is destroyed and fibrovascular regeneration is present.[198]

Of particular concern is that an update of the Memorial Sloan-Kettering experience with presurgical chemotherapy suggests that a modification of the Huvos system is in order because the implications of “favorable” and “unfavorable” response to presurgical chemotherapy have changed somewhat. It is apparent that grade IV response is predictive of favorable outcome; however, the outcome of patients with grade III response is not significantly superior to that of patients with grade II response.[199] Thus, only patients who experience a grade IV response to presurgical chemotherapy might be considered as being in the most favorable prognostic group.

Perhaps most problematic are the differences among studies conducted to date in the timing of surgery relative to the initiation of chemotherapy, and especially the variable duration of exposure to chemotherapy *before* definitive surgery and histologic evaluation of the response of the primary tumor. It appears that presurgical chemotherapy regimens of longer duration are associated with a higher proportion of “favorable” responders.[199,200] However, as the duration of presurgical chemotherapy increases, the predictive value of response for outcome may be lost; longer, more intensive presurgical regimens may achieve a greater proportion of favorable responders, but the favorable responses achieved with such regimens may not translate into more favorable outcomes. An analysis from the Memorial Sloan-Kettering Cancer Center suggests that this is indeed the case.[199]

TAILORING THERAPY

One of the most compelling rationales for presurgical chemotherapy is its use as an *in vivo* drug trial to determine the sensitivity of an individual tumor and to customize postoperative chemotherapy. As noted above, results of studies from the Memorial Sloan-Kettering Cancer Center and elsewhere suggest that patients whose tumors are responsive to presurgical therapy are destined to do well when the same therapy is continued postoperatively. Patients whose tumors are unresponsive to the presurgical regimen have a much less favorable outlook and might benefit from a change in chemotherapeutic agents. This strategy was pioneered at Memorial Sloan-Kettering in the T-10 protocol[51,98] (see Fig. 39.2-4*A*). Patients were treated preoperatively with HDMTX, the BCD combination, and doxorubicin. Those with favorable (grades III and IV) histologic responses continued to receive the same agents postoperatively (T-10B regimen). Patients demonstrating unfavorable (grades I and II) histologic responses were treated on regimen T-10A, consisting of doxorubicin and cisplatin along with the BCD combination (without HDMTX) postoperatively (see Fig. 39.2-4*B*). Although only 39% of patients achieved a favorable histologic response to presurgical chemotherapy (51% if only patients younger than 21 years were analyzed), virtually all of the favorable responders were projected to survive free of recurrence.[51,98] The patients whose primary tumors demonstrated an unfavorable histologic response were switched to the cisplatin-containing regimen, and almost 85% were initially projected to remain relapse-free at 3 years. Overall, in preliminary reports, 90% of patients treated on the T-10 regimen with tailored therapy were projected to remain disease-free at 3 years. Moreover, a significant difference in outcome could no longer be detected between those who did and did not respond to presurgical chemotherapy, supporting the contention that poor responders were "salvaged" by the administration of alternative chemotherapy postoperatively. Because of these very favorable preliminary results, the T-10 protocol served as a model for many of the osteosarcoma treatment studies launched in the 1980s and 1990s, virtually all of which featured presurgical chemotherapy and tailoring of treatment on the basis of responsiveness of the primary tumor.

NEOADJUVANT CHEMOTHERAPY

Results reported from representative trials using presurgical chemotherapy are summarized in Table 39.2-7. Responses in the primary tumor have been variable, with favorable responses observed in 30% to 85% of patients. The overall results are excellent but are comparable to adjuvant studies that used regimens of equal intensity without any preoperative chemotherapy (see Table 39.2-6). Furthermore, the importance of custom tailoring of therapy in this strategy remains to be defined. Several trials are pertinent in this regard. The CCG attempted to duplicate the T-10 regimen in a multiinstitutional setting (CCG 782).[192] Results were not as favorable as those initially reported from Memorial Sloan-Kettering Cancer Center; only 28% of the patients demonstrated favorable responses in the primary tumor. These patients fared extremely well (projected 5-year event-free survival, 87%). The remaining poor-responding patients did not benefit from a change in therapy postoperatively and had a less favorable outcome (projected 5-year event-free survival, 49%). Overall, only 56% of patients in the CCG study were projected to remain free of recurrent disease at 5 years—a disappointing result when compared with the initial results reported from Memorial Sloan-Kettering. The COSS 82 trial of the GPO[191] also tested the strategy of tailoring treatment. As in the CCG trial, results suggest that patients demonstrating poor response of the primary tumor are destined to do poorly and that treatment of poor responders with "salvage regimens" (as in the T-10 protocol) does not improve their prognosis. Investigators of the GPO concluded that active agents should not be withheld from the initial therapy of newly diagnosed patients. At the Rizzoli Institute,[177,201] overall results have improved over time, concurrent with the adoption of the strategy of presurgical chemotherapy. However, the Rizzoli investigators conclude that the improvement in prognosis more likely reflects increased effectiveness of the agents used rather than the use of presurgical chemotherapy *per se*, because a group of patients treated concurrently at the same institution without the benefits of presurgical chemotherapy fared just as well as patients treated with presurgical chemotherapy.[201] As in most trials of presurgical chemotherapy, an early trial of presurgical chemotherapy reported from the Rizzoli Institute demonstrated that favorable responders had a better overall outcome; change in the postoperative chemotherapy for poor responders did not alter their unfavorable prognosis. However, in a more recent Rizzoli trial[202] conducted between 1986 and 1990, patients were treated initially with HDMTX, doxorubicin, and intraarterial cisplatin preoperatively. Favorable responders (more than 90% necrosis in their primary tumors) were treated postoperatively with 21 additional weeks of the same agents, whereas unfavorable responders received 30 weeks of chemotherapy, including ifosfamide and etoposide in addition to doxorubicin, cisplatin, and HDMTX. Seventy-one percent of patients in this study achieved a favorable response to presurgical chemotherapy, and 71% of these patients were projected to be disease-free survivors at 5 years. Of note, the poorly responding patients had a projected disease-free survival equal to that of good responders if only patients receiving adequate therapy were considered. This is one of the few studies in which the strategy of salvage chemotherapy for poorly responding patients has been shown to be of benefit.

Perhaps of greatest significance, an update of results of the Memorial Sloan-Kettering Cancer Center studies[199,203] indicates that the very promising preliminary results have eroded with further follow-up. Moreover, no difference in overall disease-free survival is apparent, regardless of whether patients received presurgical chemotherapy. Although histologic response to preoperative chemotherapy strongly predicted subsequent disease-free survival and overall survival, with longer follow-up the Memorial Sloan-Kettering investigators were unable to demonstrate an improvement in disease-free survival for poor responders who received a modification of their postoperative chemotherapy compared with a similar group of patients treated without such tailoring of treatment.[199] In support of these findings, members of the Pediatric Oncology Group reported preliminary results of a randomized trial designed to test the impact of presurgical chemotherapy on outcome of patients with extremity osteosarcoma.[204] The overall event-free survival was identical whether patients were treated with chemotherapy *before* definitive surgery of the primary tumor. Moreover, the overall results of this study were identical to those achieved in a predecessor study (Multi-Institutional Osteosarcoma Study) in which all patients were treated with immediate surgery followed by conventional adjuvant chemotherapy. Thus, it does not appear that the administration of presurgical chemotherapy (with or without individualizing of therapy based on tumor response) *per se* has led to an improvement in the outcome of children with osteosarcoma, at least in terms of rate of cure. Rather, improvements in outcome probably reflect the increasing intensity of the chemotherapy regimens used.

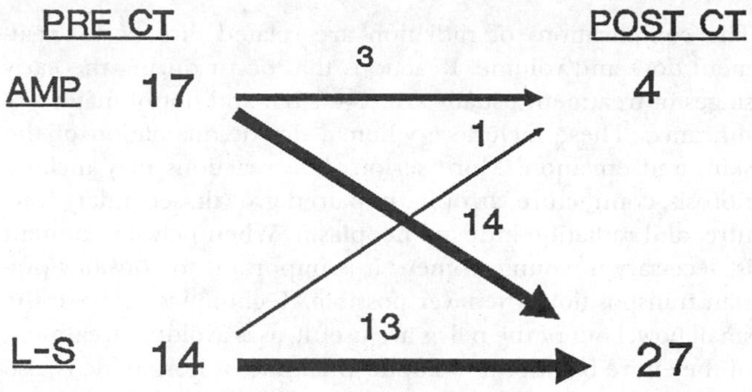

FIGURE 39.2-5. The impact of neoadjuvant chemotherapy on the choice of surgical procedure: surgical decisions made before receiving chemotherapy (PRE CT) compared with actual surgical procedure [amputation (AMP) vs. limb-sparing surgery (L-S)] performed after induction with intraarterial chemotherapy (POST CT). Initially, 17 of 31 patients (55%) would have required amputation, compared with only 4 of 31 amputations (13%) actually performed (limb salvage rate of 87%). Notice that 14 of 17 patients (82%) were converted from an amputative decision to a limb-sparing procedure. (From Malawer MM, Buch R, Reaman G, et al. Impact of two cycles of preoperative chemotherapy with intraarterial cisplatin and intravenous doxorubicin on the choice of surgical procedure for high-grade bone sarcomas of the extremities. *Clin Orthop* 1991:270:214, with permission.)

Although responsiveness of the primary tumor to presurgical chemotherapy is a powerful predictor of outcome, the likelihood that an individual patient will respond favorably cannot be predicted at the time of diagnosis. Because a majority of poor responders relapse and modifications of postsurgical chemotherapy do not have an impact on this unfavorable outcome, strategies are needed to predict favorably and poorly responding patients *before* the initiation of therapy, and markers that predict poor overall prognosis independent of response to chemotherapy, so that more aggressive approaches can be used for poor-prognosis patients earlier in treatment. Analysis of tumor DNA content,[205] tumor expression of P glycoprotein [product of the multidrug-resistant (MDR) gene[206]], and other resistance-related proteins[207]; expression of mutant p53[208]; and loss of heterozygosity of the retinoblastoma gene[209] in primary tumors before therapy have been examined as prognostic factors, but results have been inconclusive. Tumor expression of high levels of HER2/erbB-2 has been associated with unfavorable histologic response to chemotherapy and inferior event-free survival.[208,210] If confirmed, these findings suggest a possible intervention with anti-HER2 monoclonal antibodies (Herceptin) for patients whose tumors express high levels of this unfavorable molecular marker.

INTRAARTERIAL CHEMOTHERAPY

Presurgical chemotherapy may be administered directly into the arterial supply of the tumor to maximize drug delivery to the tumor vasculature (Fig. 39.2-5).[120,177,193,198,211] Doxorubicin and cisplatin, in particular, have been delivered by prolonged intraarterial infusion to the extremities, and high local drug concentrations have been achieved.[120] However, the rationale for the use of intraarterial therapy is not self-evident for several reasons. Even in the prechemotherapy era, control of the primary tumor in patients with extremity primaries was rarely a problem. Rather, micrometascopic disease present in the lung ultimately killed the patient. Improvements in the outcome of patients with osteosarcoma have resulted directly from improvements of systemic chemotherapy for micrometastatic disease rather than from better local control measures. Thus, strategies that improve drug delivery to the primary tumor at the expense of drug delivery to micrometastatic disease are counterintuitive. Little evidence suggests that responses to intraarterial administration of chemotherapy are superior to those seen with systemic intravenous administration of the same agents, nor has intraarterial chemotherapy improved the proportion of patients suitable for limb-sparing surgery. Finally, the administration of intraarterial chemotherapy in resectable osteosarcoma has waned, and the strategy cannot be recommended for most patients.

RADIOTHERAPY FOR BONE TUMORS

In keeping with the multidisciplinary, multimodality approach to the treatment of bone tumors, all patients should be evaluated by a radiation oncologist and by an orthopedic and medical (or pediatric) oncologist before decisions are made concerning therapy. Close communication between members of the care team is crucial. Tumors of the axial skeleton and facial bones are treated by a combination of limited surgery and radiotherapy. Ewing's sarcoma and peripheral primitive neuroectodermal tumors of bone may be managed by definitive radiation treatment, complete surgical excision, or combined surgical and radiotherapy approaches and are discussed in Chapter 39.1. In general, radiation therapy is not used in the primary treatment of osteosarcoma. Radiation therapy is used for patients who have refused definitive surgery, require palliation, or have lesions in axial locations.

TREATMENT PLANNING

Optimal radiotherapy of bone tumors requires careful planning (Table 39.2-10). Such planning begins with tumor localization and accurate definition of the clinical and radiographic extent of tumor as well as of all tissue at risk for microscopic involvement. Precise, three-dimensional definition is required. This evaluation is identical to that done for surgical evaluation (see Preoperative Evaluation, earlier in this chapter). Using these composite studies, the maximal tumor dimensions are established.

With the clinical physicist, decisions are then made concerning the optimal choice of radiation beam (e.g., photon, electron), technique (external beam, brachytherapy, intraop-

TABLE 39.2-10. Guidelines for Optimal Radiation Therapy in the Treatment of Bone Sarcomas

Tumor localization
Simulation
Patient immobilization
Megavoltage irradiation
High radiation dose
Large treatment fields, with use of shrinking and cone-downed fields
Beam-shaping devices
Beam modifiers—compensators, wedges
Multiple fields treated each day

erative therapy), beam modifiers (compensators, wedge filters), and immobilization system. All patients should undergo simulation and be treated with megavoltage therapy units. No role for orthovoltage (low-kilovoltage x-ray) exists in the management of primary tumors of bone.

Patient immobilization is essential to optimal radiotherapy. The patient should be placed in a comfortable position on the treatment table. The precise patient set-up should be planned using three points for reproducibility.[212] Immobilization devices, such as casts, shells, vacuum pillows, and sandbags, are frequently necessary.[213] Molding techniques that require a cast of the anatomic site to be treated are generally preferred when treatment fields are complex and the radiation course is lengthy.

DOSE AND VOLUME CONSIDERATIONS

Large treatment volumes that include the entire clinical and radiographic extent of tumor plus a generous margin for microscopic or subclinical extension of disease are needed. For tumors that tend to spread along the medullary canal (lymphoma, Ewing's sarcoma), the standard radiation field in the past included the entire bone, with a boost of radiation to the area of bulky disease. However, current practice suggests that radiation confined to the involved area may be sufficient for small round cell bone tumors that have responded to induction chemotherapy. If large fields are needed, it is desirable to use an extended source-to-skin distance to enable the entire radiation field to fit into one portal. If extended distances are not possible and two radiation fields must abut, the abutment must pass through areas of microscopic, rather than gross, disease. Match lines should be routinely moved every 10 Gy.

The irradiated field should encompass at least the volume of tissue that would be resected, plus an allowance of approximately 2 cm for patient movement and dose fall-off at the margin of the field. Extremity fields should be planned with a strip of tissue deliberately out of the beam to allow for lymphatic and venous return and to decrease morbidity. This nonirradiated strip should overlie the lymphatic drainage, which is located medially in the extremity.

Because large doses often are necessary for treatment of malignant bone tumors, a shrinking field technique is recommended, which allows treatment to a large volume of tissue involved by subclinical disease with a moderate radiation dosage, whereas the area of gross tumor is treated with a larger, sterilizing dose.

Additional principles involve using multiple beam-shaping devices so that shaped fields can be designed to conform to individual tumor volume and anatomy. Multiple fields should be used to optimize the radiation dosage, and all fields must be treated every day. Beam modifiers, including compensating filters and wedge filters, should be used to account for individual variations in patient thickness. Three-dimensional conformal radiation techniques using multiple fields, multileaf collimation, and intensity-modulated beams are useful aids to optimize the homogeneity of the dose within the target volume while sparing adjacent, critical normal structures. When chemotherapy, such as Adriamycin and dactinomycin, and radiotherapy are used, it is important to avoid concomitant administration of drugs that may act as radiation sensitizers to normal tissue.

COMPLICATIONS OF RADIATION

The complications of radiation are related directly to treatment dose and volume. Reactions that occur during the early stages of treatment usually are reversible and not of major significance. These include erythema, dry desquamation of the skin, and epilation. More serious late reactions may include fibrosis, contracture, atrophy, impaired growth, secondary fracture, and radiation-induced neoplasm. When pelvic treatment is necessary in young women, it is important to consider ovarian transposition whenever possible. Techniques to move the small bowel out of the pelvis are useful, as is avoiding treatment of the entire bladder if cyclophosphamide or ifosfamide is also being used. Fibrosis and contracture can be minimized—or possibly avoided—by embarking on an active physical therapy program during radiation therapy; such a program should be continued in the postradiation therapy follow-up period. Whenever possible, treating across a joint space and treating an open epiphysis should be avoided. For tumors of weight-bearing bones, partial weight bearing and protective bracing are important until reossification occurs.

BENIGN BONE TUMORS

SOLITARY AND MULTIPLE OSTEOCHONDROMAS (EXOSTOSIS)

Osteochondroma is the most common benign bone tumor. The tumors characteristically are sessile or pedunculated, arising from the cortex of a long tubular bone adjacent to the epiphyseal plate. Osteochondromas are usually solitary, except in multiple hereditary exostosis. Plain radiographs are usually diagnostic, and no further tests are required. Sessile osteochondromas are difficult to diagnose, especially when they occur in unusual sites, such as the distal posterior femur, where they must be differentiated from a parosteal osteosarcoma. Bone scintigraphy and CT are helpful in distinguishing between the two.

Osteochondromas grow with the individual until skeletal maturity is reached. Growth of an osteochondroma during adolescence does not, therefore, signify malignancy. Pain is not a sign of malignancy in childhood or adolescence, although in adulthood it is a significant warning sign. Pain in a child may be due to local bursitis, mechanical irritation of adjacent muscles, or pathologic fracture.

Between 1% and 2% of solitary osteochondromas undergo malignant transformation; patients with multiple hereditary exostosis are at higher risk.[2,4,57,58] Malignant tumors arising from a benign osteochondroma are usually low-grade chondrosarcomas. Proximal osteochondromas are more likely than distal ones to undergo malignant transformation. In general, surgical removal is recommended only for symptomatic osteochondromas and for those arising along the axial skeleton or pelvic or shoulder girdle.

SOLITARY AND MULTIPLE ENCHONDROMAS

Enchondromas are composed of mature hyaline cartilage that arises within a bone. They may be solitary or multiple (Ollier's disease) and have been reported in most bones.[3,4] Their bio-

TABLE 39.2-11. Radiation Guidelines for Benign Bone Lesions

Tumor	*Radiation Dose*	*Comments*
Osteoblastoma/osteoid osteoma	50 Gy	Role of radiation is limited and controversial.
Aneurysmal bone cyst	20–30 Gy	Megavoltage radiation in conventional fractionation and low total doses is effective in reducing recurrence and unlikely to be associated with long-term complications.
Langerhans' cell histiocytosis	6–10 Gy in 150-cGy fractions	Low doses of radiation have a high likelihood of local control of osseous and soft tissue lesions.
Gorham's massive osteolysis	40–45 Gy	A rare vascular abnormality that may be managed by surgery or radiotherapy.

logic potential is often over- or underestimated. In general, pathologic interpretation of cartilage tumors is more difficult than that of other bone tumors; it is particularly difficult to differentiate a benign enchondroma from a grade I chondrosarcoma.[10,11,214] Malignant transformations do occur, but the rate is difficult to determine.[215] Lesions of the pelvis, femur, and ribs are generally at higher risk for malignant transformation than are lesions at more distal sites.

Pain is a sign of local aggressiveness and possible malignancy. Enchondromas of the hands and feet are benign, irrespective of pathology,[3] whereas cartilage tumors of the pelvic or shoulder girdle are often malignant, even though the histology appearance is benign. Plain radiographs may be helpful in making this distinction. Radiographic scalloping is a sign of local aggressiveness. Bone scintigraphy is not helpful in differentiating a low-grade chondrosarcoma from an active enchondroma. Patient age is an important indicator of possible malignancy; enchondromas rarely undergo malignant transformation *before* skeletal maturity. Painful, histologically benign-looking proximal enchondromas in adults are often malignant, despite their histology. Thus, correlation of symptoms, plain radiographic findings, and histology is crucial.

CHONDROBLASTOMA, OSTEOBLASTOMA, AND OSTEOID OSTEOMA

Chondroblastoma and osteoblastoma are characterized by immature but benign chondroid or osteoid production, respectively. Both may undergo malignant transformation in rare cases.[59,216] Osteoid osteomas are smaller than 1 cm, painful, bone-forming tumors that are always benign. It is essential that the oncologist be aware of these entities and be able to differentiate them from their malignant counterparts, chondrosarcoma and osteosarcoma. Chondroblastomas appear radiographically in the epiphysis of a child; conversely, primary chondrosarcomas are rarely epiphyseal and occur in adults. Although osteoblastomas may be found in any bone, one-half of them are in the spine and skull. Osteoblastomas must be differentiated from osteosarcomas and osteoid osteoma.

Both chondroblastomas and osteoblastomas are considered aggressive, benign lesions with a high recurrence rate after simple curettage.[2–4,216] Local control can be achieved by primary resection; however, routine resection cannot be recommended for tumors adjacent to a joint. Marcove et al.[131] report a 5% to 10% local recurrence rate when curettage is combined with cryosurgery. This method has obviated resection and extensive reconstruction in select patients. Osteoid osteoma is treated by simple excision. In a few cases, nonsteroidal antiinflammatory drugs have proven curative when continued for a minimum of 1 year. Because surgical removal is the treatment of choice for these benign bone lesions, the role of radiotherapy is limited. For nonresectable tumors, radiotherapy has been associated with long-term control (Table 39.2-11), but most radiation oncologists do not believe that radiation plays a role in the management of these conditions.[214,217]

ANEURYSMAL BONE CYSTS

Aneurysmal bone cysts (ABCs) are benign tumors of childhood, occurring typically *before* skeletal maturity.[2–4] They never become malignant. They often involve the metaphyseal regions of the long bones or the vertebrae. Radiographically, ABCs are eccentric, lytic, and expansile, characterized by cortical destruction and periosteal elevation. They can grow rapidly and appear extremely aggressive, and distinguishing them from a primary malignancy may be difficult. Differential diagnosis includes GCT and telangiectatic osteosarcoma. ABCs contain some osteoid; however, careful examination reveals this to be reactive and not neoplastic. Approximately one-third arise in conjunction with another bony neoplasm.[216,218] The classic treatment is simple curettage and bone graft, which has a recurrence rate of 20% to 35%.[4] Wide curettage may decrease the recurrence rate to approximately 10%. Marcove and colleagues[130–132] recommend curettage and cryosurgery as the primary treatment. Primary resection of tumors involving weight-bearing bones is not warranted. Expandable bones, especially the ribs and fibula, may be treated by primary resection. The Mayo Clinic reviewed its experience of 238 patients with ABCs.[219] Eighty percent of those lesions involved long bones. The investigators noted that CT and MRI may show characteristic septations or fluid-fluid levels. Of 153 patients treated, 19% had recurrence after curettage. The high-risk period for local recurrence was the first 2 years. The most significant clinical problem is deciding whether a lesion is an ABC or a telangiectatic osteosarcoma.

Radiation therapy is recommended in surgically inaccessible sites.[3,217,218] Megavoltage doses (25 to 30 Gy in 18 to 24 days) have been associated with a decrease in local recurrence from 32% to 8% and are generally recommended.[98,214,218,220–222]

DESMOPLASTIC FIBROMA

Desmoplastic fibroma is an extremely rare bone tumor; only 80 cases have been reported.[216] It is characterized by abundant collagen formation and a fibrous stroma without evidence of mitosis or pleomorphism. It presents radiographically as an osteolytic lesion with well-defined margins. Most important in differential diagnosis is primary fibrosarcoma of bone. Treatment is *en bloc* resection; curettage has a significant rate of local recurrence. Radiation therapy has been suggested when surgery is not a reasonable option, but dose-response data are not available.[223]

LANGERHANS' CELL HISTIOCYTOSIS

Langerhans' cell histiocytosis is a more descriptive and recently accepted term to describe the disease commonly referred to as *histiocytosis X*. The solitary or multifocal osseous lesions (Greenberger stage IA and B) were formerly referred to as *eosinophilic granuloma*.[224] This condition can be difficult to diagnose and may mimic radiographically a primary bone malignancy.

Almost any bone can be involved. Radiographically, the lesions appear as lytic, destructive defects, with ill-defined margins. Periosteal elevation occurs in one-half of all cases. This combination of characteristics strongly resembles that of Ewing's sarcoma or osteomyelitis. When the disease arises in a flat bone, specifically the pelvis, there may be a large soft tissue component. Solitary lesions are treated by surgical curettage.

MALIGNANT BONE TUMORS

CLASSIC OSTEOSARCOMA

Osteosarcoma is a high-grade, malignant spindle cell tumor that arises within a bone. Its distinguishing characteristic is the production of "tumor" osteoid or immature bone directly from a malignant spindle cell stroma.[2,3,60,225]

Clinical Characteristics

Osteosarcoma typically occurs during childhood and adolescence. An epidemiologic study from the Swedish Cancer Institute documented that the mean and median age of patients with osteosarcoma has increased since 1971.[226] Investigators evaluated 227 patients from 1971 to 1984 and reported the peak incidence to be between 10 and 19 years of age but noted the mean and median values to be 29 and 20 years, respectively. The overall incidence—2.1 cases per million people per year—has not changed. When osteosarcoma occurs in patients older than 40 years, it is usually associated with a preexisting condition, such as Paget's disease, irradiated bones, multiple hereditary exostosis, or polyostotic fibrous dysplasia.[2,225–230] Bones of knee joint and the proximal humerus are the most common sites, accounting for 50% and 25%, respectively, of all osteosarcomas.[216] In general, 80% to 90% of osteosarcomas occur in the long tubular bones[2,4,57,227,231–233]; the axial skeleton is rarely affected. Fewer than 1% are found in the hands and feet.[2]

With the exception of serum AP levels, which are elevated in 45% to 50% of patients, laboratory findings are usually not helpful.[231] Furthermore, elevated AP per se is not diagnostic, because it is also found in association with other skeletal disease. Pain is the most common complaint. Physical examination demonstrates a firm, soft tissue mass fixed to the underlying bone with slight tenderness. No effusion is noted in the adjacent joint, and motion is normal. Incidence of pathologic fracture is less than 1%. Systemic symptoms are rare.

Radiographic Characteristics

Typical findings are increased intramedullary radiodensity (due to tumor bone or calcified cartilage), an area of radiolucency (due to nonossified tumor), a pattern of permeative destruction with poorly defined borders, cortical destruction, periosteal elevation, and extraosseous extension with soft tissue ossification.[231–233] This combination of characteristics is not seen in any other lesion. Wilner classified 600 radiographs of osteosarcoma seen at the Memorial-Sloan Kettering Cancer Center into three broad categories[233]: sclerotic (32%), osteolytic (22%), and mixed (46%). Although no statistically significant difference was found in overall survival rates among these types, the patterns are important to recognize. The sclerotic and mixed types offer few diagnostic problems. Errors of diagnosis most often occur with pure osteolytic tumors. The differential diagnosis of osteolytic osteosarcoma includes GCT, ABC, fibrosarcoma, and MFH.[234] In a series of 305 osteosarcoma cases, DeSantos and Edeiken[234] reported that 42 (13.5%) were purely lytic. Most commonly, they presented as ill-defined lesions with a moderate to large soft tissue component. Nine of the lesions had benign radiographic features.

Clinical and Prognostic Considerations

Before the era of adjuvant chemotherapy, treatment consisted of amputation. Metastasis to lungs and other bones generally occurred within 24 months. A large number of series shows an overall survival of 5% to 20% at 2 years[72–75] (Fig. 39.2-6). This pattern has been altered by adjuvant chemotherapy and aggressive thoracotomy for pulmonary disease.[46,103,235] Metastases may now appear at less common sites, and disease-free intervals are longer.[235] In 1968, Lockshin and Higgins[236] reviewed the experience of 100 authors over 50 years and concluded that there was no significant difference between survival rates of patients with the three histiogenic subtypes (osteoblastic, chondroblastic, and fibroblastic) or between patients whose lesions had a different radiographic appearance (sclerotic, osteolytic, or mixed).[236] Likewise, tumor size, patient age, and degree of malignancy did not correlate with survival. The most significant variable was

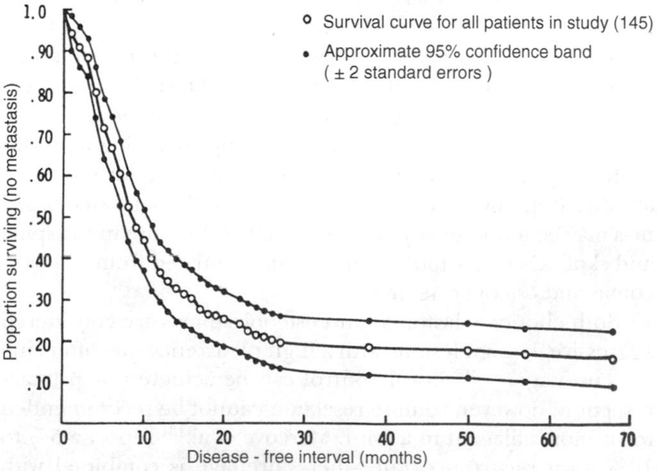

FIGURE 39.2-6. The historical survival curve for 145 patients with osteosarcoma treated by surgery alone at Memorial Sloan-Kettering Cancer Center as reported by Marcove and associates. (From Marcove RC, Mike V, Hajek JV, et al. Osteogenic sarcoma under the age of 21. *J Bone Joint Surg Am* 1966;48:1, with permission.)

anatomic site. Patients with pelvic and axial lesions had a lower survival rate than those with tumors of the extremities, probably due to surgical inaccessibility and incomplete removal. Patients with tumors of the tibia had a significantly higher survival rate than those with tumors of the distal femur (35% vs. 16%). Larsson and colleagues,[237] using a multifactorial analysis of all patients from the Swedish Cancer Registry between 1958 and 1968, similarly concluded that patients with tibial lesions had a better survival rate than those with femoral lesions (38.1% vs. 15.1%), due to the fact that the former were less advanced at the time of treatment.

Marcove et al.,[72] reviewing 145 patients younger than 21 years of age who underwent surgery without adjuvant chemotherapy at Memorial Sloan-Kettering, noted no statistically significant differences with regard to race, gender, or duration of symptoms (see Fig. 39.2-6). Younger patients developed metastases sooner, but this made no difference in overall survival. Location had no impact on the 5-year survival rate. Brostrom and coworkers[238] evaluated 52 patients treated by surgery alone. They studied tumor size and site and reported that patients with distal lesions measuring smaller than 10 cm had a significantly higher survival ($P < .01$) than those with proximal lesions larger than 10 cm (43% vs. 12%, respectively). More recently, Hudson and associates[239] reported on 98 patients treated at the M. D. Anderson Cancer Center with three different protocols. Tumor size ($P = .04$) and the percentage of tumor necrosis induced by induction therapy ($P = .01$) were the most important prognostic factors.

Baldini et al.[240] from the Rizzoli Institute have reviewed the prognostic factors of osteosarcoma patients treated with preoperative chemotherapy. This is one of the more recent studies that attempts to determine prognostic factors when chemotherapy is administered, in contrast to older studies, which evaluated prognostic factors *before* chemotherapy. Baldini et al. evaluated 160 patients with stage II high-grade osteosarcomas at a single institution. One hundred forty-two patients were treated by a limb-sparing procedure, and 18 underwent amputation. Tumor size was not found to be associated with a histologic response to chemotherapy. One-hundred fifteen patients had a good response (more than 90% necrosis), and 40 had a poor response. Larger tumors were not found to be associated with a lower likelihood of response to chemotherapy. No association was found between the size of the tumor and the event-free survival of the patients, as determined by univariate and multivariate analysis.

Changing Pattern of Metastasis

The classic pattern and time frame of metastatic dissemination of osteosarcoma has been somewhat modified by the use of adjuvant chemotherapy and thoracotomy. Bacci and coworkers[241] evaluated the pattern of metastatic spread of osteosarcoma in 193 patients at the Rizzoli Institute. Thirty patients who were treated with surgery alone were compared to 163 patients who underwent adjuvant chemotherapy. No difference was found in sites of first relapse; approximately 90% of cases in both groups occurred in the lungs. After chemotherapy, extrapulmonary spread occurred in 10% of cases, usually to bony sites. Simultaneous bone and lung metastases occurred in approximately 2%. The time to metastases differed (surgery alone was 13 months vs. adjuvant chemotherapy at 8 months), and the number of metastatic nodules were reduced. In general, lung metastases appeared later and were fewer in number after adjuvant chemotherapy but with variable difference on extrapulmonary or bony spread. The authors of this study concluded that the alteration of metastatic spread permitted surgical resection of pulmonary metastases in a larger number of patients (51% vs. 29%).

Alkaline Phosphatase

Serum AP level is an important biologic marker of tumor activity in patients with osteosarcoma.[242,243] The early studies of the relationship of AP activity and survival were evaluated in several studies *before* the introduction of adjuvant chemotherapy (i.e., in patients treated with surgery alone).

The prognostic significance of AP has more recently been evaluated in conjunction with neoadjuvant chemotherapy. Bacci and coworkers evaluated patients treated for osteosarcoma between 1972 and 1989.[244] The study demonstrated that for patients with osteosarcoma of the extremities, presurgical serum AP levels are useful prognostic markers in patients treated with adjuvant or neoadjuvant chemotherapy. Specifically, the study demonstrated that patients presenting with nonmetastatic osteosarcoma and an elevated serum AP level had a worse prognosis than those with normal values (55% of relapses versus 26%). Among those patients determined to have elevated pretreatment serum AP levels, there was a correlation showing that the higher the serum levels of AP, the greater the risk was for relapse. Patients with elevated pretreatment serum AP who experienced relapse or recurrence had a poorer disease-free survival when compared with individuals who relapsed and had normal pretreatment serum AP levels.

Surgical Resection of Localized Extremity Osteosarcoma

Before the early 1980s, treatment for localized osteosarcoma was amputation one joint above the tumor-containing bone or, occasionally, transmedullary amputation.[2,3,72–74] Since the early 1980s, parallel developments in radiology, orthopedics, and oncology have made limb-sparing procedures an option in 50% to 80% of patients.[20–34] A significant impetus for these developments was the introduction of effective chemotherapeutic agents in the early 1970s.[48–53]

Springfield and coworkers[245] from the University of Florida compared limb-sparing surgery with amputation in 53 patients with stage IIB osteosarcoma. For ethical reasons, the patients were not randomized. No difference in survival was found between amputation and resection or between radical resection and a wide surgical margin. Three local recurrences were reported. The investigators concluded that a wide surgical resection was adequate for local control. In general, they recommended amputation if the major neurovascular bundle was involved. They concluded that local recurrence was due to an extremely aggressive tumor or to skip metastases.

Rougraff and colleagues[142] updated a combined study from the Musculoskeletal Tumor Society of 227 patients from 26 institutions treated for osteosarcoma of the distal femur. One hundred nine patients (48%) were alive at an average of 11 years after surgery. No differences in local recurrence, overall survival, or duration of disease-free survival were noted between amputation and limb-sparing groups. The local recur-

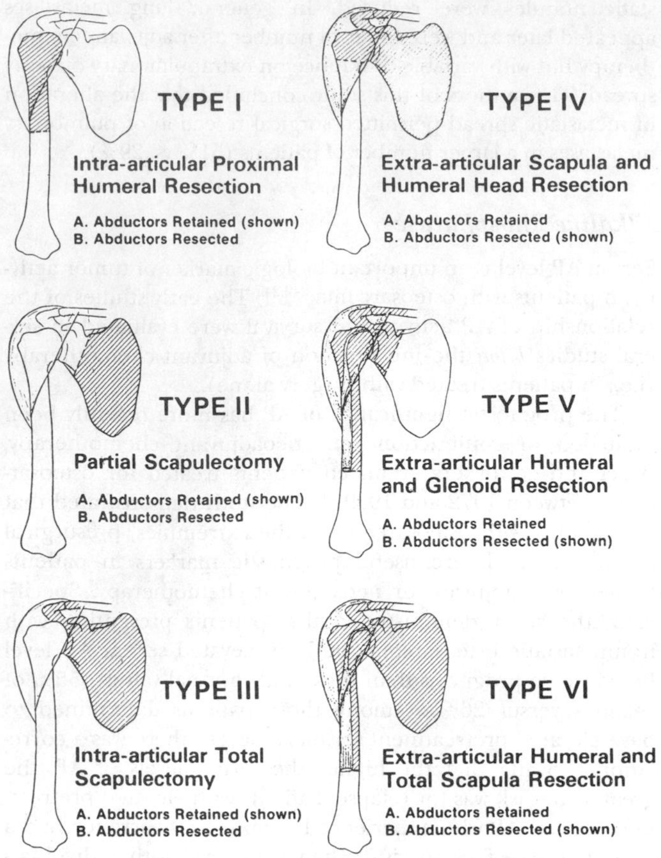

FIGURE 39.2-7. Schematic of proposed surgical classification of shoulder girdle resections. In general, types I to III are for benign or low-grade tumors, and types IV to VI are for high-grade tumors. A and B denote the status of the abductor mechanism: A is intact, and B is partially or completely excised. Types I to III and types IV to VI are intraarticular and extraarticular resections, respectively.

rence rate (10%) was identical for above-knee amputation and limb-sparing surgery. The most common causes of failed limb-sparing procedures were infection and local recurrence. Rougraff et al. concluded that the type of surgery did not affect outcomes. No difference was noted among patients treated with endoprostheses, allografts, composites, rotationplasties, and arthrodesis; however, the numbers of patients in those categories were small.

Local Recurrence, Tumor Necrosis, and Surgical Margins

During the 1990s, many surgeons intuitively believed that a patient with a good response to neoadjuvant chemotherapy was more likely to undergo a limb-sparing procedure safely than a patient with a poor response. A relationship appears to exist between the safety of limb-sparing resection and the surgical margins achieved with neoadjuvant chemotherapy. Patients whose lesions respond well to chemotherapy are less likely to develop local recurrence than those whose lesions respond poorly.[246] Picci and coworkers[246] from the Rizzoli Institute analyzed the relationship between local recurrence after neoadjuvant chemotherapy, surgical margin obtained, and tumor response as demonstrated by percentage of tumor necrosis. Of 355 patients, 7% developed local recurrences. The mean time

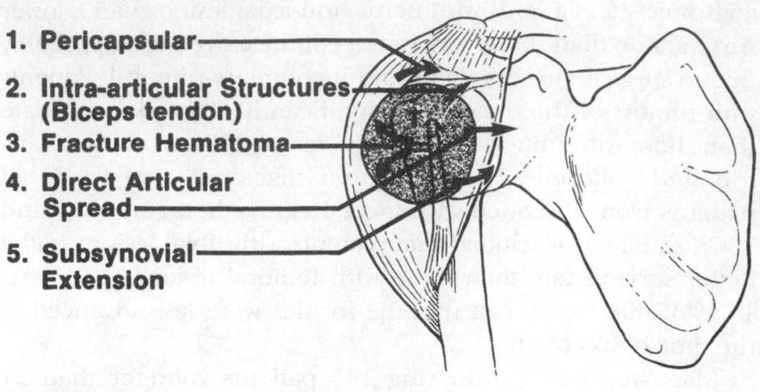

FIGURE 39.2-8. Mechanisms of local tumor spread for sarcomas of the shoulder. (From Malawer MM, Buch R, Reaman G, et al. Impact of two cycles of preoperative chemotherapy with intraarterial cisplatin and intravenous doxorubicin on the choice of surgical procedure for high-grade bone sarcomas of the extremities. *Clin Orthop* 1991;270:214, with permission.)

to local recurrence was 13 months from diagnosis (range, 2 to 56 months). Eighty-nine percent of the local recurrences developed within 18 months of the diagnosis. Of 237 patients in the group who had undergone a limb-sparing procedure, 23 (10%) developed a local recurrence. The types of surgical margins obtained and their respective local recurrence rates were as follows: wide margin, 3%; marginal margin, 29%; intralesional margin, 36%; contaminated margin, 15%.

When the type of surgical margin and the response to chemotherapy were analyzed together, differences in outcome were dramatic. The patients with poor necrosis (<60%) and wide margins had ten times the risk of local recurrence. The worst combination was poor necrosis and less than wide margins.

Treatment by Anatomic Site

The unique features of evaluation, management, and resection of tumors of the most common anatomic areas, the shoulder and knee, are described and illustrated in this section.

SHOULDER GIRDLE. A surgical classification for shoulder girdle resections has been described and is shown schematically in Figure 39.2-7.[247,248] This classification is useful for all limb-sparing procedures of the shoulder girdle. It is recommended that osteosarcomas arising from the proximal humerus be treated by a type VB resection (see Fig. 39.2-7). Figure 39.2-8 illustrates the various means by which a sarcoma may involve the shoulder joint.

PROXIMAL HUMERUS. Adequate resection of the proximal humerus requires removal of 15 to 20 cm of the humerus and shoulder joint with the deltoid, rotator cuff, and portions of the biceps and triceps muscles[249] (Fig. 39.2-9). The procedure involves suspension of the arm, motor reconstruction, and provision of adequate soft tissue coverage.

Proximal humeral lesions should not be biopsied through the deltopectoral interval. Biopsy under fluoroscopy through the anterior one-third of the deltoid by a trocar is preferred. Angiography is the most useful preoperative study. If the neurovascular bundle is clear, resection is feasible.

Extraarticular resection of the glenohumeral joint by medial scapulosteotomy is safer than intraarticular resection. A custom

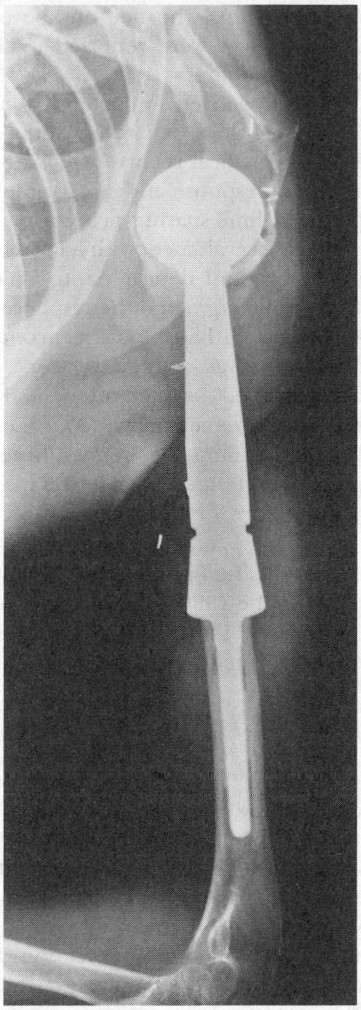

FIGURE 39.2-9. Osteosarcoma of the proximal humerus. This patient was placed in a shoulder splint and given three cycles of chemotherapy in the hope of avoiding a forequarter amputation. Due to the good clinical and radiographic response, this patient underwent a limb-sparing resection (type V).

prosthesis is used for reconstruction. Soft tissue reconstruction and suspension are essential to avoid postoperative pain, instability, and fatiguability.[249] Suspension by Dacron tape and muscle transfer is effective. Hand and wrist function is normal after resection. Shoulder motion is minimal, but stable, and scapulothoracic motion provides some internal and external rotation. Cosmesis is acceptable and can be enhanced with use of a shoulder pad.

Alternatively, resection of the proximal humerus for osteosarcomas can be performed by an intraarticular resection that preserves the glenoid and the adjacent deltoid muscle. The problems associated with this procedure include significant local recurrence rates and instability of the reconstructed prosthesis or allograft. When the glenoid and deltoid are preserved in this procedure, minimum margins are obtained along the shoulder joint, the deltoid muscle, and the axillary nerve. Because of this serious inherent drawback, this technique is not recommended by the senior author (M. M.).

DISTAL FEMUR. Adequate *en bloc* resection includes 15 to 20 cm of the distal femur and proximal tibia and portions of the adjacent quadriceps.[134] Biplane angiography is crucial to determine popliteal vessel involvement. Biopsy must avoid the sartorial canal and the knee joint. Contraindications to resection are popliteal vessel involvement, massive soft tissue contamination from previous biopsy, and fracture. Large tumors requiring removal of the entire quadriceps or hamstrings can be adequately reconstructed by an arthrodesis.

PROXIMAL TIBIA. Today, limb-sparing procedures often are feasible for tumors of the proximal tibia after induction chemotherapy.[250] It is more difficult to obtain an adequate margin of resection and a good functional result with lesions of the proximal tibia, which tend to have a higher incidence of local complications than do distal femoral tumors. These problems are directly related to the anatomic constraints: minimal adjacent soft tissue and the normal subcutaneous location of the medial tibial border. It is extremely important that the biopsy be small and that it avoid the knee joint. A core biopsy of medial flare is preferred to avoid contamination of the anterior musculature and peroneal nerve.

The popliteus muscle adjacent to the posterior aspect of the tibia prevents direct tumor involvement of the neurovascular bundle.[250,251] Lateral angiography is essential to demonstrate this interval. Tumor extension often involves the tibiofibular capsule.[250] Extraarticular resection of the proximal tibiofibular joint *en bloc* with the tibia is required to obtain a safe margin. The average resection length is 15 to 18 cm. Reconstruction is achieved by prosthetic replacement, arthrodesis, or allograft. The medial gastrocnemius is routinely transferred to provide soft tissue coverage of the reconstructed area.[252] Postoperative management consists of a long leg cast for 2 to 4 weeks to allow the extensor muscles to heal. Rehabilitation emphasizes knee extension, but not flexion, for a maximum of 2 to 3 months.[250]

PROXIMAL FIBULA. Tumors of the proximal fibula require the same evaluation as do proximal tibial lesions.[253] Unique considerations are early soft tissue extension, proximity to the lateral tibial condyle, necessity of ligation of the anterior and peroneal arteries, sacrifice of the peroneal nerve, and tumor infiltration of the tibiofibular joint capsule. Contraindications to resection are direct tibial involvement, an anomalously absent posterior tibial artery, and intraarticular knee joint extension. Adequate resection includes the fibula, the tibiofibular joint, the anterior and lateral muscle compartments, and a portion of the lateral gastrocnemius muscle. After surgery, the only functional deficit is footdrop, which is treated by an orthosis. Knee function is normal.[253]

OSTEOSARCOMA OF THE PELVIS AND PROXIMAL FEMUR

Osteosarcomas of the pelvis and proximal femur are less common than those occurring at other anatomic areas. They account for 10% and 5%, respectively, of all osteosarcomas.[216] Tumors arising from these structures are often large, involve important structures, and are difficult to resect. Hemipelvectomy often is required for pelvic tumors, whereas modified hemipelvectomy is used for tumors of the proximal femur.[145] The limb-sparing options, when feasible, are all functionally superior to amputation at this level.[254,255] A poorly planned biopsy often contaminates the extrapelvic structures, typically making a hemipelvectomy the only safe option. Detailed anatomic and surgical considerations are discussed in the section on chondrosarcomas (see Chondrosarcoma, later in this chapter), which often arise in these sites.

Fahey and Spanier[256] reviewed 25 patients with osteosarcoma of the pelvis treated at the University of Florida between 1967 and 1990 and described their biologic behavior, growth, and histologic and vascular findings. Common problems included delay in diagnosis, widespread invasion into major pelvic veins, microscopic foci of tumor in otherwise normal tissue, and extension into adjacent (and other) pelvic structures. They noted marked differences in obtaining tumor-free margins with surgery. Eighteen patients underwent surgery (ten hemipelvectomies and eight limb-sparing resections). Only two of ten hemipelvectomy patients obtained wide margins, and only two of the eight limb-sparing patients obtained negative margins. Major intraoperative complications occurred in 11 patients. Intraoperative blood loss exceeded 10 L in six patients. An unexpected intraoperative finding was obvious tumor invasion into the large veins in nine patients: the iliac veins in two patients, the inferior vena cava in three patients, and unnamed veins in four patients.

The high incidence of venous invasion requires that the iliac vessels be evaluated preoperatively and intraoperatively. Radiographic staging studies should include a thorough evaluation of the iliac vessels. This can best be performed by CT, MRI with contrast, and pelvic venography. Survival for patients with pelvic osteosarcoma is dismal. Only 1 of 25 patients remained disease-free. The five patients that lived the longest were all treated with chemotherapy. Innovative treatment strategies are needed for pelvic osteosarcomas.

Clinical Analysis of Limb-Sparing Surgery

The most recent comparison of the results of limb-sparing surgery and amputation were reported by Sluga and colleagues[257] from the University of Vienna. They evaluated 130 consecutive patients younger than 21 years of age treated for osteosarcoma of the extremity. Ninety percent (116 patients) were treated by a limb-sparing procedure. Fourteen amputations, 32 rotationplasties, and 84 resections with subsequent reconstruction were performed. The 5-year metastasis-free survival rate was 60% for patients treated by amputation or rotationplasty and 71% for patients treated by limb-sparing surgery. The surgical margins were classified as wide in 109 cases and radical in ten cases. The overall local recurrence rate was 2.3%: 4.3% for amputation and/or rotationplasty and 1.2% for limb-sparing surgery. The overall survival rate was significantly influenced by tumor volume (P = .0018), response to chemotherapy (P = .039), and presence of metastases at the time of diagnosis (P= .0001). The authors emphasize that there was no selection bias by tumor volume for the type of surgical procedure performed. The authors warn that limb-sparing is not suitable for every patient; patients with large tumors and close margins may require amputation. They emphasize the importance of wide margins to a successful limb-sparing procedure. This study, as well as previous studies, showed no difference in patient survival or local recurrence in patients treated by a limb-sparing procedure and those undergoing an amputation.

Rougraff and colleagues[142] evaluated 227 patients with non-metastatic osteosarcoma of the distal femur treated at 26 institutions. They reported eight (11%) local recurrences in 73 patients with a limb salvage procedure, and nine (8%) local recurrences in 115 patients who had an above-knee amputation. No local recurrences were reported in the 39 patients who had a hip disarticulation.

Bacci et al.[258] retrospectively evaluated 540 patients treated over 10 years in three multicenter studies with 63 participating institutions. The rate of local recurrence was 8% for patients with a poor histologic response and 3% for those with a good histologic response. A limb-sparing procedure was performed on 84% of the 540 cases evaluated, with a local recurrence rate of 6%. The most important determinant of local recurrence was the type of surgical margin and the response to chemotherapy. Of the 540 patients, 31 had a local recurrence. The overall outcome of this group was extremely poor. All local recurrences were accompanied by metastases, and despite treatment, only one patient remains alive (3%). Local recurrence did not correlate with patient age, gender, histologic type, site and volume, pathologic fracture incidence, chemotherapy, or type of surgical procedure.

It appears, in summary, that the safety and efficacy of limb-sparing procedures for high-grade bone sarcomas have been well answered during the 1990s.[259] The senior author (M. M.) would like to emphasize that these procedures are demanding and must be performed by surgeons experienced in limb-sparing procedures.

Allograft Replacement

Allograft (cadaver bone) replacement was popular in the 1970s and mid-1980s, which were the early days of limb-sparing surgery. Allograft was used for replacement of large bony segments after limb-sparing surgery. When used in patients in conjunction with chemotherapy, allografts have a significant complication rate, including infection, fracture, nonunion, and local recurrence, which may lead to secondary amputation.[260]

The most recent authors to evaluate the use of allografts for reconstruction of the distal femur (the most common site for osteosarcoma) were Powell et al.[261] They evaluated their experience over a 13-year period. A total of 37 osteoarticular allografts were used to reconstruct the distal femur of 34 patients who underwent tumor resection. Twenty-one patients with sarcoma received chemotherapy. Average follow-up was 86 months. Eighty-five percent of patients had postoperative complications, and 21 of 33 patients (73%) required further surgery. The most common complications were joint instability (55%), degenerative joint disease (44%), nonunion (36%), allograft fracture (28%), and infection (17%). Only 13 of the 36 of the allografts (36%) remained intact. A steady decline in actuarial survivorship of the reconstruction was noted over time: 83.2% at 2 years, 42.3% at 5 years, and 14.3% at 10 years.

Allograft replacement remains popular at some institutions but is reserved for low-grade tumors that do not require chemotherapy. The use of allografts has become less common with the development of reliable prosthetic replacements, especially the modular replacement systems.

Prosthesis Survival and Complications

Prosthetic replacement is commonly used for reconstruction after resection of the proximal humerus, proximal femur, distal femur (Fig. 39.2-10), and proximal tibia. Several studies have

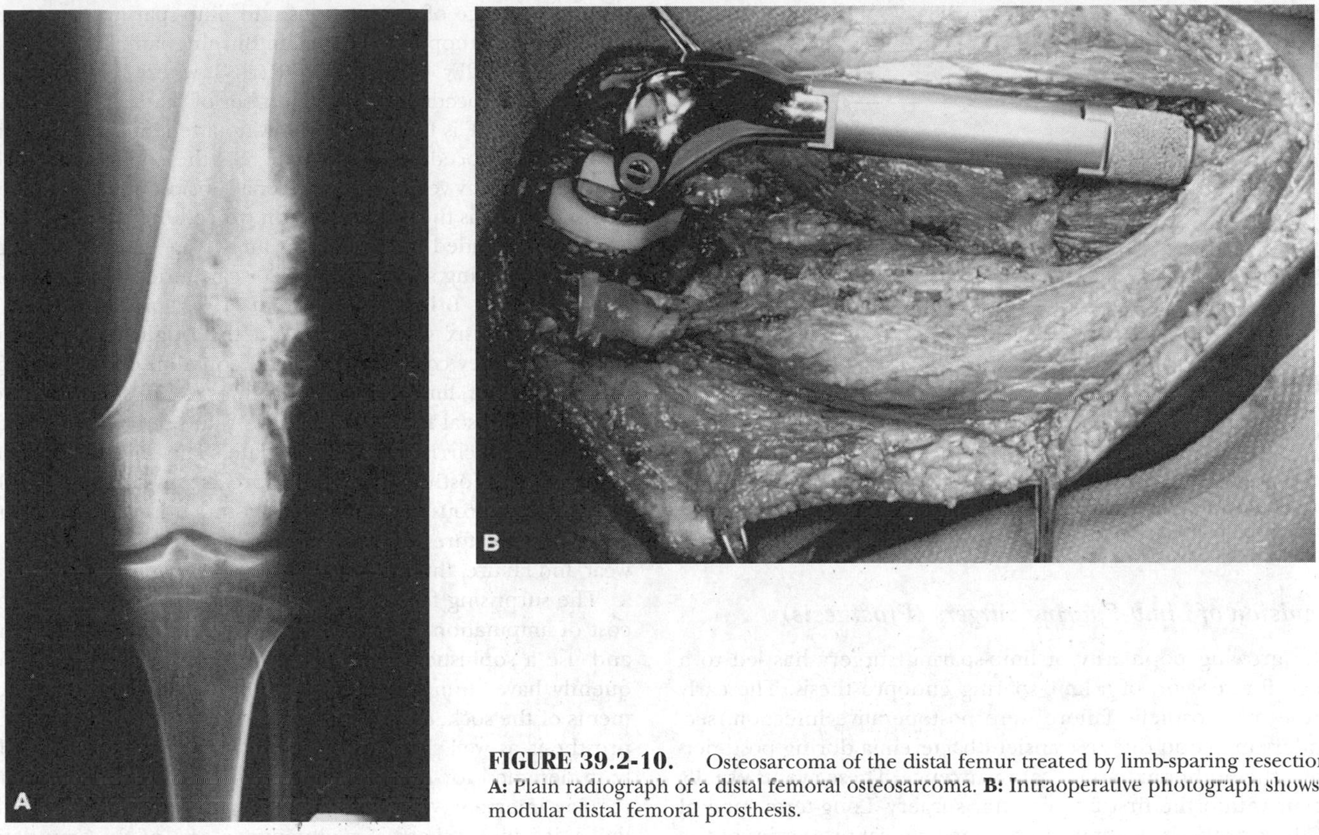

FIGURE 39.2-10. Osteosarcoma of the distal femur treated by limb-sparing resection. **A:** Plain radiograph of a distal femoral osteosarcoma. **B:** Intraoperative photograph shows a modular distal femoral prosthesis.

evaluated the long-term results, prosthetic survivorship, and complications associated with prosthetic replacement.[262–265] Ruggieri and associates[264] reported on 133 cases of nonmetastatic osteosarcoma of the extremities treated with neoadjuvant chemotherapy and limb-sparing surgery. Sixty-three percent of the patients had one or more complications. Twenty-eight complications were considered minor (i.e., no surgery was required), and 77 complications were major. The infection rate was 6.2%. Mechanical problems occurred in seven patients (5%). The average number of complications per patient was 1.3. The authors thought that the most serious problems resulting from a complication were those that required the delay of chemotherapy or deviation from the recommended dose, either of which could jeopardize survival. Such consequences were not, however, demonstrable statistically.

Campanna and colleagues[265] from the Rizzoli Institute reported on 95 distal femoral resections performed between 1983 and 1989 (average follow-up, 51 months). The overall complication and infection rates were 55% and 5%, respectively. The most common complication was failure of the polyethylene bushings used with the knee component, which occurred at an average of 5.3 years after the procedure. They reported an overall local recurrence rate of 5% (average, 15 months). Mechanical stem breakage was rare (6%) and was associated with two factors—the use of a narrow stem and extensive quadriceps excision. The results were not related to patient age or length of resection. The tibia component caused no problems. All revisions done for infections were unsatisfactory. The incidence of infection correlated with the extent of soft tissue resection of the quadriceps. No revisions were needed because of loosening.

Malawer and Chou[262] evaluated the prosthetic survivorship of large-segment prostheses in 89 patients with high-grade bone sarcomas. The overall limb survival and infection rates were 90% and 7%, respectively. The infection rate resulting in amputation was 7%. The 5- and 10-year prosthetic survival rates (no need for revision or amputation) were 83% and 67%, respectively. Age, gender, and diagnosis were not related to prosthetic survival. The authors of this study suggested that infection was related to periods of bacteremia and neutropenia associated with postoperative chemotherapy and to episodes of line sepsis.

In 1999, Henshaw et al.[266] reported the long-term prosthetic survival analysis of the 100 patients treated with the American-designed modular replacement system (Howmedica and Osteonics, Inc., Allendale, NJ). The minimum follow-up period was 2 years. *Prosthetic failure* was defined as removal of the implant for any reason. Kaplan-Meier survival analysis was performed for all implants and for each site of reconstruction. The authors reported no mechanical failures of the stem, body, or taper components. No clinically significant prosthetic loosening was reported. The infection rate was 8% (four in distal femurs, three in proximal tibias, and one in proximal humerus), leading to six amputations and one prosthetic removal. The amputation rate was 7% (six infections and one local recurrence). The Kaplan-Meier survival analysis (Fig. 39.2-11) for all sites was 88% at 10 years, with a median follow-up of 64.4 months. The estimates of 10-year survival for the distal femur, proximal humerus, proximal femur, and proximal tibia were 90%, 98%, 100%, and 78%, respectively. Today, modular prostheses are forged by several manufacturers and are the standard prostheses used for most limb-sparing procedures.[266]

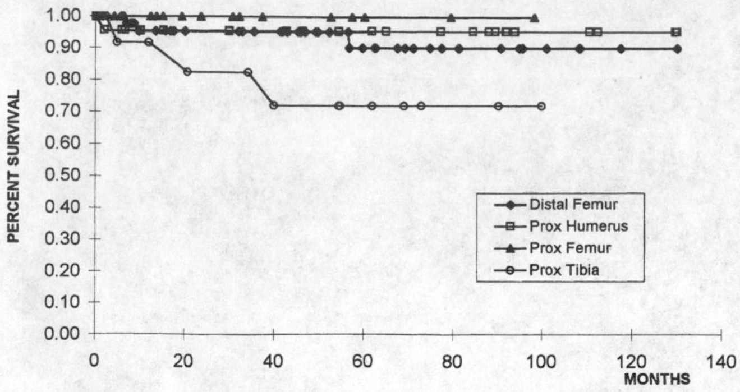

FIGURE 39.2-11. Kaplan-Meier curve showing the survival of prosthetic replacements according to anatomic site in 100 patients treated by limb-sparing surgery for high-grade bone sarcomas. The anatomic site was the most significant predictor of survival of the prosthesis. Distal Femur, distal or mid-part of the femur; Prox Humerus, proximal part of the humerus; Prox Femur, proximal portion of the femur; Prox Tibia, proximal portion of the tibia. (From ref. 266, with permission.)

Revision of Limb-Sparing Surgery (Prosthesis)

The growing popularity of limb-sparing surgery has led to a need for revision of a limb-sparing endoprosthesis. The early causes of prosthetic failure were postoperative infection, secondary infection due to transient bacteremia during postoperative chemotherapy, and local recurrence. These events usually occur within the first 2 years after surgery. Long-term survival of the prosthesis depends on the mechanical properties of the prosthesis and on the host response to the polyethylene, methylmethacrylate, and metallic components. The most common causes of late failure of a prosthesis necessitating revision (i.e., removal and replacement of the prosthesis) are aseptic loosening of the prosthesis, mechanical breakage, or polyethylene component failure.

Renard et al.[267] evaluated 26 revision procedures. The most common reasons for a revision were polyethylene wear (nine cases) and aseptic loosening (eight cases). The follow-up after the last revision ranged from 6 months to 12 years, with a median of 3 years. All patients retained their extremity, and approximately 75% incurred no functional loss after prosthetic revision.

Cost of Limb-Sparing Surgery versus Amputation

The question of the cost effectiveness of limb-salvage surgery for bone tumors has arisen in the face of managed care, especially within the United States. The only published report on this subject is by Grimer et al.,[268] who compared the cost of a limb-sparing procedure in lieu of an amputation. They developed a formula for the cost of the limb-salvage procedure versus an above-knee amputation with subsequent prosthetic replacement over the predicted life of the patient. This was calculated for tumors around the knee. They excluded tumors of the proximal humerus and of the proximal femur, because, whatever difference in cost there might be, there was a tremendous advantage of replacing the proximal femur rather than performing a hemipelvectomy or hip disarticulation. Similarly, there is a tremendous advantage in preserving the upper extremity and a functioning hand in lieu of a forequarter amputation for a proximal humeral sarcoma. Their study is based on large experience of amputations and limb-sparing procedures at the Royal Orthopedic Hospital in Birmingham, England. The formula is $E + 2Fy + sSy + rRy + 3R(rRy)$, where E is the cost of the original procedure, y is the number of years since the original operation, F is the cost of follow-up attendance, s is the risk of a service procedure in any year, S is the cost of a servicing procedure in any year, r is the risk of a revision procedure being needed, and R is the cost of revision procedure.

They concluded the savings for an average patient undergoing a limb-sparing surgery over a 20-year period to be approximately 70,000 British pounds (at 1977 prices), which is approximately six times the cost of the original limb-sparing procedure. They concluded that the equation can be used for any method of limb-salvage procedure. This study was performed with distal femoral resections that used a simple hinge prosthesis, which is now out of date. The modern rotating hinged-knee prosthesis, with an improved surface and a collar coated with porous beads, provides a much longer rate of survival. These features should provide a significantly lower rate of wear and failure, thus increasing cost-effectiveness.

The surprising feature of these findings is the considerable cost of amputation. Most active young people would demand and use a sophisticated artificial limb. These individuals frequently have stump problems and require multiple replacements of the socket and prosthesis. They often require a spare prosthesis as well. Many request and use a sports limb and a limb designed for swimming. A new prosthesis is required at regular intervals. With the increasing complexity of artificial limbs, it is likely that the maintenance cost of the amputated extremity will increase.[268]

Limb-Sparing Surgery and Pathologic Fracture

Traditionally, a fracture through an osteosarcoma was treated by amputation. As experience with induction chemotherapy and limb-sparing surgery has increased, however, several centers have attempted limb-sparing surgery in this high-risk patient population. The assumption has been that if the fracture can be immobilized during the induction period and the tumor shows clear signs of necrosis and secondary fracture healing, an amputation may be avoided. The earlier strategy, immediate amputation, was based on the presumed high risk of local recurrence after a limb-sparing procedure. A limb-sparing procedure may now be safely performed if the response to induction chemotherapy is good, as evidenced by fracture healing.

Steadman et al.[269] evaluated their experience with patients with osteosarcoma-induced pathologic fractures between 1970 and 1995. Nine primary instances of limb salvage in patients with preoperative chemotherapy and eight primary cases of amputation with postoperative chemotherapy were studied. No significant difference in survival was found. One local recurrence occurred in the limb-salvage group, and none in the amputation group. This retrospective analysis, combined with other reported results, makes a convincing case that a pathologic fracture does not indicate the need for an immediate amputation. The strategy today is to immobilize the extremity and proceed with induction chemotherapy. If the fracture heals and the tumor appears to respond to chemotherapy, a limb-sparing operation is warranted. Repeat staging studies after induction chemotherapy and close serial observation during the induction period are essential.

CLINICAL PRESENTATIONS OF OSTEOSARCOMA AND TREATMENT CONSIDERATIONS

Treatment Considerations

LOCALIZED EXTREMITY DISEASE. Management of osteosarcoma requires the expertise of a multidisciplinary team familiar with the various management options. Patients with a suspected diagnosis of osteosarcoma (based on radiographic findings) should be referred to centers with treatment programs before biopsy. The biopsy should be performed by an orthopedic surgeon familiar with the management of malignant bone tumors and experienced in the required techniques.[270] Whenever possible, this individual should be the surgeon who will ultimately perform the definitive surgical procedure, because the biopsy must be planned carefully with a consideration of subsequent definitive surgery. A poorly conceived and poorly placed biopsy may jeopardize the subsequent treatment, especially a subsequent limb-salvage procedure.

The patient with a primary tumor of the extremity without evidence of metastases requires surgery to control the primary tumor and chemotherapy to control micrometastatic disease. The choice between amputation and limb-sparing resection must be made by an experienced orthopedic oncologist, taking into account tumor location, size, or extramedullary extent; the presence or absence of distant metastatic disease; and patient factors such as age, skeletal development, and lifestyle preference. Routine amputations are no longer performed, all patients should be evaluated for limb-sparing options. Intensive, multiagent chemotherapeutic regimens have provided the best results to date (see Tables 39.2-6 and 39.2-7). Patients who are judged unsuitable for limb-sparing options may be candidates for presurgical chemotherapy; those with a good response may then become suitable candidates for limb-sparing operations. The management of these patients mandates close cooperation between the medical oncologist and surgeon.

PELVIC TUMORS AND UNRESECTABLE DISEASE. In some pelvic and most vertebral primary tumors, complete resection often is not possible. Most pelvic osteosarcomas can be treated by hemipelvectomy; more centrally located pelvic tumors, especially those involving the sacrum, are unresectable. Only a few pelvic osteosarcomas can be treated by limb-sparing resection (internal hemipelvectomy). Contraindications to resection are unusually large extraosseous extensions with sacral plexus or major vascular involvement. On rare occasions, vertebral and sacral resections have been attempted.[271–273] In general, these tumors cannot be resected with negative margins and are best treated by radiotherapy and chemotherapy. Some success has been achieved with systemic or intraarterial chemotherapy, which is administered to convert apparently inoperable tumors into lesions that can be ablated surgically.[89,90] Patients with primary tumors of the axial skeleton have had a poor outcome, because local control was rare. The prognosis for these patients may improve with a more aggressive surgical approach and more effective chemotherapy.[274] Patients whose tumors can be completely resected should be approached with curative intent; radiotherapy provides significant palliation in patients with unresectable primary tumors.

METASTATIC PULMONARY DISEASE AT DIAGNOSIS. Metastatic disease detected at initial diagnosis does not preclude a curative treatment strategy, although the presence of extrathoracic metastases makes cure extremely unlikely. In general, the surgical principles outlined for the treatment of relapsing patients apply equally to the patient presenting with macroscopic metastases. Newly diagnosed patients have not been exposed to chemotherapy and are, thus, less likely to have drug-resistant tumors. Therefore, several options are available to them.

For the patient presenting with resectable disease (i.e., usually fewer than 15 pulmonary nodules and a primary tumor of the extremity), the traditional approach has been resection of all evidence of macroscopic disease by median sternotomy and limb amputation or resection, followed by intensive adjuvant chemotherapy. The tumor burden is thereby reduced to a minimum before the application of adjuvant therapy. Some investigators have favored treatment with chemotherapy, followed weeks or months later by definitive surgery for residual macroscopic disease in primary and metastatic sites.[92,93] Arguments advanced to justify this approach are similar to those used to support preoperative chemotherapy in general, and the theoretical advantages and disadvantages of this strategy as discussed for patients with nonmetastatic osteosarcoma apply here as well. The risk for the patient with metastases is that growth of tumor nodules in the face of chemotherapy may render small, operable metastases unresectable and prevent cure. Although the timing of the surgery of the primary tumor and metastatic sites has been variable, most modern approaches entail alternating chemotherapy and surgery. The initial treatment is usually a course of chemotherapy, followed by surgical resection of the primary tumor, followed by a second course of chemotherapy and surgical ablation of metastatic sites, followed by the remaining courses of chemotherapy. Patients with tumors that respond to presurgical chemotherapy are more likely to be cured. In patients with inoperable metastases, primary treatment with chemotherapy is probably appropriate; metastases may respond sufficiently to allow complete resection. Because these patients usually require surgery for the primary tumor as a palliative procedure, early surgery may be recommended, despite unresectable pulmonary disease. Although improving, the outlook for patients presenting with metastatic disease remains poor.[275,276]

RECURRENT DISEASE AFTER CURATIVE ATTEMPT. Historically, patients developing recurrent disease had a poor prognosis and were treated palliatively; most died within 1 year of the development of metastatic disease. Because more than 85% of metastases occur in the lung, surgical resection of tumor nodules can be readily accomplished. With the advent of thoracic CT scanning, metastatic nodules can be detected when quite small and more easily resectable, although in most cases the surgeon discovers more lesions at thoracotomy than anticipated on the basis of the CT scan.[277–279] In many patients, the lungs are likely to be the only site of metastasis, especially in cases in which recurrences appear more than 1 year after diagnosis and in which the metastatic lesion is solitary. In such cases, the recurrent tumors are likely to behave more indolently and may not further metastasize. These patients have been cured by thoracotomy alone.

Surgical resection of all overt metastatic disease is a prerequisite for long-term salvage after relapse.[278–281] Patients not treated by thoracotomy have little hope for cure, because complete responses of macroscopic metastases to chemotherapy are rare.[279–281] The completeness of surgical resection is an important determinant of outcome, because patients left with measurable or microscopic disease at the resection margins are unlikely to be cured.[279]

Many investigators have recommended adjuvant chemotherapy after thoracotomy for the management of metastatic osteosarcoma to destroy residual microscopic tumor deposits.[92,102,103] For patients who develop recurrent disease within 1 year of initial surgery, the possibility of additional microscopic metastatic disease is quite high, and further chemotherapy is indicated. Long-term survival has been reported for some patients with recurrent osteosarcoma who were treated only with surgery.[98–100] These survivors were more likely to be patients experiencing late relapses with solitary pulmonary nodules.

If overt metastatic disease is discovered, a thorough search for all metastatic lesions is essential. The discovery of unresectable extrathoracic metastases or unresectable pulmonary disease is a contraindication to aggressive thoracotomy, and the patient should be treated palliatively. Radiotherapy may be particularly useful in this context. In some patients with unresectable disease, an aggressive approach with curative intent may still be indicated. Chemotherapy, with or without radiotherapy, rarely eradicates all metastatic disease; nonetheless, some patients with inoperable metastases may respond sufficiently to allow for complete resection of disease at a later date. Occasionally, patients with unresectable pulmonary metastases are cured with chemotherapy or high-dose radiotherapy alone.

Patients with resectable lung disease should undergo thoracotomy to remove all evidence of disease. Bilateral disease may be approached by staged bilateral thoracotomies or a median sternotomy. The role of adjuvant chemotherapy after thoracotomy should be studied; it is probably indicated for patients with more than three lesions appearing 6 months to 1 year after initial surgery, for patients whose metastatic disease has not been completely resected, or for those with evidence of pleural disruption by tumor. Repeat thoracotomies may be required for subsequent recurrence and should be performed if all disease can be resected.

Survival after relapse has undeniably been enhanced by approaches designed with curative intent that incorporate repeated aggressive surgery to remove overt disease. With such treatment, 30% to 40% of patients have been reported to survive beyond 5 years after relapse,[92,98,100,101,282–285] although not all of these patients are ultimately cured. Such considerations emphasize the value of close follow-up, with frequent chest radiographs and thoracic CT scans, to detect recurrent disease when it is still resectable. Thus, for the patient with osteosarcoma, the development of metastases is not a hopeless situation; aggressive systematic treatment offers prolonged survival for many patients and the possibility of cure for a significant fraction. Ironically, as adjuvant regimens used in front-line therapy of patients are intensified and the number of patients surviving without ever developing recurrence increases, the proportion who are likely to be salvageable after relapse may decrease, because relapsing patients are more likely to have drug-resistant recurrences.

Radiation Therapy in the Treatment of Osteosarcoma

BACKGROUND. Significant experience with primary radiotherapy for osteosarcomas was obtained in the 1950s and early 1960s. Primary radiotherapy with delayed amputation gained acceptance in 1955, when Cade[286] advocated initial therapy with radiation and delayed amputation for patients in whom there was no evidence of metastasis 4 to 6 months after radiotherapy. This approach was designed to circumvent amputation in the majority of patients who were destined to develop an early relapse. Radiation doses were 7000 to 8000 cGy administered over 7 to 9 weeks at 1000 cGy/week. A few patients in Cade's series who were not subjected to delayed amputation were controlled with irradiation alone, and amputation was eventually performed. The 5-year survival rate was 21.8%. Other investigators followed a similar regime, using various radiation doses and schemes (Table 39.2-12). Subsequent surgical specimens of many of the patients managed in this fashion were found to have no histologic evidence of tumor. The ability of high radiation doses to sterilize some tumors, however, was associated with significant necrosis of normal tissue.[287–292]

Results of preoperative radiation were subsequently evaluated. Overall success with preoperative radiation followed by ablative surgery was, in general, suboptimal; most patients relapsed shortly after treatment. This led Jenkin et al.[260] at Princess Margaret Hospital to recommend limiting radiation to patients who had unresectable tumors or who were being treated for palliation only. Beck et al.[293] observed no survival advantage for preoperative radiation followed by surgery over surgery alone; furthermore, only 43% of their patients obtained any palliative benefit from radiotherapy.

Radiotherapy has, however, been shown to be successful in several distinct clinical situations—facial lesions, palliation and, possibly, as a postoperative adjuvant. High-dose combination photon and proton radiation using three-dimensional treatment planning may improve long-term local control. Guidelines for

TABLE 39.2-12. Series of Primary Radiation Followed by Delayed Surgery for Osteosarcoma

Number of Patients	*Dose*	*Machine*	*Survival (%)*
133	7000–8000 cGy in 7–9 wk, 1000 cGy/wk	2 MV	21.8
10	10,000 cGy, in 180-cGy fractions	Cobalt 60 or 2 MV	60
92	6000–8000 cGy in 230-cGy fractions		21.8
16	1600–10,500 cGy in 200-cGy fractions	Orthovoltage and 2 MV	75 (1–16 y follow-up)
54	Variable	Variable	27.5
23	1800–12,000 cGy in 2–29 wk	Orthovoltage and 2 MV	26
27	5000–6000 cGy in 25- to 30-cGy fractions		0
27	5000–6000 cGy in 5–6 wk repeated once	Orthovoltage or 1–4 MV	23

TABLE 39.2-13. Radiation Guidelines for Malignant Bone Lesions

Tumor	*Radiation Dose*	*Comments*
Osteosarcoma	70–80 Gy	See Table 39.2-12.
Chondrosarcoma	50–70 CGE	Radiation indicated for unresectable or inoperable tumors.
Giant cell tumor (osteoclastoma)	30–55 Gy	Sarcomatous transformation occurs in 10% of cases.
Hemangioendothelioma	50–60 Gy	—
Chordoma	74–75 CGE	Mixed proton photon beam.
Lymphoma	40–50 Gy	High local control with chemotherapy. Radiation may not be needed in pediatric patients.

CGE, cobalt Gy equivalent.

the use of radiotherapy for osteosarcoma and other malignant bone tumors are shown in Tables 39.2-12 and 39.2-13.

PALLIATION. Radiation therapy is extremely beneficial in patients requiring palliation of metastatic bony sarcomas; tumors at axial sites, which are unresectable; and advanced, inoperable lesions of the pelvis or extremities. A novel approach using high-dose-per-fraction radiation and intraarterial 5'-bromodeoxyuridine (BUdR) as a radiosensitizer was undertaken by the Stanford Group.[294] Pulsed 48-hour BUdR infusions were performed before each 600-cGy radiation fraction, with a total radiation dose to the primary site of 4200 to 4800 cGy in 5 weeks (seven to eight fractions). Infusions of methotrexate-leucovorin were administered simultaneously. Local control was achieved in seven of the nine patients (78%) treated.[295] However, local tissue toxicity was excessive and included subcutaneous fibrosis, nonhealing traumatic fractures, peroneal neuropathy, and atrophy. Because the patients were treated with an unusual fractionation scheme using large fractions as well as intravenous chemotherapy, the specific role of the BUdR in both the local control and the excessive toxicity was not established.

Kinsella and Glatstein[296] have used intravenous radiosensitizers of BUdR, iododeoxyuridine, or misonidazole with high-dose radiotherapy, with various fractionation schemes and usually with chemotherapy, in patients with large, unresectable primary or metastatic sarcomas. Twenty-one of 29 patients (75%) achieved local control, which was defined as freedom from symptoms and absence of growth.

These studies demonstrated the efficacy of radiation therapy in obtaining long-term local control and palliation. They lend support to further clinical investigations using radiation sensitizers with high-dose radiotherapy.

VARIANTS OF CLASSIC OSTEOSARCOMA

Dahlin and Unni[60] have identified 11 variants of the classic osteosarcoma. These accounted for 268 of 1021 (28%) cases reviewed at the Mayo Clinic. Osteosarcoma arising in the jawbone, the most common variant, is characterized by well-differentiated cells with a low metastatic potential.[60] Excluding tumors arising secondary to Paget's disease, irradiation, or dedifferentiation of a chondrosarcoma, parosteal and periosteal osteosarcomas are the most common variants of classic osteosarcoma arising in the extremities. In contrast to classic osteosarcoma, which arises within a bone, both parosteal and periosteal osteosarcomas arise on the surface of the bone (juxtacortical).

The three types of surface osteosarcomas are parosteal osteosarcoma, periosteal osteosarcoma, and high-grade surface osteosarcoma. The Mayo Clinic reported 518 surface osteosarcomas seen between 1926 and 1996. The incidence was 335 parosteal osteosarcomas (64.7%), 137 periosteal osteosarcomas (26.4%), and 46 high-grade surface osteosarcomas (8.9%). These 518 surface osteosarcomas were from a pool of 4365 osteosarcoma tumors (i.e., a ratio of 1:8.4 cases).[297]

Parosteal Osteosarcoma

Parosteal osteosarcoma is a distinct variant of conventional osteosarcoma that accounts for 4% of all osteosarcoma.[60] It arises from the cortex of a bone and generally occurs in older individuals. It has a better prognosis than classical osteosarcoma.

CLINICAL CHARACTERISTICS. There is a slight predominance of parosteal osteosarcoma in women. The distal posterior femur is involved in 72% of all cases; the proximal humerus and proximal tibia are the next most frequent sites. Parosteal osteosarcoma metastasizes slowly and has an overall survival rate of 75% to 85%.[60,298] Unni and colleagues[62] noted that all patients who died of tumor lived longer than 5 years. The natural history of parosteal osteosarcoma is progressive enlargement and late metastasis. Parosteal osteosarcoma presents a mass and occasionally is associated with pain. In contrast to conventional osteosarcoma, duration of symptoms varies from months to years. Unni et al.[298] reported that 50 of 79 patients had complaints of longer than 1 year, and one-third of this group had pain for more than 5 years. Tumor size, location, and duration of symptoms did not correlate with survival.[60]

RADIOGRAPHIC FINDINGS. Roentgenograms characteristically show a large, dense, lobulated mass broadly attached to the underlying bone without involvement of the medullary canal. If old enough, the tumor may encircle the entire bone. The periphery of the lesion is characteristically less mature than the base. Ahuja and coworkers[61] emphasized that intramedullary extension is difficult to determine from plain radiographs. Unni et al.[298] emphasized that high-grade foci did not usually alter the roentgenographic appearance of these tumors.

PATHOLOGY AND GRADING. Parosteal osteosarcoma is characterized by well-formed lamellar or woven bone with a mature spindle cell stroma with few signs of malignancy. The cellularity of the spindle cell components varies; generally, it is not anaplastic, with few mitoses.[2,3,4,59,60] The differential diagnosis is osteochondroma, myositis ossificans, and conventional osteosarcoma. Cortical tumors of the posterior femur should always be suspected of malignancy; this is a rare location for a benign osteochondroma. In contrast to sarcoma, myositis ossificans is rarely attached to the underlying bone. In addition, the periphery is more mature, both radiographically and histologically. Ahuja and colleagues[60] reviewed all cases of parosteal osteosarcoma at Memorial Sloan-Kettering Cancer Center from 1934 to 1975 and described three grades: grade I (low grade), grade II (intermediate), and grade III (high grade). They emphasized the importance of evaluating the fibroblastic, cartilaginous, and osseous components independently. Of 24 patients, eight were grade I, ten grade II, and six grade III. Unni et al.[298] reviewed 79 patients and reported that 18 were grade II (23%), and seven had high-grade foci (9%). Neither group of researchers could distinguish the three grades on plain radiographs. The survival rate of patients with grade III tumors is similar to that of patients with conventional osteosarcoma.

Jelinek et al.[299] reviewed the records of the Armed Forces Institute of Pathology and evaluated 60 patients with parosteal osteosarcomas for tumor size, location, and presence of cleavage plane; intramedullary extension; soft tissue mass; and the presence and pattern of ossification. Tumors were classified as low grade or high grade. The average maximal length for low- and high-grade tumors was 7.7 and 15.0 cm, respectively. A cleavage plane was present in 20 low-grade (62%) and 19 high-grade (68%) lesions. On cross-sectional imaging, intramedullary extension was present in 13 low-grade (41%) and 14 high-grade (50%) lesions. They concluded that a poorly defined soft tissue component distinct from the ossified matrix is the most distinctive feature of high-grade parosteal osteosarcoma and may be the optimal site to perform a biopsy.

Intramedullary involvement does not necessarily imply a worse prognosis, although this may be the case in patients with high-grade lesions.[60] Eleven of 24 patients (46%) reviewed by Ahuja[61] had medullary involvement; moreover, the patients with medullary involvement who had a local resection all had a local recurrence.

Okada and associates[297] has updated the experience of the Mayo Clinic. They reviewed the records of 226 patients. Dedifferentiation was more common (16% of patients) than previously reported. They emphasized the usefulness of cross-sectional imaging in planning surgical resection. The tumor often had extensive intramedullary, extraosseous, and adjacent soft tissue components. Medullary involvement was present in 22% of the patients, and extraosseous, unmineralized soft tissue peripheral to the mineralized cortical mass was noted in 51% of the patients. Adjacent soft tissue extension occurred in 46% of patients. In contrast to their previous studies, intramedullary involvement was not a poor prognostic factor. The authors stressed the need for long-term follow-up. Eleven of the 67 patients managed at their institution died at an average of 14 years (range, 2 to 41 years). Ten of the 11 patients died from a dedifferentiated tumor.

TREATMENT. Wide excision of the tumor is the treatment of choice. This may be accomplished either by an amputation or a limb-sparing procedure. No experience with preoperative chemotherapy or radiotherapy has been reported. Parosteal osteosarcomas are often amenable to limb preservation due to their distal location, low grade, and lack of local invasiveness. If the adjacent neurovascular bundle is free of tumor, resection is feasible. Vascular displacement is not a contraindication for resection. The major surgical decision usually is whether to remove the entire end of the bone and the adjacent joint or to preserve the joint. Small lesions can be resected with joint preservation. If the medullary canal is involved, the joint usually cannot be preserved. A second factor mitigating against joint preservation is extensive cortical involvement. Techniques of resection and reconstruction are similar to those described for conventional osteosarcoma. The major difference is that only a small amount of soft tissue usually must be resected; consequently, a good functional result is obtained. Grade III parosteal lesions warrant systemic therapy because of the risk of metastasis.

Periosteal Osteosarcoma

Periosteal osteosarcoma is a rare cortical variant of osteosarcoma that arises superficially on the cortex, most often on the tibia shaft.[61] Radiographically, it is a small, radiolucent lesion with some evidence of bone spiculation. The cortex is characteristically intact, with a scooped-out appearance and a Codman's triangle (Fig. 39.2-12). Histologically, periosteal osteosarcomas are relatively high-grade chondroblastic osteosarcoma composed of a malignant cartilage with areas of anaplastic spindle cells and osteoid production. Unni and colleagues,[60] in a report of 23 cases, found periosteal osteosarcomas to be one-third as frequent as the parosteal variant. The largest tumor measured 2.5 × 3.5 cm. Four of the 23 patients died of metastatic disease.

One of the largest reported series was by Okada et al.[297] from the Mayo Clinic. They evaluated 46 patients and described their radiographic, clinical, and pathologic evaluation. All the tumors were broad based and attached to the underlying cortex. Nineteen of the 46 tumors (41%) showed infiltration into the cortex of the underlying bone. Medullary involvement was documented on gross or radiologic examination in 13 tumors and by microscopic examination only in six tumors. They attempted to evaluate the effectiveness of chemotherapy in this very rare subtype of osteosarcoma. Fifteen of the 21 patients receiving systemic treatment showed no response to chemotherapy. Among those 15 patients, only one patient remains alive. All six patients who showed a good response to chemotherapy are alive. Medullary involvement did not affect prognosis. The survival rate was 57.5% at 3 years and 46.1% at 5 years.

Treatment is similar to that of other high-grade lesions. *En bloc* resection should be performed when feasible; amputation is rarely indicated. Table 39.2-12 compares the significant characteristics of periosteal tumors with those of conventional osteosarcoma.

Paget's Sarcoma

Approximately 1% of patients with Paget's disease will develop a primary bone sarcoma.[229,230] Greditzer and colleagues[230] reported 41 sarcomas among 4415 patients with Paget's disease followed at the Mayo Clinic; 35 were osteosarcomas and six were fibrosarcomas. The average patient age was 64 years old, and the most common sites were the pelvis, femur, and humerus. One-half of these lesions were osteolytic; the remainder had a mixed pattern. Cortical destruction and a soft tissue component were the most common signs noted; periosteal ele-

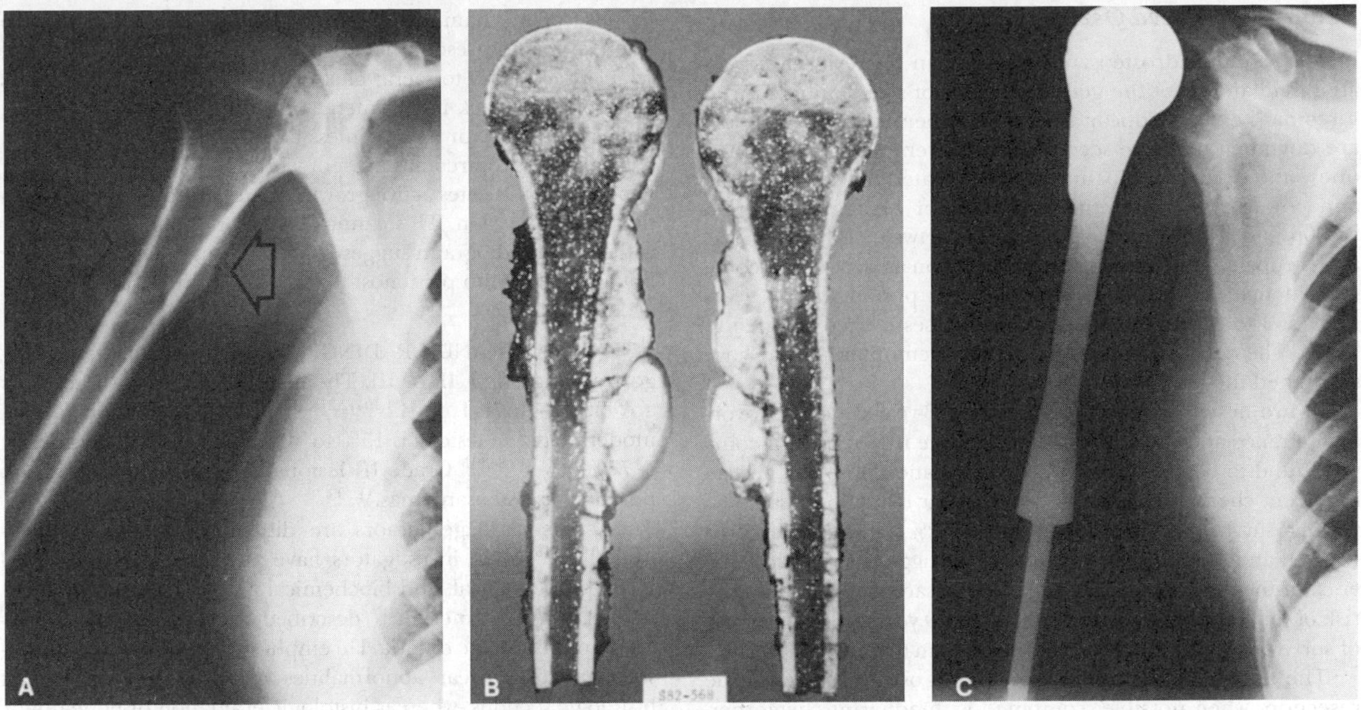

FIGURE 39.2-12. Periosteal osteosarcoma. **A:** Typical radiograph of a periosteal osteosarcoma of the humerus. Notice the cortical location with a scooped-out defect of the lateral aspect of the shaft and the diaphyseal location. **B:** Longitudinal section of the gross specimen after a limb-sparing resection. The tumor seems to arise on the outer cortex without any evidence of cortical involvement. **C:** Postoperative radiograph. A custom prosthesis was used to reconstruct the defect. (From Hall RB, Robinson LH, Malawar MM, Dunham WK. Periosteal osteosarcoma. *Cancer* 1985;55:165, with permission.)

vation was rare. Most patients with this condition present with pain; thus, a patient with known Paget's disease who complains of increasing pain, especially when it is well localized, should be evaluated radiographically. The diagnosis is usually made by plain radiography and confirmed by biopsy. Traditionally, fewer than 8% of patients survive, and most deaths occur within 2 years.[230] Treatment is similar to that recommended for adolescent patients with osteosarcoma without metastatic disease.

High-Grade Surface Osteosarcoma

High-grade surface osteosarcoma (peripheral conventional osteosarcoma) is the rarest variant of surface osteosarcoma.[300] The parosteal and periosteal osteosarcomas have a better prognosis, whereas the high-grade surface variant has the same prognosis as the conventional, intramedullary lesion. This variant was previously called *type III parosteal osteosarcoma.* Schajowicz and coworkers[300] studied the different surface osteosarcomas. They reported that only 7 of 80 surface osteosarcomas (9%) were considered to be the high-grade variant. Clinically, the median age was 13.5 years (younger than that of patients with other surface lesions), and almost all were located in the diaphyseal region of the bone. The femur was the most common site. These tumors may show extensive intramedullary involvement. Radiographically, it appears as a small or moderate-size lesion with slight to heavy calcification. The broad base of the lesion abuts the cortex. The radiographic features often are misleading and may suggest the periosteal variant; thus, the preoperative diagnosis may be difficult. But the young age, diaphyseal location and, most important, the highly malignant histologic features indicate the correct diagnosis. Wide excision with limb preservation has been reported. Adjuvant chemotherapy is warranted due to the high rate of metastases.

Small Cell Osteosarcoma

The small cell osteosarcoma, a rare variant of osteosarcomas, resembles a Ewing's sarcoma and is often classified as an "atypical" Ewing's sarcoma.[301,302] Characteristically, areas of osteoid and, on occasion, chondroid formation are present. The differential diagnosis includes Ewing's sarcoma, atypical Ewing's sarcoma, primitive neuroectodermal tumor, mesenchymal chondrosarcoma, lymphoma, and Askin's tumor. Differentiation from Ewing's sarcoma and the typical osteosarcoma is important, because the response of small cell osteosarcoma to treatment is poorly defined.

Devaney and colleagues[303] from the Bone Branch of the Armed Forces Institute of Pathology evaluated 79 round cell tumors of bone with immunohistochemistry in an attempt to distinguish small cell osteosarcoma from the other round cell tumors of bone. They noted that none reacted with cytokeratin, epithelial membrane antigen, factor VIII–related antigen, synaptophysins, or Leu-M1-positive. Thus, a strong positivity of any of these studies should rule out small cell osteosarcoma. Vimentin was seen in the majority of the various tumor types. They concluded that immunohistochemical stains alone could not make the diagnosis.

Sim et al.[301] recommend surgery, whereas at the Pediatric Branch of the National Cancer Institute, these tumors, like other pediatric round cell tumors, are treated by a combination of radiation therapy and chemotherapy.

Radiation-Induced Osteosarcoma

Radiation-induced osteosarcomas arise in a previously irradiated field and meet the general criteria of a radiation-induced sarcoma [i.e., they appear after a latent period of 5 to 20 years, are documented to be secondary (different from the original one), and occur in a documented irradiated field]. Amendola and coworkers[304] from the University of Michigan reviewed 22,306 patients treated with radiation between 1934 and 1983 and reported 23 patients with radiation-associated sarcoma (prevalence, 0.1%). The median latent period was 13 years (range, 3 to 34 years). The radiation doses ranged from 25 to 72 Gy. The data suggest that intensive chemotherapy may have shortened the latency period.

In two nested case-control studies of 3-year cancer survivors from France and the United Kingdom, the risk of osteosarcoma was found to be a linear function of radiation dose and alkylating agent chemotherapy.[305,306] The 20-year risk of osteosarcoma among survivors of retinoblastoma (7.2%), Ewing's sarcoma (5.4%), and other bone tumors (2.2%) suggests a genetic influence in the induction of secondary osteosarcoma. However, the risk of developing bone sarcoma within 20 years for the majority of survivors of childhood cancer is less than 0.9%.

The treatment of radiation-associated osteosarcoma is wide resection, when possible, combined with adjuvant chemotherapy.[307] A previously irradiated field presents a unique challenge for the surgeon—choosing the best local option. The likelihood of local complications is greater in such cases.

CHONDROSARCOMA

Chondrosarcoma is the second most common primary malignant spindle cell tumor of bone.[2] Chondrosarcomas form a heterogeneous group of tumors whose basic neoplastic tissue is cartilaginous without evidence of direct osteoid formation.[329] Occasionally, bone formation occurs from differentiation of cartilage. If evidence is found of direct osteoid or bone production, the lesion is classified as an osteosarcoma. The five types of chondrosarcomas are central, peripheral, mesenchymal, differentiated, and clear cell.[2–4,10] The classic chondrosarcomas are central (arising within a bone) or peripheral (arising from the surface of a bone). The other three are variants and have distinct histologic and clinical characteristics.

Both central and peripheral chondrosarcomas can arise as primary tumors or secondary to underlying neoplasm. Seventy-six percent of primary chondrosarcomas arise centrally.[2,10–12,308] Secondary chondrosarcomas most often arise from benign cartilage tumors. The multiple forms of benign osteochondromas or enchondromas have a higher rate of malignant transformation than the corresponding solitary lesions.[11,12,58,215]

Central and Peripheral Chondrosarcomas

CLINICAL CHARACTERISTICS. One-half of all chondrosarcomas occur in persons older than 40 years of age.[2,216] Only 3.8% occur in those younger than 20 years.[2] The most common sites are the pelvis (31%), femur (21%), and shoulder girdle (13%).[11,12,215–216] Chondrosarcomas are the most common malignant tumors of the sternum and scapula. The clinical presentation varies. Peripheral chondrosarcomas may become large without causing pain, and local symptoms develop only because of mechanical irritation. Pelvic chondrosarcomas are often large and present with referred pain to the back or thigh, sciatica secondary to sacral plexus irritation, urinary symptoms from bladder neck involvement, unilateral edema due to iliac vein obstruction, or as a painless abdominal mass. Conversely, central chondrosarcomas present with dull pain; a mass is rare. Pain, which indicates active growth, is an ominous sign of a central cartilage lesion. This cannot be overemphasized. An adult with a plain radiograph suggestive of a "benign" cartilage tumor but associated with pain most likely has a chondrosarcoma.

HISTOLOGY AND GRADING. Chondrosarcomas are categorized as grade I, II, or III. The majority of chondrosarcomas are either grade I or II.[1,10–12,215,216,308] The metastatic rate of moderate-grade lesions is 15% to 40%; in high-grade lesions, it is 75%.[1,10,11,12,86,215] Grade III lesions have the same metastatic potential as osteosarcomas.[11,308]

Because cartilage tumors are difficult to grade histologically,[10,215,216] some investigators have attempted to apply cytologic, histochemical, and biochemical analysis to evaluate these lesions.[215,309,310] Sanerkin[215] described a combination of cytologic and histologic criteria. He emphasized that cytologic analysis evaluates nuclear abnormalities better than conventional histologic sections, whereas histologic evaluation of bone-tumor interface is the best predictor of local aggressiveness. Krocberg and colleagues[311] performed a retrospective study of DNA content of 45 chondrosarcomas as an indicator of malignancy by evaluating diploid (normal DNA content) and hyperploid (abnormal increase in DNA) cells and correlating the findings to 10-year survival. Regardless of tumor grade, size, and location, patients with diploid cells had a better prognosis than those with hyperploid cells. A preliminary report assessing the malignancy of cartilage tumor by flow cytometry to determine the percentage of diploid, tetraploid, and aneuploid cells indicates that it may be a promising method of grading chondrosarcomas.[311]

RADIOGRAPHIC DIAGNOSIS AND EVALUATION. Central chondrosarcomas have two distinct radiologic patterns.[312] One is a small, well-defined lytic lesion with a narrow zone of transition and surrounding sclerosis with faint calcification. This is the most common malignant bone tumor that may appear radiographically benign. The second type has no sclerotic border and is difficult to localize. The key sign of malignancy is endosteal scalloping. It is difficult to diagnose on plain radiographs and may go undetected for a long period. In contrast, peripheral chondrosarcoma is recognized easily as a large, calcified mass protruding from a bone. Its differential diagnosis includes large benign osteochondroma, parosteal osteosarcoma, and juxtacortical myositis ossificans. Correlation of clinical, radiographic, and histologic data is essential for accurate diagnosis and evaluation of the aggressiveness of cartilage tumor. Proximal or axial location, skeletal maturity, and pain point toward malignancy, even though the cartilage may appear benign.

PROGNOSIS. Metastatic potential tends to correlate with the histologic grade of the lesions.[10,11,12,308] Marcove et al.[308] reported on long-term follow up of 113 chondrosarcomas of the proximal femur and the pelvis. The survival rates in patients with grade I, II, or III lesions were 47%, 38%, and 15%, respectively; the overall survival rate was 52%. No significant difference was noted between grades I and II; however, the mortality rate for grade III was significantly higher ($P<.02$) than for the other two. Eleven of 59 deaths occurred after 5 years. The authors emphasized that the meaningful survival interval should be considered 10 or 15 years. No relationship between grade, age, gender, or location was found, and there was no statistical difference between primary and secondary chondrosarcomas. Adequacy of surgical removal was the main determinant of recurrence. In general, chondrosarcomas occurring during childhood have a worse prognosis than those of adult onset.[313]

In a review of 125 chondrosarcomas at the Rizzoli Institute, Gitellis and colleagues[13] reported that adequacy of treatment was the main determinant of local recurrence, length of survival, and length of disease-free interval. Patients adequately treated had a 6% local recurrence rate, whereas the recurrence rate among those inadequately treated was 69%. The 10-year survival rates were 78% (adequately treated) versus 61% (inadequately treated). No relation between local recurrence and grade was determined.

In the largest reported series of chondrosarcomas from one institution, Bjornsson et al.[314] from the Mayo Clinic reported the experience and the clinical pathologic profiles of 344 patients with chondrosarcomas over 80 years. They analyzed the anatomic site, clinical history, and overall survival. Survival analysis was limited to 233 patients whose primary tumors were treated at the Mayo Clinic. The minimum follow-up was 5 years. The overall 5-year survival rate was 77%. Local recurrence developed in 19.7% of patients, and metastatic lesions in 13.7%. The recurrence rate was higher for tumors of the shoulder and pelvis than for tumors of long bones. Histologic tumor grade was an important predictor of local recurrence and metastases.

In general, peripheral chondrosarcomas have a lower grade than central lesions. Gitellis et al.[13] reported that 43% of peripheral lesions, compared with 13% of central lesions, were grade I. The 10-year survival rate among those with peripheral lesions was 77%, and among those with central lesions was 32%. Secondary chondrosarcomas arising from osteochondromas also have a low malignant potential. Eighty-five percent are grade I. Garrison and associates[58] reported that only 3% of 75 patients with secondary chondrosarcomas from an osteochondroma developed metastases, although 12% died of local recurrence.

TREATMENT. The treatment of chondrosarcomas is surgical removal.[10,12,308,313,315] No reports of effective adjuvant chemotherapy have been published. Resection guidelines for high-grade chondrosarcomas are similar to those for osteosarcoma. The shoulder and pelvic girdle are the most common sites for chondrosarcomas. This, combined with the fact that chondrosarcomas tend to be low grade, make them amenable to limb-sparing procedures. Lesions of the ribs and sternum are treated by wide excision. Cryosurgery, a technique using liquid nitrogen after thorough curettage of the lesion, has been used for central, low-grade chondrosarcomas.[131,132] There have been a few reports of effective radiation therapy for axial chondrosarcomas and, more recently, encouraging reports using fractionated proton radiation therapy for the low-grade chondrosarcomas arising at the base of the skull.[316] The Massachusetts General Hospital group report a 5-year local control rate of 82% and a 10-year local control rate of 58% among 28 patients with low-grade base-of-skull chondrosarcomas treated to approximately 69 CGE (cobalt Gy equivalent) using the proton beam.[317] High-grade chondrosarcomas warrant consideration of adjuvant chemotherapy.

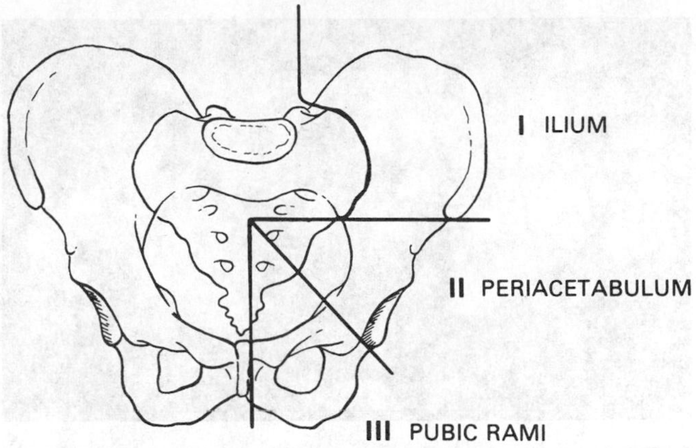

FIGURE 39.2-13. Segmental resection for pelvic tumors.

Limb-Sparing Procedures: Specific Anatomic Sites

The four most common sites of chondrosarcomas are the pelvis, proximal femur, shoulder girdle, and diaphyseal portions of long bones. The unique characteristics of each are described in the following sections.

PELVIS. The pelvis consists of three areas: ilium, periacetabulum, and pubic rami (Fig. 39.2-13). Each site may be resected independent of the others.[30,316] Resections are classified as type I (iliac wing), type II (acetabulum), or type III (public rami, pelvic floor). Bone scan most accurately determines specific bony involvement, whereas CT and MRI delineate the extraosseous component. Contraindications to resection are vascular (iliac artery and vein), peritoneal, and sacroiliac joint and/or sarcoplexus involvement.

The retroperitoneal space is explored first to determine resectability. Type I resection is performed by a supraacetabular osteotomy and disarticulation of the sacroiliac joint. Type II resection may require removal of the femoral head; intraarticular involvement of the hip joint by tumor is evaluated by arthrotomy before finalizing the surgical plan. Type II and III resections require mobilization of the iliac vessels and femoral nerve. Care must be taken to protect these structures. Type III procedure requires mobilization of the bladder and urethra before resection. Bilateral pelvic floor resection may be used for chondrosarcomas arising from the midline of the symphysis pubis, in which case urethral resection and reconstruction may be required. Partial cystectomy may be necessary.

Long-term results of these procedures have been published by Enneking and Dunham,[30] who reported that local recurrence was only 4% if adequate margins were obtained. Function was nearly normal if the hip joint was preserved. If the hip joint was removed and fusion was obtained, results were good. A saddle prosthesis (Fig. 39.2-14) has been developed, permitting reconstruction after periacetabular resections with minimal morbidity.[318]

Treatment of malignant tumors of the pelvis is one of the greatest challenges in musculoskeletal oncology. Kawai and coworkers[319] reviewed 102 patients with localized pelvic sarco-

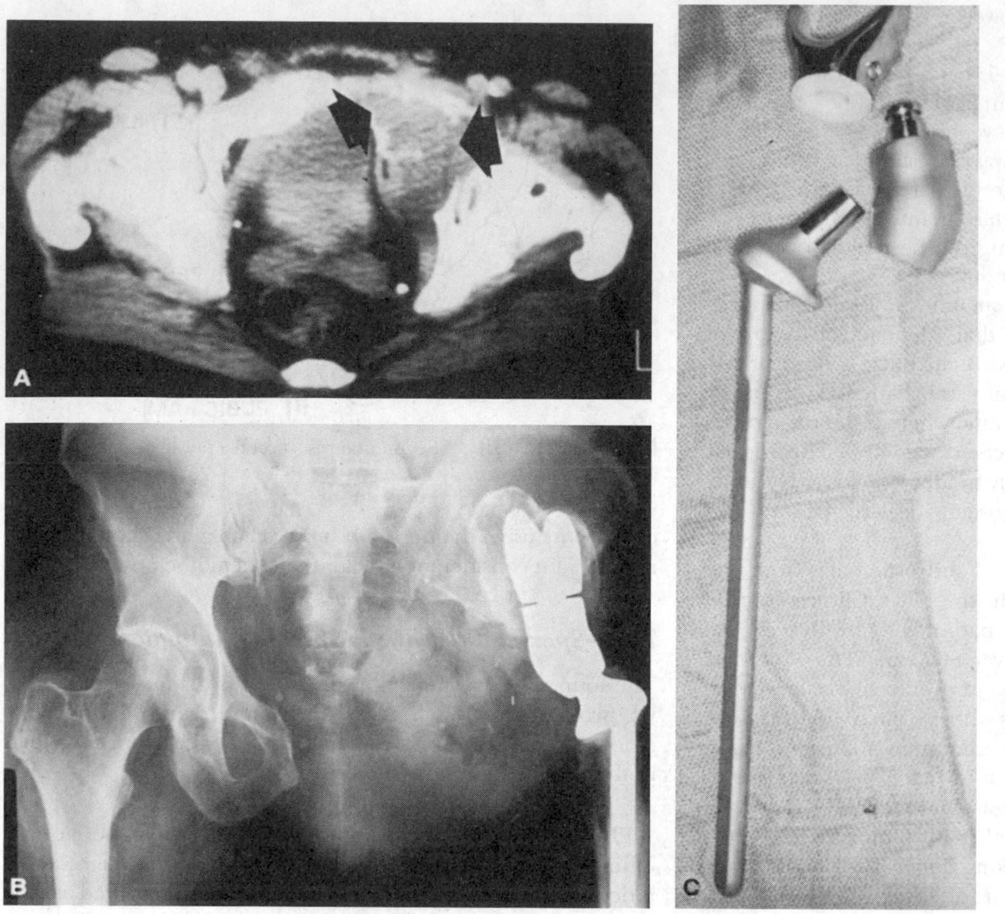

FIGURE 39.2-14. Limb-sparing resection for a large periacetabular chondrosarcoma involving the pelvic floor. **A:** Computed tomography shows acetabular destruction by a large tumor mass (*arrows*) with involvement of the pubic rami. **B:** The patient was treated by an internal hemipelvectomy (type II and III resection). **C:** A custom-made saddle prosthesis was used for the reconstruction. This is a new type of pelvic prosthesis that has made pelvic reconstruction more reliable with less morbidity than other techniques.

mas who underwent surgical excision at Memorial Sloan-Kettering Cancer Center. Chondrosarcoma was the most common diagnosis. They evaluated the prognostic factors for local recurrence, metastasis, and survival. The 5-year survival rate for sarcomas of pelvic chondrosarcomas was 65%. An inadequate surgical margin was the only independent prognostic factor for local recurrence. For distant metastases, surgical stage (i.e., histologic grade and site) is an independent prognostic factor.

PROXIMAL FEMUR. Chondrosarcoma of the proximal femur can often be treated successfully by resection and prosthetic replacement. A lateral trephine biopsy is recommended. Care must be taken to avoid intraarticular contamination. A posterior approach should be avoided because of potential contamination of the posterior flap in the event a hemipelvectomy is required.

SHOULDER. The technique of resection of chondrosarcomas of the proximal humerus and scapula is similar to that described for osteosarcomas. In low-grade, intracompartmental (stage IA) tumors, preservation of the deltoid, rotator cuff musculature, and glenoid is possible, and alternatives for reconstruction are more variable. Endoprostheses, fibula autografts, and allografts all have a high rate of success.[35–40,139–141,254,255]

DIAPHYSEAL SEGMENTS OF THE TIBIA, FEMUR, AND HUMERUS. Central diaphyseal chondrosarcomas can be adequately treated by segmental resection without sacrificing the adjacent joint. Because the ends of the bones are not involved, function is excellent. Reconstruction is performed by allografts or autografts combined with internal fixation.

CRYOSURGERY. Marcove et al.[130–132] pioneered the technique of cryosurgery for bone tumors. This method involves thorough curettage and cryotherapy of the cavity with liquid nitrogen. With increasing experience, the indications were expanded to low-grade intramedullary cartilage tumors as well as to some high-grade lesions. With these indications, they have treated 30 chondrosarcomas with only one local recurrence. The major advantages of cryosurgery are preservation of bone stock and the avoidance of resection.

Schreuder et al.[320] reported the experience of 26 benign and low-grade intramedullary chondrosarcomas treated with curettage and cryosurgery. Fourteen enchondromas and nine grade I chondrosarcomas were treated with curettage, cryosurgery, and bone grafting. After a follow-up of 26 months, no recurrences were observed. The most common complication was postoperative fracture (two cases). All bone grafts had incorporated, resulting in full weight-bearing capacity and excellent functional results. These authors emphasized that the preoperative assessment of these lesions is essential and that only low-grade cartilage tumors should be treated with a cryosurgical technique.

Variants of Chondrosarcoma

CLEAR CELL CHONDROSARCOMA. Clear cell chondrosarcoma, the rarest form of chondrosarcoma, is a slow-growing, locally recurrent tumor resembling a chondroblastoma but with some malignant potential.[321] It generally occurs in adults. The most difficult clinical problem of this entity is early recognition. It is often confused with chondroblastoma. Metastases occur only after multiple local recurrences. Primary treatment is wide excision. Systemic therapy is not required.

MESENCHYMAL CHONDROSARCOMA. Mesenchymal chondrosarcoma is a rare, aggressive variant of chondrosarcoma characterized by a biphasic histologic pattern (i.e., small, compact cells intermixed with islands of cartilaginous matrix).[322–324] It has a predilection for flat bones; long, tubular bones are rarely affected.[216] It tends to occur in younger individuals and has high rates of metastatic potential. Harwood and colleagues[322] reported that 8 of 17 patients died within 1 year of diagnosis. The 10-year survival rate is 28%.[322] This entity responds favorably to radiotherapy. It is hypothesized that the round cell component, similar to other round cell sarcomas, is relatively radiosensitive. Treatment is surgical removal combined with adjuvant chemotherapy. Radiotherapy is recommended if the tumor cannot be completely removed.[324]

Approximately 10% of chondrosarcomas may be dedifferentiated into a fibrosarcoma or osteosarcoma.[2,10,11,57] This occurs in older individuals and is highly fatal. Surgical treatment is similar to that described for other high-grade sarcomas. Adjuvant therapy is warranted.

Radiation Therapy in the Treatment of Chondrosarcoma

Unresectable or inoperable chondrosarcomas arising within the axial skeleton and pelvic and/or shoulder girdle can be controlled, and in some cases cured, by radiation therapy. A unique situation is chondrosarcomas of the facial bones and skull, in which a combination of radiotherapy and surgery has been shown to be successful.

Although chondrosarcomas have generally been considered radioresistant, data exist to show that some are radiocurable.[324] Among 38 patients undergoing radical irradiation, with or without concurrent chemotherapy, at the Princess Margaret Hospital, 5- and 10-year actuarial survival rates of 41% and 36%, respectively, were achieved. Median survival was 46 months.[324] The best results, a 48% 5-year actuarial survival rate, were obtained in the group with favorable (well and moderately differentiated) histology. Conversely, for those with unfavorable (mesenchymal and poorly differentiated) histology, the 5-year survival rate was only 22%. Radical radiotherapy was defined as a minimum of 40 Gy in 4 or more weeks of megavoltage therapy. Of the 38 patients treated, 17 developed local recurrence. The authors recommend 50 Gy in 4 weeks with treatment to the whole bone if possible and, if not, at least a 5-cm margin of normal bone. These authors noted tumor regression continued slowly for 2 to 3 years after therapy.

McNaney et al.,[325] from the M. D. Anderson Cancer Center, reported 20 patients with chondrosarcoma treated with photons and/or neutrons, with or without chemotherapy. The doses of radiation administered ranged from 4000 to 7000 cGy. Thirteen of 20 (65%) were surviving at 30 months' median follow-up. Among the 11 patients treated with radiotherapy alone, six survived (54%). Six patients, all of whom had received photon therapy alone, developed local failure. No local failures were reported among the four patients treated with a mixed beam of photons and neutrons. Similarly, Hug et al.[326] reported 100% local control and disease-free status for six patients with axial skeleton chondrosarcoma treated with a mean target dose of 73.9 CGE delivered using a 160 MeV proton beam and 23 MV megavoltage beam.

After radical irradiation, clinical regression of tumor is slow and may take months to complete. Radiographically, the affected bone never returns to normal. The combination of extremely slow regression of tumor with a persistent radiologic defect makes follow-up and assessment of response difficult. No rebiopsy data are available to document long-term sterilization of these tumors. Radiotherapy for chondrosarcoma can provide palliation. In such cases, high doses (in the range of 5000 cGy in 4 to 5 weeks, or its equivalent) are necessary; low doses for symptomatic relief are ineffective.[327]

Ryall et al.[328] used radiation and the radiosensitizer razoxane (ICRF 159) in eight patients with 12 chondrosarcomas. Seven tumors in five patients achieved complete or partial remission after 4500 to 6000 cGy. Two or the responders were disease-free 2.5 years after treatment.

GIANT CELL TUMOR OF BONE

GCT is an aggressive, locally recurrent tumor with a low metastatic potential.[14–16,64–65,216,336] It consists of spindle-shaped and ovoid cells uniformly interspersed with multinucleated giant cells. *Giant cell sarcoma of bone* is a term that refers to the *de novo*, malignant GCT, not the tumor that arises from the transformation of a GCT previously thought to be benign. These two lesions are separate clinical entities.

Clinical Characteristics

GCTs occur slightly more often in females than in males. Pain, mass, local tenderness, and decreased motion in the adjacent joint are the most common clinical symptoms. Eighty percent of GCTs in the long bones occur after skeletal maturity, and 75% of these develop around the knee joint.[3,63] An effusion or pathologic fracture, uncommon with other sarcomas, is common with GCTs. GCTs occasionally occur in the vertebrae (2% to 5%) and the sacrum (10%).[2–4]

Grading and Pathologic Characteristics

Jaffe[4] attempted to grade GCTs as grade I (completely benign), grade II (borderline), and grade III (frankly sarcomatous). In general, grades I and II do not correlate well with biologic behavior. There is also a poor correlation between the histologic pattern and the tendency for recurrence or malignant transformation.[14,15,64,216] Nineteen percent to 25% of GCTs have some osteoid production.[216] When osteoid formation is noted, care must be exercised in differentiating a GCT from an osteosarcoma. Conversely, an osteosarcoma with giant cells may be misinterpreted as a benign GCT. No correlation has been found between osteoid formation and increased risk of recurrence or metastasis. Necrosis or hemorrhage is often noted. Neither has a relationship to malignant potential or local recurrence rate.[64]

Natural History

Although GCTs are rarely malignant *de novo* (2% to 8%),[14,330] they may undergo transformation and demonstrate malignant potential histologically and clinically after multiple local recurrences.[14–16] Between 8.6% and 22% of known GCTs become malignant after local recurrence.[14–16,216,330] This rate decreases to less than 10% if patients who have undergone radiotherapy are excluded from the series. Hutter noted that 40% of malignant GCTs were malignant at the first recurrence[15]; the remainder had become malignant by the second or third recurrence. Thus, each recurrence increases the risk of malignant transformation of typical GCT, especially if the transformation occurs after radiation therapy. Local recurrence of a GCT is determined by the adequacy of surgical removal rather than histologic grade.

Radiographic and Clinical Evaluation

Giant cell tumors are eccentric lytic lesions without matrix production. They have poorly defined borders with a wide area of transition. They are juxtaepiphyseal with a metaphyseal component. Although the cortex is expanded and appears destroyed at surgery, it is usually found to be attenuated but intact. Periosteal elevation is rare; soft tissue extension is common.

Treatment

Treatment of GCT of bone is surgical removal. Resection is curative in 90% of these tumors,[14,15] whereas curettage, with or without bone grafts, has a recurrence rate of 40% to 75%.[14–16,64,331] Johnson and Dahlin[16] reported a recurrence rate of 29% within 1 year of curettage and of 54.1% within 5 years. O'Donnell and colleagues[332] reviewed the literature from 1970 to 1990 and reported an overall recurrence rate of approximately 40%.

Although *en bloc* excision offers a reliable cure, routine resection is not recommended.[331–333] Primary resection of a joint has a significant morbidity. It is recommended for GCT of the proximal radius and fibula, distal ulna, tubular bones of the hand and foot, coccyx, sacrum, and pelvic bones. Under certain situations, a curettage is reasonable. If the lesion heals, resection is avoided. In general, curettage does not rule out a later curative resection. Today, the technique of curettage is more extensive than previously performed. Curettage is accomplished through a large cortical window, equal to the length of the bony defect, using both mechanical curettage and a mechanical burr. This extensive technique has been termed *curettage/resection* and has decreased the rate of local recurrence to approximately 15% to 25%. Bone graft and PMMA are used to reconstruct the surgical defect.

O'Donnell et al.[332] reviewed the experience at the Massachusetts General Hospital of 60 patients with GCTs treated by curettage and packing with PMMA. The overall rate of local recurrence was 25% (15 of 60 patients) occurring at an average of 4 years. Risk factors for local recurrence were pathologic fracture, stage III disease, anatomic site, and the use of adjuvant treatment. The distal radius and the proximal tibia had the highest rate of local recurrence: 50% (five of ten patients) and 28% (7 of 25 patients), respectively. These authors emphasized that adjuvant treatment with a high-speed burr or PMMA, or both, after curettage decreased the local recurrence rate from 42% (8 of 19 patients) to 17% (7 of 41 patients). They concluded that PMMA alone did not reduce the rate of local recurrence, but that the use of a wide curettage combined with additional curettage with a high-speed burr is necessary.

Malawer et al.,[334] in a multicenter study of 100 cases of GCTs of the extremities (treated with wide curettage, high-speed burr, and either a single or double cycle of cryosurgery with liquid nitrogen), reported a local recurrence rate of 9% (9 of 100 patients). They used the direct-pour technique as described by Marcove.[131,132] Reconstruction of the surgical defect was performed with PMMA (combined with internal fixation in most cases). The secondary fracture rate was 5%. Only two patients required a secondary resection and prosthetic replacement. These authors recommend liquid nitrogen adjuvant after curettage in the treatment of GCTs.

Amputation is reserved for massive recurrence, malignant transformation, or infection. Because of the biologic propensity for malignant transformation, radiation is reserved for specific lesions, usually lesions of the spine, that cause bone destruction in a confined area and can lead to spinal cord compression and severe deformity.[335] Thus, treatment of GCT of the vertebrae and sacrum must be individualized. A combination of surgical excision and cryosurgery or radiotherapy is required to eradicate the tumor and prevent neurologic impairment.[117]

Cryosurgery

Cryosurgery has been used more successfully for GCTs than for any other type of bone tumor.[130–132,334] Marcove[131,132] developed the technique of cryosurgery because of the high recurrence rates after curettage and the significant risk of sarcomatous degeneration in GCTs treated by irradiation. He found cryosurgery effective in eradicating the tumor while preserving joint motion and avoiding resection or amputation. He reported a 17-year experience of 100 GCTs treated by thorough curettage and cryosurgery.[131] He noted a recurrence rate of 16% in the first 50 cases and 2% in the following 50 cases. The major complications of cryosurgery are necrosis of the adjacent bones, which are liable to develop a late pathologic fracture, and delayed union. The rate of secondary pathologic fracture has been decreased by a combination of PMMA, augmentation, bone graft, internal fixation of the cavity, and postoperative use of a long-leg brace with a quadrilateral socket.[336,337] Persson and Wouters[338] have reported curettage with PMMA augmentation of the bony defect with bony necrosis due to the heat of polymerization. This technique may provide better local control than curettage alone.

Bickels and colleagues[333] reported 102 patients treated by curettage and cryosurgery at two institutions between 1983 and 1993. The surgical stage was I in 15 cases, II in 47 cases, and III in 40 cases. Sixteen percent of the patients had presented with local recurrences. The local recurrence rate among 86 patients treated primarily with cryosurgery was 2.3%. There were six local recurrences among 16 patients who were referred with recurrent disease. The overall recurrence rate was 7.9%. The most common complication was pathologic fracture (5.9%). No pathologic fractures occurred when internal fixation was used along with PMMA. This study emphasized that the overall function was good to excellent in 92% of the patients. All 102 patients were free of disease at final follow-up.

Cryosurgery is a powerful physical adjunct to curettage in the treatment of GCTs of bone. Bickels and colleagues[333] recommend routine use of cryosurgery for all GCTs of long bones.

Giant Cell Tumors of the Sacrum

Giant cell tumors of the sacrum are difficult to treat. Patients often present with back pain, neurologic deficits, and rectal symptoms. The diagnosis is often delayed. CT, MRI, and bone scintigraphy are required for accurate local anatomic staging. Turcotte et al.[339] reviewed the treatment of 26 patients treated at the Mayo Clinic between 1960 and 1986 with an average follow-up of 7.8 years. Neurologic deficit was present in 88%. The local recurrence rate for patients treated by curettage was 33%. Twenty-one patients had radiation therapy; malignant transformation occurred in three. They suggested initial treatment is complete curettage. Radiation therapy is recommended for incomplete resection and local recurrence. Resection of the sacrum should be reserved for extensive recurrences. The technique of surgical resection of the sacrum is similar to the combined anterior and posterior approach described for chordomas.

RADIATION THERAPY. The specific indications for radiation include inoperable and incompletely resected lesions, and lesions that occur locally despite definitive surgery. These situations are most likely to occur in the spine.[335] Doses of 35 to 50 Gy in 4 to 5.5 weeks using megavoltage equipment is recommended.

Although concern has been raised about malignant transformation after radiotherapy.[340–349] transformation also occurs independent of radiation, most often after multiple local recurrences, suggesting that this observation is best explained by the natural history of the disease.[350]

Giant cell tumor is not radioresistant, as was once believed. Local control rates range from 75% to 85% in more recent series.[339,342–344] The Princess Margaret Hospital group has reported that local control was achieved in 13 of 14 patients with GCT treated with one course of megavoltage radiation. The disease in 12 patients was controlled for longer than 5 years.[342] The researchers observed no instance of malignant transformation. Larsson and colleagues[335] reported three patients with GCT of the spine and sacrum treated by moderate doses of radiotherapy; all have done well. Similarly, the Gainesville group reports 12 of 16 tumors (75%) controlled locally with 35 to 54 Gy, with no untoward complications or sccondary sarcomas.[343] Several authors now suggest curettage, followed by planned megavoltage radiation, as a good alternative to complex and difficult surgery.

MALIGNANT FIBROUS HISTIOCYTOMA

Clinical Characteristics

MFH is a high-grade bone tumor histologically similar to its soft tissue counterpart.[7–9] It is a disease of adulthood. The most common sites are the metaphyseal ends of long bones, especially around the knee. AP values are normal. Pathologic fracture is common. Huvos[9] emphasized that a lytic metaphyseal lesion with a pathologic fracture in an adult with a normal serum AP level suggests a primary MFH rather than an osteosarcoma or fibrosarcoma. MFH disseminates rapidly. Spanier and colleagues[7] reported that 9 of 11 patients died of the tumor. The average disease-free survival was 6 months. One-third of patients (three of nine) with pulmonary metastasis had lymph node dissemination. The author hypothesized that lymphatic spread was due to the histiocytic component of the tumor.

Radiographic Characteristics

MFH is an osteolytic lesion associated with marked cortical disruption, minimal cortical or periosteal reaction, and no evidence of matrix formation.[9] The extent of the tumor routinely exceeds plain radiographic signs. McCarthy et al.,[8] reporting on 35 patients with MFH, noted that four tumors were multicentric and four were associated with bone infarcts.

Treatment

Today, MFH and osteosarcoma of bone are treated in much the same way. Data demonstrate that results of limb-sparing surgery for MFH of bone, as well as responses to chemotherapy among MFH patients, are very similar to those of patients with primary osteosarcoma. Picci et al.,[351] in the largest review to date, evaluated the effects of neoadjuvant chemotherapy of MFH of bone and extremity osteosarcomas. They reported 51 patients treated with high-grade MFH of bone and 390 patients with high-grade osteosarcoma treated with identical regimens of neoadjuvant chemotherapy at the Rizzoli Institute between 1982 and 1994. All tumors were located in the limbs. Preoperative chemotherapy was performed according to three successively activated regimens consisting of methotrexate and *cis*-diamminedichlorplatinum II (CDP): MTX/CDP intraarterially, MTX/CDP plus Adriamycin, and MTX/CDP plus Adriamycin and ifosfamide). Rates of limb salvage were approximately the same for MFH (92%) and osteosarcoma (85%). Although MFH showed a statistically significantly lower rate of good histologic response, the rate of tumor necrosis for MFH was 90% or more [27% vs. 67% for osteosarcoma (P <.001)] for all three regimens. Despite this low chemosensitivity, the disease-free survival rates for the two neoplasms were similar (67% vs. 65%). Nevertheless, the two tumors had similar prognoses when treated with chemotherapy regimens based on methotrexate, cisplatinum, Adriamycin, and ifosfamide. The surgical procedures were both similar limb-sparing procedures. This study emphasized that induction chemotherapy, followed by limb-sparing surgery and subsequent postoperative chemotherapy, was just as effective for MFH of bone as for the osteosarcomas.[339]

Bacci et al.,[352,353] also from the Rizzoli Institute, reported on 65 patients treated with MFH of bonc in the extremities with neoadjuvant chemotherapy. The limb-salvage rate was 89% (58 patients) and amputation rate was 11% in seven patients. The histiologic response to preoperative chemotherapy was good (90% or more tumor necrosis) in 16 patients (25%) and poor in 49 patients (75%). At a median follow-up of 7 years, 40 patients (69%) remained free of disease and 20 patients experienced relapse (18 metastases and two local recurrences followed by metastases). The rate of disease-free survival was significantly higher for patients who had a good response than for those who had a poor response (94% vs. 61%). Similarly, these authors concluded that a high percentage of patients with MFH of the extremities can be cured with neoadjuvant chemotherapy and that it is usually possible to avoid amputation. Similarly, Nishida and colleagues[354] from the Mayo Clinic reviewed their experience with MFH of the extremities and reported that the overall prognosis for patients with MFH was not significantly different from that of patients with osteosarcoma. The primary approach to the treatment of MFH of bone is similar to that of osteosarcoma—wide surgical resection (usually limb-sparing surgery) combined with pre- and postoperative chemotherapy. Similar chemotherapeutic regimens are recommended.

FIBROSARCOMA OF BONE

Clinical Characteristics

Fibrosarcoma of bone is a rare entity characterized by interlacing bundles of collagen fibers (herringbone pattern) without any evidence of tumor bone or osteoid formation.[5] Fibrosarcoma occurs in middle age. The long bones are most affected. Fifteen percent of tumors are found in the bones of the head and neck.[216] Fibrosarcomas occasionally arise in conjunction with an underlying disease, such as fibrous dysplasia, Paget's disease, bone infarcts, osteomyelitis, and postirradiation bone and GCT.[5] Fibrosarcoma may be either central or cortical (periosteal). The histologic grade is a good prognosticator of metastatic potential. Huvos and Higinbotham[5] reported overall survival rates of 27% and 52% for central and peripheral lesions, respectively. Late metastases do occur, and 10- and 15-year survival rates vary. In general, periosteal tumors have a better prognosis than central lesions.

Radiographic Features

Fibrosarcoma is a radiolucent lesion that shows minimal periosteal and cortical reaction. The radiographic appearance closely correlates with the histologic grade of the tumor.[5] Low-grade tumors are well-defined, whereas high-grade lesions demonstrate indistinct margins and bone destruction similar to that of osteolytic osteosarcoma. In general, plain radiographs underestimate the extent of the lesion. Pathologic fracture is common (30%) owing to the lack of matrix formation. Differential diagnosis includes GCT, ABC, MFH, and osteolytic osteosarcoma.[5,6]

Fibrosarcoma of bone is primarily managed surgically. Irradiation is recommended for inoperable tumors, for patients with postsurgical residual disease, and for palliation.

MALIGNANT HEMANGIOENDOTHELIOMA OF BONE

Malignant hemangioendothelioma of bone (also referred to as *epithelioid hemangioepitheliod sarcoma* or *histiocytoid hemangioma*) comprises only 0.5% to 1.0% of primary malignant bone tumors.[355–358] More than one-third of these lesions arise in the long, tubular bones, especially those of the lower extremity.[356,358] Incidence peaks in the third decade of life, but the tumor can present at any age. Multicentric lesions are common. The treatment of choice has been surgery, often in combination with radiotherapy.[358] In rare cases, radiotherapy has been the sole modality of treatment.[355,357,358] Radiation doses in the range of 50 to 60 Gy are associated with long-term local control. Chemotherapy plays no significant role in treatment.

CHORDOMA

Chordoma is a rare neoplasm arising from notochordal remnants in the midline of the neural axis and involving the adjacent bone. The ends of the spine are the most common sites. The sacrococcus and the base of the skull (35%) near the spheno-occipital area are most commonly involved, accounting for 50% and 35%, respectively, of all chordomas.[216] Histologically, the physaliferous cell is pathognomonic. Large areas of syncytial strands of cells lying in a mass of mucus are typically present. Myxoid chondrosarcoma and metastatic carcinoma must be differentiated. This tumor is highly fatal because of the high rate of local recurrence and local complications.[359–362] Death is most commonly due to local disease.[359] Gray and colleagues[362] reviewed 222 cases from the literature and noted that only two patients were disease-free at 10 years. Average survival was 5.7 years. Mindell[359] emphasized that the main malignant potential of chordomas resides in their critical locations adjacent to important structures, their locally aggressive nature, and their extremely high rate of recurrence. Chordomas at the base of the skull are often described as chondroid chordomas. Patients with these lesions at this site tend to survive longer than those with the sacrococcygeal tumors.

The most common complaint of patients with sacrococcygeal tumors is dull pain; constipation is an occasional symptom. Bladder and sensory loss are late complaints. Clinical suspicion is the key to early diagnosis. Rectal examination characteristically reveals a large presacral mass. Spheno-occipital tumors present with signs of cranial nerve or pituitary dysfunction, or both. CT and MRI are essential for accurate evaluation. Myelography is used to determine intraspinal extension. A transrectal biopsy should not be performed because of potential contamination. A small midline posterior incision or trocar biopsy is recommended.

Treatment

The first surgical procedure has the best chance of cure.[361,362] Inadequate surgery results in local recurrence, with little chance of subsequent surgical removal. Sacrococcygeal tumors are best removed by a combined abdominosacral approach, as described by Localio and colleagues.[360,361] They emphasized wide excision of the sacrum one level higher than the lesion. A lateral position is used. The rectum can be mobilized and the iliac vessels controlled anteriorly. The rectum may be removed with the sacrum if necessary. Guterberg et al.[364] reported that if only one-half of the first sacral vertebra remains bilaterally, the pelvic girdle is still stable enough to allow immediate mobilization. DeVries and associates[363] reported two long-term survivors (7 years and 10 years) after cryosurgery of sacral chordomas.

Radiation Therapy

Because local recurrence is common with chordomas, radiation therapy is an integral treatment modality, particularly for tumors of the base of skull and spheno-occipital region. Results of conventional radiation therapy have been disappointing. Heffelfinger et al.[365] reported on 36 patients with nonchondroid varieties of chordomas of the base of skull, none of whom were rendered free of disease by surgery, radiation, or a combination thereof. However, the chondroid variant is more sensitive; of 19 patients with chondroid chordomas, seven were alive and six were disease-free.

Amendola et al.,[366] reported on 21 patients with a 5-year survival rate of 50% but a disappointing 10-year survival rate of only 20%. This is not surprising, because chordomas are relatively slow-growing. In fact, long-term survival free of tumor regrowth over 10 years is relatively rare. Amendola et al. emphasized the importance of using CT in planning the radiation field, administration of high radiation doses (i.e., 5500 to 7000 cGy with megavoltage equipment), and use of irradiation immediately after surgery to prolong local control, rather than reserving it until recurrence. The Massachusetts General Hospital experience of 48 patients is similar to that reported by others; 50% of the patients survived years or more.[367] Radiation doses varied from

4500 to 8040 cGy, but even with high doses, a 45% incidence of local recurrence was reported. The Princess Margaret Hospital group investigated various fraction schedules in an effort to impact local control. They used conventionally fractionated radiation at a median dose of 50 Gy in 25 fractions over 5 weeks, and a hyperfractionated course of 1 Gy over 4 hours four times per day, with a median dose of 40 Gy in 44 fractions over 14 days. No difference was found between the conventional or hyperfractionated regimen with respect to symptomatic response or progression-free interval. With a median survival of 65 months, the authors concluded that external-beam radiation provided useful palliation but was rarely curative.[368,369]

Investigators now advocate using precision heavy-charged particle irradiation, particularly for chordoma of the basisphenoid region and cervical spine. The Massachusetts General Hospital experience now includes 68 patients, 40 with chordomas and 28 with low-grade chondrosarcomas of the basosphenoid region and cervical spine, who have been treated with proton-beam radiation therapy at a median tumor dose of 69 CGE. The actuarial 5-year disease-free survival rate is 76%, whereas the local control rate is 82%.[370,371] No difference was found in local control between those patients with low-grade chondrosarcoma and those with either chondroid or nonchondroid chordoma.[370] Hug and the Massachusetts General Hospital investigators[326] have reported axial skeleton chordoma treated with a myxoid proton and photon beam (mean dose of 73.9 CGE). Five of 14 patients (36%) had local recurrence, and two of the five developed distant metastases. The 5-year actuarial local control and overall survival rates were 53% and 50%, respectively, for the chordoma patients. Other groups also report local control and reversal of neurologic symptoms and signs using 75.5 Gy proton therapy for chordoma of the clivus.[372] Proton therapy should be considered after initial surgical removal for inoperable clivus chordoma.

Stereotactic radiosurgery has been tried for skull-based tumors and is a potential means to provide symptomatic relief for small-volume (4 cm or smaller) tumors.[373,374]

SMALL ROUND CELL SARCOMAS OF BONE

Round cell sarcomas of bone behave differently than spindle cell sarcomas and require different therapeutic management.[375,376] These tumors consist of poorly differentiated small cells without matrix production. They present radiographically as osteolytic lesions. These lesions are best treated with radiation and chemotherapy; surgery is reserved for special situations. Non-Hodgkin's lymphoma and Ewing's sarcoma are the two most common small cell sarcomas. The differential diagnosis of all round cell sarcomas includes metastatic neuroblastoma, metastatic undifferentiated carcinoma, histiocytosis, small cell osteosarcoma, osteomyelitis, and multiple myeloma.

LYMPHOMAS OF BONE (DIFFUSE LARGE CELL LYMPHOMA)

Lymphoma of bone (previously called *reticulum cell sarcoma of bone*) accounts for only 5% of the primary bone tumors. In general, lymphoma presenting in bone is a sign of disseminated (stage IV) disease; occasionally, it may be a true solitary lesion defined as "involvement of single extralymphatic organ or site" (stage IE).[375,376] Reimer and coworkers[375] at the National Cancer Institute reported that only 1 of 12 patients presenting with bone lymphomas had a true solitary lesion. Sweet and colleagues[376] from the University of Chicago reported that 50% of so-called "solitary" lesions were associated with disease elsewhere. Sweet et al. presented a useful algorithm for the evaluation and treatment of bone lymphomas. They emphasized that all patients with a presumed solitary lymphoma of bone should undergo a thorough evaluation for other involvement.[376]

Treatment is based on extent of disease. Stage IE lesions have traditionally been treated with radiotherapy, with a reported 90% cure rate.[375] The role of surgery is limited to obtaining adequate tissue for diagnosis and treatment of pathologic fracture. The technique of biopsy is important to avoid secondary fracture through potentially irradiated bone. Biopsy for a suspected round cell tumor should always include a frozen section and additional material for electron microscopy, tissue culture, and immunophenotyping. Patients presenting with pathologic fractures require fixation. To prevent late fractures, all patients treated with radiotherapy should be protected with a brace until reossification occurs.

Radiation Therapy

Local control of the primary tumor with retention of good function of the affected part is commonly achieved after radiation therapy. Radiation therapy is administered to the entire bone and soft tissue extent with a dose of 4000 cGy and a boost to the original tumor area of 500 cGy. Regional lymph nodes should be included in the radiation port if they are adjacent to the area treated or if clinically involved. Mendenhall et al.[377] from the University of Florida achieved local and regional control in all irradiated sites among 21 patients with primary bone lymphomas. Two patients relapsed in apparently uninvolved regional lymph node sites that had not been included in the primary treatment portal.

Patients with lymphoma of the bone should be considered to have systemic disease; accordingly, they require chemotherapy. Patients treated with radiation and Adriamycin-based chemotherapy have long-term survival in the 90% to 100% range. The Dana Farber Cancer Center reported 90% lymphoma-free survival at 8 years, with radiation and the Adriamycin, prednisone, and Oncovin combination regimen.[378] Similarly, the Bone Tumor Center in Bologna, Italy, reports 88% disease-free survival at 7.5 years with radiation and Adriamycin, vincristine, and cyclophosphamide.[379] Patients presenting with monostotic disease have a better outcome than those with polystoic disease.[380,381] Although a randomized controlled clinical trial testing radiation therapy and chemotherapy versus radiation therapy alone has not been performed, combined modality is commonly used in adults with primary and non-Hodgkin's lymphoma of the bone.[383,384] The international index parameters of age 60 years or younger, normal lactate dehydrogenase, and Eastern Cooperative Oncology Group performance status of 0 are prognostic factors for good outcome.[382] The Dana Farber investigators reported second bone tumors 5 and 7.5 years after combined modality therapy. Because of this concern and the success of intensive combination chemotherapy, investigators have begun to question the need for primary radiation therapy among children responding to multiagent chemotherapy.[385,386] The Pediatric Oncology Study Group[387] studied the impact of localized bone radiotherapy in children with early-stage primary non-Hodgkin's lymphoma, all of whom received multiagent chemotherapy. Thirty of 31 were disease-free and all survived, thus leading these investigators to recommend a 9-week chemotherapy regimen of modest intensity without radiation therapy as definitive treatment of children with localized primary lymphoma of the bone.

REFERENCES

1. Landis SH, Murray T, Bolden S, et al. Cancer statistics, 1999. *CA Cancer J Clin* 1999;49:8.
2. Dahlin DC. *Bone tumors: general aspects and data on 6221 cases,* 3rd ed. Springfield, IL: Charles C Thomas Publisher, 1978.
3. Lichtenstein L. *Bone tumors,* 5th ed. St. Louis: Mosby, 1977.
4. Jaffe HL. *Tumors and tumorous conditions of the bone and joints.* Philadelphia: Lea & Febiger, 1958.
5. Huvos AG, Higinbotham NL. Primary fibrosarcoma of bone. A clinicopathologic study of 130 patients. *Cancer* 1975;35:837.
6. Wilner D. Fibrosarcoma. In: Wilner D, ed. *Radiology of bone tumors and allied disorders.* Philadelphia: WB Saunders, 1982:2291.
7. Spanier SS, Enneking WF, Enriquez P. Primary malignant fibrous histiocytoma of bone. *Cancer* 1975;36:2084.
8. McCarthy EF, Matsuno T, Dorfman HD. Malignant fibrous histiocytoma of bone: a study of 35 cases. *Hum Pathol* 1979;10:57.
9. Huvos AG. Primary malignant fibrous histiocytoma of bone: clinicopathologic study of 18 patients. *N Y State J Med* 1976;76:552.
10. Shives TS, Wold LE, Dahlin DC, Beaubout JW. Chondrosarcoma and its variants. In: Sim FH, ed. *Diagnosis and treatment of bone tumors: a team approach.* Mayo Clinic Monograph. Thorofare, NJ: Slack Inc., 1983:211.
11. Marcove RC. Chondrosarcoma: diagnosis and treatment. *Orthop Clin North Am* 1977;8:811.
12. Pritchard DJ, Lunke RJ, Taylor WF, et al. Chondrosarcoma: a clinicopathologic statistical analysis. *Cancer* 1980;45:149.
13. Gitellis S, Bertoni F, Chieti PP, et al. Chondrosarcoma of bone. *J Bone Joint Surg Am* 1981;63:1248.
14. Dahlin DC, Cupps RE, Johnson EW Jr. Giant cell tumor: a study of 195 cases. *Cancer* 1970;25:1061.
15. Hutter VP, Worcester JN Jr, Francis KC, et al. Benign and malignant giant cell tumor of bone. A clinicopathological analysis of the natural history of the disease. *Cancer* 1962;15:653.
16. Johnson EW Jr, Dahlin DC. Treatment of giant cell tumor of bone. *J Bone Joint Surg Am* 1959;41:895.
17. Nascimento AG, Huvos AC, Marcove RC. Primary malignant giant cell tumor of bone: a study of eight cases and review of the literature. *Cancer* 1979;44:1393.
18. Weingard DN, Rosenberg SA. Early lymphatic spread of osteogenic and soft tissue sarcomas. *Surgery* 1978;84:231.
19. Enneking WF, Spanier SS, Goodman MA. A system for the surgical staging of musculoskeletal sarcoma. *Clin Orthop* 1980;153:106.
20. Marcove RC, Rosen G. *En bloc* resection for osteogenic sarcoma. *Cancer* 1980;45:3040.
21. Malawer MM. Distal femoral osteogenic sarcoma, principles of soft tissue resection and reconstruction in conjunction with prosthetic replacement (adjuvant surgery). In: Chao EYS, ed. *Design and application of tumor prosthesis for bone and joint reconstruction.* New York: Thieme-Stratton, 1983:297.
22. Morton DL, Eilber FR, Townsend CM Jr, et al. Limb salvage from a multidisciplinary treatment approach for skeletal and soft tissue sarcomas of the extremity. *Ann Surg* 1976;184:268.
23. Enneking WF, Dunham WK. Resection and reconstruction for primary neoplasms involving the innominate bone. *J Bone Joint Surg Am* 1978;60:731.
24. Marcove RC, Lewis MM, Rosen G, et al. Total femur and total knee replacement: a preliminary report. *Clin Orthop* 1977;126:147.
25. Eilber FR, Morton DL, Eckardt J, Grant T, Weisenburger T. Limb salvage for skeletal and soft tissue sarcomas. Multidisciplinary preoperative therapy. *Cancer* 1984;53:2579.
26. Eilber FR, Eckhardt J, Morton DL. Advances in the treatment of sarcomas of the extremities. Current status of limb salvage. *Cancer* 1984;54:2695.
27. Weisenberg TH, Eilber FR, Grant TT, et al. Multidisciplinary "limb salvage" treatment of soft tissue and skeletal sarcomas. *Int J Radiat Oncol Biol Phys* 1981;7:1495.
28. Simon MA, Aschliman MA, Thomas N, et al. Limb salvage treatment versus amputation for osteosarcoma of the distal end of the femur. *J Bone Joint Surg Am* 1986;68:1331.
29. Enneking WF. Modification of the system for functional evaluation of surgical management of musculoskeletal tumors. In: Enneking WF, ed. *Limb-sparing surgery for musculoskeletal tumors.* New York: Churchill Livingstone, 1987:626.
30. Enneking WF, Dunham WK. Resection and reconstruction for primary neoplasms involving the innominate bone. *J Bone Joint Surg Am* 1978;60:731.
31. Marcove RC, Lewis MM, Rosen G, et al. Total femur and total knee replacement. A preliminary report. *Clin Orthop* 1977;126:147.
32. Mankin HJ, Fogelson FS, Thrasher AZ, et al. Massive resection and allograft transplantation in the treatment of malignant bone tumors. *N Engl J Med* 1976;294:1247.
33. Watts HG. Introduction to resection of musculoskeletal sarcomas. *Clin Orthop* 1980; 153:31.
34. Enneking WF, Shirley PD. Resection-arthrodesis for malignant and potentially malignant lesions about the knee using an intramedullary rod and local bone graft. *J Bone Joint Surg Am* 1977;59:223.
35. Janeck CJ, Nelson CL. *En bloc* resection of shoulder girdle: technique and indications. Report of a case. *J Bone Joint Surg Am* 1972;54:1754.
36. Francis KC, Worcester JN Jr. Radical resection for tumors of the shoulder with preservation of a functional extremity. *J Bone Joint Surg Am* 1962;44:1423.
37. Marcove RC, Lewis MM, Huvos AG. *En bloc* upper humeralinterscapular resection, the Tikhoff-Linberg procedure. *Clin Orthop* 1977;124:219.
38. Chaos EYS, Ivins JC. *Design and application of tumor prosthesis for bone and joint reconstruction. The design and application.* New York: Theime-Stratton, 1983.
39. Malawer MM, Sugarbaker PH, Lambert M, et al. Limb salvage surgery for tumors of the proximal humerus and shoulder girdle. The Tikhoff-Linberg procedure and its modifications. *Surgery* 1955;97:518.
40. Sim FH, Bowman WE, Chao EYS. Limb salvage surgery and reconstructive techniques. In: Sim FH, ed. *Diagnosis and treatment of bone tumors: a team approach.* Mayo Clinic Monograph 75-105. Thorofare, NJ: Slack, Inc., 1983.
41. DeSantos LA, Bernardino ME, Murry JA. Computed tomography in the evaluation of osteosarcoma: experience with 25 cases. *AJR Am J Roentgenol* 1979;132:535.
42. Destouet JM, Gilula LA, Murphy W. Computed tomography of long bone osteosarcoma. *Radiology* 1979;131:439.
43. McKillop JH, Etcubanas E, Goris ML. The indications for and limitations of bone scintigraphy in osteogenic sarcoma: a review of 55 patients. *Cancer* 1981;48:1133.
44. Levine E. Computed tomography of musculoskeletal tumors. *Crit Rev Diagn Imaging* 1981;16:279.
45. Rosenthal DI. Computed tomography in bone and soft tissue neoplasm: application and pathologic correlation. *Crit Rev Diagn Imaging* 1982;18:243.
46. Goldstein H, McNeil BJ, Zufall E, et al. Changing indications for bone scintigraphy in patients with osteosarcoma. *Radiology* 1980;135:177.
47. Bacci G, Picci P, Calderoni P, et al. Full lung tomograms and bone scanning in the initial workup of patients with osteogenic sarcoma. A review of 126 cases. *Eur J Cancer Clin Oncol* 1982;18:1967.
48. Jaffe N, Link MP, Cohen D, et al. High-dose methotrexate in osteogenic sarcoma. *Natl Cancer Inst Monogr* 1981;56:201.
49. Cortes EP, Holland JF, Wang JJ, et al. Amputation and Adriamycin in primary osteosarcoma. *N Engl J Med* 1974;291:998.
50. Rosen G, Marcove RC, Caparros B, et al. Primary osteogenic sarcoma. The rationale for preoperative chemotherapy and delayed survey. *Cancer* 1979;43:2163.
51. Rosen G, Caparros B, Huvos AC, et al. Preoperative chemotherapy for osteogenic sarcoma: selection of postoperative adjuvant chemotherapy based upon the response of the primary tumor to preoperative chemotherapy. *Cancer* 1982;49:1221.
52. Muggia F, Catani R, Lee YJ, et al. Factors responsible for therapeutic success in osteosarcoma. In: Jones S, Salmon S, eds. *Adjuvant therapy for cancer,* 2nd ed. New York: Grune & Stratton, 1979.
53. Cortes EP, Holland JP. Adjuvant chemotherapy for primary osteogenic sarcoma. *Surg Clin North Am* 1981;61:1391.
54. Rosen G, Murphy ML, Huvos AG, et al. Chemotherapy, *en bloc* resection and prosthetic replacement in the treatment of osteogenic sarcoma. *Cancer* 1976;37:1.
55. Goorin AM, Frei E II, Abelson HT. Adjuvant chemotherapy for osteosarcoma: a decade of experience. *Surg Clin North Am* 1981;61:1379.
56. Lichenstein L. Classification of primary tumors of bone. *Cancer* 1951;4:335.
57. Spjut HJ, Dorfman HD, Fechner DE, Ackerman LV. *Tumors of bone and cartilage.* Atlas of Tumor Pathology Fasc. 5, 2nd series. Washington, DC: Armed Forces Institute of Pathology, 1971.
58. Garrison RC, Unni KK, McLeod RA, Pritchard DJ, Dahlin DC. Chondrosarcoma arising in osteochondroma. *Cancer* 1982;49:1890.
59. Merryweather R, Middlemiss JH, Sanerkin NG. Malignant transformation of osteoblastoma. *J Bone Joint Surg (Br)* 1980;62:381.
60. Dahlin DC, Unni KK. Osteosarcoma of bone and its important recognizable varieties. *Am J Surg Path* 1977;1(1):61.
61. Ahuja SC, Villacin AB, Smith J, et al. Juxtacortical (parosteal) osteogenic sarcoma. *J Bone Joint Surg Am* 1977;59:632.
62. Unni KK, Dahlin DC, Beaubout SW. Periosteal osteogenic sarcoma. *Cancer* 1976;37:2476.
63. Unni KK, Dahlin DC, McLeod RA, Pritchard DJ. Interosseous well-differentiated osteosarcoma. *Cancer* 1977;40:1337.
64. Goldenberg RR, Campbell CJ, Bongfiglio M. Giant cell tumor of bone. An analysis of two hundred and eighteen cases. *J Bone Joint Surg Am* 1970;52:619.
65. Johnson EW, Dahlin DC. Treatment of giant cell tumor of bone: an evaluation of 24 cases treated at the Johns Hopkins hospital between 1925–1955. *Clin Ortho* 1969;62:187.
66. Madewell JE, Ragsdale BD, Sweet DE. Radiographic and pathologic analysis of solitary bone lesions. *Radiol Clin North Am* 1981;19:715.
67. Johnson LC. A general theory of bone tumors. *Bull N Y Acad Med* 1953;19:164.
68. Lodwick GS. The bone and joints. In: *Atlas of tumor radiology.* Chicago: Year Book Medical Publishers, 1971.
69. Enneking WF. *Musculoskeletal tumor surgery,* Vol I. New York: Churchill Livingstone, 1983:1.
70. Jeffree GM, Price CHG, Sissins HA. The metastatic spread of osteosarcoma. *Br J Cancer* 1975;32:87.
71. McKenna RJ, Schwinn CP, Soong KY, Higinbotham NL. Sarcoma of the osteogenic series (osteosarcoma, fibrosarcoma, chondrosarcoma, parosteal osteosarcoma and sarcomata) arising in abnormal bone: an analysis of 552 cases. *J Bone Joint Surg Am* 1966;48:1.
72. Marcove RC, Mike V, Hajack JV, et al. Osteogenic sarcoma under the age of 21. *J Bone Joint Surg Am* 1970;52:411.
73. Sweetnam R. Surgical management of primary osteosarcoma. *Clin Orthop* 1975;111:57.
74. Campanacci M, Bacci G, Bertoni F, et al. The treatment of osteosarcoma of the extremities: twenty years' experience at the Instituto Ortopedico Rizzoli. *Cancer* 1981;48:1569.

75. Campanacci M, Bacci G, Bertoni F, et al. The treatment of osteosarcoma of the extremity: twenty years' experience at the Instituto Orthopedico Rizzoli. *Cancer* 1981;48:1569.
76. Brostrom LA. On the natural history of osteosarcoma. Aspects of diagnosis, prognosis and endocrinology. *Acta Orthop Scand (Suppl)* 1980;183:1.
77. Enneking WF, Kagan A. Intramarrow spread of osteosarcoma. In: *Management of primary bone and soft tissue tumors.* Chicago: Year Book Medical Publishers, 1976:171.
78. Malawer MM, Dunham WF. Skip metastases in osteosarcoma: recent experience. *J Surg Oncol* 1983;22:236.
79. Enneking WF, Spanier SS, Malawer MM. The effect of the anatomic setting on the results of surgical procedure for soft parts sarcoma of the thigh. *Cancer* 1981;47:1005.
80. Simon MA, Spanier SS, Enneking WF. The management of soft tissue tumors of the extremities. *J Bone Surg (Am)* 1976;60:317.
81. Simon MA. Intraarticular extension of adult primary bone sarcomas: implications for limb-sparing surgical procedures. In: Chao EYS, Ivins JS, eds. *Design and application of tumor prosthesis for bone and joint reconstruction.* New York: Thieme-Stratton, 1983.
82. Bohndorf K, Reiaer M, Lochner B, et al. Magnetic resonance imaging of primary tumours and tumourlike lesions of bone. *Skeletal Radiol* 1986;15:511.
83. Cohen MD, Weetman RM, Provisor AJ, et al. Efficacy of magnetic resonance imaging in 139 children with tumors. *Arch Surg* 1986;121:522.
84. Turner DA. Nuclear magnetic resonance in oncology. *Semin Nucl Med* 1985;15:210.
85. Zimmer WD, Berquist TH, McLeod RA, et al. Bone tumors: magnetic resonance imaging versus computed tomography. *Radiology* 1985;155:709.
86. Powers JA. Magnetic resonance imaging in marrow diseases. *Clin Orthop* 1985;206:79.
87. Sundaram M, McGuire MH, Herbold DR. Magnetic resonance imaging of osteosarcoma. *Skeletal Radiol* 1987;16:23.
88. Easton EJ, Powers JA. *Musculoskeletal magnetic resonance imaging.* Thorofare, NJ: Slack, Inc., 1986.
89. Pettersson H, Springfield DS, Enneking WF. Radiologic management of musculoskeletal tumors. Philadelphia, Springer, 1999.
90. Link MP. Adjuvant therapy in the treatment of osteosarcoma. In: DeVita VT, Hellman S, Rosenberg SA, eds. *Important advances in oncology.* Philadelphia: JB Lippincott Co, 1986:193.
91. Link MP, Goorin AM, Miser AW, et al. The effect of adjuvant chemotherapy on relapse-free survival in patients with osteosarcoma of the extremity. *N Engl J Med* 1986;314:1600.
92. Eilber F, Guiliano A, Eckardt J, et al. Adjuvant chemotherapy for osteosarcoma: a randomized prospective trial. *J Clin Oncol* 1987;5:21.
93. Edmonson J, Creagan E, Gilchrist G. Phase II study of high dose methotrexate in patients with unresectable metastatic osteosarcoma. *Cancer Treat Rep* 1981;65:5438.
94. Rosen G, Nirenberg A. Chemotherapy for osteogenic sarcoma: an investigative method, not a recipe. *Cancer Treat Rep* 1982;66:1687.
95. Dahlin DC. The problems in assessment of new treatment regimens of osteosarcoma. *Clin Orthop* 1980;153:81.
96. Goorin A, Perez-Atayde A, Gebhardt M, et al. Weekly high-dose methotrexate and doxorubicin for osteosarcoma: the Dana Farber Cancer Institute/the Children's Hospital—study III. *J Clin Oncol* 1987;5:1178.
97. Ettinger LJ, Douglas HO, Mindell ER, et al. Adjuvant Adriamycin and cisplatin in newly diagnosed, nonmetastatic osteosarcoma of the extremity. *J Clin Oncol* 1986;4:353.
98. Rosen G, Marcove RC, Huvos AG, et al. Primary osteogenic sarcoma: 8-year experience with adjuvant chemotherapy. *J Cancer Res Clin Oncol* 1983;106[Suppl]:55.
99. Winkler K, Beron G, Kotz R, et al. Neoadjuvant chemotherapy for osteogenic sarcoma. Results of a cooperative German/Austrian study. *J Clin Oncol* 1984;2:617.
100. Winkler K, Beron G, Delling G, et al. Neoadjuvant chemotherapy of osteosarcoma: results of a randomized cooperative trial (COSS82) with salvage chemotherapy based on histological tumor response. *J Clin Oncol* 1988;6:329.
101. Enneking WF, Spanier SS, Goodman MA. A system for the surgical staging of musculoskeletal sarcoma. *Clin Orthop* 1980;153:106.
102. Tobias JD, Pratt CB, Parham DM, et al. The significance of calcified regional lymph nodes at the time of diagnosis of osteosarcoma. *Orthopedics* 1985;8:49.
103. Giuliano AE, Feig S, Eilber F. Changing metastatic patterns of osteosarcoma. *Cancer* 1984;54:2160.
104. Jaffe N, Smith E, Abelson H, Frei E. Osteogenic sarcoma. Alterations in the pattern of pulmonary metastases with adjuvant chemotherapy. *J Clin Oncol* 1983;1:251.
105. Fleming ID, Cooper JS, Henson DE, et al. (eds). *American Joint Committee on Cancer Staging Manual,* 5th ed. Philadelphia: JB Lippincott, 1997.
106. Iwasawa T, Tanaka Y, Aida N, et al. Microscopic intraosseous extension of osteosarcoma: assessment on dynamic contrast enhanced MRI. *Skeletal Radiol* 1997;26:214.
107. Hudson TM, Hass G, Enneking WF, Hawkins EF. Angiography in the management of musculoskeletal tumors. *Surg Gynecol Obstet* 1975;141:21.
108. Malawer MM, McHale KA. Limb-sparing surgery for high-grade malignant tumors of the proximal tibia: surgical technique and a new method of extensor mechanism reconstruction. Fourth International Symposium on Limb-Salvage Surgery in Musculoskeletal Oncology, Kyoto, Japan, 1987.
109. Menendez LR, Fideler BM, Mirra J. Thallium-201 scanning for the evaluation of osteosarcoma and soft-tissue sarcoma. *J Bone Joint Surg Am* 1993;75:526.
110. Rosen G, Loren GJ, Brien EW, et al. Serial thallium-201 scintigraphy in osteosarcoma. Correlation with tumor necrosis after preoperative chemotherapy. *Clin Orthop* 1993;293:302.
111. Springfield D. Thallium-201 scanning for the evaluation of osteosarcoma and soft-tissue sarcoma. *J Bone Joint Surg Am* 1999;75:1880.
112. Tokuumi Y, Tsuchiya H, Sunayama C, et al. Thallium-201 scintigraphy for diagnosis, evaluation of chemotherapy effects and detection of local recurrence in musculoskeletal neoplasms. *Abstract Book* 1995:175.
113. Bloem JL, Taminiau AHM, Eulderink F, Hermans J, Pauwels EKJ. Radiologic staging of primary bone sarcoma: MR imaging, scintigraphy, angiography and CT correlated with pathologic examination. *Radiology* 1988;169:805.
114. Enneking WF. The issue of the biopsy. *J Bone Joint Surg Am* 1982;64:1119.
114a. Ayala AG, Raymond AK, Ro JY, et al. Needle biopsy of primary bone lesions. M. D. Anderson experience. *Pathol Annu* 1989;24(1):219.
115. Mankin HJ, Lange TA, Spanier S. The hazards of biopsy in patients with malignant primary bone and soft-tissue tumors. *J Bone Joint Surg Am* 1982;64:1121.
116. Moore TM, Meyers MH, Patzakis MJ, et al. Closed biopsy of musculoskeletal lesions. *J Bone Joint Surg Am* 1999;61:375.
117. Savino R, Gherlinzoni F, Morandi M, et al. Surgical treatment of giant cell tumor of the spine. *J Bone Joint Surg Am* 1983;65:1283.
118. Schajowicz F, Derqui JC. Puncture biopsy in lesions of the locomotor system. Review and results in 4050 cases, including 941 vertebral punctures. *Cancer* 1968;21:5331.
119. Mail JT, Cohen MD, Mirkin LD, Provisor AJ. Response of osteosarcoma to preoperative intravenous high-dose methotrexate chemotherapy: CT evaluation. *AJR Am J Roentgenol* 1985;144:89.
120. Jaffe N, Knapp J, Chuang VP, et al. Osteosarcoma: intraarterial treatment of the primary tumor with cis-diamminedichlorplatinum II (CDP): angiographic, pathologic, and pharmacologic studies. *Cancer* 1983;51:402.
121. Chuang VP, Benjamin R, Jaffe N, et al. Radiographic and angiographic changes in osteosarcoma after intraarterial chemotherapy. *AJR Am J Roentgenol* 1982;139:1065.
122. Carrasco CH, Charnsangavel C, Raymond AK, et al. Osteosarcoma: angiographic assessment of response to preoperative chemotherapy. *Radiology* 1989;170:839.
123. Hogeboom WR, Hhoekstra HJ, Mooyaart EL, et al. Magnetic resonance imaging (MRI) in evaluating *in vivo* response to neoadjuvant chemotherapy for osteosarcomas of the extremities. *Eur J Surg Oncol* 1989;15:424.
124. Smith J, Heelan RT, Huvos AG, et al. Radiographic changes in primary osteogenic sarcoma following intensive chemotherapy. *Radiology* 1982;143:355.
125. Sommer HJ, Knop J, Heise U, Winkler K, Delling G. Histomorphometric changes of osteosarcoma after chemotherapy. Correlation with 99Tc methylene diphosphonate functional imaging. *Cancer* 1987;59:252.
126. Holscher HC, van der Woude HJ, Hermans J, et al. Magnetic resonance relaxation times of normal tissue in the course of chemotherapy: a study in patients with bone sarcoma. *Skeletal Radiol* 1994;23:181.
127. de Beare T, Vanel D, Shapeero LG, et al. Osteosarcoma after chemotherapy: evaluation with contrast material enhanced subtraction MR imaging. *Radiology* 1992;185:587.
128. Conrad EU, Bruckner JD III, Miser J, et al. Surgical imaging and staging of osteosarcoma. Eighth annual meeting of the International Society of Limb Salvage, Florence, Italy, 1995.
129. Lampreave JL, Benard F, Alavi A, Jimenez-Hoyuela J, Fraker D. PET evaluation of therapeutic limb perfusion in Merkel's cell carcinoma. *J Nucl Med* 1998;39:2087.
130. Marcove RC, Lyden JP, Huvos AC, Bullough PB. Giant cell tumor treated by cryosurgery. Report of 25 cases. *J Bone Joint Surg Am* 1973;55:1633.
131. Marcove RC, Stovell P, Huvos AC, Bullough P. The use of cryosurgery in the treatment of low and medium grade chondrosarcoma: a preliminary report. *Clin Orthop* 1977;122:147.
132. Marcove RC. A 17-year review of cryosurgery in the treatment of bone tumors. *Clin Orthop* 1982;163:231.
133. Marcove RC, Rosen G. *En bloc* resection for osteogenic sarcoma. *Cancer* 1980;45:3040.
134. Malawer MM. Distal femoral osteogenic sarcoma, principles of soft tissue resection and reconstruction in conjunction with prosthetic replacement (adjuvant surgery). In: Chao EYS, ed. *Design and application of tumor prothesis for bone and joint reconstruction.* New York: Thieme-Stratton, 1983:297.
135. Morton DL, Eilber FR, Townsend CM Jr, et al. Limb salvage from a multidisciplinary treatment approach for skeletal and soft tissue sarcomas of the extremity. *Ann Surg* 1976;184:268.
136. Enneking WF. Section 8: concluding material. In: Enneking WF, ed. *Limb-sparing surgery for musculoskeletal tumors.* New York: Churchill Livingstone, 1987:624.
137. Malawer MM, Meller I. Porous coated segmental prosthesis for large tumor defects. A prosthesis based upon immediate fixation (PMA) and extracortical bone fixation: analysis of 20 consecutive patients. Annual meeting of the Musculoskeletal Tumor Society, Toronto, 1987.
138. Heck DA, Chao EY, Sim FH, et al. Titanium fibermetal segmental replacement prostheses and radiographic analysis and review of current status. *Clin Orthop* 1987;204:266.
139. Mankin HJ, Fogelson FS, Thrasher AZ, et al. Massive resection and allograft transplantation in the treatment of malignant bone tumors. *N Engl J Med* 1976;294:1247.
140. Malawer MM. Personal experience.
141. Makley JT, Krailo M, Ertel IJ, et al. The relationship of various aspects of surgical management to outcome in childhood nonmetastatic osteosarcoma: a report from the Children's Cancer Study Group. *J Pediatr Surg* 1988;23:146.
142. Rougraff BT, Simon MA, Kneisl JS, Greenberg DB, Mankin HJ. Limb salvage compared with amputation for osteosarcoma of the distal end of the femur. A long term oncological, functional, and quality of life study. *J Bone Joint Surgery Am* 1994;76:649.
143. Greenberg DB. Quality of life in osteosarcoma survivors. *Oncology (Huntingt)* 1994;8:19.
144. Christ GH, Lane JP, Christ AE, Marcove R, Glasser D. Long term psychosocial adaptation of osteosarcoma survivors. *Oncology* 1993;335:1.
145. Malawer MM, Baker A. Amputations for tumor. In: Evarts CM, ed. *Surgery of the musculoskeletal system,* 2nd ed. New York: Churchill Livingstone, 1990.
146. Marcove RC, Mike V, Hajek JV, Levin AG, Hutter RVP. Osteogenic sarcoma under the age of twenty-one. A review of one hundred and forty-five operative cases. *J Bone Joint Surg Am* 1970;52:411.
147. Gehan EA, Sutow WW, Uribe-Botero G, Romsdahl M, Smith TL. Osteosarcoma: the M. D. Anderson experience, 1950–1974. In: Terry WD, Windhorst D, eds. Immunotherapy of cancer: present status of trials in man. *Prog Cancer Res Ther* 1978;6:271.

148. Uribe-Botero G, Russell W, Sutow W, Martin R. Primary osteosarcoma of bone: a clinicopathologic investigation of 243 cases, with necropsy studies in 54. *Am J Clin Pathol* 1977;67:427.
149. Friedman MA, Carter SK. The therapy of osteogenic sarcoma: current status and thoughts for the future. *J Surg Oncol* 1972;4:482.
150. Taylor WF, Ivins JC, Dahlin DC, Edmonson JH, Pritchard DJ. Trends and variability in survival from osteosarcoma. *Mayo Clinic Proc* 1978;53:695.
151. Taylor WF, Ivins JC, Dahlin DC, Pritchard DJ. Osteogenic sarcoma experience at the Mayo Clinic, 1963–1974. In: Terry WD, Windhorts D, eds. Immunotherapy of cancer: present status of trials in man. *Prog Cancer Res Ther* 1978;6:257.
152. Taylor WF, Ivins J, Pritchard D, et al. Trends and variability in survival among patients with osteosarcoma: a 7-year update. *Mayo Clin Proc* 1985;60:91.
153. Strander H, Adamson U, Aparisi T, et al. Adjuvant interferon treatment of human osteosarcoma. Recent results. *Cancer Res* 1979;68:40.
154. Rab GT, Ivins JC, Childs DS, Cupps RE, Pritchard DJ. Elective whole lung irradiation in the treatment of osteogenic sarcoma. *Cancer* 1976;38:939.
155. Breur K, Cohen P, Schweisguth O, Hart A. Irradiation of the lungs as an adjuvant therapy in the treatment of osteosarcoma of the limbs: an EORTC randomized study. *Eur J Cancer* 1978;14:461.
156. Edmonson JH, Green SJ, Ivins JC, et al. A controlled pilot study of high-dose methotrexate as post surgical adjuvant treatment for primary osteosarcoma. *J Clin Oncol* 1984;2:152.
157. Link MP, Goordin AM, Miser AW, et al. The effect of adjuvant chemotherapy on relapse-free survival in patients with osteosarcoma of the extremity. *N Engl J Med* 1986;314:1600.
158. Link MP, Shuster JJ, Goorin AM, et al. Adjuvant chemotherapy in the treatment of osteosarcoma: results of the Multi-Institutional Osteosarcoma Study. In: Ryan J, Baker LO, eds. *Recent concepts in sarcoma treatment.* Proceedings of the International Symposium on Sarcomas, Tarpon Springs, Florida, October 8–10, 1987. Dordrecht, The Netherlands: Kluwer Academic Publishers, 1988:283.
159. Link MP, Goorin AM, Horowitz M, et al. Adjuvant chemotherapy of high grade osteosarcoma of the extremity: updated results of the Multi-Institutional Osteosarcoma Study. *Clin Orthop* 1991;270:8.
160. Eilber F, Giuliano A, Eckardt J, et al. Adjuvant chemotherapy for osteosarcoma: a randomized prospective trial. *J Clin Oncol* 1987;5:21.
161. Laster WR Jr, Mayo JG, Simpson-Herren L, et al. Success and failure in the treatment of solid tumors. II. Kinetic parameters and "cell cure" of moderately advanced carcinoma. *Cancer Chemother Rep* 1969;53:169.
162. Schabel FM Jr. Rationale for adjuvant chemotherapy. *Cancer* 1977;39:2875.
163. Schabel FM Jr. The use of tumor growth kinetics in planning "curative" chemotherapy of advanced solid tumors. *Cancer Res* 1969;29:2384.
164. Cortes EP, Holland JF, Wang JJ, Sinks LF. Doxorubicin in disseminated osteosarcoma. *JAMA* 1972;221:1132.
165. Nitschke R, Starling KA, Vats T, Bryan H. *Cis*-diamminedichloroplatinum (NSC119875) in childhood malignancies: a Southwest Oncology Group study. *Med Pediatr Oncol* 1978;4:127.
166. Ochs JJ, Freeman AL, Douglass HO, et al. *Cis*-dichlorodiammineplatinum (II) in advanced osteogenic sarcoma. *Cancer Treat Rep* 1978;62:239.
167. Baum ES, Gaynon P, Greenberg L, Krivitt W, Hammond D. Phase II study of *cis*-dichlorodiammineplatinum (II) in childhood osteosarcoma: Children's Cancer Study Group Report. *Cancer Treat Rep* 1979;63:1621.
168. Gasparini M, Rouesse J, van Oosterom A, et al. Phase II study of cisplatin in advanced osteogenic sarcoma. *Cancer Treat Rep* 1985;69:211.
169. Jaffe N, Farber S, Traggis D, et al. Favorable response of metastatic osteogenic sarcoma to pulse high dose methotrexate with citrovorum rescue and radiation therapy. *Cancer* 1973;31:1367.
170. Pratt C, Howarth C, Ransom J, et al. High dose methotrexate used alone and in combination for measurable primary and metastatic osteosarcoma. *Cancer Treat Rep* 1980;64:11.
171. Jaffe N, Frei E, Traggis D, Watts H. Weekly high-dose methotrexate-citrovorum factor in osteogenic sarcoma. Presurgical treatment of primary tumor and overt pulmonary metastases. *Cancer* 1977;39:45.
172. Marti C, Kroner T, Remagen W, et al. High-dose ifosfamide in advanced osteosarcoma. *Cancer Treat Rep* 1985;69:115.
173. Frei E, Jaffe N, Skipper HE, Gero MG. Adjuvant chemotherapy of osteogenic sarcoma: progress and perspectives. In: Salmon SE, Jones SE, eds. *Adjuvant therapy of cancer.* Amsterdam: Elsevier/North Holland Biomedical Press, 1977:49.
174. Grem J, King S, Wittes R, Leyland Jones B. The role of methotrexate in osteosarcoma. *J Natl Cancer Inst* 1988;80:626.
175. Edmonson J, Creagan E, Gilchrist G. Phase II study of high dose methotrexate in patients with unresectable metastatic osteosarcoma. *Cancer Treat Rep* 1981;65:538.
176. Krailo M, Ertel I, Makley J, et al. A randomized study comparing high-dose methotrexate with moderate dose methotrexate as components of adjuvant chemotherapy in childhood nonmetastatic osteosarcoma: a report from the Children's Cancer Study Group. *Med Pediatr Oncol* 1987;15:69.
177. Bacci G, Picci P, Ruggieri P, et al. Primary chemotherapy and delayed surgery (neoadjuvant chemotherapy) for osteosarcoma of the extremities. The Instituto Rizzoli experience in 127 patients treated preoperatively with intravenous methotrexate (high versus moderate doses) and intraarterial cisplatin. *Cancer* 1990;65:2539.
178. Bramwell VHC, Burgers M, Sneath R, et al. A comparison of two short intensive adjuvant chemotherapy regimens in operable osteosarcoma of limbs in children and young adults: the first study of the European Osteosarcoma Intergroup. *J Clin Oncol* 1992;10:1579.
179. Winkler K, Beron G, Kotz R, et al. Neoadjuvant chemotherapy for osteogenic sarcoma: results of a cooperative German/Austrian study. *J Clin Oncol* 1984;2:617.
180. Rosen G, Nirenberg A. Chemotherapy for osteogenic sarcoma: an investigative method, not a recipe. *Cancer Treat Rep* 1982;66:1687.
181. Smith MA, Ungerleider RS, Horowitz ME, Simon R. Influence of doxorubicin dose intensity on response and outcome for patients with osteogenic sarcoma and Ewing's sarcoma. *J Natl Cancer Inst* 1991;83:1460.
182. Mosende C, Gutierrez M, Caparros B, Rosen G. Combination chemotherapy with bleomycin, cyclophosphamide and dactinomycin for the treatment of osteogenic sarcoma. *Cancer* 1977;40:2779.
183. Pratt CB, Epelman S, Jaffe N. Bleomycin, cyclophosphamide, and dactinomycin in metastatic osteosarcoma: lack of tumor regression in previously treated patients. *Cancer Treat Rep* 1987;71:421.
184. Harris MB, Gieser P, Goorin AM, et al. Treatment of metastatic osteosarcoma at diagnosis: a Pediatric Oncology Group Study. *J Clin Oncol* 1998;16:3641.
185. Souhami RL, Craft AW, Van der Eijken JW, et al. Randomised trial of two regimens of chemotherapy in operable osteosarcoma: a study of the European Osteosarcoma Intergroup. *Lancet* 1997;350:911.
186. Miser J, Arndt C, Smithson W, et al. Treatment of high grade osteosarcoma (OGS) with ifosamide (Ifos), MESNA, Adriamycin (ADR), and high dose methotrexate (HDMTX). *Proc Am Soc Clin Oncol* 1991;10:310.
187. Harris M, Gieser P, Goorin A, et al. Treatment of metastatic osteosarcoma at diagnosis: a Pediatric Oncology Group study. *J Clin Oncol* 1998;16:3641.
188. Huvos A, Rosen G, Marcove RC. Primary osteogenic sarcoma. Pathologic aspects in 20 patients after treatment with chemotherapy, *en bloc* resection and prosthetic bone replacement. *Arch Pathol Lab Med* 1977;101:14.
189. Winkler K, Beron G, Kotz R, et al. Neoadjuvant chemotherapy for osteosarcoma: results of a cooperative German/Austrian study. *J Clin Oncol* 1984;2:617.
190. Winkler K, Beron G, Kotz R, et al. Adjuvant chemotherapy in osteosarcoma effects of cisplatinum, BCD, and fibroblast interferon in sequential combination with HDMTX and Adriamycin. Preliminary results of the COSS 80 study. *J Cancer Res Clin Oncol* 1983;106[Suppl]:1.
191. Winkler K, Beron G, Delling G, et al. Neoadjuvant chemotherapy of osteosarcoma: results of a randomized cooperative trial (COSS82) with salvage chemotherapy based on histological tumor response. *J Clin Oncol* 1988;6:329.
192. Provisor AJ, Ettinger LJ, Nachman JB, et al. Treatment of nonmetastatic osteosarcoma of the extremity with preoperative and postoperative chemotherapy: a report from the Children's Cancer Group. *J Clin Oncol* 1997;15:76.
193. Hudson M, Jaffe MR, Jaffe N, et al. Pediatric osteosarcoma: therapeutic strategies, results and prognostic factors derived from a 10-year experience. *J Clin Oncol* 1990;8:1988.
194. Davis AM, Bell RS, Goodwin PJ. Prognostic factors in osteosarcoma: a critical review. *J Clin Oncol* 1994;12:423.
195. Goldie JH, Coldman AJ. A mathematical model for relating the drug sensitivity of tumors to their spontaneous mutation rate. *Cancer Treat Rep* 1979;63:1727.
196. DeVita VT. The relationship between tumor mass and resistance to chemotherapy. *Cancer* 1983;51:1209.
197. Salzer-Kuntschik M, Delling G, Beron G, Sigmund R. Morphological grades of regression in osteosarcoma after polychemotherapy. Study COSS 80. *J Cancer Res Clin Oncol* 1983;106[Suppl]:21.
198. Jaffe N, Prudich J, Knapp J, et al. Treatment of primary osteosarcoma with intra-arterial and intravenous high-dose methotrexate. *J Clin Oncol* 1983;1:428.
199. Meyers PA, Heller G, Healey J, et al. Chemotherapy for non-metastatic osteogenic sarcoma: the Memorial Sloan Kettering experience. *J Clin Oncol* 1992;10:5.
200. Jaffe N, Raymond AK, Ayala A, et al. Effect of cumulative courses of intraarterial *cis*-diamminedichloroplatin-II on the primary tumor in osteosarcoma. *Cancer* 1989;63:63.
201. Avella M, Bacci G, McDonald DJ, et al. Adjuvant chemotherapy with six drugs (Adriamycin, methotrexate, cisplatinum, bleomycin, cyclophosphamide, and dactinomycin) for nonmetastatic high-grade osteosarcoma of the extremities. Results of 32 patients and comparison to 127 patients concomitantly treated with the same drugs in a neoadjuvant form. *Chemioterapia* 1988;7:133.
202. Gherlinzoni F, Mercuri M, Monti C. Primary chemotherapy and delayed surgery for nonmetastatic osteosarcoma of the extremities. Results in 164 patients preoperatively treated with high doses of methotrexate followed by cisplatin and doxorubicin. *Cancer* 1993;72:3227.
203. Glasser DB, Lane JM, Huvos AG, Marcove RC, Rosen G. Survival, prognosis, and therapeutic response in osteogenic sarcoma. The Memorial Hospital experience. *Cancer* 1992;69:698.
204. Goorin A, Baker A, Gieser P, et al. No evidence for improved event-free survival [EFS] with presurgical chemotherapy [PRE] for non-metastatic extremity osteogenic sarcoma [OGS]: preliminary results of randomized Pediatric Oncology Group [POG] trial 8651. *Proc Am Soc Clin Oncol* 1995;14:444.
205. Baldini N, Scotlandi K, Barbanti-Brodano G, et al. Expression of P-glycoprotein in high-grade osteosarcomas in relation to clinical outcome. *N Engl J Med* 1995;333:1380.
206. Chan HSL, Grogan TM, Haddad G, et al. P-glycoprotein expression: critical determinant in the response to osteosarcoma chemotherapy. *J Natl Cancer Inst* 1997;89:1706.
207. Uozaki H, Horiuchi H, Ishida T, et al. Overexpression of resistance-related proteins (metallothioneins, glutathione-S-transferase O, heat shock protein 27, and lung resistance–related protein) in osteosarcoma: relationship with poor prognosis. *Cancer* 1997;79:2336.
208. Gorlick R, Huvos AG, Heller G, et al. Expression of HER2/erbB-2 correlates with survival in osteosarcoma. *J Clin Oncol* 1999;17:2781.
209. Feugeas O, Guriec N, Babin-Boilletot A, et al. Loss of heterozygosity of the RB gene is a poor prognostic factor in patients with osteosarcoma. *J Clin Oncol* 1996;14:467.
210. Onda M, Matsuda S, Higaki S, et al. ErbB-2 expression is correlated with poor prognosis for patients with osteosarcoma. *Cancer* 1996;77:71.
211. Jaffe N, Robertson R, Ayala A, et al. Comparison of intraarterial *cis*-diamminedichloroplatinum II with high dose methotrexate and citrovorum factor rescue in the treatment of primary osteosarcoma. *J Clin Oncol* 1985;3:1101.

212. Martinez A, Donaldson SS, Bagshaw MA. Special set up and treatment techniques for the radiotherapy of pediatric malignancies. *Int J Radiat Oncol Biol Phys* 1977;2:1007.
213. Watkins DMB. *Radiation therapy mold technology.* Toronto: Pergamon Press, 1981.
214. Order SE, Donaldson SS. *Radiation therapy for benign disease,* 2nd ed. Berlin: Springer-Verlag, 1997.
215. Sanerkin NG. The diagnosis and grading of chondrosarcoma of bone. A combined cytologic and histologic approach. *Cancer* 1980;45:582.
216. Huvos AG. *Bone tumors. Diagnosis, treatment and prognosis.* Philadelphia: WB Saunders, 1979.
217. Singer JM, Deutsch GP. The successful use of radiotherapy for osteoblastoma. *Clin Oncol* 1993;5:124.
218. Nobler MP, Higinbotham NL, Phillips RF. The cure of aneurysmal bone cyst: irradiation superior to surgery in an analysis of 33 cases. *Radiology* 1968;90:1185.
219. Vergel DD, Bond JR, Shives TC, McLeod RA, Unni KK. Aneurysmal bone cyst. A clinicopathologic study of 238 cases. *Cancer* 1992;69:2921.
220. Cassady JR. Radiation therapy in less common primary bone tumors. In: Jaffe N, ed. *Solid tumors in childhood.* Littleton, MA: PSG Publishing, 1979:205.
221. Kamikonya N, Hishikawa Y, Kurisu K, et al. Aneurysmal bone cyst treated by high-energy, low-dose radiation therapy: a case report. *Radiat Med* 1991;9:54.
222. Madea N, Tateishi H, Takaiwa H, et al. High-energy, low-dose therapy for aneurysmal bone cyst. Report of a case. *Clin Orthop* 1989;243:200.
223. Sanfilippo NJ, Wang GJ, Larner JM. Desmoplastic fibroma: a role for radiotherapy? *South Med J* 1995;88:1267.
224. Greenberger JS, Crocker AC, Vawter G, et al. Results of treatment of 127 patients with systemic histiocytosis (Letterer-Siwe syndrome, Schuller-Christian syndrome and multifocal eosinophilic granuloma). *Medicine (Baltimore)* 1981;60:311.
225. Dahlin DC, Coventry MB. Osteosarcoma, a study of 600 cases. *J Bone Joint Surg Am* 1967;49:101.
226. Stark A, Kricbergs S, Nilsonne U, Silfversward C. The age of osteosarcoma patients is increasing. An epidemiological study of osteosarcoma in Sweden 1971 to 1984. *J Bone Joint Surg Am* 1990;72B:89.
227. Richter MP, D'Angio GJ. The role of radiation therapy in the management of children with histiocytosis X. *Am J Pediatr Hematol Oncol* 1981;3:161.
228. Selch MT, Parker RG. Radiation therapy in the management of Langerhans cell histiocytosis. *Med Pediatr Oncol* 1990;8:151.
229. Wick MR, Siegal GP, Unni KK, et al. Sarcomas of bone complicating osteitis deformas (Paget's disease), 50 years' experience. *Am J Surg Pathol* 1981;5:47.
230. Greditzer HG, McLeod RA, Unni KK, et al. Bone sarcomas in Paget's disease. *Radiology* 1983;146:337.
231. Francis KC, Kohn H, Malawer MM. Osteogenic sarcoma. *J Bone Joint Surg Am* 1976;55:754.
232. Scranton PE Jr, DeCicco FA, Totten RS, Yunis EJ. Prognostic factors in osteosarcoma. A review of 20 years experience at the University of Pittsburgh Health Center Hospitals. *Cancer* 1975;36:2179.
233. Wilner D. Osteogenic sarcoma (osteosarcoma). In: *Radiology of bone tumors and allied disorders.* Philadelphia: WB Saunders, 1982:1897.
234. DeSantos LA, Edeiken B. Purely lytic osteosarcoma. *Skeletal Radiol* 1982;9:1.
235. Jaffe N, Smith E, Abelson HT, et al. Osteogenic sarcoma: alterations in the pattern of pulmonary metastases with adjuvant chemotherapy. *J Clin Oncol* 1983;1:251.
236. Lockshin MD, Higgins TT. Prognosis in osteogenic sarcoma. *Int Orthop* 1981;5:305.
237. Larsson SE, Lorentzon R, Wedren H, Boquist L. The prognosis in osteosarcoma. *Int Orthop* 1981;5:305.
238. Brostrom L, Strander H, Nisonne U. Survival in osteosarcoma in relation to tumor size and location. *Clin Orthop* 1982;167:250.
239. Hudson M, Jaffe MR, Jaffe N, et al. Pediatric osteosarcoma: therapeutic strategies results and prognostic factors derived from a 10-year experience. *J Clin Oncol* 1990;8:1988.
240. Baldini N, Scotlandi K, Barbanti-Brodano G, et al. Expression of P-glycoprotein in high-grade osteosarcomas in relation to clinical outcome. *N Engl J Med* 1995;333:1380.
241. Bacci G, Avella M, Picci P, et al. Metastatic patterns in osteosarcoma. *Tumori* 1988;74:421.
242. Levine AM, Rosenberg SA. Alkaline phosphatase levels in osteosarcoma tissue are related to prognosis. *Cancer* 1979;44:2291.
243. Levine AM, Trich T, Rosenberg SA. Osteosarcoma cells in tissue culture. II. Characterization and location of alkaline phosphatase activity. *Clin Orthop* 1975;3:33.
244. Bacci G, Picci P, Ferrari S, et al. Prognostic significance of serum alkaline phosphatase measurements in patients with osteosarcoma treated with adjuvant or neoadjuvant chemotherapy. *Cancer* 1993;71(4):1224.
245. Springfield DS, Schmidt R, Grahm-Pole J, et al. Surgical treatment for osteosarcoma. *J Bone Joint Surg Am* 1988;70:1124.
246. Picci P, Ferrari S, Bacci G, Gherlinzoni F. Treatment recommendations for osteosarcoma and adult soft tissue sarcomas. *Drugs* 1994;47:82.
247. Malawer MM, Meller I, Dunham WK. A new surgical classification system for shoulder-girdle resections. Analysis of 38 patients. *Clin Orthop* 1991;267:33.
248. Malawer MM, Meller I, Dunham WK. *Proposed surgical classification of shoulder girdle resections for bone and soft tissue tumors: description of a new system and analysis of 38 patients.* New Orleans: American Society of Shoulder and Elbow Surgery, 1987.
249. Malawer MM, Sugarbaker PH, Lambert M, et al. The Tikhoff-Linberg procedure and its modifications. In: Sugarbaker PH, ed. *Atlas of sarcoma surgery.* Philadelphia: JB Lippincott Co, 1984.
250. Malawer MM, McHale KA. Limb-sparing surgery for high grade tumors of the proximal tibia and a new method of extensor mechanism reconstruction. Fourth International Symposium on Limb-Salvage in Musculoskeletal Oncology, Kyoto, Japan, 1987.
251. Hudson TM, Springfield DS, Schiebler M. Popliteus muscle as a barrier to tumor spread: computer tomography and angiography. *J Comput Assisted Tomogr* 1984;8:498.
252. Malawer MM, Price WM. Gastrocnemius transposition flaps in conjunction with limb-sparing surgery for primary sarcomas around the knee. *Plast Reconstr Surg* 1984;73:741.
253. Malawer MM. Surgical management of aggressive malignant tumors of the proximal tibia and fibula. *Clin Orthop* 1984;186:172.
254. Enneking WF. A system for the functional evaluation of the surgical management of musculoskeletal tumors. In: Enneking WF, ed. *Limb-sparing surgery for musculoskeletal tumors.* New York: Churchill Livingstone, 1987:5.
255. Miller G. Opening remarks. In: Enneking WF, ed. *Limb-sparing surgery for musculoskeletal tumors.* New York: Churchill Livingstone, 1987:5.
256. Fahey M, Spanier SS. Osteosarcoma of the pelvis. A clinical and histopathological study of twenty-five patients. *J Bone Joint Surg Am* 1992;74:321.
257. Sluga M, Windhager R, Lang S, et al. Local and systemic control after ablative and limb-sparing surgery in patients with osteosarcoma. *Clin Orthop Rel Res* 1999;358:120.
258. Bacci G, Ferrari S, Mercuri M, et al. Predictive factors for local recurrence in osteosarcoma: 540 patients with extremity tumors followed for a minimum 2.5 years after neoadjuvant chemotherapy. *Acta Orthop Scand* 1998;69:230.
259. Malawer MM. Personal experience.
260. Jenkin RDT, Allt WEC, Fitzpatrick PJ. Osteosarcoma. An assessment of management with particular reference to primary irradiation and selective delayed amputation. *Cancer* 1972;30:393.
261. Powell GJ, Scarborough MT, Enneking WF. Osteoarticular allografts for reconstruction of the distal femur following tumor resection. Tenth International Symposium on Limb Salvage, Cairns, Australia, 1999.
262. Malawer MM, Chou L. Prosthetic survival and clinical results with the use of large segment replacements in the treatment of high-grade bone sarcomas. *J Bone Joint Surg Am* 1995;77:1154.
263. Unwin PS, Walker PS, Briggs TW. Aseptic loosening in 1001 cases of cemented custom-made bone tumor replacements: tumor replacements of the lower limb. Eighth annual meeting of the International Society of Limb Salvage, Florence, Italy, May 1995.
264. Ruggieri P, De Cristofaro R, Picci P, et al. Complications and surgical indications in 144 cases of nonmetastatic osteosarcoma of the extremities treated with neoadjuvant chemotherapy. *Clin Orthop* 1993;295:226.
265. Campanna R, Manfrini M, Ceruso M, Bertoni F, Nomtanari N. Intraepiphyseal resection in high grade bone sarcomas. Eighth annual meeting of the International Society of Limb Salvage, Florence, Italy, May 1995.
266. Henshaw R, Jones V, Malawer MM. Endoprosthetic reconstruction with the modular replacement system. Survival analysis of the first 100 implants with a minimum 2 year follow-up. Fourth combined meeting of the American and European Musculoskeletal Tumor Societies, Washington, DC, May 1998.
267. Renard AJ, Veth RP, Schreuder HW, et al. Revisions of endoprosthetic reconstructions after limb salvage in musculoskeletal oncology. *Arch Orthop Trauma Surg* 1998;117(3):125.
268. Grimer RJ, Carter SR, Pynsent PB. The cost-effectiveness of limb salvage for bone tumours. *J Bone Joint Surg (Br)* 1997;79:558.
269. Steadman PB, Pritchard DJ, Larson D. Pathological fractures in osteosarcoma—a descriptive study 1970–1985. Tenth International Symposium on Limb Salvage, Cairns, Australia, 1999.
270. Mankin HJ, Lange TA, Spanier S. The hazards of biopsy in patients with malignant primary bone and soft-tissue tumors. *J Bone Joint Surg Am* 1982;64:1121.
271. Martin NS, Williamson J. The role of surgery in the treatment of malignant tumors of the spine. *J Bone Joint Surg Am* 1970;52B:227.
272. Sterner B. Total spondylectomy in chondrosarcoma arising in the seventh thoracic vertebra. *J Bone Joint Surg Am* 1971;53B:288.
273. Sterner BL, Johnson OE. Complete removal of three vertebra for giant cell tumor. *J Bone Joint Surg Am* 1971;53B:278.
274. Estrada-Aguilar J, Greenberg H, Walling A, et al. Primary treatment of pelvic osteosarcoma. Report of five cases. *Cancer* 1992;69:1137.
275. Marina NM, Pratt CB, Rao BN, et al. Improved prognosis of children with osteosarcoma metastatic to the lung(s) at the time of diagnosis. *Cancer* 1992;70:2722.
276. Meyers PA, Heller G, Healy JH. Osteogenic sarcoma with clinically detectable metastasis at initial presentation. *J Clin Oncol* 1993;11:449.
277. Cregan E, Frytak S, Pairolero P, et al. Surgically proven pulmonary metastases not demonstrated by computed chest tomography. *Cancer Treat Rep* 1978;62:1404.
278. Telander R, Pairolero P, Pritchard D, et al. Resection of pulmonary metastatic osteogenic sarcoma in children. *Surgery* 1978;84:335.
279. Putnam JB, Roth J, Wesley M, et al. Survival following aggressive resection of pulmonary metastases from osteogenic sarcoma: analysis of prognostic factors. *Ann Thorac Surg* 1983;36:516.
280. Goorin A, Delorey M, Lack E, et al. Prognostic significance of complete surgical resection of pulmonary metastases in patients with osteogenic sarcoma: analysis of 32 patients. *Clin Oncol* 1984;2:425.
281. Meyer WH, Schell MJ, Kumar APM, et al. Thoracotomy for pulmonary metastatic carcinoma. *Cancer* 1987;59:374.
282. Han MT, Telander R, Pairolero P, et al. Aggressive thoracotomy for pulmonary metastatic osteogenic sarcoma in children and young adolescents. *J Pediatr Surg* 1981;16:928.
283. Saeter G, Hoie J, Stenwig AE, et al. Systemic relapse of patients with osteogenic sarcoma. Prognostic factors for long-term survival. *Cancer* 1995;75:1084.
284. Tabone MD, Kalifa C, Rodary C, et al. Osteosarcoma recurrences in pediatric patients previously treated with intensive chemotherapy. *J Clin Oncol* 1994;12:2614.
285. Ward WG, Mikaelian K, Dorey F, et al. Pulmonary metastases of stage IIB extremity osteosarcoma and subsequent pulmonary metastases. *J Clin Oncol* 1994;12:1849.
286. Cade S. Osteogenic sarcoma. A study based on 133 patients. *J Royal Coll Surg (Edinb)* 1955;1:79.
287. Lee ES, Mackenzie DH. Osteosarcoma: a study of the value of preoperative megavoltage radiotherapy. *Br J Surg* 1964;51:252.

288. Farrell C, Reventos A. Experience in treating osteosarcoma at the University of Pennsylvania. *Radiology* 1964;83:1080.
289. Sweetnan R, Knowelden J, Seedon H. Bone sarcoma treatment by irradiation, amputation, or a combination of the two. *BMJ* 1971;2:363.
290. Phillips TL, Sheline GE. Radiation therapy of malignant bone tumors. *Radiology* 1969;92:1537.
291. Allen CV, Stevens KR. Preoperative irradiation for osteogenic sarcoma. *Cancer* 1973;31:1365.
292. Gaitan-Yanguas M. A study of the response of osteogenic sarcoma and adjacent normal tissues to radiation. *Int J Radiat Oncol Biol Phys* 1981;7:593.
293. Beck JC, Wara WM, Bovill EG, et al. The role of radiation therapy in the treatment of osteosarcoma. *Radiology* 1976;120:163.
294. Goffinet DR, Kaplan HS, Donaldson SS, et al. Combined radiosensitizer infusion and irradiation of osteogenic sarcoma. *Radiology* 1975;117:211.
295. Martinez A, Goffinet DR, Donaldson SS, et al. Intra-arterial infusion of the radiosensitizer (BudR) combined with hypofractionated irradiation and chemotherapy for primary treatment of osteogenic sarcoma. *Radiology* 1975;117:211.
296. Kinsella TJ, Glatstein E. Clinical experience with intravenous radiosensitizers in unresectable sarcomas. *Cancer* 1987;59:908.
297. Okada K, Frassica FJ, Sim FH, et al. Parosteal osteosarcoma. A clinicopathic study. *J Bone Joint Surg Am* 1994;76:366.
298. Unni KK, Dahlin CC, Beaubout SW. Parosteal osteogenic sarcoma. *Cancer* 1976;37:2466.
299. Jelinek JS, Murphey MD, Kransdorf MJ, et al. Parosteal osteosarcoma, value of MR imaging and CT in the prediction of histologic grade. *Radiology* 1996;201:837.
300. Schajowicz F, McGuire MH, Araujo S, Muscolo DL, Gitelis S. Osteosarcoma arising on the surfaces of long bones. *J Bone Joint Surg Am* 1988;70:555.
301. Sim FH, Unni KK, Beaubout JW, et al. Osteosarcoma with small cells simulating Ewing's tumor. *J Bone Joint Surg Am* 1979;61:207.
302. Martin SE, Dwyer A, Kissane JM, et al. Small-cell osteosarcoma. *Cancer* 1982;50:990.
303. Devaney K, Vinh TN, Sweet DE. Small cell osteosarcoma of bone: an immunohistochemical study with differential diagnosis considerations. *Hum Pathol* 1993;24:1211.
304. Amendola BE, Amendola MA, McClatchey KD, et al. Radiation-associated sarcoma: a review of 23 patients over a 50-year period. *Am J Clin Oncol* 1989;12:411.
305. Le Vu B, de Vathaire F, Shamsaldin A, et al. Radiation dose, chemotherapy, and risk of osteosarcoma after solid tumors during childhood. *Int J Cancer* 1998;77:370.
306. Hawkins MM, Wilson LM, Burton HS, et al. Radiotherapy, alkylating agents, and risk of bone cancer after childhood cancer. *J Natl Cancer Inst* 1996;88:270.
307. Huvos AG, Wooard HQ, Cahan WG, et al. Postradiation osteogenic sarcoma of bone and soft-tissues, a clinicopathologic study of 66 patients. *Cancer* 1982;55:1244.
308. Marcove RC, Mike V, Hutter RVP, et al. Chondrosarcoma of the pelvis and upper end of femur. *J Bone Joint Surg Am* 1972;54:561.
309. Mankin HJ, Cantley KD, Lipielo L, et al. The biology of human chondrosarcoma. I. Description of the cases, grading, and biochemical analyses. *J Bone Joint Surg Am* 1980;62:160.
310. Mankin HJ, Cantley KD, Schiller AL, et al. The biology of human chondrosarcoma. II. Variations in chemical composite among types and subtypes of benign and malignant cartilage tumors. *J Bone Joint Surg Am* 1980;62:176.
311. Krocberg A, Zelterberg A, Soderberg G. A comparative study of cellular DNA content and clinicopathologic features. *Cancer* 1982;50:577.
312. Edeiken J. Bone tumors and tumor-like conditions. In: Edeiken J, ed. *Roentgen diagnosis and disease of bone,* 3rd ed. Baltimore: Williams & Wilkins, 1981:30.
313. Aprin H, Riserborough EJ, Hall JE. Chondrosarcoma in children and adolescents. *Clin Orthop* 1982;166:226.
314. Bjornsson J, McCleod RA, Unni K, et al. Primary chondrosarcoma of long bones and limb girdles. *Cancer* 1998;83:2105.
315. Steel HH. Partial or complete resection of the hemipelvis: an alternative to hindquarter amputation for periacetabular chondrosarcoma of the pelvis. *J Bone Joint Surg Am* 1978;60:719.
316. Austin-Seymour M. Fractionated proton radiation therapy of chordoma and low grade chondrosarcoma of the base of the skull. *J Neurosurg* 1999;30:13.
317. Scanlon PW. Split dose radiotherapy for radioresistant bone and soft tissue sarcoma: ten years' experience. *AJR Am J Roentgenol* 1972;114:544.
318. Aboulafia AJ, Faulks C, Li W, et al. Reconstruction using the saddle prosthesis following excision of malignant periacetabular tumors. In: Brown KLB, ed. *Complications of limb salvage, prevention, management and outcome.* Montreal: International Society of Limb Salvage, 1991.
319. Kawai A, Healey JH, Boland PJ, et al. Prognostic factors for patients with sarcomas of the pelvic bones. *Cancer* 1998;82:851.
320. Schreuder HW, Pruszczynski M, Veth RP, Lemmens JA. Treatment of benign and low-grade malignant intramedullary chondroid tumours with curettage and cryosurgery. *Eur J Surg Oncol* 1998;24:120.
321. Unni KK, Dahlin DC, Beaubout JW, Sim FH. Chondrosarcoma: clear cell variant. A report of 16 cases. *J Bone Joint Surg Am* 1976;57:676.
322. Harwood AR, Krajbich JI, Fornasier VL. Mesenchymal chondrosarcoma: a report of 17 cases. *Clin Orthop* 1981;158:144.
323. Huvos AG, Rosen G, Dabska M, Marcove RC. Mesenchymal chondrosarcoma: a clinicopathologic analysis of 35 patients with emphasis on treatment. *Cancer* 1983;51:1230.
324. Krochak R, Harwood AR, Cummings BJ, et al. Results of radical radiation for chondrosarcoma of bone. *Radiat Oncol* 1983;1:109.
325. McNaney D, Lindberg RD, Ayala AG, et al. Fifteen year radiotherapy experience with chondrosarcoma of bone. *Int J Radiat Oncol Biol Phys* 1982;8:187.
326. Hug EB, Fitzek MM, Liebsch NJ, Munzenrider JE. Locally challenging osteo- and chondrogenic tumors of the axial skeleton: results of combined proton and photon radiation therapy using three-dimensional treatment planning. *Int J Radiat Oncol Biol Phys* 1995;31:467.
327. Harwood AR, Krajbich JI, Fornasier VL. Radiotherapy of chondrosarcoma of bone. *Cancer* 1980;45:2769.
328. Ryall RDH, Bates T, Newton KA, et al. Combination of radiotherapy and razoxane ICRF 159 for chondrosarcoma. *Cancer* 1979;44:891.
329. Marcove RC. *The surgery of tumors of bone and cartilage,* 2nd ed. New York: Grune and Stratton, 1984.
330. Nascimento AG, Huvos AC, Marcove RC. Primary malignant giant cell tumor of bone study of eight cases and review of the literature. *Cancer* 1979;44:1393.
331. Campanacci M, Giunti A, Olmi R. Giant-cell tumors of bone: a study of 209 cases with long-term follow-up in 130. *Ital J Orthop Traumatol* 1977;1:249.
332. O'Donnell RJ, Springfield DS, Motwani HK. Recurrence of giant cell tumors of the long bones after curettage and packing with cement. *J Bone Joint Surg Am* 1994;76:1827.
333. Bickels J, Malawer MM, Meller I, et al. Cryosurgery in the treatment of giant cell tumor of bone: a multi-institutional study of 102 cases with a follow-up period of 4–15 years. Combined Meeting of the American and European Musculoskeletal Tumor Societies, Washington, DC, 1998.
334. Malawer M, Bickels J, Meller I, et al. Cryosurgery in the treatment of giant cell tumor: a long-term followup study. *Clin Orthop* 1999;359:176.
335. Larsson SE, Lorenzton R, Boquist L. Giant cell tumors of the spine and sacrum causing neurological problems. *Clin Orthop* 1975;111:201.
336. Marcove RS, Weiss L, Vaghaiwall M. Cryosurgery in the treatment of giant cell tumor of bone: a report of 52 consecutive cases. *Clin Orthop* 1978;143:275.
337. Malawer MM, Dunham WK, Zaleski T, Zielinski CJ. The management of aggressive and low grade malignant bone tumors by cryosurgery: analysis of 40 consecutive cases. In: Enneking WF, ed. *Limb-sparing surgery for musculoskeletal tumors.* New York: Churchill Livingstone, 1987:498.
338. Persson BM, Wouters HW. Curettage and acrylic cementation in surgery of giant cell tumor of bone. *J Bone Joint Surg Am* 1976;120:125.
339. Turcotte RE, Sim FH, Unni KK. Giant cell tumor of the sacrum. *Clin Orthop* 1993;291:215.
340. Cassady JR. Radiation therapy in less common primary bone tumors. In: Jaffe N, ed. *Solid tumors in childhood.* Littleton, MA: PSG Publishing, 1979:205.
341. Amendola BE, Amendola MA, McClatchey KD, Miller CH Jr. Radiation associated sarcoma: a review of 23 patients with postradiation sarcoma over a 50 year period. *Am J Clin Oncol* 1989;12:411.
342. Bell RS, Harwood AR, Goodman SB, et al. Supervoltage radiotherapy in the treatment of difficult giant cell tumors of bone. *Clin Orthop* 1983;174:208.
343. Bennett CJ, Marcus RB, Million RR, et al. Radiation therapy for giant cell tumor of bone. *Int J Radiat Oncol Biol Phys* 1993;26:299.
344. De Groof E, Verdonk R, Vercauteren M, et al. Giant-cell tumor involving a lumbar vertebra. Long-term follow-up after radiotherapy. *Spine* 1990;15:835.
345. Harwood AR, Fornasier VL, Rider WD. Supervoltage irradiation in the management of giant-cell tumor of bone. *Radiology* 1977;125:223.
346. Nair MK, Jyothami R. Radiation therapy in the treatment of giant cell tumor of bone. *Int J Radiat Oncol Biol Phys* 1998;41:59.
347. Malone S, O'Sullivan B, Catton C, et al. Long-term follow-up of efficacy and safety of megavoltage in high-risk giant cell tumors of bone. *Int J Radiat Oncol Biol Phys* 1995: 33;689.
348. Schwartz LH, Okunieff PG, Rosenberg A, et al. Radiation therapy in the treatment of difficult giant cell tumors. *Int J Radiat Oncol Biol Phys* 1989;17:1085.
349. Singhal RM, Mukopadhyaya S, Tanwar RK, et al. Case report: giant cell tumour of metacarpals: report of three cases. *Br J Radiol* 1994;67:408.
350. Brien EW, Mirra JM, Kessler S, et al. Benign giant cell tumors of bone with osteosarcomatous transformation (dedifferentiated primary malignant GCT): report of two cases. *Skeletal Radiol* 1996;41:246.
351. Picci P, Bacci G, Ferrari S, Mercuri M. Neoadjuvant chemotherapy in malignant fibrous histiocytoma of bone and in osteosarcoma located in the extremities: analogies and differences between the two tumors. *Ann Oncol* 1997;8:1107.
352. Bacci G, Springfield D, Picci P, et al. Adjuvant chemotherapy for malignant fibrous histiocytoma in the femur and tibia. *J Bone Joint Surg Am* 1985;67:620.
353. Bacci G, Mercuri M, Ruggieri P, et al. Neoadjuvant chemotherapy for malignant fibrous histiocytoma of bone and for osteosarcoma of the limbs: a comparison between the results obtained for 21 and 144 patients, respectively, treated during the same period with the same chemotherapy protocol. *Chir Organi Mov* 1996;81:139.
354. Nishida J, Sim FH, Wenger DE, Unni KK. Malignant fibrous histiocytoma of bone. A clinicopathologic study of 81 patients. *Cancer* 1997;79:482.
355. Larsson S, Lorentzon R, Boquist L. Malignant hemangioendothelioma of bone. *J Bone Joint Surg Am* 1975;57:84.
356. Campanacci M, Boriani S, Giunti A. Hemangioendothelioma of bone: a study of 29 cases. *Cancer* 1980;46:804.
357. Welles L, Dorfman H, Valentine ES, et al. Low grade malignant hemangioendothelioma of bone: a disease potentially curable with radiotherapy. *Med Pediatr Oncol* 1994;23:144.
358. Wold LE, Ivins JC, Dahlin DC, et al. Hemangioendothelial sarcoma of bone. *Am J Surg Pathol* 1982;6:59.
359. Mindell ER. Current concept review. Chordoma. *J Bone Joint Surg Am* 1981;63:501.
360. Localio AS, Eng K, Ranson JHC. Abdominosacral approach for retrorectal tumors. *Am Surg* 1980;179:555.
361. Localio AS, Francis KC, Rossano PC. Abdominosacral resection of sacrococcygeal chordoma. *Ann Surg* 1980;166:394.
362. Gray SW, Singhabhandhu B, Smith RA, Skandalakis JE. Sacrococcygeal chordoma: report of a case and review of the literature. *Surgery* 1975;78:573.
363. DeVries J, Oldhoff J, Hadders HN. Cryosurgery treatment for sacrococcygeal chordoma: report of 4 cases. *Cancer* 1986;58:2348.

364. Guterberg B, Romanus B, Sterner BL. Pelvic strength after major amputation of the sacrum. An experimental study. *Acta Orthop Scand* 1976;47:635.
365. Heffelfinger MJ, Dahlin DC, MacCarthy CS, et al. Chordomas and cartilaginous tumors of the skull base. *Cancer* 1973;32:410.
366. Amendola BE, Amendola MA, Oliver E, et al. Chordoma: role of radiation therapy. *Radiology* 1986;158:839.
367. Rich TA, Schiller A, Suit HD, et al. Clinical and pathologic review of 48 cases of chordoma. *Cancer* 1985;56:182.
368. Cummings BJ, Hodson ID, Bush RS. Chordoma: the results of megavoltage radiation therapy. *Int J Radiat Oncol Biol Phys* 1986;9:633.
369. Catton C, O'Sullivan B, Bell R, et al. Chordoma: long-term follow-up after radical proton irradiation. *Radiother Oncol* 1996;41:67.
370. Austin-Seymour M, Munzenrider J, Goitein M, et al. Proton radiation therapy of chordoma and low-grade sarcoma of the base of the skull and cervical spine. *Int J Radiat Oncol Biol Phys* 1986;12[Suppl 1]:98.
371. Raffel C, Wright DC, Gutin PH, et al. Cranial chordomas: clinical presentation and results of operative and radiation therapy in twenty-six patients. *Neurosurgery* 1985;17:703.
372. Yoshii Y, Tsunoda T, Hyodo A, et al. Proton radiation therapy for clivus chordoma—case report. *Neurol Med Chir (Tokyo)* 1993;33:173.
373. Muthukumar N, Kondziolka D, Lunsford LD, Flickinger JC. Stereotactic radiosurgery for chondroma and chondrosarcoma: further experiences. *Int J Radiat Oncol Biol Phys* 1998;39:387.
374. Miller RC, Foote RL, Coffey RJ, et al. The role of stereotactic radiosurgery in the treatment of malignant skull base tumors. *Int J Radiat Oncol Biol Phys* 1997;39:977.
375. Reimer RR, Chabner BAC, Young RC, et al. Lymphoma presenting in bone. Results of histopathology, staging, and therapy. *Ann Intern Med* 1977;87:50.
376. Sweet DL, Moss DP, Simon MA, et al. Histiocytic lymphoma (reticulum-cell sarcoma) of bone. Current strategy for orthopedic surgeons. *J Bone Joint Surg Am* 1987;63:79.
377. Mendenhall NP, Jones JJ, Kramer BS, et al. The management of primary lymphoma of bone. *Radiother Oncol* 1987;9:137.
378. Loeffler JS, Tarbell NJ, Kozakewich H, et al. Primary lymphoma of bone in children: analysis of treatment results with Adriamycin, prednisone, Oncovin (APO), and local radiation therapy. *J Clin Oncol* 1986;4:496.
379. Bacci G, Jaffe N, Emiliani E, et al. Therapy for non-Hodgkin's lymphoma of bone and a comparison of results with Ewing's sarcoma. *Cancer* 1986;57:1468.
380. Ferreri AJ, Reni M, Ceresoli JL, Villa E. Therapeutic management with Adriamycin-containing chemotherapy and radiotherapy of monostoic and polystoic non-Hodgkin's lymphoma of bone in adults. *Cancer Invest* 1998;16:554.
381. Rapoport AP, Constine LS, Packman CH, et al. Treatment of multifocal lymphoma of bone and intensified ProMACE-CytaBOM chemotherapy and involved field radiotherapy. *Am J Hematol* 1998;58:1.
382. Dubey P, Ha CS, Besa PC, et al. Localized primary lymphoma of bone. *Int J Radiat Oncol Biol Phys* 1997;37:1087.
383. Baar J, Burkes RL, Gospodarowicz M. Primary non-Hodgkin's lymphoma of bone. *Semin Oncol* 1999;26:270.
384. Christie DR, Barton MB, Bryant G, et al. Osteolymphoma (primary bone lymphoma): an Australian review of 70 cases. Australasian Radiation Oncology Lymphoma Group (ARLOG). *Aust N Z J Med* 1999;29:214.
385. Coppes MJ, Patte C, Couanet D, et al. Childhood malignant lymphoma of bone. *Med Pediatr Oncol* 1991;19:22.
386. Furman WL, Fitch S, Hutsu HO, et al. Primary lymphoma of bone in children. *J Clin Oncol* 1989;7:1275.
387. Suryanarayan K, Shuster JJ, Donaldson SS, et al. Treatment of localized primary non-Hodgkin's lymphoma of bone in children: a Pediatric Oncology Group study. *J Clin Oncol* 1999;17:456.
388. Jaffe N, Frei E, Traggis D, Watts H. Adjuvant methotrexate and citrovorum factor treatment of osteogenic sarcoma. *N Engl J Med* 1974;291:994.
389. Rosenberg SA, Chabner BA, Young RC, et al. Treatment of osteogenic sarcoma. I. Effect of adjuvant high dose methotrexate after amputation. *Cancer Treat Rep* 1979;63:739.
390. Cortes E, Necheles TF, Holland JF, et al. Adjuvant therapy of operable primary osteosarcoma: a Cancer and Leukemia Group B experience. In: Salmon S, Jones S, eds. *Adjuvant therapy of cancer,* vol 3. New York: Grune & Stratton, 1981:201.
391. Sutow WW, Sullivan WP, Fernbach DJ, et al. Adjuvant chemotherapy in primary treatments of osteogenic sarcoma. A Southwest Oncology Group study. *Cancer* 1975;36:1598.
392. Sutow WW, Gehan EA, Dyment PG, et al. Multidrug adjuvant chemotherapy for osteosarcomas of the extremity: interim report of a Southwest Oncology Group study. *Cancer Treat Rep* 1978;62:265.
393. Herson J, Sutow WW, Elder K, et al. Adjuvant chemotherapy in nonmetastatic osteosarcoma: a Southwest Oncology Group study. *Med Pediatr Oncol* 1980;8:343.
394. Van der Scheuren E, Breur K. Role of lung irradiation in the adjuvant treatment of osteosarcoma. *Recent Results Cancer Res* 1982;80:98.
395. Pratt CB, Champion JE, Fleming ID, et al. Adjuvant chemotherapy for osteosarcoma of the extremity. Long-term results of two consecutive prospective protocol studies. *Cancer* 1990;65:439.
396. Ettinger LJ, Douglass HO, Higby DJ, et al. Adjuvant Adriamycin and *cis*-diamminedichloroplatinum (cisplatinum) in primary osteosarcoma. *Cancer* 1981;47:248.
397. Weiner M, Harris M, Lewis M, et al. Neoadjuvant high dose methotrexate, cisplatin, and doxorubicin for the management of patients with nonmetastatic osteosarcoma. *Cancer Treat Rep* 1986;70:1431.
398. Bacci G, Picci P, Ferrari S, et al. Primary chemotherapy and delayed surgery for nonmetastatic osteosarcoma of the extremities. Results in 164 patients preoperatively treated with high doses of methotrexate followed by cisplatin and doxorubicin. *Cancer* 1993;72:3227.

CHAPTER 40

Benign and Malignant Mesothelioma

SECTION 1

JOSEPH R. TESTA
HARVEY I. PASS
MICHELE CARBONE

Molecular Biology of Mesothelioma

Malignant mesotheliomas (MMs) are highly aggressive neoplasms that arise primarily from the surface serosal cells of the pleural, peritoneal, and pericardial cavities. Epidemiologic studies have established that exposure to asbestos fibers is the primary cause of MM,[1] and more recent investigations have implicated simian virus 40 (SV40) in the etiology of some MMs.[2–4] MM is characterized by a long latency from the time of exposure to asbestos to the onset of disease, suggesting that multiple somatic genetic events are required for tumorigenic conversion of a normal mesothelial cell. Early evidence in support of this notion was provided by karyotypic analyses, which revealed multiple clonal cytogenetic alterations in most human MMs.[5] Although a specific chromosomal change is not shared by all MMs, several prominent sites of chromosome loss have been identified in this malignancy. Tumor suppressor genes (TSGs) residing in these deleted chromosome regions may be responsible for the tumorigenic conversion of mesothelial cells, and studies have begun to identify the specific TSGs that contribute to the development and progression of MM. In this chapter, we provide an overview of recurrent chromosome deletions and molecular genetic alterations characteristic of MM. We also review the mechanistic role of asbestos and SV40 in this malignancy.

MECHANISM OF ASBESTOS-INDUCED ONCOGENESIS

Presently, it is not known whether asbestos fibers act directly on mesothelial cells or if they act indirectly via formation of reactive oxygen species (ROS) and growth factors.[6,7] In tissue culture, asbestos can physically interact with the mitotic spindle apparatus, which can result in aneuploidy and other forms of chromosome damage.[8] *In vivo,* iron-rich crocidolite asbestos fibers may lead to the release of ROS when hydrogen peroxide and superoxide react to form hydroxyl radicals. Asbestos has been shown to induce the expression and enzymatic activity of the mammalian DNA repair enzyme, apurinic/apyrimidinic (AP) endonuclease, suggesting that ROS generated by asbestos may induce DNA damage.[9] Furthermore, the inflammatory response to asbestos leads to the generation of several cytokines that are responsible for the well-known local and systemic immunosuppressive activity of asbestos.[10] Asbestos can also induce autophosphorylation of the epidermal growth factor (EGF) receptor, leading to increased expression of the protooncogenes c-*fos* and c-*jun*, which encode transcription factors that activate various genes critical in the initiation of DNA synthesis.[6] Persistent induction of these transcription activators by asbestos may enhance cellular proliferation and could render cells more susceptible to subsequent mutations in TSGs. Such enhanced expression of protooncogenes and inactivation of TSGs may cooperate in a multistep process that leads to MM.

CYTOGENETIC ASSESSMENT OF MALIGNANT MESOTHELIOMAS

Chromosome banding analyses have revealed that most MMs have complex karyotypes.[5] Among 20 MMs karyotyped by one of us (J. R. T.), all but one displayed more than ten clonal chromosome alterations.[11] Deletions of specific regions in the short (p) arms of chromosomes 1, 3, and 9 and long (q) arm of 6 were repeatedly observed in these tumors. Loss of a copy of chromosome 22 is the single most consistent numerical change seen in MMs. In the series by Taguchi et al.,[11] deletions and unbalanced rearrangements accounted for overlapping losses from the chromosome region 1p21-22 in 17 of 20 cases (85%). Thirteen of 20 MMs (65%) had interstitial deletions or other rearrangements that resulted in losses from 3p21. Ten cases (50%) showed losses from 6q, with a shortest region of overlap (SRO) at 6q15-21. Losses involving 9p were observed in 16 cases (80%), with the SRO being 9p21-p22. Monosomy 22 was documented in 13 cases (65%). These recurrent losses of 1p, 3p, 6q, 9p, and 22q frequently occurred in combination in a given tumor. All five of these aberrations were found in 5 of our 20 MMs. Losses of 1p, 3p, 9p, and 22q coexisted in another three cases, and various combinations of three of these four abnormalities were seen in seven other cases. It is not known if this multistep cascade evolves slowly during the course of tumor formation or in rapid succession at some critical stage of the disease. In any case, the accumulated loss of DNA sequences from chromosomes 1p, 3p, 6q, 9p, and 22q appears to play a critical role in the pathogenesis of MM.

More recent molecular cytogenetic studies, using comparative genomic hybridization (CGH), also have documented recurrent genomic imbalances in MM. CGH is a fluorescence *in situ* hybridization technique that permits the identification of chromosome gains and losses in the entire tumor genome in a single experiment. Balsara et al.[12] performed CGH analyses on 24 MM cell lines derived from patients seen in the United States; each of these cell lines exhibited multiple (6 to 25) genomic imbalances. Losses involving 22q, documented in 14 of 24 cell lines (58%), was the most prominent alteration. Also in agreement with earlier karyologic findings, losses of 1p, 3p, 6q, and 9p were common, with each being observed in approximately 30% to 40% of cell lines. In addition, CGH analysis uncovered other recurrent chromosome losses not highlighted in previous karyotypic studies. In particular, 13 of 24 MMs (54%) showed losses of part or all of 15q, with the SRO being 15q11.1-21. In addition, losses involving 14q24.2-qter and 13q12-14 were each observed in 42% of the cell lines. The most frequently overrepresented chromosomal arm was 5p (54% of cases), suggesting the involvement of a putative oncogene(s) at this location.

Many of the recurrent genomic imbalances identified in U.S. cases were also detected in MM specimens examined by Finnish investigators.[13] However, three prominent imbalances in the series from the United States (i.e., losses of 15q11.1-21.1, 8p21-pter, and 3p21) were each observed in only 1 of 42 cases from Finland. Discrepancies between the data from Finland and the United States could reflect dissimilarities in the type of asbestos exposure or genetic differences in the study populations. Alternatively, they may be related to the presence of SV40 in MMs from the United States and the absence of SV40 in MMs from Finland.[14]

DELETION MAPPING

The recurrent genomic losses just described are consistent with a recessive mechanism of oncogenesis and can be viewed as indicators of the locations of putative TSGs important in the development and progression of MM. As a prelude to the isolation of these genes, the critically deleted regions in 1p, 3p, 6q, 9p, and 15q defined by cytogenetic studies of MM have been mapped at the molecular genetic level by loss of heterozygosity (LOH) analysis using polymorphic DNA markers. Results of these investigations have been reviewed in detail elsewhere,[5] but are briefly summarized here.

CHROMOSOME 1p22

To map the critically deleted region of 1p, Lee et al.[15] performed LOH analyses of 50 MMs using a large panel of DNA markers located throughout the entire short arm of chromosome 1. Allelic losses at 1p21-22 were observed in 36 cases (72%), and we were able to localize the SRO of deletions to a 4-centimorgan segment within 1p22. Currently, candidate TSGs mapped to this region are being assayed for possible mutations and altered expression in MMs.

CHROMOSOME 3p21

Research groups led by two of us (J. R. T., H. I. P.) have independently demonstrated that 3p is a common site of allelic loss in MM. In one of these investigations, for example, 15 of 24 cases (62.5%) exhibited losses from 3p, with the highest frequency being at 3p21.3. Losses from this region also have been reported in many other malignancies, particularly lung cancers, suggesting that perturbation of a TSG(s) located in this region may play a role in the development of multiple tumor types.

CHROMOSOME 6q

LOH analysis of 6q has revealed a complex pattern of allelic loss. LOH at 6q occurs in approximately 60% of MMs, and deletions fall into several discrete regions involving markers mapped within 6q14-21, 6q16.6-21, 6q21-23.2, and 6q25. Multiple nonoverlapping regions of 6q loss also have been described in other types of malignancy, such as non-Hodgkin's lymphoma.

CHROMOSOME 9p21

To map the minimal region of 9p deletion in MMs, one of us (J. R. T.) initially performed gene dosage studies on a series of MM cell lines, 83% of which showed homozygous or hemizygous deletions involving an approximately 1-megabase segment located between the interferon gene cluster and the marker D9S171 in 9p21. The *CDKN2A* locus, which encodes the alternative TSG products p16 and $p14^{ARF}$ is located within this region. The cellular function of p16 and $p14^{ARF}$ and their potential role in MM are discussed in the following section, Alterations of Tumor Suppressor Genes in Mesothelioma.

CHROMOSOME 15q11.1-15

CGH analyses performed by Balsara et al.[12] revealed losses from 15q in 13 of 24 MM cell lines (54%) examined, and subsequent LOH analyses showed allelic losses from one or more 15q loci in 10 of these 13 lines. The extent of overlap of 15q deletions was used to define a minimal region of chromosome loss within 15q11.1-15. Losses overlapping this region also have been observed in several other types of malignancy, such as metastatic tumors of the breast, lung, and colon, suggesting that this region harbors a TSG that may contribute to the progression of diverse cancer types.

ALTERATIONS OF TUMOR SUPPRESSOR GENES IN MESOTHELIOMA

One of the protein products of the *CDKN2A* locus, p16, is capable of binding to the cyclin-dependent kinase CDK4, thereby inhibiting the catalytic activity of the CDK4/cyclin D enzymes. Several months after its initial cloning, the *p16* gene was identified as the 9p21 putative TSG by using a positional cloning approach, and homozygous deletions of *p16* were detected at high frequencies in cell lines derived from many different kinds of cancer.[16]

Because of its location within the region we previously determined as the SRO of 9p deletions in MMs and because of its involvement in many other cancer types, *p16* emerged as the prime candidate for the 9p TSG in MM. Among 40 MM cell lines studied by Cheng et al.,[17] 34 (85%) had homozygous deletions of one or more *p16* exons and another had a point mutation in *p16*. Down-regulation of *p16* was observed in four of the remaining cell lines. Homozygous deletions of *p16* were identified in 5 of 23 MM specimens (22%). The finding of a much higher incidence of *p16* alterations in MM cell lines than in tumor tissues may be associated with a selective growth advantage provided by *p16* deletion during the culturing process. On the other hand, MM samples often contain a significant amount of contaminating normal stroma, which can mask the existence of a homozygous deletion in the malignant cell population. Down-regulation of *p16* in MM cells may result from 5' CpG island hypermethylation, as has been demonstrated in other types of cancer.[18] At the protein level, Kratzke et al.[19] reported abnormal expression of p16 in 12 of 12 MM specimens and 15 of 15 MM-derived cell lines examined by immunohistochemistry. Moreover, in xenograft experiments, reexpression of p16 in MM cells resulted in cell-cycle arrest and cell death, as well as inhibition of tumor formation or diminished tumor size.[20]

It is important to note that homozygous deletions of the *CDKN2A* locus would in many cases also lead to the inactivation of another putative TSG, $p14^{ARF}$ (the mouse homologue is $p19^{ARF}$), because *p16* and $p14^{ARF}$ share exons 2 and 3, although their reading frames differ. $p14^{ARF}$ is essential for the activation of p53 in response to the action of oncogenes such as Ras.[21] On the other hand, p16 induces a G_1 cell-cycle arrest by inhibiting the phosphorylation of the retinoblastoma protein, pRb. Thus, homozygous loss of $p14^{ARF}$ and *p16* would collectively affect both p53- and pRb-dependent growth regulatory pathways. However, there is evidence that retention of exon 1β, which encodes the active domain of $p14^{ARF}$, may produce a peptide containing a functional, or partly functional, protein.[21] Moreover, unlike the response to oncogenic Ras, $p14^{ARF}$ is not required for activation of p53 in response to DNA damage by agents such as asbestos, suggesting that *p16* could be the critical TSG targeted by 9p21 deletions in MM.

Extensive LOH analysis of chromosome 22 losses in MM has not been performed because an entire copy of chromosome 22 is lost in most cases. Although the neurofibromatosis type 2 TSG, *NF2*, predisposes affected individuals primarily to tumors of neuroectodermal origin, somatic mutations of *NF2* have occasionally been identified in seemingly unrelated malignancies.[22] Thus, two groups independently embarked on mutational studies of *NF2* in MM. Bianchi et al.[22] identified nucleotide mutations in 8 of 15 MM cell lines (53%). The mutations, which included deletions and insertions and one nonsense mutation, predicted truncated forms of the NF2 protein, known as *merlin* or *schwannomin*. Similar results were also reported by Sekido et al.,[23] who detected somatic mutations in one MM specimen and in 7 of 17 MM cell lines (41%). In the study by Bianchi et al.,[22] the mutations observed in complementary DNAs from MM cell lines were confirmed in genomic DNA from six matched primary tumor specimens. It is intriguing that the two complementary DNA alterations that could not be confirmed by genomic analysis were both splicing-related—that is, deletion of exon 10 in one cell line and a 49-base-pair insertion between exons 13 and 14 in the other. This finding suggests that aberrant splicing, either by mutations of cis elements or by changes in the splicing machinery regulating the processing of *NF2* transcripts, may constitute an additional mechanism for *NF2* inactivation in MM.

In a subsequent report, mutations in the *NF2* coding region were detected in 12 of 23 new MM cell lines.[24] Western blot analyses revealed high levels of NF2 in 11 MM cell lines lacking *NF2* mutations, whereas NF2 protein was not detectable in the 12 cell lines that exhibited alterations of the *NF2* gene. In addition, two cell lines with *NF2* mutations reported in an earlier study were also examined, and both of these cell lines showed no NF2 expression. LOH analyses were performed on the entire 25 MM cell lines using two polymorphic DNA markers residing at or near the *NF2* locus in chromosome 22q12. Eighteen of the 25 cell lines (72%) showed losses at one or both of these loci. All cases exhibiting mutation or aberrant expression of *NF2* showed allelic losses, implying that inactivation of *NF2* in MM occurs via a two-hit mechanism.

SIMIAN VIRUS 40

SV40 is a DNA tumor virus that has been associated with MM. Although SV40 is endogenous to the rhesus monkey, the virus infected the human population through contaminated polio- and adenovaccines, both attenuated and killed, between 1955 and 1963.[2–4] Poliovaccines were prepared in cell cultures grown as monolayers of infected rhesus monkey kidney cells. Because the virus produces no cytopathic effects in these cells, their infection went unrecognized until 1960, when high titers of the virus were found in some lots of the vaccine. As a result of this contamination, it is estimated that up to 96 million adults and children in the United States alone may have been injected with poliovaccines containing SV40. After 1963, slow-replicating strains of SV40, which are difficult to detect using cytopathic tests, may have infected humans exposed to products produced with monkey cells.[25] This hypothesis is supported by the observation that individuals born after 1962 with minimal risk of exposure to contaminated vaccines had an approximately 10% positive rate for SV40-neutralizing antibodies.[3] In addition, horizontal transmission is also possible because SV40 sequences have been detected in sperm, in circulating mononuclear phagocytes, and in cells obtained from the milk of a healthy woman.[2–4] Regardless of its method of introduction into humans, SV40 appears to be presently transmitted among humans similarly to other papovaviruses.

A link between SV40 and tumor development was first recognized in hamsters, when, in 1960, Bernice Eddy found that subcutaneous injection of rhesus monkey kidney cells into newborn hamsters led to the formation of sarcomas at the injection site. In 1991, it was found that 60% of hamsters injected intracardially with SV40 developed pleural MMs.[4] When SV40 was injected into the pleural spaces of these animals, 100% developed pleural MMs in 3 to 6 months.[4] Interestingly, in hamsters, SV40 is a much more potent carcinogen in the induction of MMs than asbestos. For example, in a study by Smith and Hubert,[26] hamsters were injected intrapleurally with varying doses of chrysotile, amosite, and tremolite. Of 50 hamsters, 13 developed MMs on injection with chrysotile. In a separate group of 50 animals, four developed MMs when injected with amosite. No tumors were observed in those injected with tremolite. Among all tumors that developed, the earliest was observed after 151 days in a hamster injected intrapleurally with 25 mg of chrysotile. In contrast, MMs developed in 100% of hamsters injected intrapleurally with SV40 in only 3 to 6 months.[4]

The discovery that SV40 produced MMs in hamsters subsequently led to the polymerase chain reaction analysis of human MM specimens for the presence of the virus.[27] It was found that 29 of 48 human MMs (60%) contained and expressed SV40 DNA. Sequence analysis revealed that these DNA sequences were homologous to SV40. These results were confirmed by many laboratories[3,4] and by an independent multilaboratory study organized by the International Mesothelioma Interest Group.[28] This study found that 83% of the MMs tested contained SV40 DNA sequences.[28] More recently, using a microdissection technique, Schivapurkar et al. demonstrated that SV40 is specifically present in neoplastic MM cells and not in the surrounding reactive stromal cells or in lung cancer cells.[29] It should be noted, however, that Finnish MM specimens consistently tested negative for SV40.[14] This finding, together with the observation of a different incidence of SV40 in bone tumors from different regions of the world, suggest geographic differences for SV40 in human tumors.[2–4] It has been hypothesized that these differences may be related either to the use of contaminated poliovaccines (because Finnish poliovaccines were not contaminated by SV40) or to other factors presently unknown.[14]

The ability of SV40 to transform human cells *in vitro* is well established. The SV40 genome is a double-stranded circular DNA molecule containing 5243 base pairs, which can be divided into two regions, early and late, according to the order in which they are transcribed.[2–4] The early region encodes three proteins—large T antigen (Tag), small t antigen (tag), and 17kT—and is responsible for the transforming ability of the virus. The late region encodes viral coat proteins. Only the early region is necessary for transformation to occur, so immortalization experiments have been done with both the whole viral genome and the early-region DNA alone.[2–4] Tag binds to viral and cellular DNA, inducing their replication, and has mutagenic and clastogenic function, as it can cause chromosome rearrangements, point mutations, and aneuploidy. Tag is also capable of binding and inactivating the products of several TSGs, including p53, pRb, pRb2/p130, p107, p400, and p300, which are necessary to prevent cells with DNA damage from cycling.[2–4] In addition, through inhibition of p53, Tag inactivates an essential cell checkpoint at which DNA alterations are repaired before the cell is allowed to continue into the S phase of the cell cycle. If the cell does not repair the mutations, normally apoptosis occurs. Tag inhibition of p53 allows the cell to undergo mitosis even in the presence of mutations. Whether continuous expression of Tag is necessary to maintain the transformed phenotype is currently unclear.[2–4] Experiments in hamsters indicate that continuous expression of Tag is necessary to induce and maintain transformation. In contrast, more recent experiments in SV40 transgenic mice and human cells *in vitro*[2,4] and in rats[30] suggest that continuous expression of Tag is not always needed for maintenance of the transformed phenotype.

A 19-kD protein, tag is found predominantly in the cytoplasm of infected or transformed cells and performs several functions to increase the transforming potential of Tag.[2–4] It increases production of Tag, causes mitosis in quiescent cells through stimulation of mitogen-activated protein (MAP) kinase and AP-1, and contributes to the complete inactivation of p53 by stimulating cellular phosphatase 2A (PP2A) to indirectly alter the phosphorylation state of p53.

After infection with SV40, some human cells die and others are transformed. Many of the transformed cells eventually reach crisis and die, but a few become immortal.[31] Although human cells immortalized by SV40 do not produce tumors in nude mice, these same cells may become oncogenic if they are transfected with an oncogene, mutated by carcinogens, or if they are passed enough times to allow a significant number of mutations to accrue.[2–4,31]

Through the actions of Tag and tag, human mesothelial cells, fibroblasts, bronchial epithelium, and breast epithelium have been transformed *in vitro*.[31] Human cells transformed by SV40 in tissue culture, when injected into human volunteers, have induced subcutaneous tumors.[4] Analysis of p53 and retinoblastoma family members demonstrated that Tag complexes and inactivates these gene products in human MM.[32,33] p53, pRb, p107, and pRb2/p130 are present in detectable quantities in human mesothelial cells, and their expression is also significantly associated with Tag expression.[32,33] Their absence of mutations, their unusually high level of expression in tumor cells, and the ability of Tag to co-precipitate with each of these tumor suppressors supports the assertion that SV40 Tag binds, stabilizes, and inactivates p53 and retinoblastoma proteins, which may allow for MM development.[32,33] This hypothesis has been supported by experiments in which transfection of antisense SV40 inhibited Tag expression, restored the p53-p21 pathway, and caused growth arrest and apoptosis of SV40-positive human MM cell lines.[34] These findings suggest that antisense SV40 strategies may be useful in the treatment of SV40-positive MM patients.[34]

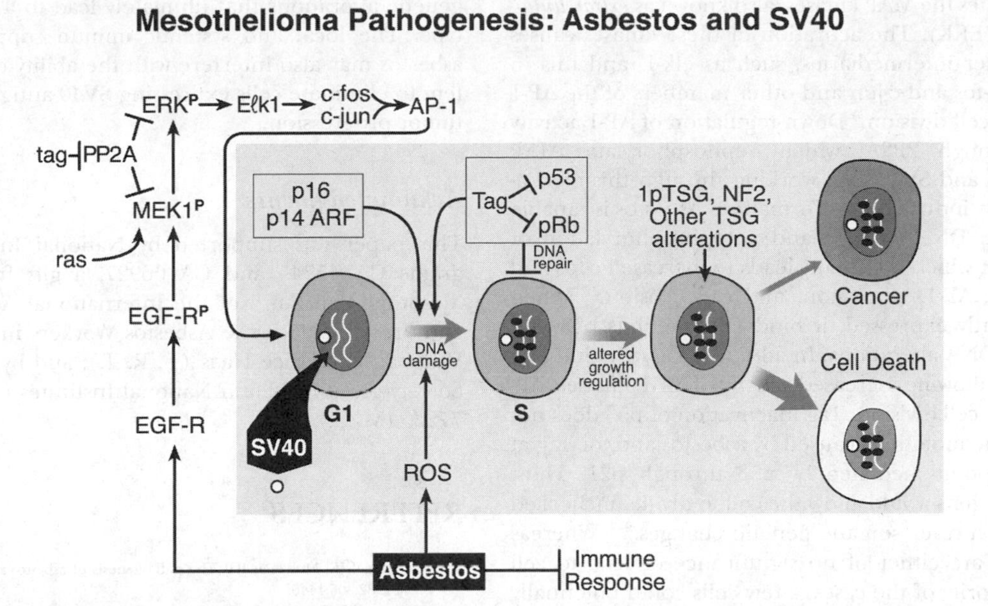

FIGURE 40.1-1. Diagram illustrating mesothelioma pathogenesis. Increased levels of activator protein 1 (AP-1) stimulate cell division.[36] The activity of AP-1 is regulated through a delicate balance between phosphorylation and dephosphorylation. Autophosphorylation of the epidermal growth factor receptor (EGF-R), or activation of ras and others, leads to phosphorylation of MEK1 kinase, which in turn phosphorylates the mitogen-activated protein (MAP) kinases also known as *extracellular-regulated kinases* (ERK). The activation of these kinases leads through other intermediaries, such as elk-1 (Elk1), to the activation of c-*fos*, c-*jun*, and other members of the AP-1 family (not shown), which through their transcriptional activity stimulate cell division.[36] Phosphatase 2A (PP2A) down-regulates AP-1 activity by dephosphorylating the MAP kinases; therefore, PP2A plays an important role in preventing asbestos-mediated cancerogenesis. Crocidolite asbestos induces both DNA mutations and autophosphorylation of the EGF-R, which leads to increased levels of c-*fos* and c-*jun* expression, AP-1 activation, and cell division.[36] When simian virus 40 (SV40) large T antigen (Tag) is expressed in this system, it binds and inhibits p53 and the retinoblastoma protein pRb, and it contributes to the development of DNA alterations.[32,33] In addition, Tag is known to be directly and indirectly (through p53 inactivation) mutagenic.[2,4] When SV40 small t antigen (tag) is also expressed in this system, it binds and inactivates PP2A and contributes to cellular transformation. This leads to increased activity of the MAP kinases, increased activity of AP-1, and cell division.[36] In this scenario, crocidolite may increase the amount of c-*fos* and c-*jun* and, to some extent, their activity, whereas tag, by removing PP2A, further increases their activity. If the dividing cells have developed DNA alterations (such as *p16* and $p14^{ARF}$) through the mutagenic effects of asbestos—mediated through the production of reactive oxygen species (ROS) created by alveolar macrophages during phagocytosis of asbestos fibers[5,36]—and/or Tag, these mutations may not be repaired because of the Tag inactivation of the G_1/S checkpoint mediated by p53 through p21.[32–34] In this scenario, the cell may complete division and possibly continue to divide.[34] Cells with unrepaired DNA damage are prone to develop additional DNA alterations that usually result in cell death but occasionally may result in immortalization, which may be followed by transformation and tumor development. Therefore, the combined effects of asbestos and SV40 may overwhelm the cell-cycle regulatory mechanisms and result in cell division and occasionally in cellular transformation, which may lead to mesothelioma development. Because asbestos depresses both the local and systemic immune responses,[10] asbestos may help mesothelial cells expressing SV40 antigens to escape immune surveillance. Arrowheads indicate a stimulatory effect, and crossed bars indicate an inhibitory effect. The circle indicates nonintegrated SV40; in some tumors, however, SV40 has been found integrated in the host cell DNA. NF2, neurofibromatosis type 2; TSG, tumor suppressor genes.

CONCLUSIONS

Multiple genetic alterations are involved in the development of most malignancies. Many MM patients who expressed SV40-Tag contained asbestos in their lungs.[8,35] Both SV40 and asbestos cause genetic damage. Thus, SV40 may act with asbestos to cause MM. Cells of patients with preexisting genetic alterations have been found to be more susceptible to SV40 transformation than normal control cells.[2–4] For instance, the transformation frequency by SV40 of fibroblasts from a lung cancer patient with Klinefelter's syndrome was three to ten times higher than that of fibroblasts from normal individuals with no history of cancer. Furthermore, fibroblasts from individuals with Down syndrome and Fanconi's anemia also have increased susceptibility to transformation by SV40 *in vitro*. Thus, it is possible that because cells with preexisting genetic alterations are more easily transformed by SV40, cells harboring DNA alterations caused by asbestos would also be more prone to SV40 transformation.

In a normal cell, mitosis is controlled through a delicate balance of phosphorylation and dephosphorylation events. Increased levels of AP-1 are ultimately responsible for cell division, and the activity of AP-1 is normally regulated through phosphorylation and dephosphorylation events (Fig. 40.1-1). Autophosphorylation of the EGF receptor, or activation of ras and others, leads to phosphorylation of MEK1 kinase, which in turn phosphorylates the MAP kinases, also known as *extracellular-regulated kinases* (ERK). The activation of these kinases causes activation of other intermediaries, such as elk-1, and this in turn stimulates c-fos and c-jun and other members of the AP-1 family, inducing cell division.[6] Down-regulation of AP-1 activity is achieved through PP2A, which dephosphorylates MAP kinases. Asbestos and SV40 Tag, working through this mechanism, may actually induce tumor formation. Asbestos is capable of inducing both DNA damage and autophosphorylation of the EGF-receptor, which eventually leads to increased c-fos and c-jun expression, AP-1 expression, and cell division.[36] When Tag is concurrently expressed, it binds and inhibits p53 and pRb and causes DNA alterations. In addition, tag can bind and inactivate PP2A, allowing increased activity of MAP kinases, AP-1 and, ultimately, cell division. Tag inactivation of p53 does not allow repair of the mutations caused by asbestos and/or Tag at the G_1/S checkpoint mediated by p53 through p21. Thus, these two carcinogens would allow the cell to divide unchecked and accumulate further somatic genetic changes.[2–4] Whereas DNA alterations are either of no significance or lead to cell death in the majority of the cases, a few cells could potentially develop perturbations of key cell-cycle regulatory genes[5] and become immortalized, transformed, and tumorigenic. Therefore, we propose that the combined effects of asbestos and SV40 overwhelm cell-cycle regulatory mechanisms, result in unchecked cell division, and occasionally allow transformation and MM development. Evidence in support of this assertion comes from experiments with p53-deficient mice.[37] These studies demonstrate that p53-deficient animals are more susceptible to the induction of MM on exposure to asbestos. Similarly, human mesothelial cells positive for SV40 have Tag-mediated inhibition of p53[33] and may be more susceptible to asbestos carcinogenicity. The finding that, in MM cells, restoration of the p53 pathway with antisense Tag causes growth arrest and apoptosis supports this scenario.[34] It should be noted that SV40 is a very strong immunogen and that cells expressing SV40 viral antigens are usually efficiently recognized and killed by the host immune system.[2–4] In other words, SV40 is a very potent carcinogen, capable of fully transforming human cells in tissue culture.[2–4] At the same time, SV40 is a strong immunogen; therefore, SV40-transformed cells should be killed by the immune system. It is possible that the local and systemic immunosuppressive activity of asbestos[10] may favor the growth of cells expressing SV40 antigens and may partly explain the strong association of SV40 with MM.

SUMMARY

A large body of experimental and epidemiologic data support the notion that asbestos, or at least amphibole asbestos, causes MM. The same data also support the notion that exposure to asbestos is usually not sufficient for MM development and that other factors, including radiation, genetic predisposition, and SV40, may render some individuals more susceptible to asbestos carcinogenicity. At this time, the involvement of radiation and genetic predisposition in MM development is speculative. On the other hand, SV40 is present in most human MMs. In these neoplasms, SV40 interferes with key cell-cycle regulatory genes and may contribute with asbestos or alone (in non–asbestos-associated tumors) to the development of molecular genetic alterations that ultimately lead to a malignant phenotype. The local and systemic immunosuppressive activity of asbestos may also interfere with the ability of the immune system to eliminate cells expressing SV40 antigens and thus favor tumor progression.

Acknowledgments

This paper was supported by National Institutes of Health grants CA 45745 and CA 06927, a gift from the Local 14 Mesothelioma Fund of the International Association of Heat and Frost Insulators & Asbestos Workers in memory of Hank Vaughan and Alice Haas (J. R. T.); and by American Cancer Society grant 8632 and National Institutes of Health grant CA 77220 (M. C.).

REFERENCES

1. Craighead JE, Mossman BT. The pathogenesis of asbestos-associated diseases. *N Engl J Med* 1982;306:1446.
2. Carbone M, Fisher S, Powers A, Pass HI, Rizzo P. New molecular and epidemiological issues in mesothelioma: role of SV40. *J Cell Physiol* 1999;180:167.
3. Butel J, Lednicky J. Cell and molecular biology of SV40: implications for human infections and disease. *J Natl Cancer Inst* 1999;91:119.
4. Carbone M, Rizzo P, Pass HI. Simian virus 40, poliovaccines, and human tumors: a review of recent developments. *Oncogene* 1997;15:1877.
5. Murthy SS, Testa JR. Asbestos, chromosomal deletions, and tumor suppressor genes in human malignant mesothelioma. *J Cell Physiol* 1999;180:150.
6. Mossman BT, Kamp DW, Weitzman SA. Mechanisms of carcinogenesis and clinical features of asbestos-associated cancers. *Cancer Invest* 1996;14:466.
7. Pache JC, Janssen YM, Walsh ES, et al. Increased epidermal growth factor-receptor protein in a human mesothelial cell line in response to long asbestos fibers. *Am J Pathol* 1998;152:333.
8. Ault JG, Cole RW, Jensen CG, et al. Behavior of crocidolite asbestos during mitosis in living vertebrate lung epithelial cells. *Cancer Res* 1995;55:792.
9. Fung H, Kow YW, Van Houten B, et al. Asbestos increases mammalian AP-endonuclease gene expression, protein levels, and enzyme activity in mesothelial cells. *Cancer Res* 1998;58:189.
10. Rosenthal GJ, Simeonova P, Corsini E. Asbestos toxicity: an immunologic perspective. *Rev Environ Health* 1999;14:11.
11. Taguchi T, Jhanwar SC, Siegfried JM, Keller SM, Testa JR. Recurrent deletions of specific chromosomal sites in 1p, 3p, 6q, and 9p in human malignant mesothelioma. *Cancer Res* 1993;52:4349.
12. Balsara BR, Bell DW, Sonoda G, et al. Comparative genomic hybridization and loss of heterozygosity analyses identify a common region of deletion at 15q11.1-15 in human malignant mesothelioma. *Cancer Res* 1999;59:450.
13. Bjorkqvist AM, Tammilehto L, Anttila S, Mattson K, Knuutila S. Recurrent DNA copy number changes in 1q, 4q, 6q, 9p, 13q, 14q, and 22q detected by comparative genomic hybridization in malignant mesothelioma. *Br J Cancer* 1997;75:523.
14. Hirvonen A, Mattson K, Karjalainen A, et al. Simian virus 40 (SV40)-like DNA sequences not detectable in Finnish mesothelioma patients not exposed to SV40 contaminated polio vaccines. *Mol Carcinog* 1999;26:93.
15. Lee WC, Balsara B, Liu Z, Jhanwar SC, Testa JR. Loss of heterozygosity analysis defines a critical region in chromosome 1p22 commonly deleted in human malignant mesothelioma. *Cancer Res* 1996;56:4297.
16. Kamb A, Gruis NA, Weaver-Feldhaus J, et al. A cell cycle regulator potentially involved in the genesis of many tumor types. *Science* 1994;264:436.
17. Cheng JQ, Jhanwar SC, Klein WM, et al. *p16* alterations and deletion mapping of 9p21-p22 in malignant mesothelioma. *Cancer Res* 1994;54:5547.
18. Merlo A, Herman JG, Mao L, et al. 5' CpG island methylation is associated with transcriptional silencing of the tumor suppressor p16/CDKN2/MTS1 in human cancers. *Nature Med* 1995;1:686.
19. Kratzke RA, Otterson GA, Lincoln CE, et al. Immunohistochemical analysis of the p16INK4 cyclin-dependent kinase inhibitor in malignant mesothelioma. *J Natl Cancer Inst* 1995;87:1870.
20. Frizelle SP, Grim J, Zhou J, et al. Re-expression of p16INK4a in mesothelioma cells results in cell cycle arrest, cell death, tumor suppression and tumor regression. *Oncogene* 1998;16:3087.
21. Palmero I, Pantoja C, Serrano M. p19ARF links the tumour suppressor p53 to Ras. *Nature* 1998;395:125.
22. Bianchi AB, Mitsunaga SI, Cheng JQ, et al. High frequency of inactivating mutations in the neurofibromatosis type 2 gene (*NF2*) in primary malignant mesotheliomas. *Proc Natl Acad Sci U S A* 1995;92:10854.
23. Sekido Y, Pass HI, Bader S, et al. Neurofibromatosis type 2 (*NF2*) gene is somatically mutated in mesothelioma but not in lung cancer. *Cancer Res* 1995;55:1227.
24. Cheng JQ, Lee WC, Klein MA, et al. Frequent alterations of *NF2* and allelic loss from chromosome band 22q12 in malignant mesothelioma: evidence for a two-hit mechanism of *NF2* inactivation. *Genes Chromosomes Cancer* 1999;24:238.

25. Rizzo P, Di Resta I, Powers A, Rattner H, Carbone M. Unique strains of SV40 in commercial poliovaccines from 1955 not readily identifiable with current testing for SV40 infection. *Cancer Res* 1999;59:6103.
26. Smith WE, Hubert DD. The intrapleural route as a means for estimating carcinogenicity. In: Karbe E, Park JF. *Experimental lung cancer. Carcinogenesis and bioassays.* New York: Springer-Verlag New York, 1974:92.
27. Carbone M, Pass HI, Rizzo P, et al. Simian virus 40–like DNA sequences in human pleural mesothelioma. *Oncogene* 1994;9:1781.
28. Testa JR, Carbone M, Hirvonen A, et al. A multi-institutional study confirms the presence and expression of simian virus 40 in human malignant mesotheliomas. *Cancer Res* 1998;58:4505.
29. Schivapurkar N, Wiethege T, Wistuba II, et al. Presence of simian virus 40 sequences in malignant mesotheliomas and mesothelial cell proliferations. *J Cell Biochem* 1999;76:181.
30. Salewski H, Bayer TA, Eidhoff U, et al. Increased oncogenicity of subclones of SV40 large T-induced neuroectodermal tumor cell lines after loss of large T antigen expression and concomitant mutation of p53. *Cancer Res* 1999;59:1980.
31. Bryan TM, Reddel RR. SV40-induced immortalization of human cells. *Crit Rev Oncog* 1994;5:331.
32. Carbone M, Rizzo P, Grimely PM, et al. Simian virus 40 large T antigen binds p53 in human mesotheliomas. *Nature Med* 1997;8:908.
33. De Luca A, Baldi A, Esposito V, et al. The retinoblastoma gene family pRb/p105, p107, pRb2/p130, and simian virus 40 large T antigen in human mesotheliomas. *Nature Med* 1997;3:913.
34. Waheed I, Guo ZS, Chen GA, et al. Antisense to SV40 early gene region induces growth arrest and apoptosis in T-antigen positive human pleural mesothelioma cells. *Cancer Res* 1999;15:6068.
35. Mayall FG, Jacobson G, Wilkins R. Mutations of p53 gene and SV40 sequences in asbestos associated and non-asbestos-associated mesotheliomas. *J Clin Pathol* 1999;4:291.
36. Robledo R, Mossmann B. Cellular and molecular mechanisms of asbestos induced fibrosis. *J Cell Physiol* 1999;180:158.
37. Marsella JM, Liu BL, Vaslet CA, Kane AB. Susceptibility of p53 deficient mice to induction of mesothelioma by crocidolite asbestos fibers. *Environ Health Perspect* 1998;141:1069.

KAREN H. ANTMAN
HARVEY I. PASS
PETER B. SCHIFF

SECTION 2
Management of Mesothelioma

EPIDEMIOLOGY

Asbestos is the predominant cause of pleural, peritoneal, and probably epididymal mesothelioma in humans. The resistance of asbestos to heat and combustion was recognized by ancient civilizations. Although Pliny had observed that asbestos miners were less healthy than other slaves, the health hazards of asbestos exposure were generally not recognized until this century.[1]

The Industrial Revolution greatly expanded demand for asbestos as insulating and packing material for machines and power generators. In 1898, pulmonary scarring and eventual death from respiratory failure was noted in asbestos workers from French and English asbestos textile mills.[2] However, the cause of the pulmonary fibrosis remained uncertain because tuberculosis and other respiratory infections were often epidemic among poor laborers. The two World Wars further increased the use of asbestos in ships and other equipment of combat and transport. The availability, durability, and low cost of asbestos additionally expanded its range of uses in industrial and consumer products. In 1930, the causal association between asbestos and asbestosis was firmly established by Merewether and Price at the London Chest Hospital.[3] When limits were set on allowable industrial levels of asbestos exposure in England, many thought the asbestos problem had been solved.[1] However, case reports of lung cancer in patients with asbestosis appeared as early as 1935.[4,5]

In 1955, Doll[6] reported a case-control study that established the association between asbestos and lung cancer. The attitudes and opinions of scientists between 1935 and 1965 reveal early agreement on the carcinogenesis of asbestos by 1943 in Germany, but rejection of German scientific thought during and after World War II and the lack of epidemiologic and experimental evidence delayed a consensus elsewhere.[7]

Up to 8 million living persons in the United States have been occupationally exposed to asbestos over the last five decades during mining and milling of asbestos and in diverse manufacturing processes that use the material. Today, many public and private buildings contain asbestos, including 10% to 15% of schools in the United States that were insulated or sprayed on interior surfaces with asbestos between 1946 and 1972. The public health significance of exposure in such buildings and the cost-effectiveness of asbestos removal are controversial.[8] However, one study suggested risk from such incidental exposures. For 9 of 12 schoolteachers with mesothelioma, the only potential asbestos exposure was that derived from asbestos-containing building materials in schools.[9]

ASBESTOS-ASSOCIATED MESOTHELIOMA

The existence of mesothelioma as a distinct pathologic entity was debated by pathologists before 1960.[10] In the late 1940s, case reports of mesotheliomas in patients with asbestosis began to appear. In 1960, Wagner et al.[11] in South Africa reported 33 cases of mesothelioma diagnosed between ages 31 and 68 years in a South African crocidolite mining community. An additional 14 cases were added in an addendum to the paper. A substantial proportion of these patients were exposed in childhood through living in the vicinity of asbestos mills and mines; a few had occupational contact. This study was followed by reports of mesotheliomas in asbestos workers in other parts of the world.

Mechanisms of Asbestos Carcinogenicity

Two major forms of asbestos exist: curly pliable serpentine asbestos (chrysotile) and rod-like amphiboles (crocidolite, amosite, anthophyllite, tremolite, and actinolyte). The first three of these are mined for their commercial utility; the latter three are usually contaminants. Asbestos fibers tend to separate readily and form numerous individual strands, which often are less than 1 μm in diameter.

Carcinogenic effects of asbestos appear to result from its physical properties, rather than chemical structure.[12] In one animal experiment, other fiber types produced mesothelioma more efficiently than amosite asbestos.[13] Long rod-like fibers of narrow diameter are more likely to induce tumors in laboratory animals.[14] Although serpentine asbestos (chrysotile) is generally considered less carcinogenic than the rod-like amphiboles (crocidolite, amosite, anthophyllite, tremolite, and actinolyte), debate continues over whether cases associated with chrysotile asbestos are actually caused by amphibole contamination[15] or are caused by chrysotile itself.[16] Long, needle-like amphibole fibers lodge more readily in the distal respiratory area, where they persist longer and are transported to the pleura and peritoneum.[14]

After inhalation most asbestos is expectorated or swallowed and subsequently excreted in the feces. The remainder can be cleared from the tracheal and bronchial tree via multiple mechanisms, including ciliary action in the trachea, ingestion by macrophages, or penetration through the endothelial lining into interstitial tissues.[17] Short fibers are cleared more readily than long fibers. Fibers that remain preferentially accumulate in the lower third of the lungs adjacent to the visceral pleura. Fibers can be counted visually or using electron microscopy and correlate with asbestos exposure,[18] although visual counting provides substantially lower estimates of fibers per gram of lung.[19]

Asbestos results in an inflammatory and fibrotic process, mediated in part by cytokines released by activated alveolar macrophages.[20] At a molecular level, protooncogenes such as c-sis (platelet-derived growth factor-β chain) are up-regulated in alveolar macrophages from fibrotic lungs, a factor that enhances mesothelial cell proliferation. In addition, asbestos can transfect DNA into cells.[20] Epidermal growth factor–positive cells have been found in 68% of mesotheliomas examined and correlate with improved survival.[21] Chrysotile fiber has been shown to be a strong mutagen in mammalian cells.[22] Asbestos fibers can cause persistent expression of early response genes, such as c-fos and c-jun in tissue culture.[23] The oxidative stress response gene product, heme oxygenase, can be induced by asbestos fibers.[24] These findings suggest that reactive oxygen species produced by asbestos fibers are responsible for the expression of cytotoxicity, DNA damage, mutation, gene expression, or carcinogenesis. Asbestos fibers have also been shown to enhance gamma ray–induced oncogenicity in mammalian cells.[22]

Risk Rates

The annual incidence of mesothelioma is not known with certainty.[25] The neoplasm can be difficult to diagnose, even by expert pathologists. Data from death certificates are unreliable for estimating disease frequency despite the usually rapidly fatal outcome of malignant mesothelioma. Cancer deaths are not coded by morphology (mesothelioma). Rather, the cause of mortality is assigned by primary site of the neoplasm (primary neoplasms of pleura and peritoneum). In a study of the Surveillance, Epidemiology, and End Results program of the National Cancer Institute, only 274 of 1130 white decedents with mesothelioma (approximately 95% diagnosed by microscopy) were recorded as having died of a primary neoplasm of pleura or peritoneum.[26] The majority of these mesothelioma cases were coded as having malignant neoplasm of the lung or unknown site.

A reasonable estimate is that 2200 new cases of mesothelioma occur annually in the United States (range, 1000 to more than 3000 cases)[26,27] or approximately 12.1 per million white men. In the United States, mesothelioma is approximately threefold more common in men than in women.[25,26] Incidence rises steadily with age and is approximately tenfold higher in men aged 60 to 64 years as compared with those aged 30 to 34.

Because of local asbestos industries, some locations in the United States have incidences as high as 636 male cases and 96 female cases per year per million population.[28] Whether risk in such communities extends to the population at large who are not employed in the asbestos industry remains controversial. The standardized incidence of mesothelioma in Wittenoom, Australia, was 260 per million for both men and women once residents employed in the crocidolite industry were excluded.[29] Purely residential exposure accounted for only 3% of incident cases in Yorkshire, England,[30] but at least 18% of the cases in South Africa.[31]

The incidence of mesothelioma appears to be increasing perhaps by as much as 50% in the last decade.[25,26] Projections of future incidence for the United States suggest that the numbers of cases will peak at the turn of the twentieth century[32] or rise moderately in the twenty-first century,[27] and then decline as a result of legislation to reduce asbestos exposure in the workplace and the ambient environment. In the Netherlands, the peak in annual male mesothelioma deaths is expected later, in approximately the year 2018. Pleural mesothelioma may account for 0.87% of all deaths in the 1943 to 1947 birth cohort of Dutch men.[33] Peto et al. project that the risk of dying of mesothelioma in Western Europe will double over the next 20 years, with the highest risk of approximately 1 in 150 men in the 1945 to 1950 birth cohort.[34]

High-Risk Individuals

Persons at high risk of mesothelioma can be identified by tracing the processing and commercial uses of asbestos. The mineral is mined, milled, and incorporated into a wide range of industrial and commercial products, including insulation, textiles, heat protectors, filters, and construction materials (spackling, roofing, siding, and floor and ceiling tiles).[1,25] Workers with high levels of asbestos exposure, therefore, are miners, millers, producers of asbestos products, and laborers who install plumbing, boilers, and heating equipment in ships, factories, and homes. The risk extends to workers who may not handle asbestos directly but are in proximity to the material, such as carpenters, electricians, and welders in shipyards.

The risk of mesothelioma associated with occupational exposure to asbestos has been examined in case-control studies and cohort studies. In case-control studies, up to 75% of cases had asbestos exposure, as compared with a small fraction of controls.[25] In cohort studies, up to 10% of asbestos workers have died of mesothelioma.[35] However, mesothelioma risk is difficult to quantitate for several reasons. First, ambient levels of asbestos in most workplaces have not been measured. A *high* level in one study might be called *moderate* or *low* in another. Duration of employment has been used as another surrogate measure of exposure. Second, the time from exposure to the development of mesothelioma is long, usually three to four decades in most reported studies. Mathematical modeling suggests that risk of mesothelioma increases exponentially by the third to fourth power of time from first exposure, but few cohorts have been followed to the end of life. Third, the composition of the inspired asbestos differed among exposed workers.

Despite the obstacles to quantifying risk of mesothelioma, several consistent observations have emerged from studies worldwide. Crocidolite is associated with high risk of mesothelioma in miners, manufacturers, and workers who install asbestos products.[36] Another amphibole, amosite, appears to carry an intermediate risk. Chrysotile, currently the major form of asbestos in production, shows the weakest association with mesothelioma.[14] Occupations with highest risk appear to be insulators, asbestos producers and manufacturers, and heating and construction tradespeople. The projected lifetime risk among these workers exposed from early adulthood ranges up to 20%. Working in proximity to these occupational groups in construction sites confers a relatively lower risk. In addition, some patients with mesothelioma have reported only isolated or brief occupational exposures to asbestos.

In a cohort study of 248 insulation workers in Sweden where exposure to asbestos had almost ended in the mid-1970s, 84 deaths occurred between 1970 and 1994 compared with 46 expected mainly due to an increased cancer mortality (approximately 50%). The morbidity was increased for lung cancer (11.0 cases vs. 2.5 expected), peritoneal mesothelioma (7 vs. 0), cancer in pancreas (5.0 vs. 0.7). No pleural mesotheliomas were found. The risk of lung cancer did not reach normal levels despite decreased asbestos exposure. Mesothelioma in insulation workers seems to be peritoneal more often than pleural.[37]

Malignant mesothelioma is rarely curable at present, so screening of asbestos workers for mesothelioma is inappropriate. However, smoking greatly increases the risk of lung cancer (but not mesothelioma) in asbestos workers and smoking cessation efforts are needed in this high-risk group.[38] Clinicians considering the diagnosis of malignant mesothelioma should take a detailed exposure history emphasizing the period 20 to 50 years before diagnosis and including possible household contact exposure. Brief exposures may be long forgotten.[39]

Exposure in the Home

Mesothelioma in wives and children of asbestos workers has prompted studies that show increased asbestos levels in their homes.[40,41] Presumably, asbestos was brought into the home on hair and on clothing to be washed in the family laundry. Asbestos workers have been required to shower and change clothing before leaving the workplace only since 1972. Asbestos-related neoplasms have been reported in multiple members of some families, but genetic predisposition to the neoplasm remains to be shown. The risk of mesothelioma in household contacts of asbestos workers has been estimated to be as high as 0.4 to 1.0%,[38] but clearly varies with the level of household contamination, and may be overestimated in the reported data. More than one-half of women with mesothelioma in one series were household contacts of asbestos workers.[42]

A high incidence of mesothelioma (22 per 10,000 persons of age greater than 25) observed in the Anatoli region of Turkey has been attributed to zeolite, a silicate ubiquitous in the soil and to tremolite[43] and sometimes sprayed onto homes. Erionite found in Karain, Turkey, is also associated with a high incidence of mesothelioma.[44] In a cohort of 162 Karain immigrants to Sweden, 18 cases of mesothelioma had occurred, accounting for 14 of the 18 deaths (78%).[45] Although human herpes virus (HHV) is associated with body cavity lymphomas, HHV-8 amplification products were absent by polymerase chain reaction in 13 diffuse malignant mesotheliomas.[46]

MESOTHELIOMAS WITHOUT A HISTORY OF ASBESTOS EXPOSURE

No asbestos exposure can be documented in approximately 30% to 50% of cases of mesothelioma. Quantitation of asbestos fibers in some of these patients has documented background pulmonary fiber levels consistent with the absence of a substantial asbestos exposure.[47] Two cases of peritoneal mesothelioma were associated with familial Mediterranean fever.[48]

Approximately 25 published cases of pleural and peritoneal mesothelioma have developed following therapeutic radiation[49,50] or in two patients, arising adjacent to deposits of thorium dioxide (thorotrast) still visible on chest radiographs after extravasation during diagnostic procedures years earlier. Patients with a history of Hodgkin's disease may have an increased risk of developing mesothelioma. All five of the mesotheliomas in one series occurred in the field of prior radiation therapy with an average interval between radiation treatment and diagnosis of mesothelioma of 15 years.[51] Three of the five patients also received chemotherapy. No patients recalled exposure to asbestos or had evidence of asbestosis on chest radiography. In reported cases a median of 16 years (range, 7 to 36 years) had elapsed between radiation and detection of mesothelioma.

BIOLOGY OF MESOTHELIOMA: PLOIDY STUDIES

Ploidy status and the percentage of cells actively synthesizing DNA have been analyzed by flow cytometry in almost 200 malignant mesotheliomas.[52–54] Ploidy and S-phase fraction seem to be consistent in different sections from the same tumor and were not associated with histologic subtype.[53] In the various studies, 60% to 78% were diploid and 27% were near diploid. In contrast, 85% to 88% of lung cancer are aneuploid.[52] Significantly shorter survival is associated with a high percentage of S-phase cells (but not aneuploidy).[53,54]

DIAGNOSIS OF MESOTHELIOMA

Initial misdiagnosis is common. Pathologic opinion appears particularly diverse when litigation is involved. Because a substantial percentage of mesotheliomas develops in patients with no known asbestos exposure and other malignancies are common in asbestos workers, asbestos exposure should not influence the diagnosis of mesothelioma. Because of the poor current prognosis of pleural mesothelioma, a major role of establishing the diagnosis is to exclude the possibility of a more treatable illness. Accurate diagnosis is also important in the event of subsequent litigation and for epidemiologic and therapeutic studies.

HUMORAL FACTORS

Hyaluronic acid has been reported to be useful in diagnosis or for following response but is relatively nonspecific.[55] The level of hyaluronic acid was studied in the pleural fluid of 19 patients with malignant mesothelioma, 27 with lung cancer, 1 with breast cancer, 1 with mediastinal tumor, and 51 with benign diseases. The pleural fluid concentration of hyaluronic acid was greater than 100 μg/mL in 37% of (7 of 19) mesotheliomas and 1.3% of (1 of 80) lung cancers and other malignant and benign diseases.[56] A markedly elevated serum or pleural fluid carcinoembryonic antigen, however, suggests a diagnosis other than mesothelioma.

Hematopoietic growth factors[57–59] and blood group antigens[60,61] have been produced by normal and malignant mesothelial cell lines. Serum levels of interleukin-6 (IL-6), C-reactive protein, α_1-acid glycoprotein, and fibrinogen were significantly higher in 25 mesothelioma patients than in patients with lung adenocarcinoma with cytology-positive pleural effusions. Serum IL-6 levels correlated with the levels of the acute-phase proteins and significantly with platelet counts. The level of IL-6 in the pleural fluid of patients with mesothelioma was approximately 60 to 1400 times higher than in the serum. Even higher levels of IL-6 in the pleural fluid and of thrombocytosis were found in patients with tuberculous pleurisy. High cytokine levels were not specific to mesothelioma (similar profiles were found in patients with tuberculous pleurisy). However, the detection of a markedly increased level of IL-6 in pleural fluid argues against a diagnosis of adenocarcinoma.[62]

PATHOLOGY

Benign inflammatory and reactive processes producing mesothelial hyperplasia or other malignant tumors may mimic mesothelioma[63] but do not invade normal tissues and lack cytologic atypia and hyperchromatism. Repeated cytologic examination or biopsy results may be negative despite active tumor. When tumor tissue is obtained, light microscopy often provides documentation of malignancy, but usually does not distinguish adenocarcinoma from mesothelioma. Electron microscopy of either needle biopsy or cytocentrifuge specimens from pleural fluid may establish the mesothelial origin of the malignant tumor. Sputum cytology and bronchoscopy may be helpful in documenting an occult bronchogenic adenocarcinoma. The Cancer Committee of the College of American Pathologists has established a checklist protocol for the examination of specimens from patients with malignant pleural mesothelioma.[64]

Adenocarcinomas from primary lung, breast, ovary, stomach, kidney, or prostate cancer frequently metastasize to the pleura and can be extremely difficult to distinguish from epithelial mesothelioma cytologically or histologically. Metastatic adenocarcinoma with extensive pleural involvement may grossly resemble mesothelioma and has been called *pseudomesothelioma.*[65]

Sarcomatous mesotheliomas must be distinguished from fibrosarcoma, malignant fibrous histiocytoma, malignant schwannoma, and hemangiopericytoma. Synovial sarcoma and carcinosarcomas, which may also have mixed sarcomatous and epithelial components, usually present as a localized mass in the lung.

Autopsy requires skilled performance and experienced interpretation to reliably exclude other occult primary carcinomas. Advanced malignant mesothelioma tends to form peripheral visceral masses mimicking primary carcinomas.[66] Asbestos counts and postmortem examinations may have legal as well as epidemiologic value.

Cytology

In one study of 21 cases of epithelial malignant mesothelioma (15 pleural, 6 peritoneal) diagnosed by effusion cytology, 13 were of the cohesive cell type and 8 were of the noncohesive cell type. Because of its resemblance to florid reactive mesothelial hyperplasia and the general lack of awareness of the existence of the single-cell pattern of mesothelioma, the noncohesive cell type can often be missed.[67]

For 29 patients with at least one cytologic pleural fluid examination, cytology was positive for mesothelioma in 32%. The median time from initial symptoms to the diagnosis of mesothelioma was 8 weeks (4 weeks for patients with positive or suspicious cytology results, and 12 weeks for those with negative cytology results). Cytogenetic analysis of pleural fluid had a sensitivity of 56% and was positive in one case in which results of cytologic examination were negative. Patients in whom the time from presentation to diagnosis was greater than 1 year all had negative cytologic results followed by long periods without further workup, despite a history of exposure to asbestos. Because the sensitivity of cytologic examination for mesothelioma is so low, patients in whom mesothelioma is suspected should undergo immediate pleural biopsy if the pleural fluid cytology result is negative.[68]

Fine-Needle Aspirations

Cytomorphologic features (amount of cytoplasm and the degree of nuclear pleomorphism and cellular cohesion) on fine-needle aspiration of primary mesothelioma and of metastatic lesions varies greatly among individual cases. However, numerous distinct, uniformly small intracytoplasmic vacuoles, believed to represent intracellular fat and glycogen, were consistently present in metastatic lesions.[69]

GROSS DESCRIPTION. Discrete nodules and plaques of firm, grayish tumor coalesce, eventually obliterating the parietal and visceral surfaces. A rind of up to 5 cm in thickness may encase and constrict the lung with only superficial invasion. The chest wall, pericardium, and diaphragm as well as the interlobar fissures are involved relatively early.[66] At autopsy, tumor invades thoracic lymph nodes in up to 70% of patients with occasional extension to cervical nodes.[63] Small hematogenous metastases are documented to liver and lung and less commonly to kidney, adrenal, and bone in 33% to 67% of cases.[63,70] Without careful postmortem examination, hematogenous metastases may be missed.

MICROSCOPIC DESCRIPTION. Extensive sampling of biopsy, laparotomy, pleurectomy, or pneumonectomy specimens is required. A *small* piece should be fixed in glutaraldehyde for electron microscopy and the remainder promptly fixed in neutral buffered formalin. There are three histologic variants: epithelial, sarcomatoid, and mixed.[66,71] Fifty percent to 60% are epithelial, characterized by tubular, papillary, solid, or vacuolated patterns. The sarcomatoid variant is composed of ovoid to spindle-shaped cells with cellularity and hyperchromatism similar to that of a fibrosarcoma. A biphasic pattern with mixed epithelial and sarcomatoid elements is virtually pathognomonic of malignant mesothelioma although extensive sampling may be required to demonstrate the minor component.

Histochemical Methods

Three methods are in common use to distinguish metastatic adenocarcinomas from epithelial mesotheliomas. The periodic acid–Schiff stain used before and after diastase digestion, is the single most reliable histochemical method generally available.[66] *Neutral* mucopolysaccharides that are strongly positive for periodic acid–Schiff diastase are found in intracellular secretory vacuoles and in intraacinar vacuoles in most adenocarcinomas, but are rarely found in mesotheliomas. Their presence is strong but not unequivocal evidence for a diagnosis of adenocarcinoma. Appropriate controls for diastase activity and to distinguish staining of vacuoles from stroma and other structures are essential. Alcian blue at pH 2.5 and colloidal iron stain acid mucopolysaccharides are present in mesothelioma and many adenocarcinomas.[63] Disappearance after digestion with hyaluronidase, which removes hyaluronic acid in intracellular and secretory vacuoles and intercellular lumens, is characteristic of mesothelioma. *Stromal* hyaluronic acid is a nonspecific finding in many tumors, however. Under most staining conditions, Mayer's mucicarmine method (which stains neutral and weakly acidic mucopolysaccharides in intracellular and intercellular secretory vacuoles pink or red) is strongly positive in many adenocarcinomas. Mesotheliomas are usually negative but occasionally may stain strongly in some laboratories possibly due to fixation or technical conditions. Thus, the method is not completely reliable.

Immunohistochemistry

Immunoperoxidase stains using various antibodies may be effectively applied to paraffin-embedded tumor tissue. Monoclonal antibodies against keratin proteins are strongly reactive in mesothelioma with diffuse cytoplasmic staining,[72] and perinuclear accentuation with ring formation. Both epithelial and spindle-shaped tumor cells of mixed and sarcomatoid variants are often stained, reflecting transitional patterns of differentiation also observed on electron microscopy.[73] This reactivity is helpful in distinguishing mesothelioma from fibrosarcoma, malignant fibrous histiocytoma (MFH), and schwannoma; however, carcinosarcomas and synovial sarcomas, which also have biphasic histology, also express keratin proteins. Adenocarcinomas also stain positively, usually with localization to the periphery of the tumor cell. Immunoperoxidase staining for Leu M1 is usually absent in mesotheliomas but positive in most adenocarcinomas. Staining for carcinoembryonic antigen is moderate to strong in most adenocarcinomas, but often weak or absent in renal, prostate, and some ovarian and endometrial carcinomas as well as mesotheliomas.[74–76] Unfortunately, there is marked variability among available monoclonal and polyclonal antibodies.[77]

Electron Microscopy

The epithelial variant is composed of polygonal cells with numerous long, slender branching surface microvilli, desmosomes, abundant tonofilaments, and intracellular lumen formation.[73,78] Primary lung, breast, and upper gastrointestinal tract adenocarcinomas have short stubby surface microvilli, fewer tonofilaments, and microvillous rootlets or lamellar bodies.[79,80] Ovarian and endometrial carcinomas lack intracytoplasmic lumens, but have few tonofilaments and may express features of intestinal metaplasia (abundant mucin droplets, numerous cilia, and dense core granules).[79,80] Elongated nuclei, and abundant rough endoplasmic reticulin are found in the sarcomatoid variant. Stromal cells separated by matrix containing collagen fibers appear spindle or ovoid with both sarcomatoid and epithelial features, characteristic of the biphasic nature of mesothelioma.[73,78]

Prognostic Correlations

Serum concentrations of two cytokeratin markers, CYFRA 21-1 and tissue polypeptide antigen, were elevated in 26 (50%) and 30 (58%) of 52 patients, respectively, and were highly correlated (r = .98). Univariate analysis of data from 51 patients showed a relation with survival for performance status (P = .010), thoracic pain (P = .014), platelet count (P = .027), CYFRA 21-1 (P = .002), and tissue polypeptide antigen (P = .003). Multivariate analysis identified independent prognostic significance for performance status, platelet count, and CYFRA 21-1. In addition to performance status, the cytokeratin markers identified patients with good prognosis in a log rank test.[81]

Microvascular quantification by staining for the antigens CD34 and CD31 in 25 mesotheliomas counted manually or on a computerized image analysis system significantly correlated with each other and with shorter survival independent of patient age and histologic type or grade of mesothelioma. No association was noted with p53 immunoexpression.[82]

MALIGNANT PLEURAL MESOTHELIOMA

PRESENTATION

Malignant pleural mesothelioma most commonly develops in the fifth to seventh decade (median age, 60 years), typically 20 to 50 or more years since first documented asbestos exposure. The risk has been estimated to be linearly proportional to the intensity and duration of exposure, and to the time since first exposure to a power of between 3 and 4. Latency periods between first exposure to asbestos and a diagnosis of mesothelioma may vary by occupation, with shorter latencies for insulators and dock workers and longer intervals for shipyard and maritime workers, as well as domestic exposures.[83] A significant proportion of patients with mesothelioma diagnosed between the ages of 20 and 40 report household or neighborhood exposure during childhood.[11,84] Children who present with the disease generally have no apparent asbestos exposure.[85–88]

A ratio of five men to one woman is affected. Dyspnea, nonpleuritic chest wall pain, or both bring 90% of patients to medical attention. Examination is generally remarkable for dullness at one base, and chest radiography reveals a large freely movable unilateral pleural effusion. Occasional patients are asymptomatic, an effusion found incidentally on chest radiography. Five patients in one series presented with spontaneous pneumothorax with the unsuspected diagnosis of mesothelioma made at pleurectomy.[89] Sixty percent have right-sided lesions, and less than 5% have bilateral involvement at the time of diagnosis.

Pulmonary function test results may document restrictive lung disease resulting from encasement of the lung and assess the potential tolerance for pneumonectomy. Obstructive spirometric changes are unrelated to mesothelioma or asbestosis. Laboratory evaluation is otherwise generally unremarkable except for an elevated platelet count and erythrocyte sedimentation rate.

STAGING

As described by Rusch and Venkatraman, the five staging systems before the International Mesothelioma Interest Group (IMIG) Staging System have been "to some extent imprecise and incompletely validated."[90] The Butchart classification (Table 40.2-1) suffers from an absence of tumor, node, metastasis (TNM) descriptors and vague statements regarding lymph node involvement and degrees of chest wall invasion.[95] Mattson's classification recognizes contralateral involvement as stage II rather than stage III and has largely been abandoned. Chahinian was the first to devise a TNM-based mesothelioma staging system, with an attempt to qualify the influence of such parameters as locoregional lymph node involvement as well as specific sites and extent of invasion.

The Union International Contra le Cancrum proposed a TNM staging system that evolved into the presently described International Mesothelioma Interest Group Staging System. The IMIG staging system has only been available for a short time, but it has been validated in two large surgical series of mesothelioma.[91,92] Sugarbaker et al. have proposed the alternative but complementary Brigham Staging System based on tumor, resectability, and nodal status.[93] In any evaluation for the patient with mesothelioma, careful attention must be paid to the diaphragmatic extent of the tumor with suspicious scans confirmed by laparoscopic evaluation for transdiaphragmatic extension.[94]

The most important preoperative prognostic indicator may be tumor status of the patients. Tumor volumes associated with malignant pleural mesothelioma patients who have no spread to lymph nodes are significantly smaller than in those patients with positive nodes. Moreover, progressively higher IMIG stage is associated with higher median preoperative solid volume of tumor.[92] Further studies verifying that preresection tumor volume is representative of tumor status in malignant pleural mesothelioma and can predict overall and progression-free survival, as well as postoperative IMIG stage, are needed to complement metabolic imaging studies.

Noninvasive Studies to Determine Stage

The major role of noninvasive procedures is to determine isolated hemithorax disease. Despite a history of asbestos contact in 50% to 70% of patients, pleural plaques or interstitial fibrosis are apparent on chest radiography in only approximately 20%, but pleural calcifications are evident on almost one-half of computed tomographic (CT) scans[96] and in up to 87% at autopsy. Scoliosis with contracture of the ipsilateral hemithorax is visible even on chest radiography with advanced disease.

A CT scan or magnetic resonance imaging (MRI) of the primary tumor to assess the extent of disease is indicated if treatment is contemplated. Characteristic CT findings in almost 100 patients are pleural thickening in 92% (and of the intralobar fissures in 86%), effusions in 74%, and pleural calcifications in 20% to 50%.[96,97] CT scan is helpful in differentiating benign from malignant pleural thickening, but does not reliably distinguish primary from metastatic malignancy.

Coronal MRI is particularly helpful to evaluate the diaphragm. In a study of 26 mesothelioma patients evaluated with sequential paired CT and MRI scans, MRI showed tumor spread into the interlobar fissures, tumor invasion of and through the diaphragm, and invasion of bony structures better than CT. Invasion of the chest wall and mediastinal soft tissue and tumor growth into the lung parenchyma were equally well seen on both imaging methods. CT was better for detecting pleural calcifications.[98]

Twenty-eight consecutive patients referred for the evaluation of suspected malignant mesothelioma were evaluated by positron emission tomography (PET) with 2-fluoro-2-deoxy-D-glucose (FDG) imaging. Video-assisted thoracoscopy or surgical biopsies provided a malignant diagnosis in 24 patients (22 with mesothelioma) and benign processes in the remaining four. The uptake of FDG was significantly higher in malignant than in benign lesions ($P = .0001$). FDG-PET images identified active tumor sites. Hypermetabolic lymph nodes were noted on FDG-PET images in 12 patients, 9 of which appeared normal on CT scans. Histologic examination in six patients confirmed malignant nodal disease in five cases and granulomatous lymphadenitis in one. Standardized uptake values were inversely correlated with duration of survival after the PET study ($P = .05$).[99] These important data require verification in larger numbers of patients but could be useful in deciding which patient may be a candidate for an aggressive approach since a high FDG uptake in these tumors may indicate a shorter patient survival.

Mesotheliomas are reported to take up gallium 67.[100] Gallium 67 scans in seven cases obtained before resection were compared with pathology. When the involved pleural thickness was over 6 mm, gallium 67 uptake correlated with the macroscopic thickness of mesothelioma in resected specimens. Thickness of the pleura on CT images was only reliable for thick involvement. No definite correlation was found between gallium 67 uptake and the histologic type, extent of tumor parenchyma, interstitial volume, and tumor vascularity.[101]

Planar ^{201}Tl scintigraphy in a single mesothelioma patient revealed diffuse pleural tumor accumulation. Single photon emission CT demonstrated exact tumor location.[102]

Brain, bone, and liver metastases or extension into other serosal surfaces, although present in more than one-half of patients at autopsy, are sufficiently uncommon at presentation to obviate the need for extensive baseline studies in the absence of symptoms or laboratory abnormalities. However, such studies may identify an occult adenocarcinoma of the lung, a pattern of widespread metastases, or a markedly elevated serum or pleural fluid carcinoembryonic antigen suggesting a diagnosis other than mesothelioma.[63,103]

Although there are no definitive biomarkers for mesothelioma, future studies investigating serial serum levels of tissue polypeptide antigen[104] or thrombomodulin[105] may be of interest.

Diagnostic Surgery

Although obtaining an accurate histologic confirmation of mesothelioma from pleural fluid cytology or needle biopsy

TABLE 40.2-1. Two of the Five Published Staging Systems for Pleural Malignant Mesothelioma

BUTCHART STAGING CLASSIFICATION[95]	
I	Tumor confined within the capsule of the parietal pleura, involving only ipsilateral pleura, lung, pericardium, and diaphragm
II	Tumor invading chest wall or involving mediastinal structures, such as esophagus, heart, opposite pleura
III	Tumor penetrating diaphragm to involve peritoneum; involvement of opposite pleura; lymph node involvement outside the chest
IV	Distant blood-borne metastases
UNION INTERNATIONAL CONTRA LE CANCRUM STAGING PROPOSAL[a]	
I	T1, N0, M0
	T2, N0, M0
II	T1, N1, M0
	T2, N1, M0
III	T3, N0, M0
	T3, N1, M0
	T1, N2, M0
	T2, N2, M0
	T3, N2, M0
IV	Any T, N3, M0
	T4, any N, M0
	Any T, any N, M1
T	Primary tumor and extent
Tx	Primary tumor cannot be assessed
T0	No evidence of primary tumor
T1	Primary tumor limited to ipsilateral parietal, visceral, or both pleura
T2	Tumor invades any of the following: ipsilateral lung, endothoracic fascia, diaphragm, pericardium
T3	Tumor invades any of the following: ipsilateral chest wall muscle, ribs, mediastinal organs or tissues
T4	Tumor extends to any of the following: contralateral pleura or lung by direct extension, peritoneum or intraabdominal organs by direct extension, cervical tissues
N	Lymph nodes
Nx	Regional lymph nodes cannot be assessed
N0	No regional lymph node metastases
N1	Metastases in ipsilateral bronchopulmonary of hilar lymph nodes
N2	Metastases in ipsilateral mediastinal lymph nodes
N3	Metastases in contralateral mediastinal internal mammary, supraclavicular, or scalene lymph nodes
M	Metastases
Mx	Presence of distant metastases cannot be assessed
M0	No (known) distant metastases
M1	Distant metastasis present

[a]Staging solely on clinical measures is designated *cTNM.* Staging that can be done on clinical pathologic information is designated as *pTNM.* Clinical and pathologic groups are identical.

specimens is often difficult, the diagnosis of mesothelioma has such a poor prognosis that an unequivocal tissue diagnosis is mandatory. Surgical intervention is usually required, either a thoracoscopy or thoracotomy, despite the risk of seeding the biopsy site or surgical scar with tumor. For patients who are not candidates for radical surgery, thoracoscopy usually obtains sufficient tissue for histochemical analysis.[106] The later development of chest wall masses from seeding of the biopsy site or surgical scar is an uncommon complication (approximately 10%) of any diagnostic procedure, but can usually be avoided by radiotherapy to the scar if appropriate (see Surgery, later in this chapter). Tumor nodules seeded from fluids rich in tumor cells may develop in the subcutaneous tissue surrounding Denver shunts and intrapleural ports.[107]

If preoperative studies suggest stage I mesothelioma in good-risk patients with asbestos exposure, most surgeons combine the diagnostic and therapeutic surgical interventions in one stage.[108] Generous biopsies can be performed at the inception of the exploration, using frozen sections to differentiate mesothelioma from adenocarcinoma. A sample of uninvaded lung should be obtained for counting asbestos fibers.[39]

Bronchoscopy should be performed in all patients suspected of mesothelioma to rule out endobronchial disease, rare in mesothelioma.[109] The role of mediastinoscopy in patients with suspected mesothelioma is undefined. Some surgeons believe it is unnecessary because nodes can be removed with the lung. Other surgeons believe that, because positive nodes indicate stage III disease, surgery would be contraindicated. Nevertheless, if radical extrapleural pneumonectomy (EPP) is contemplated, mediastinoscopy is recommended, because 20% of patients with mesothelioma have mediastinal lymph node involvement.[109]

NATURAL HISTORY

Shortness of breath and chest pain can be controlled initially by repeated thoracenteses and minor narcotics. Although chest tube drainage and sclerosis is generally unsuccessful, pleural fluid eventually becomes loculated as the tumor obliterates the pleural space.[70] With advanced disease, fatigue and dyspnea increase out of proportion to radiographic findings or pulmonary function values. Because hypoxia results from shunting of desaturated blood through a poorly aerated lung, therapeutic oxygen provides little symptomatic relief.

Mesothelioma tends to be locally invasive. Chest wall masses develop in approximately 10% of patients, generally over thoracentesis, chest tube drainage, or thoracotomy tracts.[70,110] Direct involvement of esophagus, ribs, vertebrae, nerves, and the superior vena cava cause dysphagia, pain, cord compression, brachial plexopathy, Horner's syndrome, or superior vena cava syndromes, respectively.[111] Fevers and sweats with no documented source of infection are common and often accompanied by significant weight loss, poor performance status, and an early death. Thrombocytosis and other clotting abnormalities occur in 10% to 20% (more frequently in peritoneal mesothelioma).[112,113] Disseminated intravascular coagulation, thrombophlebitis, pulmonary emboli, and Coombs' positive hemolytic anemia have been reported,[114] as well as hypercalcemia associated with elevated levels of a parathyroid hormone–like peptide.[115]

The median survival is 4 to 18 months in various series (range, weeks to 16 years). Patients generally die of respiratory failure or pneumonia. Small bowel obstruction from direct extension through the diaphragm develops in approximately one-third, and 10% die of pericardial or myocardial involvement.[84,111]

Prognostic variables at presentation are shown in Table 40.2-2. Poor prognostic variables in 180 patients in one single institution series included chest pain, older age, pleural site, and sarcomatous or mixed histology.[116]

In the European Organization for Research and Treatment of Cancer experience in 204 adults with malignant pleural mesothelioma on five consecutive phase II clinical trials, the median survival was 13 months from diagnosis and 8 months from trial entry. In the multivariate analysis, poor prognosis was associated with a poor performance status, a high white blood cell count, male gender, and the sarcomatous histologic subtype.[117]

Factors predictive of poorer survival among 337 patients with mesothelioma on Cancer and Leukemia Group B studies included poor performance status, chest pain, dyspnea, platelet count greater than 400,000/μL, weight loss, serum lactate dehydrogenase level greater than 500 IU/L, pleural involvement, low hemoglobin level, high white blood cell count, and increasing age over 75 years.

TABLE 40.2-2. Poor Prognostic Variables at Presentation

Sarcomatous histology
Poor performance
Pleural primary
Weight loss
Lactate dehydrogenase level >500
Older age
Advanced stage
Elevated platelet count
Chest pain at diagnosis

Data from refs. 116–119.

With decreasing risk ratio, a multivariate Cox analysis showed that pleural involvement, lactate dehydrogenase greater than 500 IU/L, poor performance, chest pain, platelets greater than 400,000/μL, nonepithelial histology, and increasing age older than 75 years jointly predict poor survival. Performance was the most important prognostic split in the regression tree.[118]

Localized malignant fibrous tumors of the pleura that may resemble sarcomatous mesotheliomas histologically have also been described. Of 82 malignant localized tumors, 45% were cured by simple excision.[120] If the nature of the lesion is ambiguous, involvement of the pleura on random biopsy would establish a diagnosis of diffuse (malignant) disease.

SURGICAL TREATMENT

The role of surgery in managing diffuse pleural mesothelioma remains controversial, but there are an increasing number of thoracic oncologic surgeons who are operating for this disease. Nevertheless, overwhelming pessimism for *curative* surgical options continues in most centers that do not routinely deal with the disease since the combination of effusive disease and bulky tumor renders surgical eradication virtually impossible. The disappointing long-term overall survival results, the historically high morbidity and mortality, as well as the propensity for local recurrences have forced many centers to abandon radical operations except for the rare localized situation. The arguments regarding appropriate management of mesothelioma can have geographic differences. In a United Kingdom poll of chest physicians, only 46% of the physicians surveyed would consider referral to a thoracic surgeon for radical resection (E. G. Butchart, personal communication). The French approach to the disease has been a concentration on detection of early stage I disease that is treated with intrapleural therapy, including interferon-γ with or without cisplatin.[121] Surgery is performed after this therapy only to improve local control, either by pleurectomy or EPP. In patients with stage II or III mesothelioma, Boutin et al. recommend surgery and postoperative radiation therapy. In the United States a cohort of specialized cancer centers have evolved that have maintained an interest in the surgical management of the disease. As a new cohort of aggressively trained, specialized thoracic oncologists enters practice, the necessity for such referrals may be diminished. At the present time, however, the evolution of the use of surgery with or without intraoperative, postoperative innovative adjuvant therapies is being defined by these centers. In general, innovative, multimodality protocols that incorporate surgery as part of the package are being explored in larger numbers of patients.

History of Surgical Management

Eiselberg[122] is credited with the earliest resection of mesothelioma in a 46-year-old man in whom he removed chest wall and a portion of lung. Much of the original interest in *en bloc* resection for diffuse malignant mesothelioma originated in Germany between 1920 and 1960. With advances both in surgery and anesthetic management, a more extensive resection that included lung, pleura, and diaphragm became technically feasible.

Rationale

Diffuse pleural mesotheliomas are rarely amenable to *en bloc* removal. A small proportion of tumors called *mesotheliomas* may present as an encapsulated mass, not associated with pleural effusion, and these may be amenable to surgical extirpation with negative margins of resection. The majority of diffuse malignant mesotheliomas, however, cannot be surgically removed *en bloc* with truly negative histologic margins because many of the patients have had a previous biopsy and there is invasion of the endothoracic fascia and intercostal muscles at that site, or pleural effusion, which, although cytologically negative, may be breached, or both leading to local permeation of tumor cells either into the residual cavity or into the abdomen. Nevertheless, in the largest series of EPP performed for mesothelioma from the Boston group, 66 of 183 patients were defined as having negative resection margins after EPP. Patients with this finding who had epithelial mesothelioma were found to have 2- and 5-year survival rates of 68% and 46%, if the node dissection did not reveal tumor.[93]

The operation of choice, especially for early pleural mesothelioma, has yet to be defined. There is no doubt that EPP is a more extensive dissection and may serve to remove more bulk disease than a pleurectomy, chiefly in the diaphragmatic and visceral pleural surfaces. Some surgeons, however, include diaphragmatic resection and pericardial resection with their pleurectomies to accomplish removal of "all gross disease." For EPP, it is almost a necessity to include pericardiotomy with or without resection, for the maneuver aids in the exposure of the vessels and allows intrapericardial control to prevent a surgical catastrophe. There are no real guidelines preoperatively that one can use to assure the patient which operation will accomplish tumor removal. The presence of irregular, bulky disease that on the CT infiltrates into the fissures probably dictates the necessity for EPP; a large effusion with minimal bulk disease may call for pleurectomy decortication. Moreover, the philosophy of the surgeon regarding the operation may affect his or her choice, because some surgeons reserve EPP for those patients with bulk disease that presents simple pleurectomy, whereas others believe that the greatest chance for complete gross excision is via EPP performed in the patient with minimal disease. This important factor, preoperative quantitative bulk of disease, may not only influence the choice of resection, but may be an important preoperative prognostic factor in any patient with malignant pleural mesothelioma.[92]

Indications for Surgical Management

Surgery is involved in the management of pleural mesothelioma either for diagnosis, palliative therapy, or as part of a multimodal therapeutic plan. The operations involved in this management include thoracoscopy, pleurectomy and decortication, or EPP. The indications for each of these operations depend on the extent of disease, performance and functional status of the patient, and the philosophy of the treating institution. Basically, operative intervention in mesothelioma is for primary effusion control, cytoreduction before multimodal therapy, or to deliver and monitor innovative intrapleural therapies.

Functional Evaluation of the Patient Being Considered for Surgical Intervention

The majority of patients seeking treatment for mesothelioma are middle-aged to older individuals with a long latency period between asbestos exposure and tumor development. If surgical intervention is to be considered, a detailed physiologic and functional workup directed chiefly at the cardiopulmonary axis must be performed.

PULMONARY EVALUATION. Poor underlying pulmonary function in patients with malignant mesothelioma usually reflects the burden of asbestos exposure, concomitant smoking history (up to 70% of the patients have had a heavy tobacco intake), degree of lung trapped by tumor or fluid, and patient age. Decreases in the forced vital capacity correlate with the degree of costophrenic angle involvement, width, and length of pleural fibrosis, and the presence of either circumscribed plaque or diffuse pleural thickening. The extent of fibrosis correlates with the amount of dyspnea on exertion, and the diffusion capacity of carbon dioxide is reduced in these patients. There is restriction of chest wall motion resulting in reduced lung volumes. Such changes may be bilateral and thus the extent of surgical therapy is influenced by the patient's respiratory functional reserve. Generally accepted criteria for tolerance of an EPP can be assessed by pulmonary function testing including the patients' response to bronchodilators. Patients with a forced expiratory volume in 1 second (FEV_1) of greater than 2 L/second usually are able to withstand a pneumonectomy. In general, an FEV_1 of less than 1 L/second, a PO_2 less than 55, or a pCO_2 greater than 45 are relative contraindications to performance of EPP.[93] If the patient presents with an FEV_1 of less than 2 L/second, or if the predicted FEV_1 is less than 1.2 L/minute after pneumonectomy, quantitative ventilation-perfusion scanning should be performed.

CARDIAC EVALUATION. Operations for malignant pleural mesothelioma are associated with profound blood loss and potentially significant cardiac demands. The patient should be carefully screened for a history of hypertension, angina, and previous myocardial infarction, and routine electrocardiography should reveal no signs of previous injury. Any patient sustaining a myocardial infarction within the past 3 months or having an arrhythmia requiring medication should not be considered for EPP. Patients without objective evidence of cardiac injury who have a history of chest pain compatible with angina or remote myocardial infarction should have dobutamine thallium screening to investigate reversible perfusion defects indicative of myocardium at risk. In general, patients with an ejection fraction of less than 45% are not considered to be candidates for EPP.[93] This may also affect their enrollment in innovative multimodality programs using potentially cardiotoxic drugs. These patients may then be considered for angioplasty before operative intervention for their disease, and indeed, may be better candidates if a multimodality approach is being contemplated.

Other Preoperative Evaluation

Preoperative medications must be carefully scrutinized, specifically any nonsteroidal antiinflammatory drugs that could affect platelet function. Patients should have complete extrathoracic staging evaluation including bone scan, abdominal CT, and head CT to rule out systemic involvement. If patients are to participate in multimodality programs that use drugs with potential renal toxicity (i.e., cisplatin), a preoperative creatinine clearance should be performed.

Effusion Control

In general, the indications for palliative surgery include the control or prevention of effusion that results in disabling dyspnea. The most efficacious and least invasive of the surgical procedures to accomplish effusion control is thoracoscopy with talc pleurodesis. Two to 5 g of asbestos-free, sterile talc can be insufflated over the lung and the parietal surfaces. Success rates in effusion control with talc, used either via thoracoscopy or via slurry, approach 90%. Failure of these techniques are usually associated with mesothelioma with entrapped lung, a large solid tumor mass, a long history of effusion with multiple thoracenteses leading to loculations, or age older than 70 years. This technique is widely used once the diagnosis of mesothelioma is made. Primary care physicians, however, should carefully deliberate before using sclerosants and consider the extent of visceral and parietal pleural disease. The use of talc or other sclerosants could affect the suitability for patients to enter innovative trials that incorporate either pleurectomy or EPP and could jeopardize the ability of the surgeon to spare a lung that may not have visceral pleural implants. Table 40.2-3 reviews the results of videothoracoscopic talc pleurodesis specifically for mesothelioma. Patients who were able to have a successful pleurodesis had a significantly longer survival than those who did not, and success depended on presence of trapped lung or degree of invasion of the pleura.

Effusion control via palliative surgery is occasionally attempted after lesser procedures (including sclerotherapy) have failed because of the inability of the lung to expand. Generally, the procedure of choice for such palliation is a pleurectomy with or without decortication of the underlying lung. The use of EPP for palliative intent is only rarely described in the literature and because of its morbidity and mortality some surgeons state that EPP should never be used for palliative purposes.[1]

TABLE 40.2-3. Videothoracoscopic Talc Pleurodesis for Malignant Pleural Mesothelioma

Author	*No.*	*Success[a] (%)*	*Median Survival (mo)*
Viallet[123]	88	84	9.0
Canto[124]	46	80	9.4
Charvat[125]	13	100	6.8

[a]Success defined as no further need for tapping after 1 month in patients with a resulting normal radiographic result or less than 500 mL of residual fluid remaining.

Pleurectomy

MORBIDITY AND MORTALITY. When performed routinely pleurectomy for mesothelioma can be associated with few major complications (Fig. 40.2-1). In the series that specify postoperative morbidity, the most common complication was prolonged air leak (i.e., greater than 7 days), occurring in 10% of the patients. On average the chest tubes can be removed in approximately 5.5 days with greater than 50% of the patients having the chest tube removed within 4 days. Pneumonia and respiratory insufficiency may occur and are usually related to the burden of disease and preoperative functional status. Empyema is a rare occurrence (2%) and is managed by prolonged chest tube drainage and antibiotics. Hemorrhage requiring reexploration is rare (i.e., less than 1%).

Earlier studies in patients requiring pleurectomy (but not having mesothelioma) had an inhospital or operative mortality of 10% to 18% in the 1960s.[126,127] The modern-day

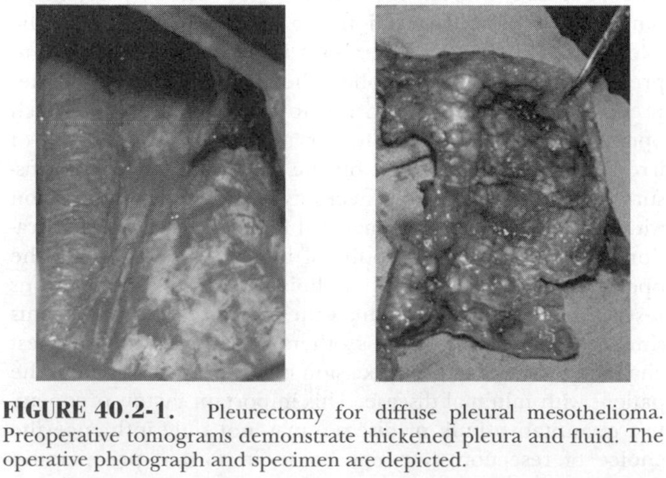

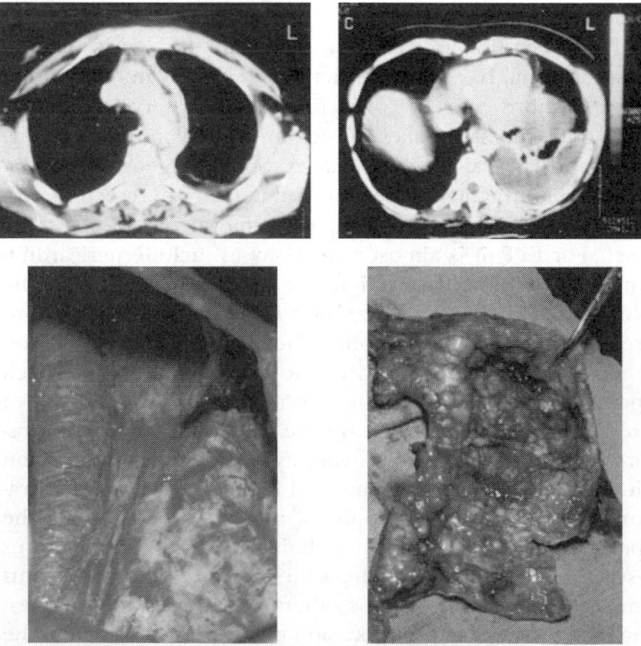

FIGURE 40.2-1. Pleurectomy for diffuse pleural mesothelioma. Preoperative tomograms demonstrate thickened pleura and fluid. The operative photograph and specimen are depicted.

mortality from pleurectomy has decreased and is generally considered to be 1.5% to 2.0%, with death either from respiratory insufficiency or hemorrhage. Most recently, total pleurectomy in 50 patients performed for mesothelioma had a 30-day mortality of 2%.[6] In a series of 39 pleurectomies, the hospital mortality was 0%.[128]

SHORT- AND LONG-TERM RESULTS. Pleurectomy and decortication are effective in controlling malignant pleural effusion. Law et al. report effusion control in 88% of patients having decortication for mesothelioma.[129] In 63 patients having partial decortication and pleurectomy Ruffie et al.[119] reported 86% control of effusion, and Brancatisano et al. reported a 98% control of effusion after pleurectomy in 50 cases of pleural mesothelioma.[130]

Many of the published series using pleurectomy for palliative management have added therapies postoperatively in an uncontrolled, institution-related fashion (Table 40.2-4). The majority have no sampling of the mediastinal nodes, little less a mediastinal dissection. Nevertheless, the overall median survival for patients having pleurectomy alone is approximately 13 months. The patients who receive pleurectomy and decortication alone usually have early effusive disease with minimal bulk tumor. If these patients have epithelial mesothelioma and are not found to have nodal involvement, survival rates can be significantly longer than that quoted previously.

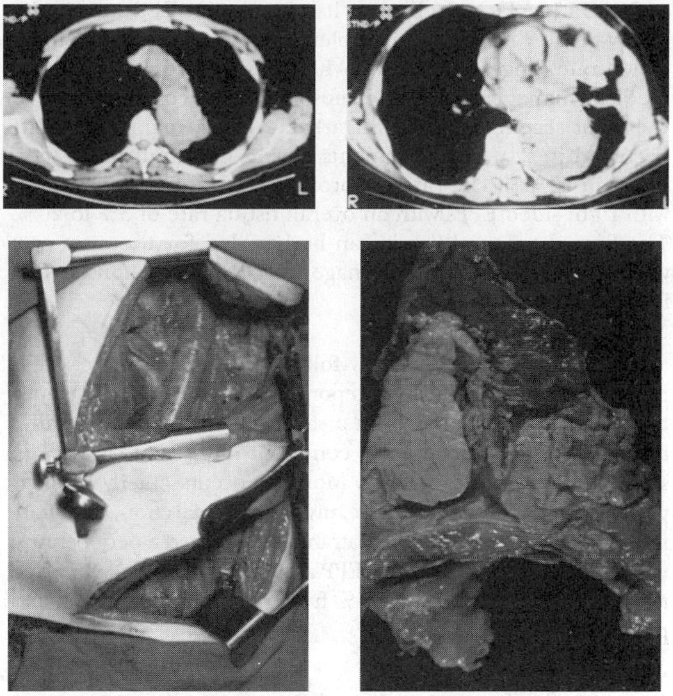

FIGURE 40.2-2. Left-sided diffuse mesothelioma. Two computed tomographic cuts show chest wall, fissure involvement, and aortic arch abutment. The surgical photograph demonstrates the skeletonized aorta, partial pericardiectomy, and partial diaphragmatic removal via a counter-incision. The surgical specimen is demonstrated in the lower right.

Radical Curative Surgery: Extrapleural Pneumonectomy

INDICATIONS. Radical EPP classically has been described for pure epithelial tumor, stage I that is technically resectable and encapsulated by the parietal pleura (Fig. 40.2-2). Due to sampling error it is impossible to clarify with 100% certainty whether the tumor is a pure epithelial type or mixed tumor based on the preoperative or intraoperative biopsy.

The centers that are able to attract large numbers of mesothelioma patients due to ongoing prospective trials may be relaxing the so-called classic indications based on stage, age, and histology. Surgeons at these institutions are chiefly concerned with the patients' functional ability to tolerate the operation, and the ability to accomplish maximal tumor debulking. If, indeed, higher stage patients can undergo the operation with risks equal to pleurectomy and decortication, enthusiasm for its general incorporation in more aggressive adjunctive trials would be justified.

TABLE 40.2-4. Results of Pleurectomy Alone for Mesothelioma

Author	*Year*	*No. of Patients*	*Percentage Mortality*	*Median Survival (mo)*
Brenner[131]	1981	69	NA	5
Chahinian[132]	1982	30	0	13
Law[129]	1984	28	11	20
DaValle[108]	1986	23	13	11
Chailleux[133]	1988	29	NA	14
Ruffie[119]	1989	63	0	10
Harvey[134]	1990	9	NA	12
Brancatisano[130]	1991	50	2	16
Rusch[135]	1991	26	NA	10
Total		327	5	13

NA, not applicable.

There are few patients who actually qualify for exploration outside the research setting. In Butchart's review, 29 of 46 or 63% of patients were eligible for EPP.[95] The only other series that reveals this percentage is DaValle's in which 33 of 56 patients over a 27-year period had EPP (59%).[136] Sugarbaker reported 50% of the patients seen at his institution are not eligible for EPP and adjuvant therapy. Unfortunately, these series really do not define why one patient may have a pleurectomy while another would have EPP, and it is obvious, however, that some institutions have simply never adopted the operation as feasible for treatment of the disease.

Probably the most enlightening study on eligibility was the Lung Cancer Study Group malignant mesothelioma pilot study from 1985 through 1988.[135] To be eligible for entry into the study the patient was required to have disease limited to the hemithorax by roentgenographic evaluation, a residual FEV_1 after resection of at least 1 L/second, and no significant cardiovascular illness, clearly more lenient criteria than those that limited eligibility due to age, histologic type, or presumed stage. Even with these relaxed criteria only 20 of the 83 evaluated patients were resected with an EPP. The reasons that EPP could not be performed were chiefly extent of disease not allowing complete gross resection (54%), inadequate respiratory reserve (33%), stage IV disease (11%), and concurrent medical illness (10%) (Table 40.2-5).

COMPLICATIONS. Due to its magnitude, EPP has significantly greater morbidity than pleurectomy. The major complication rate ranges from 20% to 40%, and arrhythmia requiring medical management is the most common complication. In the most recent report of Sugarbaker et al., major morbidity occurred in 24% of the patients having EPP and minor morbidity in 41%.[93] The rate for bronchopleural fistula is greater with right-sided EPPs with an overall fistula rate of 3% to 20%. The bronchopleural fistula can be handled for the most part with open thoracostomy drainage with or without muscle flap interposition.

MORTALITY. The mortality following EPP was unacceptably high in the 1970s, with 31% reported by Butchart et al.[95] Since then, however, there has been a steady decline in the operative mortality for the operation to consistent rates less than 10% in series of 20 or more patients. Mortality occurs chiefly in older patients from respiratory failure, myocardial infarction, or pulmonary embolus. Rusch and Venkatraman[91] reported a perioperative mortality of 6% (3 of 50) after EPP and Sugarbaker et al. reported a perioperative mortality of 3.8% from myocardial infarction and presumed pulmonary emboli.[93]

Recurrence after Extrapleural Pneumonectomy

Rusch et al.[135] described sites of recurrence after EPP to be distant areas compared with biopsy only or pleurectomy and decortication, and the local control was superior to that of the other modalities. Pass et al. also found a higher proportion of first sites of local recurrence seen in the pleurectomy population compared with the patients having EPP.[128] In the series of patients reported by Sugarbaker et al., Baldini et al. have reported that the sites of first recurrence were local in 35% of patients, abdominal in 26%, the contralateral thorax in 17%, and other distant sites in 8%.[140]

SURVIVAL. Long-term survival rates after EPP remain disappointing, with the median survivals ranging from 9.3 to 17.0 months for the majority series. Rusch and Venkatraman reported a median survival of 10 months in their series of 50 EPP,[91] and the median survival of malignant pleural mesothelioma patients having EPP (all histologies) in the National Cancer Institute series is 9.4 months. The majority of patients were pathologic stage II or III in these two series. Most recently, Sugarbaker et al.[93] reported a 17-month median survival in a series heavily weighted with stage I, epithelial patients (52 of 183), using a multimodality approach (see Combined Modality Approaches, later in this chapter) whose 2- and 5-year survivals were 68% and 46%. In the series by Rusch and Venkatraman, the 2- and 5-year survivals of stage I patients (16 of 131) were 65% and 30%, respectively.

TABLE 40.2-5. Extrapleural Pneumonectomy: Results

Author	*Year*	*No. of Patients*	*Percentage Mortality*	*Median Survival (mo)*
Wörn[137]	1974	62	20–25	19.0
Bamler[138]	1976	17	23	NA
Butchart[95]	1978	29	31	10.0
DaValle[108]	1986	33	9	13.5
Ruffie[119]	1989	23	13	9.3
Probst[139]	1990	55	5.5	10.2
Rusch[135]	1995	50	6	9.9
Sugarbaker[93, a]	1999	180	4.8	21.0
Total		291	15.5	11.1

[a]Multimodality series performed over 14 years.
NA, not applicable.

RADIATION THERAPY

The efficacy of irradiation, like that of other treatment modalities, remains uncertain in the definitive treatment of patients with pleural mesothelioma. While there are no prospective randomized clinical trials that define a role for radiation therapy, several studies suggest benefit. However, the variable clinical course of the disease and the frequent use of radiation in conjunction with either surgery or chemotherapy make assessment of its contribution to an overall treatment program difficult. One report suggests prolonged patient survival among patients with malignant pleural mesothelioma receiving combined modality treatment versus supportive care alone or single modality therapy.[141]

Mesothelioma cell lines seem to be more sensitive to radiation (as assessed by the surviving fraction after 2 Gy) than non–small cell lung cancer cell lines, but less sensitive than small cell lung cancer cells.[142] The results of a more recent study suggest that mesothelioma cell lines from different patients exhibit remarkable differences in radiosensitivity.[143] The use of radiation for mesothelioma, however, differs considerably from its use in lung cancer because of the extensive pleural involvement seen in mesothelioma. If radiation is to be used for definitive treatment of malignant mesothelioma, treatment of the entire ipsilateral pleura is indicated. This target volume is extremely difficult to radiate to tumoricidal doses without exposing patients to a risk of normal tissue injury to adjacent lung, heart, spinal cord, and liver.[144]

Most reports from the literature document occasional regressions of gross disease with modest doses of radiation, but do not indicate that survival is significantly altered by irradiation compared with supportive care (Table 40.2-6). Between 1971 and 1980, 116 patients with good performance status and without evidence of extrathoracic disease were evaluated at the Brompton and Royal Marsden Hospitals in London.[129,146] Fifty-two patients underwent active treatment, whereas the other 64 received supportive care. No difference in survival was seen between the two groups at 2 (33%) and 4 years (0% to 11%). Active treatment consisted of nonradical parietal pleurectomy and decortication of the lung in 28 patients, radiation therapy in 12 patients (following surgery in 8), and chemotherapy in the remaining 12 patients (8 of whom also underwent operation). Radiation therapy consisted of 50 to 55 Gy using rotating arc fields designed to treat the pleura and spare underlying lung. One patient showed a dramatic response to radiotherapy, with resolution of effusion, pain, and dyspnea. She was doing well 4 years after completion of treatment. Two other patients experienced sustained regression of recurrent pleural effusions after radiation therapy. Thus, although the treatment volume and adjuvant normal tissue limit radiation dose, radiation therapy to

TABLE 40.2-6. Radiation Series

Institution	*No. of Patients*	*Dose (Gy)*	*Outcome*
University of Iowa[145]	3	20–25	Symptomatic improvement
Brompton/Royal Marsden[129,146]	12	50–55	1 asymptomatic for 4 y; 2 with effusions controlled until demise
Joint Center for Radiation Therapy[110]	6	>40	4 with significant symptomatic relief
	23	<40	1 with significant symptomatic relief
Institut Gustave-Roussy[147]	14	35–50	4 alive at 1–41 mo; 10 dead at 1–37 (median, 15) mo
Thomas Jefferson Medical School[148]	9	60	2 with local control, 20 and 40 mo
Beatson Oncology Centre, Glasgow[149]	22	30	13 symptomatic improvement; median survival, 4 mo
Peter MacCallum Cancer Institute[150]	111	8–60	66 symptomatic improvement; median survival, 5 mo
University Hospital Rotterdam[151]	24	20–40	13 symptomatic improvement

bulky tumors occasionally produces significant regression and palliation.

Because of the variable course of the disease, different radiation treatment techniques used (anteroposterior and posteroanterior, rotational arc, combined photon electron), and normal tissue constraints on radiation dose, the relationship between treatment response and radiation dose is not well established. The series from the Joint Center for Radiation Therapy in Boston included 29 treatment courses for palliation between 1968 and 1980.[110] Relief of dyspnea, pain, and other symptoms was seen in four of six patients treated with doses of greater than or equal to 40 Gy, whereas only 1 of 23 treatment courses at lower doses of radiation achieved palliation of symptoms. Doses of 15 to 20 Gy (the normal tissue tolerance dose of whole lung irradiation) did not control disease in patients with diffuse involvement of the visceral pleura with 1- to 2-mm nodules.

A series from the Peter MacCallum Cancer Institute in Australia described good palliation in 17 of 26 (65%) evaluable palliative radiation courses.[152] Short-course treatment for palliation with 20 Gy in five fractions appeared to give similar results with more protracted courses (30 to 40 Gy in 10 to 15 fractions). Fifteen patients were given high-dose radiotherapy with radical intent. Twelve completed treatment to 50 Gy. The median survival of the 12 patients completing treatment was 17 months, with an estimated 2-year survival of 17%.[152] A more recent study from the Peter MacCallum Cancer Institute on 111 patients showed that 60% of the patients obtained successful palliation, with a median survival of 5 months. No dose-response curve for palliation could be identified.

In a series from Thomas Jefferson Medical School in Philadelphia, two of nine patients had local control at 20 and 40 months after 60 Gy to the entire ipsilateral pleura, mediastinum, and involved areas of lung.[148] Radiation was delivered in three courses of 20 Gy over a total of 10 weeks by a split-course technique.

While the volume of disease can influence radiotherapeutic outcome in many other tumors, its effect on the radiation response of pleural mesothelioma is not well characterized. The combination of radiation therapy with debulking surgery can be rationalized if only microscopic disease on the majority of the pleural surfaces remains after surgery. Radiation is more effective at a given dose level when treating microscopic compared with gross disease. Higher doses of boost irradiation with either a shrinking-field technique or brachytherapy can be used on sites of residual gross disease. Such a strategy likely maximizes local control while minimizing the normal tissue complications from irradiation.

Radiation therapy can be used to prevent seeding of biopsy tracts and surgical wounds. In a series from Marseilles, France, radiation treatment of 21 Gy in three fractions prevented wound seeding after thoracoscopy or thoracotomy in 24 patients.[153] Before initiation of an adjuvant irradiation policy in this setting, wound seeding occurred in 17 of 33 (61%) patients. None of the patients who developed growth of nodules in an incision site responded to subsequent irradiation.

When considering the use of radical radiation therapy in this disease, the potential complications of high-dose irradiation to a large volume should also be weighed in the treatment decision. The frequency, type, and severity of radiation complications depends on volume, dose, fractionation, technique, and normal tissue in the field, as well as type and timing of any other treatment, such as chemotherapy. Remarkably, some earlier series reported no acute or chronic complications from the use of radiotherapy alone.[110,147] This may have been the result of limited volume treatment or short survival. One series noted few complications with radiotherapy when 50 to 55 Gy were delivered with an off-axis rotational technique. Among 12 patients, complications included nausea and malaise in six, transient radiation hepatitis in one, and mild esophagitis in another.[129,146] No case of radiation pneumonitis was noted. However, in cases in which no attempt has been made to shield lung or when the organ tolerance of other tissues such as the liver has been exceeded, significant complications have been seen. Ball and Cruickshank reported a case of fatal radiation hepatitis in a patient treated for a right pleural mesothelioma and one case of radiation myelitis (after 40 Gy) in their series of 12 patients treated with radical irradiation.[152] Maasilta et al. reported deterioration in lung function after high-dose irradiation (55 to 71 Gy) given with chemotherapy.[154,155] Indeed, forced vital capacity and diffusing capacity showed a significant decline at 1.5 to 2.0 months following radiotherapy and continued to decline over the year following the end of radiation. By radiologic assessment, treatment essentially obliterated lung function on the affected side. Of note, hypoxemia and pathologic and physiologic shunting increased in two of six patients monitored. Hence, lung function should be evaluated to assess potential tolerance before undertaking hemithorax irradiation. Liver position and volume should be determined, and adequate hepatic shielding should be used. Maasilta and Hallman et al. have reported the association of bronchoalveolar lavage plasmin and surfactant in mesothelioma patients with radiation pulmonary injury.[155,156]

The use of radioactive colloids such as ^{198}Au or chromic phosphate-^{32}P instilled into the pleural space has also been studied. Pleural effusions have been reported to disappear for up to 3.5 years.[157] The exact response rate and duration to this approach is not known. In a series from Hahnemann Medical College, all six patients were alive at 12 months or longer after instillation of isotopes.[158] The extent of other treatment and exact length of survival, however, was not reported. Because of the physical characteristics of these isotopes, their effect on gross disease is limited. ^{32}P is a pure beta (electron) emitter with maximum tissue penetration of 8 mm, and the bulk of energy deposited in the first 2 mm. ^{198}Au emits 90% of its energy as beta particles (electrons) with an energy of 0.96 MeV. These have tissue penetration of less than 5 mm, although the emitted photons have energies of 0.412 to 1.099 MeV and would penetrate several centimeters. An equally important limitation on the use of radiocolloids is the problem of obtaining optimal distribution of isotope throughout the pleural space. Gordon and colleagues reported an attempt at radioisotope instillation in three patients, but fluoroscopy or gamma camera measurements indicated that the distribution was suboptimal.[110] Hence, both agents may have a limited role in patients with low-volume disease or in conjunction with surgery in patients with an adequate pleural distribution. The distribution of a radiotracer or contrast material should be tested before a therapeutic administration of these agents is considered.

Radiation Therapy Techniques

Different radiotherapy techniques have been used to irradiate the pleura to high doses. Because of the extensive pleural involvement, the target volume is large and includes the pleural surface, diaphragm, and mediastinum. Attempts at radical radiation should be limited to those patients with disease confined to one hemithorax. Field borders must extend above the first rib superiorly, below the diaphragmatic reflection of the pleura inferiorly, which is usually at about the lower border of the twelfth thoracic vertebra, laterally to clear the bony rib cage, and include the full width of the mediastinum. The field size can be increased to include masses extending into the chest wall or diaphragm, or to include the whole heart when the pericardium is involved. The identification of sites of residual gross disease with surgical clips at thoracotomy greatly facilitates radiation planning by allowing accurate, well-defined high-dose boost volumes and lessens the likelihood of normal tissue injury. CT scanning can also help delineate sites of gross disease, but may miss invasion of tumor into the mediastinum or through the diaphragm, as well as areas of miliary seeding of the pleura.[96,159] MRI has been reported to delineate mediastinal invasion by mesothelioma[160] and may have a role in radiologic assessment and treatment planning.

Radical irradiation commonly delivers 40 to 55 Gy to the entire pleural surface (with the exception of the reflections extending into the fissures in the lung) and the mediastinum. Other structures, such as the heart, are included as clinically indicated. This has been followed by boosts to focal areas of gross disease through reduced portals to doses of 55 to 71 Gy. While some have chosen to irradiate the entire hemithorax with opposed anterior and posterior photon fields to doses of 40 to 50 Gy without lung shielding followed by a cone-down to smaller fields,[144,152] such techniques are associated with irreversible pulmonary injury.[144] Hence, techniques have been developed to spare the lung. One involves the use of an off-axis beam rotational technique to irradiate the pleural space to high dose while shielding underlying lung.[129,146] Several others involve matching photon and electron beams.[148,161] These involve the use of large, opposed anterior and posterior external-beam portals with central lung blocking. The pleural areas underneath the blocks are treated with electron beams of appropriate energy (generally 10 to 15 MeV). CT scans are used to define the thickness of the chest wall, delineate patient contour, and plan treatment. Tissue compensators may improve dose distribution. None of these techniques are ideal. Even careful photon and electron techniques deliver substantial doses to the lung because of the penetrating ability of the electron beams in the lung and contribution from side-scattered electrons set in motion during photon irradiation.[161]

Advances in sophisticated conformal radiotherapy may improve the available dose distribution.[162] A single report using fast neutrons describes a complete regression of bulk disease without evidence of recurrence 78 months after treatment.[163] However, a portion of the disease was treated with cobalt 60 irradiation with similar response. Because of the poor depth dose characteristics of the available neutron beams, only thin patients could be treated with a pure neutron technique. However, these or other particles may have a role in selected patients in delivering boost treatment to sites of gross disease. Other particles, such as protons, may have a role in selected patients in delivering boost treatment to sites of gross disease.

Intensity modulated radiation therapy techniques permit higher doses of radiation to be delivered to target tissue while limiting radiation dose to the lung and other normal tissues (Fig. 40.2-3).

When conventional fractions of 1.8 to 2.0 Gy are given daily five times per week, reasonable treatment precautions would limit the spinal cord dose to 40 Gy, the esophagus to 45 to 50 Gy, the whole lung to 20 Gy, a functional portion of the liver to 30 Gy, and 50% of the heart to 40 Gy. Radiation tolerances may be lowered when radiation is given in conjunction with chemotherapy, especially doxorubicin, despite temporal separation of the two modalities by weeks or even months.

CHEMOTHERAPY

Single-Agent Studies

Before the wide availability of CT scans, most mesotheliomas were not strictly measurable. Measurable masses on chest radiography were frequently obscured by effusions that are totally unreliable in determining response to therapy. Response rates to standard agents remain difficult to define. Relatively small positive studies are reported promptly, whereas larger series with lower response rates may never be published. Nevertheless, data from single-agent studies are shown in Table 40.2-7. Response rates are included in the table when the number of evaluable patients exceeds ten.

Doxorubicin appears to have some activity against mesothelioma although response rates vary considerably. Methotrexate

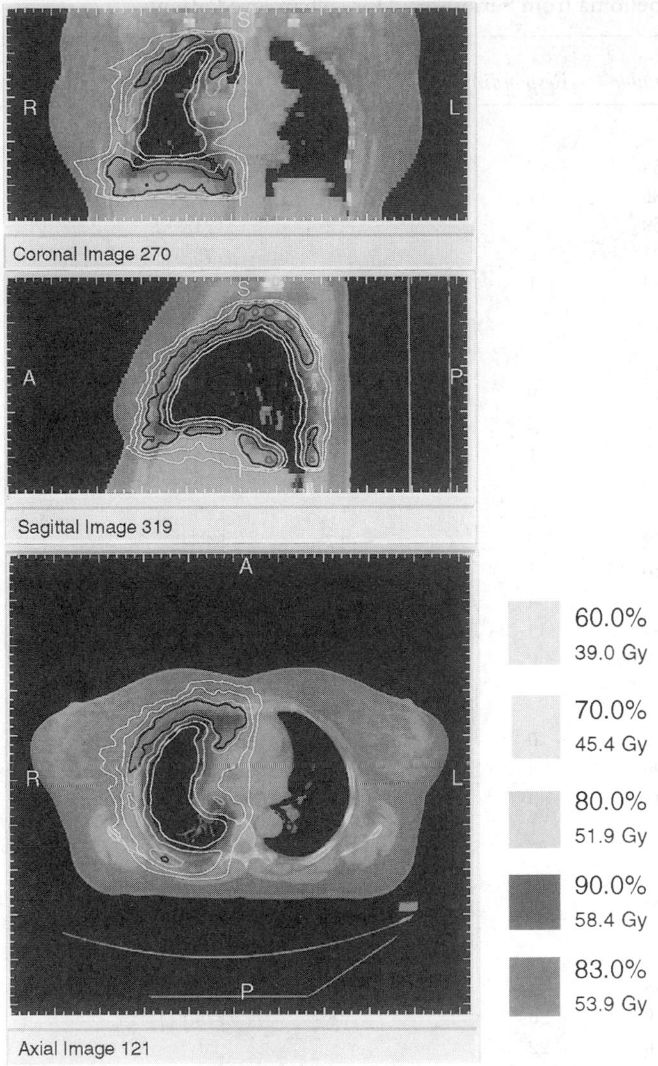

FIGURE 40.2-3. Coronal (top), sagittal (middle), and axial (bottom) views of an intensity-modulated radiation therapy treatment plan for a patient with malignant pleural mesothelioma. In this patient the target tissue surrounds the lung. In this plan the target tissue receives 54 Gy while limiting the dose to the majority of the lung to less than 20 Gy. The spinal cord, heart, and contralateral lung also receive acceptable low doses of radiation. (Courtesy of the Department of Radiation Oncology, Columbia University, New York.) (See Color Fig. 40.2-3 in the CD-ROM and on the Web at www.LWWoncology.com.)

with rescue, 5-azacitidine, and 5-fluorouracil may also have single-agent activity. Neither cisplatin nor paclitaxel as single agents appear to be significantly active.

Intrapleural Cytokine Therapy

Interferon-γ has had intriguing results by the intrapleural route as documented by Boutin et al.[230] Interferon was administered at a dose of 40 million U twice a week for 8 weeks intrapleurally via a catheter or an implantable port for 89 patients over 46 months. Thoracoscopic or surgical biopsy was performed if CT scan 2 weeks after the end of treatment demonstrated a reduction in tumor size. Eight histologically confirmed complete responses and nine partial responses with at least a 50% reduction in tumor size were obtained. The overall response rate was 20%. The response rate for patients with stage I disease was 45, with the main side effects being hyperthermia, liver toxicity, neutropenia, and catheter-related infection.

IL-2–based regimens have also been exploited in mesothelioma. The largest experience to date with *intrapleural* IL-2–based therapy has been reported by Astoul et al.[233] Of 22 patients with mesothelioma (19 epithelial, 2 mixed, 1 sarcomatous) treated with intrapleural IL-2 (21×10^6 IU/m^2/day for 5 days) 11 responded partially and 1 completely. The median survival was 18 months. The 24- and 36-month survival rates for responders were 58% and 41%, respectively.[233]

Combination Chemotherapy

Response rates for combination regimens range from 0% to 48% (Table 40.2-8). The highest response rate reported is for cisplatin and gemcitabine (48% in 21 patients). Nine of ten responders and three of nine with stable disease has symptomatic improvement, and three responders had improved vital capacity on functional testing.[234]

Randomized Trials in Mesothelioma

Doxorubicin and cyclophosphamide with or without dacarbazine yielded response rates of 7% in both arms of a large randomized trial that accrued advanced patients concurrently with a second study for stage I and II mesothelioma.[235] Thus, the response rates may be artificially low in this study because better prognosis patients were treated on a competing study.

The Cancer and Leukemia Group B randomized 79 patients with measurable mesothelioma to cisplatin and doxorubicin versus cisplatin and mitomycin C. The objective response rates in patients with measurable disease (24%) were similar but time to treatment failure (4.8 vs. 3.6 months) and survival (8.8 vs. 7.7 months) were slightly longer for the doxorubicin and cisplatin combination compared with mitomycin and cisplatin.[236]

Intrapleural Chemotherapy

Based on the activity of intraperitoneal cisplatin (see Intraperitoneal Chemotherapy, below), the Lung Cancer Study Group completed a trial of 47 patients treated with intrapleural cisplatin and cytarabine. Of the 37 patients evaluated, 49% had at least 75% decrease in the size of their effusion.[135]

Pharmacokinetic data in 12 patients treated with intrapleural cisplatin and mitomycin showed three- to fivefold higher pleural to plasma levels of both drugs.[237] In an Italian pharmacokinetic study of four patients treated with 90 mg/m^2 intrapleurally compared with seven patients treated with the same dose intravenously, the mean area under the concentration versus time curve was 50 times greater than that detected in plasma. Intrapleural cisplatin resulted in significantly lower plasma mean area under the concentration versus time curve and prolonged plasma levels of filterable platinum compared with intravenous administration.[238]

The use of an implantable port facilitates repetitive intrapleural administration and probably decreases the risk of infection.[239]

TABLE 40.2-7. Single-Agent Response Rates in Malignant Mesothelioma from Series with More Than Five Patients

Agent	*No. Evaluable*	*No. Responding*	*Percentage*	*References*
ANTHRACYCLINES AND RELATED COMPOUNDS				
Doxorubicin	164	29	18	148,164–167
Pirarubicin	85	11	14	168–170
Epirubicin	69	8	12	171,172
Detorubicin	21	9	43	173
Mitoxantrone	34	1	3	174
ALKYLATING AGENTS				
Cyclophosphamide	14	4	28	165,167,175,176
Ifosfamide	111	9	8	177–180
Mechlorethamine	6	2		167,181–183
Thiotepa	7	1		164,175,181,182,184
Melphalan	3	2		176,184
Procarbazine	6	2		185
Mitomycin C	12	2	17	84,186
Cisplatin	56	8	14	187–193
Cisplatin (weekly)	9	4	44	194
Carboplatin	97	11 (2 CRs)	11	195–200
Iproplatin	7	0		198,199
VINCAS AND RELATED COMPOUNDS				
Vincristine	23	0		201
Etoposide (IV)	100	5	5	202–206
Etoposide (daily oral)	45	3	7	206
Vindesine	37	1	3	207,208
TAXANES				
Paclitaxel	60	3	5	209,210
ANTIMETABOLITES				
5-Fluorouracil	28	4	14	165–167
Methotrexate, high dose	69	26	38	175,211
	60	22		
5-Azacitidine	7	0		212,213
Dihydro-5-azacitidine	55	4 (1 CR)	7	214,215
Gemcitabine	27	2	7	216
Bleomycin	6	1		132,217
Trimetrexate	52	6	12	218
MISCELLANEOUS				
AMSA	19	1	5	219
Topotecan	22	0		220
BIOLOGICS				
Bacille Calmette-Guérin (after surgery)	30		Inevaluable	221
Granulocyte-macrophage colony-stimulating factor (intralesional)	14	1	7	222
RNA (intrapleural)	10	8	80	223
Interferon-α	38	4	11	224,225
Interferon-β	14	0		226
Interferon-γ (intrapleural)	99	24 (7 CRs)	24	227–229
Interferon-γ (intrapleural)	89	17	20	230
Interleukin-2 (intrapleural)	46	22	48	228,231–233

CR, complete response.

TABLE 40.2-8. Reported Combinations in Series with More Than 15 Patients

Agents Used	*No. Evaluable*	*No. Responding*	*Response Rate*	*References*
DOXORUBICIN CONTAINING COMBINATIONS WITH				
5-Azacitidine	36	8	27	132,240
Ifosfamide	49	12	24	178,241,242
Cisplatin	60	17	28	236,243–246
Cisplatin, mitomycin	23	5	21	247
Cisplatin, bleomycin, mitomycin	25	11 (1 CR)	44	248
Cyclophosphamide ± dacarbazine	81	6	7	235,249
Cyclophosphamide, dacarbazine, vincristine	30	8	21	182,250,251
Interferon	25	4	16	252
CISPLATIN-CONTAINING COMBINATIONS WITH				
Etoposide	26	3	12	253
Pirarubicin	39	6	15	170,254
Irinotecan	15	4	27	255
Gemcitabine	21	10	48	234
Vinblastine	20	5	25	256
Dihydro-5-azacitidine	29	5	17	257
Interferon-α_{2a}	42	13	31	258,259
Mitomycin C	32	10	31	236,260
Mitomycin C, vinblastine	39	8	20	261
Mitomycin C, etoposide, 5-fluorouracil–leucovorin	45	17	38	262
Mitomycin C, interferon-α	43	10 (2 CRs)	23	263
Mitomycin C, interferon-α	19	2	11	264
OTHER COMBINATIONS				
Epirubicin, ifosfamide	17	1	6	265
Epirubicin, interleukin-2	21	1	5	266
Carboplatin and interferon-α_{2a}	15	1	7	267
Methotrexate (3 g) and interferon-α and -γ	26	7	27	268

CR, complete response.

MULTIMODALITY TREATMENT

COMBINED RADIOTHERAPY AND CHEMOTHERAPY

Theoretically, cisplatin or doxorubicin could be used as a radiosensitizer and may be more effective than radiotherapy or chemotherapy alone. A small group of South African patients treated with doxorubicin and radiation of 10 Gy every 6 weeks for four courses survived a median of 23 months.[269] Paclitaxel has been described as a radiation sensitizer.[270] A phase I report from the National Cancer Institute combining a 120-hour (5-day) continuous infusion of paclitaxel every 3 weeks during thoracic radiation therapy (57.6 to 63.0 Gy) has been shown to be safe in 27 patients with malignant pleural mesothelioma.[271] Many patients achieved local control; however, only four patients were alive with a median follow-up of 15 months. One of these patients is without evidence of disease at 14 months.

A nonrandomized phase II study from University Hospital in Lund, Sweden, compared the effect of hemithorax radiation (40 Gy) alone or combined with doxorubicin and cyclophosphamide in 47 patients with biopsy only.[272] No significant difference was detected between the two groups of patients with regard to tumor response, survival, or palliation of tumor-related pain.

SURGERY WITH POSTOPERATIVE ADJUVANT THERAPY

The majority of patients with mesothelioma, independent of staging, cannot be rendered free of disease with surgical therapy alone. In a Memorial Sloan-Kettering Cancer Center report of 41 patients who underwent parietal pleurectomy between 1976 and 1982, disease at the completion of surgery remained on the diaphragm (49%), visceral pleura (51%), mediastinum (49%), chest wall (27%), and lung (5%).[273] Seventy-eight percent had residual gross disease after surgery. Radical pleuropneumonectomy can remove more disease in selected patients, but many still have residual microscopic or gross tumor after even the most aggressive surgical resection.

Alberts et al.,[269] in a series of 26 selected patients (10% of a total of 262 patients), reported an 11-month median survival after maximal pleural cytoreduction, 4500 cGy postoperative radiation therapy, and doxorubicin, cyclophosphamide, and procarbazine. The results, however, may reflect a generally poor risk group as the duration of symptoms was usually less than 6 months.

A nonrandomized prospective study from Helsinki University Central Hospital[274] reported on 100 patients treated between 1977 and 1989 with debulking surgery, chemotherapy, and hemithorax irradiation. The median survival time was increased from 8 to 12 months for those patients who completed one of five protocols. The first protocol (1977 to 1981, 16 patients) was 20-Gy hemithorax irradiation in ten fractions over 2 weeks and a variable number of courses of cyclophosphamide, vincristine, doxorubicin, and dacarbazine. The second study (1982 to 1984, 26 patients) was a split-course radiation therapy program consisting of 55 Gy in 25 fractions over 7 weeks with a midway 2-week rest. Major tumor areas were boosted with 15 Gy in six fractions. Chemotherapy was as described for the first protocol. The third protocol (1985 to 1986, 15 patients) was hemithorax irradiation using a hyperfractionation schedule to 70 Gy (1.25 Gy twice daily) over 7 weeks with a 10-day rest halfway through. Radiation was preceded by single-agent chemotherapy with mitoxantrone for a maximum of six cycles. The fourth protocol (1986 to 1988, 24 patients) included 35-Gy hyperfractionated into 28 fractions over 3 weeks and hypofractionation of 36 Gy into nine fractions every other day over 3 weeks. This schedule was preceded with 4-epirubicin for a maximum of six cycles. The fifth and final protocol (1988 to 1989, 19 patients) included hemithorax irradiation using 38.5 Gy in 11 fractions over 15 days. A maximum of six cycles of etoposide preceded the radiation therapy. None of the protocols prevented progression of local disease or spread of tumor outside the hemithorax. Significant lung injury (radiation pneumonitis and fibrosis) occurred in regimens 2, 3, 4, and 5.

Pleurectomy, Intraoperative Brachytherapy, and Postoperative Radiation

Memorial Sloan-Kettering Cancer Center has been the leading proponent of this technique, which includes as complete a parietal pleurectomy as possible to remove the bulk of the tumor followed by permanent (^{125}I) or temporary (^{192}Ir) implantation to deliver 3000 rads in 3 days to a 1-cm distance from the implant plane.[273] Radioactive ^{32}P is selectively instilled intrapleurally 5 to 7 days after thoracotomy, followed by external-beam radiation therapy commencing 4 to 6 weeks postoperatively using electrons and photons to deliver 4500 rads in 4.5 weeks. They report minimum morbidity in the 41 patients discussed, and the median survival was 21 months at the time of their report. The majority of patients had recurrences at distant sites (54%) with or without local recurrence. Unfortunately, there has been little follow-up information with regard to the ongoing status of these patients, as the median follow-up in 40% of the patients was 12 months or less at the time of the first report in 1984.

PLEURECTOMY, INTRAPLEURAL CHEMOTHERAPY, WITH OR WITHOUT POSTOPERATIVE CHEMOTHERAPY

Few studies of combining debulking surgery with intracavitary treatment of pleural mesothelioma have appeared since the first reports of intrapleural chemotherapy alone for malignant mesothelioma. In a report describing intrapleural chemotherapy without surgery for malignant pleural mesothelioma in 1987, 21 patients received 20 to 30 mg of doxorubicin weekly for 4 weeks and then monthly.[275] The average survival was 21 months, but the indications for the therapy and the monitoring of responses and recurrence data were difficult to extract from the report. Kirmani et al.[276] treated 17 patients with intrapleural cisplatin (90 to 100 mg/m^2) weekly for 3 weeks followed by a 3-week rest. Only 2 of 12 evaluable patients with pleural mesothelioma responded, with a median survival of 4 months. The 2 responders survived 9 months.

Rusch et al.[277] combined the elements of intrapleural chemotherapy with cisplatin and cytarabine after surgical debulking followed by systemic chemotherapy in ten patients. One patient died postoperatively, but the chemotherapy complications were reversible, making such an approach feasible. They followed this regimen with an even more aggressive regimen of pleurectomy, immediate intracavitary cisplatin and mitomycin C, followed by two cycles of cisplatin and mitomycin C systemically.[278] Toxicity was acceptable. The overall survival rate of the 27 patients was 68% at 1 year and 44% at 2 years, with a median survival of 17 months. Recurrences, however, were chiefly locoregional.

A similar regimen combining cisplatin and mitomycin C has been attempted at the Cleveland Clinic Foundation of 14 patients.[279] The projected 18-month survival was 31%, yet patients' tolerance permitted delivery of only 50% of the chemotherapy treatments adjuvantly.

In an Italian study, pleurectomy and diaphragmatic or pericardial resection was combined with intrapleural cisplatin and cytarabine for 4 hours immediately after pleurectomy and systemic epirubicin and mitomycin C. The median time to disease progression was 7.4 months, and median survival was 11.5 months in 20 patients.[280]

Pleurectomy with intrapleural chemotherapy with or without radiation therapy remains an intriguing strategy, but its efficacy is not established. Further investigation should include standard debulking with definition of the extent of residual disease, a tolerable but effective intrapleural regimen, and compulsive follow-up to document recurrence patterns.

EXTRAPLEURAL PNEUMONECTOMY, INTRAVENOUS CHEMOTHERAPY, AND POSTOPERATIVE RADIOTHERAPY

An ongoing interest in a multimodal approach to malignant mesothelioma was developed at the Dana Farber Cancer Institute beginning in 1980.[111] The program has evolved with regard to the chemotherapy, and presently consists of EPP, followed by two cycles of paclitaxel and carboplatin. Concurrent radiation to a dose of 40.5 Gy is given with weekly paclitaxel. Over a 19-year period, 183 patients were treated, with a perioperative mortality of 3.8%. The median survival in this group of patients is approximately 17 months, which is a significant improvement over other trials. Favorable subgroups include those with no mediastinal nodal involvement and epithelial histology.[93,281]

A series of 93 patients from Hamburg who chose either multimodal treatment or best supportive care has also shown some prolongation of life expectancy with multimodal treatment.[282] The treated patients, however, were younger, had a better performance status at presentation, and had no medical contraindications to surgery. Surgery consisted of pleurectomy decortication or EPP followed by systemic chemotherapy with doxorubicin, cyclophosphamide, and vindesine. Patients in remission at the end of the chemotherapy (16 of the 57 accrued) received 45 to 60 Gy of radiation therapy to the hemithorax. Median survival was

13 months compared with 7 months for those receiving best supportive care.

NOVEL MULTIMODAL APPROACHES

Intrapleural Photodynamic Therapy

Photodynamic therapy (PDT) involves the light-activated sensitization of malignant cells.[283] Photofrin II, the sensitizer, is retained by malignant tissue *in vivo* in comparison with normal tissue. The sensitizer is activated by 630-nm light and then interacts with molecular oxygen to produce an excited reactive oxygen species. Singlet oxygen forms the basis of PDT cytotoxicity. The potential for minimal normal tissue toxicity due to the selective retention of the sensitizer within tumors has prompted an interest in studying PDT for the treatment of a variety of tumors including skin, bladder, lung, head and neck, brain, and esophagus. From July 1993 to June 1996, 63 patients at the National Cancer Institute, National Institutes of Health, with localized malignant pleural mesothelioma were randomized to surgery, with or without intraoperative PDT. All patients received postoperative immunochemotherapy with cisplatin, tamoxifen, and interferon. Median survival (14.4 vs. 14.1 months), median progression-free time (8.5 vs. 7.7 months), and sites of first recurrence were similar. Thus, aggressive multimodal therapy incorporating PDT can be delivered for patients with higher stage malignant pleural mesothelioma, but first-generation PDT does not prolong survival or increase local control for malignant pleural mesothelioma.

Pleural Perfusion

There has been a resurgence of interest in the delivery of intrapleural cytotoxic chemotherapy at the time of operation for pleural mesothelioma. Using hyperthermic pleural space perfusion, Ratto et al. delivered cisplatin to the pleural space after pleurectomy or EPP in 10 patients.[284] This study has recorded the pharmacokinetics, but has no data as of yet on survival or recurrences.

Gene Therapy

A tumor cell infected with an adenovirus construct TK gene (AdHSVtk) containing the herpes simplex thymidine kinase (TK) gene can be killed with ganciclovir. The goals of phase I trial at the University of Pennsylvania were to assess the safety, toxicity, and maximally tolerated dose of intrapleural AdHSVtk, to examine patient inflammatory response to the viral vector, and to evaluate the efficiency of intratumoral gene transfer. Twenty-one previously untreated patients were enrolled in this viral titer dose-escalation study. A replication-incompetent recombinant adenoviral vector containing the HSVtk gene under control of the Rous sarcoma virus promoter-enhancer was introduced into the pleural cavity of patients with malignant mesothelioma followed by 2 weeks of systemic therapy with 5 mg/kg twice a day of ganciclovir. The initial 15 patients underwent thoracoscopic pleural biopsy before and 3 days after vector delivery. The last six patients underwent only the postvector instillation biopsy. Dose-limiting toxicity was not reached. Side effects were minimal and included fever, anemia, transient liver enzyme elevations, and bullous skin eruptions, as well as a temporary systemic inflammatory response in those receiving the highest dose. Strong intrapleural and intratumoral immune responses were generated. Using RNA polymerase chain reaction, *in situ* hybridization, immunohistochemistry, and immunoblotting, HSVtk gene transfer was documented in 11 of 20 evaluable patients in a dose-related fashion.[285,286]

A similar approach is under investigation by the group at Louisiana State University.[287,288] In *in vitro* mixing experiments, gene-modified tumor ovarian tumor cells killed both mouse and human mesothelioma cells in a dose-dependent manner. Use of the ovarian HSVtk ovarian cells also prolonged survival of mice with mesothelioma in a dose-dependent fashion. These data have served as the basis for an ongoing phase I clinical gene therapy trial to determine the maximal tolerated dose of an HSVtk-transduced ovarian cancer cells infused into the pleural cavities of mesothelioma patients followed by systemic administration of ganciclovir.

MALIGNANT PERITONEAL MESOTHELIOMA

PRESENTATION

Patients usually present with symptoms and signs of advanced disease including pain, ascites, weight loss, or an abdominal mass.[289–291] A cake of tumor in the omentum may be palpable as an epigastric mass. No satisfactory staging system has been proposed for peritoneal mesotheliomas, which are usually confined to the abdomen at diagnosis. Chest radiography reveals pleural plaques in approximately 50% of patients with peritoneal primaries, compared with 20% in patients with pleural mesothelioma, reflecting the higher level of asbestos exposure in patients with peritoneal disease. Classic findings on CT scan include mesenteric thickening, peritoneal studding, hemorrhage within the tumor mass, and ascites; however, patients may have advanced disease with relatively normal CTs.[292,293] MRI offers the possibility of improved resolution. Given the low incidence of bone, brain, or liver metastasis at presentation, extensive evaluation for metastatic disease is inappropriate in the absence of laboratory abnormalities. Adrenal, intrapulmonary, or bony metastasis should raise the possibility of an alternative diagnosis.

Peritoneal fluid from malignant ascites may be a watery transudate or a viscous fluid rich in mucopolysaccharides. No diagnostic significance has been attached to the character of the fluid, although a viscous ascites (with high fluid hyaluronidase levels) may suggest the diagnosis. Massive ascites may result in confusion of mesothelioma with severe cirrhosis. Cytology establishes the diagnosis in only 5% to 10% of cases.[291] Ultimately, definitive diagnosis requires adequate tissue sampling, preferably from peritoneoscopy or an open directed biopsy. A generous biopsy specimen is required to perform immunohistochemical stains, as well as electron microscopy. Open biopsy also permits inspection of the abdominal cavity for extent of disease with particular attention to the bowel and ovaries to distinguish mesothelioma from other more common causes of peritoneal carcinomatosis. Peritoneal mesotheliomas can be confused with adenocarcinomas arising from any abdominal organ, but the pattern of spread and tendency to accumulate in the pelvis readily leads to confusion with adenocarcinoma of the ovary or carcinoma arising from Müllerian duct remnants in the peritoneum.

The tumor generally remains confined to the abdomen until late in the course and even then is more likely to spread to one or both pleural cavities than to disseminate hematogenously. Thrombocytosis is common and associated with high levels of IL-6 and a poor prognosis. Other common clotting abnormalities include phlebitis, emboli, hemolytic anemia, and disseminated intravascular coagulation. Most patients die without metastases or involvement of the chest.[291] Esophageal achalasia, secondary amyloidosis, and dermatomyositis have been reported.[294–296] The median survival of untreated patients in most series is short, 4 to 12 months.[114,289,290,297]

WELL-DIFFERENTIATED PAPILLARY MESOTHELIOMA OR CYSTIC MESOTHELIOMAS OF THE PERITONEUM

Rare, well-differentiated papillary variants and a syndrome of recurrent peritoneal mesothelial cysts have both been found predominantly in younger women associated with a prolonged survival despite bulky disease.[298] Rarely, the disease progresses over time to a typical malignant mesothelioma.[299] Approximately 130 cases of multiloculated peritoneal inclusion cysts (also called *benign cystic peritoneal mesotheliomas*) have been described, mainly in the pathologic and surgical literature.[300] Some authors have advocated classifying this lesion as reactive proliferation rather than as malignant.[301] The radiologic differential diagnosis has been reviewed.[300]

Frequently associated with prior surgery, endometriosis, or pelvic inflammatory disease,[301] they occur predominantly in women,[302] but can occur in men.[300,303]

Treatment should be provided for palliation of symptoms or for clearly documented progression.[299,304] Despite initial surgical resection, approximately one-half recur locally. Neither lesion size nor proliferation correlates with outcome.[301] Tamoxifen resulted in a prolonged response in a 19-year-old woman.[305] Permanent transvaginal catheter drainage in a patient with recurrent cysts resulted in infection and obliteration of the cyst.[306] The potassium titanyl phosphate laser has also been used in treatment of benign multicystic peritoneal mesothelioma.[307]

THERAPY

Surgery

Surgical and autopsy series have shown that peritoneal mesothelioma involves all peritoneal surfaces, often with masses of 5 cm or more. Sites of local invasion included the liver, abdominal wall, diaphragm, retroperitoneum, gastrointestinal tract, and bladder. Seeding of laparotomy scars and biopsy tracts has also been observed. The tumor is most often confined to the peritoneal cavity at the time of initial diagnosis and remains there for much or all of the subsequent clinical course.[114] Hence, effective local therapy may have a substantial effect on the survival of patients with this disease. Complete surgical resection is rarely, if ever, feasible, and has not been shown to afford survival benefit in the absence of additional therapy. Nevertheless, surgical intervention can provide palliation for small bowel obstruction and relief of massive ascites by peritovenous shunting or paracentesis via Tenckhoff's catheter.[308]

Radiation

Despite its use in the few reported survivors in this disease, the role of radiation therapy remains unclear. Megavoltage external radiotherapy can deliver a homogeneous dose to the entire abdominal cavity and its contents, although critical organ tolerance limits dose in several areas. Several techniques have been described and used predominantly for the therapy of ovarian carcinoma.[309] The first report was the *moving strip* technique, which was necessary because of limited field size and dose rate with cobalt 60 units but that was shown to have a higher morbidity than the *open field* techniques.[310] The technique reported from the Joint Center for Radiation Therapy uses open fields with a 67% transmission block to attenuate the dose given to the abdomen superior to the L-5 to S-1 interspace.[311] The superior border of the field is placed above the maximum excursion of the diaphragm by 1 to 2 cm as observed by fluoroscopy. The inferior border is placed at the ischial tuberosities. Laterally, the field extends 1 to 2 cm beyond the properitoneal fat stripe. Daily fractions of 1.2 Gy in the upper abdomen and 1.8 Gy in the pelvis are given five times weekly to opposed anterior and posterior fields, with both fields treated daily. Doses are prescribed to midplane on the central axis. Total doses of 30 Gy in the upper abdomen and 45 Gy in the pelvis are given in 5 weeks. Full-thickness kidney blocks are added to both anterior and posterior fields at 18 Gy. When intraperitoneal chemotherapy is used, the transmission block is omitted and a uniform daily dose of 1.2 Gy is given to a total dose of 30 Gy. Blocks are also placed over a portion of the heart and the inferior pelvis lateral to the abdominal cavity to protect the femoral heads and soft tissue. Treatment breaks are given when the total leukocyte count drops to 1500 to 2000/μL or the platelet count drops below 75 to 100,000/μL.

Intraperitoneal instillation of radioactive colloidal gold (^{198}Au) was first reported to improve the symptoms of peritoneal mesothelioma in 1955.[312] Nine other patients treated by the administration of colloidal ^{198}Au have been reported.[183] Two of nine were free of disease for 3.5 and 5.0 years, respectively. Four other patients were reported to have clinical improvement of symptoms. The concentration of radiocolloid is generally greatest in the pelvis and lateral gutters, but adhesions from prior surgery and tumor can cause adherence of loops of bowel that may result in inhomogeneous spread of the radiocolloid.[182,313] Neither ^{198}Au nor ^{32}P give substantial dose to tumor cells within gross tumor masses. The estimated dose from 20 mCi of ^{32}P is 180 Gy at 0.04 mm, but only 43 Gy at 1 mm and 17 Gy at 2 mm.[314] The distribution of a radiotracer or contrast material should be tested before the therapeutic administration of these agents. The major complication associated with intraperitoneal instillation of radiocolloids is small bowel obstruction, which occurs in 2% to 10% of patients.[315,316] When external-beam irradiation is also given to the pelvis, as many as 33% of patients may develop bowel complications.[311,317]

Intraperitoneal Chemotherapy

Because the results of intravenous chemotherapy in patients with malignant mesothelioma have been disappointing, and given the tendency of the disease to remain confined to the peritoneum, interest has focused on the use of intraperitoneal chemotherapy. The primary theoretical obstacle to this form of treatment is the shallow depth of drug penetration into tumor nodules. Advantages include greatly enhanced drug concentrations in the peritoneal cavity and decreased systemic toxicity. In addition, substantial intravenous drug concentrations are obtained from peritoneal absorption of some drugs such as cisplatin. Thus, the combination of free surface diffusion and intracapillary drug flow may be potentially more efficacious than intravenous treatment alone.

Intraperitoneal cisplatin and intravenous thiosulfate protection have resulted in a 59% complete response rate. However, many patients in this study have relapsed quickly after treatment, implying incomplete eradication of tumor using cisplatin alone.[318] Mitomycin C, doxorubicin, and epidoxorubicin have also been used intraperitoneally.[290,319,320]

Intraperitoneal cisplatin in 19 patients (with mitomycin in as well in 18) resulted in 2 (10%) disease free more than 5 years from therapy.[321] Cisplatin and etoposide resulted in one complete response in five patients with measurable disease.[322]

Of four patients receiving cisplatin-based intraperitoneal therapy in a Dutch study, two responded, one completely. At 2 years he developed intestinal obstruction. Laparotomy revealed only adhesions.[323] A case report noted continuing complete response at 53 months in a patient treated with intraperitoneal cisplatin and cytarabine.[324]

Combined Modality Approaches

Because surgery or radiotherapy alone has resulted in only a few anecdotal long-term mesothelioma survivors, intensive combined modality approaches are being studied at several institutions. One of four patients treated at Seattle with surgery, radiotherapy, and chemotherapy had no tumor by follow-up CT scan at the time of publication.[325]

In a retrospective review of 15 women with peritoneal mesothelioma, clinical features included abdominal or pelvic masses in 93%, abdominal distention in 73%, ascites in 60%, abdominal pain in 40%, thrombocytosis in 27%, thromboembolic manifestations in 20%, and elevated CA-125 in four of four. The response rate to first-line chemotherapy regimens was 30% overall, but 67% to paclitaxel and cisplatin. The median survival of all patients was 12 months. The median survival was longer for patients who underwent cytoreductive surgery versus biopsy only (14 vs. 6 months, $P = .24$), and chemotherapy versus none (29 vs. 1 month, $P = .03$).[326]

In three sequential studies by Antman and colleagues of patients with peritoneal mesothelioma treated with surgery, radiotherapy, and chemotherapy, one of three patients treated in the first trial with surgery, whole abdominal radiotherapy, and cyclophosphamide, doxorubicin, and dacarbazine remains alive more than 15 years from diagnosis.[290] Of seven patients treated on a second phase I trial between 1982 and 1985 with debulking of all lesions greater than 1 cm, and intraperitoneal doxorubicin (20 to 50 mg) alternating every 2 weeks with intraperitoneal cisplatin (20 to 100 mg/m^2) for a total of 8 to 12 treatments. At the time of second laparotomy for removal of the access device, all six patients had at least an objective 50% decrease in the size of the tumor. Chemotherapy was followed by whole abdominal irradiation in four patients. (One patient refused and a second had had prior irradiation for Hodgkin's disease.) Four of the six patients (including three of the four who received irradiation) remain disease free more than 14 years after diagnosis.[290,297] One patient requires chronic intravenous hyperalimentation due to malabsorption; the remaining three patients have normal performance status. In the third (phase II) trial begun in 1986,[297] 20 patients have completed debulking, intraperitoneal doxorubicin, and cisplatin and radiation as above. The median survival for the entire treated group is 16.4 months. Thus, intensive multimodality therapy produces a high response rate and may ultimately prolong survival for this otherwise rapidly fatal disease.

Of 18 patients with primary peritoneal mesothelioma who underwent tumor debulking followed by a 90-minute continuous hyperthermic peritoneal profusion with cisplatin as part of three consecutive phase I trials conducted at the National Cancer Institute, 13 had associated ascites. One patient had a symptomatic, multiply recurrent, benign, cystic peritoneal mesothelioma. Three patients who had a recurrence after a progression-free interval of more than 6 months after continuous hyperthermic peritoneal profusion underwent reperfusion. Two patients had superficial wound infections, and one patient each had atrial fibrillation, pancreatitis, fascial dehiscence, ileus, line sepsis, and *Clostridium difficile* colitis, but no toxic deaths occurred. Renal toxicity occurred at cisplatin doses above the recommended phase II dose. Nine of ten patients had resolution of their ascites postoperatively. Three patients with recurrent ascites at 10, 22, and 27 months after initial treatment had resolution of their ascites with ongoing responses at 4, 6, and 24 months after the second perfusion. The median progression-free survival is 26 months, and the overall 2-year survival is 80%.[327]

MALIGNANT MESOTHELIOMA OF THE TUNICA VAGINALIS TESTIS

Approximately 75 cases have been reported in the literature,[328] most often in patients between ages 55 and 75 years, although approximately 10% of the patients were younger than 25 years and occasional children are affected.[329]

Asbestos exposure was documented in approximately one-half of the more recently reported cases.[330]

Patients generally present with a hydrocele or *hernia.* An accurate preoperative diagnosis was reported in only two cases.[331] Diffuse peritoneal or abdominal lymph node involvement may be present at the time of diagnosis.

Mesotheliomas arising in the tunica vaginalis testes appear to have a more indolent disease course.[330,332] The overall recurrence rate (local and disseminated) was 52%, and 38% died of disease progression.[328] Local recurrence occurred in 36% of patients who underwent local resection of the hydrocele wall, 10% after scrotal orchiectomy, and 12% after inguinal orchiectomy.[328] More than 60% of recurrences developed within the first 2 years of the follow-up. The median survival of the patients was 23 months, but was 14 months after recurrence.

In some cases of disseminated mesothelioma, adjuvant chemotherapy or radiotherapy was given. Survival correlated significantly with younger patient's age ($P = .01$), and with localized as opposed to disseminated disease ($P = .05$) in univariate analysis. A multivariate Cox regression model of prognostic parameters concerning survival did not yield statistically significant results.[328]

MALIGNANT MESOTHELIOMA OF THE PERICARDIUM

There are approximately just over 100 cases reported in the literature in adults[333] and children.[334] Asbestos exposure has not been documented in most reported cases. Patients generally present with a pericardial effusion,[333,334] congestive heart failure,[335] an anterior mediastinal mass,[336] or tamponade.[337] Diffuse pericardial involvement is found at surgery. The diagnosis is often unsuspected before surgery or autopsy.

BENIGN MESOTHELIOMA

Benign tumors involving mesothelium arise with some frequency in the pleura and peritoneum, the tunica vaginalis testis,[338] the atrioventricular node of the heart,[339] and rarely in the mediastinum,[340] liver,[341] and adrenal.[342] Those of peritoneum, including tunica vaginalis testis and adrenal, are mesothelial derived, but the others are of disputed histogenesis (atrioventricular node) or appear to arise from submesothelial mesenchymal cells that do not exhibit mesothelial differentiation.

BENIGN FIBROUS TUMORS OF THE PLEURA

Benign fibrous tumors of the pleura are approximately one-third as common as diffuse malignant mesotheliomas[343] and are most common from age 40 to 70 years. Because they appear to arise from subsurface fibrous tissue, rather than from the mesothelial lining, they have also been called submesothelial fibromas, localized fibrous mesothelioma, or solitary fibrous tumor of the pleura.[343–345] Few patients have been exposed to asbestos, approximating the incidence of exposure in the general population. CT scan and MRI are useful but nonspecific. The differential diagnosis between benign and malignant lesions is based on histologic study.[346] Lesions have ranged in size from 1 to 36 cm. Associated effusions can be serosanguineous. Hypertrophic pulmonary osteoarthropathy has occurred in approximately one-third of patients, particularly associated with lesions more than 10 cm in size. Hypoglycemia has also been associated with large lesions, associated in some cases with tumor production of insulin-like growth factor.[347,348]

Mesotheliomas are often pedunculated and 80% arise from but usually do not invade the visceral pleura.[120] Thus, benign pleural mesotheliomas usually have a sharp separation between tumor and compressed lung, and resection can be performed without pulmonary resection. Others may require a limited chest wall resection. While generally cured if completely resected, recurrences have occurred after several decades[349] and 12% of patients eventually die of extensive local tumor.[343] Localized *malignant* fibrous tumors of the pleura have also been described. Of 82 malignant localized tumors, 45% were cured by simple excision.[120] If the nature of the lesion is ambiguous, involvement of the pleura on random biopsy would establish a diagnosis of diffuse (i.e., malignant) disease.

BENIGN FIBROUS MESOTHELIOMAS OF THE GENITAL TRACTS

Called *benign mesotheliomas* in the past, these neoplasms are probably more accurately designated *adenomatoid tumors*.[350,351] They generally arise in the scrotum and epididymis. Similar tumors histologically also are occasionally described in women. Talc granulomas have been described in proximity to the tumor in one case.[352]

BENIGN MESOTHELIOMA OF THE CARDIAC ATRIOVENTRICULAR NODE

The histologic origin of benign mesotheliomas of the atrioventricular node is disputed.[353] Patients with benign mesotheliomas of the atrioventricular node have ranged in age from newborn[354] to elderly, and present most frequently with heart block.[355] The diagnosis is often made at autopsy,[356] although clinical excision has been reported.[357] Sudden death has sometimes occurred despite the implantation of a pacemaker.

REFERENCES

1. Lee DHK, Selikoff IJ. Historical background to the asbestos problem. *Environ Res* 1979;18:300.
2. Women Inspectors of Factories. *Annual report for 1898.* Her Majesty's Stationery Office, London, 1899.
3. Merewether ERA, Price CV. *Report on effects of asbestos dust in the lungs and dust suppression in the asbestos industry.* Her Majesty's Stationery Office, London, 1930.
4. Lynch KM, Smith WA. Pulmonary asbestosis III: carcinoma of lung in asbestosilicosis. *Am J Cancer* 1935;14:56.
5. Gloyne SR. Two cases of squamous carcinoma of the lung occurring in asbestosis. *Tubercle* 1935;17:5.
6. Doll R. Morality from lung cancer in asbestos workers. *BJM* 1955;12:81.
7. Enterline PE. Changing attitudes and opinions regarding asbestos and cancer 1934–1965 [see comments]. *Ind Med* 1992;22:2591; comment in *Am J Ind Med* 1991;20:685.
8. Mossman BT, Bignon J, Corn M, et al. Asbestos: scientific developments and implications for public policy. *Science* 1990;247:294.
9. Anderson HA, Hanrahan LP, Schirmer J, et al. Mesothelioma among employees with likely contact with in-place asbestos-containing building materials. *Ann NY Acad Sci* 1991;643:550.
10. Robertson HE. Endothelioma of the pleura. *Cancer Res* 1924;8:317.
11. Wagner JC, Sleggs EA, Marchand P. Diffuse pleural mesothelioma and asbestos in the North Western Cape Province. *Br J Ind Med* 1960;17:260.
12. Timbrell V. Physical factors as etiological mechanisms, in biological effects of asbestos. *Int Agency Res Cancer (Lyon)* 1973.
13. Miller BG, Searl A, Davis JM, et al. Influence of fibre length, dissolution and biopersistence on the production of mesothelioma in the rat peritoneal cavity. *Ann Occup Hyg* 1999;43:155.
14. Stanton MF, Layard M, Tegeris A, et al. Carcinogenicity of fibrous glass: pleural response in relation to fiber dimension. *J Natl Cancer Inst* 1977;58:589.
15. Gibbs AR, Griffiths DM, Pooley FD, Jones JS. Comparison of fibre types and size distributions in lung tissues of paraoccupational and occupational cases of malignant mesothelioma. *Br J Ind Med* 1990;47:621.
16. Rogers AJ, Leigh J, Berry G, et al. Relationship between lung asbestos fiber type and concentration and relative risk of mesothelioma. A case-control study. *Cancer* 1991;67:1912.
17. Lee KP, Barras CE, Griffith FD, Waritz RD. Pulmonary response and transmigration of inorganic fibers by inhalation exposure. *Am J Pathol* 1981;102:314.
18. Kayser K, Becker C, Seeberg N, Gabius HJ. Quantitation of asbestos and asbestos-like fibers in human lung tissue by hot and wet ashing, and the significance of their presence for survival of lung carcinoma and mesothelioma patients. *Lung Cancer* 1999;24:89.
19. Dodson RF, O'Sullivan M, Corn CJ, et al. Analysis of asbestos fiber burden in lung tissue from mesothelioma patients. *Ultrastruct Pathol* 1997;21:321.
20. Rom WN, Travis WD, Brody AR. Cellular and molecular basis of the asbestos-related diseases. *Am Rev Respir Dis* 1991;143:408.
21. Dazzi H, Hasleton PS, Thatcher N, et al. Malignant pleural mesothelioma and epidermal growth factor receptor (EGF-R). Relationship of EGF-R with histology and survival using fixed paraffin embedded tissue and the F4, monoclonal antibody. *Br J Cancer* 1990;61:924.
22. Hei TK, Piao CQ, He ZY, et al. Chrysotile fiber is a strong mutagen in mammalian cells. *Cancer Res* 1992;52:6305.
23. Heintz NH, Janssen YM, Mossman BT. Persistent induction of c-fox and c-jun expression by asbestos. *Proc Natl Acad Sci U S A* 1993;90:3299.
24. Suzuki K, Hei TK. Induction of heme oxygenase (HO) in mammalian cells by mineral fibers: distinctive effect of reactive oxygen species. *Carcinogenesis* 1996;17:661.
25. McDonald AD, McDonald JC. Epidemiology of malignant mesothelioma. In: K Antman, Aisner J, ed. *Asbestos-related malignancy.* Orlando, FL: Grune & Stratton, 1987:31.
26. Connelly RR, Spirtas R, Myers MH, et al. Demographic patterns for mesothelioma in the United States. *J Natl Cancer Inst* 1987;78:1053.

27. Walker AM, Loughlin JE, Freidlander ER, et al. Projections of asbestos-related disease 1980–2009. *J Occup Med* 1983;25:409.
28. Berry M. Mesothelioma incidence and community asbestos exposure. *Environ Res* 1997;75:34.
29. Hansen J, de Klerk NH, Musk AW, Hobbs MS. Environmental exposure to crocidolite and mesothelioma: exposure-response relationships. *Am J Respir Crit Care Med* 1998;157:69.
30. Howel D, Arblaster L, Swinburne L, et al. Routes of asbestos exposure and the development of mesothelioma in an English region. *Occup Environ Med* 1997;54:403.
31. Rees D, Goodman K, Fourie E, et al. Asbestos exposure and mesothelioma in South Africa. *S Afr Med J* 1999;89:627.
32. Price B. Analysis of current trends in United States mesothelioma incidence. *Am J Epidemiol* 1997;145:211.
33. Burdorf A, Barendregt JJ, Swuste PH, Heederik D . [Future increase of the incidence of mesothelioma due to occupational exposure to asbestos in the past (see comments)]. *Ned Tijdschr Geneeskd* 1997;141:1093.
34. Peto J, Decarli A, La Vecchia C, et al. The European mesothelioma epidemic. *Br J Cancer* 1999;79:666.
35. Selikoff IJ, Hammond EC, Seidman H. Latency of asbestos disease among insulation workers in the United States and Canada. *Cancer* 1980;46:2736.
36. Wagner JC, Berry G, Polley FD. Mesotheliomas and asbestos type in asbestos textile workers: a study of lung contents. *BMJ* 1982;285:603.
37. Jarvholm B, Sanden A. Lung cancer and mesothelioma in the pleura and peritoneum among Swedish insulation workers. *Occup Environ Med* 1998;55:766.
38. Selikoff IJ, Churg J, Hammond EC. Asbestos exposure and neoplasia. *JAMA* 1964;188:22.
39. Churg A. Fiber counting and analysis in the diagnosis of asbestos-related disease. *Hum Pathol* 1982;13:381.
40. Risberg B, Nickels J, Wagermark J. Familial clustering of malignant mesothelioma. *Cancer* 1980;45:2422.
41. Vianna NJ, Polan AK. Non-occupational exposure to asbestos and malignant mesothelioma in females. *Lancet* 1978;i:1061.
42. Roggli VL, Oury TD, Moffatt EJ. Malignant mesothelioma in women. *Anat Pathol* 1997;2:147.
43. Metintas M, Ozdemir N, Hillerdal G, et al. Environmental asbestos exposure and malignant pleural mesothelioma. *Respir Med* 1999;93:349.
44. Gardner MJ, Saracci R. Effects on health of non-occupational exposure to airborne mineral fibres. *IARC Sci Publ* 1989;90:375.
45. Metintas M, Hillerdal G, Metintas S. Malignant mesothelioma due to environmental exposure to erionite: follow-up of a Turkish emigrant cohort. *Eur Respir J* 1999;13:523.
46. Ascoli V, Nardi F, Carnovale Scalzo C, et al. Absence of HHV-8 DNA sequences in malignant mesothelioma. *Mol Pathol* 1998;51:113.
47. Gibbs AR, Jones JS, Pooley FD, et al. Non-occupational malignant mesotheliomas. *IARC Sci Publ* 1989;90:219.
48. Gentiloni N, Febbraro S, Barone C, et al. Peritoneal mesothelioma in recurrent familial peritonitis. *J Clin Gastroenterol* 1997;24:276.
49. Antman KH, Corson JM, Li FP, et al. Malignant mesothelioma following radiation exposure. *J Clin Oncol* 1983;1:695.
50. Hofmann J, Mintzer D, Warhol MJ. Malignant mesothelioma following radiation therapy. *Am J Med* 1994;97:379.
51. Weissman LB, Corson JM, Neugut AI, Antman KH. Malignant mesothelioma following treatment for Hodgkin's disease. *J Clin Oncol* 1996;14:2098.
52. Burmer GC, Rabinovitch PS, Kulander BG, et al. Flow cytometric analysis of malignant pleural mesotheliomas. *Hum Pathol* 1989;20:777.
53. Dazzi H, Thatcher N, Hasleton PS, et al. DNA analysis by flow cytometry in malignant pleural mesothelioma: relationship to histology and survival. *J Pathol* 1990;162:51.
54. Pyrhonen S, Laasonen A, Tammilehto L, et al. Diploid predominance and prognostic significance of S-phase cells in malignant mesothelioma. *Eur J Cancer* 1991;27:197.
55. Hillerdal G, Lindqvist U, Engstrom AL. Hyaluronan in pleural effusions and in serum. *Cancer* 1991;67:2410.
56. Atagi S, Ogawara M, Kawahara M, et al. Utility of hyaluronic acid in pleural fluid for differential diagnosis of pleural effusions: likelihood ratios for malignant mesothelioma. *Jpn J Clin Oncol* 1997;27:293.
57. Demetri GD, Zenzie BW, Rheinwald JG, Griffin JD. Expression of colony-stimulating factor genes by normal human mesothelial cells and human malignant mesothelioma cell lines in vitro. *Blood* 1989;74:940.
58. Nakamura Y, Ozaki T, Yanagawa H, et al. Eosinophil colony-stimulating factor induced by administration of interleukin-2 into the pleural cavity of patients with malignant pleurisy. *Am J Respir Cell Mol Biol* 1990;3:291.
59. Okazaki H, Kano S, Hatake K, et al. [A case of malignant pleural mesothelioma producing colony-stimulating factor (CSF)]. *Nippon Naika Gakkai Zasshi* 1989;78:506.
60. Jordon D, Jagirdar J, Kaneko M. Blood group antigens, Lewisx and Lewisy in the diagnostic discrimination of malignant mesothelioma versus adenocarcinoma. *Am J Pathol* 1989;135:931.
61. Kawai T, Suzuki M, Torikata C, Suzuki Y. Expression of blood group-related antigens and Helix pomatia agglutinin in malignant pleural mesothelioma and pulmonary adenocarcinoma. *Hum Pathol* 1991;22:118.
62. Nakano T, Chahinian AP, Shinjo M, et al. Interleukin 6 and its relationship to clinical parameters in patients with malignant pleural mesothelioma. *Br J Cancer* 1998;77:907.
63. Kannerstein M, Churg J. A critique of the criteria for the diagnosis of diffuse malignant mesothelioma. *Mt Sinai J Med* 1977;44:485.
64. Nash G, Otis CN. Protocol for the examination of specimens from patients with malignant pleural mesothelioma: a basis for checklists. Cancer Committee, College of American Pathologists. *Arch Pathol Lab Med* 1999;123:39.
65. Harwood TR, Grecey DR, Yokoo H. Pseudomesotheliomatous carcinoma of the lung. A variant of peripheral lung carcinoma. *Am J Clin Pathol* 1976; 65:159.
66. Kannerstein M, Churg C, McCaughery WTE. Asbestos and mesothelioma: a review. *Pathol Annu* 1978;13:81.
67. Kho-Duffin J, Tao LC, Cramer H, et al. Cytologic diagnosis of malignant mesothelioma, with particular emphasis on the epithelial noncohesive cell type. *Diagn Cytopathol* 1999;20:57.
68. Renshaw AA, Dean BR, Antman KH, et al. The role of cytologic evaluation of pleural fluid in the diagnosis of malignant mesothelioma. *Chest* 1997;111:106.
69. Yu GH, Baloch ZW, Gupta PK. Cytomorphology of metastatic mesothelioma in fine-needle aspiration specimens. *Diagn Cytopathol* 1999;20:328.
70. Elmes PC, Simpson M. The clinical aspects of mesothelioma. *Q J Med* 1976;45:427.
71. Winslow DJ, Taylor HB. Malignant peritoneal mesotheliomas. *Cancer* 1960;13:127.
72. Corson J, Pinkus G. Cellular localization patterns of keratin proteins in pleural mesothelioma and metastatic adenocarcinomas: a diagnostic discriminant. *Lab Invest* 1991;64:114A.
73. Suzuki Y, Churg C, Kannerstein M. Ultrastructure of human malignant diffuse mesothelioma. *Am J Pathol* 1976; 85:241.
74. Corson JM, Pinkus GSS. Mesothelioma: profile of keratin proteins and carcinoembryonic antigen; an immunoperoxidase study of 20 cases and comparison with pulmonary adenocarcinomas. *Am J Pathol* 1982;108:80.
75. Said J, Nash G, Lee M. Immunoperoxidase localization of keratin, proteins, carcinoembryonic antigen, and factor VIII in adenomatoid tumors: evidence for a mesothelial derivation. *Hum Pathol* 1982;13:1106.
76. Dejmek A, Hjerpe A. Immunohistochemical reactivity in mesothelioma and adenocarcinoma: a stepwise logistic regression analysis. *APMIS* 1994;102:255.
77. Dejmek A, Hjerpe A. Carcinoembryonic antigen-like reactivity in malignant mesothelioma. A comparison between different commercially available antibodies. *Cancer* 1994;73:464.
78. Bolen JW, Thorning D. Mesotheliomas: a light and electron microscopical study concerning the histogenic relationships between the epithelial and the mesenchymal variants. *Am J Surg Pathol* 1980;4:451.
79. Warhol WJ, Hickey WF, Corson J. Malignant mesothelioma: ultrastructural distinction from adenocarcinoma. *Am J Surg Pathol* 1982;6:307.
80. Warhol MJ, Hunter NJ, Corson JM. An ultrastructural comparison of mesotheliomas and adenocarcinomas of the ovary and endometrium. *Int J Gynecol Pathol* 1982;1:125.
81. Schouwink H, Korse CM, Bonfrer JM, et al. Prognostic value of the serum tumour markers Cyfra 21-1 and tissue polypeptide antigen in malignant mesothelioma. *Lung Cancer* 1999,25.25.
82. Kumar-Singh S, Vermeulen PB, Weyler J, et al. Evaluation of tumour angiogenesis as a prognostic marker in malignant mesothelioma. *J Pathol* 1997;182:211.
83. Bianchi C, Giarelli L, Grandi G, et al. Latency periods in asbestos-related mesothelioma of the pleura. *Eur J Cancer Prev* 1997;6:162.
84. Antman K, Blum R, Greenberger J, et al. Multimodality therapy for mesothelioma based on a study of natural history. *Am J Med* 1980;68:356.
85. Cooper SP, Fraire AE, Buffler PA, et al. Epidemiologic aspects of childhood mesothelioma. *Pathol Immunopathol Res* 1989;8:276.
86. Geary WA, Mills SE, Frierson HJ, Pope TL. Malignant peritoneal mesothelioma in childhood with long-term survival. *Am J Clin Pathol* 1991;95:493.
87. Lin CM, Lee Y, Ho MY. Malignant mesothelioma in infancy. *Arch Pathol Lab Med* 1989;113:409.
88. Tewari SC, Kurian G, Jayaswal R, et al. Malignant mesothelioma in the young (with prosthetic aortic valve an unusual association). *J Assoc Physicians India* 1989;37:187.
89. Sheard JD, Taylor W, Soorae A, Pearson MG. Pneumothorax and malignant mesothelioma in patients over the age of 40. *Thorax* 1991;46:584.
90. Rusch VW. A proposed new international TNM staging system for malignant pleural mesothelioma. *Chest* 1995;108:1122.
91. Rusch VW, Venkatraman E. The importance of surgical staging in the treatment of malignant pleural mesothelioma. *J Thorac Cardiovasc Surg* 1996;111:815; discussion, 825.
92. Pass HI, Temeck BK, Kranda K, et al. Preoperative tumor volume is associated with outcome in malignant pleural mesothelioma. *J Thorac Cardiovasc Surg* 1998;115:310; discussion, 317.
93. Sugarbaker DJ, Flores RM, Jaklitsch MT, et al. Resection margins, extrapleural nodal status, and cell type determine postoperative long-term survival in trimodality therapy of malignant pleural mesothelioma: results in 183 patients. *J Thorac Cardiovasc Surg* 1999;117:54; discussion, 63.
94. Conlon KC, Rusch VW, Gillern S. Laparoscopy: an important tool in the staging of malignant pleural mesothelioma. *Ann Surg Oncol* 1996;3:489.
95. Butchart EG, Ashcroft T, Barnsley WC, et al. Pleuropneumonectomy in the management of diffuse malignant mesothelioma of the pleura: experience with 29 patients. *Thorax* 1976;31:15.
96. Grant DC, Seltzer SE, Antman KH, et al. Computer tomography of malignant pleural mesothelioma. *J Comput Assist Tomogr* 1983;7:626.
97. Leung AN, Muller NL, Miller RR. CT in differential diagnosis of diffuse pleural disease. *Am J Roentgenol* 1990;154:487.
98. Knuuttila A, Halme M, Kivisaari L, et al. The clinical importance of magnetic resonance imaging versus computed tomography in malignant pleural mesothelioma. *Lung Cancer* 1998;22:215.
99. Benard F, Sterman D, Smith RJ, et al. Prognostic value of FDG PET imaging in malignant pleural mesothelioma. *J Nucl Med* 1999;40:1241.
100. Nakano T, Maeda J, Iwahashi N, et al. Gallium-67 scanning in patients with malignant pleural mesothelioma. *Jpn J Med* 1990;29:255.
101. Yoshida S, Fukumoto M, Motohara T, et al. Ga-67 tumor scan in malignant diffuse mesothelioma—comparison with CT and pathological findings. *Ann Nucl Med* 1999;13:49.

102. Watanabe N, Shimizu M, Kameda K, et al. Thallium-201 scintigraphy in malignant mesothelioma. *Br J Radiol* 1999;72:308.
103. McDonald AD, Magner D, Eyssen G. Primary malignant mesothelial tumors in Canada, 1960–1968. *Cancer* 1973;31:869.
104. Pluygers E, Badewyns P, Minette P, et al. Biomarker assessments in asbestos-exposed workers as indicators for selective prevention of mesothelioma or bronchogenic carcinoma: rationale and practical implications. *Eur J Cancer Prev* 1992;1:129.
105. Collins CL, Ordonez NG, Schaefer R, et al. Thrombomodulin expression in malignant pleural mesothelioma and pulmonary adenocarcinoma. *Am J Pathol* 1991;141:827.
106. Boutin C, Rey F. Thoracoscopy in pleural malignant mesothelioma: a prospective study of 188 consecutive patients. *Cancer* 1993;72:389.
107. van Ooijen B, Eggermont AM, Wiggers T. Subcutaneous tumor growth complicating the positioning of Denver shunt and intrapleural port-a-cath in mesothelioma patients. *Eur J Surg Oncol* 1992;18:638.
108. DaValle MJ, Faber LP, Kittle CF. Extrapleural pneumonectomy for diffuse, malignant mesothelioma. *Ann Thorac Surg* 1986;42:612.
109. Martini N, McCormach PM, Baines MS, et al. Pleural mesothelioma. *Ann Thorac Surg* 1987;43:113.
110. Gordon W, Antman K, Breenberger J, et al. Radiation therapy in the management of patients with mesothelioma. *Int J Radiat Oncol Biol Phys* 1982;8:19.
111. Antman KH. Malignant mesothelioma. *N Engl J Med* 1980;303:200.
112. Wojtukiewicz MZ, Zacharski RL, Memoli VA, et al. Absence of components of coagulation and fibrinolysis pathways in situ in mesothelioma. *Thromb Res* 1989;55:279.
113. De Pangher, Manzini V, Brollo A, Bianchi C. Thrombocytosis in malignant pleural mesothelioma. *Tumori* 1990;76:576.
114. Antman K, Pomfret E, Aisner J, et al. Peritoneal mesothelioma: natural history and response to chemotherapy. *J Clin Oncol* 1983;1:386.
115. McAuley P, Asa SL, Chiu B, et al. Parathyroid hormone-like peptide in normal and neoplastic mesothelial cells. *Cancer* 1990;66:1975.
116. Antman K, Shemin R, Ryan L, et al. Malignant mesothelioma: prognostic variables in a registry of 180 patients, the Dana-Farber Cancer Institute and Brigham and Women's Hospital experience over two decades:1965–1985. *J Clin Oncol* 1988;6:147.
117. Curran D, Sahmoud T, Therasse P, et al. Prognostic factors in patients with pleural mesothelioma: the European Organization for Research and Treatment of Cancer experience. *J Clin Oncol* 1998;16:145.
118. Herndon JE, Green MR, Chahinian AP, et al. Factors predictive of survival among 337 patients with mesothelioma treated between 1984 and 1994 by the Cancer and Leukemia Group B. *Chest* 1998;113:723.
119. Ruffie P, Feld R, Minkin S, et al. Diffuse malignant mesothelioma of the pleura in Ontario and Quebec: a retrospective study of 332 patients. *J Clin Oncol* 1989;7:1157.
120. England DM, Hochholzer L, McCarthy MJ. Localized benign and malignant fibrous tumors of the pleura. A clinicopathologic review of 223 cases. *Am J Surg Pathol* 1989;13:640.
121. Boutin C, Schlesser M, Frenay C, Astoul P. Malignant pleural mesothelioma. *Eur Respir J* 1998;12:972.
122. Eiselberg AV. Im protokoll der Gesellschaft der Artze in Wein. *Wein Klin Wochenschr* 1922;1922:509.
123. Viallat JR, Boutin C. [Malignant pleural effusions: recourse to early use of talc]. *Rev Med Interne* 1998;19:811.
124. Canto A, Guijarro R, Arnau A, et al. Videothoracoscopy in the diagnosis and treatment of malignant pleural mesothelioma with associated pleural effusions. *Thorac Cardiovasc Surg* 1997;45:16.
125. Charvat JC, Brutsche M, Frey JG, Tschopp M. [Value of thoracoscopy and talc pleurodesis in diagnosis and palliative treatment of malignant pleural mesothelioma]. *Schweiz Rundsch Med Prax* 1998;87:336.
126. Beattie JE. The treatment of malignant pleural effusions by partial pleurectomy. *Surg Clin North Am* 1963;43:99.
127. Jensik R, Cagle JE, Milloy F, et al. Pleurectomy in the treatment of pleural effusion due to metastatic malignancy. *J Thorac Cardiovasc Surg* 1963;46:322.
128. Pass HI, Kranda K, Temeck BK, et al. Surgically debulked malignant pleural mesothelioma: results and prognostic factors. *Ann Surg Oncol* 1997;4:215.
129. Law MR, Gregor A, Hodson ME, et al. Malignant mesothelioma of the pleura: a study of 52 treated and 64 untreated patients. *Thorax* 1984;39:255.
130. Brancatisano RR, Joseph MG, McCaughan BC. Pleurectomy for mesothelioma. *Med J Aust* 1991;154:455.
131. Brenner J, Sordillo PP, Magill GB, Golbey RB. Malignant mesothelioma of the pleura. *Cancer* 1982;49:2431.
132. Chahinian AP, Pajak T, Holland J, et al. Diffuse malignant mesothelioma: prospective evaluation of 69 patients. *Ann Intern Med* 1982;96:746.
133. Chailleux E, Dabouis G, Pioche D, et al. Prognostic factors in diffuse malignant pleural mesothelioma. *Chest* 1988;93:159.
134. Harvey JC, Fleischman EH, Kagan R, Streeter OE. Malignant pleural mesothelioma: a survival study. *J Surg Oncol* 1990;45:40.
135. Rusch VW, Piantadose S, Holmes EC. The role of extrapleural pneumonectomy in malignant pleural mesothelioma. A Lung Cancer Study Group trial. *J Thorac Cardiovasc Surg* 1991;102:1.
136. Faber LP. 1986: Extrapleural pneumonectomy for diffuse, malignant mesothelioma. Updated in 1994. *Ann Thorac Surg* 1994;58:1782.
137. Wörn HW. Moglichkeiten und Ergebnisse der chirurgischen Behandlung des malignen Pleuramesothelioms. *Thoraxchirurgie* 1974;22:339.
138. Bamler KJ, Maassen W. Malignant pleura mesotheliomas. *Thoraxchirurgie* 1974;22:386.
139. Probst G, Buelzebruck H, Bauer H, et al. The role of pleuropneumonectomy in the treatment of diffuse malignant mesothelioma of the pleura. In: Deslauriers J, Lacquet LK, ed. *Thoracic surgery: surgical management of pleural diseases.* St. Louis: Mosby, 1990:344.
140. Baldini EH, Recht A, Strauss GM, et al. Patterns of failure after trimodality therapy for malignant pleural mesothelioma. *Ann Thorac Surg* 1997;63:334.
141. Huncharek M, Kelsey K, Mark EJ, et al. Treatment and survival in diffuse malignant pleural mesothelioma; a study of 83 cases from the Massachusetts General Hospital. *Anticancer Res* 1996;16:1265.
142. Carmichael J, Degraff WG, Gamson J, et al. Radiation sensitivity of human lung cancer cell lines. *Eur J Cancer Clin Oncol* 1989;25:527.
143. Hakkinen AM, Laasonen A, Linnainmaa K, et al. Radiosensitivity of mesothelioma cell lines. *Acta Oncol* 1996;35:451.
144. Maasilta P. Deterioration in lung function following hemithorax irradiation for pleural mesothelioma. *Int J Radiat Oncol Biol Phys* 1991;20:433.
145. Ehrenhaft JL, Sensenig DM, Lawrence MS. Mesotheliomas of the pleura. *J Thorac Cardiovasc Surg* 1960;40:393.
146. Law MR, Hodson ME, Turner-Warurch M. Malignant mesothelioma of the pleura: clinical aspects and symptomatic treatment. *Eur J Respir Dis* 1984;65:162.
147. Eschwege F, Schlienger M. La Radiotherapie des mesotheliomes pleuraux malins: a propos de 14 cas irradies a dose elevees. *J Radiol Electrol* 1973;54:255.
148. Dobelbower RR, Strubler KA, Vaisman I. *Clinical applications of high energy electron beams: the pancreas, pleura, and spine.* Berlin: Springer-Verlag, 1980:91.
149. Bissett D, Macbeth FR, Cram I. The role of palliative radiotherapy in malignant mesothelioma. *Clin Oncol* 1991;3:315.
150. Davis SR, Tan L, Ball DL. Radiotherapy in the treatment of malignant mesothelioma of the pleura, with special reference to its use in palliation. *Aust Radiol* 1994;38:212.
151. de Graaf-Strukowska L, van der Zee J, van Putten W, Senan S. Factors influencing the outcome of radiotherapy in malignant mesothelioma of the pleura—a single-institution experience with 189 patients. *Int J Radiat Oncol Biol Phys* 1999;43:511.
152. Ball DL, Cruickshank DG. The treatment of malignant mesothelioma of the pleura: review of a 5-year experience, with special reference to radiotherapy. *Am J Clin Oncol* 1990;13:4.
153. Boutin C, Irrisson M, Rathelot P, Petite JM. L'extension parietale des mesotheliomas pleu raux malins diffus apres biopsies: prevention par radiotherapie locale. *Presse Med* 1983;12:1823.
154. Maasilta P, Kivisaari L, Holsti LR, et al. Radiographic chest assessment of lung injury following hemithorax irradiation for pleural mesothelioma. *Eur Respir J* 1991;4:76.
155. Maasilta P, Salonen EM, Vaheri A, et al. Procollagen-III in serum, plasminogen activation and fibronectin in bronchoalveolar lavage fluid during and following irradiation of human lung. *Int J Radiat Oncol Biol Phys* 1991;20:973.
156. Hallman M, Maasilta P, Kivisaari L, Mattson K. Changes in surfactant in bronchoalveolar lavage fluid after hemithorax irradiation in patients with mesothelioma. *Am Rev Respir Dis* 1990;141:998.
157. Richart R, Sherman CD. Prolonged survival in diffuse pleural mesothelioma treated with Au198. *Cancer* 1959;12:799.
158. Brady LW. Mesothelioma the role for radiation therapy. *Semin Oncol* 1981;8:329.
159. Rusch VW, Godwin JD, Shuman WP. The role of computed tomography scanning in the initial assessment and the follow-up of the malignant pleural mesothelioma. *J Thorac Cardiovasc Surg* 1988;96:171.
160. Shimojo M, Tsuda N, Kamihata H, et al. [Magnetic resonance imaging for cardiovascular masses]. *J Cardiol* 1989;19:583.
161. Soubra M, Dunscombe PB, Hodson DI, et al. Physical aspects of external beam radiotherapy for the treatment of malignant pleural mesothelioma. *Int J Radiat Oncol Biol Phys* 1990;18:1521.
162. Takahashi K, Purdy J, Liu YY. Work in progress: treatment planning system for conformation radiotherapy. *Radiology* 1983;147:567.
163. Blake PR, Catterall M, Emerson PA. Pleural mesothelioma treated by fast neutron therapy. *Thorax* 1985;40:72.
164. Bonadonna G, Beretta G, Tancini G, et al. Adriamycin studies at the Instituto Nazionale Tumori, Milan. *Cancer Chemother Rep III* 1975;6:231.
165. Gerner RE, Moore GE. Chemotherapy of malignant mesothelioma. *Oncology* 1974;30:152.
166. Harvey VJ, Slevin ML, Ponder BA, et al. Chemotherapy of diffuse malignant mesothelioma: phase II trials of single-agent 5-fluorouracil and adriamycin. *Cancer* 1984;54:961.
167. Antman KH, Pass HI, Schiff P. Benign and malignant mesothelioma. In: DeVita VT, Hellman S, Rosenberg SA, eds. *Cancer: principles and practice of oncology.* Philadelphia: Lippincott, 1997:1853.
168. Kaukel E, Koschel G, Gatzemeyer U, Salewski E. A phase II study of pirarubicin in malignant pleural mesothelioma. *Cancer* 1990;66:651.
169. Sridhar KS, Hussein AM, Feun LG, Zubrod CG. Activity of pirarubicin (4'-0-tetrahydropyranyladriamycin) in malignant mesothelioma. *Cancer* 1989;63:1084.
170. Koschel G, Calavrezos A, Kaukel E, et al. Phase III randomized comparison of pirarubicin vs. pirarubicin and cisplatin for treatment of pleural mesotheliomas. *Proc Eur Congress Contra Oncol* 1991;6:
171. Magri MD, Veronesi A, Foladore S, et al. Epirubicin in the treatment of malignant mesothelioma: a phase II cooperative study. The North-Eastern Italian Oncology Group—Mesothelioma Committee. *Tumori* 1991;77:49.
172. Mattson K, Giaccone G, Kirkpatrick A, et al. Epirubicin in malignant mesothelioma: a phase II study of the E.O.R.T.C. Lung Cancer Cooperative Group. *J Clin Oncol* 1992;10:824.
173. Colbert N, Izrael V, Vannetzel JM, et al. A prospective study of detorubicin in malignant mesothelioma. *Cancer* 1985;56:2170.
174. van Breukelen FJ, Mattson K, Giaccone G, et al. Mitoxantrone in malignant pleural mesothelioma: a study by the EORTC Lung Cancer Cooperative Group. *Eur J Cancer* 1991;27:1627.
175. Butt WO. Mesothelioma of the pleura. *J Can Assoc Radiol* 1962;13:40.

176. Yap BS, Benjamin RS, Burgess MA, et al. The value of Adriamycin in the treatment of diffuse malignant pleural mesothelioma. *Cancer* 1978;42:1692.
177. Zidar BL, Metch B, Balcerzak SP, et al. A phase II evaluation of ifosfamide and mesna in unresectable diffuse malignant mesothelioma: a South West Oncology Group study. *Cancer* 1992;70:2547.
178. Alberts AS, Falkson G, Van ZL. Ifosfamide and mesna with doxorubicin have activity in malignant mesothelioma [letter; comment]. *Eur J Cancer* 1990;26:1002.
179. Falkson G, Hunt M, Borden EC, et al. An extended phase II trial of ifosfamide plus mesna in malignant mesothelioma. *Invest New Drugs* 1992;10:337.
180. Andersen MK, Krarup-Hansen A, Martensson G, et al. Ifosfamide in malignant mesothelioma: a phase II study. *Lung Cancer* 1999;24:39.
181. Jara F, Takita H, Rao UN. Malignant mesothelioma: clinicopathologic observation. *NY State J Med* 1977;77:1885.
182. Kaplan WD, Zimmerman RE, Bloomer WD, Knapp RC. Therapeutic intraperitoneal 32P: a clinical assessment of the dynamics of distribution. *Radiology* 1981;138:683.
183. Legha SS, Muggia FM. Pleural mesothelioma: clinical features and therapeutic implications. *Ann Intern Med* 1977;87:613.
184. McGowan L, Bunnag B, Arias LF. Mesothelioma of the abdomen in women; monitoring of therapy by peritoneal fluid study. *Gynecol Oncol* 1975;3:10.
185. Falkson G, DeVilliers PC, Falkson HC. (N-isopropyl-L-2-methylhydrazino)-p-toluamide hydrochloride (NSC 77213) for the treatment of cancer patients. *Cancer Chemother Rep* 1965;46:7.
186. Kelsen D, Bajorin D, Mintzer D. Phase II trial of mitomycin C in malignant mesothelioma. *Am Soc Clin Oncol* 1985; 4:146(abst).
187. Dabouis G, LeMevel B, Corroller J. Treatment of diffuse pleural malignant mesothelioma by cis dichloro diammine platinum in nine patients. *Cancer Chemother Pharmacol* 1981;5:209.
188. Daboys G, Delajartre MB, LeMevel BP. Treatment of diffuse pleural malignant mesothelioma by cis-diaminedichloroplatinum: preliminary results in eleven patients. *Med Oncol Soc* 1979;52:98.
189. Glatstein E, Fuks Z, Bagshaw M. Diaphragmatic treatment in ovarian carcinoma: a new radiotherapeutic technique. *Int J Radiat Oncol Biol Phys* 1977;2:357.
190. Hayes DM, Cvitkovic E, Golbey RB, et al. High dose cisplatinum diaminedichloride. *Cancer* 1977;39:1372.
191. Mintzer D, Kelson D, Frimmer D, et al. Phase II trial of high dose cisplatin in patients with malignant mesothelioma. *Proc Am Soc Clin Oncol* 1984;3:258.
192. Rossoff AH, Slayton RE, Perlia CP. Preliminary clinical experience with cisdiamine dichloroplatinum (II) (NSC 119875 CACO). *Cancer* 1972;30:1451.
193. Samson MK, Baker LH, Benjamin RS, et al. Cis dichlorodiammineplatinum (III in advanced soft tissue and bony sarcomas: a South West Oncology Group study. *Cancer Treat Rep* 1979;63:11.
194. Planting AS, Schellens JH, Goey SH, et al. Weekly high-dose cisplatin in malignant pleural mesothelioma. *Ann Oncol* 1994;5:373.
195. Raghavan D, Gianoutsos P, Bishop J, et al. Phase II trial of carboplatin in the management of malignant mesothelioma. *J Clin Oncol* 1990;8:151.
196. Vogelzang NJ, Goutsou M, Corson JM, et al. Carboplatin in malignant mesothelioma: a phase II study of the Cancer and Leukemia Group B. *Cancer Chemother Pharmacol* 1990;27:239.
197. Mbidde EK, Harland SJ, Calvert AH, Smith IE. Phase II trial of carboplatin (JM8) in treatment of patients with malignant mesothelioma. *Cancer Chemother Pharmacol* 1986;18:284.
198. Cantwell BMJ, Harris AL, Ghani S. Phase II studies of a novel antifolate CB3717, and the platinum analogues JM8 and JM9, in mesothelioma of pleura and peritoneum. *Cancer Treat Rep* 1986;70:1335.
199. Cantwell BMJ, Franks CR, Harris AL. A phase II study of the platinum analogues JM8 and JM9. *Cancer Chemother Pharmacol* 1986;18:286.
200. Rebattu P, Riou R, Pacheco Y, et al. Phase II study of very high dose cisplatin in the treatment of malignant mesothelioma. *Proc. 1st International Mesothelioma Conference*, Paris: 1991:36.
201. Martensson G, Sorenson S. A phase II study of vincristine in malignant mesothelioma—a negative report. *Cancer Chemother Pharmacol* 1989;24:133.
202. Falkson G, Falkson H. Clinical trial of the oral form 4'-dimethylepipodophyllotoxin-p-D ethylidene glucoside and VP-16. *Am Assoc Cancer Res* 1978;1:160.
203. Nissen NI, Larsen V, Pederson H, et al. Phase I clinical trial of a new antitumor agent, 4'dimethylepipodophyllotoxin-9-(4,6-O-ethylidene-beta-D-glucopyranoside) (NSC 141540). *Cancer Chemother Rep* 1972;56:769.
204. Nissen NI, Dombernowsky P, Hansen HH, et al. Phase I clinical trial of an oral solution of VP16-213. *Cancer Treat Rep* 1976;60:943.
205. Smit EF, Berendsen HH, Postmus PE. Etoposide and mesothelioma [letter]. *J Clin Oncol* 1990;8:1281.
206. Sahmoud T, Postmus PE, van Pottelsberghe C, et al. Etoposide in malignant pleural mesothelioma: two phase II trials of the EORTC Lung Cancer Cooperative Group. *Eur J Cancer* 1997;33:2211.
207. Boutin C, Irisson M, Guerin J, et al. Phase II trial of vindesin on malignant pleural mesothelioma. *Cancer Treat Rep* 1987;71:205.
208. Kelsen D, Gralla R, Chang E. Vindesine in the treatment of malignant mesothelioma: a phase II study. *Cancer Treat Rep* 1983;67:821.
209. van Meerbeeck J, Debruyne C, van Zandwijk N, et al. Paclitaxel for malignant pleural mesothelioma: a phase II study of the EORTC Lung Cancer Cooperative Group. *Br J Cancer* 1996;74:961.
210. Vogelzang NJ, Herndon JE, 2nd, Miller A, et al. High-dose paclitaxel plus G-CSF for malignant mesothelioma: CALGB phase II study 9234. *Ann Oncol* 1999;10:597.
211. Solheim OP, Saeter G, Finnanger AM, Stenwig AE. High-dose methotrexate in the treatment of malignant mesothelioma of the pleura. A phase II study. *Br J Cancer* 1992;65:956.
212. Vogler WR, Arkun S, Velez-Garcia E. Phase I study of twice-weekly azacytidine. *Cancer Chemother Rep* 1974;58:895.
213. Vogler WR, Miller DS, Keller JW. 5-Azacytidine: a new drug for the treatment of myeloblastic leukemia. *Blood* 1976;48:331.
214. Dhingra HM, Murphy WK, Winn RJ, et al. Phase II trial of 5, 6-dihydro-5-azacytidine in pleural malignant mesothelioma. *Invest New Drugs* 1991;9:69.
215. Vogelzang NJ, Herndon JE, 2nd, Cirrincione C, et al. Dihydro-5-azacytidine in malignant mesothelioma. A phase II trial demonstrating activity accompanied by cardiac toxicity. Cancer and Leukemia Group B. *Cancer* 1997;79:2237.
216. van Meerbeeck JP, Baas P, Debruyne C, et al. A phase II study of gemcitabine in patients with malignant pleural mesothelioma. European Organization for Research and Treatment of Cancer Lung Cancer Cooperative Group. *Cancer* 1999;85:2577.
217. Lerner H, Schoenfeld D, Martin A, et al. Malignant mesothelioma: the Eastern Cooperative Oncology Group experience. *Cancer* 1983; 52:1981.
218. Vogelzang NJ, Weissman LB, Herndon JN, et al. Trimetrexate in malignant mesothelioma: a Cancer and Leukemia Group B Phase II study. *J Clin Oncol* 1994;12:1436.
219. Falkson G, Vorobiof DA, Lerner JH. A phase II study of M-AMSA in patients with malignant mesothelioma with cyclophosphamide, adriamycin and vincristin. *Cancer Chemother Pharmacol* 1983;11:94.
220. Maksymiuk AW, Marschke RF Jr, Tazelaar HD, et al. Phase II trial of topotecan for the treatment of mesothelioma. *Am J Clin Oncol* 1998;21:610.
221. Webster I, Cochrane JWC, Burkhardt KR. Immunotherapy with BCG vaccine in 30 cases of mesothelioma. *SA Med J* 1982;81:277.
222. Davidson JA, Musk AW, Wood BR, et al. Intralesional cytokine therapy in cancer: a pilot study of GM-CSF infusion in mesothelioma. *J Immunother* 1998;21:389.
223. Esposito S. RNA therapy for pleural mesothelioma. *Lancet* 1969;ii:1203.
224. Christmas TI, Manning LS, Garlepp MJ, et al. Effect of interferon-alpha 2a on malignant mesothelioma. *J Interferon Res* 1993;13:9.
225. Ardizzoni A, Pennucci MC, Castagneto B, et al. Recombinant interferon alpha-2b in the treatment of diffuse malignant pleural mesothelioma. *Am J Clin Oncol* 1994;17:80.
226. Von Hoff DD, Metch B, Lucas JG, et al. Phase II evaluation of recombinant interferon-beta (IFN-beta ser) in patients with diffuse mesothelioma: a Southwest Oncology Group study. *J Interferon Res* 1990;10:531.
227. Boutin C, Viallat JR, Astoul P. Treatment of mesothelioma with interferon gamma and interleukin 2. *Rev Pneumol Clin* 1990;46:211.
228. Boutin C. Treatment of malignant mesothelioma using intrapleural gamma interferon. *Bull Acad Natl Med* 1990;174:421; discussion, 427.
229. Boutin C, Viallat JR, Zandwijk NV, et al. Activity of intrapleural recombinant gamma-interferon in malignant meosthelioma. *Cancer* 1991;67:2033.
230. Boutin C, Nussbaum E, Monnet I, et al. Intrapleural treatment with recombinant gamma-interferon in early stage malignant pleural mesothelioma. *Cancer* 1994;74:2460.
231. Stoter G, Goey SH, Slingerland R, et al. Intrapleural interleukin-2 in malignant pleural mesothelioma: a phase I-II study. *Proc Am Assoc Cancer Res* 1990;31:275(abst 1630).
232. Robinson BWS, Bowman RV, Christmas TI, et al. Clinical experience using immunotherapy (IL-2/LAK cells or interferon alpha 2a) in malignant mesothelioma. *Proc. 1st International Mesothelioma Conference*, Paris: 1991:38.
233. Astoul P, Picat-Joossen D, Viallat JR, Boutin C. Intrapleural administration of interleukin-2 for the treatment of patients with malignant pleural mesothelioma: a phase II study [see comments]. *Cancer* 1998;83:2099.
234. Byrne MJ, Davidson JA, Musk AW, et al. Cisplatin and gemcitabine treatment for malignant mesothelioma: a phase II study. *J Clin Oncol* 1999;17:25.
235. Samson MK, Wasser LP, Borden EC, et al. Randomized comparison of cyclophosphamide, imidazole carboxamide, and adriamycin versus cyclophosphamide and adriamycin in patients with advanced stage malignant mesothelioma: a Sarcoma Intergroup Study. *J Clin Oncol* 1987;5:86.
236. Chahinian AP, Antman K, Goutsou M, et al. Randomized phase II trial of cisplatin with mitomycin or doxorubicin for malignant mesothelioma by the Cancer and Leukemia Group B. *J Clin Oncol* 1993;11:1559.
237. Rusch VW, Niedzwiecki D, Tao Y, et al. Intrapleural cisplatin and mitomycin for malignant mesothelioma following pleurectomy: pharmacokinetic studies. *J Clin Oncol* 1992;10:1001.
238. Bogliolo GV, Lerza R, Bottino GB, et al. Regional pharmacokinetic selectivity of intrapleural cisplatin. *Eur J Cancer* 1991;27:839.
239. Driesen P, Boutin C, Viallat JR, et al. Implantable access system for prolonged intrapleural immunotherapy. *Eur Respir J* 1994;7:1889.
240. Chahinian AP, Holland JF. Treatment of diffuse malignant mesothelioma: a review. *Mt Sinai J Med* 1978;45:54.
241. Carmichael J, Cantwell BM, Harris AL. A phase II trial of ifosfamide/mesna with doxorubicin for malignant mesothelioma. *Eur J Cancer Clin Oncol* 1989;25:911.
242. Dirix LY, van Meerbeeck J, Schrijvers D, et al. A phase II trial of dose-escalated doxorubicin and ifosfamide/mesna in patients with malignant mesothelioma. *Ann Oncol* 1994;5:653.
243. Zidar B, Pugh R, Schiffer L, et al. Treatment of six cases of mesothelioma with doxorubicin and cis-platinum. *Cancer* 1983;52:1788.
244. Ardizzoni A, Rosso R, Salvati F, et al. Activity of doxorubicin and cisplatin combination chemotherapy in patients with diffuse malignant pleural mesothelioma. An Italian Lung Cancer Task Force phase II study. *Cancer* 1991;67:2984.
245. Niki Y, Nakayama S, Soga T, et al. [A case of remission induced in diffuse pleural malignant mesothelioma by the treatment with cisplatin and doxorubicin]. *Gan To Kagaku Ryoho* 1989;16:3635.
246. Stewart DJ, Gertler SZ, Tomiak A, et al. High dose doxorubicin plus cisplatin in the treatment of unresectable mesotheliomas: report of four cases. *Lung Cancer* 1994;11:251.
247. Pennucci MC, Ardizzoni A, Pronzato P, et al. Combined cisplatin, doxorubicin, and mitomycin for the treatment of advanced pleural mesothelioma: a phase II FONICAP trial. Italian Lung Cancer Task Force. *Cancer* 1997;79:1897.

248. Breau JL, Boaziz C, Morere JJF, et al. Combination chemotherapy with cisplatinum, adriamycin, bleomycin and mitomycin C, plus systemic and intrapleural hyaluronidase in 25 consecutive cases of stages II, III pleural mesothelioma. *Proc. 1st International Mesothelioma Conference*, Paris: 1991:5.
249. Dhingra H, Valdivieso M, Tannir N, et al. Combined modality treatment for mesothelioma with cytoxan, adriamycin, and DTIC (CYADIC) and adjuvant surgery. *Proc Am Soc Clin Oncol* 1983;2:205(abst C-800).
250. Spremulli E, Wampler G, Regelson E, et al. Chemotherapy of malignant mesothelioma. *Cancer* 1977;40:2038.
251. Gottlieb JA, Bodney GP, Sinkovics JG, et al. An effective new four-drug combination regimen (CY-VA-DIC) for metastatic sarcomas. *AACR/ASCO* 1974;15:162.
252. Upham JW, Musk AW, van Hazel G, et al. Interferon alpha and doxorubicin in malignant mesothelioma: a phase II study. *Aust N Z J Med* 1993;23:683.
253. Eisenhauer EA, Evans WK, Murray N, et al. A phase II study of VP-16 and cisplatin in patients with unresectable malignant mesothelioma. An NCI Canada clinical trials group study. *Invest New Drugs* 1988;6:327.
254. Niki Y, Soga T, Nishimura A, et al. [A diffuse, pleural, malignant mesothelioma kept in long remission by chemotherapy combining pirarubicin and cisplatin]. *Gan No Rinsho* 1990;36:2463.
255. Nakano T, Chahinian AP, Shinjo M, et al. Cisplatin in combination with irinotecan in the treatment of patients with malignant pleural mesothelioma: a pilot phase II clinical trial and pharmacokinetic profile. *Cancer* 1999;85:2375.
256. Tsavaris N, Mylonakis N, Karvounis N, et al. Combination chemotherapy with cisplatin-vinblastine in malignant mesothelioma [see comments]. *Lung Cancer* 1994;11:299.
257. Samuels BL, Herndon JE, 2nd, Harmon DC, et al. Dihydro-5-azacytidine and cisplatin in the treatment of malignant mesothelioma: a phase II study by the Cancer and Leukemia Group B. *Cancer* 1998;82:1578.
258. Purohit A, Moreau L, Dietemann A, et al. Weekly systemic combination of cisplatin and interferon alpha 2a in diffuse malignant pleural mesothelioma. *Lung Cancer* 1998;22:119.
259. Trandafir L, Ruffie P, Borel C, et al. Higher doses of alpha-interferon do not increase the activity of the weekly cisplatin-interferon combination in advanced malignant mesothelioma. *Eur J Cancer* 1997;33:1900.
260. Chahinian AP, Norton L, Szrajer L, et al. Mitomycin C and cisplatin in human malignant mesothelioma xenografts in nude mice: clinical correlation. *Proc AACR* 1983;24:151(abst 597).
261. Middleton GW, Smith IE, O'Brien ME, et al. Good symptom relief with palliative MVP (mitomycin-C, vinblastine and cisplatin) chemotherapy in malignant mesothelioma. *Ann Oncol* 1998;9:269.
262. Kasseyet S, Astoul P, Boutin C. Results of a phase II trial of combined chemotherapy for patients with diffuse malignant mesothelioma of the pleura. *Cancer* 1999;85:1740.
263. Metintas M, Ozdemir N, Ucgun I, et al. Cisplatin, mitomycin, and interferon-alpha2a combination chemoimmunotherapy in the treatment of diffuse malignant pleural mesothelioma. *Chest* 1999;116:391.
264. Tansan S, Emri S, Selcuk T, et al. Treatment of malignant pleural mesothelioma with cisplatin, mitomycin C and alpha interferon. *Oncology* 1994;51:348.
265. Magri MD, Foladore S, Veronesi A, et al. Treatment of malignant mesothelioma with epirubicin and ifosfamide: a phase II cooperative study. *Ann Oncol* 1992;3:237.
266. Bretti S, Berruti A, Dogliotti L, et al. Combined epirubicin and interleukin-2 regimen in the treatment of malignant mesothelioma: a multicenter phase II study of the Italian Group on Rare Tumors. *Tumori* 1998;84:558.
267. O'Reilly EM, Ilson DH, Saltz LB, et al. A phase II trial of interferon alpha-2a and carboplatin in patients with advanced malignant mesothelioma. *Cancer Invest* 1999;17:195.
268. Halme M, Knuuttila A, Vehmas T, et al. High-dose methotrexate in combination with interferons in the treatment of malignant pleural mesothelioma. *Br J Cancer* 1999;80:1781.
269. Alberts AS, Falkson G, Goedhals L, et al. Malignant pleural mesothelioma: a disease unaffected by current therapeutic maneuvers. *J Clin Oncol* 1988;6:527.
270. Tishler RB, Geard CR, Hall EJ, Schiff PB. Taxol sensitizes human astrocytoma cells to radiation. *Cancer Res* 1992;52:3495.
271. Herscher LL, Hahn SM, Kroog G, et al. Phase I study of paclitaxel as a radiation sensitizer in the treatment of mesothelioma and non-small-cell lung cancer. *J Clin Oncol* 1998;16:635.
272. Linden CJ, Mercke C, Albrechtsson U, et al. Effect of hemithorax irradiation alone or combined with doxorubicin and cyclophosphamide in 47 pleural mesotheliomas: a nonrandomized phase II study. *Eur Respir J* 1996;9:2565.
273. Hilaris BS, Dattatreyudu NK, Wong E, et al. Pleurectomy and intraoperative brachytherapy and postoperative radiation in the management of malignant pleural mesothelioma. *Int J Radiat Oncol Biol Phys* 1984;10:325.
274. Mattson K, Holsti LR, Tammilehto L, et al. Multimodality treatment programs for malignant pleural mesothelioma using high-dose hemithorax irradiation. *Int J Radiat Oncol Biol Phys* 1992;24:643.
275. Markman M, Cleary S, Pfeifle C, Howell SB. Cisplatin administered by the intracavitary route as treatment for malignant mesothelioma. *Cancer* 1986;58:18.
276. Kirmani S, Cleary SM, Mowry J, Howell SB. Intracavitary cisplatin for malignant mesothelioma; an update. *Proc Am Soc Clin Oncol* 1988;5:273.
277. Rusch V, Saltz L, Venkatraman E, et al. A phase II trial of plurectomy, docortication followed by intrapleural and systemic chemotherapy for malignant pleural mesothelioma. *J Clin Oncol* 1994;12:1156.
278. Figlin R, Mendoza E, Piantadosi S, Rusch V. Intrapleural chemotherapy without pleurodesis for malignant pleural effusions. LCSG Trial 861. *Chest* 1994;106:363S.
279. Rice TW, Adelstein DJ, Kirby TJ, et al. Aggressive multimodality therapy for malignant pleural mesothelioma. *Ann Thorac Surg* 1994;58:24.
280. Colleoni M, Sartori F, Calabro F, et al. Surgery followed by intracavitary plus systemic chemotherapy in malignant pleural mesothelioma. *Tumori* 1996;82:53.
281. Sugarbaker D, Harpole D, Healey E, et al. Multimodality treatment of malignant pleural mesothelioma. *Proc Am Soc Clin Oncol* 1995;14:356(abst 1083).
282. Calavrezos A, Koschel G, Husselmann H, et al. Malignant mesothelioma of the pleura. *Klin Wochenschr* 1988;66:607.
283. Pass HI, Donington JS. Use of photodynamic therapy for the management of pleural malignancies. *Semin Surg Oncol* 1995;11:360.
284. Ratto GB, Civalleri D, Esposito M, et al. Pleural space perfusion with cisplatin in the multimodality treatment of malignant mesothelioma: a feasibility and pharmacokinetic study. *J Thorac Cardiovasc Surg* 1999;117:759.
285. Sterman DH, Treat J, Litzky LA, et al. Adenovirus-mediated herpes simplex virus thymidine kinase/ganciclovir gene therapy in patients with localized malignancy: results of a phase I clinical trial in malignant mesothelioma. *Hum Gene Ther* 1998;9:1083.
286. Molnar-Kimber KL, Sterman DH, Chang M, et al. Impact of preexisting and induced humoral and cellular immune responses in an adenovirus-based gene therapy phase I clinical trial for localized mesothelioma. *Hum Gene Ther* 1998;9:2121.
287. Schwarzenberger P, Harrison L, Weinacker A, et al. The treatment of malignant mesothelioma with a gene modified cancer cell line: a phase I study. *Hum Gene Ther* 1998;9:2641.
288. Schwarzenberger P, Lei D, Freeman SM, et al. Antitumor activity with the HSV-tk-gene-modified cell line PA-1-STK in malignant mesothelioma. *Am J Respir Cell Mol Biol* 1998;19:333.
289. Moertel C. Peritoneal mesothelioma. *Gastroenterology* 1972;63:346.
290. Antman K, Osteen R, Klegar K, et al. Early peritoneal mesothelioma: a treatable malignancy. *Lancet* 1985;ii:977.
291. van Gelder T, Hoogsteden HC, Versnel MA, et al. Malignant peritoneal mesothelioma: a series of 19 cases. *Digestion* 1989;43:222.
292. Whitley NO, Brenner DE, Antman KH, et al. Computed tomographic evaluation of peritoneal mesotheliomas: an analysis of eight cases. *AJR Am J Roentgenol* 1982;138:531.
293. Fukuda T, Hayashi K, Mori M, et al. [Radiologic manifestations of peritoneal mesothelioma]. *Nippon Igaku Hoshasen Gakkai Zasshi* 1991;51:643.
294. Nensey YM, Ibrahim MA, Zonca MA, Ma CK. Peritoneal mesothelioma: an unusual cause of esophageal achalasia. *Am J Gastroenterol* 1990;85:1617.
295. Rashchupkina ZP, Karmilov VA, Iudina LI, Burtsev VI. [Malignant mesothelioma of the peritoneum with secondary amyloidosis of the internal organs]. *Klin Med (Mosk)* 1990;68:99.
296. von Hirschhausen R, Clemens M. [Paraneoplastic dermatomyositis in peritoneal mesothelioma]. *Med Klin* 1990;1:113.
297. Weissman L, Osteen R, Corson J, et al. Combined modality therapy for intraperitoneal mesothelioma. *Proc Am Soc Clin Oncol* 1988;7:274(abst 1063).
298. Katsube Y, Mukai K, Silverberg SG. Cystic mesothelioma of the peritoneum: a report of five cases and review of the literature. *Cancer* 1982;50:1615.
299. Burrig KF, Pfitzer P, Hort W. Well-differentiated papillary mesothelioma of the peritoneum: a borderline mesothelioma. Report of two cases and review of literature. *Virchows Arch* 1990;417:443.
300. Ozgen A, Akata D, Akhan O, et al. Giant benign cystic peritoneal mesothelioma: US, CT, and MRI findings. *Abdom Imaging* 1998;23:502.
301. Ross MJ, Welch WR, Scully RE. Multilocular peritoneal inclusion cysts (so-called cystic mesotheliomas). *Cancer* 1989;64:1336.
302. Villaschi S, Autelitano F, Santeusanio G, Balistreri P. Cystic mesothelioma of the peritoneum. A report of three cases. *Am J Clin Pathol* 1990;94:758.
303. Datta RV, Paty PB. Cystic mesothelioma of the peritoneum. *Eur J Surg Oncol* 1997;23:461.
304. Daya D, McCaughey WT. Well-differentiated papillary mesothelioma of the peritoneum. A clinicopathologic study of 22 cases. *Cancer* 1990;65:292.
305. Letterie GS, Yon JL. The antiestrogen tamoxifen in the treatment of recurrent benign cystic mesothelioma. *Gynecol Oncol* 1998;70:131.
306. van der Klooster JM, Lambers MD, van Bommel EF, Scholten PC. Successful catheter drainage of recurrent benign multicystic mesothelioma of the peritoneum. *Neth J Med* 1997;50:246.
307. Rosen DM, Sutton CJ. Use of the potassium titanyl phosphate (KTP) laser in the treatment of benign multicystic peritoneal mesothelioma. *Br J Obstet Gynaecol* 1999;106:505.
308. Lomas DA, Wallis PJ, Stockley RA. Palliation of malignant ascites with a Tenckhoff catheter. *Thorax* 1989;44:828.
309. Einhorn N, Hamos KV, Hindmarsh T, et al. Radiation therapy of ovarian carcinoma: presentation of a six-field technique. *Radiother Oncol* 1986;7:125.
310. Fazekas J, Maier JG. Irradiation of ovarian carcinomas: a prospective comparison of the open-field and moving strip techniques. *AJR Am J Roentgenol* 1974;120:118.
311. Lederman GS, Recht A, Herman T, et al. Long-term survival in peritoneal mesothelioma. The role of radiotherapy and combined modality treatment. *Cancer* 1987;59:1882.
312. Rose RG, Palmer JD, Lougheed MN. Treatment of peritoneal mesothelioma with radioactive colloidal gold. *Cancer* 1955;8:478.
313. Leichner PK, Rosenshein N, Leibel SA, Order SE. Distribution and tissue dose of intraperitoneal administered radioactive chromic phosphate (32P) in New Zealand white rabbits. *Radiology* 1980;134:729.
314. Cross WG. *Table of beta-ray dose distributions in water.* Chalk River, Ontario; Chalk River Laboratories, 1967.
315. Piver SM. Radioactive colloids in the treatment of stage IA ovarian cancer. *Obstet Gynecol* 1972;40:42.
316. Pezner RD, Stevens KR, Tong D, Allen CV. Limited epithelial carcinoma of the ovary treated with curative intent by the intraperitoneal installation of radiocolloids. *Cancer* 1978;42:2563.
317. Klaassen D, Starreveld A, Shelly W, et al. External beam pelvic radiotherapy plus intraperitoneal radioactive chromic phosphate in early stage ovarian cancer: a toxic combination. *Int J Radiat Oncol Biol Phys* 1985;11:1801.
318. Howell SB, Pfeifle CL, Wung WE, et al. Intraperitoneal cisplatin with systemic thiosulfate protection. *Ann Intern Med* 1982;97: 845.

319. Hayashi T, Nasu Y, Aramaki K, et al. [A case of peritoneal malignant mesothelioma with disappearance of ascites result of intraperitoneal instillation of mitomycin C and oral administration of UFT]. *Gan To Kagaku Ryoho* 1989;16:2449.
320. Sugarbaker PH, Cunliffe WJ, Graves T, et al. Phase I and pharmacologic studies with early postoperative intraperitoneal epiadriamycin. Fourth International Conference on Advances in Regional Cancer Therapy. Berchtesgaden, Germany, 1989.
321. Markman M, Kelsen D. Efficacy of cisplatin-based intraperitoneal chemotherapy as treatment of malignant peritoneal mesothelioma. *J Cancer Res Clin Oncol* 1992;118:547.
322. Langer CJ, Rosenblum N, Hogan M, et al. Intraperitoneal cisplatin and etoposide in peritoneal mesothelioma: favorable outcome with a multimodality approach. *Cancer Chemother Pharmacol* 1993;32:204.
323. Vlasveld LT, Taal BG, Kroon BB, et al. Intestinal obstruction due to diffuse peritoneal fibrosis at 2 years after the successful treatment of malignant peritoneal mesothelioma with intraperitoneal mitoxantrone [published erratum appears in *Cancer Chemother Pharmacol* 1992;30:249]. *Cancer Chemother Pharmacol* 1992;29:405.
324. Garcia Moore ML, Savaraj N, Feun LG, Donnelly E. Successful therapy of peritoneal mesothelioma with intraperitoneal chemotherapy alone. A case report. *Am J Clin Oncol* 1992;15:528.
325. Taylor RA, Johnson LP. Mesothelioma: current perspectives. *West J Med* 1981;134:379.
326. Eltabbakh GH, Piver MS, Hempling RE, et al. Clinical picture, response to therapy, and survival of women with diffuse malignant peritoneal mesothelioma. *J Surg Oncol* 1999;70:6.
327. Park BJ, Alexander HR, Libutti SK, et al. Treatment of primary peritoneal mesothelioma by continuous hyperthermic peritoneal perfusion (CHPP) [In Process Citation]. *Ann Surg Oncol* 1999;6:582.
328. Plas E, Riedl CR, Pfluger H. Malignant mesothelioma of the tunica vaginalis testis: review of the literature and assessment of prognostic parameters. *Cancer* 1998;83:2437.
329. Khan MA, Puri P, Devaney D. Mesothelioma of tunica vaginalis testis in a child. *J Urol* 1997;158:198.
330. Antman K, Cohn S, Green M. Malignant mesothelioma of the tunica vaginalis testis. *J Clin Oncol* 1984; 2:447.
331. Gupta SC, Gupta AK, Misra V, Singh PA. Pre-operative diagnosis of malignant mesothelioma of tunica vaginalis testis by hydrocele fluid cytology. *Eur J Surg Oncol* 1998;24:153.
332. Kamiya M, Eimoto T. Malignant mesothelioma of the tunica vaginalis. *Pathol Res Pract* 1990;186:680.
333. Asoh Y, Nakamura M, Maeda T, et al. [Brain metastasis from primary pericardial mesothelioma. Case report]. *Neurol Med Chir (Tokyo)* 1990;30:884.
334. Eker R, Cantez T, Dogan O, et al. Pericardial mesothelioma. A pediatric case report. *Turk J Pediatr* 1989;31:305.
335. Taguchi T, Fujiwara Y, Ichiki H, et al. [A case of malignant pericardial mesothelioma detected by gallium-67 scintigraphy]. *Kaku Igaku* 1991;28:281.
336. Aggarwal P, Wali JP, Agarwal J. Pericardial mesothelioma presenting as a mediastinal mass. *Singapore Med J* 1991;32:185.
337. Pascual MA, Povar J, Munoz J, et al. [Pericardial mesothelioma: apropos of a case]. *Rev Esp Cardiol* 1989;42:559.
338. DeKlerk DP, Nime F. Adenomatoid tumors (mesothelioma) of testicular and paratesticular tissue. *Urology* 1975; 6:635.
339. Scully R, Mark EJ, McNeeley BU. Case record of the Massachusetts General Hospital. *N Engl J Med* 1982;306:32.
340. Balassiano M, Reichert N, Rosenman Y, et al. Localized fibrous mesothelioma of the mediastinum devoid of pleural connections. *Postgrad Med J* 1989;65:788.
341. Kottke MK, Hart WR, Broughan T. Localized fibrous tumor (localized fibrous mesothelioma) of the liver. *Cancer* 1989;64:1096.
342. Simpson PR. Adenomatoid tumor of the adrenal gland. *Arch Pathol Lab Med* 1990;114:725.
343. Briselli M, Mark EJ, Dickersin GR. Solitary fibrous tumors of the pleura: eight new cases and review of 360 cases in the literature. *Cancer* 1981;47:2678.
344. Scharifker D, Kaneko M. Localized fibrous "mesothelioma" of pleura (sub-mesothelial fibroma). A clinicopathologic study of 18 cases. *Cancer* 1979;43:627.
345. Dalton WT, Zolliker AS, McCaughey WTE, et al. Localized primary tumors of the pleura. An analysis of 40 cases. *Cancer* 1979;44:1465.
346. Majoulet JF, Millant P, Bouillet P, et al. [Radiologic aspect of benign pleural fibrous mesothelioma. Reports of 4 cases]. *Ann Radiol (Paris)* 1990;33:229.
347. Strom EH, Skjorten F, Aarseth LB, Haug E. Solitary fibrous tumor of the pleura. An immunohistochemical, electron microscopic and tissue culture study of a tumor producing insulin-like growth factor I in a patient with hypoglycemia. *Pathol Res Pract* 1991;187:109.
348. Scotte M, Bessou JP, Andro JF, et al. [Hypoglycemic pleural mesothelioma. A case report]. *Ann Chir* 1990;44:688.
349. DeLaria G, Jensik R, Faber LP, Kittle CF. Surgical management of malignant mesothelioma. *Ann Thorac Surg* 1978;26:375.
350. Davies JH, Notley RG. Adenomatoid tumours of the male genital tract. Review of 5 men presenting with an intrascrotal swelling subsequently diagnosed as an adenomatoid tumour. *Eur Urol* 1989;16:393.
351. Lopez JI, Aranda FI. Absence of estrogen immunoreactivity in adenomatoid tumors of male reproductive system. *Pathol Res Pract* 1990;186:395.
352. Kupryjanczyk J. Adenomatoid tumour of the ovary and uterus in the same patient. *Zentralbl Allg Pathol* 1989;135:437.
353. Monma N, Satodate R, Tashiro A, Segawa I. Origin of so-called mesothelioma of the atrioventricular node. An immunohistochemical study. *Arch Pathol Lab Med* 1991;115:1026.
354. Fontaliran F, Guillois B, Colin A, et al. Congenital atrioventricular block and maternal lupus erythematosus. Histologic discovery of tumor of the atrioventricular node. *Arch Mal Coeur* 1989;82:609.
355. Corbi P, Jebara V, Fabiani JN, et al. [Benign tumors of the heart (excluding myxoma). Experience with 9 surgically treated cases]. *Ann Cardiol Angeiol (Paris)* 1990;39:433.
356. Subramanian R, Flygenring B. Mesothelioma of the atrioventricular node and congenital complete heart block. *Clin Cardiol* 1989;12:469.
357. Balasundaram S, Halees SA, Duran C. Mesothelioma of the atrioventricular node: first successful follow-up after excision. *Eur Heart J* 1992;13:718.

CHAPTER 41

Cancer of the Skin

SECTION 1

DOUGLAS E. BRASH
ALLEN E. BALE

Molecular Biology of Skin Cancer

In skin cancer, the interaction between genes and the environment figures prominently. At the molecular level, skin tumors appear to result from a succession of genetic alterations; many of these changes are caused by carcinogens, such as sunlight. At the cellular level, one of the mutant genes, *p53*, causes a deficiency in the programmed cell death of damaged keratinocytes. Without such apoptosis, large numbers of precancerous cells accumulate in the sun-exposed skin of normal individuals. A second gene, *PTCH*, affects skin development and is mutated in basal cell carcinomas (BCC). Various aspects of these advances have been reviewed.[1–5]

SKIN CARCINOGENS

Nonmelanoma skin cancer is associated with exposure to chimney soot in chimney sweeps, burn scars, arsenic ingestion, and exposure to sunlight.[6] Sunlight is the principal skin carcinogen in humans and the human carcinogen whose mechanism is clearest. Basal and squamous cell carcinomas are most frequent at low latitudes, in outdoor workers, on exposed regions of the body, and in light-skinned individuals with blonde or red hair who have a tendency to burn rather than tan.[7] Many BCCs that occur on body sites not chronically exposed to sunlight, such as the trunk and legs, seem related to intermittent sun exposure.[8] In experimental animals, the most effective wavelengths are the ultraviolet B (UVB) region of the solar spectrum; the UVA used in tanning parlors can cause skin tumors as well.[5] UVB's effectiveness is due to its ability to partially penetrate the ozone layer and stratum corneum and then be absorbed by DNA.[9] Nonmelanoma skin cancers exceed the incidence of all other cancers combined in the southern United States, Hawaii, and Australia.[10,11]

The first molecular step in sunlight-induced carcinogenesis is the induction of DNA photoproducts by UVB photons. The most frequent photoproducts involve adjacent pyrimidines.[1] UV photons tend to be absorbed at the 5-6 double bond of pyrimidines, allowing the bond to open. The result is either the cyclobutane dimer or a pyrimidine-pyrimidone (6-4) photoproduct (Fig. 41.1-1).[2] Both lead to abnormal DNA structures. When DNA is copied during subsequent DNA replication, the DNA polymerase often incorrectly inserts an adenine opposite a damaged cytosine. At the next round of replication, the adenine correctly codes for thymine opposite. After UV, these C→T mutations occur only where a cytosine lies next to a thymine or another cytosine, reflecting the specificity of the sites at which UV photoproducts occur. If two adjacent cytosines mutate, the result is CC→TT. These distinctive patterns of mutation are pathognomonic for UV radiation.[12]

Mutations are prevented by DNA repair systems that excise UV photoproducts from DNA.[13,14] A transcription-coupled repair system rapidly removes lesions from the transcribed strand of active genes, whereas a slower global excision system removes lesions from inactive genes and from the nontran-

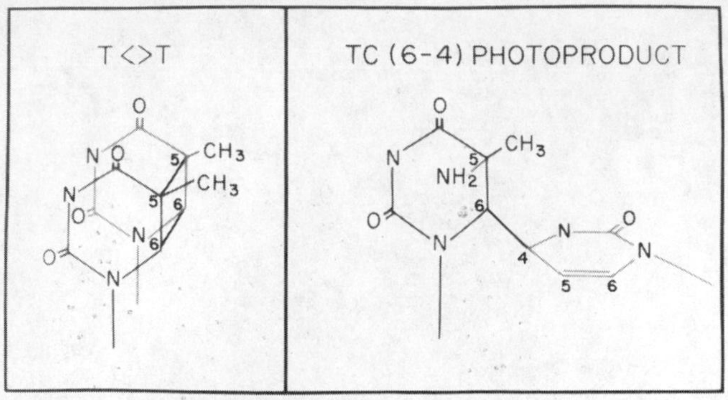

FIGURE 41.1-1. Ultraviolet light photoproducts. TT cyclobutane pyrimidine dimer (left) and TC pyrimidine-pyrimidone (6-4) photoproduct (right).

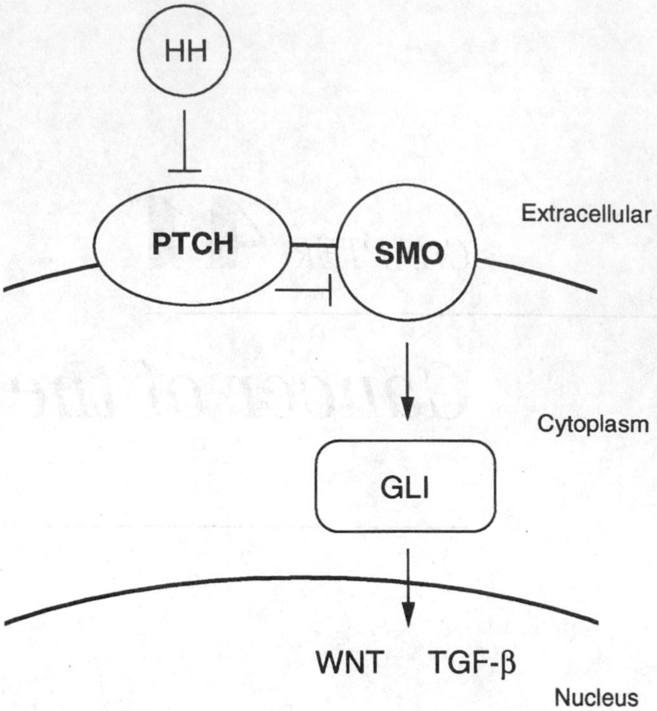

FIGURE 41.1-2. Interactions among patched (PTCH), smoothened (SMO), and hedgehog (HH) proteins. Patched represses transcription of hedgehog target genes by inactivating smoothened. Hedgehog binds to patched, thereby activating smoothened and causing increased transcription of GLI, itself a transcription factor, and its downstream targets, such as WNT and transforming growth factor-β (TGF-β). In the absence of patched, smoothened may be constitutively activated, resulting in the overexpression of these genes.

scribed strand of active ones. Individuals with xeroderma pigmentosum group A (XPA) are defective in both pathways, resulting in acute sun sensitivity and a 2000-fold elevated incidence of skin cancer.[15] The XPC subtype is defective in only the global system, yet has similar clinical features. Cockayne's syndrome is defective in only the transcription-coupled pathway and, though sun-sensitive, does not have an increased skin cancer incidence. Most genes corresponding to the XP and Cockayne's syndrome subtypes have been cloned, and their protein products successively recognize and excise not only UV photoproducts but other forms of DNA damage as well.

GENETIC EVENTS

PTCH

Two genes normally prevent cancers but are inactivated in skin tumors. *PTCH,* a component of a cellular signaling pathway, is mutated in perhaps 90% of BCCs. *p53,* which encodes a regulator of the cell cycle and cell death, is mutated in half of BCCs and more than 90% of squamous cell carcinomas (SCC).

PTCH was discovered as the gene mutated in nevoid basal cell carcinoma syndrome, an autosomal dominant disorder characterized by multiple BCCs, jaw cysts, and pits of the palms and soles. It is a human homologue of the *Drosophila* gene *patched.*[16,17] Most sporadic BCCs have inactivating *PTCH* mutations,[18] and almost all tumors without *PTCH* mutations have activating mutations in its partner, smoothened.[19]

Patched is important in establishing anterior-posterior relationships of the segments of developing *Drosophila* embryos. It encodes a large transmembrane protein that, in a complex with smoothened, another transmembrane molecule, is believed to serve as the receptor for the secreted molecule hedgehog.[20] In hedgehog's absence, smoothened and patched form an inactive complex. On hedgehog binding, smoothened is released from inhibitory effects of patched and transduces a signal (Fig. 41.1-2). Mutations that inactivate patched switch on the hedgehog pathway without hedgehog.[18] Smoothened functions as an oncogene when switched on in mouse skin, and some BCCs result from activating mutations of smoothened instead of inactivating mutations of patched.[19] GLI1, a downstream transcription factor in the hedgehog pathway, is an oncogene in brain tumors, and its overexpression causes epidermal proliferation in frogs.[21] Activating GLI turns on transcription of *WNT,* which is known to act as an oncogene in mammary tumors in mice, as well as members of the tumor growth factor-β family. The latter genes have complex roles in regulating differentiation and cell growth.

Mutating the hedgehog pathway is an early step in tumor development because minute BCCs are as likely as large tumors to have patched mutations, and all histologic subtypes have a high frequency of loss of patched. A congenital lesion that can progress to BCC, the sebaceous nevus, has allelic loss in the *PTCH* region in 40% of cases.[22] No tumors have loss on other chromosomes without involvement of the *PTCH* locus,[23] so *PTCH* appears to function as a "gatekeeper gene" in basal cell carcinogenesis. Inactivating this function seems to be necessary before clonal expansion and accumulation of other genetic hits can lead to BCC formation.[24]

Nearly all hereditary BCCs have allelic loss as their second, somatic hit. This allelic loss is usually related to sunlight, since nevoid BCC syndrome tumors are most frequent on sun-exposed skin and are rare in African Americans.[25] However, UVB causes this type of gross rearrangement of genetic material only rarely, so other wavelengths, such as UVA, may be important. Sporadic BCCs from XP group A patients contain *PTCH* mutations that are UVB-like, with CC→TT mutations predominating.[26] However, in typical patients, approximately one-third of BCCs have mutations that are clearly not UVB-induced.[18] These may reflect factors such as UVA, oxidative damage, or arsenicals. Sunscreens may need to block both UVB and UVA to be completely protective against BCC.

p53

The distinctive mutations caused by UVB radiation identify a tumor suppressor gene critical for both BCC and SCC: *p53*. More than 90% of SCC of the skin in U.S. patients contain mutations in *p53*.[4,27] These are predominantly C→T and CC→TT base substitutions at sites of adjacent pyrimidines, directly implicating cytosine-containing cyclobutane dimers or (6-4) photoproducts and sunlight UVB as the mutagen. Each *p53* mutation changes the amino acid, indicating that the mutation was selected for and contributed to tumor development, rather than being solely an indicator of sun exposure. *p53* is a transcription factor that turns on or off the expression of other genes involved in the cell cycle, programmed cell death, and DNA repair.[28,29] Most mutations inactivate *p53*'s transcriptional activator function. The gene is mutated in approximately one-half of all human cancers and is considered a tumor suppressor gene because these mutations inactivate the gene's ability to suppress growth of tumor cells in culture.[30]

BCCs, though usually diploid and nonmetastasizing, also contain UV-induced *p53* mutations.[4] Approximately one-third of BCCs occur on body sites that are relatively sun-shielded, *p53* mutations from these tumors resemble those seen with UVA, ionizing radiation, or oxidative damage, rather than UVB.[31] UVB-induced *p53* mutations are frequent in skin cancers from XP patients, with CC→TT mutations being prominent, and in carcinoma *in situ*.[32–34] Aggressive tumors from patients with exposure to both sun and tobacco or agricultural chemicals contain multiple unrelated *p53* mutations, as if multiple tumors arising in an abnormal field had merged.[35] In Taiwanese arsenic-induced BCC and SCC, *p53* mutations are not UV-like.[36] Non-UV *p53* mutations are common in keloids, results of dysregulated wound healing.[37]

The *p53* mutations in skin cancers tend to cluster at nine mutation hot spots.[38] DNA photoproducts are not particularly frequent at these sites,[38] but excision of UV photoproducts is slower than at surrounding nucleotides.[39] Excision repair of UV photoproducts is reduced in T lymphocytes from patients with BCC or a family history of skin cancer.[40]

Sunlight mutates *p53* quite early. UVB-induced mutations are found in actinic keratoses, which occasionally progress to SCC; each lesion has a different *p53* mutation.[41,42] Strikingly, some 60,000 tiny clones of *p53*-mutant cells are found in sun-exposed skin from normal individuals (Fig. 41.1-3).[43,44] Thus, precancerous cells are not only made early in life but begin to proliferate early. The molecular evidence supports migration studies indicating that sunlight exposure critical for skin cancer occurs before age 15 to 20.[45,46]

CELLULAR EVENTS

The contribution of a *p53* mutation to tumorigenesis is partially understood. The p53 protein is not required for normal development but is elevated in cells treated with DNA-damaging agents and in cells with cell-cycle abnormalities.[28,29] The signal

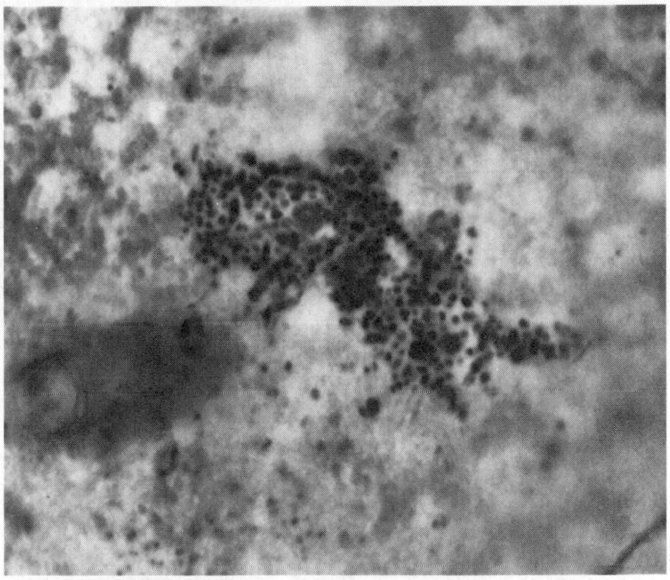

FIGURE 41.1-3. *p53*-mutant clone in whole-mount preparations of human epidermis. Sun-exposed skin from normal individuals contains 60,000 such clones. (From ref. 43, with permission.)

for UV induction of p53 originates from active genes whose transcription has been blocked.[17] Elevated p53 protein has two effects on cells. In the "guardian of the genome" pathway, DNA damage induces the p53 protein. p53 then leads to cell-cycle arrest at a G_1-phase checkpoint by inducing p21, an inhibitor of cell-cycle–dependent protein kinases. In keratinocytes, however, UV induces p21 without p53.[48] p53 facilitates DNA repair by transcriptionally activating the p48 protein, which is required for global excision repair and is defective in XPE.[49] In the "cellular proofreading" pathway,[4] inducing p53 in an aberrant cell leads to apoptosis, a form of programmed cell death.[41,50,51]

In the epidermis, cellular proofreading is operative after DNA damage. UVB and UVA induce p53 by reducing its degradation rate.[52–54] p53 then causes irradiated keratinocytes to become the apoptotic "sunburn cells" familiar to dermatologists.[55] Inactivating the *p53* gene prevents sunburn cell formation.[41] Some point mutations in *p53* do not block apoptosis,[56] so different *p53* mutations may have different effects on tumor development. Mice inactivated for the *p53* gene develop more and earlier skin cancers after UV.[57,58] Cells defective in *p53*, or mice defective in UV-induced apoptosis due to a defect in the fas ligand, accumulate mutations at a rapid rate.[59,60] Skin evidently uses the strategy that killing a damaged cell prevents it from becoming cancerous. Thus, if the *p53* gene itself is mutated by a previous sunlight exposure, the cell will be apoptosis-resistant. This cancer-prone cell will survive even if badly UV-damaged.

The situation can grow worse, due to a second consequence of death-resistance. Because the cancer-prone cell's normal neighbors undergo apoptosis when damaged, their death provides an opportunity for the *p53*-mutated cell to clonally expand. Sunlight exposure can thus act as a selection pressure favoring the clonal expansion of *p53*-mutated cells (Fig. 41.1-4). Indeed, transgenic mice carrying a *p53* point mutation that does not affect apoptosis have more tumors after UVB but no shortening of tumor latency.[61] Sunlight can thus act several times in skin carcinogenesis: first to mutate the *p53* or *PTCH*

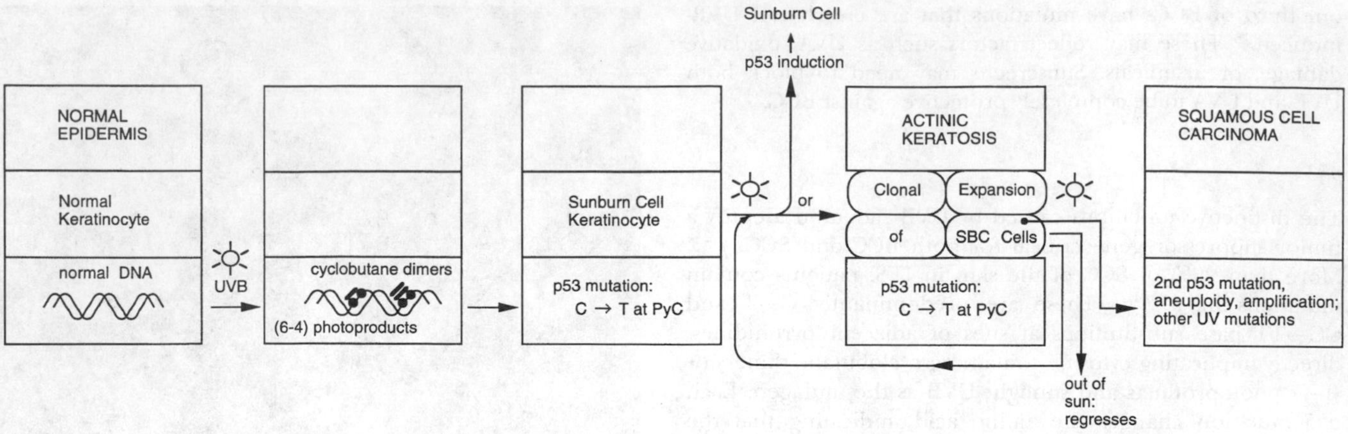

FIGURE 41.1-4. A model for genetic and cellular events in the onset of human skin cancer. Mutation of the *p53* tumor suppressor gene and selection for apoptosis-resistant *p53*-mutant cells by repeated sunlight exposure are described in the text. SBC, sunburn cells; UV, ultraviolet; UVB, ultraviolet B. (From ref. 41, with permission.)

gene and then afterward to select for clonal expansion of a *p53*-mutated cell. These two actions correspond to tumor initiation and tumor promotion. UVB is known to have tumor-promoting activity in mouse skin.[62,63]

Progression of a single mutant cell to a clone of precancerous or cancerous cells can be traced long after the fact. Taking advantage of *p53* mutations as lineage markers, it has been found that when an SCC is adjacent to carcinoma *in situ*, the two lesions carry the identical mutation.[44] Similarly, microdissecting BCCs into regions of 50 to 100 cells reveals that a BCC contains a dominant cell clone accompanied by subclones containing a second or even a third mutation.[64]

THERAPEUTICS

The foregoing molecular findings are beginning to impact the clinic, first in the realm of diagnostics. Sunscreens of SPF 15 reduce cyclobutane dimers, p53 protein induction, sunburn cells, and *p53* gene mutations nearly tenfold.[65–69] Tumors in mice are reduced up to 50-fold,[70,71] consistent with simultaneous protection of several genes. This is reassuring, since some common sunscreen ingredients are mutagenic,[72] and protection against actinic keratoses in humans is only twofold.[73,74]

Molecular therapeutics is in its infancy. A gene therapy strategy is to restore p53 to render cells more sensitive to radiotherapy- or chemotherapy-induced apoptosis.[75] Obtaining a useful therapeutic index depends on apoptosis being greater in the tumor cells than in normal tissue. In fact, many treatments leading to apoptosis in transformed fibroblasts only growth-arrest their untransformed counterparts.[76,77] Since p53 is also sensitive to cell-cycle aberrations or other aberrations of tumor cells,[28,29] an alternative therapeutic strategy introduces p53 without adjunct treatment to induce apoptosis in transformed but not normal cells.[78] *In vivo* intraperitoneal delivery of a retroviral *p53* vector leads to a 75% reduction in peritoneal metastatic cells from murine pancreatic cancer.[79] Pharmacologic approaches include activation of latent normal p53 protein with small peptides[80] and destabilizing mutant p53 using modifiers of its interaction with heat-shock protein.[81] Several chemoprevention regimens increase apoptosis of premalignant cells, including dietary antioxidants[77,82,83] and caloric restriction.[84,85]

For additional information and color images, see Chapter 41.3: Atlas of Skin Cancer, at www.LWWoncology.com.

REFERENCES

1. Brash DE. UV mutagenic photoproducts in *E coli* and human cells: a molecular genetics perspective on human skin cancer. *Photochem Photobiol* 1988;48:59.
2. Mitchell DL, Nairn RS. The biology of the (6-4) photoproduct. *Photochem Photobiol* 1989;49:805.
3. Ananthaswamy HN, Pierceall WE. Molecular mechanisms of ultraviolet radiation carcinogenesis. *Photochem Photobiol* 1990;52:1119.
4. Brash DE, Ziegler A, Jonason A, et al. Sunlight and sunburn in human skin cancer: p53, apoptosis, and tumor promotion. *J Invest Dermatol Symp Proc* 1996;1:136.
5. Black HS, deGruijl FR, Forbes D, et al. Photocarcinogenesis: an overview. *J Photochem Photobiol B* 1997;40:29.
6. Fitzpatrick TB, Eisen AZ, Wolff K, Freedberg IM, Austen KF, eds. *Dermatology in general medicine*, 4th ed, vol 1. New York: McGraw-Hill, 1993:1812.
7. Urbach F. Ultraviolet radiation and skin cancer. In: Smith KC, ed. *Topics in photomedicine.* New York: Plenum Publishing, 1984:67.
8. Bastiaens MT, Hoefnagel JJ, Bruijn JA, et al. Differences in age, site distribution, and sex between nodular and superficial basal cell carcinoma indicate different types of tumors. *J Invest Dermatol* 1998;110:880.
9. Freeman SE, Hacham H, Gange RW, Maytum DJ, Sutherland JC. Wavelength dependence of pyrimidine dimer formation in DNA of human skin irradiated *in situ* with ultraviolet light. *Proc Natl Acad Sci U S A* 1989;86:5605.
10. Glass AG, Hoover RN. The emerging epidemic of melanoma and squamous cell skin cancer. *JAMA* 1989;262:2097.
11. Parker SL, Tong T, Bolden S, Wingo PA. Cancer statistics, 1997. *CA Cancer J Clin* 1997; 47:5.
12. Hutchinson F. Induction of tandem base change mutations. *Mutat Res* 1994;309:11.
13. Wood RD. Nucleotide excision repair in mammalian cells. *J Biol Chem* 1997;272:23465.
14. de Laat WL, Jaspers NG, Hoeijmakers JH. Molecular mechanism of nucleotide excision repair. *Genes Dev* 1999;13:768.
15. Cleaver JE, Kraemer KH. Xeroderma pigmentosum and Cockayne syndrome. In: Scriver CR, Beaudet AL, Sly WS, Valle D, eds. *The metabolic and molecular bases of inherited disease,* 7th ed, vol 3. New York: McGraw-Hill, 1995:4393.
16. Hahn H, Wicking C, Zaphiropoulos PG, et al. Mutations in the human homologue of *Drosophila* patched in the nevoid basal cell carcinoma syndrome. *Cell* 1996;85:841.
17. Johnson RL, Rothman AL, Xie J, et al. Human homolog of *patched*, a candidate gene for the basal cell nevus syndrome. *Science* 1996;272:1668.
18. Gailani MR, Stahle-Backdahl M, Leffell DJ, et al. The role of the human homologue of *Drosophila patched* in sporadic basal cell carcinomas. *Nat Genet* 1996;14:78.
19. Xie J, Murone M, Luoh SM, et al. Activating smoothened mutations in sporadic basal-cell carcinoma. *Nature* 1998;391:90.
20. Gailani MR, Bale AE. Developmental genes and cancer: role of patched in basal cell carcinoma of the skin. *J Natl Cancer Inst* 1997;89:1103.
21. Dahmane N, Lee J, Robins P, Heller P, Ruiz i Altaba A. Activation of the transcription factor Gli1 and the sonic hedgehog signaling pathway in skin tumors. *Nature* 1997;389:876.
22. Xin H, Matt D, Qin JZ, Burg G, Boni R. The sebaceous nevus: a nevus with deletions of the PTCH gene. *Cancer Res* 1999;59:1834.

23. Gailani MR, Bale SJ, Leffell DJ, et al. Developmental defects in Gorlin syndrome related to a putative tumor suppressor gene on chromosome 9. *Cell* 1992;69:111.
24. Sidransky D. Is human patched the gatekeeper of common skin cancers? *Nat Genet* 1996;14:7.
25. Howell JB. Nevoid basal cell carcinoma syndrome. *J Am Acad Dermatol* 1984;11:98.
26. Bodak N, Queille S, Avril MF, et al. High levels of patched gene mutations in basal-cell carcinomas from patients with xeroderma pigmentosum. *Proc Natl Acad Sci U S A* 1999;96:5117.
27. Brash DE, Rudolph JA, Simon JA, et al. A role for sunlight in skin cancer: UV-induced p53 mutations in squamous cell carcinoma. *Proc Natl Acad Sci U S A* 1991;88:10124.
28. Ko LJ, Prives C. p53: puzzle and paradigm. *Genes Dev* 1996;10:1054.
29. Levine AJ. p53, the cellular gatekeeper for growth and division. *Cell* 1997;88:323.
30. Greenblatt MS, Bennett WP, Hollstein M, Harris CC. Mutations in the *p53* tumor suppressor gene: clues to cancer etiology and molecular pathogenesis. *Cancer Res* 1994;54:4855.
31. Matsumura Y, Nishigori C, Yagi T, Imamura S, Takebe H. Characterization of p53 gene mutations in basal-cell carcinomas: comparison between sun-exposed and less-exposed skin areas. *Int J Cancer* 1996;65:778.
32. Dumaz N, Drougard C, Sarasin A, Daya-Grosjean L. Specific UV-induced mutation spectrum in the p53 gene of skin tumors from DNA repair deficient xeroderma pigmentosum patients. *Proc Natl Acad Sci U S A* 1993;90:10529.
33. Sato M, Nishigori C, Zghal M, Yagi T, Takebe H. Ultraviolet-specific mutations in p53 gene in skin tumors in xeroderma pigmentosum patients. *Cancer Res* 1993;53:2944.
34. Campbell C, Quinn AG, Ro Y-S, Angus B, Rees JL. p53 Mutations are common and early events that precede tumor invasion in squamous cell neoplasia of the skin. *J Invest Dermatol* 1993;100:746.
35. Kanjilal S, Strom SS, Clayman GL, et al. p53 Mutations in nonmelanoma skin cancer of the head and neck: molecular evidence for field cancerization. *Cancer Res* 1995;55:3604.
36. Hsu CH, Yang SA, Wang JY, Yu HS, Lin SR. Mutational spectrum of p53 gene in arsenic-related skin cancers from the blackfoot disease endemic area of Taiwan. *Br J Cancer* 1999;80:1080.
37. Saed GM, Ladin D, Olson J, et al. Analysis of p53 gene mutations in keloids using polymerase chain reaction-based single-strand conformational polymorphism and DNA sequencing. *Arch Dermatol* 1998;1324:963.
38. Ziegler A, Leffell DJ, Kunala S, et al. Mutation hotspots due to sunlight in the p53 gene of non-melanoma skin cancers. *Proc Natl Acad Sci U S A* 1993;90:4216.
39. Tornaletti S, Pfeifer GP. Slow repair of pyrimidine dimers at *p53* mutation hotspots in skin cancer. *Science* 1994;263:1436.
40. Grossman L. Epidemiology of ultraviolet-DNA repair capacity and human cancer. *Environ Health Perspect* 1997;105:927.
41. Ziegler A, Jonason AS, Leffell DJ, et al. Sunburn and p53 in the onset of skin cancer. *Nature* 1994;372:773.
42. Taguchi M, Watanabe S, Yashima K, et al. Aberrations of the tumor suppressor *p53* gene and p53 protein in solar keratosis in human skin. *J Invest Dermatol* 1994;103:500.
43. Jonason AS, Kunala S, Price GJ, et al. Frequent clones of p53-mutated keratinocytes in normal human skin. *Proc Natl Acad Sci U S A* 1996;93:14025.
44. Ren ZP, Hedrum A, Ponten F, et al. Human epidermal cancer and accompanying precursors have identical p53 mutations different from p53 mutations in adjacent areas of clonally expanded non-neoplastic keratinocytes. *Oncogene* 1996;12:765.
45. Kricker A, Armstrong BK, English DR, Heenan PJ. Pigmentary and cutaneous risk factors for non-melanocytic skin cancer—a case-control study. *Int J Cancer* 1991;48:650.
46. Marks R, Jolley D, Lectsas S, Foley P. The role of childhood exposure to sunlight in the development of solar keratoses and non-melanocytic skin cancer. *Med J Aust* 1990;152:62.
47. Ljungman M, Zhang F. Blockage of RNA polymerase as a possible trigger for UV light-induced apoptosis. *Oncogene* 1996;13:823.
48. Liu M, Wikonkal NM, Brash DE. UV induces p21WAF1/CIP1 protein in keratinocytes without p53. *J Invest Dermatol* 1999;113:283.
49. Hwang BJ, Ford JM, Hanawalt PC, Chu G. Expression of the p48 xeroderma pigmentosum gene is p53-dependent and is involved in global genomic repair. *Proc Natl Acad Sci U S A* 1999;96:424.
50. Evan G, Littlewood T. A matter of life and cell death. *Science* 1998;281:1317.
51. Green DR, Reed JC. Mitochondria and apoptosis. *Science* 1998;281:1309.
52. Hall PA, McKee PH, Menage H, Dover R, Lane DP. High levels of p53 protein in UV-irradiated normal human skin. *Oncogene* 1993;8:203.
53. Campbell C, Quinn AG, Angus B, Farr PM, Rees JL. Wavelength specific patterns of *p53* induction in human skin following exposure to UV radiation. *Cancer Res* 1993;53:2697.
54. Liu M, Dhanwada KR, Birt DF, Hecht S, Pelling JC. Increase in p53 protein half-life in mouse keratinocytes following UV-B irradiation. *Carcinogenesis* 1994;15:1089.
55. Danno K, Horio T. Sunburn cell: factors involved in its formation. *Photochem Photobiol* 1987;45:683.
56. Li G, Mitchell DL, Ho VC, Reed JC, Tron VA. Decreased DNA repair but normal apoptosis in ultraviolet-irradiated skin of p53-transgenic mice. *Am J Pathol* 1996;148:1113.
57. Li G, Tron V, Ho V. Induction of squamous cell carcinoma in p53-deficient mice after ultraviolet irradiation. *J Invest Dermatol* 1998;110:72.
58. Jiang W, Ananthaswamy HN, Muller HK, Kripke ML. p53 protects against skin cancer induction by UV-B radiation. *Oncogene* 1999;18:4247.
59. Griffiths SD, Clarke AR, Healy LE, et al. Absence of p53 permits propagation of mutant cells following genotoxic damage. *Oncogene* 1997;14:523.
60. Hill LL, Ouhtit A, Loughlin SM, et al. Fas ligand: a sensor for DNA damage critical in skin cancer etiology. *Science* 1999;285:898.
61. Li G, Ho VC, Berean K, Tron VA. Ultraviolet radiation induction of squamous cell carcinomas in p53 transgenic mice. *Cancer Res* 1995;55:2070.
62. Epstein JH, Epstein WL. Cocarcinogenic effect of ultraviolet light on DMBA tumor initiation in albino mice. *J Invest Dermatol* 1962;39:455.
63. Blum HF. Quantitative aspects of cancer induction by ultraviolet light: including a revised model. In: Urbach F, ed. *The biologic effects of ultraviolet radiation.* Oxford: Pergamon, 1969:543.
64. Pontén F, Berg C, Ahmadian A, et al. Molecular pathology in basal cell cancer with p53 as a genetic marker. *Oncogene* 1997;15:1059.
65. Pontén F, Berne B, Ren ZP, Nister M, Pontén J. Ultraviolet light induces expression of p53 and p21 in human skin: effect of sunscreen and constitutive p21 expression in skin appendages. *J Invest Dermatol* 1995;105:402.
66. Wolf P, Cox P, Yarosh DB, Kripke ML. Sunscreens and T4N5 liposomes differ in their ability to protect against ultraviolet-induced sunburn cell formation, alterations of dendritic epidermal cells, and local suppression of contact hypersensitivity. *J Invest Dermatol* 1995;104:287.
67. Ley RD, Fourtanier A. Sunscreen protection against ultraviolet radiation–induced pyrimidine dimers in mouse epidermal DNA. *Photochem Photobiol* 1997;65:1007.
68. Ananthaswamy HN, Loughlin SM, Cox P, et al. Sunlight and skin cancer: inhibition of *p53* mutations in UV-irradiated mouse skin by sunscreens. *Nature Med* 1997;3:510.
69. Freeman SE, Ley RD, Ley KD. Sunscreen protection against UV-induced pyrimidine dimers in DNA of human skin in situ. *Photodermatology* 1998;5:243.
70. Bestak R, Halliday GM. Sunscreens protect from UV-promoted squamous cell carcinoma in mice chronically irradiated with doses of UV radiation insufficient to cause edema. *Photochem Photobiol* 1996;64:188.
71. Ananthaswamy HN, Ullrich SE, Mascotto RE, et al. Inhibition of solar simulator-induced *p53* mutations and protection against skin cancer development in mice by sunscreens. *J Invest Dermatol* 1999;112:763.
72. Gasparro FP, Mitchnick M, Nash JF. A review of sunscreen safety and efficacy. *Photochem Photobiol* 1998;68:243.
73. Thompson SC, Jolley D, Marks R. Reduction of solar keratoses by regular sunscreen use. *N Engl J Med* 1993;329:1147.
74. Naylor MF, Boyd A, Smith DW, et al. High sun protection factor sunscreen in the suppression of actinic neoplasia. *Arch Dermatol* 1995;131:170.
75. Fujiwara T, Grimm EA, Mukhopadhyay T, et al. Induction of chemosensitivity in human lung cancer cells *in vivo* by adenovirus-mediated transfer of the wild-type *p53* gene. *Cancer Res* 1994;54:2287.
76. Lowe SW, Ruley HE, Jacks T, Houseman DE. p53-dependent apoptosis modulates the cytotoxicity of anticancer agents. *Cell* 1993;74:957.
77. Liu M, Pelling JC, Ju J, Chu E, Brash DE. Antioxidant action via p53-mediated apoptosis. *Cancer Res* 1998;58:1723.
78. Fujiwara T, Grimm EA, Mukhopadhyay T, et al. A retroviral wild-type *p53* expression vector penetrates human lung cancer spheroids and inhibits growth by inducing apoptosis. *Cancer Res* 1993;53:4129.
79. Hwang RF, Gordon EM, Anderson WF, Parekh D. Gene therapy for primary and metastatic pancreatic cancer with intraperitoneal retroviral vector bearing the wild-type p53 gene. *Surgery* 1998;124:143.
80. Hupp TR, Sparks A, Lane DP. Small peptides activate the latent sequence-specific DNA binding function of p53. *Cell* 1995;83:237.
81. Blagosklonny MV, Toretsky J, Neckers L. Geldanamycin selectively destabilizes and conformationally alters mutated p53. *Oncogene* 1995;11:933.
82. Yano H, Mizoguchi A, Fukuda K, et al. The herbal medicine sho-saiko-to inhibits proliferation of cancer cell lines by inducing apoptosis and arrest at the G_0/G_1 phase. *Cancer Res* 1994;54:448.
83. Chiao C, Crothers AM, Grunberger D, et al. Apoptosis and altered redox state induced by caffeic acid phenethyl ester (CAPE) in transformed rat fibroblast cells. *Cancer Res* 1995;55:3576.
84. James SJ, Muskhelishvili L. Rates of apoptosis and proliferation vary with caloric intake and may influence incidence of spontaneous hepatoma in C57BL/6 x C3H F_1 mice. *Cancer Res* 1994;54:5508.
85. Grasl-Kraupp B, Bursch W, Ruttkay-Nedecky B, et al. Food restriction eliminates preneoplastic cells through apoptosis and antagonizes carcinogenesis in rat liver. *Proc Natl Acad Sci U S A* 1994;91:9995.

SECTION **2**

DAVID J. LEFFELL
JOHN A. CARUCCI

Management of Skin Cancer

In 1999, approximately 1 million nonmelanoma skin cancers (NMSCs) were diagnosed in the United States.[1,2] One in five Americans will develop skin cancer during life, and more than 97% of these will be NMSCs.[3] Some studies suggest that development of NMSC, including basal cell (BCC) and squamous cell carcinoma (SCC), may indicate increased risk for internal malignancy.[3] However, the precise relationship between skin cancer and the risk of internal malignancy is not yet completely defined. The approach to diagnosis and management of common skin cancers, including BCC and SCC and other, less common tumors of follicular, neuroendocrine, and fibrohistiocytic origin, is discussed in this chapter.

DIAGNOSIS

Although many NMSCs present with classic clinical findings such as nodularity and erythema, definitive diagnosis can be made only by biopsy. Adequate tissue obtained in a nontraumatic fashion is critical to histopathologic diagnosis.

Skin biopsies may be performed by shave, punch, or fusiform excision. The type of biopsy performed should be based on the morphology of the primary lesion.[4] A shave biopsy usually is adequate for raised lesions such as nodular BCC, SCC, or tumors of follicular origin. Punch biopsy is effective for sampling flat, broad lesions for which shave or fusiform excision would be technically inappropriate. An excisional biopsy may be used to sample deep dermal and subcutaneous tissue. Excision is appropriate when it is necessary to distinguish between a benign lesion such as a dermatofibroma and a malignant tumor such as a dermatofibrosarcoma protuberans.

SHAVE BIOPSY

The basic techniques involved in performing skin biopsies are demonstrated in Figure 41.2-1. A shave biopsy is performed under clean conditions. Local anesthetic (lidocaine 1% with epinephrine 1:100,000, unless contraindicated) is injected with a 30-gauge needle. The use of a sterilized razor blade, which can be precisely manipulated by the operator to adjust the depth of the biopsy, often is superior to the use of a No. 15 scalpel. After the procedure, adequate hemostasis is achieved with topical application of aqueous aluminum chloride (20%) or electrocautery.

PUNCH BIOPSY

A punch biopsy is performed under local anesthesia, using a trephine or biopsy punch. The operator makes a circular incision to the level of the superficial fat, using a rotating motion of the trephine. Traction applied perpendicularly to the relaxed skin tension lines minimizes redundancy at closure. Hemostasis is achieved by placement of simple, nonabsorbable sutures that can be removed in 7 to 14 days depending on anatomic site. If the punch biopsy is small and not in a cosmetically important area, the wound will likely heal very well by second intention.

EXCISIONAL BIOPSY

After local anesthesia has been achieved under sterile conditions, a scalpel is used to incise a fusiform ellipse to the level of deep fat. Hemostasis is obtained with cautery as needed, and the wound is closed in a layered fashion using absorbable and nonabsorbable sutures. In most cases, postoperative care involves daily cleansing with mild soap and water followed by application of antibiotic ointment and a nonstick dressing. Though popular in the past, it is now known that hydrogen peroxide may not have a favorable effect on wound healing. The toxicity of hydrogen peroxide to keratinocytes has been well described,[5,6] and its use as an adjuvant to wound care is, in our opinion, contraindicated.

GENERAL APPROACH TO MANAGEMENT OF SKIN CANCER

The management of skin cancer depends on the histologic nature of the tumor, the anatomic site, the underlying medical status of the patient, and whether the tumor is primary or recurrent. Because specific management varies with histologic diagnosis, an accurate interpretation of biopsy specimens is essential. Though the majority of BCCs and SCCs are straightforward, identification of the histologic subtypes is important because it can guide proper treatment. Depending on the aggressiveness of the tumor, cancers of the skin may be excised or, in some cases of superficial tumors or precancerous lesions, destroyed in a nonexcisional fashion. Electrodesiccation and curettage is the most common nonexcisional approach. If a cancer requires excision, the two options are conventional excisional surgery or extirpation by Mohs micrographic surgery (MMS).

EXCISION

Excisional surgery involves removal of the cancer and a margin of clinically uninvolved tissue, followed by layered closure or second-intention healing, as indicated. Frozen or permanent sections interpreted by the pathologist determine adequacy of margins. Margins are assessed from representative sections of the specimen in "breadloaf" fashion, allowing for examination of approximately 3% of the excisional margin of the specimen. This degree of examination may occasionally result in a false-negative assessment of clear margins in cases of infiltrating or aggressive-growth cancers. Similar misdiagnosis may result when one relies on vertically cut frozen specimens for intraoperative margin control. Excision, especially that performed in a physician's office rather than a hospital operating room, is effective and cost-efficient when the cancer is small (<1 cm), nonrecurrent, or noninfiltrative.

MOHS MICROGRAPHIC SURGERY

MMS facilitates optimal margin control and conservation of normal tissue in the management of NMSC.[7–9] Individuals specially trained in the technique perform MMS in an office setting under local anesthesia. Briefly, after gentle curettage, a tangential specimen of tumor with a minimal margin of clinically normal-

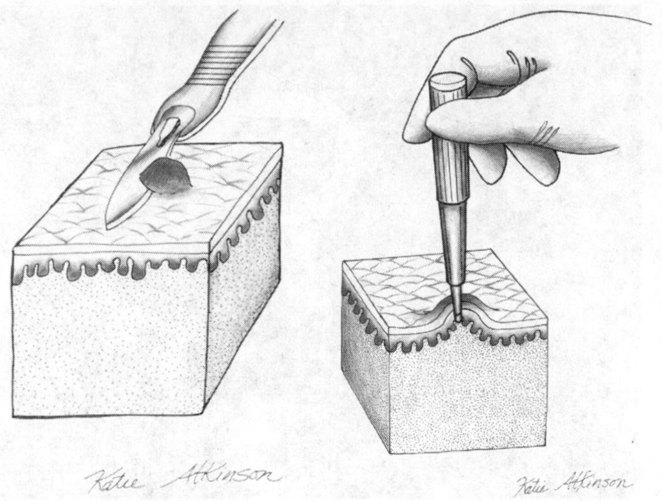

A,B

FIGURE 41.2-1. Biopsy techniques. **A:** Shave biopsy. A scalpel blade is precisely manipulated by the operator to adjust the depth of the biopsy, and hemostasis is achieved with topical application of aqueous aluminum chloride (20%), ferric chloride (25%), or electrocautery. **B:** Punch biopsy. The operator makes a circular incision to the level of the superficial fat using a rotating motion of the trephine. Traction applied perpendicularly to the relaxed skin tension lines minimizes redundancy at closure. Hemostasis is achieved by placement of sutures.

appearing tissue is obtained, precisely mapped, and processed immediately by frozen section for microscopical examination (Fig. 41.2-2). Optimal margin control is obtained by examination of the entire perimeter of the specimen and contiguous deep margin. Meticulous mapping allows for directed extirpation of any remaining tumor. A key defining feature of MMS is that the surgeon excises, maps, and reviews the specimen personally, minimizing the chance of error in tissue interpretation and orientation. MMS has gained acceptance as the treatment of choice for recurrent skin cancers as well as for primary skin cancers located on anatomic sites that require maximal tissue conservation for preservation of function and cosmesis.[10–13]

CURETTAGE AND ELECTRODESSICATION

Common methods of skin cancer destruction include curettage and electrodesiccation (C&D) and cryotherapy using liquid nitrogen.[14–19] C&D is performed under clean conditions with local anesthesia. Visible tumor is first removed by curettage. Curettage is extended for a margin of 2 to 4 mm beyond the clinical borders of the cancer. Electrodesiccation then is performed to destroy another 1 mm of tissue at the lateral and deep margins. Salasche[20] recommended that C&D be performed for three cycles. Others report satisfactory results after a single cycle of C&D for tumors smaller than 1 cm. Although this leads to decreased scarring, it may lead to higher rates of recurrence, as suggested by Robins and Albom,[21] who attributed to insufficiently aggressive treatment the higher rates of recurrence observed in young women with BCC. Tangential shave excision followed by gentle curettage and cauterization is an effective treatment approach for destruction of superficial BCCs.

CRYOSURGERY

Cryosurgery exposes skin cancers to subzero temperatures, which causes tissue destruction (Fig. 41.2-3). Heat transfer occurs from the skin, which acts as a heat sink. Tissue damage is caused by direct effects initially and, subsequently, by vascular stasis, ice crystal formation, cell membrane disruption, pH changes, and thermal shock. Successful cryosurgery requires that temperatures reach –50° to –60°C, including deep and lateral margins. The subsequent thaw leads to vascular stasis and failure of local microcirculation. The open-spray technique is used most often and requires liquid nitrogen spray delivery from a distance of 1 to 3 cm. With the confined-spray technique, liquid nitrogen is delivered through a cone that is open at both ends. With the closed-cone technique, one end of the cone is closed and a shorter delivery time is required. With the cryoprobe technique, a prechilled metal probe is applied to the tumor. Delivery time is determined via a depth-dose estimation, which takes into account freeze time, lateral spread, and halo thaw time. Immediately after cryosurgery, local erythema and edema are apparent. An exudative phase ensues in 24 to 72 hours, which is followed by sloughing at approximately day 7. Complete healing usually is seen with facial lesions at 4 to 6 weeks and in nearly 12 to 14 weeks in lesions on the trunk and extremities.

Temporary complications may include extensive drainage, edema, bulla formation, and hypertrophic scarring. Rarely, delayed hemorrhage can occur suddenly approximately 2 weeks after the procedure, most commonly after treatment on the nose, temple, and forehead. Paresthesia may occur if superficial nerves are frozen. Other less common side effects may include headache, syncope, febrile reaction, cold urticaria, pyogenic granuloma, milia formation, or hyperpigmentation. Permanent complications may include tissue contraction, hypopigmentation, and scarring. Other less frequently reported complications are neuropathy, ulceration, tendon rupture, alopecia, and ectropion. Cryosurgery is not considered the standard of care for recurrent NMSC or any tumor other than very small, superficial BCC or SCC.

Cryosurgery and C&D both are limited by the inability to evaluate thoroughness of tumor eradication. The absence of margin control and the development of dense scar, which might obscure recurrence, make these methods valuable primarily in the care of histologically superficial NMSC. Close follow-up of the patient is necessary.

RADIATION THERAPY

Radiation therapy (RT) is a treatment option for NMSC but is also limited by the inability to confirm the tumor margins definitively. In addition, treatment of an excessively large area around the tumor carries risk. RT, in properly fractionated doses, generally is indicated when the patient's health or size or extent of the tumor precludes surgical extirpation. Consideration of the permanent tissue effects of RT must include anticipation and management of recurrence.

After treatment for BCC or SCC, patients should be evaluated on an annual basis for the presence of skin cancers. In the case of a more aggressive tumor, evaluation should be more frequent and, in the case of squamous cell cancer, should include examination of draining lymph nodes. Laboratory evaluation, generally not indicated in uncomplicated cases of BCC and SCC, may be necessary for other types of particularly aggressive tumors. Imaging studies may be necessary in the case of aggressive tumors or in cases of long-neglected tumors

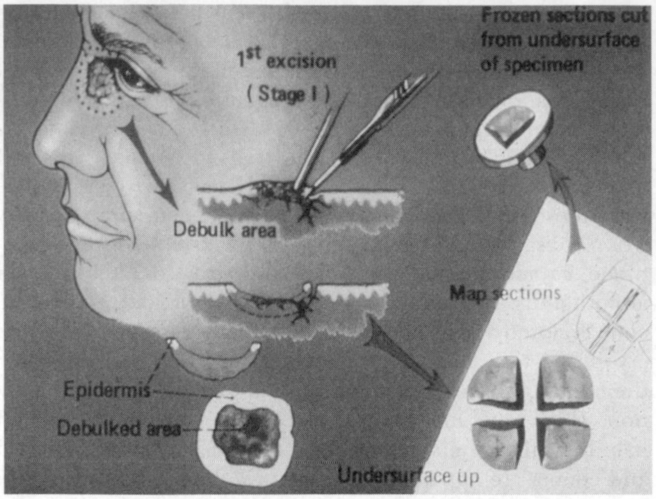
Frozen sections cut
from undersurface
of specimen
1st excision
(Stage I)
Debulk area
Map sections
Epidermis
Debulked area
Undersurface up
A

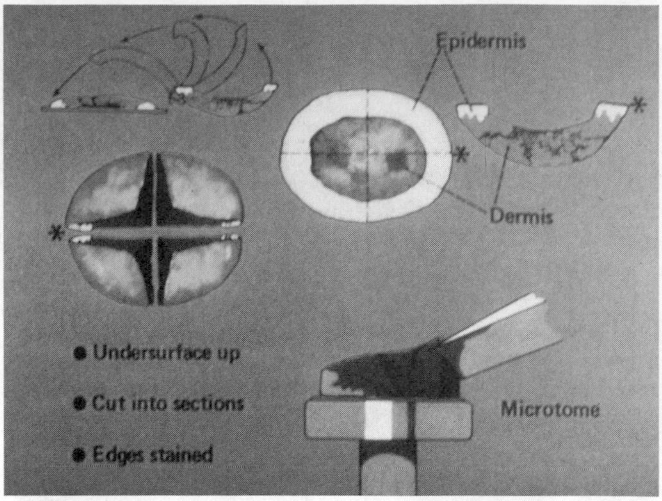
Epidermis
Dermis
Undersurface up
Cut into sections
Edges stained
Microtome
B

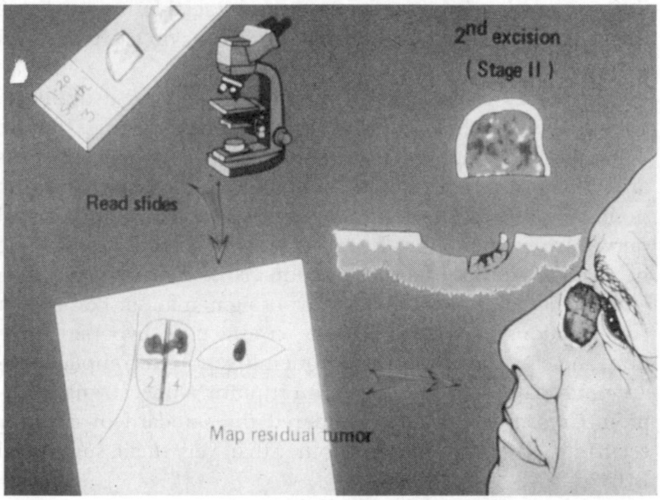
2nd excision
(Stage II)
Read slides
Map residual tumor
C

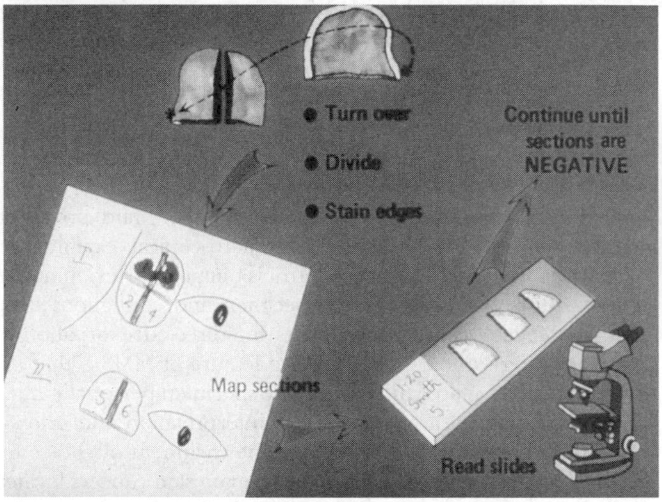
Turn over
Divide
Stain edges
Continue until
sections are
NEGATIVE
Map sections
Read slides
D

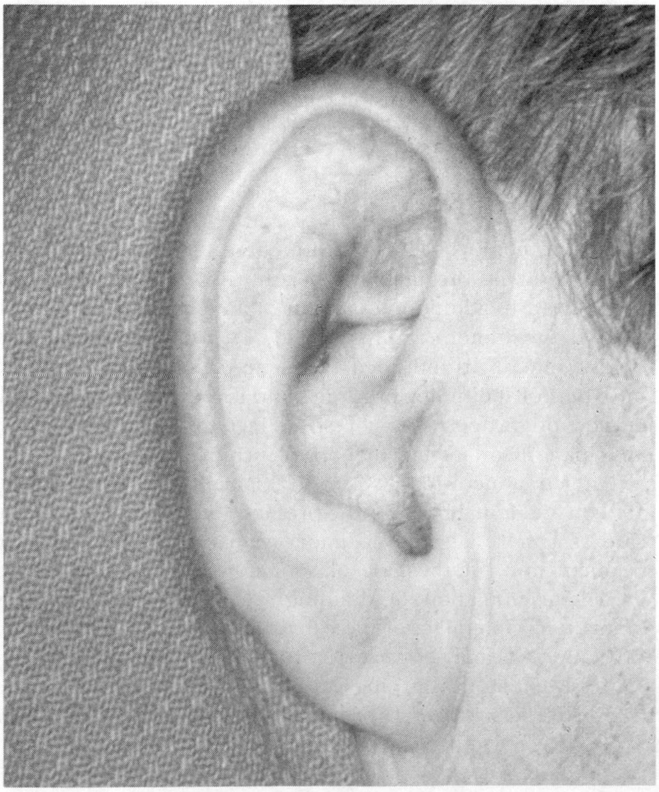
E

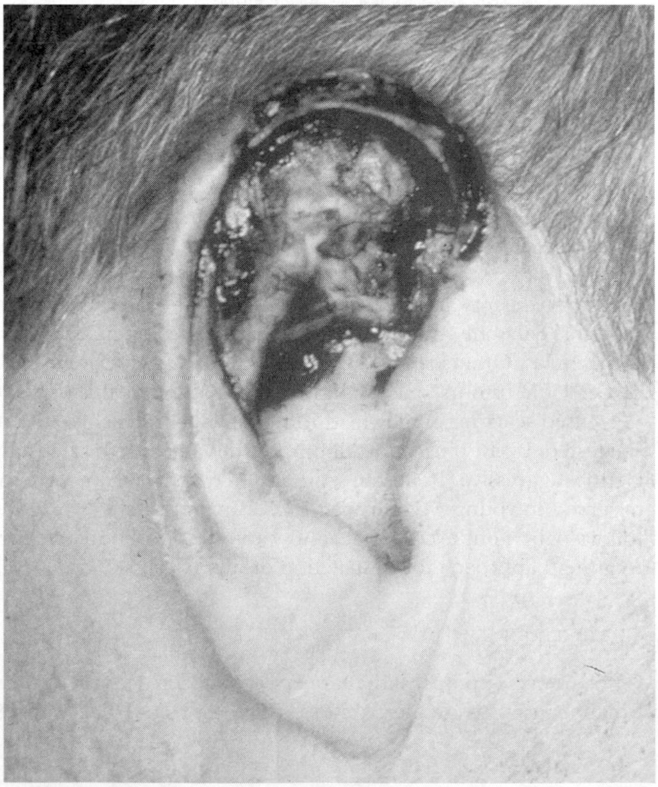
F

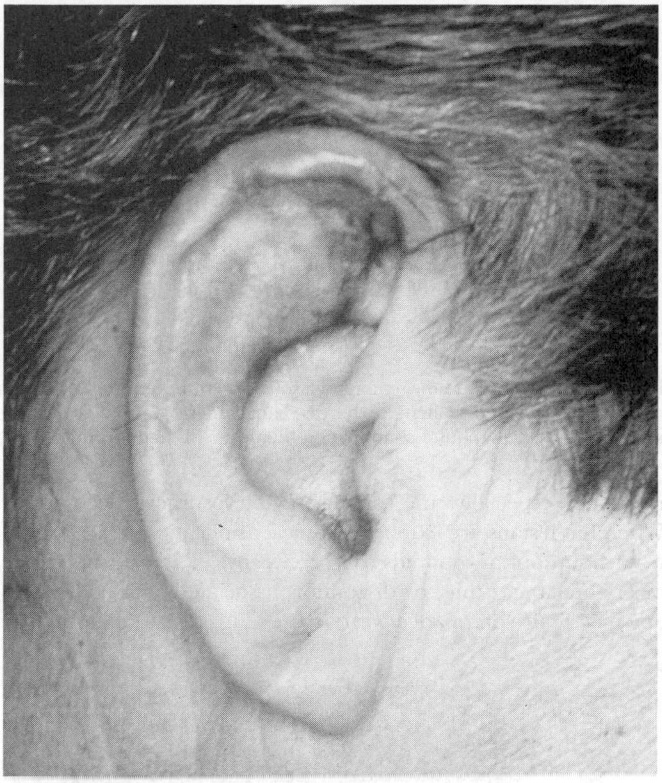

G

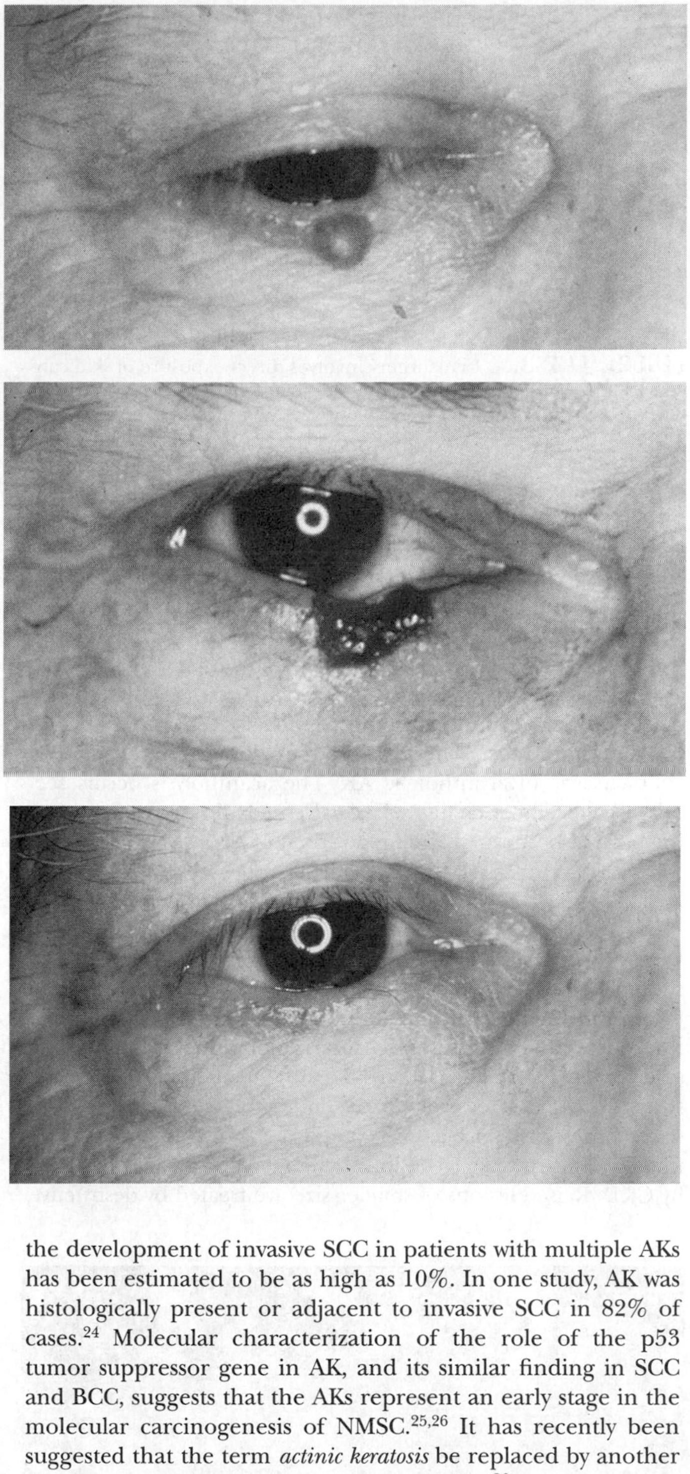

H

I

J

FIGURE 41.2-2. Mohs micrographic surgery. **A–D:** After gentle curettage, a tangential specimen of tumor with a minimal margin of clinically normal-appearing tissue is obtained, precisely mapped, and processed immediately by frozen section for microscopical examination. Superior margin control is obtained through examination of the entire perimeter of the specimen. Precise mapping allows for directed extirpation of any remaining tumor. (Courtesy of Neil A. Swanson, M.D.) **E–G:** Conservation of cartilage allowed for retention of normal contour after healing in this case of basal cell carcinoma involving the ear, which was treated by Mohs micrographic surgery. **H–J:** In tumors involving the eyelid, conservation of normal tissue and superior margin control are essential. Note second intention healing. (See Color Fig. 41.2-2 in the CD-ROM and on the Web at www.LWWoncology.com.)

impinging on vital structures. Magnetic resonance imaging allows visualization of the soft tissues, while computed tomography (CT) scan may be used to evaluate involvement of bone. In general, imaging studies have not proven helpful in definitively evaluating the presence of perineural invasion by NMSC.

NONMELANOMA SKIN CANCER AND PRECANCEROUS LESIONS

ACTINIC KERATOSIS

Actinic keratoses (AKs) are very common lesions that tend to occur on sun-exposed areas in blond or red-haired, fair-skinned, individuals with green or blue eyes.[22] Although not invasive, AKs are considered by some dermatopathologists to be SCC *in situ.*

AKs are caused by exposure to ultraviolet B light (UVB), and the possibility for progression to invasive SCC exists.[22] The risk for transformation of a single AK has been estimated to be as low as 1 per 1000 per year.[23] However, the long-term risk of the development of invasive SCC in patients with multiple AKs has been estimated to be as high as 10%. In one study, AK was histologically present or adjacent to invasive SCC in 82% of cases.[24] Molecular characterization of the role of the p53 tumor suppressor gene in AK, and its similar finding in SCC and BCC, suggests that the AKs represent an early stage in the molecular carcinogenesis of NMSC.[25,26] It has recently been suggested that the term *actinic keratosis* be replaced by another term, such as *solar keratotic intraepidermal SCC.*[26]

Clinical Features

AKs are red, pink, or brown papules with a scaly to hyperkeratotic surface (Fig. 41.2-4). They occur on sun-exposed areas and are especially common on the balding scalp, forehead, face, and dorsal hands. A hypertrophic, indurated variant [hyperplastic AK (HAK)] exists and may be difficult to distinguish from SCC.

The microscopical spectrum of AK includes hyperplastic, atrophic, bowenoid, acantholytic, and pigmented subtypes.[27] In

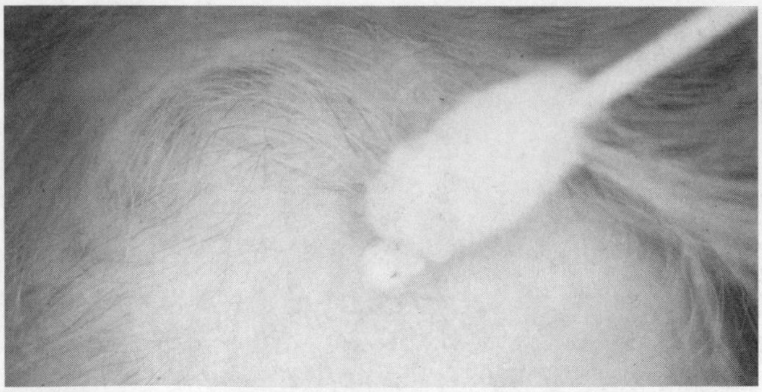

FIGURE 41.2-3. Cryosurgery involves direct exposure of skin cancers to subzero temperatures to cause destruction. (See Color Fig. 41.2-3 in the CD-ROM and on the Web at www.LWWoncology.com.)

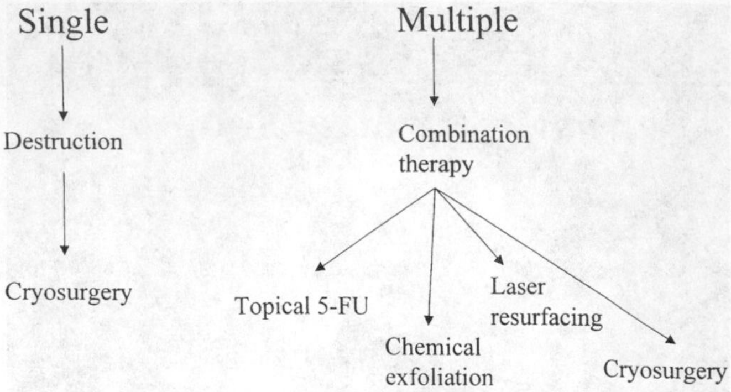

FIGURE 41.2-5. Management of a solitary actinic keratosis does not present a therapeutic challenge, whereas management of multiple actinic keratoses is likely to require combination therapy. 5-FU, 5-fluorouracil.

each subtype, disordered, atypical keratinocytes with nuclear atypia are seen. In the hyperplastic variant, pronounced hyperkeratosis is intermingled with parakeratosis. Epidermal hyperplasia and downward displacement without dermal invasion are present. A thin epidermis devoid of rete ridges characterizes the atrophic variant. Atypical cells predominate in the basal layer. The bowenoid AK is indistinguishable from Bowen's disease, also known as SCC *in situ*. In this variant, considerable epidermal cell disorder and clumping of nuclei exist, giving a windblown appearance. The presence of suprabasal lacunae is characteristic of acantholytic AK. The acantholysis occurs secondarily to cellular changes. Excessive melanin is present within the basal layer in the pigmented variant of AK.

Treatment

Due to their potential to develop into invasive SCC, AKs usually should be treated. Numerous destructive options are available for the treatment of AKs, including cryosurgery, C&D, topical 5-fluorouracil (5-FU), chemical cauterization using trichloroacetic acid, or excision (Fig. 41.2-5). Treatment of solitary lesions is straightforward. However, management of patients with hundreds of lesions can become complicated. In this situation, we initially treat the largest lesions by tangential excision followed by C&D. Raised lesions of smaller size are treated by destructive methods, especially the open-spray cryosurgery technique. When flat lesions are extensive, topical application of 5-FU with or without topical retinoids can be effective. The clinical effects of erythema, crusting, or discomfort associated with 5-FU therapy may limit compliance with its use (Fig. 41.2-6). Alternative

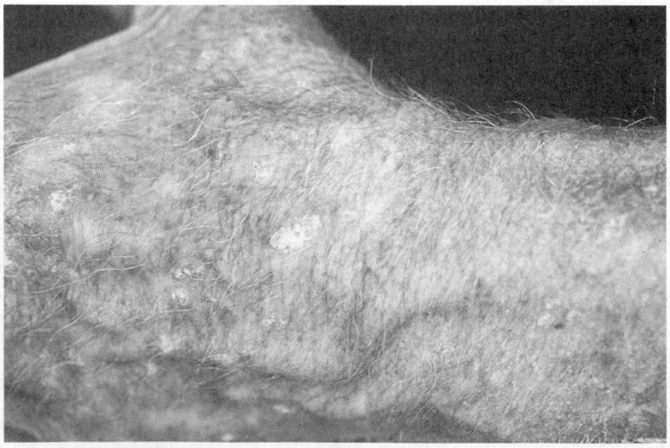

FIGURE 41.2-4. Actinic keratoses are characterized by erythema and rough surface. (See Color Fig. 41.2-4 in the CD-ROM and on the Web at www.LWWoncology.com.)

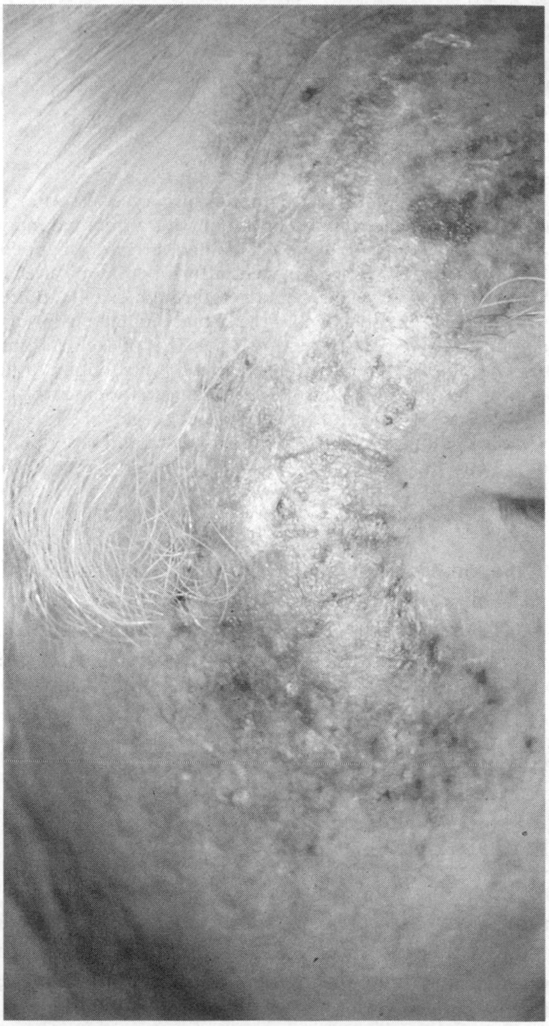

FIGURE 41.2-6. Erythema, crusting, and discomfort secondary to the use of topical 5-fluorouracil limit compliance with its use. (See Color Fig. 41.2-6 in the CD-ROM and on the Web at www.LWWoncology.com.)

specialized deepithelializing techniques, such as laser and chemical exfoliation, may be helpful in the patient with severe solar damage and extensive AKs. Regardless of the treatment used, because AK is a clonal disease that results from exposure to UVB, the chance for developing new lesions over time is clinically significant.

BASAL CELL CARCINOMA

BCC is a neoplasm of nonkeratinizing cells originating in the basal cell layer of the epidermis.[28] BCC is the most common human cancer, accounting for approximately 75% of all NMSCs and almost one-fourth of all cancers diagnosed in the United States.[29,30] Characteristically, BCC develops on sun-exposed areas of lighter-skinned individuals, with 30% of lesions occurring on the nose. Men are affected only slightly more often than are women and, although once rare before the age of 50, BCCs are becoming more common in younger individuals.[1,31]

The pathogenesis of BCC most commonly involves exposure to ultraviolet light (UVL),[32] particularly rays in the UVB spectrum (290 to 320 nm), which triggers mutations in tumor suppressor genes.[25,32–40] Other factors that appear to be involved in the pathogenesis include mutations in regulatory genes, exposure to ionizing radiation, and alterations in immune surveillance.[41–50]

BCC is a feature of inherited conditions. Included among these are the nevoid basal call carcinoma syndrome (NBCCS), Bazex syndrome, Rombo syndrome, and unilateral basal cell nevus syndrome.[42,47,51] Patients with NBCCS may exhibit a broad nasal root, borderline intelligence, jaw cysts, palmar pits, and multiple skeletal abnormalities in addition to hundreds of BCCs (Fig. 41.2-7).[52] In one case, bilateral cystic adrenal lymphangiomas have been reported in association with NBCCS.[53] Recently, studies have indicated an association with mutations in the PTCH regulatory gene.[42,54–56] In addition, mutations in the PTCH gene have been identified in sporadic nonfamilial BCC.[55]

Bazex syndrome is transmitted in an X-linked dominant fashion. Patients present with multiple BCCs, follicular atrophoderma, dilated follicular ostia with ice-pick scars, hypotrichosis, and hypohidrosis.

In contrast, Rombo syndrome is transmitted in an autosomal dominant fashion. Patients present with vermiculate atrophoderma, milia, hypertrichosis, trichoepitheliomas, BCCs, and peripheral vasodilation. Hypohidrosis is not a feature of Rombo syndrome. Patients with unilateral basal cell nevus syndrome present with a congenital, unilateral lesion of comedones and epidermoid cysts, with basal cell proliferations that are thought to be basaloid follicular hamartomas.

The role of the immune system in the pathogenesis of skin cancer that is not completely understood.[46,57] Immunosuppressed patients with lymphoma or leukemia[58,59] and patients who have undergone transplants[60–64] experience a marked increase in the incidence of SCC but only a slight increase in BCC development. A potential link between UVL and immune surveillance has been suggested by Gutierrez-Steil et al., who demonstrated that UVL-induced BCC tumor cells express Fas ligand (CD95L) and further showed that these cells were associated with CD95-bearing T cells undergoing apoptosis.[63] This represents a potential mechanism by which UVL might mediate the tumor cells' avoidance of cytotoxic T lymphocytes. Patients with depressed cellular immunity secondary to human immunodeficiency virus (HIV) infection show a higher frequency of infiltrative BCC.[64,65]

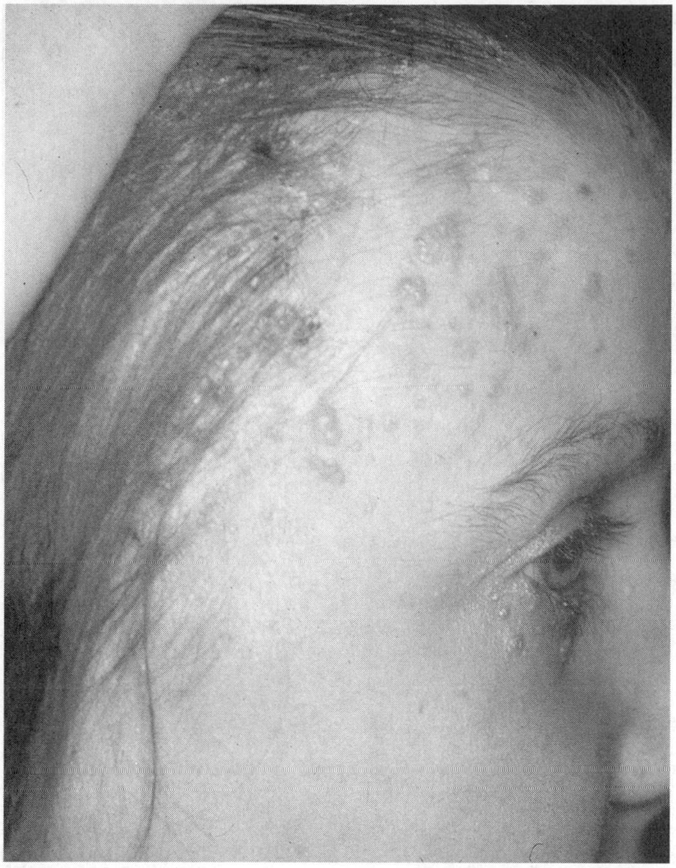

FIGURE 41.2-7. Nevoid basal cell carcinoma syndrome. Patients with this syndrome can present with hundreds of superficial basal cell carcinomas. (See Color Fig. 41.2-7 in the CD-ROM and on the Web at www.LWWoncology.com.)

Clinical Behavior of Basal Cell Cancer

BCC is associated with extremely low metastatic potential, but it does invade locally. This biologic behavior depends upon angiogenic factors, stromal conditions, and the propensity for the cancer to follow anatomic paths of least resistance.[66] BCCs can elicit angiogenic factors that account for the telangiectatic vessels characteristically seen on the tumor's surface.[68] Necrosis occurs in tumors that have outgrown their blood supply. Recently, tumor microcirculation was examined *in vivo* in 12 BCCs from the head and neck by Bedlow et al.[67] Mean blood vessel size, density, and length per unit area were increased in BCC in comparison to normal tissue. An earlier study showed that mean vessel counts were increased in SCCs versus BCCs,[68] suggesting that angiogenesis may be linked to biologic aggressiveness and that antiangiogenic factors may play a potential therapeutic role in the treatment of aggressive BCCs.

Tumor stroma is critical for both initiating and maintaining the development of BCC.[66] Transplants of neoplasms devoid of stroma usually are unsuccessful. In one study, Hernandez et al.[69] demonstrated that cultured BCC tumor cells stimulated collagenase production by fibroblasts. The concept of stromal dependence is supported by the low incidence of metastatic BCC.

BCC has a tendency to grow along the path of least resistance. Invasive BCC can migrate along the perichondrium, periosteum, fascia, or tarsal plate.[66] This type of spread accounts for higher recurrence rates noted in tumors involving the eyelid, nose, and

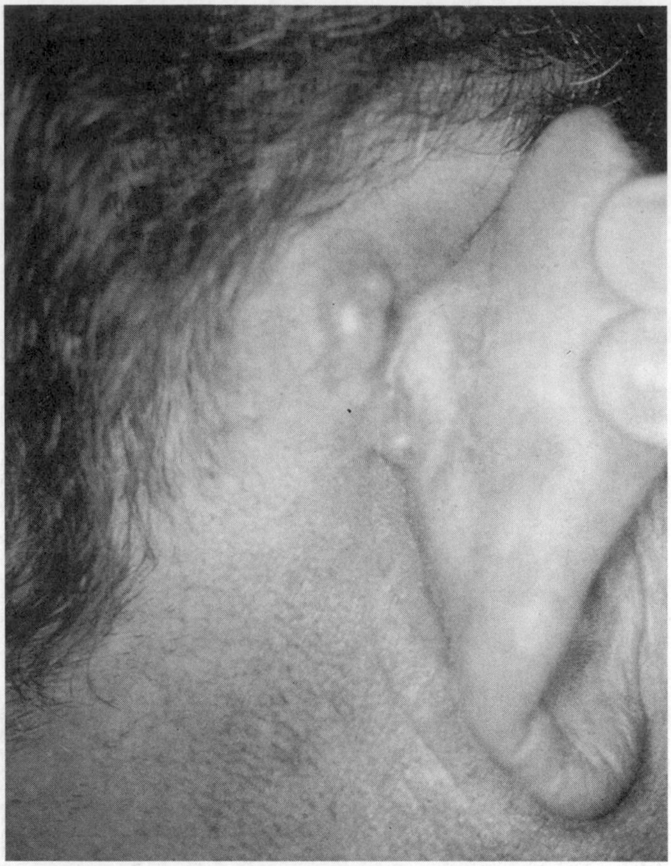

FIGURE 41.2-8. Recurrent nodular basal cell carcinoma. Embryonic fusion planes offer little resistance to tumor spread. (See Color Fig. 41.2-8 in the CD-ROM and on the Web at www.LWWoncology.com.)

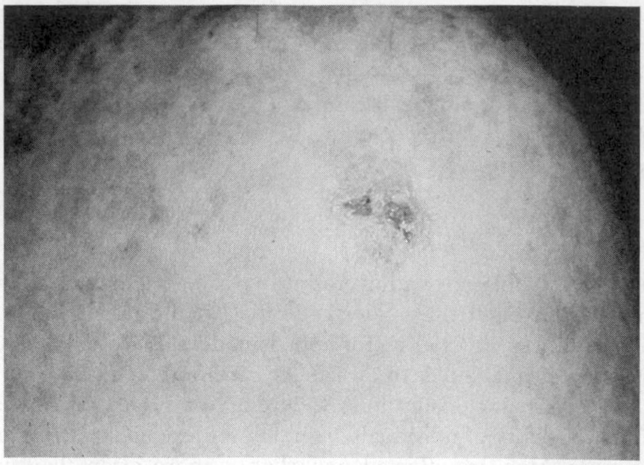

FIGURE 41.2-9. Superficial basal cell carcinoma presents as an erythematous patch and may be difficult to distinguish from dermatitis. (See Color Fig. 41.2-9 in the CD-ROM and on the Web at www.LWWoncology.com.)

scalp not treated by MMS. Embryonic fusion planes offer little resistance and can lead to deep invasion and tumor spread, with very high rates of recurrence, if complete tumor extirpation is not achieved (Fig. 41.2-8). The most susceptible areas include the inner canthus, philtrum, middle to lower chin, nasolabial groove, preauricular area, and the retroauricular sulcus.[66]

Perineural spread is uncommon and occurs most often in recurrent, aggressive lesions.[70–74] In one series, Niazi and Lamberty[74] noted perineural invasion in 0.178% of BCC. In all cases, perineural extension was associated with recurrent tumors that were most often located in the periauricular and malar areas. Perineural invasion may present with paresthesia, pain, and weakness or, in some cases, paralysis.[74,76,77] Involvement of the cranial nerves and, in one case, thoracic spine has been reported.[71,75–77] Metastatic BCC is rare, with incidence rates varying from 0.0028% to 0.1%.[78–80] Metastases, when reported, have involved lung, lymph nodes, esophagus, oral cavity, and skin.[80–86] Although long-term survival has been reported, the prognosis for metastatic BCC is generally poor, survival of 8 to 10 months after diagnosis being the norm.[86] Platinum-based chemotherapy appears to have some effect in the treatment of metastatic BCC.[87,88]

Basal Cell Carcinoma Subtypes

Clinical variants of BCC include nodular, superficial, morpheaform (also termed *aggressive-growth BCC* or *infiltrative BCC*), pigmented, and cystic BCC, and fibroepithelioma of Pinkus (FEP) (Figs. 41.2-9 through 41.2-15).[28–30,89,90] Nodular BCC presents as a raised, translucent papule or nodule, with telangiectasia, and has a propensity for involving sun-exposed areas of the face. Superficial BCC commonly presents as an erythematous scaly or eroded macule on the trunk and may be difficult to differentiate clinically from AK, SCC *in situ*, or a benign inflammatory lesion. Not uncommonly, superficial BCC may be mistakenly treated without response as eczema or even psoriasis. Biopsy in such cases is definitive. Morpheaform BCC presents as a flat, slightly firm lesion, without well-demarcated borders, and may be difficult to differentiate from a scar. The aggressive growth pattern of this subtype is highlighted by the fact that the actual size of the cancer is usually much greater than the clinical extent of the tumor. Pigmented BCC is a variant of nodular BCC and may be difficult to differentiate from nodular melanoma. The presence of pigment may be of value in determining adequate margins for excision. FEP usually presents as a pink papule on the lower back.[91] It may be difficult to distinguish clinically from amelanotic melanoma.

Histologic subtypes of BCC include superficial, nodular, and infiltrative BCC.[89,92] All BCC subtypes tend to share certain histologic characteristics. These include peripheral palisading of large, basophilic cells, nuclear atypia, and retraction from surrounding stroma. Nodular BCC accounts for approximately 50% of BCCs and is characterized by the presence of tumor cells in rounded masses within the dermis (see Fig. 41.2-14). Peripheral palisading of nuclei is prominent, and surrounding retraction artifact may be present. Groups of cells may be solid, or there may be dermal necrosis or degradation, with formation of cysts or microcysts. The stroma is characteristically coarse and myxoid. If nodules measure less than 15 µm, the tumor may be called *micronodular.* Infiltrative histology is seen in 15% to 20% of BCCs and represents that subclass of BCCs referred to as *aggressive-growth* tumors. Tumor cells manifest irregular outlines with a spiky appearance. Palisading is characteristically absent. The stroma is less myxoid than in the nodular form. In the morpheaform variant, which accounts for approximately 5% of BCCs, small groups or cords of tumor cells infiltrate a dense, collagenous stroma parallel to the skin surface (see Fig. 41.2-11*B*). Superficial multifocal BCC accounts for approximately 15% of

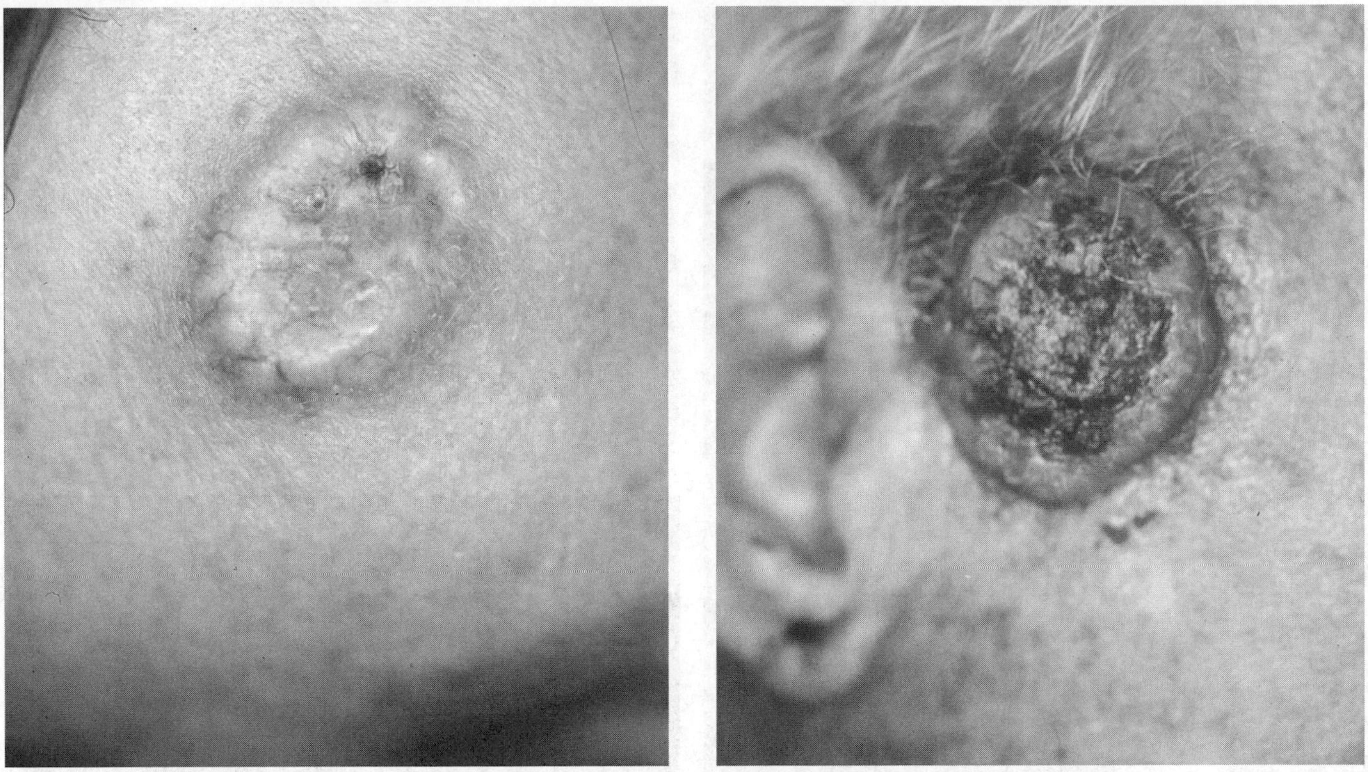

A B

FIGURE 41.2-10. Nodular basal cell carcinoma. **A:** A red, translucent nodule with rolled border, as seen here, is a classic presentation of nodular basal cell carcinoma. **B:** Nodular basal cell carcinoma demonstrating ulceration. (See Color Fig. 41.2-10 in the CD-ROM and on the Web at www.LWWoncology.com.)

BCCs and is characterized by basophilic buds extending from the epidermis. Retraction artifact is present, as is peripheral palisading within the buds. FEP, which accounts for 1% of BCCs, is characterized by a polypoid lesion in which basaloid cells grow downward from the surface in a network of anastomoses of cords of cells in loose connective tissue. Mixed histology is apparent in approximately 15% of BCCs.

The significance of histologic subtype lies in the correlation with biologic aggressiveness. The infiltrative and micronodular types are the most likely to be incompletely removed by conventional excision. Rates of incomplete excision vary from 5% to 17%. Incompletely excised infiltrative and micronodular BCCs may recur at rates of 33% to 39%. Recurrences after RT show a tendency toward infiltrative histology and evidence of squamous transformation, and even recurrent BCC after excision or C&D may become metatypical. In general, recurrences are more frequent in BCCs with infiltrative and micronodular histology, when clear margins are less than 0.38 mm, and in the presence of squamous differentiation. Although historical reports in the literature[66] suggested that 60% of incompletely excised BCCs will not recur, none of these studies provided an appraisal of recurrence rates as a function of histologic subtype. In general, incompletely excised BCCs should be removed completely, preferably by MMS, especially if they occur in anatomically critical areas such as the central zone of the face, retroauricular sulcus, or periocular area.

Adequate treatment of BCC requires appreciation of the histopathologic pattern of the neoplasm. Though some BCCs are small and superficial and behave in essentially a "biologically benign" manner as long as they are conservatively removed, others behave more aggressively and thus require more aggressive treatment. Examples of the latter include clinical BCCs that ulcerate and those located in the central face or on the ear. Furthermore, BCCs that show an aggressive growth pattern histologically require definitive treatment with confirmation of histologically negative margins.

Occasionally, it may appear that a BCC has been adequately removed by biopsy alone, leading to the question of whether to render further treatment. In one study, 41 consecutive patients with 42 BCCs apparently removed by biopsy were treated by MMS, and blocks of tissue, sectioned consecutively until exhausted, were examined for the presence of residual tumor.[93] In 28 of 42 cases (66%), residual cancer was identified. The presence of residual cancer was not related to age, site, histologic subtype, or extent of surrounding inflammation. The results indicate that patients with small BCCs that appear to be completely removed by initial biopsy may be at risk for recurrence if not treated further.

Characteristics Related to Anatomic Site

BCCs may demonstrate unique characteristics based on anatomic site. The nose is the most common site for cutaneous malignancies (30%), and BCCs involving the nose may be aggressive. A study of 193 cases of infiltrative BCC involving the nose confirmed that the majority of infiltrating and recurrent BCCs affect the ala.[94] Analysis of the recurrences' aggressive local behavior indicated that recurrent lesions were subjected to inadequate therapy initially. In one study, 26 recurrences were identified in 71 nasal skin cancers at an average of 36 months after non-MMS excision.[95] This suggests that MMS may

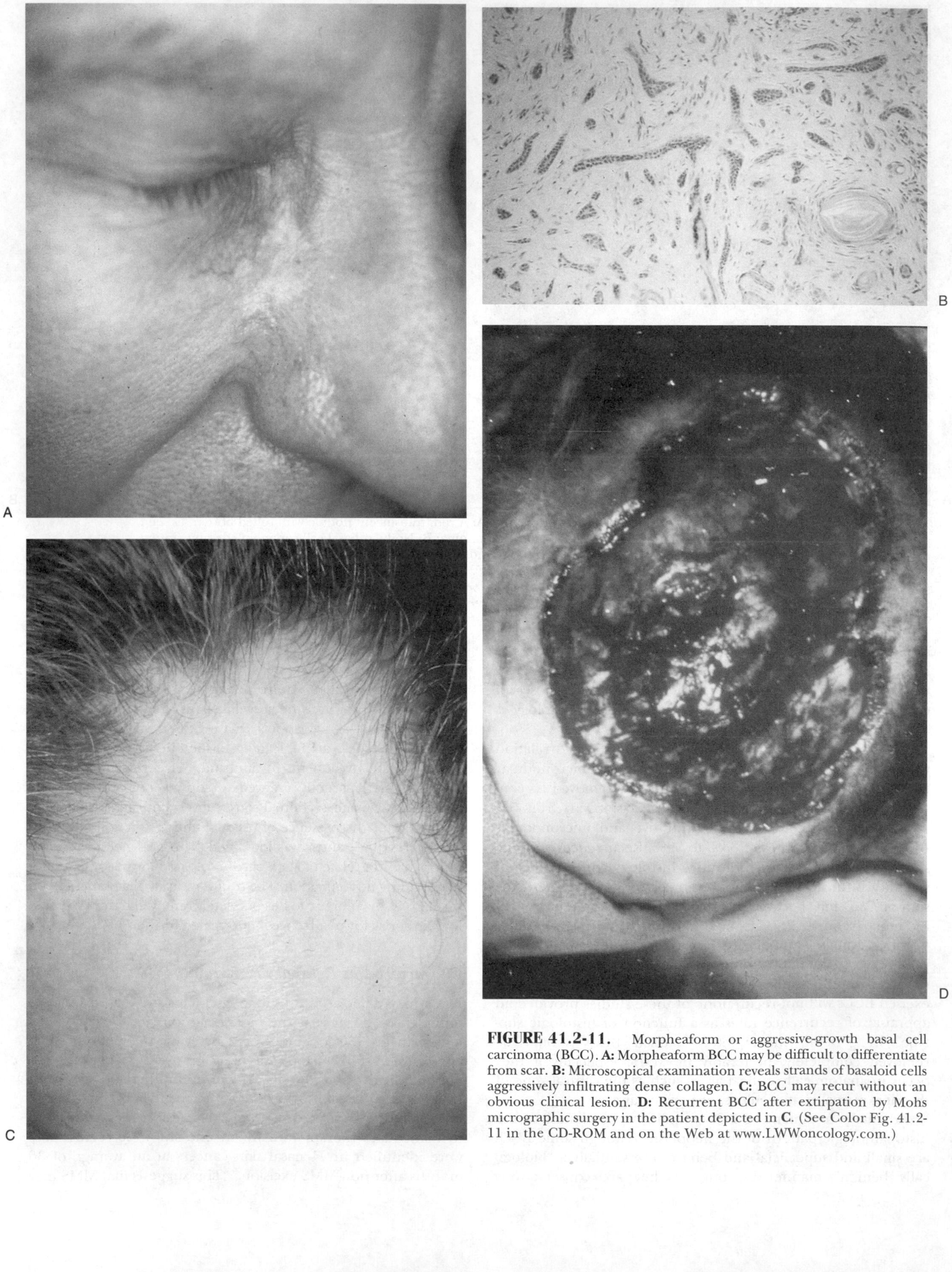

FIGURE 41.2-11. Morpheaform or aggressive-growth basal cell carcinoma (BCC). **A:** Morpheaform BCC may be difficult to differentiate from scar. **B:** Microscopical examination reveals strands of basaloid cells aggressively infiltrating dense collagen. **C:** BCC may recur without an obvious clinical lesion. **D:** Recurrent BCC after extirpation by Mohs micrographic surgery in the patient depicted in **C**. (See Color Fig. 41.2-11 in the CD-ROM and on the Web at www.LWWoncology.com.)

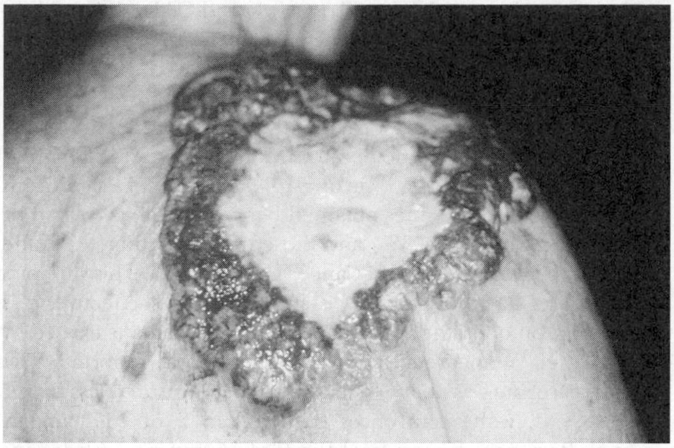

FIGURE 41.2-12. If neglected, basal cell carcinoma invades locally with devastating results. (Courtesy Neil A. Swanson, M.D.) (See Color Fig. 41.2-12 in the CD-ROM and on the Web at www.LWWoncology.com.)

be the treatment of choice for all BCCs involving the nose, especially those exhibiting aggressive growth characteristics.

Periocular BCC represents a significant therapeutic challenge. In one study, periocular BCC accounted for 7.3% of 3192 BCCs treated over a 10-year period.[10] Of these, 48.5% involved the medial canthus, 22.35% involved the lower eyelid, 10.7% involved the upper eyelid, and 5.6% involved the lateral canthus. BCC is the most common tumor affecting the eyelid. In a series of 97 cases of BCC involving the eyelid, 69% were nodular, 13% were infiltrative, 1% were ulcerated, and 12% were mixed (defined as having a significant nodular or ulcerative component in addition to an infiltrative component). Follow-up of 8 of 12 patients with mixed tumors revealed three recurrences. In one patient, orbital exenteration was required. This suggests that mixed tumors of the eyelid with aggressive growth histology warrant thorough treatment with complete margin control.

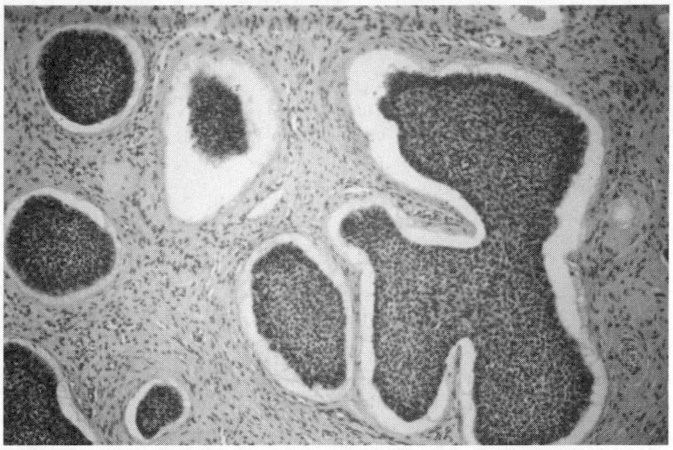

FIGURE 41.2-14. Nodular basal cell carcinoma (BCC). Microscopical examination of nodular BCC reveals islands of basophilic cells exhibiting typical BCC morphology. (See Color Fig. 41.2-14 in the CD-ROM and on the Web at www.LWWoncology.com.)

In a review of 24 eyelid tumors treated by MMS, high clearance rates were shown (100%), although follow-up was short (14.6 months).[11] In addition, 50% of patients were left with intact posterior lamellae, highlighting conservation of normal tissue. The results suggest that MMS followed by oculoplastic reconstruction, if necessary, is the preferred strategy in the management of periocular BCC.

Approximately 6% of BCCs involve the ear, a site notable for high rates of recurrence. In a recent study, nine patients with

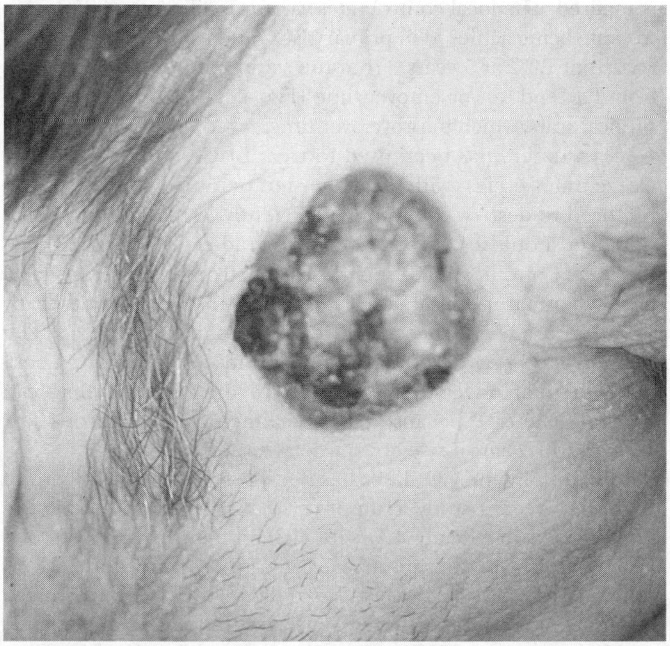

FIGURE 41.2-13. Pigmented basal cell carcinoma may be difficult to differentiate clinically from melanoma. (See Color Fig. 41.2-13 in the CD-ROM and on the Web at www.LWWoncology.com.)

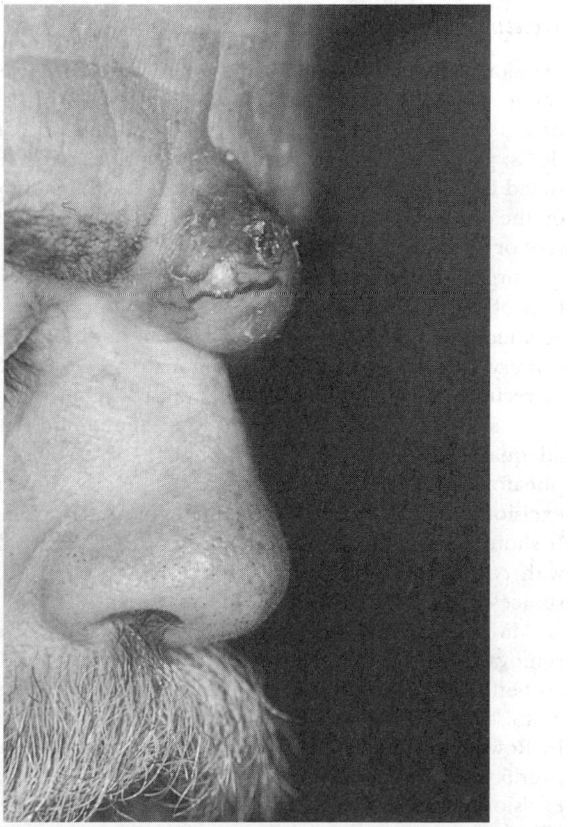

FIGURE 41.2-15. Cystic basal cell carcinoma. This variant may resemble an epidermal inclusion cyst. (See Color Fig. 41.2-15 in the CD-ROM and on the Web at www.LWWoncology.com.)

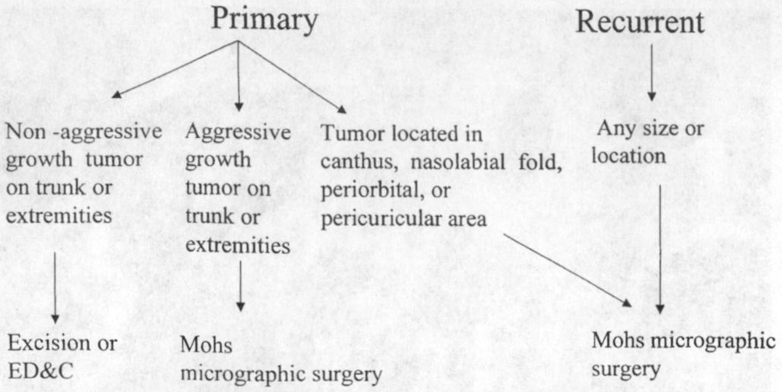

FIGURE 41.2-16. Primary basal cell carcinomas may be managed by electrodessication curettage (ED&C), excision or Mohs micrographic surgery, depending on histology, size, and anatomic location. Recurrent basal cell carcinomas should be treated by Mohs micrographic surgery.

BCC involving the conchal bowl were treated by an interdisciplinary approach.[96] In each case, tumor extirpation was accomplished by MMS, and an otolaryngologist was available in the event of temporal bone involvement. There were no cases of recurrence at mean follow-up of 1 year.

It must be stressed that BCC can occur anywhere, even in non–sun-exposed areas, and has been reported to occur on the vulva, penis, scrotum, and perianal area.[97–101] In one series of vulvar BCC, mean age at presentation was 74 years. Patients have been seen with a history of local irritation that had been present for a few months to several years.

Treatment

Excisional surgery, C&D, and cryosurgery have been used to treat circumscribed, noninfiltrating BCCs (Fig. 41.2-16).[102] MMS is the treatment method of choice for all recurrent and infiltrative BCCs, particularly if a tumor is located on the face.[103] RT is best suited for older patients, particularly those with extensive lesions on the ear, lower limbs, or eyelids.[104] RT is not indicated for recurrent or morpheaform lesions.

Surgical excision offers the advantage of histologic evaluation of the excised specimen. Although appropriate for management of most BCCs, cure rates for traditional excisional surgery are inferior to those for tumors treated by MMS in cases of recurrent BCC, infiltrative BCC, and BCC in high-risk anatomic sites.[16] It has been demonstrated that 4-mm margins are adequate for removal of BCC in 98% of cases of nonmorpheaform BCC of less than 2 cm in diameter.[105] Extending the excision into fat generally is adequate for a small primary BCC. It should be noted that the majority of BCCs are well treated with conventional excision or C&D. However, in the circumstances just outlined, MMS is especially helpful.

MMS permits superior histologic verification of complete removal, allows maximum conservation of tissue, and remains cost-effective as compared to traditional excisional surgery for NMSCs.[7,12,102,106] In a large study of treatment of primary BCC by Rowe et al.,[107] MMS demonstrated a recurrence rate of 1% over 5 years. This was superior to all other modalities including excision (10%), C&D (7.7%), RT (8.7%), and cryotherapy (7.5%). In a similar study of treatment of recurrent BCC, treatment with MMS demonstrated a long-term recurrence rate of 5.6%.[108] Once again, this was superior to all other modalities including excision (17.4%), RT (9.8%), and C&D (40%). MMS is the preferred treatment for morpheaform, recurrent, poorly delineated, high-risk, and incompletely removed BCC, and for those sites in which tissue conservation is imperative.[7,8,31,109,110]

C&D is the method most frequently used by dermatologists in the treatment of BCC. Knox et al.[111] noted cure rates as high as 98.3%, whereas Kopf et al.,[112] in an earlier study, cited a significant difference in the cure rates obtained between patients treated by private practitioners (94.3%) and those treated by trainees in the New York University Skin and Cancer Unit (81.2%). This supports the premise that though C&D is simple and cost-effective, it is dependent on operator skill. In a series of 233 patients treated by Spiller et al.,[113] an overall cure rate of 97% was reported. The highest cure rate was obtained in lesions that measured less than 1 cm (98.8%), with recurrences observed in 2 of 165 patients treated. Recurrences were noted in 2 of 45 patients with lesions that measured between 1 and 2 cm, for an overall cure rate of 95.5%. Recurrences were significantly higher in patients with lesions larger than 2 cm, for whom the overall cure rate was 84%. In this series, as in others, recurrences were most commonly noted on the forehead, temple, ears, nose, and shoulders. Some practitioners advocate that the procedure be repeated for three cycles,[16,19,114] but we believe that the histology, location, and behavior of the tumor should dictate the number of cycles.

When surgery is contraindicated, RT is an option for treating primary BCC.[104] RT may be indicated postoperatively if margins are ambiguous. Advantages of RT include minimal to no discomfort for the patient and avoidance of an invasive procedure in a patient who may not be able to tolerate or is unwilling to undergo surgery. Disadvantages include lack of margin control, poor cosmesis over time, a drawn-out course of therapy, and possible increased risk of future skin cancers. In one series, control rates of 95% were achieved in BCC involving the eyelid treated with RT. The recurrence rate for primary BCC treated by RT approaches 5% to 10% over 5 years. In one study by Wilder et al.[115] local control rates among 85 patients with 115 biopsy-proven BCCs were compared. The local control rates varied significantly, a 95% control rate being achieved in primary BCC and a 56% control rate in recurrent BCC at 5 years. From the standpoint of cosmesis, scars from RT tend to worsen over time (Fig. 41.2-17), as contrasted to surgical scars, which improve over time.

Cryosurgery has been used to treat BCC.[14,16,17,114,116,117] Two freeze-thaw cycles with a tissue temperature of –50°C are required to destroy the tumor sufficiently. A margin of normal skin also should be frozen to ensure eradication of subclinical disease. Complications include hypertrophic scarring and postinflammatory pigmentary changes. Fractional cryotherapy has been used with success in treating eyelid lesions.[116,118] The method has been described as quick and cost-effective. A serious potential adverse outcome is recurrent BCC that can become extensive because of concealment by the fibrous scar created when aggressive cryosurgery is used.

Ablation by the CO_2 laser has been used in the treatment of BCC. In a recent study, Humphreys et al.[119] reported ablation of primary superficial BCC with the high-energy, pulsed CO_2 laser. Because of the absence of margin control and lack of large series studies, physicians familiar with laser and tumor biology should use this method only in unique circumstances.

Management of BCC must be directed by the histologic nature of the tumor and the clinical context in which it presents. We recommend MMS for BCCs showing aggressive

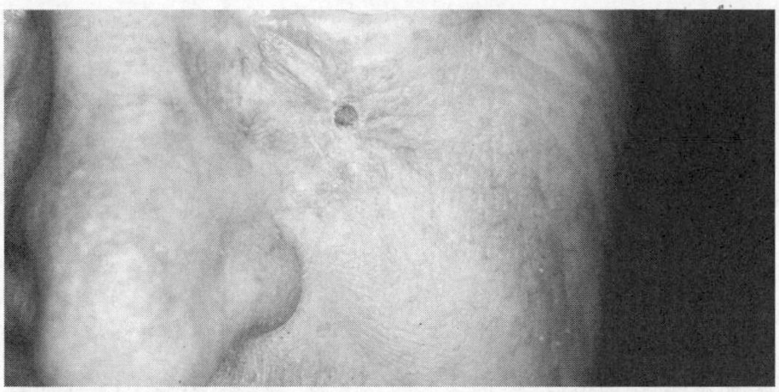

FIGURE 41.2-17. After radiation therapy, scar and hypopigmentation can result. (See Color Fig. 41.2-17 in the CD-ROM and on the Web at www.LWWoncology.com.)

growth patterns and for BCCs occurring in high-risk anatomic sites or sites that require maximum conservation of normal tissue. For non-aggressive-growth BCCs on the trunk and extremities, fusiform excision with margins of 4 mm or C&D are appropriate. For patients with numerous BCCs, including patients with NBCCS, tangential excision followed by gentle curettage and cauterization for smaller, superficial lesions is effective. Cryosurgery can be helpful in the management of multiple, small BCCs of NBCCS.

It is imperative that patients with a history of BCC receive annual full-body skin examinations. Although most recurrences appear within 1 to 5 years, they can develop later.[30] Rowe et al.[106] found that 30% of recurrences developed within the first year after therapy, 50% within 2 years, and 66% within 3 years. Subsequent new primary BCC can present at rates of approximately 40%, with 20% to 30% of these developing within 1 year of treatment of the original lesion.[30]

SQUAMOUS CELL CARCINOMA

SCC is a neoplasm of keratinizing cells that shows malignant characteristics, including anaplasia, rapid growth, local invasion, and metastatic potential.[16,120] Approximately 100,000 cases of SCC are diagnosed in the United States each year, making it the second most common human cancer after BCC. As with BCC, affected men tend to outnumber affected women.[121,122] People of Celtic descent, individuals with fair complexions, and those with poor tanning ability and a predisposition to sunburn are at increased risk for developing SCC (Fig. 41.2-18).[123] Patients taking immunosuppressive medications after organ transplantation are also at increased risk.[48,124] Another high-risk group includes patients treated with psoralens and ultraviolet A light (PUVA) for psoriasis.[125–129] Patients exposed to arsenic are at increased risk for SCC, particularly Bowen's disease.[130–133]

Pathogenesis

Factors involved in the pathogenesis of SCC are similar to those for BCC and include exposure to UVL, genetic mutations, immunosuppression, and viral infection. The evidence for an association with UVL is even stronger for SCC than for BCC.[25,33,134] UVL may mediate development of SCC through several mechanisms.[25,36] Exposure to UVB appears to interfere with the density and antigen-processing capability of Langerhans' cells and may suppress production of the T helper 1 (Th1) cytokines interleukin-2 and interferon-γ.[135–138] Recent studies have demonstrated that UVL may introduce mutations into the tumor suppressor gene p53.[25,36,39,139,140] This allows UVL to act as both tumor initiator and promoter. Development of SCC has been associated with radiation exposure, burn scars, chronic inflammatory dermatoses, ulcers, osteomyelitis, and arsenic ingestion.[48,50,141–145] Heritable conditions associated with SCC include xeroderma pigmentosum and oculocutaneous albinism. Immunosuppression also may play a role in pathogenesis. Skin cancers in immunosuppressed patients appear primarily on sun-exposed sites.[60,62] This correlation suggests that immunosuppression and UVL act as cofactors in the development of SCC. HIV patients tend to have a higher incidence of SCC than the general population.[66,67] However, the exact nature of the relationship between HIV and SCC has not yet been determined. The role of human papillomavirus (HPV) in the development of SCC has been studied. Eliezri et al.[146] found a direct correlation between the venereal spread of

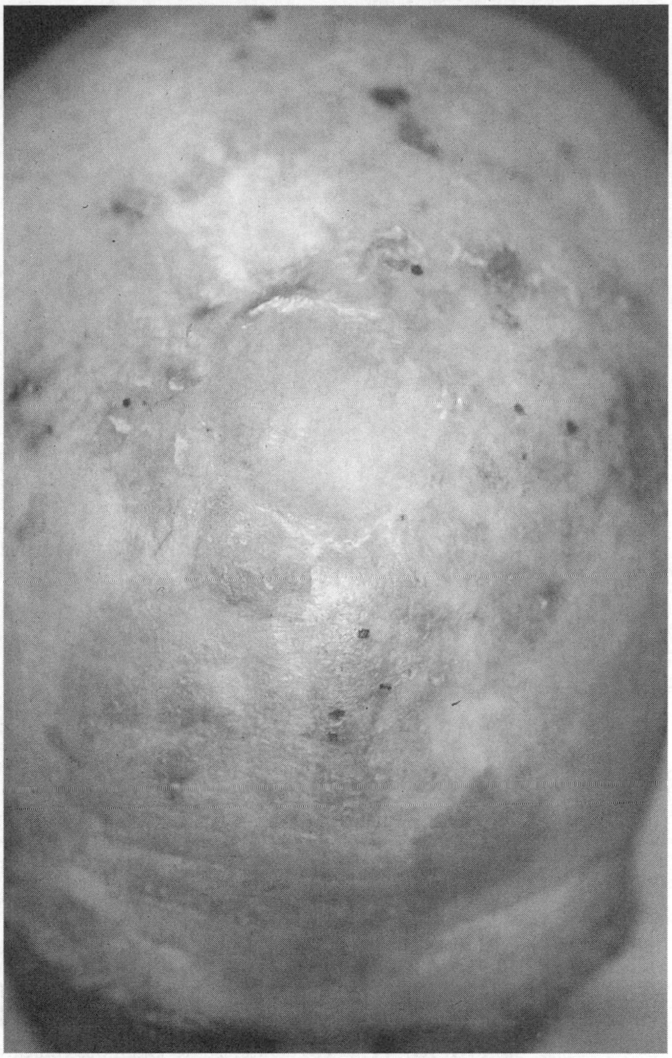

FIGURE 41.2-18. Extensive solar damage. Patients with this degree of solar damage are at increased risk for squamous cell carcinoma. (See Color Fig. 41.2-18 in the CD-ROM and on the Web at www.LWWoncology.com.)

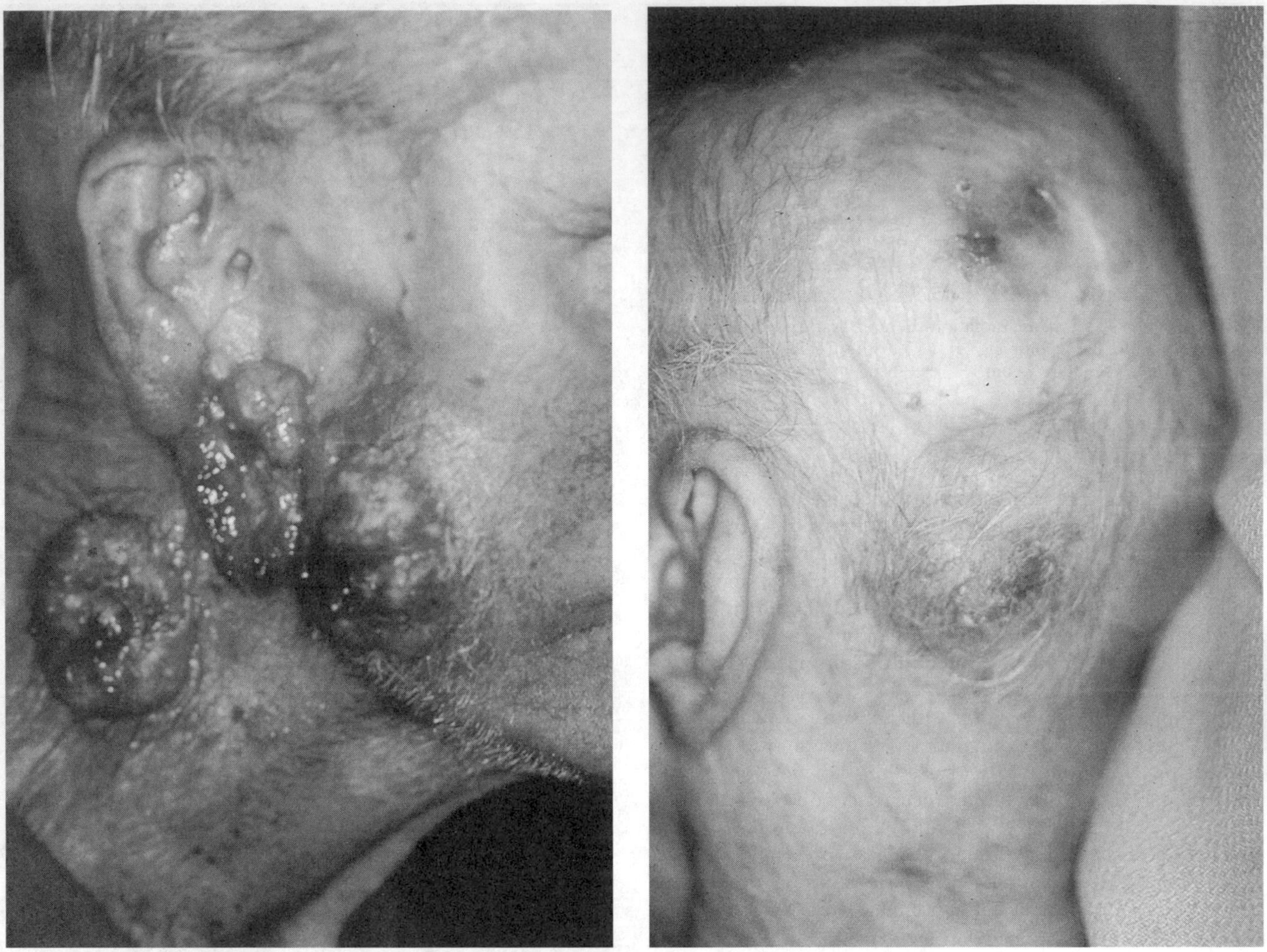

A B

FIGURE 41.2-19. Metastatic squamous cell carcinoma (SCC). **A:** In this patient, primary cutaneous SCC metastasized to the parotid gland and draining lymph nodes. **B:** Metastatic SCC after multiple excisions. (See Color Fig. 41.2-19 in the CD-ROM and on the Web at www.LWWoncology.com.)

HPV-16 and the initiation of SCC, and others have demonstrated an association of HPV-16 with periungual SCC.[147]

Biologic Behavior

The biologic behavior of SCC is determined by a number of variables.[148–150] The overall invasiveness and depth of the neoplasm is significant when determining the risk of recurrence. SCCs that invade the reticular dermis and subcutis tend to recur if not properly treated. Immerman et al.[151] observed a 20% incidence of recurrence in 86 patients with invasive SCC. Degree of cellular differentiation is an important factor in recurrence also, with poorly differentiated neoplasms showing increased rates of recurrence.

SCC *in situ* tends to arise in association with preexisting AK. Arsenical keratoses are rarely seen nowadays but are associated with SCC. These lesions are considered to be at low risk for metastasis. While SCC *in situ* carries no risk of metastasis, invasive SCC can metastasize[148–150] and can originate in neglected SCC *in situ* (Fig. 41.2-19). The most common type arises on sun-damaged skin. The incidence of metastasis of such lesions is 3% to 5%. A higher incidence (10% to 30%) is associated with SCC arising on a mucosal surfaces (lip, genitalia) and in sites of prior injury (scars, chronic ulcers).

The tendency for regional lymph node metastasis is variable. Tumors arising in areas of chronic inflammation have a 10% to 30% rate of metastasis, whereas the incidence of metastasis from SCC that is not due to preexisting inflammatory or degenerative conditions varies from 0.05% to 16%.[148–150] Although tumors that arise on sun-damaged skin may behave less aggressively than *de novo* SCC, all lesions have the potential to become invasive locally and to metastasize to draining lymph nodes. The large number of sun-mediated SCCs makes this clinical potential a concern. Friedman et al.[152] demonstrated that all trunk and extremity primary SCCs that later developed local or nodal recurrence were at least 4 mm deep and penetrated into the reticular dermis or subcutis. The extent of cellular differentiation also influences the metastatic potential in that tumors that invade regional lymph nodes tend to be more anaplastic than those that have not metastasized. Tumors are more likely to disseminate to regional lymph nodes than to distant sites, although intravascular metastases to viscera have appeared in as many as 5% to 10% of SCCs metastatic from skin.

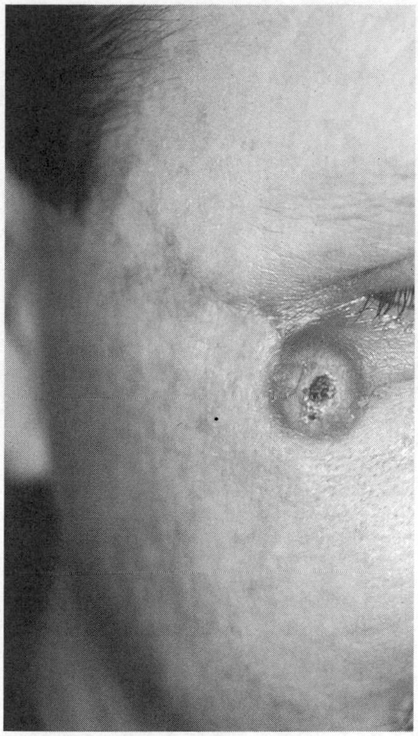

FIGURE 41.2-20. Recurrent squamous cell carcinoma, keratoacanthoma type, successfully treated by Mohs micrographic surgery. (See Color Fig. 41.2-20 in the CD-ROM and on the Web at www.LWWoncology.com.)

Invasive SCC has the potential to involve nerves.[72,148] Regional lymph node and distant metastases may increase with perineural involvement. SCCs on the skin of the head and neck may metastasize to cervical lymph nodes and distantly to the central nervous system, the latter either hematogenously or via the perineural space, which directly connects to the subarachnoid space. SCCs on the midface and lip are prone to neural involvement. These patients show a lower 10-year survival (23% vs. 88%) and a higher local recurrence rate (47% vs 7.3%) than do those without neural involvement.

Clinical Features

On the skin, SCC appears as a slightly raised, red, hyperkeratotic macule or papule on sun-exposed sites but may occur anywhere (Figs. 41.2-20, 41.2-21, 41.2-22, 41.2-23, 41.2-24. It can be

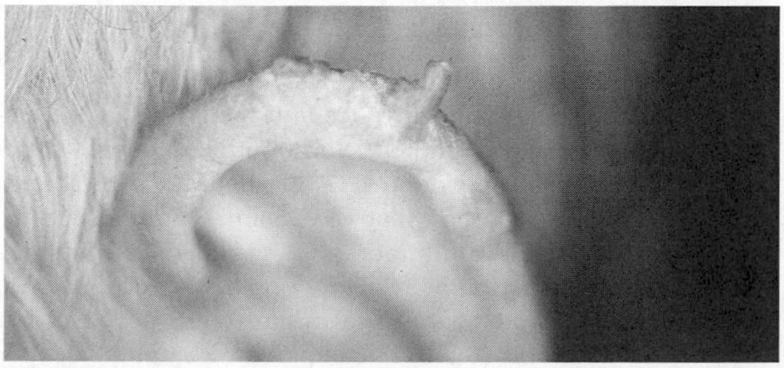

FIGURE 41.2-21. Squamous cell carcinoma can arise within a cutaneous horn. (See Color Fig. 41.2-21 in the CD-ROM and on the Web at www.LWWoncology.com.)

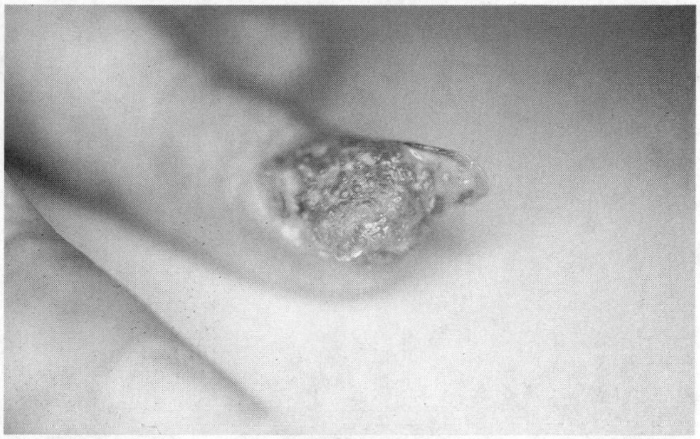

FIGURE 41.2-22. Periungual squamous cell carcinoma treated by Mohs micrographic surgery can result in sparing of a digit that otherwise may have been amputated. (See Color Fig. 41.2-22 in the CD-ROM and on the Web at www.LWWoncology.com.)

difficult to clinically distinguish an invasive SCC from a HAK, a benign seborrheic keratosis, or a benign inflammatory lesion. Appropriate biopsy should be performed on any lesion suspicious for SCC, considering the potential for invasive disease.

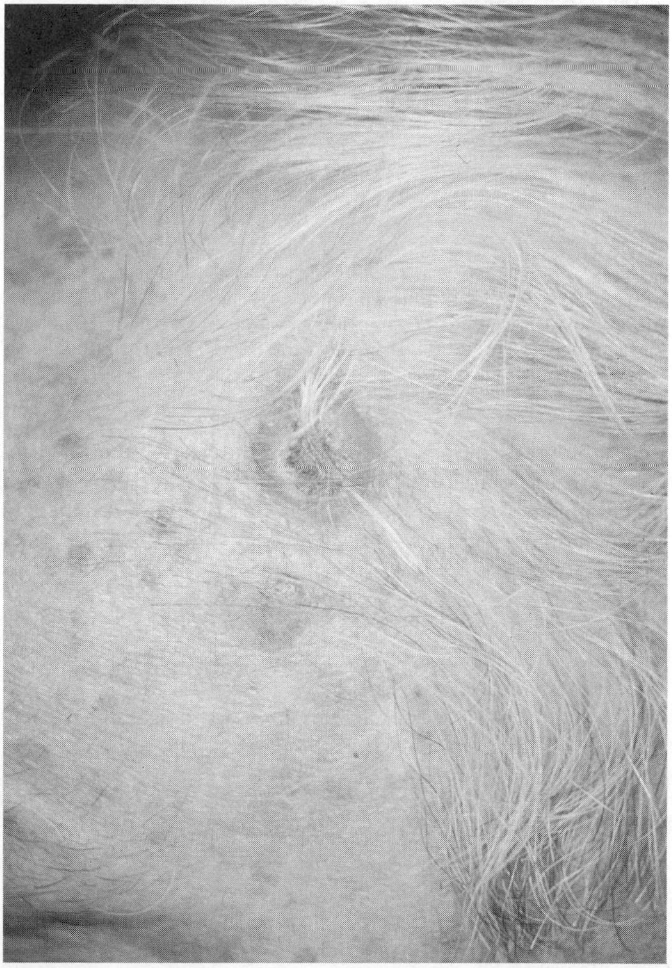

FIGURE 41.2-23. Squamous cell carcinoma, keratoacanthoma type. This variant of squamous cell carcinoma presents as a rapidly growing nodule. (See Color Fig. 41.2-23 in the CD-ROM and on the Web at www.LWWoncology.com.)

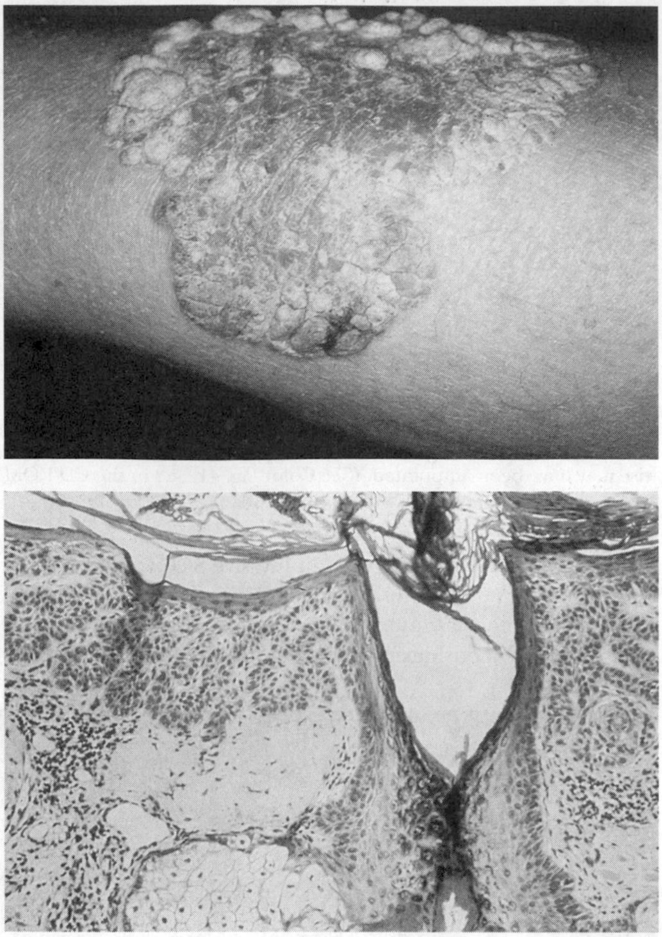

A

B

FIGURE 41.2-24. **A:** Bowen's disease presents as an erythematous macule or patch and can be difficult to differentiate from a benign inflammatory process. **B:** Bowen's disease is characterized by proliferation of atypical cells arranged in such a way as to suggest a windblown appearance. (See Color Fig. 41.2-24 in the CD-ROM and on the Web at www.LWWoncology.com.)

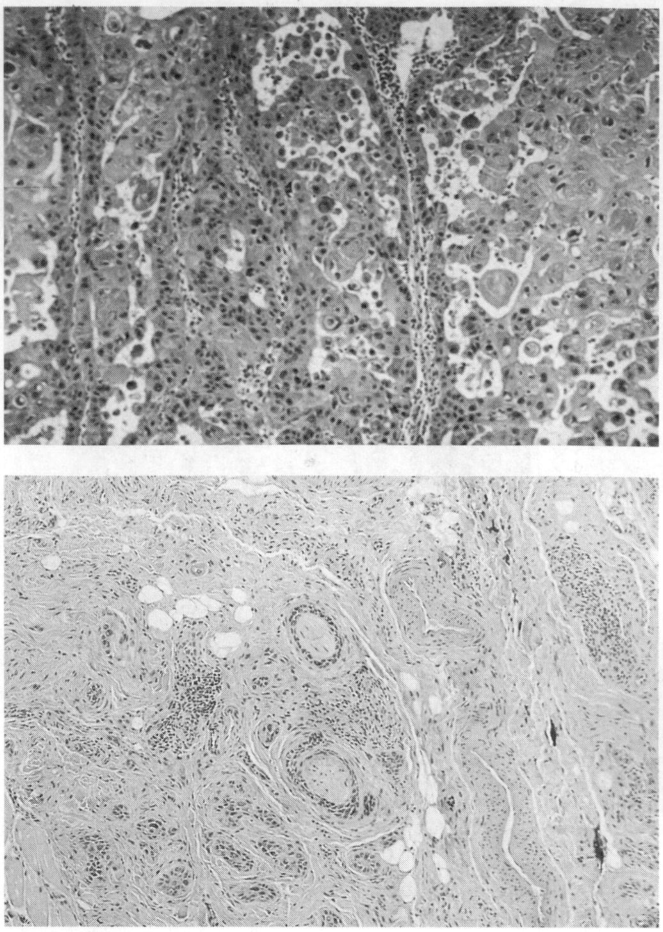

A

B

FIGURE 41.2-25. Squamous cell carcinoma (SCC), microscopical view. **A:** Infiltrative SCC. Note large cellular size and nuclear atypia. **B:** SCC demonstrating perineural invasion on microscopical examination. (See Color Fig. 41.2-25 in the CD-ROM and on the Web at www.LWWoncology.com.)

Shave biopsy is sufficient and will not lead to spread of the cancer. Verrucous carcinoma, a variant of SCC, includes oral florid papillomatosis, giant condyloma of Buschke-Löwenstein, and epithelioma cuniculatum.[153–155] A biopsy should be performed on an atypical wart or one that is unresponsive to therapy to rule out the presence of verrucous carcinoma.

Bowen's disease represents SCC *in situ* with a distinctive microscopical appearance (see Fig. 41.2-24).[156] Erythroplasia of Queyrat is simply Bowen's disease occurring on the penis.[157] Bowenoid papulosis classically presents as a reddish brown verrucous papule and is associated with HPV-16.[158] Bowenoid papulosis usually involves the genitals but may present elsewhere.[159]

SCC is characterized histologically by relatively large cellular size, lack of maturation, nuclear atypia, and the presence of mitotic figures (see Fig. 41.2-24; Fig. 41.2-25).[148] Lack of dermal invasion separates SCC *in situ* from histologically invasive SCC. Verrucous carcinoma is characterized microscopically by an endophytic epidermal proliferation with atypia sufficient to distinguish it from verruca vulgaris, or common wart.[160] Variants of Bowen's disease are characterized by proliferation of atypical cells arranged in such a way as to suggest a windblown appearance.[157] A grading system was devised to classify SCC with respect to percentage of differentiated cells. Grade 1 tumors are described as having more than 75% well-differentiated cells, whereas in grade 2 SCC, 50% to 75% of cells are described as well-differentiated and, in grade 3 SCC, 25% to 50% of cells are described this way. Primary cutaneous SCC with fewer than 25% well-differentiated cells is termed *grade 4 SCC*. Prognosis worsens with decreased degree of differentiation.[148,161]

Recurrence and Metastatic Risk

In a review of studies of SCCs from 1940 to 1992, Rowe et al.[148] correlated risk for local recurrence and metastasis with treatment modality, prior treatment, location, size, depth, histologic differentiation, evidence of perineural involvement, precipitating factors other than UVL, and immunosuppression. They found that with tumors greater than 2 cm in diameter, recurrence rates double from 7.4% to 15.2%. In addition, they demonstrated that tumors less than 4 mm deep were at low risk for metastasis (6.7%) as compared with tumors deeper than 4 mm (45.7%). Locally recurrent SCCs showed an overall metastatic rate of 30%, with high rates of metastasis in the context of local recurrence in skin (25%), lip (31.5%), and ear

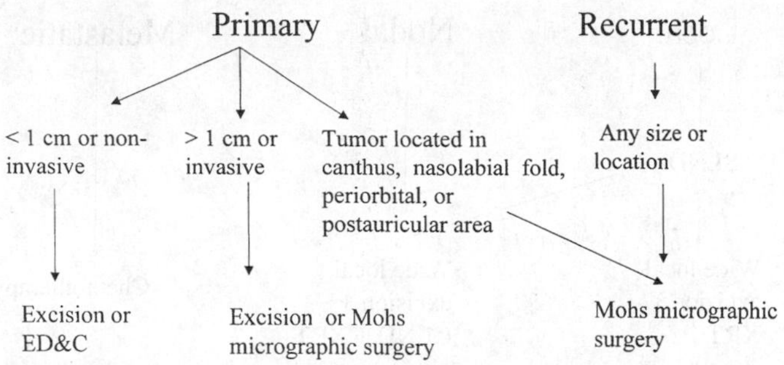

FIGURE 41.2-26. Primary squamous cell carcinoma may be managed by electrodessication and curettage (ED&C), excision, or Mohs micrographic surgery, depending on histology, tumor size, and anatomic location. Recurrent squamous cell carcinomas should be treated by Mohs micrographic surgery.

(45%). Immunosuppressed patients showed a 5- to 20-fold increase in the incidence of SCCs, with a reversal of the SCC/BCC ratio from 0.25:1 to 3:1. The number of SCCs per patient was increased, and the age at initial presentation was decreased. In immunosuppressed patients, SCCs metastasized at a rate of 12.9%. Poorly differentiated SCC metastasized more frequently (32.9%) than did well-differentiated SCC (9.2%). SCC arising on sun-exposed skin recurred at a rate of 7.9% and metastasized at a rate of 5.2%. Recurrence rates were increased in SCC on the lip (10.5%) and ear (18.7%), as were metastatic rates from the lip (13.7%) and ear (11%). SCCs with perineural invasion recurred in almost one-half of cases (47.2%) and showed a similar rate of metastasis (47.3%).

Treatment

Many of the treatments for BCC are appropriate for SCC (Fig. 41.2-26). The type of therapy should be selected on the basis of size of the lesion, anatomic location, depth of invasion, degree of cellular differentiation, and history of previous treatment.[162] There are three general approaches to treatment of SCC: (1) destruction by C&D or cryosurgery, (2) removal by traditional excisional surgery or MMS, and (3) RT.

C&D can be used for small lesions arising on sun-damaged skin. Well-differentiated, primary SCCs measuring less than 1 cm in diameter are amenable to this form of therapy. Honeycutt and Jansen[163] reported a 99% cure rate for 281 SCCs after a 4-year follow-up. In this study, two recurrences were noted in lesions less than 2 cm in diameter.

SCC *in situ* may be treated by cryotherapy. As with BCC, two freeze-thaw cycles with a tissue temperature of −50°C are required to destroy the tumor sufficiently. A margin of normal skin also should be frozen to ensure eradication of subclinical disease. Complications include hypertrophic scarring and postinflammatory pigmentary changes. Concealment of recurrence within dense scar tissue presents a danger.

Surgical excision is another well-accepted treatment modality for SCC. Brodland et al.[164] demonstrated that lesions of less than 2 cm in diameter are best treated by excision, with margins of 4 mm, whereas high-risk SCC requires 6-mm margins. These investigators found that certain characteristics were associated with a greater risk of subclinical tumor extension, thus qualifying such tumors as high-risk. These included size of 2 cm or larger, histologic grade higher than 2, invasion of the subcutaneous tissue, and location in high-risk areas. Carcinomas of the penis, vulva, and anus usually are treated by excision because of the poor tolerance of these areas to irradiation.[100,165,166] Surgical excision is the treatment of choice for verrucous carcinoma.[153]

MMS is indicated in cases of large primary or recurrent SCC, as this modality allows conservation of normal tissue with preservation of function and enhanced cosmesis. MMS is also superior to other forms of treatment with regard to local recurrence.[103,162] Recurrence rates with Mohs surgery are superior to those obtained with traditional excisional surgery in primary SCC of the ear (3.1% vs. 10.9%), primary SCC of the lip (5.8% vs. 18.7%), recurrent SCC (10% vs. 23.3%), SCC with perineural invasion (0% vs. 47%), SCC larger than 2 cm (25.2 vs. 41.7%), and poorly differentiated SCC (32.6% vs. 53.6%).[148] MMS has proven useful in SCC involving the nail unit[110] and has been used as a limb-sparing procedure in cases of SCC arising in osteomyelitis.[144]

RT may be used for head and neck cutaneous SCC in which there is no spread to bone or cartilage and there is no evidence of metastasis.[167] As with BCC, RT may be indicated for elderly patients with SCC who are unwilling or unable to undergo surgery.[104] In one series, 108 patients with SCC of the lower vermilion lip were stratified into stage T1 (82.4%), T2 (15.7%), or T3 (1.9%) disease and were treated with RT. Recurrences occurred in 12.4% of patients with T1 disease and 6.7% of patients with T2 disease.[168] Radiation therapy often is used as an adjuvant modality after treatment of SCC in which perineural involvement is identified, although no controlled studies have proven its usefulness.

MMS is indicated for invasive lesions, poorly differentiated lesions, and lesions occurring in high-risk anatomic sites or sites in which conservation of normal tissue is essential for preservation of function or cosmesis.

Invasive SCC can be a potentially lethal neoplasm and warrants close follow-up. In one study, approximately 30% of patients with SCC developed a subsequent SCC, with more than one-half of these occurring within the first year of follow-up.[169] In another study, the median time to recurrence was 15 months.[142] Thus, it is recommended that patients with SCC be examined every 3 months during the first year following treatment, every 6 months during the second year after treatment, and annually thereafter. Evaluation should include total body cutaneous examination and palpation of draining lymph nodes. Currently, roentgenography, magnetic resonance imaging, and CT play no role in the routine workup of uncomplicated cutaneous SCC.

MERKEL CELL CARCINOMA

Merkel cell carcinoma (MCC) is a potentially aggressive tumor of neuroendocrine cell origin. Though it primarily affects the head and neck, other areas may be involved.[170] MCC affects more men than women and most often occurs between the seventh and ninth decades of life.[171,172]

The pathogenesis of MCC is incompletely characterized. UVL has been indirectly implicated in its development, as 36% of such cancers arise on the face.[173] More than 50% of tumors occur on the head and neck, while 35% develop on the extremities. Mixed MCC/SCC[174] and, recently, MCC/BCC[175] have been reported, thus supporting the role of UVL exposure as a risk factor. Immunosuppression may play a role in the development of MCC, as rapid progression has been reported

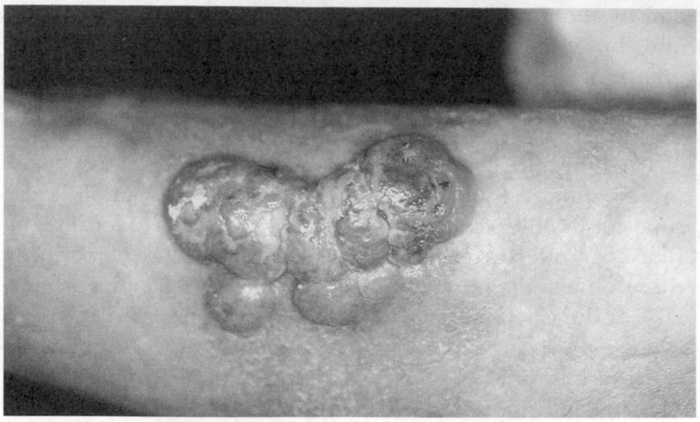

FIGURE 41.2-27. Merkel cell carcinoma presenting as a red to violaceous, dome-shaped papule or plaque on the sun-exposed skin of an elderly person. (See Color Fig. 41.2-27 in the CD-ROM and on the Web at www.LWWoncology.com.)

in the setting of immunosuppressive therapy after organ transplantation.[176,177] An association with arsenic-induced Bowen's disease has been reported, implicating arsenic exposure as a risk factor for development of MCC.[132]

Lymph node metastases have been identified in up to 20% of cases of MCC at initial presentation. Approximately 50% of patients experience nodal disease at some point in the disease course. Distant metastases have been reported in up to 30% of patients at presentation. Metastases have been noted in skin, lymph nodes, lung, liver, brain, intestine, bladder, and abdominal wall.[178–183] Although MCC is a highly aggressive and potentially lethal cancer, spontaneous regression has been reported.[184] The significance of this phenomenon is unknown.

MCC usually appears as a red, violaceous, dome-shaped papule or plaque on sun-exposed skin (Fig. 41.2-27).[170] It may develop on the extremities and can involve the trunk. Clinical differential diagnosis includes leukemia cutis, amelanotic melanoma, metastatic carcinoma, pyogenic granuloma, and SCC.

Microscopical examination reveals sheets and cords of atypical cells in the dermis, extending to the subcutaneous layer, that sometimes form an interlacing trabecular or pseudoglandular pattern.[170,185] A grenz zone often is present, separating tumor from epidermis. Cell membranes often are indistinct, giving a syncytial appearance. Cells are round to oval and generally noncohesive. Cytoplasm tends to be scant, with round to oval nuclei containing two to three nucleoli. Foci of squamous differentiation resembling SCC have occasionally been noted. Special stains may prove useful in the histologic diagnosis of MCC. Cytokeratin-20 (CK-20) staining gives a characteristic paranuclear dot pattern.[185] Histologic differential diagnosis includes lymphoma, BCC, metastatic oat cell carcinoma, or noncutaneous neuroendocrine tumors. Lymphoma cells are differentiated in that they are CD45-positive and CK-20-negative. Melanoma can be differentiated in that melanocytes are strongly S-100-positive. In addition to CK-20, MCC stains positively for chromogranin neuron-specific enolase and may be weakly positive for S-100 protein.

MCC warrants aggressive therapy (Fig. 41.2-28). Evaluation of a patient with histologically confirmed MCC must include full-body skin examination and lymph node evaluation. A complete blood cell count and liver function tests should be performed as

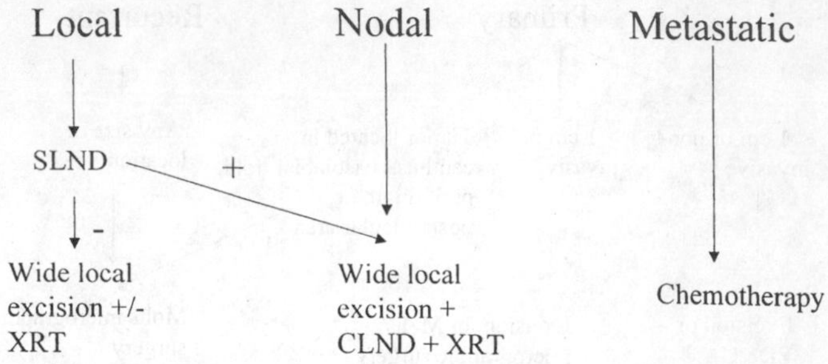

FIGURE 41.2-28. Merkel cell carcinoma should be treated by wide local excision followed by sentinel or complete lymph node dissection (SLND, CLND), radiation therapy (XRT), or chemotherapy, depending on stage.

well. CT scanning of the chest, pelvis, and abdomen may be indicated to rule out the presence of small cell carcinoma of the lung. CT scanning of the head and neck may prove valuable in detection of nodal disease. MCC tends to spread in a cascade pattern, first affecting local, then regional lymph nodes and finally progressing to fatal distant metastatic disease.[186]

Management of MCC follows staging of patients according to local, regional, or metastatic disease. Current recommendations support wide local excision (WLE) with lymph node dissection and adjuvant RT, if indicated.[187] In cases of local disease, sentinel lymph node dissection may be advisable, if available. In a recent study, 18 patients with stage I MCC underwent sentinel lymph node dissection. In two patients, involvement of the sentinel node was identified, resulting in complete lymph node dissection. Sentinel node–negative patients received no therapy other than wide and deep excision.[188] All patients remained free of recurrence at 7 months. Patients with negative sentinel nodes may be treated by WLE with margins of up to 3 cm and, possibly, adjunctive RT. Patients with positive sentinel nodes should be treated as patients with regional disease. The combination of WLE, therapeutic lymph node dissection, and RT has been suggested for treatment of regional disease.[189,190] Metastatic disease is treated with chemotherapy. The most common regimens used in the treatment of metastatic MCC include cytoxan, doxorubicin, and vincristine, and cisplatin and etoposide. However, brief responses were reported recently in a small series of patients treated with carboplatin and etoposide.[191] In a review by Voog et al.,[192] overall response to first-line chemotherapy for MCC was 61%, with a 57% response in metastatic disease and a 69% response in locally advanced disease. The 3-year survival rate was 17% in metastatic disease and 35% in locally advanced disease. In a recent series of nine patients with neuroendocrine tumors, complete response in a patient with inoperable MCC was reported using 5-FU, dacarbazine, and epirubicin. Patients with MCC must be followed up aggressively for potential local recurrence and development of metastatic disease.

MICROCYSTIC ADNEXAL CARCINOMA

Microcystic adnexal carcinoma (MAC) was first described as a distinct entity in 1982 by Goldstein et al.[193] In this study, six cases of MAC were described. In each case, the tumor was originally misdiagnosed on initial biopsy as benign. MAC originates from pluripotent adnexal cells capable of eccrine and follicular differentiation. Synonyms for MAC include *sclerosing sweat duct*

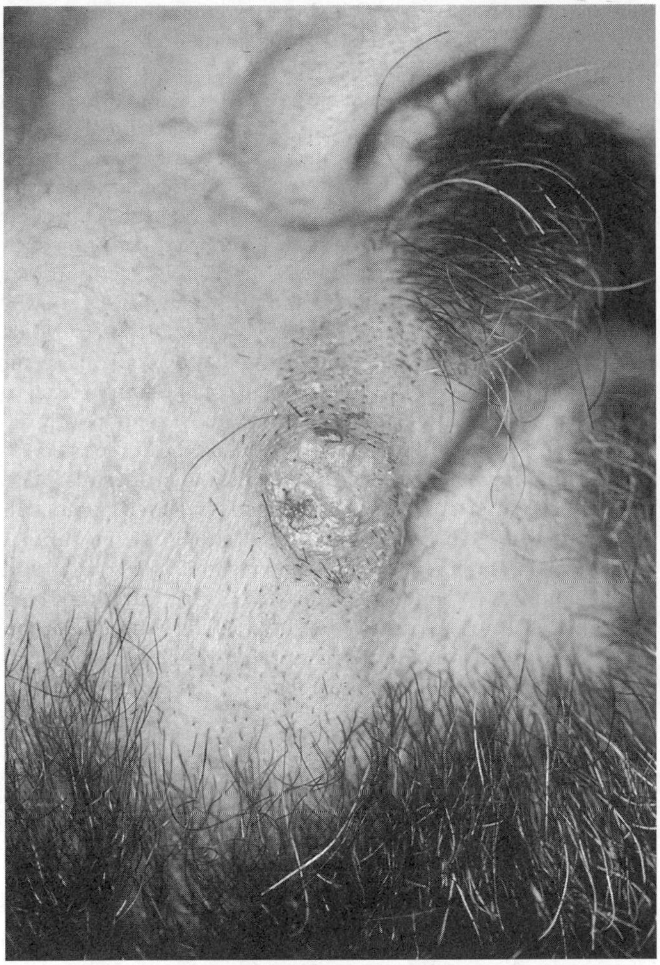

A

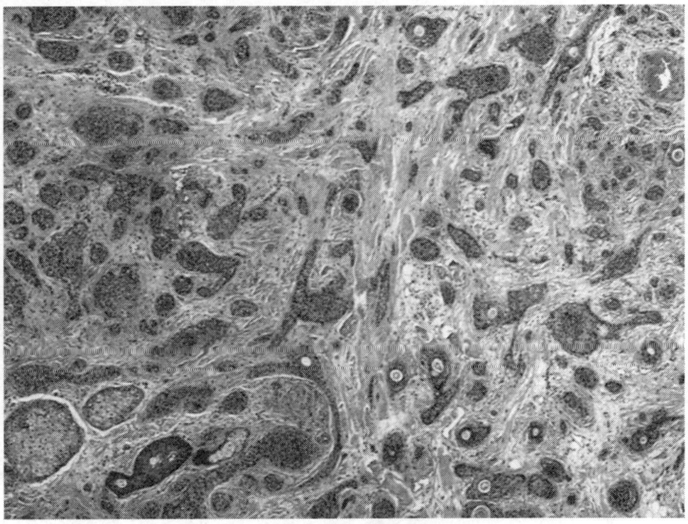

B

FIGURE 41.2-29. Microcystic adnexal carcinoma. **A:** Classic presentation is as an indurated plaque with intact epidermis and yellow hue. **B:** On microscopical examination, the dermis shows numerous basaloid cells forming cords, nests, small ducts, and horn microcysts. (See Color Fig. 41.2-29 in the CD-ROM and on the Web at www.LWWoncology.com.)

carcinoma, sweat duct carcinoma with syringomatous features, and *combined adnexal tumor of the skin.*

MAC is a tumor that primarily affects middle-aged individuals,[194] though it has been reported in an 11-year-old boy.[195] Unlike the other primary cutaneous malignancies considered thus far, affected women outnumber affected men.[194] The pathogenesis of MAC is not completely understood but may involve exposure to ionizing radiation. In many cases, patients with MAC have received RT. In general, these patients were treated with RT for conditions ranging from tinea capitis to thyroid carcinoma.[196,197] Treatment may precede development of MAC by as long as 40 years.

MAC is a locally aggressive tumor with low metastatic potential. It has been demonstrated that the increased stromal collagen observed in MAC is not due to soluble factors excreted by MAC cells.[198] Perineural invasion is common with MAC, as are involvement of muscle, perichondrium, and vascular adventitia.[199,200] Birkby et al.[200a] reported MAC on the face of a 51-year-old man that invaded the bone marrow of the mandible and spread along the inferior alveolar and mental nerves. Recently, the first case of MAC metastatic to lymph node was reported.[201]

MAC classically presents as a sclerotic or indurated plaque with intact epidermis and yellow hue (Fig. 41.2-29*A*).[193] The tumor usually involves the central face and lip but is not limited to those anatomic sites.[193,202,203] MAC involvement of the eyelid,[204] scalp,[205] tongue,[206] and eyebrow[207] have been reported.

On microscopical examination, MAC may be misdiagnosed as a benign adnexal process.[208] The epidermis is normal, although mild hyperkeratosis may be present. The dermis contains numerous basaloid cells forming cords, nests, small ducts, and horn microcysts (see Fig. 41.2-29*B*). Horn microcysts usually are present superficially, containing laminated keratin and, occasionally, small vellus hairs. Cysts may be calcified. Small ducts, either empty or filled with eosinophilic material composed of sialomucin, commonly are present. Ducts may be well-differentiated, with two rows of cuboidal cells, or less differentiated, with single strands without lumina. A dense sclerotic stroma is present. Immunohistochemical analysis may be useful in differentiating MAC from desmoplastic trichoepithelioma (DTE). Wick et al. reported that MACs were reactive to hard keratin subclasses AE13 and AE14, epithelial membrane antigen, carcinoembryonic antigen, and LeuM1.[209] DTEs were positive for AE14, epithelial membrane antigen, and LeuM1 only focally and were, in contrast, negative for carcinoembryonic antigen. Correct diagnosis of MAC is imperative, as the tumor can be highly invasive and may involve adipose, muscle, perichondrium, or bone.

MAC has been treated by WLE as well as MMS.[194] In a recent series, 11 cases of MAC treated by MMS remained free of tumor for a median of 5 years.[210] This suggests that extirpation by Mohs technique may prove beneficial in the management of MAC. However, these findings must be interpreted cautiously, as recurrences have been reported up to 30 years after surgical excision.[208] Non-Mohs surgical excision is associated with recurrence rates of 47% to 59%.[201] It appears that the tumor is resistant to RT, thus presenting difficulties in the management of MAC with perineural invasion.

After surgery for MAC, patients must be evaluated regularly for recurrence and for development of other skin cancers. Evaluation should include examination of skin and lymph nodes and, due to the potential for recurrence long after treatment, continue indefinitely.

SEBACEOUS CARCINOMA

Sebaceous carcinoma (SC) is a malignant adnexal tumor with variable sites of origin, histologic growth patterns, and clinical presentations.[211,212] Ocular SC is more common and may arise from meibomian glands and, less frequently, from the glands of Zeis. The upper eyelids are most frequently involved. Approximately 50% of SCs are initially incorrectly diagnosed histologically and, in some series, all have been initially misdiagnosed clinically.[211,212] SC is the second most common eyelid malignancy after BCC[213] and is the second most lethal after melanoma.[214]

In SC, women are affected more commonly than men, at a ratio of approximately 2:1.[211–213, 215] SC classically presents in the seventh to ninth decade.[211,212] SC is associated with sebaceous adenomas, radiation exposure, Bowen's disease, and Muir-Torre syndrome. In Muir-Torre syndrome, an autosomal dominant heritable condition, SC and (more commonly) sebaceous adenoma (or sebaceous epithelioma) are associated with a second internal malignancy, usually a carcinoma of the colon or urogenital tract. SC may be associated with a history of RT. SC has been reported after RT for retinoblastoma,[216] eczema,[217] and cosmetic epilation.[218] In one study, SC was associated with thiazide diuretic use.[213] In addition, recent studies have identified HPV DNA[219] and overexpression of p53 protein in some SCs.[220]

Commonly, SC presents as a slowly growing, deeply seated nodule of the eyelid and may present as chronic diffuse blepharoconjunctivitis or keratoconjunctivitis.[211–214] Upper eyelid involvement is more common. Approximately 25% of cases of SC involve extraocular sites, which may include head and neck, trunk,[221–223] and external genitalia.[219] A case of SC has occurred within a benign dermoid cyst of the ovary.[224]

SC can spread by lymphatic or hematogenous routes or by direct extension.[211,212] Distant metastases are reported in up to 20% of cases and may involve the lungs, liver, brain, bones, and lymph nodes.[211,212] The parotid gland may be involved secondarily.[225] Ocular SC may spread via the lacrimal secretory and excretory systems.[213]

On microscopical examination, SC shows nonencapsulated tumors within the dermis.[211] Sebaceous cells exhibiting varying degrees of differentiation, nuclear pleomorphism, hyperchromatism, and locally infiltrating surrounding tissues and neurovascular spaces are observed. Poor prognostic indicators in SC have been reviewed.[226] These include multicentric origin, poor differentiation, infiltrative pattern, pagetoid changes, vascular invasion, lymphatic channel involvement, and orbital spread.

Treatment options for SC include traditional excisional surgery and extirpation by MMS. In one study of 14 cases of SC excised with frozen-section margin control, 5 recurrences were observed in cases with surgical margins of 1 to 3 mm, whereas no recurrences were seen with margins of 5 mm.[227] Potential difficulties arise because tumors are often multicentric, and pagetoid spread is difficult to determine even on high-quality, paraffin-embedded sections. Extirpation of SC by Mohs has thus far yielded varying results. Folberg et al.[228] reported recurrences in two of three patients treated by the Mohs technique, with tumor noted at reconstruction in one of the three patients. Dzubow[229] reported two patients with recurrent SC who underwent MMS. One patient who underwent MMS followed by oculoplastic repair was tumor-free at 6 months. In the other patient, tumor distal to the Mohs defect was noted at reconstruction. A case of poorly differentiated SC successfully treated with RT has been reported.[230]

Patients with SC should be evaluated by an internist, and routine screening for internal malignancy (stool for occult blood, analysis of urine, colonoscopy) should be current. A family history for internal malignancy should be sought and family members screened, if indicated, to rule out Muir-Torre syndrome.[231] After treatment for SC, patients should be followed up for recurrence or progression through regular examination of skin and lymph nodes.

ATYPICAL FIBROXANTHOMA

Atypical fibroxanthoma (AFX) is a spindle cell tumor that occurs on the head and neck of sun-exposed individuals and on the trunk and extremities of younger patients.[232–234] Tumors of the head and neck characteristically present during the eighth decade, whereas tumors involving the extremities often present during the fourth decade.[231] The ratio of affected men to affected women appears to be equal.[232]

The pathogenesis of AFX may involve exposure to UVL, ionizing radiation, or aberrant host response. In one study of ten cases of AFX, seven cases showed mutation in p53. Of the seven, all showed abnormal single-strand conformation polymorphism, with four of those showing C→T mutations characteristically induced by UVL.[235] Exposure to ionizing radiation may play a role in the development of the tumor, as AFX after RT has been demonstrated.[236] An increased incidence of AFX was shown in a study of 642 renal transplant patients,[237] and invasive AFX has been reported in a heart transplant patient.[238] Finally, metastatic AFX has been reported in a patient with null cell variant chronic lymphocytic leukemia.[239]

AFX usually presents as an asymptomatic papule or nodule. There may be hyperpigmentation or ulceration.[240] The clinical appearance is not distinctive, and the lesion may be confused with pyogenic granuloma, SCC, or BCC.[241,242] The tumor characteristically presents on the head and neck of the elderly or the trunk or extremities of younger individuals but is not limited to these sites. Occurrences on the eyelid[243] and within the ethmoid sinus[244] and oral cavity[236] have been reported.

Although AFX rarely metastasizes, it is a locally aggressive tumor with metastatic potential.[245] Metastases to parotid gland,[246] lymph nodes,[247] and lung[248] have been reported. In a series of eight cases of metastatic AFX, poor prognostic indicators included vascular invasion, recurrence, deep tissue penetration, necrosis, and impaired host resistance.[246]

On microscopical examination, there is a dermal nodule with a dense infiltrate of bizarre spindle cells arranged in hap-

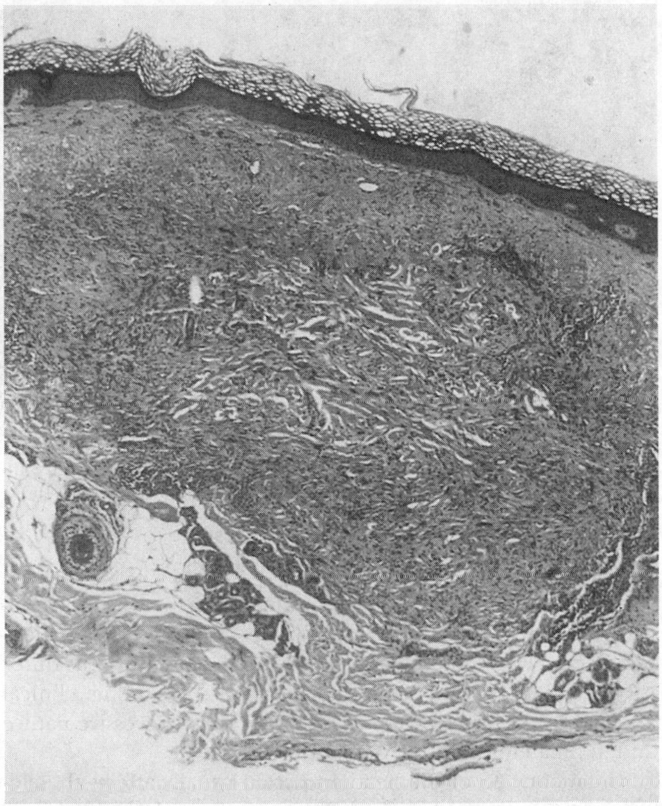

FIGURE 41.2-30. Atypical fibroxanthoma. On microscopical examination, there is a dermal nodule with a dense infiltrate of atypical spindle cells arranged in haphazard fashion and associated with bizarre giant cells. (See Color Fig. 41.2-30 in the CD-ROM and on the Web at www.LWWoncology.com.)

hazard fashion (Fig. 41.2-30).[240] Often, bizarre giant cells are present, and there is no connection to the epidermis.[240] Special stains for vimentin are positive and for CD68 are weakly positive, while stains for HMB-45 and S-100 are negative, distinguishing this lesion from spindle cell melanoma.[249,250] Differentiation from malignant fibrous histiocytoma (MFH) may be aided by special stains, as AFX stains negatively for LN-2, a marker present on B cells, Reed-Sternberg cells, and macrophages, and MFH cells are positive for LN-2 in 90% of cases.[251]

Treatment options for AFX include WLE and MMS. In one large series comparing WLE with MMS,[232] recurrences were observed during a mean follow-up period of 73.6 months in 12% of 25 cases treated by WLE. Metastatic involvement of the parotid gland occurred in one of these patients, for an overall regional metastatic rate of 4%. In contrast, no recurrences or metastases were observed over a mean follow-up period of 29.6 months in any patient treated by MMS. Others have reported similarly favorable outcomes after treatment of AFX by MMS, albeit with smaller numbers of cases.[252,253] The authors favor the use of MMS for AFX because of the superior margin control and conservation of normal tissue.

MALIGNANT FIBROUS HISTIOCYTOMA

MFH is an aggressive spindle cell cancer and is the most common soft tissue tumor in the elderly, primarily affecting the extremities.[254,255] Peak incidence is during the seventh decade.[253]

Though the pathogenesis of MFH is incompletely understood, there appears to be a predilection for development in scar tissue. Inoshita et al.[256] report development of MFH in an amputation site in one patient and in a hernioplasty scar in another. In both patients, the initial clinical diagnosis was subcutaneous abscess. MFH in a burn scar has also been reported.[257] A case of MFH associated with discoid lupus erythematosis has also been described.[258] Decreased immune surveillance may play a role in the development of MFH. A significant increase in the incidence of MFH (158 per 100,000) has been reported in a large series of renal transplant patients.[237]

MFH is aggressive, with high metastatic potential. In one series, a higher percentage of histologically infiltrative tumors (83% vs. 24%) were observed in subcutaneous MFH as opposed to intramuscular MFH.[259] An increased percentage of local recurrences (17% vs. 0%) were observed in the subcutaneous variant. However, infiltrative growth pattern was not predictive of metastatic potential. In one large series, the local recurrence rate was 44%, and the rate of metastasis was 42%.[254] Metastasis, in this series, occurred most commonly in lung (82%) and lymph nodes (32%). Factors that appeared to influence metastasis included depth and size of tumor and inflammatory response. Small, superficially located tumors and tumors with a prominent inflammatory component metastasized less frequently.

Clinically, MFH may present as a subcutaneous mass[256] or ulcerative nodule.[255] In one large series, MFH occurred principally as a mass on an extremity (lower extremity, 49%; upper extremity, 19%) or in the abdominal cavity or retroperitoneum (16%) of adults.[254] Deep fascial involvement was typical (19%), as was involvement of skeletal muscle (59%). Fascial involvement was absent in only a small percentage of cases (7%).

On microscopical examination, morphologic features vary, and MFH may show transitions from areas with a highly ordered, storiform pattern to less differentiated areas with a pleomorphic appearance. Differentiation from AFX may be aided by staining with LN-2, a marker present in 90% of MFHs in one series but absent or only weakly present in AFX.[251]

Treatment options for MFH include WLE, although recurrence rates of up to 40% have been reported with this approach.[254] Some authors have reported successful treatment of subcutaneous MFH with MMS.[251,259] Brown and Swanson[260,261] reported no recurrences over a 3-year follow-up period among 17 patients with 20 tumors treated by MMS. Hafner et al.[252] reported successful treatment of MFH by MMS with margin control achieved using paraffin-embedded tissue sections. After treatment for MFH, patients should be followed up aggressively for development of recurrent and metastatic disease.

DERMATOFIBROSARCOMA PROTUBERANS

Dermatofibrosarcoma protuberans (DFSP) is a low-grade cutaneous sarcoma with well-characterized clinical and histopathologic features. The lesion frequently appears as a plaque on the trunk and, less commonly, on the extremities of middle-aged adults.[262,263] Gender distribution of DFSP tends to vary in published series.[262]

The pathogenesis of DFSP is incompletely understood but may involve factors as diverse as aberrant tumor suppressor genes or history of local trauma. In one study, increased p53 protein immunoreactivity was found in DFSP but not in dermatofibrosarcoma, suggesting that expression of the protein may be important in the pathogenesis of DFSP.[264] In addition, DFSP has been reported to occur at previously traumatized sites.[265]

DFSP has a tendency to recur locally, with an overall rate of 50%. However, metastases are rare. In one series of 19 cases of DFSP, there were 20 local recurrences in 8 patients.[266] Recurrences in this series followed narrow excision. No recurrences were noted during a mean follow-up period of 13.2 years after WLE with margins greater than 2 cm. Lymph node metastases occur in approximately 1% of cases and distant metastases, principally to lung, occur in approximately 4% of DFSP cases.[266] A fibrosarcomatous variant, FS-DFSP, represents an uncommon form of DFSP.[267] In a series of 41 patients with FS-DFSP, follow-up in 34 patients for a mean period of 90 months revealed a local recurrence rate of 58%. Metastases were observed at a rate of 14.7%. Thus, fibrosarcomatous change in DFSP is indicative of a more aggressive clinical course.[267] A case of acral DFSP with fibrosarcomatous change and pulmonary parenchymal metastases was reported recently.[268]

DFSP classically presents as a plaque on the trunk and, less frequently, on the extremities but may occur anywhere.[262] The tumor may be difficult to differentiate clinically from a dermatofibroma or a keloid.[270] The tumor most commonly presents during early or middle adulthood, though it can occur during childhood.[271,272] The Bednar tumor is a rare pigmented variant of DFSP.[273]

Microscopically, the tumor is composed of monomorphous spindle cells arranged in a storiform pattern and embedded in a sparse to moderately dense fibrous stroma.[262] The distinction between deep penetrating dermatofibroma (DPDF), which involves the subcutis, and DFSP may be challenging. In most instances, attention to the cytologic constituency of the lesions and the overall architecture is sufficient for differentiation. DPDF is typified by cellular heterogeneity. DPDF includes giant cells and lipidized histiocytes and extends deeply, using the interlobular subcuticular fibrous septa as scaffolds, or in the form of broad fronts. In contrast, DFSP tends to be monomorphous, surrounding adipocytes diffusely or extending in stratified horizontal plates. Immunostaining for factor XIIIa and CD34 may be helpful in distinguishing DPDF from DFSP. Characteristically, DPDF is diffusely factor XIIIa–positive and CD34-negative, whereas DFSP is factor XIIIa–negative and CD34-positive.[274,275]

Treatment options for DFSP include WLE and MMS. Some authors advocate surgical excision with a minimal margin of 2 to 3 cm of surrounding skin, including the underlying fascia, without elective lymph node dissection.[266] Although WLE has been the standard treatment of DFSP, recurrence rates approach 50%. In one series, 58 patients with DFSP treated by MMS at three institutions showed a local recurrence rate of 2%.[277] There were no cases of regional or distant metastases. Other studies support MMS as the treatment of choice for DFSP, based on low recurrence rate and maximal conservation of normal tissue.[269,276,277] Caution is advised in attempting to interpret immunostains on frozen sections of DFSP since, in one study, microscopical examination of paraffin-embedded sections showed CD34-negative DFSP tumor cells with positive staining of endothelial cells.[278] The authors favor extirpation of tumor by MMS, using frozen sections with confirmation by examination of paraffin-embedded sections. Patients with DFSP should be followed up closely for evidence of local or regional recurrence or metastatic disease.

ANGIOSARCOMA

Angiosarcoma (AS) is an aggressive, usually fatal neoplasm of vascular cells.[279] Four variants of cutaneous AS currently are recognized, including AS of the scalp and face, AS in the context of lymphedema (Stewart-Treves syndrome), radiation-induced AS, and epithelioid AS. Although these variants differ in presentation, they share key features, including clinical appearance of primary lesions, a biologically aggressive nature and, ultimately, poor outcome.

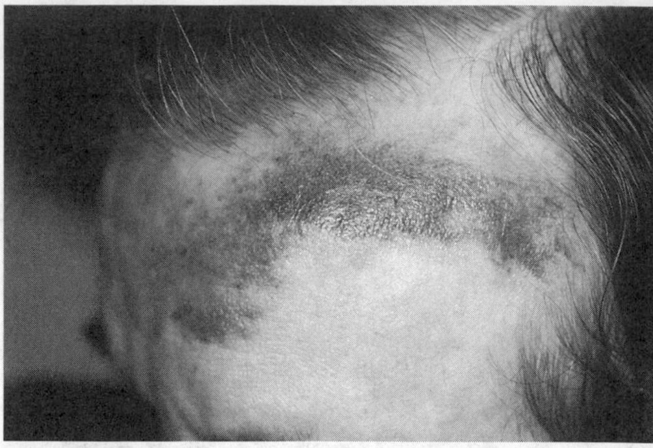

FIGURE 41.2-31. Angiosarcoma may present as a violaceous, ill-defined plaque on the scalp. (See Color Fig. 41.2-31 in the CD-ROM and on the Web at www.LWWoncology.com.)

Cutaneous AS of the head and scalp usually affects the elderly, with men being affected more often than women.[280] Although no predisposing factors have been identified, exposure to UVL has been suggested as a risk factor due to the propensity for the tumor to affect sun-exposed sites of the scalp and face. Other researchers have questioned this connection because, in several series, AS has presented on scalps protected by hair as frequently as on bald scalps. Others have demonstrated that patients with AS show no significant increase in numbers of BCCs and SCCs, thus arguing against increased UVL exposure.

AS presents as a violaceous to red ill-defined plaque, often initially resembling a bruise (Fig. 41.2-31). The differential diagnosis may include benign vascular tumors, hematoma secondary to trauma, or an inflammatory dermatosis. Unexplained facial edema may be a presenting sign as well. As AS progresses, lesions increase in size, become indurated, and may eventually ulcerate. Satellite lesions are common.

On microscopical examination, it becomes evident that AS extends far beyond clinical margins. In well-differentiated lesions, histology shows irregularly dilated vascular channels lined by flattened endothelial cells.[278] Less differentiated tumors show proliferation of polygonal or spindle-shaped, pleomorphic endothelial cells and anastomosing vascular channels. The state of cellular differentiation has not been shown to correlate with prognosis. Special stains may be of value in histologic diagnosis of AS, as cells stain positively for *Ulex europeaus* I lectin and factor VIII–related antigen. *Ulex* I is considered to be more sensitive for AS. In addition, AS cells express stem cell antigen CD34 and endothelial cell surface antigen CD31.

AS is a biologically aggressive tumor with high metastatic potential. Metastases to lymph nodes, lung, and brain are common. Prognosis for metastatic disease is poor. Although prognosis does not correlate with degree of cellular differentiation, there appears to a correlation with lesion size at presentation:

Increased survival has been demonstrated in lesions smaller than 5 cm at time of presentation.

Owing to the aggressiveness and poor prognosis of AS, treatment options are limited. Radical excision is currently the treatment of choice and may be difficult to accomplish in tumors involving the face. Amputation with shoulder disarticulation or hemipelvectomy are recommended for tumors involving the extremities. As stated, AS tends to extend far beyond clinically appreciated margins, thus complicating excision. Several cases of AS have been treated by MMS in an attempt to control margins; however, the difference between AS and normal vasculature may be difficult to interpret on frozen sections, even with the use of immunohistochemical stains. Prognosis of AS is poor, with a mortality rate of 50% at 15 months after diagnosis. The 5-year survival rate is approximately 12%.

Lymphedema-associated AS (LAS) was first reported by Stewart and Treves[281–283] in 6 patients with postmastectomy lymphedema. In each case, AS developed in the ipsilateral arm and occurred several years after mastectomy. Subsequently, LAS was reported after axillary node dissection for melanoma and in the context of congenital lymphedema, filarial lymphedema, and chronic idiopathic lymphedema. The risk for developing LAS 5 years after mastectomy is approximately 5%. The most common site is the medial aspect of the upper arm.

LAS presents as a violaceous plaque or nodule superimposed on brawny, nonpitting edema. Ulceration may develop rapidly. The pathogenesis of LAS is incompletely understood and may be related to imbalances in local immune regulation or angiogenesis, leading to proliferation of neoplastic cells. The prognosis is poor, and survival rates are comparable to AS involving the scalp and face. Long-term survival has been reported after amputation of the affected limb.

Radiation-induced AS has been reported to occur after RT for benign or malignant conditions.[279,284–286] AS may occur from 4 to 40 years after RT for benign conditions, including acne and eczema, or from 4 to 25 years after RT for malignancies. Lesions appear at sites treated with radiation and are clinically and histologically similar to AS involving the scalp and face. Prognosis is poor and comparable to that observed in other forms of AS.

Epithelioid AS (EAS) is a rare, recently described variant of AS. It tends to involve the lower extremities.[278] On microscopical examination, the tumor may mimic an epithelial neoplasm, with sheets of rounded, epithelioid cells intermingled with irregularly lined vascular channels. Epithelioid AS results in widespread metastases within 1 year of presentation. Prognosis, as in other forms of AS, is poor.

KAPOSI'S SARCOMA

Kaposi's sarcoma (KS) is an indolent vascular tumor that has been subdivided into epidemiologic variants including classic KS, African endemic KS, iatrogenic KS, and epidemic, acquired immunodeficiency syndrome–associated (AIDS-associated) KS.[62,279,287–289] Classic KS affects elderly men, with increased incidence in Ashkenazi Jews and in persons of Mediterranean descent. Classic KS typically presents with violaceous macules on the lower extremities. Slow progression with coalescence to plaques is observed. Eventually, the disease enters a nodular phase and may ultimately progress to a hyperkeratotic or even ulcerative phase.

African endemic KS can be further subdivided into a generally benign nodular disease, predominantly affecting young adults, and a fulminant lymphadenopathic disease, predominantly affecting children.[289] Nodular African endemic KS also presents with violaceous macules that eventually progress to form plaques and nodules. Cutaneous and mucous membrane involvement are rare in lymphadenopathic endemic KS.

Iatrogenic KS occurs in the context of immunosuppressive drug therapy.[62] Iatrogenic KS is usually chronic but may be somewhat more aggressive than classic KS. Iatrogenic KS presents with lesions similar to those observed in classic KS. The lesions may regress on withdrawal of the immunosuppressive agent.

Epidemic KS appears in approximately 21% of homosexual men with AIDS.[287] It is considered to be a sexually transmitted disease, and the etiologic agent appears to be human herpesvirus-8 (HHV-8). Epidemic KS presents with violaceous macules involving the face, chest, and oral mucosa. The hard palate and ocular conjunctiva are frequently involved.

KS, for the most part, behaves in an indolent fashion, with some variance according to epidemiologic subtype. Patients with long-standing classic KS may show visceral involvement, but this is usually asymptomatic. The adult variant of endemic KS tends to follow an indolent course as well. In contrast, lymphadenopathic endemic KS progresses to fulminant, fatal disease. Iatrogenic KS is somewhat more aggressive than classic KS; however, lesions usually regress on discontinuation of immunosuppressive therapy. In epidemic KS, extracutaneous involvement is commonly encountered in lymph nodes, gastrointestinal tract, and lungs. Disseminated disease accounts for death in 10% to 20% of patients with epidemic KS.

On microscopical examination, KS varies according to patch, plaque, and nodular subtypes. The histologic changes in early patch-stage KS are inconspicuous, leading to misdiagnosis of a benign inflammatory process. A superficial and deep perivascular infiltrate with increased numbers of jagged vascular spaces is observed in the dermis. The thin-walled vessels surround normal vessels and adnexal structures, resulting in the so-called promontory sign. Plasma cells may be seen surrounding the newly formed vessels. In plaque-stage KS, the entire dermis and superficial fat may be involved, with an increase in the number of spindle cells arranged in small fascicles between collagen bundles centered around proliferating vascular channels. The spindle cells outline irregular slit-like vascular spaces that contain erythrocytes. In nodular KS, the number of spindle cells increases. They are arranged in interwoven fascicles with erythrocytes scattered in the interstices. Although nuclear atypia, mitotic figures, and pleomorphism may be observed, these are not prominent. Cells that stain positively for factor VIII–related antigen and spindle cells that stain positively for *Ulex europeaus* I lectin line well-formed vessels within KS lesions.

Both local and systemic therapies have been used in the management of KS, depending on epidemiologic context, extent of disease, and concomitant disease.[279,290–294] KS has been treated successfully using cryosurgery, RT, laser ablation, and intralesional injection of cytotoxic agents. Local infiltration with vincristine has been particularly effective in the treatment of oral lesions in epidemic AIDS-associated KS. Other, more aggressive approaches have included systemic therapy with interferon or with single- or multiagent chemotherapy. Tur and Brenner[293] treated 11 classic KS patients with low-dose subcutaneous interferon-α for 6 months. Initial response,

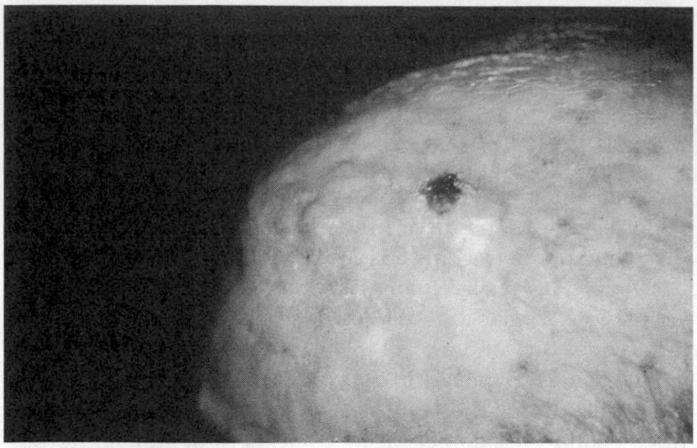

FIGURE 41.2-32. The scalp is a common site for cutaneous metastatic disease. (See Color Fig. 41.2-32 in the CD-ROM and on the Web at www.LWWoncology.com.)

defined as reduction of lesion size and fading of color, was noted in 9 of the 11 patients after 3 to 13 weeks of treatment. Maximum response was noted in 4 to 6 months, with remission lasting from 4 to 72 months. Experimental therapies including antiangiogenesis agents TNP-470 and thalidomide, 9-*cis* retinoic acid, and human chorionic gonadotropin may prove useful in management of KS in the future.[295]

CARCINOMA METASTATIC TO SKIN

The relative frequencies of cutaneous metastases are similar to those observed with primary cancers.[296] The most frequently observed cutaneous metastatic cancers are breast, colon, and melanoma in women and lung, colon, and melanoma in men. Cutaneous metastases may represent an opportunity to detect a potentially treatable cancer before other evidence of it is present, to modify therapy as appropriate to the tumor stage or, possibly, to use the cutaneous lesion as a source of easily accessible tumor cells for specific therapy. Cutaneous metastatic disease as the first sign of internal cancer is most commonly seen with cancer of the lung, kidney, and ovary. Cutaneous involvement is also seen in the leukemias, with a wide variation in morphology of lesions.[296] The scalp is a common site for cutaneous metastatic disease (Fig. 41.2-32). Perhaps the most widely known cutaneous manifestation of an internal carcinoma is the Sister Mary Joseph nodule.[297] Dr. William Mayo's surgical assistant, Sister Mary Joseph, noted the association of the presence of an indurated umbilical nodule in the setting of gastric cancer with poor prognosis. The discovery of cutaneous metastatic disease should result in prompt consultation with an oncologist for staging and management (Fig. 41.2-33).

MAC	MMS
Sebaceous carcinoma	Excision or MMS
AFX	MMS
MFH	WLE or MMS
DFSP	MMS with permanent section confirmation
Angiosarcoma	WLE or MMS with permanent section confirmation
Kaposi's sarcoma	Cryosurgery, intralesional, or systemic chemotherapy

FIGURE 41.2-33. The appropriate management of less common skin cancers may include wide local excision (WLE), Mohs micrographic surgery (MMS), cryosurgery, or intralesional or systemic chemotherapy. AFX, atypical fibroxanthoma; DFSP, dermatofibrosarcoma protuberans; MAC, microcystic adnexal carcinoma; MFH, malignant fibrous histiocytoma.

CONCLUSION

The discovery of an atypical skin lesion should result in consultation with a dermatologist for evaluation. It is necessary that skin biopsy specimens be sent to a dermatopathologist for interpretation to minimize misdiagnosis and delayed treatment of skin cancers. Management of skin cancer is based on histopathologic analysis of a given lesion; hence, accurate interpretation of skin biopsy specimens is essential. After treatment for skin cancer, patients should be followed up regularly, through full-body skin examinations performed by a dermatologist, for the development of recurrences as well as new primary skin cancers.

For additional information and color images, see Chapter 41.3: Atlas of Skin Cancer, at www.LWWoncology.com.

REFERENCES

1. Strom SS, Yamamura Y. Epidemiology of nonmelanoma skin cancer. *Clin Plast Surg* 1997;24(4):627.
2. Karagas MR, et al. Increase in incidence rates of basal cell and squamous cell skin cancer in New Hampshire, USA. New Hampshire Skin Cancer Study Group. *Int J Cancer* 1999;81(4):555.
3. Spratt JS Jr. Cancer mortality after nonmelanoma skin cancer. *JAMA* 1999;281(4):325.
4. Arpey CJ. Biopsy of the skin: thoughtful selection of technique improves yield. *Postgrad Med* 1998;103(3):179.
5. O'Toole EA, Goel M, Woodley DT. Hydrogen peroxide inhibits human keratinocyte migration. *Dermatol Surg* 1996;22(6):525.
6. Vessey DA, Lee KH, Blacker KL. Characterization of the oxidative stress initiated in cultured human keratinocytes by treatment with peroxides. *J Invest Dermatol* 1992;99(6):859.
7. Lawrence CM. Mohs micrographic surgery for basal cell carcinoma. *Clin Exp Dermatol* 1999;24(2):130.
8. Bernstein PE. Mohs '98: single-procedure Mohs surgery with immediate reconstruction. *Otolaryngol Head Neck Surg* 1999;120(2):184.
9. Shriner DL, et al. Mohs micrographic surgery. *J Am Acad Dermatol* 1998;39(1):79.
10. Arlette JP, et al. Basal cell carcinoma of the periocular region. *J Cutan Med Surg* 1998;2(4):205.
11. Kumar B, et al. A review of 24 cases of Mohs surgery and ophthalmic plastic reconstruction. *Aust NZ J Ophthalmol* 1997;25(4):289.
12. Nelson BR, Railan D, Cohen S. Mohs micrographic surgery for nonmelanoma skin cancers. *Clin Plast Surg* 1997;24(4):705.
13. Skouge JW. Mohs micrographic surgery for the treatment of difficult skin cancers. *Md Med J* 1997;46(5):231.
14. Nordin P. Curettage-cryosurgery for non-melanoma skin cancer of the external ear: excellent 5-year results. *Br J Dermatol* 1999;140(2):291.
15. Nordin P, Larko O, Stenquist B. Five-year results of curettage-cryosurgery of selected large primary basal cell carcinomas on the nose: an alternative treatment in a geographical area underserved by Mohs surgery. *Br J Dermatol* 1997;136(2):180.
16. Kibarian MA, Hruza GJ. Nonmelanoma skin cancer. Risks, treatment options, and tips on prevention. *Postgrad Med* 1995;98(6):39.
17. Sinclair RD, Dawber RP. Cryosurgery of malignant and premalignant diseases of the skin: a simple approach. *Australas J Dermatol* 1995;36(3):133.
18. Motley RJ, et al. Treatment of basal cell carcinoma by dermatologists in the United Kingdom. British Association of Dermatologists Audit Subcommittee and the British Society for Dermatological Surgery. *Br J Dermatol* 1995;132(3):437.

19. Crouch E. Curettage and cautery of skin conditions [Letter]. *Br J Gen Pract* 1992;42(362):398.
20. Salasche SJ. Status of curettage and desiccation in the treatment of primary basal cell carcinoma [Editorial]. *J Am Acad Dermatol* 1984;10(2):285.
21. Robins P, Albom MJ. Recurrent basal cell carcinomas in young women. *J Dermatol Surg* 1975;1(1):49.
22. Schwartz RA. The actinic keratosis: a perspective and update. *Dermatol Surg* 1997;23(11):1009.
23. Kuflik AS, Schwartz RA. Actinic keratosis and squamous cell carcinoma. *Am Fam Physician* 1994;49(4):817.
24. Mittelbronn MA, et al. Frequency of pre-existing actinic keratosis in cutaneous squamous cell carcinoma. *Int J Dermatol* 1998;37(9):677.
25. Brash DE, et al. Sunlight and sunburn in human skin cancer: p53 apoptosis and tumor promotion. *J Invest Dermatol Symp Proc* 1996;1(2):136.
26. Cockerell CJ. Histopathology of incipient intraepidermal squamous cell carcinoma ("actinic keratosis"). *J Am Acad Dermatol* 2000;42(1):11.
27. Picascia DD, Robinson JK. Actinic cheilitis: a review of the etiology, differential diagnosis, and treatment. *J Am Acad Dermatol* 1987;17(2):255.
28. Burns T. Basal cell carcinoma. *Practitioner* 1998; 242(1591):718.
29. Lear JT, et al. Basal cell carcinoma [see comments]. *J R Soc Med* 1998;91(11):585.
30. Lear JT, Smith AG. Basal cell carcinoma. *Postgrad Med J* 1997;73(863):538.
31. Leffell DJ, et al. Aggressive-growth basal cell carcinoma in young adults. *Arch Dermatol* 1991;127(11):1663.
32. Leffell DJ, Brash DE. Sunlight and skin cancer. *Sci Am* 1996;275(1):52.
33. English DR, et al. Sunlight and cancer. *Cancer Causes Control* 1997;8(3):271.
34. Quinn AG. Ultraviolet radiation and skin carcinogenesis. *Br J Hosp Med* 1997;58(6):261.
35. Brash DE. Sunlight and the onset of skin cancer. *Trends Genet* 1997;13(10):410.
36. Grossman D, Leffell DJ. The molecular basis of nonmelanoma skin cancer: new understanding. *Arch Dermatol* 1997;133(10):1263.
37. Ziegler A, et al. Tumor suppressor gene mutations and photocarcinogenesis. *Photochem Photobiol* 1996;63(4):432.
38. Ziegler A, et al. Sunburn and p53 in the onset of skin cancer [see comments]. *Nature* 1994;372(6508):773.
39. Walsh DS. Molecular genetics of skin cancer. *Adv Dermatol* 1997;13:167.
40. Ingham PW. The patched gene in development and cancer. [Published erratum appears in *Curr Opin Genet Dev* 1998;8(3):371.] *Curr Opin Genet Dev* 1998;8(1):88.
41. Cohen MM Jr. Nevoid basal cell carcinoma syndrome: molecular biology and new hypotheses. *Int J Oral Maxillofac Surg* 1999;28(3):216.
42. Bale SJ, Falk RT, Rogers GR. Patching together the genetics of Gorlin syndrome. *J Cutan Med Surg* 1998;3(1):31.
43. Wong ST, Chan HL, Teo SK. The spectrum of cutaneous and internal malignancies in chronic arsenic toxicity. *Singapore Med J* 1998;39(4):171.
44. Strickland FM, Kripke ML. Immune response associated with nonmelanoma skin cancer. *Clin Plast Surg* 1997;24(4):637.
45. Wicking C, Bale AE. Molecular basis of the nevoid basal cell carcinoma syndrome. *Curr Opin Pediatr* 1997;9(6):630.
46. Ron E, et al. Skin tumor risk among atomic-bomb survivors in Japan. *Cancer Causes Control* 1998;9(4):393.
47. Davis MM, et al. Skin cancer in patients with chronic radiation dermatitis [see comments]. *J Am Acad Dermatol* 1989;20(4):608.
48. Karagas MR, et al. Risk of basal cell and squamous cell skin cancers after ionizing radiation therapy. For the Skin Cancer Prevention Study Group. *J Natl Cancer Inst* 1996;88(24):1848.
49. Hahn H, et al. The patched signaling pathway in tumorigenesis and development: lessons from animal models. *J Mol Med* 1999;77(6):459.
50. Moles JP. [The gene of Gorlin's syndrome (basocellular nevomatosis) and the revival of the developmental genes in human carcinogenesis.] *Bull Cancer* 1998;85(3):207.
51. Mortele KJ, et al. Bilateral adrenal cystic lymphangiomas in nevoid basal cell carcinoma (Gorlin-Goltz) syndrome: US CT and MR findings. *J Comput Assist Tomogr* 1999;23(4):562.
52. Hahn H, et al. Mutations of the human homolog of *Drosophila* patched in the nevoid basal cell carcinoma syndrome. *Cell* 1996;85(6):841.
53. Gailani MR, et al. The role of the human homologue of *Drosophila* patched in sporadic basal cell carcinomas [see comments]. *Nat Genet* 1996;14(1):78.
54. Bale AE, Gailani MR, Leffell DJ. The Gorlin syndrome gene: a tumor suppressor active in basal cell carcinogenesis and embryonic development. *Proc Assoc Am Physicians* 1995;107(2):253.
55. Meunier L, Raison-Peyron N, Meynadier J. [UV-induced immunosuppression and skin cancers.] *Rev Med Interne* 1998;19(4):247.
56. Ramsay HM, et al. Multiple basal cell carcinomas in a patient with acute myeloid leukaemia and chronic lymphocytic leukaemia. *Clin Exp Dermatol* 1999;24(4):281.
57. Levi F, et al. Non-Hodgkin's lymphomas, chronic lymphocytic leukaemias, and skin cancers. *Br J Cancer* 1996;74(11):1847.
58. Ong CS, et al. Skin cancer in Australian heart transplant recipients. *J Am Acad Dermatol* 1999;40(1):27.
59. van Zuuren EJ, de Visscher JG, Bouwes Bavinck JN. Carcinoma of the lip in kidney transplant recipients. *J Am Acad Dermatol* 1998;38(3):497.
60. Montagnino G, et al. Cancer incidence in 854 kidney transplant recipients from a single institution: comparison with normal population and with patients under dialytic treatment. *Clin Transplant* 1996;10(5):461.
61. Leigh IM, Glover MT. Skin cancer and warts in immunosuppressed renal transplant recipients. *Recent Results Cancer Res* 1995;139:69.
62. Bouwes Bavinck JN, et al. Relation between skin cancer and HLA antigens in renal-transplant recipients [see comments]. *N Engl J Med* 1991;325(12):843.
63. Gutierrez-Steil C, et al. Sunlight-induced basal cell carcinoma tumor cells and ultraviolet-B-irradiated psoriatic plaques express Fas ligand (CD95L). *J Clin Invest* 1998;101(1):33.
64. Smith KJ, et al. Cutaneous neoplasms in a military population of HIV-1-positive patients. Military Medical Consortium for the Advancement of Retroviral Research. *J Am Acad Dermatol* 1993;29(3):400.
65. Lobo DV, et al. Nonmelanoma skin cancers and infection with the human immunodeficiency virus. *Arch Dermatol* 1992;128(5):623.
66. Miller SJ. Biology of basal cell carcinoma (part I). *J Am Acad Dermatol* 1991;24(1):1.
67. Bedlow AJ, et al. Basal cell carcinoma—an in-vivo model of human tumour microcirculation? *Exp Dermatol* 1999;8(3):222.
68. Weninger W, et al. Differences in tumor microvessel density between squamous cell carcinomas and basal cell carcinomas may relate to their different biologic behavior. *J Cutan Pathol* 1997;24(6):364.
69. Hernandez AD, Hibbs MS, Postlewaite AE, et al. Establishment of basal cell carcinoma in culture: evidence for a basal cell carcinoma-derived factor(s) which stimulates fibroblasts to proliferate and release collagenase. *J Invest Dermatol* 1985;85:470.
70. McCord MW, et al. Skin cancer of the head and neck with incidental microscopic perineural invasion. *Int J Radiat Oncol Biol Phys* 1999;43(3):591.
71. Di Gregorio C, et al. Mental nerve invasion by basal cell carcinoma of the chin: a case report. *Anticancer Res* 1998;18(6B):4723.
72. Terashi H, et al. Perineural and neural involvement in skin cancers. *Dermatol Surg* 1997;23(4):259.
73. Carlson KC, Roenigk RK. Know your anatomy: perineural involvement of basal and squamous cell carcinoma on the face. *J Dermatol Surg Oncol* 1990;16(9):827.
74. Niazi ZB, Lamberty BG. Perineural infiltration in basal cell carcinomas. *Br J Plast Surg* 1993;46(2):156.
75. Silbert PL, et al. Enigmatic trigeminal sensory neuropathy diagnosed by facial skin biopsy. *Clin Exp Neurol* 1992;29:234.
76. ten Hove MW, Glaser JS, Schatz NJ. Occult perineural tumor infiltration of the trigeminal nerve. Diagnostic considerations. *J Neuroophthalmol* 1997;17(3):170.
77. Morselli P, et al. Recurrent basal cell carcinoma of the back infiltrating the spine. *J Dermatol Surg Oncol* 1993;19(10).917.
78. Berti JJ, Sharata HH. Metastatic basal cell carcinoma to the lung. *Cutis* 1999;63(3):165.
79. Christian MM, Murphy CM, Wagner RF Jr. Metastatic basal cell carcinoma presenting as unilateral lymphedema. *Dermatol Surg* 1998;24(10):1151.
80. Berardi RS, et al. Pulmonary metastasis in nevoid basal cell carcinoma syndrome. *Int Surg* 1991;76(1):64.
81. Lo JS, et al. Metastatic basal cell carcinoma: report of twelve cases with a review of the literature [see comments]. *J Am Acad Dermatol* 1991;24(5):715.
82. Degner RA, et al. Metastatic basal cell carcinoma: report of a case presenting with respiratory failure. *Am J Med Sci* 1991;301(6):395.
83. Blinder D, Taicher S. Metastatic basal cell carcinoma presenting in the oral cavity and auditory meatus. A case report and review of literature. *Int J Oral Maxillofac Surg* 1992;21(1):31.
84. Cruse CW, O'Neill W, Rayhack J. Metastatic basal cell carcinoma of the upper extremity. *J Hand Surg [Am]* 1992;17(6):1093.
85. Mizushima J, Ohara K. Basal cell carcinoma of the vulva with lymph node and skin metastasis—report of a case and review of 20 Japanese cases. *J Dermatol* 1995;22(1):36.
86. Raszewski RL, Guyuron B. Long-term survival following nodal metastases from basal cell carcinoma. *Ann Plast Surg* 1990;24(2):170.
87. Pfeiffer P, Hansen O, Rose C. Systemic cytotoxic therapy of basal cell carcinoma A review of the literature. *Eur J Cancer* 1990;26(1):73.
88. Moeholt K, et al. Platinum-based cytotoxic therapy in basal cell carcinoma—a review of the literature. *Acta Oncol* 1996;35(6):677.
89. Rippey JJ. Why classify basal cell carcinomas? *Histopathology* 1998;32(5):393.
90. Bastiaens MT, et al. Differences in age, site distribution, and sex between nodular and superficial basal cell carcinoma indicate different types of tumors. *J Invest Dermatol* 1998;110(6):880.
91. Scherbenske JM, et al. A solitary nodule on the chest: fibroepithelioma of Pinkus. *Arch Dermatol* 1990;126(7):955.
92. Skidmore RA Jr, Flowers FP. Nonmelanoma skin cancer. *Med Clin North Am* 1998;82(6):1309.
93. Holmkvist KA, Rogers GS, Dahl PR. Incidence of residual basal cell carcinoma in patients who appear tumor free after biopsy. *J Am Acad Dermatol* 1999;41(4):600.
94. Salgarello M, Seccia A, Vricella M, Farallo E. Analysis of infiltrating epitheliomas of the nose examined from 1986 to 1995. *J Otolaryngol* 1998;27:288.
95. Evans GR, Williams JZ, Ainslie NB. Cutaneous nasal malignancies: Is primary reconstruction safe? *Head Neck* 1997;3:182.
96. Glied M, Berg D, Witterick I. Basal cell carcinoma of the conchal bowl: interdisciplinary approach to treatment. *J Otolaryngol* 1998;27(6):322.
97. Esquivias Gomez JI, et al. Basal cell carcinoma of the scrotum. *Australas J Dermatol* 1999;40(3):141.
98. Nehal KS, Levine VJ, Ashinoff R. Basal cell carcinoma of the genitalia. *Dermatol Surg* 1998;24(12):1361.
99. Ladocsi LT, et al. Basal cell carcinoma of the penis [see comments]. *Cutis* 1998;61(1):25.
100. Grossman HB. Premalignant and early carcinomas of the penis and scrotum. *Urol Clin North Am* 1992;19(2):221.
101. Paterson CA, Young-Fadok TM, Dozois RR. Basal cell carcinoma of the perianal region: 20-year experience. *Dis Colon Rectum* 1999;42(9):1200.
102. Goldberg DP. Assessment and surgical treatment of basal cell skin cancer. *Clin Plast Surg* 1997;24(4):673.
103. Leslie DF, Greenway HT. Mohs micrographic surgery for skin cancer. *Australas J Dermatol* 1991;32(3):159.
104. Halpern JN. Radiation therapy in skin cancer: a historical perspective and current applications. *Dermatol Surg* 1997;23(11):1089.
105. Wolf DJ, Zitelli JA. Surgical margins for basal cell carcinoma. *Arch Dermatol* 1987;123(3):340.
106. Cook J, Zitelli JA. Mohs micrographic surgery: a cost analysis [see comments]. *J Am Acad Dermatol* 1998;39(5):698.
107. Rowe DE, Carroll RJ, Day CL Jr. Long-term recurrence rates in previously untreated (primary) basal cell carcinoma: implications for patient follow-up. *J Dermatol Surg Oncol* 1989;15(3):315.

108. Rowe DE, Carroll RJ, Day CL Jr. Mohs surgery is the treatment of choice for recurrent (previously treated) basal cell carcinoma. *J Dermatol Surg Oncol* 1989;15(4):424.
109. Aliseda D, Vazquez J, Munuera JM. Medial canthus tumor surgery: a prospective study of microscopically controlled excision. *Eur J Ophthalmol* 1997;7(3):216.
110. Goldminz D, Bennett RG. Mohs micrographic surgery of the nail unit. *J Dermatol Surg Oncol* 1992;18(8):721.
111. Knox JM. Treatment of skin cancer. *J Am Acad Dermatol* 1985;12(3):589.
112. Kopf AW, et al. Curettage-electrodesiccation treatment of basal cell carcinomas. *Arch Dermatol* 1977;113(4):439.
113. Spiller WF, et al. Treatment of basal cell epithelioma by curettage and electrodesiccation. *J Am Acad Dermatol* 1984;11(5):808.
114. Morganroth GS, Leffell DJ. Nonexcisional treatment of benign and premalignant cutaneous lesions. *Clin Plast Surg* 1993;20(1):91.
115. Wilder RB, Kittelson JM, Shimm DS. Basal cell carcinoma treated with radiation therapy. *Cancer* 1991;68(10):2134.
116. Kuflik EG. Cryosurgery for cutaneous malignancy. An update. *Dermatol Surg* 1997;23(11):1081.
117. Zitelli JA. Cryosurgery for skin cancer [Letter]. *J Am Acad Dermatol* 1992;26(2):283.
118. Goncalves JC. Fractional cryosurgery. A new technique for basal cell carcinoma of the eyelids and periorbital area. *Dermatol Surg* 1997;23(6):475.
119. Humphreys TR, et al. Treatment of superficial basal cell carcinoma and squamous cell carcinoma in situ with a high-energy pulsed carbon dioxide laser. *Arch Dermatol* 1998;134(10):1247.
120. Katz MH. Nonmelanoma skin cancer. *Md Med J* 1997;46(5):239.
121. Gloster HM Jr, Brodland DG. The epidemiology of skin cancer. *Dermatol Surg* 1996;22(3):217.
122. Marks R. The epidemiology of non-melanoma skin cancer: who, why, and what can we do about it? *J Dermatol* 1995;22(11):853.
123. Healy E, Collins P, Barnes L. Nonmelanoma skin cancer in an Irish population: an appraisal of risk factors [see comments]. *Ir Med J* 1995;88(2):58.
124. Espana A, et al. Skin cancer in heart transplant recipients. *J Am Acad Dermatol* 1995;32(3):458.
125. Kirby B, Chalmers RJ. Multiple squamous cell carcinomas following photochemotherapy for atopic eczema [Letter]. *Clin Exp Dermatol* 1999;24(4):337.
126. Stern RS, Lunder EJ. Risk of squamous cell carcinoma and methoxsalen (psoralen) and UV-A radiation (PUVA). A meta-analysis. *Arch Dermatol* 1998;134(12):1582.
127. Lindel B, et al. PUVA and cancer risk: the Swedish follow-up study. *Br J Dermatol* 1999;141(1):108.
128. Stern RS, Liebman EJ, Vakeva L. Oral psoralen and ultraviolet-A light (PUVA) treatment of psoriasis and persistent risk of nonmelanoma skin cancer. PUVA Follow-up Study. *J Natl Cancer Inst* 1998;90(17):1278.
129. Takeda H, Mitsuhashi Y, Kondo S. Multiple squamous cell carcinomas in situ in vitiligo lesions after long-term PUVA therapy. *J Am Acad Dermatol* 1998;38(2):268.
130. Col M, et al. Arsenic-related Bowen's disease, palmar keratosis, and skin cancer. *Environ Health Perspect* 1999;107(8):687.
131. Yu HS, et al. Defective IL-2 receptor expression in lymphocytes of patients with arsenic-induced Bowen's disease. *Arch Dermatol Res* 1998;290(12):681.
132. Tsuruta D, et al. Merkel cell carcinoma Bowen's disease and chronic occupational arsenic poisoning. *Br J Dermatol* 1998;139(2):291.
133. Karagas MR, et al. Design of an epidemiologic study of drinking water arsenic exposure and skin and bladder cancer risk in a US population. *Environ Health Perspect* 1998;106[Suppl 4]:1047.
134. Brash DE, Ponten J. Skin precancer. *Cancer Surv* 1998;32:69.
135. Streilein JW, Alard P, Niizeki H. A new concept of skin-associated lymphoid tissue (SALT): UVB light impaired cutaneous immunity reveals a prominent role for cutaneous nerves. *Keio J Med* 1999;48(1):22.
136. Dandie GW, et al. Effects of UV on the migration and function of epidermal antigen presenting cells. *Mutat Res* 1998;422(1):147.
137. Goettsch W, et al. Comparative immunotoxicology of ultraviolet B exposure: I. Effects of in vitro and in situ ultraviolet B exposure on the functional activity and morphology of Langerhans cells in the skin of different species. *Br J Dermatol* 1998;139(2):230.
138. Denfeld RW, et al. Further characterization of UVB radiation effects on Langerhans cells: altered expression of the costimulatory molecules B7-1 and B7-2. *Photochem Photobiol* 1998;67(5):554.
139. Ziegler A, et al. Mutation hot-spots due to sunlight in the p53 gene of nonmelanoma skin cancers. *Proc Natl Acad Sci USA* 1993;90(9):4216.
140. Wang XM, et al. An unexpected spectrum of p53 mutations from squamous cell carcinomas in psoriasis patients treated with PUVA. *Photochem Photobiol* 1997;66(2):294.
141. Wong SS, Tan KC, Goh CL. Cutaneous manifestations of chronic arsenicism: review of seventeen cases. *J Am Acad Dermatol* 1998;38(2):179.
142. Eroglu A, Camlibel S. Risk factors for locoregional recurrence of scar carcinoma. *Br J Surg* 1997;84(12):1744.
143. Harland DL, Robinson WA, Franklin WA. Deletion of the p53 gene in a patient with aggressive burn scar carcinoma. *J Trauma* 1997;42(1):104.
144. Kirsner RS, et al. Squamous cell carcinoma arising in osteomyelitis and chronic wounds. Treatment with Mohs micrographic surgery vs amputation. *Dermatol Surg* 1996;22(12):1015.
145. Edwards MJ, et al. Squamous cell carcinoma arising in previously burned or irradiated skin. *Arch Surg* 1989;124(1):115.
146. Eliezri YD, Silverstein SJ, Nuovo GJ. Occurrence of human papillomavirus type 16 DNA in cutaneous squamous and basal cell neoplasms. *J Am Acad Dermatol* 1990;23(5):836.
147. Moy RL, et al. Human papillomavirus type 16 DNA in periungual squamous cell carcinomas [see comments]. *JAMA* 1989;261(18):2669.
148. Rowe DE, Carroll RJ, Day CL Jr. Prognostic factors for local recurrence metastasis and survival rates in squamous cell carcinoma of the skin, ear, and lip. Implications for treatment modality selection. *J Am Acad Dermatol* 1992;26(6):976.
149. Barksdale SK, O'Connor N, Barnhill R. Prognostic factors for cutaneous squamous cell and basal cell carcinoma. Determinants of risk of recurrence, metastasis, and development of subsequent skin cancers. *Surg Oncol Clin North Am* 1997;6(3):625.
150. Brodland DG, Zitelli JA. Mechanisms of metastasis. *J Am Acad Dermatol* 1992;27(1):1.
151. Immerman SC, et al. Recurrent squamous cell carcinoma of the skin. *Cancer* 1983;51(8):1537.
152. Friedman HI, Cooper PH, Wanebo HJ. Prognostic and therapeutic use of microstaging of cutaneous squamous cell carcinoma of the trunk and extremities. *Cancer* 1985;56(5):1099.
153. Spiro RH. Verrucous carcinoma then and now. *Am J Surg* 1998;176(5):393.
154. Bouquot JE. Oral verrucous carcinoma. Incidence in two US populations. *Oral Surg Oral Med Oral Pathol Oral Radiol Endod* 1998;86(3):318.
155. Casanova D, et al. Plantar verrucous carcinoma: a case report and literature review. *Ann Chir Plast Esthet* 1997;42(1):56.
156. Bell HK, Rhodes LE. Bowen's disease—a retrospective review of clinical management [Letter]. *Clin Exp Dermatol* 1999;24(4):338.
157. Fitzgerald DA. Cancer precursors. *Semin Cutan Med Surg* 1998;17(2):108.
158. Liu Y, et al. [Detecting HPV DNA in tissue of epidermal neoplasms.] *Chung Kuo I Hsueh Ko Hsueh Yuan Hsueh Pao* 1997;19(1):64.
159. Olhoffer IH, et al. Facial bowenoid papulosis secondary to human papillomavirus type 16. *Br J Dermatol* 1999;140(4):761.
160. Dogan G, et al. Three cases of verrucous carcinoma. *Australas J Dermatol* 1998;39(4):251.
161. Johnson TM, et al. Squamous cell carcinoma of the skin (excluding lip and oral mucosa). *J Am Acad Dermatol* 1992;26(3):467.
162. Goldman GD. Squamous cell cancer: a practical approach. *Semin Cutan Med Surg* 1998;17(2):80.
163. Honeycutt WM, Jansen GT. Treatment of squamous cell carcinoma of the skin. *Arch Dermatol* 1973;108(5):670.
164. Brodland DG, Zitelli JA. Surgical margins for excision of primary cutaneous squamous cell carcinoma. *J Am Acad Dermatol* 1992;27(2):241.
165. Wilson SM, Beahrs OH, Manson R. Squamous cell carcinoma of the anus. *Surg Annu* 1976;8:297.
166. Haberthur F, Almendral AC, Ritter B. Therapy of vulvar carcinoma. *Eur J Gynaecol Oncol* 1993;14(3):218.
167. Geisse JK. Comparison of treatment modalities for squamous cell carcinoma. *Clin Dermatol* 1995;13(6):621.
168. de Visscher JG, et al. Surgical treatment of squamous cell carcinoma of the lower lip: evaluation of long-term results and prognostic factors—a retrospective analysis of 184 patients. *J Oral Maxillofac Surg* 1998;56(7):814.
169. Frankel DH, Hanusa BH, Zitelli JA. New primary nonmelanoma skin cancer in patients with a history of squamous cell carcinoma of the skin. Implications and recommendations for follow-up. *J Am Acad Dermatol* 1992;26(5):720.
170. Haag ML, Glass LF, Fenske NA. Merkel cell carcinoma. Diagnosis and treatment. *Dermatol Surg* 1995;21(8):669.
171. Cook TF, Fosko SW. Unusual cutaneous malignancies. *Semin Cutan Med Surg* 1998;17(2):114.
172. Bose A. Nine cases of Merkel cell tumour. *J R Soc Med* 1997;90(8):439.
173. Miller RW, Rabkin CS. Merkel cell carcinoma and melanoma: etiological similarities and differences. [Published erratum appears in *Cancer Epidemiol Biomarkers Prev* 1999;8(5):485.] *Cancer Epidemiol Biomarkers Prev* 1999;8(2):153.
174. Iacocca MV, et al. Mixed Merkel cell carcinoma and squamous cell carcinoma of the skin. *J Am Acad Dermatol* 1998;39(5):882.
175. Simstein NL, Sduggs NK. Merkel cell tumor: two cases. *Int Surg* 1998;83(1):60.
176. Williams RH, et al. Merkel cell carcinoma in a renal transplant patient: increased incidence? *Transplantation* 1998;65(10):1396.
177. Veness MJ. Aggressive skin cancers in a cardiac transplant recipient. *Australas Radiol* 1997;41(4):363.
178. Marks S, Radin DR, Chandrasoma P. Merkel cell carcinoma. *J Comput Tomogr* 1987;11(3):291.
179. Olivero G, et al. [A rare case of Merkel's tumor with intestinal metastases.] *Ann Ital Chir* 1990;61(3):277.
180. Woo HH, Kencian JD. Metastatic Merkel cell tumour to the bladder. *Int Urol Nephrol* 1995;27(3):301.
181. Helm KF, et al. Localized limb cutaneous metastases. *J Surg Oncol* 1998;67(4):261.
182. Ikawa F, et al. Brain metastasis of Merkel cell carcinoma. Case report and review of the literature. *Neurosurg Rev* 1999;22(1):54.
183. Dunlop P, et al. Merkel cell carcinoma of the abdominal wall. *Skeletal Radiol* 1998;27(7):396.
184. Yanguas I, et al. Spontaneous regression of Merkel cell carcinoma of the skin. *Br J Dermatol* 1997;137(2):296.
185. Skelton HG, et al. Merkel cell carcinoma: analysis of clinical histologic and immunohistologic features of 132 cases with relation to survival *J Am Acad Dermatol* 1997;37(5):734.
186. Yiengpruksawan A, et al. Merkel cell carcinoma. Prognosis and management. *Arch Surg* 1991;126(12):1514.
187. Kokoska ER, et al. Early aggressive treatment for Merkel cell carcinoma improves outcome. *Am J Surg* 1997;174(6):688.
188. Hill AD, Brady MS, Coit DG. Intraoperative lymphatic mapping and sentinel lymph node biopsy for Merkel cell carcinoma. *Br J Surg* 1999;86(4):518.
189. Allen PJ, Zhang ZF, Coit DG. Surgical management of Merkel cell carcinoma. *Ann Surg* 1999;229(1):97.
190. Gray LN. Aggressive surgical management for Merkel cell carcinoma [Letter; comment]. *Plast Reconstr Surg* 1995;96(1):237.
191. Pectasides D, et al. Chemotherapy for Merkel cell carcinoma with carboplatin and etoposide. *Am J Clin Oncol* 1995;18(5):418.
192. Voog E, et al. Chemotherapy for patients with locally advanced or metastatic Merkel cell carcinoma. *Cancer* 1999;85(12):2589.
193. Goldstein DJ, Barr RJ, Santa Cruz DJ. Microcystic adnexal carcinoma: a distinct clinicopathologic entity. *Cancer* 1982;50(3):566.

194. Sebastien TS, et al. Microcystic adnexal carcinoma. *J Am Acad Dermatol* 1993;29(5):840.
195. McAlvany JP, et al. Sclerosing sweat duct carcinoma in an 11-year-old boy. *J Dermatol Surg Oncol* 1994;20(11):767.
196. Borenstein A, et al. Microcystic adnexal carcinoma following radiotherapy in childhood. *Am J Med Sci* 1991;301(4):259.
197. Lober CW, Larbig GG. Microcystic adnexal carcinoma (sclerosing sweat duct carcinoma). *South Med J* 1994;87(2):259.
198. Moy RL, Tahery DP, Howe K. Microcystic adnexal carcinoma: in vitro growth characteristics and effect on stromal collagen production. *Int J Dermatol* 1993;32(5):341.
199. Billingsley EM, Fedok F, Maloney ME. Microcystic adnexal carcinoma. Case report and review of the literature. *Arch Otolaryngol Head Neck Surg* 1996;122(2):179.
200. Yuh WT, et al. Bone marrow invasion of microcystic adnexal carcinoma. *Ann Otol Rhinol Laryngol* 1991;100(7):601.
200a. Birkby, CS, Argenvi, ZB, Whitaker, DC. Microcystic adnexal carcinoma with mandibular invasion and bone marrow replacement. *J Dermatol Surg Oncol* 1989;15:308.
201. Bier-Lansing CM, et al. Microcystic adnexal carcinoma: management options based on long-term follow-up. *Laryngoscope* 1995;105(11):1197.
202. Newman L. Microcystic adnexal carcinoma—a case report and review of the literature. *Br J Oral Maxillofac Surg* 1986;24(6):418.
203. Rongioletti F, Grosshans E, Rebora A. Microcystic adnexal carcinoma. *Br J Dermatol* 1986;115(1):101.
204. Brookes JL, et al. Microcystic adnexal carcinoma masquerading as a chalazion [Letter]. *Br J Ophthalmol* 1998;82(2):196.
205. Chow WC, Cockerell CJ, Geronemus RG. Microcystic adnexal carcinoma of the scalp. *J Dermatol Surg Oncol* 1989;15(7):768.
206. Schipper JH, Holecek BU, Sievers KW. A tumour derived from Ebner's glands: microcystic adnexal carcinoma of the tongue. *J Laryngol Otol* 1995;109(12):1211.
207. Kumar K, McGregor JC, Watson JD. Microcystic adnexal carcinoma: a report of three cases. *J R Coll Surg Edinb* 1998;43(6):412.
208. Lupton GP, McMarlin SL. Microcystic adnexal carcinoma. Report of a case with 30-year follow-up. *Arch Dermatol* 1986;122(3):286.
209. Wick MR, Cooper PH, Swanson PE, et al. Microcystic adnexal carcinoma: an immunohistochemical comparison with other cutaneous appendage tumors. *Arch Dermatol* 1990;162:189.
210. Friedman PM, et al. Microcystic adnexal carcinoma: collaborative series review and update. *J Am Acad Dermatol* 1999;41(2):225.
211. Wolfe JT, et al. Sebaceous carcinoma of the eyelid. Errors in clinical and pathologic diagnosis. *Am J Surg Pathol* 1984;8(8):597.
212. Khan JA, Doane JF, Grove AS Jr. Sebaceous and meibomian carcinomas of the eyelid. Recognition diagnosis and management. *Ophthal Plast Reconstr Surg* 1991;7(1):61.
213. Khan JA, et al. Sebaceous carcinoma. Diuretic use, lacrimal system spread, and surgical margins. *Ophthal Plast Reconstr Surg* 1989;5(4):227.
214. Tan KC, Lee ST, Cheah ST. Surgical treatment of sebaceous carcinoma of eyelids with clinico-pathological correlation. *Br J Plast Surg* 1991;44(2):117.
215. Zurcher M, et al. Sebaceous carcinoma of the eyelid: a clinicopathological study. *Br J Ophthalmol* 1998;82(9):1049.
216. Rundle P, et al. Sebaceous gland carcinoma of the eyelid seventeen years after irradiation for bilateral retinoblastoma [Letter]. *Eye* 1999;13:109.
217. Rumelt S, et al. Four-eyelid sebaceous cell carcinoma following irradiation. *Arch Ophthalmol* 1998;116(12):1670.
218. Hood IC, et al. Sebaceous carcinoma of the face following irradiation. *Am J Dermatopathol* 1986;8(6):505.
219. Carlson JW, et al. Sebaceous carcinoma of the vulva: a case report and review of the literature. *Gynecol Oncol* 1996;60(3):489.
220. Gonzalez-Fernandez F, et al. Sebaceous carcinoma. Tumor progression through mutational inactivation of p53. *Ophthalmology* 1998;105(3):497.
221. Antuna SA, et al. Metastatic lesion of the cervical spine secondary to an extraocular sebaceous carcinoma. *Acta Orthop Belg* 1996;62(4):229.
222. Bailet JW, et al. Sebaceous carcinoma of the head and neck. Case report and literature review. *Arch Otolaryngol Head Neck Surg* 1992;118(11):1245.
223. Jensen ML. Extraocular sebaceous carcinoma of the skin with visceral metastases: case report. *J Cutan Pathol* 1990;17(2):117.
224. Changchien CC, Chen L, Eng HL. Sebaceous carcinoma arising in a benign dermoid cyst of the ovary. *Acta Obstet Gynecol Scand* 1994;73(4):355.
225. Mandreker S, Pinto RW, Usgaonkar U. Sebaceous carcinoma of the eyelid with metastasis to the parotid region: diagnosis by fine needle aspiration cytology [Letter]. *Acta Cytol* 1997;41(5):1636.
226. Nelson BR, et al. Sebaceous carcinoma. *J Am Acad Dermatol* 1995;33(1):1.
227. Dogru M, et al. Management of eyelid sebaceous carcinomas. *Ophthalmologica* 1997;211(1):40.
228. Folberg R, et al. Recurrent and residual sebaceous carcinoma after Mohs excision of the primary lesion. *Am J Ophthalmol* 1987;103(6):817.
229. Dzubow LM. Sebaceous carcinoma of the eyelid: treatment with Mohs surgery. *J Dermatol Surg Oncol* 1985;11(1):40.
230. Matsumoto CS, et al. Sebaceous carcinoma responds to radiation therapy. *Ophthalmologica* 1995;209(5):280.
231. Schwartz RA, Torre DP. The Muir-Torre syndrome: a 25-year retrospect [see comments]. *J Am Acad Dermatol* 1995;33(1):90.
232. Dahl I. Atypical fibroxanthoma of the skin A clinico-pathological study of 57 cases. *Acta Pathol Microbiol Scand [A]* 1976;84(2):183.
233. Davis JL, et al. A comparison of Mohs micrographic surgery and wide excision for the treatment of atypical fibroxanthoma. *Dermatol Surg* 1997;23(2):105.
234. Fish FS. Soft tissue sarcomas in dermatology. *Dermatol Surg* 1996;22(3):268.
235. Dei Tos AP, et al. Ultraviolet-induced p53 mutations in atypical fibroxanthoma. *Am J Pathol* 1994;145(1):11.
236. High AS, Hume WJ, Dyson D. Atypical fibroxanthoma of oral mucosa: a variant of malignant fibrous histiocytoma. *Br J Oral Maxillofac Surg* 1990;28(4):268.
237. Hafner J, Kirzi W, Weinreich T. Malignant fibrous histiocytoma and atypical fibroxanthoma in renal transplant recipients. *Dermatology* 1999;198(1):29.
238. Paquet P, Pierard GE. Invasive atypical fibroxanthoma and eruptive actinic keratoses in a heart transplant patient. *Dermatology* 1996;192(4):411.
239. Kemp JD, et al. Metastasizing atypical fibroxanthoma. Coexistence with chronic lymphocytic leukemia. *Arch Dermatol* 1978;114(10):1533.
240. Heintz PW, White CR Jr. Diagnosis: atypical fibroxanthoma or not? Evaluating spindle cell malignancies on sun damaged skin: a practical approach. *Semin Cutan Med Surg* 1999;18(1):78.
241. Fretzin DF, Helwig EB. Atypical fibroxanthoma of the skin. A clinicopathologic study of 140 cases. *Cancer* 1973;31(6):1541.
242. Goette DK, Odom RB. Atypical fibroxanthoma masquerading as pyogenic granuloma. *Arch Dermatol* 1976;112(8):1155.
243. Boynton JR, Markowitch W Jr, Searl SS. Atypical fibroxanthoma of the eyelid. *Ophthalmology* 1989;96(10):1480.
244. Lesica A, Harwood TR, Yokoo H. Atypical fibroxanthoma of ethmoid sinus. *Arch Otolaryngol* 1975;101(8):506.
245. Dzubow LM. Mohs surgery report: spindle cell fibrohistiocytic tumors: classification and pathophysiology. *J Dermatol Surg Oncol* 1988;14(5):490.
246. Helwig EB, May D. Atypical fibroxanthoma of the skin with metastasis. *Cancer* 1986;57(2):368.
247. Grosso M, et al. Metastatic atypical fibroxanthoma of skin. *Pathol Res Pract* 1987;182(3):443.
248. Glavin FL, Cornwell ML. Atypical fibroxanthoma of the skin metastatic to a lung. Report of case features by conventional and electron microscopy and a review of relevant literature. *Am J Dermatopathol* 1985;7(1):57.
249. Diaz-Cascajo C, Borghi S, Bonczkowitz M. Pigmented atypical fibroxanthoma. *Histopathology* 1998;33(6):537.
250. Ma CK, Zarbo RJ, Gown AM. Immunohistochemical characterization of atypical fibroxanthoma and dermatofibrosarcoma protuberans. *Am J Clin Pathol* 1992;97(4):478.
251. Lazova R, et al. LN-2 (CD74): a marker to distinguish atypical fibroxanthoma from malignant fibrous histiocytoma. *Cancer* 1997;79(11):2115.
252. Hafner J, et al. Micrographic surgery ('slow Mohs) in cutaneous sarcomas. *Dermatology* 1999;198(1):37.
253. Limmer BL, Clark DP. Cutaneous micrographic surgery for atypical fibroxanthoma. *Dermatol Surg* 1997;23(7):553.
254. Weiss SW, Enzinger FM. Malignant fibrous histiocytoma: an analysis of 200 cases. *Cancer* 1978;41(6):2250.
255. Fletcher CD, McKee PH. Sarcomas—a clinicopathological guide with particular reference to cutaneous manifestation. I: Dermatofibrosarcoma protuberans, malignant fibrous histiocytoma, and the epithelioid sarcoma of Enzinger. *Clin Exp Dermatol* 1984;9(5):451.
256. Inoshita T, Youngberg GA. Malignant fibrous histiocytoma arising in previous surgical sites. Report of two cases. *Cancer* 1984;53(1):176.
257. Yamamura T, et al. Malignant fibrous histiocytoma developing in a burn scar. *Br J Dermatol* 1984;110(6):725.
258. Farber JN, Koh HK. Malignant fibrous histiocytoma arising from discoid lupus erythematosus. *Arch Dermatol* 1988;124(1):114.
259. Fanburg-Smith JC, et al. Infiltrative subcutaneous malignant fibrous histiocytoma: a comparative study with deep malignant fibrous histiocytoma and an observation of biologic behavior. *Ann Diagn Pathol* 1999;3(1):1.
260. Stadler FJ, Scott GA, Brown MD. Malignant fibrous tumors. *Semin Cutan Med Surg* 1998;17(2):141.
261. Brown MD, Swanson NA. Treatment of malignant fibrous histiocytoma and atypical fibrous xanthomas with micrographic surgery. *J Dermatol Surg Oncol* 1989;15(12):1287.
262. Diaz-Cascajo C, Weyers W, Borghi S. Sclerosing dermatofibrosarcoma protuberans. *J Cutan Pathol* 1998;25(8):440.
263. Garcia C, Clark RE, Buchanan M. Dermatofibrosarcoma protuberans. *Int J Dermatol* 1996;35(12):867.
264. Lee CS, Chou ST. p53 protein immunoreactivity in fibrohistiocytic tumors of the skin. *Pathology* 1998;30(3):272.
265. Bashara ME, Jules KT, Potter GK. Dermatofibrosarcoma protuberans: 4 years after local trauma. *J Foot Surg* 1992;31(2):160.
266. Rutgers EJ, et al. Dermatofibrosarcoma protuberans: treatment and prognosis. *Eur J Surg Oncol* 1992;18(3):241.
267. Mentzel T, et al. Fibrosarcomatous ("high-grade") dermatofibrosarcoma protuberans: clinicopathologic and immunohistochemical study of a series of 41 cases with emphasis on prognostic significance. *Am J Surg Pathol* 1998;22(5):576.
268. Skoll PJ, Hudson DA, Taylor DA. Acral dermatofibrosarcoma protuberans with metastases. *Ann Plast Surg* 1999;42(2):217.
269. Parker TL, Zitelli JA. Surgical margins for excision of dermatofibrosarcoma protuberans. *J Am Acad Dermatol* 1995;32(2):233.
270. Mbonde MP, Amir H, Kitinya JN. Dermatofibrosarcoma protuberans: a clinicopathological study in an African population. *East Afr Med J* 1996;73(6):410.
271. Bouyssou-Gauthier ML, et al. Dermatofibrosarcoma protuberans in childhood. *Pediatr Dermatol* 1997;14(6):463.
272. Pappo AS, et al. Dermatofibrosarcoma protuberans: the pediatric experience at St. Jude Children's Research Hospital. *Pediatr Hematol Oncol* 1997;14(6):563.
273. Elgart GW, et al. Bednar tumor (pigmented dermatofibrosarcoma protuberans) occurring in a site of prior immunization: immunochemical findings and therapy. *J Am Acad Dermatol* 1999;40(2):315.
274. Wick MR, et al. The pathological distinction between "deep penetrating" dermatofibroma and dermatofibrosarcoma protuberans. *Semin Cutan Med Surg* 1999;18(1):91.

275. Abenoza P, Lillemoe T. CD34 and factor XIIIa in the differential diagnosis of dermatofibroma and dermatofibrosarcoma protuberans [see comments]. *Am J Dermatopathol* 1993;15(5):429.
276. Ratner D, et al. Mohs micrographic surgery for the treatment of dermatofibrosarcoma protuberans. Results of a multiinstitutional series with an analysis of the extent of microscopic spread. *J Am Acad Dermatol* 1997;37(4):600.
277. Gloster HM Jr, Harris KR, Roenigk RK. A comparison between Mohs micrographic surgery and wide surgical excision for the treatment of dermatofibrosarcoma protuberans. *J Am Acad Dermatol* 1996;35(1):82.
278. Garcia C, et al. Dermatofibrosarcoma protuberans treated with Mohs surgery. A case with CD34 immunostaining variability. *Dermatol Surg* 1996;22(2):177.
279. Requena L, Sangueza OP. Cutaneous vascular proliferations: III. Malignant neoplasms, other cutaneous neoplasms with significant vascular component, and disorders erroneously considered as vascular neoplasms. *J Am Acad Dermatol* 1998;38(2):143.
280. el-Sharkawi S. Angiosarcoma of the head and neck. *J Laryngol Otol* 1997;111(2):175.
281. Kirova YM, et al. [Radiation-induced sarcoma after breast cancer. Apropos of 8 cases and review of the literature.] *Cancer Radiother* 1998;2(4):381.
282. Bisceglia M, et al. [Early stage Stewart-Treves syndrome: report of 2 cases and review of the literature.] *Pathologica* 1996;88(6):483.
283. Stewart NJ, et al. Lymphangiosarcoma following mastectomy. *Clin Orthop* 1995;320:135.
284. Kim MK, et al. Secondary angiosarcoma following irradiation—case report and review of the literature. *Radiat Med* 1998;16(1):55.
285. Cafiero F, et al. Radiation-associated angiosarcoma: diagnostic and therapeutic implications—two case reports and a review of the literature. *Cancer* 1996;77(12):2496.
286. Perin T, et al. Radiation-associated angiosarcoma: diagnostic and therapeutic implications—two case reports and a review of the literature. *Cancer* 1997;80(3):519.
287. Cianfrocca M, Roenn JH. Epidemic Kaposi's sarcoma. *Oncology (Huntingt)* 1998;12(9):1375.
288. Fenig E, et al. Classic Kaposi sarcoma: experience at Rabin Medical Center in Israel. *Am J Clin Oncol* 1998;21(5):498.
289. Matondo P, Zumla A. The spectrum of African Kaposi's sarcoma: Is it consequential upon diverse immunological responses? *Scand J Infect Dis* 1996;28(3):225.
290. McGarvey ME, et al. Emerging treatments for epidemic (AIDS-related) Kaposi's sarcoma. *Curr Opin Oncol* 1998;10(5):413.
291. Shepherd FA, et al. Treatment of Kaposi's sarcoma after solid organ transplantation. *J Clin Oncol* 1997;15(6):2371.
292. Stein ME, et al. Radiation therapy for non-AIDS associated (classic and endemic African) and epidemic Kaposi's sarcoma. *Int J Radiat Oncol Biol Phys* 1994;28(3):613.
293. Tur E, Brenner S. Classic Kaposi's sarcoma: low-dose interferon alfa treatment. *Dermatology* 1998;97(1):37.
294. Jie C, et al. Treatment of epidemic (AIDS-related) Kaposi's sarcoma. *Curr Opin Oncol* 1997;9(5):433.
295. Yarchoan R. Therapy for Kaposi's sarcoma: recent advances and experimental approaches. *J Acquir Immune Defic Syndr Hum Retrovirol* 1999;21[Suppl 1]:S66.
296. Schwartz RA. Cutaneous metastatic disease [see comments]. *J Am Acad Dermatol* 1995;33(2):161.
297. Quaglino D, et al. Cutaneous involvement in leukaemic patients. A review of the literature and personal experience. *Recent Prog Med* 1997;88(9):415.

CHAPTER **42**

Melanoma

SECTION 1 Molecular Biology of Cutaneous Melanoma

MEENHARD HERLYN
KAPAETTU SATYAMOORTHY

The normal human melanocyte adheres singly to the basement membrane of the epidermis with five to six keratinocytes between each cell. Despite normally resting, melanocytes maintain a lifelong proliferation potential. With their dendrites, they reach to keratinocytes in the upper layers of the epidermis to distribute the pigment melanin. Melanin is packaged in melanosomes and provides protective coloration against the damaging effects of ultraviolet (UV) irradiation. Developmentally, melanocytes arise from pluripotent cells of the neural crest. Their survival, migration to the skin, and differentiation is related to spatial and temporal expression of molecules, not only on the migrating cells, but also on juxtaposed other cell types and the extracellular matrix. Defects during development in genes associated with melanocyte migration lead to complete or partial loss of pigment-producing cells in the skin, whereas defects in genes of the pigmentation pathways lead to presence of melanocytes but absence of pigmentation.[1] Genes specific for either melanocyte development or pigmentation are potentially important determinants for melanoma, but a causal relationship has not yet been established. Growth factor receptor genes such as c-kit or endothelin receptor-B (ENDRB) could have a potential role in the pathogenesis of melanoma. Stem cell factor, the ligand for c-kit, is a strong mitogen for normal melanocytes, but has little effect on melanoma cells because expression of c-kit is down-regulated through as yet unknown mechanisms.

The type of pigment, eumelanin versus pheomelanin, present in the melanosomes appears to be related to susceptibility for development of melanoma.[2,3] Those individuals who produce pheomelanin instead of eumelanin are at higher risk for developing melanoma. Preliminary investigations have revealed mutations in the gene for the receptor for melanocyte-stimulating hormone (MC1R). Apparently specific point mutations in the MC1R gene correlate with high susceptibility for melanoma,[4] but not all studies came to the same conclusions.[5,6]

The incidence of melanoma has increased in the United States from 3 cases per 100,000 in 1950 to 13 cases in 2000 with annual increases of 2.5%. This yearly increase is among the highest of all human cancers. In 1999, 44,000 new cases are expected in the United States, with approximately 9000 deaths from the disease. There are no indications that the rate of increase will be slowing in the near future. Fortunately, diagnosis of melanoma in more recent years occurs at an earlier stage, resulting in higher cure rates than two decades ago. Thus, mortality has not increased as steeply as incidence rates.

ETIOLOGY OF MELANOMA

Knowledge of the etiology of melanoma comes predominantly from epidemiologic, less from genetic, studies. UV exposure at the ultraviolet B (UVB) (290 to 320 nm) and ultraviolet A (UVA) (320 to 400 nm) range is the most important, if not the only, causative agent for sporadic melanoma development.

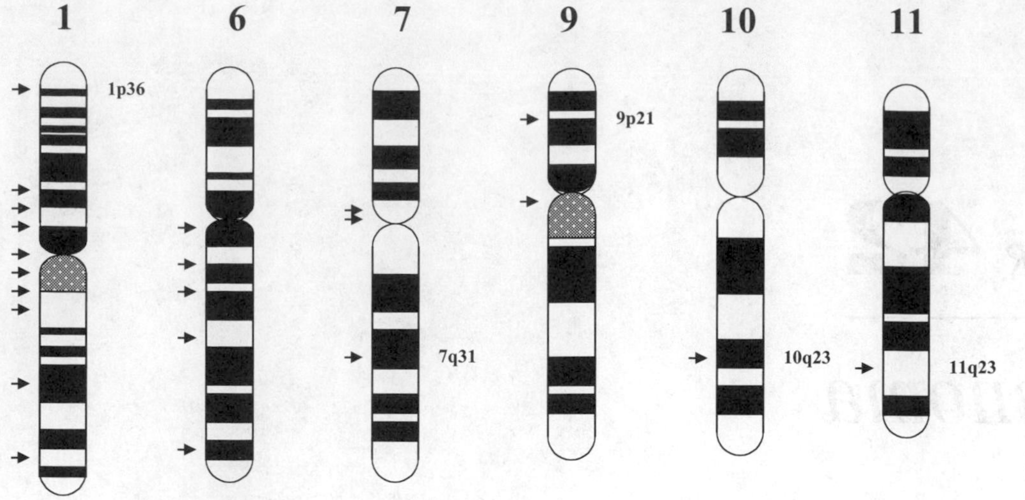

FIGURE 42.1-1. Identification of regions in human chromosomes with melanoma-specific abnormalities.

Predisposition for poor tanning in combination with high sun exposure provides the largest accumulative risk factor for melanoma development. Risk factors for melanoma development over a lifetime are, in decreasing order from less than tenfold to less than twofold: presence of over ten dysplastic nevi, presence of over 100 common acquired nevi, fair skin (types I and II), red hair, and high intermittent sun exposure (i.e., blistering sunburns as a child).[7–10] Excessive intermittent sun exposure is more prevalent in individuals from higher socioeconomic classes.

The melanoma-inducing effects of UV light have been demonstrated in experimental animal systems. Irradiation with UV light sources in the B range induced melanomas in *Xiphophorus* fish and *Monodelphus domestica*.[11–13] UVA could also transform melanocytes in the highly susceptible *Xiphophorus* fish.[14] Preliminary experimental evidence of melanoma induction by UVB comes also from a human skin/mouse chimera model, in which the human skin was grafted to severe combined immunodeficient (SCID) or recombinase activating gene (RAG) knockout mice and then treated with the carcinogen 7,12-dimethylbenz[a]anthracene followed by chronic UVB irradiation over 9 months.[15,16] In this model, which comes closest to the conditions in humans, melanocytic hyperplasia is seen after 4 to 5 months, followed 2 to 3 months later by atypia in lentiginous lesions. Human melanomas have developed but rarely.

GENETICS OF MELANOMA

Cytogenetic analyses over the last two decades have identified in melanoma cells at least six different chromosomes with loci showing nonrandom deletions, translocations (rarely), or amplifications (rarely). Extensive research efforts in the late 1980s and early 1990s focused on chromosomes 1, 6, 7, 9, 10, and 11 (Fig. 42.1-1). The severe aneuploidy of melanoma cells has made it difficult to identify specific regions because each chromosome showed several affected regions. Whereas few laboratories have continued their efforts on the cytogenetic analysis of melanoma cells, most are currently concentrating on screening specific loci or on genome-wide scans. Cytogenetic studies have helped to identify the 9p21 locus, which is frequently affected in melanoma. Intensive research efforts have identified mutations in the $p16^{INK4a}$ gene, which localizes in this region. The $p16^{INK4a}$ is affected through germline mutations or deletions in patients with familial melanoma,[9] which represent 8% to 10% of all melanoma cases. Approximately 50% of familial melanoma patients have germline abnormalities at chromosome 9p21,[17] making this the most frequently abnormal locus. Of these, approximately 50% have mutations or deletions in the $p16^{INK4a}$ gene. Thus, $p16^{INK4a}$ abnormalities represent approximately 5% of all melanomas. They are also significant in sporadic melanomas, in which 25% to 40% of all lesions have mutations or deletions or in which the gene is functionally silenced (Table 42.1-1). Besides $p16^{INK4a}$,[9] only the cyclin-dependent kinase (CDK4) gene has been found mutated in familial melanoma, but only two families have been identified to date.[18]

Among sporadic melanomas, mutations have been found in ras genes with the frequency ranging between 5% and 25%. The wide range is due to differences in the site of the lesions among the studied patients' cohorts. Melanomas in the sun-exposed face have relatively higher proportions of

TABLE 42.1-1. Gene Abnormalities in Lesions of Patients with Sporadic Melanomas

Gene	*Abnormalities*	*Frequency (%)*
$p16^{INK4}$	Mutation/deletion/silencing	25–40
Ras	Mutation	5–25
PTEN	Mutation/deletion	6
p53	Mutation	5
β-Catenin	Mutation	3
Fas	Mutation	3
Others		<1
PKC-α	Mutation	
c-myb	Mutation	
CDK4	Mutation	
NF-1	Mutation/deletion	
EWS-ATF	Translocation	

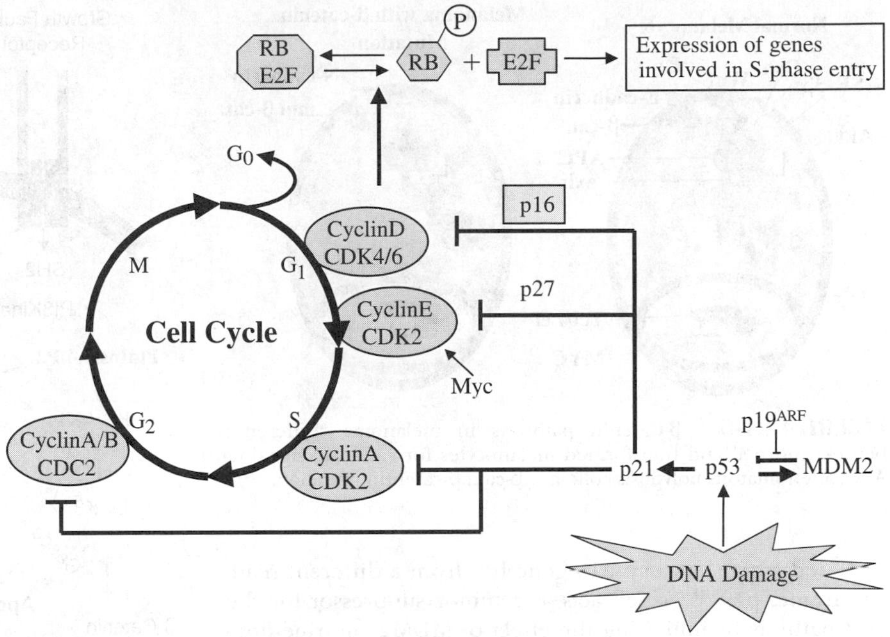

FIGURE 42.1-2. Cell-cycle regulatory proteins in melanoma. Regulation by p53, Rb, cyclins, cyclin-dependent kinases (CDKs), and CDK inhibitors during the melanoma cell cycle. MDM2, murine double minute 2.

ras mutation than those in sun-protected areas.[19] p53, phosphatase and tensin homologue deleted on chromosome 10 (PTEN) and β-catenin mutations are each around 5% of melanoma cases.[2–24] Further studies are needed to determine for each lesion the relative frequency of each of the six major genes listed in Table 42.1-1. Some lesions may accumulate several abnormalities to account for a lower overall percentage of melanomas with defined genetic aberrations. Little is also known about the sequence of gene defect accumulations in melanomas. With the exception of ras mutations, all abnormalities appear to occur in late stages of progression. Nevertheless, the aberrations have important biologic implications for melanoma progression.

FUNCTIONAL SIGNIFICANCE OF SPECIFIC GENE MUTATIONS IN MELANOMA

CELL-CYCLE–REGULATING GENES IN MELANOMA

Proliferation in melanocytes is tightly controlled in the late G_1 phase of the cell cycle through a number of checkpoint-modulating proteins. These include cyclins (cyclins A, B, D, and E),[25] CDKs such as CDK2, CDK4, CDK6, CDC2, CDK8,[26] CDK inhibitors such as $p16^{INK4a}$, $p15^{INK4b}$, $p21^{WAF1/CIP1}$, $p27^{KIP1}$,[27–29] pocket proteins of the retinoblastoma (Rb) family (p107, p130, p105),[30] E2F transcription factors (E2F 1 through 6),[31] and other regulatory proteins (Fig. 42.1-2). A clear definition of the restriction point in the cell cycle has enabled further characterization of each protein in relation to its effects on the cell cycle. Separation of pre–S phase G_1 cells from postmitotic G_1 phase by the restriction point relays the mitogenic signals from growth factors to cell-cycle regulatory proteins. In melanoma, growth factors such as basic fibroblast growth factor (bFGF) and insulin-like growth factor-1 (IGF-1) can stimulate the cells to progress from the restriction point interface to the pre–S phase. Combined with their ability to act as survival and maintenance factors, growth factors can stimulate the expression of positive regulators such as cyclins and CDKs or suppress CDK inhibitors and pocket proteins.

D-type cyclins (D1, D2, and D3) are induced in response to the presence of growth factors and, unlike other cyclins, do not oscillate during cell-cycle.[32] This growth factor–sensing ability allows the cells to synthesize D-type cyclins and interact with their CDK partners such as CDK4 and CDK6, and initiates autonomous cell-cycle entry. The main function of cyclin D–dependent kinases is phosphorylation of Rb in mid G_1 phase and at least cyclin D is required for the import of CDK4 into the nucleus. Subsequently, cyclin E-CDK2 becomes active and phosphorylates Rb on other sites. The main role of cyclins A and B–dependent cdc2 kinase appears to be the maintenance of Rb in its hyperphosphorylated form during the cell division before its hypophosphorylation during the next G_1 cycle. Hyperphosphorylated Rb in late G_1 phase does not associate with the various E2F family members, thereby allowing efficient transcription of a number of target genes, especially those involved in DNA synthesis during S phase of the cell cycle.[28,33]

The CDK inhibitors belong to two classes: the Cip/Kip and INK4 families. The most prominent protein among Cip/Kip family proteins is $p21^{WAF1/CIP1}$; others include $p57^{kip2}$ and $p27^{kip1}$. $p21^{WAF1/CIP1}$ is able to associate primarily with CDK2, in addition to other CDKs, and can interact with proteins involved in DNA repair and replication. It also has been identified as a protein induced by the p53 tumor suppressor protein. On DNA damage, p53 is stabilized and acts as a transcription factor, which, in turn, stimulates expression of $p21^{WAF1/CIP1}$. This induction of $p21^{WAF1/CIP1}$ inhibits cell-cycle progression by inhibiting cyclin-CDK complexes and by inhibiting DNA synthesis through proliferating cell nuclear antigen.[34,35] The INK4 family members consist of $p16^{INK4a}$, $p15^{INK4b}$, $p18^{INK4c}$, and $p19^{INK4d}$. The hallmark of this group of proteins is that they are able to inhibit specifically the assembled cyclin D/CDK4/6 activity, and expression directly correlates with the Rb phosphorylation status. Another protein is

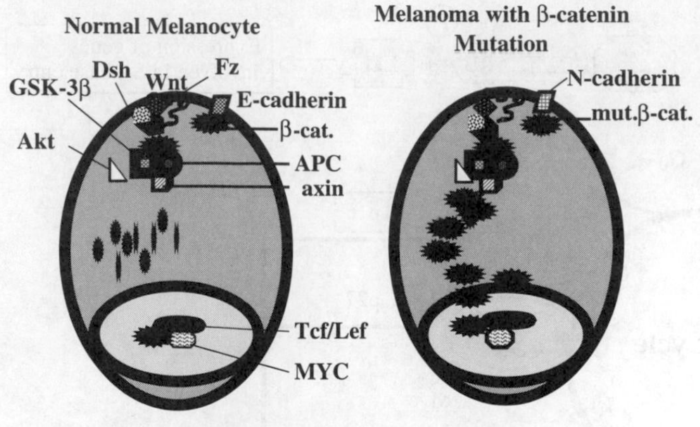

FIGURE 42.1-3. β-Catenin pathways in melanoma. Differences between normal and transformed melanocytes for cadherin signaling. APC, adenomatous polyposis coli; mut.β-cat., β-catentin mutation.

encoded from the same p16 gene but from a different reading frame, $p19^{ARF}$, which acts as a tumor suppressor for the p53 pathway by inhibiting the effect of MDM2 (murine double minute 2) on p53. At this time, there are no known abnormalities in the $p19^{ARF}$ gene in melanoma or other cancers.[36]

β-CATENIN PATHWAY

β-Catenin is a multifunctional protein that is involved in cell-cell adhesion during tissue morphogenesis and tumor growth.[37,38] Its expression levels and subcellular localization are tightly regulated.[39] In the absence of a Wnt signal or when not associated with adherens junctions, β-catenin is present as a large multiprotein complex that consists of glycogen synthase kinase 3β (GSK3β), adenomatous polyposis coli (APC), and axin (Fig. 42.1-3). Phosphorylation in this complex targets β-catenin for proteolytic degradation by the ubiquitin-protesome system.[40,41] When the Wnt signaling pathway is activated via ligand binding to *frizzled* receptors, GSK3β function is inhibited. β-Catenin then accumulates, interacts with TCF/LEF-1 (T-cell factor/lymphoid enhancer factor-1) transcription factors, and activates transcription of promoters of genes containing TCF/LEF-1 binding sites.[42] Posttranscriptionally, β-catenin's fate is regulated by at least two proteins that control GSK3β. Akt/protein kinase B (PKB), which is activated by growth factor receptors and integrins through phosphoinositide 3 kinase (PI3), phosphorylates GSK3β, thereby inhibiting its ability to phosphorylate β-catenin, leading to its degradation.[40,41,43] *Dishevelled*, which is a predominantly cytoplasmic protein, is regulated by *frizzled*.[44] *Dishevelled* contains an axin-like domain, a PDZ (three proteins) domain (involved in protein interactions), and the DEP domain (implicated in G protein regulation)[45,46] and it interacts with axin to regulate GSK3β, thereby influencing β-catenin. In addition, overexpression of axin can suppress the effect of β-catenin in cells. Mutations in the β-catenin gene in melanoma would lead to an endogenous activation without degradation.

PHOSPHATASE AND TENSIN HOMOLOGUE DELETED ON CHROMOSOME 10 PATHWAY

PTEN has emerged as a major component in regulating survival of tumor cells through its involvement in intricate cas-

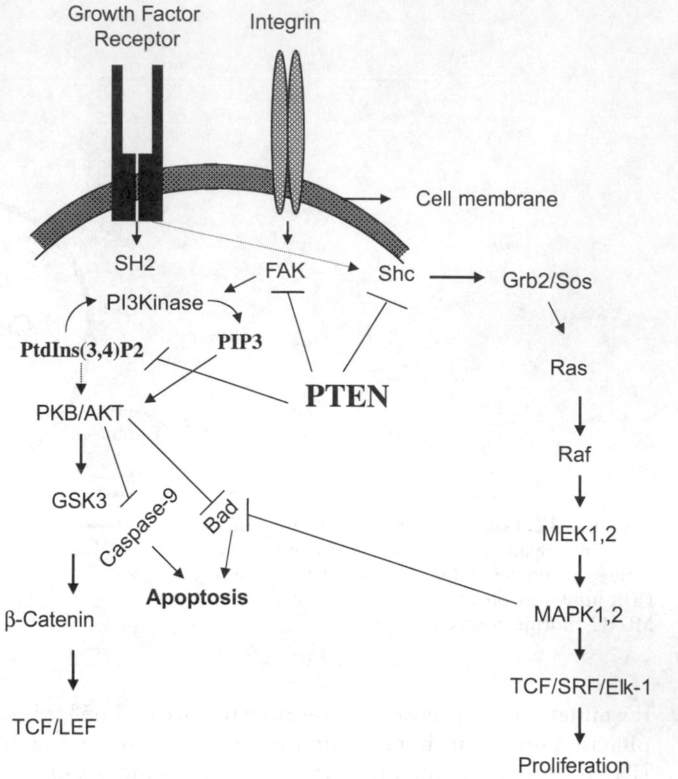

FIGURE 42.1-4. PTEN (phosphatase and tensin homologue deleted on chromosome 10) pathways in melanoma. Schematic representation of PTEN as a central molecule influencing PI3 kinase-dependent Ras and Akt signaling.

cading pathways for growth and adhesion signaling. Both the growth factor and the adhesion receptor (integrin) signaling pathways work in tandem, and signaling is initiated from PI3 kinase, which acts as a relay station (Fig. 42.1-4).[47] PI3 kinase activity is associated with the transformation ability of oncoproteins and stimulation by growth factors. Akt/PKB, an oncogene initially discovered in retroviruses, binds to phosphatidylinositol 3,4-diphosphate (PtdIns-3,4-P_2), and phosphatidylinositol 3,4-triphosphate (PtdIns-3,4,5-P_3), and is then transported to the membrane where it activates PI3 kinase. Activation of Akt/PKB in melanoma cells by IGF-1 provides survival signal by phosphorylating Bad and caspase 9. PTEN dephosphorylates PtdIns phosphates, thereby depriving the PI3 kinase of its substrate. Thus, a mutated PTEN can constitutively activate Akt/PKB to influence downstream genes. Cells accumulate in the G_1 phase of the cell cycle through up-regulation of p27. However, it is unknown whether the phosphatase activity is involved in this process and whether it is necessary for dephosphorylation of FAK leading to inhibition of integrin-mediated signaling of cell spreading.

It is not yet clear how the PTEN may signal to regulate the ras pathway.[48,49] One evidence is the involvement of Shc phosphorylation, which affects its association with Grb2. Shc and Grb2 interactions are necessary for subsequent activation of the ras/raf/MEK1/MAPK pathways, providing a central role for PTEN in controlling cellular responses to growth factor– and integrin-mediated signaling.

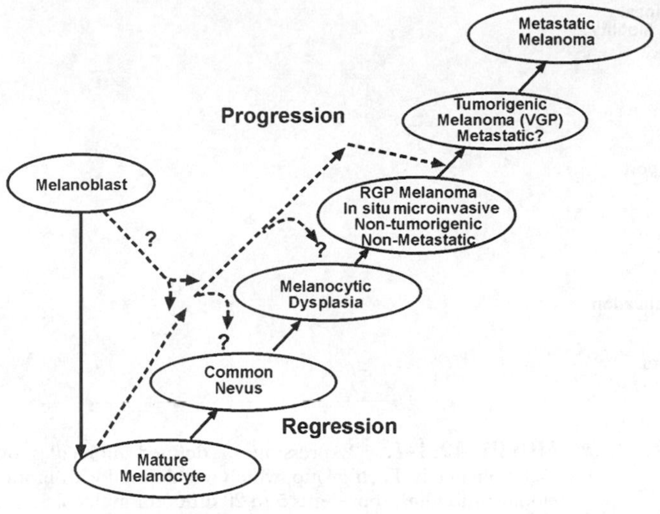

FIGURE 42.1-5. Melanoma development and progression. The model implies that melanomas develop and progress in a sequence of steps. However, malignancy can also develop *de novo*. RGP, radial growth phase; VGP, vertical growth phase.

BIOLOGY OF MELANOMA DEVELOPMENT AND PROGRESSION

PROGRESSION MODEL

Clinical and histologic studies have resulted in defining distinct steps of melanoma development and progression (Fig. 42.1-5): step 0, melanocytes; step 1, common acquired and congenital nevi with structurally normal melanocytes; step 2, dysplastic nevi with structural and architectural atypia; step 3, radial growth phase (RGP), nontumorigenic primary melanomas without metastatic competence; step 4, vertical growth phase (VGP), tumorigenic primary melanomas with competence for metastasis; and step 5, metastatic melanoma.[50–52] A refinement by Elder et al. of this classification of nevi and primary melanomas[51] divides lesions into three classes: class I represents *precursor* nevi; class II lesions are *intermediates,* confined to the epidermis or with microinvasion into the dermis and represented by *in situ* and microinvasive RGP melanomas; class III are VGP tumorigenic melanomas. As in any neoplastic system, individual melanomas can skip steps in their development, appearing without identifiable intermediate lesions. It remains to be experimentally verified that melanoma cells can develop from a melanocyte precursor cell, which appears to be present not only in murine but also in human skin.

The progression from each stage to the next is associated with specific biologic changes, which are based on experimental models and clinical and histopathologic observations (Fig. 42.1-6). The transition from the mature melanocyte to the formation of a nevus is characterized by a disruption of cell-cell cross-talk between melanocytes and keratinocytes, which leads to an escape of the melanocyte from the regulatory control of keratinocytes. Nevus cells show limited proliferation because common acquired nevi have no apparent chromosomal aberrations. Thus, nevi can develop not just through a stimulatory event, but also through loss of control of keratinocytes over melanocytes.

Progression from the melanocyte or common acquired nevus cell to a dysplastic nevus or RGP melanoma most likely

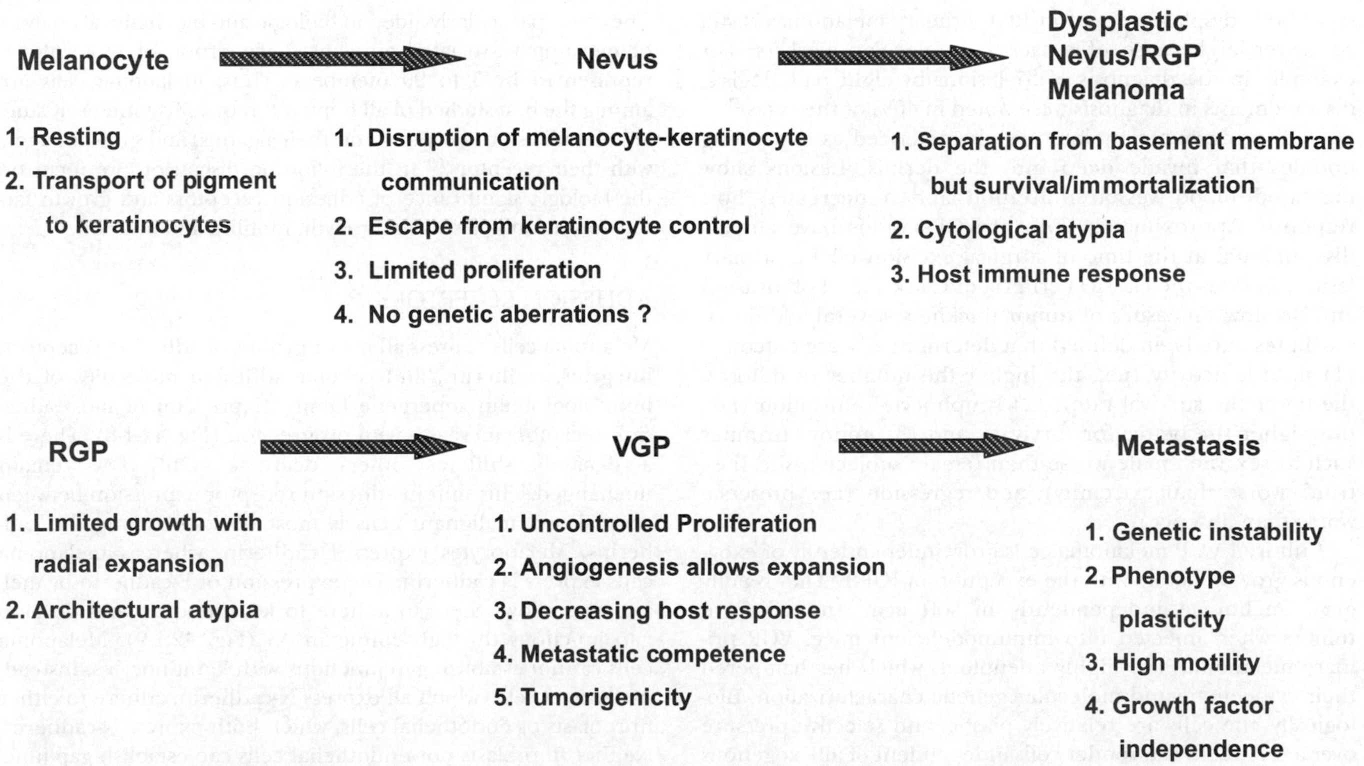

FIGURE 42.1-6. Biologic events during melanoma progression. Each transition is marked by characteristic changes in the cells. RGP, radial growth phase; VGP, vertical growth phase.

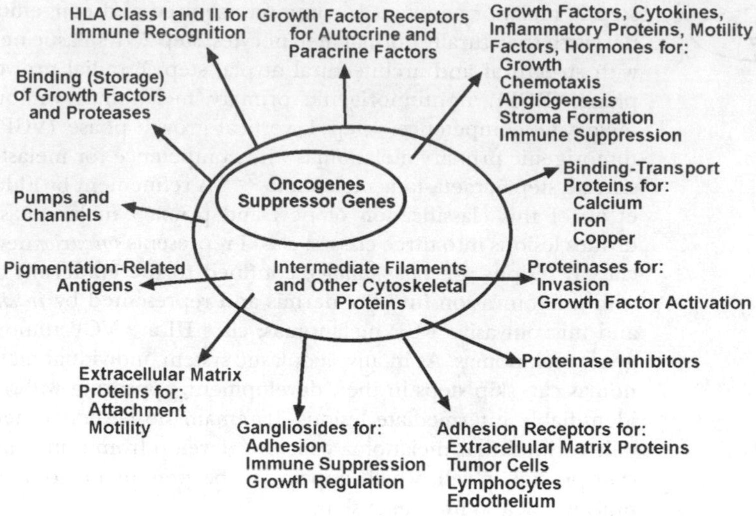

FIGURE 42.1-7. Expression of defined molecules on melanoma cells. Each group, which was defined with monoclonal antibodies, represents 5 to 20 different molecules.

involves the beginning of genetic aberrations. The cells show cytologic atypia, they can separate from the basement membrane without undergoing apoptosis, and the entire lesion shows architectural atypia. Cells from RGP lesions have biologic properties *in vitro* that are intermediate between benign and malignant. They require several growth factors for proliferation, do not grow anchorage independently in soft agar and are nontumorigenic in mice. At this time, a local immune response is observed, which could be critical for long-term disease outcome. Specificity and nature of infiltrating lymphocytes in dysplastic nevi or RGP melanoma have not yet been determined. Surgical excision of dysplastic nevi and RGP melanomas leads to a cure from the disease. The histologic diagnosis of both dysplastic nevi and RGP primary melanomas is still controversial because of a lack of molecular markers. For example, in the diagnosis of 37 lesions by eight pathologists, disagreements in diagnosis were noted in 40% of the cases.[53]

VGP primary melanomas are characterized as expanding nodules that invade deep into the dermis. Lesions show increased blood vessel infiltration and a decreased host response. Approximately 35% of VGP lesions have already disseminated at the time of surgical excision of the primary lesion. Besides the classical criteria of Clark's level of invasion and Breslow's measure of tumor thickness, several additional attributes have been defined that determine disease outcome: (1) mitotic activity (i.e., the higher the number of mitoses, the lower the survival rate); (2) lymphocyte infiltration (i.e., the higher the better for survival); and (3) minor attributes such as sex (i.e., male worse than female subjects), site (i.e., trunk worse than extremity), and regression (i.e., presence worse than absence).[54]

Cultured VGP melanoma cells grow independently of exogenous growth factors with the exception of IGF-1. They readily grow anchorage independently in soft agar and all form tumors when injected into immunodeficient mice. VGP primary melanomas are highly aneuploid, which has hampered their cytogenetic and molecular genetic characterization. Biologically, the cells are relatively plastic, and selective pressure over a few weeks can render cells independent of all exogenous growth factors[55] or they become highly invasive.[56–59] Some also acquire metastatic competence.

The metastatic phenotype of melanoma cells isolated from metastatic lesions of patients is unstable. Injection of these cells into an immunodeficient host rarely produces metastases. Metastatic cells also show a high level of phenotypic plasticity, depending on the environment and any selective pressure placed on the cells.

BIOLOGIC BASIS OF MELANOMA PROGRESSION

Monoclonal antibodies have been used for the last 20 years to characterize molecules expressed by melanoma cells (Fig. 42.1-7). They have particularly aided in biologic and biochemical analyses of melanoma-associated antigens. Each group of molecules is represented by 5 to 20 members. Thus, melanoma cells are among the best studied of all human tumors. Most intensely studied are adhesion receptors and their ligands, and growth factors with their receptors.[60] In the following discussion, we focus on the biologic significance of adhesion receptors and growth factors for melanoma survival, growth, motility, and invasion.

ADHESION RECEPTORS

Melanoma cells express all major groups of adhesion receptors: integrins, cadherins, and cellular adhesion molecules of the immunoglobulin supergene family. Expression of most adhesion receptors increases with progression (Fig. 42.1-8). There is a dynamic shift as others decrease. Only few remain unchanged. This shift in adhesion receptor expression between normal and malignant cells is most obvious among the cadherins. Melanocytes express E-cadherin, whereas melanoma cells express N-cadherin. The expression of E-cadherin by melanocytes allows them to adhere to keratinocytes and develop gap junctions through connexin 43 (Fig. 42.1-9). Melanoma cells cannot establish gap junctions with keratinocytes. Instead, melanoma cells, which all express N-cadherin, adhere to either fibroblasts or endothelial cells, which both express N-cadherin. Neither fibroblasts nor endothelial cells can establish gap junctions to keratinocytes. The biologic consequences of gap junction formation are not clear.

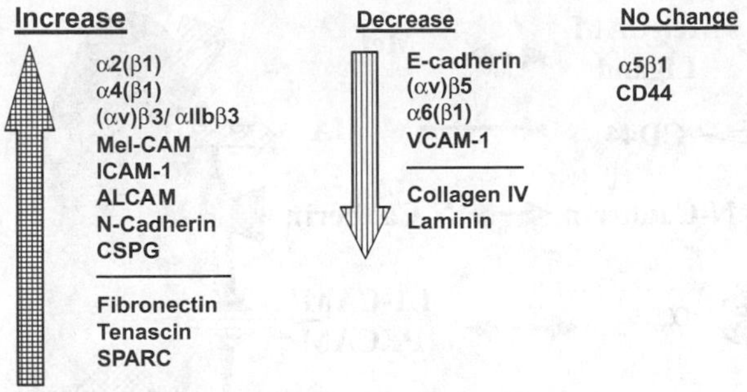

FIGURE 42.1-8. Dynamic shifts in the expression of adhesion receptors and their matrix proteins by melanoma cells. The increase or decrease in expression may already start in nevi or only in vertical growth phase melanomas.

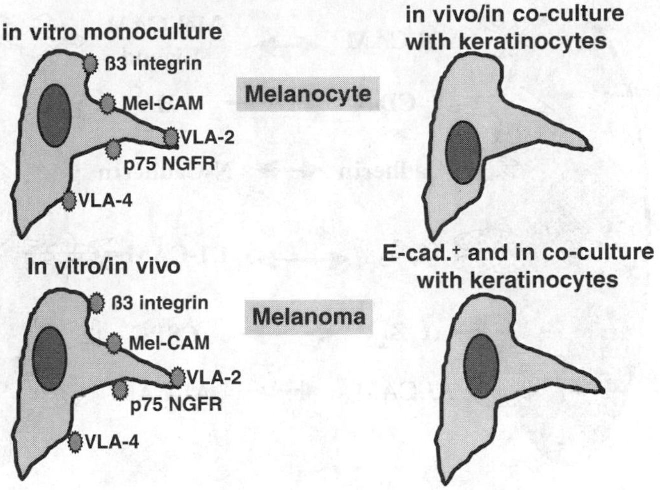

FIGURE 42.1-10. Expression of tumor-associated antigens on melanocytes and melanoma cells is dependent on the presence of E-cadherin (E-cad.) and adhesion to keratinocytes. Keratinocytes can regulate antigen expression on melanoma cells only when E-cadherin is expressed by melanoma cells.

Keratinocytes can control the phenotype of normal melanocytes but not melanoma cells. They can regulate melanocyte growth and the expression of cell surface adhesion receptors. Figure 42.1-10 illustrates that melanocytes in culture in the absence of any other cell (monoculture) express melanoma-associated antigens. However, the expression of these molecules disappears within 3 to 4 days when the cells are cocultured with normal keratinocytes to allow cell-cell contact. Melanoma cells are refractory to keratinocytes. However, if the melanoma cells are transduced with E cadherin, they can adhere to keratinocytes and establish gap junctions. At this time, cell surface molecules are down-regulated, gap junctions are established with keratinocytes, and growth of cells is controlled by keratinocytes. Highly metastatic melanoma cells are no longer invasive.[56,61,62] Little is currently known about the signaling mechanisms between keratinocytes and E-cadherin–expressing melanoma cells.

Besides N-cadherin–mediated interactions, melanoma cells can adhere through other adhesion receptor systems (see Fig. 42.1-10). Most notable is adhesion through Mel–cellular adhesion molecules and a yet unidentified ligand, also found on melanoma cells. Melanoma cells and activated endothelial cells share a number of adhesion molecules that allow heterophilic adhesion between these two cell types in a similar manner as homophilic adhesion between the malignant cells. The similarities in adhesion receptor expression could have functional consequences (Fig. 42.1-11). Maniotis and coworkers demonstrated that melanoma cells could establish tubule-like structures for blood flow, which can connect to bona fide blood vessels.[63]

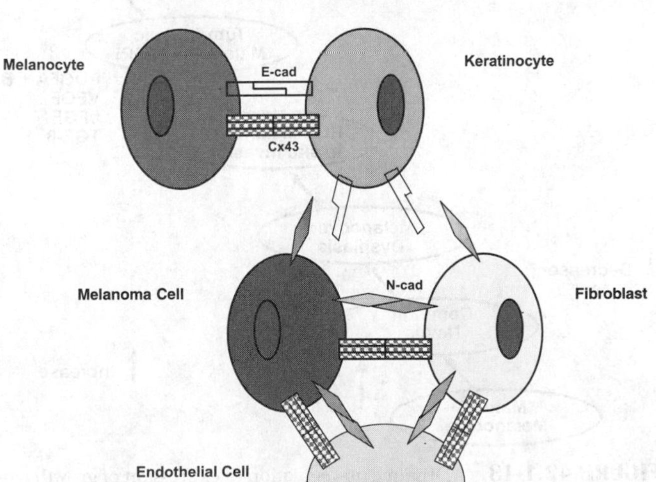

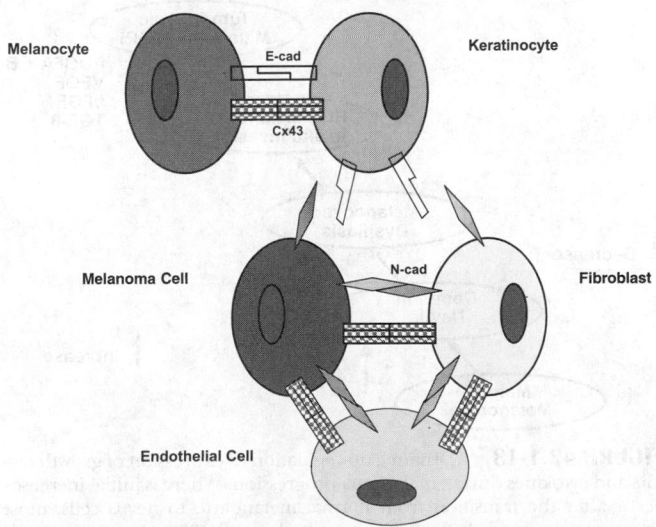

FIGURE 42.1-9. Melanocyte and melanoma cell interactions with juxtaposed cells in their environment. Adhesions occur through either E-cadherin (E-cad) or N-cadherin (N-cad) and gap junctional communication is mediated through connexin 43 hexamers.

β_3 is present on almost all VGP primary and metastatic melanomas, but not on cells of earlier stages of progression. One of the most specific markers that characterizes VGP and metastatic cells is the β_3 subunit of the vitronectin receptor $\alpha_v\beta_3$ (Fig. 42.1-12). When the β_3 gene was transduced to RGP melanoma cells, there were no changes in growth properties *in vitro.*[64] On the other hand, the cells became highly invasive in a skin reconstruction model and were now tumorigenic in mice, two attributes of VGP melanoma cells. Apparently, β_3 integrin expression triggers the up-regulation of a variety of genes associated with invasion and tumor growth. The β_3 integrin subunit is also up-regulated by tumor-infiltrating endothelial cells, and several clinical studies have been initiated to target β_3 on endothelial cells, melanoma cells, or both for therapy.

GROWTH FACTORS

With progression, melanoma cells show an increase in production of growth factors and cytokines (Fig. 42.1-13). Normal melanocytes are relatively inactive in growth factor production, even after stimulation. Nevus cells may produce bFGF and chemoattractive cytokines such as interleukin-8 or MCP-1 (monocyte chemoattractant protein-1). The strongest increase in growth factor expression, most notably a further increase in production of bFGF, and of expression of platelet-derived growth factor (PDGF) and transforming growth fac-

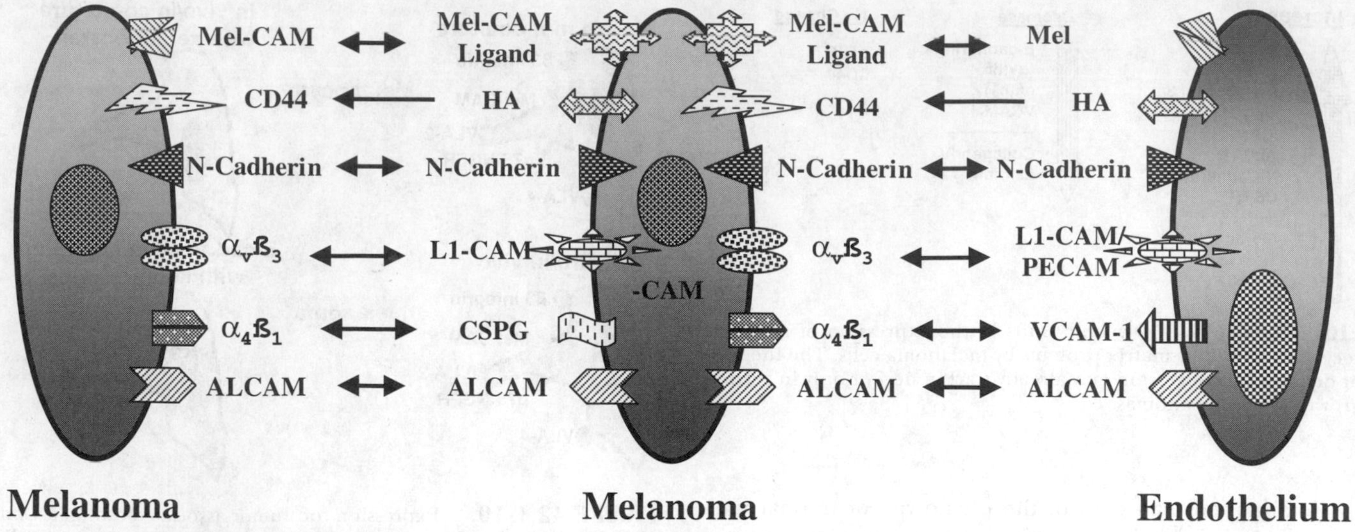

FIGURE 42.1-11. Melanoma-melanoma and melanoma-endothelial cell adhesion. Both cell types use similar molecules for cell-cell adhesion.

tor-β, can be found in VGP melanomas. Vascular endothelial growth factor (VEGF) can be triggered in VGP and metastatic cells by hypoxic growth conditions or by chemokines and growth factors. bFGF, PDGF, and VEGF act in concert with each other (see Fig. 42.1-13). bFGF is the most significant autocrine growth factor in melanoma. Blocking of bFGF production with antisense oligonucleotides stops melanoma cell proliferation.[65] Despite its lack of a signal sequence, it can be released from cells through yet unknown mechanisms. When released from cells, bFGF binds to matrix proteins such as heparan sulfate proteoglycan, and it can then stimulate both fibroblasts and endothelial cells. bFGF is not only a survival factor and a growth stimulator for melanoma cells but also a motility factor. Its role in invasion comes from up-regulation of serine proteinases (urokinase and plasminogen activator), and metalloproteinases (gelatinase A and B). Potentially, a variety of other genes are activated as well, which still need to be identified.

The biologically most significant stimulating growth factor for tumor-infiltrating fibroblasts is PDGF (Fig. 42.1-14). Melanoma cells produce both A and B isoforms. PDGF is not only mitogenic for fibroblasts, but it also induces the production of matrix proteins such as fibronectin and collagen, which provide the melanoma cells a scaffolding to which to adhere. Activated fibroblasts produce IGF-1, one of the most signifi-

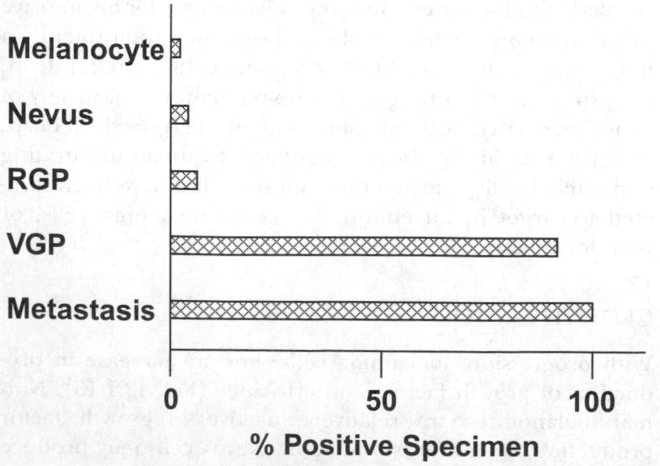

FIGURE 42.1-12. Expression of the integrin subunit β_3 of the $\alpha_v\beta_3$ vitronectin receptor in melanocytic cells from different stages of tumor progression. Expression was tested with monoclonal antibodies on both frozen and fixed tissue sections. RGP, radial growth phase; VGP, vertical growth phase.

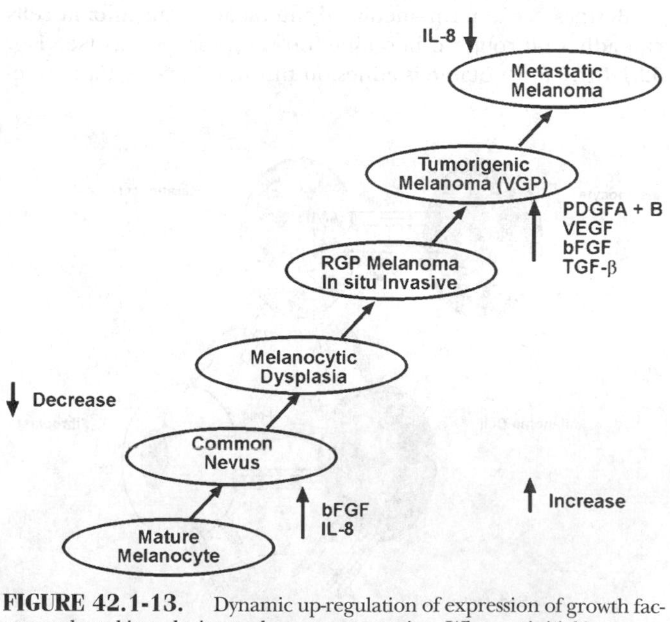

FIGURE 42.1-13. Dynamic up-regulation of expression of growth factors and cytokines during melanoma progression. Whereas initial increases occur after the transition from normal melanocyte to nevus cells, most changes occur between the radial growth phase (RGP) and vertical growth phase (VGP) of primary melanomas. Metastatic cells generally show the highest production levels. bFGF, basic fibroblast growth factor; IL-8, interleukin-8; PDGFA + B, platelet-derived growth factor-A and-B; TGF-β, transforming growth factor-β; VEGF, vascular endothelial growth factor.

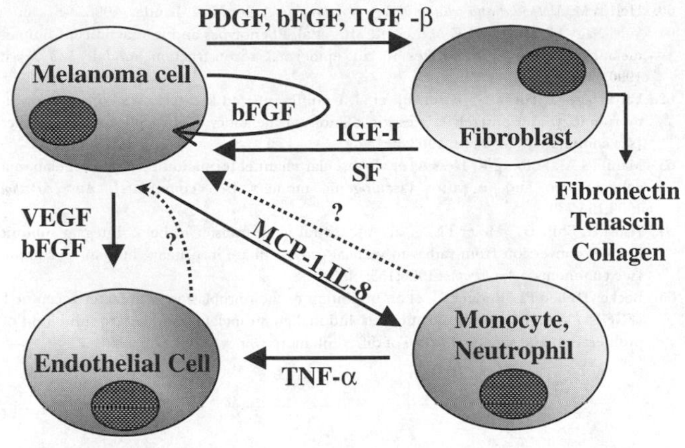

FIGURE 42.1-14. Melanoma to stroma cross-talk. Production of growth factors and cytokines by melanoma cells that affect normal host cells in the environment. A positive feedback may also occur, when the stromal cells produce stimulants for the malignant cells. bFGF, basic fibroblast growth factor; IGF-I, insulin-like growth factor 1; IL-8, interleukin-8; MCP-1, monocyte chemoattractant protein-1; PDGF, platelet-derived growth factor; SF, scatter factor; TGF-β, transforming growth factor-β; TNF-α, tumor necrosis factor-α; VEGF, vascular endothelial growth factor.

cant exogenous growth factors for melanoma cells because they do not produce it on their own. IGF-1 is highly mitogenic for melanoma cells but is also a motility factor and stimulates survival by stabilization of β-catenin. Melanoma cells are strong producers of chemoattractive proteins such as interleukin-8 (neutrophil attractant) or MCP-1 (monocyte attractant). In early malignant lesions, infiltrating neutrophils and monocytes may have a stimulatory role for tumors by producing angiogenic cytokines such as tumor necrosis factor-α or by inducing stroma formation. High production of these chemokines can lead to a strong infiltration of the inflammatory cells, which then kills the malignant cells. Thus, tumor cells must maintain a fine balance of chemokine production for biggest growth advantage. Inflammatory cell infiltrates diminish with metastasis apparently due to a breakdown of the gradient when the chemokine levels are increased to be elevated in serum.

REFERENCES

1. Spritz RA. Multi-organellar disorders of pigmentation: tied up in traffic. *Clin Genet* 1999;55:309.
2. Valverde P, Healy E, Jackson I, et al. Variants of the melanocyte-stimulating hormone receptor gene are associated with red hair and fair skin in humans [see comments]. *Nat Genet* 1995;11:328.
3. Rees JL, Healy E. Melanocortin receptors, red hair, and skin cancer. *J Invest Dermatol Symp Proc* 1997;2:94.
4. Valverde P, Healy E, Sikkink S, et al. The Asp84Glu variant of the melanocortin 1 receptor (MC1R) is associated with melanoma. *Hum Mol Genet* 1996;5:1663.
5. Sturm RA, Box NF, Ramsay M. Human pigmentation genetics: the difference is only skin deep. *Bioessays* 1998;20:712.
6. Ichii-Jones F, Lear JT, Heagerty AH, et al. Susceptibility to melanoma: influence of skin type and polymorphism in the melanocyte stimulating hormone receptor gene [see comments]. *J Invest Dermatol* 1998;111:218.
7. Dubin N, Pasternack BS, Moseson M. Simultaneous assessment of risk factors for malignant melanoma and non-melanoma skin lesions, with emphasis on sun exposure and related variables. *Int J Epidemiol* 1990;19:811.
8. Carli P, Biggeri A, Nardini P, et al. Epidemiology of atypical melanocytic naevi: an analytical study in a Mediterranean population [see comments]. *Eur J Cancer Prev* 1997;6:506.
9. Carli P, Biggeri A, Nardini P, et al. Sun exposure and large numbers of common and atypical melanocytic naevi: an analytical study in a southern European population. *Br J Dermatol* 1998;138:422.
10. Goldstein AM, Tucker MA. Etiology, epidemiology, risk factors, and public health issues of melanoma. *Curr Opin Oncol* 1993;5:358.
11. Ley RD, Applegate LA, Padilla RS, et al. Ultraviolet radiation-induced malignant melanoma in *Monodelphis domestica*. *Photochem Photobiol* 1989;50:1.
12. Moan J, Dahlback A, Setlow RB. Epidemiological support for an hypothesis for melanoma induction indicating a role for UVA radiation. *Photochem Photobiol* 1999;70:243.
13. Setlow RB. Relevance of in vivo models in melanoma skin cancer. *Photochem Photobiol* 1996;63:410.
14. Setlow RB, Woodhead AD, Grist E. Animal model for ultraviolet radiation-induced melanoma: platyfish-swordtail hybrid. *Proc Natl Acad Sci U S A* 1989;86:8922.
15. Soballe PW, Montone KT, Satyamoorthy K, et al. Carcinogenesis in human skin grafted to SCID mice. *Cancer Res* 1996;56:757.
16. Atillasoy ES, Seykora JT, Soballe PW, et al. UVB induces atypical melanocytic lesions and melanoma in human skin. *Am J Pathol* 1998;152:1179.
17. Chin L, Merlino G, DePinho RA. Malignant melanoma: modern black plague and genetic black box. *Genes Dev* 1998;12:3467.
18. Platz A, Hansson J, Ringborg U. Screening of germline mutations in the CDK4, CDKN2C and TP53 genes in familial melanoma: a clinic-based population study. *Int J Cancer* 1998;78:13.
19. Herlyn M, Satyamoorthy K. Activated ras. Yet another player in melanoma? [comment]. *Am J Pathol* 1996;149:739.
20. Rimm DL, Caca K, Hu G, et al. Frequent nuclear/cytoplasmic localization of beta-catenin without exon 3 mutations in malignant melanoma. *Am J Pathol* 1999;154:325.
21. Robbins PF, El-Gamil M, Li YF, et al. A mutated beta-catenin gene encodes a melanoma-specific antigen recognized by tumor infiltrating lymphocytes. *J Exp Med* 1996;183:1185.
22. Albino AP, Vidal MJ, McNutt NS, et al. Mutation and expression of the p53 gene in human malignant melanoma. *Melanoma Res* 1994;4:35.
23. Weiss J, Schwechheimer K, Cavenee WK, et al. Mutation and expression of the p53 gene in malignant melanoma cell lines. *Int J Cancer* 1993;54:693.
24. Tsao H, Zhang X, Benoit E, et al. Identification of PTEN/MMAC1 alterations in uncultured melanomas and melanoma cell lines. *Oncogene* 1998;16:3397.
25. Johnson DG, Walker CL. Cyclins and cell cycle checkpoints. *Annu Rev Pharmacol Toxicol* 1999;39:295.
26. Morgan DO. Cyclin-dependent kinases: engines, clocks, and microprocessors. *Annu Rev Cell Dev Biol* 1997;13:261.
27. Elledge SJ, Harper JW. Cdk inhibitors: on the threshold of checkpoints and development. *Curr Opin Cell Biol* 1994;6:847.
28. Serrano M. The tumor suppressor protein p16INK4a. *Exp Cell Res* 1997;237:7.
29. Sherr CJ, Roberts JM. CDK inhibitors: positive and negative regulators of G1-phase progression. *Genes Dev* 1999;13:1501.
30. Bartek J, Bartkova J, Lukas J. The retinoblastoma protein pathway in cell cycle control and cancer. *Exp Cell Res* 1997;237:1.
31. Black AR, Azizkhan-Clifford J. Regulation of E2F: a family of transcription factors involved in proliferation control. *Gene* 1999;237:281.
32. Elledge SJ. Cell cycle checkpoints: preventing an identity crisis. *Science* 1996;274:1664.
33. Nasmyth K. Viewpoint: putting the cell cycle in order. *Science* 1996;274:1643.
34. el-Deiry WS. p21/p53, cellular growth control and genomic integrity. *Curr Top Microbiol Immunol* 1998;227:121.
35. Ko LJ, Prives C. p53: puzzle and paradigm. *Genes Dev* 1996;10:1054.
36. Sherr CJ. Tumor surveillance via the ARF-p53 pathway. *Genes Dev* 1998;12:2984.
37. Willert K, Nusse R. Beta-catenin: a key mediator of Wnt signaling. *Curr Opin Genet Dev* 1998;8:95.
38. Polakis P. The oncogenic activation of beta-catenin. *Curr Opin Genet Dev* 1999;9:15.
39. Arias AM, Brown AM, Brennan K. Wnt signalling: pathway or network? *Curr Opin Genet Dev* 1999;9:447.
40. Dierick H, Bejsovec A. Cellular mechanisms of wingless/Wnt signal transduction. *Curr Top Dev Biol* 1999;43:153.
41. Eastman Q, Grosschedl R. Regulation of LEF-1/TCF transcription factors by Wnt and other signals. *Curr Opin Cell Biol* 1999;11:233.
42. Shulman JM, Perrimon N, Axelrod JD. Frizzled signaling and the developmental control of cell polarity. *Trends Genet* 1998;14:452.
43. Cox RT, Peifer M. Wingless signaling: the inconvenient complexities of life. *Curr Biol* 1998;8:R140.
44. Axelrod JD, Miller JR, Shulman JM, et al. Differential recruitment of Dishevelled provides signaling specificity in the planar cell polarity and Wingless signaling pathways. *Genes Dev* 1998;12:2610.
45. Li L, Yuan H, Xie W, et al. Dishevelled proteins lead to two signaling pathways. Regulation of LEF- 1 and c-Jun N-terminal kinase in mammalian cells. *J Biol Chem* 1999;274:129.
46. Lee JS, Ishimoto A, Yanagawa S. Characterization of mouse dishevelled (Dvl) proteins in Wnt/Wingless signaling pathway. *J Biol Chem* 1999;274:21464.
47. Besson A, Robbins SM, Yong VW. PTEN/MMAC1/TEP1 in signal transduction and tumorigenesis. *Eur J Biochem* 1999;263:605.
48. Cantley LC, Neel BG. New insights into tumor suppression: PTEN suppresses tumor formation by restraining the phosphoinositide 3-kinase/AKT pathway. *Proc Natl Acad Sci U S A* 1999;96:4240.
49. Maehama T, Dixon JE. PTEN: a tumour suppressor that functions as a phospholipid phosphatase. *Trends Cell Biol* 1999;9:125.
50. Clark WH Jr, Elder DE, Guerry DT, et al. A study of tumor progression: the precursor lesions of superficial spreading and nodular melanoma. *Hum Pathol* 1984;15:1147.
51. Elder DE, Clark WH Jr, Elenitsas R, et al. The early and intermediate precursor lesions of tumor progression in the melanocytic system: common acquired nevi and atypical (dysplastic) nevi. *Semin Diagn Pathol* 1993;10:18.
52. Valyi-Nagy I, Rodeck U, Kath R, et al. The human melanocyte system as a model for studies on tumor progression. *Basic Life Sci* 1991;57:315.

53. Farmer ER, Gonin R, Hanna MP. Discordance in the histopathologic diagnosis of melanoma and melanocytic nevi between expert pathologists [see comments]. *Hum Pathol* 1996;27:528.
54. Clemente CG, Mihm MC Jr, Bufalino R, et al. Prognostic value of tumor infiltrating lymphocytes in the vertical growth phase of primary cutaneous melanoma. *Cancer* 1996;77:1303.
55. Kath R, Jambrosic JA, Holland L, et al. Development of invasive and growth factor-independent cell variants from primary human melanomas. *Cancer Res* 1991;51:2205.
56. Meier F, Satyamoorthy K, Nesbit M, et al. Molecular events in melanoma development and progression. *Front Biosci* 1998;3:D1005.
57. Valyi-Nagy IT, Herlyn M. Regulation of growth and phenotype of normal human melanocytes in culture. *Cancer Treat Res* 1991;54:85.
58. Valyi-Nagy I, Shih IM, Gyorfi T, et al. Spontaneous and induced differentiation of human melanoma cells. *Int J Cancer* 1993;54:159.
59. Satyamoorthy K, DeJesus E, Linnenbach AJ, et al. Melanoma cell lines from different stages of progression and their biological and molecular analyses. *Melanoma Res* 1997;7(Suppl 2):S35.
60. Herlyn M. *Molecular and cellular biology of melanoma.* Austin: R.G. Landes, 1993.
61. Valyi-Nagy IT, Murphy GF, Mancianti ML, et al. Phenotypes and interactions of human melanocytes and keratinocytes in an epidermal reconstruction model. *Lab Invest* 1990;62:314.
62. Valyi-Nagy IT, Hirka G, Jensen PJ, et al. Undifferentiated keratinocytes control growth, morphology, and antigen expression of normal melanocytes through cell-cell contact [see comments]. *Lab Invest* 1993;69:152.
63. Maniotis AJ, Folberg R, Hess A, et al. Vascular channel formation by human melanoma cells in vivo and in vitro: vasculogenic mimicry [see comments]. *Am J Pathol* 1999;155:739.
64. Hsu MY, Shih DT, Meier FE, et al. Adenoviral gene transfer of beta3 integrin subunit induces conversion from radial to vertical growth phase in primary human melanoma [see comments]. *Am J Pathol* 1998;153:1435.
65. Becker D, Lee PL, Rodeck U, et al. Inhibition of the fibroblast growth factor receptor 1 (FGFR-1) gene in human melanocytes and malignant melanomas leads to inhibition of proliferation and signs indicative of differentiation. *Oncogene* 1992;7:2303.

MICHAEL T. LOTZE
RAMSEY M. DALLAL
JOHN M. KIRKWOOD
JOHN C. FLICKINGER

SECTION 2

Cutaneous Melanoma

Cutaneous melanoma is a readily curable neoplasm, with 85% of diagnosed patients enjoying long-term survival following simple surgical excision. In its disseminated state, however, it is a devastating illness with limited effective treatment options prompting the evolution of efforts designed to identify metastatic disease early and to develop novel biologic therapies.[1] The application of immunotherapy has so far provided benefit to only a small percentage of patients. In the majority of patients with metastatic disease, many in their youth, treatment with chemotherapy or biologic therapy is unsuccessful, and they ultimately succumb to their disease. In the United States, melanoma is diagnosed in at least 47,000 people a year, more than double the reported incidence in 1970. There has been a steady increase in melanoma incidence over the last century. In 1935, for example, the incidence of melanoma in the United States was approximately 1 in 100,000. Now, the incidence approaches 15 in 100,000. Although the basis for this increase is incompletely understood, the localized degradation of the ozone layer, the increase in solar exposure as a recreational activity, and the immigration of fair-skinned populations into equatorial latitudes each appears to play some causative role. Because of the effectiveness of early surgical treatment, the international community has focused extensively on preventive measures and screening efforts with some success. The diagnosis of the majority of melanoma occurs at thin and easily cured depths of invasion.

Large prospective, randomized, multicenter trials have answered some basic management questions, improved the care of melanoma patients, and expanded our understanding of the disease. However, many aspects of the treatment of melanoma, such as the therapeutic role of sentinel node dissection, isolated limb perfusion (ILP), and cytotoxic, biologic, or both therapies remain controversial and inconclusive. The field of melanoma is rapidly evolving with new techniques and therapeutics becoming standard care, even before substantial evidence of benefit exists. Not surprisingly, many physicians still find the enormous amount of conflicting data confusing. The changing framework of surgical, radiologic, and even pathologic assessment demands additional randomized, prospective, controlled trials to arrive at meaningful conclusions to serve as the foundation for future progress. Many of these are currently ongoing without results available at the time of preparation of this chapter.

Melanoma has been one of the most successful targets for immunotherapy, especially as biologic therapies. Interleukin-2 (IL-2) and interferon (IFN) therapy have now become routine and new peptide or protein vaccines as well as cellular and genetic therapies are being aggressively developed. Melanoma has attracted the attention of immunotherapists for many reasons. Spontaneous regression of melanoma associated with evidence supporting a specific cellular immune response occurs more frequently in patients with melanoma than with other solid tumors. The lack of effective alternatives has allowed the implementation and evolution of new treatments since, as yet, no systemic therapy has been shown to prolong survival significantly for treated cohorts in properly randomized studies. The identification of tumor rejection antigens recognized by CD4 and CD8 T cells as well as prognostically significant roles of antibody response to melanoma antigens has spawned a renaissance of immunotherapy. Occasional patients with advanced disease have been apparently *cured* by immunotherapy, surviving as long as 15 years without disease, something essentially unheard of for systemic therapy of metastases of any other major solid tumor.

The advances made in melanoma treatment have moved into other areas of oncology. Sentinel node biopsies are increasingly applied in the treatment of breast and colon cancer. The rapid advances in understanding melanocyte biology and the immunologic community's interest in studying the disease has propelled the development of novel biologic therapies for other tumors. Melanoma trials have demonstrated the importance of multidisciplinary approaches in confronting the difficult problems faced in the treatment of cancer patients.

EPIDEMIOLOGY

In 1956, Lancaster observed an association between sun exposure and the development of melanoma. He described the relationship between disease incidence and latitude among people of European background. The closer to the equator, the greater the rate of melanoma mortality and incidence of melanoma in whites.[2]

Since 1973, the Surveillance, Epidemiology and End Results (SEER) program has sampled hospital-based cancer registries

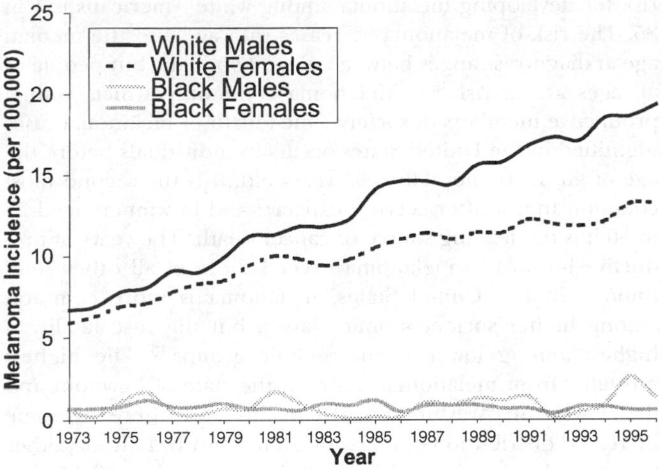

FIGURE 42.2-1. Age-adjusted incidence of melanoma in the United States from 1973 to 1996. The incidence has increased for the white population substantially and is rising faster in male than female subjects. This increase in melanoma incidence has not discernibly affected the black population. (Data from the Surveillance, Epidemiology and End Results program, 2000.)

in 11 different regions accounting for a total of 10% of the U.S. population. Even with this surveillance system, underreporting is common as numerous thin melanomas are treated in an office setting and not reported in this hospital-based system. For example up to 19% of melanomas were not reported in the Massachusetts Cancer Registry. Using national surveys of community practices, some believe the incidence of melanoma in the United States to be 2.5 times SEER estimates.[3,4]

In 2000, an estimated 7700 Americans will die of malignant melanoma.[5] The incidence of melanoma in the white U.S. population has increased alarmingly from 1 per 100,000 in 1935 to 15 per 100,000 in 1996 (Fig. 42.2-1).[6] In 2000, at least 47,000 cases are expected. However, the overall melanoma mortality has not increased nearly as dramatically over the last several decades (Fig. 42.2-2). Since 1973 the mortality only increased from 1.6 to 2.3 per 100,000 individuals in the 1996 survey (Fig. 42.2-3).[7] During the same time period, overall 5-year survival in patients with melanoma has increased significantly, possibly due to the thinner depth at diagnosis of lesions and the adoption of improved surgical techniques (Fig. 42.2-4). The increase in melanoma mortality over the last 50 years has only recently shown signs of slowing.[8] Some argue that the increased incidence of melanoma may be secondary to the detection of neoplasms that never would have acquired metastatic potential and were destined for regression. Others question whether a lead-time bias may account for the relative differences in rates of mortality and incidence changes. However, one analysis demonstrates rather clearly that the increase in incidence is only partly associated with earlier detection.[9]

Currently, melanoma is the sixth and seventh most common cancer in American men and women, respectively. The lifetime

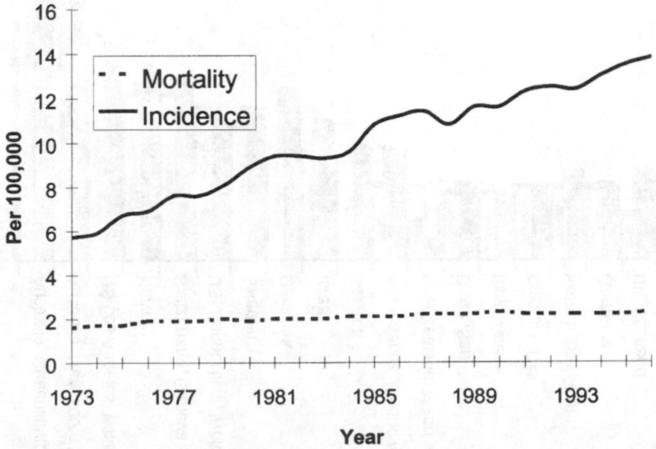

FIGURE 42.2-2. The incidence of melanoma has increased disproportionately faster than mortality. This is at least in part due to the increase in superficial lesions diagnosed relative to thicker ones. (Data from the Surveillance, Epidemiology and End Results program, 2000.)

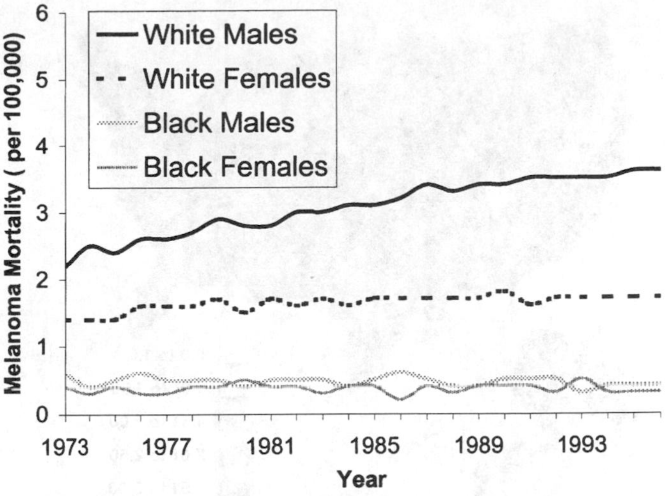

FIGURE 42.2-3. Age-adjusted U.S. mortality from melanoma from 1973 to 1996. Note the increasing mortality among white male subjects. (Data from the Surveillance, Epidemiology and End Results program, 2000.)

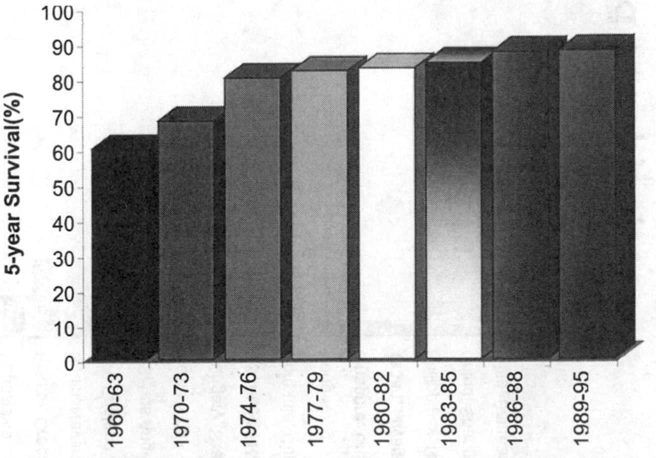

FIGURE 42.2-4. Five-year survival rates after the diagnosis of melanoma in the United States. These have improved from 1960, the earliest time period for which reliable data are available. The difference between the earliest and latest time periods are statistically significant. This increase in survival may be due to the increase in thinner melanomas compared with thicker ones. (Data from the Surveillance, Epidemiology and End Results program, 2000.)

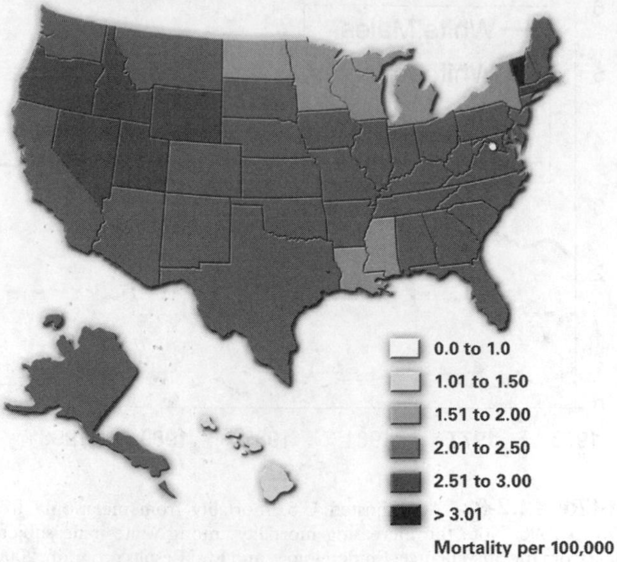

FIGURE 42.2-5. Substantial geographic variation in the incidence of melanoma. Interestingly, the U.S. mortality for melanoma is highest in Vermont (3.2 per 100,000) and lowest in Washington, DC (0.8 per 100,000) and Hawaii (1.2 per 100,000). Factors other than latitude, such as ethnic background, significantly influence the geographic risk of overall melanoma mortality. (Data from the Surveillance, Epidemiology and End Results program, 2000.)

risk for developing melanoma among white Americans is 1 in 85. The risk of melanoma increases with age and the median age at diagnosis ranges between 45 and 55 years, but people of all ages are at risk.[10,11] Melanoma commonly afflicts young, productive members of society. One-fourth of melanoma cases identified in the United States occurs in individuals before the age of 40. In women 20 to 35 years old, it is the second most common tumor after cervical cancer[12] and in women aged 25 to 30 it is the leading source of cancer death. The years of productive life lost to melanoma exceed those of all other solid tumors. In the United States, melanoma is more common among higher socioeconomic classes, but the case fatality is highest among lower socioeconomic groups.[13] The highest mortality from melanoma occurs in the state of Vermont and the lowest in Washington, DC. Although there is some increased distribution of melanoma mortality by latitude, other factors such as race are additionally important (Fig. 42.2-5).

Racial differences in susceptibility are apparent, and melanoma is most prevalent among white, European populations. For example, the incidence of cutaneous melanoma among African Americans is approximately 1/20 that of the U.S. white population and behaves differently at presentation. Among African Americans, melanoma occurs predominantly in acral sites rather than in areas of pigmented integument.[14] The worldwide incidence of melanoma varies considerably as well (Fig. 42.2-6). Rates of 0.2 per 100,000 in parts of Japan to nearly 40 per 100,000 in Queen-

FIGURE 42.2-6. Worldwide incidence of melanoma. Note the wide variation in incidence depending on race, sex, and latitude. (Data from refs. 549 and 550.)

sland have been reported. Despite these wide variations, the increase in overall melanoma incidence has increased globally.[15] Worldwide, race is the predominant risk factor for the development of melanoma, with white populations having the highest risk and Asian the lowest risk.

In the United Kingdom, trends have been similar to those in the United States. The incidence and mortality of melanoma has increased 50% during the last decade.[12] In Australia, where the incidence rates are the highest in the world, the increase in mortality is only now showing signs of slowing. However, mortality is increasing in many countries that had not previously reported increases such as France, Italy, Spain, and Hungary.[16]

RISK FACTORS, PREVENTION, AND SCREENING

With the increase in melanoma incidence over the last 40 years, effective screening strategies have become increasingly important.[17] The biologic and clinical behavior of melanoma supports the broad pursuit of screening programs. Effective screening for melanoma can be accomplished using noninvasive skin examinations since 93% of all primary melanomas are grossly visible. The remaining balance arises in mucosal, ocular, and unknown primary sites.[18] Many primary cutaneous lesions have a distinct radial growth phase that may persist for months to years, giving physicians, family, and patients ample opportunity for early recognition and appropriate excision before progressive vertical tumor invasion.[19] As melanomas less than 0.76 mm deep have a 10-year survival rate of more than 95%, the goal of screening is to identify lesions before the development of the so-called vertical growth phase associated with a worsened prognosis.[20] Furthermore, screening for melanoma can be accomplished in just minutes by trained physicians, and diagnostic biopsies are relatively inexpensive and simple to perform in the office setting.

RISK FACTORS FOR THE DEVELOPMENT OF MELANOMA IN POPULATIONS AT HIGHEST RISK FOR DEVELOPING MELANOMA

Education and screening programs should especially focus on populations that are at high risk for the development of melanoma. Many known risk factors can be used by physicians to improve the efficiency of screening programs (Table 42.2-1). Typical risk factors associated with carcinogenesis such as use of tobacco, alcohol, and estrogens do not affect the risk of melanoma. Instead, factors such as patient phenotype (hair, skin, and eye color), sun exposure, family history, and genetics play key roles.

Common Nevi

The role of moles or melanocytic nevi in the genesis of melanoma has been suspected since Norris' first description of melanoma in the English language in 1857. Small, common nevi are pigmented lesions that are often raised, symmetric in outline, and delimited with discrete regular borders. Clearly, the number of moles is an important predictor of melanoma risk and is surprisingly genetically determined, with monozygous twins having almost identical mole counts in contrast with dizygotic twins.[21] A threefold increase in melanoma risk is associated with the presence of five nevi more than 5 mm in diameter, or for those patients with more than 50 nevi greater than 2 mm in diameter.[22]

TABLE 42.2-1. Known Risk Factors for the Development of Melanoma[a]

Congenital nevi >5% body surface area
Previous melanoma
Family history
Dysplastic nevi syndrome
Dysplastic nevi
5 nevi >5 mm diameter
50 nevi >2 mm diameter
Sunburns during childhood
Poor tanning ability
White race
Red hair
Blond hair
Blue eyes
Freckles
Tanning salons
Equatorial latitudes
Psoralen sunscreen
Xeroderma pigmentosa

[a]Many risk factors have been identified for the development of melanoma. Patients with a previous history of melanoma, a family history of melanoma or dysplastic nevi, or large congenital nevi are at highest risk. Although all patients should be screened for melanoma by a trained physician, identifying risk factors can allow physicians to focus on especially high-risk patients.

Atypical Nevi

Atypical melanocytic nevi that exhibit histopathologic features of dysplasia were initially described by Reimer et al. in the setting of familial melanoma.[23] These lesions when clinically defined but not pathologically examined are classified as *atypical nevi*,[24] and lesions defined histologically with specific architectural and cytologic features are called *dysplastic nevi*.[25] An atypical nevus is defined clinically as a flat macule greater than 5 mm. At least two of the following features are also necessary to distinguish atypical nevi from banal nevi: variable pigmentation; irregular, asymmetric outline; and indistinct borders.[26] Atypical lesions in patients without familial syndromes are more commonly found on sun-exposed areas.

The majority of melanoma is sporadic, and in this setting, the role of atypical nevi has become more clearly apparent. Atypical nevi among patients with sporadic melanoma are clinically indistinguishable from those of patients with familial melanoma. Atypical nevi occur in 2% to 7% of the white population and can be identified in 25% to 40% of patients with melanoma.[22,25,27–29] Atypical nevi are a significant risk factor for the development of melanoma. Their presence may indicate a general instability in melanocyte growth. Estimating the risk incurred by the presence of atypical nevi has been difficult and ranges widely in the literature. The risk of new primary melanoma among individuals with atypical nevi was calculated according to the presence of a family or personal history of prior melanoma by Kraemer et al.[27] This risk relates both to the presence of atypical nevi, melanoma, or both in the balance of the family of a given individual. In cases in which atypical nevi are isolated in an individual, the risk is lowest (27 times population risk). When atypical nevi are found in multiple members of a family or there is a history of melanoma in additional members of the family, the risk rises. Those patients with multiple family members exhibiting atypical nevi and a having a history of melanoma have the highest risk (148 times population risk).[27,30,31] Unfortunately, the history of atypical nevi and of melanoma itself is often difficult to elicit. Crijns et al. reported that more than one-half of patients without an elicited history of melanoma or atypical nevi on initial family history are later found to have familial patterns of atypical nevi, melanoma, or both.[32] Still the identification of atypical nevi even among skilled clinicians and pathologists is problematic, and some find the distinction from conventional nevi unconvincing.[33]

The risk incurred by the presence of atypical nevi has been difficult to accurately establish. In one series, 716 patients with melanoma were compared with a group of matched controls. In the absence of atypical nevi, increased numbers of small nevi were associated with an approximately twofold elevated risk of melanoma, and increased numbers of both small and large nonatypical nevi were associated with a fourfold greater risk. The presence of a single clinically atypical nevus was associated with a twofold greater risk, while ten or more conferred a 12-fold greater risk of developing primary melanoma.[26] Another smaller series suggested the risk of developing melanoma might be as high as 37 times greater in those individuals who have atypical nevi.[34]

Congenital Nevi

Childhood melanomas are rare, but even infants have been reported with the disease, especially in association with giant congenital nevi.[35] Patients with large congenital melanocytic nevi, those that appear at birth or during early childhood, are at high risk for developing melanomas (Fig. 42.2-7). The lesions are elevated, with discrete borders and stippled pigmentation.[26] Large congenital nevi occur in 1 in 1000 to 1 in 20,000 newborns, and giant nevi involving large body surfaces (i.e., the entire trunk) occur in 1 in 500,000 newborns.[36] One-half of all cases of melanoma within large congenital nevi occur in the first decade of life so screening, surgical excision, or both should be planned early.[37] In a series of 265 patients with congenital nevi, patients with congenital nevi that covered more than 5% of their total body surface area had a risk of developing melanoma 1000-fold higher than the general population. No patients with congenital nevi that involved less than 4% of their total body surface area developed melanomas, but the study size could not exclude a small increase in risk.[38] In another series of 46 patients with large congenital nevi, two individuals developed three melanomas arising from nevi after a mean of 7.3 years of routine screening. Although the study was small, it confirms that these patients are a high-risk population.[39] Furthermore, detecting early melanoma in these lesions is difficult since malignant transformation usually evolves in the deeper layers of the nevus, and visible surface alterations are late manifestations.

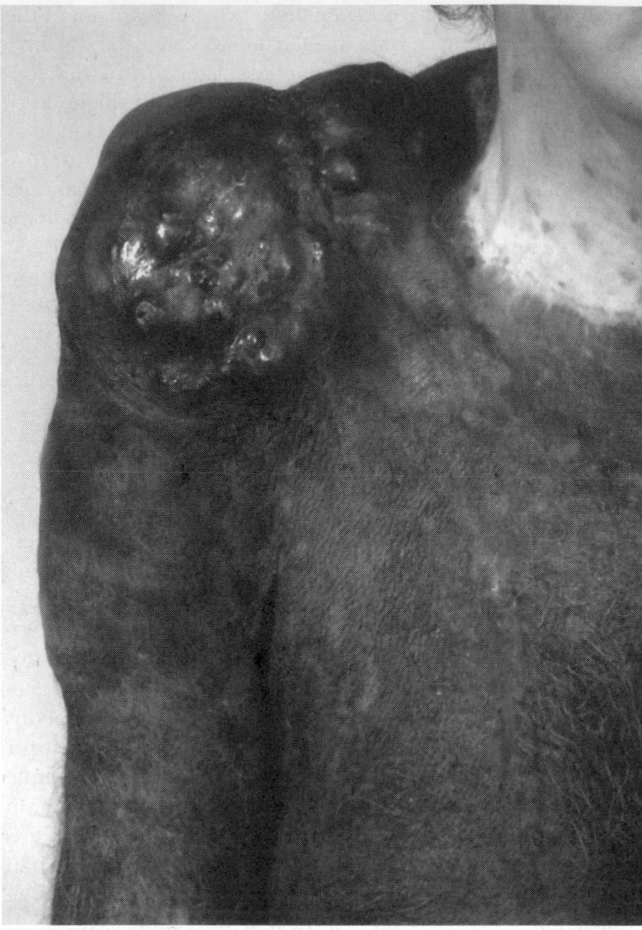

FIGURE 42.2-7. Giant congenital nevus with malignant degeneration. This melanoma developed on the shoulder of a patient with a giant congenital nevus. Patients with large congenital nevi have a 1000-fold increased risk for developing melanoma. Frequent surveillance is necessary to diagnose these lesions early. For nevi that encompass more than 5% of total body surface area, resection may prevent the development of melanoma.

Spitz Nevi

Spitz nevi are benign lesions that occur in children, and their importance stems from the difficulty in distinguishing them from melanoma. Whereas Spitz nevi are usually under 1 cm in diameter and may resemble verrucae or small hemangiomas, melanomas in children tend to be larger and quite striking clinically.[40] All children diagnosed with melanoma or Spitz nevi should have the lesions reviewed by experienced pathologists. Parameters suggesting malignancy are age of diagnosis greater than 10 years, presence of ulceration, diameter greater than 1 cm, involvement of subcutaneous fat, and a mitotic activity of at least 6/mm^2.[41]

Familial Atypical Nevus Syndromes

Melanoma is divisible into familial and sporadic patterns. Our understanding of the role of melanocytic precursor lesions in the genesis of melanoma has been clarified over the past 30 years based on pioneering studies involving familial clusters of patients with melanoma, many of whom are observed to have nevi exhibiting atypical features.[42–44]

Patients with the dysplastic nevus syndrome, a disease of autosomal dominant inheritance with incomplete penetrance, are at increased risk for developing melanoma.[22] In familial syndromes, the atypical moles of patients with the familial atypical mole-melanoma syndrome were named according to the initials of the probands (B-K nevus syndrome).[23,43] These atypical nevi were also notable for their location on the skin of the trunk that was not necessarily sun-exposed. The presence of atypical nevi identifies patients with a high risk of melanoma among family members with this syndrome.[44] The risk conferred by the presence of multiple atypical nevi in such individuals approaches 100% by age 70.[30,44–46] This risk is more complex than that of a discrete precursor lesion that progresses stepwise into malignancy. Although many melanomas have been identified to arise within atypical nevi, most occur in areas of skin that show neither gross nor histologic evidence of an antecedent atypical nevic lesion. This observation suggests that removal of atypical lesions is not akin to the reduction in carcinoma risk after resection of adenomatous polyps of the colon as most melanomas arise *de novo*. In patients with familial melanomas, it is clear that atypical nevi may serve as nonobligate precursors and markers of melanocyte dyscrasia.

Careful molecular, genetic, and pathologic studies in patients with familial atypical mole-melanoma syndrome may define the molecular basis of progression and identify markers for adequate surveillance and ultimate disease prevention. A few apparently important genetic mutations have already been identified in the cyclin-dependent kinase genes, some of which serve as inhibitors of cell-cycle progression. An enhanced incidence of melanoma is associated with a single mutation in CDK4 (12q14) as well as mutations in the CDKN2A (9p21) and CDKN2B genes.[47] There is a correlation between CDKN2A mutations in family members with atypical nevus syndromes. Clinical findings associated with this germline mutation involve nevi in abnormal locations and abnormal numbers. These include nevi on the buttocks, nevi on the feet, total nevi greater than 100, and two or more atypical nevi.[48] Germline mutations of CDKN2A have been identified in approximately 20% of melanoma-prone families, and CDK4 has been described in three families.[49] Polymorphisms occurring in the melanocyte-stimulating hormone receptor predict skin coloration, risk of developing nevi, and independently and synergistically with p16 mutations, ultimately the development of melanoma. Although familial melanoma provides important insights into the disease, the number of cases of familial melanoma are limited. They represent an estimated 10% of patients with melanoma.

History of Previous Melanoma

A significant number of patients with a past history of melanoma develop a second, metachronous lesion.[22] A study of 3310 patients from a prospective database with stage I and II melanoma showed that 3.4% developed a second primary melanoma. The 5- and 10-year risk of developing a second primary melanoma was 2.8% and 3.6%, respectively.[50] Patients with a past history of melanoma should undergo frequent cutaneous examinations to screen for such metachronous lesions. Patients who are at especially high risk for metachronous lesion are those with atypical nevi or family history.[51]

Transplant and Other Immunosuppressed Patients

Patients who have had a solid organ transplant are at increased risk for developing melanoma, and the risk is directly related to the degree of immunosuppression. Although the risk for nonmelanomatous cutaneous tumors is estimated at approximately 65-fold that of the general population, the risk for developing melanoma is increased by a more modest threefold.[52] Children who have had a renal transplantation demonstrate higher benign nevus counts than controls, and the duration and degree of immunosuppression correlates positively with these counts. Such nevi are found most commonly on the back and acral sites.[53] Interestingly, in normal adults, nevus counts increase in number, peaking in the early 20s and then progressively decreasing with time.[54] Children with genetically determined immunodeficiencies have a three- to sixfold risk of developing melanoma.[55] Of the few patients reported to have melanoma and human immunodeficiency virus in the literature, approximately one-third had metastatic disease at the time of initial examination, and systemic symptoms correlate with decreased CD4+ cell counts. Melanomas among patients with human immunodeficiency virus infection are often atypical in appearance, multiple, and metastatic.[56] The number of nevi less than 5 mm in diameter was found be greater in patients with human immunodeficiency virus than in the general population. Immunodeficiency may promote or permit the development of nevi and raises the question of whether sun-induced immunosuppression plays a role in the development of nevi.[57] The development of melanoma may relate directly to the suppression of cellular immunity. Melanoma in immunosuppressed patients may evolve from precursor nevi that are unable to elicit cellular immune recognition. The detection of dysplastic nevi offers an opportunity to identify those immunosuppressed patients who are at greatest risk of melanoma.[58–60]

Phenotypic, Solar, and Other Risk Factors

Risk factors for melanoma apart from the presence of acquired and congenital melanocytic nevi include easily identifiable phenotypic characteristics of pigmentation such as pale skin, poor tanning ability, light hair and eyes, and the presence of freckles. Compared with individuals with brown and black hair, the relative risk for developing melanoma for those with blonde and red hair is 1.8 and 2.4, respectively. Individuals with blue eyes have a risk 1.2 times that of individuals with brown eyes.[22,61] Episodic exposure to intense sunlight and a history of blistering sunburns, especially in childhood (ages 10 to 19), is strongly associated with the development of melanoma.[51,62] Childhood sunburn with blistering is also associated with increased numbers of atypical nevi.[22,63] Unlike other nonmelanoma skin cancers, recreational intermittent exposure to sunlight is more strongly associated with risk of melanoma than lifetime continuous exposure.[64]

One might expect a much higher incidence of melanoma in patients with albinism since they have minimal natural solar protection and the development of melanoma is dependent on the presence of melanocytes, not on melanin. However, only 23 cases of melanoma have been documented in the literature in patients with oculocutaneous albinism. They were all, of course, amelanotic.[65,66] Patients with xeroderma pigmentosum are another group that have little natural solar protection; however, 5% of patients develop melanoma at a median age of 19 years. They are a rare high-risk subgroup that needs close screening for cutaneous malignancies.[67]

Ultraviolet (UV) exposure is the most easily modified risk factor for the development of melanoma, but a causative role of UV exposure only partially explains observational data. Exposure to UV radiation is not obligatory for the development of melanoma. Melanomas are commonly found on the soles of the feet and in mucosal areas that never are exposed to daylight, and geographic susceptibility to melanoma does not consistently increase with the amount of UV exposure. Melanoma occurs in children and young adults who frequently have had relatively little sun exposure. UV radiation frequently initiates the development of melanoma either directly or indirectly, but patient susceptibility is a much more important risk factor.

Role of Pregnancy and Estrogens in Melanoma

As pregnancy is associated with an increase in melanocyte-stimulating hormone levels and an increase in pigmentation in some patients, the theoretical concern for stimulation of melanoma has prompted concern. Although various case reports initially suggested an adverse outcome in pregnant patients with melanoma, six well-controlled studies have evaluated the effect pregnancy has on survival. No difference in survival between patients diagnosed during pregnancy and controls has been substantiated.[68–72] Interestingly, one study implied that prior pregnancy was in fact protective by demonstrating improved survival in women under 50 who had more than five children before the diagnosis of melanoma.[73] Neither is there evidence that pregnancy occurring after the diagnosis of melanoma worsens prognosis.[70,74] In women with a history of melanoma, it may be reasonable to suggest waiting 2 years after initial diagnosis before becoming pregnant since two-thirds of recurrences occur within this time period. However, the stage and depth at diagnosis and the age and desires of the mother factor heavily into these decisions.

There is no evidence that estrogen use increases the risk of melanoma. Much of the confusion concerning estrogens results from the expression of estrogen receptors on some melanomas. The presence or absence of these receptors neither predicts prognosis nor hormone responsiveness. Tamoxifen has been suggested to have effects on melanoma; however, its actions may be indirect, through the potentiation of the cytotoxic chemotherapy or enhancing natural killer (NK) function, rather than directly affecting melanoma.[74,75] More recent randomized controlled trials failed to corroborate a significant benefit of tamoxifen with dacarbazine or multidrug therapy. Well-designed epidemiologic studies have not shown an increased rate of melanoma in patients who have used exogenous estrogens.[76,77] No studies have specifically examined the risks of hormonal replacement therapy in postmenopausal women with melanoma, but no data exist to suggest that hormonal replacement therapy is harmful.[74] The well-characterized beneficial effects of hormonal replacement therapy likely outweigh any theoretical, unsubstantiated risks of estrogens.

DIAGNOSIS: CHARACTERISTICS OF MELANOMA

Identification of features that may mark lesions suspicious for melanoma can be simply recalled using the mnemonic ABCDE. *A* stands for asymmetry, *B* for borders that are irregular or diffuse, *C* for color variegation, *D* for diameter more than 5 mm, and *E* signifies enlargement or evolution.[78] Bleeding and ulceration occurs in 10% of localized melanomas and 54% of late melanomas and is a poor prognostic finding.[79]

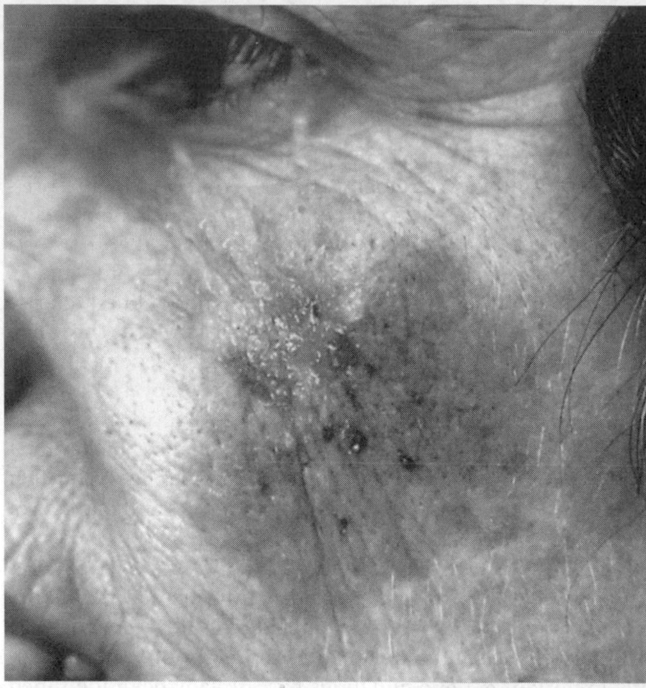

FIGURE 42.2-8. Lentigo maligna melanoma. These lesions commonly occur on the face in older patients. These lesions may require considerable planning for reconstruction.

Morphotypes

Although specific morphotypes of melanoma have been used for prognostic information, the Breslow depth of the lesion and presence or absence of ulceration are the most significant predictors of biologic behavior of the primary lesion. Morphology does not predict prognosis independently of these well-defined risk factors. The classic morphotypes now serve as descriptive tools that aid in the recognition of these lesions and as historic references (Figs. 42.2-8, 42.2-9, 42.2-10, 42.2-11, and 42.2-12). Physicians should recognize that many less dangerous (and more common) skin lesions may exhibit features similar to melanoma such as seborrheic keratosis, pigmented basal cell cancer, solar lentigines, and atypical nevi.[80]

Superficial spreading melanoma presents as an asymptomatic, flat macule or barely raised plaque with color variations that may include shades of black and brown. Areas of regression (depigmentation) are common. It is the most common growth pattern and accounts for 60% to 70% of all melanomas.[81,82] These lesions may exist for years before a rapid growth phase is identified.[22] Notching and scalloping are common, with enlargement during the radial growth phase of melanoma. They can occur at any site, although they most commonly can be seen on the lower extremities of women and on the trunk of men.[79]

Nodular melanoma typically presents as a uniform lesion that is dark black-blue or bluish-red, although 5% are amelanotic.[22,79] This is the second most common morphotype, occurring in 15% to 30% of patients, and usually exhibits a more rapid onset.[82] Nodular melanomas are associated with deeper Breslow depths because they quickly establish a vertical growth phase. Most commonly, nodular melanomas are located on the

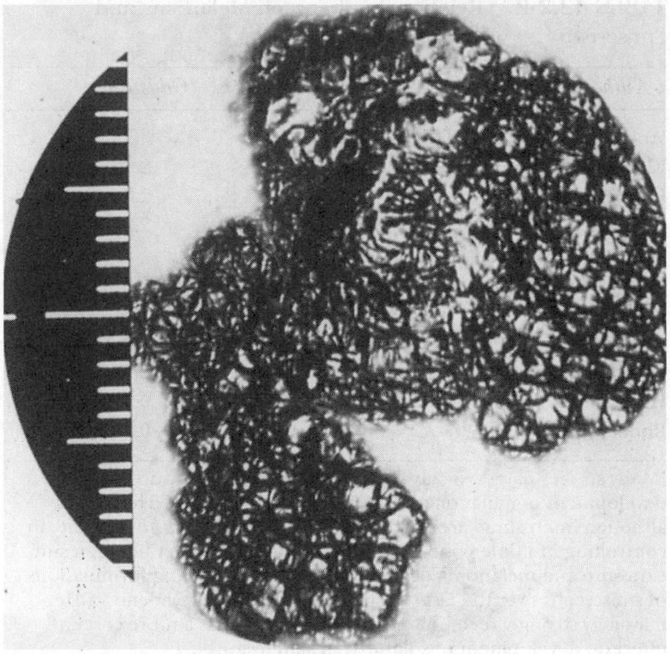

FIGURE 42.2-9. Nodular melanoma. The second most common melanoma morphotype. It is associated with the so-called vertical growth phase, manifesting a more aggressive biologic phenotype and worsened prognosis.

trunk or head and neck and are observed in men more frequently than women.

Lentigo maligna melanomas (LMM) are typically located on the face and are generally large, flat lesions that are tan colored, with differing shades of brown. Rarely, LMM can be amelanotic. Up to one-half of lentigo maligna (LM), a precursor lesion that is characterized by atypical melanocytic proliferation, degenerate into melanoma over a period of many years. The diagnosis requires the presence of sun-related changes in both the epidermis and dermis. They are found in approximately 5% of patients with melanoma.[82]

Acral lentiginous melanomas are uncommon and typically occur on the palms, soles, or beneath the nail (subungual). However, not all lesions in these locations are acral lentiginous melanomas. Melanoma in the hands or feet account for less than 5% of all melanomas, but they are much more common in dark-complexioned individuals.[83,84] These lesions tend to present late and thus are associated with a poorer prognosis. They represent up to 70% of melanomas in African Americans and up to 46% in Asians.[79] They are usually tan, brown to black macular lesions with variegation in color and an irregular border.[22] In a Japanese series of 62 plantar melanomas, 82% were acral lentiginous, 3% were superficial spreading, and 14% were nodular. The lesions most commonly affected the heel. Acral melanomas are strongly associated with high total body nevus counts [relative risk (RR) = 6.3] and with nevi on the soles. There is also an association with penetrating injuries to the feet or hands (RR = 5.0) and heavy exposure to agricultural chemicals (RR = 3.6).[85] Subungual melanomas account for only 1% to 3% of all melanomas. They commonly are diagnosed late because of their close resemblance to many benign lesions of the nail. If a nail bed lesion has not changed significantly in 4 to 6 weeks, a biopsy should be performed, accompanied by removal of the nail. Some clinical parameters that should arouse suspicion of subungual melanoma are lesions occurring in patients greater than 50 years old, a width greater than 3 mm with variegated borders, extension of pigment into the lateral or proximal nail fold, and lesions occurring in individuals of African American, Asian, or Native American ancestry.[86] Seventy percent occur on the great toe or thumb. These tumors are associated with a 5-, 10-, and 20-year median survival of 59%, 44%, and 29%, respectively. One-half have associated nail destruction and 70% ulcerate. Twenty-five percent present with metastases and 74% are greater than 1.5 mm thick.[87]

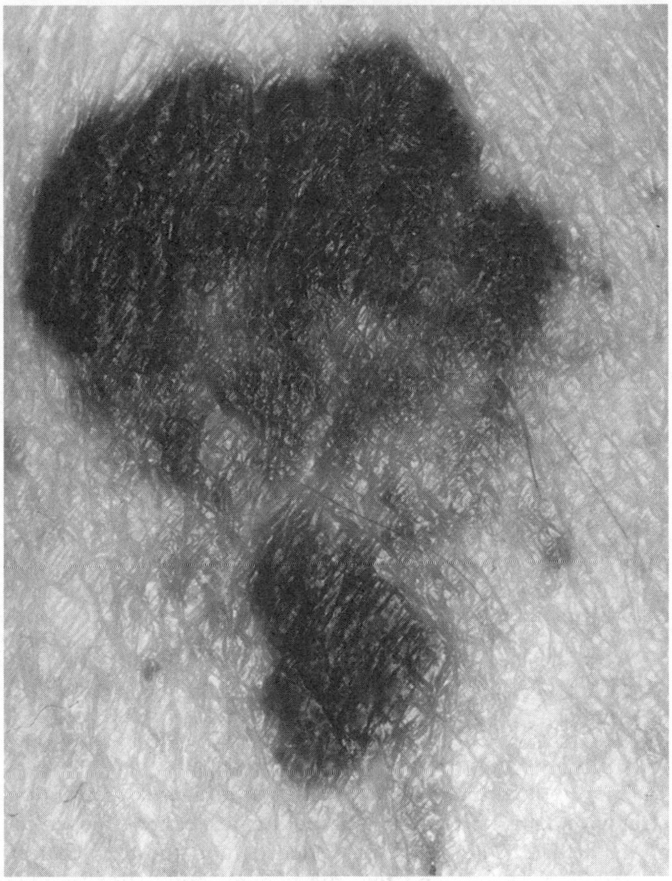

FIGURE 42.2-10. Superficial spreading melanoma. This typical example exemplifies the most common melanoma morphotype. Note the irregular borders, large size, color variegation, and asymmetry. Radial growth at the dermal-epidermal junction for prolonged periods is associated with a better prognosis.

Desmoplastic melanoma is a rare and locally aggressive variant of malignant melanoma that is difficult to diagnose clinically and microscopically. It represents approximately 1.7% of melanomas. The majority of these tumors occur on the head and neck of elderly patients and one-half are amelanotic.[88] Desmoplastic tumors are aggressive locally and behave more like mesenchymal neoplasms. These tumors stain intensely with S-100. The most reliable and characteristic histologic features of an early lesion of desmoplastic melanoma are aggregates of lymphocytes, tumor cell cytologic atypia, stromal myxoid change, and poor circumscription of the dermal infiltrate.[89] The risk of local recurrence increases when neurotropism is present.[90]

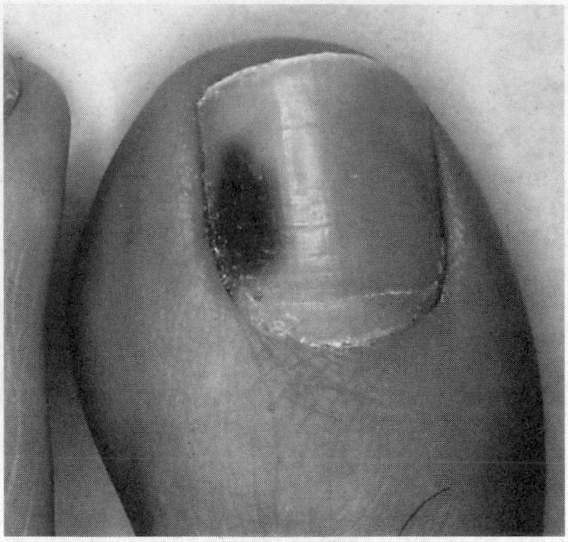

FIGURE 42.2-11. Subungual melanoma. All nail bed lesions that have grown or remained unchanged over 4 to 6 weeks should undergo an incisional biopsy and removal of the nail.

TABLE 42.2-2. Relationship between Melanoma and Sunscreen Use: Case-Controlled Studies[a]

Author	*Odds Ratio*
Wolf, 1998[577]	3.5
Klepp and Magnus, 1979[578]	2.8
Herzfeld, 1993[579]	2.6
Graham, 1985[93]	2.2
Westerdahl, 1995[580]	1.8
Autier, 1995[581]	1.8
Beitner, 1990[582]	1.8
Holman, 1986[583]	1.1
Osterlind, 1988[584]	1.1
Holly, 1995[585]	0.5
Rodenas, 1996[586]	0.2

[a]Many studies paradoxically show an increased odds ratio for the development of melanoma with the use of sunscreens. These data, although interesting, are hard to interpret because of the difficulty in controlling multiple patients variables, the long latency between sun exposure and melanoma occurrence, and the changing formulations of sunscreens over the last decades. The American Academy of Dermatology strongly recommends sunscreen that has a more certain effect on development of solar-driven skin lesions.

PREVENTION

With the assumption that the prime modifiable risk factor in the development of melanoma is UV radiation, prevention strategies focus on reducing the public's excessive exposure to sunlight. The American Cancer Society and the Skin Cancer Foundation recommend that the general population employ "sun-smart" practices. This includes the avoidance of direct midday sun exposure between the hours of 10 a.m. and 4 p.m. and the use of sunscreens, protective clothing, and appropriate shade (e.g., sun umbrellas). The increased risk of melanoma incurred through sun exposure is strongly associated with blistering sunburns between the ages of 10 and 19; thus, special attention should focused on teaching children these sun-smart practices. While the use of sunscreens of sun protection factor (SPF) of at least 15 is recommended, sunscreens have been largely shown to reduce the nonmelanoma skin cancer incidence. There is much controversy regarding the effectiveness of sunscreen for prevention of melanoma, with the epidemiologic data inconclusive at present.[91]

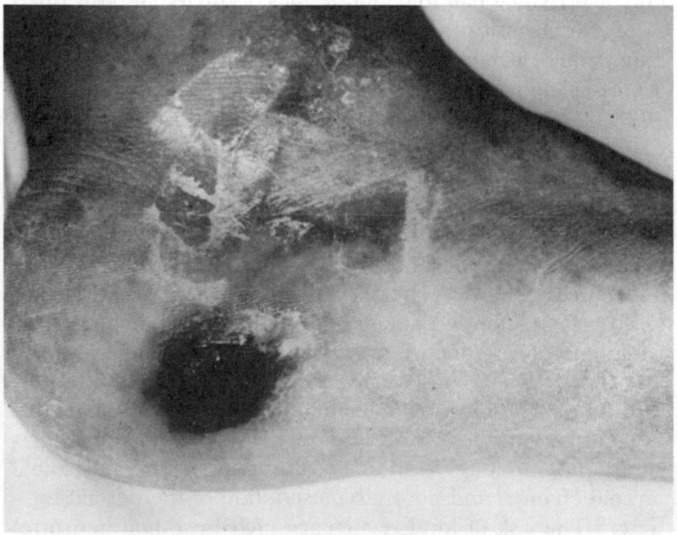

FIGURE 42.2-12. Acral lentiginous melanoma. These lesions, located in the extremity, are more common in Asians and African Americans.

Sunscreens and Sunlight

Claims of a reduction in melanoma risk from the use of sunscreens have been controversial and difficult to substantiate. In fact, most studies show an increased risk for the development of melanoma with the use of sunscreens, probably because of their ability to delay or avoid sunburn episodes, which may allow prolonged exposure to unfiltered UV radiation (Table 42.2-2). Many criticize these epidemiologic studies, for many confounding factors may contribute to these negative results. Individuals who sunbathe frequently are more likely to use sunscreens. In addition, many studies had focused on older preparations that were either less effective at blocking UVB light (low SPF) or contained psoralens, potent tanning activators. People with a poor tanning ability who have used psoralen sunscreen in the past have a risk of developing melanoma 4.5 times that of regular sunscreen users.[15] The risk reduction from newer, high SPF sunscreens is difficult to assess due to the long latency from sun exposure to the development of melanoma.[92,93] However, increases in benign nevus counts are clearly associated with the use of sunscreens. In a large, randomized, placebo-controlled study of more than 600 European children, the number of nevi increased in those who used sunscreens even when controlling for factors such as skin type and eye color.[91] A theoretical basis exists for the lack of efficacy of sunscreens. Most sunscreens offer greater protection from UVB (290 nm) than UVA (375 nm) radiation, thereby reducing the risk of sunburn while not blocking UVA radiation, which efficiently induces tanning. However, UVA penetrates more deeply and causes more DNA damage than UVB. Although the ozone layer filters UVA more effectively than UVB light, approximately 1000 times more UVA than UVB bathes the earth's surface.[94] Thus, the depletion of the ozone layer may significantly affect the incidence of melanoma. An estimated 1% increase in melanoma incidence occurs with each percentage decrease in the ozone layer.[15]

Several studies show that the excessive use of tanning salons is associated with an increased risk of developing melanoma. No study demonstrates that tanning is protective against subsequent sunburns or melanoma.[95,96] Long-term use of tanning salons is associated with premature skin aging, cataract development, and nonmelanoma skin cancers. Prevention strategies should discourage the use of tanning salons.

Self-Examination

Patients at increased risk of melanoma should be informed how to perform regular self-examinations of their skin. Most patients who develop melanoma would have alerted their physicians much earlier if they had used a simple checklist that helps identify high-risk lesions.[97] Self-examination is currently underused even in high-risk populations. Only one in five patients with melanoma practices self-screening and only 6% of patients follow recommendations for self-examination, sun protection, and yearly professional examinations.[98,99] Screening by trained physicians currently cannot be replaced by self-screening until national efforts at public education are more broadly undertaken.

Excision of Nevi

Evidence supports the removal of atypical nevi in patients with a prior history of melanoma as a preventative strategy. The excision of atypical lesions decreases the expected incidence of melanomas in high-risk cohorts, but it is unclear whether a broader population-based strategy supporting the excision of these nevi can be extrapolated.[100] Wholesale removal of unsuspicious nevi should be condemned as a surgical practice. Indiscriminant excisions are associated with unnecessary scarring and little effect on the development of melanoma. Most melanomas, even in patients with familial atypical mole-melanoma syndrome, arise *de novo*; thus, the excision of all atypical lesions may not eliminate the risk of developing melanoma. Large congenital nevi should be excised if feasible, and frequent screening should be preformed in these patients until excision is performed. If the lesion is too large for excision, surgery may be limited to biopsies of the most worrisome sites in combination with observation and photographic documentation. Dermabrasion and other superficial excisions may not decrease the risk of developing melanoma and are not recommended.

SCREENING

Prevention and screening for melanoma are reasonable objectives to restrain the rising incidence of this silent epidemic. Cancer screening for melanoma fulfills many of the requirements necessary for effectiveness. First, early detection appears to result in improved outcomes. Second, the screening process is easy to perform by primary care physicians, and third, the screening is cost effective.

Efficacy

Randomized trials to determine efficacy and cost effectiveness of screening programs would require thousands of people and prolonged (greater than 10-year) follow-up; however, there is sufficient evidence to assume the validity and efficacy of current screening programs, especially in high-risk populations. Although the true effectiveness of screening programs can only be determined by noting an increased survival in screened populations, many reports demonstrate that thinner lesions are found in screened compared with unscreened cohorts. Since the thickness of the melanoma correlates linearly with survival in stage I and II patients, screening programs can measure their effectiveness through this intermediate end-point instead of waiting 10 years (or more) for survival data.[101] Numerous studies have been published from Australia, Europe, and the United States demonstrating the effectiveness of screening programs. Many have focused on high-risk populations in order to attain a high number of events with much fewer patients.

Many of the published screening trials studied high-risk populations with either a strong family history of melanoma, a previous personal history of melanoma, or a diagnosis of the dysplastic nevus syndrome. In one series of 555 high-risk patients, screening reduced the average thickness of diagnosed melanomas to 0.52 mm compared with an average tumor thickness of 1.44 mm before the screening program was instituted. None of the 138 patients diagnosed with melanoma on screening developed metastatic disease.[102] In another series from the Netherlands, in which high-risk patients were screened, the thickness of primary lesions decreased from 1.75 mm before the screening process to 0.8 mm at the start of the screening process and then to 0.54 mm during routine follow-up.[103]

In Australia, the incidence of melanoma is the highest in the world due to an equatorial climate, a fair-skinned immigrant population, and localized depletion of the ozone layer. The decrease in average tumor Breslow depth in Australia has been attributed to extensive screening. In 1960 the average thickness of melanoma lesions was greater than 2.5 mm. By 1986, after the establishment of a comprehensive screening program in the 1960s, the mean tumor thickness dropped to 0.80.[104] In France, a unique situation exists as occupational medicine specialists examine the entire working population yearly. In a study involving 65,000 people, 273 patients examined by occupational medicine specialists were thought to have suspicious lesions. Of these patients only 172 followed up with their primary care physicians and five melanomas were found. This translates to in an incidence of 7.7 per 100,000, close to the 9 per 100,000 found in the general French population.[105]

The American Academy of Dermatology has provided more than 1 million free skin cancer screenings from 1985 to 1997. Of all the biopsies performed for suspicious lesions, 17% were found to be melanomas on histology. More than 90% of histologically confirmed melanomas were less than 1.5 mm thick, and the median thickness of all melanomas was 0.30 mm. The 8.3% of cases with advanced melanoma is a lower proportion than that reported by the 1990 SEER registry. The rate of thickest lesions (greater than 4 mm) and late-stage melanomas among all participants was 2.83 per 100,000 population. Thirty-nine percent of screened patients who had melanoma claimed they would not have sought examination otherwise and more than 30% of these melanomas were located on areas not readily visible on self-examination.[106]

Examination

Although dermatologists have superior accuracy compared with nondermatologists in the diagnosis of melanoma and dysplastic nevi, there are too few dermatologists for all routine screening.[107] Dermatologists are generally more qualified in identifying these lesions. Screening for melanoma by a dermatologist has a sensitivity and positive predictive value of 89% to 97% and 17% to 75%, respectively.[108] The use of epiluminescence microscopy by an experienced dermatologist can greatly increase the sensitivity and specificity of the examination.[109] Further, only 12% of nondermatologists were able to correctly identify five out of six melanomas, whereas 69% of dermatologists did.[101,110] A viable health strategy for reducing the mortality of melanoma involves educating primary care providers to incorporate skin examinations as part of their routine physical examinations. With education, primary care physicians should successfully incorporate skin screenings in their physical examinations as they have with breast examinations, digital examinations, and fecal occult blood testing.

Screening examinations are quick, painless, inexpensive and readily accepted by patients. Complete examination of the skin should be performed systematically, with the patient fully undressed. Care should be taken not to ignore the scalp, nails, palms, soles, ears, and beneath the breasts. Since most melanomas occur on the trunk and lower extremities in women and on the trunk and proximal upper extremities in men, these areas should be carefully examined. Lesions of the perineum are uncommon and may be excluded unless the patient has a specific lesion in question. Problems do exist with screening protocols as some melanomas may have an uncharacteristically benign appearance and a radial growth phase shorter than the screening interval.

Cost-Effectiveness

The cost of screening includes practitioner time spent with patients and the cost of biopsy and pathology. Since the ratio of positive to negative biopsy results ranges from 1:70 to 1:250, the number of biopsies subsequent to mass screenings may be considerable.[105,106] In a cost-effectiveness model of screening high-risk patients, $29,000 would be spent per year of life saved. This is less than what is currently spent on prostate-specific antigen testing, Pap smears, or annual mammography.[111]

STAGING OF MELANOMA

The staging of cutaneous melanoma involves segregation by local, regional, or distant disease and strongly correlates with survival (Fig. 42.2-13). The vast majority of patients who present with primary melanoma have localized tumors, and for this reason stage I and II have been used to designate early (low-risk) and later (intermediate-risk) tumors, even though both represent localized disease. The features of melanoma that influence the risk of relapse are encapsulated in current and proposed staging systems of the American Joint Committee on Cancer (AJCC) (Tables 42.2-3 and 42.2-4). The last formal edition of this system (1992) is currently in revision, so the features of the prior system will be contrasted to those of the proposed new system of 2000.[112] In both systems, distant metastases (M1) define stage IV disease, whereas regional lymph node metastases (N1 to N3) define stage III disease

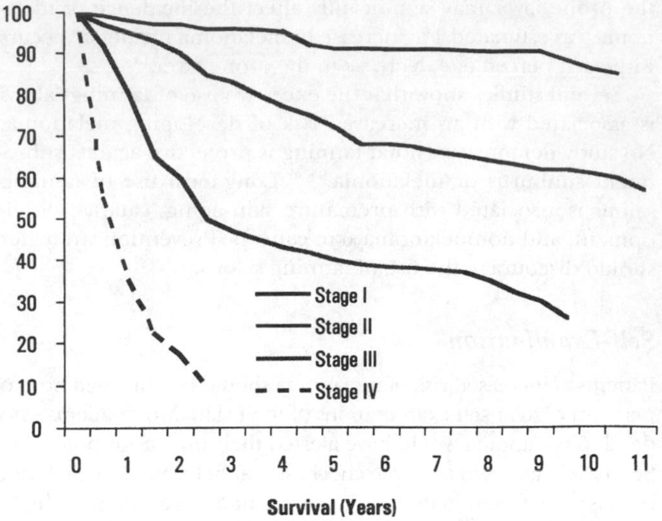

FIGURE 42.2-13. Melanoma survival correlates strongly with stage. Fifteen-year survival results are shown for over 4000 melanoma patients. (From Ketcham AS, Balch CM. Classification and staging systems. In: Balch CM, Milton GW, eds. *Cutaneous melanoma: clinical management and treatment results worldwide.* Philadelphia: JB Lippincott, 1985:55, with permission.)

and are cardinal prognostic variables for patients with melanoma of the skin. Most patients present with neither distant nor regional disease apparent, so the features of local prognostic significance assume a predominant role in defining the prospect for relapse-free survival and overall survival in patients with melanoma.

STAGE I MELANOMA

The microstage or Breslow depth and presence or absence of ulceration are the most important variables in those without regional or distant metastases.[113] Patients with localized disease apparent only at the primary site make up by far the largest category of those presenting with melanoma. The division between stages I and II has been arbitrary, in part reflecting an effort to separate low-risk from intermediate-risk disease.[114–117] The staging system adopted by the AJCC in 1992 moved from a dependence on prognostic assessment based on the levels of skin through which a tumor had penetrated, to a duality of thickness measured in millimeters according to Breslow, and levels according to Clark.[118,119] The role of the Breslow thickness has been recognized as more predictive of prognosis. A secondary importance of the Clark level, especially in thinner tumors, has been identified. The Breslow depth is the primary predictor of prognosis, even when it predicts a more favorable prognosis than the level of invasion. Although the AJCC 1992 system allowed for either thickness or level (whichever was worse) to be taken as the basis for risk assessment, thickness appears to be considerably more reproducible in predicting prognosis than the Clark level.[112,118,120,121] Thus, in the proposed new classification system[112] stage I and II melanoma prognostic assessment will be based on Breslow thickness and ulceration. The Clark

TABLE 42.2-3. American Joint Committee on Cancer Tumor (T), Node (N), Metastasis (M) Classification System for Melanoma[a]

	Current 1992	*Proposed 2000*	
T STAGE			
T0	Tis	Tis	
T1	<0.76	<1.0	A: No ulceration; B: ulceration or level IV or V
T2	0.76–1.5	1–2	
T3	1.5–4.0	2–4	
T4	>4	>4	
N STAGE			
N1	1	One lymph node	A: Micrometastasis; B: macrometastasis
N2	2–4	2–3 lymph nodes	A: Micrometastasis; B: macrometastasis; C: in-transit disease without positive nodes
N3	5 or more	4 or more metastatic lymph nodes, matted nodes, ulcerated melanoma, and metastatic lymph node(s), or nodal disease and in-transit or satellite lesions	
M STAGE			
M1	Any systemic metastasis	Any systemic metastasis	A: Distant skin, soft tissue, or nodal metastasis; B: pulmonary metastasis; C: all other visceral involvement or any patient with elevated blood levels of lactic dehydrogenase

Tis, tumor *in situ.*

[a]Proposed year 2000 version and current version. Micrometastases are diagnosed after elective or sentinel lymphadenectomy. Macrometastases are defined as clinically detectable lymph node metastases confirmed by therapeutic lymphadenectomy or when any lymph node metastasis exhibits extracapsular extension.[118]

level of the primary lesion enters multivariate analyses only as a secondary feature when the Breslow depth is less than 1 mm. Patients with T1 lesions and a Clark stage of IV or more have a 10% chance of nodal disease compared with only a 2% risk in those with T1 lesions and Clark stages less than IV. Because of the importance of Clark stage in thin tumors, lesions less than 1 mm in Breslow depth that are level IV or V are designated as T1b lesions.

TABLE 42.2-4. American Joint Committee on Cancer Tumor (T), Node (N), Metastasis (M) Stage Grouping for Cutaneous Melanoma[a]

Pathologic Stage	*T*	*N*	*M*	*Clinical Stage*	*T*	*N*	*M*
0	Tis	N0	M0	0	Tis	N0	M0
IA	T1a	N0	M0	IA	T1a	N0	M0
IB	T1b	N0	M0	IB	T1b	N0	M0
	T2a	N0	M0		T2a	N0	M0
IIA	T2b	N0	M0	IIA	T2b	N0	M0
	T3a	N0	M0		T3a	N0	M0
IIB	T3b	N0	M0	IIB	T3b	N0	M0
	T4a	N0	M0		T4a	N0	M0
IIC	T4b	N0	M0	IIC	T4b	N0	M0
IIIA	T1–4a	N1a	M0	IIIA	Any T1–4a	N1b	M0
IIIB	T1–4a	N1b	M0	IIIB	Any T1–4a	N2b	M0
	T1–4a	N2a	M0				
IIIC	Any T	N2b, N2c	M0	IIIC	Any T	N2c	M0
	Any T	N3	M0		Any T	N3	M0
IV	Any T	Any N	M1	IV	Any T	Any N	M1

[a]Clinical staging includes microstaging of the primary melanoma and clinical and radiologic evaluation. It should be used after complete excision of the primary melanoma with clinical assessment for regional and distant metastasis. Pathologic staging includes microstaging of the primary melanoma and pathologic information about the regional nodes after partial or complete lymphadenectomy, except for pathologic stage 0 or stage 1A patients, who do not need pathologic evaluation of their lymph nodes.[118]

Breslow Depth

The Breslow depth of a primary melanoma is the cardinal prognostic factor for clinically localized disease (stages I and II).[119] The risk of relapse and death due to melanoma rises incrementally with each millimeter of depth (Breslow thickness) for primary melanoma, and the relationship between primary tumor thickness and the relapse rate is linear between 1 and 6 mm (Fig. 42.2-14). Beyond 6 mm of depth, the incremental risk of relapse and death for each millimeter of invasion is less than for lesions below that thickness.

Melanoma thickness is therefore a continuous variable, for which there are no natural breakpoints, so the choice of dichotomization between stages I and II (and within stage I between substage A and substage B, or in stage II between substages A and B) is somewhat arbitrary. The designation of T1/stage IA (less than 0.76 mm), T2/stage IB (from 0.77 to 1.50 mm), T3/stage IIA (1.51 to 4.00 mm), and T4/stage IIB (greater than 4.0 mm) has been based in part on data from early series in which it appeared there might be biologically determined breakpoints at these depths. The risk for patients in these categories rises in direct relation to the Breslow depth, without any evident breakpoints, to justify the previous divisions at 0.76 and 1.50 mm. The staging system proposed for adoption by AJCC in 2000 therefore adopts integer breakpoints at 1, 2, and 4 mm in place of the previous 0.76, 1.50, and 4 mm.[112,116,118,122,123]

Ulceration

Ulceration is found in 21% to 60% of localized primary melanomas.[115,117] The presence of ulceration reduces the 5- to 10-year relapse-free survival by more than one-third and is important in both univariate and multivariate analyses. Ulceration is more common with deeper tumors, although melanomas of any depth can ulcerate. The median thickness of nonulcerated melanomas is 0.8 mm whereas that of ulcerated melanomas is 2.6 mm. Ulceration independently predicts local recurrence, regional disease, and worse overall survival.[122] In tumors with associated ulceration, the risk of regional lymph node dissemination is increased by 10% compared with nonulcerated tumors.[112,116,118,123] Adding back the depth of an ulcer crater does not correct for the decrease in survival associated with ulceration, and the width of ulceration is more significant than the depth in predicting prognosis.[124] The AJCC revision of melanoma staging for 2000 proposes the incorporation of ulceration as the major independent factor for prognostic assessment of stage I and II melanomas after the Breslow depth. The suffix *a* will indicate nonulcerated and *b* ulcerated primary melanoma.

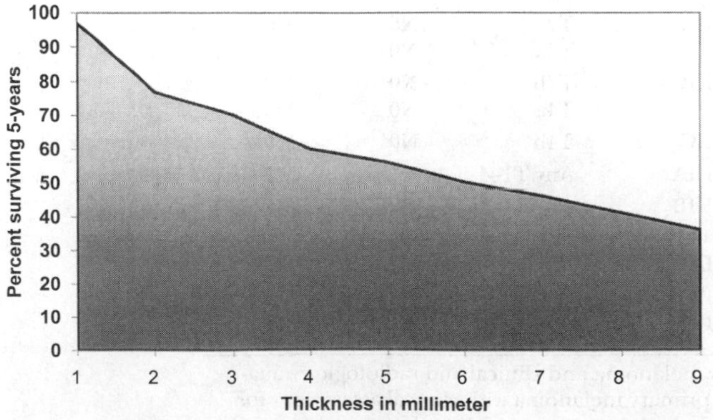

FIGURE 42.2-14. The relationship between primary melanoma thickness and survival is nearly a linear function. The American Joint Committee on Cancer breakpoints between T stages is not based on defined biologic mortality differences, but for convenience and general prognostic grouping.

Morphotype

The morphotype of the primary melanoma historically was used to predict prognosis. Nodular melanomas have a higher risk and shorter latency than superficial spreading melanomas because of their tendency toward a vertical growth pattern. The less frequent acral lentiginous melanoma similarly has been associated with increased risk when compared with that of LMM. The latter morphotype is distinctive in its occurrence at a median age of more than decade later than that of the more common superficial spreading and nodular, as well as acral lentiginous, morphotypes. The site of origin is also distinctive for LMM, which is typically found on the chronically sun-exposed areas of the head and neck, and for acral lentiginous melanoma. These descriptive terms, although helpful in pattern recognition for clinicians, are less frequently used based on more modern staging systems.

Lymphoid and Dendritic Cell Host Response

Infiltration of the primary melanoma site by lymphocytes has been correlated with an improved outcome in studies performed over the past several decades. The Boston Collaborative Melanoma Study has demonstrated a more favorable prognosis of melanomas infiltrated densely with lymphocytes.[125] The immunologic target of the lymphoid response frequently observed in primary melanomas, and less often in metastatic sites of disease, has led to intense efforts with each of the emerging therapeutic tools of immunology. There has also been a correlation with the infiltration of other immune mediators and prognosis. Dendritic cells (DC), potent antigen-presenting cells, are also found in melanoma specimens, and DC infiltrate is inversely related to tumor thickness in melanoma. DCs mediate several biologic roles including regulation of angiogenesis and the active uptake of apoptotic tumor, processing of nominal antigens and migration to local nodal basins where a specific T-cell response is capable of being stimulated.[126,127]

Regression

Historically, lesional regression characterized by the histologic presence of fibrosis and centralized depigmentation has been suggested as an ominous sign. Many interpret regression as an invalidation of the Breslow depth because the tumor may have once extended deeper than measured at the time of excision. Thus, actual prognosis would be worse than predicted since the patient would be understaged. The studies of the University of Alabama and Sydney Melanoma Unit have not borne this out; in fact, complete regression of primary as well as metastatic lesions has been well documented, and rarely, spontaneous cures occur.[128,129] Melanomas with undetermined primary sites presumably originate from regressed lesions. These patients have the same if not a slightly better prognosis than equally matched patients whose primary is known. Other evidence suggests that melanoma regression is not a negative prognostic factor. Gershenwald et al. reported that no patient with melanomas less than 1 mm thick with evidence of regression had a positive sentinel node.[130] Tumor regression indicates an active specific tumor response may have beneficial systemic effects. Tumor immunologists have tried to augment this immune response through various vaccine strategies to treat melanoma.

Site of Origin

Patients with melanoma of acral, subungual, and head and neck sites have a worse prognosis than those with melanoma arising on the extremities. Multivariate analysis from one mature series from the University of Pennsylvania (n = 488) and a multicenter German database (n = 5246) have shown that the site of tumor origin is an independent and significant prognostic variable.[131–133] In general, patients with primary lesions of the extremities have a significantly better prognosis than those with primary lesions of the trunk and head. Lesions of the upper and lower extremities do not differ in prognosis, but those found distally on the hands and feet fare worse than those with more proximal lesions.[10,131,134] The use of a model that incorporated four variables (i.e., site of origin, gender, age, and Breslow thickness) has been reported; the prognostic variables increased prediction of survival by up to 50%.[131] In patients with positive regional lymph nodes, the site of origin, gender of the patient, and age become unimportant in predicting prognosis.

STAGE II

A large and relatively heterogeneous population is the group previously designated as stage II, composed of stage IIA (T3) melanomas between 1.5 and 4.0 mm in depth, and stage IIB (T4) melanomas of more than 4 mm in depth. Relapse risk for this group lies between 10% and 40% and is directly related to the primary Breslow depth. Beyond the Breslow depth in this category, the most consistent and powerful prognostic factor identified over the past 20 years has been the presence or absence of ulceration. The presence of ulceration is significantly associated with an increase in the likelihood of nodal metastasis and reduces the prognosis for relapse-free survival by nearly 10% for any given Breslow depth.

Elective lymph node dissection (ELND) has previously been the only available means to demonstrate the presence of regional lymph node involvement and proved to be positive in 20% of these patients with lesions greater than 1 mm in depth. The development of more precise techniques of lymph node mapping has significantly affected the ability to predict prognoses for this group of patients. Many large adjuvant trials have been conducted in patients for whom the pathologic status of the regional draining lymph nodes has either not been assessed at all, or in whom this has only been assessed using anatomically guided elective regional lymphadenectomy, not isotopically or dye-guided sentinel lymph node (SLN) mapping. Thus, the surgical and pathologic assessment of melanoma at the primary site has now been coupled with techniques that have demonstrated improved precision at the regional lymph node basin(s). Consequently, the assessment of relapse and mortality risk for primary melanoma patients with intermediate risk is in substantial flux. In patients for whom SLN mapping is not feasible, the previously defined risk algorithms and factors are still of use. For those in whom SLN mapping is appropriately performed and whose results are negative, the prognosis appears to be substantially improved.[135] The series of patients that have been assessed by SLN mapping have to date less than 5 years of median follow-up. The limited follow-up in these series qualifies interpretation of the data at this time, since it is possible that the identification of nodal disease using refined pathologic, immunohistochemical, and in some cases, molecular [reverse transcriptase-polymerase chain reaction (RT-PCR)] assays for melanosomal antigens such as tyrosinase may simply have improved lead time for the diagnosis of metastatic disease.

STAGE III

In patients with nodal disease, only three variables independently affect overall prognosis: the number of lymph nodes, the presence of ulceration of the primary tumor, and whether the nodal disease is macroscopic or microscopic. In patients with macroscopic disease, more than one positive lymph node, and an ulcerated primary lesion, the 5-year survival is only 16%. In patients with only one microscopically positive node and without ulceration in the primary tumor, the overall 5-year survival is 71%. This large difference in survival demonstrates the inadequacies of previous staging systems and the heterogeneity of supposedly matched patients in previous clinical trials.[136]

Sentinel Lymph Node Mapping

The detection of lymph node metastases previously relied on crude clinical or regional ELND, which has not improved survival in several large randomized controlled trials. Currently, SLN mapping and selective lymphadenectomy directed by isotopic lymphoscintigraphy or blue dye lymphography has been shown to identify lymph node metastases more precisely and with less surgical morbidity, hospitalization time, and cost than elective dissection.[135,137,138] All of the observations reported from series attempting to refine the prognostic assessment of patients based on Breslow depth and Clark's level, with or without ulceration, has been in many ways supplanted by the availability of pathologic assessment of SLNs mapped using isotopic and dye techniques. A study of 580 patients whose sentinel draining lymph nodes localized using dye and scintigraphic techniques (e.g., SLN) and found to be pathologically negative has demonstrated that the status of the SLN is the single most powerful prognostic factor after Breslow depth ($P < .00001$ for each).[135,137,139] Sentinel node status remains a significant prognostic factor in multivariate analyses of disease-specific survival in this model after adjustment for other previously identified prognostic factors. Once SLN status is accounted for, a number of factors that have previously been considered as independent prognostic factors lose their significance. The primary site of origin, age of the patient, and sex of the patient are all nonsignificant after incorporation of SLN status in a prognostic model for outcome of stage I and II patients.[135,139] The multidisciplinary procedure of SLN evaluation requires attentive radiology and meticulous pathology as well as expert surgery for optimal outcome.[140,141] Whether the information attained from SLN biopsy allows treatment decisions that alter outcome remains a question currently being addressed in a number of prospective trials. Even though it has been widely adopted by most centers in the United States, it is less widely applied elsewhere and the results of seminal prospective studies should be available within the next few years to assess its utility in improving patient outcome. It is conceivable that strategies to quantitatively identify tumor in the peripheral blood using molecular analysis or serologic assays may supplant this surgical staging procedure.

Number of Nodes

Regional lymph node involvement defined stage III in the AJCC system in 1992 as it does currently. The size of involved lymph nodes had previously served as the basis for characterization of patients within stage III (TNM N1, N2, N3). Multiple studies have been performed using Cox regression analysis to identify the most important predictors of outcome for patients with stage III disease.[116] In all of these studies, the number of lymph nodes found to be involved with tumor (whether macroscopic or microscopic) has been the cardinal factor identified (Fig. 42.2-15). The advent of sentinel node mapping has increased the precision with which regional lymph node dissemination can be identified, but even in studies that have patients evaluated by SLN mapping, the number of involved lymph nodes has been a significant prognostic factor.[135,142] The prognosis for patients with one involved regional lymph node is significantly better than for patients with two or more involved regional lymph nodes.[112,116,143–145] The recommended AJCC 2000 staging system will adopt the number of nodes involved with tumor as the principal basis for prognostic assessment of patients with regional disease. N1 will signify one node involved, N2 will signify two to three nodes involved, and N3 will signify four or more nodes involved with tumor. N3 includes matted nodes and ulcerated melanoma with any number of metastatic lymph nodes. A secondary criterion for classification of patients with nodal metastatic disease is that of nodal bulk of disease (microscopic versus macroscopic). The former is invisible to the gross surgical or pathologic evaluation, nonpalpable, and designated (a). The N1(a)/N2(a) category of microscopic involvement represent a significant and increasing fraction of patients identified through sentinel node mapping procedures, for whom the prognosis appears to be improved. Previous data suggested a more favorable prognosis of patients with microscopic disease identified at ELND as compared with those with clinically manifest recurrence subjected to therapeutic node dissection.[146,147] Although the sentinel node is meticulously examined using immunohistochemistry and fine sections, for practical reasons, nodes from the completion lymphadenectomy specimen are not. The prognostic importance of rigorously characterizing the number of sub-micrometastatic positive nodes after completion lymphadenectomy using thin sections and immunohistochemical staining is unclear.

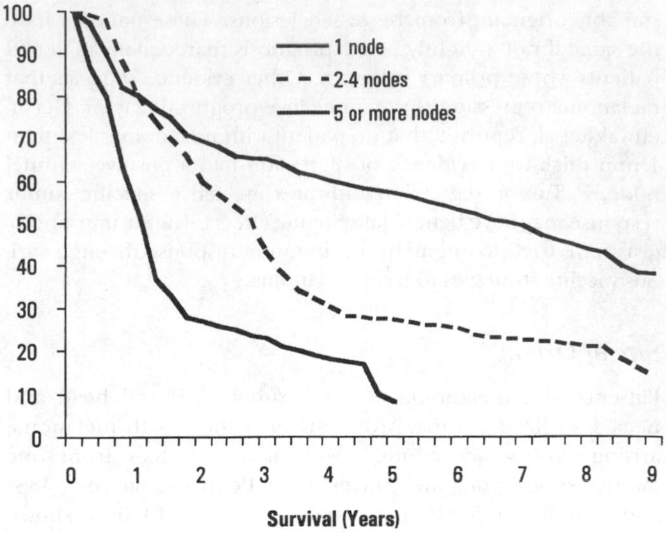

FIGURE 42.2-15. Survival for stage III patients according to the number of nodal metastases. Survival correlates strongly with increasing numbers of positive lymph nodes. (From ref. 222, with permission.)

Satellitosis and In-Transit Disease

The stage III category has also been designated for patients with forms of regional extranodal disease. Satellite involvement, *satellitosis*, is a form of tumor extension that may be manifested by deep or aggressive primary melanomas, often with intervening areas of apparently tumor-free skin. Satellite involvement signifies a poor prognosis for patient outcomes; prognosis has been shown to resemble that of patients with regional lymph node involvement. A second category of metastatic melanoma that has long been recognized to have a more ominous prognostic significance than localized primary disease is known as *in-transit disease.* In-transit melanoma does not differ from more typical nodal metastatic disease. The more indolent course of in-transit melanoma, particularly when associated with paraneoplastic hypopigmentation, has led to substantial immunologic interest in this form of melanoma, and its location has lent itself to regional isolated perfusion chemotherapy and biologic therapy.[148,149] For these reasons, both satellite involvement in the region of the primary, and in-transit melanoma between the primary and regional nodal basin have been assigned to a category N2C. Patients with both manifestations of satellite involvement or in-transit involvement with regional lymph node metastases have been assigned to the N3 category, due to their more ominous prognosis, regardless of the number of involved regional lymph nodes.[112,116,118,147,150]

STAGE IV: M1

Distant disease that has spread beyond the regional draining lymph nodes is generally denoted as M1 in the TNM system and stage IV in the AJCC and Union International Contra le Cancrum systems. The prognosis of patients with stage IV M1 disease is poor, with median survivals of less than 1 year.[151] The AJCC Subcommittee on Melanoma has reviewed criteria for this disease category, which represents the smallest fraction of patients of any stage at presentation, but a significant fraction of the patients with melanoma who will die each year. For these patients, the identification of important prognostic factors may guide treatment selection or decisions whether to pursue therapy. An analysis of the clinical factors associated with a favorable prognosis in patients with stage IV disease entering therapeutic trials of the Eastern Cooperative Oncology Group (ECOG) has demonstrated that patient factors including a normal appetite, absence of nausea and vomiting or fever, unimpaired performance status, and female gender are significant. Disease-related factors of prognostic importance included limited numbers of sites of disease, disease limited to soft tissues and lymph nodes, a time interval more than 1 year to therapy for metastasis, and the occurrence of a clinical response to treatment.[152] A current reassessment of important factors in 1325 patients with stage IV melanoma treated in eight clinical trials over 25 years in ECOG has identified many of the same factors to be significant, including the number of metastatic sites, unimpaired performance status, and female gender. A number of multivariate analyses of factors that bear on survival in stage III or IV have been reported.[153–157] The median survival in all studies has been 6 to 8 months, except for one case record analysis of the European Organization for Cancer Research and Treatment Group of Cancer (EORTC).[158] In a large metaanalysis of patients with disseminated melanoma that included 83 studies and 6322 patients, the median survival for patients diagnosed after 1985 was 8.9 months. The 2-, 3-, and 5-year survival rates were 13.6%, 9.7%, and 2.3%. Survival for patients before 1985 was 5.9 months. The study provides important information that will allow survival results from current and future trials to be compared with expected survival.[158] The number of sites or organs involved with metastatic disease appears to be of significance in most models and is unquestionably important in determining prognosis. However, the AJCC has presently chosen not to incorporate a measure of the number or volume of tumor metastases, due to the variability of imaging techniques employed to assess the presence of metastatic disease, and the state of flux of radiologic assessment for melanoma at present. The 1992 formulation of stage IV disease dichotomized metastatic disease according to its location in nonvisceral (M1a) or visceral (M1b) locations. A review of data from JWCI (John Wayne Cancer Institute),[157] the ECOG,[159,160] and other series has shown that metastatic disease involving the lung but no other viscera has a prognosis that is intermediate between that of nonvisceral distant metastasis and other visceral sites of metastasis. The proposed reformulation of the AJCC for 2000[112,118] proposes classification of nonvisceral metastatic disease limited to skin, soft tissue, and nodes be designated as M1a, and that involvement of lung sites be considered as M1b, with the M1c category left to designate all other visceral sites of disease.

Biochemical and Serologic Markers

Many studies have evaluated biochemical, immunologic, or other quantitative blood assays that might reflect the prognosis of patients with melanoma. One of the earliest was the level of the enzyme lactic dehydrogenase (LDH), assessed as a marker of metastatic disease, particularly within the liver.[161] Several multivariable proportional hazards models have evaluated the importance of an elevated LDH level (either elevated above the mean value for a laboratory or above the upper limit of normal for the laboratory). In each case in which LDH was assessed, it proved to be a significant prognostic factor. Additional factors included melanoma inhibitory activity (MIA)[162] and the level of the polypeptide S-100β.[163] The AJCC Subcommittee for Melanoma has taken a significant step in a new direction in the proposed 2000 revision of the melanoma staging system[112,118] by including LDH measurement as a factor to be employed to define a more ominous prognosis and to downstage patients with known metastatic disease who have an elevated LDH value, assigning these patients with stage IV disease to stage IV M1c.

A number of studies have proposed the prognostic utility of S-100β measured by radioimmunoassay or a more recent luminometric immunoassay.[164] A prospective, observational study evaluated the clinical and prognostic value of S-100 protein in patients with metastasis-free disease versus patients with newly occurring lymph node, visceral, brain metastases, or all three. In this series that included 570 patients and 52 normal controls, the sensitivity and specificity of S-100 measured by an immunoluminometric assay was 64% and 91%. False-negative results occurred in those with amelanotic melanoma. The negative predictive value was 99%, but the positive predictive value was only 65%.

S-100β was examined prospectively in the peripheral blood of patients undergoing surgical procedures for resection of high-risk primaries or lymph node metastases. Of the patients who were S-100β positive by luminometric immunoassay, 47% developed metastatic disease after at least 2 years of follow-up. Kaplan Meier analysis showed that patients who were S-100β positive had approximately 2.7 times shorter disease-free survival than patients negative for S-100β. This difference was statistically significant, and multivariate analysis showed that S-100β was an independent prognostic determinant of disease-free survival.[164]

RT-PCR has also been used to gain prognostic information by attempting to detect small numbers of blood-borne melanoma cells. The technique is generally limited by its extreme sensitivity. The use of tyrosinase has been somewhat problematic because tyrosinase is also present in nonmalignant cells including melanocytes in the dermis picked up by phlebotomy. Up to 10% of healthy people may have blood tyrosinase-positive cells in this assay.[165] However, tyrosinase has been used to detect circulating melanoma cells in patients with melanoma with intriguing results. Positive tyrosinase results are seen in stage I, II, III, and IV melanoma patients at a frequency of 11%, 18%, 31%, and 67%, respectively. In stage IV patients, median overall survival was 8 months compared with 12 months in those patients with a negative test result.[166] Tyrosinase is present in a proportion of long-term clinically disease-free melanoma patients, and the late presence of circulating melanoma cells predicts a subsequent high risk of relapse and death. Some studies have correlated tyrosinase positivity with increasing stage, survival, presence of visceral metastases, and higher LDH levels.[167,168] Actuarial 2-year survival is 97% for the tyrosinase-negative patients versus 72% for the tyrosinase-positive patients.[169] The use of true real-time quantitative PCR (Taqman) may improve on the prognostic utility of these melanoma assays.

MIA, a novel molecular marker, has been examined as a potential prognostic marker. One hundred sixty-six patients with melanoma were examined for expression of MIA. A correlation between positive blood sample results and tumor burden in stage III and IV patients was detected and 73% of stage I and II patients were negative for the MIA RNA. Five of 24 patients who were RT-PCR positive progressed to systemic disease within the follow-up period of 6 months. The predictive values were low and the study was too small to deduce prognostic significance.[165] MIA, as currently examined, is limited in its utility as a prognostic marker.

Immunosorting of melanoma cells using magnetic cell separation has been used to isolate, in a specific fashion, viable melanocytes from patient's blood. This technique does not have suitable sensitivity for early detection of metastasis, but may prove a valuable tool in the isolation and identification of circulating autologous melanoma cells. No patients with stage I primary melanoma were found to have circulating melanoma cells, whereas 13.6% and 15.2% of patients with stage III and IV disease were found to have them. The prognostic significance of these circulating cells is unknown.[170]

IMAGING OF MALIGNANT MELANOMA

Conventional evaluation of the patient with primary melanoma involves chest radiography for all patients with primary lesions deeper than 1 mm. In the setting of established stage II or III disease, radiologic evaluation may be indicated with the use of magnetic resonance imaging of the brain and computed tomography (CT) of the chest, abdomen, and pelvis. In the setting of known metastatic disease, thorough evaluation may be required to allow the participation in clinical trials and in planning therapy. Advances in imaging techniques have improved the ability to identify and localize primary and metastatic melanoma. The most notable advances have been positron emission tomography (PET), radionuclide agents with affinity for melanoma, and the resurgence of lymphoscintigraphy. Lymphoscintigraphy can provide valuable assistance in localizing SLNs for biopsy.[171] It is particularly helpful for tumor locations with variable lymphatic drainage and has identified previously unsuspected drainage patterns for some regions.[171]

Improvements in PET have made it a valuable staging study for melanoma. Rinne et al. prospectively compared whole body ^{18}F-fluorodeoxyglucose PET with conventional imaging (CT, magnetic resonance imaging, and so forth) in 100 consecutive patients (52 at diagnosis, 48 at follow-up).[172] At initial staging, PET was 100% sensitive and 94% specific, whereas conventional imaging did not identify any of the nine lymph node metastases and was 84% specific. In the 48 follow-up patients, the sensitivity, specificity, and accuracy of PET per metastasis was 92%, 94%, and 92%, respectively, compared with 58%, 45%, and 56% with conventional imaging. While PET was better at detecting cervical lymph node metastases (100% vs. 67%) and abdominal metastases (100% vs. 27%), CT was better for small lung metastases (87% vs. 70%). With the exception of brain imaging, where magnetic resonance imaging is superior, these authors suggested that a single whole body PET scan could replace all other imaging performed in melanoma patients. This will need to be evaluated in other series.

Other imaging techniques that show promise in melanoma are technetium 99m (^{99m}Tc)-sestamibi (MIBI), ^{99m}Tc-tetrofosmin, and iodine 123 iodobenzamide (for melanotic tumors).[173–175] Of these, ^{99m}Tc-MIBI has undergone the most thorough evaluation and appears to be a reasonably inexpensive substitute for whole body PET scans in staging melanoma patients.

RADIOBIOLOGY OF MELANOMA

Early experiences with conventional radiotherapy of melanoma led some clinicians to believe that this tumor was so radioresistant that radiotherapy was of little use. This erroneous deduction was based on experience with treating melanomas with conventional low-dose fractions (approximately 2 Gy per fraction) and moderate total overall doses. Radiobiologic studies of melanoma have subsequently altered the clinical approach to treating melanoma. Some investigators identified wide *shoulders* for *in vivo* cell survival curves for melanoma, suggesting a large capacity for repair of sublethal damage that prompted a number of investigators to treat patients with malignant melanoma with large-dose fractions.[176–182] There is some intrinsic variability within various melanoma cell cultures, and these models differ in many respects from tumors found in patients. Analyses of clinical experiences with various radiotherapy treatment schedules provided important data. Melanoma can be responsive to radiotherapy when large-dose fractions are used.

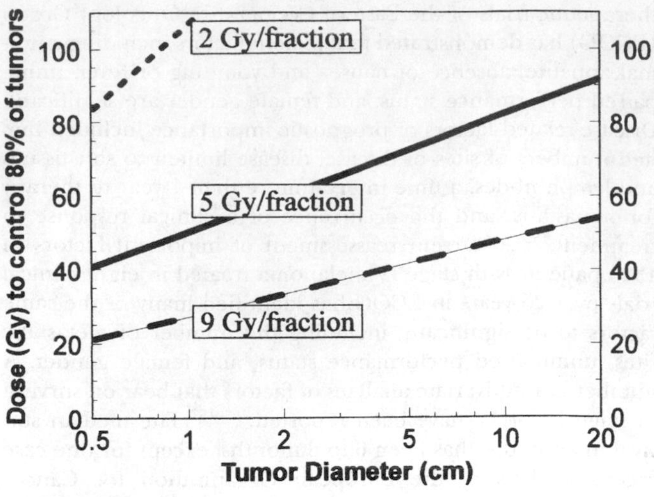

FIGURE 42.2-16. Radiosensitivity of melanoma. Total dose (Gy) necessary to control 80% of malignant melanoma tumors as a function of tumor size and dose per fraction as estimated from 239 tumors in 121 patients. (Redrawn by permission from ref. 179.)

An important study of the clinical radiobiology of melanoma is the analysis by Bentzen et al. of tumor control in 121 patients with 239 histologically proven recurrent or metastatic malignant melanomas.[179] They identified an alpha to beta ratio of 0.57 (95% confidence interval, –1.07 to 2.5 Gy). The rationale for standard fractionation is that small-dose fractions preferentially spare late reacting normal tissues with lower alpha to beta ratios (1.8 for subcutaneous) than malignant tumors, which usually have alpha to beta ratios closer to 10.[183,184] With melanoma, these clinical data indicate the reverse situation. In cases in which the larger individual dose fraction is used, more normal tissue is spared the effects of radiation compared with tumor. There is little treatment time effect (negligible repopulation during a treatment schedule) indicating that treatment may be administered with large-dose fractions twice a week rather than conventional application five times per week schedule. The subsequent protraction of the overall treatment time allows normal cell populations that determine acute radiation reactions (such as moist skin erythema and mucositis) to repopulate to a greater degree between fractions to minimize acute side effects. The dose response is markedly influenced by tumor size in radiotherapy of melanoma. Figure 42.2-16 shows the estimated total doses necessary for 80% control probability in tumors of different sizes with different dose fractions derived from their data. In contrast with these findings, the Radiation Therapy Oncology Group trial 83-05 found largely identical responses in 137 patients with measurable melanoma lesions randomized between 32 Gy in four weekly 8-Gy fractions (24% complete response, 35% partial response) compared with 40 Gy with daily 2.5-Gy fractions (23% complete response, 34% partial response).[185]

Several factors have been postulated to contribute to the relative radioresistance of melanoma including tumor hypoxia, loss or dysfunction of the p16 DNA locus, and decreased cell membrane gangliosides.[186–189] A number of different innovative techniques are being investigated to improve radiotherapy of malignant melanoma. Hypoxic cell sensitizers such as tirapazamine and gadolinium texaphyrin show promise in preferentially killing radioresistant hypoxic cells within melanoma tumors.[190] Hyperthermia combined with radiotherapy is another approach to optimize killing of hypoxic tumor cells.[191,192] Approaches that combine radiotherapy with radiosensitizing chemotherapy such as topoisomerase I targeting drugs (topotecan, camptothecin) or taxanes, which arrest cells in the most radiosensitive phase (G_2/S), also could improve radioresponsiveness.[188,193] Boron neutron capture therapy, which depends on selective drug uptake in tumor (as does gadolinium texaphyrin), also holds potential in treatment of melanoma.[194] Gene therapy including application of N-Ras or Myc transfection is another promising approach to increase radiosensitivity.[194a] The specific use of radiotherapy on primary tumors, in-transit disease, recurrences, and metastatic disease are discussed in the following sections.

STAGE I AND II DISEASE: MANAGEMENT OF PRIMARY MELANOMA

All lesions with characteristics suggestive of melanoma should be biopsied. Suspicious lesions may have irregular raised surfaces; ulceration, bleeding, or both; variegations; or recent changes in color or size. As sampling error may occur with incisional biopsies, a full-thickness excisional biopsy is the preferred diagnostic technique since the depth of the lesion determines the extent of resection. Shave biopsies are contraindicated since they may not encompass the full depth of the lesion and make pathologic interpretation of Breslow depth impossible.

PREOPERATIVE WORKUP

The most important staging information obtained from patients with melanoma is the Breslow depth, presence of ulceration, and nodal status. The 1992 National Institutes of Health Consensus conference indicated that asymptomatic patients with T1 lesions do not appear to benefit from any diagnostic staging including computed tomography, magnetic resonance imaging, or nuclear scans. A chest radiograph is performed in patients with stage IB disease or greater.[195] Liver function tests, especially LDH, and other radiologic tests are indicted in stage III and IV disease or otherwise symptomatic patients.

EXCISIONAL BIOPSY

Performing an excisional biopsy is preferable over an incisional biopsy. Sampling error may limit the reliability of assessing the Breslow depth of incisional biopsies. In most instances, a biopsy can be done in an office setting under local anesthesia with minimal morbidity. An excisional biopsy removes the lesion *en toto.* No effort is made to obtain a wide margin, but a small margin (1 to 2 mm) of normal skin is taken with the elliptical specimen and primary closure performed on most lesions. The specimen is sent to pathology for permanent section. Some surgeons suggest that a single-stage procedure is possible using frozen sections to characterize tumor depth, but this has not been validated.[196]

INCISIONAL BIOPSY

Wide excision after incisional biopsy was initially thought to be associated with a higher recurrence rate. Those studies were poorly designed and retrospective, and no evidence in the recent literature suggests a worse outcome from incisional biopsy. However, incisional biopsy has a higher rate of inaccurate microstaging[197] and should be reserved for large or subungual lesions to confirm diagnosis. Incisional biopsies may be used in areas such as the face where cosmesis and skin coverage are an issue. The biopsy should be a wedge of tissue including normal skin, the center of the lesion, and subcutaneous fat.

SURGICAL MARGINS OF RESECTION

The depth of melanoma resection does not require inclusion of the underlying muscular fascia, although this was initially suggested. Biopsies should go down to, but not include the fascia.[198] For years, no clear standard existed that guided the amount of margin to resect around the primary tumor. The margin is defined as the radial distance from the visible edge of the lesion or scar. Only relatively recently have randomized trials examined the width of surgical margin in relation to local recurrence and overall survival. Pathologists have long observed malignant cells separated by some distance from the primary lesion. Wide excisions minimize the risk of leaving behind these cells that may locally recur or metastasize. Rests of malignant cells can be found distances of 1 cm from the visible edge of the tumor, and their presence outside 1 cm is directly proportional to the depth of the primary lesion.[199,200] Some histopathologic data show morphologically bizarre melanocytes in normal skin upward of 5 cm from the primary site.[201] The extent of excision necessary should depend of the thickness of the primary tumor. Since large resections risk functional deficits, disfigurements, and increased cost, determining the minimal excision margin has been extensively studied.

Appropriate initial resection remains crucial in the management of primary melanoma since almost all patients with a local recurrence die of metastatic disease. Locally recurrent disease may be just a surrogate for more aggressive biologic behavior, but an adequate surgical resection should never be compromised.[202] Local recurrence, defined as tumor relapse within 3 to 5 cm of the primary closure or skin graft, is a relatively rare event, making the design of trials difficult. In a retrospective series of 3569 patients, local recurrences were found in only 3.2% of patients.[203] Some factors have been identified that are associated with the probability of local recurrence. One large study found that the probability of local recurrence depends on only ulceration of the primary tumor (1.5% without ulceration vs. 10.6% with ulceration) and tumor thickness (2.3%, 4.2%, 11.7% for 1 to 2 mm, 2 to 3 mm, 3 to 4 mm lesions, respectively).[204] Another large prospective series found that the site of primary tumor also

TABLE 42.2-5. Current U.S. Recommendations for Excision of Primary Melanoma

Stage	*Margin*
Melanoma *in situ*	0.5 cm
T1 (<1 mm)	1 cm
T2 (2–3 mm) or greater	2 cm
Subungual	Amputation just proximal to distal interphalangeal joint

predicted recurrence. In the 10-year reassessment of the Intergroup trial, multivariate analysis showed that the only variables that predicted local recurrence were ulceration and a head and neck primary site. The proximal extremity was least likely to have a local recurrence, followed by the trunk, distal extremity, and head and neck. When ulceration was present, the relative risk of local recurrence was 6.3 compared with nonulcerated melanomas. In patients with head and neck primaries, the relative risk for local recurrence was 9.4 compared with all sites. Both of these risks were highly significant.[136]

Although the risk of recurrence increases with more narrow margins, wide incisions can be quite morbid. A more radical excision is associated with the morbidity of cosmetic defects, functional losses, and the need for skin grafting. Wide excisions for melanoma were first popularized by Handley in 1907 who described a 1-inch skin margin with further undermining of 2 more inches laterally.[205] In 1947 Urteaga and Pack compared radiation therapy to surgical excision with an 8-cm margin and found resection to have a superior 5-year survival.[206] Others proposed routine amputations or huge 15-cm margins with *en bloc* lymphadenectomy. Until more recent randomized trials, a 3- to 5-cm excision, which frequently required skin grafting, was the standard treatment. Even as late as the 1980s, there were no national guidelines for the extent of excision necessary and much variation between surgeons existed. Although the rate of recurrence was known to depend on tumor depth, there was no correlation between the extent of operation and tumor thickness.[207] Three well-designed, randomized prospective trials and various retrospective trials supports the use of a 1-cm margin for melanomas less than 1 mm thick and a 2-cm margin for deeper lesions deeper (Table 42.2-5).

Thin and Intermediate Thickness Lesions

Breslow and Macht first questioned the need for excessively wide (3 to 5 cm) resection margins for thin melanomas in 1970.[119] The World Health Organization (WHO) designed a trial to answer the question of resection margins in thin lesions (less than 2.0 mm). In the WHO trial, 612 patients with melanomas less than 2 mm thick were randomly assigned to either receive wide excision (3 cm) or narrow excision (1 cm). The results, reported in 1988, showed that the 12-year survival rates were not significantly different at 87.2% and 85.1%, respectively. There was a 1.8% recurrence rate in the 612 patients. There were four local recurrences in patients with lesions 1.1 to 2.0 mm deep who received a narrow excision and none of the patient who had had the 3-cm excision. Although this difference was not statistically significant and there was no difference in survival between the two groups, the WHO reserved judgment on the safety of narrow excisions for intermediate-thickness lesions. They concluded that in melanomas less than 1.0 mm in depth, a 1-cm margin is to be recommended.[208]

The Melanoma Intergroup trial was designed to examine intermediate-thickness lesions and reported its initial data in 1993. The Intergroup trial entered 468 patients with lesions 1 to 4 mm in thickness and randomized patients to undergo either a 2-cm or a 4-cm wide local excision. After a median follow-up time of 8 years, the overall survival rates were 79.5% and 83.7%, respectively (no significant difference). The local recurrence rates were not significantly different at 0.8% and 1.7% in patients with 2- and 4-cm margins, respectively. With a narrow margin, the rate of skin grafting decreased from 46% to 11%, with a resultant decrease in hospital stay and cost.[209] In 1996, the Swedish Melanoma Study group subsequently reported their series of 769 randomized patients with thin and intermediate-thickness melanoma to a 2- versus a 5-cm margin. Again, there was no difference in local or regional recurrence or survival.[210] The current standard of care for lesions between 1 and 4 mm is a margin of 2 cm.

In Situ *and Thick Melanomas*

For treatment of patients with melanoma *in situ*, retrospective data supports the use of 0.5-cm margins. There have not been any reported local recurrences using this as a guideline.[195] For thick primaries, no randomized trial exists comparing different resection margins; however, a retrospective review of 278 patients compared excisions greater than 2 cm with excisions less than 2 cm in thick lesions. With a median tumor thickness of 6 mm, no correlation between the width of marginal resection and local recurrence or overall survival was found. The local recurrence rates were 11% and 13% in the less than 2-cm and greater than 2-cm excision groups, respectively.[211] Thick tumors do not require a margin greater than 2 cm since patient outcome is dictated more by the presence of regional and systemic disease. Currently, a prospective trial is accruing patients with melanomas greater than 2 mm thick and randomizing them to 1-cm versus a 2-cm margin. Outside of this trial, resection margins of 2 cm are recommended for all lesions greater than 1 mm deep.

Technique

The surgeon should mark the appropriate resection margin from the visible edge of the tumor or scar. If primary closure is desired, an elliptical incision should be performed. The minor axis of the ellipse should encompass the resection margins and the major axis should be approximately three times the minor axis. The long axis of the ellipse should be parallel to the axis of the extremity, or, if on the trunk, along Langers' lines. Care must be taken not to bevel the dissection inward, and the excision should not include the fascia. Generous undermining of the lateral flaps allows for a tension-free closure. Rotational flaps may be required for large lesions or lesions on the face.

SPECIAL SITES

Subungual Tumors

If a nail bed lesion has not changed significantly in 4 to 6 weeks, a biopsy should be performed accompanied by removal of the nail. An incisional biopsy, taking a representative wedge that

TABLE 42.2-6. Mean Age at Diagnosis for 496 Patients with Melanoma of the Head and Neck[a]

Region	*No.*	*Age (Median) (y)*
Face	316	68
Eyelid	15	66
Auricle	54	66
Neck	88	58
Scalp	23	58

[a]The mean age at diagnosis of head and neck melanoma is 15 years older than those found at other sites. These melanomas should be excised without compromise of appropriate margins. Head and neck melanomas tend to have a higher recurrence rate, have a more complicated nodal drainage, and often require tissue transfer for closure. The most common site of these melanomas is on the face.[537]

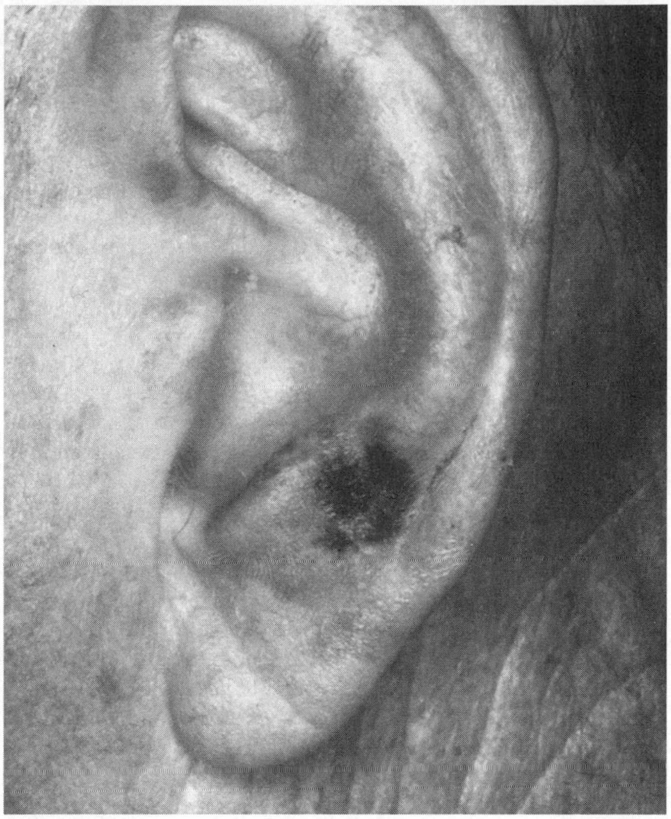

FIGURE 42.2-17. Melanoma of the external ear. These patients should be treated by a full-thickness wedge excision of the helix. Primary, three-layer closure can easily be performed with good cosmetic results. (Courtesy of H. Edington, M.D., University of Pittsburgh Cancer Institute.)

includes the middle of the lesion, is recommended to establish a diagnosis and prevent needless amputation. The biopsy should include the nail plate and should be oriented longitudinally.[84] The level of amputation does not seem to affect the incidence of recurrence or patient survival, so especially in lesions of the thumb, maintenance of function is important. For disease confined to the nail bed, amputation through the distal interphalangeal joint is recommended, and for bulky disease, a more proximal amputation through the base of the phalanx may be required.[212,213] Toe amputations should be performed more proximally as the loss of a toe at the metatarsal-phalangeal joint does not result in decreased function. Some surgeons advocate ILP, sentinel node biopsy, or both in patients with these high-risk lesions. There are few data showing a survival benefit in any patient with melanoma using adjuvant ILP.

Acral and Lentiginous Melanoma

Due to functional concerns, there is a tendency to use smaller margins, perhaps accounting for the two- to fivefold higher incidence of local recurrence in this area.[214] Excisions often require split-thickness skin grafting for closure or tissue transfer, especially in wounds involving weight-bearing areas such as the heel of the foot that may require flap transfer.[215] In most instances, skin grafts may be applied successfully to weight-bearing areas.[216]

Head and Neck

Melanoma of the face and scalp represent sites where local recurrence, nodal, and in-transit disease occur more frequently perhaps due to the extensive lymphatic drainage. Melanoma of the head and neck usually occurs in an age group 10 years older than truncal and extremity melanoma. The lesions most commonly involve the face (Table 42.2-6). LMM, a common morphotype of head and neck melanomas, is historically associated with an improved prognosis. However, appropriate excision margins for Breslow depth should not be compromised solely on cosmetic bases.[217] LM, a benign precursor lesion, can be treated through a number of techniques that do not require a wide margin of resection. Since up to one-half degenerate into malignancy, the treatment of these lesions is warranted. Multiple techniques have successfully been used to treat these lesions including excision, micrographic Moh's surgery, cryosurgery, radiotherapy, electrodesiccation and curettage, 5-fluorouracil, azelaic acid, and retinoic acid.[218] A Wood's lamp examination often helps to define the extent of pigmentation better than room light.[219] Full-thickness wedge resections are indicated for melanomas arising on helix of the ear (Fig. 42.2-17).

MOHS MICROGRAPHIC SURGERY

Mohs micrographic surgery (MMS) has been used for some time by dermatologists for nonmelanomatous lesions. The technique reduces scarring and may spare normal tissues by shaving involved tissues until a histologically negative margin. MMS employs repeated shallow (3-mm) resections, each examined histologically by frozen section. Some specialized centers have proposed the use of Mohs surgery in melanoma to minimize loss of normal tissue, especially in area such as the face, hands, and feet. Margins are generally taken somewhat less than the WHO and Intergroup trials found appropriate, which has generated much criticism from most melanoma experts. There have been no randomized trials comparing the standard surgical excision with MMS, but in some uncontrolled centers, rates of local recurrence and overall survival have not been found to be inferior to matched historic controls. Interesting differences exist between traditional surgical resection and micrographic surgery. For instance, the diameter and location of the primary tumor are prime determinants of the expected extent of excision in the MMS literature. Proponents of Mohs surgery claim that repeated frozen sectioning is accurate and saves normal tissues. Opponents cite the fact that satellite lesions may be missed using the Mohs technique and that pathologists do not generally examine the specimens. Critics also claim that frozen section is notoriously inaccurate for identification of melanoma.[220] Appropriate controlled multicenter trials are essential before this technique can be accepted by the surgical community for the treatment of melanoma.

RADIOTHERAPY OF PRIMARY SKIN TUMORS

Radiotherapy is rarely indicated in the management of primary invasive melanoma except in patients who refuse surgical excision or who are poor medical candidates. Treatment is usually administered with 6- to 9-MeV electron beams or 100- to 280-kilovolt (peak) x-rays using wide margins. Seegenschmiedt et al. reported tumor control in all 11 patients with residual (n = 6) or recurrent (n = 4) stage IIB melanoma (one patient with primary disease refused surgical excision).[180] They found better tumor control in these patients compared with control achieved through radiotherapy in patients with skin and lymph node metastases. Radiotherapy is a noninvasive alternative to surgical resection in the management of LM. This therapy may be appropriate for patients who cannot undergo or refuse surgery. Harwood reported 40 cases of LM and LMM managed with radiotherapy alone at Princess Margaret Hospital.[175] Radiotherapy doses were 45 to 50 Gy in 10 to 15 fractions with orthovoltage beams. Fourteen of 17 patients with LM and 34 of 37 with LMM were alive without tumor progression after 1 month to 7 years. Four patients with local recurrent or persistent tumor (two LM and two LMM) were salvaged by surgery (one LM, two LMM) or further radiotherapy (one LM). One LM patient died of intercurrent illness. Lesions can take up to 2 years to disappear after radiotherapy and the follow-up of available series remains short.[175]

STAGE I AND II DISEASE: EXAMINATION OF THE LYMPH NODE BASIN

Although prophylactic nodal dissection has never clearly been demonstrated to be of survival value in any other tumor, the Halstedian belief of radical lymphadenectomy has, and still dominates the treatment of melanoma. Physicians have believed that a survival benefit exists after the early removal of nodes that are subclinically involved with tumor compared with removal once obvious nodal disease develops because the longer melanoma grows in the lymphatics, the more likely it is to metastasize systemically. This concept was tested in numerous trials by comparing ELND, a complete lymphadenectomy (LND) in those at risk for nodal disease but without clinical evidence, with therapeutic lymph node dissection (TLND), LND in those with clinically positive nodes. Although no clear survival benefits have yet been demonstrated by ELND, many confounding factors may have contributed to the generally negative results. After years of controversy surrounding the potential benefit of elective nodal dissection and numerous trials, it is ironic that, regardless of the conclusions reached, the new technique of sentinel node mapping, has cast a shadow on all the answers recently obtained. The complexity of nodal drainage, the relatively low frequency of nodal disease, inadequate staging, and slight, if any, therapeutic benefit are clear obstacles in attempting to demonstrate any benefit of elective nodal dissection for melanoma. In previous texts, a detailed discussion of ELND was mandatory. Now the wholesale removal of entire nodal basins that may harbor metastatic disease based on inadequate descriptions of drainage patterns, and insensitive pathologic techniques should no longer be performed. With the advent of sentinel node mapping, ELND is only discussed as an historic reference. Regardless of possible therapeutic benefit, sentinel node biopsies efficiently predict prognosis with low morbidity. Current trials are assessing therapeutic benefit of selective nodal dissection. Unlike in breast cancer, there is no clearly beneficial adjuvant therapy available for high-risk patients, but as various new melanoma therapies are being developed, risk stratification by nodal status will become increasingly important. In the future sophisticated assays such as quantitative PCR (Taqman), which can measure melanoma antigens in the peripheral blood, may prove more important than nodal status for predicting prognosis and obviate the need for invasive procedures.

ELECTIVE LYMPH NODE DISSECTION

ELND has been an extremely controversial subject and its theoretical value hinges on the biology of melanoma metastasis. Does melanoma spread stepwise through the draining lymph nodes before reaching other more distant sites, or, as in breast cancer, does a Fisherian theory of nodal disease exist in which positive nodes are only a marker for systemic disease? Selecting patients who may be candidates for ELND has been based on the depth of the primary tumor. Patients with tumor less than 1 mm deep have a 98% cure rate and would not benefit from a relatively morbid operation. Patients with thick lesions (greater than 4 mm) at the time of diagnosis did not undergo ELND. Initial studies of ELND in this group of patients could not show any benefit and data erroneously suggested that this was due to a high percent (70%) of patients with occult metastatic disease.[221] Numerous trials have tried to understand the role of nodal dissection for intermediate-thickness lesions, but, unfortunately, many of the data are conflicting. Although sentinel node mapping has not yet proven therapeutic, the knowledge gained has helped elucidate the reasons for failure in multiple ELND trials and given much insight to the biology of nodal disease in melanoma.

Proponents of ELND advocate the use of ELND for its prognostic information since, in patients with regional disease, the actual number of nodes involved is the most important predictor of overall survival.[222] Advocates also cite retrospective studies that demonstrate a 5-year survival rate increase of up to 10% to 27% when patients with clinically occult disease have their nodal basins resected compared with delayed resection of gross disease.[223] As well, regional node disease may determine candidacy for adjuvant treatment such as IFN-α.

Opponents point out the morbidity of the operation, the lack of clear therapeutic benefit of ELND, and a controversial advantage to IFN-α treatment. One of the most important criticisms was that up to 80% of patients had negative nodes on pathology. This large percentage of patients received no benefit from the procedure. Many believe that lymph node metastases are a manifestation rather than a predecessor of distant spread. In a retrospective review of 4682 patients, only 16% of patients had positive nodes at ELND. Ten percent of metastases were positive in the contralateral node, and 6% were positive in nodal basins not classically predicted. At Breslow depths of less than 0.76 mm, 0.76 to 1.5 mm, 1.5 to 2.5 mm, 2.5 to 4.0 mm, and greater than 4 mm, the regional nodal basin was positive in 0%, 5%, 16%, 24%, and 36% of cases, respectively.[224] LND has substantial potential morbidity that includes chronic lymphedema, pain, paresthesias, cosmetic deformity, and, especially in the groin, wound complications. Lesions of the head and neck are especially problematic. As is true for squamous cell cancers of the head and neck, evidence arising from randomized prospective trials is not available to confirm the value of prophylactic nodal dissection for melanoma arising in the head and neck.[225,226]

The usefulness of ELND has been debated for decades because of conflicting trials of various quality (Table 42.2-7). Multiple trials suggest that TLND does not jeopardize the probability of cure and prevents the need for difficult toilet operations. Most trials are retrospective and mixed in conclusions. In one from Duke University and another from the Sydney Melanoma Unit, initial analysis showed a survival advantage in patients with intermediate-thickness lesions, but both, after 10 years of further data accrual, showed no advantage to ELND. This demonstrated the lack of reliability of retrospective trials and the length of time needed for adequate data accrual.

Two prospective trials from the WHO in 1977 and Mayo Clinic in 1986 showed no benefit of ELND.[227,228] Both these trials included what we now recognize as many low-risk patients and their negative results have been criticized. Both the Intergroup and WHO trunk trials are contemporary prospective randomized trials that were developed to address much of the conflicting information. Although long-term data are still accruing, results have been published.

In 1998, the WHO published a series of 252 patients randomized to immediate or delayed node dissection. All patients had truncal melanoma of at least 1.5 mm thickness. The 5-year survival observed in patients who had delayed node dissection was 51.3% compared with 61.7% in patients who had had immediate resection ($P = .09$). Multivariate analysis showed that routine use of immediate node dissection had no effect on survival.[229] The WHO study, in contrast to the Intergroup Melanoma trial, was much smaller in patient accrual, assessed patients who generally had thicker melanomas, and did not use lymphoscintigraphy to determine the appropriate drainage basins to resect.

In 1996, initial results of the Intergroup Melanoma trial were reported. The trial randomized 740 patients with intermediate-thickness lesions to ELND, and, although there was no difference in survival for the entire group, an apparent survival benefit was seen in a post hoc analysis of a subgroup of patients. Male patients younger than the age of 60, with tumors 1.1 to 2.0 mm thick, and without ulceration had a significant improvement in 5-year survival of 96% versus 84% ($P = .007$) which was confirmed in multivariate analysis. The subgroup of patients with tumor thickness 1.1 to 2.0 mm of any age who underwent an ELND also had a significantly better 5-year survival compared with the observation group (92 vs. 84%, $P = .05$).[230]

Cascinelli et al. suggest a role of prophylactic dissection in a randomized study of patients with trunk melanoma comparing elective versus delayed dissection, noting that only patients with positive lymph nodes benefited from lymphadenectomy.[229] These data become important with the advent of sentinel node biopsy and subsequent selective nodal dissection. Now a large percentage (80%) of patients who may not benefit from LND may be spared the procedure while identifying patients who may most benefit. SLN biopsy followed by dissection in patients with positive nodes eliminates the indications for prophylactic dissection, and future studies can focus on a homogenous group of patients in order to establish the true therapeutic role of lymphadenectomy.

SENTINEL NODE BIOPSY

Even before the results of the WHO and Intergroup Melanoma trials, the use of sentinel node biopsy was widely adopted as a means to minimize procedural morbidity of LND. The sentinel node is the most likely lymph node to contain metastatic dis-

TABLE 42.2-7. Results of Elective Lymph Node Dissection Trials[a]

Trial	*Design*	*Results*
Memorial Sloan-Kettering, 1975	Retrospective	Benefit for intermediate thickness
University of Alabama, 1982	Retrospective	Benefit for intermediate thickness
Duke University, 1983	Retrospective	Benefit for intermediate thickness
Sydney Melanoma Unit, 1985	Retrospective	Benefit for intermediate thickness
University of Pennsylvania, 1985	Retrospective	No benefit
Drepper, 1993	Retrospective	Benefit for intermediate thickness
Duke University, 1994	Retrospective	No benefit
Romple, 1995	Retrospective	Benefit for intermediate thickness
Sydney Melanoma Unit, 1995	Retrospective	No benefit
World Health Organization, 1977	Prospective	No benefit
Mayo Clinic, 1986	Prospective	No benefit
Intergroup Melanoma, 1996	Prospective	No benefit overall; benefit for 1–2 mm and patients <60 y
World Health Organization, 1998	Prospective	No benefit

[a]Elective lymph node dissection has been extensively examined for benefit with mixed results. Most prospective trials show no benefit, but these have been criticized. The Intergroup trial showed survival benefit in post hoc analysis for patients under the age of 60 and with lesions between 1 and 2 mm. Regardless of trial outcome, with the advent of sentinel node biopsy, patients should no longer routinely undergo lymph node dissection.

ease. The concept of sentinel node biopsy is based on the presumption of an orderly progression of disease through the lymphatic system. A negative SLN would suggest more upstream metastatic disease has not occurred, whereas a positive SLN would indicate potential involvement of other nodes in the same basin.[231] A lymphadenectomy after intraoperative lymphatic mapping and sentinel node biopsy has been termed a *completion lymph node dissection.*[232] The importance of a positive sentinel node is underscored by multivariate analyses, which show that the SLN status is the most important prognostic factor influencing disease-free and distant disease-free survival in patients with stage I and II melanoma.[233]

SLN biopsies have clarified the natural progression of melanoma metastasis.[234] The data from initial trials using sentinel node mapping demonstrate an apparent orderly progression of disease with failure to observe lymph node metastases in nodes adjacent to a negative sentinel node.[235] Cabanas was the first to describe the technique of sentinel node biopsy for penile cancer as a means to prevent the morbidity of bilateral inguinal LND.[236] This concept is that discrete areas of skin drain initially to specific node(s) within lymph node basin(s) that may or may not be proximate anatomic basins. The identification of such initially draining nodes allows for pathologic assessment in far greater detail than is possible otherwise.

Although many surgeons believe SLN biopsy is the current standard of care, the true role and benefit of sentinel node mapping is still to be determined. Undoubtedly, sentinel node status is extremely valuable in staging. Clinical trials of melanoma have been hampered by the heterogeneity of patient populations due to suboptimal staging. Accurate knowledge of the lymph node status (macroscopic, microscopic, immunohistochemical, and molecular) enables appropriate comparisons to be made between treatment groups. There is still debate whether a positive sentinel node biopsy with subsequent lymphadenectomy of clinically negative basins and adjuvant therapy is efficacious. Data suggest that the early removal of positive lymph nodes may improve survival. The Intergroup trial suggests that the benefit of elective LND may be meaningful in patients whose tumors are nonulcerated, extremity primaries, of thickness between 1 and 2 mm, and whose age is less than 60 years. Current trials are attempting to determine the efficacy of early LND guided by sentinel node mapping. Although the efficacy of adjuvant treatment for melanoma is less than desired, the ongoing studies of IFNs, chemotherapy, vaccines, and combinations will be improved by a greater precision in prognostic assessment.

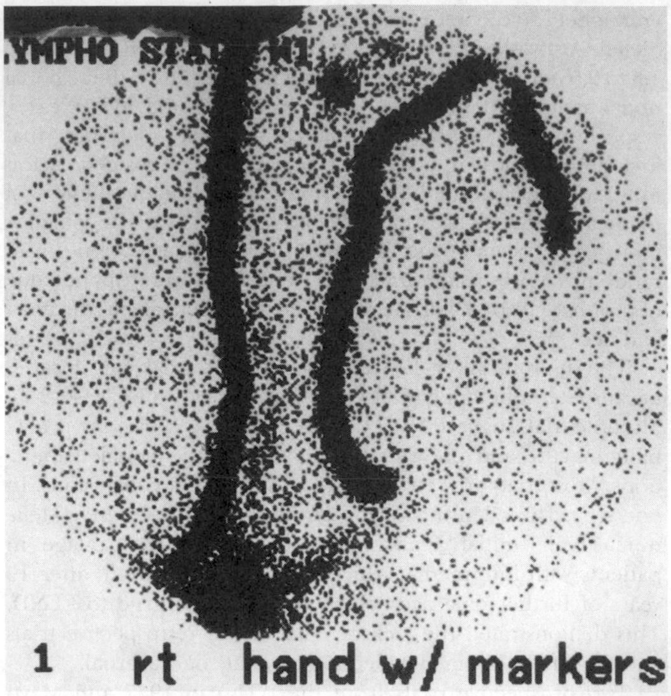

FIGURE 42.2-18. Lymphoscintigram. This patient had a biopsy-proven melanoma on the right hand (note the high area of radioactive tracer around the injection site) and was noted to have an epitrochlear sentinel node. Five percent of patients with distal extremity lesions have popliteal or epitrochlear nodes. Using classical guidelines for lymphadenectomy, a potential positive lymph node may be overlooked, which may result in incorrect staging.

Lymphoscintigraphy

In 1977 Robinson et al. described the use of cutaneous lymphoscintigraphy in the nodal basin for truncal melanomas using colloidal gold scanning.[237] In 1985, Morton began the first clinical trials using both lymphoscintigraphy and vital dye injection for the identification of sentinel nodes in melanoma patients. In 1993, Alex introduced the use of technetium 99m sulfur colloid, a radioactive tracer, injected intradermally around a primary melanoma site, followed by imaging and subsequent intraoperative use of a gamma probe to localize the sentinel node.[238]

The day before the operation, lymphoscintigraphy is performed using ^{99m}Tc (0.5 to 0.8 mCi), which is injected around the tumor site (Figs. 42.2-18 and 42.2-19). The colloidal isotopes are phagocytosed by macrophages within the lymph node. This keeps tracer in the draining node and prevents further passage through the nodal basin.[239] Immediately afterward, dynamic images are obtained, and after 2 hours static scintigrams are taken. Dynamic imaging helps differentiate between multiple sentinel nodes and spillover to nonsentinel node. The choice of tracer is also important. The ^{99m}Tc sulfur colloid has a particle size in the micrometer range, and transport may be too slow to be suitable for dynamic imaging. ^{99m}Tc colloidal albumin and technetium 99m human serum albumin appear to be the most favorable as the sentinel node becomes positive within 20 minutes in 97% of patients and is retained for up to 24 hours without an increase in the number of sentinel nodes.[240] ^{99m}Tc human serum albumin demonstrated faster washout rates from injection sites and better definition of lymph channels than either particulate agent, whereas particulate agents were retained longer in nodes and demonstrated more nodes in delayed images than in early images. Early dynamic imaging is important, as sentinel nodes cannot be distinguished reliably from nonsentinel nodes in delayed images alone.[241] The radiologist should mark the position of the sentinel node on the skin, although the surgeon must be wary that relaxation during surgery and positioning may change the position of the lymph node relative to the skin marker.

The surgeon should reexamine the SLN in the operating room with the hand-held gamma counter and make the skin incision directly over the most radioactive point. As only 1% of

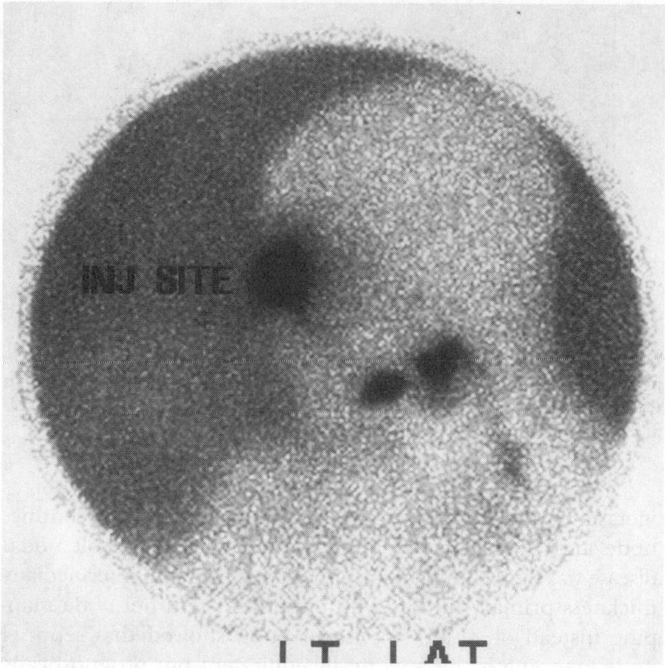

FIGURE 42.2-19. Lymphoscintigram. This patient had a primary tumor on the nose. Sentinel node mapping in the head and neck can be difficult secondary to the increased number of nodes (3.8 vs. 1.3), the overshadowing of pertinent lymph nodes by the primary injection site, the difficult dissections, and cosmetic concerns. Note, the multiple sentinel nodes suggested during early imaging. In this patient, no sentinel nodes in the parotid gland were identified. (Courtesy of H. Edington, M.D., University of Pittsburgh Cancer Institute.)

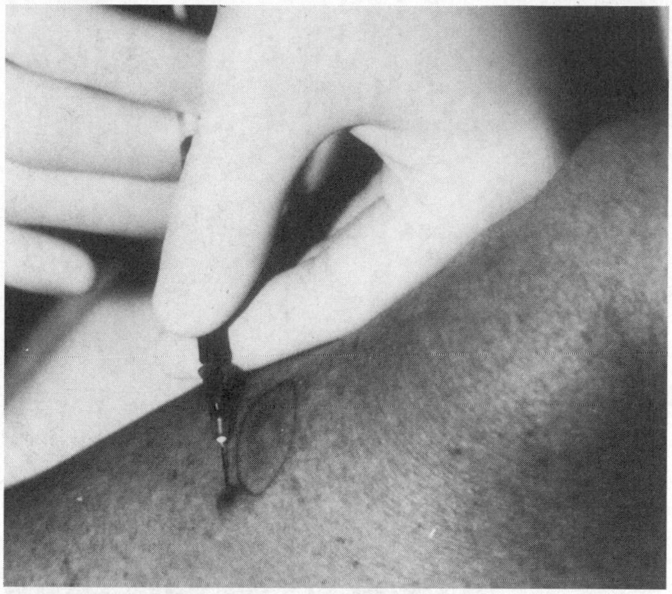

FIGURE 42.2-20. Vital blue dye injected around a primary melanoma. The patient had undergone lymphoscintigraphy before injection of the vital blue dye. (Courtesy of H. Edington, M.D., University of Pittsburgh Cancer Institute.)

the injected dose of radioactive colloid reaches the SLN, a primary site close to the nodal basin may preclude effective use of the gamma probe, even if the primary site is excised initially.[242] This shadowing becomes especially important in head and neck melanomas where nodes and the primary site overlap. After the sentinel node is removed, the wound is explored with the gamma probe for additional *hot*, blue nodes.

Sappey had originally injected mercury into the skin of cadavers and showed that a line drawn just above the umbilicus would differentiate inguinal versus axillary drainage. Lesions within 2 cm of this line had bidirectional drainage. With the use of these techniques, lymphatic drainage not predicted by Sappey's original description of the cutaneous watershed of lymph drainage has been frequently observed.[243] Only more recently, with the use of lymphoscintigraphy, has Sappey's guide to lymphatic flow been modifies by modern means of assessment.

Discordance from classical drainage patterns is especially common in the head, neck, and truck. Sixty percent of head and neck and 32% of the trunk tumors drain in unpredicted sites. Operative intervention is changed in almost one-half of patients when lymphoscintigraphy is used.[244,245] Lymphoscintigraphy may also identify patients with lymphatic drainage in two separate basins. Patients who have positive nodes in two basins have a worse prognosis when compared with patients with nodal disease in one basin, even when controlling for the total number of positive nodes.[246] Even in distal extremity lesions in which lymphatic drainage is seemingly obvious, lymphoscintigraphy may identify popliteal or epitrochlear nodes.[247]

The unpredictability of lymphatic drainage based on anatomic guidelines basins, especially in the head, neck, and trunk, make the use of routine ELND based on classic anatomy inappropriate without preoperative lymphoscintigraphy. The examination of incorrect lymphatic basins, the lack of appropriate immunohistochemical techniques, and the inclusion of patients with a relatively low likelihood of nodal involvement accounts for the difficulty in interpreting the various results of prior trials studying the role of ELND.

Vital Dye

After induction of anesthesia, vital blue dye (1.0 mL of isosulfan blue or patent blue V) is injected intradermally around the primary tumor or scar (Fig. 42.2-20). The gamma counter is more accurate than vital dyes in locating sentinel nodes, especially in the axilla or in deep fatty tissue. Techniques using dye alone require a longer learning curve to achieve success rates of only 80%. The blue dye is still helpful in visual confirmation of a hot node (Figs. 42.2-21 and 42.2-22), but up to 15% of radiolabeled sentinel nodes lack any blue dye. Conversely, 8% of blue nodes are not hot, and some of these nodes will be the only site of metastasis.[248] Complications of the technique are infrequent and minor including dye-stained urine and prolonged tattooing of the skin lasting several months.

Results of Sentinel Lymph Node Biopsy

After nodal mapping, regional recurrence rates are acceptably low and the sensitivity and specificity are quite high. Reintgen, in 1997, reported that after 600 mappings and 5 years of follow-up, no patient developed a recurrence in any basins not predicted at risk by lymphoscintigraphy.[242] In another series, the sensitivity of lymphatic mapping and SLN biopsy for extremity melanoma was

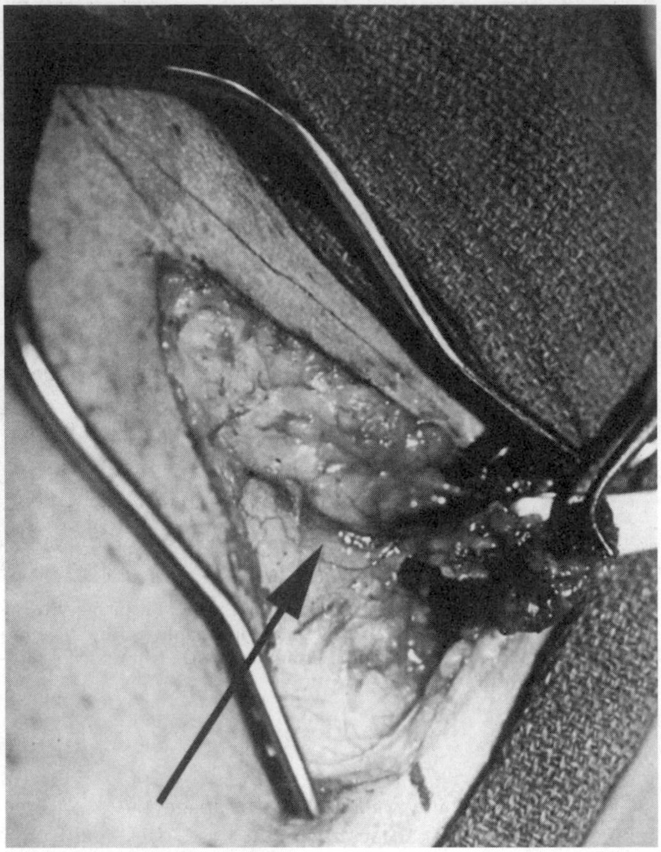

FIGURE 42.2-21. Vital blue dye leading to superficial inguinal sentinel lymph node. Arrow points to blue lymphatic channel. (Courtesy of H. Edington, M.D., University of Pittsburgh Cancer Institute.) (See Color Fig. 42.2-21 in the CD-ROM and on the Web at www.LWWoncology.com.)

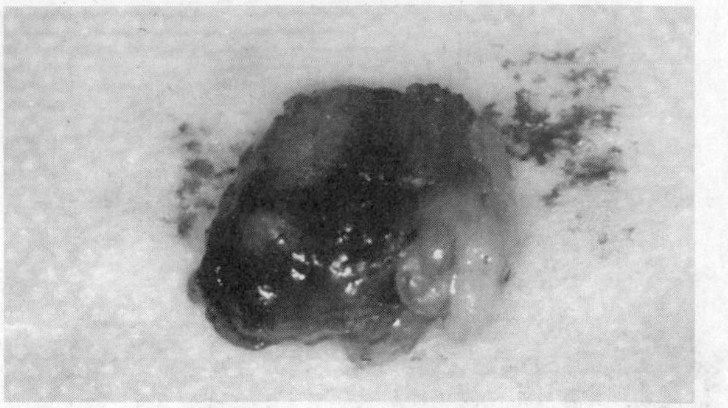

FIGURE 42.2-22. Vital blue dye staining the sentinel lymph node after removal. (Courtesy of H. Edington, M.D., University of Pittsburgh Cancer Institute.) (See Color Fig. 42.2-22 in the CD-ROM and on the Web at www.LWWoncology.com.)

100% and the specificity was 97%. Only 3% of patients with histologically negative SLNs developed inguinal nodal metastases during a mean 2-year follow-up.[249] Lenisa et al. described their series of 580 sentinel node biopsies, 15% of which had nodes involved with tumor. Positive cases were distributed according to thickness as shown in Table 42.2-8. In 77% of the patients, only a single positive node was identified after completion LND. Only eight patients (1%) had a local relapse after a negative sentinel node biopsy.[250] Using multivariate analysis, the probability of a positive sentinel node depends only on tumor thickness, ulceration, and truncal location. Although tumor thickness and ulceration influenced survival in SLN-negative patients, they provided no additional prognostic information in SLN-positive patients. Sentinel nodes are positive in 15% to 26% of patients in various series.[234,248,251] Of patients with positive sentinel nodes, 24% to 33% demonstrate lymph nodes to be involved at completion lymphadenectomy. A single SLN is found in 59% of patients, two SLNs in 37%, and three SLN in 3%.[240] The median number of sentinel nodes found in several series ranges from 1.3 to 1.8.

Essner et al. were the first to show that sentinel node biopsy followed by completion lymphadenectomy did not decrease survival compared with patients undergoing ELND. They described a series of 534 matched patients with clinical stage I melanoma; one-half of the patients were treated with lymphatic mapping and sentinel lymphadenectomy and the other half were treated with ELND. The overall incidences of nodal metastases and survival were no different between the sentinel node and ELND groups, but the incidence of occult nodal disease was significantly higher among patients with intermediate-thickness primary tumors who underwent sentinel node mapping instead of ELND.[240a] Essner et al. showed that sentinel node mapping is therapeutically equivalent but prognostically more accurate than ELND.[252]

Whether previous wide excision affects the ability to map the sentinel node by changing local lymphatic drainage has been debated. The likelihood of appropriate dye uptake is decreased by one-half if a wide excision has been previously done.[234,253] Most surgeons strongly recommend the use of lymphoscintigraphy before wide local excision to avoid disruption, artifactual drainage of the lymphatic drainage, or both.[254] Morton et al. retrospectively examined 47 patients who had SLN mapping after wide local excision and concluded that SLN biopsy can be cautiously performed in patients who have undergone previous wide local excision if the primary resection margin was no greater than 2.0 cm and the primary was not in a region of ambiguous drainage. Another retrospective review of 142 patients concluded that previous wide excision does not affect the reliability of sentinel node biopsy unless a rotational flap has been used.[255] Further study is needed before firm conclusions can be made on the timing of SLN biopsy.

SLNs of the head and neck behave somewhat differently. Sentinel node biopsy has been less consistently successful in the head and neck due to the frequent alterations in lymphatic draining; likewise, prophylactic nodal dissection has not proven

TABLE 42.2-8. Thickness of Melanoma and Sentinel Lymph Node Positivity[a]

Thickness (mm)	*No.*	*Percentage Positive Sentinel Lymph Node*
1.0–1.99	27	5
2.0–2.99	97	18
>3.0	146	27

[a]The probability of a sentinel node demonstrating metastatic disease depends on tumor thickness. Careful selection is necessary before the use of sentinel node mapping in patients with T1 melanomas. Even in patients with thin ulcerated tumors, the chance of nodal disease is less than 10%. A positive sentinel node in multivariate analysis is the single most important variable in determining long-term survival.[250]

useful. Series reports between a 90% and a 95% success rate in identifying the sentinel node, somewhat less than the success rate for sentinel nodes at other sites.[226,250,256–259] Many differences in head and neck lesions make sentinel node biopsy more difficult. Whereas most patients with extremity melanomas have a median of 1.3 to 1.8 SLNs, a median of 3.8 sentinel nodes is found in patients with intermediate-thickness head and neck lesions. Difficulties in mapping strategies are seen in nonclassical and especially parotid nodes, which may be *shadowed* by the radioisotope injected in the primary site. Furthermore, only 67% of lesions stain with vital dyes. One-half of sentinel nodes are located in nonadjacent nodal basins. One-fourth are in nonclassical sites and one-half in the parotid gland. Often, a functional node dissection with *ex vivo* dissection using the gamma probe is necessary to find small sentinel nodes.[260] Furthermore, the patients must be warned that prolonged tattooing may occur from injected dyes in cosmetically sensitive areas of the face.

In 1994, the Multicenter Selective Lymphadenectomy Trial was begun to evaluate the therapeutic role of lymphatic mapping and SLN biopsy with and without wide excision in patients with localized melanoma. This trial has just closed with 1800 patients accrued, and long-term results are awaited. The Multicenter Selective Lymphadenectomy Trial has a 99.1% success rate in obtaining sentinel node(s) using both dye and radiolabeling.[232] In centers participating in the Multicenter Selective Lymphadenectomy Trial, a minimum of 30 procedures must be performed before patients can be entered. After performing 30 cases, there was no difference in success of sentinel node biopsies between any of the centers.[261]

Pathologic Interpretation

Frozen sections do not have a place in sentinel node mapping because micrometastatic disease cannot be determined, and thus permanent pathologic interpretation is crucial to success of sentinel node staging. Hematoxylin-eosin (H&E) staining is performed with negative samples undergoing immunohistochemical staining with the antibodies reactive with melanoma including S-100 and HMB-45. Ninety percent of melanomas are positive for S-100. HMB-45 is more specific but less sensitive than S-100, which also stains neurons, melanocytes, and DCs.[22] The importance of immunostaining is exemplified in a study by Gershenwald. Of 243 patients with a histologically negative SLN on routine H&E staining, 27 (11%) developed local, in-transit, regional nodal, distant, or both nodal and distant metastases after a median follow-up of 35 months. Ten patients (4.1%) developed a nodal recurrence in the previously mapped basin. Reexamination of the original cassettes using S-100 and HMB-45 demonstrated that 80% of these patients had evidence of occult metastases by serial sectioning or immunohistochemical staining.[141] In another large series of 357 patients and 838 sentinel nodes, 45% of positive nodes were only positive by S-100 staining, again confirming the importance of immunostaining for H&E-negative nodes.[262] At a minimum, all negative SLNs should undergo immunohistochemical staining for melanoma markers.

The Multicenter Selective Lymphadenectomy Trial uses strict guidelines in handling nodal tissue. The Trial recommends cutting the lymph node in two halves through its longest diameter and fixing the specimen. Ten serial 8- to 10-μm sections are then made. Sections 1, 3, 5, and 10 are used for H&E staining, section 2 for S-100, section 4 for HMB-45, and sections 6 and 7 are negative controls for immunoperoxidase studies. Sections 8 and 9 are used to repeat any needed studies.[248]

The use of RT-PCR, or potentially in the future, Taqman analysis to examine nodes for mRNA of melanosomal proteins may be valuable as this could reduce sampling error and increase sensitivity. Its extreme sensitivity, however, may result in the inappropriate upstaging of patients and overtreatment of patients falsely termed positive. In one study of RT-PCR of 124 patients, 58% of patients with histologically negative nodes were upstaged. This group of patients had a worse overall prognosis than patients who were RT-PCR negative and histologically negative. Twenty percent of these patients developed either locoregional or systemic disease, whereas only 5% of the PCR-negative patients developed signs of disease. One melanoma cell in 1 million background cells can be detected.[263] Since approximately 80% of sentinel nodes will be negative, a quick screening of H&E-negative nodes using PCR may identify patients in whom the more labor-intensive immunostaining may be performed.[264] One aim of the current Sunbelt trial is to examine the importance of PCR-positive lymph nodes and the effect of adjuvant therapy in patients with histologically negative nodes. The introduction of Taqman analysis may allow more accurate antigen quantitation and further insight.[265]

SENTINEL LYMPH NODE RESULTS IN THIN AND THICK MELANOMAS

Only rarely are sentinel nodes found positive in patients with thin melanomas (T1). The use of sentinel node biopsy is controversial in this group of patients, and many have looked for risk factors that may predict a higher incidence of nodal metastases. Less than 2% of patients with nonulcerated primary lesions less than 1 mm (T1) and less than Clark level IV have positive sentinel nodes. No lymph node involvement has been reported in lesions less than 0.73 mm. Thus, there is no role for sentinel mapping in these patients. The two most significant risk factors for positive sentinel nodes in thin primary lesions are ulceration and Clark level greater or equal to IV. Even in patients with T1b lesions, the risk for nodal disease is less than 10%. Patients with T1b tumors have the same risk for nodal disease as T2a patients. In a series of 254 patients reported by Gershenwald, no patient with T1 lesions and a positive sentinel node had positive nodes on completion lymphadenectomy. Regression by itself was not found a risk factor for nodal disease in thin lesions.[130] Careful selection and patient education is necessary before the employment of SLN biopsies in these patients with thin lesions.

No trial has shown benefit for elective nodal dissection in patients with tumors greater than 4 mm, and, in fact, ELNDs were not performed in this group of patients. However, many centers perform sentinel node mapping in this group of patients. Perhaps the subgroup of patients that has deep lesions and negative sentinel nodes may have improved survival compared with stage III patients and would be spared adjuvant therapy.

STAGE III DISEASE: MANAGEMENT OF THE CLINICALLY POSITIVE NODAL BASIN

THERAPEUTIC NODE DISSECTION

The development of clinically palpable nodes in the draining basins of a primary melanoma requires TLND to control local disease. Although there are no randomized trials clearly demonstrating a survival difference after TLND, a significant number of patients attain 5-year survival. Furthermore, the palliative benefits of TLND are considerable. Untreated nodal metastasis can be expected to ulcerate, impinge on neural structures, and cause pain in patients whose life expectancy is more than 1 year. Even in some patients with metastasis to distant nodal regions, TLND has a role in palliation. In addition, prognostic information is obtained after TLND since the number of positive nodes correlates with survival and may guide adjuvant therapy.[143]

In patients with a prior history of melanoma but without evidence of infection, 90% of lymphadenopathy is associated with tumor.[266] Tumor-involved nodes tend to be firm and spherical. Five-year survival rates following TLND range from 19% to 38% in retrospective series.[222,266–271] In one series of 133 patients undergoing iliac and inguinal nodal dissection, those with one, two, three, or more than four lymph nodes positive for tumor had median survivals of 90, 78, 49, and 15 months, respectively. The median survival was significantly worse for those with deep nodes positive with survival of 53, 42, 14, and 9 months, respectively.[272]

Inguinal Dissection

The extent of surgical management in patients with clinically palpable inguinal nodes is a controversial topic in the treatment of melanoma. An inguinal groin dissection can be either superficial, including all nodes below the inguinal ligament, or complete, including the deep iliac and obturator nodes accessed through retroperitoneal exposure. The superficial dissection is carried out through a longitudinal incision with the removal of subcutaneous tissues, lymphatics, and the anterior portion of the femoral sheath. A sartorius muscle flap is used in closure to protect the femoral vessels and decrease wound complications.[273]

Of patients with palpable inguinal nodes, up to 37% have histologically positive deep iliac nodes. Some believe that the routine removal of all deep nodes in patients with palpable inguinal disease is indicted, whereas others believe patients with radiologically positive pelvic nodes should not undergo TLND given the likelihood of distant disease. There are currently no randomized data comparing complete and superficial LND. Case series suggest that performing a deep inguinal dissection increases the morbidity of the operation and does not to offer an obvious survival advantage in a radiologically negative pelvis. In comparing patients who undergo deep TLND for known positive iliac disease with those who have no apparent pelvic disease and only positive inguinal disease, overall survival is equivalent. For some, this is evidence that pelvic dissections are beneficial. They argue that those with grossly positive pelvic nodes should have a predictably worse prognosis since those patients had significantly more positive lymph nodes of generally larger size.[274] There is some suggestion that the probability of a groin recurrence decreased with the inclusion of a deep iliac dissection.[272] In a retrospective review of 362 therapeutic groin dissections, 20% had positive deep inguinal nodes. The 5- and 10-year survival for those patients was 24% and 20%, respectively, with the number of positive iliac nodes an independent prognostic factor. The authors suggest that deep lymph node dissection may be of benefit as up to 20% of patients are long-term survivors who would otherwise would have had residual disease if treated only by a superficial dissection.[275] A prospective trial is currently testing the value of deep iliac dissection in patients who will all have superficial dissection.

Axillary Dissections

Therapeutic axillary nodal dissection for melanoma involves the complete removal of levels I and II nodes, and some advocate the removal of level III nodes including skeletonizing the axillary vein and brachial plexus. Rarely, in patients without evidence of distant disease and with positive supraclavicular nodes, a lower cervical node dissection may be performed by resection of the middle third of the clavicle.[273] As with inguinal dissections, survival after axillary dissection correlates with the number of positive nodes. The 5-year survival rate is 80% in patients with histologically negative nodes. With one, two, three, or more than four nodes, the 5-year survival was 62%, 51%, 28%, and 5%, respectively. Patients with recurrent lymph nodes or nodes that are fixed have a 5-year survival of 13%.[276]

Neck Dissections

A functional neck dissection is indicated with the preservation of the jugular vein, sternocleidomastoid, and spinal accessory nerve unless directly involved with tumor. Modification of the extent of dissection is appropriate relative to the site of the primary tumor.[273] Patients treated with node positivity in head and neck cancer have a substantially lower survival than in patients with truncal or extremity melanoma. Superficial, nerve-sparing parotidectomy is indicated for palpable metastatic lesions for local tumor control.[277] These parotid nodes should be removed by superficial parotidectomy. Although controversial, some advocate the use of adjuvant radiotherapy for high-risk lesions because of the higher rate of recurrence in head and neck lesions.[260] This is the topic of an ongoing randomized controlled trial, E3697, by ECOG.

Popliteal and Antecubital Nodal Dissection

Infrequently, the popliteal nodes become involved with metastatic disease and cause palpable enlargement. The popliteal nodes only drain a small area of skin of the posterior calf. In the absence of distant unresectable disease, popliteal nodal dissection should be performed through an S-shaped incision. There are no data demonstrating survival benefit of this operation as there are only small case series in the literature.[273,278] Epitrochlear node involvement occurred in 18% of patients with forearm or hand lesions, and only when the primary melanoma was within 5 cm of the elbow or in the ulnar distribution.[279]

Complications of Nodal Dissection

In inguinal dissections, necrosis of the skin flap occurs to some degree in 7% of patients. Wound infection occurs in 10% of patients.[280] The most devastating long-term complication is lymphedema. This occurs in up to 24% of patients and may be upward of 40% with prolonged follow-up. A strict regimen of daily leg elevation and routine use of elastic stockings decreases the severity of symptoms. The lateral femoral cutaneous nerve is commonly sacrificed with resultant numbness of the lateral thigh. The Intergroup Melanoma Trial reports a 50% wound complication rate in inguinal lymphadenectomies. In 112 patients there were

23 wound breakdowns, 24 cases of lymphedema, one deep vein thrombosis, and one pulmonary embolism.[230]

Necrosis is rare in axillary dissection. Neuropraxia secondary to brachial plexopathy is also a rare event that is usually resolved within 3 to 6 months. Proper positioning, careful placement of retractors and careful dissection minimize this event. Lymphocele rates are 7%, and the incidence of arm edema is much lower than nodal dissection for breast cancer.[281] Mobilization after axillary dissection should be limited until after surgical drains are removed.[282]

MELANOMA OF UNKNOWN PRIMARY SITE

Melanomas presenting as regional or distant disease without an obvious primary site occur uncommonly and may represent a completely regressed primary tumor. A vigorous search for suspicious lesions is mandatory in these patients with a low threshold for biopsy. In a large series of more than 84,000 patients with melanoma, 2.2% of all melanoma presented without signs of a primary lesion. In patients with unknown primary melanomas, the distribution of metastases as localized to a region or multiple sites at presentation was 43% and 57%, respectively.[283] These patients are younger than other melanoma patients and tend to be male. The most common presenting nodal site is the axilla.[284] In patients with lymph node metastasis without a known primary site, survival is equal or better than for patients with known primaries. The clinical disease course of patients with metastatic melanoma of unknown primary origin is similar to that of patients with primary cutaneous melanoma when the same clinical stages of the disease are compared, and they should be treated accordingly.[285]

MANAGEMENT OF LOCOREGIONAL DISEASE BY RADIOTHERAPY

Radiotherapy may be useful in the management of unresectable lymph node metastases from melanoma and possibly as adjuvant therapy after repeat resection in patients with recurrent lymph node metastases. The role of adjuvant radiotherapy to regional lymphatics is presently being investigated in an ECOG protocol that randomizes patients with high-risk disease between IFN-α_{2b} with or without regional radiotherapy to 30 Gy in five biweekly 6-Gy fractions. This study was undertaken because of the favorable experience with adjuvant radiotherapy reported by Ang et al.[176,182] For 118 previously untreated patients with melanomas greater than 1.5 mm in thickness or Clark's level IV and V, with no palpable nodes managed with wide local excision and adjuvant radiotherapy to 30 Gy in five fractions, 5-year local regional control was 86% and survival was 63%. In 39 patients with clinically positive nodes and 67 patients with recurrent local regional tumor who received postoperative local regional radiotherapy, 5-year local regional control rates were 92% and 88%, respectively, while survival rates were 41% and 45%, respectively. Arm or leg edema and brachial neuropathy associated with radiation fibrosis are concerns with high-dose fraction radiotherapy of lymph node regions. Ang et al. reported mild to moderate late radiation sequelae in only 3 of 224 patients.[181,182] Arm or leg edema is managed with limb compression therapy. Radiation fibrosis with or without extremity edema appears to improve with treatment following therapy with pentoxifylline (400 mg twice a day) and vitamin E (500 IU twice a day) for 6 months.[286]

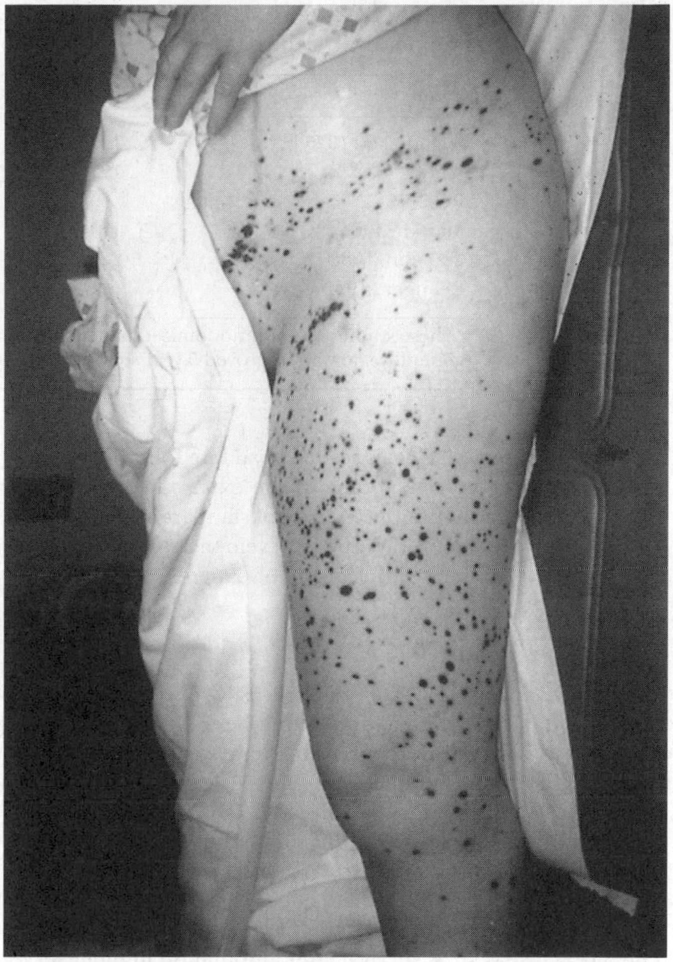

FIGURE 42.2-23. In-transit disease most often is found between the primary lesion and the draining lymph nodes but in advanced instances is able to track beyond these sites, presumably through lymphatic connections.

STAGE III DISEASE: MANAGEMENT OF IN-TRANSIT DISEASE

In-transit disease is defined as dermal or subcutaneous recurrent melanoma located in the skin or subcutaneous tissue of the lymphatic drainage of the primary tumor and found greater than 5 cm from the origin of the primary tumor (Fig. 42.2-23). If observed surrounding the site of the primary tumor, the term *satellitosis* is sometimes used. In-transit disease occurs in an estimated 2% to 10% of all melanoma patients. The probability of developing locoregional cutaneous relapse is highly associated with histologic evidence of lymphatic invasion seen in the initial primary lesion.[287] Seventy percent of in-transit disease occurs in the lower extremity, the majority originating from thick primaries.[288] The lower extremity has the highest incidence of in-transit disease perhaps due to the higher density of lymphatics. Regional nodal metastases are common and seen in up to two-thirds of patients with in-transit disease.[289] Patients with in-transit disease without regional lymph node involvement have similar disease progression as patients with two to four positive nodes, thus the proposed stage designation of N2C. Patients with nodal involvement and in-transit disease

TABLE 42.2-9. Five-Year Survival after Isolated Limb Perfusion Compared with Historic Controls[a]

Author	*No.*	*Isolated Limb Perfusion*	*Control*
Sugarbaker, 1976[562]	199	88	68
Janoff, 1982[563]	122	81	55
Rege, 1983[564]	39	91	63
Martijn, 1986[565]	120	65	40
Franklin, 1988[566]	227	77	77
Reintgen, 1992[567]	11	95	75

[a]These studies use nonrandomized patients compared with historical controls. Although these trials generally show an improved 5-year survival, randomized prospective trials have shown mixed results.

will be designated N3. The 5-year survival rate following locoregional recurrence of melanoma of the extremities is approximately 20%. Treatment options are not standardized, and until more effective systemic therapy is developed, aggressive local treatment is indicated for this group of patients.

SURGICAL EXCISION

Resection is indicated for small, easily excised recurrent tumors and patients with a limited number of in-transit lesions. Simple resection may delay or even eliminate the need for ILP. Wide excisions are unnecessary and excessively morbid in patients whose lymphatics are already contaminated. Amputation should only be considered if the limb is nonfunctional or hygiene cannot be maintained. When amputations are necessary, they should be performed as either a hip disarticulation or hemipelvectomy as distal amputations usually fail locally. The 5-year disease-free survival after amputation in older series is approximately 20% to 35%.[290]

ISOLATED LIMB PERFUSION

ILP for the introduction of chemotherapeutic agents to control regional malignant disease was first described in 1958 by Winblad. Approximately 50% of primary melanomas occur in the extremities, and approximately 10% of those patients have a recurrence as in-transit disease.[291] As only rare patients respond to systemic therapy, ILP was developed as a means of limb salvage that would enable the delivery of cytotoxic drugs locoregionally at doses many-fold higher than would be tolerable systemically. No clear agreement exists on which patients benefit most from ILP and which regimens are most active. Prospective randomized trials that examine regimen, toxicity, dosage, and response are in development. Currently, melphalan is the gold standard reagent for use in ILP. Melphalan can be safely delivered locally at doses ten times higher than systemically tolerated.[292] One-half of patients exhibit a complete response and 75% at least have a partial response to melphalan.[293] Melphalan delivered at maximal systemic doses has negligible activity against melanoma. The use of hyperthermia has also become standard during ILP since Stehlin, in 1969, described improved response rates using perfusate at temperatures of 38.8 to 40°C.[294] Current randomized studies seek to demonstrate that combination therapy using melphalan and TNF is superior to melphalan alone in treatment of patients with in-transit disease and the combination has been reported to have a 100% response rate.[295]

Indications

ILP is useful in two groups of patients. Those with locoregionally advanced melanoma such as satellitosis and in-transit metastasis and those in need of palliation who have bulky regional disease and limited systemic metastasis. Prophylactic ILP for use as an adjunct to wide local excision in patients with a high-risk primary or recurrent melanoma cannot be recommended since no improvement in survival can be shown in prospective trials.

Prophylactic (Adjuvant) Isolated Limb Perfusion

A well-designed multiinstitutional prospective trial of ILP with melphalan was conducted by the consortium of the EORTC, the WHO, and the North American Perfusion Group. In 1998, the results of this multicenter randomized phase III trial of ILP in patients with primary cutaneous melanoma greater than 1.5 mm in thickness were published. A total of 832 patients were randomized to have wide local excision or wide local excision plus ILP with melphalan and hyperthermia. Median follow-up was 6.4 years. There was no difference in survival. Patients who had not undergone ELND had a nonsignificant trend for a longer disease-free interval. In a subset of patients with melanoma of 1.5 to 2.99 mm thickness, in-transit metastasis was reduced from 6.6% to 3.3% and regional lymph node metastasis was reduced from 16.7% to 12.6%. In thicker lesions, patients succumbed to distant disease.[296]

Other retrospective series demonstrate the lack of benefit for prophylactic ILP. A series of 111 patients compared with 111 historical controls with subungual melanoma demonstrated no difference in survival after ILP with melphalan alone.[297] Prophylactic ILP with melphalan cannot be recommended as an adjunct to standard surgical therapy in high-risk melanoma patients.

Therapeutic Isolated Limb Perfusion

The role of ILP in prolonging overall survival has some support in the literature. Multiple randomized studies suggest improved survival in a subgroup of patients that undergoes ILP. ILP also is quite effective at ameliorating symptoms from bulky disease such as pain, edema, decreased mobility, and skin breakdown.[298] Numerous nonrandomized series claim survival advantages with melphalan-based ILP, but only two prospective randomized trials, with unfortunately conflicting and criticized results, exist in the literature (Tables 42.2-9, 42.2-10, and 42.2-11).

TABLE 42.2-10. Prospective Therapeutic Trials of Isolated Limb Perfusion[a]

		Recurrence Rate		
Author	*No.*	Stage I	Stage II	Stage III
Ghussen, 1984[568]	53 (treatment)	5.6	5.5	12.5
	54 (control)	27.8	31.6	58.8
		Median Tumor-Free Survival	Locoregional Recurrence	Median Overall Survival
Hafstrom, 1991[300]	36 (treatment)	17[b]	15[c]	57[c]
	33 (control)	10	24	35

[a]The significant results of the earlier trial have not been replicated. The later study was able to demonstrate an improved disease-free survival, but no overall survival benefit was established. Isolated limb perfusion should be performed in the setting of randomized trials before it can be widely recommended.
[b]$P = .04$.
[c]Not significant.

Ghussen et al. reported results in 107 patients in which wide excision and regional lymph nodes dissection were compared with hyperthermic (42°C) perfusion with melphalan at a mean follow-up period of 554 days. The recurrence rate in the control group was 27.8% in stage I, 31.6% in stage II, and 58.8% in stage III compared with 5.6% in stage I, 5.5% in stage II, and 12.5% in stage III, suggesting improved survival for stage II and III patients. However, there has been wide skepticism regarding the results of this small study.[299] Hafstrom et al. reported a prospective randomized trial in 69 patients testing application of regional hyperthermic perfusion with melphalan after surgery to one-half of patients following excision. Median disease-free survival was 17 months in the perfusion group and 10 months in the control group. There were 15 locoregional recurrences in the perfusion group and 24 in the control group. The disease-free survival was better for the perfusion group than for the control group, but no significant difference in overall survival was noted.[300] Of note, Hafstrom et al. used a lower dose of melphalan than currently standard. Patients developing recurrence after ILP may undergo repeat ILP, but there is a high limb recurrence rate and diminished response and disease control interval with increased toxicity.[301]

Patient factors that have been associated with therapeutic benefits include minimal total tumor surface area, absence of regional node involvement, number of lesions, and lack of previous recurrence.[301a]

Technique and Dosing

ILP of the lower extremity is performed via cannulation of the external iliac artery and vein through a suprainguinal retroperitoneal dissection. All venous and arterial branches including the hypogastric artery are ligated to prevent systemic leak syndrome.[302] Cannulation of the upper extremity is similarly performed through the axillary vessels. A proximal tourniquet aids in limiting systemic exposure to the perfusate. The extracorporeal perfusion circuit is primed with 700 mL saline, 1 U of packed red blood cells, and 1500 U of heparin, and flow is maintained in the range of 50 mL/L limb volume per minute (Fig. 42.2-24). The amount of systemic leak is measured using ^{131}I radiolabeled albumin or ^{99m}Tc-labeled red blood cells with the gamma counter over the precordium.[303,304]

Melphalan is an alkylating agent that is the mustard derived from phenylalanine, an essential precursor used in melanin synthesis by melanocytes. Weiberdink developed a regional toxicity scoring system to grade the reaction based on actual measurement of limb volume (Table 42.2-12). Based on this dosing regimen, a dose of 10 mg/L for the lower extremity and a dose of 13 mg/L for the upper extremities were developed to limit severe toxicities and optimize response.[305]

The use of hyperthermia has become standard with the use of ILP, as it seems to augment tissue concentrations of melphalan.[306] True hyperthermia is defined as greater than 41.5°C, mild hyperthermia as 38.5° to 41.5°C and controlled normothermia as 36° to 38°C. Temperatures above 42°C are directly cytotoxic to tumor but result in excessive adverse effects.[307] Stehlin suggested an improvement in the 5-year survival rate from 22% to 76% after introduction of hyperthermia to ILP, but others have demonstrated conflicting data. In one series of 136 patients with recurrent extremity melanoma, a minimum temperature of 41.5°C was an independent factor predictive of complete response.[308] By contrast, hyperthermia was not a significant factor related to complete response in an equally large series (n = 120).[309] The optimal duration of therapy, which has ranged from 45 minutes to 2 hours, is unknown.

TABLE 42.2-11. Tumor Response after Isolated Limb Perfusion with Melphalan Alone

Author	*No.*	*Complete Response (%)*	*Partial Response (%)*
Storm, 1985[559]	26	81	—
Santinami, 1989[560]	85	46	48
Di Filippo, 1989[308]	69	39	44
Klaase, 1994[561]	120	54	25

Other Agents

A number of other agents in addition to melphalan have been administered by ILP including cisplatin, etoposide, actinomycin D, dacarbazine, thiotepa, mitoxantrone, IL-2, IFN-γ, TNF-α, and lymphokine-activated killer (LAK) cells alone or in various combinations.[309a,309b] Although dacarbazine requires systemic hepatic conversion to its active metabolite, it has been shown, when administered by ILP, to generate an overall response rate

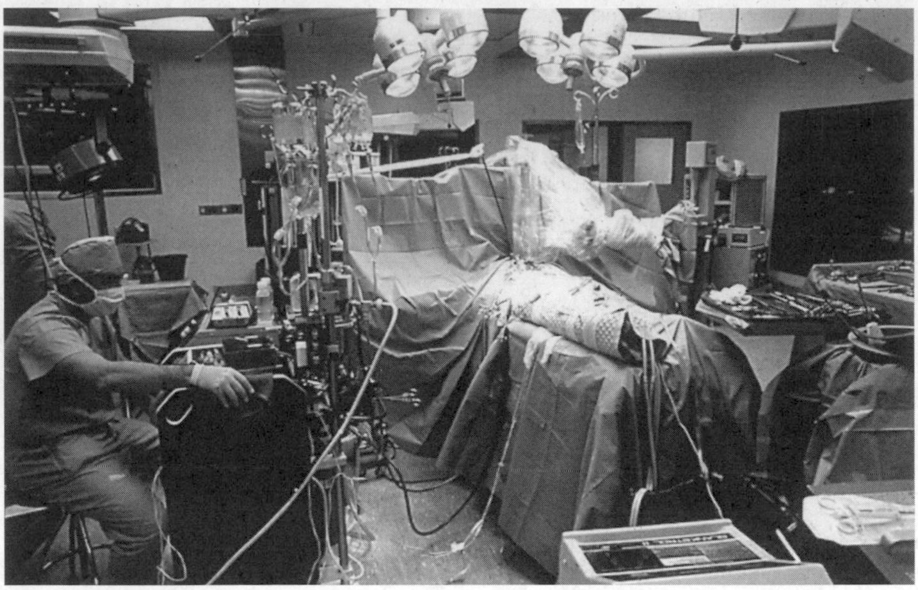

FIGURE 42.2-24. Operating room setup of isolated limb perfusion. Note the cumbersome apparatus. If clinical trials are performed demonstrating similar efficacy using isolated limb infusion, the simplification of the treatment of regional disease may enable a more widespread treatment.

of 76%.[310] Cisplatin has an overall response rate of over 50%, but the median response duration is only 5 months.[311] ILP using drugs other than melphalan and TNF is less effective and often associated with increased toxicity.[312]

In murine systems, TNF is capable of significant antitumor effects with a single intravenous injection, but effective doses cannot be achieved systemically in patients because of hemodynamic collapse. Immunohistochemical analysis of biopsies from patients treated with ILP with TNF demonstrates intravascular platelet aggregation, endothelial activation, and neutrophil invasion. Specific tumoral vasculature destruction with sparing of the normal vessels is also seen.[313]

The initial study of regional administration of high-dose TNF in conjunction with melphalan and low doses of IFN-γ was reported in 1992, demonstrating a complete response rate of 90%.[295] Many other case series corroborate the apparently enhanced activity of combination therapy (Table 42.2-13). IFN-γ induces the up-regulation of TNF receptors on tumor cells and has *in vitro* synergism with TNF in antitumor activity.[314,315] A randomized trial comparing TNF and melphalan alone or in combination with IFN-γ has shown no benefit with the addition of IFN-γ.[316]

A dose of 4 mg of TNF, more than ten times the maximal tolerable systemic dosage, is well tolerated during perfusion, and adverse effects are reportedly no greater than with melphalan alone. Subsequent clinical trials demonstrate no benefit for doses above 4 mg.[317] The melphalan and TNF regimen has been successfully applied in patients who historically do not respond to melphalan ILP treatment alone. Patients with bulky disease, who historically are less likely to respond to melphalan alone, may have an improved outcome with the addition of TNF.[317] In addition, those who have failed treatment or had recurrences after prior ILP with melphalan or other chemotherapeutics are candidates for TNF therapy.[318] Phase III randomized studies evaluating ILP and melphalan with or without TNF in patients with localized, advanced, extremity involvement are currently underway.

Toxicity

Perioperative toxicity is common but generally tolerable and reversible. Acute regional toxicity after ILP includes pain within the first 48 hours and edema that usually resolves within 14 days. Erythema associated with the procedure fades over a period of 3 to 6 months. Melanomatous lesions soften and flatten, and biopsies show melanin pigment within macrophages without evidence of melanoma cells. Patient age is not an absolute contraindication for perfusion as adverse effects do not appear to be significantly greater in patients greater than 70 years of age.[319] Vrouenraets et al. evaluated 425 patients for treatment-related toxicities after ILP, finding grade I and II toxicities in 85%, grade III and IV toxicities in 15%, and grade V toxicities in 0.5% (Table 42.2-14). The degree of limb toxicity, since it has no correlation with tumor response, should be avoided.[320] Creatinine kinase levels greater than 1000 U after the first postoperative day and temperatures higher than 40°C are both strongly associated with development of severe toxicities.[321] Although some centers recommend prophylactic fasciotomies during ILP, many surgeons simply monitor compartment pressures postoperatively. Renal failure secondary to myoglobinuria can be pre-

TABLE 42.2-12. Wieberdink Grading System for Regional Tissue Toxicity after Isolated Limb Perfusion

Grade I	No subjective evidence of reaction
Grade II	Slight erythema, edema, or both
Grade III	Considerable erythema, edema, or both with some blistering; slightly disturbed motility permissible
Grade IV	Extensive epidermolysis, obvious damage to the deep tissue, or both; causing definite functional disturbances; threatening or manifest compartment syndromes
Grade V	Reaction that may necessitate amputation

(From ref. 538, with permission.)

TABLE 42.2-13. Tumor Response after Isolated Limb Perfusion with Tumor Necrosis Factor and Melphalan[a]

Author	No.	*Complete Response (%)*	*Partial Response (%)*	*Response Rate (%)*
Lienard, 1992[554]	19	84	16	100
Vaglini, 1994[555]				
(4 mg tumor necrosis factor)	11	64	—	64
(1 mg tumor necrosis factor)	10	70	30	100
Lienard, 1994[316]	53	91	9	100
Fraker, 1996[556]	25	76	16	92
Kettelhack, 1997[557]	20	65	15	90
Lienard, 1999[558]	64	75	20	95

[a]Note the much improved response compared with melphalan alone.
Note: No randomized survival data exist directly comparing melphalan and tumor necrosis factor with melphalan alone.

vented by maintaining adequate urine output (greater than 4 L/d) and alkalization (pH greater than 7.5) during the first 2 to 3 postoperative days.[322] Serious long-term sequelae of ILP are uncommon. Mild neuropathies are noted in up to 20% to 40% of patients (possibly from the tourniquet) after perfusion (Table 42.2-15).[323,324] Some advocate the use of drugs other than melphalan to prevent wound complications and edema. The use of dacarbazine, cisplatin, or carboplatin may have less adverse effects but no trial has directly compared the therapeutic and toxic effects of these various regimens.[325] Some evidence suggests that nonmelphalan regimens have more rapid recurrence rates. The incidence of wound complications increases significantly in patients who undergo concurrent lymphadenectomy.[326] Some surgeons opt to perform a lymphadenectomy as a staged procedure after 6 to 8 weeks, whereas others routinely perform them in order to avoid a difficult operation in a previously explored site.

Almost all patients develop hypotension and tachycardia during ILP with TNF. Furthermore, patients undergoing ILP with a TNF with measured leaks of greater than 1% develop mild and transient postoperative hypotension. Prevention of systemic leak and fluid loading before tourniquet release may help prevent the need for vasopressors. The use of a perioperative Swan-Ganz catheter is strongly recommended.[327] Disturbances in pulmonary function are common with TNF but resolve to baseline in 8

TABLE 42.2-14. Regional Toxicity of Isolated Limb Perfusion[a]

		Wieberdink Grade (%)				
Author	*No.*	I	II	III	IV	V
Lejeune, 1989[551]	206	5	57	36	2	—
Klaase, 1994[552]	166	3	84	11	1	1
Van Geel, 1989[539]	57	8	72	16	2	2
Kettelhack, 1990[553]	113	13	67	18	2	—

[a]Limb toxicity is not a predictor of tumor response.

TABLE 42.2-15. Late Morbidity of Isolated Limb Perfusion[a]

Symptom	*Frequency (%)*
Edema	28
Neuropathy	3
Decreased motility	20–50
Pain	8

[a]Most of these complications are not significantly life altering.[539,540]

weeks.[328] Fever, nausea, and reversible hepatic toxicity are also common with TNF protocols.[329] Acute vascular complications are rare (2.1%) and consist mainly of arterial thrombosis for which urgent embolectomy is required.[330]

ISOLATED LIMB INFUSION

Thompson et al. have reported an alternative approach called *isolated limb infusion* with the percutaneous insertion of venous and arterial catheters in the axial vessels followed by proximal tourniquet limb vessel occlusion. The procedure is preformed under normothermic and hypoxic conditions for 30 minutes without an oxygenator, thus avoiding much of the cost and complexity of ILP. Long-term survival results are still pending, but complete response rates comparable with ILP are reported.[331] More investigation of this technique is necessary before wide acceptance.

INTRAARTERIAL THERAPY

Intraarterial cisplatin combined with systemic therapy has been used with only modest success. Fifteen patients treated with systemic vinblastine and dacarbazine and intraarterial cisplatin were observed to have a 67% response rate. Only 45% were complete responses and one was pathologically positive at subsequent biopsy. Given the significant toxicities of this regimen, it is necessary to have more experience before any recommendations can be made.[332]

LOCAL ABLATION

Hill and Thomas reported the use of the ablation of multiple melanoma nodules using a CO_2 laser. Their initial series had a surprising recurrence rate of only 2%.[333] Another small series treated 19 patients with CO_2 laser ablation. After a mean follow-up of 15 months, five patients died from the disease. Among the 14 survivors, 8 have had no limb recurrence and the remaining required further treatments to control disease.[334] In larger European trials, higher recurrence rates with this technique are reported. The use of electrical pulses directly applied to cutaneous metastases after administration of local or systemic bleomycin may have activity against melanoma. In one series, a 91% response rate was noted without any significant reported side effects.[335] The use of photodynamic therapy may have some use in the treatment of patients with in-transit disease. Photodynamic therapy can specifically ablate malignant cells at depths up to 1 cm. There are yet no series of melanoma patients using this technique.[336] These treatments may offer reasonable local control using a minimally invasive approach of nonbulky regional disease.

LOCAL IMMUNOTHERAPY

Local injection of bacille Calmette-Guérin (BCG),[337] IFN-α, and other agents has been occasionally locally effective, but has not shown systemic effect on noninjected metastases and has been occasionally associated with significant toxicity (e.g., Pott's disease with systemic BCG infection).[338,339] For those reasons, BCG is little used at present for local therapy.

RADIOTHERAPY

Radiotherapy can be useful in managing in-transit metastases that are too extensive for surgical resection and as an adjuvant therapy after reresection of recurrent in-transient disease. Treatment techniques and outcome are similar to those for management of lymph node metastases and remote subcutaneous metastases and are discussed in the sections Stage III Disease: Management of the Clinically Positive Nodal Basin and Stage I and II Disease: Management of Primary Melanoma.[180–182,340]

SYSTEMIC THERAPY

The use of dacarbazine and other systemic chemotherapy, biologic agents, or both benefits patients with in-transit disease at rates equivalent to patients with systemic disease. Immunotherapies including IFN and IL-2 have shown benefit in a small number of patients. Patients with in-transit disease may be ideal candidates for immunobiologic intervention because of their low tumor burden. The use of IL-2 and other novel immunotherapies such as IL-12, IL-18, peptide, or DC-based vaccines may prove effective in the future to control in-transit disease. Morton from the John Wayne Cancer Institute has used the CancerVax vaccine for patients with in-transit disease, and in nonrandomized patients suggests an approximate 50% 5-year survival.

ADJUVANT MEDICAL THERAPY

The prognosis of melanoma predicted from staging information allows the designation of low-, intermediate-, high-, and very high-risk groups that serve as guideposts for the potential consideration of adjuvant therapy. Patients previously enrolled in trials of adjuvant therapy have been those at high risk, in whom relapse and mortality risk exceed 50% at 5 years. The entry criteria for patients in high-risk trials has previously included both locally advanced, surgically curable (AJCC stage IIB), and regionally metastatic node-positive melanoma.

The adjuvant therapy of melanoma using IFN and other related agents is here considered separately under the previously defined categories of high-risk for recurrence melanoma (AJCC stage IIB and III), and with intermediate-risk melanoma (AJCC stage IIA). Patients with AJCC stage I disease have a low relapse risk and an excellent overall and relapse-free survival. For this reason, stage I patients are unlikely to benefit from such therapy and have not been the focus of any adjuvant therapy trials.

IMMUNOSTIMULANTS

A number of approaches for postsurgical adjuvant therapy have been tested since 1970. These have included systemic chemotherapy, immunostimulation with crude microbial agents such as BCG,[341] *Corynebacterium parvum*,[342,343] and picibanil, derived from *Streptococcus pyogenes*.[344,345] The antihelminthic chemical immunomodulator levamisole has undergone intensive evaluation.[346–350] Unfortunately, randomized controlled trials have not demonstrated reproducible increases in relapse-free or overall-survival with any of these modalities.

TABLE 42.2-16. Summary of Interferon Trials for Adjuvant Therapy of Melanoma

HIGH-DOSE TRIALS
High-risk melanoma
With induction phase
E1684
E1690 intergroup
E1694 intergroup
Without induction phase
North Central Cancer Treatment Group Trial 837052
LOW-DOSE TRIALS
High-risk melanoma
World Health Organization 16
European Organization for Research and Treatment of Cancer 18871
Intermediate-risk melanoma
French
Austrian
British
INTERMEDIATE-DOSE TRIALS
High-risk melanoma
European Organization for Research and Treatment of Cancer 18952

INTERFERONS

More recently, the use of individual cytokines obtained and partially purified from human cells or synthesized by recombinant DNA technology have demonstrated an effect on the natural history of this disease. The IFNs have been the most intensely studied agents for the adjuvant therapy of intermediate- and high-risk melanoma. Results of randomized controlled clinical trials in the United States National Cooperative Groups have now yielded both positive and negative results using high- and low-dose IFN-α_{2b}. A summary of IFN trials for the adjuvant treatment of melanomas is shown in Table 42.2-16.

The IFNs are a complex family of proteins with diverse functions that are divided into type I (IFN-α, IFN-β, IFN-τ, IFN-ω), type II (IFN-γ) and type III (IL-10, IL-19, IL-20, and IL-21). The IFNs have shown potent immunomodulatory effects *in vivo* and *in vitro* including induction of major histocompatibility antigen expression of both class I (ABC) and class II (DR, DP, and DQ) molecules. Modulation of the number and function of effector cells (NK cell, T cells, monocytes, and DCs) have been well defined, and their function in responding to nominal tumor antigens is now under intense study.[351] The type I IFNs are structurally related species derived from genes on chromosome 9 that are classically induced by exposure of cells to virus or nucleic acids. Type II IFN is produced mainly by T lymphocytes and NK cells, bears little homology to type I IFN, and is coded for by genes located on chromosome 12. The type III members of this family are produced by several lymphoid and myeloid cell types and appear to modify immunity by promoting a humoral immune response, enhancing cytolytic activity, and in some instances, having direct antitumor effects. The types of IFN differ in terms of the receptors with which they interact. IFN-α and INF-β share a common receptor distinct from the receptor that binds IFN-γ and induce a unique intracellular signal transduction cascade. Mixed results of trials examining IFN-α may be due to frequent down-regulation of IFN receptors and responsiveness to IFN after prolonged IFN-α administration. Recombinant DNA technology has allowed the production of virtually unlimited quantities of recombinant IFN, which has facilitated their testing both in the laboratory and in the clinic. In melanoma, IFN-α_2 has been the most extensively evaluated agent, of which three subspecies are commercially available: IFN-α_{2a} (Hoffman LaRoche), INF-α_{2b} (Schering Plough), and IFN-α_{2c} (Boehringer Ingelheim) that differ minimally in amino acid sequence and apparent biologic effects.

Adjuvant Therapy for High-Risk (American Joint Committee on Cancer Stage IIB and III) Melanoma

IFN-α has been widely tested for the adjuvant therapy of melanoma, and the most extensively evaluated IFN-α subspecies has been IFN-α_2. Other agents currently undergoing evaluation in randomized trials include the chemically defined ganglioside vaccines: GM2, keyhole limpet hemocyanin, plus QS 21 (Progenics) and allogeneic whole tumor cell–derived vaccines for which trials are incomplete or inconclusive [Melacine (Corixa) and CancerVax (John Wayne Cancer Institute)]. Regimens using IFN-α_2 for high-risk melanoma can be divided into high-dose regimens given for 1 year, high-dose regimens given for periods of shorter duration (3 months), and low-dose regimens given for longer intervals (of 2 to 3 years). Results of adjuvant IFN trials are shown in Table 42.2-17.

High-Dose Interferon-α_2 for 1 Year: Eastern Cooperative Oncology Group Trial E1684

The ECOG initiated a trial in 1984 (1684) for patients with melanoma at high risk for relapse following surgical resection of primary tumor, regional lymph node metastasis, or both. Twenty-nine centers contributed 287 (280 evaluable) patients who were randomized to treatment with IFN-α_{2b} or observation. Eligibility criteria included the presence of a T4 primary lesion with or without regional lymph node involvement or primary lesions of any depth with pathologically proven regional lymph node involvement. Patients with cutaneous melanoma of any thickness, but with the regional lymph nodes as the site of initial and only relapse were also eligible. All patients underwent regional lymph node dissection and were stratified with respect to clinical and pathologic stage of disease. Maximally tolerable doses of IFN-α_{2b} were used: an initial induction phase of 20 MU/m^2 intravenously daily for 5 to 7 days for 4 weeks was followed by a maintenance phase at 10 MU/m^2 subcutaneously, three times a week for 48 weeks (total treatment duration of 52 weeks). The rationale for the initial high-dose intravenous treatment phase was to provide maximal

TABLE 42.2-17. Trials for Adjuvant Interferon-α_2 for Melanoma

Trial	*Year*	*No.*	*Agent*	*Dose*	*Treatment Duration*	*Outcome Analysis*
ECOG E1684[587]	1984–1989	287	IFN-α_{2b}	20 MU/m^2 IV daily × 5/7 d/wk 10 MU/m^2 SC t.i.w.	4 wk 48 wk	OS $P = .047$ RFS $P = .004$
North Central Cancer Treatment Group 83-7052[588]	1984–1989	262	IFN-α_{2a}	20 MU/m^2 IM t.i.w.	12 wk	OS, RFS P = NS
World Health Organization 16[589]	1990–1993	444	IFN-α_{2a}	3 MU SC t.i.w.	36 mo	OS, RFS P = NS
Southwest Oncology Group 8942[590]	1988–1989	134	IFN-γ	0.1 mg SC t.i.w.	12 mo	OS, RFS P = NS
ECOG E1690	1990–1995	642	IFN-α_{2b}	A. 20 MU/m^2 IV daily × 5/7 d/wk 10 MU/m^2 SC t.i.w. (HDI) or B. 3 MU SC daily t.i.w. (LDI)	4 wk 48 wk 24 mo	HDI RFS $P = .03$ OS = NS LDI: RFS = NS OS = NS
ECOG E1694	1995–1998	880	IFN-α_{2b}vs. GMK vaccine	A. 20 MU/m^2 IV daily × 5/7 d/wk or 10 MU/m^2 SC t.i.w. B. GMK SC 1 wk/3 mo	12 mo 96 wk	HDI RFS = .007 OS = .009
European Organization for Research and Treatment of Cancer 18-871	1987–1994	800	IFN-α_{2b}	A. 1 MU t.i.w. B. 0.2 mg SC t.i.w. C. Observation	1 y 1 y	OS, RFS P = NS
European Organization for Research and Treatment of Cancer	1995–2000	1300	IFN-α_{2b}	A. 10 MU SC daily × 5/7 d/wk × 4 5 MU SC t.i.w. × 23 mo B. 10 MU SC daily × 5/7 d/wk × 4 10 MU SC t.i.w. × 11 mo C. Observation		
E1697	1998	1420	IFN-α_{2b}	20 MU/m^2/d × 5/7 d/wk	4 wk	Ongoing

ECOG, Eastern Cooperative Oncology Group; GMK, keyhole limpet hemocyanin, plus QS 21; HDI, high-dose interferon-α_{2b}; IFN, interferon; LDI, low-dose interferon-α_{2b}; NS, not significant; OS, overall survival; RFS, relapse-free survival.

dose intensity and minimize the induction of anti-IFN antibodies. At a median follow-up of 7 years, a significant improvement in both median relapse-free survival (1.72 vs. 0.98 years) and overall survival (OS) (3.82 vs. 2.78 years) was noted in an intent-to-treat analysis. Patients with established lymph node involvement, *de novo* or recurrent, appeared to derive the greatest benefit from treatment. Only a limited number of patients (31) who were clinically and pathologically node-negative (T4 pN0) entered the study, and an imbalance in the distribution of the important prognostic variable, ulceration, made it difficult to draw firm conclusions for this subset. At five years the 40% improvement in relapse-free survival (26% vs. 37%) and 25% improvement in overall survival (37% vs. 45%) led the Food and Drug Administration to approve the use of IFN-α_{2b} given for 1 year by this intravenous and subcutaneous schedule for patients with stage IIB/T4-N0 and stage III node-positive disease in 1995.

As expected, this regimen was associated with substantial toxicity, and grade 3 and 4 (ECOG toxicity scale) events were noted in the majority of recipients. Dose-modification or delays were required at least once in 50% of patients during the intravenous induction phase and in 48% of patients during the subcutaneous maintenance phase. Most treatment delays occurred in the first 4 months of the regimen. A retrospective quality-of-life (Q-TWiST) analysis revealed a mean gain of 8.9 months without relapse ($P = .03$) and 7 months of overall survival time ($P = .02$) for the IFN-treated patients after 84 months of follow-up as compared with the observation group.[352,353] The treated group experienced severe treatment-related toxicity for an average of 5.8 months. The net result was that the IFN-treated group had more quality-of-life-adjusted survival time than the observation group, regardless of the relative valuations placed on time with toxicity and time with relapse. An economic analysis of the E1684 regimen was also published.[354] The incremental cost of IFN per life-year gained ranged from $13,700 after a projected 35 years to $32,600 at 7 years (the median follow-up of E1684). The benefits of IFN projected over a lifetime yielded incremental cost per life-year or quality-adjusted life-year that are less than $16,000. This compares favorably with the rigorous Canadian benchmark of $20,000 per quality-of-life-year gained and is comparable with other accepted adjuvant therapies of breast and colorectal cancer.

To evaluate the observations regarding the results of trial E1684 and to evaluate concurrently the high-dose regimen and a low-dose IFN-α_{2b} regimen against observation, Intergroup trial E1690 was initiated in 1991. This trial was designed and implemented before the availability of mature data from the E1684 trial. Eligibility criteria for E1690 were similar to those for E1684 but dropped the requirement for regional lymphadenectomy for patients with deep (T4, greater than 4 mm) primary lesions. Six hundred forty-two (95% eligible) patients were randomized to either high-dose IFN-α_{2b} as in E1684, low-dose IFN-α_{2b} for 2 years (IFN-α_{2b} 3 MU subcutaneously, TIW), or observation. At a median follow-up of 52 months, the 5-year estimated relapse-free survival for high-dose IFN-α_{2b}, low-dose IFN-α_{2b}, and observation were 44%, 40%, and 35%, respectively. High-dose IFN-α_{2b} showed a significant effect on relapse-free survival as compared with observation in a Cox analysis ($P_2 = .03$), prolonging median time to relapse by 10 months. There was no significant effect of low-dose IFN-α_{2b} on relapse-free survival, and neither high-dose IFN-α_{2b} nor low-dose IFN-α_{2b} demonstrated a benefit in overall survival.

Of note, the median overall survival for patients assigned to observation in E1690 was 6 years as compared with only 2.8 years for observed patients on E1684. The question has arisen whether the use of systemic IFN-α_{2b} among one-third of patients who relapsed (n = 38), who were originally assigned to observation, may have been in part responsible for the large gain in postrelapse survival seen in E1690. The postrelapse survival for patients originally assigned to observation who subsequent to relapse received IFN, versus those who never received IFN, was significantly prolonged (median 2.2 years vs. 0.8 years; $P = .0024$). Other factors that could potentially account for the improved outcome for patients on this trial randomized to observation include the use of more accurate staging techniques or more modern surgical intervention at initial treatment, subsequent relapse, or both.

High-Dose Regimens of IFN-α of Intermediate Duration

The North Central Cancer Treatment Group (NCCTG) performed a randomized trial of high-dose IFN-α_{2a} given for 3 months (intramuscular, TIW) versus observation in 262 patients with primary melanomas of thickness greater than 1.69 mm deep or with presenting or recurrent regional lymph node involvement. The dose of IFN-α_{2a} used was 20 MU/m^2 given intramuscularly TIW for 12 weeks and reached a total dose approximately one-half that of the E1684 high-dose regimen. At a median follow-up of 6.1 years, the median relapse-free and overall survival were not significantly different for the two arms of the study. For patients with regional lymph node involvement, the improvement in median recurrence-free survival was significant by Cox analysis ($P_2 = .03$) for the IFN-α_{2a}–treated patients (17 months vs. 10 months), without a significant difference in overall survival. The limited number of patients in this subset does not permit a firm conclusion regarding the benefit of this regimen on either relapse-free or overall survival or the treated population as a whole.

Low-Dose Interferon-α_{2a} for 2 to 3 Years

The use of lower, nontoxic doses of IFN-α_{2a} for high-risk melanoma has been studied both in the United States and in Europe. Between 1990 and 1993, the WHO Melanoma Program entered 444 patients to a randomized trial comparing 3 years of treatment with IFN-α_{2a} (3 MU subcutaneously, TIW) or observation. This trial differed from the ECOG and NCCTG trials in regard to eligibility: Only patients with regional lymph node metastases were eligible for randomization after lymphadenectomy. One-half of the patients studied had extracapsular extension with lymph node involvement, a feature that was excluded from ECOG studies 1684, 1690, and the NCCTG 837052 trials. A preliminary report at 22 months median follow-up suggested prolongation of recurrence-free survival among women younger than 50 years and men older than 50 years, while a somewhat more mature interim report at 39 months median follow-up revealed no durable benefit in terms of either relapse-free interval or overall survival; a final publication is pending.[355,356] The negative results of the low-dose arm of the Intergroup trial E1690 discussed previously[357] confirm the results of WHO 16, both in terms of recurrence rates and overall survival for patients with high-risk melanoma.

The EORTC Trial 18952 is currently testing two intermediate doses of IFN-α_{2b} in high-risk melanoma patients. The study design incorporates two treatment arms and an observation arm. Treatment comprises a *modified induction* phase of IFN-α_{2b},

10 MU subcutaneously injected, five times per week, followed either by 10 MU subcutaneously injected three times per week, for 1 year or 5 MU subcutaneously injected, TIW for 2 years. This study will accrue 1200 patients with high-risk resected melanoma, including patients with nodal disease with or without extracapsular extension, of whom 200 will be randomized to observation and 400 to each of the IFN arms (1:2:2 unbalanced assignment) to evaluate the role of dose intensity. The Nordic Melanoma Trial group are investigating the efficacy of two intermediate dosages of IFN-α_{2b} administered for 2 years, using a similar subcutaneous daily induction treatment. While the induction phase and the maintenance phase are modeled on the pivotal E1684 trial, it is important to note that the peak levels of IFN-α_2 attained by the intravenous administration of 20 MU/m^2/d are orders of magnitude higher than the levels that can be detected following the administration of 10 MU/d, especially when given by the subcutaneous route (10,000 μ/mL vs. less than 100 μ/mL peak).

Vaccines in the Adjuvant Therapy of Stage IIB and III Melanoma

A number of vaccine approaches are being evaluated in the adjuvant treatment of patients with melanoma. Biochemical analysis has shown the presence of gangliosides of several series in melanoma, including GD3, GD3, GM1, GM2, and GM3, among others. In general, the purified gangliosides have not been shown to be immunogenic, and it has been difficult to induce antibody responses to these molecules with the exception of the ganglioside GM2, to which antibody responses have been detected spontaneously in up to 5% of patients with melanoma. Two studies have demonstrated that the presence of anti-GM2 antibodies confers a relapse-free survival advantage for patients with melanoma.[358,359] This led to the conduct of a randomized controlled trial of GM2 plus BCG versus BCG alone (both with cyclophosphamide pretreatment) in 122 patients with AJCC stage III melanoma, at the Memorial Sloan-Kettering Cancer Center in New York. GM2 antibody was detected in 50 of 58 patients treated with GM2/BCG and in only 7 of 64 patients treated with BCG alone. Patients with anti-GM2 antibodies, either preexisting or induced by treatment, had a significantly longer relapse-free survival than antibody-negative patients. A nonsignificant increase in disease-free interval (18%) and overall survival (11%) was found for the GM2/BCG-treated group as a whole. However, exclusion of patients with preexisting anti-GM2 antibodies from the analysis suggested a benefit in terms of disease-free interval for those who developed an antibody response to GM2.

A range of efforts to improve the immunogenicity of the GM2 molecule were tested, including conjugation to immunogenic carrier molecules, and admixture with potent new immunologic adjuvant agents. These have subsequently been found to induce more frequent and higher titer antibody responses to the GM2 molecule. The most potent combination tested uses the GM2 molecule coupled with a carrier protein derived from the keyhole limpet hemocyanin with an immunoadjuvant, QS21, a potent immunologic adjuvant of the saponin class. This vaccine induces qualitatively improved antibody responses of the IgG as well as IgM isotype, of higher titer than obtained by GM2 plus BCG. The GM2, keyhole limpet hemocyanin, plus QS21 vaccine has been developed for clinical evaluation (Progenics, New York, NY; Bristol Myers Squibb) and is currently being compared with high-dose IFN-α_{2b} in the Intergroup U.S. Trial E1694 for patients with AJCC stage IIB and III melanoma. This trial initiated in 1996 completed accrual of 880 patients in 1999, and its results have recently been unblinded due to the significant relapse-free interval and overall survival advantage of HDI, substantially confirming both RFS ($P = .007$) and OS ($P = .009$) benefits of HDI observed in E1684.

The John Wayne Cancer Institute has performed a series of phase II trials employing cultured tumor cell–derived vaccines (CancerVax) administered with the immunostimulant BCG for patients with metastatic disease as well as intermediate- and high-risk resected melanoma.[138,360] Encouraging phase II results have led to the initiation of two ongoing phase III randomized trials of adjuvant therapy for high-risk melanoma and resected metastatic disease patients believed to be at very high risk of recurrence. The first of these is comparing CancerVax plus BCG to BCG alone for the postsurgical treatment of AJCC stage III melanoma. The second is a randomized trial of CancerVax versus placebo for patients with stage IV melanoma rendered clinically disease free with surgery. Firm conclusions will only be possible regarding the therapeutic benefit of these vaccines as these first randomized controlled trials are completed and mature.

On the basis of evidence that cellular immune responses to melanosomal antigens may be of therapeutic value, peptide antigens that represent the immunodominant and subdominant melanosomal antigens have been brought into multicenter adjuvant trial for patients with resectable stage IV (M1) or advanced stage III melanoma in an ECOG study E4697. E4697 will investigate treatment with a multiepitope three-peptide vaccine composed of Melan-A/MART-1, gp100, and tyrosinase antigens that have been studied previously in the National Cancer Institute Surgery Branch and the University of Pittsburgh Melanoma Center/Biologics Program.[361,362]

Adjuvant Therapy for Intermediate-Risk Melanoma

Patients with T3, Breslow depth 1.5 to 4.0 mm (S1992 AJCC stage IIA) melanoma account for a substantial fraction of patients at presentation and represent a heterogeneous group with 5-year survival greater than 72%. This category is historically twice as frequent as the stage III category, representing 31% of new melanomas. With 47,000 new cases of melanoma in the United States, approximately 19,000 represent stage II melanoma and from this group 5400 deaths are anticipated. This group of patients has been the focus of several completed European and newly initiated North American cooperative group studies.

Low-Dose Interferon-α for 18 Months

Adjuvant therapy trials for high-risk melanoma have generally excluded patients with stage IIA melanoma, although a subset of patients in the NCCTG trial 83-7052 (100 patients) had stage II disease. Austrian, French, and Scottish trial groups have evaluated the low-dosage regimen tested in E1690 and WHO 16 in regimens of IFN-α administered for shorter periods of 12 to 18 months for patients with stage II melanoma (defined by clinical examination alone). The results of these trials are therefore difficult to apply to patients for whom more precise staging, by means of sentinel node mapping, is available.

The French Cooperative Group on Melanoma randomized 499 patients with AJCC stage II melanoma to IFN-α_{2a}, 3 MU subcutaneous TIW injections for 18 months, or observation. After a median follow-up of 5 years, a significant improvement in relapse-free survival ($P = .038$) but not in overall survival ($P = .059$) was noted.[363] The Austrian Malignant Melanoma Cooperative Group has reported a smaller trial that is somewhat less mature, at a mean follow-up of only 41 months.[364] Three hundred eleven patients were randomized to observation or treatment with IFN-α_{2a}, 3 MU subcutaneous daily injections for 3 weeks, followed by 3 MU subcutaneous TIW injections for 1 year. The prolongation of relapse-free survival noted in this trial ($P = .02$) must be qualified given the short follow-up period; and the absence as yet of any overall survival data for this trial.[365,366]

Patients entering these trials included those with stage IIA and stage IIB, but neither elective lymph node staging (as in E1684) nor sentinel node mapping were pursued in any participants. This stage grouping therefore represents a heterogeneous population for which multicenter sentinel lymphadenectomy trials suggest that SLNs would be positive in 20% to 28% of patients with T3, T4 melanomas, respectively. The sentinel node mapping technique has had its greatest effect in refining the prognosis for these nominal stage II patients. Sentinel node mapping is an established method for staging these patients, which defines node-negative subgroups at lower risk. These results of the reported studies of low-dose IFN-α_{2a} show prolonged relapse-free interval for patients with intermediate-risk melanoma during treatment, with loss of this benefit over time following discontinuation of therapy. These results differ from the results of the high-dose regimens described previously in showing no durable effect on continuous relapse-free survival. Indeed, one of the conclusions that may be drawn from the Austrian and French experience, is that indefinite therapy may be required to achieve durable relapse-free benefit with low dosage IFN-α_2.

High-Dose Interferon-α for 4 Weeks

The high-dose IFN regimens used in E1684 and E1690 were unique in their incorporation of an induction phase of intravenous therapy for the initial 4 weeks, at maximal tolerable dosages. The rationale for the induction phase was to provide peak levels of IFN-α_{2b} sufficient to inhibit tumor growth directly, as well as antivascular, and immunomodulatory effects on antigen-presenting and T-cell responses against melanoma antigens while avoiding the potential for induction of anti-IFN antibodies. The relative importance of the induction phase is suggested by the early effect of E1684 and E1690 regimens, in which hazard functions for relapse-free survival demonstrate early suppression of relapse risk with high-dose IFN-α_{2b} that is sustained for years after discontinuation of treatment. This has led to the hypothesis that peak dose exposure during induction may represent the critical component of the E1684/1690 regimens. Patient acceptance and tolerance for the intravenous induction phase is excellent. Dose modifications were required in one-half of patients during this phase (a fraction equivalent to the portion requiring dose modification during the subsequent maintenance phase). Removal from treatment was rarely necessary during this interval.

To help clarify the role of high-dose induction intravenous therapy, the ECOG and National Cancer Institute of Canada are currently conducting a randomized trial of intravenous therapy for 4 weeks alone, for patients with intermediate-risk stage IIA and IIB or microscopic nodal stage III N1A disease. Pathologic staging with SLN mapping and biopsy (or ELND) is encouraged but not mandatory, and patients are stratified according to the method of staging. Patients are randomized to receive either the intravenous induction therapy administered as in the first month of E1684 (IFN-α_{2b} 20 MU/m^2 5/week) or observation. To demonstrate a 7.5% improvement in relapse-free survival for the treated population with 80% power will require 1420 patients in this trial.

Sunbelt Trial

A multicenter adjuvant trial that has been designated the Sunbelt Trial tests the role of high-dose IFN-α_{2a} in patients who are staged by SLN mapping procedures and in which both routine (H&E and immunohistochemical) and molecular assays (RT-PCR for multiple markers including tyrosinase, MAGE, and gp100) are conducted. One goal is to assess the significance of molecular markers in contrast to immunohistochemistry and standard H&E. This study will require 3000 patients to have a power to assess its multiple goals.

Vaccine Trial for Intermediate-Risk Melanoma

A commercial vaccine preparation from cultured tumor cell lines (Melacine, Corixa) given together with the proprietary adjuvant agent Detox (monophosphoryl lipid A) has also been shown to induce antitumor responses in patients with metastatic melanoma.[367–369] A pilot experience suggests improved responses in recipients who have been administered IFN-α_{2b}. The Melacine-cultured melanoma tumor cell vaccine administered with the monophosphoryl lipid A adjuvant Detox has been tested by the Southwest Oncology Group for the adjuvant therapy of patients with T3 melanoma (SWOG 9035). This trial was conducted between 1990 and 1996, with 700 patients having received either the vaccine with Detox, or observation, after primary melanoma resection. Results of this trial have been preliminarily reported, showing no significant prolongation of relapse-free and overall survival in a primary efficacy analysis, but a significant effect in an intention-to-treat analysis that has yet to be clarified.[370]

TREATMENT OF STAGE IV DISEASE

Metastatic melanoma has a median survival of only 6 to 9 months and current systemic therapy has been shown to induce complete durable responses in only a small minority of patients.[371] Most common sites of initial presentation with metastatic disease are the skin, lungs, liver, brain, and bone. Chemotherapy agents, biologic agents individually and in various combinations, and surgery have been used in the treatment of these patients.

RADIOGRAPHIC ROLE IN THE DIAGNOSIS OF STAGE IV DISEASE

Weiss et al. performed a retrospective study on 261 malignant melanoma patients with resected local (greater than or equal to 1.69 mm) and regional nodal disease. Follow-up consisted of physical examination, complete blood cell count, blood chemistry panel, and chest radiography and was performed every 2 and 4 months for the first 1 and 2 years, respectively, followed by every 6 months for the subsequent 3 years. Out of 145 evaluable patients with recurrent disease, 32% were asymptomatic. Physical examination detected 37 of 45 (82%) of the asymptomatic recurrences. Chest radiography detected the other 9 of 45 (22%) recurrences, while no recurrences were detected by blood tests alone.[372] Bassares et al. studied 115 relapses in follow-up of 528 stage I melanoma patients. History and physical examination detected 90% of relapses, with chest radiography and abdominal ultrasound detecting the rest. Only two recurrences were resectable.[373] Roth et al. evaluated bone, brain, and liver scans in the follow-up of 58 patients with node-positive melanoma. Only one patient with a true positive bone scan was found, thus calling into question its utility in patients with melanoma.[374]

METASTASECTOMY AND RADIOTHERAPY

Surgical treatment of asymptomatic, distant metastatic lesions remains controversial because of the likelihood of widespread disease at other sites. However, a subgroup of patients exists that may benefit from surgical resection of metastatic lesions, and some surgeons have advocated the more widespread application of surgery in stage IV disease. Unfortunately, no randomized trials exist to support the use of metastasectomy. Retrospective reviews, largely from single institutions, have reported a survival difference in selected operated melanoma patients compared with historic controls. Although, metastatic melanoma has a worse prognosis (by a factor of two) after resection than other carcinomas, prolonged 5-year survival in some patients has been reported following complete resection of melanoma metastases of the lung, soft tissue, and even gastrointestinal tract.[375–380] Metastasectomy in melanoma has also been advocated because of the absence of a demonstrable survival effect with currently available systemic therapies in more rigorous randomized controlled trials. However, the rigor with which systemic therapy has been tested is far greater than that with which surgical approaches have been evaluated to date. Although numerous series show survival benefits for metastasectomy compared with historic controls, selection bias may account for these differences. Unfortunately, randomized trials to determine the efficacy of surgery in this setting are not likely.

Metastasectomy should be considered in the absence of locoregional disease and when metastatic disease is confined to a single site that is amenable to complete resection. Before the application of metastasectomy with therapeutic intent, patients must be able to tolerate the operation and have appropriate staging studies demonstrating limited disease. The paradigm for optimal staging includes the use of brain magnetic resonance imaging, whole body CT, and PET scanning. The use of immunotherapy following metastasectomy may afford a more suitable setting for demonstration of the potential benefits of vaccine immunotherapy, as researchers at the John Wayne Cancer Institute are attempting to demonstrate.[381]

Nonvisceral Metastasis

More than one-half of patients who have recurrent melanoma manifest disease initially at nonvisceral sites, and one-half of these lesions may be solitary.[382,383] Adequate data predicting prognosis in patients with nonvisceral metastasis range wildly, making the assessment of metastectomy's efficacy difficult. Following complete resection, median survivals of 8 to 50 months have been reported with 5-year survival between 10% and 61% of patients.[382,384–388] Radiotherapy is an alternative to surgery for managing symptomatic skin metastases not responding to systemic therapy. Impending skin breakdown and pain at the tumor site are relative indications for local ablative therapy. Lesions may respond to radiotherapy using high-dose fractions and high total doses. Commonly used fractionation schemes are 20 Gy/5 fractions and 30 Gy/10 fractions given in conventional daily fractions, or by means of hypofractionated schedules such as 21 Gy/3 fractions and 30 to 36 Gy/5 to 6 fractions.

Pulmonary Metastasis

The lung is the sole site of initial recurrence in 7% to 21% of melanoma patients and is the most common initial visceral site of metastatic disease. Lung metastases are usually detected as asymptomatic lesions on screening chest radiographs.[376,389] Up to one-third of these are benign or represent a new primary neoplasm, suggesting the importance of biopsy and pathologic confirmation.[390,391] There is conflicting information concerning prognostic factors such as rapidity of tumor growth, the disease-free interval, the number of lesions, and survival after metastasectomy. One factor that clearly correlates with median survival after resection is the ability to completely remove all metastatic disease.

The rapidity of tumor growth may affect survival after metastasectomy. The average melanoma has a tumor-doubling time of 30 days. Patients with a tumor-doubling time of greater than 60 days have a median survival of 23 months with a 5-year survival rate of 16%. Patients with a tumor doubling time less than 60 days had a median survival of 16 months and no 5-year survivors were reported. In a multivariate analysis, the number of pulmonary lesions, bilateral location, disease-free interval before diagnosis of pulmonary metastases, and size of the nodules did not significantly affect survival.[390,392]

Five-year survival after pulmonary metastasectomy is 20% to 27%.[375,376] Historic data suggest a median survival of 10 months in patients with disease confined to the lungs alone who were treated with dacarbazine, and the 1-year survival rate for patients receiving nonsurgical treatment was reported to be 36%.[382,393] In a retrospective study, improved survival was found when a second resection was performed after localized recurrence from a previous metastasectomy. Twenty percent of patients who had a second complete metastasectomy for melanoma were alive at 5 years.[394]

Although no randomized trials exist, the resection of pulmonary metastases has been suggested in patients with melanoma whose preoperative radiographic workup showed no evidence of extrapulmonary disease. Almost all of these resections can be done using minimally invasive techniques, and even bilateral procedures can be undertaken with low morbidity. Following patients' chest radiographs serially for a sufficient period may be a reasonable option in order to measure tumor-doubling time and reassess tumor burden when such therapy is considered. The rationale for such heroic surgical approaches may increase if adjuvant trials with IFNs, vaccines, or combinations are found to have a benefit in operable stage IV disease. These resected patients are ideal candidates for adjuvant immunotherapy trials as patients with limited tumor burden may respond better.

Gastrointestinal Metastasis

Only 5% of all patients who die of melanoma develop symptoms from gastrointestinal disease.[389] Most have multiple lesions and the goal of surgery has been palliation of obstruction, perforation, or bleeding. Median survival after palliative surgery is only 10 months.[395] The diagnosis of a solitary gastrointestinal lesion is quite uncommon; nonetheless, after resection of solitary gastrointestinal lesions, 5-year survival rates have been reported to be as high as 28% to 41% from some centers.[377,378]

There is no evidence that invasive procedures for the treatment of hepatic metastasis benefits patients. There are occasional case reports of long-term survival after resections of isolated hepatic melanoma metastasis, but no substantial series exists in the literature. Hepatic metastasectomy cannot be recommended outside an investigational protocol setting.[396] A series examining the use of isolated hepatic perfusion for hepatic melanoma metastasis has also only reported limited response rates in a small number of patients.[397] At the University of Pittsburgh, hepatic metastasis from ocular melanoma demonstrates no advantage for cisplatin via hepatic artery administration and embolic occlusion of the hepatic artery over systemic administration, even with doses beyond the limits of systemic tolerance.

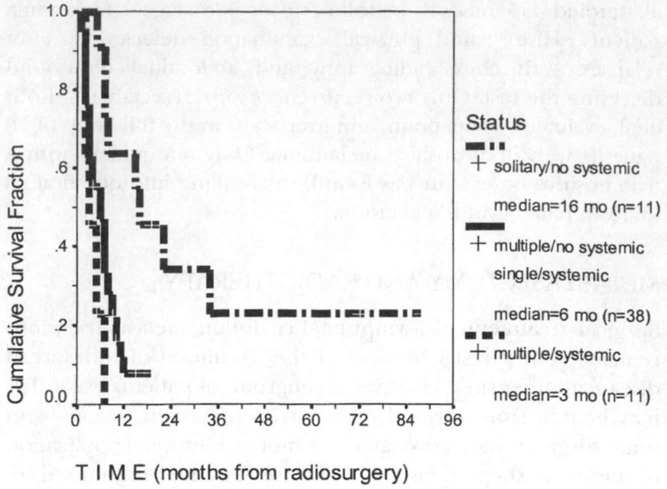

FIGURE 42.2-25. Actuarial survival curves for 60 patients with malignant melanoma treated by gamma knife radiosurgery. Survival is compared for patients with solitary brain metastasis and no active systemic disease (solitary/no systemic) at radiosurgery (n = 11), multiple brain metastases and active systemic disease (multiple/systemic) at radiosurgery (n = 11), and the remaining patients with either solitary brain metastasis and active systemic disease (single/systemic) or multiple brain metastases without active systemic disease (multiple/no systemic) at radiosurgery (n = 38). Some patients with limited brain disease and no systemic disease are able to enjoy prolonged survival. (From ref. 409, with permission.)

Adrenal Metastasis

Isolated adrenal metastases are uncommon; however, a large retrospective series of 83 patients suggested a benefit for surgical excision. Twenty-seven patients underwent surgical exploration and 18 were rendered clinically free of disease at surgery. There was a median survival of 25.7 months for patients rendered disease free compared with only 9.2 months after a palliative resection. Removal of resectable lesions is a reasonable option if other approaches are unavailable, although there is a substantial likelihood of selection bias rather than surgery *per se* accounting for the suggested benefits.[398]

Bone Metastasis

Melanoma metastasizes to the bone relatively late in the disease course. Median survival is just 4 months after diagnosis. Truncal melanomas have a higher percentage of bony metastases compared with melanomas found at other sites.[399] Of those with bone metastases, 67% responded to palliative radiotherapy or decompression with good pain relief.[400] Bone metastases from melanoma respond in a similar fashion to bone metastases from other tumors, with doses of 8 Gy/1 fraction, 20 Gy/5 fractions, or 30 Gy/10 fractions.

Brain Metastasis

Brain metastases are detected clinically in 8% to 46% of patients and at autopsy in 55% to 75% of melanoma patients.[401–403] Brain metastases usually require treatment to relieve symptoms, and available options depend on the number and location of lesions. Corticosteroid treatment often reduces symptoms by ameliorating swelling in many patients and may provide palliation. Melanoma metastatic to the brain is reasonably treated by gamma knife irradiation or surgically, if the lesion is solitary, symptomatic, and can be treated without major neurologic injury.

A series of patients with symptomatic, solitary, intracranial lesions showed a median survival after craniotomy of only 10 months.[404] Patients who responded to previous immunotherapy and subsequently relapsed with intracranial disease seem to enjoy more significant benefit after craniotomy. Forty patients with melanoma or renal cell cancer metastasis involving the brain were reported in a study by the NCI. Thirty-six were rendered free of disease after resection of a single metastasis. The median survival after craniotomy for patients exhibiting complete response, partial response, and no response to previous immunotherapy was 23, 17, and 7 months, respectively. Of the ten patients who had achieved a prior complete response, eight remained disease free in the brain at last follow-up and some have had long-term survival. Twenty-five patients experienced neurologic symptoms before craniotomy, and all had complete resolution of their symptoms after surgical excision. The benefits of resection include palliation of symptoms and the potential for a prolonged disease-free interval in the brain.[405]

The role of conventional radiation for multiple lesions or unresectable disease is controversial.[406] Possibly, because of the sensitivity of the brain to large-dose fractions, studies of whole brain radiotherapy with high-dose fractions have shown little survival improvement.[407] Whole brain radiotherapy (30 Gy/10 fractions) is standard therapy for multiple brain metastases with initial radiosurgery beneficial for cases with two to four metastases.[408] Radiosurgery alone is recommended for patients with solitary brain metastases less than 3 cm in diameter (Figs. 42.2-25 and 42.2-26). Resection followed by whole brain irradiation is recommended for larger lesions with significant mass effect unrelieved by corticosteroids. The local control rates with stereotactic radiosurgery employing single-fraction minimum tumor doses of 16 to 20 Gy are excellent. Mori reported the University of Pittsburgh experience with gamma knife radiosurgery (median marginal dose, 16 Gy; range, 10 to 20 Gy) in 118 brain melanoma brain metastases (median volume, 2.95 mL; range, 0.1 to 25.5 mL) in 60 patients.[409] Median survival was 7 months after radiosurgery and 10 months after the initial diagnosis of brain metastasis, with a 90% local control rate. Local tumor progression developed in seven patients and subsequent remote brain metastases developed in 14 patients. Multivariate analysis demonstrated improved survival was associated with solitary brain metastases and for patients with no other active systemic disease.

CYTOTOXIC CHEMOTHERAPY

Chemotherapeutic agents that have been most widely applied in metastatic disease are dacarbazine, the platinum analogs, nitrosoureas, and microtubular toxins (Table 42.2-18). Dacarbazine is considered the reference agent for melanoma, with a response rate of 14% to 20% in multiple series and a median response durations of 4 to 6 months.[410] Long-term follow-up of patients treated with dacarbazine alone indicates that less than 2% of patients survive 6 years. Although early limited phase II and III trials suggested a benefit of tamoxifen, IFN-α_{2b}, or cisplatin when added to dacarbazine for patients with metastatic disease, these benefits have not been confirmed in large-scale multicenter phase III trials. More recently completed phase III trials using dacarbazine-based combinations are summarized in Table 42.2-19.

The role of dacarbazine combinations involving either tamoxifen or IFN-α_{2b} has been carefully evaluated. In 1992, a prospective randomized trial of dacarbazine and tamoxifen versus dacarbazine alone indicated that the combination therapy might be more effective.[75,411] A 28% response rate and 41-week median survival was reported for patients receiving dacarbazine plus tamoxifen versus only a 12% response rate and 23-week median survival for patients treated with dacarbazine alone. The benefit of tamoxifen in this setting was attributed to the potentiation of the cytotoxic chemotherapy rather than to direct antitumor hormonal (antiestrogenic) effects. In a small, randomized trial that compared dacarbazine with dacarbazine and high-dose IFN-α_2, the combination therapy produced 12 complete and four partial responses in 30 patients compared with only two complete and four partial responses among 30 patients treated with dacarbazine alone.[412,413] Median response duration and survival were significantly prolonged when dacarbazine was combined with IFN-α_2. Unfortunately, a large-scale four-arm two-by-two factorial phase III ECOG trial has reexamined the benefit of both tamoxifen and IFN-α_{2b} using the same protocol and failed to confirm the initial encouraging observations.[154,414] The overall response rate in this trial (ECOG 3690) was 18% (range, 12% to 21% for the four arms), and median time to treatment failure was 2.6 months. Median survival was identical for all four arms tested at 9.1 months. There was no advantage in terms of response or survival attributable to the addition of IFN-α_{2b}, tamoxifen, or both agents, to dacarbazine. There is no evidence, based on this trial and the cumulative observations from prior studies to support the use of IFN-α or tamoxifen in combination with dacarbazine in metastatic melanoma. Unfortunately, we also have no clear indication that dacarbazine itself provides any substantial survival benefit, although it represents conventional therapy at this time.

Many chemotherapy combinations have produced response rates ranging from 30% to 50% in single-institution phase II trials for metastatic melanoma. Two of the most active combinations reported are the three-drug combination of cisplatin/vinblastine/dacarbazine (CVD) developed by Legha and the group at M. D. Anderson and the four-drug combination of cisplatin/dacarbazine/carmustine and tamoxifen (CDBT) developed by Del Prete at Dartmouth and known commonly as the Dartmouth combination.[415–417] The CVD regimen produced responses in 40% of 50 patients with 4% complete response and a median response duration of 9 months.[418] In a randomized multicenter trial comparing CVD with dacarbazine alone encompassing approximately 150 patients, the CVD arm produced a 19% response rate compared with 14% for dacarbazine alone with no differences in either response duration or survival.[419]

The four-drug CDBT or Dartmouth regimen produced responses in 46% of 141 patients (16 complete response and 49 partial responses).[420] Median response duration for this large population was more than 7 months. The inclusion of tamoxifen was suggested to be essential with response rates of 10% when tamoxifen was omitted.[420] However, a randomized phase III NCI Canada Melanoma Trial comparing CDBT with CDB alone showed a response rate of 30% for the CDBT arm and no added value resulting from tamoxifen.[421] In 1999, a randomized phase III trial

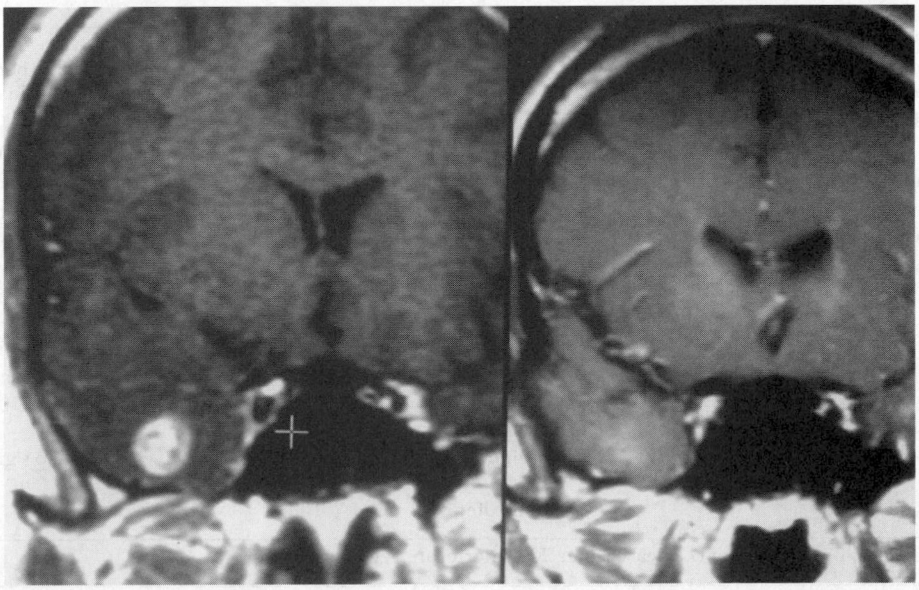

FIGURE 42.2-26. Radiosurgery of melanoma. Solitary right temporal metastasis from malignant melanoma treated by radiosurgery alone to a dose of 20 Gy at the 50% isodose volume (*left*) and at follow-up 17 months later (*right*).

TABLE 42.2-18. Single Agents with Activity Against Melanoma

Agent	*No.*	*Response Rate (Complete Response + Partial Response (%)*
Alkylators		
Dacarbazine	1868	20
Dibromodulcitol	144	20
Nitrosoureas		
Carmustine	122	13
Lomustine	270	16
Semustine	347	16
Fotemustine	226	25
Stathmokinetic agents		
Vincristine	52	12
Vinblastine	62	13
Vindesine	273	14
Taxol	71	17
Platinum analogues		
Cisplatin/carboplatin	137	15
Cytokines		
Interferon-α_2	332	15.4
Interleukin-2	283	17

performed by a consortium including ECOG and Memorial Sloan-Kettering Cancer Center showed no benefit for the CDBT combination relative to dacarbazine alone. This trial involved 240 patients, and the response rate with dacarbazine was 10.2% compared with 18.5% for the CDBT regimen ($P = .09$). The median survival time from randomization was 7 months, with no difference between the two treatment arms. Toxicity was substantially greater, with bone marrow suppression, nausea, vomiting, and fatigue significantly more frequent with the CDBT treatment regimen than with dacarbazine. Taken together, current controlled trials to date have shown no compelling evidence to support the value of combination chemotherapy.

Temozolomide is a nonclassical prodrug of MTIC (5-(3-N-methyltriazen-l-yl)-imidazole-4-carboxamide), the alkylating agent that is the active metabolite of dacarbazine. Temozolomide spontaneously converts into its active metabolite and in several trials has shown antitumor activity against melanoma that is at least equivalent to that of dacarbazine. A randomized phase III study of temozolomide versus dacarbazine was published in which patients with advanced melanoma were randomly assigned to receive either oral temozolomide at a starting dose of 200 mg/m^2/d for 5 days every 28 days or intravenous dacarbazine at a starting dose of 250 mg/m^2/d for 5 days every 21 days. Median survival was 7.7 months for patients treated with temozolomide and 6.4 months for those treated with dacarbazine. No major differences in toxicity were seen. Systemic levels of the active metabolite MTIC were higher than with the intravenous dosing of dacarbazine, and overall quality of life was improved with temozolomide.[422] Temozolomide also has been examined in phase I trials for use in conjunction with cisplatin and has been shown to be safe at the studied dosages.[423] The most attractive advantage of temozolomide is the well-documented penetration of third spaces such as the central nervous system (CNS) and ascites fluid. Approximately one-half of the circulating levels in the blood has been documented in the CNS, and temozolomide has been shown to be an active agent against CNS melanoma, as well as glioblastoma multiforme. Failure to demonstrate improvements

TABLE 42.2-19. Pivotal Phase III Trials of Chemotherapy Combinations for Stage IV Melanoma

Protocol/Principal Investigator	*Treatment*	*No.*	*Response (%)*	*Comments*
GOIRC Italian Group	Dacarbazine	52	12	Improved response and survival for dacarbazine and tamoxifen (not significant in women)
Cocconi[595]	Dacarbazine/tamoxifen	60	28	
Pretoria-South Africa	Dacarbazine	31	20	Improved response and survival for dacarbazine and IFN-α_2
Falkson[154]	Dacarbazine/IFN-α_2	30	53	
National Cancer Institutes–Canada Melanoma Group	CBD	100	21	No benefit from addition of tamoxifen to combination
Rusthoven[596]	CBD/tamoxifen	104	30	
M. D. Anderson Cancer Center	CVD	75	19	No significant difference
Buzaid[597]	Dacarbazine	75	14	
Eastern Cooperative Oncology Group E3690	Dacarbazine	69	15	No benefit from addition of IFN, tamoxifen, or both to dacarbazine
Falkson[598]	Dacarbazine/IFN-α_2	68	21	
	Dacarbazine/tamoxifen	66	18	
	Dacarbazine/IFN-α_2/tamoxifen	68	19	
North Central Cancer Treatment Group	CBD	92	33	No benefit from addition of tamoxifen
Creagan[588]	CBD/tamoxifen	92	27	
M91-140	Dacarbazine	118	10	No significant difference in response rate or survival; toxicity greater with CBD/tamoxifen
Chapman[417]	CBD/tamoxifen	108	18.5	

C, cisplatin; B, carmustine; D, dacarbazine; IFN, interferon; V, vinblastine.

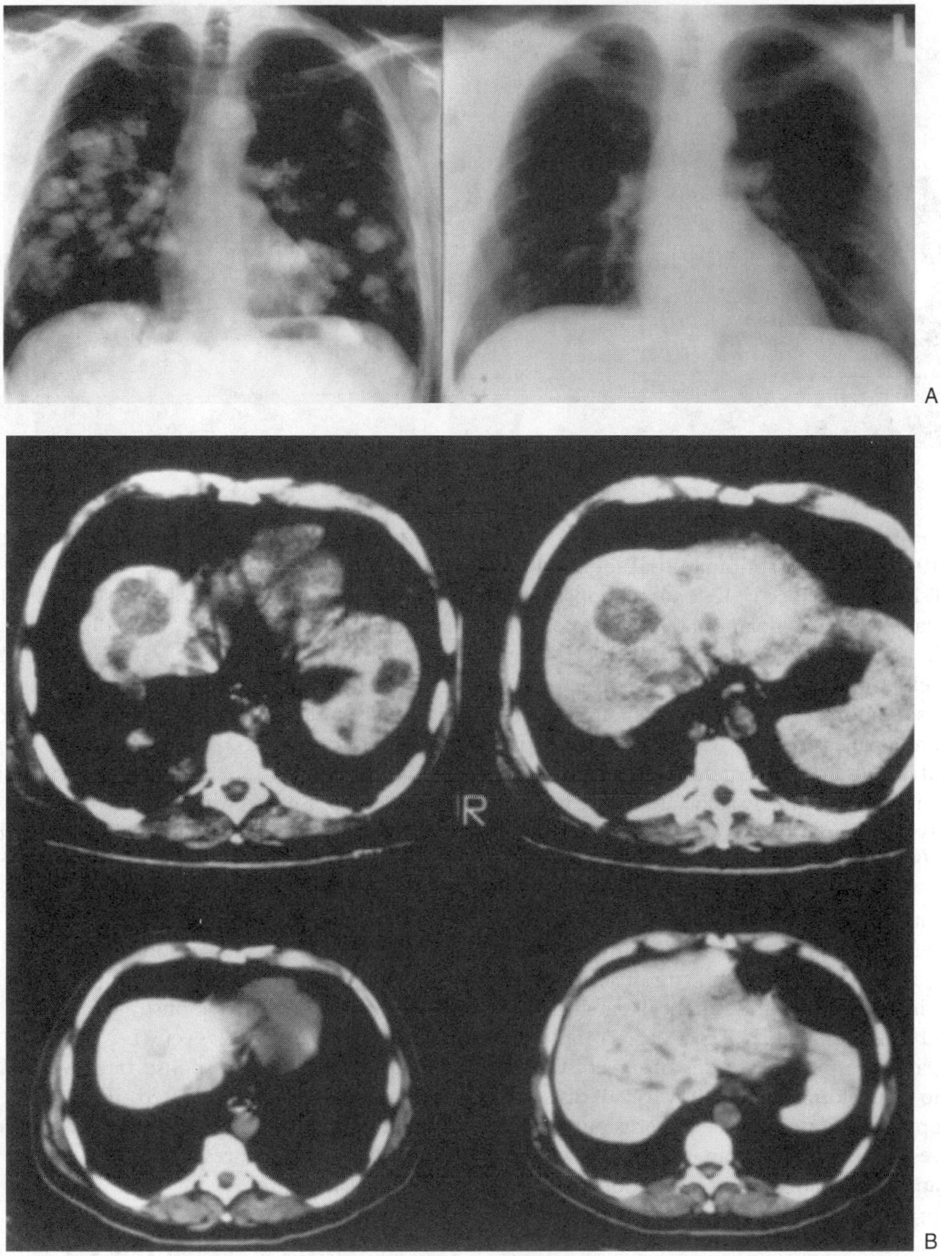

FIGURE 42.2-27. Complete response in a patient with disseminated melanoma using high-dose interleukin-2. Chest radiograph **(A)** and abdominal computed tomographic scan **(B)** showing complete regression of disease.

in survival has led to denial of licensure for melanoma, although this agent has been licensed by the U.S. Food and Drug Administration for glioblastoma multiforme.

IMMUNOTHERAPY OF METASTATIC DISEASE

Although immunotherapy currently is effective in only a small percentage of patients, the results can be quite dramatic. Six percent of patients have a complete response to IL-2, but two-thirds of patients with complete responses are disease-free survivors at a median follow-up of more than 5 years (Figs. 42.2-27 and 42.2-28).[424] These infrequent responses suggest that with a better understanding of the immune mechanisms of IL-2, a greater proportion of patients might be benefited and perhaps serve as a more effective model for developing therapies for patients with other neoplasms.

One fascinating aspect of melanoma is the evidence of tumor regression at the primary tumor site, and less commonly, at regional or distant metastatic sites. One of the hallmarks of primary melanoma is the appearance of subjacent lymphocytic infiltrate and pigment phagocytosis in monocytes associated with lesional depigmentation. Some patients develop patches of cutaneous depigmentation, remote from the primary lesion: This is known as leukoderma or paraneoplastic vitiligo, presumably secondary to a specific immune response directed toward melanocyte antigens.[425,426] Some patients who develop responses after immunotherapy, and in particular after IL-2, IFN-α_{2b}, or vaccines composed of melanosomal proteins or peptide therapy, develop marked paraneoplastic vitiligo. The presence of vitiligo predicts response to immunotherapy.

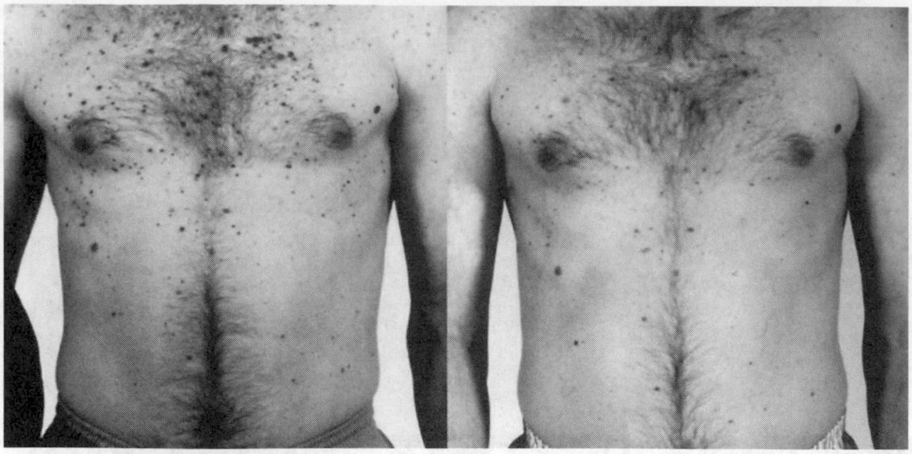

FIGURE 42.2-28. Partial response in a patient with multiple cutaneous metastatic lesions after interleukin-2 (before, *left*; after, *right*). In general, partial responses are limited in their duration to 6 to 18 months, but some can be sustained for prolonged periods (greater than 10 years).

IL-2, originally termed *T-cell growth factor*, was first identified in 1976 and the first human trials of its antitumor effects were published in 1985.[427–429] IL-2 has no apparent direct cytotoxic or cytostatic effect on melanoma. IL-2 promotes T-cell proliferation and, in high doses, like IL-4, IL-7, IL-10, IL-12, and IL-18, induces LAK cells from NK precursors. These LAK cells can nonspecifically lyse tumor *in vitro*, and in particular, those failing to express class I molecules. In some instances, IL-2 can promote apoptotic death of T cells and its targeted deletion (or that of its alpha and beta chain receptors) is associated with inflammatory bowel disease. Typical high-dose IL-2 protocols involve the administration of 600,000 to 720,000 IU/kg IL-2 every 8 hours up to a maximum of 15 doses. This is administered in two cycles of up to 5 days separated by a 10-day rest period. Numerous single-institutional case series have been published on the efficacy of IL-2 (Table 42.2-20). The NCI published the largest series of 283 consecutive patients with melanoma and renal cell carcinoma treated with high doses of IL-2 (720,000 IU/kg). A 7% complete response rate and 10% partial response rate was observed. Complete responses tended to be prolonged with many free of disease 15 years following therapy. An update of these patients published in 2000 demonstrated response durations ranging from 1.5 to greater than 122 months and a median response duration of at least 59 months. Disease progression was not observed in any patient responding for longer than 30 months.[430]

Relapse after IL-2 usually occurs within 1 to 2 years (97%) in partial responders but much less frequently (41%) in complete responders. In patients who relapse, repeat administration of IL-2 is rarely effective following IL-2 treatment.[431] Surgical resection following recurrence following IL-2 therapy is associated with a rapid relapse with a median time of 5 months before progression, and resection in such patients should be used only as palliative therapy.[432]

Considerable toxicity from IL-2 administration is observed since IL-2 is given in each patient to maximally tolerated doses on the basis of evidence that efficacy is directly related to dose intensity. Capillary leak syndrome resulting in pulmonary edema as well as renal and cardiac dysfunction, hypotension, fever, and malaise are all common side effects of administration. In these early studies, a 1% mortality was reported, although more recent reports, with careful selection of patients, suggests mortality of less than 0.1%. There has been considerable debate concerning the dosage and regimen of IL-2 necessary to optimize response and minimize toxicity. A large experience supports the application of three daily IL-2 doses of 720,000 IU/kg or as more commonly applied outside of the NCI, 600,000 IU/kg of IL-2.[433] Low-dose IL-2 appears to be markedly less effective.[434,435] Identification of patients most likely to respond to IL-2 therapy has generally not been effective, although good performance status, low pretreatment serum IL-6 levels, postinfusion thrombocytopenia, and expression of certain HLA antigens have been suggested to be helpful.[436,437]

IL-2 has been used in numerous trials alone, in combination with other cytokines, with the infusion of autologous immune effector cells, with other chemotherapeutic agents, and with radiation therapy (Tables 42.2-21 and 42.2-22).[438–440] None of these combinations has been associated with enhanced survival. The enhanced toxicity and absence of long-term survival advantage compared with IL-2 alone has led to their discontinuation.[441,442] The Extratumoral IL-2 Working Group also failed to demonstrate improved response rates of high-dose IL-2 and IFN-α over IL-2 alone in patients with melanoma in which the response rates were 10% and 5%, respectively.[443] The EORTC evaluated IFN-α and IL-2 with or without cisplatin in 138 patients with advanced metastatic melanoma. The overall response rate was 18% for patients receiving IFN-α and IL-2 and

TABLE 42.2-20. Clinical Trials Using Interleukin-2 as Monotherapy for Melanoma[a]

Author	*No.*	*Response Rate (%)*	*Duration (mo)*
Rosenberg, 1989[569]	42	24	2 to >41
Thatcher, 1989[570]	31	3	NR
Parkinson, 1990[571]	46	22	4 to >20
Whitehead, 1991[572]	42	10	NR
Dorval, 1991[573]	27	22	4 to >45
Sparano, 1993[574]	44	5	10 to >14
Legha, 1996[575]	33	33	NR
Atkins, 1999[576]	283	17	1.5 to >122

NR, not reported.
[a]These trials have shown variable response rates and durations of response; in general, patients with the highest doses have enjoyed the highest response rates. Some patients with diffusely metastatic disease enjoy complete responses and prolonged (greater than 15-year) survival.

TABLE 42.2-21. Phase II Results for Chemotherapy with Interleukin-2 Infusion and Interferon-α and Interferon-α_2 Subcutaneously

Principal Investigator	*Regimen/Dose*	*No.*	Response: Complete Response (%)	Partial Response (%)	Total (%)	*Comments*
IL-2 INFUSION AND IFN-α_2						
Legha[415]	Concurrent CVD/IL-2 infusion/ IFN-α_2 SC	53	11 (21)	23 (43)	64	Survival for concurrent and sequential therapy equivalent
McDermott[599]	Modified concurrent CVD/IL-2 infusion/IFN-α_2 SC	40	8 (20)	11 (28)	48	Response rate equivalent in patients with prior IFN; frequent CNS relapse
O'Day[600]	Concurrent CVD/tamoxifen "decrescendo" IL-2/IFN-α_2 SC	45	10 (23)	15 (34)	57	14% disease-free from 10–36 mo
Total		138	29 (21)	49 (36)	57	
IL-2 SC AND IFN-α SC						
Thompson[601]	CBDT/IL-2 (SC)/IFN-α_2	53	10 (19)	12 (23)	42	2 complete responses ongoing >2 y
Flaherty[594]	CD/IL-2 (SC)/IFN-α_2	38	1 (3)	6 (16)	19	Randomized phase II study; results suggesting improved results with IV IL-2
	CD/IL-2 (IV)/IFN-α_2	44	5(12)	11 (25)	37	
Total		135	16 (12)	29 (21)	33	

B, carmustine; C, cisplatin; CNS, central nervous system; D, dacarbazine; IFN, interferon-α ; IL-2, interleukin-2; T, tamoxifen; V, vinblastine.

increased to 35% with the addition of cisplatin. In a subset analysis considering patients with normal pretherapy LDH levels, the response rate was 23%, and with cisplatin improved to 38%. Overall survival was 9 months without any significant differences between the various groups. Although results are still early to determine the true effect IL-2 has on survival, a 5-year survival rate of 13% has been shown in patients receiving IL-2 and IFN-α regardless of the inclusion of chemotherapy.[444] Efforts to reduce toxicity associated with IL-2 administration, including the use of corticosteroids and anti-TNF antibodies, have generally been ineffective or limited the antitumor effects of IL-2.[445]

A prospective randomized trial in patients with metastatic melanoma, comparing treatment with chemobiotherapy in relation to chemotherapy was carried out at the NCI. One hundred two patients with metastatic melanoma were prospectively randomized to receive chemotherapy consisting of tamoxifen, cisplatin, and dacarbazine or this same chemotherapy followed by IFN-α_{2b} and IL-2 using a schedule that has not been explored by others. No increase in survival was seen with the addition of immunotherapy and toxicity was increased. From previous patients treated with immunotherapy alone it was suggested that the chemotherapy might have

TABLE 42.2-22. Phase III Trials of Biochemotherapy for Stage IV Melanoma

Principal Investigator	*Design*	*Status*
European Organization for Cancer Research and Treatment Group of Cancer Keilholz[591]	Decrescendo IL-2 + IFN-α_2 vs. IL-2/IFN-α_2 + C	Higher response rate IL-2/IFN-α_2 + C, without overall survival difference
National Cancer Institutes, Surgery Branch Rosenberg[362]	CD/tamoxifen vs. CD/tamoxifen + high-dose IL-2 and IFN-α_2	No significant difference in response rate or survival between the two groups
European Organization for Cancer Research and Treatment of Cancer Keilholz[592]	C/dacarbazine/IFN-α_2 vs. C/dacarbazine/IFN-α_2 + IL-2	Pending
M. D. Anderson Cancer Center Legha[593]	CVD vs. sequential CVD + IL-2/IFN-α_2	Pending
Eastern Cooperative Oncology Group/Southwest Oncology Group E3695 Flaherty[594]	CVD vs. concurrent CVD + IL-2/IFN-α_2	Pending

C, cisplatin; D, dacarbazine; IFN, interferon; IL-2, interleukin-2; V, vinblastine.

negatively affected the efficacy of the immunotherapy component of the regimen.[446]

The addition of immune effectors such as LAK cells, tumor-infiltrating lymphocytes (TILs), or activated T cells combined with IL-2 has not improved response or survival rates substantially over IL-2 alone and greatly increases cost and complexity. TILs can be demonstrated to contain some cells that are specific for known melanosomal lineage antigens of melanoma, as well as the patient's own autologous tumor. It has been suggested that the major targets of T cells in melanoma patients may be unique to each individual. Concomitant infusion of IL-2 may act as a survival factor for the infused TILs, may enhance the recruitment of T cells into the tumor site, and augment the specific cytotoxic T-cell response. In one study, 86 consecutive patients were treated with a combination of TILs and IL-2. An objective response was observed in 34% of patients, including some patients who had previously failed treatment with high-dose IL-2 alone. These T cells were also demonstrated to localize to the site following radiolabeling.[447,448] From both TILs as well as T cells derived from the peripheral blood and sensitized *in vitro*, genes encoding target antigens as well as the major histocompatibility complex (MHC)-specific peptide epitopes derived from them have been identified. These peptides are being used as vaccine antigens to enhance T-cell response and function against melanoma. Numerous clinical protocols have been initiated based on these new findings.[449] Other therapies applying cytokines that have been tested in this disease including IL-1, IL-4, IL-12, TNF, IFN-γ, and FLT3L have not been successful. In the future, they may play a role in combination with IL-2 or IFN-α.[450–455]

MANAGEMENT OF MELANOMA IN THE PREGNANT PATIENT

Appropriate surgical management should not be delayed in a pregnant patient with melanoma. The cornerstone of fetal viability is maternal health, and a delay in surgery only jeopardizes the lives of both the mother and the child. Adjuvant treatment such as high-dose IFN-α, an abortifactant, should be delayed until after delivery. Patients who have been treated with IFNs while pregnant also have had babies of low birth weight. Only rarely do situations arise in which a woman with melanoma should be advised to terminate pregnancy. In patients with stage IV disease, fetal termination should only be considered for the use of chemotherapeutic or biologic agents with the understanding that only a few percent may experience a survival benefit. Managing a pregnant patient with disseminated melanoma can be difficult, but because the prognosis is so poor in these patients and treatment options are lacking, the patient may reasonably decide to attempt a full-term gestation without therapy. Cases of women receiving chemotherapy and focused spinal radiation without subsequent harm to the fetus have been reported. Uncommonly, melanoma can pass through the placenta, but usually in only far-advanced disease. Melanomas account for only 8% of the cancers that affect pregnant women but for 46% of fetal tumors acquired transplacentally.[456] In a gestational patient with melanoma, the placenta should be specifically examined histologically for occult melanoma metastasis.[457]

FUTURE PROSPECTS FOR THE BIOLOGIC THERAPY OF PATIENTS WITH MELANOMA

Some of the goals of the tumor immunologist are (1) the development of a specific T cell response to tumor, (2) delivery of T cells across the endothelial barrier to the tumor, (3) maintenance of the T-cell survival within the tumor microenvironment, (4) the induction of long-lasting immune memory to an individual's tumor, and (5) regulation of the local angiogenic response mediated by development of a T-cell response in concert with tumor resident DCs. Future directions in immunotherapy promise more directed stimulation of a specific immune response using vaccines derived from autologous tumor, DCs, and application of known tumor antigens.

ANTIGENS OF MELANOMA

Specific cellular immune responses to melanoma antigens classically occur through the recognition of a foreign peptide on a self-MHC molecule by the T-cell receptor.[458] These peptides, generated through the processing of either exogenous (extracellular) or endogenous (intracellular) antigens, are presented by DCs to specific T cells in regional lymph nodes. Proteins are cleaved to short amino acid sequences of 8 to 10 aa for MHC class I molecules and 13 to 18 aa for MHC class II molecules. MHC class I molecules interact with CD8 cells to stimulate a cytotoxic T-cell response to melanoma, whereas MHC class II molecules activate appropriate helper CD4 cells to induce a humoral immune response.[459] Single amino acid differences in these small peptides have enormous effects on this interaction as alterations in the anchoring of the peptide in the MHC grove may occur and recognition by the T-cell receptor of the MHC/peptide complex may no longer occur with minute changes in spatial conformation and charge.[460] Escape from immune recognition can occur in a variety of ways, but evidence for defects in the peptide transporter into the endoplasmic reticulum, loss of expression of individual melanoma antigens, and loss of class I molecules (limited to single alleles or globally, often due to loss of β_2 microglobulin expression) has been associated with progression of this tumor.[461]

DCs are uniquely required for priming naive T and B cells and probably play a major role in driving the effector phase of the immune response. DCs, which express high levels of costimulatory molecules and efficiently secrete Th1 cytokines, select, activate, and expand specific T cells. Through positive and negative selection of T cells during maturation, autoreactivity should be minimized. Proteins produced from tumor cells that induce a specific T-cell response are called *tumor-associated antigens.* Those that are sufficiently potent at stimulating reactivity, demonstrated by a clinical rejection of tumor, are called *tumor-rejection antigens.* As cancer is a genetic disease, the production of mutated proteins occurs, and these proteins were thought to be prime candidates for the development of peptide vaccines. Of course, this concept is much more complicated as T cells are, in fact, quite capable of recognizing self, and, conversely, are able to develop tolerance or anergy to foreign peptides. In fact, although some mutated self-proteins have been identified in patients that can stimulate an antitumor T-cell response, most peptides thus far identified derive from normal proteins either overexpressed in melanoma or

TABLE 42.2-23. Major Histocompatibility Class I–Restricted Human Melanoma Peptide Antigens Used in Clinical Trials

Antigen	*Amino Acids*	*HLA Restriction*	*Comments*
DIFFERENTIATION ANTIGENS			
Melan-A/MART-1	27–35	A2	Naturally processed but has less than optimal anchor residue at position 2
	26–35	A2	
	32–40	A2	
	26–35	A2	27L
gp100	280–288	A2	
	154–162	A2	
	209–217	A2	
	209–217	A2	210M substitution
	280–288	A2	
	280–288	A2	288V substitution
	17–25	A2	
Tyrosinase	1–9	A2	Leader sequence
	368–376	A2	Internal sequence 370D
	240–251	A1	Cysteines may cross-link
	240–251	A1	244S substitution
	206–214	A24	
TRP-1 (ORF3)	1–9	A31/A33	Translated from alternative open reading frame
CANCER TESTIS ANTIGENS			
MAGE-1	27–35	A1	
MAGE-3	168–176	A1	A2 peptide may not be naturally processed by proteasome; also expressed in lung and head and neck carcinomas
NY-ESO-1	157–167	A2	Cysteines may cross-link
	157–167		
	155–163		

restricted to cells of melanocytic lineage.[462] Understanding the mechanisms of tolerance and the means to stimulate enhanced self-reactivity has been a goal of the tumor immunologist. By identifying antigens present in tumors (the processed epitopes express in concert with MHC class I and II molecules, which can bind with sufficient affinity to the T-cell receptor), therapeutic vaccines may be developed that induce a long-lived antitumor response.

Unique Tumor Antigens

Unique antigens, those expressed usually as a result of mutation, only occur in a single patient's melanoma and not in other patients; those may be the most important target. Techniques to sample the antigenic repertoire of autologous tumors and to express them on autologous DCs have been developed. Several sources of antigen have been applied to DCs, including the use of synthetic peptides, peptides stripped from the surface of the tumor cell by means of acid elution, and cDNA or cRNA preparations encoding genes expressed by the tumor. The creation of antigen-presenting cells by fusing autologous DCs with tumor, incubating with tumor lysates or apoptotic bodies, also has been shown to elicit an antitumor response in murine and some human studies.[463]

Shared Tumor Antigens

A number of proteins providing a source of peptide epitopes, some of them synthetically altered to improve MHC binding, have been identified and used in clinical trials. These epitopes bind either to class I (Table 42.2-23) or class II (Table 42.2-24) MHC molecules. One technique that enabled the rapid detection and identification of antigens of cancer was the technique known as serologic expression cloning.[464] This has been now shown to detect both antibody-recognized and T-cell–recognized antigens of melanoma.

Differentiation Antigens

A broad group of antigens is known as the *cancer testis* group was initially identified in melanoma as MAGE 1, 2, and 3.[465] These antigens are now known to be expressed in cancers of different histologic types, but also in only normal testis and occasionally ovary of adults. The cells in the testis expressing these antigens are immunologically privileged by their anatomic localization and their frequent lack of HLA class I molecules. Thus, cancer testis antigens are restricted to malignant cells in the adult. The identification in melanoma and melanocytes of the cancer testes MAGE genes,[466] which occur naturally in several human cancers, were

TABLE 42.2-24. Major Histocompatibility Class II Human Melanoma Peptides Used in Clinical Trials

Antigen	*Amino Acids*	*HLA Restriction*
DIFFERENTIATION ANTIGENS		
CDC27	760–771	DR4
gp100	44–59	DR4
Tyrosinase	56–70	DR4
	188–208	DR4
	386–406	DR15
	488–462	DR4
CANCER TESTIS ANTIGENS		
NY-ESO-1	115–132	DR53
	121–138	DR53
	139–156	DR53
	119–143	DR4
MAGE-3	114–127	DR13
	119–134	DR13
	281–295	DR11

(Prepared by Walter Storkus, Ph.D.[541–548])

the first identifiable tumor antigen in human solid tumors. Many more such antigens have been subsequently described.

Melanocyte and Melanoma Tumor Antigens

The predominant melanocytic antigens include Melan-A/MART-1, tyrosinase, and gp100. These gene products are expressed in both normal and malignant melanocytes, and immune responses against these targets have been associated with the development of autoimmune reactions against normal melanocytes.[467] However, these genes are not expressed in tumors derived from other cell types. Therefore, vaccination against these targets should allow a relatively tissue-specific response to be elicited.

CLINICAL APPLICATIONS

Active Immunotherapy

CELLULAR ADJUVANTS. DCs are specialized APC that have the unique ability to stimulate naive T cells.[468,469] They are also capable of presenting exogenous antigens either by the MHC class I or II pathways.[470–478] DCs can per se mediate antitumor effects[479]; however, current trials use DCs that have been manipulated through various techniques to express tumor antigen on self-restricted MHC molecules (Table 42.2-25). For example, animal studies using synthetic[480] or stripped[481] peptides pulsed onto DCs have shown potent inhibition of tumor growth. DCs can be generated easily from peripheral blood monocytes,[482] CD34+ progenitors,[483,484] or by direct purification from blood[485] and have entered clinical trials in a variety of malignant diseases including melanoma.[486–489]

Nestle et al. performed a clinical trial involving 30 patients with melanoma in which DCs were used to mediate vaccination.[487,490] Patients of HLA serotype HLA-A1 were treated with appropriate peptides derived from the MAGE-1 and MAGE-3 antigens; those who were HLA-A2+ were treated with peptides from Melan-A/MART-1, gp100, and tyrosinase; and those who expressed HLA-B44 received treatment with peptides derived from MAGE-3 and tyrosinase. Clinical responses were noted in 27% (8 of 30) of patients, including three complete remissions and five partial remissions. This study is the most mature of current DC and peptide studies in melanoma and has indicated the feasibility, safety, as well as the tolerance of such therapy. The meaningful clinical responses induced in a group of patients with poor prognosis disease is encouraging but needs further evaluation.

TABLE 42.2-25. Uses of Dendritic Cells in Immunotherapy[a]

TUMOR DELIVERED INTO DCS
DCs "fed"
- Apoptotic bodies
- Tumor lysates
- Known recombinant tumor antigens
- RNA-encoding known tumor antigens
- DNA-encoding known tumor antigens
- RNA subtraction library

Tumor-DC fusion heteroconjugates
Tumor peptide-pulsed DC-derived exosomes

DC DELIVERY INTO TUMOR
Mobilization of DC *in vivo* using
- Granulocyte-macrophage colony-stimulating factor and IL-4
- FLT3L ligand

Autologous DC injection into tumor
Adoptive transfer of autologous DCs
DCs transduced with
- IL-12
- Granulocyte-macrophage colony-stimulating factor
- IL-18

DC, dendritic cell; IL, interleukin.
[a]Specific T cells require appropriate stimulation by dendritic cells in order to activate and proliferate. By loading dendritic cells with tumor antigens, a specific antitumor response can be induced.

A University of Pittsburgh Cancer Institute trial initiated in 1996 has also shown encouraging evidence of activity in 23 patients.[491] The first patient treated exhibited a relapsing and remitting course of her melanoma over several years and multiple trials. After DC vaccination, this patient developed a complete remission and has remained free of disease for more than 20 months. Another patient on this study attained a complete remission sustained for over 3 years, and a third has had a partial remission.

New adjuvants are also becoming available. Cytokines of great potential interest are FLT3L and CD40L, which preferentially expands or activates DC in the peripheral blood and many tissues.[492–494] A major difficulty in conducting trials of cancer immunotherapy is the selection of appropriate end points. Most patients on such studies are heavily pretreated and immunosuppressed. It is logical to apply these treatments to patients with a much lower burden of disease such as in the adjuvant setting, where all obvious disease is removed, but there is a high chance of relapse due to microscopic residual or metastatic disease. Performing such studies using the clinical end points of time to tumor progression or survival involves studying large numbers of patients over a long period. This is justifiable if phase II studies in patients with advanced disease indicate that there is significant clinical activity, but for most strategies, this has not yet been shown to be the case.

CYTOKINE ADJUVANTS. Granulocyte-macrophage colony-stimulating factor (GM-CSF) is an important cytokine promoting survival and expansion of DCs.[482,483,495] In gene transfer models, GM-CSF gene transfer into poorly immunogenic tumors leads to rejection of those tumors in animal models[496] or to clinical and immunologic responses in humans.[497,498] Direct injection of GM-CSF into subcutaneous melanoma metastases may also lead to regression of injected and noninjected tumor deposits.[499] A study using GM-CSF together with peptides derived from Melan-A/MART-1, tyrosinase, and gp100 in HLA-A2 melanoma patients was reported in 1996.[500] Immunologic responses were observed, consisting of development of skin reactions to intradermal injections of peptide, infiltration of injection site by CD4 and CD8 lymphocytes, and detectable cytotoxic T lymphocytes in peripheral blood without apparent toxicity. Three patients were reported in whom tumor regressions were seen despite having progressive melanoma at the time of entry into the study: One patient showed complete regression of tumor and the others displayed partial regressions. In a study using modified gp100 HLA-A2 peptides, 13 of 31 patients receiving the peptide plus systemic IL-2 showed regression of metastatic melanoma, with an additional four patients showing minor or mixed responses. Immunologic responses could be generated in 91% of patients using blood lymphocytes stimulated *in vitro* before assay.[501]

Another approach to the enhancement of immune response to tumor cells consists of introducing genes encoding costimulatory molecules or alloantigens. In human clinical trials, tumor cells (autologous or allogeneic) or normal cells such as fibroblasts, have been transfected with individual cytokine gene(s) and have been used to induce tumor immunity. So far, only early toxicity results from phase I trials have been reported using this approach in advanced disease patients. Current efforts are underway involving the evaluation of IL-4 or IL-12 gene therapy in patients with melanomas. A human clinical trial using this approach was reported using IFN-γ gene modified and irradiated autologous melanoma cells. The preparation was given every 2 weeks for a total of six doses. Twenty stage III and IV melanoma patients were treated. Two complete responses were observed and two patients had a decrease in the size and number of their subcutaneous nodules. The vaccinated population showed an increased IgG response dominated by IgG-2, suggesting the development of an effective T-helper cell response.[502] Palmer et al. reported on 12 patients who were treated with autologous irradiated tumor engineered to secrete IL-2 by infection with recombinant retrovirus. No clinical responses were seen, but three patients had stable disease for 7 to 15 months.[503]

Arienti et al. reported the vaccination of 12 patients with metastatic melanoma with an allogeneic human melanoma line genetically modified to release IL-4. Only two mixed responses were recorded, without objective clinical responses by conventional criteria. However, induction of a specific immune response was demonstrated by *in vitro* studies. Antibodies to alloantigens could be detected in 2 of 11 patients tested. A significant increase in IFN-γ release was detected in 7 of 11 cases when postvaccination lymphocytes were stimulated by the untransduced allomelanoma cells. However, induction of a specific recognition of autologous melanoma cells by peripheral blood lymphocytes was obtained after vaccination in only one of six cases studied. This response involved the melanoma peptide Melan-A/MART-1[501,504–511] that was recognized in an HLA-A2–restricted fashion. These results, although modest, show that the induction of a specific immune response is possible in a few patients through novel vaccination strategies.[451]

The feasibility of using melanosomal proteins for the immunotherapy of patients with melanoma is now being addressed. Immunization using peptides or recombinant viruses containing genes encoding the melanosomal antigens MART-1 or gp100, with or without coadministration of cytokines such as IL-2, IL-12, or GM-CSF, are ongoing at the National Institutes of Health, as well as in the ECOG.[512]

PEPTIDES ALONE. Initial studies using melanoma peptides were performed using peptides alone. One of the first involved the use of a MAGE-3 HLA-A1–restricted peptide without of any immunologic adjuvant.[355] In this study, 6 of 19 patients with melanoma displayed tumor regression, and toxicity was minimal. In one patient, tumor regression occurred several months after completing peptide vaccination, although the tumor had progressed while on treatment, leading to the initiation of vaccination. Eventually four of five lung metastases in this patient disappeared entirely.[513] This initial study demonstrated that synthetic peptides derived from self-tumor antigens were safe and that clinical responses could be obtained in some individuals in the absence of any other adjuvant. Cytotoxic T-lymphocyte responses against melanoma differentiation antigens correlate inversely with expression of the antigen in melanoma tissues: Patients with progressing disease have been shown in several experiences to displayed antigen-loss variants, implying *in vivo* immunoselection under the pressure of peptide vaccination.[513a,513b]

A series of studies was performed at the NCI involving peptides derived from the melanoma differentiation antigen gp100.[501,506,507] Initially, HLA-A2+ patients were treated with the native peptide, and subsequent patients were treated with a version of this peptide containing a single modified amino acid.[507] This substituted peptide has a higher binding affinity for HLA-A*0201 than the native peptide and has been pursued in the hopes that there will be correspondingly greater induction of *in vivo*, as well as *in vitro* cytotoxic T lymphocytes.[507] Patients treated with the substituted peptide developed cytotoxic T lymphocytes recognizing both native and modified peptide-pulsed target cells, as well as HLA-A2+ tumor cell lines expressing gp100 in almost all cases. Following administration of IL-2 many of these T cells were not found in the peripheral blood, but a substantial number of patients were observed to respond. Presumably, reactive T cells migrated to the site of antigen.

Considerable work has been done in relation to several HLA class I subtypes to map binding pockets and to determine preferential anchor residues for binding peptides.[509] To improve the stability of the class I complex, some investigators have produced modified class I peptides with amino acid variations designed to introduce residues that improve the binding to individual class I molecules. This has enhanced the generation of cytotoxic T lymphocytes with specificity not only for the modified peptide-pulsed target cells, but also for unmodified peptide and for naturally processed peptide.[507,510] Vaccination using modified peptides has now entered evaluation in clinical trials, and cytotoxic T lymphocytes have clearly been demonstrated in patients vaccinated in these studies.[501]

Allogeneic tumor vaccines are based on the presumption that same cell type tumors from different individuals share several common antigens that are capable of inducing an immunologic response. One vaccine based on this approach, CancerVax, has been developed at John Wayne Cancer Institute. CancerVax is a whole cell irradiated vaccine developed from three allogeneic melanoma cell lines that were subsequently demonstrated to express several known immunogenic tumor-associated antigens. Phase II nonrandomized trials have shown impressive results in a select group of patients. Stage IV patients received CancerVax after resection of all evident metastatic disease and were compared with a matched set of controls. The 5-year overall survival and median survival for patients who received the vaccine appears to be improved, but it is well recognized that historic controls have great liabilities. Forty-two percent of patients who received the vaccine were alive at 5 years and the median survival was 42 months. The historic reference had a 19% 5-year survival and an 18-month median survival. After multivariate analysis, CancerVax therapy was suggested to be a significant predictor of survival.[360] It is believed that prior surgery enabled success of the vaccine by reducing tumor load and identifying a better group of patients. Prospective randomized studies are now needed, and underway, to appropriately evaluate this therapy in patients with resected stage III and stage IV melanoma.[514] Use of peptides fused to heat-shock protein hsp70 has been shown to be rapidly taken up by DCs and to bypass the need for T-cell help in murine models.[515] *In vivo* immunization with these hybrid peptides caused rejection of tumors expressing antigen and may represent important strategies to be taken into clinical trials.

Lysate vaccines are produced by mechanical disruption of whole tumor cells. Vaccine preparations have been evaluated in which nonpathogenic viruses such as vaccinia virus and Newcastle disease virus, are used to lyse cells to enhance their immunogenicity (viral melanoma oncolysate). They contain multiple tumor-associated antigens and are capable of stimulating a polyvalent immune response. Wallack et al. compared a vaccinia melanoma oncolysate with vaccinia virus alone in AJCC stage III melanoma patients. This phase III, randomized, multicenter trial demonstrated no significant difference in either disease-free or overall survival at a median follow-up of 46 months.[516] Similar studies by Hersey from Australia have also failed to show either relapse-free survival or overall survival benefit.[517]

CELLULAR ADJUVANTS

Passive Immunotherapy

Passive immunotherapy is a term generally applied to agents that are thought to have direct antitumor activity themselves. Most specifically, this would include the adoptive transfer of cells or antibodies. Application of the adoptive transfer of T cells and LAK cells has been discussed previously (see Immunotherapy of Metastatic Disease, earlier in this chapter). Although responses have been observed in conjunction with delivery of IL-2, the general sense is that these responses are inferior in quality and duration to those of IL-2 alone and provide no long-term benefit. With an improved understanding of the so-called central (CCR7+ vs. CCR7–) memory T cells that could provide long-term benefit, it would be worthwhile to reevaluate these approaches with these cells as opposed to the effector memory T cells (CCR7+), which are most likely to provide only short-term responses.[518,519] Application of gene therapies using gene-marked TILs, IL-4, or IL-12 may also enhance induction of a melanoma-specific immune response.[520–522]

The application of antibodies in melanoma was first evaluated with the notion that such antibodies could confer complement or antibody-dependent cellular cytotoxicity on tumor cells.[523,524] The subsequent genetic engineering of monoclonal antibodies (MAB), resulting in human molecules, and successes with antibodies targeting breast cancer and lymphoma in clinical trials has led to a reevaluation of these reagents alone or in combination with molecularly defined cytokines and growth factors for the immunotherapy of melanoma. The development of a human IgG anti-mouse antibody (HAMA) has been observed in virtually every patient and limited the effectiveness of these early approaches in treated patients. However, first-generation murine MABs have been developed that have been used to effectively map melanosomal, melanocyte, and melanoma antigens.[525] One of these antibodies, R24, an IgG3 murine monoclonal antibody that recognizes GD3, a ganglioside present on melanoma cells and a subset of T cells, was reported initially to mediate 3 of 12 responses in patients with melanoma.[526] Evidence of immune reactivity with inflammatory reactions (urticaria, pruritus, erythema, subcutaneous ecchymoses) were observed at tumor sites in some patients treated at doses greater than or equal to 80 mg/m^2. Tumor biopsies during and after treatment showed lymphocyte and mast cell infiltration, mast cell degranulation, and complement deposition. Subsequent studies with this antibody have failed to confirm this level of response.[527] As a single agent, R24 induced responses in 10 of 103 patients two of which were complete. Combining R24 with cytotoxic drugs or cytokines did not increase the response rate. An alternative approach was to develop strategies to immunize with the antiidiotype (so-called Ab2) to induce a host immune response to the original antigen (Ab3).[528,529] BEC2, an antiidiotypic MAB mimics GD3 has been tested with two immunologic adjuvants, BCG and QS21, administered with BEC2 in melanoma patients free of disease after surgical resection. All patients developed high-titer IgG antibodies against BEC2. Anti-GD3 antibodies were induced in 3 of 14 patients immunized with BEC2/BCG; no patient immunized with BEC2/QS21 developed such antibodies. Conjugation of BEC2 to keyhole limpet hemocyanin did not increase the immunogenicity of BEC2 when administered with BCG. Prolonged disease-free intervals were noted in a majority of treated patients in these adjuvant studies. Two clinical trials with the mouse antiidiotypic MAB MF11-30, which is an Ab2 of human high-molecular-weight melanoma-associated antigen was administered subcutaneously to patients with advanced melanoma.[530,531] In the first phase I trial in 16 patients, minor responses were observed in three patients. In a second clinical trial MAB MF11-30 was administered to 21; 17 of 19 evaluable patients had increased levels of anti-mouse Ig antibodies and 16 developed antibodies that inhibit the binding of antiidiotypic MAB MF11-30 to the immunizing anti–high-molecular-weight melanoma-associated antigen MAB 225.28. One patient had increased levels of anti–high-molecular-weight melanoma-associated antigen antibodies. One patient achieved a complete remission with disappearance of multiple abdominal lymph nodes for a duration of 95 weeks. Minor responses were observed in three patients. These collective results suggest that such antiidiotype antibodies may be useful in patients with melanoma. Additional antibodies including those directed against the cell surface high-molecular-weight antigen or a transferrin-like molecule have been used in experimental studies of imaging or therapy with cytokines including IL-2.[527,532–535] MABs with tumor specificity are able to enhance the immunologic specificity of IL-2–activated LAK cells. MAB 3F8 and 14.G2a, which are specific for neuroblastoma and melanoma and recognize ganglioside GD2, were able to mediate antibody-dependent cell-mediated cytotoxicity with fresh effector cells and antibody-binding targets. Use of cross-linked antibodies or humanized antibodies has yet to be clinically explored in this disease but may represent promising approaches.[536]

REFERENCES

1. Lotze MT. Keystone symposium. Melanoma and biology of the neural crest. *Melanoma Res* 1992;2:131.
2. Lancaster HO. Some geographical aspects of the mortality from melanoma in Europeans. *Med J Aust* 1956;1:1082.
3. Kopf AW, Salopek TJ, Slade J, et al. Management of cutaneous malignant melanoma by dermatologists in the USA. The Sixth World Congress on Cancers of the Skin, Buenos Aires, Argentina, 2000.
4. Koh HK, Clapp RW, Barnett JM, et al. Systematic underreporting of cutaneous malignant melanoma in Massachusetts. Possible implications for national incidence figures. *J Am Acad Dermatol* 1991;24:545.
5. Greenlee RT, Murray T, Bolden S, Wingo P. Cancer statistics 2000. *CA Cancer J Clin* 2000;50:7.
6. Polednak AP, Flannery JT. Cancer Incidence in Connecticut, 1935–1991. Hartford, Connecticut, Department of Public Health, 1996.
7. National Cancer Institute DoCPaC. Surveillance, Epidemiology, and End Results Program Public Use CD-ROM (1973–1994). National Cannocer Institute, Surveillance Program, Statistics Branch, 1997.
8. Roush GC, McKay L, Holford TR. A reversal in the long-term increase in deaths attributable to malignant melanoma. *Cancer* 1992;69:1714.
9. Dennis LK. Analysis of the melanoma epidemic, both apparent and real: data from the 1973 through 1994 Surveillance, Epidemiology, and End Results program registry. *Arch Dermatol* 1999;135:275.
10. Balch CM, Soong SJ, Shaw HS, Urist MM, McCarthy WH. An analysis of prognostic factors in 8500 patients with cutaneous melanoma. In: *Cutaneous melanoma.* Philadelphia: Lippincott, 1992:165.
11. Koh HK. Cutaneous melanoma. *N Engl J Med* 1991;325:171.
12. Jackson A, Wilkinson C, Ranger M, Pill R, August P. Can primary prevention or selective screening for melanoma be more precisely targeted through general practice? A prospective study to validate a self administered risk score. *BMJ* 1998;316:34.
13. Geller AC, Miller DR, Lew RA, et al. Cutaneous melanoma mortality among the socioeconomically disadvantaged in Massachusetts. *Am J Pub Health* 1996;86:538.
14. American Cancer Society. *American Cancer Society facts and figures—1998.* American Cancer Society, Atlanta, 1998.
15. Liu T, Soong SJ. Epidemiology of malignant melanoma. *Surg Clin North Am* 1996;76:1205.
16. Berwick M, Halpern A. Melanoma epidemiology. *Curr Opin Oncol* 1997;9:178.
17. Glass AG, Hoover RN. The emerging epidemic of melanoma and squamous cell skin cancer. *JAMA* 1989;262:2097.
18. Reintgen DS, McCarty KS, Woodard B, Cox E, Seigler HF. Metastatic malignant melanoma with an unknown primary. *Surg Gynecol Obstet* 1983;156:335.
19. Mihm MC Jr, Fitzpatrick TB. Early detection of malignant melanoma. *Cancer* 1976;37:597.
20. Balch CM, Soong SJ, Shaw HM, et al. An analysis of prognostic factors in 4000 patients with cutaneous melanoma. In: Balch CM, Milton GW, eds. *Cutaneous melanoma: clinical management and treatment results worldwide.* Philadelphia: Lippincott, 1985:321.
21. Lotze MT, Heyward N. Personal communication, 2000.
22. Mansfield PF, Lee JE, Balch CM. Cutaneous melanoma: current practice and surgical controversies. *Curr Probl Surg* 1994;31:253.
23. Reimer RR, Clark WH Jr, Greene MH, Ainsworth AM, Fraumeni JF Jr. Precursor lesions in familial melanoma. A new genetic preneoplastic syndrome. *JAMA* 1978;239:744.
24. Nordlund JJ, Kirkwood J, Forget BM, et al. Demographic study of clinically atypical (dysplastic) nevi in patients with melanoma and comparison subjects. *Cancer Res* 1985;45:1855.
25. Elder DE, Goldman LI, Goldman SC, Greene MH, Clark WH Jr. Dysplastic nevus syndrome: a phenotypic association of sporadic cutaneous melanoma. *Cancer* 1980;46:1787.
26. Tucker MA, Halpern A, Holly EA, et al. Clinically recognized dysplastic nevi. A central risk factor for cutaneous melanoma. *JAMA* 1997;277:1439.
27. Kraemer KH, Greene MH, Tarone R, et al. Dysplastic naevi and cutaneous melanoma risk. *Lancet* 1983;2:1076.
28. Elder DE, Goldman LI, Goldman SC, Greene MH, Clark WH Jr. Dysplastic nevus syndrome: a phenotypic association of sporadic cutaneous melanoma. *Cancer* 1980;46:1787.
29. Bondi EE, Clark WH Jr, Elder D, Guerry D, Greene MH. Topical chemotherapy of dysplastic melanocytic nevi with 5% fluorouracil. *Arch Dermatol* 1981;117:89.
30. Kraemer K. Dysplastic nevi as precursors to hereditary melanoma. *J Dermatol Surg Oncol* 1983;9:619.
31. Kraemer KH, Greene MH. Dysplastic nevus syndrome. Familial and sporadic precursors of cutaneous melanoma. *Dermatol Clin* 1985;3:225.
32. Crijns MB, Vink J, van Hees CL, Bergman W, Vermeer RJ. Dysplastic nevi. Occurrence in first- and second-degree relatives of patients with "sporadic" dysplastic nevus syndrome. *Arch Dermatol* 1991;127:1346.
33. Ackerman AB. What naevus is dysplastic, a syndrome and the commonest precursor of malignant melanoma? A riddle and an answer. *Histopathology* 1988;13:241.
34. Snels DG, Hille ET, Gruis NA, Bergman W. Risk of cutaneous malignant melanoma in patients with nonfamilial atypical nevi from a pigmented lesions clinic. *J Am Acad Dermatol* 1999;40:686.
35. Mehregan AH, Mehregan DA. Malignant melanoma in childhood. *Cancer* 1993;71:4096.
36. Kopf AW, Bart RS, Hennessey P. Congenital nevocytic nevi and malignant melanomas. *J Am Acad Dermatol* 1979;1:123.
37. Ruiz-Maldonado R, Tamayo L, Laterza AM, Duran C. Giant pigmented nevi: clinical, histopathologic, and therapeutic considerations. *J Pediatr* 1992;120:906.
38. Swerdlow AJ, English JS, Qiao Z. The risk of melanoma in patients with congenital nevi: a cohort study. *J Am Acad Dermatol* 1995;32:595.
39. Egan CL, Oliveria SA, Elenitsas R, Hanson J, Halpern AC. Cutaneous melanoma risk and phenotypic changes in large congenital nevi: a follow-up study of 46 patients. *J Am Acad Dermatol* 1998;39:923.
40. Ceballos PI, Ruiz-Maldonado R, Mihm CM Jr. Melanoma in children. *N Engl J Med* 1995;332:656.
41. Spatz A, Calonje E, Handfield-Jones SE, Barnhill RL. Spitz tumors in children: a grading system for risk stratification. *Arch Dermatol* 1999;135:282.
42. Lynch HT, Fusaro RM, Pester J, Lynch JF. Familial atypical multiple mole melanoma (FAMMM) syndrome: genetic heterogeneity and malignant melanoma. *Br J Cancer* 1980;42:58.
43. Clark WH, Reimer RR, Greene M. Origin of familiar malignant melanomas from heritable melanocytic lesions. *Arch Dermatol* 1978;114:732.
44. Greene MH, Clark WH Jr, Tucker MA, et al. High risk of malignant melanoma in melanoma-prone families with dysplastic nevi. *Ann Intern Med* 1985;102:458.
45. Perera MIR, Um K, Greene MH, et al. Hereditary dysplastic nevus syndrome: lymphoid cell ultraviolet hypermutability in association with increased melanoma susceptibility. *Cancer Res* 1986;46:1005.
46. Barnhill RL, Mihm MC Jr. Hstopathology of malignant melanoma and its precursor lesions. In: Balch CM, Houghton AN, Milton GW, eds. *Cutaneous melanoma.* Philadelphia: Lippincott, 1992:234.
47. Flores JF, Pollock PM, Walker GJ, et al. Analysis of the CDKN2A, CDKN2B and CDK4 genes in 48 Australian melanoma kindreds. *Oncogene* 1997;15:2999.
48. Aitken J, Welch J, Duffy D, et al. CDKN2A variants in a population-based sample of Queensland families with melanoma. *J Natl Cancer Inst* 1999;91:446.
49. Greene MH. The genetics of hereditary melanoma and nevi: 1998 update. *Cancer* 1999;86:1644.
50. DiFronzo LA, Wanek LA, Elashoff R, Morton DL. Increased incidence of second primary melanoma in patients with a previous cutaneous melanoma. *Ann Surg Oncol* 1999; 6:705.
51. Titus-Ernstoff L, Mansson-Brahme E, Thorn M, et al. Factors associated with atypical nevi: a population-based study. *Cancer Epidemiol Biomarkers Prev* 1998;7:207.
52. Jensen P, Hansen S, Moller B, et al. Skin cancer in kidney and heart transplant reciepients and different long-term immunosuppresive therapy regimens. *J Am Acad Dermatol* 1999;40:177.
53. Smith CH, McGregor JM, Barker JN, et al. Excess melanocytic nevi in children with renal allografts. *J Am Acad Dermatol* 1993;28:51.
54. Szepietowski J, Wasik F, Szepietowski T, et al. Excess benign melanocytic naevi in renal transplant recipients. *Dermatology* 1997;194:17.
55. Greene MH. Dysplastic nevus syndrome. *Hosp Pract* 1984;19:91.
56. Aboulafia DM. Malignant melanoma in an HIV-infected man: a case report and literature review. *Cancer Invest* 1998;16:217.
57. Grob JJ, Bastuji-Garin S, Vaillant L, et al. Excess of nevi related to immunodeficiency: a study in HIV-infected patients and renal transplant recipients. *J Invest Dermatol* 1996;107:694.
58. Greene MH, Young TI. Malignant melanoma in renal transplant recipients. *Lancet* 1981;318:1196.
59. Stern RS, Nichols KT, Vakeva LH. Malignant melanoma in patients treated for psoriasis with methoxsalen (psoralen) and ultraviolet A radiation (PUVA). The PUVA Follow-Up Study. *N Engl J Med* 1997;336:1041.
60. Veness MJ, Quinn DI, Ong CS, et al. Aggressive cutaneous malignancies following cardiothoracic transplantation: the Australian experience. *Cancer* 1999;85:1758.
61. Bliss JM, Ford D, Swerdlow AJ, et al. Risk of cutaneous melanoma associated with pigmentation characteristics and freckling: systemic overview of 10 case-control studies. *Int J Cancer* 1995;62:367.
62. Evans RD, Kopf AW, Lew RA, et al. Risk factors for the development of malignant melanoma—I: Review of case-control studies. *J Dermatol Surg Oncol* 1988;14:393.
63. Titus-Ernstoff L, Ernstoff MS, Duray PH, et al. A relation between childhood sun exposure and dysplastic nevus syndrome among patients with nonfamilial melanoma. *Epidemiology* 1991;2:210.
64. Elwood JM, Jopson J. Melanoma and sun exposure: an overview of published studies. *Int J Cancer* 1997;73:198.
65. Levine EA, Ronan SG, Shirali SS, Das Gupta TK. Malignant melanoma in a child with oculocutaneous albinism. *J Surg Oncol* 1992;51:138.
66. Ihn H, Nakamura K, Abe M, et al. Amelanotic metastatic melanoma in a patient with oculocutaneous albinism. *J Am Acad Dermatol* 1993;28:895.
67. Kraemer KH, Lee MM, Scotto J. Xeroderma pigmentosum: cutaneous, ocular, and neurologic abnormalities in 830 published cases. *Arch Dermatol* 1987;123:241.
68. Smith MA, Fine JA, Barnhill RL, Berwick M. Hormonal and reproductive influences and risk of melanoma in women. *Int J Epidemiol* 1998;27:751.

69. McManamny DS, Moss AL, Pocock PV, Briggs JC. Melanoma and pregnancy: a long-term follow-up. *Br J Obstet Gynaecol* 1989;96:1419.
70. MacKie RM, Bufalino R, Morabito A, Sutherland C, Cascinelli N. Lack of effect of pregnancy on outcome of melanoma. For The World Health Organisation Melanoma Programme. *Lancet* 1991;337:653.
71. Reintgen DS, McCarty KS Jr, Vollmer R, Cox E, Seigler HF. Malignant melanoma and pregnancy. *Cancer* 1985;55:1340.
72. Slingluff CL Jr, Reintgen DS, Vollmer RT, Seigler HF. Malignant melanoma arising during pregnancy. A study of 100 patients. *Ann Surg* 1990;211:552.
73. Bork K, Brauninger W. Prior pregnancy and melanoma survival. *Arch Dermatol* 1986;122:1097.
74. MacKie RM. Pregnancy and exogenous hormones in patients with cutaneous malignant melanoma. *Curr Opin Oncol* 1999;11:129.
75. Cocconi G, Bella M, Calabresi F, et al. Treatment of metastatic malignant melanoma with dacarbazine plus tamoxifen. *N Engl J Med* 1992;327:516.
76. Grin CM, Driscoll MS, Grant-Kels JM. The relationship of pregnancy, hormones, and melanoma. *Semin Cutan Med Surg* 1998;17:167.
77. Gefeller O, Hassan K, Wille L. Cutaneous malignant melanoma in women and the role of oral contraceptives. *Br J Dermatol* 1998;138:122.
78. Friedman RJ, Rigel DS, Kopf AW. Early detection of malignant melanoma: the role of physician examination and self-examination of the skin. *CA Cancer J Clin* 1985;35:130.
79. Langley R, Sober AJ. Clinical recognition of melanoma and its precursors. *Hematol Oncol Clin North Am* 2000;12:699.
80. Muglia JJ, Pesce K, McDonald CJ. Skin cancer screening: a growing need. *Surg Oncol Clin North Am* 1999;8:735.
81. Clark WH Jr, Ainsworth AM, Bernardino EA, et al. The developmental biology of primary human malignant melanomas. *Semin Oncol* 1975;2:83.
82. Averbook BJ, Russo LJ, Mansour EG. A long-term analysis of 620 patients with malignant melanoma at a major referral center. *Surgery* 1998;124:746.
83. Crombie IK. Racial differences in melanoma incidence. *Br J Cancer* 1979;40:185.
84. Tseng JF, Tanabe KK, Gadd MA, et al. Surgical management of primary cutaneous melanomas of the hands and feet. *Ann Surg* 1997;225:544.
85. Green A, McCredie M, MacKie R, et al. A case-control study of melanomas of the soles and palms (Australia and Scotland). *Cancer Cause Control* 1999;10:21.
86. Levit EK, Kagen MH, Scher RK, Grossman M, Altman E. The ABC rule for clinical detection of subungual melanoma. *J Am Acad Dermatol* 2000;42:269.
87. Heaton KM, el Naggar A, Ensign LG, Ross MI, Balch CM. Surgical management and prognostic factors in patients with subungual melanoma. *Ann Surg* 1994;219:197.
88. Eng W, Tschen JA. Comparison of S-100 versus hematoxylin and eosin staining for evaluating dermal invasion and peripheral margins by desmoplastic malignant melanoma. *Am J Dermatopathol* 2000;22:26.
89. Wharton JM, Carlson JA, Mihm MC Jr. Desmoplastic malignant melanoma: diagnosis of early clinical lesions. *Hum Pathol* 1999;30:537.
90. Quinn MJ, Crotty KA, Thompson JF, et al. Desmoplastic and desmoplastic neurotropic melanoma: experience with 280 patients. *Cancer* 1998;83:1128.
91. Autier P, Dor JF, Grier N, et al. Sunscreen use and duration of sun exposure: a double-blind, randomized trial. *J Natl Cancer Inst* 1999;91:1304.
92. Urbach F. Ultraviolet radiation and skin cancer of humans. *J Photochem Photobiol B* 1997;40:3.
93. Graham S, Marshall J, Haughey B, et al. An inquiry into the epidemiology of melanoma. *Am J Epidemiol* 1985;122:606.
94. Hill L, Ferrini RL. Skin cancer prevention and screening: summary of the American College of Preventive Medicine's practice policy statements. *CA Cancer J Clin* 1998;48:232.
95. Autier P, Dore JF, Lejeune F, et al. Cutaneous malignant melanoma and exposure to sunlamps or sunbeds: an EORTC multicenter case-control study in Belgium, France and Germany. EORTC Melanoma Cooperative Group. *Int J Cancer* 1994;58:809.
96. Rossi CR, Foletto M, Vecchiato A, et al. Management of cutaneous melanoma M0: state of the art and trends. *Eur J Cancer* 1997;33:2302.
97. Healsmith MF, Bourke JF, Osborne JE, Graham-Brown RA. An evaluation of the revised seven-point checklist for the early diagnosis of cutaneous malignant melanoma. *Br J Dermatol* 1994;130:48.
98. Koh HK, Miller DR, Geller AC, et al. Who discovers melanoma? Patterns from a population-based survey. *J Am Acad Dermatol* 1992;26:914.
99. Lee G, Massa MC, Welykyj S, Choo J, Greaney V. Yield from total skin examination and effectiveness of skin cancer awareness program. Findings in 874 new dermatology patients. *Cancer* 1991;67:202.
100. Cohen MH, Cohen BJ, Shotkin JD, Morrison PT. Surgical prophylaxis of malignant melanoma. *Ann Surg* 1991;213:308.
101. Reintgen D, Ross M, Bland K, Seigler HF, Balch C. Prevention and early detection of melanoma: a surgeon's perspective. *Semin Surg Oncol* 1993;9:174.
102. Masri GD, Clark WH Jr, Guerry D, et al. Screening and surveillance of patients at high risk for malignant melanoma result in detection of earlier disease. *J Am Acad Dermatol* 1990;22:1042.
103. Vasen HFA, Bergman W, Van Haeringen A, Scheffer E, Van Slooten EA. The familial dysplastic nevus syndrome. *Eur J Cancer Clin Oncol* 1989;25:337.
104. Roush GC, Berwick M, Koh HK, MacKie RM. Screening for melanoma. In: CM Balch. *Cutaneous melanoma*. Philadelphia: Lippincott, 1992:70.
105. Guibert P, Mollat F, Ligen M, Dreno B. Melanoma screening: report of a survey in occupational medicine. *Arch Dermatol* 2000;136:199.
106. Koh HK, Norton LA, Geller AC, et al. Evaluation of the American Academy of Dermatology's National Skin Cancer Early Detection and Screening Program. *J Am Acad Dermatol* 1996;34:971.
107. Whited JD, Hall RP, Simel DL, Horner RD. Primary care clinicians' performance for detecting actinic keratoses and skin cancer. *Arch Intern Med* 1997;157:985.
108. Koh HK, Caruso A, Gage I, et al. Evaluation of melanoma/skin cancer screening in Massachusetts. Preliminary results. *Cancer* 1990;65:375.
109. Rajadhyaksha M, Grossman M, Esterowitz D, et al. In vivo confocal scanning laser microscopy of human skin: melanin provides strong contrast. *J Invest Dermatol* 1995;104:946.
110. Ramsay DL, Fox AB. The ability of primary care physicians to recognize the common dermatoses. *Arch Dermatol* 1981;117:620.
111. Freedberg KA, Geller AC, Miller DR, Lew RA, Koh HK. Screening for malignant melanoma: a cost-effectiveness analysis. *J Am Acad Dermatol* 1999;41:738.
112. Balch CM. A new AJCC staging system for cutaneous melanoma. *Cancer* 2000;88:1484.
113. Stephenson EM, Stephenson NG. Invasive locomotory behaviour between malignant human melanoma cells and normal fibroblasts filmed in vitro. *J Cell Sci* 1978;32:389.
114. Melanoma of the skin. In: Beahrs OH, Myers MH, eds. *Manual for staging of cancer, American Joint Committee on Cancer*. Philadelphia: Lippincott, 1983:117.
115. Stadelmann WK, Rapaport DP, Soong SJ, et al. Prognostic clinical and pathologic features. In: Balch CA, Houghton AN, Sober AJ, Soong SJ, eds. *Cutaneous melanoma*. St. Louis: Quality Medical Publishing, 1998:11.
116. Buzaid AC, Ross MI, Balch CM, et al. Critical analysis of the current American Joint Committee on Cancer staging system for cutaneous melanoma and proposal of a new staging system. *J Clin Oncol* 1997;15:1039.
117. Stadelman WK, Rapaport DP, Soong SJ, et al. Prognostic clinical and pathologic features. In: Balch CM, Houghton AN, Sober AJ, Soong SJ, eds. *Cutaneous melanoma*. St. Louis: Quality Medical Publishing, 1998:11.
118. Balch CM, Buzaid AC, Atkins MB, et al. A new American Joint Committee on Cancer staging system for cutaneous melanoma. *Cancer* 2000;88:1484.
119. Breslow A. Thickness, cross-sectional areas and depth of invasion in the prognosis of cutaneous melanoma. *Ann Surg* 1970;172:902.
120. Corona R, Mele A, Amini M, et al. Interobserver variability on the histopathologic diagnosis of cutaneous melanoma and other pigmented skin lesions. *J Clin Oncol* 1996;14:1218.
121. Lock-Andersen J, Hou-Jensen K, Hansen JP, et al. Observer variation in histological classification of cutaneous malignant melanoma. *Scand J Plast Reconstruc Surg Hand Surg* 1995; 29:141.
122. Balch CM, Murad TM, Soong SJ, et al. A multifactorial analysis of melanoma: prognostic histopathological features comparing Clark's and Breslow's staging methods. *Ann Surg* 1978;188:732.
123. Buttner P, Garbe C, Bertz J, et al. Primary cutaneous melanoma. Optimized cutoff points of tumor thickness and importance of Clark's level for prognostic classification. *Cancer* 1995;75:2499.
124. Balch CM, Wilkerson JA, Murad TM, et al. The prognostic significance of ulceration of cutaneous melanoma. *Cancer* 1980;45:3012.
125. Day CL, Sober AJ, Kopf AW. A prognostic model for clinical stage I melanoma of the lower extremity: location on foot as independent risk factor for recurrent disease. *Surgery* 1981;89:599.
126. Toriyama K, Wen DR, Paul E, Cochran AJ. Variations in the distribution, frequency, and phenotype of Langerhans cells during the evolution of malignant melanoma of the skin. *J Invest Dermatol* 1993;100:269S.
127. Lotze MT. *Dendritic cells: biology and clinical applications*. San Diego: Academic, 1999.
128. Kang S, Barnhill RL, Mihm MC Jr, Sober AJ. Histologic regression in malignant melanoma: an interobserver concordance study. *J Cutan Pathol* 1993;20:126.
129. Blessing K, McLaren KM. Histological regression in primary cutaneous melanoma: recognition, prevalence and significance. *Histopathology* 1992;20:315.
130. Gershenwald J, Berman R, Mansfield P, Lee J, Ross M. *Role of sentinel lymph node biopsy in patient with thin (<1 mm) cutaneous melnoma*. Presented at the Society of Surgical Oncology Annual Meeting, New Orleans, LA, March 2000.
131. Schuchter L, Schultz DJ, Synnestvedt M, et al. A prognostic model for predicting 10-year survival in patients with primary melanoma. The Pigmented Lesion Group. *Ann Intern Med* 1996;125:369.
132. Garbe C, Buttner P, Bertz J, et al. Primary cutaneous melanoma. Prognostic classification of anatomic location. *Cancer* 1995;75:2492.
133. Garbe C, Büttner P, Bertz J, et al. Primary cutaneous melanoma. *Cancer* 1995;75:2484.
134. Balch CM, Houghton AN, Milton GW, eds. *Cutaneous melanoma*. Philadelphia: Lippincott, 1992.
135. Gershenwald JE, Thompson W, Mansfield PF, et al. Multi-institutional melanoma lymphatic mapping experience: the prognostic value of sentinel lymph node status in 612 stage I or II melanoma patients. *J Clin Oncol* 1999;17:976.
136. Balch CM, Soong S. *Long-term results of a prospective surgical trial comparing 2 vs 4 cm excision margins for patients with 1–4 mm melanomas*. Presented at the Society of Surgical Oncology Annual Meeting, New Orleans, LA, March 2000.
137. Reintgen D, Rapaport D, Tanabe KK, Ross M. Lymphatic mapping and sentinel node biopsy in patients with malignant melanoma. *J FL Med Assoc* 1997;84:188.
138. Morton DL, Foshag LJ, Hoon DS, et al. Prolongation of survival in metastatic melanoma after active specific immunotherapy with a new polyvalent melanoma vaccine. *Ann Surg* 1992;216:463.
139. Nocks BN, Olsson CA, Prout GR Jr, et al. Abdominal mass in 43-year-old man. *J Urol* 1981;125:80.
140. Strickland D, Lee JA. Melanomas of eye: stability of rates. *Am J Epidemiol* 1981;113:700.
141. Gershenwald JE, Colome MI, Lee JE, et al. Patterns of recurrence following a negative sentinel lymph node biopsy in 243 patients with stage I or II melanoma. *J Clin Oncol* 1998;16:2253.
142. Bonfrer JM, Korse CM, Nieweg OE, Rankin EM. The luminescence immunoassay S-100: a sensitive test to measure circulating S-100B: its prognostic value in malignant melanoma. *Br J Cancer* 1998;77:2210.
143. Balch CM, Soong SJ, Shaw HS, Urist MM, McCarthy WH. An analysis of prognostic factors in 8500 patients with cutaneous melanoma. In: Balch CM, Houghton AN, Milton GW, eds. *Cutaneous melanoma*. Philadelphia: Lippincott, 1992:165.
144. Morton DL, Wanek L, Nizze JA, Elashoff RM, Wong JH. Improved long-term survival

after lymphadenectomy of melanoma metastatic to regional nodes. Analysis of prognostic factors in 1134 patients from the John Wayne Cancer Clinic. *Ann Surg* 1991;214:491.
145. Drepper H, Biess B, Hofherr B, et al. The prognosis of patients with stage III melanoma. Prospective long-term study of 286 patients of the Fachklinik Hornheide. *Cancer* 1993;71:1239.
146. Cascinelli N, Morabito A, Santinami M, MacKie R, Belli F. Immediate or delayed dissection of regional nodes in patients with melanoma of the trunk: a randomized trial. *Lancet* 1998;351:793.
147. Coit DG, Rogatko A, Brennan MF. Prognostic factors in patients with melanoma metastatic to axillary or inguinal lymph nodes. A multivariate analysis. *Ann Surg* 1991;214:627.
148. Nordlund JJ, Kirkwood JM, Forget BM, et al. Vitiligo in patients with metastatic melanoma: a good prognostic sign. *J Am Acad Dermatol* 1983;9:689.
149. Keilholz U, Goey SH, Punt CJA, et al. Interferon alfa-2a and interleukin-2 with or without cisplatin in metastatic melanoma: a randomized trial of the European organization for research and treatment of cancer melanoma cooperative group. *J Clin Oncol* 1997;15:2579.
150. Bevilacqua RG, Coit DG, Rogatko A, Younes RN, Brennan MF. Axillary dissection in melanoma. Prognostic variables in node-positive patients. *Ann Surg* 1990;212:125.
151. Lee ML, Tomsu K, Von Eschen KB. Duration of survival for disseminated malignant melanoma: results of a meta analysis. *Melanoma Res* 2000;10:81.
152. Ryan L, Kramar A, Borden E. Prognostic factors in metastatic melanoma. *Cancer* 1993;71:2995.
153. Ilson DH, Sirott M, Saltz L, Kelsen DP. A Phase II trial of interferon alpha-2A, 5-fluorouracil, and cisplatin in patients with advanced esophageal carcinoma. *Cancer* 1995;75:2197.
154. Falkson CI, Ibrahim J, Kirkwood J, Blum R. A randomized phase III trial of dacarbazine (DTIC) versus DTIC + interferon alfa-2b (IFN) versus DTIC + tamoxifen (TMX) versus DTIC + IFN + TMX in metatastic malignant melanoma: an ECOG trial. *Proc Am Soc Clin Oncol* 1996;15:435.
155. Sirott MN, Bajorin DF, Wong GY, et al. Prognostic factors in patients with metastatic malignant melanoma. A multivariate analysis. *Cancer* 1993;72:3091.
156. Falkson CI, Falkson HC. Prognostic factors in metastatic malignant melanoma. An analysis of 236 patients treated on clinical research studies at the Department of Medical Oncology, University of Pretoria, South Africa from 1972–1992. *Oncology* 1998;55:59.
157. Brand CU, Ellwanger U, Stroebel W, et al. Prolonged survival of 2 years or longer for patients with disseminated melanoma. An analysis of related prognostic factors. *Cancer* 1997;79:2345.
158. Keilholz U, Conradt C, Legha SS, et al. Results of interleukin-2-based treatment in advanced melanoma: a case record-based analysis of 631 patients. *J Clin Oncol* 1998;16:2921.
159. Kirkwood JM, Nordlund JJ, Lerner AB, et al. Favorable prognosis of melanoma associated with hypopigmentation (HYP) in a randomized adjuvant trial comparing DTIC-BCG (DB) vs monobenzyl ether of hydroquininone (HQ) vs null (NL) treatment. *Proc Am Soc Clin Oncol* 1985;4:149.
160. Harris JE, Ryan L, Hoover HC Jr, et al. Adjuvant active specific immunotherapy for stage II and III colon cancer with an autologous tumor cell vaccine: Eastern Cooperative Oncology Group Study E5283. *J Clin Oncol* 2000;18:148.
161. Finck SJ, Giuliano AE, Morton DL. LDH and melanoma. *Cancer* 1983;51:840.
162. Bosserhoff AK, Kaufmann M, Kaluza B, et al. Melanoma-inhibiting activity, a novel serum marker for progression of malignant melanoma. *Cancer Res* 1997;57:3149.
163. Berd D, Maguire HC Jr, McCue P, Mastrangelo MJ. Treatment of metastatic melanoma with an autologous tumor-cell vaccine: clinical and immunologic results in 64 patients. *J Clin Oncol* 1990;8:1858.
164. Curry BJ, Farrelly M, Hersey P. Evaluation of S-100 beta assays for the prediction of recurrence and prognosis in patients with AJCC stage I-III melanoma. *Melanoma Res* 1999;9:557.
165. Muhlbauer M, Langenbach N, Stolz W, et al. Detection of melanoma cells in the blood of melanoma patients by melanoma-inhibitory activity (MIA) reverse transcription-PCR. *Clin Cancer Res* 1999;5:1099.
166. Proebstle TM, Jiang W, Hogel J, et al. Correlation of positive RT-PCR for tyrosinase in peripheral blood of malignant melanoma patients with clinical stage, survival and other risk factors. *Br J Cancer* 2000;82:118.
167. Battayani Z, Grob JJ, Xerri L, et al. Polymerase chain reaction detection of circulating melanocytes as a prognostic marker in patients with melanoma. *Arch Dermatol* 1995;131:443.
168. Curry BJ, Myers K, Hersey P. Polymerase chain reaction detection of melanoma cells in the circulation: relation to clinical stage, surgical treatment, and recurrence from melanoma. *J Clin Oncol* 1998;16:1760.
169. Mellado B, Gutierrez L, Castel T, et al. Prognostic significance of the detection of circulating malignant cells by reverse transcriptase-polymerase chain reaction in long-term clinically disease-free melanoma patients. *Clin Cancer Res* 1999;5:1843.
170. Benez A, Geiselhart A, Handgretinger R, Schiebel U, Fierlbeck G. Detection of circulating melanoma cells by immunomagnetic cell sorting. *J Clin Lab Anal* 1999;13:229.
171. Thompson JF, Uren RF, Shaw HM, et al. Location of sentinel lymph nodes in patients with cutaneous melanoma: new insights into lymphatic anatomy. *J Am Coll Surg* 1999;189:195.
172. Rinne D, Baum RP, Hor G, Kaufmann R. Primary staging and follow-up of high risk melanoma patients with whole-body 18F-fluorodeoxyglucose positron emission tomography: results of a prospective study of 100 patients. *Cancer* 1998;82:1664.
173. Alonso O, Martinez M, Mut F, et al. Detection of recurrent malignant melanoma with ^{99m}Tc-MIBI scintigraphy. *Melanoma Res* 1998;8:355.
174. Alonso O, Martinez M, Mut F, et al. Scintigraphic evaluation of malignant melanoma lesions with Tc-99m tetrofosmin. *Clin Nucl Med* 1998;23:683.
175. Harwood AR. Conventional radiotherapy in the treatment of lentigo maligna and lentigo maligna and lentigo maligna melanoma. *J Am Acad Dermatol* 1982;6:310.
176. Ang KK, Peters LJ, Weber RS, et al. Postoperative radiotherapy for cutaneous melanoma of the head and neck region. *Int J Radiat Oncol Biol Phys* 1994;30:795.
177. Hornsey S. The relationship between total dose, number of fractions and fractions size in the response of malignant melanoma in patients. *Br J Radiol* 1978;51:905.
178. Overgaard J. Radiation treatment of malignant melanoma. *Int J Radiat Oncol Biol Phys* 1980;6:41.
179. Bentzen SM, Overgaard J, Thames HD, et al. Clinical radiobiology of malignant melanoma. *Radiother Oncol* 1989;16:169.
180. Seegenschmiedt MH, Keilholz L, Altendorf-Hofmann A, et al. Palliative radiotherapy for recurrent and metastatic malignant melanoma: prognostic factors for tumor response and long-term outcome: a 20-year experience. *Int J Radiat Oncol Biol Phys* 1999;44:607.
181. Geara FB, Ang KK. Radiation therapy for malignant melanoma. *Surg Clin North Am* 1996;76:1383.
182. Balch CM, Reintgen DS, Kirkwood JM, et al., eds. Cutaneous melanoma. In: *Cancer principles & practices of oncology*. Philadelphia: Lippincott–Raven, 1997:1947.
183. Bentzen SM, Juul Christensen J, Overgaard J, Overgaard M. Some methodological problems in estimating radiobiological parameters from clinical data. Alpha/beta ratios and electron RBE for cutaneous reactions in patients treated with postmastectomy radiotherapy. *Acta Oncol* 1988;27:105.
184. Williams MV, Denekamp J, Fowler JF. Review of alpha/beta ratios for experimental tumors: implications for clinical studies of altered fractionation. *Int J Radiat Oncol Biol Phys* 1985;11:87.
185. Sause WT, Cooper JS, Rush S, et al. Fraction size in external beam radiation therapy in the treatment of melanoma. *Int J Radiat Oncol Biol Phys* 1991;20:429.
186. Matsumura Y, Yamagishi N, Miyakoshi J, Imamura S, Takebe H. Increase in radiation sensitivity of human malignant melanoma cells by expression of wild-type p16 gene. *Cancer Lett* 1997;115:91.
187. Thomas CP, Buronfosse A, Combaret V, et al. Gangliosides protect human melanoma cells from ionizing radiation-induced clonogenic cell death. *Glycoconjugate Journal* 1996;13:377.
188. Ng CE, Cybulski SE, Bussey AM, Aubin RA, Raaphorst GP. DNA topoisomerase I content of a pair of human melanoma cell lines with very different radiosensitivities correlates with their in vitro sensitivities to camptothecin. *Anticancer Res* 1998;18:3119.
189. Rofstad EK, Maseide K. Fraction of radiobiologically hypoxic cells in human melanoma xenografts measured by using single-cell survival, tumour growth delay and local tumour control as end points. *Br J Cancer* 1998;78:893.
190. Zhang M, Stevens G. Effect of radiation and tirapazamine (SR-4233) on three melanoma cell lines. *Melanoma Res* 1998;8:510.
191. Emami B, Perez CA, Konefal J, et al. Thermoradiotherapy of malignant melanoma. *Int J Hypertherm* 1988;4:373.
192. Engin K, Tupchong L, Waterman FM, et al. Hyperthermia and radiation in advanced malignant melanoma. *Int J Radiat Oncol Biol Phys* 1993;25:87.
193. Lamond JP, Wang M, Kinsella TJ, Boothman DA. Concentration and timing dependence of lethality enhancement between topotecan, a topoisomerase I inhibitor, and ionizing radiation. *Int J Radiat Oncol Biol Phys* 1996;36:361.
194. Utsumi H, Tano K, Mizuma N, Kobayashi T, Ichihashi M. Cellular effect of thermal neutron capture treatment using 10B1-para-boronophenylalanine: lethal effect on melanoma cells with different degrees of X-ray sensitivity. *J Radiat Res* 1996;37:193.
194a. Pomp J, Ouwerkerk IJ, Hermans J, et al. The influence of the oncogenes NRAS and MYC on the radiation sensitivity of cells of a human melanoma cell line. *J Radiat Res* 1996;146(4):374.
195. NIH Consensus conference. Diagnosis and treatment of early melanoma. *JAMA* 1992;268:1314.
196. Kiehl P, Matthies B, Ehrich K, Volker B, Kapp A. Accuracy of frozen section measurements for the determination of Breslow tumour thickness in primary malignant melanoma. *Histopathology* 1999;34:257.
197. Griffiths RW, Briggs JC. Biopsy procedures, primary wide excisional surgery and long-term prognosis in primary clinical stage I invasive cutaneous malignant melanoma. *Ann R Coll Surg* 1985;67:75.
198. Da Costa ML, Redmond P, Bouchier-Hayes DJ. The effect of laparotomy and laparoscopy on the establishment of spontaneous tumor metastases. *Surgery* 1998;124:516.
199. Breuninger H, Schlagenhauff B, Stroebel W, et al. Patterns of local horizontal spread of melanomas: consequences for surgery and histopathologic investigation. *Am J Surg Pathol* 1999;23:1493.
200. Kelly JW, Sagebiel RW, Calderon W, et al. The frequency of local recurrence and microsatellites as a guide to reexcision margins for cutaneous malignant melanoma. *Ann Surg* 1984;200:759.
201. Wong CK. A study of melanocytes in the normal skin surrounding malignant melanomata. *Dermatologica* 1970;141:215.
202. Dong XD, Tyler D, Johnson JL, DeMatos P, Seigler HF. Analysis of prognosis and disease progression after local recurrence of melanoma. *Cancer* 2000;88:1063.
203. Urist MM, Balch CM, Soong S, et al. The influence of surgical margins and prognostic factors predicting the risk of local recurrence in 3445 patients with primary cutaneous melanoma. *Cancer* 1985;55:1398.
204. Karakousis CP, Balch CM, Urist MM, et al. Local recurrence in malignant melanoma: long-term results of the multiinstitutional randomized surgical trial. *Ann Surg Oncol* 1996;3:446.
205. Handley S. The Hunterian lectures: the pathology of melanotic growths in relation to their operative treatment. *Lancet* 1907;1:927.
206. Urteaga O, Pack GT. On the antiquity of melanoma. *Cancer* 1966;19:607.
207. Balch CM, Karakousis C, Mettlin C, et al. Management of cutaneous melanoma in the United States. *Surg Gynecol Obstet* 1984;158:311.
208. Veronesi U, Cascinelli N, Adamus J, et al. Thin stage I primary cutaneous malignant melanoma. Comparison of excision with margins of 1 or 3 cm. *N Engl J Med* 1988;318:1159.
209. Balch CM, Urist MM, Karakousis CP, et al. Efficacy of 2-cm surgical margins for intermediate-thickness melanomas (1 to 4 mm). Results of a multi-institutional randomized surgical trial. *Ann Surg* 1993;218:262.
210. Ringborg U, Andersson R, Eldh J, et al. Resection margins of 2 versus 5 cm for cutaneous malignant melanoma with a tumor thickness of 0.8 to 2.0 mm: randomized study by the Swedish Melanoma Study Group. *Cancer* 1996;77:1809.

211. Heaton KM, Sussman JJ, Gershenwald JE, et al. Surgical margins and prognostic factors in patients with thick (>4mm) primary melanoma. *Ann Surg Oncol* 1998;5:322.
212. Park KG, Blessing K, Kernohan NM. Surgical aspects of subungual malignant melanomas. The Scottish Melanoma Group. *Ann Surg* 1992;216:692.
213. Krementz ET, Feed RJ, Coleman WP III, et al. Acral lentiginous melanoma. A clinicopathologic entity. *Ann Surg* 1982;195:632.
214. Balch CM, Houghton AN, Milton GW, eds. *Cutaneous melanoma. Clinical management and treatment results worldwide.* Philadelphia: Lippincott, 1998.
215. Fortin PT, Freiberg AA, Rees R, Sondak VK, Johnson TM. Malignant melanoma of the foot and ankle. *J Bone Joint Surg Am* 1995;77:1396.
216. Schnur PL. Volar foot skin grafts do work! *Ann Plastic Surg* 1994;33:572.
217. Geraghty PJ, Johnson TM, Sondak VK, Chang AE. Surgical therapy of primary cutaneous melanoma. *Semin Surg Oncol* 1996;12:386.
218. Gaspar ZS, Dawber RP. Treatment of lentigo maligna. *Aust J Dermatol* 1997;38:1.
219. Cohen LM. Lentigo maligna and lentigo maligna melanoma. *J Am Acad Dermatol* 1995;33:923.
220. Zitelli JA, Brown C, Hanusa BH. Mohs micrographic surgery for the treatment of primary cutaneous melanoma. *J Am Acad Dermatol* 1997;37:236.
221. Balch CM, Murad TM, Soong SJ, et al. Tumor thickness as a guide to surgical management of clinical stage I melanoma patients. *Cancer* 1979;43:883.
222. Balch CM, Soong SJ, Murad TM, Ingalls AL, Maddox WA. A multifactorial analysis of melanoma: III. Prognostic factors in melanoma patients with lymph node metastases (stage II). *Ann Surg* 1981;193:377.
223. Link EM, Michalowski AS, Rosch F. 211At-methylene blue for targeted radiotherapy of disseminated melanoma: microscopic analysis of tumour versus normal tissue damage. *Eur J Cancer* 1996;32A:1986.
224. Slingluff CL Jr, Stidham KR, Ricci WM, Stanley WE, Seigler HF. Surgical management of regional lymph nodes in patients with melanoma. Experience with 4682 patients. *Ann Surg* 1994;219:120.
225. Van d V, Eggermont AM, Van Putten WL, Wiggers T. Therapeutic lymphadenectomy in melanomas of the head and neck. *Head Neck* 1993;15:377.
226. Peralta EA, Yarington CT, Glenn MG. Malignant melanoma of the head and neck: effect of treatment on survival. *Laryngoscope* 1998;108:220.
227. Veronesi U. Regional lymph node dissection in melanoma of the limbs. Stage I. A cooperative international trial (WHO Collaborating Centers for diagnosis and treatment of melanoma). *Rec Res Cancer Res* 1977;80:8.
228. Sim FH, Taylor WF, Pritchard DJ, Soule EH. Lymphadenectomy in the management of stage I malignant melanoma: a prospective randomized study. *Mayo Clin Proc* 1986; 61:697.
229. Cascinelli N, Morabito A, Santinami M, MacKie RM, Belli F. Immediate or delayed dissection of regional nodes in patients with melanoma of the trunk: a randomised trial. WHO Melanoma Programme. *Lancet* 1998;351:793.
230. Balch CM, Soong SJ, Bartolucci AA, et al. Efficacy of an elective regional lymph node dissection of 1 to 4 mm thick melanomas for patients 60 years of age and younger. *Ann Surg* 1996;224:255.
231. Reintgen D, Cruse CW, Wells K, et al. The orderly progression of melanoma nodal metastases. *Ann Surg* 1994;220:759.
232. Morton DL, Thompson JF, Essner R, et al. Validation of the accuracy of intraoperative lymphatic mapping and sentinel lymphadenectomy for early-stage melanoma. *Ann Surg* 1999;230:453.
233. Gershenwald J, Thompson W, Mansfield P, et al. Patterns of failure in melanoma patients after successful lymphatic mapping and negative sentinel node biopsy. *Soc Surg Oncol* 1996;20.
234. Morton DL, Wen DR, Wong JH, et al. Technical details of intraoperative lymphatic mapping for early stage melanoma. *Arch Surg* 1992;127:392.
235. Veronesi U. Delayed node dissection in stage one malignant melanoma: justification and advantages. *Cancer Invest* 1987;5:47.
236. Cabanas RM. An approach for the treatment of penile carcinoma. *Cancer* 1977;39:456.
237. Robinson DS, Sample WF, Fee HJ, Holmes C, Morton DL. Regional lymphatic drainage in primary malignant melanoma of the trunk determined by colloidal gold scanning. *Surg Forum* 1977;28:147.
238. Alex JC, Weaver DL, Fairbank JT, Rankin BS, Krag DN. Gamma-probe-guided lymph node localization in malignant melanoma. *Surg Oncol* 1993;2:303.
239. Hung JC, Wiseman GA, Wahner HW, et al. Filtered technetium-99m-sulfur celloid evaluated for lymphoscintigraphy. *J Nucl Med* 1995;36:1895.
240. Pijpers R, Borgstein PJ, Meijer S, et al. Sentinel node biopsy in melanoma patients: dynamic lymphoscintigraphy followed by intraoperative gamma probe and vital dye guidance. *World J Surg* 1997;21:788.
240a. Essner R, Conforti A, Kelley MC, et al. Efficacy of lymphatic mapping, sentinel lymphadenectomy, and selective complete lymph node dissection as a therapeutic procedure for early-stage melanoma. *Ann Surg Oncol* 1999;6(5):442.
241. Glass EC, Essner R, Morton DL. Kinetics of three lymphoscintigraphic agents in patients with cutaneous melanoma. *J Nucl Med* 1998;39:1185.
242. Reintgen D. Lymphatic mapping and sentinel node harvest for malignant melanoma. *J Surg Oncol* 1997;66:277.
243. Sappey MP. *Injection, preparation, et conservation des vaisseaux lymphatique. These pour le doctorat en medecine.* No 24. Paris: Rignoux, Imprimeur de la Faculte de Medecine, 1843.
244. Norman J, Wells K, Kearney R, et al. Identification of lymphatic drainage basins in patients with cutaneous melanoma. *Semin Surg Oncol* 1993;9:224.
245. McCarthy WH, Shaw HM, Milton GW. Efficacy of elective lymph node dissection in 2,347 patients with clinical stage I malignant melanoma. *Surg Gynecol Obstet* 1985;161:575.
246. Dale PS, Foshag LJ, Wanek LA, Morton DL. Metastasis of primary melanoma to two separate lymph node basins: prognostic significance. *Ann Surg Oncol* 1997;4:13.
247. Uren RF, Howman-Giles R, Thompson JF, et al. Lymphoscintigraphy to identify sentinel lymph nodes in patients with melanoma. *Melanoma Res* 1994;4:395.
248. Bostick P, Essner R, Glass E, et al. Comparison of blue dye and probe-assisted intraoperative lymphatic mapping in melanoma to identify sentinel nodes in 100 lymphatic basins. *Arch Surg* 1999;134:43.
249. Pu LL, Cruse CW, Wells KE, et al. Lymphatic mapping and sentinel lymph node biopsy in patients with melanoma of th elower extremity. *Plast Reconstruct Surg* 1999; 104:964.
250. Lenisa L, Santinami M, Belli F, et al. Sentinel node biopsy and selective lymph node dissection in cutaneous melanoma patients. *J Exp Clin Cancer Res* 1999;18:69.
251. Krag DN, Meijer SJ, Weaver DL, et al. Minimal-access surgery for staging of malignant melanoma. *Arch Surg* 1995;130:654.
252. Essner R, Conforti A, Kelley MC, et al. Efficacy of lymphatic mapping, sentinel lymphadenectomy, and selective complete lymph node dissection as a therapeutic procedure for early-stage melanoma. *Ann Surg Oncol* 1999;6:442.
253. Morton DL, Wen DR, Foshag LJ, Essner R, Cochran A. Intraoperative lymphatic mapping and selective cervical lymphadenectomy for early-stage melanomas of the head and neck. *J Clin Oncol* 1993;11:1751.
254. Glass FL, Cottam JA, Reintgen DS, Fenske NA. Lymphatic mapping and sentinel node biopsy in the management of high-risk melanoma. *J Am Acad Dermatol* 1998;39:603.
255. Karakousis CP, Grigoropoulos P. Sentinal node biopsy before and after wide excision of the primary melanoma. *Ann Surg Oncol* 1999;6:785.
256. Jansen L, Koops HS, Nieweg OE, et al. Sentinel node biopsy for melanoma in the head and neck region. *Head Neck* 2000;22:27.
257. Uren RF, Howman-Giles RB, Thompson JF, Roberts J, Bernard E. Variability of cutaneous lymphatic flow rates in melanoma patients. *Melanoma Res* 1998;8:279.
258. Pitman KT, Johnson JT, Edington H, et al. Lymphatic mapping with isosulfan blue dye in squamous cell carcinoma of the head and neck. *Head Neck Surg* 1998;124:790.
259. Wells KE, Rapaport DP, Cruse CW, et al. Sentinel lymph node biopsy in melanoma of the head and neck. *Plast Reconstruct Surg* 1997;100:591.
260. Clayman G. *Sentinel node mapping for the head and neck.* Presented at the Society of Surgical Oncology Annual Meeting, New Orleans, LA, March 2000.
261. Morton DL, Thompson JF, Essner R, et al. Validation of the accuracy of intraoperative lymphatic mapping and sentinel lymphadenectomy for early-stage melanoma: a multicenter trial. Multicenter Selective Lymphadenectomy Trial Group. *Ann Surg* 1999; 230:453.
262. Messina JL, Glass LF, Cruse CW, et al. Pathologic examination of the sentinel lymph node in malignant melanoma. *Am J Surg Pathol* 1999;23:686.
263. Reintgen DS, et al. Accurate nodal staging of malignant melanoma: cancer control. *Journal of the Moffitt Cancer Center* 1995;1995:405.
264. van der Velde-Zimmermann D, Schipper ME, De Weger RA, Hennipman A, Borel Rinkes IH. Sentinel node biopsies in melanoma patients: a protocol for accurate, efficient, and cost-effective analysis by preselection for immunohistochemistry on the basis of Tyr-PCR. *Ann Surg Oncol* 2000;7:51.
265. Wang T, Brown MJ. mRNA quantification by real time TaqMan polymerase chain reaction: validation and comparison with RNase protection. *Ann Biochem* 1999;269:198.
266. Karakousis CP, Emrich LJ, Driscoll DL, Rao U. Survival after groin dissection for malignant melanoma. *Surgery* 1991;109:119.
267. McNeer G, Das Gupta T. Prognosis in malignant melanoma. *Surgery* 1964;56:512.
268. Das Gupta TK. Results of treatment of 269 patients with primary cutaneous melanoma: a five-year prospective study. *Ann Surg* 1977;186:201.
269. Roses DF, Provet JA, Harris MN, Gumport SL, Dubin N. Prognosis of patients with pathologic stage II cutaneous malignant melanoma. *Ann Surg* 1985;201:103.
270. Callery C, Cochran AJ, Roe DJ, et al. Factors prognostic for survival in patients with malignant melanoma spread to the regional lymph nodes. *Ann Surg* 1982;196:69.
271. Cohen MH, Ketcham AS, Felix EL, et al. Prognostic factors in patients undergoing lymphadenectomy for malignant melanoma. *Ann Surg* 1977;186:635.
272. Kissin MW, Simpson DA, Easton D, White H, Westbury G. Prognostic factors related to survival and groin recurrence following therapeutic lymph node dissection for lower limb malignant melanoma. *Br J Surg* 1987;74:1023.
273. Karakousis CP. Therapeutic node dissections in malignant melanoma. *Semin Surg Oncol* 1998;14:291.
274. Mann GB, Coit DG. Does the extent of operation influence the prognosis in patients with melanoma metastatic to inguinal nodes? *Ann Surg Oncol* 1999;6:263.
275. Strobbe LJ, Jonk A, Hart AA, Nieweg OE, Kroon BB. Positive iliac and obturator nodes in melanoma: survival and prognostic factors. *Ann Surg Oncol* 1999;6:255.
276. Karakousis CP, Hena MA, Emrich LJ, Driscoll DL. Axillary node dissection in malignant melanoma: results and complications. *Surgery* 1990;108:10.
277. Wells KE, Stadelmann WK, Rapaport DP, et al. Parotid selective lymphadenectomy in malignant melanoma. *Ann Plast Surg* 1999;43:1.
278. Karakousis CP. The technique of popliteal lymph node dissection. *Surg Gynecol Obstet* 1980;151:420.
279. Smith TJ, Sloan GM, Baker AR. Epitrochlear node involvement in melanoma of the upper extremity. *Cancer* 1983;51:756.
280. Karakousis CP, Goumas W, Rao U, Driscoll DL. Axillary node dissection in malignant melanoma. *Am J Surg* 1991;162:202.
281. Karakousis CP, Hena MA, Emrich LJ, Driscoll DL. Axillary node dissection in malignant melanoma: results and complications. *Surgery* 1990;108:10.
282. Lotze MT, Duncan MA, Gerber LH, Woltering EA, Rosenberg, SA. Early versus delayed shoulder motion following axillary dissection: a randomized prospective study. *Ann Surg* 1981;193:288.
283. Chang AE, Karnell LH, Menck HR. The National Cancer Data Base report on cutaneous and noncutaneous melanoma: a summary of 84,836 cases from the past decade. The American College of Surgeons Commission on Cancer and the American Cancer Society. *Cancer* 1998;83:1664.

284. Sutherland CM, Chmiel JS, Bieligk S, Henson DE, Winchester DP. Patient characteristics, treatment, and outcome of unknown primary melanoma in the United States for the years 1981 and 1987. *Am Surg* 1996;62:400.

285. Schlagenhauff B, Stroebel W, Ellwanger U, et al. Metastatic melanoma of unknown primary origin shows prognostic similarities to regional metastatic melanoma: recommendations for initial staging examinations. *Cancer* 1997;80:60.

286. Delanian S, Balla-Mekias S, Lefaix J-L. Striking regression of chronic radiotherapy damage in a clinical trial of combined pentoxifylline and tocopherol. *J Clin Oncol* 1999;17:3283.

287. Borgstein PJ, Meijer S, van Diest PJ. Are locoregional cutaneous metastases in melanoma predictable? *Ann Surg Oncol* 1999;6:315.

288. Wong JH, Cagle LA, Kopald KH, Swisher SG, Morton DL. Natural history and selective management of in transit melanoma. *J Surg Oncol* 1990;44:146.

289. Stehlin JS Jr, Smith JL Jr, Jing BS, Sherrin D. Melanomas of the extremities complicated by in-transit metastases. *Surg Gynecol Obstet* 1966;122:3.

290. Jaques DP, Coit DG, Brennan MF. Major amputation for advanced malignant melanoma. *Surg Gynecol Obstet* 1989;169:1.

291. Coit DG. Hyperthermic isolation limb perfusion for malignant melanoma: a review. *Cancer Invest* 1992;10:277.

292. Briele HA, Walker MJ, Das Gupta TK. Melanoma of the head and neck. *Clin Plastic Surg* 1985;12:495.

293. Lejeune FJ, Deloof T, Ewalenko P, et al. Objective regression of unexcised melanoma in-transit metastases after hyperthermic isolation perfusion of the limbs with melphalan. *Rec Res Cancer Res* 1983;86:268.

294. Stehlin JS Jr. Hyperthermic perfusion with chemotherapy for cancers of the extremities. *Surg Gynecol Obstet* 1969;129:305.

295. Lienard D, Lejeune FJ, Ewalenko P. In transit metastases of malignant melanoma treated by high dose rTNF alpha in combination with interferon-gamma and melphalan in isolation perfusion. *World J Surg* 1992;16:234.

296. Koops HS, Vaglini M, Suciu S, et al. Prophylactic isolated limb perfusion for localized, high-risk limb melanoma: results of a multicenter randomized phase III trial. European Organization for Research and Treatment of Cancer Malignant Melanoma Cooperative Group Protocol 18832, the World Health Organization Melanoma Program Trial 15, and the North American Perfusion Group Southwest Oncology Group-8593. *J Clin Oncol* 1998;16:2906.

297. Lingam MK, McKay AJ, MacKie RM, Aitchison T. Single-centre prospective study of isolated limb perfusion with melphalan in the treatment of subungual malignant melanoma. *Br J Surg* 1995;82:1343.

298. Fraker DL, Alexander HR, Andrich M, Rosenberg SA. Palliation of regional symptoms of advanced extremity melanoma by isolated limb perfusion with melphalan and high-dose tumor necrosis factor. *Cancer Journal from Scientific American* 1995;1:122.

299. Ghussen F, Kruger I, Groth W, Stutzer H. Randomized melanoma study of perfusion of the extremities. Results of treament 2 1/2 years after premature discontinuation. *Chirurg* 1986;57:619.

300. Hafstrom L, Rudenstam CM, Blomquist E, et al. Regional hyperthermic perfusion with melphalan after surgery for recurrent malignant melanoma of the extremities. Swedish Melanoma Study Group. *J Clin Oncol* 1991;9:2091.

301. Klop WM, Vrouenraets BC, van Geel BN, et al. Repeat isolated limb perfusion with melphalan for recurrent melanoma of the limbs. *J Am Coll Surg* 1996;182:467.

301a. Klaase JM, Kroon BB, van Geel AN, et al. Limb recurrence-free interval and survival in patients with recurrent melanoma of the extremities treated with normothermic isolated perfusion. *J Am Coll Surg* 1994;178(6):564.

302. Klaase JM, Kroon BB, van Geel AN, Eggermont AM, Franklin HR. Systemic leakage during isolated limb perfusion for melanoma. *Br J Surg* 1993;80:1124.

303. Barker WC, Andrich MP, Alexander HR, Fraker DL. Continuous intraoperative external monitoring of perfusate leak using iodine-131 human serum albumin during isolated perfusion of the liver and limbs. *Eur J Nucl Med* 1995;22:1242.

304. Hoekstra HJ, Naujocks T, Schraffordt KH, et al. Continuous leaking monitoring during hyperthermic isolated regional perfusion of the lower limb: techniques and results. *Reg Cancer Treat* 1992;4:301.

305. Wieberdink J. Dosimetry in isolated perfusion of the limbs by assessment of perfused tissue volume and grading of toxic tissue reactions. *Eur J Cancer Clin Oncol* 1982;18:905.

306. Scott RN, Blackie R, Kerr DJ, et al. Melphalan concentration and distribution in the tissues of tumour-bearing limbs treated by isolated limb perfusion. *Eur J Cancer* 1992;28A:1811.

307. Cavaliere R, Ciocatto EC, Giovanella BC, et al. Selective heat sensitivity of cancer cells: biochemical and clinical studies. *Cancer* 1967;20:1351.

308. Di Filippo F, Calabro A, Giannarelli D, et al. Prognostic variables in recurrent limb melanoma treated with hyperthermic antiblastic perfusion. *Cancer* 1989;63:2551.

309. Klaase JM, Kroon BB, van Geel AN, et al. Limb recurrence-free interval and survival in patients with recurrent melanoma of the extremities treated with normothermic isolated perfusion. *J Am Coll Surg* 1994;178:564.

309a. Lienard D, Lejeune FJ, Ewalenko P. In transit metastases of malignant melanoma treated by high dose rTNF alpha in combination with interferon-gamma and melphalan in isolation perfusion. *World J Surg* 1992;16(2):234.

309b. Belli F, Arienti F, Rivoltini L, et al. Treatment of recurrent in transit metastases from cutaneous melanoma by isolation perfusion in extracorporeal circulation with interleukin-2 and lymphokine activated killer cells. A pilot study. *Melanoma Res* 1992;2(4):263.

310. Cavaliere R, Cavaliere F, Deraco M, et al. Hyperthermic antiblastic perfusion in the treatment of stage IIIA-IIIAB melanoma patients. Comparison of two experiences. *Melanoma Res* 1994;4(Suppl 1):5.

311. Hoekstra HJ, Schraffordt KH, de Vries LG, van Weerden TW, Oldhoff J. Toxicity of hyperthermic isolated limb perfusion with cisplatin for recurrent melanoma of the lower extremity after previous perfusion treatment. *Cancer* 1993;72:1224.

312. Vrouenraets BC, Klaase JM, Nieweg OE, Kroon BB. Toxicity and morbidity of isolated limb perfusion. *Semin Surg Oncol* 1998;14:224.

313. Renard N, Lienard D, Lespagnard L, et al. Early endothelium activation and polymorphonuclear cell invasion precede specific necrosis of human melanoma and sarcoma treated by intravascular high-dose tumour necrosis factor alpha (rTNF alpha). *Int J Cancer* 1994;57:656.

314. Lejeune FJ. High dose recombinant tumour necrosis factor (rTNF alpha) administered by isolation perfusion for advanced tumours of the limbs: a model for biochemotherapy of cancer. *Eur J Cancer* 1995;31A:1009.

315. Sugarman BJ, Palladino MA Jr, Figari IS, Palladino MA, Shepard HM. Recombinant human tumor necrosis factor-alpha: effects on proliferation of normal and transformed cells in vitro. *Science* 1985;230:943.

316. Lienard D, Eggermont AM, Schraffordt KH, et al. Isolated perfusion of the limb with high-dose tumour necrosis factor-alpha (TNF-alpha), interferon-gamma (IFN-gamma) and melphalan for melanoma stage III. Results of a multi-centre pilot study. *Melanoma Res* 1994;4(Suppl)1:21.

317. Alexander HR Jr, Fraker DL, Bartlett DL. Isolated limb perfusion for malignant melanoma. *Semin Surg Oncol* 1996;12:416.

318. Bartlett DL, Ma G, Alexander HR, Libutti SK, Fraker DL. Isolated limb reperfusion with tumor necrosis factor and melphalan in patients with extremity melanoma after failure of isolated limb perfusion with chemotherapeutics. *Cancer* 1997;80:2084.

319. Ariyan S, Poo WJ. Safety and efficacy of isolated perfusion of extremities for recurrent tumor in elderly patients. *Surgery* 1998;123:335.

320. Vrouenraets BC, Hart GA, Eggermont AM, et al. Relation between limb toxicity and treatment outcomes after isolated limb perfusion for recurrent melanoma. *J Am Coll Surg* 1999;188:522.

321. Vrouenraets BC, Kroon BB, Klaase JM, et al. Value of laboratory tests in monitoring acute regional toxicity after isolated limb perfusion. *Ann Surg Oncol* 1997;4:88.

322. Hohenberger P, Kettelhack C. Clinical management and current research in isolated limb perfusion for sarcoma and melanoma. *Oncology* 1998;55:89.

323. Vrouenraets BC, Eggermont AM, Klaase JM, et al. Long-term neuropathy after regional isolated perfusion with melphalan for melanoma of the limbs. *Eur J Surg Oncol* 1994;20:681.

324. Drory VE, Lev D, Groozman GB, Gutmann M, Klausner JM. Neurotoxicity of isolated limb perfusion with tumor necrosis factor. *J Neurol Sci* 1998;158:1.

325. Ariyan S, Poo WJ, Bolognia J. Regional isolated perfusion of extremities for melanoma: a 20-year experience with drugs other than L-phenylalanine mustard. *Plast Reconstruct Surg* 1997;99:1023.

326. Klaase JM, Kroon BB, van Geel BN, et al. Patient- and treatment-related factors associated with acute regional toxicity after isolated perfusion for melanoma of the extremities. *Am J Surg* 1994;167:618.

327. Sigurdsson GH, Nachbur B, Lejeune FJ. Anesthesiologists' management of isolated limb perfusion with "high-dose" tumor necrosis factor alpha. *Anesthesiology* 1993;79:1433.

328. Sleijfer S, van Ginkel RJ, van der Mark TW, et al. Effects of hyperthermic isolated limb perfusion with tumor necrosis factor-alpha and melphalan on pulmonary function assessments. *J Immunother* 1997;20:202.

329. Vrouenraets BC, Kroon BB, Ogilvie AC, et al. Absence of severe systemic toxicity after leakage-controlled isolated limb perfusion with tumor necrosis factor-alpha and melphalan. *Ann Surg Oncol* 1999;6:405.

330. Klicks RJ, Vrouenraets BC, Nieweg OE, Kroon BB. Vascular complications of isolated limb perfusion. *Eur J Surg Oncol* 1998;24:288.

331. Thompson JF, Kam PC, Waugh RC, Harman CR. Isolated limb infusion with cytotoxic agents: a simple alternative to isolated limb perfusion. *Semin Surg Oncol* 1998;14:238.

332. Eton O, East M, Legha SS, et al. Pilot study of intra-arterial cisplatin and intravenous vinblastine and dacarbazine in patients with melanoma in-transit metastases. *Melanoma Res* 1999;9:483.

333. Hill S, Thomas JM. Use of the carbon dioxide laser to manage cutaneous metastases from malignant melanoma. *Br J Surg* 1996;83:509.

334. Lingam MK, McKay AJ. Carbon dioxide laser ablation as an alternative treatment for cutaneous metastases from malignant melanoma. *Br J Surg* 1995;82:1346.

335. Heller R, Jaroszeski MJ, Reintgen DS, et al. Treatment of cutaneous and subcutaneous tumors with electrochemotherapy using intralesional bleomycin. *Cancer* 1998;83:148.

336. Keller SM. Photodynamic therapy. Biology and clinical application. *Chest Surg Clin North Am* 1995;5:121.

337. Morton DL, Malmgren RA, Holmes EC, Ketcham AS. Demonstration of antibodies against human malignant melanoma by immunofluorescence. *Surgery* 1968;64:233.

338. von Wussow P, Block B, Hartmann F, Deicher H. Intralesional interferon-alpha therapy in advanced malignant melanoma. *Cancer* 1988;61:1071.

339. Morton DL, Eilber FR, Holmes EC, et al. BCG immunotherapy of malignant melanoma: summary of a seven-year experience. *Ann Surg* 1974;180:635.

340. Overgaard J, von der MH, Overgaard M. A randomized study comparing two high-dose per fraction radiation schedules in recurrent or metastatic malignant melanoma. *Int J Radiat Oncol Biol Phys* 1985;11:1837.

341. Cascinelli N, Rumke P, MacKie R, Morabito A, Bufalino R. The significance of conversion of skin reactivity to efficacy of bacillus Calmette-Guerin (BCG) vaccinations given immediately after radical surgery in stage II melanoma patients. *Cancer Immunol Immunother* 1989;28:282.

342. Wallack MK, McNally K, Michaelides M, et al. A phase I/II SECSG (Southeastern Cancer Study Group) pilot study of surgical adjuvant immunotherapy with vaccinia melanoma oncolysates (VMO). *Am Surg* 1986;52:148.

343. Balch CM, Smalley RV, Bartolucci AA, et al. A randomized prospective clinical trial of adjuvant C. parvum immunotherapy in 260 patients with clinically localized melanoma (stage I): prognostic factors analysis and preliminary results of immunotherapy. *Cancer* 1982;49:1079.

344. Kirkwood JM, Wilson J, Whiteside TL, Donnelly S, Herberman RB. Phase IB trial of picibanil (OK-432) as an immunomodulator in patients with resected high-risk melanoma. *Cancer Immunol Immunother* 1997;44:137.

345. Kirkwood J. Interferon alpha to be as adjuvant therapy for high risk melanoma. *Melanoma Res* 1997;7:S23.

346. Yeilding NM, Gerstner C, Kirkwood JM. Analysis of two human monoclonal antibodies against melanoma. *Int J Cancer* 1992;52:967.
347. Heredia A, Villena J, Romaris M, Molist A, Bassols A. Transforming growth factor beta 1 increases the synthesis and shedding of the melanoma-specific proteoglycan in human melanoma cells. *Arch Biochem Biophys* 1996;333:198.
348. Spitler LE, Sagebiel R. A randomized trial of levamisole versus placebo as adjuvant therapy in malignant melanoma. *N Engl J Med* 1980;303:1143.
349. Spitler LE. A randomized trial of levamisole versus placebo as adjuvant therapy in malignant melanoma. *J Clin Oncol* 1991;9:736.
350. Quirt IC, Shelley WE, Pater JL, et al. Improved survival in patients with poor-prognosis malignant melanoma treated with adjuvant levamisole: a phase III study by the National Cancer Institute of Canada Clinical Trials Group. *J Clin Oncol* 1991;9:729.
351. Abramowitz J, Chavin W. In vitro effects of hormonal stimuli upon tyrosinase and peroxidase activities in murine melanomas. *Biochem Biophys Res Comm* 1978;85:1067.
352. Cole BF, Gelber RD, Kirkwood JM, et al. Quality-of-life-adjusted survival analysis of interferon alfa-2b adjuvant treatment of high-risk resected cutaneous melanoma: an Eastern Cooperative Oncology Group study. *J Clin Oncol* 1996;14:2666.
353. Cole BF, Gelber RD, Kirkwood JM, et al. A quality-of-life adjusted survival analysis of interferon alfa-2b (IFNa2b) adjuvant treatment for high-risk resected cutaneous melanoma: an Eastern Cooperative Oncology Group (ECOG) study. *Proc Am Soc Clin Oncol* 1996;15:437.
354. Hillner BE, Kirkwood JM, Atkins MB, Johnson ER, Smith TJ. Economic analysis of adjuvant interferon alfa-2b in high-risk melanoma based on projections from Eastern Cooperative Oncology Group 1684. *J Clin Oncol* 1997;15:2351.
355. Marchand M, Weynants P, Rankin E, et al. Tumor regression responses in melanoma patients treated with a peptide encoded by gene MAGE-3. *Int J Cancer* 1995;63:883.
356. Cascinelli N. Evaluation of efficacy of adjuvant rIFNa 2A in melanoma patients with regional node metastases. *Proc Am Soc Clin Oncol* 1995;14:A1296.
357. Kirkwood JM, Ibrahim J, Sondak VK, et al. High- and low-dose interferon alfa-2b in high-risk melanoma: first analysis of Intergroup Trial E1690/S9111/C9190. *J Clin Oncol* 2000; 18(12):2444.
358. Livingston PO, Wong GY, Adluri S, et al. Improved survival in stage III melanoma patients with GM2 antibodies: a randomized trial of adjuvant vaccination with GM2 ganglioside. *J Clin Oncol* 1994;12:1036.
359. Livingston PO, Adluri S, Helling F, et al. Phase 1 trial of immunological adjuvant QS-21 with a GM2 ganglioside-keyhole limpet haemocyanin conjugate vaccine in patients with malignant melanoma. *Vaccine* 1994;12:1275.
360. Hsueh EC, Famatiga E, Gupta RK, Qi K, Morton DL. Enhancement of complement-dependent cytotoxicity by polyvalent melanoma cell vaccine (CancerVax): correlation with survival. *Ann Surg Oncol* 1998;5:595.
361. Restifo NP, Rosenberg SA. Developing recombinant and synthetic vaccines for the treatment of melanoma. *Curr Opin Oncol* 1999;11:50.
362. Rosenberg SA, Yang JC, Schwartzentruber DJ, et al. Prospective randomized trial of the treatment of patients with metastatic melanoma using chemotherapy with cisplatin,dacarbazine, and tamoxifen alone or in a combination with interleukin-2 and interferon alfa-2b. *J Clin Oncol* 1999;17:968.
363. Grob JJ, Dreno B, de la SP, et al. Randomised trial of interferon alpha-2a as adjuvant therapy in resected primary melanoma thicker than 1.5 mm without clinically detectable node metastases. French Cooperative Group on Melanoma. *Lancet* 1998;351:1905.
364. Pehamberger H, Soyer HP, Steiner A, et al. Adjuvant interferon alfa-2a treatment in resected primary stage II cutaneous melanoma. Austrian Malignant Melanoma Cooperative Group. *J Clin Oncol* 1998;16:1425.
365. Kirkwood JM. Adjuvant IFNa2 therapy of melanoma. *Lancet* 1998;351:1901.
366. Kirkwood JM. Adjuvant IFN alpha2 therapy of melanoma. *Lancet* 1998;351:1901.
367. Quan WD Jr, Dean GE, Spears L, et al. Active specific immunotherapy of metastatic melanoma with an antiidiotype vaccine: a phase I/II trial of I-Mel-2 plus SAF-m. *J Clin Oncol* 1997;15:2103.
368. Eton O, Kharkevitch DD, Gianan MA, et al. Active immunotherapy with ultraviolet B-irradiated autologous whole melanoma cells plus DETOX in patients with metastatic melanoma. *Clin Cancer Res* 1998;4:619.
369. Mitchell MS. Perspective on allogeneic melanoma lysates in active specific immunotherapy. *Semin Oncol* 1998;25:623.
370. Sondak VK, Liu PY, Flaherty LE, et al. A phase II evaluation of all-*trans*-retionic acid plus interferon alfa-2a in stage IV melanoma: a Southwest Oncology Group Study. *Cancer J from Scientific American* 1999;5:41.
371. Atkins MB. The treatment of metastatic melanoma with chemotherapy and biologics. *Curr Opin Oncol* 1997;9:205.
372. Weiss M, Loprinzi CL, Creagan ET, et al. Utility of follow-up tests for detecting recurrent disease in patients with malignant melanomas. *JAMA* 1995;274:1703.
373. Basseres N, Grob JJ, Richard MA, et al. Cost-effectiveness of surveillance of stage I melanoma. A retrospective appraisal based on a 10-year experience in a dermatology department in France. *Dermatology* 1995;191:199.
374. Roth JA, Eilber FR, Bennett LR, Morton DL. Radionuclide photoscanning. Usefulness in preoperative evaluation of melanoma patients. *Arch Surg* 1975;110:1211.
375. Tafra L, Dale PS, Wanek LA, Ramming KP, Morton DL. Resection and adjuvant immunotherapy for melanoma metastatic to the lung and thorax. *J Thorac Cardiovasc Surg* 1995;110:119.
376. Harpole DH Jr, Johnson CM, Wolfe WG, George SL, Seigler HF. Analysis of 945 cases of pulmonary metastatic melanoma. *J Thorac Cardiovasc Surg* 1992;103:743.
377. Ricaniadis N, Konstadoulakis MM, Walsh D, Karakousis CP. Gastrointestinal metastases from malignant melanoma. *Surg Oncol* 1995;4:105.
378. Ollila DW, Essner R, Wanek LA, Morton DL. Surgical resection for melanoma metastatic to the gastrointestinal tract. *Arch Surg* 1996;131:975.
379. Karakousis CP, Velez A, Driscoll DL, Takita H. Metastasectomy in malignant melanoma. *Surgery* 1994;115:295.
380. Pastorino U, Buyse M, Friedel G, et al. Long-term results of lung metastasectomy: prognostic analysis based on 5206 cases. *J Thorac Cardiovasc Surg* 1999;113:137.
381. Hsueh EC, Gupta RK, Qi K, Morton DL. Correlation of specific immune responses with survival in melanoma patients with distant metastases receiving polyvalent melanoma cell vaccine. *J Clin Oncol* 1998;16:2913.
382. Balch CM, Soong SJ, Murad TM, et al. A multifactorial analysis of melanoma. IV. Prognostic factors in 200 melanoma patients with distant metastases (stage III). *J Clin Oncol* 1983;1:126.
383. Feun LG, Gutterman J, Burgess MA, et al. The natural history of resectable metastatic melanoma (stage IVA melanoma). *Cancer* 1982;50:1656.
384. Amer MH, Al Sarraf M, Vaitkevicius VK. Clinical presentation, natural history and prognostic factors in advanced malignant melanoma. *Surg Gynecol Obstet* 1979;149:687.
385. Markowitz JS, Cosimi LA, Carey RW, et al. Prognosis after initial recurrence of cutaneous melanoma. *Arch Surg* 1991;126:703.
386. Overett TK, Shiu MH. Surgical treatment of distant metastatic melanoma. Indications and results. *Cancer* 1985;56:1222.
387. Hena MA, Emrich LJ, Nambisan RN, Karakousis CP. Effect of surgical treatment on stage IV melanoma. *Am J Surg* 1987;153:270.
388. Wornom IL III, Smith JW, Soong SJ, et al. Surgery as palliative treatment for distant metastases of melanoma. *Ann Surg* 1986;204:181.
389. Calabro A, Singletary SE, Balch CM. Patterns of relapse in 1001 consecutive patients with melanoma nodal metastases. *Arch Surg* 1989;124:1051.
390. Pogrebniak HW, Stovroff M, Roth JA, Pass HI. Resection of pulmonary metastases from malignant melanoma: results of a 16-year experience. *Ann Thorac Surg* 1988;46:20.
391. Mathisen DJ, Flye MW, Peabody J. The role of thoracotomy in the management of pulmonary metastases from malignant melanoma. *Ann Thorac Surg* 1979;27:295.
392. Ollila DW, Stern SL, Morton DL. Tumor doubling time: a selection factor for pulmonary resection of metastatic melanoma. *J Surg Oncol* 1998;69:206.
393. Einhorn LH, Burgess MA, Vallejos C, et al. Prognostic correlations and response to treatment in advanced metastatic malignant melanoma. *Cancer Res* 1974;34:1995.
394. Ollila DW, Hsueh EC, Stern SL, Morton DL. Metastasectomy for recurrent stage IV melanoma. *J Surg Oncol* 1999;71:209.
395. Caputy GG, Donohue JH, Goellner JR, Weaver AL. Metastatic melanoma of the gastrointestinal tract. Results of surgical management. *Arch Surg* 1991;126:1353.
396. Mondragon-Sanchez R, Barrera-Franco JL, Cordoba-Gutierrez H, Meneses-Garcia A. Repeat hepatic resection for recurrent metastatic melanoma. *Hepato-Gastroenterology* 1999;46:459.
397. Lindner P, Fjalling M, Hafstrom L, et al. Isolated hepatic perfusion with extracorporeal oxygenation using hyperthermia, tumor necrosis factor alpha and melphalan. *Eur J Surg Oncol* 1999;25:179.
398. Haigh PI, Essner R, Wardlaw JC, Stern SL, Morton DL. Long-term survival after complete resection of melanoma metastatic to the adrenal gland. *Ann Surg Oncol* 1999;6:633.
399. Gokaslan ZL, Aladag MA, Ellerhosrt JA. Melanoma metastatic to the spine: a review of 133 cases. *Melanoma Res* 2000;10:78.
400. Kirova YM, Chen J, Rabarijaona LI, Piedbois Y, Le Bourgeois JP. Radiotherapy as palliative treatment for metastatic melanoma. *Melanoma Res* 1999;9:11.
401. Bullard DE, Cox EB, Seigler HF. Central nervous system metastases in malignant melanoma. *Neurosurgery* 1981;8:26.
402. Amer MH, Al Sarraf M, Baker LH, Vaitkevicius VK. Malignant melanoma and central nervous system metastases: incidence, diagnosis, treatment and survival. *Cancer* 1978;42:660.
403. Patel JK, Didolkar MS, Pickren JW, Moore RH. Metastatic pattern of malignant melanoma. A study of 216 autopsy cases. *Am J Surg* 1978;135:807.
404. Brega K, Robinson WA, Winston K, Wittenberg W. Surgical treatment of brain metastases in malignant melanoma. *Cancer* 1990;66:2105.
405. Hurst R, White DE, Heiss J, et al. Brain metastasis after immunotherapy in patients with metastatic melanoma or renal cell cancer: is craniotomy indicated? *J Immunother* 1999;22:356.
406. Hagen NA, Cirrincione C, Thaler HT, DeAngelis LM. The role of radiation therapy following resection of single brain metastasis from melanoma. *Neurology* 1990;40:158.
407. Vlock DR, Kirkwood JM, Leutzinger C, Kapp DS, Fischer JJ. High-dose fraction radiation therapy for intracranial metastases of malignant melanoma: a comparison with low-dose fraction therapy. *Cancer* 1982;49:2289.
408. Kondziolka D, Patel A, Lunsford LD, Kassam A, Flickinger JC. Stereotactic radiosurgery plus whole brain radiotherapy versus radiotherapy alone for patients with multiple brain metastases. *Int J Radiat Oncol Biol Phys* 1999;45:427.
409. Mori Y, Kondziolka D, Flickinger JC, et al. Stereotactic radiosurgery for cerebral metastatic melanoma: factors affecting local disease control and survival. *Int J Radiat Oncol Biol Phys* 1998;42(3):581.
410. Kirkwood JM, Agarwala S. Systemic cytotoxic and biologic therapy melanoma. *PPO Updates* 1993;7:1.
411. Cocconi G, Bella M, Calabresi F, et al. Treatment of metastatic malignant melanoma with dacarbazine plus tamoxifen. *N Engl J Med* 1992;327:516.
412. Falkson CI, Falkson G, Falkson HC. Improved results with the addition of interferon alfa-2b to dacarbazine in the treatment of patients with metastatic malignant melanoma. *J Clin Oncol* 1991;9:1403.
413. Falkson CI, Falkson G, Falkson HC. Improved results with the addition of interferon alfa-2b to dacarbazine in the treatment of patients with metastatic malignant melanoma. *J Clin Oncol* 1991;9:1403.
414. Falkson CI, Ibrahim J, Kirkwood JM, et al. Phase III trial of dacarbazine versus dacarbazine with interferon a-2b versus dacarbazine with tamoxifen versus dacarbazine with interferon a-2b and tamoxifen in patients with metastatic malignant melanoma: an Eastern Cooperative Oncology Group study (E3690). *J Clin Oncol* 1998;16:1743.
415. Legha SS, Ring S, Eton O, et al. Development of a biochemotherapy regimen with concurrent administration of cisplatin, vinblastine, dacarbazine, interferon alfa, and interleukin-2 for patients with metastatic melanoma. *J Clin Oncol* 1998;16:1752.

416. Lattanzi SC, Tosteson T, Chertoff J, et al. Dacarbazine, cisplatin and carmustine, with or without tamoxifen, for metastatic melanoma: 5-year follow-up. *Melanoma Res* 1995;5:365.
417. Chapman PB, Einhorn LH, Meyers ML, et al. Phase III multicenter randomized trial of the Dartmouth regimen versus dacarbazine in patients with metastatic melanoma. *J Clin Oncol* 1999;17:2745.
418. Heinemann D, Smith PJB, Symes MO. Expression of histocompatibility antigens and characterization of mononuclear cell infiltrates in human renal cell carcinomas. *Br J Cancer* 1987;56:433.
419. Agarwala SS, Atkins MB, Kirkwood JM. Current approaches to advanced and high-risk melanoma. *Proc Am Soc Clin Oncol* 2000 *(in press)*.
420. Oster W, Lindemann A, Horn S, Mertelsmann R, Herrmann F. Tumor necrosis factor (TNF)-alpha but not TNF-beta induces secretion of colony stimulating factor for macrophages (CSF-1) by human monocytes. *Blood* 1987;70:1700.
421. Klostergaard J. Role of tumor necrosis factor in monocyte/macrophage tumor cytotoxicity in vitro. *Nat Immun Cell Growth Reg* 1987;6:161.
422. Middleton MR, Grob JJ, Aaronson N, et al. Randomized phase III study of temozolomide versus dacarbazine in the treatment of patients with advanced metastatic malignant melanoma. *J Clin Oncol* 2000;18:158.
423. Britten CD, Rowinsky EK, Baker SD, et al. A phase I and pharmacokinetic study of temozolomide and cisplatin in patients with advanced solid malignancies. *Clin Cancer Res* 1999;5:1629.
424. Atkins MB, Lotze M, Wiernick P, et al. High-dose IL-2 therapy alone results in long-term durable complete responses in patients with metastatic melanoma. *Proc Am Soc Clin Oncol* 1997;16:494a.
425. Nathanson L. Spontaneous regression of malignant melanoma: a review of the literature on incidence, clinical features, and possible mechanisms. Conference on spontaneous regression of cancer. *Natl Cancer Inst Monogr* 1976;44:67.
426. Rosenberg SA, White DE. Vitiligo in patients with melanoma: normal tissue antigens can be targets for cancer immunotherapy. *Journal of Immunotherapy with Emphasis on Tumor Immunology* 1996;19:81.
427. Rosenberg SA, Lotze MT, Muul LM. Observations on the systemic administration of autologous lymphokine-activated killer cells and recombinant interleukin-2 in patients with metastatic melanoma. *N Engl J Med* 1985;313:1485.
428. Mier JW, Gallo RC. Purification and some characteristics of human T-cell growth factor from phytohemagglutinin-stimulated lymphocyte-conditioned media. *Proc Natl Acad Sci U S A* 1980;77:6134.
429. Donohue JH, Rosenstein M, Change AE, et al. The systemic administration of purified interleukin 2 enhances the ability of sensitized murine lymphocytes to cure a disseminated syngeneic lymphoma. *J Immunol* 1984;132:2123.
430. Atkins MB, Kunkel L, Sznol M, Rosenberg SA. High-dose recombinant interleukin-2 therapy in patients with metastatic melanoma: long-term survival update. *Cancer J from Scientific American* 2000;6:S11.
431. Lee DS, White DE, Hurst R, Rosenberg SA, Yang JC. Patterns of relapse and response to retreatment in patients with metastatic melanoma or renal cell carcinoma who responded to interleukin-2-based immunotherapy. *Cancer J from Scientific American* 1998;4:86.
432. Sherry RM, Pass HI, Rosenberg SA, Yang JC. Surgical resection of metastatic renal cell carcinoma and melanoma after response to interleukin-2-based immunotherapy. *Cancer* 1992;69:1850.
433. Ettinghausen SE, Rosenberg SA. Immunotherapy of murine sarcomas using lymphokine activated killer cells: optimization of the schedule and routine of administration of recombinant interleukin-2. *Cancer Res* 1986;46:2784.
434. Legha SS, Gianan MA, Plager C, Eton OE, Papadopoulos NE. Evaluation of interleukin-2 administered by continuous infusion in patients with metastatic melanoma. *Cancer* 1996;77:89.
435. Tagliaferri P, Barile C, Caraglia M, et al. Daily low-dose subcutaneous recombinant interleukin-2 by alternate weekly administration: antitumor activity and immunomodulatory effects. *Am J Clin Oncol* 1998;21:48.
436. Rubin JT, Day R, Duquesnoy R, et al. HLA-DQ1 is associated with clinical response and survival of patients with melanoma who are treated with interleukin-2. *Ther Immunol* 1995;2:1.
437. Marincola FM, Venzon D, White D, et al. HLA association with response and toxicity in melanoma patients treated with interleukin 2-based immunotherapy. *Cancer Res* 1992;52:6561.
438. Lange JR, Raubitschek AA, Pockaj BA, et al. A pilot study of the combination of interleukin-2-based immunotherapy and radiation therapy. *J Immunother* 1992;12:265.
439. Rosenberg SA. Adoptive cellular therapy: clinical applications. In: De Vita VT, Hellman S, Rosenberg SA, eds. *Biological therapy of cancer.* Philadelphia: Lippincott, 1991:214.
440. Kirkwood JM, Agarwala SS. Systemic cytotoxic and biologic therapy of melanoma. In: DeVita VT, Hellman S, Rosenberg SA, eds. *PPO Updates.* Philadelphia: Lippincott, 1993:1.
441. Lotze MT. The future role of interleukin-2 in cancer therapy. *Cancer J from Scientific American* 2000;6:S58.
442. Rosenberg SA, Lotze MT, Yang JC, et al. Combination therapy with interleukin-2 and alpha-interferon for the treatment of patients with advanced cancer. *J Clin Oncol* 1989;7:1863.
443. Sparano JA, Fisher RI, Sunderland M. Randomized phase III trial of treatment with high-dose interleukin-2 either alone or in combination with interferon-alfa-2a in patients with advanced melanoma. *J Clin Oncol* 1993;11:1969.
444. Keilholz U, Eggermont AM. The role of interleukin-2 in the management of stage IV melanoma: the EORTC melanoma cooperative group program. *Cancer J from Scientific American* 2000;6:S99.
445. Margolin K, Atkins M, Sparano J, et al S. Prospective randomized trial of lisofylline for the prevention of toxicities of high-dose interleukin 2 therapy in advanced renal cancer and malignant melanoma. *Clin Cancer Res* 1997;3:565.
446. Rosenberg SA, Yang JC, Schwartzentruber DJ, et al. Prospective randomized trial of the treatment of patients with metastatic melanoma using chemotherapy with cisplatin, dacarbazine, and tamoxifen alone or in combination with interleukin-2 and interferon alfa-2b. *J Clin Oncol* 1999;17:968.
447. Rosenberg SA, Yannelli JR, Yang JC, et al. Treatment of patients with metastatic melanoma with autologous tumor-infiltrating lymphocytes and interleukin-2. *J Natl Cancer Inst* 1994;86:1159.
448. Fisher B, Packard BS, Read EJ, et al. Tumor localization of adoptively transferred indium-111 labeled tumor infiltrating lymphocytes in patients with metastatic melanoma. *J Clin Oncol* 1989;7:250.
449. Rosenberg SA. Keynote address: perspectives on the use of interleukin-2 in cancer treatment. *Cancer J from Scientific American* 1997;3(Suppl 1):S2.
450. Veltri S, Smith JW. Interleukin 1 trials in cancer patients: a review of the toxicity, antitumor and hematopoietic effects. *Oncologist* 1996;1:190.
451. Arienti F, Belli F, Napolitano F, et al. Vaccination of melanoma patients with interleukin 4 gene-transduced allogeneic melanoma cells. *Hum Gene Ther* 1999;10:2907.
452. Janik JE, Miller LL, Kopp WC, et al. Treatment with tumor necrosis factor-alpha and granulocyte-macrophage colony-stimulating factor increases epidermal Langerhans' cell numbers in cancer patients. *Clin Immunol Immunopathol* 1999;93:209.
453. Fernandez N, Duffour MT, Perricaudet M, et al. Active specific T-cell-based immunotherapy for cancer: nucleic acids, peptides, whole native proteins, recombinant viruses, with dendritic cell adjuvants or whole tumor cell-based vaccines. Principles and future prospects. *Cytokines, Cellular & Molecular Therapy* 1998;4:53.
454. Nemunaitis J, Fong T, Robbins JM, et al. Phase I trial of interferon-gamma (IFN-gamma) retroviral vector administered intratumorally to patients with metastatic melanoma. *Cancer Gene Ther* 1999;6:322.
455. Atkins MB, Robertson MJ, Gordon M, et al. Phase I evaluation of intravenous recombinant human interleukin 12 in patients with advanced malignancies. *Clin Cancer Res* 1997;3:409.
456. Freedman WL, McMahon FJ. Placental metatasis: review of the literature and report of a case of metastatic melanoma. *Obstet Gynecol* 1960;16:550.
457. Sober AJ, Day CL Jr, Fitzpatrick TB, et al. Factors associated with death from melanoma from 2 to 5 years following diagnosis in clinical stage I patients. *J Invest Dermatol* 1983;80(Suppl 6):53s.
458. Maeurer MJ, Hurd S, Martin D, Storkus WJ, Lotze MT. Cytolytic T-cell clones define HLA-A2 restricted human cutaneous melanoma peptide epitopes—correlation with T-cell receptor usage. *Cancer J* 1995;2:162.
459. Maeurer MJ, Lotze MT. Immune responses to melanoma antigens. In: Balch CM, Houghton AN, Sober AJ, Soong SJ, eds. *Cutaneous melanoma.* St Louis: Quality Medical Publishing, 1998:517.
460. Maeurer MJ, Martin DM, Storkus WJ, Lotze MT. Evidence for shared T-cell receptor usage in cytolytic T-cells recognizing HLA-A2 presented antigens shared by melanoma and melanocytes. *Immunol Today* 1995;16:603.
461. Maeurer MJ, Martin DM, Gollin SM, et al. Recurrent melanoma exhibiting downregulation of the peptide transporter protein, TAP-1 and antigen-loss of the immunodominant antigen MART-1/Melan-A recognized by CD8+ cytotoxic T-lymphocytes. *J Clin Invest* 1996;98:1633.
462. Maeurer MJ, Storkus WJ, Kirkwood JM, Lotze MT. Immunization with melanoma derived peptide T-cell epitopes represents a new treatment option for patients with melanoma. *Melanoma Res* 1996;6:11.
463. Kugler A, Stuhler G, Walden P, et al. Regression of human metastatic renal cell carcinoma after vaccination with tumor cell-dendritic cell hybrids. *Nat Med* 2000;6:332.
464. Chen YT, Scanlan MJ, Sahin U, et al. A testicular antigen aberrantly expressed in human cancers detected by autologous antibody screening. *Proc Natl Acad Sci U S A* 1997;94:1914.
465. Gure AO, Tureci O, Sahin U, et al. SSX: a multigene family with several members transcribed in normal testis and human cancer. *Int J Cancer* 1997;14:173.
466. Knuth A, Wolfel T, Klehmann E, Boon T, Meyer zum Buschenfelde KH. Cytolytic T-cell clones against an autologous human melanoma: specificity study and definition of three antigens by immunoselection. *Proc Natl Acad Sci U S A* 1989;86:2804.
467. Kawakami Y, Rosenberg SA. Immunobiology of human melanoma antigens MART-1 and gp100 and their use for immuno-gene therapy. *Int Rev Immunol* 1997;14:173.
468. Inaba K, Metlay JP, Crowley MT, Witmer-Pack M, Steinman RM. Dendritic cells as antigen presenting cells in vivo. *Int Rev Immunol* 1990;6:197.
469. Takamizawa M, Rivas A, Fagnoni F, et al. Dendritic cells that process and present nominal antigens to naive T lymphocytes are derived from CD2+ precursors. *J Immunol* 1997;158:2134.
470. Reimann J, Kaufmann SH. Alternative antigen processing pathways in anti-infective immunity. *Curr Opin Immunol* 1997;9:462.
471. Brossart P, Bevan MJ. Presentation of exogenous protein antigens on major histocompatibility complex class I molecules by dendritic cells: pathway of presentation and regulation by cytokines. *Blood* 1997;90:462.
472. Shen Z, Reznikoff G, Dranoff G, Rock KL. Cloned dendritic cells can present exogenous antigens on both MHC class I and class II molecules. *J Immunol* 1997;158:2723.
473. Norbury CC, Chambers BJ, Prescott AR, Ljunggren HG, Watts C. Constitutive macropinocytosis allows TAP-dependent major histocompatibility complex class I presentation of exogenous soluble antigen by bone marrow-derived dendritic cells. *Eur J Immunol* 1997;27:280.
474. Harding CV. Class I MHC presentation of exogenous antigens. *J Clin Immunol* 1996;16:90.
475. Bohm W, Schirmbeck R, Elbe A, et al. Exogenous hepatitis B surface antigen particles processed by dendritic cells or macrophages prime murine MHC class I-restricted cytotoxic T lymphocytes in vivo. *J Immunol* 1995;155:3313.
476. Rock KL, Rothstein L, Gamble S, Fleischacker C. Characterization of antigen-presenting cells that present exogenous antigens in association with class I MHC molecules. *J Immunol* 1993;150:438.
477. Albert ML, Sauter B, Bhardwaj N. Dendritic cells acquire antigen from apoptotic cells and induce class I-restricted CTLs. *Nature* 1998;392:86.
478. Ingulli E, Mondino A, Khoruts A, Jenkins MK. In vivo detection of dendritic cell antigen presentation to CD4+ T cells. *J Exp Med* 1997;185:2133.
479. Knight SC, Hunt R, Dore C, Medawar PB. Influence of dendritic cells on tumor growth. *Proc Am Soc Clin Oncol* 1985;82:4495.

480. Mayordomo JI, Zorina T, Storkus WJ, et al. Bone marrow-derived dendritic cells pulsed with synthetic tumor peptides elecit protective and therapeutic antitumor immunity. *Nat Med* 1995;1:1297.
481. Zitvogel L, Mayordomo JI, Tjandrawan T, et al. Therapy of murine tumors with tumor peptide-pulsed dendritic cells: dependence on T cells, B7 costimulation, and T helper cell 1-associated cytokines. *J Exp Med* 1996;183:87.
482. Sallusto F, Lanzavecchia A. Efficient presentation of soluble antigen by cultured human dendritic cells is maintained by granulocyte/macrophage colony-stimulating factor plus interleukin 4 and down-regulated by tumor necrosis factor α. *J Exp Med* 1994;179:1109.
483. Luft T, Pang KC, Thomas E, et al. A serum-free culture model for studying the differentiation of human dendritic cells from adult CD34+ progenitor cells. *Exp Hematol* 1998;26:489.
484. Luft T, Pang KC, Thomas E, et al. Type I IFNs enhance the terminal differentiation of dendritic cells. *J Immunol* 1998;161:1947.
485. McLellan AD, Sorg RV, Williams LA, Hart DNJ. Human dendritic cells activate T lymphocytes via a CD40:CD40 ligand-dependent pathway. *Eur J Immunol* 1996;26:1204.
486. Mukherji B, Chakraborty NG, Yamasaki S, et al. Induction of antigen-specific cytolytic T cells in situ in human melanoma by immunization with synthetic peptide-pulsed autologous antigen presenting cells. *Proc Natl Acad Sci U S A* 1995;92:8078.
487. Nestle FO, Alijagic S, Gilliet M, et al. Vaccination of melanoma patients with peptide- or tumor lysate-pulsed dendritic cells. *Nat Med* 1998;4:328.
488. Lotze MT, Shurin M, Davis I, Amoscato A, Storkus WJ. Dendritic cell based therapy of cancer. *Adv Exp Med Biol* 1997;417:551.
489. Lotze MT, Hellerstedt B, Stolinski L, et al. The role of interleukin-2, interleukin-12, and dendritic cells in cancer therapy. *Cancer J from Scientific American* 1997;3(Suppl 1):S109.
490. Nestle FO. DC vaccination: clinical trial in melanoma. In: Lotze MT, Steinman R, Banchereau J, eds. *5th International symposium on dendritic cells in fundamental and clinical immunology.* Pittsburgh, PA: Society for Leukocyte Biology, 1998.
491. Lotze MT, Elder E, Whiteside TL. Dendritic cell therapy of cancer—not just an antigen presenting cell. In: Lotze MT, Steinman R, Banchereau J, eds. *5th International symposium on dendritic cells in fundamental and clinical immunology.* Pittsburgh, PA: Society for Leukocyte Biology, 1998.
492. Chen K, Braun S, Lyman S, et al. Antitumor activity and immunotherapeutic properties of Ftl3-ligand in a murine breast cancer model. *Cancer Res* 1997;57:3511.
493. Fields RC, Osterholzer JJ, Fuller JA, et al. Comparative analysis of murine dendritic cells derived from spleen and bone marrow. *J Immunother* 1998;21:323.
494. Rosenzwajg M, Camus S, Guigon M, Gluckman JC. The influence of interleukin (OL)-4, IL-13, and Flt3 ligand on human dendritic cell differentiation from cord blood CD34+ progenitor cells. *Exp Hematol* 1998;26:63.
495. Caux C, Dezutter-Dambuyant C, Schmitt D, Banchereau J. GM-CSF and TNF-alpha cooperate in the generation of dendritic Langerhans cells. *Nature* 1992;360:258.
496. Dranoff G, Jaffee E, Lazenby A, et al. Vaccination with irradiated tumor cells engineered to secrete murine granulocyte-macrophage colony-stimulating factor stimulates potent, specific, and long-lasting anti-tumor immunity. *Proc Natl Acad Sci U S A* 1993;90:3539.
497. Ellem KA, O'Rourke MG, Johnson GR, et al. A case report: immune responses and clinical course of the first human use of granulocyte/macrophage-colony-stimulating-factor-transduced autologous melanoma cells for immunotherapy. *Cancer Immunol Immunother* 1997;44:10.
498. Simons JW, Jaffee EM, Weber CE, et al. Bioactivity of autologous irradiated renal cell carcinoma vaccines generated by ex vivo granulocyte-macrophage colony-stimulating factor gene transfer. *Cancer Res* 1997;57:1537.
499. Si Z, Hersey P, Coates AS. Clinical responses and lymphoid infiltrates in metastatic melanoma following treatment with intralesional GM-CSF. *Melanoma Res* 1996;6:247.
500. Jager E, Ringhoffer M, Dienes HP, et al. Granulocyte-macrophage-colony-stimulating factor enhances immune responses to melanoma-associated peptides in vivo. *Int J Cancer* 1996;67:54.
501. Rosenberg SA, Yang JC, Schwartzentruber DJ, et al. Immunologic and therapeutic evaluation of a synthetic peptide vaccine for the treatment of patients with metastatic melanoma. *Nat Med* 1998;4:321.
502. Abdel-Wahab Z, Weltz C, Hester D, et al. A phase I clinical trial of immunotherapy with interferon-gamma gene-modified autologous melanoma cells: monitoring the humoral immune response. *Cancer* 1997;80:401.
503. Palmer K, Moore J, Everard M, et al. Gene therapy with autologous, interleukin 2-secreting tumor cells in patients with malignant melanoma. *Hum Gene Ther* 1999;10:1261.
504. Jager E, Ringhoffer M, Altmannsberger M, et al. Immunoselection in vivo: independent loss of MHC class I and melanocyte differentiation antigen expression in metastatic melanoma. *Int J Cancer* 1997;71:142.
505. Jager E, Bernhard H, Romero P, et al. Generation of cytotoxic T cell responses with synthetic melanoma associated peptides in vivo: implications for tumor vaccines with melanoma associated antigens. *Int J Cancer* 1996;66:162.
506. Kawakami Y, Eliyahu S, Jennings C, et al. Recognition of multiple epitopes in the human melanoma antigen gp100 by tumor-infiltrating T lymphocytes associated with in vivo tumor regression. *J Immunol* 1995;154:3961.
507. Parkhurst MR, Salgaller ML, Southwood S, et al. Improved induction of melanoma-reactive CTL with peptides from the melanoma antigen gp100 modified at HLA-A*0201-binding residues. *J Immunol* 1996;157:2539.
508. Sette A, Vitiello A, Reherman B, et al. The relationship between class I binding affinity and immunogenicity of potential cytotoxic T cell epitopes. *J Immunol* 1994;153:5586.
509. Ruppert J, Sidney J, Celis E, et al. Prominent role of secondary anchor residues in peptide binding to HLA-A2.1 molecules. *Cell* 1993;74:929.
510. Valmori D, Fonteneau JF, Lizana CM, et al. Enhanced generation of specific tumor-reactive CTL in vitro by selected Melan-A/MART-1 immunodominant peptide analogues. *J Immunol* 1998;160:1750.
511. Gervois N, Guilloux Y, Diez E, Jotereau F. Suboptimal activation of melanoma infiltrating lymphocytes (TIL) due to low avidity of TCR/MHC-tumor peptide interactions. *J Exp Med* 1996;183:2403.
512. Kawakami Y, Robbins PF, Wang RF, et al. The use of melanosomal proteins in the immunotherapy of melanoma. *J Immunother* 1998;21:237.
513. Davis ID. Cytokine therapy in meatstatic renal cancer [letter]. *N Engl J Med* 1998;339:199.
513a. Jager E, Ringhoffer M, Karbach J, et al. Inverse relationship of melanocyte differentiation antigen expression in melanoma tissues and CD8+ cytotoxic-T-cell responses: evidence for immunoselection of antigen-loss variants in vivo. *Int J Cancer* 1996;66(4):470.
513b. Jager E, Ringhoffer M, Altmannsberger M, et al. Immunoselection in vivo: independent loss of MCH class I and melanocyte differentiation antigen expression in metastatic melanoma. *Int J Cancer* 1997;71(2):142.
514. Hsueh EC, Foshag L, Essner R, Stern S, Morton D. *A new paradigm for the management of metastatic melanoma.* Presented at Society of Surgical Oncology Annual Meeting, New Orleans, LA, March 2000.
515. Moroi Y, Mayhew M, Trcka J, et al. An induction of cellular immunity by immunization with novel hybrid peptides complexed to heat shock protein 70. *Proc Natl Acad Sci U S A* 2000;97:3485.
516. Wallack MK, Sivanandham M, Balch CM, et al. Surgical adjuvant active specific immunotherapy for patients with stage III melanoma: the final analysis of data from a phase III, randomized, double-blind, multicenter vaccinia melanoma oncolysate trial. *J Am Coll Surg* 1998;187:69.
517. Hersey P. Evaluation of vaccinia viral lysates as therapeutic vaccines in the treatment of melanoma. *Ann NY Acad Sci* 1993;690:167.
518. Sallusto F, Lenig D, Forster R, Lipp M, Lanzavecchia A. Two subsets of memory T lymphocytes with distinct homing potentials and effector functions. *Nature* 1999;401:708.
519. Reisfeld RA. Monoclonal antibodies in cancer immunotherapy. *Clin Lab Med* 2000;12:201.
520. Rosenberg SA, Aebersold P, Cornetta K, et al. Gene transfer into humans—immunotherapy of patients with advanced melanoma, using tumor-infiltrating lymphocytes modified by retroviral gene transduction. *N Engl J Med* 1990;323:570.
521. Lotze MT. Clinical protocol: the treatment of patients with melanoma using IL-2, IL-4, and tumor infiltrating lymphocytes. *Hum Gene Ther* 1992;3:167.
522. Tahara H, Zeh HJ III, Storkus WJ, et al. Fibroblasts genetically engineered to secrete interleukin 12 can suppress tumor growth and induce antitumor immunity to a murine melanoma in vivo. *Cancer Res* 1994;54:182.
523. Houghton AN, Scheinberg DA. Monoclonal antibody therapies —a "constant" threat to cancer. *Nat Med* 2000;6:373.
524. Steffens TA, Bajorin DF, Houghton AN. Immunotherapy with monoclonal antibodies in metastatic melanoma. *World J Surg* 1992;16:261.
525. Herlyn M, Koprowski H. Melanoma antigens: immunological and biological characterization and clinical significance. *Ann Rev Immunol* 1988;6:283.
526. Houghton AN, Mintzer D, Cordon-Cardo C, et al. Mouse monoclonal IgG3 antibody detecting GD3 ganglioside: a phase I trial in patients with malignant melanoma. *Proc Natl Acad Sci U S A* 1985;82:1242.
527. Kirkwood JM, Mascavi RA, Edington HD. Analysis of therapeutic and immunologic effects of R(24) anti-GD3 monoclonal antibody in 37 patients with metastatic melanoma. *Cancer* 2000;88:2693.
528. Yao TJ, Meyers M, Livingston PO, Houghton AN, Chapman PB. Immunization of melanoma patients with BEC2-keyhole limpet hemocyanin plus BCG intradermally followed by intravenous booster immunizations with BEC2 to induce anti-GD3 ganglioside antibodies. *Clin Cancer Res* 1999;5:77.
529. McCaffery M, Yao TJ, Williams L, et al. Immunization of melanoma patients with BEC2 anti-idiotypic monoclonal antibody that mimics GD3 ganglioside: enhanced immunogenicity when combined with adjuvant. *Clin Cancer Res* 1996;2:679.
530. Mittelman A, Chen ZJ, Kageshita T, et al. Active specific immunotherapy in patients with melanoma. A clinical trial with mouse antiidiotypic monoclonal antibodies elicited with syngeneic anti-high-molecular-weight-melanoma-associated antigen monoclonal antibodies. *J Clin Invest* 1990;86:2136.
531. Mittelman A, Wang X, Matsumoto K, Ferrone S. Antiantiidiotypic response and clinical course of the disease in patients with malignant melanoma immunized with mouse antiidiotypic monoclonal antibody MK2-23. *Hybridoma* 1995;14:175.
532. Lotze MT, Carrasquillo JA, Weinstein JN, et al. Monoclonal antibody imaging of human melanoma. Radioimmunodetection by subcutaneous or systemic injection. *Ann Surg* 1986;204:223.
533. Del Vecchio S, Reynolds JC, Carrasquillo JA, et al. Local distribution and concentration of intravenously injected 131I-9.2.27 monoclonal antibody in human malignant melanoma. *Cancer Res* 1989;49:2783.
534. Lotze MT. Interleukin-2 based immunotherapy of malignant melanoma. In: Rumke P, Karger S, eds. *Therapy of advanced melanoma.* Basel: Kager, 1990:163.
535. Hank JA, Robinson RR, Surfus J, et al. Augmentation of antibody dependent cell mediated cytotoxicity following in vivo therapy with recombinant interleukin 2. *Cancer Res* 1990;50:5234.
536. Lotze MT, Roberts K, Custer MC, Segal DA, Rosenberg SA. Specific binding and lysis of human melanoma by IL-2-activated cells coated with anti-T3 or anti-Fc receptor cross-linked to antimelanoma antibody: a possible approach to the immunotherapy of human tumors. *J Surg Res* 1987;42:580.
537. Gillgren P, Mansson-Brahme E, Frisell J, et al. Epidemiological characteristics of cutaneous malignant melanoma of the head and neck. *Acta Oncol* 1999;38:1069.
538. Wieberdink J, Benckhuysen C, Braat RP, Van Slooten EA, Olthuis GA. Dosimetry in isolation perfusion of the limbs by assessment of perfused tissue volume and grading of toxic tissue reactions. *Eur J Cancer Clin Oncol* 1982;18:905.
539. van Geel AN, van Wijk J, Wieberdink J. Functional morbidity after regional isolated perfusion of the limb for melanoma. *Cancer* 1989;63:1092.
540. Vrouenraets BC, Klaase JM, Kroon BB, et al. Long-term morbidity after regional isolated perfusion with melphalan for melanoma of the limbs. The influence of acute regional toxic reactions. *Arch Surg* 1995;130:43.
541. Zavour HM, Storlans WJ, Brusic V, et al. NY-ESO-1 encodes DRB*0401–restricted epitopes recognized by melanoma-reactive CD4 T cells. *Cancer Res* 2000;60:1.

542. Zarour HM, Kirkwood JM, Kierstead LS, et al. Melan-A/MART-1_{51-73} represents an immunogenic HLA-DR4-restricted epitope recognized by melanoma-reactive CD4+ T cells. *Proc Natl Acad Sci U S A* 2000;97:400.
543. Reintgen D, Rapaport D, Tanabe KK, Ross M. Lymphatic mapping and sentinel node biopsy in patients with malignant melanoma. *J Fl Med Assoc* 1997;84:188.
544. Jager E, Jager D, Karbach J, et al. Identification of NY-ESO-1 epitopes presented by human histocompatibility antigen (HLA)-DRB4*0101-0103 and recognized by CD4+ T lymphocytes of patients with NY-ESO-1-expressing melanoma. *J Exp Med* 2000;191:625.
545. Topalian SL, Gonzales MI, Parkhurst M, et al. Melanoma-specific CD4+ T cells recognize nonmutated HLA-DR-restricted tyrosinase epitopes. *J Exp Med* 1996;183:1965.
546. Kobayashi H, Kokubo T, Sato K, et al. CD4+ T cells from peripheral blood of a melanoma patient recognize peptides derived from nonmutated tyrosinase. *Cancer Res* 1998;58:296.
547. Chaux P, Vantomme V, Stroobant V, et al. Identification of MAGE-3 epitopes presented by HLA-DR molecules to CD4(+) T lymphocytes. *J Exp Med* 1999;189:767.
548. Mancini S, Sturniolo T, Imro MA, et al. Melanoma cells present a MAGE-3 epitope to CD4+ cytotoxic T cells in association with histocompatibility leukocyte antigen DR11. *J Exp Med* 1999;189:871.
549. Whelan SL, Parkin DM, Masoyer E. *Patterns of cancer in five continents.* International Agency for Research on Cancer, 1990.
550. Liu T, Soong, S-J. Epidemiology of malignant melanoma. *Surg Clin North Am* 1996;76:1205.
551. Lejeune FJ, Lienard D, el Douaihy M, Seyedi JV, Ewalenko P. Results of 206 isolated limb perfusions for malignant melanoma. *Eur J Surg Oncol* 1989;15:510.
552. Klaase JM, Kroon BB, van Geel AN, et al. Is there an indication for a double perfusion schedule with melphalan for patients with recurrent melanoma of the limbs? *Melanoma Res* 1994;4(Suppl 1):13.
553. Kettelhack C, Kraus T, Hupp T, Manner M, Schlag P. Hyperthermic limb perfusion for malignant melanoma and soft tissue sarcoma. *Eur J Surg Oncol* 1990;16:370.
554. Lienard D, Ewalenko P, Delmotte JJ, Renard N, Lejeune FJ. High-dose recombinant tumor necrosis factor alpha in combination with interferon gamma and melphalan in isolation perfusion of the limbs for melanoma and sarcoma. *J Clin Oncol* 1992;10:52.
555. Vaglini M, Santinami M, Manzi R, et al. Treatment of in-transit metastases from cutaneous melanoma by isolation perfusion with tumour necrosis factor-alpha (TNF-alpha), melphalan and interferon-gamma (IFN-gamma). Dose-finding experience at the National Cancer Institute of Milan. *Melanoma Res* 1994;4(Suppl 1):35.
556. Fraker DL, Alexander HR, Andrich M, Rosenberg SA. Treatment of patients with melanoma of the extremity using hyperthermic isolated limb perfusion with melphalan, tumor necrosis factor, and interferon gamma: results of a tumor necrosis factor dose-escalation study. *J Clin Oncol* 1996;14:479.
557. Kettelhack C, Hohenberger P, Schlag PM. Die isolierte extremitatenperfusion min tumornekrsefaktor alpha und melphalan beim malignen melanom. *Dtsch Med Wochenschr* 1997;122:177.
558. Lienard D, Eggermont AM, Koops HS, et al. Isolated limb perfusion with tumor necrosis factor-alpha and melphalan with or without interferon-gamma for the treatment of in-transit melanoma metastases: a multicenter randomized phase II study. *Melanoma Res* 1999;9:491.
559. Storm FK, Morton DL. Value of therapeutic hyperthermic limb perfusion in advanced recurrent melanoma of the lower extremity. *Am J Surg* 1985;150:32.
560. Santinami M, Belli F, Cascinelli N, Rovini D, Vaglini M. Seven years experience with hyperthermic perfusions in extracorporeal circulation for melanoma of the extremities. *J Surg Oncol* 1989;42:201.
561. Klaase JM, Kroon BB, van Geel AN, et al. Prognostic factors for tumor response and limb recurrence-free interval in patients with advanced melanoma of the limbs treated with regional isolated perfusion with melphalan. *Surgery* 1994;115:39.
562. Sugarbaker EV, McBride CM. Survival and regional disease control after isolation-perfusion for invasive stage I melanoma of the extremities. *Cancer* 1976;37:188.
563. Janoff KA, Moseson D, Nohlgren J, et al. The treatment of state I melanoma of the extremities with regional hyperthermic isolation perfusion. *Ann Surg* 1982;196:316.
564. Rege VB, Leone LA, Soderberg CH Jr, et al. Hyperthermic adjuvant perfusion chemotherapy for stage I malignant melanoma of the extremity with literature review. *Cancer* 1983;52:2033.
565. Martijn H, Schraffordt KH, Milton GW, et al. Comparison of two methods of treating primary malignant melanomas Clark IV and V, thickness 1.5 mm and greater, localized on the extremities. Wide surgical excision with and without adjuvant regional perfusion. *Cancer* 1986;57:1923.
566. Franklin HR, Schraffordt KH, Oldhoff J, et al. To perfuse or not to perfuse? A retrospective comparative study to evaluate the effect of adjuvant isolated regional perfusion in patients with stage I extremity melanoma with a thickness of 1.5 mm or greater. *J Clin Oncol* 1988;6:701.
567. Reintgen DS, Cruse CW, Wells KE, Saba HI, Slingluff CL Jr. Isolated limb perfusion for recurrent melanoma of the extremity. *Ann Plast Surg* 1992;28:50.
568. Ghussen F, Nagel K, Groth W, Muller JM, Stutzer H. A prospective randomized study of regional extremity perfusion in patients with malignant melanoma. *Ann Surg* 1984;200:764.
569. Rosenberg SA, Lotze MT, Yang JC, et al. Experience with the use of high-dose interleukin-2 in the treatment of 652 cancer patients. *Ann Surg* 1989;210:474.
570. Thatcher N, Dazzi H, Johnson RJ, et al. Recombinant interleukin-2 (rIL-2) given intrasplenically and intravenously for advanced malignant melanoma. A phase I and II study. *Br J Cancer* 1989;60:770.
571. Parkinson DR, Abrams JS, Wiernik PH, et al. Interleukin-2 therapy in patients with metastatic malignant melanoma: a phase II study. *J Clin Oncol* 1990;8:1650.
572. Whitehead RP, Kopecky KJ, Samson MK, et al. Phase II study of intravenous bolus recombinant interleukin-2 in advanced malignant melanoma: Southwest Oncology Group study. *J Natl Cancer Inst* 1991;83:1250.
573. Dorval T, Mathiot C, Brandely M. Lack of effect of tumour infiltrating lymphocytes in patients with metastatic melanoma who failed to respond to interleukin 2 [letter]. *Eur J Cancer* 1991;27:599.
574. Sparano JA, Fisher RI, Sunderland M, et al. Randomized phase III trial of treatment with high-dose interleukin-2 either alone or in combination with interferon alfa-2a in patients with advanced melanoma. *J Clin Oncol* 1993;11:1969.
575. Legha SS, Gianan MA, Plager C, Eton OE, Papadopoulous NE. Evaluation of interleukin-2 administered by continuous infusion in patients with metastatic melanoma. *Cancer* 1996;77:89.
576. Atkins MB, Lotze MT, Dutcher JP, et al. High-dose recombinant interleukin 2 therapy for patients with metastatic melanoma: analysis of 270 patients treated between 1985 and 1993. *J Clin Oncol* 1999;17:2105.
577. Wolf P, Quehenberger F, Mullegger R, Stranz B, Kerl H. Phenotypic markers, sunlight-related factors and sunscreen use in patients with cutaneous melanoma: an Austrian case-control study. *Melanoma Res* 1998;8:370.
578. Klepp O, Magnus K. Some environmental and bodily characteristics of melanoma patients. A case-control study. *Int J Cancer* 1979;23:482.
579. Herzfeld PM, Fitzgerald EF, Hwang SA, Stark A. A case-control study of malignant melanoma of the trunk among white males in upstate New York. *Cancer Detect Prev* 1993;17:601.
580. Westerdahl J, Olsson H, Masback A, Ingvar C, Jonsson N. Is the use of sunscreens a risk factor for malignant melanoma? *Melanoma Res* 1995;5:59.
581. Autier P, Dore JF, Schifflers E, et al. Melanoma and use of sunscreens: an Eortc case-control study in Germany, Belgium and France. The EORTC Melanoma Cooperative Group. *Int J Cancer* 1995;61:749.
582. Beitner H, Norell SE, Ringborg U, Wennersten G, Mattson B. Malignant melanoma: aetiological importance of individual pigmentation and sun exposure. *Br J Dermatol* 1990;122:43.
583. Holman CD, Armstrong BK, Heenan PJ. Relationship of cutaneous malignant melanoma to individual sunlight-exposure habits. *J Natl Cancer Inst* 1986;76:403.
584. Osterlind A, Tucker MA, Stone BJ, Jensen OM. The Danish case-control study of cutaneous malignant melanoma. II. Importance of UV-light exposure. *Int J Cancer* 1988;42:319.
585. Holly EA, Aston DA, Cress RD, Ahn DK, Kristiansen JJ. Cutaneous melanoma in women. *Am J Epidemiol* 1995;141:923.
586. Rodenas JM, Delgado-Rodriguez M, Herranz MT, Tercedor J, Serrano S. Sun exposure, pigmentary traits, and risk of cutaneous malignant melanoma: a case-control study in a Mediterranean population. *Cancer Cause Control* 1996;7:275.
587. Kirkwood JM, Strawderman MH, Ernstoff MS, et al. Interferon alfa-2b adjuvant therapy of high-risk resected cutaneous melanoma: the Eastern Cooperative Oncology Group Trial EST 1684. *J Clin Oncol* 1996;14:7.
588. Creagan ET, Dalton RJ, Ahmann DL, et al. Randomized, surgical adjuvant clinical trial of recombinant interferon alfa-2a in selected patients with malignant melanoma. *J Clin Oncol* 1995;13:2776.
589. Cascinelli N, Bufalino R, Morabito A, MacKie R. Results of adjuvant interferon study in WHO melanoma programme. *Lancet* 1994;343:913.
590. Kirkwood JM, Sosman J, Ernstoff M, et al. E2690: A study of the mechanism of IFN alfa-2b in high risk melanoma in the ECOG/intergroup trial E1690. *Proc Am Assoc Cancer Res* 1995;36:641.
591. Keilholz U, Goey SH, Punt CJ, et al. Interferon alfa-2a and interleukin-2 with or without cisplatin in metastatic melanoma: a randomized trial of the European Organization for Research and Treatment of Cancer Melanoma Cooperative Group. *J Clin Oncol* 1997;15:2579.
592. Keilholz U, Goey SH, Punt CJA, et al. A randomized trial if IFNa/IL-2 with or without CDDP in advanced melanoma: an eortic melanoma cooperatie group trial. *Proc Am Soc Clin Oncol* 1996;15.
593. Legha S, Ring S, Bedikian A. Treatment of metastatic melanoma with combined chemotherapy containing cisplatin, vinblastin and dacarbazine (CVD) and biotherapy using interleukin-2 and interferon-a. *Ann Oncol* 1996;7:827.
594. Flaherty LE, Atkins M, Sosman J, et al. Randomized phase II trial of chemotherapy and outpatient biotherapy with inteleukin-2 (IL-2) and interferon alpha (IFN) in metastatic malignant melanoma (MMM). *Proc Am Soc Clin Oncol* 1999;18:536a.
595. Cocconi G, Bella M, Calabresi F, et al. DTIC versus DTIC plus tamoxifen in metastatic malignant melanoma. *Proc Am Soc Clin Oncol* 1990;9:278.
596. Rusthoven J, Quirt I, Iscoe N, et al. A randomized, placebo-controlled trial comparing BCNU (B), decarbazine, and cisplatin (P) versus BDP and high-dose tamoxifen in the treatment of metastic melanoma. *Proc Am Soc Clin Oncol* 1995;14:413.
597. Buzaid AC, Legha S, Winn R, et al. Cisplatin(C), vinblastine(V), and dacarbazine(D) (CVD) versus dacarbazine alone in metastatic melanoma: preliminary results of a phase III cancer community oncology program (CCOP) trial. *Proc Am Soc Clin Oncol* 1993;12:389.
598. Falkson CI, Ibrahim J, Kirkwood JM, et al. Phase III trial of dacarbazine versus dacarbazine with interferon alpha-2b versus dacarbazine with tamoxifen versus dacarbazine with interferon alpha-2b and tamoxifen in patients with metastatic malignant melanoma: an Eastern Cooperative Oncology Group study. *J Clin Oncol* 1998;16:1743.
599. McDermott DF, Mier JW, Lawrence DP, et al. A phase II pilot trial of concurrent biochemotherapy with cisplatin, vinblastine, and dacarbazine (CVD), interleukin-2 (IL-2) and interferon alpha-2b (IFN) in patients with metastatic melanoma. *Proc Am Soc Clin Oncol* 1997;16:490a.
600. O'Day SJ, Gammon G, Boasberg PD, et al. Advantages of concurrent biochemotherapy modified by decrescendo interleukin-2, granulocyte colony-stimulating factor, and tamoxifen for patients with metastatic melanoma. *J Clin Oncol* 1999;17:2752.
601. Thompson JA, Gold PJ, Fefer A. Outpatient chemoimmunotherapy for the treatment of metastatic melanoma. *Semin Oncol* 1997;24:S44.

JOSÉ A. SAHEL
ARTHUR S. POLANS
MINESH P. MEHTA
RICHARD M. AUCHTER
DANIEL M. ALBERT

SECTION 3

Intraocular Melanoma

Melanomas are the most common primary intraocular malignancy in whites. They arise from uveal melanocytes (i.e., mature melanin-producing and melanin-containing cells) residing in the uveal stroma and originating from the neural crest. Whereas reactive or neoplastic proliferations of pigmented cells can occur in the epithelia of the iris, ciliary body, and retina, forming adenomas or adenocarcinomas, this chapter deals exclusively with uveal melanomas. A particular emphasis is given to the current therapeutic concerns and issues since (1) the appropriate treatment of the primary tumor remains in many instances controversial and (2) management of metastatic disease is essentially palliative.

EPIDEMIOLOGY

The annual age-adjusted incidence of nonskin melanomas as reported in the Surveillance, Epidemiology, and End Results program during 1973 to 1977 was 0.7 per 100,000 population in the United States. Similar figures were reported from epidemiologic studies conducted in New England (0.65 per 100,000 residents from 1984 to 1985), the Swedish west coast (0.72 per 100,000 over the period 1956 to 1975), and Iceland (0.7 per 100,000 in male patients and 0.5 per 100,000 in female patients over the period 1955 to 1979). In the Third National Cancer Survey, conducted from 1969 to 1971, the annual age-adjusted incidence in the United States was estimated at 0.6 per 100,000. The precise anatomic origin of ocular melanomas was unspecified in approximately 25% of cases. Seventy-three percent of the tumors arose within the globe (mainly from the choroid), and 2% developed from the conjunctiva. Melanoma accounted for 70% of all primary ocular malignancies, followed in frequency by the childhood tumor retinoblastoma (13%). In persons older than 20, melanoma was the reported diagnosis for 80% of all primary ocular cancers. Data from the Missouri Department of Health; China; the Surveillance, Epidemiology, and End Results program; New England; Iceland; Finland; and the Ocular Melanoma Task Force are similar to those reported by the Third National Cancer Survey.[1] A French study in 1992 provided accurate data on the incidence of this condition in the French population: 0.73 per 100,000.[2] The annual age-adjusted incidence of ocular melanomas is approximately one-eighth that of skin melanomas in the United States. The recently observed increase in the incidence of cutaneous melanomas has not been observed for uveal melanomas.[3]

Although the incidence increases steadily by decade, with a peak in the seventh decade, uveal melanoma cases occur before the age of 20, as illustrated by 101 of the 6359 cases on file at the Registry of Ophthalmic Pathology at the Armed Forces Institute of Pathology (AFIP), 40 of 3706 consecutive patients seen at Wills Eye Hospital, and by several other reports. Most studies show a median age at diagnosis of approximately 55, with rates dropping after age 70.[3,13]

RACE

The lower incidence of uveal melanoma in African Americans has been noticed in several large series. Only 10 African American patients were identified among more than 3586 patients with uveal melanoma (0.39%) from the oncology service at Wills Eye Hospital between 1974 and 1989.[3] Findings from the Florida Cancer Data System showed a 32-fold greater risk of uveal melanoma in whites than in African Americans.[4] White men had 72 times the risk of developing uveal melanoma as compared with that of African American men. For white women, this risk was 22 times that of African American women.[4] According to the Florida Cancer Data System, the risk of uveal melanoma in Hispanics is 62% less than that of white non-Hispanics. These findings may support at least in part the hypothesis that the sunlight effect on the causation of melanoma is primarily a direct one, since this is not found for visceral melanomas.[5] A study of the initial clinical manifestations and pathologic characteristics in Hispanic patients enucleated for choroidal melanomas showed an earlier onset, a larger tumor diameter, and a heavier pigmentation in this population than in other groups.[6] An epidemiologic study of posterior uveal melanoma in Israel over the period 1961 to 1989 shows that the incidence rates have been stable over this 30-year period. The incidence rate is lowest in Jews from Asia and Africa (2.2) and in non-Jews (1.5) and is highest in Jews born in Israel (6.8), Europe, and the Americas (7.5). The significance of these figures with regard to the role of constitutional factors and timing of sunlight irradiation remains conjectural.[7]

GENDER

Although Scotto et al. found that the overall risk of ocular melanomas did not vary by gender, Jensen, Gislason et al., and others noted a predominance of male patients.[8–10] Ocular and skin melanoma show similar age patterns, with more women affected at younger ages and more men later in life. The Third National Cancer Survey indicated a left-sided excess of 18% for ocular melanomas in men and a right-sided excess in women.[1]

MORTALITY

As emphasized by Markowitz et al.[11] in a review of mortality from choroidal melanoma, very few reports are complete enough to be informative. Diener-West et al.,[12] using selected data published during the period from 1966 to 1988, performed a pooled analysis (metaanalysis) of 5-year mortality rates among enucleated patients, providing weighed estimates of 5-year mortality after enucleation: 16% for small tumors [95% confidence interval (CI), 14% to 18%], 32% for medium-size tumors (95% CI, 29% to 34%), and 53% for large tumors (95% CI, 50% to 56%). The most complete long-term survival studies after enucleation were performed in Denmark by Jensen[9] et al. and in Finland by Raivio.[13] In the Finnish study, the 5-, 10-, and 15-year survival rates were 65%, 52%, and 46%,[13] respectively. In the Danish study, survival rates were similar; at the end of the 25-year period, 51% patients had died from metastasis.[9] A French study of survival of patients with uveal melanomas treated by enucleation with a long-term follow-up reported similar figures.[14] Rates of survival after radiation therapy appear comparable in the short term and mean term. Yet, as the following discussion shows, both the validity of these data and the long-term predictability of prognosis after conservative treatment remain a matter of controversy. The median survival of patients with metastatic disease is reportedly very short: 2 to 5 months.[11,12]

ETIOLOGY AND HISTOGENESIS OF OCULAR MELANOMAS

As is the case for most human cancers, the specific causes of ocular melanomas are unknown. However, epidemiologic, electron-microscopical, and experimental data allow characterization of risk factors, predisposing conditions, and hypothetical genetic or oncogenic causes.

GENETICS AND IMMUNOHISTOCHEMISTRY

There is now considerable evidence that, like many cancers, a subset of uveal melanomas is caused by an inherited predisposition. The familial occurrence of uveal melanomas was first mentioned by Silcock[15] in 1892 and reported since several times.[16–18] Despite the rare occurrence of uveal melanoma in a family and the presence of many skips in these pedigrees, the occurrence of familial uveal melanoma is not caused by fortuitous familial aggregation of sporadic cases.[18] Because of an insufficient number of families with more than two affected individuals, it is impossible to distinguish between polygenic inheritance, single-gene inheritance with reduced penetrance, and the role of environmental factors as causes of this familial aggregation. A few cytogenetic studies argue for the putative role of a recessive oncogene on chromosome 2, 3, or 6q[19,20] and showed abnormalities again on chromosomes 6 and 8q.[19,21–23] Other studies emphasize the possible relationship of monosomy 3 and multiplication of chromosome 8q to uveal melanoma,[24,25] suggesting monosomy 3 as an early, if not primary, event and supporting a role for chromosome 8q multiplication in the proliferation of cloned tumor cells *in vitro*. A role for the c-*myc* oncogene, located in the region 8q2.1-qter, in uveal melanoma formation and progression, probably linked to the regulation of cell proliferation, has been hypothesized. This is partly supported by cytogenetic[21] as well as immunohistochemical studies.[26] Abnormalities of the p53 gene have also been demonstrated.[27,28] The coexistence of ocular and cutaneous melanoma in some patients suggests a predisposition to both types and may imply mutations in the CDKN2A gene on chromosome 9 in a proportion of these cases.[29] An association between ocular melanoma and breast or ovarian cancer (or both) has also been reported, and BRCA2 on chromosome 13 may also be involved.[29]

Additional molecular genetic studies are necessary to understand the pathogenesis of familial uveal melanoma. In several studies,[30–33] investigators have demonstrated a close link between oncogenesis and the cell-cycle machinery. Progression through the cell cycle is orchestrated by sequential activation of a series of cyclin-dependent kinases (CDKs). The CDKs' activity is primarily dependent on the association with their activating cyclin subunits (Ds, E, G_1). CDK activity is counterbalanced by a variety of CDK-inhibitory proteins (CKIs), such as p21, p27, p16, and the like. Deregulated expression of G_1 cyclins p21, p27, p16 CKIs, and alteration in the interaction of CKIs with CDKs may be implicated in the neoplastic transformation of human ocular melanocytes to malignant melanoma cells.[30,31,33]

MDR1 gene and its gene product, P glycoprotein, which are known to cause drug resistance in cancer cells, are expressed in ocular melanoma.[32] Dunne et al.[32] reported a statistically significant association between MDR1 expression by tumor cells and shorter survival times, which was most striking at grade III.[32] Whether P glycoprotein is a marker for tumor aggressiveness, for clinical chemotherapy resistance, or perhaps for both remains to be clarified.

PREDISPOSING CONDITIONS

Ocular and oculodermal melanocytosis (i.e., nevus of Ota) predispose to the development of uveal melanomas. In 4.6% of reported cases of nevus of Ota, malignant transformation was reported[34] and, except for a single anecdotal case, the melanoma occurred in the pigmented eye. In the vast majority (90%) of patients with oculodermal melanosis and uveal melanoma, the uveal melanoma was diagnosed between the ages of 31 years and 80 years.[34] Rare cases of uveal melanomas have been reported in patients with type 1 neurofibromatosis,[35] a neurocristopathy. The tumor cells in neurofibromatosis have their origin in the neural crest, in common with melanocytes.[35]

Evidence that nevi are the origin of most choroidal melanomas has been provided by Yanoff and Zimmerman.[36] Yet a nevus-like configuration associated with choroidal melanoma may, in some cases, be explained by other mechanisms, such as (1) flattening of normal uveal melanocytes or of tumor cells, (2) a secondary proliferative effect of the malignancy, or (3) common oncogenic stimuli. The last two mechanisms have been postulated in a few cases of bilateral diffuse melanocytic tumors of the uvea in patients with systemic carcinoma.[36]

In some instances (as discussed), a familial increased occurrence of uveal melanoma has been recorded.[16,17,18] Data on the occurrence of uveal melanocytic tumors in patients with the dysplastic nevus syndrome are controversial[36] but generally support the value of periodic ophthalmoscopic examination of patients with atypical nevi.[37] A recent case-control study by Bataille et al.[38] demonstrated that (1) numerous common nevi (i.e., 100) were present in 10% of cases versus 3% of controls; (2) four or more atypical nevi were present in 7% of cases versus 0.4% controls; (3) pigmented iris nevi were significantly more common in cases than in controls (odds ratio, 3.1); and (4) the atypical mole syndrome was a strong risk factor (odds ratio, 7.3).

The association between uveal melanomas and other cancers is still a matter of controversy. Turner et al.[39] showed that the overall prevalence of non–basal cell cancers in uveal melanoma patients was twice the expected prevalence based on an age- and gender-matched population.[39] Anecdotal cases of uveal melanomas associated with various cancers exist, including breast cancer[28] and lymphomas.[40] A link between cutaneous and uveal melanoma was suspected on the basis of the association, in three cases (among 333 patients), of primary uveal and cutaneous melanomas. A family history of cutaneous or uveal melanoma was present in 14 of the primary uveal melanoma patients and 2 of the cutaneous melanoma patients.[41] Bataille et al.[41] reported five cases of primary ocular and cutaneous melanoma occurring in the same individual. Lischko et al. conducted a case-control study among 197 New England cases with 385 matched controls and 337 cases (from the United States) with 800 controls. They concluded that the association of prior malignancies with uveal melanomas is weak.[42] Holly et al., in a similar study of 407 uveal melanoma patients from the western United States with 870 control subjects, found no excess prior cancer.[43]

ONCOGENIC STIMULI

Certain electron-microscopical and biomolecular studies of ocular melanomas suggest an etiologic role of viruses. Viruses such as the feline sarcoma have been used successfully in the induction of animal ocular melanoma models.[53,54]

In a study of a single population of chemical workers, a statistically significant and higher-than-expected incidence of ocular melanomas was found. Nicotine has been incriminated in the unusual incidence of uveal melanomas in male patients but does not appear to increase the risk for metastasis.[44] Various chemicals, including nickel bisulfamide, platinum, methylcholanthrene, ethionine, N-2-fluorenylacetamide, radium, and N-methyl-N-nitrosourea have been reported to induce ocular melanocytic tumors in animals.[55] An exploratory study of various occupational associations provided elevated odds ratios for agriculture and farming work, several industrial operations, and exposure to inks, insecticides, gases, radioactive substances, polybromated phenyls, and chemical solvents.[33,45] A possible connection between Parkinson's disease, levodopa therapy, and malignant melanoma has been mentioned. The role of hormonal factors and pregnancy has been suggested in some reports. Hartge et al.[46a] reported a case-control study comparing 238 women with uveal melanoma with 223 matched control women. They showed that women with a history of pregnancy or hormonal substitutive treatment with estrogens had an increased risk, whereas a history of oophorectomy had a decreasing influence on relative risk (risk ratio, 0.6), and oral contraceptives had no influence on relative risk.[46] Seddon et al. and Shields et al.[44a,45a] have documented the role of pregnancy in the growth of uveal melanomas. Whether the growth observed clinically is secondary to cellular growth or other factors (e.g., fluid retention or vascular engorgement) is unclear.[55,57,58] Foss et al.[46] failed to detect any estrogen or progesterone receptors in 27 choroidal melanomas and questioned the role of these hormones in the development or progression of these tumors.

A case-control study lends support to the etiologic role of sunlight exposure.[49] A study of host factors (Northern ancestry, light skin color, 10 or more cutaneous nevi), ultraviolet radiation, and risk of uveal melanoma indicated that personal attributes are strong independent risk factors.[48] Holly et al.[43] showed that light skin color and easily sunburned skin increase by twofold the risk of uveal melanoma, while ultraviolet exposure increases this risk by fourfold, and sevenfold if intensive.[49] These data, contradicting previous studies, confirm the high association between light iris color and the presence of melanocytic lesions.[50] More recent evidence of an association between light iris color and melanocytic lesions has come from cases of melanomas associated with xeroderma pigmentosum[47,48,56] as well as a case-control study of patients with uveal melanoma. It has been suggested that cutaneous freckles (25 or more) or iris freckles and nevi may be risk factors for uveal melanomas.[49] Also, a relationship has been suggested between cutaneous or iris nevi and ocular melanomas.[38] Paraneoplastic uveal melanocytic proliferations have been observed in association with various systemic malignancies, such as ovary and lung.[50,51] These appear as diffuse multinodular infiltration of the uveal tract by predominantly diploid nevoid cells as well as more anaplastic cells; in addition, an association between bilateral uveal melanoma and a proliferation associated antigen (Ki-67) has been described.[52] The pathogenesis of paraneoplastic uveal melanocytic proliferation remains speculative. Hamartomatous paraneoplastic proliferation or stimulation of a preexisting tumor are possible underlying factors.[50]

HISTOPATHOLOGY, PROGNOSTIC PARAMETERS, AND NATURAL HISTORY

CYTOLOGIC AND HISTOLOGIC CLASSIFICATION

Experienced pathologists generally make the accurate microscopical diagnosis of uveal melanoma easily, but it is still occasionally difficult to differentiate between primary and metastatic choroidal melanomas.[71,72] In rare cases, differentiation from metastatic carcinoma may be facilitated by immunohistochemical labeling with monoclonal antibodies to S-100 protein.[72] This technique is not helpful in differentiating other neural crest–derived tumors (schwannomas, neurofibromas, and leiomyomas).[73] The S-100 immunophenotypes of uveal melanomas differ considerably from cutaneous melanomas.[74–77] S-100β is not helpful for distinguishing between primary and metastatic choroidal melanoma. HMB-45 immunostaining appears to be a useful adjunct in the differentiation between nonmelanocytic and melanocytic tumors but serves as a marker of melanocytic activation rather than a tool to differentiate uveal melanomas from nevi.[72,75,76] Studies of the immunocytochemistry of uveal melanomas using antibodies against cutaneous melanomas or anti-HLA antibodies have not yet provided a clinically useful characterization of the ocular tumors.[77,78] Cytometry can phenotype cells in suspension from ocular melanoma tissue.[73] Lawry et al.[73] described antibody binding for MHC antigens, the adhesion molecule ICAM-1, and the oncoproteins c-erb B-2, c-myc, and bcl-2. Further studies should be undertaken to question whether there are any relationships between traditional clinical and pathologic parameters (tumor cell type, volume, location, the tissue origin) and the flow cytometric measurement of cell surface protein or cytoplasmic-nuclear oncoprotein expression in cells taken from samples of primary uveal melanomas.

In 1931, Callender recognized major cell types in the spectrum of cells composing uveal melanomas, and this provided a cytologic classification clearly correlated with prognosis after enucleation. The different cell types are based on cell size and shape, cytoplasmic features, nuclear and nucleolar characteristics, evidence of loss of cohesion, and relative number of various cell types as outlined in Table 42.3-1.

According to Callender's cytologic characterization, uveal melanomas are divided into three categories:

- Spindle cell melanomas type A, B, or both, accounting for 30% of intraocular tumors, composed of spindle cells
- Mixed cell melanomas, when fewer than one-half of the tumor sections examined are composed of epithelioid cells
- Epithelioid cell melanomas (accounting for 5% of intraocular tumors), when greater than one-half is composed of epithelioid cells

TABLE 42.3-1. Designation of the Cell Type Based on the Armed Forces Institute of Pathology Modification of the Callender Classification

Callender Cell Type	*Cell Size and Description*	*Cytoplasm*	*Nucleus*	*Nucleolus*	*Other*
Spindle A	Elongated spindle or small and round, depending on plane of section; cell membrane not distinct; may appear more distinct in cross section	Usually sparse but may be relatively abundant	Elongated, fine chromatin pattern; chromatin line characteristic but not necessary for diagnosis; plumper than in nevus cells	Indistinct or none	Cohesive; mitoses extremely rare
Spindle B	Plumper spindle or round depending on plane of section; cell membrane not typically distinct (syncytial) but may be identified in cross section	Relatively sparse	Larger, plumper than spindle A; coarser chromatin pattern; chromatin clumping	Sharper definition; deeply stained, small, and round; often eccentric	Less cohesive than spindle A; may form fascicular arrangements; occasional mitoses
Epithelioid	Larger, more pleomorphic, often polygonal; distinct cell border	Abundant; may be eosinophilic	Largest, round; pleomorphic; chromatin margination, often marked; can be multinucleated	Largest, may be multiple; eosinophilic; usually central; distinct	Loss of cohesiveness; cells possibly separated easily in sectioning; more mitoses

(From ref. 74, with permission.)

Based on Callender classification, spindle cell tumors carry the best prognosis and epithelioid cell tumors the worst. In the Collaborative Ocular Melanoma Study (COMS) series,[74] large tumors contain more epithelioid cells than small tumors do; small tumors contain a higher percentage of spindle cell types. In their series, a more malignant cell type was observed more commonly in tumors with large size and anterior location.

Paul et al. reviewed 2652 cases accessioned at the AFIP by 1959 and found that 95% of patients with spindle A tumors, 85% of those with spindle B tumors, 60% of those with mixed tumors, and 83% of those with epithelioid tumors were alive 5 years after enucleation.[43a] At 15 years after enucleation, the survival rates were 85% for spindle A, 80% for spindle B, 46% for mixed, and 34% for epithelioid.[74] McLean et al.,[79a] in a review of 3432 cases from the AFIP, found that the overall mortality from metastasis 15 years after enucleation was 46%. The mortality of patients with mixed cell melanomas was three times that of patients with pure spindle cell lesions.[74]

In Jensen's series of 302 cases reported from Denmark that had been observed for 25 years, 150 patients (50%) died of metastatic melanoma. Fewer than 1% of patients with spindle A tumors died of metastatic disease; 63% with mixed tumors died of this cause; and the cause of death in 71% with epithelioid tumors was metastatic melanoma.[9]

Works by Sorenson et al. and Gamel et al.[80,81] and others have corroborated the well-documented prognostic value of Callender's classification, especially as to the pejorative significance of a high epithelioid cell content.[82] Yet, the major cell types described by Callender are part of a continuous spectrum, and the pathologist's identification of a particular cell type involves subjective judgment.

In the COMS report number 6,[74] balloon cells were associated with epithelioid tumors but not with tumor size. Metastases containing balloon cells have been reported. These lipid-laden cells are thought to be metabolically less active than spindle or epithelioid cells.[74]

This issue was addressed by Sorenson et al. and Gamel et al.,[80,81] who described a more objective method of assessing uveal melanomas histopathologically. This technique uses computed cytomorphometry and entails evaluating the inverse of the standard deviation of the nucleolar area with measurements made of the mean of the 10 largest nucleoli and stereologic estimates produced of the volume-weighted mean nucleolar volume.[79,80] This, in conjunction with tumor size as estimated by largest tumor diameter, is among the best objective cytologic measures of a tumor's malignant potential (P >.001).[81] Marcus et al.,[84] counting nucleolar organizing regions, reached similar figures.

Folberg et al.,[82,83] Pe'er et al.,[85] and Rummelt et al.,[86] using sections stained with periodic acid–Schiff, described nine vascular patterns that they observed in ×10 objective fields of uveal malignant melanomas:

- Normal vessels
- Silent-avascular zones
- Straight with randomly distributed vessels
- Parallel-oriented straight vessels without cross-linking
- Parallel with cross-linking between vessels
- Arcs that are incomplete loops
- Arcs with branching
- Loops that represent fibrovascular septa that completely surround lobules of tumor
- Networks that are composed of at least three back-to-back loops

The detection of these patterns in histologic sections is highly reproducible between observers,[87] and more than one pattern can exist in a tumor.[88] Foss et al.[88] showed that the avascular zones contain large numbers of small blood vessels as demonstrated by factor VIII staining.

Two of these microvascularization patterns (networks, parallel with cross-linking) showed a very strong correlation with metastatic disease; two other microvascularization patterns (silent, parallel without cross-linking) were correlated with a more favorable outcome for the patient.[82,83,85,86,89–91] The survival rate was 80% at 20 years in the absence of loops, networks, or parallel with cross-linking vascular patterns and only 40% when these patterns were present.[82,83,85,86] The presence of epithelioid cells is associated with the presence of networks, and the absence of epithelioid cells is associated with avascular zones.[87] These microcirculatory patterns of primary uveal melanomas appear also in foci of metastasis, regardless of the site of dissemination.[92]

The Callender classification cell typing is highly subjective because it is based on multiple cytoplasmic, nuclear, and nucleolar features. Loops and mean of the largest nucleoli (MLN) should be less subjective than cell type, because these variables are based on only one feature and MLN is measured objectively.[93]

Several attempts to evaluate the growth and malignant potential of uveal melanomas have been made recently using DNA cell-cycle studies (e.g., bromodeoxyuridine uptake or Ki-67 antibody as a marker of cycling cells,[96] proliferating cell nuclear antigen,[94,95] DNA or RNA content by flow cytometry).[96] Several reports of DNA ploidy analysis in uveal melanomas showed a progressive predominance of diploid over aneuploid tumors moving from spindle to epithelioid cell type and worsening prognosis.[96–98] The value of this technique as a diagnostic and prognostic tool in combination with fine-needle aspiration biopsy needs further confirmation.[97,99]

After the works of Rosenberg et al. on the prognostic and therapeutic value of tumor-infiltrating lymphocytes (TIL), a reappraisal of the lymphocytic infiltration of some uveal melanomas has been undertaken.[100] Whelchel et al.[101] and other authors[102] unexpectedly showed that T-lymphocytic infiltration is associated with death from metastasis. T cells appear predominant among TIL. Attempts to generate TIL cytotoxic for ocular melanoma cells showed that after interleukin-2 addition, cells expressing natural killer (NK) cells, lymphokine-activated killer cells, and tumor-specific cytotoxic properties were obtained.[100] Moreover, allogeneic melanomas could substitute for autologous tumors in active specific immunotherapy with CD8+ cytotoxic T lymphocytes.[103] A few studies suggest a link between host-immune responses to the tumor and gangliosides profile (e.g., GM3 vs. GD2 and 3).[104,105] The role of infiltrating lymphocytes in the regression of animal models of tumors was shown in nude mice for NK cell-mediated lysis[106,107] and for CD8+ cytotoxic T lymphocytes in the rejection of tumors from transgenic mice.[106,107]

TISSUE CULTURE AND ANIMAL MODELS OF UVEAL MELANOMAS

Several cell lines of human ocular melanomas have been established and characterized.[53–58] These vary greatly regarding doubling times or morphology and are mostly used for genetic studies and the development of animal models.

The most commonly used model of uveal melanoma is the Greene melanoma, which represents a transplantable hamster amelanotic melanoma. When injected into a rabbit eye, this tumor grows rapidly with marked spontaneous necrosis and is, therefore, not reflective of the clinical situation.[59,60] Other models of either induced or spontaneous pigmented intraocular tumors are available arising from the retinal pigment epithelium or representing atypical nevi.[61–64] Yet, to date, the most clinically relevant model to the human situation appears to be the heterotransplantation of human uveal melanomas into the choroid of rabbits,[65–69] and the newer transgenic mouse models.[70] These transgenic models are based on using the promoter region of the tyrosinase gene to target the expression of oncogenes to pigment-producing cells of different origins. Most of the models have been successful in producing intraocular pigmented tumors, including retinal pigment epithelium tumors, carcinomas, and ocular melanosis.[70] These models might provide better understanding of uveal malignant melanoma pathobiology.

HISTOPATHOLOGIC EFFECTS OF RADIATION

The histopathology of radiation-treated globes is of value in understanding the therapeutic mode of action.[108–113] The aim of treatment is to kill all tumor cells or to render them incapable of sustained proliferation. It is postulated that this result can be achieved through indirect tumor necrosis and hypoxia secondary to blood supply damage.[108] Most studies are biased by the small size of the sample and by the complicated nature of cases examined in the pathology laboratory. Changes in eyes enucleated for radiation-induced complications or poor tumor control may not reflect the radiation response of most treated cases. Using conventional light-microscopy methods, it was difficult in most studies to characterize histopathologically the radiation response aside from radiation-induced damage (radiation retinopathy, rubeosis iridis, cataract, vitreous hemorrhage). In the COMS,[74] preenucleation radiation significantly reduced, but did not eliminate, mitotic activity. Not surprisingly, tumor regrowth is correlated with significant mitotic activity,[112] whereas good tumor response is linked with fewer mitotic figures and tumor and blood vessel damage.[113] It seems likely that loss of replicative capacity through DNA damage is a major mode of action of this method. Other significant features of irradiated tumors include necrosis, fibrosis, and balloon cell formation.[109,111,113]

Further studies of the sequence of changes after proton beam treatment of uveal melanomas indicates progressive changes with decreased inflammation and increased fibrosis. In successfully treated tumors, mitotic figures persist only for the first 30 months after treatment.[114,115]

NATURAL HISTORY

Doubling Time

Little is known about the natural history of uveal melanomas. Until recent decades, all patients underwent enucleation immediately after the diagnosis.[113] Data on the growth pattern of small melanomas from series of patients observed by Gass and others have contributed to our knowledge of the rate of intraocular tumor growth prior to treatment.[50] These findings and other selected reports suggest a gompertzian (exponential) growth curve, as postulated by Manschot et al.[129] The doubling time of uveal tumors may vary from 2 months or less to several years. In rapidly growing tumors, a high mitotic activity and the presence of epithelioid cells have been documented. Spontaneous regression of a choroidal melanoma has been described.[116]

Intraocular Spread

Small melanomas grow from a discoid to a hemispheric shape. They progressively obliterate the choriocapillaris and displace

Bruch's membrane and the retina inward. When Bruch's membrane is disrupted, the tumor usually grows in the subretinal space in a mushroom configuration.[118–120] The retinal pigment epithelium overlying the tumors undergoes early changes called *tumor-associated retinal pigment epitheliopathy,* which includes drusen formation and orange pigment (lipofuscin) accumulation.[120] The neurosensory retina is frequently detached and, in some instances, infiltrated by tumor cells, which can seed into the vitreous. Most often, but not exclusively, this is a late finding.

Anterior tumors are more likely to affect the lens and to involve the posterior chamber. The zonules, lens, iris, anterior chamber, and angle may be affected by the tumor. A secondary glaucoma may result from obstruction of the outflow pathways by tumor cells, cell debris, and phagocytic cells swollen with ingested cell debris (melanomalytic glaucoma). The tumor may infiltrate through the scleral spur into the anterior chamber.

Although the sclera is thought to be an effective barrier against extraocular extension, scleral infiltration by tumor cells along ciliary vessels and nerves and along the vortex veins is frequent (32.3% of large melanomas in a series reported by Shammas and Blodi).[122] Approximately 5% of melanomas grow diffusely in the plane of the uvea or circumferentially along the root of the iris. They induce a slight thickening of the uvea (approximately 3 to 5 mm) and are often unsuspected or diagnosed late when secondary glaucoma or extraocular spread occurs. Extraocular spread may occur adjacent to or within the optic nerve or can occur anteriorly about the limbus.[124]

Extraocular Extension

Although extrascleral extension may be observed with small tumors, it is more likely to occur when the tumor has reached a larger size.[125] In a study by Shammas and Blodi,[122] extrascleral extension was observed in 18% of tumors exceeding 10 mm in diameter. The overall incidence of transscleral extension was determined to be approximately 13% among 1842 malignant melanomas studied by Starr and Zimmerman.[125] Other series arrive at similar data. Starr and Zimmerman noted a tenfold increase in the incidence of postoperative recurrence if the tumor extended to the surgical margin. The depth of scleral extension may have a prognostic significance. Other less common paths of extraocular spread include the optic nerve and the lumen of the vortex veins.[124]

Metastases

Lymphatic spread has not been demonstrated, as would be expected from the absence of lymphatics in the eye. This is in contrast to cutaneous melanomas. Hematogenous dissemination to the liver is a frequent form of metastatic spread. The respective roles of nonspecific trapping and of cell surface antigens in the invasiveness and dissemination of uveal melanomas are not yet fully established.[117] Plasminogen activator function[118] and the epidermal growth factor receptor[119] may play a role in the occurrence and progression of metastases. Metastases to other sites (lung, heart, gastrointestinal tract, lymph nodes, pancreas, skin, central nervous system, bones, spleen, adrenal, kidneys, ovaries, thyroid) generally occur in association with liver metastases.[120] In a survey of metastases from proton beam–treated melanomas, liver involvement was documented in almost all patients (136 of 145); the overall 1-year survival was 13%.[120]

In a series of studies, McLean et al. found that most deaths from metastatic disease occurred in the first 5 years after enucleation, with a peak mortality in the second and third years (approximately 8% per year). They compared these data with the natural course of untreated melanomas[126] and reached a conclusion that remains controversial: McLean et al.[126] incriminated enucleation as a risk factor and suggested two principal mechanisms: (1) dissemination of tumor cells during traumatic operations, as demonstrated experimentally by Fraunfelder et al.,[127] and (2) decreased host resistance to disseminated tumor cells. This latter mechanism has been called by Niederkorn et al.[61] the "loss of intraocular induced concomitant immunity" mediated by cytotoxic T lymphocytes. Zimmerman and McLean's assumptions have been challenged by several investigators. Seigel et al.[128] concluded that the statistical data can be interpreted differently and that no evidence suggested that the existing pattern of treatment be altered.[128] Manschot and Van Peperzeel,[129] Kersten and Blodi,[130] and Davidorf[131] pointed out that most melanomas are diagnosed only when they have reached a relatively large size and concomitantly given rise to metastases, and only then are enucleated. The clinical consequences of these controversies are the use of less traumatic techniques for enucleation and new impetus to the search for alternative treatments.[132]

Multiple Choroidal Malignant Melanoma

It has been estimated that only one person will develop bilateral choroidal melanomas in a population of 50 million.[121] There is no clinical evidence of an inherited genetic predisposition for bilateral primary uveal melanoma, and it may be associated with ocular melanocytosis.[123] Unilateral multifocal intraocular malignant melanoma appears to be even rarer than bilateral intraocular melanoma.[121] To eliminate the possibility of a multinodular tumor, serial sections of the enucleated eye are useful to exclude continuity between the two tumors. Intraocular multifocal melanoma has been associated with ocular melanocytosis, iris melanoma with invasion of the ciliary body, iris or choroidal nevus (or both), and with systemic malignant neoplasm.[121,124] However, other cases of double melanoma do not show any such associations. It is also unknown whether the prognosis for life differs in patients with multiple versus unifocal primary uveal melanoma.

DIAGNOSIS OF UVEAL MELANOMAS: CHOROIDAL AND CILIARY BODY MELANOMAS

The diagnosis of choroidal and ciliary body melanomas has reached a high degree of accuracy at eye centers where experienced clinicians and modern ancillary testing facilities are available.[134] This is well illustrated by a comparison of the misdiagnosis rates among the eyes on file at the AFIP: 19% (of 529 eyes) until 1962; 20% (of 208 eyes) between 1963 and 1970; and 6.4% (of 744 eyes) between 1970 and 1980. During the 11-year period of the last study, the rate of misdiagnosis declined from 12.5% to 1.4%. Between 1954 and 1977, the misdiagnosis rate was 2.6% (of 224 eyes) at the Mayo Clinic. In the Mayo

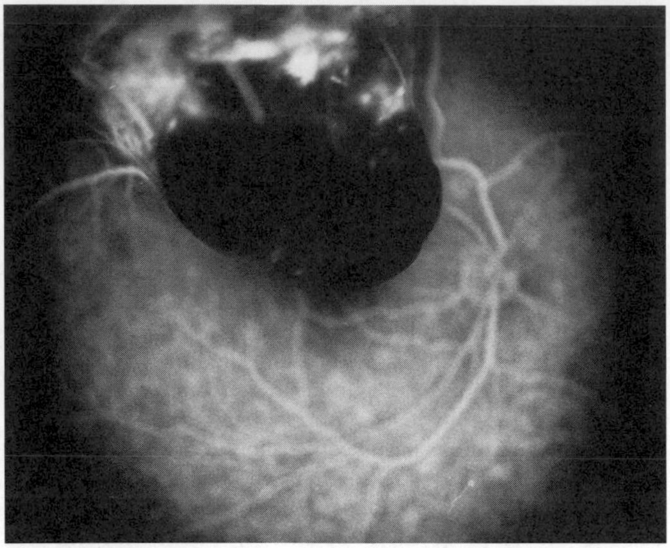

FIGURE 42.3-1. Fluorescein angiogram showing characteristic pattern of choroidal melanoma.

series, in addition, six clinically unsuspected melanomas were found.[132]

This high rate of correct clinical diagnosis is particularly impressive because only outpatient procedures (including clinical examination, ultrasonography, and fluorescein angiography) were used. No biopsies were performed, as is used for many other tumors. A review of 395 eyes enucleated during a 50-year period, drawn from the pathology files of Ohio State University, revealed a misdiagnosis rate of 10.9% in the period 1931 to 1959 that decreased to 1.7% in the period 1960 to 1981. Nine percent of choroidal melanomas were unsuspected preoperatively; all were in eyes with opaque media. In a series of 400 consecutive patients referred to the oncology unit of the Wills Eye Hospital with an incorrect diagnosis of melanoma (i.e., patients who proved to have a so-called pseudomelanoma), the correct diagnosis was reached through clinical evaluation in 397 cases (99%). In that series, the most commonly encountered conditions mimicking a melanoma included suspicious choroidal nevi (26.5%), peripheral disciform degeneration (11%), congenital hypertrophy of the retinal pigment epithelium (9.5%), and choroidal hemangioma (8%). Most metastatic carcinomas had been correctly diagnosed by the referring ophthalmologists. The diagnostic accuracy of 99.7% in the COMS exceeds previously documented rates.[132] It reflects the value of rigorous and standardized ophthalmic and systemic evaluations.

The cornerstone of diagnosis of posterior uveal melanoma remains clinical examination and, in particular, indirect ophthalmoscopy through a dilated pupil. Fundus contact lens examination and the use of a three-mirror lens can be extremely helpful.[142] Scleral transillumination as advocated by Reese is also a useful aid.[182a] Pigmented conjunctival lesions, such as conjunctival melanoma, staphylomas, scleral ectasia, hematoma, cellular blue nevi, and ocular melanocytosis, may mimic extraocular extension of uveal melanomas. Visual field studies are of little help, especially in distinguishing melanomas from choroidal nevi. Although clinical examination by an experienced observer remains the most important test in establishing the presence of an ocular melanoma, ancillary diagnostic testing can be extremely valuable.[142–145]

Fluorescein angiography and monochromatic photography have proved useful in differentiating subretinal or choroidal hemorrhage and hemangioma from melanoma (Fig. 42.3-1). Although no angiographic pattern is pathognomonic, features of value include early mottling fluorescence, orange pigment over the margin of the tumor, progressive fluorescence of the lesion with late staining, and multiple pinpoint leaks that increase in size. Breaks in Bruch's membrane and retinal invasion can be detected from abnormalities, such as a double or tumor circulation pattern (simultaneous visualization of retinal and choroidal circulation).[134–137] However, this double circulation pattern is often difficult to recognize, particularly when the overlying retinal pigment epithelium is completely intact. An *in vitro* study of endogenous fluorescence[133] emphasized the differences between low tumor autofluorescence and bright retinal pigment epithelium autofluorescence due to lipofuscin deposits.

Indocyanine green angiography was formerly used as a tool to differentiate melanomas from nevi, but early photographs had a rather poor resolution.[134] Since the introduction of videoangiography and high-resolution fundus digital imaging systems, this technique has proven useful in documenting retinal vascular and choroidal diseases.[135,136] It can also be useful to further differentiate amelanotic choroidal tumors, such as some nevi or melanomas from hemangiomas or metastases, the latter appearing almost invariably hyperfluorescent on early or late frames (or both). This imaging system might also better delineate tumor borders. Indocyanine green angiography using a confocal scanning laser ophthalmoscope is superior to fluorescein angiography in imaging microvascularization patterns.[89,90,137] The angiographically seen microvascularization patterns appear to be identical to patterns identified histologically that have prognostic significance in choroidal melanomas.[89,90,138] *In vivo* imaging of these microvascularization patterns may offer the possibility of improving the prognostic assessment of choroidal melanomas.

The combined use of A- and B-mode ultrasonographic techniques is of great value in confirming the clinical diagnosis of choroidal melanoma, especially in the presence of opaque media.[139,140] The B-mode ultrasonographic characteristics useful in differentiating melanomas from metastases or hemangiomas are acoustic hollowness, choroidal excavation,[141] and orbital shadowing (Fig. 42.3-2). Small tumors elevated less than 2 mm to 3 mm cannot be evaluated accurately. In large tumors, ultrasonography provides valuable size data for serial measurements.[146] However, a difference between ultrasonographic and histopathologic measurements of tumor thickness was demonstrated, probably consecutive to tumor shrinkage after laboratory preparation. Extrascleral extension can be detected by contact B-mode ultrasonography. Ultrasonic tissue characterization and tumor volume determination might bear prognostic information.[141–147] Ultrasonography is also a very important follow-up tool after conservative treatment of uveal melanoma.[145]

Three-dimensional ultrasonography is a promising imaging technique for evaluating the accurate position of radioactive plaques secured beneath intraocular tumors.[148] It can also be used to observe extrascleral extension of a choroidal melanoma,[149] to quantify the tumor volume, and for posttreatment follow-up.

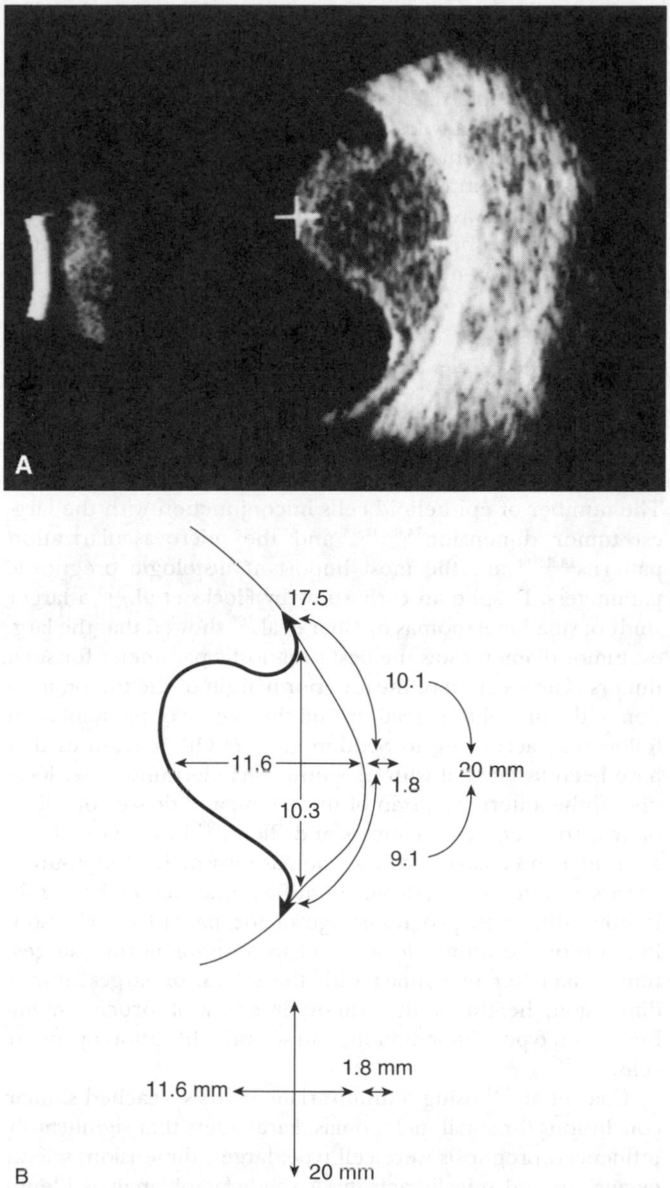

FIGURE 42.3-2. **A:** Ultrasonographic appearance of choroidal tumor. **B:** Tumor dimensions correspond to schematic drawing showing dimensions.

Direct observation by indirect ophthalmoscopy or the use of a three-mirror lens is useful to display the anterior border of these tumors. Clinical transillumination is helpful but is dependent on tumor characteristics and can be more difficult in those patients with amelanotic tumors,[74,150] with ocular melanocytosis, and with dark pigmentation, or tumors complicated with paratumoral hemorrhage. Transillumination may provide an inaccurate assessment of the anterior tumor margins of the peripheral choroid. Anatomic features evident on ultrasonographic biomicroscopy before enucleation were correlated with pathologic examination: supraciliary choroidal effusions, ciliary body rotation, anterior tumor margin position, and angle involvement.[150]

The clinical need to define the anterior borders of peripheral choroidal melanomas clearly is related mainly to decisions regarding treatment options. Secondarily, the pattern of ciliary body involvement can help differentiate tumors of ciliary origin from those of choroidal origin.

Recent reports on the usefulness of color-coded Doppler imaging in the characterization and follow-up of melanomas are promising, particularly for detection of pulsatile ocular blood flow (POBF) at the tumor base.[151–156] The tumor blood flow can also be quantified indirectly by ocular blood flow tonography. The higher POBF values observed in eyes with choroidal melanoma indicate that the pulsatile component of choroidal blood flow is increased.[151] At present, these techniques must be interpreted with caution. Fundamental studies to validate the theoretically derived POBF values and clinical studies to determine reference ranges are required before any meaningful interpretation of these parameters can be made.

The usefulness of radioactive phosphorus (^{32}P) in determining malignancy remains controversial, and this is little used at present. It has limited indications for use in routine cases in which adequate support for a diagnosis of ocular melanoma can be obtained with less complicated procedures.[157]

Radiologic examination, including computed tomography (CT), is useful in evaluating the presence and size of extraocular extension of tumor. It does not, however, add significant information to ultrasonography and implies low doses of radiation.[145]

Images of uveal melanoma have been obtained by magnetic resonance imaging (MRI). This imaging modality has become more useful with employment of thin-section imaging, surface coils, and contrast material (gadolinium). Typically, due to the postulated paramagnetic properties of melanin, pigmented melanomas are hyperintense on T1-weighted images with enhancement by gadolinium and hypointense on T2-weighted images when compared to the brightness of the vitreous.[158,159] This method is, therefore, promising in the detection and characterization of tumors in difficult cases as well as in the differentiation of associated serous retinal detachments.[159] ^{31}P magnetic resonance spectroscopy may be helpful in this respect in the near future.[158] Nevertheless, to this date, ultrasonography is by far the main diagnostic modality in intraocular melanomas. Ocular ultrasonography is also more sensitive than MRI or CT for the detection of extraocular extension of choroidal malignant melanomas.[160] Ultrasonography and fluorescein angiography are together very useful in patients' follow-up (Fig. 42.3-3).

Immunologic testing does not yet offer reliable results.[161,162] Using the indirect immunoperoxidase method, Folberg et al.[162a] found that 78% of patients with uveal malignancy had tumor-associated antibodies (TAA), whereas 24% of controls tested positive for TAA. However, TAA assays could not be used to separate primary from secondary uveal tumors. Studies with monoclonal antibodies (discussed earlier in Cytologic and Histologic Classification) are still in the experimental phase. Radioimmunoscintigraphy using technetium 99m–labeled monoclonal antibodies are still too preliminary to be considered as reliable diagnostic tools, even after pretargeting techniques.[161] However, surveillance of melanoma-associated antigens and carcinoembryonic antigens may be useful for monitoring recurrence or metastatic disease.[162]

In a review of 51 consecutive patients who had undergone enucleation for a choroidal melanoma and 50 patients with simulating lesions, Char et al. found that the ophthalmoscopic

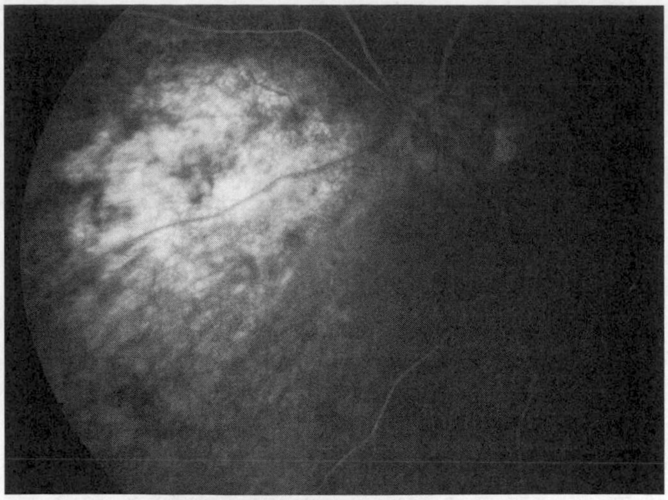

FIGURE 42.3-3. Angiographic appearance of choroidal melanoma during follow-up.

examination was the most accurate diagnostic modality, allowing correct diagnosis of choroidal melanomas in all patients with clear media.[163] Subretinal fluid, orange pigmentation, and collar-button configuration occurred more often with melanomas than with other lesions. In 63% of melanoma patients, fluorescein angiography was diagnostic; in 82%, A- and B-mode ultrasonography was diagnostic.[163]

In some problematic cases, fine-needle aspiration biopsy has been proposed. However, the interpretation of aspirates may be difficult even in the hands of an experienced pathologist, and subsequent tumor cell seeding in the needle track has been reported. Nonetheless, in selected cases, this technique has proven useful in differentiating benign lesions or lymphoid infiltrates from melanoma. Such biopsies obtained through a transocular approach with a 22-gauge needle provided informative specimens in almost 90% of cases, with an accuracy of approximately 98%.[164] It should be emphasized that the lack of histologic data prior to conservative treatment of most uveal melanomas represents a major limitation to our understanding of tumor response to radiation, accurate adaptation of conservative approaches, and establishment of prognosis.

Despite ancillary examinations, the differential diagnosis of small tumors may be difficult. Careful follow-up of such patients at short intervals with photography, fluorescein angiography, and ultrasonography is advocated to demonstrate tumor growth.[165,166] Buttler et al.[165] showed that the presence of symptoms, tumor thickness, orange pigment, acoustic hollowness, and hot spots on fluorescein angiography was a significant predictor of growth.

Patients with suspected intraocular melanoma should undergo a physical examination and metastatic workup. Clinical laboratory studies should include routine blood work, chest radiography, and liver enzyme measurements. CT should be performed if other tests suggest liver involvement.[165–168] Detection of circulating melanocytes using reverse transcriptase-polymerase chain reaction amplification of the tyrosinase gene is a promising approach.[67,167,168] Nevertheless, even though it is known that the detection of melanoma cells in blood cannot automatically be taken as a definitive sign for the presence of metastatic disease, polymerase chain reaction might help in interpreting the result of conventional markers for metastasis in the near feature. Haynie et al.[169] noted significant differences in the peripheral blood lymphocytes in two subgroups of patients with clincially less favorable choroidal melanoma; ciliary body involvement was related to reduction in NK cells and, in patients with extrascleral extension, an increased number of activated T cells was noted. Liver ultrasonography, liver-spleen scans, CT of the head, and MRI appear useful in the initial workup and follow-up.[158]

MANAGEMENT

PROGNOSTIC ASSESSMENT OF CHOROIDAL AND CILIARY BODY MELANOMAS

The number of epithelioid cells in conjunction with the largest tumor dimension[74,90,91,93] and the microvascularization patterns[14,82–86] are the most important histologic prognostic parameters. Despite an early study by Flocks et al.,[170] a larger study of small melanomas by Char et al.[163] showed that the largest tumor diameter was the best prognostic parameter for such tumors. The location of the anterior margin of the tumor, invasion of the line of transsection, and the degree of pigmentation follow this, according to Seddon et al.[215] Other features that have been associated with prognosis include tumor size, location of the anterior margin of the tumor, and degree of ciliary body involvement.[74] Shammas and Blodi,[122] in a study of 253 choroidal and ciliary body melanomas for which a follow-up of 5 years or more was available, identified nine factors that significantly influenced prognosis: age of the patient enucleation; location of the tumor; location of its anterior border; largest tumor diameter in contact with the sclera, or largest tumor dimension; height of the tumor; integrity of Bruch's membrane; cell type; pigmentation; and scleral infiltration by tumor cells.[171,173]

Char et al.,[163] using a multivariate analysis, reached similar conclusions for small melanomas. Parameters that significantly influenced prognosis were cell type, largest dimension, scleral extension, and mitotic activity. A single-factor analysis identified three additional factors of significance: degree of scleral invasion, optic nerve invasion, and pigmentation. In most studies, increased pigmentation has been associated with increased mortality.[174] However, in a multivariate analysis, these last three parameters appear statistically related to cell type and tumor size.[171] Regan et al.[172] described iris color as a prognostic factor in ocular melanoma and concluded that patients with blue or gray irises show light to moderate tumor pigmentation and appear to be at increased risk of metastatic death from choroidal melanoma, independent of other risk factors. Maximum tumor size is believed to be an important predictor of outcome.[74] In the COMS report number 6,[74] anterior location was observed more commonly with large tumor size and more malignant cell type. In many studies, tumors involving the ciliary body have a worse prognosis than those located entirely in the choroid.[74,87] Microvascular networks tend to develop more commonly in the ciliary body relative to the choroid.[87] This observation is important, because deletion of chromosome 3 may be characteristic of ciliary body melanomas and has been associated with their aggressive behavior.[87]

TABLE 42.3-2. Classification of Tumor Size According to Boundary Lines

Type	*Apical Height*	*Largest Basal Diameter*
Small	1.0–2.5 mm	5 mm
Medium	2.5–10.0 mm	5–16 mm
Large	10 mm	16 mm

(Adapted from ref. 174.)

A matter of concern in the present classification of posterior uveal melanomas is the lack of an accurate, consistent, and clinically pertinent size classification.[173] This question is not purely theoretic, since size classification is most often the only available prognostic parameter; a clinically relevant size classification should assign tumors to currently accepted elective treatment modality, or at least to groups of significantly different life prognosis; and a comparison of results using various therapeutic approaches is required. The current TNM staging by the American Joint Committee on Cancer[174] draws boundary lines for small, medium, and large tumors. According to this classification, many tumors considered medium in the current conservative management would belong to the large-tumor category. Whereas a classification according to the largest tumor dimension would appear best suited to predict patient survival, a size classification taking into account tumor thickness and basal diameter is currently in use in most centers and in the COM study (Table 42.3-2).[74] Data from retrospective evaluations,[173] as well as recommendations from the COM Study group,[174] tend to classify tumors as in Table 42.3-2. In COMS report number 6,[74] larger tumor size was related more commonly with anterior location and more malignant cell type. Large tumors invaded the retina, the vitreous, and vortex veins and ruptured Bruch's membrane more often than medium tumors.[74]

It has been shown that certain histologically identified microvascularization patterns are an independent risk factor for the growth and metastatic behavior of choroidal melanomas. The microvascularization patterns that are networked and parallel with cross-linking indicate a high probability for metastatic disease, whereas the presence of microvascular patterns that are silent and parallel without cross-linking indicates a better prognosis.[14,82–86,90,91] A Cox proportional hazards model was generated with the conventional prognostic factors (including the largest tumor dimension in contact with the sclera, cell type, tumor-infiltrating lymphocytes, mitotic figures, gender, and location of the tumor within the eye) and the presence or absence of each of the nine microcirculatory patterns. The most important variable was the network pattern (back-to-back loops). Other significant factors in the model include (in decreasing order of importance) largest tumor dimension, mitoses, parallel with cross-linking vascular patterns, age, the presence of tumor-infiltrating lymphocytes, and male gender.[87,175] However, in the Foss et al. series,[88] the parallel with cross-linking pattern did not carry a poor prognosis; in this series, a poor prognosis was associated with absence of the normal pattern and the presence of arcs, arcs with branches, loops, and networks. Foss et al.[88] suggested that the periodic acid–Schiff patterns are based on three underlying factors that have been identified as (1) presence of disordered growth, (2) presence of rapidly growing subclones, and (3) sectioning orientation. The first two of these factors carried prognostic significance in a multivariate Cox model that included tumor size and microvessel density.[88]

Mehaffey et al.[91] observed that larger areas of these microcirculatory patterns (tumors with >2% occupied) imply a worse prognosis than small isolated foci (tumors with <0.5% occupied). This study also showed that it is possible to separate choroidal melanomas into three prognostic groups by cross-sectional area measured from histologic sections: small (tumor area <16.0 mm^2); medium (tumor area >16.0 mm^2 but <61.4 mm^2); and large (>61.4 mm^2).

The estimation of tumor volume was related to outcome, but the relation between estimated volume and outcome did not hold for relatively small tumors (measuring <1.344 mm^3).[175] In a series of 217 small tumors (measuring <1.400 mm^3), the largest tumor dimension in contact with the sclera was more strongly associated with outcome than estimated volume, possibly because diffuse melanomas may have a relatively small volume but follow an aggressive clinical course.[169]

Technologic advances have implemented the assessment of nucleolar area, nucleolar organized regions, tumor vascular patterns, and tumor vascular density as potential prognostic factors. Cell type, however, remains the most potent single predictor of outcome.[74,93]

Seregard et al. have shown that the MLN and PC10 immunostaining counts retain a prognostic value in uveal melanoma when adjusting for the effect of the mean of the diverse vascular patterns.[176] In recent studies,[177,178] high expression of HLA-A (and, to a lesser extent, of HLA-B) antigens on the primary uveal melanoma was strongly correlated with poor patient survival. High HLA-B expression was significantly correlated with the presence of epithelioid cells in the tumor.[172] The primary uveal melanomas showed a high expression of monomorphic and polymorphic HLA-A antigens, while metastases showed a high expression of monomorphic and a lower expression of polymorphic antigens.[173]

In summary, all studies show that the prognosis of a patient with a choroidal or ciliary body melanoma is adversely affected by the following factors:

- Tumor containing loops, networks, or parallel with cross-linking vascular patterns[91,93,172]
- Largest tumor dimension exceeding 10 mm
- Presence of numerous mitotic figures (mean count per 40 high-power field)
- Patient age older than 56[81]
- Presence of tumor-infiltrating lymphocytes[87]
- Male gender[87]
- Tumor containing epithelioid cells (or related cytologic features, such as nucleolar parameters and vascular architecture, as discussed earlier in Cytologic and Histologic Classification)
- Anterior tumor border anterior to equator[174]
- Tumor extending to the scleral surface

In the COMS report number 4,[174] older patients with a history of diabetes and patients with more anteriorly located tumors were at increased risk for death. Yet a close interval-by-interval analysis of the prognostic value of size and cell type in a series of 3680 patients shows a decline over time after tumor excision.[175] Gamel et al.,[179] applying the log-normal survival model[175,179] to 2892 patients treated by enucleation, demonstrated that the probability that the patient is cured by tumor resection is not modulated by the same biologic factors as those determining survival time among patients. Their analysis showed that mixed cell type and advanced patient age are associated only with a short median survival time. In contrast, pleomorphic nucleoli and large tumor size were independently associated with both a low probability of curative resection and short median survival time. Many of these prognostic parameters are lacking in patients treated conservatively. Furthermore, due to a shorter follow-up, bias in patient selection and size of samples, and the use of different survival analysis models, comparison of survival rates between conservative approaches or between conservative approaches and enucleation remains a subject of intense controversy.[163,179–181] To date, the survival rates in large series after 5 years do not differ significantly. The reported tumor-related mortality 5 years after radiation therapy ranges from 11% to 25%,[181,183] whereas preliminary assumptions based on a log-normal model may indicate a poorer life prognosis after 10 years for patients treated conservatively. The COMS, a prospective multicenter study, should provide answers to this most crucial and controversial issue.[209]

Several studies have established a correlation between rapid tumor regression after radiation therapy and a poorer life prognosis.[175] Rapid regression of tumor height after radiation therapy appears as a risk factor for metastasis. Rapid regression can possibly be correlated with a less differentiated cell type of fast-regressing tumors. However, such a hypothesis is difficult to ascertain for several reasons: (1) Cytologic study of melanomas is rarely performed before radiation therapy; (2) when needle biopsy is obtained, it often does not provide a reliable characterization of the cell type; and (3) study of enucleated eyes after radiation therapy for any reason may not accurately reflect features of the tumor prior to radiation therapy, particularly in mixed or epithelioid tumors.

PRETREATMENT CLINICAL STAGING

In light of current knowledge, it is useful to discuss the treatment of choroidal and ciliary body melanomas in terms of tumor size, following the size classification discussed previously in Management. In contrast with the Reese-Ellsworth classification[182a] of retinoblastoma, the current classifications are of marginal help in predicting the visual outcome of conservative approaches, since such factors as the distance to the optic nerve and macula are important in estimating final visual acuity.

Another problem is related to the rarity of detectable metastases, particularly lymphatic, at the time of diagnosis. Attempts to detect and treat subclinical metastases should develop in the near future to address appropriately this major clinical problem. Moreover, the lack of histopathologic data in most cases managed conservatively has given emphasis to clinical patterns of tumor growth prior to treatment and histologic analysis of tumor regression after radiation therapy based on enucleated eyes. The results of comparisons of data from retrospective studies have been a source of confusion and controversy.

TREATMENT OF CHOROIDAL AND CILIARY BODY MELANOMAS

In the late nineteenth century, enucleation became the standard and almost universally accepted treatment for all choroidal or ciliary body melanomas. Even today, early enucleation continues to have its ardent advocates.[181] However, in the last two decades, enucleation has been reassessed as the standard means of treating malignant melanomas of the choroid and ciliary body. This reassessment has resulted from (1) the development of newer and more precise diagnostic tests for recognizing malignant melanomas and the serial documentation of their size; (2) more information about clinical and pathologic features that determine survival; (3) additional observations about the natural course of untreated ciliary body and choroidal melanomas; (4) therapeutic developments other than enucleation to treat these tumors without destroying the eye; and (5) disagreements as to the value and risks of enucleation.[183]

Most authors today agree that the goals of an ophthalmologist treating a uveal melanoma should be to destroy or inactivate the neoplasm, to maintain useful vision in the involved eye, to employ a treatment with as few side effects as possible but, most important, to provide the patient with the best prognosis for life possible.[175,176] Regarding which treatment can best achieve these goals, controversies will continue until results from prospective randomized treatment trials are collected.[183] In the absence of these data, the selection of treatment is based on the specific findings in each case with regard to tumor size, location, and growth rate; the preferences of the ophthalmologist; and the desires of the patient. Recently, Cruickshanks et al. showed that treatment choice does not seem to be associated with large differences in quality of life (as assessed by the Medical Outcome Study Short Form 36 and the National Eye Institute Visual Function Questionnaire).[184]

Small Melanomas

The choices open to the physician treating a small choroidal or ciliary body melanoma include (1) observation; (2) some method of local treatment, such as radiation therapy, photoradiation, cryotherapy, ultrasonic hyperthermia, or local resection; and (3) enucleation.

OBSERVATION. An accumulating body of evidence indicates that the risks in observing most melanomas are generally low.[184] Serial examination every 3 months without intervention seems appropriate if the tumor is asymptomatic and appears *dormant*, the diagnosis is equivocal, and no growth is seen on serial ophthalmoscopic, photographic, and ultrasonographic examinations. Observation is also indicated for elderly or seriously ill patients or for tumors in the patient's only useful eye, particularly where the tumor is growing slowly. If the tumor shows progression, especially rapid growth or an increase in size beyond 10 mm in diameter and 3 mm in elevation, or if the lesion results in significant impairment of vision, treatment is indicated.

PHOTOCOAGULATION. In the photocoagulation method, the xenon arc, the argon laser, photoradiation with red light after photosensitization with hematoporphyrin derivatives, or dye laser after phthalocyanine photosensitization can be used.[185] Some success with photocoagulation has been documented histologically in small series.[186–189] The following criteria[188,189] for selecting patients with melanoma for photocoagulation treatment were suggested by Meyer-Schwickerath[188] and Vogel[189] and adapted by Shields[186]:

1. The diagnosis of melanoma and evidence of growth should be documented thoroughly.
2. The tumor should not be greater than 5 diopters in elevation and 6 disc diameters at its greatest diameter.

3. The tumor must be surrounded completely without damaging the fovea or the optic disc.
4. The patient must have clear ocular media and a sufficient mydriasis to enable photocoagulation to be performed.
5. The tumor surface should not have large retinal vessels.

Photocoagulation requires several outpatient treatment sessions and is carried out after mydriasis and, in the case of xenon photocoagulation, use of retrobulbar anesthesia. A double confluent row of heavy coagulation is repeated three times at monthly intervals to encircle the tumor and to obliterate the choroidal vasculature supplying the lesion. The tumor subsequently becomes necrotic, with gray discoloration and a surrounding chorioatrophic scar.

Long-term complications of photocoagulation include retinal vascular obstruction, visual field defect, macular pucker, cystoid macular edema, choroid neovascularization, vitreous hemorrhage, and retinal detachment.[186] Recurrences may appear, usually within 2 years of treatment. In a 20-year follow-up of 54 patients with uveal melanoma, Vogel[189] reported that 63% were alive, although only 46% were considered cured by photocoagulation. Twenty percent of patients subsequently underwent enucleation. Of the 20 patients (37%) who died, 8 did so as a result of metastatic disease, 3 died of other causes and, in 9 patients, the cause of death was undetermined.[166] Shields[186] reported that among 35 patients treated between 1976 and 1979, 25 retained useful vision, 5 had poor vision, and 5 subsequently underwent enucleation. There were no tumor-related deaths. Effects of laser phototherapy are strongly correlated with tumor pigmentation.[185] Comparison of xenon arc and argon laser photocoagulation in 38 consecutive patients with a minimal follow-up of 58 months showed that recurrences were less frequent and appeared later after xenon radiation therapy.[190a] Moreover, primary photocoagulation of small posterior choroidal melanoma with argon laser is not recommended in view of a risk of immediate visual loss.[189]

Photocoagulation seems best suited for small posterior melanomas located within 3 mm of the optic disc or fovea. In such lesions, radiation-induced retinopathy may cause visual loss.[186,187] The patient's wish to avoid radiation therapy or enucleation may be the deciding factor. Phototherapy could also be used as an adjunct to brachytherapy.[190–192] Photocoagulation can be helpful in the treatment of secondary serous macular detachments. Reports on hematoporphyrin, benzoporphyrin derivative monoacid and phthalocyanine, and indocyanine green–enhanced phototherapy are still preliminary.[191–193]

Transpupillary thermotherapy is a technique that employs infrared light (diode laser, 810 mm) delivered as heat to induce necrosis in tumor tissues. Transpupillary thermotherapy offers very promising results in the management of retinoblastoma. It also may be an effective treatment for small choroidal melanomas, theoretically reducing radiation-induced complications.[194,195] In a 14-month follow-up of 100 patients with posterior choroidal melanomas, Shields et al.[195] reported tumor control in 94% of the cases but worsening of visual acuity in 42%. A longer follow-up is necessary to assess the actual rate of local recurrence, survival, and visual outcome.

OTHER LOCAL NONSURGICAL TECHNIQUES. Lincoff et al. obtained discouraging results with cryotherapy of ocular melanomas in four patients. Anecdotal reports of successful treatments for small peripheral melanomas exist.[196] Even more than with radiation therapy, the efficacy of these alternative approaches lacks unequivocal evidence.

LOCAL RESECTION. Peyman et al. developed a technique of local sclerochorioretinal resection for choroidal melanomas.[197–201] After a series of photocoagulation treatments around the tumor to create a firm chorioretinal adhesion or an area of bare sclera, the tumor is surgically removed, along with the adjacent sclera and retina. The defect is replaced by a scleral graft. Peyman has suggested that surgical candidates should exhibit the following criteria: (1) no evidence of metastatic disease; (2) the ability to tolerate general anesthesia; (3) a tumor base no larger than 12 mm and tumor location at least 3 disc diameters from the optic disc; (4) exudative retinal detachment no larger than one-third of the fundus; and (5) clear media.

After local resection, one-third of the eyes required enucleation because of complications, including vitreous hemorrhage and retinal detachment. Shields et al.[195] advocate, in selected cases, the use of partial lamellar sclerouvectomy.[200,201] Damato et al.,[202] reporting the large experience of a skilled team, concluded that with a technique combining lamellar scleral flap for eye closure, hypotensive anesthesia for homeostasis[202,203] and, more recently, ocular decompression by pars plana vitrectomy, good visual results can be obtained in nasal tumors and for tumors located more than 1 disc diameter from the optic nerve and fovea. Yet, most authors note that patients treated by local resection are also amenable to radiation therapy and that early visual loss is far more frequent after surgical resection than with radiation.[204] The risk of leaving some viable tumor cells after treatment is also a matter of major concern. Local resection has not been widely adopted. Recently Damato et al.[202] recommended to adjunct systematically ^{106}Ru brachytherapy to prevent tumor recurrence after local resection.[204]

Iridocyclectomy has proven useful in the treatment of ciliary body melanomas in several series.[205] In the report by Forrest et al.[206] of 107 iridocyclectomies for ciliary body melanoma, 6% of the patients had subsequent enucleation. The majority of problems related to surgical management occurred within 4 years of surgery.[206] Damato et al. have promoted and employed this method for many years with good results.[202] A surprising feature is the low incidence of recurrence even when tumor extends to the margins of the resection. In contrast to resection of choroidal melanomas, iridocyclectomy is widely accepted for the treatment of ciliary body melanomas.[204] Endoresection of choroidal melanoma is technically challenging but may bear some interest for the conservation of central vision after removal of juxtapapillary tumors. Preliminary results are encouraging in terms of visual outcome despite a high rate of complication, including retinal detachment (40%), and cataract (65%).[205,207] The risk of tumor cell release during surgery warrants long-term assessment of this procedure.

ENUCLEATION. In the case of patients with a healthy second eye, enucleation is advised if the tumor shows evidence of rapid progression and invasion of the optic nerve or extraocular extension is suspected.[208,209] Other considerations, including loss of central vision, failure of previous conservative treatment, and the patient's desire for complete surgical removal of the tumor, may make enucleation a reasonable choice.

Large Melanomas

There is at present general agreement that it would be inadvisable to treat cases of large melanoma by methods other than enucleation.[208] Possible exceptions include patients with only one sighted eye, rare patients in whom vision can be salvaged, and patients who refuse enucleation. Abramson et al.[182] recommended local radiation therapy in these latter difficult cases. Some authors recommend external radiation therapy prior to enucleation. Only experimental evidence in animal models exists for the usefulness of this therapy. This method is currently being evaluated in the COMS.[174] This randomized trial reported initial mortality findings that showed no survival difference in the preenucleation irradiated group.[208,209]

Zimmerman et al. have suggested that when enucleation is carried out, the "no-touch" technique of Fraunfelder should be considered.[210] This method was designed to minimize the possibility of seeding of tumor cells into the blood vessels during enucleation. The authors claim that this technique avoids intraocular pressure elevations above 15 mm before complete freezing occurs around the tumor. Cryotherapy is used to minimize the flow of fluid and blood to or from the tumor during the manipulation necessary for enucleation. Although most surgeons do not use the no-touch technique, it is increasingly recognized that enucleation should be carried out by a person skilled and experienced in the procedure and that surgery should be done with a minimum of manipulation.[210]

Medium-Sized Melanomas

Treatment of medium-sized tumors is the subject of current controversy. Although general agreement exists that the observation of small melanomas carries little risk and that large melanomas should be treated by enucleation, there is less consensus regarding the treatment of medium-sized melanomas.

Nonsurgical Techniques

RADIATION THERAPY FOR OCULAR MELANOMA. Ocular melanomas have been successfully treated by a variety of radiotherapeutic modalities, including external-beam techniques using photons or charged particles (protons and helium ions); stereotactic radiosurgery with modified linear accelerators and multisource cobalt units; brachytherapy (plaque) techniques using a wide variety of isotopes; hyperthermia in combination with brachytherapy; and, at least experimentally, boron neutron capture therapy (BNCT). Techniques with the most widely reported clinical experience to date include charged-particle beam therapy and plaque therapy.

CHARGED-PARTICLE BEAM THERAPY. Charged-particle beams (protons or helium ions) have specific dosimetric advantages in the delivery of high radiation dose to very precisely localized targets. Treatment of ocular melanoma requires pinpoint accuracy to limit dose to the adjacent retina, optic nerve, lens, and brain. Charged-particle beams are produced by a cyclotron or synchrotron available at only a few sites around the world. High-energy charged particles travel a fixed distance in tissue that varies with the energy of the particle and the nature of the tissue. Near the end of their path, they deposit the bulk of their energy within a well-defined volume, referred to as the *Bragg peak*. A high and relatively uniform dose can be achieved within a small volume, thereby sparing adjacent normal tissues.[211]

Proton beam therapy is available at only 16 facilities in nine countries and helium and other ion beams at even fewer sites.[212] Charged-particle beam therapy is generally delivered in four or five treatment sessions over 1 to 2 weeks. The treatment requires sophisticated planning techniques, precise tumor mapping, immobilization of the head, and fixation of the eye at a reproducible and verifiable gaze angle. Surgical placement of inert radiopaque rings on the sclera assists in identifying the target volume. Patients are treated in a seated position, with a face mask and bite block to immobilize the head. The correct gaze angle, chosen so that the beam enters the sclera and minimizes radiation therapy of the anterior chamber, is verified by an infrared camera with the patient's vision focused on a fixation light. The treatment portal (beam diameter) ranges from 1 to 4 cm. Daily setup of the patient is accomplished in 10 minutes, and the duration of radiation therapy is only 1 to 2 minutes.[213] Long-term data on the experience with helium ion therapy for ocular melanoma have recently been updated.[214] Three hundred forty-seven patients were reported, with local tumor control achieved in 96%. Although rare cases of tumor regrowth were identified as late as 5 years after treatment, 85% of local regrowth was detected within 3 years. The total enucleation rate was 19% (3% for local regrowth and 16% for complications of radiation therapy, including neovascular glaucoma). The 10-year overall survival is 76%, with 24% of patients manifesting distant metastasis. Risk of metastasis was related to previously known negative prognostic factors, such as large tumor size or unfavorable location.

Proton beam treatment centers report similar local control rate of 90% to 95%.[213] Risk of distant metastasis also appears comparable to the helium ion–treated patients, approximately 20% at 5 years. Randomized studies comparing proton beam therapy and enucleation have not been reported, and retrospective comparisons are difficult because of the need to balance the known prognostic factors (tumor size, tumor location and ocular structures involved, patient age) between the treatment groups. A large and statistically well-balanced comparison of proton-treated patients with enucleated patients from the same institution has shown no apparent difference in long-term survival.[216]

Visual preservation is one of the goals of eye-conserving therapies for ocular melanoma. Radiation maculopathy and papillopathy are major causes of visual loss after successful treatment of melanoma with charged-particle beams. Although preservation of peripheral vision and ambulatory vision has been satisfactory, visual acuity of 20/100 or better was observed in only 32% of patients treated at one major center for proton radiation therapy[218] and was 20/200 or better in only 36% of patients treated with helium ion therapy.[214] These studies concur in the finding that posttreatment visual acuity is greatly effected by tumor location (in relation to optic disc and fovea), tumor size, pretreatment visual acuity, and treatment parameters. In proton beam–treated patients with tumor edge more than 3 mm from the optic disc and fovea, 67% retained useful vision (20/200 or better); with tumors located within 3 mm of these structures, only 39% maintained useful vision.[213]

EPISCLERAL PLAQUE RADIATION THERAPY. Episcleral plaque therapy, a highly specialized multidisciplinary treatment approach, is more widely available than charged-particle beam therapy for ocular melanoma. A concave plaque is con-

TABLE 42.3-3. Retrospective Data on Radioactive Episcleral Plaque Therapy

	Gunduz[222]	*Finger*[218]	*Seregard*[224]	*Petrovich*[223]	*Beitler*[225]
No. of eyes treated	630	80	266	85	116
Isotope	^{125}I (61%), ^{60}Co, ^{192}Ir	^{103}Pd	^{106}Ru	^{192}Ir, ^{125}I	^{60}Co
Follow-up (y)	Minimum = 7	Median = 3.2	Median = 3.6	Median = 5	Mean = 3.8
Enucleation	11%	8%	17%	15%	6%[a]
Local control	5 y = 91% 10 y = 88%	3 y = 94%	82%	—	83%
Overall survival	5 y = 87%	3 y = 92%	5 y = 83%	5 y = 88%, 8 y = 84%	—
Metastatic disease	5 y = 12%, 10 y = 22%	3 y = 5%	5 y = 14%	5 y = 11%	5 y = 12%

[a]Includes enucleations for complications only; excludes enucleation for tumor recurrence.

structed to house several small radioactive sources based on preoperative tumor measurements. This requires integration of data from clinical examination, ultrasonography, CT, or MRI scan. The specially designed plaque containing multiple radioactive sources is temporarily sutured to the sclera overlying the tumor under general or retrobulbar anesthesia. Operative localization of the plaque placement is guided by transillumination, ophthalmoscopic observation, or ultrasonography. The plaque remains in place for 2 to 5 days, depending on the type and activity of the radioactive source, and is then removed under similar operative conditions.

Iodine 125 is the most commonly used radioisotope in the United States and is the only isotope permitted in the COMS trial. Ruthenium 106 is frequently used in Europe; other isotopes include cobalt 60 and palladium 103. Isotopes with lower photon and electron radiation (^{125}I, ^{106}Ru, ^{103}Pd) are more easily shielded to reduce the exposure to adjacent normal tissues in the patient and the potential exposure to medical personnel. The choice of radioisotope has been based historically on availability and experience. Newer isotopes have been used after detailed dosimetric study and computer modeling. ^{103}Pd has dosimetric advantages based on its lower photon energy as compared to ^{125}I.[217] Phase I trials of ^{103}Pd have been favorable.[218] A nonrandomized comparison of ^{125}I and ^{106}Ru plaques showed better tumor control with the ^{125}I.[219]

The COMS group recently completed accrual to a randomized trial comparing standardized ^{125}I plaque therapy to enucleation for medium-sized melanomas. A review of factors considered in selecting ^{125}I plaque therapy for this trial has been published.[220] In comparison to ^{60}Co plaque, ^{125}I results in a significantly reduced exposure of normal tissue to high radiation dose. Each plaque consists of a flexible inner plastic plaque and a rigid outer gold plaque that is sutured in place. Six different plaque sizes are available, and the size selected covers a 2- to 3-mm margin around the base of the tumor. ^{125}I seeds are sandwiched between the gold and plastic plaques. The activity and number of seeds are selected to achieve an apical dose rate between 42 and 105 cGy/h. Treatment duration for the plaque therapy is calculated to deliver a total dose of 85 Gy to the prescription point.

Study end points include survival, freedom from melanoma metastasis, as well as useful vision retained. The accrual objective was reached in July 1998, when 43 clinical centers enrolled a total of 1317 patients. Published data will be available when reliable 5-year survival estimates are known. The COMS data will have a major influence on the choice of treatments. No other randomized trial has been published comparing enucleation with any radiotherapeutic approach. As with proton beam therapy, retrospective comparisons between plaque therapy and enucleation require careful analysis and balancing of prognostic factors. A large retrospective series comparing ^{60}Co plaque therapy to enucleation identified no significant difference in long-term survival.[221]

Table 42.3-3 summarizes some of the retrospective data available for a variety of plaque therapies. Survival rates at 5 years range from 80% to 88%. The rate of metastatic disease is approximately 10% at 5 years but appears to increase to close to 20% for studies reporting 10-year data. Enucleation has been required for either tumor progression or severe radiation complication (neovascular glaucoma, vitreous hemorrhage) in 10% to 17% of patients. In Table 42.3-4, clinical outcomes for charged-particle beam treatments and plaque therapy are com-

TABLE 42.3-4. Clinical Outcomes from Three Different Radiation Therapy Techniques

Treatment	*Local Control (%)*	*Enucleation (%)*	*5-Y Overall Survival (%)*	*Distant Metastasis Rate (%)*	*Visual Acuity ≥20/200 (%)*
Proton beam (Munzenrider[213])	95	10	80	16	49
Helium ion beam (Castro[214])	96	19	80	24	36
Plaque therapy (see refs. 218, 222, 223)	82–94	6–17	83–87	5–22	44

TABLE 42.3-5. Collaborative Ocular Melanoma Study Randomized Trial of Preenucleation Radiation Therapy for Large Choroidal Melanomas

	Enucleation	*Preenucleation Radiation Therapy*	*Probability Value*
No. of patients randomly assigned	506	497	—
Acute complications	4%	8%	$P = .03$
Severe ptosis	10%	5%	$P = .007$
Orbital recurrence (no. of patients)	5	0	$P = .03$
Overall 5-y survival	57% (CI 52%–62%)	62% (CI 57%–66%)	—
Death from metastatic melanoma (at 5 y)	26%	28%	—

CI = 95% confidence interval.
(From refs. 209 and 226, with permission.)

pared, with no apparent significant differences between any of the modalities.

Preservation of useful vision is one of the anticipated benefits of plaque therapy. However, the documentation and analysis of visual outcomes after eye-conserving therapies have been limited by a number of factors. Acuity may decrease with time after radiation therapy, and follow-up data may be incomplete for patients referred to distant tertiary eye care centers. Data from the various retrospective series are not always directly comparable. Visual acuity has been expressed as useful vision, reading vision, ambulatory vision, Snellen chart line decrement, and other measures. As noted with particle beam treatment, loss of acuity is a complex interaction of tumor size, location, and treatment effects. In the recently updated report by Gunduz et al.,[222] final visual acuity was better than 20/200 for 44% of patients, but visual decrement of 3 or more Snellen lines was seen in 82% of patients at 10 years.[224] The initial report of patients treated with ^{103}Pd shows more favorable visual preservation with 77% of patients at 20/200 or better, but follow-up has been only 3 years.[218] For tumors with favorable size and location, the rate of useful vision preservation is encouraging.

PREENUCLEATION ORBITAL RADIATION THERAPY. For the treatment of larger melanomas, where enucleation is the accepted standard treatment, COMS has reported initial results of a randomized comparison of preoperative orbital radiation therapy (20 Gy in 5 fractions) followed immediately by enucleation versus enucleation alone. The hypothesis tested was that preoperative orbital radiation might reduce the risk of seeding of viable tumor cells during surgery and thereby improve survival through the reduction in the incidence of distant metastasis.

With the sponsorship of the National Eye Institute of the National Institutes of Health, the COMS Group enrolled 1003 patients from 1986 through closure in December 1994. Five-year outcome data on the first 800 patients have been published.[209,226]

As shown in Table 42.3-5, no advantage in overall survival or prevention of melanoma metastasis was seen with the use of preenucleation orbital radiation therapy at the dose and fractionation studied. The trial had the statistical power of 90% to detect a 20% relative difference in survival between the two arms. Acute complications (occurring 1 to 6 weeks after enucleation) were slightly more common in irradiated patients, but all complications were minor. For late complications (>6 months after enucleation), no increase in cosmetic or functional complications was seen after radiation therapy. In fact, severe ptosis was observed less frequently in patients receiving radiation therapy (5% vs. 10%).

Preoperative radiation did appear to lower the risk of orbital recurrence, although this was a rarely noted event (<1% of the total study population developed local relapse). No recurrences were noted in the preenucleation radiation therapy arm, and five biopsy-proven recurrences were documented in the enucleation-only arm. The five patients with orbital recurrence had metastatic melanoma diagnosed prior to diagnosis of the orbital recurrence and died less than 1 year after presentation of the local recurrence.

With no survival benefit noted from the COMS trial, routine preoperative orbital radiation therapy, as administered in this trial, would not be considered standard therapy. The COMS patients will continue to have follow-up assessments, but any late difference in survival is unlikely, as 46% of patients on study have died at time of this analysis. Preoperative or postoperative orbital radiation therapy may still be considered for selected patients who are at high risk for incomplete tumor excision or perioperative tumor seeding.

INVESTIGATIONAL RADIOTHERAPEUTIC TECHNIQUES. *Radiosurgery and Fractionated Stereotactic Radiation Therapy.* High-dose, highly focused radiation therapy for small target lesions (<2 cm) can be accomplished by either gamma knife radiosurgery (multiple fixed, precisely aimed cobalt teletherapy beams) or stereotactic radiation therapy (multiple rotational arcs of photon beams from a linear accelerator). Both techniques are similar in their use of standard energy proton beams for treatment and rely on meticulous patient immobilization to deliver treatment to a precisely localized target within a coordinate mapping system. These techniques have been widely used and well described for the treatment of intracranial neoplasms (meningiomas, acoustic neuromas, and metastatic tumors) and for the ablation of arteriovenous malformations. Several recent retrospective series have examined the application of these techniques for the treatment of ocular melanomas.

The use of high-dose single-fraction Leksell gamma knife radiosurgery has been reported in a few small retrospective series.[227,228] This technique has been marked by significant adverse radiation reactions, including retinopathy, optic neuropathy, and glaucoma after treatment with 50 to 70 Gy in a single fraction. Optimal dose and technique have not yet been defined for this approach.

Linear accelerator (photon) fractionated stereotactic radiosurgery has been studied to use the radiobiologic advantage of multiple- rather than single-fraction treatment.[229,230] Reproducible immobilization of the head and eye is required, and active optical fixation systems, similar to proton beam techniques, have been described.[231] In these studies, 35 to 70 Gy has been delivered in 2 to 8 fractions. Outcome data and toxicity reports will require additional follow-up time, and further refinement of treatment technique will be necessary.[232] The preliminary data indicate a risk of significant adverse treatment effects with the techniques and radiation doses reported to date. The use of these techniques outside of the investigational setting is not recommended, except for patients who cannot be treated with proton beam or plaque therapy.

Hyperthermia and Episcleral Plaque Radiation Therapy. Hyperthermia has been investigated in conjunction with radiation therapy to treat a variety of tumors. Preclinical experiments have demonstrated that neoplastic cell lethality is proportional to temperature increase in the target tissue and that the combination of hyperthermia and radiation produces enhanced antitumor effects.[233,234] Ocular tumor heating has been achieved by a variety of techniques, including microwave applicators,[235] ultrasonic applicators, or ferromagnetic seeds.[236]

One of the primary objectives for combining hyperthermia and radiation is to reduce the radiation dose, which is expected to result in fewer visual complications with a comparable rate of tumor control. An initial report of combined hyperthermia and episcleral plaque therapy employed a 30% reduction in radiation dose (72 Gy, as compared to the prior standard dose of 100 Gy).[237] In this phase I study of 25 patients, 22 showed decrease in tumor height, and ambulatory vision (>5/200) was maintained in 20 patients. Two patients had severe complications (hemorrhagic retinal detachment and vitreous hemorrhage). Evaluation of long-term efficacy and late effects will require additional follow-up.

Boron Neutron Capture Radiation Therapy. BNCT is a specialized form of radiation therapy in which a neutron beam is targeted against a tumor that has been pretreated with a boron-containing compound. The boron nucleus is 10,000 times more likely than a hydrogen atom to capture a thermal neutron; therefore, preferential localization of boron in the tumor would result in precise and focal radiation delivery. The capture of the slow neutron by the boron nucleus leads to an energetic fission reaction with the formation of a lithium ion and an alpha particle (helium ion), accompanied by 2.4 MV of energy. The lithium and helium ions travel a distance of only 10 mm, limiting the lethal effect of the radiation to a radius approximately the diameter of one cell.[238]

The administration of boron-containing compounds and neutron radiation therapy has shown efficacy in the Greene melanoma-rabbit model.[239] Boronated compounds have been administered experimentally to human subjects with ocular melanoma prior to enucleation. Increased uptake of boron within the melanoma cells, compared to vitreous body, retina, and sclera was observed.[240] The use of BNCT in humans with melanoma, for the treatment of skin nodules, has been reported.[241,242] This approach for the treatment of ocular melanoma is at an early experimental stage, and further technical refinement will be required before clinical trials can be considered.

FUTURE DIRECTIONS FOR RESEARCH

Uveal melanoma, like retinitis pigmentosa, may not constitute a single disease; it may instead consist of an assortment of maladies with multiple genetic origins that simply culminate in a limited phenotype. In the case of retinitis pigmentosa, varying proportions of rod and cone photoreceptor cells degenerate owing to a variety of genetic mutations within the same or different genes.[243] In contrast to a phenotype associated with cell death, uveal melanoma is characterized by uncontrolled proliferation. Fundamentally different mechanisms can lead to unwarranted cell growth, supported in the case of uveal melanoma by cytogenetic[19,25,244–250] and biochemical[33,234,251] findings that disparate genetic events likely initiate the transformation of normal uveal melanocytes.

Cancer, as a multistage process, has an impact on a large number of genes and their related cellular pathways. Recent advances in both biochemical and molecular methods render it possible to study the cellular pathways that comprise this multistage process, endowing tumor cells with properties related to their malignant and metastatic capabilities. Such studies can provide significant information about the course of the disease and about effective treatments, independent of knowing the genetic mutations that cause the disease. It may, in fact, be more prudent to study the common cellular pathways that define the properties of these cells and to develop treatments based on these findings rather than attempting to "fix" a diverse array of genetic mutations.

Many features of ocular melanoma can be studied initially using established cell lines derived from biopsies of human tissues.[53,100,252] Normal uveal melanocytes also can be passaged in culture.[253] They are nonmalignant, neither growing in soft agar or athymic nude mice and, therefore, differ from uveal melanomas that can grow in either circumstance as well as alter the structure of the uvea and metastasize to other sites. Comparisons between *uveal melanocytes* and *uveal melanomas* can reveal the biochemical pathways that promote malignancy and metastatic disease. It is important to note, however, that the results obtained from *in vitro* studies need to be confirmed using primary tumor tissue.

In addition, although several properties associated with transformation can be studied *in vitro*, animal models are essential, since the most general and accepted definition of malignancy requires demonstrating the formation of invasive or metastasizing tumors *in vivo*. Cells derived from human uveal melanomas, for example, have been shown to grow in athymic nude mice after intraocular or subcutaneous inoculation; migration to the liver ensues, resulting in metastatic lesions and death.[254,255] An animal model, therefore, can be used to grade the malignant and metastatic properties of different cell lines; these cell lines then can be modified to alter the expression of a gene suspected of being involved in tumor progression, and the consequences for growth and dissemination of the tumor then can be measured in the animal.

As a first step, how can *in vitro* comparisons be made between uveal melanocytes and uveal melanomas? Genes and their products (proteins) that are uniquely expressed in one cell type can be identified by one of several new approaches, including differential display,[256,257] suppression subtractive hybridization,[258] two-dimensional gel electrophoresis–mass spectrometry[259,260] and, most recently, by using cDNA chip arrays.[261] As an example, sub-

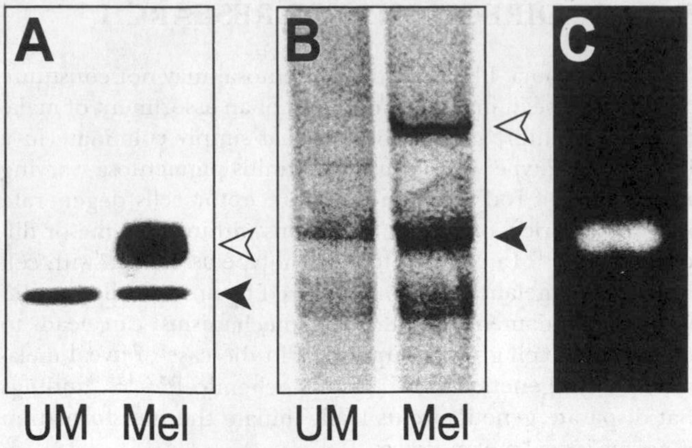

FIGURE 42.3-4. **A:** Tissue Factor (*open arrowhead*) was compared by Western blot analysis using protein from cultured uveal melanocytes (UM) and a uveal melanoma cell line (Mel). GAPDH immunostaining (*filled arrowhead*) served as a control for loading artifact. **B:** Tissue Factor mRNA was detected by RNase protection assay (symbols are the same as in **A**). **C:** Reverse transcriptase-polymerase chain reaction detection of Tissue Factor using specific primers and RNA isolated from a paraffin-embedded section of human uveal melanoma.

tractive cDNA hybridization recently was used to identify differences in mRNA species obtained from normal uveal melanocytes and an epithelioid melanoma cell line. Tissue Factor was among the genes identified and suspected of elevated expression in the melanoma cell line. Tissue Factor has angiogenic properties, contributing to the formation of new vessels associated with solid tumors,[257,258,262–264] perhaps including uveal melanoma. The expression of angiogenic factors is an example of one of the cellular events contributing to the cancer phenotype but which has little to do with the initial genetic mutation underlying transformation. Also, treatments based on antiangiogenic strategies are a prime example of how studying cellular pathways can be beneficial.[265]

The differential expression of Tissue Factor was confirmed by Western blot analysis (detecting levels of protein) and by RNase protection assay (measuring levels of mRNA), as illustrated in Figure 42.3-4*A* and *B*. Thus, multiple techniques support *in vitro* findings that Tissue Factor is expressed at elevated levels in a uveal melanoma cell line compared to normal uveal melanocytes.

To avoid *in vitro* artifacts stemming from culture conditions, however, differential expression must be confirmed in primary ocular tissues. Biopsies from primary uveal melanomas and normal tissues derived from human donor eyes can be compared by Western blot analysis and by immunohistochemistry using specific antibodies. The expression of the corresponding genes also can be compared by Northern blot hybridization using the same ocular tissues. In addition, archival specimens can be used for case-corroborative purposes by employing such techniques as *in situ* hybridization, immunohistochemistry, and reverse transcriptase-polymerase chain reaction. As illustrated in Figure 42.3-4*C*, RNA isolated from a 6-mm paraffin section of an enucleated eye with a uveal melanoma was used for reverse transcriptase-polymerase chain reaction with primers specific for Tissue Factor. Tissue Factor was detected in the primary tumor tissue, thus corroborating *in vitro* studies. In the near future, it will be especially informative to compare these sorts of detailed molecular findings with outcome data for patients made available through the collection of archival specimens.

Further correlations can be established between specific biochemical events and the malignant properties of an ocular tumor by genetic manipulation using established cell lines. Transfection experiments can be conducted to alter the level of expression of interesting genes (e.g., Tissue Factor); the consequences of altered expression on division, growth, and progression of the transfected cells then can be determined both *in vitro* and *in vivo*. In some cases, the biochemical function of the protein can be ascertained, and this provides further clues about additional portions of a cellular pathway that might be useful for targeted intervention. The promoters for melanocyte-specific genes also may be useful for targeting oncogenic expression in a transgenic animal, thereby creating an important model of uveal melanoma.

Oncogenes, such as the SV40 transgene producing the large T and small t antigens, can be used to generate pigmented tumors of the eye. To obtain models more representative of uveal melanoma, however, the transgene apparently needs to be driven by a promoter specific for uveal melanocytes rather than one common to multiple cell types.[266,267] Again, this can be accomplished by comparing normal uveal melanocytes with related ocular tissues and skin. Once the identification has been successful and an appropriate model of uveal melanoma available, the efficacy of different treatments can be evaluated more fully.

However, there is a general misconception that ocular melanoma and cutaneous melanoma are essentially the same disease and that research of the more prevalent skin disorder will satisfy needs within the ophthalmology community. This is not the case. The two diseases differ in their systemic symptoms, metastatic patterns, and susceptibility to treatments.[268] Clearly, the study of ocular melanoma remains within the purview of the vision scientist. Further, the advent of new molecular and biochemical techniques coupled with the availability of tissue specimens and established cell lines now renders it possible to advance our understanding and treatment of ocular tumors. Additionally, as has often been the case, studies of ocular tissues have enhanced our understanding of other tissue types and associated pathologies; delineating the cellular pathways contributing to cancer phenotypes in the eye should be no exception.

Acknowledgments

Drs. Laurent Meyez, Jean-Louis Uzel, and Fernande Porto. Ghislaine Hirth.

REFERENCES

1. Cutler SJ, Young JL, eds. Third National Cancer Survey: incidence data. NCI Monogr 1975;41:1.
2. Vidal JL, Bacin F, Albuisson E, et al. "Mélanome 1992." Etude épidémiologique des mélanomes uvéaux en France. *J Fr Ophtalmol* 1995;18:520.
3. Phillpotts BA, Sanders RJ, Shields JS, et al. Uveal melanomas in black patients: a case series and comparative review. *J Natl Med Assoc* 1995;87:709.
4. Margo CE, Mulla Z, Billiris K. Incidence of surgically treated uveal melanoma by race and ethnicity. *Ophthalmology* 1998;105:1087.
5. Neugut AI, Kizelnik-Freilich S, Ackerman C. Black-white differences in risk for cutaneous, ocular, and visceral melanomas. *Am J Public Health* 1994;84:1828.
6. Hudson HL, Valluri S, Rao NA. Choroidal melanomas in Hispanic patients. *Am J Ophthalmol* 1994;18:57.

7. Iscovich J, Ackerman C, Andreev H, Peter J, Steinitz R. An epidemiological study of posterior uveal melanoma in Israel, 1961–1989. *J Cancer* 1995;61:291.
8. Scotto J, Fraumeni JF, Lee JAH. Melanoma of the eye and other noncutaneous sites. *JNCI* 1976;56:489.
9. Jensen QA, Prause JU. Malignant melanomas of the human uvea in Denmark: incidence and a 25-year follow-up of cases diagnosed between 1943 and 1952. In: Lommatzsch PK, Blodi FC, eds. *Intraocular tumors.* Berlin: Springer-Verlag, 1983:85.
10. Gialason I, Magnussen G, Tulinius H. Malignant melanoma of the uvea in Iceland, 1955–1979. *Acta Ophthalmol (Copenh)* 1985;63, 385, 394.
11. Markowitz JA, Hawkins BS, Diener-West M, Schachat AP. A review of mortality from choroidal melanoma: I. Quality of published reports, 1966 through 1988. *Arch Ophthalmol* 1992;110:239.
12. Diener-West M, Hawkins BS, Markowitz JA, Schachat AP. A review of mortality from choroidal melanoma: II. A meta-analysis of 5-year mortality rates following enucleation, 1966 through 1988. *Arch Ophthalmol* 1992;110:245.
13. Raivio I. Uveal melanoma in Finland: an epidemiological, clinical, histological and prognostic study. *Acta Ophthalmol* 1977;133(Suppl):3.
14. Panigel K, Speeg-Schatz C, Schaffer P, Brini A, Sahel J. Facteurs pronostiques des mélanomes choroïdiens. *J Fr Ophtalmol* 1992;15:410.
15. Silcock A. Hereditary sarcoma of the eyeball in three generations. *Br Med J* 1892;1:1079.
16. Singh AD, Donoso LA. Genetic aspects of uveal melanoma. *Int Ophthalmol Clin* 1993;33:47.
17. Young LH, Egan KM, Walsh SM, Gragoudas ES. Familial uveal melanoma. *Am J Ophthalmol* 1994;117:516.
18. Singh AD, Wang MX, Donoso LA, et al. Familial uveal melanoma: III. *Arch Ophthalmol* 1996;114:1101.
19. Singh AD, Boghosian-Sell L, Wary KK, et al. Cytogenetic findings in primary uveal melanoma. *Cancer Genet Cytogenet* 1994;72:109.
20. Copeman MC. The putative melanoma tumor-suppressor gene on human chromosome 6q. *Pathology* 1992;24:307.
21. Prescher G, Bornfeld N, Becher R. Nonrandom chromosomal abnormalities in primary uveal melanoma. *J Natl Cancer Inst* 1990;82:1765.
22. Dahlenfors R, Tornqvist G, Wettrell K, Mark J. Cytogenetical observations in nine ocular malignant melanomas. *Anticancer Res* 1993;13:1415.
23. Sisley K, Cottam DW, Rennie IG, et al. Non-random abnormalities of chromosomes 3, 6 and 8 associated with posterior uveal melanoma. *Genes Chromosomes Cancer* 1992;5:197.
24. Gordon KB, Thompson CT, Char DH, et al. Comparative genomic hybridization in the detection of DNA copy number abnormalities in uveal melanoma. *Cancer Res* 1994;54:4764.
25. Prescher G, Bornfeld N, Becher R. Two subclones in a case of uveal melanoma. Relevance of monosomy 3 and multiplication of chromosome 8q. *Cancer Genet Cytogenet* 1994;77:144.
26. Royds JA, Sharrard RM, Parsons MA, et al. C-myc oncogene expression in ocular melanomas. *Graefes Arch Clin Exp Ophthalmol* 1992;230:366.
27. Tobal K, Warren W, Cooper CS, McCartney A, Hungerford J, Lightman S. Increased expression and mutation of p53 in choroidal melanoma. *Br J Cancer* 1992;66:900.
28. Jay M, McCartney AC. Familial malignant melanoma of the uvea and p53: a Victorian detective story. *Surv Ophthalmol* 1993;37:457.
29. Houlston RS, Damato BE. Genetic predisposition to ocular melanoma. *Eye* 1999;13:43.
30. Mouriaux F, Maurage CA, Labalette P, Casagrande F, Malecaze F, Darbon JM. Les inhibiteurs des CDK cyclines dans les mélanocytes choroidiens normaux et transformés *J Fr Ophtalmol* 1999;22:339.
31. Mouriaux F, Casagrande F, Pillaire MJ, Manenti S, Malecaze F, Darbon JM. Differential expression of G_1 cyclins and cyclin-dependent kinase inhibitors in normal and transformated melanocytes. *Invest Ophthalmol Vis Sci* 1998;39:876.
32. Dunne BM, McNamara M, Clynes M, et al. MDR1 expression is associated with adverse survival in melanoma of the uveal tract. *Hum Pathol* 1998;27(6):594.
33. Coupland SE, Bechrakis N, Schüler A, et al. Expression patterns of cyclin D1 and related proteins regulating G_1-S phase transition in uveal melanoma and retinoblastoma. *Br J Ophthalmol* 1998;82:961.
34. Singh AD, De Potter P, Fijal BA, Shields CL, Shields JA, Elston RC. Lifetime prevalence of uveal melanoma in white patients with oculo (dermal) melanocytosis. *Ophthalmology* 1998;105:195.
35. Rehany U, Rumelt S. Iridocorneal melanoma associated with type 1 neurofibromatosis—a clinicopathologic study. *Ophthalmology* 1999;106:614.
36. Yanoff M, Zimmerman LE. Histogenesis of malignant melanomas of the uvea III. The relationship of congenital ocular melanocytosis and neurofibromatosis to uveal melanomas. *Arch Ophthalmol* 1967;77:331.
37. Van Hees CL, De Boer A, Jager MJ, et al. Are atypical nevi a risk factor for uveal melanoma? A case-control study. *J Invest Dermatol* 1994;103:202.
38. Bataille V, Sasieni P, Cuzick J, Hungerford JL, Swerdlow A, Newton Bishop JA. Risk of ocular melanoma in relation to cutaneous and iris naevi. *Int J Cancer* 1995;60:622.
39. Turner BJ, Statkowski RM, Ausberger JJ, et al. Other cancers in uveal melanoma patients and their families. *Am J Ophthalmol* 1989;107:601.
40. Kuchle M, Tiemann M, Holbach L, Naumann GO. Necrotic malignant melanoma of the choroid and concurrent intraocular manifestation of malignant non-Hodgkin's B cell lymphoma. *Ophthalmologica* 1994;208:65.
41. Bataille V, Pinney E, Hungerford JL, Cuzick J, Bishop DT, Newton JA. Five cases of coexistent primary ocular and cutaneous melanoma. *Arch Dermatol* 1993;129:198.
42. Lischko AM, Seddon JM, Gragoudas ES, et al. Evaluation of prior primary malignancy as a determinant of uveal melanoma: a case-control study. *Ophthalmology* 1989;96:1716.
43. Holly EA, Ashton DA, Ahn DK, et al. No excess prior cancer in patients with uveal melanoma. *Ophthalmology* 1991;98:608.
43a. Paul EV, Parnell BL, Fraker M. Prognosis of malignant melanomas of the choroid and ciliary body. *Int Ophthalmol Clin* 1968;5:387.
44. Egan KM, Gragoudas ES, Seddon JM, Walsh SM. Smoking and the risk of early metastases from uveal melanoma. *Ophthalmology* 1992;99:537.
44a. Seddon JM, MacLaughlin DT, Albert DM, et al. Uveal melanomas presenting during pregnancy and the investigation of estrogen receptors in melanomas. *Br J Ophthalmol* 1982;66:695.
45. Ajani UA, Seddon JM, Hsieh CC, Egan KM, Albert DM, Gragoudas ES. Occupation and risk of uveal melanoma. An exploratory study. *Cancer* 1992;70:2891.
45a. Shields CL, Shields JA, Eagle RC Jr. et al. Uveal melanoma and pregnancy. *Ophthalmology* 1991;98:1667.
46. Foss AJE, Alexander RA, Phil M, et al. Estrogen and progesterone receptor analysis in ocular melanomas. *Ophthalmology* 1995;102:431.
46a. Hartge P, Tucker MA, Shields JA, et al. Case-control study of female hormones and eye melanoma. *Cancer Res* 1989;49:4622.
47. Kraemer KH, Lee MM, Scotto J. Xeroderma pigmentosum: cutaneous, ocular, and neurologic abnormalities in 830 published cases. *Arch Dermatol* 1987;123:241.
48. Kraemer KH, Lee MM, Andrews AD, Lambert WC. The role of sunlight and DNA repair in melanoma and non-melanoma skin cancer. The xeroderma pigmentosum paradigm. *Arch Dermatol* 1994;130:1018.
49. Horn EP, Hartge P, Shields JA, Tucker MA. Sunlight and risk of uveal melanoma. *J Natl Cancer Inst* 1994;86:1476.
50. Gass JDM, Gieser RG, Wilkinson CP, Beahm DE, Pautler SE. Bilateral diffuse uveal melanocytic proliferation in patients with occult carcinoma. *Arch Ophthalmol* 1990;108:527.
51. Leys AM, Dierick HG, Sciot RM. Early lesions of bilateral diffuse melanocytic proliferation. *Arch Ophthalmol* 1991;109:1590.
52. Mooy CM, De Jong PTVM, Strous C. Proliferative activity in bilateral paraneoplastic melanocytic proliferation and bilateral uveal melanoma. *Br J Ophthalmol* 1994;78:483.
53. Albert DM, Ruzzo MA, McLaughlin MA, Robinson NL, Craft JL, Epstein J. Establishment of cell lines of uveal melanoma. *Invest Ophthalmol Vis Sci* 1984;25:1284.
54. Belkhou R, Abbé JCh, Pham P, et al. Uptake and metabolism of boronophenylalanine in human uveal melanoma cells in culture. Relevance to boron neutron capture therapy of cancer cells. *Amino Acids* 1995;8:217.
55. Belkhou R, Mykita S, Meyer L, et al. Effet létal de la réaction de capture neutronique du bore sur des cellules de mélanome uvéal humain en culture incubées avec la borophénylalanine. *C R Acad Sci Paris* 1992;315(3):485.
56. Benathan M, Alvero-Jackson H, Mooy AM, Scaletta C, Frenk E. Relationship between melanogenesis, glutathione levels and melphalan toxicity in human melanoma cells. *Melanoma Res* 1992;2:305.
57. Aubert C, Rouge F, Reillaudou M, Metge P. Establishment and characterization of human ocular melanoma cell lines. *Int J Cancer* 1993;54:784.
58. Goodal T, Buffey JA, Rennie IG, et al. Effect of melanocyte stimulating hormone on human cultured choroidal melanocytes, uveal melanoma cells, and retinal epithelial cells. *Invest Ophthalmol Vis Sci* 1994;35:826.
59. Olsen KR, Blumkranz M, Hernandez E, Hajek A, Hartzer M. Fluorouracil therapy in intraocular Greene melanoma in the rabbit. *Arch Ophthalmol* 1988;106:812.
60. Waard-Siebinga, van Delft JL, Wolff-Rouendaal D, Jager M. Hamster Greene melanoma in the rabbit eye: immunosuppressive treatment to improve this tumor model. *Graefes Arch Clin Exp Ophthalmol* 1994;232: 683.
61. Niederkorn J, Sanborn GE, Scarbrough EE. Mouse model of brachytherapy in consort with enucleation for treatment of malignant intraocular melanoma. *Arch Ophthalmol* 1990;108:865.
62. Pe'er J, Folberg R, Massicotte SJ, et al. Clinicopathologic spectrum of primary uveal melanocytic lesions in an animal model. *Ophthalmology* 1992;99:977.
63. Mintz B, Klein-Szanto AJ. Malignancy of eye melanomas originating in the retinal pigment epithelium of transgenic mice after genetic ablation of choroidal melanocytes. *Proc Natl Acad Sci U S A* 1992;89:11421.
64. Anand R, Ma D, Alizadeh H, et al. Characterization of intraocular tumors arising in transgenic mice. *Invest Ophthalmol Vis Sci* 1994;35:3533.
65. Liggett PE, Lo G, Pince KJ, Rao NA, Pascal SG, Kan-Mitchel J. Heterotransplantation of human uveal melanoma. *Graefes Arch Clin Exp Ophthalmol* 1994;232(31):15.
66. Pignol JP, Abbé JC, Lefebvre O, Stampfler A, Methlin G, Sahel J. Thérapie par capture de neutrons des mélanomes oculaires : approches dosimétrique et microdosimétrique. *C R Acad Sci* 1994;317:543.
67. Kan-Mitchell J, Mitchell MS, Rao N, Liggett PE. Characterization of uveal melanoma cell lines that grow as xenografts in rabbit eyes. *Invest Ophthalmol Vis Sci* 1989;30:829.
68. Hu LK, Huh K, Gragoudas ES, Young LH. Establishment of pigmented choroidal melanomas in a rabbit model. *Retina* 1994;14:264.
69. Mueller AJ, Folberg R, Freeman WR, et al. Evaluation of human choroidal melanoma rabbit model for studying microcirculation patterns with confocal ICG and histology. *Exp Eye Res* 1999;68:671.
70. Kramer TR, Powell MB, Wilson MM, Salvatore J, Grossniklaus HE. Pigment uveal tumors in a transgenic mouse. *Br J Ophthalmol* 1998;82:953.
71. Scull JJ, Alcocer CE, Deschênes J, Burnier MN Jr. Primary choroidal melanoma in a patient with previous cutaneous melanoma. *Arch Ophthalmol* 1997;115:796.
72. Grossniklaus HE, Albert DM, Green R, Conway BP, Hovland KR, for the Collaborative Ocular Melanoma Study Group. Clear cell differentiation in choroidal melanoma: COMS Report No. 8. *Arch Ophthalmol* 1997;115:894.
73. Lawry J, Smith MO, Parsons AJ, Rennie IG. Simultaneous cell cycle and phenotypic analysis of primary uveal melanoma by flow cytometry. *Eye* 1998;12:431.
74. Collaborative Ocular Melanoma Study Group. Histopathologic characteristic of uveal melanomas in eyes enucleated: COMS Report No. 6. *Am J Ophthalmol* 1998;125:745.
75. Beckenkamp G, Schäfer HJ, Von Domarus D. Immunocytochemical parameters in ocular malignant melanomas. *Eur J Cancer Clin Oncol* 1988;24[suppl2]:542.
76. Steuhl KP, Rohrbach JM, Knorr M, Thiel HJ. Significance, specificity, and ultrastructural localization of HMB-45 antigen in pigmented ocular tumors. *Ophthalmology* 1993;100:208.

77. Berge PJ, Danen EH, Van Muijen GN, Jager MJ, Ruiter DJ. Integrin expression in uveal melanoma differs from cutaneous melanoma. *Invest Ophthalmol Vis Sci* 1993;34:3635.
78. Wang MX, Earley JJ Jr, Shields JA, Donoso LA. An ocular melanoma-associated antigen. Molecular characterization. *Arch Ophthalmol* 1992;110:399.
79. McCurdy J, Gamel JW, McLean I. A simple, efficient, and reproducible method for estimating the malignant potential of uveal melanoma from routine H and E slides. *Pathol Res Pract* 1991;187:1025.
79a. McLean IW, Foster WD, Zimmerman LE. Prognostic factors in small malignant melanomas of the choroid and ciliary body. *Arch Ophthamol* 1977;95:48.
80. Sorensen FB, Gamel JW, McCurdy J. Stereologic estimation of nucleolar volume in ocular melanoma: a comparative study of size estimators with prognostic impact. *Hum Pathol* 1993;24:513.
81. Gamel JW, McCurdy JB, McLean IW. A comparison of prognostic covariates for uveal melanomas. *Invest Ophthalmol Vis Sci* 1992;33:1919.
82. Folberg R, Pe'er J, Gruman LM, et al. The morphologic characteristics of tumor blood vessels as a marker of tumor progression in primary human uveal melanoma. *Hum Pathol* 1992;23:1298.
83. Folberg R, Rummelt V, Parys-Van Ginderdeuren R, et al. The prognostic value of tumor blood vessel morphology in primary uveal melanoma. *Ophthalmology* 1993;100:1389.
84. Marcus DM, Minokovitz JB, Wardwell SD, et al. The value of nucleolar organizer regions in uveal melanoma. *Am J Ophthalmol* 1990;100:527.
85. Pe'er J, Rummelt V, Mawn L, Hwang T, Woolson RF, Folberg R. Mean of the ten largest nucleoli, microcirculation architecture, and prognosis of ciliochoroidal melanomas. *Ophthalmology* 1994;101:1227.
86. Rummelt V, Folberg R, Rummelt C, et al. Microcirculation architecture of melanocytic nevi and malignant melanomas of the ciliary body and choroid. A comparative histopathologic and ultrastructural study. *Ophthalmology* 1994;101:718.
87. Folberg R, Mehaffey MG, Gardner LM, Meyer M, Rummelt V, Pe'er J. The microcirculation of choroidal and ciliary body melanomas. *Eye* 1997;11:227.
88. Foss AJE, Alexander RA, Hungerford JL, Harris AL, Cree IA, Lightman S. Reassessment of the PAS patterns in uveal melanoma. *Br J Ophthalmol* 1997;81:240.
89. Mueller AJ, Freeman WR, Folberg R, et al. Evaluation of microvascularization pattern visibility in human choroidal melanomas: comparison of confocal fluorescein with indocyanine green angiography. *Graefes Arch Clin Exp Ophthalmol* 1999;237:448.
90. Mueller AJ, Bartsch DU, Folberg R, et al. Imaging the microvasculature of choroidal melanoma with confocal indocyanine green scanning laser ophthalmoscopy. *Arch Ophthalmol* 1998;116:31.
91. Mehaffey MG, Folberg R, Meyer M, et al. Relative importance of quantifying area and vascular patterns in uveal melanomas. *Am J Ophthalmol* 1997;123:798.
92. Rummelt V, Mehaffey MG, Campbell J, et al. Microcirculation architecture of metastases from primary ciliary body and choroidal melanoma. *Am J Ophthalmol* 1998;126:303.
93. McLean IW, Keefe KS, Burnier MN. Uveal melanoma. Comparison of the prognostic value of fibrovascular loops, mean of the ten largest nucleoli, cell type, and tumor size. *Ophthalmology* 1997;104:777.
94. Ward TP, McLean IW, Raberts AO. Expression of proliferating cell nuclear antigen (PCNA) in primary uveal melanoma. *Invest Ophthalmol Vis Sci* 1994;35[Suppl]:1926(abst).
95. Pe'er J, Gnessin H, Shargal Y, Livni N. PC-10 immunostaining of proliferating cell nuclear antigen in posterior uveal melanoma. Enucleation versus enucleation postirradiation groups. *Ophthalmology* 1994;101:56.
96. Karlsson M, Boeryd B, Carstensen J, Kagedal B, Wingren S. DNA ploidy and S-phase fraction as prognostic factors in patients with uveal melanomas. *Br J Cancer* 1995;71:177.
97. Coleman K, Baak JP, van Diest PJ, et al. DNA ploidy status in 84 ocular melanomas: a study of DNA quantitation in ocular melanomas by flow cytometry and automatic and interactive static image analysis. *Hum Pathol* 1995;26:99.
98. Mooy C, Vissers K, Luyten G, et al. DNA flow cytometry in uveal melanoma: the effect of pre-enucleation irradiation. *Br J Ophthalmol* 1995;79:174.
99. Char DH, Kroll SM, Stoloff A, et al. Cytomorphometry of uveal melanoma. Comparison of fine needle aspiration biopsy samples with histologic sections. *Anal Quant Histol* 1991;13:293.
100. Ksander BR, Rubsamen PE, Olsen KR, Cousins SW, Streilein JW. Studies of tumor-infiltrating lymphocytes from a human choroidal melanoma. *Invest Ophthalmol Vis Sci* 1991;32:3198.
101. Whelchel JC, Farah SE, McLean IW, Burnier MN. Immunohistochemistry of infiltrating lymphocytes in uveal malignant melanoma. *Invest Ophthalmol Vis Sci* 1993;34:2603.
102. de la Cruz PO, Specht CS, McLean IW. Lymphocytic infiltration in uveal malignant melanoma. *Cancer* 1990;65:112.
103. Huang XQ, Mitchell MS, Liggett PE, Murphree AL, Kan-Mitchell J. Non-fastidious, melanoma specific CD8+ cytotoxic T lymphocytes from choroidal melanoma patients. *Cancer Immunol Immunother* 1994;38:399.
104. Kanda S, Cochran AJ, Lee WR, Morton DL, Irie RF. Variations in the ganglioside profile of uveal melanoma correlate with cytologic heterogeneity. *Int J Cancer* 1992;52:682.
105. Tardif M, Coulombe J, Soulieres D, Rousseau A, Pelletier G. Gangliosides in human uveal melanoma process. *Int J Cancer* 1996;68:97.
106. Ma D, Luyten GP, Luider TM, Niederkorn JY. Relationship between natural killer cell susceptibility and metastasis of human uveal melanoma cells in a murine model. *Invest Ophthalmol Vis Sci* 1995;36:435.
107. Ma D, Alizadeh H, Comerford SA, et al. Rejection of intraocular tumors from transgenic mice by tumor-infiltrating lymphocytes. *Curr Eye Res* 1994;13:361.
108. MacFaul PA, Morgan G. Histopathological changes in malignant melanomas of the choroid after cobalt plaque therapy. *Br J Ophthalmol* 1977;61:221.
109. Klaus H, Lommatzsch PK, Fuchs U. Histopathology studies in human malignant melanomas of the choroid after unsuccessful treatment with 106Ru/106Rh ophthalmic applicators. *Graefes Arch Clin Exp Ophthalmol* 1991;229:480.
110. Fuchs U, Kivela T, Tarkkainen A, Laatikanen L. Histopathology of enucleated intraocular melanomas irradiated with cobalt and ruthenium plaques. *Acta Ophthalmol* 1988;66:255.
111. Crawford JB, Char DH. Histopathology of uveal melanomas treated with charged particle radiation. *Ophthalmology* 1987;94:639.
112. Shields CL, Shields JA, Karlsson U, Menduke H, Brady LW. Enucleation after plaque radiotherapy for posterior uveal melanoma. Histopathologic findings. *Ophthalmology* 1990;97:1665.
113. Saornil MA, Egan KM, Gragoudas ES, Seddon JM, Walsh S, Albert DM. Histopathology of proton beam irradiated versus enucleated uveal melanomas. *Arch Ophthalmol* 1992;110:1112.
114. Gragoudas ES, Egan KM, Saornil MA, Walsh SM, Albert DM, Seddon JM. The time course of irradiation changes in proton beam-treated uveal melanomas. *Ophthalmology* 1993;100:1555.
115. Schilling H, Bornfeld N, Friedrichs W, Pauleikhoff D, Sauerwein W, Wessing A. Histopathologic findings in large uveal melanomas after brachytherapy with iodine 125 ophthalmic plaques. *Germ J Ophthalmol* 1994;3:232.
116. Hardman Lea SJ, Levesey SJ, Lowe J, Rothwell I, Haworth SM. Disappearance of ocular malignant melanoma on computerized scan after spontaneous necrosis: clinical, radiological and pathological features. *Eye* 1991;5:748.
117. Rennie I. Melanomas, metastases, and survival. *Br J Ophthalmol* 1993;77:685.
118. Ma D, Gerard RD, Li XY, Alizadeh H, Niederkorn JY. Inhibition of metastasis of intraocular melanomas by adenovirus-mediated gene transfer of plasminogen activator inhibitor type 1 (PAI-1) in an athymic mouse model. *Blood* 1997;90:2738.
119. Ma D, Niederkorn JY. Role of epidermal growth factor receptor in the metastasis of intraocular melanomas. *Invest Ophthalmol Vis Sci* 1998;39:1067.
120. Gragoudas ES, Egan KM, Seddon JM, et al. Survival of patients with metastases from uveal melanoma. *Ophthalmology* 1991;98:383.
121. Dithmar S, Völcker HE, Grossniklaus HE. Multifocal intraocular malignant melanoma: report of two cases and review of the literature. *Ophthalmology* 1999;106:1345.
122. Shammas HF, Blodi FC. Prognostic factors in choroidal and ciliary body melanomas. *Arch Ophthalmol* 1977;95:63.
123. Singh AD, Shields CL, Shields JA, De Potter P. Bilateral primary uveal melanoma: bad luck or bad genes? *Ophthalmology* 1996;103:256.
124. Blumenthal EZ, Pe'er J. Multifocal choroidal malignant melanoma: at least 3 melanomas in one eye. *Arch Ophthalmol* 1999;117:255.
125. Starr HJ, Zimmerman LE. Extrascleral extension and orbital recurrence of a malignant melanoma of the choroid and ciliary body. *Int Ophthalmol Clin* 1962;2:369.
126. McLean IW, Foster MD, Zimmerman LE. Uveal melanoma: location, size, cell type and enucleation as risk factors in metastasis. *Hum Pathol* 1981;13:123.
127. Fraunfelder FT, Boozman FW, Wilson RS, et al. No-touch technique for intraocular malignant melanomas. *Arch Ophthalmol* 1977;95:1616.
128. Seigel D, Myers M, Ferris F III, et al. Survival rates after enucleation of eyes with malignant melanomas. *Am J Ophthalmol* 1979;87:761.
129. Manschot WA, van Peperzeel HA. Choroidal melanoma: enucleation or observation? A new approach. *Arch Ophthalmol* 1980;98:71.
130. Kersten RC, Blodi FC. Prognosis of choroidal melanomas. *Ophthal Forum* 1983;1:21.
131. Davidorf FH. The melanoma controversy: a comparison of choroidal, cutaneous, and iris melanomas. *Surv Ophthalmol* 1981;25:373.
132. Collaborative Ocular Melanoma Study Group. Accuracy of diagnosis of choroidal melanoma in the collaborative ocular melanoma study. COMS report. *Arch Ophthalmol* 1990;108:1268.
133. Lohmann W, Wiegand W, Stolwijk TR, van Delft JL, Best JA. Endogenous fluorescence of ocular malignant melanomas. *Ophthalmologica* 1995;209:7.
134. Bischoff PM, Flower RW. Ten years' experience with choroidal angiography using indocyanin green dye: a new routine examination or an epilogue? *Doc Ophthalmol* 1985;60:235.
135. Harino S, Miyamoto K, Ogawa K, et al. Indocyanine green videoangiographic findings in choroidal metastatic tumor. *Graefes Arch Exp Ophthalmol* 1995;233:339.
136. Shields CL, Shields JA, De Potter P. Patterns of indocyanine green videoangiography of choroidal tumours. *Br J Ophthalmol* 1995;79:237.
137. Meyer K, Augsburger JJ. Independent diagnostic value of fluorescein angiography in the evaluation of intraocular tumors. *Graefes Arch Exp Ophthalmol* 1999;237:489.
138. Rummelt V, Naumann GO. Reassessment of the PAS patterns in uveal melanoma. *Br J Ophthalmol* 1998;82:101.
139. Gosbell AD, Barry WR, Favilla I, Burgess F. Volume measurement of intraocular tumours by cross-sectional ultrasonographic scans. *Aust NZ J Ophthalmol* 1991;19:327.
140. Berger RW, Guthoff R, Helmke K, Winkler P. Doppler ultrasonography in the follow-up of malignant melanoma of the choroid. *Doc Ophthalmol Proc Ser* 1990;53:327.
141. Van Gool CA, Thijssen JM, Verbeek AM. B-mode echography of choroidal melanoma; echographic and histological aspects of choroidal excavation. *Int Ophthalmol* 1991;15:327.
142. Coleman DJ, Lizzi FL, Silvermann RH, Woods SM, Rondeau MJ. Three-dimensional acoustic tissue staining of uveal melanoma for monitoring of treatment. *Invest Ophthalmol Vis Sci Suppl* 1992;33:1440.
143. Damms T, Schäfer HJ, Guthoff R, et al. Histological determination of tumor-vascularization and their correlation with Doppler sonography in patients with malignant melanoma of the choroid. *Invest Ophthalmol Vis Sci Suppl* 1992;33:2750.
144. Jensen PK, Hansen MK. Ultrasonographic, three-dimensional scanning for determination of intraocular tumor volume. *Acta Ophthalmol* 1991;69:178.
145. Jensen PK. Ultrasonographic three-dimensional scanning for determination of intraocular tumour volume. *Acta Ophthalmol* 1992;[Suppl 204]:23.
146. Thijssen JM, Verbeek AM, Romijn RL, de Wolf-Rouendaal D, Oosterhuis JA. Echographic differentiation of intraocular melanomas by computer analysis. *Acta Ophthalmol* 1992;[Suppl 204]:26.

147. Coleman DJ, Silverman RH, Rondeau MJ, et al. Ultrasonic tissue characterization of uveal melanoma and prediction of patient survival after enucleation and brachytherapy. *Am J Ophthalmol* 1991;112:682.
148. Finger PT, Romero JM, Rosen RB, et al. Three-dimensional ultrasonography of choroidal melanoma: localization of radioactive eye plaques. *Arch Ophthalmol* 1998;116:305.
149. Romero JM, Finger PT, Iezzi R, Rosen RB, Cocker RS. Tri-dimensional ultrasonography of choroidal melanoma: extrascleral extension. *Am J Ophthalmol* 1998;126:842.
150. Maberly DAL, Pavlin CJ, McGowan HD, Foster FS, Simpson ER. Ultrasound biomicroscopic imaging of the anterior aspect of peripheral choroidal melanomas. *Am J Ophthalmol* 1997;123:506.
151. Yang YC, Kent D, Fenerty CH, Kosmin AS, Damato BE. Pulsatile ocular blood flow in eyes with untreated choroidal melanoma. *Eye* 1997;11:331.
152. Guthoff RF, Berger RW, Winkler P, Helmke K, Chumbleu LC. Doppler ultrasonography of malignant melanomas of the uvea. *Arch Ophthalmol* 1992;109:537.
153. Guthoff R, Winkler P, Helmke K, Berger R. Diagnosis and treatment control of choroidal melanomas—the role of B-scan and Doppler-technique. *Acta Ophthalmol* 1992;[Suppl 59]:204.
154. Wolff-Kormann PG, Kormann BA, Hasenfratz GC, Spengel FA. Duplex and color Doppler ultrasound in the differential diagnosis of choroidal tumors. *Acta Ophthalmol* 1992;[Suppl 204]:66.
155. Wolff-Kormann PG, Kormann BA, Riedel KG, Hasenfratz GC, Spengel FA. Quantitative duplex and color Doppler ultrasound in the follow-up of beta-irradiated (106Ru/106Rh) choroidal melanomas. A prospective study. *Germ J Ophthalmol* 1992;1:151.
156. Gulani AC, Morparia H, Bhatti SS, Jehangir RP. Colour Doppler sonography: a new investigative modality for intraocular space-occupying lesions. *Eye* 1994;8:307.
157. Schaling DF, Oosterhuis JA, Jager MJ, Kakebeeke-Kemme H, Pauwels EK. Possibilities and limitations of radioimmunoscintigraphy and conventional diagnostic modalities in choroidal melanoma. *Br J Ophthalmol* 1994;78:244.
158. Lashkari K, Garrido L, Hughes MS, et al. Magnetic resonance microscopy of eyes with uveal melanoma and retinoblastoma. *Invest Ophthalmol Vis Sci Suppl* 1992;33:925.
159. Ferris JD, Bloom PA, Goddard PR, Collins C. Quantification of melanin and iron content in uveal malignant melanomas and correlation with magnetic resonance image. *Br J Ophthalmol* 1993;77:297.
160. Scott IU, Murray TG, Randall Hughes J. Evaluation of imaging technics for detection of extraocular extension of choroidal melanoma. *Arch Ophthalmol* 1998;116:897.
161. Modorati G, Brancato R, Paganelli G, et al. Immunoscintigraphy with three step monoclonal pretargeting technique in diagnosis of uveal melanoma: preliminary results. *Br J Ophthalmol* 1994;78:19.
162. Modorati G, Paganelli G, Magnani P, et al. Radioimmunoscintigraphy with three-step monoclonal pretargeting technique in diagnosis of uveal melanoma: preliminary results. *Invest Ophthalmol Vis Sci Suppl* 1992;33:2749.
162a. Folberg R, Rummelt V, Parys-Van Ginderdeuren R, et al. The prognostic value of tumor blood vessel morphology in uveal melanoma. *Ophthalmology* 1993;100:1389.
163. Char DH, Stone RD, Irvine AR, et al. Diagnosis modalities in choroidal melanoma. *Am J Ophthalmol* 1980;89:223.
164. Shields JA, Shields CL, Ehya H, Eagle RC Jr, De Potter P. Fine-needle aspiration biopsy of suspected intraocular tumors. The 1992 Urwick Lecture. *Ophthalmology* 1993;100:1677.
165. Buttler P, Char DH, Zarbin M, Kroll S. Natural history of indeterminate pigmented choroidal tumors. *Ophthalmology* 1994;101:710.
166. Augsburger JJ, Vrabec TR. Impact of delayed treatment in growing posterior uveal melanomas [published erratum appears in *Arch Ophthalmol* 1994;112(3):335]. *Arch Ophthalmol* 1993;111:1382.
167. Tobal K, Sherman LS, Foss AJ, Lightman SL. Detection of melanocytes from uveal melanoma in peripheral blood using the polymerase chain reaction. *Invest Ophthalmol Vis Sci* 1993;34:2622.
168. Wang MX, Shields JA, Donoso LA. Subclinical metastasis of uveal melanoma. *Int Ophthalmol Clin* 1993;33:119.
169. Haynie GD, Shen TT, Gragoudas ES, Young LUH. Flow cytometric analysis of peripheral blood lymphocytes in patients with choroidal melanoma. *Am J Ophthalmol* 1997;124:357.
170. Flocks M, Gerende JH, Zimmerman LH. The size and shape of malignant melanomas of the choroid and ciliary body in relation to prognosis and histologic characteristics. A statistical study of 210 tumors. *Trans Am Acad Ophthalmol Otolaryngol* 1955;59:740.
171. Coleman K, Baak JPA, van Diest P, Mullaney J, Farrel M, Fenton M. Prognostic factors following enucleation of 111 uveal melanomas. *Br J Ophthalmol* 1993;77:688.
172. Regan S, Judge HE, Gragoudas ES, Egan KM. Iris color as a prognostic factor in ocular melanoma. *Arch Ophthalmol* 1999;117:811.
173. Augsburger JJ. Size classification of posterior uveal malignant melanomas. *Year Book Ophthalmol* St. Louis: Mosby, 1993;155.
174. Collaborative Ocular Melanoma Study Group. Mortality in patients with small choroidal melanoma: COMS report no. 4. *Arch Ophthalmol* 1997;115:886.
175. McLean IW. Prognostic features of uveal malignant melanoma. *Ophthalmol Clin North Am* 1995;8:143.
176. Seregard S, Spangberg B, Juul C, Oskarsson M. Prognostic accuracy of the mean of the largest nucleoli, vascular patterns and PC-10 in posterior uveal melanoma. *Ophthalmology* 1998;105:485.
177. Blom DJR, Luyten GPM, Mooy C, et al. Human leucocyte antigen class I expression: marker of poor prognosis in uveal melanoma. *Invest Ophthalmol Vis Sci* 1997;38:1865.
178. Blom DJR, Schurmans LRHM, De Waard-Siebinga I, et al. HLA expression ina primary uveal melanoma, its cell line, and four of its metastases. *Br J Ophthalmol* 1997;81:989.
179. Gamel JW, McLean IW, McCurdy JB. Biologic distinctions between cure and time to death in 2892 patients with intraocular melanoma. *Cancer* 1993;71:2299.
180. Potter P, Shields CL, Shields JA, Cater JR, Tardio DJ. Impact of enucleation versus plaque radiotherapy in the management of juxtapapillary choroidal melanoma on patient survival. *Br J Ophthalmol* 1994;78:109.
181. Manschot WA, Van Strik R. Choroidal melanoma: analysis of published therapeutic results. *Fortschr Ophthalmol* 1987;84:183.
182. Adams KS, Abramson DH, Ellsworth RM, et al. Cobalt plaque versus enucleation for uveal melanoma: comparison of survival rates. *Br J Ophthalmol* 1988;72:494.
182a. Reese AB. *Tumors of the eye.* 3rd ed. Hagerstown, MD: Harper & Row, 1976:174.
183. Apple D, Blodi FC. Pathologic observations and clinical approach to uveal melanomas. In: Nicholson D, ed. *Ocular pathology update.* New York: Masson, 1980:213.
184. Cruickshanks KJ, Fryback DG, Nondahl DM, et al. Treatment choice and quality of life in patients with choroidal melanoma. *Arch Ophthalmol* 1999;117:461.
185. Favilla I, Barry WR, Gosbell A, Ellims P, Burgess F. Phototherapy of posterior uveal melanomas. *Br J Ophthalmol* 1991;75:718.
186. Shields JA. The expanding role of laser photocoagulation for intraocular tumors. The 1993 H. Christian Zweng Memorial Lecture. *Retina* 1994;14:310.
187. Eide N. Primary laser photocoagulation of small choroidal melanomas. *Acta Ophthalmol Scand* 1999;77:351.
188. Meyer-Schwickerath G. The preservation of vision by treatment of the intraocular tumors with light coagulation. *Arch Ophthalmol* 1961;66:458.
189. Vogel MH. The application of photocoagulation in the treatment of the choroid. *Ophthalmic Forum* 1983;1:46.
190. Augsburger JJ, Kleineidam M, Mullen D. Combined iodine-125 plaque irradiation and indirect ophthalmoscope laser therapy of choroidal malignant melanomas: comparison with iodine-125 and cobalt-60 plaque radiotherapy alone. *Graefes Arch Clin Exp Ophthalmol* 1993;231:500.
190a. Shields JA, Glazer LC, Mieler WF, Shields CL, Gottlieb MS. Comparison of xenon ard and argon laser photocoagulation in the treatment of choroidal melanomas. *Am J Ophthalmol* 1990;109:647.
191. Gonzalez VH, Hu LK, Theodossiadis PG, et al. Photodynamic therapy of pigmented choroidal melanomas. *Invest Ophthalmol Vis Sci* 1995;36:871.
192. Chong LP, Ozler SA, de Queiroz JM Jr, Liggett PE. Indocyanine green–enhanced diode laser treatment of melanoma in a rabbit model. *Retina* 1993;13:251.
193. Schmidt-Erfurth U, Bauman W, Gragoudas E, et al. Photodynamic therapy of experimental choroidal melanoma using lipoprotein-delivered benzoporphyrin. *Ophthalmology* 1994;101:89.
194. Oosterhuis JA, Journée-de Korver HG, Keunen JEE. Transpupillary thermotherapy: results in 50 patients with choroidal melanoma. *Arch Ophthalmol* 1998;116:157.
195. Shields CL, Shields JA, Cater J, et al. Transpupillary thermotherapy for choroidal melanoma: tumor control and visual results in 100 consecutive cases. *Ophthalmology* 1998;105:581.
196. Lincolff H, McLean T, Long R. The cryosurgical treatment of intraocular tumors. *Am J Ophthalmol* 1977;63:389.
197. Peyman GA, Ericson ES, Axelrod AJ, et al. Full-thickness eyewall resection in primates: an experimental approach to the treatment of choroidal melanoma. *Arch Ophthalmol* 1973;89:410.
198. Peyman GA, Apple DJ. Local excision of a choroidal malignant melanoma: full-thickness eyewall resection. *Arch Ophthalmol* 1974;92:216.
199. Peyman GA. Eyewall resection. *Ophthalmic Forum* 1983;4:38.
200. Peyman GA, Juarez CL, Diamond FG, et al. Ten-year experience with eyewall resection for uveal malignant melanomas. *Ophthalmology* 1984;91:1720.
201. Peyman GA, Gremillon CM. Eyewall resection in the management of uveal neoplasms. *Jpn J Ophthalmol* 1989;33:458.
202. Damato BE, Paul J, Foulds WS. Predictive factors of visual outcome after local resection of choroidal melanoma. *Br J Ophthalmol* 1993;77:616.
203. Chaudhri S, Colvin JR, Todd JG, Kenny GN. Evaluation of closed loop control of arterial pressure during hypotensive anaesthesia for local resection of intraocular melanoma. *Br J Anaesth* 1992;69:607.
204. Rennie IG. From the outside in, or the inside out. Resecting uveal melanomas. *Br J Ophthalmol* 1998;82:209.
205. Reese AB, Jones IS, Cooper WC. Surgery for tumors of the iris and ciliary body. *Am J Ophthalmol* 1968;60:173.
206. Forrest AW, Keyser RB, Spencer WH. Iridocyclectomy for melanomas of the ciliary body: a follow-up study of pathology and surgical mortality. *Trans Am Acad Ophthalmol* 1978;85:1237.
207. Damato B, Groenewald C, McGalliard J, Wong D. Endoresection of choroidal melanoma. *Br J Ophthalmol* 1998;82:213.
208. The Collaborative Ocular Melanoma Study (COMS) randomized trial of pre-enucleation radiation of large choroidal melanoma: I. Characteristics of patients enrolled and not enrolled. COMS report no. 9. *Am J Ophthalmol* 1998;125:767.
209. The Collaborative Ocular Melanoma Study Group (COMS) randomized trial of pre-enucleation radiation of large choroidal melanoma: II. Initial mortality findings, COMS report no. 10. *Am J Ophthalmol* 1998;125:779.
210. Fraunfelder FT, Boozman FW, Wilson RS, et al. No-touch technique for intraocular malignant melanomas. *Arch Ophthalmol* 1977;95:1616.
211. Lamond JP, Auchter RM, Harari PM. Radiation therapy of ocular and orbital disease. In: Albert DM (ed), *Ophthalmic surgery principles and techniques.* Malden, MA: Blackwell Science, 1999:1653.
212. Phillips MH, Griffin TW. Physics of high LET particles and protons. In: Perez CA, Brady LW, eds. *Principles and practice of radiation oncology.* Philadelphia: Lippincott-Raven Publishers, 1998:593.
213. Munzenrider JE. Proton therapy for uveal melanomas and other eye lesions. *Strahlenther Onkol* 1999;175:68.

214. Castro JR, Char DH, Petti PL, et al. 15 years experience with helium ion radiotherapy for uveal melanoma. *Int J Radiat Oncol Biol Phys* 1997;39:989.
215. Seddon JM, Gragoudas ES, Egan KM, et al. Relative survival rates after alternative therapies for uveal melanoma. *Ophthalmology* 1990;97:769.
216. Gragoudas ES, Wenjun L, Lane AM, Munzenrider J, Egan KM. Risk factors for radiation maculopathy and papillopathy after intraocular irradiation. *Ophthalmology* 1999;106:1571.
217. Finger PT, Lu D, Buffa A, DeBlasio DS, Bosworth JL. Palladium-103 versus iodine-125 for ophthalmic plaque radiotherapy. *Int J Radiat Oncol Biol Phys* 1993;27:849.
218. Finger PT, Berson A, Szechter A. Palladium-103 plaque radiotherapy for choroidal melanoma. *Ophthalmology* 1999;106:606.
219. Wilson MW, Hungerford JL. Comparison of episcleral plaque and proton beam radiation therapy for the treatment of choroidal melanoma. *Ophthalmology* 1999;106:1579.
220. Earle J, Kline RW, Robertson DM. Selection of iodine 125 for the Collaborative Ocular Melanoma Study. *Arch Ophthalmol* 1987;105:763.
221. Augsburger JJ, Correa ZM, Freire J, Brady LW. Long-term survival in choroidal and ciliary body melanoma after enucleation versus plaque radiation therapy. *Ophthalmology* 1998;105:1670.
222. Gunduz K, Shields CL, Shields JA, et al. Radiation complications and tumor control after plaque radiotherapy of choroidal melanoma with macular involvement. *Am J Ophthalmol* 1999;127:579.
223. Petrovich Z, Luxton G, Langholz B, Astrahan MA, Liggett PE. Episcleral plaque radiotherapy in the treatment of uveal melanomas. *Int J Radiat Oncol Biol Phys* 1992;24:247.
224. Seregard S, Trampe E, Lax I, Kock E, Lundell G. Results following episcleral ruthenium plaque radiotherapy for posterior uveal melanoma. The Swedish experience. *Acta Ophthalmol Scand* 1997;75:11.
225. Beitler JJ, McCormick B, Ellsworth RM, et al. Ocular melanoma: total dose and dose rate effects with Co-60 plaque therapy. *Radiology* 1990;176:275.
226. Collaborative Ocular Melanoma Study Group. The Collaborative Ocular Melanoma Study Group (COMS) randomized trial of pre-enucleation radiation of large choroidal melanoma III: local complications and observations following enucleation. COMS report no. 11. *Am J Ophthalmol* 1998:126:362.
227. Rennie I, Forster D, Kemeny A, Walton L, Kunkler I. The use of single fraction Leksell stereotactic radiosurgery in the treatment of uveal melanoma. *Acta Ophthalmol Scand* 1996;74:558.
228. Marchini G, Gerosa M, Piovan E, et al. Gamma knife stereotactic radiosurgery for uveal melanoma: clinical results after 2 years. *Stereotact Funct Neurosurg* 1996;66:208.
229. Tokuuye K, Akine Y, Sumi M, et al. Fractionated stereotactic radiotherapy for choroidal melanoma. *Radiother Oncol* 1997;43:87.
230. Zehetmayer M, Dieckmann K, Kren G, et al. Fractionated stereotactic radiotherapy with linear accelerator for uveal melanoma—preliminary Vienna results. *Strahlenther Onkol* 1999;175:74.
231. Dieckmann K, Zehetmayer M, Poetter R. Fractionated stereotactic radiotherapy for choroidal melanoma [Comment]. *Radiother Oncol* 1998;49:197.
232. Buatti JM, Parsons JT, Mendenhall WM, Meeks SL. Fractionated stereotactic radiotherapy for choroidal melanoma [Comment]. *Radiother Oncol* 1997;45:99.
233. Mieler WF. Concurrent versus sequential application of ferromagnetic hyperthermia and ^{125}I brachytherapy of melanoma in an animal model. *Trans Am Ophthalmol Soc* 1997;95:611.
234. Burgess SE, Chang S, Svitra P, et al. Effect of hyperthermia on experimental choroidal melanoma. *Br J Ophthalmol* 1985;69:854.
235. Finger PT. Microwave thermoradiotherapy for uveal melanoma: results of a 10-year study. *Ophthalmology* 1997;104:1794.
236. Steeves RA, Murray TG, Moros EG, et al. Concurrent ferromagnetic hyperthermia and ^{125}I brachytherapy in a rabbit choroidal melanoma model. *Int J Hyperthermia* 1992;8:443.
237. Petrovich Z, Pike M, Astrahan MA, et al. Episcleral plaque thermoradiotherapy of posterior uveal melanomas. *Am J Clin Oncol* 1996;19:207.
238. Hawthorne MF. New horizons for therapy based on the boron neutron capture reaction. *Mol Med Today* 1998;4:174.
239. Packer S, Coderre J, Saraf S, et al. Boron neutron capture therapy of anterior chamber melanoma with p-boronophenylalanine. *Invest Ophthalmol Vis Sci* 1992;33:395.
240. Wadabayashi N, Honda C, Mishima Y, Ichihashi M. Selective boron accumulation in human ocular melanoma vs surrounding eye components after 10B1-p-boronophenylalanine administration. *Melanoma Res* 1994;4:185.
241. Laramore GE, Risler R, Griffin TW, Wootton P, Wilbur DS. Fast neutron radiotherapy and boron neutron capture therapy: application to a human melanoma test system. *Bull Cancer Radiother* 1996;83[Suppl]:191s.
242. Mishima Y, Ichihashi M, Tsuji M, et al. Treatment of malignant melanoma by selective thermal neutron capture therapy using melanoma-seeking compound. *J Invest Dermatol* 1989;92:321s.
243. Farber DB, Danciger M. Identification of genes causing photoreceptor degenerations leading to blindness. *Curr Opin Neurobiol* 1997;7:666.
244. Speicher MR, Prescher G, Du Manoir S, et al. Chromosomal gains and losses in uveal melanomas detected by comparative genomic hybridization. *Cancer Res* 1994;54:3817.
245. Prescher G, Bornfeld N, Friedrichs W, Seeber S, Becher R. Cytogenetics of twelve cases of uveal melanoma and patterns of nonrandom anomalies and isochromosome formation. *Cancer Genet Cytogenet* 1995;80:40.
246. Luyten GPM, Mooy CM, Post J, et al. Metastatic uveal melanoma—a morphologic and immunohistochemical analysis. *Cancer* 1996;78:1967.
247. McNamara M, Kennedy SM. Successful establishment of uveal and conjunctival melanoma *in vitro*. *In Vitro Cell Dev Biol Anim* 1997;33:236.
248. McNamara M, Felix C, Davison EV, Fenton M, Kennedy SM. Assessment of chromosome 3 copy number in ocular melanoma using fluorescence *in situ* hybridization. *Cancer Genet Cytogenet* 1997;98:4.
249. Mitelman F, Mertens F, Johansson B. A breakpoint map of recurrent chromosomal rearrangements in human neoplasia. *Nature Genet* 1997;15:417(abst).
250. White VA, Chambers JD, Courtright PD, Chang WY, Horsman DE. Correlation of cytogenetic abnormalities with the outcome of patients with uveal melanoma. *Cancer* 1998;83:354.
251. Mourizux F, Casagrande F, Pillaire M, et al. Differential expression of G_1 cyclins and cyclin-dependent kinase inhibitors in normal and transformed melanocytes. *Invest Ophthalmol Vis Sci* 1998;39:876.
252. De Waard-Siebinga I, Blom D-JR, Griffioen M, et al. Establishment and characterization of an uveal-melanoma cell line. *Int J Cancer* 1995;62:155.
253. Hu D, McCormick SA, Ritch R, Pelton-Henrion K. Studies of human uveal melanocytes *in vitro*: isolation, purification and cultivation of human uveal melanocytes. *Invest Ophthalmol Vis Sci* 1993;34:2210.
254. Niederkorn JY, Mellon J, Pidherney M, Mayhew E, Anand R. Effect of anti-ganglioside antibodies on the metastatic spread of intraocular melanomas in a nude mouse model of human uveal melanoma. *Curr Eye Res* 1993;12:3423.
255. Ma D, Luyten GP, Luider TM, Jager MJ, Niederkorn JY. Association between nm23-H1 gene expression and metastasis of human uveal melanoma in an animal model. *Invest Ophthalmol Vis Sci* 1996;37:2293(abst).
256. Liang P, Zhu W, Zhang X, et al. Differential display using one-base anchored oligo-dT primers. *Nucleic Acids Res* 1994;22:5763(abst).
257. Liang P, Pardee AB. Differential display of eukaryotic messenger RNA by means of the polymerase chain reaction. *Science* 1992;257:967(abst).
258. Diatchenko L, Lau YC, Campbell AP, et al. Suppression subtractive hybridization: a method for generating differentially regulated or tissue-specific cDNA probes and libraries. *Proc Natl Acad Sci USA* 1996;93:6025(abst).
259. Clauser KR, Hall SR, Smith DM, et al. Rapid mass spectrometric peptide sequencing and mass matching for characterization of human melanoma proteins isolated by two-dimensional PAGE. *Proc Natl Acad Sci U S A* 1995;92:5072(abst).
260. Matsui NM, Smith DM, Clauser KR, et al. Immobilized pH gradient two-dimensional gel electrophoresis and mass spectrometric identification of cytokine-regulated proteins in ME-180 cervical carcinoma cells. *Electrophoresis* 1997;18:409.
261. Brown PO, Botstein D. Exploring the new world of the genome with DNA microarrays. *Nature Genet* 1999;21:33.
262. Zhang Y, Deng Y, Luther T, et al. Tissue factor controls the balance of angiogenic and antiangiogenic properties of tumor cells in mice. *J Clin Invest* 1994;94:1320.
263. Carmeliet P, Collen D. Molecules in focus: Tissue Factor. *Int J Biochem Cell Biol* 1998;30:661.
264. Nakagawa K, Zhang Y, Tsuji H, et al. The angiogenic effect of tissue factor on tumors and wounds. *Semin Thromb Hemost* 1998;24:207.
265. Molema G, Meijer DKF, deLeij LFMH. Tumor vasculature targeted therapies. *Biochem Pharmacol* 1998;55:1939.
266. Zetter BR. Angiogenesis and tumor metastasis. *Annu Rev Med* 1998;49:407.
267. Syed NA, Windle JJ, Darjatmoko SR, et al. Characterization of transgenic mice with pigmented intraocular tumors: tissue of origin and treatment. *Invest Ophthalmol Vis Sci* 1998;39:2800.
268. Albert DM, Ryan LM, Borden EC. Metastatic ocular and cutaneous melanoma: a comparison of patient characteristics and prognosis. *Arch Ophthalmol* 1996;114:107.

CHAPTER **43**

Neoplasms of the Central Nervous System

SECTION **1**

DAVID N. LOUIS
WEBSTER K. CAVENEE

Molecular Biology of Central Nervous System Neoplasms

Neoplastic transformation appears to be a multistep process in which the normal controls of cell proliferation and cell-cell interaction are lost, thus transforming a normal cell into a tumor cell. This tumorigenic process involves an interplay between different classes of genes, including oncogenes, tumor suppressor genes, DNA repair genes, and cell death genes. Alterations of these types of genes in turn underlie human brain tumor formation. In addition, such molecular genetic information has begun to have clinical significance, in both the classification and management of brain tumors. The following chapter reviews the molecular basis of brain tumorigenesis, covering primary tumors of the brain as well as other primary intracranial neoplasms that commonly affect the central nervous system.

DIFFUSE, FIBRILLARY ASTROCYTOMAS

FORMATION OF LOW-GRADE ASTROCYTOMA

Diffuse, fibrillary astrocytomas are the most common type of primary brain tumor in adults. These tumors are divided histopathologically into three grades of malignancy: World Health Organization (WHO) grade II astrocytoma, WHO grade III anaplastic astrocytoma, and WHO grade IV glioblastoma multiforme (GBM). WHO grade II astrocytomas are the most indolent of the diffuse astrocytoma spectrum. Nonetheless, these low-grade tumors are infiltrative and have a marked potential for malignant progression, and any biologic model for astrocytomas must account for these cardinal features of malignant progression and invasion.[1]

p53, a tumor suppressor encoded by the TP53 gene on chromosome 17p, has an integral role in a number of cellular processes, including cell-cycle arrest, response to DNA damage, apoptosis, angiogenesis, and differentiation. The TP53 gene is involved in the early stages of astrocytoma tumorigenesis.[2] TP53 mutations and allelic loss of chromosome 17p are observed in at least one-third of all three grades of adult astrocytomas, suggesting that inactivation of p53 is important in the formation of the grade II tumors. Moreover, high-grade astrocytomas with homogeneous TP53 mutations evolve clonally from subpopulations of similarly mutated cells present in initially low-grade tumors.[3] Such mutation studies are complemented by functional studies that have recapitulated the role of the p53 inactivation in the early stages of astrocytoma formation. For instance, cortical astrocytes from mice without functional p53 appear immortalized when grown *in vitro* and rapidly acquire a transformed phenotype. Cortical astrocytes from mice with one functional copy of TP53 behave more like wild-type astrocytes and only show signs of immortalization and transformation after they have lost the one functional TP53 copy.[4,5] Interestingly, those cells without functional p53 become markedly aneuploid,[4] confirming prior work showing that p53 loss results in genomic instability and that astrocytomas with mutant TP53 are often aneuploid.[6] Thus, the abrogation of astrocytic p53 function appears to facilitate some events integral to neoplastic transformation, setting the stage for further malignant progression.

Many growth factors and their receptors are overexpressed in astrocytomas, including platelet-derived growth factor (PDGF), fibroblast growth factors, and vascular endothelial growth factor (VEGF). PDGF ligands and receptors are expressed approximately equally in all grades of astrocytoma, suggesting that such overexpression is also important in the initial stages of astrocytoma formation. Tumors often overexpress cognate PDGF ligands and receptors in an autocrine stimulatory fashion.[7] The mechanisms for PDGF overexpression in most cases have not been elucidated, although rare astrocytomas display amplification of the PDGF-α receptor gene. Significantly, loss of chromosome 17p in the region of the TP53 gene is closely correlated with PDGF-α receptor overexpression, in that 17p loss is most often seen in those astrocytomas that have PDGF-α receptor overexpression.[8] These observations may imply that TP53 mutations have an oncogenic effect only in the presence of PDGF-α receptor overexpression. This interdependence is highlighted by observations that mouse astrocytes without functional p53 become transformed only in the presence of specific growth factors.[5]

Astrocytomas display a remarkable tendency to infiltrate the surrounding brain, confounding therapeutic attempts at local control. These invasive abilities are often apparent in low-grade as well as high-grade tumors, implying that the invasive phenotype is acquired early in tumorigenesis. Investigations into astrocytoma invasion have highlighted the complex nature of cell-cell and cell-extracellular matrix interactions.[9,10] A variety of cell surface and extracellular matrix molecules such as CD44 glycoproteins, gangliosides, and integrins are differentially expressed in astrocytomas. Many of the growth factors expressed in astrocytomas, such as fibroblast growth factor, epidermal growth factor (EGF), and VEGF, also stimulate migration.[9] Such growth factors, cell surface receptors, and extracellular molecules most likely reflect a dynamic interplay between cell-cell adhesion, remodeling of the extracellular matrix, and cell motility.[10]

Less common molecular changes also occur in grade II astrocytomas. Loss of chromosome 22q, for instance, suggests the presence of a chromosome 22q glioma tumor suppressor gene.[11] Comparative genomic hybridization studies have also demonstrated common gains of chromosome 7q in low-grade astrocytomas.[12] Finally, methylation of critical growth regulatory genes has been noted in some astrocytomas and may be another mechanism for gene alteration (W. Cavenee, unpublished data).

PROGRESSION TO ANAPLASTIC ASTROCYTOMA

The transition from WHO grade II astrocytoma to WHO grade III anaplastic astrocytoma is accompanied by a marked increase in malignant behavior. Although many patients with grade II astrocytomas survive for 5 or more years, patients with anaplastic astrocytomas often die within 2 or 3 years and frequently show transformation to GBM. Histologically, the major differences between grade II and grade III tumors are increased cellularity and the presence of mitotic activity, implying that higher proliferative activity is the hallmark of the progression to anaplastic astrocytoma.

A number of molecular abnormalities have been associated with anaplastic astrocytoma, and some studies have suggested that most of these abnormalities converge on one critical cell-cycle regulatory complex that includes the p16, cyclin-dependent kinase-4 (cdk4), cdk6, cyclin D1, and retinoblastoma (RB) proteins. The simplest schema suggests that p16 inhibits the cdk6/cyclin D1 or cdk4/cyclin D1 complex, preventing these complexes from phosphorylating pRB, and so ensuring that pRB maintains its brake on the cell cycle. Individual components in this pathway are altered in up to 50% of anaplastic astrocytomas and in the majority of GBM.

Chromosome 9p loss occurs in approximately 50% of anaplastic astrocytomas and GBMs, with 9p deletions primarily affecting the region of the CDKN2A gene,[13] which encodes the p16 protein and the p14ARF protein. The CDKN2A gene is inactivated either by homozygous deletion or, less commonly, by point mutations or hypermethylation, thereby affecting p16 and p14ARF expression.[14–16] Moreover, replacement of CDKN2A/p16 into GBM cell lines lacking the gene results in growth suppression.[17]

Loss of chromosome 13q occurs in one-third to one-half of high-grade astrocytomas, with the RB gene preferentially targeted by losses and inactivating mutations.[18] Overall, analysis of chromosome 13q loss, RB gene mutations and RB protein expression suggests that the RB gene is inactivated in approximately 20% of anaplastic astrocytomas and 35% of GBM.[14,18] Interestingly, RB and CDKN2A/p16 alterations in primary gliomas are inversely correlated, rarely occurring together in the same tumor.[13]

Amplification of the CDK4 gene provides an alternative to subvert cell-cycle control and facilitate progression to GBM.[19] CDK4, located on chromosome 12q13-14, is amplified in 15% of malignant gliomas,[20] although this frequency may be higher among cases without CDKN2A/p16 loss, perhaps reaching 50% of GBMs without CDKN2A/p16 loss.[19] CDK4 amplification and CDKN2A/p16 deletions do not occur together in GBM cell lines and some GBM cell lines overexpress cyclin D1.[21] On the other hand, in some GBMs and GBM cell lines, CDK4 amplification and cyclin D1 overexpression appear to represent alternative events to CDKN2A/p16 deletions, because these genetic changes only rarely occur in the same tumors.[19,21] CDK6 amplification also occurs, although not as commonly as CDK4 amplification.[22]

Allelic losses on 19q have been observed in up to 40% of anaplastic astrocytomas and GBMs, indicating a progression-associated glial tumor suppressor gene on chromosome 19q.[23] This tumor suppressor gene may be unique to glial tumors[24] and is involved in all three major types of diffuse cerebral gliomas (astrocytomas, oligodendrogliomas, and oligoastrocytomas). This gene maps to a region of chromosome 19q13.3, telomeric to the marker D19S412 and centromeric to the STD locus gene,[25,26] but is yet to be identified.

PROGRESSION TO GLIOBLASTOMA MULTIFORME

GBM is the most malignant stage of astrocytoma, with survival times of less than 2 years for most patients. Histologically, these tumors are characterized by dense cellularity, high proliferation indices, microvascular proliferation, and focal necrosis. The highly proliferative nature of these lesions is no doubt the result of multiple mitogenic effects. As mentioned previously, at least one such effect is deregulation of the p16-cdk4-cyclin D1-pRB pathway of cell-cycle control. The vast majority, if not all, GBMs have alterations of this system, whether it be inactivation of p16 or pRB or overexpression of cdk4.[13,19]

Chromosome 10 loss is a frequent finding in GBM, occurring in 60% to 95% of GBMs but far less commonly in anaplastic astrocytomas.[27,28] At least two tumor suppressor loci are present on the long arm of chromosome 10, and there may be a third locus on the short arm. The PTEN/MMAC1/TEP-1 gene at 10q23.3 has been implicated as one of these genes, with PTEN mutations identified in approximately 20% of GBM.[29–31] PTEN functions as a protein tyrosine phosphatase and has 3' phosphoinositol phosphatase activity; in addition, PTEN has an amino-terminal domain with homologies to tensin and auxilin.[10] Thus, PTEN may regulate cell migration via affecting focal adhesion kinase and may regulate cell proliferation via control of the AKT serine/threonine kinase. Indeed, introduction of wild-type PTEN into glioma cells with mutant PTEN leads to growth suppression.[32] Nonetheless, given the remarkably high frequency of chromosome 10 loss in GBM, it is likely that other glioma tumor suppressors reside on this chromosome; one candidate is the DBMT1 gene.[33]

EGFR is a transmembrane receptor tyrosine kinase, whose ligands include EGF and transforming growth factor-α. The EGFR gene is the most frequently amplified oncogene in astrocytic tumors,[34] being amplified in approximately 40% of all GBM[27] but in few anaplastic astrocytomas.[35] Those GBMs that exhibit EGFR gene amplification have almost always lost genetic material on chromosome 10[27] and often have CDKN2A deletions.[36] GBMs with EGFR gene amplification display overexpression of EGFR at both the mRNA and protein levels, suggesting that activation of this growth signal pathway is integral to malignant progression to GBM.[35,37] Approximately one-third of those GBM with EGFR gene amplification also have specific EGFR gene rearrangements, which produce truncated molecules similar to the v-erbB oncogene.[10] These truncated receptors are capable of conferring dramatically enhanced tumorigenicity to GBM cells.[38] The downstream targets of EGFR activation in GBMs include the Shc-Grb2-ras pathway, involving EGFR in a cascade that facilitates mitogenesis and decreases apoptosis in tumor cells.[39] Less commonly amplified oncogenes include N-*myc*, *gli*, PDGF-α receptor, c-*myc*, *myb*, K-*ras*, CDK4, and MDM2.

As mentioned previously, one of the hallmarks of GBM is microvascular proliferation. A host of angiogenic growth factors and their receptors are found in GBMs.[10] For example, VEGF and PDGF are expressed by tumor cells while their tyrosine kinase receptors, VEGF receptors 1 and 2 for VEGF and the PDGF-β receptor for PDGF, are expressed on endothelial cells. VEGF and its receptors, in particular, appear to play a major role in GBM angiogenesis.[40–42] A paracrine mechanism has been suggested in which VEGF is secreted by tumor cells and bound by the VEGF receptors on endothelial cells. Interestingly, VEGF is preferentially up-regulated by tumor cells surrounding regions of necrosis, perhaps as a result of necrosis-induced hypoxia, since hypoxia can up-regulate VEGF. In addition, PDGF may up-regulate VEGF expression by endothelial cells, thereby providing an early stimulus for angiogenesis.[43] A link between p53 and tumor angiogenesis has been suggested by the observations that some mutant p53 molecules can enhance VEGF expression[40] and that wild-type p53 regulates the secretion of a glioma-derived angiogenesis inhibitory factor.[44] Related mechanisms may also be responsible for tumoral edema in GBM, because some of these angiogenic molecules, such as VEGF, may also cause vascular permeability and hence tumoral edema.

SUBSETS OF GLIOBLASTOMA MULTIFORME

The assumption that all astrocytomas progress through distinct genetic stages in a linear fashion is most likely an oversimplification. Indeed, it appears as if there are biologic subsets of astrocytomas that may reflect the clinical heterogeneity observed in these tumors[45] (Fig. 43.1-1). For instance, approximately one-third of GBM have TP53/chromosome 17p alterations, one-third have EGFR gene amplification, and one-third have neither change[46] (i.e., TP53 mutations and EGFR amplification are mutually exclusive). Experimental data also support this distinction by showing that p53-deficient cells are not transformed when cultured in the presence of EGF, whereas they are transformed in the presence of other growth factors.[5] Primary GBMs with TP53 mutations may therefore not be expected to acquire EGFR gene amplification, if activation of the EGF-EGFR system does not produce a growth advantage in such cells.

The genetic pathway involving TP53 mutations often involves progression from a lower grade astrocytic lesion, so-called secondary GBM.[46–48] On the other hand, those GBM with EGFR amplification may arise either *de novo* or rapidly from a preexisting tumor, without a clinically evident, preceding lower-grade astrocytoma.[46,47] Interestingly, younger age at initial diagnosis has been an important prognostic parameter among patients with GBM, with younger patients faring better than older patients. In turn, those GBMs with loss of chromosome 17p occur in patients younger than those characterized by EGFR gene amplification.[49,50] The predominance of tumors with 17p loss in a younger population of astrocytoma patients may therefore reflect the age-based difference in prognosis. The data suggest that genetic analysis may begin to explain the clinical observations concerning age differences in astrocytic tumors. However, convincing differences in prognosis have not been found in a variety of retrospective studies of either TP53 or EGFR alterations in GBM. Nonetheless, because effective therapies do not exist for GBM, possible clinical differences may be obscured by the universally grim prognosis of these tumors (see Oligodendrogliomas and Oligoastrocytomas, later in this chapter).

OTHER GLIOMAS

OTHER ASTROCYTOMAS

Pilocytic astrocytoma is the most common astrocytic tumor of childhood and differs clinically and histopathologically from the diffuse, fibrillary astrocytoma that affects adults. Pilocytic astrocytomas do not have the same genomic alterations as diffuse, fibrillary astrocytomas. Because pilocytic astrocytomas frequently affect patients with neurofibromatosis type 1 (NF1), it would not be surprising if the NF1 gene on chromosome 17q were altered in pilocytic astrocytomas; in fact, allelic loss occurs on chromosome 17q in one-fourth of cases.[51] Unfortunately, detailed mutational analysis of the NF1 gene in pilocytic tumors has not yet been performed, because of the large size of the gene.

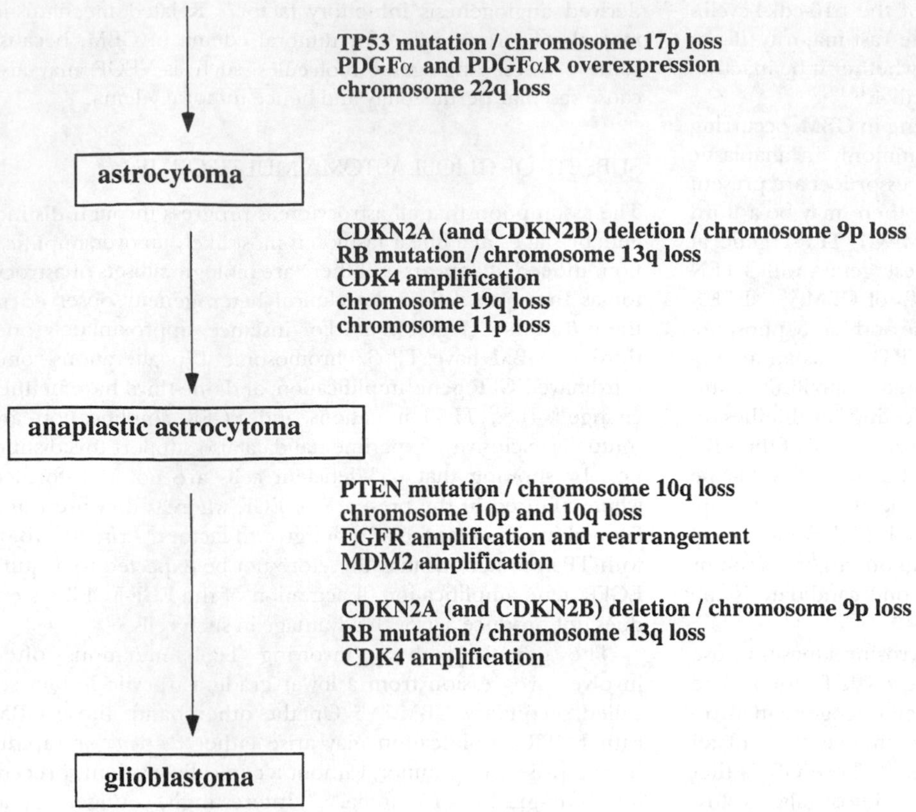

FIGURE 43.1-1. Molecular alterations characteristic of different stages of astrocytoma progression. EGFR, epidermal growth factor receptor; PDGFα(R), platelet-derived growth factor-α (receptor)

Other pediatric astrocytic tumors are histologically similar to the astrocytomas, anaplastic astrocytomas, and GBMs that occur in adults. Some of these are associated with similar genetic alterations, such as TP53 mutations. For instance, brain stem gliomas have frequent TP53 gene and chromosome 17p alterations without EGFR gene amplification,[52] as do those diffuse cerebral astrocytic tumors that occur in children older than 4 years of age.[53] Desmoplastic cerebral astrocytoma of infancy and desmoplastic infantile ganglioglioma are large, superficial, usually cystic, benign astrocytomas that affect children in the first year or two of life. Allelic loss of chromosomes 10 or 17 have not been detected in these lesions.[54] In adult gangliogliomas, another benign form of astrocytic glioma, EGFR gene amplification or allelic loss on chromosomes 10, 13q, 17p, 19q, and 22q has not been detected (A. von Deimling and D. N. Louis, unpublished data).

Pleomorphic xanthoastrocytoma (PXA) is a superficial, low-grade astrocytic tumor that predominantly affects young adults. While these tumors have a bizarre histologic appearance, they are typically slow-growing tumors that may be amenable to surgical cure. Some PXAs, however, may recur as GBM. Nonetheless, the genetic events that underlie PXA formation and progression differ from those involved in diffuse astrocytoma tumorigenesis.[55] PXAs may have TP53 mutations, but the few documented mutations have been somewhat different from those usually found in diffuse, fibrillary astrocytomas.[55] EGFR gene amplification does not occur in PXAs, but GBMs that arise from PXAs may display EGFR gene amplification. On the other hand, allelic losses of chromosomes 9, 10, and 19q are not observed in PXA.

Subependymal giant cell astrocytomas (SEGA) are periventricular, low-grade astrocytic tumors that are usually associated with tuberous sclerosis (TS) and are histologically identical to the so-called candle-gutterings that line the ventricles of TS patients. Similar to the other tumorous lesions in TS, these are slowly growing and may be more akin to hamartomas than true neoplasms. The association of SEGA with TS leads to the prediction that the TS genes, TSC1 on chromosome 9q and TSC2 on chromosome 16p (see Neurologic Tumor Syndromes, later in this chapter), are involved in SEGA formation. Loss of heterozygosity studies have shown allelic loss of chromosome 9q and 16p loci in some SEGAs, particularly of the TSC2 locus on 16p, suggesting that the TS genes act as tumor suppressors.[56–58]

OLIGODENDROGLIOMAS AND OLIGOASTROCYTOMAS

Oligodendrogliomas and oligoastrocytomas (mixed gliomas) are diffuse, usually cerebral, tumors that are clinically and biologically most closely related to the diffuse, fibrillary astrocytomas. The tumors, however, are less common than astrocytomas and have generally better prognoses than the diffuse astrocytomas; patients with WHO grade II oligodendrogliomas, for instance, may have mean survival times of 10 years. In addition, oligodendroglial tumors appear to be differentially chemosensitive,[59] when compared with the diffuse astrocytomas.

Allelic losses in oligodendrogliomas and oligoastrocytomas occur preferentially on chromosomes 1p and 19q, affecting 40% to 80% of these tumor types.[23,60,61] Because of the frequent loss of these loci in low-grade as well as anaplastic oligodendrogliomas and oligoastrocytomas, the 1p and 19q tumor suppressors are probably important early in oligodendroglial tumorigenesis. Mapping of the chromosome 19q locus has demonstrated that the gene resides in the same vicinity as the astrocytoma gene and

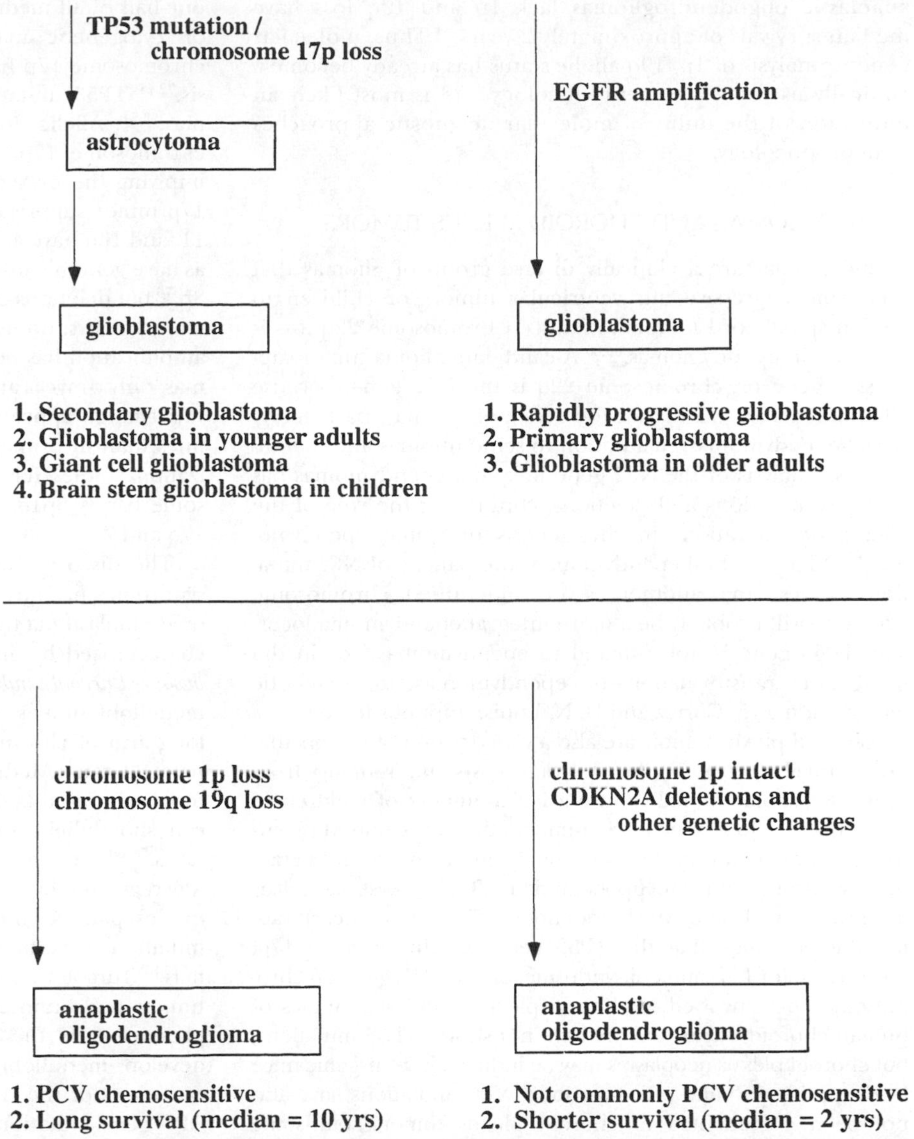

FIGURE 43.1-2. Molecular genetic subsets of glioblastoma (top) and anaplastic oligodendroglioma (bottom) (see text for details). PCV, procarbazine, CCNU, and vincristine

is likely the same gene.[25,62] Similar mapping of chromosome 1p has implicated the telomeric region of 1p.[61,62] Interestingly, chromosome 1p and 19q losses are closely associated; oligodendroglial tumors with 1p loss typically also have loss of 19q, suggesting that these two putative tumor suppressor genes may be involved in biologically distinct pathways.[60,61] In fact, microdissection of the oligodendroglial and astrocytic components in oligoastrocytomas has shown that, despite the histologic differences, the molecular changes are identical in these two components.[61] Oligoastrocytomas may also suffer allelic losses of chromosome 17p,[60] although these losses are not often associated with TP53 mutations,[60,63] perhaps implying a second chromosome 17p glioma gene. Oncogene amplification has only rarely been noted in oligodendroglial tumors.[34,60]

Oligodendrogliomas and oligoastrocytomas may progress, either to WHO grade III anaplastic oligodendroglioma or anaplastic oligoastrocytoma, and sometimes to higher-grade tumors with histologic features similar to GBM (Fig. 43.1-2). Anaplastic oligodendrogliomas and oligoastrocytomas may display allelic losses of chromosomes 9p involving the CDKN2A gene and chromosome 10.[60,64] Thus, allelic loss of chromosome 10 may be a common finding in high-grade malignant gliomas, whether they are astrocytic or oligodendroglial in original lineage.[28]

Anaplastic oligodendrogliomas have proven to be the first brain tumor for which molecular genetic analysis has had practical clinical ramifications: Anaplastic oligodendrogliomas that have allelic losses of chromosomes 1p and 19q follow different clinical courses from those tumors that do not have these genetic changes. Anaplastic oligodendrogliomas that have 1p and 19q loss are essentially always sensitive to procarbazine, lomustine, and vincristine chemotherapy, with nearly 50% of such tumors demonstrating complete neuroradiologic responses; correspondingly, patients whose tumors have 1p and 19q loss have median survivals of approximately 10 years.[64] On the other hand, anaplastic oligodendrogliomas that lack 1p and 19q loss are only chemosensitive approximately 25% of the time and only rarely have complete neuroradiologic responses; as a result, patients whose anaplastic oligodendrogliomas lack 1p and 19q loss have median survivals of approximately 2 years.[64] Thus, molecular genetic analysis of 1p/19q allelic status has already become a clinically useful test in neurooncology and is most likely an indication of the utility of molecular diagnostic approaches in neurooncology.

EPENDYMOMAS AND CHOROID PLEXUS TUMORS

Ependymomas are a clinically diverse group of gliomas that vary from aggressive intraventricular tumors of children to benign spinal cord tumors in adults. Chromosome 22q loss is common in ependymomas.[65,66] A candidate glioma tumor suppressor gene on chromosome 22q is the NF2 gene, because NF2 patients have a higher incidence of gliomas, particularly spinal ependymomas, in addition to schwannomas and meningiomas. Analysis of the NF2 gene in spinal ependymomas has revealed mutations and deletions, confirming the role of the NF2 gene alterations in the genesis of spinal ependymomas.[67,68] For cerebral ependymomas, the paucity of NF2 mutations suggests that another, as yet unidentified, chromosome 22q gene will probably be a more integral ependymoma locus. The TP53 gene is not mutated in ependymomas[63] or in the malignant transformation of ependymomas to anaplastic ependymoma (S. Cortez and D. N. Louis, unpublished data).

Choroid plexus tumors are also a varied group of tumors that preferentially occur in the ventricular system, ranging from aggressive supratentorial intraventricular tumors of children to benign cerebellopontine angle tumors of adults. Choroid plexus tumors have been reported occasionally in patients with Li-Fraumeni syndrome and von Hippel-Lindau (VHL) disease (as well as in Aicardi's syndrome, which does not predispose to cancer), raising the possibility that the TP53 gene on chromosome 17p, responsible for Li-Fraumeni syndrome, or the VHL gene on chromosome 3p is involved in choroid plexus neoplasia. Studies of human choroid plexus tumors have not shown TP53 mutations, but choroid plexus neoplasms may be induced in transgenic mice by disrupting p53 and pRB function.[69] VHL mutations have also not been documented in choroid plexus tumors, but some reported choroid plexus tumors in VHL patients may instead reflect papillary tumors of the middle ear (endolymphatic sac tumors), which occur in higher frequency in VHL patients and which histologically resemble choroid plexus neoplasms.

Oncogenic viruses may cause human cancer, particularly those viruses whose products interfere with tumor suppressor gene functions, such as the human papillomaviruses implicated in cervical carcinoma. One study has identified sequences similar to SV40 virus, an oncogenic virus that has the ability to inactivate both the RB and p53 proteins in human ependymomas and choroid plexus papillomas.[70] This observation raised considerable excitement since SV40 has been implicated as an oncogenic factor in transgenic models of choroid plexus neoplasia.[69] However, SV40-like sequences have not been found in other choroid plexus papillomas or ependymomas and the role of oncogenic viruses in these tumors remains undefined.

MEDULLOBLASTOMAS

Medulloblastomas are highly malignant, primitive tumors that arise in the posterior fossa, primarily in children. One-third to one-half of all medulloblastomas have an isochromosome 17q on cytogenetic analysis,[71] and corresponding allelic loss of chromosome 17p has been noted on molecular genetic analysis.[72,73] TP53 mutations, however, are rare in medulloblastomas.[63,74] Allelic losses occur preferentially at regions of chromosome 17p that are telomeric to the TP53 locus,[73,75] implying the presence of a second, more distal chromosome 17p tumor suppressor gene. Allelic losses of chromosome 6q, 11, and 16q have also been noted frequently in these tumors,[72] as have genomic losses on chromosomes 10q, 11, 16q, 17p, and 8p,[76] but deletions of the CDKN2A gene, which are common in many tumors, do not occur in medulloblastomas.[77] Oncogene amplification has not been found frequently in medulloblastomas; only c-myc is amplified in significant numbers of cases and this change appears more common in medulloblastoma cell lines than in primary tumors.[71] Comparative genomic hybridization studies have demonstrated amplification of chromosome bands 5p15.3 and 11q22.3 and gains of chromosomes 17q and 7.[76]

The discovery of genes underlying two hereditary tumor syndromes has directed attention to two pathways involved in medulloblastoma tumorigenesis. Gorlin syndrome, a condition characterized by multiple basal cell carcinomas (also termed *basal cell nevoid syndrome*), bone cysts, dysmorphic features, and medulloblastomas arises from defects in the PTCH gene on the long arm of chromosome 9, a homologue of the Drosophila patched gene. Medulloblastomas, particularly the nodular desmoplastic variants that are characteristic of Gorlin syndrome, can show allelic loss of chromosome 9q and PTCH mutations.[78–80] The protein encoded by PTCH functions in the pathway regulated by the Sonic hedgehog protein; other molecules in this pathway include smoothened, and rare smoothened mutations have been documented in sporadic medulloblastomas.[81] Turcot syndrome, a condition characterized by colonic tumors and brain tumors, is also linked to medulloblastoma; patients with the adenomatous polyposis phenotype may develop medulloblastomas, and these patients often have mutations of the APC gene on chromosome 5q.[82] Curiously, APC gene mutations and loss of chromosome 5q are rare in sporadic medulloblastomas.[83] The APC protein operates in a molecular pathway that includes the β-catenin protein, and rare mutations of β-catenin have now been noted in sporadic medulloblastomas.[84] It is likely that other components of these two pathways will also be implicated in medulloblastoma tumorigenesis.

The question of whether molecular analyses can provide ancillary information for the management of medulloblastoma patients remains open. Some papers have suggested that patients whose tumors have loss of chromosome 17p may follow a more aggressive course,[85] but this has not been a universal finding. Others have provided intriguing evidence that the level of expression of the trkC receptor may relate to prognosis, with those tumors showing high trkC expression following a more favorable course.[86]

MENINGIOMAS

Meningiomas are common intracranial tumors that arise in the meninges and compress the underlying brain. Meningiomas are usually benign, but some atypical meningiomas may recur locally, and some meningiomas are frankly malignant. Monosomy 22 is common in meningiomas, with the NF2 gene on chromosome 22q frequently mutated in meningiomas, clearly implicating it in meningothelial tumorigenesis.[87–89] In sporadic meningiomas, both chromosome 22q allelic loss and NF2 gene mutations are more common in fibroblastic and transitional subtypes than in meningothelial forms.[88] As in schwannomas (see Peripheral Nerve Tumors, later in this chapter), NF2 gene alterations result predominantly in immediate truncation, splicing abnormalities, or altered reading frames, producing grossly truncated proteins.

Approximately 40% of meningiomas have neither NF2 gene mutations nor allelic loss of chromosome 22q. For these tumors, it is likely that a second meningioma tumor suppressor gene is involved. This putative second gene is probably not on chromosome 22q, since NF2 gene mutations in meningiomas correlate fairly closely with chromosome 22q loss. Nonetheless, a few meningiomas have been described with loss of portions of chromosome 22q that do not include the NF2 gene, suggesting the possibility of a second meningioma locus on chromosome 22.[90] Furthermore, a family with multiple meningiomas but without vestibular schwannomas does not show linkage to the NF2 locus on chromosome 22q, suggesting yet another meningioma predisposition gene.[91] One study has suggested that alternative meningioma genes may reside on chromosomes 1p and 3p.[92] Allelic losses in meningiomas have been noted on a variety of other chromosomes, including 1p, 3p, 5p, 5q, 11, 13, and 17p.[93,94]

Atypical and malignant meningiomas are not as common as benign meningiomas. Atypical meningiomas often show allelic losses of chromosomal arms 1p, 6q, 9q, 10q, 14q, 17p, and 18q, suggesting that progression-associated genes may lie at these loci.[94–96] More frequent losses of chromosomes 6q, 9p, 10, and 14q also occur in anaplastic meningiomas.[94] Chromosomal gains have also been noted in higher-grade meningiomas, with gains of chromosomes 20q, 12q, 15q, 1q, 9q, and 17q most commonly observed.[94] Chromosome 10 loss, in particular, has been associated with those meningiomas with morphologic features of malignancy, rather than those meningiomas that are designated as malignant on the basis of brain invasion alone.[96] Interestingly, brain invasion used to be considered a histologic indicator of malignancy in meningiomas; molecular genetic inquires have, however, shown that histologically benign meningiomas that invade the brain do not have the molecular hallmarks of higher-grade meningiomas.[94,96] These observations provide another example of how molecular genetic investigations have clarified grading issues in neurooncology.

PERIPHERAL NERVE TUMORS

Schwannomas are benign tumors that arise on peripheral nerves. Schwannomas may arise on cranial nerves, particularly the vestibular portion of the eighth cranial nerve (vestibular schwannomas, acoustic neuromas) where they present as cerebellopontine angle masses. NF2 patients are defined by the presence of bilateral vestibular schwannomas,[97] although unilateral vestibular schwannomas are common in the general population as well. Therefore, like meningiomas, schwannomas occur frequently in NF2 patients, have frequent loss of chromosome 22q, and harbor NF2 gene mutations in at least 50% of cases, in vestibular tumors as well as schwannomas from other sites.[97] The majority of the somatic changes are small deletions or insertions that create either frameshifts and premature stop codons or altered splicing. Inactivating mutations are relatively evenly distributed across the first 15 exons with no outstanding hot spots. Furthermore, loss of the NF2 gene–encoded merlin protein occurs in all schwannomas, consistent with an integral and universal role for NF2 gene inactivation in schwannoma formation.[98] Thus, inactivation of NF2 is a common feature underlying both inherited and sporadic forms of schwannoma.

Neurofibromas are also benign tumors of peripheral nerve that most often arise on distal, superficial nerves. Multiple neurofibromas are associated with NF1, suggesting that the NF1 gene on chromosome 17q is involved in the genesis of these benign nerve sheath lesions. Unfortunately, the large size of the NF1 gene has precluded extensive mutation analysis in these lesions. Neurofibromas, particularly the plexiform variants associated with NF1, have the potential for malignant progression to malignant peripheral nerve sheath tumors, a transition that is associated with inactivation of the NF1, TP53, and CDKN2A genes.[99–101]

MISCELLANEOUS TUMORS

HEMANGIOBLASTOMAS

Hemangioblastomas are tumors of uncertain origin that are composed of endothelial cells, pericytes, and so-called stromal cells. These benign tumors most frequently occur in the cerebellum and spinal cord of young adults. Multiple hemangioblastomas are characteristic of VHL, an inherited tumor syndrome in which patients have a tendency to develop tumors, particularly hemangioblastomas, retinal angiomas, renal cell carcinomas, and pheochromocytomas.[102] Allelic loss occurs in hemangioblastomas in the region of the VHL gene on chromosome 3p[103] and the VHL gene is mutated in sporadic hemangioblastomas.[104] These observations suggest that the VHL gene acts as a classical tumor suppressor and is involved in both sporadic hemangioblastomas and familial tumors. The mechanism of action of the VHL protein appears complex, with evidence suggesting that it may stabilize mRNA of angiogenic compounds such as VEGF,[105] as well as extracellular matrix components such as fibronectin.[106] These actions at least begin to explain the highly vascular nature of hemangioblastomas.

HEMANGIOPERICYTOMAS

Hemangiopericytomas (HPCs) are dural tumors that may display locally aggressive behavior and may metastasize. The histogenesis of dural-based HPC has long been debated, with some authors classifying it as a distinct entity and others classifying it as a subtype of meningioma. Molecular genetic studies have greatly clarified this issue. Meningiomas contain frequent mutations of the NF2 gene, whereas HPCs do not, suggesting that HPC is genetically distinct from meningioma.[107] In addition, homozygous deletions of the CDKN2A gene are common in HPCs but not in meningiomas and suggest that alterations of the p16-mediated cell-cycle regulatory pathway may underlie the malignant potential of some HPCs.[108] Rearrangements of chromosome 12q13 are common in peripherally located, soft tissue HPCs and have been reported in meningeal HPCs, implying that an oncogene or tumor suppressor gene at this locus is important in HPC formation. A number of oncogenes reside in this region, including MDM2, CDK4, and CHOP/GADD153.

NEUROLOGIC TUMOR SYNDROMES

Hereditary neurologic tumor syndromes, in which patients are at risk for developing multiple nervous system tumors, have provided important clues to the genetic basis of brain tumors. These tumor syndromes provide unique insights into tumor suppressor genes. For instance, the hereditary RB syndrome, which provided much of the impetus for current tumor suppressor gene research, results from a mutation in both RB tumor suppressor alleles.[109] In the case of familial RB, the patient inherits one mutant, inactive copy of the RB gene and thus carries a germline mutation in every cell,[110] which is unveiled when the second copy of the gene is inactivated, either by mutation or by loss of a portion of chromosome 13q. A patient with sporadic RBs does not carry the germline mutation and must acquire both inactivating hits in the same cell during his or her life. Therefore, a familial RB patient, in which every cell contains a mutation, is much more likely to develop a second RB than a sporadic RB patient. This same paradigm appears to hold true for most, but not all,[111] of the hereditary brain tumor syndromes.

Neurologic tumor syndromes include the so-called neurocutaneous syndromes, such as NF1, NF2, TS, and VHL, and other tumor conditions such as Li-Fraumeni, Turcot, Gorlin, and Cowden syndromes.[97,102,111–113] Each syndrome is accompanied by a characteristic panoply of tumors, both neurologic and non-neurologic. A catalogue of only the gliomas would feature optic nerve gliomas and other astrocytomas in NF1; ependymomas and astrocytomas in NF2; SEGAs in TS; and various malignant gliomas in Li-Fraumeni syndrome, Turcot syndrome, and the hereditary glioma pedigrees. Linkage studies have provided powerful means for tracking down the genes associated with these tumor syndromes and have assigned the NF1 gene to chromosome 17q; the NF2 gene to chromosome 22q; the TS genes to chromosome 9q and 16p; and Turcot syndrome genes to chromosome 5q (APC gene) and to the DNA mismatch repair genes on various chromosomes. The NF1 gene codes for a guanosine triphosphatase–activating protein termed *neurofibromin.* Neurofibromin interacts with the p21 product of the *ras* oncogene and is most likely important in growth factor-mediated signal transduction. The NF2 gene codes for a protein, termed *merlin,* which most likely functions by facilitating signal transduction from the cell surface via the cytoskeleton. One of the TS genes, TSC2 on chromosome 16p, TSC2 encodes a guanosine triphosphatase activating protein–related protein, tuberin; whereas the TSC1 gene on 9q encodes a protein known as *hamartin* that has no known homology to other proteins. Nonetheless, tuberin and hamartin appear to bind one another and function in a single cellular pathway, consistent with a similar phenotype for patients with either TSC1 or TSC2 gene mutations. For the Li-Fraumeni syndrome, mutational analyses have implicated the TP53 gene on 17p.

SUMMARY

Human brain tumors have molecular alterations that are characteristic of each type of tumor and of most stages of progression. For instance, the formation of low-grade astrocytoma and the subsequent progression to anaplastic astrocytoma and GBM involve alterations of distinct tumor suppressor genes and oncogenes. Furthermore, molecular genetic analysis has been used to distinguish subsets of astrocytomas. For instance, one type of GBM, characterized by TP53 gene mutations, is more common in younger patients and may be associated with slower progression from lower-grade astrocytoma; another type of GBM, characterized by EGFR gene amplification, is more common in older patients and may be associated with more rapid progression or *de novo* growth. In the case of anaplastic oligodendrogliomas, molecular genetic subtyping has already provided practical information for the management of patients, since tumors with chromosome 1p and 19q loss are differentially chemosensitive and more indolent.

For the less common gliomas and for other primary tumors such as medulloblastomas, molecular genetic studies have defined sets of genetic alterations. For meningiomas and schwannomas, the NF2 gene has been clearly implicated, although other genetic alterations must underlie the formation of some meningiomas as well. For some tumors, such as HPC and brain-invasive meningiomas, molecular investigations have clarified classification and grading issues. For those tumors associated with hereditary tumor syndromes, such as the SEGAs in TS and the hemangioblastomas in VHL, the same genes appear responsible for the syndromes when mutated in the germline, and for sporadic tumors when mutated on a somatic basis. At present, however, these molecular data are incomplete. Once the molecular pathways are completely understood, such knowledge will no doubt contribute to the development of more effective therapies for many of these tumors.

REFERENCES

1. Louis DN. A molecular genetic model of astrocytoma histopathology. *Brain Pathol* 1997;7:755.
2. Louis DN. The p53 gene and protein in human brain tumors. *J Neuropathol Exp Neurol* 1994;53:11.
3. Sidransky D, Mikkelsen T, Schwechheimer K, et al. Clonal expansion of p53 mutant cells is associated with brain tumor progression. *Nature* 1992;355:846.
4. Yahanda AM, Bruner JM, Donehower LA, et al. Astrocytes derived from p53-deficient mice provide a multistep in vitro model for development of malignant gliomas. *Mol Cell Biol* 1995;15:4249.
5. Bogler O, Huang H-JS, Cavenee WK. Loss of wild-type p53 bestows a growth advantage on primary cortical astrocytes and facilitates their in vitro transformation. *Cancer Res* 1995;55:2746.
6. van Meyel DJ, Ramsay DA, Casson AG, et al. p53 mutation, expression, and DNA ploidy in evolving gliomas: evidence for two pathways of progression. *J Natl Cancer Inst* 1994;86:1011.
7. Hermanson M, Funa K, Hartman M, et al. Platelet-derived growth factor and its receptors in human glioma tissue: expression of messenger RNA and protein suggests the presence of autocrine and paracrine loops. *Cancer Res* 1992;52:3213.
8. Hermanson M, Funa K, Westermark B, et al. Association of loss of heterozygosity on chromosome 17p with high platelet-derived growth factor a receptor expression in human malignant gliomas. *Cancer Res* 1996;56:164.
9. Pilkington GJ. Tumour cell migration in the central nervous system. *Brain Pathol* 1994;4:157.
10. Cavenee WK, Furnari FB, Nagane M, et al. Diffuse astrocytomas. In: Kleihues P, Cavenee PK, eds. *Pathology and genetics of tumours of the nervous system.* Lyon: International Agency for Research on Cancer, 2000.
11. Ino Y, Silver JS, Blazejewski L, et al. Common regions of deletion on chromosome 22q12.3-13.1 and 22q13.2 in human astrocytomas appear related to malignancy grade. *J Neuropathol Exp Neurol* 1999;58:881.
12. Schrock E, Blume C, Meffert MC, et al. Recurrent gain of chromosome arm 7q in low-grade astrocytic tumors studied by comparative genomic hybridization. *Genes Chromosomes Cancer* 1996;15:199.
13. Ueki K, Ono Y, Henson JW, et al. CDKN2/p16 or RB alterations occur in the majority of glioblastomas and are inversely correlated. *Cancer Res* 1996;56:150.
14. Burns KL, Ueki K, Jhung SL, et al. Molecular genetic correlates of p16, cdk4 and pRb immunohistochemistry in glioblastomas. *J Neuropathol Exp Neurol* 1998;57:122.

15. Nishikawa R, Furnari F, Lin H, et al. Loss of $p16^{INK4}$ expression is frequent in high grade gliomas. *Cancer Res* 1995;55:1941.
16. Merlo A, Herman JG, Mao L, et al. 5'CpG island methylation is associated with transcriptional silencing of the tumor suppressor p16/CDKN2/MTS1. *Nature Med* 1995;1:686.
17. Arap W, Nishikawa R, Furnari FB, et al. Replacement of the p16/CDKN2 gene suppresses human glioma cell growth. *Cancer Res* 1995;55:1351.
18. Henson JW, Schnitker BL, Correa KM, et al. The retinoblastoma gene is involved in malignant progression of astrocytomas. *Ann Neurol* 1994;36:714.
19. Schmidt EE, Ichimura K, Reifenberger G, et al. CDKN2 (p16/MTS1) gene deletion or CDK4 amplification occurs in the majority of glioblastomas. *Cancer Res* 1994;54:6321.
20. Reifenberger G, Reifenberger J, Ichimura K, et al. Amplification of multiple genes from chromosomal region 12q13-14 in human malignant gliomas: preliminary mapping of the amplicons shows preferential involvement of CDK4, SAS, and MDM2. *Cancer Res* 1994;54:4299.
21. He J, Allen JR, Collins VP, et al. CDK4 amplification is an alternative mechanism to p16 gene homozygous deletion in glioma cell lines. *Cancer Res* 1994;54:5804.
22. Costello JF, Plass C, Arap W, et al. Cyclin-dependent kinase 6 (CDK6) amplification in human gliomas identified using two-dimensional separation of genomic DNA. *Cancer Res* 1997;57:1250.
23. von Deimling A, Louis DN, von Ammon K, et al. Evidence for a tumor suppressor gene on chromosome 19q associated with human astrocytomas, oligodendrogliomas and mixed gliomas. *Cancer Res* 1992;52:4277.
24. Seizinger BR, Klinger HP, Junien C, et al. Report of the committee on chromosome and gene loss in human neoplasia. *Cytogenet Cell Genet* 1991;58:1080.
25. Rubio M-P, Correa KM, Ueki K, et al. The putative glioma tumor suppressor gene on chromosome 19q maps between APOC2 and HRC. *Cancer Res* 1994;54:4760.
26. Rosenberg JE, Lisle DK, Burwick JA, et al. Refined deletion mapping of the chromosome 19q glioma tumor suppressor gene to the D19S412-STD interval. *Oncogene* 1996;13:2483.
27. von Deimling A, Louis DN, von Ammon K, et al. Association of epidermal growth factor receptor gene amplification with loss of chromosome 10 in human glioblastoma multiforme. *J Neurosurg* 1992;77:295.
28. James CD, Carlblom E, Dumanski JP, et al. Clonal genomic alterations in glioma malignancy stages. *Cancer Res* 1988;48:5546.
29. Dürr E-M, Rollbrocker B, Hayashi Y, et al. PTEN mutations in gliomas and glioneuronal gliomas. *Oncogene* 1998;16:2259.
30. Li J, Yen C, Liaw D, et al. PTEN, a putative protein tyrosine phosphatase gene mutated in human brain, breast and prostate cancer. *Science* 1997;275:1943.
31. Steck PA, Pershouse MA, Jasser SA, et al. Identification of a candidate tumour suppressor gene, MMAC1, at chromosome 10q23.3 that is mutated in multiple advanced cancers. *Nature Genet* 1997;15:356.
32. Furnari FB, Lin H, Huang HS, et al. Growth suppression of glioma cells by PTEN requires a functional phosphatase catalytic domain. *Proc Natl Acad Sci U S A* 1997;94:12479.
33. Mollenhauer J, Wiemann S, Scheurlen W, et al. DMBT1, a new member of the SRCR superfamily, on chromosome 10q25.3-26.1 is deleted in malignant brain tumours. *Nature Genet* 1997;17:32.
34. Fuller GN, Bigner SH. Amplified cellular oncogenes in neoplasms of the human central nervous system. *Mutat Res* 1992;276:299.
35. Ekstrand AJ, James CD, Cavenee WK, et al. Genes for epidermal growth factor receptor, transforming growth factor a, and epidermal growth factor and their expression in human gliomas in vivo. *Cancer Res* 1991;51:2164.
36. Hayashi Y, Ueki K, Waha A, et al. Association of EGFR gene amplification and CDKN2 (p16/MTS1) gene deletion in glioblastoma multiforme. *Brain Pathol* 1997;7:871.
37. Wong AJ, Bigner SH, Bigner DD, et al. Increased expression of the epidermal growth factor receptor gene in malignant gliomas is invariably associated with gene amplification. *Proc Natl Acad Sci U S A* 1987;84:6899.
38. Nishikawa R, Ji XD, Harmon RC, et al. A mutant epidermal growth factor receptor common in human glioma confers enhanced tumorigenicity. *Proc Natl Acad Sci U S A* 1994;91:7727.
39. Nagane M, Coufal F, Lin H, et al. A common mutant epidermal growth factor receptor confers enhanced tumorigenicity on human glioblastoma cells by increasing proliferation and reducing apoptosis. *Cancer Res* 1996;56:5079.
40. Plate KH, Breier G, Risau W. Molecular mechanisms of developmental and tumor angiogenesis. *Brain Pathol* 1994;4:207.
41. Plate KH, Breier G, Weich HA, et al. Vascular endothelial growth factor is a potential tumour angiogenesis factor in human gliomas in vivo. *Nature* 1992;359:845.
42. Cheng SY, Huang HJ, Nagane M, et al. Suppression of glioblastoma angiogenicity and tumorigenicity by inhibition of endogenous expression of vascular endothelial growth factor. *Proc Natl Acad Sci U S A* 1996;93:8502.
43. Wang D, Huang HJ, Kazlauskas A, et al. Induction of vascular endothelial growth factor expression in endothelial cells by platelet-derived growth factor through the activation of phosphatidylinositol 3-kinase. *Cancer Res* 1999;59:1464.
44. Van Meir EG, Polverini PJ, Chazin VR, et al. Release of an inhibitor of angiogenesis upon induction of wild type p53 expression in glioblastoma cells. *Nature Genet* 1994;8:171.
45. Louis DN, Gusella JF. A tiger behind many doors: multiple genetic pathways to malignant glioma. *Trends Genet* 1995;11:412.
46. von Deimling A, von Ammon K, Schoenfeld D, et al. Subsets of glioblastoma multiforme defined by molecular genetic analysis. *Brain Pathol* 1993;3:19.
47. Watanabe K, Tachibana O, Sato K, et al. Overexpression of the EGF receptor and p53 mutations are mutually exclusive in the evolution of primary and secondary glioblastomas. *Brain Pathol* 1996;6:217.
48. Reifenberger J, Ring GU, Gies U, et al. Analysis of p53 mutation and epidermal growth factor receptor amplification in recurrent gliomas with malignant progression. *J Neuropathol Exp Neurol* 1996;55:822.
49. Louis DN, von Deimling A, Chung RY, et al. Comparative study of p53 gene and protein alterations in human astrocytomas. *J Neuropathol Exp Neurol* 1993;52:31.
50. Rasheed BKA, McLendon RE, Herndon JE, et al. Alterations of the TP53 gene in human gliomas. *Cancer Res* 1994;54:1324.
51. von Deimling A, Louis DN, Menon AG, et al. Deletions on the long arm of chromosome 17 in pilocytic astrocytoma. *Acta Neuropathol* 1993;86:81.
52. Louis DN, Rubio M-P, Correa K, et al. Molecular genetics of pediatric brain stem gliomas. Application of PCR techniques to small and archival brain tumor specimens. *J Neuropathol Exp Neurol* 1993;52:507.
53. Pollack IF, Hamilton RL, Finkelstein SD, et al. The relationship between TP53 mutations and overexpression of p53 and prognosis in malignant gliomas of childhood. *Cancer Res* 1997;57:304.
54. Louis DN, von Deimling A, Dickersin G, et al. Desmoplastic cerebral astrocytoma of infancy: a histopathological, immunohistochemical, ultrastructural and molecular genetic study. *Hum Pathol* 1992;23:1402.
55. Paulus W, Lisle DK, Tonn JC, et al. Molecular genetic alterations in pleomorphic xanthoastrocytoma. *Acta Neuropathol* 1996;91:293.
56. Green AJ, Smith M, Yates JRW. Loss of heterozygosity on chromosome 16p13.3 in hamartomas from tuberous sclerosis patients. *Nature Genet* 1994;6:193.
57. Green AJ, Johnson PH, Yates JR. The tuberous sclerosis gene on chromosome 9q34 acts as a growth suppressor. *Hum Mol Genet* 1994;3:1833.
58. Henske EP, Scheithauer BW, Short MP, et al. Allelic loss is frequent in tuberous sclerosis kidney lesions but rare in brain lesions. *Am J Hum Genet* 1996;59:400.
59. Cairncross JG, Macdonald DR, Ramsay DA. Aggressive oligodendroglioma: a chemosensitive tumor. *Neurosurgery* 1992;31:78.
60. Reifenberger J, Reifenberger G, Liu L, et al. Molecular genetic analysis of oligodendroglial tumors shows preferential allelic deletions on 19q and 1p. *Am J Pathol* 1994;145:1175.
61. Kraus JA, Koopman J, Kaskel P, et al. Shared allelic losses on chromosomes 1p and 19q suggest a common origin of oligodendroglioma and oligoastrocytoma. *J Neuropathol Exp Neurol* 1995;54:91.
62. Smith JS, Alderete B, Minn Y, et al. Localization of common deletion regions on 1p and 19q in human gliomas and their association with histological subtype. *Oncogene* 1999;18:4144.
63. Ohgaki H, Eibl RH, Wiestler OD, et al. p53 mutations in nonastrocytic human brain tumors. *Cancer Res* 1991;51:6202.
64. Cairncross JG, Ueki K, Zlatescu MC, et al. Specific chromosomal losses predict chemotherapeutic response and survival in patients with anaplastic oligodendrogliomas. *J Natl Cancer Inst* 1998;90:1473.
65. Ransom DT, Ritland SR, Kimmel PJ, et al. Cytogenetic and loss of heterozygosity studies in ependymomas, pilocytic astrocytomas, and oligodendrogliomas. *Genes Chromosomes Cancer* 1992;5:348.
66. James CD, He J, Carlbom E, et al. Loss of genetic information in central nervous system tumors common to children and young adults. *Genes Chromosomes Cancer* 1990;2:94.
67. Rubio M-P, Correa KM, Ramesh V, et al. Analysis of the neurofibromatosis 2 (NF2) gene in human ependymomas and astrocytomas. *Cancer Res* 1994;54:45.
68. Birch BD, Johnson JP, Parsa A, et al. Frequent type 2 neurofibromatosis gene transcript mutations in sporadic intramedullary spinal cord ependymomas. *Neurosurgery* 1996;39:135.
69. Van Dyke TA. Tumors of the choroid plexus. In: Levine AJ, Schmidek HH, eds. *Molecular genetics of nervous system tumors.* New York: Wiley-Liss, 1993:287.
70. Bergsagel DJ, Finegold MJ, Butel JS, et al. DNA sequences similar to those of simian virus 40 in ependymomas and choroid plexus tumors of childhood. *N Engl J Med* 1992;326:988.
71. Bigner SH, Vogelstein B. Cytogenetics and molecular genetics of malignant gliomas and medulloblastoma. *Brain Pathol* 1990;1:12.
72. Thomas GA, Raffel C. Loss of heterozygosity on 6q, 16q, and 17p in human central nervous system primitive neuroectodermal tumors. *Cancer Res* 1991;51:639.
73. Cogen PH, Daneshvar L, Metzger AK, et al. Deletion mapping of the medulloblastoma locus on chromosome 17p. *Genomics* 1990;8:279.
74. Saylors RL, Sidransky D, Friedman HS, et al. Infrequent p53 gene mutations in medulloblastomas. *Cancer Res* 1991;51:4721.
75. Biegel JA, Burk CD, Barr FG, et al. Evidence for a 17p tumor related locus distinct from p53 in pediatric primitive neuroectodermal tumors. *Cancer Res* 1992;52:3391.
76. Reardon DA, Michalkiewicz E, Boyett JM, et al. Extensive genomic abnormalities in childhood medulloblastoma by comparative genomic hybridization. *Cancer Res* 1997;57:4042.
77. Raffel C, Ueki K, Harsh GR, et al. The multiple tumor suppressor 1/cyclin dependent kinase inhibitor 2 gene (MTS1/CDKN2) in human central nervous system primitive neuroectodermal tumor. *Neurosurgery* 1995;36:971.
78. Schofield D, West DC, Anthony DC, et al. Correlation of loss of heterozygosity at chromosome 9q with histologic subtype in medulloblastomas. *Am J Pathol* 1995;146:472.
79. Raffel C, Jenkins RB, Frederick L, et al. Sporadic medulloblastomas contain PTCH mutations. *Cancer Res* 1997;57:842.
80. Pietsch T, Waha A, Koch A, et al. Medulloblastomas of the desmoplastic variant carry mutations of the human homologue of *Drosophila* patched. *Cancer Res* 1997;57:2085.
81. Reifenberger J, Wolter M, Weber RG, et al. Missense mutations in SMOH in sporadic basal cell carcinomas of the skin and primitive neuroectodermal tumors of the central nervous system. *Cancer Res* 1998;58:1798.
82. Hamilton SR, Liu B, Parsons RE, et al. The molecular basis of Turcot's syndrome. *N Engl J Med* 1995;332:839.
83. Yong WH, Raffel C, von Deimling A, et al. Lack of allelic loss at APC in sporadic medulloblastomas [Letter]. *N Engl J Med* 1995;333:524.
84. Zurawel RH, Chiappa SA, Allen C, et al. Sporadic medulloblastomas contain oncogenic β-catenin mutations. *Cancer Res* 1998;58:896.
85. Scheurlen WG, Schwabe GC, Joos S, et al. Molecular analysis of childhood primitive neuroectodermal tumors defines markers associated with poor outcome. *J Clin Oncol* 1998;16:2478.
86. Segal RA, Goumnerova LC, Kwon YK, et al. Co-expression of neurotrophin-3 and trkC

linked to a more favorable prognosis in medulloblastoma. *Proc Natl Acad Sci U S A* 1994;91:12867.
87. Ruttledge MH, Sarrazin J, Rangaratnam S, et al. Evidence for the complete inactivation of the NF2 gene in the majority of sporadic meningiomas. *Nature Genet* 1994;6:180.
88. Wellenreuther R, Kraus JA, Lenartz D, et al. Analysis of the neurofibromatosis 2 gene reveals molecular variants of meningioma. *Am J Pathol* 1995;146:827.
89. Lekanne Deprez RH, Bianchi AB, Groen NA, et al. Frequent NF2 gene transcript mutations in sporadic meningiomas and vestibular schwannomas. *Am J Hum Genet* 1994;54:1022.
90. Ruttledge MH, Xie YG, Han FY, et al. Deletions on chromosome 22 in sporadic meningioma. *Genes Chromosomes Cancer* 1994;10:122.
91. Pulst S-M, Rouleau GA, Marineau C, et al. Familial meningioma is not allelic to neurofibromatosis 2. *Neurology* 1993;43:2096.
92. Carlson KM, Bruder C, Nordenskjold M, et al. 1p and 3p deletions in meningiomas without detectable aberrations of chromosome 22 identified by comparative genomic hybridization. *Genes Chromosomes Cancer* 1997;20:419.
93. Schneider G, Lutz S, Henn W, et al. Search for the putative suppressor genes in meningiomas: significance of chromosome 22. *Hum Genet* 1992;53:579.
94. Weber RG, Bostrom J, Wolter M, et al. Analysis of genomic alterations in benign, atypical, and anaplastic meningiomas: toward a genetic model of meningioma progression. *Proc Natl Acad Sci U S A* 1997;94:14719.
95. Lindblom A, Ruttledge M, Collins VP, et al. Chromosomal deletions in anaplastic meningiomas suggest multiple regions outside chromosome 22 as important in tumor progression. *Int J Cancer* 1994;56:354.
96. Rempel SA, Schwechheimer K, Davis RL, et al. Loss of heterozygosity for loci on chromosome 10 is associated with morphologically malignant meningioma progression. *Cancer Res* 1993;53:2387.
97. Louis DN, Ramesh V, Gusella JF. Neuropathology and molecular genetics of neurofibromatosis 2 and related tumors. *Brain Pathol* 1995;5:163.
98. Stemmer-Rachamimov AO, Xu L, Gonzalez-Agosti C, et al. Universal absence of merlin, but not other ERM family members, in schwannomas. *Am J Pathol* 1997;152:1649.
99. Legius E, Marchuk DA, Collins FS, et al. Somatic deletion of the neurofibromatosis type 1 gene in a neurofibrosarcoma supports a tumor suppressor gene hypothesis. *Nature Genet* 1993;3:122.
100. Menon AG, Anderson KM, Riccardi VM, et al. Chromosome 17p deletions and p53 gene mutations associated with the formation of malignant neurofibrosarcomas in Recklinghausen neurofibromatosis. *Proc Natl Acad Sci U S A* 1990;87:5435.
101. Nielsen GP, Stemmer-Rachamimov AO, Ino Y, et al. Malignant transformation of neurofibromas in neurofibromatosis 1 is associated with CDKN2A/p16 inactivation. *Am J Pathol* 1999;155:1879.
102. Neumann HPH, Lips CJM, Hsia YE, et al. Von Hippel-Lindau syndrome. *Brain Pathol* 1995;5:181.
103. Crossey PA, Foster K, Richards FM, et al. Molecular genetic investigations of the mechanism of tumourigenesis in von Hippel-Lindau disease: analysis of allele loss in VHL tumours. *Hum Genet* 1994;93:53.
104. Kanno H, Kondo K, Ito S, et al. Somatic mutations of the von Hippel-Lindau tumor suppressor gene in sporadic central nervous system hemangioblastomas. *Cancer Res* 1994;54:4845.
105. Gnarra JR, Zhou S, Merrill MJ, et al. Post-transcriptional regulation of vascular endothelial growth factor mRNA by the product of the VHL tumor suppressor gene. *Proc Natl Acad Sci U S A* 1996;93:10589.
106. Ohh M, Yauch RL, Lonergan KM, et al. The von Hippel-Lindau tumor suppressor protein is required for proper assembly of extracellular fibronectin matrix. *Mol Cell* 1998;1:959.
107. Joseph JT, Lisle DK, Jacoby LB, et al. NF2 gene analysis distinguishes hemangiopericytoma from meningioma. *Am J Pathol* 1995;147:1450.
108. Ono Y, Ueki K, Joseph JT, et al. Homozygous deletions of the CDKN2/p16 gene in dural hemangiopericytomas. *Acta Neuropathol* 1996;91:221.
109. Cavenee WK, Dryja TP, Phillips RA, et al. Expression of recessive alleles by chromosomal mechanisms in retinoblastoma. *Nature* 1983;305:779.
110. Cavenee WK, Murphree AL, Shull MM, et al. Prediction of familial predisposition to retinoblastoma. *N Engl J Med* 1986;314:1201.
111. Louis DN, von Deimling A. Hereditary tumor syndromes of the nervous system: overview and rare syndromes. *Brain Pathol* 1995;5:145.
112. Short MP, Richardson EP, Haines JL, et al. Clinical, neuropathological, and genetic aspects of the tuberous sclerosis complex. *Brain Pathol* 1995;5:173.
113. von Deimling A, Krone W, Menon AG. Neurofibromatosis type 1: pathology, clinical features, and molecular genetics. *Brain Pathol* 1995;5:153.

VICTOR A. LEVIN
STEVEN A. LEIBEL
PHILIP H. GUTIN

SECTION 2
Neoplasms of the Central Nervous System

INCIDENCE AND CLASSIFICATION

Available registry data from Surveillance, Epidemiology, and End Results for 1973 to 1990 indicate that the combined incidence of all recorded primary intracranial and spinal axis tumors is between 2 and 19 in 100,000 per year, depending on age.[1] There is an early peak (3.1 in 100,000) between 0 and 4 years, a trough (1.8 in 100,000) between 15 and 24 years, and then a steady rise in incidence that reaches a plateau (17.9 to 18.7 in 100,000) between 65 and 79 years of age. In general, the incidence of primary brain tumors is more common in whites than blacks and the mortality is higher in male than female subjects.

The diversity in primary intracranial and spinal axis tumors partly results from the diversity of phenotypically distinct cells capable of transformation into tumors. Table 43.2-1 shows the hypothetical 15 cell types that can give rise to these tumors. Because of changes in classification and reporting of these tumors, the tumor registry data are not completely accurate. The relative frequency of 15 families of intracranial tumors is given in Table 43.2-2, and the distribution of spinal tumors is shown in Table 43.2-3.[2,3] The most common tumors are those that are derived from glial precursors (astrocytes, ependymocytes, and oligodendrocytes). The existence of histologically mixed astrocytoma-oligodendroglioma and the extremely uncommon astrocytoma-ependymoma implies that astrocytomas, oligodendrogliomas, and ependymomas may arise from common stem or progenitor cells. The facts that these tumors arise in different locales within the cranium and the spinal axis and that various types predominate at different ages suggest that differing molecular and genetic mechanisms may underlie tumorigenesis at different times in the life span.

Central nervous system (CNS) tumors are the most prevalent solid neoplasms of childhood, the second leading cancer-related cause of death in children younger than 15 years of age, and the third leading cancer-related cause of death in adolescents and adults between the ages of 15 and 34 years. However, most intracranial tumors occur in people older than 45 years. Glioblastoma rarely occurs in people younger than 15 years, but dramatically increases after the age of 45. The incidence of most glial tumors, other than glioblastoma multiforme, actually decreases with increasing age. There is some concern that the incidence of glioblastoma multiforme is increasing in the elderly population,[4] although incorrect ascertainment preceding the widespread availability of computed tomography (CT) scans in the late 1970s and magnetic resonance imaging (MRI) in the 1980s may account for some of the presumed increase in incidence.[5,6] A similar age-related increase in prevalence occurs with differentiated or *benign* meningiomas that increase from 0.2% of all primary intracranial tumors in patients younger than 24 years of age to 39% of tumors in patients older than 65 years.

The overall incidence of primary spinal cord tumors is approximately 15% of that of brain tumors. For gliomas, the age-adjusted incidence is 0.11% to 0.14%; for meningiomas,

TABLE 43.2-1. Classification of Primary Intracranial Tumors by Cell of Origin

Normal Cell	*Tumor*
Astrocyte	Astrocytomas, glioblastoma multiforme
Ependymocyte	Ependymoma, ependymoblastoma
Oligodendrocyte	Oligodendroglioma
Arachnoidal fibroblasts	Meningioma
Nerve cell or neuroblast retinoblastoma	Ganglioneuroma, neuroblastoma
External granular cell or neuroblast	Medulloblastoma
Schwann cell	Schwannoma (neurinoma)
Melanocyte	Melanotic carcinoma
Chorioid epithelial cell	Choroid plexus papilloma or carcinoma
Pituitary	Adenoma
Endothelial cell or stromal cell	Hemangioblastoma
Primitive germ cells	Germinoma, pinealoma, teratomas, cholesteatoma
Pineal parenchymal cells	Pinealcytoma
Notochordal remnants	Chordoma

0.08% to 0.28%, depending on sex (female higher than male subjects); and for nerve sheath tumors, 0.07% to 0.13%.[3] As shown in Table 43.2-3, the frequency of specific spinal cord tumors is strikingly different from that of the brain tumors. Gliomas constitute 46% of primary intracranial tumors while only 23% of spinal tumors. Unlike brain gliomas, most spinal

TABLE 43.2-2. Frequency of Primary Intracranial Central Nervous System (CNS) Tumors

Histopathology	*Primary Brain Tumors (%)*	*Gliomas (%)*
Glioblastoma multiforme	21.7	47
Malignant astrocytomas	16.6	36
All oligodendroglioma	3.1	6.7
All ependymomas	2.3	5.1
Low-grade astrocytoma	1.8	3.9
Meningioma and other mesenchymal tumors	26.7	—
Pituitary	9.7	—
Nerve sheath (e.g., schwannoma)	7.3	—
CNS lymphoma	3.5	—
Medulloblastoma and other primitive neuroectodermal tumors	1.7	—
All neuron and neuron/glial tumors	1.0	—
Craniopharyngioma	1.0	—
Germ cell	0.5	—
Choroid plexus	0.3	—
Other tumors	2.7	—

(Data from ref. 1.)

TABLE 43.2-3. Distribution of Primary Spinal Tumors[a]

Histology	*Sloof et al.[2]*	*Preston-Martin[3]*
Schwannoma	29.0	22.0
Meningioma	25.5	42.0
Ependymoma	12.8	15.1
Sarcomas	11.9	—
Astrocytoma	6.5	11.2
Other gliomas	—	1.9
Vascular tumors	6.2	—
Chordomas	4.0	—
Epidermoids	1.4	—
Other	2.7	5.6

[a]Lipoma and subarachnoid seeding from primary intracranial tumor.

cord gliomas are ependymomas with a predilection for the cauda equina. Schwannomas and meningiomas account for approximately 60% of spinal tumors, with schwannomas being slightly more frequent; both types occur most often in adult life. Other less common spinal tumors are the lipomas, dermoids, and hemangioblastomas.

GENETIC, MOLECULAR, ENVIRONMENTAL, VIRAL, AND OTHER FACTORS ASSOCIATED WITH CENTRAL NERVOUS SYSTEM NEOPLASIA

In Chapter 43.1, the contribution of genetics and molecular biology to the understanding of CNS tumorigenesis is covered in detail. Less important associations of CNS neoplasia are those associated with viruses, chemicals, and physical forces.

The epidemiology of primary CNS tumors has provided hints but few definitive observations with respect to environmental or occupational causes. Although brain tumors can be experimentally induced in a high proportion of rodents by the use of certain chemicals, the association of chemical exposure and brain tumors is limited to a few occupations. A higher than expected increase in the incidence of brain tumors has been observed as a result of purported exposure to pesticides, herbicides, and fertilizers,[7] various petrochemical industries,[8] and health professions.[9] Whether these statistical observations are credible is difficult to determine. Aside from a known association between vinyl chloride and gliomas, there are no common chemical or environmental threads among these observations.[8] There has also been concern that electromagnetic fields could account for some glial tumors, although the majority of studies do not support such a conjecture.[10–12]

Viruses have been implicated directly in the development of gliomas only in rats, dogs, and monkeys. In all cases, direct CNS injection of the virus is required. In rats, the avian sarcoma virus produces glial tumors[13]; in dogs, Rous sarcoma virus leads to gliosarcomas[14]; in owl monkeys, a human polyoma virus (JC virus) produces glial neoplasms[15]; and in hamsters, JC virus produces medulloblastomas.[16] Although a direct association between virus exposure and CNS tumors has not been established in humans, patients with primary CNS lymphoma have been observed to have a high incidence of infection with Epstein-Barr virus and evidence of Epstein-Barr virus in their tumor tissue.[17] Common viral exposure could explain the occasional glioma cluster observed in schools and communities. However, it is extremely difficult to pinpoint mutations due to a virus to validate this hypothesis.

CNS neoplasia, like most cancers, appears to be unassociated with prior trauma. It has been suggested that the incidence of meningiomas is higher in patients with a prior history of head trauma, but this hypothesis was not supported by a prospective study.[18] Trauma could be a progression event; however, this theory would be difficult to prove.

The incidence of CNS tumors after treatment for a prior malignancy is small. The literature contains examples of astrocytomas occurring 3 to 7 years after craniospinal axis irradiation and chemotherapy for acute lymphocytic leukemia and craniopharyngioma[19–21]; unfortunately, none of the reports contains sufficient information to determine risk assessment. In non-Hodgkin's lymphoma, 2% of 44 second malignancies were an astrocytoma.[22] As in the cases discussed previously, no measure of risk assessment is possible, although such infrequent reporting would suggest that these are uncommon or rare events. Meningiomas have been reported in association with scalp irradiation for tinea capitis, the risk for meningiomas being as high as 21% in one study.[23,24]

For unknown reasons, transplant recipients and patients with acquired immunodeficiency syndrome have substantially increased risks for primary CNS lymphoma but not gliomas.

ANATOMIC AND CLINICAL CONSIDERATIONS

The clinical presentation of the various tumors is best appreciated by considering the relation of signs and symptoms to anatomy.[25]

INTRACRANIAL TUMORS

Intracranial tumors produce symptoms primarily by two mechanisms: mass effect (and increased intracranial pressure), due entirely to the tumor or to the tumor and surrounding edema, or infiltration and destruction of normal tissue.

General Signs and Symptoms

Typical infiltrative intracerebral tumors, such as the various grades of astrocytoma and oligodendroglioma and some of the more primitive neuroectodermal tumors, can produce headache, gastrointestinal upset such as nausea and vomiting, personality changes, and slowing of psychomotor function. These may be the only clinical indications of tumor.

Because headache is a common presenting symptom in patients with intracranial tumor, clinical patterns and their localizing value must be appreciated. Brain parenchyma does not have pain-sensitive structures, and tumor pain (headache) has been attributed to local swelling and distortion of pain-sensitive nerve endings associated with blood vessels, primarily in the meninges. Tumors grow at different rates and, therefore, achieve variable size before signs and symptoms occur. But once a tumor has achieved a critical volume causing compression and displacement of brain, the onset and demise of headache seem to correlate with changes in intracranial pressure.

Headaches can vary in severity and quality; they often occur in the early morning hours or on first awakening. Patients sometimes complain of an uncomfortable feeling in the head rather than headache. Although there is not an exact relation between the location of tumor headache and the location of the tumor, some rules are worth remembering. More often than not, frontal and temporal tumors produce headache in frontal, retroorbital, or temporal regions, whereas infratentorial tumors tend to produce occipital and retroauricular headache. Occasionally, however, retroorbital headaches are observed with infratentorial tumors.

Gastrointestinal symptoms are common. Patients complain of loss of appetite, queasiness, nausea, and, occasionally, vomiting. Vomiting appears more commonly in children and in patients harboring infratentorial rather than supratentorial tumors. Although textbooks discuss projectile vomiting as an infrequent generalized symptom of brain tumors, in these authors' experience, it is common in children but rare in adults. From reports in the literature and discussions with experienced neurosurgeons, it seems as though there is a lower incidence of vomiting currently compared with past years; this may reflect the fact that patients are diagnosed earlier than in previous years and receive glucocorticoids that can modify dramatically many of the generalized signs and symptoms of brain tumors.

Sometimes the only presenting symptoms are changes in personality, mood, mental capacity, and concentration. Occasionally, merely a slowing of psychomotor activity is the antecedent symptom of intracranial tumor. Patients with brain tumors tend to sleep longer at night and nap during the day. These changes in function and activity often are apparent to the family and the examiner but not to the patient; in other instances, only the patient recognizes the changes in mental function. None of these symptoms are unique to brain tumors; they could easily be confused with depression, neurasthenia, or other psychological problems.

Focal Cerebral Syndromes

Although fewer than 10% of patients presenting with seizures have a brain tumor as the cause of the seizure, seizures are a presenting symptom in approximately 20% of patients with supratentorial brain tumors. With rapidly growing infiltrative malignant gliomas, they are likely to take the form of focal motor or sensory seizures, although generalized seizures are also common. In patients with slowly growing astrocytomas, oligodendrogliomas, or meningiomas, generalized seizures may antedate the clinical diagnosis by months to years. The value of the focal seizure as a means of tumor localization is high, sufficiently so that tumor should be considered causative until proven otherwise.

The distribution of infiltrative parenchymal tumors in the brain is directly related to the mass of the lobe or region. Frontal tumors occur more commonly than parietal tumors, which, in turn, occur more often than temporal lobe tumors, and so forth. Anatomic or regional involvement by tumors, although not completely stereotypic as it is with CNS vascular disease, nonetheless has certain features that distinguish them and help the clinician localize the tumor or, at least, to consider the diagnosis.

The frontal lobe syndrome varies markedly from patient to patient. It can range from personality change to headache and mild slowing of contralateral hand movements and to contralateral spastic hemiplegia, marked elevation in mood, or loss of initiative and dysphasia (if it is the dominant lobe). Assuming the normal pattern of left hemisphere dominance, unilateral tumors affecting the right frontal lobe can cause left hemiplegia, slight elevation in mood, difficulty in adapting to new situations, loss of initiative, and even occasional primitive grasp and sucking reflexes. Left frontal lobe tumors can cause right hemiplegia and nonfluent dysphasia with or without some apraxia of lip, tongue, or hand movements.

Bifrontal disease, a condition usually associated with infiltrative gliomas and primary CNS lymphomas, can cause varying degrees of bilateral hemiplegia, spastic bulbar palsy, severe impairment of intellect, lability of mood, dementia, and prominent primitive grasp, suck, and snout reflexes.

Temporal lobe syndromes, like frontal lobe syndromes, can range from symptoms that are detectable only on careful testing of perception and spatial judgment to severe impairment of recent memory. Homonymous quadrantanopsia, auditory hallucinations, and even aggressive behavior can occur as a result of tumors of either temporal lobe. Involvement of the nondominant temporal lobe can also result in minor perceptual problems and spatial disorientation. Dominant temporal lobe involvement can lead to dysnomia, impaired perception of verbal commands, and even a full-blown, fluent Wernicke-like aphasia. Bilateral disease, involving both temporal lobes, is rare in comparison with the bilaterality of frontal lobe tumors that readily cross through the corpus callosum. This is fortunate, because bitemporal tumor involvement is devastating. It produces impairment of memory, especially recent memory, and can lead to dementia.

Parietal lobe syndromes affect sensory and perceptual functions more than motor modalities, although mild hemiparesis is sometimes seen with extensive parietal lobe tumors. Tumors impinging on either parietal lobe can produce a decrease in the perception of cortical sensory stimuli that may vary from mild sensory extinction, observable only by testing, to a more severe sensory loss with deep tumors that leads to hemianesthesia or other hemisensory abnormalities. Homonymous hemianopsia or visual inattention also may occur. In addition, involvement of the nondominant parietal lobe can lead to perceptual abnormalities and, in severe cases, to anosognosia and apraxia for self-dressing. Unilateral dominant parietal lobe tumors lead to alexia, dysgraphia, and certain types of apraxia.

Occipital lobe tumors can produce contralateral homonymous hemianopsia or visual aberrations that take the form of imperception of color, object size, or object location. Bilateral occipital disease can produce cortical blindness.

The classic disconnection syndromes associated with corpus callosum lesions are seen rarely in patients with brain tumors. Even though infiltrative gliomas often cross the corpus callosum in the region of the genu or the splenium, the involvement of additional structures complicates neurologic interpretation, obscuring classic disconnection syndromes. With respect to partial lesions, interruption of association fibers in the anterior part of the corpus callosum usually causes a failure of the left hand to carry out spoken commands. Lesions in the splenium of the corpus callosum interrupt visual fibers connecting the right occipital lobe and left angular gyrus, resulting in an inability of patients to read or name colors.

Symptoms related to thalamic tumors vary as a function of tumor size and whether the tumor produces secondary blockage of cerebrospinal fluid (CSF) flow and hydrocephalus. Occasionally, tumors in the thalamus and, less commonly, in the basal ganglia, can reach 3 to 4 cm in diameter before the patient has symptoms severe enough to seek medical attention. Patients typically present with headaches resulting from hydrocephalus and increased intracranial pressure secondary to trapping of the lateral horn of one of the ventricles. In addition or independently, patients can present with a mild sensory abnormality on the contralateral side, which is detected only by testing of sensory extinction or, rarely, severe neuropathic pain syndrome. Patients may complain of intermittent paresthesias on the contralateral side; because they are episodic and seizure-like, anticonvulsant drugs are used sometimes and actually may be beneficial. With more involvement of the basal ganglia, contralateral intention tremor and hemiballistic-like movement disorders can be observed. Thalamic tumors usually do not present in a manner typical of thalamic strokes, unless bleeding into the tumor has occurred.

Focal Infratentorial Syndromes

The brain stem, composed of the medulla oblongata and the pons, has both nuclear groups and traversing axons. Tumors invading or compressing the brain stem can produce dire consequences; even a small increase in size (e.g., 1 to 2 mm) may lead to death or devastating signs and symptoms. Tumors can be primarily intrinsic or intrinsic with exophytic components in the fourth ventricle, peripontine cisterns, or in both locations. Cranial nerve involvement, therefore, can be at the nuclear level or of the cranial nerve as it leaves the brain stem.

The most common tumor of the brain stem is an astrocytoma (glioma), the initial clinical manifestations of which are palsies involving cranial nerves VI and VII on one side in 90% of patients. These usually are followed by involvement of long tracts resulting in hemiplegia, unilateral limb ataxia, ataxia of gait, paraplegia, hemisensory syndromes, gaze disorders, and, occasionally, hiccups. Less commonly, long tract signs precede the cranial nerve abnormalities; this is more likely with confined intrinsic brain stem lesions.

The midbrain, juxtaposed between the pons and the cerebral hemispheres, encompasses the tectum, the cerebral peduncles, and the cerebral aqueduct. If the midbrain is involved, obstructive hydrocephalus can occur, producing vomiting, drowsiness, and cerebellar signs. Patients with medullary tumors have a more rapidly progressive course and are more likely to have deficits in cranial nerves VI (usually late), VII, IX, and X, and dysarthria, personality change, and head tilt. Unlike the expansive posterior fossa tumors, headache, vomiting, and papilledema occur late. Fourth ventricular tumors, because of their location, tend to produce obstructive hydrocephalus early in their development. This produces profound headache and vomiting and associated disturbances of gait and balance. With rapidly progressing lesions, cerebellar herniation may develop.

Tumors of the cerebellum have valuable localizing signs and symptoms. In slowly growing tumors, the initial symptoms may be headache and nausea, which are caused by increased intracranial pressure, and mild imbalance in gait or ataxia of a limb. In more rapidly growing cerebellar tumors, there may be prominent morning headache; vomiting; a stumbling gait with frequent falling, nystagmus, and dizziness; and visual symptoms caused by papilledema. Abnormal posturing of the head is seen often in children but not in adults. In children, the head is tilted back and away from the side of the tumor. Posturing of the head

TABLE 43.2-4. Differential Diagnosis of Tumors at the Base of the Skull

Site of Lesion	*Associated Tumors*	*Clinical Findings*
Anterior parts	Carcinomas invasive from frontal and ethmoid sinuses; meningiomas	Unilateral anosmia, frontal lobe syndrome, seizures
Superior orbital	Meningiomas, carcinoma of nasopharynx	III, IV, V1, VI nerve lesions with ophthalmoplegia and pain and hypesthesia in V1 distribution
Cavernous sinus	Chondromas, meningiomas, sellar and parasellar tumors	III, IV, VI, and sometimes V nerve involvement with ophthalmoplegia
Apex of the petrous temporal bone	Cholesteatoma, chondroma meningioma, neurinoma sarcoma	V and VI nerve involvement with sensory and motor findings and diplopia
Sphenoid and petrous bones	Meningioma, chondroma, nasopharyngeal carcinoma, metastasis	III, IV, VI nerve lesions result in ophthalmoplegia; V may be associated with trigeminal neuralgia syndrome
Jugular foramen	Glomus jugular tumors, neurinomas, chondromas cholesteatoma, meningioma, nasopharyngeal carcinoma	IX, X, XI nerves producing difficulty with swallowing, speaking, and weakness of strap muscles of neck
Cerebellopontine	Neurinoma, meningioma, cholesteatoma, metastasis cerebellar tumors	VII nerve lesions causing angle loss of hearing, vertigo, and nystagmus; cerebellar lesions producing ataxia of limbs and gait; V, VII, and occasionally IX and XII nerve lesions; brain stem symptoms and signs of increased intracranial pressure

(Adapted from ref. 26.)

is curious in that it indicates unilateral cerebellum-foramen magnum herniation. Bilateral sixth cranial nerve palsies are uncommon. Midline lesions in and around the cerebellar vermis lead to truncal and gait ataxia, whereas lesions in a cerebellar hemisphere lead to unilateral appendicular ataxia, most readily observed in upper extremity movements.

Tumors of the base of the skull, although not particularly common, nevertheless are important because many are curable by surgery. Table 43.2-4[26] summarizes the salient clinical features of seven of the more common clinical syndromes.

A classic base of skull tumor presentation is that associated with vestibular schwannomas, the most frequent cause of the cerebellopontine angle syndrome. Almost all such patients have involvement of the auditory or vestibular portions of cranial nerve VIII; fortunately, most patients have little morbidity from surgery. Potential postoperative complications depend on size of tumor and surgical approach used. The morbidity of surgery can be facial weakness, hypoesthesia of cornea, disturbance of taste, sensory loss of the face, ataxia of gait, and unilateral appendicular ataxia. Deafness and vestibular dysfunction due to damage to the auditory and vestibular nerve branches are characteristic of these tumors. Finally, these tumors can attain an extremely large size before they are discovered.

Another group of tumors that present with distinct signs and symptoms is that which occurs in or near the sella turcica. Table 43.2-5 summarizes the location, tumors, and some of the salient features of sellar and parasellar tumors.[27]

Many patients present with defects of the visual field, less commonly with blindness and optic atrophy. The visual field abnormality is usually a partial or complete bitemporal hemianopsia associated with intrasellar tumors such as pituitary adenomas. With lesions that expand from below the optic chiasm, the upper temporal quadrants are affected first. Patients can also present with scotomata in either eye. With long-standing, slowly progressive disease, unilateral or bilateral optic atrophy can be observed. Expansion of tumor may involve the hypothalamus and compression of the third ventricle, leading to obstructive hydrocephalus and signs of increased intracranial pressure, such as headache and nausea and vomiting.

Some of the pituitary tumors produce secondary signs and symptoms, because they elaborate hormones that create various syndromes of endocrine hyperactivity (Table 43.2-6). A few pituitary tumors produce no detectable hormones or produce hormones in quantities that assume no clinical significance. Currently, it is uncommon for patients with endocrine-active tumors to present with large tumors; it is more common for patients with endocrine-inactive tumors to seek medical attention because of optic chiasmal compression hypopituitarism as a consequence of a large mass. Compression leads to detectable hyposecretion of specific cells, with production of growth hormone being the most sensitive, followed closely by gonadotropins. Cells producing thyroid-stimulating hormone and corticotrophin are much more resistant, and their function is impaired only at a later stage of growth.

Table 43.2-7 summarizes the differential diagnosis of tumors by location in children and adults.[28]

Acute and Life-Threatening Syndromes Caused by Intracranial Tumors

Because the brain and the spinal cord are surrounded by a rigid skull and dural membranes, expanding lesions within or abutting the brain or spinal cord can cause displacement of vital structures. This can lead, in the brain, to respiratory arrest and death and, in the spinal cord, to paraplegia or quadriplegia.

To understand the sequence of events leading to temporal lobe-tentorial (uncal) herniation and cerebellar-foramen magnum herniation, a visual image of intracranial anatomy is needed. The tentorium cerebelli forms a rigid tissue partition between the cerebral hemispheres above and the cerebellum and brain stem below. Through this opening passes the midbrain centrally and cranial nerve III anterolaterally. Immediately lateral to cranial nerve III lies the medial portion of the temporal lobe called the *uncus.* An expanding mass lesion situated above the tentorium may displace the uncus medially and

TABLE 43.2-5. Clinical Syndromes Associated with Tumors of Sellar Region

	Disorders			
Tumor	Anterior Pituitary Gland	Hypothalamus	*Incidence and Degree*	*Syndromes*
IN THE SELLA				
Adenoma				
Active	+			Cushing's disease, acromegaly, gigantism
Inactive	+	±		Forbes-Albright syndrome, hypopituitarism
Chondroma	+			
Metastasis	+			
Craniopharyngioma			Regular	
Intrasellar	+		Clinical	
Intrasellar and suprasellar	+	+		
CLOSE TO SELLA				
Suprasellar craniopharyngioma	+	+	Regular clinical	Adiposogenital dystrophy (Fröhlich's syndrome)
Suprasellar meningioma		±		
Suprasellar epidermoid				
Optic pathway glioma		±	Rare	Russell's syndrome
Hypothalamic glioma		+	Frequent	Precocious puberty
Hypothalamic hamartoma		+	Clinical	
Pineal tumors		+	Frequent clinical	
Tumors with aqueductal obstruction and hydrocephalus		+		Cushingoid
REMOTE FROM SELLA				
Cerebral hemispheres	±	±	Rare	
Meningioma glioma			Latent	

(From ref. 27, with permission.)

inferiorly beneath the tentorium. Table 43.2-8 summarizes the neurologic findings and pathologic causes for the events that constitute the temporal lobe-tentorial herniation syndrome.[29]

A rapid increase in the volume of the supratentorial compartment leading to herniation can be caused by many different factors. A rapidly growing glioblastoma can present in this manner, although it is more usual for it to occur as a terminal or near terminal event after ineffective therapy for the tumor. It can also occur when there is a dramatic increase in the amount of edema associated with metastasis to the brain or with hyponatremia and hypoosmolar syndromes. The injudicious use of parenteral hypoosmolar 5% dextrose in water often is sufficient to produce an abrupt increase in brain edema and temporal lobe herniation. The authors of this chapter also have seen temporal lobe herniation follow a group of shortly spaced seizures. Presumably, the seizures, which are associated with hypoventilation, produce local hypoxia around the tumor with a resultant increase in brain edema.

Mass lesions in the infratentorial compartment can displace brain tissue upward through the tentorium, but more commonly force brain tissue downward through the foramen magnum. In this situation, the cerebellar tonsils move caudally through the foramen magnum, and in doing so, wedge against the medulla, causing the findings summarized in Table 43.2-9.[29]

Cerebellar-foramen magnum herniation frequently results from, or is contributed to by, obstructive hydrocephalus. In such instances, emergency removal of fluid from the more cephalad ventricular system may relieve symptoms and be life saving. Surgical intervention is indicated only if the reason for the herniation is treatable. In the instance of cerebellar-foramen magnum herniation aggravated by acute obstructive hydrocephalus, ventriculoperitoneal shunting is often necessary. Care must be taken, however, because too rapid a change in the CSF dynamics can lead to a rapid and damaging move-

TABLE 43.2-6. Clinical Syndromes Produced by Endocrine-Activity Pituitary Adenomas

Hormone Produced	*Clinical Syndrome*
Prolactin	Amenorrhea and galactorrhea, impotence
Growth hormone	Gigantism and acromegaly
Adrenocorticotropic hormone	Cushing's disease, Nelson's syndrome (following adrenalectomy)
Thyroid-stimulating hormone (rare)	Hyperthyroidism

TABLE 43.2-7. Differential Diagnosis of Tumors by Location and Age at Onset of Symptoms

Location	Child	Adult
Supratentorial	Astrocytoma	Metastatic
	Glioblastoma multiforme	Glioblastoma multiforme
	Oligodendroglioma	Astrocytoma
	Sarcoma	Meningioma
	Neuroblastoma	Oligodendroglioma
	Oligoastrocytoma	Oligoastrocytoma
Infratentorial	Astrocytoma	Metastatic
	Medulloblastoma	Astrocytoma
	Ependymoma	Glioblastoma multiforme
	Brain stem glioma	Ependymoma
		Brain stem glioma
Sellar and parasellar	Craniopharyngioma	Pituitary
	Optic glioma	Meningioma
	Epidermoid	
Base of the skull	—	Neurinoma
		Meningioma
		Chordoma
		Carcinoma
		Dermoid, epidermoid

TABLE 43.2-9. Cerebellar Foramen Magnum Herniation

Neurologic Findings	Pathologic Cause
Head tilt, stiff neck, posturing of neck, or paresthesias over the neck	Downward displacement of inferior hemispheres through the foramen magnum; may be unilateral or bilateral
Tonic extensor spasms of limbs and body (cerebellar fits) and later coma	Compressive effects of cerebellum or hydrocephalus on the upper brain stem
Respiratory arrest	Medullary compression

ment of the brain, which can lead to occlusion of posterior cerebral arteries and brain stem injury.

These two herniation syndromes lead to death, unless there is prompt intervention. The immediate intravenous administration of hyperosmotic agents, such as mannitol or urea, and large doses of synthetic glucocorticoids, such as dexamethasone or methylprednisolone, should be given promptly to reduce intracranial pressure and to avert impending death.

Hemorrhage into a tumor is not as common as might be expected, although the incidence of intratumor hemorrhage may increase because of iatrogenic thrombocytopenia associated with the current use of chemotherapy in the treatment of brain tumors. Primary tumors that most commonly bleed *de novo* are glioblastoma and oligodendrogliomas; of the metastatic tumors, those from the lung, melanoma, hypernephroma, and choriocarcinoma are most likely to be associated with intratumoral hemorrhage. Signs and symptoms of intratumoral hemorrhage may be temporized by the use of osmotic agents and glucocorticoids, but if extensive and life-threatening, operation and decompression are indicated. Under no circumstances should a lumbar puncture be performed in any of the acute herniation syndromes. In fact, lumbar puncture should never be done indiscriminately. The indications for lumbar puncture are discussed in another section of this chapter (see Neurodiagnostic Tests, later in this chapter).

SPINAL AXIS

To understand the clinical presentation of tumors of the spinal axis, the local anatomy (Fig. 43.2-1) and how tumors might present with respect to anatomy must be appreciated. The cranial dura is firmly adherent to the skull (with the exception of dural duplications of the falx and tentorium), and no extradural space normally exists between dura and skull. An entirely different anatomic relation in the spinal canal accounts for a well-defined extradural space containing epidural fat and blood vessels. By way of the intervertebral foramina, this extradural space communicates with adjacent extraspinal compartments (e.g., the mediastinum and the retroperitoneal space). With rare exceptions, extradural tumors are metastatic, reaching the extradural space through intervertebral foramina.

TABLE 43.2-8. Temporal Lobe-Tentorial (Uncal) Herniation

Neurologic Findings	Pathologic Cause
Pupillary dilation and ptosis	Compression of ipsilateral oculomotor nerve between herniating tissue and petroclinoid ligament
Ipsilateral hemiplegia	Compression of contralateral cerebral peduncle against tentorium (Kernohan's notch)
Contralateral hemiplegia	Compression of ipsilateral cerebral peduncle; when associated with compression of contralateral peduncle, bilateral corticospinal tract signs will be present
Homonymous hemianopia	Compression of posterior cerebral artery against the tentorium can lead to occipital ischemia or infarction and contralateral homonymous hemianopia; occasionally bilateral field cuts occur
Midbrain syndrome: Cheyne-Stokes respirations, stupor or coma, bipyramidal signs, decerebrate rigidity, dilated fixed pupils, gaze paresis, altered oculocephalic reflexes	Crushing of midbrain between herniating temporal lobe and leaf of tentorium associated with vascular occlusion and perivascular hemorrhage
Coma, rising blood pressure, and bradycardia	These late signs occur from rising intracranial pressure and hydrocephalus as the aqueduct is compressed and subarachnoid space compromised

(Adapted from ref. 29.)

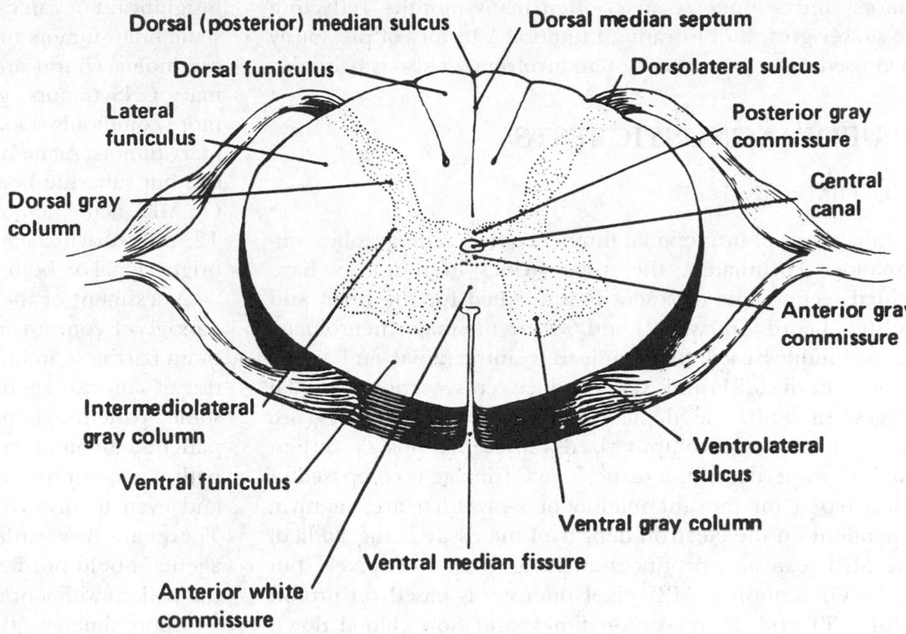

FIGURE 43.2-1. Cross-section of thoracic spinal cord shows relation of spinal nerves to intraspinal tracts.

Tumors arising inside of the dural tube (intradural tumors) may originate within the spinal cord (intramedullary), or they may take origin outside the spinal cord (extramedullary). The two common extramedullary intradural tumors, neurilemmoma (schwannoma) and meningioma, are attached, respectively, to sensory nerve roots and to dura and involve the spinal cord by compression.

Neurology of Spinal Cord Tumors

A spinal tumor produces two effects: local (focal) and distal (remote). Local effects indicate the tumor's location along the spinal axis, and distal effects reflect involvement of motor and sensory long tracts within the spinal cord. Table 43.2-10 summarizes the clinical findings useful in localizing a spinal cord tumor.

Distal effects are common to all spinal tumors sooner or later, and symptoms and signs are confined to structures innervated below the spinal cord level of involvement. Although neurologic manifestations commonly begin unilaterally, a full-blown Brown-Séquard syndrome of cord hemisection can occur but is rare. More characteristic are motor changes: weakness and spasticity, if the tumor lies above the conus medullaris, or weakness and flaccidity, if at or below the conus. Typically, sensory impairment begins distally in the feet. Impairment of bladder function occurs later in tumors above the conus, but may be an early manifestation of tumors in or below the conus. The upper level of impaired long tract function usually is several segments below the actual site of tumor involvement.

Local manifestations may reflect involvement of bone, with pain constituting the cardinal symptom of metastatic tumors. Involvement of spinal roots produces pain, sensory impairment, and weakness with atrophy in the appropriate radicular distribution. Less often, involvement of spinal gray matter produced by extensive pressure from extramedullary tumors or direct damage by intramedullary tumors causes segmental sensory and motor changes.

Historically, tumors at or near the foramen magnum have been diagnosed incorrectly more often than have spinal tumors at any other site, because foramen magnum tumors can mimic such diverse conditions as multiple sclerosis, amyotrophic lateral sclerosis, and cervical disk disease. The frequency of delayed diagnoses of these tumors justifies the dictum that MRI is indicated as a diagnostic measure in any neurologic disease that can be accounted for by a lesion at or below the foramen magnum.

Occasionally, a cervical intramedullary tumor mimics syringomyelia, with dissociated sensory loss, weakness, and wasting in the arms and hands and variable long tract involvement. In most instances, the clinical presentation of a spinal tumor does not indicate if it is extradural or intradural.

The rate at which symptoms develop can be helpful in distinguishing extradural from intradural tumor, with a history of

TABLE 43.2-10. Clinical Manifestations of Spinal Cord Tumors

Location	*Findings*
Foramen magnum	11th and 12th cranial nerve palsies; ipsilateral arm weakness early; cerebellar ataxia; and neck pain
Cervical	Ipsilateral arm weakness with leg and opposite arm in time; wasting and fibrillation of ipsilateral neck, shoulder girdle, and arm; decreased pain and temperature sensation in upper cervical regions early; and pain in cervical distribution
Thoracic	Weakness of abdominal muscles; sparing of arms; unilateral root pains; sensory level with ipsilateral changes early and bilateral with time
Lumbosacral	Root pain in groin region, sciatic distribution, or both; weakened proximal pelvic muscles; impotence; bladder paralysis; and decreased knee jerk and brisk ankle jerks
Cauda equina	Unilateral pain in back and leg becoming bilateral when the tumor is quite large; bladder and bowel paralysis

days to a few weeks characterizing metastatic extradural tumors, and a longer course, often many months, reflecting the slower growth of intradural tumors. A history of previously diagnosed cancer or other system involvement also is helpful.

NEURODIAGNOSTIC TESTS

NEUROIMAGING

The diagnosis of intracranial tumor requires radiographic confirmation. Fortunately, the great strides in radiology have yielded technologic advances best adapted for the brain and the spinal cord. Today MRI and CT are the major neuroimaging techniques used to demonstrate intracranial and spinal lesions. Both MRI and CT produce cross-sectional digital images. In both, the depicted anatomy and pathology are based on numeric computerized representations of certain physical properties of the tissue. The CT image is composed of pixels based on the attenuation of x-rays that are, in turn, dependent on the electron density of the tissue being studied. The MRI scan also produces an image based on pixels, but unlike CT scanning, MRI pixel intensity is based on proton density, T1 and T2 relaxation times, and flow (blood flow). The MRI scan, therefore, represents a complex interrelation of four parameters. Data acquisition also can be manipulated by the operator to a greater degree than can be done with CT scans. CT and MRI also differ in that MRI data can be acquired in any plane desired, including oblique planes, in a primary fashion such that there is no compromise of spatial or contrast detail. CT scans can be acquired only in the axial or half-axial planes. Computer-generated reformations are required to generate alternative views, such as orthogonal and off-axis images, all of which have degradation of both spatial and contrast detail. Because MRI scanning can generate images in any plane and offers high resolution and contrast without associated bone artifact, it has been shown to be superior to CT scan in detecting and localizing brain tumors and evaluating edema, hydrocephalus, or hemorrhage.

Intraaxial CNS tumors normally produce edema that is partially correlated with the rapidity of tumor growth. An exception is the benign cerebral meningioma, a slow-growing tumor that can produce profound edema. The so-called vasogenic edema associated with brain tumors is fluid that has leaked through an incompetent blood–brain barrier and is seen on the CT scan as relatively low attenuation compared with normal brain. On MRI, edema appears as an area of low-signal intensity on T1-weighted images and high-signal intensity on T2-weighted images.

Mass lesions in the brain can obstruct the ventricular system, resulting in hydrocephalus. MRI is superior to CT in evaluating hydrocephalus and its causes, because more planes of view are available to the radiologist. Dilation of one or both of the lateral ventricles and not the rest of the ventricular system suggests obstruction at the foramen of Monro as is seen with colloid cysts or gliomas in this region. Dilatation of a temporal horn of the ventricular system suggests a tumor in the ventricular atrium *trapping* the temporal horn. Dilation of only the lateral and third ventricles points to a lesion of the aqueduct; when all the ventricles are dilated, communicating hydrocephalus caused by tumor seeding to the meninges or by the reaction to previous therapy should be considered.

Brain tumors occasionally bleed, and this bleeding can be insignificant or can cause dramatic clinical consequences. Metastatic brain tumors that tend to bleed are melanoma, renal cell carcinoma, choriocarcinoma, and thyroid carcinoma. Of the primary CNS tumors, glioblastoma and oligodendrogliomas are more commonly associated with hemorrhage than are other primary tumors. Acute hemorrhage appears as high attenuation on CT, but subacute hemorrhage may be harder to detect by CT. On MRI, acute hemorrhage is of low-signal intensity on T1 and T2; the subacute hemorrhage poorly seen on CT produces a bright signal on both T1- and T2-weighted MRI scans.

Assessment of the disruption of tumor endothelia and the passage of contrast material compared with the intact blood–brain barrier is an important step in radiologic evaluation. The use of contrast agents in CT and MRI scanning provides, in some patients, improved tumor visualization and, in all patients, an improved ability to discern tumors from other pathologic entities, to discern one tumor type from another, and even to discern higher from lower grade malignancies. There are few situations when administration of contrast agents should not be included in the radiologic evaluation of the patient with a brain tumor.

Approximately 50% of patients with low-grade gliomas may present with tumors that do not exhibit contrast enhancement on CT scan. Some may not be detected on CT because they are isodense with brain. It is in these patients that the differential sensitivity of MRI can be seen clearly, even in the absence of a paramagnetic contrast agent. Figure 43.2-2 shows an example of a CT scan in a patient with a seizure disorder that was interpreted prospectively and retrospectively as normal before and after contrast agent administration. The MRI scan is clearly abnormal. Stereotactic biopsy demonstrated a well-differentiated astrocytoma.

The possibility of obtaining high-quality coronal images without artifact associated with beam hardening through bone makes MRI particularly attractive for evaluating the base of the skull and the posterior fossa. Figure 43.2-3 is an example of a high-quality MRI scan in a patient with pituitary adenoma. Although this lesion would be identified readily on CT, the relation to the optic chiasm and infundibulum would certainly not be identified as clearly.

In the posterior fossa, the lack of artifact and the availability of sagittal and coronal planes make MRI uniquely suited for detecting and characterizing neoplasms. Both intraaxial and extraaxial masses are distinguished easily, and their relation to the ventricular cisternal systems is assessed easily.

In the evaluation of intracranial tumors, cerebral angiography is used much less frequently than in the past. For many cases MR angiography suffices. Angiography may be used to confirm an impression gained by MRI or CT that the lesion in question is a vascular malformation or an aneurysm rather than a neoplasm. In certain situations (e.g., with large meningiomas) angiography may be useful before surgery to determine the blood supply so that it can be embolized during the angiographic procedure or obliterated during the surgical procedure, or both.

In the evaluation of intramedullary and extramedullary spinal cord lesions, high-quality MRI is the diagnostic study of choice. Indications for myelography currently are extremely limited, because multiplanar MRI can provide superb delineation of the spinal cord contour, and the addition of gadolinium-diethylenetri-

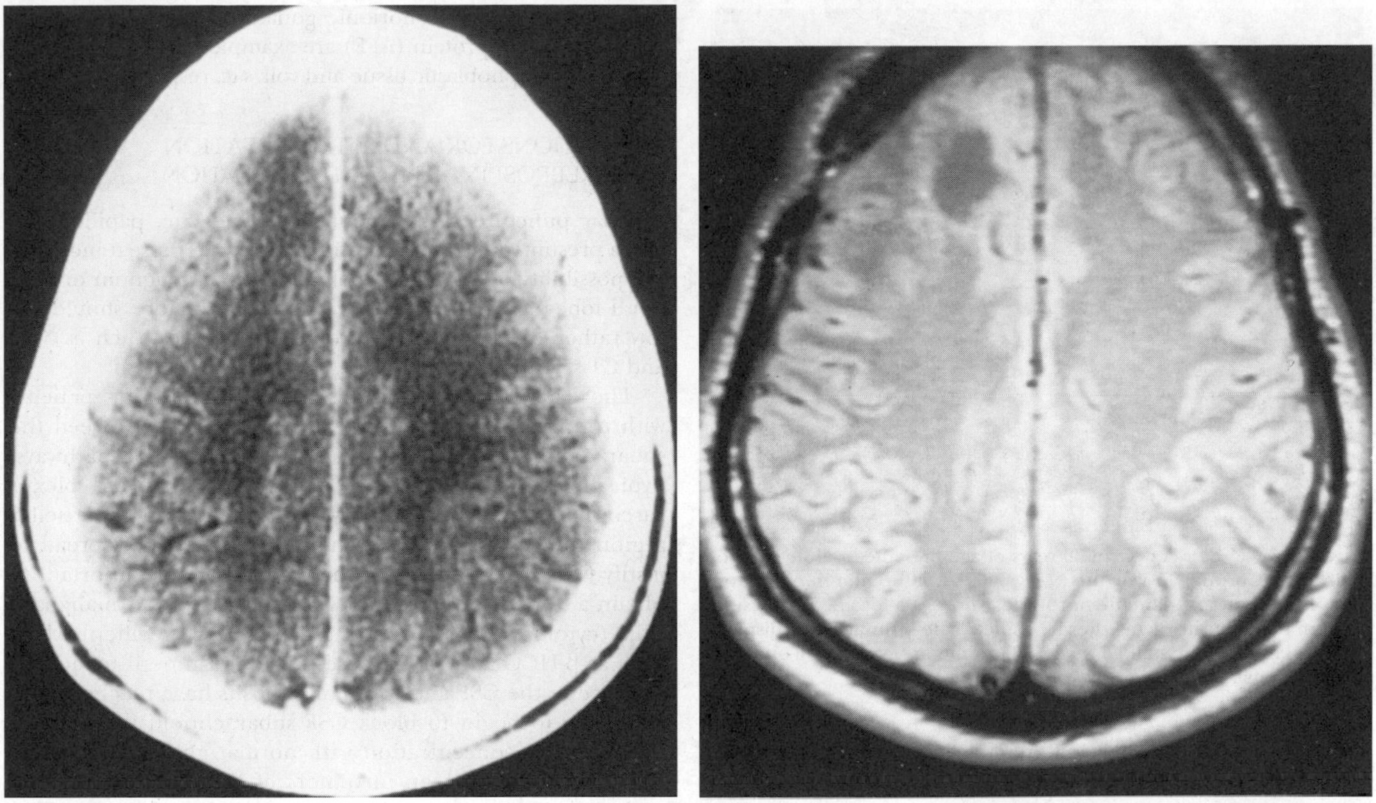

A B

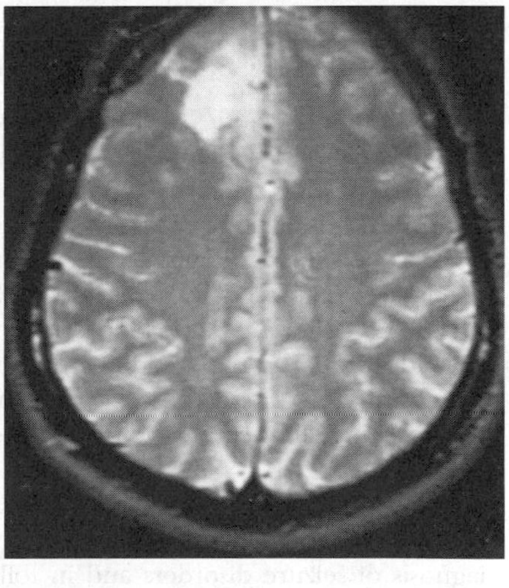

C

FIGURE 43.2-2. A young man presented with a single focal seizure that generalized into a major motor seizure. **A:** A postcontrast axial computed tomographic scan demonstrates a poorly defined area of low density involving the most anterior portion of the corona radiate extending anteriorly to the gray matter on the right. No contrast enhancement, sulcal effacement, or mass effect is present. **B:** After this computed tomographic scan, a T2-weighted (TR 2000, TE 20) axial magnetic resonance imaging scan was performed that shows an area of decreased signal intensity at the gray-white junction at the most anterior medial aspect of the right frontal lobe. **C:** On the second echo (TR 2000, TE 60), the lesion exhibits high signal intensity. On biopsy, the tumor was found to be a well-differentiated astrocytoma.

aminepenta-acetic acid provides enhancement and visualization of almost all intrinsic tumors (such as ependymomas, astrocytomas, meningiomas, and schwannomas) and facilitates the diagnosis of leptomeningeal disease. Tumor cysts are readily identified on MRI, and currently spinal cord tumors can be distinguished much more reliably from syringomyelia (Fig. 43.2-4).

Another unique and particularly important application of MRI is the use of the sagittal image in radiation treatment planning. The MRI sagittal image can be superimposed on radiographic simulator films so that the tumor can be localized accurately for appropriate port design. The use of the MRI scan is now routine in treatment planning of brain and spinal cord tumors.

Newer MRI techniques such as MR spectroscopy, dynamic contrast-enhanced MRI, functional MRI, and diffusion-perfusion MRI can provide additional information. MR spectroscopy can evaluate the regional distribution of chemicals associated with energy metabolism in the tumor. Dynamic contrast-enhanced MRI, by quantitating the uptake of gadolinium contrast agents into the lesion, can distinguish the slow rate of uptake of radiation injury from the rapid rate of uptake commonly seen in highly malignant primary CNS tumors. Functional MRI reflects small localized changes in blood flow that occur in response to cortical localization of various neurologic functions. Thus, for instance, dominance of cerebral function or importance of a supplementary motor area can be quickly determined before surgery to enable the surgeon to better protect normal brain function during a surgical resection of a tumor. Diffusion-perfusion MRI can provide better information regarding free and restricted water dif-

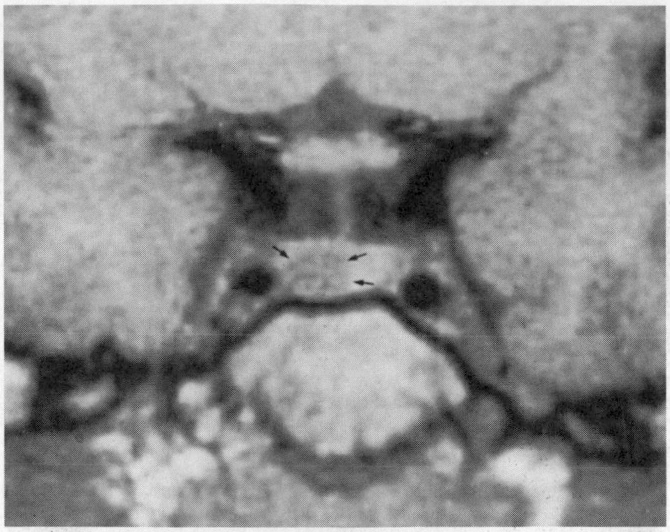

FIGURE 43.2-3. A woman 30 years of age presented with hyperprolactinemia. Coronal T1-weighted (TR 600, TE 20) 3-mm-thick section scan of the pituitary gland demonstrates (*arrows*) a low-intensity lesion 9 mm in diameter involving the right side of the pituitary fossa displacing the gland and the stalk to the left. Findings are typical of a pituitary microadenoma.

fusion in the brain to help differentiate tumor malignancy and secondary effects of treatment on the tumor.

TANGENT SCREEN, PERIMETRY, AUDIOMETRY, AND ELECTROENCEPHALOGRAPHY

Testing for abnormalities of the visual system is part of the neurologic examination. However, the results of confrontation visual field testing need quantitation to provide greater accuracy and to follow the effects of treatment. Formal visual field testing is done using tangent screens, and scotomas and field defects are diagnosed with perimetry. Schematic representation of the common visual field abnormalities and their anatomic localization can be readily found in any neurology text.

Quantitation of deafness is performed by formal audiometric testing. This can be helpful in the diagnosis of acoustic neurinomas.

Electroencephalography once had a place in the diagnosis and follow-up study of intracranial neoplasms. Its major value is in the diagnosis of seizure disorders and in following the rare patient whose neurologic deterioration may be related to subclinical seizures rather than tumor growth. Visual-evoked potentials measured over the visual cortex after visual stimuli are less valuable in the evaluation or follow-up study of patients with brain tumors, but can help distinguish multiple sclerosis from tumor.

TUMOR AND CEREBROSPINAL FLUID MARKERS

For patients with intracranial and spinal tumors, examination of peripheral blood and CSF has been found to be helpful for diagnosis and for therapy monitoring. Pituitary tumors often produce endocrinologic abnormalities measurable by sensitive radioimmunoassays. Polycythemia associated with a tumor of the posterior fossa (cerebellum) may be useful as presumptive evidence for the diagnosis of hemangioblastoma. Some parasellar and pineal region embryonal tumors secrete unique hormones and proteins; human chorionic gonadotropin-β hormone (β-HCG) and α-fetoprotein (AFP) are examples of hormones associated with trophoblastic tissue and yolk sac, respectively.

INDICATIONS FOR AND INTERPRETATION OF CEREBROSPINAL FLUID EXAMINATION

Lumbar puncture in a patient with headache, papilledema, and a presumed diagnosis of tumor is risky, because it increases the possibility of a fatal cerebellum-foramen magnum or temporal lobe-tentorial herniation. Lumbar puncture should follow rather than precede neuroimaging studies, such as MRI and CT scanning.

The examination of CSF is useful in following patients with intracranial tumors that have a propensity to seed the subarachnoid space and spread through the CSF pathways. Typically, medulloblastoma, ependymoma, choroid plexus carcinoma, and some embryonal pineal and suprasellar region tumors have a high enough likelihood of spread to justify CSF examinations. In these patients, it is important to obtain a lumbar puncture for CSF to examine for malignant cells (cytology), protein, and glucose, and specific markers such as β-HCG and AFP. These tests determine if malignant cells are in the CSF and if tumor deposits have reached sufficient size to begin to block CSF subarachnoid pathways. A high protein concentration with normal glucose levels and normal cytology is seen in tumors of the base of the skull, such as acoustic neurinoma, and in spinal cord tumors. The appearance of xanthochromic CSF, due to high protein content, with an absence of erythrocytes is characteristic of spinal cord tumors obstructing the subarachnoid space and producing stasis of the CSF in the caudal lumbar sac.

Evaluation of Patients with Intracranial Tumors during Therapy

Critical to the evaluation of the efficacy of any therapy for brain tumors is the reliability of the measurement of tumor growth (deterioration) or tumor regression (response). Today, contrast-enhanced MRI and, to a lesser extent, CT are used as the primary measure of response to treatment. The extreme sensitivity of the MRI to changes in brain water content and small enhancing lesions can be confusing in the evaluation of tumor regrowth and progression, especially following radiotherapy. The use of MR spectroscopy, diffusion-perfusion algorithms, and dynamic contrast-enhanced MRI may improve the ability to assess tumor regrowth in the postirradiation period.

To interpret the results of therapy correctly and to improve patient care, understanding factors other than cell division is important.

FACTORS THAT MAY PRODUCE CLINICAL DETERIORATION

The most common causes of neurologic deterioration in brain tumor patients undergoing radiation therapy or chemotherapy, or both, are growth of the tumor or increased peritumoral edema. Both cause increased pressure in the cranial cavity that is transmitted primarily to the adjacent brain; in turn, hydrostatic pressure on the brain can lead to impairment of cerebral blood flow. The clinical result can be progressive impairment

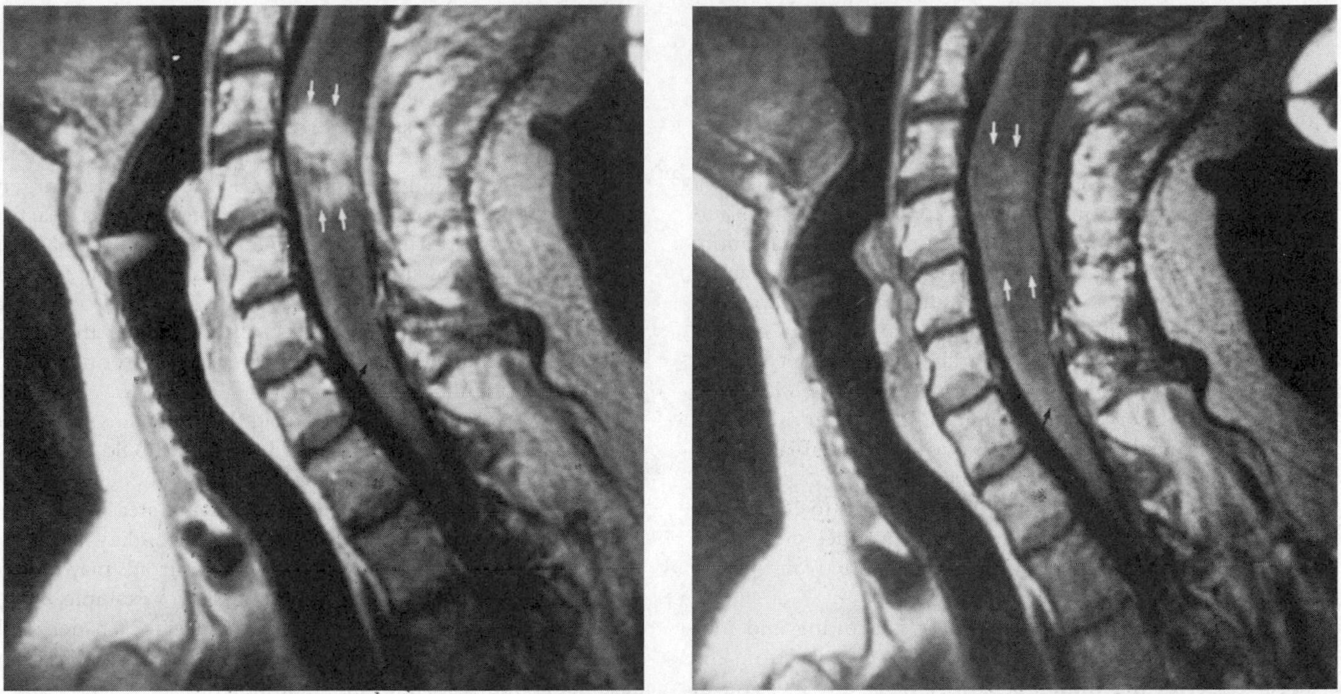

A B

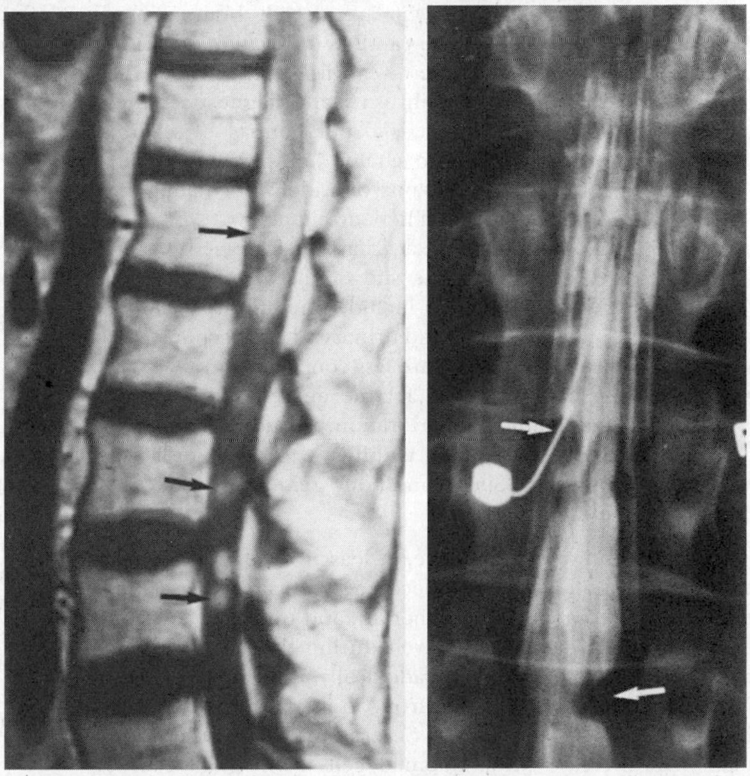

C, D

FIGURE 43.2-4. A 39-year-old man with a known cerebral glioblastoma multiforme developed spinal cord symptoms. **A:** A T1-weighted (TR 600, TE 20) sagittal scan of the thoracolumbar spine shows mild heterogeneity of signal near the conus, but is otherwise normal. **B:** A T2-weighted (TR 2000, SE 35, 70) sagittal scan provides no additional information. **C:** A T1-weighted (TR 600, SE 20) image after gadolinium-diethylenetriaminepenta-acetic acid administration clearly shows high signal-enhancing tumor (*black arrows* show some of lesions) immediately caudad to the conus resulting in a high-grade partial block and multiple additional drop metastases. **D:** A water-soluble contrast myelogram demonstrates the drop metastases (*white arrows* show some of lesions) and incompletely delineates the mass adjacent to the conus. (Courtesy of Gordon Sze, Department of Radiology, Yale University School of Medicine, New Haven, CT.)

of functioning brain with resultant neurologic deficits. These manifestations may include signs and symptoms of increased intracranial pressure and temporal lobe or cerebellar herniation (see Tables 43.2-9 and 43.2-10).

Neurologic deterioration, without neuroimaging evidence of tumor growth, can occur for any of the following reasons:

- Obstructive hydrocephalus can occur secondary to tumor in the ventricular system at the aqueduct of Sylvius, fourth ventricle, or foramen of Monro or communicating hydrocephalus due to infiltrative tumor (carcinomatosis, CNS leukemia, and arachnoiditis).
- Hemorrhage into a tumor may occur.

- Fluid imbalance, particularly hyponatremia caused by excessive administration of parenteral dextrose in water solutions, may develop.
- Hypertension can accentuate intratumoral and peritumoral edema.
- Reactive peritumoral edema (or demyelination) may develop early in the course of radiation therapy.
- An *early delayed* syndrome, observed in approximately 15% to 40% of patients completing a course of cranial irradiation, can be distinguished from tumor regrowth only by waiting and finding that the patient's condition improves without further treatment.[41] This encephalopathy responds to corticosteroids and resolves within several weeks without specific sequelae. This syndrome is not unique to patients with brain tumors and is observed in leukemic children after prophylactic cranial irradiation and in those with extracranial tumors who receive incidental radiation to the brain.
- Radiation necrosis can occur within 3 months to 13 years or longer after radiation therapy and can produce neurologic impairment that may be indistinguishable from tumor recurrence.
- Seizures may suggest that the tumor is growing and may result in an increase in the neurologic deficit apart from any direct effect of the tumor. Recovery from any increase in weakness and mental dullness may take several hours to a week in postictal patients who are already brain injured. Even subclinical seizures can cause deterioration, persisting for hours to days, which resolves with control of the seizures. Electroencephalography is usually diagnostic in these patients, and the treatment is better control of seizures. Patients receiving long-term chemotherapy often require higher doses of anticonvulsants or widely fluctuating dosages caused by drug-induced hepatic changes.
- Infection and fever often exacerbate neurologic signs and symptoms, regardless of the site of infection. The more common causes of infection include pneumonia secondary to aspiration or atelectasis and urinary tract infections; meningitis and cerebral abscess are less common.
- Metabolic disorders, anemia, fatigue, and emotional depression can cause clinical deterioration, including increase in focal deficit on testing, that is difficult to distinguish from tumor progression. Such conditions generally produce no alteration of neuroimages.

In these authors' experience, at least 10% of patients who eventually respond to therapy become significantly worse at the end of a first course of chemotherapy, and transient deterioration is observed occasionally even during the second year of continuous chemotherapy. Paradoxically, this clinical worsening early in therapy may result from an increase in tumor bulk resulting from *effective* therapy. Several factors contribute: cell mass may increase when doomed cells form giant cells or undergo one or more successful cell divisions before dying; the CNS also has an inefficient mechanism for disposing of dead cells produced by chemotherapy or irradiation; and edema, probably caused by irritative products of cell lysis, may be present within the tumor mass and in adjacent brain.

GLUCOCORTICOID USE

Administration of glucocorticoids is usually begun before surgery for brain tumor. If an adequate surgical decompression is achieved, the corticosteroid dose can be tapered off rapidly and discontinued within the first week or two after the operation. Some patients require corticosteroid maintenance because a large volume of tumor remains, because tumor occupies the brain stem or spinal cord, or because of corticosteroid dependence resulting from long-term prior usage.

Patients who no longer require corticosteroids after surgery may need them during or after radiation therapy. Reactive edema may occur during irradiation, and there may be a transient period of drowsiness and increased deficit for 6 to 16 weeks after treatment. In both instances, signs and symptoms usually resolve within a few weeks; observation of the subsequent clinical course is often the only way to differentiate these reactions from tumor progression.

The lowest dosage of glucocorticoid that maintains patients at their maximum levels of comfort and function should be sought. Ordinarily, this is determined by decreasing the dosage until symptoms increase or become apparent, then increasing the dosage until they subside. If deterioration is secondary to tumor growth or treatment-induced effects, glucocorticoids may have to be increased to keep the patient comfortable. For example, 3 mg/d of dexamethasone may have the desired effect for a patient with stabilized disease; however, a deteriorating patient may require dexamethasone doses of 64 mg/d or more.

The efficacy of chemotherapy and radiation therapy can be affected by glucocorticoid dosage. A decrease in corticosteroid requirement suggests improvement, assuming that the previous dosage was actually required. An increase in dosage suggests deterioration. Because increased glucocorticoid dosage may improve neurologic status and reduce the image size on CT scan, an attempt should be made to document tumor recurrence before increasing glucocorticoid dosage. The ability of glucocorticoids to reduce the size of primary brain tumors as measured by MRI is well established.

SURGERY

GENERAL CONSIDERATIONS

No other modality can reduce tumor bulk as quickly as surgery, and advances in imaging, computerized navigation, pharmacologic agents for brain edema, neuroanesthesia, and surgical magnification, illumination, and instrumentation such as ultrasonic aspirators have made operative approaches to tumors in even the most remote corners of the CNS possible and reasonably safe. The goal of brain tumor surgery is to resect and cure the tumor completely. If surgical cure is not possible, such as in most gliomas, tumor bulk reduction and consequent decompression of the brain is the next goal and, when possible, should be the first therapeutic modality for the tumor.

An extremely important by-product of cytoreductive surgery is the acquisition of adequate tissue for histopathologic examination. Only rarely should brain tumors be treated with radiation or chemotherapy without a definitive tissue diagnosis. In patients with tumors that are believed to be inaccessible by open craniotomy or in patients for whom open craniotomy would not be helpful, a needle biopsy should be performed with guidance from CT, MRI, or ultrasound. CT-guided stereotaxy is the easiest method for obtaining tissue with a needle.

SURGICAL PLANNING

The intrinsic characteristics of a tumor's appearance and its relative position in the brain as shown on a technically adequate MRI scan can most often narrow the diagnostic possibilities to one or two choices, and a view of the tumor in several planes simplifies surgical planning.

For tumors that appear to be located in critical motor or language areas, functional MRI is becoming an important preoperative screening test to determine the feasibility of the surgery. If the surgery is deemed possible, the functional MRI scans are used in conjunction with intraoperative electrophysiologic mapping (see Craniotomy for Supratentorial Tumors, later in this chapter) to plan a safe approach to an intraaxial tumor.[30]

Cerebral angiography is sometimes useful in surgical planning for tumors that may encircle critical cerebral blood vessels, such as basal meningiomas, or for tumors that can be extremely vascular, such as hemangioblastomas, glomus tumors, and certain meningiomas. Angiography done in temporal proximity (24 to 96 hours) to the planned surgical procedure can be combined with embolization of the tumor's blood supply, in many instances making the surgical procedure technically easier.

The final selection of a surgical approach is made after adequate imaging, after developing a differential diagnosis, and after assessing the patient's general condition. In the era of modern neuroanesthesia, it is rare that a craniotomy must not be done because of poor general medical status. The design of an appropriate scalp incision and bone flap is the final preoperative decision.

PREOPERATIVE AND ANESTHETIC MANAGEMENT

Patients undergoing surgery for supratentorial tumors should be placed on anticonvulsants except in the case of surgery for brain metastasis without prior history of seizures. Corticosteroids (commonly dexamethasone) should be administered for a few days preoperatively, when possible, to reduce cerebral edema and thereby facilitate cerebral retraction for perfect exposure. Blood levels of anticonvulsants should be monitored to ensure that the therapeutic range has been achieved. Anticonvulsants should also be continued for at least 1 year. Corticosteroids should be continued into the postoperative period and then tapered, when possible. The anesthetic agents are selected for their lack of effect on intracranial pressure. In general, the head is held rigidly with pin fixation to minimize movement as the surgeon is looking through the operating microscope, where the slightest movement is dramatically amplified. As the procedure is about to commence, mannitol (1 g/kg body weight) is administered and hyperventilation to a pCO_2 of 25 to 30 mm Hg is accomplished for definitive reduction of the intracranial pressure in preparation for brain retraction.

CRANIOTOMY FOR SUPRATENTORIAL TUMORS

The bony opening is designed so that it is generous enough to facilitate surgery. The bone flap is centered over the tumor or positioned to provide access to the route of approach. In all instances, the scalp flap is designed to accommodate the bone flap fully, and the vascular supply to the scalp is given careful consideration in the design.

After the scalp incision is made and the scalp flap reflected, burr holes are drilled and connected with a power saw. The bone flap can be turned back, attached to the temporal muscle (osteoplastic flap) or its blood supply, or removed completely (free flap). The dura is opened only after the brain has been softened completely by mannitol diuresis and intraoperative hyperventilation. Sometimes a few minutes' wait is necessary to secure maximum decompression, and this brief pause can be critical to the success of the subsequent surgical approach.

The dura is reflected back, and the approach to the tumor is made. The surgeon can be confronted by a field of normal appearing and, in some areas, potentially critical functional cortical structures when seeking to resect a subcortical lesion. In this situation, mapping of cortical motor and speech function can be carried out intraoperatively using electrical stimulation of the cortex.[31] The preoperative functional MRI scan can serve as a guide. Motor mapping can be done in the anesthetized patient when muscle relaxants are not used during surgery, and an increasing number of glioma resections in the dominant hemisphere are being done under local anesthesia for the purpose of speech mapping.[31] Localization of subcortical tumors can be accomplished using intraoperative ultrasonography, but more recently, frameless image-guided interactive surgical systems have been developed.[32] With these systems, a preoperative MRI scan is done with markers on the patient's scalp, which at the time of surgery allow computer digitization of the images onto the patient's head. Placement of the system's probe at the time of surgery gives immediate feedback as to localization as visualized on the MRI. This sort of guidance is invaluable for the design of the craniotomy flap, the localization of the subcortical tumor, and even determination of the extent of tumor resection.

Tumor removal is usually done with grasping instruments, bipolar coagulation, and suction, but removal of firm, adherent, or calcified tumor tissue can be difficult and is simplified by use of the Cavitron ultrasonic aspirator (CUSA), which ultrasonically disrupts the tumor at its tip and sucks it away. Tumor in locations where access is limited (e.g., the third ventricle) and space to use graspers and other equipment is not available sometimes can be dealt with best by use of the CO_2 laser, which can vaporize tumor tissue with a hands-off technique. Tumor removal with a laser is slow, however, and is reserved for special circumstances.

In the rare situations in which brain swelling is worrisome at the time of closure, a catheter is left in the subdural space to measure the intracranial pressure. All patients are monitored in the intensive care unit for at least 1 night after surgery, and an MRI scan is done within 48 hours to evaluate the success of the tumor resection. Serum electrolyte levels and osmolality are measured frequently in the postoperative period to ensure that the patient is relatively dehydrated through the first several days and to detect the possible onset of inappropriate secretion of antidiuretic hormone or diabetes insipidus.

CRANIOTOMY FOR POSTERIOR FOSSA TUMORS

The occiput and, commonly, the dorsal aspects of C-1 and C-2 are exposed. A generous craniotomy is done unilaterally or bilaterally to accommodate an approach through the vermis or through, over, or around the cerebellar hemisphere. A laminectomy of C-1 and sometimes C-2 is done in certain midline approaches to improve tumor exposure or extend the decompression. The cisterna magna is opened to drain CSF and decompress the cerebellum before initiating retraction.

STEREOTACTIC TUMOR BIOPSY

For intrinsic tumors of the deep midline (e.g., pontine or corpus callosum gliomas), for deep tumors of the dominant hemisphere, or for diffuse nonfocal tumors, surgical resection is not practical. In these situations, needle biopsy for diagnosis is essential. There is no longer any reason to perform a full craniotomy for the purpose of biopsy only. Tissue can be obtained through a needle directed by hand through a burr hole under CT or MRI scan guidance or a needle directed by many devices that incorporate ultrasound images. However, in these authors' opinion, nothing is as simple or accurate as CT- or MRI-directed stereotactic biopsy.

A number of image-guided stereotactic systems are available.[33,34] Typically, the patient undergoes a CT or MRI scan with a rigid array of bars affixed tightly to the skull to minimize movement. In adults, local anesthesia usually is used; children usually require general anesthesia. The CT scan image demonstrates the lesion in which the biopsy will be performed and also the localizing rods, thereby relating the target to a volume encompassed by the rods. By digitizing the position of the target and the position of the rods, this relation is formalized, and the coordinates for a trajectory to the target are created in a way specific to the individual stereotactic system used.

The target is approached through a burr hole or a (smaller) twist drill hole. The biopsy instrument is guided to the target by use of an adjustable stereotactic arc that is placed on the head in fixed relation to the former position of the localizing rods used for the CT scan. A fragment of tissue is aspirated or grasped for removal, and a frozen section confirms the acquisition of diagnostic material and most often also suggests a working diagnosis. Experienced surgeons obtain diagnostic tissue in more than 95% of patients, and these patients stay only 1 night in the hospital.[34] The principal risk of the surgery, hemorrhage at the biopsy site, occurs in few patients. Occasionally, cerebral edema is exacerbated by the procedure.

RADIATION THERAPY

GENERAL CONSIDERATIONS

Most primary CNS neoplasms are unifocal; however, the more common brain tumors, such as the low-grade and malignant astrocytomas, are infiltrative into surrounding *normal* brain tissue for a distance of 1 to 3 cm or more. Radiotherapeutic approaches for these brain tumors generally consist of an initial dose to the enhancing disease (which contains solid tumor tissue) plus surrounding edema (which is comprised of normal brain infiltrated by microscopic tumor) plus a 2-cm margin of normal brain tissue followed by a boost dose to the enhancing tumor plus a 2-cm margin. Because of the penetrating nature of the high-energy radiation beams used in current practice, and the presence of a large amount of normal brain tissue in the edema and margin, substantial amounts of normal tissue are often irradiated in the typical patient receiving high-dose radiation with curative intent. The tolerance of the normal brain (and spinal cord in the case of cord tumors) may then be a limiting factor to achieving local control and cure of a CNS neoplasm.

TOLERANCE OF THE BRAIN

Adverse reactions associated with cranial irradiation differ in their pathogenesis and can be temporally classified into (1) acute reactions that occur during or shortly after radiation therapy; (2) early delayed reactions that appear within a few weeks to 4 months after irradiation; and (3) late delayed injuries that develop several months to years after treatment.[35]

Acute reactions are thought to be caused by radiation-induced edema. Within a few hours after the first fraction of radiation, patients may develop headache, nausea, vomiting, somnolence, fever, and worsening neurologic symptoms. Symptoms occur most commonly after large dose fractions (3.0 to 6.0 Gy) are delivered to a large volume of the brain in patients with increased intracranial pressure from primary or metastatic brain tumors. Thus, if symptoms of increased intracranial pressure are present, patients undergoing cranial irradiation should be protected with corticosteroids, administered for at least 48 to 72 hours before beginning treatment.[36] When larger fractions (7.5 Gy or more) are used, this disorder may culminate in abrupt neurologic deterioration or death.[35] However, with conventional daily fractions of 1.8 to 2.0 Gy, the acute radiation reaction most commonly presents as mild headache and nausea, becoming progressively less severe with each succeeding fraction.[36] Treatment with hyperfractionated irradiation schedules of 0.9 to 1.2 Gy, two or three times daily and accelerated fractionation programs of 1.6 to 2.0 Gy given two or three times daily delivered to a portion of the brain are also well tolerated.[35]

The early delayed reaction is thought to result from temporary demyelination caused by the effects of radiation on oligodendroglial cells[37] or radiation-induced changes in capillary permeability.[36] It is characterized by transient neurologic deterioration, somnolence, and an exacerbation of tumor-associated signs and symptoms depending on the presence or absence of an underlying brain tumor, the volume of brain irradiation, and the dose delivered.[35] In patients with brain tumors, perilesional vascular abnormalities and tumor necrosis may induce clinical and radiographic changes that are indistinguishable from tumor progression. Although signs and symptoms are usually mild, corticosteroid therapy and intensive medical support may be required. The appearance of new findings during this early posttreatment interval does not always indicate that the tumor has recurred or that a change in therapy is needed; observation is often the only way to distinguish this situation from tumor progression.

Late delayed radiation injuries make up the most serious complications of therapeutic irradiation on the brain and vary in their appearance and severity from asymptomatic white matter changes to potentially fatal necrosis. Late radiation injury has been attributed to vascular endothelial injury or to a direct effect on oligodendroglial cells, and multiple mechanisms are probably involved.[35] The late delayed reaction presents as a focal or as a diffuse white matter injury that may occur together in the same patient. The clinical presentation depends on the site and volume of the brain exposed. Patients with focal radiation necrosis present with localizing neurologic signs, often accompanied by symptoms of increased intracranial pressure. Focal hypodensity or a contrast-enhancing mass

TABLE 43.2-11. Factors Associated with Radiation Tolerance of the Normal Central Nervous System (CNS) Tissues

Factor[a]	*Factors for Increased Risk of Injury*	*Tolerance Increased by*
Total dose	Higher total dose	Decreasing total dose, hyperfractionation,[b] radiosensitizers
Dose per fraction	Dose per fraction >180–200 cGy	Decreasing dose/fraction to <180–200 cGy
Volume	Increased volume (e.g., whole organ radiation)	Decreasing volume (e.g., partial organ radiation)
Host factors	Medical illness (e.g., hypertension, diabetes)	Unknown, possibly radioprotectors
Beam quality	High LET radiation beams (e.g., neutrons)	Low LET beams (e.g., photons)
Adjunctive therapy	Concomitant use of CNS toxic drugs (e.g., methotrexate)	Avoid concomitant use of CNS toxic drugs or use sequentially

LET, linear energy transfer.
[a]Total time is not a major determinant of normal CNS tissue tolerance.
[b]Defined as multiple daily fractions, usually two with doses per fraction of less than or equal to 180 to 200 cGy, usually 100 to 120 cGy, separated by 4 to 8 hours, to total doses higher than those given with standard fractionation.
(Data from refs. 35 and 38.)

with surrounding vasogenic edema may be seen on CT scan. MRI shows a contrast-enhancing mass with focal and confluent white matter alterations on T2-weighted images. Diffuse white matter injury typically occurs after large-volume or whole brain irradiation. Clinical features range from seizure disorders and varying degrees of neuropsychological impairment to incapacitating dementia. Diffuse white matter hypodensity is seen on CT scan, often accompanied by a focal enhancing mass, whereas T2-weighted MRI shows diffuse periventricular white matter hyperintensity. Cerebral cortical atrophy, probably a late finding related to diffuse white matter injury, is observed in 17% to 39% of patients who receive whole brain irradiation with chemotherapy for malignant gliomas. Enlarged cerebral sulci and ventricles are seen in neuroimaging studies.[36] The pathogenesis of this formal radiation damage is uncertain.[36] Rarely, therapeutic irradiation causes an intracranial vessel occlusive vasculopathy or secondary neoplasia.

The tolerance of the brain depends on the size of the dose per fraction, total dose administered, overall treatment time, volume of brain irradiated, host factors, and adjunctive therapies. The probability of injury increases with larger daily doses (2.2 Gy per fraction) and doses in excess of 60 Gy delivered in 30 fractions over approximately 6 weeks. Table 43.2-11 defines the role of these factors in radiation tolerance and injury to the normal CNS tissues, as well as ways they might be modified to increase tolerance (i.e., reduce injury).[35,38] Sheline and associates suggested that the threshold doses for brain injury are approximately 35 Gy for 10 fractions, 60 Gy for 35 fractions, and 76 Gy for 60 fractions.[39] They further demonstrated that the isoeffective dose (termed *neuret*) formula should have an exponent of N = 0.41 and an exponent of T = 0.03 (where N is the number of fractions and T is the total time in days). This formula may not be applicable to extremely small or large numbers of fractions or to extremely short or long overall treatment times. Based on models such as these, the TD 5/5 (a 5% complication rate in 5 years) for the whole brain is between 40 and 60 Gy, for part of the brain is 50 to 10 Gy, and for a 10-cm segment of spinal cord is 45 to 50 Gy (see discussion of spinal cord tolerance in this section), as shown in Table 43.2-12. Although the TD 50/5 (a 50% complication rate in 5 years) for spinal cord is reportedly lower than that of brain, there are not good data to support this difference. Rather, the sequelae of spinal cord radiation injury are perceived as greater than those of brain injury, therefore tolerance doses have been arbitrarily lowered. In clinical practice, TD 5/5's of 60 Gy for partial brain and 50 Gy for a limited segment of spinal cord are commonly used.

The TD 5/5's given for brain and spinal cord tolerance assume a *standard* fraction size of 180 to 200 cGy/d. For primary CNS tumor patients being treated with curative intent, fraction size should rarely exceed 200 cGy daily, and in most situations, should be 150 to 200 cGy. Fraction sizes greater than 200 cGy daily (usually 250 to 300 cGy) are commonly used for

TABLE 43.2-12. Tolerance Doses (TD) for Normal Central Nervous System Tissues at 2 Gy Per Fraction over 5 Days per Week

Central Nervous System Tissue	*TD 5/5 (Gy)*	*TD 50/5 (Gy)*	*End Point*
RUBIN ET AL.[40]			
Brain			Infarction, necrosis
Whole	60	70	
Partial (25%)	70	80	
Spinal cord			Infarction, necrosis
Partial (10-cm length)	45	55	
EMAMI ET AL.[447]			
Brain			Infarction, necrosis
One-third	60	75	
Two-thirds	50	65	
Whole	40	60	
Brain stem			Infarction, necrosis
One-third	60	—	
Two-thirds	53	—	
Whole	50	65	
Spinal cord			Myelitis, necrosis
5 cm	50	70	
10 cm	50	70	
20 cm	47	—	
Cauda equina damage	60	75	Clinically apparent nerve
Brachial plexus damage			Clinically apparent nerve
One-third	62	77	
Two-thirds	61	76	
Whole	60	75	

TABLE 43.2-13. Tolerance Doses (TD) for Miscellaneous Normal Tissues of the Cranium

Normal Tissue	*TD 5/5 (Gy)*	*TD 50/5 (Gy)*	*Manifestations of Severe Injury*
Ear (middle/ external)	30–55	40–65	Acute or chronic serous otitis
Eye			
Retina	45	65	Blindness
Lens	10	18	Cataract formation
Optic nerve or chiasm	50	65	Blindness

(Data from refs. 41–43 and 447.)

palliation of brain metastases and spinal cord compression, but only because such patients are not expected to live long enough to manifest normal tissue injury.

Table 43.2-13 shows the tolerance doses for other normal tissues of the CNS, including the brain stem, eye, ear, optic chiasm, optic nerve, and pituitary gland. The clinical manifestations of severe injury to these structures is listed.[40–43]

Approximately 4% to 9% of patients treated to 50 to 60 Gy with conventional fractionated radiation for brain tumors develop clinically detectable focal radiation necrosis, but this form of injury may be found in as many as 10% to 22% of patients at autopsy. A review by Marks and colleagues of 139 patients who received irradiation for primary brain tumors with at least 45 Gy in daily dose fractions of 1.8 to 2.0 Gy disclosed 7 patients (5%) with brain necrosis.[44] A recalculation of their data, assuming a daily dose of 1.8 Gy given five times per week, demonstrated that the incidence of necrosis was directly related to dose. Of 51 patients who received total doses of 57.6 Gy or less, there were no cases of necrosis. Two of 60 patients (3%) who received between 57.6 and 64.8 Gy developed necrosis, and 5 of 28 patients (18%) who received 64.8 to 75.6 Gy developed necrosis.[45]

Several additional factors may affect the radiation tolerance of the brain. Children younger than 2 to 3 years of age are thought to be more susceptible to injury than are adults because of incomplete development of the CNS.[39] Vasculopathy associated with endocrine disorders, CNS infection, and cerebral edema also appear to potentiate the effects of radiation.

The risk of injury may be amplified by some chemotherapeutic agents. The most dramatic illustration of the toxicity of combined modality therapy was observed in children with acute lymphoblastic leukemia treated with prophylactic brain irradiation and methotrexate administered intravenously and intrathecally. Two delayed syndromes, necrotizing leukoencephalopathy and mineralizing microangiopathy, have been recognized in children who received 24 Gy in 1.5 to 2.0 Gy daily increments, which without chemotherapy are well below tolerance levels. Although necrotizing leukoencephalopathy has not been reported with a dose of 24 Gy in the absence of chemotherapy and occurs in fewer than 1% to 2% of patients receiving intrathecal and high-dose intravenous methotrexate, the incidence with all three therapies combined is as high as 45%.[46] It is currently recognized that methotrexate is most toxic when given during or after radiation therapy, and attention to this detail has reduced the frequency of this complication significantly.

Radiation and chemotherapy-induced changes are often indistinguishable from tumor recurrence on CT. By MRI the changes are better defined and can be more easily anticipated, nevertheless, at time the radiographic diagnosis of radiation necrosis may be difficult to confirm. Thallium 201 single-photon emission CT, ^{18}F fluorodeoxyglucose positron emission tomography, and dynamic contrast-enhanced MRI[47] studies may help separate patients with radiation and chemotherapy necrosis from those with recurrent tumor. However, because most patients have a mixture of necrosis and tumor, a biopsy may be required to confirm the diagnosis, especially when the injury occurs at or near the tumor site.

Corticosteroids may improve or stabilize the neurologic symptoms associated with the effects of radiation and radiation with chemotherapy injury. Surgical resection is often beneficial to patients with favorably situated, focal radiation-induced lesions who deteriorate neurologically and become dependent on corticosteroids.[48] While anticoagulation has been suggested as a therapeutic alternative when surgery is not feasible, a clinical trial that demonstrates real benefit to the patient is lacking at present. In unpublished trials, we and others have tried vitamin E, pentoxifylline (Trental), aspirin, *cis*-retinoic acid, heparin, coumadin, and enoxaparin (Lovenox) without conclusive evidence of reproducible benefit. As an anecdote, the occasional patient appears to benefit from anticoagulation,[49] *cis*-retinoic acid, or both.

Decreased levels of intellectual function have been observed after cranial irradiation in children and adults with acute lymphoblastic leukemia, small cell lung carcinoma, and primary brain tumors. IQ decrements and perceptual and learning disabilities seen after CNS prophylaxis in children with acute lymphoblastic leukemia have long been attributed to cranial irradiation. However, a study comparing the long-term cognitive outcome of children treated with 18 or 24 Gy and intrathecal methotrexate or intrathecal and intravenous methotrexate without cranial irradiation failed to demonstrate an overall decline in verbal, performance, or full-scale IQ in any of the three groups, although 22% to 30% of children in each group showed at least a 15-point decline in IQ during the study period. The authors proposed that ecologic factors or continuation phase chemotherapy rather than radiation therapy might account for the IQ changes.[50]

Neuropsychological deterioration has been recognized in long-term surviving patients with small cell lung carcinoma who receive prophylactic cranial irradiation. These patients are treated with a variety of chemotherapeutic agents that may enhance the effects of radiation on the CNS. The risk and severity of impairment appear to be related to radiation dose and fraction size and to the type, sequence, and dose intensity of the chemotherapeutic agents used.

Children irradiated for brain tumors have IQ decrements and behavioral disturbances. Most require formal psychological intervention and special education programs. Young age at treatment, supratentorial tumor sites, the use of whole brain irradiation, poorly controlled seizure disorders, the presence of sensorimotor deficits, and the addition of chemotherapy have a negative influence on IQ.[51] The risk and severity of neuropsychological dysfunction are also affected by psychological stress, reduced school attendance, and the adequacy of rehabilitative efforts.[52]

Cranial irradiation also leads to intellectual impairment in adults. Unlike in children, however, only a limited amount of quantitative information is available, especially for patients treated with radiation therapy alone. Patients in whom a substantial portion of the brain is irradiated frequently develop recent memory loss and difficulty with attending to tasks that may prevent their return to gainful employment. Impairment is most pronounced in those patients who have had chemotherapy and whole brain irradiation.[52] We found that approximately 60% of long-term survivors irradiated for gliomas were able to be employed at occupations comparable with those they held before treatment.[53] As expected, patients irradiated with partial brain fields had superior memory function and better employment histories than those treated with whole brain fields. Decrements in tests of new learning ability, recent memory, abstraction, and problem solving have been observed in patients who fail to retain their premorbid social or occupational level of function.[51] Early return to work after treatment may lead to improvement or recovery of neuropsychological function.

Radiation therapy may cause hypothalamic-pituitary dysfunction, and the incidence and degree of hormone suppression appear to be dose related.[41] Growth hormone deficiency, the most frequent endocrine dysfunction observed after radiation therapy, can occur after doses as low as 18 Gy. Deficiencies of gonadotrophins, thyroid-stimulating hormone, and adrenocorticotrophins as well as hyperprolactinemia can be seen with doses in excess of 40 Gy.[41] Patients at risk for neuroendocrinologic sequelae should be evaluated for pituitary function before, and periodically after, irradiation. Early detection of a deficiency permits appropriate hormonal replacement therapy before irreversible damage has occurred.

TOLERANCE OF THE SPINAL CORD

Radiation myelopathy may present as a transient early delayed or as a more ominous late delayed reaction. Transient radiation myelopathy is clinically manifested by momentary, electrical shock-like paresthesias or numbness radiating from the neck to the extremities, precipitated by neck flexion (Lhermitte's sign). The syndrome develops after an average latent period of 3 to 4 months and gradually resolves over the ensuing 3 to 6 months without the need for specific therapy. These findings have been attributed to transient demyelination caused by radiation-induced inhibition of myelin-producing oligodendroglial cells in the irradiated cord segment. An alternative hypothesis suggests that radiation induces a transient disruption of the blood-spinal cord barrier, resulting in vasogenic edema, which in turn leads to demyelination.[5]

Radiation myelopathy is one of the most feared complications in clinical radiotherapy. In addition to its obvious neurologic sequelae, nearly 50% of patients die from secondary complications.[54] The latent period between the completion of radiation therapy and the onset of symptoms is bimodal in distribution, with the first peak occurring at 12 to 14 months and the second occurring at 24 to 28 months. Demyelination and white matter necrosis due to a direct effect on oligodendroglial cells and intramedullary microvascular injury each play a role in the pathogenesis of radiation myelopathy. In addition, microglia, astrocytes, and the release of cytokines are also involved.[38] It is probable that multiple mechanisms exist and that the relative contribution of each depends on radiation dose and other factors. The signs and symptoms that accompany radiation myelopathy are irreversible. They may be partial in some patients, whereas in others there is progressive functional loss that becomes complete over several months. Less commonly, radiation myelopathy is manifested by the acute onset of paraplegia or quadriplegia that evolves over several hours or a few days, resulting from infarction of the cord. Myelopathy may also be heralded by lower motor neuron dysfunction due to selective injury to anterior horn cells.

The diagnosis of radiation myelopathy requires a history of radiation therapy in doses sufficient to result in injury. The portion of the cord irradiated must be slightly above the dermatome level of expression of the lesion, and the latent period from the completion of treatment to the onset of injury must be consistent with that observed in radiation myelopathy. There are no confirmatory laboratory tests or imaging studies that distinguish radiation myelopathy from other spinal cord lesions. MRI findings include swelling of the cord with decreased intensity in T1-weighted and hyperintensity in T2-weighted images.[55] The diagnosis is often one of exclusion.

The medical and legal consequences of radiation myelopathy are such that treatment with radiation therapy is often compromised to keep the spinal cord dose within a safe level.[56] A dose of 45 Gy in 22 fractions over 5 weeks usually is considered to be safe, the risk of myelopathy being less than 0.2%,[38,56] well below the steep portion of the dose-response curve.[56] It is estimated that with conventionally fractionated irradiation (1.8 to 2.0 Gy per fraction, five fractions per week), the incidence of myelopathy is 5% for doses in the range of 57 to 61 Gy and 50% for doses of 68 to 73 Gy.[38] There is no convincing evidence that the cervical and thoracic cord differ in their radiosensitivity. The belief that the cervical cord is more tolerant than the thoracic cord probably arose from differences in biologic dose resulting from the practice of treating with one field per day, which was common through the mid-1970s.[57] There appears to be little change in tolerance with variations in the length of cord irradiated.[38]

Various isoeffect formulas have been proposed for the spinal cord. Wara and coworkers, for example, derived a formula with an exponent of $N = -0.377$ and an exponent of $T = -0.058$.[58] These formulas suggest that in addition to the total dose given, radiation myelopathy is related to the size of the individual daily dose and predict that spinal cord tolerance will continue to increase with decreasing fraction size. However, data indicate that reducing the fraction size to lower than 2 Gy does not alter the dose response significantly. Furthermore, because radiation damage is not completely repaired between multiple daily fractions, extrapolating from a conventionally fractionated cord dose to an equivalent hyperfractionated cord dose using any biomathematical formula should be approached with caution. A dose of 45 Gy in twice daily fractions of 1.2 Gy with an interfraction interval of 6 hours appears safe.[38] Interestingly, experimental animal studies suggest that the majority of occult lesions caused by a dose of 44 Gy in 20 fractions is revealed within 2 years. This may have implications on treatment recommendations for previously treated patients.[38]

CENTRAL NERVOUS SYSTEM RADIOTHERAPY TOXICITY SCORING SYSTEMS

The most commonly used system for scoring radiation-associated acute and chronic CNS toxicity is that of the Radiation Therapy Oncology Group (RTOG) and its European counterpart, the European Organization for the Research and Treatment of Cancer (EORTC), and is shown in Table 43.2-14.[59] Pavy et al. have proposed a more sophisticated system for scor-

TABLE 43.2-14. Central Nervous System (CNS) Toxicity Levels of the Radiation Therapy Oncology Group and the European Organization for the Research and Treatment of Cancer[a]

ACUTE TOXICITY GRADE, BRAIN			
1: Fully functional status (i.e., able to work) with minor neurologic findings; no medication needed	2: Neurologic findings sufficient to require home care; nursing assistance may be required; medications including corticosteroids and antiseizure agents may be required	3: Neurologic findings requiring hospitalization for initial management	4: Serious neurologic impairment that includes paralysis, coma, or seizures >3 per week despite medication and/or hospitalization required
CHRONIC TOXICITY GRADE, BRAIN			
1: Mild headache; slight lethargy	2: Moderate headache; great lethargy	3: Severe headaches; severe CNS dysfunction (partial loss of power or dyskinesia)	4: Seizure or paralysis; coma
CHRONIC TOXICITY GRADE, SPINAL CORD			
1: Mild Lhermitte's syndrome	2: Severe Lhermitte's syndrome	3: Objective neurologic findings at or below cord level treated	4: Monoplegia, paraplegia, or quadriplegia

[a]Grade 0 toxicity, none; grade 1, mild; grade 2, moderate; grade 3, severe; grade 4, life threatening; grade 5, fatal.
(From ref. 59, with permission.)

ing radiation toxicity, called Late Effects on Normal Tissues (LENT), in which they describe four components for each toxicity, including the subjective, objective, management, and analytical (SOMA) components.[60] The LENT/SOMA system is currently being validated by the RTOG and may eventually replace the RTOG/EORTC system.

TUMOR TARGET VOLUME AND TREATMENT TECHNIQUES

The appropriate volume to encompass within the radiation treatment portal varies according to the specific histopathologic tumor type and, with certain histologies, is a topic of considerable controversy. Because their tendency to infiltrate beyond the lesional borders visualized by neuroimaging studies is limited, certain tumors, such as benign meningiomas, pituitary adenomas, craniopharyngiomas, and acoustic neurilemmomas, may be treated with narrow margins of surrounding normal tissue. In contrast, the astrocytic gliomas require larger margins for uncertainty because of their tendency to infiltrate beyond the identifiable tumor periphery. Improved imaging techniques and a better understanding of recurrence patterns have fostered the use of limited radiation portals rather than whole brain irradiation for malignant gliomas. Comparisons of CT and MRI studies with clinical and pathologic findings have shown that (1) malignant gliomas are localized, and microscopic invasion of the perilesional brain is limited at the time of initial diagnosis[61]; (2) only 1.1% of patients present with multiple lesions[62]; (3) after initial treatment, most of these lesions, when they recur, do so at their original location[63]; and (4) isolated tumor cell infiltration may extend to the periphery of T2-weighted MRI abnormalities.[64] Clinical studies have failed to demonstrate that irradiating the whole brain is superior to treating more limited fields,[45] and patients surviving for extended periods after whole brain irradiation, especially in combination with chemotherapy, may experience considerable treatment-related morbidity.[52] Until the primary tumor can be controlled with greater frequency, and the patterns of failure in such patients suggest that local fields are unjustified, there is little rationale for treating the whole brain.

The radiation beam energy and field arrangements are selected after consideration of the location of the tumor within the brain and the geometry of the target volume. The across target volume is defined as a three-dimensional reconstruction of the tumor contour based on operative findings and data from CT and MRI studies. The planning target volume consists of the volume of tissue that must be irradiated to encompass the tumor volume with a margin of surrounding tissue considered to be at risk for microscopic tumor spread and to account for patient movement and daily set-up uncertainties. Depending on tumor size and location, treatment portals may be coaxially opposed or designed in a more complex fashion, using multiple or rotational fields with wedge filters. Three-dimensional conformal radiation therapy and the advanced technique of intensity modulated radiation therapy (see Chapter 29.4) are new methods of treatment planning and delivery designed to enhance the conformation of the dose to the target volume, while maximally restricting the dose delivered to the normal tissue outside the treatment volume. In the future, these techniques may improve the outcome of patients with brain tumors by allowing higher than traditional radiation doses to be administered safely. Megavoltage equipment with energies ranging from cobalt 60 to 15 MV photons is used to administer radiation therapy. Treatment is generally given in daily fractions of 1.8 to 2.0 Gy/d five times per week. In this chapter, the total doses referred to assume that a *conventional* fractionation scheme is used unless otherwise specified.

Certain neoplasms, such as medulloblastomas and other primitive neuroectodermal tumors as well as some ependymomas and germ cell tumors, require treatment to the entire craniospinal axis. Patients are treated prone in an immobilization cast to ensure daily positional reproducibility. The intracranial contents, including the upper one or two segments of the cervical cord, are treated through parallel opposed lateral fields. The spine is treated through one or two posterior fields, depending on the size of the patient. The collimator for the lateral cranial fields is angled to match the divergence of the upper border of the adjacent spinal field, and the treatment couch is angulated so that the inferior border of the cranial field is perpendicular to the superior edge of the spinal field. Individualized focused blocks protect the normal extracranial head and neck tissues from the primary radiation beam. The cranial and posterior spine fields may be abutted, but a gap of 0.5 to 1.0 cm is often left between the fields. When two posterior spinal fields are used, as is usually the case, a gap is calculated so that the 50% isodose lines meet at the level of the spinal cord. All junction lines are moved 0.5 to 1.0 cm daily or at least every 10 Gy to avoid overdosing or underdosing segments of the cord. This is accomplished by expanding the lateral cranial fields and moving the posterior spine fields caudally without changing their dimensions. A fixed block is placed at the inferior margin of the caudal spinal field to keep the lower margin of the irradiated volume at the same location. Several modifications of this approach are used in clinical practice.

Radiosurgery is being used to treat a diverse group of intracranial lesions, including small arteriovenous malformations, pituitary adenomas, acoustic neurinomas, meningiomas, gliomas, and brain metastases. Radiosurgery is a method of highly focal, closed skull external irradiation that uses an imaging-compatible stereotactic device for precise target localization. The relationship between the stereotactic coordinate system and the radiation source(s) allows accurate delivery of radiation to the target volume. Radiosurgery can be administered by gamma knife units, made up of multiple cobalt beams, and by modified linear accelerators. This technique is designed to deliver a high radiation dose to an intracranial target in a single session without delivering significant radiation to adjacent normal tissues. The dose that can be safely administered in a single fraction is limited by the volume irradiated, and to maintain a steep dose gradient at the edge of the field, the application of radiosurgery is restricted to lesions measuring 4 cm or less in diameter.

Radiosurgery may be delivered in a fractionated dose schedule using stereotactic radiosurgery hardware and software and head frames that can be relocalized daily in a reproducible fashion. This approach is referred to as *stereotactic radiotherapy* or *fractionated radiosurgery*. Because fractionating the radiation dose improves the therapeutic ratio, larger tumors and those located within or adjacent to critical intracranial structures are suitable for this treatment technique. This approach is being applied to the treatment of malignant gliomas, craniopharyngiomas, pituitary adenomas, small optic tract tumors, and as a boost for medulloblastomas.

CHEMOTHERAPY

GENERAL PHARMACOLOGIC CONSIDERATIONS

The use of anticancer agents in the treatment of intracranial and spinal tumors is established for many primary tumors. For parenchymal CNS tumors, however, controversy surrounds the concept of limited antitumor efficacy for agents with restricted blood–brain barrier permeability,[65] supporting the concept is the fact that many infiltrative primary CNS tumors (e.g., gliomas) have cellular regions within the brain with apparently intact normal-appearing brain capillaries. In addition, the actual extent of capillary breakdown accounting for the leakage responsible for positive-contrast CT and MRI as well as radionuclide brain scans is small.[66] Although drug delivery to portions of any primary tumor would be expected to occur to the same extent as with non-CNS tumors, delivery (by diffusion) to infiltrative regions distant from leaky tumor capillaries would be expected to be compromised. Diffusion, being a slow process, cannot achieve significant drug concentrations, unless plasma drug levels are sustainable for prolonged periods, and the diffusing drug is relatively stable in the tumor tissue as it diffuses.

A secondary supporting argument is that most agents with antitumor activity against CNS tumors readily cross the blood–brain barrier.[67] For example, all of the non–sugar-containing chloroethylnitrosoureas such as bischloroethylnitrosourea (BCNU), lomustine (CCNU), [1-(2-chloroethyl)-3-(2,5-dioxo-3-piperidyl)-1-nitrosourea] (PCNU), and nimustine (ACNU) have shown efficacy as single agents, whereas sugar-containing chloroethylnitrosoureas are less effective.[25] Procarbazine and a new agent, temozolomide (Temodar), also cross the blood–brain barrier and are active. Agents such as bleomycin, doxorubicin, cisplatin, vincristine (VCR), and mithramycin do not readily cross the blood–brain barrier and have shown limited activity against gliomas and have limited activity against primitive childhood and embryonal tumors.

Whether ease of blood–brain barrier passage constitutes an absolute or relative advantage is somewhat academic, given the paucity of chemotypes with demonstrable antitumor activity. Even a small pharmacokinetic disadvantage takes on disproportionate importance when the selective cytotoxicity of a drug is small. This may well be the case with many of the drugs used, because they share narrow therapeutic indices because of dose-limiting systemic toxicity.

Finally, with respect to drugs for CNS tumors, many of the available anticancer drugs can be toxic to the CNS if given at extremely high doses or when given in a manner to circumvent the blood–brain barrier.[68,69] The blood–brain barrier exists to protect the brain from many potentially toxic compounds. If the blood–brain barrier did not exist, CNS toxicity rather than myelotoxicity or gastrointestinal toxicity would be dose limiting for most drugs.

Pharmacokinetic considerations for intracranial nonparenchymal tumors and extramedullary spinal tumors are less dependent on the ability to cross the blood–brain barrier readily, because many of these tumors gain blood supply from meningeal blood vessels that are significantly more permeable than those of the brain.

REGIONAL DRUG DELIVERY CONSIDERATIONS

Under most circumstances regional drug delivery produces greater drug exposure than does systemic intravenous or oral administration. With respect to intracranial and spinal tumors, the regional delivery takes the form of intra-CSF therapy, intraarterial infusion, and intratumoral therapy.

Therapy by the CSF route (usually by ventricular reservoir) is a form of regional drug delivery that is used to treat meningeal neoplasia resulting from primary or secondary tumor invasion of the subarachnoid space and, less commonly, one of the ventricular cavities. It is often, but not always, associated with malignant cells floating in the CSF.

The advantages of intra-CSF therapy are high local drug levels; low systemic toxicity; and the ability to increase the frequency of treatments. However, delivery of drugs through the CSF can be dangerous and is associated with a high morbidity. The drugs commonly used are methotrexate, cytarabine, and thiotepa. All three drugs have been reported to produce CNS damage ranging from fever and chills to leukoencephalopathy and myelitis. Efficacy is limited when gross lesions exist (greater than or equal to 5 mm diameter) or when CSF pathways are blocked and CSF flows are diverted.

Of concern in the use of CSF therapy is that slow clearance of drug can lead to increased neurotoxicity. Normally, these authors find, after injection into a ventricular reservoir and pumping the reservoir five times, the CSF distribution and flow of radionuclide-labeled albumin in the ventricle is well distributed and the half-time from ventricle to cisterna magnum is approximately 60 minutes. In many instances, obvious hydrocephalus is not apparent by neuroimaging, but a physiologic slowing of CSF flow (and presumably CSF absorption) is present. This slowing of CSF flow can lead to poor distribution in the subarachnoid CSF for drugs with high capillary clearance, such as cytarabine, and a greater likelihood of serious CNS toxicity for a drug such as methotrexate.

Another form of regional therapy is the intraarterial administration of anticancer drugs through carotid or vertebral arteries. The advantage of this approach is an increased uptake during the first passage of drug through tumor capillaries. Increased efficacy would be expected for patients whose tumors reside within the perfusion territory of the infused artery. Contrary to what may be thought, systemic toxicity is not reduced unless the total administered dose is reduced, because the actual amount of drug taken up into the tumor is a small fraction of the injected dose. On the other hand, focal brain and retinal morbidity are increased, as was demonstrated by the clinical trials with BCNU[70] and cisplatin.[71] Controversial results of clinical trials do not commend this form of treatment, except under controlled experimental conditions.

Intratumoral therapy is regional therapy that is applicable for cystic tumors or postsurgical cavities with a narrow rim of surrounding tumor. Pharmacokinetic considerations implicate problems with maintenance of tumor cavity drug levels if the goal is to maintain a concentration in the cavity as a drug source for diffusion into the surrounding tumor and brain. These problems relate to conservation of mass, diffusion distances from the cavity to the outer margin of tumor, nonspecific biodegradation and binding of drug or drug products, and the need for repeat treatments. Modern clinical trials evaluating this form of regional therapy have not been published.

Another intratumoral approach uses a biodegradable drug-containing polymer that allows zero order release of drug that can diffuse into the surrounding tumor and brain. This approach, using BCNU (the Gliadel wafer system) has received approval by the Food and Drug Administration for use in patients with glioblastoma multiforme at recurrence. Patient survival benefit is modest in published clinical trials.[72]

CEREBRAL ASTROCYTOMAS

PATHOLOGY CLASSIFICATION

This section deals primarily with the classification of astrocytomas of varying degrees of aggressiveness, ranging from juvenile pilocytic astrocytoma to glioblastoma multiforme. The slower growing or less aggressive lesions are often referred to as low grade or benign and the more rapidly progressive neoplasms are referred to as high grade or malignant. With the exception of juvenile pilocytic astrocytomas, subependymomas, and the limited number of astrocytomas that can be completely resected, even *benign* astrocytomas are highly lethal. For instance, median 5-year survival for low-grade infiltrating astrocytomas ranges between 21% and 55% following surgery and the 10-year survival between 10% and 43%. For patients with residual tumor after surgery, irradiation increases survival from an average 30% at 5 years to 49%.[73] Median survival for glioblastoma multiforme, on the other hand, ranges between 42 and 60 weeks (Table 43.2-15 for later studies).

Many classification systems for astrocytomas have been advanced that have advocated the presumed cell of origin, the degree of malignancy, or both. Most common classification schemas in use over the past two decades have been modifications of that developed by Ringertz.[74] A slightly different approach was proposed by Daumas-Duport and colleagues. Their grading system assigned a point system to nuclear atypia, mitoses, endothelial proliferation, and necrosis.[75] Grade I tumors had none of these features, grade II had one feature, grade III had two features, and grade IV had three or more features. While in their initial evaluation, this grouping led to distinct and separate median survival curves, a subsequent review of 251 cases at the Massachusetts General Hospital found no

TABLE 43.2-15. Survival for Adult Glioblastoma Multiforme Patients with Karnofsky Performance Scores Greater Than or Equal to 60 Treated on Protocols Published Since 1990

Radiation Therapy	*Chemotherapy during Radiation*	*Postradiation Chemotherapy*	*50% Survival (wk)*	*25% Survival (wk)*	*Reference*
60 Gy WB	Hydroxyurea	BCNU	57	71	448
60 Gy WB	Hydroxyurea	PCV	53	94	448
60 Gy LF	—	PCB/VCR-BCNU/FU	50	na (59)[a]	449
60 Gy LF	Bromodeoxyuridine	PCV	62	104	103
57 Gy AF-LF	Carboplatin	PCV	55	91	450
57 Gy AF-LF	Bromodeoxyuridine	PCV	57	79	115
60 Gy LF	Hydroxyurea	6TG/BCNU	56	120	149
60 Gy LF	Hydroxyurea or none	DFMO/PCV	58	78	451
		PCV	60	82	
Radiation therapy followed by brachytherapy	None	PCV[b]	88	142	126

AF, accelerated fractionated irradiation; BCNU, bischloroethylnitrosourea; CDDP, *cis*-diaminedichloroplatinum; DFMO, difluoromethylornithine; FU, fluorouracil; LF, limited field radiation; PCB, procarbazine; PCV, lomustine, procarbazine, vincristine; 6TG, 6-thioguanine; na, not available; VCR, vincristine; WB, whole brain irradiation.
[a]Only time to tumor progression available.
[b]Of the 106 patients, the majority received PCV following combined external beam and brachytherapy; tumor size and location selection bias differed from the other studies cited.

statistical difference in survival between grades II and III.[76] Necrosis was found to be a significant predictor of short survival, in agreement with previous studies.[77] The most recent grading system is that proposed by the World Health Organization.[74] For practical purposes, a three-tier system is generally satisfactory for infiltrative adult astrocytomas:

- Astocytoma (includes fibrillary, protoplasmic, gemistocytic)
- Astic (malignant) astrocytoma
- Glioblastoma multiforme (includes gliosarcoma and giant cell glioblastoma)

RATIONALE FOR SURGERY

Data from animal experiments suggest, and a large clinical experience with tumors at many sites would confirm, that maximal surgical resection improves the results of subsequent radiation therapy and chemotherapy. This principle is transferable to the treatment of astrocytomas. Gross total surgical resection was among the dominant factors favoring longer survival in patients with grade I or II astrocytomas treated at the Mayo Clinic[78] and in patients with the more malignant astrocytomas.[79,80] If one takes a different perspective and looks at the amount of tumor present on the postoperative CT scan and compares it with survival it can be shown that the two are inversely related even comparing for other variables.[81–83]

A number of factors might be responsible for the improved clinical outcome when astrocytomas are aggressively resected. An assiduous resection can remove 90% of a typical astrocytoma (1-log cell-kill) and thereby decompress the brain as well as substantially reducing the tumor cell burden. In addition, a large tumor mass left in the brain can serve as a nidus for cerebral edema after radiation therapy because of the indolent removal of dead cells from the brain.[84,85]

SURGICAL PRINCIPLES FOR CEREBRAL ASTROCYTOMAS

The goal of every craniotomy for a cerebral astrocytoma is gross total resection, and adequate exposure should be accomplished for this purpose, although sometimes aggressive resection proves impossible at the time of the operation. Tumors are approached through an incision in the crest of an overlying gyrus or through a sulcus. The selection of the entry site is aided by intraoperative ultrasound images and the frameless image-guided stereotactic system. Self-retaining retractors are placed to retract gently both sides of the cortical incision (generally approximately 3 cm in length), and then the operating microscope is brought in for the approach through the subcortical white matter to the tumor. The tumor is resected with suction, two-point coagulation forceps, grasping instruments, the CO_2 laser, or the CUSA, the resection proceeding from the inside out, so that surrounding normal white matter is disturbed minimally. The glistening peritumoral white matter is seen easily through the microscope as each of the tumor's margins are reached, and it is at this interface that the resection is stopped. Hemostasis is sometimes difficult but must be perfect. Hemispheric tumor cysts can be drained and, when possible, fenestrated into an adjacent ventricle to prevent reaccumulation. Tumors not amenable to resection because of their location or their diffuseness should be biopsied stereotactically. Again, there is no indication for a craniotomy when the purpose is merely to biopsy (and not resect) a tumor.

The introduction of cortical mapping procedures into brain tumor surgery has made feasible the extensive resection of tumors in functionally critical areas. By use of intraoperative cortical stimulation, motor- and speech-associated cortex can be mapped, and safe routes to deep-lying tumors and safe resection limits determined.[31] A principal disadvantage of surgery that incorporates mapping of speech is that the patient cannot be given general anesthesia, and the surgeon must, therefore, anticipate unexpected patient movement and possibly inferior brain relaxation during the operation.

REOPERATION FOR CEREBRAL ASTROCYTOMAS

Evidence is accumulating that reoperation for resection of cerebral astrocytomas at the time of their recurrence can be efficacious.[80,86,87] The rationale cited earlier for the aggressive initial resection of cerebral astrocytomas seems to fit equally well the prospect for reresection at recurrence. This is only true, however, if there is some treatment modality (e.g., chemotherapy and brachytherapy) that the patient can receive after the reoperation, and most often there is.

Salcman proposes from experience with reoperation of all patients who were to receive further therapy for recurrence of malignant glioma that a relatively nonselective approach might be rational, given that reoperation is safe and of potential benefit despite the patient's age, performance status, tumor grade, or interval between initial surgery and recurrence.[80] Young and coworkers argue for more rigid selection criteria when choosing candidates for reoperation on recurrent malignant gliomas.[86] They found that patients with a Karnofsky performance score (KPS) higher than 60 and an interval between the initial surgery and recurrence of at least 6 months had the longest survival times after reoperation. Harsh and associates looked at the effect of reoperation on the subsequent high-quality survival (KPS of at least 70) of patients with recurrent malignant gliomas.[87] Age and preoperative KPS have effects on the duration of high-quality survival in this study, with relative youth and high performance scores being advantageous. Because their data suggest that reoperation can significantly enhance the effects of chemotherapy on recurrent brain tumors, Harsh and associates would not suggest confining reoperation to young patients in excellent condition, but would suggest instead simply using these factors as guidelines in the broader therapeutic picture. Barker and his coworkers updated the experience from the same institution [University of California, San Francisco (UCSF)] and found that while the number of patients with *high quality* survival after reoperation had increased, the overall survival remained poor.[472] In this series the KPS was the single significant determinant for longer survival after reoperation.

RADIATION THERAPY

Astrocytoma

Differentiated or low-grade astrocytomas constitute a heterogenous group of tumors. Median survival times may vary from 1 to 12 years depending on the patient's age, performance status, and the presence or absence of tumor enhancement on neuroimaging studies.[88] The variability in their behavior has led to uncertainties regarding their therapy and prognosis. Fortunately, randomized trials are being performed to clarify many of the issues surrounding the treatment of these tumors.

Approximately 10% to 35% of astrocytomas are amenable to total surgical resection.[89] The local control rate for completely resected cystic cerebellar astrocytomas approaches 100%, and postoperative irradiation is not recommended.[90] Similarly, the 5- and 10-year survival rates for patients with juvenile pilocytic astrocytomas are almost 100% after complete or *radical subtotal* resection and radiation.[89,91] Wallner and coworkers reported 10- and 20-year progression-free survival rates of 74% and 41%, respectively, for incompletely resected and irradiated juvenile pilocytic astrocytomas.[91] The authors had no data relative to incompletely resected and nonirradiated lesions. Shaw and associates found that patients with supratentorial pilocytic astrocytomas who underwent subtotal resection or biopsy and irradiation survived longer than nonirradiated patients.[89] However, the number of patients treated with surgery alone was small, and, therefore, the efficacy of radiotherapy for this tumor is uncertain. Based on these data, postoperative irradiation is not indicated for pilocytic astrocytomas when a complete or near complete resection has been performed. After subtotal resection, either immediate irradiation or close follow-up, reserving treatment for those patients with symptomatic, progressive, nonresectable tumors may be recommended.[92]

The 5-year recurrence-free survival rates of patients with infiltrative (nonpilocytic) astrocytomas or mixed oligoastrocytomas who undergo total or radical subtotal tumor resection range from 52% to 95%.[93] The variation in outcome may reflect prognostic differences related to age, the inclusion of patients with radical subtotal resections, and the reliance on retrospective evaluations of operative reports to determine the completeness of resection in the era before CT and MRI studies. Because recurrences are infrequent in children with completely resected astrocytomas, postoperative irradiation is generally not recommended. The outcome of adult patients after total or radical subtotal resection, has been found in some series to be similar to that of patients undergoing less extensive surgery.[93] Thus, in adults, postoperative irradiation has been recommended after complete resection by some authors,[93] whereas others advise that radiation therapy be withheld until there is evidence of tumor recurrence.[94]

Retrospective reviews published between 1956 and 1990 suggested that postoperative irradiation is beneficial for incompletely resected infiltrative low-grade astrocytomas. For irradiated patients, 5-year survival rates varied from 36% and 55%, and 10-year rates ranged from 26% to 43%. In contrast, 5-year survival rates for subtotally resected, nonirradiated tumors varied from 19% to 32% and 10-year rates were approximately 10%.[92,93] Many series that report the outcome of irradiated patients do not include a comparable control group, whereas others have presented results for selected groups of irradiated and nonirradiated patients. Further, marked changes in the quality of surgery, radiation therapy, and patient management occurred over the long time intervals spanned by these studies. Indeed, survival rates in these reports increase directly as a function of the time period in which the patients were treated.[95] Most of these data precede the era of modern neuroimaging techniques. The outcome of patients diagnosed and treated in the CT/MRI era is notably better than that reported in the older literature. Median survival times in more recent series are in the range of 7.2 to 10.0 years,[95,96] raising concerns over the value of the older literature in making treatment decisions today. The improved outcome appears to be related to the earlier diagnosis of tumors in neurologically intact patients who exhibit only seizures at the time of diagnosis.[96] In addition, CT and MRI may assist in operative planning, allowing a greater percentage of patients to undergo complete resections.[94,97]

The earlier diagnosis of patients with low-grade astrocytomas raised new questions regarding the timing of therapeutic intervention. Is it better to intervene early, or to wait until there is disease progression? Recht and colleagues[96] reported 26 patients with suspected low-grade supratentorial gliomas (based on clinical and radiologic features only) who were monitored without other treatment except anticonvulsants. Of these patients, 58% subsequently required intervention (surgery alone or with radiotherapy) within a median of 29 months (range, 4 to 123 months) because of increased size of the radiographic abnormality, refractory seizures, new symptoms, or malignant transformation. When compared with 20 patients who had similar characteristics but in whom the decision was made for immediate intervention, there was no difference in the outcome of patients who received immediate or deferred treatment and no difference in the time to neoplastic transformation. Arguments for performing an immediate biopsy are to confirm the diagnosis and to identify patients with nonenhancing anaplastic tumors. Further, complete surgical resection may improve survival, obviate the need for irradiation, and decrease the risk of malignant transformation, the most common cause of death in low-grade astrocytoma patients,[95–97] by reducing the tumor burden.[97]

The timing of postoperative irradiation is another area of controversy. Although it is generally agreed that patients with unfavorable astrocytomas with radiographic evidence of tumor growth, intractable seizures, progressive neurologic impairment, or malignant transformation of the tumor should undergo radiotherapy, this treatment is commonly deferred in patients with well-controlled seizures who present with asymptomatic, indolent tumors. Proponents of this approach argue that with CT and MRI, the disease is diagnosed much earlier in its natural history than in the past and that it is unclear whether early irradiation provides an outcome advantage over delayed irradiation, can delay or prevent tumor dedifferentiation, or whether radiation therapy even alters the prognosis.[92]

This issue was clarified in a randomized trial conducted by the EORTC and British Medical Research Council Brain Tumor Working Party. Patients with low-grade astrocytomas (65%), oligodendrogliomas (25%), or mixed tumors (10%) were randomized to receive immediate postoperative irradiation to a dose of 54 Gy or no further treatment until neurologic and CT scan evidence of disease progression. Among those in the control arm, 65% of patients received subsequent radiotherapy, 19% underwent surgery, chemotherapy, or both, and the remainder received only supportive care. A preliminary analysis of the study demonstrated that although immediate irradiation improved the 5-year progression-free survival (44% vs. 37%, $P = .02$), there was no improvement in overall 5-year survival (63% vs. 66%).[98] The outcome of patients with astrocytomas strongly correlates with the proliferative potential of the tumor as measured by bromodeoxyuridine (BUdR) and Ki67. The use of immunohistochemical and molecular markers may provide an opportunity for earlier intervention and improvement in the outcome for the prognostically more unfavorable subsets of patients.

Because radiotherapy is likely to lead to unacceptable sequelae in children younger than 3 to 5 years of age, treatment in this age group is postponed for as long as possible, provided that no significant neurologic deficits and no neuroimaging changes indicative of rapid tumor progression are present. Management decisions are also individualized in older children with incompletely resected astrocytomas who, compared with adults, have a better prognosis, a less pronounced survival improvement with postoperative irradiation, and a greater risk of late radiation sequelae.[93]

Limited radiation fields are used in the treatment of low-grade astrocytomas. The lesion defined by CT scan is encompassed with a 2-cm margin of normal tissue, whereas the T2-weighted MRI abnormality, which tends to be larger than the CT-defined lesion is given a margin of 1 to 2 cm. Complex treatment planning should be used whenever appropriate to minimize the risk of long-term sequelae. The standard dose is 54 Gy, administered using daily fractions of 1.8 to 2.0 Gy. The dose is reduced to 50.4 Gy for children younger than 5 years of age.

Two studies indicate that higher radiation doses do not improve the outcome (at least at 5 years) and suggest that lower doses may be preferable. In a trial conducted by the EORTC, patients were randomized to receive 45 Gy in 25 fractions or 59.4 Gy in 33 fractions. No difference in survival was observed between the two dose levels. The 5-year survival rates were 58% for 45 Gy and 59% for 59.4 Gy. Progression-free rates were also similar (47% vs. 50%). Minimal surgery, poor neurologic status, large tumors, advanced age, and unfavorable histologic features were adverse prognostic factors.[99] Similarly, a combined North Central Cancer Treatment Group, RTOG, and Eastern Cooperative Oncology Group trial randomized adult patients with supratentorial astrocytomas to receive 50.4 Gy in 28 fractions or 64.8 Gy in 36 fractions. As in the EORTC study, the 5-year survival rates were similar for the two dose levels studied, 73% for 50.4 Gy and 68% for 64.8 Gy ($P = .57$). Age 40 or older and astrocytoma-dominant histology were poor prognostic features.[100] An increase in functional sequelae[101] and radiation necrosis[100] was observed in patients treated in the high dose arms of these studies.

There have been few studies evaluating combined chemotherapy and radiation therapy for low-grade astrocytomas. In a Southwest Oncology Group trial, adult patients with incompletely excised low-grade gliomas were randomized to receive radiation therapy alone or radiation therapy and CCNU. The median survival time for all patients was 4.45 years with no difference between the two treatment arms.[102] A trial by the RTOG is studying whether the addition of PCV to radiotherapy improves the outcome over radiotherapy alone.

Levin and coworkers[103] treated 22 adult patients with contrast-enhancing astrocytomas with the halopyrimidine analogue BUdR and radiation therapy. BUdR was given in weekly 96-hour infusions throughout the course of irradiation. This was followed by 1 year of PCV chemotherapy. The estimated 6-year progression-free and overall survival rates were 63% and 79%, respectively, comparing favorably with survival rates for enhancing low-grade gliomas reported by others.[97] These results require further confirmation.

Malignant Gliomas

Prospective clinical trials conducted by the Brain Tumor Cooperative Group provided seminal evidence supporting the efficacy of radiation therapy in the treatment of malignant gliomas. The Brain Tumor Cooperative Group trial demonstrated a significant survival advantage for patients who received radiotherapy alone or with BCNU, as compared with those treated with resection and supportive care or with BCNU alone. The median survival time for patients receiving supportive care alone was 14 weeks, whereas those treated with radiation therapy had a median survival time of 36 weeks ($P = .001$).[104] Patients with anaplastic astrocytomas and glioblastoma multiforme were treated to a dose of 60 Gy in single daily fractions of 1.8 to 2.0 Gy, five times per week. With this schedule, 25% of patients with glioblastoma multiforme and 50% of those with anaplastic astrocytoma exhibit a significant radiographic response by the completion of radiation therapy. Only 5% of patients have a complete tumor response, and a delayed response after irradiation is uncommon.[105]

Partial brain fields (also called *limited field*), defined by the extent of tumor on neuroimaging studies, are used for the treatment of malignant gliomas.[106] The target volume is defined as a 2- to 3-cm margin of tissue surrounding the perimeter of the CT- and MRI-defined contrast-enhancing lesion. RTOG protocols use a shrinking field approach. Initially, the treatment volume includes the contrast-enhancing lesion and surrounding edema on the preoperative CT or MRI study with a 2-cm margin. Subsequently (after 46 Gy of a 60-Gy course), the target volume is reduced to include the enhancing lesion only (without edema) with a 2.5-cm margin.

With conventional radiation therapy the median survival time for patients with anaplastic astrocytoma is 36 months, and the 3-year survival rate is approximately 55%.[107] In contrast, the median survival time for patients with glioblastoma multiforme is 10 months, whereas the 3-year survival rate is only 6%.[106] The response of malignant gliomas to standard radiation therapy techniques is limited by their striking inherent radioresistance and the radiosensitivity of the surrounding normal brain tissue. Thus, research in the treatment of malignant gliomas has been directed at improving the efficacy of radiotherapy. In addition to pursuing more effective chemotherapy programs (see Chemotherapy section), areas of investigation have included the use of chemical modifiers of the radiation response, altered fractionation schemes, dose escalation with interstitial brachytherapy, radiosurgery and three-dimensional conformal radiotherapy, and the use of heavy particle irradiation.

Two different classes of radiation-sensitizing agents have been investigated in malignant gliomas. The combination of the hypoxic cell radiation sensitizer, misonidazole, and radiation was compared with radiation alone in ten randomized trials. No survival improvement was observed in any of the dose-fractionation or drug schedules tested.[108] In addition, two halopyrimidine analogues, BUdR[103,109,110] and iododeoxyuridine,[111] have been tested. In a phase II study conducted by the Northern California Oncology Group, patients with malignant gliomas received BUdR in six weekly 96-hour infusions during the course of radiation therapy. This was followed by 1 year of PCV chemotherapy. The median survival times for patients with glioblastoma multiforme and anaplastic astrocytoma were 64 and 272 weeks, respectively.[103,109] Compared with historical controls, the survival of patients with anaplastic astrocytoma using this regimen was particularly encouraging. Based on these results, a randomized trial comparing radiotherapy alone or with BUdR plus PCV chemotherapy in patients with anaplastic astrocytoma was conducted by the RTOG, North Central Cancer Treatment Group, and Southwest Oncology Group. Enrollment into the study was discontinued before it reached its full accrual when it was estimated that there would be no difference between the two treatment arms.[110]

Hyperfractionated irradiation is the use of two or more treatments per day with fraction sizes smaller than conventional dose fractions to deliver a higher dose in the same overall treatment time as conventionally fractionated therapy. With hyperfractionation, tumor control probabilities should improve without increasing the risk of late complications. Further, with a 6-hour interval between doses, there is greater probability that rapidly proliferating tumor cells will be irradiated during more radiosensitive phases of the cell cycle and become *self-sensitized* by redistribution. Target cells for late sequelae proliferate slowly, and, therefore, for these tissues little redistribution or self-sensitization occurs.

The RTOG conducted a randomized phase II dose-escalation study in which patients were given 64.8, 72.0, 76.8, or 81.6 Gy in 1.2-Gy twice-daily fractions. Patients receiving 72 Gy had the longest median survival time, and no further improvement in outcome was observed at the higher dose levels.[112] A randomized trial comparing 72-Gy hyperfractionated irradiation with conventionally fractionated 60-Gy radiotherapy (BCNU given in both arms) was subsequently conducted by the RTOG. The median survival times for patients with glioblastoma multiforme were similar (10.2 months with hyperfractionation and 11.2 months with conventional fractionation). Likewise, for patients with anaplastic astrocytoma, the median survival was 44 months with hyperfractionation and 50 months with conventional fractionation ($P = .81$).[113]

Another fractionation option, accelerated fractionation, attempts to reduce the overall treatment time by giving conventional sized dose fractions two or three times daily. This treatment schedule may improve the therapeutic ratio by reducing the opportunity for tumor cell repopulation during treatment, thereby increasing the probability of tumor control for a given dose level. Several trials using accelerated regimens have been conducted, but none has shown a survival benefit over conventional irradiation.[114] These studies indicated that although rapid regeneration does not appear to explain the radioresistance of malignant gliomas, the overall treatment time can be shortened. Altered fractionation schedules also provide an opportunity to integrate chemosensitizers and hypoxic cell sensitizers in a novel fashion. Trials applying this approach, however, have yet to demonstrate a benefit.[115] On the other hand, the use of accelerated fractionation and other short-course fractionation schemes may be especially appropriate in patients with relatively short survival expectancies.

Most gliomas are localized to a single area of the brain,[62,63] and they should be controllable if sufficiently high radiation doses can be delivered without damaging the surrounding normal brain tissue. One approach to augmenting the radiation dose is with interstitial brachytherapy. Iodine 125 and iridium 192 sources have been used in clinical practice, and stereotactic techniques have been devised for the placement of afterloading catheters that are removed after the prescribed dose has been accrued. Well-circumscribed, peripheral, solitary supratentorial lesions measuring as large as 5 cm are best suited for implantation. Further, candidates must have good neurologic function and a KPS of at least 70. Based on these criteria, approximately one-third of patients with newly diagnosed malignant gliomas are candidates for this procedure.[116]

Several phase II studies have demonstrated survival improvements in patients with glioblastoma multiforme when external irradiation is combined with brachytherapy. Gutin and coworkers evaluated brachytherapy as an adjunct to external irradiation and chemotherapy in patients with newly diagnosed supratentorial malignant gliomas.[117] Patients received involved field external irradiation to 60 Gy with concomitant hydroxyurea (300 mg/m^2 orally every other day) followed by an iodine 125 implant to deliver an additional minimum tumor dose of 50 to 60 Gy. Following removal of the implants, they were given PCV chemotherapy every 6 to 8 weeks for 1 year. Although the median survival time of patients with glioblastoma multiforme (22 months) compared favorably with that of historical controls, there was no apparent gain observed in performing implantation at diagnosis in patients with anaplastic gliomas (median survival time, 39 months). Loeffler and associates reported the outcome of 35 patients with glioblastoma multiforme who underwent partial brain external irradiation (59.4 Gy in 33 fractions) followed by an additional 50 Gy given by interstitial implantation.[118] Survival rates at 1 and 2 years were 87% and 57%, respectively, for patients receiving brachytherapy compared with 40% and 12%, respectively, for a control group matched by radiographic and patient characteristics ($P > .001$). Reoperation for brachytherapy-induced symptomatic radiation injury is required in approximately 40% of patients.[117,118]

The Brain Tumor Cooperative Group compared interstitial implantation (60 Gy at 10 Gy/d) preceding external irradiation (60.2 Gy at 1.72 Gy per fraction) and BCNU with external irradiation and BCNU alone in a randomized trial. Implanted patients experienced improvement in median survival (16 months vs. 13 months) and 18-month survival (47% vs. 32%) compared with those who did not receive brachytherapy.[119] However, in another randomized trial, Laperriere and colleagues found no difference in outcome in patients randomized to receive external beam irradiation alone to 50 Gy (median survival, 14 months) or external beam irradiation and an iodine 125 implant delivering a minimum tumor dose of 60 Gy (13 months).[120] A randomized trial testing the addition of interstitial microwave hyperthermia to the brachytherapy boost after external irradiation in newly diagnosed patients with glioblastoma multiforme was conducted at the UCSF. Median survival was 85 weeks versus 76 weeks and the 2-year survival was 31% versus 15%, favoring patients receiving hyperthermia compared with those treated with external beam irradiation and brachytherapy alone ($P = .045$ and $P = .02$, respectively).[121] Brachytherapy has also been shown to improve the survival and quality of life of patients with recurrent malignant gliomas who meet the criteria of implantation.[122]

Stereotactic radiosurgery has also been used to augment the dose of external beam irradiation in initial treatment of patients with malignant gliomas. Shrieve and colleagues[123] used radiosurgery as a boost after standard external beam irradiation (59.4 Gy) in 78 patients with newly diagnosed glioblastoma multiforme. Patients with discrete, geometrically spherical lesions measuring 4 cm or less in diameter and a KPS of 70 or higher were selected for radiosurgery. The median minimum tumor dose was 12 Gy. The median survival was 20 months, and the 1- and 2-year survival rates were 88% and 36%, respectively. Similar to brachytherapy, 50% of the patients required reoperation for symptomatic radiation necrosis or recurrent tumor. Based on tumor size, geometry and functional status guidelines proposed for radiosurgery, only 12% of patients with malignant gliomas met the criteria for radiosurgery. The median survival time for radiosurgery-eligible glioblastoma multiforme patients was 12.5 months, compared with 10.5 months for ineligible patients (P = .07).[124] A comparison of these data with those cited previously suggests that for glioblastoma multiforme a survival advantage of approximately 7 months is conferred when radiosurgery is actually given. Unfortunately, the benefit of radiosurgery diminishes when broader selection criteria are used.[125]

Radiosurgery may also be used to retreat patients with small previously irradiated tumors. In one series the median survival time of 86 patients with recurrent glioblastoma multiforme was 10 months from the time of radiosurgery, similar to the published experience for brachytherapy at recurrence.[126,127]

Three-dimensional conformal photon radiation therapy is a mode of treatment planning and delivery designed to enhance the conformation of the radiation dose to the target volume, while maximally restricting the dose delivered to the normal tissue outside the treatment volume. Conformal treatment planning techniques when applied to cerebral tumors have permitted a 30% to 50% reduction in the volume of normal brain tissue irradiated to high doses.[128] This new approach to treatment planning may not only decrease the risk of normal tissue injury, but also allow higher than traditional radiation doses to be safely administered to patients with malignant gliomas. In an ongoing study at the University of Michigan, doses as high as 80 Gy have been administered using three-dimensional techniques, and escalation to higher dose levels is planned.[129] Fitzek and colleagues used conformal techniques to plan combined treatment with photons and proton beams using an accelerated fractionation regimen to escalate the tumor dose to 90 cobalt gray equivalent (CGE). Twenty-three patients were treated with this approach. The median survival time was 20 months (a 5- to 11-month improvement compared with patients with comparable risk factors treated with conventional radiotherapy) and the 2- and 3-year actuarial survival rates were 34% and 18%, respectively. Tumor regrowth, demonstrated by histologic tissue examination, occurred most commonly in areas that received 70 CGE or less, whereas tumor was found in the 90 CGE volume in only one case.[130]

CHEMOTHERAPY

The era of controlled clinical trials for malignant astrocytomas began with the inception of the Brain Tumor Study Group in 1967. The European Organization for Research on Treatment of Cancer then established a comparable group. In addition, other national and regional cooperative groups have conducted controlled chemotherapy trials. Tables 43.2-12 and 43.2-13[103,131–133] summarize selected data from some of these groups. Differences in reports are sometimes confusing, for instance, some groups report survival or time to tumor progression (TTP) from initiation of therapy, whereas others use the original surgery date for untreated patients. Some groups define histologic groups and separate glioblastoma multiforme from anaplastic astrocytoma, and others combine the two groups under the heading of malignant glioma. For more detail, see a published review of chemotherapy for gliomas in the 1990s.[134]

In addition to histology, other factors influence the likelihood and duration of response. Major known factors are age, performance status, and extent of surgical resection at onset of therapy. For instance, younger patients are more likely to respond and for a longer period; better performance status patients do best; and patients who have more extensive surgical resection do better than those who do not have surgery or who have biopsy only.[80,135]

With consideration for these covariates, it is still clear that adjuvant chemotherapy after surgery and radiation therapy for glioblastoma and anaplastic astrocytomas increases both TTP and survival, more so for the patients with anaplastic gliomas than for glioblastoma. There is less precise information with respect to response because of differing criteria used by the various groups. However, most investigators agree on the definition of deterioration or tumor progression: TTP and survival are more universal measures for controlled clinical trials. TTP is a more pure measure of efficacy, because at time of initial progression, many patients receive other forms of therapy. Survival, however, is a better measure of the social usefulness of the life attained by the therapy.

Clinical trials have demonstrated the efficacy of a number of drugs when combined with irradiation as adjuvant therapy for patients with glioblastoma multiforme and anaplastic astrocytoma. Table 43.2-15 summarizes some of the trials of adjuvant chemotherapy for glioblastoma.[126,128,131,136–149] The data are disappointing in that evidence-based survival gains for adjuvant chemotherapy have not occurred over the past 25 years. Chemotherapy appears to benefit modestly those patients that are in the 25th percentile of survivors. This is reasonable, because *in vitro* tumor drug-sensitivity assays suggest that approximately 60% of patients are resistant to the cytotoxic anticancer drugs used in those studies.[150,151] From Table 43.2-15 it would appear that nitrosourea-based drug combinations may be modestly superior to monotherapy[131,132,149] in that the 25% survival for BCNU is 71 weeks, whereas it is 91 to 120 weeks for drug combinations.

For anaplastic astrocytoma and other anaplastic gliomas, the benefits of combination chemotherapy appear to be greater and better accepted. The first study to open this door was the randomized study of postradiation BCNU to the PCV combination. In that study the survival at the 50th percentile was 157 weeks for PCV compared with only 82 weeks for BCNU-treated patients (P = .009). Even better was the 25th percentile survival, which was greater than 7.7 years for PCV patients compared with 4.1 years for BCNU patients. Jeremic and coauthors found similar results with their combination of CCNU, procarbazine, and vincristine.[132] The study with bromodeoxyuridine together with irradiation and then followed by PCV appears similar for anaplastic astrocytoma patients in whom the median survival is actually higher (4 years vs. 3 years), although it offers no advantage for glioblastoma patients.[103,109] Another nitrosourea combination, 6-thioguanine and BCNU, appears to be at least as active against anaplastic astrocytoma (and other anaplastic gliomas) with an anticipated median survival of more than 5 years.[149]

More approaches need to be considered to improve the results cited in Tables 43.2-15 and 43.2-16. The status of phase II chemotherapy trials is summarized in Table 43.2-17. These studies are dis-

TABLE 43.2-16. Survival for Adult Anaplastic Glioma Patients with Karnofsky Performance Scores Greater Than or Equal to 60 Treated on Protocols Published Since 1990

Radiation Therapy	*Chemotherapy during Radiation*	*Postradiation Chemotherapy*	*50% Survival (wk)*	*25% Survival (wk)*	*Reference*
60 Gy WB	Hydroxyurea	BCNU	82	157	131
60 Gy WB	Hydroxyurea	PCV	157[a]	na (>317 progression-free survival)	131
60 Gy WB	None	mPCV	148	na	132
60 Gy LF	None	PCNU or BCNU	74–88[b]	204–208	133
60 Gy LF	Bromodeoxyuridine	PCV	208	na	452
60 Gy LF	Hydroxyurea	6TG/BCNU	>284[c]	na	149

BCNU, bischloroethylnitrosourea; LF, limited field radiation; mPCV, different schedule of procarbazine, lomustine, and vincristine; na, not attained or reported; PCNU, [1-(2-chloroethyl)-3-(2,5-dioxo-3-piperidyl)-1-nitrosourea); PCV, procarbazine, lomustine, and vincristine; 6TG, 6-thioguanine; WB, whole brain irradiation.
[a]$P = .009$ compared with BCNU.
[b]P not significant for either PCNU or BCNU.
[c]Not attained with lower confidence interval of 284 weeks.

appointing and show that response rate (response plus stable disease) does not correlate with durability of response. Table 43.2-17[67,128,145,152–180] shows that even though the number of patients benefiting from chemotherapy is high in some studies, nevertheless, among the response and stable tumor patients, the duration of benefit has shown only modest gains during the last decade. This failure of chemotherapy is probably a function of *de novo* and emergent resistance of tumor cell subclones. It is disappointing that drugs designed specifically for gliomas, such as diaziquone and spiromustine, were only mediocre agents in the clinic.[158–160,162]

The use of the combination of polyamine inhibitors for anaplastic astrocytomas was somewhat encouraging, and one of the authors has spent many years in pursuit of better drug combinations with little positive gain to date. Alpha-difluoromethyl ornithine (eflornithine; DFMO) has been studied alone,[181] with methyl-bisguanylhydrazone,[175] with BCNU,[174] and most recently with PCV (glioblastoma multiforme [GBM] study submitted). As a single agent, DFMO appears to have similar activity to the DFMO–methyl-bisguanylhydrazone combination. In both instances, the median time to progression (MTP) for recurrent anaplastic gliomas achieving response and stable disease was almost 1 year. The difference in response rates (72% vs. 46%) may reflect too lenient entry requirements for the DFMO patients and a subsequent high number of patients who went off therapy before the first evaluation at 8 weeks.[182]

It has long been known that some alkylating agents such as the nitrosoureas have their DNA damage repaired by an alkyltransferase. Tumors with high alkyltransferase levels are able to repair nitrosourea-inflicted DNA damage and are thus considered *resistant* to the chemotherapy. This can reflect itself in decreased survival.[183,184] We have conducted some uncontrolled phase II studies in an attempt to overcome tumor resistance to nitrosoureas. In one study, 6-thioguanine, dibromodulcitol, and procarbazine were given before CCNU to enhance tumor cell kill by interfering with DNA repair.[176] The results were dramatic for the anaplastic gliomas, when 95% of patients who had failed radiation therapy responded or stabilized for an MTP of 15 months, and 25% did not fail until 33 months; 61% of glioblastoma patients with response or stable disease had an MTP of 9.3 months. Of those who failed earlier nitrosourea therapies, 38% of anaplastic glioma patients and 58% of glioblastoma patients benefited, with MTPs of 10.6 and 5.1 months, respectively. Using a modification of this protocol, we combined 6-thioguanine, procarbazine, CCNU, and hydroxyurea and found that in the anaplastic glioma group, 23% of patients had a partial response and 53% had stable disease. This included 77% of 30 patients who had not received prior chemotherapy and 76% of 17 who had undergone previous chemotherapy. The median time to disease progression was 50 weeks for patients responding who had not undergone previous chemotherapy and 25 weeks for those who had undergone previous chemotherapy. More careful controlled studies with drugs that block alkyltransferase levels are indicated, but expectations should not be too high as these early data remain discouraging.

Intravenous cisplatin and carboplatin have shown only modest activity with respect to TTP, although response and stable rates appear high.[163,185] This may reflect poor tumor and adjacent brain penetration of these drugs and their inability to kill tumor cells at a distance from the main tumor mass. Compounding this pharmacokinetic disadvantage is recent experimental data in rodent tumors that show that dexamethasone can reduce cisplatin penetration into the brain adjacent to tumor where infiltrative tumor cells reside.[186]

Paclitaxel studies have shown acceptable toxicity but only modest antitumor activity in the treatment of recurrent malignant gliomas. Against recurrent anaplastic astrocytoma, Chamberlain and Kormanik found a remarkable 80% response and stabilization rate for a median of 7.5 months.[187] Experience with paclitaxel was summarized in a review article where it was shown to have modest activity.[188] Evaluation of paclitaxel has been complicated by accelerated plasma clearance in patients on anticonvulsants.[189]

The newest alkylating agent to be approved by the European and American regulatory authorities is temozolomide. It has been approved for anaplastic astrocytoma in the United States and also for glioblastoma multiforme in Europe. The drug has been shown to be modestly active in glioblastoma and moderately active against anaplastic astrocytoma.[190,191] Temozolomide is oral, better tolerated than procarbazine by patients, and has a predictable and short nadir period. These features make it a popular choice for drug combination regimens. Currently, trials have been completed or are underway to evaluate temozolomide with interferon-α, *cis*-retinoic acid, BCNU, and Marimastat to name a few trials.

Betaseron, an interferon-β, attained 50% response and stable rates in a cooperative study; however, the duration of benefit is

TABLE 43.2-17. Chemotherapy of Recurrent and Progressive Supratentorial Astrocytomas

Treatment	Responders + Stable/Total % (MTP, wk)[a] GM	AA
SINGLE AGENTS		
BCNU[67,153]	29 (22)	64 (22)
PCNU[155]	33 (8)	60 (28)
Procarbazine[152,453,b]	27–32 (17–30)	28 (40)
BIC[454]	20 (na)	23 (22)
AZQ, 24 hr[158]	50 (18)	47 (16)
Melphalan (oral)[161]	0 (na)	7 (na)
Melphalan (IV)	0 (na)	0 (na)
Cisplatin[163]	73 (8)	83 (12)
Carboplatin[185]	43 (14)	54 (16)
Eflornithine (DFMO)[455,c]	21 (na)	44 (48)
Betaseron[165]	51 (18)	50 (16)
Trans-retinoic acid[166]	33 (na)	67 (na)
Cis-retinoic acid[456,457]	43.2–53.0 (19–40)	47 (na)
Temozolomide[190,191,b]	46 (20)	58 (41)
Tamoxifen[195]		63 (78)
Irinotecan[458]	71 (na)	70 (na)
COMBINATIONS		
BCNU/PCB[168]	46 (17)	56 (23)
CCNU/PCB/VCR[169,459]	45 (15)	65 (27)
BCNU/FU[460]	—	89 (32)
BCNU/FU/HU/MP[172]	55 (23)	71 (46)
BCNU/INF-α[173]	0 (na)	30 (na)
DFMO/BCNU[174]	30 (8)	57 (76)
DFMO/MGBG[461]	—	72 (49)
6TG/PCB/DBD/CCNU/FU/HU[462]	61 (40)	92 (65)
PCB/FU/HU/MP[a]	33 (16)	50 (20)
AZQ/BCNU[132,133]	0–28 (9)	80 (37)
AZQ/PCB[132]	31 (25)	53 (42)
Cytoxan/VCR[179]	60 (15)	78 (35)
Carboplatin/FU/PCB[180]	45 (27)	53 (29)
6TG/PCB/CCNU/HU[463]	33 (21)	77 (38)
Nitrogen mustard/VCR/PCB[464]	4 (11)	18 (16–19)
Carboplatin/*cis*-retinoic acid[465]	52 (30)	—

AA, anaplastic astrocytoma; AZQ, aziridinylbenzoquinone; BCNU, bischloroethylnitrosourea; BIC, 5-[3,3-bis(2-chloroethyl) 1 triazeno]-imidazole-4-carboxamide; CCNU, lomustine; DBD, dibromodulcitol; DFMO, difluoromethylornithine; FU, fluorouracil; GM, glioblastoma; HU, hydroxyurea; INF, interferon; MGBG, methyl-bisguanylhydrazone; MP, 6-mercaptopurine; MTP, median time to progression; PCB, procarbazine; PCNU, (1-(2-chloroethyl)-3-(2,5-dioxo-3-piperidyl)-1-nitrosourea); 6TG, 6-thioguanine; VCR, vincristine.
[a]MTP is for only the stable and responding patients when available.
[b]Also from Schering Plough Research Institute data on file.
[c]VA Levin et al., unpublished observations, 1987 and 1991.

low, with MTPs of 16 to 18 weeks.[165] Tamoxifen, an antiestrogen with the ability to reduce protein kinase C levels and possibly interfere with angiogenesis, has taken on almost cult status as a brain tumor agent.[192–195]

Autologous bone marrow transplantation has had few practitioners, generally because of a low rate of observed complete responses to any form of chemotherapy. Single-agent BCNU was used years ago with no definable gains over conventional dose nitrosourea therapy.[196] Other researchers have used thiotepa[236] and etoposide.[197,198] Although neither thiotepa nor etoposide alone has shown remarkable activity against gliomas, various combinations of the three agents are being evaluated.[199,200] It is currently unclear whether autologous bone marrow transplantation has a place in the management of cerebral gliomas.

BRAIN STEM GLIOMAS

CLINICAL AND PATHOLOGIC CONSIDERATIONS

Tumor involvement of the brain stem is caused by, in order of decreasing frequency, astrocytoma, glioblastoma, and ependymoma. These tumors can be primarily central, diffuse, and infiltrative or focally infiltrative with or without an exophytic; the latter carry a better prognosis. Cranial nerve involvement can be at the nuclear level or of the cranial nerve as it leaves the brain stem. The initial manifestations of a brain stem glioma are unilateral palsies of cranial nerves VI and VII in approximately 90% of patients. Cranial nerve involvement is usually followed by long tract signs, such as hemiplegia, unilateral limb ataxia, ataxia of gait, paraplegia, hemisensory syndromes, gaze disorders, and, occasionally, hiccups. Less commonly, long tract signs precede the cranial nerve abnormalities; this is more likely with confined central intrinsic lesions.

If the tumor is a well differentiated or an anaplastic astrocytoma, it is likely to involve the midbrain and produce hydrocephalus, vomiting, drowsiness, and cerebellar signs; if the tumor is a glioblastoma, it more often involves the medulla. Children with glioblastoma characteristically have a rapidly progressive course and are likely to have deficits in cranial nerves VI, VII, IX, and X, and dysarthria, personality change, and head tilt. Unlike expansive posterior fossa tumors, headache, vomiting, and papilledema occur late.

As a group, the prognosis is poor, with 5-year survival rates varying between 0% and 38% and a median survival of less than 1 year in most series.[201–203] Certain patients do better than others. For instance, patients with type II tumors do better than those with infiltrative type I tumors. Moderately anaplastic exophytic tumors do better than higher grade anaplastic tumors. Landolfi and others reported a small series of 19 brain stem glioma patients between 17 and 70 years of age with a median survival of 54 months.[204] In their group were 2 tectal, 4 cervicomedullary, and 13 pontine gliomas; three pontine tumors had an exophytic component. Surprisingly, only 12 were treated initially with radiotherapy and 3 were treated at recurrence.

SURGERY

Modern imaging of the CNS with MRI has improved the capability for definitive diagnosis of brain stem tumors. Lesions previously difficult to distinguish from brain stem glioma (e.g., clivus tumors, foramen magnum meningiomas, multiple sclerosis, occult arteriovenous malformations, and brain stem abscesses) usually can now be excluded. Still, biopsy of brain stem gliomas for confirmation of the diagnosis and for definite tumor grading should be performed when possible. Biopsy of brain stem gliomas accessible through the floor of the fourth ventricle or presenting on the lateral surface of the pons can be accomplished safely, and associated symptomatic cysts can be drained. Attempt at complete resection of these tumors is contraindicated. Stereotactic needle biopsy of brain stem gliomas using CT and MRI guidance seems to have a low complication rate, so this method is being used increasingly, with the consequence that fewer patients are being treated without a tissue diagnosis.[205]

RADIATION THERAPY

Radiation therapy, the primary treatment for brain stem tumors, improves survival and can stabilize or reverse neurologic dysfunction in 75% to 90% of patients.[203] Traditionally, brain stem gliomas have been treated with doses of 54 Gy, administered in daily fractions of 1.8 Gy, through parallel opposed portals with the tumor dose calculated at the midline on the central axis of the beam. According to a multiinstitutional survey by Freeman and Suissa,[202] the 1-, 2-, and 5-year survival rates of children treated with conventional radiation therapy techniques were 50%, 29%, and 23%, respectively.

Because of the relatively poor results obtained with conventional radiation dose-fractionation schedules and the observation that these tumors recur locally, hyperfractionated irradiation, designed to deliver higher tumor doses, was evaluated by several investigators.[206–209] Early reports demonstrating consistent, although modest, improvements in outcome have been observed when patients treated with hyperfractionation regimens of up to doses of 70.2 to 72.0 Gy (1.0 to 1.17 Gy twice daily) were compared with historical control patients treated with conventional or low-dose hyperfractionated irradiation.[250,253] There was no outcome improvement when the dose was increased to 75.6 Gy and 78 Gy,[208] but considerable morbidity was observed at these higher dose levels.[210] The Pediatric Oncology Group (POG) conducted a dose-escalation trial of 66.0, 70.2, and 75.6 Gy in twice-daily fractions of 1.1, 1.17, and 1.26 Gy, respectively, in children with diffuse brain stem gliomas. No difference in the median time to progression (7 to 8 months) and median survival time (10 months) between the three dose schedules was found. The highest dose was associated with steroid dependency in 62% of patients and a 45% incidence of intralesional necrosis.[209] Thus, the 70.2-Gy dose level was considered to have the best therapeutic ratio, and was tested by POG in a randomized trial comparing hyperfractionated radiotherapy with 54 Gy given with conventional fractionation. Children in both treatment arms received cisplatin during radiotherapy.[209] Hyperfractionation did not improve event-free survival ($P = .96$) or overall survival ($P = .65$) over that of the conventional dose fractionation regimen. For patients receiving the conventional fractionation regimen, the median time to progression was 6 months, the median survival time was 8.5 months, and the 1- and 2- year survival rates were 30.9% and 7.1%, respectively. For those receiving the hyperfractionated irradiation regimen, the median time to progression was 5 months, the median survival time was 8 months, and the 1- and 2- year survival rates were 27% and 6.7%, respectively.[211]

Based on the results of the POG trial, the current standard for the treatment of diffuse intrinsic brain stem gliomas consists of conventionally fractionated radiotherapy given to a dose of 54.0 to 59.4 Gy. The availability of MRI and three-dimensional conformal radiotherapy treatment planning approaches offers improved target definition and allows the high-dose radiation volume to be better tailored to the contour of the lesion. The irradiated volume includes a margin of normal tissue of approximately 2 cm around the tumor. Smaller margins may be used for more focal lesions.[210] Dorsal exophytic and cervicomedullary tumors that are completely resected do not require routine postoperative irradiation.[210]

CHEMOTHERAPY

As with cerebral astrocytomas, chemotherapy is primarily nitrosourea based.[212] The use of chemotherapy, adjuvant to irradiation, has been infrequent. The Children's Cancer Group (CCG) randomly compared radiation therapy with radiation therapy followed by CCNU, PCV, and prednisone.[170] The mean survival was 11 months, and there was no difference between the two groups. In another trial, 5-fluorouracil and CCNU before radiation therapy and hydroxyurea and misonidazole during radiation therapy were evaluated[258]; in that study, TTP (32 weeks) and survival (44 weeks) were not better than the initial CCG study. A pilot study evaluating oral etoposide during and after radiotherapy was closed to accrual by the CCG; analysis of the data has not yet been reported.

For recurrent or progressive brain stem gliomas, few therapies have been evaluated.[213] Some benefit has been demonstrated, but the extent of benefit has not been well established. In one study, 5-fluorouracil, CCNU, hydroxyurea, and 6-mercaptopurine were used to treat children and adults with recurrent or progressive brain stem gliomas.[214] Sixty-nine percent of 13 patients had response or stabilization, with a relapse-free survival of 25 weeks; the overall survival was 27 weeks. This finding is somewhat worse than would be expected for supratentorial gliomas. These authors conducted a phase II study of recurrent malignant gliomas with a combination of BCNU and DFMO. In that study, three of five patients benefited, with the three continuing to benefit at 1 to 3 years.[174] Although not curative, some of these chemotherapeutic leads should be exploited.

CEREBELLAR ASTROCYTOMAS

CLINICAL AND PATHOLOGIC CONSIDERATIONS

Astrocytomas arising in the cerebellum are considered separately, because their prognosis is consistently better than astrocytomas arising in the cerebrum or brain stem. These tumors, which occur most often during the first two decades of life, arise in the vermis or more laterally in a cerebellar hemisphere. Cerebellar astrocytomas usually are well circumscribed; they can be cystic, solid, or an admixture of polycystic and solid.

Histologically, most astrocytomas are low grade and lack features commonly associated with anaplasia; many are pilocytic in appearance and, histologically, some are juvenile pilocytic astrocytomas. In a series on 451 children reported from the Hospital for Sick Children of Toronto, cerebellar astrocytomas accounted for 25% of all posterior fossa tumors; 99 of 111 (89%) of the cerebellar astrocytomas were low grade, with nearly all vermian in origin.[215] Approximately 75% of these tumors are located only in the cerebellum, with the remainder involving the brain stem as well.[216]

Because most of these tumors arise in the vermis, the clinical presentation is similar to medulloblastoma, with truncal ataxia, headache, nausea and vomiting, and in the young, split cranial sutures and head enlargement from increased intracranial pressure.

SURGERY

Cystic cerebellar astrocytomas are exposed through a posterior fossa craniectomy. The cyst is located with ultrasound, cannulated, and then exposed by an incision through the cerebellar folia. Self-retaining retractors are placed into the cyst and then, with the aid of the operating microscope, the cyst is examined and the vascular, firm mural module identified, dissected, and removed. The nonneoplastic cyst wall is not excised.

Solid cerebellar astrocytomas are separated carefully from surrounding cerebellar white matter, again using the improved visualization offered by the operating microscope. The texture and appearance of the tumor are usually distinct and the separation from white matter usually is not difficult, so the only barrier to complete resection becomes deep penetration of the tumor into the dentate nucleus, cerebellar peduncles, or brain stem.

TABLE 43.2-18. Chemotherapy for Recurrent Cerebellar Astrocytomas

Parameter	*Adjuvant Chemotherapy*	*Chemotherapy at Progression*
Total number	5	10
Glioblastoma	3	1
Anaplastic glioma	2	7
Low-grade gliomas	—	2
Median age (y; range)	13 (8–25)	30 (4–42)
Therapies	RT-BUdR-PCV, RT-8422, RT-PCV, RT-CYCLE	BCNU, CCNU, PCB, PCV, BTRC-8522, BTRC-8422, BFHM, CYCLE
Outcome	75% alive at 1 y	Median progression-free survival 24 wk

BCNU, bischloroethylnitrosourea; BFHM, bischloroethylnitrosourea, 5-fluorouracil, hydroxyurea, 6-mercaptopurine; BTRC 8422, 6-thioguanine, procarbazine, dibromodulcitol, lomustine, vincristine; BTRC 8522, 6-thioguanine, procarbazine, dibromodulcitol, lomustine, 5-fluorouracil, hydroxyurea; BUdR, bromodeoxyuridine; CCNU, lomustine; CYCLE, bischloroethylnitrosourea, 5-fluorouracil, lomustine, procarbazine; PCB, procarbazine; PCV, lomustine, procarbazine, vincristine; RT, radiation therapy.
(Data from ref. 217.)

RADIATION THERAPY

See the discussion in the section on Cerebral Astrocytomas; the same principles apply. Completely resected cerebellar astrocytomas do not require postoperative radiation therapy. The remainder receive total doses of 50 to 60 Gy, depending on the histologic features and the age of the patient.

CHEMOTHERAPY

Because surgery alone or surgery and irradiation is often curative, chemotherapy has been limited to cases of recurrence or if the tumor is histologically highly anaplastic. For these tumors, the authors' approach has been to use nitrosourea-based therapies.

Chemotherapy adjuvant to surgery and radiation has not been commonly advocated for these tumors. The authors' experience is anecdotal (Table 43.2-18), but appears consistent with chemotherapy results for cerebral gliomas.[217] All patients received a nitrosourea; however, the chemotherapy combinations varied depending on which program was being used at the time for supratentorial gliomas. For patients at recurrence, chemotherapy provided palliation, with a median TTP of 24 weeks and 25% of patients surviving longer than 32 months.[217] As with the adjuvant chemotherapy patients, all were treated on a protocol being used at the time for cerebral gliomas. Among these patients, 5 of 18 (28%) developed metastases to the leptomeninges (three of five) or intracranial extracerebellar parenchymal sites (two of five). All leptomeningeal disseminations occurred in conjunction with locoregional recurrences. In many patients, therefore, combined systemic and intraventricular therapy may be needed for tumor control.

Other chemotherapy agents have been used on an ad hoc basis to treat recurrent cerebellar gliomas primarily in children. One report cited the palliative potential of oral etoposide in the treatment of juvenile pilocytic astrocytoma with 50% (6 of 12) of responding and stable patients achieving a median 7 months' progression-free survival.[218] It is safe to assume that temozolomide will be used alone and in combination for recurrent cerebellar gliomas in the future.

OPTIC, CHIASMAL, AND HYPOTHALAMIC GLIOMAS

CLINICAL AND PATHOLOGIC CONSIDERATIONS

Nearly all gliomas of the optic nerve and chiasm are discovered in patients before the age of 20 years, and most before the age of 10 years.[219] In some patients there is a family kindred of neurofibromatosis. Lewis and colleagues prospectively evaluated 217 patients with neurofibromatosis and found that gliomas along the anterior visual pathway occurred in 15% and were occasionally bilateral.[220] Sixty-seven percent of these tumors were not suspected clinically or obvious on ophthalmologic examination.

With respect to tumor location, Housepian and associates reported that 25% involved one optic nerve, 73% the chiasm, and 3% the optic tracts.[221] In another series, 25% involved the chiasm alone, 33% the chiasm and hypothalamus, and 42% the chiasm and optic nerves or tracts.[265] Clinically, these tumors produce loss of visual acuity (70%), strabismus and nystagmus (33%), visual field impairment (bitemporal hemianopsia, 8%), developmental delay, macrocephaly, ataxia, hemiparesis, proptosis, and precocious puberty. Funduscopic evaluation demonstrates a range of findings from normal optic disks through venous engorgement to disk pallor due to atrophy. Tumors involving the chiasm often grow to involve the hypothalamus, causing a diencephalic syndrome that is characterized by emaciation (especially in children between 3 months and 2 years of age), motor overactivity, and euphoria.

Pathologically, these tumors range from primarily piloid and stellate astrocytes (most common), with or without oligodendroglia, through the gamut of malignant astrocytomas to glioblastoma multiforme (rare). Typically, optic gliomas appear as fusiform expansions of any part of the nerve; they tend to bridge through the optic foramen and expand as dumbbell-shaped tumors within the skull. The nerve can be infiltrated by tumor originating in the chiasm, the walls of the third ventricle, or the hypothalamus. The tumors found in patients with neurofibromatosis often affect a single optic nerve and are grossly normal in appearance, although infiltrated by tumor and surrounded by a fibrous stroma.

Diagnosis is best made by MRI scan and should use images in the sagittal plane. The CT scan is satisfactory for diagnosis but is not as sensitive or descriptive as the MRI scan. The MRI also shows hypothalamic involvement more clearly.

SURGERY

Unilateral tumors of the optic nerve (as opposed to the chiasm) should be resected, particularly when there is profound vision loss or when proptosis is disfiguring. A transcranial approach to the orbit is preferred, permitting complete resection of the tumor-infiltrated nerve from the chiasm to the globe and sparing the globe for an optimal cosmetic effect.[222] The involved nerve is inspected through a unilateral craniotomy, and the nerve is sectioned at the chiasm. The orbit is then unroofed, and the optic nerve's attachment to the globe is exposed and divided, allowing the tumor to be removed.

Biopsy of smaller tumors of the optic nerve, tumors involving the nerve and chiasm, and tumors of the chiasm alone must sometimes be done when radiographic studies cannot exclude meningioma, craniopharyngioma, or other diagnoses definitively. Subtotal resection of such tumors, particularly if exophytic, can sometimes be done for decompression before radiation or chemotherapy.[223] Resection of the chiasm with resultant blindness is never indicated.

RADIATION THERAPY

Treatment of optic nerve and chiasmal gliomas is controversial, because some patients with incomplete surgical resections have been followed for 10 to 20 years without progression.[219] The literature suggests, however, that untreated optic gliomas, especially those involving the chiasm or extending into the hypothalamus or optic tracts, progress locally or are fatal in 75% of patients. Tenny and coworkers found that only 21% of patients who were followed after biopsy or exploration survived compared with 64% of those who received radiation therapy.[224] In general, optic nerve gliomas have a better prognosis than those involving the chiasm, and tumors confined to the anterior chiasm have a better outcome than those that involve adjacent structures (posterior chiasmal tumors).[225–227]

Routine postoperative irradiation is not indicated for most gliomas confined to the optic nerve.[227] In contrast, radiation therapy can prevent tumor progression, improve disease-free survival, and stabilize or improve vision in patients with chiasmal lesions. Wong and colleagues reported that 6 of 27 (22%) chiasmal gliomas that did not receive radiation therapy progressed locally, whereas 9 of 20 (45%) that received radiation therapy failed.[226] Three of these recurrences were seen in the adults with extremely aggressive, nonresponsive tumors. Further, 87% of the irradiated patients who received a dose of 50 to 55 Gy were controlled compared with 55% of those who received 46 Gy or less. Radiation therapy significantly improved the relapse-free survival but not the overall survival. Tao and colleagues concluded that radiotherapy was effective in the majority of patients with progressive chiasmal gliomas. The 10-year progression-free and overall survival rates after radiotherapy were 89% and 100%, respectively. Stabilization or improvement in vision was achieved in 81% of the evaluable treated patients. The authors drew attention to the fact that the median time for a radiographic response of 50% or more was 62 months. Hypopituitarism was common after radiotherapy, underscoring the need for life-long endocrine follow-up with appropriate replacement after treatment.[228] Jenkin and colleagues[227] found that for posterior optic gliomas irradiation was more effective in preventing subsequent relapse than subtotal resection alone. The 10-year relapse-free survival rate was 70% for irradiated patients, compared with 41% for those who did not receive primary radiotherapy ($P = .03$). However, there was no difference in overall survival between these two patient groups due largely to the efficacy of radiation therapy in previously nonirradiated relapsed patients. Erkal and colleagues also reported a progression-free survival rate of 77% in children irradiated for optic nerve and chiasmal hypothalamic gliomas.[229] The prognosis for patients with optic pathway tumors and chiasmatic hypothalamic lesions was similar. In a series collected from the literature, local control was achieved in 154 of 189 (81%) irradiated anterior chiasmal tumors, whereas 92 of 142 (65%) posterior tumors were controlled. Vision improved in 61 of 210 (29%) evaluable patients and remained stable in 118 of 210 (56%) patients.[225] For hypothalamic tumors, radiation therapy produced radiographic improvement in 11 of 24 (46%) with a median progression-free survival of 70 months compared with 30 months for those patients who did not receive radiation therapy.[230]

Although some clinicians advocate deferring irradiation in asymptomatic patients or in those with lesser visual disturbance until there are signs of disease progression,[227] others recommend that radiation therapy be given early in the course of the disease to minimize the risk of visual deterioration.[226] The radiation portals are tailored to the tumor volume and designed to avoid irradiation of the lens of the eye. Three-dimensional conformal, intensity-modulated radiotherapy and stereotactic radiotherapy techniques are used to minimize the dose to adjacent structures. A dose of 50 to 54 Gy in daily 1.8-Gy fractions is recommended.

CHEMOTHERAPY

The published chemotherapy trials for this group of patients represent small series. Chemotherapy has been used successfully to delay the initiation of radiation therapy in young children.[231,232] Packer and associates treated 24 children (median age, 1.6 years) with a combination of dactinomycin and vincristine.[233] Six of the cases involved the chiasm, eight involved the chiasm and hypothalamus, and ten involved the chiasm and visual pathways. At a median follow-up period of 4.3 years, 38% of patients had disease that progressed.

Petronio and coworkers reported on 19 infants or children with chiasmatic and hypothalamic gliomas treated with chemotherapy after diagnosis.[234] Of the 12 tumors in which a biopsy was obtained, there were 7 juvenile pilocytic astrocytomas, 2 astrocytomas, 2 anaplastic astrocytomas, and 1 subependymal giant cell astrocytoma. The children were between 3 months and 15 years of age when treated. The chemotherapy included one of three regimens: one with dactinomycin and vincristine; one with the combination of BCNU, 5-fluorouracil, hydroxyurea, and 6-mercaptopurine; and 15 with the combination of 6-thioguanine, procarbazine, dibromodulcitol, CCNU, and vincristine (BTRC 8422 protocol). Fifteen of 18 initially treated with chemotherapy responded or stabilized; the median follow-up period exceeded 1.5 years (range, 1.4 months to 5.8 years). Rodriguez and colleagues reported a series of 33 patients with hypothalamic gliomas,[230] some of whom were included in the Petronio series.[234] Chemotherapy at presentation or recurrence was beneficial in 10 of 16 (62%) patients.

In another study, Prados and colleagues treated 42 children with low-grade gliomas who had either progressive neurologic symptoms or radiographic tumor enlargement with a combination of 6-thioguanine, procarbazine, dibromodulcitol, CCNU, and vincristine (TPDCV).[235] In that group were 33 patients with hypothalamic chiasmatic gliomas. Multivariate analysis demonstrated no difference between this group and those with low-grade gliomas elsewhere; for the entire group of 42 patients the median progression-free survival was 2.5 years and the 5-year median survival was 78%, reflecting the value of secondary chemotherapy regimens and radiotherapy.

OLIGODENDROGLIOMAS

CLINICAL AND PATHOLOGIC CONSIDERATIONS

Oligodendrogliomas have a relatively flat peak incidence between 25 and 49 years. Although they are most common (80%) in the cerebral hemispheres, approximately 15% occur in the third or lateral ventricles or protrude into a ventricle from the thalamus.[236] Grossly, these tumors are often well demarcated, and in 20% they are cystic. They have a 10% likelihood of spreading through the CSF pathways. Like astrocytomas, they vary in malignancy. Attempts have been made to grade oligodendrogliomas on an A through D scale[236]; however, grades A through C vary little, and B and C are virtually identical with respect to survival such that these subdivisions seem unnecessary; a designation of differentiated or highly anaplastic may be sufficient. These tumors often have both astrocytic or ependymal elements seen at biopsy; such tumors are called *mixed gliomas.*

Clinically, these tumors present in the typical fashion of hemispheral astrocytomas. However, two features distinguish them from astrocytomas: the antecedent history, averaging 7 to 8 years, tends to be longer, and seizures are more common, occurring in 70% to 90% of patients by the time of diagnosis. Provisional diagnosis may be made by MRI or CT neuroimaging, but histologic confirmation is necessary and almost always possible. Approximately 50% of oligodendrogliomas have scattered calcification, usually related to intrinsic blood vessels, which are evident by CT scan.

At recurrence or autopsy, approximately 60% of oligodendroglioma and most mixed oligoastrocytoma patients demonstrate histologically an anaplastic astrocytoma or glioblastoma multiforme. This may belie a common origin of both types of tumors to the O2A progenitor cell.

SURGERY

The surgical resection of hemispheric oligodendrogliomas follows the same principles as discussed earlier for cerebral astrocytomas, with gross total removal being the goal when this is consistent with good neurologic outcome. The margins of oligodendrogliomas can appear to be more distinct than those of astrocytomas, but generally they are infiltrative. Because of this, surgical cure remains unlikely; but the indolent course of these tumors allows for a long progression-free interval after an aggressive resection in some patients. Oligodendrogliomas often recur in the previous operative site. Under these circumstances, reoperation may be advisable, particularly when followed by chemotherapy.

RADIATION THERAPY

The infrequency of oligodendrogliomas and their variable and often long prediagnosis and posttreatment natural history make it difficult to evaluate the effect of radiation therapy in patients with differentiated oligodendrogliomas. Data from Mirk and colleagues[237] indicate that the behavior of these tumors may be more unpredictable and their prognosis less favorable than previously believed. The problems in evaluating retrospective reports for oligodendrogliomas are similar to those previously discussed for low-grade astrocytomas. Conclusions regarding the value of radiotherapy are contradictory, and the lack of randomized trials precludes the statement of firm recommendations. Five-year survival rates for irradiated patients range from 36% and 83% and 10-year rates vary from 30% to 46%. In contrast, 5-year survival rates for subtotally resected, nonirradiated tumors range from 25% to 55% and 10-year rates vary from 13% to 25%.[92,93,238–241] Some authors recommend immediate postoperative irradiation for patients with incompletely resected lesions,[238–241] whereas others have been unable to show that postoperative irradiation is of benefit.[242] It has also been suggested that radiation therapy be deferred until there is evidence of tumor progression or recurrence or that only patients with anaplastic tumors or mixed oligoastrocytomas should receive treatment.[92]

Most retrospective studies comparing surgery alone with surgery and radiation therapy do not contain analyses to ensure that the distribution of patients in the two treatment groups are comparable with respect to prognostic variables such as age,[242] completeness of resection,[237,243] neurologic signs and symptoms,[239,242] and histopathologic features.[236,239,242,243] Furthermore, treatment selection criteria are either not stated or unknown.[241] It is likely that many retrospective studies in which the pathology material was not independently reviewed contain patients with both differentiated and anaplastic oligodendrogliomas. This has been considered to be an important distinction because on average patients with low-grade oligodendroglioma tumors survive 9 years, as compared with 2.2 years for those with high-grade tumors.[93,236,244] Our own data compiled at the University of Texas M. D. Anderson Cancer Center and the University of California Brain Tumor Center (San Francisco) found that median survival was comparable and greater than 7 years.

Although there is some controversy, most neurooncology specialists find that the outcome of patients with pure oligodendroglioma is significantly better than those with mixed oligoastrocytomas. Shaw and colleagues found that the 5- and 10-year survival rates for patients with oligodendrogliomas were 72% and 46%, respectively, whereas for mixed oligoastrocytomas the survival rates were 63% and 33%.[244]

Taken together, the data suggest that there may be a benefit to radiation therapy for patients with incompletely resected tumors during the first 5 years after treatment, but this effect appears to diminish over time. Gannett and colleagues found a significant improvement in survival with postoperative irradiation. Patients treated with surgery alone had 5- and 10-year survival rates of 51% and 36%, respectively, compared to 83% and 46% for irradiated patients (P = .032). Lindegaard and colleagues found that radiation therapy prolonged the median survival time (38 months vs. 26.5 months, P = .039) but did not influence the overall cure rate when given after subtotal resection, whereas it did not appear to be indicated after total resection.[241] Wallner and associates reviewed the outcome of 42 patients and observed 5- and 10-year survival rates of 61% and 33%, respectively; relapse-free survival rates were only 33% and 25%.[240] The 10-year survival rate for patients with pure oligodendrogliomas who received at least 45 Gy was 56% compared with 18% for nonirradiated patients (P = .092). Wallner and coworkers concluded that adjunctive radiation therapy increased the time to tumor recurrence and the number of long-term survivors.[240] Shaw and colleagues[244] also found a survival advantage in irradiated patients with incompletely resected tumors who received at least 50 Gy. However, the survival differences between the irradiated and the nonirradiated groups did not reach statistical significance. The 10-year survival rate for patients treated with subtotal resection alone was 25%, compared with 31% for those treated with surgery and radiation therapy to at least 50 Gy. Shimizu and colleagues performed a metaanalysis on reports from the current literature and concluded that postoperative irradiation conferred a 14% improvement in 5-year survival (P <.01).[238] The data presented in these studies suggest that more effective therapies are needed to improve the long-term outcome of patients with oligodendrogliomas.

As in the case in low-grade astrocytomas, it is difficult to take a categorical position regarding the role of radiation therapy in the treatment of low-grade oligodendrogliomas.[92] Some small asymptomatic (except for controlled seizures) tumors can be carefully observed, delaying surgical or radiotherapeutic intervention until there is tumor progression or uncontrolled neurologic symptoms. If feasible, large, symptomatic or progressive tumors should be resected. Patients with completely resected or small asymptomatic incompletely resected low-grade oligodendrogliomas can be observed, delaying radiotherapy until the time of recurrence.[92] Because of the poor long-term prognosis associated with some of these tumors and data that suggest that radiotherapy may improve survival, at least up to 5 years, patients with large, symptomatic unresectable or incompletely resected tumors should receive radiation therapy.[92] As in the case of low-grade astrocytomas, proliferation markers such as the MIB-1 labeling index may help to distinguish patients who require aggressive treatment from those who can be observed.

Radiation therapy is given using fields that encompass the tumor volume with a 2-cm margin. A dose of 54 to 60 Gy is used in adults, and the dose is reduced to 50 Gy in children. PCV chemotherapy (see following Chemotherapy section) may be useful in some patients as initial treatment, as combined therapy or to reduce the size of large tumors before beginning radiotherapy.[245,246] In the latter situation, reducing the volume of brain irradiated may decrease risk of treatment-related adverse effects.

Patients with pure or mixed anaplastic oligodendrogliomas have a poorer outcome than those with low-grade tumors. Winger and colleagues reported median survival times of 1.3 years and 5.3 years, respectively, for patients with mixed anaplastic oligoastrocytomas and pure anaplastic oligodendrogliomas treated with radiotherapy and chemotherapy.[83] Shaw and coworkers found that patients with high-grade mixed oligoastrocytomas and oligodendrogliomas (based on the St. Anne-Mayo system had similar outcomes with a median survival of 4.5 years, and 5- and 10-year survival rates of 45% and 25%, respectively.[247] Patients with pure and mixed anaplastic oligodendrogliomas receive postoperative irradiation to a dose of 60 Gy in conventional daily fractions of 1.8 to 2.0 Gy using an approach similar to that used for malignant gliomas. Clinical trials are currently testing whether the combination of PCV with radiotherapy improves the outcome of anaplastic lesions.[248] Others are using high-dose chemotherapy with stem cell rescue to defer radiotherapy until there is evidence of tumor progression.

CHEMOTHERAPY

Prospective clinical chemotherapy trials of oligodendroglioma patients are underway; until they are completed and reported, we

TABLE 43.2-19. Status of Phase II Studies of Lomustine, Procarbazine, and Vincristine for Recurrent Oligodendroglioma and Oligoastrocytoma

Reference	*Complete Response % (MTP, mo)*	*Partial Response % (MTP, mo)*	*Stable Disease % (MTP, mo)*
466	17 (25)	46 (12)	19 (7)
467	12 (45)	50 (24)	31 (32)
468	33 (25)	40 (16)	20 (7)
Total	18 (31)[a]	46 (16)[a]	23 (14)[a]

[a]Weighted mean of three medians.

have two sources of information: individual patients reported within trials for malignant astrocytomas and some PCV trials that led up to the randomized studies currently in progress. In those reports, chemotherapy was limited to the treatment of recurrent, well-differentiated, and moderately anaplastic oligodendrogliomas and the primary treatment of the highly anaplastic oligodendrogliomas with surgery, radiation therapy, and chemotherapy. Adjuvant chemotherapy following surgery and irradiation yields 58% 5-year survival for oligodendroglioma patients, a 50% 3-year survival for anaplastic oligodendroglioma patients, and an 80% 2-year relapse-free survival for oligoastrocytoma patients.

Table 43.2-19 summarizes the status of PCV chemotherapy for recurrent oligodendroglioma from three contemporary publications. The complete response rate was 19% for a MTP of 31 months, the partial response rate was 45% for a MTP of 14 months, and the stable disease rate was 22% for a MTP of 8 weeks. Thus, the majority (86%) of patients treated with PCV at recurrence are expected to either respond or stabilize for a period in excess of 1 year.

For anaplastic oligodendrogliomas, Kyritsis and coworkers found a median 1.3 years relapse-free survival after chemotherapy (mostly PCV therapy).[249] For recurrent oligoastrocytoma, the median relapse-free survival is 1.0 to 1.2 years.[249,250] To test the efficacy of this chemotherapy regimen in newly diagnosed patients, the RTOG is coordinating an intergroup randomized trial that compares neoadjuvant intensive PCV chemotherapy followed by radiation therapy with radiation therapy alone.

EPENDYMOMA

CLINICAL AND PATHOLOGIC CONSIDERATIONS

Ependymoma tumors arise from cells of ependymal lineage and, therefore, have a propensity for occurring in the obliterated central canal of the spinal cord, the filum terminale, and white matter adjacent to a ventricular surface (usually a highly angulated surface).[28] Sixty percent of intracranial ependymomas are infratentorial, and 40% are supratentorial.[251] Of infratentorial sites, the fourth ventricle is the most common site. Extension into the subarachnoid space occurs in 50% of these cases, and encasement of the medulla and upper cervical cord can occur. Of supratentorial ependymomas, 50% are primarily intraventricular, and the remainder are parenchymal, arising from ependymal rests. Most of the intraventricular tumors arise in the lateral ventricles, and fewer (25%) occur in the third ventricle.

Ependymomas can be classified in various ways. Ependymomas are either differentiated (ependymoma or myxopapillary ependymoma) and, therefore, low-grade or, less commonly, they are anaplastic and higher grade and more likely to disseminate through the CSF pathways.

Clinical presentations are dependent on the location of tumor. Intraventricular tumors often cause increased intracranial pressure and hydrocephalus. As a result, headache, nausea and vomiting, papilledema, ataxia, and vertigo are found in most patients at presentation. Focal neurologic signs and symptoms are more often seen with extraventricular supratentorial ependymomas.

Either MRI or CT scanning is sufficient to make the anatomic diagnosis before surgery. The presence of calcium in a fourth ventricular tumor is highly suggestive but not diagnostic of an ependymoma. Surgical exploration and biopsy are essential for the selection of appropriate treatment. For anaplastic ependymomas, staging myelography and examination of the CSF for cytologic evidence of malignancy are essential.

The inclusion of ependymoblastomas, which are known for their propensity to disseminate throughout the CNS, tends to overestimate the risk of seeding.[252,253] In a literature review, Vanuytsel and Brada found that the overall incidence of spinal seeding was 6.9%.[254] It was 1.6% for supratentorial tumors, 9.7% for infratentorial lesions, 8.4% for high-grade tumors, and 4.5% for low-grade lesions. No patient with high-grade supratentorial lesions developed spinal seeding, whereas 15.7% of those with high-grade infratentorial tumors developed spinal dissemination. For low-grade tumors, 2.7% of patients with supratentorial lesions developed seeding compared with 5.5% for those with infratentorial lesions. The incidence of spinal seeding was related directly to local tumor control, regardless of tumor grade. The incidence of spinal dissemination was 3.3% in locally controlled patients and 9.5% in those with uncontrolled primary lesions ($P<.05$).

SURGERY

Approximately one-half of hemispheric ependymomas arise from the wall of the lateral ventricle, and one-half appear to be intraparenchymal, arising perhaps from remote fetal ependymal cell rests.[255] Hemispheric ependymomas tend to be cystic and, even when not, are often well circumscribed from surrounding brain, allowing gross total resection. A wide craniotomy permits a transcortical exposure of the tumor through a cortical incision placed to avoid injury to vital brain tissue. The tumor is removed using the operating microscope, and every effort is made to minimize bleeding into the ventricular cavity. At the end of the resection, the ventricular system is gently irrigated free of blood and blood clots to prevent mechanical obstruction to CSF flow, to prevent the blockage of the CSF absorptive bed (arachnoid granulations), and to reduce the irritation of bloody CSF to the brain.

Ependymomas arising from the floor of the fourth ventricle are approached through a wide bilateral suboccipital craniectomy and laminectomy of C-1. The tumor is exposed by retracting the cerebellar tonsils laterally and splitting the inferior aspect of the vermis, although often a tongue of tumor is visible over the dorsal aspect of the medulla and upper cervical spinal cord before the tonsils are retracted. The dorsal convexity of the tumor comes into view as the cerebellar vermis is divided, and its attachment to the floor of the fourth ventricle can then be exposed progressively and evaluated. Firm attachment precludes a complete resection, as does infiltration of the tumor into the cranial nerves of the cerebellopontine angle through the foramen of Luschka. Tumor is removed to the extent possible using illumination and magnification afforded by the operating microscope.

There would appear to be a relation between residual ependymoma left by the surgeon and a poorer outcome after radiation therapy.[256] In ependymomas, as in most of the gliomas, a maximal surgical resection should be carried out when possible.

RADIATION THERAPY

It is well established that postoperative irradiation improves the survival of patients with intracranial ependymomas, and 5-year survival rates with doses of 45 Gy or more range from 40% to 87%.[45] Tumor grade has been considered to be the most important determinant of tumor behavior and prognosis. The 5-year survival for patients with low-grade tumors ranges from 60% to 80%, whereas for anaplastic ependymomas it is only 10% to 47%.[45] Most series fail to distinguish patients with malignant ependymomas from those with ependymoblastomas that are classified as primitive neuroectodermal tumors and have an especially poor prognosis. Analysis of these data when these lesions are excluded suggested that tumor grade may have less prognostic value.[252]

The amount of normal CNS tissues to include in the treatment volume and the need for prophylactic irradiation to the entire craniospinal axis are major areas of controversy. The differences of opinion are based on the potential for ependymomas to spread into the ventricular system and to disseminate into the spinal subarachnoid space. In their literature review, Vanuystel and Brada found that risk of seeding was independent of whether prophylactic spinal irradiation was given.[254] For high-grade lesions, spinal dissemination occurred in 9.4% of patients receiving craniospinal irradiation and in 6.7% of those treated with local radiation therapy only. Similarly, for low-grade tumors, spinal seeding occurred in 9.3% after craniospinal irradiation, whereas 2.2% developed seeding without prophylactic treatment.

The treatment volumes recommended for low-grade supratentorial ependymomas vary from generous local fields to fields encompassing the whole brain, whereas for low-grade infratentorial tumors they include local fields, the whole brain with cervical spine extension, and the craniospinal axis. Wallner and coworkers reviewed the outcome of 20 patients with supratentorial and infratentorial low-grade ependymomas treated with partial or whole brain irradiation after surgery; only 1 in 16 patients, who was eventually found to have a local recurrence, developed spinal dissemination.[257] The 5- and 10-year survival rates for those who received more than 45 Gy (approximately 50 Gy in most instances) were 67% and 57%, respectively. As nearly all recurrences were limited to the original primary tumor site, it was concluded that treatment of the whole brain was unnecessary. Based on this series and data from others[253,254,258] and the greater precision in determining tumor extent currently available through high-quality diagnostic imaging, low-grade supratentorial ependymomas are treated using partial brain fields with a dose of at least 54 Gy. Spinal MRI and CSF evaluation are not obtained unless there is evidence of ventricular involvement or signs of subarachnoid metastases. Low-grade infratentorial ependymomas are also treated with limited fields. The craniospinal axis is irradiated only if pretreatment CSF cytology studies reveal malignant cells or if radiographic studies show evidence of tumor spread.

Many authors recommend inclusion of the entire craniospinal axis in the treatment of anaplastic ependymomas[257,259,260]; the entire craniospinal axis should be treated, although some recommend whole brain irradiation with an additional boost for high-grade supratentorial lesions located away from the CSF pathways, if there is no evidence of leptomeningeal spread.[253] A dose of 54 Gy is given to the primary tumor site and 36 Gy to the remainder of the axis. If spread within the brain is demonstrated, the entire brain receives 54 Gy. Spinal imaging studies are routinely performed, and any area of gross involvement is boosted to 50 Gy. However, despite the apparent superiority of craniospinal irradiation in some series,[259] local recurrence is the primary pattern of failure with high-grade ependymomas,[253,257,258,261] and subarachnoid seeding is uncommon in the absence of local recurrence.[45] Furthermore, the patterns of failure are similar in patients treated with local fields or with craniospinal axis irradiation,[253,258,260] and prophylactic treatment may not prevent spinal metastases.[253,254] Merchant and colleagues reviewed the outcome of 28 patients with anaplastic ependymomas.[261] Twelve patients received craniospinal irradiation, 2 were treated to the whole brain, and 14 received treatment to limited fields. The actuarial 5- and 10-year survival rates were 56% and 38%, respectively. All 19 patients who failed radiotherapy had relapses at the primary site, and one of these also developed subarachnoid dissemination. A benefit from craniospinal irradiation could not be demonstrated. Based on these data and the findings in other reported series, craniospinal irradiation is generally not recommended for patients with anaplastic (high-grade) ependymomas unless evidence of leptomeningeal spread is pathologically or radiographically documented.[253,258,261] Others, however, suggest that prophylactic craniospinal irradiation be reserved for those with infratentorial high-grade lesions.[258]

Because the inability to eradicate the primary tumor remains the single most important factor leading to treatment failure,[260] clinical trials are examining more aggressive local therapies to improve local tumor control, both in low- and high-grade ependymomas. These include the use of boosts with stereotactic radiotherapy or conformal radiotherapy techniques as well as hyperfractionated dose schedules.[258] There is no evidence thus far that the addition of chemotherapy to radiotherapy improves the outcome.[262]

CHEMOTHERAPY

Because ependymomas are uncommon tumors and before MRI these tumors were difficult to assess, there are few chemotherapeutic trials. For instance, the only trial for initial treatment of anaplastic ependymomas is one the authors started in 1984. It combined craniospinal axis irradiation with oral hydroxyurea followed by six courses of polydrug chemotherapy TPDCV.[263] Since 1984 17 consecutive children and adults were treated. At publication 11 of 17 patients had failed with an MTP of 141 weeks; the median follow-up for the eight who had not died was 469 weeks, whereas nine patients who died had a median survival of 183 weeks.

Table 43.2-20[163,264–267] summarizes some published and unpublished series of chemotherapy for recurrent differentiated or anaplastic ependymomas. The therapies range from

TABLE 43.2-20. Chemotherapy for Recurrent Ependymoma and Anaplastic Ependymomas

Treatment	*No.*	*Responding and Stable (%)*	*Median Time to Progression (mo)*
Bischloroethylnitrosourea[a]	14	78	13
Dibromodulcitol[469]	12	75	16
AZQ[265]	12	42	10
Carboplatin[266]	14	28	14
Cisplatin[163]	8	75	3.8
VCR-CDDP-CCNU-PCB-VP16-IFSO combinations[267,b]	16	22	9
6TG-PCB-DBD-CCNU-VCR[c]	11	82	21.6 16

AZQ, aziridinylbenzoquinone; CCNU, lomustine; CDDP, cis-platin; DBD, dibromodulcitol IFSO, ifosfamide; PCB, procarbazine; 6TG, 6-thioguanine; VCR, vincristine VP16, etoposide.
[a]VA Levin, et al., unpublished observations, 1987.
[b]Sixteen patients were treated on 37 different trials.
[c]M Prados, VA Levin, MSB Edwards, unpublished observations, 1991.

TABLE 43.2-21. Sites of Predilections of Meningiomas within the Intracranial Regions

Site	*No.*
Parasagittal	65
Convexity	54
Sphenoidal ridge	53
Olfactory groove	29
Suprasellar	28
Posterior fossa	23
Spinal	18
Peritorcular	12
Temporal fossa	8
Falx	7
Choroidal	6
Gasserian	5
Multiple	2
Combined with neurinomas	2
Intraorbital	1

(From ref. 268, with permission.)

single-agent therapies to the five-drug protocol, TPDCV. The best single agents were BCNU and dibromodulcitol, with combined response plus stable disease rates of 75% to 78% and MTP of 13 to 16 months.[264] Results are somewhat better than those achieved for anaplastic astrocytomas. With a variety of drug combinations the best response plus stable disease rate was 82% with an MTP of 21 months for TPDCV.

Goldwein and colleagues retrospectively analyzed 16 recurrent ependymoma patients treated with a variety of agents alone and in combination (VCR, cisplatin, CCNU, procarbazine, VP-16, and ifosfamide).[267] Approximately 20% of patient trials led to a partial response or stable disease (more common 7:1), for an approximate median of 6 to 10 months.

Gaynon and associates of the CCG used carboplatin every 4 weeks and found a response and stable disease rate of 28% (4 in 14) with a duration of 6+, 17+, 12, and 15 months.[266] Those who did not receive prior cisplatin were more likely to respond to carboplatin. Bertolone and coworkers evaluated cisplatin and found 6 of 8 (75%) benefiting, with an MTP of 3.8 months.[163] Ettinger and colleagues, also of the CCG, used diaziquone on a 5-day schedule every 3 weeks in 12 children with recurrent or metastatic disease. One response more than 35 months was reported.[265]

If the 87 patients cited in the studies presented in Table 43.2-20 are weighted for the number of patients in each trial, the mean TTP was 16 months.

MENINGIOMAS

CLINICAL AND PATHOLOGIC CONSIDERATIONS

Meningiomas arise from arachnoidal cells in the meninges, especially in areas of the arachnoid villi. In some series, meningiomas constitute 39% of primary CNS tumors.[24] The most frequent locations of these tumors are along the sagittal sinus and over the cerebral convexity. Table 43.2-21 summarizes the frequency of these tumors according to location.[268] Meningiomas are extraaxial, intracranial (and sometimes spinal) tumors that produce symptoms and signs through compression of adjacent brain tissue and cranial nerves. They often also produce hyperostosis. Table 43.2-22 summarizes the symptoms and signs associated with these tumors.

Histologically, most meningiomas are differentiated, with low proliferative capacity and limited invasiveness. Less commonly, meningiomas are more anaplastic with a higher proliferative capacity and are invasive. Even though the difference in the 30-minute bromodeoxyuridine labeling index *in situ* for the differentiated meningiomas may be less than 1% versus 3% to 4% for anaplastic meningiomas,[269] biologically, the anaplastic meningiomas behave considerably differently than the more differentiated meningiomas. MIB-1, an antibody to the

TABLE 43.2-22. Neurologic Findings Associated with Meningiomas as a Function of Their Location

Site	*Presentation*
Sphenoidal ridge	Nonpulsating, painless unilateral exophthalmos; unilateral vision loss; ophthalmoplegia; ICP
Cerebral convexity	Altered mentation; ICP; seizures
Intraventricular	Hydrocephalus; headache; mental changes; visual field abnormalities
Olfactory groove	Central scotoma; ipsilateral optic atrophy; contralateral papilledema; ipsilateral loss of smell; altered mentation; focal motor abnormalities
Tuberculum sellae	Loss of vision; bitemporal hemianopsia; papilledema or optic atrophy
Other basilar sites	See Table 43.2-5
Cerebellar convexity	ICP; cerebellar findings
Cerebellar-pontine angle	Cerebellar findings; hearing loss
Foramen magnum	No findings; spastic paresis and sensory findings in upper extremities

ICP, increased intracranial pressure.

Ki-67 protein, has been used as a proliferative marker in meningioma patients and found to correlate closely with the bromodeoxyuridine labeling index.[315]

SURGERY

The perception that meningiomas are surgically resectable gives these tumors an undeserved reputation of benignity. Although meningiomas usually are well circumscribed and do not invade adjacent brain, they can occur virtually anywhere in the CNS, and access is sometimes only by deep retraction. In addition, these tumors may be extremely vascular and can surround important structures such as cranial nerves and major arteries at the skull base. Such characteristics can preclude a smooth operation, and a total removal is commonly not possible. Simpson reported on a large series of surgically resected meningiomas and documented that even when there was a perceived total resection, the recurrence rate was 9%.[270] A more modern series from Massachusetts General Hospital shows that a *total resection* is followed by 7% recurrence rate at 5 years, 20% at 10 years, and 32% at 15 years.[271]

Since many meningiomas are surgically resectable, the neurosurgeon is usually more favorably disposed toward operating on them than another glioma. The neurosurgeon's zeal must be tempered, however, with an understanding of the risks of removing a meningioma in a particular location and an understanding of the effect of this meningioma on the well-being of the patient, because these tumors are often exceedingly slow growing and the patients are often elderly. When surgery is undertaken in an elderly patient, partial removal is sometimes adequate.

Preoperative Planning

The preoperative preparation of the patient, surgical planning, and intraoperative anesthetic management are as described in the earlier Surgery section. However, the planning of surgery for meningiomas must be extremely assiduous, because a detailed knowledge of surgical anatomy is necessary in these tumors. A preoperative angiogram to assess overall tumor vascularity and to identify arterial feeders is often important. In many instances, the angiography procedure is combined with embolization of the tumor's blood supply. The angiogram is done within 24 to 96 hours of the operative procedure, so that alternative vascular routes to the tumor do not have time to develop.

Surgical Principles

Those feeding arteries that could not be occluded by embolization are addressed first at the operation, if they are accessible. These arteries are meningeal and cerebral in origin. The tumor is retracted from surrounding normal brain progressively as the tumor bulk is reduced by the use of the CUSA or, for extremely vascular tumors, the cutting loop of the electrocoagulation unit or the CO_2 laser. Meningiomas at individual sites pose special surgical problems.

At the cerebral convexity, a large bone flap is made around the tumor, a dural incision circumscribes the tumor, and the dura attached to the tumor is used to retract the tumor from the brain as microdissection frees the adhesions between the tumor and surrounding brain.

Parasagittal meningiomas abut the midline; difficulties in removal are related to critical draining veins, to involvement of the sagittal sinus with tumor, and to the occasionally massive overlying bony erosion or hyperostosis or both. A patent sagittal sinus cannot be transected for a complete tumor removal except in its anterior one-third, so a careful study of the preoperative arteriogram looking for the patency of the sinus and for the position of the draining veins in the region is critical. Some clinicians advocate opening the sagittal sinus for removal of tumor that has grown through its wall, and others advocate resecting and grafting the involved sagittal sinus wall. In the authors' opinion, these dangerous maneuvers are not usually indicated, because recurrence-free survivals after subtotal resection of these lesions are extended,[271] and because the tumor may grow to occlude the sinus completely, thereby making complete resection possible later with a lesser risk to life.

Falx meningiomas do not involve the sagittal sinus but occupy the falx below the sinus, often becoming bilateral. Major complications of resection of falx meningiomas relate to interruption of draining veins and consequent cerebral edema and venous infarction.

Olfactory groove meningiomas grow extremely large before their neurologic sequelae lead to their discovery. Surgery is carried out through a large frontal bone flap based low on the forehead. The broad sessile base of the tumor is attacked first so that its blood supply can be interrupted. The tumor's bulk is then reduced by internal coring and dissection, with attention to protection of the optic nerves, carotid artery, and anterior cerebral arteries on the tumor's posterior aspect.

Tuberculum sellae meningiomas are smaller at presentation because of their proximity to the optic apparatus. Attention to the safety of the optic apparatus and the anterior cerebral and carotid arteries is equally critical.

The approach to sphenoid ridge meningiomas varies according to whether they occupy the outer, middle, or inner third of the sphenoid bone. Outer third tumors can be a problem purely of tumor mass, purely of massive temporal hypertosis from en plaque tumor invading bone, or a combination of both. When it is present, the tumor mass insinuates itself in the sylvian tissue, and its removal through a frontotemporal craniotomy is complicated by the tumor's adherence (on its medial aspect) to sylvian veins. Surgical cure is not possible. Middle third tumors grow into both the frontal and temporal fossae in a globular fashion. The approach is through a frontotemporal craniotomy, with the base of the tumor approached first to eliminate the blood supply. Surgical cure is likely. Inner third tumors arise from the anterior clinoid process and compress the optic nerve and encase the carotid and middle cerebral arteries. In addition, medial sphenoid ridge meningiomas can grow diffusely into the cavernous sinus and optic canal. Only in those situations in which the tumor presents early because of optic nerve compression is total removal feasible, with the surgeon stopping when the risk of the surgery exceeds potential benefits.

Tentorial meningiomas arise from the broad surface or free edge of the tentorium and are approached under the temporal lobe or under the occipital lobe, depending on their placement. In all instances, the principle of removal is incision of the tentorium around the tumor and gradual bulk reduction and separation of the tumor from surrounding brain. Venous sinuses and critical draining veins, particularly the vein of Labbe, must be protected.

Cerebellopontine angle meningiomas arise from the petrous bone and if small and dorsolaterally situated are exposed through a posterior fossa craniectomy by retracting the cerebellum medially. More ventrally situated tumors arising at the junction of the petrous bone and the clivus or from the clivus itself are exposed through a combined approach above and below the tentorium, which allows a better angle to work medially and more generous exposure with less brain retraction.[272] Posterior fossa meningiomas may engulf critical blood vessels and cranial nerves and may be characterized by extreme adherence to the brain stem, so attempts at complete removal must proceed cautiously. In younger patients, particularly, these tumors should be completely resected during the first attempt if possible as subsequent operations are complicated by scarring, with obliteration of surgical planes and increased adherence to the brain stem.

RADIATION THERAPY

The need for adjunctive radiation therapy is determined by the extent of surgical resection and the histopathologic features of the tumor (benign vs. malignant). The risk of recurrence for completely resected benign meningiomas is small, and postoperative irradiation is not usually recommended. In contrast, the risk of relapse after subtotal resection ranges from 33% to 60% at 5 years to more than 90% at 15 years.[271,273,274] Several reports provide evidence that postoperative irradiation prolongs the interval to recurrence, prevents tumor regrowth in some patients, and improves the survival of patients with incompletely resected meningiomas. Barbaro and associates compared the outcome of 54 patients who were treated with subtotal resection and radiation therapy with a group of 30 patients who underwent subtotal resection alone.[275] Sixty percent of the nonirradiated patients developed recurrence, whereas 32% of the irradiated patients recurred. The median time to recurrence was 10.4 years for the irradiated patients compared with 5.5 years for the nonirradiated group ($P < .05$). Irradiated patients had a more favorable outcome than nonirradiated patients, despite the fact that they more frequently had tumors located in surgically unfavorable sites. This series was recently updated by Goldsmith and colleagues who reported the results of 140 patients (117 benign and 23 malignant) treated at UCSF with subtotal resection and postoperative irradiation. The median tumor dose was 54 Gy.[276] For patients with benign meningiomas, the 5- and 10-year progression-free survival rates were 89% and 77%, respectively. Patients who received at least 52 Gy had a 20-year progression-free survival of more than 90%. The 5-year progression-free survival of patients treated after 1980 was 98%, compared with 77% of those treated before 1980. This improvement was attributed to the availability of CT scanning and MRI for tumor localization and treatment planning.

A multivariate analysis identified that for benign meningiomas, improved progression-free survival was not related to tumor size but was associated with younger age ($P = .01$) and treatment after 1980 with innovative technologies ($P = .002$).[277] Condra and coworkers found that at 15 years 70% of their patients relapsed after subtotal excision alone, whereas only 13% of those treated with subtotal excision and postoperative irradiation recurred ($P = .0001$). The 15-year cause-specific survival rate was 86% for patients treated with combined therapy compared with 51% for nonirradiated patients ($P = .0003$). For patients undergoing complete resection, 24% relapsed after 15 years, and the 15-year cause-specific survival was 88%.[278] The actuarial 5-, 10-, and 15-year relapse-free survival rates for patients undergoing subtotal resection and irradiation reported by Graholm and colleagues were 78%, 67%, and 56%, respectively.[279] These results and those of Goldsmith and coworkers[276] compare favorably with the relapse-free survival rates of 63%, 45%, and 9% reported by Mirimanoff and associates for incompletely resected, nonirradiated patients.[271]

The size of the residual meningioma affects the outcome of radiotherapy. Connell and colleagues showed that for tumors of 5 cm or larger, the 5-year progression-free survival rate was 40%, significantly less than the 93% observed for smaller tumors.[280] Among patients irradiated for unresectable tumors and in those with residual disease, the volume of visible tumor on imaging studies rarely decreases by more than 15% and often only after many years.[277]

It is controversial whether patients should be treated with radiation therapy after their initial subtotal resection or when signs of disease progression appear. Some clinicians have found that patients with benign meningiomas do equally well with either approach[281]; others suggest that initial postoperative irradiation is preferable,[277] because recurrence has an adverse influence on outcome, and many patients who recur after initial subtotal excision alone may not be salvaged by subsequent treatment.[278] Postoperative irradiation often is deferred in elderly patients and in those in poor medical condition until there is evidence of symptomatic progression. When a surgical resection is not feasible, radiation therapy may relieve symptoms and substantially decrease the rate of tumor progression.[279]

Malignant meningiomas behave in a more aggressive manner than their benign counterparts. Chan and Thompson found that the median survival of six patients treated with surgery alone was only 7.2 months, compared with 5.1 years for 12 patients treated with surgery and postoperative irradiation.[282] Six of the nine patients with malignant histology reported by Graholm and coworkers died within 5 years.[279] Goldsmith and colleagues reported a 5-year progression-free survival of 48% for 23 patients treated by subtotal resection and irradiation.[277] The recurrence rate among 53 patients with malignant meningiomas collected from six series in the literature was 49%. The recurrence rates were 33% for patients treated with complete resection alone, 12% for those undergoing complete resection and radiation therapy, 55% for patients treated by subtotal resection and irradiation, and 100% for those treated by subtotal resection alone.[273] These data support the recommendation that all patients with atypical and malignant meningiomas should be offered postoperative irradiation, regardless of the extent of resection.[277,283]

For benign meningiomas, the planning target volume consists of the residual tumor with a 1 to 2 cm margin of normal tissue, defined by CT scan or MRI and modified by the neurosurgeon's description of the site of residual disease. Extensive tumors of the base of the skull and malignant meningiomas require more generous margins. The preoperative tumor volume is used for planning completely resected malignant lesions. A dose of 54 Gy in daily fractions of 1.8 to 2.0 Gy is recommended for benign meningiomas, whereas the dose is increased to 60 Gy for atypical and malignant tumors. Complex three-dimensional conformal treatment planning and delivery techniques and intensity modulated radiotherapy are used to restrict the dose to normal tissues.

Radiosurgery is another option for the treatment of meningiomas. Kondziolka and colleagues reported that 93% of their patients treated with radiosurgery and followed for 5 to 10 years required no further therapy for their tumors.[284] Nearly 85% of patients treated by Hakim and coworkers were controlled with a median follow-up time of 22.9 months.[285] Complications, including cranial neuropathies, transient neurologic deficits, radiation necrosis, and malignant edema, have been reported 6% to 42% of radiosurgically treated patients.[286,287] Complications have been observed most frequently in patients with large or deep-seated tumors and those treated with high single doses.[288] These data suggest that treatment with radiosurgery should be limited to small lesions, whereas fractionated radiotherapy may be preferable for other subsets of tumors. Although tumor control rates for small meningiomas appear promising, several more years of patient accrual and follow-up will be required to fully evaluate the efficacy of radiosurgery in comparison with surgery and conventional radiotherapy.

CHEMOTHERAPY

There is currently no defined role for chemotherapy for newly diagnosed and nonirradiated meningiomas. Chemotherapy has been used for the most intransigent recurrences. For patients with histologically malignant meningiomas or recurrent, surgically inaccessible, more differentiated meningiomas, the situation is only slightly different. Because of the potentially lethal consequences of these two situations, the authors have been treating with aggressive surgery, focal irradiation, and chemotherapy.

The authors have evaluated primarily sarcoma regimens such as the combinations of cyclophosphamide, doxorubicin, and vincristine (VCR) (nine patients); dacarbazine (DTIC) and doxorubicin (five patients); and high-dose ifosfamide with mesna (two patients). Little objective activity was noted for the first, one in five responses in the second, and one in two in the third. Grunberg and colleagues reported on the use of mifepristone, an antiprogesterone, in 14 patients with recurrent meningiomas; 5 in 14 showed objective response after 6 to 12 months of daily oral therapy.[289] A randomized trial for incompletely resected meningiomas is active through Southwest Oncology Group to better determine the efficacy of mifepristone (RU-486).

Kaba and colleagues reported on six patients with either a recurrent malignant meningioma or an unresectable meningioma who were treated with interferon-α at a dosage of 4 mU/m^2/d, 5 days per week.[290] Five of six patients exhibited positive response to treatment with stabilization of the size of the tumor in four patients and slight regression in one for 6 to 14 months. A larger study has been opened at the University of Texas M. D. Anderson Cancer Center.

Lastly, there are preliminary data suggesting that hydroxyurea may provide treatment in patients with unresectable and recurrent meningiomas.[291]

PRIMITIVE NEUROEPITHELIAL TUMORS

CLINICAL AND PATHOLOGIC CONSIDERATIONS

The treatment of primitive neuroepithelial tumors is controversial and complex. Much of the controversy is based on the failure to understand that there are multiple entities included within this pathologic diagnosis. Controversy surrounds the classification of these tumors.[292] Primitive cells that remain undifferentiated or exhibit varying degrees of neuronal or glial differentiation, or both, are the hallmark of these tumors. Conceptually, these tumors can be viewed as developmentally aberrant brain cells. Therefore, primitive neuroepithelial tumors can be divided into the following classification schema: medulloepithelioma, neuroblastoma, spongioblastoma, ependymoblastoma, pineoblastoma, and medulloblastoma. With the exception of medulloblastoma, primitive neuroepithelial tumors are rare.

It has been proposed that all neoplasms showing primitive poorly differentiated neuroepithelial cells be called primitive neuroectodermal tumors, regardless of location or cell type. Because of the infrequency of these tumors and the controversy surrounding an all-inclusive classification schema currently, it is best to refer to each histiotype separately.

Clinically, however, these tumors share some common and disquieting features. Primarily, they are proliferative and malignant tumors that tend to spread throughout the neuraxis like medulloblastoma. As a result, a complete evaluation of the CNS, including contrast-enhanced CT scans of the entire brain, CSF cytology, and metrizamide myelography, must be performed before the initiation of treatment.

SURGERY

The initial therapy for primitive neuroectodermal tumors is surgical bulk reduction whenever feasible. Surgical principles are the same as those for cerebral astrocytoma described earlier.

RADIATION THERAPY

There is general consensus that patients with primitive neuroectodermal tumors should receive postoperative irradiation. Although radiation therapy appears to improve survival time, the outcome is generally poor, and most patients develop local or regional recurrences. Because of their propensity to spread throughout the subarachnoid space, primitive neuroectodermal tumors are treated with craniospinal axis irradiation. The primary tumor is given 54 to 56 Gy and the remainder of the axis receives 36 Gy. The dose is reduced in very young children. Chemotherapy is usually a part of the treatment program. Primitive neuroectodermal tumors are less radiocurable than medulloblastomas. Whereas in some series 1-year survival rates are as low as 10%,[293] others report 5-year survival rates of 20% to 25%.[294] The disparity in outcome data reflects the heterogeneity of malignancies that are classified under the term of primitive neuroectodermal tumors.[295] For example, in a series of 14 patients reported by Gaffney and coworkers the 3-year survival rate was 29%. None of the patients with tumors containing more than 90% undifferentiated elements were alive at 3 years, whereas 60% of those with less primitive tumors survived 3 years.[296] In another study, Mikaeloff and colleagues reported on 30 patients with CNS primitive neuroectodermal tumors other than medulloblastoma treated with gross tumor resection (16 of 30) who were considered good risk who had a 37% 3-year survival.[297] In a more recent series, Paulino and Melian reported a 5-year survival rate of 47% in a small group of patients treated for supratentorial primitive neuroectodermal tumors.[298]

Cerebral neuroblastomas are biologically distinct from other primitive neuroectodermal tumors. They tend to be less malignant, have a better outcome, and are less likely to disseminate throughout the craniospinal axis.[299] These tumors may present as a cystic lesion with a peripheral nodule or as a solid mass, and their morphologic appearance is related to prognosis. Berger and colleagues found that 7 of the 11 patients treated with local irradiation to an average of 52 Gy were alive with no evidence of tumor progression.[300] Of the six patients with cystic tumors, none had recurrent disease, whereas four of the five patients with solid tumors had recurrences. The only patient with a solid lesion who did not have a recurrence received adjuvant chemotherapy. Although subarachnoid dissemination is found in autopsied cases,[301] this pattern of spread does not represent a significant clinical problem. Thus, localized cerebral neuroblastomas are treated with involved field irradiation to 54 Gy. The craniospinal axis is included only if there is evidence of tumor dissemination beyond the site of origin by imaging studies or CSF cytology.

CHEMOTHERAPY

Because primitive neuroectodermal tumors are an uncommon type of tumor, there are no controlled chemotherapy trials. Reports of isolated cases and small series indicate that drugs active against medulloblastoma have activity in primitive neuroectodermal tumors (see medulloblastoma Chemotherapy section, later in this chapter).

MEDULLOBLASTOMA

CLINICAL AND PATHOLOGIC CONSIDERATIONS

Medulloblastoma appears more similar to the primitive neuroectodermal tumors of childhood than to the gliomas. Although the cell of origin of these tumors is controversial, it is probable that medulloblastoma takes its origin from germinative neuroepithelial cells in the roof of the fourth ventricle.[28] Consistent with its embryonal nature is the fact that the peak incidence occurs in the first decade of life; 50% to 60% of medulloblastomas occur in the first decade, with a peak between 5 and 9 years. A second but lesser peak occurs between 20 and 30 years. The typical location for childhood medulloblastoma is in the cerebellum, mostly in the midline and posterior vermis (Fig. 43.2-5); many encroach on the cisterna magna and the fourth ventricle. In adolescents and adults, there is an increasing tendency for tumors to be laterally placed in the cerebellar hemispheres. Regardless of where in the cerebellum they occur, the tendency for metastatic spread (within craniospinal intradural axis) of medulloblastoma is relatively high. At presentation, as many as 30% of patients have positive cytology or myelographic evidence of spinal metastasis.[302,303] Extra-CNS metastasis is less common and occurs in fewer than 5% of patients; most metastases are to long bones.[302]

Based on bromodeoxyuridine 30-minute labeling indices, medulloblastoma would be considered a highly proliferative tumor because its labeling index is approximately 14%, as opposed to gliomas, which range between less than 1% to 10%.[269]

The overall disease-free 5-year survival for medulloblastoma is approximately 50%.[212,302,304–307] However, the extent of disease at initial diagnosis defines risk. When risk factors are considered, survival is altered dramatically. Poor risk is defined as

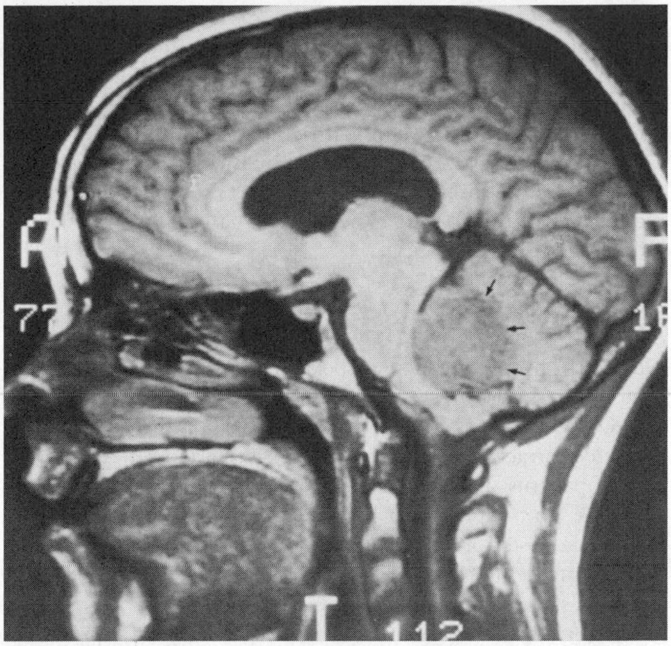

FIGURE 43.2-5. This young girl presented with headache and gait ataxia. A T1-weighted sagittal magnetic resonance imaging scan (TR 600, TE 20) demonstrated a large, low-intensity mass involving the inferior aspect of the cerebellum in the midline and extending to and filling the fourth ventricle. There is arcuate stretching and displacement of the medulla and secondary hydrocephalus. The well-circumscribed nature and location of the tumor is fairly characteristic for medulloblastoma.

less than a 75% resection (probably greater than 1 cc residual); invasion of the brain stem (less clearly established); metastasis to the spinal cord, cerebrum, and leptomeninges or seeding of the cerebellum; positive CSF cytology 2 weeks after surgery; and age younger than 4 years.[212,304,305] Of the poor risk factors, two need explanation. Resection of less than 75% is an imprecise measure of remaining tumor; CT and MRI measurement of residual tumor volume would be better. However, in most patients, if the surgeon can remove more than 75% of tumor, the resection is usually a gross total resection. Poor risk associated with age 4 years and younger may relate more to the restricted irradiation to the developing CNS and its negative effect on tumor control. Most radiation therapists do not treat with full doses of craniospinal irradiation at 4 years of age.

The disease-free survival of poor-risk patients with craniospinal irradiation with or without chemotherapy is approximately 25% to 30%.[306] Good-risk patients, on the other hand, have 5-year disease-free survivals of 66% to 70%.[307,308]

At relapse, the major site of first recurrence is the posterior fossa in more than 50% of patients, the frontal lobe in nearly 20%, bone in 10% to 15%, and other cerebral and suprasellar regions in 10% to 15%.[302,308]

The incidence of systemic metastasis varies between 10% and 30%,[305,306] although the 10% incidence is most similar to the authors' experience. Most extra-CNS metastases are to long bones and ribs, with lymph nodes being a distant second site. In the series by Park and associates[305] and Lowery and colleagues,[306] the median time to the development of extra-CNS metastasis was 10 to 12 months; in the authors' more recent study, it was 18 months.[309] In the Park study, 17% of ventriculoperitoneal-shunted patients developed systemic metastases, whereas only 4% in unshunted patients did so. In Lowery's series, 30% of patients developed systemic metastases, and none had been shunted previously. These authors' experience is that, except in patients with rampant disease, they did not find an association between ventriculoatrial or ventriculoperitoneal shunting, with or without an in-line filter, and systemic metastases. Bone metastases can occur as the only evidence of recurrence in unshunted patients years after their initial presentation with CNS disease.

SURGERY

Although hydrocephalus associated with medulloblastoma obstructing the fourth ventricle can be relieved with a preresection CSF shunt, it is more usual to defer shunting and control increased intracranial pressure with corticosteroids. In as many as 60% of patients, aggressive resection of the tumor relieves hydrocephalus. An occipital burr hole is commonly placed at surgery, before the posterior fossa exposure is done, to allow cannulation of the ventricles for drainage of CSF to lower the increased intracranial pressure so that the dura can be opened safely.

Surgery for medulloblastoma is carried out in the prone or the sitting position. The prone position is preferred, especially in children. The incision and bony exposure are usually in the midline, but a paramedian incision and unilateral bony removal are done when the tumor is limited to one hemisphere, particularly in adults. The more commonly used midline craniectomy extends down through the foramen magnum, and a laminectomy of C-1 (and rarely, C-2) is performed to decompress herniated cerebellar tonsils or to remove a caudally extending tongue of tumor over the dorsum of the spinal cord.

After the dura is opened, the cerebellar tonsils are retracted laterally, and it is in the foramen of Magendie that the purplish-gray tumor usually is first seen. The floor of the fourth ventricle is separated from the tumor by a cottonoid pledget. The pledget is advanced to protect the floor of the fourth ventricle as the tumor is resected.

The thinned cerebellar vermis is progressively incised in the midline until the dorsum of the tumor is exposed. The tumor is usually soft and moderately vascular and is readily removed with suction irrigation, the CUSA, or laser, using the operating microscope for magnification and illumination. Clinical studies of cooperative groups show that an aggressive (gross total) removal is associated with an improved prognosis for the patient.[305] Dissection is continued laterally to remove tumor from the cerebellar hemispheres and ventrally to remove tumor from the fourth ventricle. When the obstructive hydrocephalus has been relieved, the CSF can be seen flowing from the aqueduct of Sylvius superiorly. It is rare for medulloblastoma to invade the floor of the fourth ventricle. Closure is carried out in multiple layers, with particular attention to a tight dural closure to decrease the risk for pseudomeningocele (bulging wound) formation and the risk for aseptic meningitis and consequent communicating hydrocephalus from spilled blood products. Postoperative CSF shunting for hydrocephalus remains necessary in approximately 30% to 40% of patients.

RADIATION THERAPY

Medulloblastomas commonly infiltrate the subarachnoid space and have a striking propensity to spread throughout the CSF. As many as 25% to 30% of patients have clinically unsuspected cytologic and radiographic evidence of CNS dissemination at the time of diagnosis,[303] and for this reason, radiation therapy is directed to the entire craniospinal axis. Doses of 54 to 55 Gy to the primary tumor site and 35 to 36 Gy to the remainder of the craniospinal axis are generally recommended. These doses usually are reduced by approximately 10 Gy for children younger than 2 or 3 years of age. Five-year survival rates in more recent series range from 50% to 65% or higher.[45] The prognosis is affected by local tumor extent, completeness of surgical resection, presence of CSF dissemination, and age at diagnosis.[307] Survival and patterns of relapse in adults with medulloblastoma are similar to those reported for children.[310] Although medulloblastoma is considered to be one of the most radiosensitive tumors of the CNS, local recurrence remains the primary cause of failure.[311,312]

Although modern radiation therapy techniques have greatly improved the prognosis for patients with medulloblastoma, the maximum benefit that can be achieved with conventional radiation therapy has probably been reached. Adjunctive chemotherapy programs are being pursued actively to further improve the outcome. Randomized trials have been conducted by the International Society of Pediatric Oncology[307] and the CCG.[308] Each study compared radiation therapy plus chemotherapy with radiation therapy alone. The International Society of Pediatric Oncology study used a regimen of weekly VCR during radiation therapy followed by eight courses of VCR and CCNU, cycled every 6 weeks. Patients in the CCG study received similar chemotherapy plus prednisone. Neither trial demonstrated an overall improvement in outcome with the addition of chemotherapy. The 5-year disease-free survival rates in the CCG and International Society of Pediatric Oncology studies were 59% and 55%, respectively, for radiation therapy plus chemotherapy, and 50% and 43%, respectively, for radiation therapy alone. Chemotherapy did, however, appear to benefit certain patients with more advanced stages of disease, including those having only partial or subtotal tumor excision, those with brain stem involvement, and those with advanced T (T3 and T4) and M (M1 to M3) stages. Based on these findings, patients with medulloblastoma have been separated into low-stage or good-risk and high-stage or poor-risk subgroups, and different study questions are being examined in each group.

Clinical studies in good-risk patients have been directed at decreasing treatment-related morbidity, including neuropsychological dysfunction, impaired growth of the spine, and hypothalamic-pituitary dysfunction, by reducing the dose of prophylactic irradiation to areas remote from the primary tumor site. A randomized trial conducted by CCG and POG, which compared 23.4 Gy with the standard 36 Gy craniospinal prophylactic dose in good-risk patients, demonstrated an excessive number of overall treatment failures and isolated neuraxis recurrences in the low-dose arm.[313] In a pilot study conducted by the CCG, the survival rates of patients treated with a combination of low-dose craniospinal axis irradiation and chemotherapy in the form of VCR, CCNU, and cisplatin were found to compare favorably with those in studies of full-dose radiotherapy alone or conventional radiation therapy and chemotherapy.[314]

Studies are also being directed at improving local tumor control. Wara and colleagues used a hyperfractionation schedule (1.0 Gy twice a day) to treat the craniospinal axis to 30 Gy and to boost the posterior fossa to 72 Gy.[315] Poor-risk patients also received chemotherapy. An excess of failures occurred outside of the primary site in good-risk patients, and there was no improvement in survival over that observed with conventional regimens in either risk group.[316] Investigators are currently exploring the use of stereotactic radiosurgery and three-dimensional conformal radiotherapy techniques to deliver an incremental increase in dose to the primary tumor site.[312,315]

CHEMOTHERAPY

Medulloblastomas are responsive to a variety of antineoplastic agents, including VCR, nitrosoureas, procarbazine, dibromodulcitol, cyclophosphamide, methotrexate, platinum compounds, and various drug combinations. Table 43.2-23[128,152,160,167,201,264,266,299,317–338] summarizes some of the single agents and their observed response rates for CNS medulloblastoma when treated at recurrence or for progressive disease. For extra-CNS disease, these same agents have activity, although drugs such as cyclophosphamide, methotrexate, doxorubicin, and VCR may be more active than the nitrosoureas and procarbazine.

Table 43.2-24[339–347,406] summarizes some of the drug combinations that have been used for recurrent or progressive CNS medulloblastoma. It is not possible to compare the durability of these responses, because some reports pool the primitive neuroectodermal tumor patients with medulloblastoma, whereas others do not provide individual lengths of response, an MTP, or Kaplan-Meier curves. This is unfortunate, because those studies suggest an MTP range of 10 to 19 months among the better single agent and combination chemotherapy programs.[346] It is clear, however, that better treatments are needed for recurrent and progressive disease. Whether well-founded or not, current emphasis appears to be with drug combinations such as cyclophosphamide, teniposide, and cisplatin or CCNU, VCR, and cisplatin. Whether these approaches provide long-standing benefit or short term gain awaits more careful adjuvant studies. Problems with drug delivery of these agents to the CNS and inherent drug resistance may compromise long-term benefits and ultimate cure.

TABLE 43.2-23. Efficacy of Single-Agent Chemotherapy for Recurrent and Progressive Central Nervous System Medulloblastoma

Treatment (Reference)	*No.*	*Response Rate[a] (%)*
Doxorubicin[317]	6	0
PCNU[318]	4	0
Etoposide[319]	4	0
AZQ[160,201]	21	28
Bischloroethylnitrosourea[167,320]	6	33
Carboplatin[266,321]	34	35
Methotrexate, IV[322–324]	13	38
Cisplatinum[325–327]	27	40
Melphalan, IV[328]	12	50
Dibromodulcitol[469]	29	51
Vincristine[329–334]	15	73
Procarbazine[152]	4	75
Lomustine[153,335–337,470]	15	80
Cyclophosphamide[338]	7	100

AZQ, aziridinylbenzoquinone; CR, complete response; PCNU, [1-(2-chloroethyl)-3-(2,5-dioxo-3-piperidyl)-1-nitrosourea]; PR, partial response; SD, stable disease.
[a]Response = (CR + PR + SD)/total patients.

TABLE 43.2-24. Efficacy of Combination Chemotherapy for Recurrent and Progressive Central Nervous System Medulloblastoma

Treatment (Reference)	*No.*	*Response Rate[a] (%)*
Vincristine-prednisone-procarbazine[339]	12	25
Vincristine-cyclophosphamide[340]	4	50
6-Thioguanine-procarbazine-dibromodulcitol-lomustine-vincristine[b]	10	60
Lomustine-procarbazine-vincristine[341]	16	62
Etoposide-lomustine-prednisone[342]	3	67
8-drugs-in-1-day[343]	9	67
Nitrogen mustard-vincristine-procarbazine[344]	19	73
Vincristine-methotrexate-bischloroethylnitrosourea[345]	8	100
Vincristine-bischloroethylnitrosourea-dexmethotrexate, IV[345]	8	100
Lomustine-vincristine-cisplatinum[471]	6	100
Carboplatin-teniposide[347]	25	72

CR, complete response; PR, partial response; SD, stable disease.
[a]Response = (CR + PR + SD)/total patients.
[b]M Prados, VA Levin, MSB Edwards, unpublished observations, 1991.

As adjuvant therapy to surgery and irradiation, chemotherapy has shown inconsistent but sometimes dramatic benefit. Part of the problem resides with an agreement for the definition of good and poor risk and the tendency of some investigators to pool data from medulloblastoma with other primitive neuroectodermal tumors. Another constraint is that patients who receive craniospinal irradiation do not tolerate high-dose aggressive chemotherapy protocols well because of reduced bone marrow reserves. In an attempt to improve the tolerance to cytotoxic agents, these authors and others conducted trials to evaluate reduced craniospinal radiation therapy doses. Packer et al. 1994[348,473] reported a 10-year experience with medulloblastoma treated with craniospinal local-boost radiotherapy and adjuvant chemotherapy with vincristine weekly during radiotherapy followed by eight 6-week cycles of cisplatin, lomustine, and vincristine. To be eligible, children had to have a subtotal resection, evidence of metastatic disease, brain stem involvement, or all three. Of the 63 eligible patients, 42 had brain stem involvement, 15 had metastatic disease at the time of diagnosis, and 19 had a subtotal resection. Progression-free survival for the entire group at 5 years was 85%. Progression-free survival was not adversely affected by younger age at diagnosis, brain stem involvement, or subtotal resection. Patients with metastatic disease at the time of diagnosis had a 5-year progression-free survival rate of 67%, as compared with 90% for those children with localized disease at the time of diagnosis ($P = .037$).

The authors conducted a nonrandomized trial of preradiation procarbazine and hydroxyurea during reduced craniospinal irradiation.[304] In that study they found that after 2 weeks of oral procarbazine and irradiation with hydroxyurea, reducing the craniospinal radiation dose to 25 Gy to the spinal axis and 25 to 35 Gy to the whole brain was not detrimental with respect to dis-

TABLE 43.2-25. Classification of Pineal Region Tumors and Tumor Markers

Tumor	*α-Fetoprotein*	*Human Chorionic Gonadotropin-β*	*Lactic Dehydrogenase Isoenzyme*	*Placental Alkaline Phosphatase*
TUMORS OF GERM CELL ORIGIN				
Germinoma (atypical teratoma, dysgerminoma, seminoma)		±	++	++
Embryonal carcinoma				
Extraembryonic structures	+	++		
Endodermal sinus tumors (yolk sac tumor)	+++			
Choriocarcinoma		+++		
Embryonic endoderm, mesoderm, ectoderm				
Immature (malignant) teratoma	±			
Mature teratoma				
TUMORS OF PINEAL PARENCHYMAL CELLS				
Pineoblastoma				
Pineocytoma				
TUMORS OF GLIAL AND OTHER CELL ORIGIN				
NONNEOPLASTIC CYSTS AND MASSES				

(Data from refs. 355 and 356.)

ease-free survival or recurrence patterns in good- and poor-risk patients. When this group was compared with historical controls treated with conventional doses, Halberg and associates[349] found no increase in tumor recurrence in the brain or spinal axis. The 5-year disease-free survival rates for good- and poor-risk patients were 77% and 39%, respectively. In both groups, 70% of recurrences were in the posterior fossa only.

A randomized postoperative trial with postirradiation nitrogen mustard, PCV, procarbazine, and prednisone versus radiation therapy alone for newly diagnosed medulloblastoma found that patients treated with irradiation plus nitrogen mustard, PCV, procarbazine, and prednisone had a statistically significant increase in overall survival rate at 5 years compared with patients treated with radiation therapy alone (74% vs. 56%; $P = .06$).[350]

The authors presented preliminary results of a study that opened in 1984.[232] In that study, they gave combination chemotherapy with TPDCV before and for as many as eight cycles every 6 weeks after radiation therapy in children and adults with high-risk (more than 25% residual tumor, brain stem invasion, positive CSF cytology, positive myelogram) medulloblastoma. Radiation therapy consisted of 54 Gy to the posterior fossa and 24 Gy to the craniospinal axis. Of the 30 patients evaluable (25 children and 5 adults), there were 17 failures, a 5-year disease-free survival of 30%, and an MTP of 4.3 years. Seven pineoblastomas were also treated, with four failures to date, an MTP of 1.6 years, and 38% 5-year disease-free survival.

Hyperfractionated radiation therapy regimens, although potentially less damaging to the CNS, may lead to more bone marrow damage and less tolerance to systemic chemotherapy. One approach that is being evaluated consists of aggressive preradiation therapy chemotherapy. The advantage of this approach is that it unequivocally defines response; the disadvantage is that some drugs may fail to achieve adequate levels in patients with poor risk due to CSF spread of tumor cells.

Eight-in-1-day therapy has also been evaluated before radiation therapy.[343] Of 21 eligible medulloblastoma patients who received at least two courses of chemotherapy, 12 (57%) responded (including three complete responses and three partial responses). The MTP for the combined medulloblastoma primitive neuroectodermal tumor group was 2 years.

In another study, Kovnar and associates treated 11 newly diagnosed children with measurable residual disease and characteristics indicative of poor prognosis with preradiation therapy cisplatin and etoposide.[474] There were 2 of 11 complete responses, 8 partial responses, and 1 stable disease determined radiographically in the series.

For extracranial metastases, the best results appear with aggressive combination chemotherapy. In this situation, issues of CNS drug delivery are not important, and many drugs are active. Initially, these authors evaluated the combination of cyclophosphamide, doxorubicin, and VCR; seven patients treated responded for a median duration of 17 months, and two continue at 34 and 62 months without evidence of disease.[308] Other combinations with good activity are cyclophosphamide and VCR[351]; VCR, dactinomycin, and cyclophosphamide[352]; cisplatin, cyclophosphamide, and VP-16; and DTIC and doxorubicin.[181]

PINEAL REGION TUMORS

CLINICAL AND PATHOLOGIC CONSIDERATIONS

The pineal gland is located in the posterior portion of the third ventricle. Tumors in this region are rare, accounting for fewer than 1% of intracranial tumors, although in children they constitute 3% to 8% of intracranial tumors.[353] The peak incidence of germ cell tumors is the second decade, and few present after the third decade.[354] Table 43.2-25 summarizes the types of tumors found in the pineal region and their tumor markers.[355,356] In all

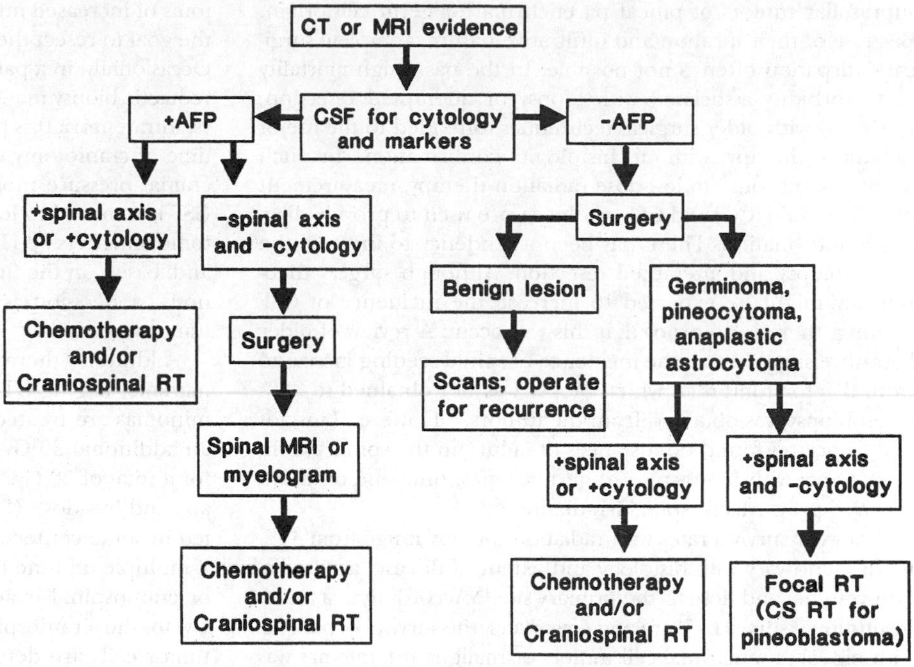

FIGURE 43.2-6. Treatment and evaluation schema for pineal region tumors. AFP, α-fetoprotein; CS, craniospinal; CT, computed tomography; MRI, magnetic resonance imaging; RT, radiation therapy. (Modified from Edwards MSB, Hudgins RJ, Wilson CB, et al. Pineal region tumors in children. *J Neurosurg* 1988;68:689.)

series, germinomas are the most common histology, accounting for 33% to 50% of pineal tumors (the higher frequencies are seen in Japan). Gliomas are the second most common, accounting for approximately 25% of pineal tumors; astrocytomas are the most common of the glial neoplasms arising at this site.

Neurologic signs and symptoms are caused by obstructive hydrocephalus and involvement of ocular pathways. Major symptoms are headache, nausea and vomiting, lethargy, and diplopia. Signs are primarily ocular but can include ataxia and hemiparesis. The major ocular manifestation is paralysis of conjugate upward gaze (Parinaud's syndrome), although pupillary and convergence abnormalities are seen, as are skew deviation and papilledema.

Determination of tumor histology, tumor cell markers, and extent of disease is critical for optimal management of pineal region tumors. Figure 43.2-6 is a schema the authors use to evaluate end-stage patients with pineal region tumors.

The prognosis for these tumors varies depending on the histology and size of tumor and the extent of disease at presentation. Typically, patients with mature teratomas do well with surgery alone; germinomas do best with radiation, although preradiation therapy chemotherapy may increase the cure rate and reduce the total radiation dose; gliomas respond to therapy in a manner discussed in earlier sections; and the remaining tumors respond variably to chemotherapy and radiation therapy, leading to survivals ranging from months to years before recurrence.

SURGERY

Because pineal tumors are near the center of the brain, they are among the most difficult brain tumors to remove, and it is this factor that has created some controversy in their management. However, the application of modern surgical technology, with superb illumination, magnification, surgical guidance, and neuroanesthesia to microsurgical approaches to the pineal region have made this region much more accessible. Surgeons choose from several accepted approaches depending on personal preference and the tumor's position and extent.[357] The current recommendation is to obtain a tissue diagnosis when a diagnosis is not forthcoming from CSF markers, cytology, or both. When possible a gross total resection of the tumor is performed. Resection is particularly important for pineal masses that are relatively radioresistant or that do not require radiation therapy, such as teratomas, arachnoid cysts, and meningiomas.

Many surgical approaches to the pineal region have been described: (1) through the dilated lateral ventricle; (2) through the posterior corpus callosum; (3) under the occipital lobe; and (4) through the posterior fossa over the cerebellum.[358] The most commonly used microsurgical approaches are currently the infratentorial supracerebellar approach described first by Horsley, later by Krause, and resurrected and modernized by Stein, and the supratentorial approach under the occipital lobe described by Poppen and popularized by Clark.[358] Both have been associated with low morbidity and mortality in experienced hands.

The place of image-guided (stereotactic) biopsy in the diagnosis of pineal region tumors is unclear. Although such biopsies have been described as relatively safe, particularly in large tumors, there is a risk that tissue sampling of these heterogenous tumors may not depict accurately the correct histologic nature of the tumor.[359] Without an accurate histologic diagnosis, treatment planning may be erroneous or inadequate. In its favor is the advantage of rapid tissue diagnosis and shortened hospital stay.

RADIATION THERAPY

With certain exceptions, such as benign teratomas, radiation therapy has an established role in the treatment of pineal and suprasellar tumors of pineal parenchymal or germ cell origin. Because of their location and infiltrative nature, complete surgical extirpation often is not possible. In the past, high mortality and morbidity associated with biopsy or attempted resection, especially with older surgical techniques, often led to the use of radiation therapy without histologic confirmation. In such instances, response to low-dose radiation therapy, measurement of AFP and β-HCG, and CSF cytology were used to provide diagnostic information. There has been a tendency to increase the use of biopsy and attempted resection. Although surgery theoretically might be expected to increase the incidence of CSF seeding, there is no proof that this will occur. A review of older literature suggests that the incidence of spinal seeding increased from 3% for tumors in which biopsy was not obtained to 23% when biopsy was obtained from the tumors.[45] However, Linstadt and associates found no instances of failure in the spinal axis in 13 patients with biopsy-proved germinomas, only one of whom received prophylactic spinal irradiation.[360]

Five-year survival rates with radiation therapy range from 44% to 78% and vary with histology and extent of disease, age, radiation volume, and dose to the primary site.[45] According to a multi-institutional survey by Wara and coworkers, the survival of patients with pineal parenchymal cell tumors or malignant teratomas was 21% (3 of 14) compared with 72% (26 of 36) for those with germinomas.[361] More recently, Wolden and colleagues reported 5-year disease-free survival rates of 91% for germinomas, 63% for unbiopsied tumors and 60% for nongerminoma germ cell tumors irradiated to doses of 50 to 54 Gy to the local tumor site with or without additional treatment to the whole brain or ventricular system.[362] Patients younger than 25 to 30 years of age have survival rates of 65% to 80% compared with 35% to 40% for older patients.[361,363] This finding may reflect the increased incidence of true germinomas in younger patients.

Germinomas are infiltrative tumors that tend to spread along the ventricular walls or throughout the leptomeninges. The incidence of CSF seeding ranges from 7% to 12%. Because of these features, the use of fields encompassing the entire ventricular system, the whole brain, and even the entire craniospinal axis has been recommended. In a literature review, Salazar and colleagues found a recurrence-free survival rate of 76% for patients with whole brain irradiation compared with 61% for irradiation to the ventricular system and 51% for smaller volumes.[364] Further analysis of those data showed a 90% survival rate for patients treated with whole brain irradiation and a tumor dose of at least 50 Gy. If smaller fields were used or the dose to the primary tumor site was less than 50 Gy, the survival was 33%. With less than whole brain irradiation, recurrences at the margin of the irradiated volume were reported in the older literature. However, the frequency of such recurrences has been reduced with the availability of CT and MRI for treatment planning. Linstadt and associates concluded that the risk for spinal metastases from germinomas was too small to justify routine prophylactic spinal irradiation, but recommended its use when there is tumor spill at surgery or in those patients with malignant CSF cytology or known subependymal or leptomeningeal metastases.[360]

The paradigm described by Edwards and Levin for management of pineal region tumors differs somewhat from the approach just discussed and is outlined in Figure 43.2-6.[365] If hydrocephalus is present, patients are placed on corticosteroids. A shunt is placed only if corticosteroids fail to relieve the symptoms of increased intracranial pressure. An open operation with the goal to resect the tumor is preferred to a stereotactic biopsy. Occasionally, in a patient with widely disseminated disease, a stereotactic biopsy may be indicated. The approach (supratentorial vs. infratentorial) is planned on the basis of the MRI scan. At the time of craniotomy, an external ventricular drain with an intracranial pressure monitor is placed in the lateral ventricle and CSF is removed to lower intracranial pressure and measure CSF tumor markers (β-HCG and AFP). A tumor biopsy is obtained, and, based on the findings at operation and the histologic diagnosis, a decision is reached regarding the aggressiveness of tumor resection.

Additional therapy is planned based on the histology, CSF markers, staging CT and MRI, and myelography; localized germinomas are treated with 20 Gy to the ventricular system and an additional 30 Gy to the tumor with a 1.5- to 2.0-cm margin for a total of 50 Gy.[362] Treatment with neoadjuvant chemotherapy and low-dose (30 to 40 Gy) focal irradiation is being studied in some centers.[366,367] If the germinoma is disseminated or if multiple midline tumors are present, systemic chemotherapy or craniospinal irradiation is administered. Doses of 20 to 35 Gy to the craniospinal axis have been recommended when tumor cells are detected in the CSF.[368] Patients given chemotherapy as their primary treatment but who have an incomplete response or subsequently recur can be successfully treated with radiotherapy.[369]

Nongerminomatous malignant germ cell tumors, whether localized or disseminated, are treated with systemic chemotherapy (for six courses), followed by restaging studies. After restaging, localized tumors receive focal radiation therapy (20 to 24 Gy to the ventricular system with a tumor boost to 54 to 60 Gy), and disseminated tumors receive craniospinal irradiation (54 to 60 Gy to the primary tumor, 45 Gy to the ventricular system, 35 Gy to the spinal cord, and 45 Gy to any localized spinal cord lesions).[362]

Biopsy-verified tumors with little or no tendency to metastasize to the spinal cord, such as teratomas, pineocytomas, and low-grade gliomas, are treated by resection or with local field irradiation.[370] Craniospinal axis irradiation is reserved for tumors that have a strong tendency toward cord involvement (such as pineoblastoma), for those with positive CSF cytology, or for those with radiographic evidence of spinal cord involvement.

CHEMOTHERAPY

Chemotherapy for glial neoplasms is similar to that covered in earlier sections. The chemotherapy for germ cell tumors is in flux but is encouraging. Adjuvant multidrug therapy with agents such as cisplatin, etoposide, and bleomycin together with high-dose radiotherapy have produced encouraging disease-free and overall survival rates.[371] Finaly and coworkers have used high-dose chemotherapy alone (carboplatin, etoposide, and bleomycin) with deferral of radiotherapy.[372] These results also appear promising.

For germinomas, complete responses before radiation therapy or at recurrence have been observed with cisplatin and bleomycin[373]; carboplatin[374]; cyclophosphamide[375,376]; the combination of cyclophosphamide, vinblastine, and bleomycin[375]; the combination of cisplatin and etoposide[377]; and dactinomycin, methotrexate, vinblastine, and cisplatin.[354,365] This has led to attempts to reduce or defer radiotherapy.[378] Following surgical diagnosis of germinoma, two courses of high-dose cyclophosphamide produced complete response in 91%.[375] Because of this, Allen and coworkers reduced the radiation dose and volume. Of the 10 complete response patients treated with reduced radiation, only 10% of patients have failed 5 years later. A comparable approach using carboplatin produced an 88% response rate and a radiation dose-reduction in five of eight patients.[374] More recently, Bouffet and colleagues reported on a Societe Francaise d'Oncologie Pediatrique study of four courses of alternating etoposide-carboplatin and etoposide-ifosfamide followed by 40 Gy localized radiation therapy for nonmetastatic cases and craniospinal radiation therapy for metastatic cases.[366] Of the 57 patients registered, 47 had biopsy proof of germinoma. Median follow-up was 42 months. The estimated 3-year event free survival was 96%.

For nongerminoma malignant germ cell tumors (e.g., embryonal, endodermal sinus, and mixed tumors), the benefits of chemotherapy are far less impressive, with partial rather than complete responses and recurrence within months to years being the norm. Chemotherapies with activity include combinations of cyclophosphamide, vinblastine, and bleomycin[375]; cisplatin, VCR, and bleomycin[379]; cisplatin and etoposide[380]; and cisplatin, bleomycin, and teniposide.[381] Occasional patients with recurrent germ cell tumors who have failed the combination of cisplatin, bleomycin, and vinblastine therapies have responded to chemotherapy with TPDCV.

The results with chemotherapy have appeared paradoxical, because patients with systemic seminoma treated with cisplatin, bleomycin, and vinblastine have developed brain metastases while receiving chemotherapy. Using nonseminomatous testicular germ cell lines, Pera and colleagues found that temozolomide was quite cytotoxic and they predict that temozolomide will be active against intracranial metastases from testicular seminomas as well as primary germ cell tumors in the CNS.[382]

Given the rarity of CNS germ cell tumors and the similarity of small trials reported in the literature, it is obvious that cooperative group trials are necessary to determine which of the existing chemotherapy combinations are most active. Second-generation studies could then address modifications based on a reasonable database rather than the few anecdotal studies in the literature. Much study needs to be done to elucidate the best drug combinations and use of chemotherapy in these patients.

PITUITARY ADENOMAS

CLINICAL AND PATHOLOGIC CONSIDERATIONS

Pituitary gland tumors tend to produce neuroendocrine or neurologic symptoms and signs. Anatomically, tumors arising from the pituitary gland can compress the pituitary, grow out of the sella to compress and invade the optic chiasm, and, if growth is unabated, extend into the temporal lobe, third ventricle, and the posterior fossa. The chief finding in most patients is vision loss initially characterized by a bitemporal hemianopia. Headache occurs in approximately 20%. Less frequent are ocular palsies due to compression or invasion of the cavernous sinus.

Neuroendocrine abnormalities can be associated with tumor compression of the pituitary gland or hypersecretion of hormones, or both. Table 43.2-6 summarizes some of the more common syndromes and their endocrine abnormalities. Sexual impotence in men and amenorrhea and galactorrhea in women are commonly associated with hyperprolactinemia. Growth hormone hypersecretion is associated with acromegaly or gigantism, depending on the age of the patient. Corticotropin hypersecretion results in Cushing's disease. Elements of hypothyroidism, adrenal insufficiency, and growth hormone deficiency may follow compression of the pituitary gland by growth of an adenoma.

The diagnosis of a pituitary tumor is based on sensitive radioimmunoassays, CT scans, and, most recently, MRI. Figure 43.2-3 shows an MRI scan of a pituitary adenoma before surgery. Pituitary adenomas are classified as endocrine inactive or endocrine active. Most secrete one or, occasionally, two hormones. The reported incidence of the various types of pituitary adenomas depends on the institution's referral patterns. Of 800 patients operated on at UCSF between 1970 and 1981, 630 of 800 (79%) were endocrine active; of these, 331 of 630 (52%) were prolactin secreting, 27% growth hormone secreting, 20% corticotropin secreting, and only 0.3% were thyroid-stimulating hormone secreting.[383] Undifferentiated cell adenomas are considered to be nononcocytic (null) or oncocytic (oncocytoma) tumors.

Of prognostic importance are the functional status of the tumor and how large or invasive it is. Table 43.2-6 is the grading and staging system used at UCSF.[383]

SURGERY

The goal of surgery for the larger (usually, but not always, endocrine inactive) pituitary tumors is to decompress the visual pathways and reduce tumor bulk, whereas the goal for hypersecreting adenomas is normalization of the hypersecretion with preservation of remaining normal pituitary function. For larger nonsecreting pituitary adenomas, surgical cure is often not possible or even necessary, because radiation therapy adjuvant to surgery is usually curative. However, radiation therapy is often withheld until regrowth is suspected on postoperative surveillance scans. In contrast, the hypersecreting adenoma should be resected in its entirety, whenever possible, because the effects of hypersecretion can be devastating, and response to radiation therapy is slow and less predictable.

The operative approach of choice for most pituitary tumors is transsphenoidal, because it is safer and better tolerated than the alternative transcranial (frontal craniotomy) approach.[384] The transsphenoidal approach is possible for tumors occupying the sella turcica and even in those with generous suprasellar extension as long as the tumor is soft (the usual case) and can drop into the sella with progressive resection. Tough, woody suprasellar tumors and those with extension laterally into the middle fossa or anteriorly beneath the frontal lobes must be resected by craniotomy.

RADIATION THERAPY

Microadenomas of the pituitary, usually diagnosed because of endocrine hypersecretion, may be totally resected. There is no indication for radiation therapy, unless there is persistent hormone elevation. Radiation therapy is also indicated for hormone-secreting adenomas that are refractory to pharmacologic management. Macroadenomas, particularly the endocrine inactive lesions, may invade into adjacent structures, such as the cavernous sinus, the optic chiasm, or the third ventricle.

Subtotal resection and postoperative irradiation can relieve mass effect, shrink the remaining tumor, prevent regrowth, and lower hormone levels. Further, radiation therapy alone or medical treatment for patients with hormone-secreting tumors are effective alternatives to resection for patients who are medically inoperable or who refuse surgery.

Breen and colleagues found that for irradiated nonfunctioning adenomas the actuarial tumor control rate was 87.5% at 10 years, 77.6% at 20 years, and 64.7% at 30 years. The oncocytic variant of pituitary adenoma appears to be less sensitive to control by radiotherapy than the nononcocytic form of undifferentiated cell adenoma.[385] Sheline demonstrated that patients with large, nonfunctioning adenomas or prolactin-secreting adenomas associated with visual field deficits had a 60% recurrence rate (using visual field changes as an end point) within 5 years after incomplete resection alone.[386] The recurrence rate was reduced to approximately 4% by the addition of radiation therapy, whereas 7% treated with radiation therapy alone recurred. Approximately two-thirds of patients who presented with modest visual field defects, involving not more than one quadrant, who were treated by surgery or radiation therapy alone had return of normal vision in the involved eyes. With larger visual field defects, restoration of vision was better in patients who received preirradiation therapy and surgical decompression than in those treated by radiation therapy alone. Normal vision was achieved by irradiation alone in approximately two-thirds of patients with acromegaly and visual field defects.

Radiation therapy is less effective in controlling endocrine hypersecretion than in controlling the growth of pituitary adenomas. Radiation therapy decreases serum growth hormone concentrations to normal levels (defined as basal growth hormone levels of less than 5 ng/mL and glucose-suppressed growth hormone levels of less than 2 ng/mL) in 80% to 85% of acromegalic patients.[387] Growth hormone levels decrease at a rate of 10% to 30% per year. Thus, several years may be required for the levels to normalize.[387] The probability of normalization is related to the pretreatment growth hormone level. Radiation therapy is most effective in tumors with relatively small preradiation therapy growth hormone elevations (30 to 50 ng/mL), whereas the response is less predictable with higher growth hormone levels.[386] In contrast, serum insulin-like growth factor-1 levels remain elevated after radiotherapy,[388] and long-term treatment with somatostatin or its analogues may be required.[389] Radiation therapy controls hypercortisolism in 50% to 75% of adults and 80% of children with Cushing's disease. Response occurs within 6 to 9 months of treatment.[390]

Data on control of prolactin secretion by conventional radiation therapy are difficult to interpret. When radiation therapy is used as primary treatment or after incomplete surgical resection, the rate of prolactin normalization varies from 30% to 70%.[391,392] The response occurs over several years, and the probability of cure (defined as prolactin less than 25 ng/mL) is inversely related to the baseline prolactin level. In some cases persistent hyperprolactinemia after treatment may be caused by damage to the hypothalamic prolactin inhibitory pathway.[393] Dopamine agonist therapy with agents such as cabergoline is often part of the initial management of prolactinomas.[394] Radiation therapy in such cases is reserved for patients who fail to respond to this treatment.

Pituitary adenomas may be treated using several different techniques. One approach is to use bilateral coronal arcs with moving wedge filters. The usual treatment plan includes two 110-degree arcs with 30-degree wedge filters. The field size is chosen to include the target volume in the 95% isodose line. The neck is placed in the flexed position so that the plane of rotation is behind the eyes. During simulation, markers are placed on the eyelids. Three tattoo marks are placed on the skin and used for alignment with laser beams to ensure daily positional reproducibility. For large tumors, a three-field technique with lateral opposed wedged portals and a superior or vertex field may be used. Three-dimensional conformal radiotherapy approaches as well as stereotactic radiosurgery and radiotherapy and charged particle beams have also been advocated.[395,396] With conventional radiotherapy techniques, the total dose is carried to 45 Gy in 25 fractions of 1.8 Gy, calculated at the 95% isodose line. This combination of fraction size and total dose controls tumor growth in 90% of cases at 10 years, and, therefore, a larger dose is not indicated.[397–399] Further, radiation-induced injury to optic apparatus or adjacent brain with this dose-fractionation scheme is rare, whereas larger fractions or greater total doses lead to a higher incidence of injury. The optic chiasm appears especially sensitive to radiation injury in patients with acromegaly.[39] Hypopituitarism, however, may develop as a late complication years after completion of radiation therapy.[397] It is more likely to occur in patients who have had surgery and postoperative radiation therapy than in those who have been treated by radiation therapy or surgery alone.[397] Because hypopituitarism is largely correctable by hormone replacement therapy, patients treated for pituitary adenomas should be observed by an endocrinologist for the remainder of their lives. The risk of developing a radiation-induced brain tumor after treatment is 1.3% to 2.7% at 10 years and 2.7% at 30 years.[385,400]

Reirradiation can be considered for patients with recurrent pituitary adenomas when there has been a long interval after the first course of radiotherapy and when other therapeutic methods have been unsuccessful. Schoenthaler and colleagues reported the outcome of 15 patients who were retreated (median dose, 42 Gy) after a median of 9 years from their initial course of radiation therapy (median dose, 40.8 Gy). With a median follow-up time of 10 years, 80% of patients were locally controlled. Although no visual complications were observed, all patients developed hypopituitarism and two sustained temporal lobe injury.[401]

CRANIOPHARYNGIOMAS

CLINICAL AND PATHOLOGIC CONSIDERATIONS

Craniopharyngiomas occur primarily in children. These tumors arise from cell rests that are remnants of Rathke's pouch at the juncture of the infundibular stalk and the pituitary gland. Most of these tumors become symptomatic only after they have attained a diameter of approximately 3 cm. They are usually cystic at the time of presentation. They may compress the optic chiasm or pituitary gland and extend up into the third ventricle. The cyst is high in proteinaceous material and calcium and is seen easily by CT scan or MRI.

Clinically, craniopharyngiomas produce increased intracranial pressure and hypopituitary-hypothalamic-chiasmal dysfunction. Symptoms vary and, in children, may include obesity, delayed development, decreased vision and optic atrophy, field defects, and papilledema.

SURGERY

Craniopharyngiomas usually are approached by a microsurgical procedure done through a frontal or frontotemporal craniotomy. Large craniopharyngioma cysts that enter and enlarge the sella turcica can be drained and resected through a transsphenoidal procedure.

The goal of most surgeons in the surgery of craniopharyngioma is total removal, but some do a more conservative operation and depend on the excellent results with radiation therapy. Aggressive removal nearly guarantees some injury to the pituitary stalk, with subsequent temporary or permanent diabetes insipidus and elements of hypopituitarism. Patients injured in this manner must take replacement hormones and use inhaled desmopressin acetate spray for the control of diabetes insipidus for life. However, patients whose vision was affected by the craniopharyngioma can expect improvement after surgery. The mortality of craniopharyngioma resection should be extremely low.

In Europe, a few centers are treating craniopharyngioma cysts with stereotactic puncture and the instillation of colloidal therapeutic radioisotopes, particularly yttrium 90.[402] Such treatments are being tried in this country also with colloidal phosphorus 32.[403] Intracystic therapy may be a good treatment for craniopharyngioma cysts recurring after conventional external beam irradiation.

RADIATION THERAPY

Although debate exists regarding the extent to which total excision should be attempted, numerous reports demonstrate that local tumor control and survival after subtotal removal, consisting of extensive resection or of limited biopsy and cyst aspiration and irradiation, is comparable with that achieved by radical excision.[404–406] The local control rates after complete resection, subtotal resection alone, and incomplete resection and postoperative irradiation are 70%, 26%, and 75%, respectively.[406] Ten-year survival rates range from 24% to 100% for complete resection, 31% to 52% for subtotal resection, 62% to 86% for incomplete resection and irradiation,[404,405,407] and 100% after radiotherapy alone.[407] The latter group are comprised of patients with small tumors at presentation. Patients undergoing conservative treatment including biopsy and cyst drainage and irradiation appear to enjoy a better quality of life and demonstrate less psychosocial impairment than those initially treated with more extensive resections.[405] Further, conservative therapy is associated with less hypothalamic and pituitary dysfunction and a lower incidence of persistent diabetes insipidus than when a total or near total excision is attempted.[408] More extensive resections using a subfrontal approach may be associated with frontal lobe and visual perceptual dysfunction.[409]

The radiation therapy target volume is based largely on CT and MRI scanning using relatively small margins around demonstrated tumor. The technique varies according to size and location of residual tumor, but most patients are treated by bicoronal arcs with moving wedge filters, similar to the method used for pituitary adenomas. More sophisticated three-dimensional conformal radiotherapy and intensity-modulated radiotherapy approaches and stereotactic radiotherapy techniques using relocatable immobilization devices may further spare surrounding normal tissues.[407] The use of radiosurgery is limited because of the proximity of most lesions to the optic chiasm and brain stem. The total dose is 50 to 55 Gy, given in daily 1.8-Gy increments. In children younger than 3 years of age, it is recommended that, if possible, irradiation be delayed until the child is older.

CEREBELLOPONTINE VESTIBULAR SCHWANNOMAS

CLINICAL AND PATHOLOGIC CONSIDERATIONS

The major tumors occurring in this region are the acoustic nerve tumors and meningiomas. Meningiomas have been discussed previously (see Meningiomas, earlier in this chapter); therefore, the discussion that follows is limited to vestibular schwannomas (acoustic neuromas). These tumors originate on cranial nerve VIII, almost always on the vestibular division, at the point where the nerve acquires its reticulin and Schwann cell investment. Within the skull, this transition zone occurs in the internal auditory foramen and causes local erosion of the internal auditory meatus. Slow growth characterizes these tumors; therefore, they can grow to substantial size before clinical symptoms lead to diagnosis. They often occupy the posterior fossa at the angle between the cerebellum and the pons. By compression, they can affect cranial nerves VII, V, and, less often, IX and X, alone or in various combinations. When large enough, they can compress the medulla and obstruct the CSF, leading to hydrocephalus.

Vestibular schwannomas are most common in the fifth decade and can be associated with familial neurofibromatosis. In the latter instance they occur earlier, in late childhood and adolescence, and may be bilateral.

In a series from the Massachusetts General Hospital, auditory and vestibular branch involvement was found to occur in 98% of patients, facial weakness with disturbances of taste in 56%, sensory loss over the face in 56%, gait abnormality in 41%, and appendicular ataxia in 20%.[29] Diagnosis by skull radiographic examination is suggestive, but definitive diagnosis is most effectively made with MRI or CT scan done in conjunction with the CSF administration of metrizamide contrast.

SURGERY

The aim of surgery for vestibular schwannomas is complete resection, with the surgical approach chosen after consideration of the patient's age, residual hearing, and the size and location of the tumor.[410] When useful hearing is present, the suboccipital approach is taken because of the possibility of hearing preservation postoperatively, particularly in smaller tumors. In patients with poor hearing, the translabyrinthine approach, which produces deafness in the ear operated on, is used for its lower overall morbidity. Occasionally, tumors that reside purely within lateral portions of the internal acoustic canal are approached through the middle cranial fossa.[410]

The translabyrinthine route requires only a small incision behind the ear through which the petrous bone is gradually removed with a high-speed drill until the facial nerve is identified and exposed to the point where it can be separated from the tumor and protected. The dura of the posterior fossa is seen easily and can be opened to gain access to the intradural component of the tumor.

The transoccipital approach requires a unilateral posterior fossa craniectomy, after which the dura is opened and the cerebellum is retracted medially to expose the cerebellopontine angle. The lower cranial nerves are protected while tumor is removed, and the porus acousticus is unroofed in an effort to identify the facial nerve, and in smaller tumors, the acoustic nerve as well. Once the facial nerve is identified, the remainder of the tumor is removed in a usually lengthy and involved operation that fully exploits the surgeon's microsurgical skill.

Complete removal of vestibular schwannomas through the posterior fossa can be predicted in almost every instance, and life-threatening complications are rare except in patients with extremely large tumors. While preservation of the acoustic nerve is uncommon in even small tumors, the facial nerve is in continuity at the end of most acoustic tumor resections. Therefore, any postoperative paresis or paralysis tends to be temporary. When the facial nerve is divided during surgery, it is sutured together when possible, or a nerve graft is placed between the stumps. Facial paralysis with no evidence of recovery within a few months is treated by surgical reinnervation, wherein another cranial nerve, usually the hypoglossal nerve, is joined to the facial nerve peripherally. Bilateral acoustic tumors are seen with neurofibromatosis type 2 and present difficult problems in surgical decision making.[411] In general, a conservative approach is taken, treating the largest tumor when symptoms absolutely require it. Bilateral aggressive tumor resections lead to complete deafness and confer the possibility of bilateral facial nerve paralysis, a cosmetic and functional problem.

RADIATION THERAPY

There have been few reports on the role of conventional radiation therapy for treatment of acoustic neurilemmomas. A review by Wallner and colleagues disclosed 62 patients who were thought to have had a total resection and did not receive irradiation.[412] The recurrence rate in this group was only 3% (2 of 62). The 15-year actuarial survival and relapse-free survival rates were 98% and 94%, respectively. Thirty patients underwent subtotal resection, defined as removal of less than 90% of the tumor. Six of the 13 (46%) patients with subtotally resected lesions recurred, whereas only 1 of 17 (6%) of those treated with subtotal resection and postoperative irradiation to a dose higher than 45 Gy relapsed. The 15-year relapse-free survival rate for patients treated with subtotal resection and radiation therapy (greater than 45 Gy) was 94% compared with 41% for nonirradiated patients ($P = .01$); the corresponding 15-year survival rates were 100% and 67%, respectively ($P = .016$). There were no recurrences among three patients in whom biopsy was obtained at the time of surgery that was followed by irradiation. On the other hand, four of seven patients who were irradiated for disease progression after having had resection alone subsequently developed a second recurrence. Based on these data, it was concluded that postoperative irradiation should be given after subtotal resection to reduce the risk of local tumor progression. The target volume includes a narrow margin around the residual tumor. Maire and colleagues reported a local control rate of 88% among 24 patients with large tumors, the majority of whom were irradiated without initial surgical resection. Hearing was maintained in three of five patients with bilateral neurilemmomas after contralateral tumor resection. No patient developed facial or trigeminal neuropathy.[413] Treatment is given using a homolateral pair of angled beams with wedge filters in daily increments of 1.8 to 2.0 Gy to a total of 50 to 55 Gy.

Stereotactic radiosurgery and stereotactic radiotherapy have been used as an alternative to surgery in selected patients with small acoustic neurilemmomas. In a long-term follow-up study Kondziolka and colleagues reported that 98% of 162 patients treated to a median dose of 16 Gy were controlled.[414] Only four patients required subsequent surgical treatment. Normal facial function was preserved in 79% of patients after 5 years, and normal trigeminal function was preserved in 73%. Patients may develop new incomplete trigeminal and facial cranial neuropathies within a median of 6 to 7 months after radiosurgery. These tend to be mild and usually improve within 8 to 13 months of onset. Approximately, 45% to 50% of patients with useful hearing before radiosurgery maintain their pretreatment hearing level, whereas patients with hearing deficits before treatment generally do not improve after radiosurgery.[393,414,415] The risk of treatment-induced cranial neuropathy is directly related to the volume of the lesion, the dose administered, and the length of nerve irradiated.[416] Efforts are being directed at decreasing the complication rates while maintaining the high control rates with more sophisticated planning and treatment techniques and reducing dose levels.[417]

GLOMUS JUGULARE TUMORS

CLINICAL AND PATHOLOGIC CONSIDERATIONS

Glomus jugulare tumors arise from glomus tissue in the adventitia of the jugular bulb (glomus jugulare) or along Jacobson's nerve in the temporal bone, sometimes multifocally. The tumor invades temporal bone diffusely, but growth is characteristically slow. Sometimes they are endocrine active, with a carcinoid or pheochromocytoma-like syndrome.[418] Because glomus jugulare tumors occur in the jugular foramen, they commonly cause lower cranial nerve palsies and early symptoms of hoarseness and difficulty swallowing. Later, facial weakness, hearing loss, and atrophy of the tongue become prominent. Pulsating tinnitus also may be a presenting symptom, and a pulsating mass can sometimes be seen behind the eardrum. A presumptive radiologic diagnosis of glomus tumor can be made by CT or MRI scanning, with jugular neurilemmoma being the main differential diagnosis. Because glomus tumors incite a tremendous blood supply, particularly by way of the ascending pharyngeal artery, cerebral angiography provides the definitive diagnosis. Because preoperative tumor embolization is essential to surgical removal of glomus tumors, the diagnostic angiogram should be performed just before surgery when possible.

Histopathologically, numerous vascular channels are distinctive. The background is composed of clear cells clumped in a fibrous matrix. A small percentage of glomus tumors are malignant.

SURGERY

The treatment of glomus jugulare tumors is controversial, with advocates for radiation,[419] surgery, and the combination.[420]

Most clinicians would agree that a resection should be attempted and that in most instances gross surgical resection, if not a cure, is a realistic goal. Surgery on glomus tumors is most often performed by a neurosurgeon and a head and neck surgeon together after preoperative embolization. The base of the skull in the region of the jugular foramen is first exposed, and neurovascular structures are identified and mobilized through a high transverse cervical incision. When the incision is extended behind the pinna and a mastoidectomy is completed, the facial nerve can be protected, and the entire tumor bulb, jugular bulb, and internal jugular vein can be seen passing through the base of the skull. Finally, after a suboccipital craniectomy, the sigmoid sinus above and the jugular vein below can be ligated, and the segment between them excised with the attached tumor. Complications of this procedure include CSF leak and cranial nerve (particularly facial) palsy.

RADIATION THERAPY

Even though glomus tumors are histologically benign, radiation therapy is effective and has been recommended for symptomatic lesions that cannot be totally resected or as primary treatment.[421,422] These tumors regress slowly after irradiation, and the success of radiation therapy is measured by the amelioration of symptoms and the absence of disease progression. In their review of the literature, Springate and Weichselbaum found a 94% local control rate for temporal bone glomus tumors treated with radiotherapy alone and a 91% local control rate for glomus tympanicum and jugulare tumors treated with radiotherapy alone or with preoperative or postoperative irradiation.[421] The dose required for control is relatively modest. Kim and associates reported a series of 40 patients with such lesions and added a literature survey.[423] The control rate with subtotal resection and postoperative irradiation was 85%. When radiation therapy only was used for inoperable or recurrent tumors, control was achieved in 88%. Their composite data, including cases from the literature, showed a 25% recurrence rate for doses lower than 40 Gy, whereas only 1.4% recurred with doses of 40 Gy or higher.

Based on these data, a dose of 45 Gy in 5 weeks is recommended. Although a dose of 50 Gy has been advocated for more advanced tumors, there is no evidence that such lesions require higher doses.[422] Treatment is usually delivered through a homolateral pair of angled, wedged portals, depending on the precise location of the lesion. More sophisticated three-dimensional conformal techniques may be used to reduce the dose to surrounding normal tissue structures.

CHORDOMAS

CLINICAL AND PATHOLOGIC CONSIDERATIONS

Chordomas occur along the pathway of the primitive notochord, which extends, in human embryos, from the tip of the dorsum sellae to the coccyx. Chordomas are extradural, multilobulated tumors, varying in consistency from extremely soft to woody and cartilaginous. They are pseudoencapsulated and may invade through the basal dura.

The typical chordoma is composed of cord-like rows of distended, vacuolated (physaliferous) cells. A variant, the chondroid chordoma, has distinctly chondroid elements and may be less aggressive.[424] None of the histopathologic characteristics of tumor aggressiveness (cellularity, pleomorphism, and mitoses) seems to be predictive in chordoma.

The diagnosis of clivus chordomas cannot be made without radiologic tests and often is delayed because symptoms are nonspecific and vague. At onset there is usually headache and intermittent diplopia. These vague symptoms often are not reported, allowing the tumor to grow to an enormous size before the diagnosis is made. Gradually, headache (upper clivus tumors) and neck pain (lower clivus tumors) worsen. Superiorly placed tumors proceed to cause diplopia and facial numbness as the cavernous sinus and Meckel's cave are invaded. Lower clivus tumors compress the lower cranial nerves and later the brain stem.

The differential diagnosis of cranial chordoma includes basal meningioma, neurilemmoma (schwannoma), nasopharyngeal carcinoma, pituitary adenoma, and craniopharyngioma. MRI scanning usually results in a working diagnosis of chordoma, but surgical biopsy (and resection) is mandatory.

SURGERY

Surgery for cranial chordomas is obligatory to obtain diagnostic tissue, to enhance the effectiveness of subsequent radiation therapy, and to improve the patient's clinical condition. With an aggressive surgical resection, a favorable effect on the severe headaches and neurologic deficits associated with chordomas can be anticipated.

Intracranial chordomas occur at the base of the skull, a region relatively remote from surgical access. Consequently, a variety of innovative approaches have been developed by neurosurgeons and head and neck surgeons, and these procedures are commonly done with both types of specialist in attendance.

For midline lesions of the upper clivus that extend into the sella or sphenoid sinus, or both, a transseptal, transsphenoidal approach (as for pituitary tumors) is best. Large, compressive, transdural extensions of these upper clivus tumors into the interpeduncular cistern must be removed through a transcranial, subtemporal, intradural approach. For the more lateralized upper clival tumor and some lateralized midclival tumors, an approach through a sphenoethmoidectomy (to which may be added a maxillectomy) is useful. For midline tumors of the midclivus and lower clivus, a transoral resection is commonly used. A combination of exposures sometimes is necessary for extremely large tumors.

A potentially serious complication of the transsphenoidal, transsphenoethmoid, and transoral approaches is CSF leakage and consequent meningitis. Therefore, every attempt must be made to keep the dura intact during these procedures. Because dural invasion by cranial chordomas may occur 50% of the time, inadvertent entry of the dura during tumor resection is sometimes unavoidable. Careful intraoperative patching of the leak with fat and muscle grafts followed by postoperative spinal CSF drainage is essential.

Cranial chordomas often recur after surgery and radiation therapy. In this situation, reoperation directed toward symptomatic improvement is the only treatment option. Reoperations are complicated by surgical scarring and tissue compromise from irradiation.

RADIATION THERAPY

Chordomas and low-grade chondrosarcomas of the base of skull, clivus, and axial skeleton are not amenable to complete surgical resection. With conventional megavoltage irradiation (median dose of 50 Gy), the local control rate for these lesions is only 27%.[425] Although higher doses appear to improve the local control rate, the proximity of dose-limiting critical structures, such as the optic nerves, chiasm, other cranial nerves, brain stem, temporal lobes, and spinal cord, limit the dose that can be delivered safely to these lesions. Charged particle beams such as protons and helium ions, which feature sharp lateral beam edges and a finite range in tissue, may be used to deliver higher doses than are possible with conventional photon irradiation while keeping the dose to neighboring critical structures at a safe level. The depth of penetration can be tailored to the clinical situation by varying the energy of the beam or by interposing bolus material in the beam path. Charged particle beams can be made to stop in front of a critical structure, such as the spinal cord, and in combination with other lateral or oblique beams, a target volume may be *wrapped* around a critical structure. Precise tumor and normal tissue identification and beam delivery techniques, highly reproducible patient positioning, and accurate compensation for tissue inhomogeneities in the beam path are required.

Available data suggest that the higher doses that are achievable with charged particle irradiation result in higher local control rates than have been observed with conventional radiation therapy techniques. Munzenrider and coworkers reported the outcome of 132 patients with nonchondroid and chondroid skull base chordomas treated postoperatively at the Harvard Cyclotron Laboratory at Massachusetts General Hospital with a 160-MeV proton beam. Patients received a median dose of 69 cobalt Gy equivalent (CGE; the dose in proton Gy multiplied by 1.1, the relative biologic effectiveness for protons compared with cobalt 60), with a range of 36 to 79 CGE, and 95% received 67 CGE (70% to 100% of dose given with proton beam). Follow-up ranged from 2 to 158 months (median, 46 months). Local control was achieved in 70% of patients (93 of 132). Local control was more common in men than women (77% vs. 40%) and more frequent in those with chondroid chordomas than in nonchondroid tumors (83% vs. 66%). The 5-year actuarial local control and disease-specific survival rates were 59% and 80%, respectively.[426] Treatment was complicated by functional and anatomic abnormalities in the brain and brain stem, visual and auditory deficits, and pituitary insufficiency requiring hormone replacement. Skull base chondrosarcomas treated with proton therapy have a better prognosis than chordomas. Rosenberg and colleagues reported a 5- and 10-year local control rate of 99% and 98%, respectively, whereas the disease-specific survival rates at 5 and 10 years were both 99%.[427]

Berson and colleagues reviewed the results of 45 patients with chordomas and chondrosarcomas of the base of skull and cervical spine treated at the University of California Lawrence Berkeley Laboratory with helium ion or neon beams.[428] Total doses ranged from 59.4 to 80.0 Gy equivalent (the physical dose multiplied by the relative biologic effectiveness; 1.2 to 1.3 for helium and 2.0 to 3.3 for neon). After initial subtotal resection, 23 patients were treated with charged particles alone, and 13 were treated with photons and particles combined. Nine patients were treated for recurrent disease. Similar to the findings of Munzenrider and coworkers,[426] the 5-year actuarial local control and survival rates were 59% and 62%, respectively. The 2-year actuarial local control rate for patients treated at initial diagnosis was 78% compared with 33% for those with recurrent tumors ($P < .01$). The 2-year local control rate for tumor volumes of less than 20 mL was 80%, whereas it was 33% for larger lesions ($P < .05$). Complications included unilateral or bilateral blindness in five patients, and four patients developed brain stem injury.

HEMANGIOBLASTOMAS AND HEMANGIOMAS

CLINICAL AND PATHOLOGIC CONSIDERATIONS

Hemangioblastoma accounts for approximately 2% of intracranial tumors, arising most often in the cerebellar hemispheres and vermis. Usually solitary, these tumors can be multiple and may also occur in the brain stem, spinal cord, and supratentorial compartment. Cerebellar hemangioblastoma can be sporadic or occur as a familial disorder as part of the von Hippel-Lindau complex that is transmitted as an autosomal dominant disorder with varying degrees of penetrance. Other entities associated with familial hemangioblastoma are hypernephroma, polycystic kidneys, pancreatic cysts, pheochromocytoma, and erythrocytosis.

Cerebellar hemangioblastomas usually are recognized in the third decade, causing symptoms of increased intracranial pressure and symptoms and signs of cerebellar dysfunction. Gait disturbance and imbalance are particularly common. Clinical progression is slow because these tumors enlarge extremely slowly.

The hemangioblastoma probably arises during embryonic life from primitive endothelial cells around the fourth ventricle. The tumor is composed of numerous capillary and sinusoidal channels lined with endothelial cells. Interspersed are nests of lipid-laden pseudoxanthoma cells. The tumor is usually cystic and contains proteinaceous, xanthochromic fluid. The cyst contains a red (vascular) firm mural nodule, the apparent source of the fluid. The cyst wall is a glial nonneoplastic reaction to the secreted fluid. Occasional hemangioblastomas (brain stem and spinal cord, particularly) are without cysts.

SURGERY

In most instances, the diagnosis can be made by CT scan or MRI. Angiography, to confirm the diagnosis and map the tumor's blood supply, is usually done before surgery. Cerebellar hemangioblastoma tumors are readily approached and excised, with the cyst drained and the entire solid portion carefully dissected and removed. Solid hemangioblastomas of the brain stem are exceedingly vascular, and their removal is associated with high mortality. Such tumors are sometimes irradiated with or without a confirmatory biopsy.

RADIATION THERAPY

Radiation therapy is recommended for patients with unresectable, incompletely excised, and recurrent hemangioblastomas and for those patients who are medically inoperable. Smalley and associates reported the outcome of 25 patients treated with radiation therapy for hemangioblastoma.[429] Nineteen patients had gross residual disease after initial surgery or recurrent tumors, whereas six had only microscopic disease. The overall 5-, 10-, and 15-year survival rates were 85%, 58%, and 58%, respectively, and the recurrence-free survival rates were 76%, 52%, and 42%, respectively. Eight of the 19 patients with gross disease were locally controlled. In-field disease control rates were significantly higher in patients who received at least 50 Gy ($P = .06$) than in those who received lower doses. Five of the six patients treated for microscopic disease had the disease controlled. Based on these data, doses of at least 50 to 55 Gy in 5.5 to 6.0 weeks appear to be warranted.

Radiosurgery has also been applied to the treatment of hemangioblastomas. Patrice and colleagues summarized the outcome of 38 lesions in 22 patients (eight patients with multifocal tumors) who received radiosurgery as definitive treatment or in relapsed patients after surgery or surgery and conventional radiotherapy. The median tumor volume was 0.97 cc (range, 0.05 to 12.0 cc), and the median dose was 15.4 Gy (range, 12 to 20 Gy). With a median follow-up time of 24.5 months (range, 6 to 77 months), 31 of 36 evaluable tumors (86%), including all tumors treated definitively with radiosurgery, remained locally controlled. All five lesions that relapsed after radiosurgery were among the tumors that were treated for recurrence after initial surgery. Better control rates were associated with higher doses and smaller tumor volumes. The 3-year actuarial progression-free survival rate was 86%, and the 2-year actuarial survival rate was 88%.[430] Among 29 hemangioblastomas treated by Chang and coworkers, only one (3%) progressed. Five tumors (17%) regressed completely, 16 (55%) partially regressed, and 7 (24%) remained unchanged in size.[431] Radiosurgery should be considered for surgically unresectable hemangioblastomas, as adjuvant treatment for incompletely excised tumors, as definitive treatment of multifocal disease, and for salvage therapy for discrete recurrences after surgical relapse.[430,431]

CHOROID PLEXUS PAPILLOMA AND CARCINOMA

CLINICAL AND PATHOLOGIC CONSIDERATIONS

Choroid plexus papilloma and carcinoma are rare tumors that occur most often in children younger than 12 years of age, although they can occur at any age. Nearly one-half of these tumors are found in patients younger than 20 years of age. The tumor is an irregularly lobulated reddish mass, which on histopathologic examination is apparently normal choroid plexus. Rarely, these tumors show malignant features and are then classified as choroid plexus carcinoma.

In children, choroid plexus papillomas most often occur in the lateral ventricles. In adults, the fourth ventricular papilloma is most common. Third ventricle tumors are exceedingly rare. Because papillomas tend to grow slowly within ventricles, they expand to fill the ventricle and block CSF flow. In addition, papillomas are thought to secrete CSF. Choroid plexus papillomas (and carcinomas) can produce hydrocephalus secondary to obstruction of the CSF; by CSF overproduction by the tumor; or by damage to the CSF resorptive bed from recurrent hemorrhages. As a result, increased intracranial pressure without focal findings is the most common presentation; fourth ventricular tumors can also be associated with focal findings of ataxia and nystagmus.

Although choroid plexus papillomas and carcinomas extensively seed throughout the ventricular and subarachnoid spaces, seeding from papillomas is usually subclinical, whereas that from carcinomas is frequent and dramatically symptomatic. These tumors are seen easily by CT scan and MRI. For patients with anaplastic changes, the authors advocate staging by myelography and examination of the CSF.

Therapy for anaplastic tumors should be approached in a manner similar to medulloblastoma and malignant ependymomas. Because of the aggressive nature of the more anaplastic tumors, therapy must be equally aggressive, requiring radiation therapy and, in some instances, intraventricular chemotherapy.

SURGERY

The treatment of choroid plexus papillomas is total surgical excision. Choroid plexus tumors of the lateral ventricle are approached through a high parietal cortical incision and transcortical approach to the ventricular trigone. The predilection of these tumors for the left (often dominant) side makes this approach worrisome. Hydrocephalus is the rule and simplifies the exposure when retraction into the ventricle is established. Tumor arteries and veins are identified by use of the operating microscope and then coagulated, after which smaller tumors are removed intact and larger tumors are removed piecemeal. In one-half of the patients, hydrocephalus is relieved by tumor resection, but persistent hydrocephalus requires shunting.

Choroid plexus papillomas of the third ventricle are exceedingly rare but can be approached through various surgical exposures of the third ventricle. The problems of removal of fourth ventricular choroid plexus tumors are similar to those associated with suboccipital removal of medulloblastomas or ependymomas, as discussed in surgery sections for those tumors.

RADIATION THERAPY

Because choroid plexus papillomas are often cured by complete surgical resection, there is little information regarding their response to radiation.[299] The studies that are available do not provide sufficient detail to allow an assessment of the value of radiotherapy for these tumors. Pathology specimens from patients who received low-dose preoperative radiation therapy (approximately 30 Gy) demonstrated a marked reduction in tumor size, obliteration of the capillary bed, and necrosis, although at this dose level there was little change in the neoplastic choroidal cells. Naguib and coworkers reported a case of an inoperable choroid plexus papilloma with extensive involvement of the mastoid bone.[432] This patient received 49.5 Gy in 32 treatments during a 33-day period. Serial CT scans showed that 16 months after completion of the radiation therapy, the mass was markedly reduced in size. Such anecdotal reports suggest that it is reasonable to offer local radiation therapy to patients with inoperable or recurrent choroid plexus papillomas.[299]

Radiation therapy may be beneficial in patients with choroid plexus carcinomas even after gross total resection.[433,434] Because ventricular and subarachnoid tumor seeding may occur in up to 44% of cases,[435] consideration must be given to treating the entire craniospinal axis. However, data to support this approach are unavailable. Chow and colleagues recommend that patients with completely excised localized choroid plexus carcinomas be treated with either chemotherapy or limited field irradiation if their spinal MRI and CSF cytology study results are negative. They advise both chemotherapy and craniospinal axis irradiation for those with incompletely excised tumors or evidence of leptomeningeal spread.[434] Infants and young children may be successfully treated initially with postoperative chemotherapy and delayed radiation.[436]

CHEMOTHERAPY

Usually, chemotherapy is not used for choroid plexus papillomas. For the more anaplastic tumors, however, the authors have increasingly used chemotherapy adjuvant to surgery and irradiation to prevent the inevitable recurrence and CSF dissemination common to the choroid plexus carcinomas. As with many of the less common tumors discussed, there are no chemotherapeutic guidelines and few reports to guide the therapist.

Initially, the authors used chemotherapy only for recurrent disease. They have used combinations of cyclophosphamide, doxorubicin, and VCR and nitrosourea-based combinations. They have seen transient responses and disease control with both. They have also used intraventricular chemotherapy with low-dose methotrexate (2 to 3 mg/d for 5 days) or cytosine arabinoside (30 mg/d for 3 days), or both, to stave subarachnoid spread. As a result of this experience, the authors currently advocate the use of adjuvant chemotherapy with a nitrosourea-based combination after irradiation and the use of concomitant intraventricular chemotherapy. During irradiation, they have used intraventricular cytosine arabinoside and methotrexate after irradiation. Further study and additional approaches should be considered.

SPINAL AXIS TUMORS

CLINICAL AND PATHOLOGIC CONSIDERATIONS

Some of the clinical features of spinal axis tumor localization and diagnosis have been discussed previously. Most primary spinal axis tumors produce symptoms and signs as a result of spinal cord and nerve root compression rather than because of parenchymal invasion.

The reported frequency of primary spinal cord tumors is between 10% and 19% of all primary CNS tumors.[437] Although most spinal axis tumors are extradural, most primary spinal axis tumors are intradural. Of intradural tumors, the intradural extramedullary neurilemmomas and meningiomas are the most common (see Table 43.2-3). Neurilemmomas and meningiomas are normally intradural, but occasionally they may present as extradural tumors. Other intradural extramedullary tumors are vascular tumors, chordomas, and epidermoids.

Intramedullary tumors have the same cellular origins as the other CNS tumors discussed previously. In terms of frequency, ependymomas occur in approximately 40% of patients with intramedullary tumors; next most common are the astrocytomas of low- and mid-anaplasia. These are followed in frequency by less common histologies such as oligodendroglioma, ganglioglioma, medulloblastoma, and various hemangiomas and hemangioblastomas.

Table 43.2-26 classifies spinal axis tumors by location. Although different tumor types exhibit a predilection for certain spinal regions, taken altogether, spinal tumors are distributed almost evenly along the spinal axis. Approximately 50% of spinal tumors involve the thoracic spinal canal, 30% involve the lumbosacral spine, and the remainder involve the cervical spine, including the foramen magnum. Some tumors, such as the neurilemmomas, occur with greatest frequency in the thoracic region, although they can be found throughout the spine and often extend through an intervertebral foramen to acquire a dumbbell configuration.

TABLE 43.2-26. Classification of Spinal Tumors by Their Location in Relation to the Spinal Cord and Dura Mater

Location	*Usual Tumor Histologies*
Extradural	Metastatic (carcinoma, lymphoma, melanoma, sarcoma), chordoma
Intradural	
Extramedullary	Schwannoma,[a] meningioma[a]
Intramedullary	Astrocytoma, ependymoma[b]

[a]May extend along nerve root into extradural and extraspinal spaces.
[b]Ependymomas originating from the filum terminale and involving the cauda equina, not intramedullary in the strictest sense, are included here by custom.

Meningiomas are dural based and arise preferentially at the foramen magnum and in the thoracic spine. Astrocytomas are distributed throughout the spinal cord, and most ependymomas involve the conus medullaris and the cauda equina. Spinal chordomas are characteristically sacral.

Clinically, patients with spinal axis tumors present with a sensorimotor spinal tract syndrome, a painful radicular spinal cord syndrome, or a central syringomyelic syndrome. In the sensorimotor presentation, symptoms and signs are in response to compression of the spinal cord. The onset is gradual over weeks to months, initial presentation is asymmetric, and motor weakness predominates. The level of impairment determines the muscle groups involved. Because of external compression, dorsal column involvement occurs with paresthesia and abnormalities of pain and temperature on the side contralateral to the motor weakness.

Radicular spinal cord syndromes occur because of external compression and infiltration of spinal cord roots. The main symptom is sharp, knife-like pain in the distribution of a sensory nerve root. The intense pain is often of short duration, with pain that is more aching in nature persisting for longer periods. The pain typically is exacerbated by coughing and sneezing or other maneuvers that increase intracranial pressure. Local paresthesia and impairment of sensations of pain and touch are common, as are weakness and muscle wasting. These findings commonly antedate cord compression by months.

Spinal tumors, particularly intramedullary tumors, can produce syringomyelic dysfunction by destruction and cavitation within the central gray matter of the cord. This produces lower motor neuron destruction and attendant segmental muscle weakness, wasting, and loss of reflexes. There is also a dissociated sensory loss of pain and temperature sensation with preservation of touch. With extension of the lesion, however, touch, vibration, and position sense are affected.

Finally, many patients with spinal axis tumors or supratentorial tumors that show a tendency toward drop metastases tend to lead to leptomeningeal neoplasia. Choucair and colleagues found that 1.2% of glioblastomas and 1.5% of anaplastic gliomas had metastatic spread of their supratentorial tumors to the spinal cord at some time during the course of their disease.[62]

SURGERY

General Considerations

The use of the operating microscope is as essential for spinal cord tumor surgery as it is for brain tumor surgery. In addition, other surgical adjuncts, such as intraoperative ultrasound, the CO_2 laser, and the CUSA, are equally valuable for the resection of spinal cord tumors. The ultrasound is particularly useful for examining the spinal cord through an intact or open dura to assess the level of maximum tumor involvement or to differentiate tumor cysts from solid tumor masses.

Surgical Planning

MRI scanning is invaluable for the diagnosis, localization, and characterization of spinal tumors (see Fig. 43.2-4). In all but vascular tumors (e.g., hemangioblastoma), in which angiography is needed, or tumors that cause extensive bony destruction (e.g., metastasis), where CT scanning might be helpful, a technically excellent MRI scan is most often sufficient for preoperative planning for spinal tumors. Determination of the spinal level of the tumor and its exact relation to the spinal cord is important in localization. Corticosteroids are given before, during, and after spinal cord tumor surgery to help control spinal cord edema.

Removal of Intradural Extramedullary Tumors

Meningiomas and neurilemmomas (schwannomas) occur in the intradural extramedullary spinal compartment. Most of these tumors can be completely resected (cured), because through a laminectomy exposure they can be easily separated and rotated away from the spinal cord, which is already displaced, but not invaded, by tumor.

Neurilemmomas arise from spinal rootlets (most often dorsal rootlets), and their removal includes sections of those rootlets involved. Neurilemmomas can grow along the nerve root in a dumbbell fashion through a neural foramen; and although some of these extraspinal tumor extensions can be removed by extending the initial laminectomy exposure laterally, some must be resected at a separate operation through a thoracotomy, a costotransversectomy, or a retroperitoneal approach.

Meningiomas in most patients can be removed through a posterior (laminectomy) approach, because they are commonly lateral or anterolateral, and even the more anteriorly placed tumors cause enough lateral displacement of the spinal cord to allow access for resection without traction on the spinal cord. The uncommon tumor directly anterior to the spinal cord must sometimes be approached anteriorly, anterolaterally, or posterolaterally. Anteriorly situated meningiomas at the foramen magnum are sometimes unresectable because of their encasement of the vertebral artery.

Removal of Intramedullary Tumors

The most common intramedullary tumors are ependymoma and astrocytoma. Hemangioblastoma is another (infrequent) tumor occurring in the spinal intramedullary compartment. Surgery is the principal treatment for all these tumors, with the exception of anaplastic astrocytomas.

Intramedullary tumors are approached through a laminectomy exposure, and after the dura is opened, a longitudinal myelotomy is made over the widened region of spinal cord and the incision deepened several millimeters to the tumor surface. Dissection planes around the tumor are sought microsurgically and, in the case of ependymomas, usually found and extended gradually around the tumor's surface, because removal of the central tumor bulk (by CO_2 laser or CUSA) causes the tumor to collapse. Usually, such tumors are completely removed. Tumors with indefinite dissection planes (usually low-grade astrocytomas) cannot be removed completely, but bulk reduction can cause long-term palliation. If frozen section shows a tumor to be malignant, surgery is aborted, and radiation therapy is the treatment.

Hemangioblastomas are extremely vascular tumors, so the tumor margins are addressed first where feeding arteries are coagulated, and the tumor is dissected and removed *en bloc*. The dorsal location of most of these tumors and the commonly associated cyst simplifies the removal to some extent.

RADIATION THERAPY

Radiation therapy is recommended for unresectable and incompletely resected neoplasms of the spinal axis. As a rule, doses of 50 to 54 Gy are used so that the risk of radiation injury to the cord is less than that from the neoplasm itself. Low-grade tumors and meningiomas are treated at the lower dose level and malignant tumors to the higher level.[438] For lesions involving only the cauda equina and in situations in which irreversible and complete transverse myelopathy already has occurred, higher doses are permissible. The tumor usually is treated with a margin of 2 to 3 cm or two vertebral bodies above and below the lesion. Extension of the portals to include the thecal sac has been suggested for ependymomas that are removed piecemeal[439] and for those arising in the distal spinal canal.[440] Ependymomas of the cord have a longer natural history than astrocytomas. Although most astrocytomas that recur do so within 3 years of treatment, recurrence of ependymomas may be delayed for as long as 12 years.[440,441]

Adjunctive radiation therapy is not necessary when ependymomas are removed completely in an *en bloc* fashion. However, 75% of patients (three of four) reported by Wen and associates recurred locally or with spread to the thecal sac after complete resection alone when the tumor was excised piecemeal.[439] All seven nonirradiated patients with incompletely excised lesions reported by Barone and Elvidge[442] and Schuman and coworkers[443] recurred. In contrast, postoperative radiation therapy appears to improve tumor control and disease-free survival in patients with incompletely resected ependymomas. Sloof and colleagues found their irradiated patients survived nearly twice as long as those who were not irradiated.[2] Five- and 10-year survival rates in irradiated patients with localized ependymomas range from 60% to 100% and 68% to 95%, respectively, whereas 10-year relapse-free survival rates vary from 43% to 61%.[440,444] Tumor grade has a significant effect on outcome. Waldron and colleagues found that for well-differentiated tumors the 5-year cause-specific survival was 97% as compared with 71% for intermediate or poorly differentiated tumors ($P = .005$).[440] Myxopapillary ependymomas that arise exclusively in the conus medullaris have a better prognosis than the cellular ependymomas that arise in the cord.[439] Local recurrence is the predominate pattern of treatment failure, occurring in 25% of irradiated patients.[440]

The 5- and 10-year survival rates for irradiated patients with low-grade astrocytomas of the spinal cord vary from 60% to 90% and 40% to 90%, respectively; 5- and 10-year relapse-free survival rates range from 66% to 83% and 53% to 83%, respectively.[438,441] Approximately 50% to 65% of astrocytomas are controlled locally. Patients with malignant gliomas have a much poorer prognosis; none of the patients with anaplastic astrocytoma or glioblastoma multiforme reported by Linstadt and colleagues survived longer than 8 months.[441]

CHEMOTHERAPY

There have been no reports of controlled clinical trials of chemotherapy for primary spinal axis tumors. Drugs active against intracranial astrocytomas, oligodendrogliomas, ependymomas, medulloblastoma, and germ cell tumors logically may be assumed to be equally efficacious against these same histologies in the spinal cord. Along with reports of chemotherapy activity against intracranial tumors, anecdotal patient reports have been included.

The authors' experience suggests that palliation is possible for astrocytomas using nitrosourea-based chemotherapy regimens. No therapy is clearly superior. For drop metastases from ependymomas, they have used BCNU and dibromodulcitol as single agents and various combinations with some benefit.[181,445] For drop metastases from medulloblastoma, various drugs have been found to be beneficial. Specifically, cyclophosphamide, carboplatin, methotrexate, procarbazine, teniposide, and VCR have been used alone or in various combinations. These drugs would be expected to produce palliation for weeks to many months.

Although leptomeningeal spread is a common complication of primary spinal axis tumors, the use of intraventricular and intrathecal chemotherapy is limited to the treatment of microscopic deposits. Biodistribution in the subarachnoid CSF can be limited in the face of intradural extramedullary tumors. In addition, deposits of 5 mm in diameter or larger are not likely to benefit because of limitations in diffusion coupled with transcapillary loss of drug in the tumor.[446]

REFERENCES

1. Davis FG, Preston-Martin S. Epidemiology. Incidence and survival. In: Bigner DD, McLendon RE, Bruner JM, eds. *Russell and Rubinstein's pathology of tumors of the nervous system.* London: Arnold, 1999:7.
2. Sloof JL, Kernohan JW, MacCarty CS. *Primary intramedullary tumors of the spinal cord and filum terminale.* Philadelphia: WB Saunders, 1964.
3. Preston-Martin S. Descriptive epidemiology of primary tumors of the spinal cord and spinal meninges. *Neuroepidemiology* 1990;9:106.
4. Davis DL, Hoel D, Percy C, et al. Is brain cancer mortality increasing in industrial countries? *Ann NY Acad Sci* 1990;609:791.
5. Boyle P, Maisonneuve P, Saracci R, et al. Is the increased incidence of primary malignant brain tumors in the elderly real? *JNCI* 1990;82:1594.
6. Greig NH, Ries LG, Yancik R, et al. Increasing annual incidence of primary malignant brain tumors in the elderly. *JNCI* 1990;82:1621.
7. Musicco M, Filippini G, Bordo BM, et al. Gliomas and (occupational) exposure to carcinogens: case-control study. *Am J Epidemiol* 1982;116:782.
8. Moss AR. Occupational exposure and brain tumors. *J Toxicol Environ Health* 1985;16:703.
9. McLaughlin JK, Malker HS, Blot WJ, et al. Occupational risks for intracranial gliomas in Sweden. *JNCI* 1987;78:253.
10. Wrensch M, Yost M, Miike R, et al. Adult glioma in relation to residential power frequency electromagnetic field exposures in the San Francisco Bay area. *Epidemiology* 1999;10:523.
11. Kheifets LI, Sussman SS, Preston-Martin S. Childhood brain tumors and residential electromagnetic fields (EMF). *Rev Environ Contam Toxicol* 1999;159:111.
12. Higashikubo R, Culbreth VO, Spitz DR, et al. Radiofrequency electromagnetic fields have no effect on the in vivo proliferation of the 9L brain tumor. *Radiat Res* 1999;152:665.
13. Copeland DD, Bigner DD. Glial-mesenchymal tropism of in vivo avian sarcoma virus neuro-oncogenis in rats. *Acta Neuropathol* 1978;41:23.
14. Wodinski I, Kensler CJ, Rall DP. The induction and transplantation of brain tumors in neonate beagles. *Proc Am Assoc Cancer Res* 1969;99.
15. Beutler AS, Banck MS, Wedekind D, et al. Tumor gene therapy made easy: allogeneic major histocompatibility complex in the C6 rat glioma model. *Hum Gene Ther* 1999;10:95.
16. Toki S, Tanaka T, Uosaki Y, et al. RP-1551s, a family of azaphilones produced by *Penicillium* sp., inhibit the binding of PDGF to the extracellular domain of its receptor. *J Antibiot (Tokyo)* 1999;52:235.
17. Hochberg FH, Miller G, Scholley RT, et al. Central nervous system lymphoma ralated to Epstein-Barr virus. *N Engl J Med* 1983;309:745.
18. Annegers JF, Laws ER Jr, Kurland LT, et al. Head trauma and subsequent brain tumors. *Neurosurgery* 1979;4:203.
19. Relling MV, Rubnitz JE, Rivera GK, et al. High incidence of secondary brain tumors after radiotherapy and antimetabolites. *Lancet* 1999;354:34.
20. Malone M, Lumley H, Erdohazi M. Astrocytoma as a second malignancy in patients with acute lymphoblastic leukemia. *Cancer* 1986;57:979.
21. Sogg RL, Donaldson SS, Yorke CH. Malignant astrocytoma following radiotherapy of a craniopharyngioma. *J Neurosurg* 1978;48:622.
22. Poster DS, Bruno S. The occurrence of second primary neoplasms in patients with non-Hodgkin's lymphomas. *IRCS Med Sci Cancer* 1980;8:554.
23. Rubinstein AB, Shalit MN, Cohen M, et al. Radiation-induced cerebral meningioma: a recognizable entity. *J Neurosurg* 1984;61:966.
24. Spallone A, Gagliardi FM, Vagnozzi R, et al. Intracranial meningiomas related to external cranial irradiation. *Surg Neurol* 1979;12:153.
25. Levin VA, Wilson CB. Clinical characteristics of cancer in the brain and spinal cord. In: Crook ST, Prestaydo A, eds. *Cancer and chemotherapy: introduction to neoplasia and antineoplastic chemotherapy.* New York: Academic Press, 1981:167.
26. Bingas B. Tumors of the base of the skull. In: Vinken PJ, Bruyn GW, eds. *Handbook of clinical neurology: tumors of the brain and skull.* Amsterdam: North Holland, 1974:136.
27. Fahlbusch R, Marguth F. Endocrine disorders associated with intracranial tumors. In: Vinken PJ, Bruyn GW, eds. *Handbook of clinical neurology: tumors of the brain and skull.* Amsterdam: North Holland, 1974:345.
28. Russell DJ. *Pathology of tumors of the nervous system.* Baltimore: Williams & Wilkins, 1977.
29. Adams R, Victor M. *Principles of neurology.* New York: McGraw-Hill, 1977.
30. Fandino J, Kollias SS, Wieser HG, et al. Intraoperative validation of functional magnetic resonance imaging and cortical reorganization patterns in patients with brain tumors involving the primary motor cortex. *J Neurosurg* 1999;91:238.
31. Berger MS, Kincaid J, Ojemann GA, et al. Brain mapping techniques to maximize resection, safety and seizure control in children with brain tumors. *Neurosurgery* 1999;25:786.
32. McDermott MW, Gutin PH. Image-guided surgery for skull base neoplasms using the ISG viewing wand. Anatomic and technical considerations. *Neurosurg Clin North Am* 1996;7:285.
33. Heilbrun MP. Computed tomography-guided stereotactic systems. *Clin Neurosurg* 1984;31:564.
34. Apuzzo ML, Chandrasoma PT, Cohen D, et al. Computed imaging stereotaxy: experience and perspective related to 500 procedures applied to brain masses. *Neurosurgery* 1987;20:930.
35. Leibel SA, Sheline GE. Tolerance of the brain and spinal cord to conventional irradiation. In: Gutin PH, Leibel SA, Sheline GE, eds. *Radiation injury to the nervous system.* New York: Raven Press, 1991:211.
36. Posner JB. Side effects of radiotherapy. In: *Neurologic complications of cancer.* Philadelphia, PA: FA Davis, 1995:311.
37. Hoffman WF, Levin VA, Wilson CB. Evaluation of malignant glioma patients during the postirradiation period. *J Neurosurg* 1979;50:624.
38. Schultheiss TE, Kun LE, Ang KK, et al. Radiation response of the central nervous system. *Int J Radiat Oncol Biol Phys* 1995;31:1093.
39. Sheline GE, Wara WM, Smith V. Therapeutic irradiation and brain injury. *Int J Radiat Oncol Biol Phys* 1980;6:1215.
40. Rubin P. Radiation biology and radiation pathology syllabus. 1975.
41. Sklar CA, Constine LS. Chronic neuroendocrinological sequelae of radiation therapy. *Int J Radiat Oncol Biol Phys* 1995;31:1113.
42. Gordon KB, Char DH, Sagerman RH. Late effects of radiation on the eye and ocular adnexa. *Int J Radiat Oncol Biol Phys* 1995;31:1123.
43. Cooper JS, Fu K, Marks J, et al. Late effects of radiation therapy in the head and neck region. *Int J Radiat Oncol Biol Phys* 1995;31:1141.
44. Marks JE, Baglan RJ, Prassad SC, et al. Cerebral radio-necrosis: incidence and risk in relation to dose, time, fractionation and volume. *Int J Radiat Oncol Biol Phys* 1981;7:243.
45. Leibel SA, Sheline GE. Radiation therapy for neoplasms of the brain. *J Neurosurg* 1987;66:1.
46. Bleyer WA, Griffin TW. White matter necrosis, mineralizing microangiopathy, and intellectual abilities in surviovors of childhood leukemia. In: Gilbert HA, Kagan AR, eds. *Radiation damage to the nervous system.* New York: Raven Press, 1980:155.
47. Hazle JD, Jackson EF, Schomer DF, et al. Dynamic imaging of intracranial lesions using fast spin-echo imaging: differentiation of brain tumors and treatment effects. *J Magn Reson Imaging* 1997;7:1084.
48. Gutin PH. Treatment of radiation necrosis of the brain. In: Gutin PH, Leibel SA, Sheline GE, eds. *Radiation injury to the nervous system.* New York: Raven Press, 1991:271.
49. Glantz MJ, Burger PC, Friedman AH, et al. Treatment of radiation-induced nervous system injury with heparin and warfarin. *Neurology* 1994;44:2020.
50. Mulhern RK, Fairclough D, Ochs J. A prospective comparison of neuropsychologic performance of children surviving leukemia who received 18- Gy, or no cranial irradiation. *J Clin Oncol* 1991;9:1348.
51. Mulhern RK, Ochs J, Kun LE. Changes in intellect associated with cranial radiation therapy. In: Gutin PH, Leibel SA, Sheline GE, eds. *Radiation injury to the nervous system.* New York: Raven Press, 1991:325.
52. Eiser C. Intellectual abilities among survivors of childhood leukemia as a function of CNS irradiation. *Arch Dis Child* 1978;53:391.

53. Kleinberg L, Wallner K, Malkin MG. Good performance status of long-term disease-free survivors of intracranial gliomas. *Int J Radiat Oncol Biol Phys* 1993;26:129.
54. Schultheiss TE, Stephens LC, Peters LJ. Survival in radiation myelopathy. *Int J Radiat Oncol Biol Phys* 1986;12:1765.
55. Wang PY, Shen WC, Jan JS. Magnetic resonance imaging in radiation myelopathy. *Am J Neuroradiol* 1992;13:1049.
56. Marcus RB Jr, Million RR. The incidence of myelitis after irradiatin of cervical spinal cord. *Int J Radiat Oncol Biol Phys* 1990;19:3.
57. Schultheiss TE. Spinal cord radiation "tolerence" doctrine versus data. *Int J Radiat Oncol Biol Phys* 1990;19:219.
58. Wara WM, Phillips TL, Sheline GE, et al. Radiation tolerance of the spinal cord. *Cancer* 1975;35:1558.
59. Cox JD, Stetz J, Pajak TF. Toxicity criteria of the Radiation Therapy Oncology Group (RTOG) and the European Organization for Research and Treatment of Cancer (EORTC). *Int J Radiat Oncol Biol Phys* 1995;31:1341.
60. Pavy JJ, Denekamp J, Letschert J, et al. EORTC Late Effects Working Group. Late effects toxicity scoring: the SOMA scale. *Radiother Oncol* 1995;35:11.
61. Burger PC, Dubis PJ, Schold SC Jr, et al. Computerized tomographic and pathologic studies in untreated, quiescent, and recurrent glioblastoma multiforme. *J Neurosurg* 1983;58:159.
62. Choucair AK, Levin VA, Gutin PH, et al. Development of multiple lesions during radiation therapy and chemotherapy in patients with gliomas. *J Neurosurg* 1986;65:654.
63. Hochberg FH, Pruitt A. Assumptions in the radiotherapy of glioblastoma. *Neurology* 1980;30:907.
64. Kelly PJ, Daumas-Duport C, Kispert DB, et al. Imaging-based stereotaxic serial biopsies in untreated intracranial glial neoplasms. *J Neurosurg* 1987;66:865.
65. Levin VA. Pharmacokinetics and CNS chemotherapy. In: Hellmann K, Carter SK, eds. *Fundamentals of cancer chemotherapy.* New York: McGraw-Hill, 1986:28.
66. Levin VA, Patlak CS, Landahl HD. Heuristic modeling of drug delivery to malignant brain tumors. *J Pharmacokinet Biopharm* 1980;8:257.
67. Levin VA. Chemotherapy of primary brain tumors. *Neurol Clin North Am* 1985;3:855.
68. Weiss HD, Walker MD, Wiernik PH. Neurotoxicity of commonly used antineoplastic agents. *N Engl J Med* 1974;291:75.
69. Shapiro WR, Young DF. Neurological complications of antineoplastic therapy. *Acta Neurol Scand* 1984;100:125.
70. Feun LG, Wallace S, Yung WK, et al. Phase I trial of intrcarotid BCNU and cisplatin in patients with malignant intracerebral tumors. *Cancer Drug Deliv* 1984;1:239.
71. Stewart DJ, Grahovac Z, Benoit B et al. Intracarotid chemotherapy with a combination of 1,3-bis(2-chloroethyl)-1-nitrosourea (BCNU), cis-diaminedichloroplatinum (cisplatin), and 4'-o-demethyl-1-o-(4,6-o-2-thenylidene-beta-d-glucopyranosyl) epipodophyllotoxin (vm-26) in the treatment of primary and metastatic brain tumors. *Neurosurgery* 1984;15:828.
72. Brem H, Piantadosi S, Burger PC, et al. Placebo-controlled trial of safety and efficacy of intraoperative controlled delivery by biodegradable polymers of chemotherapy for recurrent gliomas. The Polymer-brain Tumor Treatment Group. *Lancet* 1995;345:1008.
73. Levin VA. Management of gliomas, medulloblastoma and CNS germ cell tumors. In: Cavalli F, Hansen HH, Kaye SB, eds. *Textbook of medical oncology.* London: Martin Dunitz, 1997:309.
74. Kleihues P, Burger PC, Scheithauer BW. *Histological typing of tumors of the central nervous system.* Berlin: Springer-Verlag, 1993.
75. Daumas-Duport C, Scheithauer B, O'Fallon J, et al. Grading of astrocytomas, a simple and reproducible method. *Cancer* 1988;62:2152.
76. Kim TS, Halliday AL, Hedley-Whyte ET, et al. Correlates of survival and the Daumas-Duport grading system of astrocytomas. *J Neurosurg* 1991;74:27.
77. Nelson JS, Tsukada Y, Schoenfeld D, et al. Necrosis as a prognostic criterion in malignant supratentorial, astrocytic gliomas. *Cancer* 1983;52:550.
78. Laws ER Jr, Taylor WF, Clifton MB, et al. Neurosurgical management of low-grade astrocytoma of the cerebral hemispheres. *J Neurosurg* 1984;61:665.
79. Waller MD, Alexander E Jr, Hunt WE, et al. Evaluation of BCNU and/or radiotherapy in the treatment of anaplastic gliomas: a cooperative clinical trial. *J Neurosurg* 1978;49:333.
80. Salcman M. Malignant glioma management. *Neurosurg Clin North Am* 1990;1:49.
81. Levin VA, Hoffman WF, Heilbron DC, et al. Prognostic significance of the pretreatment CT scan on time to progression for patients with malignant gliomas. *J Neurosurg* 1980;52:642.
82. Wood JR, Green SB, Shapiro WR. The prognostic importance of tumor size in malignant gliomas: a computed tomographic scan study by the Brain Tumor Cooperative Group. *J Clin Oncol* 1988;6:338.
83. Winger MJ, Macdonald DR, Cairncross JG. Supratentorial anaplastic gliomas in adults: the prognostic importance of extent of resection and prior low-grade glioma. *J Neurosurg* 1989;71:487.
84. Kumar ARV, Hoshino T, Wheeler KT, et al. Comparative rates of dead tumor cell removal from brain, muscle, subcutaneous tissue, and peritonal cavity. *JNCI* 1974;52:1751.
85. Gutin PH, Leibel SA, Wara WM, et al. Recurrent malignant gliomas: improved survival following interstitial brachytherapy with high-activity iodine-125 sources. *J Neurosurg* 1987;67:864.
86. Young B, Oldfield EH, Markesbery WR, et al. Reoperation for glioblastoma. *Neurosurgery* 1981;55:917.
87. Harsh GR IV, Levin VA, Gutin PH, et al. Reoperation for recurrent glioblastoma and anaplastic astrocytoma. *Neurosurgery* 1987;21:615.
88. Bauman G, Lote K, Larson D, et al. Pretreatment factors predict overall survival for patients with low- grade glioma: A recursive partitioning analysis. *Int J Radiat Oncol Biol Phys* 1999;45:923.
89. Shaw EG, Daumas-Duport C, Scheithauer B, et al. Radiation therapy in the management of low-grade supratentorial astrocytomas. *J Neurosurg* 1989;70:853.
90. Leibel SA, Sheline GE, Wara WM, et al. The role of radiation therapy in the treatment of astrocytomas. *Cancer* 1975;35:1551.
91. Wallner KE, Gonzales MF, Edwards MS, et al. Treatment results of juvenile pilocytic astrocytoma. *J Neurosurg* 1988;69:171.
92. MacDonald DR. Low-grade gliomas, mixed gliomas, and oligodendrogliomas. *Semin Oncol* 1994;21:236.
93. Berger MS, Leibel SA, Bruner JM, et al. Primary central nervous system tumors of the supratentorial compartment. In: Levin VA, ed. *Cancer in the nervous system.* New York: Churchill Livingstone, 1995:57.
94. Berger MS, Deliganis AV, Dobbins J, et al. The effect of extent of resection on recurrence in patients with low grade cerebral hemisphere gliomas. *Cancer* 1994;74:1784.
95. Vertosick FT, Selker RG, Arena VC. Survival of patients with well-differentiated astrocytomas diagnosed in the era of computer tomography. *Neurosurgery* 1991;28:496.
96. Recht LD, Lew R, Smith TW. Suspected low-grade glioma: Is deferring treatment safe? *Ann Neurol* 1992;31:431.
97. McCormack BM, Miller DC, Budzilovich GN, et al. Treatment and survival of low-grade astrocytoma in adults 1977–1988. *Neurosurgery* 1992;31:636.
98. Karim ABMF, Cornu P, Bleehan N, et al. Immediate postoperative radiotherapy in low grade glioma improves progression free survival but not overall survival: preliminary results of an EORTC/MRC randomized phase III trial. *Proc Am Soc Clin Oncol* 1998;17:400a.
99. Karim AB, Maat B, Hatlevoll R, et al. Randomized trial on dose-response in radiation therapy of low-grade cerebral glioma: European Organization for Research and Treatment of Cancer (EORTC) Study 22844. *Int J Radiat Oncol Biol Phys* 1996;36:549.
100. Shaw E, Arusell R, Scheithauer B, et al. A prospective randomized trial of low versus high-dose radiation therapy in adults with supratentorial low-grade glioma: initial report of a NCCG-RTOG-ECOG study. *Proc Am Soc Clin Oncol* 1998;17:401a.
101. Kiebert GM, Curran D, Aaronson NK, et al. Quality of life after radiation therapy of cerebral low-grade gliomas of the adult: results of a randomised phase III trial on dose response (EORTC trial 22844). EORTC Radiotherapy Co-operative Group. *Eur J Cancer* 1998;34:1902.
102. Eyre HJ, Crowley JJ, Townsend JJ, et al. A randomized trial of radiotherapy versus radiotherapy plus CCNU for incompletely resected low-grade gliomas: a Southwest Oncology Group Study. *J Neurosurg* 1993;78:909.
103. Levin VA, Prados MD, Wara WM, et al. Radiation therapy and bromodeoxyuridine chemotherapy followed by procarbazine, lomustine, and vincristine for the treatment of anaplastic gliomas. *Int J Radiat Oncol Biol Phys* 1995;32:75.
104. Walker MD, Alexander E, Hunt WE, et al. Evaluation of BCNU and /or radiotherapy in the treatment of anaplastic gliomas. *J Neurosurg* 1978;49:333.
105. Gaspar LE, Fisher BJ, MacDonald DR, et al. Malignant glioma-timing of response to radiation therapy. *Int J Radiat Oncol Biol Phys* 1993;25:877.
106. Leibel SA, Scott CB, Loeffler JS. Contemporary approaches to the treatment of malignant gliomas with radiation therapy. *Semin Oncol* 1994;21:198.
107. Prados MD, Scott C, Curran WJ, et al. Procarbazine, CCNU, and vincristine (PCV) chemotherapy for anaplastic astrocytoma: a retrospective review of Radiation Therapy Oncology Group protocols comparing survival with carmustine or PCV adjuvant chemotherapy. *J Clin Oncol* 1999;17:3389.
108. Leibel SA, Scott CB, Loeffler J. Contemporary approaches to the treatment of malignant gliomas with radiation therapy. *Semin Oncol* 1994;21:198.
109. Phillips TL, Levin VA, Ahn DK, et al. Evaluation of bromodeoxyuridine in glioblastoma multiforme: a Northern California Cancer Center Phase II study. *Int J Radiat Oncol Biol Phys* 1991;21:709.
110. Prados MD, Scott C, Sandler H, et al. A phase 3 randomized study of radiotherapy plus procarbazine, CCNU, and vincristine (PCV) with or without BUdR for the treatment of anaplastic astrocytoma: a preliminary report of RTOG 9404. *Int J Radiat Oncol Biol Phys* 1999;45:1109.
111. Sullivan FJ, Herscher LL, Cook JA, et al. National Cancer Institute (phase II) study of high-grade glioma treated with accelerated hyperfractionated radiation and iododeoxyuridine: results in anaplastic astrocytoma. *Int J Radiat Oncol Biol Phys* 1994;30:583.
112. Nelson DF, Curran WJ, Nelson JS, et al. Hyperfractionation in malignant glioma, report on a dose-searching phase I/II protocol of the radiation therapy oncology group (RTOG). *Am Soc Clin Oncol* 1990;9:A350.
113. Scott CB, Curran W, Yung WKA, et al. Long term results of RTOG 9006: randomized trial of hyperfractionated radiotherapy (RT) to 72 Gy & carmustine vs. standard RT & carmustine for malignant glioma patients with emphasis on anaplastic astrocytoma patients. *Am Soc Clin Oncol* 1998;17:40a.
114. Keim H, Potthoff PC, Schmidt K, et al. Survival and quality of life after continuous accelerated radiotherapy of glioblastomas. *Radiother Oncol* 1987;9:21.
115. Groves MD, Maor MH, Meyers C, et al. A phase II trial of high-dose bromodeoxyuridine with accelerated fractionation radiotherapy followed by procarbazine, lomustine, and vincristine for glioblastoma multiforme. *Int J Radiat Oncol Biol Phys* 1999;45:127.
116. Florell RC, Macdonald DR, Irish WD, et al. Selection bias, survival, and brachytherapy for glioma. *J Neurosurg* 1992;76:179.
117. Gutin PH, Prados MD, Phillips TL, et al. External irradiation followed by an interstitial high activity iodine-125 implant "boost" in the initial treatment of malignant gliomas: NCOG study 6G-82-2. *Int J Radiat Oncol Biol Phys* 1991;21:601.
118. Loeffler JS, Alexander E, Wen PY, et al. Results of stereotactic brachytherapy used in the initial management of patients with glioblastoma. *J Natl Cancer Inst* 1990;82:1918.
119. Green SB, Shapiro WR, Burger PC, et al. A randomized trial of interstitial radiotherapy (RT) boost for newly diagnosed malignant glioma: Brain Tumor Cooperative Group (BTCG) trial 8701. *Am Soc Clin Oncol* 1994;13:A486.
120. Laperriere NJ, Leung PM, McKenzie S, et al. Radomized study of brachytherapy in the initial management of patients with malignant astrocytoma. *Int J Radiat Oncol Biol Phys* 1998;41:1005.
121. Sneed PK, Stauffer PR, McDermott MW, et al. Survival benefit of hyperthermia in a prospective randomized trial of brachytherapy boost +/- hyperthermia for glioblastoma multiforme. *Int J Radiat Oncol Biol Phys* 1998;40:287.
122. Leibel SA, Gutin PH, Wara WM, et al. Survival and quality of life after interstitial implantation of removable high-activity iodine-125 sources for the treatment of patients with recurrent malignant gliomas. *Int J Radiat Oncol Biol Phys* 1989;17:1129.

123. Shrieve DC, Alexander E III, Black PM, et al. Treatment of patients with primary glioblastoma multiforme with standard postoperative radiotherapy and radiosurgical boost: prognostic factors and long-term outcome. *J Neurosurg* 1999;90:72.
124. Tang XM, Beesley JS, Grinspan JB, et al. Cell cycle arrest induced by ectopic expression of p27 is not sufficient to promote oligodendrocyte differentiation. *J Cell Biochem* 2000;76:270.
125. Mehta MP, Masciopinto J, Rozental J, et al. Stereotactic radiosurgery for glioblastoma multiforme: report of a prospective study evaluating prognostic factors and analyzing long-term survival advantage. *Int J Radiat Oncol Biol Phys* 1994;30:541.
126. Scharfen CO, Sneed PK, Wara WM, et al. High activity iodine-125 interstitial implant for gliomas. *Int J Radiat Oncol Biol Phys* 1992;24:583.
127. Shrieve DC, Alexander E, Wen PY, et al. Comparison of stereotactic radiosurgery and brachytherapy in the treatment of recurrent glioblastoma multiforme. *Neurosurgery* 1995;36:275.
128. Thornton AF. Three-dimensional treatment planning of astrocytomas, a dosimetric study of cerebral irradiation. *Int J Radiat Oncol Biol Phys* 1991;20:1309.
129. Lee SW, Fraass BA, Marsh LH, et al. Patterns of failure following high-dose 3-D conformal radiotherapy for high-grade astrocytomas: a quantitative dosimetric study. *Int J Radiat Oncol Biol Phys* 1999;43:79.
130. Fitzek MM, Thornton AF, Rabinov JD, et al. Accelerated fractionated proton/photon irradiation to 90 cobalt gray equivalent for glioblastoma multiforme: results of a phase II prospective trial. *J Neurosurg* 1999;91:251.
131. Levin VA, Silver P, Hannigan J, et al. Superiority of post-radiotherapy adjuvant chemotherapy with CCNU, procarbazine, and vincristine (PCV) over BCNU for anaplastic gliomas: NCOG 6G61 Final Report. *Int J Radiat Oncol Biol Phys* 1990;18:321.
132. Jeremic B, Jovanovic D, Djuric LJ, et al. Advantage of post-radiotherapy chemotherapy with CCNU, procarbazine, and vincristine (mPCV) over chemotherapy with VM-26 and CCNU for malignant gliomas. *J Chemother* 1992;4:123.
133. Dinapoli RP, Brown LD, Arusell RM, et al. Phase III comparative evaluation of PCNU and carmustine combined with radiation therapy for highy2Dgrade glioma. *J Clin Oncol* 1993; 11:1316.
134. Levin VA. Chemotherapy for brain tumors of astrocytic and oligodendroglial lineage: the past decade and where we are heading. *Neuro-Oncology* 1999;1:69.
135. Byar DP, Green SB, Strike TA. Prognostic factors for malignant glioma. In: Walker MD, ed. *Oncology of the nervous system.* Boston: Martinus Nijhoff, 1983:379.
136. Walker MD, Green SB, Byar DP, et al. Randomized comparison of radiotherapy and nitrosoureas for the treatment of malignant glioma after surgery. *N Engl J Med* 1980;303:1323.
137. Green SB, Byar DP, Walker MD, et al. Comparison of carmustine, procarbazine, and high-dose methylprednisolone as additions to surgery and radiotherapy for the treatment of malignant glioma. *Cancer Treat Rep* 1983;67:1.
138. Paoletti P, Cuna GRD, Knerich R, et al. Multidisciplinary treatment for central nervous system tumors with nitrosourea compounds. *Acta Neurochir* 1978;41:287.
139. Eyre HJ, Quagliana JM, Eltringham JR, et al. Randomized comparisons of radiotherapy and CCNU versus radiotherapy, CCNU plus procarbazine for the treatment of malignant gliomas following surgery. *J Neurooncol* 1983;1:171.
140. Adinolfi DBP, Casotto A, et al. Multidiscriplinary treatment for brain tumors. *J Neurosurg* 1978;22:111.
141. EORTC Brain Tumor Group. Effect of CCNU on survival rate of objective remission and duration of free interval in patients with malignant brain glioma—final evaluation. *Eur J Cancer* 1978;14:851.
142. Deutsch MGS, Strike TA, et al. Results of a randomized trial comparing BCNU plus radiotherapy, streptozotocin plus radiotherapy, BCNU plus hyperfractionated radiotherapy, and BCNU following misonidazole plus radiotherapy in the postoperative treatment of malignant glioma. *Int J Radiat Oncol Biol Phys* 1989;16:1389.
143. Feun LG, Steward DJ, Maor M, et al. A pilot study of MD+UL, cis MD-UL-diaminedichloroplatinum and radiation therapy in patients with high-grade astrocytomas. *J Neurooncol* 1983;1:109.
144. Shapiro WR, Green SB, Burger PC, et al. Randomized trial of three chemotherapy regimens and two radiotherapy regimens in postoperative treatment of malignant glioma: Brain Tumor Cooperative Group Trial 8001. *J Neurosurg* 1989;71:1.
145. Yung WK, Janus TJ, Maor M, et al. Adjuvant chemotherapy with carmustine and cisplatin for patients with malignant gliomas. *J Neurooncol* 1992;12:131.
146. Grossman SA, Wharam M, Sheidler V, et al. BCNU/cisplatin (B/C) followed by radiation in poor-prognosis patients with high-grade astrocytomas (HGA). *Proc Am Soc Clin Oncol* 1992;11:A418.
147. Rozental JM, Robins HI, Finlay J, et al. Eight-in-one-day chemotherapy administered before and after radiotherapy to adult patients with malignant gliomas. *Cancer* 1989;63:2475.
148. Levin VA, Wara WM, Davis RL, et al. NCOG Protocol 6G91: seven drug chemotherapy and irradiation for patients with glioblastoma multiforme. *Cancer Treat Rep* 1986;70:739.
149. Prados MD, Larson DA, Lamborn K, et al. Radiation therapy and hydroxyurea followed by the combination of 6-thioguanine and BCNU for the treatment of primary malignant brain tumors. *Int J Radiat Oncol Biol Phys* 1998;40:57.
150. Rosenblum ML, Gerosa MA, Wilson CB, et al. Stem cell studies of human brain tumors. *J Neurosurg* 1983;58:170.
151. Thomas DGT, Darling JL, Paul EA, et al. Assay of anti-cancer drugs in tissue culture: relationship of relapse free interval (RFI) and in vitro chemosensitivity in patients with malignant cerebral glioma. *Br J Cancer* 1985;51:525.
152. Kumar ARV, Renaudin J, Wilson CB, et al. Procarbazine hyudrochloride in the treatment of brain tumors. *J Neurosurg* 1974;40:365.
153. Wilson CB, Gutin P, Boldrey EB, et al. Single-agent chemotherapy of brain tumors. A five-year review. *Arch Neurol* 1976;33:739.
154. Rosenblum ML, Reynolds AF, Smith KA, et al. Chloroethyl-cyclohexyl-nitrosourea (CCNU) in the treatment of malignant brain tumors. *J Neurosurg* 1973;39:306.
155. Levin VA, Resser K, McGrath L, et al. PCNU treatment for recurrent malignant gliomas. *Int J Radiat Oncol Biol Phys* 1984;68:969.
156. Nelson DF, Schoenfeld D, Weinstein AS, et al. A randomized comparison of misonidazole sensitized radiotherapy plus BCNU and radiotherapy plus BCNU for treatment of malignant glioma after surgery: preliminary results of an RTOG study. *Int J Radiat Oncol Biol Phys* 1983;9:1143.
157. Levin VA, Crafts DC, Wilson CB, et al. Imidazole carboxamides: relationship of lipophilicity to activity against intracerebral murine glioma 26 and preliminary phase II clinical trial of 5-(3,3-bis chlorethyl)-1-troazeno)-imidazole-4-carboxamide (NSC-82196) in primary and secondary brain tumors. *Cancer Chemother Rep* 1975;59:107.
158. Chamberlain MC, Prados MD, Silver P, et al. A phase I/II study of 24 hour intravenous AZQ in recurrent primary brain tumors. *J Neurooncol* 1988;6:319.
159. Decker DA, Al Sarraf M, Kresge C, et al. Phase II study of Aziridinylbenzoquinone (AZQ: NSC-182986) in the treatment of malignant gliomas recurrent after radiation. *J Neurooncol* 1985;3:19.
160. Schold SC Jr, Friedman HS, Bjornsson TD, et al. Treatment of patients with recurrent primary brain tumors with AZQ. *Neurosurgery* 1984;34:615.
161. Chamberlain MC, Prados MD, Silver P, et al. A phase II trial of oral melphalan in recurrent primary brain tumors. *Am J Clin Oncol* 1988;11:52.
162. Prados M, Rodriguez L, Seager M, et al. Phase II study of spirohydantoin mustard for the treatment of recurrent malignant gliomas. *Cancer Treat Rep* 1987;71:1105.
163. Bertolone SJ, Baum ES, Krivit W, et al. A phase II study of cisplatin therapy in recurrent childhood brain tumors. *J Neurooncol* 1989;7:5.
164. Yung WK, Mechtler L, Gleason MJ. Intravenous carboplatin for recurrent malignant glioma: a phase II study. *J Clin Oncol* 1991;9:860.
165. Yung WK, Prados M, Levin VA, et al. Intravenous recombinant interferon beta in patients with recurrent malignant gliomas: a phase I/II study. *J Clin Oncol* 1991;9:1945.
166. Kaba SE, Kyritsis AP, Conrad C, et al. The treatment of recurrent cerebral gliomas with all-trans-retinoic acid (tretinoin). *J Neurooncol* 1997;34:145.
167. Fewer D, Wilson CB, Boldrey EB, et al. Chemotherapy of brain tumors: clinical experience with carmustine and vincristine. *JAMA* 1972;222:549.
168. Levin VA, Crafts DC, Wilson CB, et al. BCNU and procarbazine treatment for malignant brain tumors. *Cancer Treat Rep* 1979;60:243.
169. Gutin PH, Wilson CB, Kumar AR, et al. Phase II study of procarbazine, CCNU, and vincristine combination chemotherapy in the treatment of malignant brain tumors. *Cancer* 1975;35:1398.
170. Levin VA, Edwards MS, Wright DC, et al. Modified procarbazine, CCNU, and vincristine (PCV 3) combination chemotherapy in the treatment of malignant brain tumors. *Cancer Treat Rep* 1980;64:237.
171. Levin VA, Hoffman WF, Pischer TL, et al. BCNU 5 fluorouracil combination in the treatment of recurrent malignant brain tumors. *Cancer Treat Rep* 1978;62:2071.
172. Levin VA, Phuphanich S, Liu H-C, et al. Phase II study of combined BCNU, 5-fluorouracil, hydroxyurea, and 6-mercaptopurine (BFHM) for the treatment of malignant gliomas. *Cancer Treat Rep* 1986;70:1271.
173. Buckner JC, Brown LD, Kugler JW, et al. Phase II evaluation of recombinant interferon alpha and BCNU in recurrent glioma. *J Neurosurg* 1995;82:430.
174. Prados MD, Rodriguez L, Chamberlain MC, et al. Treatment of recurrent gliomas with 1,3 (2-chloroethyl)-1-nitrosourea and difluoromethylornithine. *Neurosurgery* 1989;24:806.
175. Levin VA, Chamberlain MC, Prados MD, et al. Phase I - II study of eflornithine and mitoguazone combined in the treatment of recurrent primary brain tumors. *Cancer Treat Rep* 1987;71:459.
176. Levin VA, Prados MD, Davis RL, et al. Treatment of recurrent gliomas with a polydrug protocol designed to combat nitrosourea resistance. *J Clin Oncol* 1992;10:766.
177. Schold SC Jr, Mahaley MS Jr, Vick NA, et al. Phase II diaziquone-based chemotherapy trials in patients with anaplastic supratentorial astrocytic neoplasms. *J Clin Oncol* 1987;5:464.
178. Yung WK, Harris MI, Bruner JM, et al. Intravenous BCNU and AZQ in patients with recurrent malignant gliomas. *J Neurooncol* 1989;7:237.
179. Longee DC, Friedman HS, Albright RE, et al. Treatment of patients with recurrent gliomas with cyclophosphamide and vincristine. *J Neurosurg* 1990;72:583.
180. Flowers A, Gleason MJ, Levin VA, et al. Combination chemotherapy with carboplatin, 5-fluorouricil, and procarbazine for recurrent malignant gliomas. *Am Assoc Cancer Res* 1993; 12:180.
181. Levin VA, et al. Unpublished observations. 1987 and 1991.
182. Levin VA, Prados MD, Yung WK, et al. Treatment of recurrent gliomas with eflornithine. *JNCI* 1992;84:1432.
183. Mason W, Louis DN, Cairncross JG. Chemosensitive gliomas in adults—which ones and why. *J Clin Oncol* 1997;15:3423.
184. Jaeckle KA, Eyre HJ, Townsend JJ, et al. Correlation of tumor O6 methylguanine-DNA methyltransferase levels with survival of malignant astrocytoma patients treated with bis-chloroethylnitrosourea: a Southwest Oncology Group study. *J Clin Oncol* 1998;16:3310.
185. Yung WK, Mechtler L, Gleason MJ. Intravenous carboplatin for recurrent malignant glioma: a phase II study. *J Clin Oncol* 1991;9:860.
186. Straathof CS, van den Bent MJ, Ma J, et al. The effect of dexamethasone on the uptake of cisplatin in 9L glioma and the area of brain around tumor. *J Neurooncol* 1998;37:1.
187. Chamberlain MC, Kormanik P. Salvage chemotherapy with taxol for recurrent anaplastic astrocytomas. *J Neurooncol* 1999;43:71.
188. Glantz MJ, Chamberlain MC, Chang S, et al. The role of paclitaxel in the treatment of primary and metastatic brain tumors. *Semin Radiat Oncol* 1999;9:27.
189. Fetell MR, Grossman SA, Fisher JD, et al. Preirradiation paclitaxel in glioblastoma multiforme: efficacy, pharmacology, and drug interactions. New Approaches to Brain Tumor Therapy Central Nervous System Consortium. *J Clin Oncol* 1997;15:3121.
190. Yung WKA, Prados MD, Yaya-Tur R, et al. Multicenter phase II trial of temozolomide in patients with anaplastic astrocytoma or anaplastic oligoastrocytoma at first relapse. *J Clin Oncol* 1999;17:2762.
191. Yung WKA, Albright RE, Olson J, et al. Randomized, multicenter, open-label, phase II,

comparative study of temozolomide and procarbazine in the treatment of patients with glioblastoma multiforme at first relapse. *Br J Cancer (in press).*
192. Ben Arush MW, Postovsky S, Goldsher D, et al. Clinical and radiographic response in three children with recurrent malignant cerebral tumors with high-dose tamoxifen. *Pediatr Hematol Oncol* 1999;16:245.
193. Couldwell WT, Weiss MH, DeGiorgio CM, et al. Clinical and radiographic response in a minority of patients with recurrent malignant gliomas treated with high-dose tamoxifen. *Neurosurgery* 1993;32:485.
194. Couldwell WT, Hinton DR, Surnock AA, et al. Treatment of recurrent malignant gliomas with chronic oral high-dose tamoxifen. *Clin Cancer Res* 1996;2:619.
195. Chamberlain MC, Kormanik PA. Salvage chemotherapy with tamoxifen for recurrent anaplastic astrocytomas. *Arch Neurol* 1999;56:703.
196. Goodwin W, Crowley J. A retrospective comparison of high-dose BCNU with antologous marrow rescue plus radiotherapy vs IV BCNU plus radiation therapy in high grade gliomas: a Southwest ONcology Group review. *Am Soc Clin Oncol* 1989;8:A352.
197. Long J, Leff R, Daly M, et al. Phase II trial of high-dose etoposide (E) and autologous bone marrow transplantation for treatment of progressive glioma. *Am Soc Clin Oncol* 1989;8:A360.
198. Glannone L, Wolff SN. Phase II treatment of central nervous system gliomas with high-dose etoposide and autologous bone marrow transplantation. *Cancer Treat Rep* 1987;71:759.
199. Finlay JL, August C, Packer R, et al. High-dose multi-agent chemotherapy followed by bone marrow 'rescue' for malignant astrocytomas of childhood and adolescence. *J Neurooncol* 1990;9:239.
200. Finlay JL. The role of high-dose chemotherapy and stem cell rescue in the treatment of malignant brain tumors. *Bone Marrow Transplant* 1996;18(Suppl 3):S1.
201. Allen JC, Bloom J, Ertel I, et al. Brain tumors in children: current cooperative and institutional chemotherapy trials in newly diagnosed and recurrent disease. *Semin Oncol* 1986;13:110.
202. Freeman CR, Suissa S. Brain stem tumors in children: results of a survey of 62 patients treated with radiotherapy. *Int J Radiat Oncol Biol Phys* 1986;12:1823.
203. Eifel PJ, Cassady JR, Belli JA. Radiation therapy of tumors of the brainstem and midbrain in children: experience of the Joint Center For Radiation Therapy and Children's Hospital Medical Center (1971–1981). *Int J Radiat Oncol Biol Phys* 1987;13:847.
204. Landolfi JC, Thaler HT, DeAngelis LM. Adult brainstem gliomas. *Neurology* 1998;51:1136.
205. Coffey RJ, Lunsford LD. Stereotactic surgery for mass lesions of the midbrain and pons. *Neurosurgery* 1985;17:12.
206. Edwards MS, Wara WM, Urtasun RC, et al. Hyperfractionated radiation therapy for brain-stem glioma: a phase I-II trial. *J Neurosurg* 1989;70:691.
207. Packer RJ, Boyett JM, Zimmerman RA, et al. Hyperfractionated radiation therapy (72 Gy) for children with brain stem gliomas. A Childrens Cancer Group Phase I/II Trial. *Cancer* 1993;72:1414.
208. Prados MD, Wara WM, Edwards MS, et al. The treatment of brain stem and thalamic gliomas with 78 Gy of hyperfractionated radiation therapy. *Int J Radiat Oncol Biol Phys* 1995; 32:85.
209. Freeman CR, Krischer JP SR, et al. Final results of a study of escalating doses of hyperfractionated radiotherapy in brain stem tumors in children: a Pediatric Oncology Study. *Int J Radiat Oncol Biol Phys* 1993;27:197.
210. Freeman CR, Farmer JP. Pediatric brain stem gliomas: a review. *Int J Radiat Oncol Biol Phys* 1998;40:265.
211. Mandell LR, Kadota R, Freeman C, et al. There is no role for hyperfractionated radiotherapy in the management of children with newly diagnosed diffuse intrinsic brainstem tumors: results of a pediatric oncology group phase III trial comparing conventional vs. hyperfractionated radiotherapy. *Int J Radiat Oncol Biol Phys* 199;43:959.
212. Jenkin D. Posterior fossa tumors in childhood: radiation treatment. *Clin Neurosurg* 1983;30:203.
213. Fulton DS, Levin VA, Wara WM, et al. Chemotherapy of pediatric brain-stem tumors. *J Neurosurg* 1981;54:721.
214. Rodriguez LA, Prados M, Fulton D, et al. Treatment of recurrent brain stem gliomas and other central nervous system tumors with 5-fluorouracil, CCNU, hydroxyurea, and 6-mercaptopurine. *Neurosurgery* 1988;22:691.
215. Humphreys RP. Posterior cranial fossa brain tumors in children. In: Appuzzo M, ed. *Third ventricular tumors.* Baltimore: Williams & Wilkins, 1987:838.
216. Pencalet P, Maixner W, Sainte-Rose C, et al. Benign cerebellar astrocytomas in children. *J Neurosurg* 1999;90:265.
217. Chamberlain MC, Silver P, Levin VA. Poorly differentiated gliomas of the cerebellum. A study of 18 patients. *Cancer* 1990;65:337.
218. Chamberlain MC. Recurrent cerebellar gliomas: salvage therapy with oral etoposide. *J Child Neurol* 1997;12:200.
219. Walsh FB, Hoyt WF. *Clinical neuro-opthalmology.* Baltimore: Williams & Wilkins, 1969:2076.
220. Lewis RA, Gerson LP, Axelson KA, et al. von Recklinghausen neurofibromatosis: II Incidence of optic gliomata. *Ophthalmology* 1984;91:929.
221. Housepian EM, Trokel SL, Jakobiec FO, et al. Tumors of the orbit. In: Youman JR, ed. *Neurological surgery.* Philadelphia: WB Saunders, 1982:3024.
222. Housepian EM. Surgical treatment of unilateral optic nerve glimas. *J Neurosurg* 1969;31:604.
223. Sutton LN, Molloy PT, Sernyak H, et al. Long-term outcome of hypothalamic/chiasmatic astrocytomas in children treated with conservative surgery. *J Neurosurg* 1995;83:583.
224. Tenny RT, Laws ER, Young BR, et al. The neurosurgical management of optic gliomas: results in 104 patients. *J Neurosurg* 1982;57:452.
225. Bataini JP, Delanian S, Ponvert D. Chiasmal gliomas: results of irradiation management and review of literature. *Int J Radiat Oncol Biol Phys* 1991;21:615.
226. Wong JYC, Uhl V, Wara WM, et al. Optic gliomas: a re-analysis of the University of California, San Francisco experience. *Cancer* 1987;60:1847.
227. Jenkin D, Angyalfi S, Beckler L, et al. Optic glioma in children: surveillance, resection, or irradiation? *Int J Radiat Oncol Biol Phys* 1993;25:215.
228. Tao ML, Barnes PD, Billett AL, et al. Childhood optic chiasm gliomas: radiographic response following radiotherapy and long-term clinical outcome. *Int J Radiat Oncol Biol Phys* 1997;39:579.
229. Erkal HS, Serin M, Cakmak A. Management of optic pathway and chiasmatic-hypothalamic gliomas in children with radiation therapy. *Radiother Oncol* 1997;45:11.
230. Rodriguez LA, Edwards MS, Levin VA. Management of hypothalamic gliomas in children: an analysis of 33 cases. *Neurosurgery* 1990;26:242.
231. Rosenstock JG, Packer RJ, Bilaniuk LT. Chiasmatic optic glioma treated with chemotherapy. *J Neurosurg* 1985;63:862.
232. Prados MD, Levin VA, Edwards MS, et al. Combined chemotherapy/radiotherapy for pediatric brain tumors: the UCSF experience. *International symposium on Pediatric Neuro-Oncology*, Seattle, WA, 1989.
233. Packer RJ, Sutton LN, Bilaniuk LT, et al. Treatment of chiasmatic/hypothalamic gliomas of childhood with chemotherapy: an update. *Ann Neurol* 1988;23:79.
234. Petronio J, Edwards MS, Prados MD, et al. Management of chiasmal and hypothalamic gliomas of infancy and childhood with chemotherapy. *J Neurosurg* 1990;74:701.
235. Prados MD, Edwards MS, Rabbitt J, et al. Treatment of pediatric low-grade gliomas with a nitrosourea-based multiagent chemotherapy regimen. *J Neurooncol* 1997;32:235.
236. Ludwig CL, Smith MT, Godfrey AD, et al. A clinicopathologic study of 323 patients with oligodendrogliomas. *Ann Neurol* 1986;19:15.
237. Mirk SJ, Lindegaard K-F, Halvorsen TB, et al. Oligodendroglioma: incidence and biological behavior in a defined population. *J Neurosurg* 1985;63:881.
238. Shimizu KY, Tran LM, Mark RJ, et al. Management of oligodendrogliomas. *Radiology* 1993;186:569.
239. Gannett DE, Wisbeck WM, Silbergeld DL, et al. The role of postoperative irradiation in the treatment of oligodendroglioma. *Int J Radiat Oncol Biol Phys* 1994;30:567.
240. Wallner KE, Gonzales M, Sheline GE. Treatment of oligodendrogliomas with or without postoperative irradiation. *J Neurosurg* 1988;68:684.
241. Lindegaard K-F, Mork SJ, Eide GE, et al. Statistical analysis of clinicopathological features, radiotherapy, and survival in 170 cases of oligodendroglioma. *J Neurosurg* 1987;67:224.
242. Buckner JC, Brown LD, Kugler JW, et al. Oligodendroglioma: an analysis of the value of radiation therapy. *Cancer* 1987;60:2179.
243. Mirk SJ, Halvorsen TB, Lindegaard K-F, et al. Oligodendroglioma: histologic evaluation and prognosis. *J Neuropath Exp Neurol* 1986;45:65.
244. Shaw EG, Scheithauer BW, O'Fallon JR, et al. Oligodendrogliomas: the Mayo Clinic Experience. *J Neurosurg* 1992;76:428.
245. Allison RR, Schulsinger A, Vongtama V, et al. Radiation and chemotherapy improve outcome in oligodendroglioma. *Int J Radiat Oncol Biol Phys* 1997;37:399.
246. Mason WP, Krol GS, DeAngelis LM. Low-grade oligodendroglioma responds to chemotherapy. *Neurology* 1996;46:203.
247. Shaw EG, Scheithauer B, O'Fallon JR. Astrocytomas (A), oligo-astrocytomas (OA), and oligodendrogliomas (O): a comparative survival study. *Neurology* 1992;42:342.
248. Jeremic B, Shibamoto Y, Grujicic D, et al. Combined treatment modality for anaplastic oligodendroglioma: a phase II study. *J Neurooncol* 1999;43:179.
249. Kyritsis AP, Yung WK, Bruner J, et al. The treatment of anaplastic oligodendrogliomas and mixed gliomas. *Neurosurgery* 1993;32:365.
250. Cairncross JG, Macdonald DR. Chemotherapy for oligodendroglioma: progress report. *Arch Neurol* 1991;48:225.
251. Kernohan JW, Sayre GP. *Tumors of the central nervous system. Atlas of tumor pathology.* Washington, DC: Armed Forces Institute of Pathology, 1952.
252. Ross GW, Rubinstein LJ. Lack of histopathological correlation of malignant ependymomas with postoperative survival. *J Neurosurg* 1989;70:31.
253. Goldwein JW, Corn BW, Finlay JL, et al. Is craniospinal irradiation required to cure children with malignant (anaplastic) intracranial ependymomas? *Cancer* 1991;67:2766.
254. Vanuytsel L, Brada M. The role of prophylactic spinal irradiation in localized intracranial ependymoma. *Int J Radiat Oncol Biol Phys* 1991;21:825.
255. Svien HJ, Mabon RF, Kernohan JW, et al. Ependymoma of the brain: pathologic aspects. *Neurology* 1953;3:1.
256. Healey EA, Barnes PD, Kupsky WJ, et al. The prognostic significance of postoperative residual tumor in ependymoma. *Neurosurgery* 1991;28:666.
257. Wallner KE, Wara WM, Sheline GE, et al. Intracranial ependymomas: results of treatment with partial or whole brain irradiation without spinal irradiation. *Int J Radiat Oncol Biol Phys* 1986;12:1937.
258. McLaughlin MP, Marcus RB Jr, Buatti JM, et al. Ependymoma: results, prognostic factors and treatment recommendations. *Int J Radiat Oncol Biol Phys* 1998;40:845.
259. Salazar OM, Castro-Vita H, Van Houtte P, et al. Improved survival in cases of intracranial ependymoma after radiation therapy: late report and recommendations. *J Neurosurg* 1983;59:652.
260. Vanuytsel LJ, Bessell EM, Ashley SE, et al. Long-term results of a policy of surgery and radiotherapy. *Int J Radiat Oncol Biol Phys* 1992;23:313.
261. Merchant TE, Haida T, Wang MH, et al. Anaplastic ependymoma: treatment of pediatric patients with or without craniospinal radiation therapy. *J Neurosurg* 1997;86:943.
262. Robertson PL, Zeltzer PM, Boyett JM, et al. Survival and prognostic factors following radiation therapy and chemotherapy for ependymomas in children: a report of the Children's Cancer Group. *J Neurosurg* 1998;88:695.
263. Levin VA, Lamborn K, Wara W, et al. Phase II study of 6-thioguanine, procarbazine, lomustine, dibromodulcitol, and vincristine chemotherapy (TPDCV) with radiotherapy for the treatment of malignant gliomas in children. *Neuro-Oncology* 1999;2:22.
264. Levin VA, Edwards MS, Gutin PH, et al. Phase II evaluation of dibromodulcitol in the treatment of recurrent medulloblastoma, ependymoma, and malignant astrocytoma. *J Neurosurg* 1984;61:1063.

265. Ettinger LJ, Ru N, Krailo MD, et al. A phase II study of diaziquone in children with recurrent or progressive primary brain tumors; a report from the Children's Cancer Study Group. *J Neurooncol* 1990;9:69.
266. Gaynon PS, Ettinger LJ, Baum ES, et al. Carboplatin in childhood brain tumors. A Children's Cancer Study Group phase II trial. *Cancer* 1990;66:2465.
267. Goldwein JW, Leahy JM, Packer RJ, et al. Intracranial ependymomas in children. *Int J Radiat Oncol Biol Phys* 1990;19:1497.
268. Cushing H, Eisehardt L. *Meningiomas: their classification, regional behavior, life history and surgical end results.* Springfield, IL: Charles C Thomas, 1938:73.
269. Hoshino T, Nagashima T, Murovic J, et al. Cell kinetic studies of in situ human brain tumors with bromodeoxyuridine. *Cytometry* 1985;6:627.
270. Simpson D. The recurrence of intracranial meningiomas after surgical treatment. *J Neurol Neurosurg Psychiatry* 1957;20:22.
271. Mirimanoff RO, Dosoretz DE, Linggood RM, et al. Meningioma: analysis of recurrence and progression following neurosurgical resection. *J Neurosurg* 1985;62:18.
272. Jackler RK, Sim DW, Gutin PH, et al. Systematic approach to intradural tumors ventral to the brainstem. *Am J Otol* 1995;16:39.
273. Karlsson UL, Leibel SA, Wallner K, et al. Brain tumors. In: Perez CA, Brady LW, eds. *Principles and practice of radiation oncology.* 2nd ed. Philadelphia: Lippincott, 1992:515.
274. Stafford SL, Perry A, Suman VJ, et al. Primarily resected meningiomas: outcome and prognostic factors in 581 Mayo Clinic patients, 1978–1988. *Mayo Clin Proc* 1998;73:936.
275. Barbaro NM, Gutin PH, Wilson CB, et al. Radiation therapy in the treatment of partially resected meningiomas. *Neurosurgery* 1987;20:525.
276. Goldsmith BJ, Wara WM, Wilson CB, et al. Postoperative irradiation for subtotally resected meningiomas. A retrospective analysis of 140 patients treated from 1967 to 1990. *J Neurosurg* 1994;80:195.
277. Wilson C. Meningiomas: genetics, malignancy, and the role of radiation in induction and treatment. *J Neurosurg* 1994;81:666.
278. Condra KS, Buatti JM, Mendenhall WM, et al. Benign meningiomas: treatment selection affects survival. *Int J Radiat Oncol Biol Phys* 1997;39:427.
279. Graholm J, Bloom HJG, Crow JH. The role of radiotherapy in the management of intracranial meningiomas: the Royal Marsden Hospital experience with 186 patients. *Int J Radiat Oncol Biol Phys* 1990;18:755.
280. Connell PP, Macdonald RL, Mansur DB, et al. Tumor size predicts control of benign meningiomas treated with radiotherapy. *Neurosurgery* 1999;44:1194.
281. Solan MJ, Kramer S. The role of radiation therapy in the management of intracranial meningiomas. *Int J Radiat Oncol Biol Phys* 1985;11:675.
282. Chan RC, Thompson GB. Morbidity, mortality, and quality of life following surgery for intracranial meningiomas. *J Neurosurg* 1984;60:52.
283. Milosevic MF, Frost PJ, Laperriere NJ, et al. Radiotherapy for atypical or malignant meningioma. *Int J Radiat Oncol Biol Phys* 1996;34:817.
284. Kondziolka D, Levy EI, Niranjan A, et al. Long-term outcomes after meningioma radiosurgery: Physician and patient perspectives. *J Neurosurg* 1999;91:44.
285. Hakim R, Alexander E, Loeffler JS, et al. Results of linear accelerator-based radiosurgery for intracranial meningiomas. *Neurosurgery* 1998;42:446.
286. Engenhart R, Kimming BN, Hover KH, et al. Stereotactic single high dose radiation therapy of benign intracranial meningiomas. *Int J Radiat Oncol Biol Phys* 1990;19:1021.
287. Kondiziolka D, Lunsford LD, Coffey RJ, et al. Stereotactic radiosurgery for meningiomas. *J Neurosurg* 1991;74:552.
288. Morita A, Coffey RJ, Foote RL, et al. Risk of injury to cranial nerves after gamma knife radiosurgery for skull base meningiomas: experience in 88 patients. *J Neurosurg* 1999;90:42.
289. Grunberg SM, Weiss MH, Spitz IM, et al. Treatment of unresectable meningiomas with the antiprogesterone agent mifepristone. *J Neurosurg* 1991;74:861.
290. Kaba SE, DeMonte F, Bruner JM, et al. The treatment of recurrent unresectable and malignant meningiomas with interferon alpha-2B. *Neurosurgery* 1997;40:271.
291. Schrell UM, Rittig MG, Anders M, et al. Hydroxyurea for treatment of unresectable and recurrent meningiomas. II. Decrease in the size of meningiomas in patients treated with hydroxyurea. *J Neurosurg* 1997;86:840.
292. McComb RD, Burger PC. Pathologic analysis of primary brain tumors. *Neurol Clin North Am* 1985;3:711.
293. Kosnik EJ, Boesel CP, Bay J, et al. Primitive neuroectodermal tumors of the central nervous system in children. *J Neurosurg* 1978;48:741.
294. Humphrey GB, Dehner LP, Kaplan RJ, et al. Overview on the management of primitive neuroectodermal tumors. In: Humphrey GB, Dehner LP, eds. *Pediatric oncology I.* The Hague: Martinus Nijhoff, 1981:289.
295. Rubinstein LJ. Embryonal central neuroepithelial tumors and their differentiation potential. *J Neurosurg* 1985;62:795.
296. Gaffney CC, Sloane JP, Bradley NJ, et al. Primitive neuroectodermal tumors of the cerebrum: pathology and treatment. *J Neurooncol* 1985;4:63.
297. Mikaeloff Y, Raquin MA, Lellouch-Tubiana A, et al. Primitive cerebral neuroectodermal tumors excluding medulloblastomas: a retrospective study of 30 cases. *Pediatr Neurosurg* 1998;29:170.
298. Paulino AC, Melian E. Medulloblastoma and supratentorial primitive neuroectodermal tumors: an institutional experience. *Cancer* 1999;86:142.
299. Cohen ME. Primitive neuroectodermal tumors, oligodendrogliomas, choroid plexus papillomas. In: *Brain tumors of childhood: principles of diagnosis and treatment.* New York: Raven Press, 1984:273.
300. Berger MS, Edwards MS, Wara WM, et al. Primary cerebral neuroblastoma. Long-term follow-up review and therapeutic guidelines. *J Neurosurg* 1983;59:418.
301. Horten BC, Rubinstein LJ. Primary cerebral neuroblastoma: a clinicopathological study of 35 cases. *Brain* 1976;99:735.
302. Bloom HJG. Medulloblastoma in children: increasing survival rates and further prospects. *Int J Radiat Oncol Biol Phys* 1982;8:2023.
303. Deutsch M. The impact of myelography on the treatment results for medulloblastoma. *Int J Radiat Oncol Biol Phys* 1984;10:999.
304. Levin VA, Rodriguez LA, Edwards MS, et al. Treatment of medulloblastoma with procarbazine hydroxyurea, and reduced radiation doses to whole brain and spine. *J Neurosurg* 1988;68:383.
305. Park TS, Hoffman HJ, Hendrick EB, et al. Medulloblastoma: clinical presentation and management experience at the hospital for sick children Toronto, 1950–1980. *J Neurosurg* 1983;58:543.
306. Lowery GS, Kimball JC, Patterson RB, et al. Extraneural metastases from cerebellar medulloblastoma. *Am J Pediatr Hematol Oncol* 1982;4:259.
307. Tait DM, Thornton-Jones H, Bloom HJG, et al. Adjuvant chemotherapy for medulloblastoma: the first multi-centre control trial of the International Society of Pediatric Oncology (SIOP I). *Eur J Cancer* 1990;26:464.
308. Evans AE, Jenkin RD, Sposto R, et al. The treatment of medulloblastoma: results of a prospective randomized trial of radiation therapy with and without CCNU, vincristine and prednisone. *J Neurosurg* 1990;72:572.
309. Chamberlain MC, Silver P, Edwards MS, et al. Treatment of extraneural metastatic medulloblastoma with a combination of cyclophosphamide, adriamycin, and vincristine. *Neurosurgery* 1988;23:476.
310. Prados MD, Warnick RE, Wara WM, et al. Medulloblastoma in adults. *Int J Radiat Oncol Biol Phys* 1995;32:1145.
311. Leibel SA, Sheline GE. Radiation therapy for neoplasms of the brain. *J Neurosurg* 1987;66:1.
312. Merchant TE, Wang MH, Haida T, et al. Medulloblastoma: long-term results for patients treated with definitive radiation therapy during the computed tomography era. *Int J Radiat Oncol Biol Phys* 1996;36:29.
313. Deutsch M, Thomas P, Boyett J, et al. Low-stage medulloblastoma: a Children's Cancer Study Group (CCSG) and Pediatric Oncology Group (POG) randomized study of standard vs reduced neuraxis irradiation. *Proc Am Soc Clin Oncol* 1991;10:124.
314. Packer RJ, Goldwein J, Nicholson HS, et al. Treatment of children with medulloblastomas with reduced-dose craniospinal radiation therapy and adjuvant chemotherapy: a Children's Cancer Group study. *J Clin Oncol* 1999;17:2127.
315. Wara WM, Le Q-Tx, Sneed PK, et al. Pattern of recurrence of medulloblastoma after low-dose craniospinal radiotherapy. *Int J Radiat Oncol Biol Phys* 1994;30:551.
316. Prados MD, Edwards MS, Chang SM, et al. Hyperfractionated craniospinal radiation therapy for primitive neuroectodermal tumors: results of a phase II study. *Int J Radiat Oncol Biol Phys* 1999;43:279.
317. Benjamin RS, Wiernik PH, Bachur NR. Adriamycin chemotherapy: efficacy, safety, and pharmacologic basis of an intermittent single high-dose schedule. *Cancer* 1974;74:1784.
318. Hancock C, Allen J, Tan CTC. Phase II trial of PCNU in children with recurrent brain tumors and Hodgkin's disease. *Cancer Treat Rep* 1984;68:441.
319. Bleyer WA, Krivit W, Chard RL. Phase II study of VM26 in leukemia, neuroblastoma, and other refractory childhood malignancies: a report from the Children's Cancer Study Group. *Cancer Treat Rep* 1979;63:977.
320. Shapiro WR. Chemotherapy of primary malignant brain tumors. *Cancer Child* 1975;35:965.
321. Allen JC, Walker R, Luks E, et al. Carboplatin and recurrent childhood brain tumors. *J Clin Oncol* 1987;5:459.
322. Rosen G, Ghavimi F, Nirenberg A, et al. High-dose methotrexate with citrovorum factor rescue for the treatment of central nervous system tumors in children. *Cancer Treat Rep* 1977;61:681.
323. Djerassi I, Kim JS, Shulman K. High-dose methotrexate-citrovorum factor rescue in the management of brain tumors. *Cancer Treat Rep* 1977;61:691.
324. Mooney C, Souhami R, Pritchard J. Recurrent medulloblastoma: lack of response to high-dose methotrexate. *Cancer Chemother Pharmacol* 1983;10:135.
325. Walker RW, Allen JC. Treatment of recurrent primary intracranial childhood tumors with cis-diamine-dichloroplatinum. *Ann Neurol* 1983;14:371.
326. Bertolone SJ, Baum E, Krivit W, et al. Phase II trial of cisplatinum diaminodichloride (CPDD) in recurrent childhood brain tumors: a CCSG trial. *Proc Annu Meet Am Assoc Cancer Res* 1983;2:72.
327. Sexauer CL, Kahn A, Burger PC, et al. MD+UL-platinum in recurrent pediatric brain tumors: a POG phase II study. *Cancer* 1985;56:1497.
328. Friedman HS, Schold SC Jr, Mahaley MS Jr, et al. Phase II treatment of medulloblastoma and pineoblastoma with melphalan: clinical therapy based on experimental models of human medulloblastoma. *J Clin Oncol* 1989;7:904.
329. Haddy TB, Ferbach DJ, Watkins WL, et al. Vincristine in uncommon malignant disease in children. *Cancer Chemother Rep* 1964;41:41.
330. Lassman LP, Pearce GW, Gang J. Effect of vincristine sulfate on the intracranial gliomata of childhood. *Br J Surg* 1966;53:774.
331. Lampkin BC, Maurer AM, McBride BH. Response of medulloblastoma to vincristine sulfate: a case report. *Pediatrics* 1967;39:761.
332. Smart CR, Ottoman RE, Rochlin DB, et al. Clinical experience with vincristine in tumors of the central nervous system and other malignant diseases. *Cancer Chemother Rep* 1968;52:733.
333. Afra D. Vincristine therapy in malignant glioma recurrencies. *Neurochirurgia* 1973;16:189.
334. Rosenstock JG, Evans AE, Schut L. Response to vincristine of recurrent brain tumors in children. *J Neurosurg* 1976;45:135.
335. Ward HWC. Central nervous system tumors of childhood treated with CCNU, vincristine and radiation. *Med Pediatr Oncol* 1978;4:315.
336. Garrett MJ, Hughs HJ, Ryall RDH. CCNU in brain tumors. *Clin Radiol* 1974;25:183.
337. Ward HWC. CCNU in the treatment of recurrent medulloblastoma. *BMJ* 1974;1:642.
338. Allen JC, Helson L. High-dose cyclophosphamide chemotherapy for recurrent CNS tumors in children. *J Neurosurg* 1981;55:749.
339. Cangir A, Ragab AH, Steubner P, et al. Combination chemotherapy with vincristine, procarbazine, prednisone with or without nitrogen mustard (MOOP vs OPP) in children with recurrent brain tumors. *Med Pediatr Oncol* 1984;12:1.

340. Friedman HS, Mahaley MS, Schold SC Jr, et al. The efficacy of vincristine and cyclophosphamide in the therapy of recurrent medulloblastoma. *Neurosurgery* 1986;18:335.
341. Crafts DC, Levin VA, Edwards MS, et al. Chemotherapy of recurrent medulloblastoma with combined procarbazine, CCNU, and vincristine. *J Neurosurg* 1978;49:589.
342. Seiler RW. Combination chemotherapy with VM26 and CCNU in primary malignant brain tumors of children. *Helv Peadiatr Acta* 1980;35:51.
343. Pendergrass TW, Milstein JM, Geyer JR, et al. Eight drugs in 1 day chemotherapy for brain tumors: experience in 107 children and rationale for preirradiation chemotherapy. *J Clin Oncol* 1987;5:1221.
344. van Eys J, Baram TZ, Cangir A, et al. Salvage chemotherapy for recurrent primary brain tumors in children. *J Pediatr* 1988;113:601.
345. Thomas P, Duffner PK, Cohen ME, et al. Multimodality therapy for medulloblastoma. *Cancer* 1980;45:666.
346. Lefkowitz IB, Packer RJ, Siegel KR, et al. Results of treatment of children with recurrent medulloblastoma/primitive neuroectodermal tumors with lomustine, cisplatin, and vincristine. *Cancer* 1990;65:412.
347. Gentet JC, Doz F, Bouffet E, et al. Carboplatin and VP 16 in medulloblastoma: a phase II Study of the French Society of Pediatric Oncology (SFOP). *Med Pediatr Oncol* 1994;23:422.
348. Packer RJ, Sutton, L, Goldwein JW, et al. Improved survival with the use of adjuvant chemotherapy in the treatment of medulloblastoma. *J Neurosurg* 1991;74:433.
349. Halberg FE, Wara WM, Fippin LF, et al. Low-dose craniospinal radiation therapy for medulloblastoma. *Int J Radiat Oncol Biol Phys* 1991;20:651.
350. Krischer J, Ragab AH, Kun LE, et al. Nitrogen mustard, vincristine, procarbazine, and prednisone as adjuvant chemotherapy in the treatment of medulloblastoma: a Pediatric Oncology Group Study. *J Neurosurg* 1991;74:905.
351. Christ WM, Ragab AH, Vietti TJ, et al. Chemotherapy of childhood medulloblastoma. *Am J Dis Child* 1976;13:639.
352. Nathanson L, Kovacs SG. Chemotherapeutic response in metastatic: report of two cases and review of the literature. *Med Pediatr Oncol* 1978;4:105.
353. Hoffman HJ. Pineal region tumors. *Prog Exp Tumor Res* 1987;30:281.
354. Matsutani M, Takakura K, Sano K. Primary intracranial germ cell tumors: pathology and treatment. *Prog Exp Tumor Res* 1987;30:307.
355. Herrick MK. Pathology of pineal tumors. In: Neuwelt EA, ed. *Diagnosis and treatment of pineal region tumors.* Baltimore: Williams & Wilkins, 1984:31.
356. Allen JC, Bruce J, Kun LE, et al. Pineal region tumors. In: Edwards MS, Levin V, eds. *Cancer in nervous system.* New York: Churchill Livingstone, 1995:421.
357. Rhoton AL Jr, Yamamoto I, Peace DA. Microsurgery of the third ventricle: part 2. Operative approaches. *Neurosurgery* 1981;8:357.
358. Schmidek HH, Waters A. Pineal masses: clinical features and management. In: Wilkins RH, Rengachary SS, eds. *Neurosurgery.* New York: McGraw-Hill, 1985:688.
359. Pecker J, Scarabin JM, Vallee B, et al. Treatment in tumor of the pineal region: value of stereotaxic biopsy. *Surg Neurol* 1979;12:341.
360. Linstadt D, Wara WM, Edwards MS, et al. Radiotherapy of primary intracranial germinomas: the case against routine craniospinal irradiation. *Int J Radiat Oncol Biol Phys* 1988;15:291.
361. Wara WM, Evans A, et al. Tumors of the pineal and supreasellar region: Children's Cancer Study Group. *Cancer* 1979;43:698.
362. Wolden SL, Wara WM, Larson DA, et al. Radiation therapy for primary intracranial germcell tumors. *Int J Radiat Oncol Biol Phys* 1995;32:943.
363. Jenkin RDT, Simpson WJK, Keen CW, et al. Pineal and suprasellar germinomas: results of radiation treatment. *J Neurosurg* 1978;48:99.
364. Salazar OM, Castro-Vita H, Bakos RS, et al. Radiation therapy for tumors of the pineal region. *Int J Radiat Oncol Biol Phys* 1979;5:491.
365. Edwards MSB LV. Chemotherapy of third ventricle tumors. In: Appuzzo M, ed. *Third ventricular tumors.* Baltimore: Williams & Wilkins, 1987:838.
366. Bouffet E, Baranzelli MC, Patte C, et al. Combined treatment modality for intracranial germinomas: results of a multicentre SFOP experience. *Br J Cancer* 1999;79:1199.
367. Buckner JC, Peethambaram PP, Smithson WA, et al. Phase II trial of primary chemotherapy followed by reduced-dose radiation for CNS germ cell tumors. *J Clin Oncol* 1999;17:933.
368. Shibamoto Y, Oda Y, Yamashita J, et al. The role of cerebrospinal fluid cytology in radiotherapy planning for intracranial germinoma. *Int J Radiat Oncol Biol Phys* 1994;29:1089.
369. Merchant TE, Davis BJ, Sheldon JM, et al. Radiation therapy for relapsed CNS germinoma after primary chemotherapy. *J Clin Oncol* 1998;16:204.
370. Fuller BG, Kapp DS, Cox R. Radiation therapy of pineal region tumors: 25 new cases and a review of 208 previously reported cases. *Int J Radiat Oncol Biol Phys* 1993;28:229.
371. Patel SR, Buckner JC, Smithson WA, et al. Cisplatin-based chemotherapy in primary central nervous system germ cell tumors. *J Neurooncol* 1992;12:47.
372. Finlay J, Walker R, Balmaceda, et al. Chemotherapy without irradiation (XRT) for primary central nervous system (CNS) germ cell tumors (GCT): a report of international study. *Am Soc Clin Oncol* 1992;11:A420.
373. Matsukado Y, Abe H, Tanaka R, et al. Cisplatin, vinblastine and bleomycin (PVB) combination chemotherapy in the treatment of intracranial malignant germ cell tumors; a preliminary report of a phase II study. The Japanese Intracranial Germ Cell Tumor Study Group. *Gan No Rinsho* 1986;32:1387.
374. Allen JC, DaRosso RC, Donahue B, et al. A phase II trial of preirradiation carboplatin in newly diagnosed germinoma of the central nervous system. *Cancer* 1994;74:940.
375. Allen JC, Kim JH, Packer RJ. Neoadjuvant chemotherapy for newly diagnosed germ-cell tumors of the central nervous system. *J Neurosurg* 1987;67:65.
376. Jereb B, Zupancic N, Petric J. Report of seven cases. *Pediatr Hematol Oncol* 1990;7:183.
377. Mizuno M, Yoshida J, Noda S. Combined chemotherapy of CDDP and etoposide in intracranial germinomas. *Gan To Kagaku Ryoho* 1989;16:3457.
378. Balmaceda C, Heller G, Rosenblum M et al. Chemotherapy without irradiation—a novel approach for newly diagnosed CNS germ cell tumors: results of an international cooperative trial. The First International Central Nervous System Germ Cell Tumor Study. *J Clin Oncol* 1996;14:2908.
379. Miyamachi K, Aida T, Abe H. Five cases of primary intracranial germ cell tumors treated by combination chemotherapy with cisplatin. *No Shinkei Geka* 1989;16:1053.
380. Kobayashi T, Yoshida J, Sugita K, et al. Combination chemotherapy with cisplatin and etoposide for intracranial germ cell tumors. International Symposium on Pediatric Neuro-Oncology. Seattle, WA, 1989(abst A5).
381. Ablin A, Isaacs H Jr. Pediatric oncology: germ cell tumors. In: Pizzo PA, Poplack DG, eds. *Principles and practice of pediatric oncology.* Philadelphia: Lippincott, 1989:713.
382. Pera MF, Koberle B, Masters JR. Exceptional sensitivity of testicular germ cell tumour cell lines to the new anti-cancer agent, temozolomide. *Br J Cancer* 1995;71:904.
383. Wilson CB. Surgical management of endocrine-active pituitary adenomas. In: Walker MD, ed. *Oncology of the nervous system.* Boston: Martinus-Nijhoff, 1983:117.
384. Eastman RC, Gorden P, Roth J. Conventional supervoltage irradiation is an effective treatment for acromegaly. *J Clin Endocrinol Metab* 1979;48:931.
385. Breen P, Flickenger JC, Kondziolka D, et al. Radiotherapy for nonfuctional pituitary adenomas: analysis of long-term tumor control. *J Neurosurg* 1998;89:933.
386. Sheline GE TJ. Pituitary tumors. In: Perez CA BL, ed. *Principles and practice of radiation oncology.* Philadelphia: Lippincott, 1987:1108.
387. Malmed S. Acromegaly. *N Engl J Med* 1990;322:966.
388. Barkan AL, Halasz I, Dornfeld KJ, et al. Pituitary irradiation is ineffective in normalizing plasma insulin-like growth factor I in patients with acromegaly. *J Clin Endocrinol Metab* 1997;82:3187.
389. Suliman M, Jenkins R, Ross R, et al. Long-term treatment of acromegaly with somatostatin analogue SR-lanreotide. *J Endocrinol Invest* 1999;22:409.
390. Jennings AS, Liddle GW, Orth DN. Results of treating childhood Cushing's disease with pituitary irradiation. *N Engl J Med* 1977;297:957.
391. Sheline GE, Grossman A, Jones AH, et al. Radiation therapy of prolactinomas. In: Black PM, Zervas NT, Ridgeway ED, Martin JB, eds. *Secretory tumors of the pituitary gland.* New York: Raven Press, 1984:1.
392. Littley MD, Shalet SM, Reid H, et al. The effect of extenal pituitary irradiation on elevated serum prolactin levels in patients with pituitary microadenomas. *Q J Med* 1991;81:985.
393. Tsao MN, Wara WM, Larson DA. Radiation therapy for benign central nervous system disease. *Semin Oncol* 1999;9:120.
394. Cannavo S, Curto L, Squadrito S, et al. Cabergoline: a first choice treatment in patients with previously untreated prolactin-secreting pituitary adenoma. *J Endocrinol Invest* 1999;22:354.
395. Mitsumori M, Schrieve DC, Alexander E 3rd, et al. Initial clinical results of LINAC-based sterotactic radiosurgery and sterotactic radiotherapy for pituitary adenomas. *Int J Radiat Oncol Biol Phys* 1998;42:573.
396. Levy RP, Schulte PWM, Slater JD, et al. Stereotactic radiosurgery-the role of charged particles. *Acta Oncol* 1999;38:165.
397. Zierhut D, Flentje M, Adolph J, et al. External radiotherapy of pituitary adenomas. *Int J Radiat Oncol Biol Phys* 1995;33:307.
398. McCord MW, Buatti JM, Fennell EM, et al. Radiotherapy for pituitary adenoma: long term outcome and sequelae. *Int J Radiat Oncol Biol Phys* 1997;39:437.
399. Tsang RW, Brierley JD, Panzarella T, et al. Role of radiation therapy in clinical hormonally-active pituitary adenomas. *Radiother Oncol* 1996;41:45.
400. Bradra M, Ford, Ashely S, et al. Risk of second brain tumor after conservative surgery and radiotherapy for pituitary adenoma. *BMJ* 1992;304:1343.
401. Schoenthalar R, Albright NW, Wara WM, et al. Reirradiation of pituitary adenoma. *Int J Radiat Oncol Biol Phys* 1992;24:307.
402. Coffey RJ, Lunsford LD. The role of stereotactic techniques in the management of craniopharyngiomas. In: Rosanblum ML, ed. *The role of surgery in brain tumor management.* Philadelphia: Saunders, 1991:161.
403. Pollock BE, Lunsford LD, Kondziolka D, et al. Phosphorus-32 intracavitary irradiation of cystic craniopharyngiomas: current technique and long-term results. *Int J Radiat Oncol Biol Phys* 1995;33:437.
404. Richmond IL, Wara WM, Wilson CB. Role of radiation therapy in the management of craniopharyngiomas in children. *Neurosurgery* 1980;6:513.
405. Fischer EG, Welch K, Belli JA, et al. Treatment of craniopharyngiomas in children, 1972–1981. *J Neurosurg* 1985;62:496.
406. Wen B-C, Hussey DH, Staples J, et al. A comparison of the roles of surgery and radiation therapy in the management of craniopharyngiomas. *Int J Radiat Oncol Biol Phys* 1989;16:17.
407. Hetelekidis S, Barnes PD, Tao ML, et al. 20 year experience in childhood carniopharyngioma. *Int J Radiat Oncol Biol Phys* 1993;27:189.
408. Thomsett MJ, Conte FA, Kaplan SL, et al. Endocrine and neurologic outcome in childhood craniopharyngioma: review of effect of treatment in 42 patients. *J Pediatr* 1980;97:728.
409. Cavazzuti V, Fischer EC, Welch K, et al. Neurological and psychophysiological sequelae following different treatments of craniopharyngiomas in children. *J Neurosurg* 1983;59:409.
410. Jackler RK, Pitts LH. Acoustic neuroma. *Neurosurg Clin North Am* 1990;1:199.
411. Martuza RL, Ojemann RG. Bilateral acoustic neuromas: clinical aspects, pathogenesis, and treatment. *Neurosurgery* 1982;10:1.
412. Wallner KE, Sheline GE, Pitts LH, et al. Efficacy of irradiation for incompletely excised acoustic neurilemomas. *J Neurosurg* 1987;67:858.
413. Maire JP, Caudry M, Darrouzet V, et al. Fractionated radiation therapy in the treatment of stage III and IV cerebello-pontine angle neruinomas: long-term results in 24 cases. *Int J Radiat Oncol Biol Phys* 1995;32:1137.

414. Kondziolka D, Lunsford LD, McLaughlin MR, et al. Long-term outcomes after radiosurgery for acoustic neuromas. *N Engl J Med* 1998;339:1426.
415. Flickinger JC, Lunsford LD, Linskey ME, et al. Gamma knife radiosurgery for acoustic tumors: multivariate analysis of 4-year results. *Radiother Oncol* 1993;27:91.
416. Linskey ME, Flickinger JC, Lunsford LD. Cranial nerve length predicts the risk of delayed facial and trigeminal neuropathies after acoustiv tumor stereotactic radiosurgery. *Int J Radiat Oncol Biol Phys* 1993;25:227.
417. Miranjan A, Lunsford LD, Flickenger JC, et al. Dose reduction improves hearing preservation rates after intercanalicular acoustic tumor radiosurgery. *Neurosurgery* 1999;45:762.
418. Farriro JB III, Hymas VL, Benke RH, et al. Carcinoid apudoma arising in glomus jugulare tumors. *Laryngoscope* 1980;90:110.
419. Simko TG, Griffin TW, Gerdes AJ, et al. The role of radiation therapy in the treatment of glomus jugulare tumors. *J Neurol Neurosurg Psychiatry* 1957;20:22.
420. Gardner G, Cocke EW Jr, Robertson JT, et al. Glomus jugulare tumors: combined treatment. *J Laryngol Otol* 1981;95:437.
421. Springate SC, Weichselbaum RR. Radiation or surgery for chemodectoma of the temporal bone: a review of local control and complications. *Head Neck* 1990;12:303.
422. Million RR, Cassisi NJ, Mancuso AA, et al. Chemodectomas (glomus body tumors). In: Million RR, Cassisi NJ, eds. *Management of head and neck cancer.* Philadelphia: Lippincott, 1994:765.
423. Kim JA, Elkon D, Lim ML, et al. Optimum dose of radiotherapy for chemodectomas of the middle ear. *Int J Radiat Oncol Biol Phys* 1980;6:815.
424. Heffelfinger MJ, Dahlin DC, MacCarty CS, et al. Chordomas and cartilaginous tumors at the skull base. *Cancer* 1973;32:410.
425. Phillips T, Newman H. Chordomas. In: Deeley T, ed. *Modern radiotherapy and oncology: central nervous system tumors.* Boston: Butterworths, 1974:184.
426. Munzenrider JE, Hug E, McManus P, et al. Skull base chordomas: treatment outcome and prognostic factors in adult patients following conformal treatment with 3D planning and high dose fractionated combined proton and photon radiation therapy. *Int J Radiat Oncol Biol Phys* 1995;32:209.
427. Rosenberg AE, Nielsen GP, Keel SB, et al. Chondrosarcoma of the base of the skull: a clinicopathologic study of 200 cases with emphasis on its distinction from chordoma. *Am J Surg Pathol* 1999;23:1370.
428. Berson AM, Castro JR, Petti P, et al. Charged particle irradiation of chordoma and chondrosarcoma of the base of the skull and cervical spine: the Lawrence Berkeley Laboratory Experience. *Int J Radiat Oncol Biol Phys* 1988;15:559.
429. Smalley SR, Schomberg PJ, Earle JD, et al. Radiotherapeutic considerations in the treatment of hemangioblastomas of the central nervous system. *Int J Radiat Oncol Biol Phys* 1990;18:1165.
430. Patrice SJ, Sneed PK, Flickinger JC, et al. Radiosurgery for hemangioblastoma: results of a multiinstitutional experience. *Int J Radiat Oncol Biol Phys* 1996;35:493.
431. Chang SD, Meisel JA, Hancock SL, et al. Treatment of hemangioblastomas in von Hippel-Lindau disease with linear accelerator-based radiosurgery. *Neurosurgery* 1998;43:28.
432. Naguib MG, Chou SH, Mastri A. Radiation therapy of a choroid plexus papilloma of the cerebellopontine angle with bone involvement. *J Neurosurg* 1981;54:245.
433. Wolff JE, Sajedi M, Coppes MJ, et al. Radiation therapy and survival in choroid plexus carcinoma. *Lancet* 1999;353:2126.
434. Chow E, Reardon DA, Shah AB, et al. Pediatric choroid plexus neoplasms. *Int J Radiat Oncol Biol Phys* 1999;44:249.
435. Ausman JI, Schrontz C, Chason J, et al. Aggressive choroid plexus papilloma. *Surg Neurol* 1984;22:472.
436. Duffner PK, Kun LE, Burger PC, et al. Postoperative chemotherapy and delayed radiation in infants and very young children with choroid plexus carcinomas. The Pediatric Oncology Group. *Pediatr Neurosurg* 1995;22:189.
437. Connolly ES. Spinal cord tumors in adults. In: Youman JR, ed. *Youmans' neurological surgery.* Philadelphia: WB Saunders, 1982:3196.
438. Linstadt DE. Spinal cord. In: Leibel SA, Phillips TL, eds. *Textbook of radiation oncology.* Philadelphia: WB Saunders, 1998:401.
439. Wen B-C, Hussey DH, Hitchon PW, et al. The role of radiation therapy in the management of ependymomas of the spinal cord. *Int J Radiat Oncol Biol Phys* 1991;20:781.
440. Waldron JN, Laperriere NJ, Jaakkimainen L, et al. Spinal cord ependymomas: a retrospective analysis of 59 cases. *Int J Radiat Oncol Biol Phys* 1993;27:223.
441. Linstadt D, Wara WM, Leibel SA, et al. Postoperative radiotherapy of primary spinal cord tumors. *Int J Radiat Oncol Biol Phys* 1989;16:1397.
442. Barone B, Elvidge A. Ependymomas: a clinical survey. *J Neurosurg* 1970;33:428.
443. Schuman R, Alvord E, Leech R. The biology of childhood ependymomas. *Arch Neurol* 1975;32:731.
444. Whitaker SJ, Bessell EM, Ashley SE, et al. Postoperative radiotherapy in the management of spinal cord ependymoma. *J Neurosurg* 1991;74:720.
445. Cairncross JG, Laperriere N. Low-grade glioma: to treat or not to treat? *Arch Neurol* 1989;46:1238.
446. Forman AD, Levin VA. Intraventricular therapy. In: Perry MC, ed. *The chemotherapy source book.* Baltimore: Williams & Wilkins, 1991:213.
447. Emami B, Lyman J, Brown A, et al. Tolerance of normal tissue to therapeutic irradiation. *Int J Radiat Oncol Biol Phys* 1991;21:109.
448. Levin VA, Silver P, Hannigan J, et al. Superiority of post-radiotherapy adjuvant chemotherapy with CCNU, procarbazine, and vincristine (PCV) over BCNU for anaplastic gliomas: NCOG 6G61 final report. *Int J Radiat Oncol Biol Phys* 1990;18:321.
449. Levin VA, Wara WM, Davis RL, et al. Northern California Oncology Group protocol 6G91: response to treatment with radiation therapy and seven-drug chemotherapy in patients with glioblastoma multiforme. *Cancer Treat Rep* 1986;70:739.
450. Levin VA, Maor MH, Thall PF, et al. Phase II study of accelerated fractionation radiation therapy with carboplatin followed by vincristine chemotherapy for the treatment of glioblastoma multiforme. *Int J Radiat Oncol Biol Phys* 1995;33:357.
451. Levin VA, Uhm JH, Jaeckle KA, et al. Phase III randomized study of post-radiotherapy chemotherapy with DFMO-PCV versus PCV for glioblastoma multiforme. *Clin Cancer Res* 2000 *(in press).*
452. Levin VA, Prados MD, Wara WM, et al. Radiation therapy and bromodeoxuruidine chemotherapy followed by procarbazine, lomustine,and vincristine for the treatment of anaplastic gliomas. *Int J Radiat Oncol Biol Phys* 1995;32:75.
453. Rodriguez L, Prados M, Silver P, et al. Re-evaluation of procarbazine for the treatment of recurrent malignant CNS tumors. *Cancer* 1989;64:2420.
454. Levin VA, Crafts D, Wilson CB, et al. Imidazole carboxamides: relationship of lipophilicity to activity against intracerebral murine glioma 26 and preliminary phase II clinical trial of 5-[3,3-bis(2-chloroethyl)-1-triazeno]imidazole-4-carboxamide (NSC-82196) in primary and secondary brain tumors. *Cancer Chemother Rep* 1975;59:327.
455. Levin VA, Prados MD, Yung WK, et al. Treatment of recurrent gliomas with eflornithine. *J Natl Cancer Inst* 1992;84:1432.
456. Yung WK, Kyritsis AP, Gleason MJ, et al. Treatment of recurrent malignant gliomas with high-dose 13-cis-retinoic acid. *Clin Cancer Res* 1996;2:1931.
457. Groves MD, Jaeckle KA, Kyritsis AP, et al. *Cis*-retinoic acid for the treatment of recurrent glioblastoma multiforme. *Neuro-Oncology* 1999;1:314.
458. Friedman HS, Petros WP, Friedman AH, et al. Irinotecan therapy in adults with recurrent or progressive malignant glioma. *J Clin Oncol* 1999;17:1516.
459. Levin VA, Edwards MS, Wright DC, et al. Modified procarbazine, CCNU, and vincristine (PCV 3) combination chemotherapy in the treatment of malignant brain tumors. *Cancer Treat Rep* 1980;64:237.
460. Levin VA, Hoffman WF, Pischer TL, et al. BCNU-5-fluorouracil combination therapy for recurrent malignant brain tumors. *Cancer Treat Rep* 1978;62:2071.
461. Levin VA, Chamberlain MC, Prados MD, et al. Phase I-II study of eflornithine and mitoguazone combined in the treatment of recurrent primary brain tumors. *Cancer Treat Rep* 1987;71:459.
462. Levin VA, Prados MD. Treatment of recurrent gliomas and metastatic brain tumors with a polydrug protocol designed to combat nitrosourea resistance. *J Clin Oncol* 1992;10:766.
463. Kyritsis AP, Yung WK, Jaeckle KA, et al. Combination of 6-thioguanine, procarbazine, lomustine, and hydroxyurea for patients with recurrent malignant gliomas. *Neurosurgery* 1996;39:921.
464. Galanis E, Buckner JC, Burch PA, et al. Phase II trial of nitrogen mustard, vincristine, and procarbazine in patients with recurrent glioma: North Central Cancer Treatment Group results. *J Clin Oncol* 1998;16:2953.
465. Kunschner LJ, Yung WKA, Levin VA, et al. Carboplatin and 13-*cis*-retinoic acid for recurrent glioblastoma multiforme. *Neuro-Oncology* 1999;1:320.
466. van den Bent MJ, Kros JM, Heimans JJ, et al. Response rate and prognostic factors of recurrent oligodendroglioma treated with procarbazine, CCNU, and vincristine chemotherapy. Dutch Neuro-Oncology Group. *Neurology* 1998;51:1140.
467. Soffietti R, Ruda R, Bradac GB, et al. PCV chemotherapy for recurrent oligodendrogliomas and oligoastrocytomas. *Neurosurgery* 1998;43:1066.
468. Cairncross G, Macdonald D, Ludwin S et al. Chemotherapy for anaplastic oligodendroglioma. National Cancer Institute of Canada Clinical Trials Group. *J Clin Oncol* 1994;12:2013.
469. Levin VA, Edwards MS, Gutin PH et al. Phase II evaluation of dibromodulcitol in the treatment of recurrent medulloblastoma, ependymoma, and malignant astrocytoma. *J Neurosurg* 1984;61:1063.
470. Fewer D, Wilson CB, Boldrey EB, et al. Phase II study of 1-(2-choloroethyl)-3-cyclohexyl-1-nitrosourea (CCNU) in the treatment of brain tumors. *Cancer Chemother Rep* 1972;56:421.
471. Lefkowitz IB, Packer RJ, Siegel KR, et al. Results of treatment of children with recurrent medulloblastoma/primitive neuroectodermal tumors with lomustine, cisplatin, and vincristine. *Cancer* 1990;65:412.
472. Barker FG, Chang SM, Gutin PH, et al. Survival and functional status after resection of recurrent glioblastoma multiforme. *Neurosurgery* 1998;42:709.
473. Packer RJ, Sutton LN, Elterman R, et al. Outcome for children with medulloblastoma treated with radiation and cisplatin, CCNU, and vincristine chemotherapy. *J Neurosurg* 1994;81:690.
474. Kovnar EH, Kellie SJ, Horowitz ME, et al. Preirradiation cisplatin and etoposide in the treatment of high-risk medulloblastoma and other malignant embryonal tumors of the central nervous system: a phase II study. *J Clin Oncol* 1990;8:330.

CHAPTER **44**

Cancers of Childhood

SECTION **1**

LEE J. HELMAN
DAVID MALKIN

Molecular Biology of Childhood Cancers

The biologic nature of tumors of childhood is clinically, histopathologically, and biologically distinct from that of adult-onset malignancies. Childhood cancers tend to have short latency periods, are often rapidly growing and aggressively invasive, are rarely associated with exposure to carcinogens implicated in adult-onset cancers, and are generally more responsive to standard modalities of treatment, in particular chemotherapy. Most childhood tumors occur sporadically in families with at most a weak history of cancer. In approximately 10% to 15% of cases,[1,2] however, a strong familial association is recognized, or the child has a congenital or genetic disorder that imparts a higher likelihood of specific cancer types. Examples of genetic disorders that render a child at increased risk of tumor development include xeroderma pigmentosa, Bloom's syndrome, or ataxia-telangiectasia, which predispose to skin cancers, leukemias, or lymphoid malignancies, respectively. In all three cases, constitutional gene alterations that disrupt normal mechanisms of genomic DNA repair are blamed for the propensity to cell transformation. Other hereditary disorders including Beckwith-Wiedemann syndrome (BWS) and the multiple endocrine neoplasias types 1 and 2 are thought to be associated with their respective tumor spectra through constitutional activation of molecular pathways of deregulated cellular growth and proliferation. The cancers that occur in these syndromes are generally secondary phenotypic manifestations of disorders that have distinctive recognizable physical stigmata. On the other hand, some cancer predisposition syndromes are recognized only by their malignant manifestations, with nonmalignant characteristics being virtually absent. These include hereditary retinoblastoma, the Li-Fraumeni syndrome (LFS), familial Wilms' tumor (WT), and familial adenomatous polyposis coli. Each of these presents with distinct cancer phenotypes, and for each the identified molecular defect is unique (Table 44.1-1).

The study of pediatric cancer and rare hereditary cancer syndromes and associations has led to the identification of numerous cancer genes including dominant oncogenes and tumor suppressor genes. These have proved to be important not only in hereditary predisposition, but also as major players in the normal growth, differentiation, and proliferation pathways of all cells. Alterations of these genes have been consistently found in numerous sporadic tumors of childhood and led to studies of their functional role in carcinogenesis. The numerous properties of transformed malignant cells in culture or *in vivo* can be explained by the complex abnormal interaction of numerous positive and negative growth regulatory genes. Pediatric cancers offer unique models in which to study these pathways in that they are less likely to be disrupted by nongenetic factors. The embryonic ontogeny of many childhood cancers suggests that better understanding of the nature of the genetic events leading to these cancers will also augment the understanding of normal embryologic growth and development. This chapter begins with an outline of tumor suppressor genes, the most frequently implicated class of cancer genes in childhood malignancy. This leads into discussion of molecular features of retinoblastoma, the paradigm of cancer genetics, followed by

TABLE 44.1-1. Hereditary Syndromes Associated with Childhood Cancers

Hereditary Syndrome	*Predominant Pediatric Neoplasms*
Hereditary retinoblastoma	Retinoblastoma, osteosarcoma
Familial Wilms' tumor	Wilms' tumor
Beckwith-Wiedemann syndrome	Wilms' tumor, hepatoblastoma, rhabdomyosarcoma, adrenocortical carcinoma
Li-Fraumeni syndrome	Sarcomas, brain tumor, leukemia, adrenocortical carcinoma, choroid plexus carcinoma
Ataxia-telangiectasia	Lymphoma, brain tumors, leukemia
Neurofibromatosis type 1	Sarcoma, glioma
Neurofibromatosis type 2	Meningioma, acoustic neuroma
Multiple endocrine neoplasia, types 1 and 2	Adenomas/carcinomas of endocrine organs
Familial polyposis coli	Intestinal polyps, colon carcinoma, hepatoblastoma
Gorlin syndrome	Medulloblastoma, basal cell nevi
Bloom's syndrome	Leukemia

analysis of the molecular understanding of other common pediatric cancers. Evaluation of the importance of molecular alterations in familial cancers, as well as new approaches in molecular therapeutics, are also addressed.

TUMOR SUPPRESSOR GENES

Faulty regulation of cellular growth and differentiation leads to neoplastic transformation and tumor initiation. Many inappropriately activated growth-potentiating genes, or *oncogenes*, have been identified through the study of RNA tumor viruses and the transforming effects of DNA isolated from malignant cells. However, activated dominant oncogenes themselves do not readily explain a variety of phenomena related to transformation and tumor formation. Among these is the suppression of tumorigenicity by fusion of malignant cells with their normal counterparts. If these malignant cells carried an activated dominant oncogene, it would be expected that such a gene would initiate transformation of the normal cells, likely leading to either embryonic or fetal death. The observation is more readily explained by postulating the existence of a factor in the normal cell that acts to suppress growth of the fused malignant cells. Malignant cells commonly exhibit specific chromosomal deletions (Table 44.1-2). The best example of this occurs in retinoblastoma, a rare pediatric eye tumor in which a small region of the long arm of chromosome 13 is frequently missing.[3,4] The presumed loss of genes in specific chromosomal regions argues strongly against the concept of a dominantly acting gene being implicated in the development of the tumor. Hereditary forms of cancer are also not readily explained by altered growth-potentiating genes. Comparisons between the frequencies of familial tumors and their sporadic counterparts led Knudson to suggest that the familial forms of some tumors could be explained by constitutional mutations in growth-limiting genes.[5] The resulting inactivation of these genes would facilitate cellular transformation.[6] Such growth-limiting genes were termed *tumor suppressor genes.*

Unlike dominant oncogenes, mutant tumor suppressor genes may be found either in germ cells or somatic cells. In the former, they may arise *de novo* or be transmitted from generation to generation within a family. Despite many similarities among the various cloned tumor suppressors, it has become evident that this family of genes is heterogeneous in many respects. The diversity of functions, cellular locations, and tissue-specific expression of the tumor suppressor genes suggests the existence of a complex, yet coordinated, cellular pathway that limits cell growth by linking nuclear processes with the intracytoplasmic and extracytoplasmic environment. This discussion is limited to those genes for which pediatric tumors are frequently associated.

RETINOBLASTOMA: THE PARADIGM

Retinoblastoma is the prototype cancer caused by mutations of a tumor suppressor gene. It is a malignant tumor of the retina that occurs in infants and young children, with an incidence of approximately 1 in 20,000.[7] Approximately 40% of retinoblastoma cases are of the heritable form[8] in which the child inherits one mutant allele at the retinoblastoma susceptibility locus (RB1) through the germline. A somatic mutation in a single retinal cell causes loss of function of the remaining normal allele, leading to tumor formation. Tumors are often bilateral and multifocal. The disease is inherited as an autosomal dominant trait, with a penetrance approaching 100%.[9] The remaining 60% of retinoblastoma cases are sporadic (nonheritable).[10] Both RB1 alleles in a single retinal cell have been inactivated by somatic mutations. As one can imagine, such an event is rare, and these patients usually have only one tumor that presents later than in infants with the heritable form. Fifteen percent of unilateral retinoblastoma is heritable,[9] but by chance develops in only one eye. Survivors of heritable retinoblastoma have a several-hundred-fold increased risk of developing mesenchymal tumors such as osteogenic sarcoma, fibrosarcomas, and melanomas later in life.[10,11] It is thought that several genetic mechanisms may be involved in elimination of the second wild-type RB1 allele in an evolving tumor. These include chromosomal duplication or nondisjunction, mitotic recombination, or gene conversion.[12]

The RB1 gene was eventually mapped to chromosome 13q14.[13] Using Southern blot analysis, it was then possible to

TABLE 44.1-2. Common Cytogenetic Rearrangements in Solid Tumors of Childhood

Solid Tumor	*Cytogenetic Rearrangement*
Ewing's sarcoma	t(11;22)(q24;q12), +8
Neuroblastoma	del1p32-36, double-minute chromosomes, homogeneous staining regions, +17q21-qter
Retinoblastoma	del13q14
Wilms' tumor	del11p13, t(3;17)
Synovial sarcoma	t(X;11)(p11;q11)
Osteogenic sarcoma	del13q14
Rhabdomyosarcoma	t(2;13)(q35;q14), t(1;13), (q36;q14), 11p-
Peripheral neuroepithelioma	t(11;22)(q24;q12), +8
Astrocytoma	i(17q)
Meningioma	delq22, -22
Atypical teratoid/rhabdoid tumor	delq22.11
Germ cell tumor	i(12p)

demonstrate that the second target gene that led to disease was actually the second copy of the RB1 locus. Reduction to homozygosity of the mutant allele [or loss of heterozygosity (LOH) of the wild-type allele] would lead to the loss of functional RB1 and account for tumor development.

Using classic cloning techniques, a 4.7-kb cDNA fragment was isolated from retinal cells.[14] This gene, RB1, consisted of 27 exons and encoded a 105 kD nuclear phosphoprotein. As well as being altered in retinoblastoma, this gene and its protein product have also been found to be altered in osteosarcomas, small cell lung carcinomas, and bladder, breast, and prostate carcinomas.[14,15]

Although it is clear that RB1 and its protein product play some role in growth regulation, the precise nature of this role remains obscure. In the developing retina, inactivation of the RB1 gene is both necessary and sufficient for tumor formation.[16] Although the RB1 gene is expressed in virtually all mammalian tissues, only in the retina is its inactivation sufficient for tumor initiation. Outside the retina, RB1 inactivation is often a rate-limiting step in tumorigenesis generated by multiple genetic events. The molecular characteristics and potential functional activities of RB1 are outlined in detail elsewhere in this volume.

The patterns of inheritance and presentation of retinoblastoma have been well described, and the responsible gene identified. Although the basic mechanisms by which the gene is inactivated are understood, much still remains to be determined about the biologic function of the gene and its protein product.

WILMS' TUMOR: THREE DISTINCT LOCI

WT, or nephroblastoma, is an embryonal malignancy of the kidney that arises from remnants of immature kidney. It affects approximately 1 in 10,000 children, usually before the age of 6 years (median age at diagnosis, 3.5 years). Some 5% to 10% of children present with either synchronous or metachronous bilateral tumors.[17] A peculiar feature of WT is its association with nephrogenic rests, foci of primitive but nonmalignant cells whose persistence suggests a defect in kidney development. These precursor lesions are found within the normal kidney tissue of 30% to 40% of children with WT. Nephrogenic rests may persist, regress spontaneously, or grow into a large mass that simulates a true WT and presents a difficult diagnostic challenge.[18] Another interesting feature of this neoplasm is its association with specific congenital abnormalities, including genitourinary anomalies, sporadic aniridia, mental retardation, and hemihypertrophy. The WT1 tumor suppressor gene is homozygously deleted, at least in part, in a small but highly informative set of sporadic WTs. In addition, both sporadic and hereditary WTs have been described in which WT1 is specifically altered.

A genetic predisposition to WT is observed in two distinct disease syndromes with urogenital system malformations (the WAGR syndrome and the Denys-Drash syndrome)[19] as well as in an overgrowth syndrome characterized by visceromegaly, macroglossia, and hyperinsulinemic hypoglycemia (BWS).[20] These congenital disorders have now been linked to abnormalities at specific genetic loci implicated in Wilms' tumorigenesis.

The WAGR syndrome, the association of WT (W) with congenital aniridia (A), genitourinary malformations (G), and mental retardation (R), has been correlated with constitutional deletions of band q13 of chromosome 11.[21] Whereas it is now known that the WAGR deletion encompasses a number of contiguous genes, including the aniridia gene *Pax6*,[22] the cytogenetic observation in patients with WAGR was also important in the cloning of WT1 at chromosome 11p13.[23–25] Characterization of WT1 demonstrated that this gene spans approximately 50 kb of DNA and contains 10 exons. The WT1 protein is a transcription factor.[26] However, the identity of the gene(s) targeted by WT1 during normal kidney development is not known.

The second syndrome closely associated with this locus was initially described by Denys in 1967 and recognized as a syndrome by Drash 3 years later.[27,28] Denys-Drash syndrome is a rare association of WT, intersex disorders, and progressive renal failure.[28] It has been demonstrated that virtually all patients with Denys-Drash syndrome carry WT1 point mutations in the germline.[29]

WT1 is altered in only 10% of WTs. This observation implies the existence of alternative loci in the etiology of this childhood renal malignancy. One such locus also resides on the short arm of chromosome 11, telomeric of WT1, at 11p15. This gene, designated WT2, is associated with BWS. Patients with BWS are at increased risk of developing WT, as well as other embryonic malignancies including rhabdomyosarcoma (RMS), neuroblastoma, and hepatoblastoma. The putative BWS gene maps to chromosome 11p15[30,31] and is tightly linked to the Ha-*ras* oncogene homologue *HRAS-I* and the insulin growth factor-2 gene (*IGF-2*). Whether the BWS gene and *WT2* are one and the same or two distinct yet closely linked genes remains to be determined.

Although linkage studies have indicated that the gene for familial WT must be distinct from WT1 and WT2, and from the gene that predisposes to BWS, to date, this gene has been neither cytogenetically localized nor isolated. Whether, of course, the gene for familial WT interacts with the gene product of either of the two WT suppressor genes has yet to be determined.

Finally, loss of the long arm of chromosome 16 has been observed in approximately 20% of WT specimens.[32] This observation implicates yet another genetic locus in WT. Since linkage studies have also excluded this locus as the *familial* WT gene,[33] a total of four loci have thus far been associated with this pediatric malignancy. However, it is not known whether alterations at 16q can initiate tumorigenesis or simply reflect subsequent steps in the progression of malignancy.

It is apparent that the influence of the genetic alterations in WT is quite different from those of the retinoblastoma gene. In the latter, there is strong evidence that a single gene is involved, whereas a series of genetic alterations, or at least distinct genetic events, is required for Wilms' tumorigenesis.

NEUROFIBROMATOSES

The neurofibromatoses (NF) comprise two similar entities. NF1 is one of the most common autosomal dominantly inherited disorders, affecting approximately 1 in 3500 people,[34] one-half of which arise from new spontaneous mutations. Carriers of mutant NF1 are predisposed to a variety of tumors including optic nerve glioma, neurofibroma and neurofibrosarcoma, malignant schwannoma, astrocytoma, and pheochromocytoma.[35,36] Occurring with less frequency are leukemias, osteosarcoma, RMS, and WT.

Using standard linkage analysis, the NF1 gene was mapped to chromosomal band 17q11 and subsequently cloned.[37,38] The NF1 gene is unusual in that it contains three embedded genes, OMGP, EV12A, and EV12B, in a single intron.[39] This gene encodes a 2818 amino acid protein, termed *neurofibromin,* that is ubiquitously expressed. One region of the gene shows extensive structural homology to the GTPase activating domain of mammalian guanosine triphosphatase-activating proteins: Loss of the protein's activity results in failure of hydrolysis of guanosine triphosphate to guanosine diphosphate by the ras oncoprotein. Loss of neurofibromin function usually results from mutations in one allele of the gene leading to premature truncation of the protein, followed by absence or mutations of the second allele in tumors. This loss of function is thought to lead to elevated levels of the guanosine triphosphate–bound RAS protein that transduces signals for cell division. There appears to be more than one mechanism whereby malignant tumors develop in NF patients. In addition to structural alterations of both alleles of the NF1 gene, alternative splicing leading to dysregulation at the level of transcription has also been demonstrated. It appears that the two types of resulting protein may modify the modulation of RAS-regulated signal transduction.

NF2 is much less frequent than NF1, occurring in only 1 in 1 million persons. Although it is also inherited as an autosomal dominant disorder with high penetrance, the new mutation rate in NF2 is low.[40] It is clinically characterized by bilateral acoustic neuromas, spinal nerve root tumors, and meningiomas.

The NF2 locus was mapped to chromosome 22, band q12,[41] and its 69-kD encoded protein, termed *merlin,* has been shown to be expressed in various tissues, including brain, although not as ubiquitously as NF1.[42,43] The mechanism of tumor formation in NF2 appears to be in concordance with the Knudson two-hit model, although the mechanism of action of the NF2 protein has not yet been elucidated. It is, however, postulated that a defect in such a molecule may dysregulate normal cell growth by disrupting a signal transduction pathway, anchorage dependence, or cell-cycle regulation.[43]

NEUROBLASTOMA

Nonrandom chromosomal abnormalities are observed in more than 75% of neuroblastomas,[44] and many of these are also found in neuroblastoma-derived cell lines. The most common of these is deletion or rearrangement of the short arm of chromosome 1, although loss, gain, and rearrangements of chromosomes 10, 14, 17, and 19 have also been reported. The allelic losses indicate loss of function of as yet unknown tumor suppressor genes in these regions. It is believed that a tumor suppressor gene that lies on band p36 of chromosome 1 is critically important in the pathogenesis and aggressive nature of neuroblastoma. It has been shown that the loss of chromosome 1p is a strong prognostic factor in patients with neuroblastoma, independent of age and stage.[45,46] Two other unique cytogenetic rearrangements are highly characteristic of neuroblastoma.[47,48] These structures, homogeneous staining regions and double-minute chromosomes, contain regions of gene amplification. The N-myc gene, an oncogene with considerable homology to the cellular protooncogene c-myc, is amplified within homogeneous staining regions and double-minute chromosomes. Virtually all neuroblastoma tumor cell lines demonstrate amplified and highly expressed N-myc,[49] and N-myc amplification is thought to be associated with rapid tumor progression. Expression of N-myc is increased in undifferentiated tumor cells compared with much lower (or single copy) levels in more differentiated cells (ganglioneuroblastoma and ganglioneuroma). N-myc expression is diminished in association with the *in vitro* differentiation of neuroblastoma cell lines.[50] This observation formed the basis for current therapeutic trials demonstrating a survival advantage to patients treated with *cis*-retinoic acid.[51] Furthermore, a close correlation exists between N-myc amplification and advanced clinical stage.[52]

Although it is clear that altered expression of N-myc contributes to the development of malignancy, it is not yet apparent which cellular functions are altered. The molecular mechanisms underlying regulation of neuroblastoma differentiation may be explained in part through the contribution of other genes and proteins.

Neuroblastoma cells that express the high-affinity nerve growth factor receptor trkA[53] can be terminally differentiated by nerve growth factor and may demonstrate morphologic changes typical of ganglionic differentiation. Tumors showing ganglionic differentiation and trk gene activation have a favorable prognosis.[53] As noted previously, resistance to multidrug chemotherapeutic regimens (multidrug resistance) is characteristic of aggressive, poorly responsive N-myc amplified neuroblastomas. It is interesting to note that expression of the multidrug-resistance-associated protein, found to confer multidrug resistance *in vitro*, is increased in neuroblastomas with N-myc amplification and decreased after differentiation of tumor cells *in vitro*.[54] It has been demonstrated in fact that high levels of multidrug-resistance-associated protein expression are significantly associated with poor outcome, independent of N-myc amplification.[54] Gain of chromosome segment 17q21-qter has been shown to be the most powerful prognostic factor yet.[55] However, no gene has yet been implicated at this site.

Finally, insulin growth factor-2 (IGF-2) is a developmentally regulated gene that may play a role in the pathogenesis of neuroblastoma. IGF-2 is expressed in embryonic adrenal cortex, as well as adult adrenal medulla. It is a stimulatory ligand for neuroblastoma cell growth. IGF-2 is highly expressed in tumor cell lines that express a pattern of developmentally regulated genes found late in the chromaffin lineage and functions in an autocrine growth pathway.[56] Cell lines that express markers corresponding to more immature cells are responsive to IGF-2, but do not produce the mitogen itself. This paracrine growth-mediating effect is consistent with observations of IGF-2 expression in infiltrating tumor specimens and adjacent normal tissues.[57]

EWING'S SARCOMA FAMILY OF TUMORS

Ewing's sarcoma is one of the first examples in which the application of molecular diagnostics led to improved tumor classification. Ewing's sarcoma was first described by James Ewing as a bone tumor characterized by small blue round cells and minimal mitotic activity.[58] Turc-Carel identified a recurring reciprocal t(11;22) chromosomal translocation in these tumors in 1983.[59] Investigators subsequently demonstrated a cytogenetically identical t(11;22) in adult neuroblastoma or peripheral primitive neuroectodermal tumor, so named because of its histologic similarity to neuroblastoma.[60] Based on the presence of the identical translocation, it was hypothesized that peripheral primitive neuroectodermal tumor was related to Ewing's sarcoma. This translocation breakpoint has been molecularly characterized as an in-frame fusion between a new Ewing's sarcoma gene, EWS, on chromosome 22 and an ETS transcription family member, FLI-1, on chromosome 22.[61–63]

In addition to this fusion transcript being identified in peripheral primitive neuroectodermal tumor, other variants, notably the chest wall Askin's tumor and soft tissue Ewing's sarcoma, previously treated as a RMS because of its location in soft tissue, were also shown to bear the identical fusion transcript. Several variant translocations have also been identified, invariably fusing the EWS gene to an ETS family member.[64,65] Greater than 90% of Ewing's sarcoma family of tumors carry the EWS-ETS fusion gene, and a search for EWS-ETS by either reverse transcriptase polymerase chain reaction or fluorescence *in situ* hybridization should be considered standard practice in the diagnostic evaluation of suspected Ewing's sarcoma family of tumors. The nature of the novel fusion transcription factor and its downstream targets are currently under intense investigation. Interestingly, it has been suggested that the specific fusion protein expressed in the Ewing's sarcoma family of tumors has prognostic significance.[66,67]

RHABDOMYOSARCOMA

The two major histologic subtypes of RMS, embryonal and alveolar, have both unique histologic appearance as well as distinctive molecular genetic abnormalities, while sharing a common myogenic lineage. Embryonal tumors make up two-thirds of all RMS and are histologically characterized by a stroma-rich, spindle-cell appearance. Alveolar tumors make up approximately one-third of RMS and are histologically characterized by densely packed small round cells often lining a septation reminiscent of a pulmonary alveolus, giving rise to its name. Both histologic subtypes express muscle-specific proteins including α-actin, myosin, desmin, and MyoD,[68–70] and they virtually always express high levels of IGF-2.[71,72]

At the molecular level, embryonal tumors are characterized by LOH at the 11p15 locus, which is of particular interest since this region harbors the IGF-2 gene.[73,74] The loss of heterozygosity (LOH) at 11p15 occurs by loss of maternal and duplication of paternal chromosomal material.[75] While LOH is normally associated with loss of tumor suppressor gene activity, in this instance LOH with paternal duplication may result in activation of IGF-2. This occurs because IGF-2 is now known to be normally imprinted (i.e., this gene is normally transcriptionally silent at the maternal allele, with only the paternal allele being transcriptionally active).[76,77] Thus, LOH with paternal duplication potentially leads to a twofold gene-dosage effect of the IGF-2 locus. Furthermore, in alveolar tumors where LOH does not occur, the normally imprinted maternal allele has been shown to be reexpressed.[78,79] Thus, LOH and loss of imprinting may in this case lead to the same functional result, namely, biallelic expression of the normally monoallelically expressed IGF-2. However, loss of an as yet unidentified tumor suppressor gene due to LOH also remains a possibility.

Alveolar RMS is characterized by a t(2;13)(q35;q14) chromosomal translocation.[80,81] Molecular cloning of this translocation has identified the generation of a fusion transcription factor, fusing the 5' DNA-binding region of PAX-3 on chromosome 2 to the 3' transactivation domain region of FKHR gene on chromosome 13.[82,83] A variant t(1;13)(q36;q14) has been identified in a small number of alveolar RMS tumors that fuses the 5' DNA-binding region of the PAX 7 gene on chromosome 1 with the identical 3' transactivation domain of the FKHR gene.[84] Fluorescence *in situ* hybridization or reverse transcriptase polymerase chain reaction can be used to identify these PAX-FKHR fusions in approximately 90% of tumors and are diagnostic of alveolar RMS. As noted previously, the fusion protein generated by the translocation leads to a novel transcription factor. The nature of this transcription factor and its downstream targets are the subject of active investigation. Of particular interest is the association of the PAX3-FKHR fusion with increased expression of c-met.[85,86] Met is the receptor tyrosine kinase for hepatocyte growth factor/scatter factor and is overexpressed in both embryonal and alveolar RMS.[87] It has also been suggested that, like the Ewing's sarcoma family of tumors, where the specific expressed fusion transcript has prognostic significance, the PAX3-FKHR and the PAX7-FKHR fusions lead to distinct clinicopathologic entities.[88]

Other frequently reported genetic alterations that may be common to both embryonal and alveolar RMS include activated forms of N-RAS and K-RAS,[89,90] inactivating p53 mutations,[91] as well as amplification and overexpression of MDM2, CDK4, and N-MTC.[92]

HEREDITARY SYNDROMES ASSOCIATED WITH TUMORS OF CHILDHOOD

LI-FRAUMENI SYNDROME

A few hereditary cancer syndromes are associated with the occurrence of both childhood and adult-onset neoplasms. The paradigm Li-Fraumeni familial cancer syndrome was originally described in 1969 from an epidemiologic evaluation of more than 600 medical and family history records of childhood sarcoma patients.[93,94] The original description of kindred with a spectrum of tumors that includes soft tissue sarcomas, osteosarcomas, breast cancer, brain tumors, leukemia, and adrenocortical carcinoma has been overwhelmingly substantiated by numerous subsequent studies,[95] although other cancers are also observed. Germline alterations of the *p53* tumor suppressor gene are associated with LFS.[96–98] These are primarily missense mutations that yield a stabilized mutant protein. The spectrum of mutations of p53 in the germline are indistinct from somatic mutations found in a wide variety of tumors. Carriers are heterozygous for the mutation, and in tumors derived from these individuals, the second (wild-type) allele is frequently deleted or mutated, leading to functional inactivation.[99–101] Only 60% to 80% of *classic* LFS families have detectable alterations of the gene. It is not yet determined whether the remainder are associated with the presence of modifier genes, promoter defects yielding abnormalities of p53 expression, or simply the result of weak genotype-phenotype correlations. Other candidate predisposition genes, such as p16, p15, p21, BRCA1, BRCA2, and PTEN, associated with multisite cancer associations have generally been ruled out as potential targets.

Germline p53 alterations have also been reported in some patients with cancer phenotypes that resemble the classic LFS phenotype. Between 3% and 10% of children with apparently sporadic RMS or osteosarcoma have been shown to carry germline p53 mutations.[102,103] These patients tend to be younger than those who harbor wild-type p53. It appears as well that more than 75% of children with apparently sporadic adrenocortical carcinoma carry germline p53 mutations, although in some of these cases, a family history develops that is not substantially distinct from LFS.[104,105] These observations suggest that germline p53 alterations may be associated with early-onset development of the childhood component tumors of the syndrome. It is not clear what clinical significance these findings have in that no studies of prognostic significance or potential impact on anticancer treatment modalities are reported. Nevertheless, in light of the critical role played by p53 in the initiation and potentiation of gamma irradiation or chemotherapy-induced DNA damage repair, studies into the effect of such germline mutations on the potentiation of tumor development related to therapeutic interventions would be important.

BECKWITH-WIEDEMANN SYNDROME

BWS occurs with a frequency of 1 in 13,700 births. More than 450 cases have been documented since the original reported associations of exomphalos, macroglossia, gigantism, and other congenital anomalies. With increasing age, phenotypic features of BWS become less pronounced. Laboratory findings may include, at birth, hypoglycemia (extremely common), polycythemia, hypocalcemia, hypertriglyceridemia, hypercholesterolemia, and high serum α-fetoprotein levels. Early diagnosis of the condition is crucial to avoid deleterious neurologic effects of neonatal hypoglycemia and to initiate an appropriate screening protocol for tumor development. The increased risk for tumor formation in BWS patients is estimated at 7.5% and is further increased to 10% if hemihyperplasia is present. Tumors occurring with the highest frequency include WT, hepatoblastoma, neuroblastoma, and adrenocortical carcinoma.[20,106]

The genetic basis of BWS is complex. Various 11p15 chromosomal or molecular alterations have been associated with the BWS phenotype and its tumors.[107] It is unlikely that a single gene is responsible for the BWS phenotype. Because it appears that abnormalities in the region affect imprinted domain, it is more likely that normal gene regulation in this part of chromosome 11p15 occurs in a regional manner and may depend on various interdependent factors or genes. Chromosomal abnormalities associated with BWS are extremely rare, with only 20 cases having been associated with 11p15 translocations or inversions. The chromosomal breakpoint in each of these cases is always found on the maternally derived chromosome 11.[108] This parent-of-origin dependence in BWS suggests that the chromosome translocations disrupt imprinting of a gene in the 11p15 region. On the other hand, BWS-associated 11p15 duplications (approximately 30 reported cases) are always paternally derived, and the duplication breakpoints are heterogeneous.[109] Paternal uniparental disomy, in which there are two alleles inherited from one parent (the father), has been reported in approximately 15% of sporadic BWS patients.[110] It is interesting that the insulin/IGF-2 region is always represented in the uniparental disomy, although the extent of chromosomal involvement is highly variable. Alterations in allele-specific DNA methylation of IGF-2 and H19 reflect this paternal imprinting phenomenon.[111] Although there are associated cytogenetic and molecular findings for some patients, no single diagnostic test exists for BWS. This observation is not unlike that described for LFS, or perhaps for other multisite cancer phenotypes, in which the clarity of the phenotype is often weak, making the genetic link cloudy and the likelihood of multiple pathways to tumor formation strong.

GORLIN SYNDROME

Nevoid basal cell carcinoma syndrome, or Gorlin syndrome, is a rare autosomal dominant disorder characterized by multiple basal cell carcinomas, developmental defects including bifid ribs and other spine and rib abnormalities, palmar and plantar pits, odontogenic keratocysts, as well as generalized overgrowth.[112] This syndrome appears to be caused by germline mutations of the tumor suppressor gene PTCH, a receptor for sonic hedgehog.[113,114] Approximately 5% of patients with Gorlin syndrome develop medulloblastoma. Furthermore, approximately 10% of patients diagnosed with medulloblastoma by the age of 2 years are found to have other phenotypic features consistent with Gorlin syndrome and also harbor germline PTCH mutations.[115] Of further note, mice with heterozygous PTC deletions develop RMS.[116] Although RMS is not associated with Gorlin syndrome, the mouse studies suggest a possible link between PTC signaling and RMS.[117]

MALIGNANT RHABDOID TUMORS

These unusual pediatric tumors occur as primary renal tumors, but have also been described in lung, liver, soft tissues, and the CNS, where it is often termed *atypical and teratoid rhabdoid tumor.*[118,119] Recurrent chromosomal translocations of chromosome 22 involving a breakpoint at 22q11.2, as well as complete or partial monosomy 22, have been observed, strongly suggesting the presence of a tumor suppressor gene in this area. The hSNF5/INI1 gene has been isolated and shown to be the target for biallelic, recurrent, inactivating mutations.[120] The encoded gene product is thought to be involved in chromatin remodeling. Studies have not only demonstrated the presence of inactivating mutations in the majority of malignant rhabdoid tumors (renal or extrarenal), but also in chronic myeloid leukemia,[121] as well as in a wide variety of other childhood and adult-onset malignancies.[122,123] An intriguing feature in some individuals with malignant rhabdoid tumors is the observation of germline mutations, suggesting that this family of tumors may occur as a result of a primary inherited defect in one allele of the INI1 gene.[124] Further studies of the function of this gene will be important in determining its role in tumorigenesis of this wide spectrum of neoplasms.

PREDICTIVE TESTING FOR GERMLINE MUTATIONS AND CHILDHOOD CANCERS

Several important issues have arisen as a result of the identification of germline mutations of tumor suppressor genes in cancer-prone individuals and families. These include ethical questions of predictive testing in such families and in unaffected relatives, and selection of patients to be tested, as well as the development of practical and accurate laboratory techniques, development of pilot testing programs, and the role of clinical intervention based on test results. This chapter was not meant to discuss these problems in detail, but one would be remiss to ignore their significance.

For several reasons, testing cannot as yet be offered to the general pediatric population, particularly in light of the demonstrably low carrier rate of the abnormal tumor suppressor genes and the general lack of standardized methods of preclinical screening of carriers. Exceptions to these limitations include screening of gene carriers in RB, BWS, multiple endocrine neoplasia, and multiple melanoma families. Whether predictive testing studies are initiated in high-risk families or surveys are carried out in cancer populations likely to harbor germline mutations in tumor suppressor genes, the investigations should be undertaken in a research setting involving expertise in oncology, psychiatry, psychology, genetics and genetic counseling, medical ethics, and molecular genetics. The development of screening programs should address aspects of cost, informed consent (particularly where it affects children), socioeconomic impact on the individual tested, consistency in providing results, and counseling.[125,126]

MOLECULAR THERAPEUTICS

With the identification of alterations in a variety of molecular signaling pathways, including activated growth factor signaling pathways (e.g., IGF-2) and altered tumor suppressor pathways (e.g., RB), it has become increasingly apparent that these alterations may potentially represent the Achilles heel for these tumors. New agents targeting the tyrosine kinase enzymes that transduce growth factor signals are at various stages of development in early clinical studies. Agents blocking the growth hormone IGF-1 pathway are currently being tested in clinical trials in osteosarcoma and breast cancer. Farnesyl transferase inhibitors, blockers of the RAS pathway, have been developed and are also currently in clinical testing. Of note, the activity of farnesyl transferase inhibitors against NF is under investigation, since activation of RAS signaling has been observed in NF-associated tumors (see previous discussion). As targets of mutant transcription factors generated are identified, it is hoped that they may represent additional targets for therapeutic intervention.

Finally, fusion proteins derived from tumor-specific translocations may themselves represent potential neoantigens that could be targeted by cytotoxic T cells. It is likely that the molecular characterization of pediatric tumors will lead to novel and perhaps more effective treatment approaches in the near future. It is likely that some of these innovative approaches will at least initially be integrated into standard therapeutic protocols.

REFERENCES

1. Knudson AG. Hereditary cancers disclose a class of cancer genes. *Cancer* 1988;63:1888.
2. Li FP. Cancer families: human models of susceptibility to neoplasia. *Cancer Res* 1988;48:5381.
3. Balaban G, Gilbert F, Nichols W, et al. Abnormalities of chromosome #13 in retinoblastoma from individuals with normal constitutional karyotypes. *Cancer Genet Cytogenet* 1982;6:213.
4. Benedict WF, Banerjee A, Mark C, et al. Nonrandom chromosomal changes in untreated retinoblastoma. *Cancer Genet Cytogenet* 1983;10:311.
5. Knudson AG. Mutation and cancer: statistical study of retinoblastoma. *Proc Natl Acad Sci U S A* 1971;68:820.
6. Comings DE. A general theory of carcinogenesis. *Proc Natl Acad Sci U S A* 1973:70:3324.
7. Devesa SS. The incidence of retinoblastoma. *Am J Opthalmol* 1975;80:263.
8. Francois J, Matton M-Th, De Bie S, et al. Genesis and genetics of retinoblastoma. *Ophthalmologica* 1975;170:405.
9. Knudson AG, Hethcote HW, Brown BW. Mutation and childhood cancer: a probabilistic model for the incidence of retinoblastoma. *Proc Natl Acad Sci U S A* 1975;72:5116.
10. Abramson DH, Ellsworth RM, Kitchin FD, et al. Second nonocular tumors in retinoblastoma survivors: are they radiation induced? *Ophthalmology* 1984;91:1351.
11. Smith LM, Donaldson SS, Egbert PR, et al. Aggressive management of second primary tumors in survivors of hereditary retinoblastoma. *Int J Radiat Oncol Biol Phys* 1989;17:499.
12. Cavenee WK, Dryga TP, Phillips RA, et al. Expression of recessive alleles by chromosomal mechanisms in retinoblastoma. *Nature* 1983;305:779.
13. Squire J, Dryja TP, Dunn J, et al. Cloning of the esterase D gene: a polymorphic gene probe closely linked to the retinoblastoma locus on chromosome 13. *Proc Natl Acad Sci U S A* 1986;83:6573.
14. Friend SH, Bernards R, Rogelj S, et al. A human DNA segment with properties of the gene that predisposes to retinoblastoma and osteosarcoma. *Nature* 1986;323:643.
15. Bookstein R, Shew J-Y, Chen P-L, et al. Suppression of tumorigenicity of human prostate carcinoma cells by replacing a mutated RB gene. *Science* 1990;247:643.
16. Gonzalez FF, Lopes MB, Garcia FJM, et al. Expression of developmentally defined retinal phenotypes in the histogenesis of retinoblastoma. *Am J Pathol* 1992;141:363.
17. Montgomery BT, Ketalis PP, Blute ML, et al. Extended follow-up of bilateral Wilms' tumor: results of the National Wilms Tumor Study. *J Urol* 1991;146:514.
18. Beckwith JB, Kiviat NB, Bonadio JF. Nephrogenic rests, nephroblastomatosis, and the pathogenesis of Wilms tumor. *Pediatr Pathol* 1990;10:1.

19. Mueller RF. The Denys-Drash syndrome. *J Med Genet* 1994;31:471.
20. Wiedemann HR. Tumors and hemihypertrophy associated with Wiedemann-Beckwith syndrome. *Eur J Pediatr* 1983;141:129.
21. Riccardi VM, Sujansky E, Smith AC, et al. Chromosomal imbalance in the aniridia-Wilms' tumor association: 11p interstitial deletion. *Pediatrics* 1978;61:604.
22. Ton CC, Hirvonen H, Miwa H, et al. Positional cloning and characterization of a paired box and homeobox-containing gene from the aniridia region. *Cell* 1991;67:1059.
23. Call KM, Glaser T, Ito CY, et al. Isolation and characterization of a zinc finger polypeptide gene at the human chromosome 11 Wilms' tumor locus. *Cell* 1990;60:509.
24. Gesler M, Poustka A, Cavenee W, et al. Homozygous deletion in Wilms tumors of a zinc-finger gene identified by chromosome jumping. *Nature* 1990;343:774.
25. Bonetta L, Kuehn S, Huang A, et al. Wilms tumor locus on 11p13 defined by multiple CpG island-associated transcripts. *Science* 1990;250:994.
26. Rauscher FJ III. The WT1 Wilms tumor gene product: a developmentally regulated transcription factor in the kidney functions as a tumor suppressor. *FASEB J* 1993;7:896.
27. Drash A, Sherman F, Hartmann WH, et al. A syndrome of pseudohermaphroditism, Wilms tumor, hypertension and degenerative renal disease. *J Pediatr* 1970;76:585.
28. Jadresic L, Leake J, Gordon I, et al. Clinicopathologic review of twelve children with nephropathy, Wilms tumor, and genital abnormalities (Drash syndrome). *J Pediatr* 1990;117:717.
29. Coppes M, Liefers GJ, Higuchi M, et al. Inherited WT1 mutations in Denys-Drash syndrome. *Cancer Res* 1992;52:6125.
30. Koufos A, Grundy P, Morgan K, et al. Familial Wiedemann-Beckwith syndrome and a second Wilms tumor locus both map to 11p15.5. *Am J Hum Genet* 1989;44:711.
31. Ping AJ, Reeve AE, Law DJ, et al. Genetic linkage of Beckwith-Wiedemann syndrome to 11p15. *Am J Hum Genet* 1989;44:720.
32. Maw MA, Grundy PE, Millow LJ, et al. A third Wilms tumor locus on chromosome 16q. *Cancer Res* 1992;52:3094.
33. Huff V, Reeve AE, Leppert M, et al. Nonlinkage of 16q markers to familial predisposition to Wilms tumor. *Cancer Res* 1992;52:6117.
34. Stumpf GR, Alkane JF, Annegers JF, et al. Neurofibromatosis. *Arch Neurol* 1987;45:575.
35. Riccardi VM, Eichner JE. *Neurofibromatosis: phenotype, natural history, and pathogenesis.* Baltimore, MD: Johns Hopkins, 1986.
36. Halliday AL, Sobel RA, Martuza RL. Benign spinal nerve sheath tumors: their occurrence sporadically and in neurofibromatosis types 1 and 2. *J Neurosurg* 1991;74:248.
37. Marchuk DA, Saulino AM, Tavakkol R, et al. cDNA cloning of the type 1 neurofibromatosis gene: complete sequence of the NF1 gene product. *Genomics* 1991;11:931.
38. DeClure JE, Cohen BD, Lowy DR. Identification and characterization of the neurofibromatosis type 1 protein product. *Proc Natl Acad Sci U S A* 1991;88:9914.
39. Viskochil D, Buchberg AM, Xu G, et al. Deletions and a translocation interrupt a cloned gene at the neurofibromatosis type 1 locus. *Cell* 1990;62:187.
40. Martuza RL, Eldridge R. Neurofibromatosis 2 (bilateral acoustic neurofibromatosis). *N Engl J Med* 1988;318:684.
41. Trofatter JA, MacCollin MM, Rutter JL, et al. A novel moesin-, ezrin-, radixin-like gene is a candidate for the neurofibromatosis 2 tumor suppressor. *Cell* 1993;73:791.
42. Rouleau GA, Merel P, Lutchman M, et al. Alteration in a new gene encoding a putative membrane-organizing protein causes neurofibromatosis type 2. *Nature* 1993;363:515.
43. Hara T, Bianchi AB, Seizinger BR, et al. Molecular cloning and characterization of alternatively spliced transcripts of the mouse neurofibromatosis 2 gene. *Cancer Res* 1994;54:330.
44. Brodeur G, Sekhon G, Goldstein M. Chromosomal aberrations in human neuroblastoma. *Cancer* 1977;40:2256.
45. Maris JM, White PS, Beltinger CP, et al. Significance of chromosome 1p loss of heterozygosity in neuroblastoma. *Cancer Res* 1995;55:4664.
46. Caron H, van Sluis P, de Kraker J, et al. Allelic loss of chromosome 1p is a predictor of unfavorable outcome in patients with neuroblastoma. *N Engl J Med* 1996;334:225.
47. Biedler J, Ross R, Sharske S, et al. Human neuroblasotma cytogenetics: search for significance of homogeneously staining regions in double minute chromosomes. In: Evans A, ed. *Advances in neuroblastoma research.* New York: Raven Press, 1980:81.
48. Biedler JL, Spengler BA. A novel chromosome abnormality on human neuroblastoma and anti-folate resistant Chinese hamster cell lines in culture. *J Natl Cancer Inst* 1976;57:683.
49. Schwab M, Alitalo K, Lempnauer K, et al. Amplified DNA with limited homology to myc cellular oncogene is shared by human neuroblasotoma cell lines and a neuroblastoma tumor. *Nature* 1983;305:245.
50. Thiele CJ, Reynolds PC, Israel MA. Decreased expression of N-myc precedes retinoic acid induced phenotypic differentiation of human neuroblastoma. *Nature* 1985;313:404.
51. Matthay KK, Villablanca JG, Seeger RC, et al. Treatment of high-risk neuroblastoma with intensive chemotherapy, radiotherapy, autologous bone marrow transplantation, and 13-cis-retinoic acid. *N Engl J Med* 1999;341:1165.
52. Schwab M, Ellison J, Busch M, et al. Enhanced expression of the human N-myc gene consequent to amplification of DNA may contribute to malignant progression of neuroblastoma. *Proc Natl Acad Sci U S A* 1984;81:4940.
53. Nakagawara A, Arima-Nakagawara M, Scavarda NJ, et al. Association between high levels of expression of the TRK gene and favorable outcome in human neuroblastoma. *N Engl J Med* 1993;328:847.
54. Norris MD, Bordow SB, Marshall GM, et al. Expression of the gene for multidrug-resistance-associated protein and outcome in patients with neuroblastoma. *N Engl J Med* 1996;334:231.
55. Bown N, Cotterill S, Lastowska M, et al. Gain of chromosome arm 17q and adverse outcome in patients with neuroblastoma. *N Engl J Med* 1999;340:1954.
56. El-Badry OM, Romanous JA, Helman LJ, et al. Autonomous growth of a human neuroblastoma cell line is mediated by insulin-like growth factor II. *J Clin Invest* 1989;84:829.
57. El-Badry OM, Israel MA. Growth regulation of human neuroblastoma. *Cancer Treat Res* 1992;63:105.
58. Ewing J. Diffuse endothelioma of bone. *Proc NY Pathol Soc* 1921;21:17.
59. Turc-Carel C, Philip I, Berger M, et al. [Chromosomal translocation (11;22) in cell lines of Ewing's sarcoma]. *C R Seances Acad Sci III* 1983;296:1101 [French].
60. Whang-Pheng J, Triche T, Knutesen T, et al. Chromosome translocation in peripheral neuroepithelioma. *N Engl J Med* 1984;311:584.
61. Delattre O, Zucman J, Ploustagel B, et al. Gene fusion with an ETS DNA-binding domain caused by chromosome translocation in human tumours. *Nature* 1992;359:162.
62. Zucman J, Delattre O, Desmaze C, et al. Cloning and characterization of the Ewing's sarcoma and peripheral neuroepithelioma t(11;22) translocation breakpoints. *Genes Chromosome Cancer* 1992;5:271.
63. May WA, Gishizky ML, Lessnick SL, et al. Ewing sarcoma 11;22 translocation produces a chimeric transcription factor that requires the DNA-binding domain encoded by FLI1 for transformation. *Proc Natl Acad Sci U S A* 1993;90:5752.
64. Desmaze C, Brizard F, Turc-Carel C, et al. Multiple chromosomal mechanisms generate an EWS/FLI1 or an EWS/ERG fusion gene in Ewing tumors. *Cancer Genet Cytogenet* 1997;97:12.
65. Jeon IS, Davis JN, Braun BS, et al. A variant Ewing's sarcoma translocation (7;22) fuses the EWS gene to the ETS gene ETV1. *Oncogene* 1995;10:1229.
66. Zoubek A, Dockhorn-Dworniczak B, Delattre O, et al. Does expression of different EWS chimeric transcripts define clinically distinct risk groups of Ewing tumor patients? *J Clin Oncol* 1996;14:1245.
67. de Alava E, Kawai A, Healey JH, et al. EWS-FLI1 fusion transcript structure is an independent determinant of prognosis in Ewing's sarcoma. *J Clin Oncol* 1998;16:1248.
68. Parham DM, Webber B, Holt H, et al. Immunohistochemical study of childhood rhabdomyosarcomas and related neoplasms. Results of an Intergroup Rhabdomyosarcoma study project. *Cancer* 1991;67:3072.
69. Dodd S, Malone M, McCulloch W. Rhabdomyosarcoma in children: a histological and immunohistochemical study of 59 cases. *J Pathol* 1989;158:13.
70. Dias P, Parham DM, Shapiro DN, et al. Myogenic regulatory protein (MyoD1) expression in childhood solid tumors: diagnostic utility in rhabdomyosarcoma. *Am J Pathol* 1990;137:1283.
71. El-Badry OM, Minniti C, Kohn EC, et al. Insulin-like growth factor II acts as an autocrine growth and motility factor in human rhabdomyosarcoma tumors. *Cell Growth Diff* 1990;1:325.
72. Minniti CP, Tsokos M, Newton WA, et al. Specific expression of insulin-like growth factor-II in rhabdomyosarcoma tumor cells. *Am J Pathol* 1994;101:198.
73. Scrable H, Witte D, Lampkin B, et al. Chromosomal localization of the human rhabdomyosarcoma locus by mitotic recombination mapping. *Nature* 1987;329:645.
74. Scrable H, Witte D, Shimada H, et al. Molecular differential pathology of rhabdomyosarcoma. *Genes Chromosome Cancer* 1989;1:23.
75. Scrable H, Cavenee W, Ghavimi F, et al. A model for embryonal rhabdomyosarcoma tumorigenesis that involves genome imprinting. *Proc Natl Acad Sci U S A* 1989;86:7480.
76. Rainier S, Johnson LA, Dobry CJ, et al. Relaxation of imprinted genes in human cancer. *Nature* 1993;362:747.
77. Ogawa O, Eccles MR, Szeto J, et al. Relaxation of insulin-like growth factor II gene imprinting implicated in Wilms' tumour. *Nature* 1993;362:749.
78. Zhan S, Shapiro DN, Helman LJ. Activation of an imprinted allele of the insulin-like growth factor II gene implicated in rhabdomyosarcoma. *J Clin Invest* 1994;94:445.
79. Zhan S, Shapiro D, Zhang L, et al. Concordant loss of imprinting of the human insulin-like growth factor II gene promoters in cancer. *J Biol Chem* 1995;270:27983.
80. Turc-Carel C, Lizard-Nacol S, Justrabo E, et al. Consistent chromosomal translocation in alveolar rhabdomyosarcoma. *Cancer Genet Cytogenet* 1986;19:361.
81. Douglass EC, Valentine M, Ectubanas E, et al. A specific chromosomal abnormality in rhabdomyosarcoma. *Cytogenet Cell Genet* 1987;45:148.
82. Barr FG, Galili N, Holick J, et al. Rearrangement of the PAX3 paired box gene in the paediatric solid tumour alveolar rhabdomyosarcoma. *Nat Genet* 1993;3:113.
83. Shapiro DN, Sublett JE, Li B, et al. Fusion of PAX3 to a member of the forkhead family of transcription factors in human alveolar rhabdomyosarcoma. *Cancer Res* 1993;53:5108.
84. Davis RJ, D'Cruz CM, Lovell MA, et al. Fusion of PAX7 to FKHR by the variant t(1;13)(p36;q14) translocation in alveolar rhabdomyosarcoma. *Cancer Res* 1994;54:2869.
85. Epstein J, Shapiro D, Cheng J, et al. Pax3 modulates expression of the c-Met receptor during limb muscle development. *Proc Natl Acad Sci U S A* 1996;93:4213.
86. Ginsberg JP, Davis RJ, Bennicelli JL, et al. Up-regulation of MET but not neural cell adhesion molecule expression by the PAX3-FKHR fusion protein in alveolar rhabdomyosarcoma. *Cancer Res* 1998;58:3542.
87. Ferracini R, Olivero M, Di Renzo MF, et al. Retrogenic expression of the MET proto-oncogene correlates with the invasive phenotype of human rhabdomyosarcomas. *Oncogene* 1996;12:1697.
88. Kelly KM, Womer RB, Sorensen PH, et al. Common and variant gene fusions predict distinct clinical phenotypes in rhabdomyosarcoma. *J Clin Oncol* 1997;15:1831.
89. Chardin P, Yeramian P, Madaule P, et al. N-ras gene activation in the RD human rhabdomyosarcoma cell line. *Int J Cancer* 1985;35:647.
90. Stratton MR, Fisher C, Gusterson BA, et al. Detection of point mutations in N-ras and K-ras genes of human embryonal rhabdomyosarcomas using oligonucleotide probes and the polymerase chain reaction. *Cancer Res* 1989;49:6324.
91. Felix CA, Kappel CC, Mitsudomi T, et al. Frequency and diversity of p53 mutations in childhood rhabdomyosarcoma. *Cancer Res* 1992;52:2243.
92. Merlino G, Helman LJ. Rhabdomyosarcoma—working out the pathways. *Oncogene* 1999;18:5340.
93. Li FP, Fraumeni JF. Rhabdomyosarcoma in children: epidemiologic study and identification of a familial cancer syndrome. *J Natl Cancer Inst* 1969;43:1365.

94. Li FP, Fraumeni JF. Prospective study of a family cancer syndrome. *JAMA* 1982;247:2692.
95. Li FP, Fraumeni JF, Mulvihill JJ, et al. A cancer family syndrome in 24 kindreds. *Cancer Res* 1988;48:5358.
96. Malkin D, Li FP, Strong LC, et al. Germline p53 mutations in a familial syndrome of breast cancer, sarcomas, and other neoplasms. *Science* 1990;250:1233.
97. Srivastava S, Zou Z, Pirollo K, et al. Germline transmission of a mutated p53 gene in a cancer-prone family with Li-Fraumeni syndrome. *Nature* 1990;348:747.
98. Malkin D. Li-Fraumeni syndrome. In: Vogelstein B, Kinzler KW, eds. *The genetic basis of human cancer.* 1st ed. New York: McGraw-Hill, 1998:393.
99. Sedlacek Z, Kodet R, Seemanova E, et al. Two Li-Fraumeni syndrome families with novel germline p53 mutations: loss of the wild-type allele in only 50% of tumors. *Br J Cancer* 1998;77:1034.
100. Varley JM, Thorncroft M, McGown G, et al. A detailed study of loss of heterozygosity on chromosome 17 in tumours from Li-Fraumeni patients carrying a mutation of the TP53 gene. *Oncogene* 1997;14:65.
101. Frebourg T, Kassel J, Lam KT, et al. Germline mutations of the p53 tumor suppressor gene in patients with high risk for cancer inactivate the protein. *Proc Natl Acad Sci U S A* 1992;89:6413.
102. Diller L, Sexsmith E, Gottlieb A, et al. Germline p53 mutations are frequently detected in young children with rhabdomyosarcoma. *J Clin Invest* 1994;95:1606.
103. McIntyre JF, Smith-Sorensen B, Friend SH, et al. Germline mutations of the p53 tumor suppressor gene in children with osteosarcoma. *J Clin Oncol* 1994;12:925.
104. Wagner J, Portwine C, Rabin K, et al. High frequency of germline p53 mutations in childhood adrenocortical cancer. *J Natl Cancer Inst* 1994;86:1707.
105. Varley JM, McGown G, Thorncroft M, et al. Are there low-penetrance TP53 alleles? Evidence from childhood adrenocortical tumors. *Am J Hum Genet* 1999;65:995.
106. Clericuzio CL, Johnson C. Screening for Wilms tumor in high-risk individuals. *Hematol Oncol Clin North Am* 1995;9:1255.
107. Weksberg R, Teshima I, Williams B, et al. Molecular characterization of cytogenetic alterations associated with the Beckwith-Wiedemann syndrome phenotype refines the localization and suggests the gene for BWS is imprinted. *Hum Mol Genet* 1993;2:549.
108. Mannens M, Hoovers JMN, Redeker E, et al. Parental imprinting of human chromosome region 11p15.2-pter involved in the Beckwith-Wiedemann syndrome and various human neoplasia. *Eur J Hum Genet* 1994;2:3.
109. Henry I, Jeanpierre M, Barichard F, et al. Duplication of HRAS1, INS and IGF2 is not a common event in Beckwith-Wiedemann syndrome. *Annal Genetique* 1988;31:216.
110. Henry I, Bonaiti-Pellie C, Chehensse V, et al. Uniparental paternal disomy in a genetics cancer-predisposing syndrome. *Nature* 1991;351:665.
111. Reik W, Brown KW, Schneid H, et al. Imprinting mutations in the Beckwith-Wiedemann syndrome suggested by an altered imprinting pattern in the IGF2-H19 domain. *Hum Mol Genet* 1995;265:464.
112. Gorlin RJ. Nevoid basal-cell carcinoma syndrome. *Medicine (Baltimore)* 1987;66:98.
113. Gailani MR, Stahle-Backdahl M, Leffell DJ, et al. The role of the human homologue of *Drosophila* patched in sporadic basal cell carcinomas. *Nat Genet* 1996;14:78.
114. Hahn H, Wicking C, Zaphiropoulous PG, et al. Mutations of the human homolog of *Drosophila* patched in the nevoid basal cell carcinoma syndrome. *Cell* 1996;85:841.
115. Cowan R, Hoban P, Kelsey A, et al. The gene for the naevoid basal cell carcinoma syndrome acts as a tumour-suppressor gene in medulloblastoma. *Br J Cancer* 1997;76:141.
116. Hahn H, Wojnowski L, Zimmer AM, et al. Rhabdomyosarcomas and radiation hypersensitivity in a mouse model of Gorlin syndrome. *Nat Med* 1998;4:619.
117. Zhan S, Helman LJ. Glimpsing the cause of rhabdomyosarcoma. *Nat Med* 1998;4:559.
118. Parham DM, Weeks DA, Beckwith JB. The clinicopathologic spectrum of putative extrarenal rhabdoid tumors. *Am J Surg Pathol* 1994;18:1010.
119. Rorke LB, Packer R, Biegel J. Central nervous system atypical teratoid/rhabdoid tumors of infancy and childhood: definition of an entity. *J Neurosurg* 1996;85:56.
120. Versteege I, Sevenet N, Lange J, et al. Truncating mutations of hSNF5/INI1 in aggressive pediatric cancer. *Nature* 1998;394:203.
121. Grand F, Kulkarni S, Chase A, et al. Frequent deletion of hSNF5/INI1, a component of the SWI/SNF complex, in chronic myeloid leukemia. *Cancer Res* 1999;59:3870.
122. Sevenet N, Sheridan E, Amram D, et al. Constitutional mutations of the hSNF5/INI1 gene predispose to a variety of cancers. *Am J Hum Genet* 1999;65:1342.
123. Sevenet N, Lellouch-Tubiana A, Schofield D, et al. Spectrum of hSNF5/INI1 somatic mutations in human cancer and genotype-phenotype correlations. *Hum Mol Genet* 1999;8:2359.
124. Biegel JA, Zhou JY, Rorke LB, et al. Germ-line and acquired mutations in INI1 in atypical teratoid and rhabdoid tumors. *Cancer Res* 1999;59:74.
125. Knoppers BM, Chadwick R. The Human Genome Project: under and international ethical microscope. *Science* 1995;265:464.
126. Malkin D, Knoppers BM. Genetic predisposition to cancer: issues to consider. *Semin Cancer Biol* 1996;7:49.

SECTION **2**

DAVID H. EBB
DANIEL M. GREEN
ROBERT C. SHAMBERGER
NANCY J. TARBELL

Solid Tumors of Childhood

Malignant solid tumors account for 30% of all cases of childhood cancer. Collaborative, multimodality treatment efforts undertaken in the context of pediatric cooperative group clinical trials have produced a remarkable improvement in survival since the 1970s. In addition to improvements in survival and functional outcome, the cooperative group studies have also facilitated a rapid growth in our understanding of cancer genetics and tumor biology. Prospective studies are currently underway to validate new risk group stratification schemes that integrate classical tumor staging information with prognostically significant features of tumor biology detectable with molecular diagnostics. We review the epidemiology, pathology, clinical presentation, evaluation, treatment, and prognosis of the common malignant solid tumors of children and adolescents.

EPIDEMIOLOGY

Approximately 12,400 children and adolescents younger than 20 years of age were diagnosed with cancer in 1998.[1] Malignant neoplasms are a major cause of mortality in children between 1 and 14 years of age. In 1998, the most recent year for which statistics are available, accidents, congenital anomalies, and homicide were responsible for more deaths in the age group 1 to 4 years, whereas only accidents were a more frequent cause of death in the age group 5 to 14 years.[2]

The most common malignant neoplasms diagnosed in pediatric patients are acute leukemia, non-Hodgkin's lymphoma, Hodgkin's disease, and primary tumors of the central nervous system. The most common malignant solid tumors are neuroblastoma, Wilms' tumor, rhabdomyosarcoma (RMS), and retinoblastoma[1] (Table 44.2-1).

Insights into the etiology of malignant solid tumors of childhood have been suggested by well-designed case-control studies[3-13] (Table 44.2-2).

Some childhood solid tumors occur in association with well-recognized single gene defects. Examples of these include the association of Wilms' tumor with Denys-Drash syndrome [Wilms' tumor suppressor gene (WT1) mutation],[13] bilateral retinoblastoma [retinoblastoma tumor suppressor gene (RB1) mutation],[14] hepatoblastoma and adenomatous polyposis coli (APC gene mutation),[15] RMS or malignant peripheral nerve sheath tumor and neurofibromatosis type 1 (NF1 gene mutation),[16] RMS and Li-Fraumeni syndrome (p53 gene mutation).[17,18]

The etiology of most childhood tumors is unknown. Knudson proposed the two-event model to explain the pattern of retinoblastoma, in which approximately 10% of patients with sporadic unilateral tumors and all patients with bilateral tumors carry a germline mutation of RB1.[19] This mutation could be either a new germinal mutation transmitted from the father[20] or a mutation transmitted from a carrier or affected parent.[21] The interstitial deletion occurs preferentially in the paternally derived allele of RB1,[22] as is the case for new germinal mutations of WT1,[23]

TABLE 44.2-1. Annual Incidence Rates and Percentage Distribution of Malignant Diseases in U.S. Children

	Incidence[a]	
Disease	White	African American
Acute lymphoblastic leukemia	32.9 (23.6%)	16.9 (15.6%)
Astrocytoma	17.9 (12.8%)	14.3 (13.2%)
Neuroblastoma	10.2 (7.3%)	7.8 (7.2%)
Non-Hodgkin's lymphoma	9.1 (6.5%)	5.4 (5.0%)
Wilms' tumor	8.3 (5.9%)	9.4 (8.7%)
Hodgkin's disease	7.3 (5.2%)	4.7 (4.3%)
Primitive neuroectodermal	6.8 (4.9%)	5.9 (5.4%)
Acute myeloid leukemia	5.8 (4.2%)	4.8 (4.4%)
Rhabdomyosarcoma	4.7 (3.4%)	4.1 (3.8%)
Retinoblastoma	3.9 (2.8%)	4.5 (4.1%)
Osteosarcoma	3.4 (2.4%)	3.9 (3.6%)
Ewing's sarcoma	3.3 (2.4%)	0.3 (0.3%)
All histologic types	139.5 (100.0%)	108.3 (100.0%)

[a]Per million children younger than 15 years of age.

resulting in the loss of function of one of the alleles of the RB1 or WT1 gene. A tumor arises only if a second event occurs, resulting in the loss of function of the remaining normal allele. This loss occurs via one of several mechanisms (Fig. 44.2-1), recognized by loss of heterozygosity for markers of specific chromosomal regions, all of which result in complete absence of the normal gene product.[21] This mechanism has been demonstrated in tumor tissue derived from embryonal RMS, hepatoblastoma, retinoblastoma, and Wilms' tumor.[24]

The genetics of some childhood solid tumors may be more complex. Analysis of the epidemiologic and clinicopathologic features suggest, for example, some cases of bilateral and multicentric Wilms' tumor may arise from somatic mosaicism rather than germline mutation.[25,26]

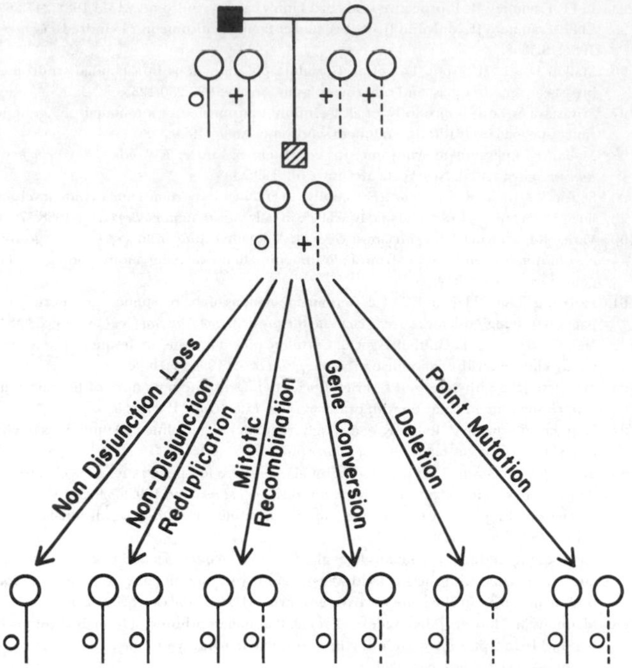

FIGURE 44.2-1. Loss of heterozygosity may occur by a variety of mechanisms. (From Cavenee WK, Dryja TP, Phillips RA, et al. Expression of recessive alleles by chromosomal mechanisms in retinoblastoma. *Nature* 1983;305:779, with permission.)

MANAGEMENT OF CHILDHOOD CANCER

Childhood malignant solid tumors are unique due to their responsiveness to many chemotherapeutic agents. Effective combination chemotherapy regimens have been identified and evaluated through cooperative group multiinstitutional trials. The cooperative groups' membership includes multidisciplinary treatment teams consisting of pediatric oncologists, radiologists, surgeons, and surgical subspecialists, as well as pediatric pathologists, pediatric radiation oncologists, and allied pediatric health professionals. The dramatic improvements in survival of pediatric patients with cancer are the result of treatment by such teams with experience in the evaluation, staging, surgical management, radiation treatment, and administration of intensive chemotherapy regimens to these children.

Surgery plays two roles in the management of solid tumors. The first role is establishing a histologic diagnosis and staging the tumor; the second is resection of the primary site of disease. It is increasingly important that the surgeon work in a collaborative fashion with the pediatric oncologist and radiation oncologist, since resection may be best accomplished after initial chemotherapy and radiotherapy. These initial treatments may decrease both

TABLE 44.2-2. Risk of Solid Tumors Following Parental Preconception Exposures

	Maternal		*Paternal*	
Histology	Exposure	Relative Risk	Exposure	Relative Risk
Wilms' tumor	Hair coloring product	3.6	Machinists, welders	5.3
Neuroblastoma	Diuretics, high blood pressure	4.1		
	Tranquilizer, analgesia	3.2		
	Alcohol (daily)	12.0		
Retinoblastoma	Morning sickness medication	2.8		
Hepatoblastoma	Metals	7.0	Metals	3.0
	Petroleum products	3.7		
	Paints or pigments	3.7		
Rhabdomyosarcoma	Marijuana use	3.0	Marijuana use	2.0
	Cocaine use	5.1	Cocaine use	2.1

the potential risks of resection and the long-term morbidity. Similarly, it is critical that the surgeon be involved from the outset in the care of a child presenting with a solid tumor since an inappropriately performed biopsy of the tumor may complicate later resection efforts. Questions regarding timing and feasibility of resection should only be considered by surgeons who are facile in reconciling the sometimes competing demands of durable local control and optimal functional outcome in a growing child. In light of the exquisite radiosensitivity of most pediatric solid tumors, all deliberations concerning timing and extent of resection efforts must recognize the importance of radiotherapy as an effective adjunct in efforts to secure local control.

Advances in anesthetic management of infants and children have contributed greatly to the surgical resection of solid tumors. Procedures that were performed in the past with a significant mortality, such as hepatectomy and extensive retroperitoneal resections, are now accomplished on a routine basis with limited risk. The duration of a procedure with modern anesthetic techniques is also rarely a consideration. Although the length of anesthesia was once a major determinant of operative morbidity and mortality, duration of a procedure is now rarely an issue.

Significant advances have also been achieved in postoperative pain management. Epidural catheters and continuous intravenous infusions of narcotics by mechanical pumps have greatly limited the severity of pain following extensive resections. Improvements in pain management have permitted more rapid mobilization of postoperative patients, with a corresponding decrease in the risk of pneumonia.

These advances in surgical management have been complemented by substantial improvements in radiation planning and delivery. Conformal radiotherapy using three-dimensional treatment planning to spare normal tissues has had a salutary effect on functional outcome. Advances in our knowledge of radiation dosing and planning techniques are discussed separately under each specific tumor type.

WILMS' TUMOR

Wilms' tumor is the most common primary malignant renal tumor of childhood. The striking success of national cooperative studies in improving survival and decreasing treatment-related morbidity mark this disease as the paradigm for multimodal treatment of a pediatric malignant solid tumor.

EPIDEMIOLOGY AND GENETICS

The incidence rate of Wilms' tumor is 7.9 cases per 1 million in white children younger than 15 years of age.[1] The incidence rate is approximately three times higher for African Americans in the United States and blacks in Africa than for East Asians, with rates for white populations in Europe and North America between these extremes.[27]

Wilms' tumor in the United States is slightly less frequent in boys than in girls. The tumor presents at an earlier age among boys, with the mean age at diagnosis for those with unilateral tumors being 41.5 months compared with 46.9 months among girls. The mean age at diagnosis for those who present with bilateral tumors is 29.5 months for boys and 32.6 months for girls.[28]

Children with Wilms' tumor may have associated anomalies, including aniridia, hemihypertrophy (as an isolated abnormality, or as a component of the Beckwith-Wiedemann syndrome), cryptorchidism, and hypospadias.[29–31] Children with pseudohermaphroditism and renal disease (glomerulonephritis or nephrotic syndrome) who develop Wilms' tumor may have the Denys-Drash syndrome,[32,33] which is associated with mutations within the same gene implicated in the Wilms' tumor, aniridia, genitourinary malformations, mental retardation (WAGR) syndrome.[34]

Wilms' tumor has become an important model for the study of fundamental mechanisms of tumorigenesis. The etiology of Wilms' tumor was thought to follow the two-event model proposed by Knudson to explain the pattern of retinoblastoma. Case reports of the familial occurrence of Wilms' tumor, however, remain uncommon. Approximately 1.5% of National Wilms' Tumor Study Group (NWTSG) cases have one or more family members with the disease.[26,35] In the absence of a history of parental consanguinity in such families, the mode of inheritance is generally thought to be autosomal dominant, with variable penetrance and expressivity. The rate of synchronous and metachronous bilaterality among NWTSG familial cases is significantly higher than for the NWTSG population as a whole. In addition, the mean age at diagnosis for familial unilateral or familial bilateral cases is significantly lower than the corresponding group of sporadic cases.[35]

Predicting the outcome in multicentric disease is likely to be more complex than previously imagined because of the emerging evidence for genetic heterogeneity. Mechanisms other than an inherited mutation may account for at least some of the bilateral and multicentric cases. Analysis of the epidemiologic and clinicopathologic features of Wilms' tumor patients led NWTSG investigators to suggest that some bilateral and multicentric tumors may arise from somatic mosaicism rather than germline mutation.[25,26] They also suggested that the disease comprises at least two pathogenetic entities that are identifiable on the basis of distinct precursor lesions.[36]

PATHOLOGY

Wilms' tumor is characterized by tremendous histologic diversity and is thought to be composed of, or derived from, primitive metanephric blastema. Most Wilms' tumors are unicentric lesions, although a substantial number arise multifocally in the kidney. Among 1905 NWTSG cases, approximately 5% involved both kidneys either at initial presentation or subsequent to diagnosis. An additional 7% of reported cases were multicentric unilateral tumors.[26] There is no predilection or either side. The tumor may arise anywhere within the kidney, which is usually markedly distorted by the neoplasm.

The most distinctive microscopic feature of Wilms' tumor is its structural diversity. The classic nephroblastoma is made up of varying proportions of three cell types (i.e., blastemal, stromal, and epithelial), but they are not all present in every case.[37] Anaplasia is marked by the presence of gigantic polyploid nuclei within the tumor sample. The new definition of focal anaplasia emphasizes distribution, requiring that cells with anaplastic nuclear changes be confined to sharply restricted foci within the primary tumor. By definition, focally anaplastic disease must not be identifiable in any site outside the renal parenchyma.[38]

Clear cell sarcoma of the kidney is an important primary renal tumor associated with a significantly higher rate of relapse and death than favorable histology Wilms' tumor.[39,40] Clear cell sarcoma of the kidney has a wider distribution of metastases than favorable histology Wilms' tumor. Most clear cell sarcomas of the kidney specimens have a distinct histologic appearance, although a number of variant patterns, such as epithelioid, spindling, myxoid, and cystic patterns, invite confusion with Wilms' tumor or other tumor types.[41,42]

Rhabdoid tumor of the kidney was identified for the first time in 1978 by NWTSG pathologists.[39] The neoplasm, previously confused with Wilms' tumor, is a monomorphous tumor like clear cell sarcoma of the kidney. The cell of origin for this distinctive tumor remains unknown.[43] Rhabdoid tumor of the kidney tends to metastasize to the lung and brain. Several studies have reported that separate primary neuroectodermal tumors of the brain have apparently developed in children with this neoplasm.[44] Primary rhabdoid tumors of the kidney and brain (atypical teratoid/rhabdoid tumors) share deletions of chromosome band 22q11.2.[45] This deleted locus appears to be the site of INI1, a putative tumor suppressor gene.[46,47]

The existence of precursor lesions to Wilms' tumor has been recognized for many years.[48,49] They take the form of small, usually microscopic clusters of blastemal cells, tubules, or stromal cells that are generally situated at the periphery of the renal lobe. The lesion that occurs within the deeper cortex of medulla has been termed an *intralobar nephrogenic rest* in contrast with the more commonly encountered *perilobar nephrogenic rest.* One or both of these variants are encountered in the renal parenchyma of approximately 30% of Wilms' tumor cases.[36] These nephrogenic rests are present in approximately 1% of random perinatal postmortem examinations.[49]

Congenital mesoblastic nephroma is important to recognize since it is usually curable by nephrectomy alone.[50] These tumors are typically identified in the first months of life, with a median age at diagnosis of 2 months.

CLINICAL PRESENTATION AND NATURAL HISTORY

Most children with Wilms' tumor come to medical attention because of abdominal swelling or the presence of an abdominal mass. This feature is usually noticed by a parent while bathing or dressing the child. Abdominal pain, gross hematuria, and fever may be present at diagnosis. Hypertension, present in approximately 25% of cases, has been attributed to an increase in renin activity.[51]

During the physical examination, it is important to note the location and size of the abdominal mass and its movement with respiration. A varicocele secondary to obstruction of the spermatic vein may be associated with the presence of a tumor thrombus in the renal vein or inferior vena cava. It is also important to note specifically any signs of the Wilms' tumor-associated syndromes marked by the presence of aniridia, partial or complete hemihypertrophy, and genitourinary abnormalities, such as hypospadias and cryptorchidism.

STAGING

The staging system currently employed by the NWTSG is shown in Table 44.2-3.

TABLE 44.2-3. National Wilms' Tumor Study Group Staging System for Renal Tumors

Stage	*Description*
I	The tumor was limited to the kidney and was completely excised. The renal capsule has an intact outer surface. The tumor was not ruptured or biopsied before removal (fine-needle aspiration biopsies are excluded from this restriction). The vessels of the renal sinus are not involved. There is no evidence of tumor at or beyond the margins of resection.
II	The tumor extended beyond the kidney, but was completely excised. There may be regional extension of tumor (i.e., penetration of the renal capsule or extensive invasion of the renal sinus). The blood vessels outside the renal parenchyma, including those of the renal sinus, may contain tumor. The tumor was biopsied (except for fine-needle aspiration), or there was spillage of tumor before or during surgery that is confined to the flank and does not involve the peritoneal surface. There must be no evidence of tumor at or beyond the margins of resection.
III	Residual nonhematogenous tumor is present and confined to the abdomen. Any one of the following may occur:
	1. Lymph nodes within the abdomen or pelvis are found to be involved by tumor (renal hilar, paraaortic, or beyond). (Lymph node involvement in the thorax or other extraabdominal sites would be a criterion for stage IV.)
	2. The tumor has penetrated through the peritoneal surface.
	3. Tumor implants are found on the peritoneal surface.
	4. Gross or microscopic tumor remains postoperatively (e.g., tumor cells are found at the margin of surgical resection on microscopic examination).
	5. The tumor is not completely resectable because of local infiltration into vital structures.
	6. Tumor spill not confined to the flank occurred either before or during surgery.
IV	Hematogenous metastases (lung, liver, bone, brain, and so forth) or lymph node metastases outside the abdominopelvic region are present.
V	Bilateral renal involvement is present at diagnosis. An attempt should be made to stage each side according to the previously mentioned criteria on the basis of the extent of disease before biopsy or treatment.

EVALUATION

Laboratory evaluation should include a complete blood cell count, differential white blood cell count, platelet count, liver function tests, renal function tests, serum calcium, and urinalysis. Elevation of the serum calcium may occur in children with rhabdoid tumor of the kidney or congenital mesoblastic nephroma.[52]

DIAGNOSTIC IMAGING

Imaging studies initially should be restricted to those necessary to establish the presence of an intrarenal space-occupying lesion. These studies should also be directed at identifying the presence of a contralateral kidney, which must be assessed for possible tumor involvement. In addition, imaging of the affected kidney must look for evidence of tumor thrombus in the renal vein and measure its proximal extent.

The initial radiographic study often selected is an abdominal ultrasound examination. This demonstrates whether the abdominal mass is solid or cystic and may allow identification of the mass's organ of origin and measurement of the maxi-

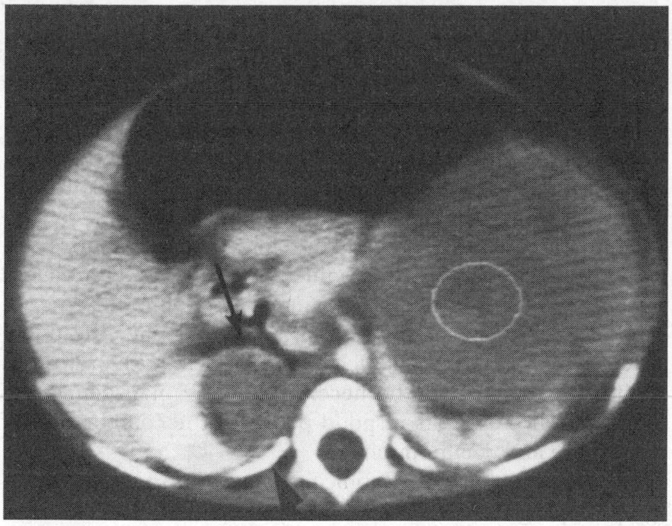

FIGURE 44.2-2. Computed tomography scan of abdomen demonstrating bilateral renal tumors (*arrows*).

mum diameter of the mass. Contrast-enhanced computed tomography (CT) of the abdomen, performed to further evaluate the nature and extent of the mass, may suggest apparent extension of the tumor into adjacent structures such as the liver, spleen, and colon (Fig. 44.2-2). However, most children believed to have invasion of the liver on CT are found to have hepatic compression at the time of surgery, rather than hepatic invasion.[53] The examination also may demonstrate small lesions that may be nephrogenic rests or Wilms' tumor in the opposite kidney. Small superficial or intrarenal lesions are frequently not identified even when CT is employed.[54]

The patency of the inferior vena cava may be demonstrated relatively inexpensively using real-time ultrasonography. When tumor is identified within that vessel, the proximal extent of the thrombus must be established before operation. Extension of the thrombus to the right atrium may produce few, if any, clinical signs and may not be suspected preoperatively.[55,56]

The results of the radiographic studies and real-time ultrasonography provide sufficient information to support proceeding with a laparotomy in most children, although no imaging study unequivocally establishes the histologic diagnosis of Wilms' tumor.

Plain chest radiographs should be obtained to determine if pulmonary metastases are present. Insufficient data are currently available to firmly establish the need for CT of the chest in the initial evaluation of children with Wilms' tumor. Substantial interobserver variation exists in the interpretation of chest CT scans of children with Wilms tumor.[57] The available data suggest that, in many cases, nodules identified are not metastatic tumor. Thus, at least one nodule should be biopsied to confirm the stage.

A radionuclide bone scan and skeletal survey should be obtained postoperatively on all children with clear cell sarcoma of the kidney and all children, regardless of histologic type, with pulmonary or hepatic metastases who have suggestive symptomatology. Both studies are necessary due to the potential of clear cell sarcoma of the kidney to cause lytic bony lesions, which may be evident on plain radiographs but undetectable on bone scan.[58,59]

In light of the association of intracranial metastases with both clear cell sarcoma and rhabdoid tumor of the kidney, children with either of these histologies should undergo brain imaging.[43,60]

TREATMENT

Surgery

Resection is the primary means of achieving local control in Wilms' tumor, with radiotherapy reserved for locally advanced or metastatic disease. Accurate surgical staging is critical as it determines subsequent requirements for chemotherapy and radiotherapy based on penetration of renal capsule by tumor, regional lymph node involvement, and residual tumor. These factors cannot be determined radiographically with sufficient sensitivity for treatment planning. A review of children treated in NWTS-4 demonstrated an increased incidence of local recurrence in those cases in which lymph node biopsies were not obtained.[61] Presumably, these children were understaged and thus, undertreated. The increased incidence of local recurrence in these cases highlights the need for complete surgical staging.

Initial resection of the tumor has been the policy supported by the NWTSG through all of its protocols. Despite the presentation of most Wilms' tumors as a large mass, resection is generally feasible. In contrast to neuroblastoma, attempted resections of Wilms' tumors are less likely to be complicated by tumor invasion of surrounding organs. Close surveillance of children undergoing initial nephrectomy in the NWTS-3 cohort demonstrated an operative complication rate of 19.8% in a group closely followed and evaluated.[62] The most frequent complication was intestinal obstruction, occurring in 6.9%, followed by extensive intraoperative hemorrhage in 5.8% of cases.[63] Injuries to other visceral organs (1%) and extensive vascular injuries (1.4%) were much less frequent. Factors that correlated with increased risk of surgical complications included advanced local stage, intravascular extension of the tumor, and resection of other organs. Resected adjacent organs were often found to be merely compressed or distorted by the tumor rather than directly infiltrated. Extensive resection involving removal of other organs or procedures that may carry a high risk of morbidity or mortality should be avoided. In such cases of extensive disease, initial surgery should be limited to a biopsy, followed by administration of chemotherapy. Resection can be more readily performed after the tumor has regressed.

The International Society of Pediatric Oncology (SIOP) has promoted the use of preoperative treatment of children with Wilms' tumor with radiotherapy or chemotherapy, without histologic confirmation of the diagnosis before therapy is initiated. They report a lower surgical complication rate of 8% by following this policy.[64] This approach has several risks, including (1) the potential for administration of chemotherapy for benign disease; (2) modification of the tumor histology; (3) loss of staging information; and (4) delivering treatment that is inappropriate for a particular histology (e.g., rhabdoid tumor of the kidney). Treatment without an initial diagnosis is difficult to support when NWTSG and SIOP studies have both demonstrated a 7.6% to 9.9% rate of benign or other malignant diagnosis in children with a prenephrectomy diagnosis of Wilms' tumor.[65,66]

A major driving factor for the use by SIOP of preoperative therapy was the high rate of operative tumor rupture in their early series. This rate decreased from 33% to 4% in the SIOP series when prenephrectomy abdominal radiation was given. However, 33% is an extremely high frequency of this complication.[66] Operative rupture occurred in NWTS-1 and NWTS-2 in 22% and 12% of children, respectively. In NWTS-4, operative rupture occurred in 14% of cases.[65,67,68] A subsequent randomized SIOP study reported that the rate of rupture was essentially the same for children receiving abdominal radiation and dactinomycin (8%) and those receiving vincristine and dactinomycin (6%).[69,70] In two consecutive nonrandomized studies, the proportion of stage II lymph node–negative children versus stage II lymph node–positive and stage III changed from 45% to 32% and 33% to 19%, suggesting that the preoperative treatments significantly decreased the apparent stage of the children's disease.[71] Evaluation of NWTS-4 clearly demonstrates that operative rupture, whether localized to the renal fossa or diffuse in the peritoneal cavity, is associated with an increased incidence of local recurrence.[68] This supports the need to avoid rupture by use of an adequate abdominal or thoracoabdominal incision to safely remove the tumor.

Adequate biopsy of lymph nodes in the renal hilum and along the vena cava or aorta is critical for staging. The surgeon must always consider the possibility of stage III disease, and obtain adequate tissue for its diagnosis. While grossly involved lymph nodes are generally resected, this approach should not be extrapolated into a recommendation for an extensive retroperitoneal lymph node dissection since this has not been shown to improve local control.[72]

The histologic diagnosis following preoperative treatment in a group of children followed by the NWTSG did not appear to have been distorted by treatment. It is less certain, however, that the pathologic findings that would determine staging were not altered by preoperative therapy.[73] A SIOP study randomized the use of local radiotherapy (20 Gy) in children treated preoperatively with chemotherapy who had stage II node-negative disease at resection. The study was terminated after randomization of 123 children because of an increased incidence of abdominal recurrence during the first year of follow-up in the children not receiving radiation (six vs. zero).[70] This difference in outcome suggested that prenephrectomy treatment altered the pathologic findings that would otherwise have led to a diagnosis of stage III disease (i.e., lymph node involvement or capsular penetration) and inclusion of local radiation.

Preoperative treatment of Wilms' tumor is generally accepted in certain circumstances. These include the occurrence of Wilms' tumor in children with a solitary kidney, bilateral renal tumors, tumor in a horseshoe kidney, and respiratory distress from extensive pulmonary metastases. In most instances, pretreatment biopsy should be obtained. In children with bilateral disease or involvement of a solitary kidney, preoperative chemotherapy is intended to permit maximal conservation of uninvolved renal parenchyma. Studies on pretreatment of children with unilateral tumors have demonstrated that in most instances a complete nephrectomy is still required due to extensive involvement with the kidney at presentation.[74]

In the bilateral cases, preservation of normal renal tissue is a more critical issue. In these children the contralateral tumor often is smaller and more amenable to a partial nephrectomy after treatment with chemotherapy. Concerns about long-term renal impairment following removal of more than one-half of the renal parenchyma have resulted in a less radical surgical approach to the treatment of these children.[75]

The goal of therapy in bilateral cases is first, to eradicate all tumor, and second, to preserve as much renal tissue as possible to minimize the frequency of chronic renal failure.[76,77] The management presently recommended is initial bilateral renal biopsy and staging. Children then receive combination chemotherapy based on the stage and histology. A reevaluation is performed after 5 weeks to determine if there has been sufficient response of the tumors to allow tumor resection, with preservation of a substantial amount of normal renal tissue. Additional chemotherapeutic agents, such as doxorubicin, with or without radiation therapy, may be necessary for the management of children whose tumors respond poorly to the combination of vincristine and dactinomycin.

The absence of radiographic response or evidence of radiographic progression does not always imply lack of histologic response. Fetal rhabdomyomatous nephroblastoma is being recognized with increasing frequency as an entity with a favorable prognosis that may be misinterpreted as chemotherapy-resistant tumor in the absence of histologic confirmation.[78,79] This potential lack of concordance between radiographic and histologic response mandates that changes in chemotherapy, the addition of radiation therapy, or both in the management of children with bilateral or inoperable tumors should only be made after evaluation of a posttreatment biopsy.

In the most recent NWTSG series (NWTS-4), 98 children with bilateral Wilms' tumors underwent a partial nephrectomy.[80] One hundred thirty-four kidneys were managed with renal salvage procedures (120 partial nephrectomies and 14 enucleations). Definitive surgical resection was performed at initial operation in 58 kidneys (34 were salvage procedures). Complete resection of gross disease was accomplished in 118 (88%) of the 134 kidneys. The higher incidence of positive surgical margins (21%) and local tumor recurrence (8.2%) seen in this group of children compared with children with unilateral tumors was justified by the attempts to maximize renal preservation. Local recurrence occurred in only one of the children with gross residual disease or positive margins. Overall, 72% of the kidneys were preserved, and the 4-year survival rate was 81.7%. In a similar effort, the United Kingdom Children's Cancer Study Group reported on 70 children with bilateral Wilms' tumor.[81] The majority (57) had initial biopsy and chemotherapy with delayed resection, whereas the rest had initial surgical resection. Overall survival of 69% was similar in both groups (initial vs. delayed resection), as was the 80% incidence of normal renal function. Only the estimated mean preserved renal mass differed between the two groups, with 45% preservation when surgery was delayed versus 35% in patients with surgery at initial diagnosis.

Intracaval or intraatrial extension of a tumor thrombus is an uncommon event, occurring in 4% of children with Wilms' tumor. Identification of vascular extension by preoperative radiographic studies or by palpation early in the surgical exploration is critical to avoid embolization during mobilization of the kidney. Traditionally, vascular extension has been managed by resection during nephrectomy. Cardiopulmonary bypass is used for atrial extension. This approach has been associated with a significant risk of complications. In one NWTSG report, 23 children with vascular extension were treated initially with chemotherapy after biopsy of the renal mass. Complete resolution of the tumor thrombus occurred in seven children, and all lesions except one decreased in size.[56] Of the 14 children with tumor initially extending into the atrium, only 4 had residual atrial involvement at resection requiring sternotomy and bypass. Tumor embolism did not occur during chemotherapy. This study suggests that children with atrial or caval involvement generally require less extensive resection after preliminary treatment with combination chemotherapy.

Gross hematuria in children with Wilms' tumor is infrequent, but should lead to suspicion of extensive involvement of the renal pelvis with possible extension into the ureter. Cystoscopy should be considered in these children to identify extension of the tumor into the bladder and avoid transection of the tumor with division of the ureter. Ureteral extension that is recognized and entirely resected does not increase the stage of the tumor.

Exploration of the contralateral kidney has been recommended by the NWTSG based on the 5% occurrence of synchronous lesions. Exploration of the renal fossa by opening Gerota's fascia to directly examine the anterior and posterior aspects of the kidney is suggested. A review of children with bilateral tumors treated on NWTS-4 identified 9 of 122 children in whom the diagnosis of bilateral disease was missed by the preoperative imaging studies [CT, ultrasonography, or magnetic resonance imaging (MRI)].[54] All but one of these lesions were small, with five being less than 1 cm and three being 1 to 3 cm in diameter. CT was found to be more sensitive for diagnosing contralateral disease than ultrasonography. Thus, 7% of the 5% of children presenting with bilateral disease would have been missed if exploration had not been performed, or an incidence of 0.35% among children with Wilms' tumor. This low frequency explains why more recent studies with smaller numbers of children have reached other conclusions.

The role of surgery in the treatment of pulmonary relapse has been evaluated by the NWTSG in 211 patients. While diagnostic confirmation of relapse may be required, there was no therapeutic benefit identified to resection of a solitary pulmonary metastasis in addition to pulmonary radiotherapy and chemotherapy alone.[82] Four-year survival rates were identical in the two groups.

Radiation Therapy

Pioneering radiation oncologists noted that Wilms' tumors were responsive to radiation therapy. This modality then became routine postoperative treatment at Children's Hospital, Boston, where many of the initial observations concerning the management of these children were made.[83] First, the treatment volume was extended across the midline to include the entire circumference of the implicated vertebral bodies.[84] This was done to equalize the growth suppression; irradiation of only one side of a vertebra had been shown to lead to an obligatory scoliosis convex away from the irradiated side.

The original radiation therapy concepts have been modified as the result of the clinical trials conducted by the NWTSG. For example, the age-adjusted dosages were shown to be unnecessary in tumors of favorable histology. The advent of effective drugs had a profound effect, not only on the general management of these children, but also on the indications for the administration of postnephrectomy abdominal irradiation. Presumed microscopic residual disease in the tumor bed of children with stage I favorable histology Wilms' tumor can be successfully treated with combination chemotherapy rather than flank irradiation. This was demonstrated in the first two NWTSG randomized clinical trials that indicated the overall relapse-free survival rate in all patients, regardless of age, was similar to that of irradiated patients in NWTS-1 who had received chemotherapy with only dactinomycin. Retrospective analyses of the data accumulated in NWTS-1 and NWTS-2 were conducted to determine the patterns of relapse and to evaluate the relationship between abdominal radiation therapy dose and intraabdominal tumor recurrence.[85–87] In NWTS-3, the unirradiated and the irradiated (20 Gy) stage II, favorable histology patients had similar relapse-free survival percentages, as did those with stage III, favorable histology, who received nominal doses of 10 versus 20 Gy. Meanwhile, excellent results continued to be recorded for stage I, favorable histology patients, none of whom received radiation therapy.[88] In summary, NWTS-1, NWTS-2, and NWTS-3 demonstrated that stage I and II patients with favorable histology tumors who receive vincristine and dactinomycin do not require postoperative irradiation. A dose of 1000 cGy is sufficient for local control in stage III, favorable histology patients if they also received chemotherapy with vincristine, dactinomycin, and doxorubicin.[89]

Whole lung irradiation (12 Gy) is recommended for patients who present with pulmonary metastases visible on plain chest radiography. Chemotherapy doses given immediately after the completion of whole lung irradiation are decreased by 50%.

A pilot study conducted by investigators from SIOP produced results similar to those of the NWTSG in stage IV, favorable histology patients following treatment with nephrectomy and chemotherapy only.[90] Patients with persistent or recurrent lung nodules received whole lung radiation therapy or surgical removal of the metastatic lesions or both. Using a similar approach, the United Kingdom Children's Cancer Study Group reported results inferior to those of the NWTSG in this group of patients.[91]

The potential adverse effects of whole lung irradiation and chemotherapy (which includes vincristine, dactinomycin, and doxorubicin as employed in the NWTSG treatment regimens) include radiation pneumonitis or *Pneumocystis carinii* pneumonitis, or both. These complications are an important cause of morbidity and mortality in patients with stage IV Wilms' tumor.[92]

Patients with pulmonary lesions identified only on CT of the chest should undergo biopsy of one or more lesions to confirm that they are due to metastatic Wilms' tumor if treatment with whole lung irradiation and doxorubicin is planned. A report from St. Jude Children's Research Hospital suggested that such patients have an increased risk of pulmonary recurrence following treatment with chemotherapy only.[93] A review of the experience with such patients treated on NWTS-3 and NWTS-4 did not demonstrate a clear benefit of whole lung irradiation for such patients. The 4-year relapse-free survival rate was 89% among 53 irradiated patients and 80% among 37 unirradiated patients.[94,95] This improvement in relapse-free survival must be balanced against the increase in potential side effects of therapy, leaving the use of whole lung irradiation as a continued source of debate.

Chemotherapy

Wilms' tumor was the first pediatric malignant solid tumor found to be responsive to the systemic chemotherapeutic agent dactinomycin.[96] Other active agents were subsequently identified, including vincristine, doxorubicin, and cyclophosphamide.[51]

FAVORABLE HISTOLOGY WILMS' TUMOR

NATIONAL WILMS' TUMOR STUDY-3

Patients with stage I Wilms' tumor were successfully treated using an 11-week regimen composed of vincristine and dactinomycin without abdominal irradiation. The 4-year relapse-free percentage and overall survival percentage with this regimen were 89.0% and 95.6%, respectively.[88]

Patients with stage II Wilms' tumor were randomized to receive vincristine and dactinomycin or these two drugs and doxorubicin. They were also randomized to receive tumor bed irradiation (20 Gy) or no radiation therapy. The 4-year relapse-free percentage and overall survival percentage for patients who were treated with vincristine and dactinomycin and no abdominal irradiation were 87.4% and 91.1%, respectively. There was no statistically significant difference between these results and those for the remaining three treatment regimens for patients with stage II, favorable histology tumors.[88]

Patients with stage III Wilms' tumor were randomized to treatment with vincristine and dactinomycin or these two drugs and doxorubicin. They were also randomized to receive 10 or 20 Gy of abdominal irradiation. This study demonstrated that these patients benefited from the addition of doxorubicin to the two-drug combination of vincristine and dactinomycin. There was no statistically significant difference in the frequency of intraabdominal relapse among those treated with 10 Gy compared with 20 Gy. Although there was no statistically significant difference in the frequency of intraabdominal relapse in any of the subgroups, there appeared to be a higher frequency among those treated with vincristine and dactinomycin with 10 Gy (7 of 61), compared with those receiving vincristine and dactinomycin with 20 Gy (3 of 68) or vincristine, dactinomycin, and doxorubicin with 10 Gy (3 of 70).[89] The 4-year relapse-free percentage and overall survival percentage of those children treated with vincristine, dactinomycin, doxorubicin, and 10 Gy of abdominal irradiation were 82.0% and 90.9%, respectively.[88]

Patients with stage IV Wilms' tumor were randomized to receive vincristine, dactinomycin, and doxorubicin or these three drugs and cyclophosphamide. All underwent immediate nephrectomy, and all received abdominal irradiation (20 Gy) and whole lung irradiation (12 Gy). The 4-year relapse-free percentage and overall survival percentage for the patients treated with vincristine, dactinomycin, and doxorubicin were 79.0% and 80.9%, respectively. There was no statistically significant improvement in the 4-year relapse-free percentage or overall survival percentage from the addition of cyclophosphamide to the three-drug regimen.[88]

NATIONAL WILMS' TUMOR STUDY-4

Previous success in treatment strategies allowed the design of a unique study, NWTS-4, with the primary aims of continuing to improve treatment results while decreasing the cost of therapy through modification of the schedule of drug administration. This study was based on experimental and clinical data[97,98] demonstrating the safety and efficacy of dactinomycin when administered in a single, moderately high dose.

The design of NWTS-4 (Fig. 44.2-3) allowed the results of pulse-intensive chemotherapy regimens employing single doses of dactinomycin and doxorubicin to be compared with treatment regimens using divided dose regimens of each drug. In addition, treatment durations of 6 and 15 months were compared in patients with stages II to IV, favorable histology tumors.

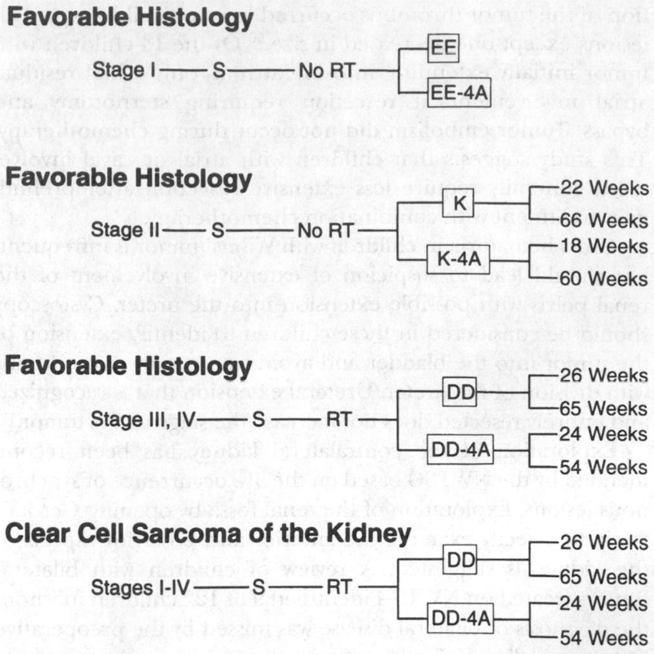

FIGURE 44.2-3. Treatment randomization for patients entered on National Wilms' Tumor Study-4. Doxorubicin and radiation therapy (RT) are included in the treatment regimen only for patients with stage III or IV Wilms' tumor. EE, K, and DD are regimen designations; RT, radiotherapy; S, surgery.

Toxicity analyses confirmed that the pulse-intensive regimens produce less hematologic toxicity than the standard regimens, and the administered drug dose intensity is greater on the pulse-intensive regimens.[99] Also, an analysis of the cost of chemotherapy treatment suggested that at least $728,000 per year could be saved if all U.S. children with stages I to IV, favorable histology Wilms' tumor were treated using the pulse-intensive regimens.[100] In addition, there were no statistically significant differences in the 2-year or 4-year relapse-free percentages or overall survival percentage of patients treated with pulse-intensive, compared with standard, modes of chemotherapy administration.[101]

TREATMENT

These recommendations are based on the results of the NWTSG, which advocates early surgery without preoperative therapy and modulates therapy according to stage and histology. For stage I, favorable or anaplastic histology, stage II, favorable histology, combination chemotherapy with vincristine and dactinomycin is recommended; no abdominal radiation therapy is necessary. For stage III, favorable histology, combination chemotherapy with vincristine, dactinomycin, and doxorubicin and postnephrectomy abdominal radiation therapy are recommended. For stage IV, favorable histology, combination chemotherapy with vincristine, dactinomycin, and doxorubicin and postnephrectomy abdominal radiation therapy if renal tumor is stage III are recommended; all patients with pulmonary metastases receive whole lung radiation therapy. For stages II through IV, anaplastic histology, combination chemotherapy with dactinomycin, vincristine, doxorubicin, and cyclophosphamide is recommended; all patients receive abdominal radiation therapy; and all patients with pulmonary metastases receive whole lung radiation therapy. For stages I through IV, clear cell sarcoma of the kidney, combination chemotherapy with vincristine, dactinomycin, and doxorubicin is recommended; all patients receive abdominal radiation therapy; and all patients with pulmonary metastases receive whole lung radiation therapy.

Prognostic Factors

Tumor size, age of the patient, histology, lymph node metastases, and local features of the tumor, such as capsular or vascular invasion, have been predictive of outcome. Modern treatments have been so successful that some of these factors no longer pertain.

The results of the first three NWTS were evaluated using logistic regression analysis. Children entered on NWTS-1 who were younger than 24 months of age had a significantly better prognosis than those who were older. The relapse rate was 14.8% for those younger than 2 years of age, compared with 34.7% for those between 2 and 4 years old, and 27.6% for those older than 4 years.[102]

The histology of Wilms' tumor was identified as the most important determinant of prognosis. More recent analyses have confirmed the importance of histopathology and lymph node involvement, whereas the prognostic significance of other factors, such as age and tumor size, changes as treatment efficacy improves.[102–104]

NEUROBLASTOMA

EPIDEMIOLOGY AND GENETICS

Neuroblastoma is the most common malignant intraabdominal tumor in children. Based on the most recent epidemiologic survey compiled in 1995, neuroblastoma (including ganglioneuroblastoma) occurs at an annual rate of 9.1 cases per 1 million U.S. children younger than 15 years of age.[1] Neuroblastoma occurs more frequently in boys than in girls. The median age at diagnosis was 2 years for both boys and girls.[51]

Neuroblastoma has been pathologically documented in additional members of immediate and extended families, including parents, siblings, twins, and cousins.[51] Mediastinal or cervical neuroblastoma is associated with heterochromia and Horner's syndrome.[105] Patients with neuroblastoma have been diagnosed with several other conditions, including neurofibromatosis, Beckwith-Wiedemann syndrome, and Hirschsprung's disease.[51]

Neuroblastoma *in situ* was identified in 0.37% to 2.58% of infants younger than 3 months of age who died of other causes and underwent autopsy examination.[51] This finding suggests that the frequency of neuroblastoma may be higher than indicated by figures derived from death certificate diagnoses or clinical (pathologic) diagnoses. Many *in situ* neuroblastomas may undergo involution or maturation or both.

PATHOLOGY

The microscopic features of a typical neuroblastoma include the presence of nests of tumor cells, separated by fibrovascular septa, with additional areas of hemorrhage, calcification, and necrosis. The tumor cells are uniform round cells with a round hyperchromatic or densely speckled nucleus. Mitoses are not frequent. Homer-Wright rosettes, with a central fibrillar core, may be present.[106] Lymphocytic infiltration may be observed. Neuroblastoma may contain mature elements, including ganglion cells.

Histochemical stains may aid in the differentiation of neuroblastoma from other common pediatric solid tumors. The periodic acid–Schiff stain result is generally negative, and neuron-specific enolase is generally positive.[107]

Shimada and colleagues developed a histologic classification of neuroblastomas based on the separation of tumors into two large groups: stroma-rich and stroma-poor tumors based on the presence or absence of schwannian spindle cell stroma. Stroma-poor tumors were further subdivided into those that were differentiated and those that were undifferentiated. Stroma-rich tumors were subdivided into those that were nodular, well-differentiated, or mixed. These histopathologic features were evaluated along with other characteristics, including patient age and the mitotic-karyorrhexis index for their importance in predicting prognosis. Patients with nodular, stroma-rich histology and undifferentiated, stroma-poor histology had a poor prognosis. This histologic classification was based on an examination of 295 pathologic specimens from a population of patients, of whom only 25% had stage IV (Evans') disease.[108] This stage distribution is not representative of unselected series of neuroblastoma patients. Several subsequent reports have evaluated the Shimada classification in case series that included patients with advanced disease.[109,110] There may be a high degree of overlap between classification as a ganglioneuroblastoma and stroma-rich tumors.[111] The International Neuroblastoma Pathology Committee has developed a modification of the Shimada system[112] that was validated in a case-cohort sample of 227 neuroblastic tumors.[113] The International Neuroblastoma Pathology Classification (the Shimada system) is proposed for international use in assessing neuroblastic tumors. Further statistical evaluation of this histopathologic classification and its correlation with other prognostic variables, such as age at diagnosis, stage, primary tumor site, and biologic variables (i.e., N-myc copy number and DNA ploidy), is necessary to establish the importance of histopathologic grading for the management of children with neuroblastoma.

CLINICAL PRESENTATION AND NATURAL HISTORY

Neuroblastoma may originate from any sympathetic nervous system tissue in the body (Fig. 44.2-4). The most common site of origin of neuroblastoma is within the abdomen. The adrenal gland is the primary tumor site in 38% of cases. Other intraabdominal sites include the paravertebral sympathetic ganglia, celiac ganglion, superior mesenteric ganglion, and inferior mesenteric ganglion. The remaining patients with neuroblastoma have tumors that originate in the thorax or neck.[51]

Infants and children with neuroblastoma come to medical attention with a variety of signs and symptoms, most commonly the presence of abdominal swelling or an abdominal mass. Abdominal or thoracic paravertebral tumors frequently cause symptoms referable to the central nervous system. Children with hematogenous metastases may complain of pain in one or more bones or present with periorbital swelling or ecchymoses. Fever is present in 23% of patients at diagnosis. Uncommon clinical presentations include hydrops fetalis,[51] chronic diarrhea due to secretion of vasoactive intestinal polypeptide by the tumor,[51,114] and myoclonus-opsoclonus.[51] Jones and coworkers

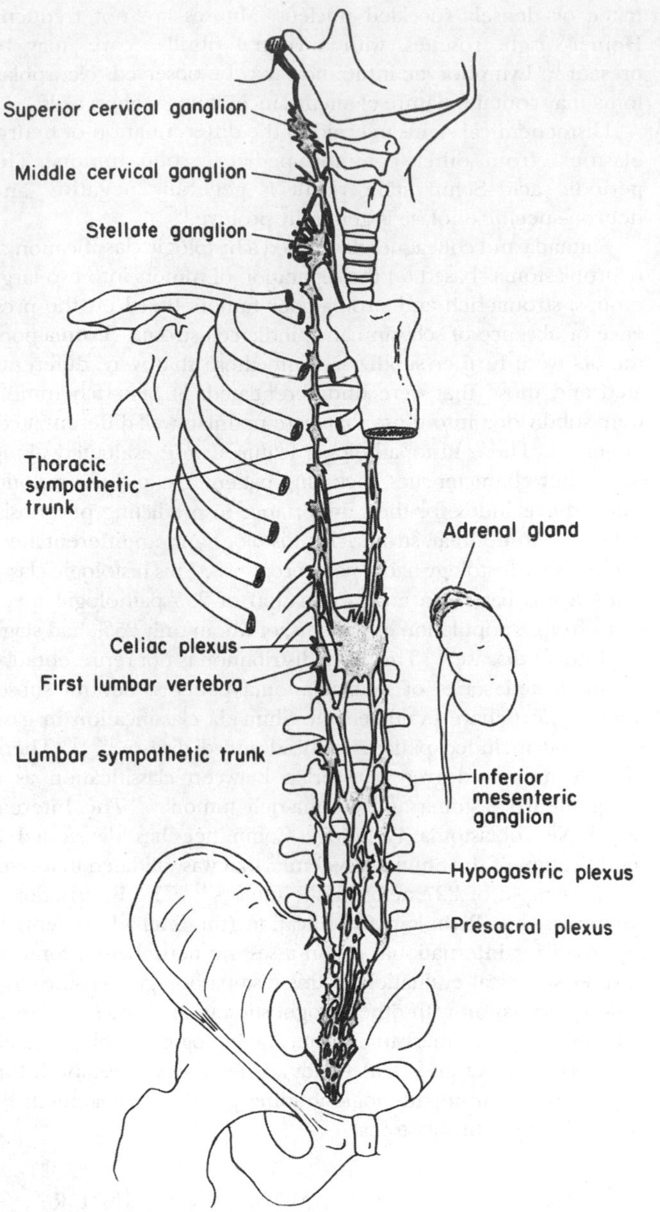

FIGURE 44.2-4. Neuroblastoma may originate from the adrenal gland or any sympathetic nervous system plexus. (From House EL, Pansky B. General visceral efferent system. In: *A functional approach to neuroanatomy*, 2nd ed. New York: McGraw-Hill, 1967:281, with permission.)

reported that 50% (8 of 16) of patients evaluated for acute cerebellar encephalopathy were found to have neuroblastoma.[115] Although the prognosis for complete recovery from the movement disorder is poor,[116–118] treatment with intravenous gamma globulin[119] has been effective in some patients, supporting an autoimmune etiology for this disorder.[120] Hypertension is an uncommon presenting sign in children with neuroblastoma.[121]

Infants and children with neuroblastoma frequently present with hematogenous metastases. These were identified in 62% of patients. The most frequently involved sites were bones, liver, bone marrow, lung, and skin.[51]

Normal sympathetic tissues secrete the catecholamines epinephrine and norepinephrine. Most patients with neuroblastoma have increased urinary excretion of vanillylmandelic acid, homovanillic acid, dihydroxyphenylalanine, dopamine, and norepinephrine at the time of diagnosis.[51]

Mass screening of infants at 4 months of age has been employed in Kyoto, Japan, since 1974, and throughout Japan since 1985. Data from both Kyoto and Sapporo suggest that mass screening has resulted in a decrease in the incidence of neuroblastoma among older children and a decrease in the percentage of patients who have metastatic disease at diagnosis.[122,123] However, the absence of adequate data have precluded the demonstration that screening in Japan has altered the mortality due to neuroblastoma. Population-based screening of 3-week-old infants has been conducted in Quebec province, Canada.[124] Because excellent population-based data on incidence, survival, and mortality are available,[125] these studies address the questions raised by the studies from Japan. Unfortunately, the Canadian experience has paralleled the outcome of the Japanese efforts. Mass screening in both countries has led to the preclinical identification of increased numbers of infants with favorable tumor biology. Most of these infants would have had an excellent prognosis with little, if any, therapy. Neither screening effort has had any effect on the number of children identified with clinically advanced disease and unfavorable tumor biology. To date, newborn screening has had a negligible effect on survival and may have led to overtreatment of children with good prognostic features.[126,127]

STAGING

Local features of neuroblastoma that can be related to treatment success include the extent of the primary tumor and the presence or absence of lymph node metastases. Dissemination of tumor to the liver, subcutaneous tissue, bone marrow, and bones can also influence prognosis.

Evans and colleagues developed a staging system, first reported in 1971, that considered the extent of the primary tumor, the presence or absence of regional lymph node tumor metastases, and the presence or absence of hematogenous metastases in determining the tumor stage. This system recognized the existence of a unique group of infants with small primary tumors and liver, skin, and bone marrow metastases, but without positive findings in the skeletal survey (stage IVS). This system demonstrated the favorable prognosis of patients with localized primary tumors, but did not consider the possible independent effects of lymph node involvement or surgical excision on prognosis.[128]

A new staging system, the International Neuroblastoma Staging System, was proposed in 1988.[129] Because of ambiguity regarding the classification of tumors originating near the midline and having a favorable prognosis,[130] the staging system was revised in 1993.[131] This staging system, recommended for adoption by the Children's Cancer Group (CCG) and the Pediatric Oncology Group (POG), is shown in Table 44.2-4.

CLINICAL EVALUATION

The evaluation of a child suspected to have neuroblastoma begins with a careful history. The maternal history should be examined for the use of tranquilizers, anticonvulsant medications, and the abuse of alcohol. The review of systems should include careful questioning regarding symptoms such as diarrhea and ataxia. The physical examination should include a careful examination of the skin. Subcutaneous metastases from neuroblastoma are reddish-

TABLE 44.2-4. International Neuroblastoma Staging System

Stage	*Description*
I	Localized tumor with complete gross excision, with or without microscopic residual disease; representative ipsilateral lymph nodes negative for tumor microscopically (nodes attached to and removed with the primary tumor may be positive).
IIA	Localized tumor with incomplete gross excision; representative ipsilateral nonadherent lymph nodes negative for tumor microscopically.
IIB	Localized tumor with or without complete gross excision, with ipsilateral nonadherent lymph nodes positive for tumor. Enlarged contralateral lymph nodes must be negative microscopically.
III	Unresectable unilateral tumor infiltrating across the midline (defined as the vertebral column), with or without regional lymph node involvement; or localized unilateral tumor with contralateral lymph node involvement; or midline tumor with bilateral extension by infiltration (unresectable) or by lymph node involvement.
IV	Any primary tumor with dissemination to distant lymph nodes, bone, bone marrow, liver, skin, or other organs (except as defined for stage IVS).
IVS	Localized primary tumor (as defined for stage I, IIA or IIB), with dissemination limited to skin, liver, or bone marrow (less than 10% of nucleated cells identified as malignant), limited to infants younger than 1 year of age.

purple, raised lesions that may be solitary. Periorbital ecchymoses are a frequent finding in children with disseminated tumor. The color of the irises and the location and consistency of the abdominal mass should be noted. A careful neurologic examination should be performed. Occasionally, the tumor mass in a child with paraplegia can be detected only on rectal examination.

The laboratory examination of a child suspected to have a neuroblastoma should include a complete blood cell count, urinalysis, liver and renal function tests, sedimentation rate, serum ferritin, and a urine sample for quantitation of the excretion of vanillylmandelic acid and total catecholamines.

The radiographic evaluation of a child with an abdominal mass suspected to be a neuroblastoma begins with a plain supine examination of the abdomen that may demonstrate the presence of a soft tissue mass frequently having calcification. Abdominal ultrasonography demonstrates the presence of a solid mass that may contain cystic areas.[132] CT provides information regarding the extent of intraabdominal disease that is not obtained with the plain radiography or abdominal ultrasound. However, there is a substantial difference between findings using CT and surgical findings.[133,134] Patients with thoracic neuroblastomas typically have a posterior mediastinal mass demonstrated on plain chest radiography. Calcification is present within this mass less frequently than within primary intraabdominal neuroblastomas. Detailed films of the ribs and vertebral bodies may demonstrate erosion of the adjacent ribs, transverse processes, and widening of the intervertebral foramina.

Patients with paraspinal primary tumors may have asymptomatic extension of the tumor through the spinal foramina. Armstrong and coworkers reported symptoms suggestive of spinal cord or nerve root compression by tumor were present in only 55% of patients with paraspinal neuroblastoma subsequently shown to have such compression at myelography.[135] Due to the increased risk of neurologic compromise with paraspinal tumors, patients with tumors in this location should undergo careful evaluation of the spinal canal using MRI with gadolinium.

All patients should have a conventional skeletal survey, including the long bones, spine, ribs, and skull, and a technetium 99m methylene diphosphonate bone scan. Although most bone metastases are identified using the radionuclide bone scan, occasional lesions, especially in the metaphyses of long bones, are identified only on the conventional skeletal survey.[136]

Bilateral trephine bone marrow biopsies and bone marrow aspirates should be performed. The biopsy is positive in 11% to 30% of children with negative bone marrow aspirate results.[137,138] Bone marrow replacement by tumor is occasionally so extensive that the microscopic picture resembles acute leukemia.[51]

TREATMENT

Surgery

Surgery plays a major role in the treatment of low-stage neuroblastoma. The surgical approach varies depending on the stage and site of the primary. It is increasingly recognized that the biologic characteristics of the tumor should also contribute to therapeutic decision making. Most thoracic, pelvic, and cervical primaries and limited abdominal lesions that do not extend across the midline to involve the great vessels are resectable at presentation. Surgery alone is curative in many children with low-stage disease. The need for postresection chemotherapy is now frequently determined by the biologic markers of the resected tumor. Reports suggest that even subtotal resection in infants and children with neuroblastoma with favorable biologic features results in a correspondingly favorable outcome and constitutes adequate therapy.[139,140]

Improved survival has been identified in children with more extensive primary tumors (stage III disease) whose tumors were completely resected at initial exploration or during subsequent surgeries following administration of chemotherapy.[141] This improvement in outcome may be more a reflection of favorable biology than a product of skillful surgery. Children previously treated on CCG protocols were reclassified using the International Neuroblastoma Staging System. This study demonstrated a strong correlation between survival and the extent of residual tumor after resection.[142] Histologically, viable neuroblastoma is found in most tumors resected following preliminary chemotherapy, supporting the important role of resection in achieving local control.[143] No difference in survival was found between those children undergoing resection at presentation versus those receiving preliminary chemotherapy.

Neuroblastoma arising in the posterior mediastinum appears to have a favorable prognosis when compared with other primary sites.[144] This has been correlated with a higher incidence of favorable biologic markers in mediastinal tumors.[145] Large tumors are also more readily resected in the chest than in the abdomen where they may surround the aorta, vena cava, renal vessels, celiac axis, and the superior mesenteric artery.[146]

Regrettably, the majority of infants and children present with metastatic disease. In these cases, the initial role of surgery is obtaining diagnostic tissue. Traditionally, surgical diagnosis has employed either a laparotomy or thoracotomy. Improved methods have been developed for percutaneous biopsy with radiographic imaging or biopsy via laparoscopic or thoracoscopic techniques. If these latter methods are used, it is critical that adequate tissue be obtained for evaluation of biologic markers.

Most children with widely disseminated disease have large primaries. Abdominal primaries arising from adrenal or paravertebral sites often encircle the celiac axis and the superior mesenteric vessels. Several studies have demonstrated that resection of these extensive lesions can be best accomplished after initial treatment with chemotherapy. In addition to reducing tumor volume, preoperative chemotherapy decreases the vascularity and friability of the tumor. This neoadjuvant approach has also contributed to decreased operative morbidity,[143] including a lower complication ratio with nephrectomy.[147]

Postoperative diarrhea may complicate resections of extensive tumors surrounding the superior mesenteric or celiac arteries.[148] This increased stool output is presumably produced by disruption of the autonomic nerve supply to the gut and not related to the timing of surgery. Several studies have demonstrated an apparent decrease in the frequency of local recurrences following resection of the primary in stage IV tumors.[149–151] Improved survival, however, has not been achieved since the majority of these advanced stage patients ultimately succumb to relapse at distant sites.[152] As systemic therapy improves, local control will become more critical. Use of radiolabeled metaiodobenzylguanidine[153] and a hand-held gamma detector to identify sites of neuroblastoma in extensive or recurrent cases has been described. Whether use of these techniques will result in better outcomes has yet to be established.

Attempts should be made to preserve the ipsilateral kidney during resection of the primary tumor in children with stage IV neuroblastoma.[154] Many of these children receive either a bone marrow transplant or nephrotoxic agents, making maximal preservation of maximum renal function an important goal. Children with adrenal or paravertebral primaries generally have metastatic tumor in lymph nodes that wraps around the renal vessels. These must be dissected free to preserve the kidney. The risk of nephrectomy is greatest in children undergoing resection before the administration of chemotherapy.[143]

Infants with stage IVS disease require exploration or a percutaneous biopsy for diagnosis. In most cases resection is not necessary unless the most readily obtained tissue for diagnosis is a small, easily resected primary.[155] There is no convincing evidence that resection of the primary will accelerate or ensure resolution of metastatic disease.[156,157] In fact, one review of 110 infants with stage IVS disease treated by members of the POG showed that there was no statistical difference in survival rate for patients with complete resection of their primary tumor compared with those who underwent partial resection or biopsy only.[158] Decreased survival was associated with age less than 2 months, diploid ploidy, amplification of the N-myc protooncogene, or tumors with unfavorable histology. If a mass remains at the primary site after resolution of the distant disease, resection is often performed and frequently demonstrates a ganglioneuroma or neuroblastoma with extensive maturation. Surgical techniques have been developed for abdominal expansion for infants presenting with extensive hepatomegaly that impairs respiratory function. The abdominal fascia is divided and prosthetic material is inserted to increase the volume of the abdominal cavity.[159,160]

Antenatal diagnosis of neuroblastoma appears to identify a particularly good risk population of infants. The biologic markers on these tumors are favorable. In keeping with their less aggressive biology, infants have done well following resection of the primary tumor.[161] It is not known whether spontaneous regression would occur if these infants were observed, but a report of four infants with antenatal diagnosis of adrenal masses (two solid and two cystic) demonstrated resolution of the abnormalities by 2.5 to 8.0 weeks of age.[162]

Radiation Therapy

Radiation therapy has been used in the treatment of patients with neuroblastoma both to decrease the frequency of local tumor recurrence and to eradicate microscopic or macroscopic distant metastases.[49] Wyatt and Farber systematically treated patients with neuroblastoma with local irradiation. They suggested radiation therapy should be instituted in every case once the diagnosis is established.[163]

Rosen and colleagues reported local control in 100% (14 of 14) of patients with stage I to stage III (Evans') neuroblastoma treated with 10 to 20 Gy, and in 87.5% (21 of 24) of patients treated with 20 to 40 Gy. One patient had recurrence in the treatment volume, whereas two others were considered marginal misses, occurring outside of high-dose boost volumes.[164]

Reports have demonstrated patients with stage I (International Neuroblastoma Staging System) neuroblastoma have a 4-year relapse-free survival percentage of 89% when treated with surgery only.[165] Children with stage II (Evans') neuroblastoma with microscopic residual disease may benefit from local irradiation.[166] The POG randomized patients with stage C neuroblastoma to treatment with postoperative chemotherapy or postoperative chemotherapy and local irradiation (24 to 30 Gy). The 3-year event-free survival percentage was 32% for patients with stage III (Evans') randomized to treatment with combination chemotherapy, compared with 59% for those randomized to the same chemotherapy and local radiation therapy (P = .009).[167] Thus, in patients with residual disease or positive lymph nodes, the addition of radiation therapy appears to improve the prognosis. Refinements of these recommendations may be necessary in the future as newer studies that use biologic markers for treatment stratification identify subsets that do or do not benefit from local radiation therapy.

Chemotherapy

Although two published studies offer a glimmer of hope for metastatic patients treated with dose-intensive regimens incorporating stem cell support,[169,173] prospects for long-term survival in advanced stage disease remain poor despite increasingly toxic therapies. At the other end of the spectrum, trials conducted in patients without evidence of gross residual disease have not demonstrated a survival advantage for adjuvant chemotherapy. A retrospective analysis of patients with *locally* unresected disease, however, demonstrated a clear survival advantage for children treated with teniposide and cisplatin (93%) versus those whose treatment did not include these two drugs (42%; P= .02).[170] The role of chemotherapy in these patients must be addressed in future randomized trials.

The poor response of patients with metastatic neuroblastoma to aggressive combination chemotherapy programs stimulated clinical trials that incorporated autologous bone marrow transplantation (ABMT) or peripheral blood stem cell rescue. Event-free survival 2 years after ABMT was reported to be 6% to 64% [171–173] among progression-free patients with advanced neuroblastoma who received a bone marrow transplant. The spectrum of results may reflect patient selection. A retrospective analysis by the POG showed no significant prognostic benefit of changing, in remission, from conventional therapy to bone marrow transplant.[174] The CCG reported the results of a randomized trial comparing the outcome following intensive chemotherapy without bone marrow transplant to that following ABMT. The 3-year event-free survival was 34% ± 4% for those randomized to ABMT, compared with 22% ± 4% for those randomized to continuation chemotherapy ($P = .034$). However, 32% of patients randomized to ABMT did not receive the randomized therapy, whereas 21% of those randomized to continuation chemotherapy did not receive the randomized treatment. ABMT did not improve overall survival compared with continuation chemotherapy. A secondary randomization involving a 6-month course of 13-*cis* retinoic acid following completion of treatment produced a 3-year relapse-free survival rate of 46% ± 6% for those who received the drug. This outcome compared favorably with the 29% ± 5% relapse-free survival for patients who were not randomized to treatment with *cis*-retinoic acid ($P = .027$).[168] Current treatment protocols employed by the POG and the CCG stratify patients by stage, age, N-myc status, Shimada histology, and DNA ploidy (Table 44.2-5).

Low-Risk Patients

Children with stage I neuroblastoma have an excellent prognosis following excision of the primary tumor without adjuvant therapy. Children with stage II disease with a single copy of N-myc, regardless of histology, have an excellent prognosis following tumor excision alone. Stage II patients with greater than ten copies of N-myc and favorable Shimada histology also have a good prognosis following tumor resection. Despite the amplification of N-myc in this subset of children with localized disease, the favorable Shimada histology has sufficient predictive power that radiation and chemotherapy are not recommended unless recurrence is documented. Perhaps the most unique cohort of low-risk patients consists of asymptomatic infants with disseminated stage IVS neuroblastoma and hyperdiploidy (DNA index greater than 1.0). Since many of these infants spontaneously improve, they should be observed without treatment.

Intermediate-Risk Patients

Among children without N-myc amplification, those with stage III neuroblastoma who are younger than 12 months of age, stage III patients with favorable Shimada histology who are more than 12 months of age, and those with stage IV neuroblastoma who are less than 12 months of age all have a moderate risk of disease recurrence. Their treatment may include local radiation therapy and combination chemotherapy. As noted previously, infants with stage IVS neuroblastoma require supportive care only. Those younger than 6 weeks of age at diagnosis may have feeding intolerance or respiratory insufficiency due to massive hepatomegaly, mandating a brief course of chemotherapy.

High-Risk Patients

All children with N-myc amplification, regardless of stage, and all children older than 1 year of age with stage IV neuroblastoma have a substantial risk of disease progression. These children should be treated using study regimens being evaluated by the national or international pediatric clinical trials groups. The role of ABMT is being evaluated in the subgroup of patients who have a favorable response to combination chemotherapy.

TABLE 44.2-5. Risk Group and Protocol Assignment Schema: Pediatric Oncology Group and Children's Cancer Group

International Neuroblastoma Staging System Stage	*Age (y)*	*N-myc Status*	*Shimada Histology*	*DNA Ploidy*	*Risk Group/Study*
1	0–21	Any	Any	Any	Low
2A and 2B	<1	Any	Any	Any	Low
	≥1–21	Nonamplified[a]	Any	NA	Low
	≥1–21	Amplified[b]	Favorable	NA	Low
	≥1–21	Amplified	Unfavorable	NA	High
3	<1	Nonamplified	Any	Any	Intermediate
	<1	Amplified	Any	Any	High
	≥1–21	Nonamplified	Favorable	NA	Intermediate
	≥1–21	Nonamplified	Unfavorable	NA	High
	≥1–21	Amplified	Any	NA	High
4	<1	Nonamplified	Any	Any	Intermediate
	<1	Amplified	Any	Any	High
	≥1–21	Any	Any	NA	High
4S	<1	Nonamplified	Favorable	>1	Low
	<1	Nonamplified	Any	1	Intermediate
	<1	Nonamplified	Unfavorable	Any	Intermediate
	<1	Amplified	Any	Any	High

NA, not applicable.
[a]N-myc copy number ≤10.
[b]N-myc copy number >10.

PROGNOSTIC FACTORS

Breslow and McCann evaluated the interaction between age at diagnosis, stage (Evans'), and probability of survival. These investigators confirmed the adverse effect of both increasing age at diagnosis and advanced stage on the probability of survival.[175]

Other clinical investigators have reported lower survival percentages in stage IV (Evans') patients with a vanillylmandelic acid to homovanillic acid ratio of less than 1.5.[176] A poorer prognosis has also been ascribed to stage III and IV (Evans') patients with a neuron-specific enolase level greater than 100 ng,[177] and for stage IV patients (Evans') with serum lactate dehydrogenase greater than 1000 IU.[178]

Look and coworkers reported that patients with hyperdiploid tumor cells had a more favorable response to combination chemotherapy than did patients with diploid tumor cells.[179] Brodeur and colleagues demonstrated the relationship between advanced tumor stage and increased copy number of N-myc,[180] and Nakagawara and associates reported that increased expression of TRK-A was associated with a favorable prognosis.[181] Although several reports have documented the prognostic effect of several of these markers,[181–183] the retrospective design of the published analyses and the small number of patients with all markers evaluated has prevented an adequate multivariate analysis from being performed. A prospective study in which treatment was not a variable would facilitate this important analysis.

RETINOBLASTOMA

EPIDEMIOLOGY AND GENETICS

Retinoblastoma is the most frequent malignant ocular tumor in pediatric patients. The incidence rate per year is 3.8 cases per 1 million U.S. children younger than 15 years of age.[1] Approximately 70% to 75% of all cases are unilateral. Among children with unilateral disease, 10% to 15% have hereditary germline deletions of chromosome 13, band q14, which contains the RB1 tumor suppressor gene locus. Germline mutations of 13q14 uniformly affect the 25% to 30% of children with bilateral disease.[19] Retinoblastoma occurs slightly more frequently in boys than girls, especially among those who have bilateral retinoblastoma. The median age at diagnosis was 2 years for boys and 1 year for girls with unilateral retinoblastoma. In cases of bilateral disease, the median age at diagnosis is less than 12 months for both boys and girls.[51]

Retinoblastoma may occur in children with other anomalies, including congenital cardiovascular defects, cleft palate, Bloch-Sulzberger syndrome, infantile cortical hyperostosis, dentinogenesis imperfecta, incontinentia pigmenti, and familial congenital cataracts.[51]

Although most children with retinoblastoma have normal intellectual function, some patients have been reported who had mental retardation in addition to a constellation of features associated with the deletion of the more distal portion of 13q.[184,185] These features include a broad nasal bridge, hypertelorism, microphthalmos, micrognathia, and variable foot and toe anomalies.[51]

While the majority of new cases of retinoblastoma arise spontaneously from new somatic mutations, a significant, and possibly increasing, fraction of retinoblastoma cases are hereditary. The familial pattern may demonstrate direct transmission of retinoblastoma from parent to child, or the presence of two or more affected offspring from unaffected parents who have affected first-degree relatives. Retinoblastoma is transmitted in each of these situations as a highly penetrant, autosomal dominant trait.[186] An analysis of the offspring of patients with sporadic, bilateral retinoblastoma demonstrated that 49.2% of the offspring developed the disease. This suggests that essentially all patients with sporadic, bilateral retinoblastoma had a germinal mutation that was transmitted in an identical manner as in families with a positive history of retinoblastoma. Approximately 5.5% of the offspring of patients with sporadic, unilateral retinoblastoma developed the disease, suggesting that 9.9% to 12.3% of patients with sporadic, unilateral retinoblastoma actually have a germinal mutation that may be transmitted to their offspring.[187]

A more complex problem in genetic counseling arises when one is asked to estimate the risk of an unaffected member of a sibship with a positive family history for retinoblastoma who carries the retinoblastoma gene. It is also difficult to estimate the risk for recurrence of retinoblastoma in a sibship from unaffected parents with one affected sibling. Nussbaum and Puck have analyzed these situations and developed equations for estimating these various probabilities.[188]

The parents and siblings of all patients with retinoblastoma should have a thorough ophthalmoscopic examination. Retinoblastomas may undergo spontaneous regression, leaving characteristic retinal changes.[189] Margo and associates suggested such lesions were benign at their outset. These lesions indicated the presence of the same mutation found in patients with retinoblastoma, although they occurred in a more mature retinal cell.[190]

PATHOLOGY

The gross appearance of retinoblastoma is that of a chalky white, friable tumor with dense foci of calcification. Those arising from cells in the internal nuclear layer, nerve fiber layer, ganglion cell layer, or external, nuclear layer grow toward the subretinal space, pushing the retina inward and frequently causing retinal detachment. Such tumors are called the *exophytum type.* Those tumors arising from the inner layers of the retina grow toward the vitreous and are called the *endophytum type.* Multiple foci of tumor are usually present.[191]

Retinoblastoma is composed of uniform small, round, or polygonal cells, which have scanty, poorly staining cytoplasm. The sparse cytoplasm is located at one side of the cell, suggesting the appearance of an embryonal retinal cell. The nucleus is large and deeply staining. Three types of cellular arrangements may be identified: the Homer-Wright rosette (a radial arrangement of cells surrounding a tangle of fibrils), the Flexner-Wintersteiner rosette (a radial arrangement of cuboidal to short columnar cells about a lumen, with the nuclei displaced basally, away from the lumen), and the fleurette (areas composed of pale-appearing cells, with abundant, pale eosinophilic cytoplasm and small, hyperchromatic nuclei; the cells are arranged in a fleur-de-lis pattern). Calcification and necrosis are often observed in retinoblastomas.[192]

CLINICAL PRESENTATION

Patients with retinoblastoma come to medical attention most frequently because of the presence of leukokoria. Strabismus, conjunctival erythema, or decreased visual acuity are other common presenting complaints. The tumor may be diagnosed during a routine examination performed because of a family history of retinoblastoma or during an examination for an unrelated complaint in patients without a family history of retinoblastoma.[51]

The history obtained during the evaluation of a child with leukokoria should include questions regarding the administration of oxygen following birth, the eating of dirt, or the close association of the patient with a dog. Prolonged administration of oxygen is associated with the occurrence of retrolental fibroplasia. Domestic animals, particularly young puppies, may be infested with *Toxocara canis*, a parasite that may cause an ocular lesion resembling retinoblastoma in some of its clinical features. The family history should be examined for other cases of eye and bone tumors.

The physical examination reveals the presence of a white pupillary reflex. Tumors located near the macula may be readily apparent with direct ophthalmoscopy, whereas those located at the periphery of the retina may not be detected unless the patient looks in a particular direction. Esotropia or exotropia may be identified. The eye may be red and painful due to uveitis following spontaneous necrosis of a retinal tumor or due to glaucoma. Decreased visual acuity may be due to involvement of the macula by the tumor or the presence of cells and debris in the vitreous.[191]

EVALUATION

The laboratory evaluation of a child suspected of having retinoblastoma should include a complete blood cell count with white blood cell differential, tests of renal and hepatic function, and a urinalysis. An enzyme-linked immunoabsorbent assay for the detection of *Toxocara* antibody is available. An antibody was detected in the serum of 65% of patients with ocular toxocariasis, indicating this determination may be helpful in differential diagnosis when an antibody is present.[193]

Radiographic evaluation of a child with suspected retinoblastoma may include CT of the orbit or orbital ultrasonography.[194] CT may be used both to define the extent of the intraocular tumor and to determine the presence and extent of extraocular disease. Calcification was identified in orbital CT scans of 48% of patients with retinoblastoma confined to the globe, compared with 13% of patients with tumor extension beyond the globe.[195] Head CT or MRI may identify intracranial extension in patients who have normal plain radiographs of the bones adjacent to the orbit. Retinoblastoma may metastasize to the central nervous system, bones, or bone marrow.[196] The risk of such dissemination is related to the extent of the ocular tumor. A diagnostic lumbar puncture with examination of the cerebrospinal fluid following cytocentrifugation should be performed on all patients with involvement of the choroid, ora serrata, ciliary body, or anterior chamber. It should also be performed on patients with involvement of other extraocular structures, including the orbit or optic nerve, or when symptoms, signs, or diagnostic imaging studies suggest involvement of bones, soft tissues, or the central nervous system.[197]

Radionuclide bone scans should be obtained only for patients with extensive ocular involvement, symptoms suggesting the presence of a bone metastasis, and bone marrow involvement by retinoblastoma.[198]

TABLE 44.2-6. Staging System for Retinoblastoma (Reese and Ellsworth)

Group	*Description*
Group I	
A	Solitary tumor, less than 4 disc diameters in size, at or behind the equator
B	Multiple tumors, 4 to 10 disc diameters in size, all at or behind the equator
Group II	
A	Solitary tumor, 4 to 10 disc diameters in size, at or behind the equator
B	Multiple tumors, 4 to 10 disc diameters in size, behind the equator
Group III	
A	Any lesion anterior to the equator
B	Solitary tumors larger than 10 disc diameters behind the equator
Group IV	
A	Multiple tumors, some larger than 10 disc diameters
B	Any lesion extending anteriorly to the ora serrata
Group V	
A	Massive tumors involving over half the retina
B	Vitreous seeding

STAGING

Martin and Reese proposed the first staging system for patients with retinoblastoma in 1942. The classification segregated patients into large treatment groups and established four categories: (1) unilateral tumors not extending outside of globe; (2) bilateral tumors; (3) residual tumors in the optic nerve or orbit at the time of enucleation or recurrent tumors following enucleation; and (4) widely disseminated retinoblastoma.[199] These investigators recognized the more favorable prognosis of patients with a small flat tumor and the ominous nature of tumors that extended toward the vitreous or into the choroid.[200] Subsequently, those patients with anteriorly located tumors were shown to have an unfavorable prognosis.[201] These factors were considered in developing a more detailed staging system (Table 44.2-6).

A useful staging system for patients with retinoblastoma must incorporate those features known to influence prognosis, therapy, or both. Simplicity would allow easy adoption of the system by investigators at many treatment centers. The system adopted by the St. Jude Children's Research Hospital incorporates many of these features (Table 44.2-7).[202,203]

TREATMENT

The diagnosis of retinoblastoma is based on the clinical history of the patient (including the family history) and the results of an examination of both eyes under general anesthesia. Ellsworth suggested the pupils must be maximally dilated and the examination be performed with the binocular indirect ophthalmoscope.[191] Scleral indentation must be performed around the entire circumference of the ora serrata to ensure detection of all anteriorly located tumors. Using scleral indentation, retinoblastoma may be identified in the periphery of the fundus in approximately 65% of patients. These tumors either originated

TABLE 44.2-7. Staging System for Retinoblastoma (St. Jude Children's Research Hospital)

Stage	*Description*
Stage I	Tumor (unifocal or multifocal) confined to retina
A	Occupying one quadrant or less
B	Occupying two quadrants or less
C	Occupying more than 50% of retinal surface
Stage II	Tumor (unifocal or multifocal) confined to globe
A	With vitreous seeding
B	Extending to optic nerve head
C	Extending to choroid
D	Extending to choroid and optic nerve head
E	Extending to emissaries
Stage III	Extraocular extension of tumor (regional)
A	Extending beyond cut end of optic nerve (including subarachnoid extension)
B	Extending through sclera into orbital contents
C	Extending to choroid and beyond cut end of optic nerve (including subarachnoid extension)
D	Extending through sclera into orbital contents and beyond cut end of optic nerve (including subarachnoid extension)
Stage IV	Distant metastases
A	Extending through optic nerve to brain
B	Blood-borne metastases to soft tissues and bones
C	Bone marrow metastases

posterior to the equator of the globe (82%) or were of small to moderate size and located anterior to the equator, where they could only be seen with indentation of the sclera.[204] The examination of the retinal surface is not completed when the first tumor is identified. The entire retinal surface of both eyes must be evaluated and the locations of tumors noted on a diagram.

SURGICAL CONSIDERATIONS

The indications for enucleation include (1) unilateral retinoblastoma that completely fills the globe or that has damaged and disrupted the retina so extensively that restoration of useful vision is not possible; (2) bilateral retinoblastoma in which the previously mentioned conditions exist in only one eye; (3) a tumor present in the anterior chamber; (4) painful glaucoma with loss of vision following rubeosis iridis; (5) extensive bilateral retinoblastoma in which there is no potential for restoration of useful vision; (6) retinoblastoma unresponsive to other forms of local therapy; and (7) cases with permanent visual loss in which intraocular tumor is suspected.[205]

ADVANCED UNILATERAL DISEASE

Patients with suspected retinoblastoma should be referred to a pediatric ophthalmologist experienced with the treatment of retinoblastoma. The standard surgical technique is modified to allow excision of the longest possible segment of optic nerve in continuity with the globe. The surgeon must be careful not to perforate the globe when the extraocular muscles are divided. The globe and optic nerve are inspected for evidence of extraocular extension of the tumor. Orbital biopsies should be obtained when extraocular extension is suspected to be present. After the globe is enucleated, a plastic implant is placed in the muscle funnel. Although the presence of the ocular prosthesis may prevent early detection of an orbital recurrence of tumor, the cosmetic result and promotion of normal development of the bony orbit are considerably improved with the use of a prosthesis.[204]

The importance of including a sufficient (10 to 15 mm) length of optic nerve in the surgical specimen is emphasized by reports of inferior survival rates among patients with extension of retinoblastoma to the margin of the excised optic nerve.[206,207]

The survival rate reported for patients with retinoblastoma confined to one or both globes, treated only with enucleation, was 86% for those with unilateral disease and 97% for those with bilateral disease.[51]

LIMITED UNILATERAL OR LIMITED BILATERAL DISEASE

Patients with limited unilateral or bilateral residual or recurrent disease after radiation therapy may benefit from photocoagulation or cryotherapy. Photocoagulation was reported to have successfully eradicated retinoblastomas in 80% of the patients treated. Hopping and Meyer-Schwickerath stated that suitable cases for this technique included solitary or multiple tumors, less than 4 to 5 disc diameters in size, situated at or posterior to the equator. Tumors located near the macula or papillary area and those with a mushroom shape should not be treated with photocoagulation.[208]

Cryotherapy was first employed for the treatment of a patient with retinoblastoma in 1963.[209,210] Subsequent reports that included some patients treated sequentially with local irradiation and cryotherapy suggested long-term control of retinoblastoma was possible using this technique.[211] Abramson and colleagues reported long-term control of retinoblastoma with one cryotherapy session in 80% of patients with previously untreated tumors, 59% of new postirradiation tumors, and 56% of recurrent tumors following irradiation. Tumors arising from the vitreous base were not responsive to cryotherapy. These investigators stated that previously untreated patients with tumors located anterior to the equator and those with recurrent or new tumors following irradiation were candidates for cryotherapy.[212] Cryotherapy is generally effective for tumors up to 2.5 mm in diameter and 1.0 mm thick that are confined to the sensory retina.[213]

BILATERAL DISEASE

Historically, external-beam irradiation was used for the treatment of the less involved eye, following enucleation of the more involved eye of a patient with bilateral retinoblastoma. The decision to irradiate or enucleate the remaining eye was based on consideration of the location of the tumor, the presence of multiple foci of tumor or vitreous seeding with tumor, and the size of the tumor.

The development of megavoltage radiation allowed the design of treatment plans that could irradiate the retinal surface to a uniform dose, while relatively sparing the posterior surface of the lens. All current techniques require meticulous attention to daily field placement. Treatment can be administered reproducibly with the use of general anesthesia.[214] Many radiation oncologists prefer to use a single, temporal field, moving the edge of the field anteriorly in patients who are at high risk of anterior recurrence of tumor.[215]

Many new techniques have been proposed for a more conformal dose distribution in retinoblastoma.[216] Proton beam therapy or stereotactic techniques offer significant advantages in sparing normal tissues. For example, even with the conventional small fields used, the posterior field edge frequently encompasses the hypothalamic and pituitary area. This may lead to the late occurrence of endocrine dysfunction. Proton beam techniques avoid such an exit dose to normal structures.[217]

Several patterns of tumor regression following irradiation have been described, including the following patterns. In type I (*cottage cheese* calcium) the tumor shrinks in size and assumes an irregular, glistening white appearance similar to cottage cheese. In type II, the tumor shrinks in size to one-half to three-fourths of the initial volume and loses the pink color of capillary injection. The surface is gray and homogeneous, and some areas may be markedly translucent. An annulus of pigment disturbance may be exposed at the border of the tumor. In type III, a glistening white nidus of calcium, or DNA, is present in the center of an amorphous, translucent gray mass. The lesion loses its pink, solid appearance. It may be possible to see through the translucent tumor and identify normal choroidal markings. A pigment disturbance is frequently noted at the periphery of this lesion.[191]

Increased awareness of the risk of retinoblastoma among the siblings and offspring of retinoblastoma patients resulted in the diagnosis of tumors when they were small. Abramson and coworkers reported on the treatment of patients with early, bilateral retinoblastoma using bilateral irradiation. The radiation dose used for the treatment of the majority of the patients was 35 Gy. Residual tumors were present in 37% of the eyes when treatment was completed, and additional tumors developed in 16% of the eyes treated. All patients had group I, II, or III tumors. The risk of developing a second, nonocular malignancy in this group of irradiated patients is significant.[218]

Patients presenting with group IV and V bilateral retinoblastoma have been treated with radiation doses of 35 to 60 Gy. Enucleation was subsequently required for persistent or recurrent tumors in 67% of the treated eyes. The survival rate of the combined series of patients treated with bilateral irradiation was 82% compared with a survival rate of 71% among a group of patients treated only with bilateral enucleation.[219] Although the risk of a radiation-related second malignant tumor developing in a patient with bilateral retinoblastoma is considerable, the data available suggest the long-term survival of patients treated with bilateral irradiation is not worse than that of patients treated with bilateral enucleation only. The preservation of some useful vision in these patients is an obvious advantage of such a treatment approach, but prolonged follow-up of patients so treated will be necessary to thoroughly evaluate the effect of radiation-related second malignant tumors on long-term survival.[220]

Local irradiation, after enucleation, is recommended for all patients with extension of retinoblastoma into the orbit. Presentation with exophthalmos or a palpable mass through the eyelids suggests the presence of orbital extension of the tumor. The identification of an encapsulated or unencapsulated extraocular mass, enlargement of the cut end of the optic nerve at the time of enucleation, or rupture of the globe during removal are associated with orbital contamination with the tumor. These findings are confirmed histologically by the identification of an episcleral mass of tumor tissue or tumor at the margin of the cut end of the optic nerve.[221] The presence of tumor cells in the choroid and scleral emissaria, in the tissue between the choroid and optic nerve, or the presence of significant scleral necrosis, are highly suggestive of orbital contamination with the tumor. Patients with orbital retinoblastoma should receive irradiation to a volume, including the entire orbit and the optic nerve to the optic chiasm, as indicated. The recommended dose is 44 Gy in 4 weeks to 50 Gy in 4.5 to 5.0 weeks.[222]

CHEMOTHERAPY

The role of adjuvant single-agent or combination chemotherapy in the management of patients with retinoblastoma is not well defined. Wolff and associates reported the results of a randomized study of adjuvant chemotherapy with cyclophosphamide (40 mg/kg) and vincristine (0.05 mg/kg) administered every 3 weeks for 57 weeks to patients with unilateral group V retinoblastoma following enucleation. The control patients received no adjuvant chemotherapy. The relapse rates of 7.4% among those randomized to receive adjuvant chemotherapy and 11.1% among those randomized to receive no adjuvant chemotherapy did not differ statistically.[223] Subsequently, Pratt and his colleagues[224,225] and others[226,227] reported successful treatment of some patients with advanced or recurrent retinoblastoma using various combinations of etoposide, cisplatinum, doxorubicin, and cyclophosphamide.

The combination of etoposide and carboplatin was evaluated in patients with extraocular retinoblastoma, 85% of whom had partial or complete responses following treatment.[228] These two drugs, in combination with vincristine, doxorubicin, and cyclophosphamide, have been recommended for treatment of children with orbital involvement from retinoblastoma.[229]

The demonstration that combination chemotherapy can produce responses in children with advanced or recurrent tumors has led to pilot studies of combination chemotherapy for reduction of tumor bulk in previously untreated patients. The goal of these trials has been preservation of vision, primarily in children with bilateral disease. Tumor shrinkage may decrease the need for enucleation or external-beam radiation therapy for local control. Unfortunately, the use of different end points, particularly for the definition of treatment failure, has complicated interpretation of the outcomes of these studies. Responses to chemotherapy have been sufficiently provocative, however, that a multiinstitution, randomized trial of chemotherapy has been undertaken. This trial is intended to assess the therapeutic value of chemotherapy combined with cyclosporin for multidrug resistance reversal in managing advanced stage retinoblastoma.[230–236]

RHABDOMYOSARCOMA

EPIDEMIOLOGY AND GENETICS

RMS is the most common malignant tumor of the soft tissues in infants and children. The incidence rate per year is 4.6 cases per 1 million U.S. children younger than 15 years of age.[1] The annual incidence is lower for Asian children than for whites or

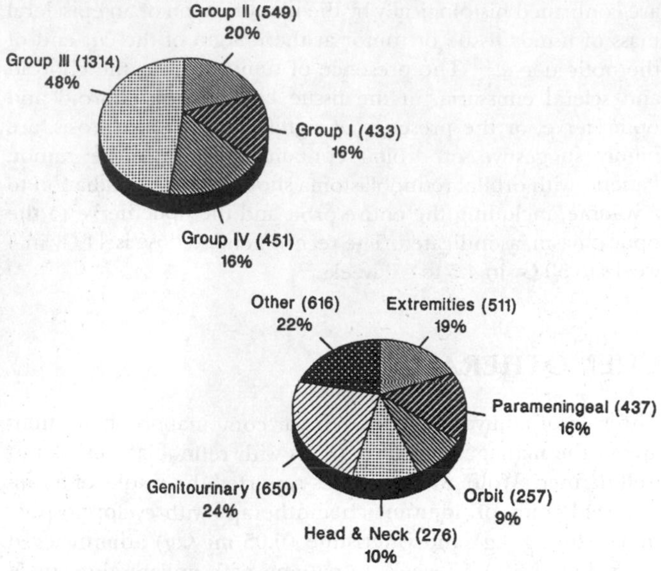

FIGURE 44.2-5. Overall distribution of patients in major Intergroup Rhabdomyosarcoma Study clinical trials according to clinical group and primary site. (From ref. 241, with permission.)

African American children.[27] RMS occurs slightly more frequently in boys.[51] The median age at diagnosis of children with RMS is approximately 4 years, with girls presenting at slightly older ages than boys.[51]

RMS has been pathologically documented in siblings and cousins of patients[51] and is a frequent tumor in families affected by the Li-Fraumeni syndrome.[17] This syndrome is defined by familial clustering of cancers that include RMS and adrenocortical carcinoma in children and breast cancer in young adults. Affected relatives share germline mutations in the p53 tumor suppressor gene, which maps to chromosome 17p13.[237] In addition to p53 mutations, which have been associated with nearly 50% of RMS cases, mutations in the NF1 gene occurring in children with neurofibromatosis confer an increased risk for developing RMS.[238–240]

RMS may arise anywhere in the body, although the head and neck region is most frequently involved, accounting for 35% of all cases[241] (Fig. 44.2-5). The most common primary site for RMS is the orbit, accounting for 29% of the RMS in the head and neck, and 13% of all RMS in children.[51]

The remaining primary tumor sites in the head and neck are divided into parameningeal and nonparameningeal locations. The parameningeal sites, including the nasopharynx, paranasal sinuses, middle ear, mastoid, pterygopalatine fossa, and infratemporal fossa, account for 40% of the RMS that originate in the head and neck. Additional primary tumor sites in the head and neck include the scalp, oral cavity, oropharynx, larynx, parotid gland, and neck.[51]

The second most frequently involved regions include the abdomen and genitourinary tract, which account for the location of 29% of primary tumor sites in children with RMS. These tumors originate most frequently from the paratesticular tissues. Other primary tumor sites include the bladder, prostate, vagina, uterus, cervix, and bile ducts.[51] RMS arising in the genitourinary tract tends to affect young children, particularly the vaginal botryoid variant, which commonly presents in infancy.

The third group of tumor sites for RMS originates within the thorax or from the soft tissues of the trunk or extremities. The most common sites involve the lower extremities, with 22% originating in the thigh or groin.[51] In contrast to the predilection for genitourinary tumors to develop in young children, RMS arising in the extremities is more likely to be identified in the second decade of life. Almost one-half of these extremity primaries contain alveolar elements that are associated with a more aggressive tumor biology (see Pathology, later in this chapter).

Overall, nearly 25% of all newly diagnosed cases of RMS are metastatic at initial presentation. The most common sites of dissemination include lung, bone marrow, bone, and lymph nodes, in approximate order of frequency.[242]

PATHOLOGY

RMS has been traditionally classified into three histologies, consisting of embryonal (including botryoid), alveolar, and pleomorphic subtypes. As noted previously, tumor histology is strongly correlated with the primary tumor site. Alveolar histology is uncommon except in primary tumors of the trunk and extremity, whereas embryonal histology is most common in RMS of the head and neck and those of the genitourinary system.[51] Slightly over one-half of all cases are characterized by favorable embryonal histology, with an additional 6% demonstrating the uniquely favorable botryoid architecture. The prognostically unfavorable alveolar histology constitutes only 21% of all cases of RMS.[242]

Various histologic classification schemes have been proposed since Horn and Enterline first categorized RMS as either embryonal or alveolar in 1958.[243–247] A revised classification of childhood RMS was proposed in 1995, based on the results of an international collaborative study. This system recognizes six subtypes: botryoid RMS, spindle cell RMS, embryonal RMS, alveolar RMS, undifferentiated sarcoma, and RMS with rhabdoid features. Application of this system has been shown to have greater reproducibility than prior classification schemes, separating patients into prognostically significant groups.[248] Histologic classification of childhood RMS can be difficult, however, since individual tumors may have areas consistent with two or more histologic subtypes. Although immunohistochemical staining for desmin may be useful for the identification of RMS, some tumors lack distinguishing microscopic characteristics and cannot be further categorized.

In light of the limitations of immunohistochemical assessment, molecular diagnostics may prove to be important in identifying biologically less favorable subsets of patients for stratification to more intensive treatment regimens. Embryonal RMS is characterized by loss of heterozygosity at the chromosome 11p15 locus. Although chromosomal translocations are rarely associated with embryonal histology, alveolar tumors are characterized by rearrangement of the PAX3 gene on the long arm of chromosome 2 with the FKHR gene on the long arm of chromosome 13. Rearrangement of these genes produces the characteristic translocation t(2;13)(q35;q14).[249] The fusion transcript of this chimeric gene is thought to contribute to dysregulated transcriptional activation, culminating in transformation.[241] Employing reverse transcriptase polymerase chain reaction methodology, this signature translocation can now be identified with great sensitivity.

TABLE 44.2-8. Tumor (T), Node (N), Metastasis (M) Pretreatment Staging for Rhabdomyosarcoma

Stage	*Sites*	*T*	*Size*	*N*	*M*
1	Orbit Head and neck (excluding parameningeal) Genitourinary: nonbladder/nonprostate	T1 or T2	a or b	N0 or N1 or N2	M0
2	Bladder/prostate Extremity Cranial parameningeal Other	T1 or T2	a	N0 or Nx	M0
3	Bladder/prostate Extremity Cranial parameningeal Other	T1 or T2	a b	N1 N0 or N1 or Nx	M0 M0
4	All	T1 or T2	a or b	N0 or N1	M1

Notes:
T1: confined to anatomic site of origin
a: less than 5 cm in diameter
b: greater than 5 cm in diameter
T2: extension, fixation, or both to surrounding tissue
a: less than 5 cm in diameter
b: greater than 5 cm in diameter
N0: regional lymph nodes not clinically involved
N1: regional lymph nodes clinically involved by tumor
Nx: clinical status of regional lymph nodes unknown
M0: no distant metastases
M1: metastases present

CLINICAL PRESENTATION AND EVALUATION

Because RMS may originate from so many sites, the radiographic examination of the primary tumor must be individualized. Evaluation of children with RMS requires expert radiographic interpretation, competent pathologic examination of surgical specimens, and knowledge of distant sites to which RMS may spread.

The lungs should be evaluated with plain chest radiography and CT of the chest. Pulmonary nodules identified in children with RMS are frequently benign,[250] suggesting that solitary nodules identified on a chest radiograph of a child with RMS should be examined pathologically.

The skeleton may be evaluated using conventional radiography and radionuclide scanning.[251,252]

The bone marrow may be involved by RMS in the absence of bone or pulmonary metastases. Potential bone marrow involvement that may produce hypercalcemia[253,254] is assessed by bilateral bone marrow aspiration and biopsy. The bone marrow aspirate was positive at the time of diagnosis in approximately 10% of patients and may be the only definite site of identifiable disease.[255]

In addition to the aforementioned sites of hematogenous dissemination, lymph node involvement has been documented in 10% to 20% of cases of RMS.[256] These nodal sites may be evaluated radiographically or pathologically.

STAGING

Staging and risk-group stratification of children with RMS is complicated by the many potential sites from which the tumor may originate and the correspondingly different prognoses for affected children depending on site, resectability, and histology. Recognizing these difficulties, an international panel of experts evaluated two staging systems and concluded that the TNM system (Table 44.2-8) best defined the pretreatment extent of the disease, facilitating patient management based on the extent of the disease and comparisons of treatment outcome between studies.[257] Treatment decisions for patients treated using the Intergroup Rhabdomyosarcoma Study Group protocols are based on both TNM stage and clinical group, as shown in Table 44.2-9.

TREATMENT

Surgery

Surgical considerations for RMS are site specific. Although biopsy is required of tumors in all locations, progressive improvements in the response to chemotherapy and radiotherapy have obviated the need for immediate surgical resection, particularly of orbital primaries. Surgery is more frequently employed at other sites where resection does not produce major functional impairment (e.g., paratesticular and extremity lesions).

In most cases an initial incisional biopsy should be performed. The biopsy site and direction of the incision should always be planned with future excision in mind. Unsuccessful attempts at initial resection of an extremity lesion, leaving positive margins, can greatly complicate future resection.

Lymph node biopsy should be considered based on the primary site. Children presenting without distant metastases have an overall 10% incidence of lymphatic spread. Lymph node involvement is most frequent for tumors arising in the prostate (41%), paratesticular (26%), and genitourinary sites (24%). Extremity lesions had an intermediate frequency of 12%, whereas orbit (0%), nonorbital head and neck sites (7%), and truncal sites (3%) had the lowest frequency of lymphatic dissem-

TABLE 44.2-9. Intergroup Rhabdomyosarcoma Study Group Grouping System for Rhabdomyosarcoma

Group	*Description*
Group I	Localized disease, completely resected. Regional lymph nodes not involved; lymph node biopsy or dissection is required except for head and neck lesions.
A	Confined to muscle or organ of origin.
B	Contiguous involvement; infiltration outside the muscle or organ of origin, as through fascial planes. This includes both gross inspection and microscopic confirmation of complete resection. Any lymph nodes that may be inadvertently removed with the specimen must be negative. If the lymph nodes are involved microscopically, the patient is placed in group IIb or IIc (see following discussion).
Group II	Total gross resection with evidence of regional spread.
A	Grossly resected tumor with microscopic residual disease. Surgeon believes that all of the tumor has been removed, but the pathologist finds tumor at the margin of resection *and* additional resection to achieve a negative margin is not feasible. No evidence of gross residual tumor. No evidence of regional lymph node involvement. Once radiotherapy or chemotherapy have been started, reexploration and removal of the area of microscopic residual does not change the patient's group.
B	Regional disease with involved lymph nodes, completely resected with no microscopic residual.
C	Regional disease with involved lymph nodes, grossly resected but with evidence of microscopic residual and histologic involvement of the most distal regional lymph node (from the primary site) in the dissection.
Group III	Incomplete resection with gross residual disease.
A	After biopsy only.
B	After gross or major resection of the primary (less than 50%).
Group IV	Metastatic disease present at onset (lung, liver, bones, bone marrow, brain, and distant muscle and lymph nodes). The presence of positive cytology in the cerebrospinal fluid, pleural, or peritoneal fluid as well as implants on the pleural or peritoneal surfaces are regarded as indications for placing the patient in group IV.

ination.[256] In the extremity and genitourinary sites, assessment of lymph node involvement is essential to ensure that radiation fields are appropriately designed and sufficiently inclusive.

Radiation Therapy

Cassady and colleagues demonstrated in 1968 that embryonal RMS of the orbit could be controlled locally with irradiation.[258] In fact, orbital irradiation was proven to be superior to exenteration for the treatment of orbital RMS.[259]

Local irradiation is necessary for patients with known microscopic or gross residual disease. The role of local irradiation in the treatment of patients with group I disease was examined in the first Intergroup Rhabdomyosarcoma Study (IRS).[260] All patients had gross and microscopic complete tumor excisions, and all received adjuvant chemotherapy with vincristine, dactinomycin, and cyclophosphamide (VAC). One-half of these patients were randomized to receive tumor bed irradiation. Relapse-free survival was 86% for those who did not receive local irradiation compared with 80% for stage I patients who were irradiated. The incidence of local failure was 6.3% (3 of 47) for those who did not receive local irradiation versus 7.6% (2 of 26) for those patients randomized to receive irradiation.[261,262] These findings indicated that radiation did not confer a survival advantage to clinical group I patients (i.e., patients who had undergone complete resections with negative margins). In light of these findings, radiation was not included in the treatment of group I patients enrolled on IRS-II.

IRS-III accrued 1062 patients from 1984 through 1991. All patients received postoperative radiation therapy except those with group I, favorable histology tumors and selected special pelvic sites, who had pathologic confirmation of complete remission after primary chemotherapy. The dose for microscopic residual disease was 41.4 Gy and 50.4 Gy for gross residual disease. The overall survival in IRS-III improved to 73%, a significant improvement from the results of IRS-I and -II[263] (Fig. 44.2-6).

IRS-IV opened in 1991, completing accrual in 1997. This study used the TNM staging system to determine the chemotherapy regimen, and the IRS clinical group system to determine radiation therapy. Group III patients were randomized between hyperfractionated radiation therapy (110 cGy twice a day to a total dose of 59.4 Gy) and conventional radiation therapy (180 cGy once a day to a total dose of 50.4 Gy).[264]

Chemotherapy

The development of combination chemotherapy programs for children with RMS paralleled the identification of new chemotherapeutic agents with significant activity. The first combination reported to be active included VAC.[51]

IRS-I was initiated in 1972 to answer questions suggested by the results of the prior pilot studies in children with RMS.[261,262] Three additional studies have been completed (IRS-II, IRS-III, and IRS-IV). The results of these studies suggest the following points: (1) The addition of cyclophosphamide to the combination of vincristine and dactinomycin does not improve the relapse-free survival percentage of children with group I RMS (excluding alveolar RMS of the extremity).[263,265] (2) The addition of cyclophosphamide to the combination of vincristine and dactinomycin did not improve the relapse-free survival percentage of children with group II RMS (excluding alveolar RMS of the extremity).[265] The addition of doxorubicin to the combination of vincristine and dactinomycin improved the relapse-free survival of children with group II RMS (excluding alveolar histology and excluding primary tumors of the orbit, head, and paratesticular tissues) from 63% to 77%.[263] Analysis of histiotypes among group II patients on IRS-II and IRS-III revealed a disproportionate number of patients with favorable histologies on IRS-III. Thus, the better outcome on IRS-III with the addition doxorubicin may have reflected a more favorable patient cohort, rather than more effective therapy. In light of the uncertainty around the therapeutic value of doxorubicin in this setting, the current recommendations for nonalveolar group II disease remains vincristine plus dactinomycin, without doxorubicin.[241] (3) The addition of doxorubicin to the combination of VAC did not improve the relapse-free survival percentage of children with group III RMS (excluding primary

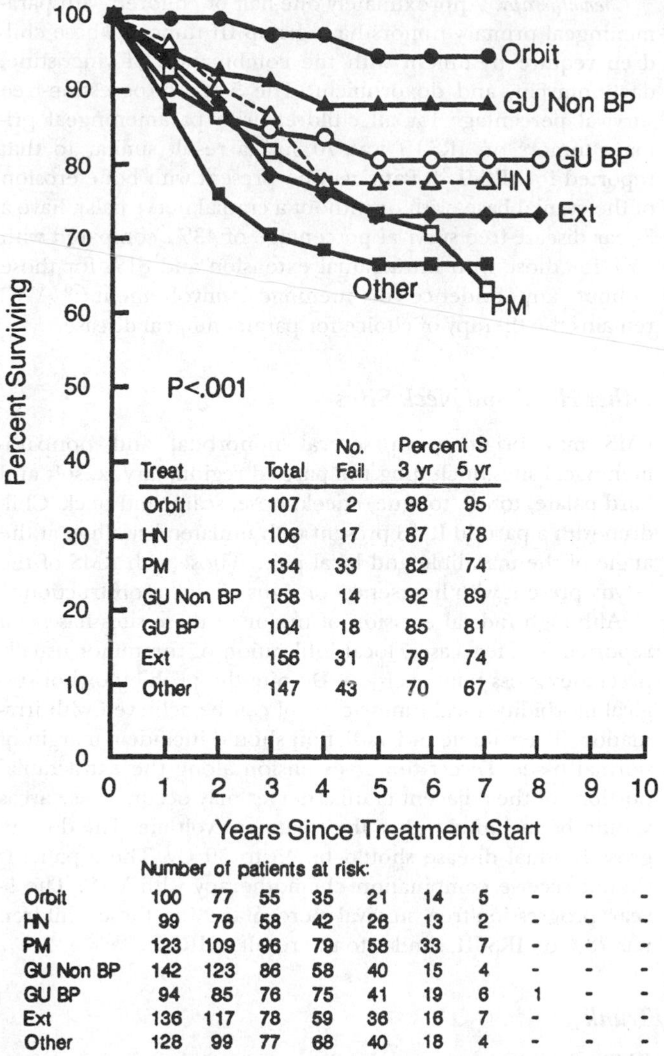

FIGURE 44.2-6. Survival (S) by primary site for all patients treated in Intergroup Rhabdomyosarcoma Study-III. BP, bladder/prostate; Ext, extremities; GU, genitourinary tract; HN, head and neck; PM, parameningeal sites. (From ref. 263, with permission.)

tumors of the bladder, prostate, vagina, and uterus).[265] The addition of cisplatin with or without etoposide to the combination of VAC did not improve the relapse-free survival of children with group III RMS (excluding primary tumors of the bladder, prostate, vagina, uterus, orbit, scalp, parotid gland, oral cavity, larynx, oropharynx, and cheek).[263] (4) The addition of doxorubicin to the combination of VAC did not improve the relapse-free survival of children with group IV RMS.[265] The addition of doxorubicin and cisplatin, with or without etoposide, to the combination of VAC did not improve the relapse-free survival of children with group IV RMS.[263]

From 1991 to 1997, 894 patients were enrolled on IRS-IV. This study randomized patients between VAC, VAI (vincristine, actinomycin-D, ifosfamide), and VIE (vincristine, ifosfamide, etoposide). The 3-year failure-free survival for all three groups was approximately 75% for nonmetastatic disease. There were no statistically significant differences in outcome between the randomized treatment groups. In light of the therapeutic parity of the three regimens, VAC remains the gold standard due to the lesser risk of renal damage compared with the two regimens containing ifosfamide.[266]

The current IRS-V study, which was first started in 1995, focuses on improving survival in the intermediate- and high-risk subsets of patients. An attempt at dose-escalating cyclophosphamide (Cytoxan) in one of these pilots was proven to be prohibitively toxic. Since all three agents in the VAC regimen are currently delivered at maximal dose intensity, improvements in survival will require identification of new active agents. Based on encouraging pilot data from treatment of metastatic patients with VAC plus topotecan, a phase III study is now being conducted in intermediate-risk patients. Eligible patients are being randomized to VAC alone versus VAC alternating with vincristine, topotecan, and Cytoxan.

Survival for metastatic (stage IV) patients has only marginally improved from 20% to 32% since the inception of the IRS in 1972. In an effort to improve survival in this very high-risk subset of children, a series of phase II window studies have been undertaken. Patients with metastatic RMS are now being treated with an induction regimen that combines vincristine with irinotecan. Like topotecan, irinotecan is a camptothecin analogue that exerts its cytotoxic effect by inhibition of topoisomerase I. Irinotecan has demonstrated impressive antitumor activity in preclinical studies with murine xenografts. Subsequent pilot studies for metastatic patients may revisit the therapeutic potential of anthracyclines in the form of Doxil, a liposomally encapsulated analogue of doxorubicin, currently in phase I studies. It is hoped that the liposomal delivery system will minimize cardiotoxicity, permitting more dose-intensive application of anthracyclines to sarcoma therapy.

SPECIFIC PRIMARY TUMOR SITES

Head and Neck

ORBIT. Children with orbital RMS present with proptosis, due to a retrobulbar tumor, or swelling of the eyelid. The radiographic evaluation must demonstrate whether the tumor is confined to the orbit or has extended inferiorly into the maxillary sinus or posteriorly into the ethmoid sinus and cranial cavity. CT provides excellent definition of the soft tissue mass and can demonstrate the presence of bone destruction.[267]

Surgery. Biopsy is required before beginning treatment of orbital tumors. Due to the excellent response to radiation and chemotherapy, orbital exenteration is not indicated except for the unusual cases of recurrent disease in this site.

Radiation Therapy. The technique of local irradiation should include treatment of a volume that includes the entire soft tissue mass, demonstrated radiographically, with a margin of normal tissue. The dose given to the macroscopic tumor should be 45 to 55 Gy, administered over 5 to 6 weeks. Historically, a wedged lateral and anterior or three-field treatment plan was used. Three-dimensional treatment planning yields a superior dose distribution and can potentially avoid irradiation of the pituitary gland. Children with RMS of the orbit are at a small risk of developing disease recurrence in the meninges.[258,268,269]

Chemotherapy. Children with group II or III RMS of the orbit have a 5-year progression-free survival of approximately 90% when treated with local radiation therapy and chemotherapy that includes vincristine and dactinomycin.[263,265] These patients do not benefit from the addition of either doxorubicin or cyclophosphamide to the chemotherapy regimen.

PARAMENINGEAL SITES. The parameningeal sites include the middle ear, nasopharynx, and adjacent areas. Children with a primary tumor in the middle ear present with a peripheral facial nerve palsy or a mass in the external auditory canal and may have been misdiagnosed as having chronic otitis media or Bell's palsy.[270] Those with a RMS of the nasopharynx present with signs of upper airway obstruction, which is frequently associated with cranial nerve palsies. On examination, they are found to have a soft tissue mass that is depressing the palate and extending into the retropharyngeal space.

The radiographic evaluation of a patient with a parameningeal RMS must document the presence and extent of bone destruction and identify local or intracranial extension of the tumor. The temporal bone, petrous bone, mastoid, and infratemporal fossa can be adequately evaluated using CT. Coronal sections obtained either by rescanning the patient or reprocessing the data obtained from the axial scan of the head allow identification of tumor extension into the floor of the middle and posterior cranial fossae.[51]

Surgery. Surgical resection is infrequently required at this site because of the excellent response to chemotherapy and radiotherapy. In children who have persistent disease after completion of radiotherapy or who have tumor recurrence, surgery should be considered.[271] Modern methods of resection and reconstruction of these sites make surgery much less mutilating than in the past, with improved long-term functional outcomes. Before the initiation of therapy, a lumbar puncture should be performed. A cytocentrifuge preparation of the cerebrospinal fluid should be examined for tumor cells.

Radiation Therapy. Parameningeal RMS progresses locally by destruction of the adjacent bones and by growth along nerves.[272,273] To achieve local control of this tumor, a generous margin of these tissues must be included within the volume of irradiation.[274,275] The tumor mass must receive a radiation dose of at least 50 Gy. Meticulous treatment planning is necessary to deliver adequate therapy to the tumor without causing excessive or unnecessary damage to adjacent normal tissues including the brain and eye.[275]

RMS of the middle ear may recur as diffuse meningeal disease. This occurred in 17.5% of patients with a parameningeal primary tumor entered on IRS-I.[276] The high rate of primary meningeal relapse in this study may have been related to inadequate radiation technique. Although these investigators recommended the administration of craniospinal irradiation to prevent meningeal recurrence, others reported isolated meningeal relapse in 5.4% to 7.4%[274,277,278] of patients with parameningeal RMS.

This suggests that the rate of meningeal recurrence is related to the adequacy of the volume and dose of irradiation to the primary tumor. Current guidelines in IRS-V for parameningeal disease do not recommend craniospinal irradiation. Treatment is confined to the tumor volume plus a 2-cm margin for parameningeal tumors without intracranial extension. In cases of documented intracranial extension, the skull is included in the radiated target volume.

Chemotherapy. Approximately one-half of children with parameningeal primary tumors have group III tumors. These children require treatment with the combination of vincristine, dactinomycin, and doxorubicin. The 5-year progression-free survival percentage for all children with parameningeal primary tumors on IRS-III was 70%,[263] a result similar to that reported for IRS-II.[265] Patients who present with bone erosion of the cranial base, with or without a cranial nerve palsy, have a 3-year disease-free survival percentage of 43%, compared with 65% for those with intracranial extension and 81% for those without any evidence of meningeal involvement.[279] VAC remains the therapy of choice for parameningeal disease.

Other Head and Neck Sites

RMS may originate in several nonorbital and nonparameningeal sites, including the parotid region, larynx, soft and hard palate, tonsil, tongue, cheek, nose, scalp, and neck. Children with a parotid RMS present with unilateral swelling at the angle of the mandible and local pain. Those with RMS of the larynx present with hoarseness or signs of airway obstruction.

Although radical excision of tumor in these sites has been reported in a few cases, local infiltration of the tumor usually precludes gross total excision. Despite the prohibitions of surgical morbidity, local tumor control can be achieved with irradiation. The volume of irradiation should include a margin of normal tissue. Direct tumor extension along the extracranial portions of the adjacent cranial nerves may occur. These areas should be included within the treatment volume. The dose to gross residual disease should be 45 to 50 Gy. These patients should receive combination chemotherapy with VAC. The 5-year progression-free survival percentage for these children was 78% on IRS-III, similar to the result of IRS-II.[263,265]

Trunk

RMS of the thorax may arise from the soft tissues of the chest wall or within the thoracic cavity. Primary tumors of the chest wall present as a localized swelling.

The radiographic evaluation of a patient with a primary tumor of the chest wall should include plain chest radiography and CT.

SURGERY. Lesions in the trunk, arising in the chest or abdominal wall and paraspinal or retroperitoneal sites, are best resected if possible because of their less favorable response to chemotherapy and radiotherapy. Complete surgical removal is limited by the frequently large size of these lesions at diagnosis as well as their involvement of vital structures within the abdomen or chest. Resections of the chest or abdominal wall often require prosthetic mesh reconstruction. Primary reexcision should be considered if pathologic examination of the initial specimen demonstrates microscopic residual disease.[280] In a review of IRS studies II and III, there were 84 patients with thoracic sarcomas.[281] Although 71% (60 patients) achieved an initial complete response, 39 suffered a local relapse, whereas an additional 22 patients developed distant relapse. Fifty-eight percent (49 patients) have died, with an average survival of 1.1 years. Survival was significantly associated with clinical group, size, and local or distant recurrence.

RMS arising in the abdominal wall is rare, accounting for only 1% of all cases of this disease. A review of patients with abdominal wall primaries treated on IRS I through IV demonstrated a substantial advantage to complete versus partial resection of localized tumors (100% vs. 62%).[282]

Biliary tract primaries appear to be more responsive to chemotherapy than other truncal sites.[283] Affected children typically present with symptoms of biliary tract obstruction. Diagnostic biopsy followed by chemotherapy is appropriate, with resection reserved for those children with persistent disease.

Initial biopsy followed by chemotherapy and radiation has also been standard therapy for bulky tumors of the retroperitoneum and nongenitourinary pelvic sites. These tumors make up approximately 10% of all RMS. The treatment outcome for these tumors on IRS-III and -IV has been reviewed. All of the 138 eligible patients with tumors in these locations were either group III (gross residual) or group IV (metastatic). Nearly one-half of these patients were metastatic at diagnosis. Children with embryonal histology had a 4-year failure-free survival of 56% versus only 33% for children with alveolar or undifferentiated histology. Nearly all of the patients with alveolar tumors underwent biopsy only, followed by chemotherapy and radiation. In contrast, 40% of patients with embryonal tumors underwent extensive debulking at initial surgery. Among the embryonal patients, the failure-free survival at 4 years was 72% for those who underwent debulking versus only 48% for those embryonal patients who underwent biopsy followed by chemotherapy and radiation. The apparent advantage to debulking will be prospectively analyzed in IRS-V.[284]

RADIATION THERAPY. When complete tumor excision is not possible, local control is established with the use of radiation therapy. The volume must include the grossly apparent tumor with a margin of normal tissue. A radiation dose of 40 Gy is adequate for microscopic residual disease, while 50 Gy is required for gross residual disease. The pleural space is considered contaminated if there is a malignant pleural effusion, or if the tumor is cut across and the pleural space is opened at the time of surgery. The entire pleural surface must be irradiated when pleural contamination with tumor cells has occurred. Failure to do so may result in disease recurrence on the pleural surface not included within the volume of irradiation.

CHEMOTHERAPY. Embryonal RMS of the trunk should be treated using the chemotherapy regimens appropriate for the clinical group. Group I tumors are treated with the combination of vincristine and dactinomycin,[263,265] whereas groups II, III, and IV are managed with the combination of VAC.[263,265] Primary tumors of the trunk frequently consist of alveolar elements.[285] As in other sites, alveolar tumors in the trunk do not respond to chemotherapy as favorably as embryonal disease. Children with intermediate- or high-risk disease arising in these sites are currently being evaluated for response to VAC plus one of the camptothecin analogues.

Extremity

Patients with RMS of an extremity usually present with localized swelling. Occasionally, a child with RMS of an extremity comes to medical attention due to symptoms caused by metastases, such as spinal cord compression secondary to vertebral body metastases, or pain due to other bone metastases. Nearly 25% of extremity primaries are metastatic at the time of diagnosis.

Radiographic evaluation of a patient with an RMS of the extremity should include plain radiographs of the primary tumor site and a bone scan. The presence of increased radionuclide uptake in the adjacent bone, although generally not associated with frank invasion of the bone by tumor, is correlated with the presence of inflammatory adhesions between the tumor and adjacent bone. Local recurrence of the tumor is likely if the tumor is not removed *en bloc* with the adjacent bone.[286] CT and MRI are useful for defining the extent of the soft tissue mass and the presence of bone destruction. Arteriography may be necessary to evaluate the relationship between the tumor, contiguous muscle compartments, and their vascular supply.

SURGERY. Complete resection of the tumor with negative microscopic margins is the goal in extremity sarcomas.[287] There is no advantage to amputation or muscle group excision compared with local excision with an adequate surrounding rim of normal tissue, provided the resection results in negative microscopic margins. The extent of the resection is often tempered by attempts to minimize functional impairment. In extremity tumors, consideration of the initial biopsy site and the direction of the incision are particularly important, because an inappropriate biopsy can greatly complicate later resection. Extremity lesions should rarely be resected without an initial biopsy because the surgical approach when resecting a malignant lesion will be quite different from the approach for a benign lesion.

Extensive local lesions with invasion of vital structures are often treated first with chemotherapy and subjected to delayed surgical resection. The goal of delayed resection is to render the child free of gross residual disease and accept microscopic residual disease that can be controlled with a lower dose of radiotherapy than the dose required for gross residual disease (40 vs. 55 Gy). This multidisciplinary approach results in good local control, while minimizing the potential morbidity of a more extensive initial resection or amputation.

Lymph node sampling is important in extremity RMS due to the significant risk of lymphatic involvement. Nearly 25% of all extremity tumors demonstrated regional nodal infiltration.[242] A representative sample of lymph nodes from the draining nodal group should be biopsied. A lymph node resection should not be performed because of the risks of producing lymphedema, which complicate radiotherapy and subsequent surgical resection of the primary lesion.

Analysis of data from IRS-III has shown that estimated 5-year survival was directly related to the clinical group, with a 95% survival in group I, versus 67% in group II, 58% in group III, and 33% in group IV. Survival was independent of histology or site. Multivariate analysis of pretreatment factors showed that lymph node metastasis, age over 10 years, and distant metastasis predicted worse survival. The difference between the survival percentage of 51 group II and III patients with lymph node–negative distal extremity lesions who could have been made group I with extensive resection and that of patients with group I distal extremity tumors approached statistical significance in univariate analysis ($P < .06$).[288] All four group II patients who had reexcision of margins survived, whereas only 18 of 31 without reexcision survived. In IRS-IV, the failure-free survival rate was 55%, with an overall survival rate of 70%. Again, the 3-year failure-free survival was closely related to group (group I, 91%; II, 72%; III, 50%; IV, 23%). In this cohort, clinical group and stage were both highly predictive of outcome. None of the other variables were predictors of failure-free survival by multivariate analysis.[289]

RADIATION THERAPY. Postoperative irradiation must be to a volume that includes a generous margin around the tumor. The radiation dose should be 50 Gy to areas of gross residual disease. Patients with histologic confirmation of regional lymph node involvement should receive similar treatment to a volume that includes the involved lymph nodes.

CHEMOTHERAPY. Embryonal RMS of the extremity should be treated using the chemotherapy regimens described earlier for RMS of the trunk. Approximately one-half of extremity RMS have alveolar histology and require chemotherapy appropriate for this histologic subtype with a poorer prognosis.[285]

Genitourinary

Patients with RMS of the paratesticular tissue present with painless enlargement of the testis. The age distribution is bimodal, with peaks at 5 and 16 years of age.[51] Children with RMS of the prostate present most frequently with acute urinary retention or with difficulty in voiding. Hematuria, dysuria, and abdominal swelling are also observed. Those with RMS of the bladder usually present because of hematuria, urinary frequency, or dysuria.[51] The physical examination of children with a prostate tumor is unremarkable except for the presence of a mass between the bladder and rectum that is palpable on rectal examination. Radiographic evaluation should include a voiding cystourethrogram or CT of the abdomen and pelvis. These studies demonstrate displacement of the bladder, in the case of a prostatic primary tumor, or the presence of multiple polypoid masses within the bladder, with thickening of the bladder wall in the case of a bladder primary tumor.[290]

Children with sarcoma botryoids of the vagina frequently present with a polypoid mass protruding from the vaginal orifice or with vaginal bleeding. These children should have an α-fetoprotein (AFP) level obtained before tumor biopsy or excision, since yolk sac tumor may also present as a vaginal mass.

SURGERY. Anterior pelvic exenteration is rarely required today. Bladder, prostate, and vaginal primaries are first biopsied, and lymph node extension is defined. Chemotherapy and radiotherapy are then used to eradicate residual disease. In the IRS-I and -II studies there were 28 vaginal and 10 uterine lesions.[291] Vaginal lesions generally arise from the anterior vaginal wall in the area of the embryonic vesicovaginal septum. The mean age of children with vaginal tumors was under 2 years. Over the course of the first four IRS studies spanning 25 years, the percentage of children undergoing resections of vaginal tumors has steadily decreased from 90% to 13%. Despite the limitation of surgical intervention to biopsy, survival in this group remains excellent, exceeding 90% with minimal surgical morbidity.[292]

In contrast to vaginal lesions, uterine primary tumors arise in older children demonstrate a greater propensity for local recurrence. As with vaginal lesions, initial surgical intervention is limited to biopsy in most cases. Hysterectomy is reserved for those patients who fail to achieve a complete response to chemotherapy and radiation. Survival in children with uterine disease approaches 90%.[293]

Preservation of the bladder and prostate was one of the primary goals of the IRS-II study in which surgical therapy was shifted from initial resection to primary biopsy with subsequent radiotherapy or surgery.[294] The 3-year survival rate of patients on IRS-II (70%) was similar to that of IRS-I (78%), but the 3-year disease-free survival rate was lower (52% vs. 70%). The percentages of 95 children with bladder and prostate tumors in IRS-II who retained their bladder and were alive at 2 and 3 years of age were 33% and 22%, respectively, compared with 26% and 23% in the 66 children with bladder or prostate tumors in IRS-I. Sequential treatment on this protocol failed to improve bladder salvage. The rate of retention of a functional bladder at 4 years from diagnosis was 60%. Excluding children who presented with disseminated disease, mortality was only 10% among children treated on IRS-III for bladder or prostate tumors.[295]

Successful treatment of paratesticular RMS first requires a transinguinal radical orchiectomy. Testicular masses should never be approached through the scrotum due to the risk of inducing spread into the pelvis via the inguinal lymphatics. In addition, the desired high inguinal ligation of the spermatic cord cannot be accomplished by the scrotal approach. A total of 121 boys with paratesticular RMS treated on IRS-III had retroperitoneal lymph node dissection to evaluate nodal status.[296] Lymph nodes were radiographically negative based on CT in 81% of the boys, 14% of whom had positive nodes when biopsy or retroperitoneal lymph node dissection was performed. Among the boys with abnormal nodes by radiographic criterion, 94% had pathologic confirmation of lymph node involvement. Retroperitoneal relapse occurred in only 2 of the 121 boys, one of whom had pathologically negative lymph nodes and did not receive radiotherapy. While CT was accurate if lymph node abnormalities were identified, it was not extremely sensitive in identifying nodal involvement.

RADIATION THERAPY. The IRS reported that there was no obvious benefit from prophylactic retroperitoneal lymph node irradiation among patients with paratesticular RMS, who had negative pathologic staging of retroperitoneal nodes.[297]

Tumors of the bladder and prostate were initially managed with radical resections including cystectomy.[298] Although excellent survival was achieved with this approach, the extensive surgical morbidity of this strategy prompted subsequent efforts at tissue-sparing treatment designs. Current IRS guidelines now recommend early introduction of radiation in combination with chemotherapy following a minimally invasive biopsy.[299] Employing this multimodal approach on IRS-III produced improved progression-free survival of approximately 75%, while maintaining partial or complete bladder function.[263]

CHEMOTHERAPY. Patients with group II paratesticular primary tumors of embryonal histology have an excellent prognosis when treated with the combination of vincristine and dactinomycin, with a 5-year progression-free survival percentage of 81%.[263] All patients with group III (biopsy only) genitourinary tumors are treated with VAC.

PROGNOSTIC FACTORS

As noted previously, the favorable prognostic factors for children and adolescents with RMS include tumor status (T1, tumor localized in the organ or tissue of origin) and primary tumor site (orbit, genitourinary nonbladder, or prostate).[300] Although alveolar histology predicts a poorer outcome with standard therapy, the difference in survival between alveolar and embryonal cases resolves when more intensive therapy is applied to alveolar tumors. Despite improvements in therapy, however, children with metastatic disease still fare poorly, with a 5-year survival between 20% and 30%. Most of these metastatic patients have alveolar tumors. In a noteworthy departure from the dismal prognosis for children with disseminated RMS, there is a subset of younger children with embryonal histology with a 50% rate of failure-free survival. Identification of this relatively favorable subset of metastatic patients reinforces the importance of histology in predicting the behavior of this disease. Unfortunately, efforts at maximal dose intensification of chemotherapy with stem cell support have failed to improve the prognosis for children with metastatic disease.[301] Improved survival will require identification of new active cytotoxic agents in conjunction with efforts to target the unique genetic perturbations that are ubiquitous features of alveolar disease.

EWING'S SARCOMA AND PERIPHERAL PRIMITIVE NEUROECTODERMAL TUMOR

EPIDEMIOLOGY AND GENETICS

Ewing's sarcoma and primitive neuroectodermal tumor are closely related, if not identical, malignancies that may occur as osseous or soft tissue tumors.[302,303] Ewing's sarcoma is the second most common primary bone tumor in pediatric patients. The incidence rate per year is 3.4 cases per 1 million U.S. white children less than 15 years of age. The corresponding figure for African American children is only 0.6 per 1 million.[1] The rarity of Ewing's sarcoma in African American and Asian populations has been confirmed by several investigators.[27] Ewing's sarcoma occurs more frequently in boys than girls and has been reported in three pairs of female siblings.[51]

The femur is the most frequent primary site for Ewing's sarcoma, accounting for approximately 20% to 25% of all cases. Lower extremity tumors may also arise in the tibia, fibula, or the bones of the feet. Combining all potential sites of lower extremity disease, these tumors account for 45% of newly diagnosed Ewing's sarcomas.[304] The pelvis is the second most common primary site for Ewing's sarcoma, accounting for an additional 20% of new cases. Pelvic tumors may arise in the ilium, ischium, pubic bone, or sacrum. Upper extremity sites comprise another 12% to 16% of new diagnoses, with the humerus accounting for the majority of these cases. The remainder of Ewing's sarcomas originate from the vertebrae, ribs, clavicle, mandible, and skull.[51] These axial lesions account for nearly 13% of all newly diagnosed cases.[304]

PATHOLOGY

Ewing's sarcoma and primary neuroectodermal tumors are counted among the small blue round cell tumors of childhood. Based on readily apparent features noted on light microscopy, this grouping includes neuroblastoma, RMS, and non-Hodgkin's lymphoma. Tumors of the Ewing's sarcoma family are characterized by the presence of highly cellular aggregates of tumor cells compartmentalized by widely separated strands of fibrous tissue. The tumor cells are regular in shape, with round to oval nuclei. The slightly granular cytoplasm is often framed by indistinct cellular outlines. The nuclei contain finely dispersed chromatin, giving the nucleus a ground glass appearance. Inconspicuous nucleoli may be present with occasional mitotic figures.[305]

Within the Ewing's family of tumors, primary neuroectodermal tumors are characterized by significant neuroectodermal differentiation. These tumors typically demonstrate Homer-Wright pseudorosettes on light microscopy and positive immunohistochemical staining for synaptophysin and neuron-specific enolase. In contrast to primary neuroectodermal tumors, Ewing's sarcomas are poorly differentiated tumors that do not form pseudorosettes and do not stain positively for neural markers.[306,307] Regardless of the extent of neural differentiation, nearly all tumors within the Ewing's sarcoma family express the MIC2 gene product (CD99) on their cell membranes.[308] Approximately 95% of all Ewing's family tumors contain translocations consisting of either t(11;22) or t(21;22). These gene rearrangements combine the N-terminal region of the EWS gene on chromosome 22 with the C-terminal region of one of two closely related genes on chromosome 11 (FLI1) or chromosome 21 (ERG). Both FLI1 and ERG are members of the Ets gene family of transcriptional activators. The majority of these translocations involve EWS and FLI1, t(11;22), producing a fusion transcript that is presumed to contribute to dysregulated cell growth and transformation.[309] Although the mechanism of tumorigenesis mediated by EWS-FLI1 remains uncertain, one study implicates the transforming growth factor-β (TGF-β) type II receptor as a target. TGF-β is a putative tumor suppressor gene. Levels of TGF-BR2 are reduced when EWS-FLI1 is introduced into embryonic stem cells. Antisense oligonucleotides to EWS-FLI1 restore TGF-β sensitivity and block tumorigenicity in cell lines containing the fusion gene.[310]

Studies of EWS-FLI1 have demonstrated a variety of genomic breakpoints within the rearranged genes. Differences in the resulting fusion transcripts are thought to contribute to the clinical heterogeneity of Ewing's sarcoma. The most common rearrangement, designated *type 1*, consists of the first seven exons of EWS fused to exons 6 to 9 of FLI1. This fusion gene accounts for nearly two-thirds of all cases. The type 2 rearrangement, constituting an additional 25% of cases, fuses EWS to exon 5 of FLI1. Type 2 appears to be a more potent transactivator, which may account for the poorer prognosis associated with this fusion product.[311–313]

Rapid identification of EWS gene rearrangement using fluorescent *in situ* hybridization on frozen section specimens has been described.[314] Application of this diagnostic tool may facilitate prompt discrimination between the Ewing's family tumors and other morphologically similar small round cell tumors, expediting the initiation of appropriate therapy.

CLINICAL PRESENTATION AND NATURAL HISTORY

Localized pain is typically the first symptom reported by pediatric patients with bone tumors. The pain progresses from intermittent to more constant, often awakening the patient from sleep. Depending on the location of the tumor, the patient may develop a limp, complain of pain that increases with respiration, or experience pain that is radicular in character. Local swelling is often noticed by the patient. This finding is more readily identified when the tumor is located in an extremity. Paraplegia secondary to vertebral disease is present at the time of diagnosis in approximately 3% of patients.

The clinical presentation of patients with Ewing's sarcoma is similar to that of patients with osteomyelitis.[315] Fever is present in 28% of patients with Ewing's sarcoma at the time of diagnosis.[51]

Metastases are present in approximately 26% of patients at initial diagnosis. The most frequent sites of metastases are the lungs and other bones. Patients may seek medical attention because of symptoms related to metastatic disease, rather than the primary tumor. Multiple pulmonary metastases may produce respiratory insufficiency, or paraplegia may develop secondary to a vertebral body metastasis.

Evaluation of a patient suspected of having Ewing's sarcoma includes radiographic examinations of the primary tumor site, documentation of the presence or absence of hematogenous metastases, and additional laboratory studies that correlate with prognosis or exclude the presence of other possible diagnoses.

Lesions that originate in the long bones characteristically involve the diaphysis, with extension toward the metaphases. A lytic or mixed lytic-sclerotic lesion is identified in the bone. Parallel, lamellated periosteal new bone formation (onion skin) or, less frequently, radiating bone spicules may be present. A soft tissue mass is frequently identified on CT or gadolinium-enhanced MRI.

Plain radiographs of tumors that originate in the pelvic bones frequently demonstrate a mixed lytic and blastic lesion. CT and MRI of the pelvis are required to adequately delineate the presence and extent of any associated soft tissue mass.

Radionuclide bone scans should be obtained, both to define more precisely the extent of disease at the primary site and to determine whether bone metastases are present.

The sedimentation rate and serum lactate dehydrogenase level are frequently elevated in patients with Ewing's sarcoma.[316,317]

STAGING

Ewing's sarcoma can metastasize to the lungs, other bones, and bone marrow. As with other sarcomas, nodules identified on plain chest radiography or CT of the chest in patients with Ewing's sarcoma are not always malignant. Cohen and colleagues reported that 60% (three of five) of nodules identified in such radiographs were benign.[250] A solitary nodule identified only on the CT scan of one patient was shown pathologically to be secondary to histoplasmosis.[318]

Radionuclide bone scans demonstrated disease in additional bones in approximately 10% of patients with Ewing's sarcoma.[319,320]

Patients with Ewing's sarcoma may have disseminated bone marrow disease in the absence of radiographically detectable bone metastases.[321] Bilateral bone marrow sampling is required to complete the staging of all patients regardless of primary site or tumor size.

TREATMENT

Surgery

Local control must be achieved by either high-dose radiotherapy or resection. Larger tumor size (more than 8 cm) or volume (more than 100 cm^3) has correlated with decreased success in achieving durable local control.[322–324] No randomized study has been performed to define whether local control is better accomplished with surgical resection or radiotherapy. In nonrandomized trials, the improved survival in the surgical resection group has been attributed to the allocation of larger tumors with correspondingly poorer prognosis to the radiation group.[325–327] Not all series have reported better survival among patients treated surgically than among those treated with radiation therapy.[328] In the German Cooperative Ewing's Sarcoma Study, survival with resection was better, although this relative advantage of surgery lost statistical significance when tumor size was considered.[329] The 3-year relapse-free survival was 78% for patients whose tumor volume was less than 100 mL, compared with 17% for patients with tumor volumes greater than 100 mL. Extraosseous extension has also been associated with an increased risk of distant relapse.[330]

The long-term morbidity produced by radiotherapy versus surgery is often the deciding factor when selecting the most appropriate modality for local control. In addition to analyses of resectability and functional outcome, deliberations about local control must also consider the risk of late-onset second malignancies in tissues treated with intensive radiotherapy. Central pelvic or spinal lesions are frequently treated with radiation alone. Extremity lesions amenable to limb-sparing resections are treated predominantly with resection after an initial 12- to 15-week phase of induction chemotherapy. It is critical for the surgeon performing the diagnostic biopsy to place the incision appropriately to avoid complicating future resection.

Chest wall lesions make up 6.5% of primary Ewing's sarcomas, representing the most frequent chest wall tumor in children. They frequently present with large lesions extending into the thoracic cavity. Traditionally, these have been biopsied by open techniques that can be difficult because of the extremely vascular nature of this tumor and the limited surgical exposure. Percutaneous biopsy, which can provide adequate material for histologic and cytogenetic testing, may be a preferable approach in many cases.[331]

Preoperative chemotherapy can greatly reduce the size, vascularity, and friability of the tumor, facilitating resection and decreasing the risk of intraoperative tumor rupture.[332] Analysis of the 53 patients with nonmetastatic chest wall primaries treated on the first intergroup Ewing's Sarcoma Study (POG/CCG) demonstrated a decreased incidence of residual tumor in those patients resected after induction chemotherapy, in contrast to those who underwent resections before treatment with chemotherapy.[333] Current practice mandates the addition of radiotherapy for all patients with microscopic or gross residual disease after resection. Since surgical outcome was improved in patients receiving preoperative chemotherapy, they were less likely to require postoperative chest wall radiotherapy with its well-established risks of cardiac and pulmonary damage. As noted previously, the inclusion of 12 to 15 weeks of systemic chemotherapy before introduction of local control measures has become standard practice, regardless of tumor size, location, or stage.

Radiation Therapy

Radiation responsiveness was one of the cardinal diagnostic features of the bone tumor first described by Ewing in 1921.[304] Unfortunately, the long-term survival rate of patients with

Ewing's sarcoma following treatment with local radiation alone was only 9%. The vast majority of these patients ultimately succumbed to metastatic disease, suggesting the presence of occult metastatic tumor foci in most affected children.[51] These findings presaged the routine inclusion of systemic chemotherapy in the treatment of this disease, leading to a marked improvement in survival over the past three decades.

Local control of Ewing's sarcoma with radiation is dependent on the delivery of a sufficient dose of irradiation to an adequate volume of tissue. Both the requisite minimum dose and the optimal treatment volume continue to be debated. Although dose-response information is limited for modern studies that employ adjuvant chemotherapy, local control rates have been fairly similar, ranging from 75% to 90% at radiation doses varying from 45 to 65 Gy.[334]

Local control rates have improved with the introduction of adjuvant chemotherapy. Chan and colleagues[505] reported local tumor recurrence in only 2.8% of patients treated with 60 Gy and adjuvant chemotherapy. Local disease recurrence was identified in 33.3% of patients who received identical local irradiation, but no adjuvant chemotherapy.

The Intergroup Ewing's Sarcoma Study (IESS) examined the relation of primary tumor site, radiation therapy dose, treatment volume, and adjuvant chemotherapy regimen to local tumor control. Local tumor recurrence occurred in 22.6% of patients with primary tumors in the humerus, 15.3% of those with tumors originating in the pelvis, 10.3% of patients with tibial primaries, and 6.7% of those whose tumor originated in the femur. A dose-response relationship was not apparent when local control was evaluated in patients who had received treatment to an adequate volume.[335]

Minor or major violations of radiation therapy technique, resulting in treatment of an insufficient volume, yielded inferior local control rates among patients who did not receive doxorubicin as part of the adjuvant chemotherapy program.[335] Local recurrence occurred in 21.4% of patients who had a margin of less than 5 cm of normal tissue included within the treatment volume. This compared with 7.9% of patients who had a margin of 5 or more centimeters of normal tissue within the treatment volume.[336] There was no improvement of the local control rate in patients with a pelvic primary tumor from the addition of doxorubicin when an adequate volume of tissue was irradiated.[337]

Local control percentages that are derived from series in which the majority of patients who died of disease did not have an autopsy may overestimate the frequency of local control.[338]

Studies from the National Cancer Institute confirmed the importance of autopsy examination for the identification of locally recurrent Ewing's sarcoma. Telles and colleagues identified recurrent or persistent tumor at the primary site in 13 of 20 patients at autopsy.[339] Tepper and coworkers reported that local tumor recurrence was clinically apparent in 5 of 20 autopsied patients, but was identified histologically in an additional 6 of 20 patients.[340] Since many of these patients had widespread metastatic disease, the possibility that the primary tumor site was reseeded with tumor cells derived from metastatic disease cannot be excluded. These results suggest that local failure rates in irradiated patients may be higher than suggested by the clinical determination of locally recurrent tumor.

Improved local control of tumor with irradiation followed the identification of a target volume encompassing the entire medullary cavity to moderately high-dose levels.[341,342] Suit summarized the experience of the 1950s and 1960s in recommending irradiation to the entire involved bone with a higher dose boost to the primary tumor site, noting few instances of marginal or distant intramedullary recurrence with such treatment.[343]

Assessment of the primary target volume requires detailed attention to both intraosseous and adjacent soft tissue tumor extent. Prior treatment recommendations included a 3- to 5-cm margin beyond the known soft tissue extension and inclusion of the entire intramedullary cavity. The radiation therapy results of IESS-I demonstrated an overall increase in local recurrence with fields that had not included the opposite epiphysis.[337] Although local failure increased from 7% to 20% with marginal or inadequate treatment fields, the differences were not statistically significant. Subsequent studies have reported comparable irradiation results using treatment techniques that have not included the opposite epiphysis.[326,344]

The results of the German Cooperative Ewing Sarcoma Study indicated an excessive rate of local recurrence attributed to poor quality control for radiation therapy. Protocol modifications, which included central planning for radiation therapy, diminished the frequency of local treatment failure.[344,345]

Local or tailored fields encompassing the primary tumor with a 3- to 5-cm margin, rather than treatment of the entire bone, have been evaluated.[346,347] Marcus et al. reported excellent local control using tailored fields, noting the ability to spare a component of the long bones in tumors less than 8 cm in diameter, while frequently requiring whole bone irradiation to achieve a 4-cm margin around larger tumors.[347]

The POG prospectively evaluated whole bone (conventional) irradiation compared with tailored treatment fields, ultimately collapsing a planned randomized study to a single arm trial using only tailored fields. A published analysis of this trial supports the efficacy of more limited treatment volume as defined by prechemotherapy tumor extent.[291] There was no difference in local control rates between patients receiving whole bone versus involved field radiation. This more tailored field has become the standard strategy used in the most recent CCG and POG Ewing's sarcoma trials.

The data available in the literature, and those accumulated by the IESS, have not demonstrated a strong relationship between the radiation dose and the local control rate when doses greater than 40 Gy were employed. Radiation doses greater than 60 Gy did not appear to significantly increase the local control rate and were associated with considerable long-term morbidity. Although the available data did not suggest that doses exceeding 40 Gy were essential for adequate local control rates in patients treated with adjuvant chemotherapy, comparisons between this dose and higher doses should be conducted in controlled trials. The current standard for the open POG and CCG trial is 55.8 Gy for gross and 45 Gy for microscopic residual disease.

The comparable outcome achieved with smaller, tailored fields is most provocative when considered in the context of the late sequelae of radiation therapy. The risk of secondary sarcomas arising in irradiated bone is variously reported as ranging from 5% to 10% at 20 years from diagnosis. Although no clear therapeutic advantage can be attributed to radiation doses in excess of 60 Gy, analysis of the long-term outcome in patients treated with doses greater than or equal to 60 Gy demonstrated an unacceptable excess risk of secondary bone sarcomas. In marked contrast to the late complications seen in patients receiving very high-dose radiation, the risk of developing a secondary bone tumor in the irradiated field was negligible at doses below 48 Gy.[348]

Chemotherapy

The availability of chemotherapeutic agents active against macroscopic deposits of Ewing's sarcoma suggested that improved relapse-free survival rates might be achieved with the use of these agents in patients with microscopic residual disease.

In 1973, the IESS initiated a trial (IESS-I) to evaluate the potential additional benefit of adding doxorubicin and prophylactic whole lung irradiation to standard treatment of patients with nonmetastatic Ewing's sarcoma with vincristine, dactinomycin, and cyclophosphamide. The patients treated with the four-drug regimen that included doxorubicin had superior relapse-free survival.[349,350] In a subsequent study (IESS-II), the efficacy of administration of high-dose (1400 mg/m^2) cyclophosphamide every 6 weeks was compared with administration of cyclophosphamide (500 mg/m^2) weekly for 6 weeks. The regimen that included high-dose cyclophosphamide also included a higher dose of doxorubicin (75 mg/m^2) than did the weekly cyclophosphamide schema. The 5-year relapse-free survival was 73% for the high-dose cyclophosphamide, high-dose doxorubicin regimen, compared with 56% for the weekly cyclophosphamide regimen ($P = .03$),[351] a finding supported by the analysis by Smith and colleagues.[352]

The POG and CCG completed an intergroup study comparing the combination of vincristine, doxorubicin, cyclophosphamide, and dactinomycin to the combination of these four drugs plus ifosfamide and etoposide. The 5-year event-free survival was 68% for those who received the six-drug regimen, compared with 52% for those who received the four-drug regimen ($P = .0005$).[353] Similar improvements in survival with the addition of ifosfamide have been reported in studies by the National Cancer Institute and multiple European cooperative groups.[354–356]

Standard chemotherapy for nonmetastatic disease currently consists of a five-drug regimen including the three-drug combination of vincristine, doxorubicin, and cyclophosphamide, alternating with the two-drug combination of ifosfamide and etoposide for a total of 48 weeks. The intergroup POG/CCG study for nonmetastatic Ewing's sarcoma compared this 48-week five-drug combination with a dose-intensified 30-week schedule employing the same agents at identical cumulative doses. The experimental arm in this study increased the dose intensity of alkylating agents by 25%. Preliminary statistical analysis of this study reveals no evidence of improved event-free survival with the dose-intensified regimen.[357] Although the Kaplan-Meier plots for event-free survival may yet diverge, current data from this randomized study suggest that new treatment strategies will be required if further improvements in survival are to be achieved.

In contrast to the improvement in survival for nonmetastatic patients treated with the addition of ifosfamide and etoposide, no comparable benefit could be demonstrated for metastatic patients. Previous studies, however, had shown improved survival with the addition of radiation to metastatic sites of disease. Patients with hematogenous metastases entered on IESS-II were treated with irradiation to the primary tumor, in addition to whole lung radiation (18 Gy) for patients with pulmonary metastases and local bone irradiation for bone metastases. This strategy yielded a progression-free survival of 39%, demonstrating that some patients with hematogenous metastases can be successfully treated.[358]

Several groups have explored the feasibility and efficacy of maximally dose intensive chemotherapy regimens in combination with total body irradiation and peripheral blood stem cell rescue in an effort to improve the prognosis for high-risk patients.[359–364] Analysis of these studies is complicated by the nonstandardized inclusion of both metastatic and nonmetastatic patients in some of the high-risk cohorts. One study reported a 3-year relapse-free survival of 43% following megatherapy with chemotherapy, total body irradiation and stem cell rescue.[365] Unfortunately, longer follow-up of this cohort revealed a disappointing decline in event-free survival to 27%.[366] Another study reported a 6-year event-free survival of 34% with similar high-dose chemoradiotherapy.[367] None of these results is clearly superior to the outcome reported for similar patients treated on IESS-II without intensive chemotherapy or total body irradiation. While the early response data from several of these dose-intensive regimens appears promising, their small size and short follow-up mandate a guarded approach to their therapeutic potential. Further substantial improvements in survival for both metastatic and nonmetastatic patients will require identification of new non–cross-resistant cytotoxic agents and translation of our growing understanding of the unique molecular derangements of this disease into targeted biologic therapies.[368]

PROGNOSTIC FACTORS

Historically, the prognosis for children and young adults with Ewing's family tumors has been assessed based on tumor size, location, and extent. Aside from the poor prognosis associated with metastatic disease, large tumor size (greater than 8 cm in diameter) and volume (greater than 100 mL) have correlated with adverse outcome. Children with nonmetastatic pelvic primary sites also have a poorer prognosis than children with extremity primaries, although this difference may be related to the larger size and more difficult resectability of pelvic tumors. High serum lactate dehydrogenase levels at diagnosis have been shown to predict a poorer prognosis in several studies.

Although not true prognostic factors assessable at the time of diagnosis, radiographic and histologic response to initial chemotherapy appear to be strong predictors of treatment outcome. Poor histologic response correlates with a poor prognosis, while complete or near complete tumor necrosis strongly correlates with good outcome, with a 5-year event-free survival of 84% to 95%.[369,370] Researchers in Vienna and New York have independently identified the type of EWS-FLI1 fusion transcript as a strong predictor of outcome in nonmetastatic patients. Both studies reported remarkably congruent results, with a predicted 5-year event-free survival of approximately 70% for type 1 transcripts versus 20% for all other types of fusion transcripts.[311,312] Nearly two-thirds of all patients in both studies were found to have type 1 fusion transcripts. Although the prognostic significance of this finding appears to be substantial, these findings must be prospectively validated before they are used to stratify patients for therapeutic purposes. All upcoming north American pediatric cooperative group studies conducted by the Children's Oncology Group (POG/CCG) will require submission of diagnostic tissue for molecular analyses that will include determination of EWS-FLI1 gene rearrangement status.

PRIMARY HEPATIC TUMORS

EPIDEMIOLOGY AND GENETICS

Approximately 60% to 70% of all primary liver tumors in children are malignant, with hepatoblastoma and hepatocellular carcinoma (HCC) representing the vast majority of malignancies arising in this location. Hemangiomas and hamartomas constitute the majority of nonmalignant liver tumors in the pediatric population.[371]

Hepatoblastoma accounts for slightly more than one-half of hepatic malignancies, occurring at an annual rate of 1.3 cases per 1 million children less than 15 years of age. In contrast, HCC occurs less frequently in children, accounting for one-third of all malignant hepatic tumors, with an annual incidence of 0.4 cases per 1 million.[27] In addition to the significant difference in incidence, hepatoblastoma and HCC are distinguished by age at diagnosis. Hepatoblastoma tends to affect young children, with a median age at diagnosis of 1 year. HCC is typically identified in older children, with a median age of 12 years. Both tumors demonstrate a male predominance.[372]

Children diagnosed with hepatoblastoma have had additional anomalies, including hemihypertrophy, Meckel's diverticulum, congenital absence of the kidney, congenital absence of the adrenal gland, and umbilical hernia.[371] Infants and children with incomplete or complete forms of the Beckwith-Wiedemann syndrome have an increased risk of developing hepatoblastoma, suggesting a linkage between loss of heterozygosity at chromosome 11p15.5 and the pathogenesis of both diseases.[373] Familial adenomatous polyposis has been identified in the mothers and maternal relatives of several patients with hepatoblastoma.[374] The risk of hepatoblastoma arising in children from kindreds with the adenomatous polyposis coli (APC) gene on the long arm of chromosome 5 is 1000 to 2000 times higher than the risk in sporadic cases with no family history of familial adenomatous polyposis.[375] Other karyotypic abnormalities associated with the pathogenesis of hepatoblastoma include trisomy 1 or 1q,[376] trisomy 2 or 2q, and trisomy of chromosome 20.[377] In addition to these chromosomal derangements, children with a history of prematurity and very low birth weight appear to be at increased risk for hepatoblastoma.[378,379] In a study based on the Japanese Children's Cancer Registry, hepatoblastoma accounted for 58% of the cancer diagnoses in children with a history of extremely low birth weight (less than 1000 g).[378] The authors suggest that this association points to a combination of aberrant genetic endowments and prenatal events or exposures that contribute to disruptions in normal organogenesis, culminating in transformation of hepatocytes.

HCC is strongly associated with infection with hepatitis B virus, both in the presence and absence of pathologic evidence of cirrhosis in nontumorous hepatic tissue. Hepatitis B virus can be acquired via vertical transmission from seropositive mothers or through exposure to contaminated blood products.[380,381] Several studies have documented a near 100% rate of seropositivity for HBsAg in children who develop HCC.[382] Efforts to reduce the incidence of hepatitis B infection with universal hepatitis B vaccination in Taiwan have produced a corresponding decrease in the risk of developing HCC.[380–382]

In addition to the association with hepatitis B, HCC has been diagnosed in pediatric patients with several other underlying diseases, including tyrosinemia, galactosemia, biliary atresia, progressive familial cholestatic cirrhosis, giant cell hepatitis of infancy, Fanconi's anemia, type I glycogen storage disease, hepatic glycogenosis with Fanconi's syndrome, α_1-antitrypsin deficiency (MZ phenotype), Soto's syndrome, and neurofibromatosis.[51,383] Hemochromatosis has not been associated with HCC in pediatric patients, although it is frequently associated with this disease in adult populations. Determinations of iron reserves, as estimated by serum iron, unsaturated iron-binding capacity, and serum ferritin, might clarify the relationship between hemochromatosis and HCC in children.[384,385]

PATHOLOGY

Hepatoblastoma may be divided into two broad histologic subsets of uncertain prognostic significance. The pure epithelial type consists of either fetal or embryonal elements or a combination of both cell types. Alternatively, the tumor may consist of a mixture of epithelial cells with mesenchymal elements.[386] Pure fetal histology is prognostically favorable in patients with completely resected hepatoblastoma.[387] Hepatoblastoma tends to occupy a single site within the liver, most commonly arising in the right lobe.

Two types of HCC are frequently recognized in pediatric patients: microtrabecular and fibrolamellar.[388,389] The fibrolamellar histology is most commonly seen in older children and young adults. In contrast to hepatoblastoma, HCC is often multicentric at diagnosis, substantially limiting the feasibility of complete resection.[372]

CLINICAL PRESENTATION

Infants and children with hepatoblastoma are most frequently identified by the discovery of an abdominal mass or abdominal distention. Symptoms such as weight loss, anorexia, or fever may also be present, although jaundice is infrequent. A rare but interesting presentation of patients with hepatoblastoma occurs in young boys with isosexual precocious puberty due to production of human chorionic gonadotropin (HCG) by the tumor cells.[390]

The presenting physical findings in children with HCC are quite similar to the characteristic features of hepatoblastoma. Children with HCC typically present with an abdominal mass or abdominal distention. Abdominal pain, anorexia, and weight loss are less frequent complaints. Jaundice is infrequently present at the time of diagnosis, although it is a more common finding in HCC than hepatoblastoma. Occasionally, a patient with HCC presents with acute abdominal pain due to tumor rupture, with intraabdominal hemorrhage.[51]

EVALUATION AND STAGING

The history of pediatric patients suspected of having a malignant hepatic tumor should be reviewed for any history of jaundice or hepatitis. Laboratory data obtained in the perinatal period for the evaluation of hyperbilirubinemia should be reviewed. The maternal prenatal history should be evaluated for the use of steroidal hormones. Previous exposures to hepatotoxic agents should be recorded. The family history should be reviewed for prior cases of hepatic or biliary disease in siblings or parents.

The physical examination may reveal a solitary or multiple hepatic nodules. The presence of dilated collateral vessels on the anterior thorax and abdomen should be noted. Hemihypertrophy or stigmata of the Beckwith-Wiedemann syndrome, such as macroglossia or omphalocele, may be present.

Laboratory evaluation should include a complete blood count, white blood cell differential, tests of renal and hepatic function, and a urinalysis. The serum levels of total bilirubin, alkaline phosphatase, and glutamic-oxaloacetic acid transaminase are not generally useful for the differential diagnosis of malignant hepatic tumors in children.

The serum level of AFP is increased in approximately 90% of patients with hepatoblastoma[391,392] and 78% of adult patients with HCC. The increase of AFP in 51% of white and 81% of African American patients with HCC suggests the presence of ethnic variability in the production of this protein by malignant hepatocytes.[393] Once the diagnosis of hepatocellular carcinoma is established, additional studies should include hepatitis B surface antigen, hepatitis B antibody, serum iron, total iron-binding capacity, serum ferritin, and α_1-antitrypsin phenotyping. The serum level of HCG should be determined if the clinical presentation included precocious puberty. Several authors reported the excretion of increased amounts of cystathionine in the urine of patients with hepatoblastoma.[394] This finding has also been reported in patients with neuroblastoma, decreasing the utility of this determination for the differential diagnosis of hepatomegaly.

Abdominal radiographic examination may demonstrate the presence of a homogeneous density in the upper abdomen. Malignant hepatic tumors are rarely calcified.[395]

Abdominal ultrasonography demonstrates the presence and extent of a solid mass. Sonography assesses both kidneys and the inferior vena cava, providing information useful for differential diagnosis and surgical management. The proximal extent of tumor thrombus within the inferior vena cava may be determined by echocardiography or cardiac angiography.

A radionuclide liver and spleen scan may demonstrate solitary or multiple defects in the liver. Transient, early perfusion of the defect is frequently observed in hepatic adenomas, hepatoblastomas, and HCCs. Persistent perfusion is found in hepatic hemangiomas and hepatic adenomas.[396]

Pulmonary metastases are identified on plain chest radiography in approximately 10% of patients with hepatoblastoma[391] and HCC.[389] The additional yield of CT in pediatric patients with hepatoblastoma or HCC has not been evaluated.

The grouping system employed in the therapeutic studies of children with malignant hepatic tumors conducted by the CCG and POG segregates patients according to the resectability of the primary tumor, a criterion that may vary among treatment centers. This staging system also accounts for the presence of lymph node or hematogenous metastases (Table 44.2-10).[397]

TABLE 44.2-10. Clinical Staging System for Childhood Hepatic Tumors

Stage	*Description*
Stage I	Patient had complete resection of tumor by wedge resection, lobectomy, or extended lobectomy, as the initial procedure.
Stage II	Patient has microscopic residual disease after surgical resection. There is no evidence of regional lymph node involvement by tumor. There was no spillage of tumor.
Stage III	Gross residual disease or regional lymph node involvement by tumor or tumor spilled.
A	Regional lymph node involvement by tumor or tumor spill, but primary tumor completely resected.
B	Gross tumor not completely resected.
Stage IV	Distant metastases are present.
A	Primary tumor completely resected.
B	Primary tumor not completely resected.

TREATMENT

Surgery

Resection is the cornerstone of treatment for hepatoblastoma and HCC. Long-term survival is rare for patients who have not undergone a successful resection.[397] Hepatoblastoma is generally unifocal, arising at one site within the liver parenchyma, whereas HCC is frequently multifocal. HCC has an invasive pattern of spread across anatomic planes and is generally unresponsive to current forms of chemotherapy.[398] Complete resection of HCC is frequently difficult due to its multifocality and invasiveness. Approximately one-half of all hepatoblastomas are resectable at initial presentation, whereas only 30% of HCCs can be fully resected at diagnosis.[371]

The resectability of a primary liver tumor is determined by its anatomic location within the liver and by its size. Surgical considerations are complex and best addressed by surgeons intimately familiar with hepatic anatomy and resection. For successful resection, perfusion and drainage for an anatomic segment of the liver must be preserved. The liver lobes are perfused by the two divisions of the hepatic artery and the portal vein, with one branch to each lobe. The left and right lobes are divided along a plane between the bed of the gallbladder and the anterior aspect of the vena cava. The liver is drained by three veins into the vena cava at the most superior aspect of the liver. The right hepatic vein drains the major portion of the right lobe (the posterior segment and a portion of the anterior segment of the lobe).[399] The middle hepatic vein, which courses along the plane anterior to the vena cava between the right and left lobes, drains one-third of the liver (a large portion of the anterior segment of the right lobe and all of the medial segment of the left lobe). The left hepatic vein, arising from a short common trunk with the middle vein in 50% of cases, travels along the umbilical fissure of the liver and primarily drains the lateral segment of the left lobe. In a right or left lobectomy, the left or right branches of the hepatic artery and portal vein are preserved, along with the left and middle or right and middle hepatic veins. In an extended right or left hepatectomy (also referred to as a *trisegmentectomy*), the same inflow vessels are removed, along with the middle and left or right hepatic veins. A much greater portion of the hepatic parenchyma is removed in this type of resection (Fig. 44.2-7).

Radiographic imaging before surgical exploration is critical to the surgeon. It defines the critical relationship between the tumor and associated vasculature. Historically, most children underwent angiography to facilitate surgical planning before hepatic resection. In view of the remarkable anatomic detail afforded by current radiographic techniques including MRI and spiral CT, angiography is less frequently required.[400] Ulti-

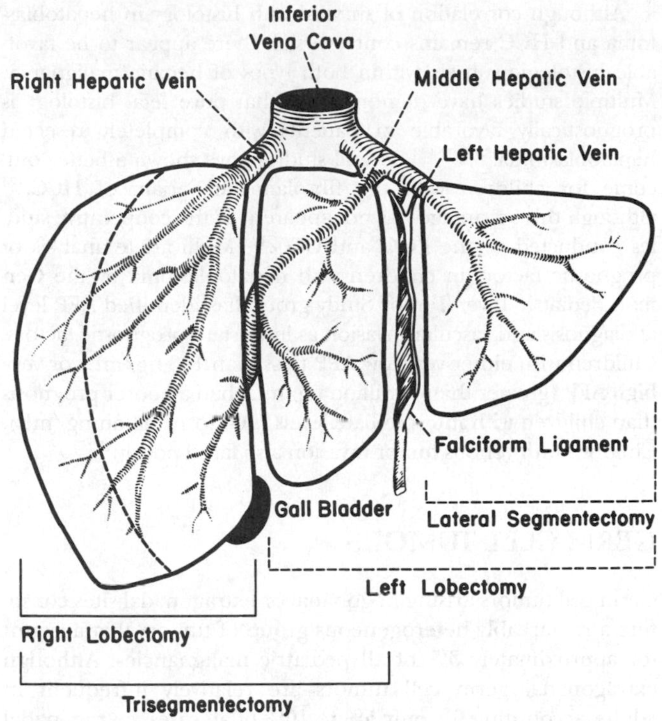

FIGURE 44.2-7. Relation between hepatic anatomy and nomenclature for various types of hepatic resection. (From Iwatsuki S, Starzl TE. Hepatectomy in children. *Int Adv Surg Oncol* 1982;5:163, with permission.)

mately, the feasibility of resection can only be determined by direct surgical exploration. When angiography is not performed, the surgeon must be aware of the frequent anomalies of the hepatic artery. The right hepatic artery may arise from the superior mesenteric artery, while the left hepatic artery may arise from the celiac axis. These variations, if present, must be identified before division of any vessels in the hepatic porta. Factors that render a liver tumor unresectable include involvement of both lobes of the liver and lymph node involvement in the porta hepatis or mediastinum. Additional features that preclude resection include direct extension into the inferior vena cava, a central lesion that involves both the left and right hepatic arteries or the portal vein, or lesions that involve all branches of the hepatic vein.

A large hepatoblastoma grossly distorts the normal anatomy and relationships of the vessels. Hepatoblastoma, in contrast with HCC, does not invade surrounding liver segments as much as it distorts them. It is as if a balloon is placed within the liver parenchyma and is progressively inflated. The vessels to the uninvolved segments may be tightly drawn over a massively enlarged segment, making safe dissection and preservation difficult. As the tumor responds to chemotherapy, it does not regress from areas of involvement, although its decreased volume permits identification of the normal uninvolved segments. Treatment with chemotherapy before definitive surgery has permitted complete resections in children whose hepatoblastomas were initially deemed unresectable.[101,402] Regrettably, HCC has been much less responsive to chemotherapy, limiting the effectiveness of preoperative pharmacologic intervention. When feasible, aggressive attempts at initial resection of HCC should be pursued.

Although complications from hepatectomy persist, perioperative mortality has significantly decreased. Bile leaks, strictures, subphrenic or subhepatic abscesses, and intraoperative hemorrhage are the most frequent complications. Major postoperative complications have occurred more frequently in children undergoing resection after chemotherapy (25%) than in children resected at presentation (8%).[403] In a series published by King et al. in 1991, the increased frequency of complications in the group resected following chemotherapy did not appear to be explained by disproportionate numbers of more extensive resections being performed in that subset. The distribution between lobectomies and trisegmentectomies was similar for children undergoing primary resections and resections following several course of induction chemotherapy.[403]

Hepatic transplantation has been used by several centers for children with unresectable liver tumors, with a survival rate of 50.0% to 87.5% reported for children with hepatoblastoma.[404,405] Success with this treatment approach for patients with hepatocellular carcinoma has been extremely limited and is difficult to justify. Disease must be limited to the liver for efforts to be successful. Lymph node involvement is a contraindication for efforts at resection and transplantation.

Cryoablation or radiofrequency ablation of hepatic malignancies has been increasingly used in adults, particularly for metastatic lesions in the liver.[406] While these techniques have been employed in treatment of recurrent disease, their overall role in treatment of pediatric neoplasms remains to be defined.

Long-term evaluation of infants and children following hepatic resection has demonstrated normal synthetic and degradative function of the liver. Liver volumes assessed by MRI are near normal, despite prior anatomic lobectomies or trisegmentectomies. Sequential studies have shown that hepatic volumes continue to increase as the children grow following completion of their treatment.[407]

Radiation Therapy

Radiation therapy has a limited role in the treatment of hepatoblastoma or HCC. Generally, combination chemotherapy is given preoperatively to patients with large, unresectable tumors. Postoperative radiation therapy may be valuable in the treatment of children with residual disease following resection.[408] Generally, doses of 25 to 40 Gy are recommended for treatment of limited volumes.

Chemotherapy

Following initial biopsy, combination chemotherapy has been administered to children with malignant hepatic tumors to facilitate subsequent surgical excision. In addition to its role in reducing the size of tumors before attempted resections, chemotherapy has been employed as a postoperative adjuvant following complete excision of the primary tumor. Initially reported by single institutions,[409–413] these results led to the design of much larger cooperative group trials of combination chemotherapy in children with hepatoblastoma and HCC.

Evans and coworkers reported the results of sequential studies conducted by two pediatric cooperative groups in patients with malignant hepatic tumors. Patients with hepatoblastoma and HCC were evaluated together. Those patients with completely resected disease (group 1) entered on the first study received no therapy following surgery. Those entered on the second study received adjuvant chemotherapy consisting of doxorubicin, cyclophosphamide, vincristine, and 5-fluorouracil. Comparison of these sequential studies demonstrated a significant survival advantage for those patients who received adjuvant chemotherapy compared with patients treated only with surgery.[397]

Based on pilot data that demonstrated the activity of the combination of doxorubicin and cisplatin[408] and of the combination of cisplatin, vincristine, and 5-fluorouracil[414] in patients with malignant liver tumors, the CCG and POG conducted a randomized comparison of these two combinations. The results of this trial demonstrated that the two combinations produced similar relapse-free and overall survival percentages within stages. The combination of cisplatin, vincristine, and 5-fluorouracil produced substantially less severe myelosuppression, less need for prolonged hyperalimentation, and fewer toxic deaths. Event-free survival rates for patients treated with the three-drug regimen were 85% for stage I, 100% for stage II, 62% for stage III, and 23% for stage IV.[415] Similar results have been reported by investigators in Toronto,[416] Japan,[417] and Germany.[418] These studies have consistently demonstrated that a substantial number of initially unresectable tumors can be surgically removed at second exploration following treatment with variations on either of the two drug combinations.[403,419] Despite the remarkable similarity in outcomes between these various studies, there was a significant difference in survival for children who underwent initial complete resection, corresponding to postoperative management. The Toronto group reported a 100% event-free survival for children with complete resections treated with postoperative chemotherapy, versus 72% survival for a similar group of children on the POG/CCG study who received no chemotherapy following definitive surgery.[416] Although the numbers in the comparison groups are small, the more favorable outcome with inclusion of chemotherapy suggests that this approach should be prospectively examined.

Japanese investigators have reported successful application of transarterial chemoembolization using cisplatinum and doxorubicin in combination with iodized oil in treatment of a small number of children with inoperable hepatoblastoma.[420] Although the results of this limited series are provocative, the role of this more invasive technique is uncertain given the efficacy of systemic, intravenous administration of the same chemotherapeutic agents.

PROGNOSIS

For both hepatoblastoma and HCC, resectability of the primary tumor and disease extent at diagnosis remain the strongest predictors of survival. Prospects for long-term survival are extremely poor for both histologies in cases of widely metastatic disease. Despite aggressive efforts at surgical management of HCC, long-term survival remains dismal even for patients with fully resected tumors. A North American Pediatric Cooperative Group study demonstrated only 13% survival for children with totally resected HCC.[421] This outcome sharply contrasts with the good survival documented for children with localized, completely resected hepatoblastoma, as described previously (see Surgery, earlier in this chapter).

Although correlation of survival with histology in hepatoblastoma and HCC remains controversial, there appear to be favorable histologic subsets within both types of hepatic malignancy. Multiple studies have demonstrated that pure fetal histology is prognostically favorable in patients with completely resected hepatoblastoma.[387,422,423] Several studies have shown a better outcome for children with the fibrolamellar variant of HCC,[424] although this advantage was not apparent in the cooperative studies conducted by the POG and CCG.[423] Multivariate analysis of prognostic factors in children with hepatoblastoma by the German Pediatric Liver Tumor Study group has identified AFP level at diagnosis and vascular invasion as important prognostic factors. Children with either very low AFP (less than 100 ng/mL) or very high AFP (greater than 1 million ng/mL) had a poorer prognosis than children with intermediate levels (100 to 1 million ng/mL). Children with venous tumor invasion also fared poorly.[422]

GERM CELL TUMORS

Germ cell tumors arising in gonadal or extragonadal sites constitute a remarkably heterogeneous group of tumors that account for approximately 3% of all pediatric malignancies. Although extragonadal germ cell tumors are relatively infrequent in adults, accounting for only 5% to 10% of all cases, extragonadal tumors make up nearly two-thirds of all germ cell tumors in children.[425] The sacrococcygeal region represents the most common site for germ cell tumors in children, constituting 40% of all childhood germ cell tumors,[426] and 78% of all extragonadal disease.[427] Less commonly, extragonadal disease arises in the mediastinum, retroperitoneum, vagina, and pineal region. Biologic behavior among this diverse grouping of tumors varies from the benign mature teratoma to the highly malignant embryonal carcinoma and choriocarcinoma. Fortunately, the introduction of platinum-based chemotherapy by Einhorn and Donahue in the 1970s has greatly improved survival for most children affected by these highly chemosensitive tumors[428] (Table 44.2-11).

EMBRYOLOGY

Primordial germ cells arise in the embryonic yolk sac endoderm. These cells migrate through the wall of the midgut to the genital ridge at 4 to 5 weeks' gestation. Migration along this paravertebral gonadal ridge proceeds in a caudal to cranial direction. Arrested migration of these germ cells along this pathway has been proposed as an explanation for the near midline location of most extragonadal germ cell tumors, including the sacrococcygeal region, retroperitoneum, mediastinum, and intracranial sites, which primarily consist of the pineal and suprasellar regions.[425,427,429]

PATHOLOGY

Pediatric germ cell tumors include an enormously diverse array of histologies. The majority of extragonadal tumors arising in infancy are benign teratomas. Similarly, most ovarian germ cell tumors are benign lesions. In contrast, the vast majority of germ cell tumors developing in the testis contain malignant yolk sac elements. While many of these tumors contain a mixture of benign and malignant elements, their clinical behavior and therapeutic management are determined by the most

TABLE 44.2-11. Relative Incidence According to Age and Pathology

Site	Relative Incidence (%)	Age	Pathology
Sacrococcyx	35	Neonate	Teratoma: mature 65%, immature 5%, malignant 10–30%
Ovary	25	Early teens	Teratoma: mature 65%, immature 5%, malignant 30% (pure yolk sac 30%, mixed 30%)
Testis	20	Infant and adolescent	Teratoma: mature 20%, malignant 80% (yolk sac 90%, germinoma 10%, embryonal carcinoma 1–5%)
Cranium	5	Child	Germinoma: 20–50%, embryonal carcinoma 20–50%, mature teratomas 20–30%
Mediastinum	5	Adolescent	Teratoma: mature 60%, mixed 20%, embryonal carcinoma 20%
Retroperitoneum	5	Infant	Teratoma: mature or immature, rarely malignant
Head and neck	3	Infant and neonate	Usually mature teratoma, immature rarely malignant
Vagina	2	Infant	Usually yolk sac

(From ref. 429, with permission.)

malignant component identified on extensive sectioning.[427] This section reviews the various histopathologic subtypes of germ cell tumors most frequently seen in children.

TERATOMA

Teratomas contain elements derived from more than one of the three primary germ layers (ectoderm, mesoderm, entoderm), frequently arranged in a haphazard manner. The tissues are immature to well differentiated and foreign to the anatomic site. Mature teratomas are either cystic or solid, although the cystic presentation predominates in gonadal sites. Immature teratomas are graded according to the amount of immature tissue present on light microscopic assessment of sampled tissue. Grade 1 immature teratomas have neuroepithelium or other immature elements limited to only one low-power field per slide. Grade 3 immature teratomas contain abundant immature tissue that is identifiable on greater than or equal to four low-power fields per slide.[430] Nearly all mature teratomas are diploid with normal karyotypes. In contrast, chromosomal derangements are frequently identified in immature teratomas. Ploidy may correlate with clinical behavior in immature ovarian teratomas. Grade 1 and 2 immature teratomas are typically diploid, whereas grade 3 tumors are often aneuploid.[431]

YOLK SAC TUMOR (ENDODERMAL SINUS TUMOR)

Intracellular and intercellular hyaline droplets are present in typical yolk sac tumors. This material is periodic acid–Schiff-positive and resists digestion with diastase. Several groups of investigators have shown that these droplets contain AFP as well as other proteins.[51,432] Teilum and colleagues suggested that the presence of AFP in these tumors supported the theory that such tumors contained or originated from the yolk sac endoderm.[433]

The polyvesicular vitelline tumor is a variant of the yolk sac tumor that is composed predominantly of cystic structures.[434,435] Such evidence of differentiation has been associated with a more favorable prognosis for patients with this histologic subtype of yolk sac tumor.

A cytogenetic study of childhood endodermal sinus tumors employing fluorescent *in situ* hybridization demonstrated deletions of the distal portion of the short arm of chromosome 1 (1p36) in eight of ten cases. This deletion maps to the same locus identified in neuroblastoma, another embryonal malignancy that typically affects young children.[436] The prognostic importance of this finding remains uncertain. Several putative tumor suppressor genes have been mapped within or adjacent to this locus, however, suggesting a role of this deletion in the pathogenesis of these tumors.

EMBRYONAL CARCINOMA

Embryonal carcinoma is composed of cells that resemble epithelial cells. There is considerable variation in their size, shape, and arrangement. They may be large and pleomorphic without distinct cell borders. The cytoplasm may be homogeneously amphophilic or vacuolated. The nuclei are irregular, oval, or round, with an irregular and coarse nuclear membrane, and one or more large nucleoli. The cells may occur as solid sheets. Frequently, small or large acinar, tubular, and papillary structures are formed. Hemorrhage and necrosis are frequent.[437]

SEMINOMA

Seminomas arising outside the testis are referred to as germinomas or dysgerminomas (ovarian). Typical seminoma is composed of uniform cells supported by a delicate connective tissue stroma. Characteristically, the seminoma cell is large, polyhedral, or round, with a distinct cell border. It has clear or granular cytoplasm and a large, centrally located, spherical hyperchromatic nucleus, an irregular nuclear membrane, distinct and granular chromatin distribution, and one or two basophilic nucleoli. Tumor giant cells may be seen. Lymphocytic infiltration is present in most seminomas, with a granulomatous reaction identifiable in approximately one-half of cases.[437] As is commonly found in adult testicular tumors, isochrome 12p (two copies of the short arm of chromosome 12) is frequently identified in adolescent testicular germinomas.[438,439] This chromosomal abnormality is rarely seen in malignant testicular tumors of infancy in which yolk sac tumor is the predominant histology.

CHORIOCARCINOMA

Choriocarcinoma consists of two distinct cell types: syncytiotrophoblast and cytotrophoblast. The syncytiotrophoblast is a large, multinucleated cell with many hyperchromatic, irregular nuclei and cytoplasm usually eosinophilic or amphophilic. Cytotrophoblast cells are medium sized and closely packed with clear cytoplasm, distinct cell borders, and a single, uniform, moderate-sized vesicular nucleus.[437]

TERATOCARCINOMA

Teratocarcinomas contain derivatives of more than one of the three primary germ cell layers (entoderm, mesoderm, ectoderm) consistent with the diagnosis of teratoma, and areas of embryonal carcinoma. In addition, areas of seminoma, endodermal sinus tumor, and choriocarcinoma may be identified within the tumor.[437]

LABORATORY MARKERS

AFP and the β subunit of HCG (β-HCG) are oncofetoproteins that are found at elevated serum levels in association with a variety of germ cell tumors. These proteins are clinically useful both as diagnostic tools and in surveillance of children on or off treatment for tumors that secrete these markers. AFP is a glycoprotein that is produced in the liver, gastrointestinal tract, and yolk sac of the human fetus. The serum concentration of AFP reaches a maximum at 13 weeks of gestation.[440] It is readily detectable at birth, when high physiologic levels confound its diagnostic utility in infants with suspected germ cell tumors. Due to its long serum half-life of 7 days, the level of AFP may remain elevated in normal infants as old as 6 months of age.[441,442] Abelev and colleagues reported in 1967 that patients with testicular tumors that contained elements of embryonal carcinoma had elevated levels of AFP in their serum.[443] Other investigators have reported that children with embryonal carcinomas and malignant teratomas have elevated serum levels of AFP. Most commonly, high serum levels of AFP are identified in pediatric patients with testicular, ovarian, presacral, and vaginal primary yolk sac tumors.[51,444]

HCG is a glycoprotein that is secreted by the placenta. Patients with a pure yolk sac tumor do not have detectable serum levels of HCG. Patients with malignant germ cell tumors of the ovary or embryonal carcinoma of the ovary or testis may have elevated serum HCG levels.[445] HCG has a much shorter serum half-life than AFP, lasting only 24 to 36 hours. Thus, a decline in the serum level of this marker occurs much more rapidly with successful therapeutic intervention than is seen in management of tumors that secrete AFP.

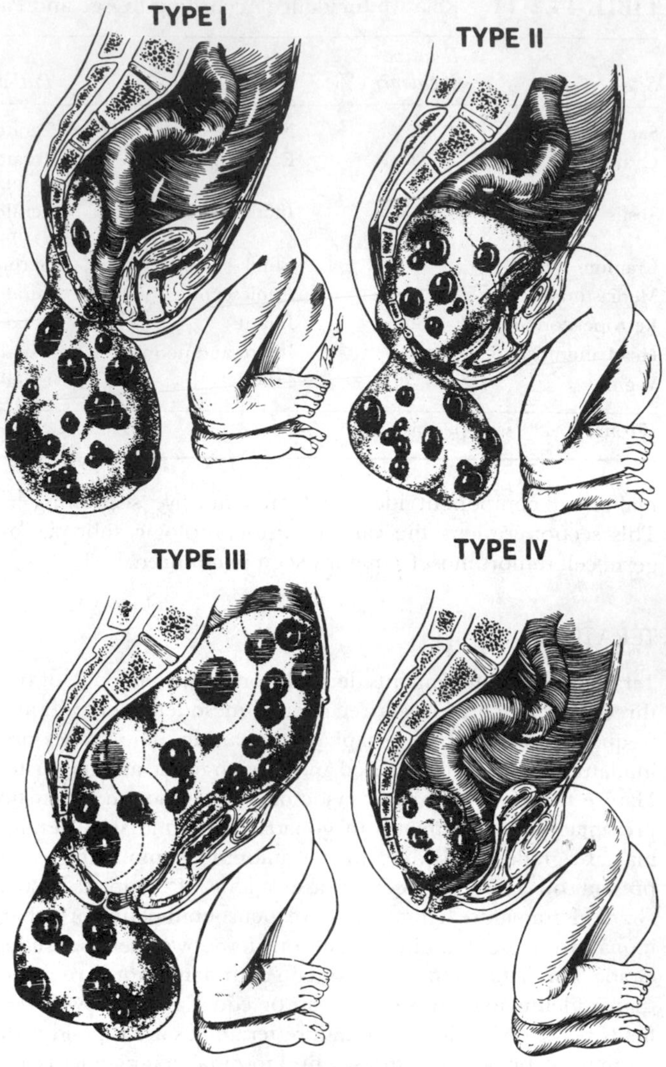

FIGURE 44.2-8. The types of presacral teratomas. Malignancy rates are as follows: type 1, 8%; type II, 21%; type III, 34%; type IV, 38%. (From ref. 446, with permission.)

CLINICAL PRESENTATION AND TREATMENT BY ANATOMIC SITE

SACROCOCCYGEAL TUMORS

Presacral and sacrococcygeal teratomas are usually diagnosed at birth or during the first month of life. Four types have been defined on the basis of the extent of pelvic and abdominal extension of the teratoma, and the presence or absence of external extension of the teratoma (Fig. 44.2-8).[446]

Only 2% of presacral and sacrococcygeal teratomas diagnosed before 6 months of age were malignant, compared with 65% of those diagnosed after 6 months of age. Both benign and malignant teratomas are more frequent in girls.[426] Children with presacral or sacrococcygeal teratomas frequently have congenital anomalies of the vertebrae, genitourinary system, or anorectum.[446,447]

Malignant presacral or sacrococcygeal teratomas may arise *de novo* or at the site of a previously excised benign teratoma.[448,449] The frequency of malignancy depends on the type of teratoma, varying from 8% for patients with type I, to 21% for those with type II, 34% for those with type III, and 38% for those with type IV lesions.[446] The much higher rate of malignancy in type IV tumors may reflect inadequate or delayed treatment of infants with foci of endodermal sinus tumor within a mature or immature sacrococcygeal teratoma.[450]

Clinical Presentation and Evaluation of Sacrococcygeal Teratomas

Children with malignant pelvic teratomas present with an abdominal or buttock mass or signs of urinary and fecal obstruction. Rectal examination reveals the presence of a mass between the rectum and the sacrum. The mass may extend through the sciatic notch deep into the gluteal muscles.

Staging of the patient with a sacrococcygeal teratoma requires a radionuclide bone scan, plain radiographs of any positive area on the scan and any symptomatic bone, plain chest radiography and CT of the chest, abdomen, and pelvis (Table 44.2-12).

TABLE 44.2-12. Pediatric Oncology Group/Children's Cancer Group Staging for Malignant Extragonadal Germ Cell Tumors

Stage	*Description*
I	Complete resection at any site; coccygectomy for sacrococcygeal site; negative tumor margins; tumor markers positive or negative
II	Microscopic residual; lymph nodes negative; tumor markers positive or negative
III	Gross residual or biopsy only; retroperitoneal nodes negative or positive; tumor markers positive or negative
IV	Distant metastases, including liver

(From ref. 425, with permission.)

TABLE 44.2-13. Management Schema for Pediatric Germ Cell Tumors

Group	*Treatment*
Low risk	Surgery and observation
Stage I gonadal	
Stage I extragonadal	
All immature teratomas	
Intermediate risk	Surgery and PEB × 3 cycles[a]
Stage II–IV gonadal	
Stage II extragonadal	
High risk	Surgery and PEB-C × 4 cycles[a]
Stage III–IV extragonadal	

B, bleomycin; C, cyclophosphamide; E, etoposide; P, cisplatin.
[a]Patients with initial biopsy or incomplete resection have surgical resection of residual disease after completion of initial therapy. Patients who are complete responders (no viable tumor) receive no further therapy, and those with partial response receive additional chemotherapy. Patients with progressive disease receive alternative chemotherapy.
(From ref. 425, with permission.)

Yolk sac tumor accounts for the vast majority of malignant presacral and sacrococcygeal teratomas.[451] In marked contrast to the predominance of benign teratomas in neonates with type I tumors, nearly 90% of children with type IV anatomy have tumors consisting of malignant elements.[451] Before the inclusion of cisplatinum in chemotherapy regimens for pelvic yolk sac tumors, survival was poor, barely exceeding 10%.[452] Since the advent of modern, platinum-based chemotherapy in the late 1970s, however, more than 80% of patients with malignant sacrococcygeal teratomas are survivors.[425]

Surgery

Before surgical resection, the upper limit of the tumor should be assessed by both rectal examination and either ultrasonography or MRI. In the vast majority of cases, the tumor can be resected by a perineal approach in which an incision is placed around the periphery of the protruding teratoma, preserving the maximum amount of skin. In approximately 10% of infants, a combined perineal and abdominal approach is required.[446] The plane between a benign teratoma and the normal anatomic structures can be readily defined. All normal structures should be preserved, accepting a narrow margin of resection. In light of a much higher recurrence rate when the adjacent coccyx is spared, the coccyx should routinely be removed with the tumor. The sacrum, however, can be preserved. Caution must be taken when resecting the anterior aspect of the teratoma to preserve the anal musculature, which may be directly adherent, and to avoid injury to the rectum that is draped over the anterior aspect of the tumor. If the tumor is identified in an older child or there is suspicion of malignancy, a preliminary biopsy should be performed. Preoperative chemotherapy should be administered if malignancy is confirmed. A complete resection of malignant teratomas can rarely be achieved without prior treatment with combination chemotherapy. This approach allows maximum preservation of normal structures including the rectum, anus, and the sacral plexus, which is critical for bladder and bowel function. If significant abdominal extension of the tumor is present, initial abdominal exploration allows control of the vascular supply to the tumor before the perineal dissection.[453]

Radiation Therapy

Radiation therapy is not necessary for those children who undergo a complete excision or who have a complete response to combination chemotherapy.[454] In patients who have residual disease after treatment with chemotherapy and second-look surgery, local control with irradiation is poor.[455] If irradiation is indicated, the dose required for extragonadal germ cell tumors is 45 to 50 Gy.

Chemotherapy

As noted previously, malignant pelvic yolk sac tumors are highly responsive to chemotherapy regimens that include cisplatinum.[456–458] Children with pelvic yolk sac tumors should be treated aggressively, with the expectation that such an approach will result in long-term tumor control. Table 44.2-13 contains an algorithm for the inclusion of chemotherapy in the treatment of germ cell tumors based on the risk-group stratification currently employed by North American pediatric cooperative groups (POG/CCG).[425]

TESTICULAR TUMORS

Testicular tumors make up approximately 10% of all pediatric germ cell tumors. The vast majority of these tumors are malignant (80%), characteristically containing yolk sac elements. In contrast to adult testicular tumors, which are frequently metastatic at initial diagnosis, 90% of pediatric testicular germ cell tumors are localized.[427] Malignant germ cell tumors of the testis occur at an annual incidence of 1.1 cases per 1 million U.S. white children younger than 15 years of age. The corresponding figure for African American children is only slightly lower at 0.9 cases per 1 million.[459] Testicular germ cell tumors follow a bimodal age distribution, occurring in very young children and adolescent boys. Yolk sac tumor, or endodermal sinus tumor, is the most common malignant germ cell tumor of the testis in prepubertal boys, with a median age at diagnosis of 24 months. Testicular tumors in adolescent boys have histologic features similar to those of adults.[429]

Children with yolk sac tumors of the testis have been diagnosed with additional anomalies including inguinal hernia, double ureter, ectopic kidney, hypospadias, and renal agenesis.[460]

Clinical Presentation and Evaluation

Most children with primary testicular tumors present with painless testicular enlargement. In the relatively infrequent cases of metastatic disease, patients present with abdominal swelling due to malignant ascites, inguinal lymphadenopathy, or acute abdominal pain.

Physical examination reveals testicular enlargement. Transillumination is usually negative, but the presence of a hydrocele should not decrease the index of suspicion that a testicular tumor is present. Yolk sac tumor occurs with equal frequency in the right and left testis. Less than 1% of cases had bilateral testicular involvement at the time of initial presentation.[51]

The preoperative evaluation of a child suspected to have a malignant tumor of the testis should include a plain chest radiograph and serum AFP and HCG levels. Additional studies, including CT of the abdomen, pelvis, and chest, are not necessary before orchiectomy, although they are ultimately required for complete staging of testicular tumors containing malignant elements.

Management of the Undescended Testis

Patients with an undescended testis have an increased risk of developing testicular cancer, although most associated tumors are diagnosed well beyond 15 years of age, often arising in the fourth decade.[461–463] The undescended testis occupies an intraabdominal location in 14.2% of patients. Cryptorchid testes in intraabdominal sites account for 51.5% of the cases of cancer diagnosed in patients with undescended testes, suggesting these patients are at the greatest risk of malignancy.[462,464]

Orchiopexy has been recommended both to preserve testicular function and to facilitate the identification of malignancy in the abnormally located testis. Several authors have reported the occurrence of testicular cancer in maldescended testes following orchiopexy.[465] Most patients were more than 6 years of age when orchiopexy was performed.[466] While orchiopexy permits identification of tumors, it does not uniformly prevent their occurrence. Normal testicular function is unlikely in boys who undergo orchiopexy after 2 years of age.[467,468] Children with an undescended testis and a normal contralateral testis should undergo orchiectomy if the undescended testis is not recognized until puberty. Orchiopexy is the treatment of choice for younger patients with cryptorchidism. Preservation of normal testicular function is most likely if surgical repair is performed before 2 years of age.[469]

Staging

Once the histologic diagnosis is established, the patient must be staged. Although the majority of pediatric testicular germ cell tumors are nonmetastatic, the tumors may spread to retroperitoneal lymph nodes, liver, lungs, and rarely to bones or brain.

As noted previously, staging must include CT of the chest, abdomen, and pelvis, in addition to a radionuclide bone scan.

The retroperitoneal lymph nodes may be evaluated by CT or MRI. Absence of significant retroperitoneal fat in these young children and the inability of CT to identify normal sized lymph nodes that contain tumor may limit the sensitivity of CT for staging these patients. Since 90% of malignant testicular germ cell tumors in young children elaborate AFP, adjuvant chemotherapy is reserved for advanced stage disease and the small percentage of children with occult metastatic disease whose AFP fails to decline following orchiectomy (Table 44.2-14).

TABLE 44.2-14. Pediatric Oncology Group/Children's Cancer Group Staging System for Testicular Germ Cell Tumors

Stage	*Description*
I	Limited to testis: tumor markers normal after appropriate half-life decline (α-fetoprotein, 5 days; human chorionic gonadotropin, 16 hours)
II	Transscrotal orchiectomy: microscopic disease in scrotum or high in spermatic cord (<5 cm from proximal end); retroperitoneal lymph node involvement (>2 cm), increased tumor markers after appropriate half-life decline, or both
III	Retroperitoneal lymph node involvement (>2 cm) but no visceral or extraabdominal involvement
IV	Distant metastases, including liver

(From ref. 425, with permission.)

Treatment Planning

SURGERY. Preoperative diagnostic studies of a scrotal mass may include ultrasonography that can define the solid or cystic nature of the mass and its relationship to the testicle. All scrotal masses should be explored through an inguinal incision. A transcrotal biopsy contaminates the scrotum and its lymphatic drainage to the inguinal lymph nodes and prevents high ligation of the spermatic cord. If the tumor is clearly malignant, high ligation of the spermatic cord should be performed at the internal ring.

Increasingly, effective cisplatin-based chemotherapy for nonseminomatous germ cell tumors has decreased the role of surgical resection of the retroperitoneal lymph nodes as a therapeutic modality. Infants have a predominance of early-stage lesions that are primarily endodermal sinus tumors (yolk sac tumors), in contrast with teenage boys in whom the embryonal carcinoma or mixed germ cell tumors predominate. Teenagers frequently delay seeking medical attention, resulting in a higher proportion of advanced stage disease at initial presentation.[470] In most series, infants with clinical stage I (Table 44.2-15) endodermal sinus tumors are treated by radical orchiectomy and then close follow-up. In the United Kingdom Children's Cancer Group Study of malignant germ cell tumors, 87% of the boys presented with stage I testicular tumors that were treated by orchiectomy alone.[471] The pathology of these lesions was predominantly yolk sac tumors (57 of 61). In seven boys, a rising serum AFP was the only evidence for incomplete resection. All responded well to chemotherapy. Survival using this protocol was 100%. A smaller series from the Institute Gustave-Roussy reported recurrence in 2 of 12 boys followed without adjuvant chemotherapy or retroperitoneal lymph node dissection. Both were cured by surgery and chemotherapy.[472]

The clinical behavior of testicular embryonal carcinomas is similar in teenagers and adults. Studies have demonstrated that adults with clinical stage I embryonal carcinoma of the testes have positive retroperitoneal lymph nodes in approximately 30% of cases.[473] This earlier finding is supported by reports of a 28% relapse rate in adults with stage I disease who were initially observed after radical orchiectomy.[474] A similar approach to

TABLE 44.2-15. Staging System for Yolk Sac Tumor of the Testis

Stage	*Description*
Stage I	Tumor limited to one (or both) testes, which are removed by high inguinal orchiectomy; no clinical, radiographic, or histologic evidence of residual disease beyond the testis; serum α-fetoprotein negative postoperatively.
Stage II	Transscrotal tumor aspiration, biopsy of tumor within the scrotal sac or scrotal orchiectomy; microscopic residual disease within the scrotum or high in the spermatic cord (less than 5 cm from the proximal end); microscopic retroperitoneal lymph node involvement (lymph nodes less than 2 cm in diameter, but histologically positive for tumor) or serum α fetoprotein positive more than 4 weeks after orchiectomy.
Stage III	Gross retroperitoneal lymph node involvement (lymph nodes more than 2 cm in diameter and histologically positive for tumor).
Stage IV	
A	Extraabdominal lymph node metastases.
B	Extranodal metastases are present (e.g., liver, lung, peritoneum, bones, bone marrow, or brain).

localized disease in children was employed at the St. Jude Children's Research Hospital where relapse with a pulmonary metastasis was seen in one of eight boys.[475] In many current protocols, children with clinical stage I disease (i.e., no radiographically identifiable retroperitoneal tumor and falling serum markers) are followed after radical orchiectomy. Children with identifiable retroperitoneal tumor frequently receive initial chemotherapy, with surgery reserved for residual masses or persistently elevated markers. Resection of postchemotherapy residual masses in adults demonstrated that 45.0% had necrosis, 42.5% had teratoma, and 12.5% had viable germ cell tumor.[476] Both the North American and European pediatric cooperative groups currently employ this strategy of surgery alone followed by close surveillance in children with stage I germ cell tumors, regardless of site or histology.

Children with yolk sac tumors of the testis rarely require bilateral retroperitoneal lymph node dissection for adequate staging. The procedure results are usually negative, but the procedure carries a substantial risk of producing impotence and retrograde ejaculation. In one series, only 2 of 49 bilateral retroperitoneal lymph node dissections and 4 of 29 unilateral retroperitoneal lymph node dissections performed in children with yolk sac tumor of the testis were positive.[51] The percentage of positive retroperitoneal lymph node dissections was not influenced by the age of the patient. Since this diagnostic procedure carries substantial potential morbidity and infrequently provides information that will change the stage or influence therapy, retroperitoneal lymphadenectomy should be avoided.

CHEMOTHERAPY. Current therapeutic practice reserves chemotherapy for children with either advanced stage disease, recurrent localized tumors, or children with stage I disease whose tumor markers fail to decline following orchiectomy. Inclusion of chemotherapy in the treatment of children with stage I disease has not provided a statistically significant advantage in relapse-free survival.

The application of combination chemotherapy to the treatment of children with advanced stage or recurrent yolk sac tumor has proceeded from the use of similar programs for the management of adults with nonseminomatous germ cell tumors of the testis. The first effective combinations included dactinomycin, chlorambucil, and methotrexate or dactinomycin, vincristine, and cyclophosphamide.[51] Unfortunately, neither of these regimens significantly increased the number of patients with advanced abdominal or pulmonary metastatic disease who achieved long-term, disease-free survival.

Subsequent identification of bleomycin and cisplatinum as active agents against testicular germ cell tumors, however, has substantially improved survival for patients with disseminated disease. The Einhorn regimen, consisting of cisplatin, vinblastine, and bleomycin (PVB), was developed at the Indiana University Medical Center in 1974. It has been active against embryonal carcinoma, teratocarcinoma, choriocarcinoma, and yolk sac tumor of the testis.[428] The addition of doxorubicin did not increase the complete response rate. The activity of this three-drug combination has been confirmed by several groups of investigators. Increasing the dose intensity of cisplatin does not improve the response rate or survival rate, but does increase the toxicity of the PVB regimen.[477] Substitution of etoposide for vinblastine in the PVB regimen did not change the response rate and substantially decreased the toxicity of the chemotherapy regimen.[478,479] In light of the pulmonary toxicity of bleomycin, multiple studies have been conducted to assess the value of continued inclusion of this agent in platinum-based regimens. Although several randomized adult studies suggest that bleomycin may be deleted from the cisplatin, etoposide, and bleomycin combination based on comparable response rates with and without this agent, there were sufficient differences in overall and relapse-free survival to recommend its continued use.[480–482] In view of impressive responses to alternative regimens using ifosfamide and etoposide and a United Kingdom study that effectively substituted carboplatinum for cisplatinum, there are now several potentially less toxic chemotherapy options that need to be prospectively tested.[483–486]

The same guidelines for management of young children with yolk sac tumors of the testis should be applied to adolescents with malignant germ cell tumors. Teenagers with stage I nonseminomatous germ cell tumors may be managed with close surveillance.[487] Those with more advanced stage disease should receive platinum-based combination chemotherapy.

OVARY

Ovarian tumors account for approximately 25% of all pediatric germ cell tumors. The majority of these tumors arise later in childhood, with a peak incidence at 10 years of age. Most of these tumors are benign mature cystic teratomas, although nearly one-third contain malignant elements. In contrast to adult ovarian tumors, malignancies of epithelial or stromal cell origin are uncommon in children. The most common pediatric ovarian neoplasias are dysgerminomas and yolk sac tumors. Immature teratomas account for approximately 10% of ovarian masses.[426,429,488,489]

Clinical Presentation

Patients with ovarian tumors present with abdominal pain or an abdominal mass. The pain may be severe due to torsion of the ovarian pedicle by the ovary and tumor.[490] Fever is present in 24% of patients at the time of diagnosis.

Preoperative radiographic evaluation should include studies that localize the mass to the ovary. A plain abdominal radiograph should be obtained and examined for the presence of calcification. Abdominal ultrasonography demonstrates whether the mass is cystic in nature. CT provides more detailed information about the site of origin of the tumor. In patients with suspected ovarian germ cell tumors, serum levels of AFP and HCG should be assayed before diagnostic or therapeutic surgical intervention. Once the tissue diagnosis is established, the potential sites of metastatic disease should be examined. Possible sites of dissemination include peritoneal implants, retroperitoneal lymph nodes, lung, liver, and bone. There has been considerable controversy regarding the proper risk group stratification and treatment of patients with immature teratomas and gliomatosis peritonei (peritoneal seeding with mature glial tissue). In general, immature teratomas are treated with surgery alone. The controversy resides in questions about the appropriateness of surgery alone for immature teratomas that have extensively seeded the omentum and peritoneal surfaces. In a report by POG/CCG documenting 135 cases of childhood immature teratomas, 22 of 86 cases of ovarian immature teratoma were characterized by gliomatosis peritonei. Investigators on this study found that this feature had no adverse effect on outcome in patients treated with surgery alone.[491] Only the finding of microscopic foci of malignant yolk sac tumor in immature teratomas correlated with poor prognosis, mandating inclusion of adjuvant chemotherapy for this small subset of children. These same authors note that while modest elevations of AFP (less than 60) may be recorded in children with immature teratomas without malignant elements, nearly all patients with AFP greater than 100 have occult foci of malignant yolk sac tumor.[491]

Staging

Staging evaluation should include CT of the chest, abdomen, and pelvis, in addition to bone scintigraphy with technetium 99m pertechnetate. Ovarian tumors are staged using the POG/CCG staging system, which represents a simplified derivation of the International Federation of Gynecology and Obstetrics staging system[425,492] (Table 44.2-16).

Table 44.2-16. Pediatric Oncology Group/Children's Cancer Group Staging System for Pediatric Ovarian Germ Cell Tumors

Stage	*Description*
I	Limited to ovary (ovaries) peritoneal washings negative; tumor markers normal after appropriate half-life decline (α-fetoprotein, 5 days; human chorionic gonadotropin, 16 hours)
II	Microscopic residual or positive lymph nodes (<2 cm); peritoneal washings negative for malignant cells, tumor markers positive or negative
III	Lymph node involvement (>2 cm); gross residual or biopsy only; contiguous visceral involvement (omentum, intestine, bladder); peritoneal washings positive for malignant cell; tumor markers positive or negative
IV	Distant metastases, including liver

Treatment Planning

SURGERY. Surgical exploration of an ovarian mass must accomplish two goals: resection of the primary tumor and adequate staging. Peritoneal fluid should be aspirated for cytology. If no fluid is present, peritoneal washings should be obtained. Any peritoneal seeding should be biopsied and a partial or complete omentectomy performed. Ipsilateral lymph nodes should be examined and biopsies taken from the iliac, low periaortic, or pericaval nodes and the periaortic or pericaval nodes at the level of the renal vessels. The contralateral ovary should be examined closely, and if nodules are present, particularly in dysgerminomas or teratomas, a biopsy should be obtained. With current techniques available for *in utero* fertilization, increasing efforts are taken to preserve the fallopian tube and uterus in cases in which both ovaries must be resected.[493]

CHEMOTHERAPY. Combination chemotherapy with VAC was employed in the 1970s in two small series of pediatric patients with ovarian yolk sac tumor. These early studies demonstrated that improved survival could be achieved with inclusion of chemotherapy in treatment of patients with stage I and II disease.[494,495] Results of these pediatric trials were consistent with the outcomes of studies in adults with ovarian yolk sac tumor that documented similar improvements in survival with adjuvant VAC chemotherapy.[496,497] Neither study reported the response rate of women with advanced ovarian yolk sac tumor to VAC.

Closely paralleling the chronology and evolution of chemotherapy for testicular germ cell tumors, subsequent clinical trials for ovarian germ cell tumors employed the combination of PVB in the treatment of women with advanced ovarian germ cell tumors. In one series, the response rate was 91%, with six women achieving a complete response.[498] Several other investigators have reported activity of the PVB combination against a variety of ovarian germ cell tumor histologies.[499,500] Current pediatric practice uses the cisplatin, etoposide, and bleomycin regimen for treatment of primary nonlocalized or recurrent ovarian germ cell tumors. This regimen has produced survival rates exceeding 90% for localized and advanced stage ovarian germ cell tumors in children.[425]

RADIATION THERAPY. With the advent of such effective chemotherapy for ovarian germ cell tumors, the current role of radiation therapy is uncertain. No radiation therapy is given for histologies other than dysgerminoma if surgery and chemotherapy render the child free of disease.[434] In the unusual situation in which there is persistent disease after initial surgery, chemotherapy, and a second-look operation, 40 Gy is recommended.

Treatment options for ovarian dysgerminoma are more complex. Dysgerminomas are curable with irradiation, with one small pediatric study documenting a 5-year overall survival of 94%. Unfortunately, this same study described extensive late sequelae to radiation therapy, including infertility, dysmenorrhea, hypogonadism, and pelvic fibrosis.[501] Given the morbidity of pelvic irradiation and the exquisite chemosensitivity of this tumor, radiation should be reserved for second-line therapy in patients who have relapsed following surgery and chemotherapy. In those rare cases in which radiation therapy is indicated, doses required for dysgerminoma are 20 to 25 Gy, with a boost to gross residual disease to a total dose of 35 to 40 Gy.[493]

MEDIASTINUM

Germ cell tumors of the thoracic cavity typically arise in the anterior mediastinum of adolescent boys. While the majority of these tumors are benign teratomas, malignant yolk sac tumor and choriocarcinoma have been identified in this location.[502,503] Several patients with Klinefelter's syndrome have developed yolk sac tumors.[504] The clinical presentation is characterized by a brief history of cough, dyspnea, and chest pain due to tracheobronchial compression.

Routine chest radiographs may demonstrate an incidental anterior mediastinal mass. The diagnosis is established by biopsy of the primary tumor at thoracotomy or mediastinoscopy, or by biopsy of an involved supraclavicular lymph node. Staging studies, including a bone scan, skeletal survey, bone marrow aspirate, and biopsy, should be performed immediately after tissue diagnosis is established.

The results of therapy have improved with the use of cisplatin-containing chemotherapy regimens, with approximately 40% of patients being relapse-free survivors.[454,498,502]

There are insufficient data available to evaluate the relative importance of surgical excision, local irradiation, and combination chemotherapy in the management of patients with yolk sac tumor of the mediastinum. Frequently, therapeutic failure is due to local progression of the tumor. Since achieving complete surgical excision in this site may be difficult, therapeutic morbidity may be minimized by treating malignant tumors with neoadjuvant chemotherapy followed by delayed resection. Treatment outcomes have improved with the application of cisplatinum-based chemotherapy regimens.[454,499,503]

REFERENCES

1. Ries LAG, Smith MA, Gurney JG, et al., eds. *Cancer incidence and survival among children and adolescents: United States SEER Program 1975–1995.* National Cancer Institute, SEER Program. NIH Publication No. 99-4649, Bethesda, MD, 1999.
2. Guyer B, Hoyert DL, Martin JA, et al. Annual summary of vital statistics—1998. *Pediatrics* 1999;104:1229.
3. Buckley JD, Sather H, Ruccione K, et al. A case-control study of risk factors for hepatoblastoma. A report from the Children's Cancer Study Group. *Cancer* 1989;64:1169.
4. Grufferman S, Schwartz AG, Ruymann FB, Maurer HM. Parents' use of cocaine and marijuana and increased risk of rhabdomyosarcoma in their children. *Cancer Causes Control* 1993;4:217.
5. Grufferman S, Wang HH, DeLong ER, et al. Environmental factors in the etiology of rhabdomyosarcoma in childhood. *J Natl Cancer Inst* 1982;68:107.
6. Bunin GR, Kramer S, Marrero O, Meadows AT. Gestational risk factors for Wilms' tumor: results of a case-control study. *Cancer Res* 1987;47:2972.
7. Olshan AF, Breslow NE, Falletta JM, et al. Risk factors for Wilms' tumor. Report from the National Wilms' Tumor Study. *Cancer* 1993;72:938.
8. Olshan AF, Breslow NE, Daling JR, et al. Wilms' tumor and paternal occupation. *Cancer Res* 1990;50:3212.
9. Bunin GR, Petrakova A, Meadows AT, et al. Occupation of parents of children with retinoblastoma. A report from the Children's Cancer Study Group. *Cancer Res* 1990;50:7129.
10. Bunin GR, Meadows AT, Emanuel BS, et al. Pre- and postconception factors associated with sporadic heritable and nonheritable retinoblastoma. *Cancer Res* 1989;49:5730.
11. Schwartzman JA. Influence of the mother's prenatal drug consumption on risk of neuroblastoma in the child. *Am J Epidemiol* 1992;135:1358.
12. Kramer S, Ward E, Meadows AT, Malone KE. Medical and drug risk factors associated with neuroblastoma: a case-control study. *J Natl Cancer Inst* 1987;78:797.
13. Coppes MJ, Higuchi M, Liefers GJ, et al. Inherited WT1 mutation in Denys-Drash syndrome. *Cancer Res* 1992;52:1.
14. Yandell DW, Campbell TA, Dayton SH, et al. Oncogenic point mutations in the human retinoblastoma gene: their application to genetic counseling. *N Engl J Med* 1989;321:1689.
15. Kurahashi H, Takami K, Oue T, et al. Biallelic inactivation of the APC gene in hepatoblastoma. *Cancer Res* 1995;55:5007.
16. Cawthon RM, Weiss R, Xu G, et al. A major segment of the neurofibromatosis type 1 gene: cDNA sequence, genomic structure, and point mutations. *Cell* 1990;62:193.
17. Li FP, Fraumeni JF Jr, Mulvihill JJ, et al. A cancer family syndrome in twenty-four kindreds. *Cancer Res* 1988;48:5358.
18. Santibanez-Koref MF, Birch JM, Hartley AL, et al. p53 germline mutations in Li-Fraumeni syndrome. *Lancet* 1991;338:1490.
19. Knudson AG. Mutation and cancer: statistical study of retinoblastoma. *Proc Natl Acad Sci U S A* 1971;68:820.
20. Ejima Y, Sasaki MS, Kaneko A, Tanooka H. Types, rates, origin and expressivity of chromosome mutations involving 13q14 in retinoblastoma patients. *Hum Genet* 1988;79:118.
21. Cavenee WK, Dryja TP, Phillips RA, et al. Expression of recessive alleles by chromosomal mechanisms in retinoblastoma. *Nature* 1983;305:779.
22. Dryja TP, Mukai S, Petersen R, et al. Parental origin of mutations of the retinoblastoma gene. *Nature* 1989;339:556.
23. Huff V, Meadows A, Riccardi VM, Strong LC, Saunders GF. Parental origin of de novo constitutional deletions of chromosomal band 11p13. *Am J Hum Genet* 1990;47:155.
24. Koufos A, Hansen MF, Copeland NG, et al. Loss of heterozygosity in three embryonal tumors suggests a common pathogenetic mechanism. *Nature* 1985;316:330.
25. Breslow NE, Beckwith JB. Epidemiological features of Wilms tumor: results of the National Wilms Tumor Study. *J Natl Cancer Inst* 1982;68:429.
26. Breslow NE, Beckwith JB, Ciol M, Sharples K. Age distribution of Wilms tumor: report from the National Wilms Tumor Study. *Cancer Res* 1988;48:1653.
27. Parkin DM, Stiller CA, Draper GJ, et al., eds. *International incidence of childhood cancer.* Lyon: International Agency for Research on Cancer, 1988.
28. Breslow N, Olshan A, Beckwith JB, Green DM. Epidemiology of Wilms tumor. *Med Pediatr Oncol* 1993;21:172.
29. Miller RW, Fraumeni JF Jr, Manning MD. Association of Wilms' tumor with aniridia, hemihypertrophy and other congenital malformations. *N Engl J Med* 1964;270:922.
30. Franco EL, de Camargo B, Saba L, Marques LA. Epidemiological and clinical correlations with genetic characteristics of Wilms' tumor: results of the Brazilian Wilms' Tumor Study Group. *Int J Cancer* 1991;48:641.
31. Bonaiti-Pellie C, Chompret A, Tournade MF, et al. Genetics and epidemiology of Wilms' tumor: the French Wilms' Tumor Study. *Med Pediatr Oncol* 1992;20:284.
32. Drash A, Sherman F, Hartmann WH, Blizzard RM. A syndrome of pseudohermaphroditism, Wilms tumor, hypertension and degenerative renal disease. *J Pediatr* 1970;76:585.
33. Denys P, Malvaux P, Van Den Berghe H, Tanghe W, Proesmans W. Association d'un syndrome anatomo-pathologique de pseudohermaphroditism masculin, d'une tumeur de Wilms, d'une nephropathie parenchymateuse et d'un mosaicism XX hXY. *Arch Fr Pediatr* 1967;24:729.
34. Coppes MJ, Huff V, Pelletier J. Denys-Drash syndrome: relating a clinical disorder to genetic alterations in the tumor suppressor gene WT1. *J Pediatr* 1993;123:673.
35. Breslow N, Olson J, Moksness J, Beckwith JB, Grundy P. Familial Wilms tumor: a descriptive study. *Med Pediatr Oncol* 1996;27:398.
36. Beckwith JB, Kiviat NB, Bonadio J. Nephrogenic rests, nephroblastomatosis and the pathogenesis of Wilms tumor. *Pediatr Pathol* 1990;10:1.
37. Murphy WM, Beckwith JB, Farrow GM. *Atlas of tumor pathology.* 3rd Series. Fascicle 11. Tumors of the kidney, bladder, and related urinary structures. Washington, DC: Armed Forces Institute of Pathology, 1994.
38. Faria P, Beckwith JB, Kishra K, et al. Focal versus diffuse anaplasia in Wilms tumor: new definitions with prognostic significance. A report from the National Wilms Tumor Study Group. *Am J Surg Pathol* 1996;20:909.
39. Beckwith JB, Palmer NF. Histopathology and prognosis of Wilms tumor. Results of the National Wilms Tumor Study. *Cancer* 1978;41:1937.
40. Marsden HB, Lawler W, Kumar PM. Bone metastasizing renal tumor of childhood. *Cancer* 1978;42:1922.
41. Haase HE, Bonadio JF, Beckwith BJ. Clear cell sarcoma of the kidney with emphasis on ultrastructural studies. *Cancer* 1984;54:2978.
42. Schmidt D, Harms D, Evers KG, Bliesener JA, Beckwith JB. Bone metastasizing renal tumor (clear cell sarcoma) of childhood with epithelioid elements. *Cancer* 1985;56:609.
43. Weeks DA, Beckwith JB, Mierau GW, Luckey DW. Rhabdoid tumor of kidney. *Am J Surg Pathol* 1989;13:439.
44. Bonnin JM, Rubinstein LJ, Palmer NF, Beckwith JB. The association of embryonal tumors originating in the kidney and in the brain. *Cancer* 1984;54:2137.
45. White FV, Dehner LP, Belchis DA, et al. Congenital disseminated malignant rhabdoid tumor: a distinct clinicopathologic entity demonstrating abnormalities of chromosome 22q11. *Am J Surg Pathol* 1999;23:249.
46. Rousseau-Merck MF, Versteege I, Couturier J, et al. hSNFS/INI1 inactivation is mainly associated with homozygous deletions and mitotic recombinations in rhabdoid tumors. *Cancer Res* 1999;59:3152.
47. Biege JA, Zhou JY, Rourke LB, et al. Germline and acquired mutations of INI1 in atypical teratoid and rhabdoid tumors. *Cancer Res* 1999;59:74.
48. Bove KE, McAdams AJ. The nephroblastomatosis complex and its relationship to Wilms' tumor: a clinicopathological treatise. *Perspect Pediatr Pathol* 1976;3:185.
49. Shanklin DR, Sotelo-Avila C. In situ tumors in fetuses, newborns and young infants. *Biol Neonate* 1969;14:286.
50. Bolande RP, Brough AJ, Izant RJ Jr. Congenital mesoblastic nephroma of infancy. *Pediatrics* 1967;40:272.
51. Green DM. *Diagnosis and management solid tumors in infants and children.* Boston: Martinus Nijhoff, 1985.
52. Jayabose S, Iqbal K, Newman L, et al. Hypercalcemia in childhood renal tumors. *Cancer* 1988;61:788.

53. Ng YY, Hall-Graggs MA, Dicks-Mireaux C, Pritchard J. Wilms' tumor: pre- and post-chemotherapy CT appearances. *Clin Radiol* 1991;43:255.
54. Ritchey ML, Green DM, Breslow N, Moksness J, Norkool P. Accuracy of current imaging modalities in the diagnosis of synchronous bilateral Wilms tumor: a report from the National Wilms Tumor Study Group. *Cancer* 1995;75:600.
55. Nakayama DK, deLorimier AA, O'Neill JA, Norkool P, D'Angio GJ. Intracardiac extension of Wilms' tumor. A report of the National Wilms' Tumor Study. *Ann Surg* 1986;204:693.
56. Ritchey ML, Kelalis PP, Haase GM, et al. Preoperative therapy for intracaval and atrial extension of Wilms tumor. *Cancer* 1993;71:4104.
57. Wilimas JA, Kaste SC, Kauffman WM, et al. Use of chest computed tomography in the staging of pediatric Wilms' tumor: interobserver variability and prognostic significance. *J Clin Oncol* 1997;15:2631.
58. Feusner JH, Beckwith JB, D'Angio GJ. Clear cell sarcoma of the kidney: accuracy of imaging methods for detecting bone metastases. Report from the National Wilms' Tumor Study. *Med Pediatr Oncol* 1990;18:225.
59. Gururangan S, Wilimas JA, Fletcher BD. Bone metastases in Wilms' tumor—report of three cases and review of literature. *Pediatr Radiol* 1994;24:85.
60. Green DM, Breslow NE, Beckwith JB, et al. The treatment of children with clear cell sarcoma of the kidney. A report from the National Wilms Tumor Study Group. *J Clin Oncol* 1994;12:2132.
61. Shamberger RC, Guthrie KA, Ritchey ML, et al. Surgery-related factors and local recurrence of Wilms' tumor in National Wilms' Tumor Study 4. *Ann Surg* 1999;229:292.
62. Ritchey ML, Etzioni R, Breslow N, et al. Surgical complications following nephrectomy for Wilms' tumor. A report of NWTS-3. *Surg Gynecol Obstet* 1992;175:507.
63. Ritchey ML, Kelalis PP, Etzioni R, et al. Small bowel obstruction following nephrectomy for Wilms tumor: a report of NWTS-3. *Ann Surg* 1993;218:654.
64. Godzinski J, Tournade MF, deKraker J, et al. Rarity of surgical complications after postchemotherapy nephrectomy for nephroblastoma. Experience of the International Society of Paediatric Oncology—trial and study "SIOP-9." *Eur J Pediatr Surg* 1998;8:83.
65. D'Angio GJ, Evans AE, Breslow N, et al. The treatment of Wilms' tumor. *Cancer* 1976;38:633.
66. Lemerle J, Voute PA, Tournade MF, et al. Preoperative versus post-operative radiotherapy, single versus multiple courses of actinomycin D in the treatment of Wilms' tumor. *Cancer* 1976;38:647.
67. D'Angio GJ, Evans AE, Breslow N, et al. The treatment of Wilms' tumor: results of the second national Wilms' tumor study. *Cancer* 1981;47:2302.
68. Shamberger RC, Guthrie KA, Ritchey ML, et al. Surgery related factors and local recurrence of Wilms' tumor in National Wilms' Tumor Study 4.6. *Ann Surg* 1999;229:292.
69. Lemerle J, Voute PA, Tournade MF, et al. Effectiveness of preoperative chemotherapy in Wilms' tumor: results of an International Society of Paediatric Oncology (SIOP) clinical trial. *J Clin Oncol* 1983;1:604.
70. Tournade MF, Com-Hougue C, Voute PA, et al. Results of the sixth International Society of Pediatric Oncology Wilms tumor trial and study: a risk-adapted therapeutic approach in Wilms tumor. *J Clin Oncol* 1993;11:1014.
71. Godzinski J, Tournade MF, deKraker J, et al. The role of preoperative chemo in the treatment of nephroblastoma: the SIOP experience. *Semin Urol Oncol* 1998;17:28.
72. Othersen HB Jr, DeLorimier A, Hrabovsky E, et al. Surgical evaluation of lymph node metastases in Wilms' tumor. *J Pediatr* Surg 1990;25:330.
73. Zuppan CW, Beckwith JB, Weeks DA, Luckey DW, Pringle KC. Effect of preoperative therapy on the histologic features of Wilms' tumor. An analysis of cases from the Third National Wilms' Tumor Study. *Cancer* 1991;68:385.
74. Moorman-Voestermans CGM, Staalman CR, Delamarre JFM. Partial nephrectomy in unilateral Wilms tumor is feasible without local recurrence. *Med Pediatr Oncol* 1994;23:218(abst).
75. Novick AC, Gephardt G, Guz B, Steinmuller D, Tubbs RR. Long-term follow-up after partial removal of a solitary kidney. *N Engl J Med* 1991;325:1058.
76. Montgomery BT, Kelalis P, Blute ML, et al. Extended follow-up of bilateral Wilms' tumor: results of the National Wilms' Tumor Study. *J Urol* 1991;146:514.
77. Ritchey ML, Green DM, Thomas PRM, et al. Renal failure in Wilms tumor patients: a report from the National Wilms Tumor Study Group. *Med Pediatr Oncol* 1996;26:75.
78. Maes P, Delamarre J, deKraker J, Ninane J. Fetal rhabdomyomatous nephroblastoma: a tumor of good prognosis but resistant to chemotherapy. *Eur J Cancer* 1999;35:1356.
79. Saba LMB, deCamargo B, Gabriel-Arana M. Experience with six children with fetal rhabdomyomatous nephroblastoma: review of the clinical, biologic, and pathologic features. *Med Pediatr Oncol* 1998;30:152.
80. Horwitz J, Ritchey M, Moksness J, et al. Renal salvage procedures in patients with synchronous bilateral Wilms' tumors: a report from the National Wilms' Tumor Study Group. *J Pediatr Surg* 1996;8:1020.
81. Kumar R, Fitzgerald R, Breatnach F. Conservative surgical management of bilateral Wilms' tumor: results of the United Kingdom Children's Cancer Study Group. *J Urol* 1998;160:1450.
82. Green DM, Breslow N, Ii Y, et al. The role of surgical excision in the management of relapsed Wilms' tumor patients with pulmonary metastases. *J Pediatr Surg* 1991;26:728.
83. Gross RE, Neuhauser EBD. Treatment of mixed tumors of the kidney in childhood. *Pediatrics* 1950;6:843.
84. Neuhauser EBD, Wittenborg MH, Berman CZ, Cohen J. Irradiation effects of roentgen therapy on the growing spine. *Radiology* 1952;59:637.
85. Tefft M, D'Angio GJ, Grant W III. Postoperative radiation therapy for residual Wilms' tumor. *Cancer* 1976;37:2768.
86. D'Angio GJ, Tefft M, Breslow N, Meyer JA. Radiation therapy of Wilms' tumor: results according to dose, field, post-operative timing and histology. *Int J Radiat Oncol Biol Phys* 1978;4:769.
87. Thomas PRM, Tefft M, Farewell VT, et al. Abdominal relapses in irradiated second national Wilms' tumor study patients. *J Clin Oncol* 1984;2:1098.
88. D'Angio GJ, Breslow N, Beckwith JB, et al. The treatment of Wilms' tumor. Results of the Third National Wilms' Tumor Study. *Cancer* 1989;64:349.
89. Thomas PRM, Tefft M, Compaan PJ, et al. Results of two radiation therapy randomizations in the third National Wilms' Tumor Study. *Cancer* 1991;68:1703.
90. de Kraker J, Lemerle J, Voute PA, et al. Wilms' tumor with pulmonary metastases at diagnosis. The significance of primary chemotherapy. *J Clin Oncol* 1990;8:1187.
91. Pritchard J, Imeson J, Barnes J, et al. Results of the United Kingdom Children's Cancer Study Group (UKCCSG) first Wilms' tumor study (UKW-1). *J Clin Oncol* 1995;13:124.
92. Green DM, Finkelstein JZ, Tefft M, Norkool P. Diffuse interstitial pneumonitis after pulmonary irradiation for metastatic Wilms' tumor. A report from the National Wilms' Tumor Study. *Cancer* 1989;63:450.
93. Wilimas JA, Douglass EC, Magil HL, Fitch S, Hustu HO. Significance of pulmonary computed tomography at diagnosis in Wilms' tumor. *J Clin Oncol* 1988;6:1144.
94. Green DM, Fernbach DJ, Norkool P, Kollia G, D'Angio GJ. Treatment of Wilms' tumor patients with pulmonary metastases detected only with computerized tomography. *J Clin Oncol* 1991;9:1776.
95. Meisel JA, Guthrie KA, Breslow NE, Donaldson SS, Green DM. Significance and management of computed tomography detected pulmonary nodules: a report from the National Wilms' Tumor Study Group. *Int J Radiat Oncol Biol Phys* 1999;44:579.
96. Farber S. Chemotherapy in the treatment of leukemia and Wilms' tumor. *JAMA* 1966;198:826.
97. Green DM, Sallan SE, Krishan A. Actinomycin D in childhood acute lymphocytic leukemia. *Cancer Treat Rep* 1978;62:829.
98. Green DM. Evaluation of single-dose vincristine, actinomycin D and cyclophosphamide in childhood solid tumors. *Cancer Treat Rep* 1978;62:1517.
99. Green DM, Breslow NE, Evans I, et al. The effect of chemotherapy dose intensity on the hematological toxicity of the treatment for Wilms tumor. A report from the National Wilms' Tumor Study. *Am J Pediatr Hematol Oncol* 1994;16:207.
100. Green DM, Breslow NE, Beckwith JB, et al. Effect of duration of treatment outcome and cost of treatment for Wilms' tumor: a report from the National Wilms' Tumor Study Group. *J Clin Oncol* 1998;16:3744.
101. Green D, Breslow N, Beckwith J, et al. Comparison between single-dose and divided-dose administration of dactinomycin and doxorubicin for patients with Wilms' tumor: a report from the National Wilms' Tumor Study Group. *J Clin Oncol* 1998;16:237.
102. Breslow NE, Palmer NF, Hill LR, Buring J, D'Angio GJ. Wilms' tumor: prognostic factors for patients without metastases at diagnosis. *Cancer* 1978;41:1577.
103. Breslow N, Churchill G, Beckwith JB, et al. Prognosis for Wilms' tumor patients with nonmetastatic disease at diagnosis—results of the Second National Wilms' Tumor Study. *J Clin Oncol* 1985;3:521.
104. Breslow N, Sharples K, Beckwith JB, et al. Prognosis in nonmetastatic, favorable histology Wilms' tumor: results of the Third National Wilms' Tumor Study. *Cancer* 1991;68:2345.
105. Jaffe N, Cassady JR, Filler RM, Petersen R, Traggis D. Heterochromia and Horner syndrome associated with cervical and mediastinal neuroblastoma. *J Pediatr* 1975;87:75.
106. Triche TJ, Askin FB. Neuroblastoma and the differential diagnosis of small-, round-, blue cell tumors. *Hum Pathol* 1983;14:569.
107. Tsokos M, Linnoila RL, Chandra RS, Triche TJ. Neuron-specific enolase in the diagnosis of neuroblastoma and other small, round-cell tumors in children. *Hum Pathol* 1984;15:575.
108. Shimada H, Chatten J, Newton WA Jr, et al. Histopathologic prognostic factors in neuroblastic tumors. Definition of subtypes of ganglioneuroblastoma and an age-linked classification of neuroblastomas. *J Natl Cancer Inst* 1984;73:405.
109. Joshi VV, Chatten J, Sather HN, Shimada H. Evaluation of the Shimada classification in advanced neuroblastoma with a special reference to the mitosis-karyorrhexis index. A report from the Children's Cancer Study Group. *Mod Pathol* 1991;4:139.
110. Chatten J, Shimada H, Sather HN, et al. Prognostic value of histopathology in advanced neuroblastoma. A report from the Children's Cancer Study Group. *Hum Pathol* 1988;19:1187.
111. Joshi VV, Cantor AB, Altshuler G, et al. Recommendations for modification of terminology of neuroblastic tumors and prognostic significance of Shimada classification. A clinicopathologic study of 213 cases for the Pediatric Oncology Group. *Cancer* 1992;69:2183.
112. Shimada H, Ambros IM, Dehner LP, et al. Terminology and morphologic criteria of neuroblastic tumors. Recommendations by the International Neuroblastoma Pathology Committee. *Cancer* 1999;86:349.
113. Shimada H, Abros IM, Dehner LP, et al. The International Neuroblastoma Pathology Classification (the Shimada system). *Cancer* 1999;86:364.
114. Schiebel E, Rechnitzer C, Fahrenkrug J, Hertz H. Vasoactive intestinal polypeptide (VIP) in children with neutral crest tumours. *Acta Paediatr Scand* 1982;71:721.
115. Jones A, Groover R, Smithson W. Acute cerebellar encephalopathy (ACE): its natural history and relationship to neuroblastoma (NB). *Proc Am Soc Clin Oncol* 1984;3:86(abst).
116. Telander RL, Smithson WA, Groover RV. Clinical outcome in children with acute cerebellar encephalopathy and neuroblastoma. *J Pediatr Surg* 1989;24:11.
117. Koh PS, Raffensperger JG, Berry S, et al. Long-term outcome in children with opsoclonus-myoclonus and ataxia and coincident neuroblastoma. *J Pediatr* 1994;125:712.
118. Hiyama E, Yokoyama T, Ichikawa T, et al. Poor outcome in patients with advanced stage neuroblastoma and coincident opsomyoclonus syndrome. *Cancer* 1994;74:1821.
119. Petruzzi MJ, de Alarcon PA. Neuroblastoma-associated opsoclonus-myoclonus treated with intravenously administered immune globulin G. *J Pediatr* 1995;127:328.
120. Fisher PG, Wechsler DS, Singer HS. Anti-Hu antibody in a neuroblastoma-associated paraneoplastic syndrome. *Pediatr Neurol* 1994;10:309.
121. Weinblatt ME, Heisel MA, Siegel SE. Hypertension in children with neurogenic tumors. *Pediatrics* 1983;71:947.
122. Nishi M, Miyake H, Takeda T, et al. Mass screening of neuroblastoma in Sapporo City, Japan. *Am J Pediatr Hematol Oncol* 1992;14:327.
123. Sawada T, Matsumura T, Kawakatsu H, et al. Long-term effects of mass screening for neuroblastoma in infancy. *Am J Pediatr Hematol Oncol* 1991;13:3.
124. Woods WG, Tuchman M, Bernstein ML, et al. Screening for neuroblastoma in North America. 2-year results from the Quebec project. *Am J Pediatr Hematol Oncol* 1992;14:312.

125. Bernstein ML, Leclerc JM, Bunin G, et al. A population-based study of neuroblastoma incidence, survival and mortality in North America. *J Clin Oncol* 1992;10:323.
126. Brossard J, Bernstein M, Lemieux B. Neuroblastoma: an enigmatic disease. *Br Med Bull* 1996;52:787.
127. Besho F. Is there a future for neuroblastoma mass screening? *Med Pediatr Oncol* 1998;31:106.
128. Evans AE, D'Angio GJ, Randolph J. A proposed staging for children with neuroblastoma. *Cancer* 1971;27:374.
129. Brodeur GM, Seeger RC, Barrett A, et al. International criteria for diagnosis, staging, and response to treatment in patients with neuroblastoma. *J Clin Oncol* 1988;6:1874.
130. Evans AE, D'Angio GJ, Sather HN, et al. A comparison of four staging systems for localized and regional neuroblastoma: a report from the Children's Cancer Study Group. *J Clin Oncol* 1990;8:678.
131. Brodeur GM, Pritchard J, Berthold F, et al. Revisions of the international criteria for neuroblastoma diagnosis, staging, and response to treatment. *J Clin Oncol* 1993;11:1466.
132. White SJ, Stuck KJ, Blane CE, Silver TM. Sonography of neuroblastoma. *Am J Roentgenol* 1983;141:465.
133. Ng YY, Kingston JE. The role of radiology in the staging of neuroblastoma. *Clin Radiol* 1993;47:226.
134. Foglia RP, Fonkalsrud EW, Feig SA, et al. Accuracy of diagnostic imaging as determined by delayed operative intervention in advanced neuroblastoma. *J Pediatr Surg* 1989;24:708.
135. Armstrong EA, Harwood-Nash DCF, Ritz CR, et al. CT of neuroblastomas and ganglioneuromas in children. *Am J Roentgenol* 1982;139:571.
136. Kaufman RA, Thrall JH, Keyes JW Jr, Brown ML, Zakem JF. False negative bone scans in neuroblastoma metastatic to the ends of long bones. *Am J Roentgenol* 1978;130:131.
137. Cozzutto C, De Bernardi B, Comelli A, Guarino M. Bone marrow biopsy in children: a study of 111 patients. *Med Pediatr Oncol* 1979;6:57.
138. Franklin IM, Pritchard J. Detection of bone marrow invasion by neuroblastoma is improved by sampling at two sites with both aspirates and trephine biopsies. *J Clin Pathol* 1983;36:1215.
139. Kushner BH, Cheung NKV, LaQuaglia MP, et al. Survival from locally invasive or widespread neuroblastoma without cytotoxic therapy. *J Clin Oncol* 1996;14:373.
140. Kaneko M, Iwakawa M, Ikebukuro K, et al. Complete resection is not required in patients with neuroblastoma under 1 year of age. *J Pediatr Surg* 1998;33:1690.
141. Haase GM, Wong KY, deLorimier AA, Sather HN, Hammond GD. Improvement in survival after excision of primary tumor in stage III neuroblastoma. *J Pediatr Surg* 1989;24:194.
142. Haase GM, Atkinson JB, Stram DO, Lukens JN, Matthay KK. Surgical management and outcome of locoregional neuroblastoma: comparison of the Children's Cancer Group and the International staging systems. *J Pediatr Surg* 1995;30:289.
143. Shamberger RC, Allarde-Segundo A, Kozakewich HPW, Grier HE. Surgical management of stage III and IV neuroblastoma: resection before or after chemotherapy? *J Pediatr Surg* 1991;26:1113.
144. Adams GA, Shochat SJ, Smith EI, et al. Thoracic neuroblastoma: a Pediatric Oncology Group study. *J Pediatr Surg* 1993;28:372.
145. Morris JA, Shochat SJ, Smith EI, et al. Biological variables in thoracic neuroblastoma: a Pediatric Oncology Group study. *J Pediatr Surg* 1995;30:296.
146. Azizkhan RG, Shaw A, Chandler JG. Surgical complications of neuroblastoma resection. *Surgery* 1985;97:514.
147. Shamberger RC, Smith EI, Joshi VV, et al. The risk of nephrectomy during local control in abdominal neuroblastoma. *J Pediatr Surg* 1998;33:161.
148. Rees H, Markley MA, Kiely EM, et al. Diarrhea after resection of advanced abdominal neuroblastoma: a common management problem. *Surgery* 1998;123:568.
149. Ikeda H, August CS, Goldwein JW, et al. Sites of relapse in patients with neuroblastoma following bone marrow transplantation in relation to preparatory "debulking" treatments. *J Pediatr Surg* 1992;27:1438.
150. Tsuchida Y, Yokoyama J, Kaneko M, et al. Therapeutic significance of surgery in advanced neuroblastoma: a report from the Study Group of Japan. *J Pediatr Surg* 1992;27:616.
151. Haase GM, O'Leary MC, Ramsay NKC, et al. Aggressive surgery combined with intensive chemotherapy improves survival in poor-risk neuroblastoma. *J Pediatr Surg* 1991;26:1119.
152. Kiely EM. The surgical challenge of neuroblastoma. *J Pediatr Surg* 1994;29:128.
153. Heij HA, Rutgers EJTH, Kraker J, Vos A. Intraoperative search for neuroblastoma by MIBG and radioguided surgery with the gamma detector. *Med Pediatr Oncol* 1997;28:171.
154. Hata Y, Uchino J, Sasaki F, et al. Kidney-preserving radical tumor resection in advanced neuroblastoma. *J Pediatr Surg* 1989;24:382.
155. Evans AE, Chatten J, D'Angio GJ, et al. A review of 17 IV-S neuroblastoma patients at the Children's Hospital of Philadelphia. *Cancer* 1980;45:833.
156. Martinez DA, King DR, Ginn-Pease ME, Haase GM, Wiener ES. Resection of the primary tumor is appropriate for children with stage IV-S neuroblastoma: an analysis of 37 patients. *J Pediatr Surg* 1992;27:1016.
157. Gugielmi M, DeBernardi B, Rizzo A, et al. Resection of primary tumor at diagnosis in stage IV-S neuroblastoma: does it affect the clinical course? *J Clin Oncol* 1996;14:1537.
158. Katzenstein HM, Bowman LC, Brodeur GM, et al. Prognostic significance of age, MYCN oncogene amplification, tumor cell ploidy, and histology in 110 infants with stage D(S) neuroblastoma: the Pediatric Oncology Group experience—a Pediatric Oncology Group study. *J Clin Oncol* 1998;16:2007.
159. Lee EW, Applebaum H. Abdominal expansion as a bridging technique in stage IV-S neuroblastoma with massive hepatomegaly. *J Pediatr Surg* 1994;29:1470.
160. McGahren Ed, Rodgers BM, Waldron PE. Successful management of stage 4S neuroblastoma and severe hepatomegaly using absorbable mesh in an infant. *J Pediatr Surg* 1998;33:1554.
161. Ho PTC, Estroff JA, Kozakewich H, et al. Prenatal detection of neuroblastoma: a ten year experience from the Dana Farber Cancer Institute and Children's Hospital. *Pediatrics* 1993;92:358.
162. Holgersen LO, Subramaniam S, Kirpekar M, Mootabar H, Marcus JR. Spontaneous resolution of antenatally diagnosed adrenal masses. *J Pediatr Surg* 1996;31:153.
163. Wyatt GM, Farber S. Neuroblastoma sympatheticum. *Am J Roentgenol* 1941;46:485.
164. Rosen EM, Cassady JR, Frantz CN, et al. Neuroblastoma: the Joint Center for Radiation Therapy Dana-Farber Cancer Institute Children's Hospital experience. *J Clin Oncol* 1984;2:719.
165. Nitschke R, Smith EI, Shochat S, et al. Localized neuroblastoma treated by surgery: a Pediatric Oncology Group study. *J Clin Oncol* 1988;6:1271.
166. Matthay KK, Sather HN, Seeger RC, Haase GM, Hammond GD. Excellent outcome of stage II neuroblastoma is independent of residual disease and radiation therapy. *J Clin Oncol* 1989;7:236.
167. Castleberry RP, Kun LE, Shuster JJ, et al. Radiotherapy improves the outlook for patients older than 1 year with Pediatric Oncology Group stage C neuroblastoma. *J Clin Oncol* 1991;9:789.
168. Matthay KK, Villablanca JG, Seeger RC, et al. Treatment of high-risk neuroblastoma with intensive chemotherapy, radiotherapy, autologous bone marrow transplantation, and 13-cis-retinoic acid. *N Engl J Med* 1999;341:1165.
169. Frappaz D, Michou J, Coze C, et al. LMCE3 treatment strategy: results in 99 consecutively diagnosed stage 4 neuroblastomas in children older than 1 year at diagnosis. *J Clin Oncol* 2000;18:468.
170. Bowman LC, Hancock ML, Santana VM, et al. Impact of intensified therapy on clinical outcome in infants and children with neuroblastoma: the St. Jude Children's Research Hospital Experience, 1962 to 1988. *J Clin Oncol* 1991;9:1599.
171. Sawaguchi S, Kaneko M, Uchino J-I, et al. Treatment of advanced neuroblastoma with emphasis on intensive induction chemotherapy. A report from the Study Group of Japan. *Cancer* 1990;66:1879.
172. Kushner BH, Gulati SC, Kwon J-H, et al. High-dose melphalan with 6-hydroxydopamine-purged autologous bone marrow transplantation for poor-risk neuroblastoma. *Cancer* 1991;68:242.
173. Matthay KK, Seeger RC, Reynolds CP, et al. Allogeneic versus autologous purged bone marrow transplantation for neuroblastoma: a report from the Children's Cancer Group. *J Clin Oncol* 1994;12:2382.
174. Shuster JJ, Cantor AB, McWilliams N, et al. The prognostic significance of autologous bone marrow transplant in advanced neuroblastoma. *J Clin Oncol* 1991;9:1045.
175. Breslow N, McCann B. Statistical estimation of prognosis for children with neuroblastoma. *Cancer Res* 1971;31:2098.
176. Laug WE, Siegel SE, Shaw KNF, et al. Initial urinary catecholamine metabolite concentrations and prognosis in neuroblastoma. *Pediatrics* 1978;62:77.
177. Zeltzer PM, Marangos PJ, Parma AM, et al. Raised neuron-specific enolase in serum of children with metastatic neuroblastoma. *Lancet* 1983;2:361.
178. Shuster JJ, McWilliams NB, Castleberry R, et al. Serum lactate dehydrogenase in childhood neuroblastoma. A Pediatric Oncology Group recursive partitioning study. *Am J Clin Oncol* 1992;15:295.
179. Look AT, Hayes FA, Nitschke R, McWilliams NB, Green AA. Cellular DNA content as a predictor of response to chemotherapy in infants with unresectable neuroblastoma. *N Engl J Med* 1984;311:231.
180. Brodeur GM, Seeger RC, Schwab M, Varmus HE, Bishop JM. Amplification of N-myc in untreated human neuroblastomas correlates with advanced disease stage. *Science* 1984;224:1121.
181. Nakagawara A, Arima-Nakagawara M, Scavarda NJ, et al. Association between high levels of expression of the TRK gene and favorable outcome in human neuroblastoma. *N Engl J Med* 1993;328:847.
182. Look AT, Hayes FA, Shuster JJ, et al. Clinical relevance of tumor cell ploidy and N-myc gene amplification in childhood neuroblastoma: a Pediatric Oncology Group study. *J Clin Oncol* 1991;9:581.
183. Joshi VV, Cantor AB, Brodeur GM, et al. Correlations between morphologic and other prognostic markers of neuroblastoma. A study of histologic grade, DNA index, N-myc gene copy number, and lactic dehydrogenase in patients in the Pediatric Oncology Group. *Cancer* 1993;71:3173.
184. Allderdice PW, Davis JG, Miller OJ, et al. The 13q–deletion syndrome. *Am J Hum Genet* 1969;21:499.
185. Noel B, Quack B, Rethore MO. Partial deletions and trisomies of chromosome 13. Mapping of bands associated with particular malformations. *Clin Genet* 1976;9:593.
186. Matsunaga E. Hereditary retinoblastoma. Penetrance, expressivity and age at onset. *Hum Genet* 1976;33:1.
187. Vogel F. Genetics of retinoblastoma. *Hum Genet* 1979;51:1.
188. Nussbaum R, Puck J. Recurrence risks for retinoblastoma: a model for autosomal dominant disorders with complex inheritance. *J Pediatr Ophthalmol* 1976;13:89.
189. Sanborn GE, Augsburger JJ, Shields JA. Spontaneous regression of bilateral retinoblastoma. *Br J Ophthalmol* 1982;66:685.
190. Margo C, Hidayat A, Kopelman J, Zimmerman LE. Retinocytoma. A benign variant of retinoblastoma. *Arch Ophthalmol* 1983;101:1519.
191. Ellsworth RM. The practical management of retinoblastoma. *Trans Am Ophthalmol Soc* 1969;67:462.
192. Sang DN, Albert DM. Retinoblastoma: clinical and histopathologic features. *Hum Pathol* 1982;13:133.
193. Schantz PM, Meyer D, Glickman LT. Clinical, serologic and epidemiologic characteristics of ocular toxocariasis. *Am J Trop Med Hyg* 1979;28:24.
194. Shields JA, Leonard BC, Michelson JB, Sarin LK. B-scan ultrasonography in the diagnosis of atypical retinoblastomas. *Can J Ophthalmol* 1976;11:42.
195. Danziger A, Price HI. CT findings in retinoblastoma. *Am J Roentgenol* 1979;133:783.
196. Freeman CR, Esseltine D-L, Whitehead VM, Chevalier L, Little JM. Retinoblastoma: the case for radiotherapy and for adjuvant chemotherapy. *Cancer* 1980;46:1913.
197. Pratt CB, Meyer D, Chenaille P, Crom DB. The use of bone marrow aspirations and lumbar punctures at the time of diagnosis of retinoblastoma. *J Clin Oncol* 1989;7:140.

198. Pratt CB, Crom DB, Magill L, Chenaille P, Meyer D. Skeletal scintigraphy in patients with bilateral retinoblastoma. *Cancer* 1990;65:26.
199. Martin H, Reese AB. Treatment of retinoblastoma (retinal glioma) surgically and by irradiation. *Arch Ophthalmol* 1942;27:40.
200. Martin H, Reese AB. Treatment of bilateral retinoblastoma (retinal glioma) surgically and by irradiation. *Arch Ophthalmol* 1945;33:429.
201. Reese AB, Ellsworth RM. The evaluation and current concept of retinoblastoma therapy. *Trans Am Acad Ophthalmol Otolaryngol* 1963;67:164.
202. Howarth C, Meyer D, Hustu HO, et al. Stage-related combined modality treatment of retinoblastoma. *Cancer* 1980;45:851.
203. Pratt CB, Fontanesi J, Lu X, et al. Proposal for a new staging scheme for intraocular and extrocular retinoblastoma based on an analysis of 103 globes. *Oncologist* 1997;2:1.
204. Howard RD, Ellsworth RM. Findings in the peripheral fundi of patients with retinoblastoma. *Am J Ophthalmol* 1966;62:243.
205. Cassady JR. Retinoblastoma: questions in management. In: Carter SK, Glatstein E, Livingston RB, eds. *Principles of cancer treatment.* New York: McGraw-Hill, 1982:891.
206. Brown DH. The clinicopathology of retinoblastoma. *Am J Ophthalmol* 1966;61:508.
207. Stannard C, Lipper S, Sealy R, Sevel D. Retinoblastoma: correlation of invasion of the optic nerve and choroid with prognosis and metastasis. *Br J Ophthalmol* 1979;63:560.
208. Hopping W, Meyer-Schwickerath G. Light coagulation treatment in retinoblastoma. In: Boniuk M, ed. *Ocular and adnexal tumors.* St Louis: Mosby, 1964:192.
209. Lincoff H. A report on the freezing of intraocular tumors. *Mod Probl Ophthalmol* 1968;7:348.
210. Lincoff H, McLean J, Long R. The cryosurgical treatment of intraocular tumors. *Am J Ophthalmol* 1967;63:389.
211. Faris BM, Tarakji MS, Baghdassarian SA, To'mey KF. The role of cryotherapy in the management of early lesions of retinoblastoma. *Ann Ophthalmol* 1978;10:1005.
212. Abramson DH, Ellsworth RM, Rozakis GW. Cryotherapy for retinoblastoma. *Arch Ophthalmol* 1982;100:1253.
213. Shields JA, Parsons H, Shields CL, Giblin ME. The role of cryotherapy in the management of retinoblastoma. *Am J Ophthalmol* 1989;108:260.
214. Weiss DR, Cassady JR, Petersen R. Retinoblastoma: a modification in radiation therapy technique. *Radiology* 1975;114:705.
215. Donaldson SS. Retinoblastoma. In: Levine AS, ed. *Cancer in the young.* New York: Masson, 1982:683.
216. McCormick B, Ellsworth R, Abramson D, et al. Radiation therapy for retinoblastoma: comparison of results with lens-sparing versus lateral beam techniques. *Int J Rad Oncol Biol Phys* 1988;15:567.
217. Kooy HM, Dunbar SF, Tarbell NJ, et al. Adaptation and verification of the relocatable Gill-Thomas-Cosman frame in stereotactic radiotherapy. *Int J Radiat Oncol Biol Phys* 1994;30:685.
218. Abramson DH, Ellsworth RM, Tretter P, Javitt J, Kitchin FD. Treatment of bilateral groups I through IV retinoblastoma with bilateral radiation. *Arch Ophthalmol* 1981;99:1761.
219. Abramson DH, Ronner HJ, Ellsworth RM. Second tumors in nonirradiated bilateral retinoblastoma. *Am J Ophthalmol* 1979;87:624.
220. Wong FL, Boice JD, Abramson D, et al. Cancer incidence after retinoblastoma. Radiation dose and sarcoma risk. *JAMA* 1997;278:1262.
221. Rootman J, Ellsworth RM, Hofbauer J, Kitchin D. Orbital extension of retinoblastoma: a clinicopathologic study. *Can J Ophthalmol* 1978;13:72.
222. Halperin EC, Constine LS, Tarbell NJ, Kun LE. *Pediatric radiation oncology,* 2nd ed. New York: Raven Press, 1994:140.
223. Wolff JA, Boesel CP, Dyment PG, et al. Treatment of retinoblastoma. A preliminary report. In: Raybaud C, Clement R, Lebreuil G, Bernard JL, eds. *Pediatric oncology.* Amsterdam: Excerpta Medica, 1982:364.
224. Pratt CB, Crom DB, Howarth C. The use of chemotherapy for extraocular retinoblastoma. *Med Pediatr Oncol* 1985;13:330.
225. Pratt CB, Fontanesi J, Chenaille P, et al. Chemotherapy for extraocular retinoblastoma. *Pediatr Hematol Oncol* 1994;11:301.
226. Advani SH, Rao SR, Iyer RS, et al. Pilot study of sequential combination chemotherapy in advanced and recurrent retinoblastoma. *Med Pediatr Oncol* 1994;22:125.
227. Schvartzman E, Chantada G, Fandino A, et al. Results of a stage-based protocol for the treatment of retinoblastoma. *J Clin Oncol* 1996;14:1532.
228. Doz F, Neuenschwander S, Plantaz D, et al. Etoposide and carboplatin in extraocular retinoblastoma: a study by the Société Franscaise d'Oncologie Pediatrique. *J Clin Oncol* 1995;13:902.
229. Doz F, Khelfaoui F, Mosseri V, et al. The role of chemotherapy in orbital involvement of retinoblastoma. The experience of a single institution with 33 patients. *Cancer* 1994;74:722.
230. Shields CL, DePotter P, Himelstein BP, et al. Chemoreduction in the initial management of intraocular retinoblastoma. *Arch Ophthalmol* 1996;114:1330.
231. Gallie BL, Budning A, DeBoer G, et al. Chemotherapy with focal therapy can cure introcular retinoblastoma. *Arch Ophthalmol* 1996;114:1321.
232. Kingston JE, Hungerford JL, Madreperla SA, Plowman PN. Results of combined chemotherapy and radiotherapy for advanced intraocular retinoblastoma. *Arch Ophthalmol* 1996;114:1339.
233. Murphree AL, Villablanca JG, Deegan WF III, et al. Chemotherapy plus local treatment in the management of intraocular retinoblastoma. *Arch Ophthalmol* 1996;114:1348.
234. Friedman DL, Himelstein B, Shields CL, et al. Chemoreduction and local ophthalmic therapy for intraocular retinoblastoma. *J Clin Oncol* 2000;18:12.
235. Chan HSL, DeBoer G, Thiessen JJ, et al. Combining cyclosporin with chemotherapy controls intraocular retinoblastoma without requiring radiation. *Clin Cancer Res* 1996;2:1499.
236. Greenwald MJ, Strauss LC, Correspondence RE, et al. Combining cyclosporin with chemotherapy controls intraocular retinoblastoma without requiring radiation. *Clin Cancer Res* 1997;3:491.
237. Rubnitz JE, Crist WM. Molecular genetics of childhood cancer: implications for pathogenesis, diagnosis and treatment. *Pediatrics* 1997;100:101.
238. Felix CA, Kappel CC, Mitsudo I. Frequency and diversity of p53 mutations in childhood rhabdomyosarcoma. *Cancer Res* 1992;52:2247.
239. Matsui I, Tanimura M, Kobayashi N, et al. Neurofibromatosis type 1 and childhood cancer. *Cancer* 1993;72:2746.
240. Shearer P, Parham DI, Kovnar E, et al. Neurofibromatosis type 1 and malignancy: review of 32 pediatric cases treated at a single institution. *Med Pediatr Oncol* 1994;22:78.
241. Pappo AS, Shapiro DN, Crist WM, et al. Biology and therapy of pediatric rhabdomyosarcoma. *J Clin Oncol* 1995;13:2123.
242. Wexler LH, Helman LJ. Rhabdomyosarcoma and the undifferentiated sarcomas. In: Pizzo PA, Poplack DG, eds. *Principles and practice of pediatric oncology,* 3rd ed. Philadelphia: Lippincott, 1987:799.
243. Horn RC Jr, Enterline HT. Rhabdomyosarcoma: a clinicopathological study and classification of 39 cases. *Cancer* 1958;11:181.
244. Tsokos M, Webber BL, Parham DM, et al. Rhabdomyosarcoma. A new classification scheme related to prognosis. *Arch Pathol Lab Med* 1992;116:847.
245. Palmer NG, Sachs N, Foulkes M. Histopathology and prognosis in rhabdomyosarcomas (IRS-1). *Proc Am Soc Clin Oncol* 1982;1:170(abst).
246. Caillaud JM, Gerard-Marchant R, Marsden HB, et al. Histopathological classification of childhood rhabdomyosarcoma: a report from the International Society of Pediatric Oncology Pathology Panel. *Med Pediatr Oncol* 1989;17:391.
247. Asmar L, Gehan EA, Newton WA, et al. Agreement among and within groups of pathologists in the classification of rhabdomyosarcomas and related childhood sarcomas. *Cancer* 1994;74:2579.
248. Newton WA Jr, Gehan EA, Webber BL, et al. Classification of rhabdomyosarcomas and related sarcomas. Pathologic aspects and proposal for a new classification—an Intergroup Rhabdomyosarcoma Study. *Cancer* 1995;76:1073.
249. Arndt CA, Crist WM. Medical progress: common musculoskeletal tumors of childhood and adolescence. *N Engl J Med* 1999;341:342.
250. Cohen M, Smith WL, Weetman R, Provisor A. Pulmonary pseudometastases in children with malignant tumors. *Radiology* 1981;141:371.
251. Quddus FF, Espinola D, Kramer SS, Leventhal BG. Comparison between x-ray and bone scan detection of bone metastases in patients with rhabdomyosarcoma. *Med Pediatr Oncol* 1983;11:125.
252. Weinblatt ME, Miller JH. Radionuclide scanning in children with rhabdomyosarcoma. *Med Pediatr Oncol* 1981;9:293.
253. Hutchinson RJ, Shapiro SA, Raney RB Jr. Elevated parathyroid hormone levels in association with rhabdomyosarcoma. *J Pediatr* 1978;92:780.
254. Ruymann FB, Newton WA Jr, Ragab AH, Donaldson MH, Foulkes M. Bone marrow metastases at diagnosis in children and adolescents with rhabdomyosarcoma. *Cancer* 1984;53:368.
255. Kuttesch JF Jr, Parham DM, Kaste SC, et al. Embryonal malignancies of unknown primary origin in children. *Cancer* 1995;75:115.
256. Lawrence W Jr, Hays DM, Moon TE. Lymphatic metastases with childhood rhabdomyosarcoma. *Cancer* 1977;39:556.
257. Rodary C, Flamant F, Donaldson SS. An attempt to use a common staging system in rhabdomyosarcoma: a report from an international workshop initiated by the International Society of Pediatric Oncology (SIOP). *Med Pediatr Oncol* 1989;17:210.
258. Cassady JR, Sagerman RH, Tretter P, Ellsworth RM. Radiation therapy for rhabdomyosarcoma. *Radiology* 1968;91:116.
259. Loeffler JS, Leslie NT, Cassady JR. Case 10-1984: orbital rhabdomyosarcoma [Letter]. *N Engl J Med* 1984;311:262.
260. Tefft M, Lindberg RD, Gehan EA. Radiation therapy combined with systemic chemotherapy of rhabdomyosarcoma in children: local control in patients enrolled in the Intergroup Rhabdomyosarcoma Study. *Monogr Natl Cancer Inst* 1981;56:75.
261. Maurer HM. The Intergroup Rhabdomyosarcoma Study: update, November 1978. *Monogr Natl Cancer Inst* 1981;56:61.
262. Maurer HM, Moon T, Donaldson M, et al. The Intergroup Rhabdomyosarcoma Study. *Cancer* 1977;40:2015.
263. Crist W, Gehan EA, Ragab AH, et al. The third Intergroup Rhabdomyosarcoma Study. *J Clin Oncol* 1995;13:610.
264. Donaldson S, Asmar L, Breneman J, et al. Hyperfractionated radiation in children with rhabdomyosarcoma—results of the Intergroup Rhabdomyosarcoma pilot study. *Int J Radiat Oncol Biol Phys* 1995;32:903.
265. Maurer HM, Gehan EA, Beltangady M, et al. The Intergroup Rhabdomyosarcoma Study-I. *Cancer* 1993;71:1904.
266. Crist WM, Anderson J, Maurer H, et al. Preliminary results for patients with local/regional tumors treated on the Intergroup Rhabdomyosarcoma Study-IV (1991–1997). *Proc Am Soc Clin Oncol* 1999;18:555(abst).
267. Forbes GS, Ernest F IV, Waller RR. Computed tomography of orbital tumors, including late-generation scanning techniques. *Radiology* 1982;142:387.
268. Weichselbaum RR, Cassady JR, Albert DM, Gonder JR. Multimodality management of orbital rhabdomyosarcoma. *Int Ophthalmol Clin* 1980;20:247.
269. Fuesner JE, Pizzo PA, Poplack DG, Freeman C. Meningeal relapse of orbital rhabdomyosarcoma. *Med Pediatr Oncol* 1978;4:247.
270. Pratt CB, Smith JW, Woerner S, et al. Factors leading to delay in diagnosis and affecting survival of children with head and neck rhabdomyosarcoma. *Pediatrics* 1978;61:30.
271. Weiner ES. Head and neck rhabdomyosarcoma. *Semin Pediatr Surg* 1994;3:203.
272. Dodd GD, Dolan PA, Ballantyne AJ, Ibanez ML, Chau P. The dissemination of tumors of the head and neck via the cranial nerves. *Radiol Clin North Am* 1970;8:445.
273. Gerson JM, Jaffe N, Donaldson MH, Tefft M. Meningeal seeding from rhabdomyosar-

coma of the head and neck with base of skull invasion: recognition of the clinical evolution and suggestions for management. *Med Pediatr Oncol* 1978;5:137.
274. Berry MP, Jenkin RDT. Parameningeal rhabdomyosarcoma in the young. *Cancer* 1981;48:281.
275. Martinez A, Donaldson SS, Bagshaw MA. Special set-up and treatment techniques for the radiotherapy of pediatric malignancies. *Int J Radiat Oncol Biol Phys* 1977;2:1007.
276. Tefft M, Fernandez C, Donaldson M, Newton W, Moon TE. Incidence of meningeal involvement by rhabdomyosarcoma of the head and neck in children. *Cancer* 1978;42:253.
277. Chan RC, Sutow WW, Lindberg RD. Parameningeal rhabdomyosarcoma. *Radiology* 1979;131:211.
278. Tarbell NJ, Schwenn M, Delorey M, et al. Extent of bone erosion predicts survival in nonorbital rhabdomyosarcoma of the head and neck in children. *Proc Am Soc Clin Oncol* 1987;6:222(abst).
279. Raney RB Jr, Tefft M, Newton WA, et al. Improved prognosis with intensive treatment of children with cranial soft tissue sarcomas arising in nonorbital parameningeal sites. A report from the Intergroup Rhabdomyosarcoma Study. *Cancer* 1987;59:147.
280. Hays DM, Lawrence W Jr, Wharam M, et al. Primary reexcision for patients with "microscopic residual" tumor following initial excision of sarcomas of the trunk and extremity sites. *J Pediatr Surg* 1989;24:5.
281. Andrassy RJ, Wiener ES, Raney RB, et al. Thoracic sarcomas in children. *Ann Surg* 1998;227:170.
282. Beech TR, Moss RL, Anderson JA, et al. What constitutes appropriate therapy for children/adolescents with rhabdomyosarcoma in the abdominal wall? A report from the IRS. *J Pediatr Surg* 1999;34:668.
284. Blakely ML, Lobe TE, Anderson JR, et al. Does debulking improve survival rate in advanced-stage retroperitoneal embryonal rhabdomyosarcoma? *J Pediatr Surg* 1999; 34:736.
285. Newton WA Jr, Soule EH, Hamoudi AB, et al. Histopathology of childhood sarcomas, Intergroup Rhabdomyosarcoma Studies I and II: clinicopathologic correlation. *J Clin Oncol* 1988;6:67.
286. Simon MA, Enneking WF. The management of soft-tissue sarcomas of the extremities. *J Bone Joint Surg Am* 1976;58A:317.
287. LaQuaglia MP. Extremity rhabdomyosarcoma. Biological principles, staging, and treatment. *Semin Surg Oncol* 1993;9:510.
288. Andrassy RJ, Corpron CA, Hays D, et al. Extremity sarcomas: an analysis of prognostic factors from the Intergroup Rhabdomyosarcoma Study (IRS) III. *J Pediatr Surg* 1996;31:191.
289. Neville HL, Andrassy RJ, Lobe TE, et al. Preoperative staging, prognostic factors and outcome in extremity rhabdomyosarcoma: a preliminary report from the Intergroup Rhabdomyosarcoma study IV (1991–97). *J Pediatr Surg* 2000;35:317.
290. Lee FA. Rhabdomyosarcoma. In: Parker BR, Castellino RA, eds. *Pediatric oncologic radiology*. St Louis: Mosby, 1977:417.
291. Hays DM, Shimada H, Raney RB, et al. Clinical staging and treatment results in rhabdomyosarcoma of the female genital tract among children and adolescents. *Cancer* 1988;61:1893.
292. Andrassy RJ, Wiener ES, Raney RB, et al. Progress in surgical management of vaginal rhabdomyosarcoma: a 25 year review from the Intergroup Rhabdomyosarcoma Study Group. *J Pediatr Surg* 1999;34:731.
293. Corpron CA, Andrassy RJ, Hays DM, et al. Conservative management of uterine pediatric rhabdomyosarcoma: a report of the Intergroup Rhabdomyosarcoma Study III and IV pilot. *J Pediatr Surg* 1995;30:942.
294. Raney RB Jr, Gehan EA, Hays DM, et al. Primary chemotherapy with or without radiation therapy and/or surgery for children with localized sarcoma of the bladder, prostate, vagina, uterus, and cervix. *Cancer* 1990;66:2072.
295. Hays DM. Bladder/prostate rhabdomyosarcoma: results of the multi-institutional trials of the Intergroup Rhabdomyosarcoma Study. *Semin Surg Oncol* 1993;9:520.
296. Wiener ES, Lawrence W, Hays D, et al. Retroperitoneal node biopsy in paratesticular rhabdomyosarcoma. *J Pediatr Surg* 1994;29:171.
297. Tefft M, Hays D, Raney RB Jr, et al. Radiation to regional nodes for rhabdomyosarcoma of the genitourinary tract in children: is it necessary? *Cancer* 1980;45:3065.
298. Hays DM, Raney RB Jr, Lawrence W, et al. Bladder and prostatic tumors in the Intergroup Rhabdomyosarcoma Study (IRS-I). *Cancer* 1982;50:1472.
299. Hays DM, Raney RB Jr, Lawrence W, et al. Primary chemotherapy in the treatment of children with bladder-prostate tumors in the Intergroup Rhabdomyosarcoma Study (IRS-II). *J Pediatr Surg* 1982;17:812.
300. Rodary C, Gehan EA, Flamant F, et al. Prognostic factors in 951 nonmetastatic rhabdomyosarcoma in children: a report from the International Rhabdomyosarcoma Workshop. *Med Pediatr Oncol* 1991;19:89.
301. Walterhouse DO, Hoover ML, Marymount MA, Kletzel M. High-dose chemotherapy followed by peripheral blood stem cell rescue for metastatic rhabdomyosarcoma: the experience at Chicago Children's Memorial Hospital. *Med Pediatr Oncol* 1999;32:88.
302. Dehner LP. Primitive neuroectodermal tumor and Ewing's sarcoma. *Am J Surg Pathol* 1993;17:1.
303. Tsokos M. Peripheral primitive neuroectodermal tumors. Diagnosis, classification, and prognosis. In: Garvin AJ, O'Leary TJ, Bernstein J, Rosenberg HS, eds. *Pediatric molecular pathology: quantitation and applications. Perspectives in pediatric pathology.* Basel: Karger, 1992:27.
304. Grier HE. The Ewing family of tumors. *Pediatr Clin North Am* 1997;44:991.
305. Dahlin DC. *Bone tumors,* 3rd ed. Springfield, IL: Charles C Thomas, 1978:274.
306. Kissane JM, Askin FB, Foulkes M, Stratton LB, Shirley SF. Ewing's sarcoma of bone: clinicopathologic aspects of 303 cases from the Intergroup Ewing's Sarcoma Study. *Hum Pathol* 1983;14:773.
307. Dekner LP. Primitive neuroectodermal tumor and Ewing's sarcoma. *Am J Surg Pathol* 1993;17:1.
308. Ambros IM, Ambros PF, Strehl S, et al. MIC2 is a specific marker for Ewing's sarcoma and peripheral primitive neuroectodermal tumors. Evidence for a common histogenesis of Ewing's sarcoma and peripheral primitive neuroectodermal tumors from MIC2 expression and specific chromosome aberration. *Cancer* 1991;67:1886.
309. Delattre O, Zucman J, Melot T, et al. The Ewing family of tumors—a subgroup of small-round-cell tumors defined by specific chimeric transcripts. *N Engl J Med* 1994;331:294.
310. Hahm KB, Cho K, Lee C, et al. Repression of the gene encoding the TGF-beta type II receptor is a major target of the EWS-FLI1 oncoprotein. *Nature Genet* 1999;23:222.
311. Zoubek A, Dockhorn-Dwarniak B, Delattre O, et al. Does expression of different EWS chimeric transcripts define clinically distinct risk groups of Ewing tumor patients? *J Clin Oncol* 1996;14:1245.
312. deAlva E, Kawai A, Healey JH, et al. EWS-FLI1 fusion transcript structure is an independent determinant of prognosis in Ewing's sarcoma. *J Clin Oncol* 1998;16:1248.
313. Lin PP, Brody RI, Hamelin AC, et al. Differential transactivation by alternative EWS-FLI1 fusion proteins correlates with clinical heterogeneity in Ewing's sarcoma. *Cancer Res* 1999;59:1428.
314. Monforte-Munoz H, Lopez-Terrada D, Affendie H, et al. Documentation of EWS gene rearrangements by fluorescence in-situ hybridization (FISH) in frozen sections of Ewing's sarcoma—peripheral primitive neuroectodermal tumor. *Am J Surg Pathol* 1999;23:309.
315. Durbin M, Randall RL, James M, et al. Ewing's sarcoma masquerading as osteomyelitis. *Clin Orthop* 1998;357:176.
316. Glaubiger DL, Makuch R, Schwarz J, Levine AS, Johnson RE. Determination of prognostic factors and their influence on therapeutic results in patients with Ewing's sarcoma. *Cancer* 1980;45:2213.
317. Rosen G, Caparros B, Nirenberg A, et al. Ewing's sarcoma: ten-year experience with adjuvant chemotherapy. *Cancer* 1981;47:2204.
318. Cohen M, Grosfeld J, Baehner R, Weetman R. Lung CT for detection of metastases: solid tumor neoplasms in children. *Am J Roentgenol* 1982;139:895.
319. Reiman RE, Rosen G, Gelbard AS, Benua RS, Laughlin JS. Imaging of primary Ewing's sarcoma with (13) N-glutamate. *Radiology* 1982;142:495.
320. Goldstein H, McNeil BJ, Zufall E, Treves S. Is there still a place for bone scanning in Ewing's sarcoma? *J Nucl Med* 1980;21:10.
321. Delta BG, Pinkel D. Bone marrow aspiration in children with malignant tumors. *J Pediatr* 1964;64:542.
322. Evans R, Nesbit M, Askin F, et al. Local recurrence, rate and sites of metastases, and time to relapse as a function of treatment regimen, size of primary and surgical history in 62 patients presenting with non-metastatic Ewing's sarcoma of the pelvic bones. *Int J Radiat Oncol Biol Phys* 1985;11:129.
323. Hayes FA, Thompson EI, Meyer WH, et al. Therapy for localized Ewing's sarcoma of bone. *J Clin Oncol* 1989;7:208.
324. Arai Y, Kun LE, Brooks MT, et al. Ewing's sarcoma: local tumor control and patterns of failure following limited volume radiation therapy. *Int J Radiat Oncol Biol Phys* 1991;21:1501.
325. Pritchard DJ, Dahlin DC, Dauphine RT, Taylor WF, Beabout JW. Ewing's sarcoma: a clinicopathological and statistical analysis of patients surviving five years or longer. *J Bone Joint Surg Am* 1975;57A:10.
326. Brown AP, Fixsen JA, Plowman PN. Local control of Ewing's sarcoma: an analysis of 67 patients. *Br J Radiol* 1987;60:261.
327. Thomas PRM, Foulkes MA, Gilula LA, et al. Primary Ewing's sarcoma of the ribs. *Cancer* 1983;51:1021.
328. Scully SP, Temple HT, O'Keefe RJ, et al. Role of surgical resection in pelvic Ewing's sarcoma. *J Clin Oncol* 1995;13:2336.
329. Göbel V, Jürgens H, Etspuler G, et al. Prognostic significance of tumor volume in localized Ewing's sarcoma of bone in children and adolescents. *J Cancer Res Clin Oncol* 1987;113:187.
330. Mendenhall CM, Marcus RB Jr, Enneking WF, et al. The prognostic significance of soft tissue extension in Ewing's sarcoma. *Cancer* 1983;51:913.
331. Hoffer FA, Kozakewich H, Shamberger RC. Percutaneous biopsy of thoracic lesions in children. *Cardiovasc Intervent Radiol* 1990;13:32.
332. Shamberger RC, Tarbell NJ, Perez-Atayde AR, Grier HE. Malignant small round cell tumor (Ewing's-PNET) of the chest wall in children. *J Pediatr Surg* 1994;29:179.
333. Shamberger RC, LaQuaglia MP, Krailo MD, et al. Ewing's sarcoma of the rib: results of an intergroup study with analysis of outcome by timing of resection. *J Thorac Cardiovasc Surg* 2000;119:1154.
334. Horowitz ME, Malawer MM, Woo SY, et al. Ewing's sarcoma family of tumors: Ewing's sarcoma of bone. In: Pizzo PA, Poplack DG, eds. *Principles and practice of pediatric oncology,* 3rd ed. Philadelphia: Lippincott-Raven, 1997:831.
335. Perez CA, Tefft M, Nesbit M, et al. The role of radiation therapy in the management of non-metastatic Ewing's sarcoma of bone. Report of the intergroup Ewing's sarcoma study. *Int J Radiat Oncol Biol Phys* 1981;7:141.
336. Razek A, Perez CA, Tefft M, et al. Intergroup Ewing's sarcoma study. *Cancer* 1980;46:516.
337. Tefft M, Razek A, Perez CA, et al. Local control and survival related to radiation dose and volume and to chemotherapy in non-metastatic Ewing's sarcoma of pelvic bones. *Int J Radiat Oncol Biol Phys* 1978;4:367.
338. Fernandez CH, Lindberg RD, Sutow WW, Samuels ML. Localized Ewing's sarcoma—treatment and results. *Cancer* 1974;34:143.
339. Telles NC, Rabson AS, Pomeroy TC. Ewing's sarcoma: an autopsy study. *Cancer* 1978; 41:2321.
340. Tepper J, Glaubiger D, Lichter A, Wackenhut J, Glatstein E. Local control of Ewing's sarcoma of bone with radiotherapy and combination chemotherapy. *Cancer* 1980;46:1969.
341. Phillips TL, Sheline GE. Radiation therapy of malignant bone tumors. *Radiology* 1969;92:1537.

342. Vietti TJ, Gehan EA, Nesbit ME Jr, et al. Multimodal therapy in metastatic Ewing's sarcoma: an intergroup study. *Natl Cancer Inst Monogr* 1981;56:279.
343. Suit HD. Role of therapeutic radiology in cancer of bone. *Cancer* 1975;35:930.
344. Prindull G, Jurgens H, Jentsch F, Sauer R, Lasson U. Radiotherapy of non-metastatic Ewing's sarcoma. *J Cancer Res Clin Oncol* 1985;110:127.
345. Sauer R, Jurgens H, Burgers JMV, et al. Prognostic factors in the treatment of Ewing's sarcoma. *Radiother Oncol* 1987;10:101.
346. Donaldson S, Shuster J, Andreozzi C. The Pediatric Oncology Group (POG) experience in Ewing's sarcoma of bone. *Med Pediatr Oncol* 1989;17:283(abst).
347. Marcus RB Jr, Graham-Pole JR, Springfield DS, et al. High-risk Ewing's sarcoma: end-intensification using autologous bone marrow transplantation. *Int J Radiat Oncol Biol Phys* 1988;15:53.
348. Kuttesch JF, Wexler LH, Marcus RB, et al. Second malignancies after Ewing's sarcoma: radiation dose-dependency of secondary sarcomas. *J Clin Oncol* 1996;14:2818.
349. Nesbit ME Jr, Perez CA, Tefft M, et al. Multimodal therapy for the management of primary, non-metastatic Ewing's sarcoma of bone: an intergroup study. *Monogr Natl Cancer Inst* 1981;56:255.
350. Nesbit ME Jr, Gehan EA, Burgert EO, et al. Multimodal therapy for the management of primary, nonmetastatic Ewing's sarcoma of bone: a long-term follow-up of the first intergroup study. *J Clin Oncol* 1990;8:1664.
351. Burgert EO Jr, Nesbit ME, Garnsey LA, et al. Multimodal therapy for the management of nonpelvic, localized Ewing's sarcoma of bone: Intergroup Study IESS-II. *J Clin Oncol* 1990;8:1514.
352. Smith MA, Ungerleider RS, Horowitz ME, Simon R. Influence of doxorubicin dose intensity on response and outcome for patients with osteogenic sarcoma and Ewing's sarcoma. *J Natl Cancer Inst* 1991;83:1460.
353. Grier H, Krailo M, Tarbell N, et al. Adding ifosfamide and etoposide to vincristine, cyclophosphamide, adriamycin and actinomycin improves outcome in non-metastatic Ewing's and PNET: update of CCG/POG study. *Med Pediatr Oncol* 1996;27:259.
354. Wexler LH, Delaney TF, Tsokos M, et al. Ifosfamide and etoposide plus vincristine, doxorubicin, and cyclophosphamide for newly diagnosed Ewing's sarcoma family of tumors. *Cancer* 1996;78:901.
355. Craft A, Cotterill S, Malcolm A, et al. Ifosfamide-containing chemotherapy in Ewing's sarcoma: the second United Kingdom Children's Cancer Study Group and the Medical Research Council Ewing's tumor study. *J Clin Oncol* 1998;16:3628.
356. Rosito P, Mancini AF, Rondell R, et al. Italian cooperative study for the treatment of children and young adults with localized Ewing sarcoma of bone. *Cancer* 1999;86:421.
357. Granowetter L. Personal communication, April 2000.
358. Cangir A, Vietti TJ, Gehan EA, et al. Ewing's sarcoma metastatic at diagnosis. Results and comparisons of two Intergroup Ewing's Sarcoma Studies. *Cancer* 1990;66:887.
359. Madero L, Munoz A, Sanchez deToledo J, et al. Megatherapy in children with high risk Ewing's sarcoma in first complete remission. *Bone Marrow Transplant* 1998;21:795.
360. Ozkaynek MF, Matthay K, Cairo M, et al. Double alkylator non-total-body irradiation regimen with autologous hematopoietic stem-cell transplantation in pediatric solid tumors. *J Clin Oncol* 1998;16:937.
361. Boulad F, Kernan NA, LaQuaglia MP, et al. High-dose induction chemoradiotherapy followed by autologous bone marrow transplantation as consolidation therapy in rhabdomyosarcoma, extrosseous Ewing's sarcoma, and undifferentiated sarcoma. *J Clin Oncol* 1998;16:1697.
362. Thomson B, Hawkins D, Felgenhauer J, Radick JP. RT-PCR evaluation of peripheral blood, bone marrow and peripheral blood stem cells in children and adolescents undergoing VACIME chemotherapy for Ewing's sarcoma and alveolar rhabdomyosarcoma. *Bone Marrow Transplant* 1999;24:527.
363. Marina NM, Pappo AS, Parham DM, et al. Chemotherapy dose-intensification for pediatric patients with Ewing's family of tumors and desmoplastic small round-cell tumors: a feasibility study at St. Jude Children's Research Hospital. *J Clin Oncol* 1999;17:180.
364. Perentesis J, Katsanis E, DeFor T, et al. Autologous stem cell transplantation for high-risk pediatric solid tumors. *Bone Marrow Transplant* 1999;24:609.
365. Burdach S, Jurgens H, Peters C, et al. Myeloablative radiochemotherapy and hematopoietic stem-cell rescue in poor-prognosis Ewing's sarcoma. *J Clin Oncol* 1993;11:1482.
366. Paulusseu M, Ahrens S, Burdach S, et al. Primary metastatic (stage IV) Ewing tumor: survival analysis of 171 patients from the EICESS studies. *Ann Oncol* 1998;9:275.
367. Horowitz ME, Kinsella TJ, Wexler LH, et al. Total-body irradiation and autologous bone marrow transplant in the treatment of high-risk Ewing's sarcoma and rhabdomyosarcoma. *J Clin Oncol* 1993;11:1911.
368. Tanaka K, Iwakuma T, Harimaya K, et al. EWS-FLI1 antisense oligodeoxynucleotide inhibits proliferation of human Ewing's sarcoma and primitive neuroectodermal tumor cells. *J Clin Invest* 1997;99:239.
369. Picci P, Bohling T, Bacci G, et al. Chemotherapy-induced tumor necrosis as a prognostic factor in localized Ewing's sarcoma of the extremities. *J Clin Oncol* 1997;15:1553.
370. Wunder JS, Paulian G, Huvos AG, et al. The histological response to chemotherapy as a predictor of the oncological outcome of operative treatment of Ewing sarcoma. *J Bone Surg Am* 1998;80:1020.
371. Reynolds M. Pediatric liver tumors. *Semin Surg Oncol* 1999;16:159.
372. Greenberg H, Filler RM. Hepatic tumors. In: Pizzo PA, Poplack DG, eds. *Principles and practice of pediatric oncology*, 3rd ed. Philadelphia: Lippincott-Raven, 1997.
373. Sotelo-Avila C, Gonzalez-Crussi F, Fowler JW. Complete and incomplete forms of Beckwith-Wiedemann syndrome: their oncogenic potential. *J Pediatr* 1980;96:47.
374. Kingston JE, Herbert A, Draper GJ, Mann JR. Association between hepatoblastoma and polyposis coli. *Arch Dis Child* 1983;58:959.
375. Oda H, Imai Y, Nakatsura Y, et al. Somatic mutations of the APC gene in sporadic hepatoblastomas. *Cancer Res* 1996;56:3320.
376. Kraus JA, Albrecht S, Wiestler OD, et al. Loss of heterozygosity of chromosome 1 in human hepatoblastoma. *Int J Cancer* 1996:67:467.
377. Nagata T, Mugiskima H, Shickino H, et al. Karyotypic analyses of hepatoblastoma. *Cancer Genet Cytogenet* 1999;114:42.
378. Ideda H, Matsuyama S, Tauimura M. Association between hepatoblastoma and very low birth weight: a trend or a chance? *J Pediatr* 1997;130:557.
379. Ross JA. Hepatoblastoma and birth weights: too little, too big or just right? *J Pediatr* 1997;130:516.
380. Ohaki Y, Misugi K, Sasaki Y, Tsunoda A. Hepatitis B surface antigen positive hepatocellular carcinoma in children. *Cancer* 1983;51:822.
381. Leuschner I, Harms D, Schmidt D. The association of hepatocellular carcinoma in childhood with hepatitis B virus infection. *Cancer* 1988;62:2363.
382. Chang M-H, Chen C-J, Lai M-S, et al. Universal hepatitis B vaccination in Taiwan and the incidence of hepatocellular carcinoma in children. *N Engl J Med* 1997;336:1855.
383. Eriksson S, Carlson J, Velez R. Risk of cirrhosis and primary liver cancer in alpha$_1$-antitrypsin deficiency. *N Engl J Med* 1986;314:736.
384. Beaumont C, Simon M, Fauchet R, et al. Serum ferritin as a possible marker of the hemochromatosis allele. *N Engl J Med* 1979;301:169.
385. Cartwright GE, Edwards CQ, Kravitz K, et al. Hereditary hemochromatosis. *N Engl J Med* 1979;301:175.
386. Weinberg AC, Finegold MJ. Primary hepatic tumors in childhood. In: Finegold M, ed. *Pathology of neoplasia in children and adolescents*. Philadelphia: WB Saunders, 1986.
387. Haas JE, Muczynski KA, Krailo M, et al. Histopathology and prognosis in childhood hepatoblastoma and hepatocarcinoma. *Cancer* 1989;64:1082.
388. Farhi DC, Shikes RH, Murari PJ, Silverberg SG. Hepatocellular carcinoma in young people. *Cancer* 1983;52:1516.
389. Lack EE, Neve C, Vawter GF. Hepatocellular carcinoma. Review of 32 cases in childhood and adolescence. *Cancer* 1983;52:1510.
390. McArthur JW, Toll GD, Russfield AB, et al. Sexual precocity attributable to ectopic gonadotropin secretion by hepatoblastoma. *Am J Med* 1973;54:390.
391. Lack EE, Neave C, Vawter GF. Hepatoblastoma. A clinical and pathologic study of 54 cases. *Am J Surg Pathol* 1982;6:693.
392. Pritchard J, da Cunha A, Cornbleet MA, Carter CJ. Alpha feto (AFP) monitoring of response to adriamycin in hepatoblastoma. *J Pediatr Surg* 1982;17:429.
393. Alpert E, Hershberg R, Schur P II, Isselbacher KJ. Alpha-fetoprotein in human hepatoma: improved detection in serum, and quantitative studies using a new sensitive technique. *Gastroenterology* 1971;61:137.
394. Geiser CF, Shih VE. Cystathionuria and its origin in children with hepatoblastoma. *J Pediatr* 1980;96:72.
395. Miller JH, Gates GH, Stanley P. The radiographic investigation of hepatic tumors in childhood. *Radiology* 1977;124:451.
396. Gates GF, Miller JH, Stanley P. Scintiangiography of hepatic masses in childhood. *JAMA* 1978;239:2667.
397. Evans AE, Land VJ, Newton WA, et al. Combination chemotherapy (vincristine, adriamycin, cyclophosphamide and 5-fluorouracil) in the treatment of children with malignant hepatoma. *Cancer* 1982;50:821.
398. Ni Y-H, Chang M-H, Hsu H-Y, et al. Hepatocellular carcinoma in childhood. *Cancer* 1991;68:1737.
399. Goldsmith NA, Woodburne RT. The surgical anatomy pertaining to liver resection. *Surg Gynecol Obstet* 1957;105:310.
400. Boechat MI, Kangarloo H, Ortega J, et al. Primary liver tumors in children: comparison of CT and MR imaging. *Radiology* 1988;169:727.
401. Stringer MD, Hennayake S, Howard ER, et al. Improved outcome for children with hepatoblastoma. *Br J Surg* 1995;82:386.
402. Takahiko S, Ando H, Watanabe Y, et al. Treatment of hepatoblastoma: less extensive hepatectomy after effective preoperative chemotherapy with cisplatin and adriamycin. *Surgery* 1998;123:407.
403. King DR, Ortega J, Campbell J, et al. The surgical management of children with incompletely resected hepatic cancer is facilitated by intensive chemotherapy. *J Pediatr Surg* 1991;26:1074.
404. Koneru B, Flye MW, Busuttil RW, et al. Liver transplantation for hepatoblastoma: the American experience. *Ann Surg* 1991;213:118.
405. Bilik R, Superina R. Transplantation for unresectable liver tumors in children. *Transplant Proc* 1997;29:2834.
406. Curley SA, Izzo F, Delrio P, et al. Radiofrequency ablation of unresectable primary and metastatic hepatic malignancies. *Ann Surg* 1999;230:1.
407. Shamberger RC, Leichtner AM, Jonas MM, LaQuaglia MP. Long-term hepatic regeneration and function in infants and children following liver resection. *J Am Coll Surg* 1996;182:515.
408. Ortega JA, Krailo MD, Haas JE, et al. Effective treatment of unresectable or metastatic hepatoblastoma with cisplatin and continuous infusion doxorubicin chemotherapy: a report from the Children's Cancer Study Group. *J Clin Oncol* 1991;9:2167.
409. Quinn JJ, Altman AJ, Robinson HT, et al. Adriamycin and cisplatin for hepatoblastoma. *Cancer* 1985;56:1926.
410. Heifetz SA, French M, Correa M, Grossfeld JL. Hepatoblastoma: the Indiana experience with preoperative chemotherapy for inoperable tumors. *Pediatr Pathol Lab Med* 1997;17:857.
411. Weinblatt ME, Siegel SE, Siegel MM, Stanley P, Weitzman JJ. Preoperative chemotherapy for unresectable primary hepatic malignancies in children. *Cancer* 1982;50:1061.
412. Filler RM, Ehrlich PF, Greenberg ML, Babyn PS. Preoperative chemotherapy in hepatoblastoma. *Surgery* 1991;110:591.
413. Ninane J, Perilongo G, Stalens J-P, et al. Effectiveness and toxicity of cisplatin and doxo-

rubicin (PLADO) in childhood hepatoblastoma and hepatocellular carcinoma: a SIOP pilot study. *Med Pediatr Oncol* 1991;19:199.

414. Douglass EC, Reynolds M, Finegold M, Cantor AB, Glicksman A. Cisplatin, vincristine, and fluorouracil therapy for hepatoblastoma: a Pediatric Oncology Group study. *J Clin Oncol* 1993;11:96.
415. Ortega JA, Douglass E, Feusner J, et al. A randomized trial of cisplatin (DDP)/vincristine (VCR) h5-fluorouracil (5FU) versus DDP /doxorubicin (DOX) I.V. continuous infusion (CI) for the treatment of hepatoblastoma (HB). Results from the Pediatric Intergroup Hepatoma Study (CCG-8881 hPOG-8945). *Proc Am Soc Clin Oncol* 1994;13:416(abst).
416. Ehrlich PF, Greenberg ML, Filler RM. Improved long-term survival with preoperative chemotherapy for hepatoblastoma. *J Pediatr Surg* 1997;32:999.
417. Uchiyama M, Iwafuchi M, Naito M, et al. A study of therapy for pediatric hepatoblastoma: prevention and treatment of pulmonary metastasis. *Eur J Pediatr Surg* 1999;9:142.
418. von Schweinitz D, Byrd DJ, Hecker H, et al. Efficiency and toxicity of ifosfamide, cisplatin and doxorubicin in the treatment of childhood hepatoblastoma. *Eur J Cancer* 1997; 33:1243.
419. Reynolds M, Douglass EC, Finegold M, Cantor A, Glicksman A. Chemotherapy can convert unresectable hepatoblastoma. *J Pediatr Surg* 1992;27:1080.
420. Han Y-M, Park H-H, Lee J-M, et al. Effectiveness of preoperative transarterial chemoembolization in presumed inoperable hepatoblastoma. *J Vasc Intervent Radiol* 1999;10;1275.
421. Douglas E, Ortega J, Feusner J, et al. Hepatocellular carcinoma in children and adolescents. Results from the Pediatric Intergroup Study (CCG 8881/POG 8945). *Proc Am Soc Clin Oncol* 1994;13:420(abst 1439).
422. von Schweinitz D, Hecker H, Schmidt-von-Arndt G, et al. Prognostic factors and staging systems in childhood hepatoblastoma. *Int J Cancer* 1997;74:593.
423. Haas JE, Muczynski KA, Krailo M, et al. Histopathology and prognosis in childhood hepatoblastoma and hepatocarcinoma. *Cancer* 1989;64:1082.
424. Giacomantonio M, Ein SH, Mancer K, Stephens CA. Thirty years of experience with pediatric primary malignant liver tumors. *J Pediatr Surg* 1984;19:523.
425. Rescorla FJ. Pediatric germ cell tumors. *Semin Surg Oncol* 1999;16:144.
426. Göbel V, Calaminus G, Engert J, et al. Teratomas of infancy and childhood. *Med Pediatr Oncol* 1998;31:8.
427. Castleberry RP, Cushing B, Perlman E, Hawkins EP. Germ cell tumors. In: Pizzo PA, Poplack DG, eds. *Principles and practice of pediatric oncology*, 3rd ed. Philadelphia: Lippincott-Raven, 1997:921.
428. Einhorn LH, Donohue J. Cis-diamminedichloroplatinum, vinblastine and bleomycin combination chemotherapy in disseminated testicular cancer. *Ann Intern Med* 1977; 87:293.
429. Pinkerton CR. Malignant germ cell tumors in childhood. *Eur J Cancer* 1997;33:895.
430. Dehner LP. Gonadal and extragonadal germ cell neoplasms: teratomas in childhood. In: Finegold MJ, Bennington J, eds. *Pathology of neoplasia in children and adolescents*. Philadelphia: WB Saunders, 1986:282.
431. Silver SA, Wiley JM, Perlman EJ. DNA ploidy analysis of pediatric germ cell tumors. *Mod Pathol* 1994;7:951.
432. Shirai T, Itoh T, Yoshiki T, et al. Immunofluorescent demonstration of alpha-fetoprotein and other plasma proteins in yolk sac tumors. *Cancer* 1976;38:1661.
433. Teilum G, Albrechtsen R, Norgaard-Pedersen B. The histogenetic-embryologic basis for reappearance of alpha-fetoprotein in endodermal sinus tumors (yolk sac tumors) and teratomas. *Acta Pathol Microbiol Scand* 1975;83:80.
434. Kurman RJ, Norris HJ. Malignant germ cell tumors of the ovary. *Hum Pathol* 1977;8:551.
435. Teilum G. The concept of endodermal sinus (yolk sac) tumour. *Scand J Immunol* 1978;8(Suppl):75.
436. Perlman EJ, Valentine MB, Griffin CA, Look AT. Deletion of 1p36 in childhood endodermal sinus tumors by two-color fluorescence in situ hybridization: a Pediatric Oncology Group study. *Genes Chromosomes Cancer* 1996;16:15.
437. Mostofi FK, Price EB Jr. *Atlas of tumor pathology*. Second Series. Fascicle 8. Tumors of the male genital system. Washington, DC: American Registry of Pathology, 1973.
438. Bosl GJ, Dmitrovsky E, Reuter VE, et al. Isochrome of chromosome 12: clinically useful marker for male germ cell tumors. *J Natl Cancer Inst* 1989;81:1874.
439. Hoffner L, Deka R, Chakravarti A, Surti V. Cytogenetics and origins of pediatric germ cell tumors. *Cancer Genet Cytogenet* 1994;74:54.
440. Gitlin D, Boesman M. Serum alpha feto-protein, albumin and gamma G-globulin in the human conceptus. *J Clin Invest* 1966;45:1826.
441. Tsuchida Y, Endo Y, Saito S, et al. Evaluation of alpha-fetoprotein in early infancy. *J Pediatr Surg* 1978;13:155.
442. Wu JT, Book L, Sudar K. Serum alpha fetoprotein (AFP) levels in normal infants. *Pediatr Res* 1981;15:50.
443. Abelev GI, Assecritova IV, Kraevsky NA, Perova SD, Perevodchikova NI. Embryonal serum alpha-globulin in cancer patients: diagnostic value. *Int J Cancer* 1967;2:551.
444. Mann JR, Lakin GE, Leonard JC, et al. Clinical applications of serum carcinoembryonic antigen and alpha-fetoprotein levels in children with solid tumors. *Arch Dis Child* 1978;53:366.
445. Morinaga S. Ojima M, Sasano M. Human chorionic gonadotropin and alpha-fetoprotein in testicular germ cell tumors: an immunohistochemical study in comparison with tissue concentrations. *Cancer* 1983;52:1281.
446. Altman RP, Randolph JG, Lilly JR. Sacrococcygeal teratoma: American Academy of Pediatrics Surgical Section survey—1973. *J Pediatr Surg* 1974;9:389.
447. Fraumeni JF Jr, Li FP, Dalager N. Teratomas in children: epidemiologic features. *J Natl Cancer Inst* 1973;51:1425.
448. Ein SH, Adeyeimi SD, Mancer K. Benign sacrococcygeal teratomas in infants and children. A 25 year review. *Ann Surg* 1980;191:382.
449. Gross RE, Clatworthy HW Jr, Meeker IA. Sacrococcygeal teratomas in infants and children. A report of 40 cases. *Surg Gynecol Obstet* 1951;92:341.
450. Hawkins E, Isaacs H, Cushing B, Rogers P. Occult malignancy in neonatal sacrococcygeal teratomas. A report from a combined Pediatric Oncology Group and Children's Cancer Group study. *Am J Pediatr Hematol Oncol* 1993;15:406.
451. Ein SH, Mancer K, Adeyemi SD. Malignant sacrococcygeal teratoma—endodermal sinus, yolk sac tumor—in infants and children. A 32 year review. *J Pediatr Surg* 1985;20:473.
452. Schropp KP, Lobe TE, Rao B, et al. Sacrococcygeal teratoma: the experience of four decades. *J Pediatr Surg* 1992;27:1075.
453. Teitelbaum D, Teich S, Cassidy S, et al. Highly vascularized sacrococcygeal teratoma: description of this atypical variant and its operative management. *J Pediatr Surg* 1994;29:98.
454. Ablin AR, Krailo MD, Ramsay NKC, et al. Results of treatment of malignant germ cell tumors in 93 children. A report from the Children's Cancer Study Group. *J Clin Oncol* 1991;9:1782.
455. Kersh CR, Constable WC, Hahn SS, et al. Primary malignant extragonadal germ cell tumors. An analysis of the effect of radiotherapy. *Cancer* 1990;65:2681.
456. Green DM, Brecher ML, Grossi M, et al. The use of different induction and maintenance chemotherapy regimens for the treatment of advanced yolk sac tumors. *J Clin Oncol* 1983;1:111.
457. Pinkerton CR, Pritchard J, Spitz L. High complete response rate in children with advanced germ cell tumors using cisplatin-containing combination chemotherapy. *J Clin Oncol* 1986;4:194.
458. Hawkins EP, Finegold MJ, Hawkins HK, et al. Nongerminomatous malignant germ cell tumors in children. A review of 89 cases from the Pediatric Oncology Group, 1971–1984. *Cancer* 1986;58:2579.
459. Young JL Jr, Ries LG, Silverberg E, Horm JW, Miller JW. Cancer incidence, survival, and mortality for children younger than age 15 years. *Cancer* 1986;58:598.
460. Birch JM, Marsden HB, Swindell R. Pre-natal factors in the origin of germ cell tumours of childhood. *Carcinogenesis* 1982;3:75.
461. Gilbert JB, Hamilton JB. Studies in malignant testis tumors. III. Incidence and nature of tumors in ectopic testes. *Surg Gynecol Obstet* 1940;71:731.
462. Campbell HE. Incidence of malignant growth of the undescended testicle. *Arch Surg* 1942;44:353.
463. Giwercman A, Grindsted J, Hansen B, Jensen OM, Skakkebaek NE. Testicular cancer risk in boys with maldescended testis: a cohort study. *J Urol* 1987;138:1214.
464. Batata MA, Chu FCH, Hilaris BS, Whitmore WF, Golbey RB. Testicular cancer in cryptorchids. *Cancer* 1982;49:1023.
465. Pike MC, Chilvers C, Peckham MJ. Effect of age at orchiopexy on risk of testicular cancer. *Lancet* 1986;i:1246.
466. Martin DC. Malignancy in the cryptorchid testis. *Urol Clin North Am* 1982;9:371.
467. Lipschultz LI, Caminos-Torres R, Greenspan CS, Snyder PJ. Testicular function after orchiopexy for unilaterally undescended testis. *N Engl J Med* 1976;295:15.
468. Werder EA, Illig R, Torresani T, et al. Gonadal function in young adults after surgical treatment for cryptorchidism. *BMJ* 1976;2:1357.
469. Johnson DE, Woodhead DM, Pohl DR, Robison JR. Cryptorchidism and testicular tumorigenesis. *Surgery* 1968;63:919.
470. Fernandes ET, Etcubanas E, Rao BN, et al. Two decades of experience with testicular tumors in children at St. Jude Children's Research Hospital. *J Pediatr Surg* 1989;24,677.
471. Mann JR, Pearson D, Barrett A, et al. Results of the United Kingdom Children's Cancer Study Group's malignant germ cell tumor studies. *Cancer* 1989;63:1657.
472. Flamant F, Nihoul-Fekete C, Patte C, Lemerle J. Optimal treatment of stage I yolk sac tumor of the testis in children. *J Pediatr Surg* 1986;21:108.
473. Staubitz WJ. Surgical treatment of nonseminomatous germinal testis tumors. In: Johnson DE, Samuels ML, eds. *Cancer of the genitourinary tract*. New York: Raven Press, 1979:135.
474. Hoskin P, Dilly S, Easton D, et al. Prognostic factors in stage I non-seminomatous germ-cell testicular tumors managed by orchiectomy and surveillance: implications for adjuvant chemotherapy. *J Clin Oncol* 1986;4:1031.
475. Marina N, Fontanesi J, Kun L, et al. Treatment of childhood germ cell tumors: review of the St. Jude experience from 1979 to 1988. *Cancer* 1992;70:2568.
476. Aprikian AG, Herr HW, Bajorin DF, Bosl GJ. Resection of postchemotherapy residual masses and limited retroperitoneal lymphadenectomy in patients with metastatic testicular nonseminomatous germ cell tumors. *Cancer* 1994;74:1329.
477. Nichols CR, Williams SD, Loehrer PJ, et al. Randomized study of cisplatin dose intensity in poor-risk germ cell tumors. A Southwestern Cancer Study Group and Southwest Oncology Group protocol. *J Clin Oncol* 1991;9:1163.
478. Wozniak AJ, Samson MK, Shah NT, et al. A randomized trial of cisplatin, vinblastine, and bleomycin versus vinblastine, cisplatin, and etoposide in the treatment of advanced germ cell tumors of the testis: a Southwest Oncology Group study. *J Clin Oncol* 1991;9:70.
479. Williams SD, Birch R, Einhorn LH, et al. Treatment of disseminated germ-cell tumors with cisplatin, bleomycin, and either vinblastine or etoposide. *N Engl J Med* 1987;316:1435.
480. Levi JA, Raghavan D, Harvey V, et al. The importance of bleomycin in combination chemotherapy for good-prognosis germ cell carcinoma. *J Clin Oncol* 1993;11:1300.
481. Loehrer PJ Sr, Johnson D, Elson P, Einhorn LH, Trump D. Importance of bleomycin in favorable-prognosis disseminated germ cell tumors: an Eastern Cooperative Oncology Group trial. *J Clin Oncol* 1995;13:470.
482. Stoter G, Kaye S, Jones W, et al. Cisplatin (P) and VP16 (E) +/- bleomycin (B), (BEP) versus (EP) in good risk patients with disseminated non-seminomatous testicular cancer; a randomized EORTC GU Group study. *Onkologie* 1991;14(Suppl 4):17(abst).
483. Wheeler BM, Loehrer PJ, Williams SD, Einhorn LH. Ifosfamide in refractory male germ cell tumors. *J Clin Oncol* 1986;4:28.
484. Bokemeyer C, Kohrman O, Tischler J, et al. A randomized trial of cisplatin, etoposide and bleomycin (PEB) versus carboplatin, etoposide and bleomycin (CEB) for patients with "good risk" metastatic non-seminomatous germ cell tumors. *Ann Oncol* 1996;7:1015.

485. Mann JR, Raafat F, Robinson K, et al. The UKCCSG's germ cell tumor (GCT) studies: carboplatin, etoposide, and bleomycin are as effective as and less toxic than previous regimens for malignant extracranial non-gonadal tumors. *Med Pediatr Oncol* 1996, SIOP XXVIII (abst).
486. Frazier AL, Grier HE, Green DM. Treatment of endodermal sinus tumor in children using a regimen that lacks bleomycin. *Med Pediatr Oncol* 1996;27:69.
487. Fung CY, Garnick MB. Clinical stage I carcinoma of the testis. *J Clin Oncol* 1988;6:734.
488. Scully RE. *Atlas of tumor pathology.* Second Series. Fascicle 16. Tumors of the ovary and maldeveloped gonads. Washington, DC: Armed Forces Institute of Pathology, 1978.
489. Norris HJ, Zirkin HJ, Benson WL. Immature (malignant) teratoma of the ovary. A clinical and pathologic study of 58 cases. *Cancer* 1976;37:2359.
490. Breen JL, Maxson WS. Ovarian tumors in children and adolescents. *Clin Obstet Gynecol* 1977;20:607.
491. Heifetz SA, Cushing B, Giller R, et al. Pathologic considerations: a report from the combined Pediatric Oncology Group/Children's Cancer Group. *Am J Surg Pathol* 1998;22:1115.
492. Kottmeier HL. Classification and staging of malignant tumors in the female pelvis. *Int J Obstet Gynecol* 1971;9:172.
493. Buskirk SJ, Schray MF, Podratz KC, et al. Ovarian dysgerminoma: a retrospective analysis of results of treatment, sites of treatment failure and radiosensitivity. *Mayo Clin Proc* 1987;62:1149.
494. Cangir A, Smith J, van Eys J. Improved prognosis in children with ovarian cancers following modified VAC (vincristine sulfate, dactinomycin and cyclophosphamide) chemotherapy. *Cancer* 1978;42:1234.
495. Ungerleider RS, Donaldson SS, Warnke RA, Wilbur JR. Endodermal sinus tumor. The Stanford experience and the first reported case arising in the vulva. *Cancer* 1978;41:1627.
496. Gershenson DM, del Junco G, Herson J, Rutledge FN. Endodermal sinus tumor of the ovary: the MD Anderson experience. *Obstet Gynecol* 1983;61:194.
497. Slayton RE, Hreshchyshyn MM, Silberberg SG, et al. Treatment of malignant ovarian germ cell tumors. *Cancer* 1978;42:390.
498. Williams S, Clayton R, Silberberg S, et al. Response of malignant ovarian germ cell tumors to cis-platinum, vinblastine and bleomycin (PVB). *Proc Am Assoc Cancer Res* 1981;22:463(abst).
499. Gershenson DM, Kavanagh JJ, Copeland LJ, et al. Treatment of malignant nondysgerminomatous germ cell tumors of the ovary with vinblastine, bleomycin, and cisplatin. *Cancer* 1986;57:1731.
500. Taylor MH, Depetrillo AD, Turner AR. Vinblastine, bleomycin, and cisplatin in malignant germ cell tumors of the ovary. *Cancer* 1985;56:1341.
501. Teinturier C, Gelez J, Flamant F, et al. Pure dysgerminoma of the ovary in childhood: treatment results and sequelae. *Med Pediatr Oncol* 1994;23:1.
502. Norohna PA, Noronha R, Rao DS. Primary anterior mediastinal endodermal sinus tumors in childhood. *Am J Pediatr Hematol Oncol* 1985;7:312.
503. Kuzur ME, Vobleigh MA, Greco FA, Einhorn LH, Oldham RK. Endodermal sinus tumor of the mediastinum. *Cancer* 1982;50:766.
504. Flamant F, Schwartz L, Delons E, et al. Nonseminomatous malignant germ cell tumors in children. Multidrug therapy in stages III and IV. *Cancer* 1984;54:1687.
505. Chan RC, Sutow WW, Lindberg RD, et al. Management and results of localized Ewing's sarcoma. *Cancer* 1979;43:1001.

CHAPTER 45

Lymphomas

SECTION 1

RICCARDO DALLA-FAVERA
GIANLUCA GAIDANO

Molecular Biology of Lymphomas

The term *lymphoma* identifies two distinct groups of neoplasms: non-Hodgkin's lymphoma (NHL) and Hodgkin's lymphoma (HL).[1,2] Since the late 1970s, significant progress has been made in the elucidation of the pathogenesis of NHL as a clonal malignant expansion of B or T cells. The molecular characterization of the most frequent cytogenetic abnormalities associated with NHL has led to the identification of a number of genes that are altered in B-cell or T-cell NHL. The pathogenicity of most of these alterations has been confirmed by their ability to cause tumors in transgenic animal models. In addition, it has been established that most of these genetic lesions selectively associate with specific NHL types, thus representing specific markers of possible diagnostic significance for various NHL subtypes.[1,2] In contrast to NHL, the molecular pathogenesis of HL is less well understood, and until the advent of single-cell molecular analysis, genetic studies of HL had been hampered by the paucity of the neoplastic population within HL biopsies.

This chapter outlines the main types of genetic lesions in lymphomas and their distribution among the various clinicopathologic subtypes of these disorders, with major emphasis on NHL. The last section of the chapter briefly discusses the present and future applications of molecular genetic analysis in the clinical management of lymphomas.

HISTOGENETIC PATHWAYS OF LYMPHOMA

The histogenesis of lymphoma can be assessed by identifying the precise cellular subset from which a given lymphoma category derives (Fig. 45.1-1). This is achieved by defining the lineage and the precise differentiation stage of the various types of lymphoma and by comparing them with the features proper of the different maturation stages of normal lymphocytes. To date, the histogenesis of lymphoma has been clarified to a sizable extent in the case of lymphomas derived from B cells, whereas it is still poorly understood in the case of lymphomas originating from T cells.

B lymphocytes are generated in the bone marrow as a result of a multistep differentiation process.[3–5] Precursor B cells usually begin immunoglobulin (Ig) gene rearrangements of the heavy-chain locus followed by rearrangements of the light-chain locus.[3–5] If precursor B cells express a functional surface antibody acting as antigen receptor, they are positively selected into the peripheral B-cell pool comprising naive B cells.[3–5] Cells failing to express a functional antigen receptor are eliminated within the bone marrow.[3–5] For many B cells, the subsequent maturation steps are linked to the histologic structure of the germinal center.[3–5] The germinal center is constituted by a dark zone, characterized by a dominant growth of rapidly proliferating B cells, and by a light zone, in which nonproliferating B cells are selected and induced to differentiate through interactions with follicular dendritic cells and T helper cells. Within the germinal center, antigen-activated B cells accumulate somatic point mutations within their rearranged heavy- and light-chain genes (a phenomenon known as *somatic hypermutation*), which modify the affinity of their surface antibody to the antigen.[3–8] Only B cells that have acquired mutations leading to high-affinity binding are positively selected and differentiate

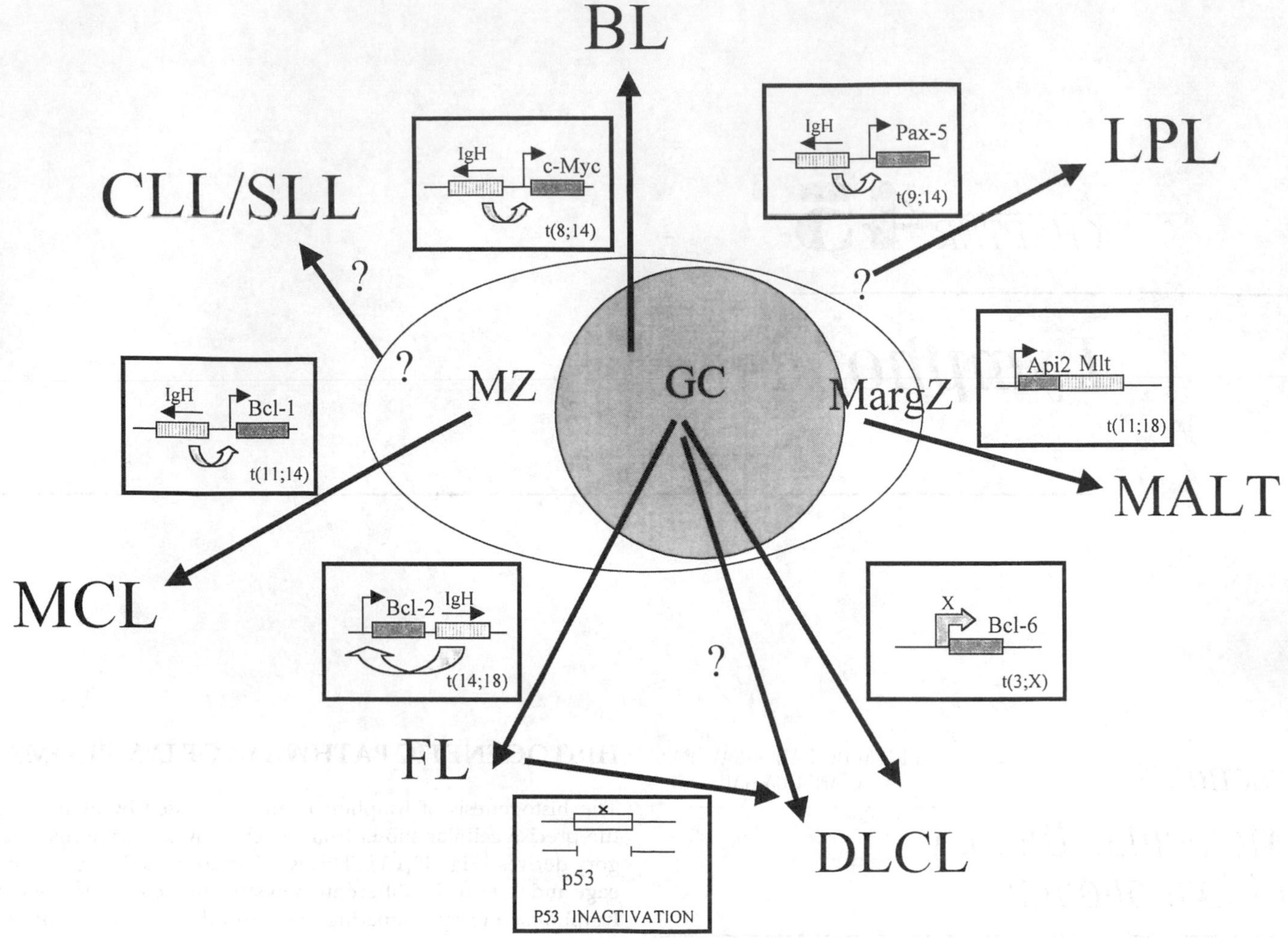

FIGURE 45.1-1. Model of B-cell non-Hodgkin's lymphoma (NHL) histogenesis and pathogenesis. A lymphoid follicle, constituted by the germinal center (GC) and the mantle zone (MZ), is represented together with the surrounding marginal zone (MargZ). On entering the GC, B cells activate into centroblasts, proliferate, and mature into centrocytes. These events are coupled to somatic hypermutation of immunoglobulin (Ig) genes and isotype switch of the Ig produced. Only GC B cells that are positively selected by antigen survive and exit the GC successfully. Cells that have exited the GC (post-GC B cells) have two fates: differentiation into plasma cells or memory B cells. Based on the absence or presence of somatic Ig hypermutation, B-cell NHL may be distinguished into two broad histogenetic categories: (1) B-cell NHL derived from pre-GC B cells and devoid of Ig mutations, represented in the figure by mantle cell lymphoma (MCL) and a fraction of chronic lymphocytic leukemia/small lymphocytic lymphoma (CLL/SLL); and (2) B-cell NHL derived from B cells that have transited through the GC and harbor Ig mutations, represented in the figure by follicular lymphoma (FL), lymphoplasmacytoid lymphoma (LPL), mucosa-associated lymphoid tissue lymphoma (MALT), diffuse large cell lymphoma (DLCL), and Burkitt's lymphoma (BL). For each lymphoma category, the arrow indicating the histogenetic origin is flanked by the genetic lesion associated with the lymphoma. In the case of CLL/SLL, as well as in a subset of DLCL, the relevant cancer related gene has not been identified.

into memory B cells or plasmablasts, whereas the majority of B cells are eliminated by apoptosis within the germinal center.[3–8]

The use of somatic hypermutation as a specific marker of B-cell transition through the germinal center allows for the definition of two broad histogenetic categories of B-cell lymphoma[9,10]:

1. Lymphomas devoid of somatic Ig hypermutation, which may derive from either pre–germinal center B cells or from B cells that have achieved maturation without transiting through the germinal center. Lymphomas generally devoid of somatic Ig hypermutation include mantle cell lymphoma and a substantial percentage of B-cell chronic lymphocytic leukemia/small lymphocytic lymphoma.[9,10]
2. Lymphomas associated with somatic Ig hypermutation and thus putatively derived from germinal center or post–germinal center B cells. Among the NHLs, lymphomas generally associated with somatic Ig hypermutation include follicular lymphoma, lymphoplasmacytoid lymphoma, mucosa-associated lymphoid tissue (MALT) lymphoma, diffuse large cell lymphoma (DLCL), Burkitt's lymphoma, and primary effusion lymphoma.[9–16] In addition, a fraction of B-cell chronic lymphocytic leukemia/small lymphocytic lymphoma, approximating 50%

of cases, is thought to originate from germinal center–related B cells.[17,18] Most, if not all, HL cases also are thought to derive from germinal center or post–germinal center B cells.[10,19–23] Extranodal lymphomas associated with somatic Ig hypermutation are postulated to originate from B cells that have transited through the germinal center and subsequently migrated to the involved extranodal site.

GENERAL MECHANISMS OF GENETIC LESIONS IN LYMPHOMA

Analogous to most cancer types, the pathogenesis of lymphoma represents a multistep process involving the progressive and clonal accumulation of multiple genetic lesions affecting protooncogenes and tumor suppressor genes. However, several important features distinguish the mechanism and type of genetic alterations associated with lymphoma from those associated with solid tumors. Extensive cytogenetic studies have shown that, during most stages of the disease, the genome of lymphoma cells is relatively stable and is not affected by the generalized random instability typical of many solid tumors, particularly those of epithelial origin.[24] Lymphoma also appears devoid of microsatellite instability, the hallmark of molecular defects in DNA mismatch repair genes observed in some hereditary cancer predisposition syndromes as well as in most sporadic tumor types.[25–27] Conversely, the genome of lymphoma cells is characterized by few, sometimes single, nonrandom chromosomal abnormalities, commonly represented by chromosomal translocations.[28]

At the molecular level, the genetic lesions identified so far in lymphomas include activation of oncogenes by chromosomal translocations, as well as inactivation of tumor suppressor loci by chromosomal deletion and mutation. In addition, the genome of certain lymphoma subtypes can be altered by the introduction of exogenous genes by various oncogenic viruses.

CHROMOSOMAL TRANSLOCATIONS

Chromosomal translocations represent the genetic hallmark of lymphoid malignancies, including NHL. As in other types of malignancies, NHL-associated translocations represent reciprocal and balanced recombinations between two specific chromosomes that are recurrently associated with a given tumor type and clonally represented in each tumor case.

The precise mechanisms leading to chromosomal translocations in hematopoietic neoplasms are not clearly understood. However, data suggest that the translocation process most likely occurs during Ig gene and T-cell receptor gene rearrangements in B and T cells, respectively, as a consequence of errors of the VDJ recombination machinery or the class switch machinery. This evidence is supported by the following observations:

1. A significant number of translocations involve chromosomal breakpoints within the Ig or T-cell receptor loci.[24]
2. In B-cell NHL, breakpoints within the Ig loci are often located precisely within sequences that normally mediate Ig gene rearrangement in B cells, such as the J and switch sequences.[29] Moreover, N-nucleotides, which are template-independent nucleotide additions generated at the site of VDJ recombination by terminal deoxynucleotidyl transferase, can be detected at certain breakpoint junctions, suggesting the action of the recombinase.[30]
3. Similarity has been shown between the sequences surrounding the breakpoints and recombination targeting motifs, such as the heptamer/nonamers and the bp45 nuclease binding sequence.[31]

Not all the chromosomal translocations are due to errors of the recombination machinery of the immune system. A defect in the DNA damage repair mechanism may be responsible in at least some translocations.[32] For example, based on sequence analysis of reciprocal chromosomal breakpoints, the chromosomal translocation t(4;11) seen in acute leukemias of B lineage appears to be initiated by several DNA strand breaks on both participating chromosomes and by subsequent DNA repair by an "error-prone" DNA repair mechanism. Similarly, analysis of the breakpoint junction sequence at *TEL* in t(12;21)(p13;q22) supports the occurrence of staggered DNA double-strand breaks followed by DNA repair.[33] Therefore, the generation of DNA double-strand breaks by exogenous and endogenous sources (e.g., chemicals and oxygen-free radicals) and faulty DNA repair can lead to chromosomal rearrangements.[34,35] These models have been validated by mouse models but have yet to be proven in humans.[36]

The suggestion also has been made that some translocations, namely those occurring in lymphoid malignancies derived from germinal center B cells, such as Burkitt's lymphoma and DLCL, may be a result of somatic hypermutation that takes place in the germinal center B cells.[37] It has been shown that deletions and duplications can be introduced into the rearranged variable $(V)_H$ genes in a substantial portion of germinal center cells during somatic hypermutation. Because the formation of these deletions and duplications is intrinsically associated with DNA double-strand breaks, they may provide a potential source for chromosomal translocations in germinal center B cells. Somatic hypermutation may be the underlying mechanism of the chromosomal translocations between the Ig_H locus and c-*MYC* in the endemic form of Burkitt's lymphoma, and these translocations are generally believed to be a result of errors of the VDJ recombination machinery. This theory is supported by the observation that the breakpoints at the Ig_H loci in endemic Burkitt's lymphoma are not usually directly adjacent to the recombination signal sequence that mediates VDJ recombination, but are located in the J intron or within rearranged VJ genes (i.e., the target region for hypermutation).[38] It remains to be seen if somatic hypermutation also plays a role in the generation of chromosomal translocations at the *BCL*-6 locus, which also is a target for somatic hypermutation, in B-cell DLCL (see Diffuse Large Cell Lymphoma, later in this chapter).

The common feature of all chromosomal translocations associated with NHL is the presence of protooncogenes in proximity to the chromosomal recombination sites. In most cases, the structure of the protooncogene and, in particular, its coding domain is not affected by the translocation, but the pattern of expression of the gene is altered as a consequence of the juxtaposition of heterologous regulatory sequences derived from the

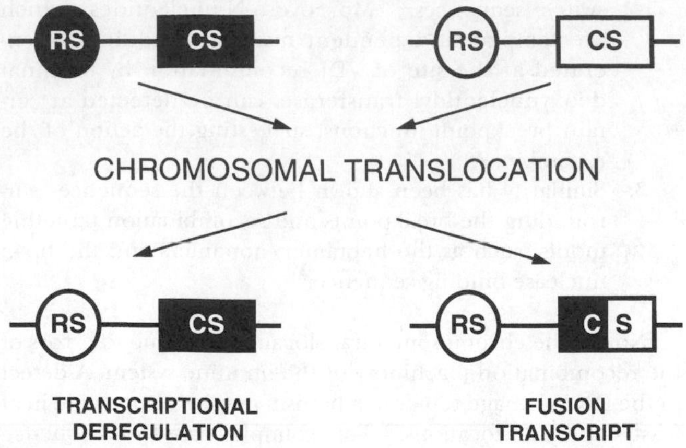

FIGURE 45.1-2. Models of chromosomal translocations in non-Hodgkin's lymphoma (NHL). The two genes involved in the translocation event are represented by their coding sequences (CS), which are represented by the rectangles, and by their regulatory sequences (RS), which are represented by the circles. The two genes are identified by different colors (black or white). **Top:** Germline configuration of the two genes involved in the translocation. The coding sequence of each of the two genes is proximal to its physiologic regulatory sequences, which coordinate the normal expression of the gene. **Bottom:** Chromosomal translocations may lead to two different consequences. In the case of transcriptional deregulation, the normal regulatory sequences of the protooncogene are removed and substituted with regulatory sequences derived from the partner chromosome. The protooncogene coding sequence (*black rectangle*) is thus juxtaposed to heterologous regulatory sequences (*white circle*). In NHL, most commonly the novel regulatory regions are derived from the immunoglobulin gene loci, which are consistently expressed at high levels in mature B cells. In the case of fusion transcript formation, part of the coding sequence of the two genes involved is fused together, generating a novel fusion protein with biochemical properties distinct from the native proteins.

partner chromosome (protooncogene deregulation) (Fig. 45.1-2). Two distinct types of protooncogene deregulation may occur, including homotopic and heterotopic deregulation. Homotopic deregulation occurs when the protooncogene is expressed constitutively in the lymphoma, whereas its expression is tightly regulated in normal lymphoid cells. Conversely, heterotopic deregulation occurs when the protooncogene, which is normally not expressed in lymphoid cells, undergoes ectopic expression in the lymphoma. In most types of NHL-associated translocations, the heterologous regulatory regions responsible for protooncogene deregulation are derived from antigen receptor loci, which are expressed at high levels in the target tissue.

An alternative mechanism of oncogene activation by chromosomal translocation is the juxtaposition of two genes to form a chimeric gene coding for a novel chimeric protein. This mechanism, which is common in chromosomal translocations associated with acute leukemias, is rarely associated with NHL. Examples are the t(11;18) of MALT lymphoma and the t(2;5) of T-cell anaplastic lymphoma.

The molecular cloning of the genetic loci involved in the translocations most frequently associated with NHL has led to the identification of a number of protooncogenes involved in lymphomagenesis (Table 45.1-1). The majority of these protooncogenes code for nuclear molecules belonging to major families of transcription factors, although regulators of programmed cell death and signal transducers may also be involved. The structural and functional consequences of each chromosomal translocation associated with NHL are described in each section of this chapter dedicated to the molecular pathogenesis of the various NHL subtypes.

OTHER MECHANISMS OF PROTOONCOGENE ALTERATION

In addition to chromosomal translocations, other mechanisms of protooncogene activation can also occur in NHL. Protooncogene amplification is substantially less common than in epithelial cancers, yet it occurs in some cases of high-grade NHL, as exemplified by the instance of *REL* amplifications in DLCL.[39] Amplification may involve many other unknown chromosomal sites, which are likely to be revealed by the extensive use of advanced cytogenetic techniques, such as comparative genomic hybridization. Point mutations can alter the coding sequence of the protooncogene, as in the case of c-*MYC* and *BCL*-2, and thus alter the biologic properties of the protooncogene product.[40,41] Alternatively, mutations may affect the protooncogene regulatory sequences, as in the case of c-*MYC* and *BCL*-6, thus altering their sensitivity to factors normally regulating the expression of the protooncogene through binding to its regulatory sequences.[42–45] Mutations of the *RAS* genes, which represent a frequent protooncogene alteration in human neoplasia, are virtually always absent in NHL.[46] Mutations activating unknown oncogenes may be a frequent event in NHL, and the search for these oncogenes is the focus of current investigations.

INACTIVATION OF TUMOR SUPPRESSOR GENES

Deletions and mutations of the *p53* tumor suppressor gene, which are thought to represent the most common genetic alteration in human cancer,[47] are restricted to specific subsets of NHL, including late stages of follicular lymphoma and Burkitt's lymphoma.[48–50] The mechanisms of *p53* inactivation in NHL is similar to that detected in human neoplasia in general and occurs through point mutation of one allele, chromosomal deletion of the second allele, or both.[47]

In addition, NHLs are associated with specific chromosomal deletions, suggesting the loss of presently unknown tumor suppressor genes. The most frequent of these deletions involves the long arm of chromosome 6 (6q).[24,51] The observations that 6q deletions may occur as the sole cytogenetic abnormality in some NHL cases[24] and are associated with poor prognosis[28] strongly support a pathogenetic role for these alterations. Deletions of chromosome 13q14 represent the most frequent lesion in B-cell chronic lymphocytic leukemia/small lymphocytic lymphoma, occurring in more than 50% of cases.[24] Mapping studies have ruled out the involvement of the *RB1* tumor suppressor gene, which is also located on chromosome 13q14, and have suggested the presence of a distinct tumor suppressor gene in the same region.[52–58]

ONCOGENIC VIRUSES

The infection of tumor cells by oncogenic viruses must be considered as a mechanism of genetic lesion because viruses introduce foreign genes into their target cells. Three distinct viruses are associated with the pathogenesis of specific NHL subtypes: Epstein-Barr virus (EBV), human herpesvirus-8 (HHV-8), and human T-cell leukemia virus type I (HTLV-I).

TABLE 45.1-1. Chromosomal Translocations of Non-Hodgkin's Lymphomas

Non-Hodgkin's Lymphoma Histologic Type	*Translocation*	*Protooncogene Involved*	*Mechanism of Protooncogene Activation*	*Protooncogene Function*
Lymphoplasmacytoid lymphoma	t(9;14)(p13;q32)	*PAX-5*	Transcriptional deregulation	Transcription factor regulating B-cell proliferation and differentiation
Follicular lymphoma	t(14;18)(q32;q21); t(2;18)(p11;q21); t(18;22)(q21;q11)	*BCL-2*	Transcriptional deregulation	Negative regulator of apoptosis
Mucosa-associated lymphoid tissue lymphoma	t(11;18)(q21;q21)	*API2/MLT*	Fusion protein	Negative regulator of apoptosis
	t(1;14)(p22;q32)	*BCL-10*	Transcriptional deregulation and truncation of caspase recruitment domain	Regulator of apoptosis
Mantle cell lymphoma	t(11;14)(q13;q32)	*BCL-1*/cyclin D1	Transcriptional deregulation	Regulator of the early phases of the cell cycle
B-lineage diffuse large cell lymphoma	der(3)(q27)	*BCL-6*	Transcriptional deregulation	Transcriptional repressor implicated in formation and function of germinal centers
Burkitt's lymphoma	t(8;14)(q24;q32); t(2;8)(p11;q24); t(8;22)(q24;q11)	c-*MYC*	Transcriptional deregulation	Transcription factor regulating cell proliferation, differentiation, and apoptosis
T-cell anaplastic large cell lymphoma	t(2;5)(p23;q35)	*NPM/ALK*	Fusion protein	*ALK* is a tyrosine kinase

EBV was initially identified in cases of endemic Burkitt's lymphoma from Africa; subsequently, EBV also was detected in a fraction of sporadic forms of Burkitt's lymphomas, acquired immunodeficiency syndrome (AIDS)–associated lymphomas, and primary effusion lymphomas.[49,59–68] With infection of a B lymphocyte, the EBV genome is transported into the nucleus, where it exists predominantly as an extrachromosomal circular molecule (episome).[59] The formation of circular episomes is mediated by the cohesive terminal repeats, which are represented by a variable number of tandem repeats sequence.[59,69] Because of this termini heterogeneity, the number of variable number of tandem repeats sequences enclosed in newly formed episomes may differ considerably, thus representing a constant clonal marker of the episome and, consequently, of a single infected cell.[69] Evidence for a pathogenetic role of the virus in NHL infected by EBV is at least twofold. On one side, it is well recognized that EBV is able to significantly alter the growth of B cells.[59] On the other side, EBV-infected lymphomas usually display a single form of fused EBV termini, suggesting that the lymphoma cell population represents the clonally expanded progeny of a single infected cell.[49,61]

HHV-8 is a gamma herpesvirus initially identified in tissues of patients with AIDS-related Kaposi's sarcoma, and it subsequently was found to infect a peculiar type of lymphoma known as *primary effusion lymphoma*[70–75] as well as a substantial fraction of multicentric Castleman's disease.[76] Phylogenetic analysis has shown that the closest relative of HHV-8 is herpesvirus saimiri, a gamma-2 herpesvirus of primates associated with T-cell lymphoproliferative disorders.[77,78] Like the other gamma herpesviruses, HHV-8 is lymphotropic, because it can be found in lymphocytes both *in vitro* and *in vivo*.[67,70–76,79,80] Lymphoma cells naturally infected by HHV-8 harbor the viral genome in its episomal configuration and display a marked restriction of viral gene expression, suggesting a pattern of latent infection.[78] HHV-8 carries several genes that may behave as oncogenes, including a gene homologous to the cellular D-type cyclins, a G protein–coupled receptor displaying constitutive activation, and several genes encoding for molecules displaying high homology with cellular cytokines [viral interleukin (IL)-6] and chemokines [viral macrophage inflammatory protein (MIP)-1α, MIP-2].[81–83] However, because primary effusion lymphoma cells carry latent HHV-8 infection, only a restricted subset of viral genes are expressed *in vivo*, including viral cyclin D and viral IL-6.[81,84]

HTLV-I is a member of the lentivirus group, which can immortalize normal T cells *in vitro* and can cause adult T-cell leukemia/lymphoma.[85–87] Unlike acutely transforming retroviruses, the HTLV-I genome does not encode a viral oncogene.[85–87] Furthermore, this retrovirus does not transform T cells by *cis*-activation of an adjacent cellular protooncogene, because the provirus appears to integrate randomly within the host genome.[85–87] Rather, the pathogenetic effect of HTLV-I seems to be due to viral production of a transregulatory protein (HTLV-I tax) that markedly increases expression of all viral gene products and transcriptionally activates the expression of certain host genes, including IL-2, the α chain of the IL-2 receptor (CD25), c-sis, c-fos, and granulocyte-macrophage colony-stimulating factor.[88–92] The central role of these genes in normal T-cell activation and growth, coupled to direct experimental evidence, support the notion that tax-mediated activation of these host genes represents an important mechanism by which HTLV-I initiates T-cell transformation.[93] In addition, it has been suggested that tax may mediate DNA damage as a consequence of either inactivation of the *p53* checkpoint or a repression of DNA repair functions.[94,95] It has been shown that tax may abrogate a mitotic checkpoint by targeting the TXBP181 cellular gene, a homologue of the yeast mitotic checkpoint MAD1 protein.[96] These features of tax are consistent with the fact that adult T-cell leukemia/lymphoma cells are karyotypically abnormal and frequently present as pleomorphic multinucleated giant cells.[97,98]

MOLECULAR PATHOGENESIS OF B-CELL NON-HODGKIN'S LYMPHOMA

The following section describes the detailed genetic lesions and the molecular pathways presently identified in association with distinct B-cell NHL categories classified according to the World Health Organization (WHO) system of lymphoid neoplasia.[2] B-cell NHL categories known to associate with specific genetic lesions include B-cell chronic lymphocytic leukemia/small lymphocytic lymphoma, lymphoplasmacytoid lymphoma, mantle cell lymphoma, follicular lymphoma, MALT lymphoma, DLCL, and Burkitt's lymphoma among B-cell NHL. The molecular pathogenesis of AIDS-related NHL also is addressed. The precise molecular pathogenesis of all other B-cell NHL types has not yet been elucidated.

B-CELL CHRONIC LYMPHOCYTIC LEUKEMIA/SMALL LYMPHOCYTIC LYMPHOMA

The molecular pathogenesis of B-cell chronic lymphocytic leukemia/small lymphocytic lymphoma is still largely unknown (see Fig. 45.1-1). Mutations of the *p53* gene and loss of heterozygosity at 17p, the *p53* site, are found in a small number (10% to 15%) of cases.[48,99] A higher frequency of *p53* alterations is observed after transformation of B-cell chronic lymphocytic leukemia/small lymphocytic lymphoma to Richter's syndrome, a highly aggressive lymphoma with a poor clinical outcome,[48] suggesting that *p53* may be involved in the genetic mechanisms underlying B-cell chronic lymphocytic leukemia/small lymphocytic lymphoma progression. Despite initial suggestions, it is now well established that "true" cases of B-cell chronic lymphocytic leukemia/small lymphocytic lymphoma (i.e., CD5+, CD23+, according to the WHO and the Revised European-American Lymphoma classification[1,2]) are consistently devoid of *BCL-1* and *BCL-2* rearrangements[99] (Table 45.1-2). Because high levels of *bcl-2* expression are consistently seen in B-cell chronic lymphocytic leukemia/small lymphocytic lymphoma,[100] it is conceivable that they result from mechanisms other than chromosomal translocation. A small fraction of B-cell chronic lymphocytic leukemia/small lymphocytic lymphoma harbor mutations of the *a*taxia-*t*elangiectasia *m*utated (*ATM*) gene.[101–103] Because these mutations may occur in the patient germline, *ATM* mutations may account, at least in part, for the familial cases of the disease.

Despite the paucity of information regarding the molecular lesions associated with B-cell chronic lymphocytic leukemia/small lymphocytic lymphoma, cytogenetic studies have revealed several recurrent chromosomal abnormalities.[24,104] Trisomy 12 is found in approximately 35% of B-cell chronic lymphocytic leukemia/small lymphocytic lymphoma cases evaluated by interphase fluorescence *in situ* hybridization and correlates with a poor survival.[105–107] Based on karyotypic and deletion mapping studies, it is likely that the 13q14 chromosomal region harbors a novel tumor suppressor gene that is involved at high frequency in B-cell chronic lymphocytic leukemia/small lymphocytic lymphoma.[52–58] In fact, deletions of 13q14 occur in approximately 60% of cases when analyzed by sensitive molecular tools, but the relevant gene has not been identified.[52–58] Deletions of 6q define a subset of B-cell chronic lymphocytic leukemia/small lymphocytic lymphoma cases displaying prolymphocytic features.[108]

Studies of B-cell chronic lymphocytic leukemia/small lymphocytic lymphoma have revealed novel insights into the disease histogenesis. It is now apparent that the clinical heterogeneity of B-cell chronic lymphocytic leukemia/small lymphocytic lymphoma might be related to heterogeneity in the disease histogenesis. Although B-cell chronic lymphocytic leukemia/small lymphocytic lymphoma has been traditionally viewed as a tumor of naive, pre–germinal center B cells, more recent data have suggested that a fraction of cases derives from germinal center–related B cells. In fact, the malignant cells of approximately 50% of B-cell chronic lymphocytic leukemia/small lymphocytic lymphoma harbor mutations of Ig genes, with or without *BCL-6* mutations,[17,18,45,109] which are well-established markers of germinal center transit. The molecular spectrum of Ig and *BCL-6* mutations in B-cell chronic lymphocytic leukemia/small lymphocytic lymphoma is superimposable to that of germinal center–derived lymphomas.[17,18,45,109] Intriguingly, the histogenetic heterogeneity of B-cell chronic lymphocytic leukemia/small lymphocytic lymphoma appears to carry prognostic relevance, because cases with mutations of Ig genes are associated with a significantly longer survival.[110,111]

LYMPHOPLASMACYTOID LYMPHOMA

Lymphoplasmacytoid lymphoma is typically CD5-negative and associates in a large fraction of cases with a monoclonal serum IgM-type paraprotein, causing the clinical syndrome known as *Waldenström's macroglobulinemia*.[1,2] Approximately 50% of these lymphomas associate with the t(9;14)(p13;q32) translocation, a recurrent chromosomal abnormality in B-cell NHL[112] (see Table 45.1-1 and Fig. 45.1-1). The chromosomal breakpoints of t(9;14)(p13;q32) involve the Ig_H locus on chromosome 14q32 and, on chromosome 9p13, a genomic region containing the paired homeobox-5 (*PAX-5*) gene.[113] *PAX-5* encodes a B-cell–specific transcription factor involved in the control of B-cell proliferation and differentiation.[114] Presumably, the juxtaposition of *PAX-5* to the Ig_H locus in NHL carrying t(9;14)(p13;q32) causes the deregulated expression of the gene, thus contributing to tumor development.[113] Apart from t(9;14)(p13;q32), no other genetic lesion has been detected at significant frequencies in lymphoplasmacytoid lymphoma (see Table 45.1-2).

MANTLE CELL LYMPHOMA

Mantle cell lymphoma constitutes 25% of nonfollicular small B-cell lymphomas and is typically associated with t(11;14)(q13;q32)[1,2,115–117] (see Fig. 45.1-1). The t(11;14)(q13;q32) translocation juxtaposes the *BCL-1* locus at 11q13 with Ig_H[118–120] (see Table 45.1-1). Although early characterization of the *BCL-1* locus did not identify a putative oncogene implicated in the translocation, it is now evident that t(11;14) consistently leads to homotopic deregulation of *BCL-1* (also known as *CCND1* or *PRAD1*), a gene located in proximity to the breakpoint region and encoding for cyclin D1, a member of the D-type G_1 cyclins that regulate the early phases of the cell cycle.[121–125] The consistent and selective clustering of *BCL-1* overexpression with NHLs carrying t(11;14) strongly suggests that this gene is indeed the critical component of t(11;14)(q13;q32).[121–125]

The precise contribution of cyclin D1 to cell-cycle regulation is still under investigation. As for other D-type cyclins, cyclin D1 is thought to act primarily as a growth factor sensor, integrating extracellular signals with the cell-cycle clock.[126] The pathogenetic role of *BCL-1* activation in human neoplasia is

TABLE 45.1-2. Frequency of Genetic Lesions in B-Cell Non-Hodgkin's Lymphoma[a]

Histology	*BCL-1*	*BCL-2*	*BCL-6 R*[b]	*BCL-6 M*[b]	*c-MYC*	*PAX-5*	*API2/ MLT*	*BCL-10*	*p53*	*p16*	*Epstein-Barr Virus*
Small lymphocytic lymphoma	—	—	—	30%	—	—	—	—	10%	—	—
Lymphoplasmocytoid lymphoma	—	—	—	30%	—	50%	—	—	—	—	—
Mantle cell lymphoma	70%	—	—	—	—	—	—	—	20%[c]	50%[c]	—
Mucosa-associated lymphoid tissue lymphoma	—	—	—	50%	—	—	50%	Rare			
Follicular lymphoma	—	90%	Rare	50%	—	—	—	—	—	—	—
Diffuse large cell lymphoma											
De novo	—	30%	35%	70%	—	—	—	—	—	—	—
Transformed	—	90%	—	—	Rare	—	—	—	90%	30%	—
Burkitt's lymphoma	—	—	—	40%	100%	—	—	—	30%	30%	30–100%[d]

[a]Dashes indicate molecular lesion or viral infection not involved; where positive, the percentage of positive cases is indicated.
[b]R indicates rearrangement, and M indicates mutations, of the 5' noncoding region.
[c]Fifty percent in aggressive mantle cell lymphoma variant.
[d]Thirty percent in sporadic Burkitt's lymphoma; 100% in endemic Burkitt's lymphoma.

suggested by the ability of cyclin D1 overexpression to transform cells *in vitro* and contribute to B-cell lymphomagenesis in transgenic mice.[197–199]

The application of strict phenotypic criteria to the classification of B-cell lymphoproliferations has defined that the distribution of *BCL-1* rearrangements and activation are restricted to mantle cell lymphoma (see Table 45.1-2).[130–132] The frequency and specificity of this genetic lesion provide an excellent marker for diagnosis of mantle cell lymphoma.[117] The precise identification of mantle cell lymphoma among nonfollicular small B-cell lymphomas is clinically relevant because mantle cell lymphoma is a far more aggressive disease and displays a significantly shorter survival than other histologically related forms.[115,116]

Other genetic alterations may be also involved in mantle cell lymphoma. Inactivation of *p53* occurs in approximately 20% of cases and is a marker of poor prognosis.[133] Inactivation of *p16* by deletion, mutation, or hypermethylation is detectable in approximately one-half of cases belonging to the aggressive mantle cell lymphoma variant characterized by a blastoid cell morphology.[134]

FOLLICULAR LYMPHOMA

The genetic hallmark of follicular lymphoma is represented by chromosomal breaks at 18q21 and rearrangements of *BCL-2*, which are detected in 80% to 90% of the cases independent of cytologic subtype[135–139] (see Table 45.1-2 and Fig. 45.1-1). Other genetic lesions may also occur, especially in follicular lymphoma cases that have undergone histologic progression to a high-grade NHL.[50,134,140]

Chromosomal Translocations Involving the BCL-2 Gene

The t(14;18)(q32;q21) translocation is the most common translocation in human lymphoid malignancies[135–139] (see Table 45.1-1). The rare variant translocations t(2;18)(p11;q21) and t(18;22)(q21;q21) represent biologic equivalents. Virtually all follicular lymphomas and a fraction of DLCLs carry breaks at 18q21[135–139,141] (see Table 45.1-2). In t(14;18), the rearrangement joins the *BCL-2* gene at its 3' untranslated region to an Ig_H J segment (Fig. 45.1-3), resulting in homotopic deregulation of *BCL-2* expression.[135–139] The consequence of the translocation is the presence within the cells of constitutively high levels of *BCL-2* protein resulting from both enhanced transcription and, possibly, more efficient RNA processing.[142,143] Approximately 70% of the chromosome 18 breakpoints cluster within the major breakpoint region, and the remaining cases usually break in the more distant minor cluster region.[135–139]

The *BCL-2* gene encodes a 26-kD integral membrane protein that has been localized to mitochondria, endoplasmic reticulum, and perinuclear membrane.[144] In contrast to most protooncogenes of lymphoid neoplasia, *BCL-2* has little or no ability to promote cell-cycle progression or cell proliferation, but rather controls the cellular apoptotic threshold by preventing programmed cell death.[144–148] In normal cells, the topographic restriction of *BCL-2* expression to germinal center zones of surviving B cells suggests that *BCL-2* drives the emergence of long-surviving memory B cells.[149] Indeed, *BCL-2*–trangenic animals show markedly protracted secondary immune responses and an extended lifetime for memory B cells in the absence of antigen.[150]

The precise molecular mechanisms by which *BCL-2* regulates cell death stem from the observation that *BCL-2* is only one member of a family of apoptotic regulators, which also includes *BAX* and *BCL-X*.[151–153] It is now clear that *BCL-2* exists as part of a high-molecular-weight complex generated through heterodimerization with *BAX*.[152,153] The inherent ratio of *BCL-2* to *BAX* determines the functional activity of *BCL-2*.[152,153] When *BAX* is in excess, *BAX* homodimers dominate and cell death is accelerated; conversely, when *BCL-2* is in excess, as in NHL carrying *BCL-2* rearrangements, *BCL-2*/

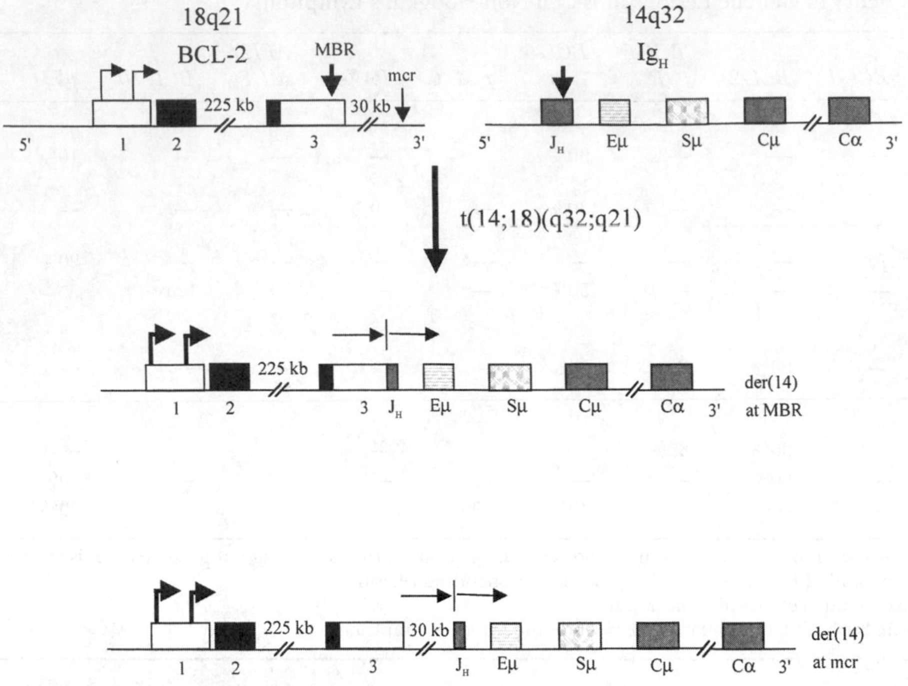

FIGURE 45.1-3. Schematic representation of BCL-2 translocations. The germline configuration of the BCL-2 gene, mapping to 18q21, is shown in the upper panel of the figure. In its germline configuration, BCL-2 is composed of three exons with a large intron between exon 2 and exon 3. The coding region of the BCL-2 gene is indicated by black boxes, whereas noncoding exons (or portions of exons) are indicated by white boxes. The BCL-2 promoters within exon 1 are shown by arrows. The location of the major breakpoint region (MBR) and minor cluster region (mcr), where most BCL-2 breakpoints fall, is indicated by an arrow. The germline configuration of Ig_H on chromosome 14q32 is also shown in the upper panel of the figure. Boxes indicate the joining (J), switch (S), and constant (C) regions of Ig_H. The 14q32 breakpoint (indicated by an arrow) falls within J_H. The bottom panels of the figure depict the molecular consequences of t(14;18)(q32;q21), which causes the juxtaposition of BCL-2 to the Ig_H locus. Both the MBR and mcr type of translocations are shown. Within the Ig_H locus, the breakpoint involves J_H sequences. Notably, the BCL-2 coding sequence of the translocated BCL-2 allele is intact. Because the BCL-2 coding region is preserved, the hybrid BCL-2/Ig_H transcript gives rise to a wild-type and normal-size BCL-2 protein. The reader is referred to the text for a description of the functional consequences of BCL-2 translocations on the transcriptional regulation of BCL-2.

BAX heterodimers are the prevalent species and cell death is repressed. The biochemistry of the *BCL-2* antiapoptotic function has been elucidated to a certain extent and relies on activation of an antioxidant pathway at sites of free radical generation or regulation of endoplasmic reticulum–associated Ca^{2+} fluxes.[154,155]

The precise role of *BCL-2* activation in follicular lymphoma pathogenesis is complex. Despite the fact that follicular lymphoma is comprised of mature B cells, the translocation appears to occur earlier in ontogeny at a pre-B cell stage.[156] In contrast to other genetic lesions occurring in pre-B cells and leading to B-cell lineage acute lymphoblastic leukemia through a differentiative block of the target cells, *BCL-2* rearrangements are permissive of B-cell maturation to the stage of surface $sIgM^+/sIgD^+$ B cells.[156] The pathogenetic contribution of *BCL-2* lesions to follicular lymphoma development is documented by the observation that the growth of human B-cell NHL bearing *BCL-2* translocations is specifically and efficiently inhibited *in vitro* by antisense oligonucleotides targeted against the *BCL-2* gene.[157] Furthermore, *BCL-2* transgenic mice develop a pattern of polyclonal hyperplasia of mature, long-lived B cells resting in G_0, which, despite morphologic similarities, contrasts with the consistent monoclonality of human follicular lymphoma.[158] Hence the view that *BCL-2* activation is not sufficient for follicular lymphoma development and that other genetic lesions or host factors are required. A strong candidate is represented by chronic antigen stimulation and selection that would synergize with *BCL-2* in driving follicular lymphoma expansion.[156,159] With time, and analogous to the human disease, a fraction of *BCL-2* transgenic mice progresses to develop aggressive, clonal large cell lymphomas that have acquired additional genetic lesions[160] (see the following section, Other Genetic Lesions).

Other Genetic Lesions

Other cancer-related genes involved in lymphomagenesis, such as c-*MYC* and *p53*, do not appear to be involved in follicular lymphoma. Deletions of chromosome 6 are present in 20% of cases.[51] Over time, follicular lymphomas tend to convert into an aggressive lymphoma with a diffuse large cell architecture[1,2] (see Fig. 45.1-1). This histologic shift is generally accompanied by the accumulation of *p53* mutations and, in approximately 40% of cases, by mutations of *BCL-6* or inactivation of *p16* (or both).[45,50,134] Rearrangements of c-*MYC* may also accompany the histologic transformation of follicular lymphoma in rare cases.[140]

MUCOSA-ASSOCIATED LYMPHOID TISSUE LYMPHOMAS

The majority of gastric MALT lymphomas are associated with *Helicobacter pylori* infection.[161] It has been suggested that gastric MALT lymphomas may be dependent on antigen stimulation by *H pylori* because malignant lymphoid cells respond to *H pylori* antigens and because the lymphoma may regress, at least partially, when the infection is eradicated.[162] The potential role of antigen in MALT lymphoma pathogenesis is further supported by the observation that MALT lymphoma cells harbor the genotypic clue of antigen-experienced B cells (i.e., somatic hypermutation of Ig genes).[9,10,13] Whether the development of MALT lymphoma arising in body sites other than the stomach is also dependent on antigen stimulation and selection remains an open question. In this respect, it is remarkable that thyroid MALT lymphoma is generally a sequela of Hashimoto thyroiditis, an autoimmune process causing the exposure of B cells to thyroid-derived autoantigens.

Cytogenetic studies have pointed to several abnormalities selectively and recurrently involved in these tumors. The most common of these abnormalities is t(11;18)(q21;q21).[24] The t(11;18)(2;33) translocation occurs in approximately 50% of cytogenetically abnormal MALT lymphomas, independent of the site of origin.[163,164] The genes involved by t(11;18) are *API2* on 11q21 and *MLT* (for *M*ALT *l*ymphoma *t*ranslocation) on 18q21. *API2* belongs to the family of *i*nhibitor of *a*poptosis *p*roteins that plays an evolutionary conserved role in regulating programmed cell death in diverse species. Although the function of *MLT* is currently unknown, it has been hypothesized that the *API2/MLT* fusion protein resulting from t(11;18)(q21;q21) may lead to increased inhibition of apoptosis and, therefore, confer a survival advantage to MALT lymphomas.[163,164]

Other recurrent chromosomal abnormalities of MALT lymphomas are trisomy 3 and t(1;14). The genes involved by trisomy 3 are not presently known.[165] Recurrent abnormalities of chromosomal band 1p22, generally represented by t(1;14)(p22;q32), occur in a small percentage of MALT lymphomas and cause alterations of the *BCL*-10 gene.[166,167] *BCL*-10 is a cellular homologue of the equine herpesvirus-2 E10 gene and encodes an amino-terminal caspase recruitment domain homologous to that found in several apoptotic molecules.[166,167] The wild-type *BCL*-10 gene activates the NF-κB signaling cascade and is able to induce apoptosis in different cell types. Two distinct types of *BCL*-10 aberrations are observed in MALT lymphomas carrying t(1;14)(p22;q32).[166,167] First, *BCL*-10 is overexpressed. Second, *BCL*-10 genes from t(1;14)-positive MALT lymphomas harbor truncations either in, or carboxy-terminal to, the caspase recruitment domain. *BCL*-10 mutants lose the proapoptotic ability of wild-type *BCL*-10 and, in some cases, also fail to activate NF-κB.[166,167] Therefore, it is conceivable that overexpression of *BCL*-10–translocated alleles might have a twofold effect on lymphomagenesis: Loss of *BCL*-10 proapoptosis may confer a survival advantage to MALT B cells, and constitutive NF-κB activation may provide both antiapoptotic and proliferative signals mediated via its transcriptional targets.

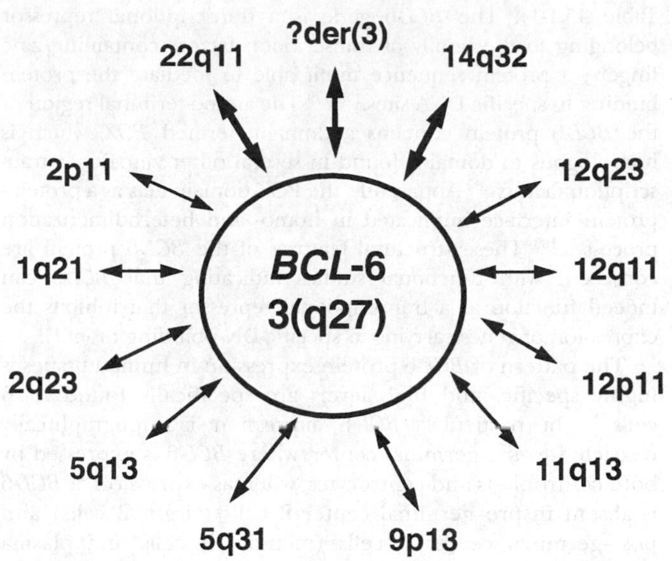

FIGURE 45.1-4. Chromosomal sites implicated in der(3)(q27) and leading to rearrangement of BCL-6. The variability of the partner chromosome juxtaposed to 3q27 in B-lineage diffuse large cell lymphoma suggests that these chromosomal abnormalities belong to the group of "promiscuous" translocations. The thick arrows point to some sites that are involved more frequently than others. In many cases, indicated by *?der(3)* in the figure, the partner chromosomal site cannot be identified with precision by conventional cytogenetics.

Other genetic alterations commonly involved in other lymphoma types also have been observed in MALT lymphomas, including *BCL*-6 alterations and *p53* mutations.[45,168–170]

DIFFUSE LARGE CELL LYMPHOMA

B-lineage DLCL is a potentially curable disease that accounts for approximately 40% of NHLs of adulthood.[1,2] The molecular pathogenesis of DLCL is complex and includes both genetic lesions specific for this disease (i.e., rearrangements of *BCL*-6) and molecular alterations common to other NHL categories (see Fig. 45.1-1).

Chromosomal Translocations Involving the BCL-6 Gene

Cytogenetic studies of NHL have demonstrated that chromosomal alterations affecting band 3q27 are a frequent recurrent abnormality in B-lineage DLCL.[171,172] These alterations are predominantly represented by reciprocal translocations between the 3q27 region and several alternative partner chromosomes, including, though not restricted to, the sites of the Ig genes at 14q32 (Ig_H), 2p11 (Ig_k), and 22q11 (Ig_l)[171,172] (Fig. 45.1-4). The variability of the partner chromosomes juxtaposed to 3q27 in B-lineage DLCL translocations suggests that these abnormalities belong to the group of "promiscuous" translocations, which involve a fixed chromosomal breakpoint on one side and, on the other side, have different chromosomal partners in different cases.

The cloning of the 3q27 chromosomal breakpoints revealed the *BCL*-6 gene, which is involved in the overwhelming majority of B-lineage DLCL cases harboring 3q27 breaks, irrespective of the partner chromosome participating in the translocation[173–177] (see

Table 45.1-1). The *BCL-6* gene is a transcriptional repressor belonging to the family of transcription factors containing zinc fingers, a protein sequence motif able to mediate the protein binding to specific DNA sites.[173–179] The amino-terminal region of the *BCL-6* protein contains a domain, termed *POZ*, which is homologous to domains found in several other zinc-finger transcription factors.[180] Apparently, the POZ domain acts as a protein-protein interface implicated in homo- and heterodimerization processes.[180] These structural features of the *BCL-6* protein are consistent with functional studies indicating that *BCL-6* can indeed function as a transcriptional repressor that inhibits the expression of genes carrying its specific DNA-binding motif.[181]

The pattern of *BCL-6* protein expression in human tissues is highly specific, and high levels are specifically found in B cells.[182] In particular, *BCL-6* expression is topographically restricted to the germinal center, where *BCL-6* is expressed by both centroblasts and centrocytes, whereas expression of *BCL-6* is absent in pre–germinal center B cells (virgin B cells) and post–germinal center B cells (memory B cells and plasma cells).[182] The observation that *BCL-6* is expressed within the germinal center, but not before entrance into or after exit from the germinal center, led to the postulation that *BCL-6* may be needed for germinal center development and sustainment, whereas its down-regulation may be necessary for further differentiation of B cells.[182–185]

The precise role of *BCL-6* in physiologic immune processes has been further clarified by knockout animal models carrying biallelically disrupted *BCL-6* genes.[186,187] Mice carrying the *BCL-6*–/– phenotype consistently fail to form germinal centers. Consistent with lack of germinal center formation, *BCL-6*–/– mice also display impairments in the T-cell–dependent antigen-specific IgG response. Overall, these animal models unequivocally demonstrate that *BCL-6* is a key regulator of germinal center formation and B-cell immune response.

Chromosomal translocations involving band 3q27 truncate the *BCL-6* gene within its 5' flanking region or within the first exon or intron (Fig. 45.1-5), making these alterations readily detectable as rearrangements by Southern blot hybridization analysis of tumor DNA.[173–177] By conventional molecular assays, *BCL-6* rearrangements are detectable in 35% of B-lineage DLCL cases and in a small fraction of follicular lymphomas.[188,189] Conversely, *BCL-6* rearrangements are virtually absent in all other types of lymphoid neoplasms.[188,189] The coding domain of the *BCL-6* gene is left intact in all cases displaying *BCL-6* rearrangements, whereas the 5' regulatory sequences, which contain the *BCL-6* promoter, are either truncated or, alternatively, completely removed.[173–177] In all *BCL-6* rearrangements, the entire coding sequence of *BCL-6* is juxtaposed downstream to heterologous sequences that, based on cytogenetic data, may originate from different chromosomal sites in different patients (see Figs. 45.1-4 and 45.1-5). The common functional consequence of *BCL-6* translocations is the juxtaposition of heterologous promoters to the *BCL-6* coding domain, a mechanism called *promoter substitution*[190,191] (see Fig. 45.1-5). The substitution of the *BCL-6* promoter by heterologous regulatory sequences causes deregulated *BCL-6* expression in B-lineage DLCL carrying *BCL-6* rearrangements. One feature shared by the heterologous promoters linked to rearranged *BCL-6* alleles is that they are physiologically active in normal B cells and are not down-regulated during the late stages of B-cell differentiation.[190,191] Thus, *BCL-6* rearrangements may prevent down-regulation of *BCL-6* and, in turn, block the differentiation of germinal center B cells toward the stage of plasma cells. According to this model, B-lineage DLCL cells carrying *BCL-6* rearrangements would thus be "frozen" at the stage of germinal center cells.

Beside promoter substitution, the *BCL-6* gene can also be altered by somatic hypermutation at its 5' noncoding region. Hypermutation of *BCL-6* can be found in normal germinal center cells.[44,192] It is also found in B-cell NHLs that are also characterized by somatic IgV hypermutation,[43–45,193,194] suggesting a common mechanism of mutation. Functional analysis of *BCL-6* mutated alleles indicates that some mutations derived from DLCL but not from normal germinal center cells may deregulate the basal level of *BCL-6* transcription (unpublished results). This finding indicates that *BCL-6* can also be deregulated by somatic hypermutation of its promoter, which further supports the role of *BCL-6* deregulation in the pathogenesis of DLCL.

Molecular Heterogeneity of Diffuse Large Cell Lymphoma

The WHO classification has established that, with current knowledge and methods, it is impractical to histologically subclassify DLCL into its morphologic variants (i.e., diffuse centroblastic lymphoma and diffuse immunoblastic lymphoma).[1,2] However, both clinicians and pathologists reach consensus in suggesting that DLCL is in fact a heterogeneous disease.[1] Most likely, diversity does not depend on cytologic features, but rather on the tumor genotype. The biologic diversity of DLCL has been validated by the identification of at least three distinct genetic types of the disease[50,141,195,196] (Fig. 45.1-6). The first type, accounting for approximately 40% of cases, associates with rearrangements of *BCL-6* in the absence of other known genetic lesions. DLCLs harboring *BCL-6* rearrangements are *de novo* lymphomas, presenting without a previous history of follicular lymphoma. The second genetic type of DLCL involves activation of *BCL-2* in combination with *p53* mutations. DLCLs harboring *BCL-2* rearrangements and *p53* mutations derive from the histologic transformation of a previous follicular lymphoma. Finally, the third genetic group of DLCL displays germline *BCL-2* and *BCL-6* genes. The genotypic configuration of DLCL is thought to be of prognostic relevance. For example, some studies suggested that DLCLs associated with *BCL-6* rearrangements display the most favorable prognosis, whereas cases carrying *BCL-2* translocations have the poorest outcome.[195,197,198] The exact prognostic relevance of *BCL-6* rearrangements, however, still remains a controversial issue.[188,199,200]

The application of novel DNA technologies to DLCL is likely to refine the biologic heterogeneity of this disease. One study using DNA microarrays demonstrated diversity in gene expression among DLCL cases, allowing for the distinction between a germinal center–like variant of the disease and a variant resembling peripheral blood B cells activated *in vitro*.[201] This distinction has been proposed to be of prognostic value, because patients with the germinal center–like variant of the disease display a better overall survival.[201]

BURKITT'S LYMPHOMA

Burkitt's lymphoma includes two clinical variants: sporadic Burkitt's lymphoma and endemic Burkitt's lymphoma.[1,2] Some cases may present as acute leukemias with Burkitt's tumor cells and are termed *L3 acute lymphoblastic leukemias*.[1,2] All Burkitt's lymphoma

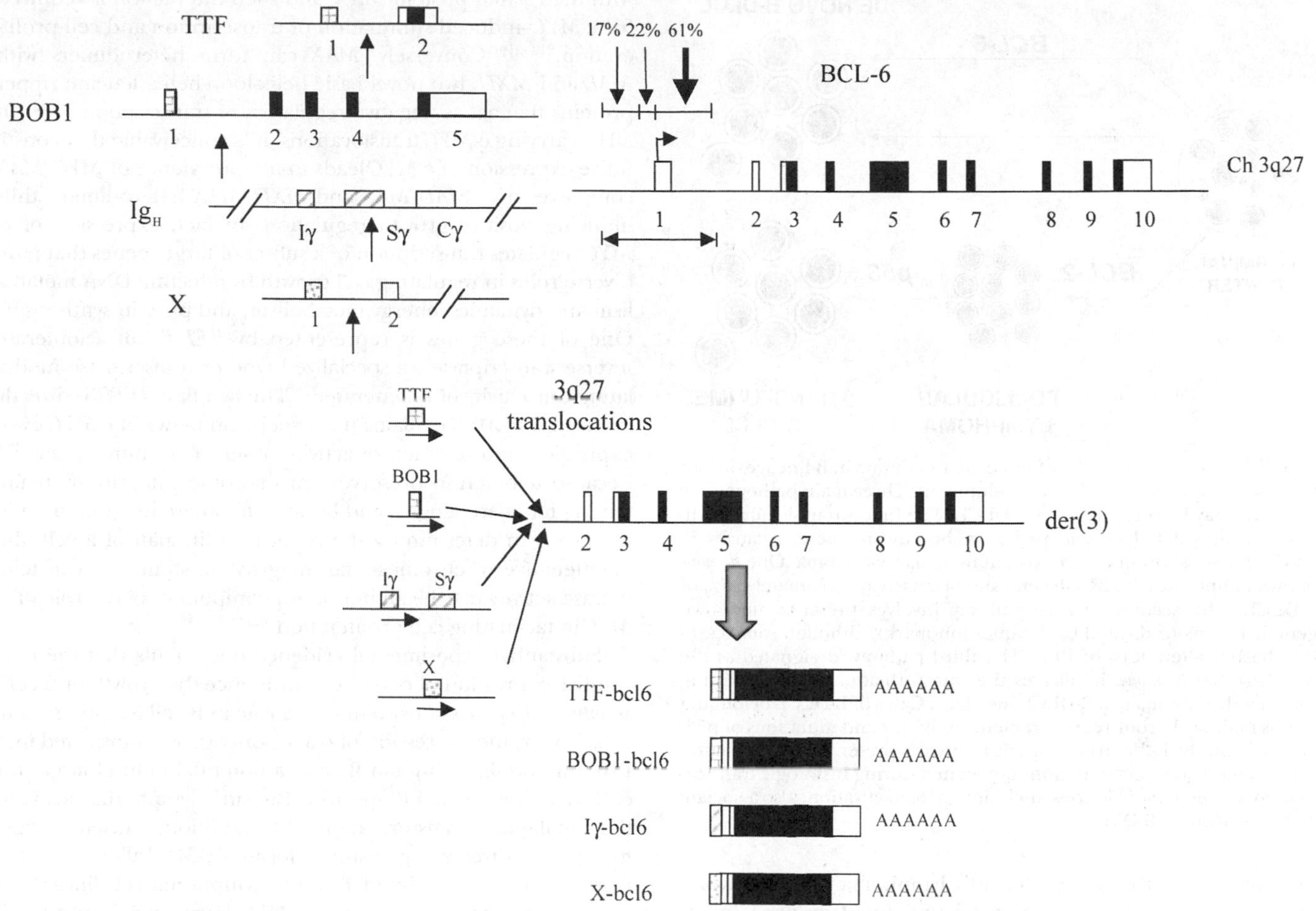

FIGURE 45.1-5. Schematic representation of BCL-6 translocations. The germline configuration of the BCL-6 gene, mapping to 3q27, is shown in the upper right panel of the figure. In its germline configuration, BCL-6 is composed of ten exons. The coding region of the BCL-6 gene is indicated by black boxes, whereas the noncoding exons (or portions of exons) are indicated by white boxes. The physiologic BCL-6 promoter within exon 1 is shown by an arrow. The frequency of BCL-6 breakpoint locations is also shown. The germline configuration of several BCL-6 translocation partners (TTF, BOB1, Ig_H, and other hypothetical genes designated as *X*) is shown in the upper left panel of the figure. The bottom panel of the figure depicts the molecular configuration of representative translocated BCL-6 alleles. Independent of the partner chromosome involved, all translocated BCL-6 alleles are deprived of their exon 1 and, consequently, of their physiologic promoter. The novel sequences derived from the partner chromosomes are thus juxtaposed 5' to the intron 1 of BCL-6. These novel sequences provide a heterologous promoter to BCL-6, such as the Ig_H germline transcript promoter Iγ (or, alternatively, Iμ) in the case of t(3;14); the TTF promoter in the case of t(3;4); and the BOB1 promoter in the case of t(3;11). The genomic configuration of the BCL-6 gene downstream to the breakpoint site is preserved, thus leaving intact the BCL-6 coding sequence. The transcripts resulting from representative BCL-6 translocations are also shown in the lower part of the bottom panel of the figure. In all cases, the translocation gives rise to a fusion transcript, exemplified by TTF/BCL-6, BOB1/BCL-6, Iγ/BCL-6, and X/BCL-6. These transcripts initiate from the heterologous promoter provided by the chromosomal site juxtaposed to BCL-6, and they retain the entire normal BCL-6 coding domain, which translates into a normal-size BCL-6 protein.

cases, including the leukemic variants, share one common genetic lesion (chromosomal translocations involving region 8q24 and one of the Ig loci) and, at variable frequency, other genetic lesions, including inactivation of *p53* and *p16*, deletions of 6q, and infection by EBV[48,51,59–63,134,202] (see Fig. 45.1-1).

Chromosomal Translocations Involving the c-MYC Gene

Translocations of region 8q24 involve the c-*MYC* locus and have provided the first example of the involvement of protooncogenes in tumor-associated chromosomal abnormalities.[202] The c-*MYC* locus can be involved in three distinct translocations with one of the Ig loci, including Ig_H, Ig_k, or Ig_λ[202–207] (see Table 45.1-1). Ig_H is involved in 80% of the cases leading to t(8;14)(q24;q32). The remaining 20% is composed of t(2;8)(p11;q24), which involves Ig_k (15%), and t(8;22)(q24;q11), which involves Ig_λ (5%).

Although fairly homogeneous at the microscopic level, these translocations display a high degree of molecular heterogeneity. The t(8;14) breakpoints are located 5' and centromeric to c-*MYC*, whereas they map 3' to c-*MYC* in t(2;8) and t(8;22).[202–207] Further molecular heterogeneity derives from the exact breakpoint sites of chromosomes 8 and 14 of t(8;14) (Fig. 45.1-7).

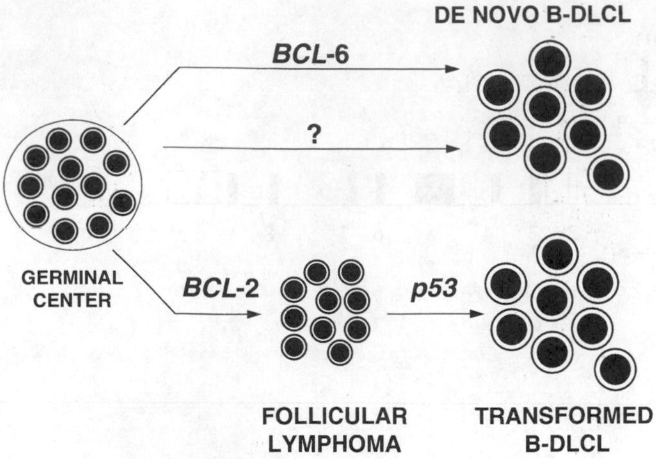

FIGURE 45.1-6. Model of molecular pathways in B-lineage diffuse large cell lymphoma (B-DLCL) development. Three main pathogenetic pathways may be recognized in B-DLCL. The first two molecular pathways are designated *de novo* pathways, because in these instances B-DLCL develops without a preexistent follicular lymphoma. One *de novo* pathway implicates the BCL-6 gene and occurs in approximately 35% of B-DLCL. The second *de novo* pathway involves presently unknown genetic lesions (indicated by the question mark), although some cases may harbor alterations of REL. The third pathway, designated as the *transformation pathway*, implicates the transformation of a preexisting follicular lymphoma to a B-DLCL histology. Cases of B-DLCL belonging to this pathway harbor rearrangements of BCL-2 and mutations of p53. Whereas the BCL-2 rearrangement is already present in the follicular lymphoma phase, p53 mutations are gained during histologic transformation. Other genetic lesions, including p16 inactivation, also associate with transformed B-DLCL.

Translocations of endemic Burkitt's lymphoma tend to involve sequences on chromosome 8 at an undefined distance (more than 1000 kilobases) 5' to c-*MYC*, and sequences on chromosome 14 within or in proximity to the Ig J_H region.[38,208] In sporadic Burkitt's lymphoma, t(8;14) preferentially involves sequences within or immediately 5' (fewer than 3 kilobases) to c-*MYC* on chromosome 8, and sequences on chromosome 14 within the Ig switch regions.[38,208]

The common effect of t(8;14), t(2;8), and t(8;22) is that c-*MYC*–translocated alleles are expressed constitutively in tumor cells, as opposed to the tight regulation of c-*MYC* levels in normal B cells.[209–211] At least two distinct mechanisms may be responsible for c-*MYC* deregulation. These include (1) juxtaposition of c-*MYC* to heterologous enhancers derived from Ig loci; and (2) structural alterations in the 5' regulatory regions of c-*MYC*, putatively altering their responsiveness to cellular factors regulating c-*MYC* expression. In fact, the c-*MYC* exon 1–intron 1 border, where c-*MYC* regulatory sequences are located, is either decapitated by the translocation or undergoes selective and consistent mutations in translocated alleles[42,203–207] (see Fig. 45.1-7). In addition to homotopic deregulation, oncogenic conversion of c-*MYC* is also thought to be due to amino acid substitutions in c-*MYC* exon 2 corresponding to the transactivation domain of the c-*MYC* protein.[41,212] These mutations would abolish the physiologic ability of *p107*, a nuclear protein related to *RB1*, to suppress the transactivation domain of c-*MYC*.[213]

The product of c-*MYC* is a ubiquitously expressed nuclear phosphoprotein that functions as a transcriptional regulator controlling cell proliferation, differentiation, and apoptosis.[202] *In vivo*, c-*MYC* is found mainly in heterodimeric complexes with the related protein *MAX*, and such interaction is required for c-*MYC*–induced stimulation of transcription and cell proliferation.[214–219] Conversely, *MAX* can form heterodimers with *MAD* and *MXI1*, two novel basic helix-loop-helix/leucine zipper proteins that act as negative regulators of transcription.[220,221] In NHL carrying c-*MYC* translocations, it is conceivable that constitutive expression of c-*MYC* leads to the prevalence of *MYC/MAX* complexes over *MAD/MAX* and *MXI1/MAX* heterodimers, thus inducing positive growth regulation. In fact, expression of c-*MYC* regulates transcription of a subset of target genes that have diverse roles in regulating cell growth by affecting DNA metabolism and dynamics, energy metabolism, and protein synthesis.[222] One of these genes is represented by *TERT* (for *t*elomerase *r*everse *t*ranscriptase), a specialized type of transcriptase modulating the activity of telomerase.[223] The fact that *TERT* is directly induced by c-*MYC* explains the association between c-*MYC* overexpression and telomerase activity observed in human cells.[223] Because telomerase preserves chromosome integrity by maintaining telomere length, and because telomere length is a limiting factor in determining the replicative lifespan of a cell, the maintenance of chromosomal integrity via stimulation of telomerase activity may be an important component of the role of c-*MYC* in facilitating cell proliferation.[223,224]

Substantial experimental evidence documents that the constitutive expression of c-*MYC* can influence the growth of B cells *in vitro* and *in vivo*, consistent with a role in B-cell lymphomagenesis. *In vitro*, the expression of c-*MYC* oncogenes transfected into EBV immortalized human B cells, a potential natural target for c-*MYC* activation in EBV-positive Burkitt's lymphoma, leads to their malignant transformation.[225] In addition, antisense oligonucleotides directed against translocated c-*MYC* alleles are able to revert tumorigenicity of Burkitt's lymphoma cell lines.[226] *In vivo*, the targeted expression of c-*MYC* oncogenes in the B-cell lineage of transgenic mice leads to the development of B-cell malignancy at relatively high frequency.[227]

Other Genetic Lesions

In addition to c-*MYC* activation in 100% of Burkitt's lymphoma cases, disruption of *p53* occurs in 30% of sporadic and endemic Burkitt's lymphoma[48] (see Table 45.1-2). Deletions of 6q are detected in approximately 30% of the Burkitt's lymphoma cases independent of the clinical variant.[51] Inactivation of *p16* also has been reported in a fraction of cases.[228] Another lesion that contributes to the development of this malignancy is monoclonal EBV infection, present in virtually all cases of endemic Burkitt's lymphoma and in approximately 30% of sporadic Burkitt's lymphoma[60–64] (see Table 45.1-2). Because EBV infection in Burkitt's lymphoma displays a peculiar latent infection phenotype characterized by negativity of both EBV-transforming antigens, LMP-1 and EBNA-2, the precise pathogenetic role of the virus has remained elusive. However, it has been proposed that a class of small RNA molecules, termed *EBER* and consistently expressed by all Burkitt's lymphomas, may mediate the transforming potential of EBV in Burkitt's lymphoma.[229]

ACQUIRED IMMUNODEFICIENCY SYNDROME–RELATED NON-HODGKIN'S LYMPHOMA

The association between an immunodeficiency state and the development of lymphoma has been long since recognized in

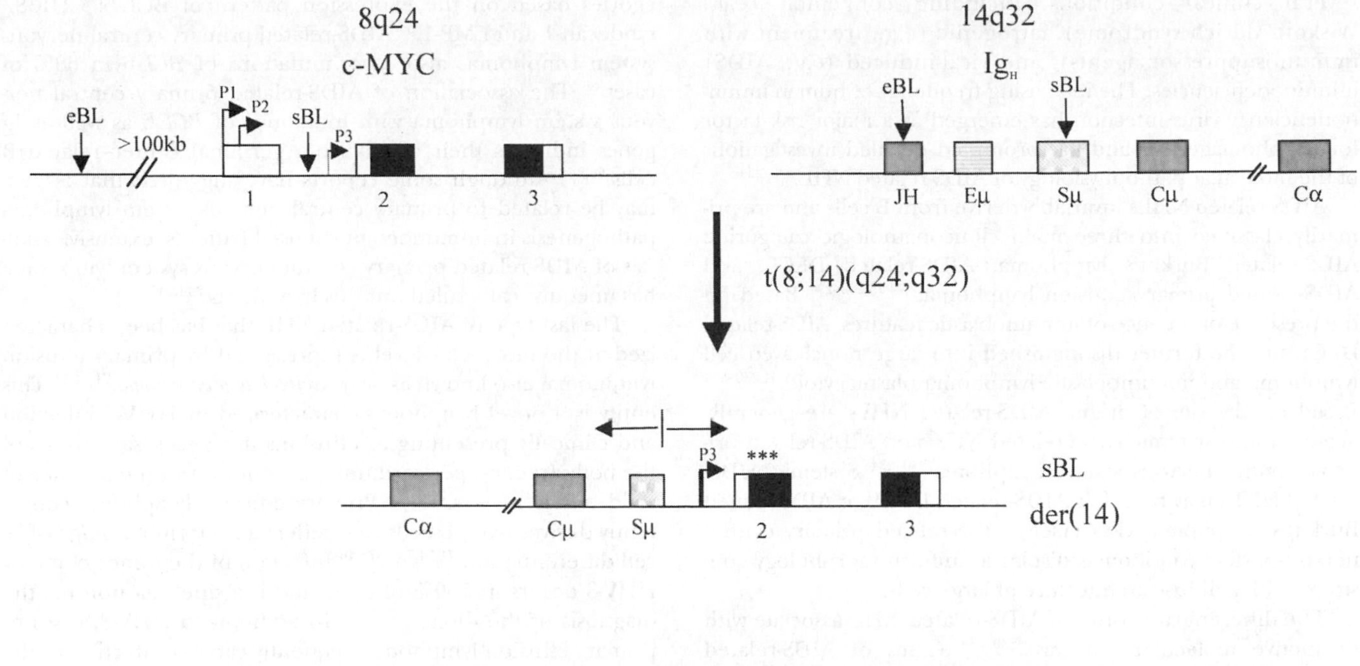

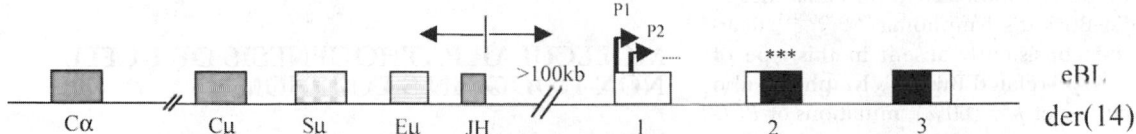

FIGURE 45.1-7. Schematic representation of c-MYC translocations. The germline configuration of the c-MYC gene, mapping to 8q24, is shown in the upper panel of the figure. In its germline configuration, c-MYC is composed of three exons. The coding region of the c-MYC gene is indicated by black boxes, whereas noncoding exons (or portions of exons) are indicated by white boxes. The c-MYC promoters within exon 1 are indicated by arrows. The 8q24 breakpoint regions of sporadic Burkitt's lymphoma (sBL) and endemic Burkitt's lymphoma (eBL) also are indicated. The germline configuration of Ig$_H$ on chromosome 14q32 also is shown in the upper panel of the figure. Boxes indicate the joining (J), switch (S), and constant (C) regions of Ig$_H$. The 14q32 breakpoint regions of sBL and eBL also are indicated. The bottom panels of the figure depict the molecular consequences of t(8;14)(q24;q32), which causes the juxtaposition of c-MYC to the Ig$_H$ locus. Two molecularly distinct types of translocations are recognized, which preferentially associate with either sBL or eBL. In the case of t(8;14) of sBL, the c-MYC breakpoint involves sequences within c-MYC, which is thus decapitated of its exon 1. Because the physiologically active promoters of c-MYC are removed by t(8;14) of sBL, a novel transcriptional initiation site (P3), located within c-MYC intron 1 and otherwise silent in physiologic conditions, is activated in c-MYC alleles involved by t(8;14) of sBL. Within the Ig$_H$ locus, the breakpoint falls in the proximity of the switch μ (Sμ) region. Notably, the gross configuration of the coding sequence of the translocated c-MYC allele is left intact. At the nucleotide level, however, translocated c-MYC alleles frequently harbor point mutations within the exon 2 coding sequence, leading to alteration in the amino acid sequence of the c-MYC protein. The complementary DNA (cDNA) resulting from t(8;14) of sBL includes c-MYC exons 2 and 3, which, on their 5' side, are preceded by an abnormally transcribed sequence of intron 1, starting from the novel transcriptional initiation site within c-MYC intron 1. Because the c-MYC coding region is intact, a normal-size c-MYC protein is translated by t(8;14) of sBL. The reader is referred to the text for a description of the functional consequences of t(8;14) of sBL in terms of deregulation of translocated c-MYC.

In the case of t(8;14) of eBL, the c-MYC breakpoint involves sequences on chromosome 8 at an undefined distance (more than 100 kilobases) 5' to c-MYC and sequences on chromosome 14 within or in proximity to the immunoglobulin J$_H$ region. The internal genomic configuration of the translocated c-MYC allele is thus apparently preserved. However, c-MYC alleles involved by t(8;14) of eBL consistently harbor small mutations clustered around the exon 1–intron 1 border, where c-MYC regulatory regions are located. In addition, and in common with t(8;14) of sBL, point mutations within the exon 2 coding sequence, leading to alteration in the amino acid sequence of the c-MYC protein, also are frequently detected in c-MYC alleles affected by t(8;14) of eBL. The cDNA transcribed by t(8;14) of eBL includes c-MYC exons 1 through 3 and gives rise to a normal-size c-MYC protein. The reader is referred to the text for a description of the functional consequences of t(8;14) of eBL on the transcriptional regulation of c-MYC.

several clinical conditions, including congenital (e.g., Wiskott-Aldrich syndrome), iatrogenic (e.g., treatment with immunosuppressor agents), and viral-induced (e.g., AIDS) immunodeficiencies. The increasing frequency of human immunodeficiency virus infection has emerged as a major risk factor for lymphomagenesis and has prompted detailed investigations of the molecular pathophysiology of AIDS-related NHL.[230–234]

AIDS-related NHLs invariably derive from B cells and are primarily classified into three main clinicopathologic categories: AIDS-related Burkitt's lymphoma, AIDS-related DLCL, and AIDS-related primary effusion lymphoma.[2,74,75,230–234] Based on the presence or absence of immunoblastic features, AIDS-related DLCL may be further distinguished into large noncleaved cell lymphoma and immunoblastic lymphoma plasmacytoid.[64,230–234] Based on the site of origin, AIDS-related NHLs are generally grouped into systemic AIDS-related NHL and AIDS-related primary central nervous system lymphoma.[230–234] Systemic AIDS-related NHLs may be either AIDS-related DLCL or AIDS-related Burkitt's lymphoma. Conversely, AIDS-related primary central nervous system lymphomas display a uniform morphology consistent with a diffuse architecture of large cells.

The different categories of AIDS-related NHL associate with distinctive molecular pathways.[230–234] Cases of AIDS-related Burkitt's lymphoma consistently display activation of c-*MYC* by chromosomal translocations that show structural similarities to those found in sporadic Burkitt's lymphoma.[49,62,230–235] Rearrangements of *BCL-6* are consistently absent in this type of AIDS-related NHL.[235,236] AIDS-related Burkitt's lymphoma also frequently harbors mutations of *p53* (60%), mutations of *BCL-6* 5' noncoding regions (60%) and, in 30% of cases, infection of the tumor clone by EBV.[49,64,68,193,235,236] The EBV-encoded antigens LMP-1 and EBNA-2 are not expressed by AIDS-related Burkitt's lymphoma.[64,238,239] In addition to genetic lesions and EBV infection, stimulation and selection by antigens, frequently represented by autoantigens, appear to be a prominent feature of AIDS-related Burkitt's lymphoma.[240,241]

AIDS-related DLCL displays several genotypic differences when compared with AIDS-related Burkitt's lymphoma.[230–234] First, the most frequent genetic alteration detected in AIDS-related DLCL is infection by EBV, which occurs in approximately 60% to 70% of cases and associates frequently, although not always, with expression of LMP-1.[49,64,68] Second, AIDS-related DLCL displays rearrangements of *BCL-6* in 20% of cases.[236] Mutations of *BCL-6* 5' noncoding regions occur in 70% of AIDS-related DLCL cases.[193] AIDS-related DLCL can be segregated into two distinct histogenetic categories based on the expression pattern of the *BCL-6* protein: the EBV-encoded LMP-1; and the CD138/syndecan-1 antigen, a proteoglycan associated with the terminal phases of B-cell differentiation.[64,239] AIDS-related DLCL associated with the BCL-6$^+$/syndecan-1$^-$/LMP-1$^-$ phenotype tend to display a large noncleaved cell morphology and closely reflect the phenotype of germinal center B cells.[64,239] Conversely, BCL-6$^-$/syndecan-1$^+$/LMP-1$^+$ AIDS-related DLCLs are morphologically consistent with immunoblastic lymphoma plasmacytoid and reflect a post–germinal center stage of B-cell differentiation.[64,239]

All AIDS-related primary central nervous system lymphomas harbor EBV infection.[66,242] However, only a fraction of AIDS-related primary central nervous system lymphomas, namely those with immunoblastic plasmacytoid morphology, express the LMP-1–transforming protein of EBV.[66] As for systemic AIDS-related DLCL, AIDS-related primary central nervous system lymphomas may be distinguished into two phenotypic categories based on the expression pattern of BCL-6: CD138/syndecan-1 and LMP-1.[66] AIDS-related primary central nervous system lymphomas also carry mutations of *BCL-6* in 60% of cases.[66] The association of AIDS-related primary central nervous system lymphoma with mutations of *BCL-6* as well as Ig genes indicates their origin from germinal center–related B cells.[66,243] Although some reports have suggested that HHV-8 may be related to primary central nervous system lymphoma pathogenesis in immunocompromised patients, extensive analysis of AIDS-related primary central nervous system lymphoma has unequivocally ruled out this hypothesis.[244,245]

The last type of AIDS-related NHL that has been characterized at the molecular level is represented by primary effusion lymphoma, also known as *body cavity–based lymphoma.*[71,74,75] This entity is a novel lymphoma characterized by HHV-8 infection and clinically presenting as effusions in the serosal cavities of the body (pleura, pericardium, peritoneum) in the absence of solid tumor masses.[71,74,75] Primary effusion lymphoma consistently derives from B cells that reflect a preterminal stage of B-cell differentiation.[71,74,75,237,246] Infection of the tumor clone by HHV-8 occurs in 100% of cases and is a sine qua non for the diagnosis of the disease.[71,74,75] In addition to HHV-8, cases of primary effusion lymphoma frequently carry coinfection of the tumor clone by EBV.[65,67,71,74,75]

MOLECULAR PATHOGENESIS OF T-CELL NON-HODGKIN'S LYMPHOMA

Malignancies of mature T cells are a highly heterogeneous group of diseases.[1,2] These malignancies greatly differ in clinical behavior, immunophenotypic features, and genetic lesions involved in their pathogenesis.[1,2] In Western countries, mature T-cell malignancies overall represent only 15% to 20% of tumors derived from mature lymphocytes and are relatively uncommon when compared to mature B-cell malignancies.[247] A higher frequency of mature T-cell malignancies is reported in other parts of the world, namely Japan and the Caribbean.[247]

Only a few categories of mature T-cell malignancies have been investigated in detail at the molecular level. These include Ki-1$^+$ (CD30$^+$) anaplastic large cell lymphoma, adult T-cell leukemia/lymphoma, T-cell prolymphocytic leukemia and, to a lesser extent, cutaneous T-cell lymphoma. CD30$^+$ anaplastic large cell lymphoma tends to occur in childhood and young adults.[1,2] The term *adult T-cell leukemia/lymphoma* encompasses a spectrum of lymphoproliferative diseases associated with the human retrovirus HTLV-1 and characteristically expressing large amounts of IL-2 receptors (CD25). The geographic distribution of adult T-cell leukemia/lymphoma is mainly restricted to Southwestern Japan and the Caribbean basin, although cases also have been reported in the United States and Europe in long-term immigrants from the affected geographic areas.[1,2] T-cell prolymphocytic leukemia represents a rare T-cell malignancy that presents predominantly as a leukemic disease.[1,2] An intrinsic tropism for the skin is displayed by cutaneous T-cell lymphoma, which includes mycosis fungoides and its leukemic manifestation, known as *Sézary syndrome.*[1,2]

T-CELL ANAPLASTIC LARGE CELL LYMPHOMA

Anaplastic large cell lymphoma is a specific category of T-cell NHL composed of large pleomorphic cells that usually express the CD30 antigen.[1,2] Anaplastic large cell lymphoma is characterized by frequent cutaneous and extranodal involvement.[1,2] Conventional karyotyping analysis of anaplastic large cell lymphoma cases has shown a unique translocation involving bands 2p23 and 5q35 in a substantial fraction of cases.[24] The cloning of the t(2;5)(p23;q35) translocation has demonstrated that it involves the fusion of the nuclephosmin/B23 (*NPM*) gene on 5q35 to a novel *a*naplastic *l*ymphoma *k*inase (*ALK*) on 2p23 (see Table 45.1-1).[248] As a consequence of this translocation, the *NPM* and *ALK* genes are fused to form a chimeric transcript that encodes a hybrid protein (p80) in which the aminoterminus of *NPM* is linked to the catalytic domain of *ALK*.[248] Two distinct oncogenic effects are thought to be caused by the t(2;5) translocation. First, the *ALK* gene, which is not physiologically expressed in normal T lymphocytes, undergoes heterologous expression in lymphoma cells, conceivably because of its juxtaposition to the promoter sequences of *NPM*, which are physiologically expressed in T cells. Second, based on the activation model of other tyrosine kinase oncogenes, one would predict that the truncated *ALK* constitutively phosphorylates intracellular targets to trigger malignant transformation.

The pathogenetic role of *NPM/ALK* rearrangements is supported by studies *in vitro* and *in vivo*. First, overexpression of the p80 hybrid protein induces neoplastic transformation of target cells in *in vitro* models, substantiating the notion that the p80 kinase is in fact aberrantly activated.[249] Second, retroviral-mediated gene transfer of *NPM/ALK in vivo* causes T-cell lymphoid malignancies in mice.[250] In such animal models, *NPM/ALK* selectively transforms lymphoid cells of T-cell lineage, whereas the growth properties of other hematopoietic cells remain unaffected.[250]

The distribution of *NPM/ALK* rearrangements throughout the spectrum of NHL is highly selective, being virtually restricted to T-cell lineage anaplastic large cell lymphoma.[251–253] Within this category, *NPM/ALK* rearrangements seem to preferentially associate with cases of childhood (more than 85% positivity), although they are also detected in a large fraction of cases of adulthood (60%).[251–253]

ADULT T-CELL LEUKEMIA/LYMPHOMA

The molecular pathogenesis of adult T-cell leukemia/lymphoma has been elucidated to a wider extent in comparison with other mature T-cell tumors. Adult T-cell leukemia/lymphoma is associated with HTLV-I infection of the tumor cells in 100% of cases, although the rate of adult T-cell leukemia/lymphoma development among seropositive individuals is relatively low (less than 5% lifetime risk).[85–87,254–260] The period between infection and onset of clinical disease is typically quite long, varying between 10 and 30 years.[260] Unlike acutely transforming animal retroviruses, the HTLV-I genome does not encode a known oncogene.[85–87,254–260] Furthermore, this retrovirus does not transform T cells by *cis*-activation of an adjacent protooncogene, because this provirus appears to integrate randomly within the host genome.[85–87,254–260] Rather, the pathogenetic effect of HTLV-I in adult T-cell leukemia/lymphoma seems to be due to the viral production of a transregulatory protein (HTLV-I tax) that markedly increases expression of all viral gene products and transcriptionally activates the expression of certain host genes, including IL-2, the α chain of the IL-2 receptor (CD25), c-sis, c-fos, and granulocyte-macrophage colony-stimulating factor.[88–92] Indeed, a property of adult T-cell leukemia/lymphoma cells is the constitutive high level expression of IL-2 receptors. The central role of these genes in normal T-cell activation and growth, together with the results of *in vitro* studies, support the notion that tax-mediated activation of these host genes represents an important mechanism by which HTLV-I initiates T-cell transformation.[89] In addition, tax interferes at multiple sites with DNA damage repair functions and with mitotic checkpoints, consistent with the fact that adult T-cell leukemia/lymphoma cells harbor a high frequency of karyotypic abnormalities.[94–96]

The long period of clinical latency that precedes the development of adult T-cell leukemia/lymphoma, the small percentage of infected patients that develop this malignancy, and the observation that leukemic cells from adult T-cell leukemia/lymphoma are monoclonal suggest that HTLV-I is not sufficient to cause the full malignant phenotype.[85–87] An attractive model for adult T-cell leukemia/lymphoma would therefore include an early period of tax-induced polyclonal T-cell proliferation that, in turn, would facilitate the occurrence of additional genetic events leading to the monoclonal outgrowth of a fully transformed cell. In this respect, a recurrent genetic lesion in adult T-cell leukemia/lymphoma is represented by mutations of the *p53* tumor suppressor gene, which is inactivated in 40% of cases.[261,262]

T-CELL PROLYMPHOCYTIC LEUKEMIA

T-cell prolymphocytic leukemia frequently carries cytogenetic abnormalities of chromosome 11, the most common abnormalities being monosomy 11, partial or terminal deletions of 11q, and unbalanced translocations involving the 11q arm.[24] The gene relevant to these abnormalities has been identified and has been shown to correspond to *ATM*, a gene that is also responsible for the hereditary disorder ataxia-telangiectasia.[263,264] Whereas *ATM* is mutated in the germline of ataxia-telangiectasia patients, it is altered somatically in cases of T-cell prolymphocytic leukemia.[263,264] Mutations of *ATM* in T-cell prolymphocytic leukemia associate with the deletion of the other allele and lead to the absence, premature truncation, or alteration of the *ATM* gene product, consistent with the inactivation model of tumor suppressor genes.[263,264] Circumstantial evidence suggests that *ATM* might be involved in cell-cycle regulation and DNA repair, which in fact have been shown to be defective in cells with biallelic *ATM* inactivation.[265]

CUTANEOUS T-CELL LYMPHOMA

Rearrangements of the *lyt*-10/*NFKB*-2 gene at 10q24 have been demonstrated in a sizable fraction of cutaneous T-cell lymphoma tumors. The *lyt*-10 gene (also called *NFKB*-2) is a novel member of the NF-κB rel family of transcription factors.[266,267] The normal products of these genes have structural homologies within the DNA-binding rel domain and share the ability to bind to specific (κB) target sequences found in various inducible enhancer and promoter elements. In addition to the DNA-binding domain, the *lyt*-10/*NFKB*-2 gene harbors an ankyrin motif, which is thought to regulate the physiologic nuclear/cytoplasm distribution of the *lyt*-10/*NFKB*-2 protein.[266,267] The translocation breaks observed in NHL consistently disrupt the ankyrin domain, separating it from the DNA-binding domain. It is therefore conceivable that an intact DNA-binding domain, once separated from the regulatory ankyrin portion of the gene, might be constitutively activated and act as an oncogene to T cells.

MOLECULAR PATHOGENESIS OF HODGKIN'S LYMPHOMA

HL, also known as *Hodgkin's disease,* is characterized by scattered large atypical cells residing in a complex admixture of inflammatory cells.[1,2] Two different biologic entities have been recognized within HL: nodular lymphocyte predominance HL (NLPHL) and classic HL comprising the nodular sclerosis, mixed cellularity, and lymphocyte depletion variants. Historically, biologic studies of HL have been hampered by the paucity of HL diagnostic cells [i.e., Reed-Sternberg (RS) or Hodgkin's cells] in HL biopsies. More recently, however, the availability of sophisticated laboratory techniques that enable the isolation and enrichment of HL neoplastic cells has been instrumental in the understanding of HL histogenesis.

The neoplastic cells of both classic HL and NLPHL typically represent clonal populations of B-lineage cells, as documented by the presence of clonal rearrangements of Ig genes.[268–274] The consistent occurrence of somatic mutations and their pattern within (V) region genes amplified from neoplastic cells of both classic HL and NLPHL indicate that both types of HL are derived from B cells that reside in, or have transited through, the germinal center.[268–274] Neoplastic cells of NLPHL display ongoing mutation of IgV genes, suggesting derivation from centroblasts residing in the germinal center. Also, neoplastic cells of NLPHL show the typical clues of antigen selection, indicating a putative pathogenetic role of stimulation by antigen molecules. Conversely, no ongoing mutation of IgV genes is observed in RS cells of classic HL, consistent with derivation from centrocytes or post–germinal center B cells. In some cases, RS cells of classic HL harbor stop codons in in-frame V_H gene rearrangements (crippling mutations). Because IgV crippling mutations prevent antigen selection, it is likely that RS cells of classic HL have escaped apoptosis through a mechanism not linked to antigen stimulation, possibly represented by a transforming event, such as that mediated by the EBV LMP-1. The differences in the histogenesis of NLPHL and classic HL revealed by molecular studies also have been confirmed at the phenotypic level. In fact, the neoplastic cells of NLPHL consistently display the BCL-6$^+$/syndecan-1$^-$ profile typical of germinal center B cells, whereas RS cells of classic HL frequently, although not always, display the BCL-6$^-$/syndecan-1$^+$ phenotype of post–germinal center B cells.[275–277] Although the overwhelming majority of HL cases derive from the B lineage, occasional cases have been formally proved to be of T-cell origin.[278]

The truly neoplastic nature of RS cells has been debated since the description of HL. The detection of heterogeneous clonal karyotypic changes in HL lymph nodes and in cells identifiable as RS cells suggested that HL may indeed represent a clonal malignancy.[279–282] Many chromosomal breaks detected in HL are also shared by other lymphoid malignancies, whereas a cytogenetic abnormality specifically associated with HL has yet to be found.

The *p53* pathway is thought to be altered in HL. RS cells express abnormal levels of the MDM2 protein,[283] which, in turn, conceals functional domains of the wild-type *p53,* thus blocking the physiologic activity of the tumor suppressor gene.[284] Despite initial observations,[285,286] it appears that the *p53* gene itself is not affected by mutations in HL.[287]

A number of epidemiologic features of HL suggest that the disease might result also from infectious cofactors. HL lesions express EBV antigens, carry EBV DNA demonstrable by conventional Southern blot or *in situ* hybridization techniques, and contain EBV-encoded RNA.[288–302] EBV infection of RS cells is virtually always absent in NLPHL, whereas it occurs in approximately 50% of classic HL and in 100% of AIDS-related HL.[1,277,288–302] Notably, the EBV infection of RS cells is monoclonal, suggesting that infection precedes clonal expansion and further confirming the monoclonal nature of RS cells. Of the two B-cell transforming antigens encoded by the EBV genome, infected RS cells most commonly express LMP-1 but not EBNA-2.[288–302] The latent infection protein phenotype of RS cells (LMP-1–positive, EBNA-2–negative) is distinct from that of Burkitt's lymphoma (LMP-1–negative, EBNA-2–negative) or B-lymphoblastoid cell lines (LMP-1–positive, EBNA-2–positive) and is similar to the EBV expression pattern detected in nasopharyngeal carcinoma and a fraction of AIDS-related DLCL. The reason for these alternative EBV expression patterns is not known with precision, but it is likely influenced by the developmental stage of the infected cells as well as by the host's immune function.

GENETIC LESIONS AS CLINICAL TOOLS IN THE MANAGEMENT OF LYMPHOMA

From a clinical standpoint, NHL genetic lesions represent molecular markers of disease serving four purposes: (1) They assist morphologic diagnosis, (2) they provide a prognostic indicator in some cases, (3) they allow evaluation of minimal residual disease by highly specific and highly sensitive technologies, and (4) they provide targets for molecular therapy.

With respect to diagnosis, the use of genetic lesions as markers for NHL diagnosis is justified by the selective association between a given genetic alteration and a specific NHL category[1,2] (see Fig. 45.1-1 and Table 45.1-1). For example, the detection of *BCL-1* activation in nonfollicular small cell NHL is considered the most specific clue to the diagnosis of mantle cell lymphoma.[1,2] The growing knowledge of the molecular pathogenesis of lymphoma will progressively refine the way we classify these disorders. Ideally, genetically distinct groups of lymphomas should be considered as distinct diseases requiring distinct therapeutic options.

The prognostic relevance of genetic lesions of lymphoma is a growing field of investigation that may provide significant improvement in the therapeutic stratification of lymphoma. Although several genetic alterations have been proposed to influence the prognosis of specific lymphoma categories, the application of novel DNA technologies, namely DNA microarrays, is likely to rapidly expand the molecular markers available for prognostic studies. On these grounds, the application of DNA microarrays to DLCL has allowed the recognition of distinct disease variants with different response to therapy and survival.[201]

Genetic lesions of lymphoma also represent the most specific and the most sensitive marker for evaluation of minimal residual disease by polymerase chain reaction (PCR). Examples are the PCR assay for *BCL-2* in follicular lymphoma and for *BCL-1* in mantle cell lymphoma. Overall, the sensitivity of PCR analysis is several-fold higher than that of standard diagnostic techniques and allows the detection of one tumor cell among 10^6 normal cells. To date, most studies of minimal residual disease in lymphoma have centered on follicular lymphoma and have demonstrated a survival advantage in cases achieving PCR negativity compared to cases that remained positive for minimal residual disease.[303]

Finally, the study of the molecular pathogenesis of lymphoma may provide molecular targets for therapeutic strategies aimed at reversing the very genetic lesions that are responsible for tumor development. Such therapy should, by definition, be largely specific for the lymphoma cells and, hence, devoid of the major side effects presently encountered with antineoplastic therapy.

REFERENCES

1. Harris NL, Jaffe ES, Stein H, et al. A revised European-American classification of lymphoid neoplasms: a proposal from the International Lymphoma Study Group. *Blood* 1994;84:1361.
2. Harris NL, Jaffe ES, Diebold J, et al. World Health Organization classification of neoplastic diseases of the hematopoietic and lymphoid tissues: report of the Clinical Advisory Committee meeting, Airlie House, Virginia, November 1997. *J Clin Oncol* 1999;17:3835.
3. Burrows PD, Cooper MD. B cell development and differentiation. *Curr Opin Immunol* 1997;9:239.
4. Liu YJ, Arpin C. Germinal center development. *Immunol Rev* 1997;156:1115.
5. Gordon J, Gregory CD, Grafton G, Pound JD. Signals for survival and apoptosis in normal and neoplastic B lymphocytes. *Adv Exp Med Biol* 1996;406:139.
6. Kosko-Vilbois MH, Zentgraf H, Gerdes J, Bonnefoy JY. To "B" or not to "B" a germinal center? *Immunol Today* 1997;18:2257.
7. Liu YJ, de Bouteiller O, Fugier-Vivier I. Mechanisms of selection and differentiation in germinal centers. *Curr Opin Immunol* 1997;9:256
8. Berek C. Somatic mutation and memory. *Curr Opin Immunol* 1993;5:218.
9. Muller-Hermelink HK, Greiner A. Molecular analysis of human immunoglobulin heavy chain variable genes (IgV_H) in normal and malignant B cells. *Am J Pathol* 1998;153:1341.
10. Kuppers R, Klein U, Hansmann ML, Rajewsky K. Cellular origin of human B-cell lymphomas. *N Engl J Med* 1999;341:1520.
11. Bahler DW, Levy R. Clonal evolution of a follicular lymphoma: evidence for antigen selection. *Proc Natl Acad Sci U S A* 1992;89:6770.
12. Tamaru J, Hummel M, Marafioti T, et al. Burkitt's lymphomas express V_H genes with a moderate number of antigen-selected somatic mutations. *Am J Pathol* 1995;147:1398.
13. Bertoni F, Cazzaniga G, Bosshard G, et al. Immunoglobulin heavy chain diversity genes rearrangement pattern indicates that MALT-type gastric lymphoma B cells have undergone an antigen selection process. *Br J Haematol* 1997;97:830.
14. Kuppers R, Rajewsky K, Hansmann ML. Diffuse large cell lymphomas are derived from mature B cells carrying V region genes with a high load of somatic mutation and evidence of selection for antibody expression. *Eur J Immunol* 1997;27:1398.
15. Sahota SS, Garand R, Bataille R, Smith AJ, Stevenson FK. V_H gene analysis of clonally related IgM and IgG from human lymphoplasmacytoid B-cell tumors with chronic lymphocytic leukemia features and high serum monoclonal IgG. *Blood* 1998;91:238.
16. Fais F, Gaidano G, Capello D, et al. Immunoglobulin V region gene use and structure suggest antigen selection in AIDS-related primary effusion lymphomas. *Leukemia* 1999;13:1093.
17. Fais F, Ghiotto F, Hashimoto S, et al. Chronic lymphocytic leukemia B cells express restricted sets of mutated and unmutated antigen receptors. *J Clin Invest* 1998;102:1515.
18. Capello D, Fais F, Vivenza D, et al. Identification of three subgroups of B cell chronic lymphocytic leukemia based upon mutations of BCL-6 and IgV genes. *Leukemia* 2000;14:811.
19. Kuppers R, Rajewsky K. The origin of Hodgkin and Reed/Sternberg cells in Hodgkin's disease. *Annu Rev Immunol* 1998;16:471.
20. Kuppers R, Kanzler H, Hansmann ML, Rajewsky K. Immunoglobulin V genes in Reed-Sternberg-cells. *N Engl J Med* 1996;334:405.
21. Kuppers R, Kanzler H, Hansmann ML, Rajewsky K. Single cell analysis of Hodgkin/Reed-Sternberg cells. *Ann Oncol* 1996;7[Suppl 4]:27.
22. Kuppers R, Rajewsky K, Zhao M, et al. Hodgkin's disease: clonal Ig gene rearrangements in Hodgkin and Reed-Sternberg cells picked from histological sections. *Ann N Y Acad Sci* 1995;764:523.
23. Marafioti T, Hummel M, Foss HD, et al. Hodgkin and Reed-Sternberg cells represent an expansion of a single clone originating from a germinal center B-cell with functional immunoglobulin gene rearrangements but defective immunoglobulin transcription. *Blood* 2000;95:1443.
24. Mitelman F, Mertens F, Johansson B. A breakpoint map of recurrent chromosomal rearrangements in human neoplasia. *Nat Genet* 1997;[Special issue]:417.
25. Bedi GC, Westra WH, Farzadegan H, Pitha PM, Sidransky D. Microsatellite instability in primary neoplasms from HIV+ patients. *Nat Med* 1995;1:65.
26. Gamberi B, Gaidano G, Parsa N, et al. Lack of microsatellite instability is rare in B-cell non-Hodgkin's lymphoma. *Blood* 1997;89:975.
27. Eshleman JR, Markowitz SD. Microsatellite instability in inherited and sporadic neoplasms. *Curr Opin Oncol* 1995;7:83.
28. Offit K, Wong G, Filippa DA, Tao Y, Chaganti RSK. Cytogenetic analysis of 434 consecutively ascertained specimens of non-Hodgkin's lymphoma: clinical correlations. *Blood* 1991;77:1508.
29. Tycko B, Sklar J. Chromosomal translocations in lymphoid neoplasia: a reappraisal of the recombinase model. *Cancer Cells* 1990;2:1.
30. Tycko B, Reynolds TC, Smith SD, Sklar J. Consistent breakage between consensus recombinase heptamers of chromosome 9 DNA in a recurrent chromosomal translocation of human T cell leukemia. *J Exp Med* 1989;169:369.
31. Jaeger U, Karth GD, Knapp S, et al. Molecular mechanism of the t(14;18)—a model for lymphoid-specific chromosomal translocations. *Leuk Lymphoma* 1994;14:197.
32. Gillert E, Leis T, Repp R, et al. A DNA damage repair mechanism is involved in the origin of chromosomal translocations t(4;11) in primary leukemic cells. *Oncogene* 1999;18:4663.
33. Romana S, Poirel H, Della Valle V, et al. Molecular analysis of chromosomal breakpoints in three examples of chromosomal translocation involving the TEL gene. *Leukemia* 1999;13:1754.
34. Richardson C, Moynahan ME, Jasin M. Homologous recombination between heterologs during repair of a double-strand break. Suppression of translocations in normal cells. *Ann N Y Acad Sci* 1999;886:183.
35. Morgan WF, Corcoran J, Hartmann A, et al. DNA double-strand breaks, chromosomal rearrangements, and genomic instability. *Mutat Res* 1998;404:125.
36. Difilippantonio MJ, Zhu J, Chen HT, et al. DNA repair protein Ku80 suppresses chromosomal aberrations and malignant transformation. *Nature* 2000;404:510.
37. Goossens T, Klein U, Kuppers R. Frequent occurrence of deletions and duplications during somatic hypermutation: implications for oncogene translocations and heavy chain disease. *Proc Natl Acad Sci U S A* 1998;95:2463.
38. Neri A, Barriga F, Knowles DM, Magrath IT, Dalla-Favera R. Different regions of the immunoglobulin heavy-chain locus are involved in chromosomal translocations in distinct pathogenetic forms of Burkitt lymphoma. *Proc Natl Acad Sci U S A* 1988;85:2748.
39. Houldsworth J, Mathew S, Rao PH, et al. REL proto-oncogene is frequently amplified in extranodal diffuse large cell lymphoma. *Blood* 1996;87:25.
40. Tanaka S, Louie DC, Kant JA, Reed JC. Frequent incidence of somatic mutations in translocated bcl2 oncogenes of non-Hodgkin's lymphomas. *Blood* 1992;79:229.
41. Bhatia K, Huppi K, Spangler G, et al. Point mutations in the c-MYC transactivation domain are common in Burkitt's lymphoma and mouse plasmacytoma. *Nat Genet* 1993;5:56.
42. Cesarman E, Dalla-Favera R, Bentley D, Groudine M. Mutations in the first exon are associated with altered transcription of c-myc in Burkitt lymphoma. *Science* 1987;238:1272.
43. Migliazza A, Martinotti S, Chen W, et al. Frequent somatic hypermutation of the 5' noncoding region of the BCL-6 gene in B-cell lymphoma. *Proc Natl Acad Sci U S A* 1995;92:12520.
44. Pasqualucci L, Migliazza A, Fracchiolla N, et al. BCL-6 mutations in normal germinal center B cells: evidence of somatic hypermutation acting outside Ig loci. *Proc Natl Acad Sci U S A* 1998;95:11816.
45. Capello D, Vitolo U, Pasqualucci L, et al. Distribution and pattern of BCL-6 mutations throughout the spectrum of B-cell neoplasia. *Blood* 2000;95:651.
46. Neri A, Knowles DM, Greco A, McCormick F, Dalla-Favera R. Analysis of RAS oncogene mutations in human lymphoid malignancies. *Proc Natl Acad Sci U S A* 1988;85:9268.
47. Hollstein M, Sidransky D, Vogelstein B, Harris CC. p53 mutations in human cancers. *Science* 1991;253:49.
48. Gaidano G, Ballerini P, Gong JZ, et al. p53 mutations in human lymphoid malignancies: association with Burkitt lymphoma and chronic lymphocytic leukemia. *Proc Natl Acad Sci U S A* 1991;88:5413.
49. Ballerini P, Gaidano G, Gong JZ, et al. Multiple genetic lesions in acquired immunodeficiency syndrome–related non-Hodgkin's lymphoma. *Blood* 1993;81:166.
50. Lo Coco F, Gaidano G, Louie DC, et al. p53 mutations are associated with histologic transformation of follicular lymphoma. *Blood* 1993;82:2289.
51. Gaidano G, Hauptschein RS, Parsa NZ, et al. Deletions involving two distinct regions of 6q in B-cell non Hodgkin lymphoma. *Blood* 1992;80:1781.
52. Brown AG, Ross FM, Dunne EM, Steel CM, Weir-Thompson EM. Evidence for a new tumor suppressor locus (DBM) in human B-cell neoplasia telomeric to the retinoblastoma gene. *Nat Genet* 1993;3:67.
53. Devilder MC, François S, Bosic C, et al. Deletion cartography around the D13S25 locus in B cell chronic lymphocytic leukemia and accurate mapping of the involved tumor suppressor gene. *Cancer Res* 1995;55:1355.
54. Liu Y, Hermanson M, Grandér D, et al. 13q deletions in lymphoid malignancies. *Blood* 1995;86:1911.
55. Garcia-Marco JA, Caldas C, Price CM, et al. Frequent somatic deletion of the 13q12.3 locus encompassing BRCA2 in chronic lymphocytic leukemia. *Blood* 1996;88:1568.
56. Kalachikov S, Migliazza A, Cayanis E, et al. Cloning and gene mapping of the chromosome 13q14 region deleted in chronic lymphocytic leukemia. *Genomics* 1997;42:369.
57. Migliazza A, Cayanis E, Bosch-Albareda F, et al. Molecular pathogenesis of B-cell chronic lymphocytic leukemia: analysis of 13q14 chromosomal deletions. *Curr Top Microbiol Immunol* 2000 (*in press*).
58. Cuneo A, Bigoni R, Rigolin GM, et al. 13q14 deletion in non-Hodgkin's lymphoma: correlation with clinicopathologic features. *Haematologica* 1999;84:589.
59. Kieff E, Leibowitz D. Oncogenesis by herpesvirus. In: Weinberg RA, ed. *Oncogenes and the molecular origin of cancer.* Cold Spring Harbor, NY: Cold Spring Harbor Laboratory Press, 1989:259.
60. zur Hausen H, Schulte-Holthausen H, Klein G, et al. EBV DNA in biopsies of Burkitt tumors and anaplastic carcinomas of the nasopharynx. *Nature* 1970;228:1056.

61. Neri A, Barriga F, Inghirami G, et al. Epstein-Barr virus infection precedes clonal expansion in Burkitt's and acquired immunodeficiency–associated lymphoma. *Blood* 1991;77:1092.
62. Pelicci PG, Knowles DM II, Arlin ZA, et al. Multiple monoclonal B cell expansions and c-myc oncogene rearrangements in acquired immunodeficiency syndrome–related lymphoproliferative disorders. Implications for lymphomagenesis. *J Exp Med* 1986;164:2049.
63. Hamilton-Dutoit SJ, Pallesen G. A survey of Epstein-Barr virus gene expression in sporadic non-Hodgkin's lymphomas. *Am J Pathol* 1992;140:1315.
64. Carbone A, Gaidano G, Gloghini A, et al. Differential expression of BCL-6, CD138/syndecan-1 and EBV-encoded latent membrane protein-1 identifies distinct histogenetic pathways of AIDS-related non-Hodgkin's lymphomas. *Blood* 1998;91:747.
65. Horenstein MG, Nador RG, Chadburn A, et al. Epstein-Barr virus latent gene expression in primary effusion lymphomas containing Kaposi's sarcoma–associated herpesvirus/human herpesvirus-8. *Blood* 1997;90:1186.
66. La Rocca LM, Capello D, Rinelli A, et al. The molecular and phenotypic profile of primary central nervous system lymphoma identifies distinct categories of the disease and is consistent with histogenetic derivation from germinal center–related B-cells. *Blood* 1998;92:1011.
67. Fassone L, Bhatia K, Gutierrez M, et al. Molecular profile of Epstein-Barr virus infection in HHV-8 positive primary effusion lymphoma. *Leukemia* 2000;14:271.
68. Cingolani A, Gastaldi R, Fassone L, et al. Epstein-Barr virus infection is predictive of central nervous system involvement in systemic AIDS-related non-Hodgkin's lymphomas. *J Clin Oncol* 2000 (*in press*).
69. Raab-Traub N, Flynn K. The structure of the termini of the Epstein-Barr virus as a marker of clonal cellular proliferation. *Cell* 1986;47:883.
70. Chang Y, Cesarman E, Pessin MS, et al. Identification of herpesvirus-like DNA sequences in AIDS-associated Kaposi's sarcoma. *Science* 1994;266:1865.
71. Cesarman E, Chang Y, Moore PS, Said JW, Knowles DM. Kaposi's sarcoma–associated herpesvirus-like DNA sequences in AIDS-related body-cavity-based lymphomas. *N Engl J Med* 1995;332:1186.
72. Carbone A, Gloghini A, Vaccher E, et al. Kaposi's sarcoma–associated herpesvirus DNA sequences in AIDS-related and AIDS-unrelated lymphomatous effusions. *Br J Haematol* 1996;94:533.
73. Gaidano G, Pastore C, Gloghini A, et al. Distribution of human herpesvirus-8 sequences throughout the spectrum of AIDS-related neoplasia. *AIDS* 1996;10:941.
74. Carbone A, Gaidano G. HHV-8 positive body cavity based lymphoma: a novel lymphoma entity. *Br J Haematol* 1997;97:515.
75. Gaidano G, Carbone A. Primary effusion lymphoma. A liquid phase lymphoma of fluid-filled body cavities. *Adv Cancer Res* 2000 (*in press*).
76. Soulier J, Grollet L, Oksenhendler E, et al. Kaposi's sarcoma–associated herpesvirus-like DNA sequences in multicentric Castleman's disease. *Blood* 1995;86:1276.
77. Roizman B, Desrosiers RC, Fleckenstein B, et al. The family herpesviridae: an update. *Arch Virol* 1992;123:425.
78. Moore PS, Gao SJ, Dominguez G, et al. Primary characterization of a herpesvirus agent associated with Kaposi's sarcoma. *J Virol* 1996;70:549.
79. Gaidano G, Cechova K, Chang Y, et al. Establishment of AIDS-related lymphoma cell lines from lymphomatous effusions. *Leukemia* 1996;10:1237.
80. Mesri EA, Cesarman E, Arvanitakis L, et al. Human herpesvirus-8/Kaposi's sarcoma–associated herpesvirus is a new transmissible virus that infects B cells. *J Exp Med* 1996;183:2385.
81. Chang Y, Moore PS, Talbot SJ, et al. Cyclin encoded by KS herpesvirus. *Nature* 1996;382:410.
82. Moore PS, Boshoff C, Weiss RA, Chang Y. Molecular mimicry of human cytokine and cytokine response pathway genes by KSHV. *Science* 1996;274:1739.
83. Arvanitakis L, Geras-Raaka E, Varma A, Gershengorn MC, Cesarman E. Human herpesvirus KSHV encodes a constitutively active G-protein-coupled receptor linked to cell proliferation. *Nature* 1997;385:347.
84. Carbone A, Gloghini A, Bontempo D, et al. Proliferation in HHV-8-positive primary effusion lymphomas is associated with expression of HHV-8 cyclin but independent of p27(kip1). *Am J Pathol* 2000;156:1209.
85. Ferreira OC Jr, Planelles V, Rosenblatt JD. Human T-cell leukemia viruses: epidemiology, biology, and pathogenesis. *Blood Rev* 1997;11:91.
86. Uchiyama T. Human T cell leukemia virus type I (HTLV-I) and human diseases. *Annu Rev Immunol* 1997;15:15.
87. Yoshida M. Howard Temin memorial lectureship. Molecular biology of HTLV-1: deregulation of host cell gene expression and cell cycle. *Leukemia* 1997;11:14.
88. Inoue J, Seiki M, Taniguchi T, Tsuru S, Yoshida M. Induction of interleukin-2 receptor gene expression by p40 encoded by human T-cell leukemia virus type I. *EMBO J* 1987;5:2883.
89. Cross SL, Feinberg MB, Wolf JB, et al. Regulation of the human interleukin-2 α chain promoter: activation of a non-functional promoter by the transactivator gene of HTLV-I. *Cell* 1987;49:47.
90. Fujii M, Sassone-Corsi P, Verma IM. c-fos promoter transactivation by the tax1 protein of human T-cell leukemia virus type I. *Proc Natl Acad Sci U S A* 1988;85:8526.
91. Wano Y, Feinberg M, Hosking JB, Bogerd H, Greene WC. Stable expression of the tax gene of type I human T-cell leukemia virus in human T-cell activates specific cellular genes involved in growth. *Proc Natl Acad Sci U S A* 1988;85:9733.
92. Nimer SD, Gasson JC, Hu K, et al. Activation of the GM-CSF promoter by HTLV-I and -II tax proteins. *Oncogene* 1989;4:671.
93. Arima N. Autonomous and interleukin-2-responsive growth of leukemic cells in adult T-cell leukemia (ATL): a review of the clinical significance and molecular basis of ATL cell growth. *Leuk Lymphoma* 1997;26:479.
94. Uittenbogaard MN, Giebler HA, Reisman D, Nyborg JK. Transcriptional repression of p53 by human T-cell leukemia virus type I Tax protein. *J Biol Chem* 1995;270:28503.
95. Jeang KT, Widen SG, Semmes OJ IV, Wilson SH. HTLV-I trans-activator protein, tax, is a trans-repressor of the human beta-polymerase gene. *Science* 1990;247:1082.
96. Jin DY, Spencer F, Jeang KT. Human T cell leukemia virus type 1 oncoprotein Tax targets the human mitotic checkpoint protein MAD1. *Cell* 1998;93:81.
97. Poiesz BJ, Ruscetti FW, Gazdar AF, et al. Detection and isolation of type C retrovirus particles from fresh and cultured lymphocytes of a patient with cutaneous T-cell lymphoma. *Proc Natl Acad Sci U S A* 1980;77:7415.
98. Kikuchi M, Mitsui T, Takeshita M, et al. Virus associated adult T-cell leukemia (ATL) in Japan: clinical, histological and immunological studies. *Hematol Oncol* 1986;4:67.
99. Gaidano G, Newcomb EW, Gong JZ, et al. Analysis of alterations of oncogenes and tumor suppressor genes in chronic lymphocytic leukemia. *Am J Pathol* 1994;144:1312.
100. Schena M, Larsson LG, Gottardi D, et al. Growth- and differentiation-associated expression of BCL-2 in B-chronic lymphocytic leukemia cells. *Blood* 1992;79:2981.
101. Starostik P, Manshouri T, O'Brien S, et al. Deficiency of the ATM protein expression defines an aggressive subgroup of B-cell chronic lymphocytic leukemia. *Cancer Res* 1998;58:4552.
102. Bullrich F, Rasio D, Kitada S, et al. ATM mutations in B-cell chronic lymphocytic leukemia. *Cancer Res* 1999;59:24.
103. Stankovic T, Weber P, Stewart G, et al. Inactivation of ataxia telangiectasia mutated gene in B-cell chronic lymphocytic leukemia. *Lancet* 1999;353:26.
104. Autio K, Aalto Y, Franssila K, et al. Low number of DNA copy number changes in small lymphocytic lymphoma. *Haematologica* 1998;83:690.
105. Juliusson G, Oscier DG, Fitchett M, et al. Prognostic subgroups in B-cell chronic lymphocytic leukemia defined by specific chromosomal abnormalities. *N Engl J Med* 1990;323:720.
106. Anastasi J, Le Beau MM, Vardiman JW, et al. Detection of trisomy 12 in chronic lymphocytic leukemia by fluorescence *in situ* hybridization to interphase cells: a simple and sensitive method. *Blood* 1992;79:1796.
107. Hjalmar V, Kimby E, Matutes E, et al. Trisomy 12 and lymphoplasmacytoid lymphocytes in chronic leukemic B-cell disorders. *Haematologica* 1998;83:602.
108. Offit K, Louie DC, Parsa NZ, et al. Clinical and morphologic features of B-cell small lymphocytic lymphoma with del(6) (q21q23). *Blood* 1994;83:2611.
109. Sahota SS, Davis Z, Hamblin TJ, Stevenson FK. Somatic mutation of bcl-6 genes can occur in the absence of V(H) mutations in chronic lymphocytic leukemia. *Blood* 2000;95:3534.
110. Damle RN, Wasil T, Fais F, et al. Ig V gene mutation status and CD138 expression as novel prognostic indicators in chronic lymphocytic leukemia. *Blood* 1999;94:1840.
111. Hamblin TJ, Davis Z, Gardiner A, Oscier DG, Stevenson FK. Unmutated Ig V(H) genes are associated with a more aggressive form of chronic lymphocytic leukemia. *Blood* 1999;94:1848.
112. Offit K, Parsa NZ, Filippa D, Jhanwar SC, Chaganti RSK. t(9;14)(p13;q32) denotes a subset of low-grade non-Hodgkin's lymphoma with plasmacytoid differentiation. *Blood* 1992;80:2594.
113. Iida S, Rao PH, Nallasivam P, et al. The t(9;14)(p13;q32) chromosomal translocation associated with lymphoplasmacytoid lymphoma involves the PAX-5 gene. *Blood* 1996;88:4110.
114. Neurath MF, Stuber ER, Strober W. BSAP: a key regulator of B-cell development and differentiation. *Immunol Today* 1995;16:564.
115. Berger F, Felman P, Sonet A, et al. Nonfollicular small B-cell lymphomas: a heterogeneous group of patients with distinct clinical features and outcome. *Blood* 1994;83:2829.
116. Fisher RI, Dahlberg S, Nathwani BN, et al. A clinical analysis of two indolent lymphoma entities: mantle cell lymphoma and marginal zone lymphoma (including the mucosa-associated lymphoid tissue and monocytoid B subcategories): a Southwest Oncology Study Group. *Blood* 1995;85:1075.
117. Raffeld M, Jaffe ES. bcl-1, t(11;14), and mantle zone lymphomas. *Blood* 1991;78:259.
118. Tsujimoto Y, Yunis J, Onorato-Showe L, et al. Molecular cloning of the chromosomal breakpoint on chromosome 11 in human B-cell neoplasms with the t(11;14) chromosome translocation. *Science* 1984;224:1403.
119. Tsujimoto Y, Jaffe ES, Cosman J, Gorham J, Croce CM. Clustering of breakpoints on chromosome 11 in human B-cell neoplasms with the t(11;14) chromosome translocation. *Nature* 1985;315:340.
120. Erikson J, Finan J, Tsujimoto Y, Nowell PC, Croce CM. The chromosome 14 breakpoint in neoplastic B cells with the t(11;14) translocation involves the immunoglobulin heavy chain locus. *Proc Natl Acad Sci U S A* 1984;81:4144.
121. Motokura T, Bloom T, Goo KH, et al. A novel cyclin encoded by a bcl-1 linked candidate oncogene. *Nature* 1991;350:512.
122. Withers DA, Harvey RC, Faust JB, et al. Characterization of a candidate bcl-1 gene. *Mol Cell Biol* 1991;11:4846.
123. Rosenberg CL, Wong E, Petty EM, et al. PRAD1, a candidate BCL1 oncogene: mapping and expression in centrocytic lymphoma. *Proc Natl Acad Sci U S A* 1991;88:9638.
124. Seto M, Yamamoto K, Iida S, et al. Gene rearrangement and overexpression of PRAD-1 in lymphoid malignancy with t(11;14)(q13;q32) translocation. *Oncogene* 1992;7:1401.
125. Rimokh R, Berger F, Delsol G, et al. Rearrangement and overexpression of the BCL-1/PRAD-1 gene in intermediate lymphocytic lymphomas and in t(11q13)-bearing leukemias. *Blood* 1993;81:3063.
126. Murakami MS, Strobel MJ, Vande Woude JF. Cell cycle regulation, oncogenes, and antineoplastic drugs. In: Mendelsohn J, Howley PM, Israel MA, Liotta LA, eds. *The molecular basis of cancer.* Philadelphia: WB Saunders, 1995:3.
127. Jiang W, Kahn SM, Zhou P, et al. Overexpression of cyclin D1 in rat fibroblasts causes abnormalities in growth control, cell cycle progression and gene expression. *Oncogene* 1993;8:3447.
128. Bodrug S, Warner B, Bath M, et al. Cyclin D1 transgene impedes lymphocyte maturation and collaborates with the myc gene. *EMBO J* 1994;13:2124.
129. Lovec H, Grzeschiczek A, Möröy T. Cyclin D1/bcl-1 cooperates with myc genes in the generation of B-cell lymphomas in transgenic mice. *EMBO J* 1994;13:3487.
130. Williams ME, Meeker TC, Swerdlow SH. Rearrangement of the chromosome 11 bcl-1 locus in centrocytic lymphoma: analysis with multiple breakpoint probes. *Blood* 1991;78:493.
131. Williams ME, Swerdlow SH. Cyclin D1 overexpression in non-Hodgkin's lymphoma with chromosome 11 bcl-1 rearrangement. *Ann Oncol* 1994;5:S71.

132. Rimokh R, Berger F, Delsol G, et al. Detection of the chromosomal translocation t(11;14) by polymerase chain reaction in mantle cell lymphomas. *Blood* 1994;83:1871.
133. Louie DC, Offit K, Jaslow R, et al. p53 overexpression as a marker of poor prognosis in mantle cell lymphomas with t(11;14)(q13;q32). *Blood* 1995;86:2892.
134. Pinyol M, Cobo F, Bea S, et al. p16(INK4a) gene inactivation by deletions, mutations, and hypermethylation is associated with transformed and aggressive variants of non-Hodgkin's lymphomas. *Blood* 1998;91:2977.
135. Bakshi A, Jensen JP, Goldman P, et al. Cloning the chromosomal breakpoint of t(14;18) of human lymphomas: clustering around J_H on chromosome 14 and near a transcriptional unit on 18. *Cell* 1985;41:889.
136. Tsujimoto Y, Finger LR, Yunis J, Nowell PC, Croce CM. Cloning of the chromosome breakpoints of neoplastic B cells with the t(14;18) chromosomal translocation. *Science* 1984;226:1097.
137. Cleary ML, Sklar J. Nucleotide sequence of a t(14;18) chromosomal breakpoint in follicular lymphoma and demonstration of a breakpoint cluster region near a transcriptionally active locus on chromosome 18. *Proc Natl Acad Sci U S A* 1985;82:7439.
138. Cleary ML, Smith SD, Sklar J. Cloning and structural analysis of cDNAs for bcl-2 and a hybrid bcl-2/immunoglobulin transcript resulting from the t(14;18) translocation. *Cell* 1986;47:19.
139. Cleary ML, Galili N, Sklar J. Detection of a second t(14;18) breakpoint cluster region in human follicular lymphomas. *J Exp Med* 1986;164:315.
140. Yano T, Jaffe ES, Longo DL, Raffeld M. MYC rearrangements in histologically progressed follicular lymphomas. *Blood* 1992;80:758.
141. Volpe G, Vitolo U, Carbone A, et al. Molecular heterogeneity of B-lineage diffuse large cell lymphoma. *Genes Chromosomes Cancer* 1996;16:21.
142. Graninger WB, Seto M, Boutain B, Goldman P, Korsmeyer SJ. Expression of BCL-2 and BCL-2-Ig fusion transcripts in normal and neoplastic cells. *J Clin Invest* 1987;80:1512.
143. Ngan BY, Chen-Levy Z, Weiss LM, Warnke RA, Cleary ML. Expression in non-Hodgkin's lymphoma of the bcl-2 protein associated with the t(14;18) chromosomal translocation. *N Engl J Med* 1988;318:1638.
144. Korsmeyer SJ. Bcl-2 initiates a new category of oncogenes: regulators of cell death. *Blood* 1992;80:879.
145. Chao DT, Korsmeyer SJ. BCL-2 family: regulators of cell death. *Annu Rev Immunol* 1998;16:395.
146. Hockenberry D, Nunez G, Milliman C, Schreiber RD, Korsmeyer SJ. Bcl-2 is an inner mitochondrial membrane protein that blocks programmed cell death. *Nature* 1990;348:334.
147. Nuñez G, Seto M, Seremetis S, et al. Growth- and tumor-promoting effects of deregulated BCL2 in human B-lymphoblastoid cells. *Proc Natl Acad Sci U S A* 1989;86:4589.
148. Vaux DL, Cory S, Adams JM. Bcl-2 gene promotes hematopoietic cell survival and cooperates with c-MYC to immortalize pre-B cells. *Nature* 1988;335:440.
149. Hockenbery DM, Zutter M, Hickey W, Nahm M, Korsmeyer SJ. Bcl-2 protein is topographically restricted in tissues characterized by apoptotic cell death. *Proc Natl Acad Sci U S A* 1991;88:6961.
150. Nuñez G, Hockenbery D, McDonnel TM, Sorensen CM, Korsmeyer SJ. Bcl-2 maintains B cell memory. *Nature* 1991;353:71.
151. Boise LH, González-García M, Postema CE, et al. bcl-x, a bcl-2-related gene that functions as a dominant regulator of apoptotic cell death. *Cell* 1993;74:597.
152. Oltvai ZN, Milliman CL, Korsmeyer SJ. Bcl-2 heterodimerizes *in vivo* with a conserved homolog, Bax, that accelerates programmed cell death. *Cell* 1993;74:609.
153. Yin XM, Oltvai ZN, Korsmeyer SJ. BH1 and BH2 domains of Bcl-2 are required for inhibition of apoptosis and heterodimerization with Bax. *Nature* 1994;369:321.
154. Hockenbery DM, Oltvai ZN, Yin XM, Milliman CL, Korsmeyer SJ. Bcl-2 functions in an antioxidant pathway to prevent apoptosis. *Cell* 1993;75:241.
155. Lam M, Dubyak G, Chen L, et al. Evidence that BCL-2 represses apoptosis by regulating endoplasmic reticulum–associated Ca^{2+} fluxes. *Proc Natl Acad Sci U S A* 1994;91:6569.
156. Zelenetz AD, Chen TT, Levy R. Clonal expansion in follicular lymphoma occurs subsequent to antigenic selection. *J Exp Med* 1992;176:1137.
157. Reed JC, Stein C, Subasinghe C, et al. Antisense-mediated inhibition of bcl-2 protooncogene expression and leukaemic cell growth and survival: comparisons of phosphodiester and phosphorothioate oligodeoxynucleotides. *Cancer Res* 1990;50:6565.
158. McDonnel TJ, Deane N, Platt FM, et al. bcl-2-immunoglobulin transgenic mice demonstrate extended B cell survival and follicular lymphoproliferation. *Cell* 1989;57:79.
159. Bahler DW, Levy R. Clonal evolution of a follicular lymphoma: evidence for antigen selection. *Proc Natl Acad Sci U S A* 1992;89:6770.
160. McDonnel TJ, Korsmeyer SJ. Progression from lymphoid hyperplasia to high-grade malignant lymphoma in mice transgenic for the t(14;18). *Nature* 1991;349:254.
161. Parsonnet J, Hansen S, Rodriguez L, et al. *Helicobacter pylori* infection and gastric lymphoma. *N Engl J Med* 1994;330:1267.
162. Wotherspoon AC, Doglioni C, Diss TC, et al. Regression of primary low-grade B-cell gastric lymphoma of mucosa-associated lymphoid tissue after eradication of *Helicobacter pylori*. *Lancet* 1993;342:575.
163. Dierlamm J, Baens M, Wlodarska I, et al. The apoptosis inhibitor gene API2 and a novel 18q gene, MLT, are recurrently rearranged in the t(11;18)(q21;q21) associated with mucosa-associated lymphoid tissue lymphoma. *Blood* 1999;93:3601.
164. Akagi T, Motegi M, Tamura A, et al. A novel gene, MALT1 at 18q21, is involved in t(11;18)(q21;q21) found in low-grade B-cell lymphoma of mucosa-associated lymphoid tissue. *Oncogene* 1999;18:5785.
165. Ott G, Kalla J, Steinhoff A, et al. Trisomy 3 is not a common feature in malignant lymphomas of mucosa-associated lymphoid tissue type. *Am J Pathol* 1998;153:689.
166. Willis TG, Jadayel DM, Du MQ, et al. Bcl10 is involved in t(1;14)(p22;q32) of MALT B cell lymphoma and mutated in multiple tumor types. *Cell* 1999;96:35.
167. Zhang Q, Siebert R, Yan M, et al. Inactivating mutations and overexpression of BCL-10, a caspase recruitment domain-containing gene, in MALT lymphoma with t(1;14)(p22;q32). *Nat Genet* 1999;22:63.
168. Du M, Peng H, Singh N, Isaacson PG, Pan L. The accumulation of p53 abnormalities is associated with progression of mucosa-associated lymphoid tissue lymphoma. *Blood* 1995;86:4587.
169. Gaidano G, Volpe G, Pastore C, et al. Detection of BCL-6 rearrangements and p53 mutations in Malt-lymphomas. *Am J Hematol* 1997;56:206.
170. Gaidano G, Capello D, Gloghini A, et al. Frequent mutation of BCL-6 proto-oncogene in high grade, but not low grade, MALT lymphomas of the gastrointestinal tract. *Haematologica* 1999;84:582.
171. Offit K, Jhanwar S, Ebrahim SAD, et al. t(3;22)(q27;q11), a novel translocation associated with diffuse non-Hodgkin's lymphoma. *Blood* 1989;74:1876.
172. Bastard C, Tilly H, Lenormand B, et al. Translocations involving band 3q27 and Ig gene regions in non-Hodgkin's lymphoma. *Blood* 1992;79:2527.
173. Baron BW, Nucifora G, McNabe N, et al. Identification of the gene associated with the recurring chromosomal translocations t(3;14)(q27;q32) and t(3;22)(q27;q11) in B-cell lymphomas. *Proc Natl Acad Sci U S A* 1993;90:5262.
174. Kerckaert JP, Deweindt C, Tilly H, et al. LAZ3, a novel zinc-finger encoding gene, is disrupted by recurring chromosome 3q27 translocations in human lymphoma. *Nat Genet* 1993;5:66.
175. Ye BH, Lista F, Lo Coco F, et al. Alterations of BCL-6, a novel zinc-finger gene, in diffuse large cell lymphoma. *Science* 1993;262:747.
176. Ye BH, Rao PH, Chaganti RSK, et al. Cloning of BCL-6, the locus involved in chromosome translocations affecting band 3q27 in B-cell lymphoma. *Cancer Res* 1993;53:2732.
177. Miki T, Kawamata N, Arai A, et al. Molecular cloning of the breakpoint for 3q27 translocation in B-cell lymphomas and leukemias. *Blood* 1994;83:217.
178. Nelson HC. Structure and function of DNA-binding proteins. *Curr Opin Genet Dev* 1995;5:180.
179. Mackay JP, Crossley M. Zinc fingers are sticking together. *Trends Biochem Sci* 1998;23:1.
180. Bardwell VJ, Treisman R. The POZ domain: a conserved protein-protein interaction motif. *Genes Dev* 1994;8:1664.
181. Chang CC, Ye BH, Chaganti RSK, et al. BCL-6, a POZ/Zinc-finger protein, is a sequence specific transcriptional repressor. *Proc Natl Acad Sci U S A* 1996;93:6947.
182. Cattoretti G, Chang C, Cechova K, et al. BCL-6 protein is expressed in germinal-center B cells. *Blood* 1995;86:45.
183. Dalla-Favera R, Ye BH, Cattoretti G, et al. BCL-6 in diffuse large-cell lymphomas. *Important Adv Oncol* 1996;139.
184. Allman D, Jain A, Dent A, et al. BCL-6 expression during B-cell activation. *Blood* 1996;87:5257.
185. Niu H, Ye BH, Dalla-Favera R. Antigen receptor signaling induces MAP kinase–mediated phosphorylation and degradation of the BCL-6 transcription factor. *Genes Dev* 1998;12:1953.
186. Dent AL, Shaffer AL, Yu X, et al. Control of inflammation, cytokine expression, and germinal center formation by BCL-6. *Science* 1997;276:589.
187. Ye BH, Cattoretti G, Shen Q, et al. The BCL-6 proto-oncogene controls germinal-centre formation and Th2-type inflammation. *Nat Genet* 1997;16:161.
188. Bastard C, Deweindt C, Kerckaert JP, et al. LAZ3 rearrangements in non-Hodgkin's lymphoma: correlation with histology, immunophenotype, karyotype, and clinical outcome in 217 patients. *Blood* 1994;83:2423.
189. Lo Coco F, Ye BH, Lista F, et al. Rearrangements of the BCL-6 gene in diffuse large cell non-Hodgkin's lymphoma. *Blood* 1994;83:1757.
190. Ye BH, Chaganti S, Chang CC, et al. Chromosomal translocations cause deregulated BCL6 expression by promoter substitution in B cell lymphoma. *EMBO J* 1995;14:6209.
191. Dallery E, Galiegue-Zouitina S, Collyn-d'Hoohge M, et al. TTF, a gene encoding a novel small G protein, fuses to the lymphoma-associated LAZ3 gene by t(3;4) chromosome translocation. *Oncogene* 1995;10:2171.
192. Shen HM, Peters A, Baron B, Zhu X, Storb U. Mutation of BCL-6 gene in normal B cells by the process of somatic hypermutation of Ig genes. *Science* 1998;280:1750.
193. Gaidano G, Carbone A, Pastore C, et al. Frequent mutation of the 5' noncoding region of the BCL-6 gene in acquired immunodeficiency syndrome–related non-Hodgkin's lymphomas. *Blood* 1997;89:3755.
194. Capello D, Carbone A, Pastore C, et al. Point mutations of the BCL-6 gene in Burkitt's lymphoma. *Br J Haematol* 1997;99:168.
195. Offit K, Lo Coco F, Louie DC, et al. Rearrangements of the bcl-6 gene as a prognostic marker in diffuse large-cell lymphoma. *N Engl J Med* 1994;331:74.
196. Dalla-Favera R, Ye BH, Lo Coco F, et al. Identification of genetic lesions associated with diffuse large-cell lymphoma. *Ann Oncol* 1994;5:S55.
197. Yunis JJ, Mayer MG, Arnesen MA, et al. Bcl-2 and other genomic alterations in the prognosis of large-cell lymphoma. *N Engl J Med* 1989;320:1947.
198. Tang SC, Visser L, Hepperle B, Hanson J, Poppema S. Clinical significance of bcl-2 MBR gene rearrangement and protein expression in diffuse large-cell non-Hodgkin lymphoma: an analysis of 83 cases. *J Clin Oncol* 1994;12:149.
199. Vitolo U, Gaidano G, Botto B, et al. Rearrangements of BCL-6, BCL-2, c-MYC and 6q deletion in B-diffuse large cell lymphoma: clinical relevance in 71 patients. *Ann Oncol* 1998;9:55.
200. Pescarmona E, Lo Coco F, Pacchiarotti A, et al. Analysis of the BCL-6 gene configuration in diffuse B-cell non-Hodgkin's lymphomas and Hodgkin's disease. *J Pathol* 1995;177:21.
201. Alizadeh AA, Eisen MB, Davis RE, et al. Distinct types of diffuse large B-cell lymphoma identified by gene expression profiling. *Nature* 2000;403:503.
202. Dalla-Favera R. Chromosomal translocations involving the c-myc oncogene in lymphoid neoplasia. In: Kirsch IR, ed. *The causes and consequences of chromosomal aberrations.* Boca Raton, FL: CRC Press, 1993:312.
203. Dalla-Favera R, Bregni M, Erickson J, et al. Human c-myc oncogene is located on the region of chromosome 8 that is translocated in Burkitt lymphoma cells. *Proc Natl Acad Sci U S A* 1982;79:7824.
204. Dalla-Favera R, Martinotti S, Gallo RC, Erikson J, Croce CM. Translocation and rearrangements of the c-myc oncogene in human undifferentiated B-cell lymphomas. *Science* 1983;219:963.
205. Taub R, Kirsch I, Morton C. Translocation of c-myc gene into the immunoglobulin heavy chain locus in human Burkitt lymphoma and murine plasmacytoma cells. *Proc Natl Acad Sci U S A* 1982;79:7837.

206. Davis M, Malcolm S, Rabbits TH. Chromosome translocations can occur on either side of the c-myc oncogene in Burkitt lymphoma cells. *Nature* 1984;30:286.
207. Hollis GF, Mitchell KF, Battey J, et al. A variant translocation places the lambda immunoglobulin genes 3' to the c-myc oncogene in Burkitt's lymphoma. *Nature* 1984;307:752.
208. Pelicci PG, Knowles DK, Magrath I, Dalla-Favera R. Chromosomal breakpoints and structural alterations of the c-myc locus differ in endemic and sporadic forms of Burkitt lymphoma. *Proc Natl Acad Sci U S A* 1986;83:2984.
209. Hayday AC, Gillies SD, Saito H, et al. Activation of a translocated human c-myc gene by an enhancer in the immunoglobulin heavy chain locus. *Nature* 1984;307:334.
210. Rabbits TH, Forster A, Baer R, Hamlin PH. Transcriptional enhancer identified where the human Cμ immunoglobulin heavy chain gene is unavailable to the translocated c-myc gene in a Burkitt's lymphoma. *Nature* 1983;306:806.
211. ar-Rushdi A, Nishikura K, Erikson J, et al. Differential expression of the translocated and untranslocated c-myc oncogene in Burkitt's lymphoma. *Science* 1983;222:390.
212. Bhatia K, Spangler G, Gaidano G, et al. Mutations in the coding region of c-myc occur frequently in acquired immunodeficiency syndrome–associated lymphomas. *Blood* 1994;84:883.
213. Gu W, Bhatia K, Magrath IT, Dang CV, Dalla-Favera R. Binding and suppression of the c-Myc transcriptional activation domain by p107. *Science* 1994;264:251.
214. Blackwood EM, Eisenman RN. Max: a helix-loop-helix zipper protein that forms a sequence-specific DNA-binding complex with Myc. *Science* 1991;251:1211.
215. Blackwood EM, Lüscher B, Eisenman RN. Myc and Max associate *in vivo*. *Genes Dev* 1992;6:71.
216. Kretzner L, Blackwood EM, Eisenman RN. Myc and Max proteins possess distinct transcriptional activities. *Nature* 1992;359:426.
217. Amati B, Dalton S, Brooks MW, et al. Transcriptional activation by the human c-Myc oncoprotein in yeast requires interaction with Max. *Nature* 1992;359:423.
218. Gu W, Cechova K, Tassi V, Dalla-Favera R. Differential regulation of target gene expression by Myc/Max ratio. *Proc Natl Acad Sci U S A* 1993;90:2935.
219. Amati B, Brooks MW, Levy N, et al. Oncogenic activity of the c-Myc protein requires dimerization with Max. *Cell* 1993;72:233.
220. Ayer DE, Kretzner L, Eisenman RN. Mad: a heterodimeric partner for Max that antagonizes Myc transcriptional activity. *Cell* 1993;72:211.
221. Zervos AS, Gyuris J, Brent R. Mxi1, a protein that specifically interacts with Max to bind Myc-Max recognition sites. *Cell* 1993;72:223.
222. Dang CV. c-Myc target genes involved in cell growth, apoptosis, and metabolism. *Mol Cell Biol* 1999;19:1.
223. Wu KJ, Grandori C, Amacker M, et al. Direct activation of TERT transcription by c-MYC. *Nat Genet* 1999;21:220.
224. Cerni C. Telomeres, telomerase, and myc. An update. *Mutat Res* 2000;462:31.
225. Lombardi L, Newcomb EW, Dalla-Favera R. Pathogenesis of Burkitt lymphoma: expression of an activated c-myc oncogene causes the tumorigenic conversion of EBV-infected human B lymphoblasts. *Cell* 1987;49:161.
226. McManaway ME, Neckers LM, Loke SL, et al. Tumor-specific inhibition of lymphoma growth by an antisense oligodeoxy-nucleotide. *Lancet* 1990;335:808.
227. Adams JM, Harris AW, Pinkert CA, et al. The c-myc oncogene driven by immunoglobulin enhancers induces lymphoid malignancy in transgenic mice. *Nature* 1985;318:533.
228. Klangby U, Okan I, Magnusson KP, et al. p16/INK4a and p15/INK4b gene methylation and absence of p16/INK4a mRNA and protein expression in Burkitt's lymphoma. *Blood* 1998;91:1680.
229. Komano J, Maruo S, Kurozumi K, Oda T, Takada K. Oncogenic role of Epstein-Barr virus–encoded RNAs in Burkitt's lymphoma cell line Akata. *J Virol* 1999;73:9827.
230. Gaidano G, Carbone A. AIDS-related lymphomas: from pathogenesis to pathology. *Br J Haematol* 1995;90:235.
231. Knowles DM. Molecular pathology of acquired immunodeficiency syndrome–related non-Hodgkin's lymphoma. *Semin Diagn Pathol* 1997;14:67.
232. Gaidano G, Carbone A, Dalla-Favera R. Pathogenesis of AIDS-related lymphomas: molecular and histogenetic heterogeneity. *Am J Pathol* 1998;152:623.
233. Gaidano G, Carbone A, Dalla-Favera R. Genetic basis of acquired immunodeficiency syndrome–related lymphomagenesis. *J Natl Cancer Inst Monogr* 1998;23:95.
234. Gaidano G, Capello D, Carbone A. The molecular basis of AIDS-related lymphomagenesis. *Semin Oncol* 2000;24(4):431.
235. Gaidano G, Pastore C, Gloghini A, et al. Genetic heterogeneity of AIDS-related small noncleaved cell lymphoma. *Br J Haematol* 1997;98:726.
236. Gaidano G, Lo Coco F, Ye BH, et al. Rearrangements of the BCL-6 gene in acquired immunodeficiency syndrome–associated non-Hodgkin's lymphoma: association with diffuse large-cell subtype. *Blood* 1994;84:397.
237. Gaidano G, Capello D, Cilia AM, et al. Genetic characterization of HHV-8/KSHV positive primary effusion lymphoma reveals frequent mutations of BCL-6: implications for disease pathogenesis and histogenesis. *Genes Chromosomes Cancer* 1999;24:16.
238. Carbone A, Gloghini A, Gaidano G, et al. AIDS-related Burkitt's lymphoma. Morphologic and immunophenotypic study of biopsy specimens. *Am J Clin Pathol* 1995;103:561.
239. Carbone A, Gaidano G, Gloghini A, et al. BCL-6 protein expression in AIDS-related non-Hodgkin's lymphomas. Inverse relationship with Epstein-Barr virus–encoded latent membrane protein-1 expression. *Am J Pathol* 1997;150:155.
240. Riboldi P, Gaidano G, Schettino EW, et al. Two acquired immunodeficiency syndrome–associated Burkitt's lymphomas produce specific anti-i IgM cold agglutinins using somatically mutated V_H4-21 segments. *Blood* 1994;83:2952.
241. Jain R, Roncella S, Hashimoto S, et al. A potential role for antigen selection in the clonal evolution of Burkitt's lymphoma. *J Immunol* 1994;153:45.
242. MacMahon EME, Glass JD, Hayward SD, et al. Epstein-Barr virus in AIDS-related primary central nervous system lymphoma. *Lancet* 1991;338:969.
243. Julien S, Radosavljevic M, Labouret N, et al. AIDS primary central nervous system lymphoma: molecular analysis of the expressed V_H genes and possible implications for lymphomagenesis. *J Immunol* 1999;162:1551.
244. Gaidano G, Capello D, Pastore C, et al. Analysis of human herpesvirus type 8 infection in AIDS-related and AIDS-unrelated primary central nervous system lymphoma. *J Infect Dis* 1997;175:1193.
245. Antinori A, Larocca LM, Fassone L, et al. HHV-8/KSHV is not associated with AIDS-related primary central nervous system lymphoma. *Brain Pathol* 1999;9:199.
246. Gaidano G, Gloghini A, Gattei V, et al. Association of Kaposi's sarcoma–associated herpesvirus-positive primary effusion lymphoma with expression of the CD138/syndecan-1 antigen. *Blood* 1997;90:4894.
247. Lin AY, Tucker MA. Epidemiology of Hodgkin's disease and non-Hodgkin's lymphoma. In: Canellos GP, Lister TA, Sklar JL, eds. *The lymphomas*. Philadelphia: WB Saunders, 1998:43.
248. Morris SW, Kirstein MN, Valentine MB, et al. Fusion of a kinase gene, ALK, to a nucleolar protein gene, NPM, in non-Hodgkin's lymphoma. *Science* 1994;263:1281.
249. Fujimoto J, Shiota M, Iwahara T, et al. Characterization of the transforming activity of p80, a hyperphosphorylated protein in a Ki-1 lymphoma cell line with chromosomal translocation t(2;5). *Proc Natl Acad Sci U S A* 1996;93:4181.
250. Kuefer MU, Look AT, Pulford K. Retrovirus-mediated gene transfer of NPM/ALK causes lymphoid malignancy in mice. *Blood* 1997;90:2901.
251. Lamant L, Meggetto F, al Saati T, et al. High incidence of the t(2;5)(p23;q35) translocation in anaplastic large cell lymphoma and its lack of detection in Hodgkin's disease: comparison of cytogenetic analysis, reverse transcriptase-polymerase chain reaction, and p-80 immunostaining. *Blood* 1996;87:284.
252. Sarris AH, Luthra L, Papadimitracopoulou V, et al. Amplification of genomic DNA demonstrates the presence of the t(2;5)(p23;q35) in anaplastic large cell lymphoma, but not in other non-Hodgkin's lymphomas, Hodgkin's disease, or lymphomatoid papulosis. *Blood* 1996;88:1771.
253. Yee HT, Ponzoni M, Merson A, et al. Molecular characterization of the t(2;5)(p23;q35) translocation in anaplastic large cell lymphoma (Ki-1) and Hodgkin's disease. *Blood* 1996;87:1081.
254. Poiesz BF, Ruscetti FW, Gazdar AF, et al. Detection and isolation of type C retrovirus particles from fresh cultured lymphocytes of a patient with cutaneous T-cell lymphoma. *Proc Natl Acad Sci U S A* 1980;77:7415.
255. Catovsky D, Rose M, Goolden AWG, et al. Adult T-cell lymphoma-leukaemia in blacks from the West Indies. *Lancet* 1982;1:639.
256. Yoshida M, Miyoshi I, Hinuma Y. Isolation and characterization of retrovirus from cell lines of adult T-cell leukemia and its implication in the disease. *Proc Natl Acad Sci U S A* 1982;79:2031.
257. Gallo RC, Kalyanaraman VS, Sarngadharan MG, et al. Association of the human type of C retrovirus with a subset of adult T-cell cancers. *Cancer Res* 1983;43:3892.
258. Wong-Staal F, Hahn B, Manzari V, et al. A survey of human leukemias for sequences of a human retrovirus. *Nature* 1983;302:626.
259. Yoshida M, Seiki M, Yamaguchi K, et al. Monoclonal integration of human T-cell leukemia provirus in all primary tumors of adult T-cell leukemia suggests causative role of human T-cell leukemia virus in the disease. *Proc Natl Acad Sci U S A* 1984;81:2534.
260. Smith MR, Green W. Molecular biology of the type I human T-cell leukemia virus (HTLV-I) and adult T-cell leukemia. *J Clin Invest* 1991;87:761.
261. Sakashita A, Hattori T, Miller CW, et al. Mutations of the p53 gene in adult T-cell leukemia. *Blood* 1992;79:477.
262. Cesarman E, Chadburn A, Inghirami G, et al. Structural and functional analysis of oncogenes and tumor suppressor genes in adult T-cell leukemia/lymphoma shows frequent p53 mutations. *Blood* 1992;80:3205.
263. Stilgenbauer S, Schaffner C, Litterst A, et al. Biallelic mutations in the ATM gene in T-prolymphocytic leukemia. *Nature Med* 1997;3:1155.
264. Vorechovsky I, Luo L, Dyer MJ, et al. Clustering of missense mutations in the ataxia-telangiectasia gene in a sporadic T-cell leukemia. *Nat Genet* 1997;17:96.
265. Westphal CH. Cell-cycle signaling: Atm displays its many talents. *Curr Biol* 1997;7:R789.
266. Neri A, Chang CC, Lombardi L, et al. B cell lymphoma–associated chromosomal translocation involves candidate oncogene lyt-10, homologous to NF-κB p50. *Cell* 1991;67:1075.
267. Lenardo MJ, Baltimore D. NF-κB: a pleiotropic mediator of inducible and tissue-specific gene control. *Cell* 1989;58:227.
268. Kanzler H, Kuppers R, Hansmann ML, Rajewsky K. Hodgkin and Reed-Sternberg cells in Hodgkin's disease represent the outgrowth of a dominant tumor clone derived from (crippled) germinal center B cells. *J Exp Med* 1996;184:1495.
269. Braeuninger A, Kuppers R, Strickler JG, et al. Hodgkin and Reed-Sternberg cells in lymphocyte predominant Hodgkin disease represent clonal populations of germinal center derived tumor B cells. *Proc Natl Acad Sci U S A* 1997;94:9337.
270. Hummel M, Marafioti T, Stein H. Immunoglobulin V genes in Reed-Sternberg cells. *N Engl J Med* 1996;334:405.
271. Ohno T, Stribley JA, Wu G, et al. Clonality in nodular lymphocyte-predominant Hodgkin's disease. *N Engl J Med* 1997;337:459.
272. Marafioti T, Hummel M, Anagnastopoulos I, et al. Origin of nodular lymphocyte-predominant Hodgkin's disease from a clonal expansion of highly mutated germinal-center B cells. *N Engl J Med* 1997;337:453.
273. Kuppers R, Rajewsky K, Zhao M, et al. Hodgkin disease: Hodgkin and Reed-Sternberg cells picked from histological sections show clonal immunoglobulin gene rearrangements and appear to be derived from B cells at various stages of development. *Proc Natl Acad Sci U S A* 1994;91:10962.
274. Brauninger A, Hansmann ML, Strickler JG, et al. Identification of common germinal-center B-cell precursors in two patients with both Hodgkin's disease and non-Hodgkin's lymphoma. *N Engl J Med* 1999;340:1239.
275. Carbone A, Gloghini A, Gattei V, et al. Reed-Sternberg cells of classical Hodgkin's disease react with the plasma cell specific monoclonal antibody B-B4 and express human synde-

can-1. *Blood* 1997;89:3787.
276. Carbone A, Gloghini A, Gaidano G, et al. Expression status of BCL-6 and syndecan-1 identifies distinct histogenetic subsets of Hodgkin's disease. *Blood* 1998;92:2220.
277. Carbone A, Gloghini A, Larocca LM, et al. HIV-associated Hodgkin's disease derives from post-germinal center B-cells. *Blood* 1999;93:2319.
278. Seitz V, Hummel M, Marafioti T, et al. Detection of clonal T-cell receptor gamma-chain gene rearrangements in Reed-Sternberg cells of classic Hodgkin disease. *Blood* 2000;95:3020.
279. Rowley J. Chromosomes in Hodgkin's disease. *Cancer Treat Rep* 1982;66:639.
280. Teerenhovi L, Lindholm C, Pakkala A, et al. Unique display of a pathologic karyotype in Hodgkin's disease by Reed-Sternberg cells. *Cancer Genet Cytogenet* 1988;34:305.
281. Schouten H, Sanger W, Duggan M, et al. Chromosomal abnormalities in Hodgkin's disease. *Blood* 1989;73:2149.
282. Tilly H, Bastard C, Delastre T, et al. Cytogenetic studies in untreated Hodgkin's disease. *Blood* 1991;77:1298.
283. Chilosi M, Doglioni C, Menestrina F, et al. Abnormal expression of the p53-binding protein MDM2 in Hodgkin's disease. *Blood* 1994;84:4295.
284. Momand J, Zambetti GP, Olson DC, George D, Levine AJ. The MDM2 oncogene product forms a complex with the p53 protein and inhibits p53-mediated transactivation. *Cell* 1992;691:1237.
285. Gupta RK, Patel K, Bodmer WF, Bodmer JG. Mutation of p53 in primary biopsy material and cell lines from Hodgkin's disease. *Proc Natl Acad Sci U S A* 1993;90:2817.
286. Trumper LH, Brady G, Bagg A, et al. Single-cell analysis of Hodgkin and Reed-Sternberg cells: molecular heterogeneity of gene expression and p53 mutations. *Blood* 1993;81:3097.
287. Montesinos-Rongen M, Roers A, Kuppers R, et al. Mutation of the p53 gene is not a typical feature of Hodgkin and Reed-Sternberg cells in Hodgkin's disease. *Blood* 1999;94:1755.
288. Pallesen G, Hamilton-Dutoit SJ, Rowe M, Young LS. Expression of Epstein-Barr virus latent gene products in tumour cells of Hodgkin's disease. *Lancet* 1991;337:320.
289. Weiss L, Strickler J, Warnke R, Purtillo D, Sklar J. Epstein-Barr viral DNA in tissues of Hodgkin's disease. *Am J Pathol* 1987;129:86.
290. Weiss L, Mohaved L, Warnke R, Sklar J. Detection of Epstein-Barr viral genomes in Reed-Sternberg cells of Hodgkin's disease. *N Engl J Med* 1989;320:502.
291. Herbst H, Dallenbach F, Hummel M, et al. Epstein-Barr virus latent membrane protein expression in Hodgkin and Reed-Sternberg cells. *Proc Natl Acad Sci U S A* 1991; 88:4766.
292. Boiocchi M, De Re V, Gloghini A, et al. High incidence of monoclonal EBV episomes in Hodgkin's disease and anaplastic large-cell Ki-1-positive lymphomas in HIV-1-positive patients. *Int J Cancer* 1993;54:895.
293. Vasef MA, Kamel OW, Chen YY, Medeiros LJ, Weiss LM. Detection of Epstein-Barr virus in multiple sites involved by Hodgkin's disease. *Am J Pathol* 1995;147:1408.
294. Carbone A, Dolcetti R, Gloghini A, et al. Immunophenotypic and molecular analyses of acquired immune deficiency syndrome–related and Epstein-Barr virus–associated lymphomas: a comparative study. *Hum Pathol* 1996;27:133.
295. Alkan S, Ross CW, Hanson CA, Schnitzer B. Epstein-Barr virus and bcl-2 protein overexpression are not detected in the neoplastic cells of nodular lymphocyte predominance Hodgkin's disease. *Mod Pathol* 1995;8:544.
296. Stein H, Hummel M, Marafioti T, Anagnostopoulos I, Foss HD. Molecular biology of Hodgkin's disease. *Cancer Surv* 1997;30:107.
297. Oudejans JJ, Jiwa NM, Meijer CJ. Epstein-Barr virus in Hodgkin's disease: more than just an innocent bystander. *J Pathol* 1997;181:353.
298. Dolcetti R, Zancai P, De Re V, et al. Epstein-Barr virus strains with latent membrane protein-1 deletions: prevalence in the Italian population and high association with human immunodeficiency virus–related Hodgkin's disease. *Blood* 1997;89:1723.
299. Chapman AL, Rickinson AB. Epstein-Barr virus in Hodgkin's disease. *Ann Oncol* 1998;9[Suppl 5]:S5.
300. Enblad G, Sandvej K, Sundstrom C, Pallesen G, Glimelius B. Epstein-Barr virus distribution in Hodgkin's disease in an unselected Swedish population. *Acta Oncol* 1999;38:425.
301. Jarret RF, MacKenzie J. Epstein-Barr virus and other candidate viruses in the pathogenesis of Hodgkin's disease. *Semin Hematol* 1999;36:260.
302. Harris NL. Hodgkin's disease: classification and differential diagnosis. *Mod Pathol* 1999;12:159.
303. Corradini P, Ladetto M, Pileri A, Tarella C. Clinical relevance of minimal residual disease monitoring in non-Hodgkin's lymphomas: a critical reappraisal of molecular strategies. *Leukemia* 1999;13:1691.

SECTION **2**

HOWARD J. WEINSTEIN
NANCY J. TARBELL

Leukemias and Lymphomas of Childhood

LEUKEMIAS

The development of successful therapy for most children with acute lymphoblastic leukemia (ALL) can be attributed to a series of prospective clinical studies that clarified the pathophysiology of ALL and showed the importance of combination chemotherapy, sanctuary-specific treatment, and supportive care measures.[1] On the other hand, the relative resistance of acute myelogenous leukemia (AML) to chemotherapy led to the development of treatment strategies that include dose-intensified chemotherapy and bone marrow transplantation (BMT).[2] During the 1990s, we have also greatly advanced our knowledge of leukemia cell biology, most notably in the area of molecular pathogenesis. Molecular biologists have developed powerful diagnostic tools, sensitive methods for detecting minimal residual leukemia, and potential new therapeutic targets.[3] The improvement in long-term survival for children with acute leukemia has been gratifying but also has been associated with significant late effects that underscore the need for vigilant follow-up and for designing risk-adapted therapies.

EPIDEMIOLOGY

Leukemia is the most common form of cancer in children. Approximately 2500 new cases of childhood leukemia are diagnosed each year in the United States.[4] ALL and AML are diagnosed in 75% and 20% of the cases, respectively, and chronic myeloid leukemia in fewer than 5%. The well-established peak incidence of childhood leukemia at age 4 years is due to ALL. ALL affects males and whites more often than females and African Americans. Nearly a threefold higher incidence of ALL at 2 to 3 years of age occurs for white children compared to black children. The incidence of AML is constant during childhood, except for a slight peak in infancy and late adolescence.[4]

It is likely that the majority of acute leukemias in children are initiated by acquired mutations within the hematopoietic tissues.[5] Intriguing results of molecular genetic studies using stored neonatal blood spots from children who eventually developed ALL suggest a prenatal origin in some patients.[6] In studies of monozygotic twins who both developed acute leukemia (approximately 5% concordance rate), it appears that the initial chromosome translocation occurred *in utero* with subsequent transfer of the leukemia clone from one twin to the other via the shared blood supply. Because the concordance rate for leukemia is low in identical twins, it follows that an additional event or environmental exposure is required postnatally.

A small number of children are at increased risk to develop leukemia because of an inherited predisposition.[5] For example, children with Down syndrome have a 10- to 20-fold increased risk of leukemia during the first 10 years of life.[7] The types of leukemia in children with Down syndrome follow the usual distribution of childhood leukemia, except at younger than 3 years of age when AML (mostly FAB M7) is more likely to occur than ALL. Neonates with Down syndrome or trisomy 21 mosaicism may also develop a "transient myeloproliferative disorder" (TMD) that is indistinguishable from congenital AML. This disorder is usually diagnosed within the first 2 weeks of life, and the incidence is unknown. Peripheral blood or bone marrow blasts from infants with TMD have features of the megakaryocytic and erythroid lineages and, in some cases, have been shown to be

TABLE 45.2-1. French-American-British Classification of Acute Myelogenous Leukemia in Children

Morphology	*Frequency (%)*	*Associations*
M0: large agranular blasts; negative myeloperoxidase	2	Blasts may express CD34 and TdT
M1: poorly differentiated myeloblasts	13	
M2: myeloblasts with differentiation and frequent Auer rods	28	Granulocytic sarcomas (myeloblastomas) with t(8;21)
M3: hypergranular abnormal promyelocytes with multiple Auer rods	6	Disseminated intravascular coagulation
M4: myeloblastic and monoblastic differentiation (>20% monoblasts); $M4E_0$ variant associated with dysplastic eos	19	Age less than 2 y, EM (especially leukemia cutis)
M5: monoblastic	21	Age less than 2 y, EM (especially leukemia cutis)
M6: erythroleukemia with bizarre dyserythropoiesis and megaloblastic features	1	
M7: megakaryoblastic (occasional myelofibrosis)	10	Down syndrome

EM, extramedullary leukemia; TdT, terminal deoxynucleotidyl transferase.
(Based on 180 cases of AML in children studied at St. Jude Children's Research Hospital from 1984 to 1992.)

clonal in origin. In more than 90% of these infants, however, the blasts spontaneously disappear and normal blood counts recover within the first several weeks to months after diagnosis of TMD. One retrospective study reported that up to 30% of infants with TMD eventually developed either a myelodysplastic syndrome or AML before the age of 3 years.[8] Because the majority of these infants appear never to develop leukemia, neonates with Down syndrome and a hematologic picture consistent with AML should be observed for 4 to 10 weeks before cytotoxic therapy is initiated. If therapy is eventually needed, the outcome for these children has been surprisingly favorable.[9]

Children with neurofibromatosis are predisposed to develop myeloid malignancies, especially myelodysplastic and myeloproliferative syndromes.[10] In patients with neurofibromatosis who develop leukemia, evidence indicates loss of both neurofibromatosis (NF-1) alleles in bone marrow cells. These data provide evidence that NF-1 may function as a tumor-suppressor gene in children with NF-1.

Some epidemiologic studies suggest that maternal reproductive history of previous fetal loss and maternal alcohol consumption during pregnancy is associated with an increased risk of AML in infants.[11] In general, most studies have not found a consistent association between common infectious or environmental exposures and an increased risk of childhood leukemia.[5,12] On the other hand, AML has been observed as a secondary leukemia in both children and adults who were treated with alkylating agents or topoisomerase II inhibitors (e.g., epipodophyllotoxins).[13,14]

CLONALITY AND CELL OF ORIGIN

Normal blood cell production is polyclonal, whereas leukemia is a clonal disorder. The return of polyclonal hematopoiesis in remission and the reappearance of the original clone at relapse suggests that the leukemic clone was suppressed but not eradicated by chemotherapy. This also implies that normal bone marrow stem cells repopulate the marrow during remission. In rare situations, patients with AML in remission have had persistent clonal hematopoiesis.[15] The significance of this observation remains unknown.

Within the hierarchy of hematopoietic development, there are many potential targets for leukemic transformation. Characterization of the leukemic blast population by morphology, genetics, and immunologic methods has helped to establish a revised classification system that may or may not reflect the nature of the leukemic "stem cell." The detection of lymphoid lineage–associated determinants on the surface of lymphoblasts plus an analysis of immunoglobulin (Ig) and T-cell receptor gene rearrangements suggest that ALL derives from either a precursor T or precursor B cell.[16] The cell of origin for AML has been postulated to be either a multipotent or committed myeloid progenitor (e.g., CFU-GEMM or granulocyte-macrophage colony-forming unit), but more recent data indicate that the AML stem cell may be more primitive than previously postulated.[17,18]

CLASSIFICATION

Morphology

In the 1970s, a morphologic classification system was developed for the acute leukemias by a French-American-British (FAB) Cooperative Working Group and has since gained wide acceptance.[19] The FAB system divides ALL into three morphologic subtypes (L1, L2, and L3). L1 lymphoblasts, the most common FAB type in children, have scanty cytoplasm and inconspicuous nucleoli. Blasts in the L2 category account for 10% of cases; they are larger and more pleomorphic in size, with abundant cytoplasm and prominent nucleoli, and they may be difficult to distinguish by morphology alone from FAB subtype M0 AML.

L3 is the rarest subtype (1% to 2%) of ALL, and these blasts have very basophilic vacuolated cytoplasm. These L3 blasts have the same immunophenotype as well as karyotype and molecular genetic abnormalities as the tumor cells in small noncleaved or Burkitt lymphomas[3] (see Non-Hodgkin's Lymphoma, later in this chapter).

The FAB classification recognizes eight subtypes of AML (M0 to M7). Table 45.2-1 presents a distribution of FAB subtypes for 180 cases of AML in children younger than 18 years of age studied at St. Jude Children's Research Hospital from 1984 to 1992. Most children younger than 2 years of age with AML have either the M4 or M5 subtypes.[2] Although the M7 subtype may have several characteristic morphologic features, the diagnosis of M7 AML requires confirmation either by ultrastructural histochemistry (platelet peroxidase granules on electron microscopy) or monoclonal antibody positivity for specific megakaryocyte or platelet glycoproteins (e.g., IIB\IIIA or IB).[20]

TABLE 45.2-2. Percentage Distribution of Immunophenotypes of Acute Lymphoblastic Leukemia by Age Group

Immunophenotype	*Infants (<1.5 y)*	*Children (1.5 to 10.0 y)*	*Adolescents (>10 y)*
Early pre-B	64	68	58
CD10 (CALLA)	49	94	87
Pre-B (cIgM)	26	18	18
T	6	13	23
B	4	1	1

cIgM, cytoplasmic immunoglobulin M.
Numbers shown are weighted means from eight different studies.
(Modified from Rivera G, Crist W. Blood: principles and practice of hematology. In: Handin R, Stossel T, Lux S, eds. *Acute lymphoblastic leukemia.* Philadelphia: JB Lippincott, 1995:747.)

The FAB M7 subtype most often is seen in children younger than 3 years of age with Down syndrome.[7]

Immunophenotype

By using a panel of lineage-associated monoclonal antibodies, most cases of ALL can be broadly divided into precursor B- and precursor T-cell subgroups.[16] Precursor B-cell ALL is further subdivided into early pre-B and pre-B, and the T-cell cases are subtyped according to level of thymocyte differentiation (e.g. early, mid-, or late thymocyte).[21] The expression of several antigens, such as CD10 (CALLA) and CD34, are not lineage-specific and, in some studies, were of prognostic importance. The CALLA antigen is expressed in most cases of precursor B ALL, hence the derivation of the term *common ALL* previously used to define this large subgroup of childhood ALL. Most infants with ALL have a CALLA-negative, early pre-B immunophenotype.[22] The proportion of children with specific immunophenotypes of ALL is shown in Table 45.2-2 according to age group.

Compared to early pre-B-cell ALL, the pre-B (cytoplasmic Ig) immunophenotype develops more often in African Americans, is associated with a higher initial leukocyte count and hemoglobin level, and is more likely to have a DNA index lower than 1.16 and a pseudodiploid karyotype.[23] The previously known adverse outcome associated with pre-B ALL was due to the subgroup with the t(1:19)(q23;p13). The clinical features of T-cell ALL have long been recognized and include an adolescent male with a high leukocyte count, bulky lymphadenopathy (especially mediastinal), and extramedullary leukemia [central nervous system (CNS), skin, testes].[24,25] In the past, these children had a poor prognosis. However the prognostic distinctions among ALL immunophenotypes have been lost by improvements in therapy with risk-directed protocols.[1]

B-cell (surface Ig) ALL is associated with L3 morphology, male predominance, and bulky extramedullary disease (e.g., intraabdominal masses).[1] Many children with B-cell ALL come to medical attention because of a "primary tumor mass," which on biopsy is a small noncleaved or Burkitt lymphoma and on further staging is found to have extensive replacement of the bone marrow with L3 blasts. If more than 25% marrow blasts are present, these children are considered to have mature B-cell ALL rather than advanced-stage Burkitt's lymphoma, but they are treated on identical protocols and now enjoy a favorable prognosis.[26]

There has been limited clinical use for a classification of AML based on immunophenotype.[27] The primary value of cell surface antigen analysis in most cases of AML is distinguishing between AML and ALL (L2 versus M0) and diagnosing FAB M7 AML.

Hybrid or Acute Mixed-Lineage Leukemias

Blasts from approximately 5% to 20% of children with acute leukemia have either morphologic, cytochemical, immunophenotypic, or genetic markers suggesting derivation from both myeloid and lymphoid lineages.[28] In these biphenotypic, hybrid, or acute mixed lineage leukemias, individual blasts usually co-express markers of more than one lineage, but in rare instances, two distinct populations of blasts are present. Whether these cases represent aberrant gene expression or transformation of a multipotent stem cell is unknown. Hybrid leukemias appear to be more common in patients with prior myelodysplastic syndromes, secondary leukemias, leukemias associated with 11q23 [especially t(4;11)] translocations and the Philadelphia (Ph) chromosome.

Myeloid-antigen expression (blasts reactive with two or more myeloid-specific monoclonal antibodies) is detected in fewer than 10% of cases of childhood ALL, and lymphoid-antigen expression is noted in approximately 15% of AML.[28] Mixed-lineage expression in AML lacks prognostic significance, and patients should be treated on AML protocols.[27,29] Myeloid-antigen–positive ALL is not associated with a poor prognosis if patients are treated on intensive, risk-adapted ALL protocols.[30,31] Leukemias with two distinct leukemic clones (one lymphoid and the other myeloid) are rare. No specific treatment recommendations have been established for these patients, but most oncologists favor a hybrid ALL/AML protocol in this situation.

CYTOGENETICS AND MOLECULAR GENETICS

The combination of cytogenetics, fluorescence *in situ* hybridization, and molecular methods identify chromosomal abnormalities in approximately 80% of cases of childhood acute leukemia.[3,32] Identification of numerous chromosomal abnormalities in leukemia blasts, including translocations, deletions, and inversions, have enabled molecular geneticists to clone the genes that ultimately have been shown to be important in the malignant transformation of hematopoietic cells. The genetic abnormalities also have been proved valuable as diagnostic and prognostic tools. For example, TEL-AML1, or ETV6-CBFA2, is a newly identified fusion gene that is detected in approximately 25% of children with precursor B ALL. The fusion gene results from a cryptic t(12;21) translocation and identifies a group of patients with a favorable prognosis[33,34] (Fig. 45.2-1).

Many of the chromosomal translocations in ALL involve Ig or T-cell receptor genes and transcription factors. The prototype translocation is the t(8;14) in L3 ALL and Burkitt's lymphoma [see Small Noncleaved Cell (Burkitt's) Lymphoma, later in this chapter].[1,3] The t(1;19) is seen in approximately one-fourth of patients with pre-B-cell ALL and fuses the E2A gene on chromosome 19 with the PBX1 gene on chromosome 1.[35] Approximately 2% to 5% of children with ALL have the t(9;22)(9q34;q11) or Ph chromosome.[1,3] In Ph-positive chronic myelogenous leukemia, the translocation results in a bcr-abl fusion gene product of 210-kD, whereas in most cases of Ph-positive ALL, the breakpoint within the bcr region is more cen-

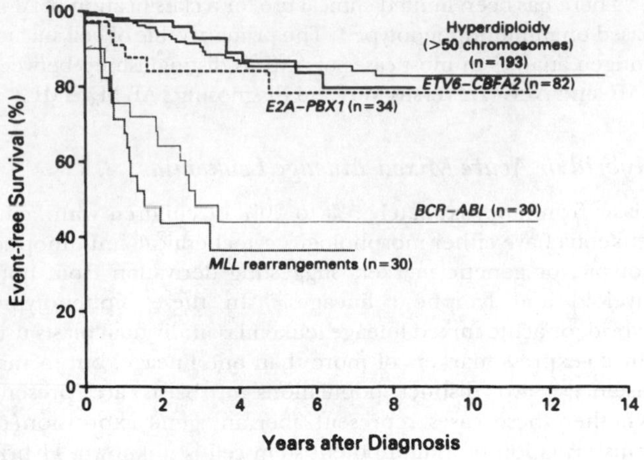

FIGURE 45.2-1. Kaplan-Meier analysis of event-free survival according to genetic features of blast cells in 369 children with acute lymphoblastic leukemia treated at St. Jude Children's Research Hospital from 1984 to 1997. The relatively good survival of patients with *BCR-ABL* fusion reflects successful treatment of a subgroup with low leukocyte counts at diagnosis. The *E2A-PBX1* abnormality, once associated with poor survival, now is associated with the same favorable prognosis as the *ETV6-CBFA2 (TEL-AML1)* abnormality. (From ref. 1, with permission.)

tromeric, yielding a smaller fusion protein (185 kD). The presence of the Ph chromosome in ALL usually indicates high-risk leukemia warranting a stem cell transplantation in first remission, except for those children presenting with a low leukocyte count or good early response to prednisone.[36,37] The genetic abnormalities associated with T-cell ALL are discussed in the section Lymphoblastic Lymphoma, later in this chapter.[25] Genes involved in cell-cycle control (e.g., p53, p16) also have been implicated in the pathogenesis of ALL.[38–40]

Childhood ALL can also be classified by the number of chromosomes (or DNA content) per leukemic cell.[41] Hyperdiploidy with a DNA index greater than 1.16 (greater than 50 chromosomes) is associated with the precursor B-cell phenotype and a highly favorable prognosis, especially if there are trisomies of chromosomes 4 and 10.[42] It is not known why patients with a DNA index greater than 1.16 respond well to chemotherapy, but it may be related either to a favorable intracellular metabolism of methotrexate or the marked propensity for hyperdiploid blasts to undergo apoptosis.[43,44] On the other hand, hypodiploidy (less than 45 chromosomes) is associated with a poor prognosis.[45]

Many of the chromosomal abnormalities in AML are associated with specific FAB subtypes.[46,47] These include t(8:21)(q22:q22) and FAB M2; t(15;17)(q22;q11-21) and acute promyelocytic leukemia (FAB M3); translocations involving chromosome band 11q23 and various partner chromosomes [e.g., t(9;11) and FAB M4 and M5]; and inv(16)(p13;q22) and FAB M4eo. The t(8;21) and t(15;17) translocations are extremely rare in patients younger than 2 years of age, whereas translocations involving 11q23 are quite common in this age group.[48] Translocations of 11q23 almost always involve the MLL gene and are also the most frequent karyotypic change in infants with ALL. Infants with t(4;11)(q21;q23) or molecular rearrangements of MLL have an almost fivefold higher risk of relapse compared with other infants.[49] The MLL gene is also rearranged in most cases of secondary AML induced by topoisomerase II inhibitors.[14] The t(1;22)(p13,q13), a unique but rare chromosomal translocation, has been detected in infants with FAB M7 AML.[50] Monosomies or partial deletions of chromosomes 5 or 7 are commonly observed in adults with AML and patients with secondary AML (postalkylating agent therapy or myelodysplastic syndromes) but are unusual in *de novo* childhood AML.[46] The critical genes involved in leukemic transformation on chromosomes 5 and 7 have not yet been identified.

CLINICAL AND LABORATORY MANIFESTATIONS AND DIAGNOSIS

The most common presenting signs and symptoms in children with acute leukemia are fever or infection, fatigue, pallor, and bleeding. These symptoms result from decreased normal hematopoiesis secondary to bone marrow infiltration by leukemic blasts, leading to neutropenia, anemia, and thrombocytopenia. Bone or joint pain (or both) are initial complaints in approximately 25% of children with acute leukemia and are more commonly observed in ALL than AML.[51] Bone pain is usually due to periosteal elevation but may be secondary to microfractures or bone necrosis. The classic radiologic findings in acute leukemia include metaphyseal lucent bands (growth arrest lines), periosteal elevation, and lytic lesions. These changes are best seen in the long bones near the knees, ankles, or wrists.

Moderate to massive lymphadenopathy and hepatosplenomegaly are associated with T-cell ALL and infant acute leukemias.[21,52] Nonspecific abdominal pain is relatively common and may be secondary to organomegaly, gastrointestinal bleeding or, rarely, leukemic infiltration of the bowel wall. Most of the gastrointestinal lesions encountered in patients with leukemia are secondary to complications of treatment and include oral mucositis, esophagitis, gastritis, typhlitis or neutropenic enterocolitis, lactose malabsorption, and hepatitis or cholestasis.

Extramedullary Leukemia

Extramedullary spread of leukemia at either the time of diagnosis or relapse is important because it can cause local problems, represent a sanctuary site of disease, or herald bone marrow relapse. At diagnosis, clinically detectable extramedullary leukemia of the central nervous system (CNS), skin, and testes is rare, except in infants. Therefore, the major treatment strategies are aimed at eradication of subclinical disease.[1] In the past, the most common sites of extramedullary relapse included the CNS and testes.[53]

Symptomatic CNS leukemia (e.g., increased intracranial pressure or cranial nerve palsies) is extremely rare, but between 4% and 10% of children with acute leukemia have blasts present in the cerebrospinal fluid (CSF) at diagnosis.[54,55] The diagnosis of CNS leukemia is made by examining a cytocentrifuged preparation of CSF. Traditionally, CNS leukemia was defined by the presence of at least five leukocytes per microliter of CSF with blasts. However, more recent data indicates that the presence of blasts in CSF samples with fewer than five leukocytes per microliter may be of prognostic significance. The most common signs of CNS leukemia include headache, nausea and vomiting, lethargy, or cranial nerve palsies (sixth and seventh being most common). Neurologic symptoms in children with acute leukemia may also be due to epidural masses causing cord compression or myeloblastomas of the cerebral cortex or cerebellum, hemorrhage, or leukostasis (plugging of vessels by aggregates of leukemic blasts). Patients with AML and initial leukocyte counts greater than 200,000 cells per microliter are at highest risk for leukostasis.[56]

Leukemia cutis is a rare finding seen most often in AML (FAB M4 and M5) and T-cell ALL. Infants with AML are at particularly high risk for leukemia cutis.[57] The lesions of leukemia cutis are typically subcutaneous nodules that are blue-gray or salmon in color. The skin nodules in babies with AML have been observed to spontaneously regress for short periods before progressive leukemia ensues.

Overt testicular leukemia is extremely unusual at diagnosis, and with current effective chemotherapy regimens, it is rarely encountered as a site of relapse.[1] Clinically it presents as a firm, painless, unilateral or bilateral testicular swelling. The diagnosis should be confirmed by testicular biopsy. Enlarged kidneys from infiltration of leukemia is not uncommon but is usually asymptomatic. The rare cases of renal failure in newly diagnosed children with acute leukemia are either secondary to uric acid nephropathy or ureteral obstruction from retroperitoneal lymphadenopathy.

Leukemic infiltration of the pericardium/myocardium or lungs is also extremely rare at diagnosis or during treatment. Congestive heart failure during therapy is much more likely due to sepsis or anthracycline cardiac toxicity rather than leukemic infiltration. Diffuse pulmonary infiltrates are most often secondary to an infection, but leukemic infiltration, diffuse alveolar hemorrhage, and pulmonary leukostasis should be considered in the differential diagnosis.

The most common ocular findings in patients with acute leukemia include retinal hemorrhages secondary to either thrombocytopenia or vessel infiltration, or papilledema from CNS leukemia. Leukemic involvement of the anterior chamber (hypopyon) or retinal infiltration are both infrequent.

Myeloblastomas are also referred to as *chloromas* or *granulocytic sarcomas* and occur in fewer than 5% of children with AML.[2,57,58] These solid tumors of myeloid leukemia cells can appear simultaneously with bone marrow infiltration or may be the initial clinical manifestation of leukemia, occurring weeks to months before an increase in bone marrow blasts occurs. Myeloblastomas have a predilection for the CNS (brain or epidural) and the bones and soft tissues of the head and neck (especially the orbits).

Laboratory Features and Differential Diagnosis

The peripheral blood findings in patients with acute leukemia often include a normocytic anemia with teardrop or nucleated red blood cells, thrombocytopenia with platelet counts averaging between 20,000 and 50,000 cells per microliter, and leukocyte counts between 5000 and 50,000 cells per microliter (Table 45.2-3).[51] Approximately 20% of patients, however, have leukocyte counts greater than 100,000 cells per microliter. The white blood cell (WBC) differential usually reveals neutropenia (absolute neutrophil count <1000 cells per microliter) and circulating blasts, especially if the leukocyte count is greater than 5000 cells per microliter.

The bone marrow biopsy in most cases of acute leukemia is hypercellular, with blasts accounting for the majority of nucleated cells. The numbers of normal granulocyte/monocyte, erythroid, and megakaryocytic precursors are markedly decreased. To establish the diagnosis of acute leukemia, the

TABLE 45.2-3. Initial Clinical and Laboratory Features in Children with Acute Lymphoblastic Leukemia According to Major Immunophenotypes

	Precursor B (%)	*T Cell (%)*
Leukocyte count/mm³		
<10,000	50	20
10,000–50,000	35	30
>50,000	15[a]	50
Platelet count/mm³		
<20,000	25	15
Hemoglobin (g/dL)		
<7.5	50	25
Hepatomegaly	8	13
Splenomegaly	10	20
Mediastinal mass	1–2	50
Lymphadenopathy (moderate/ marked)	25	50

[a]Twenty-five percent of patients with pre-B subtype of precursor B acute lymphoblastic leukemia have leukocytes greater than 50,000.
(Data from Crist W, Rivera G, Pullen J, Weinstein H. The leukemias of childhood. In: Rosenthal DS, Feinstein DI, Goodnight S, McArthur JR, eds. *Hematology, 1985*. Washington, DC: American Society of Hematology, 1985.)

bone marrow aspirate or biopsy must have more than 25% and 30% blasts, respectively, in ALL and AML. Most cases of childhood acute leukemia can be readily diagnosed and classified by routine bone marrow morphology and histochemistry. Additional laboratory tests, such as genetics and immunophenotyping, are important for risk assignment and are sometimes necessary for distinguishing ALL from AML.

Other significant laboratory findings at diagnosis may include metabolic derangements [see Small Noncleaved Cell (Burkitt's) Lymphoma, later in this chapter] and disseminated intravascular coagulation or fibrinolysis. Disseminated intravascular coagulation usually is associated with acute promyelocytic leukemia (FAB M3) or FAB M5 AML, but it may be seen in other children with newly diagnosed acute leukemia.[59,60]

The differential diagnosis in a child suspected of having acute leukemia includes juvenile myelomonocytic leukemia, myelodysplastic syndromes, metastatic tumors with marrow involvement (neuroblastoma and rhabdomyosarcoma), idiopathic thrombocytopenic purpura, juvenile rheumatoid arthritis, aplastic anemia, sepsis and other conditions that might result in neutropenia, infectious diseases associated with lymphocytosis, and the TMD in neonates with Down syndrome.[7]

TREATMENT

Acute Lymphoblastic Leukemia

Most children with acute leukemia are referred to tertiary care hospitals, where they are treated by pediatric oncologists according to institutional or cooperative group protocols [e.g., Pediatric Oncology Group (POG), Children Cancer Group (CCG), Berlin-Frankfort-Munster (BFM), Medical Research Council].[61] Therapy for childhood ALL has been based on risk classification systems because it has become clear that outcome of treatment varies substantially among different subsets of children with the disease. The philosophy behind this approach has been to use less toxic therapy for children with a lower risk of relapse and to treat high-risk patients with experimental and potentially more aggressive regimens. Because no single best protocol has been established for either low- or high-risk patients with ALL, enrollment in clinical trials is still encouraged.

PROGNOSTIC FACTORS. Numerous prognostic factors (Table 45.2-4) have been identified for children with ALL, and some of these have been incorporated into risk classification systems used to assign treatment. These prognostic factors include combinations of presenting clinical and laboratory parameters, biologic features of the leukemia blast, and early response to chemotherapy. Because prognostic factors are treatment-dependent, improvements in therapy may abrogate a previously accepted prognostic variable. In an effort to compare the results of various clinical trials worldwide, a uniform risk classification for treatment assignment was accepted at a National Cancer Institute workshop.[62] The agreed on standard risk category includes patients 1 to 9 years of age with precursor B ALL and a WBC count at diagnosis of less than 50,000 cells per microliter. The remaining patients are classified as high risk. The event-free survival rate for children in the standard-risk category is approximately 80% at 4 years and approximately 65% for the high-risk patients.

Some investigators continue to classify T-cell ALL as an independent high-risk feature, and others assign risk to these children based on age and WBC criteria.[1,21,25] The prognosis for patients with T-cell ALL has significantly improved during the 1990s with the advent of multiagent dose-intensified ALL protocols.[25,63] Children with mixed lineage or myeloid antigen–positive ALL are no longer considered high risk based on immunophenotype alone.[30,31]

In addition to age and WBC count, other important prognostic variables established in the workshop include hyperdiploidy, cytogenetics, early response to treatment, and CNS status. The prognosis for patients with blasts with additional copies of whole chromosomes (hyperdiploidy) has been very favorable, as reported by several groups.[41,42,44] Hyperdiploidy can be measured by DNA content (DNA index) of leukemic cells and by karyotyping. A DNA index of more than 1.16, especially if blasts contain extra copies of chromosomes 4 and 10, is associated with an extremely favorable prognosis. The majority of children with hyperdiploid blasts have standard-risk age and WBC features. In some studies, DNA index and trisomies of chromosomes 4 and 10 are used to change risk assignment independent of age and WBC criteria.[42]

TABLE 45.2-4. Acute Leukemia: Adverse Prognostic Factors

Acute lymphoblastic leukemia
Age younger than 1 or older than 10 y
White blood cell count >50,000/µL
DNA index <1.16
Chromosomal translocation t(9;22); t(4;11) in infants
Central nervous system leukemia at diagnosis
Slow response to induction chemotherapy
Acute myelogenous leukemia
White blood cell count >100,000/µL
Monosomy 7
Translocations involving 11q23 (controversial)
Secondary acute myelogenous leukemia or prior myelodysplastic syndromes
More than one course to complete response

Early response to chemotherapy as measured by bone marrow findings within 7 to 14 days of induction or peripheral blood blast response to corticosteroids on day 8 of treatment is associated with outcome. A more rapid clearing of blasts from either the blood or bone marrow confers a more favorable prognosis.[64,65] In one study, an augmented postinduction therapy for children with high-risk ALL and a slow response to induction has improved their long-term outcome.[66]

Patients with the Ph chromosome [t(9;22)] and a high initial WBC count or slow early response to prednisone, and infants with t(4;11), continue to be at high risk for treatment failure.[37,67] Experimental therapies, such as allogeneic stem cell transplantation in first remission, are recommended for these very high-risk patients. Studies have shown that the poorer response associated with t(1:19) can be overcome by more intensive therapy.[35]

New genetic abnormalities are continuing to be identified in patients with ALL. For example, the TEL/AML1 fusion gene occurs in approximately 25% to 30% of cases of pediatric precursor B ALL and defines a subgroup with a favorable prognosis.[33,34] Molecular studies also are identifying genetic changes (e.g., MLL, TAL, TEL/AML1) in leukemic blasts that are undetectable at the routine cytogenetic level.[1,68]

Other factors that have been shown to independently affect prognosis include race, gender, blast cell morphology, lymphomatous presentations, and serum lactic dehydrogensase.[69–71] African Americans have a poorer prognosis than whites for reasons that cannot be totally explained based on known prognostic factors.[71] In several studies, males had a higher risk of bone marrow relapse compared to females.[70,72] Long-term follow-up data also indicate that females have an increased risk for some late effects, especially CNS and cardiac effects.[73,74]

REMISSION INDUCTION. The achievement of a complete remission is a prerequisite for the long-term survival of patients with acute leukemia. In 1948, Sidney Farber demonstrated the first remissions in ALL using aminopterin, an analogue of methotrexate.[75] Vincristine and prednisone are effective in inducing remissions in 85% to 90% of children with ALL, without unduly suppressing normal bone marrow function. Daunorubicin and L-asparaginase were subsequently identified as active drugs in the treatment of ALL. The addition of either one of these drugs to vincristine and prednisone increased the complete remission rate in childhood ALL to more than 95%. The combination of vincristine, prednisone, and L-asparaginase is one of the standard remission induction regimens in childhood ALL.[1,76] The use of additional drugs, such as the anthracyclines (daunorubicin or doxorubicin) or cyclophosphamide, are often reserved for children with high-risk ALL.[66,76]

Data from both experimental models and human clinical trials indicate that maximum leukemia cell kill during induction decreases the likelihood for the emergence of drug-resistant clones and results in higher cure rates. Therefore, maximum tolerated doses of all active agents are delivered as early as possible during treatment. As previously discussed, a more rapid response to induction chemotherapy as measured by day 8 peripheral blast count or day 14 marrow aspirate is a favorable prognostic sign.[64] New technologies, including polymerase chain reaction and multiparameter flow cytometry, are able to quantitate "minimal residual leukemia" at the end of induction.[77,78] The results of this type of analysis may be predictive for risk of subsequent relapse, although the best assay and optimal timing for testing are not known.

CONTINUATION THERAPY. It has been estimated that approximately two to three logs of leukemic blasts are killed during the induction phase of therapy, leaving a residual leukemic burden of approximately 100 million cells. Therefore, additional treatment is necessary to prevent relapse. In the past, children with ALL relapsed within a median of 4 to 6 months when treatment was not continued beyond the remission induction phase. In the late 1960s, investigators at St. Jude Children's Research Hospital developed a "total therapy" approach for the treatment of children with ALL.[1] The model included remission induction, continuation chemotherapy with or without intensification, and preventive CNS therapy. The choice of continuation therapy was empiric. The early St. Jude studies evaluated 6-mercaptopurine, methotrexate, cyclophosphamide, and cytarabine in various doses and combinations. The best outcome was achieved in patients who received 2 to 3 years of daily oral 6-mercaptopurine and weekly methotrexate. Long-term follow-up of patients treated with this latter combination show a 42% disease-free survival rate for children with initial WBC counts of fewer than <25,000 cells per microliter, whereas it was only 16% for all other patients.[79]

Before the observation that the intensity of treatment required for a successful outcome varied substantially among subsets of patients, investigators in the BFM group, at Memorial Sloan-Kettering Cancer Center and the Dana Farber Cancer Institute treated all children with ALL with up-front intensive multiagent chemotherapy. The Memorial Sloan-Kettering Cancer Center protocols used a cell kinetic rationale that combined eight cell-cycle specific and nonspecific agents.[80] The Dana Farber Cancer Institute protocols emphasized the intensive use of L-asparaginase and doxorubicin, and the BFM group used 4 months of intensive multidrug therapy (induction, consolidation, and intensification).[63,76] CNS prophylaxis varied between the groups (see Central Nervous System Prophylaxis, later in this chapter). Children with high-risk ALL benefited most from these protocols. The advantage of these regimens compared to antimetabolite-based protocols for children with lower risk ALL was less obvious. However, more recent BFM and POG randomized trials have shown the importance of intensive reinduction therapy or dose intensified antimetabolite therapy, even for patients with favorable risk features.[72,76]

Other successful approaches for patients with high-risk ALL have included the use of alternating non–cross-resistant pairs of active agents. For example, investigators at St. Jude Children's Research Hospital reported encouraging results with the combination of VM-26 and cytarabine in refractory ALL and subsequently introduced those drugs into front-line protocols.[1,79] Most protocols for high-risk patients include the use of four or more drugs during remission induction, followed by intensification therapy for a brief period, CNS prophylaxis, and continuation therapy. With this approach, the cure rates for these very high-risk patients have reached levels of 65% to 75%. The use of bone marrow transplant (BMT) from a related or unrelated histocompatible donor for select groups of very high-risk patients in first remission is being investigated.[81]

Several groups treat infants with ALL and those with T-cell ALL on separately designed protocols.[21,80,82] The results of these studies have been comparable to therapies used to treat a more inclusive group of patients with high-risk ALL. On the other hand, because children with B-cell ALL (Burkitt's or L3 type) had such a dismal prognosis after treatment with classic ALL protocols, an entirely different treatment approach was developed. These children were treated according to regimens that were designed for patients with advanced-stage Burkitt's lymphoma. The protocols for B-cell ALL and advanced-stage Burkitt's lymphoma included short but dose-intensive chemotherapy cycles that include cyclophosphamide, methotrexate, and cytarabine plus intensive intrathecal (IT) chemotherapy. The long-term disease-free survival rates increased from less than 10% to more than 60% with this approach.[26,83] As more is learned about the biologic, pharmacologic, and other factors that distinguish the various "genotypic species" or subtypes of ALL, we will hopefully be able to select our therapies accordingly.

The duration of continuation therapy for children with ALL has been empiric. Chemotherapy has not been given for indefinite periods because of its short- and long-term toxicities. Because of our new techniques for quantifying minimal residual leukemia, we may soon be able to adjust the length of treatment based on more objective measures.[77,78] The duration of continuation chemotherapy has gradually been shortened from 5 to approximately 2 years without undue risk of relapse.[1,79] The risk of relapse after cessation of therapy is highest in the first year and tapers off to 2% to 3% in the second and third years.[79] Very late relapse, after 5 or more years in remission, is rare but reported. There appears to be an increased risk of relapse off therapy for males compared to females.

PREVENTIVE OR PROPHYLACTIC CENTRAL NERVOUS SYSTEM THERAPY. CNS relapse in children with ALL became clinically apparent as bone marrow remissions became more durable. Before the use of preventive CNS therapy, CNS relapse heralded bone marrow relapse in almost 60% of patients. It was postulated by investigators at St. Jude Children's Research Hospital that leukemia blasts were already present in the CNS by the time ALL was diagnosed and that the drugs used to treat leukemia did not penetrate the meninges in therapeutic concentrations. The CNS was considered a "sanctuary site," requiring site-specific therapy for subclinical disease. This concept proved to be correct and led to major increments in cure rates for childhood ALL. Clinical trials at St. Jude Children's Research Hospital established that the risk for CNS relapse could be reduced to less than 5% by the early use of 24 Gy of craniospinal irradiation (CSI) or 24 Gy of cranial irradiation plus IT methotrexate.[84] Cranial irradiation plus IT methotrexate replaced craniospinal irradiation because of the toxicities of CSI. CSI was myelosuppressive and also caused impaired growth of vertebral bodies.

The target volume for cranial irradiation includes the entire intracranial subarachnoid space. By convention, the caudal margin of the field extends to the bottom of the second cervical vertebra. Standard guidelines for preventive cranial irradiation also include the posterior retina and orbital apex, encompassing the extension of the subarachnoid space along the optic nerves. A subacute somnolence syndrome that follows cranial irradiation has been well described.[85] Approximately 50% of children develop some degree of lethargy, irritability, or low-grade fever at a median onset of 4 to 8 weeks after cranial irradiation.

The neurologic and cognitive sequelae of 24-Gy cranial irradiation led to treatment modifications.[86–88] The CCG safely reduced the dose of cranial irradiation to 18 Gy.[89] In an effort to further reduce toxicity, the Dana Farber ALL consortium compared 18 Gy given in a single daily fraction with a hyperfractionated schedule (twice daily), and the BFM reduced the dose to 12 Gy.[90,91]

An alternative strategy for preventing CNS relapse has been the use of IT chemotherapy alone, starting during induction and continuing for an extended period throughout therapy.[92,93] Protocols using repetitive doses of IT chemotherapy also include multiple cycles of intravenous moderate- to high-dose methotrexate. This approach has been successful in preventing CNS relapse in children with standard-risk ALL, as well as intermediate- and high-risk patients in some studies, but it is also associated with neurotoxicity.[94]

IT methotrexate has the same efficacy as triple IT therapy (methotrexate, hydrocortisone, and cytarabine) and may be less neurotoxic. The risk of a CNS event was gender-dependent in the CCG trials. Boys were at greater risk for relapse, whereas girls were more vulnerable than boys to cognitive and growth dysfunction after cranial irradiation and IT chemotherapy.[95] Similar findings have been observed by the Nordic and Dana Farber groups.[90]

In some protocols, select subgroups of children with ALL at high risk of CNS relapse (e.g., WBC count higher than 50,000 cells per microliter, T-cell ALL, Ph-positive ALL, and infants) continue to be treated with cranial irradiation (12 to 18 Gy) plus IT chemotherapy.[90,91] The percentage of children with ALL who currently receive cranial irradiation as part of CNS prophylaxis ranges from 15% to 60% depending on the protocol.

OVERT CENTRAL NERVOUS SYSTEM LEUKEMIA AT DIAGNOSIS. Fewer than 5% of children with ALL have leukemic blasts detected in the CSF at diagnosis. The definition of CNS leukemia has been revised.[54] Three categories have been defined according to CSF findings: CNS-1 (no blasts), CNS-2 (fewer than 5 WBCs per microliter with blasts), and CNS-3 (more than 5 WBCs per microliter with blasts or cranial nerve palsy). Patients with CNS-3 status have a higher frequency of isolated CNS relapse and a lower long-term survival rate than patients with CNS-1 status, but the significance of CNS-2 status is not clear. Some investigators treat patients with CNS-2 status with additional doses of IT chemotherapy but give a risk assignment based on age and WBC criteria.

The management of patients with overt CNS leukemia (CNS-3) is less controversial than is the choice of preventive or prophylactic CNS therapy. After inducing a complete hematologic and CNS remission with IT and systemic chemotherapy, most investigators give CNS irradiation toward the latter part of the first year of treatment. Doses of 24 to 30 Gy of radiation have been given to these children.

THERAPY AFTER RELAPSE. The two most important factors relating to prognosis after relapse are the length of the initial remission and the site of relapse.[96,97] Children with late relapse have a better prognosis than those with early relapse, but the definition of early and late relapse is variable. An initial remission duration of less than 3 years is considered to represent an early relapse. Relapse in extramedullary sites compared to bone marrow is also more favorable in terms of survival.[97]

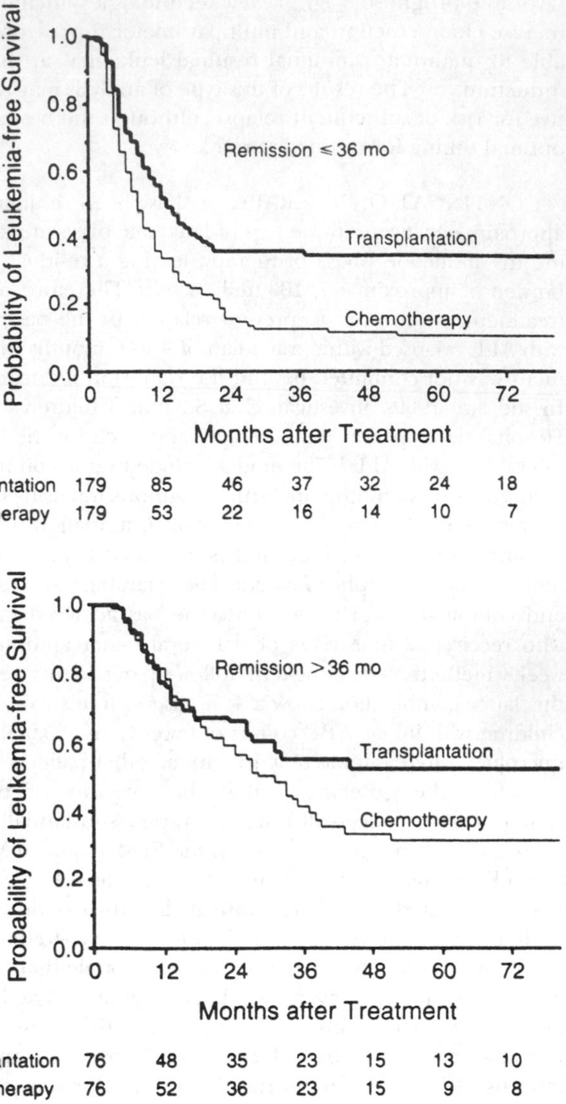

FIGURE 45.2-2. Actuarial probability of leukemia-free survival in matched cohorts of children receiving chemotherapy or undergoing transplantation, according to the duration of the first remission. The numbers below the figure indicate the numbers of children at risk. (From ref. 98, with permission.)

The second complete remission rate is more than 80%. The question of whether to perform a BMT or to continue chemotherapy has been one of the most controversial issues in second remission.[98,99] The likelihood of long-term survival after chemotherapy alone is less than 10% to 15% for patients with early relapse. This finding is in contrast to a 40% to 50% leukemia-free survival rate for children whose first remission was longer than 3 years.[96] These children also require a second course of CNS-directed therapy. BMTs from HLA-identical sibling donors compared with chemotherapy result in fewer relapses and better leukemia-free survival rates for the early-relapse group and, in some studies, for all risk groups[98,99] (Fig. 45.2-2).

Some investigators recommend autologous BMT for children with ALL in second remission who lack histocompatible family donors.[100,101] Various methodologies have been developed to purge or remove contaminating leukemia cells present in the patient's harvested marrow, but the merits of this approach are unknown. The relapse rates are higher after autologous BMT compared to allogeneic BMT because of the lack of a graft-versus-leukemia effect. It remains controversial as to whether autologous BMT is superior to chemotherapy for children with ALL in second remission. The value of matched unrelated stem cell transplantation in the therapy of children with recurrent ALL is under investigation.[102]

Isolated CNS relapse occurs in 5% to 10% of children treated for ALL on current protocols despite CNS-directed therapy. In the past, CNS relapse was associated with a very poor long-term prognosis, and the few survivors had serious long-term neurotoxicity. Salvage therapies included cranial or craniospinal irradiation plus IT or intraventricular chemotherapy. In the early trials, hematologic relapse rather than a subsequent CNS event was the main obstacle to a long-term second remission. Current approaches for these children include intensified reinduction and consolidation chemotherapy, IT chemotherapy, and delayed craniospinal irradiation to 6 months in remission.[103] The delay in craniospinal irradiation allows for intensive chemotherapy to be administered during the early phases of therapy. The 5-year disease-free survival estimates are approximately 70% with this strategy. However, a very high rate of relapse still occurs in children whose initial duration of remission was less than 18 months. The neurologic toxicity with this type of therapy has been acceptable. BMT should be considered for the very high-risk patients with an isolated CNS relapse.

Reports of ALL treatment in the 1970s indicated that 5% to 16% of boys had a testicular relapse during hematologic remission.[79,104] Males with T-cell ALL were at highest risk for testicular leukemia. The time of testicular relapse was early for patients with T-cell ALL and usually was after cessation of therapy for most others. These data led to trials of prophylactic testicular irradiation in T-cell ALL and testicular biopsies at completion of chemotherapy for patients with precursor B ALL. Prophylactic testicular irradiation significantly reduced the incidence of testicular relapse but did not influence overall survival. As therapy for children with ALL has improved, testicular relapse has become a rare event. As with other sites of relapse, patients who develop early testicular relapse have a worse prognosis than those with a late relapse. Treatment includes both local radiation (24 Gy to both testes) and systemic chemotherapy. The target volume for radiation therapy includes the entire scrotal region, encompassing both the testes and epididymis bilaterally. Patients with late isolated testicular relapse have a 75% long-term disease-free survival rate.[104] However, hormonal dysfunction usually is seen after these doses of gonadal irradiation.

COMPLICATIONS. The most concerning late complications of leukemia therapy include second cancers, adverse effects on growth and development, cardiotoxicity, and neuropsychological dysfunction.[105–107] In a retrospective review of children treated for ALL, a sevenfold excess of all cancers and a 22-fold excess of CNS tumors were found compared with the prevalence rate in the general population.[107] Children who received cranial irradiation before the age of 5 years had the highest incidence of brain tumors. Patients treated intensively for ALL with the epipodophyllotoxins are at high risk for developing secondary AML.[108]

Short stature and obesity are common in children who received cranial irradiation, especially girls who were treated at a very young age.[105] Many of these patients, however, have had satisfactory growth after growth hormone replacement therapy. The chemotherapeutic agents used in the treatment of the acute leukemias have been associated with many acute and chronic toxicities. The prolonged use of corticosteroids may induce osteoporosis and pathologic fractures. Avascular necrosis of long bones and foot bones also has been observed in patients with ALL who have received steroid treatment. The antimetabolites (e.g., methotrexate, 6-mercaptopurine, and cytarabine) induce cholestatic and hepatotoxic changes in the liver but are associated with few documented long-term toxicities in this population of patients. L-Asparaginase is associated with significant acute toxicity, including allergy, pancreatitis, and deep venous thrombosis, but has not been associated with long-term complications. The anthracycline antibiotics, doxorubicin and daunorubicin, have been associated with cardiomyopathy, especially when the cumulative doses administered are more than 300 mg per square meter of body surface area. Studies indicate that a very high percentage of long-term survivors of childhood cancer who received doxorubicin have subclinical echocardiographic abnormalities, including impaired contractility and increased afterload. Risk factors for doxorubicin cardiac toxicity include female gender, young age at treatment, cumulative dose, and dose intensity.[73] The clinical significance of these findings remains to be determined, but late congestive heart failure and death have been reported. ALL regimens that do not include alkylating agents appear not to impair reproductive function.

The neurologic and cognitive sequelae of CNS-directed therapy for children with acute leukemia have been a major concern and a highly controversial subject.[74,88,94] It was once thought that cranial irradiation produced a greater impairment in cognitive function (e.g., impairment of verbal memory and coding and IQ declines) than did chemotherapy. Because of those concerns, many investigators eliminated cranial radiation from therapeutic protocols. However, studies indicate that prednisone and high doses of intravenous or IT methotrexate are associated with neurotoxicity and that 18 Gy of cranial irradiation may not be an independent toxic agent for cognitive outcome.[90,94] High-dose intravenous methotrexate is particularly toxic if it follows cranial irradiation.[74]

Acute Myelogenous Leukemia

In contrast to ALL, only a modest improvement has been made in the long-term survival of children with AML since the late 1970s.[2,109] The complete remission rate has increased from less than 50% to approximately 85%, but only 30% to 50% of patients are long-term survivors.[110–114] The survival rate is somewhat better for those children with HLA-matched family donors who receive an allogeneic BMT early in first remission.[111,112,114]

INDUCTION. The most commonly used remission induction regimen for children with AML, excluding those with Down syndrome and FAB M3, includes a 5- to 7-day course of cytosine arabinoside, plus 2 to 3 days of daunorubicin, with or without thioguanine or etoposide.[2,109] The high complete remission rate with all-*trans*-retinoic acid (ATRA) in patients with acute promyelocytic leukemia (FAB M3) led to prospective randomized trials testing the value of ATRA in the overall treatment plan.[115,116] Results of these studies clearly show that the combined use of ATRA and chemotherapy is superior to chemotherapy alone for patients with acute promyelocytic leukemia.[115,116] Therefore, induction therapy for all patients with acute promyelocytic leukemia should include ATRA combined with an anthracycline (daunorubicin or idarubicin) and cytarabine. Chemotherapy for children with Down syndrome and AML needs to be less intensive than standard AML therapy because of the increased risk of toxicity in these patients. Despite dose modifications, the outcome of children with Down syndrome and AML is excellent.[9]

CENTRAL NERVOUS SYSTEM PROPHYLAXIS. Isolated CNS relapse occurs in approximately 20% of children with AML.[2,109] IT chemotherapy in combination with high-dose systemic cytosine arabinoside is effective in lowering the CNS relapse rate. Data from the BFM studies using historical comparisons suggests that cranial irradiation plus IT chemotherapy in children with standard-risk AML improves outcome.[117]

POSTREMISSION THERAPY. The intensity and duration of postremission chemotherapy and the role of allogeneic and autologous BMT in first remission have been under active investigation. The improvement in overall survival rates to approximately 40% to 50% at 5 years is a result of more effective remission induction and postremission chemotherapy.[2,113,118,119] There is no proven role for maintenance chemotherapy if it follows several courses of high-dose cytarabine–based consolidation chemotherapy.[119] Most pediatric AML protocols include one to three cycles of high-dose cytarabine after remission is achieved.

BONE MARROW TRANSPLANTATION IN FIRST REMISSION. Allogeneic BMT was first applied to children and young adults with AML in first remission as an alternative to continued chemotherapy in the mid-1970s.[112,120,121] The early results were favorable compared with chemotherapy, but the transplantations were done in a selected group of patients. The CCG initiated the first cooperative group study comparing allogeneic BMT to chemotherapy in children with AML in first remission.[112] Long-term follow-up of that study, plus data from POG and Associazione Italiana Ematologia ed Ongologia Pediatrica, all show a survival advantage for allogeneic BMT compared to chemotherapy.[111,112,114] However, fewer than one-fourth of children have a fully histocompatible family donor. Because of improving results of chemotherapy and the morbidity and mortality associated with BMT, the German BFM and Medical Research Council cooperative groups are not recommending allogeneic BMT in first remission for patients with favorable prognostic factors.[110,113] BMTs are reserved for second remission in this group of patients.

For patients who lack histocompatible family donors, autologous BMT became an attractive option in first remission after it was reported to be efficacious (30% to 40% survival) in second remission of AML.[122] The results of the early studies were controversial because they were not prospectively controlled. Beginning in the mid-1980s, both the adult and pediatric AML cooperative groups initiated prospective randomized studies to compare autologous BMT and intensive postremission chemotherapy.[111,114,118] In the pediatric trials, no event-free or survival advantage was found for autologous BMT compared with chemotherapy. The majority of failures after autologous BMT are due to recurrent leukemia.

PROGNOSTIC FACTORS. In contrast to childhood ALL, very few clinical or laboratory factors are consistently related to prognosis[2,46,47,110] (see Table 45.2-4). A leukocyte count of more than 100,000 cells per microliter, karyotype with monosomy 7, and secondary AML are associated with lower remission rates. The lower remission rates associated with hyperleukocytosis are only partially accounted for by early deaths secondary to leukostasis. In the German BFM AML studies, two risk groups were identified.[110] Standard-risk patients included FAB subtypes M1 or M2 with Auer rods, M3 or M4eo, rapid response to initial induction chemotherapy, and Down syndrome. The standard-risk group includes patients with "favorable chromosomal abnormalities" [t(8;21), t(15;17), and inv 16].[47] All other patients are high risk and include approximately 70% of the entire group. Event-free survival rates for standard-risk versus high-risk patients was 65% and 34%, respectively.

MANAGEMENT OF THE RELAPSED PATIENT. The prognosis for children with AML who do not enter complete remission or who relapse is poor.[2,123] BMT offers these patients a chance for long-term survival.[102,123,124] A variety of chemotherapy regimens have been evaluated in children with refractory or relapsed AML.[2,109,123,125] The second remission rates range from approximately 30% to 50% and are highest for children whose first remission duration was longer than 1 year. However, the length of chemotherapy-maintained second remissions are very brief. On the other hand, 5-year event-free survival ranges from 30% to 50% for those patients who receive an allogeneic (related or unrelated marrow donor) marrow transplantation.[124] Autologous BMT in second remission for patients who lack suitable marrow donors offers some hope for long-term survival, but it has become a less attractive option because of the expanding unrelated marrow and cord blood banks and the opportunity to find a matched unrelated donor for an allogeneic transplantation.[102,126]

FUTURE DIRECTIONS

The major challenge for the future is to develop effective therapy for patients who have a poor prognosis and to minimize toxicity for those children who are successfully treated. Strategies are being developed to target drug doses to achieve predetermined serum or intracellular concentrations to improve the therapeutic index.[1] The use of recombinant human hematopoietic growth factors may reduce the myelosuppressive complications from chemotherapy and allow dose intensification to proceed safely.

Mechanisms of drug resistance are beginning to be elucidated.[127] For example, increased expression of the multidrug resistance gene (mdr1) or its protein product (P glycoprotein) has been demonstrated in blasts from 20% to 40% of newly diagnosed patients with AML, and it increases approximately twofold at the time of relapse. High *in vitro* expression of mdr1 correlates with resistance to multiple drugs (e.g., etoposide, anthracyclines, vincristine) by promoting their cellular efflux. A number of biologically active agents, including verapamil and cyclosporine, are capable of reversing the mdr1 phenotype *in vitro*. To date, only limited evidence indicates that this strategy works *in vivo*, but controlled clinical trials are under way.

The wider availability of stem cell transplantations from unrelated marrow or cord blood donors has enabled many more patients to successfully undergo marrow transplantation.[102,126] Studies are testing nonmyeloablative marrow transplantations in an effort to achieve mixed chimerism that will hopefully achieve a more favorable balance of the graft-versus-host and graft-versus-leukemia reactions.[128] Biologic response modifiers, such as interleukin-2 and -12, are under study for their potential to enhance the host response to tumor. It is now possible to target the genetic lesions of leukemia cells, as exemplified by the successful use of ATRA in acute promyelocytic leukemia and a specific bcr-abl tyrosine kinase inhibitor in Ph-positive leukemias.[115,129]

NON-HODGKIN'S LYMPHOMA

The lymphomas are the third most common childhood malignancy and account for approximately 10% of cancers in children.[4,26] Approximately two-thirds of the lymphomas diagnosed in children are non-Hodgkin's lymphoma (NHL) and the remainder are Hodgkin's disease. The spectrum of NHL seen in pediatric patients differs significantly from that seen in adults. The three major histologic categories of NHL in children are lymphoblastic, small noncleaved cell (Burkitt's), and large cell lymphoma (Table 45.2-5).[26] In adults, Burkitt's and lymphoblastic lymphoma are rare, but follicular center cell lymphoma, a histologic type exceedingly rare in children, predominates.[130] No sharp age peak (median age, 11 years) occurs in children with NHL, and the male to female ratio approaches 3:1.

Therapy is best delivered by a team of pediatric oncologists, surgeons, and radiation oncologists at a major medical center with expertise in treating children. Before the use of multiagent leukemia regimens for children with all stages and histologic subtypes of NHL, fewer than 20% of children were cured.[131] The survival of children with NHL, especially those with advanced-stage disease, has markedly improved during the 1990s. The 5-year survival rate is approximately 90% for children with early-stage NHL and 70% for those with advanced-stage disease.[26,132,133]

RISK FACTORS

Numerous factors have been linked to an increased risk of NHL. Children with severe combined immunodeficiency syndrome, Wiskott-Aldrich syndrome, common variable immunodeficiency, ataxia-telangiectasia, and the X-linked lymphoproliferative syndrome are at increased risk for developing a lymphoma.[26,134,135] Acquired immunodeficiency secondary to human immunodeficiency virus infection or immunosuppressive therapy, especially after solid organ transplantation or BMT, also places individuals at greater risk for developing a lymphoproliferative disorder or malignant lymphoma.[136,137] Most of the lymphomas that occur in these high-risk groups are B-lineage large cell or small noncleaved (Burkitt's). Monoclonal Epstein-Barr virus (EBV) DNA has been identified in tumor tissue from many of these patients, indicating an important and early role for the virus in tumor development.[138] It has been postulated that the immunodeficient host does not generate an adequate T-lymphocyte response (EBV-specific cytotoxic T cells) against B cells that are latently infected with EBV.

EBV has long been associated with endemic Burkitt's lymphoma, and more recently with hairy leukoplakia, nasopharyngeal carcinoma, and leiomyosarcomas in children with human immunodeficiency virus.[139] The role of EBV in the pathogenesis of Burkitt's lymphoma and other malignancies is unknown [see Small Noncleaved Cell (Burkitt's) Lymphoma, later in this chapter].

CLASSIFICATION

In the Working Formulation, the major categories of childhood NHL are lymphoblastic, small noncleaved cell (Burkitt's and non-Burkitt's), diffuse large cell, and large cell immunoblastic.[140] The pediatric NHLs in the Revised European-American Lymphoma classification include precursor B and precursor T lymphoblastic lymphoma/leukemia, Burkitt's lymphoma, diffuse large B-cell lymphoma, and anaplastic large cell lymphoma (ALCL) (T- and null cell types).[141]

STAGING

The Ann Arbor staging classification is not well suited for childhood NHL for several reasons. It does not adequately reflect prognosis, because there is early widespread, noncontiguous dissemination of disease despite the limited initial sites of involvement (e.g., mediastinal lymphoblastic lymphoma). In addition, extranodal involvement is common, whereas stage III nodal disease is rare. In view of these deficiencies, an alternative staging system (Table 45.2-6) was developed at St. Jude Children's Research Hospital.[131] The St. Jude system considers

TABLE 45.2-5. Pediatric Non-Hodgkin's Lymphoma: Correlation of Histology, Presenting Sites, and Immunophenotype

Histology	*Frequency*	*Major Anatomic Sites by Stage*	*Immunophenotype*
Lymphoblastic	30%	Stage 1/2: neck nodes, Waldeyer's ring, scalp or other cutaneous	Precursor B
		Stage 3/4: anterior mediastinum, pleural effusions, bone marrow, bone, peripheral lymphadenopathy, meninges	Precursor T
Small noncleaved cell (Burkitt's)	40–50%	Stage 1/2: Waldeyer's ring, neck nodes, jaw, epidural, "limited ileocecal"	B cell
		Stage 3/4: Unresectable abdominal, ascites, ovary, kidney, bone marrow, central nervous system, and bone	B cell
Diffuse large cell	25%	Stage 1/2: Waldeyer's ring, cervical nodes, cutaneous, bone	B-cell null T cell
		Stage 3/4: Anterior mediastinum, gastrointestinal tract, bone, peripheral lymphadenopathy, cutaneous, and brain	B-cell null T cell

TABLE 45.2-6. St. Jude Children's Research Hospital Staging System for Pediatric Non-Hodgkin's Lymphoma

Stage	*Description*
I	A single tumor (extranodal) or single anatomic area (nodal), with the exclusion of mediastinum or abdomen
II	A single tumor (extranodal) with regional node involvement
	Two or more nodal areas on the same side of the diaphragm
	Two single (extranodal) tumors with or without regional node involvement on the same side of the diaphragm
	A primary gastrointestinal tract tumor, usually in the ileocecal area, with or without involvement of associated mesenteric nodes only[a]
III	Two single tumors (extranodal) on opposite sides of the diaphragm
	Two or more nodal areas above and below the diaphragm
	All the primary intrathoracic tumors (mediastinal, pleural, thymic)
	All extensive primary intraabdominal disease[a]
	All paraspinal or epidural tumors, regardless of other tumor sites
IV	Any of the above with initial central nervous system or bone marrow involvement[b]

[a]Stage II abdominal disease typically is limited to a segment (usually distal ileum) of the gut plus or minus the associated mesenteric nodes only, and the primary tumor can be completely removed grossly by segmental excision. Stage III abdominal disease typically exhibits spread to paraaortic and retroperitoneal areas by implants and plaques in mesentery or peritoneum, or by direct infiltration of structures adjacent to the primary tumor. Ascites may be present, and complete resection of all gross tumor is not possible.
[b]If bone marrow involvement is present at diagnosis, the percent blasts or abnormal cells must be 25% or less to be classified as stage 4 non-Hodgkin's lymphoma. If there are more than 25% blasts, the patient is classified as having acute leukemia (either precursor B or T acute lymphoblastic leukemia or L3 acute lymphoblastic leukemia).

both primary site and extent of tumor in assigning a clinical stage, and it has been widely accepted. Pathologic staging is not helpful in the overall management of children with NHL because the mainstay of treatment is systemic chemotherapy with a very limited role for irradiation of involved sites of disease.[25,133]

LYMPHOBLASTIC LYMPHOMA

Lymphoblastic lymphomas account for 30% of childhood NHL and share many clinical and biologic features with ALL.[21,25,142] The distinction between lymphoblastic lymphoma and ALL is arbitrary (see Table 45.2-2) and has not been based on clinical presentation. If the bone marrow has more than 25% lymphoblasts, the patient is considered to have ALL rather than stage 4 lymphoblastic lymphoma.

The tumor cells of lymphoblastic lymphoma are morphologically indistinguishable from the lymphoblasts of precursor B and precursor T ALL.[141] They have round or convoluted nuclei, finely dispersed chromatin, inconspicuous nucleoli, and scant cytoplasm.[142] Lymphoblastic lymphomas in the anterior mediastinum have a precursor T cell immunophenotype that most often correlates with the middle or late stage of thymocyte maturation.[21] The cells express various combinations of the CD1, CD2, CD5, and CD7 antigens and, in many cases, express both CD4 and CD8. The CD3 antigen and associated T-cell receptor molecule are not commonly expressed. The CD10 or CALLA antigen is variably present. Significant overlap of the immunophenotype is found in many cases of lymphoblastic lymphoma and T-cell ALL, suggesting a common cell of origin.[142] The early-stage lymphoblastic lymphomas have the phenotype of an early B-cell precursor, identical to that seen in most children with ALL.[1,143]

In more than one-half of the cases of T-cell lymphoblastic lymphoma/leukemia, recurrent nonrandom chromosomal translocations involving the α, β, and γ chains of the T-cell receptor have been identified. Many of these translocations arise in error during the normal process of rearrangement of the T-cell receptor genes, a situation that is analogous to the Ig rearrangements noted in Burkitt's lymphoma.[25,144] Several of the partner genes involved in these translocations include the transcription factors TAL1 and HOX11, and the cysteine-rich (LIM) proteins RHOMB1 and RHOMB2. In the t(1;14)(p32;q11), detected in 3% of patients with T ALL, the TAL1 gene is rearranged in its 5' regular sequence by its translocation into the T-cell receptor α/δ chain locus. A submicroscopic deletion in the same region of TAL1 is detected in up to 25% of patients with T-cell ALL/lymphoblastic lymphoma, making it the most common genetic change in this disease.[25,145]

Clinical Presentation and Staging

Most children with lymphoblastic lymphoma present with rapidly enlarging neck and mediastinal lymphadenopathy, although subdiaphragmatic nodal presentations are occasionally seen.[26] The classic presentation is that of an adolescent male with respiratory distress due to a large anterior mediastinal mass with or without pleural effusions. Cough, wheezing, or shortness of breath and facial swelling (evidence of superior vena cava syndrome) are frequent complaints in these patients. Other common presenting sites of disease include cervical nodes, Waldeyer's ring, cutaneous lesions, bone marrow, and single- or multiple-site bone disease. The majority of children have advanced-stage disease (see Table 45.2-5).

Because the pace of the disease is usually rapid, diagnostic studies and institution of therapy should proceed quickly. The least invasive procedure should be used to establish the diagnosis. Because bone marrow is frequently involved and patients with T-cell ALL often present with an anterior mediastinal mass, a close examination of the peripheral blood and bone marrow should be undertaken before proceeding to a more invasive procedure. Pleural effusions should be tapped because they are often positive for malignant cells. If the bone marrow and pleural fluid are nondiagnostic, a lymph node outside of the mediastinum should be biopsied, if possible. Sufficient tissue should be obtained for histopathology, genetic studies, and immunophenotyping. Biopsy under general anesthesia should be avoided if at all possible, especially if there is significant airway narrowing or symptoms of respiratory distress.[146,147] The prebiopsy use of mediastinal irradiation or steroids for respiratory distress results in rapid disappearance of the mass and jeopardizes the likelihood of establishing a tissue diagnosis. The remainder of the workup should include a lumbar puncture with a cytocentrifuged examination of cerebral spinal fluid, and a computed tomographic (CT) scan or magnetic resonance imaging of the primary site. Bone and liver-spleen scans are not necessary.

Routine blood chemistries and liver function tests should be obtained before starting therapy.

Treatment

Historically, children with lymphoblastic lymphoma had less than a 10% survival rate after careful pathologic staging followed by extended-field radiotherapy.[148,149] Within several months from the start of radiation therapy, disease progression to a leukemic phase that was indistinguishable from ALL was noted in most patients. This finding suggested that widespread dissemination of lymphoma already existed at the time of diagnosis, especially to the bone marrow and meninges. Based on these observations, investigators at St. Jude Children's Research Hospital added chemotherapy that was effective against childhood ALL to local irradiation.[149] This systemic treatment approach dramatically improved the outcome for children with lymphoblastic lymphoma. Similar treatment strategies were adopted for the other histologic types of childhood NHL.

The combined use of ALL therapy with local irradiation was very effective for children with early-stage lymphoblastic lymphoma (80% survival).[150,151] Despite the favorable outcome, the toxicity of combined modality therapy led to attempts to reduce the intensity and duration of treatment without compromising survival. Several single-institution and cooperative group protocols were successful in maintaining excellent survival rates (85% to 90%) while reducing the morbidity and mortality of therapy. The CCG protocols demonstrated the equal efficacy of 6 and 18 months of the cyclophosphamide, Oncovin, methotrexate, and prednisone (COMP) combination.[151] However, all children also received radiotherapy to involved fields. A POG study demonstrated that the omission of radiotherapy from the treatment of localized NHL in children did not jeopardize survival.[133] The POG chemotherapy regimen included three cycles of cyclophosphamide, doxorubicin, Oncovin, and prednisone (CHOP) followed by 24 weeks of 6-mercaptopurine and methotrexate. The CCG and POG protocols included IT methotrexate for patients with primary tumors in the head and neck region. Treatment with either CHOP or COMP results in 65% event-free survival for children with localized lymphoblastic lymphoma, but survival is 90% because of the successful treatment of relapse with salvage chemotherapy.

Fewer than 40% of patients with advanced-stage (stages 3 and 4) lymphoblastic lymphoma were cured with standard-risk ALL regimens (e.g., vincristine, steroid, L-asparaginase, methotrexate, and 6-mercaptopurine) or COMP therapy.[131,150] The addition of drugs such as the anthracyclines, cyclophosphamide, cytosine arabinoside, or the epipodophyllotoxins to ALL regimens substantially improved the prognosis for these children.

The vincristine, doxorubicin (Adriamycin), and prednisone (APO) and LSA2L2 regimens were two of the early successful protocols for children with high-risk ALL or advanced-stage lymphoblastic lymphoma. LSA2L2 included ten drugs, and the APO protocol featured intensification with doxorubicin and L-asparaginase (Table 45.2-7).[150,152,153] Both protocols included preventive CNS therapy. Radiation therapy to the mediastinum was generally limited to emergency situations. These regimens resulted in approximately 65% survival for children with advanced-stage lymphoblastic lymphoma. The use of more intensive ALL chemotherapy regimens appears to further improve the outcome for these children.[25,132] Although radiotherapy has been omitted from most of the protocols, a small percentage of patients have local tumor failure.[154]

TABLE 45.2-7. Recommended Protocols by Histology and Stage for Pediatric Non-Hodgkin's Lymphoma

Histology	*Protocol*	*5-Y EFS (%)*	*References*
Lymphoblastic			
Stages 1 and 2	CHOP	60	133
	COMP	67	150,151
Stages 3 and 4	APO	60	153
	LSA2L2	65	150
	NHL-BFM 90	90	154
Small noncleaved cell (Burkitt's)			
Stages 1 and 2	CHOP	88	133
	COMP	85	150,151
Stage 3	NHL-BFM 90	73	83
	POG	81	160
	LMB 89	87	159
Stage 4/B ALL	NHL-BFM 90	78	83
	LMB 89	85	159
Large cell			
Stages 1 and 2	CHOP	86	133
	COMP	84	150,151
Stages 3 and 4	APO	65	176
	St. Jude	75	181
	ACOP+	67	178

ACOP+, Adriamycin, Cytoxan, Oncovin, and prednisone; ALL, acute lymphoblastic leukemia; APO, vincristine, doxorubicin (Adriamycin), and prednisone; CHOP, cyclophosphamide, doxorubicin, Oncovin, and prednisone; COMP, cyclophosphamide, Oncovin, methotrexate, and prednisone; EFS, event-free survival; LMB 89, French Pediatric Oncology Society B Non-Hodgkin's Lymphoma Trials; LSA2L2, Wollner's protocol; NHL-BFM 90, Non-Hodgkin's Lymphoma Berlin-Frankfort-Munster 90 trial; POG, Pediatric Oncology Group; St. Jude, St. Jude Children's Research Hospital trial.

Early preventive CNS therapy is critical in the treatment for children with advanced-stage lymphoblastic lymphoma. IT chemotherapy alone or combined with cranial irradiation has been the mainstay of CNS preventive therapy.[154]

Relapse at any site is a significant obstacle to cure in children with advanced-stage lymphoblastic lymphoma. Most of the relapses occur within 2 years from diagnosis, but occasional late relapse is observed. In contrast to relapse for early-stage disease, the outcome after a second course of chemotherapy is poor. However, these patients have a 30% to 50% survival rate after allogeneic BMT from a histocompatible sibling donor.[155]

SMALL NONCLEAVED CELL (BURKITT'S) LYMPHOMA

The small noncleaved cell lymphomas (Burkitt's type) were initially described by Dennis Burkitt in equatorial Africa where the tumor is endemic.[156] These lymphomas were subsequently recognized worldwide and account for approximately 40% of childhood NHL. The endemic form is common (100 per 1 million children) and is nearly always associated with EBV (95%), whereas the sporadic form is rare (1 to 2 per 1 million children) and uncommonly associated with EBV (15%). In endemic areas, involvement of the jaw and other facial bones is frequent, whereas extensive intraabdominal disease and bone marrow involvement are commonly seen in sporadic cases.[157]

Histologically, the small noncleaved cell lymphomas include the Burkitt's and non-Burkitt's types. The Burkitt's type was defined by the World Health Organization in 1969. It is characterized by homogeneous cells with round to oval nuclei with multiple nuclei and intensely basophilic vacuolated cytoplasm that contains neutral fat. The non-Burkitt's type has a greater degree of nuclear pleomorphism compared to the Burkitt's type. The non-Burkitt's type may be difficult to distinguish on a morphologic basis from some large B-cell lymphomas. In children, no obvious differences are found between the Burkitt's and non-Burkitt's lymphomas, and therefore they are considered the same for treatment purposes.[158]

Burkitt's lymphoma is a B-cell tumor based on expression of cell surface Ig heavy chains (usually IgM) and either κ or λ light chains.[11] Approximately 50% of cases are also CD10 (CALLA)-positive. L3 lymphoblasts have a similar immunophenotype and are cytologically indistinguishable from Burkitt's cells. Because many patients with L3 ALL also have primary tumor masses, it is likely that the essential difference in these diseases lies in their extent at presentation. Cure rates of 75% to 85% have been achieved for children with B-cell ALL (FAB L3) using treatment programs developed for advanced-stage Burkitt's lymphoma.[83,159,160]

Chromosomal translocations involving the c-myc locus on chromosome 8q24 and Ig receptor genes are characteristic of Burkitt's lymphoma.[3,26,161] These translocations appear to result from errors in the normal process of recombination that drives Ig gene rearrangement during B-cell development. The majority of cases have a t(8;14)(q24;q32) translocation in which c-myc is translocated into the Ig heavy-chain gene on chromosome 14q32. Two variant translocations, t(2;8)(p12;q24) and t(8;22)(q24;q11), occur with less frequency. In these translocations, c-myc is fused with the κ or λ light-chain genes located on chromosome 2 and 22, respectively. These translocations juxtapose Ig transcriptional regulatory sequences adjacent to the c-myc gene, leading to its dysregulated activity. In endemic and sporadic cases, the breakpoints on chromosome 14 involve the Ig heavy-chain joining region and switch region, respectively, suggesting that the translocation in the sporadic cases occurs at a later stage of B-cell development.[162] Up-regulation of c-myc influences the ratio between myc/max complexes in favor of transcriptional activation and B-cell proliferation.[163] In transgenic mice, the translocation-induced dysregulation of c-myc has been shown to directly induce B-cell lymphomas.[164]

The role of EBV in the pathogenesis of endemic Burkitt's lymphoma is unknown.[165] Studies of EBV gene expression in lymphoblastoid cell lines and in human tumor biopsy specimens have identified three distinct forms of virus latency. EBV gene expression is more restricted in Burkitt's lymphoma (EBNA1 and EBERs) compared with lymphoblastoid cell lines, posttransplantation lymphoproliferative processes, and some cases of EBV-positive Hodgkin's disease and nasopharyngeal cancer.[166] Tumor cells of endemic Burkitt's lymphoma are not susceptible to killing by EBV-specific cytotoxic T cells, which may be due to the lack of the EBNA3 family of proteins. Furthermore, Burkitt's cells display down-regulated expression of adhesion molecules and HLA class I alleles, further impairing the action of cytotoxic T cells. The role of malarial infection remains unknown but may also result in a relative T-cell immunodeficiency.

Clinical Presentation

The abdomen is the most common presenting site in sporadic cases of Burkitt's lymphoma (see Table 45.2-5).[26] Approximately one-third of children with an abdominal primary tumor present with a right lower quadrant mass or with signs and symptoms of either acute appendicitis or intestinal obstruction secondary to an ileocecal intussusception.[157,167] This presentation is typically seen in boys between 5 and 10 years of age. An exploratory laparotomy is indicated for diagnostic purposes. If a tumor is discovered, it is invariably a small noncleaved Burkitt's lymphoma that is limited in extent to the distal ileum or cecum. Complete surgical resection of the involved segment of gut with its associated mesentery, followed by an end-to-end anastomosis, is the proper treatment. Children with completely resected Burkitt's lymphoma (stage 2) of the intestinal tract have an excellent prognosis after treatment with a limited course of chemotherapy (discussed later, in the section Treatment). The majority of patients with Burkitt's lymphoma of the abdomen, however, have unresectable disease that may involve the mesentery, retroperitoneum, kidneys, ovaries, and peritoneal surfaces (often associated with malignant ascites). Surgical debulking is not feasible or appropriate for this latter group of patients.[167]

The head and neck region is the second most common site of disease presentation. Patients in nonendemic areas present with tonsillar enlargement, cervical lymphadenopathy and, occasionally, a soft tissue facial mass associated with involvement of the jaw or other facial bones.[133,157] Less common presenting sites include an epidural mass, skin nodules, bone, and bone marrow.

The least invasive procedure should be used to establish the diagnosis, and the staging evaluation should be expedited because these patients usually have rapidly growing tumors with significant electrolyte imbalance as well as impaired renal function. This is especially true for children with massive abdominal disease. Effusions are usually malignant in these children and contain sufficient numbers of tumor cells for cytology and biology studies. Imaging should include a CT scan or magnetic resonance imaging of the primary site and a bone scan. Patients with head and neck primary tumors may have clinically nondetectable disease in the abdomen (especially of the kidneys) and therefore should also have abdominal imaging studies.

Particular attention to kidney function, and the serum levels of uric acid, potassium, calcium, and phosphorus, is critical in children with advanced-stage Burkitt's lymphoma. These patients are at high risk for the "tumor lysis syndrome" and uric acid nephropathy.[168] Measures should be taken to reduce the likelihood of uric acid nephropathy, including vigorous intravenous hydration, alkalinization of urine with either sodium bicarbonate or Diamox, administration of allopurinol, and careful monitoring of serum electrolytes. Hemodialysis is required in a small percentage of cases.[160]

Treatment

Complete remissions were induced in 80% of African children with Burkitt's lymphoma with cyclophosphamide administered as a single agent.[169] Patients with facial tumors (early stage) had sustained remissions with single- or multiple-dose cyclophosphamide, whereas the majority of children with abdominal tumors relapsed with systemic and CNS disease. Successor protocols used combination chemotherapy and IT methotrexate. The use of cyclophosphamide and vincristine with methotrexate or cytarabine was associated with higher remission rates and more durable remissions compared to single-agent cyclophosphamide.[170] The most important prognostic factor was the extent of tumor at diagnosis.

Clinical trials in the United States demonstrated that the complete response rate, relapse frequency, and survival in American patients were similar to results in Africa.[171] Approximately 85% of patients with early-stage Burkitt's lymphoma were cured using as little as 9 weeks of CHOP chemotherapy.[133] Similar results were achieved after 6 months of COMP therapy.[151] A POG study demonstrated that the addition of involved-field radiation therapy did not influence outcome.[133] Treatment for patients with head and neck primary sites of disease also included IT methotrexate.

COMP therapy, however, resulted in only a 40% survival rate for patients with advanced-stage disease,[150] which was similar to the African experience.[170] Relapses occurred in systemic and CNS sites at a median of 3 months from the beginning of therapy. Protocols that were highly effective for children with ALL and lymphoblastic lymphoma (e.g., LSA2L2 and APO) were less effective than COMP for advanced-stage Burkitt's lymphoma or L3 ALL.[150] These poor results were most likely due to the omission or limited use of cyclophosphamide.

Several groups of investigators began to evaluate dose-intensified systemic and IT chemotherapy for these high-risk patients.[83,159,160] Cyclophosphamide, methotrexate, and cytarabine were administered in high doses with or without anthracyclines and the epipodophyllotoxins. Treatment courses were repeated at early signs of bone marrow recovery in an attempt to prevent regrowth of tumor between cycles of chemotherapy. Hematopoietic growth factors were used in some protocols to enhance bone marrow recovery. CNS prophylaxis included systemic chemotherapy that penetrated the CNS (high-dose methotrexate and cytarabine) and intensive IT chemotherapy. Radiation therapy was usually reserved for patients who presented with initial CNS involvement. The duration of treatment ranged from 2 months to 1 year. The results of these studies were impressive. Event-free survival increased from 50% to 80% for stage 3 and from less than 20% to more than 80% for patients with stage 4 Burkitt's lymphoma and L3 ALL (see Table 45.2-7).

The management of patients with recurrent Burkitt's lymphoma is problematic. Relapse tends to occur early, while the patient is still on therapy. BMT offers the only realistic hope of long-term survival for these children.[26,172] The outcome is more favorable for patients who achieve a second remission before proceeding to BMT. However, second remissions are difficult to induce in these patients, especially for those with advanced-stage disease.

LARGE CELL LYMPHOMA

The large cell lymphomas constitute approximately 30% of childhood NHL.[26] Approximately 30% of pediatric large cell lymphomas are classified as ALCL in the Revised European-American Lymphoma classification.[141] The remainder are diffuse large B-cell lymphoma, primary mediastinal large B-cell lymphoma, and the rare peripheral T-cell lymphoma. ALCL in children tends to involve lymph nodes and extranodal sites, including the skin, soft tissues, lung, and bone.[173] Lymphomatoid papulosis and the primary cutaneous form of ALCL are rare in childhood. The majority of the cases of ALCL studied in children have had a T-cell phenotype. The t(2;5)(p23;q35) translocation has been associated with Ki-1+ or CD30+ lymphomas in both children and adults.[174] The chromosomal breakpoints involved in the t(2;5) have been cloned and involve the gene that encodes nucleophosmin (NPM), a nonribosomal nuclear phosphoprotein on chromosome 5, and a gene that encodes a novel transmembrane tyrosine-specific protein kinase (ALK) located on chromosome 2.[175] The translocation results in the fusion of these genes, producing a chimeric NPM-ALK gene and message. Reverse transcriptase–polymerase chain reaction assays for this translocation have been positive in all cases with cytogenetic evidence of the t(2;5) and in several cases of ALCL with a normal karyotype.

Clinical Presentation

The clinical presenting features of large cell lymphoma in children are more varied than those for lymphoblastic or Burkitt's lymphoma. Also, a relatively equal distribution is seen between early- and advanced-stage disease. The most common primary sites of disease include the nasopharynx, cervical nodes, skin, soft tissues, mediastinum, bone, and abdomen. The bone marrow and CNS are rarely infiltrated (see Table 45.2-5).

Evaluation and Treatment

The workup and staging of the child with large cell lymphoma are similar to that recommended for children with the other histologic subtypes of NHL. The treatment of large cell lymphoma in children has evolved from local radiotherapy to primarily combination chemotherapy.[26,176] Because of the relative rarity of large cell lymphoma in children, many of the treatment strategies and protocols derive from adult studies.[177]

Children with localized large cell lymphoma have a very favorable prognosis. The COMP and CHOP regimens that are effective in early-stage lymphoblastic and Burkitt's lymphoma also result in 85% survival for these children (see Table 45.2-7).[133,150] The results of CHOP with or without involved-field irradiation were similar.

CHOP has not been systematically evaluated in children with advanced-stage large cell lymphoma. The results of COMP therapy for these children were disappointing (approximately 50% event-free survival).[150] However, the use of the APO and Adriamycin, Cytoxan, Oncovin, and prednisone (ACOP+) regimens resulted in approximately 70% event-free survival for children with stage 3 or 4 large cell lymphoma.[176,178] These latter protocols include up-front vincristine, prednisone, doxorubicin, and cyclophosphamide (ACOP+ only). Because of the similar outcomes after APO and ACOP+ therapy and the concerns of secondary malignancy and gonadal failure after cyclophosphamide, POG investigators prospectively compared APO to ACOP+ in children with advanced-stage large cell lymphoma.[179] The event-free survival rate is approximately 70% in both arms at 5 years, thereby questioning the value of the addition of an alkylating agent to an Adriamycin-containing regimen. Conclusions about the safety of omitting cyclophosphamide await confirmatory studies and a detailed analysis of various subsets of patients.

The most important prognostic factor in children with large cell lymphoma is stage. Children with ALCL do not have an adverse prognosis compared with other subgroups of patients with large cell lymphoma. In a retrospective POG study, B-cell phenotype was associated with superior survival.[180]

Most protocols for children with advanced-stage large cell lymphoma do not include involved-field radiotherapy, but no controlled trials have addressed this issue.[181] The risk of an isolated CNS relapse is rare, but nevertheless, pediatric protocols include IT chemotherapy for these patients.

HODGKIN'S DISEASE

Approximately 10% to 15% of all cases of Hodgkin's disease occur in patients younger than 16 years.[182,183] The natural history of Hodgkin's disease and outcome of treatment is similar in children and young adults 20 to 45 years of age.[184–187] Fully grown adolescents generally are evaluated and managed in the same way as adults. Treatment decisions are more complex in young children because of the adverse effects of irradiation on growth of bone and soft tissues and the risk of secondary malignancies.[189,190] The preceding concerns led to the development in the 1970s of combined modality therapy with reduced doses and volumes of irradiation for children with both early and advanced stages of Hodgkin's disease.[191,192] The following section focuses on the unique aspects of the treatment of Hodgkin's disease in children.

EPIDEMIOLOGY

In industrialized countries, the age of Hodgkin's incidence is bimodal, with a first peak in adults 20 to 30 years of age and a second peak in late adulthood. Hodgkin's is uncommon before age 5 years, and the majority of pediatric cases are in children older than 11 years.[4,182] Before age 10, the male to female ratio is approximately 3:1; this ratio approaches 1:1 by adolescence.

The etiology of Hodgkin's disease remains unknown. An increased risk of Hodgkin's disease is noted in children with inherited immunodeficiency syndromes. Genetic susceptibility and environmental factors probably both play a role in the pathogenesis of Hodgkin's disease (discussed in detail in Chapters 45.1 and 45.6). Although rare, Hodgkin's can be familial. Evidence is increasing for the role of EBV in some subgroups of patients with Hodgkin's disease, especially children with mixed-cellularity histology.[193]

CLINICAL PRESENTATION, STAGING, AND WORKUP

Hodgkin's disease usually presents in supradiaphragmatic lymph nodes, with cervical, anterior mediastinal, and axillary nodes occurring in decreasing frequency. Mediastinal adenopathy may produce symptoms such as dyspnea, cough, or superior vena cava syndrome. Approximately 90% of children present with painless neck adenopathy, and 60% have involvement of anterior mediastinal, paratracheal, or hilar lymph nodes. Isolated infradiaphragmatic Hodgkin's disease is rare. Approximately one-third of children have B symptoms [unexplained fever (exceeding 100.4°F), drenching night sweats, more than 10% weight loss]. The Ann Arbor staging system is used for all age groups of patients with Hodgkin's disease and is described in detail in Chapter 45.6.

Although not included in the staging system, a precise measurement of the size of the anterior mediastinal mass is important. If the ratio of the width of the mediastinal mass over the maximum transthoracic diameter is greater than one-third, this is considered large mediastinal adenopathy and is an adverse prognostic variable.[194] The diagnosis of Hodgkin's disease must be established by lymph node or tissue biopsy. The lymphocyte-predominant subtype is closely associated with stage I and II Hodgkin's disease, and lymphocyte depletion is extremely rare in children.[183] Despite the unique biology and natural history of lymphocyte-predominant Hodgkin's disease, most pediatric oncologists recommend the same stage-appropriate treatment as given to other children with Hodgkin's disease.[195] The pathology and immunobiology of Hodgkin's disease is reviewed in detail in Chapter 45.6.

Once the diagnosis is established, the pretherapy evaluation begins with "clinical" staging.[196,197] Clinical staging should include a history and physical examination with particular emphasis on defining lymphadenopathy by palpating the major lymph node chains. The size of the nodes should be measured and recorded for staging and follow-up. Laboratory studies include complete blood cell count with platelets, erythrocyte sedimentation rate, and kidney and liver function studies. Patients with B symptoms or stage III or IV disease should have bone marrow biopsies from two separate sites.

Imaging studies should include a chest radiograph with a posteroanterior and lateral view, and thoracic and abdominal CT scans. Lower extremity lymphangiography is no longer routinely performed in most centers because it does not visualize the upper abdominal nodes and spleen and sometimes require general anesthesia in children. High-dose gallium scanning in children with Hodgkin's disease, similar to the situation in adults, is most helpful for following response to therapy if the tumor is gallium-avid.[198]

The thoracic CT scan is useful for detecting minimal mediastinal disease, pulmonary parenchymal and hilar disease, pericardial involvement, paracardiac nodes, and chest wall extension. No optimal method has been developed for detecting abdominal involvement of Hodgkin's disease. The false-positive and false-negative rates for abdominal CT scans were 14% and 22%, respectively, in a pediatric series.[196] More than 90% of children who are upstaged by laparotomy have evidence of splenic involvement that is not detected by CT scanning or lymphangiograms.[197] In a POG study, models based on clinical and radiographic findings were developed to predict for splenic involvement and upstaging with laparotomy. Risk factors, such as B symptoms, an erythrocyte sedimentation rate of more than 70, histology other than nodular sclerosis or lymphocyte predominant, more than four sites of involvement, and an enlarged spleen (based on spleen CT index), were predictive for abdominal disease but still were associated with 25% to 30% false-negative and false-positive rates, respectively.[196]

The merits of staging laparotomy remain a source of controversy.[185,196] Although information provided by a staging laparotomy and splenectomy may be unobtainable by other means, surgical staging is recommended only if the information provided will influence treatment planning. If radiation therapy alone is used for stage I and II disease, pathologic staging will more accurately define appropriate patients and, in certain cases, spare them paraaortic and splenic irradiation. However, staging laparotomy is no longer routinely performed in children because of the increasing use of combined modality therapy for all stages of disease.

In the era of staging laparotomy in children, a concern existed for the risk of overwhelming postsplenectomy sepsis from encapsulated pathogens.[193,197] With the use of pneumococcal, meningococcal, and *Haemophilus influenzae* vaccinations before surgery and prophylactic antibiotics, this risk appears to have decreased.[199]

Among 2238 consecutive patients with Hodgkin's disease treated at Stanford University, 4% were 10 years old or younger and 11% were 11 to 16 years old. Stage I and II disease was present in approximately 60% of children. Stage I disease was slightly more common in younger children (18%) than in adolescents (8%); stage II disease occurred in 40% to 50% of all age groups; and stage IV disease was less common in younger children (3%) than in adolescents (15%). B symptoms occurred in 19% of younger children and in 30% of adolescents.[200]

As the treatment of Hodgkin's disease has improved, previously identified prognostic factors have diminished in importance. However, stage, tumor bulk, and constitutional symptoms continue to influence the success and certainly the choice of therapy.[192,200,201] Because prognostic factors are similar for adults and children with Hodgkin's disease, the reader is referred to Chapter 45.6 for an in-depth discussion of this topic.

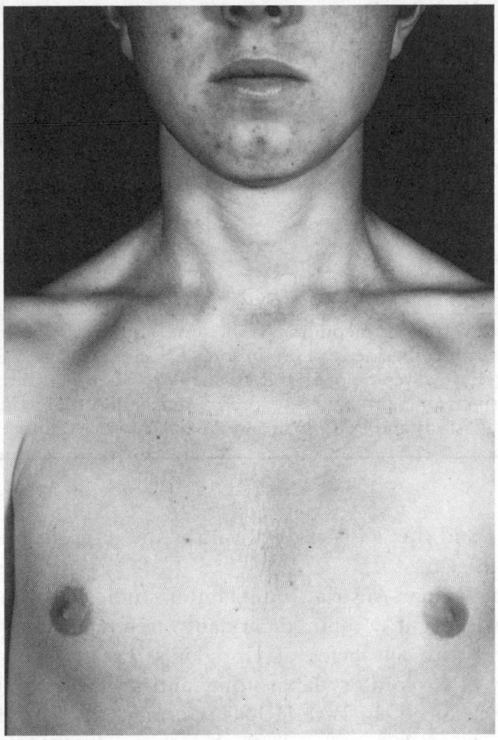

FIGURE 45.2-3. Frontal view of patient several years after mantle irradiation with 4-MeV linear accelerator for Hodgkin's disease. Note the intraclavicular narrowing and hypodevelopment of neck musculature.

SELECTION OF THERAPY

The cure rate for children with all stages of Hodgkin's disease is approximately 90%. As the cure rate has increased, an increasing focus has been placed on the late complications of therapy. In the pediatric patient, especially the prepubescent child, treatment decisions must be weighed in view of the toxicities of radiation therapy on growth and development. For example, the use of high-dose (40 Gy) extended-field radiotherapy alone in children and adults with pathologic stage I or II Hodgkin's disease results in 85% to 90% 10-year survival.[185,202] However, this therapy has serious late effects on musculoskeletal growth in the prepubescent child.[185,188] In this young age group, the effect on bone and soft tissue is manifest by intraclavicular narrowing, shortened sitting height, decreased mandibular growth, and decreased muscle development in the treated volume (Fig. 45.2-3). Other well-known late complications of irradiation, including hypothyroidism and second neoplasms, are not unique in patients treated for Hodgkin's disease in childhood (discussed later in the section Complications).[189,203,204]

In an attempt to decrease the late effects of high-dose extended-field irradiation, alternative treatments have been developed. These have included chemotherapy combined with both lower doses and less extensive fields of irradiation and chemotherapy alone (Table 45.2-8).

A Stanford study was one of the first to demonstrate that combined modality therapy with Mustargen, Oncovin, procarbazine, and prednisone (MOPP) and low-dose radiation to involved regions was highly effective and associated with fewer adverse effects on musculoskeletal growth and development than had been observed with high-dose radiation alone.[191] In this study, patients were surgically staged and treated with six cycles of MOPP chemotherapy and an age-adjusted radiation dose of 15 to 25 Gy. Boost doses of 10 Gy were used in select patients. The projected 10-year survival rate was 89% for all patients. However, the long-term side effects included a 10-year risk of 6.5% for the development of secondary leukemia, as well as azoospermia in all males tested. The Princess Margaret Hospital team in Toronto used a similar combined modality approach, but avoided staging laparotomy.[192] In an effort to maintain efficacy while decreasing the occurrence of secondary leukemia and male infertility, the Stanford successor study alternated MOPP with doxorubicin, bleomycin, vinblastine, and dacarbazine (ABVD) for six cycles in combination with a 15- to 25-Gy radiation dose to involved fields.[186] The projected 10-year survival rates are 96%, and growth and development have progressed normally. At the time of the report, no patient had developed a second leukemia, but one solid tumor in a radiation field was noted. Approximately one-third of patients had asymptomatic changes noted on pulmonary function tests. Azoospermia is documented in approximately one-third of patients treated with ABVD, but it appears transitory in almost all patients.[205]

Similar treatment strategies with the goal of decreasing the risk of secondary leukemia, solid tumors, and gonadal failure have been reported by other groups. The French Society of Pediatric Oncology randomized patients with clinical stage I and IIA Hodgkin's disease to four cycles of ABVD, or two cycles of MOPP and two cycles of ABVD, plus low-dose (20-Gy) involved-field radiation therapy.[206] Children with advanced disease (stages IB, IIIB, III, and IV) were given three cycles of MOPP and three cycles of ABVD plus extended-field low-dose radiotherapy. Patients with a poor response to chemotherapy received full doses of irradiation. The disease-free survival rate

TABLE 45.2-8. Representative Combined Modality Trials for Pediatric Hodgkin's Disease

Center	*Number of Patients*	*Stage*	*Chemotherapy*	*Radiotherapy*	*5-Y EFS (%)*
Stanford University[186]	57	PS I–IV	3 ABVD/3 MOPP	15–25 Gy IF	100 (I–III); 69 (IV)
FSOP[206]	132	CS I–IIA	2 ABVD/2 MOPP vs. 4 ABVD	20–40 Gy IF	90 vs. 87
German HD 90[207]	588	CS/PS I–IIA	2 OPPA or 2 OEPA	30–35 Gy IF	94 (I–IIA)
		IIB–IV	2 OPPA or 2 OEPA		86–93 (IIB–IV)
POG protocol 8625[209]	244	PS I–IIA	2–3 MOPP/2–3 ABVD	±25 Gy IF	86 vs. 89
St. Jude[211]	85	CS/PS II–IV	4–5 COPP/3–4 ABVD	20 Gy IF	96 (I–IIB); 93 (III–IV)
POG protocol 8725[210]	183	CS/PS IIB–IV	4 MOPP/4 ABVD	±21 Gy TNI	80 (CMT); 79 (C)

ABVD, doxorubicin, bleomycin, vinblastine, and dacarbazine; C, chemotherapy only; CMT, combined modality trial; COPP, cyclophosphamide, Oncovin, procarbazine, and prednisone; CS, clinical stage; EFS, event-free survival; FSOP, French Society of Pediatric Oncology; HD, Hodgkin's Disease; IF, involved field; MOPP, Mustargen, Oncovin, procarbazine, and prednisone; OEPA, vincristine, etoposide, prednisone, and Adriamycin; OPPA, vincristine, procarbazine, prednisone, and Adriamycin; POG, Pediatric Oncology Group; PS, pathologic stage; TNI, total nodal irradiation. The FSOP study and POG 8625 and POG 8725 were randomized trials.

is 88%, and the actuarial survival for the entire group is 95% (see Table 45.2-8).

The German-Austrian multicenter studies also have developed successful combined modality treatment programs for children with all stages of Hodgkin's disease.[205,207] The frequency of exploratory laparotomy and splenectomy has been greatly reduced. In DAL-HD-90 (German-Austrian Hodgkin's trials), chemotherapy was limited to two cycles for stages I and IIA. Boys received vincristine, etoposide, prednisone, and Adriamycin (OEPA), and girls were given two cycles of vincristine, procarbazine, prednisone, and Adriamycin (OPPA). Radiation was applied to involved sites (25 Gy). The 5-year event-free survival rate is 95%. Patients with more advanced-stage disease received two cycles of OPPA or OEPA and an additional two cycles (stages IIB and IIIA) or four cycles (stages IIIB and IV) of cyclophosphamide, Oncovin, procarbazine, and prednisone (COPP) plus involved-field irradiation. Five-year event-free survival rates were 90% to 95% for intermediate stages and 84% to 89% for stages IIIB and IV. Testicular function was normal in the regimens without procarbazine.[207]

In the past, there had been only limited experience using chemotherapy as the only treatment modality in children with Hodgkin's disease. The early experience was reported by the investigators from the Royal Children's Hospital in Melbourne, Australia.[208] After clinical staging, they treated children with stage I to IV Hodgkin's disease with either MOPP or chlorambucil, vinblastine, procarbazine, and prednisone (ChlVPP) therapy. The event-free survival rate was 92% at a median follow-up of 45 months. Twenty-eight of 32 patients with stage I or II disease and 14 of 15 patients with stage III or IV were disease-free. Although the outcome was excellent, these children were exposed to multiple cycles of alkylating agents with the high risk of secondary leukemia and infertility in males.

The POG investigators have completed two large randomized trials in early-stage and advanced-stage Hodgkin's disease. The first POG study compared six cycles of MOPP alternating with ABVD to four cycles of the same chemotherapy followed by involved-field irradiation (25 Gy) in surgically staged children with stage I to IIIA Hodgkin's disease.[209] The event-free survival rate was 90% at 6 years, with no difference noted in the two arms of the study (see Table 45.2-8). These children were exposed to less alkylating agent than in the Australian study because of the alternating use of MOPP and ABVD.

In the second randomized study, POG showed that no benefit existed for low-dose total nodal or subtotal nodal radiation after eight cycles of MOPP alternating with ABVD in children with advanced-stage Hodgkin's disease.[210] Results of CCG study 5942 indicate inferior results in patients with advanced-stage disease or B symptoms who were randomized to receive chemotherapy only (J. Nachman, personal communication). Further investigations are needed before radiation therapy is omitted in the treatment of children with Hodgkin's disease, especially for unfavorable subgroups.

The combined modality approach using limited doses of both radiation (15 to 30 Gy) and alkylating agents for children with all stages of Hodgkin's disease produces an excellent outcome with significant reduction in the risk of serious late effects. As the doses of irradiation are safely lowered in combined modality treatments, future studies will undoubtedly test whether chemotherapy alone can achieve these excellent results. In addition, less toxic and equally effective chemotherapy regimens are being tested.

COMPLICATIONS

The risk of infertility, secondary cancers, and late cardiopulmonary complications of newer generation combined modality therapies in young children with Hodgkin's disease remains to be determined.[207] Several reports provide evidence that the risk of a second neoplasm is increased approximately 18 times in long-term survivors of childhood Hodgkin's disease.[190,204] Breast cancer and thyroid cancer were the most common solid tumors. The actuarial risk of a solid tumor at 20 years after the diagnosis of Hodgkin's disease was significantly higher among women (12.6%) than men (3.9%). The actuarial risk of breast cancer among women approached 35% at 40 years of age. An age of more than 10 years at the diagnosis of Hodgkin's disease and a higher dose of mantle radiation were independently associated with increased risk. The relative risk for a dose between 20 Gy and 40 Gy was 5.9 and 23.7 for a dose exceeding 40 Gy.

The cumulative risk of leukemia was highest in patients receiving chemotherapy alone (7.9%) and rose with an increase in the alkylating agent score. Based on these data, efforts to lower the doses and volumes of radiation and limit exposure to alkylating agents and anthracyclines are steps in the right direction.

REFERENCES

1. Pui CH, Evans WE. Acute lymphoblastic leukemia. *N Engl J Med* 1998;339:605.
2. Ebb DH, Weinstein HJ. Diagnosis and treatment of childhood acute myelogenous leukemia. *Pediatr Clin North Am* 1997;44:847.
3. Rubnitz JE, Look AT. Molecular genetics of childhood leukemias. *J Pediatr Hematol Oncol* 1998;20:1.
4. Smith MA, Ries LAG, Gurney JG, Ross JA. Cancer incidence and survival among children and adolescents: United States SEER Program 1975–1995. In: Ries L, Smith M, Gurney J, et al. eds. *Leukemia (ICCC I)*. National Institutes of Health Pub. No. 99-4649. Bethesda, MD: National Cancer Institute SEER Program, 1999:17.
5. Greaves M. A natural history for pediatric acute leukemia. *Blood* 1993;82:1043.
6. Wiemels JL, Daniotti M, Eden OB, et al. Prenatal origin of acute lymphoblastic leukemia in children. *Lancet* 1999;354:1499.
7. Zipursky A, Poon A, Doyle J. Leukemia in Down syndrome: a review. *Pediatr Hematol Oncol* 1992;9:139.
8. Homans AC, Verissimo AM, Vlacha V. Transient abnormal myelopoiesis of infancy associated with trisomy 21. *Am J Pediatr Hematol Oncol* 1993;15:392.
9. Ravindranath Y, Abella E, Krischer J, et al. Acute myeloid leukemia (AML) in Down's syndrome is highly responsive to chemotherapy: experience of Pediatric Oncology Group AML Study 8498. *Blood* 1992;80:2210.
10. Shannon K, O'Connell P, Martin G, et al. Loss of the normal NFI allele from the bone marrow of children with type 1 neurofibromatosis and malignant myeloid disorders. *N Engl J Med* 1994;330:597.
11. Shu XO, Ross J, Pendergrass T, et al. Parental alcohol consumption, cigarette smoking, and risk of infant leukemia: Children's Cancer Group study. *J Natl Cancer Inst* 1996;88:24.
12. Linet MS, Hatch EE, Kleinerman RA, et al. Residential exposure to magnetic fields and acute lymphoblastic leukemia in children. *N Engl J Med* 1997;337:1.
13. Tucker MA, Meadows AT, Boice JD, et al. Leukemia after therapy with alkylating agents for childhood cancer. *J Natl Cancer Inst* 1987;78:459.
14. Pui CH, Ribeiro R, Hancock M, et al. Acute myeloid leukemia in children treated with epipodophyllotoxins for acute lymphoblastic leukemia. *N Engl J Med* 1991;325:1682.
15. Busque L, Gilliland DG. Clonal evolution in acute myeloid leukemia. *Blood* 1993;82:337.
16. Pui CH, Behm FG, Crist WM. Clinical and biologic relevance of immunologic marker studies in childhood acute lymphoblastic leukemia. *Blood* 1993;82:343.
17. Faikow PJ, Singer JW, Raskind W, et al. Clonal development, stem-cell differentiation, and clinical remissions in acute nonlymphocytic leukemia. *N Engl J Med* 1987;317:468.
18. Lapidot T, Sirard C, Vormoor J, et al. A cell initiating human acute myeloid leukemia after transplantation into SCID mice. *Nature* 1994;367:645.
19. Bennett JM, Catovsky D, Daniel MT, et al. Proposed revised criteria for the classification of acute myeloid leukemia. *Ann Intern Med* 1985;103:626.
20. Bennett JM, Catovsky D, Daniel M, et al. Criteria for the diagnosis of acute leukemia of megakaryocyte lineage (M7). *Ann Intern Med* 1985;103:450.
21. Uckun FM, Gaynon PS, Sensel MG, et al. Clinical features and treatment outcome of childhood T-lineage acute lymphoblastic leukemia according to the apparent maturational stage of T-lineage leukemic blasts: a Children's Cancer Group study. *J Clin Oncol* 1997;15:2214.
22. Felix CA, Lange BJ. Leukemia in infants. *Oncologist* 1999;4:225.
23. Pui CH, Raimonde SC, Hancock ML, et al. Immunologic cytogenetic, and clinical characterization of childhood acute lymphoblastic leukemia with the t(1;19)(q23:p13) or its derivative. *J Clin Oncol* 1994;12:2601.
24. Pui CH, Behm FG, Singh B, et al. Heterogeneity of presenting features and their relation to treatment outcome in 120 children with T-cell acute lymphoblastic leukemia. *Blood* 1990;75:174.
25. Uckun FM, Sensel MG, Sun L, et al. Biology and treatment of childhood T-lineage acute lymphoblastic leukemia. *Blood* 1998;91:735.
26. Sandlund JT, Downing JR, Crist WM. Non-Hodgkin's lymphoma in childhood. *N Engl J Med* 1996;334:1238.
27. Creutzig U, Harbott J, Sperling C, et al. Clinical significance of surface antigen expression in children with acute myeloid leukemia: results of study AML-BFM-87. *Blood* 1995;86:3097.
28. Pui CH, Raimondi SC, Head DR, et al. Characterization of childhood acute leukemia with multiple myeloid and lymphoid markers at diagnosis and at relapse. *Blood* 1991;78:1327.
29. Smith FO, Lampkin BC, Bersteeg C, et al. Expression of lymphoid-associated cell surface antigens by childhood acute myeloid leukemia cells lacks prognostic significance. *Blood* 1992;79:2415.
30. Putti MC, Rondelli R, Cocito MG, et al. Expression of myeloid markers lacks prognostic impact in children treated for acute lymphoblastic leukemia: Italian experience in AIEOP-ALL 88-91 studies. *Blood* 1998;92:795.
31. Pui CH, Rubnitz JE, Hancock ML, et al. Reappraisal of the clinical and biologic significance of myeloid-associated antigen expression in childhood acute lymphoblastic leukemia. *J Clin Oncol* 1998;16:3768.
32. Rabbitts TH. Chromosomal translocations in human cancer. *Nature* 1994;372:143.
33. McLean TW, Ringold S, Neuberg D, et al. TEL/AML-1 dimerizes and is associated with a favorable outcome in childhood acute lymphoblastic leukemia. *Blood* 1996;88:4252.
34. Rubnitz JE, Shuster JJ, Land VJ, et al. Case-control study suggests a favorable impact of TEL rearrangement in patients with B-lineage acute lymphoblastic leukemia treated with antimetabolite-based therapy: a Pediatric Oncology Group study. *Blood* 1997;89:1143.
35. Uckun FM, Sensel MG, Sather HN, et al. Clinical significance of translocation t(1;19) in childhood acute lymphoblastic leukemia in the context of contemporary therapies: a report from the Children's Cancer Group. *J Clin Oncol* 1998;16:527.
36. Schrappe M, Arico M, Harbott J, et al. Philadelphia chromosome–positive (Ph+) childhood acute lymphoblastic leukemia: good initial steroid response allows early prediction of a favorable treatment outcome. *Blood* 1998;92:2730.
37. Ribeiro RC, Broniscer A, Rivera GK, et al. Philadelphia chromosome–positive acute lymphoblastic leukemia in children: durable responses to chemotherapy associated with low initial white blood cell counts. *Leukemia* 1997;11:1493.
38. Rowley JD. The critical role of chromosome translocations in human leukemias. *Annu Rev Genet* 1998;32:495.
39. Hartwell LH, Kastan MB. Cell cycle control and cancer. *Science* 1994;266:1821.
40. Quesnel B, Preudhomme C, Philippe N, et al. p16 Gene homozygous deletions in acute lymphoblastic leukemia. *Blood* 1995;85:657.
41. Trueworthy R, Shuster J, Look T, et al. Ploidy of lymphoblasts is the strongest predictor of treatment outcome in B-progenitor cell acute lymphoblastic leukemia of childhood: a Pediatric Oncology Group study. *J Clin Oncol* 1992;10:606.
42. Harris MB, Shuster JJ, Carroll A, et al. Trisomy of leukemic cell chromosomes 4 and 10 identifies children with B-progenitor cell acute lymphoblastic leukemia with a very low risk of treatment failure: a Pediatric Oncology Group study. *Blood* 1992;79:3316.
43. Whitehead VM, Vuchich MJ, Laver SJ, et al. Accumulation of high levels of methotrexate polyglutamates in lymphoblasts from children with hyperdiploid (greater than 50 chromosomes) B-lineage acute lymphoblastic leukemia: a POG study. *Blood* 1992;80:1316.
44. Ito C, Kumagai M, Manabe A, et al. Hyperdiploid acute lymphoblastic leukemia with 51 to 65 chromosomes: a distinct biological entity with a marked propensity to undergo apoptosis. *Blood* 1999;93:315.
45. Heerema NA, Nachman JB, Sather HN, et al. Hypodiploidy with less than 45 chromosomes confers adverse risk in childhood acute lymphoblastic leukemia: a report from the Children's Cancer Group. *Blood* 1999;94:4036.
46. Grimwade D, Walker H, Oliver F, et al. The importance of diagnostic cytogenetics on outcome in AML: analysis of 1,612 patients entered into the MRC AML 10 trial. *Blood* 1998;92:2322.
47. Raimondi SC, Chang MN, Ravindranath Y, et al. Chromosomal abnormalities in 478 children with acute myeloid leukemia: clinical characteristics and treatment outcome in a cooperative Pediatric Oncology Group study—POG 8821. *Blood* 1999;94:3707.
48. Sorensen P, Chen CS, Smith F, et al. Molecular rearrangements of the MLL gene are present in most cases of infant acute myeloid leukemia and are strongly correlated with monocytic or myelomonocytic phenotypes. *J Clin Invest* 1994;93:429.
49. Johansson B, Moorman AV, Haas OA, et al. Hematologic malignancies with t(4;11)(q21;q23)—a cytogenetic, morphologic, immunophenotypic and clinical study of 183 cases. European 11q23 Workshop participants. *Leukemia* 1998;12:779.
50. Carroll A, Civin C, Schneider N, et al. The t(1:22) (p13,q13) is nonrandom and restricted to infants with acute megakaryoblastic leukemia: a Pediatric Oncology Group study. *Blood* 1991;78:748.
51. Choi S, Simone JV. Acute nonlymphocytic leukemia in 171 children. *Med Pediatr Oncol* 1976;2:119.
52. Pui CH, Frankel LS, Carroll AJ, et al. Clinical characteristics and treatment outcome of childhood acute lymphoblastic leukemia with the t(4;11)(q21;q23): a collaborative study of 40 cases [See comments]. *Blood* 1991;77:440.
53. Bleyer WA, Poplack DG. Prophylaxis and treatment of leukemia in the central nervous system and other sanctuaries. *Semin Oncol* 1985;12:131.
54. Mahmoud HH, Rivera GK, Hancock ML, et al. Low leukocyte counts with blast cells in cerebrospinal fluid of children with newly diagnosed acute lymphoblastic leukemia. *N Engl J Med* 1993;329:314.
55. Gelber R, Sallan SE, Cohen HJ, et al. Central nervous system treatment in childhood acute lymphoblastic leukemia: long-term follow-up for patients diagnosed 1973–1985. *Cancer* 1993;72:261.
56. Bunin NJ, Pui CH. Differing complications of hyperleukocytosis in children with acute lymphoblastic or acute nonlymphoblastic leukemia. *J Clin Oncol* 1985;3:1590.
57. Pui CH, Kalwinsky D, Schell M, et al. Acute nonlymphoblastic leukemia in infants: clinical presentation and outcome. *J Clin Oncol* 1988;6:1008.
58. Tallman MS, Hakimian D, Shaw JM, et al. Granulocytic sarcoma is associated with the 8;21 translocation in acute myeloid leukemia. *J Clin Oncol* 1993;11:690.
59. Creutzig U, Ritter J, Buddle M, et al. Early deaths due to hemorrhage and leukostasis in childhood acute myelogenous leukemia. *Cancer* 1987;60:3071.
60. Warrell RP Jr, de The H, Wang ZY, Degos L. Acute promyelocytic leukemia. *N Engl J Med* 1993;329:177.
61. Bleyer WA. The U.S. pediatric cancer clinical trials programmes: international implications and the way forward. *Eur J Cancer* 1997;33:1439.
62. Smith M, Arthur D, Camitta B, et al. Uniform approach to risk classification and treatment assignment for children with acute lymphoblastic leukemia. *J Clin Oncol* 1996;14:18.
63. Clavell LA, Gelber RD, Cohen HJ, et al. Four agent induction and intensive asparaginase therapy for treatment of childhood acute lymphoblastic leukemia. *N Engl J Med* 1986;315:657.
64. Gaynon PS, Desai AA, Bostrom BC, et al. Early response to therapy and outcome in childhood acute lymphoblastic leukemia: a review. *Cancer* 1997;80:1717.
65. Gajjar A, Ribeiro R, Hancock ML, et al. Persistence of circulating blasts after 1 week of multiagent chemotherapy confers a poor prognosis in childhood acute lymphoblastic leukemia. *Blood* 1995;86:1292.
66. Nachman JB, Sather HN, Sensel MG, et al. Augmented post-induction therapy for children with high-risk acute lymphoblastic leukemia and a slow response to initial therapy [See comments]. *N Engl J Med* 1998;338:1663.
67. Reaman GH, Sposto R, Sensel MG, et al. Treatment outcome and prognostic factors for infants with acute lymphoblastic leukemia treated on two consecutive trials of the Children's Cancer Group [See comments]. *J Clin Oncol* 1999;17:445.
68. Bash RO, Crist WM, Shuster JJ, et al. Clinical features and outcome of T-cell acute lymphoblastic leukemia in childhood with respect to alterations at the TAL1 locus: a Pediatric Oncology Group study. *Blood* 1993;81:2110.
69. Shuster JJ, Camitta BM, Pullen J, et al. Identification of newly diagnosed children with acute lymphocytic leukemia at high risk for relapse. *Cancer Res Ther Control* 1999;9:101.

70. Chessells JM, Richards SM, Bailey CC, et al. Gender and treatment outcome in childhood lymphoblastic leukaemia: report from the MRC UKALL trials. *Br J Haematol* 1995;89:364.
71. Pui CH, Boyett JM, Hancock ML, et al. Outcome of treatment for childhood cancer in black as compared with white children. The St. Jude Children's Research Hospital experience, 1962 through 1992 [See comments]. *JAMA* 1995;273:633.
72. Shuster JJ, Wacker P, Pullen J, et al. Prognostic significance of sex in childhood B-precursor acute lymphoblastic leukemia: a Pediatric Oncology Group study. *J Clin Oncol* 1998;16:2854.
73. Lipshultz S, Lipsitz S, Mone S, et al. Female sex and higher drug dose as risk factors for late cardiotoxic effects of doxorubicin therapy for childhood cancer. *N Engl J Med* 1995;33:1738.
74. Waber D, Tarbell N, Fairclough D, et al. Cognitive sequelae of treatment in childhood acute lymphoblastic leukemia: cranial radiation requires an accomplice. *J Clin Oncol* 1995;13:2490.
75. Farber S, Diamond LK, Mercer RD, Sylvester RF, Wolff JA. Temporary remission in acute leukemia in children produced by folic acid antagonist, 4 amino pteroylglutamic acid (Aminopterin). *N Engl J Med* 1948;238:787.
76. Reiter A, Schrappe M, Ludwig WD, et al. Chemotherapy in 998 unselected childhood acute lymphoblastic leukemia patients: results and conclusions of the multicenter trial ALL-BFM 86. *Blood* 1994;84:3122.
77. Cave H, van der Werff ten Bosch J, Suciu S, et al. Clinical significance of minimal residual disease in childhood acute lymphoblastic leukemia. European Organization for Research and Treatment of Cancer—Childhood Leukemia Cooperative Group [See comments]. *N Engl J Med* 1998;339:591.
78. Dibenedetto SP, Lo NL, Mayer SP, et al. Detectable molecular residual disease at the beginning of maintenance therapy indicates poor outcome in children with T-cell acute lymphoblastic leukemia. *Blood* 1997;90:1226.
79. Pui C, Crist W. Biology and treatment of acute lymphoblastic leukemia. *J Pediatr* 1994;124:491.
80. Gaynon PS, Steinherz PG, Bleyer WA, et al. Improved therapy for children with acute lymphoblastic leukemia and unfavorable presenting features: a follow-up report of the Children's Cancer Group Study CCG-106. *J Clin Oncol* 1993;11:2234.
81. Hongeng S, Krance R, Bowman L, et al. Outcomes of transplantation with matched-sibling and unrelated-donor bone marrow in children with leukemia. *Lancet* 1997;350:767.
82. Frankel LS, Ochs J, Shuster JJ, et al. Therapeutic trial for infant acute lymphoblastic leukemia: the Pediatric Oncology Group experience (POG 8493). *J Pediatr Hematol Oncol* 1997;19:35.
83. Reiter A, Schrappe M, Tiemann M, et al. Improved treatment results in childhood B-cell neoplasms with tailored intensification of therapy: a report of the Berlin-Frankfurt-Munster Group Trial NHL-BFM 90. *Blood* 1999;94:3294.
84. Aur RJA, Hustu HO, Verzosa MS, Wood A, Simone JV. Comparison of two methods of preventing central nervous system leukemia. *Blood* 1973;42:349.
85. Freeman AI, Johnston PG, Voke JM. Somnolence after prophylactic cranial irradiation in children with acute lymphoblastic leukemia. *BMJ* 1973;4:523.
86. Pinkel D, Woo S. Prevention and treatment of meningeal leukemia in children. *Blood* 1994;84:355.
87. Ochs JJ. Neurotoxicity due to central nervous system therapy for childhood leukemia. *Am J Pediatr Hematol Oncol* 1989;11:93.
88. Smibert E, Anderson V, Godber T, et al. Risk factors for intellectual and educational sequelae of cranial irradiation in childhood acute lymphoblastic leukaemia. *Br J Cancer* 1996;73:825.
89. Nesbit ME Jr, Robison LL, Littman PS, et al. Presymptomatic central nervous system therapy in previously untreated childhood acute lymphoblastic leukemia: comparison of 1800 rad and 2400 rad: a report for Children's Cancer Study Group. *Lancet* 1981;28:461.
90. Waber DP, Tarbell NJ, Fairclough D, et al. Cognitive sequelae of treatment in childhood acute lymphoblastic leukemia: cranial radiation requires an accomplice [See comments]. *J Clin Oncol* 1995;13:2490.
91. Schrappe M, Reiter A, Riehm H. Prophylaxis and treatment of neoplastic meningeosis in childhood acute lymphoblastic leukemia. *J Neurooncol* 1998;38:159.
92. Tubergen DG, Gilchrist GS, O'Brien RT, et al. Prevention of CNS disease in intermediate-risk acute lymphoblastic leukemia: comparison of cranial radiation and intrathecal methotrexate and the importance of systemic therapy: a Childrens Cancer Group report. *J Clin Oncol* 1993;11:520.
93. Pullen J, Boyett J, Shuster J, et al. Extended triple intrathecal chemotherapy trial for prevention of CNS relapse in good-risk and poor-risk patients with B-progenitor acute lymphoblastic leukemia: a Pediatric Oncology Group study. *J Clin Oncol* 1993;11:839.
94. Mahoney DH Jr, Shuster JJ, Nitschke R, et al. Acute neurotoxicity in children with B-precursor acute lymphoid leukemia: an association with intermediate-dose intravenous methotrexate and intrathecal triple therapy—a Pediatric Oncology Group study. *J Clin Oncol* 1998;16:1712.
95. Bleyer A. CNS chemoradiotherapy of childhood leukemia: the plot thickens but the ending bodes well. *J Clin Oncol* 1995;13:2480.
96. Chessells J, Leiper A, Richards S. A second course of treatment for childhood acute lymphoblastic leukemia: long term follow-up is needed to assess results. *Br J Hematol* 1994;86:48.
97. Gaynon PS, Qu RP, Chappell RJ, et al. Survival after relapse in childhood acute lymphoblastic leukemia: impact of site and time to first relapse—the Children's Cancer Group Experience. *Cancer* 1998;82:1387.
98. Barrett AJ, Horowitz MM, Pollock BH, et al. Bone marrow transplants from HLA-identical siblings as compared with chemotherapy for children with acute lymphoblastic leukemia in a second remission. *N Engl J Med* 1994;331:1253.
99. Wheeler K, Richards S, Bailey C, Chessells J. Comparison of bone marrow transplant and chemotherapy for relapsed childhood acute lymphoblastic leukaemia: the MRC UKALL X experience. Medical Research Council Working Party on Childhood Leukaemia. *Br J Haematol* 1998;101:94.
100. Billett A, Kornmehl E, Tarbell N, et al. Autologous bone marrow transplantation after a long first remission for children with recurrent acute lymphoblastic leukemia. *Blood* 1993;81:1651.
101. Weisdorf DJ, Billett AL, Hannan P, et al. Autologous versus unrelated donor allogeneic marrow transplantation for acute lymphoblastic leukemia. *Blood* 1997;90:2962.
102. Casper J, Camitta B, Truitt R, et al. Unrelated bone marrow donor transplants for children with leukemia or myelodysplasia. *Blood* 1995;85:2354.
103. Kumar P, Kun LE, Hustu HO, et al. Survival outcome following isolated central nervous system relapsed treated with additional chemotherapy and craniospinal irradiation in childhood acute lymphoblastic leukemia [See comments]. *Int J Radiat Oncol Biol Phys* 1995;31:477.
104. Wofford MM, Smith SD, Shuster JJ, et al. Treatment of occult or late overt testicular relapse in children with acute lymphoblastic leukemia: a Pediatric Oncology Group study. *J Clin Oncol* 1992;10:624.
105. Katz JA, Pollock BH, Jacaruso D, Morad A. Final attained height in patients successfully treated for childhood acute lymphoblastic leukemia. *J Pediatr* 1993;123:546.
106. Ochs J, Mulhern R, Fairclough D, et al. Comparison of neuropsychologic functioning and clinical indicators of neurotoxicity in long-term survivors of childhood leukemia given cranial radiation or parenteral methotrexate: a prospective study. *J Clin Oncol* 1991;9:145.
107. Neglia JP, Meadows AT, Robinson LL, et al. Second neoplasms after acute lymphoblastic leukemia in childhood. *N Engl J Med* 1991;325:1330.
108. Pui CH, Relling MV, Rivera GK, et al. Epipodophyllotoxin-related acute myeloid leukemia: a study of 35 cases. *Leukemia* 1995;9:1990.
109. Hurwitz CA, Mounce KG, Grier HE. Treatment of patients with acute myelogenous leukemia: review of clinical trials of the past decade. *J Pediatr Hematol Oncol* 1995;17:185.
110. Creutzig U, Ritter J, Schellong G. Identification of two risk groups in childhood acute myelogenous leukemia after therapy intensification in study AML-BFM-83 as compared with study AML-BFM-78. *Blood* 1990;75:1932.
111. Amadori S, Testi AM, Arico M, et al. Prospective comparative study of bone marrow transplantation and postremission chemotherapy for childhood acute myelogenous leukemia. *J Clin Oncol* 1993;11:1046.
112. Nesbit M, Buckley J, Feig S, et al. Chemotherapy for induction of remission of childhood acute myeloid leukemia followed by marrow transplantation or multiagent chemotherapy: a report from the Children's Cancer Group. *J Clin Oncol* 1994;12:127.
113. Stevens RF, Hann IM, Wheatley K, et al. Marked improvements in outcome with chemotherapy alone in paediatric acute myeloid leukemia: results of the United Kingdom Medical Research Council's 10th AML trial. MRC Childhood Leukemia Working Party. *Br J Haematol* 1998;101:130.
114. Ravindranath Y, Yeager AM, Chang MN, et al. Autologous bone marrow transplantation versus intensive consolidation chemotherapy for acute myeloid leukemia in childhood. *N Engl J Med* 1996;334:1428.
115. Tallman MS, Andersen JW, Schiffer CA, et al. ALL-trans-retinoic acid in acute promyelocytic leukemia. *N Engl J Med* 1997;337:1021.
116. Castaigne S, Chomienne C, Daniel MT, et al. ALL-trans-retinoic acid as a differentiation therapy for acute promyelocytic leukemia. I. Clinical results. *Blood* 1990;76:1704.
117. Creutzis U, Ritter J, Zimmermann M, et al. Does cranial irradiation reduce the risk for bone marrow relapse in acute myelogenous leukemia? Unexpected results of the childhood acute myelogenous leukemia study BFM-87. *J Clin Oncol* 1993;11:279.
118. Woods WG, Kobrinsky N, Buckley JD, et al. Timed-sequential induction therapy improves postremission outcome in acute myeloid leukemia: a report from the Children's Cancer Group. *Blood* 1996;87:4979.
119. Woods WG, Ruyman FB, Lampkin B, et al. The role of timing of high-dose cytosine arabinoside intensification and of maintenance therapy in the treatment of children with acute nonlymphocytic leukemia. *Cancer* 1990;66:1106.
120. Sanders JE, Thomas ED, Buckner CE, et al. Marrow transplantation of children in first remission of acute nonlymphoblastic leukemia: an update. *Blood* 1985;66:460.
121. Brochstein JA, Kornan NA, Groshen S, et al. Allogeneic bone marrow transplantation versus intensive consolidation chemotherapy for acute myeloid leukemia in childhood. *N Engl J Med* 1996;334:1428.
122. Yaeger AM, Kaizer H, Santos GW, et al. Autologous bone marrow transplantations in patients with acute nonlymphocytic leukemia, using *ex vivo* marrow treated with 4-hydroperoxycyclophosphamide. *N Engl J Med* 1986;315:141.
123. Webb D, Wheatley K, Harrison G, et al. Outcome for children with relapsed acute myeloid leukemia following initial therapy in the Medical Research Council (MRC) AML 10 trial. *Leukemia* 1999;13:25.
124. Clift RA, Buckner CD, Thomas ED, et al. The treatment of acute non-lymphoblastic leukemia by allogeneic marrow transplantation. *Bone Marrow Transplant* 1987;2:243.
125. Steuber C, Krischer J, Holbrook T, et al. Therapy of refractory or recurrent acute myeloid leukemia using amsacrine and etoposide with or without azacytidene: a Pediatric Oncology Group randomized phase II study. *J Clin Oncol* 1996;14:1521.
126. Wagner JE, Rosenthal J, Sweetman R, et al. Successful transplantation of HLA-matched and HLA mismatched umbilical cord blood from unrelated donors: analysis of engraftment and acute graft versus host disease. *Blood* 1996;88:795.
127. Arceci RJ. Clinical significance of P-glycoprotein in multidrug resistance malignancies. *Blood* 1993;81:2215.
128. Wekerle T, Sykes M. Mixed chimerism as an approach for the induction of transplantation tolerance. *Transplantation* 1999;68:459.
129. Druker B, Resta M, Peng B, et al. Clinical efficacy and safety of an abl specific tyrosine kinase inhibitor as targeted therapy for chronic myelogenous leukemia. *Blood* 1999;94[Suppl 1]:368a(abst 1639).
130. Murphy SB. Classification, staging and end results of treatment in childhood non-Hodgkin's lymphoma: dissimilarities from lymphomas in adults. *Semin Oncol* 1980;7:332.
131. Murphy S, Fairclough D, Hutchison R, et al. NHL of childhood. An analysis of the histology, staging and response to treatment of 338 cases at a single institution. *J Clin Oncol* 1989;7:186.

132. Reiter A, Schrappe M, Parwasesch R, et al. Non-Hodgkin's lymphomas of childhood and adolescence: results of a treatment stratified for biologic subtypes and stage—a report of the Berlin-Frankfort-Munster Group. *J Clin Oncol* 1995;13:359.
133. Link MP, Shuster JJ, Donaldson SS, et al. Treatment of children and young adults with early-stage non-Hodgkin's lymphoma. *N Engl J Med* 1997;337:1259.
134. Filipovich AH, Mathur A, Kamat D, Shapiro RS. Primary immunodeficiencies: genetic risk factors for lymphoma. *Cancer Res* 1992;52[Suppl]:5465S.
135. Taylor A, Metcalfe J, Thick J, Mak Y. Leukemia and lymphoma in ataxia telangiectasia. *Blood* 1996;87:423.
136. Fischer A, Blanche S, LeBidois J, et al. Anti-B cell monoclonal antibodies in the treatment of severe B-cell lymphoproliferative syndrome following bone marrow and organ transplantation. *N Engl J Med* 1991;324:1451.
137. McClain KL, Joshi VV, Murphy SB. Cancers in children with HIV infection. *Hematol Oncol Clin North Am* 1996;10:1189.
138. Anagnostopoulos I, Herbst H, Niedobitek G, Stein H. Demonstration of monoclonal EBV genomes in Hodgkin's disease and Ki-1-positive anaplastic large cell lymphoma by combined Southern blot and *in situ* hybridization. *Blood* 1989;74:810.
139. McClain K, Leach C, Jenson H, et al. Association of Epstein-Barr virus with leiomyosarcomas in young people with AIDS. *N Engl J Med* 1995;332:12.
140. The Non-Hodgkin's Lymphoma Pathologic Classification Project. National Cancer Institute sponsored study of classifications of non-Hodgkin's lymphomas: summary and description of a working formulation for clinical usage. *Cancer* 1982;49:2112.
141. Harris N, Jaffe E, Stein H, et al. A revised European-American classification of lymphoid neoplasms: a proposal from the International Lymphoma Study Group. *Blood* 1994;84:1361.
142. Nathwani B, Diamond L, Windberg C, et al. Lymphoblastic lymphoma: a clinical pathologic study of 95 patients. *Cancer* 1981;48:2347.
143. Link MP, Roper M, Dorfman RF, et al. Cutaneous lymphoblastic lymphoma with pre-B markers. *Blood* 1983;61:838.
144. Finger L, Harvey R, Moore R, et al. A common mechanism of chromosomal translocation in T and B cell neoplasia. *Science* 1986;234:982.
145. Brown L, Gheng JT, Chen Q, et al. Site-specific recombination of the tal-1 gene is a common occurrence in human T cell leukemia. *EMBO J* 1990;9:3343.
146. King DR, Patrick LE, Ginn-Pease ME, et al. Pulmonary function is compromised in children with mediastinal lymphoma. *J Pediatr Surg* 1997;32:294.
147. Shamberger RC, Holzman RS, Griscom NT, et al. Prospective evaluation by computed tomography and pulmonary function tests of children with mediastinal masses. *Surgery* 1995;118:468.
148. Glatstein E, Kim H, Donaldson S, et al. Non-Hodgkin's lymphomas. VI. Results of treatment in childhood. *Cancer* 1974;34:204.
149. Aur R, Hustu H, Simone J, et al. Therapy of localized and regional lymphosarcoma of childhood. *Cancer* 1971;27:1328.
150. Anderson JR, Jenkin RD, Wilson JF, et al. Long-term follow-up of patients treated with COMP or LSA2L2 therapy for childhood non-Hodgkin's lymphoma: a report of CCG-551 from the Children's Cancer Group. *J Clin Oncol* 1993;11:1024.
151. Meadows A, Sposto R, Jenkin R, et al. Similar efficacy of 6 and 18 months of therapy with four drugs (COMP) for localized non-Hodgkin's lymphoma of children: a report from the Childrens Cancer Study Group. *J Clin Oncol* 1989;7:92.
152. Wollner N, Burchenal J, Liebermann P, et al. Non-Hodgkin's lymphoma in children: a comparative study of two modalities of therapy. *Cancer* 1976;37:123.
153. Weinstein HJ, Cassady JR, Levey R. Long-term results of the APO protocol (vincristine, doxorubicin (adriamycin), and prednisone) for treatment of mediastinal lymphoblastic lymphoma. *J Clin Oncol* 1983;1:537.
154. Reiter A, Schrappe M, Ludwig WB, et al. Intensive ALL type therapy without local radiotherapy provides a 90% event free survival for children with T-cell lymphoblastic lymphoma: a BFM Group report. *Blood* 2000;95:416.
155. Chopra R, Goldstone A, Pearce R, et al. Autologous versus allogeneic bone marrow transplantation for non-Hodgkin's lymphoma: a case controlled analysis of the European Bone Marrow Transplant Group registry data. *J Clin Oncol* 1992;10:1690.
156. Burkitt D. The discovery of Burkitt's lymphoma. *Cancer* 1983;51:1777.
157. Ziegler JL. Burkitt's lymphoma. *N Engl J Med* 1981;30:735.
158. Hutchinson R, Murphy S, Fairclough D, et al. Diffuse small noncleaved cell lymphoma in children, Burkitt versus non-Burkitt's types. *Cancer* 1989;64:23.
159. Patte C, Phillip T, Rodary C, et al. High survival rate in advanced stage B-cell lymphomas and leukemias without CNS involvement with a short intensive polychemotherapy. Results from the French Pediatric Oncology Society of a randomized trial of 216 children. *J Clin Oncol* 1991;9:123.
160. Bowman WP, Shuster JJ, Cook B, et al. Improved survival for children with B-cell acute lymphoblastic leukemia and stage IV small noncleaved-cell lymphoma: a Pediatric Oncology Group study. *J Clin Oncol* 1996;14:1252.
161. Abshire TC, Buchanan GR, Jackson JF, et al. Morphologic, immunologic and cytogenetic studies in children with acute lymphoblastic leukemia at diagnosis and relapse: a Pediatric Oncology Group study. *Leukemia* 1992;6:357.
162. Shiramizu B, Barriga F, Neeguaye J, et al. Patterns of chromosomal breakpoint locations in Burkitt's lymphoma: relevance to geography and Epstein-Barr virus association. *Blood* 1991;77:1516.
163. Zervos AS, Gyuris J, Brent R. Mxi1, a protein that specifically interacts with Max to bind Myc-Max recognition sites. *Cell* 1993;72:223.
164. Adams JM, Harris AW, Pinkert CA, et al. The c-myc oncogene driven by immunoglobulin enhancers induces lymphoid malignancy in transgenic mice. *Nature* 1985;318:533.
165. Strauss S, Cohen J, Tosado G. et al. Epstein-Barr virus infections: biology, pathogenesis, and management. *Ann Intern Med* 1993;118:45.
166. Niedobitek G, Agathanggelou A, Rowe M, et al. Heterogeneous expression of Epstein-Barr virus latent proteins in endemic Burkitt's lymphoma. *Blood* 1995;86:659.
167. Shamberger R, Weinstein HJ. The role of surgery in abdominal Burkitt's lymphoma. *J Pediatr Surg* 1992;27:236.
168. Cohen LF, Balow JE, Magrath IT, Poplack DG, Ziegler JL. Acute tumor lysis syndrome. A review of 37 patients with Burkitt's lymphoma. *Am J Med* 1980;68:486.
169. Ziegler JL. Chemotherapy of Burkitt's lymphoma. *Cancer* 1972;30:1534.
170. Olweny C, Keatongole-Mbidde E, Kaddu-Mukasa A, et al. Treatment of Burkitt's lymphoma: randomized clinical trial of single agent versus combination chemotherapy. *Int J Cancer* 1976;17:436.
171. Ziegler JL. Treatment results of 54 American patients with Burkitt's lymphoma are similar to the African experience. *N Engl J Med* 1977;297:75.
172. Ladenstein R, Pearce R, Hartmann O, et al. High-dose chemotherapy with autologous bone marrow rescue in children with poor-risk Burkitt's lymphoma: a report from the European Lymphoma Bone Marrow Transplantation Registry. *Blood* 1997;90:2921.
173. Sandlund J, Pui C, Santana V, et al. Clinical features and treatment outcome for children with CD30+ large cell NHL. *J Clin Oncol* 1994;12:895.
174. Sandlund J, Pui CH, Roberts M, et al. Clinicopathologic features and treatment outcome of children with large cell lymphoma and the t(2;5) (p23,q35). *Blood* 1994;84:2467.
175. Morris SW, Kirstein MN, Valentine MB, et al. Fusion of a kinase gene ALK, to a nucleolar protein gene, NPM, in non-Hodgkin's lymphoma. *Science* 1994;263:1281.
176. Weinstein HJ, Lack E, Cassady JR. APO therapy for malignant lymphoma of large cell "histiocytic" type of childhood: analysis of treatment results for 29 patients. *Blood* 1984;64:422.
177. Santana VM, Abromowitch M, Sandlund JT, et al. MACOP-B treatment in children and adolescents with advanced diffuse large-cell non-Hodgkin's lymphoma. *Leukemia* 1993;7:187.
178. Hvizdala EV, Berard C, Calihan T. Nonlymphoblastic lymphoma in children—histology and stage-related response to therapy: a pediatric oncology group study. *J Clin Oncol* 1991;9:1189.
179. Pick T, Weinstein HJ, Schwenn M, et al. Treatment of advanced stage large cell non-Hodgkin's lymphoma in childhood. A Pediatric Oncology Group study (8615). *Blood* 1993;82:333a.
180. Hutchinson R, Berard C, Shuster J, et al. B-cell lineage confers a favorable outcome among children and adolescents with large cell lymphoma: a Pediatric Oncology Group study. *J Clin Oncol* 1995;13:2023.
181. Sandlund JT, Santana V, Abromowitch M, et al. Large cell non-Hodgkin lymphoma of childhood: clinical characteristics and outcome. *Leukemia* 1994;8:30.
182. Cleary S, Link M, Donaldson S. Hodgkin's disease in the very young. *Int J Radiat Oncol Biol Phys* 1994;28:77.
183. Donaldson SS, Link MP. Hodgkin's disease: treatment of the young child. *Pediatr Clin North Am* 1991;38:457.
184. Mauch PM. Controversies in the management of early stage Hodgkin's disease. *Blood* 1994;83:318.
185. Mauch PM, Weinstein H, Botnick L, Belli J, Cassady JR. An evaluation of long-term survival and treatment complications in children with Hodgkin's disease. *Cancer* 1988;51:925.
186. Hunger S, Link M, Donaldson S. Long-term results of ABVD/MOPP and low dose involved field radiotherapy (LDFRT) in pediatric Hodgkin's disease: the Stanford Experiences. *J Clin Oncol* 1993;12:386.
187. Horning SJ, Rosenberg SA, Hoppe RT. Brief chemotherapy (Stanford V) and adjuvant radiotherapy for bulky or advanced Hodgkin's disease: an update. *Ann Oncol* 1996;7[Suppl 4]:105.
188. William K, Cox R, Donaldson S. Radiation induced height impairment in pediatric Hodgkin's disease. *Int J Radiat Oncol Biol Phys* 1994;28:85.
189. Tarbell NJ, Gelber RD, Weinstein HJ, Mauch P. Sex differences in risk of second malignant tumors after Hodgkin's disease in childhood. *Lancet* 1993;341:1428.
190. Bhatig S, Robison L, Oberlin O, et al. Breast cancer and other second neoplasms after childhood Hodgkin's disease. *N Engl J Med* 1996;334:745.
191. Donaldson SS, Link MP. Combined modality treatment with low-dose radiation and MOPP chemotherapy for children with Hodgkin's disease. *J Clin Oncol* 1987;5:742.
192. Jenkin D, Doyle J, Berry M, et al. Hodgkin's disease in children: treatment with MOPP and low-dose, extended field irradiation without laparotomy. Late results and toxicity. *Med Pediatr Oncol* 1990;18:265.
193. Amblinder RF, Browning PJ, Lorenzana I, et al. Epstein-Barr virus and childhood Hodgkin's disease in Honduras and the United States. *Blood* 1993;81:462.
194. Mauch P, Tarbell NJ, Weinstein HJ, et al. Stage IA–IIA supradiaphragmatic Hodgkin's disease: prognostic factors in surgically staged patients. *J Clin Oncol* 1988;6:1576.
195. Karayalcin G, Behm FG, Gieser PW, et al. Lymphocyte predominant Hodgkin's disease: clinico-pathologic features and results of treatment—the Pediatric Oncology Group experience. *Med Pediatr Oncol* 1997;29:519.
196. Mendenhall N, Cantor A, Williams J, et al. With modern techniques, is staging laparotomy necessary in pediatric Hodgkin's disease? A Pediatric Oncology Group study. *J Clin Oncol* 1993;11:2218.
197. Breuer CK, Tarbell NJ, Mauch PM, et al. The importance of staging laparotomy in pediatric Hodgkin's disease. *J Pediatr Surg* 1994;29:1085.
198. Zinzani PL, Zompatori M, Bendandi M, et al. Monitoring bulky mediastinal disease with gallium-67, CT-scan and magnetic resonance imaging in Hodgkin's disease and high-grade non-Hodgkin's lymphoma. *Leuk Lymphoma* 1996;22(1–2):131.
199. The Advisory Committee on Immunization Practices (ACIP). Recommendations of the Advisory Committee on Immunization Practices (ACIP): use of vaccines and immune globulins for persons with altered immunocompetence. *MMWR Morb Mortal Wkly Rep* 1993;42(RR-4):1.
200. Donaldson SS, Whitaker SJ, Plowman PN, et al. Stage I–II pediatric Hodgkin's disease: long-term follow-up demonstrates equivalent survival rates following different management schemes. *J Clin Oncol* 1990;8:1128.
201. Shah AB, Hudson MM, Poquette CA, et al. Long-term follow-up of patients treated with primary radiotherapy for supradiaphragmatic Hodgkin's disease at St. Jude Children's Research Hospital. *Int J Radiat Oncol Biol Phys* 1999;44:867.

202. Maity A, Goldwein JW, Lange B, D'Angio JG. Comparison of high-dose and low-dose radiation with and without chemotherapy for children with Hodgkin's disease: an analysis of the experience at the Children's Hospital of Philadelphia and the Hospital of the University of Pennsylvania. *J Clin Oncol* 1992;10:929.
203. Constine LS, Donaldson SS, McDougall IR, et al. Thyroid dysfunction after radiotherapy in children with Hodgkin's disease. *Cancer* 1984;53:878.
204. Sankila R, Garwicz S, Olsen JH, et al. Risk of subsequent malignant neoplasms among 1,641 Hodgkin's disease patients diagnosed in childhood and adolescence: a population-based cohort study in the five Nordic countries. *J Clin Oncol* 1996;14:1442.
205. Schellong G. The balance between cure and late effects in childhood Hodgkin's lymphoma: the experience of the German-Austrian Study Group since 1978. German-Austrian Pediatric Hodgkin's Disease Study Group. *Ann Oncol* 1996;7[Suppl 4]:67.
206. Oberlin O, Leverger G, Pacquement H, et al. Low dose radiation therapy and reduced chemotherapy in childhood Hodgkin's disease: the experience of the French Society of Pediatric Oncology. *J Clin Oncol* 1992;10:1602.
207. Schellong G, Potter R, Bramswig J, et al. High cure rate and reduced long-term toxicity in pediatric Hodgkin's disease: the German-Austrian Multicenter Trial DAL-HD-90. *J Clin Oncol* 1999;17:3736.
208. Ekert H, Waters KD, Smith PF, Toogood I, Mauger D. Treatment with MOPP and CHIVPP chemotherapy only for all stages of childhood Hodgkin's disease. *J Clin Oncol* 1988;6:1845.
209. Kung F, Behm F, Cantor A, et al. Abbreviated chemotherapy versus chemoradiotherapy in early stage Hodgkin's disease. *Proc Am Soc Clin Oncol* 1993;12:414.
210. Weiner MA, Leventhal B, Brecher ML, et al. Randomized study of intensive MOPP-ABVD with or without low dose total-nodal radiation therapy in the treatment of stages IIB, IIIA2, IIIB, and IV Hodgkin's disease in pediatric patients: a Pediatric Oncology Group study. *J Clin Oncol* 1997;15:2769.
211. Hudson MM, Greenwald C, Thompson E, et al. Efficacy and toxicity of multiagent treatment with chemotherapy and low-dose involved-field radiotherapy in children and adolescents with Hodgkin's disease. *J Clin Oncol* 1993;11:100.

JAMES O. ARMITAGE
PETER M. MAUCH
NANCY LEE HARRIS
PHILIP BIERMAN

SECTION 3

Non-Hodgkin's Lymphomas

Neoplasms of lymphoid cells can present clinically as leukemia, lymphoma, and myeloma. Leukemia and myeloma are dealt with in separate chapters in this text (see individual Chapters 46.1, 46.2, 46.3, 46.4, and 46.5). Lymphomas (i.e., the solid tumors of lymphoid cells) are typically subdivided into Hodgkin's disease (see Chapter 45.6) and non-Hodgkin's lymphomas (NHL), the topic of this chapter.

Our knowledge of the biology of NHLs has increased dramatically over the last decade. This is reflected in an improved system of classification that categorizes patients in a more clinically relevant way. New insights into the immunology and genetics of lymphomas have offered new therapeutic opportunities. Some of these, such as monoclonal antibodies directed against specific proteins on the surface of malignant lymphoma cells, have already become widely applied.

It has been known for more than 30 years that some patients with NHL can be cured using chemotherapy. Those clinical factors that predict curability are now well known. The prognostic effect of clinical variables such as age, stage, performance status, serum lactic dehydrogenase level, and specific sites of involvement must be mediated through expression of certain genes. The next improvement in lymphoma classification, improved prognostic categories, and new opportunities for therapy will come as the patterns of gene expression that underlie clinical variables become increasingly apparent.

EPIDEMIOLOGY

In 2000 it is estimated that there will be 54,900 new cases of NHL diagnosed in the United States, and that 26,100 people will die with this diagnosis.[1] NHL accounts for 5% of new cancers in men and 4% of new cancers in women each year in the United States and is responsible for 5% of deaths. In 1997, NHL was reported to be the leading cause of death from cancer in men between the ages of 20 and 39.

According to the Surveillance, Epidemiology, and End Results program of the National Cancer Institute, the U.S. age-adjusted incidence rate for NHL was 15.5 per 100,000 in 1996.[2] International NHL incidence rates vary as much as fivefold. The highest reported incidence rates are in the United States, and also Europe and Australia, while the lowest rates have generally been reported in Asia.[3–5]

NHL is more common in male subjects, with a reported incidence of 19.2 per 100,000 as compared with 12.2 per 100,000 for women.[2] In some sites, such as the thyroid, NHL incidence may be higher in women, however.[6] The incidence rate for whites is 15.9 per 100,000 as compared with 12.0 per 100,000 for African Americans. The NHL incidence rate for white male subjects is approximately 54% higher than Japanese Americans and 27% higher than Chinese Americans.[3] Incidence rates are also lower among Native Americans and Hispanics.[2]

The median age of NHL diagnosis was 65 years in the American College of Surgeons' National Cancer Data Base.[7] NHL incidence increases with age and peaks in the 80 to 84 age group (Fig. 45.3-1). In the period between 1992 and 1996, the incidence rate for white men in this age group was 131.5 per 100,000.[2] Incidence rates have tripled for patients older than 65 years of age.[8]

There has been a striking increase in NHL incidence rates over the last four decades that has been referred to as an epidemic of NHL. The lifetime risk of being diagnosed with NHL is 2.08%.[2] The incidence rate for white men and women increased 150% between the late 1940s to the late 1980s.[3] The incidence rate is increasing approximately 3% per year and has increased

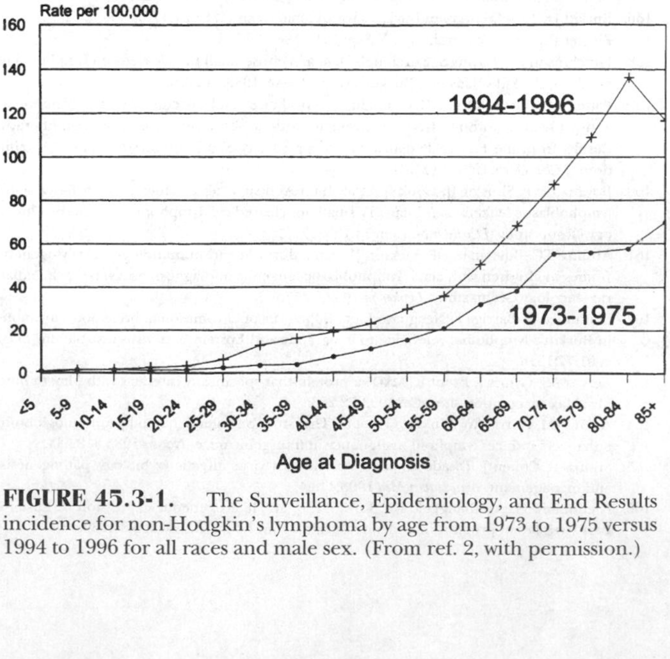

FIGURE 45.3-1. The Surveillance, Epidemiology, and End Results incidence for non-Hodgkin's lymphoma by age from 1973 to 1975 versus 1994 to 1996 for all races and male sex. (From ref. 2, with permission.)

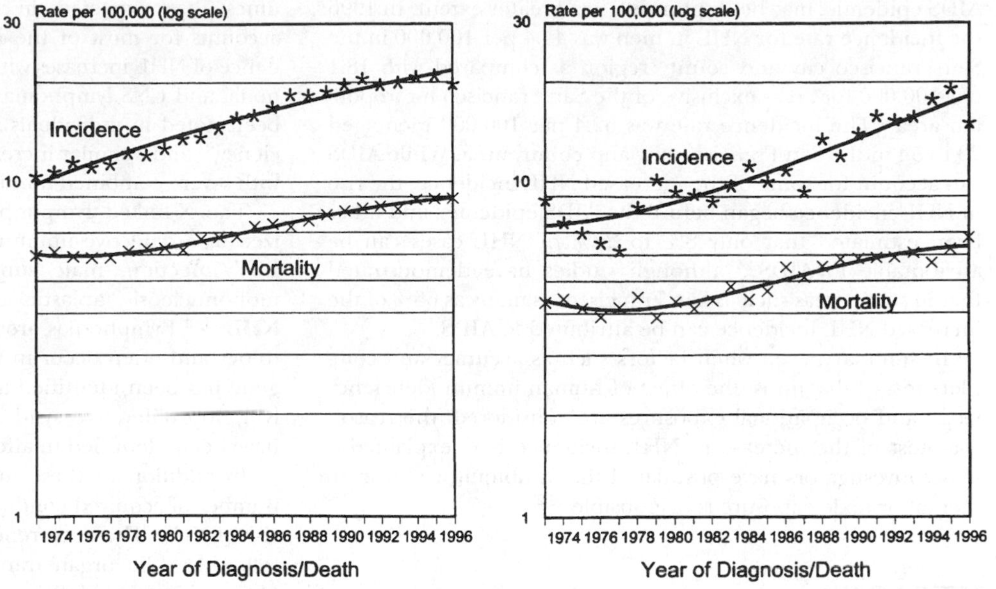

A,B

FIGURE 45.3-2. Surveillance, Epidemiology, and End Results incidence and U.S. mortality for non-Hodgkin's lymphoma for male sex and by race. **A:** White. **B:** Black. (From ref. 2, with permission.)

more than 80% since 1973 (Fig. 45.3-2). An increase in incidence has been observed in all geographic areas of the United States, although the largest increase has been from the San Francisco area.[2,9] A registry analysis from seven European countries showed that the incidence rate for NHL increased 4.8% each year between 1985 and 1992.[10] Similar increases in NHL incidence have been noted in international cancer registries in addition to well-defined population-based registries.[5,8,11]

There has been an increase in all histologic types of NHL except for diffuse small cleaved histology.[2,6] The decreasing incidence of this histology probably reflects the reclassification of most of these biopsies to a diagnosis of mantle cell histology. The largest increases have occurred in patients with high-grade lymphomas.[2,3] The incidence of extranodal lymphomas has increased more rapidly than nodal disease in some reports,[3,6,8] whereas others have noted similar increases in the incidence of nodal and extranodal disease.[4] The incidence of primary CNS lymphoma in the United States increased more than tenfold between 1973 and 1991 to 1992.[12] This increase is undoubtedly related to the occurrence of primary CNS lymphomas in patients with acquired immunodeficiency syndrome (AIDS),[13] although the increase in incidence began before the AIDS epidemic, and incidence rates have increased in non-AIDS populations.[8,12] Furthermore, some studies have failed to show evidence of an increasing incidence of primary CNS lymphoma in non-AIDS populations.[14,15]

Geographic differences in histologic subtypes of NHL have been noted. Examples include the endemic form of Burkitt's lymphoma, which is seen most commonly in children in equatorial Africa.[16] Higher rates of gastric lymphoma have been reported to occur in Northern Italy.[17] Other examples include nasal T-cell lymphomas, which are most common in China, certain small intestinal lymphomas, which are most common in the Middle East, and adult T-cell leukemia/lymphoma (ATL), which is most common in southern Japan and the Caribbean. Several reports have shown a lower incidence of follicular lymphomas in Asia and in developing countries.[18–20] The incidence of follicular lymphomas is lower in Asian immigrants to the United States as compared with later generations, suggesting an environmental influence.[21] Geographic differences in the distribution of mantle cell lymphoma, certain T-cell lymphomas, and in the incidence of primary extranodal lymphomas have also been described.[4,20]

The mortality for NHL has also increased steadily over the last four decades, although mortality increased more slowly than incidence (see Fig. 45.3-2). Increasing mortality suggests that increased incidence rates cannot be entirely due to artifacts of improved detection.[8,22] Between 1973 and 1996 the U.S. mortality increased from 4.7 per 100,000 to 6.9 per 100,000.[2] Mortality for NHL is approximately 20% higher in urban areas when compared with rural areas, and rates are higher in counties with higher median education levels among residents.[3]

Several hypotheses have been used to explain the increasing incidence of NHL. Some of the increase may be artifactual. For example, new NHL classification systems and techniques such as gene rearrangement studies have led to a diagnosis of NHL in some patients who would have previously had other diagnoses such as pseudolymphoma or atypical lymphoid hyperplasia.[3] This is especially true for entities such as lymphomas of mucosa-associated lymphoid tissue (MALT) as well as certain T-cell lymphomas that might have previously been given diagnoses such as angioimmunoblastic lymphadenopathy. However, these changes in diagnosis can only account for a small fraction of the increase in incidence.[8,23] In addition, improved imaging techniques have undoubtedly led to more NHL diagnoses, particularly for primary CNS lymphoma, and less invasive biopsy techniques have led to more vigorous attempts at establishing a diagnosis than before.[3] Finally, some increase in NHL incidence can be attributed to reclassification of cases that would have previously been called Hodgkin's disease.[3,5,8,23] It has been estimated that this may account for 10% to 15% of cases,[23] although in some series more than 25% of Hodgkin's disease patients were reclassified as NHL.[5] However, such large discrepancies apply mostly to cases diagnosed before the 1970s and are unlikely to be responsible for much of the later increase in incidence.[23,24] While these artifacts have undoubtedly led to some increase in the reported incidence of NHL, they can only account for a small fraction of the increase.[25]

The aging U.S. population can account for only a small increase in NHL incidence, although other factors, such as the

AIDS epidemic, may be responsible to a greater extent. In 1996 the incidence rate for NHL in men was 44.4 per 100,000 in the San Francisco city and county region as compared with 18.1 per 100,000 for areas exclusive of the San Francisco metropolitan area.[2] The incidence rate was 62.4 per 100,000 men aged 20 to 54 in the San Francisco city and county area. While AIDS can account for some of the increased NHL incidence, the rise in NHL incidence began before the AIDS epidemic, and it has been estimated that only 8% to 27% of NHL cases can be attributable to AIDS,[26] although studies have demonstrated that in some areas such as San Francisco, as many as 66% of the increased NHL incidence can be attributed to AIDS.[13]

In summary, even when factors such as accuracy and completeness of diagnosis, the effect of human immunodeficiency virus, and occupational exposures are considered, the reason for most of the increase in NHL incidence is unexplained.[24] Many investigators have postulated that a ubiquitous environmental or toxic exposure is responsible.[22,25]

ETIOLOGY

The cause of most cases of NHL is unknown, although several genetic diseases, environmental agents, and infectious agents have been associated with the development of lymphoma. Although the existence of a familial NHL risk is debated, familial aggregations of NHL have been described, and some studies have shown a higher risk of NHL in siblings or first-degree relatives of people with lymphoma or other hematologic malignancies.[27–29] Three categories of familial aggregates have been described.[28] The first consists of male preadolescents and adolescent siblings who often have extranodal lymphoma. The second category consists of adult siblings with NHL, and the third is represented by adults with NHL from two or more generations. Familial clustering may reflect a true genetic susceptibility or a shared environmental exposure.[29,30] In some cases, affected individuals in familial clusters have had well-defined or subtle immune deficiencies.[28,29] In one study, no evidence of germline p53 mutations was noted in unaffected members of lymphoma-prone kindreds.[31]

IMMUNODEFICIENCY

Several rare inherited disorders are associated with as much as a 25% risk of developing lymphoma.[32,33] These disorders include severe combined immunodeficiency, hypogammaglobulinemia, common variable immunodeficiency, Wiskott-Aldrich syndrome, and ataxia-telangiectasia. Lymphomas associated with these disorders are often associated with Epstein-Barr virus (EBV) and vary in appearance from polyclonal B-cell hyperplasia at one end of the spectrum to monoclonal lymphomas at the other end.[32,34]

Ataxia-telangiectasia is an autosomal recessive multisystem disorder associated with a risk of lymphoma that is increased more than 250-fold in affected individuals.[35] Both B-cell and T-cell NHL has been described.[36] A mutated ataxia-telangiectasia gene (ATM) has been cloned and localized to chromosome 11. Mutations are thought to inactivate or eliminate a protein involved with control of cell-cycle checkpoints responding to DNA damage.[37] Mutations and deletions of ATM have also been identified in chronic lymphocytic leukemia and mantle cell lymphoma.[38,39]

The Wiskott-Aldrich syndrome is an X-linked recessive disorder. The relative risk of developing malignancy is more than 100 times that expected in the general population.[33,40] NHL accounts for most of the increased cancer risk, and the incidence of NHL increases with age. Patients frequently have extranodal and CNS lymphomas. A 30-fold excess of lymphoma has been noted in individuals with common variable immunodeficiency,[41] and a similar increase in risk has been noted in patients with severe combined immunodeficiency syndrome.[33]

The X-linked lymphoproliferative syndrome is characterized by a defective immune response to EBV.[42] After primary EBV infection, male subjects can develop fatal infectious mononucleosis, aplastic anemia, dysgammaglobulinemia, or NHL.[43,44] Lymphomas are frequently of small noncleaved histology and often occur in the ileocecal region.[33] The SH2D1A gene has been identified as the gene responsible for X-linked lymphoproliferative syndrome, and mutations and deletions have been identified in affected individuals.[44,45]

In addition to these inherited immunodeficiency states, a number of acquired conditions are associated with an increased risk of NHL. The occurrence of NHL in patients with AIDS and following solid organ transplantation are discussed later (see Human Immunodeficiency Virus–Associated Non-Hodgkin's Lymphoma and Posttransplant Lymphoproliferative Disorders, later in this chapter). Patients with a variety of autoimmune disorders also have an increased risk of developing NHL.

Several registry-based studies and case-control studies have shown that the risk of developing NHL is increased approximately twofold in patients with rheumatoid arthritis.[46–48] Other series have failed to find an increased risk, however.[49] EBV-related lymphoproliferative disorders have also been seen in patients receiving methotrexate and other immunosuppressive drugs for rheumatoid arthritis and similar disorders.[50] These lymphomas may undergo regression on withdrawal of immunosuppression.

The risk of developing NHL in association with Sjögren's syndrome is increased approximately 30- to 40-fold.[46,51,52] These lymphomas are usually marginal zone lymphomas that most commonly occur in salivary glands and other extranodal sites such as the stomach and lung.[51,53] Another condition associated with NHL is Hashimoto's thyroiditis. Most cases of thyroid lymphoma occur in association with thyroiditis.[54] NHL may also be more common in patients with systemic lupus erythematosus.[55] Celiac sprue is associated with poor-prognosis lymphomas that are now classified as enteropathy-type intestinal T-cell lymphomas.[56,57]

INFECTIOUS AGENTS

EBV was discovered in cell lines from tumors of patients with African (endemic) Burkitt's lymphoma. EBV DNA is associated with 95% of endemic Burkitt's lymphomas, and less commonly with sporadic Burkitt's lymphoma.[58,59] Both type A and type B EBV strains are observed.[60] Since EBV is not seen in all cases of Burkitt's lymphoma, the actual relationship and the mechanism by which EBV might contribute to the development of Burkitt's lymphoma is unknown.[59,61] Burkitt's lymphoma is associated with c-myc deregulation, although different chromosome 8 breakpoints are observed in the endemic and sporadic forms, and the presence or absence of EBV DNA is related to the breakpoint location.[62] It is hypothesized that early EBV infection and environmental factors may increase the numbers of EBV-infected precursors and the risk of genetic error.[58]

EBV is also linked to posttransplant lymphoproliferative disorders (PTLDs), some AIDS-associated lymphomas, and some lymphomas associated with congenital immunodeficiency. Virtually all AIDS-associated primary CNS lymphomas have EBV in the tumor clone, although EBV is associated with other AIDS-associated lymphomas less frequently.[63] Following EBV infection, normal host immune responses mediated by T lymphocytes suppress EBV-induced proliferation.[64] In patients with depressed T-cell immunity, clones of EBV-transformed B cells can proliferate, leading to the development of lymphoma. The pattern of EBV-associated nuclear proteins in AIDS-associated Burkitt's lymphomas differs from large cell lymphomas.[63] C-myc activation in the absence of EBV infection can occur in AIDS-associated lymphomas.[65] The EBV latent membrane protein 1 is a viral analogue of the tumor necrosis factor receptor. The activity of this protein is similar to activated CD40 and is essential for *in vitro* transformation of B cells by EBV.[64,66] In EBV-positive AIDS-associated NHL and PTLD, it appears that latent membrane protein 1 binds to members of the tumor necrosis factor receptor–associated factor family and activates the NF-κB transcription factor, leading to cellular proliferation.[66] EBV is also seen in association with human-herpesvirus-8 (HHV-8) in primary effusion lymphomas.

The human T-cell lymphotropic virus type I (HTLV-I) was the first human retrovirus associated with a malignancy. HTLV-I is a type C RNA virus that is responsible for ATL in addition to HTLV-I–associated myelopathy/tropical spastic paraparesis and other disorders.[67] HTLV-I is primarily transmitted by means of breast feeding, sexual contact, and blood transfusion. The latent period between infection and development of ATL is several decades.[59,68] HTLV-I seropositivity and ATL are most prevalent in southern Japan, South America, Africa, and the Caribbean,[69] although ATL is sometimes seen in the United States.[70] In endemic areas more than 50% of all NHL cases are ATL, although the risk of developing disease is only approximately 5% in infected patients.[69] The HTLV-I genome contains the regulatory *tax* gene, whose product is a potent transcriptional activator of several genes and is thought to be responsible for the transforming features of HTLV-I.[67,68,71] The risk of ATL may be higher in patients with higher anti–HTLV-I titers and lower reactivity to *tax*.[72]

A third virus associated with NHL is HHV-8. This virus was originally discovered in Kaposi's sarcoma lesions from AIDS patients and was called *Kaposi's sarcoma–associated herpesvirus*.[73] The virus is also associated with multicentric Castleman's disease.[74] An analysis of 193 lymphoma specimens from patients with and without AIDS identified the presence of virus in only eight specimens, all of which were from patients with primary effusion lymphomas.[75] The virus was subsequently shown to be a member of the gamma herpesvirus subfamily and was named *HHV-8*.[76] Subsequent studies have shown that primary effusion lymphomas are EBV-associated, lack c-myc gene rearrangements, and have distinct clinical and phenotypic features.[77] The mechanism of HHV-8 growth stimulation is unknown, although several potential mechanisms have been proposed.[64] It has been suggested that HHV-8 may be necessary for EBV-induced transformation in these patients.[64,77]

Evidence also links hepatitis C virus (HCV) infection with NHL. Infection with HCV is strongly associated with essential mixed cryoglobulinemia, which is itself associated with low-grade NHL. Several analyses have demonstrated significantly higher rates of HCV infection when B-cell NHL patients were compared with controls.[78,79] The association appears strongest for patients with monocytoid B-cell lymphoma and lymphoplasmacytoid lymphomas. HCV has been identified in NHL cells from a patient with type II mixed cryoglobulinemia.[80,81] Although HCV is not thought to be oncogenic, chronic antigenic stimulation from circulating HCV RNA may produce clonal expansion leading to development of NHL.[82] Some studies have failed to find an association between HCV infection and NHL.[83]

Several lines of evidence link the bacteria *Helicobacter pylori* to gastric MALT lymphomas.[84] *H pylori* can be found in the gastric mucosa of patients with gastric MALT lymphoma,[85] and patients with gastric lymphoma are more likely than controls to have serologic evidence of past *H pylori* infection.[86] It is hypothesized that development of gastric MALT lymphomas is a multistep process beginning with *H pylori* colonization. This leads to chronic antigenic stimulation and gastritis and the subsequent development of malignant B-cell clones.[87,88] Stimulation by *H pylori*–associated antigens appears to be strain specific and T-cell mediated.[89]

ENVIRONMENTAL AND OCCUPATIONAL EXPOSURES

Studies of occupational and environmental NHL risk are frequently inconsistent and contradictory. Difficulties in estimating risk are often related to sample size and other methodologic difficulties in addition to difficulties in quantifying exposure. The risk of NHL has been reported to be increased in several occupations.[90–93] Occupations frequently associated with a higher risk include farmers, forestry workers, and agricultural workers. Metaanalysis has shown a slightly increased risk of NHL in farmers.[94,95] Increased risk of NHL in farmers may be related to an infectious agent or chemical exposure.

Several studies have shown an increased risk of NHL in relation to herbicide exposure, especially phenoxy herbicides such as 2,4-dichlorophenoxyacetic acid.[93,96,97] Other analyses have found less evidence for an association between 2,4-dichlorophenoxyacetic acid exposure and NHL.[98–100] The development of NHL has also been linked to hair dyes, especially darker and permanent colors,[101–103] although some studies have failed to find an association.[104,105] NHL has also been associated with organic solvents.[90,91,106,107] High levels of nitrates in drinking water have been associated with NHL in some studies,[108] but not others.[109]

DIET AND OTHER EXPOSURES

Cohort and case-control studies suggest that the risk of NHL is increased approximately twofold in association with higher intake of meats and dietary fat.[110–112] Recreational drug use has been associated with increased NHL risk,[113] and tobacco use has been associated with a higher risk in some studies, but not others.[114–116] The risk of NHL may be increased more than 20-fold after treatment for Hodgkin's disease.[117–119] Studies examining the relative risk of combined modality treatment have been inconsistent, although the risk of NHL in association with ionizing radiation is minimal.[120] Solar ultraviolet exposure has been associated with NHL in some studies.[121,122] Although some analyses have shown that the risk of NHL is increased after blood transfusion, other studies have failed to identify a significantly increased risk.[123]

BIOLOGIC BACKGROUND FOR CLASSIFICATION OF LYMPHOID NEOPLASMS

Although the normal counterpart of the neoplastic cell is not known for all types of lymphoid neoplasms, it can be postulated for many of them. Understanding the normal counterpart of neoplastic cells can provide a useful framework for understanding the morphology, immunophenotype, and to some extent, the clinical behavior of the neoplasms (Figs. 45.3-3A to C).

Anatomy and Morphology of Normal Lymphoid Tissues

Lymphoid tissues can be divided into two major categories: (1) the *central* or *primary* lymphoid tissues, which harbor lymphoid precursor cells and provide for their maturation to a stage at which they are capable of performing their function in response to antigen; and (2) the *peripheral* or *secondary* lymphoid tissue, in which antigen-specific reactions occur.

Primary (Central) Lymphoid Tissues

BONE MARROW (BURSA EQUIVALENT). Many of the early experiments that elucidated the basic biology of the lymphoid system used chickens and other avian species as experimental animals; in avians, an organ known as the bursa of Fabricius, located in the region of the cloaca, was proven to be the source of cells capable of producing antibody. Thus, these cells were termed *B cells*, for bursa-derived cells. In mammals, the bursa does not exist, and experiments have shown that the precursors of antibody-producing cells come from the bone marrow. The bone marrow is also the source of other hematopoietic cells, including T cells (so named because their crucial maturation steps cannot occur in the absence of the thymus).

THYMUS. The thymus, located in the anterior mediastinum, is the site at which immature T-cell precursors (prethymocytes) that migrate from the bone marrow undergo maturation and selection to become mature, naive T cells, which are capable of responding to antigen. The thymus is divided into a cortex and a medulla, each of which is characterized by specialized epithelium and accessory cells, which provide the milieu for T-cell maturation.

Secondary (Peripheral) Lymphoid Tissues

LYMPH NODES. Lymph nodes are located at sites throughout the body, strategically placed to process antigens present in lymph drained from most organs via the afferent lymphatics. Lymph nodes have a capsule, a cortex, a medulla, and sinuses (subcapsular, cortical, and medullary). The sinuses contain macrophages, which take up and process antigen, which may then be presented to lymphocytes. The cortex is divided into follicular and diffuse (paracortical) regions, and the medulla into medullary cords and sinuses. The paracortex contains high endothelial venules, through which both T and B lymphocytes enter the node, and specialized antigen-presenting cells (APC), the interdigitating dendritic cells, which may be related to the cutaneous Langerhans' cell, and which present antigen to T cells. Both T-cell and early B-cell reactions to antigen occur in the paracortex, while the germinal center reaction occurs in the follicular cortex. The

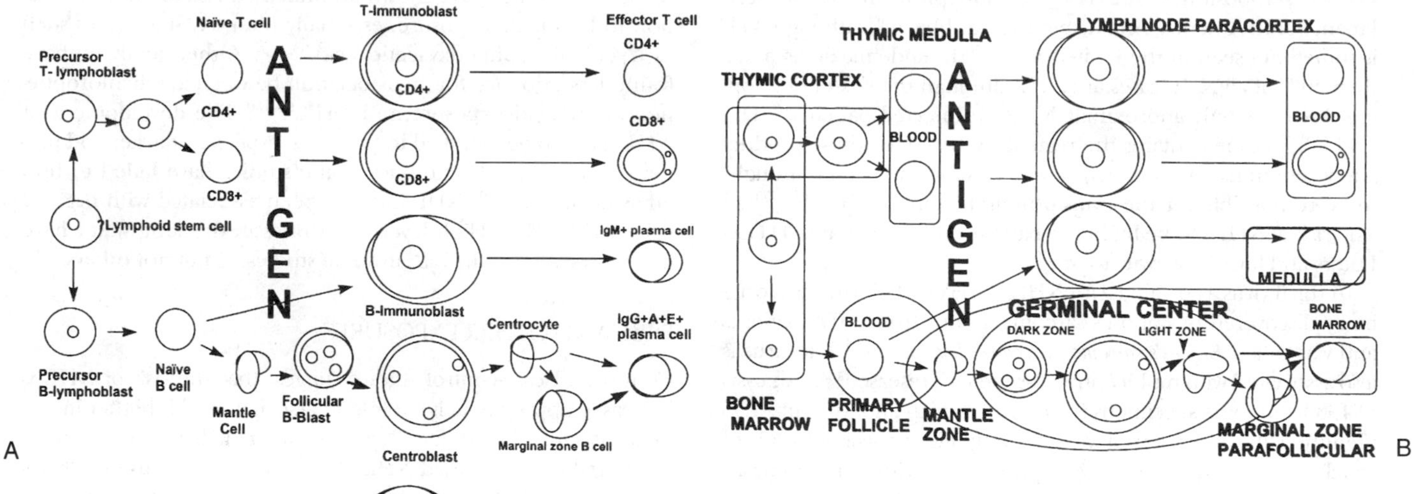

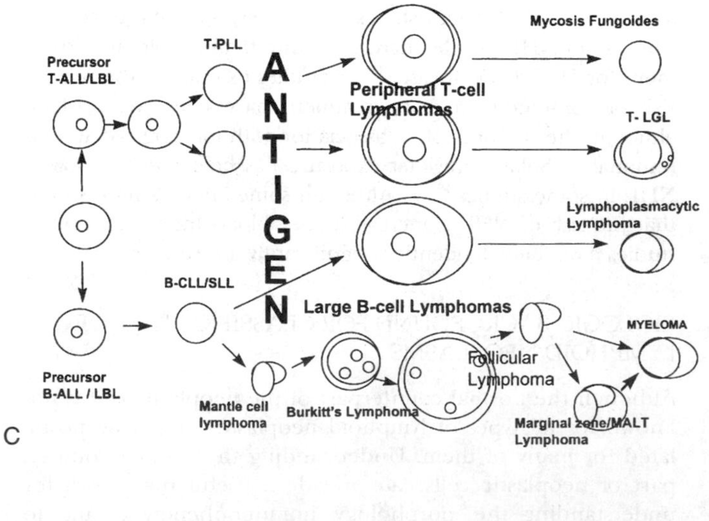

FIGURE 45.3-3. **A:** Hypothetical scheme of lymphocyte differentiation, showing anatomic locations of different stages of T- and B-cell differentiation. T cells are shown at top; B cells are at bottom. **B:** Differentiation scheme, showing nomenclature for various types of T cells (*top*) and B cells (*bottom*). **C:** Differentiation scheme, showing postulated normal counterpart of many of the T- and B-cell neoplasms that can currently be recognized. B-ALL, B-cell acute lymphoblastic leukemia; B-CLL, B-cell chronic lymphocytic leukemia; Ig, immunoglobulin; LBL, lymphoblastic lymphoma; MALT, mucosa-associated lymphoid tissue; SLL, small lymphocytic lymphoma; T-LGL, T-cell large granular lymphocyte; T-PLL, T-cell prolymphocytic leukemia.

follicular cortex also contains a specific type of accessory cell, the follicular dendritic cell (FDC); adhesion to the FDC-antigen complex is important in the differentiation of B cells in response to antigen. Plasma cells and effector T cells generated by immune reactions accumulate in the medullary cords and exit via the medullary sinuses.

SPLEEN. The spleen, located in the left upper abdomen, has two major compartments: the red pulp, which functions as a filter for particulate antigens and for the formed elements of the blood, and the white pulp, which is virtually identical in its compartments to the lymphoid tissue of the lymph node. Follicles and germinal centers are found in the Malpighian corpuscles, whereas T cells and interdigitating dendritic cells are found in the adjacent periarteriolar lymphoid sheath. Plasma cells accumulate in the red pulp.

MUCOSA-ASSOCIATED LYMPHOID TISSUE. Specialized lymphoid tissue is found in association with certain epithelia, in particular the nasopharynx and oropharynx (Waldeyer's ring: adenoids, tonsils), the gastrointestinal tract (gut-associated lymphoid tissue: Peyer's patches of the distal ileum, mucosal lymphoid aggregates in the colon and rectum), and lung (bronchus-associated lymphoid tissue). Collectively, this is known as mucosa-associated lymphoid tissue (MALT). These tissues tend to have prominent B-cell follicles, but also may have discrete T-cell zones, similar to the paracortex of lymph nodes. MALT is thought to function in response to intraluminal antigens and the generation of mucosal immunity. Lymphoid cells that respond to antigen in the MALT acquire homing properties that enable them to return to these tissues.[3]

B- and T-Cell Differentiation

In both the T- and B-cell systems, there are two major phases of differentiation: antigen-independent and antigen-dependent (see Figs. 45.3-3*A* and *B*). Antigen-independent differentiation occurs in the primary lymphoid organs [bursa equivalent (bone marrow possibly) and thymus] without exposure to antigen and produces a pool of lymphocytes that are capable of responding to antigen (naive or virgin T and B cells). The early stages are stem cells and lymphoid blasts, which are self-renewing, while the later stages are resting cells with a finite life span ranging from weeks to years. On exposure to antigen, the naive lymphocyte undergoes *blast transformation* and becomes a large, proliferating cell, which gives rise to progeny that are capable of direct activity against the inciting antigen (antigen-specific effector cells). The earlier stages of antigen-dependent differentiation are proliferating cells, while the fully differentiated effector cells are less mitotically active. Thus, neoplasms that correspond to proliferating stages of either antigen-independent or antigen-dependent differentiation are likely to be aggressive, whereas those that correspond to naive or mature effector stages are likely to be indolent.

B-Cell Differentiation

ANTIGEN-INDEPENDENT B-CELL DIFFERENTIATION

Precursor B Cells. The earliest B cells have rearranged immunoglobulin (Ig) heavy-chain genes, but lack surface immunoglobulin (SIg); the B cells at this stage are called *precursor B cells* or *pre-pre-B cells.* At the next stage, pre-B cells make cytoplasmic μ heavy-chain, but no light-chain, and do not express SIg. Both types of cells are lymphoblasts, with dispersed chromatin and small nucleoli. They contain the intranuclear enzyme, terminal deoxynucleotidyl transferase (TdT), and express CD34, a glycoprotein present on immature cells of both lymphoid and myeloid lineage, HLA-DR [class II major histocompatibility complex (MHC) antigens], and the common acute lymphoblastic leukemia (ALL) antigen (CD10). Expression of class II MHC antigens persists throughout the life of the B cell and is important in interactions with T cells. Pan-B-cell antigens are sequentially expressed on precursor B cells: CD19 and cytoplasmic CD22, followed by surface CD20. The leukocyte common antigen (CD45) does not appear until surface CD20; thus, staining for CD45 may not be useful in identifying early B-cell neoplasms. Precursor B cells also express CD79a, a molecule that is associated with SIg and is involved in transduction of signal after engagement of the SIg with antigen, analogous to CD3 and the T-cell receptor (TCR) molecule.

Fetal early B-cell development occurs in the liver, bone marrow, and spleen, whereas in adults it is restricted to the bone marrow. Cells with the morphologic and immunologic features of precursor B cells can be found in normal and regenerating bone marrow, where they correspond to the lymphocyte-like cells known as *hematogones.* Neoplasms of precursor B cells usually involve bone marrow and peripheral blood and are known as common or precursor B ALL; rarely, they present as solid tumors (precursor B lymphoblastic lymphoma).

Naive B Cells. The end stage of antigen-independent B-cell differentiation is the mature, naive (virgin) B cell, which expresses both complete surface IgM and IgD, lacks TdT and common ALL antigen, and is capable of responding to antigen. Naive B cells have rearranged but unmutated Ig genes. Each individual B cell is committed to a single light-chain, either κ or λ, and all of its progeny express the same light-chain. In contrast to precursor B cells, naive B cells lack CD10 and CD34. In addition to SIg, naive B cells express pan-B-cell antigens (CD19, CD20, CD22, CD40, and CD79a), HLA class II molecules, complement receptors (CD21 and CD35), CD44, Leu-8 (L-selectin), CD23, and the pan-T-cell antigen, CD5. Many of the surface antigens expressed by mature B cells are involved in *homing* or adhesion to vascular endothelium, interaction with APCs, and signal transduction. SIg, CD79a, CD19, and CD20, appear to be involved in signal transduction, CD22 is involved in signaling, and CD40 is involved in interaction with T cells and in further differentiation of B cells. Resting B cells also produce the bcl-2 protein, which promotes survival in the resting state. CD5-positive B cells produce Ig that often has broad specificity (cross-reactive idiotypes) and reactivity with self-antigens (autoantibodies).

Naive B cells are small resting lymphocytes. In fetal tissues, they are the predominant lymphoid cell in the spleen; in adults, they circulate in the blood and also make up a minor fraction of the B cells in primary lymphoid follicles and follicle mantle zones (so-called recirculating B cells). Studies of single cells picked from the mantle zones of reactive follicles show that they are clonally diverse and contain unmutated Ig genes, consistent with naive B cells. Tumors of these cells are usually clinically indolent and histologically low grade. In addition, they are often widespread and leukemic, consistent with the recirculating behavior of the normal naive B cell. Two neoplasms appear to correspond to CD5-positive B cells: B-cell chronic lymphocytic leukemia (B-CLL) and mantle cell (centrocytic/intermediate) lymphoma.

ANTIGEN-DEPENDENT B-CELL DIFFERENTIATION

Immunoblastic and Plasma Cell Reaction. On encountering antigen, the naive B cell transforms into a proliferating cell, which ultimately matures into an antibody-secreting plasma cell. In T-cell–independent reactions, and in the early primary immune response, naive B cells transform into IgM-positive blast cells (B blasts or immunoblasts) in the T-cell zones, proliferate, and differentiate into IgM-secreting plasma cells, producing the IgM antibody of the primary immune response. These plasma cells have largely unmutated Ig genes. Surface IgD is lost during blast transformation, as are some other antigens, such as CD21 and CD22. Other antigens associated with activation are up-regulated. With maturation to plasma cells, most surface antigens are lost, including pan-B-cell antigens HLA-DR and the leukocyte common antigen CD45, and secretory cytoplasmic IgM accumulates. The corresponding neoplasm to the IgM-producing plasma cell may be lymphoplasmacytic lymphoma (immunocytoma) or Waldenström's macroglobulinemia.

Germinal Center Reaction. Later in the primary response (within 3 to 7 days of antigen challenge in experimental animals) and in secondary responses, the T-cell–dependent germinal center reaction occurs. Each germinal center is formed from between three and ten naive B cells and ultimately contains approximately 10,000 to 15,000 B cells; thus, more than ten generations are required to form a germinal center. Proliferating IgM-positive B blasts formed from naive B cells that have encountered antigen in the T-cell zone (paracortex) migrate into the center of the primary follicle and fill the FDC mesh work by approximately 3 days after antigen stimulation, forming a germinal center. These B blasts differentiate into Ig-negative *centroblasts* (large noncleaved follicular center cells), which appear at approximately 4 days, and accumulate at one pole of the germinal center, forming the *dark zone.* Centroblasts are large proliferating cells with vesicular nuclei, one to three prominent, peripheral nucleoli, and a narrow rim of basophilic cytoplasm. They lack SIg and also switch off the gene that encodes the bcl-2 protein; thus, they and their progeny are susceptible to death through apoptosis. Germinal center cells express antigens associated with activation, most of which are involved with interaction with T cells, including CD23, CD71, CD40, and CD86, as well as antigens associated with adhesion to FDCs, including CD11a/18 and CD29/49d, and antigens that may promote apoptosis, such as CD95. An important event in germinal center development is expression of bcl-6 protein, a nuclear zinc finger transcription factor that is expressed by both centroblasts and centrocytes, but not by naive or memory B cells, mantle cells, or plasma cells. Interestingly, normal resting B cells express high levels of bcl-6 messenger RNA, while lacking the protein.

In centroblasts, a process of somatic mutation of the Ig gene variable (V) region begins, which alters the affinity for antigen of the antibody that will be produced by the cell. In addition, the cell may also switch from IgM to IgG or IgA production; through these mechanisms, the germinal center reaction gives rise to the better fitting IgG or IgA antibody of the late primary or secondary immune response. Studies on single centroblasts picked from the dark zone of germinal centers suggest that in the early stages, a germinal center may contain approximately five to ten clones of centroblasts, which show only a moderate amount of Ig gene V region mutation; later, the number of clones diminishes to as few as three, and the degree of somatic mutation increases.

Centroblasts mature to nonproliferating medium-sized cells with irregular nuclei, inconspicuous nucleoli, and scant cytoplasm, called *centrocytes* (small or large cleaved follicular center cells), which accumulate in the opposite pole of the germinal center, known as the *light zone,* which also contains a high concentration of FDCs. Centrocytes reexpress SIg, which has the same VDJ rearrangement as the parent naive B cell and the centroblast of the dark zone, but which may have undergone heavy-chain class switch and which has an altered antibody-combining site, because of the somatic mutations in the Ig V region. This process of somatic mutation thus results in marked intraclonal diversity of antibody-combining sites in a population of cells derived from only a few precursors. Also in the germinal center, the bcl-6 gene undergoes somatic mutation of the 5' noncoding promoter region, at a lower frequency than is seen in the Ig genes. Thus, both Ig gene mutation and bcl-6 mutation serve as markers of cells that have experienced the germinal center.

Centrocytes whose Ig gene mutations have resulted in *decreased* affinity for antigen rapidly die by apoptosis (programmed cell death); the prominent *starry sky* pattern of phagocytic macrophages seen in germinal centers at this stage is a result of the apoptosis of centrocytes. In contrast, centrocytes whose Ig gene mutations have resulted in *increased* affinity are able to bind to native, unprocessed antigen trapped in antigen-antibody complexes by the complement receptors on the processes of FDCs. The centrocytes are able to process the antigen and present it to T cells in the light zone of the germinal center. It is thought that this activation of T cells may induce them to express CD40 ligand (CD40L), which can engage CD40 on the B cell. Both ligation of the antigen receptor by antigen and ligation of CD40 on the surfaces of germinal center B cells can *rescue* them from apoptosis. Interaction with surface molecules expressed by FDCs, such as CD23, appears to be important in directing differentiation of the centrocytes into plasma cells, while interaction with the numerous T cells present in the light zone, through the CD40 molecule and its ligand on T cells, appears to be important in the generation of memory B cells. In addition, both antigen receptor ligation and CD40 ligation switch off bcl-6 messenger RNA production and bcl-6 protein expression.

Follicular lymphomas are tumors of germinal center B cells, in which centrocytes fail to undergo apoptosis because they have a chromosomal rearrangement, t(14;18), that prevents the normal switching off of the antiapoptosis gene, bcl-2. Most large B-cell lymphomas are composed of cells that at least in part resemble centroblasts and have mutated Ig V region genes and are therefore thought to derive from the germinal center stage of differentiation. Finally, it is possible that Burkitt's lymphoma corresponds to the early SIgM-positive B blast found in the early germinal center reaction in experimental animals.

Marginal Zone and Monocytoid (Parafollicular) B Cells. When the germinal center polarizes into a dark and a light zone, the mantle zone becomes better defined and eccentric, with the broader portion surrounding the light zone of the germinal center. Antigen-specific B cells generated in the germinal center reaction leave the follicle and reappear in the outer mantle zone, to form a *marginal zone*; these are particularly prominent in mesenteric lymph nodes, Peyer's patches, and the spleen. Marginal zone B cells have slightly irregular nuclei, resembling those of centrocytes, but with more abundant, pale cytoplasm. The term *centrocyte-like* has been applied to similar neoplastic cells. On rechallenge with antigen, splenic marginal zone B cells migrate first into the germinal center and then quickly appear in the T-cell zone as Ig-positive blast cells, which give rise to antigen-specific plasma cells; thus, they are thought to be memory B cells. Memory B cells are also detectable in the peripheral blood, where they may be IgM-positive and even CD5-positive. Studies on single marginal zone B cells from spleen and Peyer's patches show that they have mutated V region genes, may be oligoclonal, and are not clonally related to the adjacent germinal center. Cells that resemble marginal zone B cells, but with even more nuclear indentation and abundant cytoplasm, known as monocytoid B lymphocytes, are seen in clusters adjacent to subcapsular and cortical sinuses of some reactive lymph nodes, peripheral to and often continuous with the follicle marginal zone. In contrast to marginal zone B cells, the monocytoid B cells found in reactive lymph nodes appear to have either unmutated Ig V region genes or to show only a small number of randomly distributed mutations that do not suggest selection by antigen. Nodal and splenic tumors resembling normal marginal zone and monocytoid B cells have been described. Analysis of Ig V region genes suggests that most of these have mutations consistent with germinal center exposure and antigen selection.

Bone Marrow Plasma Cells. IgG-producing plasma cells accumulate in the lymph node medulla, but it appears that the immediate precursor of the bone marrow plasma cell leaves the node and migrates to the bone marrow. Plasma cells lose SIg, pan-B-cell antigens, HLA-DR, CD40, and CD45, and cytoplasmic IgG or IgA accumulates. Plasma cells also express CD38. They have rearranged and mutated Ig genes, but do not have the ongoing mutations seen in follicle center cells. Tumors of these marrow-homing plasma cells correspond to plasmacytoma and multiple myeloma.

Mucosa-Associated Lymphoid Tissue. A subset of B cells, including all the differentiation stages listed previously, are programmed for gut-associated rather than nodal lymphoid tissue. In these tissues (Waldeyer's ring, Peyer's patches, and mesenteric nodes), similar responses occur to antigen, but both the intermediate and end-stage B cells that originate in the gut or mesenteric lymph nodes preferentially return there, rather than to peripheral lymph nodes or bone marrow. Thus, the plasma cells generated in gut-associated lymphoid tissue home preferentially to the lamina propria, rather than to the bone marrow.[3] Many extranodal low-grade B-cell lymphomas are thought to arise from this MALT. Since most MALT lymphomas contain prominent marginal zone type B cells, in addition to small B lymphocytes and plasma cells, and since similar lymphomas occur in non-MALT sites, the term *extranodal marginal zone lymphoma of MALT type* has been proposed for these tumors.[124] MALT-type lymphomas have somatically mutated V region genes, consistent with an antigen-selected post–germinal center B-cell stage.

T-Cell Differentiation

ANTIGEN-INDEPENDENT T-CELL DIFFERENTIATION

Cortical Thymocytes. As in the B-cell system, the earliest stages of T-cell differentiation involve characteristic rearrangement of the DNA encoding the antigen receptor molecule. The earliest antigen-independent stages of T-cell differentiation occur in the bone marrow; later stages occur in the thymic cortex. The exact site at which precursor cells become committed to the T lineage is not known, since the thymus contains cells that can differentiate into either T cells or natural killer (NK) cells, but not B cells. Cortical thymocytes are lymphoblasts, which contain the intranuclear enzyme TdT. The earliest committed T-cell precursors are CD34+ and CD45RA+, express the CD13 and CD33 antigens usually associated with myeloid cells, and lack CD3, CD4, and CD8 (*triple negative* cells); within the thymus they sequentially acquire CD1, CD2, CD5, and cytoplasmic CD3, and first the CD4 helper and then the CD8 suppressor antigen (*double positive*). In the thymus, rearrangement of the TCR genes is initiated, beginning with the γ and δ chains, followed by the β and then the α chain genes; these proteins are then expressed on the cell surface. Surface CD3 expression appears at the same time as expression of the T-cell antigen receptor β chain, with which it is closely associated and participates in signal transduction. Cortical thymocytes express the CD45RO epitope of the leukocyte common antigen, instead of CD45RA, and lack the antiapoptosis protein bcl-2.

In addition to providing a pool of mature T cells through proliferation of precursor cells, the thymus plays a major role in the selection of T cells, so that the resulting pool of mature T cells do not react to self-antigens. Both positive and negative selection occur in the thymus at the double positive (CD4+, CD8+) stage. Thymocytes that have anti–self-specificity bind strongly via their TCR $\alpha\beta$ complex to self-antigens presented by the MHC on thymic dendritic cells and die by apoptosis. Those that lack anti–self-reactivity undergo positive selection on thymic epithelial cells; they then express increased levels of surface CD3, acquire CD27 and CD69, switch their CD45 isotype from RO back to RA, lose CD1, express bcl-2, and lose either CD4 or CD8 to become mature, naive T cells. The tumor that corresponds to the stages of T-cell differentiation in the thymic cortex is precursor T-lymphoblastic lymphoma and leukemia; the variety of immunophenotypes and antigen receptor gene rearrangements found in precursor T-cell neoplasia corresponds to the variety of stages of intrathymic T-cell differentiation.

Naive T Cells. Mature, naive (virgin) T cells have the morphologic appearance of small lymphocytes, have a low proliferation fraction, lack TdT and CD1, and express either (but not both) CD4 or CD8, as well as surface CD3 and CD5, CD45RA, and bcl-2. These cells leave the thymus and can be found in the circulation, in the paracortex of lymph nodes, and in the thymic medulla. Some cases of T-cell prolymphocytic leukemia and peripheral T-cell lymphoma may correspond to naive T cells.

ANTIGEN-DEPENDENT T-CELL DIFFERENTIATION. A complex interaction of T-cell surface molecules with molecules on the surface of APCs is required for T-cell activation in response to antigen. On the T cell, the CD4 or CD8 molecules bind to MHC class II or class I molecules, respectively, on the APC. A complex of CD3 and the T-cell antigen receptor (which may be of either γδ or αβ type and has a combining site that fits the specific peptide antigen) binds to the antigen-MHC complex on the APC. The adhesion molecule lymphocyte function-associated–1 on the T cell binds to intercellular adhesion molecule-1 on the APC; the activation-associated molecule CD40L on the T cell binds to CD40; and CD28 and CTLA4 on the T cell bind to B7-1 and B7-2 (CD86) on the APC. The binding of CD40-CD40L provides an activation stimulus for both the T cell and the APC, and binding of CD28 or CTLA4 to B7 provides a crucial second stimulus for the T cell, without which anergy develops. In addition, both the T cell and the APC release stimulatory molecules, such as interferon-γ and interleukins, which provide further mutual activation stimuli.

T Immunoblasts. On encountering antigen, mature T cells transform into immunoblasts, which are large cells with prominent nucleoli and basophilic cytoplasm, that may be indistinguishable from B immunoblasts. T immunoblasts, in contrast to T lymphoblasts (thymocytes), are TdT and CD1 negative, strongly express pan-T-cell antigens, and continue to express either CD4 or CD8, not both. Activated or proliferating T cells express HLA-DR, as well as CD25 (interleukin-2 receptor), and both CD71 and CD38. Antigen-dependent T-cell reactions occur in the paracortex of lymph nodes and the periarteriolar lymphoid sheath of the spleen, as well as at extranodal sites of immunologic reactions.

Effector T Cells. From the T-immunoblastic reaction come antigen-specific effector T cells of either CD4 or CD8 type, as well as memory T cells. Antigen-stimulated T cells switch their CD45 isotype from CD45RA to CD45RO. Effector T cells of the CD4 type typically act as helper cells, and those of the CD8 type as suppressor cells *in vitro*; however, both types can be cytotoxic. CD4 cells are cytotoxic to cells that display antigen complexed with MHC class II antigen, whereas CD8 cells are cytotoxic to cells that display it complexed with MHC class I antigen. In addition to cytotoxicity, effector T cells produce a variety of cytokines that affect the function of B cells and APCs, which modulate the immune response. Fully differentiated T-effector cells are small lymphocytes, morphologically similar to other nonproliferating lymphocytes of either T or B type. In addition to differences in subset antigen (CD4 vs. CD8 or double negative) expression, peripheral T cells may differ in their TCR expression (γδ vs. αβ). The majority of T cells in the circulation and in most lymphoid tissues are γδ+; αβ T cells are more numerous in mucosae and in the spleen.

Most cases of peripheral T-cell lymphoma are thought to correspond to stages of antigen-dependent T-cell differentiation (e.g., mycosis fungoides corresponds to a mature effector CD4+ cell; hepatosplenic γδ T-cell lymphoma to a γδ T cell; T-cell large granular lymphocyte leukemia to a mature effector CD8+ cell); however, the relationship between neoplastic and normal T cells is not nearly as well understood as in the B-cell system. The systemic symptoms such as fever, skin rashes, and hemophagocytic syndromes associated with some peripheral T-cell lymphomas may be a consequence of cytokine production by the neoplastic T cells.

Natural Killer Cells. A third line of lymphoid cells, called *NK cells* since they can kill certain targets without sensitization and without MHC restriction, appears to derive from a common progenitor with T cells. NK cells recognize self class I MHC molecules on the surfaces of cells and kill cells that lack these antigens. Immature NK cells have cytoplasmic CD3, but these cells do not rearrange their T-cell receptor genes or express T-cell receptors or surface CD3. They are characterized by certain NK cell–associated antigens (CD16, CD56, and CD57), which can also be expressed on some T cells and also express some T-cell–associated antigens (CD2, CD28, and CD8). NK cells appear in the peripheral blood as a small proportion of circulating lymphocytes; they are usually slightly larger than most normal T and B cells, with abundant pale cytoplasm containing azurophilic granules (so-called large granular lymphocytes). Angiocentric and nasal T/NK cell lymphoma and some types of large granular lymphocytes leukemia appear to correspond to immature and mature NK cells, respectively.

IMMUNOPHENOTYPING OF LYMPHOID CELLS

Individual B- and T-lymphoid cells as well as accessory cells of the mononuclear phagocyte system can be recognized in cell suspensions or tissue sections by the presence of surface or cytoplasmic molecules (antigens) that can be detected using antibodies labeled with either fluorescence or enzymatic (immunohistochemical) methods. Immunophenotyping with monoclonal antibodies can be done using viable cell suspensions, frozen tissue sections, or paraffin-embedded tissue sections. Using monoclonal antibodies and acetone-fixed cryostat sections, it has been possible to characterize many types of normal and neoplastic lymphoid cells. A series of international workshops has developed a standardized nomenclature for many of the antigens detected by more than one monoclonal antibody. For cells in body fluids, particularly the peripheral blood, flow cytometry with fluorescent-labeled antibodies is the method of choice; this method can also be applied to fine-needle aspiration biopsy specimens and to cell suspensions prepared from fresh tissue specimens, but sampling problems can occur due to selective loss of fragile neoplastic cells. Acetone-fixed frozen sections are the most reliable method for the pathologist to assess the phenotype of lymphoid cells in tissue sections. However, the technology for detecting lymphocyte-associated antigens in paraffin-embedded tissue has greatly improved, so that most clinically necessary immunophenotyping can be accomplished using only routinely processed tissue. Nonetheless, it is still advisable to prepare fresh frozen tissue in all cases of suspected lymphoma, in case a diagnosis cannot be made with certainty on paraffin tissue section analysis and also for possible molecular genetic analysis.

MOLECULAR GENETIC ANALYSIS OF LYMPHOID CELLS

Lymphocyte differentiation involves rearrangement of the genes involved in antigen recognition. This process is required for development of a functional antigen receptor gene and serves to increase the diversity of these receptors beyond what can be *hard-coded* into the genome, so that lymphoid cells can develop a repertoire large enough to respond to the majority of antigens they may encounter. Analysis of these rearrangements has provided insights into normal T- and B-cell differentiation and can also be useful in the diagnosis and classification of lymphoid neoplasms. In addition to these normal rearrangements, chromosome translocations frequently occur in lymphoid neoplasms, as they do in other tumors. In lymphomas, these translocations often involve *hot spots* in the antigen receptor genes; these translocations can also be useful in the diagnosis and classification of lymphoid neoplasms.

Antigen Receptor Gene Rearrangement

IMMUNOGLOBULIN GENE REARRANGEMENT. B-cell differentiation involves rearrangements of the genes involved in Ig production. The genes that encode the constant and variable regions of the Ig heavy and light-chain molecules are located far apart on the chromosomes in germline cells. To produce RNA for an Ig protein, many thousands of base pairs of DNA must be deleted from the genome to bring the different portions of the Ig gene together. These rearrangements change the position on the DNA of restriction sites (points at which restriction endonucleases cleave the DNA). Thus, fragments produced by digesting B-cell DNA with these enzymes are of a different size than those produced by digesting non–B-cell (germline) DNA and migrate differently in an electrophoresis gel. When radiolabeled DNA probes (cloned segments of DNA produced by bacteria) that are complementary to specific portions of the Ig gene are applied to such a gel, they specifically mark the position of the Ig gene, which can be demonstrated on an autoradiograph. The exact size, and therefore position on the gel (Southern blot), of each Ig gene fragment is unique to an individual B cell; thus, this technique provides not only a specific marker for B cells, but also a true marker for monoclonality.

T-CELL RECEPTOR GENE REARRANGEMENT. A process of gene rearrangement analogous to that seen in B cells also occurs during T-cell differentiation. This process involves the DNA encoding a T-cell–specific surface molecule that serves as the T-cell receptor for antigen, analogous to surface Ig on B cells. As in the B-cell system, the size of restriction fragments of the DNA encoding the T-cell receptor gene is specific for a single clone of T cells. Thus, T-cell receptor gene rearrangement is a specific marker for T cells and also a true marker for monoclonality in T cells.

Oncogene Rearrangements

In addition to rearrangements of antigen receptor genes, hematologic malignancies frequently have specific chromosomal translocations. Cellular oncogenes (genes that can cause malignant transformation when transfected in activated or altered form into cultured normal cells) have been identified in association with some of the more common chromosome translocations that characterize lymphoid malignancies. These translocations can be detected using DNA probes that hybridize to the breakpoint regions on the chromosome carrying the oncogene. Using a technique for amplifying unique DNA segments [polymerase chain reaction (PCR)], rare cells carrying a given translocation can be detected, using probes that span the breakpoint, or using a reverse transcriptase technique to detect RNA produced by the altered or fused gene (reverse transcriptase–PCR). Numeric abnormalities of chromosomes are also common in lymphoid malignancies; these can be detected by fluorescence *in situ* hybridization, using probes to specific chromosomes.

To the extent to which specific histologic subtypes, prognostic groups, or both of lymphomas are associated with specific gene rearrangements, detection of these rearrangements may prove useful in the characterization of lymphomas. In addition, this technique can potentially be used to detect disseminated or recurrent lymphoma on small biopsy specimens or in the blood. Finally, study of the function of the translocated oncogene is providing clues to the mechanisms of oncogenesis.

USE OF IMMUNOPHENOTYPING AND GENETIC STUDIES IN THE DIAGNOSIS OF LYMPHOID NEOPLASMS

Each of the lymphoid neoplasms has a characteristic morphology, which may be sufficient in a given case to permit diagnosis and classification on morphologic grounds alone, if well-prepared sections are available; thus, most cases of lymphoma can be diagnosed and classified with reasonable certainty on the basis of routine histologic sections alone. However, there are many pitfalls in the histologic diagnosis of malignant lymphoma, and immunophenotyping or, less often, genetic studies can be useful in resolving major differential diagnostic problems (Table 45.3-1). Problems that can be resolved by these techniques include (1) reactive versus neoplastic lymphoid infiltrates; (2) lymphoid versus nonlymphoid malignancies; and (3) subclassification of lymphoma. In a clinical study of the Revised European-American Classification of Lymphoid Neoplasms (REAL), the interobserver reproducibility of experts using the classification was tested, and the contribution of immunophenotype to reproducibility was assessed (Table 45.3-2). For most of the common entities (follicular lymphoma, MALT lymphoma, B-CLL), immunophenotyping was not necessary; however, in some diseases (mantle cell lymphoma, diffuse large B-cell lymphoma) it was helpful, and in all types of T-cell lymphoma it was essential. In a given case, if the morphology is typical of a given entity but the immunophenotypic or genetic features are unusual, the histologic sections should be reexamined; however, the case may still be accepted as an example of the entity suggested by morphologic features. If the morphology is atypical but the immunophenotype and genetic features are classic for a given entity, these features may override morphology in classification. If both the morphology and the immunophenotype are atypical, then the case is best regarded as unclassifiable or borderline.

PRINCIPLES OF CLASSIFICATION OF LYMPHOID NEOPLASM

Revised European-American Classification of Lymphoid Neoplasms from the International Lymphoma Study Group

The International Lymphoma Study Group (ILSG), an informal group of 19 hematopathologists from the United States,

TABLE 45.3-1. Cluster Designation (CD) of Leukocyte-Associated Molecules

CD	*Common Name(s)*	*Monoclonal Antibodies*	*Function/Comment*	*Major Distribution*
1a	T6, gp49	Leu6, T6, OKT6, NA1/34	γδ T-cell ligand/lipid binding	Cortical thymocytes (strong), Langerhans' cells (histiocytosis X)
2	T11, sheep erythrocyte receptor, LFA-2	Leu5b, T11, OKT11, RT11	LFA-3 receptor, adhesion, activation	T pan, thymocytes, NK cells, B cells
3	T3 e	Leu4, T3, OKT3, UCHT1, WT31	Signal transduction with T-cell receptor	T pan, T specific, thymocytes
3	T3 z	TIA-2	Signal transduction with T-cell receptor	T pan, T specific, thymocytes, NK
4	T4, gp59	Leu3a, T4, OKT4/4a, RT4.1	MHC II receptor, human immunodeficiency virus receptor, p56-lck association	T subset (MHC class II restricted), thymocytes, monocytes
5	T1, Tp67	Leu1, T1, OKT1, RT1, T101	Increases phospholipase C	T cells, thymocytes, some B cells (B-CLL, mantle cell lymphoma)
6	T12	T12, OKT17, TU33	Single-chain glycoprotein	T pan, medullary thymocytes, B cells
7	3A1	Leu9, 3A1, RT7.1, TU14	Activation?	Prethymocytes, most circulating T cells, NK subset (acute lymphoblastic leukemia)
8	T8 a/a	Leu2a, T8, OKT8a, RT8.1	MHC I receptor, a/a dimer, p56-lck	T subset (MHC class I restricted), NK subset, thymocytes, sinusoidal cells in spleen
9	BA-2, p24	CLB-thromb/8, BA-2, J2	Platelet activation	Monocytes, pre-B, platelets, activated T cells
10	CALLA	Anti-CALLA, J5, OKB-cALLa	Neutral endopeptidase	Pre-B, granulocytes, fibroblasts, kidney (acute lymphoblastic leukemia)
11a	LFA-1 a/a L integrin	LFA-1, 2H8.3, 8F2.7	Adhesion to ICAM1, ICAM2, ICAM3	Leukocytes, thymocytes
11b	MAC1, Mo1, CR3, M integrin	Leu15, Mo1, OKM1	C3bi receptor, leukocyte adhesion	Granulocytes, monocytes, NK
11c	p150/95, a X integrin	LeuM5	Monocyte and granulocyte adhesion, LPS receptor	Monocytes, granulocytes, activated CD8+ T cells, NK, B subset (HCL)
15s	X Hapten, lacto-N-fucose pentosyl III	LeuM1, MY1	Lacto-N-fucose pentosyl III; adhesion to CD62	Granulocytes, monocytes, activated T cells (Reed-Sternberg cells)
16	IgG FcR IIIA/FcR IIIB	Leu11, OK-NK	IgG FcR (low affinity), ADCC receptor	NK cells, granulocytes, macrophages
18	LFA β chain; LEU-CAM	LFA-1β, 60.3, MHM23	Adhesion with CD11 to CD54; LPS binding	Leukocytes (platelets negative)
19	B4	Leu12, B4, OKpanB, 1F1	Activation; linked to surface immunoglobulin	B pre, B pan, B activated
20	B1, Bp35	Leu16, B1, 1F5, L26	Activation, inhibition, ion transport	B cells, FDC, T cells (CLL)
21	CR2, Epstein-Barr virus receptor	Anti-CR2, B2, OKB7	C3d receptor, Epstein-Barr virus receptor, activation	B pan, C3d red cells, FDC
22	Bgp135	Leu14, OKB22, TO15, SHCL1, B3	Activation with IgM	B pan; in cytoplasm of early and mature
23	Blast-2	Leu20, B6, Blast-2	IgE FcR low affinity	Activated B, FDC (CLL)
24	BA-1; HSA/heat stable antigen	OKB2, BA1, HB8, HB9	Glycoprotein	B pan, granulocytes, monocytes
25	IL-2α receptor p55	Anti–IL-2 receptor, OKT26a, Tac, 7E11	Broad functional effects on T, B, NK cells	T, B cells, monocytes, thymocytes, basophils, eosinophils (HCL)
27	p55 (dimer)	OKT18A, S152, VIT14	Disulfide linked homodimer	T cells, thymocytes, plasma cells (cytoplasmic stain)
28	gp44	9.3, KOLT 2, 15E8, 248.23.2	Binding to B7-1 /BB1; costimulation	T subset (cytotoxic precursors), plasma cells
29	Very late antigen b-1, platelet GPIIa	4B4, K20, A-1A5	Cell adhesion	Leucocytes; weak on granulocytes, not on erythrocytes
30	Ki-1 antigen	BERH2, BERH6, BERH4, VIP1	Activation related; on cells releasing Th2 cytokines	Activated T and B cells (Reed-Sternberg cells)
40	gp50	G28-5, S2C6	B cell Ig class switching via binding to CD40L (gp39)	B and T cells, monocytes, thymic epithelium, interdigitating dendritic cells, basal epithelium, carcinomas

(continued)

TABLE 45.3-1. *(Continued)*

CD	*Common Name(s)*	*Monoclonal Antibodies*	*Function/Comment*	*Major Distribution*
43	gp95, sialophorin	Leu22, 84-3C1, G10-2, G19-1	T-cell activation	T cells, B subset, NK, monocytes, plasma and myeloid cells
44	Homing cell adhesion molecule, Hermes, Pgp-1	Leu44, A3D8, 1-173, F10-44-2	Hyaluronate receptor	Leucocytes, red cells
45	LCA/T200	HLe-1, LCA	IL-2 receptor modulation, signal transduction	Leukocyte common antigen, all leukocytes except plasma cells
45 RA	LCA-RA	Leu18, 2H4	Naive, resting cell marker	Suppressor-inducer CD4+, suppressor CD8+, monocytes, NK and B cells
45 RB	LCA-RB	PD17/26/16	Down-regulates with activation	T subset, B cell, monocytes, granulocytes
45 RO	LCA-RO	UCHL1, A7, OPD4	Memory, activated cell marker	Helper-inducer CD4+, cytotoxic CD8+, thymocytes, granulocytes, monocytes
56	Neural cell adhesion molecule, NKH-1	Leu19, NKH-1A, FP-2-11.14	Homotypic adhesion	Pan NK, activated T cells, myoblasts, lung cancer cell lines
57	HNK-1	Leu7, L183, L186	Chondroitin sulphate proteoglycan	T cell and NK cell subset, neural tissue
70	Ki-24	Ki-24, HNE 51, HNC 142	CD27– ligand	Activated B and T cells (Reed-Sternberg cells)
75w	CDw75	LN1, HH2, EBU-141	Surface sialyltransferase	Mature B cells
80	B7-1/BB1	B7/BB1	Ligand for CD28 and CTLA-4; costimulation	Activated B cells, macrophages
86	B7-2, FUN-1, BU63	BU63, FUN-1	B-cell activation antigen; CTL4 binding	B and NK cells, monocytes (lymphomas, Hodgkin's, Reed-Sternberg cells)
95	APO-1, FAS	7C11, APO-1, IPO-4	Signals apoptosis; CD4+ targeted cytotoxicity	T cells, B cells, thymocytes, liver, heart (various malignant cell lines)
100	BB18, A8; semaphorin	BB18, BD16, A8	T-cell proliferation signal, activation	T cells, germinal center B cells, NK cells, granulocytes, monocytes, platelets
103	HML-1 (human mucosal lymph)	2G5.1, F3F7, LF61, B-Ly7	Adhesion	Intraepithelial mucosal lymphocytes (HCL)
125	IL-2 receptor		T-cell signaling	Activated T cells (HCL)
138	Syndecan-1		Adhesion	Plasma cells

B, B cells; CALLA, common acute lymphoblastic leukemia antigen; CLL, chronic lymphocytic leukemia; FcR, Fc receptor; FDC, follicular dendritic cells; HCL, hairy cell leukemia; ICAM, intercellular adhesion molecule; Ig, immunoglobulin; IL-2, interleukin-2; LCA, leucocyte common antigen; LFA, lymphocyte function-associated; MHC, major histocompatibility complex; NK, natural killer.

TABLE 45.3-2. Immunohistologic and Genetic Features of Common B-Cell Neoplasms

Neoplasm	*SIG; cIg*	*CD5*	*CD10*	*CD23*	*CD43*	*CD103*	*Cyclin D1*	*Genetic Abnormality*	*Immunoglobulin Genes*
B-cell chronic lymphocytic leukemia/small lymphocytic lymphoma	+; ±	+	–	+	+	–	±	Trisomy 12; 13q	R, U
Lymphoplasmacytic lymphoma	+; +	–	–	–	±	–	–	t(9;14); del 6(q23)	R, M
Hairy cell leukemia	+; –	–	–	–	+	++	±	None known	R, M
Splenic marginal zone lymphoma	+; ±	–	–	–	–	+	–	None known	R, M
Follicle center lymphoma	+; –	–	±	±	–	–	–	t(14;18); bcl-2	R, M, O
Mantle cell lymphoma	+; –	+	–	–	+	–	+	t(11;14); bcl-1	R, U
Mucosa-associated lymphoid tissue lymphoma	+; ±	–	–	±	±	–	–	Trisomy 3, t(11;18)	R, M, O
Diffuse large B-cell lymphoma	±	–	±	NA	±	NA	–	t(14;18), t(8;14), 3q; bcl-2, myc, bcl-6	R, M
Burkitt's lymphoma	+	–	+	–	–	NA	–	t(8;14), t(2;8), t(8;22); c-myc; EBV±	R, M

NA, not applicable.

Europe, and Asia, adopted a new approach to lymphoma classification in 1993. In this approach, *all* available information (i.e., morphology, immunophenotype, genetic features, and clinical features) is used to define a disease entity. The relative importance of each of these features varies among diseases, and there is no one gold standard. Morphology is always important, and some diseases are primarily defined by morphology (e.g., follicular lymphoma, angioimmunoblastic T-cell lymphoma, nodular sclerosis Hodgkin's disease), with immunophenotype as backup in difficult cases. Some diseases have a virtually specific immunophenotype [e.g., mantle cell lymphoma, small lymphocytic lymphoma (SLL), anaplastic large cell lymphoma] such that one would hesitate to make the diagnosis in the absence of the immunophenotype. In some lymphomas a specific genetic abnormality is an important defining criterion [e.g., t(11;14) in mantle cell lymphoma, t(8;14) in Burkitt's lymphoma; t(14;18) in follicular lymphoma), whereas others lack specific genetic abnormalities (e.g., MALT lymphoma and diffuse large B-cell lymphoma). Still others require a knowledge of clinical features as well (e.g., nodal vs. extranodal presentation in marginal zone lymphoma and peripheral T-cell lymphomas, and mediastinal location in mediastinal large B-cell lymphoma). The inclusion of clinical criteria was one of the most novel aspects of the ILSG approach. The emphasis on defining *real* disease entities, rather than focusing on subtleties of morphology or immunophenotype or primarily on patient survival, represented a new paradigm in lymphoma classification.

The ILSG developed a consensus on a list of diseases that its members recognized in daily practice, using a combination of available morphologic, immunologic, and genetic information, and that appeared to be distinct clinical entities. This consensus approach represented the second major departure from previous classifications, most of which represented the work of one or a few individuals. The ILSG recognized that the complexity of the field in the 1990s made it impossible for a single person or small group to be completely authoritative, and also that broad agreement is necessary if the result is to be used by multiple pathologists, even if it requires compromise. The ILSG consensus list of well-defined, real diseases was published in 1994 (Table 45.3-3).[124] Since it represented a revision of current or prior European and American lymphoma classifications (Table 45.3-4), it was called the *Revised European-American Classification of Lymphoid Neoplasms.* Although its initial publication incited considerable controversy, experience over the intervening years has shown that it can be used by most pathologists, and that the entities it describes have distinctive clinical features, making it a useful and practical classification, despite its apparent complexity.[125–127]

TABLE 45.3-3. Revised European-American Classification of Lymphoid Neoplasms (1994)

B-CELL NEOPLASMS

I. Precursor B-cell neoplasm
  Precursor B-lymphoblastic leukemia/lymphoma
II. Peripheral B-cell neoplasms
  1. B-cell chronic lymphocytic leukemia/prolymphocytic leukemia/small lymphocytic lymphoma
  2. Lymphoplasmacytoid lymphoma/immunocytoma
  3. Mantle cell lymphoma
  4. Follicle center lymphoma, follicular
    Provisional cytologic grades: I (small cell), II (mixed small and large cell), III (large cell)
    Provisional subtype: diffuse, predominantly small cell type
  5. Marginal zone B-cell lymphoma, extranodal mucosa-associated lymphoid tissue type (with or without monocytoid B cells)
    Provisional subtype: nodal marginal zone lymphoma (with or without monocytoid B cells)
    Provisional entity: splenic marginal zone lymphoma (with or without villous lymphocytes)
  6. Hairy cell leukemia
  7. Plasmacytoma/plasma cell myeloma
  8. Diffuse large B-cell lymphoma[a]
    Subtype: primary mediastinal (thymic) B-cell lymphoma
  9. Burkitt's lymphoma
  10. Provisional entity: high-grade B-cell lymphoma, Burkitt-like[a]

T-CELL AND PUTATIVE NATURAL KILL-CELL NEOPLASMS

I. Precursor T-cell neoplasm
  Precursor T-lymphoblastic lymphoma/leukemia
II. Peripheral T-cell and natural killer-cell neoplasms
  1. T-cell chronic lymphocytic leukemia/prolymphocytic leukemia
  2. Large granular lymphocyte leukemia
    T-cell type
    Natural killer-cell type
  3. Mycosis fungoides/Sézary syndrome
  4. Peripheral T-cell lymphomas, unspecified[a]
    Provisional cytologic categories: medium-sized cell, mixed medium and large cell, large cell, lymphoepithelioid cell
    Provisional subtype: hepatosplenic γδ T-cell lymphoma
    Provisional subtype: subcutaneous panniculitic T-cell lymphoma
  5. Angioimmunoblastic T-cell lymphoma
  6. Angiocentric lymphoma
  7. Intestinal T-cell lymphoma (with or without enteropathy associated)
  8. Adult T-cell lymphoma/leukemia
  9. Anaplastic large cell lymphoma, CD30+, T- and null-cell types
  10. Provisional entity: anaplastic large cell lymphoma, Hodgkin's-like

[a]These categories are thought likely to include more than one disease entity.
(From ref. 124, with permission.)

World Health Organization Classification of Hematologic Malignancies

Since 1995, members of the European and American Hematopathology societies have been collaborating on a new World Health Organization (WHO) classification of hematologic malignancies. It will use an updated version of the REAL classification for lymphomas (Table 45.3-5) and will expand the principles of the REAL classification to the classification of myeloid and histiocytic neoplasms.[128,129] The WHO project includes over 50 pathologists from around the world, as well as a Clinical Advisory Committee of more than 30 international expert hematologists and oncologists.[130] Proponents of current classifications (e.g., Working Formulation, Kiel, REAL and French-American-British) are in agreement that the final WHO consensus will replace existing classifications. Thus, it will represent the first true international consensus on the classification of hematologic malignancies.

TABLE 45.3-4. Comparison of the Original Revised European-American Classification of Lymphoid Neoplasms with the Kiel Classification and the Working Formulation

Kiel Classification	*Revised European-American Classification of Lymphoid Neoplasms*	*Working Formulation*
B-lymphoblastic	Precursor B-lymphoblastic lymphoma/leukemia	Lymphoblastic
B-lymphocytic, CLL; B-lymphocytic; prolymphocytic leukemia; lymphoplasmacytoid immunocytoma	B-cell CLL/prolymphocytic leukemia/small lymphocytic lymphoma	*Small lymphocytic, consistent with CLL*; small lymphocytic; plasmacytoid
Lymphoplasmacytic immunocytoma	Lymphoplasmacytoid lymphoma	*Small lymphocytic, plasmacytoid*; diffuse, mixed small and large cell
Centrocytic; centroblastic, centrocytoid subtype	Mantle cell lymphoma	Small lymphocytic; *diffuse, small cleaved cell*; follicular, small cleaved cell; diffuse, mixed small and large cell; diffuse, large cleaved cell
Centroblastic-centrocytic, follicular	Follicular center lymphoma, follicular Grade 2 Grade 2 Grade 3	*Follicular, predominantly small cleaved cell; follicular, mixed small and large cell*; follicular, predominantly large cell
Centroblastic, follicular		
Centroblastic-centrocytic, diffuse	Follicular center lymphoma, diffuse, small cell (provisional)	*Diffuse, small cleaved cell*; diffuse, mixed small and large cell
—	Extranodal marginal zone B-cell lymphoma (low-grade B-cell lymphoma of mucosa-associated lymphoid tissue type)	*Small lymphocytic*; diffuse, small cleaved cell; diffuse, mixed small and large cell
Monocytoid, including marginal zone; immunocytoma	Nodal marginal zone B-cell lymphoma (provisional)	*Small lymphocytic*; diffuse, small cleaved cell; diffuse, mixed small and large cell; unclassifiable
—	Splenic marginal zone B-cell lymphoma (provisional)	*Small lymphocytic*; diffuse, small cleaved cell
Hairy cell leukemia	Hairy cell leukemia	—
Plasmacytic	Plasmacytoma/myeloma	Extramedullary plasmacytoma
Centroblastic (monomorphic, polymorphic and multilobated subtypes); *B-immunoblastic*; B-large cell anaplastic (Ki–1+)	Diffuse large B-cell lymphoma	*Diffuse, large cell*; large cell immunoblastic; diffuse, mixed small and large cell
—[a]	Primary mediastinal large B-cell lymphoma	*Diffuse, large cell*; large cell immunoblastic
Burkitt's lymphoma	Burkitt's lymphoma	Small noncleaved cell, Burkitt's lymphoma
— (some cases of centroblastic and immunoblastic?)	High-grade B-cell lymphoma, Burkitt-like (provisional)	*Small noncleaved cell, non-Burkitt's*; diffuse, large cell; large cell immunoblastic
T-lymphoblastic	Precursor T-lymphoblastic lymphoma/leukemia	Lymphoblastic
T-lymphocytic, CLL type; T-lymphocytic, prolymphocytic leukemia	T-cell CLL/prolymphocytic leukemia	*Small lymphocytic*; diffuse, small cleaved cell
T-lymphocytic, CLL type	Large granular lymphocytic leukemia: T-cell type, natural killer-cell type	*Small lymphocytic*; diffuse, small cleaved cell
Small cell cerebriform (mycosis fungoides, Sézary syndrome)	Mycosis fungoides/Sézary syndrome	Mycosis fungoides
T-zone; lymphoepithelioid; pleomorphic, small T-cell; *pleomorphic, medium-sized and large T-cell*; T-immunoblastic	Peripheral T-cell lymphomas, unspecified (including provisional subtype: subcutaneous panniculitic T-cell lymphoma)	Diffuse, small cleaved cell; *diffuse, mixed small and large cell*; diffuse, large cell; *large cell immunoblastic*
—	Hepatosplenic $\gamma\delta$ T-cell lymphoma (provisional)	—
Angioimmunoblastic (angioimmunoblastic T-cell lymphoma, large)	Angioimmunoblastic T-cell lymphoma	*Diffuse, mixed small and large cell*; diffuse, large cell; *large cell immunoblastic*
—[a]	Angiocentric lymphoma	Diffuse, small cleaved cell; *diffuse, mixed small and large cell*; diffuse, large cell; *large cell immunoblastic*
—	Intestinal T-cell lymphoma	Diffuse, small cleaved cell; diffuse, mixed small and large cell; diffuse, large cell; *large cell immunoblastic*
Pleomorphic small T-cell, human T-cell lymphotropic virus type I positive; *pleomorphic medium-sized and large T-cell, human T-cell lymphotropic virus type I positive*	Adult T-cell lymphoma/leukemia	Diffuse, small cleaved cell; diffuse, mixed small and large cell; diffuse, large cell; *large cell immunoblastic*
T-large cell anaplastic (Ki–1+)	Anaplastic large cell lymphoma, T- and null-cell types	Large cell immunoblastic

CLL, chronic lymphocytic leukemia.
[a]Not listed in classification, but discussed as rare or ambiguous type.

Principles of the Revised European-American Classification of Lymphoid Neoplasms/World Health Organization Classification of Lymphoid Neoplasms

The REAL/WHO classification is a list of distinct disease entities, which are defined by a combination of morphology, immunophenotype, and genetic features, and which have distinct clinical features. It recognizes that all of these criteria are at best approximations, and that continued research and experience will be needed to continue to improve the definition of these diseases. Morphology remains the first and most basic approach and is sufficient for both diagnosis and classification in many typical cases of lymphoma. Immunophenotyping and, particularly, molecular genetic studies are not needed in all cases; however, they are useful in difficult cases and improve interobserver reproducibility. It is the availability of these more objective methods that make a consensus on lymphoma classification possible now, while it was impossible in the 1970s, when classification was based purely on subjective morphologic features.

The classification includes all lymphoid neoplasms (i.e., Hodgkin's disease, NHLs, lymphoid leukemias, and plasma cell neoplasms). Both lymphomas and lymphoid leukemias are included, since both solid and circulating phases are present in many lymphoid neoplasms, and distinction between them is artificial. Thus, B-CLL and B-SLL are simply different manifestations of the same neoplasm, as are lymphoblastic lymphomas and ALLs. In addition, Hodgkin's disease and plasma cell myeloma are now recognized as lymphoid neoplasms of B lineage and therefore belong in a compilation of lymphoid neoplasms. Immunodeficiency-associated lymphomas are classified according to the basic lymphoma classification; a separate classification of the posttransplant lymphoid proliferations that do not fulfill criteria for lymphoma is also given (Table 45.3-6). Many of the neoplasms recognized in the classification have morphologic variants, clinical subtypes, or both.

TABLE 45.3-5. Proposed Updated Revised European-American Classification of Lymphoid Neoplasms/World Health Organization Classification of Lymphoid Neoplasms[a]

B-CELL NEOPLASMS
Precursor B-cell neoplasm
Precursor B-lymphoblastic leukemia/lymphoma (precursor B-cell acute lymphoblastic leukemia)[b]
Mature (peripheral) B-cell neoplasms[c]
B-cell chronic lymphocytic leukemia/small lymphocytic lymphoma[b]
B-cell prolymphocytic leukemia
Lymphoplasmacytic lymphoma
Splenic marginal zone B-cell lymphoma (with or without villous lymphocytes)
Hairy cell leukemia
Plasma cell myeloma[b]/plasmacytoma
Extranodal marginal zone B-cell lymphoma of mucosa-associated lymphoid tissue type[b]
Nodal marginal zone B-cell lymphoma (with or without monocytoid B cells)
Follicular lymphoma[b]
Mantle cell lymphoma[b]
Diffuse large B-cell lymphoma[b]
Mediastinal large B-cell lymphoma
Primary effusion lymphoma
Burkitt's lymphoma/Burkitt's cell leukemia[b]
T- AND NK-CELL NEOPLASMS
Precursor T-cell neoplasm
Precursor T-lymphoblastic lymphoma/leukemia (precursor T-cell acute lymphoblastic leukemia)[b]
Mature (peripheral) T-cell neoplasms[b]
T-cell prolymphocytic leukemia
T-cell granular lymphocytic leukemia
Aggressive NK-cell leukemia
Adult T-cell lymphoma/leukemia (human T-cell lymphotropic virus type I positive)
Extranodal NK/T-cell lymphoma, nasal type
Enteropathy type T-cell lymphoma
Hepatosplenic γδ T-cell lymphoma
Subcutaneous panniculitis-like T-cell lymphoma
Mycosis fungoides[b]/Sézary syndrome
Anaplastic large cell lymphoma, T/null-cell, primary cutaneous type
Peripheral T-cell lymphoma, not otherwise characterized[b]
Angioimmunoblastic T-cell lymphoma[b]
Anaplastic large cell lymphoma, T/null-cell, primary systemic type[b]

NK, natural killer.
[a]Only major categories are included. Subtypes and variants are discussed in the text and in other tables.
[b]More common entities.
[c]B- and T/NK-cell neoplasms are grouped according to major clinical presentations (predominantly disseminated/leukemic, primary extranodal, predominantly nodal).

Clinical Test of the Revised European-American Classification of Lymphoid Neoplasms

An initial criticism of the REAL was that it had not been tested in a clinical study,[131] although it only included diseases that

TABLE 45.3-6. Categories of Posttransplant Lymphoproliferative Disorders

EARLY LESIONS
Reactive plasmacytic hyperplasia
Infectious mononucleosis-like
POSTTRANSPLANT LYMPHOPROLIFERATIVE DISORDERS, POLYMORPHIC
Polyclonal (rare)
Monoclonal
POSTTRANSPLANT LYMPHOPROLIFERATIVE DISORDERS, MONOMORPHIC (CLASSIFY ACCORDING TO LYMPHOMA CLASSIFICATION)
B-cell lymphomas
Diffuse large B-cell lymphoma (immunoblastic, centroblastic, anaplastic)
Burkitt's/Burkitt-like lymphoma
Plasma cell myeloma
T-cell lymphomas
Peripheral T-cell lymphoma, not otherwise categorized
Other types (hepatosplenic γδ, T/natural killer)
OTHER TYPES (RARE)
Hodgkin's disease–like lesions (associated with methotrexate therapy)
Plasmacytoma-like lesions

TABLE 45.3-7. Reproducibility of Lymphoma Diagnosis

	Contribution of Immunophenotype (%)
REPRODUCIBILITY >85% (86% TO 96%)	
B-cell chronic lymphocytic leukemia/small lymphocytic lymphoma	3
Mantle cell lymphoma	10
Follicular lymphoma	0
Marginal zone/mucosa-associated lymphoid tissue	2
Diffuse large B-cell lymphoma	15
T-lymphoblastic lymphoma	40
Anaplastic large-cell lymphoma	30
Peripheral T-cell lymphoma, unspecified	41
Mycosis fungoides	
REPRODUCIBILITY 80%	
Angioimmunoblastic T-cell lymphoma	
Extranodal natural killer/T-cell lymphoma	
REPRODUCIBILITY <50%	
Burkitt-like lymphoma	6
Lymphoplasmacytic lymphoma	

(Data from ref. 126, with permission.)

had been previously published and for which the clinical features were known.[132] To address this issue, an international group of oncologists and pathologists devised a clinical study of the classification, in which five expert pathologists reviewed over 1300 cases of NHL at centers around the world.[126,127] The aims of the study were to (1) see whether the classification could be used in practice; (2) test its interobserver reproducibility; (3) determine the need for immunophenotyping in diagnosis; (4) determine whether the categories of disease identified in the classification were clinically distinctive either at presentation or in outcome; and (5) determine the relative frequency of these diseases in the populations studied.

This study convincingly demonstrated that the classification could be used by expert hematopathologists: Over 95% of the cases with adequate material could be classified into one or another of the categories. The interobserver reproducibility was substantially better than that for other classifications and was better than 85% for most diseases (Table 45.3-7). Immunophenotyping was helpful in some diseases, such as mantle cell lymphoma and diffuse large B-cell lymphoma, in which it improved accuracy by 10% to 15% and was essential for all types of T-cell lymphoma, improving reproducibility from approximately 50% to over 90%. It was not required for many diseases, such as follicular lymphoma, B-SLL, and MALT lymphoma.[126]

The relative frequency of the different B-cell and T/NK-cell lymphomas in the study population was similar to previous patterns reported in the literature (Table 45.3-8). The most common lymphoma was diffuse large B-cell lymphoma, followed by follicular lymphoma; together, these accounted for 50% of the lymphomas in the study. New entities not specifically recognized in the Working Formulation accounted for 27% of the cases: MALT lymphoma, 8%; mantle cell, 7%; peripheral T-cell, 6%; nodal marginal zone, 2%; mediastinal large B-cell, 2%; and anaplastic large T/null-cell, 2%. These results are reassuring, confirming that the majority of the cases that will be encountered by oncologists and pathologists will be only a few subtypes, with which they are already familiar. However, they also underscore the need for recognizing the more recently described entities, which although less common, have important clinical differences. The study also found differences in geographic distribution of the lymphoma types, with follicular lymphoma being more common in North America and western Europe, T-cell lymphomas more common in Hong Kong, and both mediastinal large B-cell lymphoma and mantle cell lymphoma more common in Ticino (the Italian-speaking canton), Switzerland.[20]

The different entities recognized by the classification had significantly different clinical presentations and survivals. For example, diffuse aggressive lymphomas, which would be lumped as intermediate or high grade in the Working Formulation, include diffuse large B-cell lymphoma, mediastinal large B-cell lymphoma, peripheral T-cell lymphoma, and anaplastic

TABLE 45.3-8. Presenting Features of Common B- and T-Cell Neoplasms

				Stage					Any			International Prognostic Index		
Neoplasm	*Frequency (%)*	*Age*	*Male*	I	II	III	IV	*B-Symptoms*	*Extranodal Site Including Bone Marrow*	*Bone Marrow*	*Gastro-intestinal*	0/1	2/3	4/5
Large B-cell	31	64	55	25	29	13	33	33	71	16	18	35	46	9
Mediastinal	2	37	34	10	56	3	31	38	56	3	0	52	37	11
Follicular	22	59	42	18	15	16	51	28	64	42	4	45	48	7
Small lymphocytic lymphoma/chronic lymphocytic leukemia	6	65	53	4	5	8	83	33	80	72	3	23	64	13
Mucosa-associated lymphoid tissue	8	60	48	39	28	2	31	19	98	14	50	44	48	8
Mantle cell	6	63	74	13	7	9	71	28	81	51	9	23	54	23
Peripheral T-cell	7	61	55	8	12	15	65	50	82	36	15	17	52	31
Anaplastic large cell lymphoma	2	34	69	19	32	10	39	53	59	13	9	61	18	21

large T/null-cell lymphoma. The clinical features at presentation were strikingly different, with a younger age group for mediastinal large T-cell lymphoma and anaplastic large T/null-cell lymphoma, and striking differences in male to female ratios, suggesting that these are distinctive biologic entities (see Table 45.3-8). When overall survivals were analyzed, entities that would have been lumped together as *low grade* or *intermediate/high grade* in the Working Formulation showed marked differences in survival, again confirming that they need to be recognized and treated as distinct entities.

A critical finding in this study was that classification is not the only predictor of clinical outcome. Patients with any of these diseases could be stratified into better and worse prognostic groups according to the International Prognostic Index.[133] For example, although patients with follicular lymphoma typically have International Prognostic Index scores of 1 to 3, those patients with scores of 4 or 5 had a predicted median overall survival of only 18 months. Thus, to plan treatment for an individual patient, the oncologist must know not only the diagnosis, but the clinical prognostic factors that influence that patient's course.

DIFFERENTIAL DIAGNOSIS OF INDOLENT DISSEMINATED LYMPHOMA

For most of the indolent lymphoid neoplasms, both the clinical and pathologic differential diagnosis includes, first, a benign lymphoid proliferation, and second, another type of indolent lymphoma or leukemia. In distinguishing B-CLL/SLL, immunocytoma, or splenic marginal zone lymphoma (SMZL) with villous lymphocytes from reactive lymphocytosis, cytologic criteria can be difficult, since cytologic atypia may be minimal; the only reliable technique is SIg analysis for clonality, usually by flow cytometry. In lymph nodes or other tissues, the most important distinguishing features include effacement of the architecture and the presence or absence of pseudofollicles. On frozen sections or flow cytometry, demonstration of monotypic SIg and CD5 expression are also useful. On paraffin sections, demonstration of a predominance of interfollicular B cells, often with coexpression of CD43, can provide suggestive evidence of B-cell lymphoma.

B-SLL/CLL, immunocytoma, and SMZL must be distinguished from one another and from MALT type lymphoma (in extranodal sites) and mantle cell lymphoma (which can involve blood, bone marrow, and spleen). The presence of pseudofollicles is diagnostic of CLL/SLL; expression of CD23 (frozen sections) and lack of cyclin D1 (paraffin sections) can exclude mantle cell lymphoma, whereas expression of CD5 argues against a diagnosis of MALT type lymphoma, lymphoplasmacytoid lymphoma, or SMZL. By flow cytometry, SIg in CLL is usually weak, whereas it tends to be stronger in the other lymphomas; CD25 or CD103 are also uncommon in B-CLL and more common in some of the other lymphoid leukemias.

Clinically and pathologically, the differential diagnosis of SMZL also includes hairy cell leukemia. Although the cells in the peripheral blood may resemble hairy cells, the nuclei are usually smaller, with more condensed chromatin, and the villi are polar and less conspicuous than those of hairy cell leukemia. The marrow infiltrate is usually sparse and nodular, in contrast to hairy cell leukemia. The cells may, however, express CD25, CD103, and even TRAP. In the past, many cases were probably diagnosed as atypical hairy cell leukemia or B-CLL. Distinction from lymphoplasmacytoid lymphoma is more problematic; both are CD5– and both may have an M component and evidence of plasmacytoid differentiation. The relationship between SMZL/splenic lymphoma with villous lymphocytes and lymphoplasmacytoid lymphoma needs further study.

DIFFERENTIAL DIAGNOSIS OF INDOLENT EXTRANODAL AND NODAL LYMPHOMAS

The most important clinical and pathologic differential diagnosis in indolent lymphomas in either lymph nodes or extranodal sites is with benign lymphoid hyperplasias. In this situation, if morphologic criteria are insufficient, staining for Ig light-chains is the most useful test to determine clonality.

In the differential diagnosis of gastric MALT type lymphomas, clinical features favoring lymphoma include evidence of a mass, enlargement of gastric folds, or a multinodular appearance to the mucosa. Histologically, the presence of a dense, diffuse infiltrate of marginal zone B cells, with destruction of glands and prominent lymphoepithelial lesions is required for a confident diagnosis. In borderline cases, paraffin section immunoperoxidase stains for cIg may be helpful in approximately 50% of the cases; frozen section immunophenotyping for detection of monotypic SIg is definitive in the rest. If gastric MALT lymphoma is suspected in a patient with *Helicobacter* infection, it is important *not* to treat with antibiotics until the diagnosis is ruled in or out by special studies, including rebiopsy if necessary. Antibiotic therapy often causes the lymphoma to regress, but the long-term outcome of these patients is not known, and therefore it is important to know *before* treatment, whether the patient has lymphoma or just gastritis.

The major differential diagnosis, both clinically and pathologically, for follicular lymphoma is with reactive follicular hyperplasia. The presence of persistent, nontender lymph nodes in an older adult should raise the suspicion of follicular lymphoma, particularly if more than one site is involved. Histologic criteria for this differential diagnosis are well established; in the minority of cases in which a confident diagnosis is not possible on routine sections, demonstration of monotypic SIg on flow cytometry or frozen section, or of bcl-2 expression within the follicles, can confirm the diagnosis. Molecular genetic studies to confirm Ig gene or bcl-2 rearrangement are rarely necessary but can be helpful.

Follicular lymphoma, mantle cell lymphoma, nodal monocytoid B-cell lymphoma, and extranodal MALT lymphoma must all be distinguished from one another. Clinically, the first three usually involve generalized lymph nodes; however, when mantle cell lymphoma presents with extranodal involvement in the form of lymphomatous polyposis of the gastrointestinal tract, it may be confused with MALT type lymphoma. The presence of widespread disease involving multiple gastrointestinal sites strongly favors mantle cell lymphoma. In other extranodal sites such as the orbit[134] and breast,[135] follicular lymphoma may be more common than MALToma and should be considered in the differential diagnosis.

Although most cases of indolent nodal lymphoma can be correctly classified by morphologic criteria if good histologic sections are available, immunophenotyping studies can be helpful and are occasionally necessary for correct subclassification (see Table 45.3-2). Expression of CD5 and CD43 and lack of CD23 and (usually) CD10 are useful in distinguishing mantle cell lymphoma from CLL and follicular center lymphoma, respectively. In extranodal sites, CD5 is useful in distinguishing mantle cell lymphoma from MALToma. Staining for cyclin D1 is potentially the most specific marker for mantle cell lymphoma; Southern blot or PCR studies can also be used to detect the t(11;14).

DIFFERENTIAL DIAGNOSIS OF MATURE (PERIPHERAL) T-CELL LYMPHOMAS

With most peripheral T-cell lymphomas, the clinical and pathologic differential diagnosis includes an atypical reactive process, such as a viral infection, and one of the more common B-cell lymphomas. Because of the great variety of clinical presentations and morphologic features, establishing a diagnosis can be difficult and may require multiple diagnostic procedures. Since there is no reliable immunophenotypic marker for clonality in T cells, molecular genetic analysis is often necessary when the differential diagnosis includes a reactive process. These studies can often be performed on cells isolated from blood or body fluids or from needle-aspiration biopsies, if the initial diagnostic biopsy has not been processed to obtain fresh tissue. An important caveat is excluding a B-cell lymphoma; many B-cell lymphomas of both low and high grade contain numerous reactive T cells in biopsy specimens. Therefore, simply demonstrating a predominance of T cells does not establish the diagnosis of a T-cell lymphoma; tissues should always be stained for B-cell–associated antigens and Ig.

PRINCIPLES OF MANAGEMENT OF NON-HODGKIN'S LYMPHOMA

The principles of the management of patients with NHL have steadily evolved. The phases of patient management include obtaining an adequate biopsy for an accurate diagnosis, a careful history and physical examination, appropriate laboratory studies, imaging studies, and possibly, further biopsies to determine an accurate stage and to plan therapy. Finally, taking into account factors related to the patient, type of lymphoma, and stage and pace of disease, a treatment recommendation must be made. Treatment choices include no initial therapy, radiotherapy, cytotoxic chemotherapy, a variety of new biologic therapies, and hematopoietic stem cell transplantation.

HISTORY AND PHYSICAL EXAMINATION

A careful history and physical examination is the basis for subsequent studies to determine the extent of the disease and key factor in the therapeutic decision. The duration of symptoms and the pace of progression of the illness should be documented. The physician should not discount the possibility that waxing and waning lymphadenopathy could be related to the lymphoma. Especially in follicular lymphomas, spontaneous regressions are frequent. The presence of specific symptoms known to have an adverse prognosis in patients with some types of lymphoma should be ascertained. These include fevers, night sweats, and unexplained weight loss. Symptoms referable to a particular organ system such as pain in the chest, abdomen, or bones might lead to identification of specific sites of involvement. History of a concurrent illness such as diabetes or congestive heart failure might modify therapeutic decisions.

A careful physical examination can lead to important observations that will direct subsequent care. Obviously, examination of all lymph node–bearing areas and a search for hepatomegaly or splenomegaly are important. Pharyngeal involvement, a thyroid mass, evidence of pleural effusion, abdominal mass, testicular mass, or cutaneous lesions are all examples of findings that might direct further investigations and subsequent therapy. Certain associations of involvement between two organ sites are worth remembering. For example, patients with involvement of Waldeyer's ring often have gastrointestinal involvement, and the converse is also true. These patients usually have mantle cell lymphoma. Patients with paranasal sinus, testicular involvement, and epidermal lymphoma are especially prone to meningeal spread and deserve a diagnostic lumbar puncture and, probably, prophylactic therapy. Patients with one testicle involved are likely to relapse on the opposite side and radiotherapy should be directed to the entire scrotum with this in mind. Patients with ocular lymphoma almost always have dissemination to other parts of the CNS in the absence of prophylactic therapy.

LABORATORY EVALUATION

Laboratory studies should include complete blood count and screening chemistry studies to include renal and hepatic function studies, serum glucose, calcium, albumin, lactate dehydrogenase (LDH), and β_2-microglobulin level. Serum protein electrophoresis is frequently appropriate. The purpose of these studies is to aid in determining the prognosis (e.g., LDH, β_2-microglobulin, albumin) and identifying abnormalities in other organ systems that might complicate therapy (e.g., renal or hepatic dysfunction).

In addition to the diagnostic biopsy, almost all patients should have a bone marrow aspirate and biopsy performed. The chances of finding bone marrow involvement varies considerably among different subtypes of lymphoma (Table 45.3-9). It is present in approximately 70% of patients with SLL, lymphoplasmacytoid lymphoma, and mantle cell lymphoma. Patients with follicular lymphoma have bone marrow involvement approximately 50% of the time, while it is seen in approximately 15% of patients with diffuse large B-cell lymphoma[126] (see Table 45.3-9). Bone marrow involvement in patients with

TABLE 45.3-9. Frequency of Extranodal Involvement by Non-Hodgkin's Lymphomas

Subtype of Non-Hodgkin's Lymphoma	*Bone Marrow (%)*	*Gastrointestinal Tract (%)*	*Any Extranodal Site (%)*
Follicular	42	4	64
Small lymphocytic	72	3	80
Mucosa-associated lymphoid tissue	14	50	98
Mantle cell	64	9	81
Diffuse large B-cell	16	18	71
Burkitt's	33	11	78
Lymphoblastic	50	4	82
Peripheral T-cell	36	15	82
Anaplastic large T/null cell	13	9	59

follicular and SLL has little prognostic import except when bone marrow is extensively involved and cytopenias or large numbers of circulating lymphoma cells are present. In patients with diffuse large B-cell lymphoma, bone marrow involvement can occur with the large cells or small B cells. Patients with large cell lymphoma in the marrow have a distinctly adverse prognosis, while marrow involvement by small cells has a much less clear effect on prognosis.[136]

IMAGING STUDIES

Chest Radiography and Computed Tomographic Scans

Chest radiography and computed tomographic (CT) scans of the chest, abdomen, and pelvis should be performed at the initial evaluation in almost all patients with NHL. Although the chest radiograph is abnormal in less than 50% of patients, identification of hilar or mediastinal adenopathy, parenchymal lesions, or pleural effusions is important and provides an easy method for reevaluation. CT scanning can identify both nodal and extranodal sites of involvement and provides an important approach to monitoring the response to therapy. This approach has largely replaced lymphangiography for the evaluation of retroperitoneal lymphadenopathy. This is partly because of the difficulty of performing lymphangiography. The abdominal and pelvic CT scan can identify mesenteric and retrocrural nodes and is more accurate than the lymphangiogram in determining the dimension of nodal disease.[137,138] Involvement of intraabdominal organs such as kidney, ovary, spleen, and liver can be identified on CT scans.

Magnetic Resonance Imaging

The value of magnetic resonance imaging (MRI) in the staging of NHL is limited. This technique can be used in lieu of CT scanning in many patients, but its higher cost makes this impractical. MRI is particularly useful in identifying bone and CNS involvement. MRI can suggest meningeal involvement when gadolinium has been used. MRI can also identify bone marrow involvement[139] and might be more sensitive than bone marrow biopsy in this regard. However, it has not yet been accepted as a substitute for bone marrow biopsy.

Nuclear Medicine Studies

The most common nuclear medicine studies used in staging patients with lymphoma are bone scans and gallium scans. Bone scans are rarely used as part of the initial staging studies. They can sometimes be useful in patients who present with or develop back pain during the course of their lymphoma, looking for vertebral involvement and potential spinal cord compression.

Gallium scans are more often used as part of the staging evaluation. This study, because it provides functional rather than purely anatomic information, has potential value in resolving difficulties in determining the response to therapy.[140] To be maximally valuable, high doses of gallium need to be administered and single photon emission CT needs to be used. Gallium scan results are more likely to be positive in patients with aggressive lymphoma such as diffuse large B-cell lymphomas than in more indolent lymphoma such as follicular lymphoma, but can be positive in any subtype. Gallium scans are more accurate in evaluating supradiaphragmatic rather than infradiaphragmatic sites because of colon uptake of the gallium. Unfortunately, this test is most often needed in determining intraabdominal sites of involvement.

On rare occasions, technetium liver spleen scans can be helpful in determining the cause of splenic involvement in the patient in whom lymphoma is suspected. One of the differential diagnoses in such patients is occult liver disease. Technetium liver spleen scans that show more uptake in the spleen than liver suggest occult liver disease, and a liver biopsy should be done before considering splenectomy.

Positron Emission Tomographic Scans

Positron emission tomographic (PET) scanning has been increasingly applied in staging patients with lymphoma. The specificity and sensitivity of PET scanning seems to be at least that of gallium scanning. The procedure has been more widely adopted in some countries in Europe than in the United States. Despite enthusiastic reports, more large comparative trials assessing the relative merits of PET scanning, gallium scanning, and CT scanning need to be completed before PET replaces previous tests. Merely adding PET scanning to all the previous studies will only increase the cost of therapy.

STAGING LAPAROTOMY

Staging laparotomies became popular in the late 1960s and 1970s for evaluating patients with Hodgkin's disease. The same approach was used in patients with NHLs. Studies showed that a large proportion of patients with apparently localized follicular lymphoma would be upstaged using staging laparotomy, but this was a less common event in diffuse large B-cell lymphoma. Because of improvements in imaging studies, and the morbidity and potential mortality associated with staging laparotomy, this procedure is rarely appropriate in the initial evaluation of a patient with NHL. However, some patients with NHL are diagnosed at laparotomy, and if the diagnosis is known during the procedure, careful evaluation of other lymph nodes sites and organs by the surgeon can be valuable.

POLYMERASE CHAIN REACTION FOR EVALUATING MINIMAL RESIDUAL DISEASE

The use of PCR to expand small numbers of cells with a particular genetic abnormality can allow identification of cells as frequent as 1 in 10^5.[141] This has usually been applied to studying blood and bone marrow, but could be applied in other sites. Studies to date have generally focused on the t(14;18) translocation and the associated bcl-2 gene. Several observations have been made. PCR positivity for bcl-2 gene rearrangements can be found in healthy individuals.[142] However, patients with lymphoma in remission who show positive results for bcl-2 gene rearrangement using PCR in the blood or bone marrow are more likely to relapse than patients who do not have this abnormality discovered.[143] Unfortunately, some patients that are positive do not relapse and some patients that are negative do relapse. At present, this approach is probably better considered a research tool. Planning further therapy based only on this abnormality appears risky, until the test is better standardized and the implications of an abnormal finding are better quantified.

TABLE 45.3-10. Ann Arbor Staging System

Stage	*Description*[a]
I	Involvement of a single lymph node region or a single extralymphatic organ or site (IE)
II	Involvement of two or more lymph node regions on the same side of the diaphragm (II) or localized involvement of an extralymphatic organ or site (IIE)
III	Involvement of lymph node regions on both sides of the diaphragm (III) or localized involvement of an extralymphatic organ or site (IIIE) or spleen (IIIS) or both (IIISE)
IV	Diffuse or disseminated involvement of one or more extralymphatic organs with or without associated lymph node involvement. Bone marrow and liver involvement are

[a]Identification of the presence or absence of symptoms should be noted with each stage designation: A, asymptomatic; B, fever, sweats, weight loss greater than 10% of body weight.

STAGING AND PROGNOSTIC SYSTEMS

The goal of the initial evaluation of a patient with lymphoma is to provide information that allows intelligent planning of therapy, imparting the prognosis to the patient, and making possible comparisons between patients in clinical trials. The studies to accomplish these goals can be aimed at identifying sites of involvement, characteristics of the patient (i.e., age, performance status, and so forth), or characteristic of the lymphoma (serum LDH, serum β_2-microglobulin, growth fraction, and so forth) that predict treatment outcome.

The Ann Arbor Staging System was developed for patients with Hodgkin's disease. This system[144] (Table 45.3-10) identifies anatomic sites of involvement by lymphoma and assigns patients into four categories based on the extent of disease dissemination. Patients are also subcategorized by the presence of unexplained fevers, night sweats, or weight loss. This system has a significant effect on prognosis and is important in treatment planning.

Other staging systems have been identified.[145–147] These have used anatomic stage as identified by the Ann Arbor System, symptoms, performance status, serum LDH, serum β_2-microglobulin, tumor size, number of sites of involvement, and bone marrow involvement. The bulk of lymphoma is an important prognostic indicator whenever it has been studied. Unfortunately, there has been no consensus on how to best measure bulk. The diameter of the largest mass has been the most common method used, but diameters of 5, 7, and 10 cm have been used by different investigators, making comparisons difficult. Even so, a greater than 10-cm mass, regardless of anatomic stage, is a serious negative prognostic factor. These patients might benefit from adjuvant radiotherapy even if the disease is disseminated.

At present, the most valuable and widely used system to stratify patients is the International Prognostic Index[148] (Table 45.3-11). It was developed by investigators throughout the world for use in predicting outcome for patients with diffuse aggressive NHLs treated with an anthracycline-containing combination chemotherapy regimen. Five features were found to have approximately an equal and independent effect on survival. These included age, serum LDH, performance status, anatomic stage, and the number of extranodal sites. Because of the approximately equal effect on outcome, the number of abnormalities were simply summed to develop the prognostic index. Thus, patients might have a score of 0 to 5. For patients under the age of 60, a simplified index can be applied that incorporates only anatomic stage, serum LDH, and performance status. This system was initially developed only for patients with diffuse aggressive lymphoma. However, it is clear that it applies to patients with almost all subtypes of NHL.[127]

RESTAGING

After patients have received three or four cycles of the planned treatment regimen or at the completion of the entire regimen, reevaluation should be done to determine the response to therapy. For patients with diffuse aggressive lymphoma, reevaluation after three or four cycles of therapy can add prognostic information. Patients who have a complete response are more likely to be cured than patients who have only achieved a partial response at this point. Achieving a complete remission to therapy is the most important single prognostic factor in patients with NHL.[149] Documenting complete remission is important. It is particularly true since salvage treatment such as high-dose therapy and autologous or allogeneic bone marrow transplantation can sometimes cure disease in patients who fail to respond to initial therapy.

TABLE 45.3-11. International Prognostic Index for Diffuse Large Cell Lymphoma

Number of Risk Factors	*Percentage of Patients*	*Complete Response Rate (%)*	*5-Y Disease-Free Survival (%)*	*5-Y Survival (%)*
All patients (adverse risk factors, age >60 y; performance status ≥2, lactate dehydrogenase greater than normal; Ann Arbor stage III or IV, ≥2 extranodal sites)				
0, 1	35	87	70	73
2	27	67	50	51
3	22	55	49	43
4, 5	16	44	40	26
Patients <60 y old (adverse risk factors, Ann Arbor stage III or IV, lactate dehydrogenase greater than normal, performance status ≥2)				
0, 1	22	92	86	83
2	32	78	66	69
3	32	57	53	46
4, 5	14	46	58	32

A restaging evaluation typically involves repeating all previous studies with abnormal results to document their current normal results. However, especially in sites of bulky disease, masses do not always completely regress. This does not necessarily mean that patients will have persisting lymphoma. Rebiopsy under these circumstances can be difficult and is not always accurate. If the patient was known to have a positive gallium scan or PET scan at the outset of treatment, a normal result of that test despite a residual mass raises the possibility that only residual fibrous tissue is present. Gallium avidity midtreatment cycle or at the end of treatment is associated with a much higher relapse rate than seen in patients who have negative results on gallium scanning.[140]

SPECIFIC DISEASE ENTITIES

B-CELL NEOPLASMS

Precursor B-Lymphoblastic Leukemia and Lymphoma (Precursor B-Cell Acute Lymphoblastic Leukemia/ Precursor B-Lymphoblastic Lymphoma)

DEFINITION. The definition is a neoplasm of lymphoblasts committed to the B-cell lineage, typically composed of small to medium-sized blast cells with scant cytoplasm, moderately condensed to dispersed chromatin and indistinct nucleoli, involving bone marrow and blood (ALL), and occasionally presenting with primary involvement of nodal or extranodal sites (lymphoblastic lymphoma).

MORPHOLOGY. On smears, lymphoblasts vary from small cells with scant cytoplasm, condensed nuclear chromatin, and indistinct nucleoli to larger cells with a moderate amount of cytoplasm, dispersed chromatin, and multiple nucleoli. Azurophilic granules may be present. In tissue sections, the cells are small to medium sized, with scant cytoplasm; round, oval, or convoluted nuclei; fine chromatin; and indistinct or small nucleoli. Occasional cases have larger cells. The pattern is infiltrative rather than destructive, with partial preservation of the subcapsular sinus and germinal centers. A *starry-sky* pattern may be present, but this is usually less prominent than in Burkitt's lymphoma.

IMMUNOPHENOTYPE. The lymphoblasts are typically positive for TdT and variably express CD19, CD22, CD20, and CD79a, as well as CD45 and CD10. The constellation of antigens defines stages of differentiation, ranging from early precursor (membrane CD19 and CD79a and cytoplasmic CD22) to common ALL (CD10+) to late pre-B ALL (CD20+, cytoplasmic μ heavy-chain). CD34 is expressed on 40%, and coexpression of myeloid antigens is seen in up to 30%, most commonly CD13 (14%), CD33(16%), or both.[150,151] Expression of CD13 and CD33 is associated with rearrangement of ETV6 [t(12;21)(p12;q22),ETV6-CBFA2 or TEL-AML1], while expression of CD68, CD15, and CD33 are seen in cases with 11q23/ MLL abnormalities.[151]

GENETIC FEATURES. Rearrangement of antigen receptor genes is variable in lymphoblastic neoplasms and may not be lineage specific; thus, precursor B-cell neoplasms may have either or both Ig heavy-chain and TCR γ or β chain gene rearrangements, or may show no rearrangements.[152–154]

POSTULATED NORMAL COUNTERPART. The postulated normal counterpart is precursor B lymphoblast at varying stages of differentiation.

CLINICAL FEATURES AND THERAPY. Precursor B-ALL/ lymphoblastic lymphoma occurs most frequently in childhood, with a second peak in the elderly. The outcome is less favorable in infants less than 1 year of age and in adults. In addition to cytogenetic features, risk groups are based on age, leukocyte count, sex, and response to therapy. In infants, many cases have translocations involving the MLL gene at 11q23, which is associated with a poor prognosis at any age[155]; older children more often have hyperdiploidy or t(12;21), which confers a better prognosis (85% to 90% long-term survival).[156] Adult precursor B-ALL is more often associated with the poor-prognosis t(9;22) or t(v11q23), and the survival is much poorer than that for childhood cases.[150,157] Myeloid antigen expression does not seem to be an independent prognostic factor in ALL.[151,158] Therapy is the same as described for T-lymphoblastic lymphoma.

B-Cell Chronic Lymphocytic Leukemia/Small Lymphocytic Lymphoma

DEFINITION. The definition of B-CLL/SLL is a neoplasm of monomorphic, small round B lymphocytes in the peripheral blood and lymph nodes, admixed with prolymphocytes and paraimmunoblasts in lymph nodes, usually expressing CD5 and CD23. B-SLL is defined as a tissue infiltrate with the morphology and immunophenotype of B-CLL.

MORPHOLOGY. The lymph node infiltrate of B-CLL/SLL is composed predominantly of small lymphocytes with condensed chromatin, round nuclei, and occasionally a small nucleolus.[159,160] Larger lymphoid cells (prolymphocytes and paraimmunoblasts) with more prominent nucleoli and dispersed chromatin are always present, usually clustered in pseudofollicles. In some cases, the cells show moderate nuclear irregularity, which can lead to a differential diagnosis of mantle cell lymphoma.[161,162] Occasional cases show plasmacytoid differentiation.

IMMUNOPHENOTYPE. The tumor cells of B-CLL have faint SIgM, and most coexpress IgD. The antigen specificity of the SIg in many cases has been shown to be against self-antigens, and these antibodies often have broad specificity, so-called cross-reactive idiotypes.[163] Cytoplasmic Ig is detectable in approximately 5% of the cases. B-cell–associated antigens (CD19, CD20, CD79a) are positive, but particularly CD20 may be weak; tumor cells characteristically express both CD5 and CD23.[164] CD23 is particularly useful in distinguishing B-CLL/SLL from mantle cell lymphoma and should be evaluated in every case, if possible.[164]

GENETIC FEATURES. Ig heavy and light-chain genes are rearranged. Most cases (75%) in early studies did not show somatic mutation of their V regions, suggesting that they corresponded to a cell that has not yet undergone antigen selection in the germinal center.[165] However, more recent studies have found up to 40% of the cases to have V region mutations, consistent with exposure to the germinal center. Cases with mutations are reported to express CD38 and to be associated with a better prognosis than cases without mutations or that are CD38–.[166,167]

Approximately 50% of cases have abnormal karyotypes.[168] Trisomy 12 is reported in one-third of the cases with cytogenetic abnormalities[169] and correlates with atypical histology and an aggressive clinical course.[162,170] Abnormalities of 13q are reported in up to 25% of the cases and are associated with long survival. t(11;14) and bcl-1 gene rearrangement have been reported,[171,172] but many of these cases may be examples of leukemic mantle cell lymphoma; however, at least two clear-cut cases of B-CLL have been reported with bcl-1 gene rearrangement, cyclin D1 overexpression, or both; in both it was associated with an unusually aggressive clinical course.[173,174] Abnormalities of 11q23 are found in a small subset of cases and are associated with lymphadenopathy and an aggressive course.[175,176]

POSTULATED NORMAL COUNTERPART. Many cases of B-CLL are thought to correspond to the recirculating CD5+ CD23+ naive B cells,[177] which are found in the peripheral blood, primary follicle, and follicle mantle zone.[178,179] It has been suggested that they are an anergic, self-reactive CD5+ B-cell subset.[180,181] Cases that show V region mutations may correspond to a subset of peripheral blood CD5+ IgM+ B cells that appear to be memory B cells.[182]

CLINICAL FEATURES. B-CLL accounts for 90% of chronic lymphoid leukemias in the United States and Europe; nonleukemic B-SLL accounts for less than 5% of NHLs. In the International Non-Hodgkin's Lymphoma Classification Project, 6.7% of 1378 cases were diagnosed as B-CLL/SLL. The median age was 65 years, and 83% had stage IV disease, 73% with bone marrow involvement. Generalized lymphadenopathy, hepatosplenomegaly, and extranodal infiltrates may occur. Sixty-four percent had an International Prognostic Index score of 2/3. The 5-year overall actuarial survival was 51%, with a failure-free survival of 25%; for those patients with an International Prognostic Index of 0/1, the overall actuarial survival was 76%, whereas for those with an International Prognostic Index of 4/5 it was only 38%. Thus, the extent of the disease at the time of the diagnosis is the best predictor of survival; however, chromosomal abnormalities and immunophenotype may also have prognostic importance.[183]

Patients with SLL can present with hypogammaglobulinemia or develop it over the course of the illness.[184,185] The presence of hypogammaglobulinemia is associated with an increased incidence of infections and can be managed in some patients with intermittent gamma globulin injections. Polyclonal or monoclonal hypergammaglobulinemia can also be seen.[185,186] Autoimmune hemolytic anemias can be seen in patients with SLL[187] and are particularly likely to develop in patients treated with fludarabine.[188] Autoimmune thrombocytopenia is not rare.[189] Autoimmune neutropenia and pure red cell aplasia are unusual.[185]

THERAPY. Localized SLL is unusual and was seen in only 4% of patients in a large series.[127] The rare patient who presents in this manner could be treated with local radiotherapy. Such patients should have their slides reviewed to make certain they do not have a MALT lymphoma.

Some patients with disseminated SLL/chronic lymphocytic leukemia have a slowly progressive or stable disorder that does not require therapy. The traditional treatment for this lymphoma has been oral chlorambucil or oral cyclophosphamide. However, it is now clear that fludarabine is the most active single agent. Several randomized trials have been completed. One study with 544 patients randomized received fludarabine, chlorambucil, or a combination of both drugs. Patients who failed to respond to an individual drug were crossed over to the other arm. The overall response rate (70% vs. 43%) and complete response rate (27% vs. 3%) favored fludarabine over chlorambucil.[190] Although progression-free survival also favored fludarabine, there was no difference in overall survival. Another randomized trial[191,192] studied 695 patients and compared fludarabine with anthracycline-containing combinations. Fludarabine had a superior response rate. It appears that combinations including fludarabine and cyclophosphamide are also active and might be more active than fludarabine alone.[193]

Patients with SLL/chronic lymphocytic leukemia can respond to monoclonal antibody therapy using rituximab (anti-CD20) and Campath-1 (anti-CD52). However, the response rate to rituximab appears to be on the order of 20%, perhaps because of the lower level of expression of CD20 than seen in follicular lymphoma.[194,195]

Combination chemotherapy using CHOP or FND produces significant response rates in SLL, but the patients almost always relapse. High-dose therapy and autologous transplantation[196] and allogeneic transplantation[197] have both been used in fairly small numbers of patients. It appears that allogeneic transplantation can probably be curative. In general, principles of therapy of SLL apply to patients with lymphoplasmacytic lymphoma.

Lymphoplasmacytic Lymphoma (with or without Waldenström's Macroglobulinemia)

DEFINITION. Lymphoplasmacytic lymphoma is defined as a neoplasm of small B lymphocytes, plasmacytoid lymphocytes, and plasma cells, involving bone marrow, lymph nodes, and spleen, lacking CD5, usually with a serum monoclonal protein with hyperviscosity or cryoglobulinemia. Plasmacytoid variants of other neoplasms are excluded. The name, lymphoplasma*cytoid* (REAL) has been changed to lymphoplasma*cytic* (WHO).

MORPHOLOGY. The tumor consists of a diffuse proliferation of small lymphocytes, plasmacytoid lymphocytes, and plasma cells, with variable numbers of immunoblasts. In lymph nodes, sinuses are often open and may contain histiocytes reacting to secreted periodic acid–Schiff-positive Ig. In the spleen, both red and white pulp may be infiltrated. The pattern is usually diffuse, without a distinct marginal zone or nodularity in the red pulp. The bone marrow infiltrate may be either diffuse or nodular and is often interstitial and rather subtle. It is usually less massive than that of B-CLL and contains plasma cells and plasmacytoid cells in addition to small lymphocytes. Peripheral blood involvement is usually less prominent than in CLL, and the cells often have a plasmacytoid appearance.

IMMUNOPHENOTYPE. The cells have surface and cytoplasmic (some cells) Ig, usually of IgM type, usually lack IgD, and strongly express B-cell–associated antigens (CD19, CD20, CD22, and CD79a). The cells are CD5–, CD10–, CD23–, CD43+/–; CD25 or CD11c may be faintly positive in some cases.[164,198–200] Lack of CD5 and CD23, strong SIg and CD20, and the presence of cytoplasmic Ig are useful in distinguishing it from B-CLL.

GENETIC FEATURES. Ig heavy and light-chain genes are rearranged, and V region genes show somatic mutations, suggesting that, in contrast to B-CLL, these cells arise from a population of B cells that have undergone antigen B–driven selection.[165,201–203] Translocation t(9;14)(p13;q32) and rearrangement of the PAX-5 gene is reported in up to 50% of the cases. PAX-5 encodes a protein, B-cell–specific activator protein, which is important in early B-cell development. Expression of B-cell–specific activator protein is restricted to B cells and appears to be independent of the translocation.[204]

POSTULATED NORMAL COUNTERPART. The postulated normal counterpart is a peripheral B lymphocyte stimulated to differentiate to a plasma cell, possibly corresponding to the primary immune response to antigen, or to a post–germinal center cell that has undergone somatic mutation but not heavy-chain class switch.

CLINICAL FEATURES AND THERAPY. Lymphoplasmacytic lymphoma made up only 1.2% (16 of 1378) of the cases in the REAL clinical study.[126] Similar to B-CLL/SLL, the median age was 63 years and 53% were men; most (73%) had bone marrow involvement. Sixty-nine percent had an International Prognostic Index of 2/3. Lymph node and splenic involvement are common. A monoclonal serum paraprotein of IgM type, with or without hyperviscosity syndrome (Waldenström's macroglobulinemia), is present in most patients[205]; as with B-CLL, the paraprotein may have autoantibody or cryoglobulin activity.

Most cases of mixed cryoglobulinemia have been shown to be related to HCV infection, even in patients who have demonstrable B-cell lymphoma in the bone marrow.[206,207] Treatment of patients with HCV and cryoglobulinemia with interferon to reduce viral load has been associated with regression of the lymphoma.[208] HCV infection has also been documented in patients with B-cell lymphoma without cryoglobulinemia, most commonly in MALT type/monocytoid B-cell lymphomas and in lymphomas of the salivary gland and liver (two sites of chronic viral infection).[79,209–211] HCV is an RNA virus that cannot integrate into the host genome, but it does infect lymphocytes, and viral proteins have been detected in lymphoid cells in these patients.[212] It is not clear at this point whether HCV has transforming potential, or whether these neoplasms are antigen driven, similar to MALT type lymphomas.

The clinical course of LPL is indolent; in some European series it has been reported to be more aggressive than typical B-CLL,[213,214] but in the REAL clinical study, 5-year overall actuarial survival (58%) and failure-free survival (25%) were identical to that of CLL/SLL.[126] The traditional therapy for this disorder has been chlorambucil with or without prednisone.[215] Anthracycline-based combination chemotherapy has not been shown to be more effective. However, fludarabine and cladribine[216,217] are active as single agents. Combinations including fludarabine are now being studied.

Extranodal Marginal Zone B-Cell Lymphoma (Low-Grade B-Cell Lymphoma of Mucosa-Associated Lymphoid Tissue)

DEFINITION. Extranodal marginal zone B-cell lymphoma is defined as an extranodal lymphoma consisting of heterogeneous small B cells, including marginal zone (centrocyte-like) cells, monocytoid cells, and small lymphocytes in varying proportions, and scattered immunoblast- and centroblast-like cells, with plasma cell differentiation in 40% of the cases. The infiltrate is in the marginal zone of reactive B-cell follicles and extends into the interfollicular region.

MORPHOLOGY. Extranodal marginal zone B-cell (MALT) lymphoma reproduces the morphologic features of normal MALT. It is characterized by a polymorphous infiltrate of small lymphocytes, marginal zone (centrocyte-like) B cells, monocytoid B cells, and plasma cells, as well as rare large basophilic blast cells (centroblast- or immunoblast-like). Reactive follicles are usually present, with the neoplastic marginal zone or monocytoid B cells occupying the marginal zone, the interfollicular region, or both; occasional follicles may be *colonized* by marginal zone or monocytoid cells. In epithelial tissues, the marginal zone B cells typically infiltrate the epithelium, forming so-called lymphoepithelial lesions.[218] While blast cells are typically present, they are by definition in the minority. Clusters or sheets of blasts sufficiently large to warrant a diagnosis of large cell lymphoma are associated with a worse prognosis. In these cases, a separate diagnosis of diffuse large B-cell lymphoma should be made. The term *high-grade MALT lymphoma* should be avoided for large B-cell lymphomas in MALT sites, since it may lead to inappropriate treatment with antibiotics instead of aggressive antilymphoma therapy.[130]

IMMUNOPHENOTYPE. The tumor cells express SIg (M greater than G greater than A), lack IgD, and 40% to 60% have monotypic cytoplasmic Ig, indicating plasmacytoid differentiation. They express B-cell–associated antigens (CD19, CD20, CD22, CD79a) and are usually negative for CD5 and CD10. Immunophenotyping studies are useful in confirming malignancy (light-chain restriction) and in excluding B-CLL (CD5+), mantle cell (CD5+), and follicle center (CD10+ CD43–, CD11c–, usually cIg–) lymphomas.[164,219]

GENETIC FEATURES. Ig genes are rearranged, and the variable region has a high degree of somatic mutation, as well as intraclonal diversity consistent with a post–germinal center stage of B-cell development.[220–222] Ig heavy-chain variable regions in the analyzed cases are those often found in autoantibodies, consistent with prior studies showing that the antibodies produced by the tumor cells have specificity against self-antigens such as endothelial cells.[222] The bcl-1 and bcl-2 genes are germline[223]; trisomy 3 (60%) and t(11;18) (25% to 40%) are the most common reported cytogenetic abnormalities.[224–226] Interestingly, neither of these abnormalities is common in primary large cell lymphomas of the gastrointestinal tract.[226,227] Analysis of the t(11;18) breakpoint has shown fusion of the apoptosis-inhibitor gene AP12 to a novel gene at 18q21, named *MLT*, in two cases of MALT lymphoma.[228] A gene involved in a breakpoint in MALT lymphomas with t(1;14) has been cloned;

named *BCL-10,* it is an apoptosis-promoting gene that in mutated form may cause cellular transformation.[229]

POSTULATED NORMAL COUNTERPART. The postulated normal counterpart is a post–germinal center B memory cell with capacity to differentiate into marginal zone, monocytoid, and plasma cells.

CLINICAL FEATURES. Extranodal marginal zone B-cell (MALT) lymphoma accounts for the majority of low-grade gastric lymphomas and almost 50% of all gastric lymphomas[230]; in other sites, such as the ocular adnexa, they make up approximately 40% of the cases,[134] and they account for the majority of low-grade pulmonary lymphomas.[231] Patients are usually older adults, although they may be in their 20s and 30s. A slight female predominance has been reported in some series.[164] The majority of patients present with localized stage I or II extranodal disease, involving glandular epithelial tissues of various sites. The stomach is the most frequent site, but most low-grade lymphomas (and former pseudolymphomas) presenting in the lung, thyroid, salivary gland, and orbit are of this type; skin and soft tissues may also be the presenting site. Many patients have a history of autoimmune disease, such as Sjögren's syndrome or Hashimoto's thyroiditis, or of *Helicobacter* gastritis in the case of gastric MALT lymphoma. *Acquired MALT* secondary to autoimmune disease or infection in these sites is thought to be the substrate for lymphoma development.[232]

Proliferation of the cells of marginal zone lymphoma at certain sites depends on the presence of activated, antigen-driven T cells; in gastric tumors, it has been shown that the T cells are driven by *Helicobacter pylori* antigens.[89] Therapy directed at the antigen (*Helicobacter pylori* in gastric lymphoma) results in regression of most early lesions.[233,234] The long-term prognosis of these patients is not known, however, and patients treated with antibiotic therapy require long and careful follow-up. The disease known as *Mediterranean abdominal lymphoma, a heavy-chain disease,* and *immunoproliferative small intestinal disease,* which occurs in young adults in eastern Mediterranean countries, is another example of a MALT type lymphoma that may respond to antibiotic therapy in its early stages.[235]

THERAPY OF MUCOSA-ASSOCIATED LYMPHOID TISSUE LYMPHOMAS

Nodal and Extranodal Marginal Zone B-Cell Non-Hodgkin's Lymphoma (Mucosa-Associated Lymphoid Tissue). The indolent extranodal lymphomas associated with MALT involve the gastrointestinal tract, salivary glands, breast, thyroid, orbit, conjunctiva, skin, lung, and less commonly other sites. As these diseases tend to remain localized for long periods of time, local treatment (surgery or local or regional irradiation) is effective at long-term control of disease and provides the opportunity for cure. In particular, low doses of radiation therapy (RT; 30 Gy) almost always control sites of disease. These doses are somewhat lower than used for patients with localized follicular grade 1 and 2 disease. Data regarding irradiation of gastric MALT suggest that doses above 30 Gy are probably not needed.[236]

The use of chemotherapy for MALT lymphomas has received limited attention as this indolent NHL does not routinely require the use of systemic treatment in patients with early-stage disease. In one study of 24 patients with low-grade MALT treated with daily cyclophosphamide or chlorambucil for 12 to 24 months, the complete response rate at 1 year was 75% and approximately 50% continued to be in remission at the time of the study.[237] Although these results are favorable, control of limited disease is superior with RT, and the use of chemotherapy should be limited to patients with advanced-stage disease.

One-half or more of patients with gastric NHL have the indolent MALT type. The optimal treatment of gastric MALT lymphoma remains to be determined. Gastric MALT lymphoma is frequently associated with chronic gastritis and *H pylori* infection. Based on clinical observations, it has been postulated that *H pylori* infection leads to the accumulation of MALT in the stomach, and that gastric MALT lymphomas arise within this *acquired MALT* tissue. This has prompted speculation that eradication of the *H pylori* infection might lead to tumor regression. Promising early results have been seen with the use of antibiotics for gastric MALT NHL. In one study from the German MALT Lymphoma Group, 33 patients with low-grade MALT were treated with antibiotics. At 1-year median follow-up more than 70% of patients remained in complete remission.[238] However, in a follow-up study, 22 of 31 patients in continuous complete remission (median follow-up, 16 months) had a monoclonal B-cell population on PCR analysis, leaving open the question of durability of complete response after antibiotics.[239] Nonetheless, the standard treatment for patients with gastric MALT who are positive for *H pylori* is antibiotics and follow-up endoscopy 3 and 6 months later. Patients who have a complete response should be followed without further treatment. Patients who have a partial response and remain *H pylori* positive should receive a second course of antibiotics before proceeding to more definitive treatment.

Patients who are negative for *H pylori* may be less likely to respond to antibiotics than *H pylori*–positive patients; initial treatment of *H pylori*–negative patients with antibiotics remains under study.[240] For patients who have persistent disease after antibiotics, local regional irradiation therapy is the treatment of choice. Good results have been obtained with total or partial gastrectomy; however, this approach has been associated with long-term morbidity. Local and regional radiation through the three-field approach (anterior and two lateral fields to minimize radiation to the left kidney) provides local control and relief of symptoms in greater than 90% of patients. Although more information is needed, 30 Gy appears sufficient to control disease in most patients.[236]

More than 80% of patients with pulmonary NHL have indolent histology; nearly 80% of these are MALT.[241] The 5-year survival of patients with pulmonary MALT is greater than 90%. Often surgery is the initial treatment for patients with pulmonary MALT; however, development of recurrent disease is common and moderately low-dose RT has the potential to provide durable remissions. Gastrointestinal MALT is less common than gastric MALT. Approximately 25% of patients with gastrointestinal NHL have MALT. Few data exist on the success of treatment of these patients. The most common sites are the jejunum and the ileocecum.

Patients with MALT in the salivary glands may have a history of Sjögren's disease. Because these patients often have symptoms of mild xerostomia and low doses of RT worsen the xerostomia, we recommend that the radiation fields be limited to the ipsilateral salivary gland region and draining nodes to spare as much of the remaining salivary tissue as possible.

Lymphomatous involvement occurs in the orbit and in the conjunctiva with approximately equal frequency, accounting for between 5% and 14% of all extranodal presentations. These locations should be considered individually as they are often histologically distinct and have different natural histories. Conjunctival lymphoma tends to be localized, but may be associated with advanced disease. Due to its infiltrative nature, conjunctival lymphoma recurs with a high frequency following surgical excision alone. Surgery is used for diagnosis, but local RT to the entire conjunctiva is the definitive treatment of choice. Treatment of conjunctival lymphoma can be accomplished with either electrons or with photons. We generally use electrons as the lens can be protected with daily placement of a tungsten eyeshield. Dunbar and colleagues from the Massachusetts General Hospital have recommended doses of 24 to 30 Gy for patients with conjunctival lymphoma. They saw no local recurrences in a series of 12 patients treated with electron-beam RT.[242]

CT scanning and MRI are useful for the evaluation of the extent of disease and important for radiation treatment planning when the orbit is involved. Various treatment field arrangements can be employed depending on the location of the disease (i.e., disease limited to the anterior portion of the orbit, involving both eyes, or involving the lacrimal glands). In treatment of orbital NHL in contrast to conjunctival NHL, it is not possible to block the lens and cataract development is more common. When disease is unilateral, a single anterior photon field can be used to avoid dose to the contralateral eye; however, this field produces a higher anterior dose and more dose than optimal to the lacrimal gland, resulting in a greater risk of some eye dryness. Alternatively, an anterior wedged pair can allow for better dose distribution within the tumor and less dose to normal tissues. Doses restricted to 30 to 36 Gy controls nearly 100% of indolent NHL of the orbit while maintaining a low risk of toxicity to the lacrimal glands and retina. With MALT lymphoma of the orbit, the dose can probably be reduced to 30 Gy.

MALT lymphomas can also be disseminated and present at an advanced stage in approximately one-third of cases.[243–245] Dissemination is usually to lymph nodes but can involve other extranodal sites. Patients with widespread MALT lymphoma should probably be treated in a manner similar to that described for follicular lymphoma.

Nodal Marginal Zone B-Cell Lymphoma

DEFINITION. Nodal marginal zone B-cell lymphoma is defined as a primary nodal lymphoma with features identical to lymph nodes involved by MALT lymphoma, but without evidence of extranodal disease. Monocytoid B cells may be prominent. This diagnosis should not be made in patients with MALT lymphoma at other sites, Sjögren's syndrome, or when another low-grade B-cell lymphoma (follicular, mantle cell) is present in the same node.

MORPHOLOGY. Tumors with morphologic features identical to those described for extranodal marginal zone (MALT type) lymphoma have occasionally been reported with isolated or disseminated nodal involvement, in the absence of extranodal disease.[246,247] Most reported cases of nodal monocytoid B-cell lymphoma have been in patients with Sjögren's syndrome and thus represent nodal involvement by a MALT type lymphoma of the salivary gland.[248,249] Others have been reported as *composite* lymphomas with other histologically low-grade lymphomas, chiefly follicular lymphoma. In these cases, however, this phenomenon represents focal differentiation to marginal zone or monocytoid B cells and not a true composite lymphoma; these cases should be classified as follicular lymphoma (see Follicular Lymphoma, later in this chapter).[250] Nonetheless, there are occasional cases that do not appear to be associated with other types of lymphoma. Two morphologic types have been described: cases that resemble MALT lymphoma and cases that more closely resemble splenic marginal zone lymphoma.[251] Those that resemble MALT lymphoma show aggregates of monocytoid B cells in a parafollicular, perivascular, and perisinusoidal distribution, with preserved germinal centers and mantle zones. Those that resemble SMZL had infiltrates of marginal zone cells surrounding reactive follicles with germinal centers, but with attenuated mantle zones.

IMMUNOPHENOTYPE AND GENETIC FEATURES. The cases that resembled splenic marginal zone lymphoma are reported to express IgD and to lack CD5, CD23, and cyclin D1. Those that resemble MALT lymphoma are IgD– and have an immunophenotype identical to those of extranodal marginal zone B-cell lymphoma (MALT).[251]

POSTULATED NORMAL COUNTERPART. The postulated normal counterpart is nodal monocytoid or marginal zone B cell.

CLINICAL FEATURES AND THERAPY. This is a rare disorder, accounting for 1% of the cases in the international study of the REAL.[126] The patients presented with isolated or generalized nodal disease; bone marrow was involved in 30%; rarely, peripheral blood may be involved.[127,252] However, when peripheral and blood involvement appears, it seems to have a poor prognosis.[253] The cases reported by Campo and associates were predominantly localized at the time of the diagnosis.[251] Although elderly women with vocalized disease have been reported much more frequently, the disease appears in both genders, and patients with advanced stage are not infrequent. Transformation to large cell lymphoma occurs and has a poor prognosis.[254] Of those that resembled MALT lymphoma, 44% of those with follow-up had an extranodal lymphoma, whereas those resembling SMZL did not. The overall and failure-free survivals appear to be similar to those of follicular or SLLs.[127] The optimal therapy for patients with monocytoid B-cell lymphoma is not known. Patients are frequently treated with regimens that are used for follicular lymphoma.

Splenic Marginal Zone Lymphoma with or without Villous Lymphocytes

DEFINITION. Splenic marginal zone lymphoma is defined as a neoplasm of small B lymphocytes that surround and replace splenic white pulp germinal centers, merging with an outer marginal zone of larger cells with pale cytoplasm admixed with large transformed blasts; both small and large cells infiltrate red pulp, often with villous lymphocytes in the peripheral blood.[255]

MORPHOLOGY. In the spleen, the neoplastic cells occupy both the mantle and marginal zone of the splenic white pulp, usually with a central residual germinal center, which may be either atrophic or hyperplastic.[219,235,256] Both the mantle and marginal zones are expanded. The cells in the mantle zone are small, with slight nuclear irregularity and scant cytoplasm, while those in the marginal zone have more dispersed chromatin and abundant pale cytoplasm, resembling marginal zone cells, and are admixed with centroblasts and immunoblasts. The red pulp is also involved, with both a diffuse and micronodular pattern and sinus infiltration. Epithelioid histiocytes may be present singly or in clusters and, particularly in the bone marrow, may give rise to the differential diagnosis of an infectious process. Splenic hilar lymph nodes are often involved; the neoplastic cells form vague nodules, often without a central germinal center, and a marginal zone pattern may or may not be present.[257] Sinuses are often open. The marrow usually contains discrete lymphoid aggregates, without a marginal zone pattern, with or without diffuse lymphoid infiltration. When tumor cells are present in the peripheral blood they often have abundant cytoplasm with small surface *villous* projections or may appear plasmacytoid.

IMMUNOPHENOTYPE. The tumor cells are IgM+, IgD+, CD5–, CD10–, CD43–, CD23–, express B-cell antigens (CD19, CD20, CD22) and bcl-2, and lack CD11c and CD25.[235,258] In the majority of cases, lack of CD5 serves to distinguish this disorder from B-CLL, and lack of CD103 and CD25 are useful in distinguishing it from hairy cell leukemia. The cells are cyclin D1 negative by immunoperoxidase staining.[259]

GENETIC FEATURES. Analysis of the Ig variable region genes indicates a high degree of somatic mutation, consistent with a post–germinal center stage of B-cell development.[260] More recently, ongoing mutations of V region genes, similar to germinal center cells, has been reported.[261] Bcl-2 is germline. Early reports that t(11;14)(q13;132), bcl-1 rearrangement, and cyclin D1 overexpression were common are now thought to have reflected inclusion of cases of leukemic mantle cell lymphoma.[262,263] Trisomy 3, found in nodal and extranodal marginal zone lymphoma, is detected in only a small number of cases.[224,264]

POSTULATED NORMAL COUNTERPART. The postulated normal counterpart is post–germinal center, memory B cell of splenic type.

CLINICAL FEATURES AND THERAPY. Splenic marginal zone lymphoma accounts for only 1% to 2% of chronic lymphoid leukemia found on bone marrow examination, but up to 25% of low-grade B-cell neoplasms in splenectomy specimens.[235,256,265,266] It may make up the majority of chronic B-cell leukemia and low-grade splenic lymphomas that do not fit the defining criteria of B-CLL, lymphoplasmacytic lymphoma, mantle cell lymphoma, follicular lymphoma, or hairy cell leukemia. Patients typically present with weakness, fatigue, or symptoms related to splenomegaly.[267] Physical examination revealed splenomegaly in almost all patients, hepatomegaly in up to 40% of patients, but lymphadenopathy is rare.[267] Lymphocytosis is a uniform finding, but extreme lymphocytosis is unusual. Anemia and thrombocytopenia are present in a minority of patients. In some series more than one-half of the patients have been shown to have a monoclonal Ig.[267] Although most commonly seen in elderly men, the disease can be seen in both genders and in young patients.[267–269] Although the disease is usually confined to the spleen, bone marrow, and blood, unusual sites of involvement such as leukemic meningitis[270] have been described.

Most patients have an indolent course and require no immediate therapy or respond to splenectomy.[267,269,271] However, transformation to a large cell lymphoma with an aggressive course can be seen in some patients.[267,272] For patients in whom splenectomy is inappropriate, splenic radiation can be an alternative.[267,269] Oral alkylating agents appear to be marginally effective.[269] One report described four patients who achieved a complete remission with fludarabine.[273]

Follicular Lymphoma

DEFINITION. Follicular lymphoma is a lymphoma of follicle center B cells (centrocytes and centroblasts), which has at least a partially follicular pattern.

MORPHOLOGY. The tumor is composed of follicle center cells, usually a mixture of centrocytes (cleaved follicle center cells) and centroblasts (large noncleaved follicle center cells). Centrocytes typically predominate; centroblasts are usually in the minority, but by definition are always present. Rare lymphomas with a follicular growth pattern consist almost entirely of centroblasts. Occasional cases may show plasmacytoid differentiation or foci of marginal zone or monocytoid B cells.[254] The proportion of centroblasts varies from case to case, and the clinical aggressiveness of the tumor increases with increasing numbers of centroblasts. Numerous criteria have been proposed for grading follicular lymphoma. The WHO Classification is adopting the cell-counting method of Mann and Berard (Table 45.3-12).[130,274] In addition to typical follicular lymphoma, two variants are recognized whose relationship to

TABLE 45.3-12. Follicular and Mantle Cell Lymphomas: Grading and Variants

FOLLICULAR LYMPHOMA
Grades
Grade 1: 0–5 centroblasts per high-power field
Grade 2: 6–15 centroblasts per high-power field
Grade 3: >15 centroblasts per high-power field
3a: >15 centroblasts, but centrocytes are still present
3b: Centroblasts form solid sheets with no residual centrocytes
Variants
Cutaneous follicle center lymphoma
Diffuse follicle center lymphoma
Grade 1: 0–5 centroblasts per high-power field
Grade 2: 6–15 centroblasts per high-power field
MANTLE CELL LYMPHOMA
Variant: blastoid

follicular lymphoma remains controversial: cutaneous follicle center lymphoma and diffuse follicle center lymphoma.

IMMUNOPHENOTYPE. The tumor cells of follicle center lymphoma are usually SIg+; approximately 50% to 60% express IgM; approximately 40% express IgG; and rare cases express IgA. The tumor cells express pan-B-cell–associated antigens, approximately 60% are CD10+, and they are CD5–, CD23–/+, CD43– (most cases), and CD11c–. Tightly organized mesh works of FDCs are present in follicular areas.[198,275] Most cases are bcl-2+, and nuclear bcl-6 is expressed by at least some of the neoplastic cells.[276,277] The Ki-67+ fraction is lower than that of reactive follicles.

GENETICS. Ig heavy and light-chain genes are rearranged, and analysis of the Ig variable region genes shows that most cases have extensive somatic mutations and a high frequency of intraclonal diversity, indicating ongoing mutations, similar to normal germinal center cells.[278,279] t(14;18) and bcl-2 gene rearrangement are present in the majority of the cases.

POSTULATED NORMAL COUNTERPART. The postulated normal counterpart is germinal center B cells, both centrocytes (small cleaved follicular center cells) and centroblasts (large noncleaved follicular center cells).

CLINICAL FEATURES. Follicular lymphoma is the second most common lymphoma in the United States and western Europe, accounting for 20% of all NHLs and up to 70% of low-grade lymphomas reported in American and European clinical trials.[7,126] Thus, our understanding of the clinical features and response to treatment of *low-grade lymphoma* is essentially that of follicular lymphoma. Follicular lymphoma affects predominantly older adults, with a slight female predominance.[126,280] Most patients have widespread disease at diagnosis, usually predominantly lymph nodes, but also spleen, bone marrow, and occasionally peripheral blood or extranodal sites. Despite the advanced stage, the clinical course is generally indolent, with median survivals in excess of 8 years; however, the disease is not usually curable with available treatment. In the international study of the REAL, the few patients (7%) with International Prognostic Index scores of 4/5 have a much worse prognosis, with a median survival of only 1 year.[126] In that study, cases with monocytoid B-cell differentiation had a worse prognosis than other cases.[250]

THERAPY OF LOCALIZED FOLLICULAR LYMPHOMA

Stage I and II, Follicular Grade 1 and 2 Non-Hodgkin's Lymphoma. There are a number of questions regarding RT and follicular grade 1 and 2 NHL. Is follicular grade 1 and 2 NHL curative with RT alone? (Yes.) What is the frequency of recurrence after 10 years? (Only approximately 10%.) Are there prognostic factors for recurrence? (Yes, age is the most influential.) What is the extent and dose of RT needed? What are the late effects of treatment? What is the role of CT in early-stage low-grade NHL? Many published studies have demonstrated the efficacy of RT in the treatment of clinically staged patients with localized follicular small cleaved cell NHL. Patients with early-stage disease are curable with local regional irradiation. The updated series from Stanford University details the results of RT in 177 patients treated from 1961 to 1994.[281] Out of 177 patients, 73 were stage I and 104 had stage II disease. Staging laparotomy was performed in 25% of patients and 20% of patients had extranodal presentations. Total nodal irradiation (TLI) and subtotal nodal irradiation were given to 41 patients, and involved-field or extended-field irradiation was delivered to 133 patients. Staging laparotomy and TLI were used in the early years of the study. Histology was follicular grade 1 in 57% of cases and follicular grade 2 to 3 in 43% of patients. The median follow-up was 7.7 years. The 10-year, 15-year, and 20-year survivals were 64%, 44%, and 35%, respectively. The 10-year, 15-year, and 20-year disease-free survivals were 44%, 40%, and 37%, respectively. Only 5 of 47 patients in remission for 10 years or longer have relapsed at longer intervals. This study demonstrates that a substantial percentage of patients with early-stage follicular small cleaved cell NHL never have recurrence of disease following local regional irradiation.

Several other series using local regional radiation demonstrate similar results and are shown in Table 45.3-13. All the series demonstrate greater than a 40% freedom from treatment failure at 10 years. Median survival ranges from 13 to 16 years in the studies. Prognostic factors for relapse were analyzed.[281–285] Age in all studies was a significant adverse factor for relapse. Although most studies use age under and over 60, the British National Lymphoma Investigation (BNLI) study found no difference in relapse for patients in their 50s or 60s and only age 70 or greater was an adverse factor.[284] Other significant but less important prognostic factors for increasing recurrence risk include extranodal disease, female gender, and stage II disease. There appears to be little difference in outcome between follicular grade 1 and follicular grade 2 disease.

The techniques of RT (field arrangement and size and dose) in the treatment of NHL are guided by the histologic subtype, the stage of disease, and the patterns of failure. Early-stage indolent lymphomas treated with RT alone have been shown to relapse in extranodal sites or in nodal sites distant from the radiation fields when involved-field or extended-field RT has been used. This observation led some to recommend TLI for patients with follicular small cleaved cell NHL. Several factors, however, argue against the use of such extensive RT for patients with early-stage indolent disease. On multivariant analysis, for patients with stage I to II disease, there is no evidence that the use of extended-field or TLI provided for a survival advantage compared with involved-field or regional irradiation in the Stanford

TABLE 45.3-13. Radiation Therapy Alone for Early-Stage, Low-Grade Follicular Non-Hodgkin's Lymphoma

Center	*No. of Patients*	*Stage*	*Freedom from Recurrence*	*Median Survival*	*Grade*
Princess Margaret Hospital	596	I–II	>40% at 10 y	15.3 y	Follicular grade 1–3
British National Lymphoma Investigation	208	I	49% at 10 y	64% at 10 y	Follicular grade 1–3
Stanford University	177	I–II	44% at 10 y	13.8 y	Follicular grade 1–2
Royal Marsden Hospital	58	I–II	43% at 10 y	79% at 10 y	Follicular grade 1–2

study. There are concerns for increased toxicity with larger RT fields and the possibility that subsequent treatment, if needed, will be compromised as more than 50% of stage I to II patients eventually develop a recurrence and require more aggressive treatment. In addition, there is a high conversion rate of follicular small cleaved cell NHL to a more aggressive histology over time, requiring treatment with chemotherapy.[286,287] Prior treatment with TLI may compromise marrow reserve and limit subsequent multiagent chemotherapy given either for recurrent indolent NHL or for NHL transformed to a more aggressive histology. Also, there appears to be an increased risk of late complications including second cancers with large-field irradiation.[281]

There are no large prospective or randomized studies evaluating the dose and field size of RT for patients with stage I to II follicular small cleaved cell NHL. However, most centers use radiation doses between 30 and 40 Gy, and either involved-field irradiation or regional fields. Current recommendations include the use of regional RT fields. This consists of irradiating the involved nodal region plus one additional uninvolved region on each side of the involved nodes. For example, the treatment field for lymphoma of the inguinal nodes would include the ipsilateral femoral, inguinal, and external iliac nodes. The treatment of a stage I lymphoma of the right supraclavicular nodes would include the ipsilateral axilla, supraclavicular, and cervical nodes. The cervical, supraclavicular, oropharyngeal, and nasopharyngeal nodes would be irradiated in patients with involvement of Waldeyer's ring. The recommended dose for patients with follicular small cleaved cell NHL is 3000 to 3600 cGy, with a boost to areas of initial involvement to 36 to 40 Gy. When there is a possibility of significant morbidity from treatment, such as long-term xerostomia from irradiation of the salivary glands, lower doses to the uninvolved nodal areas are recommended (i.e., 25 to 30 Gy).

The role of combination chemotherapy in the management of early-stage follicular lymphoma is unclear. At least three randomized studies conducted in the 1970s failed to demonstrate that non–adriamycin-containing combination chemotherapy regimens plus RT were superior to RT alone.[288–290] A more recent BNLI study randomized 148 patients to receive either RT alone or RT plus chlorambucil chemotherapy.[291] There were no differences in freedom from recurrence or survival between the groups. A single-arm study of 91 stage I and II patients treated at the M. D. Anderson Cancer Center with cyclophosphamide, vincristine, and prednisone (COP) or cyclophosphamide, doxorubicin, vincristine, and prednisone-bleomycin (CHOP-Bleo) chemotherapy in addition to RT demonstrated an improved freedom from recurrence compared with historic controls but no overall survival differences.[292,293] In part, the choice of therapy may lie in the careful assessment of prognostic factors. Most patients with Ann Arbor clinical stage I or II follicular small cleaved cell and follicular mixed lymphomas should have a good prognosis following local regional RT alone. For patients whose prognosis is less certain, such as patients with stage II disease with multiple sites of involvement or bulky nodes, or patients with follicular large cell histology, chemotherapy followed by involved-field irradiation may provide more durable remissions.

THERAPY OF DISSEMINATED FOLLICULAR LYMPHOMA. The optimal treatment strategy for patients with advanced-stage follicular lymphoma is controversial.[294] Treatment has followed one of two divergent approaches: an aggressive approach that may include extensive RT, combination chemotherapy, or both; and a conservative approach that consists of no initial treatment followed by a palliative single-agent chemotherapy or involved-field radiotherapy when treatment is needed. Although many years of clinical investigation have failed to prove that immediate aggressive therapy improves survival compared with conservative therapy,[294] the median survival of only 7 to 8 years from diagnosis in patients with stage III and IV disease has prompted the continuation of aggressive treatment approaches.[295–297] Despite the indolent nature of the follicular lymphomas, most patients ultimately die of their disease. Of 147 previously untreated patients enrolled at St. Bartholomew's Hospital in various protocols, ranging from no initial therapy to conservative treatment with single alkylating agents, only 53 of 147 patients remain alive; 94 patients have died, and only 18 patients died from causes unrelated to lymphoma.[296]

RT in the treatment of patients with stage III and IV follicular lymphoma serves two roles, as palliative treatment and as part of a potentially curative approach in clinical trials. RT has much to offer as a palliative approach. For patients with isolated disease that has returned after remission or has not responded as well as other sites to chemotherapy, involved-field irradiation can allow for patients to go significant periods of time without the need for additional combination therapy. In addition, follicular lymphoma can produce troubling symptoms through bone or spine involvement, through pressure on peripheral nerves, by disfigurement via large neck or axillary nodes, by intraorbital involvement, and through many other mechanisms. Follicular lymphoma is sensitive to RT, and often nodes resistant to chemotherapy begin to shrink after four to five radiation treatments. Sometimes even a large volume of lymph nodes can be encompassed because the low doses of radiation needed results in minimal toxicity to normal tissues.

As a curative approach, TLI combined with chemotherapy has been used for the treatment of stage III patients in past studies. McLaughlin and colleagues reported on the use of CHOP chemotherapy and TLI in 74 patients with follicular lymphomas. The relapse-free survival at 5 years was 52%. This study did not provide sufficient evidence that patients were cured with this approach.[298] The National Cancer Institute initiated a prospective randomized study comparing conservative treatment (no initial therapy) with aggressive combined modality therapy with ProMACE/MOPP chemotherapy followed by low-dose (24 Gy) total lymphoid RT.[299] Eighty-nine patients were randomized. The disease-free survival was significantly higher in the combined modality therapy group at 4 years (51% vs. 12%); however, no differences in overall survival were seen. As these studies have failed to show a survival advantage for an initial aggressive approach in the management of patients with advanced-stage indolent lymphomas, new high-dose chemotherapy approaches are being developed that for the most part do not include the use of TLI.

When a decision is made to treat a patient with disseminated follicular lymphoma using cytotoxic chemotherapeutic agents, a wide variety of choices is available. These include single-agent chlorambucil, cyclophosphamide, or fludarabine, or popular combination chemotherapy regimens such as cyclophosphamide, vincristine, and prednisone (CVP), CHOP, and fludarabine, mitoxantrone, and dexamethasone (FND). Each of these approaches produces objective responses in a high proportion of patients with previously untreated follicular lymphoma.[300–304] In general, complete responses occur more rapidly with combination chemotherapy regimens, but it is unclear that the ultimate treatment result is superior with combinations. Approximately 20% of complete responders remain in remission for longer than 10 years.[294]

Patients with follicular lymphoma who are followed without therapy sometimes have spontaneous regressions that can be complete.[305] Spontaneous regressions appear most frequently in patients with predominantly follicular small cleaved cell lymphoma and least frequently in patients with follicular large cell lymphoma.

Interferon-α has long been known to be an active drug in the treatment of patients with follicular lymphoma and has an objective response rate of 30% to 55% when used as a single agent with relapsed disease.[306–308] The value of adding interferon to standard combination chemotherapy regimens has been tested in a number of clinical trials.[309–316] The dose and duration of administration of interferon-α varied among these studies. A significant increase in remission duration was observed in several studies,[311–313,315,316] and a prolongation of survival was found in one setting.[312] A metaanalysis of eight of the randomized trials incorporating 1756 patients has been initially reported.[317] This analysis found an improvement in overall survival in patients who received an anthracycline-containing chemotherapy regimen and received a dose of interferon of at least 36 MU/month.

The activity of rituximab in patients with relapsed follicular lymphoma has led to its incorporation into the initial treatment and has produced encouraging results.[318] Use of the radiolabeled monoclonal antibody tositumomab in previously untreated patients has also been reported to produce a high complete response rate. Two trials of autologous hematopoietic stem cell transplantation incorporated in the primary therapy of patients with follicular lymphoma have reported high complete response rates, but the observation period is too short to know if a subset of these patients will be cured.[319,320]

The importance of determining what has been called a molecular response in patients receiving primary therapy for follicular lymphoma has been studied. A molecular response refers to disappearance of previously apparent bcl-2 gene rearrangements detected by the PCR in the blood or bone marrow. Most studies have found a better disease-free survival in patients achieving a molecular remission.[321–323] At the present time, determining the molecular response is an important research tool, but since prolonged remissions have been reported in patients who are persistently positive[321] the practical clinical utility of this measurement is uncertain.

The subdivision of patients with follicular lymphoma into those with predominantly small cells (follicular small cleaved cell), those with an intermediate number of small and large cells (follicular mixed), and those with more large cells (follicular large cell) is difficult.[126] However, even considering the imprecision of the distinction, patients classified as follicular large cell lymphoma have a shorter remission duration and overall survival than patients with the other subtypes.[126] The incorporation of an anthracycline into the initial treatment regimen seems to be more important in patients with follicular large cell lymphoma.[302,324,325] A subset of patients with follicular large cell lymphoma who receive an intensive chemotherapy regimen can achieve long-term disease-free survival.[326]

SALVAGE THERAPY. Most patients with follicular lymphoma, despite complete response to initial chemotherapy, relapse and are candidates for salvage treatment. However, unlike the situation with diffuse large B-cell lymphoma or other aggressive NHLs, patients with relapsed follicular lymphoma do not necessarily pursue an aggressive course. In an asymptomatic patient, particularly if the patient is elderly, observation without treatment can be an acceptable option. In a patient with follicular lymphoma who relapses with transformation to a diffuse large B-cell lymphoma, however, treatment is almost always indicated. The majority of patients with follicular lymphoma undergoes transformation to diffuse large B-cell lymphoma. This transformation is clinically recognized in approximately 40% of patients, but present in autopsy in almost 100% of patients.[327] The clinical manifestations of histologic transformation to diffuse large B-cell lymphoma typically include rapidly progressive lymphadenopathy (i.e., often localized); the development of new symptoms such as fevers, night sweats, weight loss, and pain; or both. In general, histologic transformation to diffuse large B-cell lymphoma has a poor prognosis and frequently a rapidly fatal outcome. However, some patients can have complete responses to salvage chemotherapy regimens and achieve durable complete remissions.[328] These patients are typically left with persisting follicular lymphoma.

A wide variety of second-line chemotherapy regimens has been used in patients with follicular lymphoma. In addition to repeating standard front-line regimen, purine analogues such as fludarabine[329] and cladribine[330] are often used. However, even when the initial therapy is repeated, patients with follicular lymphoma often respond. In one series using chlorambucil, the response rate was 68% for the second course of therapy in contrast to 70% in the initial treatment.[331,332]

A variety of other treatment approaches has been used in patients with relapsed follicular lymphoma. Interferon-α used as a single agent has a 30% to 55% response rate.[306–308] The monoclonal antibody rituximab produces objective responses in 35% to 50% of patients with relapsed follicular lymphoma.[333] Radiolabeled antibodies also directed against CD20 have even higher response rates in patients with relapsed follicular lymphoma.[334,335] Other treatments such as use of antisense molecules[336] and tumor vaccines[337] have also been shown to produce objective responses.

Both autologous and allogeneic hematopoietic stem cell transplantations have been used for patients with relapsed follicular lymphoma. Both purged[338,339] and unpurged[340,341] autologous stem cell products have been used. The value of purging, particularly when blood stem cell products are used, remains uncertain. Autologous transplantation in patients with relapsed follicular lymphoma produces remissions durable for 5 years in approximately 50% of patients who are transplanted at the time of initial treatment failure.[339–341] Patients transplanted after multiple treatment failures have a poorer outcome. Use of allogeneic bone marrow transplantation is associated with a much higher treatment-related mortality and a lower relapse rate.[342]

Mantle Cell Lymphoma

DEFINITION. A mantle cell lymphoma is a neoplasm of monomorphous small to medium-sized B cells with irregular nuclei, which resemble the cleaved cells (centrocytes) of germinal centers and overexpress cyclin D1; neoplastic transformed cells (centroblasts or immunoblasts) are absent. Tumor cells are typically CD5+ CD23–.

MORPHOLOGY. The pattern of mantle cell lymphoma may be either diffuse, nodular, or mantle zone, or a combination of the three. Some reports indicate a better prognosis for cases with a mantle zone pattern.[343] Most cases are composed exclusively of small to medium-sized lymphoid cells, with slightly irregular or *cleaved*, nuclei; however, the morphology in various cases can range from lymphocyte-like to large cleaved or lymphoblast-like.[160,164,344–346] Despite the small size and bland appearance, there is often more mitotic activity than in other histologically low-grade lymphomas. Single epithelioid histiocytes may be present, but clusters and granulomas are not seen. Transformed cells with basophilic cytoplasm (centroblast- or immunoblast-like cells) are extremely rare or absent.

IMMUNOPHENOTYPE. The tumor cells express strong SIgM and IgD, which is often of λ light-chain type, strongly express B-cell–associated antigens, and coexpress CD5, similar to B-CLL/SLL, but are CD23–. Rare cases may be CD5– or CD23+.[363,363a] In contrast to follicle center lymphoma, mantle cell lymphoma are usually CD10– and CD43+. A prominent, irregular mesh work of FDCs is found, even in diffuse cases.[164,198,275] The product of the cyclin D1 gene can be detected in the nuclei of neoplastic mantle cells in paraffin-embedded tissue sections with the immunoperoxidase technique and is useful in distinguishing mantle cell lymphoma from other low-grade B-cell lymphomas.[173,347]

GENETIC FEATURES. Ig heavy and light-chain genes are rearranged. The Ig V region genes lack somatic mutations, indicating a pre–germinal center stage of differentiation, consistent with an origin from the follicle mantle.[348] A t(11;14) in the majority of the cases results in overexpression of a gene known as PRAD1 or cyclin D1, which encodes a cell-cycle–associated protein that is not normally expressed in lymphoid cells.[173,349,350] The protein is overexpressed even in cases lacking the t(11;14), suggesting that point mutations may also result in overexpression.[351,352] Overexpression of this protein may explain the often high mitotic index and aggressive clinical course of this histologically low-grade lymphoma. Studies have shown abnormalities in expression of other genes associated with the cell cycle, including mutations of the cdk inhibitors p16 and p17 in blastoid variants and decreased expression of p27, another cdk inhibitor, in the majority of the cases.[353] Cases of the blastoid variant have been reported to have a high incidence of tetraploidy and p53 gene mutations.[354–356] Acquisition of a myc translocation has been reported in some fatal cases.[357]

POSTULATED NORMAL COUNTERPART. Mantle cell lymphoma corresponds to a naive B cell of follicle mantle or germinal center origin that is distinct from both the recirculating B cell of B-CLL/SLL and the later centrocyte of follicle center lymphomas.[179,198]

Clinical Features. Mantle cell lymphoma accounts for approximately 7% of adult NHLs in the United States and Europe.[126,160] In a review of 376 cases of disseminated low-grade lymphoma (Working Formulation categories A through E), mantle cell lymphoma made up 10% of the cases.[358] It is a tumor of older adults, with a marked male predominance (75%).[126] The majority (70%) of patients are in stage IV at diagnosis; sites involved include lymph nodes, spleen, Waldeyer's ring, bone marrow (greater than 60%), blood (up to 50%), and extranodal sites, especially the gastrointestinal tract (lymphomatous polyposis).[359] The course is moderately aggressive. The median overall survival in most series is 3 years, with no plateau in the curve, and failure-free survival is around 1 year.[127] The blastoid variant is reported in some studies to be more aggressive.[126,358,360–363]

THERAPY. Since mantle cell lymphoma was widely accepted as an entity in only the last decade, the number of therapeutic trials are not as extensive as for some other types of NHL. Localized mantle cell lymphoma is quite rare, seen in only 13% of unselected patients in one large series.[127] The failure-free survival of patients treated for localized mantle cell lymphoma is quite poor, suggesting that unrecognized dissemination was usually present. The optimal treatment for these patients is not known.

Most patients present with disseminated disease. Single-agent chemotherapy has been used less commonly than in other small cell lymphomas, with chlorambucil, fludarabine, and cladribine being the most commonly used agents. The most frequently used combination regimens have been CVP and CHOP. Overall response rates have ranged between 60% and 80% and complete response rates between 30% and 60%. A randomized trial comparing CVP and CHOP showed no significant difference in overall survival (84% vs. 88%) and failure-free survival (41% vs. 58%).[360] A new chemotherapy regimen that was originally used for patients with leukemia called hyper-CVAD (cyclophosphamide, vincristine, dexamethasone, and doxorubicin) has been used in mantle cell lymphoma and has a high response rate.[364] In an historic control study from M. D. Anderson Cancer Center, hyper-CVAD had a superior 3-year event-free survival to CHOP (72% vs. 28%).[364]

Because of the poor long-term outlook, patients with mantle cell lymphoma who are sufficiently young and healthy often undergo autologous or allogeneic bone marrow transplantation at best response.[365–368] The long-term benefits of autologous and allogeneic transplantation are still uncertain, although long-term survivors with both approaches are reported. Patients who relapse and are not candidates for transplantation or those who relapse can be treated with rituximab and interferon.

Monoclonal antibody therapy for patients with mantle cell lymphoma has been attempted with rituximab.[369] The antibody yielded a response rate of 33% in relapsed patients. Further trials will be necessary to define the place of rituximab in the management of patients with mantle cell lymphoma. Interferon-α has been used in the treatment of mantle cell lymphoma. In one randomized trial including 47 patients with mantle cell lymphoma, 22 patients received interferon and 25 patients did not.[370] The disease-free survival was 47% for the patients receiving interferon and 27% for the patients observed without therapy. However, the number of patients and the period of follow-up were not long enough to reach a firm conclusion.

Diffuse Large B-Cell Lymphoma

DEFINITION. Diffuse large B-cell lymphoma is defined as a neoplasm of large, transformed B cells with prominent nucle-

TABLE 45.3-14. Morphologic Variants and Subtypes of Diffuse Large B-Cell Lymphoma

DIFFUSE LARGE B-CELL LYMPHOMA, MORPHOLOGIC VARIANTS
Centroblastic
Immunoblastic
T-cell/histiocyte-rich
Lymphomatoid granulomatosis type
Anaplastic large B-cell
Plasmablastic
DIFFUSE LARGE B-CELL LYMPHOMA, SUBTYPES
Mediastinal (thymic) large B-cell lymphoma
Primary effusion lymphoma
Intravascular large B-cell lymphoma

oli and basophilic cytoplasm, with a diffuse growth pattern and a high (greater than 40%) proliferation fraction. The cells may resemble centroblasts, immunoblasts, multilobated cells, or anaplastic large cells. Rare cases contain only scattered large cells in a background of small T cells and epithelioid histiocytes (T-cell/histiocyte-rich large B-cell lymphoma).

MORPHOLOGY. Diffuse large B-cell lymphomas are probably a heterogeneous group of neoplasms. They are typically composed of large cells that resemble centroblasts or immunoblasts, most often with a mixture of the two. Several morphologic variants can be recognized, but their clinical significance is debated (Table 45.3-14).

Centroblastic Variant. The monomorphic centroblastic (large noncleaved cell) type is composed of medium to large lymphoid cells with oval to round vesicular nuclei with fine chromatin and two to four membrane-bound nucleoli. The cytoplasm is generally scanty and amphophilic to basophilic. The multilobated centroblastic type contains many large lymphoid cells with nuclei having more than three lobes. A polymorphic type shows a mixture of centroblasts and immunoblasts and may contain up to 90% immunoblasts.

Immunoblastic Variant. Approximately 10% of the cases of diffuse large B-cell lymphomas have over 90% immunoblasts with a prominent central nucleolus and abundant, basophilic cytoplasm. Plasmacytoid differentiation may be present. These cases are more common in immunosuppressed patients. In nonimmunosuppressed patients, they have been reported to carry a worse prognosis.[371]

Anaplastic Variant. In some cases of diffuse large B-cell lymphomas, the cells are identical to those of T/null anaplastic large cell lymphoma and strongly express CD30 (Ki-1) as well as T-cell antigens. Although these have been called *B-cell anaplastic large cell lymphoma* (B-ALCL), they do not have the same distinctive clinical or genetic features of T/null-ALCL and are considered a morphologic variant of large B-cell lymphoma in the REAL/WHO classifications. The most significant differential diagnostic problem presented by such cases is with classical Hodgkin's disease expressing B-cell antigens.

T-Cell–Rich/Histiocyte-Rich Large B-Cell Lymphoma. Some cases of large B-cell lymphoma have a prominent background of reactive T cells and often histiocytes, so-called T-cell or histiocyte-rich large B-cell lymphoma. They may resemble Hodgkin's disease of either lymphocyte predominance or mixed cellularity type.[372,373] In contrast to those with Hodgkin's disease, patients with T-cell/histiocyte-rich large B-cell lymphoma typically present with disseminated disease involving the liver and spleen and have a poor survival. The relationship of this disease to lymphocyte-predominance, classical Hodgkin's disease, or both remains to be elucidated.

Large B-Cell Lymphoma, Lymphomatoid Granulomatosis Type. The entity described as *lymphomatoid granulomatosis,* which had been thought to be related to nasal or angiocentric lymphoma, has been shown in most cases to be an EBV+ large B-cell lymphoma with a T-cell–rich background.[374–377] The infiltrates show extensive necrosis, often with only a few atypical large B cells in a background of lymphocytes; the infiltrate may be both angiocentric and angioinvasive. Patients typically present with extranodal disease, most commonly involving lung, brain, kidneys, or all three. Evidence of past or present immunosuppression may be found. Although the infiltrates may resemble those of nasal or angiocentric lymphoma, there is no biologic and little clinical overlap, since the latter is an NK cell or T-cell neoplasm that involves the upper airway and midfacial region, skin, and sometimes the gastrointestinal tract, and rarely the lung or CNS.

IMMUNOPHENOTYPE. Diffuse large B-cell lymphomas express one or more B-cell–associated antigens (CD19, CD20, CD22, CD79a), as well as CD45, and often but not always, surface Ig. They may coexpress CD5 or CD10.[198,378] Twenty-five percent to 80% in various studies express bcl-2 protein, and this may be associated with a worse prognosis.[379–383] Approximately 70% express bcl-6 protein, consistent with a germinal center origin[382,383]; this expression is independent of bcl-6 gene rearrangement.

GENETIC FEATURES. Most cases of diffuse large B-cell lymphomas have somatic mutations in the Ig variable region genes.[182,384] The bcl-2 gene is rearranged in 15% to 30% of diffuse large B-cell lymphomas; it is associated with nodal and disseminated disease, but is not associated with either a worse prognosis or with bcl-2 expression.[379] The c-myc gene is rearranged in 5% to 15%,[385,386] and the bcl-6 gene is rearranged in 20% to 40% of cases[386,387] and shows mutations in the 5' noncoding region in 70%.[388,389] Both the 5' noncoding mutations of the bcl-6 gene[390] and the Ig variable region gene mutations are found in normal germinal center cells[391]; their presence in diffuse large B-cell lymphomas is consistent with a germinal center or post–germinal center stage of differentiation.

POSTULATED NORMAL COUNTERPART. The postulated normal counterpart is proliferating peripheral B cells, centroblasts or immunoblasts in most cases.

DIFFERENTIAL DIAGNOSIS. For large B-cell lymphoma, as for most of the aggressive lymphomas, the major differential diagnosis is with a nonlymphoid tumor, including poorly differentiated carcinoma, germ cell tumor, glioma, melanoma, or sarcoma. Clinically, when patients present with lymphadenopathy, lymphoma is often at the top of the differential diagnosis, but in extranodal sites, lymphoma may not be suspected. Clinical features that tend to favor lymphoma in extranodal sites include the presence of multiple, noncontiguous lesions, characteristic radiographic findings (e.g., permeative lesions in bone, ring-enhancing lesions in the CNS), involvement of lymphoid organs, and systemic symptoms such as fever and weight loss.

Histologically, the most important factor in establishing the diagnosis is a high index of suspicion and a recognition of the morphologic spectrum of diffuse large B-cell lymphoma. In this differential diagnosis, immunoperoxidase stains on paraffin sections are usually definitive; however, a panel of several antibodies must be used (e.g., cytokeratin, EMA, CD45, pan-B and pan-T antigens, Ig light-chains, and if relevant, S-100 and HMB-45).

CLINICAL FEATURES. Diffuse large B-cell lymphoma was the most common lymphoma in the international study of the REAL, accounting for 31% of the cases. Patients typically present with a rapidly enlarging symptomatic mass, with B symptoms in one-third of the cases.[126,127] Localized (stage I or II) extranodal disease occurs in up to 30%; bone marrow involvement was seen in only 16%. Up to 40% of diffuse large B-cell lymphomas are extranodal; common sites include the gastrointestinal tract, bone, and CNS. The prognosis was highly associated with the International Prognostic Index score,[127] but not with histologic subclassification according to either the Working Formulation or the Kiel Classification. Large B-cell lymphoma may occur as a high-grade transformation of several low-grade B-cell lymphomas (B-CLL, lymphoplasmacytic lymphoma, follicular lymphoma, MALT lymphoma, splenic marginal zone lymphoma). Diffuse large B-cell lymphoma of certain extranodal sites, such as the CNS, may be clinically distinctive and may have specific treatment protocols.

THERAPY OF LOCALIZED DIFFUSE LARGE B-CELL LYMPHOMA. Patients with localized diffuse large B-cell lymphoma often have extranodal disease. It now appears that patients with localized extranodal lymphoma might have a better outcome than seen for patients with equal stage nodal lymphoma.[282] This might be related to an occult MALT origin of the large cell lymphoma in some of these patients. The data are clearest for gastric lymphomas.

Before 1980, RT was the primary treatment for patients with localized diffuse large cell lymphoma. Approximately 50% of patients with stage I and 20% of patients with stage II disease were alive without recurrence at 5 years.[392,393] Among the patients who had recurrences, 15% to 20% were within the radiation field; the remainder were in distant sites. Early randomized trials, published in the 1980s, compared RT alone with RT followed by CVP or BACOP chemotherapy.[288,289,394] These studies demonstrated a disease-free and overall survival advantage for combined CT and RT. This dramatically changed the treatment of localized large cell lymphoma. Staging laparotomy and large-field RT became obsolete as combination chemotherapy with or without RT produced disease-free and overall survival rates equivalent to or better than those seen even in the most selected studies reporting results with RT alone.

New clinical trials were then initiated to evaluate the role of RT as adjuvant to chemotherapy in patients with stage I or II diffuse large cell lymphoma. Small retrospective studies had advocated chemotherapy alone[395,396] or combined chemotherapy and RT.[397–399] Several centers reported excellent results using reduced chemotherapy and involved-field irradiation. At the National Cancer Institute, more than 90% of the 49 stage I or IE patients with diffuse large cell lymphoma treated with four cycles of ProMACE-MOPP (cyclophosphamide, etoposide, doxorubicin, nitrogen mustard, vincristine, procarbazine, high-dose methotrexate with leucovorin rescue and prednisone) at reduced doses (75% of normal) followed by involved-field RT to 40 Gy remained disease free.[399] In a similar study from Vancouver 78 patients were treated with three cycles of CHOP chemotherapy followed by involved-field RT to a total dose of 30 to 45 Gy; at 3 years the disease-free survival was 84%.[400] Both studies excluded patients with bulky disease (greater than 10 cm). In a third study, which included some patients with bulky disease, 183 patients treated with four cycles of CHOP and 40 to 44 Gy involved-field RT have 5-year relapse-free and overall survival rates of 83%.[401]

Two prospective randomized trials have further evaluated the role of RT in patients with early-stage diffuse large cell lymphoma. The Eastern Cooperative Oncology Group randomized 365 patients with bulky stage I and patients with stage II diffuse large cell lymphoma to eight cycles of CHOP with or without involved-field RT. Patients with complete response were randomized to 30 Gy involved-field RT or no further treatment. Patients with partial response received 40 Gy. The disease-free survival (73% vs. 58%; $P = .03$), freedom from recurrence (73% vs. 58%; $P = .04$), and survival (84% vs. 70; $P = .06$) all favored the patients who received adjuvant involved-field irradiation.[402] The Southwest Oncology Group Trial randomized 401 stage I and nonbulky stage II patients to receive either three cycles of CHOP and involved-field irradiation (40 to 55 Gy) or eight cycles of CHOP alone. The 5-year progression-free survival (77% vs. 64%; $P = .03$) and overall survival (82% vs. 72%; $P = .02$) favored the CHOP and involved-field RT treatment arm.[403] As a result of these trials, combination chemotherapy and adjuvant RT has become the standard of care for patients with stage I and II diffuse large cell lymphoma.

There are no prospective trials evaluating dose of radiation when combined with chemotherapy in patients with early-stage diffuse large cell lymphoma. In general, the dose of RT should be based on the number of cycles of chemotherapy and the bulk of disease. Patients with bulky mediastinal or abdominal disease or with multiple sites of involvement have a somewhat worse prognosis; these patients should receive six cycles of CHOP combined with RT.[397,404,405] Prior studies support the use of three to four cycles of CHOP combined with RT in patients with more limited disease.[399–401,403] With a complete response after six cycles of CHOP we recommend 30-Gy involved-field RT for patients with favorable presentations, and 35 to 40 Gy for patients with initial bulky disease. Patients with diffuse large cell lymphoma localized to the bone should receive 40 Gy.[406] With a complete response after four cycles of CHOP we recommend 40 Gy. These recommendations are derived from the studies cited previously.

THERAPY OF DISSEMINATED DIFFUSE LARGE B-CELL LYMPHOMA. The curability of disseminated diffuse large B-cell lymphoma using chemotherapeutic agents was reported in the early 1970s.[407,408] In both early reports, the majority of patients who achieved a documented complete remission at the end of planned therapy did not relapse on prolonged follow-up. These reports led to a large number of clinical trials documenting the possibility of cure for patients with disseminated diffuse large B-

TABLE 45.3-15. Combination Chemotherapeutic Regimens for Newly Diagnosed Aggressive Non-Hodgkin's Lymphoma

	Regimen	*Dose (mg/m²)*	*Days of Administration*	*Frequency*
CHOP	Cyclophosphamide	750 IV	1	q21d
	Doxorubicin	50 IV	1	
	Vincristine[a]	1.4 IV	1	
	Prednisone	100 PO	1–5	
CNOP	Cyclophosphamide	750 IV	1	q21d
	Mitoxantrone	12 IV	1	
	Vincristine[a]	1.4 IV	1	
	Prednisone	100 PO	1–5	
m-BACOD	Methotrexate	200 IV	8 and 15	q21d
	Bleomycin[a]	4 IV	1	
	Doxorubicin	45 IV	1	
	Cyclophosphamide	600 IV	1	
	Vincristine[a]	1.4 IV	1	
	Dexamethasone	6 PO	1–5	
	Leucovorin	10 PO	24 h after methotrexate, then q6h for 8 doses	
ProMACE/CytaBOM	Prednisone	60 PO	1–14	q28d
	Doxorubicin	25 IV	1	
	Cyclophosphamide	650 IV	1	
	Etoposide	120 IV	1	
	Cytarabine	300 IV	8	
	Bleomycin	5 IV	8	
	Vincristine[a]	1.4 IV	8	
	Methotrexate	120 IV	8	
	Leucovorin	25 IV	24 h after methotrexate, then q6h for 5 doses	
MACOP-B	Methotrexate	400 IV	8	q28d × 3
	Doxorubicin	50 IV	1 and 15	
	Cyclophosphamide	350 IV	1 and 15	
	Vincristine[a]	1.4 IV	8 and 22	
	Prednisone fixed dose	75 PO	Daily for 12 weeks	
	Bleomycin	10 IV	28	
	Leucovorin	15 PO	24 h after methotrexate, then q6h for 6 doses	
ACVB	Cyclophosphamide	1200 IV	1	q14d × 4 followed by consolidation therapy
	Doxorubicin	75 IV	1	
	Vindesine	2 IV	1	
	Bleomycin[b]	10 IV	1	
	Methylprednisone	60 IV	1–5	
	Methotrexate	15 mg intrathecal	1	

[a]Vincristine dose often capped at 2 mg total.
[b]Total bleomycin dose, 10 mg.

cell lymphoma. Principles of therapy that have evolved include the administration of highly active drugs given in combination for several cycles and then to restage the patient to document complete remission (Table 45.3-15). Two or more further cycles of chemotherapy are usually administered after complete remission is documented. In most series, 50% to 75% of completely responding patients do not relapse. It appears that patients who achieve remission promptly are most likely to be cured.[409]

A great deal of effort has gone into attempts to identify the best treatment regimen for patients with advanced diffuse aggressive lymphoma. Most patients in these studies had diffuse large B-cell lymphoma. More than 40 randomized clinical trials have been reported.[407,408,410–453] The majority of these trials have not found a significant treatment advantage for any particular regimen.[407,408,410–444] The most widely quoted trial was carried out in the United States comparing CHOP, m-BACOD, ProMACE/CytaBOM, and MACOP-B[410] (Table 45.3-16). This trial was carried out because of enthusiasm generated by single-arm trials showing apparent superiority of m-BACOD, ProMACE/CytaBOM, and MACOP-B over the older CHOP regimen.[419,454,455] This study of 899 patients showed no improvement in failure-free or overall survival with the newer regimen, but did find increased toxicity with m-BACOD and MACOP-B.[410] The 6-year overall survival for the four regimens were CHOP, 33%; m-BACOD, 36%; ProMACE/CytaBOM, 34%; and MACOP-B, 32%. The conclusion from the study was that the less complicated and less expensive CHOP regimen should be considered the treatment of choice. This has been

TABLE 45.3-16. Treatment of Aggressive Non-Hodgkin's Lymphoma (Approximately 80% Diffuse Large B-Cell): A Comparison of Four Regimens

Regimen	*Complete Remission (%)*	*Partial Remission (%)[a]*	*3-Y Failure-Free Survival (%)*	*Overall Survival (%)*
CHOP	44	36	41	54
m-BACOD	48	34	46	52
ProMACE/CytaBOM	56	31	46	50
MACOP-B	51	32	41	50

[a]Some patients who responded partially had only a residual mass on imaging studies and might actually have been in complete remission.
(Data from refs. 127, 281, 282, 284, 285, and 469.)

widely applied, and today most patients with diffuse large B-cell lymphoma or other aggressive lymphomas receive CHOP.

Several randomized trials have identified superiority of one chemotherapy regimen over another for the treatment of patients with diffuse large B-cell lymphoma.[414,419,424,445–453] The most consistent finding from these studies is the superiority of an anthracycline-containing chemotherapy regimen over regimens that do not contain an anthracycline.[414,446,448–450] This appears to be true in older as well as younger patients.[446,447] An anthracycline, usually doxorubicin, appears to be a key component in optimizing the chances for the cure of patients with diffuse aggressive lymphoma. Substitution of another anthracycline such as mitoxantrone or epirubicin has been controversial, with some studies finding the drugs equivalent,[420,426–429] whereas others have found an advantage for doxorubicin.[453]

The importance of duration of follow-up in interpreting comparative trials is pointed out by a study done by the Australian and New Zealand lymphoma group.[411,445] Investigators carried out a trial comparing CHOP with MACOP-B. Two hundred thirty-six patients were eligible for analysis and an initial report showed no significant difference in outcome between the two approaches, except for more severe toxicity with MACOP-B. The 4-year overall survival was 56% for MACOP-B and 51% for CHOP, with 3.2-year median follow-up. The authors reported the study again with 6.5-year median follow-up. At that point the failure-free survival (i.e., 42% vs. 30%) and overall survival (54% vs. 41%) favored the MACOP-B regimen.

Currently, there is no one superior regimen for the treatment of patients with disseminated diffuse large B-cell lymphoma. Unfortunately, this is because all the regimens are equally bad, rather than that they are all extremely effective. Patients with advanced-stage diffuse large B-cell lymphoma are cured with chemotherapy less than 50% of the time. New treatment approaches are badly needed. Attempts have been made to improve the response to CHOP by combining it with the monoclonal antibody rituximab. An early study of 33 patients showed a 97% response rate and a 73% complete response rate.[456] The place of combined chemotherapy and monoclonal antibody therapy in the management of patients with diffuse large B-cell lymphoma will be determined by subsequent comparative clinical trials.

One approach to improve treatment results in patients with disseminated diffuse large B-cell lymphoma would be the addition of adjuvant drugs, radiotherapy, high-dose therapy with transplant, immunotherapy, or antibodies after a standard chemotherapy regimen. The addition of levamisole, bacille Calmette-Guérin, or both did not improve treatment outcome.[457] Aviles et al. found an improved disease-free and overall survival with the use of adjuvant interferon-α.[451] A combination of standard chemotherapy regimens and monoclonal antibodies is currently being tested.

The most widely studied adjuvant therapy has involved high-dose therapy and autologous bone marrow transplantation. Attempts to shorten the standard chemotherapy regimens and substitute high-dose therapy and autologous bone marrow transplantation have been disappointing. One study that randomized slowly responding patients to continuing CHOP or to autologous transplantation found a superior overall survival in continuing CHOP (85% vs. 56%).[458]

Two studies have found an improved disease-free survival and overall survival in patients who underwent autologous bone marrow transplantation after achieving a remission with a standard chemotherapy regimen.[459,460] In both cases, benefits were restricted to patients who presented with a high International Prognostic Index score. In a French study, the disease-free survival (59% vs. 39%) and overall survival (65% vs. 52%) both significantly favored adjuvant autologous bone marrow transplantation. In an Italian study, the disease-free survival (87% vs. 48%) favored adjuvant autologous bone marrow transplantation, but there was no difference in overall survival. In another Italian study, sequential high doses of individual drugs followed by autotransplant yielded a better disease-free survival (76% vs. 49%), but not overall survival, than MACOP-B.[461] An international consensus conference[462] reached the conclusion that autologous high-dose therapy and autotransplantation in patients with high-risk International Prognostic Index scores seemed to provide benefit.

SALVAGE THERAPY. The phrase *salvage therapy* encompasses subsequent treatment administered to patients who failed to achieve an initial remission and the treatment administered to patients who relapse from complete remission. A major prognostic factor for patients receiving any form of salvage therapy relates to the chemotherapy sensitivity of the lymphoma (i.e., patients who achieve an initial complete remission and then relapse generally have a better prognosis than patients who are primarily resistant to chemotherapy). Patients with lymphoma that progresses on the previous chemotherapy regimen have a poorer outlook than those who have stable or partially responding disease.[463–465] Patients who have been in complete remission and then relapsed require a rebiopsy before initiating salvage therapy. Some patients who present with diffuse large B-cell lymphoma are found to have a follicular lymphoma at the time of relapse.[466]

The initial step in planning salvage chemotherapy is to determine the goal of treatment. Some patients who fail to achieve an initial remission or relapse from complete remission can be cured. This is less likely in elderly patients, those with extensive disease, and those with a poor performance status. In such patients less intensive, palliative treatments might be better pursued.

Radiotherapy can frequently be used to alleviate thc symptoms at a particular site of involvement in patients with relapsed diffuse large B-cell lymphoma. This can frequently be accomplished with minimal morbidity. However, the chance for cure with salvage radiotherapy is extremely small. Most patients receive second-line combination chemotherapy regimens. These regimens usually incorporate drugs such as cisplatin, ifosfamide, etoposide, and cytarabine.[464,465,467–472] The chances for achieving a complete remission have varied widely in different studies, but generally fall in the 20% to 40% range.[464,465,467–472] A subset of complete responding patients can be long-term survivors, with the overall *cure* rate for salvage chemotherapy in patients with relapsed diffuse large B-cell lymphoma being approximately 5% to 10%.[464,465,467–472]

Other approaches used for salvage therapy in patients with diffuse large B-cell lymphoma include the monoclonal antibody rituximab and interferon-α. In 30 patients with diffuse large B-cell lymphoma treated with rituximab, 11 (37%) had an objective response. Most responses were partial. The median time to progression had not been reached at the time of the report.[473] Responding patients were more likely to have tumors less than 5 cm in maximum diameter, and no patient with a tumor greater than 10 cm in maximum diameter responded. Occasional patients with relapsed diffuse large B-cell lymphoma respond to interferon-α.[474] These responses can be complete and durable for several years.

Because of the poor response to salvage chemotherapy in patients with relapsed refractory diffuse large B-cell lymphoma, autologous bone marrow transplantation was tested soon after its development. In a study of 100 patients with relapsed diffuse aggressive lymphoma, both complete remission and prolonged disease-free survival could be predicted by the history of previous response to chemotherapy.[475] Approximately 35% of patients who relapsed from complete remission but remained sensitive to chemotherapy at relapse achieved prolonged disease-free survival and apparent cure, in contrast to approximately 10% of those who were chemotherapy resistant at the time of relapse and no patients who were initially refractory to therapy and failed to achieve a complete remission.[476] This study formed the basis for an international randomized trial referred to as the PARMA study.[477] In this trial, 109 patients who had relapsed from complete remission and responded to two cycles of DHAP (dexamethasone, cytarabine, cisplatin) were randomly allocated to high-dose chemotherapy using BEAC regimen (carmustine, etoposide, cytarabine, cyclophosphamide) or continued treatment with DHAP. Both groups were to receive involved-field radiotherapy. Bone marrow transplantation was associated with a superior failure-free survival (51% vs. 12% at 5 years) and overall survival (53% vs. 32% at 5 years). At present, high-dose therapy and autologous bone marrow transplantation are the treatments of choice for patients with chemotherapy-sensitive relapse who are young enough and healthy enough to undergo the procedures.

Allogeneic bone marrow transplantation has been used less frequently for patients with diffuse large B-cell lymphoma. While occasional patients failing autologous transplantation can have prolonged survival with allogeneic transplantation,[478] overall results from the North American Bone Marrow Transplant Registry have favored autologous transplantation.

Primary Mediastinal (Thymic) Large B-Cell Lymphoma

MORPHOLOGY. Primary mediastinal large B-cell lymphoma usually involves the thymus at presentation.[479,480] The tumor is composed of large cells with variable nuclear features, resembling centroblasts, large centrocytes, or multilobated cells, often with pale or *clear* cytoplasm. Less often, the tumor cells resemble immunoblasts. Reed-Sternberg–like cells may be present. Many cases have fine, compartmentalizing sclerosis.

IMMUNOPHENOTYPE. The tumor cells are often Ig–, but express B-cell–associated antigens (CD19, CD20, CD22, CD79a) and CD45.[480]

GENETIC FEATURES. Ig heavy and light-chain genes are rearranged; the bcl-2 gene is usually germline.[480–482] Bcl-6 gene rearrangements are uncommon.[483] Amplification of the *REL* oncogene has been described in a minority of the cases.[484]

POSTULATED NORMAL COUNTERPART. The postulated normal counterpart is putative thymic (medullary) B cell.

DIFFERENTIAL DIAGNOSIS. The major differential diagnoses clinically are thymoma, germ cell tumor, and Hodgkin's disease. In female subjects, germ cell tumor can be confidently excluded. Involvement of lymph nodes argues against a diagnosis of thymoma. The presence of superior vena cava syndrome argues against Hodgkin's disease. Histologically, the diagnosis depends on recognition of the characteristic morphology; immunohistochemical stains, as for other diffuse large B-cell lymphomas, are helpful.

CLINICAL FEATURES AND THERAPY. Primary diffuse large B-cell lymphoma of the mediastinum is a distinct clinicopathologic entity, requiring knowledge of both morphology, immunophenotype, and presenting site for the diagnosis.[126] It accounted for 7% of diffuse large B-cell lymphomas (2.4% of all NHL) in the international REAL study.[126,127] There is a female predominance and a median age in the fourth decade; patients present with a locally invasive anterior mediastinal mass originating in the thymus, with frequent airway compromise and superior vena cava syndrome.[485] Relapses tend to be extranodal, including liver, gastrointestinal tract, kidneys, ovaries, and CNS.

Although early studies suggested an unusually aggressive, incurable tumor, others have reported cure rates similar to those for other large cell lymphomas with aggressive therapy, usually combining chemotherapy with mediastinal irradiation.[485,486] With no evidence to the contrary, we recommend treating these patients similar to other patients with localized diffuse large cell lymphoma (i.e., with four to six cycles of CHOP and involved-field RT). The prognosis of patients with localized mediastinal large cell NHL is similar to other patients with poor prognosis early-stage disease; approximately 50% of patients are alive without disease at 5 years. Patients who present with a pleural effusion or who remain gallium positive after CHOP have a worse prognosis. Patients without bulky disease have a better prognosis.[487] Patients with disseminated disease should be treated like other patients with disseminated diffuse large B-cell lymphoma.

Intravascular Large B-Cell Lymphoma

Rare cases of large cell lymphoma, usually of B-cell type, present with a disseminated intravascular proliferation of large lymphoid cells, involving small blood vessels, without an obvious extravascular tumor mass or leukemia.[488,489] This tumor has also been variously known as intravascular lymphomatosis, angiotropic lymphoma, and malignant angioendotheliomatosis. The neoplastic lymphoid cells are mainly lodged in the lumina of small vessels in many organs. The tumor cells are large with vesicular nuclei, prominent nucleoli, and frequent mitotic figures. Malignant cells are rarely seen in cerebrospinal fluid, blood, or bone marrow. The organs most commonly involved are CNS, kidneys, lungs, and skin, but virtually any site may be involved.

Patients present with a bewildering variety of symptoms related to organ dysfunction secondary to vascular occlusion, which may be transient. Patients often present with neurologic dysfunction.[490–492] Other presentations include pulmonary involvement,[493,494] syndrome of inappropriate antidiuretic hormone production,[494] skin lesions,[495] lytic bone lesions,[495] endocrine dysfunction,[496] disseminated intravascular coagulation,[497] edema and hypoalbuminemia,[498] and thrombotic thrombocytopenic purpura.[499] Because of the wide variety of presentations, diagnosis is often difficult, and many reported cases were diagnosed by autopsy. If a timely diagnosis is made and combination chemotherapy instituted, patients can attain a complete remission, and long-term survival appears to be possible.[500]

Burkitt's Lymphoma

DEFINITION. Burkitt's lymphoma is a B-cell lymphoma composed of monomorphic, medium-sized cells with basophilic cytoplasm and a high proliferation fraction, characterized by translocation and deregulation of the c-myc gene on chromosome 8, which is often extranodal and occurs most often in children (endemic, sporadic) and immunocompromised hosts.

MORPHOLOGY. Burkitt's tumor cells are monomorphic, medium-sized cells with round nuclei, multiple nucleoli, and basophilic cytoplasm. Cytoplasmic lipid vacuoles are usually evident on imprints or smears. There is an extremely high rate of proliferation as well as a high rate of spontaneous cell death. A starry-sky pattern is usually present, imparted by numerous benign macrophages that have ingested apoptotic tumor cells. Although most cases present no problem in diagnosis, some cases may have larger cells or an admixture of immunoblast-like cells, and there is morphologic overlap with diffuse large B-cell lymphoma. These borderline cases are often called *non-Burkitt*[501] or *Burkitt-like.*[124] In children and human immunodeficiency virus–positive patients, these often have a c-myc translocation and behave similarly to typical Burkitt's lymphoma, whereas in adults, so-called Burkitt-like lymphomas often have bcl-2 gene rearrangement and may represent an aggressive variant of diffuse large B-cell lymphoma.[502] In the international study of the REAL,[126] Burkitt-like lymphoma was a nonreproducible category, in which the pathologists agreed on the diagnosis only 50% of the time: Disagreements were equally split between large B-cell and Burkitt's lymphoma.

The most appropriate way to handle this borderline between Burkitt's lymphoma and diffuse large B-cell lymphoma has been the subject of debate in the WHO classification project: Should it continue to be a separate, nonreproducible category; should it be a subtype of large B-cell lymphoma; or should it be a subtype of Burkitt's lymphoma? From a clinical standpoint, it is important to identify patients who should be treated as though they had Burkitt's lymphoma, since patients with Burkitt's lymphoma do not do well with treatment that would be effective for large cell lymphoma. On the other hand, treatment for Burkitt's lymphoma is considerably more aggressive than that for large B-cell lymphoma and may have significant treatment-related morbidity,[503] so that it should not be used for usual large B-cell lymphomas. The question is how to draw the line between large cell lymphoma and Burkitt's lymphoma so that morphologically borderline cases will be assigned to the correct category?

The defining biologic feature of Burkitt's lymphoma is c-myc deregulation, as a consequence of which the tumor cells remain constantly in cycle. It is this phenomenon that results in both its morphologic homogeneity and its clinical behavior. Unfortunately, detection of c-myc translocation is not practical in all clinical specimens for technical reasons. In addition, some large B-cell lymphomas have t(8;14) and c-myc deregulation, and it is not clear if all such cases should be treated like Burkitt's lymphoma. The best practical surrogate for c-myc deregulation is proliferation fraction: In a tumor with c-myc deregulation, 100% of viable cells should be in cycle and should express Ki-67. Thus, the WHO committees concluded that a diagnosis of Burkitt-like lymphoma should only be made in *a tumor with morphologic features intermediate between Burkitt's lymphoma and diffuse large B-cell lymphoma, in which the Ki-67 fraction of viable cells is at least 99%*. This tumor will be considered a subtype of Burkitt's lymphoma in the WHO classification.[130] Cases with morphologic features of large cell lymphoma with a high proliferation fraction [or t(8;14)] and cases that are morphologically borderline between Burkitt's lymphoma and large B-cell lymphoma with a lower proliferation fraction, should be classified as diffuse large B-cell lymphoma.

IMMUNOPHENOTYPE. Burkitt's lymphoma cells express SIgM and B-cell–associated antigens (CD19, CD20, CD22, CD79a), as well as CD10 and CD43; they lack CD5 and bcl-2 and typically lack CD23.[504] They show nuclear staining for BCL-6 protein, which is independent of bcl-6 gene rearrangement.[505]

GENETIC FEATURES. Ig heavy and light-chain genes are rearranged. Studies of the Ig variable region genes show conflicting results: One study reported unmutated genes,[506] whereas others report somatic mutations and intraclonal heterogeneity, consistent with ongoing mutations.[507–509] Most cases have a translocation of c-myc from chromosome 8 to either the Ig heavy-chain region on chromosome 14 [t(8;14)] or light-chain loci on 2 [t(2;8)] or 22 [t(8;22)]. In African (endemic) cases, the breakpoint on chromosome 14 involves the heavy-chain joining region, whereas in nonendemic cases, the translocation involves the heavy-chain switch region.[510,511] Mutations in the 5' noncoding region of the bcl-6 gene, similar to those seen in large B-cell lymphoma, have been reported in 25% to 50% of the cases.[512] Most African cases contain EBV genomes, as do 25% to 40% of the cases associated with AIDS.[513]

POSTULATED NORMAL COUNTERPART. The postulated normal counterpart is peripheral B cell of unknown stage: perhaps B blast of early germinal center reaction.

DIFFERENTIAL DIAGNOSIS. Burkitt's lymphoma must be distinguished from other primary abdominal malignancies in childhood, including Wilms' tumor, neuroblastoma, and peripheral neuroectodermal tumor. In the bone marrow, it must be distinguished from B- and T-precursor and myeloid leukemias. Morphologic features are usually sufficient for the diagnosis if adequate material is available. The presence of leukocyte-associated antigens and Ig and the lack of TdT are important in distinguishing Burkitt's lymphoma from the other tumors mentioned. Among peripheral B-cell lymphomas, the major differential diagnosis is with diffuse large B-cell lymphoma; although this is usually straightforward on histologic grounds, occasional borderline cases occur; a provisional category of *high-grade B-cell lymphoma, Burkitt-like* is used for these cases. Burkitt's lymphoma is more likely to express CD10 and to have c-myc rearrangement than is diffuse large B-cell lymphoma.

CLINICAL FEATURES AND THERAPY. Three distinct clinical forms of Burkitt's lymphoma can be recognized: endemic, sporadic, and immunodeficiency-associated.[514] Although they are histologically identical and have similar clinical behavior, there are differences in epidemiology, clinical presentation, and genetic features between the three forms. Endemic and sporadic Burkitt's lymphomas are both most common in children, but the median age is younger in endemic patients. Burkitt's lymphoma accounts for 30% of nonendemic pediatric lymphomas, but less than 1% of adult NHLs; in human immunodeficiency virus–positive patients it typically affects those with a relatively high CD4 count and no opportunistic infections. In all groups, the majority of patients are male (3 to 4:1). In endemic cases, the jaws and other facial bones are often involved, as well as the mesentery and gonads. In sporadic cases, the majority are present in the abdomen, most often involving distal ileum, cecum, mesentery, or both cecum and mesentery; ovaries, kidneys, or breasts may be involved.[515] Immunodeficiency-related cases more often involve lymph nodes, and both these and sporadic cases may present as acute leukemia.

Patients typically present with rapidly growing tumor masses and often have a high serum LDH. Burkitt's lymphoma is highly aggressive but potentially curable with aggressive therapy. Because of the extremely rapid progression of Burkitt's lymphoma, patients with this disease should be approached as a medical emergency. Staging should be completed quickly and therapy initiated at the earliest possible time. Because of the risk of tumor lysis syndrome, patients should be well-hydrated, receive allopurinol, and be watched closely after the initiation of therapy. Death from hyperkalemia has been reported.[516,517] Some patients require hemodialysis to control hyperkalemia.

Burkitt's lymphoma was one of the first malignancies to be shown to be curable with chemotherapy,[518] and the majority of patients should be curable today with aggressive combination chemotherapy regimens. High-dose regimens of fairly brief duration are used to treat patients with Burkitt's lymphoma.[519–522] Patients with localized disease are cured in approximately 90% of the cases with these intensive regimens, and cure rates within excess of 50% have been reported in patients with extensive disease.[519] When treated with similar regimens, adults and children have comparable outcomes.[519] Because of the propensity for CNS metastases, treatment regimens for Burkitt's lymphoma always involve prophylactic therapy to the CNS. Salvage therapy for patients with relapsed Burkitt's lymphoma has generally been unsatisfactory. However, occasional patients can be cured with autologous bone marrow transplantation.[523] Patients with isolated CNS relapse can sometimes be cured with bone marrow transplantation[524] or a combination of systemic therapy at traditional doses and intrathecal treatment.[525]

T-CELL AND NATURAL KILLER–CELL NEOPLASMS

Precursor T-Lymphoblastic Lymphoma/Leukemia (Precursor T-Cell Acute Lymphoblastic Leukemia/ Precursor T-Cell Lymphoblastic Lymphoma)

DEFINITION. A T-cell and NK-cell neoplasm is a neoplasm of lymphoblasts committed to the T-cell lineage, typically composed of small to medium-sized blast cells with scant cytoplasm, moderately condensed to dispersed chromatin and indistinct nucleoli, variably involving bone marrow and blood (precursor T-cell ALL), thymus, lymph nodes, or all (precursor T-cell lymphoblastic lymphoma).

MORPHOLOGY. On smears, lymphoblasts vary from small cells with scant cytoplasm, condensed nuclear chromatin, and indistinct nucleoli to larger cells with a moderate amount of cytoplasm, dispersed chromatin, and multiple nucleoli. Azurophilic granules may be present. In tissue sections, the cells are small to medium-sized, with scant cytoplasm, round, oval, or convoluted nuclei, and fine chromatin and indistinct or small nucleoli. Occasional cases have larger cells. The pattern is infiltrative rather than destructive, with partial preservation of the subcapsular sinus and germinal centers. A starry-sky pattern may be present, but is usually less prominent than in Burkitt's lymphoma.

IMMUNOPHENOTYPE. The lymphoblasts are typically positive for TdT and variably express CD2, CD7, CD3, CD5, CD1a, CD4, CD8, or all of these. Only CD3 is considered lineage specific. The constellation of antigens defines stages of differentiation, ranging from early or pro-T (CD2, CD7, and cytoplasmic CD3), to *common* thymocyte (CD1a, sCD3, CD4, and CD8), to late thymocyte (CD4 or CD8). Although there is some correlation with presentation and differentiation stage (cases with bone marrow and blood presentation may show earlier differentiation stage than cases with thymic presentation),[526,527] there is overlap.[528]

GENETIC FEATURES. Rearrangement of antigen receptor genes is variable in lymphoblastic neoplasms and may not be lineage specific; thus, precursor T-cell neoplasms may have either or both TCR β or γ chain gene rearrangements and Ig heavy-chain gene rearrangements.[529]

Chromosomal translocations involving the TCR α and δ loci at chromosome 14q11 and β and γ loci at 7q34 are present in approximately one-third of the cases[150,530]; the partner genes are variable and include the transcription factors c-MYC (8q24), TAL1/SCL (1p32), RBTN1 (11p35), RBTN2 (11913), and HOX11 (10q24) and the cytoplasmic tyrosine kinase LCK (1p34). In an additional 25%, the TAL1 locus at 1p32 has deletions in the 5' regulatory region.[531] Deletions of 9p involving deletion of the p16^{INK4a} tumor suppressor gene (cdk4 inhibitor) is also seen in T-lymphoblastic neoplasms.

POSTULATED NORMAL COUNTERPART. The postulated normal counterpart is precursor T lymphoblast at varying stages of differentiation.

CLINICAL FEATURES AND THERAPY. Precursor T-cell neoplasia occurs most frequently in late childhood, adolescence, and young adulthood, with a male predominance; it accounts for 15% of childhood and 25% of adult ALL.[157] The prognosis is typically worse than that for precursor B-cell neoplasms and is not affected by immunophenotype or genetic abnormalities. Patients typically present with a high leukocyte count and often a mediastinal mass. Clinically, a case is defined as lymphoma if there is a mediastinal or other mass and less than 25% blasts in the bone marrow, and as leukemia if there are greater than 25% bone marrow blasts, with or without a mass. In children, treatment is generally more aggressive than that for precursor B-ALL and is typically the same for lymphomatous and leukemic presentations.[530]

Adults with lymphoblastic lymphoma seem to have an excellent prognosis when presenting with stage I or II disease.[532] In such patients treatment with CHOP, intrathecal methotrexate, and CNS radiotherapy, and maintenance chemotherapy with methotrexate and mercaptopurine yielded a 94% 5-year freedom from relapse rate for patients with lymph node–based disease and a normal serum LDH level.[532] Patients who presented with bone marrow involvement, CNS involvement, or a high serum LDH had a 5-year freedom from relapse rate of only 19%. Because of the propensity for CNS relapse, all patients with lymphoblastic lymphoma should receive prophylactic treatment to the CNS.

More intensive chemotherapy regimens of the type used to treat ALL appeared to yield better results in patients with lymphoblastic lymphoma.[533–535] Adjuvant autologous bone marrow transplantation in high-risk patients has been reported to improve the long-term disease-free survival rate.[536] These data have been supported by the early results from a randomized trial.[537] There is some evidence that allogeneic bone marrow transplantation might have a superior result to autologous bone marrow transplantation.[535] Some patients who relapse from remission can be cured with autologous or allogeneic bone marrow transplantation, although the overall prognosis in such patients is poor.[538]

Mature T Cell: Mycosis Fungoides

For a discussion of mycosis fungoides, see Chapter 45.4.

Adult T-Cell Lymphoma and Leukemia

DEFINITION. Adult T-cell lymphoma and leukemia is defined as a peripheral T-cell neoplasm caused by HTLV-I.

MORPHOLOGY. Cells with hyperlobated nuclei (flower cells) are common in the peripheral blood in leukemic cases. In addition, there is a small proportion of blast-like cells with a deep basophilic cytoplasm. Bone marrow infiltrates are usually patchy, ranging from sparse to moderate. In lymph nodes, the infiltrates are diffuse with architectural effacement. Neoplastic cells are usually medium to large with nuclear pleomorphism; the cytoplasm is amphophilic, basophilic, or pale. Mitotic activity is variable. Reed-Sternberg–like cells and giant cells with convoluted or cerebriform nuclei may be present. Rare cases may be composed of small atypical lymphocytes with nuclear pleomorphism or may resemble anaplastic large cell lymphoma. In the background there is a mild to moderate proliferation of high endothelial venules.

IMMUNOPHENOTYPE. Tumor cells express T-cell–associated antigens (CD2, CD3, CD5), but usually lack CD7. Most cases are CD4+ and CD8–. Rare cases are CD4–, CD8+, or CD8+ and CD4+. CD25 is expressed in a majority of the cases. Anaplastic large cell types react with CD30, but are ALK (p80) negative.

GENETICS. Clonally integrated HTLV-I genes are found in all cases. The TCR genes are clonally rearranged.

POSSIBLE NORMAL COUNTERPART. The possible normal counterpart is peripheral CD4+ T cells in various stages of transformation.

DIFFERENTIAL DIAGNOSIS. Chronic and smoldering forms must be distinguished from benign lymphocytosis. Cutaneous involvement must be distinguished from mycosis fungoides. Lymphomatous presentations may clinically and histologically resemble large B-cell or other peripheral T-cell lymphomas. The typical acute form is clinically and morphologically distinctive, with leukocytosis and the characteristic flower cells in an Asian or Caribbean patient, often with hypercalcemia. Since the disease may be mimicked by other peripheral T-cell lymphomas, and because of its highly aggressive course, serologic evaluation for HTLV-I infection is recommended in any patient with a newly diagnosed peripheral T-cell lymphoma.

CLINICAL FEATURES. ATL is one manifestation of infection by HTLV-I. Tropical spastic paraparesis and HTLV-I–associated myelopathy appear to be more common manifestations of infection than ATL. The diagnosis is established when a patient with a typical clinical and pathologic syndrome is found to have antibodies to HTLV-I. Most patients are adults, although children are occasionally seen with the disorder when they received transfusions in infancy. The virus can be acquired by vertical transmission from mother to child, sexual transmission, or via blood products. Most cases occur in Japan or the Caribbean, with sporadic cases found elsewhere in the world.

In the United States the diagnosis is frequently difficult because ATL is not considered since many clinicians are not acquainted with the syndrome. Several variants have been described depending on the clinical features: acute, lymphomatous, chronic, and smoldering. The most common *acute type* presents with neoplastic cells in the blood, skin rashes, generalized lymphadenopathy, hepatosplenomegaly, and hypercalcemia. The *lymphomatous type* is characterized by prominent lymphadenopathy but no blood involvement. The *chronic type* shows skin lesions and an increased white blood cell count with absolute lymphocytosis, but no hypercalcemia. The *smoldering type* shows normal blood lymphocyte counts with ≤5% circulating neoplastic cells. Patients frequently have skin or pulmonary lesions, but hypercalcemia is not present. Progression from chronic and smoldering to acute types eventually occurs in up to 25% of the cases. Peripheral blood and bone marrow are the most frequent sites of involvement, although essentially any organ can be involved by the disease including gastrointestinal tract, liver, lung, and CNS.

THERAPY. The treatment of ATL has been unsatisfactory. Patients with the chronic or smoldering syndromes can sometimes be followed without therapy for extended periods of time. When the disease becomes asymptomatic, combination chemotherapy regimens have usually been used.[145] Although patients frequently respond to the initial combination chemotherapy regimen, the overall survival remains poor, with less than 10% of the patients surviving 5 years after initiating therapy. A variety of the new treatment approaches has been studied including new chemotherapeutic agents, monoclonal antibodies, and allogeneic bone marrow transplantation. One case of long-term, disease-free survival with allogeneic bone marrow transplantation has been described.[539]

Peripheral T-Cell Lymphoma, Not Otherwise Categorized

DEFINITION. In peripheral T-cell lymphoma, not otherwise categorized, a number of distinct entities have been defined, which correspond to recognizable subtypes of T-cell neoplasia. There remains a large group of predominantly nodal T-cell lymphomas, which make up the largest group of T-cell neoplasms in western countries. Although a variety of morphologic subtypes has been described, no consistent immunophenotypic, genetic, or clinical features have been associated with most of them. Therefore, for the time being, these presumably diverse cases are lumped under the heading peripheral T-cell lymphoma, not otherwise categorized, or unspecified. This category includes heterogeneous diseases that require further definition.

MORPHOLOGIC FEATURES. Peripheral T-cell lymphomas typically contain a mixture of small and large atypical cells[540,541] and are classified as *diffuse small cleaved, mixed, large cell,* and *immunoblastic* in the Working Formulation.[127,542] Admixed eosinophils or epithelioid histiocytes may be numerous[543]; the term *lymphoepithelioid cell (Lennert's) lymphoma* has been used for cases rich in epithelioid cells.[543] Because of their relative rarity and heterogeneity, it has been impossible to arrive at a generally useful classification.[541,544–547] For the time being, these tumors are simply designated *peripheral T-cell lymphomas, unspecified.*

IMMUNOPHENOTYPE. T-cell–associated antigens are variably expressed (CD3+/–, CD2+/–, CD5+/–, CD7–/+), CD4 is more often expressed than CD8, and tumors may be CD4– and CD8–. B-cell–associated antigens are lacking.[540,548]

GENETIC FEATURES. The TCR genes are usually but not always rearranged; Ig genes are germline.[540,549] No specific cytogenetic or oncogene abnormality has been reported, although complex karyotypes are common in cases with larger cells.

POSTULATED NORMAL COUNTERPART. The postulated normal counterpart is peripheral T cells in various stages of transformation.

CLINICAL FEATURES. Peripheral T-cell lymphomas accounted for only 6% of lymphomas in the international study of the REAL,[126,127] reflecting their rarity in American and European populations. The median age was in the seventh decade, and 65% of the patients had stage IV disease. Blood eosinophilia, pruritus, and hemophagocytic syndromes may occur[550]; lymph nodes, skin, liver, spleen, and other viscera may be involved.[551,552] The clinical course is aggressive, and relapses are more common than in large B-cell lymphoma.[545,553–556] In the international REAL study, this group had one of the lowest overall and failure-free survival rates.[126,127]

THERAPY. Treatment regimens used for peripheral T-cell lymphoma are the same as used for diffuse large B-cell lymphoma. Because of the poorer overall survival in peripheral T-cell lymphoma as compared with diffuse large B-cell lymphoma, bone marrow transplantation is more likely to be used as part of the primary therapy. Bone marrow transplantation may be as effective in peripheral T-cell lymphoma as in diffuse large B-cell lymphoma.[557]

Angioimmunoblastic T-Cell Lymphoma

DEFINITION. Angioimmunoblastic T-cell lymphoma is a T-cell lymphoma characterized by systemic disease, a polymorphous infiltrate involving lymph nodes, and a prominent proliferation of high endothelial venules and FDCs.

MORPHOLOGY. The nodal architecture is effaced; peripheral sinuses are typically open and even dilated, but the abnormal infiltrate often extends beyond the capsule into the perinodal fat. There are prominent arborizing high endothelial venules, many of which show thickened or hyalinized periodic acid–Schiff-positive walls. Clusters of epithelioid histiocytes and numerous eosinophils and plasma cells may be present. Expanded aggregates of FDCs, visible on immunostained sections, surround the proliferating blood vessels and may have the appearance of *burnt-out* germinal centers. The lymphoid cells are a mixture of small lymphocytes, immunoblasts, plasma cells, and medium-sized cells with round nuclei and clear cytoplasm. B immunoblasts may be numerous.

IMMUNOPHENOTYPE. Tumor cells express T-cell–associated antigens and usually CD4, but many CD8+ cells are often present; expanded FDC clusters (CD21+) are present around proliferated venules.[558] The latter feature is useful in distinguishing this disorder from other T-cell lymphomas.[547] Polyclonal plasma cells and B immunoblasts may be numerous.

GENETIC FEATURES. The TCR genes are rearranged in 75%; IgH in 10%, corresponding to expanded B-cell clones.[558,559] EBV genomes are detected in many cases and may be present in either T or B cells[560,561]; trisomy 3, 5, or both may occur.[562]

POSTULATED NORMAL COUNTERPART. The postulated normal counterpart is peripheral T cell of unknown subset in various stages of transformation.

CLINICAL FEATURES. Angioimmunoblastic T-cell lymphoma is one of the more common peripheral T-cell lymphomas encountered in western countries. In the Kiel Registry, it accounted for 20% of all T-cell lymphomas and approximately 4% of all lymphomas.[547] Angioimmunoblastic T-cell lymphoma is clinically distinctive: Patients typically have generalized lymphadenopathy, fever, weight loss, skin rash, and polyclonal hypergammaglobulinemia[563] and are susceptible to infections. The course is moderately aggressive, with occasional spontaneous remissions, and is not reliably predicted by the histologic appearance.

THERAPY. Approximately 30% of the patients may have initial remission on corticosteroids alone, but most require some form of cytotoxic chemotherapy. Median survivals range from 15 to 24 months, and curability has not been well established. Some patients develop a secondary EBV+ large B-cell lymphoma. A prospective but nonrandomized trial compared an anthracycline-based combination chemotherapy regimen with prednisone followed by combination chemotherapy only if the disease progressed. Initial chemotherapy yielded a higher complete remission rate (64% vs. 29%) and median survival (19 vs. 11 months).[564]

Extranodal Natural Killer/T-Cell Lymphoma, Nasal Type (Formerly Angiocentric Lymphoma)

DEFINITION. Extranodal NK/T-cell lymphoma, nasal type, is an extranodal lymphoma, usually with an immature NK-cell phenotype and EBV+, with a broad morphologic spectrum, frequent necrosis and angioinvasion, and most commonly presenting in the midfacial region, but also in other extranodal sites. It is designated NK/T because of uncertainty regarding lineage.

MORPHOLOGIC FEATURES. Nasal NK/T-cell lymphoma is typically characterized by a polymorphous infiltrate composed of a mixture of normal appearing small lymphocytes and atypical lymphoid cells of varying size,[565,566] along with plasma cells and occasionally eosinophils and histiocytes. A characteristic feature is invasion of vascular walls and, usually, occlusion of lumina by lymphoid cells with varying degrees of cytologic atypia; however, this is not seen in all the cases. There is usually prominent ischemic necrosis of both tumor cells and normal tissue. The term *angiocentric lymphoma* has proven confusing, since angiocentricity is not evident in all cases. Since the most characteristic presentation is midfacial, and the cells have both T and NK features, the term *extranodal T/NK-cell lymphoma, nasal type,* has been proposed.[567]

Cases of pulmonary *lymphomatoid granulomatosis* were for a time considered to be part of the spectrum of angiocentric lymphoma. Studies suggest that most pulmonary cases are EBV-associated B-cell proliferations, and therefore a distinct disease category[374,377]; however, some pulmonary lymphomas with histologic features of lymphomatoid granulomatosis lack CD20+ cells and EBV and may be examples of peripheral T-cell lymphoma.[377] Thus, pulmonary lymphomas with angiocentric growth patterns and necrosis may be heterogeneous.

IMMUNOPHENOTYPE. The atypical cells in most cases are CD2+, CD56+, surface CD3–, and cytoplasmic CD3+ (Leu 4– but positive with the polyclonal anti-CD3, which detects the epsilon chain of CD3). They are typically CD4– and CD8–, but may express CD4, CD7, or both.[566,568,569] Most cases express cytotoxic granule proteins such as Granzyme B and TIA-1.[570]

GENETIC FEATURES. The TCR and Ig genes are usually germline; EBV genomes are usually present and are detectable in the majority of the cells in most cases by *in situ* hybridization for EBER-1.[569,571]

POSTULATED NORMAL COUNTERPART. The postulated normal counterpart is immature NK cell.

CLINICAL FEATURES. Nasal-type T/NK lymphoma is a rare disorder in the United States and Europe, but is more common in Asia and in native populations in Peru. It may affect children or adults. Extranodal sites are invariably involved, including nose, palate, upper airway, gastrointestinal tract, and skin.[565,566,569,572,573] The clinical course is typically aggressive, with relapses in other extranodal sites.[569,574] Hemophagocytic syndromes may occur. Some cases of the aggressive variant of NK-cell leukemia and lymphoma may be related to this disorder.[575]

THERAPY. Patients with localized NK/T-cell lymphoma in the nasal pharynx can be cured with a combination of chemotherapy and local radiotherapy.[576] With radiotherapy alone, treatment failure is frequent. Patients with disseminated NK/T-cell lymphoma have an extremely poor outlook. Occasional long-term survivors are seen using the CHOP regimen.[577] Less aggressive regimens have a uniformly poor outcome.

High-dose chemotherapy and autologous bone marrow transplantation can be curative in some patients after relapse from standard therapy.[578,579] Because of the poor results with standard chemotherapeutic approaches, incorporation of bone marrow transplantation as a primary management of patients with disseminated NK/T-cell lymphoma might improve treatment outcome.

Enteropathy Type T-Cell Lymphoma

DEFINITION. Enteropathy type T-cell lymphoma is a tumor of intraepithelial T lymphocytes, usually associated with features of gluten-sensitive enteropathy, showing varying degrees of transformation but usually presenting as a high-grade (blastic) tumor.

MORPHOLOGY. This disorder was originally termed *malignant histiocytosis of the intestine,* but has since been conclusively shown to be a T-cell lymphoma.[580] On gross examination, circumferentially oriented jejunal ulcers are present, often multiple, and often with perforation. A mass may or may not be present. The tumors contain a variable admixture of small, medium and mixed, large or anaplastic tumor cells, often with a high content of intraepithelial T cells in adjacent mucosa. The adjacent mucosa may or may not show villous atrophy[552]; this varies depending on the segment analyzed, since in sprue, villous atrophy is most prominent in the proximal small intestine and may be absent in distal jejunum or ileum. Early lesions may show mucosal ulceration with only scattered atypical cells and numerous reactive histiocytes, without formation of large masses[581]; these lesions are nonetheless clonal. Intraepithelial lymphocytes in apparently non-neoplastic mucosa may also be clonal.[582] Clonal TCR gene rearrangements have been found in cases of celiac disease unresponsive to a gluten-free diet, suggesting that these cases may represent early T-cell lymphomas.[583] The tumor may involve liver, spleen, lymph nodes, and other viscera such as the gallbladder.

IMMUNOPHENOTYPE. The tumor cells are T cells expressing pan-T antigens (CD3+, CD7+), usually CD8+ and CD4–, and expressing the mucosal lymphoid antigen CD103.[584] CD30 may be positive in some cells. Expression of cytotoxic T-cell–associated proteins (Granzyme B, TIA-1, perforin) is seen in many of the cases.[585,586]

GENETIC FEATURES. The TCRβ gene is clonally rearranged[580]; no specific cytogenetic abnormality has been described.

POSTULATED NORMAL COUNTERPART. The postulated normal counterpart is intestinal intraepithelial cytotoxic T cells in various stages of transformation.

CLINICAL FEATURES AND THERAPY. This disease occurs in adults, typically with a rather brief history of gluten-sensitive enteropathy, as the initial event in a patient found to have villous atrophy in the resected intestine, or without evidence of enteropathy but with either or both antigliadin antibodies or the typical HLA type (DQA1*0501, DQB1*0201) of patients with celiac disease.[587] It is uncommon in most areas of the United States and Europe, but is seen with increased frequency in areas in which gluten-sensitive enteropathy is common. Treatment of celiac disease with a gluten-free diet effectively prevents the development of lymphoma, so that patients diagnosed with celiac disease early in life usually do not develop lymphoma, and patients with lymphoma rarely have a long history of celiac disease.[136,588] Patients present with abdominal pain, often associated with jejunal perforation; stomach or colon are affected less often,[589] and other viscera, skin, or soft tissues may be involved.[590–592] The course is aggressive, and death usually occurs from multifocal intestinal perforation due to refractory malignant ulcers. A poor response to therapy has been reported. It is probably related to the severe nutritional and immunologic abnormalities found in patients with uncontrolled celiac disease.

Hepatosplenic γδ T-Cell Lymphoma

DEFINITION. Hepatosplenic γδ T-cell lymphoma is a neoplasm of mature γδ T cells with sinusoidal infiltration of spleen, liver, and bone marrow.

MORPHOLOGY. Hepatosplenic γδ T-cell lymphoma produces a sinusoidal infiltrate in liver and spleen, as well as bone marrow, of medium-sized lymphoid cells with round nuclei, moderately condensed chromatin, and moderately abundant, pale cytoplasm.[593] Mitotic activity is generally low.[594] The white pulp is atrophic. Erythrophagocytosis may be prominent in splenic and bone marrow sinuses.

IMMUNOPHENOTYPE. The tumor cells are CD2+, CD3+, CD5–, CD4–, CD8–, CD16+, CD56 +/–, and lack the αβ TCR protein, expressing instead the γδ complex. Cytotoxic granule protein TIA-1 is typically expressed, but Granzyme B and perforin are absent, indicating a nonactivated cytotoxic T-cell phenotype.[595–597]

GENETIC FEATURES. The TCR γ and δ genes are rearranged; the TCR β gene may be rearranged or germline. The tumor cells are EBV–. Isochromosome 7q and trisomy 8 have been reported in many cases.[598–600]

POSTULATED NORMAL COUNTERPART. The postulated normal counterpart is γδ T cell of splenic type.

CLINICAL FEATURES AND THERAPY. This is a rare neoplasm, but because it has only relatively recently been characterized, its frequency is not known; cases have probably been classified as T-CLL/prolymphocytic leukemia or peripheral T-cell lymphoma unspecified. The diagnosis is often difficult. These patients frequently present as with a multisystem disease with hepatomegaly, splenomegaly, or both.[594,601] The absence of lymphadenopathy and the sinusoidal pattern of infiltration of the liver, spleen, and bone marrow make the diagnosis difficult. Frequently, only the demonstration of a T-cell gene rearrangement leads to the correct diagnosis.

Patients have been predominantly adolescent boys and young adult men. Although most patients were previously healthy, the disease has been described in immunosuppressed, solid organ allograft recipients.[598,602] Unusual sites of involvement such as skin, nasal cavity, gastrointestinal tract, lung, mucosal, and larynx[603,604] have been described. Although circulating neoplastic cells are usually not prominent, subtle bone marrow involvement may be present.[605,606]

Despite the relatively bland appearance of the cells, this is an aggressive tumor. Complete remission can occur with combination chemotherapy,[594,606] but most patients relapse. Long-term survival has been described with autologous bone marrow transplantation.[594,606]

Subcutaneous Panniculitis-Like T-Cell Lymphoma

DEFINITION. Subcutaneous panniculitis-like T-cell lymphoma is a T-cell lymphoma that preferentially infiltrates subcutaneous tissue, with atypical cells of varying size, showing prominent tumor necrosis and karyorrhexis.

MORPHOLOGIC FEATURES. There is a variable mixture of small, medium, and large atypical cells, often containing irregular, hyperchromatic nuclei and pale cytoplasm. Reactive histiocytes with phagocytized nuclear debris, lipid, or both are numerous. Granulomas may be present. Individual adipocytes are rimmed by neoplastic cells.[551,607]

IMMUNOPHENOTYPE. Most cases express pan-T antigens and usually CD8, although they may be CD4+, express cytotoxic granule proteins TIA-1 and perforin, and in most cases, the α-β TCR.[608] Occasional cases derive from γδ T cells.[607]

GENETIC FEATURES. TCR γ genes are rearranged; usually β but occasionally δ chain genes are rearranged.[607] No specific cytogenetic abnormalities have been described.

POSTULATED NORMAL COUNTERPART. The postulated normal counterpart is the mature cytotoxic T cell.

CLINICAL FEATURES AND THERAPY. Patients present with one or more subcutaneous nodules and are often misdiagnosed as having panniculitis. Hemophagocytic syndrome is common. The disease may present in an indolent fashion but typically becomes aggressive.[551,607] Patients may respond to combination chemotherapy regimens, but the responses are usually transient. These lymphomas are generally radiosensitive, and radiotherapy can be used to control symptoms. However, the long-term outlook with this disorder is poor.

Anaplastic Large T/Null-Cell Lymphoma, Primary Systemic Type

DEFINITION. Anaplastic large T/null-cell lymphoma, primary systemic type, is a neoplasm of large lymphoid cells with pleomorphic or multiple nuclei and abundant cytoplasm, a cohesive growth pattern, and sinusoidal spread in lymph nodes, expressing CD30 and either T-cell or no lineage-specific antigens, involving lymph nodes or extranodal sites, but not limited to the skin.

MORPHOLOGIC FEATURES. The tumor is usually composed of large blastic cells with round or pleomorphic, often horseshoe-shaped or multiple nuclei with multiple or single prominent nucleoli, and abundant cytoplasm, which gives the cells an epithelial or histiocyte-like appearance. The so-called hallmark cell has an eccentric nucleus and a prominent, eosinophilic Golgi region.[609] The tumor cells grow in a cohesive pattern and often preferentially involve the lymph node sinuses or paracortex.[610] In some cases, the tumor cells may have a more monomorphous appearance, with round to oval nuclei and no Reed-Sternberg–like cells; these cases have in common with the more anaplastic cases a low nuclear to cytoplasmic ratio, with dense, abundant cytoplasm and a cohesive, often sinusoidal growth pattern.[611] Lymphohistiocytic and small cell variants have been described, again, more commonly in children.[612,613] Study of cytogenetic and molecular genetic abnormalities as well as clinical features suggests that these cases belong to the same disease entity as the more anaplastic cases.[609,614]

A variant of ALCL resembling Hodgkin's disease of nodular sclerosis type has been described,[615,616] originally called *ALCL Hodgkin's-related* and included as a provisional entity under the name *ALCL Hodgkin's-like,* in the REAL.[124] This subtype is defined as having architectural features of Hodgkin's disease (nodularity and sclerosis), but cytologic features of ALCL (sheets of neoplastic cells and sinusoidal infiltration). Many patients are young adults with mediastinal masses, and the outcome was said to be intermediate between that of typical ALCL and nodular sclerosis Hodgkin's disease. Several studies suggest that these are not true borderline cases. First, most cases of ALCL Hodgkin's-like lack the t(2;5) or ALK protein.[617,618] Second, most cases of Hodgkin's disease are now thought to be B-cell derived, based on single-cell studies showing Ig gene rearrangement,[559,619–622] while ALCL is predominantly a T-cell disease; thus, there should be no true biologic borderline. Finally, a randomized study showed that patients with ALCL Hodgkin's-like responded equally well to the ABVD regimen for Hodgkin's disease as to a MACOP-B regimen for aggressive NHL,[623] suggesting a closer relationship to Hodgkin's disease than to typical ALCL. The current consensus is that the majority of these cases can be resolved as either Hodgkin's disease (CD15+, CD30+ T-cell antigen, ALK–) or ALCL (CD15–, CD30+ T-cell antigen +/–, ALK+/–) by a combination of morphology and immunophenotype. Thus, this category will be eliminated from the WHO classification.[130]

IMMUNOPHENOTYPE. The tumor cells are CD30+ and usually express CD25 and EMA; they are typically CD45+ and CD15–; approximately 60% express one or more T-cell–associated antigens (CD3, CD43, or CD45RO). Studies have shown cytotoxic granule proteins in many of the cases.[624,625] The ALK protein can be detected in 40% to 60% of the cases using the ALK1 monoclonal antibody, showing both nuclear and cytoplasmic staining in cases with the t(2;5), since nucleophosmin is a nuclear protein. ALK+ cases are more common in children and have a better prognosis than ALK– cases.[617,618,626]

GENETIC FEATURES. The majority of the cases have TCR genes rearranged; 20% to 30% have no rearrangement of TCR or Ig genes. Between 20% and 50% of primary systemic ALCL have a t(2;5),[627,628] which results in a fusion of the nucleophosmin gene (NPM) on chromosome 5 to a novel tyrosine kinase gene on chromosome 2, called anaplastic lymphoma kinase (ALK). The specificity of this translocation for ALCL has been debated, in part because of differing criteria for the diagnosis of ALCL. Using the reverse transcriptase–PCR or an antibody to the fusion protein, the fusion gene product can be detected in approximately 50% of ALCL of T and null type; however, it is also detected in some T-cell lymphomas without obvious anaplastic morphology.[626,628,629] Based on illustrations published in some of these articles, the so-called nonanaplastic cases appear to represent examples of the monomorphic, small cell, or histiocyte-rich variants.[628] Rare cases of B-cell lymphoma with the t(2;5) have been reported.[626,630] Finally, variant translocations have been described, which also result in overexpression of ALK protein but without the nuclear localization.[631]

Based on current information, t(2;5) and ALK expression are not considered defining features of ALCL, since negative case results exist; however, the positive case results appear clinically relatively homogeneous: young patients with a relatively good prognosis.

DIFFERENTIAL DIAGNOSIS. Many cases of ALCL were previously diagnosed as nonlymphoid tumors (malignant histiocytic tumors,[627] regressing atypical histiocytosis,[632] melanoma, metastatic carcinoma, sarcoma) or as lymphocyte-depleted Hodgkin's disease. A high index of suspicion is important in recognizing the tumor as lymphoid; immunophenotyping studies on paraffin sections (CD45, CD30, pan-T antigens, lack of epithelial or melanocyte-associated antigens) usually confirm the diagnosis.

CLINICAL FEATURES. Anaplastic large cell lymphoma represents approximately 2% of all lymphomas, but approximately 10% of childhood lymphomas and 50% of large cell pediatric lymphomas.[125–127,547,633,634]

Primary systemic ALCL may involve lymph nodes or extranodal sites, including the skin, but is not localized to the skin. Tumors that present with systemic disease (with or without skin involvement) have a bimodal age distribution in children and adults and are associated with the t(2;5), particularly in children, in 20% to 40% of the cases. Patients may present with isolated lymphadenopathy or extranodal disease in any site, including gastrointestinal tract and bone.[633] Anaplastic large cell lymphoma in children is characterized by frequent high stage but a good response to therapy with overall excellent survival.[628,633,634] In adults the tumor is aggressive but potentially curable, similar to other aggressive lymphomas.[635] Cases with the t(2;5) have a significantly better prognosis than cases lacking the t(2;5).[626]

THERAPY. Treatment regimens used for anaplastic large T/null-cell lymphoma of the primary systemic type are the same as used in diffuse large B-cell lymphoma. Treatment results have been excellent, with better survival in ALK+ patients (71% to 93%) than in ALK– patients (31% to 37%).[636] Excellent results are seen in adults as well as children.[616,637] One report using autologous bone marrow transplantation early in the treatment of patients with anaplastic large cell lymphoma reported an excellent treatment outcome.[638]

SPECIAL CLINICAL SITUATIONS

CHILDREN

See Chapter 45.2 for a discussion of lymphomas and leukemias in children.

ELDERLY PATIENTS

The incidence of NHL increases with age[2] and more than 50% of patients are beyond 60 years of age at diagnosis.[7,639–641] Some studies have failed to identify age as an important prognostic factor in patients who receive aggressive therapy for NHL,[642] although the vast majority of studies have shown that elderly patients have worse outcomes than younger patients.[643–649] The International Prognostic Index demonstrated that NHL patients older than 60 years of age had a significantly lower complete remission rate, greater chance of relapsing from remission (relative risk, 1.8), and higher risk of death (relative risk, 1.96).[133]

There are several explanations for the poorer outcome in elderly adults. Some analyses have shown that older patients were more likely to have mortality from chemotherapy-related toxicity than younger patients, despite similar complete remission rates.[650] Other studies have identified higher relapse rates in elderly patients.[644] Still other analyses have shown inferior survival in elderly patients to be a result of increased deaths from cardiovascular disease and other nonrelapse causes.[645,648,651] A Non-Hodgkin's Lymphoma Classification Project demonstrated that elderly patients were more likely to have a high International Prognostic Index than younger patients.[648] Other studies have shown that older patients are more likely to have poor performance status,[647] advanced-stage disease,[652] and diffuse histology[647,653] and are more likely to have extranodal disease.[641,653] Older patients are also more likely to have comorbid conditions.[639,647] These factors have often led to arbitrary dose reductions or use of less aggressive therapy, which may reduce the possibility of cure.[639,646–648] This is exemplified by Southwest Oncology Group studies that revealed a complete remission rate of 37% in patients 65 years of age and above who received initial 50% dose reductions of cyclophosphamide and doxorubicin.[643] Complete remission rates were 52%, a rate similar to younger patients, when full-dose chemotherapy was used.

Some analyses have shown that less intensive regimens may be associated with diminished mortality and equivalent outcomes when compared with more aggressive regimens in elderly NHL patients.[654] These results have led to a multitude of phase II trials of chemotherapy regimens designed specifically for treatment of elderly patients with NHL. In general, these regimens have used anthracyclines with less cardiotoxicity than doxorubicin, have substituted mitoxantrone for doxorubicin,[447,655–658] or have used short-duration weekly therapy.[657,659–663] Although these regimens may be well-tolerated, selection bias and lack of appropriate comparisons make it difficult to determine whether these novel regimens are superior to standard regimens.

Several prospective randomized trials have examined results of NHL treatments in elderly patients. A Canadian trial compared standard CHOP administered every 3 weeks with a regimen in which CHOP was administered weekly at a one-third dose.[437] Patients were 65 years of age or older and had intermediate-grade NHL. No significant differences in complete response rate or progression-free survival were observed, although 2-year overall survival was 74% in the CHOP group and 51% in patients given weekly therapy (P = .05). A Dutch trial compared CHOP and CNOP (cyclophosphamide, mitoxantrone, vincristine, and prednisone) in patients 60 years of age and older with aggressive NHL.[453] The complete response rate was 49% in CHOP-treated patients and 31% in patients who received CNOP (P= .03). Overall survival at 3 years was 42% and 26%, respectively. A trial from the European Organization for Research and Treatment of Cancer randomized patients older than age 70 with aggressive NHL between treatment with CHOP and a regimen consisting of etoposide, mitoxantrone, and prednimustine.[446] The complete response rate was 77% in the CHOP arm and 50% in the etoposide, mitoxantrone, and prednimustine arm (P= .01). Progression-free survival was also significantly longer in the CHOP arm and overall survival at 2 years was 65% and 30%, respectively (P= .004). A Groupe d'Etude des Lymphomes de l'Adulte trial randomized patients beyond 69 years of age with aggressive NHL to treatment with cyclophosphamide, teniposide, and prednisolone or to treatment with cyclophosphamide, teniposide, prednisolone, and pirarubicin.[447] The complete remission rate was 47% in patients who received the anthracycline-containing regimen, as compared with 32% in the cyclophosphamide, teniposide, and prednisolone arm (P = .0001). Time to treatment failure was significantly longer in patients who received the more aggressive regimen, and 5-year overall survival rates were 27%

and 19%, respectively (*P* <.05). A British National Lymphoma Investigation trial studied two treatment regimens in patients older than age 60 with aggressive NHL.[664] Patients were randomized between six-drug regimens that contained either doxorubicin or mitoxantrone. Toxic deaths were significantly less common in patients who received the mitoxantrone-containing regimen, and the complete remission rate was 62%, as compared with 55% in patients who received doxorubicin (*P* = .07). Overall survival at 4 years was 55% and 35%, respectively (*P* = .0014).

Another Groupe d'Etude des Lymphomes de l'Adulte prospective randomized trial compared fludarabine versus cyclophosphamide, doxorubicin, teniposide, and prednisolone (CHVP) plus interferon in patients older than age 59 with follicular lymphoma.[665] Higher response rates were noted in patients treated with CHVP and interferon. Two-year failure-free survival was 63% in the CHVP plus interferon arm and 49% in the fludarabine arm (*P* <.05). Overall survival rates were 77% and 62%, respectively (*P*<.05).

Elderly patients who participate in clinical trials may be subject to selection bias,[647,666] although these results suggest that these patients may be able to tolerate aggressive anthracycline-containing regimens. When adverse characteristics such as poor performance status are excluded, elderly NHL patients may have outcomes similar to younger patients.[667] It seems unreasonable to arbitrarily reduce drug dosages or to withhold aggressive therapy because of chronologic age alone in NHL patients with good performance status and without significant comorbidity. These patients should be treated aggressively with CHOP or similar regimens, which can be reduced in intensity at a later time if not tolerated. Other patients may still be candidates for less aggressive therapy, or even a watch and wait approach, if disease is behaving indolently. The use of colony-stimulating factors (CSFs) may allow elderly patients to receive planned chemotherapy doses, although they may be less effective for the oldest patients and do not entirely prevent neutropenic complications.[668,669] A randomized trial showed that granulocyte-CSF (G-CSF) was able to reduce the incidence of neutropenia and infection in elderly patients receiving an aggressive NHL regimen, although response rates and survival were not significantly different.[670]

POSTTRANSPLANT LYMPHOPROLIFERATIVE DISORDERS

The risk of developing lymphoma is markedly increased following solid organ transplantation.[671] PTLDs occur in 0.8% to 20.0% of transplanted patients.[672] Although mortality of 60% to 80% is frequently reported, more favorable outcomes have been described.[673] Identical disorders are seen after allogeneic bone marrow transplantation, especially in recipients of T-cell–depleted marrow. PTLDs are almost always EBV-related, although cases unrelated to EBV have been described.[674] The development of PTLD results from proliferation of EBV-transformed B-cell clones when patients receive immunosuppressive therapy following transplantation.[672] Occasional cases of Hodgkin's disease and T-cell NHL have been reported.[675] Most PTLDs following solid organ transplants are host derived.[676]

The histologic appearance of PTLD is highly variable. Classification systems with clinical relevance have been proposed.[677–679] Lesions may be polymorphic or monomorphic. In some cases the appearance may resemble infectious mononucleosis and other cases may be indistinguishable from aggressive NHL or plasmacytomas.[677,678] Lesions may be polyclonal, oligoclonal, or monoclonal. Clinically, patients may have a syndrome similar to infectious mononucleosis with fevers, lymphadenopathy, tonsillar enlargement, and hepatitis. This presentation is more common in children and is frequently seen in the first year after transplantation. Other patients have nodal or extranodal presentations more typical of NHL. Involvement of the CNS and extranodal sites is common, as is involvement of the transplanted organ.[671]

The risk of PTLD is highest in recipients of heart-lung transplants and lowest in kidney transplant recipients, although the incidence rate is still 20 times higher than the general population.[671] Patients who receive the most aggressive immunosuppression are also more likely to develop PTLD,[680] as are patients who are EBV seronegative before transplant.[672] Disease that occurs more than 1 year after transplantation has been associated with worse outcome in most,[671,681,682] but not all, reports.[683] The presence of BCL-6 gene mutations may also correlate with histology and poor response to therapy.[684]

No prospective trials of PTLD treatment have been performed, and management decisions must be individualized. Interpretation of results is also hampered by lack of standardized histologic classification. Suggested treatment guidelines have been published.[672] Initial management should consist of reduction or cessation of immunosuppression. Patients who develop early-onset PTLD are most likely to benefit from this approach.[681] Many investigators recommend concurrent administration of acyclovir or ganciclovir, although the value of this approach has been questioned.[685] Surgical excision or RT may be curative for patients with localized PTLD.[672,683,685,686] Surgery should be considered for patients with isolated PTLD in renal transplants. Patients who fail to respond to reduction of immunosuppression can be treated with anthracycline-based combination chemotherapy. Durable remissions can be seen, although mortality is higher than nonimmunosuppressed NHL patients.[683] Interferon may also be considered for patients who are not progressing rapidly.[685]

Responses have also been reported with anti–B-cell monoclonal antibodies, including rituximab.[682,687] This modality may be considered before the use of chemotherapy. Autologous lymphokine-activated killer cell infusion has also been investigated for PTLD following solid organ transplantation,[688] and donor leukocyte infusion has become accepted therapy for patients who develop PTLD following allogeneic bone marrow transplantation.[689]

HUMAN IMMUNODEFICIENCY VIRUS–ASSOCIATED NON-HODGKIN'S LYMPHOMA

The risk of developing NHL is markedly increased in patients infected with human immunodeficiency virus type 1. Large cell lymphomas, small noncleaved cell NHL, and primary CNS lymphoma are considered AIDS-defining conditions.[690] The risk of developing NHL after another AIDS-defining diagnosis is increased 165-fold in the first 3.5 years.[13]

AIDS-related lymphomas are B-cell neoplasms. Virtually all primary CNS lymphomas and approximately 50% of other AIDS-related NHL are EBV-related.[63] Most cases are classified as small noncleaved cell histology or diffuse large cell lymphoma. The risk of low-grade NHL may also be increased, although these lymphomas are not considered to be diagnostic of AIDS. Small noncleaved cell lymphomas are associated with c-myc activation in virtually all cases and are frequently associated with p53 mutations.[63] Rearrangements of bcl-6 are detected in approximately 40% of diffuse large cell lymphomas. Primary effusion lymphoma is seen in 1% to 3% of AIDS patients and is associated with HHV-8.[63,77]

AIDS-associated NHL usually behaves aggressively. Systemic symptoms are common, along with involvement of extranodal sites.[691] Gastrointestinal tract involvement is common, as well as unusual sites such as anus and rectum, skin and soft tissues, and heart. Approximately 15% of cases are primary CNS lymphomas.[13] The prognosis for AIDS-associated NHL is poor. Median survival averages approximately 6 months and 2-year survival rates are 10% to 20%.[13,692] Factors associated with improved survival include higher CD4 counts,[692–694] EBV-negative lymphomas,[692] higher performance status,[691,693,695] younger age,[694] and low stage.[694,695] Patients with a history of drug abuse have worse outcomes,[694] and outcome is better for patients without an AIDS-defining illness before NHL diagnosis.[691,693,695]

Aggressive chemotherapy regimens are associated with significant toxicity, and the use of lower dose chemotherapy regimens have been investigated. A randomized trial comparing m-BACOD with reduced-dose m-BACOD demonstrated median survival rates of 31 weeks and 35 weeks, respectively ($P = .25$), with less toxicity in the low-dose arm.[696] Similar survival has been noted in a phase II trial of oral lomustine, etoposide, cyclophosphamide, and procarbazine.[697] Median survival was 9.3 months in AIDS-associated NHL patients who received the LNH-84 regimen, which incorporates CNS prophylaxis.[698] Median survival was 18 months using a regimen of continuous infusion cyclophosphamide, doxorubicin, and etoposide combined with didanosine,[699] and median survival was 13 months using weekly methotrexate combined with zidovudine.[700]

The lack of randomized trials makes it difficult to reach consensus on management approaches for AIDS patients with NHL. Dose-modified regimens should be considered, although many patients can tolerate full-dose chemotherapy.[696,698] Other investigators have recommended CHOP or similar regimens for low-risk patients, and dose-attenuated regimens for patients with poor performance status, low CD4 counts, or a prior AIDS-defining condition.[701] The benefits of CSFs are uncertain, and no clear survival advantages have been demonstrated, although routine use may be justified.[702,703] Antiretroviral therapy and prophylactic antibiotics should be continued during therapy.[698,701] There are differing opinions on the use of CNS prophylaxis,[698,701] although patients with small noncleaved histology and those with sinus or testicular involvement should receive prophylactic intrathecal therapy.

The prognosis for AIDS patients with primary CNS lymphoma is also poor. Standard therapy has consisted of whole brain irradiation, although median survival is 3 to 4 months.[698] Patients may respond to high-dose methotrexate, and the role of combined modality therapy is being investigated. No standardized approaches have been developed for primary effusion lymphoma and these patients should probably be treated like other patients with AIDS-related NHL.

EXTRANODAL SITES

Primary Central Nervous System Lymphoma

Primary CNS lymphoma accounts for less than 5% of all primary brain tumors and approximately 1% to 2% of all lymphomas in immunocompetent patients.[704] The incidence of primary CNS lymphoma rises with age and has increased four times as rapidly as extranodal NHL as a whole, although there is controversy as to whether this increase is entirely explained by the AIDS epidemic.[8] Most cases are large cell lymphoma, although other histologic subtypes can be observed.[705] Ocular lymphoma is common and slit-lamp examination should be performed for all patients. Leptomeningeal involvement also occurs commonly. Corticosteroid administration may lead to rapid regression of primary CNS lymphoma and make it difficult to obtain diagnostic tissue. Every effort should be made to perform biopsies before corticosteroids are administered to patients with suspected CNS lymphoma.

The median survival of untreated patients is less than 4 months. Median survival was 16 months and actuarial 5-year survival was 19% in a series of 226 patients treated heterogeneously.[705] Overall survival is not improved after surgical resection, and surgery has little role except for diagnostic purposes. The use of RT improves overall survival, although median survival after whole brain radiation is only approximately 12 months, a rate similar to glioblastoma multiforme.[706] Most patients progress locally after RT despite high rates of remission.

Conventional regimens such as CHOP have little efficacy in primary CNS lymphoma.[707,708] Several regimens designed specifically for treatment of primary CNS lymphoma have been developed. These regimens have generally employed drugs that penetrate the CNS, such as methotrexate and cytarabine, combined with intrathecal prophylaxis, and RT.[705,709–711] It is thought that RT should be administered after chemotherapy because of evidence that neurotoxicity is enhanced if radiation is administered first. Results from these phase II studies, as well as retrospective analyses, suggest that overall survival rates are improved with the use of chemotherapy regimens containing high-dose methotrexate.[708,712]

Unfortunately, the use of whole brain radiation results in rates of leukoencephalopathy that may be as high as 25% 5 years after treatment.[708] In other studies, the rate of neurotoxicity was estimated to be nearly 80% in patients over the age of 60 who survived at least 1 year after treatment.[713] Few patients return to their former functional status after treatment for primary CNS lymphoma and median survival is less than 12 months for patients who develop neurotoxicity.[708]

Analyses of patient-related prognostic factors have consistently identified age over 60 years and poor performance status as adverse prognostic characteristics for patients with primary CNS lymphoma.[706,708,712] It has been suggested that improved results associated with combined modality therapy may be due to patient selection,[714,715] and some trials have shown that regimens using chemotherapy, without whole brain radiation, may be as good as combined modality therapy.[716–718] Other investigators have reported high response rates using osmotic blood–brain barrier disruption and intraarterial chemotherapy for patients with primary CNS lymphoma.[719]

We recommend that patients receive initial therapy with a regimen that uses high-dose methotrexate. It is unknown whether this eliminates the need for intrathecal therapy, although some analyses have shown that overall survival was improved using regimens that included intrathecal chemotherapy.[712] The use of radiation as initial therapy should be avoided, except in patients who are unlikely to tolerate chemotherapy. Because of the risk of leukoencephalopathy, withholding radiation after chemotherapy may be considered, especially in older patients who achieve a complete remission with chemotherapy.

Testicle

Primary testicular NHL accounts for approximately 1% to 9% of all testicular neoplasms and is the most common testicular neoplasm in men over the age of 60.[720,721] Testicular lymphoma is frequently associated with involvement of Waldeyer's ring, skin and subcutaneous tissue, lung, and CNS. Involvement of the contralateral testis is common at diagnosis or later in the course of disease. Most tumors are classified as diffuse large cell histology or immunoblastic lymphoma, although Burkitt's lymphoma is common in children, and follicular lymphomas and other histologic subtypes have been described.[721–723]

Most series have reported poor outcomes with relatively few long-term survivors. Five-year overall survival was 17% in a Danish population-based study.[724] Median survival is less than 12 months in many series,[720] although somewhat better results have been reported in more recent series.[725–728] Nevertheless long-term disease-free survival is poor, especially for patients with advanced disease, and most series have failed to show a survival plateau. Factors reported to be associated with improved outcome have included localized disease,[723,724,729] low International Prognostic Index score,[727,730] age,[725] presence of sclerosis within biopsies,[729] tumor size,[731] and right-sided tumors.[729,732]

Orchiectomy is universally recommended as initial therapy for patients with localized disease. Although long-term disease-free survival has been described after orchiectomy alone, the vast majority of patients relapse, and this is not adequate therapy, even for patients with IE disease.[720] Furthermore, relapse rates exceeding 50% have been observed in the majority of reports in which adjuvant RT was used following orchiectomy. Relapses often occur in extranodal sites, and this suggests that testicular NHL is usually a systemic disease, even when clinically localized.[720]

These poor results have led to use of chemotherapy following orchiectomy for patients with stage IE and IIE disease. The Danish Lymphoma Study Group noted that the relapse rate was 15.4% for stage IE or IIE patients who received combination chemotherapy after orchiectomy, as compared with 63.6% for the remaining patients (P <.05).[724] Median relapse-free survival was 28 months and 14 months, respectively. An analysis of men with stage IE disease at Harvard demonstrated that 5-year relapse-free survival was 75% for men who got adjuvant chemotherapy, as compared with 50% for those who received no adjuvant therapy.[733] However, by 10 years no difference in relapse-free survival was observed. The best results in patients with stage IE and IIE disease have been reported by the Vancouver group.[734] Patients were treated with a brief course of doxorubicin-based chemotherapy followed by scrotal radiation for stage IE patients and additional pelvic and paraaortic radiation for patients with stage IIE disease. The 4-year overall survival and relapse-free survival rates were 93%, as compared with 50% in a historic control group treated with orchiectomy and radiation alone. No relapses in the contralateral testis or CNS were observed, and the routine use of CNS prophylaxis was thought to be unnecessary.

However, other groups have reported CNS relapses and contralateral testis relapse after doxorubicin-based chemotherapy and RT in stage IE patients.[727,728,730,733] The use of adjuvant radiation has been recommended by some groups,[734,735] whereas others found no apparent advantage when pelvic or paraaortic radiation was added to stage IE patients who received chemotherapy.[720,733] High rates of CNS relapse with aggressive combination chemotherapy have led some groups to recommend routine CNS prophylaxis[724–726,730,735] or to consider this for patients who achieve remission.[720] Others have questioned the value of this approach.[728,734] The high rate of contralateral testis recurrence has led some to recommend prophylactic scrotal radiation.[723,728,730,734]

Cardiac

Lymphoma involving the heart is not often recognized clinically. Cardiac involvement can be primary or secondary. Patients with mediastinal involvement by a lymphoma frequently have secondary cardiac involvement, particularly pericardial disease.[736] In one series, 64% of the patients presenting with mediastinal lymphoma were found to have cardiac involvement, with pericardial infusions or infiltration being the most common finding.[736] In one series of 150 patients undergoing autopsies after death from lymphoma, cardiac involvement was found in 9%.[737] Cardiac involvement is most often identified by echocardiography, but MRI and radionuclide studies can be helpful.[736,738] Patients with secondary cardiac involvement are most likely to present with symptoms of pericardial disease, although arrhythmias have been described[739] as well as ventricular perforation.[752]

Primary cardiac lymphoma is unusual, but several cases have been described.[740–745] Primary cardiac lymphoma is often reported in patients with AIDS,[743,744,746] but is also seen in immunocompetent patients.[743,745] Primary cardiac lymphoma is often found at autopsy because of difficulty in diagnosis. However, responses to combination chemotherapy are possible.[742]

Thyroid and Adrenal

Most cases of thyroid NHL arise in a background of Hashimoto's thyroiditis,[54,747,748] and evidence of thyroiditis is frequently detected in biopsies.[749–751] Most thyroid lymphomas are classified as diffuse large cell lymphomas and most of the remainder are MALT lymphomas.[54] These lymphomas may be difficult to distinguish from thyroiditis, especially when fine-needle aspirates are performed. Large cell lymphomas frequently have a small cell component, suggesting a MALT origin.[747,748,751,752] Factors reported to be associated with better prognosis have included lack of bulk,[750,753] stage IE disease,[753–755] and absence of mediastinal or retrosternal extension.[749,753,755]

The role of surgery in the management of thyroid NHL is controversial. Some authors have recommended complete surgical excision whenever possible,[749,756] while others have argued against the use of extensive resection, particularly for patients with large cell histology, except for rare cases in which disease is confined to the thyroid and resection can be accomplished without morbidity.[54,753,757,758] Results of RT for thyroid lymphoma vary widely, with 5-year relapse-free survival rates of 38% to 64%.[54] A retrospective BNLI study showed a 5-year cause-specific survival of 90% following RT of thyroid lymphomas of MALT origin, as compared with 55% for patients without MALT histology (P <.01).[759] Radiation therapy alone is usually inadequate for primary large cell lymphoma, and reports have shown better outcomes with the addition of chemotherapy.[750,760] Patients with localized thyroid large cell lymphoma can be successfully treated with a brief course of anthracycline-based chemotherapy followed by involved-field radiation in the same manner as other localized lymphomas.[403] Patients with disseminated disease should receive a full course of chemotherapy.

Primary adrenal lymphoma is unusual. Most patients have diffuse large B-cell lymphoma, and the disease is sometimes bilateral.[761,762] The disease might present with adrenal insufficiency, but more commonly the presenting manifestation is an adrenal mass that might be found incidentally on imaging studies.

Pancreas

Lymphoma presenting in the pancreas is rare. Lymphomas presenting in the pancreas are usually diffuse large B-cell lymphomas. Although rare, recognizing their presence is extremely important for the patient. Diffuse large B-cell lymphoma has a much better prognosis than adenocarcinoma of the pancreas, and failure to make an accurate histologic diagnosis keeps a patient from appropriate therapy and a chance for cure.

Breast

Lymphomas presenting in the breast are rare.[763] Lymphomas in this site can be MALT lymphomas, diffuse large B-cell lymphoma, and Burkitt's lymphoma. Breast involvement and Burkitt's lymphoma have been seen particularly in association with pregnancy.[764]

Kidney, Ureter, Bladder, and Prostate

Lymphomas presenting in the kidney, ureter, bladder, and prostate are rare.[765] The most common lymphoma seen involving the kidney is diffuse large B-cell lymphoma. Prostatic involvement by lymphoma is often related to SLL.

Ovary, Uterus, and Vagina

Lymphomas presenting in the female genital tract are rare.[766,767] The most common has been diffuse large B-cell lymphoma, although MALT lymphoma can be seen.[768] An accurate histologic diagnosis is important to avoid inappropriate therapy.

Eye and Orbit

Lymphomas presenting in the orbit are most often MALT lymphomas.[769–774] In the past, these tumors were often called *pseudolymphomas.* In one series, 80% were MALT lymphomas, 14% were diffuse large B-cell lymphomas, and rare cases of mantle cell lymphoma and lymphoplasmacytic lymphoma were seen.[769] Patients with MALT lymphomas in the orbit most often present with unilateral swelling and most have stage I disease. Treatments used have included observation, radiotherapy, chemotherapy, and combined modality therapy. Radiotherapy alone can produce durable remissions in the majority of patients with localized disease and is probably the treatment of choice. Patients with more aggressive subtypes of lymphoma should be treated with modalities appropriate for that subtype.

Primary ocular lymphoma most often presents with altered vision or uveitis that is refractory to therapy.[775–779] Patients might also present with photophobia, a red eye, retinal detachment, pain, glaucoma, or the symptoms of lymphoma involving other parts of the CNS. Intraocular lymphoma should be considered one presentation of primary CNS lymphoma. Treatment of these patients should include radiotherapy of the eye along with combined chemotherapy and radiotherapy to treat the entire CNS.[717]

Lung

Lymphomas presenting in the lung are unusual and have a wide variety of histologic appearances. These include MALT lymphomas, diffuse large B-cell lymphoma, lymphomatoid granulomatosis (which is usually a manifestation of diffuse large B-cell lymphoma), and intravascular lymphomatosis.[780] MALT lymphomas in the lung and at other extranodal sites have an indolent course. Surgery can sometimes be curative. Patients with diffuse large B-cell lymphoma should receive aggressive combination chemotherapy regimens.

Bone

NHL presenting primarily in the bone makes up as many as 5% of extranodal NHLs. Since the report by Parker and Jackson,[781] this has been recognized as a distinct clinical pathologic entity. The vast majority of patients have diffuse large B-cell lymphoma and present with bone pain, a palpable mass, or both.[406,782–786] As is always true in diagnosing lymphomas, an adequate biopsy is essential for accurate diagnosis.

Most patients with primary lymphoma of the bone have localized disease, often with extension to adjacent soft tissues. The masses can be quite large. Patients have been treated with radiotherapy, chemotherapy, or combined modality therapy.[406,782–785,787–790] There is a trend in these reports for better failure-free survival in patients treated with combined modality therapy. Patients should be managed in conjunction with an orthopedic surgeon because of the risk of fracture. Delayed follow-up should include observation for avascular necrosis as a consequence of the therapy.

Pleura

Pleural involvement in NHL is not rare, with a frequency as high as 20% being reported.[791] Pleural involvement can be seen at presentation of the lymphoma or develop during the course of the disease. Effusions can be seen in any subtype of NHL. Most effusions are exudative, with a few patients having chylous effusion. Cytologic examination results are often positive.[792] In SLL the diagnosis can be difficult because of the bland nature of the lymphoma cells in the fluid. In these circumstances, demonstration of a B-cell immunophenotype can be helpful, since most reactive pleural effusions have predominantly T lymphocytes.[793,794] The presence of pleural effusion at the time of diagnosis does not seem to adversely affect prognosis in comparison with other patients with similar stages.[792]

A distinct type of pleural involvement by lymphoma has been referred to as *pleural effusion lymphoma.*[77] These patients demonstrate Kaposi's sarcoma–associated herpesvirus (also known as *HHV-8*) in the lymphoma cells.[77,795,796] These tumors also have been associated with EBV infection.[797] Patients have diffuse large B-cell lymphomas, sometimes with immunoblastic or anaplastic appearance.[77] These lymphomas rarely express c-myc, bcl-2, or bcl-6 gene rearrangement. The tumors often remain confined to the pleura. These patients have a poor prognosis, probably in large part because of the frequent occurrence of this lymphoma in patients infected by the human immunodeficiency virus. However, this lymphoma has been reported in patients with negative results for human immunodeficiency virus.[798]

Skin

Following the gastrointestinal tract, the skin is the second most common extranodal site primarily involved by NHL. As opposed to lymph nodes and most other extranodal sites of presentation of lymphoma, the skin is unusual in that T-cell lymphomas occur more frequently than B-cell lymphomas. The most common cutaneous T-cell lymphoma, mycosis fungoides, is dealt with in Chapter 45.4. The most common presentation is a new or unusual skin lesion.

Skin lymphomas can be classified using the WHO classification. However, the European Organization for Research on the Treatment of Cancer[799] has also developed a classification that specifically deals with primary cutaneous lymphomas. An important feature interpreting any histologic diagnosis of a cutaneous lymphoma is to remember that the clinical behavior may be different than when the same diagnosis is identified in nodal or other extranodal sites. It is also important to realize that full-thickness biopsies usually are required for diagnosis. The diagnosis of cutaneous lymphomas can be extremely difficult, even with immunohistochemical and molecular genetics studies. Repeat biopsies are sometimes required for a definite diagnosis. In addition, the clinical history may be important in making the diagnosis. Lymphomatoid papulosis is histologically quite similar to CD30+, T/null-cell lymphomas in the skin. Often a history of chronic recurring lesions is the key to making the correct diagnosis.[800–803] There is a clinical spectrum of cutaneous CD30+ lymphoproliferative disorders ranging from the benign behavior of lymphomatoid papulosis to an aggressive anaplastic large cell lymphoma.[804] Peripheral T-cell lymphomas that are CD30– can involve the skin and typically follow an aggressive clinical course.[805] Tumors with a high proportion of large cells seem to be more aggressive. Angiocentric lymphomas can also have cutaneous presentations and are associated with a highly aggressive course.

Primary B-cell lymphomas in the skin are less common, but occur more frequently than previously appreciated. These can include marginal zone lymphoma and diffuse large B-cell lymphomas. Marginal zone lymphomas of the skin are typically of MALT type.[806–808] These lymphomas have an excellent survival with local therapy, although local recurrence sometimes occurs. Primary diffuse large B-cell lymphoma occurring on the trunk tends to behave indolently and can be managed with local therapy, in contrast to those that occur on the legs, which tend to follow a more aggressive course.[799,809,810]

Paranasal Sinuses

Paranasal sinuses represent an unusual site of presentation of NHL in North America. In North America most of these patients have diffuse large B-cell lymphoma,[811] in contrast to frequent T-cell or NK-cell lymphoma with angiocentric involvement seen in Asia.[567] Patients typically present with pain, rhinorrhea, airway obstruction, swelling, epistaxis, proptosis, or diplopia. In general, patients with disease confined to the primary site should receive combined modality therapy, with a combination chemotherapy regimen including an anthracycline followed by radiotherapy. In some patients, the radiotherapy might be not given and a longer course of chemotherapy may be used because of concerns about visual toxicity or persistently dry mouth. Because this type of lymphoma has a predilection to spread to the CNS, these patients should receive prophylactic CNS treatment with intrathecal chemotherapy.

Gastrointestinal Tract

Gastrointestinal tract represents the most frequent extranodal site of presentation of NHLs. Lymphomas can present in the oral pharynx,[812–814] esophagus,[815] stomach,[816–821] small intestine,[822,823] or rectum.[824] In North America, lymphomas in most of these sites are predominantly diffuse large B-cell lymphomas. In the stomach MALT lymphomas represent a minority of NHLs in the United States, but are more common in other areas in the world.[20] Lymphomas occurring in the small intestine can include enteropathy associated T-cell lymphomas and lymphomas arising in immunoproliferative disease of the small intestine.[825,826] In addition, Burkitt's lymphomas as well as diffuse large B-cell lymphoma can be seen in the rectum in patients affected with human immunodeficiency virus.[824] Patients presenting with multiple polyps in the colon usually have mantle cell lymphoma.[827]

Symptoms and signs of presentation reflect the site of involvement. The most serious presenting symptoms include perforation and bleeding. These can also be complications of therapy. Because of the seriousness of perforation of the colon, removal before the administration of systemic therapy is often appropriate. For patients presenting with diffuse large B-cell lymphoma in other sites, it is now clear that surgery, while associated with a modest chance for cure,[821,828] is not required for cure, and that chemotherapy with or without radiotherapy seems to yield a higher cure rate.[818–820] Patients with gastric MALT lymphoma can be treated with eradication of *H pylori* as described in the section on MALT lymphoma (see Infectious Agents, earlier in this chapter). For patients with MALT lymphoma who do not respond to this treatment but have disease confined to the stomach, radiotherapy is usually curative.

REFERENCES

1. Greenlee RT, Murray T, Bolden S, Wingo PA. Cancer statistics, 2000. *CA Cancer J Clin* 2000;50:7.
2. Ries LAG, Kosary CL, Hankey BF, et al. *SEER cancer statistics review.* Bethesda, MD, 1999.
3. Rabkin CS, Devesa SS, Zahm SH, Gail MH. Increasing incidence of non-Hodgkin's lymphoma. *Semin Hematol* 1993;30:286.
4. Newton R, Ferlay J, Beral V, Devesa SS. The epidemiology of non-Hodgkin's lymphoma: comparison of nodal and extra-nodal sites. *Int J Cancer* 1997;72:923.
5. Seow A, Lee J, Sng I, Fong CM, Lee HP. Non-Hodgkin's lymphoma in an Asian population: 1968–1992 time trends and ethnic differences in Singapore. *Cancer* 1996;77:1899.
6. Greiner TC, Medeiros LJ, Jaffe ES. Non-Hodgkin's lymphoma. *Cancer* 1995;75:370.
7. Glass AG, Karnell LH, Menck HR. The National Cancer Data Base report on non-Hodgkin's lymphoma. *Cancer* 1997;80:2311.
8. Hartge P, Devesa SS, Fraumeni JF Jr. Hodgkin's and non-Hodgkin's lymphomas. *Cancer Surv* 1994;20:423.
9. Devesa SS, Fears T. Non-Hodgkin's lymphoma time trends: United States and international data. *Cancer Res* 1992;52:5432s.
10. Cartwright R, Brincker H, Carli PM, et al. The rise in incidence of lymphomas in Europe 1985–1992. *Eur J Cancer* 1999;35:627.
11. Rolland-Portal I, Tazi MA, Milan C, Couillault C, Carli PM. Non-Hodgkin's lymphoma: time trends for incidence and survival in Cote-d'Or, France. *Int J Epidemiol* 1997;26:945.

12. Corn BW, Marcus SM, Topham A, Hauck W, Curran WJ Jr. Will primary central nervous system lymphoma be the most frequent brain tumor diagnosed in the year 2000? *Cancer* 1997;79:2409.
13. Cote TR, Biggar RJ, Rosenberg PS, et al. Non-Hodgkin's lymphoma among people with AIDS: incidence, presentation and public health burden. AIDS/Cancer Study Group. *Int J Cancer* 1997;73:645.
14. Krogh-Jensen M, D'Amore F, Jensen MK, et al. Clinicopathological features, survival and prognostic factors of primary central nervous system lymphomas: trends in incidence of primary central nervous system lymphomas and primary malignant brain tumors in a well-defined geographical area. Population-based data from the Danish Lymphoma Registry, LYFO, and the Danish Cancer Registry. *Leuk Lymphoma* 1995;19:223.
15. Hao D, DiFrancesco LM, Brasher PM, et al. Is primary CNS lymphoma really becoming more common? A population-based study of incidence, clinicopathological features and outcomes in Alberta from 1975 to 1996. *Ann Oncol* 1999;10:65.
16. Ziegler JL. Burkitt's lymphoma. *N Engl J Med* 1981;305:735.
17. Doglioni C, Wotherspoon AC, Moschini A, de Boni M, Isaacson PG. High incidence of primary gastric lymphoma in northeastern Italy [see comments]. *Lancet* 1992;339:834.
18. Shih LY, Liang DC. Non-Hodgkin's lymphomas in Asia. *Hematol Oncol Clin North Am* 1991;5:983.
19. Ortega V, Verastegui E, Flores G, et al. Non-Hodgkin's lymphomas in Mexico. A clinicopathological and molecular analysis. *Leuk Lymphoma* 1998;31:575.
20. Anderson JR, Armitage JO, Weisenburger DD. Epidemiology of the non-Hodgkin's lymphomas: distributions of the major subtypes differ by geographic locations. Non-Hodgkin's Lymphoma Classification Project. *Ann Oncol* 1998;9:717.
21. Herrinton LJ, Goldoft M, Schwartz SM, Weiss NS. The incidence of non-Hodgkin's lymphoma and its histologic subtypes in Asian migrants to the United States and their descendants. *Cancer Causes Control* 1996;7:224.
22. Dinse GE, Umbach DM, Sasco AJ, Hoel DG, Davis DL. Unexplained increases in cancer incidence in the United States from 1975 to 1994: possible sentinel health indicators? *Annu Rev Public Health* 1999;20:173.
23. Banks PM. Changes in diagnosis of non-Hodgkin's lymphomas over time. *Cancer Res* 1992;52:5453s.
24. Hartge P, Devesa SS. Quantification of the impact of known risk factors on time trends in non-Hodgkin's lymphoma incidence. *Cancer Res* 1992;52:5566s.
25. Holford TR, Zheng T, Mayne ST, McKay LA. Time trends of non-Hodgkin's lymphoma: are they real? What do they mean? *Cancer Res* 1992;52:5443s.
26. Gail MH, Pluda JM, Rabkin CS, et al. Projections of the incidence of non-Hodgkin's lymphoma related to acquired immunodeficiency syndrome [see comments]. *J Natl Cancer Inst* 1991;83:695.
27. Lynch HT, Marcus JN, Lynch JF. Genetics of Hodgkin's and non-Hodgkin's lymphoma: a review. *Cancer Invest* 1992;10:247.
28. Linet MS, Pottern LM. Familial aggregation of hematopoietic malignancies and risk of non-Hodgkin's lymphoma. *Cancer Res* 1992;52:5468s.
29. Zhu K, Levine RS, Gu Y, et al. Non-Hodgkin's lymphoma and family history of malignant tumors in a case- control study (United States). *Cancer Causes Control* 1998;9:77.
30. Siebert R, Louie D, Lacher M, Schluger A, Offit K. Familial Hodgkin's and non-Hodgkin's lymphoma: different patterns in first-degree relatives. *Leuk Lymphoma* 1997;27:503.
31. Weintraub M, Lin AY, Franklin J, et al. Absence of germline p53 mutations in familial lymphoma. *Oncogene* 1996;12:687.
32. Filipovich AH, Mathur A, Kamat D, Shapiro RS. Primary immunodeficiencies: genetic risk factors for lymphoma. *Cancer Res* 1992;52:5465s.
33. Mueller BU, Pizzo PA. Cancer in children with primary or secondary immunodeficiencies [see comments]. *J Pediatr* 1995;126:1.
34. Elenitoba-Johnson KS, Jaffe ES. Lymphoproliferative disorders associated with congenital immunodeficiencies. *Semin Diagn Pathol* 1997;14:35.
35. Morrell D, Cromartie E, Swift M. Mortality and cancer incidence in 263 patients with ataxia- telangiectasia. *J Natl Cancer Inst* 1986;77:89.
36. Taylor AM, Metcalfe JA, Thick J, Mak YF. Leukemia and lymphoma in ataxia telangiectasia. *Blood* 1996;87:423.
37. Lavin MF, Shiloh Y. The genetic defect in ataxia-telangiectasia. *Annu Rev Immunol* 1997;15:177.
38. Schaffner C, Stilgenbauer S, Rappold GA, Dohner H, Lichter P. Somatic ATM mutations indicate a pathogenic role of ATM in B-cell chronic lymphocytic leukemia. *Blood* 1999;94:748.
39. Stilgenbauer S, Schaffner C, Winkler D, et al. The ATM gene in the pathogenesis of mantle-cell lymphoma. *Ann Oncol* 2000;11:127.
40. Perry GSD, Spector BD, Schuman LM, et al. The Wiskott-Aldrich syndrome in the United States and Canada (1892–1979). *J Pediatr* 1980;97:72.
41. Kinlen LJ, Webster AD, Bird AG, et al. Prospective study of cancer in patients with hypogammaglobulinaemia. *Lancet* 1985;1:263.
42. Levine AM. Lymphoma complicating immunodeficiency disorders. *Ann Oncol* 1994;5:29.
43. Purtilo DT. Opportunistic non-Hodgkin's lymphoma in X-linked recessive immunodeficiency and lymphoproliferative syndromes. *Semin Oncol* 1977;4:335.
44. Sumegi J, Gross TG, Seemayer TA. The molecular genetics of X-linked lymphoproliferative (Duncan's) disease. *Cancer J Sci Am* 1999;5:57.
45. Yin L, Ferrand V, Lavoue MF, et al. SH2D1A mutation analysis for diagnosis of XLP in typical and atypical patients. *Hum Genet* 1999;105:501.
46. Kinlen L. Immunosuppressive therapy and acquired immunological disorders. *Cancer Res* 1992;52:5474s.
47. Gridley G, McLaughlin JK, Ekbom A, et al. Incidence of cancer among patients with rheumatoid arthritis [see comments]. *J Natl Cancer Inst* 1993;85:307.
48. Mellemkjaer L, Linet MS, Gridley G, et al. Rheumatoid arthritis and cancer risk. *Eur J Cancer* 1996;32A:1753.
49. Moder KG, Tefferi A, Cohen MD, Menke DM, Luthra HS. Hematologic malignancies and the use of methotrexate in rheumatoid arthritis: a retrospective study. *Am J Med* 1995;99:276.
50. Kamel OW, Holly EA, van de Rijn M, Lele C, Sah A. A population based, case control study of non-Hodgkin's lymphoma in patients with rheumatoid arthritis. *J Rheumatol* 1999;26:1676.
51. Royer B, Cazals-Hatem D, Sibilia J, et al. Lymphomas in patients with Sjogren's syndrome are marginal zone B-cell neoplasms, arise in diverse extranodal and nodal sites, and are not associated with viruses. *Blood* 1997;90:766.
52. Valesini G, Priori R, Bavoillot D, et al. Differential risk of non-Hodgkin's lymphoma in Italian patients with primary Sjogren's syndrome. *J Rheumatol* 1997;24:2376.
53. Mariette X. Lymphomas in patients with Sjogren's syndrome: review of the literature and physiopathologic hypothesis. *Leuk Lymphoma* 1999;33:93.
54. Ansell SM, Grant CS, Habermann TM. Primary thyroid lymphoma. *Semin Oncol* 1999;26:316.
55. Abu-Shakra M, Gladman DD, Urowitz MB. Malignancy in systemic lupus erythematosus. *Arthritis Rheum* 1996;39:1050.
56. Pricolo VE, Mangi AA, Aswad B, Bland KI. Gastrointestinal malignancies in patients with celiac sprue. *Am J Surg* 1998;176:344.
57. Gale J, Simmonds PD, Mead GM, Sweetenham JW, Wright DH. Enteropathy-type intestinal T-cell lymphoma: clinical features and treatment of 31 patients in a single center. *J Clin Oncol* 2000;18:795.
58. Magrath I. Molecular basis of lymphomagenesis. *Cancer Res* 1992;52:5529s.
59. zur Hausen H. Viruses in human cancers. *Science* 1991;254:1167.
60. Tao Q, Robertson KD, Manns A, Hildesheim A, Ambinder RF. Epstein-Barr virus (EBV) in endemic Burkitt's lymphoma: molecular analysis of primary tumor tissue [published erratum appears in *Blood* 1998;91:3091]. *Blood* 1998;91:1373.
61. Griffin BE, Xue SA. Epstein-Barr virus infections and their association with human malignancies: some key questions. *Ann Med* 1998;30:249.
62. Shiramizu B, Barriga F, Neequaye J, et al. Patterns of chromosomal breakpoint locations in Burkitt's lymphoma: relevance to geography and Epstein-Barr virus association. *Blood* 1991;77:1516.
63. Gaidano G, Carbone A, Dalla-Favera R. Genetic basis of acquired immunodeficiency syndrome-related lymphomagenesis. *J Natl Cancer Inst Monogr* 1998;23:95.
64. Kieff E. Current perspectives on the molecular pathogenesis of virus-induced cancers in human immunodeficiency virus infection and acquired immunodeficiency syndrome. *J Natl Cancer Inst Monogr* 1998;23:7.
65. Subar M, Neri A, Inghirami G, Knowles DM, Dalla-Favera R. Frequent c-myc oncogene activation and infrequent presence of Epstein-Barr virus genome in AIDS-associated lymphoma. *Blood* 1988;72:667.
66. Liebowitz D. Epstein-Barr virus and a cellular signaling pathway in lymphomas from immunosuppressed patients [see comments]. *N Engl J Med* 1998;338:1413.
67. Manns A, Hisada M, La Grenade L. Human T-lymphotropic virus type I infection [see comments]. *Lancet* 1999;353:1951.
68. Franchini G. Molecular mechanisms of human T-cell leukemia/lymphotropic virus type I infection. *Blood* 1995;86:3619.
69. Arisawa K, Soda M, Endo S, et al. Evaluation of adult T-cell leukemia/lymphoma incidence and its impact on non-Hodgkin lymphoma incidence in southwestern Japan. *Int J Cancer* 2000;85:319.
70. Blayney DW, Jaffe ES, Blattner WA, et al. The human T-cell leukemia/lymphoma virus associated with American adult T-cell leukemia/lymphoma. *Blood* 1983;62:401.
71. Mori N, Fujii M, Ikeda S, et al. Constitutive activation of NF-kappaB in primary adult T-cell leukemia cells. *Blood* 1999;93:2360.
72. Hisada M, Okayama A, Shioiri S, et al. Risk factors for adult T-cell leukemia among carriers of human T-lymphotropic virus type I. *Blood* 1998;92:3557.
73. Antman K, Chang Y. Kaposi's sarcoma. *N Engl J Med* 2000;342:1027.
74. Soulier J, Grollet L, Oksenhendler E, et al. Kaposi's sarcoma-associated herpesvirus-like DNA sequences in multicentric Castleman's disease [see comments]. *Blood* 1995;86:1276.
75. Cesarman E, Chang Y, Moore PS, Said JW, Knowles DM. Kaposi's sarcoma-associated herpesvirus-like DNA sequences in AIDS-related body-cavity-based lymphomas [see comments]. *N Engl J Med* 1995;332:1186.
76. Mesri EA, Cesarman E, Arvanitakis L, et al. Human herpesvirus-8/Kaposi's sarcoma-associated herpesvirus is a new transmissible virus that infects B cells. *J Exp Med* 1996;183:2385.
77. Nador RG, Cesarman E, Chadburn A, et al. Primary effusion lymphoma: a distinct clinicopathologic entity associated with the Kaposi's sarcoma-associated herpes virus. *Blood* 1996;88:645.
78. Silvestri F, Pipan C, Barillari G, et al. Prevalence of hepatitis C virus infection in patients with lymphoproliferative disorders. *Blood* 1996;87:4296.
79. Zuckerman E, Zuckerman T, Levine AM, et al. Hepatitis C virus infection in patients with B-cell non-Hodgkin lymphoma [see comments]. *Ann Intern Med* 1997;127:423.
80. De Vita S, Sansonno D, Dolcetti R, et al. Hepatitis C virus within a malignant lymphoma lesion in the course of type II mixed cryoglobulinemia. *Blood* 1995;86:1887.
81. Karavattathayyil SJ, Kalkeri G, Liu HJ, et al. Detection of hepatitis C virus RNA sequences in B-cell non-Hodgkin lymphoma. *Am J Clin Pathol* 2000;113:391.
82. Dammacco F, Gatti P, Sansonno D. Hepatitis C virus infection, mixed cryoglobulinemia, and non-Hodgkin's lymphoma: an emerging picture. *Leuk Lymphoma* 1998;31:463.
83. Shariff S, Yoshida EM, Gascoyne RD, et al. Hepatitis C infection and B-cell non-Hodgkin's lymphoma in British Columbia: a cross-sectional analysis. *Ann Oncol* 1999;10:961.
84. Wotherspoon AC. Gastric lymphoma of mucosa-associated lymphoid tissue and Helicobacter pylori. *Annu Rev Med* 1998;49:289.
85. Wotherspoon AC, Ortiz-Hidalgo C, Falzon MR, Isaacson PG. *Helicobacter pylori*-associated gastritis and primary B-cell gastric lymphoma [see comments]. *Lancet* 1991;338:1175.
86. Parsonnet J, Hansen S, Rodriguez L, et al. *Helicobacter pylori* infection and gastric lymphoma [see comments]. *N Engl J Med* 1994;330:1267.
87. Zucca E, Bertoni F, Roggero E, et al. Molecular analysis of the progression from *Helicobacter pylori*-associated chronic gastritis to mucosa-associated lymphoid-tissue lymphoma of the stomach. *N Engl J Med* 1998;338:804.
88. Isaacson PG. Gastric MALT lymphoma: from concept to cure. *Ann Oncol* 1999;10:637.

89. Hussell T, Isaacson PG, Crabtree JE, Spencer J. The response of cells from low-grade B-cell gastric lymphomas of mucosa-associated lymphoid tissue to *Helicobacter pylori* [see comments]. *Lancet* 1993;342:571.

90. Pearce N, Bethwaite P. Increasing incidence of non-Hodgkin's lymphoma: occupational and environmental factors. *Cancer Res* 1992;52:5496s.

91. Scherr PA, Hutchison GB, Neiman RS. Non-Hodgkin's lymphoma and occupational exposure. *Cancer Res* 1992;52:5503s.

92. Fritschi L, Siemiatycki J. Lymphoma, myeloma and occupation: results of a case-control study. *Int J Cancer* 1996;67:498.

93. Persson B, Fredrikson M. Some risk factors for non-Hodgkin's lymphoma. *Int J Occup Med Environ Health* 1999;12:135.

94. Keller-Byrne JE, Khuder SA, Schaub EA, McAfee O. A meta-analysis of non-Hodgkin's lymphoma among farmers in the central United States. *Am J Ind Med* 1997;31:442.

95. Khuder SA, Schaub EA, Keller-Byrne JE. Meta-analyses of non-Hodgkin's lymphoma and farming. *Scand J Work Environ Health* 1998;24:255.

96. Morrison HI, Wilkins K, Semenciw R, Mao Y, Wigle D. Herbicides and cancer. *J Natl Cancer Inst* 1992;84:1866.

97. Hardell L, Eriksson M. A case-control study of non-Hodgkin lymphoma and exposure to pesticides [see comments]. *Cancer* 1999;85:1353.

98. Munro IC, Cardo GL, Orr JC, et al. A comprehensive, integrated review and evaluation of the scientific evidence relating to the safety of the herbicide 2,4-D. *J Am Coll Toxicol* 1992;11:559.

99. Cantor KP, Blair A, Everett G, et al. Pesticides and other agricultural risk factors for non-Hodgkin's lymphoma among men in Iowa and Minnesota [see comments]. *Cancer Res* 1992;52:2447.

100. Dich J, Zahm SH, Hanberg A, Adami HO. Pesticides and cancer. *Cancer Causes Control* 1997;8:420.

101. Cantor KP, Blair A, Everett G, et al. Hair dye use and risk of leukemia and lymphoma. *Am J Public Health* 1988;78:570.

102. Zahm SH, Weisenburger DD, Babbitt PA, et al. Use of hair coloring products and the risk of lymphoma, multiple myeloma, and chronic lymphocytic leukemia [see comments]. *Am J Public Health* 1992;82:990.

103. La Vecchia C, Tavani A. Epidemiological evidence on hair dyes and the risk of cancer in humans. *Eur J Cancer Prev* 1995;4:31.

104. Thun MJ, Altekruse SF, Namboodiri MM, et al. Hair dye use and risk of fatal cancers in U.S. women [see comments]. *J Natl Cancer Inst* 1994;86:210.

105. Holly EA, Lele C, Bracci PM. Hair-color products and risk for non-Hodgkin's lymphoma: a population-based study in the San Francisco bay area. *Am J Public Health* 1998;88:1767.

106. Lynge E, Anttila A, Hemminki K. Organic solvents and cancer. *Cancer Causes Control* 1997;8:406.

107. Hayes RB, Yin SN, Dosemeci M, et al. Benzene and the dose-related incidence of hematologic neoplasms in China. Chinese Academy of Preventive Medicine—National Cancer Institute Benzene Study Group [see comments]. *J Natl Cancer Inst* 1997;89:1065.

108. Ward MH, Mark SD, Cantor KP, et al. Drinking water nitrate and the risk of non-Hodgkin's lymphoma. *Epidemiology* 1996;7:465.

109. Law G, Parslow R, McKinney P, Cartwright R. Non-Hodgkin's lymphoma and nitrate in drinking water: a study in Yorkshire, United Kingdom. *J Epidemiol Community Health* 1999;53:383.

110. Chiu BC, Cerhan JR, Folsom AR, et al. Diet and risk of non-Hodgkin lymphoma in older women [see comments]. *JAMA* 1996;275:1315.

111. De Stefani E, Fierro L, Barrios E, Ronco A. Tobacco, alcohol, diet and risk of non-Hodgkin's lymphoma: a case-control study in Uruguay. *Leuk Res* 1998;22:445.

112. Zhang S, Hunter DJ, Rosner BA, et al. Dietary fat and protein in relation to risk of non-Hodgkin's lymphoma among women. *J Natl Cancer Inst* 1999;91:1751.

113. Nelson RA, Levine AM, Marks G, Bernstein L. Alcohol, tobacco and recreational drug use and the risk of non-Hodgkin's lymphoma. *Br J Cancer* 1997;76:1532.

114. Freedman DS, Tolbert PE, Coates R, Brann EA, Kjeldsberg CR. Relation of cigarette smoking to non-Hodgkin's lymphoma among middle-aged men [see comments]. *Am J Epidemiol* 1998;148:833.

115. Herrinton LJ, Friedman GD. Cigarette smoking and risk of non-Hodgkin's lymphoma subtypes. *Cancer Epidemiol Biomarkers Prev* 1998;7:25.

116. Waddell BL, Blair A, Zahm SH. Re: "Relation of cigarette smoking to non-Hodgkin's lymphoma among middle-aged men" [letter; comment]. *Am J Epidemiol* 1999;150:661.

117. Abrahamsen JF, Andersen A, Hannisdal E, et al. Second malignancies after treatment of Hodgkin's disease: the influence of treatment, follow-up time, and age [see comments]. *J Clin Oncol* 1993;11:255.

118. van Leeuwen FE, Klokman WJ, Hagenbeek A, et al. Second cancer risk following Hodgkin's disease: a 20-year follow-up study. *J Clin Oncol* 1994;12:312.

119. Mauch PM, Kalish LA, Marcus KC, et al. Second malignancies after treatment for laparotomy staged IA-IIIB Hodgkin's disease: long-term analysis of risk factors and outcome. *Blood* 1996;87:3625.

120. Boice JD Jr. Radiation and non-Hodgkin's lymphoma. *Cancer Res* 1992;52:5489s.

121. McMichael AJ, Giles GG. Have increases in solar ultraviolet exposure contributed to the rise in incidence of non-Hodgkin's lymphoma? *Br J Cancer* 1996;73:945.

122. Bentham G. Association between incidence of non-Hodgkin's lymphoma and solar ultraviolet radiation in England and Wales [see comments]. *BMJ* 1996;312:1128.

123. Alexander FE. Blood transfusion and risk of non-Hodgkin lymphoma. *Lancet* 1997;350:1414.

124. Harris NL, Jaffe ES, Stein H, et al. A revised European-American classification of lymphoid neoplasms: a proposal from the International Lymphoma Study Group [see comments]. *Blood* 1994;84:1361.

125. Weisenburger D. The International Lymphoma Study Group (ILSG) Classification of non-Hodgkin's lymphoma (NHL): pathology findings from a large multicenter study. *Mod Pathol* 1997;10:136A.

126. A clinical evaluation of the International Lymphoma Study Group classification of non-Hodgkin's lymphoma. The Non-Hodgkin's Lymphoma Classification Project. *Blood* 1997;89:3909.

127. Armitage JO, Weisenburger DD. New approach to classifying non-Hodgkin's lymphomas: clinical features of the major histologic subtypes. Non-Hodgkin's Lymphoma Classification Project. *J Clin Oncol* 1998;16:2780.

128. Jaffe ES, Harris NL, Chan JKC, Stein H, Vardiman J. Proposed World Health Organization classification of neoplastic diseases of hematopoietic and lymphoid tissues. *Am J Surg Pathol* 1997;21:114.

129. Jaffe ES, Harris NL, Diebold J, Muller-Hermelink HK. World Health Organization Classification of lymphomas: a work in progress. *Ann Oncol* 1998;9:S25.

130. Harris NL, Jaffe ES, Diebold J, et al. World Health Organization classification of neoplastic diseases of the hematopoietic and lymphoid tissues: report of the Clinical Advisory Committee meeting—Airlie House, Virginia, November 1997. *J Clin Oncol* 1999;17:3835.

131. Rosenberg SA. Classification of lymphoid neoplasms [editorial; comment]. *Blood* 1994;84:1359.

132. Harris NL, Jaffe ES, Stein H, et al. Lymphoma classification proposal: clarification [letter; comment]. *Blood* 1995;85:857.

133. A predictive model for aggressive non-Hodgkin's lymphoma. The International Non-Hodgkin's Lymphoma Prognostic Factors Project [see comments]. *N Engl J Med* 1993;329:987.

134. Ferry J, White W, Grove A. Malignant lymphoma of ocular adnexa: a spectrum of B-cell neoplasia including low grade B-cell lymphoma of MALT type. *Lab Invest* 1992;66:77A.

135. Mattia AR, Ferry JA, Harris NL. Breast lymphoma. A B-cell spectrum including the low grade B-cell lymphoma of mucosa associated lymphoid tissue. *Am J Surg Pathol* 1993;17:574.

136. Conlan MG, Bast M, Armitage JO, Weisenburger DD. Bone marrow involvement by non-Hodgkin's lymphoma: the clinical significance of morphologic discordance between the lymph node and bone marrow. *J Clin Oncol* 1990;8(7):1163.

137. Castellino RA, Dunnick NR, Goffinet DR, Rosenberg SR, Kaplan HS. Predictive value of lymphography for sites of subdiaphragmatic disease encountered at staging laparotomy in newly diagnosed Hodgkin's disease and non-Hodgkin's lymphoma. *J Clin Oncol* 1983;1:532.

138. Lee JK, Stanley RJ, Sagel SS, Levitt RG. Accuracy of computed tomography in detecting intraabdominal and pelvic adenopathy in lymphoma. *AJR Am J Roentgenol* 1978;131:311.

139. Hoane BR, Shields AF, Porter BA, Shulman HM. Detection of lymphomatous bone marrow involvement with magnetic resonance imaging [see comments]. *Blood* 1991;78:728.

140. Kaplan WD, Jochelson MS, Herman TS, et al. Gallium-67 imaging: a predictor of residual tumor viability and clinical outcome in patients with diffuse large-cell lymphoma. *J Clin Oncol* 1990;8:1966.

141. Finke J, Slanina J, Lange W, Dolken G. Persistence of circulating t(14;18)-positive cells in long-term remission after radiation therapy for localized-stage follicular lymphoma. *J Clin Oncol* 1993;11:1668.

142. Limpens J, de Jong D, van Krieken JH, et al. Bcl-2/JH rearrangements in benign lymphoid tissues with follicular hyperplasia. *Oncogene* 1991;6:2271.

143. Cabanillas F, McLaughlin MSP, Hagemeister FB, et al. Early achievement of molecular complete remission assayed by PCR predicts failure free survival (FFS) in grade follicular lymphomas (LGFL). *Blood* 1995;86:604a(abst).

144. Carbone PP, Kaplan HS, Musshoff K, Smithers DW, Tubiana M. Report of the Committee on Hodgkin's Disease Staging Classification. *Cancer Res* 1971;31:1860.

145. Jagannath S, Velasquez WS, Tucker SL, et al. Tumor burden assessment and its implication for a prognostic model in advanced diffuse large-cell lymphoma. *J Clin Oncol* 1986;4:859.

146. Velasquez WS, Jagannath S, Tucker SL, et al. Risk classification as the basis for clinical staging of diffuse large-cell lymphoma derived from 10-year survival data. *Blood* 1989;74:551.

147. Coiffier B, Gisselbrecht C, Vose JM, et al. Prognostic factors in aggressive malignant lymphomas: description and validation of a prognostic index that could identify patients requiring a more intensive therapy. The Groupe d'Etudes des Lymphomes Agressifs [see comments]. *J Clin Oncol* 1991;9:211.

148. Shipp M, Harrington D, Anderson J, et al. A predictive model for aggressive non-Hodgkin's lymphoma. *N Engl J Med* 1993;329:987.

149. Salles G, Shipp MA, Coiffier B. Chemotherapy of non-Hodgkin's aggressive lymphomas. *Semin Hematol* 1994;31:46.

150. Khalidi HS, Chang KL, Medeiros LJ, et al. Acute lymphoblastic leukemia. Survey of immunophenotype, French-American-British classification, frequency of myeloid antigen expression, and karyotypic abnormalities in 210 pediatric and adult cases. *Am J Clin Pathol* 1999;111:467.

151. Pui CH, Rubnitz JE, Hancock ML, et al. Reappraisal of the clinical and biologic significance of myeloid-associated antigen expression in childhood acute lymphoblastic leukemia. *J Clin Oncol* 1998;16:3768.

152. Kitchingman GR, Rovigatti U, Mauer AM, et al. Rearrangement of immunoglobulin heavy chain genes in T cell acute lymphoblastic leukemia. *Blood* 1985;65:725.

153. Tawa A, Hozumi N, Minden M, Mak TW, Gelfand EW. Rearrangement of the T-cell receptor beta-chain gene in non-T-cell, non-B-cell acute lymphoblastic leukemia of childhood. *N Engl J Med* 1985;313:1033.

154. Felix CA, Poplack DG, Reaman GH, et al. Characterization of immunoglobulin and T-cell receptor gene patterns in B-cell precursor acute lymphoblastic leukemia of childhood. *J Clin Oncol* 1990;8:431.

155. Pui CH, Behm FG, Downing JR, et al. 11q23/MLL rearrangement confers a poor prognosis in infants with acute lymphoblastic leukemia. *J Clin Oncol* 1994;12:909.

156. Rubnitz JE, Pui CH, Downing JR. The role of TEL fusion genes in pediatric leukemias. *Leukemia* 1999;13:6.

157. Boucheix C, David B, Sebban C, et al. Immunophenotype of adult acute lymphoblastic leukemia, clinical parameters, and outcome: an analysis of a prospective trial including 562 tested patients (LALA87). French Group on Therapy for Adult Acute Lymphoblastic Leukemia. *Blood* 1994;84:1603.

158. Uckun FM, Sather HN, Gaynon PS, et al. Clinical features and treatment outcome of children with myeloid antigen positive acute lymphoblastic leukemia: a report from the Children's Cancer Group. *Blood* 1997;90:28.

159. Ben-Ezra J, Burke JS, Swartz WG, et al. Small lymphocytic lymphoma: a clinicopathologic analysis of 268 cases. *Blood* 1989;73:579.

160. Lennert K, Stein H. *Malignant lymphomas other than Hodgkin's disease: histology, cytology, ultrastructure, immunology.* New York: Springer-Verlag, 1978.
161. Perry DA, Bast MA, Armitage JO, Weisenburger DD. Diffuse intermediate lymphocytic lymphoma. A clinicopathologic study and comparison with small lymphocytic lymphoma and diffuse small cleaved cell lymphoma. *Cancer* 1990;66:1995.
162. Bonato M, Pittaluga S, Tierens A, et al. Lymph node histology in typical and atypical chronic lymphocytic leukemia. *Am J Surg Pathol* 1998;22:49.
163. Kipps TJ, Carson DA. Autoantibodies in chronic lymphocytic leukemia and related systemic autoimmune diseases. *Blood* 1993;81:2475.
164. Zukerberg LR, Medeiros LJ, Ferry JA, Harris NL. Diffuse low-grade B-cell lymphomas. Four clinically distinct subtypes defined by a combination of morphologic and immunophenotypic features [see comments]. *Am J Clin Pathol* 1993;100:373.
165. Aoki H, Takishita M, Kosaka M, Saito S. Frequent somatic mutations in D and/or JH segments of Ig gene in Waldenstrom's macroglobulinemia and chronic lymphocytic leukemia (CLL) with Richter's syndrome but not in common CLL. *Blood* 1995;85:1913.
166. Oscier DG, Thompsett A, Zhu D, Stevenson FK. Differential rates of somatic hypermutation in V(H) genes among subsets of chronic lymphocytic leukemia defined by chromosomal abnormalities. *Blood* 1997;89:4153.
167. Damle RN, Wasil T, Fais F, et al. Ig V gene mutation status and CD38 expression as novel prognostic indicators in chronic lymphocytic leukemia [see comments]. *Blood* 1999;94:1840.
168. Juliusson G, Oscier DG, Fitchett M, et al. Prognostic subgroups in B-cell chronic lymphocytic leukemia defined by specific chromosomal abnormalities. *N Engl J Med* 1990;323:720.
169. Knuutila S, Elonen E, Teerenhovi L, et al. Trisomy 12 in B cells of patients with B-cell chronic lymphocytic leukemia. *N Engl J Med* 1986;314:865.
170. Juliusson G, Merup M. Cytogenetics in chronic lymphocytic leukemia. *Semin Oncol* 1998;25:19.
171. Croce CM, Tsujimoto Y, Erikson J, Nowell P. Chromosome translocations and B cell neoplasia. *Lab Invest* 1984;51:258.
172. Tsujimoto Y, Yunis J, Onorato-Showe L, et al. Molecular cloning of the chromosomal breakpoint of B-cell lymphomas and leukemias with the t(11;14) chromosome translocation. *Science* 1984;224:1403.
173. Yang WI, Zukerberg LR, Motokura T, Arnold A, Harris NL. Cyclin D1 (Bcl-1, PRAD1) protein expression in low-grade B-cell lymphomas and reactive hyperplasia. *Am J Pathol* 1994;145:86.
174. Bosch F, Jares P, Campo E, et al. PRAD-1/cyclin D1 gene overexpression in chronic lymphoproliferative disorders: a highly specific marker of mantle cell lymphoma. *Blood* 1994;84:2726.
175. Zhu Y, Monni O, El-Rifai W, et al. Discontinuous deletions at 11q23 in B cell chronic lymphocytic leukemia. *Leukemia* 1999;13:708.
176. Sembries S, Pahl H, Stilgenbauer S, Dohner H, Schriever F. Reduced expression of adhesion molecules and cell signaling receptors by chronic lymphocytic leukemia cells with 11q deletion. *Blood* 1999;93:624.
177. Kipps TJ. The CD5 B cell. *Adv Immunol* 1989;47:117.
178. MacLennan IC, Liu YJ, Oldfield S, Zhang J, Lane PJ. The evolution of B-cell clones. *Curr Top Microbiol Immunol* 1990;159:37.
179. Inghirami G, Foitl DR, Sabichi A, Zhu BY, Knowles DM. Autoantibody-associated cross-reactive idiotype-bearing human B lymphocytes: distribution and characterization, including Ig VH gene and CD5 antigen expression. *Blood* 1991;78:1503.
180. Caligaris-Cappio F. B-chronic lymphocytic leukemia: a malignancy of anti-self B cells. *Blood* 1996;87:2615.
181. Caligaris-Cappio F, Hamblin TJ. B-cell chronic lymphocytic leukemia: a bird of a different feather. *J Clin Oncol* 1999;17:399.
182. Klein U, Rajewsky K, Kuppers R. Human immunoglobulin (Ig)M+IgD+ peripheral blood B cells expressing the CD27 cell surface antigen carry somatically mutated variable region genes: CD27 as a general marker for somatically mutated (memory) B cells. *J Exp Med* 1998;188:1679.
183. O'Brien S, del Giglio A, Keating M. Advances in the biology and treatment of B-cell chronic lymphocytic leukemia. *Blood* 1995;85:307.
184. Rozman C, Montserrat E, Vinolas N. Serum immunoglobulins in B-chronic lymphocytic leukemia. Natural history and prognostic significance. *Cancer* 1988;61:279.
185. Pangalis GA, Angelopoulou MK, Vassilakopoulos TP, Siakantaris MP, Kittas C. B-chronic lymphocytic leukemia, small lymphocytic lymphoma, and lymphoplasmacytic lymphoma, including Waldenstrom's macroglobulinemia: a clinical, morphologic, and biologic spectrum of similar disorders. *Semin Hematol* 1999;36:104.
186. Morrison WH, Hoppe RT, Weiss LM, Picozzi VJ Jr, Horning SJ. Small lymphocytic lymphoma. *J Clin Oncol* 1989;7:598.
187. Sthoeger ZM, Sthoeger D, Shtalrid M, et al. Mechanism of autoimmune hemolytic anemia in chronic lymphocytic leukemia. *Am J Hematol* 1993;43:259.
188. Myint H, Copplestone JA, Orchard J, et al. Fludarabine-related autoimmune haemolytic anaemia in patients with chronic lymphocytic leukaemia. *Br J Haematol* 1995;91:341.
189. Hamblin TJ, Oscier DG, Young BJ. Autoimmunity in chronic lymphocytic leukaemia. *J Clin Pathol* 1986;39:713.
190. Rai KR, Peterson B, Elias L, et al. A randomized comparison of fludarabine and CLB for patients with previously untreated chronic lymphocytic leukemia: a CALGB, SWOG, CTG/NCI-C and ECOG intergroup study. *Blood* 1996;88:14a(abst).
191. Johnson S, Smith AG, Loffler H, et al. Multicentre prospective randomised trial of fludarabine versus cyclophosphamide, doxorubicin, and prednisone (CAP) for treatment of advanced-stage chronic lymphocytic leukaemia. The French Cooperative Group on CLL [see comments]. *Lancet* 1996;347:1432.
192. Leporrier M, Chevret S, Cazin B, et al. Randomised comparison of fludarabine, CAP and CHOP in 695 previously untreated stage B and C CLL. *Hematology and Cell Therapy* 1997;39:S58(abst 17).
193. Hochster HS, Oken MM, Winter JN, et al. Phase I study of fludarabine plus cyclophosphamide in patients with previously untreated low-grade lymphoma: results and long-term follow-up—a report from the Eastern Cooperative Oncology Group. *J Clin Oncol* 2000;18:987.
194. Osterborg A, Dyer MJ, Bunjes D, et al. Phase II multicenter study of human CD52 antibody in previously treated chronic lymphocytic leukemia. European Study Group of CAMPATH-1H Treatment in Chronic Lymphocytic Leukemia. *J Clin Oncol* 1997;15:1567.
195. Jensen M, Winkler U, Manzke O, Diehl V, Engert A. Rapid tumor lysis in a patient with B-cell chronic lymphocytic leukemia and lymphocytosis treated with an anti-CD20 monoclonal antibody (IDEC- C2B8, rituximab). *Ann Hematol* 1998;77:89.
196. Pavletic ZS, Bierman PJ, Vose JM, et al. High incidence of relapse after autologous stem-cell transplantation for B-cell chronic lymphocytic leukemia or small lymphocytic lymphoma. *Ann Oncol* 1998;9:1023.
197. Khouri IF, Przepiorka D, van Besien K, et al. Allogeneic blood or marrow transplantation for chronic lymphocytic leukaemia: timing of transplantation and potential effect of fludarabine on acute graft-versus-host disease. *Br J Haematol* 1997;97:466.
198. Stein H, Lennert K, Feller AC, Mason DY. Immunohistological analysis of human lymphoma: correlation of histological and immunological categories. *Adv Cancer Res* 1984;42:677.
199. Harris NL, Bhan AK. B-cell neoplasms of the lymphocytic, lymphoplasmacytoid, and plasma cell types: immunohistologic analysis and clinical correlation. *Hum Pathol* 1985;16:829.
200. Lennert K, Tamm I, Wacker H-H. Histopathology and immunocytochemistry of lymph node biopsies in chronic lymphocytic leukemia and immunocytoma. *Leukemia Lymphoma* 1991;5(Suppl):157.
201. Crouzier R, Martin T, Pasquali JL. Monoclonal IgM rheumatoid factor secreted by CD5-negative B cells during mixed cryoglobulinemia. Evidence for somatic mutations and intraclonal diversity of the expressed VH region gene. *J Immunol* 1995;154:413.
202. Sahota SS, Garand R, Bataille R, Smith AJ, Stevenson FK. VH gene analysis of clonally related IgM and IgG from human lymphoplasmacytoid B-cell tumors with chronic lymphocytic leukemia features and high serum monoclonal IgG. *Blood* 1998;91:238.
203. Wagner SD, Martinelli V, Luzzatto L. Similar patterns of V kappa gene usage but different degrees of somatic mutation in hairy cell leukemia, prolymphocytic leukemia, Waldenstrom's macroglobulinemia, and myeloma. *Blood* 1994;83:3647.
204. Krenacs L, Himmelmann AW, Quintanilla-Martinez L, et al. Transcription factor B-cell-specific activator protein (BSAP) is differentially expressed in B cells and in subsets of B-cell lymphomas. *Blood* 1998;92:1308.
205. Dimopoulos MA, Alexanian R. Waldenstrom's macroglobulinemia. *Blood* 1994;83:1452.
206. Agnello V, Chung RT, Kaplan LM. A role for hepatitis C virus infection in type II cryoglobulinemia [see comments]. *N Engl J Med* 1992;327:1490.
207. Pozzato G, Mazzaro C, Crovatto M, et al. Low-grade malignant lymphoma, hepatitis C virus infection, and mixed cryoglobulinemia. *Blood* 1994;84:3047.
208. Mazzaro C, Franzin F, Tulissi P, et al. Regression of monoclonal B-cell expansion in patients affected by mixed cryoglobulinemia responsive to alpha-interferon therapy. *Cancer* 1996;77:2604.
209. Jorgensen C, Legouffe MC, Perney P, et al. Sicca syndrome associated with hepatitis C virus infection. *Arthritis Rheum* 1996;39:1166.
210. Ascoli V, Lo Coco F, Artini M, et al. Extranodal lymphomas associated with hepatitis C virus infection [see comments]. *Am J Clin Pathol* 1998;109:600.
211. De Vita S, Sacco C, Sansonno D, et al. Characterization of overt B-cell lymphomas in patients with hepatitis C virus infection. *Blood* 1997;90:776.
212. Sansonno D, De Vita S, Cornacchiulo V, et al. Detection and distribution of hepatitis C virus-related proteins in lymph nodes of patients with type II mixed cryoglobulinemia and neoplastic or non-neoplastic lymphoproliferation. *Blood* 1996;88:4638.
213. Brittinger G, Bartels H, Common H, et al. Clinical and prognostic relevance of the Kiel classification of non-Hodgkin lymphomas results of a prospective multicenter study by the Kiel Lymphoma Study Group. *Hematol Oncol* 1984;2:269.
214. Engelhard M, Brittinger G, Heinz R, et al. Chronic lymphocytic leukemia (B-CLL) and immunocytoma (LP-IC): clinical and prognostic relevance of this distinction. *Leukemia Lymphoma* 1991;5(Suppl):161.
215. Petrucci MT, Avvisati G, Tribalto M, Giovangrossi P, Mandelli F. Waldenstrom's macroglobulinaemia: results of a combined oral treatment in 34 newly diagnosed patients. *J Intern Med* 1989;226:443.
216. Dimopoulos MA, Weber D, Delasalle KB, Keating M, Alexanian R. Treatment of Waldenstrom's macroglobulinemia resistant to standard therapy with 2-chlorodeoxyadenosine: identification of prognostic factors. *Ann Oncol* 1995;6:49.
217. Kantarjian HM, Alexanian R, Koller CA, Kurzrock R, Keating MJ. Fludarabine therapy in macroglobulinemic lymphoma. *Blood* 1990;75:1928.
218. Isaacson PG, Spencer J. Malignant lymphoma of mucosa-associated lymphoid tissue. *Histopathology* 1987;11:445.
219. Schmid C, Kirkham N, Diss T, Isaacson PG. Splenic marginal zone cell lymphoma. *Am J Surg Pathol* 1992;16:455.
220. Miklos J, Swerdlow S, Bahler D. Analysis of immunoglobulin VH genes used by low grade salivary gland lymphomas of the mucosa-associated lymphoid tissues (MALT) type. *Blood* 1995;86:182a.
221. Qin Y, Greiner A, Trunk MJ, et al. Somatic hypermutation in low-grade mucosa-associated lymphoid tissue-type B-cell lymphoma. *Blood* 1995;86:3528.
222. Du M, Diss T, Xu C, et al. Somatic mutations and intraclonal variations in MALT lymphoma immunoglobulin genes. *Blood* 1995;86:181a.
223. Pan L, Diss TC, Cunningham D, Isaacson PG. The bcl-2 gene in primary B cell lymphoma of mucosa-associated lymphoid tissue (MALT). *Am J Pathol* 1989;135:7.
224. Finn T, Isaacson P, Wotherspoon A. Numerical abnormality of chromosomes 3, 7, 12, and 18 in low grade lymphomas of MALT type and splenic marginal zone lymphomas detected by interphase cytogenetics on paraffin embedded tissue. *J Pathol* 1993;170:335A.
225. Auer IA, Gascoyne RD, Connors JM, et al. t(11;18)(q21;q21) is the most common translocation in MALT lymphomas. *Ann Oncol* 1997;8:979.
226. Ott G, Katzenberger T, Greiner A, et al. The t(11;18)(q21;q21) chromosome translocation is a frequent and specific aberration in low-grade but not high-grade malignant non- Hodgkin's lymphomas of the mucosa-associated lymphoid tissue (MALT-) type. *Cancer Res* 1997;57:3944.

227. Barth TF, Dohner H, Werner CA, et al. Characteristic pattern of chromosomal gains and losses in primary large B-cell lymphomas of the gastrointestinal tract. *Blood* 1998;91:4321.
228. Dierlamm J, Baens M, Wlodarska I, et al. The apoptosis inhibitor gene API2 and a novel 18q gene, MLT, are recurrently rearranged in the t(11;18)(q21;q21)p6 associated with mucosa-associated lymphoid tissue lymphomas. *Blood* 1999;93:3601.
229. Willis TG, Jadayel DM, Du MQ, et al. Bcl10 is involved in t(1;14)(p22;q32) of MALT B cell lymphoma and mutated in multiple tumor types [see comments]. *Cell* 1999;96:35.
230. Radaszkiewicz T, Dragosics B, Bauer P. Gastrointestinal malignant lymphomas of the mucosa-associated lymphoid tissue: factors relevant to prognosis. *Gastroenterology* 1992;102:1628.
231. Cogliatti SB, Schmid U, Schumacher U, et al. Primary B-cell gastric lymphoma: a clinicopathological study of 145 patients. *Gastroenterology* 1991;101:1159.
232. Isaacson PG. Gastrointestinal lymphoma. *Hum Pathol* 1994;25:1020.
233. Wotherspoon AC, Doglioni C, Diss TC, et al. Regression of primary low-grade B-cell gastric lymphoma of mucosa-associated lymphoid tissue type after eradication of *Helicobacter pylori* [see comments]. *Lancet* 1993;342:575.
234. Pinotti G, Roggero E, Zucca E, et al. Primary low-grade gastric MALT lymphoma. *Proc Am Soc Clin Oncol* 1995;14:393.
235. Isaacson PG, Matutes E, Burke M, Catovsky D. The histopathology of splenic lymphoma with villous lymphocytes. *Blood* 1994;84:3828.
236. Schechter NR, Portlock CS, Yahalom J. Treatment of mucosa-associated lymphoid tissue lymphoma of the stomach with radiation alone. *J Clin Oncol* 1998;16:1916.
237. Hammel P, Haioun C, Chaumette MT, et al. Efficacy of single-agent chemotherapy in low-grade B-cell mucosa-associated lymphoid tissue lymphoma with prominent gastric expression. *J Clin Oncol* 1995;13:2524.
238. Bayerdorffer E, Neubauer A, Rudolph B, et al. Regression of primary gastric lymphoma of mucosa-associated lymphoid tissue type after cure of *Helicobacter pylori* infection. MALT Lymphoma Study Group [see comments]. *Lancet* 1995;345:1591.
239. Neubauer A, Thiede C, Morgner A, et al. Cure of *Helicobacter pylori* infection and duration of remission of low-grade gastric mucosa-associated lymphoid tissue lymphoma [see comments]. *J Natl Cancer Inst* 1997;89:1350.
240. Steinbach G, Ford R, Glober G, et al. Antibiotic treatment of gastric lymphoma of mucosa-associated lymphoid tissue. An uncontrolled trial. *Ann Intern Med* 1999;131:88.
241. Fiche M, Caprons F, Berger F, et al. Primary pulmonary non-Hodgkin's lymphomas. *Histopathology* 1995;26:529.
242. Dunbar SF, Linggood RM, Doppke KP, Duby A, Wang CC. Conjunctival lymphoma: results and treatment with a single anterior electron field. A lens sparing approach [see comments]. *Int J Radiat Oncol Biol Phys* 1990;19:249.
243. Berger F, Felman P, Thieblemont C, et al. Non-MALT marginal zone B-cell lymphomas: a description of clinical presentation and outcome in 124 patients. *Blood* 2000;95:1950.
244. Isaacson PG. Mucosa-associated lymphoid tissue lymphoma. *Semin Hematol* 1999;36:139.
245. Zinzani PL, Magagnoli M, Galieni P, et al. Nongastrointestinal low-grade mucosa-associated lymphoid tissue lymphoma: analysis of 75 patients. *J Clin Oncol* 1999;17:1254.
246. Sheibani K, Burke JS, Swartz WG, Nademanee A, Winberg CD. Monocytoid B-cell lymphoma. Clinicopathologic study of 21 cases of a unique type of low-grade lymphoma. *Cancer* 1988;62:1531.
247. Nizze H, Cogliatti SB, von Schilling C, Feller AC, Lennert K. Monocytoid B-cell lymphoma: morphological variants and relationship to low-grade B-cell lymphoma of the mucosa-associated lymphoid tissue. *Histopathology* 1991;18:403.
248. Ngan BY, Warnke RA, Wilson M, et al. Monocytoid B-cell lymphoma: a study of 36 cases [see comments]. *Hum Pathol* 1991;22:409.
249. Shin SS, Sheibani K, Fishleder A, et al. Monocytoid B-cell lymphoma in patients with Sjogren's syndrome: a clinicopathologic study of 13 patients [see comments]. *Hum Pathol* 1991;22:422.
250. Nathwani BN, Anderson JR, Armitage JO, et al. Clinical significance of follicular lymphoma with monocytoid B cells. Non-Hodgkin's Lymphoma Classification Project. *Hum Pathol* 1999;30:263.
251. Campo E, Miquel R, Krenacs L, et al. Primary nodal marginal zone lymphomas of splenic and MALT type. *Am J Surg Pathol* 1999;23:59.
252. Carbone A, Gloghini A, Pinto A, et al. Monocytoid B-cell lymphoma with bone marrow and peripheral blood involvement at presentation [see comments]. *Am J Clin Pathol* 1989;92:228.
253. Traweek ST, Sheibani K. Monocytoid B-cell lymphoma. The biologic and clinical implications of peripheral blood involvement [see comments]. *Am J Clin Pathol* 1992;97:591.
254. Nathwani BN, Drachenberg MR, Hernandez AM, Levine AM, Sheibani K. Nodal monocytoid B-cell lymphoma (nodal marginal-zone B-cell lymphoma). *Semin Hematol* 1999;36:128.
255. Pathology of the spleen: report on the workshop of the VIIIth meeting of the European Association for Haematopathology, Paris. *Histopathology* 1998;32:172.
256. Mollejo M, Menarguez J, Lloret E, et al. Splenic marginal zone lymphoma: a distinctive type of low-grade B-cell lymphoma. A clinicopathological study of 13 cases. *Am J Surg Pathol* 1995;19:1146.
257. Mollejo M, Lloret E, Menarguez J, Piris MA, Isaacson PG. Lymph node involvement by splenic marginal zone lymphoma: morphological and immunohistochemical features. *Am J Surg Pathol* 1997;21:772.
258. Matutes E, Morilla R, Owusu-Ankomah K, Houlihan A, Catovsky D. The immunophenotype of splenic lymphoma with villous lymphocytes and its relevance to the differential diagnosis with other B-cell disorders. *Blood* 1994;83:1558.
259. Savilo E, Campo E, Mollejo M, et al. Absence of cyclin D1 protein expression in splenic marginal zone lymphoma. *Mod Pathol* 1998;11:601.
260. Zhu D, Oscier DG, Stevenson FK. Splenic lymphoma with villous lymphocytes involves B cells with extensively mutated Ig heavy chain variable region genes. *Blood* 1995;85:1603.
261. Dunn-Walters DK, Boursier L, Spencer J, Isaacson PG. Analysis of immunoglobulin genes in splenic marginal zone lymphoma suggests ongoing mutation. *Hum Pathol* 1998;29:585.
262. Oscier DG, Matutes E, Gardiner A, et al. Cytogenetic studies in splenic lymphoma with villous lymphocytes. *Br J Haematol* 1993;85:487.
263. Jadayel D, Matutes E, Dyer MJ, et al. Splenic lymphoma with villous lymphocytes: analysis of BCL-1 rearrangements and expression of the cyclin D1 gene. *Blood* 1994;83:3664.
264. Brynes RK, Almaguer PD, Leathery KE, et al. Numerical cytogenetic abnormalities of chromosomes 3, 7, and 12 in marginal zone B-cell lymphomas. *Mod Pathol* 1996;9:995.
265. Pittaluga S, Verhoef G, Criel A, et al. "Small" B-cell non-Hodgkin's lymphomas with splenomegaly at presentation are either mantle cell lymphoma or marginal zone cell lymphoma. A study based on histology, cytology, immunohistochemistry, and cytogenetic analysis. *Am J Surg Pathol* 1996;20:211.
266. Arber DA, Rappaport H, Weiss LM. Non-Hodgkin's lymphoproliferative disorders involving the spleen. *Mod Pathol* 1997;10:18.
267. Mulligan SP, Matutes E, Dearden C, Catovsky D. Splenic lymphoma with villous lymphocytes: natural history and response to therapy in 50 cases. *Br J Haematol* 1991;78:206.
268. Bates I, Bedu-Addo G, Rutherford T, Bevan DH. Splenic lymphoma with villous lymphocytes in tropical West Africa [see comments]. *Lancet* 1992;340:575.
269. Catovsky D, Matutes E. Splenic lymphoma with circulating villous lymphocytes/splenic marginal-zone lymphoma. *Semin Hematol* 1999;36:148.
270. Yamazaki K, Shimizu S, Negami T, et al. Leukemic meningitis in a patient with splenic lymphoma with villous lymphocytes (SLVL). Meningitis as a possible initial manifestation of SLVL. *Cancer* 1994;74:61.
271. Bassan R, Amaru R, Rambaldi A, et al. The natural history of monoclonal villous lymphocytosis: a chronic lymphoproliferative disorder of CD11c+ B cells. *Leuk Lymphoma* 1996;21:181.
272. Matutes E, Catovsky D. Clinical and laboratory features of splenic lymphoma with villous lymphocytes. In: Armitage JO, Newland A, et al, eds. *Cambridge medical reviews: haematological oncology.* Cambridge, UK: Cambridge University Press, 1995:135.
273. Bolam S, Orchard J, Oscier D. Fludarabine is effective in the treatment of splenic lymphoma with villous lymphocytes [see comments]. *Br J Haematol* 1997;99:158.
274. Mann RB, Berard CW. Criteria for the cytologic subclassification of follicular lymphomas: a proposed alternative method. *Hematol Oncol* 1983;1:187.
275. Harris NL, Nadler LM, Bhan AK. Immunohistologic characterization of two malignant lymphomas of germinal center type (centroblastic/centrocytic and centrocytic) with monoclonal antibodies. Follicular and diffuse lymphomas of small- cleaved-cell type are related but distinct entities. *Am J Pathol* 1984;117:262.
276. Pittaluga S, Ayoubi TA, Wlodarska I, et al. BCL-6 expression in reactive lymphoid tissue and in B-cell non-Hodgkin's lymphomas. *J Pathol* 1996;179:145.
277. Flenghi L, Bigerna B, Fizzotti M, et al. Monoclonal antibodies PG-B6a and PG-B6p recognize, respectively, a highly conserved and a formol-resistant epitope on the human BCL-6 protein amino-terminal region. *Am J Pathol* 1996;148:1543.
278. Cleary ML, Meeker TC, Levy S, et al. Clustering of extensive somatic mutations in the variable region of an immunoglobulin heavy chain gene from a human B cell lymphoma. *Cell* 1986;44:97.
279. Bahler DW, Campbell MJ, Hart S, et al. Ig VH gene expression among human follicular lymphomas. *Blood* 1991;78:1561.
280. National Cancer Institute sponsored study of classifications of non-Hodgkin's lymphomas: summary and description of a working formulation for clinical usage. The Non-Hodgkin's Lymphoma Pathologic Classification Project. *Cancer* 1982;49:2112.
281. Mac Manus MP, Hoppe RT. Is radiotherapy curative for stage I and II low-grade follicular lymphoma? Results of a long-term follow-up study of patients treated at Stanford University. *J Clin Oncol* 1996;14:1282.
282. Gospodarowicz M, Lippuner T, Pintilie M, et al. Stage I and II follicular lymphoma: long-term outcome and pattern of failure following treatment with involved field radiation therapy alone. *Int J Radiat Biol Onocol Phys* 1999;43:217a.
283. Gospodarowicz MK, Bush RS, Brown TC, Chua T. Prognostic factors in nodular lymphomas: a multivariate analysis based on the Princess Margaret Hospital experience. *Int J Radiat Oncol Biol Phys* 1984;10:489.
284. Vaughan Hudson B, Vaughan Hudson G, MacLennan KA, Anderson L, Linch DC. Clinical stage 1 non-Hodgkin's lymphoma: long-term follow-up of patients treated by the British National Lymphoma Investigation with radiotherapy alone as initial therapy. *Br J Cancer* 1994;69:1088.
285. Pendlebury S, el Awadi M, Ashley S, Brada M, Horwich A. Radiotherapy results in early stage low grade nodal non-Hodgkin's lymphoma. *Radiother Oncol* 1995;36:167.
286. Hubbard SM, Chabner BA, DeVita VT Jr, et al. Histologic progression in non-Hodgkin's lymphoma. *Blood* 1982;59:258.
287. Acker B, Hoppe RT, Colby TV, et al. Histologic conversion in the non-Hodgkin's lymphomas. *J Clin Oncol* 1983;1:11.
288. Monfardini S, Banfi A, Bonadonna G, et al. Improved five year survival after combined radiotherapy-chemotherapy for stage I-II non-Hodgkin's lymphoma. *Int J Radiat Oncol Biol Phys* 1980;6:125.
289. Landberg TG, Hakansson LG, Moller TR, et al. CVP-remission-maintenance in stage I or II non-Hodgkin's lymphomas: preliminary results of a randomized study. *Cancer* 1979;44:831.
290. Toonkel LM, Fuller LM, Gamble JF, et al. Laparotomy staged I and II non Hodgkin's lymphomas: preliminary results of radiotherapy and adjunctive chemotherapy. *Cancer* 1980;45:249.
291. Kelsey SM, Newland AC, Hudson GV, Jelliffe AM. A British National Lymphoma Investigation randomised trial of single agent chlorambucil plus radiotherapy versus radiotherapy alone in low grade, localised non-Hodgkins lymphoma. *Med Oncol* 1994;11:19.
292. McLaughlin P, Fuller L, Redman J, et al. Stage I-II low-grade lymphomas: a prospective trial of combination chemotherapy and radiotherapy. *Ann Oncol* 1991;2(Suppl 2):137.
293. Seymour JF, McLaughlin P, Fuller LM, et al. High rate of prolonged remissions following combined modality therapy for patients with localized low-grade lymphoma. *Ann Oncol* 1996;7:157.

294. Rosenberg SA. Karnofsky memorial lecture. The low-grade non-Hodgkin's lymphomas: challenges and opportunities. *J Clin Oncol* 1985;3:299.
295. Horning SJ, Rosenberg SA. The natural history of initially untreated low-grade non-Hodgkin's lymphomas. *N Engl J Med* 1984;311:1471.
296. Lister TA. The management of follicular lymphoma. *Ann Oncol* 1991;2(Suppl 2):131.
297. Pittaluga S, Bijnens L, Teodorovic I, et al. Clinical analysis of 670 cases in two trials of the European Organization for the Research and Treatment of Cancer Lymphoma Cooperative Group subtyped according to the Revised European-American Classification of Lymphoid Neoplasms: a comparison with the Working Formulation. *Blood* 1996;87:4358.
298. McLaughlin P, Fuller LM, Velasquez WS, et al. Stage III follicular lymphoma: durable remissions with a combined chemotherapy-radiotherapy regimen. *J Clin Oncol* 1987;5:867.
299. Young RC, Longo DL, Glatstein E, et al. The treatment of indolent lymphomas: watchful waiting v aggressive combined modality treatment. *Semin Hematol* 1988;25:11.
300. Lister TA, Cullen MH, Beard ME, et al. Comparison of combined and single-agent chemotherapy in non-Hodgkin's lymphoma of favourable histological type. *BMJ* 1978;1:533.
301. Ezdinli EZ, Anderson JR, Melvin F, et al. Moderate versus aggressive chemotherapy of nodular lymphocytic poorly differentiated lymphoma. *J Clin Oncol* 1985;3:769.
302. Dana BW, Dahlberg S, Nathwani BN, et al. Long-term follow-up of patients with low-grade malignant lymphomas treated with doxorubicin-based chemotherapy or chemoimmunotherapy. *J Clin Oncol* 1993;11:644.
303. McLaughlin P, Hagemeister FB, Romaguera JE, et al. Fludarabine, mitoxantrone, and dexamethasone: an effective new regimen for indolent lymphoma. *J Clin Oncol* 1996;14:1262.
304. Solal-Celigny P, Brice P, Brousse N, et al. Phase II trial of fludarabine monophosphate as first-line treatment in patients with advanced follicular lymphoma: a multicenter study by the Groupe d'Etude des Lymphomes de l'Adulte. *J Clin Oncol* 1996;14:514.
305. Krikorian JG, Portlock CS, Cooney P, Rosenberg SA. Spontaneous regression of non-Hodgkin's lymphoma: a report of nine cases. *Cancer* 1980;46:2093.
306. Foon KA, Sherwin SA, Abrams PG, et al. Treatment of advanced non-Hodgkin's lymphoma with recombinant leukocyte A interferon. *N Engl J Med* 1984;311:1148.
307. O'Connell MJ, Colgan JP, Oken MM, et al. Clinical trial of recombinant leukocyte A interferon as initial therapy for favorable histology non-Hodgkin's lymphomas and chronic lymphocytic leukemia. An Eastern Cooperative Oncology Group pilot study. *J Clin Oncol* 1986;4:128.
308. Rohatiner AZ, Richards MA, Barnett MJ, Stansfeld AG, Lister TA. Chlorambucil and interferon for low grade non-Hodgkin's lymphoma. *Br J Cancer* 1987;55:225.
309. Price CG, Rohatiner AZ, Steward W, et al. Interferon-alpha 2b in the treatment of follicular lymphoma: preliminary results of a trial in progress. *Ann Oncol* 1991;2(Suppl 2):141.
310. Petersen B, Petroni G, Oken MM, et al. Cyclophosphamide versus cyclophosphamide plus interferon alpha-2b in follicular low-grade lymphomas: an intergroup phase III trial (CALGB 8691 and EST 7486). *Proc Am Soc Clin Oncol* 1997;14a(abst 48).
311. Arranz R, Garcia-Alfonso P, Sobrino P, et al. Role of interferon alfa-2b in the induction and maintenance treatment of low-grade non-Hodgkin's lymphoma: results from a prospective, multicenter trial with double randomization. *J Clin Oncol* 1998;16:1538.
312. Solal-Celigny P, Lepage E, Brousse N, et al. Doxorubicin-containing regimen with or without interferon alfa-2b for advanced follicular lymphomas: final analysis of survival and toxicity in the Groupe d'Etude des Lymphomes Folliculaires 86 Trial [see comments]. *J Clin Oncol* 1998;16:2332.
313. Smalley R, Weller E, Hawkins M, et al. Alpha-interferon in non-Hodgkin's lymphoma. An update of the ECOG I-COPA trial (E6484). *Blood* 1998;92:486a(abst 2004).
314. Dana B, Unger J, Fisher R, et al. A randomized study of alpha-interferon consolidation in patients with low-grade lymphoma who have responded to PRO-MACE-MOPP (day 18) (SWOG 8809). *Proc Am Soc Clin Oncol* 1998;3a(abst 10).
315. Hagenbeek A, Carde P, Meerwaldt JH, et al. Maintenance of remission with human recombinant interferon alfa-2a in patients with stages III and IV low-grade malignant non-Hodgkin's lymphoma. European Organization for Research and Treatment of Cancer Lymphoma Cooperative Group. *J Clin Oncol* 1998;16:41.
316. Unterhalt M, Hermann R, Koch P, et al. Long term interferon alpha maintenance prolongs remission duration in advanced low grade lymphomas and is related to the efficacy of initial cytoreductive chemotherapy. *Blood* 1996;88:453a(abst 1801).
317. Rohatiner A, Gregory W, Peterson B, et al. A meta-analysis of randomized trials evaluating the role of interferon as treatment for follicular lymphomas. *Proc Am Soc Clin Oncol* 1998;4a(abst 11).
318. Czuczman MS, Grillo-Lopez AJ, White CA, et al. Treatment of patients with low-grade B-cell lymphoma with the combination of chimeric anti-CD20 monoclonal antibody and CHOP chemotherapy. *J Clin Oncol* 1999;17:268.
319. Freedman AS, Gribben JG, Neuberg D, et al. High-dose therapy and autologous bone marrow transplantation in patients with follicular lymphoma during first remission. *Blood* 1996;88:2780.
320. Horning S, Negrin R, Hoppe R, et al. High dose therapy and autografting for follicular low grade lymphoma in first remission: the Stanford experience. *Blood* 1997;90:594a(abst).
321. Lopez-Guillermo A, Cabanillas F, McLaughlin P, et al. The clinical significance of molecular response in indolent follicular lymphomas. *Blood* 1998;91:2955.
322. Gribben JG, Neuberg D, Freedman AS, et al. Detection by polymerase chain reaction of residual cells with the bcl-2 translocation is associated with increased risk of relapse after autologous bone marrow transplantation for B-cell lymphoma. *Blood* 1993;81:3449.
323. Salles G, Colombat P, Soubeyran P, et al. Early molecular responses in newly diagnosed follicular lymphoma patients with rituximab as first line treatment. *Ann Oncol* 1999;34(abst 103).
324. Bartlett NL, Rizeq M, Dorfman RF, Halpern J, Horning SJ. Follicular large-cell lymphoma: intermediate or low grade? *J Clin Oncol* 1994;12:1349.
325. Kantarjian HM, McLaughlin P, Fuller LM, et al. Follicular large cell lymphoma: analysis and prognostic factors in 62 patients. *J Clin Oncol* 1984;2:811.
326. Wendum D, Sebban C, Gaulard P, et al. Follicular large-cell lymphoma treated with intensive chemotherapy: an analysis of 89 cases included in the LNH87 trial and comparison with the outcome of diffuse large B-cell lymphoma. Groupe d'Etude des Lymphomes de l'Adulte. *J Clin Oncol* 1997;15:1654.
327. Garvin AJ, Simon RM, Osborne CK, et al. An autopsy study of histologic progression in non-Hodgkin's lymphomas. 192 cases from the National Cancer Institute. *Cancer* 1983;52:393.
328. Yuen AR, Kamel OW, Halpern J, Horning SJ. Long-term survival after histologic transformation of low-grade follicular lymphoma. *J Clin Oncol* 1995;13:1726.
329. Redman JR, Cabanillas F, Velasquez WS, et al. Phase II trial of fludarabine phosphate in lymphoma: an effective new agent in low-grade lymphoma. *J Clin Oncol* 1992;10:790.
330. Kay AC, Saven A, Carrera CJ, et al. 2-Chlorodeoxyadenosine treatment of low-grade lymphomas [see comments]. *J Clin Oncol* 1992;10:371.
331. Gallagher CJ, Gregory WM, Jones AE, et al. Follicular lymphoma: prognostic factors for response and survival. *J Clin Oncol* 1986;4:1470.
332. Johnson PW, Rohatiner AZ, Whelan JS, et al. Patterns of survival in patients with recurrent follicular lymphoma: a 20-year study from a single center. *J Clin Oncol* 1995;13:140.
333. Maloney DG, Grillo-Lopez AJ, White CA, et al. IDEC-C2B8 (Rituximab) anti-CD20 monoclonal antibody therapy in patients with relapsed low-grade non-Hodgkin's lymphoma. *Blood* 1997;90:2188.
334. Kaminski MS, Zasadny KR, Francis IR, et al. Iodine-131-anti-B1 radioimmunotherapy for B-cell lymphoma. *J Clin Oncol* 1996;14:1974.
335. White CA, Halpern SE, Parker BA, et al. Radioimmunotherapy of relapsed B-cell lymphoma with yttrium 90 anti-idiotype monoclonal antibodies. *Blood* 1996;87:3640.
336. Webb A, Cunningham D, Cotter F, et al. BCL-2 antisense therapy in patients with non-Hodgkin lymphoma. *Lancet* 1997;349:1137.
337. Levy R. Karnofsky lecture: immunotherapy of lymphoma. *J Clin Oncol* 1999;17:7.
338. Freedman AS, Ritz J, Neuberg D, et al. Autologous bone marrow transplantation in 69 patients with a history of low-grade B-cell non-Hodgkin's lymphoma. *Blood* 1991;77:2524.
339. Rohatiner AZ, Johnson PW, Price CG, et al. Myeloablative therapy with autologous bone marrow transplantation as consolidation therapy for recurrent follicular lymphoma. *J Clin Oncol* 1994;12:1177.
340. Bastion Y, Brice P, Haioun C, et al. Intensive therapy with peripheral blood progenitor cell transplantation in 60 patients with poor-prognosis follicular lymphoma. *Blood* 1995;86:3257.
341. Bierman PJ, Vose JM, Anderson JR, et al. High-dose therapy with autologous hematopoietic rescue for follicular low-grade non-Hodgkin's lymphoma. *J Clin Oncol* 1997;15:445.
342. Chopra R, Goldstone AH, Pearce R, et al. Autologous versus allogeneic bone marrow transplantation for non-Hodgkin's lymphoma: a case-controlled analysis of the European Bone Marrow Transplant Group Registry data. *J Clin Oncol* 1992;10:1690.
343. Majlis A, Pugh WC, Rodriguez MA, Benedict WF, Cabanillas F. Mantle cell lymphoma: correlation of clinical outcome and biologic features with three histologic variants. *J Clin Oncol* 1997;15:1664.
344. Lardelli P, Bookman MA, Sundeen J, Longo DL, Jaffe ES. Lymphocytic lymphoma of intermediate differentiation. Morphologic and immunophenotypic spectrum and clinical correlations. *Am J Surg Pathol* 1990;14:752.
345. Ott MM, Ott G, Kuse R, et al. The anaplastic variant of centrocytic lymphoma is marked by frequent rearrangements of the bcl-1 gene and high proliferation indices. *Histopathology* 1994;24:329.
346. Banks PM, Chan J, Cleary ML, et al. Mantle cell lymphoma. A proposal for unification of morphologic, immunologic, and molecular data [see comments]. *Am J Surg Pathol* 1992;16:637.
347. Zukerberg LR, Yang WI, Arnold A, Harris NL. Cyclin D1 expression in non-Hodgkin's lymphomas. Detection by immunohistochemistry. *Am J Clin Pathol* 1995;103:756.
348. Hummel M, Tamaru J, Kalvelage B, Stein H. Mantle cell (previously centrocytic) lymphomas express VH genes with no or very little somatic mutations like the physiologic cells of the follicle mantle. *Blood* 1994;84:403.
349. Vandenberghe E, De Wolf-Peeters C, van den Oord J, et al. Translocation (11;14): a cytogenetic anomaly associated with B-cell lymphomas of non-follicle centre cell lineage. *J Pathol* 1991;163:13.
350. Rosenberg CL, Wong E, Petty EM, et al. PRAD1, a candidate BCL1 oncogene: mapping and expression in centrocytic lymphoma. *Proc Natl Acad Sci U S A* 1991;88:9638.
351. Swerdlow SH, Yang WI, Zukerberg LR, et al. Expression of cyclin D1 protein in centrocytic/mantle cell lymphomas with and without rearrangement of the BCL1/cyclin D1 gene. *Hum Pathol* 1995;26:999.
352. de Boer CJ, Vaandrager JW, van Krieken JH, et al. Visualization of mono-allelic chromosomal aberrations 3' and 5' of the cyclin D1 gene in mantle cell lymphoma using DNA fiber fluorescence in situ hybridization. *Oncogene* 1997;15:1599.
353. Quintanilla-Martinez L, Thieblemont C, Fend F, et al. Mantle cell lymphomas lack expression of p27Kip1, a cyclin-dependent kinase inhibitor. *Am J Pathol* 1998;153:175.
354. Greiner TC, Moynihan MJ, Chan WC, et al. p53 mutations in mantle cell lymphoma are associated with variant cytology and predict a poor prognosis. *Blood* 1996;87:4302.
355. Ott G, Kalla J, Ott MM, et al. Blastoid variants of mantle cell lymphoma: frequent bcl-1 rearrangements at the major translocation cluster region and tetraploid chromosome clones. *Blood* 1997;89:1421.
356. Dreyling MH, Bullinger L, Ott G, et al. Alterations of the cyclin D1/p16-pRB pathway in mantle cell lymphoma. *Cancer Res* 1997;57:4608.
357. Tirier C, Zhang Y, Plendl H, et al. Simultaneous presence of t(11;14) and a variant Burkitt's translocation in the terminal phase of a mantle cell lymphoma. *Leukemia* 1996;10:346.
358. Fisher RI, Dahlberg S, Nathwani BN, et al. A clinical analysis of two indolent lymphoma entities: mantle cell lymphoma and marginal zone lymphoma (including the mucosa-associated lymphoid tissue and monocytoid B-cell subcategories): a Southwest Oncology Group study. *Blood* 1995;85:1075.
359. Isaacson PG, MacLennan KA, Subbuswamy SG. Multiple lymphomatous polyposis of the gastrointestinal tract. *Histopathology* 1984;8:641.
360. Meusers P, Engelhard M, Bartels H, et al. Multicentre randomized therapeutic trial for advanced centrocytic lymphoma: anthracycline does not improve the prognosis. *Hematol Oncol* 1989;7:365.

361. Berger F, Felman P, Sonet A, et al. Nonfollicular small B-cell lymphomas: a heterogeneous group of patients with distinct clinical features and outcome. *Blood* 1994;83:2829.

362. Zukerberg L, Medeiros L, Ferry J, Harris N. Diffuse low grade B-cell lymphomas: identification of four major immunophenotypic subtypes. *Lab Invest* 1991;65:87a(abst).

363. Bosch F, Lopez-Guillermo A, Campo E, et al. Mantle cell lymphoma: presenting features, response to therapy, and prognostic factors. *Cancer* 1998;82:567.

363a. Dorfman DM, Pinkus GS. Distinction between small lymphocytic and mantle cell lymphoma by immunoreactivity for CD23. *Mod Pathol* 1994;7:326.

364. Khouri IF, Romaguera J, Kantarjian H, et al. Hyper-CVAD and high-dose methotrexate/cytarabine followed by stem-cell transplantation: an active regimen for aggressive mantle-cell lymphoma. *J Clin Oncol* 1998;16:3803.

365. Stewart DA, Vose JM, Weisenburger DD, et al. The role of high-dose therapy and autologous hematopoietic stem cell transplantation for mantle cell lymphoma. *Ann Oncol* 1995;6:263.

366. Freedman AS, Neuberg D, Gribben JG, et al. High-dose chemoradiotherapy and anti-B-cell monoclonal antibody-purged autologous bone marrow transplantation in mantle-cell lymphoma: no evidence for long-term remission [see comments]. *J Clin Oncol* 1998;16:13.

367. Andersen NS, Donovan JW, Borus JS, et al. Failure of immunologic purging in mantle cell lymphoma assessed by polymerase chain reaction detection of minimal residual disease. *Blood* 1997;90:4212.

368. Corradini P, Ladetto M, Astolfi M, et al. Clinical and molecular remission after allogeneic blood cell transplantation in a patient with mantle-cell lymphoma. *Br J Haematol* 1996;94:376.

369. Coiffier B, Ketterer N, Haioun C, et al. A multicenter, randomized phase II study of rituximab (chimeric anti0CD20 mAb) at two dosages in patients with relapsed or refractory intermediate or high-grade non-Hodgkin's lymphoma or in elderly patients in first-line therapy. *Blood* 1997;90:510a(abst 2271).

370. Hiddemann W. Features of presentation and treatment strategies. *Lymphoma Biology and Research* 1997;1:4.

371. Engelhard M, Brittinger G, Huhn D, et al. Subclassification of diffuse large B-cell lymphomas according to the Kiel classification: distinction of centroblastic and immunoblastic lymphomas is a significant prognostic risk factor. *Blood* 1997;89:2291.

372. Delabie J, Vandenberghe E, Kennes C, et al. Histiocyte-rich B-cell lymphoma. A distinct clinicopathologic entity possibly related to lymphocyte predominant Hodgkin's disease, paragranuloma subtype. *Am J Surg Pathol* 1992;16:37.

373. McBride JA, Rodriguez J, Luthra R, et al. T-cell-rich B large-cell lymphoma simulating lymphocyte-rich Hodgkin's disease [see comments]. *Am J Surg Pathol* 1996;20:193.

374. Guinee D Jr, Jaffe E, Kingma D, et al. Pulmonary lymphomatoid granulomatosis. Evidence for a proliferation of Epstein-Barr virus infected B-lymphocytes with a prominent T-cell component and vasculitis. *Am J Surg Pathol* 1994;18:753.

375. Haque AK, Myers JL, Hudnall SD, et al. Pulmonary lymphomatoid granulomatosis in acquired immunodeficiency syndrome: lesions with Epstein-Barr virus infection. *Mod Pathol* 1998;11:347.

376. Katzenstein AL, Peiper SC. Detection of Epstein-Barr virus genomes in lymphomatoid granulomatosis: analysis of 29 cases by the polymerase chain reaction technique. *Mod Pathol* 1990;3:435.

377. Myers JL, Kurtin PJ, Katzenstein AL, et al. Lymphomatoid granulomatosis. Evidence of immunophenotypic diversity and relationship to Epstein-Barr virus infection. *Am J Surg Pathol* 1995;19:1300.

378. Doggett RS, Wood GS, Horning S, et al. The immunologic characterization of 95 nodal and extranodal diffuse large cell lymphomas in 89 patients. *Am J Pathol* 1984;115:245.

379. Gascoyne RD, Adomat SA, Krajewski S, et al. Prognostic significance of Bcl-2 protein expression and Bcl-2 gene rearrangement in diffuse aggressive non-Hodgkin's lymphoma. *Blood* 1997;90:244.

380. Kramer MH, Hermans J, Parker J, et al. Clinical significance of bcl2 and p53 protein expression in diffuse large B-cell lymphoma: a population-based study. *J Clin Oncol* 1996;14:2131.

381. Sanchez E, Chacon I, Plaza MM, et al. Clinical outcome in diffuse large B-cell lymphoma is dependent on the relationship between different cell-cycle regulator proteins. *J Clin Oncol* 1998;16:1931.

382. Skinnider BF, Horsman DE, Dupuis B, Gascoyne RD. Bcl-6 and Bcl-2 protein expression in diffuse large B-cell lymphoma and follicular lymphoma: correlation with 3q27 and 18q21 chromosomal abnormalities. *Hum Pathol* 1999;30:803.

383. de Leval L, Shipp M, Neuberg D, et al. Nodal diffuse large B-cell lymphomas (DLB-CLs) are more likely to be derived from germinal center B-cells than extranodal DLB-CLs. *Blood* 1999;94(10).

384. Kuppers R, Rajewsky K, Hansmann ML. Diffuse large cell lymphomas are derived from mature B cells carrying V region genes with a high load of somatic mutation and evidence of selection for antibody expression. *Eur J Immunol* 1997;27:1398.

385. Yunis JJ, Mayer MG, Arnesen MA, et al. bcl-2 and other genomic alterations in the prognosis of large-cell lymphoma [see comments]. *N Engl J Med* 1989;320:1047.

386. Kramer MH, Hermans J, Wijburg E, et al. Clinical relevance of BCL2, BCL6, and MYC rearrangements in diffuse large B-cell lymphoma. *Blood* 1998;92:3152.

387. Bastard C, Deweindt C, Kerckaert JP, et al. LAZ3 rearrangements in non-Hodgkin's lymphoma: correlation with histology, immunophenotype, karyotype, and clinical outcome in 217 patients. *Blood* 1994;83:2423.

388. Migliazza A, Martinotti S, Chen W, et al. Frequent somatic hypermutation of the 5' noncoding region of the BCL6 gene in B-cell lymphoma. *Proc Natl Acad Sci U S A* 1995;92:12520.

389. Vitolo U, Gaidano G, Botto B, et al. Rearrangements of bcl-6, bcl-2, c-myc and 6q deletion in B-diffuse large-cell lymphoma: clinical relevance in 71 patients. *Ann Oncol* 1998;9:55.

390. Shen HM, Peters A, Baron B, Zhu X, Storb U. Mutation of BCL-6 gene in normal B cells by the process of somatic hypermutation of Ig genes. *Science* 1998;280:1750.

391. Kuppers R, Zhao M, Hansmann ML, Rajewsky K. Tracing B cell development in human germinal centres by molecular analysis of single cells picked from histological sections. *Embo J* 1993;12:4955.

392. Chen MG, Prosnitz LR, Gonzalez-Serva A, Fischer DB. Results of radiotherapy in control of stage I and II non-Hodgkin's lymphoma. *Cancer* 1979;43:1245.

393. Reddy S, Saxena VS, Pellettiere EV, Hendrickson FR. Early nodal and extra-nodal non-Hodgkin's lymphomas. *Cancer* 1977;40:98.

394. Nissen NI, Ersboll J, Hansen HS, et al. A randomized study of radiotherapy versus radiotherapy plus chemotherapy in stage I-II non-Hodgkin's lymphomas. *Cancer* 1983;52:1.

395. Cabanillas F, Bodey GP, Freireich EJ. Management with chemotherapy only of stage I and II malignant lymphoma of aggressive histologic types. *Cancer* 1980;46:2356.

396. Miller TP, Jones SE. Initial chemotherapy for clinically localized lymphomas of unfavorable histology. *Blood* 1983;62:413.

397. Mauch P, Leonard R, Skarin A, et al. Improved survival following combined radiation therapy and chemotherapy for unfavorable prognosis stage I-II non-Hodgkin's lymphomas. *J Clin Oncol* 1985;3:1301.

398. Rodriguez J, McLaughlin P, Hagemeister FB, et al. Follicular large cell lymphoma: an aggressive lymphoma that often presents with favorable prognostic features. *Blood* 1999;93:2202.

399. Longo DL, Glatstein E, Duffey PL, et al. Treatment of localized aggressive lymphomas with combination chemotherapy followed by involved-field radiation therapy. *J Clin Oncol* 1989;7:1295.

400. Connors JM, Klimo P, Fairey RN, Voss N. Brief chemotherapy and involved field radiation therapy for limited- stage, histologically aggressive lymphoma. *Ann Intern Med* 1987;107:25.

401. Tondini C, Giardini R, Bozzetti F, et al. Combined modality treatment for primary gastrointestinal non-Hodgkin's lymphoma: the Milan Cancer Institute experience [see comments]. *Ann Oncol* 1993;4:831.

402. Glick J, Kim K, Earle J, O'Connell M. An ECOG randomized phase III trial of CHOP vs. CHOP + radiotherapy for intermediate grade early stage non-Hodgkin's lymphoma. *Proc Am Soc Clin Oncol* 1995;391.

403. Miller TP, Dahlberg S, Cassady JR, et al. Chemotherapy alone compared with chemotherapy plus radiotherapy for localized intermediate- and high-grade non-Hodgkin's lymphoma [see comments]. *N Engl J Med* 1998;339:21.

404. Prestidge BR, Horning SJ, Hoppe RT. Combined modality therapy for stage I-II large cell lymphoma. *Int J Radiat Oncol Biol Phys* 1988;15:633.

405. Velasquez WS, Fuller LM, Jagannath S, et al. Stages I and II diffuse large cell lymphomas: prognostic factors and long-term results with CHOP-bleo and radiotherapy. *Blood* 1991;77:942.

406. Dubey P, Ha CS, Besa PC, et al. Localized primary malignant lymphoma of bone. *Int J Radiat Oncol Biol Phys* 1997;37:1087.

407. Levitt M, Marsh JC, DeConti RC, et al. Combination sequential chemotherapy in advanced reticulum cell sarcoma. *Cancer* 1972;29:630.

408. DeVita VT Jr, Canellos GP, Chabner B, et al. Advanced diffuse histiocytic lymphoma, a potentially curable disease. *Lancet* 1975;1:248.

409. Armitage JO, Weisenburger DD, Hutchins M, et al. Chemotherapy for diffuse large-cell lymphoma—rapidly responding patients have more durable remissions. *J Clin Oncol* 1986;4:160.

410. Fisher RI, Gaynor ER, Dahlberg S, et al. Comparison of a standard regimen (CHOP) with three intensive chemotherapy regimens for advanced non-Hodgkin's lymphoma [see comments]. *N Engl J Med* 1993;328:1002.

411. Cooper IA, Wolf MM, Robertson TI, et al. Randomized comparison of MACOP-B with CHOP in patients with intermediate-grade non-Hodgkin's lymphoma. The Australian and New Zealand Lymphoma Group. *J Clin Oncol* 1994;12:769.

412. Dupont J, Pavlovsky S, Woolley P, et al. A comparison of two chemotherapy regimens, C-MOPP and BACOP, for the treatment of diffuse mixed (DML) and histiocytic (DHL) lymphomas. *Proc Am Soc Clin Oncol* 1983;215(abst).

413. O'Connell M, Anderson J, Earle J, et al. Combined modality therapy of advanced unfavorable non-Hodgkin's lymphoma (NHL): an ECOG randomized clinical trial. *Proc Am Soc Clin Oncol* 1984;241(abst).

414. Hagberg H, Bjorkholm M, Glimelius B, et al. CHOP vs MEV for the treatment of non-Hodgkin's lymphoma of unfavourable histopathology: a randomized clinical trial. *Eur J Cancer Clin Oncol* 1985;21:175.

415. Gordon LI, Harrington D, Andersen J, et al. Comparison of a second-generation combination chemotherapeutic regimen (m-BACOD) with a standard regimen (CHOP) for advanced diffuse non-Hodgkin's lymphoma [see comments]. *N Engl J Med* 1992;327:1342.

416. Cooper IA, Ding JC, Matthews JP, et al. A randomized comparison of MACOP-B and CHOP in intermediate grade non-Hodgkin's lymphoma. *Proc Am Soc Clin Oncol* 1991;271(abst).

417. Garcia-Conde J, Vinolas N, Estape J. ProMACE-CytaBOM vs CHOP in the treatment of unfavorable lymphomas: a randomized trial. *Blood* 1991;78:127a(abst).

418. Tura S, Zinzani PL, Mazza P, et al. F-MACHOP versus MACOP-B in the treatment of high grade malignant non-Hodgkin's lymphomas. *Blood* 1991;78:109a.

419. Longo DL, DeVita VT Jr, Duffey PL, et al. Superiority of ProMACE-CytaBOM over ProMACE-MOPP in the treatment of advanced diffuse aggressive lymphoma: results of a prospective randomized trial [published erratum appears in *J Clin Oncol* 1991;9:710]. *J Clin Oncol* 1991;9:25.

420. Gherlinzoni F, Guglielmi C, Mazza P, et al. Phase III comparative trial (m-BACOD v m-BNCOD) in the treatment of stage II to IV non-Hodgkin's lymphomas with intermediate- or high-grade histology. *Semin Oncol* 1990;17:3; discussion 8.

421. Federico M, Moretti G, Gobbi PG, et al. ProMACE-cytaBOM versus MACOP-B in intermediate and high grade NHL. Preliminary results of a prospective randomized trial. *Leukemia* 1991;5:95.

422. Chisesi T, Santini G, Capnist G, et al. ProMACE-MOPP vs MACOP-B in high grade non-Hodgkin's lymphomas: a randomised study in a multicenter cooperative study group (NHLCSG). *Leukemia* 1991;5:107.

423. Koppler H, Pfluger KH, Eschenbach I, et al. Sequential versus alternating chemotherapy for high grade non-Hodgkin's lymphomas: a randomized multicentre trial. *Hematol Oncol* 1991;9:217.

424. Carde P, Meerwaldt JH, van Glabbeke M, et al. Superiority of second over first generation chemotherapy in a randomized trial for stage III-IV intermediate and high-grade non- Hodgkin's lymphoma (NHL): the 1980-1985 EORTC trial. The EORTC Lymphoma Group. *Ann Oncol* 1991;2:431.
425. Jerkeman M, Anderson H, Cavallin-Stahl E, et al. CHOP versus MACOP-B in aggressive lymphoma—a Nordic Lymphoma Group randomised trial. *Ann Oncol* 1999;10:1079.
426. Pavlovsky S, Santarelli MT, Erazo A, et al. Results of a randomized study of previously untreated intermediate and high grade lymphoma using CHOP versus CNOP [see comments]. *Ann Oncol* 1992;3:205.
427. Brusamolino E, Bertini M, Guidi S, et al. CHOP versus CNOP (N = mitoxantrone) in non-Hodgkin's lymphoma: an interim report comparing efficacy and toxicity. *Haematologica* 1988;73:217.
428. Bezwoda W, Rastogi RB, Erazo Valla A, et al. Long-term results of a multicentre randomised, comparative phase III trial of CHOP versus CNOP regimens in patients with intermediate- and high-grade non-Hodgkin's lymphomas. Novantrone International Study Group. *Eur J Cancer* 1995;31A:903.
429. Guglielmi C, Gherlinzoni F, Amadori S, et al. A phase III comparative trial of m-BACOD vs m-BNCOD in the treatment of stage II-IV diffuse non-Hodgkin's lymphomas. *Haematologica* 1989;74:563.
430. Mazza P, Zinzani PL, Martelli M, et al. MACOP-B vs F-MACHOP regimen in the treatment of high-grade non-Hodgkin's lymphomas. *Leuk Lymphoma* 1995;16:457.
431. Koppler H, Pfluger KH, Eschenbach I, et al. Randomised comparison of CHOEP versus alternating hCHOP/IVEP for high-grade non-Hodgkin's lymphomas: treatment results and prognostic factor analysis in a multi-centre trial. *Ann Oncol* 1994;5:49.
432. Takagi T, Sampi K, Sawada U, Sakai C, Oguro M. A comparative study of CHOP versus MEVP (mitoxantrone, etoposide, vindesine, prednisolone) therapy for intermediate-grade and high-grade non-Hodgkin's lymphoma: a prospective randomized study. *Int J Hematol* 1993;57:67.
433. Cameron DA, White JM, Proctor SJ, et al. CHOP-based chemotherapy is as effective as alternating PEEC/CHOP chemotherapy in a randomised trial in high-grade non-Hodgkin's lymphoma. Scotland and Newcastle Lymphoma Group. *Eur J Cancer* 1997;33:1195.
434. Bailey NP, Stuart NS, Bessell EM, et al. Five-year follow-up of a prospective randomised multi-centre trial of weekly chemotherapy (CAPOMEt) versus cyclical chemotherapy (CHOP-Mtx) in the treatment of aggressive non-Hodgkin's lymphoma. Central Lymphoma Group. *Ann Oncol* 1998;9:633.
435. Nair R, Ramakrishnan G, Nair NN, et al. A randomized comparison of the efficacy and toxicity of epirubicin and doxorubicin in the treatment of patients with non-Hodgkin's lymphoma. *Cancer* 1998;82:2282.
436. Zinzani PL, Martelli M, Storti S, et al. Phase III comparative trial using CHOP vs CIOP in the treatment of advanced intermediate-grade non-Hodgkin's lymphoma. *Leuk Lymphoma* 1995;19:329.
437. Meyer RM, Browman GP, Samosh ML, et al. Randomized phase II comparison of standard CHOP with weekly CHOP in elderly patients with non-Hodgkin's lymphoma. *J Clin Oncol* 1995;13:2386.
438. Silingardi V, Federico M, Cavanna L, et al. ProMECE-CytaBOM vs MACOP-B in advanced aggressive non-Hodgkin's lymphoma: long term results of a multicenter study of the Italian Lymphoma Study Group (GISL). *Leuk Lymphoma* 1995;17:313.
439. Sertoli MR, Santini G, Chisesi T, et al. MACOP-B versus ProMACE-MOPP in the treatment of advanced diffuse non-Hodgkin's lymphoma: results of a prospective randomized trial by the non-Hodgkin's Lymphoma Cooperative Study Group. *J Clin Oncol* 1994;12:1366.
440. Todd M, Cadman E, Spiro P, et al. A follow-up of a randomized study comparing two chemotherapy treatments for advanced diffuse histiocytic lymphoma. *J Clin Oncol* 1984;2:986.
441. De Lena M, Maiello E, Lorusso V, et al. Comparison of CHOP-B vs CEOP-B in "poor prognosis" non-Hodgkin's lymphomas. A randomized trial. *Med Oncol Tumor Pharmacother* 1989;6:163.
442. Somers R, Burgers JM, Qasim M, et al. EORTC trial non-Hodgkin lymphomas. *Eur J Cancer Clin Oncol* 1987;23:283.
443. Gomez GA, Barcos M, Han T, Henderson ES. Cyclophosphamide, vincristine, adriamycin, and prednisone (CHOP) with and without intermediate dose methotrexate for the treatment of non-Hodgkin's lymphomas of diffuse histology. *Cancer* 1987;60:18.
444. Gottlieb AJ, Anderson JR, Ginsberg SJ, et al. A randomized comparison of methotrexate dose and the addition of bleomycin to CHOP therapy for diffuse large cell lymphoma and other non-Hodgkin's lymphomas. Cancer and Leukemia Group B study 7851. *Cancer* 1990;66:1888.
445. Wolf M, Matthews JP, Stone J, et al. Long-term survival advantage of MACOP-B over CHOP in intermediate-grade non-Hodgkin's lymphoma. The Australian and New Zealand Lymphoma Group. *Ann Oncol* 1997;8:71.
446. Tirelli U, Errante D, Van Glabbeke M, et al. CHOP is the standard regimen in patients > or = 70 years of age with intermediate-grade and high-grade non-Hodgkin's lymphoma: results of a randomized study of the European Organization for Research and Treatment of Cancer Lymphoma Cooperative Study Group. *J Clin Oncol* 1998;16:27.
447. Bastion Y, Blay JY, Divine M, et al. Elderly patients with aggressive non-Hodgkin's lymphoma: disease presentation, response to treatment, and survival—a Groupe d'Etude des Lymphomes de l'Adulte study on 453 patients older than 69 years. *J Clin Oncol* 1997;15:2945.
448. Gams RA, Rainey M, Dandy M,et al. Phase III study of BCOP v CHOP in unfavorable categories of malignant lymphoma: a Southeastern Cancer Study Group trial. *J Clin Oncol* 1985;3:1188.
449. Jones SE, Grozea PN, Metz EN, et al. Superiority of adriamycin-containing combination chemotherapy in the treatment of diffuse lymphoma: a Southwest Oncology Group study. *Cancer* 1979;43:417.
450. Bishop JF, Wiernik PH, Wesley MN, et al. A randomized trial of high dose cyclophosphamide, vincristine, and prednisone plus or minus doxorubicin (CVP versus CAVP) with long-term follow-up in advanced non-Hodgkin's lymphoma. *Leukemia* 1987;1:508.
451. Aviles A, Calva A, Diaz-Maqueo JC, et al. Dose escalation of epirubicin in the CEOP-BLEO regimen: a controlled clinical trial comparing standard doses for the treatment of diffuse large cell lymphoma. *Leuk Lymphoma* 1997;25:319.
452. Khaled HM, Zekri ZK, Mokhtar N, et al. A randomized EPOCH vs. CHOP front-line therapy for aggressive non-Hodgkin's lymphoma patients: long-term results. *Ann Oncol* 1999;10:1489.
453. Sonneveld P, de Ridder M, van der Lelie H, et al. Comparison of doxorubicin and mitoxantrone in the treatment of elderly patients with advanced diffuse non-Hodgkin's lymphoma using CHOP versus CNOP chemotherapy. *J Clin Oncol* 1995;13:2530.
454. Klimo P, Connors JM. MACOP-B chemotherapy for the treatment of diffuse large-cell lymphoma. *Ann Intern Med* 1985;102:596.
455. Shipp MA, Yeap BY, Harrington DP, et al. The m-BACOD combination chemotherapy regimen in large-cell lymphoma: analysis of the completed trial and comparison with the M-BACOD regimen. *J Clin Oncol* 1990;8:84.
456. Vose JM, Link BK, Grossbard ML, et al. Phase II study of Rituximab in combination with CHOP chemotherapy in patients with previously untreated intermediate or high-grade non-Hodgkin's lymphoma (NHL). *Ann Oncol* 1999;10:195(abst).
457. Jones SE, Grozea PN, Miller TP, et al. Chemotherapy with cyclophosphamide, doxorubicin, vincristine, and prednisone alone or with levamisole or with levamisole plus BCG for malignant lymphoma: a Southwest Oncology Group Study. *J Clin Oncol* 1985;3:1318.
458. Verdonck LF, van Putten WL, Hagenbeek A, et al. Comparison of CHOP chemotherapy with autologous bone marrow transplantation for slowly responding patients with aggressive non-Hodgkin's lymphoma [see comments]. *N Engl J Med* 1995;332:1045.
459. Haioun C, Lepage E, Gisselbrecht C, et al. Comparison of autologous bone marrow transplantation with sequential chemotherapy for intermediate-grade and high-grade non-Hodgkin's lymphoma in first complete remission: a study of 464 patients. Groupe d'Etude des Lymphomes de l'Adulte [see comments]. *J Clin Oncol* 1994;12:2543.
460. Santini G, Salvagno L, Leoni P, et al. VACOP-B versus VACOP-B plus autologous bone marrow transplantation for advanced diffuse non-Hodgkin's lymphoma: results of a prospective randomized trial by the non-Hodgkin's Lymphoma Cooperative Study Group. *J Clin Oncol* 1998;16:2796.
461. Gianni AM, Bregni M, Siena S, et al. High-dose chemotherapy and autologous bone marrow transplantation compared with MACOP-B in aggressive B-cell lymphoma [see comments]. *N Engl J Med* 1997;336:1290.
462. Shipp MA, Abeloff MD, Antman KH, et al. International Consensus Conference on high-dose therapy with hematopoietic stem cell transplantation in aggressive non-Hodgkin's lymphomas: report of the jury. *J Clin Oncol* 1999;17:423.
463. Gribben JG, Goldstone AH, Linch DC, et al. Effectiveness of high-dose combination chemotherapy and autologous bone marrow transplantation for patients with non-Hodgkin's lymphomas who are still responsive to conventional-dose therapy. *J Clin Oncol* 1989;7:1621.
464. Cabanillas F, Hagemeister FB, Bodey GP, Freireich EJ. IMVP-16: an effective regimen for patients with lymphoma who have relapsed after initial combination chemotherapy. *Blood* 1982;60:693.
465. Cabanillas F, Hagemeister FB, McLaughlin P, et al. Results of MIME salvage regimen for recurrent or refractory lymphoma. *J Clin Oncol* 1987;5:407.
466. Hoskins PJ, Le N, Gascoyne RD, et al. Advanced diffuse large-cell lymphoma treated with 12-week combination chemotherapy: natural history of relapse after initial complete response and prognostic variables defining outcome after relapse. *Ann Oncol* 1997;8:1125.
467. Press OW, Livingston R, Mortimer J, Collins C, Appelbaum F. Treatment of relapsed non-Hodgkin's lymphomas with dexamethasone, high-dose cytarabine, and cisplatin before marrow transplantation. *J Clin Oncol* 1991;9:423.
468. Velasquez WS, Cabanillas F, Salvador P, et al. Effective salvage therapy for lymphoma with cisplatin in combination with high-dose Ara-C and dexamethasone (DHAP). *Blood* 1988;71:117.
469. Philip T, Chauvin F, Bron D, et al. PARMA international protocol: pilot study on 50 patients and preliminary analysis of the ongoing randomized study (62 patients). *Ann Oncol* 1991;2(Suppl 1):57.
470. Chao NJ, Rosenberg SA, Horning SJ. CEPP(B): an effective and well-tolerated regimen in poor-risk, aggressive non-Hodgkin's lymphoma. *Blood* 1990;76:1293.
471. Ruit JB, Lowenberg B, Hagenbeek A, et al. Phase II study of lomustine, cytarabine, mitoxantrone, and prednisone (CAMP) combination chemotherapy for doxorubicin-resistant intermediate- and high-grade malignant non-Hodgkin's lymphoma. *Semin Oncol* 1990;17:24.
472. Velasquez W, Hagemeister F, McLaughlin P, et al. E-SHAP: an effective treatment for refractory and relapsing lymphoma. A long follow-up. *Proc Am Soc Clin Oncol* 1992;A1111(abst).
473. Coiffier B, Haioun C, Ketterer N, et al. Rituximab (anti-CD20 monoclonal antibody) for the treatment of patients with relapsing or refractory aggressive lymphoma: a multicenter phase II study. *Blood* 1998;92:1927.
474. Armitage JO, Coiffier B. Activity of interferon-alpha in relapsed patients with diffuse large B-cell and peripheral T-cell non-Hodgkin's lymphoma. *Ann Oncol* 2000;11:1.
475. Philip T, Armitage JO, Spitzer G, et al. High-dose therapy and autologous bone marrow transplantation after failure of conventional chemotherapy in adults with intermediate-grade or high-grade non-Hodgkin's lymphoma. *N Engl J Med* 1987;316:1493.
476. Armitage JO. Bone marrow transplantation [see comments]. *N Engl J Med* 1994;330:827.
477. Philip T, Guglielmi C, Hagenbeek A, et al. Autologous bone marrow transplantation as compared with salvage chemotherapy in relapses of chemotherapy-sensitive non-Hodgkin's lymphoma [see comments]. *N Engl J Med* 1995;333:1540.
478. Vose JM, Bierman PJ, Anderson JR, et al. Progressive disease after high-dose therapy and autologous transplantation for lymphoid malignancy: clinical course and patient follow-up. *Blood* 1992;80:2142.
479. Addis BJ, Isaacson PG. Large cell lymphoma of the mediastinum: a B-cell tumour of probable thymic origin. *Histopathology* 1986;10:379.
480. Lamarre L, Jacobson JO, Aisenberg AC, Harris NL. Primary large cell lymphoma of the mediastinum. A histologic and immunophenotypic study of 29 cases. *Am J Surg Pathol* 1989;13:730.

481. Moller P, Moldenhauer G, Momburg F, et al. Mediastinal lymphoma of clear cell type is a tumor corresponding to terminal steps of B cell differentiation. *Blood* 1987;69:1087.
482. Scarpa A, Bonetti F, Menestrina F, et al. Mediastinal large-cell lymphoma with sclerosis. Genotypic analysis establishes its B nature. *Virchows Arch A Pathol Anat Histopathol* 1987;412:17.
483. Tsang P, Cesarman E, Chadburn A, Liu YF, Knowles DM. Molecular characterization of primary mediastinal B cell lymphoma. *Am J Pathol* 1996;148:2017.
484. Joos S, Otano-Joos MI, Ziegler S, et al. Primary mediastinal (thymic) B-cell lymphoma is characterized by gains of chromosomal material including 9p and amplification of the REL gene. *Blood* 1996;87:1571.
485. Jacobson JO, Aisenberg AC, Lamarre L, et al. Mediastinal large cell lymphoma. An uncommon subset of adult lymphoma curable with combined modality therapy. *Cancer* 1988;62:1893.
486. Lazzarino M, Orlandi E, Paulli M, et al. Treatment outcome and prognostic factors for primary mediastinal (thymic) B-cell lymphoma: a multicenter study of 106 patients. *J Clin Oncol* 1997;15:1646.
487. Kirn D, Mauch P, Shaffer K, et al. Large-cell and immunoblastic lymphoma of the mediastinum: prognostic features and treatment outcome in 57 patients. *J Clin Oncol* 1993;11:1336.
488. Ferry JA, Harris NL, Picker LJ, et al. Intravascular lymphomatosis (malignant angioendotheliomatosis). A B-cell neoplasm expressing surface homing receptors. *Mod Pathol* 1988;1:444
489. Sheibani K, Battifora H, Winberg CD, et al. Further evidence that "malignant angioendotheliomatosis" is an angiotropic large-cell lymphoma. *N Engl J Med* 1986;314:943.
490. Demirer T, Dail DH, Aboulafia DM. Four varied cases of intravascular lymphomatosis and a literature review. *Cancer* 1994;73:1738.
491. Glass J, Hochberg FH, Miller DC. Intravascular lymphomatosis. A systemic disease with neurologic manifestations. *Cancer* 1993;71:3156.
492. Fredericks RK, Walker FO, Elster A, Challa V. Angiotropic intravascular large-cell lymphoma (malignant angioendotheliomatosis): report of a case and review of the literature. *Surg Neurol* 1991;35:218.
493. Yousem SA, Colby TV. Intravascular lymphomatosis presenting in the lung. *Cancer* 1990;65:349.
494. Pellicone JT, Goldstein HB. Pulmonary malignant angioendotheliomatosis. Presentation with fever and syndrome of inappropriate antidiuretic hormone. *Chest* 1990;98:1292.
495. Stroup RM, Sheibani K, Moncada A, Purdy LJ, Battifora H. Angiotropic (intravascular) large cell lymphoma. A clinicopathologic study of seven cases with unique clinical presentations. *Cancer* 1990;66:1781.
496. Kraus MD, Jones D, Bartlett NL. Intravascular lymphoma associated with endocrine dysfunction: a report of four cases and a review of the literature. *Am J Med* 1999;107:169.
497. Stahl RL, Chan W, Duncan A, Corley CC Jr. Malignant angioendotheliomatosis presenting as disseminated intravascular coagulopathy. *Cancer* 1991;68:2319.
498. Suzumiya J, Ohshima K, Kanda M, et al. Intravascular large cell lymphoma associated with hypoalbuminemia. *Leuk Lymphoma* 1998;32:179.
499. Sill H, Hofler G, Kaufmann P, et al. Angiotropic large cell lymphoma presenting as thrombotic microangiopathy (thrombotic thrombocytopenic purpura). *Cancer* 1995;75:1167.
500. DiGiuseppe JA, Nelson WG, Seifter EJ, Boitnott JK, Mann RB. Intravascular lymphomatosis: a clinicopathologic study of 10 cases and assessment of response to chemotherapy. *J Clin Oncol* 1994;12:2573.
501. Grogan TM, Warnke RA, Kaplan HS. A comparative study of Burkitt's and non-Burkitt's "undifferentiated" malignant lymphoma: immunologic, cytochemical, ultrastructural, cytologic, histopathologic, clinical and cell culture features. *Cancer* 1982;49:1817.
502. Yano T, van Krieken JH, Magrath IT, et al. Histogenetic correlations between subcategories of small noncleaved cell lymphomas. *Blood* 1992;79:1282.
503. Sweetenham JW, Pearce R, Taghipour G, et al. Adult Burkitt's and Burkitt-like non-Hodgkin's lymphoma—outcome for patients treated with high-dose therapy and autologous stem-cell transplantation in first remission or at relapse: results from the European Group for Blood and Marrow Transplantation. *J Clin Oncol* 1996;14:2465.
504. Garcia CF, Weiss LM, Warnke RA. Small noncleaved cell lymphoma: an immunophenotypic study of 18 cases and comparison with large cell lymphoma. *Hum Pathol* 1986;17:454.
505. Falini B, Fizzotti M, Pileri S, et al. Bcl-6 protein expression in normal and neoplastic lymphoid tissues. *Ann Oncol* 1997;8:101.
506. Carroll WL, Yu M, Link MP, Korsmeyer SJ. Absence of Ig V region gene somatic hypermutation in advanced Burkitt's lymphoma. *J Immunol* 1989;143:692.
507. Chapman CJ, Mockridge CI, Rowe M, Rickinson AB, Stevenson FK. Analysis of VH genes used by neoplastic B cells in endemic Burkitt's lymphoma shows somatic hypermutation and intraclonal heterogeneity. *Blood* 1995;85:2176.
508. Chapman CJ, Zhou JX, Gregory C, Rickinson AB, Stevenson FK. VH and VL gene analysis in sporadic Burkitt's lymphoma shows somatic hypermutation, intraclonal heterogeneity, and a role for antigen selection. *Blood* 1996;88:3562.
509. Klein U, Klein G, Ehlin-Henriksson B, Rajewsky K, Kuppers R. Burkitt's lymphoma is a malignancy of mature B cells expressing somatically mutated V region genes. *Mol Med* 1995;1:495.
510. Neri A, Barriga F, Knowles DM, Magrath IT, Dalla-Favera R. Different regions of the immunoglobulin heavy-chain locus are involved in chromosomal translocations in distinct pathogenetic forms of Burkitt lymphoma. *Proc Natl Acad Sci U S A* 1988;85:2748.
511. Pelicci PG, Knowles DMD, Magrath I, Dalla-Favera R. Chromosomal breakpoints and structural alterations of the c-myc locus differ in endemic and sporadic forms of Burkitt lymphoma. *Proc Natl Acad Sci U S A* 1986;83:2984.
512. Capello D, Carbone A, Pastore C, et al. Point mutations of the BCL-6 gene in Burkitt's lymphoma. *Br J Haematol* 1997;99:168.
513. Hamilton-Dutoit SJ, Pallesen G, Franzmann MB, et al. AIDS-related lymphoma. Histopathology, immunophenotype, and association with Epstein-Barr virus as demonstrated by in situ nucleic acid hybridization. *Am J Pathol* 1991;138:149.
514. Wright DH. What is Burkitt's lymphoma? [editorial]. *J Pathol* 1997;182:125.
515. Magrath IT, Shiramizu B. Biology and treatment of small non-cleaved cell lymphoma. *Oncology (Huntingt)* 1989;3:41; discussion 53.
516. Arseneau JC, Bagley CM, Anderson T, Canellos GP. Hyperkalaemia, a sequel to chemotherapy of Burkitt's lymphoma. *Lancet* 1973;1:10.
517. Cohen LF, Balow JE, Magrath IT, Poplack DG, Ziegler JL. Acute tumor lysis syndrome. A review of 37 patients with Burkitt's lymphoma. *Am J Med* 1980;68:486.
518. Ziegler JL, Magrath IT, Olweny CL. Cure of Burkitt's lymphoma. Ten-year follow-up of 157 Ugandan patients. *Lancet* 1979;2:936.
519. Magrath I, Adde M, Shad A, et al. Adults and children with small non-cleaved-cell lymphoma have a similar excellent outcome when treated with the same chemotherapy regimen. *J Clin Oncol* 1996;14:925.
520. Patte C, Philip T, Rodary C, et al. Improved survival rate in children with stage III and IV B cell non-Hodgkin's lymphoma and leukemia using multi-agent chemotherapy: results of a study of 114 children from the French Pediatric Oncology Society. *J Clin Oncol* 1986;4:1219.
521. Murphy SB, Bowman WP, Abromowitch M, et al. Results of treatment of advanced-stage Burkitt's lymphoma and B cell (SIg+) acute lymphoblastic leukemia with high-dose fractionated cyclophosphamide and coordinated high-dose methotrexate and cytarabine. *J Clin Oncol* 1986;4:1732.
522. McMaster ML, Greer JP, Greco FA, et al. Effective treatment of small-noncleaved-cell lymphoma with high-intensity, brief-duration chemotherapy. *J Clin Oncol* 1991;9:941.
523. Philip T, Biron P, Philip I, et al. Massive therapy and autologous bone marrow transplantation in pediatric and young adults Burkitt's lymphoma (30 courses on 28 patients: a 5-year experience). *Eur J Cancer Clin Oncol* 1986;22:1015.
524. Philip T, Biron P, Maraninchi D, et al. Massive chemotherapy with autologous bone marrow transplantation in 50 cases of bad prognosis non-Hodgkin's lymphoma. *Br J Haematol* 1985;60:599.
525. Haddy TB, Adde MA, Magrath IT. CNS involvement in small noncleaved-cell lymphoma: is CNS disease per se a poor prognostic sign? *J Clin Oncol* 1991;9:1973.
526. Bernard A, Boumsell L, Reinherz EL, et al. Cell surface characterization of malignant T cells from lymphoblastic lymphoma using monoclonal antibodies: evidence for phenotypic differences between malignant T cells from patients with acute lymphoblastic leukemia and lymphoblastic lymphoma. *Blood* 1981;57:1105.
527. Gouttefangeas C, Bensussan A, Boumsell L. Study of the CD3-associated T-cell receptors reveals further differences between T-cell acute lymphoblastic lymphoma and leukemia. *Blood* 1990;75:931.
528. Quintanilla-Martinez L, Zukerberg LR, Harris NL. Prethymic adult lymphoblastic lymphoma. A clinicopathologic and immunohistochemical analysis. *Am J Surg Pathol* 1992;16:1075.
529. Szczepanski T, Pongers-Willemse MJ, Langerak AW, et al. Ig heavy chain gene rearrangements in T-cell acute lymphoblastic leukemia exhibit predominant DH6-19 and DH7-27 gene usage, can result in complete V-D-J rearrangements, and are rare in T-cell receptor alpha beta lineage. *Blood* 1999;93:4079.
530. Uckun FM, Sensel MG, Sun L, et al. Biology and treatment of childhood T-lineage acute lymphoblastic leukemia. *Blood* 1998;91:735.
531. Begley CG, Green AR. The SCL gene: from case report to critical hematopoietic regulator. *Blood* 1999;93:2760.
532. Coleman CN, Picozzi VJ Jr, Cox RS, et al. Treatment of lymphoblastic lymphoma in adults. *J Clin Oncol* 1986;4:1628.
533. Levine AM, Forman SJ, Meyer PR, et al. Successful therapy of convoluted T-lymphoblastic lymphoma in the adult. *Blood* 1983;61:92.
534. Jost LM, Jacky E, Dommann-Scherrer C, et al. Short-term weekly chemotherapy followed by high-dose therapy with autologous bone marrow transplantation for lymphoblastic and Burkitt's lymphomas in adult patients. *Ann Oncol* 1995;6:445.
535. Bouabdallah R, Xerri L, Bardou VJ, et al. Role of induction chemotherapy and bone marrow transplantation in adult lymphoblastic lymphoma: a report on 62 patients from a single center. *Ann Oncol* 1998;9:619.
536. Santini G, Pierluigi D, Congiu M, et al. Lymphoblastic lymphoma in adults: clinical aspects and therapy. *FORUM Trends in Experimental and Clinical Medicine* 1995;5:626.
537. Wilson WH, Grossbard ML, Alvarez M, et al. Dose-escalating EPOCH chemotherapy (CT) in previously untreated large cell lymphoma (LCL). *Proc Am Soc Clin Oncol* 1998;17:65(abst 65).
538. Sweetenham JW, Liberti G, Pearce R, et al. High-dose therapy and autologous bone marrow transplantation for adult patients with lymphoblastic lymphoma: results of the European Group for Bone Marrow Transplantation. *J Clin Oncol* 1994;12:1358.
539. Hall TC, Choi OS, Abadi A, Krant MJ. High-dose corticoid therapy in Hodgkin's disease and other lymphomas. *Ann Intern Med* 1967;66:1144.
540. Weiss LM, Crabtree GS, Rouse RV, Warnke RA. Morphologic and immunologic characterization of 50 peripheral T-cell lymphomas. *Am J Pathol* 1985;118:316.
541. Suchi T, Lennert K, Tu LY, et al. Histopathology and immunohistochemistry of peripheral T cell lymphomas: a proposal for their classification. *J Clin Pathol* 1987;40:995.
542. Medeiros LJ, Lardelli P, Stetler-Stevenson M, Longo DL, Jaffe ES. Genotypic analysis of diffuse, mixed cell lymphomas. Comparison with morphologic and immunophenotypic findings. *Am J Clin Pathol* 1991;95:547.
543. Patsouris E, Noel H, Lennert K. Histological and immunohistological findings in lymphoepithelioid cell lymphoma (Lennert's lymphoma). *Am J Surg Pathol* 1988;12:341.
544. Chott A, Augustin I, Wrba F, et al. Peripheral T-cell lymphomas: a clinicopathologic study of 75 cases. *Hum Pathol* 1990;21:1117.
545. Weisenburger DD, Linder J, Armitage JO. Peripheral T-cell lymphoma: a clinicopathologic study of 42 cases. *Hematol Oncol* 1987;5:175.
546. Hastrup N, Hamilton-Dutoit S, Ralfkiaer E, Pallesen G. Peripheral T-cell lymphomas: an evaluation of reproducibility of the updated Kiel classification. *Histopathology* 1991;18:99.
547. Lennert K, Feller A. *Histopathology of non-Hodgkin's lymphomas.* New York: Springer-Verlag, 1992.
548. Borowitz MJ, Reichert TA, Brynes RK, et al. The phenotypic diversity of peripheral T-cell lymphomas: the Southeastern Cancer Study Group experience. *Hum Pathol* 1986;17:567.

549. Weiss LM, Picker LJ, Grogan TM, Warnke RA, Sklar J. Absence of clonal beta and gamma T-cell receptor gene rearrangements in a subset of peripheral T-cell lymphomas [published erratum appears in *Am J Pathol* 1988;131:604]. *Am J Pathol* 1988;130:436.
550. Falini B, Pileri SA, Flenghi L, et al. Selection of a panel of monoclonal antibodies for monitoring residual disease in peripheral blood and bone marrow of interferon-treated hairy cell leukaemia patients. *Br J Haematol* 1990;76:460.
551. Gonzalez CL, Medeiros LJ, Braziel RM, Jaffe ES. T-cell lymphoma involving subcutaneous tissue. A clinicopathologic entity commonly associated with hemophagocytic syndrome. *Am J Surg Pathol* 1991;15:17.
552. Chott A, Dragosics B, Radaszkiewicz T. Peripheral T-cell lymphomas of the intestine. *Am J Pathol* 1992;141:1361.
553. Armitage JO, Greer JP, Levine AM, et al. Peripheral T-cell lymphoma. *Cancer* 1989;63:158.
554. Lippman SM, Miller TP, Spier CM, Slymen DJ, Grogan TM. The prognostic significance of the immunotype in diffuse large-cell lymphoma: a comparative study of the T-cell and B-cell phenotype. *Blood* 1988;72:436.
555. Coiffier B, Brousse N, Peuchmaur M, et al. Peripheral T-cell lymphomas have a worse prognosis than B-cell lymphomas: a prospective study of 361 immunophenotyped patients treated with the LNH-84 regimen. The GELA (Groupe d'Etude des Lymphomes Agressives). *Ann Oncol* 1990;1:45.
556. Dunn-Walters DK, Isaacson PG, Spencer J. Sequence analysis of rearranged IgVH genes from microdissected human Peyer's patch marginal zone B cells. *Immunology* 1996;88:618.
557. Vose JM, Peterson C, Bierman PJ, et al. Comparison of high-dose therapy and autologous bone marrow transplantation for T-cell and B-cell non-Hodgkin's lymphomas. *Blood* 1990;76:424.
558. Feller AC, Griesser H, Schilling CV, et al. Clonal gene rearrangement patterns correlate with immunophenotype and clinical parameters in patients with angioimmunoblastic lymphadenopathy. *Am J Pathol* 1988;133:549.
559. Weiss LM, Strickler JG, Hu E, Warnke RA, Sklar J. Immunoglobulin gene rearrangements in Hodgkin's disease [published erratum appears in *Hum Pathol* 1986;17:1106]. *Hum Pathol* 1986;17:1009.
560. Anagnostopoulos I, Hummel M, Finn T, et al. Heterogeneous Epstein-Barr virus infection patterns in peripheral T-cell lymphoma of angioimmunoblastic lymphadenopathy type. *Blood* 1992;80:1804.
561. Weiss LM, Jaffe ES, Liu XF, et al. Detection and localization of Epstein-Barr viral genomes in angioimmunoblastic lymphadenopathy and angioimmunoblastic lymphadenopathy-like lymphoma. *Blood* 1992;79:1789.
562. Schlegelberger B, Feller A, Godde E, Grote W, Lennert K. Stepwise development of chromosomal abnormalities in angioimmunoblastic lymphadenopathy. *Cancer Genet Cytogenet* 1990;50:15.
563. Frizzera G, Moran EM, Rappaport H. Angio-immunoblastic lymphadenopathy with dysproteinaemia. *Lancet* 1974;1:1070.
564. Siegert W, Agthe A, Griesser H, et al. Treatment of angioimmunoblastic lymphadenopathy (AILD)-type T-cell lymphoma using prednisone with or without the COPBLAM/IMVP-16 regimen. A multicenter study. Kiel Lymphoma Study Group. *Ann Intern Med* 1992;117:364.
565. Chan JK, Sin VC, Wong KF, et al. Nonnasal lymphoma expressing the natural killer cell marker CD56: a clinicopathologic study of 49 cases of an uncommon aggressive neoplasm. *Blood* 1997;89:4501.
566. Chan JK, Ng CS, Lau WH, Lo ST. Most nasal/nasopharyngeal lymphomas are peripheral T-cell neoplasms [published erratum appears in *Am J Surg Pathol* 1987;11:742]. *Am J Surg Pathol* 1987;11:418.
567. Jaffe ES, Chan JK, Su IJ, et al. Report of the Workshop on Nasal and Related Extranodal Angiocentric T/Natural Killer Cell Lymphomas. Definitions, differential diagnosis, and epidemiology. *Am J Surg Pathol* 1996;20:103.
568. Ho FC, Srivastava G, Loke SL, et al. Presence of Epstein-Barr virus DNA in nasal lymphomas of B and "T" cell type. *Hematol Oncol* 1990;8:271.
569. Ferry JA, Sklar J, Zukerberg LR, Harris NL. Nasal lymphoma. A clinicopathologic study with immunophenotypic and genotypic analysis. *Am J Surg Pathol* 1991;15:268.
570. Elenitoba-Johnson KS, Zarate-Osorno A, Meneses A, et al. Cytotoxic granular protein expression, Epstein-Barr virus strain type, and latent membrane protein-1 oncogene deletions in nasal T-lymphocyte/natural killer cell lymphomas from Mexico. *Mod Pathol* 1998;11:754.
571. Chan JK, Yip TT, Tsang WY, et al. Detection of Epstein-Barr viral RNA in malignant lymphomas of the upper aerodigestive tract [published erratum appears in *Am J Surg Pathol* 1994;18:1274]. *Am J Surg Pathol* 1994;18:938.
572. Ho FC, Choy D, Loke SL, et al. Polymorphic reticulosis and conventional lymphomas of the nose and upper aerodigestive tract: a clinicopathologic study of 70 cases, and immunophenotypic studies of 16 cases. *Hum Pathol* 1990;21:1041.
573. Lipford EH Jr, Margolick JB, Longo DL, Fauci AS, Jaffe ES. Angiocentric immunoproliferative lesions: a clinicopathologic spectrum of post-thymic T-cell proliferations. *Blood* 1988;72:1674.
574. Cuadra-Garcia I, Proulx GM, Wu CL, et al. Sinonasal lymphoma: a clinicopathologic analysis of 58 cases from the Massachusetts General Hospital. *Am J Surg Pathol* 1999;23:1356.
575. Soler J, Bordes R, Ortuno F, et al. Aggressive natural killer cell leukaemia/lymphoma in two patients with lethal midline granuloma. *Br J Haematol* 1994;86:659.
576. Kwong YL, Chan AC, Liang R, et al. CD56+ NK lymphomas: clinicopathological features and prognosis. *Br J Haematol* 1997;97:821.
577. Chim CS, Kwong YL, Lie AK, Lee CK, Liang R. CEOP treatment results and validity of the International Prognostic Index in Chinese patients with aggressive non-Hodgkin's lymphoma. *Hematol Oncol* 1998;16:117.
578. Liang R, Chen F, Lee CK, et al. Autologous bone marrow transplantation for primary nasal T/NK cell lymphoma. *Bone Marrow Transplant* 1997;19:91.
579. Nawa Y, Takenaka K, Shinagawa K, et al. Successful treatment of advanced natural killer cell lymphoma with high-dose chemotherapy and syngeneic peripheral blood stem cell transplantation. *Bone Marrow Transplant* 1999;23:1321.
580. Isaacson PG, O'Connor NT, Spencer J, et al. Malignant histiocytosis of the intestine: a T-cell lymphoma. *Lancet* 1985;2:688.
581. Ashton-Key M, Diss TC, Pan L, Du MQ, Isaacson PG. Molecular analysis of T-cell clonality in ulcerative jejunitis and enteropathy-associated T-cell lymphoma. *Am J Pathol* 1997;151:493.
582. Murray A, Cuevas EC, Jones DB, Wright DH. Study of the immunohistochemistry and T cell clonality of enteropathy-associated T cell lymphoma. *Am J Pathol* 1995;146:509.
583. Carbonnel F, Grollet-Bioul L, Brouet JC, et al. Are complicated forms of celiac disease cryptic T-cell lymphomas? [see comments]. *Blood* 1998;92:3879.
584. Spencer J, Cerf-Bensussan N, Jarry A, et al. Enteropathy-associated T cell lymphoma (malignant histiocytosis of the intestine) is recognized by a monoclonal antibody (HML-1) that defines a membrane molecule on human mucosal lymphocytes. *Am J Pathol* 1988;132:1.
585. Daum S, Foss HD, Anagnostopoulos I, et al. Expression of cytotoxic molecules in intestinal T-cell lymphomas. The German Study Group on Intestinal Non-Hodgkin Lymphoma. *J Pathol* 1997;182:311.
586. de Bruin PC, Connolly CE, Oudejans JJ, et al. Enteropathy-associated T-cell lymphomas have a cytotoxic T-cell phenotype [published erratum appears in *Histopathology* 1997;31:578]. *Histopathology* 1997;31:313.
587. Howell WM, Leung ST, Jones DB, et al. HLA-DRB, -DQA, and -DQB polymorphism in celiac disease and enteropathy-associated T-cell lymphoma. Common features and additional risk factors for malignancy. *Hum Immunol* 1995;43:29.
588. Egan LJ, Stevens FM, McCarthy CF. Celiac disease and T-cell lymphoma [letter; comment]. *N Engl J Med* 1996;335:1611.
589. Case records of the Massachusetts General Hospital. Weekly clinicopathological exercises. Case 15-1996. A 79-year-old woman with anorexia, weight loss, and diarrhea after treatment for celiac disease [see comments]. *N Engl J Med* 1996;334:1316.
590. Mantovani G, Esu S, Astara G, et al. Primary T cell CD30-positive anaplastic large-cell lymphoma associated with adult-onset celiac disease and presenting with skin lesions. *Acta Haematol* 1995;94:48.
591. Shiboski CH, Greenspan D, Dodd CL, Daniels TE. Oral T-cell lymphoma associated with celiac sprue. A case report. *Oral Surg Oral Med Oral Pathol* 1993;76:54.
592. Alegre VA, Winkelmann RK, Diez-Martin JL, Banks PM. Adult celiac disease, small and medium vessel cutaneous necrotizing vasculitis, and T cell lymphoma. *J Am Acad Dermatol* 1988;19:973.
593. Gaulard P, Bourquelot P, Kanavaros P, et al. Expression of the alpha/beta and gamma/delta T-cell receptors in 57 cases of peripheral T-cell lymphomas. Identification of a subset of gamma/delta T-cell lymphomas. *Am J Pathol* 1990;137:617.
594. Farcet JP, Gaulard P, Marolleau JP, et al. Hepatosplenic T-cell lymphoma: sinusal/sinusoidal localization of malignant cells expressing the T-cell receptor gamma delta. *Blood* 1990;75:2213.
595. Boulland ML, Kanavaros P, Wechsler J, Casiraghi O, Gaulard P. Cytotoxic protein expression in natural killer cell lymphomas and in alpha beta and gamma delta peripheral T-cell lymphomas. *J Pathol* 1997;183:432.
596. Salhany KE, Feldman M, Kahn MJ, et al. Hepatosplenic gamma-delta T-cell lymphoma: ultrastructural, immunophenotypic, and functional evidence for cytotoxic T lymphocyte differentiation. *Hum Pathol* 1997;28:674.
597. Cooke CB, Krenacs L, Stetler-Stevenson M, et al. Hepatosplenic T-cell lymphoma: a distinct clinicopathologic entity of cytotoxic gamma delta T-cell origin [see comments]. *Blood* 1996;88:4265.
598. Francois A, Lesesve JF, Stamatoullas A, et al. Hepatosplenic gamma/delta T-cell lymphoma: a report of two cases in immunocompromised patients, associated with isochromosome 7q. *Am J Surg Pathol* 1997;21:781.
599. Wang CC, Tien HF, Lin MT, et al. Consistent presence of isochromosome 7q in hepatosplenic T gamma/delta lymphoma: a new cytogenetic-clinicopathologic entity. *Genes Chromosomes Cancer* 1995;12:161.
600. Jonveaux P, Daniel MT, Martel V, Maarek O, Berger R. Isochromosome 7q and trisomy 8 are consistent primary, non-random chromosomal abnormalities associated with hepatosplenic T gamma/delta lymphoma. *Leukemia* 1996;10:1453.
601. Diez-Martin JL, Lust JA, Witzig TE, Banks PM, Li CY. Unusual presentation of extranodal peripheral T-cell lymphomas with multiple paraneoplastic features. *Cancer* 1991;68:834.
602. Ross CW, Schnitzer B, Sheldon S, Braun DK, Hanson CA. Gamma/delta T-cell posttransplantation lymphoproliferative disorder primarily in the spleen. *Am J Clin Pathol* 1994;102:310.
603. Arnulf B, Copie-Bergman C, Delfau-Larue MH, et al. Nonhepatosplenic gammadelta T-cell lymphoma: a subset of cytotoxic lymphomas with mucosal or skin localization. *Blood* 1998;91:1723.
604. Shapira MY, Caspi O, Amir G, Zlotogorski A, Naparstek Y. Gastric-mucocutaneous gd T cell lymphoma: possible association with Epstein-Barr virus? *Leuk Lymphoma* 1999;35:397.
605. Wong KF, Chan JK, Matutes E, et al. Hepatosplenic gamma delta T-cell lymphoma. A distinctive aggressive lymphoma type [see comments]. *Am J Surg Pathol* 1995;19:718.
606. Cooke C, Greiner T, Raffeld M, et al. T-cell lymphoma: a distinct clinicopathologic entity. *Mod Pathol* 1994;7:106A.
607. Salhany KE, Macon WR, Choi JK, et al. Subcutaneous panniculitis-like T-cell lymphoma: clinicopathologic, immunophenotypic, and genotypic analysis of alpha/beta and gamma/delta subtypes. *Am J Surg Pathol* 1998;22:881.
608. Kumar S, Krenacs L, Medeiros J, et al. Subcutaneous panniculitic T-cell lymphoma is a tumor of cytotoxic T lymphocytes. *Hum Pathol* 1998;29:397.
609. Benharroch D, Meguerian-Bedoyan Z, Lamant L, et al. ALK-positive lymphoma: a single disease with a broad spectrum of morphology. *Blood* 1998;91:2076.
610. Stein H, Mason DY, Gerdes J, et al. The expression of the Hodgkin's disease associated antigen Ki-1 in reactive and neoplastic lymphoid tissue: evidence that Reed-Sternberg cells and histiocytic malignancies are derived from activated lymphoid cells. *Blood* 1985;66:848.
611. Chan J, Ng C, Hui P, et al. Anaplastic large cell Ki-1 lymphoma: delineation of two morphological types. *Histopathology* 1989;15:11.

612. Pileri S, Falini B, Delsol G, et al. Lymphohistiocytic T-cell lymphoma (anaplastic large cell lymphoma CD30+/Ki-1 + with a high content of reactive histiocytes). *Histopathology* 1990;16:383.
613. Kinney MC, Collins RD, Greer JP, et al. A small-cell-predominant variant of primary Ki-1 (CD30)+ T-cell lymphoma. *Am J Surg Pathol* 1993;17:859.
614. Falini B, Bigerna B, Fizzotti M, et al. ALK expression defines a distinct group of T/null lymphomas ("ALK lymphomas") with a wide morphological spectrum. *Am J Pathol* 1998;153:875.
615. Pileri S, Bocchia M, Baroni CD, et al. Anaplastic large cell lymphoma (CD30 +/Ki-1+): results of a prospective clinico-pathological study of 69 cases. *Br J Haematol* 1994;86:513.
616. Zinzani PL, Bendandi M, Martelli M, et al. Anaplastic large-cell lymphoma: clinical and prognostic evaluation of 90 adult patients [see comments]. *J Clin Oncol* 1996;14:955.
617. Pulford K, Lamant L, Morris SW, et al. Detection of anaplastic lymphoma kinase (ALK) and nucleolar protein nucleophosmin (NPM)-ALK proteins in normal and neoplastic cells with the monoclonal antibody ALK1. *Blood* 1997;89:1394.
618. Pittaluga S, Wiodarska I, Pulford K, et al. The monoclonal antibody ALK1 identifies a distinct morphological subtype of anaplastic large cell lymphoma associated with 2p23/ALK rearrangements. *Am J Pathol* 1997;151:343.
619. Kanzler H, Kuppers R, Hansmann ML, Rajewsky K. Hodgkin and Reed-Sternberg cells in Hodgkin's disease represent the outgrowth of a dominant tumor clone derived from (crippled) germinal center B cells. *J Exp Med* 1996;184:1495.
620. Kuppers R, Rajewsky K, Zhao M, et al. Hodgkin disease: Hodgkin and Reed-Sternberg cells picked from histological sections show clonal immunoglobulin gene rearrangements and appear to be derived from B cells at various stages of development. *Proc Natl Acad Sci U S A* 1994;91:10962.
621. Hummel M, Ziemann K, Lammert H, et al. Hodgkin's disease with monoclonal and polyclonal populations of Reed-Sternberg cells [see comments]. *N Engl J Med* 1995;333:901.
622. Sundeen J, Lipford E, Uppenkamp M, et al. Rearranged antigen receptor genes in Hodgkin's disease [published erratum appears in *Blood* 1987;70:893]. *Blood* 1987;70:96.
623. Zinzani PL, Martelli M, Magagnoli M, et al. Anaplastic large cell lymphoma Hodgkin's-like: a randomized trial of ABVD versus MACOP-B with and without radiation therapy. *Blood* 1998;92:790.
624. Foss HD, Anagnostopoulos I, Araujo I, et al. Anaplastic large-cell lymphomas of T-cell and null-cell phenotype express cytotoxic molecules. *Blood* 1996;88:4005.
625. Krenacs L, Wellmann A, Sorbara L, et al. Cytotoxic cell antigen expression in anaplastic large cell lymphomas of T- and null-cell type and Hodgkin's disease: evidence for distinct cellular origin. *Blood* 1997;89:980.
626. Shiota M, Nakamura S, Ichinohasama R, et al. Anaplastic large cell lymphomas expressing the novel chimeric protein p80NPM/ALK: a distinct clinicopathologic entity. *Blood* 1995;86:1954.
627. Mason DY, Bastard C, Rimokh R, et al. CD30-positive large cell lymphomas ("Ki-1 lymphoma") are associated with a chromosomal translocation involving 5q35 [see comments]. *Br J Haematol* 1990;74:161.
628. Weisenburger DD, Gordon BG, Vose JM, et al. Occurrence of the t(2;5)(p23;q35) in non-Hodgkin's lymphoma. *Blood* 1996;87:3860.
629. Downing JR, Shurtleff SA, Zielenska M, et al. Molecular detection of the (2;5) translocation of non-Hodgkin's lymphoma by reverse transcriptase-polymerase chain reaction. *Blood* 1995;85:3416.
630. Sandlund JT, Pui CH, Roberts WM, et al. Clinicopathologic features and treatment outcome of children with large-cell lymphoma and the t(2;5)(p23;q35). *Blood* 1994;84:2467.
631. Wlodarska I, De Wolf-Peeters C, Falini B, et al. The cryptic inv(2)(p23q35) defines a new molecular genetic subtype of ALK-positive anaplastic large-cell lymphoma. *Blood* 1998;92:2688.
632. Headington JT, Roth MS, Schnitzer B. Regressing atypical histiocytosis: a review and critical appraisal. *Semin Diagn Pathol* 1987;4:28.
633. Reiter A, Schrappe M, Tiemann M, et al. Successful treatment strategy for Ki-1 anaplastic large-cell lymphoma of childhood: a prospective analysis of 62 patients enrolled in three consecutive Berlin-Frankfurt-Munster group studies. *J Clin Oncol* 1994;12:899.
634. Sandlund JT, Pui CH, Santana VM, et al. Clinical features and treatment outcome for children with CD30+ large-cell non-Hodgkin's lymphoma. *J Clin Oncol* 1994;12:895.
635. Greer JP, Kinney MC, Collins RD, et al. Clinical features of 31 patients with Ki-1 anaplastic large-cell lymphoma [see comments]. *J Clin Oncol* 1991;9:539.
636. Skinnider BF, Connors JM, Sutcliffe SB, Gascoyne RD. Anaplastic large cell lymphoma: a clinicopathologic analysis. *Hematol Oncol* 1999;17:137.
637. Tilly H, Gaulard P, Lepage E, et al. Primary anaplastic large-cell lymphoma in adults: clinical presentation, immunophenotype, and outcome. *Blood* 1997;90:3727.
638. Fanin R, Silvestri F, Geromin A, et al. Primary systemic CD30 (Ki-1)-positive anaplastic large cell lymphoma of the adult: sequential intensive treatment with the F-MACHOP regimen (+/- radiotherapy) and autologous bone marrow transplantation. *Blood* 1996;87:1243.
639. van Spronsen DJ, Janssen-Heijnen ML, Breed WP, Coebergh JW. Prevalence of co-morbidity and its relationship to treatment among unselected patients with Hodgkin's disease and non-Hodgkin's lymphoma, 1993–1996. *Ann Hematol* 1999;78:315.
640. Namboodiri KK, Harris RE. Hematopoietic and lymphoproliferative cancer among male veterans using the Veterans Administration Medical System. *Cancer* 1991;68:1123.
641. d'Amore F, Brincker H, Christensen BE, et al. Non-Hodgkin's lymphoma in the elderly. A study of 602 patients aged 70 or older from a Danish population-based registry. The Danish LYEO-Study Group. *Ann Oncol* 1992;3:379.
642. Grogan L, Corbally N, Dervan PA, Byrne A, Carney DN. Comparable prognostic factors and survival in elderly patients with aggressive non-Hodgkin's lymphoma treated with standard-dose adriamycin-based regimens. *Ann Oncol* 1994;5:47.
643. Dixon DO, Neilan B, Jones SE, et al. Effect of age on therapeutic outcome in advanced diffuse histiocytic lymphoma: the Southwest Oncology Group experience. *J Clin Oncol* 1986;4:295.
644. Solal-Celigny P, Chastang C, Herrera A, et al. Age as the main prognostic factor in adult aggressive non-Hodgkin's lymphoma. *Am J Med* 1987;83:1075.
645. Vose JM, Armitage JO, Weisenburger DD, et al. The importance of age in survival of patients treated with chemotherapy for aggressive non-Hodgkin's lymphoma. *J Clin Oncol* 1988;6:1838.
646. Rossini F, Mingozzi S, Pogliani EM, et al. Non-Hodgkin's lymphoma of the elderly. Prognostic factors and outcome. *Recent Prog Med* 1991;82:262.
647. Ansell SM, Falkson G, van der Merwe R, Uys A. Chronological age is a multifactorial prognostic variable in patients with non-Hodgkin's lymphoma. *Ann Oncol* 1992;3:45.
648. Effect of age on the characteristics and clinical behavior of non-Hodgkin's lymphoma patients. The Non-Hodgkin's Lymphoma Classification Project. *Ann Oncol* 1997;8:973.
649. Maartense E, Hermans J, Kluin-Nelemans JC, et al. Elderly patients with non-Hodgkin's lymphoma: population-based results in The Netherlands. *Ann Oncol* 1998;9:1219.
650. Armitage JO, Potter JF. Aggressive chemotherapy for diffuse histiocytic lymphoma in the elderly: increased complications with advancing age. *J Am Geriatr Soc* 1984;32:269.
651. Neilly IJ, Ogston M, Bennett B, Dawson AA. High grade non-Hodgkins lymphoma in the elderly—12 year experience in the Grampian Region of Scotland. *Hematol Oncol* 1995;13:99.
652. Elias L. Differences in age and sex distributions among patients with non-Hodgkin's lymphoma. *Cancer* 1979;43:2540.
653. Carbone A, Volpe R, Gloghini A, et al. Non-Hodgkin's lymphoma in the elderly. I. Pathologic features at presentation. *Cancer* 1990;66:1991.
654. Tirelli U, Zagonel V, Serraino D, et al. Non-Hodgkin's lymphomas in 137 patients aged 70 years or older: a retrospective European Organization for Research and Treatment of Cancer Lymphoma Group Study. *J Clin Oncol* 1988;6:1708.
655. Sonneveld P, Michiels JJ. Full dose chemotherapy in elderly patients with non-Hodgkin's lymphoma: a feasibility study using a mitoxantrone containing regimen. *Br J Cancer* 1990;62:105.
656. Tirelli U, Zagonel V, Errante D, et al. A prospective study of a new combination chemotherapy regimen in patients older than 70 years with unfavorable non-Hodgkin's lymphoma. *J Clin Oncol* 1992;10:228.
657. Zinzani PL, Storti S, Zaccaria A, et al. Elderly aggressive-histology non-Hodgkin's lymphoma: first-line VNCOP-B regimen experience on 350 patients. *Blood* 1999;94:33.
658. Niitsu N, Umeda M. THP-COPBLM (pirarubicin, cyclophosphamide, vincristine, prednisone, bleomycin and procarbazine) regimen combined with granulocyte colony-stimulating factor (G-CSF) for non-Hodgkin's lymphoma in elderly patients: a prospective study. *Leukemia* 1997;11:1817.
659. McMaster ML, Johnson DH, Greer JP, et al. A brief-duration combination chemotherapy for elderly patients with poor-prognosis non-Hodgkin's lymphoma. *Cancer* 1991;67:1487.
660. O'Reilly SE, Klimo P, Connors JM. Low-dose ACOP-B and VABE: weekly chemotherapy for elderly patients with advanced-stage diffuse large-cell lymphoma. *J Clin Oncol* 1991;9:741.
661. O'Reilly SE, Connors JM, Howdle S, et al. In search of an optimal regimen for elderly patients with advanced-stage diffuse large-cell lymphoma: results of a phase II study of P/DOCE chemotherapy. *J Clin Oncol* 1993;11:2250.
662. Martelli M, Guglielmi C, Coluzzi S, et al. P-VABEC: a prospective study of a new weekly chemotherapy regimen for elderly aggressive non-Hodgkin's lymphoma. *J Clin Oncol* 1993;11:2362.
663. Bertini M, Freilone R, Vitolo U, et al. P-VEBEC: a new 8-weekly schedule with or without rG-CSF for elderly patients with aggressive non-Hodgkin's lymphoma (NHL). *Ann Oncol* 1994;5:895.
664. Mainwaring PN, Cunningham D, Gregory W, et al. A BNLI randomized study of padriacebo vs. pmitcebo in patients with high-grade lymphoma (HGL) over 60 years of age. *Proc Am Soc Clin Oncol* 1998;12a.
665. Coiffier B, Neidhardt-Berard EM, Tilly H, et al. Fludarabine alone compared with CHVP plus interferon in elderly patients with follicular lymphoma and adverse prognostic parameters: a GELA study. Groupe d'Etudes des Lymphomes de l'Adulte. *Ann Oncol* 1999;10:1191.
666. Meyer RM, Chen C, Skingley P. A comparison of outcomes of elderly patients with aggressive histology lymphoma (AHL) who were entered or not entered on to a randomized phase II trial. *Proc Am Soc Clin Oncol* 1999;17a.
667. Gomez H, Hidalgo M, Casanova L, et al. Risk factors for treatment-related death in elderly patients with aggressive non-Hodgkin's lymphoma: results of a multivariate analysis. *J Clin Oncol* 1998;16:2065.
668. Gomez H, Mas L, Casanova L, et al. Elderly patients with aggressive non-Hodgkin's lymphoma treated with CHOP chemotherapy plus granulocyte-macrophage colony-stimulating factor: identification of two age subgroups with differing hematologic toxicity. *J Clin Oncol* 1998;16:2352.
669. Guerci A, Lederlin P, Reyes F, et al. Effect of granulocyte colony-stimulating factor administration in elderly patients with aggressive non-Hodgkin's lymphoma treated with a pirarubicin-combination chemotherapy regimen. Groupe d'Etudes des Lymphomes de l'Adulte. *Ann Oncol* 1996;7:966.
670. Zinzani PL, Pavone E, Storti S, et al. Randomized trial with or without granulocyte colony-stimulating factor as adjunct to induction VNCOP-B treatment of elderly high-grade non-Hodgkin's lymphoma. *Blood* 1997;89:3974.
671. Opelz G, Schwarz V, Wujciak T, et al. Analysis of non-Hodgkin's lymphomas in organ transplant recipients. *Transplant Rev* 1995;9:231.
672. Paya CV, Fung JJ, Nalesnik MA, et al. Epstein-Barr virus-induced posttransplant lymphoproliferative disorders. ASTS/ASTP EBV-PTLD Task Force and The Mayo Clinic Organized International Consensus Development Meeting. *Transplantation* 1999;68:1517.
673. Shapiro R, Nalesnik M, McCauley J, et al. Posttransplant lymphoproliferative disorders in adult and pediatric renal transplant patients receiving tacrolimus-based immunosuppression. *Transplantation* 1999;68:1851.
674. Leblond V, Davi F, Charlotte F, et al. Posttransplant lymphoproliferative disorders not associated with Epstein-Barr virus: a distinct entity? *J Clin Oncol* 1998;16:2052.
675. Bierman PJ, Vose JM, Langnas AN, et al. Hodgkin's disease following solid organ transplantation. *Ann Oncol* 1996;7:265.
676. Weissmann DJ, Ferry JA, Harris NL, et al. Posttransplantation lymphoproliferative disorders in solid organ recipients are predominantly aggressive tumors of host origin. *Am J Clin Pathol* 1995;103:748.

677. Knowles DM, Cesarman E, Chadburn A, et al. Correlative morphologic and molecular genetic analysis demonstrates three distinct categories of posttransplantation lymphoproliferative disorders. *Blood* 1995;85:552.
678. Harris NL, Ferry JA, Swerdlow SH. Posttransplant lymphoproliferative disorders: summary of Society for Hematopathology Workshop. *Semin Diagn Pathol* 1997;14:8.
679. Chadburn A, Chen JM, Hsu DT, et al. The morphologic and molecular genetic categories of posttransplantation lymphoproliferative disorders are clinically relevant. *Cancer* 1998;82:1978.
680. Swinnen LJ, Costanzo-Nordin MR, Fisher SG, et al. Increased incidence of lymphoproliferative disorder after immunosuppression with the monoclonal antibody OKT3 in cardiac-transplant recipients [see comments]. *N Engl J Med* 1990;323:1723.
681. Armitage JM, Kormos RL, Stuart RS, et al. Posttransplant lymphoproliferative disease in thoracic organ transplant patients: ten years of cyclosporine-based immunosuppression. *J Heart Lung Transplant* 1991;10:877; discussion 886.
682. Benkerrou M, Jais JP, Leblond V, et al. Anti-B-cell monoclonal antibody treatment of severe posttransplant B-lymphoproliferative disorder: prognostic factors and long-term outcome. *Blood* 1998;92:3137.
683. Swinnen LJ. Durable remission after aggressive chemotherapy for post-cardiac transplant lymphoproliferation. *Leuk Lymphoma* 1997;28:89.
684. Cesarman E, Chadburn A, Liu YF, et al. BCL-6 gene mutations in posttransplantation lymphoproliferative disorders predict response to therapy and clinical outcome. *Blood* 1998;92:2294.
685. Swinnen LJ. Overview of posttransplant B-cell lymphoproliferative disorders. *Semin Oncol* 1999;26:21.
686. Morrison VA, Dunn DL, Manivel JC, Gajl-Peczalska KJ, Peterson BA. Clinical characteristics of post-transplant lymphoproliferative disorders. *Am J Med* 1994;97:14.
687. Milpied N, Vasseur B, Antoine C, et al. Chimeric anti CD20 monoclonal antibody (Rituximab) in B posttransplant lympho-proliferative disorders (B PTLDs): A retrospective analysis on 32 patients (PTS). *Blood* 1999;89:631a (abst 2803).
688. Nalesnik MA, Rao AS, Furukawa H, et al. Autologous lymphokine-activated killer cell therapy of Epstein-Barr virus-positive and -negative lymphoproliferative disorders arising in organ transplant recipients. *Transplantation* 1997;63:1200.
689. Papadopoulos EB, Ladanyi M, Emanuel D, et al. Infusions of donor leukocytes to treat Epstein-Barr virus-associated lymphoproliferative disorders after allogeneic bone marrow transplantation [see comments]. *N Engl J Med* 1994;330:1185.
690. 1993 Revised classification system for HIV infection and expanded surveillance case definition for AIDS among adolescents and adults. *MMWR* 1992;41:961.
691. Kaplan LD, Abrams DI, Feigal E, et al. AIDS-associated non-Hodgkin's lymphoma in San Francisco. *JAMA* 1989;261:719.
692. Kaplan LD, Shiramizu B, Herndier B, et al. Influence of molecular characteristics on clinical outcome in human immunodeficiency virus-associated non-Hodgkin's lymphoma: identification of a subgroup with favorable clinical outcome. *Blood* 1995;85:1727.
693. Gisselbrecht C, Oksenhendler E, Tirelli U, et al. Human immunodeficiency virus-related lymphoma treatment with intensive combination chemotherapy. French-Italian Cooperative Group. *Am J Med* 1993;95:188.
694. Straus DJ, Huang J, Testa MA, Levine AM, Kaplan LD. Prognostic factors in the treatment of human immunodeficiency virus-associated non-Hodgkin's lymphoma: analysis of AIDS Clinical Trials Group protocol 142—low-dose versus standard-dose m-BACOD plus granulocyte-macrophage colony-stimulating factor. National Institute of Allergy and Infectious Diseases. *J Clin Oncol* 1998;16:3601.
695. Levine AM, Sullivan-Halley J, Pike MC, et al. Human immunodeficiency virus-related lymphoma. Prognostic factors predictive of survival [see comments]. *Cancer* 1991;68:2466.
696. Kaplan LD, Straus DJ, Testa MA, et al. Low-dose compared with standard-dose m-BACOD chemotherapy for non-Hodgkin's lymphoma associated with human immunodeficiency virus infection. National Institute of Allergy and Infectious Diseases AIDS Clinical Trials Group [see comments]. *N Engl J Med* 1997;336:1641.
697. Remick SC, McSharry JJ, Wolf BC, et al. Novel oral combination chemotherapy in the treatment of intermediate-grade and high-grade AIDS-related non-Hodgkin's lymphoma. *J Clin Oncol* 1993;11:1691.
698. Kaplan LD. Clinical management of human immunodeficiency virus-associated non-Hodgkin's lymphoma. *J Natl Cancer Inst Monogr* 1998;23:101.
699. Sparano JA, Wiernik PH, Hu X, et al. Pilot trial of infusional cyclophosphamide, doxorubicin, and etoposide plus didanosine and filgrastim in patients with human immunodeficiency virus-associated non-Hodgkin's lymphoma. *J Clin Oncol* 1996;14:3026.
700. Tosi P, Gherlinzoni F, Mazza P, et al. 3'-Azido 3'-deoxythymidine + methotrexate as a novel antineoplastic combination in the treatment of human immunodeficiency virus-related non-Hodgkin's lymphomas. *Blood* 1997;89:419.
701. Spina M, Vaccher E, Carbone A, Tirelli U. Neoplastic complications of HIV infection. *Ann Oncol* 1999;10:1271.
702. Errante D, Vaccher E, Tirelli U. Are hematopoietic colony-stimulating factors useful in association with chemotherapy in the treatment of HIV-related non-Hodgkin's lymphomas? *Ann Oncol* 1996;7:233.
703. Gabarre J, Lepage E, Thyss A, et al. Chemotherapy combined with zidovudine and GM-CSF in human immunodeficiency virus-related non-Hodgkin's lymphoma. *Ann Oncol* 1995;6:1025.
704. Maher EA, Fine HA. Primary CNS lymphoma. *Semin Oncol* 1999;26:346.
705. Blay JY, Bouhour D, Carrie C, et al. The C5R protocol: a regimen of high-dose chemotherapy and radiotherapy in primary cerebral non-Hodgkin's lymphoma of patients with no known cause of immunosuppression [see comments]. *Blood* 1995;86:2922.
706. Nelson DF, Martz KL, Bonner H, et al. Non-Hodgkin's lymphoma of the brain: can high dose, large volume radiation therapy improve survival? Report on a prospective trial by the Radiation Therapy Oncology Group (RTOG): RTOG 8315 [see comments]. *Int J Radiat Oncol Biol Phys* 1992;23:9.
707. Schultz C, Scott C, Sherman W, et al. Preirradiation chemotherapy with cyclophosphamide, doxorubicin, vincristine, and dexamethasone for primary CNS lymphomas: initial report of radiation therapy oncology group protocol 88-06. *J Clin Oncol* 1996;14:556.
708. Blay JY, Conroy T, Chevreau C, et al. High-dose methotrexate for the treatment of primary cerebral lymphomas: analysis of survival and late neurologic toxicity in a retrospective series. *J Clin Oncol* 1998;16:864.
709. DeAngelis LM, Yahalom J, Thaler HT, Kher U. Combined modality therapy for primary CNS lymphoma. *J Clin Oncol* 1992;10:635.
710. Bessell EM, Graus F, Punt JA, et al. Primary non-Hodgkin's lymphoma of the CNS treated with BVAM or CHOD/BVAM chemotherapy before radiotherapy. *J Clin Oncol* 1996;14:945.
711. Brada M, Hjiyiannakis D, Hines F, Traish D, Ashley S. Short intensive primary chemotherapy and radiotherapy in sporadic primary CNS lymphoma (PCL). *Int J Radiat Oncol Biol Phys* 1998;40:1157.
712. Reni M, Ferreri AJ, Garancini MP, Villa E. Therapeutic management of primary central nervous system lymphoma in immunocompetent patients: results of a critical review of the literature. *Ann Oncol* 1997;8:227.
713. Abrey LE, DeAngelis LM, Yahalom J. Long-term survival in primary CNS lymphoma. *J Clin Oncol* 1998;16:859.
714. Corry J, Smith JG, Wirth A, Quong G, Liew KH. Primary central nervous system lymphoma: age and performance status are more important than treatment modality. *Int J Radiat Oncol Biol Phys* 1998;41:615.
715. O'Neill BP, Wang CH, O'Fallon JR, et al. Primary central nervous system non-Hodgkin's lymphoma (PCNSL): survival advantages with combined initial therapy? A final report of the North Central Cancer Treatment Group (NCCTG) Study 86-72-52. *Int J Radiat Oncol Biol Phys* 1999;43:559.
716. Cher L, Glass J, Harsh GR, Hochberg FH. Therapy of primary CNS lymphoma with methotrexate-based chemotherapy and deferred radiotherapy: preliminary results. *Neurology* 1996;46:1757.
717. Sandor V, Stark-Vancs V, Pearson D, et al. Phase II trial of chemotherapy alone for primary CNS and intraocular lymphoma [see comments]. *J Clin Oncol* 1998;16:3000.
718. Cheng AL, Yeh KH, Uen WC, et al. Systemic chemotherapy alone for patients with non-acquired immunodeficiency syndrome-related central nervous system lymphoma: a pilot study of the BOMES protocol. *Cancer* 1998;82:1946.
719. Doolittle ND, Miner ME, Hall WA, et al. Safety and efficacy of a multicenter study using intraarterial chemotherapy in conjunction with osmotic opening of the blood-brain barrier for the treatment of patients with malignant brain tumors. *Cancer* 2000;88:637.
720. Shahab N, Doll DC. Testicular lymphoma. *Semin Oncol* 1999;26:259.
721. Doll DC, Weiss RB. Malignant lymphoma of the testis. *Am J Med* 1986;81:515.
722. Hyland J, Lasota J, Jasinski M, et al. Molecular pathological analysis of testicular diffuse large cell lymphomas. *Hum Pathol* 1998;29:1231.
723. Crellin AM, Hudson BV, Bennett MH, Harland S, Hudson GV. Non-Hodgkin's lymphoma of the testis. *Radiother Oncol* 1993;27:99.
724. Moller MB, d'Amore F, Christensen BE. Testicular lymphoma: a population-based study of incidence, clinicopathological correlations and prognosis. The Danish Lymphoma Study Group, LYFO. *Eur J Cancer* 1994;12:1760.
725. Linassier C, Desablens B, Yves Le Prise P, et al. Primary testicular non-lymphoblastic intermediate-high-grade non-Hodgkin's lymphoma: results of a goelams prospective study. *Proc Am Soc Clin Oncol* 1999;326a(abst 1253).
726. Niitsu N, Umeda M. Clinical features of testicular non-Hodgkin's lymphoma—focus on treatment strategy. *Acta Oncol* 1998;37:677.
727. Tondini C, Ferreri AJ, Siracusano L, et al. Diffuse large-cell lymphoma of the testis. *J Clin Oncol* 1999;17:2854.
728. Fonseca R, Habermann TM, Colgan JP, et al. Testicular lymphoma is associated with a high incidence of extranodal recurrence. *Cancer* 2000;88:154.
729. Ferry JA, Harris NL, Young RH, et al. Malignant lymphoma of the testis, epididymis, and spermatic cord. A clinicopathologic study of 69 cases with immunophenotypic analysis. *Am J Surg Pathol* 1994;18:376.
730. Touroutoglou N, Dimopoulos MA, Younes A, et al. Testicular lymphoma: late relapses and poor outcome despite doxorubicin-based therapy. *J Clin Oncol* 1995;13:1361.
731. Sussman EB, Hajdu SI, Lieberman PH, Whitmore WF. Malignant lymphoma of the testis: a clinicopathologic study of 37 cases. *J Urol* 1977;118:1004.
732. Read G. Lymphomas of the testis—results of treatment 1960–77. *Clin Radiol* 1981;32:687.
733. Zietman AL, Coen JJ, Ferry JA, et al. The management and outcome of stage IAE non-Hodgkin's lymphoma of the testis. *J Urol* 1996;155:943.
734. Connors JM, Klimo P, Voss N, Fairey RN, Jackson S. Testicular lymphoma: improved outcome with early brief chemotherapy. *J Clin Oncol* 1988;6:776.
735. Zucca E, Roggero E, Bertoni F, Cavalli F. Primary extranodal non-Hodgkin's lymphomas. Part 1: Gastrointestinal, cutaneous and genitourinary lymphomas. *Ann Oncol* 1997;8:727.
736. Tesoro-Tess JD, Biasi S, Balzarini L, et al. Heart involvement in lymphomas. The value of magnetic resonance imaging and two-dimensional echocardiography at disease presentation. *Cancer* 1993;72:2484.
737. McDonnell PJ, Mann RB, Bulkley BH. Involvement of the heart by malignant lymphoma: a clinicopathologic study. *Cancer* 1982;49:944.
738. Hamada S, Nishimura T, Hayashida K, Uehara T. Intracardiac malignant lymphoma detected by gallium-67 citrate and thallium-201 chloride. *J Nucl Med* 1988;29:1868.
739. Donnelly MS, Weinberg DS, Skarin AT, Levine HD. Sick sinus syndrome with serocon-strictive pericarditis in malignant lymphoma involving the heart: a case report. *Med Pediatr Oncol* 1981;9:273.
740. Pozniak AL, Thomas RD, Hobbs CB, Lever JV. Primary malignant lymphoma of the heart. Antemortem cytologic diagnosis. *Acta Cytol* 1986;30:662.
741. Curtsinger CR, Wilson MJ, Yoneda K. Primary cardiac lymphoma. *Cancer* 1989;64:521.
742. Nand S, Mullen GM, Lonchyna VA, Moncada R. Primary lymphoma of the heart. Prolonged survival with early systemic therapy in a patient. *Cancer* 1991;68:2289.

743. Gill PS, Chandraratna PA, Meyer PR, Levine AM. Malignant lymphoma: cardiac involvement at initial presentation. *J Clin Oncol* 1987;5:216.
744. Balasubramanyam A, Waxman M, Kazal HL, Lee MH. Malignant lymphoma of the heart in acquired immune deficiency syndrome. *Chest* 1986;90:243.
745. Ceresoli GL, Ferreri AJ, Bucci E, et al. Primary cardiac lymphoma in immunocompetent patients: diagnostic and therapeutic management. *Cancer* 1997;80:1497.
746. Holladay AO, Siegel RJ, Schwartz DA. Cardiac malignant lymphoma in acquired immune deficiency syndrome. *Cancer* 1992;70:2203.
747. Hyjek E, Isaacson PG. Primary B cell lymphoma of the thyroid and its relationship to Hashimoto's thyroiditis. *Hum Pathol* 1988;19:1315.
748. Kossev P, Livolsi V. Lymphoid lesions of the thyroid: review in light of the revised European-American lymphoma classification and upcoming World Health Organization classification. *Thyroid* 1999;9:1273.
749. Tupchong L, Hughes F, Harmer CL. Primary lymphoma of the thyroid: clinical features, prognostic factors, and results of treatment. *Int J Radiat Oncol Biol Phys* 1986;12:1813.
750. Tsang RW, Gospodarowicz MK, Sutcliffe SB, et al. Non-Hodgkin's lymphoma of the thyroid gland: prognostic factors and treatment outcome. The Princess Margaret Hospital Lymphoma Group. *Int J Radiat Oncol Biol Phys* 1993;27:599.
751. Lam KY, Lo CY, Kwong DL, Lee J, Srivastava G. Malignant lymphoma of the thyroid. A 30-year clinicopathologic experience and an evaluation of the presence of Epstein-Barr virus. *Am J Clin Pathol* 1999;112:263.
752. Pedersen RK, Pedersen NT. Primary non-Hodgkin's lymphoma of the thyroid gland: a population based study. *Histopathology* 1996;28:25.
753. Skarsgard ED, Connors JM, Robins RE. A current analysis of primary lymphoma of the thyroid. *Arch Surg* 1991;126:1199; discussion 1203.
754. Jensen MH, Davis RK, Derrick L. Thyroid cancer: a computer-assisted review of 5287 cases. *Otolaryngol Head Neck Surg* 1990;102:51.
755. Vigliotti A, Kong JS, Fuller LM, Velasquez WS. Thyroid lymphomas stages IE and IIE: comparative results for radiotherapy only, combination chemotherapy only, and multimodality treatment. *Int J Radiat Oncol Biol Phys* 1986;12:1807.
756. Shaw JH, Holden A, Sage M. Thyroid lymphoma. *Br J Surg* 1989;76:895.
757. Pyke CM, Grant CS, Habermann TM, et al. Non-Hodgkin's lymphoma of the thyroid: is more than biopsy necessary? *World J Surg* 1992;16:604; discussion 609.
758. Matsuzuka F, Miyauchi A, Katayama S, et al. Clinical aspects of primary thyroid lymphoma: diagnosis and treatment based on our experience of 119 cases. *Thyroid* 1993;3:93.
759. Laing RW, Hoskin P, Hudson BV, et al. The significance of MALT histology in thyroid lymphoma: a review of patients from the BNLI and Royal Marsden Hospital. *Clin Oncol* 1994;6:300.
760. Doria R, Jekel JF, Cooper DL. Thyroid lymphoma. The case for combined modality therapy. *Cancer* 1994;73:200.
761. Salvatore JR, Ross RS. Primary bilateral adrenal lymphoma. *Leuk Lymphoma* 1999;34:111.
762. Wang J, Sun NC, Renslo R, et al. Clinically silent primary adrenal lymphoma: a case report and review of the literature. *Am J Hematol* 1998;58:130.
763. Brogi E, Harris NL. Lymphomas of the breast: pathology and clinical behavior. *Semin Oncol* 1999;26:357.
764. Armitage JO, Feagler JR, Skoog DP. Burkitt lymphoma during pregnancy with bilateral breast involvement. *JAMA* 1977;237:151.
765. Okuno SH, Hoyer JD, Ristow K, Witzig TE. Primary renal non-Hodgkin's lymphoma. An unusual extranodal site. *Cancer* 1995;75:2258.
766. Pelstring RJ, Essell JH, Kurtin PJ, Cohen AR, Banks PM. Diversity of organ site involvement among malignant lymphomas of mucosa-associated tissues. *Am J Clin Pathol* 1991;96:738.
767. Muntz HG, Ferry JA, Flynn D, Fuller AF Jr, Tarraza HM. Stage IE primary malignant lymphomas of the uterine cervix. *Cancer* 1991;68:2023.
768. van de Rijn M, Kamel OW, Chang PP, et al. Primary low-grade endometrial B-cell lymphoma. *Am J Surg Pathol* 1997;21:187.
769. Nakata M, Matsuno Y, Katsumata N, et al. Histology according to the Revised European-American Lymphoma Classification significantly predicts the prognosis of ocular adnexal lymphoma. *Leuk Lymphoma* 1999;32:533.
770. Knowles DM, Jakobiec FA, McNally L, Burke JS. Lymphoid hyperplasia and malignant lymphoma occurring in the ocular adnexa (orbit, conjunctiva, and eyelids): a prospective multiparametric analysis of 108 cases during 1977 to 1987 [see comments]. *Hum Pathol* 1990;21:959.
771. Medeiros LJ, Harris NL. Lymphoid infiltrates of the orbit and conjunctiva. A morphologic and immunophenotypic study of 99 cases. *Am J Surg Pathol* 1989;13:459.
772. Medeiros LJ, Harmon DC, Linggood RM, Harris NL. Immunohistologic features predict clinical behavior of orbital and conjunctival lymphoid infiltrates. *Blood* 1989;74:2121.
773. Keleti D, Flickinger JC, Hobson SR, Mittal BB. Radiotherapy of lymphoproliferative diseases of the orbit. Surveillance of 65 cases. *Am J Clin Oncol* 1992;15:422.
774. Wotherspoon AC, Diss TC, Pan LX, et al. Primary low-grade B-cell lymphoma of the conjunctiva: a mucosa-associated lymphoid tissue type lymphoma. *Histopathology* 1993;23:417.
775. Char DH, Ljung BM, Miller T, Phillips T. Primary intraocular lymphoma (ocular reticulum cell sarcoma) diagnosis and management. *Ophthalmology* 1988;95:625.
776. Char DH, Margolis L, Newman AB. Ocular reticulum cell sarcoma. *Am J Ophthalmol* 1981;91:480.
777. Whitcup SM, de Smet MD, Rubin BI, et al. Intraocular lymphoma. Clinical and histopathologic diagnosis. *Ophthalmology* 1993;100:1399.
778. Peterson K, Gordon KB, Heinemann MH, DeAngelis LM. The clinical spectrum of ocular lymphoma. *Cancer* 1993;72:843.
779. Freeman LN, Schachat AP, Knox DL, Michels RG, Green WR. Clinical features, laboratory investigations, and survival in ocular reticulum cell sarcoma. *Ophthalmology* 1987;94:1631.
780. Habermann TM, Ryu JH, Inwards DJ, Kurtin PJ. Primary pulmonary lymphoma. *Semin Oncol* 1999;26:307.
781. Parker F, Jackson H Jr. Primary reticulum cell sarcoma of bone. *Surg Gynecol Obstet* 1939;68:45.
782. Susnerwala SS, Dinshaw KA, Pande SC, et al. Primary lymphoma of bone: experience of 39 cases at the Tata Memorial Hospital, India. *J Surg Oncol* 1990;44:229.
783. Baar J, Burkes RL, Bell R, et al. Primary non-Hodgkin's lymphoma of bone. A clinicopathologic study. *Cancer* 1994;73:1194.
784. Fairbanks RK, Bonner JA, Inwards CY, et al. Treatment of stage IE primary lymphoma of bone. *Int J Radiat Oncol Biol Phys* 1994;28:363.
785. Dosoretz DE, Murphy GF, Raymond AK, et al. Radiation therapy for primary lymphoma of bone. *Cancer* 1983;51:44.
786. Baar J, Burkes RL, Gospodarowicz M. Primary non-Hodgkin's lymphoma of bone. *Semin Oncol* 1999;26:270.
787. Bacci G, Jaffe N, Emiliani E, et al. Therapy for primary non-Hodgkin's lymphoma of bone and a comparison of results with Ewing's sarcoma. Ten years' experience at the Istituto Ortopedico Rizzoli. *Cancer* 1986;57:1468.
788. Mendenhall NP, Jones JJ, Kramer BS, et al. The management of primary lymphoma of bone. *Radiother Oncol* 1987;9:137.
789. Stokes SH, Walz BJ. Pathologic fracture after radiation therapy for primary non-Hodgkin's malignant lymphoma of bone. *Int J Radiat Oncol Biol Phys* 1983;9:1153.
790. Lucraft HH. Primary lymphoma of bone: a review of 13 cases emphasizing orthopaedic problems. *Clin Oncol (R Coll Radiol)* 1991;3:265.
791. Berkman N, Breuer R, Kramer MR, Polliack A. Pulmonary involvement in lymphoma. *Leuk Lymphoma* 1996;20:229.
792. Elis A, Blickstein D, Mulchanov I, et al. Pleural effusion in patients with non-Hodgkin's lymphoma: a case-controlled study. *Cancer* 1998;83:1607.
793. Katz RL, Raval P, Manning JT, McLaughlin P, Barlogie B. A morphologic, immunologic, and cytometric approach to the classification of non-Hodgkin's lymphoma in effusions. *Diagn Cytopathol* 1987;3:91.
794. Celikoglu F, Teirstein AS, Krellenstein DJ, Strauchen JA. Pleural effusion in non-Hodgkin's lymphoma. *Chest* 1992;101:1357.
795. Said W, Chien K, Takeuchi S, et al. Kaposi's sarcoma-associated herpesvirus (KSHV or HHV8) in primary effusion lymphoma: ultrastructural demonstration of herpesvirus in lymphoma cells. *Blood* 1996;87:4937.
796. Strauchen JA, Hauser AD, Burstein D, et al. Body cavity-based malignant lymphoma containing Kaposi sarcoma-associated herpesvirus in an HIV-negative man with previous Kaposi sarcoma. *Ann Intern Med* 1996;125:822.
797. Horenstein MG, Nador RG, Chadburn A, et al. Epstein-Barr virus latent gene expression in primary effusion lymphomas containing Kaposi's sarcoma-associated herpesvirus/human herpesvirus 8. *Blood* 1997;90:1186.
798. Said JW, Tasaka T, Takeuchi S, et al. Primary effusion lymphoma in women: report of two cases of Kaposi's sarcoma herpes virus-associated effusion-based lymphoma in human immunodeficiency virus-negative women. *Blood* 1996;88:3124.
799. Willemze R, Kerl H, Sterry W, et al. EORTC classification for primary cutaneous lymphomas: a proposal from the Cutaneous Lymphoma Study Group of the European Organization for Research and Treatment of Cancer. *Blood* 1997;90:354.
800. LeBoit PE. Lymphomatoid papulosis and cutaneous CD30+ lymphoma. *Am J Dermatopathol* 1996;18:221.
801. Karp D, Horn T. Lymphoid papulosis. *J Am Acad Dermatol* 1994;30:379.
802. Willemze R, Beljaards RC. Spectrum of primary cutaneous CD30 (Ki-1)-positive lymphoproliferative disorders. A proposal for classification and guidelines for management and treatment. *J Am Acad Dermatol* 1993;28:973.
803. Cabanillas F, Armitage J, Pugh WC, Weisenburger D, Duvic M. Lymphomatoid papulosis: a T-cell dyscrasia with a propensity to transform into malignant lymphoma. *Ann Intern Med* 1995;122:210.
804. de Bruin PC, Beljaards RC, van Heerde P, et al. Differences in clinical behaviour and immunophenotype between primary cutaneous and primary nodal anaplastic large cell lymphoma of T-cell or null cell phenotype. *Histopathology* 1993;23:127.
805. Beljaards RC, Meijer CJ, Van der Putte SC, et al. Primary cutaneous T-cell lymphoma: clinicopathological features and prognostic parameters of 35 cases other than mycosis fungoides and CD30-positive large cell lymphoma. *J Pathol* 1994;172:53.
806. Willemze R, Rijlaarsdam JU, Meijer CJ. Are most primary cutaneous B-cell lymphomas "marginal cell lymphomas"? [comment]. *Br J Dermatol* 1995;133:950; discussion 953.
807. Bailey EM, Ferry JA, Harris NL, et al. Marginal zone lymphoma (low-grade B-cell lymphoma of mucosa-associated lymphoid tissue type) of skin and subcutaneous tissue: a study of 15 patients [see comments]. *Am J Surg Pathol* 1996;20:1011.
808. LeBoit PE, McNutt NS, Reed JA, Jacobson M, Weiss LM. Primary cutaneous immunocytoma. A B-cell lymphoma that can easily be mistaken for cutaneous lymphoid hyperplasia. *Am J Surg Pathol* 1994;18:969.
809. Kerl H, Cerroni L. Primary B-cell lymphomas of the skin. *Ann Oncol* 1997;8:29.
810. Vermeer MH, Geelen FA, van Haselen CW, et al. Primary cutaneous large B-cell lymphomas of the legs. A distinct type of cutaneous B-cell lymphoma with an intermediate prognosis. Dutch Cutaneous Lymphoma Working Group [see comments]. *Arch Dermatol* 1996;132:1304.
811. Abbondanzo SL, Wenig BM. Non-Hodgkin's lymphoma of the sinonasal tract. A clinicopathologic and immunophenotypic study of 120 cases. *Cancer* 1995;75:1281.
812. Banfi A, Bonadonna G, Ricci SB, et al. Malignant lymphomas of Waldeyer's ring: natural history and survival after radiotherapy. *BMJ* 1972;3:140.
813. Hoppe RT, Burke JS, Glatstein E, Kaplan HS. Non-Hodgkin's lymphoma: involvement of Waldeyer's ring. *Cancer* 1978;42:1096.
814. Liang R, Ng RP, Todd D, et al. Management of stage I-II diffuse aggressive non-Hodgkin's lymphoma of the Waldeyer's ring: combined modality therapy versus radiotherapy alone. *Hematol Oncol* 1987;5:223.
815. Okerbloom JA, Armitage JO, Zetterman R, Linder J. Esophageal involvement by non-Hodgkin's lymphoma. *Am J Med* 1984;77:359.
816. Brooks JJ, Enterline HT. Primary gastric lymphomas. A clinicopathologic study of 58 cases with long-term follow-up and literature review. *Cancer* 1983;51:701.

817. Hockey MS, Powell J, Crocker J, Fielding JW. Primary gastric lymphoma. *Br J Surg* 1987;74:483.
818. Shchepotin IB, Evans SR, Shabahang M, et al. Primary non-Hodgkin's lymphoma of the stomach: three radical modalities of treatment in 75 patients. *Ann Surg Oncol* 1996;3:277.
819. Rabbi C, Aitini E, Cavazzini G, et al. Stomach preservation in low- and high-grade primary gastric lymphomas: preliminary results. *Haematologica* 1996;81:15.
820. Haim N, Leviov M, Ben-Arieh Y, et al. Intermediate and high-grade gastric non-Hodgkin's lymphoma: a prospective study of non-surgical treatment with primary chemotherapy, with or without radiotherapy. *Leuk Lymphoma* 1995;17:321.
821. Bozzetti F, Audisio RA, Giardini R, Gennari L. Role of surgery in patients with primary non-Hodgkin's lymphoma of the stomach: an old problem revisited [see comments]. *Br J Surg* 1993;80:1101.
822. Domizio P, Owen RA, Shepherd NA, Talbot IC, Norton AJ. Primary lymphoma of the small intestine. A clinicopathological study of 119 cases. *Am J Surg Pathol* 1993;17:429.
823. d'Amore F, Brincker H, Gronbaek K, et al. Non-Hodgkin's lymphoma of the gastrointestinal tract: a population-based analysis of incidence, geographic distribution, clinicopathologic presentation features, and prognosis. Danish Lymphoma Study Group. *J Clin Oncol* 1994;12:1673.
824. Freter CE. Acquired immunodeficiency syndrome-associated lymphomas. *J Natl Cancer Inst Monogr* 1990;10:45.
825. Rechavi G, Ramot B. Primary intestinal lymphoma and a-heavy-chain disease. In: Magrath IT, ed. *The non-Hodgkin's lymphomas*, 2nd ed. London: Arnold; 1997:513.
826. Salem PA, Jones DV. Treatment of malignant neoplasms of the mucosa-associated lymphoid tissues. In: Magrath IT, ed. *The non-Hodgkin's lymphomas*, 2nd ed. London: Arnold; 1997:989.
827. Zucca E, Stein H, Coiffier B. European Lymphoma Task Force (ELTF): report of the workshop on Mantle Cell Lymphoma (MCL) [see comments]. *Ann Oncol* 1994;5:507.
828. Ernst M, Stein H, Ludwig D, et al. Surgical therapy of gastrointestinal non-Hodgkin's lymphomas. *Eur J Surg Oncol* 1996;22:177.

LYNN D. WILSON
GLENN W. JONES
BARRY M. KACINSKI
RICHARD L. EDELSON
PETER W. HEALD

SECTION 4

Cutaneous T-Cell Lymphomas

Cutaneous T-cell lymphoma (CTCL) is a lymphoproliferative disorder of epidermotropic, neoplastic T cells with a wide range of clinical manifestations. Although previously considered as distinct clinical entities, mycosis fungoides (MF), Sézary syndrome (SS), reticulum cell sarcoma of the skin, and several other cutaneous lymphocytic dyscrasias are now recognized as different clinical presentations of CTCL.[1] All forms of CTCL are neoplasms of T lymphocytes, which home to skin and to the T-cell zones of lymphoid structures but generally not to bone marrow. The clinical value of the umbrella classification of CTCL is twofold. First, it highlights the relationship between distinct clinical presentations that can nevertheless evolve into one another (i.e., the plaque stage of MF can develop into the erythrodermic SS) or coexist [i.e., plaque-stage MF and lymphomatoid papulosis (LP)]. Second, the nomenclature emphasizes the clinical relevance of advances in the understanding of the biology of the malignant T cells. Recognition of the malignant clone-specific properties of the T-cell receptor (TCR) for antigen on the CTCL cells in individual patients has both provided the most sensitive diagnostic tool for the disease and offered an extraordinary target for selective immunologic attack of CTCL cells in such treatments as photopheresis. Still, it remains fairly useful for the clinician to attach the subtype of CTCL to the name (e.g., CTCL/MF), as the management scheme and prognosis for these subtypes differ.

PATHOBIOLOGY

CTCL is a clonal neoplasm[2–4] of mature CD4+ helper-inducer T cells,[5,6] which are capable of stimulating immunoglobulin synthesis by B cells,[7,8] perhaps by secretion of interleukin-4 (IL-4) or other cytokines.[9] CTCL cells also express BE-2, a molecule related to heat-shock proteins the function of which is yet unknown; the CD45RO marker characteristic of "memory" T cells[10]; and cutaneous lymphoid antigen (CLA), a glycoprotein that is expressed on the surface of only a small fraction of normal T cells in cutaneous infiltrates.[11] Both of the last two markers are simultaneously expressed on the surface of virtually all circulating CTCL cells. The deficiency of normal T cells that can accompany the systemic dissemination of lymphoma may reflect the production of IL-10, an inhibitory cytokine produced by those CTCL cells.

CLA is the physiologic ligand of endothelial cell E-selectin, a cell adhesion molecule expressed on the surface of endothelial cells of cutaneous venules during chronic inflammation.[12,13] Interactions between CLA on the surface of CTCL cells and E-selectin on endothelial cells allow CTCL cells to adhere to the walls of cutaneous venules, leave the circulation, and enter the skin.

Once CTCL cells enter into the skin, their most striking trait is their profound epidermotropism.[14] The latter may be a consequence of neoplastic and normal T-cell production of interferon-γ (IFN-γ), which stimulates keratinocytes to express the intracellular adhesion molecule-1 (ICAM-1) on their surface.[15] Because ICAM-1 is the physiologic ligand for lymphocyte function–associated antigen-1 expressed on the surface of all T cells, CTCL cells should adhere to keratinocytes exposed to IFN-γ.[16] In addition, there is evidence for avid binding of CTCL cells to keratinocytes by other, non-ICAM-1–dependent mechanisms.

In addition to producing cytokines, CTCL cells are exposed to a complex paracrine environment composed of many growth factors and cytokines elaborated by keratinocytes and stromal fibroblasts, macrophages, endothelial cells, and normal and neoplastic T lymphocytes. Preformed IL-1 may be released by proliferating keratinocytes to stimulate both keratinocytes and benign or neoplastic T cells to release granulocyte-macrophage colony-stimulating factor (GM-CSF) and macrophage colony-stimulating factor (M-CSF).[17] The latter two cytokines enhance the antigen-presenting capabilities of Langerhans' cells (LC) and activate resting macrophages, which respond by releasing a complex mix of cytokines active on keratinocytes, fibroblasts, and endothelial and lymphohematopoietic cells.[18]

In more advanced stages of disease, CTCL cells lose their dependence on epidermal cell adhesion molecules and cytokines so that their epidermotropism either is diminished (to permit the development of tumor nodules that extend deep into the dermis) or is lost completely (to permit dissemination of the neoplastic T cells to nodal and visceral sites). At this stage, the clinical presentation of CTCL may become indistinguishable from that of a peripheral T-cell lymphoma, although the broad involvement of the skin usually remains a distinguishing feature. Even at this advanced stage, the distinctive tissue distribution of the malignant cells (skin infiltration, preferential localization in interfollicular regions of lymph nodes, and avoidance of bone marrow) remains evident.

EPIDEMIOLOGY

CTCL is a relatively rare neoplasm, and the Surveillance, Epidemiology, and End Results program[19] reports that the incidence had increased 3.2-fold between 1973 and 1984. The overall incidence rate is approximately 4 per 1,000,000, according to data from that program.[22] The actual incidence rate may be an order of magnitude higher, given possible underreporting and the difficulty and confusion in making the diagnosis. The incidence of CTCL rises with age such that the majority of patients are between 40 and 60 years old. The disease is 2.2 times more common in male than in female subjects, and incidence rates are somewhat higher in African Americans than in whites.

ETIOLOGY

The inability to propagate CTCL cells *in vitro* after isolation from skin lesions, even from rapidly growing cutaneous tumors, has rendered molecular biologic studies of CTCL far less informative than they have been for many other lymphoid neoplasms; to date, the molecular etiology of CTCL remains unclear. However, at least one study has implicated rearrangements or deletions of the tal-1 and NFκB2/lyt-10 encoded transcription factors in a subset of CTCL patients with very aggressive disease.[133] In addition, transgenic mice that constitutively synthesize IL-7 develop extensive dermal infiltrates that progress to a cutaneous lymphoma resembling CTCL—results that suggest that overexpression of IL-7 might contribute to the development of CTCLs.[23,24] Such infiltrates develop even when the transgene is expressed in athymic nude mice, implying that the evolution of IL-7–induced dermal lymphoma may be dependent on the skin rather than on the thymus. Although the phenotypes of the lymphomatous T cells and their distribution in the skin are not identical with those of human CTCL, a refinement of this experimental system may ultimately provide an animal model for the human disorder.

Given the inherent immunologic nature of the neoplastic cells responsible for this disorder, it has been proposed that chronic exposure to occupational chemicals, pesticides, or tobacco may predispose to the development of CTCL; however, none of these potential associations has survived scrutiny.[20,21] The observations that the disease is more common in African Americans than in whites and that it often presents first in areas normally shielded from the sun (i.e., "bathing trunk" distribution) together suggest that actinic exposure may actually inhibit the evolution of the malignant clone from normal "cutaneous T cells." It is noteworthy that the epidermotropic collections of CTCL cells, referred to as *Pautrier microabscesses,* may represent congregation of malignant T cells around LC, the dendritic antigen-presenting cells (DC) of the epidermis, and that LC are fairly sensitive to ultraviolet (UV) damage. This observation has suggested that epidermotropic CTCL cells may receive growth signals from their contact with LC. Therefore, it is possible that UV damage of LC, more significant in whites than in African Americans (whose darker pigment shields the LC), may interrupt this growth signal and inhibit the replication of CTCL cells in UV-exposed skin sites. It is also intriguing that the often profound response of plaque-stage CTCL to UV treatment may reflect this phenomenon as well. The observation that individuals infected with the human T-cell leukemia virus type I (HTLV-I) often develop T-cell leukemias with skin involvement indistinguishable from those of CTCL has led some to hypothesize that CTCL may be a consequence of infection with HTLV-I or another unknown retrovirus, a possibility that remains the subject of active investigation.

CLINICAL PRESENTATION

MYCOSIS FUNGOIDES

The classic MF presentation of CTCL progresses through the following four distinct phases:

1. A premycotic phase with an asymptomatic, scaling erythematous macular eruption, often in sun-shielded areas (i.e., bathing trunk distribution), which lasts for months to years during which the diagnosis may be suspected but cannot be confirmed by standard clinical or histopathologic means
2. A patch phase with thin, barely palpable, erythematous and eczematous lesions the histologic features of which are at least "consistent with" the diagnosis of CTCL
3. A plaque phase with more readily palpable erythematous lesions
4. A tumor phase, in which the neoplastic infiltrate extends below the upper dermis

Painful erythroderma may arise *de novo* or during any of the earlier described phases and is not always associated with frank T-cell leukemia (SS). Infrequently, CTCL presents with cutaneous tumor nodules in the absence of patches or plaques. Patients may also present with involvement of internal organs.

RELATED CONDITIONS

The MF presentation of CTCL often manifests alongside (and can be confused with) several related, more benign cutaneous lymphoid dyscrasias. They include LP,[25–27] alopecia mucinosa–follicular mucinosis (AM-FM),[28,29] and pagetoid reticulosis (PR).[30] CTCL also has features in common with two other, clearly malignant disorders: adult T-cell leukemia-lymphoma (ATLL) and CD30+ anaplastic large cell lymphoma.

LP is a dermatologic disorder that resembles pityriasis lichenoides et varioliformis acuta. LP lesions often appear as groups of erythematous brown papules that develop a scale or crust. Resolving LP lesions may leave residual pigment or superficial atrophic scars. Depending on the clinical series, from 5% to 20% of patients with LP eventually develop a non-B-cell lymphoma, most often CTCL. Regressing atypical histiocytosis is thought to be a variant of LP.

AM is an infiltrative, cutaneous T-cell dyscrasia also known as *follicular mucinosis* (FM). AM-FM is characterized by the accumulation of acid mucopolysaccharides in the sebaceous glands and root sheaths of hair follicles. When the lesions of AM-FM develop in a hair-bearing area, patchy alopecia may be their presenting sign. Overall, 15% to 30% of AM-FM patients either have or will develop CTCL.

PR, or Woringer-Kolopp disease, presents as a solitary cutaneous lesion of long duration and is characterized histologically by significant numbers of abnormal mononuclear cells infiltrating the epidermis. The underlying dermis is involved by a mixed inflammatory cell infiltrate. Clonal T-cell gene rearrangements have been observed in PR, which, in all likelihood, represents an indolent, particularly epidermotropic variant of CTCL.

ADULT T-CELL LEUKEMIA-LYMPHOMA AND CD30+ ANAPLASTIC LARGE CELL LYMPHOMAS

ATLL is a disorder that develops in some HTLV-I-infected individuals. The clinical presentation of ATLL is often acute, with rapidly growing cutaneous lesions, hypercalcemia, marked lymphadenopathy, and infiltration of visceral organs.[100–102] Patients also present with systemic symptoms, such as drenching night sweats and weight loss and, in marked contrast to CTCL, the diagnosis of ATLL is usually made soon after presentation. Patients may present with a leukemic form of ATLL with extremely high white blood cell counts or may present a lymphomatous variant. ATLL patients are often severely immunocompromised and are susceptible to a variety of opportunistic pathogens. Peripheral blood and cutaneous lymphocytes often express high levels of IL-2 receptor. Current therapy for ATLL consists of simultaneous antiretroviral therapy (zidovudine) and IFN.[103]

Ki-1 (CD30+) anaplastic large cell lymphoma may occur primarily in the skin or with systemic involvement. Patients may present with tumor-like lesions with central ulceration, which may undergo spontaneous regression. Systemic involvement is unusual, and cutaneous lesions may be treated with radiation therapy alone. However, lesions often relapse, even though the overall clinical course may be indolent.[130] Patients with systemic disease, age older than 60 years, or whose tumors do not spontaneously regress appear to have a less favorable prognosis. Anaplastic (vs. nonanaplastic) cell histology does not imply a poorer prognosis; however, prognosis is poor for those patients whose tumors are CD30–.[131] Serum levels of CD30 may serve as a marker for response to therapy.[132]

APPROACH TO PATIENTS WITH MYCOSIS FUNGOIDES

The most important clinical prognostic variables related to CTCL are the type of lesion and the percentage of the total skin surface involved, nodal involvement, dissemination to visceral sites, and the presence of CTCL cells in the circulation. These parameters have been codified in the modified TNM staging classification (Table 45.4-1) proposed by the Cutaneous T-Cell Lymphoma Workshop in 1979.[31] Also, this staging system has yet to be modified to incorporate the many clinical, immunologic, and molecular biologic discoveries relevant to the diagnosis and treatment of CTCL.

SKIN LESIONS

Prognosis in CTCL patients depends on both the type of lesions and the extent of cutaneous involvement. All patients should have the number and distribution of each type of lesion and an estimate of the total skin surface involved by CTCL carefully recorded before initiation of therapy. Patients with patches or plaques that involve less than 10% of the body surface (stage T1) are far more likely to be palliated over the long term or cured than those with the same types of lesions occupying more than 10% of the skin surface (stage T2) (Fig. 45.4-1). Prognosis is significantly worse for patients with cutaneous tumors (T3), although it is better for patients with less than 10% of their skin surface involved by tumors than for those with more extensive involvement (Fig. 45.4-2).[128] Prognosis is poorer still for patients with erythroderma either alone or in addition to patches, plaques, and tumors.

Skin biopsies at multiple sites may be necessary to define T-stage, as lesion morphology varies from patient to patient and for different lesions from the same patient.

However, because the histopathologic criteria for the diagnosis of early CTCL are not firmly established and there is significant interobserver variability in the pathologic interpretation of

TABLE 45.4-1. TNM Classification of Cutaneous T-Cell Lymphomas

TNM DEFINITIONS	
Skin[a]	
Tumor (T)	
T0	Clinically or histopathologically suspicious lesions
T1	Limited plaques, papules, or eczematous patches covering <10% of the skin surface
T2	Generalized plaques, papules, or erythematous patches covering 10% of the skin surface
T3	Tumors
T4	Generalized erythroderma
Lymph nodes (N)[b]	
N0	No clinically abnormal peripheral lymph nodes, negative for CTCL
N1	Clinically abnormal peripheral lymph nodes, pathology negative for CTCL
N2	No clinically abnormal peripheral lymph nodes, pathology positive for CTCL
N3	Clinically abnormal peripheral lymph nodes, pathology positive for CTCL
Visceral organs	
Metastases (M)	
M0	No visceral organ involvement
M1	Visceral involvement (must have pathology confirmation and organ involved should be specified)

STAGE GROUPING			
IA	T1	N0	M0
IB	T2	N0	M0
IIA	T1–2	N1	M0
IIB	T3	N0–1	M0
III	T4	N0–1	M0
IVA	T1–4	N2–3	M0
IVB	T1–4	N0–3	M1

CTCL, cutaneous T-cell lymphoma.
[a]Pathology of T1 to T4 is diagnostic of cutaneous T-cell lymphoma. When more than one T stage exists, both are recorded, and the highest is used for staging [e.g., T4(3)].
[b]Record number of sites of abnormal nodes [e.g., cervical (left and right)].
Note: The complete classification contains a category in which the number of circulating atypical cells is noted. This category, however, has never been used for the clinical staging and is, therefore, not included here. It has not been demonstrated that it is a useful parameter in this classification.

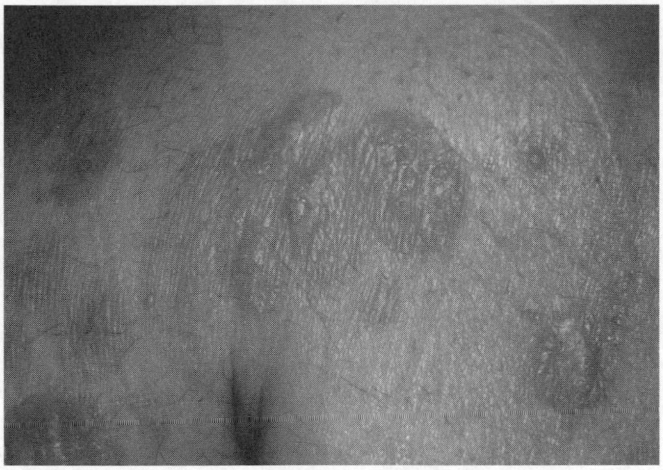

FIGURE 45.4-1. Patch-plaque (T1 to T2 disease). (See Color Fig. 45.4-1 in the CD-ROM and on the Web at www.LWWoncology.com.)

the same specimens,[32] accurate definition of T-stage and diagnostic correlation with pathologic material is far from routine. Such problems are especially evident for early patch or plaque lesions wherein only a small fraction of the infiltrating T lymphocytes (confined exclusively to the epidermis) are actually neoplastic. Most of the cells in the underlying, often much more impressive, dermal infiltrate are nonneoplastic, reactive CD4+ and CD8+ T lymphocytes and represent the host's immune response to the neoplastic clone. This typical histopathologic pattern can be significantly modified by prior therapy, as even topical steroids can significantly alter the intensity and appearance of both the neoplastic and nonneoplastic lymphoid infiltrates.

CTCL biopsy specimens should be reviewed by dermatopathologists with specific experience and interest in the study and diagnosis of CTCL. Specimens that exhibit epidermal collections of lymphocytes (i.e., Pautrier's microabscesses) with characteristic hyperchromatic, irregularly shaped nuclei without spongiosis are interpreted as "diagnostic" for CTCL, and those that exhibit at least two of these features (epidermal collections of lymphocytes, atypical nuclei, or absence of spongiosis) are judged "consistent with" CTCL. Histopathologic features of "transformation" to a high-grade lymphoma, such as an enlarged pale nucleus and prominent nucleoli or loss of normal T-cell markers, are all associated with a poorer prognosis.

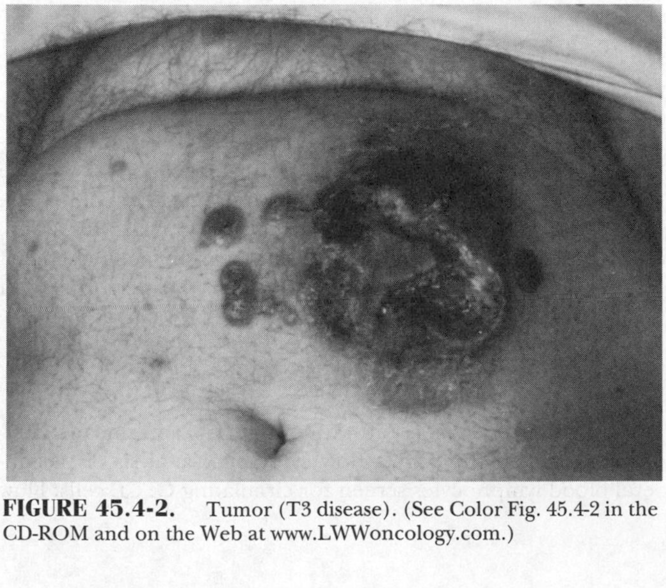

FIGURE 45.4-2. Tumor (T3 disease). (See Color Fig. 45.4-2 in the CD-ROM and on the Web at www.LWWoncology.com.)

In an attempt to quantitate more precisely the histopathologic features of CTCL, one group of investigators has attempted to use vertical measurements (analogous to the Breslow level in melanoma) to delineate the depth of the cutaneous infiltrates.[33] In their preliminary analysis, a positive correlation with morbidity was noted for the distance from the granular layer of the epidermis to the lower limit of the CTCL infiltrate. Cell density has also been found to correlate with clinical outcomes. Jones et al.[144] have demonstrated that cell density predicted remission and progression-free, overall, and cause-specific survival after total skin electron-beam therapy (TSEBT).

Skin biopsies should also be subjected to immunophenotyping to define better the identity of the benign and neoplastic cell populations present in the cutaneous lesions. Several studies have reported correlations between the immunophenotypes of the cells present in the infiltrates and stage of disease. In general, as disease progresses, fewer CD8+ cells are observed, and the relative ratio of CD4+ to CD8+ cells increases.[34,35] However, in one rare and clinically very aggressive form of CTCL, the neoplastic T cells are CD8–, CD4–, as they have undergone Γδ– but not αβ–TCR chain rearrangement.[126]

Immunogenotyping of skin biopsies can help to define whether an early lesion suggestive of CTCL actually contains a clonal T-cell population. Such analyses are best performed by polymerase chain reaction–based (PCR-based) techniques, as one rarely obtains sufficient neoplastic cell DNA from skin biopsies for routine Southern blot analyses. PCR analysis is performed with primers designed to amplify TCR Γ chain rearrangements that occur in all T cells before rearrangement of the α and β chain loci. Such PCR-based assays are able to detect clonal T-cell populations in 90% of skin biopsies that show diagnostic CTCL pathology. The 10% false-negative rate may reflect the fact that the currently available PCR primer pairs amplify only 90% of Γ chain variable regions. This high degree of sensitivity contrasts with the somewhat lower (79%) sensitivity of standard Southern blot techniques that require significantly more DNA.[36]

LYMPH NODES

The incidence of lymphadenopathy increases with T-stage and is associated with a poorer prognosis. Imaging studies (computed tomography scan or magnetic resonance imaging) are recommended at initial evaluation for those with advanced disease and during follow-up to detect enlargement of thoracic, abdominal, or pelvic nodes. In practice, biopsy of uninvolved nodal sites is uncommon; lymph nodes are subjected to biopsy either at initial staging or afterward only if they are found to be obviously enlarged on physical examination or imaging studies.

Flow cytometry, immunophenotyping, and Southern blot (or PCR-based) genotyping for clonality are recommended for all nodal samples and may detect neoplastic T cells even in so-called reactive, dermatopathic (stage N1) nodes not obviously involved by CTCL. In a study of lymph node samples from 17 patients with stage N1 disease, eight showed evidence of clonal T-cell abnormalities consistent with CTCL on Southern blotting, and these eight patients had a poorer prognosis than those whose nodes were free of CTCL.[37] Another study of lymph nodes in patients with CTCL revealed that specific histologic factors were predictive of outcome. Those patients with small cell infiltrates had a median survival of 40 months, and

TABLE 45.4-2. Peripheral Blood Values of Six Patients with Advanced Cutaneous T-Cell Lymphoma

Patient	*Total Lymphocyte Count*[a]	*CD4:CD8 Ratio*[b]	*Sézary Syndrome (%)*[c]	*Vb (%)*[d]
1	7184	50	32	67
2	794	10	10	32
3	684	13	7	74
4	3276	17	9	78
5	5160	90	13	87
6	3650	14	5	59

[a]Normal range, 1500–3000.
[b]Normal range, 0.5–3.5.
[c]Sézary cells are expressed as a percentage of lymphocytes; normal range, 0–5%.
[d]Percentage of lymphocytes expressing a particular β chain variable region; normal range, 0–5%. In patients in whom there is an identifiable Vβ region, the values in this column represent the percentage of lymphocytes that are malignant.

those with high-grade immunoblastic features had a median survival of only 9 months.[38]

PERIPHERAL BLOOD

The level of circulating neoplastic cells in CTCL patients correlates adversely with prognosis and is an important parameter to document and quantitate both at presentation and during follow-up. The application of nearly clone-specific, family-specific antibodies against the Vβ regions of TCRs has also revealed that morphologic evaluations alone often grossly underestimate the level of circulating CTCL cells.

In normal individuals, none of the more than 50 available anti-Vβ monoclonal antibodies (mAbs) react with more than 2% to 5% of the circulating peripheral T cells. As shown in Table 45.4-2, it is possible to use these mAbs to detect and quantitate precisely the levels of circulating CTCL cells. Such analyses have revealed a remarkable clinical heterogeneity within patients who present with T4 disease. In most, the level of circulating CTCL cells is actually much higher than estimated by less sensitive techniques.[39] In some, the expansion of the neoplastic T-cell clone is accompanied by depression of normal T cells to levels comparable with those observed in advanced acquired immunodeficiency syndrome. Such a *de facto* T-cell deficiency may both explain the susceptibility of erythrodermic CTCL patients to infection by bacterial, viral, and fungal pathogens[129] and contribute to the progression of the disease, which is often held in check by host immune mechanisms.

In the absence of such specific anti-CTCL mAbs, flow cytometry and Southern blot (or PCR-based) analyses of Γ chain rearrangements can be used to detect and quantitate circulating CTCL more accurately. Flow cytometry should be performed with antibodies to the CD4, CD8, CD3, CD45R0, and CD20 antigens. The ratio of CD4+ to CD8+ cells is normally 0.5:3.5; elevations in this ratio correlate with total leukocyte count and with extent of skin disease in CTCL patients. An elevated ratio of CD4+ to CD8+ cells in excess of 4.5:1 reliably indicates significant levels of circulating CTCL cells, and a routine leukocyte count, manual differential, and smear supplemented by a measurement of the CD4:CD8 ratio serve as a good initial screen for circulating CTCL cells. If flow cytometric analysis reveals a marked elevation of the CD4:CD8 ratio or an elevation in the percentage of CD45R0+ cells, it is worthwhile to perform flow cytometry with anti-Vβ mAbs to determine whether a clonal expansion of T cells is present.

If any of the aforementioned studies suggest the presence of circulating CTCL cells, the more laborious and expensive TCR gene rearrangement studies to confirm their presence are also worthwhile. Even standard Southern blot assay for TCR rearrangement can detect a neoplastic clone that represents only 1% of the total lymphocyte population and, thus, is far more sensitive in detecting circulating CTCL cells than any of the previously mentioned techniques, including flow cytometry. Nonetheless, in only approximately 10% of CTCL cases with circulating cells are Southern blots the only laboratory abnormality. In one study of 11 CTCL patients in whom circulating CTCL cells were documented by Southern blotting, ten also had CD4:CD8 ratios greater than 10:1. Only one patient's CD4:CD8 ratio was less than 2:1.[40]

PATIENT EVALUATION

HISTORY

The duration of the eruption and the evolution of its distribution should be carefully noted. The patient should also be asked about cutaneous integrity, temperature imbalance, fissuring, pruritus, and the use of moisturizers.

PHYSICAL EXAMINATION

A complete physical examination should be performed with particular attention to the skin and lymph nodes. Examination of the skin should record the number of lesions, including their type (patch, plaque, tumor, or erythroderma), distribution, and the percentage of skin surface involved by CTCL lesions (i.e., by the "rule of nines" used in the evaluation of burn patients). Evaluation of the abdomen should be performed to detect hepatosplenomegaly, and the site, size, and number of palpable peripheral lymph nodes should be recorded.

DIAGNOSTIC TESTS

Dermatopathology

At least two skin biopsies should be obtained for routine hematoxylin and eosin histopathology. Frozen specimens should be harvested for immunophenotyping for the CD2, CD3, CD4, CD5, CD7, CD8, CD19, CD20, CD25, CD30, CD45R0, CD56, βF1, and δ antigens. PCR for Γ chain rearrangements and, if available, β chain rearrangements should be performed on either the paraffin or frozen section tissue.

Peripheral Blood Evaluation

A complete blood cell count with differential and smear examination supplemented by a flow cytometric analysis of peripheral blood lymphocytes screen for circulating CTCL cells. Flow cytometric analysis can measure peripheral blood involvement by revealing an elevation of the CD4:CD8 ratio, an increase in CD4+CD7– lymphocytes, or an elevation of CD45R0+ lymphocytes. The interpretation of these findings is facilitated by the demonstration of the malignant clone by PCR testing for gene rearrangement in the peripheral blood. The latter, in turn, is facilitated by similar PCR testing on the patient's skin biopsy. If the clone is detectable in skin, the test is useful in the peripheral blood. If the clone is undetectable by PCR, this method is not interpretable when performed on the peripheral blood.

Other Studies

A posteroanterior and a lateral chest radiograph should be performed in all patients. Computed tomography or magnetic resonance scans should be carried out of the chest, abdomen, and pelvis both to evaluate mediastinal, retroperitoneal, and pelvic nodes as well as to supplement physical examination of the axillary and inguinal nodes in patients with T3 and T4 disease.[122] The location of pathologically enlarged nodes should be noted and their size recorded. Such enlarged nodes should undergo biopsy (preferably by excision rather than needle sampling) to document both the presence of neoplastic T cells and the histopathologic pattern of involvement (i.e., dermatopathic adenopathy vs. more extensive replacement). The latter can be supplemented by immunophenotypic and TCR rearrangement analyses to document the presence of neoplastic T cells. Bone marrow evaluation is not routinely performed unless abnormalities are noted on complete blood cell count or smear.

TABLE 45.4-3. General Management of Cutaneous T-Cell Lymphoma

PATIENTS WITH T1 DISEASE (PATCHES OR PLAQUES <10% OF SURFACE)
Topical chemotherapy
PUVA
Localized external-beam radiotherapy
PATIENTS WITH T2 DISEASE (PATCHES OR PLAQUES >10% OF SURFACE)
PUVA
Topical chemotherapy
TSEBT
PATIENTS WITH T3 DISEASE (TUMORS)
TSEBT
TSEBT and PUVA
TSEBT and ECP
Investigational modalities
PATIENTS WITH T4 DISEASE (ERYTHRODERMA)
ECP
TSEBT and ECP
Interferon
Investigational modalities
PALLIATION OF VISCERAL DISEASE
Systemic chemotherapy (nucleotide derivatives)
Photon irradiation

ECP, extracorporeal photochemotherapy; PUVA, psoralen and ultraviolet A therapy; TSEBT, total skin electron-beam therapy.

PRINCIPLES OF THERAPY

The therapy for CTCLs is fairly distinct from that of other lymphomas. Hence, many therapeutic strategies that have proved successful with localized and disseminated B-cell lymphomas have often been found to be inappropriate for CTCL. CTCL is first and foremost a disease of cutaneous lymphocytes. Hence, early-stage disease that is localized to the skin has an excellent chance of cure with therapies directed to the skin alone. However, disease that has disseminated and become established in lymph nodes or visceral sites (liver, lung, central nervous system) can be palliated but rarely cured, even with the most aggressive regimens of systemic chemotherapy. This result contrasts with that seen in B-cell lymphomas in which patients with extensive nodal and visceral disease are often cured by aggressive combination chemotherapy or bone marrow or stem cell transplantation.

Effective therapies for CTCL include both skin-directed and systemic therapies (Table 45.4-3). Skin-directed therapy includes topical chemotherapy with such agents as carmustine (BCNU) and nitrogen mustard (NM), systemically administered psoralens activated in the skin by psoralen and ultraviolet A light (PUVA) therapy, and local and generalized superficial ionizing radiation that includes both electron-beam and x-ray therapy.

All skin-directed therapies exert their primary effects on disease confined to the skin. All are capable of destroying CTCL cells directly, probably by triggering T-lymphocyte apoptosis,[127] and all interfere with the local production of cytokines by epithelial and stromal cells necessary for neoplastic T-cell survival and proliferation.

Photopheresis, a systemic immunologic therapy, acts both directly by killing T lymphocytes by the cytotoxic actions of UVA light/psoralen and indirectly by eliciting anti–CTCL cell immune responses. Similarly, other systemic agents, such as retinoids and the biologic response modifiers (IFN-α and -Γ) may exert their therapeutic effects by modifying production by keratinocytes and dermal fibroblasts of cytokines necessary for neoplastic T-cell survival and proliferation. This is in addition to any direct cytotoxic or cytostatic effects they exert on benign and neoplastic T lymphocytes.[41]

TOPICAL CHEMOTHERAPY

Therapy for T1 and T2 CTCL can be carried out with either topical mechlorethamine (NM) or BCNU, both potent DNA-alkylating agents. Topical NM therapy is generally administered daily with a fresh solution of 10 mg in 50 mL tap water, which is applied to the entire body surface. Because NM is a potent irritant, patients should wear protective plastic gloves while applying the solution. Topical NM therapy results in delayed hypersensitivity reactions in up to 40% of patients, who often require at least temporary cessation of therapy. Such reactions can be circumvented by induction of tolerance to NM by topical desensitization or by PUVA-induced suppression of the hypersensitivity reaction. Ointment-based NM is less likely to induce allergic reactions and, in its typical formulation of 10 mg/dL, NM in Aquaphor is stable at room temperature.

Other side effects of topical NM therapy include induction of second cutaneous malignancies (e.g., squamous cell carcinomas), hyperpigmentation, and hypopigmentation. Between 64% and 90% of NM-treated patients with T1 and T2 CTCL can achieve a complete response (CR) to therapy. In one series of 243 patients, the median survival of treated patients was 8 years, and the response rate was better in those with less extensive disease.[42] Although some patients appear to be cured by topical NM therapy, seven of eight patients experience relapse within 3 years unless a maintenance topical NM regimen has been instituted. Maintenance topical NM can also be used to prevent or delay relapse of cutaneous lesions in patients who have achieved a CR to TSEBT or to treat minimal patch or plaque recurrences after such therapy.[75,149]

Another topical chemotherapeutic agent useful in the treatment of CTCL is BCNU. Because topical BCNU is not immunologically cross-reactive with NM, this agent can be used in patients who have developed allergies to NM. Topical BCNU can be formulated either as a 10- to 40-mg/dL ointment stable indefinitely at room temperature or as a 25- to 50-mg/dL solution in dilute alcohol, which is stable for at least 3 months when refrigerated.

Cutaneous hypersensitivity reactions to topical BCNU are rare and, in one series, such reactions interfered with continuation of therapy in only 10 of 152 patients. However, significant erythema in the treated areas and posttreatment telangiectasia occur in one of three patients. Also, as a small fraction of the drug is absorbed, marrow suppression can occur but is unusual unless the total dose exceeds 600 mg (in increments of 20 to 25 mg).[43] Therefore, hematologic monitoring is necessary when using BCNU.

PSORALEN AND ULTRAVIOLET A THERAPY

Cutaneous photochemotherapy with orally administered PUVA irradiation of the skin, or PUVA therapy, kills cutaneous lymphocytes and interferes with antigen presentation and cytokine production in the skin. PUVA therapy is also able to induce complete remissions as reliably as TSEBT therapy in CTCL patients with patches or thin plaques. In patients with thicker plaques or tumors, PUVA therapy alone is unlikely to produce a CR but may be used to maintain the CRs induced by other skin-directed therapies, including TSEBT.

PUVA therapy requires the ingestion of 0.6 mg/kg of 8-methoxypsoralen (8-MOP) 1 to 2 hours before the exposure of the skin surface to UVA light (320 to 400 nm). To induce remission, treatments should begin three times per week at doses that are minimally phototoxic. After most of the lesions have cleared, the frequency of PUVA can be decreased to twice weekly until the patient has achieved a CR.[44] Such a schedule of multiple treatments per week must be maintained for a minimum of 3 months and a maximum of 6 months. If a CR has not been achieved by this time, several strategies can be used to supplement or enhance the efficacy of PUVA. We have often used local spot x-ray or electron-beam therapy to treat lesions refractory to PUVA, particularly in regions anatomically shielded from receiving the full UVA dose. Addition of such "PUVA boosters" as IFNs, retinoids, or oral methotrexate can also be considered.

INTERFERON

IFN-α at doses of 3 to 6 MU can help to clear skin lesions refractory to PUVA alone.[45] However, the systemic side effects of such therapy can be troublesome, although some patients experience no significant toxicity. Retinoids also have a role as adjunctive agents in achieving remission or palliating symptoms. Retinoids for acne and psoriasis have been used in the past. However, the ability of bexarotene to improve CTCL as monotherapy[46] suggests that it will supplant other retinoids in the adjunctive role with PUVA and other therapies. If such boosters are successful, maintenance PUVA therapy alone should be sufficient to maintain disease-free status.

Once a CR has been achieved, PUVA is administered once weekly as maintenance therapy for 1 year. If the remission is sustained, the interval between treatments can be extended to 2 weeks for a total of 26 sessions per year for an additional year. If there is still no evidence of relapse, the interval between treatments can be extended to 3 weeks and continued for another 2 years. Interruptions of maintenance PUVA due to intercurrent illness or injury can be followed by recurrence of disease, sometimes within 1 or 2 months. After 5 years of maintenance therapy, consideration can be given to cessation of therapy or to extending the interval between PUVA treatments to 4 to 6 weeks.

Patients may be free of disease at this stage, but studies of patients treated with TSEBT have noted relapses at times more than 5 years later, particularly in those with T2 disease.[64] Whether such late relapses are the consequence of the persistence and regrowth of the original neoplastic clone or are "true" second primary CTCLs has not yet been defined. It is also not known whether such "late" recurrences or second primaries will also be observed in patients who have received 5 years of maintenance PUVA. However, patients should probably not be considered "cured" until they have remained disease-free for at least 5 years after completing therapy. Some reports suggest that PUVA therapy may result in true "cures," because the mortality rate from early disease was decreased after the adoption of PUVA as the standard therapy for CTCL in Scandinavia.[47]

LOCAL EXTERNAL-BEAM IRRADIATION

Local x-ray therapy for CTCL lesions was first reported in 1902 by Scholtz, less than a decade after the discovery of x-rays by Roentgen.[48] The cutaneous lesions of CTCL are extremely radioresponsive, and a dose-response relationship has been demonstrated.[49–51] Superficial [30 to 125 kV(p)] and orthovoltage [125 to 500 kV(p)] x-rays as well as electrons can be used to treat localized primary or recurrent patches, plaques, and tumors.[52] Doses between 20 and 36 Gy are effective in fractional sizes of 1 to 2 Gy, depending on the size and location of the lesions. Such therapy is rarely first-line but can be considered for the unusual patient with very localized primary patches, plaques, or tumors. Local x-ray or electron-beam therapy in similar doses is also fairly effective in clearing isolated lesions that fail to respond to PUVA or recur after CR to PUVA or TSEBT.

Local treatment of isolated lesions is very effective, and the CR rate is in excess of 90% for both plaques and tumors. Cotter et al.[51] demonstrated that none of nine patients failed when treated with doses in excess of 30 Gy, with a minimum of 1 year follow-up. Approximately 5% of patients with stage IA disease will present with a solitary cutaneous lesion or several in close proximity. Wilson et al.[145] have found that the rate of clinical remission after local external-beam radiotherapy is 97%. A total of 21 patients were evaluated with a minimum follow-up of 1 year and treated to a median dose of 20 Gy. Seventeen of the 21 patients received 20 Gy or higher. The median follow-up was 36 months. The actuarial disease-free survival (DFS) rates at 5 and 10 years were 75% and 64%, respectively, with a local control rate of 75% at 10 years. Acute and chronic toxicities were minor, and such treatment does not preclude TSEBT in the future. For metastatic disease (e.g., nodes, central nervous system and spine and lung involvement), radiation with 4 to 20 Gy may provide a meaningful palliative response.

TOTAL SKIN ELECTRON-BEAM THERAPY

Principles of Application

Treatment of the entire cutaneous surface with TSEBT is technically much more challenging than local x-ray therapy and should be attempted only in centers with appropriate equipment and in which a close working relationship has been established between dermatologists and radiation oncologists committed to and experienced in the treatment of patients with CTCL. TSEBT is excellent treatment for patients with diffuse involvement with thick plaques or cutaneous tumors and is also suitable for patients with symptomatic erythroderma (T4 disease). TSEBT is also an excellent alternative for patients with extensive patches or thin plaques refractory to PUVA or other skin-directed therapies.

The application of TSEBT for the treatment of CTCL was first reported by Trump et al.[52] in 1953, and since that time, a variety of fractionation schedules and techniques have been implemented.[53–64] In 1960, Karzmark et al.[55] described the details of the "Stanford technique" for the administration of TSEBT, which was later modified to a six-field array to improve the homogeneity of dose delivered to the total skin surface.[65,66,67]

Electrons ranging in energy between 4 and 7 MeV are used to treat the epidermis and dermis homogeneously. Structures below the deep dermis are spared, as most of the dose (80%) is delivered within the first 1.0 cm, and less than 5% beyond 2.0 cm depth. Blood and superficial lymph nodes may receive 20% to 40% of the skin surface dose.

At Yale, treatment is offered via a Varian 6-MeV linear accelerator at a treatment distance of 7 m, with a single incident beam energy of 3.9 MeV at the skin. Therapy is delivered via six fields, and supplemental local boosts to the scalp, perineum, and soles of the feet are administered with 120-kV(p) x-rays. Treatment is delivered to the six fields over a 2-day cycle, with three of six fields (anteroposterior, left posterior oblique, right posterior oblique) treated on the first day and the remaining three (posteroanterior, left anterior oblique, right anterior oblique) on the second. External and internal eye shields are used sequentially throughout, and the hands and feet are shielded for 50% of the treatment course. Patients receive TSEBT 4 days per week for a total of 9 weeks, and the boost fields are treated concurrently.

The dose to the skin surface is 36 Gy, 4 Gy/wk and usually fractionated over 4 days and two cycles. Photon contamination to the body is 1.2% of the electron dose. Supplemental boosts to the scalp, perineum, and soles of the feet are 6 Gy (2 Gy/d), 20 Gy, and 20 Gy (1 Gy/d), respectively. Areas "shadowed" from the electron beam by large pendulous breasts, abdominal panniculi, or other deep skin folds receive similar boosts with 15 to 20 Gy (1 to 2 Gy/d) of electron-beam or orthovoltage x-ray therapy. Gross tumor lesions that have not completely regressed by the completion of TSEBT should also be evaluated for supplementary boost via x-ray or electron-beam therapy.

More commonly, a dual-beam six-field arrangement has been used.[143] Although the techniques differ between Yale and Hamilton, for example, the dosimetry is similar, as are the clinical results.[140] Regardless of technique, it should be noted that 4 MeV electron energy and more than 30 Gy to the skin surface are recommended. Jones and Thorson[146] have demonstrated (as have other investigators) that improved progression-free, cause-specific, and overall survival are related to these parameters.

Results

Clinical CR rates for patients with T1 or T2 (patch or plaque) disease range from 71% to 98% and are higher in patients with less extensive disease. Representative data on disease-free and overall survival are presented in Tables 45.4-4 and 45.4-5. In our institution, patients with T1 and T2 disease treated with TSEBT have disease-free and overall survivals of 50% to 65% and 80% to 90%, respectively, at 5 years, although patients with antecedent or coexisting LP or AM-FM appear to have shorter DFS after TSEBT than those who do not.[64] Patients with more advanced T3 and T4 disease fare significantly worse, with 5-year disease-free and overall survivals of approximately 20% and 50%, respectively. However, those T3 patients with less than 10% of the total skin surface involved by CTCL have significantly better disease-free and overall survival after TSEBT than those with more extensive disease.[128]

For patients with erythrodermic MF (T4) who are managed with TSEBT alone (32 to 40 Gy), without concomitant or neoadjuvant therapy, the CR rate is 74%. The 5-year progression-free, cause-specific, and overall survivals are 26%, 52%, and 38%, respectively.[147]

Palliation of adenopathy or visceral involvement in patients with N3 disease can be accomplished by the use of appropriate high-energy orthovoltage or megavoltage photons to doses of 20 to 30 Gy. Even 6 to 8 Gy in 3 fractions is sufficient if added during TSEBT. Combinations of TSEBT with total nodal irradiation have been investigated. Although feasible, such combinations do not appear to prolong survival and may be associated with hematologic toxicities not observed with TSEBT alone.[68,69]

TOXICITY. TSEBT is well tolerated by most patients, and acute sequelae either during or within the initial 6 months after treatment may include pruritus, desquamation, epilation, hypohidrosis, xerosis, erythema, lower-extremity edema, bullae of the feet, and onychoptosis. Chronic changes can include atrophy of the skin, telangiectasia, alopecia, hypohidrosis, and xerosis.[70] Because of the superficial penetration of the electron beam, patients do not experience gastrointestinal or hematologic toxicities. Second malignancies, such as squamous and basal cell carcinomas, as well as malignant melanomas have been observed in patients treated with TSEBT, and such risk is likely increased by other mutagenic, skin-directed therapies, such as PUVA or mechlorethamine (or both). It is interesting that additional

TABLE 45.4-4. Progression-Free Survival and Remission Rates for Mycosis Fungoides Patients after Total Skin Electron-Beam Therapy

			Progression-Free Survival		
	No. of Patients	*CR (%)*	2.5 Y (%)	5.0 Y (%)	7.5 Y (%)
ND					
IA	99	95	68	54	51
IB	58	88	41	20	9
IIA	13	85	18	18	
IIB	12	75	42	31	16
III	8	75	45	45	—
IVA	6	83	42	—	—
IVB	1	100	—	—	—
FPT					
IA	22	73	54	27	27
IB	24	83	34	34	34
IIA	13	77	50	17	—
IIB	14	43	0	—	—
III	2	50	—	—	—
IVA	7	71	—	—	—
IVB	3	67	—	—	—

CR, complete response; FPT, failed prior therapy; ND, newly diagnosed.
Note: Ascertained by stage. Data recorded at Hamilton Regional Cancer Center (282 patients).

x-ray or electron-beam irradiation after TSEBT does not appear to increase the risk of second cutaneous malignancies.[71,72]

REPEAT TREATMENT. For patients who have diffuse cutaneous recurrences after TSEBT not amenable to other skin-directed therapies, a second course of TSEBT is both feasible and worthwhile.[60,73,74] At Yale, a total of 14 patients have received two, and five patients have received three courses of TSEBT. The median total dose after these additional courses was 57 Gy, and 86% of the patients achieved a CR after the second course, with a median disease-free interval of 11.5 months. Median dose was 36 Gy for the first course, 18 Gy for the second, and 12 Gy for the third.[73] A similar experience was reported from Stanford, where 15 patients were identified who had been treated with a second course of TSEBT (median dose, 20 Gy), with a CR rate of 40%. Nine of these patients had a partial response to therapy, and the median total dose for the entire group was 56 Gy. In both series, repeat courses were relatively well tolerated, and sequelae were similar to those observed during and after the first course of therapy.[74] Both studies also support the contention that the palliative benefits of additional courses of TSEBT outweigh their risks in appropriately selected patients. Criteria for retreatment include an extended disease-free interval after the first course of TSEBT, a CR to the initial course, diffuse cutaneous involvement, and the failure of other palliative modalities.

TABLE 45.4-5. Overall Survival at 5 and 10 Years for Mycosis Fungoides Patients after Total Skin Electron-Beam Therapy

		Overall Survival	
	No. of Patients	5 Y (%)	10 Y (%)
ND			
IA	99	95	92
IB	58	91	81
IIA	13	63	63
IIB	12	55	41
III	8	50	50
IVA	6	100	100
IVB	1	—	—
FPT			
IA	22	83	—
IB	24	76	76
IIA	13	42	31
IIB	14	34	26
III	2	—	—
IVA	7	67	—
IVB	3	—	—

FPT, failed prior therapy; ND, newly diagnosed.
Note: Data recorded at Hamilton Regional Cancer Center (282 patients).

COMBINED AND SEQUENTIAL THERAPY. Several other CTCL therapies, including topical NM, systemic chemotherapy, etretinate, PUVA, and extracorporeal photochemotherapy (ECP) have been administered concomitantly with or adjuvantly after TSEBT with varying degrees of success.[75–78]

We have observed that the adjuvant use of PUVA after TSEBT in patients with T1 and T2 disease significantly decreases cutaneous relapse. Patients treated with adjuvant PUVA after TSEBT had a 5-year DFS of 85%, compared to 50% for those not receiving PUVA ($P<.02$). The median DFS for the T1 patients receiving adjuvant PUVA was not reached at 103 months, versus 66 months for the non-PUVA group ($P<.01$). For those with T2 disease, the DFS figures were 60 and 20 months, respectively ($P<.03$).[78,148] Adjuvant topical NM also appears able to delay cutaneous recurrence after TSEBT. At

Stanford, the median DFS of patients was prolonged from 29 to 37 months by the addition of topical NM therapy after TSEBT.[75] In 1999, Chinn et al.[149] from Stanford showed that TSEBT with or without NM provided improved response rates as compared to mustard alone for those patients with T2 and T3 level disease, respectively (76% vs. 39%; $P = .03$ for T2; 44% vs. 8%; $P < .05$ for T3). For those with patch-plaque (T2), adjuvant mustard offered improved freedom from relapse after TSEBT as compared to no adjuvant treatment. No significant survival difference was noted between the groups.[149]

Concurrent use of systemic chemotherapy with TSEBT was evaluated in a randomized clinical trial conducted by Kaye et al.,[79] in which a combination of TSEBT (30 Gy) and combination chemotherapy was compared with a regimen of sequential skin-directed therapies followed by TSEBT if cutaneous lesions progressed. Those patients who received concurrent TSEBT and chemotherapy experienced considerable hematologic toxicity but had a significantly higher CR rate than those who did not. However, there was no statistically significant difference between the two groups with respect to either DFS (12.9 vs. 21.3 months; $P = .19$) or overall survival (91 vs. 76 months) at 75 months.

Several nonrandomized studies have suggested that the adjuvant use of single or combination systemic therapy after TSEBT might be of benefit in the treatment of CTCL.[80–84] In a study of adjuvant doxorubicin-cyclophosphamide after TSEBT, the DFS was longer for those patients who received adjuvant chemotherapy for the first 2 to 3 years of follow-up.[85] However, this early advantage was no longer apparent after 5 years.

In contrast, ECP administered during and after TSEBT appears to improve survival ($P < .06$) for patients with T3 or T4 disease who have achieved a CR to TSEBT, but the group of treated patients is small, and the data are retrospective.[76] We currently do not administer adjuvant systemic chemotherapy after TSEBT but are developing a randomized clinical trial to evaluate the potential utility of adjuvant ECP in patients with T3 and T4 CTCL. Wilson et al.[150] have found a significant improvement in cause-specific survival for erythrodermic patients treated with the combination of TSEBT and ECP as compared to those not treated with ECP. The 2-year progression-free, cause-specific, and overall survival for those receiving TSEBT/ECP were 66%, 100%, and 88%, respectively, versus 36%, 69%, and 63% for those not managed with the combination. These data should be interpreted with caution, though, as the total number of patients was low and the series was nonrandomized.

SYSTEMIC THERAPIES

Systemic therapy for CTCL initially consisted of single- and multiple-agent cytotoxic chemotherapy regimens, often modeled after those that have been used with great success in the treatment of advanced B-cell lymphomas. In most clinical settings, however, cytotoxic chemotherapy has been supplanted by a variety of immunologically based therapies, including ECP (also known as *photopheresis*), IFNs, mAbs, and an investigational agent, the diphtheria toxin/IL-2 hybrid, DABIL-2.

Basic Principles: Photopheresis

Given the intrinsic immunologic nature of the cells responsible for CTCL, it is reasonable that agents that either directly or indirectly modulate T-cell function or other aspects of host immune response should be applied to the therapy of CTCL. The efficacy of most chemotherapeutic and topical treatments used to treat CTCL has never been directly evaluated by U.S. Food and Drug Administration advisory committees, but the agency has approved three systemic therapies for the specific indication of CTCL. The earliest, ECP, received approval in 1988 and was the first such sanctioned selective immunotherapy for any malignancy. More recently, Ontak (diphtheria toxin conjugated to IL-2) and Targretin (Bexarotene) have become available.

Development of Ontak followed Waldmann's original investigation[139] of an mAb against IL-2 that had shown efficacy in preliminary studies. Activated T cells may develop avid receptors for this growth factor. By attaching a toxin to a carrier that binds to the IL-2 receptor, targeted malignant T cells can then be destroyed, sparing non-IL-2 receptor–bearing bystander cells. Some limitations to the approach are that usually only a minority of CTCL cells, even in an actively expanding tumor, are IL-2 receptor–positive.

ECP, or photopheresis, involves systemic pretreatment with oral or parenteral psoralens, removal of a portion of the patient's blood, pheresis of white blood cells away from red blood cells, and exposure to UVA of the white blood cells that have undergone pheresis in an effort to photoactivate intercalated, DNA-bound psoralen to produce psoralen monoadducts and diadducts in DNA. The irradiated cells are then reinfused back into the patient.

The reinfusion of the killed, irradiated CTCL cells appears to stimulate host immune responses selectively against neoplastic T cells. Evidence that such clone-specific immunization actually occurs has come from several different lines of investigation.

Some observations with Vβ-family–specific antibodies have demonstrated that only a minority of infiltrating T cells in patches and plaques are actually neoplastic,[86] and of the benign T cells found in CTCL plaques, approximately 20% are CD8+ cells.[87] When studied *in vitro*, these reactive, nonneoplastic CD8+ T cells have been shown to produce large amounts of IFN-Γ and tumor necrosis factor-α.[88] Both of the last two cytokines increase benign and neoplastic T-cell surface expression of major histocompatibility complex (MHC) class I molecules and presentation of bound peptide antigens to other CD8+ cells, including cytotoxic T lymphocytes. In this context, it is interesting to note that the CD8+ T cells of several patients who underwent photopheresis were found to be cytotoxic only for autologous CTCL cells.

Similarly, others have demonstrated that exposure of murine T-cell lymphoma cells to 8-MOP and UVA in an experimental protocol analogous to photopheresis, and reinfusion of the treated cells into syngeneic mice protects them against subsequent challenge with this cell line. In theory, such anti-CTCL cell "immunization" should occur after any therapy that selectively kills a significant number of neoplastic T cells; however, certain animal studies suggest that ECP may accomplish this by a unique mechanism.

Ex vivo exposure of a lymphocytic murine tumor line to 8-MOP (at the temperature at which photopheresis is conducted) appears to block normal intracellular insertion of cytoplasmic peptides into the peptide antigen-binding groove of MHC class I molecules, resulting in the unusual expression of "empty" class I molecules at the cell surface. In theory, such empty class I molecules are free to bind any extracellular peptides that are recognized by the specific amino acid sequence of the antigen-binding groove.

If such exogenous peptides happen to be derived from protein components of other dying, neoplastic T cells (i.e., the neoplastic clone's TCR), such MHC class I–peptide antigen presentation should facilitate the expansion of clones of CD8+ "killer" and "suppressor" cells specifically directed against the neoplastic clone and immunize the host against its own CTCL cells. Evidence that such phenomena actually occur *in vivo* in patients undergoing photopheresis has come from studies of the peptide fractions eluted from the MHC class I molecules of CTCL patients who underwent photopheresis. Such peptide fractions appear to be unique and characteristic only of the patient's neoplastic T cells and are not observed on nonneoplastic T cells or B lymphoblasts.

Currently, ECP is frequently used as monotherapy for CTCL, but its combination with other therapies such as TSEBT is currently under study. ECP is initially administered on a once-a-month schedule, with therapy continued until maximal clearing is established. An additional 6 months of therapy may be administered to consolidate the clinical response. After the patient's disease has stabilized, the interval between ECP treatments is gradually prolonged by 1 week per cycle every three cycles. After the interval between treatments has reached 8 weeks for three cycles, therapy can be discontinued.

Patients may experience transient responses 1 to 2 days after photopheresis but begin to show sustained clinical improvement as early as the second month of therapy. However, some do not clear or achieve their maximal response until 12 months after starting therapy. On the average, after 4 to 6 months of therapy, a sustained decrease in erythema, scaling, and pruritus is observed. Patients often notice more subtle changes, such as the return of body hair, loss of rigors, and return of the ability to sweat.

Previous reports suggest that conventional systemic therapies are ineffective in prolonging the survival of patients with erythrodermic CTCL. A population-based estimate in one tumor registry survey revealed a 31-month median survival for patients with erythematous skin related to CTCL. A similar analysis of erythrodermic patients in the Mycosis Fungoides Cooperative Group yielded a 30-month survival. In contrast, patients in the original cohort of ECP patients were found to have a median survival of 60 months, or twice as long as had been obtained with prior conventional systemic therapies.[89–94]

No side effects of ECP that compromises its continued administration have been observed in more than 7 years of follow-up. Patients with CTCL in the original cohort treated with ECP have also been carefully studied to determine whether this therapy exerted any adverse effects on host immune response, but none were found. Lymphocyte and leukocyte counts never decreased to low levels. Lymphocyte stimulation studies showed no evidence of immunosuppression, even after years of therapy. Delayed hypersensitivity tests revealed improvement in recall responses after photopheresis; in fact, most of the patients had to experience significant improvement in their erythroderma to allow the skin testing studies to be performed.

In the treatment of T4 CTCL, particularly in patients with markedly elevated white blood cell counts and immunosuppression, ECP has been combined with a variety of other therapies, including IFNs, methotrexate, etoposide, and TSEBT. TSEBT can be particularly useful in producing prompt remissions of symptomatic erythroderma, and results suggest that T4 patients treated with TSEBT and ECP have longer survival than those treated with either modality alone.[76,150]

The mechanism of response to this immunotherapy appears to involve the simultaneous induction of large numbers of DCs and apoptotic CTCL cells. Passage through the UV exposure apparatus, at a film thickness of only 1 mm, causes blood monocytes to adhere transiently to the plastic surface, thereby activating these cells. Over the next few days, at least one-third of the treated monocytes are stimulated in this way to evolve into fully functional DC, the most efficient antigen-presenting cells in the body. This effect is UV-independent, in contrast to the induction of apoptosis of CTCL cells by the photoactivated 8-MOP. The apoptotic CTCL cells are ingested by the newly formed DC, a phenomenon that can be greatly enhanced by delaying the return of the treated blood for 1 day and cocultivating the young DC with the damaged CTCL cells. The CTCL antigens are processed by the DC through the class I MHC pathway and presented to anti-CTCL CD8 T cells, perhaps accounting for the observed enhanced antitumor responses. Trial of this variation on the conventional ECP approach has led to encouraging results in a preliminary study and merits extended study before it becomes more widely used.

Interferons

Whereas all three IFNs—Γ, β, and α—have been studied in CTCL, most clinical studies have been performed with IFN-α. Early studies have reported a CR rate of 10% to 27% with response duration of less than 6 months with doses ranging from 3 to 12 MU/m^2 three times weekly (with the lower dose being the best tolerated).[95] As with other therapies, the extent of prior treatment correlated inversely with the clinical response. With IFN-Γ, partial responses were attained in one-third of the patients, and improvements in the therapeutic response to PUVA have also been observed, as mentioned. Kuzel et al.[141] reported a series of 39 patients (stages I to IV) treated with IFN-α_{2a} in combination with phototherapy and found a 90% response rate (62% CR), with a median duration of 28 months and survival of 62 months.

All IFNs induce similar toxicities. The first week of IFN therapy may be complicated by flu-like syndrome with fever, myalgia, fatigue, and listlessness. After these acute symptoms remit, patients are often left with residual mild, chronic fatigue. Long-term toxicities of concern include neuropathy, dementia, and myelopathy. IFN therapy can also be complicated by such autoimmune phenomena as proteinuria, thrombocytopenia, and anemia.[95,96]

Retinoids (Vitamin A Derivatives)

Retinoids have found a role in the management of several malignancies, including all-*trans*-retinoic acid therapy of acute promyelocytic leukemia and topical allitretinoin in the treatment of Kaposi's sarcoma. Each retinoid has distinct binding patterns with respect to the major classes of retinoid receptors: RAR and RXR. Initial studies in CTCL demonstrated that the retinoids approved for acne and psoriasis (binding both RAR and RXR) could produce responses in CTCL.[117–119] These nonspecific retinoids had also been combined with other therapies, such as PUVA,[120] TSEBT,[121] and IFN.[123–125] Bexarotene is an oral RXR-selective retinoid. In a clinical trial of heavily pretreated, refractory CTCL, oral monotherapy with bexarotene had a 50% response rate in a group of 94 patients with plaque, tumor, or erythrodermic CTCL.[46] The ideal starting dose is 300 mg/m^2 as a single dose taken with a meal. The most frequent toxicity is hypertriglyceridemia necessitating antilipemic therapy in the majority of patients. Hypothyroidism occurred in approximately one-third of patients, and supplemental thyroid hormone was needed. In one report of nine patients with erythrodermic CTCL, there were rapid palliative and remitting responses induced (within 12 weeks) by monotherapy with oral bexarotene. The nine patients with erythrodermic CTCL included those with SS and those without circulating atypical cells. Two achieved CR, and the other seven showed partial responses.[46] As a treatment of erythroderma, this agent could be considered as monotherapy but, in the management of plaque and tumor disease, bexarotene will most likely be combined with skin-directed therapies, including topical steroids. Given the high rate of partial responses with bexarotene monotherapy, it would be anticipated that the combination treatments could achieve a CR, the desired goal of therapy.

Monoclonal Antibodies

Several forms of mAbs have been used in the treatment of CTCL. Miller and Levy[134] have studied the anti-CD5 antibody, and although preliminary study demonstrated partial responses, subsequent investigations were less promising, with no CRs in 34 patients.[135–137] Anti-CD4 therapy has been shown by Knox et al.[138] to be effective in seven of eight patients, with a mean freedom from progression of 25 weeks. Seven of the eight patients had plaque disease, and no patient had visceral or SS involvement.[142] Anti-Tac therapy has been studied by Waldmann[139] and, in an effort to enhance the effect, anti-TAC was used in concert with toxins and α and β emitters. Of 17 patients studied, 11 had a partial or CR to such therapy.

Fusion Toxin

The efficacy of fusion toxin therapy was established in a trial treating patients with refractory CTCL. Fusion toxins are a family of targeted drugs that are recombinant proteins generated by fusing the gene for the targeting factor (with CTCL, the T-cell growth factor IL-2 was used) with the gene for diphtheria toxin. The recombinant peptide is selectively toxic for IL-2 receptor–positive T cells at picometer to nanomolar concentrations. This specific killing can be blocked by the addition of excess IL-2 or mAb to the p55 portion of the IL-2 receptor. Patients are given intravenous infusions of the fusion toxin over a 30-minute period for 5 consecutive days and repeated every 3 weeks. Using doses of 9 µg/kg/d and 18 µg/kg/d, it was possible to demonstrate the dose responsiveness of the efficacy of IL-2 fusion toxin in treating CTCL. The toxicities were also dose-responsive. A vascular leak syndrome occurred at severe levels in 13% of patients. Pretreatment with systemic corticosteroids appears to minimize this complication. Overall, the response rate in heavily treated patients was 30%.[97] Almost all responses occurred within the first three infusion cycles and were maximal at eight cycles. Tumor and plaque lesions appeared to be the most responsive. Patient selection for fusion toxin therapy traditionally depends on skin biopsy or flow cytometry demonstration of lymphocytes expressing the high affinity IL-2 receptor (CD25). However, dramatic responses have occurred in CD25-negative CTCLs. The level for CD25 expression to confer toxicity from the fusion toxin is below the level of detection from immunoperoxidase. Thus, the ultimate screening test for a response to fusion toxin is to monitor the patient over two to three cycles and then continue for a full eight cycles to optimize a response. In those patients with remission, retreatment has recaptured the response.

Systemic Chemotherapy

Chemotherapy has been traditionally associated with increased toxicity in the management of CTCL.[79] Presumably, the immunosuppressive effects of advancing CTCL render patients particularly prone to the suppressive effects of chemotherapy. In addition, central lines in patients with CTCL tend to become infected, owing to the continuous seeding by bacteria from the open skin lesions. Thus, there are two strategies with chemotherapy in the management of CTCL: traditional intravenous chemotherapy and low-dose oral chemotherapy. There have not been any formal studies comparing these two distinct dosing regimens. The oral agents used in managing CTCL patients are methotrexate,[98] etoposide,[104] and chlorambucil.[105,106] Methotrexate is probably the most commonly used, at doses of 15 to 50 mg/wk.[98] If chlorambucil or etoposide is used, the peripheral blood cell count must be carefully monitored. More intense intravenous regimens with cytotoxic chemotherapy palliate patients with CTCL. Single-agent therapy can yield CRs in approximately 30% of patients, but the response durations are relatively short.[84] Commonly used agents have included cyclophosphamide, doxorubicin, vincristine, etoposide, and prednisone.

Several studies have reported that the adenine nucleotide derivatives 2'-deoxycoformycin, 2-chlorodeoxyadenosine, and fludarabine might be useful in the treatment of CTCL.[104–114, 151] Although these agents are active against T lymphocytes through their inhibition of the enzyme adenosine deaminase, their clinical utility in CTCL has been less than initially hoped. In early studies, response rates of approximately 40% were reported for both 2'-deoxycoformycin and 2-chlorodeoxyadenosine, whereas fludarabine was somewhat less effective. The duration of these responses was relatively short, however, and severe myelosuppression was often observed. Combinations of these agents with IFN have been studied, but preliminary results reveal no significant advantages over either modality alone.[115,116]

Overall, combination systemic therapy yields CR rates of 35% to 50% in CTCL, but there is no significant advantage in the use of drug combinations over single-agent therapy. Chemotherapy may be helpful for patients who are in need of symptomatic palliation when other modalities have proven ineffective or when visceral disease is symptomatic. The use of high-dose systemic chemotherapy with stem cell or bone marrow rescue is investigational, and preliminary results have been discouraging.[99]

Acknowledgment

Dr. Edelson's work was supported in part by National Institutes of Health grant RO1-CA43058.

REFERENCES

1. Edelson R. Membrane properties of the abnormal cells of cutaneous T cell lymphomas. *Ann Intern Med* 1975;83:536.
2. Edelson R, Berger C, Raafat J, Warburton D. Karyotype studies of cutaneous T cell lymphoma: evidence for clonal origin. *J Invest Dermatol* 1979;73:548.
3. Weiss LM, Hu E, Wood GS, et al. Clonal rearrangements of T-cell receptor genes in mycosis fungoides and dermatopathic lymphadenopathy. *N Engl J Med* 1985;313:539.
4. Berger CL, Eisenberg A, Soper L, et al. Dual genotype in cutaneous T cell lymphoma: immunoglobulin gene rearrangement in clonal T cell. *J Invest Dermatol* 1988;90:73.
5. Kung PC, Berger CL, Goldstein G, LoGerfo P, Edelson RL. Cutaneous T cell lymphoma: characterization by monoclonal antibodies. *Blood* 1981;57:261.
6. Haynes BF, Metzgar RS, Minna JD, Bunn PA. Phenotypic characterization of cutaneous T-cell lymphoma: use of monoclonal antibodies to compare with other malignant T cells. *N Engl J Med* 1981;304:1319.
7. Broder S, Edelson R, Lutzner M, et al. The Sézary syndrome: a malignant proliferation of helper T cells. *J Clin Invest* 1976;58:1297.
8. Berger C, Warburton D, Raafat L, LoGerfo P, Edelson R. Cutaneous T cell lymphoma: neoplasm of T cell with helper activity. *Blood* 1979;53:642.
9. Vowels BR, Cassin M, Vonderheid EC, Rook AH. Aberrant cytokine production by Sézary syndrome patients: cytokine secretion pattern resembles murine Th2 cells. *J Invest Dermatol* 1992;99:90.
10. Nickoloff BJ, Griffiths CEM. Intraepidermal but not dermal T lymphocytes are positive for a cell-cycle-associated antigen (Ki-67) in mycosis fungoides. *Am J Pathol* 1990;136:261.
11. Picker LJ, Michie SA, Rott LS, Butcher EC. A unique phenotype of skin-associated lymphocytes in humans: preferential expression of the HECA-452 epitope by benign and malignant T cells at cutaneous sites. *Am J Pathol* 1990;136:1053.
12. Picker LJ, Kishimoto TK, Smith CW, Warnock RA, Butcher EC. ELAM-1 is an adhesion molecule for skin-homing T cells. *Nature* 1991;349:796.
13. Berg EL, Yoshino T, Rott LS, et al. The cutaneous lymphocyte antigen is a skin lymphocyte homing receptor for the vascular lectin endothelial cell-leukocyte adhesion molecule-1. *J Exp Med* 1991;174:1461.
14. Lever WF, Schaumburg-Lever G. *Histopathology of the skin*. Philadelphia: JB Lippincott Co, 1990:819.
15. Nickoloff BJ, Griffiths CEM, Baadsgaard O, et al. Markedly diminished epidermal keratinocyte expression of intercellular adhesion molecule-1 (ICAM-1) in Sézary syndrome. *JAMA* 1998;261:2217.
16. Nickoloff BJ, Mitra RS, Shimuzu Y, et al. HUT 78 cells bind to noncytokine-stimulated keratinocytes using a non-CD18-dependent adhesion pathway. *Am J Pathol* 1992;140:1365.
17. Kupper TS, Lee F, Birchall N, Clark S, Dower S. Interleukin 1 binds to specific receptors on human keratinocytes and induces granulocyte macrophage colony-stimulating factor mRNA and protein. A potential autocrine role for interleukin 1 in epidermis. *J Clin Invest* 1998;82:1787.
18. Bergstresser PR, Cruz PD, Niederkorn JY, Takashima A. Third International Workshop on Langerhans Cells: discussion overview. *J Invest Dermatol* 1992;99:1S.
19. Weinstock MA, Horm J. Mycosis fungoides in the United States. Increasing incidence and descriptive epidemiology. *JAMA* 1988;260:42.
20. Tuyp E, Burgoyne A, Aitchison T, MacKie R. A case-control study of possible causative factors in mycosis fungoides. *Arch Dermatol* 1987;123:196.
21. Whittemore AS, Holly E, Lee IM, et al. Mycosis fungoides in relation to environmental exposures and immune response: a case-control study. *J Natl Cancer Inst* 1989;81:1560.
22. Wilson LD. Personal communication regarding the Surveillance, Epidemiology, and End Results (SEER) Program, National Cancer Institute. October 1995.
23. Dalloul A, Laroche L, Bagot M, et al. Interleukin-7 is a growth factor for Sézary cells. *J Clin Invest* 1992;90:1054.
24. Rich BE, Campos-Torres J, Tepper RI, Moreadith RW, Leder P. Cutaneous lymphoproliferation and lymphomas in interleukin 7 transgenic mice. *J Exp Med* 1993;177:305.
25. Macaulay WL. Lymphomatoid papulosis update. *Arch Dermatol* 1989;125:1387.
26. Weiss LM, Wood GA, Trela M, Warnke RA, Sklar J. Clonal T-cell populations in lymphomatoid papulosis: evidence of a lymphoproliferative origin for a clinically benign disease. *N Engl J Med* 1986;315:475.
27. Kardashian JL, Zachheim HS, Egbert BM. Lymphomatoid papulosis associated with plaque-stage and granulomatous mycosis fungoides. *Arch Dermatol* 1985;121:1175.
28. Mehregan D, Gibson L, Muller S. Follicular mucinosis: histopathologic review of 33 cases. *Mayo Clin Proc* 1991;66:387.
29. Buchner SA, Meier M, Rulfi T. Follicular mucinosis associated with mycosis fungoides. *Dermatologica* 1991;183:66.
30. Wood GS, Weiss LM, Hu CH, et al. T-cell antigen deficiencies and clonal rearrangement of T-cell receptor genes in pagetoid reticulosis (Woringer-Kolopp disease). *N Engl J Med* 1988;318:164.
31. Bunn PA, Lamberg SI. Report of the committee on staging and classification of cutaneous T-cell lymphomas. *Cancer Treat Rep* 1979;63:725.
32. Olerud JE, Kulin PA, Chew DE, et al. Cutaneous T-cell lymphoma: evaluation of pretreatment skin biopsy specimens by a panel of pathologists. *Arch Dermatol* 1992;128:501.
33. Marti RM, Estrach T, Reverter JC, Mascaro JM. Prognostic clinicopathologic factors in cutaneous T-cell lymphoma. *Arch Dermatol* 1991;127:1511.
34. Hoppe RT, Medeous LJ, Warnke RA, Woods GS. CD8 positive tumor infiltrating lymphocytes influence the long term survival of patients with mycosis fungoides. *J Am Acad Dermatol* 1995;32:448.
35. Vonderheid EC, Tan E, Sobel EL, et al. Clinical implications of immunologic phenotyping in cutaneous T cell lymphoma. *J Am Acad Dermatol* 1987;17:40.
36. Wood GS, Tung RM, Crooks CF, et al. Detection of early cutaneous T-cell lymphoma. *J Invest Dermatol* 1994;103:34.
37. Lynch JW, Linoilla I, Sausville EA, et al. Prognostic implications of evaluation for lymph node involvement by T-cell antigen receptor gene rearrangement in mycosis fungoides. *Blood* 1992;79:3293.
38. Vonderheid EC, Diamond LW, van Vloten WA, et al. Lymph node classification systems in cutaneous T-cell lymphoma: evidence for the utility of the working formulation of non-Hodgkin's lymphomas for clinical usage. *Cancer* 1994;73:207.
39. Heald P, Yan SL, Latkowski J, Edelson R. Profound deficiency in normal circulating T-cells in erythrodermic cutaneous T-cell lymphoma. *Arch Dermatol* 1994;130:198.
40. Bakels V, van Oostveen JW, Gorkijn RL, Walboomers JM, Meijer CJ. Diagnostic value of T cell receptor beta gene rearrangement analysis in peripheral blood lymphocytes of patients with erythroderma. *J Invest Dermatol* 1991;97:782.
41. Heald P, Rook A. The immunology of cutaneous T-cell lymphoma. *Hematol Oncol Clin* 1995;9:997.
42. Vonderheid EC, Tan ET, Cantor AF, et al. Long term efficacy, curative potential, and carcinogenicity of topical mechlorethamine chemotherapy and cutaneous T-cell lymphoma. *J Am Acad Dermatol* 1989;20:416.
43. Zackheim HS, Epstein EH, Crain WR. Topical carmustine (BCNU) for cutaneous T cell lymphoma: a 15-year experience in 143 patients. *J Am Acad Dermatol* 1990;22:802.
44. Honigsmann H, Brenner W, Rauschmeier W, Konrad K, Wolff K. Photochemotherapy for cutaneous T cell lymphoma. *J Am Acad Dermatol* 1984;10:238.
45. Mostow EN, Neckel SL, Oberhelman L, Anderson TF, Cooper KD. Complete remissions in psoralen and UV-A(PUVA)-refractory mycosis fungoides-type cutaneous T-cell lymphoma with combined interferon alfa and PUVA. *Arch Dermatol* 1993;129:747.
46. Heald PW, Duvic M. Palliative and remittive properties of oral bexarotene in the management of erythrodermic cutaneous T-cell lymphoma. *Blood* 1999 (*in press*).
47. Swanbeck G, Roupe G, Sandstrom MH. Indication of a considerable decrease in the death rate in mycosis fungoides by PUVA therapy. *Acta Dermatovener* 1994;74:465.
48. Scholtz W. Ueber den einflussder roentgenstohlen auf die haut in gesundem und krankem zustande. *Arch Dermatol Syph (Berlin)* 1902;59:421.
49. Kim JH, Nisce LZ, D'Angio GJ. Dose-time fractionation study in patients with mycosis fungoides and lymphoma cutis. *Radiology* 1976;119:439.
50. Hoppe RT, Fuks Z, Bagshaw MA. Radiation therapy in the management of cutaneous T-cell lymphomas. *Cancer Treat Rep* 1979;63:625.
51. Cotter GW, Baglan RJ, Wasserman TH, et al. Palliative radiation treatment of cutaneous mycosis fungoides: a dose response. *Int J Radiat Oncol Biol Phys* 1983;9:1477.
52. Trump JG, Wright KA, Evans WW, et al. High energy electrons for the treatment of extensive superficial malignant lesions. *AJR Am J Roentgenol* 1953;69:623.
53. Fuks Z, Bagshaw MA. Total-skin electron treatment of mycosis fungoides. *Radiology* 1971;100:145.
54. Haybittle JL. A 24 curie strontium 90 unit for whole-body superficial irradiation with beta rays. *Br J Radiol* 1964;37:297.
55. Karzmark CJ, Loevinger R, Steele RE, et al. Technique for large-field, superficial electron therapy. *Radiology* 1960;74:633.
56. Hoppe RT, Cox RS, Fuks Z, et al. Electron-beam therapy for mycosis fungoides: the Stanford University experience. *Cancer Treat Rep* 1979;63:691.
57. Jones GW, Tadros A, Hodson DJ, et al. Prognosis with newly diagnosed mycosis fungoides after total skin electron radiation of 30 of 35 Gy. *Int J Radiat Oncol Biol Phys* 1994;28:839.
58. Lo TCM, Salzman FA, Moschella SL, et al. Whole body surface electron irradiation in the treatment of mycosis fungoides. *Radiology* 1979;130:453.
59. Micaily B, Moser C, Vonderheid EC, et al. The radiation therapy of early stage cutaneous T-cell lymphoma. *Int J Radiat Oncol Biol Phys* 1990;18:1333.
60. Nisce LZ, Safai B, Kim JH. Effectiveness of once weekly total skin electron beam therapy in mycosis fungoides and the Sézary syndrome. *Cancer* 1981;47:870.
61. Reddy S, Parker CM, Shidnia H, et al. Total skin electron beam radiation therapy for mycosis fungoides. *Am J Clin Oncol* 1992;15:119.
62. Van Der Merwe DG. Total skin electron therapy: a technique which can be implemented on a conventional electron linear accelerator. *Int J Radiat Oncol Biol Phys* 1993;27:391.
63. Van Vloten WA, de Vroome H, Noordijk EM, et al. Total skin electron irradiation for cutaneous T-cell lymphoma (mycosis fungoides). *Br J Dermatol* 1985;112:692.
64. Wilson LD, Cooper DL, Goodrich AL, et al. Impact of non-CTCL dermatologic diagnoses and adjuvant therapies on cutaneous T-cell lymphoma patients treated with total skin electron beam radiation therapy. *Int J Radiat Oncol Biol Phys* 1994;28:829.
65. Bjarngard BE, Chen GTY, Piontek RW, et al. Analysis of dose distributions in whole body superficial electron therapy. *Int J Radiat Oncol Biol Phys* 1977;2:319.
66. Page V, Gardner P, Karzmark CJ. Patient dosimetry in electron treatment of large superficial lesions. *Radiology* 1970;94:635.
67. Hoppe RT, Wood GS, Abel EA. Mycosis fungoides and the Sézary syndrome: pathology, staging and treatment. *Curr Probl Cancer* 1990;14:295.
68. Micaily B, Campbell O, Moser C, et al. Total skin electron beam and total nodal irradiation of cutaneous T-cell lymphoma. *Int J Radiat Oncol Biol Phys* 1991;20:809.
69. Micaily B, Vonderheid EC, Brady LW, et al. Total skin electron beam and total nodal irradiation for treatment of patients with cutaneous T-cell lymphoma. *Int J Radiat Oncol Biol Phys* 1985;11:1111.
70. Price NM. Radiation dermatitis following electron beam therapy. *Arch Dermatol* 1978;114:63.
71. Licata AG, Wilson LD, Braverman IM, et al. Malignant melanoma and other second cutaneous malignancies in cutaneous T-cell lymphoma (the influence of additional therapy after total skin electron beam radiation). *Arch Dermatol* 1995;131:432.
72. Abel EA, Sendagorta E, Hoppe RT. Cutaneous malignancies and metastatic squamous cell carcinoma following topical therapies for mycosis fungoides. *J Am Acad Dermatol* 1986;14:1029.
73. Wilson LD, Quiros PA, Kolenik SA, et al. Additional courses of total skin electron beam therapy in the retreatment of patients with cutaneous T-cell lymphoma. *J Am Acad Dermatol* 1996;35:69.

74. Becker M, Hoppe RT, Knox SJ. Multiple courses of high-dose total skin electron beam therapy in the management of mycosis fungoides. *Int J Radiat Oncol Biol Phys* 1995;32:1445.
75. Price NM, Hoppe RT, Constantine FS, et al. The treatment of mycosis fungoides: adjuvant topical mechlorethamine after electron-beam therapy. *Cancer* 1977;40:2851.
76. Wilson LD, Licata AL, Braverman IM, et al. Systemic chemotherapy and extracorporeal photochemotherapy for T3 and T4 cutaneous T-cell lymphoma patients who have achieved a complete response to total skin electron beam therapy. *Int J Radiat Oncol Biol Phys* 1995;32:987.
77. Jones G, McLean J, Rosenthal D, et al. Combined treatment with oral etretinate and electron beam therapy in patients with cutaneous T-cell lymphoma (mycosis fungoides and Sézary syndrome). *J Am Acad Dermatol* 1992;26:960.
78. Wilson LD, Quiros P, Braverman IM, et al. Impact of prognostic factors, adjuvant therapies and retreatment on CTCL patients treated with TSEBT. Proceedings of the seventy-eighth annual meeting of the American Radium Society, Paris, France, April 29–May 3, 1995.
79. Kaye FJ, Bunn PA, Steinberg SM, et al. A randomized trial comparing combination electron-beam radiation and chemotherapy with topical therapy in the initial treatment of mycosis fungoides. *N Engl J Med* 1989;321:1784.
80. Bunn PA, Fischmann AB, Schechter GP, et al. Combined modality therapy with electron-beam irradiation and systemic chemotherapy for cutaneous T-cell lymphomas. *Cancer Treat Rep* 1979;63:713.
81. Griem ML, Tokars RP, Petras V, et al. Combined therapy for patients with mycosis fungoides. *Cancer Treat Rep* 1979;63:655.
82. Hallahan DE, Griem ML, Griem SF, et al. Combined modality therapy for tumor stage mycosis fungoides: results of a 10 year follow-up. *J Clin Oncol* 1988;6:1177.
83. Winkler CF, Sausville EA, Ihde DC, et al. Combined modality treatment of cutaneous T-cell lymphoma: results of a six year follow-up. *J Clin Oncol* 1986;4:1094.
84. Bunn PA, Hoffman SJ, Norris D, et al. Systemic therapy of cutaneous T-cell lymphomas (mycosis fungoides and the Sézary syndrome). *Ann Intern Med* 1994;121:592.
85. Braverman IM, Yager NB, Chen M, et al. Combined total body electron beam irradiation and chemotherapy for mycosis fungoides. *J Am Acad Dermatol* 1987;16:45.
86. Bagot M, Wechsler J, Lescs MC, et al. Intraepidermal localization of the clone in cutaneous T-cell lymphoma. *J Am Acad Dermatol* 1992;27:589.
87. Wood GS, Dubiel C, Mueller C, et al. Most $CD8^+$ cells in skin lesions of $CD3^+$ $CD4^+$ mycosis fungoides are $CD3^+$ T cells that lack CD11b, CD16, CD56, CD57, and human hanukah factor mRNA. *Am J Pathol* 1991;138:1545.
88. Reinhold U, Pawelec G, Fratila A, et al. Phenotypic and functional characterization of tumor infiltrating lymphocytes in mycosis fungoides: continuous growth of $CD4^+$ $CD45R^+$ T-cell clones with suppressor-inducer activity. *J Invest Dermatol* 1990;94:304.
89. Edelson RL, Berger CL, Gasparro F, et al. Treatment of cutaneous T cell lymphoma by extracorporeal photochemotherapy: preliminary results. *N Engl J Med* 1987;316:297.
90. Marks D, Rockman SP, Oziemski MA, Fox RM. Mechanisms of lymphocytotoxicity induced by extracorporeal photochemotherapy for cutaneous T cell lymphoma. *J Clin Invest* 1990;86:2080.
91. Armus S, Keyes B, Cahill C, et al. Successful treatment of cutaneous T cell lymphoma with photopheresis. *J Am Acad Dermatol* 1990;23:898.
92. Zic J, Arzubiaga C, Salhany KE, et al. Extracorporeal photopheresis for the treatment of cutaneous T-cell lymphoma. *J Am Acad Dermatol* 1992;27:729.
93. Heald PW, Rook A, Perez M, et al. Treatment of erythrodermic cutaneous T-cell lymphoma patients with photopheresis. *J Am Acad Dermatol* 1992;27:427.
94. Heald P, Laroche L, Knobler R. Photoinactivated lymphocyte therapy of cutaneous T-cell lymphoma. *Dermatol Clin* 1994;12:443.
95. Bunn PA, Foon KA, Ihde DC, et al. Recombinant leukocyte A interferon: an active agent in advanced cutaneous T-cell lymphomas. *Ann Intern Med* 1984;101:484.
96. Olsen EA, Rosen ST, Vollmer RT, et al. Interferon α2A in the treatment of cutaneous T-cell lymphomas. *J Am Acad Dermatol* 1989;203:395.
97. Olsen E, Duvic M, Frankel A, et al. Pivotal phase III trial of two dose levels of DAB-389IL-2 for the treatment of cutaneous T-cell lymphoma. *J Clin Oncol* (*in press*).
98. Zackheim HS, Epstein EH. Low dose methotrexate for the Sézary syndrome. *J Am Acad Dermatol* 1989;21:757.
99. Bigler RD, Crilly P, Micaily B, et al. Autologous bone marrow transplantation for advanced stage mycosis fungoides. *Bone Marrow Transplant* 1991;7:133.
100. Hollsberg P, Hafler DA. Pathogenesis of diseases induced by human lymphotropic virus type 1 infection. *N Engl J Med* 1993;328:1173.
101. Broder S, Bunn PA Jr. Neoplasms of T-cell origin: immunologic aspects and therapy. *Semin Oncol* 1980;7:310.
102. Bunn PA Jr, Schechter GP, Blayney D, et al. Clinical course of retrovirus-associated adult T-cell lymphoma in the United States. *N Engl J Med* 1983;309:257.
103. Gill PS, Harrington W, Kaplan M, et al. Treatment of adult T cell leukemia lymphoma with a combination of interferon alfa and zidovudine. *N Engl J Med* 1995;332:1744.
104. Rijlaarsdam JU, Huijgens PC, Beljaards RC, Bakels V, Willemze R. Oral etoposide in the treatment of cutaneous large-cell lymphomas. *Br J Dermatol* 1992;127:524.
105. Lorent A, Feermans W, Blondeel A, Meerts P, Achten G. Sezary syndrome: treatment with a prednisolone chlorambucil combination. *Dermatologica* 1982;165:464.
106. Winkelmann RK, Diaz-Perez JL, Buechner SA. The treatment of Sézary syndrome. *J Am Acad Dermatol* 1984;10:1000.
107. Cummings FJ, Kim K, Neiman RS, et al. Phase II trial of pentostatin in refractory lymphomas and cutaneous T-cell disease. *J Clin Oncol* 1991;9:565.
108. Dearden C, Matutes E, Catovsky D. Deoxycoformycin in the treatment of mature T-cell leukaemias. *Br J Cancer* 1991;64:903.
109. Kanofsky JR, Roth DG, Smyth J, et al. Treatment of lymphoid malignancies with 2´-deoxycoformycin: a pilot study. *Am J Clin Oncol* 1982;5:179.
110. Dang-VU AP, Olsen EA, Vollmer RT, Greenberg ML, Hershfield MS. Treatment of cutaneous T-cell lymphoma with 2´-deoxycoformycin (pentostatin). *J Am Acad Dermatol* 1988;19:692.
111. Lee E, Kuzel T, Samuelson E, et al. Phase II trial of 2-chlorodeoxyadenosine for the treatment of cutaneous T-cell lymphoma. Proceedings of the thirty-fifth annual meeting of the American Society of Hematology. *Blood* 1993;82[Suppl 1]:142a.
112. Saven A, Carrera CJ, Carson DA, Beutler E, Piro LD. 2-Chlorodeoxyadenosine: an active agent in the treatment of cutaneous T-cell lymphoma. *Blood* 1992;80:587.
113. Kuzel TM, Samuelson E, Roenigk HH Jr, Torp E, Rosen ST. Phase II trial of 2 chlorodeoxyadenosine for the treatment of mycosis fungoides or the Sézary syndrome. *Proc Am Soc Clin Oncol* 1992;11:A1089(abst).
114. Von Hoff DD, Dahlberg S, Hartstock RJ, Eyre HJ. Activity of fludarabine monophosphate in patients with advanced mycosis fungoides: a Southwest Oncology Group Study. *J Natl Cancer Inst* 1990;82:1353.
115. Foss F, Tingsgaard P, Jorgensen H, Vejlsgaard Gl. Interferon treatment of cutaneous T-cell lymphoma. *Eur J Haematol* 1993;51:63.
116. Foss FM, Ihde DC, Breneman DL, et al. Phase II study of pentostatin and intermittent high-dose interferon α_{2a} in advanced mycosis fungoides/Sézary syndrome. *J Clin Oncol* 1992;10:1907.
117. Molin L, Thomsen K, Volden G, et al. Oral retinoids in mycosis fungoides and Sézary syndrome: a comparison of isotretinoin and etretinate. *Acta Dermatol Venereol* 1987;67:232.
118. Thomsen K, Hammar H, Molin L, Volden G. Retinoids plus PUVA (RePUVA) and PUVA in mycosis fungoides, plaque stage: a report from the Scandinavian Mycosis Fungoides Group. *Acta Derm Venereol* 1989;69:536.
119. Kessler JF, Jones SE, Levine N, Lynch PJ, Booth AR. Isotretinoin and cutaneous helper-T-cell lymphoma (mycosis fungoides). *Arch Dermatol* 1987;123:201.
120. Thomsen K, Molin L, Volden G, Lange Wantzin G, Hellbe L. 13-*Cis*-Tretinoic acid effective in mycosis fungoides: a report from the Scandinavian Mycosis Fungoides Group. *Acta Derm Venereol* 1984;64:563.
121. Jones G, McLean J, Rosenthal D, Roberts J, Sauder DN. Combined treatment with oral etretinate and electron beam therapy in patients with cutaneous T-cell lymphoma (mycosis fungoides and Sézary syndrome). *J Am Acad Dermatol* 1992;26:960.
122. Bass JC, Korobkin MT, Cooper KD, Kane NM, Platt JF. Cutaneous T-cell lymphoma: CT in evaluation and staging. *Radiology* 1993;186:273.
123. Dreno B, Celerier P, Litoux P. Roferon-A in combination with Tigason in cutaneous T-cell lymphomas. *Acta Haematol* 1993;89[Suppl 1]:28.
124. Knobler RM, Trautinger F, Radaszkiewicz T, Kokoschka EM, Micksche M. Treatment of cutaneous T-cell lymphoma with a combination of low-dose interferon α2b and retinoids. *J Am Acad Dermatol* 1991;24:247.
125. Altomare GF, Capella GL, Pigatto PD, Finzi AF. Intramuscular low dose alpha-2B interferon and etretinate for treatment of mycosis fungoides. *Int J Dermatol* 1993;32:138.
126. Heald P, Buckley P, Gilliam A, et al. Correlations of unique clinical, immunotypic, and histologic findings in cutaneous gamma/delta T-cell lymphoma. *J Am Acad Dermatol* 1992;26:865.
127. Dewey WC, Ling CC, Meyn RE. Radiation-induced apoptosis: relevance to radiotherapy. *Int J Radiat Oncol Biol Phys* 1995;33:781.
128. Quiros PA, Kacinski BM, Wilson LD. Extent of skin involvement as a prognostic indicator of disease free and overall survival in T3 stage cutaneous T-cell lymphoma patients treated with total skin electron beam radiation therapy. *Cancer* 1996;77:1912.
129. Axelrod PI, Lorber B, Vanderheid EC. Infections complicating mycosis fungoides and Sézary syndrome. *JAMA* 1992;267:1354.
130. Beljaards RC, Kaudewitz P, Berti E, et al. Primary cutaneous CD 30–positive large cell lymphoma: definition of a new type of cutaneous lymphoma with a favorable prognosis. A European multicenter study of 47 patients. *Cancer* 1993;71:2097.
131. Pauli M, Berti E, Rosso R, et al. CD 30/Ki-1-positive lymphoproliferative disorders of the skin: clinicopathologic correlation and statistical analysis of 86 cases: a multicentric study from the European organization for research and treatment of cancer cutaneous lymphoma project group. *J Clin Oncol* 1995;13:1343.
132. Nadali G, Vinante F, Stein H, et al. Serum levels of the soluble form of CD30 molecule as a tumor marker in CD30+ anaplastic large-cell lymphoma. *J Clin Oncol* 1995;13:1355.
133. Neri A, Fracchiolla NS, Roscetti E, et al. Molecular analysis of cutaneous B- and T-cell lymphomas. *Blood* 1995;86:3160.
134. Miller RA, Levy R. Response of cutaneous T-cell lymphoma to therapy with hybridoma monoclonal antibody. *Lancet* 1981;2:226.
135. Bunn PA, Norris DA. The therapeutic role of interferons and monoclonal antibodies in cutaneous T-cell lymphomas. *J Invest Dermatol* 1990;95:209S.
136. Dillman RO, Shawler DL, Dillman JB, Royston I. Therapy of chronic lymphocytic leukemia and cutaneous T-cell lymphoma with T101 monoclonal antibody. *J Clin Oncol* 1984;2:881.
137. Bertram JH, Gill PS, Levine AM, et al. Monoclonal antibody T101 in T cell malignancies: a clinical pharmacokinetic and immunologic correlation. *Blood* 1986;68:752.
138. Knox SJ, Levy R, Hodgkinson S, et al. Observations on the effect of chimeric anti-CD4 monoclonal antibody in patients with mycosis fungoides. *Blood* 1991;77:20.
139. Waldmann TA. Anti-IL-2 receptor monoclonal antibody (anti-Tac) treatment of T-cell lymphoma. *Important Adv Oncol* 1994;[review]:131.
140. Jones GW, Hoppe RT, Glatstein E. Electron beam treatment for cutaneous T-cell lymphoma. *Hematol Oncol Clin North Am* 1995;9:1057.
141. Kuzel TM, Roenigk HH, Samuelson E, et al. Effectiveness of interferon alpha-2A combined with phototherapy for mycosis fungoides and the Sézary syndrome. *J Clin Oncol* 1995;13:257.
142. Knox S, Hoppe RT, Maloney D, et al. Treatment of cutaneous T-cell lymphoma with chimeric anti-CD4 monoclonal antibody. *Blood* 1996;87:893.
143. Jones GW. Update of the Ontario experience of TSEBT for patients with newly diagnosed CTCL. Personal communication, May 1996.
144. Jones GW, Savilo E, Roberts JT, et al. Infiltrative cell density in pre-irradiated skin as a prognostic factor in Mycosis Fungoides. *Clin Invest Med* 17S:B119(abstract 706), 1994.
145. Wilson LD, Kacinski BM, Jones GW. Local superficial radiotherapy in the management of minimal stage IA cutaneous T-cell lymphoma (mycosis fungoides). *Int J Radiat Oncol Biol Phys* 1998;40:109.

146. Jones GW, Thorson B. Cutaneous T-cell lymphoma (mycosis fungoides). *Lancet* 1999;348:130.
147. Jones GW, Rosenthal D, Wilson LD. Total skin electron radiation for patients with erythrodermic cutaneous T-cell lymphoma (mycosis fungoides and the Sézary syndrome). *Cancer* 1999;85:1985.
148. Quiros PA, Jones GW, Kacinski BM, et al. Total skin electron beam therapy followed by adjuvant psoralen/ultraviolet A light in the management of patients with T1 and T2 cutaneous T-cell lymphoma (mycosis fungoides). *Int J Radiat Oncol Biol Phys* 1997;38:1027.
149. Chinn DM, Chow S, Kim YH, et al. Total skin electron beam therapy with or without topical nitrogen mustard or nitrogen mustard alone as initial treatment of T2 and T3 mycosis fungoides. *Int J Radiat Oncol Biol Phys* 1999;43:951.
150. Wilson LD, Jones GW, Kim D, et al. Experience with total skin electron beam therapy in combination with extracorporeal photopheresis in the management of patients with erythrodermic (T4) mycosis fungoides. *J Am Acad Dermatol* 2000;43:54.
151. Kurzrock R, Pilat S, Duvic M. Pentostatin therapy of T-cell lymphomas with cutaneous manifestations. *J Clin Oncol* 1999;17:3117.

LISA M. DEANGELIS
JOACHIM YAHALOM

SECTION 5

Primary Central Nervous System Lymphoma

Primary central nervous system lymphoma (PCNSL) is the term applied to non-Hodgkin's lymphoma (NHL) arising in and confined to the central nervous system (CNS). In the past, this tumor was called *microglioma, reticulum cell sarcoma,* or *perivascular sarcoma,* but its lymphocytic origin, usually the B cell, is now well established.[1–3] How a lymphoma can develop within the CNS, which lacks lymph nodes and lymphatics, remains unanswered; however, lymphocytes do normally traffic in and out of the CNS, and these lymphocytes may be the source of PCNSL.

PCNSL was formerly a rare tumor, accounting for only 0.5% to 1.2% of all intracranial neoplasms, and usually associated with congenital, acquired, or iatrogenic immunodeficiency states such as Wiskott-Aldrich syndrome or renal transplantation.[2,4,5] The highest incidence has been reported in patients with the acquired immunodeficiency syndrome (AIDS), in whom it is seen in 1.9% to 6.0%.[6,7] One autopsy study demonstrated an overall risk of 12%, but only one-half of patients were suspected to harbor CNS disease before death.[8] There is a strong clinical impression among experienced clinicians that widespread use of highly active antiretroviral therapy has reduced the incidence of PCNSL in the AIDS population, but this has yet to be confirmed by formal epidemiologic studies. However, there has been a clear and dramatic increase in the incidence of PCNSL among apparently immunocompetent individuals. An epidemiologic study in the United States revealed a threefold increase in the incidence of PCNSL between 1973 and 1984; a tenfold increase has been observed in southeast England.[9,10] This increase far exceeds the 3% to 4% per year increase seen in systemic NHLs during the same period.[11] Not all epidemiologic studies indicate an increased incidence, and it is unclear if these geographic variations contain important etiologic clues.[12] Currently, PCNSL has an incidence of 0.31 per 100,000 person years, suggesting that approximately 800 new cases occur in the United States every year.[11] This change in incidence cannot be attributed to new diagnostic techniques or the adoption of a uniform nosology, and the reason for this marked rise in PCNSL is unknown.

CLINICAL FEATURES

GENERAL

PCNSL affects all ages, from the very young to the elderly. Its peak incidence occurs in the sixth and seventh decades in immunocompetent patients and younger in immunosuppressed patients.[13] Among apparently immunocompetent individuals, there is a 3:2 male to female ratio, but in the AIDS population, more than 90% of patients are men.[14]

By definition, PCNSL is limited to the nervous system and has not metastasized there from a systemic site. Metastatic NHL typically involves the leptomeninges, rarely the brain, and usually occurs in the setting of advanced disseminated disease.[15] Systemic staging of PCNSL patients has yielded only a 3% to 4% incidence of systemic disease.[16,17] In all patients, the systemic site was extranodal and identified by bone marrow biopsy or abdominopelvic computed tomographic scan, suggesting that these are the only tests necessary for a systemic evaluation.

BRAIN

Most PCNSLs present with symptoms of an intracranial mass lesion. The specific presenting symptoms and signs reflect the location of the tumor, with focal cerebral deficits occurring in approximately one-half of patients[13]; however, the presentation of PCNSL has some differences from that of other brain tumors. Because the frontal lobe is the most frequently involved region of the brain and multiple lesions are often seen, changes in personality and level of alertness are common presenting symptoms. Headaches and symptoms of increased intracranial pressure are also seen frequently. Seizures are less common than in patients with other types of brain tumors, occurring in approximately 10% of patients as a presenting sign, because most PCNSLs involve deep brain structures rather than seizure-prone cerebral cortex. PCNSL is a rapidly growing tumor, and symptoms are usually present for only weeks to a few months before a diagnosis is made.

- Staging for PCNSL should include the following tests:
- Cranial magnetic resonance imaging (MRI) with gadolinium
- Lumbar puncture
- Ophthalmologic examination with slit lamp
- Spinal MRI with gadolinium (when appropriate)
- Abdominal computed tomographic scan
- Bone marrow testing
- Chest radiography
- Human immunodeficiency virus-1 serology

PCNSL is often disseminated within the nervous system at diagnosis. Brain lesions are multifocal in 40% of immunocompetent patients and almost 100% of AIDS patients. Multiple lesions often cause diagnostic confusion with brain metastases, particularly as 13% of PCNSL patients have a history of a prior systemic malignancy.[18] Many lesions are periventricular, allowing tumor cells to easily gain access to the CSF. At least 42% of patients have demonstrable leptomeningeal seeding based on a positive CSF cytologic examination, pathologic leptomeningeal invasion, or unequivocal radiographic evidence of subarachnoid tumor, but patients rarely have symptoms or signs of leptomeningeal lymphoma.[19] At autopsy, 100% of patients have leptomeningeal tumor from either direct invasion into the ventricular system by periventricular tumor or local involvement of the leptomeninges overlying a cortical lesion.[20] In addition, approximately 20% of PCNSL patients have ocular involvement at diagnosis.[21]

EYE

The eye, a direct extension of the brain, is a common site of disease in PCNSL. Lymphoma can originate within the eye, and 50% to 80% of these patients eventually develop cerebral lymphoma, usually after several years of latency.[22,23] Ocular lymphoma typically involves the vitreous, retina, or choroid, but optic nerve infiltration can also occur.[22–24] Disease outside of the globe but within the orbit is not a feature of ocular lymphoma; it represents systemic NHL. Ocular lymphoma can present with blurred vision or floaters, or it may be clinically silent; it may begin unilaterally, but most patients eventually develop bilateral, but asymmetric, disease. A cellular infiltrate of the vitreous can be visualized only by slit-lamp examination, and choroidal or retinal lesions often require indirect ophthalmoscopy. Lymphoma can be identified in vitrectomy specimens[22]; false-negative biopsy results may occur when patients have too few vitreal lymphocytes for the pathologist to examine or if the patient has been given corticosteroids to treat a presumed uveitis.[24,25]

LEPTOMENINGES

Primary leptomeningeal lymphoma, in the absence of a parenchymal brain mass, is rare, accounting for approximately 7% of PCNSLs.[26–28] Patients can present with progressive leg weakness, urinary incontinence or retention, cranial neuropathies, increased intracranial pressure, confusion, or a combination of these symptoms. Symptoms are usually present for only 2 to 3 months before diagnosis, but occasionally a patient can have symptoms for 1 to 2 years before being diagnosed.[26] Diagnosis is established by demonstrating malignant lymphocytes in the CSF or on meningeal biopsy. The CSF invariably shows an elevated protein concentration and a lymphocytic pleocytosis often in excess of 100 cells/μL; CSF glucose is low in approximately one-third of patients. A gadolinium MRI scan of the head or spine reveals meningeal enhancement, hydrocephalus, or multiple intradural nodules.

SPINAL CORD

Primary spinal cord lymphoma is even less common than primary leptomeningeal lymphoma.[28–31] Lymphoma in the spinal cord parenchyma can occur in isolation or with brain lymphoma. Patients present with painless bilateral limb weakness, usually involving the legs; sensory symptoms and signs may initially follow a radicular pattern, but eventually a sensory level may be found. CSF may be normal or have a mildly elevated protein concentration with a few lymphocytes. Prognosis has been poor, with patients surviving only a few months from the onset of symptoms, but this is often because the diagnosis was not made until autopsy and no appropriate therapy was administered.

DIAGNOSTIC TESTS

CRANIAL IMAGING

MRI scanning is the standard imaging technique for any patient with a cerebral neoplasm. The MRI of PCNSL is usually quite distinctive, and the diagnosis may be suspected on the basis of the radiographic appearance alone. The tumor has an isointense signal on the pregadolinium T1 MRI, and after contrast is administered, there is dense and diffuse enhancement.[32,33] The lesions often have indistinct borders, and the amount of surrounding edema is quite variable. Unlike brain metastases or malignant gliomas, ring enhancement is rarely seen.

Prominent contrast enhancement is characteristic of PCNSL, occurring in more than 90% of patients; however, nonenhancing lesions may be seen in 10% or fewer patients, particularly at recurrence.[34] Nonenhancing tumor can occur in the absence of corticosteroid administration, particularly in immunosuppressed patients, although it is also seen in immunocompetent patients. At its extreme, nonenhancing PCNSL can rarely present as lymphomatosis cerebri, with diffuse infiltration of the entire brain, usually presenting as a progressive dementia.[35] Although it is a minor component of disease in most patients, nonenhancing PCNSL has important therapeutic implications, indicating tumor behind a relatively intact blood–brain barrier.

The radiographic features of PCNSL in the immunosuppressed patient differ from the characteristic image seen in immunocompetent individuals.[33] In the AIDS patient, ring enhancement is typical, reflecting the higher incidence of necrosis seen pathologically in this group. Consequently, it is impossible to distinguish PCNSL from more common cerebral infections, such as toxoplasmosis, on the basis of MRI. However, positron emission tomography or single photon emission computed tomographic imaging can reliably differentiate PCNSL from toxoplasmosis in most patients, frequently eliminating the need for histologic confirmation.[36–38]

LUMBAR PUNCTURE

Lumbar puncture should be part of the diagnostic evaluation of every patient with PCNSL. The protein concentration is elevated in 85% of patients, although rarely above 150 mg/dL.[19,20,39,40] The glucose concentration is usually normal, but can be low when florid leptomeningeal tumor is present. A CSF pleocytosis is seen in more than one-half of patients and always consists of lymphocytes, either reactive or malignant. An unequivocally positive CSF cytology eliminates the need for a brain biopsy. This may be particularly important in the immunosuppressed or desperately ill patient at increased risk for a surgical complication. Occasionally, immunohistochemical stains of CSF demonstrate a monoclonal population of cells establishing the neoplastic nature of the pleocytosis even if the cells appear to be cytologically benign.[41] Tumor markers, such as β_2-microglobulin, lactic acid dehydrogenase isoenzymes, and β-glucuronidase, when their levels are elevated, provide circumstantial evidence for tumor invasion of the leptomeninges.

Systemic lymphomas in immunocompromised patients are often associated with the Epstein-Barr virus (EBV); the virus is believed to be oncogenic in these patients.[42] Using *in situ* hybridization and the polymerase chain reaction, EBV has been detected in the tumor tissue of most AIDS-related PCNSLs and some non-AIDS tumors as well[43,44]; EBV may play an important role in the development of this tumor in immunosuppressed patients, comparable with its presumed role in systemic polyclonal and monoclonal lymphoid proliferations in the immunocompromised host. Regardless of its role in the genesis of the neoplasm, it may serve a useful diagnostic function. With polymerase chain reaction, EBV DNA has been detected in the CSF of AIDS patients with PCNSL, but not in the CSF of AIDS patients without PCNSL; this approach offers a simple, noninvasive diagnostic alternative to brain biopsy in the AIDS population,[37,38,45,46] and when combined with a positive positron emission tomography or single photon emission computed tomographic scan result, provides 100% specificity for a diagnosis of PCNSL.[37,38]

PATHOLOGY

PCNSL is a NHL, usually of an intermediate malignant subtype.[2,28] Most are diffuse large cell lymphomas or diffuse large cell immunoblastic lymphomas. Response to treatment or prognosis is not related to pathologic subtype; however, most series contain so few patients in any given category that a relationship may be missed. Further prospective studies with a large number of patients may reveal differences comparable with that seen for systemic lymphomas. At this time, all PCNSLs are treated in the same manner, regardless of subtype or cell of origin.

Macroscopically, PCNSL is usually a brownish space-occupying mass involving the deep white matter.[2] In some cases, only a thickened corpus callosum may occur without discoloration, and in occasional patients the brain is grossly normal, but diffuse infiltration is seen microscopically. Histologically, PCNSL can grow as sheets of cells, but a characteristic vasocentric growth pattern with tumor infiltrating the brain parenchyma between involved blood vessels is found in virtually all cases. Neither necrosis nor hemorrhage is a dominant histologic feature. In autopsy specimens, tumor is always found in multiple regions of the CNS that appeared normal on neuroimaging studies.

Several investigators have demonstrated the B-cell nature of this tumor, with immunohistochemistry showing monoclonal immunoglobulin heavy- or light-chain production or identifying B-cell markers.[3,28,47] Immunoglobulin gene rearrangement has also been shown and may be diagnostically useful in some patients.[48] A study of adhesion molecules revealed an identical pattern of expression for PCNSL and systemic lymphomas.[49] *Bcl* rearrangements have not been detected in PCNSL, and no unique molecular marker has been identified to discriminate PCNSL from its systemic counterparts.[49] Rare, T-cell PCNSLs seem to have a predisposition to develop in the leptomeninges.[50–52] Reports suggest a rising incidence in the number of T-cell PCNSLs.[53] This may be a result of newer immunohistochemical techniques, or it may be an artifact of the difficulties interpreting immunohistochemical studies. In both the CSF and the tumor itself, these neoplasms may be accompanied by a reactive lymphocytosis.[54] These reactive cells are T cells and can make interpretation of special stains difficult. For the most part, one can clearly distinguish the cytologically malignant cells, which are usually B cells, from the reactive lymphocytes, which are T cells. In lesions partially treated by corticosteroids, however, the reactive T cells may be all that is apparent on a biopsy specimen, making accurate diagnosis difficult.

MANAGEMENT

The appropriate management of a patient with PCNSL requires a correct diagnosis. This may be difficult because the clinical presentation of PCNSL is not distinctive and other primary and secondary brain tumors are much more common; however, the method outlined here can aid in the approach to a patient who harbors this tumor.

When an MRI scan reveals an intracranial mass, the radiographic appearance may strongly suggest PCNSL; multiple lesions, deep or periventricular location, diffuse and dense contrast enhancement, and poorly defined borders are common imaging characteristics. In addition, the clinical setting in which the tumor arises may point to the diagnosis (e.g., an immunocompromised patient). If PCNSL is a strong diagnostic consideration, corticosteroids should be withheld unless the patient is in imminent danger of herniation, a rare situation. Corticosteroids may alter or even eliminate the ability to establish the diagnosis pathologically. Histologic confirmation is essential, by stereotactic biopsy, lumbar puncture demonstrating leptomeningeal lymphoma, or vitreous biopsy demonstrating lymphomatous cells. If the patient requires the immediate use of corticosteroids, or if PCNSL was not considered originally and the patient was placed on corticosteroids, a repeat MRI scan should be done to evaluate for possible resolution or marked shrinkage of the lesion or lesions. Biopsy should still be considered if the lesions are reduced in size but still evident; however, nondiagnostic tissue may be obtained. Corticosteroid-induced resolution of an intracranial mass does not establish the diagnosis of PCNSL, because nonneoplastic contrast-enhancing processes such as multiple sclerosis or sarcoidosis can resolve after corticosteroid administration.

Using the clinical staging criteria developed for systemic lymphomas, PCNSL corresponds to stage IE (i.e., disease confined to a single extranodal site). Systemic stage IE disease has a 100% complete response rate and at least a 70% 10-year survival, or cure, rate with focal radiotherapy.[55] Surprisingly, the prognosis for PCNSL is poor. Despite the highly responsive nature of PCNSL to initial treatment, median survival is only 12 to 18 months with cranial radiotherapy,[21,28,39,40,56] and the 5-year survival rate is only 3% to 4%. This short survival is a result of recurrence of PCNSL after an initial response to cranial irradiation. Relapse occurs primarily in the brain, often in regions remote from the original site but within the prior radiation port; it also occurs in the leptomeninges and eye. Systemic lymphoma is found in only 7% to 8% of autopsied patients, and the vast majority of these patients have a single focus of clinically silent disease, thought to represent a systemic metastasis from recurrent nervous system tumor.[21,39]

Because of its poor prognosis, new treatment approaches have been developed. The therapeutic strategies differ, depending on the immunologic status of the patient. Most data regarding effective therapies have been accumulated in immunocompetent patients. The presence of significant immunosuppression may compromise the patient's ability to tolerate more vigorous forms of treatment. Thus, we divide the descriptions of existing and potential treatment regimens for PCNSL into treatments for the immunologically intact patient and those for patients with diminished immune systems from a preexisting condition.

IMMUNOLOGICALLY NORMAL PATIENTS

Corticosteroids

A unique feature of PCNSL compared with other brain tumors is its exquisite sensitivity to corticosteroids. In at least 40% of patients, tumor masses significantly shrink or disappear on MRI scan after corticosteroids are administered.[28,32,57] This apparent remission is a direct result of the cytotoxic effect of corticosteroids, comparable with their effect in systemic lymphoma. Experimentally, corticosteroid receptor-like molecules have been identified on mouse lymphoma cells, and their presence correlates with cell lysis after exposure to corticosteroids.[58] Clinically, disappearance of PCNSL lesions is accompanied by improvement, which may last long after the corticosteroids have been discontinued. There are isolated reports of patients being cured or having prolonged survival after treatment with corticosteroids alone.[57] Regardless of apparent tumor regression, corticosteroid-induced remission is short-lived in most patients and is not definitive treatment. Biopsy after corticosteroid administration often yields normal or nondiagnostic tissue. Occasionally, biopsy results are misleading as the corticosteroids can lyse the malignant B cells, leaving the reactive T cells behind, which may be interpreted as an inflammatory process.

Surgery

Surgery is an important means of confirming the histologic diagnosis, but it has no therapeutic role. Mean survival of patients with PCNSL with supportive care alone is 1.8 to 3.3 months.[1,4,39] Surgical resection adds little, prolonging the average survival to only 3.3 to 5.0 months.[39,59,60] Unlike malignant glioma, for which extensive resection is an important component of therapy, PCNSL's multifocal and infiltrative nature makes surgical extirpation difficult. Furthermore, the deep location of many PCNSLs leaves the patient susceptible to severe postoperative deficits if a complete resection is attempted.[32] Therefore, the diagnostic method of choice is stereotactic biopsy, which also allows for biopsy of deep lesions that cannot be approached safely by conventional surgery. If craniotomy is undertaken because the diagnosis of PCNSL is not considered preoperatively, an intraoperative frozen section often establishes the diagnosis of PCNSL; the procedure can then be terminated, because further resection is unnecessary.

Radiotherapy

Whole brain radiotherapy (WBRT), combined with corticosteroids, was the conventional treatment for PCNSL, yielding median survivals of 12 to 18 months. There is no clear radiotherapy dose-response relationship in PCNSL.[61] The Radiation Therapy Oncology Group conducted a prospective study of patients with PCNSL treated with 4000 cGy WBRT plus a 2000-cGy boost to the involved area, to assess whether dose intensification improved outcome.[56,61] Median survival was only 12.2 months, and most recurrences were in the boosted field. This is comparable with our experience at Memorial Sloan-Kettering Cancer Center, where relapses occurred with equal frequency in a boosted region receiving a total of 5440 cGy and in other areas of the brain treated with only 4000 cGy.[62] Because the added radiotherapy does not improve local control and can contribute to late neurologic sequelae, we have eliminated the boost and use 4500-cGy WBRT in our current protocol.

The primary treatment of ocular disease is radiotherapy to the globe[23,24,63]; 3500 to 4000 cGy over 4 to 5 weeks is the recommended total dose. Because ocular lymphoma is predominately a binocular process, both eyes should be irradiated, even when only monocular disease can be detected on slit-lamp examination. Most patients experience both symptomatic improvement and resolution of cells in the vitreous after radiotherapy; however, some have vitreal clearing without improved vision, and others may not respond to radiotherapy. The incidence of long-term ocular toxicity from radiotherapy in this disease is unknown, but it may increase with improved survival because many of the complications are delayed. Accelerated cataract formation is almost a certainty after these doses of radiation therapy. Conjunctivitis, dry eyes, retinal atrophy, and vitreous hemorrhage have all been reported in PCNSL patients after ocular radiotherapy.[63] However, most patients tolerate a fractionated dose of 3600 cGy to both eyes without significant acute or permanent delayed complications.

Craniospinal irradiation has been proposed as the initial therapy for PCNSL because of the high incidence of clinically evident meningeal tumor at recurrence and the invariable demonstration of leptomeningeal infiltration at autopsy. Few data exist to evaluate this approach, although results in the few patients treated with neuraxis radiotherapy suggest improved survival over WBRT alone.[64] However, irradiation of such a large portion of the bone marrow compromises the patient's ability to tolerate subsequent systemic chemotherapy that is likely to be necessary at relapse. Administration of intrathecal chemotherapy at diagnosis is an effective alternative to neuraxis radiotherapy in treating leptomeningeal lymphoma, and it is associated with less systemic toxicity.

Chemotherapy

No large prospective trials have compared chemotherapy plus radiotherapy with radiotherapy alone, but accumulating data from multiple phase II studies clearly document the chemosensitivity of PCNSL to systemic chemotherapy and superior outcomes with combined modality therapy. It is improbable that a phase III trial will ever be mounted to study this issue given the small number of patients with PCNSL and the long time needed to complete such a protocol.

Most studies have focused on the use of preradiation chemotherapy for two reasons:

1. It permits assessment of response to treatment. Almost all patients have a complete, although short-lived, response to radiotherapy; therefore, no measurable disease is present to assess adjuvant chemotherapy. This is particularly important in PCNSL because we are still trying to identify active agents and cannot simply adopt regimens effective against comparable systemic NHLs.
2. The administration of drugs, particularly methotrexate, before radiotherapy may reduce the synergistic toxicity of combining chemotherapy with cranial irradiation. Although methotrexate has been best studied, the enhanced neurotoxic potential of chemotherapy after cranial radiotherapy may apply to other agents as well. Cranial irradiation opens the blood–brain barrier, and this may persist for weeks to months after radiotherapy is completed. This enhanced permeability of the blood–brain barrier permits greater drug concentrations to accumulate in normal brain tissue. Completing chemotherapy before cranial irradiation is started should minimize brain exposure to potentially neurotoxic agents.

Several investigators have used chemotherapeutic regimens for PCNSL that were successful in treating systemic NHL. The combinations of preradiation cyclophosphamide, doxorubicin, and vincristine with prednisone (CHOP) or dexamethasone (CHOD) have been studied most extensively. Stewart and associates were the first to note responses of brain lesions to CHOP, although patients quickly developed florid leptomeningeal tumor.[65,66] Lachance and associates noted initial responses, but patients rapidly developed multifocal brain recurrence in sites distant from the original location of disease before chemotherapy could be completed.[67] In contrast to these data, isolated patients have been reported to experience prolonged survival with CHOP plus WBRT.[68,69] However, two prospective, multicentered trials clearly established the poor efficacy and high toxicity of CHOP/CHOD for PCNSL.[70,71] The Radiation Therapy Oncology Group conducted a study in which patients received three cycles of CHOD followed by cranial irradiation.[70] The median survival was only 16.1 months for the 52 patients treated. A separate multiinstitutional trial of preradiation CHOP included 46 evaluable patients with an estimated median survival of approximately 9.5 months.[71] Only 54% of patients completed two cycles of CHOP before beginning radiotherapy; in the others disease progression or toxicity occurred, with a 15% mortality. Furthermore, it appears that, when effective, CHOP is associated with a high incidence of delayed neurologic toxicity.[69] In addition to CHOP, Brada and associates studied methotrexate, 400 mg/m², with doxorubicin, cyclophosphamide, vincristine, prednisone, and bleomycin (MACOP-B) preceding cranial radiotherapy, but median survival was only 14 months.[72] When added to radiotherapy, neither CHOP nor MACOP-B improved survival over that seen with radiotherapy alone.

Although the agents in these regimens should have excellent activity against PCNSL cells, they are unable to penetrate an intact blood–brain barrier. Adequate drug concentrations are likely to be achieved in areas of bulky disease seen on MRI scan where the blood–brain barrier is disrupted by tumor, which accounts for the initial resolution of tumor masses; however, the drugs are unable to reach microscopic disease, which persists behind a relatively preserved blood–brain barrier. Drug delivery issues may only partially explain the difficulty of treating PCNSL, but these data strongly argue for the use of drugs that can permeate the blood–brain barrier (Table 45.5-1).

TABLE 45.5-1. Management of Primary Central Nervous System Lymphoma

SURGERY
Biopsy for diagnosis
Resection should be avoided
CHEMOTHERAPY
Should be considered at diagnosis for every patient
Must penetrate the blood–brain barrier
Lipophilic (e.g., procarbazine)
High-dose with central nervous system penetration (e.g., methotrexate)
Must have antilymphoma activity
Should be given before radiotherapy
RADIOTHERAPY
Must be whole brain, if used
4500 cGy, boost not necessary
3600 cGy to eyes, if indicated
May be deferred in some patients who have a complete response to chemotherapy

High-dose methotrexate has emerged as the most important drug for the treatment of PCNSL. Two large retrospective studies have convincingly demonstrated that methotrexate is the single most active agent for PCNSL.[73–75] A number of years ago, we treated PCNSL patients at Memorial Sloan-Kettering Cancer Center with systemic, 1 g/m², and intra-Ommaya methotrexate followed by radiotherapy and high-dose cytarabine.[62] An analysis of this original cohort confirms a cause-specific median survival of 42 months, with a 22% 5-year survival, a significant improvement over radiotherapy alone[76] (Fig. 45.5-1 and Table 45.5-2). Age older than 50 years was a poor prognostic factor for response and survival. Others have confirmed that age and performance status are important prognostic factors, regardless of treatment type.[56,70,71,73,74] Additional regimens using nitrosoureas, procarba-

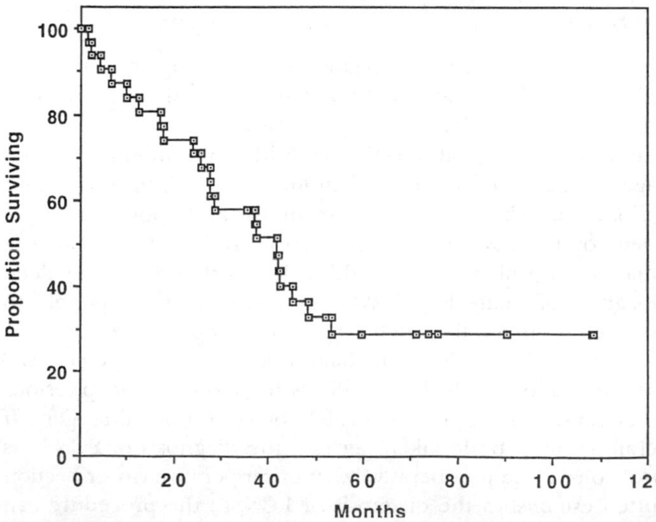

FIGURE 45.5-1. Kaplan-Meier curve demonstrating cause-specific survival for 31 patients treated with chemotherapy plus cranial irradiation. Median survival was 42 months, and the 5-year survival rate was 30%.

TABLE 45.5-2. Chemotherapy Regimens for Primary Central Nervous System Lymphoma

Regimen	*Median Survival (mo)*	*5-Y Survival Rate (%)*	*Reference*
High-dose methotrexate	42	28	76
Blood–brain barrier disruption and intraarterial methotrexate	40	30	81
Cyclophosphamide, doxorubicin, and vincristine with prednisone or dexamethasone	9.5–16.0	14[a]	70,71
Methotrexate with doxorubicin, cyclophosphamide, vincristine, prednisone, and bleomycin	14	10[a]	72
Whole brain radiotherapy alone	12–18	3	21

[a]Three-year survival.

zine, cyclophosphamide, and doxorubicin have all been used in a few patients, with reported success.[68,77–70]

The history of treatment for systemic NHL documents the superiority of combination chemotherapy over single agents. Consequently, new regimens for PCNSL are combining multiple agents that can penetrate the blood–brain barrier (Table 45.5-3). An intergroup trial with the Radiation Therapy Oncology Group and the Southwest Oncology Group, using a 10-week preradiation regimen of high-dose methotrexate, 2.5 g/m^2, procarbazine, and vincristine has just been completed. Preliminary results show a median survival of 30 months[80] (Fig. 45.5-2). This is the first multicentered trial to demonstrate an improved outcome over radiation therapy alone.

In an effort to circumvent the blood–brain barrier and deliver multiagent treatment, Dahlborg and coworkers used blood–brain barrier disruption followed by intraarterial methotrexate, combined with systemic cyclophosphamide, procarbazine, and dexamethasone without cranial irradiation.[81] Their 39 patients treated at the time of diagnosis had a median survival of 40 months; however, 31% required WBRT. Neither the rate of relapse nor failure of the regimen was reported.

Although most studies have focused on preradiation chemotherapy, the question of adjuvant chemotherapy in patients who have completed WBRT and not received prior chemotherapy often arises. It is unknown if adjuvant chemotherapy is equivalent to a preradiation drug, but preliminary data suggest it is superior to radiotherapy alone. Chamberlain and Levin followed WBRT with procarbazine, lomustine, and vincristine, achieving a 41-month median survival in 16 patients.[82] Therefore, four to six cycles of procarbazine, lomustine, and vincris-

TABLE 45.5-3. Active Chemotherapy Regimens

	Current Memorial Sloan-Kettering Cancer Center regimen								
Week	1	2	3	4	5	6[a]	11	16	20
Methotrexate	X		X		X				
Vincristine	X		X		X				
Procarbazine	X→				X→				
Intra-ommaya methotrexate		X		X		X			
Whole brain irradiation							X		
High-dose cytarabine								X	X

	Scheme for blood–brain barrier disruption with chemotherapy[b]					
Days	1	2	3–7	8–16	17–23	24–28
Cyclophosphamide	X	X				
Blood–brain barrier disruption[c]	X	X				
Intraarterial methotrexate	X	X				
Leucovorin		X	X			
Procarbazine			X	X		
Dexamethasone			X	X		
Dexamethasone taper					X	

	Harvard regimen			
Days	1	11	21	42
Methotrexate[d]	X	X	X	
Whole brain irradiation				X

[a]Repeat through week 10.
[b]This 28-day course is repeated for 12 cycles.
[c]Two arterial distributions treated per cycle (e.g., left carotid and vertebral). Infusions are rotated each cycle such that each vascular territory is treated eight times over the 1-year course of therapy.
[d]Methotrexate given for three or more cycles.

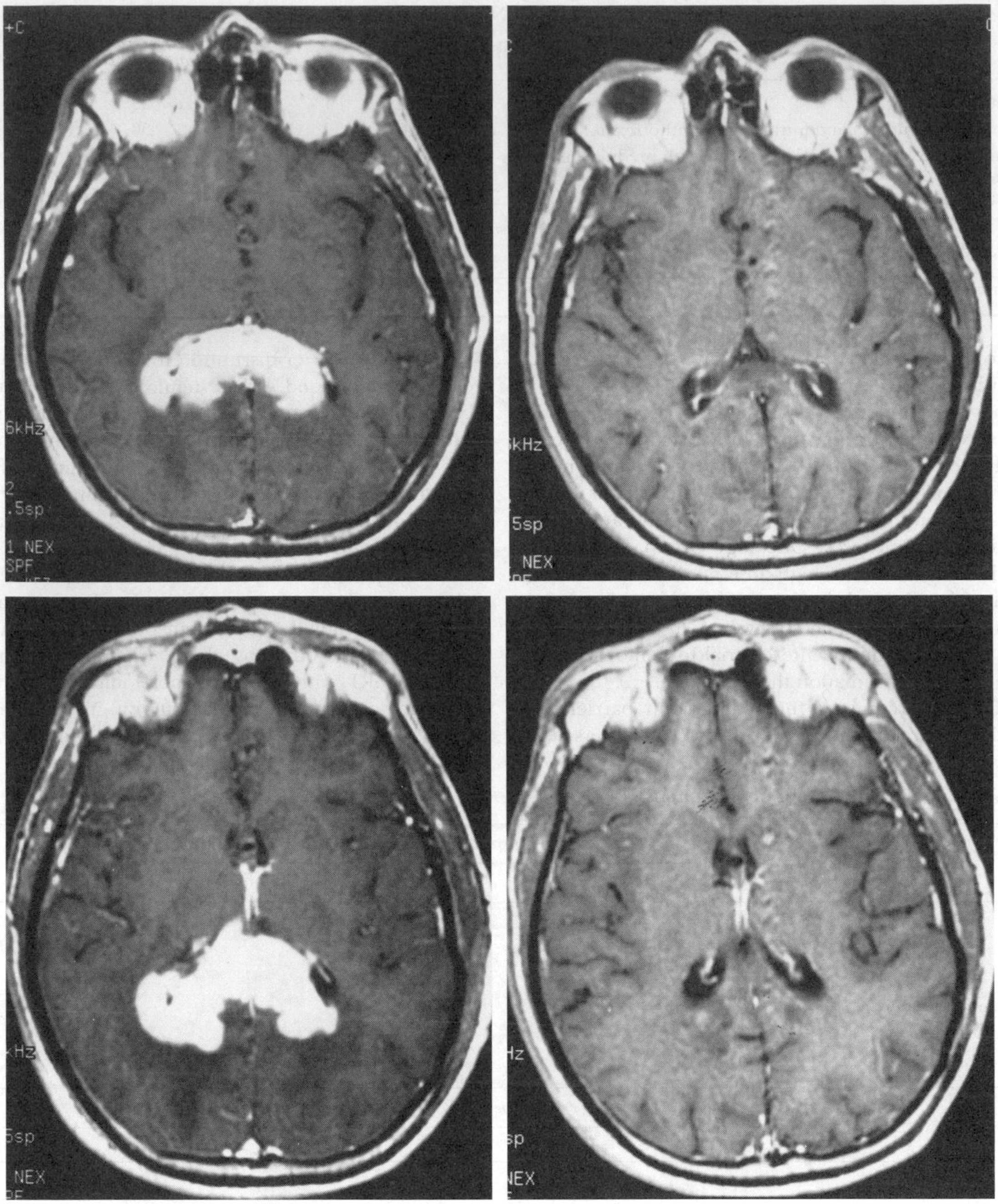

FIGURE 45.5-2. Gadolinium-enhanced magnetic resonance imaging scans demonstrating a complete response of primary central nervous system (CNS) lymphoma to high-dose methotrexate, procarbazine, and vincristine. The prominent and diffuse enhancement pattern and periventricular location are characteristic of primary CNS lymphoma.

tine after WBRT is completed seem to be reasonable in patients who have received no prior chemotherapy. We have avoided methotrexate in this setting because of potential CNS toxicity.

The prolonged survival seen with combined modality regimens has led to greater appreciation of treatment-induced late neurologic toxicity. Merchut and associates first reported radiation necrosis in a patient with PCNSL treated with radiotherapy alone.[83] Liang and associates noted a high incidence of late toxicity in survivors treated with CHOP and intrathecal methotrexate plus WBRT.[69] Long-term follow-up of our original cohort of patients reveals that almost 100% of patients older than the age of 60 years at diagnosis experience significant late sequelae within 4 years of treatment, whereas only 30% of younger patients have similar problems after a 7.5-year latency.[76] Mass and associates report no toxicity with intraarterial therapy; however, their own experimental work clearly demonstrates damage of normal brain structures when chemotherapy follows blood–brain barrier disruption.[84] These issues led to an exploration of systemic chemotherapy alone as effective treatment for PCNSL. Glass and associates reported long-term survival in a few patients treated with high-dose methotrexate alone.[85] We, and others, have treated elderly patients with a multiagent chemotherapeutic regimen.[86–88] The response rate was greater than 90%, with most patients having a complete response. Median survival for patients older than age 60 years was 33 months, superior to a median of 7.1 months for radiation therapy alone in a comparable age group.[56] Furthermore, no patient developed neurotoxicity. Similar results were observed in 14 patients treated by Sandor et al. with a high-dose methotrexate-based regimen without radiation therapy.[89] These preliminary data suggest that good disease control can be achieved by chemotherapy alone.

There are few examples of ocular lymphoma being treated with chemotherapy. Barr and associates used cyclophosphamide and then vincristine in one patient with metastatic ocular lymphoma without effect.[90] Sullivan and Dallow reported both systemic and ocular remission in a patient with a systemic histiocytic lymphoma and a ciliary body metastasis, after treatment with procarbazine, CCNU, and vincristine.[91] Baumann and coworkers reported a patient with lymphomatous uveitis who relapsed after ocular irradiation.[92] Treatment with intravenous cytarabine, 500 mg, and methotrexate, 200 mg, had no effect; however, high-dose cytarabine, 3 g/m^2, produced a complete response that was long lasting. Furthermore, therapeutic cytarabine levels were documented in both aqueous and vitreous humor 90 minutes after infusion was completed. Strauchen and associates treated six patients with primary ocular lymphoma with high-dose cytarabine, obtaining a response in five.[93] We have observed responses of ocular lymphoma to high-dose methotrexate before ocular radiotherapy. In addition, Valluri and coworkers used our original PCNSL regimen to treat three patients with ocular lymphoma, two of whom had concurrent CNS disease; these patients remained in CNS and ocular remission 30 to 40 months after diagnosis.[94] The role of chemotherapy in treating ocular involvement in PCNSL remains to be clarified; however, these reports suggest that some agents or combination regimens may prove useful in the future. Intravitreal injection of methotrexate was described as effective treatment for recurrent ocular lymphoma.[95] Although this approach eliminates systemic toxicity from intravenous chemotherapy, it requires frequent intraocular injections.

IMMUNOCOMPROMISED PATIENTS

The treatment modalities for PCNSL in immunocompetent patients are also used to treat AIDS-related PCNSL, although they are generally less effective and more toxic in immunodeficient patients. The initiation of treatment first requires a histologic diagnosis of PCNSL. In the non-AIDS immunocompromised patient a stereotactic biopsy should be performed when an intracranial mass lesion is first diagnosed. In AIDS patients, a noninvasive diagnosis can often be achieved with the use of positron emission tomography or single photon emission computed tomographic imaging and the detection of EBV DNA in CSF. In the absence of a definitive circumstantial diagnosis, biopsy should be performed. Toxoplasmosis continues to be the most common cause of an intracranial mass in an AIDS patient, but PCNSL is the second most common. However, empiric treatment with 2 to 3 weeks of antitoxoplasmosis therapy is an unacceptable diagnostic trial because most PCNSL patients markedly deteriorate during this time, severely limiting subsequent treatment options.

Corticosteroids and cranial irradiation are the mainstays of treatment for PCNSL in immunosuppressed patients. Use of corticosteroids should be limited because they can contribute to the underlying immunosuppression; however, they are still valuable for short-term control of neurologic symptoms and may be necessary during the course of WBRT. AIDS patients with PCNSL do respond to cranial irradiation, but median survival is only 2 to 5 months because most die of systemic or coexistent CNS infections.[96–99]

Chemotherapy for PCNSL has been used infrequently in immunodeficient patients. Intrathecal methotrexate for leptomeningeal lymphoma was reported to be effective in a single patient with immunoglobulin A deficiency, although the benefit was of short duration.[100] Potent intravenous chemotherapy programs are often inappropriate for immunosuppressed patients, particularly those with AIDS. However, there is a subset of AIDS patients who benefit from a vigorous approach.[101,102] Typically, these are patients with a good performance status, no active comorbid conditions, and a relatively high CD4 cell count (200/μL or more). Such patients do have prolonged survival when chemotherapy is added to WBRT, often surviving more than 1 year and occasionally for many years. Again, high-dose methotrexate is the agent of choice.[103] There are isolated reports of patients with AIDS-related PCNSL who have been successfully treated with antiviral and biologic agents or reconstitution of their immune system using highly active antiretroviral therapy.[104,105] These reports open new therapeutic avenues for what has been a virulent and deadly complication of human immunodeficiency virus-1 infection. Furthermore, monitoring the level of CSF EBV DNA may prove helpful in assessing treatment response, in addition to conventional imaging techniques.[106]

REFERENCES

1. Burstein SD, Kernohan JW, Uihlein A. Neoplasms of the reticuloendothelial system of the brain. *Cancer* 1963;16:289.
2. Rubinstein LJ. Tumors of the central nervous system. In: *Atlas of tumor pathology.* Second series, Fascicle 6. Washington, DC: Armed Forces Institute of Pathology, 1972:215.
3. Taylor CR, Russell R, Lukes RJ, Davis RL. An immunohistological study of immunoglobulin content of primary central nervous system lymphomas. *Cancer* 1978;41:2197.
4. Jellinger K, Radaskiewicz TH, Slowik F. Primary malignant lymphomas of the central nervous system in man. *Acta Neuropathol (Berl)* 1975;(Suppl VI):95.
5. Zimmerman HM. Malignant lymphomas of the nervous system. *Acta Neuropathol (Berl)* 1975;(Suppl VI):69.
6. Rosenblum ML, Levy RM, Bredesen DE, et al. Primary central nervous system lymphoma in patients with AIDS. *Ann Neurol* 1988;(Suppl) 23:S13.
7. Welch K, Finkbeiner W, Alpers CE, et al. Autopsy findings in the acquired immune deficiency syndrome. *JAMA* 1984;1152:252.
8. Goplen AK, Dunlop O, Liestol K, et al. The impact of primary central nervous system lymphoma in AIDS patients: a population-based autopsy study from Oslo. *J Acquir Immune Defic Syndr Hum Retroviral* 1997;14:351.
9. Eby NL, Grufferman S, Flannelly CM, et al. Increasing incidence of primary brain lymphoma in the US. *Cancer* 1988;62:2461.
10. Lutz JM, Coleman MP. Trends in primary cerebral lymphoma. *Br J Cancer* 1994;716:70.
11. Devesa SS, Fears T. Non-Hodgkin's lymphoma time trends: United States and international data. *Cancer Res* 1992;(Suppl)52:5432S.
12. Hao D, DiFrancesco LM, Brasher PMA, et al. Is primary CNS lymphoma really becoming more common? A population-based study of incidence, clinicopathological features and outcomes in Alberta from 1975 to 1996. *Ann Oncol* 1999;10:65.
13. DeAngelis LM, Yahalom J, Rosenblum M, Posner JB. Primary CNS lymphoma: managing patients with spontaneous and AIDS-related disease. *Oncology* 1987;52:1.
14. So YT, Choucair A, Davis RL, et al. Neoplasms of the central nervous system in acquired immunodeficiency syndrome. In: Rosenblum ML, Levy RM, Bredesen DE, eds. *AIDS and the nervous system.* New York: Raven Press, 1988:285.
15. Recht L, Straus DJ, Cirrincione C, et al. Central nervous system metastases from non-Hodgkin's lymphoma: treatment and prophylaxis. *Am J Med* 1988;84:425.
16. O'Neill BP, Dinapoli RP, Kurtin PJ, Habermann TM. Occult systemic non-Hodgkin's lymphoma (NHL) in patients initially diagnosed as primary central nervous system lymphoma (PCNSL): how much staging is enough? *J Neurooncol* 1995;67:25.
17. Herrlinger U. Primary CNS lymphoma: findings outside the brain. *J Neurooncol* 1999;43:227.
18. DeAngelis LM. Primary central nervous system lymphoma as a secondary malignancy. *Cancer* 1991;67:1431.

19. Balmaceda C, Gaynor JJ, Sun M, Gluck JT, DeAngelis LM. Leptomeningeal tumor in primary central nervous system lymphoma: recognition, significance, and implications. *Ann Neurol* 1995;38:202.
20. Schaumburg HH, Plank CR, Adams RD. The reticulum cell sarcoma-microglioma group of brain tumours: a consideration of their clinical features and therapy. *Brain* 1972;95:199.
21. DeAngelis LM. Current management of primary central nervous system lymphoma. *Oncology* 1995;63:9.
22. Char DH, Ljung B-M, Miller T, Phillips T. Primary intraocular lymphoma (ocular reticulum cell sarcoma) diagnosis and management. *Ophthalmology* 1988;95:625.
23. Rockwood EJ, Zakov ZN, Bay JW. Combined malignant lymphoma of the eye and CNS (reticulum-cell sarcoma). *J Neurosurg* 1984;61:369.
24. Whitcup SM, de Smet MD, Rubin BI, et al. Intraocular lymphoma clinical and histopathologic diagnosis. *Ophthalmology* 1993;100:1399.
25. Peterson K, Gordon KB, Heinemann MH, DeAngelis LM. The clinical spectrum of ocular lymphoma. *Cancer* 1993;72:843.
26. Lachance DH, O'Neill BP, Macdonald DR, et al. Primary leptomeningeal lymphoma: report of 9 cases, diagnosis with immunocytochemical analysis, and review of the literature. *Neurology* 1991;41:95.
27. Scott TF, Hogan EL, Carter TD, et al. Primary intracranial meningeal lymphoma. *Am J Med* 1990;89:536.
28. Hochberg FH, Miller DC. Primary central nervous system lymphoma. *J Neurosurg* 1988;68:835.
29. Bruni J, Bilbao JM, Gray T. Primary intramedullary malignant lymphoma of the spinal cord. *Neurology* 1977;27:896.
30. Hautzer NW, Aiyesimoju A, Robitaille Y. "Primary" spinal intramedullary lymphomas: a review. *Ann Neurol* 1983;62:14.
31. Mitsumoto H, Breuer AC, Lederman RJ. Malignant lymphoma of the central nervous system: a case of primary spinal intramedullary involvement. *Cancer* 1980;46:1258.
32. DeAngelis LM, Yahalom J, Heinemann M-H, et al. Primary CNS lymphoma: combined treatment with chemotherapy and radiotherapy. *Neurology* 1990;40:80.
33. Herrlinger U, Schabet M, Bitzer M, et al. Primary central nervous system lymphoma: from clinical presentation to diagnosis. *J Neurooncol* 1999;43:219.
34. DeAngelis LM. Cerebral lymphoma presenting as a non-enhancing lesion(s) on CT/MR scan. *Ann Neurol* 1993;33:308.
35. DeAngelis LM. Primary central nervous system lymphoma: curable without toxicity? *Cancer J Sci Am* 1996;2:137.
36. Hoffman JM, Waskin HA, Schifter T, et al. FDG-PET in differentiating lymphoma from nonmalignant central nervous system lesions in patients with AIDS. *J Nucl Med* 1993;34:567.
37. Castagna A, Cinque P, d'Amico A, et al. Evaluation of contrast-enhancing brain lesions in AIDS patients by means of Epstein-Barr virus detection in cerebrospinal fluid and ^{201}thallium single photon emission tomography. *AIDS* 1997;11:1522.
38. Antinori A, De Rossi G, Ammassari A, et al. Value of combined approach with thallium-201 single-photon emission computed tomography and Epstein-Barr virus DNA polymerase chain reaction in CSF for the diagnosis of AIDS-related primary CNS lymphoma. *J Clin Oncol* 1999;17:554.
39. Henry JM, Heffner RR, Dillard SH, et al. Primary malignant lymphomas of the central nervous system. *Cancer* 1974;34:1293.
40. Littman P, Wang CC. Reticulum cell sarcoma of the brain. *Cancer* 1987;35:1412.
41. Li C-Y, Witzig TE, Phyliky RL, et al. Diagnosis of B-cell non-Hodgkin's lymphoma of the central nervous system by immunocytochemical analysis of cerebrospinal fluid lymphocytes. *Cancer* 1986;57:737.
42. List AF, Greco FA, Vogler LB. Lymphoproliferative diseases in immunocompromised hosts: the role of Epstein-Barr Virus. *J Clin Oncol* 1987;5:1673.
43. Rouah E, Rogers BB, Wilson DR, et al. Demonstration of Epstein-Barr virus in primary central nervous system lymphomas by the polymerase chain reaction and in situ hybridization. *Hum Pathol* 1990;21:545.
44. DeAngelis LM, Wong E, Rosenblum M, Furneaux H. Epstein-Barr virus in AIDS and non-AIDS primary central nervous system lymphoma. *Cancer* 1992;70:1607.
45. MacMahon EME, Glass JD, Hayward SD, et al. Epstein-Barr virus in AIDS-related primary central nervous system lymphoma. *Lancet* 1991;969:338.
46. Clinque P, Brytting M, Vago L, et al. Epstein-Barr virus DNA in cerebrospinal fluid from patients with AIDS-related primary lymphoma of the central nervous system. *Lancet* 1993;398:342.
47. Nakhleh RE, Manivel JC, Hurd E, Sung JH. Central nervous system lymphomas: immunohistochemical and clinicopathologic study of 26 autopsy cases. *Arch Pathol Lab Med* 1989;1050:113.
48. Kumanishi T, Washiyama K, Nishiyama A, et al. Primary malignant lymphoma of the brain: demonstration of immunoglobulin gene rearrangements in four cases by the Southern blot hybridization technique. *Acta Neuropathol (Berl)* 1989;23:79.
49. Jellinger KA, Paulus W. Primary central nervous system lymphomas: new pathological developments. *J Neurooncol* 1995;33:24.
50. Marsh WL, Stevenson DR, Long HJ. Primary leptomeningeal presentation of T-cell lymphoma: report of a patient and review of the literature. *Cancer* 1983;51:1125.
51. Schmitt-Graff A, Pfitzer P. Cytology of the cerebrospinal fluid in primary malignant lymphomas of the central nervous system. *Acta Cytol* 1983;27:267.
52. Grant JW, Gallagher PJ, Jones PD. Primary cerebral lymphoma: a histologic and immunohistochemical study of six cases. *Arch Pathol Lab Med* 1986;110:897.
53. Morgello S, Maiese K, Petito CK. T-cell lymphoma in the CNS: clinical and pathologic features. *Neurology* 1989;39:1190.
54. Bashir R, Chamberlain M, Ruby E, Hochberg FH. T-cell infiltration of primary CNS lymphoma. *Neurology* 1996;46:440.
55. Vokes EE, Ultmann JE, Golomb HM, et al. Long-term survival of patients with localized diffuse histiocytic lymphoma. *J Clin Oncol* 1985;3:1309.
56. Nelson DF, Martz KL, Bonner H, et al. Non-Hodgkin's lymphoma of the brain: can high dose, large volume radiation therapy improve survival? Report on a prospective trial by the Radiation Therapy Oncology Group (RTOG): RTOG 8315. *Int J Radiat Oncol Biol Phys* 1992;9:23.
57. Weller M. Glucocorticoid treatment of primary CNS lymphoma. *J Neurooncol* 1999;43:237.
58. Gametchu B. Glucocorticoid receptor-like antigen in lymphoma cell membranes: correlation to cell lysis. *Science* 1987;236:456.
59. Kawakami Y, Tabuchi K, Ohnishi R, et al. Primary central nervous system lymphoma. *J Neurosurg* 1985;62:522.
60. Mendenhall NP, Thar TL, Agee OF, et al. Primary lymphoma of the central nervous system: computerized tomography scan characteristics and treatment results for 12 cases. *Cancer* 1983;52:1993.
61. Nelson DF. Radiotherapy in the treatment of primary central nervous system lymphoma (PCNSL). *J Neurooncol* 1999;241:43.
62. DeAngelis LM, Yahalom J, Thaler HT, Kher U. Combined modality treatment for primary CNS lymphoma. *J Clin Oncol* 1992;10:635.
63. Margolis L, Fraser R, Lichter A, Char DH. The role of radiation therapy in the management of ocular reticulum cell sarcoma. *Cancer* 1980;45:688.
64. Rampen RHJ, van Andel JG, Sizoo W, van Unnik JAM. Radiation therapy in primary non-Hodgkin's lymphomas of the CNS. *Eur J Cancer* 1980;16:177.
65. Stewart DJ, Russell N, Atack EA, et al. Cyclophosphamide, doxorubicin, vincristine, and dexamethasone in primary lymphoma of the brain: a case report. *Cancer Treat Rep* 1983;67:287.
66. Stewart DJ, Russell N, Dennery M, et al. Cyclophosphamide, adriamycin, vincristine and dexamethasone in the treatment of bulky central nervous system lymphomas. *J Neurooncol* 1984;2:289(abst).
67. Lachance DH, Brizel DM, Gockerman JP, et al. Cyclophosphamide, doxorubicin, vincristine, and prednisone for primary central nervous system lymphoma: short-duration response and multi-focal intracerebral recurrence preceding radiotherapy. *Neurology* 1994;44:1721.
68. Pollack IF, Lunsford LD, Flickinger JC, Dameshek HL. Prognostic factors in the diagnosis and treatment of primary central nervous system lymphoma. *Cancer* 1989;63:939.
69. Liang BC, Grant R, Junck L, et al. Primary central nervous system lymphoma: treatment with multiagent systemic and intrathecal chemotherapy with radiation therapy. *Int J Oncol* 1993;3:1001.
70. Schultz C, Scott C, Sherman W, et al. Preirradiation chemotherapy with cyclophosphamide, doxorubicin, vincristine, and dexamethasone (CHOD) for primary CNS lymphomas: Initial report of Radiation Therapy Oncology Group protocol 88-06. *J Clin Oncol* 1996;14:556.
71. O'Neill BP, O'Fallon JR, Earle JD, et al. Primary central nervous system non-Hodgkin's lymphoma: survival advantages with combined initial therapy? *Int J Radiat Oncol Biol Phys* 1995;33:663.
72. Brada M, Dearnaley D, Horwich A, Bloom HJG. Management of primary cerebral lymphoma with initial chemotherapy: preliminary results and comparison with patients treated with radiotherapy alone. *Int J Radiat Oncol Biol Phys* 1990;18:787.
73. Reni M, Ferreri AJM, Garancini MP, Villa E. Therapeutic management of primary central nervous system lymphoma in imunocompetent patients: results of a critical review of the literature. *Ann Oncol* 1997;8:227.
74. Blay J-Y, Conroy T, Chevreau C, et al. High-dose methotrexate for the treatment of primary cerebral lymphomas: analysis of survival and late neurologic toxicity in a retrospective series. *J Clin Oncol* 1998;16:864.
75. DeAngelis LM. Primary CNS lymphoma: treatment with combined chemotherapy and radiotherapy. *J Neurooncol* 1999;43:249.
76. Abrey LE, DeAngelis LM, Yahalom J. Long-term survival in primary central nervous system lymphoma. *J Clin Oncol* 1998;16:859.
77. Cohen IJ, Vogel R, Matz S, et al. Successful non-neurotoxic therapy (without radiation) of a multifocal primary brain lymphoma with a methotrexate, vincristine, and BCNU protocol (DEMOB). *Cancer* 1986;6:57.
78. Socie G, Piprot-Chauffat C, Schlienger M, et al. Primary lymphoma of the central nervous system: an unresolved therapeutic problem. *Cancer* 1990;65:322.
79. Shibamoto Y, Tsutsui K, Dodo Y, et al. Improved survival rate in primary intracranial lymphoma treated by high-dose radiation and systemic vincristine-doxorubicin-cyclophosphamide-prednisolone chemotherapy. *Cancer* 1990;65:1907.
80. DeAngelis LM, Seiferheld W, Schold SC, et al. Combined modality treatment of primary central nervous system lymphoma (PCNSL): RTOG 93-10. *Proc Am Soc Clin Oncol* 1999;18:140a.
81. Dahlborg SA, Henner WD, Crossen JR, et al. Non-AIDS primary CNS lymphoma: the first example of a durable response in a primary brain tumor using enhanced chemotherapy delivery without cognitive loss and without radiotherapy. *Cancer J Sci Am* 1996;2:166.
82. Chamberlain MC, Levin VA. Primary central nervous system lymphoma: a role for adjuvant chemotherapy. *J Neurooncol* 1992;14:271.
83. Merchut MP, Haberland C, Naheedy MH, Rubino FA. Long survival of primary cerebral lymphoma with progressive radiation necrosis. *Neurology* 1985;35:552.
84. Mass MK, Remsen L, McCormick C, et al. Neurotoxicity of chemotherapeutic agents and immunoconjugates delivered after blood-brain barrier modification: neuropathological studies. *Ann Neurol* 1995;38:342(abst).
85. Glass J, Gruber ML, Cher L, Hochberg FH. Preirradiation methotrexate chemotherapy of primary central nervous system lymphoma: long-term outcome. *J Neurosurg* 1994;81:188.
86. Freilich RJ, Delattre JY, Monjour A, DeAngelis LM. Chemotherapy without radiation therapy as initial treatment for primary central nervous system lymphoma in older patients. *Neurology* 1996;46:435.
87. Guha-Thakurta N, Damek D, Pollack C, Hochberg FH. Intravenous methotrexate as initial treatment for primary central nervous system lymphoma: response to therapy and quality of life of patients. *J Neurooncol* 1999;43:259.
88. Abrey LE, Yahalom J, DeAngelis LM. Combination chemotherapy in primary central nervous system lymphoma (PCNSL). *Proc Am Soc Clin Oncol* 1999;18:146a.

89. Sandor V, Stark-Vancs V, Pearson D, et al. Phase II trial of chemotherapy alone for primary CNS and intraocular lymphoma. *J Clin Oncol* 1998;16:3000.
90. Barr CC, Green WR, Payne JW, et al. Intraocular reticulum-cell sarcoma: clinico-pathologic study of four cases and review of the literature. *Surv Ophthalmol* 1975;19:224.
91. Sullivan SF, Dallow RL. Intraocular reticulum cell sarcoma: its dramatic response to systemic chemotherapy and its angiogenic potential. *Ann Ophthalmol* 1977;9:401.
92. Baumann MA, Ritch PS, Hande KR, et al. Treatment of intraocular lymphoma with high-dose Ara-C. *Cancer* 1986;57:1273.
93. Strauchen JA, Dalton J, Friedman AH. Chemotherapy in the management of intraocular lymphoma. *Cancer* 1989;63:1918.
94. Valluri S, Moorthy RS, Khan A, Rao NA. Combination treatment of intraocular lymphoma. *Retina* 1995;15:125.
95. Fishburne BC, Wilson DJ, Rosenbaum JT, Neuwelt EA. Intravitreal methotrexate as an adjunctive treatment of intraocular lymphoma. *Arch Ophthalmol* 1997;115:1152.
96. Gill PS, Levine AM, Meyer PR, et al. Primary central nervous system lymphoma in homosexual men: clinical, immunologic, and pathologic features. *Am J Med* 1985;78:741.
97. So YT, Beckstead LH, Davis RL. Primary central nervous system lymphoma in acquired immune deficiency syndrome: a clinical and pathological study. *Ann Neurol* 1986; 20:566.
98. Baumgartner JE, Rachlin JR, Beckstead JH, et al. Primary central nervous system lymphomas: natural history and response to radiation therapy in 55 patients with acquired immunodeficiency syndrome. *J Neurosurg* 1990;73:206.
99. Ling SM, Roach III M, Larson DA, Wara WM. Radiotherapy of primary central nervous system lymphoma in patients with and without human immunodeficiency virus. *Cancer* 1994;73:2570.
100. Gregory MC, Hughes JT. Intracranial reticulum cell sarcoma associated with immunoglobulin A deficiency. *J Neurol Neurosurg Psychiatry* 1973;36:769.
101. Forsyth PA, Yahalom J, DeAngelis LM. Combined-modality therapy in the treatment of primary central nervous system lymphoma in AIDS. *Neurology* 1994;44:1473.
102. Chamberlain MC. Long survival in patients with acquired immune deficiency syndrome-related primary central nervous system lymphoma. *Cancer* 1994;73:1728.
103. Jacomet C, Girard PM, Lebrette MG, et al. Intravenous methotrexate for primary central nervous system non-Hodgkin's lymphoma in AIDS. *AIDS* 1998;12:1725.
104. Raez L, Cabral L, Cai J-P, et al. Treatment of AIDS-related primary central nervous system lymphoma with zidovudine, ganciclovir, and interleukin 2. *AIDS Res Hum Retrovirus* 1999;15:713.
105. McGowan JP, Shah S. Long-term remission of AIDS-related primary central nervous system lymphoma associated with highly active antiretroviral therapy. *AIDS* 1998;12:952.
106. Antinori A, Cingolani A, De Luca A, et al. Epstein-Barr virus in monitoring the response to therapy of acquired immunodeficiency syndrome –related primary central nervous system lymphoma. *Ann Neurol* 1999;5:259.

SECTION 6

VOLKER DIEHL
PETER M. MAUCH
NANCY LEE HARRIS

Hodgkin's Disease

HISTORY

A great deal has been written about the life and accomplishments of Thomas Hodgkin.[1] In his historic paper entitled "On Some Morbid Appearances of the Exorbant Glands and Spleen," presented to the Medical Chirurgical Society in London on January 10, 1832, Hodgkin described the clinical history and postmortem findings of the massive enlargement of lymph nodes and spleens of six patients studied at Guy's Hospital in London and of a seventh patient who had been seen by Carswell in 1828.[2] Without a microscope, Hodgkin recognized that these patients had a disease that started in the lymph nodes located along the major vessels in the neck, chest, or abdomen, rather than from an inflammatory condition.

In 1856, Sir Samuel Wilks, a Guy's Hospital pathologist, described ten postmortem cases that had "a peculiar enlargement of the lymphatic glands frequently associated with disease of the spleen." By 1865, Dr. Wilks had collected 15 cases, which were published in a second paper entitled "Cases of the Enlargement of the Lymphatic Glands and Spleen (or Hodgkin's Disease) with Remarks."[3] This linked Hodgkin's name permanently to this newly identified disease. Wilks's initial descriptions gave us some of our earliest understanding of Hodgkin's disease (HD). He described the disease as a cancer that started and remained in the lymph nodes for a long time, perhaps years, before involving the spleen and then spreading to other organs. He also noted anemia, weight loss, and fevers in some of the patients with HD.

Although other physicians had provided descriptions of the characteristic giant cells present in the lymph nodes and spleens of patients with HD, Dr. W. S. Greenfield in 1878 was the first to contribute drawings of them from a low microscopical magnification of a lymph node specimen.[4] Despite Greenfield's findings, Dr. Carl Sternberg (in 1898) and Dr. Dorothy Reed (in 1902) are credited with the first definitive microscopical descriptions of HD.[5,6]

Both Sternberg and Reed, along with many other physicians, believed that HD was caused by an associated infection rather than by a separate malignant process of the lymph nodes. Proponents of the infectious theory cited the frequent association of HD with tuberculosis. Eight of Sternberg's thirteen cases of HD had coexistent tuberculosis, and he believed HD to be a variant of tuberculosis. Other physicians believed that HD was a cancer of the lymph nodes. Clinical and pathologic studies, available in the early twentieth century, helped to confirm their view.[7] Despite the very strong evidence for the malignant nature of HD over the last century, it has only recently been shown that Hodgkin's-Reed-Sternberg (H-RS) cells are clonal, confirming their origin from a single malignant cell.[8]

ETIOLOGY AND EPIDEMIOLOGY

Approximately 7500 new cases of HD are diagnosed each year in the United States. Slightly more men than women develop this malignancy (1.4:1). In economically developed countries, there is an age-related bimodal incidence for HD. The first peak occurs in the third decade of life, and a second rise in incidence occurs after the age of 50 years. The incidence of HD by age also differs by histologic subtype.[9]

Mycobacterium tuberculosis was first suspected of being the etiologic organism for HD because of the high coexistence of tuberculosis in these patients.[5] This theory was later discounted when it was appreciated that HD was associated with deficits in the immune system that accounted for the increased presence of associated infections.[10] Several studies in the 1970s suggested that HD might be contagious because of reports of clustering of the disease. The first reports, by Vianna and Poln,[11] noted clustering among high school students exposed to HD. However, population-based studies, using cancer registries in Connecticut and California, convincingly made the argument that the reported clusters occurred by chance alone, and a study that repeated the methodology of Vianna and Poln[11] in a different location failed to confirm their findings.[12]

A number of studies have suggested that a genetic predisposition for HD exists. There is an increased incidence in Jews and also among first-degree relatives.[13] Siblings appear to have a two- to fivefold increased risk; in siblings of the same gender, there is as much as a ninefold increased risk.[14] An increased risk among parent-child pairs but not among spouses again suggests a genetic predisposition. Also, HD has been linked with certain HLAs.[15,16]

There is less support for most other potential causes of HD. In contrast to other malignancies, HD rarely is seen as a second malignancy and does not appear to be increased in patients with illness- or treatment-related chronic immunosuppression. Although HD has been noted in patients with the acquired immunodeficiency syndrome (AIDS), evidence for a direct correlation with the immunosuppression associated with AIDS is lacking.[17]

In contrast, increasing evidence suggests a viral etiology for HD. In economically developed countries, studies report an association between HD in younger patients and increased maternal education, decreased numbers of siblings and playmates, early birth order, and single-family dwellings in childhood.[18,19] This association between HD and childhood factors that decrease exposure to infectious agents at an early age has led investigators to propose that the epidemiologic features of HD appear to mimic those of a viral illness that has an age-related host response to infection.

Epstein-Barr virus (EBV) is the leading viral candidate for HD causation.[20] There is a twofold to threefold excess in the incidence of HD among patients with a history of mononucleosis, a disease caused by EBV. In addition, there appears to be an altered antibody pattern to EBV in patients before presenting clinically with HD, with elevated titers against the viral capsid antigen and against the EBV nuclear antigen (EBNA) as compared to controls.[21] This suggests that such patients may have had more severe initial EBV infections or more frequent viral replication associated with the development of HD.

Patients in nonindustrialized countries and from lower socioeconomic groups, as well as children, who develop HD are more likely to have EBV-positive HD than are patients with high socioeconomic backgrounds in the young adult age group.[20,22] In these groups, even nodular sclerosis HD (NSHD) has a higher incidence of EBV positivity than it does in the young adult cases.

Some cellular and molecular biology data have provided additional support for the association of EBV and HD.[23] Through the use of sensitive molecular probes, including Southern blot, *in situ* hybridization, and polymerase chain reaction (PCR) assays, 30% to 50% of HD specimens have been found to contain EBV genome fragments in the diagnostic RS cells.[24] In the United States and Western Europe, the tumor cells of classic HD (CHD) are EBV-positive in approximately 50% of the cases. The positivity rate is lower in NSHD (15% to 30%) and higher in mixed-cellularity HD (MCHD) (60% to 70%) (Table 45.6-1).[25]

EBV genome status appears to be stable over time when studied in initial biopsies and at relapse. The latent gene products, latent membrane protein (LMP) and EBNA2, have important roles in EBV-induced cell transformation *in vitro*. EBV genome–positive RS cells express the phenotype LMP1 and LMP2+/EBNA1+ EBNA2–, a phenotype found in EBV genome–positive nasopharyngeal carcinoma and in a small portion of T-cell non-Hodgkin's lymphomas (NHLs). LMP1 has transforming activity for B cells, and its expression should give a survival advantage to infected cells. Because EBV is capable of immortalizing B cells, and because all the cells in infected cases carry the same clone of EBV and express the most potent transforming protein (LMP1), the obvious conclusion is that EBV must play some role in the pathogenesis of HD. However, the fact that EBV is not present in all the cases leaves open the question of the pathogenesis of EBV-negative cases and, more important, the question of whether EBV is important even in positive cases.

TABLE 45.6-1. Hodgkin's Disease: Differences in EBV Association (Approximate)

EBV-Positive Cases	*NS (%)*	*Total (%)*	*MC (%)*
Japan	—	25	—
United States-Europe	35	40	65
Mexico	50	70	80
Other Latin American	—	70–100	—
Africa	80	80	100
China	50	60	90–100
Children	—	80	—
HIV	—	80	—

EBV, Epstein-Barr virus; HIV, human immunodeficiency virus; MC, mixed cellularity; NS, nodular sclerosis.

Patients with autoimmune disease who are treated with rather mild immunosuppression with methotrexate occasionally develop a Hodgkin's-like lesion, which is EBV-positive in nearly 50% of the cases.[26] Taken together, these observations suggest that immunosuppression *per se* does not predispose to the development of HD but that, when it does develop, it is likely to be of mixed-cellularity (MC) or lymphocyte-depleted (LD) type and EBV-positive.[27]

H-RS cells show a specific expression pattern of the viral latent genes with expression of EBNA1 and LMP.[28] This pattern is identical to that found in nasopharyngeal carcinoma endemic in the southwest of China. It differs from such other EBV-associated neoplasias as endemic Burkitt's lymphoma and immunoblastic B-cell NHLs of immunocompromised patients. Except for EBNA1, all latent viral proteins represent targets for cytotoxic T lymphocytes (CTLs). Thus, EBV-infected cells either express the complete set of latent viral genes in an immunocompromised host (immunoblastic NHL) or they down-regulate these proteins except EBNA1 (Burkitt's lymphoma), possibly to escape the host's immune response. Thus far, it remains unclear how the specific latent viral gene expression pattern in HD (EBNA2- and LMP-positive) and the pronounced T-cell proliferation in affected lymph nodes relate to each other.

The functional relevance of LMP expression in H-RS cells is not understood. LMP has a transforming potential: Transformation of epithelial cells after transfection of LMP has been described. In lymphocytes, apoptoses can be prevented by LMP via up-regulation of the bcl-2 gene. LMP is also a target for CTLs. In addition, it up-regulates (partly in cooperation with EBNA2) numerous cellular genes [e.g., activation-associated antigens (CD23, CD30, CD39)] and adhesion molecules [intracellular adhesion molecule-1 (ICAM-1), lymphocyte function-associated antigen 3 (LFA-3)]. Thus it may render a cell indirectly more susceptible for a T-cell response. Knecht et al.[29] described in some HD cases mutations in the carboxy-terminal part of the LMP1 gene identical to those previously reported in LMP isolates from Chinese nasopharyngeal carcinoma. These authors discussed an association of these mutations with a clinically more aggressive HD phenotype.

At least three hypotheses can be advanced to explain EBV-negative cases of HD. First, another virus could be involved in these cases; however, studies to date have failed to identify another virus.[30] Second, EBV may be involved in all the cases but may remain undetectable in some; this has been called the *hit-and-run theory*. In this scenario, EBV infects the cell, alters the DNA in some way, and then is eliminated, leaving the cell either transformed or susceptible to transformation. Elimination of EBV, with its immunogenic proteins, might be expected to occur most commonly in patients with active immune systems, such as the young women with NSHD. However, a third possibility, and the one perhaps best supported by epidemiologic data, is that EBV is not important in the pathogenesis of any of the cases of HD and that its presence in some cases simply reflects the presence of a larger reservoir of latently EBV-infected cells in these individuals.

Examination of the epidemiology of EBV-associated HD reveals several paradoxes, which cast doubt on the causative role of EBV in many cases. First, the group in which EBV had been predicted most likely to be involved—young women from high socioeconomic groups with NSHD—proved to have the lowest incidence of EBV in tumor tissue.[20] Second, there is no correlation between a history of either infectious mononucleosis or unusually high titers of antibodies to EBV and detectable EBV in HD tissues.[31] Thus, in contrast to what one would expect if most HD cases were caused by EBV, populations in which HD is common (young women in affluent societies) have EBV-negative HD and populations in which HD is rare (young children in underdeveloped countries, older individuals, and immunosuppressed patients) have EBV-positive HD.[20] These apparent paradoxes force us to at least consider the possibility that EBV may be merely an epiphenomenon in HD, reflecting a high incidence of EBV-infected B cells in the patient, rather than an etiologic factor.

In summary, despite data that suggest an etiologic role for EBV in HD, direct evidence of a causative role is lacking . The lack of an animal model and the difficulties in studying the malignant cells in HD continue to frustrate investigators. Additional epidemiologic, serologic, and molecular data are needed to determine whether EBV is a causative agent.

BIOLOGY AND CELL OF ORIGIN

LINEAGE, ORIGIN, AND CLONALITY OF HODGKIN'S-REED-STERNBERG CELLS

Specific Morphologic Features of Hodgkin's Disease

Lymph nodes affected by HD consist of a heterogeneous mixture of lymphocytes, histiocytes, eosinophils, plasma cells, fibroblasts, and other cells. The mononuclear Hodgkin's cells and their polynucleated counterparts, the RS cells, which have long been considered to represent the malignant substrate of the disease, represent only 0.1% to 1.0% of the entire cell population in CHD [i.e., lymphocyte-rich CHD (LRCHD) and the NS, MC, and LD subtypes].[10] Similarly, in lymphocyte-predominant HD (LPHD, nodular paragranuloma), the pathognomonic lymphocytic and histiocytic (L&H) cells represent only a small minority of the total cell population. This scarcity of the putative tumor cells was one of the major obstacles for understanding the nature of these cells. Whereas in the LP subtype of HD, H-RS cells consistently express B-cell-specific surface antigens (CD19, CD20), in CHD H-RS cells express, in the majority of cases, the activation markers Ki-1 (CD30), the Leu-M1 antigen (CD15), the interleukin-2 (IL-2) receptor (CD25), the transferrin receptor (CD71), and HLA class II molecules (HLA-DR), but not surface antigens, which helped to determine their physiologic counterpart.[32] Until recently, the application of conventional molecular-genetic methods for a more detailed analysis of H-RS cells was not possible owing to their scarcity. In addition, these cells could not be enriched from tissue affected by HD, presumably due to their fragility. Thus, over decades, the cell of origin of the H-RS cells remained an enigma.

Cell Lines and Animal Models

The establishment of permanently growing cell lines permitted the biologic and genetic characterization of the tumor cell population in numerous human neoplasias. In contrast, outgrowth of a cell line is extremely rare in HD. The first two permanent cell lines (designated L428 and L540) were established in 1979 from patients with advanced-stage HD [clinical stage (CS) IVB].[33] These cell lines grew from a pleural effusion and bone marrow. With few exceptions, all subsequently established cell lines were also obtained from body fluids (bone marrow, pleural effusion, peripheral blood) of advanced-stage patients.[34] This observation may reflect an *in vivo* adaptation of the cells to the conditions of suspension culture as prerequisite for *in vitro* outgrowth. Thus far, only 15 cell lines have been established that may be regarded as HD-derived. Analysis of immunophenotype, karyotype, immunoglobulin (Ig), or T-cell receptor gene rearrangements of these cell lines revealed, in analogy to analysis of primary tissue, heterogeneous results, not allowing any conclusion to be drawn on the cell of origin of HD. In addition, their derivation from primary H-RS cells could not be determined unequivocally.[34] A novel EBV-negative cell line (L1236) has been established from the peripheral blood of a patient with advanced HD of the MC subtype.[35] Using H-RS single-cell PCR, it could be shown that the genomic sequences of the Ig gene rearrangements of the H-RS cells in the patient's bone marrow were identical to those detected in L1236 cells.[36] Thus, in this cell line, the H-RS cell origin is definitely proven on the molecular level.

HD-derived cell lines were used successfully for the discovery of H-RS cell–associated antigens, which include CD30 (Ki-1), CD70, and Ki-27,[37,38] for cloning the CD30 gene,[39] and for studying the CD30 signal transduction pathway. They also enabled the *in vitro* testing of new immunotherapeutic modalities such as Ricin A–linked anti-CD30 immunotoxins,[40] Saporin-linked anti-CD30 immunotoxins,[41] and anti-CD16/CD30 bispecific antibodies.[42]

Though none of these HD-derived cell lines could be grown reproducibly in thymus-aplastic T-cell-deficient nude mice, the HD-derived cell lines L540, HD-MyZ, and L1236 have been shown to disseminate intralymphatically after inoculation into T- and B-cell–deficient severe combined immunodeficient (SCID) mice.[35,43] The SCID mouse model is used for the preclinical *in vivo* testing of new experimental therapeutic approaches.[43] However, no reproducible growth of primary H-RS cells has been observed after transplantation of biopsy material.[44]

Results of Single-Cell Analysis: Hodgkin's-Reed-Sternberg Cells Are Clonal B Cells

A methodologic breakthrough for the biologic analysis of H-RS cells was achieved by the establishment of micromanipulation of immunophenotyped single cells from frozen sections, allowing the amplification and analysis of genes derived from a single cell. Küppers et al.[45] amplified rearranged Ig heavy-chain genes from single H-RS cells micromanipulated from two cases of CHD and one case of LPHD. Sequence analysis revealed the clonal B-cell origin of the H-RS cells in all three cases. In 14 of 15 additional cases of CHD, again clonally rearranged Ig genes were detected in the H-RS cells. Clonal Ig gene rearrangements in H-RS cells of CHD were also found by others using micromanipulation and single-cell PCR.[46] Similarly, using the new method, clonally related Ig gene rearrangements were detected in L&H cells isolated from frozen tissue sections of LPHD.[47] Thus, there is overwhelming evidence that at least a substantial proportion of cases (if not all cases) of CHD and LPHD represent monoclonal B-cell disorders.

Germinal Center Derivation of H-RS Cells

The site of physiologic contact between a specific antigen and a B lymphocyte is the germinal center (GC) of a lymph node. This contact results in somatic mutations accumulating in the Ig genes and leading to the expression of antibodies with a higher affinity due to amino acid exchanges. However, somatic mutations might also result in a lower affinity of the antibody or even in generation of a stop codon. When B cells lose their ability to express an antibody or when they express an antibody with lower affinity, they subsequently undergo apoptosis within the GC. All other B cells accumulating favorable mutations are rescued from apoptosis by expressing the bcl-2 gene. These B cells clonally expand and can accumulate further mutations to improve the affinity of their antibody. After leaving the GC, they differentiate into B memory cells or plasma cells. In a substantial proportion of LPHD cases, the clonal L&H cells revealed ongoing mutations, which provides evidence that L&H cells are GC-derived B cells that depend on antigen binding and selection.[47] In this context, L&H cells are comparable with follicular lymphoma (FL) cells. Whereas FL cells frequently harbor the chromosomal translocation t(14;18), resulting in activation of the bcl-2 gene, the transforming event in L&H cells remains unknown. H-RS cells of CHD differ from FL as well as from LPHD in that they accumulate crippling somatic mutations within potentially functional Ig gene rearrangements, which prevent further antibody expression.[36] These crippling mutations do not necessarily have to be located within the coding region of Ig genes. One case of MCHD has been described in which a somatic mutation within a regulatory element of the IgH promoter was associated with down-regulation of Ig gene expression.[48] The detection of crippling mutations rendering potential functional Ig gene rearrangements nonfunctional suggests that H-RS cells, as a rule, grow independently from antigen selection and even antibody expression. Indeed, no Ig gene expression in H-RS cells could be demonstrated by several groups. The mechanism preventing apoptosis of the H-RS cells within the GC still is unknown.

GENETIC ALTERATIONS IN HODGKIN'S DISEASE

Conventional karyotype analysis of Hodgkin's and RS cells is hampered by the low number of obtainable mitoses from lymph node suspensions and their poor chromosome-banding qualities. In addition, karyotypes cannot be unequivocally attributed to malignant cells, as the cellular compartment with the highest mitotic index in affected tissue is that of nonmalignant lymphocytes in the neighborhood of the H-RS cells. Thus, proliferating cells with a normal karyotype most probably represent reactive lymphoid cells.[49] Depending on the histologic subtype, between 75% (NS) and 42% (LP) of cases studied yielded evaluable metaphases. In karyotype analyses performed by different groups, the percentage of abnormal karyotypes varied considerably, between 22% and 83%. Although numeric and structural cytogenetic abnormalities were observed, a specific chromosomal marker of HD—as, for instance, the Burkitt's lymphoma–specific chromosomal translocations—has not yet been defined.[50] In a study of 60 lymph nodes obtained from untreated patients with HD, numeric or structural aberrations (or both) were found in approximately one-half of the analyzable cases.[51] Among HD-associated chromosomal abnormalities, aneuploidy (100%) with hyperdiploidy (70%) is the most frequent. Chromosomes 1, 2, 5, 12, and 21 are often triplicated. In a few cases, a loss of chromosomes is reported; for example, chromosomal translocations or deletions were found in two-thirds of cases.[51]

Analysis of whole tissue sections for genomic alterations or deregulated expression of the oncogenes MYC, JUN, RAF, and RAS did not reveal any characteristic pattern.[52] Because the t(14;18) translocation results in overexpression of the bcl-2 protein preventing apoptotic death of FL cells, many attempts were made using PCR to detect breakpoints in the major breakpoint region (mbr) of t(14;18) in H-RS cells. In several studies, the t(14;18) translocation was found in 0% to 39% of HD cases. Whether the translocation was localized in the H-RS cells remained unproven in these positive cases, however, particularly as the detection of the bcl-2 protein by immunohistochemistry *in situ* was not congruent with the detection of the translocation itself in all cases. In one report using micromanipulation of single H-RS cells followed by PCR, the t(14;18) was shown to be localized in nonmalignant bystander B cells and not in a single case in the H-RS cells.[53] Mutations in the p53 tumor suppressor, which are commonly found in a variety of human cancers, also could not be detected in H-RS cells using single-cell analysis.[54] In view of the derivation of H-RS cells from the GC of lymph nodes, putative mechanisms preventing apoptosis of their precursors are of special interest for understanding the transforming events. The nuclear transcription factor NFκB might be involved in prevention of apoptosis. Indeed, constitutive expression of NFκB has been found in HD-derived cell lines as well as in primary H-RS cells *in situ*.[55] It also has been suggested that defects in the inhibitory molecule IκB might underlie the overexpression of NFκB, at least in some cases of HD. So far, however, the mechanisms preventing apoptosis in H-RS cells are not understood.[56]

IMMUNOLOGY OF HODGKIN'S DISEASE

Cellular Immunodeficiencies

HD is associated with a complex deficiency in cellular immunity, including impairment of delayed cutaneous hypersensitivity, enhanced Ig production, high levels of circulating immune complexes, production of antilymphocyte and anti-Ia antibodies, decreased natural killer (NK) cell cytotoxicity, enhanced sensitivity to suppressor monocytes and T suppressor cells, and a variety of other disorders of serum factors, including high levels of circulating IL-2 receptors. *In vitro*, peripheral blood lymphocytes show spontaneous DNA and IgG synthesis and depressed proliferative response to T-cell mitogen stimulation, with impairment of lymphokine production.

Increasing numbers of long-term survivors provided the opportunity to restudy anergy and *in vitro* lymphocyte responsiveness in patients who have been successfully treated. Studies at the National Cancer Institute (NCI), in a population of uniformly staged and treated patients, showed that anergy did not influence prognosis within a given stage. After successful treatment, anergy to recall antigens was reversible, although response to neoantigens remained suppressed. This defect appears to be disease-related, as patients with other types of lymphomas did not show this defect. Unlike the defects in delayed hypersensitivity, most studies have shown that the antibody response of B cells and the B-cell numbers are normal in HD patients, except in those with advanced disease.

Antigen-Presenting Phenotype of Hodgkin's-Reed-Sternberg Cells

In affected lymph nodes, the rare H-RS cells are surrounded by a majority of nonmalignant bystander cells. The majority of lymphocytes in affected lymphatic tissue are activated T helper cells (CD4+, CD45R0+, CD45RB).[57] These lymphocytes represent the population with the highest mitotic index in affected lymph nodes. The lymph nodes often grow slowly and show fluctuations in their size in early disease stages. These observations point toward a cellular immune reaction as the primary reason for the lymph node enlargement in HD. In contrast to benign lymphoproliferative lesions (e.g., reactive lymph nodes), the immune reaction in HD is not self-limited. One reason might be the inability of the immune system to eliminate the malignant cells expressing the target antigen.[58] The recently established HD-derived cell line L1236 expresses HLA class I and II molecules, B7.1 and B7.2 (CD80, CD86), and the adhesion molecules ICAM-1 (CD54) and LFA-3 (CD58).[59] All of these molecules are essential for efficient T-cell recruitment (accessory molecules). Expression of HLA antigens and of B7.1 molecules has also been described on H-RS cells in biopsy specimens and on other HD-derived cell lines (L428, L540; unpublished observation). The expression pattern of the surface antigens on H-RS cells thus points toward an antigen-presenting functional phenotype.

Antigen-presenting cells and, in particular, dendritic cells play a major role in the recruitment and activation of antigen-specific T cells, which is mainly attributed to their ability effectively to present antigens and to provide costimulatory signals via CD40, members of the B7 family (CD80, CD86), and adhesion molecules (CD11a, CD11c, LFA-3, ICAM-1). Furthermore, immunoregulatory cytokines such as IL-12, secreted by dendritic cells, promote the development of Th1 T cells, which play a major role in tumor-specific T-cell responses (Fig. 45.6-1).

Hodgkin's Disease and Immunity against Epstein-Barr Virus

In one study, it was shown that the H-RS cell population was uniformly HLA class I–positive in at least 75% of cases of EBV genome–positive HD, whereas the figure was much lower in EBV genome–negative tumors.[60] More than one-half of the EBV genome–nega-

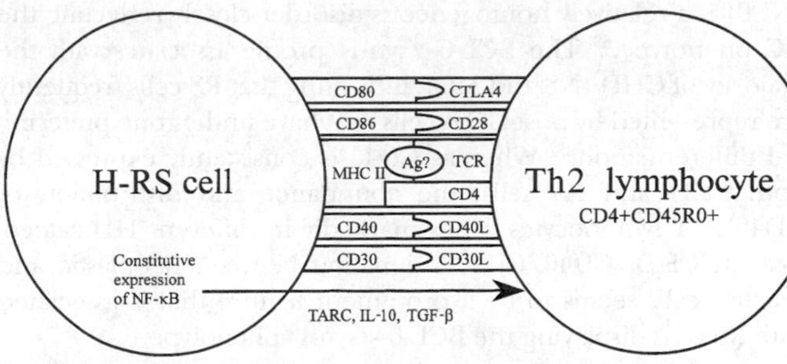

FIGURE 45.6-1. Antigen-presenting cell–like functional phenotype of a B-cell–derived tumor cell. Ag, antigen; H-RS, Hodgkin's-Reed-Sternberg; IL-10, interleukin-10; MHC, major histocompatibility complex; TARC, thymus and activation regulated chemokine; TCR, T-cell receptor; TGF-β, transforming growth factor-β; Th2, T helper cell 2.

tive tumors had no detectable HLA class I expression in tumor cells. Analyses of transporter associated with antigen processing (TAP) expression in H-RS cells found that almost all HD cases, regardless of EBV status, were positive for TAP1 and for TAP2. Furthermore, it has been shown that in the HD-derived cell line L1236, the LMP2 can be processed and presented through the HLA class I pathway. Although TAP expression in L1236 is not down-regulated, processing of the LMP2-derived target epitope might also have occurred via a TAP-independent route.

Nerve Growth Factor Superfamily: Relevant Molecules?

The CD30 antigen, a member of the nerve growth factor superfamily, has been defined by a cluster of antibodies raised first against the HD-derived cell line L428.[61] Initially, the expression of CD30 seemed to be related exclusively to H-RS cells, thus representing a tumor-specific antigen. Subsequently, the CD30 antigen was also found on activated T and B cells as well as on activated and differentiated macrophages. The highest CD30 expression is seen on HD lymphoma cells, CD30+ large cell lymphomas (LCLs) with T-cell phenotype, and acute lymphocytic leukemia T cells.

The CD30/CD30 ligand (CD30/CD30L) interaction probably plays a central role in the complex interaction between H-RS cells and their microenvironment. A CD30L has been described[39] that exerts pleiotropic effects on different lymphoma subtypes *in vitro* and is expressed only on the bystander cells (T cells, monocytes, granulocytes) but not on the H-RS cells. In tissue culture experiments, some biologic functions of the CD30/CD30L interaction have been characterized that point toward a cytokine receptor function of the CD30 antigen. It remains to be established whether the pleiotropic effects of CD30/CD30L interaction in different cell types are due to a different intracellular signaling or whether they reflect sequence differences in the CD30 gene.

The soluble form of CD30 (sCD30) is detectable in the serum of patients with advanced stages of HD. This has been considered to reflect a prognostic factor for an unfavorable outcome.[62] It has been shown *in vitro* that CD40/CD40L signaling is able to down-regulate BCL-6 in B cells with a GC phenotype. A similar effect is exerted *in vitro* also by LMP1, which is functionally homologous to CD40. It thus may be postulated that CD40 ligation is the major determinant of the phenotype of the RS cell. The BCL-6^{+}/syn-1^{-} profile associates with 100% nodular LPHD (NLPHD), thus corroborating the notion that nodular lymphocyte predominance

(NLP) is a relatively homogeneous disorder closely reflecting the GC phenotype.[63] The BCL-6–/syn-1+ profile associates with the majority of CHD (NS and MC), indicating that RS cells frequently are represented by post-GC B cells that have undergone preterminal differentiation.[64] Whereas CD40 is consistently expressed by both L&H and RS cells, the abundance and distribution of CD40L+ T lymphocytes varies markedly in different HD categories. In CHD, CD40/CD40L signaling between neoplastic and reactive cells seems to be a prominent feature that is associated with RS cells displaying the BCL-6–/syn-1+ phenotype.

Chronic Secretion of Cytokines

IL-2 receptor levels and other inflammatory cytokines are elevated in the sera of patients. The (deregulated?) expression of cytokines may at least partially explain the complex interaction between H-RS and bystander cells. For instance, eosinophilia in HD is caused by IL-5, and fibrosis may be triggered by IL-1 and transforming growth factor-β (TGF-β). IL-1, IL-6, and IL-9, which are produced by H-RS cells, may act as autocrine growth factors and as paracrine growth stimulators for T cells.[65] Vice versa, the T cells may stimulate H-RS cells via IL-2 and IL-6. Many cytokines, including IL-1, IL-5, IL-6, IL-9, IL-10, and TGF-β, are produced by RS cells, and it is suspected that constitutive nuclear expression of NFκB is responsible for this phenomenon.[58]

IL-10 is a pleiotropic cytokine with potent inhibitory effects toward Th1 cells and is mainly produced by Th2 cells, activated monocytes and macrophages, stimulated B cells, and mast cells. It has been suggested that IL-10 is involved in the pathogenesis of malignant B-cell lymphomas. HD is characterized by an abnormal or unbalanced secretion or production of cytokines, including IL-10, which supports growth of both neoplastic Hodgkin's and Reed-Sternberg (H-RS) cells and their surrounding reactive bystander cells.

In untreated HD patients, 13% were found to be seropositive for IL-10 before therapy, whereas IL-10 was not detectable in a healthy control population. HD patients whose disease was at an advanced clinical stage (stage III or IV) were found to have higher IL-10 serum levels. A univariate analysis indicated a correlation of elevated IL-10 serum levels with early relapse and reduced long-term survival. The group of IL-10-seropositive HD patients showed a significant correlation of elevated IL-10 serum level with a reduced relapse-free survival. Thus, the increased production of IL-10 in HD could be associated with a poor clinical prognosis and may serve as a prognostic factor.[66]

PATHOLOGY

DEFINITION OF HODGKIN'S DISEASE

The clinical features and responses to treatment of HD differ dramatically from those of most so-called NHLs, suggesting that a specific immunologic reaction is important not only in the definition but also in the clinical behavior of this disease. Studies in the 1980s showed that in NLPHD, the RS cell variants expressed B-cell–associated antigens,[67] whereas these cells in most cases of NSHD and MCHD lacked these antigens.[68] This difference in immunophenotype, together with the observation that NLPHD follows a more indolent clinical course,[69] led to the suggestion that NLPHD was a low-grade B-cell lymphoma and should be removed from the category of HD and placed with the NHLs. However, both immunophenotypic and, more recently, molecular genetic studies have shown that CHD of the NS and MC types can express B-cell–associated antigens and, similar to NLPHD, have rearranged Ig genes.[70,71] Furthermore, NLPHD and CHD share the feature of having a small number of neoplastic cells in a reactive background, which distinguishes both from most B-cell NHLs. Thus, although it is now known that the neoplastic cells in most cases of both LPHD and CHD are monoclonal B cells, their distinctive pathologic and clinical features still warrant placing them together in a separate category from other lymphoid neoplasms.[72] It is important for both pathologists and oncologists to recognize that HD is two distinct diseases. Therefore, current classifications include two main categories of HD: CHD (NS, MC, and LD) and NLPHD. In summary, the Hodgkin's lymphomas are defined as lymphomas containing one of the characteristic types of RS cells in a background of nonneoplastic cells; cases are subclassified according to the morphology and immunophenotype of the RS cells and the composition of the cellular background. The differences in the morphology of the RS cells and the composition of the cellular background have formed the basis for the pathologic subclassification of HD (Table 45.6-2).

CLASSIFICATIONS OF HODGKIN'S DISEASE

The early classification by Jackson and Parker[73] recognized three categories of HD: paragranuloma, granuloma, and sarcoma. The distinction among the three categories was based on the ratio of neoplastic to normal cells, which increased from paragranuloma to granuloma to sarcoma, and predicted decreasing survival. In 1966, Lukes et al.[74] recognized that the category of granuloma could be subdivided into two categories—NS and MC—which were characterized by distinctive morphology and clinical features. Lukes et al.[74] also recognized that there were two variants of what they called *lymphocytic* or *histiocytic predominance type* (replacing paragranuloma)—a nodular and a diffuse variant—which they found differed in prognosis. The Lukes and Butler classification was modified and simplified at the Rye conference in 1966.[74] The Rye classification has remained the standard classification since that time.

In 1994, the International Lymphoma Study Group introduced an updated classification, incorporating new immunologic and molecular data, as part of the Revised European-American Lymphoma (REAL) Classification.[75] These concepts have been incorporated into the new World Health Organization (WHO) classification of hematologic malignancies, a joint effort of the Society for Hematopathology and the European Association of Hematopathologists.[354]

Several major differences exist between the REAL/WHO classification of HD and older classifications. Most important is the recognition that there are two distinct diseases that have been called HD: CHD, which consists predominantly of NS and MC, and NLPHD (Table 45.6-3). Simply a predominance of lymphocytes in the background is not sufficient to classify a case as NLPHD; cases that have the RS-cell morphology and immunophenotype of CHD, even if they contain predominantly lymphocytes, are classified as *lymphocyte-rich classic Hodgkin's disease* (LRCHD). A second difference is that, in the Lukes-Butler and Rye classifications, MC was a heterogeneous category, including both typical cases and all other cases that did not fit into one of the other categories. We now recommend that MC be restricted to typical cases and that unclassifiable cases be categorized as *HD unclassifiable*. Finally, it is now clear that immunophenotype is important in the subclassification of HD, both in distinguishing

TABLE 45.6-2. Classifications of Hodgkin's Disease

Jackson and Parker[a]	*Lukes and Butler*[b]	*Rye Conference*[c]	*REAL Classification*[d]	*WHO Classification*[e]
Paragranuloma	Lymphocytic or histiocytic, nodular	Lymphocyte-predominant	Nodular lymphocyte-predominant classic HD	Lymphocyte-predominant, nodular classic HD
	Lymphocytic or histiocytic, diffuse	—	Lymphocyte-rich classic HD[f]	Lymphocyte-rich classic HD
Granuloma	Nodular sclerosis	Nodular sclerosis	Nodular sclerosis	Nodular sclerosis
	Mixed cellularity[g]	Mixed cellularity[g]	Mixed cellularity	Mixed cellularity
Sarcoma	Diffuse fibrosis	Lymphocyte-depleted	Lymphocyte-depleted	Lymphocyte-depleted
	Reticular	—	—	Unclassifiable classic HD

HD, Hodgkin's disease; REAL, Revised European-American Lymphoma; WHO, World Health Organization.
[a]Jackson JH, Parker JF. Hodgkin's disease. General considerations. *New Engl J Med* 1944;230:1.
[b]Lukes RJ, Butler JJ. The pathology and nomenclature of Hodgkin's disease. *Cancer Res* 1966;26:1063.
[c]Lukes RJ, Craver LF, Hall TC, et al. Report of the nomenclature committee. *Cancer Res* 1966;26:1311.
[d]Harris NL, Jaffe ES, Stein H, et al. A revised European-American classification of lymphoid neoplasms: a proposal from the International Lymphoma Study Group. *Blood* 1994;84:1361.
[e]Harris NL, Jaffe ES, Diebold J, et al. The World Health Organization classification of hematological malignancies report of the Clinical Advisory Committee Meeting, Airlie House, Virginia, November 1997. *Mod Pathol* 2000;13:193.
[f]Includes some lymphocytic and histiocytic nodular cases.
[g]Includes unclassifiable cases.

NLPHD from classic types and in distinguishing HD from NHL; thus, the immunophenotype is included in the definitions of HD in the REAL/WHO classification. Typical freedom-from-treatment-failure (FFTF) and survival curves for the main histologic subtypes are illustrated in Figure 45.6-2 using German Hodgkin's Lymphoma Study Group data.

Nodular Lymphocyte-Predominant Hodgkin's Disease

MORPHOLOGIC FEATURES. NLPHD is defined as having at least a partially nodular growth pattern; diffuse areas are present in a minority of cases, and it is controversial whether purely diffuse cases exist.[76] The RS-cell variants differ from mononuclear and classic RS cells: They have vesicular, polylobed nuclei and distinct but small, usually peripheral nucleoli, without perinucleolar halos; these have been called *L&H cells* (after Lukes and Butler) or *popcorn cells*, because of the resemblance of their nuclei to an exploded kernel of corn.[74] In fact, they resemble "exploded" centroblasts. Although popcorn cells may be very numerous, usually no classic, diagnostic RS cells are found. In occasional cases, however, the RS cells may resemble classic or lacunar types; in such cases, immunophenotyping is helpful in establishing the diagnosis. The background is predominantly lymphocytes; clusters of epithelioid histiocytes may be numerous; plasma cells, eosinophils, and neutrophils rarely are seen and, if present, are not numerous.[77] Occasional sclerosis may cause some cases to resemble NSHD.

PROGRESSIVE TRANSFORMATION OF GERMINAL CENTERS. A distinctive type of follicular lymphoid hyperplasia, known as *progressive transformation of germinal centers* (PTGCs), is seen focally in approximately 20% of lymph nodes involved by NLPHD and may be seen in the absence of HD in other lymph nodes in the same patient.[78] PTGCs are enlarged follicles that contain numerous small B cells of mantle zone type; these follicles may closely resemble the nodules of NLPHD. This phenomenon has given rise to speculation that NLPHD may arise from PTGCs. PTGCs usually are seen as single or only a few enlarged

TABLE 45.6-3. Morphologic and Immunophenotypic Features of Nodular Lymphocyte-Predominant and Classic Hodgkin's Disease

	Classic HD	*NLPHD*
Pattern	Diffuse, interfollicular, nodular	Nodular, at least in part
Tumor cells	Diagnostic RS cells; mononuclear or lacunar cells	L&H or "popcorn" cells
Background	Lymphocytes, histiocytes, eosinophils, plasma cells	Lymphocytes, histiocytes
Fibrosis	Common	Rare
CD15	+	–
CD30	+	–
CD20	±	+
CD45	–	+
EMA	–	+
EBV (in RS cells)	+ (~50%)	–
Background lymphocytes	T cells > B cells	B cells > T cells
CD57+ T cells	–	+
Ig genes (single-cell PCR)	Rearranged, clonal, mutated, "crippled"	Rearranged, clonal, mutated, ongoing

EBV, Epstein-Barr virus; EMA, epithelial membrane antigen; RS, Reed-Sternberg; HD, Hodgkin's disease; Ig, immunoglobulin; L&H, lymphocytes and histiocytes; NLPHD, nodular lymphocyte-predominant Hodgkin's disease; PCR, polymerase chain reaction.

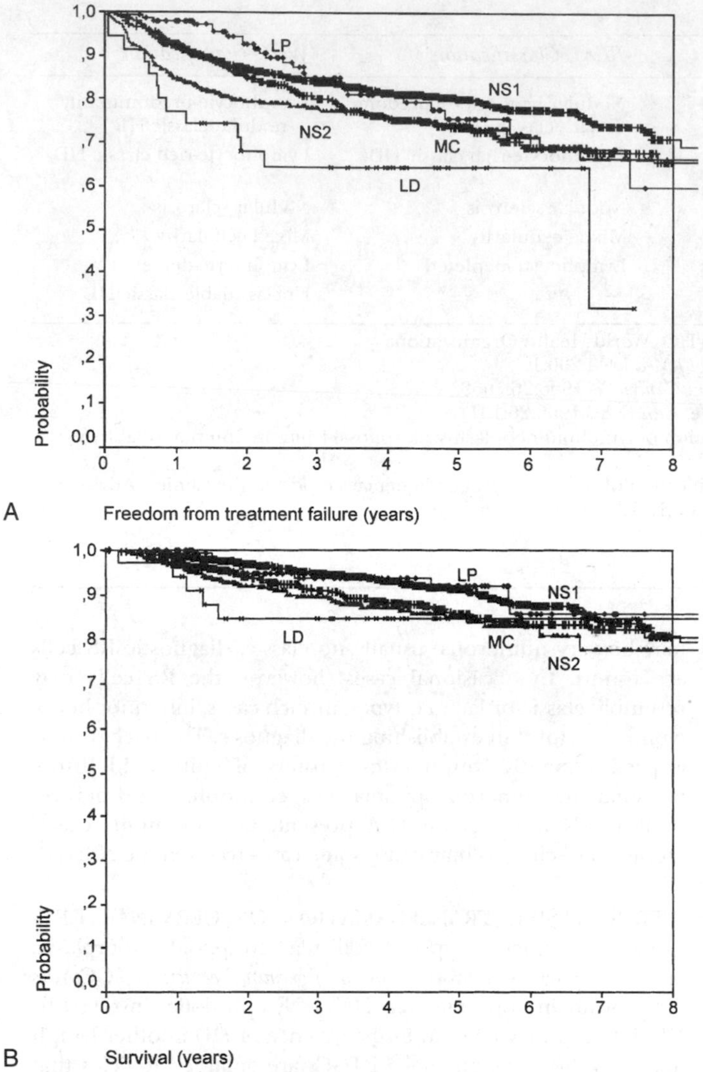

FIGURE 45.6-2. **A:** Reviewed histologic subtype: freedom from treatment failure in the German Hodgkin's Study Group trials, 1988 through 1998, all stages. Significant ($P \leq .01$) comparisons: NS1 vs. NS2, $P = .0012$; LP vs. LD, $P = .0088$; NS1 vs. LD, $P = .0017$. **B:** Reviewed histologic subtype: survival in the German Hodgkin's Study Group trials, 1988 through 1998. Significant ($P \leq .01$) comparisons: NS1 vs. NS2, $P = .0021$. LD, lymphocyte-depleted (n = 35); LP, lymphocyte-predominant (n = 144); NS1, nodular sclerosis grade 1 (n = 1397); NS2, nodular sclerosis grade 2 (n = 361); MC, mixed-cellularity (n = 596).

follicles in a setting of nonspecific reactive follicular lymphoid hyperplasia; however, on occasion, they may be numerous and associated with prominent lymph node enlargement, particularly in adolescents and young adults.[79]

NODULAR LYMPHOCYTE-PREDOMINANT HODGKIN'S DISEASE AND LARGE B-CELL LYMPHOMA. Patients with NLPHD have a slightly higher risk of developing NHL than do patients with other types of HD.[80] Transformation of NLP to LCL, usually with a B-cell phenotype and often monoclonal with respect to Ig (both phenotype and genotype), is most common. Hansmann et al.[81] reported 2.6% in a series of 537 cases, and the British National Lymphoma Investigation (BNLI) reported a 2% incidence in 182 cases[80]; the range in recent reports is from 2% to 6.5%.[82] The LCL does not necessarily consist of typical L&H cells and usually resembles other diffuse, large B-cell lymphomas (DLBCLs).[81] Most cases studied have had a B-cell immunophenotype, with B-lineage antigen expression in the majority and monotypic Ig expression in approximately 30% to 50%. In some cases, a clonal relationship between the LP and the DLBCL has been shown by molecular genetic analysis.[83]

In addition to the cases that progress to DLBCL, NLP may be composite with DLBCL in thc same lymph node, at the time of either diagnosis or relapse.[84] In reported cases, the prognosis of these patients appears to be significantly better than that for usual DLBCL, and patients who respond to treatment may later relapse with only NLP.[84]

IMMUNOPHENOTYPE. The immunophenotype is an important part of the definition of NLP. In contrast to CHD, the atypical cells are CD45+, express B-cell–associated antigens (CD19, CD20, CD22, CD79a) and epithelial membrane antigen (EMA), but lack CD15 and CD30. In contrast to typical B-cell lymphomas, however, they are usually Ig-negative by routine techniques. J-chain has been demonstrated in many cases.[85] Studies using *in situ* hybridization for light-chain messenger RNA (mRNA) have shown clonal expression in the atypical cells.[86] Popcorn cells also express the nuclear protein encoded by the bcl-6 gene, which is associated with normal GC B-cell development, and the activation-associated molecules CD40 and CD86 (B7/BB1), which are involved in B-cell interaction with T cells.[87]

The nodules of LP are actually altered follicles or GCs. The small lymphocytes in the nodules are a mixture of polyclonal B cells with a mantle zone phenotype (IgM and IgD+), and numerous T cells, many of which are CD57+, similar to the T-cell population in normal and progressively transformed GCs.[88] T cells in NLP may exhibit significant nuclear enlargement and irregularity, resembling centrocytes. In contrast to the T cells in reactive or progressively transformed follicles, which are scattered singly and often concentrated in the light zone or at the junction with the mantle zone, the T cells in NLP form small aggregates, often giving the follicle a broken-up, moth-eaten, or irregular contour. They typically surround the neoplastic B cells, forming rings, rosettes, or collarettes. Although several reports suggest that the T cells surrounding popcorn cells are mostly CD57+,[89,90] this can be difficult to demonstrate in many cases, and absence of CD57+ cells in the rosettes does not argue against the diagnosis. A prominent concentric meshwork of follicular dendritic cells (FDCs) is present within the nodules. The interfollicular region contains predominantly T cells; when there are diffuse areas, the background lymphocytes are also predominantly T cells, and the FDC meshwork is lost.[91]

CLINICAL FEATURES. NLPHD accounts for 4% to 5% of the cases of HD in most series. The median age of patients is in the mid 30s, but cases may be seen both in children and the elderly. The male-female ratio is 3:1 or greater. NLPHD usually involves peripheral lymph nodes, with sparing of the mediastinum. Nearly 80% of the patients in most series are stage I or II at the time of the diagnosis, but rare patients may present with stage III or IV disease, with a concomitantly worse prognosis. More than 90% of the patients have a complete response to therapy, and 90% are alive at 10 years. The cause of death is often NHL, other cancers, or complications of treatment, rather than HD.[82,92]

Classic Hodgkin's Disease

CHD is defined by the presence of classic, diagnostic RS cells in a background of NS, MC, or LD, with classic immunophenotype (CD15+, CD30+, T- and B-cell–associated antigens usually negative). CHD includes NS, MC, and LD, as well as the proposed new category of LRCHD. Because the immunophenotype, genetic features, and postulated normal counterpart are the same for all of the classic types, these will be discussed together at the end of this section.

NODULAR SCLEROSIS HODGKIN'S DISEASE. *Morphologic Features.* NSHD, by definition, has at least a partially nodular pattern, with fibrous bands separating the nodules in most cases; diffuse areas are common, as is necrosis. The characteristic cell is the lacunar type RS cell, which may be very numerous. These are cells with characteristically multilobed nuclei and small nucleoli, with abundant, pale cytoplasm that retracts in formalin-fixed sections, producing an empty space, or lacuna. Diagnostic RS cells also are present but may be rare. The background usually contains lymphocytes, histiocytes, plasma cells, eosinophils, and neutrophils.[74]

In some cases with characteristic lacunar cells and a nodular or diffuse pattern, fibrous bands may be absent, and differentiating this type from NLP may be difficult. These cases have been called the *cellular phase* of NS[74]; in one series, the clinical course of these cases was slightly worse than that for typical cases.[93] Another morphologic variant, syncytial NS, has been described, in which, locally, the NS pattern is lost and large sheets of cells resembling lacunar RS-cell variants are seen. The prognosis of this variant was not reported to be different from that of typical NS. However, some studies have suggested that NS with lymphocyte depletion is associated with large mediastinal masses, advanced stage, and poor response to radiotherapy alone.[94]

Grading. The BNLI developed a system for grading NSHD (grade 1 and grade 2), based on the number and atypia of the RS cells in the nodules.[95] Cases of grade 2 NS overlap with the syncytial and LD variants already described. Based on this system, approximately 75% to 85% of the cases in most series are grade 1 and 15% to 25% are grade 2. In the BNLI series, grade 2 (NS2) tumors were associated with a worse prognosis than grade 1 (NS1) tumors, with NS2 tumors having an increased rate of relapse, shorter survival, and worse response to initial therapy (see Fig. 45.6-2). The BNLI studies have been criticized because some series included patients who were not pathologically staged and because, as compared to some other series, their patients had a relatively poor outcome.

Results from American and European centers have conflicted, showing either no influence on outcome or a significantly worse outcome for NS2 patients.[96,97] In general, when a center reports either a relatively high rate of relapse or relatively poor survival, NS2 patients are found to have a significantly worse outcome than NS1 patients; conversely, when overall relapse rates are low and survival high, grade has no impact on outcome.[97] This phenomenon was illustrated most clearly in a study of 195 patients treated in the Netherlands[98]; for patients treated between 1972 and 1980, when overall survival was relatively poor, grade 2 patients had a significantly worse outcome (5-year overall survival for NS1 and NS2, 83% and 43%, respectively), whereas for those treated between 1981 and 1992, grade had no impact on outcome (5-year overall survival for NS1 and NS2, 81% and 82%, respectively).

The impact of NS2 on survival is most evident in patients who experience relapse; those with NS2 have significantly shorter survival after relapse than do those with NS1. Taken together, these results suggest that more aggressive therapy benefits grade 2 patients; they also suggest the possibility that patients with NS1 could be treated less aggressively and still do as well. It could be argued that in future studies, NS should be consistently graded and that trials of less aggressive initial treatment for NS1 might be appropriate.

Clinical Features. NSHD is the most common subtype of HD in developed countries (60% to 80% in most series). It is most common in adolescents and young adults but can occur at any age; the number of affected female individuals equals or exceeds the number of affected male persons. The mediastinum and other supradiaphragmatic sites are commonly involved.

MIXED-CELLULARITY HODGKIN'S DISEASE. *Morphologic Features.* In MCHD, the infiltrate is usually diffuse or, at best, vaguely nodular, without band-forming sclerosis, although fine interstitial fibrosis may be present. RS cells are of the classic, diagnostic type and usually are easily identified. Many mononuclear variants are also usually present; rare lacunar cells may be seen. Diagnostic RS cells are large cells with bilobed, double, or multiple nuclei, with a large, eosinophilic, inclusion-like nucleolus in at least two lobes or nuclei. The infiltrate typically contains lymphocytes, epithelioid histiocytes, eosinophils, and plasma cells.[74]

Clinical Features. MCHD is accountable for 15% to 30% of HD cases in most series; it may be seen at any age and lacks the early adult peak of NSHD. Involvement of the mediastinum is less common than in NSHD, whereas abdominal lymph node and splenic involvement are more common.

LYMPHOCYTE-DEPLETED HODGKIN'S DISEASE. *Morphologic Features.* The infiltrate in lymphocyte-depleted HD (LDHD) is diffuse and often appears hypocellular, due to the presence of diffuse fibrosis and necrosis; there are large numbers of RS cells and bizarre sarcomatous variants, with a paucity of other inflammatory cells. Confluent sheets of RS cells and variants may occur and rarely predominate (reticular variant or Hodgkin's sarcoma).[74] Before the availability of immunophenotyping studies, many cases diagnosed as LDHD were, in reality, cases of large B-cell lymphoma or T-cell lymphomas, often of the anaplastic large cell lymphoma (ALCL) type. Cases of the reticular variant of LDHD may be difficult to distinguish from ALCL.[99]

Clinical Features. LDHD is the least common variant of HD, accounting for fewer than 1% of the cases in recent reports. It is most common in older people, in human immunodeficiency virus–positive (HIV-positive) individuals,[27] and in nonindustrialized countries. LDHD frequently presents with abdominal lymphadenopathy and spleen, liver, and bone marrow involvement, without peripheral lymphadenopathy.[100] The stage is usually advanced at diagnosis; however, response to treatment is reported not to differ from that of other subtypes of comparable stage.[94]

IMMUNOPHENOTYPE OF CLASSIC HODGKIN'S DISEASE. In most cases of NSHD, MCHD, and LDHD, the tumor cells are CD15+, CD30+, and CD45–. The frequency with which CD15 and CD30 are detected varies in reported series, probably because of technical problems. With microwave antigen retrieval and use of an anti-IgM secondary antibody, the German Hodgkin's Study Group (GHSG) reported 83% of 1751 cases to be positive for CD15, 96% positive for CD30, and 5% positive for CD20. Expression of B-cell antigens has been reported in a varying number of cases, usually only weakly and in a minority of the cells.[101] Thus, expression of B-cell antigens does not exclude a diagnosis of HD if the morphologic features are typical.

The diagnosis of HD still is made on routine sections, and immunophenotyping studies are an adjunct to the diagnosis. In a morphologically typical case, immunophenotyping studies are not absolutely necessary; however, they are becoming more standard practice. Failure to detect CD15 or CD30 or expression of a B-cell–associated antigen does not preclude a diagnosis of HD; however, absence of both CD15 and CD30 and expression of CD20 should prompt reexamination of the slides and consideration of either NLPHD or LRCHD. Expression of T-cell antigens is distinctly unusual, and should prompt both re-review of the slides and molecular genetic analysis of the T-cell receptor gene.

In addition to CD15 and CD30, RS cells express CD25, HLA-DR, ICAM-1, CD95 (apo-1/fas), and both CD40 and CD86 (B7), molecules associated with B-cell activation and interaction with T cells. T cells surrounding the RS cells express both CD40L and CD28, the ligand for CD86. In contrast to NLPHD, the RS cells of CHD lack the nuclear bcl-6 protein associated with follicle center B cells.[102] In EBV-positive cases, the tumor cells express EBV LMP but not EBNA2.

CLINICAL BEHAVIOR OF CLASSIC HODGKIN'S DISEASE. Several studies have addressed the impact of immunophenotype on the survival of patients with CHD, with varying results. The GHSG study found that cases that lacked CD15 but expressed CD30 had a significantly worse freedom from relapse and overall survival than did CD15+ cases. Coexpression of CD20 with CD15 or CD30 (or both) had no impact on outcome, but cases that expressed CD20 alone had poor survival; this result is similar to that reported by McBride et al.[103] and raises the question whether these may represent cases of T-cell–rich large B-cell lymphoma (see later, in Differential Diagnosis of Classic Hodgkin's Disease).

LYMPHOCYTE-RICH CLASSIC HODGKIN'S DISEASE. *Morphologic Features.* Some cases of HD with RS cells of the classic type, both by morphology and immunophenotype, may have a background infiltrate that consists predominantly of lymphocytes, with rare or no eosinophils. The term *lymphocyte-rich classic Hodgkin's disease* was proposed for these cases in the REAL classification. Some cases of LRCHD have a nodular pattern, with remnants of regressed GCs in the nodules and RS cells and variants located within the mantle zones and interfollicular regions,[104] mimicking NLPHD. This has been termed *follicular Hodgkin's lymphoma* or *nodular LRCHD.*[105]

Of 426 cases initially diagnosed as LPHD, review and immunophenotyping by a panel formed by the European Task Force on Lymphoma (ETFL) revealed that only 51% were confirmed as NLPHD, whereas 27% were LRCHD with a nodular pattern, with RS cells in the mantles of reactive follicles and in the interfollicular regions.[105] In a study from the GHSG, a similar rate of misdiagnosis of NLPHD was found; only 44% of 208 cases considered by at least one pathologist as LPHD had the immunophenotype of LPHD, whereas 56% were CHD. When the expert panel reclassified the cases by morphology alone, only 75% of the cases classified as LPHD and 88% of the cases classified as CHD were confirmed by immunophenotyping. Thus, cases of LRCHD may very closely resemble NLPHD and require immunophenotyping for differential diagnosis.

Immunophenotype. Cases of LRCHD have the immunophenotype of CHD, with expression of CD15 and CD30 by the RS cells; similar to other types of CHD, CD20 is coexpressed in 3% to 5% of cases.[105] In nodular areas, the background lymphocytes are predominantly B cells, similar to LPHD, and follicular meshworks of FDC are seen with antibodies to CD21 or CD35. Staining for FDC often reveals a small, dense aggregate of FDC consistent with a regressed GC, associated with a broad mantle zone with more loosely spaced FDC processes. The RS cells are found within the mantle area or at the junction of the mantle and interfollicular regions. CD57+ T cells may also be present and may rim the RS cells; thus, it is actually the immunophenotype of the RS cells that distinguishes LRCHD from NLPHD.

Clinical Features. The frequency of LRCHD among cases classified as HD can be roughly calculated from the two GHSG reports.[106] Of 1959 cases of HD with immunophenotyping for CD15, CD30, and CD20, LRCHD comprised 6% of cases (116) and LPHD 5% (92). In the ETFL and GHSG series, the clinical features at presentation of LRCHD seem to be intermediate between those of LPHD and CHD: similar to those with NLPHD, patients had early-stage disease and lacked bulky disease or B-cell symptoms; as in patients with either NLPHD or MCHD and in contrast to those with NLPHD, they lacked mediastinal disease and were predominantly male and, like MCHD patients, their median age was older than either NLPHD or NSHD patients. In the ETFL series, the overall survival for both LPHD and LRCHD patients was excellent but not significantly different from that for other types of HD. However, patients with NLPHD had an increased frequency of multiple relapses and better survival after relapse, as compared with LRCHD, NSHD, and MCHD patients. In the GHSG study, the overall survival of LRCHD was significantly worse than that of NLPHD. These data do not clearly define LRCHD as a distinct entity but are consistent with either an early phase of MCHD or a novel subtype. It is suggested that this category continue to be recognized within the classification of HD, so that additional data can be collected.

ASSOCIATION OF CLASSIC HODGKIN'S DISEASE WITH OTHER LYMPHOMAS. CHD may be associated with other lymphomas, most often of the B-cell type.[107] These lymphomas may occur before, simultaneously with, or after HD. Patients treated for HD are at risk for development of high-grade B-cell lymphomas (DLBCL or Burkitt's or Burkitt-like lymphoma), which have been presumed to arise in a setting of immunosuppression secondary to therapy for HD; the estimated risk ranges from 1% to 5%. However, EBV has not been demonstrated in the secondary lymphomas, in contrast to the situation in most immunosuppression-associated NHLs. Numerous cases of CHD associated with FL or DLBCL have been reported; the HD may precede, follow, or occur simultaneously with the NHL.[107,108] Two cases of HD occurring with NHL (one case of composite HD and FL and one case of DLBCL followed by HD) have been studied by single-cell PCR; a common clone was found in HD and NHL in both cases.[109] Rare cases of B-cell chronic lymphocytic leukemia (CLL) may contain cells with the morphology and immunophenotype of classic RS cells, whereas other patients with typical CLL may go on to develop HD—a so-called HD variant of Richter's syndrome.[110] Sev-

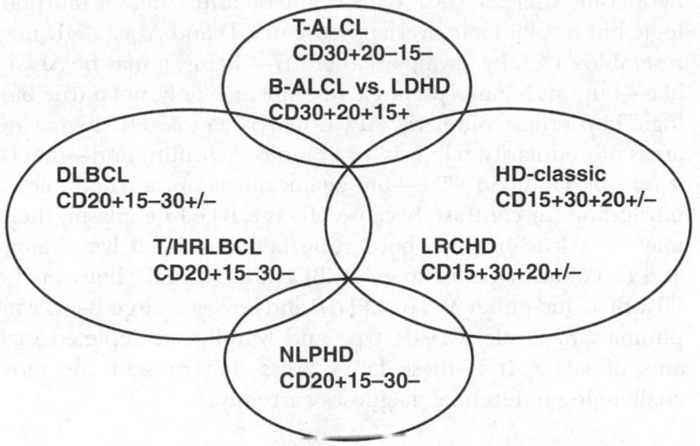

FIGURE 45.6-3. Differential diagnosis of Hodgkin's disease (HD). There is morphologic overlap between classic HD, T-cell/histiocyte-rich large B-cell lymphoma (T/HRLBCL), B-cell anaplastic large cell lymphoma (B-ALCL), and T-cell anaplastic large cell lymphoma (T-ALCL). Immunophenotyping can be useful in the differential diagnosis. DLBCL, diffuse large B-cell lymphoma; LDHD, lymphocyte depleted HD; LRCHD, lymphocyte-rich classic HD; NLPHD, nodular lymphocyte-predominant HD.

eral such cases have been studied using single-cell PCR; in the majority of the cases, the RS cells were of the same clone as the CLL cells, though in one case, they were clonally unrelated.[111] Finally, cases of mycosis fungoides or lymphomatoid papulosis associated with HD have been reported.[112] Thus, it is clear that patients with CHD are at some increased risk for development of NHL. In some patients, a single neoplastic B cell can give rise to both HD and NHL, whereas in other patients, it appears that either immunosuppression or other unknown factors can give rise to two independent malignancies.

DIFFERENTIAL DIAGNOSIS OF CLASSIC HODGKIN'S DISEASE

Two lymphomas have been described that have significant morphologic overlap with HD and may cause problems in differential diagnosis (Fig. 45.6-3): T-cell/histiocyte-rich large B-cell lymphoma (T/HRLBCL) and T-cell ALCL. In addition, DLBCLs with anaplastic cytology may be difficult to distinguish from HD with LD (Table 45.6-4).

T-Cell/Histiocyte-Rich Large B-Cell Lymphoma

In the late 1990s, several groups reported an unusual type of lymphoma with morphologic features reminiscent of diffuse LPHD or MCHD, with a predominance of small T lymphocytes and scattered large neoplastic cells that express B-cell antigens. Patients typically present with advanced-stage disease and have a poor prognosis.[103] The term *histiocyte-rich* or *T-cell–rich large B-cell lymphoma* has been used for these cases. The cases that resemble HD are different from earlier cases reported as T-cell–rich B-cell lymphoma, many of which are simply B-cell lymphomas of follicle center or large cell type in which T cells compose 50% or more of the infiltrate. Whether T/HRLBCL constitutes a distinct disease or is simply an aggressive variant of LPHD is not clear. However, it is important to distinguish it from either NLPHD or CHD because of its aggressive clinical course.

T/HRLBCL is a diffuse lymphoma with a lymphocyte-rich background, with small clusters of epithelioid histiocytes and scattered large mononuclear cells, suggesting either LPHD or CHD. The large cells may resemble popcorn cells, immunoblasts, or centroblasts, or all three.

The neoplastic cells express CD20 and other pan-B antigens, may or may not express cytoplasmic light chains, and may or may not have detectable Ig gene rearrangement by Southern blot or whole section PCR. Like LPHD, they are often EMA-positive but are CD15-, CD30-, and EBV-negative. The background lymphocytes are T cells that are CD57-negative, and FDC aggregates are not seen.

The immunophenotype of the large cells is of limited value in the differential diagnosis with LPHD, as it is similar; however, readily detectable Ig light chains would tend to favor a diagnosis of T/HRLBCL. In addition, staining for CD20 may reveal a nodular pattern and a B-cell–rich background, which would favor NLPHD. Follicular aggregates of FDC (anti-CD21) also favor NLPHD, as do large numbers of CD57+ cells. In distinguishing T/HRLBCL from CHD, immunophenotyping is essential and helpful. If the large cells express CD20 and lack CD15 and CD30, the diagnosis of T/HRLBCL is strongly favored, whereas expression of either CD15 or CD30 strongly favors a diagnosis of CHD. Furthermore, in cases diagnosed as CHD that express only CD20, the prognosis appears to be significantly worse than for cases expressing CD15 or CD30, with or without CD20.[103,106]

TABLE 45.6-4. Differential Diagnosis of Hodgkin's Disease

Diagnosis	*Morphology (Large Cells)*	*Immunophenotype (Large Cells)*	*T-Cell Rings*	*Genetics (Southern Blot)*
NLPHD	Popcorn cells	CD20+, EMA+, CD15–, CD30–	+	Ig polyclonal
Classic HD, lymphocyte-rich	Classic RS cells	CD20–, EMA–, CD15+, CD30+	+	Ig polyclonal
PTGC	Centroblasts	CD20+, EMA–, CD15–, CD30–	–	Ig polyclonal
Follicular lymphoma	Centroblasts	CD20+, EMA– (Ig monoclonal)	–	Ig monoclonal
T-cell, histiocyte-rich large B-cell lymphoma	Centroblasts, immunoblasts, popcorn cells	CD20+, EMA+, CD15–, CD30– (Ig monoclonal±)	–	Ig monoclonal
Anaplastic large-cell lymphoma (T-cell)	Horseshoe-shaped nuclei, paranuclear hof	CD20–, EMA±, CD15–, CD30+, T-Ag±	–	TCR monoclonal
Large B-cell lymphoma, anaplastic subtype	Bizzarre, large cells, RS-like cells	CD20+, EMA±, CD15–, CD30+	–	Ig monoclonal

Ag, antigen; EMA, epithelial membrane antigen; HD, Hodgkin's disease; Ig, immunoglobulin; NLPHD, nodular lymphocyte-predominant Hodgkin's disease; PTGC, progressive transformation of germinal centers; RS, Reed-Sternberg; TCR, T-cell receptor.
Note: EMA may be difficult to detect in formalin-fixed tissues. Classic HD may be CD20+ (15%) or CD15+ (15%).

Anaplastic Large-Cell Lymphoma

ALCL is a T-cell lymphoma characterized by large malignant cells with prominent nucleoli and abundant cytoplasm, which may resemble mononuclear or multinucleated RS-cell variants.[113] However, the tumor cells grow in cohesive sheets and frequently involve lymph node sinuses, a pattern that is unusual in HD. In addition, the neoplastic cells usually are smaller than RS cells, have less conspicuous nucleoli, without perinucleolar halos, and often have bean-shaped or horseshoe-shaped nuclei, with a prominent paranuclear hof, in contrast to the round nuclei of mononuclear RS cells.[114] ALCL has a bimodal age distribution, with one peak in childhood and another in adulthood.

A subtype of ALCL, called *Hodgkin's-related ACLC*, has been described (modified to *Hodgkin's-like* in the REAL classification; a provisional entity).[115] This variant was characterized by cytologic features similar to common ALCL—confluent sheets of tumor cells, a cohesive growth pattern, and sinusoidal infiltration—but with architectural features that resemble HD of the NS type, with nodular growth of tumor cells and occasional fibrous bands. The immunophenotype of ALCL-HD was reported to be similar to that of common ALCL, but some cases had CD15 expression and EBV infection. There has been an ongoing debate about whether ALCL Hodgkin's-like is a variant of HD, a variant of ALCL, a heterogeneous mixture of the two, or a distinct disease.

Analysis of the t(2;5) associated with ALCL has helped to resolve this problem. Studies of the translocation have shown that it is absent in cases of typical HD.[116,117] In immunophenotyping studies using antibodies to either the ALK protein or the p80 fusion product of the t(2;5), several groups have found the protein to be present in a subset of ALCL but not in HD. Cases diagnosed as ALCL-HD typically lack the ALK protein.[118]

Most hematopathologists now believe that cases reported in the literature as ALCL Hodgkin's-like are heterogeneous. Some represent LD variants of HD—either NSHD (syncytial, LD, or NS grade 2) type or LD (LDHD; Hodgkin's sarcoma)—whereas others are cases of ALCL with a nodular growth pattern. Most cases can be resolved as either HD (CD45–, CD15+, T-cell antigen–, CD20–/+, t(2;5)–, ALK1–, EMA–) or ALCL (CD45+, CD15–, T-cell antigen+, CD20–, t(2;5)+, ALK1+, EMA+).

In cases that are histologically borderline between HD and T-ALCL, immunophenotyping on paraffin sections with CD45, CD15, CD30, CD20, EMA, pan-T antigens, ALK1 and, if necessary, genetic studies should be undertaken to resolve the differential diagnosis. Expression of CD15 or CD20 tends to exclude a diagnosis of T-ALCL (CD20+ cases may be either HD or DLBCL), whereas expression of CD45, T-cell antigens, ALK1, or EMA tend to exclude HD. Southern blot or whole section PCR analysis showing T-cell antigen receptor gene rearrangement would tend to exclude HD and confirm the diagnosis of ALCL. Ig gene rearrangement by these techniques would not usually be detectable in HD and would favor DLBCL, but a weak band would not exclude HD. Cases that cannot be resolved by immunophenotype or genetic studies should be considered unclassifiable; clinical judgment should be used in deciding whether to perform another biopsy or to treat for either HD or ALCL. The category of ALCL Hodgkin's-like will be eliminated from the proposed WHO classification.

In summary, the data currently available suggest that there is no true borderline between HD and ALCL of the T-null type as defined in the REAL classification: HD is, in most cases, a B-cell neoplasm, whereas ALCL is a T-cell neoplasm. There is morphologic but not biologic overlap between HD and ALCL. HD may resemble ALCL by having areas of LD—that is, it may be ALCL-like—but this is a morphologic resemblance only, not a true biologic borderline. Similarly, ALCL may resemble HD by having areas of nodularity, sclerosis, or granulocyte infiltration—that is, it may be Hodgkin's-like—but again, this is not a true biologic borderline. In contrast, because HD is a B-cell neoplasm, there may be a true biologic borderline between B-cell lymphomas and HD of any type, between DLBCL and NLPHD, between T/HRLBCL and either MC or LPHD, and between large B-cell lymphoma, anaplastic, CD30+ type and lymphocyte-depleted variants of CHD. It is these latter areas that present the most challenging differential diagnoses currently.

DIAGNOSIS AND STAGING

NATURAL HISTORY AND PATTERNS OF SPREAD

The Swiss radiotherapist Gilbert is credited with first reporting that HD spread by contiguity from one lymph node chain to adjacent chains.[10,119] His work was extended by Peters,[120] Kaplan,[121] and others, who evaluated the use of prophylactic radiotherapy to lymph nodes adjacent to those involved with disease. The development of new radiographic studies and the routine use of staging laparotomy improved understanding of the presentation and evolution of HD.[121,122] Although there is strong evidence that HD begins in a single group of lymph nodes and then spreads to contiguous lymph nodes, eventually the malignant cells become more aggressive, may invade blood vessels, and spread to organs in a manner similar to other malignancies. This is more likely to occur in patients with stage III than with stage I or II HD.

Most patients with NSHD or MCHD have a central pattern of lymph node involvement (cervical, mediastinal, paraaortic). In contrast, certain nodal chains (mesenteric, hypogastric, presacral, epitrochlear, popliteal) seldom are involved. Occult adenopathy in patients with negative radiographic staging ranges from 6% to 35%. The spleen is involved more frequently in patients with adenopathy below the diaphragm, systemic symptoms, and MC histology. Involvement of the liver in an untreated patient is rare and almost always occurs with concomitant splenic involvement. Infiltration of the bone marrow is usually focal and almost invariably associated with extensive disease, systemic symptoms, and unfavorable histology. In the great majority of patients, the initial pattern of spread occurs nonrandomly and predictably via lymphatic channels to contiguous lymph node chains. This important observation, first made in the 1930s, continues to form the basis for prophylactic irradiation of adjacent lymph node–bearing regions in patients with apparently localized HD treated with radiotherapy alone.

STAGING CLASSIFICATIONS

Prior experience with staging laparotomy, the advent of new imaging modalities, and the frequent use of combined modality treatment have made staging procedures simpler and less invasive. The latest international staging classification was proposed in 1989 during a meeting held in Cotswolds, England.[123] The Cotswolds classification (Table 45.6-5) is a modification of the Ann Arbor classification using information from staging and treatment over the 1970s and 1980s.

Some of the recommended modifications include adding criteria for clinical involvement of the spleen and liver, including evidence of focal defects with two imaging techniques, eliminating consideration of abnormalities of liver function, adding the suffix *X* to designate bulky disease (larger than 10 cm maximum dimension), adding a new category of response to therapy (i.e., unconfirmed or uncertain complete remission) to accommodate the difficulty of persistent radiologic abnormalities of uncertain significance after primary therapy, and separately classifying certain selected patients with localized extranodal disease (e.g., lung, pleura, chest wall, bone) contiguous to involved nodes as the appropriate lymph node system stage followed by the subscript *E*. The *E* designation excludes multiple extranodal deposits or bilateral lung extension, which constitute stage IV disease. Recommended staging procedures are listed in Table 45.6-6. An adequate surgical biopsy, possibly of more than one intact lymph node, is required for histopathologic examination.

RADIOGRAPHIC STAGING ABOVE THE DIAPHRAGM

More than 60% of patients with newly diagnosed HD have radiographic evidence of intrathoracic involvement. Frontal and lateral chest radiographs should be routinely ordered and also represent the ideal for subsequent surveillance.

Massive mediastinal adenopathy [large mediastinal adenopathy (LMA)] has been arbitrarily defined as the ratio greater than one-third between the largest transverse diameter of the mediastinal mass over the transverse diameter of the thorax at the diaphragm on a standing posteroanterior chest radiograph.[123] Alternatively, others have defined extensive mediastinal disease as greater than 35% of the thoracic diameter at T5-6, or as measuring greater than 5 to 10 cm in width. Patients with LMA have an increased risk of relapsing in nodal and extranodal sites above the diaphragm after radiotherapy alone.[124,125] These patients make up 20% to 25% of CS I to II patients, generally present with involvement of multiple supradiaphragmatic nodal chains, and may have extension of tumor into the lung, pericardium, or chest wall.[124] Systemic symptoms frequently are present.

Staging with thoracic computed axial tomographic (CAT) scanning can more precisely identify sites of initial involvement.[126] CAT scanning is especially apt at detecting pulmonary disease, pleural or pericardial involvement, apical cardiac nodal enlargement, and extension into the chest wall, and in defining the extent of involved axillary lymph nodes. Such information has considerable potential to alter clinical management.[127] Identification of the extent of thoracic disease will help to define the use of combination chemotherapy and the dose, extent, and need for radiotherapy.

With improved gamma camera resolution, several investigators have described the ability of ^{67}Ga scanning to detect intrathoracic lymphadenopathy, though the reported sensitivities and specificities are somewhat less than those of CAT scanning. Today, the primary role for ^{67}Ga scanning in the thorax is to answer specific questions that arise after treatment (e.g., whether a residual mass represents viable tumor rather than necrosis or fibrosis). As an alternative to gallium scanning, positron emission tomography is being explored in Europe and in the United States.[128]

TABLE 45.6-5. Cotswolds Staging Classification for Hodgkin's Disease

Stage I	Involvement of a single lymph node region or lymphoid structure (e.g., spleen, thymus, Waldeyer's ring) or involvement of a single extralymphatic site.
Stage II	Involvement of two or more lymph node regions on the same side of the diaphragm (hilar nodes, when involved on both sides, constitute stage II disease); localized contiguous involvement of only one extranodal organ or site and lymph node region on the same side of the diaphragm (IIE). The number of anatomic regions involved should be indicated by a subscript (e.g., II_3).
Stage III	Involvement of lymph node regions on both sides of the diaphragm (III), which may also be accompanied by involvement of the spleen (III_S) or by localized contiguous involvement of only one extranodal organ site (IIIE) or both (III SE).
III_1	With or without involvement of splenic, hilar, celiac, or portal nodes.
III_2	With involvement of paraaortic, iliac, and mesenteric nodes.
Stage IV	Diffuse or disseminated involvement of one or more extranodal organs or tissues, with or without associated lymph node involvement.
DESIGNATIONS APPLICABLE TO ANY DISEASE STAGE	
A	No symptoms.
B	Fever (temperature, >38°C), drenching night sweats, unexplained loss of >10% body weight within the preceding 6 months.
X	Bulky disease (a widening of the mediastinum by more than one-third of the presence of a nodal mass with a maximal dimension >10 cm).
E	Involvement of a single extranodal site that is contiguous or proximal to the known nodal site.
CS	Clinical stage.
PS	Pathologic stage (as determined by laparotomy).

TABLE 45.6-6. Recommended Staging Procedures

Adequate surgical biopsy reviewed by an experienced hemopathologist
Detailed history with attention to the presence or absence of systemic symptoms
Careful physical examination, emphasizing node chains, size of liver and spleen, and Waldeyer's ring inspection
Routine laboratory tests (complete blood cell count, erythrocyte sedimentation rate, and liver function tests)
Chest radiograph (posteroanterior and lateral) with measurement of mass-thoracic ratio
Chest and abdominal computed tomography scans
Radioisotopic evaluation with ^{67}Ga or positron emission tomography when the results of other conventional diagnostic procedures are not conclusive
Core needle biopsy of bone marrow from the posterior iliac crest in patients with stage IIB–IV disease
Needle or surgical biopsy of any suspicious extranodal (e.g., hepatic, osseous, pulmonary, cutaneous) lesion
Cytologic examination of any effusion
Staging laparotomy (with splenectomy, needle and wedge biopsy of the liver, and biopsies of paraaortic, mesenteric, portal, and splenic hilar lymph nodes) in rare circumstances in early-stage Hodgkin's disease in which the use of limited radiotherapy alone depends on pathologic staging

Some investigations suggest that the ability of magnetic resonance imaging (MRI) to detect tumor in mediastinum or hilar lymph nodes is not superior to that of CAT scanning.[129] Although, MRI can probably function as an alternative to CAT scanning in the thorax, particularly at the level of chest wall involvement, its continuing high cost and lack of clinical data prevent this modality from being used routinely.

RADIOGRAPHIC STAGING BELOW THE DIAPHRAGM

CAT scanning, lymphangiography (LAG), MRI, and ^{67}Ga scanning all have limitations in the radiologic evaluation of abdominal nodes. No single study is reliable for detecting HD in normal-size nodes, and all studies have a 20% to 25% false-negative rate due to the inability to detect occult HD in the spleen.[130,131] Ninety percent of patients who are up-staged have splenic involvement either alone or in addition to other infradiaphragmatic nodal sites.[130] Head-to-head comparisons of bipedal LAG and CAT scanning suggests that LAG has a small statistical advantage over CAT, particularly in the presence of small lymphadenopathies, because it provides useful information on lymph node architecture. On the other hand, CAT scanning can better evaluate adenopathy in the celiac axis, splenic hilus, porta hepatis, and mesentery, relying almost exclusively on increases in the size of the nodes. CAT scanning can also demonstrate foci of HD in the liver and spleen; however, the false-negative results are too numerous to allow one to rely heavily on CAT assessment of these organs.

During the late 1990s, LAG gave way to CAT scanning as the examination of choice. MRI may be more sensitive than CAT scanning in the evaluation of abdominal nodes, but information on its usefulness is still limited. MRI appears to be a potentially valuable tool in investigating bone marrow involvement and can help in directing image-guided biopsies. Gallium scanning can also complement LAG or CAT scanning, but its use in the abdomen may be hampered by normal uptake in the liver, spleen, and bowel. With the infrequent use of staging laparotomy and splenectomy in the staging of HD, the risk of overstaging based on a single radiographic test of abdominal involvement (false-positive outcome) has greater potential consequences. Therefore, we recommend that two separate studies (i.e., CAT scanning and ^{67}Ga scanning) be used to assess abdominal involvement and that positive findings on both tests be required to confirm abdominal involvement for the routine radiographic staging of HD.

STAGING LAPAROTOMY

Staging laparotomy was extensively used when radiotherapy was the only potentially curative treatment for early-stage HD and when it was mandatory to define the extent of abdominal disease to help determine the extent of radiation needed below the diaphragm. With the increasing use of combination chemotherapy, staging laparotomy gradually evolved into a tool that aids in determining whether radiotherapy or chemotherapy should be selected as definitive treatment. With many groups using prognostic factors to determine treatment for HD, laparotomy has disappeared as a routine staging procedure. Its use now is reserved for patients with limited disease who are to receive limited treatment.

CLINICAL PRESENTATION

First reports about clinical manifestations of HD and patterns of its course of spreading were conducted by Gilbert,[132] Peters,[120] and others. Their findings that HD spreads by contiguity from one lymph node chain to adjacent chains were extended by the use of prophylactic radiotherapy to lymph node regions adjacent to those involved with HD. The understanding of the presentation and evolution of HD has been improved by the development of new radiographic studies and the use of staging laparotomy.[130] Although there is evidence that the course of HD is characterized by its onset in a single lymph node or group of lymph nodes, followed by spreading to contiguous lymph nodes, there are indications that the disease can spread to organs similar to other malignancies by invading blood vessels.[121] Most convincing data for contiguous spread in HD were found for NS and MC histology. In NS and MC histologic subtypes, a central pattern of lymph node involvement (cervical, mediastinal, paraaortic) was more common than nodal involvement of mesenteric, hypogastric, presacral, or popliteal regions.

In general, HD patients present with peripheral lymphadenopathy. The nodes usually are not tender, and changes in the overlying skin are not the norm. Otherwise, tenderness and skin changes are believed to reflect rapid growth with stretching of nodal capsules. In most cases, the nodes are discrete and freely movable. Occult presentation with central (chest and abdomen) lymphadenopathy, visceral involvement, or systemic symptoms of the disease is uncommon. The most characteristic clinical presentation of HD is enlarged superficial lymph nodes in young adults, the most frequent locations being cervical and supraclavicular (60% to 80%), high in the neck or axillary. Less often, such enlarged nodes are found in the inguinal-femoral region.

Mediastinal involvement is discovered often by routine staging chest radiography, and even fairly large masses may occur without producing local symptoms. Otherwise, symptoms of retrosternal chest pain, cough, or shortness of breath may be clinical signs of an intrathoracic disease presentation. A bulky mediastinal mass is not uncommonly associated with small amounts of pericardial and pleural fluid, but malignant effusions, diagnosed by thoracentesis or pleural biopsy, are rare.

Involvement of the liver in a patient with newly diagnosed HD is uncommon and occurs almost always with concomitant splenic involvement. HD limited to the spleen is rare. Patients may present with abdominal swelling secondary to hepatomegaly or splenomegaly or, rarely, with ascites. Infradiaphragmatic lymphadenopathy may give rise to discomfort and pain in the retroperitoneum or the paravertebral or loin regions, particularly in the supine position, by nodular compression of nerves or nerve roots. Advanced intraabdominal disease may be associated with obstruction of the ureters or compression of the renal vein, with or without ascites.

Bone marrow infiltration is usually focal and, in most cases, is associated with extensive disease, including systemic symptoms. Laboratory findings such as leukopenia, anemia, thrombocytopenia, and an elevated alkaline phosphatase level may give indications of bone marrow infiltration.

Involvement of the central nervous system is rare, although invasion of the epidural space can occur by nodular extension from the paraaortic region through the intervertebral foramina, presenting neurologic symptoms and pain as leading clinical features.[133] Several paraneoplastic neurologic syndromes have been reported in association with HD, but all are very rare.

Complaints due to extranodal manifestations of disease may occur, such as cough from pulmonary infiltration, jaundice from hepatic involvement, or abdominal pain from disease adjacent to the bowel. Gastrointestinal involvement is an extremely rare event and might occur as infiltration from mesenteric lymph nodes. Initial symptoms of disease limited to extranodal tissue are much rarer in HD than in NHLs.

A significant proportion of patients with undiagnosed HD present systemic symptoms before the discovery of enlarged lymph nodes. Typical symptoms are fever, drenching night sweats, and weight loss (so-called B-symptoms, relating to the Ann Arbor classification). This characteristic HD-associated fever occurs intermittently and recurs at variable intervals for several days or weeks. Fever and drenching night sweats are found in 25% of all patients at first presentation, increasing to 50% of patients with more advanced disease. Other nonspecific symptoms are pruritus, fatigue, and the development of pain shortly after drinking alcohol. This pain usually is transient at the site of nodal involvement and may be severe. Pruritus, although currently not a defined B-symptom, may be an important systemic symptom of disease but occurs infrequently, in fewer than 20% of patients. It often occurs months or even a year before HD is first diagnosed.[134] The underlying pathophysiologic mechanisms leading to pruritus are unknown but may be due to an autoimmune reaction in which a number of cytokines are activated by tumor lysis.

TREATMENT METHODS

RADIOTHERAPY

Principles

The early treatment of HD with crude x-irradiation in 1901 followed the discoveries by Roentgen, Becquerel, and the Curies at the end of the eighteenth century. The first reports of x-ray treatments that would dramatically shrink enlarged lymph nodes produced great excitement and premature predictions for the successful treatment of HD.[135,136] During the first two decades of the twentieth century, physicians mainly used two methods to treat HD with radiation. Small doses of radiation were administered to the entire trunk at weekly intervals for many weeks or were given as a single massive dose just to the tumor. Neither method controlled the HD, and both caused severe side effects.[10] Enlarged nodes usually shrank with both techniques, but recurrence and spread to previously uninvolved nodes invariably followed. After several courses of radiotherapy, the HD became more resistant to treatment, and very few patients survived 5 years from diagnosis. These multiple recurrences were not attributed to poor radiotherapeutic techniques but were viewed as inherent to the HD itself. Consequently, by 1920, most physicians had stopped using radiation as a means of curing HD. For the next 40 years, in most centers, treatment was mainly palliative, to shrink large nodes that were painful or interfered with movement, eating, or breathing.

The development of modern radiotherapeutic techniques for the treatment of HD began with the work of Gilbert,[137] a Swiss radiotherapist, in the 1920s. He advocated treatment to apparently uninvolved adjacent lymph node chains that might contain suspected microscopic disease, as well as to the evident sites of lymph node involvement. Peters also adapted this technique at the Princess Margaret Hospital in the late 1930s and early 1940s. In her historic paper published in the *American Journal of Roentgenology* in 1950, Peters[120] provided evidence that patients with limited HD could be cured with aggressive radiotherapy that treated involved nodal disease as well as adjacent nodal sites. She did this by identifying a group of patients with limited-stage HD that was cured with high-dose, fractionated radiotherapy. She reported 5-year and 10-year survival rates of 88% and 79%, respectively, for patients with disease limited to a single lymph node region, rates that were notably high for a disease in which virtually no one survived 10 years. Nevertheless, the concept that early-stage HD might be curable with radiotherapy using higher doses and larger fields was slow to be accepted. Before the 1960s, most patients with limited HD were not treated at all or with only small doses of radiation.

No one deserves more credit than Henry Kaplan for the development of successful modern treatment for HD. His accomplishments are many and include pioneering work on developing the linear accelerator,[121,138] defining radiation field sizes and doses for a curative approach for early HD,[121] refining and improving diagnostic staging techniques, developing models for translating laboratory findings into clinical practice, and promoting early randomized clinical trials in the United States.

TECHNIQUES

Excellent results in the treatment of early-stage HD have been achieved through careful delineation of disease and meticulous attention to technique.[139] Treatment-machine generated verification films should be used to ensure proper alignment. Daily doses of no more than 180 to 200 cGy to the mantle field (unless the treatment field includes the entire heart or entire lung, in which case the dose should be limited to 150 cGy/d or less) reduces risks to both the heart and lungs. Adjusting treatment on the basis of off-central axis dose calculations can reduce dose inhomogeneity from differences in patient separation within the large mantle field. Extended source-to-skin distances of 110 cm or greater, rather than a source-to-skin distance of 100 cm, also reduces tissue inhomogeneity. Proper use of megavoltage energies will ensure that superficial nodes are not underdosed in the buildup region. A 4- to 6-MeV linear accelerator should be used for mantle and pelvic fields, whereas higher energies (10 to 15 MV) can be used for treating paraaortic nodes.

The mantle field encompasses the submandibular, cervical, supraclavicular, infraclavicular, axillary, mediastinal, subcarinal, and hilar lymph nodes. A total dose of 3000 cGy to the entire mantle field is sufficient for patients with supradiaphragmatic HD when radiotherapy alone is used. Areas of initial involvement should receive a total dose of 3600 to 4000 cGy through the addition of a cone-down field. Reduction of the radiation dose to 3000 cGy to areas of initial involvement is recommended for patients receiving combined modality therapy, especially when there has been a good response confirmed by CAT scanning. When at least four cycles of chemotherapy have been given, radiation to initial uninvolved prophylactic sites probably is not needed. Further reduction to 1500 to 2500 cGy may be desirable in prepubertal patients receiving combined modality treatment or, occasionally, in patients with extensive nodal involvement who are receiving treatments to large radiation fields after chemotherapy.

There is an increasing use of involved field irradiation after chemotherapy in the treatment of early-stage HD. Involved field irradiation should encompass the entire involved lymph node region, as defined initially by Stanford University Medical School.[10] For example, the ipsilateral cervical and supraclavicular nodes and the inguinal and femoral nodes constitute single regions.

Mantle paraaortic-splenic irradiation after a negative laparotomy occasionally is used as a radiotherapy-alone approach for early-stage disease patients who have not had a staging laparotomy. The paraaortic field encompasses the paraaortic nodes down to the fourth to fifth lumbar vertebral interspace (L4-5). Without staging laparotomy and splenectomy, the entire spleen must be irradiated. A CAT scan should be used to localize the position of the spleen and enable blocking of as much of the left kidney as is possible. The dose to the paraaortic lymph nodes should be 3000 cGy when there is no known disease, and radiotherapy alone is used. Beam divergence from the mantle and paraaortic fields creates the potential for an overdose at the spinal cord. A number of different matching techniques have been published.[140]

Prophylactic pelvic irradiation is used rarely in the modern-day treatment of supradiaphragmatic HD. However, pelvic irradiation continues to be used for patients presenting with stage I or II infradiaphragmatic HD. Iliac wing blocks to spare bone marrow and a pelvic block to shield the bladder and central pelvic organs should be part of the treatment technique (which includes irradiation of inguinal and femoral nodes). Loss of fertility in both men and women is a risk with the use of pelvic irradiation for subdiaphragmatic HD, and techniques should be used to reduce this risk whenever possible.[141]

CHEMOTHERAPY

The development of chemotherapeutic programs for HD is a story of success. After the discovery of the cytotoxic effects of nitrogen mustard in the 1940s, a number of different drugs—including chlorambucil, cyclophosphamide, procarbazine, vinblastine, and vincristine—were developed and showed efficacy in HD. Response rates were approximately 50% to 60% with 10% to 30% complete response. However, relapse was seen in almost all cases, and no cure could be achieved.

On the basis of a murine leukemia cell line, Skipper et al.[141a] postulated a model of tumor cell kill based on the logarithmic cell growth and a logarithmic response to cytotoxic agents. From this model, the authors predicted that response to chemotherapy would depend on tumor burden, drug dose, and kinetics of residual tumor cells. It was further postulated that the simultaneous use of several drugs with different modes of action might yield superior results. The combination of drugs might be tolerated if the toxicities were nonoverlapping. Initial attempts with two-drug combinations revealed the potential of this approach.

However, the relevance of this model was realized in 1967, when DeVita et al.[141b] reported on a four-drug combination chemotherapy program, MOPP [mechlorethamine, vincristine (Oncovin), procarbazine, and prednisone]. This combination established the curability of more than 50% of patients with stage III or IV disease.

The development of MOPP was a milestone in oncology, demonstrating that advanced-stage HD could be cured. The differences in survival between historic controls and MOPP-treated patients were so dramatic that randomized clinical trials were not needed to validate these results. Further information on chemotherapy is provided in Advanced-Stage Disease later in this chapter.

Combined Modality Chemotherapy

In addition to the many factors that affect either chemotherapy or radiotherapy when used alone, there are several issues that arise specifically because of potential interaction and summing of effects when they are combined. It is important to remember that the purpose of adding a second modality is to overcome resistance to the first and, in the case of adding irradiation to chemotherapy for HD, it seems likely that full-dose irradiation may be needed to overcome primary resistance to chemotherapy. Of particular interest are two German trials recently summarized,[142] in which patients with stage IA+B, IIA+B, and stage IIIA disease with extensive mediastinal or splenic involvement or E lesions were treated with two-course cyclophosphamide, Oncovin, procarbazine, and prednisone (COPP) and doxorubicin (Adriamycin), bleomycin, vinblastine, and dacarbazine (ABVD) followed by irradiation. In the first trial (HD1), responders to chemotherapy then were given extended-field irradiation with a dose to nonbulky sites assigned randomly to be either 20 Gy or 40 Gy. In the second trial (HD5), a similar group of patients received 30 Gy to the nonbulky sites. Bulky sites received 40 Gy in each trial. Failure-free survival was the same in all groups, strongly implying that after optimal chemotherapy, irradiation dose, at least to nonbulky sites, can be reduced without sacrificing efficiency.

The risk of two important late complications of irradiation may be reduced by lowering the dose. Studies of late sequelae of treatment for HD suggest that the risk of second neoplasms, especially breast cancer in women, may be reduced by lower radiation dose.[143] The other late toxicity possibly associated with radiation dose is cardiovascular. Stanford University investigators found that a higher dose of irradiation to the mediastinum was associated with increased mortality from cardiac disease.[144]

An alternative approach to reduce toxicity from irradiation when used in combined modality treatment is to reduce not the dose but the extent of the field encompassed. Several trials involving patients with limited-stage HD have shown that results comparable to those achieved with irradiation alone to an extended field can be achieved when chemotherapy is combined with involved field irradiation.[125,145] The ability to preserve efficacy while limiting toxicity by reducing the size of the treatment fields is one of the most attractive aspects of using combined modality treatment.

The same theoretic considerations that apply to irradiation are relevant when one considers reduction of the dose of chemotherapy used in combined modality treatment. The section Choice of Treatment examines these results in more detail.

In theory, either the chemotherapy or the radiotherapy could come first in the sequence of combined modality treatment. In practice, it is almost always desirable for chemotherapy to precede radiotherapy. The reason for this includes early effective treatment of disseminated disease, delay in induction of irreversible loss of bone marrow function, and the opportunity to use smaller, potentially less toxic radiation treatment fields after chemotherapy has induced tumor regression.

High-Dose Chemotherapy Plus Stem Cell Support

PRINCIPLES. High-dose chemotherapy (HDCT) has been used extensively in patients with relapsed and refractory HD. Implicit in the rationale for this approach is the assumption of a steep dose-response relation for lymphoma patients subjected to chemoradiotherapy. Although care must be exercised in interpreting clinical results, both animal models and clinical studies support the existence of such a relationship.[146]

The use of autologous bone marrow or peripheral blood stem cells (PBSCs) to support intensification of chemotherapy as salvage treatment has changed the options available for relapsed patients. Autologous transplantation involves the replacement of hematopoietic stem cells that have been irreversibly injured by HDCT or radiotherapy (or both). This can be accomplished either with bone marrow cells obtained by multiple aspirations from the posterior iliac crest under anesthesia or with PBSCs collected by apheresis. The use of PBSCs has surpassed the use of bone marrow, and PBSCs may be used exclusively in the future. The advantage of using PBSCs includes avoiding general anesthesia and more rapid hematopoietic reconstitution.

CONDITIONING REGIMENS. Several conditioning regimens have been used and summarized previously.[147] The most commonly used are cyclophosphamide, etoposide (VP-16), and BCNU (CVB) or BCNU, etoposide, cytarabine (arabinoside), and melphalan (BEAM) given in different dose schedules. When BCNU-containing regimens are used, careful clinical monitoring to detect early signs of delayed lung toxicity is important, particularly when BCNU doses of 450 mg/m^2 are given. Mucositis and enterocolitis represent the most significant nonhematologic toxicities associated with high-dose melphalan. Total body irradiation has been used only in a few studies, owing to the fact that many HD patients have already received thoracic irradiation by the time they have reached the transplantation stage and to the high treatment-related mortality of patients prepared by total body irradiation–containing regimens.[148,149] Although the toxicity profiles differ with these regimens, there currently is no evidence to support the superiority of any particular regimen in HD.

Sequential HDCT is increasingly being used in the treatment of solid tumors and lymphoma. First results from phase II studies show that this kind of therapy is safe and effective.[150,151] In accordance with the Norton-Simon hypothesis, after initial cytoreduction, a few non-cross-resistant agents are given in short intervals.[152] In general, the transplantation of autologous stem cells and the use of growth factors allow application of the most effective drugs in highest doses in intervals of 1 to 3 weeks. Sequential HDCT permits the highest possible dosing in minimum time.

INCORPORATING RADIOTHERAPY IN HIGH-DOSE CHEMOTHERAPY PROGRAMS. Radiotherapy is a very effective locoregional treatment modality in HD. The rationale for incorporation of radiotherapy into HDCT programs stems from the observation that disease progression after HDCT often occurs in sites of prior involvement. Several investigators showed that in 65% to 95% of cases, the sites of failure are involved immediately before HDCT.[148,153] Retrospective analysis suggests that radiotherapy may be incorporated as cytoreductive treatment before HDCT or as a consolidative therapy after HDCT.[154,155] However, no prospective clinical trial has yet answered the questions regarding the extent of the radiation field, the timing of treatment, and the appropriate dose to use. The complementary role of radiotherapy in salvage HDCT is uncertain and remains to be investigated.

CHOICE OF TREATMENT

PROGNOSTIC FACTORS AND TREATMENT GROUPS

A prognostic factor is a measurement or classification of an individual patient, performed at or soon after diagnosis, that gives information on the likely outcome of the disease. This information will generally be phrased in terms of probabilities—for instance, the probability of cure for various values of a prognostic factor. It may be used for informing the patient or, in the context of clinical trials, for defining or describing the study population or adjusting the data analysis; however, for the clinician, the most important role of the prognostic factor is to help in selecting an appropriate treatment strategy.

In HD, patients have traditionally been divided into two or three prognostic groups, chiefly according to stage and B-symptoms but also taking various other factors into consideration. Most basically, patients with stage IIIB or IV (advanced-stage) disease have been associated with the poorest prognosis and assigned an intensive chemotherapy protocol, sometimes followed by adjuvant radiotherapy. Further prognostic factors often were used to assign stage IIIA or stage IIB patients to the advanced-stage group. Among the remaining patients with early-stage disease who had previously continued to receive radiotherapy alone, an "unfavorable" subgroup often was defined to select patients for combined modality therapy. Each group has thus been associated with a typical standard treatment strategy:

- Early stages, favorable: radiation alone (extended field)
- Early stages, unfavorable: moderate amount of chemotherapy (typically four cycles) plus radiation
- Advanced stages: extensive chemotherapy (typically eight cycles) with or without consolidating (usually local) radiation

These "typical" strategies are not uniformly applied, and the investigation of alternatives (e.g., the use of chemotherapy in favorable early stages) is continuing. In the scheme just listed, two divisions between the three prognostic groups must be noted, each division possibly being defined by a different set of factors. Furthermore, the attempt has been made to identify advanced-stage patients with a particularly high risk of failure for intensified therapy (e.g., early HDCT with stem cell support).[156] The selection of factors and the definition of the prognostic groups vary among institutions, as does the choice of treatment.

Prognostic factors are rarely the subject of specific clinical studies but are discovered and evaluated using data from large cohorts of uniformly treated, well-documented, and reliably followed-up patients, usually from large clinical trials.[157,158] The diversity of diagnostic and treatment strategies used for the early stages, as well as statistical problems caused by the low rate of treatment fail-

TABLE 45.6-7. Definition of Treatment Groups in Two Large Cooperative Trial Groups

Treatment Group	*GHSG Risk Factors*		*EORTC/GELA Risk Factors*	
	A	Large mediastinal mass	A'	Large mediastinal mass
	B	Extranodal disease	B'	Age ≥50 y
	C	Elevated ESR[a]	C'	Elevated ESR[a]
	D	≥3 Involved regions	D'	≥4 Involved regions
Lymphocyte predominance	NLPHD histology in CS I–II with no RF		NLPHD histology in supradiaphragmatic CS I–II	
Early stage favorable	CS I–II with no RF		CS I–II supradiaphragmatic with no RF	
Early stage unfavorable	CS I, CS IIA with one or more RF; CS IIB with C/D but without A/B		CS I–II supradiaphragmatic with one or more RF	
Advanced stage	CS IIB with A/B; CS III–IV		CS III–IV	

CS, clinical stage; EORTC, European Organization for Research and Treatment of Cancer; ESR, erythrocyte sedimentation rate; GELA, Groupe d'Etude des Lymphomes de l'Adulte; GHSG, German Hodgkin's Lymphoma Study Group; NLPHD, nodular lymphocyte-predominant Hodgkin's disease; RF, risk factor.
[a]Erythrocyte sedimentation rate (≥50 without or ≥30 with B-symptoms).

ure events, has led to the reporting and use of different prognostic factors by different institutions and trial groups.

In the following few sections, recognized prognostic factors are described for early stages treated with radiotherapy alone, for early stages treated with chemotherapy, and for advanced stages (treated with chemotherapy), respectively. Such factors are required to show independent prognostic value in multivariate analyses of large numbers of patients. This account refers in general to clinically staged patients, because laparotomy is now rarely performed. The use of these factors to define prognostic groups for treatment purposes, as practiced by various institutions and study groups, are described.

Prognostic Factors for Early-Stage Disease (Clinical Stage I or II) Treated with Radiotherapy Alone

For those patients with early-stage (CS I or II) disease who are to be treated by radiotherapy alone, recognized adverse factors are (1) advanced age (which correlates with the presence of occult abdominal disease and with poor results of salvage therapy and may also be associated with treatment complications, leading to reduced or delayed treatment); (2) male gender (which has a small effect only); (3) histologic subtype MC (which is associated with the presence of occult abdominal disease); (4) the presence of B-symptoms (which is associated with the presence of occult abdominal disease); (5) presence of a large mediastinal mass (LMM), for which there is some evidence of an increased relapse rate in the thorax (although there are few data, as few LMM patients were treated with radiotherapy alone); (6) the number of involved nodal regions; (7) an elevated erythrocyte sedimentation rate (ESR); (8) presence of anemia; and (9) a low serum albumin level.

These factors are relevant to the decision as to which early-stage patients should be classed as unfavorable and receive combined modality therapy because their prognosis with radiotherapy alone is relatively poor. Major study groups have used criteria as described next. Favorable patients were generally given radiation only, although the additional application of mild chemotherapy has increased.

The European Organization for the Research and Treatment of Cancer (EORTC) has, since 1982, defined CS I and II (supradiaphragmatic only) patients as unfavorable if any of the following factors applied: age older than 50 years, asymptomatic with ESR in excess of 50, B-symptoms with ESR in excess of 30, and LMM, based on the results of earlier EORTC trials H1 and H2. In previous trials, stage II, MC or LD histology, and number of involved regions also were counted as adverse factors.[159]

The GHSG has, since 1988, assigned combined modality treatment to CS I and II patients with any of the following adverse factors: (1) LMM, (2) number of regions (≥3), (3) elevated ESR, (4) localized extranodal infiltration (so-called E-lesions), or (5) massive splenic involvement.[160] Owing to the rarity of splenectomy, the last-mentioned factor was seldom reported and was abandoned for the present trial generation. It can be difficult to distinguish consistently between E-lesions and stage IV disease, and varying assessments of the prognostic value of this feature have been obtained by different investigators (Table 45.6-7). Stanford began in 1980 to give combined modality treatment to CS I and II patients with LMM or multiple E-lesions.

The EORTC has investigated the use of localized radiotherapy in a "very favorable" subgroup of early-stage patients. Inclusion criteria were a stage IA female patient younger than 40 years, with disease of NS or LP histology, without elevated ESR or LMM. A 30% long-term failure rate was observed, however, and this policy was not continued.

Prognostic Factors for Early-Stage Disease (Clinical Stage I or II) Treated with Chemotherapy

Despite the different mode of action of chemotherapy as compared with radiotherapy, similar prognostic factors have emerged from analyses of cohorts treated with radiation and with combined modality therapy. All the factors listed for radiation-treated patients have also been reliably confirmed in cohorts who also received chemotherapy,[161,162] either in early or in advanced stages. This similarity of prognostic effects is supported by the observation from a metaanalysis of radiotherapy versus combined modality treatment in early stages that the size of the difference in failure-free survival between these two treatment strategies was essentially constant over different prognostic groups.[163]

As a consequence, the prognostic factors relevant to the division between unfavorable early and advanced-stage cases (i.e., between moderate and extensive chemotherapy) are essentially the same as those listed for the division between favorable and unfavorable disease categories. However, gener-

TABLE 45.6-8. Final Cox Regression Model

Factor	*Log Hazard Ratio*	*P Value*	*Relative Risk*
Serum albumin <4 g/dL	0.40 ± 0.10	<.001	1.49
Hemoglobin <10.5 g/dL	0.30 ± 0.11	.006	1.35
Male gender	0.30 ± 0.09	.001	1.35
Stage IV disease	0.23 ± 0.09	.011	1.26
Age ≥45 y	0.33 ± 0.10	.001	1.39
White blood cell count ≥15,000/mm³	0.34 ± 0.11	.001	1.41
Lymphocyte count <600/mm³ or <8% of white blood cell count	0.31 ± 0.10	.002	1.38

(From ref. 161, with permission.)

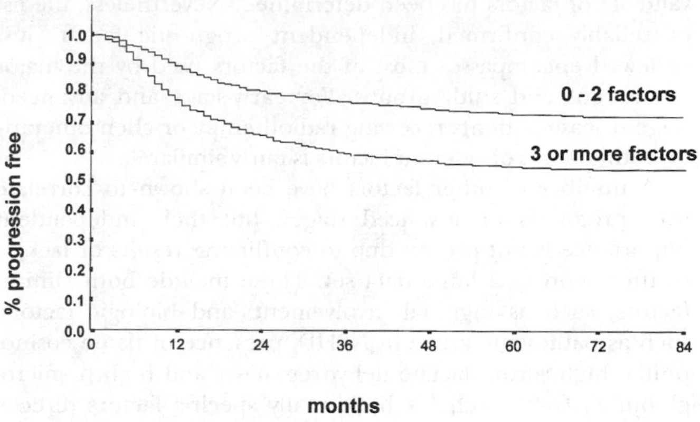

FIGURE 45.6-4. International prognostic score split at three prognostic factors.

ally only stage IIB or III patients are given "advanced-stage" treatment owing to the presence of these factors.

The EORTC includes in its advanced-stage cohorts stages III and IV only, without regard to other factors, as did the U.S. NCI and several U.S. cooperative groups.

In the GHSG, all stage III and IV patients plus stage IIB with LMM or E-lesions are included in the advanced-stage group. Earlier trials included in the unfavorable early-stage category either all stage IIIA patients or just those without any of the five GHSG factors listed. This gradual shift to use of more intensive therapy was based on prognostic factor analyses.

Certain other trial groups include further stage I and II patients in the advanced prognostic group (e.g., IB and IIB or bulky stage II disease).[164]

Prognostic Factors for Advanced-Stage Disease

The more uniform treatment modality and the greater frequency of treatment failure events has permitted more conclusive and generally applicable results for prognostic factor analyses for the advanced stages, as compared with early stages. The results of the International Prognostic Factors Project,[161] though not necessarily including all possible factors, can be taken as reliable (Table 45.6-8).

All these factors were highly significant in the multivariate analysis of data from 5141 patients treated in 25 centers, and their prognostic power was confirmed in an independent sample. Note that factors 1, 2, 4, and 5 are also prognostic for early-stage patients. All seven factors were associated with similar relative risks of between 1.26 and 1.49. Therefore, Hasenclever and Diehl[161] recommended combining these factors into a single score by simply counting the number of adverse factors, thus giving an integer prognostic score between 0 and 7. However, even patients exhibiting five or more factors (7% of cases) had a 5-year failure-free rate of more than 40%. The best failure-free rate was close to 80% for those with, at most, one factor (29% of cases), suggesting that a group of advanced-stage patients with a relatively favorable prognosis could be recognized (1618 patients included in the final analysis for FFTF, according to whether the prognostic score was 0 to 2 or 3 or higher) (Fig. 45.6-4).

A number of other factors have been shown to correlate with prognosis in advanced stages, but their independent importance is not proven due to conflicting results or lack of confirmation in a large data set. These include pathologic grade in NSHD, presence of tissue eosinophilia, elevated inguinal involvement, high serum lactate dehydrogenase level, and β_2-microglobulin.

Factors relevant to advanced-stage patients may be used to identify patients for either treatment intensification or treatment reduction. Reduction can be achieved by creating a modified protocol or by including these patients in the early-stage group. Concerning intensification, various investigators have treated a poor-prognosis subset of advanced-stage patients, who had attained a remission by conventional chemotherapy, with HDCT accompanied by hematologic stem cell support.[156,165] Proctor et al.[165] constructed a continuous numeric index for this purpose as a weighted sum of the variables age, stage, lymphocyte count, hemoglobin, and presence of bulky disease, and included patients with an index greater than 0.5 in the poor-prognosis subset. Carella et al.[231] included patients with two or more of the following factors: high lactate dehydrogenase level, very large mediastinal mass, two or more extranodal sites, inguinal involvement, low hematocrit, and bone marrow involvement. However, none of these methods could consistently select a subset with a failure rate of less than 40% with conventional therapy. This means that the early high-dose approach is unlikely to show a clinically relevant long-term survival benefit as compared with conventional treatment.[166]

Concerning treatment reduction, the short-duration, reduced-dose Stanford V chemotherapeutic regimen (mechlorethamine, Adriamycin, vinblastine, vincristine, etoposide, bleomycin, and prednisone)[194] with or without radiotherapy is currently being tested in patients with bulky stage II or advanced-stage disease who have, at most, two International Prognostic Factor Project adverse factors.[167] Stanford V is, however, not merely a reduction of therapy but rather a rescheduling with lower total doses but greater dose intensities. No data are available on the results of treatment reduction in a favorable subset of the advanced-stage patients.

In conclusion, the three-level scheme of division into early-stage favorable, early-stage unfavorable, and advanced-stage cases remains valid according to current knowledge (see Table 45.6-7). Separation of very favorable early-stage or poor-risk advanced-stage patients for especially mild or intensive therapy, respectively, does not appear justified. Several prognostic factors, other than clinical stage, are used in the divisions among favorable, unfavorable, and advanced cases, and no universally valid set of factors has been determined. Nevertheless, the list of reliably confirmed, independent prognostic factors just reviewed encompasses most of the factors used by the major institutions and study groups. For early-stage and advanced-stage disease patients receiving radiotherapy or chemotherapy or both, the set of relevant factors is fairly similar.

A number of other factors have been shown to correlate with prognosis in advanced stages, but their independent importance is not proven due to conflicting results or lack of confirmation in a large data set. These include both clinical factors, such as inguinal involvement, and biologic factors, such as pathologic grade in NSHD, presence of tissue eosinophilia, high serum lactate dehydrogenase, and high β_2-microglobulin. The search for biologically specific factors directly related to tumor activity is now an important research goal.

EARLY-STAGE FAVORABLE DISEASE

Reduction of Staging or Treatment: Ongoing and Recently Completed Trials

Increasing concern for the long-term consequences of treatment has prompted many investigators to reexamine the aggressive approaches developed for the staging and treatment of early-stage HD in the 1970s and 1980s. Many of the ongoing and recently completed studies were developed in an attempt to reduce the long-term complications of treatment without increasing mortality from HD. These include studies that look at reduction of radiation dose or reduction of field size in pure radiotherapy; seek an optimal, short, or less toxic chemotherapeutic regimen; explore an optimal radiation volume in combined modality therapy; or evaluate chemotherapy alone.

Clinical Trials of Radiotherapy Alone

RADIATION DOSE REDUCTION. Although a few studies have comprehensively reviewed dose-response data for HD, only one prospective randomized study is available.[168] This multicenter trial by the GHSG evaluated the tumoricidal doses for subclinical involvement by HD.[169] A total of 376 laparotomy-staged favorable-prognosis IA to IIB HD patients were enrolled. Only patients without risk factors were included in the trial. Any one of the following risk factors was cause for exclusion: presence of LMA, massive splenic involvement, extranodal disease, an ESR of more than 30 and B-symptoms, an ESR of more than 50 and no B-symptoms, or more than three regions of involvement. Patients were randomized to receive either 40-Gy extended-field radiotherapy or 30-Gy extended-field radiotherapy followed by an additional 10 Gy to involved lymph node regions.

The 5-year FFTF results favored the 30-Gy extended-field plus 10 Gy arm over the 40-Gy extended-field arm (81% vs. 70%, respectively; $P = .026$). The 5-year FFTF and survival rates were (nonsignificantly) higher in the reduced-dose arm, suggesting that 30 Gy is sufficient for treating subclinical involvement of HD with radiotherapy alone.[169]

RADIATION FIELD SIZE REDUCTION

Mantle Irradiation Alone in Clinical Stage IA to IIA Patients. The use of mantle irradiation alone for early-stage HD is attractive because all treatment is completed within 5 weeks, patients avoid the long-term risks of radiation to the upper abdomen, and the potential for salvage with combination chemotherapy is not compromised. Results of prospective and retrospective studies of mantle irradiation alone for unselected CS I and II patients have been disappointing. The EORTC H1 trial, one of the first studies to evaluate the role of chemotherapy in the treatment of early-stage HD, randomized clinically staged I and II patients to receive mantle irradiation alone or combined with vinblastine chemotherapy. All CS I and II patients were enrolled. Fewer recurrences were seen in patients who received both mantle irradiation and vinblastine chemotherapy. However, relapse rates were high in both groups. The freedom from recurrence was only 38% in the mantle-alone group, and the 15-year survival rate was only 58%. This suggests that mantle irradiation alone is not adequate treatment for unselected patients with CS I to II HD and that vinblastine is only partially effective in eliminating recurrences, many of which occurred below the diaphragm.[170] Similarly, the Toronto series reported a 10-year rate of freedom from recurrence of only 54%.[171] These high recurrence rates in unselected patients are not surprising, as more than 20% of CS I to II patients have occult abdominal involvement, and absence of treatment of potential abdominal disease (with radiotherapy or chemotherapy) will result in higher recurrence rates than are achieved with more extensive treatment. When mantle irradiation was restricted to clinically staged, asymptomatic patients in whom a single lymph node region was involved (CS IA), better results have been seen, with 10- to 15-year freedom-from-recurrence rates of 58% to 81%.[172]

Clinically Staged Patients with a Very Low Risk of Abdominal Involvement. Clinically staged patients with a very low risk of abdominal involvement include female patients with CS IA NSHD, patients with CS IA LP histology, and CS IA patients with interfollicular HD.[130] A similar subgroup of patients was defined by the EORTC (women <40 years of age with CS IA lymphocytic predominance or NS histology and an ESR <50 mm) and treated with mantle irradiation alone without staging laparotomy in the EORTC H7VF (very favorable) and H8VF trials. In the H7VF trial, 40 patients were treated with mantle irradiation alone; complete remission was achieved in 95%. However, 23% of patients experienced relapse, yielding a 6-year event-free survival rate of 66%, a relapse-free survival rate of 73%, and overall and cause-specific survival rates of 96%.[173] The relapse rates were thought to be unacceptably high in this selected subgroup of stage IA patients. The very favorable subgroup now is treated according to the EORTC strategy for the favorable subgroup.

Mantle Irradiation Alone in Favorable-Prognosis Stage IA and IIA Patients. To determine the role of prophylactic abdominal irradiation in early-stage HD, the EORTC H5 trial (1977 through 1982) compared the use of mantle and paraaortic-splenic pedicle irradiation to mantle irradiation alone in patients with favorable early-stage HD.[159,170] This study included only patients with NS or LP histology, aged 40 years or younger, with prognostically staged (PS) I or II disease with mediastinal adenopathy, and an ESR of less than 70. No differences were seen in disease-free survival or overall survival between the two treatment groups with or without paraaortic irradiation. A 1997 update of this trial shows no statistical difference between the two treatment arms, either for treatment failure probability ($P = .62$) or overall survival ($P = .69$).

In 1989, a single-arm prospective trial was initiated at the Harvard University Medical School Joint Center for Radiotherapy of mantle irradiation alone in laparotomy-staged IA to IIA HD patients. The objectives were to identify patients most suitable for mantle irradiation alone, to establish guidelines for follow-up after treatment, to evaluate the requirement for staging laparotomy, and to provide an assessment of risk versus gain for the reduction of treatment in early-stage HD. The eligibility criteria for the study included a negative laparotomy, the absence of LMA and B-symptoms, and NS or LP histology. Thoracic CAT scanning and ^{67}Ga scanning were required to establish the extent of thoracic involvement, and patients with HD in hilar, subcarinal, or cardiophrenic lymph node regions were not eligible for the trial. Eighty-four patients have been enrolled. The 5-year actuarial rate of freedom from recurrence exceeds 80%. These excellent results with mantle irradiation alone also have been seen in other retrospective studies.[174]

Clinical Trials of Combined Chemoradiotherapy

Some randomized trials of combined modality therapy are based on the premise that this approach results in a very high freedom from recurrence in early-stage HD and that efficacy can be maintained when using less toxic chemotherapeutic and radiotherapeutic regimens.

LESS TOXIC CHEMOTHERAPY WITH RADIATION: COMPARISON WITH RADIATION ALONE. These trials use chemotherapeutic regimens given for four or six cycles in combination with radiotherapy. The regimens are combined with involved-field or regional (mantle) radiotherapy with the premise that the drugs being tested will be able to control both adjacent prophylactic sites and occult abdominal disease in clinically staged patients without upper abdominal and splenic irradiation. Analysis of patterns and frequency of failure eventually will provide better guidelines for designing optimal regimens to control occult HD not appreciated on physical examination or radiographic evaluation. If successful, these regimens should reduce treatment-related morbidity and mortality by reducing both the amount and toxicity of chemotherapy and by using smaller radiation volumes.

With the objective of reducing acute toxicity and chronic morbidity (sterility, increased risk of leukemia), Horning et al.[175] developed a "nontoxic" chemotherapeutic regimen—vinblastine, bleomycin, and methotrexate (VBM)—which was tested in a randomized trial of PS IA to IIB and PS IIIA patients. The trial compared subtotal or total nodal irradiation to involved-field irradiation (44 Gy) followed by VBM.[175] Data on freedom from disease progression at 9 years favored involved-field irradiation and VBM (98%) over subtotal or total nodal irradiation (78%) (P = .01). No differences were seen in overall survival (P = .09). The BNLI has confirmed the efficacy of VBM with involved-field irradiation but, in that group's experience, this approach produced unacceptable pulmonary and hematologic toxicity.[176] Favorable results with VBM and extended-field radiotherapy in CS IA to IIA HD also have been reported by the Gruppo Italiano per lo Studio dei Linfomi.[177] In that study of 50 patients, the 5-year progression-free survival rate was 82%. Sixteen percent of patients in the trial experienced pulmonary toxicity.

Based on the Stanford trial results reported above,[175] a follow-up Stanford University trial has been completed.[145] Patients with CS IA to IIA HD (staging laparotomy and splenectomy were eliminated) were treated either with subtotal nodal and splenic irradiation or two cycles of VBM, followed by regional (mantle) irradiation, followed by four additional cycles of VBM (with a reduced bleomycin dose). No differences in 4-year freedom from disease progression or survival were noted between the two arms of the trial.

Epirubicin, bleomycin, vinblastine, and prednisone (EBVP) and involved-field irradiation (n = 168) versus mantle and paraaortic-splenic irradiation (n = 165) for favorable-prognosis CS IA to IIA patients was tested in the EORTC H7F trial (1988 through 1993). The EORTC EBVP II regimen (one dose per cycle) was proposed as a potentially less toxic but similarly effective regimen as compared to ABVD. In the H7F trial for patients with favorable disease, six cycles of EBVP were combined with involved-field radiation and were randomly compared with subtotal nodal and splenic irradiation in favorable CS I and II patients. At 6 years, the relapse survival rate was significantly higher for patients on the combined chemoradiotherapy arm than for those on the radiotherapy-alone arm (92% vs. 81%, respectively; P = .004). The 6-year survival rate was excellent in both treatment arms (98% vs. 96%, respectively; P = .156).[178,179] In contrast, in the H7U trial for patients with unfavorable disease, EBVP and involved-field radiotherapy was inferior to MOPP and ABV and involved-field radiotherapy, suggesting that the use of prognostic factors is crucial in selecting patients for treatment with reduced chemotherapeutic and radiotherapeutic regimens.

REDUCED NUMBER OF CHEMOTHERAPY CYCLES. The trials noted here use combination chemoradiotherapy with fewer than four cycles of chemotherapy. Although the primary goal of these trials is to evaluate the efficacy of short courses of chemotherapy, new regimens are also being tested [i.e., Stanford V; vincristine, Adriamycin, prednisolone, etoposide, cyclophosphamide, and bleomycin (VAPEC-B)]. The optimal extent of radiotherapy needed is less certain in the short-course trials. For example, there are at least limited data that four to six cycles of chemotherapy are sufficient to control occult abdominal disease in the majority of CS I to II patients.[124,180] With short-course chemotherapy, very few data are available on the effectiveness of different regimens to control HD outside of the involved regions, as defined by physical examination or radiographic evaluation. This uncertainty is reflected in some of the trial designs that use subtotal nodal and splenic irradiation rather than involved-field or mantle irradiation in combination with chemotherapy. Ongoing and recently completed short-course trials are listed in Table 45.6-9.

The GHSG HD7 trial (1994 through 1998) randomized 643 favorable CS IA to IIB HD patients to subtotal nodal and splenic irradiation alone or to two courses of ABVD and the radiotherapeutic regimen. A preliminary analysis of 365 patients showed an advantage in FFTF in the patients receiving ABVD (96%) as compared to those treated with irradiation alone (87%; P = .05) (see Table 45.6-9).[181]

Several questions are raised by this study. First, with an expected long-term FFTF in favorable CS IA to IIA HD of approximately 70% to 75% with radiotherapy alone, is the added benefit in FFTF with two cycles of ABVD worth the extra risk from the doxorubicin and bleomycin? Second, is it more difficult to salvage patients whose disease recurs after subtotal nodal and splenic irradiation and two cycles of

TABLE 45.6-9. Clinical Trials in Favorable-Prognosis Stage I–II Hodgkin's Disease: Trials to Identify the Optimal Number of Chemotherapy Cycles

Trial	*Eligibility*	*Treatment Regimens*	*No. of Patients*	*Outcome*
GHSG HD7	CS IA–IIB *without* large mediastinal mass (≥0.33 m/t); massive splenic involvement; localized extranodal involvement; ESR ≥50 mm in A, ≥30 mm in B; three or more involved areas	A: EFRT 30 Gy (IFRT 40 Gy)	180	FFTF, 87%[a]; SV (22 mo), 97%[b]
		B: 2 ABVD + EFRT 30 Gy (IFRT 40 Gy)	185	FFTF, 96%[a]; SV, 98%[b]
GHSG HD10	CS IA–IIB *without* large mediastinal mass (≥0.33 m/t); localized extranodal involvement; ESR ≥50 mm in A, ≥30 mm in B; three or more involved areas	A. 2 ABVD + IFRT (30 Gy) B: 2 ABVD + IFRT (20 Gy) C: 4 ABVD + IFRT (30 Gy) D: 4 ABVD + IFRT (20 Gy)	Open	Open
BNLI	CS IA–IIA *without* large mediastinal disease	A: 1 VAPEC-B + IFRT (30–40 Gy) B: Mantle RT 30–35 Gy (IFRT 30–40 Gy)	Open	Open
SWOG 9133/ CALGB 9391	CS IA–IIA *without* age <16; large mediastinal disease; pericardial involvement	A: 3 (doxorubicin + vinblastine) + STLI (S) (36–40 Gy) B: STLI (S) (36–40 Gy)	Open	Open
EORTC/GELA H8F	CS IA–IIB *without* age ≥50; ESR ≥50 mm in A, ≥30 mm in B; four or more sites of disease; large mediastinal disease	A: 3 MOPP/ABV + IFRT (36 Gy) B: STLI (S)	No report	No report
Stanford V for favorable CS IA–IIA HD	CS I–II *without* B-symptoms; age <16 and >60 y; large mediastinal disease; two or more extranodal sites	Stanford V for 8 wk + modified IFRT (30 Gy)	Open	Open

ABV, doxorubicin (Adriamycin), bleomycin, and vinblastine; ABVD, Adriamycin, bleomycin, vinblastine, and dacarbazine; BNLI, British National Lymphoma Investigation; CALGB, Cancer and Leukemia Group B; CS, clinical stage; EFRT, extended-field radiotherapy; EORTC, European Organization for Research and Treatment of Cancer; ESR, erythrocyte sedimentation rate; FFTF, freedom from treatment failure; FU, follow-up; GELA, Groupe d'Etude des Lymphomes de l'Adulte; GHSG, German Hodgkin's Lymphoma Study Group; HD, Hodgkin's disease; IFRT, involved-field radiotherapy; LP, lymphocyte predominance histology; MOPP, mechlorethamine, vincristine (Oncovin), procarbazine, prednisone; m/t, mass-thoracic ratio; NS, nodular sclerosis histology; RT, radiotherapy; STLI (S), subtotal nodal irradiation (splenic irradiation); SV, survival; SWOG, Southwest Oncology Group; VAPEC-B, vincristine, Adriamycin, prednisolone, etoposide, cyclophosphamide, bleomycin.
[a]$P = .05$.
[b]Not significant.
Note: Stanford V regimen consists of mechlorethamine, doxorubicin, vinblastine, prednisone, vincristine, bleomycin, VP-16.

ABVD than after subtotal nodal and splenic irradiation alone? These are questions that can be answered only with longer follow-up.

The GHSG HD10 trial (opened in 1998) has essentially the same eligibility criteria as does the GHSG HD7 trial. Patients are to be randomized to four arms, namely the four combinations of two or four cycles of ABVD followed by 20- or 30-Gy involved-field radiotherapy. This trial should help to determine the number of cycles of ABVD needed to control occult HD in the abdomen and to prevent recurrence of HD in apparently uninvolved sites adjacent to known HD (adjacent to the irradiated involved site). It should also help to determine the dose of radiation needed to control HD when combined with limited chemotherapy.

In a Manchester pilot study and a BNLI trial, VAPEC-B chemotherapy is given for 4 weeks, followed by involved-field irradiation or mantle irradiation alone. Preliminary reports from the Manchester pilot study using the relatively brief 4-week VAPEC-B regimen in early-stage HD provide background data for the ongoing BNLI trial. In the Manchester study, 111 CS IA to IIA patients without mediastinal bulk have been randomized since 1989 to receive either limited radiotherapy alone or VAPEC-B followed by local irradiation only to the involved regions. With a median follow-up time of 3.3 years, there have been only two recurrences in the VAPEC-B–plus–local irradiation arm (progression-free survival rate at 3 years, 91%).[182] The current BNLI study has a similar design; however, the radiotherapy-alone arm includes full mantle irradiation rather than a more limited field (see Table 45.6-9).

The Southwest Oncology Group–Cancer and Leukemia Group B (SWOG/CALGB) study of three cycles of adjuvant doxorubicin and vinblastine plus subtotal nodal and splenic irradiation versus subtotal nodal and splenic irradiation alone in CS IA to IIA HD patients is ongoing (see Table 45.6-9). As of June 1998, 284 patients have been enrolled in the study (information provided courtesy of Dr. Todd Wasserman, CALGB update, June 1998). Of these, 162 patients have been evaluated for short-term toxicity. The questions raised by this study are similar to those for the GHSG HD7 study, including the potential extra toxicity of the doxorubicin and vinblastine in a group of patients with an expected favorable prognosis with treatment by radiotherapy alone and the overall strategy in trial design of giving enough chemotherapy to eliminate the need for abdominal irradiation.

The EORTC H8F trial (1993 through 1998), which compares three cycles of MOPP/ABV hybrid and involved-field irradiation to mantle and paraaortic-splenic irradiation for favorable-prognosis CS IA to IIA patients, was activated in 1993 (see Table 45.6-9). This trial should answer the following important questions: Are three cycles of standard chemotherapy sufficient to control subclinical HD in favorable-prognosis CS IA to IIA patients? Can patients who experience relapse after three cycles of MOPP/ABV and involved-field radiotherapy be cured with an alternative treatment, short of HDCT and stem cell rescue? The one concern of the trial is the use of the hybrid regimen, which confers some risk of sterility and leukemogenesis in these favorable-prognosis HD patients. ABVD and EBVP are proposed for the H9 trials.

The modified Stanford V trial for early-stage favorable-prognosis HD involves a relatively short, but intensive, chemotherapeutic regimen given for 12 weeks to patients with poor-prognosis stage I to II disease.[183] A modification of this trial has been opened for favorable-prognosis CS IA to IIA patients using 8 weeks of the Stanford V regimen and modified involved-field irradiation to sites of initial involvement (identified radiographically as nodal enlargement of ≥1.5 cm). The chemotherapeutic regimen includes mechlorethamine (6 mg/m^2 in weeks 1 and 5), doxorubicin (25 mg/m^2 in weeks 1, 3, 5, and 7), vinblastine (6 mg/m^2 in weeks 1, 3, 5, and 7), prednisone (40 mg/m^2 on days 1 through 36, followed by tapering), vincristine (1.4 mg/m^2 in weeks 2, 4, 6, and 8), bleomycin (5 mg/m^2 in weeks 2, 4, 6, and 8), and VP-16 (60 mg/m^2 on days 15 and 16 and days 43 and 44). This regimen will evaluate the ability of brief but intense chemotherapy to control HD outside of initially involved sites in favorable-prognosis CS I to II patients.

RADIATION VOLUME AND DOSE. Two ongoing trials in favorable-prognosis early-stage HD are evaluating radiation dose to involved sites after chemotherapy. The GHSG initiated a trial, HD10, that compares 30-Gy with 20-Gy irradiation after two cycles of ABVD, as described previously in the section Reduced Number of Chemotherapy Cycles (see Table 45.6-9). The EORTC H9F trial is evaluating 36-Gy or 20-Gy irradiation or no radiation to involved sites in patients who have achieved a complete remission after six cycles of EBVP.

Clinical Trials of Chemotherapy Alone

Probably the first published experience of the use of MOPP chemotherapy alone in early stages of childhood HD comes from Uganda, where no radiotherapy was available.[184] Several small, retrospective studies have also reported treatment with MOPP alone.[185] On the basis of this limited experience, two randomized studies were devised to compare radiotherapy alone to MOPP chemotherapy alone in laparotomy-staged patients; both studies have median follow-up times of 7.5 to 8 years. Although both studies now are dated because of the use of the MOPP regimen and the requirement for staging laparotomy, results from these trials provide valuable information for the design of future protocols.

CHEMOTHERAPY VERSUS RADIATION. The NCI study was initially designed to include patients with intermediate-prognosis HD.[186] Although the trial included patients with favorable-prognosis PS IIA disease, the most favorable patients (PS IA patients with peripheral sites) were not included in the trial and were treated with radiotherapy alone. Patients with an unfavorable prognosis (B-symptoms, LMA, and limited stage III disease) were included in the trial. Patients were randomized to 6 months of MOPP chemotherapy alone or to subtotal nodal irradiation alone. After researchers recognized that patients with massive mediastinal involvement and PS IIIA disease were not optimal candidates for radiotherapy alone, the randomization criteria were changed while the study was ongoing. No difference in disease-free or overall survival was seen at 10 years.

The Italian prospective study randomized patients with PS IA to IIA HD to receive either 6 months of MOPP alone or subtotal nodal irradiation alone.[187] There were no differences in freedom from progression. However, the survival rate was significantly higher in patients treated with radiotherapy alone (93%) than in those treated with chemotherapy alone (56%). The difference in survival was attributed to the inability to salvage patients who experienced relapse after MOPP chemotherapy; these results are similar to the poor results of salvage ABVD in patients who experienced relapse after MOPP for advanced HD.

Both the NCI and the Italian studies demonstrated greater acute toxicities in patients who received MOPP chemotherapy. In the Longo et al.[186] study, more than 50% of patients treated with MOPP had at least one hospital admission for fever and neutropenia.

The NCIC CTG HD6 study (unpublished data) is a modification of the NCI and Italian studies, with randomization of clinically staged, rather than pathologically staged, patients and the use of ABVD as the chemotherapeutic regimen. Favorable-prognosis patients (NS or LP histology, age <40 years, ESR <50, one to three sites of involvement) are randomized to subtotal nodal irradiation and splenic irradiation versus four cycles of ABVD alone. This study will test the efficacy of four cycles of ABVD alone in favorable-prognosis early-stage HD. The study is open for accrual.

CHEMOTHERAPY VERSUS COMBINED MODALITY THERAPY. In 1977, the Grupo Argentino de Tratamiento de la Leucemia Aguda (GATLA)/Grupo Latinamericano de Trataniento de Hematopatias Malignas cooperative groups initiated a randomized study[187a] of chemotherapy with cyclophosphamide (600 mg/m^2 on day 1), vinblastine (6 mg/m^2 on day 1), procarbazine (100 mg/m^2 on days 1 through 14), and prednisone (40 mg on days 1 through 14) (CVPP) alone for six cycles versus CVPP plus radiotherapy consisting of 30 Gy to involved areas for patients with CS I to II disease. Overall, the 7-year disease-free survival rate was 71% for chemoradiotherapy as compared to 62% for chemotherapy alone (P = .01); survival rates were 89% and 81%, respectively (P = .3). In a subgroup of patients with favorable-prognosis CS I to II disease, no differences were observed in actuarial rates of disease-free survival (77% vs. 70%) or overall survival (92% vs. 91%), respectively, for CVPP plus involved-field irradiation versus CVPP alone. In comparing these results with other adult studies, one should note that in this study and in the subsequent GATLA study, nearly 50% of the patients were younger than 16 years. It is possible that treatment approaches with chemotherapy alone may be more successful in children than in adult patients.

In the subsequent GATLA study, patients with favorable prognosis were randomized to CVPP for three cycles versus six cycles.[188] At 5 years, the actuarial event-free survival (80% vs. 84%) and overall survival (91% vs. 92%) rates were not significantly different.

The ongoing EORTC three-armed trial (H9F) for favorable-prognosis CS I to II patients who achieve a complete remission after six cycles of EBVP are randomized to 36-Gy involved-field irradiation versus 20-Gy involved-field irradiation versus no radiotherapy.

The Memorial Sloan-Kettering Cancer Center trial randomizes CS I through IIIA patients without LMA or bulky disease, who have achieved a complete remission after six cycles of ABVD, to either mantle irradiation (35 Gy) or no further treatment. This trial has enrolled approximately 120 patients of a planned total of 200 patients.

Recommendations and Future Directions

Standard care currently provides a number of treatment options for patients with early-stage favorable-prognosis HD. These include the use of mantle irradiation alone for selected patients with negative laparotomy staging, mantle plus paraaortic and splenic irradiation without laparotomy staging, and combination chemotherapy and radiotherapy, often with a reduced number of cycles of chemotherapy and reduction of radiation field sizes and doses (e.g., ABVD for four cycles followed by involved-field radiation to 20 to 30 Gy).

Current clinical trials are evaluating the use of alternative chemotherapy combinations, shortened courses of chemotherapy, chemotherapy with smaller radiation fields or lower radiation doses, and chemotherapy without radiotherapy. Death from HD in favorable-prognosis early-stage patients is unusual, and mortality from other causes occurs many years later. Therefore, survival is not a useful parameter for evaluating midterm results in early-stage HD. Current trials must be judged by freedom-from-first-recurrence rates, acute morbidity, and by new criteria such as quality of life and, perhaps, cost-effectiveness. Trials aiming at high freedom-from-first-recurrence rates may show that the tested regimens do not provide the optimum treatment once long-term (10- to 20-year) data are available; treatment-related mortality may exceed HD mortality in favorable-prognosis early-stage patients. New methods in decision analysis should also help in the design of trials and in the analysis of retrospective data.

Despite the increasing availability of guidelines for the treatment of HD, there must remain room for individualization of treatment. With different treatment options, some of which may result in a higher recurrence risk at the gain of less toxic initial treatment, patient preferences must be assessed. In addition, treatment should be individualized when a particular treatment approach might result in a higher risk of a serious late complication (e.g., risk of late breast cancer in young female patients treated with large radiation fields). This is an exciting time for the development of new strategies in the treatment of early-stage HD. Many of the ongoing trials ask questions that will allow us to optimize treatment for early-stage patients and minimize long-term toxicity.

EARLY-STAGE UNFAVORABLE DISEASE

Numerous studies analyzed clinical prognostic factors for patients with stage I to II HD in the 1970s and 1980s.[163,170] On the basis of these studies, clinical investigators have defined favorable and unfavorable prognostic groups of patients with stage I to II HD in an effort to refine the design of clinical trials and to tailor treatment in accordance with prognostic factors. Although the definition of favorable- and unfavorable-prognosis early-stage HD continues to vary among different cooperative groups and institutions, three factors of poor prognostic significance are used as grouping criteria in most clinical trials: LMA or bulky disease, B-symptoms, and advanced age. For each prognostic group, the goal is to define the precise amount of treatment that will both minimize recurrence and mortality from HD and provide the least risk for long-term toxicity. Patients with unfavorable disease require, in general, more aggressive treatment than do those with favorable disease. However, the likelihood of cure of patients with unfavorable stage I to II disease is still high and, therefore, consideration of long-term toxicity remains an important issue in the treatment of these patients.

A number of clinical trials comparing radiotherapy alone to combined modality therapy for unfavorable-prognosis stage I to II HD were conducted in the 1970s and 1980s. The high recurrence rates with radiotherapy alone led to the development of strategies in current trials that use various combinations of chemotherapy and radiotherapy. To illustrate, one large trial conducted by the EORTC (H5U)[159] randomized patients with unfavorable prognostic factors to total nodal irradiation or MOPP chemotherapy (six cycles) and mantle irradiation. Although overall survival did not differ (69% in both arms at 15 years), treatment failure (35% vs. 16%; $P < .001$) strongly favored the chemotherapy arm.

Trials to Identify the Best Chemotherapy Combination

The evolution of studies to identify the best chemotherapy combination for unfavorable early-stage HD paralleled analogous trials for advanced stages. Early trials evaluated MOPP versus MOPP-like combinations, later trials compared these combinations with ABVD and, finally, the most recent trials compare new intense chemotherapy combinations with ABVD.

The first combined modality trial to test MOPP versus ABVD in unfavorable-prognosis patients was the Milan study, conducted between 1974 and 1982, using split-course treatment (three cycles of chemotherapy preceding and following subtotal nodal irradiation), which showed no significant difference in freedom from progression.[189] However, in the EORTC H6U trial (1982 through 1988) comparing split-course MOPP and ABVD, the 10-year survival was equivalent in both arms, but the FFTF rate was significantly higher with ABVD than with MOPP.[190,191]

The GATLA trial and the EORTC H7U trial (Table 45.6-10) studied modified nonalkylating agent regimens versus standard alkylating agent regimens in unfavorable-prognosis early-stage patients. All patients received combined radiotherapy and chemotherapy. In both trials, the arms using modified chemotherapy were associated with significantly higher recurrence rates.

In the EORTC trial, the recurrence rate was high enough to result in early closure of the trial. Although, in favorable-prognosis stage I to II HD, less toxic and less intense chemotherapeutic regimens have been effective in combined modality therapy programs, this does not appear to be the case for patients with unfavorable-prognosis disease. In the GATLA trial, the event-free survival was 66% for doxorubicin, vincristine, prednisone, and etoposide versus 85% for CVPP ($P =$

TABLE 45.6-10. Randomized Clinical Trials in Unfavorable-Prognosis Stage I–II Hodgkin's Disease: Trials to Identify the Optimal Chemotherapy Combination

Trial	*Eligibility*	*Treatment Regimens*	*No. of Patients*	*Outcome*
EORTC H6U 1982–1988	CS I–II *with* large mediastinal mass (≥0.33 m/t) or ESR ≥50 mm in A, ≥30 mm in B; three or more involved areas	A: 3 MOPP + mantle + 3 MOPP	165	FFTF, 68%[a]; SV (10-y), 87%[b]
		B: 3 ABVD + mantle + 3 ABVD	151	FFTF, 90%[a]; SV (10-y), 87%[b]
Istituto Nazionale Tumori, Milan, 1974–1982	PS IIB	A: 3 MOPP + STLI/TLI + 3 MOPP	33	FFP (5-y), 66%[c]
		B: 3 ABVD + STLI/TLI + 3 ABVD	36	FFP, 72%[c]
GATLA 1986–1992	Score of age, B-symptoms, stage, number of sites, and bulky disease	A: 3 CVPP + IFRT (30 Gy) + 3 CVPP	92	EFS, 85%[d]; SV (5-y), 95%[e]
		B: 3 AOPE + IFRT (30 Gy) + 3 AOPE	84	EFS, 66%[d]; SV, 87%[e]
EORTC H7U 1988–1992	CS IA–IIA *with* age >50 or ESR ≥50 mm in A, ≥30 mm in B or large mediastinal mass (≥0.33 m/t)	A: 6 EBVP II + IFRT (36 GY)	160	EFS, 68%[f]; SV (6-y), 82%[g]
		B: 6 MOPP/ABV + IFRT	156	EFS, 90%[f]; SV, 89%[g]
EORTC H9U 1988–1992	Same as H7U	A: 6 ABVD + IFRT (30 Gy)	Open	Open
		B: 4 ABVD + IFRT		
		C: 4 BEACOPP + IFRT		
GHSG HD11 1998	CS IA–IB, IIA *with* age ≥50 or ESR ≥50 mm or CS IIB and ESR ≥30 mm or large mediastinal disease	A: 4 ABVD + IFRT (30 Gy)	Open	Open
		B: 4 ABVD + IFRT (20 Gy)		
		C: 4 BEACOPP + IFRT (30 Gy)		
		D: 4 BEACOPP + IFRT (20 Gy)		
ECOG 2496 1998	Large mediastinal disease	A: 6 ABVD + IFRT (36 Gy) to bulky sites (>5 cm)	Open	Open
		B: 12 weeks Stanford V + IFRT to bulky sites		

ABV, doxorubicin (Adriamycin), bleomycin, and vinblastine; ABVD, Adriamycin, bleomycin, vinblastine, and dacarbazine; AOPE, doxorubicin, vincristine, prednisone, and etoposide; BEACOPP, bleomycin, etoposide, Adriamycin, cyclophosphamide, vincristine, procarbazine, and prednisone; CS, clinical stage; CVPP, cyclophosphamide, vinblastine, procarbazine, and prednisone; EFS, event-free survival; EBVP, epirubicin, bleomycin, vinblastine, and prednisone; ECOG, Eastern Cooperative Oncology Group; EORTC, European Organization for Research and Treatment of Cancer; ESR, erythrocyte sedimentation rate; FFP, freedom from progression; FFTF, freedom from treatment failure; GATLA, Grupo Argentino de Tratamiento de la Leucemia Aguda; GHSG, German Hodgkin's Study Group; IFRT, involved-field irradiation; LP, lymphocyte predominance histology; MOPP, mechlorethamine, vincristine (Oncovin), procarbazine, prednisone; m/t, mass-thoracic ratio; NS, nodular sclerosis histology; PS, prognostic stage; RT, radiotherapy; Stanford V, mechlorethamine, doxorubicin, vinblastine, prednisone, vincristine, bleomycin, VP-16; STLI, subtotal lymph node irradiation; TLI, total lymph node irradiation; SV, survival.

[a] $P < .0001$.
[b] $P = .52$.
[c] $P = .2$.
[d] $P = .009$.
[e] $P = .16$.
[f] $P < .0001$.
[g] $P = .18$.

.009).[188] In the EORTC trial, the event-free survival was 68% for EBVP II and involved-field radiotherapy versus 90% for MOPP/ABV ($P = .0001$).[178]

Several nonrandomized trials also have evaluated alternative chemotherapeutic regimens using a reduced number of cycles of chemotherapy or modified chemotherapeutic regimens.[192,193] It is worth noting one recent trial: At Stanford, the Stanford V regimen, administered for 3 months, was followed by involved-field irradiation to 36 Gy in 38 patients with large mediastinal disease. No patients have experienced relapse or died (median follow-up, 40 months).[194]

Based mainly on trials in advanced HD, ABVD has become the standard regimen used in patients with CS I to II disease. A number of current trials compare combined modality therapy using ABVD with more intense, novel regimens. Both the EORTC H9U and GHSG HD11 studies of combined modality therapy are comparing four cycles of ABVD with four cycles of BEACOPP.[181] In the Eastern Cooperative Oncology Group (ECOG) 2496 trial of combined modality therapy, six cycles of ABVD are being compared to 3 months of the Stanford V regimen.[194]

Trials to Identify the Optimal Number of Cycles of Chemotherapy

Two large, randomized trials are currently evaluating whether four cycles of combination chemotherapy and radiotherapy is sufficient treatment as compared to six cycles of chemotherapy and radiotherapy. The recently closed EORTC H8U study randomized patients to combined modality therapy with four or six cycles of MOPP/ABV, but the results have not yet been reported (see Table 45.6-10). The new EORTC H9U trial randomizes patients to four and six cycles of ABVD.[181] A number of retrospective or prospective single-arm studies have evaluated the role of the number of cycles of chemotherapy in patients with large mediastinal disease.[193,195,196] The results vary, and the number of patients studied is small; a more definitive answer will need to come from the large, randomized trials currently under way.

Trials to Identify the Appropriate Radiotherapy Volume

Several randomized trials have addressed the question of radiotherapy volumes in combined modality programs. The French trial reported by Zittoun et al.[197] randomized 218 stage I to II unfavorable-prognosis patients to six cycles of MOPP sandwiched around involved-field (40-Gy) or extended-field (40-Gy) irradiation. The 6-year disease-free survival rates were 87% and 93%, respectively ($P = .15$). The Milan study reported by Hoppe et al.[197a] incorporated only 4 months of chemotherapy (ABVD), followed by involved-field (36-Gy) or subtotal nodal irradiation (30 to 36 Gy). The 5-year freedom-from-progression rates were 96% and 93%, respectively (Table 45.6-11).

The three-arm EORTC/Groupe d'Etude les Lymphomes de l'Adulte H8U trial, randomized patients to four cycles of MOPP/ABV plus involved-field irradiation or subtotal nodal irradiation.[197b] The GHSG HD8 trial, conducted between 1993 and 1998, used two cycles (4 months) of COPP/ABVD followed by either involved-field or extended-field irradiation to 30 Gy (see Table 45.6-11).[197b] Preliminary evidence from these randomized trials as well as from several nonrandomized studies suggests that radiation fields may be safely limited to involved regions in most combined modality programs when chemotherapy is given over 4 months or more.[198,199]

Trials of Chemotherapy Alone versus Combined Modality Therapy

Only one prospective trial of chemotherapy alone versus combined modality therapy in unfavorable-prognosis stage I to II disease patients has been reported. The GATLA randomized 104 patients with unfavorable disease characteristics to six cycles of CVPP alone or six cycles of CVPP sandwiched around involved-field irradiation (30 Gy).[200] The 7-year survival rates were 66% and 84%, and the freedom-from-relapse rates were 34% and 75% ($P < .001$), both favoring combined modality treatment.

The ongoing NCI of Canada (NCI-C) HD6 trial evaluates patients with unfavorable disease characteristics but excludes patients with LMA or bulky disease. Patients are randomized to receive combined modality therapy with two cycles of ABVD followed by irradiation (an extended mantle plus splenic irradiation or mantle plus paraaortic and splenic irradiation) or four to six cycles of ABVD alone (depending on the rapidity of response).

Recommendations and Future Directions

The outcome of treatment for patients with unfavorable-prognosis stage I to II HD has improved dramatically since the 1970s. Mainly, this is due to the use of combined modality therapy, as historically either radiotherapy alone or chemotherapy alone was associated with recurrence rates of approximately 50%. Current clinical trials are exploring new combinations of radiotherapy and chemotherapy to try to reduce late morbidity and mortality while maintaining a high probability of freedom from first recurrence.

TABLE 45.6-11. Randomized Clinical Trials in Unfavorable Prognosis Stage I to II Hodgkin's Disease: Trials to Identify the Appropriate Radiation Volume

Trial	*Eligibility*	*Treatment Regimens*	*No. of Patients*	*Outcome*[a]
French Cooperative 1976–1981	CS I–II *and* age <45 y; ≤3 involved areas; no bulky disease	A: 3 MOPP + IFRT (40 Gy) + 3 MOPP	82	DFS, 87%; SV (6-y), 92%
		B: 3 MOPP + EFRT (40 Gy) + 3 MOPP	91	DFS, 93%; SV (6-y), 91%
Milan 1990–1997	All CS I–II	A: 4 ABVD + STLI	65	FFP (5-y), 96%
		B: 4 ABVD + IFRT	68	FFP (5-y), 93%
EORTC/GELA H8U 1993–1998	CS IA–IIB *and* age ≥50 y; ESR ≥50 mm in A; ≥30 mm in B; ≥4 involved sites; large mediastinal disease	A: 6 MOPP/ABV + IFRT (36 Gy) B: 4 MOPP/ABV + IFRT (36 Gy) C: 4 MOPP/ABV + STLI	Not reported	Not reported
GHSG HD8 1993–1998	CS IA-IIB *and* ESR ≥50 mm in A; ≥30 mm in B; ≥3 involved sites; large mediastinal disease	A: 4 COPP/ABVD + EFRT	482	FFTF, 94%; SV (26-mo.), 97%
		B: 4 COPP/ABVD + IFRT	483	FFTF, 92%; SV (26-mo.), 97%

ABV, doxorubicin (Adriamycin), bleomycin, and vinblastine; ABVD, Adriamycin, bleomycin, vinblastine, and dacarbazine; COPP, cyclophosphamide, vincristine (Oncovin), procarbazine, and prednisone; CS, clinical stage; DFS, disease-free survival; EFRT, extended-field radiotherapy; EORTC, European Organization for the Research and Treatment of Cancer; ESR, erythrocyte sedimentation rate; FFP, freedom from progression; FFTF, freedom from treatment failure; GELA, Groupe d'Etude des Lymphomes de l'Adulte; GHSG, German Hodgkin's Study Group; IFRT, involved-field radiotherapy; MOPP, mechlorethamine, Oncovin, procarbazine, and prednisone; STLI, subtotal nodal irradiation; SV, survival.
[a]All not significant.

ADVANCED-STAGE DISEASE

Basic Regimens: MOPP and ABVD

MECHLORETHAMINE, VINCRISTINE (ONCOVIN), PROCARBAZINE, AND PREDNISONE. Initially the four-drug MOPP program was administered with each drug given at full dose over 2 weeks, resulting in a complete remission rate of 81%. Complete remission rates of 73% to 81%, long-term freedom from progression of 36% to 52%, and long-term overall survival of 50% to 64% were obtained in major trials of MOPP in advanced-stage HD.[201–203]

Despite the good initial results with MOPP therapy, several groups investigated alternative regimens to improve the efficacy or reduce toxicities. The CALGB showed that omission of the alkylating agents nitrogen mustard or procarbazine from the MOPP regimen were associated with inferior complete remission rates.[204] Thus, the four-drug principle was considered a standard at that time, to which all alternative combinations had to be compared.

Modifications of the MOPP scheme included the substitution of an alkylating agent such as cyclophosphamide or chlorambucil for mechlorethamine (COPP) or a vinca alkaloid such as vinblastine or vincristine for Oncovin (MVPP), as well as alteration of the doses of procarbazine and prednisone.

The ECOG developed a five-drug regimen containing BCNU, cyclophosphamide, vinblastine, procarbazine, and prednisone (BCVPP) with MOPP.[205] Their results showed that BCVPP had a significantly higher freedom-from-progression rate (50% vs. 33%) and overall survival rate (83% vs. 75%) than did MOPP at 5 years. However, the interpretation of these results is complicated by the inclusion of previously treated patients.

In the United Kingdom, the MVPP combination was used, which revealed comparable results to MOPP, with complete remission rates of 60% to 80% and 5- year overall survival rates of 70% to 80%.[206,207] Also in the United Kingdom, the chlorambucil, vinblastine, procarbazine, and prednisone (ChlVPP) regimen was developed and showed similar efficacy with less acute toxicity as compared to MOPP, although a randomized comparison was not performed. The BNLI performed a randomized trial to compare chlorambucil (Leukeran), Oncovin, procarbazine, and prednisone (LOPP) with MOPP. No significant differences were observed in complete remission or overall survival rates.[208] Taken together, several MOPP-like regimens showed similar efficacy with less acute gastrointestinal and neurologic toxicities.

ADRIAMYCIN, BLEOMYCIN, VINBLASTINE, AND DACARBAZINE. MOPP and its derivatives had two limitations: Only approximately 50% of patients could be cured, and the alkylating agent–based combination was associated with an increased risk of sterility and acute leukemia. In an attempt to develop a regimen for patients in whom MOPP had failed, Bonadonna et al.[209] introduced the ABVD regimen. Vinblastine had demonstrated high activity as a single agent and lacked cross-resistance with vincristine in human tumors. Both doxorubicin and bleomycin were very active drugs and showed objective responses in approximately 50% of patients. Dacarbazine was added because it was active as a single agent and also showed synergism with doxorubicin.

The Milan group compared three cycles of MOPP or ABVD followed by extended-field irradiation and three additional cycles of the same chemotherapy.[210] A significant difference in favor of ABVD could be achieved, with freedom-from-progression rates of 63% for MOPP versus 81% for ABVD.

Both MOPP and ABVD were highly active regimens and had nonoverlapping toxicities. It was therefore straightforward to test combinations of MOPP and ABVD to further increase treatment results. The Milan group randomized patients with stage IV disease to MOPP or MOPP/ABVD for up to 12 cycles. The results were emphatically in favor of the alternating program, with a statistically significant difference in freedom from progression at 8 years (36% MOPP vs. 65% MOPP/ABVD; $P<.005$).[205] Subsequently, three large cooperative trial groups (ECOG,[211] CALGB,[211a] and EORTC[212]) have confirmed these results and demonstrated superior results with the combination of MOPP/ABVD over MOPP or a MOPP derivative. ECOG compared the MOPP derivative BCVPP with MOPP followed by ABVD. Both complete remission and overall survival rates were superior with the MOPP/ABVD combination.

The CALGB tested, in a three-arm trial, six to eight cycles of MOPP, six to eight cycles of ABVD, and 12 cycles of MOPP alternating with ABVD.[211] At 10 years, the failure-free survival rates were 38% for MOPP, 55% for ABVD, and 50% for MOPP/ABVD, with a probability value of .02. Overall survival was not significantly different among the three arms, although there was a trend in favor of ABVD or MOPP/ABVD as compared to MOPP alone.[211]

The EORTC compared two courses of MOPP alternating with two courses of ABVD to a total of eight courses.[212] Radiotherapy was given to initial bulk or residual masses after chemotherapy. MOPP/ABVD showed a significantly higher failure-free survival rate at 6 years (43% MOPP vs. 60% MOPP/ABVD).[212]

Thus, ABVD alone and MOPP/ABVD are more effective than MOPP alone. In addition, ABVD alone offers the advantage of less acute and long-term toxicities.

DURATION OF THERAPY. In the original NCI studies of MOPP, two additional monthly cycles were given after a complete remission was achieved.[213] Viviani et al.[164] initially applied up to 12 cycles of MOPP and later, in the alternating program, eight cycles without reduction in efficacy. The CALGB trial demonstrated that eight cycles of ABVD was comparable to 12 cycles of alternating MOPP/ABVD.[214] A total of eight to 12 cycles of chemotherapy was given in the more recent phase III trials. Thus, although the optimal duration is not known precisely, eight cycles of MOPP, ABVD, or a combination appear to be sufficient.

Hybrid Regimens

The theoretic basis for multidrug regimens is the predicted advantage of the early introduction of all active agents to avoid resistant tumor cell clones. This idea is based on a model proposed by Goldie and Coldman,[215] who related the drug sensitivity of tumors to their spontaneous mutation rate. The model formed the basis of "hybrid" schemes, which were tested by several groups in advanced-stage HD.

Groups in Vancouver and Milan independently designed two hybrids of MOPP and ABVD to test the Goldie-Coldman hypothesis prospectively.[215] The NCI-C compared the MOPP-ABV hybrid with alternating MOPP/ABVD in patients with stage IIIB or IV HD. At 5 years, there was no significant difference in the overall survival rates between both arms, although the hybrid regimen was associated with higher hematologic and nonhematologic toxicities.[216]

The Milan group compared their MOPP/ABV hybrid with alternating MOPP/ABVD. Freedom-from-progression and overall survival rates at 10 years revealed no significant difference between the hybrid and alternating arms.[164]

The GHSG compared a new hybrid scheme—COPP, ABV, and ifosfamide, methotrexate, and etoposide (IMEP) with their standard COPP/ABVD. Complete remissions, FFTF, and overall survival rates showed no statistically significant difference between the two treatment arms.[217]

A second intergroup trial[217a] that compared an MOPP/ABV hybrid with ABVD was performed in the United States, recruiting a total of 856 patients with stage III or IV HD or recurrent disease after radiotherapy. This study was prematurely stopped by the Data and Safety Monitoring Board because an excess of treatment-related deaths and second malignancies with the hybrid regimen was observed. At 3 years, similar failure-free survival rates were observed for ABVD (65%) and MOPP/ABV (67%). From this trial, it was concluded that ABVD and MOPP/ABV are equally effective but that ABVD is less toxic and should remain the standard treatment.

The potential relevance of scheduling was exemplified in a recent BNLI study in which a significant difference was found between a LOPP and etoposide, vincristine, and Adriamycin (EVA) hybrid and LOPP alternating with EVA that contained identical total doses. The complete remission was significantly less in the hybrid arm, and the trial was stopped prematurely.[218]

To summarize, the Goldie-Coldman hypothesis could not be proven in advanced-stage HD, although this could be due to the fact that the optimal hybrid regimen has not been identified thus far. ABVD has emerged as the standard against which newer treatments must be compared. With ABVD, 60% to 70% of patients will be free of disease at 5 years. ABVD is much less likely to cause severe myelotoxicity, acute leukemia, or sterility than are treatment programs that contain significant doses of alkylating agents.

New Chemotherapeutic Regimens

The success of ABVD in the CALGB and in the intergroup trials indicated that alkylating agents are not essential for curative treatment for advanced HD. However, the pulmonary toxicity of bleomycin, which is especially pronounced in children and in combination with mediastinal irradiation, remains a major concern with ABVD. A number of drugs showing high efficacy in relapsed HD have become candidates for use in first-line therapy. The topoisomerase inhibitor etoposide has gained special interest among several groups, as a 20% to 60% response rate in refractory HD was reported with single-agent etoposide.[219] On the basis of these considerations, several etoposide-containing drug regimens have been developed.

At Stanford, the five-drug regimen Stanford V was developed.[183] The program was applied weekly over a total of 12 weeks. Sophisticated consolidative radiotherapy to sites of initial bulky disease was used. In this phase II trial, 126 patients had been recruited. The estimated 5-year freedom-from-progression rate was 89%, and the overall survival was 96% at a median observation time of 4.5 years in this single-center study. Reduced long-term toxicities with preserved fertility was a major goal and could be achieved both in men and women. An intergroup trial of Stanford V versus ABVD has been initiated in selected patients with low-risk advanced HD.

Similarly, the Manchester group developed an abbreviated, 11-week chemotherapeutic program, VAPEC-B. In a randomized trial, VAPEC-B and the hybrid ChlVPP/EVA were compared with radiotherapy applied to previous bulky disease or residual disease.[220] This study was stopped after 26 months owing to a threefold increase in the rate of progression after VAPEC-B.

The Southampton group developed another abbreviated, weekly chemotherapeutic regimen consisting of PACE-BOM.[221] Radiotherapy was applied to residual disease. A 64% failure-free survival was reported after a median observation time of 5 years.

Caution should be exercised when comparing results of different trials; particularly the amount of consolidative radiation, can vary widely. Large, randomized trials provide the only reliable comparisons between regimens. Table 45.6-12 shows the doses and scheduling of polychemotherapeutic regimens in HD.

Dose and Dose Intensity

In several animal models, a clear relationship between chemotherapy dose and tumor response has been demonstrated. In HD, retrospective analyses of drug delivery with MOPP chemotherapy showed that patients receiving less than the optimal doses had inferior results.[222] Such dose effects were detected independently with mustard, procarbazine, and vincristine.

Until recently, no prospective randomized trials to analyze the role of dose intensity in the treatment of advanced HD had been conducted. There are two principal ways to test dose intensity: Doses of cytotoxic drugs can be intensified by increasing individual drug dose or by shortening the interval between treatments (or both). Gerhartz et al.[223] compared COPP/ABVD with a dose- and time-escalated COPP/ABVD regimen given with granulocyte-macrophage colony-stimulating factor support. The delivered dose intensity in the dose-intensified arm was 1.22, as compared with 0.92 in the standard arm (1.0 = standard intended dose). The preliminary analysis revealed a higher complete remission rate in the intensified arm, but definite results have not been reported yet.

The GHSG has conducted a series of clinical trials to address the role of dose intensity in advanced HD in a comprehensive way. A mathematic model of tumor growth and chemotherapeutic effects was developed and fitted to the data from 705 patients treated by the GHSG.[224] This model predicted that moderate dose escalation would increase tumor control by 10% to 15% at 5 years. The BEACOPP regimen was devised and used as a standard combination for dose escalation.[225] After establishing excellent tolerability as well as efficacy in a pilot trial, a second study of escalated BEACOPP was performed in which doxorubicin was increased to a fixed level and doses of cyclophosphamide and etoposide were increased in a stepwise fashion with granulocyte colony-stimulating factor support.[226] Maximum practicable doses were found to be 190% of cyclophosphamide and 200% of etoposide.

TABLE 45.6-12. Polychemotherapy Regimens Used in Hodgkin's Disease

Drug	*Dose (mg/m²)*	*Route*	*Schedule (days)*	*Cycle Length (days)*
MOPP				21
Mechlorethamine	6	IV	1, 8	
Oncovin (vincristine)	1.4	IV	1, 8	
Procarbazine	100	PO	1–14	
Prednisone	40	PO	1–14	
COPP				28
Cyclophosphamide	650	IV	1, 8	
Oncovin (vincristine)	1.4	IV	1, 8	
Procarbazine	100	PO	1–14	
Prednisone	40	PO	1–14	
LOPP				28
Leukeran (chlorambucil)	10 total	PO	1–10	
Oncovin (vincristine)	1.4	IV	1, 8	
Procarbazine	100	PO	1–10	
Prednisone	25	PO	1–14	
ABVD				28
Adriamycin (doxorubicin)	25	IV	1, 15	
Bleomycin	10	IV	1, 15	
Vinblastine	6	IV	1, 15	
Dacarbazine	375	IV	1, 15	
MOPP/ABV Hybrid				28
Mechlorethamine	6	IV	1	
Oncovin (vincristine)	1.4[a]	IV	1	
Procarbazine	100	PO	1–7	
Prednisone	40	PO	1–14	
Adriamycin (doxorubicin)	35	IV	8	
Bleomycin	10	IV	8	
Vinblastine	6	IV	8	
BEACOPP (baseline)				21
Bleomycin	10	IV	8	
Etoposide	100	IV	1–3	
Adriamycin (doxorubicin)	25	IV	1	
Cyclophosphamide	650	IV	1	
Oncovin (vincristine)	1.4[a]	IV	8	
Procarbazine	100	PO	1–7	
Prednisone	40	PO	1–14	
BEACOPP (escalated)				21
Bleomycin	10	IV	8	
Etoposide	200	IV	1–3	
Adriamycin (doxorubicin)	35	IV	1	
Cyclophosphamide	1250	IV	1	
Oncovin (vincristine)	1.4[a]	IV	8	
Procarbazine	100	PO	1–7	
Prednisone	40	PO	1–14	
G-CSF	+	SC	8+	
ChlVPP/EVA				21
Chorambucil	10 total	PO	1–7	
Vinblastine	10 total	IV	1	
Procarbazine	150 total	PO	1–7	
Prednisolone	50 total	PO	1–7	
Etoposide	200	IV	8	
Vincristine	2 total	IV	8	
Adriamycin (doxorubicin)	50	IV	8	
ChlVPP/PABlOE				50
Chorambucil	6	PO	1–14	
Vinblastine	6	IV	1, 8	

(continued)

TABLE 45.6-12. (Continued)

Drug	*Dose (mg/m²)*	*Route*	*Schedule (days)*	*Cycle Length (days)*
Procarbazine	100	PO	1–14, 29–43	
Prednisolone	30	PO	1–14	
Adriamycin (doxorubicin)	40	IV	29	
Bleomycin	10	IV	29, 36	
Vincristine	1.4[a]	IV	29, 36	
Etoposide	200	PO	30–32	
Stanford V				12 wk
Mechlorethamine	6	IV	Wk 1, 5, 9	
Adriamycin (doxorubicin)	25	IV	Wk 1, 3, 5, 9, 11	
Vinblastine	6	IV	Wk 1, 3, 5, 9, 11	
Vincristine	1.4[a]	IV	Wk 2, 4, 6, 8, 10, 12	
Bleomycin	5	IV	Wk 2, 4, 6, 8, 10, 12	
Etoposide	60 × 2	IV	Wk 3, 7, 11	
Prednisone	40	IV	Wk 1–10 q.o.d.	
G-CSF	—	SC	Dose reduction or delay	
VAPEC-B				11 wk
Vincristine	1.4[a]	IV	Wk 2, 4, 6, 8, 10	
Adriamycin (doxorubicin)	35	IV	Wk 1, 3, 5, 7, 9, 11	
Prednisolone	50	PO	Wk 1–6	
Etoposide	75–100 × 5	PO	Wk 3, 7, 11	
Cyclophosphamide	350	IV	Wk 1, 5, 9	
Bleomycin	10	IV	Wk 2, 4, 6, 8, 10	

G-CSF, granulocyte colony-stimulating factor.
[a]Vincristine dose capped at 2 mg.

The GHSG then designed a three-arm study comparing COPP/ABVD, standard BEACOPP, and escalated BEACOPP in patients with advanced HD.[227] Radiotherapy was prescribed for bulky disease at diagnosis or for residual disease after eight cycles of chemotherapy, and approximately two-thirds of patients received consolidative radiotherapy. In 1996, at the time of a planned interim analysis, the COPP/ABVD arm of this trial was closed to accrual because of superior outcomes in the combined BEACOPP arms.[227] In a subsequent interim analysis, with 1070 patients evaluated, superior FFTF results were seen with escalated BEACOPP (88%) versus standard BEACOPP (79%) and COPP/ABVD (69%). A major difference was observed in the rate of primary progressive disease during initial therapy, which was significantly lower with escalated BEACOPP (2%) versus BEACOPP (8%) and COPP/ABVD (12%). Although there was a trend in the overall survival rate in favor of BEACOPP, this was significant only at the time of this interim analysis.

As expected, escalated BEACOPP was associated with greater hematologic toxicity, including a greater use of both red blood cell and platelet transfusions. Second malignancies, including acute myeloid leukemia possibly related to etoposide, were reported with BEACOPP. However, the rate of secondary high-grade NHLs was similarly reduced after escalated BEACOPP. The mature data from this important study, particularly with survival as an end point, are awaited with great interest.

HDCT frequently is used in patients with first or later relapses of HD. Numerous phase II trials and two randomized trials from the BNLI and the GHSG have shown superior results with a high-dose program as compared to conventional treatment.[228–230] In advanced-stage HD, limited data concerning the role of HDCT are available. The Genua group of Carella et al.[231] conducted a phase II trial of myeloablative therapy and autografting among patients with poor-risk features as described by Straus et al.[232] Subsequently, the European Bone Marrow Transplant Registry (EBMT) initiated a prospective study in poor-risk patients comparing HDCT and autografting with additional chemotherapy after four cycles of ABVD-containing chemotherapy. Proctor et al.[165] have used their previously published model to identify patients at risk for an ongoing study in which patients are randomized to additional chemotherapy or HDCT and autografting after three cycles of a hybrid regimen and radiotherapy to bulky sites.[232] No interim results of these studies have yet been published.

Role of Radiotherapy

The ability of radiotherapy to provide local control in HD is well established. Furthermore, radiotherapy is non–cross-resistant with standard combination chemotherapy. However, the role of radiotherapy in advanced-stage HD is still controversial. Despite this uncertainty, most large trial groups include some radiotherapy as an integral part of their advanced-stage treatment strategy.

The potential contribution of radiotherapy depends on a variety of factors, including patient parameters (e.g., age, stage of the disease, and tumor mass) and the chemotherapy program. The field and dose influence efficacy and toxicity. Radiotherapy in advanced HD can be considered in three clinical settings. First, radiotherapy may be used as an adjuvant after complete remission with standard chemotherapy. Second, radiotherapy may be an integrated component of a combined modality program, possibly with reduced or brief chemotherapy. Finally, radiotherapy can serve as a non-cross-resistant treatment for patients with partial or uncertain response after chemotherapy.

There have been several reports indicating that patients treated with chemotherapy alone failed to completely respond or progressed, primarily in previously involved nodal sites. In the SWOG study, 80% of relapses after MOP-BAP chemotherapy were detected in initially involved sites.[233] A number of authors have reported that approximately 30% of selected patients who experienced relapse after chemotherapy can achieve long-term remissions with radiotherapy. However, the benefits of consolidative radiotherapy must be balanced against the risk for serious side effects, particularly second malignancy in the irradiated field.

A number of phase III trials investigated the role of consolidative radiotherapy after primary chemotherapy, with divergent results. After MOP-BAP chemotherapy, 61% of patients who achieved complete remission were randomized to low-dose involved-field radiotherapy or to no further treatment in a SWOG study.[233] In this trial, no significant differences in remission duration or overall survival were detected.

The GHSG analyzed the role of low-dose (20-Gy) involved-field radiotherapy versus two cycles of additional chemotherapy consolidation in 288 patients in complete remission after initial chemotherapy with COPP/ABVD. There was no significant difference in freedom-from-progression or overall survival rates between the treatment arms.[234]

To overcome the insufficient power of the randomized studies with too few patients to detect a relevant difference, Loeffler et al.[235] performed a metaanalysis of 14 studies involving more than 1700 patients in total. Two study designs were compared: In the additional design, the same chemotherapy with and without additional irradiation was compared, whereas in the parallel design, irradiation following chemotherapy was compared with further cycles of chemotherapy.

In the additional design, radiotherapy reduced the hazard rate by approximately 40%. The benefit of irradiation was more pronounced among patients with mediastinal involvement and provided no reduction in relapse among patients with stage IV disease. There was no survival benefit detected by radiotherapy in any subgroup analyzed. In the parallel design, there was no significant difference in disease-free survival. However, overall survival was significantly higher among patients treated with chemotherapy alone. In the combined modality group, there were more deaths from causes other than HD, including leukemia. The results of the metaanalysis should be regarded with caution, because the studies were initiated 20 or more years ago and because, in most instances, a MOPP-based chemotherapeutic regimen was used, which is not regarded as standard therapy today.

The most important issue today relates to the added efficacy of radiotherapy as adjuvant treatment to modern anthracycline-containing chemotherapy and the added late toxicity of this combined modality. Prospective, randomized trials, such as the comparison of a MOPP-ABV hybrid with or without consolidative radiotherapy by the EORTC,[236] are needed to address these questions. In this EORTC trial, patients in complete remission after MOPP/ABV receive two further chemotherapy cycles followed by randomization to involved-field radiotherapy or observation. A similar approach with a potentially more active chemotherapeutic regimen, BEACOPP, is currently being taken by the GHSG. In this trial, patients are randomized to eight cycles of escalated BEACOPP or four cycles of escalated BEACOPP plus four cycles of BEACOPP-baseline. Subsequently, patients are randomized to radiotherapy to initial bulky and residual disease or to no further treatment. These two important trials should define the role of radiotherapy applied with highly active chemotherapeutic protocols.

Conclusions

After more than 30 years of clinical research, advanced-stage HD became a curable disease in most instances. Adriamycin-containing chemotherapy has emerged as the standard against which modern strategies must be compared. With modern chemotherapy, approximately 60% to 70% of patients will be alive and free of disease at 5 years (Table 45.6-13). ABVD has a favorable toxicity profile and causes less myelotoxicity, acute leukemia, or sterility relative to many previous treatment programs

TABLE 45.6-13. Results of Polychemotherapy Regimens in Advanced-Stage Disease

Regimen	*RT (%)*	*CR (%)*	*EFS/FFP/FyaFTF* %	Years	Parameter	*Survival* %	Years	*Reference*
ABVD	0	82	61	5	FFP	73	5	211
MOPP/ABVD	0	83	65	5	FFP	75	5	211
MOPP/ABV	0	83	64	8	FFP	79	5	347
ABVD	0	71	65	5	FFS	87	5	348
MOPP/ABV	ns	73	67	5	FFS	85	5	348
MOPP/ABVD	ns	76	67	5	FFP	83	5	349
MOPP/ABV	ns	80	71	5	FFP	81	5	349
ChlVPP/EVA	ns	65	73	5	EFS	83	5	220
COPP/ABVD	63	83	69	3	FFTF	86	3	227
BEACOPP, baseline	72	88	79	3	FFTF	90	3	227
MOPP/ABV	67	95	82	5	EFS	84	5	236
Stanford V	86	99	89	5	FFP	93	5	194
BEACOPP, escalated	72	96	88	3	FFTF	91	3	227

CR, complete response; EFS, event-free survival; FFP, freedom from progression; FFTF, freedom from treatment failure; ns, not specified; RT, radiotherapy.
Note: See Table 45.6-12 for definition of the various drug regimens.

containing alkylating agents. However, 20% to 30 % of patients eventually experience relapse and then are frequently treated with high-dose programs.

The two major goals in advanced HD are to improve the cure rate and to reduce acute and late toxicities. The definition of prognostic factors identified patients who are at a higher risk for relapse as well as those for whom less toxic approaches might be tested. The optimal approach or program has not been identified yet, although new chemotherapeutic regimens (e.g., Stanford V and BEACOPP) with increased efficacies have been identified. These new drug combinations hold the promise of achieving these goals, but efficacy and toxicity data must mature before their contributions can be assessed with certainty (Table 45.6-14). Although the addition of radiotherapy improved disease control in some trials, a survival benefit was not identified and so the role of radiotherapy remains controversial.

Recommendations for primary treatment of early (favorable und unfavorable group) and advanced stages of disease outside clinical trials are given in Table 45.6-15.

PROGRESSIVE AND RELAPSED DISEASE

Diagnosis and Staging at Disease Progression or Relapse

Although late relapses more than 10 years after primary treatment have been reported in HD, relapse generally occurs within 1 to 5 years after primary therapy.[237] At relapse, a new histologic workup should be obtained, as the risk for second tumors—NHL or solid tumors—is increased.[238,239] Moreover, a proportion of NHL patients initially receive a misdiagnosis, as HD or composite lymphomas are not detected during first diagnosis.[240] Therefore, another biopsy at the time of relapse or disease progression is required.

In all patients with relapsed or primary progressive HD, clinical and radiographic restaging is recommended. Because most patients receive salvage treatment, restaging has prognostic and therapeutic importance. Isolated nodal recurrence is associated with a better prognosis than is disseminated relapse, and salvage treatment strategies vary depending on prior therapy and time of failure. The issue of how to define complete remission, partial remission, no change, or progressive disease after salvage treatment is vital, because salvage therapies generally are more intense and more toxic than are first-line regimens. In salvage therapy studies, the response criteria usually are defined as in first-line therapies. In most series reported, however, a minimum duration of response of 4 weeks after the end of a salvage therapy is required.

Prognostic Factors

The likelihood of successful salvage therapy is determined by biologic features, which may be linked to certain clinical features. Adverse prognostic factors for patients with treatment failure include the treatment modality used in first-line therapy, patient age, relapse sites, quantity of disease at relapse, and presence or absence of systemic symptoms. In addition, the duration of first remission is a major determinant of a second complete response.

It was first noted in 1979 that the length of a remission after first-line chemotherapy had a marked effect on the ability of patients to respond to subsequent salvage treatment.[241] In 1992, the NCI updated their experience with the long-term follow-up of patients who experienced relapse after polychemotherapy.[242] Derived primarily from investigations involving failures after MOPP and MOPP variants, the conclusions are relevant to other chemotherapeutic programs. On this basis, chemotherapy failures can be divided into three subgroups:

- Primary progressive HD (approximately 10% of all cases)—that is, patients who never achieved a complete remission
- Early relapses within 12 months of complete remission (approximately 15% of all cases)
- Late relapses after complete remission lasting longer than 12 months (approximately 15% of all cases)

Using conventional chemotherapies for patients with primary progressive disease, virtually no patient survives more than 8 years. In contrast, for patients with early relapse or late relapse, the projected 20-year survival was 11% and 22%, respectively.[242]

Patients in whom treatment with first-line radiotherapy, combination chemotherapy, or combined modality therapy fails can be divided into two groups and their treatment selected accordingly: relapse after irradiation for early-stage disease and relapse after primary chemotherapy.

RELAPSE AFTER IRRADIATION FOR EARLY-STAGE DISEASE. Primary radiotherapy alone has been used more extensively in the past than in current practice. The survival of patients treated with conventional chemotherapy after relapse of irradiated early-stage disease is at least equal to that of advanced-stage patients initially treated with chemotherapy. Overall survival and disease-free survival range from 57% to 71%.[163,243,244]

Patients who experience relapse after radiotherapy alone for localized HD (stage I and II) have satisfactory results with combination chemotherapy and are not considered candidates for HDCT and autologous stem cell transplantation (ASCT). The relapse rates after radiotherapy varied from 19% to 35%, the highest rates being in the series that included only clinical rather than laparotomy staging. The majority of patients in these series had salvage treatment based on MOPP or similar regimens. The range of 10-year survival was 57% to 71%, resembling the results of primary treatment with MOPP in patients with advanced disease. This suggests that prior radiotherapy does not cause drug resistance or a clinically significant compromise of chemotherapy dose intensity.

Stage at relapse is an important prognostic variable in radiotherapy failures. A study from Stanford including more than 100 patients with relapsed HD after subtotal or total nodal irradiation showed that conventional salvage chemotherapy is sufficient in patients with limited-stage disease having no systemic symptoms on recurrence (stage IA and IIA); after 10 years, 90% of these patients remained disease-free.[241] In contrast, the 10-year disease-free survival for those with stage III and IV disease or with B-symptoms (all stages) at the time of relapse was 58% and 34%, respectively. An analysis using the International Database on Hodgkin's Disease showed a worse prognosis for patients whose relapse included an extranodal site and stage IV at relapse and for those patients older than 40 years.[245]

Patients with LP or NS histology fared better than did those with MC or LD histology: Ten-year freedom from relapse for patients with favorable histologies was 67% versus 47% ($P = .04$) for patients with unfavorable histologies.[243,246,247]

TABLE 45.6-14. Randomized Clinical Trials in Advanced-Stage Hodgkin's Disease: Major Trials Currently Recruiting or Not Yet Published

Trial	*Eligibility*	*Treatment Regimens*	*No. of Patients*	*Outcome*
GHSG HD12 (V Diehl)	CS IIB with large mediastinal invasion or E-lesions; CS III and IV	A: BEACOPP (escalated × 8) ± RT (bulk/residual) B: BEACOPP (escalated × 8) C: BEACOPP (escalated × 4 + baseline × 4) ± RT (bulk/residual) D: BEACOPP (escalated × 4 + baseline × 4)	Began 1/98; planned: n = 1200	Final analysis planned for 2006
EORTC 20884 (JMM Raemaekers, JMV Burgers)	CS III and IV	6–8 MOPP/ABV + (if CR after 6 cycles): A: IFRT (24–30 Gy) B: No further treatment	Began 9/89; n = 666 (1/1999)	Recruitment to end 2/2000; 5-y OS, 84% (no arm comparison)
GELA (C Fermé, M Diviné)	IPS 0–2	A: 6 ABVD ± RT (bulk) B: intensified conventional chemo ± RT (bulk)	ne	ne
GELA/EBMT H96-1 (C Fermé, M Diviné)	IPS 3+	A: 8 ABVD ± RT (bulk) B: brief intensified chemo, then HDCT + ASCT ± RT (bulk)	ne	ne
UKLG (BNLI) LY09 (BW Hancock)	Disease requiring systemic therapy = CS I–II with bulk or >3 sites; CS III–IV	A: 6–8 ABVD ± RT (bulk/residual) B: 6–8 ChlVPP/PABlOE ± RT (bulk/residual) *or* 6–8 ChlVPP/EVA ± RT (bulk/residual)	Began 2/98; planned: n = 200–800	ne
UKLG (BNLI) phase II study (BW Hancock)	CS IIB, III, IV with large mediastinal invasion or ≥2 extranodal sites	A: 6–8 ABVD ± RT (bulk) B: Stanford V[a] ± RT (bulk)	Began 3/98; planned: n = 80	End point: response; phase III trial to follow
SNLG HDIII (S Proctor)	SNLG index <0.5 (high-risk)	3 PVACEBOP ± RT (bulk) + (if response): A. 2 PVACEBOP B: Melphalan, VP-16 then HDCT + ASCT	n = 105; randomized, n = 59 (1999)	1999: 5-y OS, 78% (all patients); arms not different
SWOG/ECOG 2496 (SJ Horning, CA Coltman)	CS II with bulk and III and IV; IPS 0–2	A: 6–8 ABVD ± RT (bulk) B: Stanford V[a] ± RT	Not yet recruiting (1999); planned: 1008	4 years' recruitment planned
SWOG/ ECOG	CS II with bulk and III and IV; IPS 3+	A: ABVD B: ABVD, then HDCT (BCNU, VP-16, cyclophosphamide) + ASCT	Not yet recruiting (1999)	ne

ABV, doxorubicin (Adriamycin), bleomycin, and vinblastine; ABVD, Adriamycin, bleomycin, vinblastine, and dacarbazine; ASCT, autologous stem cell transplantation; BEACOPP, bleomycin, etoposide, Adriamycin, cyclophosphamide, vincristine, procarbazine, and prednisone; chemo, chemotherapy; ChlVPP, chlorambucil, vinblastine, procarbazine, and prednisone; CR, complete remission; CS, clinical stage; EBMT, European Bone Marrow Transplant Registry; ECOG, Eastern Cooperative Oncology Group; EORTC, European Organization for the Research and Treatment of Cancer; EVA, etoposide, vincristine, and Adriamycin; GELA, Groupe d'Etude des Lymphomes de l'Adulte; GHSG, German Hodgkin's Study Group; HDCT, high-dose chemotherapy; IFRT, involved-field radiotherapy; IPS, International Prognostic Factors Project; MOPP, mechlorethamine, vincristine (Oncovin), procarbazine, and prednisone; ne, not evaluated; OS, overall survival; RT, radiotherapy; SNLG, Scotland and Newcastle Lymphoma Group; SWOG, Southwest Oncology Group; UKLG, United Kingdom Lymphoma Group.
[a]The Stanford V regimen consists of mechlorethamine, Adriamycin, vinblastine, vincristine, etoposide, bleomycin, and prednisone.

The original experience using systemic therapy for radiation failures was based on the use of MOPP. The likelihood of freedom from second relapse was 57% at 10 years.[248] However, sufficient data from doxorubicin-based regimens indicate that the principles for selecting a salvage regimen for a relapse after radiotherapy are the same as the principles for selecting a primary treatment for advanced disease. On the basis of the available evidence, ABVD has superior effects as compared with MOPP for radiation recurrence. The Milan Cancer Institute observed a disease-free survival rate of 81% with ABVD variants, as compared to 54% with MOPP.[249]

RELAPSE AFTER PRIMARY CHEMOTHERAPY. Treating recurrence after primary chemotherapy is a difficult issue. The choices available are salvage radiotherapy, conventional salvage chemotherapy, and HDCT followed by ASCT.

Salvage Radiotherapy. There are relatively few instances in which radiotherapy alone would be considered the standard salvage treatment because the perception is that recurrence indicates disseminated disease. However, salvage radiotherapy offers a potentially curative option with low morbidity for a subset of selected patients. Salvage radiotherapy is a valid treatment alternative in patients without B-symptoms who have not been given radiation previously or who experience relapse locally outside the initial radiation field.

This approach has been reported in series of more than 100 patients. Wirth et al.[250] reported the experience of salvage radiotherapy in 51 patients with relapsed or refractory HD. Twenty-three patients (45%) achieved a complete response after irradiation. Five-year failure-free survival and overall survival rates were 26% and 57%, respectively. Significant prognostic factors for failure-free survival were B-symptoms at the

TABLE 45.6-15. Recommendations for Primary Treatment Outside Clinical Trials

Group	*Stage*	*Recommendation*
Early stages (favorable)	CS I–II A/B no RF	EFRT (30–36Gy) *or* 4–6 cycles chemo[a] + IFRT (20–36 Gy)
Early stages (unfavorable)	CS I–II A/B + RF	4–6 cycles chemo[b] + IFRT (20–36 Gy)
Advanced stages	CS IIB + RF; CS III A/B; CS IV A/B	6–8 cycles chemo[c] + RT (20–36 Gy) to residual lymphoma and bulk

chemo, chemotherapy; CS, clinical stage; EFRT, extended-field radiotherapy; IFRT, involved-field radiotherapy; RF, risk factors (see Table 45.6-7); RT, radiotherapy.
[a]ABVD [doxorubicin (Adriamycin), bleomycin, vinblastine, and dacarbazine], EBVP (epirubicin, bleomycin, vinblastine, and prednisone), or VBM (vinblastine, bleomycin, and methotrexate).
[b]ABVD, Stanford V (mechlorethamine, Adriamycin, vinblastine, vincristine, etoposide, bleomycin, and prednisone), or MOPP/ABV [mechlorethamine, vincristine (Oncovin), procarbazine, and prednisone/Adriamycin, bleomycin, vinblastine].
[c]ABVD, MOPP/ABV, ChlVPP/EVA (chlorambucil, vinblastine, procarbazine, and prednisone/etoposide, vincristine, and Adriamycin), or BEACOPP (bleomycin, etoposide, Adriamycin, cyclophosphamide, vincristine, procarbazine, and prednisone) escalated.

time of salvage radiotherapy, extranodal involvement, and histology. For overall survival, significant factors were B-symptoms, patient age, and number of prior chemotherapeutic regimens. For patients who relapsed in supradiaphragmatic nodal sites without B-symptoms, 5-year failure-free survival and overall survival rates were 36% and 75%, respectively.

Table 45.6-16 demonstrates that selected patients who experience relapse after chemotherapy in an isolated nodal site without systemic symptoms can be salvaged by radiotherapy alone. Comparing radiotherapy with other types of salvage treatment is difficult, because the selection criteria for the different forms of treatment vary and no randomized study exists.

Conventional Salvage Chemotherapy. Since 1990, a number of new salvage chemotherapeutic regimens have been tested that incorporate drugs not used in the initial combination. Because most first-line management programs use MOPP, ABVD, or combinations of both, new salvage regimens have been designed anticipating resistance to these drugs in patients who have relapsed.[251–254]

Primary progressive disease and early relapse suggest cellular resistance to conventional doses of drugs. Patients with primary refractory HD on treatment with MOPP or alternative regimens usually respond poorly to second or third induction attempts and have a particularly poor prognosis (life expectancy <1.5 years). Fewer than 50% of patients who experience relapse after a short initial remission achieve a second complete remission, even when treated with non-cross-resistant regimens, with a median survival of 2.5 to 4.0 years. For the vast majority of these patients, second-line chemotherapy followed by HDCT is required. In contrast, more than 80% of patients with late relapse achieve a second complete remission with MOPP or alternative regimens, having a median survival of less than 4 years.[242] The Milan and NCI data suggest that late relapse does not necessarily imply resistance, as retreatment with the initial first-line regimen may result in response. An important goal for any retreatment in late relapse is the achievement of a second complete response, as nearly 50% of second complete responses will result in prolonged progression-free survival.[242,255]

Table 45.6-17 lists the second-line salvage regimens for HD published since 1985. Detailed analysis and interpretation are difficult because, in some trials, the number of patients is small, the clinical status of patients varied, the duration of first remission is heterogeneous, and a large number of these patients also received subsequent HDCT plus ASCT. No randomized trial exists comparing the effectiveness of different conventional salvage chemotherapeutic regimens.

TABLE 45.6-16. Salvage Radiotherapy Alone for Relapse after Chemotherapy

No. of Patients	*FFP*	*OS*	*Prognostic Factor for FFP*	*Reference*
53	26% (5 y)	57% (5 y)	B-symptoms, extranodal sites, histology	250
44	38% (5 y)	48% (5 y)	Extranodal sites	349
28	40% (5 y)	63% (5 y)	Duration of response	350
10	38% (5 y)	60% (5 y)	ne	351

FFP, freedom from progression; ne, not evaluated; OS, overall survival.

TABLE 45.6-17. Salvage Regimens for Hodgkin's Disease at Conventional Dosages

Regimen	*No. of Patients*	*RR (%)*	*Plus HDCT (no. of patients)*	*RFS (%)*	*Reference*
CEP	75	54	—	16	249
CEVD	32	48	—	22	253
Dexa-BEAM	56	56	19	25	251
Mini-BEAM	44	84	26	36	353
MIME	47	63	—	8	252
DHAP	19	68	—	ne	254
ASHAP	56	70	39	40	352
MINE	100	75	72	46	255

ASHAP, doxorubicin (Adriamycin), high-dose arabinoside, and cisplatin (platinum); CEP, CCNU, etoposide, and prednimustine; CEVD, CCNU, etoposide, vindesine, and dexamethasone; Dexa-BEAM, dexamethasone, BCNU, etoposide, arabinoside, and melphalan; DHAP, dexamethasone, high-dose arabinoside, and platinum; HDCT, high-dose chemotherapy; MIME, methyl-GAG, ifosfamide, methotrexate, and etoposide; MINE, methyl-GAG, ifosfamide, vinorelbine, and etoposide; Mini-BEAM, BCNU, etoposide, arabinoside, and melphalan; MOPLACE, methotrexate, vincristine (Oncovin), prednisone, leucovorin, arabinoside, cyclophosphamide, and etoposide; ne, not evaluated; RR, response rate; RFS, relapse-free survival.

High-Dose Chemotherapy Plus Stem Cell Support. Most clinical results are derived from transplantation centers where a great deal of selection is used in referral and in the decision for HDCT and ASCT. The encouraging results from numerous phase II studies and analyses using transplantation registry data, as well as the reduction of early transplant-related mortality to less than 5%, have led to widespread acceptance of HDCT as an important component in the management of progressive and relapsed HD. HDCT followed by ASCT has been shown to produce 30% to 70% long-term disease-free survival in selected patients with primary progressive and relapsed disease.[153,256,257]

Although results with HDCT have generally been better than those observed after conventional-dose salvage therapy, the validity of this comparison has been questioned because of the lack of randomized trials. The most compelling evidence for the superiority of high-dose therapy in relapsed HD comes from two reports from the BNLI and the GHSG together with the EBMT. In the BNLI trial, patients with relapsed or refractory HD were treated with a combination of BEAM at a conventional-dose level (mini-BEAM) or a high-dose level (BEAM) with autologous bone marrow transplantation. The actuarial 3-year event-free survival was significantly better in patients who received HDCT (53% vs. 10%).[258]

The largest randomized, multicenter trial was performed by the GHSG/EBMT to determine the benefit of HDCT in relapsed HD. Patients with relapse after polychemotherapy were randomized between four cycles of dexamethasone-BEAM and two cycles of the dexamethasone-BEAM regimen followed by HDCT (with BEAM) and ASCT: The interim analysis of 142 evaluable patients revealed that for 115 patients with partial or complete response after two cycles of chemotherapy, the FFTF in the HDCT group was 53%, as opposed to 39% for the patients receiving an additional two cycles of conventional chemotherapy (Table 45.6-18).[259]

High-Dose Chemotherapy in Primary Progressive Hodgkin's Disease. Patients with primary progressive disease, defined as progression during induction treatment or within 90 days after the end of treatment, have a particularly poor prognosis. Treatment of patients with primary progressive HD has consisted of salvage chemotherapy, radiotherapy, and HDCT with ASCT. Conventional salvage regimens have given disappointing results in the vast majority of patients: Response to salvage treatment is low, and the duration of response is often short. The 8-year overall survival ranges between 0% and 8%. FFTF in second remission is 0% at 4 to 8 years in small series reported.[242,260] Extensive disease often limits the use of radiotherapy.

In contrast, the data on HDCT and ASCT in these patients are more promising. The EBMT reported its analysis of 175 patients with primary progressive disease who received HDCT and ASCT.[261] The 5-year actuarial progression-free and overall survival rates were 32% and 36%, respectively. The Autologous Blood and Marrow Transplant Registry recently reported a progression-free survival of 38% and an overall survival of 50% at 3 years in 122 patients with primary induction failure.[262] In single-institution series evaluating the efficacy of HDCT exclusively in induction failures, Reece et al.[263] reported a 42% progression-free survival at a median of 3.6 years. Similarly, an updated report from Stanford University showed an event-free survival of 49% at 4 years.[229] Gianni et al.[151] reported an event-free survival of 31% at 4 years. The studies by Yuen et al.[264] and André et al.[265] reported improved outcome after HDCT and ASCT as compared with historical control groups given conventional chemotherapy for induction failures. Thus, HDCT and ASCT should be considered for HD patients with primary induction failure.

The GHSG retrospectively analyzed 206 patients with progressive disease to determine outcome after salvage therapy and to identify prognostic factors.[266] The 5-year freedom-from-second-failure and overall survival rates for all patients were 17% and 26%, respectively. As reported from transplantation centers, the 5-year freedom-from-second-failure and overall survival rates for patients treated with HDCT were 42% and 48%, respectively, but only 33% of all patients received HDCT. A high proportion of those patients will rapidly succumb to progressive disease. Life-threatening severe toxicity on salvage treatment occurred in 11% of the patients. Insufficient stem cell harvest, poor performance status, and older age had also contributed to ineligibility for HDCT. In a multivariate analysis, the Karnofsky performance score at progress ($P < .0001$), age ($P = .019$), and attainment of a temporary remission to first-line chemotherapy ($P = .0003$) were significant prognostic factors for survival. In conclusion, HDCT is an effective treatment for a proportion of patients with primary progressive HD.[267] Owing to the poor outcome of HD patients with progressive disease, future trials must aim at identifying patients at very high risk for induction failure and modifying primary treatment in this group to avoid progressive disease.

High-Dose Chemotherapy in Early and Late Relapsed Hodgkin's Disease. Patients who receive transplantation at first relapse from complete remission can often be cured with HDCT and ASCT.[257,268,269] At present, patients with early relapse are good candidates for HDCT followed by ASCT. A report from Stanford in which historical controls were used found a 4-year event-free survival of 56% for patients with early relapse, as compared to 19% in patients who received standard-dose salvage chemotherapy.[264] In addition, the HDR-1 study showed

TABLE 45.6-18. Randomized Studies in Relapsed Hodgkin's Disease: High-Dose Chemotherapy versus Conventional Salvage Therapy

No. of Patients	*Treatment*	*Outcome*	*P*	*Follow-Up*	*Reference*
40	2–3 × Mini-BEAM	10% EFS	.025	3 y	258
	BEAM	53% EFS			
142	4 × Dexa-BEAM	39% FFTF	.025	3 y	259
	2 × Dexa-BEAM + BEAM	53% FFTF			

BEAM, BCNU, etoposide, arabinoside, and melphalan; Dexa-BEAM, dexamethasone, BCNU, etoposide, arabinoside, and melphalan; EFS, event-free survival; FFTF, freedom from treatment failure.

improved FFTF for patients with early relapse after HDCT, as compared with conventional chemotherapy.[259] Although the results reported with HDCT in patients with late relapse have been superior to those reported in most series of conventional chemotherapy, the use of HDCT in late relapses has been an area of controversy. Patients with late relapse have high second complete remission rates even with conventional chemotherapies and overall survival rates ranging from 40% to 55%. The HDR-1 study of the GHSG showed improved FFTF and overall survival after HDCT as compared with conventional chemotherapy in patients with late relapses. Therefore, HDCT should be considered as standard treatment even for patients with late relapses.[259]

Several published studies have evaluated the importance of prognostic factors for patients with HD undergoing HDCT with subsequent ASCT.[228,257,270] Adverse prognostic factors identified by multivariate analysis included age, chemoresistance, disease status, poor performance status, extranodal disease, female gender, elevated lactate dehydrogenase level, and failure of more than two prior regimens. An important variable that affects outcome is the ability of conventional salvage chemotherapy to reduce tumor volume before HDCT. Patients who experience relapse after chemotherapy but respond to subsequent conventional salvage therapy make up most of the long-term survivors in transplantation programs. Nevertheless, the role of conventional salvage chemotherapy before HDCT has not been clearly defined. Several studies have confirmed that a subset of patients with disease resistant to conventional salvage therapy clearly benefit from HDCT, with reported long-term survival of 10% to 31%.[228,262,268,271] The number of patients with chemoresistant disease who benefit from HDCT and ASCT largely depends on the definition of chemoresistance or the number and intensity of courses of chemotherapy administered to reduce the tumor burden. Accordingly, chemoresistant patients should not routinely be excluded from transplantation programs.

Allogeneic stem cell transplantation has clear advantages as compared with autologous transplantation: Donor cells uninvolved by malignancy are used, avoiding the risk of infusing occult lymphoma cells, which, despite purging, may contribute to relapse in patients who undergo autologous transplantation. In addition, donor lymphoid cells can potentially mediate a graft-versus-lymphoma effect. As in all allograft studies, issues of donor availability and age constraints have limited its use. Moreover, in all reports using allogeneic stem cell transplantation, a high treatment-related mortality rate of up to 75% was observed in patients with HD, which casts doubt on the feasibility of this approach in larger series.[272–274] In most circumstances, allogeneic transplantation from HLA-identical siblings is not recommended for patients with HD. The reduced relapse rate associated with a graft-versus-tumor effect is offset by lethal graft-versus-host toxicity.

In conclusion, patients who experience relapse after radiotherapy alone for localized HD have satisfactory results with combination chemotherapy and are not considered candidates for HDCT with ASCT. Current data support the use of HDCT with ASCT for patients with relapse and refractory HD after combination chemotherapy (Table 45.6-19).

TABLE 45.6-19. Recommendations for Treatment of Relapsed and Primary Progressive Hodgkin's Disease

Relapse after first-line radiotherapy	Conventional chemotherapy
Nodal relapse (CS I + II)	Salvage radiotherapy
No B-symptoms	
No prior radiotherapy	
Primary progressive disease	HDCT + ASCT
Early relapse	HDCT + ASCT
Late relapse	HDCT + ASCT

ASCT, autologous stem cell transplantation; CS, clinical stage; HDCT, high-dose chemotherapy.

SPECIAL CASES: LYMPHOCYTE-PREDOMINANT HODGKIN'S DISEASE

The early-stage characteristics, indolent course, and relatively good prognosis of LP variants of HD have been recognized since the 1930s.[275] Earlier studies consistently demonstrated that patients with an LP variant of HD enjoyed a better prognosis than did those with other forms of the disease.[276] However, the introduction of clinical staging showed that the extent of disease was a more important prognostic factor than was histology and that the localized nature of LPHD could well account for the good prognosis of this subtype.[277] In addition, modern therapeutic strategies were able to improve survival and cure rates for all types of patients, and prognostic differences due to histology often were no longer evident.[93,278] The clinical relevance of the recent REAL[75] and WHO classifications, particularly the distinction between LPHD and LRCHD, has been clarified by the international retrospective study of the ETFL.[279] The many smaller studies of LPHD paint a similar picture.[280–282]

CLINICAL FEATURES

LPHD patients show a similar age distribution to MC patients and are somewhat older, on average, than NS patients (Table 45.6-20). Approximately 75% of patients are male, again similar to MC and different from NS (approximately 50%). Of LPHD patients, 53% had stage I and only 6% had stage IV disease. Thus, the proportion of early stages is consistently high in

TABLE 45.6-20. Characteristics of 219 Cases Confirmed as LPHD in the European Task Force on Lymphoma Project Compared with Nodular Sclerosis and Mixed-Cellularity Cases in the 1988–1994 Trials of the German Hodgkin's Study Group

	LPHD (n = 219)	*NSHD (n = 599)*	*MCHD (n = 174)*
Median age (y)	35	30	35
Male gender (%)	74	49	73
Stage I (%)	53	10	21
Stage II (%)	28	47	32
Stage III (%)	14	29	35
Stage IV (%)	6	14	13
B-symptoms (%)	10	42	35

LPHD, lymphocyte-predominant Hodgkin's disease; NSHD, nodular sclerosis Hodgkin's disease; MCHD, mixed-cellularity Hodgkin's disease.

comparison with CHD, and stage IV is consistently rare, although not negligible. B-symptoms were present in only 10% of cases, far less than in CHD. LPHD seems to favor the peripheral upper neck and inguinal node sites and to occur relatively seldom in central sites such as the mediastinum and upper abdomen.[283]

TREATMENT RESULTS

There is some evidence to support the hypothesis that certain LPHD patients do well without any therapy beyond excision. Among the 51 nodular LP cases reported by Miettinen,[284] 31 were given no treatment except possibly surgical removal of the tumor, as malignant disease was not suspected. After 7 years' median follow-up, only seven of the untreated patients died. These results must be cautiously interpreted, as it is likely that especially mild examples would predominate in this retrospective sample. Most LPHD patients have received first-line therapy similar to that prescribed for CHD patients. LPHD cases appear to relapse just as frequently as other subtypes, but the relapse is less aggressive, resulting in frequent multiple relapses and good survival rates (see Fig. 45.6-2).

TRANSFORMATION TO NON-HODGKIN'S LYMPHOMA

The possibility of occurrence of an NHL after primary LPHD is clinically important for several reasons. The treatment should be chosen to prevent development or progression of NHL; it should avoid inducing a secondary NHL; and a monitoring and diagnostic strategy should be chosen to detect and correctly identify recurrent and secondary tumors. In an analysis from the International Database on Hodgkin's Disease,[285] a significantly higher risk for secondary NHL, increased by a factor 1.8, was found for LP patients as compared with NS and MC patients. Several smaller LPHD studies report secondary NHL, indicating a rate of 2% to 3% on average. Miettinen et al.[284] reported four secondary NHLs among 31 cases of untreated LPHD, suggesting that some, if not all, such NHLs develop independently of treatment.

CONSEQUENCES FOR FUTURE TREATMENT

Although, the prognosis superiority of LPHD as compared with CHD is scarcely discernible under modern treatment, the relatively good prognosis of LPHD cases under earlier, less intensive treatment does indicate a potential for treatment reduction. Furthermore, as many LPHD patients died of fatal treatment-related secondary leukemias and solid tumors as died from HD directly. This suggests that current treatment strategies might be too intensive, particularly when other late effects, such as cardiac and pulmonary complications, are taken into account. Disadvantages of treatment reduction could include the greater risk of disease progression or of development of NHL.

Caution is needed in identifying those patients for whom treatment reduction is an option. First, immunostaining is needed for a reliable differential diagnosis among LPHD, CHD, and certain NHL variants. Second, patients with advanced-stage LPHD (20% to 25%) had an overall survival and tumor-free survival that was substantially worse than that of patients with early-stage LPHD and was similar to advanced-stage CHD patients.[279] This implies that thorough staging and, in the case of advanced-stage disease, aggressive treatment are needed irrespective of histologic subtype.

A watch-and-wait treatment strategy, in which patients are monitored without treatment until the disease shows signs of progression, has been advocated for LPHD and for other indolent lymphomas. However, most authors report only anecdotal untreated cases.[284] A prospective study with explicit inclusion criteria is required to assess the feasibility, risks, and benefits of a watch-and-wait strategy. The EORTC is currently adopting a watch-and-wait approach for stage I supradiaphragmatic LPHD after complete resection of the tumor; the involved field is to be irradiated only if the disease progresses. The GHSG is now treating CS IA LPHD without risk factors with involved-field irradiation.

Involved-field radiotherapy has been shown to be inferior to more extensive irradiation in early-stage CHD but might be adequate for the very localized, less aggressive LP subtype. Two study groups, the EORTC and the GHSG, are currently treating certain early-stage LPHD patients with involved-field irradiation.

A new development potentially relevant to LPHD is the use of immunotherapy. The monoclonal antibody Rituximab, in particular, is directed against the B-cell-restricted CD20 antigen; this antigen is expressed by the L&H cells of LPHD but rarely by the H-RS cells of CHD. First experiences with indolent follicular B-cell lymphomas have shown good results, with nearly 55% overall responses even in heavily pretreated patients.[286] This therapy is now being tested by the GHSG in relapsed and refractory LPHD.

HODGKIN'S DISEASE IN THE ELDERLY PATIENT

HD treatment results, reflected in complete remission, relapse, and survival rates, tend to worsen with increasing age of the patient at diagnosis. There is no definite threshold age for the onset of this effect, although many authors report changes appearing at approximately age 60 years and older.

HD rarely occurs in patients older than 60 years. Two basic problems in the management of elderly patients emerge as a recurrent theme: a high rate of toxicities during treatment and frequent early relapses. At least two factors are considered to contribute to this poor prognosis. First, older patients differ from younger patients in disease characteristics: Advanced clinical stage and MC histology[287] are more frequent. Second, the older patient may be more likely to experience treatment complications, which in turn influence the given intensity of therapy.

The patient's physical and mental condition, disease history, and the presence of concurrent disorders influence the treatment strategy. Age, in general, is not a contraindication for aggressive treatment. Biologically young patients in good physical and mental condition should be treated by stage-adapted regimens, analogous to conventional treatment protocols. In this subgroup, complete remission rates and relapse-free and overall survival appear to be as good as in younger cohorts.[288] Combined modality treatment with a mild chemotherapeutic regimen and limited radiation (i.e., two cycles of ABVD plus involved-field radiotherapy) is increasingly considered the standard therapy in favorable early-stage HD. If no chemotherapy can be administered, mantle or inverted-Y fields should be irradiated, possibly at a reduced dose. For the patients with intermediate-stage (unfavorable early-stage) disease, two to four cycles of chemotherapy may be administered before involved-field radiotherapy is undertaken.

In advanced-stage disease, treatment should also be given with curative intent. The well-established ABVD combination (six to eight cycles) represents a safe regimen, whereas protocols with severe hematologic toxicities should be avoided. The time-intensified BEACOPP regimen, which has proved especially effective in advanced-stage HD patients aged up to 65 years, appears to be too toxic for patients older than 65.[289] Support with hematopoietic growth factors (granulocyte colony-stimulating factor) should be given liberally, as infectious complications due to prolonged neutropenia are common. Close monitoring of toxicity (i.e., electrocardiography, echocardiography, pulmonary function tests) and response to treatment are important for adjusting treatment at an early juncture.

Treatment for those patients with impairment of lung, liver, heart, or kidney should be individually adapted. Depending on preexisting impairment of organs, single drugs with organ-specific toxicities (i.e., bleomycin, Adriamycin) may be omitted from the chemotherapeutic regimen, replaced, or modified in dose. Involved-field radiotherapy, oral combination therapy (CCNU, etoposide, prednimustine), or less aggressive drugs, such as gemcitabine[290] in the initial treatment as well as the combination of vinblastine, bleomycin, and methotrexate,[291] present possible treatment alternatives.

HODGKIN'S DISEASE DURING PREGNANCY

The peak incidence of HD occurs at female reproductive age. Therefore, the association with pregnancy is not uncommon. One case of HD has been reported per 1000 to 6000 deliveries, making it the fourth most common cancer diagnosed during pregnancy.[292] Several studies have shown that pregnancy does not worsen the clinical course of the disease and that the 20-year survival of pregnant women with HD is not different from that of nonpregnant women.[293]

The clinical presentation of HD is not influenced by pregnancy. However, there are significant limitations on staging and treatment of the pregnant patient. CAT scanning should be avoided because it exposes the fetus to ionizing radiation. Ultrasonography, which is without known adverse fetal effects, is helpful not only for assessing fetal development but also for detecting the presence of lymphadenopathy. MRI will complete the radiologic staging because it appears to be free from genetic hazards. Decisions about the need for chest radiography should be made on the basis of clinical examination.

If HD is diagnosed in the first trimester, most experts agree that a therapeutic abortion should be encouraged. If the woman wishes to continue her pregnancy, treatment should be deferred until the second trimester at least, because the options for therapy at the beginning of pregnancy are rather limited. If therapy is indicated, supradiaphragmatic irradiation with doses less than 10 Gy or vinblastine chemotherapy for more advanced disease may be commenced.

In the second or third trimester, a stage I to II disease may be closely observed, and treatment should be postponed until an early delivery, usually at approximately 32 to 34 weeks' gestation. If there is any sign of rapid disease progression, in supradiaphragmatic lymphadenopathy radiotherapy alone is recommended. Most studies indicate doses of 10 to 44 Gy to the classic mantle field or the involved field, with abdominal shielding to protect the fetus. In the second and third trimesters, the risk of adverse sequelae for the fetus by supradiaphragmatic radiation is low. In infradiaphragmatic lymphadenopathy and in stage III to IV disease, combination chemotherapy will be the choice of treatment. Because most chemotherapeutic agents freely cross the placenta and enter the fetal circulation, both the patient and the fetus must be closely monitored. Chemotherapy administered in the second and third trimester may increase the risk of intrauterine growth retardation, microcephaly, and mental retardation.[294] Application of cytotoxic drugs shortly before birth may be particularly hazardous, as the placenta is also the primary means of drug elimination, and metabolism and excretion will be delayed in the neonatus. The current concept is that antimetabolites, especially methotrexate, confer a high risk of teratogenesis, whereas alkylating agents, Adriamycin, bleomycin, etoposide, and the vinca alkaloids would appear acceptable.[294] The ABVD regimen may be used when chemotherapy is indicated beyond the first trimester. Because chemotherapeutic agents reach significant levels in milk, mothers are best advised not to breast feed during treatment.

HODGKIN'S DISEASE IN HUMAN IMMUNODEFICIENCY VIRUS–POSITIVE PATIENTS

EPIDEMIOLOGY AND CLINICAL PRESENTATION

The majority of recent studies demonstrate a slight increase in the incidence of HD in young adult and middle-aged homosexual men. They also suggest that, with regard to a certain risk behavior, HD associated with HIV infection occurs preferentially in intravenous drug users. An increased incidence of HD among such other risk groups as hemophiliacs or women with an increased risk for AIDS has not been convincingly demonstrated.

Several data support the thesis that EBV probably represents a relevant factor involved in the pathogenesis of HIV-associated HD. First, EBV is found in H-RS cells in nearly 80% to 100% of HD tissue specimens from HIV-infected patients, in contrast to the HIV-negative population with EBV in 50% to 70% of HD cases.[295] Second, a pathogenetic role of EBV in HIV-associated HD is supported by the fact that tumor cells of virtually all cases of HIV-associated HD express EBV-encoded LMP1.[296]

A characteristic of HD in HIV-infected patients is the predominance of unfavorable histologic subtypes.[297] Most studies from Europe and the United States reported MC to be the most frequent histologic subtype among HIV-infected patients (40% to 100%). NS was less frequent (0% to 40%) in the HIV population than in HIV-negative persons. The incidence of the LP subtype was rather low (0% to 4%); in contrast, more than 20% of all cases were classified as LD.[298]

At the time of diagnosis, 70% to 90% of all patients with HIV-associated HD present with advanced disease. Extranodal involvement is frequent (60%), the most common sites being bone marrow, liver, and spleen. In contrast to non–HIV-related HD in the general population, in which the involvement of contiguous lymph node groups is typical and dissemination and infiltration of extranodal sites are late occurrences, in HIV-infected patients noncontiguous spread of lymphoma, such as liver involvement without splenic disease or lung involvement without mediastinal adenopathy, can be observed. Bone marrow involvement occurs in 40% to 50% of patients and may be the first indicator of the presence of HD in nearly 20% of cases.[299] HD tends to develop as an earlier manifestation of HIV infection, presenting in patients with a median CD4+ cell count in a range of 275 to 306/µL.[17] At the time of diagnosis, the majority of patients have persistent generalized lymphadenopathy and, in 50% of cases, lymphoma may be concurrently present with persistent generalized lymphadenopathy in the same lymph node group.[300] Therefore, it is important to be aware of HIV-associated HD as a differential diagnosis.

TREATMENT

Treatment is difficult, considering the underlying immunodeficiency caused by HIV itself, and may increase the risk of opportunistic infections by inducing further immunosuppression. Survival of patients with HIV-associated HD is short, typically 12 to 18 months, and the incidence of opportunistic infections is increased owing to standard therapeutic regimens. Because most patients have advanced HD, they have been treated with combination chemotherapeutic regimens such as MOPP and ABVD, but the response was poor in comparison with HIV-unrelated HD. Retrospective evaluations show a complete response rate far below that of HIV-negative patients with HD, poor tolerance of chemotherapy, and necessity of dose reduction or delay of treatment.[301] Other prospective studies show that tailored chemotherapeutic regimens having moderate bone marrow toxicity (e.g., epirubicin, bleomycin, and vinblastine) in combination with antiretroviral treatment with zidovudine result in a substantial decrease of opportunistic infection, yet overall survival was not significantly improved.[302] Improvement of response rate and median survival could be achieved by full-dose regimens like EBVP[303] or ABVD[304] combined with antiretroviral treatment, prophylaxis of the most common opportunistic infection, *Pneumocystis carinii*, and the use of granulocyte colony-stimulating factor.[305] Preliminary data with BEACOPP showed promising results regarding complete remission, toxicity, and median survival.[306]

In summary, treatment of HIV-associated HD demands a special approach. Therefore, it will likely be the combination of unconventional chemotherapy, antiretroviral agents, prophylaxis of opportunistic infections, and hematopoietic growth factors that will lead to cure of HIV-associated HD. However, the individual components of the recipe are not yet defined.

SEQUELAE

Long-term complications of mantle irradiation include lung, heart, and thyroid dysfunction, second primary cancers, and Lhermitte's syndrome (Table 45.6-21). Complications such as transverse myelitis and constrictive pericarditis should not occur with the use of modern radiotherapeutic techniques. Other long-term toxicities are not totally avoidable but can be reduced in severity or frequency.

TABLE 45.6-21. Treatment-Related Complications after Curative Therapy for Hodgkin's Disease

Potentially fatal
Acute myelomonocytic leukemia
Diffuse, high-grade non-Hodgkin's lymphoma
Solid tumors (mostly lung and breast cancer)
Overwhelming bacterial sepsis after splenectomy or spleen irradiation (OPSI)
Serious
Myocardial damage from radiation and anthracyclines
Lung fibrosis from radiation plus bleomycin
Sterility in men and women
Growth abnormalities in children and adolescents
Opportunistic infections
Psychological problems
Minor
Chemical or clinical hypothyroidism
Long-term alteration of lymphocyte function

PULMONARY COMPLICATIONS

Radiation pneumonitis typically occurs 1 to 6 months after completion of mantle irradiation. Once it resolves, usually there are no long-term sequelae. A mild, nonproductive cough, low-grade fever, and dyspnea on exertion characterize symptomatic radiation pneumonitis. The overall incidence of symptomatic pneumonitis is less than 5% after mantle irradiation; patients with LMA or who receive combined chemotherapy and radiotherapy have a two- to threefold greater risk (10% to 15%).[307] Radiographically, pneumonitis is characterized by the formation of infiltrates confined to the original radiation fields. Infection rather than pneumonitis is more likely if the infiltrates extend into areas of the lung initially protected from radiation. Severe pneumonitis may require treatment with steroids.

Various cardiac complications, including arrhythmias, myocardial infarction, and coronary artery disease, pericarditis, myocarditis, pericardial effusion, and tamponade have been documented after radiotherapy to the mediastinum.[307,308] In many early studies, these complications were related to treatment techniques that resulted in a high radiobiologic dose to the anterior mediastinum and heart. Current practice, which limits the dose to the whole heart, blocks the subcarinal region part-way into treatment, delivers treatments equally from front and back, and uses a lower overall radiation dose and smaller treatment volumes by the use of preradiation chemotherapy, has yielded more satisfactory results. Some studies have shown a modest increase in cardiac mortality after mantle irradiation. Boivin and Hutchison[309] have demonstrated an increased, age-adjusted risk of death from myocardial infarction after mediastinal irradiation. When analyzed by year of diagnosis of HD, the risk was much greater for patients treated in 1966 or earlier (relative risk, 6.33; confidence interval, 1.73 to 23.16) as compared to 1967 or later (relative risk, 1.97; confidence interval, 0.75 to 5.17), suggesting an important role for modern treatment techniques in reducing the risk of complications.

CARDIAC COMPLICATIONS

The risk of chronic cardiomyopathy appears to increase as the cumulative dose of doxorubicin exceeds 400 to 450 mg/m^2. It is still unknown whether there is an increased risk of cardiomyopathy at lower cumulative does (as commonly given with ABVD) in patients treated with mediastinal irradiation before or after chemotherapy. Careful cardiac evaluation of patients treated with combined radiotherapy and chemotherapy is recommended because of concerns that mediastinal irradiation may predispose to accelerated coronary arteriosclerosis, and this risk may be further increased by the administration of anthracyclines. Consideration should also be given to using lower doses and blocking the lower portion of the heart whenever possible.

SECONDARY NEOPLASIA

The occurrence of second malignancies, including acute leukemia, NHL, and a variety of solid tumors, has become a well-acknowledged reality that adversely affects survival of some patients cured of HD. Some of these cases may represent chance association. However, physicians should be aware that HD patients are at higher risk of developing a second neoplasm.

A number of reports have stressed the possibility that the occurrence of acute nonlymphocytic leukemia is closely related to drug combinations containing alkylating agents. The use of ABVD in chemotherapeutic regimens for HD has reduced the risk of leukemia. In most studies, the use of radiotherapy in combination with chemotherapy does not increase the risk over chemotherapy alone, although there may be an increased risk when chemotherapy is combined with extensive irradiation (i.e., total nodal irradiation). There does not appear to be an increased risk of developing acute nonlymphoblastic leukemia after radiotherapy alone.

The total incidence of acute leukemia, which usually occurs within the first 10 years after initial treatment, is reported in most published series to range from 2% to 6%.[310,311] The classic form of treatment-related leukemia is characterized by a relatively long latency period, namely 3 to 5 years, a preceding myelodysplastic phase, trilineage bone marrow dysplasia, and abnormalities of chromosome 5 or 7 (or both). Topoisomerase II inhibitors—primarily the epipodophyllotoxins, but also anthracyclines when given in combination with alkylating agents—have been implicated in the development of a clinically and cytogenetically distinct form of secondary acute myeloid leukemia in both adult and pediatric patients.[312]

Nearly all cases of NHL occurring after HD are of intermediate-grade or high-grade histology and are similar to lymphomas seen in patients with immunodeficiency diseases or under chronic immunosuppression for organ transplantation or autoimmune disorders. These lymphomas have a cumulative risk of 1.2% to 2.1% at 15 years.[313,314]

The actual incidence of solid tumors, which have not revealed a particular histopathologic pattern, is unknown, as the full extent of the expression of risk of a second neoplasm may not be appreciated for another decade. The solid tumors tend to occur in the second decade after treatment and, thus far, appear to represent a hazard of both radiotherapy and chemotherapy. The major risks appear to be lung cancer (mostly in smokers) and breast cancer among women when irradiated young.[310,315] Other cancers include sarcomas, melanomas, connective tissue and bone tumors, and salivary, stomach, and skin cancers.[314,316]

A major argument against the use of radiotherapy as primary or adjunct therapy in HD has been its potential induction of secondary solid tumors by radiation.

The large study from the BNLI of 2846 patients included 987 patients who were treated with chemotherapy alone.[317] The BNLI study showed that the relative risk of developing a secondary solid tumor after chemotherapy alone was 5.7. This was not significantly different from the relative risk after radiotherapy alone (4.8) or after combined modality therapy (5.8). Furthermore, a case-control study from a collaborative group of population-based registries and cancer centers that maintains data on 25,665 cases of HD[318] showed that HD patients treated with chemotherapy alone were at approximately twice the risk of developing lung cancer as were those treated by radiotherapy alone or by both modalities. Most of these data are from cases involving MOPP or MOPP-like regimens; little is known of the use of ABVD and the risk of second solid tumors.

GONADAL DYSFUNCTION

Many patients who complete successful treatment for HD go on to raise normal children. However, under some circumstances, gonadal dysfunction is an important iatrogenic toxicity that considerably affects the quality of life of patients after HD. Three to six cycles of MOPP or MOPP-like chemotherapy induces azoospermia in 50% to 100% of male patients. This finding is associated with germinal hyperplasia and increased follicle-stimulating hormone levels, with normal levels of luteinizing hormone and testosterone. Only 10% to 20% of patients will eventually show recovery of spermatogenesis after a long interval. After MOPP alternated with ABVD, the incidence of permanent azoospermia is approximately 50%. With full-course MOPP chemotherapy, nearly half of women become amenorrheal, with occurrence of age-dependent premature ovarian failure (>30 years, 75% to 85%; <30 years, ~20%).

The Milan Cancer Institute has reported that the administration of ABVD chemotherapy produces only limited and transient germ cell toxicity in men and no drug-induced amenorrhea.[319] To circumvent chemotherapy-induced sterility, the use of drug regimens not containing alkylating agents, procarbazine, or nitrosourea derivatives is highly recommended. An alternative for men undergoing MOPP or MOPP/ABVD therapy is sperm storage before chemotherapy. The usefulness of the administration of analogues of gonadotropin-releasing hormone in men or oral contraceptives in premenopausal women remains to be fully defined; however, limited data have been discouraging.

OTHER COMPLICATIONS

Minor complications can be summarized as follows: Hypothyroidism is a common event (~30%) after mantle-field irradiation, typically picked up by means of an elevated thyroid-stimulating hormone level.[307] Hormone replacement therapy is required. Herpes zoster is another common complication, self-limited and usually occurring in one to two contiguous dermatomes within the first 2 years after treatment and affecting 15% to 20% of patients treated with radiotherapy or chemotherapy alone, but the incidence appears higher in patients treated with combined radiotherapy and chemotherapy. Cutaneous dissemination and visceral involvement from this virus are rare. Early treatment with antiviral agents may limit the intensity and duration of the infection. Acute transient radiation myelopathy or Lhermitte's sign (paresthesias down the dorsal portion of the extremities when the neck is flexed) occurs in approximately 10% to 15% of patients after mantle irradiation. This particular complication typically occurs 6 weeks to 3 months after radiotherapy and is self-limited, resolving in weeks to months. Xerostomia is a temporary complication of mantle irradiation; saliva returns to normal usually within 6 months of treatment. However, xerostomia may be prolonged in patients older than 40 years at treatment, or if Waldeyer's ring is treated. Fluoride supplementation and careful dental care will minimize the risks of radiation caries. The risk of postsplenectomy sepsis can occur particularly in children,[320] but it can be minimized by immunization with pneumococcal vaccine; in more recent years, vaccines have been developed against *Haemophilus* and *Neisseria* species, the other microorganisms associated with small but finite risks of overwhelming postsplenectomy sepsis.

QUALITY OF LIFE

A review of most randomized clinical trials in HD reveals that quality of life has been neglected as a primary or even a secondary outcome measure. After a review of the literature in pediatric oncology, Bradlyn et al.[321] demonstrated that only 3% of all randomized clinical trial reports reviewed (n = 70) include quality-of-life data. However, mainly retrospective analyses of long-term survivors of HD have been performed.[322,323] These analyses showed that a substantial subgroup of patients still shows serious sequelae of the disease and its treatment even many years after treatment has ended. In one study, men who have experienced serious illness since treatment and who earn less than $15,000 U.S. annually, are currently unemployed, are single, or are less educated were found to be at high risk for maladaptation years after treatment. Furthermore, 22% of the 273 patients studied met the criterion suggested for psychiatric diagnosis.[322] Currently, it remains unclear at which point in the course of the disease patients with a good coping capacity can be distinguished from those without such a capacity. To characterize phases of readaptation and maladaptation more precisely, quality-of-life assessment has to be implemented in prospective, randomized clinical trials. To obtain completeness of data, quality-of-life investigations should be a mandatory component of the clinical trial design and part of the inclusion criteria.[324]

The assessment of quality of life has become an essential tool in clinical trials, in particular in the evaluation of therapies given to patients with chronic illness such as cancer. Although survival and survival without disease have long been used as the sole end points in clinical trials, these limits are no longer accepted today because other characteristics now are considered to be as important as survival by both patients and physicians. Among these, treatment burden, treatment-related toxicity, and the psychological and social impacts of disease and treatment are of great importance.

Obviously, this change originates from the dramatic improvement in the efficacy of cancer treatments, particular in HD. Effective therapies, however, have several drawbacks that might limit their use. Chemotherapy and radiotherapy induce severe acute and late toxicities, which may diminish the long-term benefit of curative treatment. Several studies including a quality-of-life approach have highlighted the difficulties that survivors may experience even long after the treatment, such as general fatigue, poor health, and social problems.

NEW DRUGS IN HODGKIN'S DISEASE

VINORELBINE

Vinorelbine belongs to the family of vinca alkaloids and is a semisynthetic analogue of vinblastine (5'nor-anidro-vinblastine). The main side effect of vinorelbine is myelosuppression. WHO grade III to IV neutropenia occurs in up to 70% of patients but is of very short duration, with a low incidence of infectious complications.[325] Vinorelbine used as single-agent therapy in HD was administered in all studies in a weekly schedule with 30 mg/m^2. Devizzi et al.[326] report on 22 patients with HD refractory or resistant to at least two chemotherapeutic regimens, of which 50% (n = 11) showed an objective response (complete remission, n = 3; partial remission, n = 8) with a median duration of 6 months. Benchekroun et al.[327] evaluated the response to vinorelbine in untreated patients with advanced HD. Thirty-two patients received four weekly doses of vinorelbine before MOPP/ABVD chemotherapy, and 90% achieved a partial remission.

IDARUBICIN

Idarubicin is a semisynthetic drug that was first purified in 1976. Idarubicin differs from its parent drug daunorubicin only by the replacement of the C-4 methoxyl group in the D ring with a hydrogen atom. This modification has major consequences for the pharmacokinetic characteristics: Idarubicin is much more lipophilic and can be administered orally. Its main metabolite idarubicinol is as active as the parent compound. In addition, idarubicin has shown greater cytotoxicity than daunorubicin or doxorubicin *in vitro*. Idarubicin exhibits less cardiotoxicity at equieffective doses as compared with other anthracyclines, whereas hemotoxicity and mucositis appear to be more pronounced. The GHSG is currently conducting a clinical phase II study in which idarubicin (8 mg/m^2, days 1 and 2) is administered together with etoposide (60 mg/m^2, days 1 to 4), ifosfamide (1000 mg/m^2, days 1 to 4 continuous infusion), and dexamethasone (20 mg/m^2, days 1 to 4) in patients with relapsed or refractory HD.

GEMCITABINE

Gemcitabine is a new pyrimidine antimetabolite with unique metabolic and mechanistic properties among the nucleoside analogues.[328] It is a derivative of deoxycytidine, with fluorine substituted for the two hydrogen atoms in the 2'-position of the deoxyribose sugar. Although structurally similar to cytarabine, gemcitabine differs pharmacokinetically and pharmacologically. It acts as a competitive substrate for incorporation into the DNA, where it leads to chain termination. Based on the impressive results in solid tumors such as non–small cell lung cancer and pancreatic cancer, gemcitabine was given in a multicenter clinical phase II study in patients with multiple relapsed or refractory HD who had received at least two prior chemotherapeutic regimens.[290] Gemcitabine was administered in a weekly schedule of 1250 mg/m^2 on days 1, 8, and 15 of a 28-day cycle. An interim analysis of this trial showed an overall response of 39%, with 2 of 23 complete remissions and 7 of 23 partial remissions. Another ten patients had stable disease. Myelosuppression was the main toxicity.

IMMUNOTHERAPY

Tumor cells that survive intensive therapy in small quantities are defined as minimal residual disease. These partially dormant, chemoresistant lymphoma cells might be eradicated by new immunotherapeutic strategies with a different mechanism of action. Current approaches comprise passive immunotherapy with antibody-based regimens for specific targeting of malignant cells as well as active immunotherapy with modulation of the cellular immune response using cytokines, tumor vaccines, or gene transfer. The combination of immunotherapeutic strategies with standard chemotherapeutic regimens seems to be most promising: Owing to different mechanisms of action, cross-resistance of malignant cells is expected to be rare. Furthermore, the side effects of these two treatment modalities differ, so that toxicity will not usually be additive.

PASSIVE IMMUNOTHERAPY

Systemically administered chemotherapeutic agents kill all rapidly dividing cells, whereas monoclonal antibodies can target tumor cells selectively. Normal cells that lack specific tumor antigens are not harmed. For a variety of reasons, Hodgkin's lymphoma seems to be an ideal target for antibody-based therapeutic approaches: First, H-RS cells express many different cell surface antigens, such as CD15, CD25, CD30, CD40, and CD80 (B7-1), which are present on only a minority of normal human cells.[113] Due to low cross-reactivity with healthy human tissue, side effects are rare. Second, because many different markers can be detected on the surface of Hodgkin's cells, "cocktails" (i.e., a combination of various antibody conjugates targeting different Hodgkin's-specific antigens) might be useful for selective immunotherapy. If one malignant antigen-deficient cell clone is resistant to one antibody, cells might still be targeted by the second or third antibody conjugate administered at the same time. Third, the number of malignant cells that must be killed is small, as the majority of cells in the involved lymph nodes are reactive bystander cells. Fourth, lymphomas are well vascularized,[329] so that intravenously administered antibody conjugates can easily reach their target cells. Therefore, chemotherapy or radiotherapy (or both) can be used for treatment of bulky disease, whereas immunotherapeutic agents are applied thereafter to eliminate minimal residual disease and thus prevent relapses.

Native Monoclonal Antibodies

Ideally, the antibody targets with high specificity an antigen present only on the tumor cells and has no cross-reactivity with normal human tissue. The mechanisms of action of native antibodies include complement activation, antibody-dependent cellular toxicity, phagocytosis of antibody-coated target cells, inhibition of cell-cycle progression, and induction of apoptosis. In early phase I and II trials, native antibodies have exhibited moderate adverse effects, such as chills, fever, dyspnea, nausea, diarrhea, and myalgia. Toxicity usually was related to the number of circulating tumor cells and the development of human anti–mouse antibodies. New chimeric antibodies that consist of human constant and murine variable regions rarely induce human anti–mouse antibody formation.[286]

Engert et al.[330] evaluated more than 40 different monoclonal antibodies for their antitumor activity toward Hodgkin's-derived cell lines *in vitro*. Thus far, it has not been possible to identify monoclonal antibodies against Hodgkin's-associated antigens that exhibit potency *in vitro* or *in vivo* when used in native form. The chimeric monoclonal anti-CD20 antibody Rituximab (IDEC-C2B8) has been approved by the U.S. Food and Drug Administration for treatment of patients with relapsed advanced follicular NHL after a pivotal trial demonstrated response rates up to 50% in 166 patients.[331] Because the CD20 antigen is expressed on all malignant cells in paragranuloma or LPHD, this entity might be a good target for treatment with Rituximab. An international study currently is investigating the safety and efficacy of Rituximab in patients with relapsed or refractory LPHD and other multiple relapsed CD20-positive cases of CHD.

Immunotoxins

Immunotoxins generally consist of a binding moiety and a toxin moiety, which are either covalently linked via a chemical linker or generated by recombinant fusion technology. The binding domain is usually a monoclonal antibody, a Fab' fragment, a single-chain variable fragment, or a cytokine, whereas the toxin is of bacterial or plant origin. Recombinant toxins are constructed by fusing coding regions of toxins such as diphtheria toxin or *Pseudomonas* exotoxin-A to ligand genes.[332] Immunotoxins can bind selectively to their target cells. After internalization of the construct by endocytosis, the toxin is transferred to the ribosomal subunits, where it interferes with protein synthesis, thus killing the tumor cell.

Another interesting target for selective immunotherapy in HD is the IL-2 receptor (CD25), which is expressed on the majority of H-RS cells. In a phase I study, 15 patients with refractory Hodgkin's lymphoma were treated with the anti-CD25 immunotoxin RFT5.dgA.[333] All patients in this trial were heavily pretreated with a mean of five prior chemotherapeutic regimens, including autologous bone marrow transplantation. Most side effects were related to vascular leak syndrome. Clinical response included two partial remissions, one minor response, and three stable diseases. Promising approaches include deleting immunodominant epitopes and humanizing the antibody moiety of the immunotoxin.

A variety of monoclonal antibodies have been evaluated for their potential clinical use as ricin A chain immunotoxin against HD.[334] The most potent anti-CD30 immunotoxin, Ki-4.dgA, is currently being investigated in a clinical dose escalation trial.[335] In humans, sequential application of anti-CD30 antibodies linked to distinct ribosome-inactivating proteins might prevent formation of human antibodies against the individual toxins.

Radioimmunoconjugates

Radioimmunoconjugates are constructed by linking a monoclonal antibody to radioisotopes without significantly altering the immunologic specificity of the protein. The most important advantage of these constructs as compared to all other antibody-based therapeutic strategies is that β-particles emitted by radionuclides can kill adjacent tumor cells through a crossfire effect, regardless of whether cells express the target antigen. As opposed to external-beam radiotherapy, radiolabeled antibodies deliver radiation continuously at a low dose rate to the whole body, including occult micrometastases.[336] Currently, both nonmyeloablative and myeloablative strategies involving radiolabeled antibodies are investigated for imaging and treatment of HD.

Low-energy radionuclides are coupled to monoclonal antibodies either for diagnostic use (immunoscintigraphy) or for low-dose radioimmunotherapy without severe myelosuppression. A phase I trial was initiated to investigate the safety of the ^{99m}Tc-labeled anti-CD30 antibody Ber-H2 for immunoscintigraphy and possible immunotherapy in patients with refractory HD and large cell anaplastic lymphoma. Preliminary results suggest good tolerance of the therapy with no major side effects and satisfactory efficacy for imaging or detecting HD lesions. Future trials involving modern radioisotopes (^{111}In, ^{90}Y, ^{186}Rh) are warranted.[337]

Stem cell support for hematopoietic recovery might be necessary in high-dose radioimmunotherapy. A phase I to II study with ^{90}Y-labeled polyclonal antiferritin antibodies for refractory Hodgkin's lymphoma followed by autologous bone marrow transplantation was performed by Vriesendorp et al.[338] Of 17 patients, seven achieved complete remissions lasting 2 to 26 or more months, and four patients achieved partial remissions (2 to 6 months). Twelve patients received a reduced dose (20 mCi) due to bone marrow involvement or unsuccessful marrow harvest. Complete remissions were observed in two and partial remissions in five of them. For all doses, response rates were better in patients with small tumor burden. Based on these encouraging results, radioimmunotherapy appears to be a new promising option, either alone or in combination with other chemotherapy or immunotherapy (or both).

Bi-Specific Monoclonal Antibodies

Bi-specific monoclonal antibodies contain two different recognition sites, one for antigens on tumor cells and another for antigens on immunologic effector cells, such as macrophages, T lymphocytes, or NK cells. For treatment of HD with NK-cell–activating bi-specific antibodies, a CD16/CD30 bi-specific antibody was constructed using hybridoma technology.[42] Heavily pretreated patients with refractory HD received intravenous infusions of the CD16/CD30 (A9/HRS-3) antibody four times every 3 or 4 days.[339] Fifteen patients with refractory HD were treated with escalating doses. Side effects were rare and consisted of short-lasting fever, pain in involved lymph nodes, and a maculopapular rash. A total of one complete and one partial remission (lasting 16 and 3 months, respectively), three minor responses (1 to 11+ months), and one mixed response was observed.

ACTIVE IMMUNOTHERAPY

Therapeutic strategies modulating the cellular immune response have been investigated in lymphoma patients for more than 25 years. As immunotherapy with Bacillus Calmette-Guérin had suggested therapeutic effects when combined with chemotherapy in patients with acute myelocytic leukemia and breast cancer, several randomized clinical trials were initiated in patients with advanced Hodgkin's lymphoma as well.[340] Because of a documented lack of therapeutic benefit and a higher frequency of unacceptable toxicity, trials investigating Bacillus Calmette-Guérin treatment were discontinued.

IL-2 was one of the first immunotherapeutic agents used for anticancer therapy. Several clinical studies were performed to investigate the efficacy of IL-2 alone or in combination with autologous lymphokine activated killer cells (adoptive immunotherapy) in patients with refractory Hodgkin's lymphoma.[341–343] Toxicity was mild, mainly comprising fever, rash, hypotension, and anemia. In these clinical pilot trials, several transient partial remissions were achieved in heavily pretreated patients with relapsed or refractory disease. IL-2 is currently under clinical investigation as maintenance therapy alone or in combination with other cytokines after HDCT.

Case reports of a few patients who received interferon for treatment of viral infection noted minor responses of Hodgkin's lymphoma. Therefore, some pilot studies were conducted to investigate the efficacy of interferon in the salvage or maintenance therapy of HD. Preliminary results suggest a limited activity of interferon-α in patients with relapsed or refractory HD.[344]

GENE THERAPY

Modulation of EBV-directed T-cell activity might be another interesting new immunotherapeutic option: Heslop et al.[345] developed EBV-specific CTLs for treatment of EBV-associated lymphoma after bone marrow transplantation. Donors' blood samples were used for generation of EBV-transformed B-cell lines (LCLs) and for production of CTLs.[345] Incubation of activated CTLs with LCLs of the same probe induced formation of EBV-specific CTLs. In three of ten patients, elevated levels of EBV DNA after allogeneic transplantation normalized after infusion of the EBV-specific CTLs. EBV-specific CTLs were isolated for an adoptive transfer in patients with EBV-positive HD.[346] Nine patients with active, relapsed HD and four who were in complete remission after first or subsequent therapy were treated with autologous EBV-specific CTLs: A 100-fold reduction of EBV DNA was observed in all patients; in two of them, B-symptoms ceased.

REFERENCES

1. Hellman S. A brief consideration of Thomas Hodgkin and his times. In: Mauch PM, Armitage JO, Diehl V, Hoppe RT, Weiss LM, eds. *Hodgkin's disease.* Philadelphia: Lippincott Williams & Wilkins, 1999:3.
2. Hodgkin T. On some morbid appearances of the absorbent glands and spleen. *Medico-Chirurg Trans* 1832;17:68
3. Wilks S. Cases of enlargement of the lymphatic glands and spleen (or Hodgkin's disease), with remarks. *Guy's Hosp Rep* 1865;11:56.
4. Greenfield W. Specimens illustrative of the pathology of lymphadenoma and leucocythemia. *Trans Pathol Soc Lond* 1878;29:272.
5. Sternberg C. Uber eine eigenartige unter dem Bilde der Pseudoleukamie verlaufende Tuberculose des lymphatischen Apparates. *Ztschr Heilk* 1898;19:21.
6. Reed D. On the pathological changes in Hodgkin's disease, with special reference to its relation to tuberculosis. *Johns Hopkins Hosp Rep* 1902;10:133.
7. Benda C. Zur Histologie der pseudoleukamischen Geschwulste. *Verh Dtsch Ges Pathol* 1904:7.
8. Stein H, Diehl V, Marafioti T, et al. Hodgkin's disease. In: Mauch PM, Armitage JO, Diehl V, Hoppe RT, Weiss LM, eds. *Hodgkin's disease.* Philadelphia: Lippincott Williams & Wilkins, 1999:121.
9. Correa P, O'Conor G, Berard C. International comparability and reproducibility in histologic subclassification of Hodgkin's disease. *J Natl Cancer Inst* 1973;50:1429.
10. Kaplan H. *Hodgkin's disease,* vol 2. Cambridge: Harvard University Press, 1980:245.
11. Vianna J, Poln A. Epidemiological evidence for transmission of Hodgkin's disease. *N Engl J Med* 1973;289:499.
12. Grufferman S, Cole P, Levitan T. Evidence against transmission of Hodgkin's disease in high schools. *N Engl J Med* 1979;300:1006.

13. Bernard S, Cartwright R, Darwin C, et al. Hodgkin's disease: case control epidemiological study in Yorkshire. *Br J Cancer* 1987;55:85.
14. Razis DV, Diamond HD, Craver LF. Familial Hodgkin's disease: its significance and implications. *Ann Intern Med* 1959;51:933.
15. Bryden H, MacKenzie J, Andrew L, et al. Determination of HLA-A*02 antigen status in Hodgkin's disease and analysis of an HLA-A*02-restricted epitope of the Epstein-Barr virus LMP-2 protein. *Int J Cancer* 1997;72:614.
16. Poppema S, Visser L. Epstein-Barr virus positivity in Hodgkin's disease does not correlate with an HLA A2-negative phenotype. *Cancer* 1994;73:3059.
17. Lowenthal D, Straus D, Campbell S, et al. AIDS-related lymphoid neoplasia: the Memorial Hospital experience. *Cancer* 1988;61:2325.
18. Mueller N. Hodgkin's disease. In: Schnottenfeld D, Fraumeni J, eds. *Cancer epidemiology and prevention,* vol 2. New York: Oxford University Press, 1992:877.
19. Gutensohn N. Social class and age at diagnosis of Hodgkin's disease: new epidemiologic evidence for the "two-disease hypothesis". *Cancer Treat Rep* 1982;66:689.
20. Glaser S, Lin R, Stewart S, et al. Epstein-Barr virus-associated Hodgkin's disease: epidemiologic characteristics in international data. *Int J Cancer* 1997;70:375.
21. Mueller N, Evans A, Harris N, et al. Hodgkin's disease and Epstein-Barr virus. Altered antibody pattern before diagnosis. *N Engl J Med* 1989;320:689.
22. Zarate-Osorno A, Roman L, Kingma D, et al. Hodgkin's disease in Mexico. Prevalence of Epstein-Barr virus sequences and correlations with histologic subtype. *Cancer* 1995;75:1360.
23. Ambinder RF, Weiss LM. Hodgkin's disease. In: Mauch PM, Armitage JO, Diehl V, Hoppe RT, Weiss LM, eds. *Hodgkin's disease.* Philadelphia: Lippincott Williams & Wilkins, 1999:79.
24. Staal S, Ambinder R, Beschorner W, et al. A survey of Epstein-Barr virus DNA in lymphoid tissue. Frequent detection in Hodgkin's disease. *Am J Clin Pathol* 1989;91:1.
25. Brousset P, Chittal S, Schlaifer D, et al. Detection of Epstein-Barr virus messenger RNA in Reed-Sternberg cells of Hodgkin's disease by in situ hybridization with biotinylated probes on specially processed modified acetone methyl benzoate xylene (ModAMeX) sections. *Blood* 1991;77:1781.
26. Kamel O, Weiss L, van dRM, et al. Hodgkin's disease and lymphoproliferations resembling Hodgkin's disease in patients receiving long-term low-dose methotrexate therapy. *Am J Surg Pathol* 1996;20:1279.
27. Pelstring R, Zellmer R, Sulak L, et al. Hodgkin's disease in association with human immunodeficiency virus infection. Pathologic and immunologic features. *Cancer* 1991;67:1865
28. Herbst H, Anagnostopoulos J, Heinze B, et al. ALK gene products in anaplastic large cell lymphomas and Hodgkin's disease. *Blood* 1995;86:1694.
29. Knecht H, Bachmann E, Brousset P, et al. Deletions within the LMP1 oncogene of Epstein-Barr virus are clustered in Hodgkin's disease and identical to those observed in nasopharyngeal carcinoma. *Blood* 1993;82:2937.
30. Siebert J, Ambinder R, Napoli V, et al. Human immunodeficiency virus-associated Hodgkin's disease contains latent, not replicative, Epstein-Barr virus. *Hum Pathol* 1995;26:1191.
31. Armstrong A, Shield L, Gallagher A, et al. Lack of involvement of known oncogenic DNA viruses in Epstein-Barr virus-negative Hodgkin's disease. *Br J Cancer* 1998;77:1045.
32. Haluska FG, Brufsky AM, Canellos GP, et al. The cellular biology of the Reed-Sternberg cell. *Blood* 1994;84:1005.
33. Diehl V, Kirchner H, Burrichter H, et al. Characteristics of Hodgkin's disease-derived cell lines. *Cancer Treat Rep* 1982;66:615
34. Diehl V, von KC, Fonatsch C, et al. The cell of origin in Hodgkin's disease. *Semin Oncol* 1990;17:660.
35. Wolf J, Kapp U, Bohlen H, et al. Peripheral blood mononuclear cells of a patient with advanced Hodgkin's lymphoma give rise to permanently growing Hodgkin-Reed Sternberg cells. *Blood* 1996;87:3418.
36. Kanzler H, Hansmann M, Kapp U, et al. Molecular single cell analysis demonstrates the derivation of a peripheral blood-derived cell line (L1236) from the Hodgkin/Reed-Sternberg cells of a Hodgkin's lymphoma patient. *Blood* 1996;87:3429.
37. Stein H, Gerdes J, Schwab U, et al. Identification of Hodgkin and Sternberg-reed cells as a unique cell type derived from a newly-detected small-cell population. *Int J Cancer* 1982;30:445.
38. Schwab U, Stein H, Gerdes J, et al. Production of a monoclonal antibody specific for Hodgkin and Sternberg-Reed cells of Hodgkin's disease and a subset of normal lymphoid cells. *Nature* 1982;299:65.
39. Durkop H, Latza U, Hummel M, et al. Molecular cloning and expression of a new member of the nerve growth factor receptor family that is characteristic for Hodgkin's disease. *Cell* 1992;68:421.
40. Engert A, Martin G, Pfreundschuh M, et al. Antitumor effects of ricin A chain immunotoxins prepared from intact antibodies and Fab' fragments on solid human Hodgkin's disease tumors in mice. *Cancer Res* 1990;50:2929.
41. Falini B, Bolognesi A, Flenghi L, et al. Response of refractory Hodgkin's disease to monoclonal anti-CD30 immunotoxin. *Lancet* 1992;339:1195.
42. Hombach A, Jung W, Pohl C, et al. A CD16/CD30 bispecific monoclonal antibody induces lysis of Hodgkin's cells by unstimulated natural killer cells in vitro and in vivo. *Int J Cancer* 1993;55:830.
43. Winkler U, Gottstein C, Schon G, et al. Successful treatment of disseminated human Hodgkin's disease in SCID mice with deglycosylated ricin A-chain immunotoxins. *Blood* 1994;83:466.
44. Kapp U, Wolf J, Hummel M, et al. Hodgkin's lymphoma-derived tissue serially transplanted into severe combined immunodeficient mice. *Blood* 1993;82:1247.
45. Kuppers R, Rajewsky K, Zhao M, et al. Hodgkin disease: Hodgkin and Reed-Sternberg cells picked from histological sections show clonal immunoglobulin gene rearrangements and appear to be derived from B cells at various stages of development. *Proc Natl Acad Sci U S A* 1994;91:10962.
46. Vockerodt M, Soares M, Kanzler H, et al. Detection of clonal Hodgkin and Reed-Sternberg cells with identical somatically mutated and rearranged VH genes in different biopsies in relapsed Hodgkin's disease. *Blood* 1998;92:2899.
47. Marafioti T, Hummel M, Anagnostopoulos I, et al. Origin of nodular lymphocyte-predominant Hodgkin's disease from a clonal expansion of highly mutated germinal-center B cells. *N Engl J Med* 1997;337:453.
48. Jox A, Zander T, Kuppers R, et al. Somatic mutations within the untranslated regions of rearranged Ig genes in a case of classical Hodgkin's disease as a potential cause for the absence of Ig in the lymphoma cells. *Blood* 1999;93:3964.
49. Rowley J. Chromosomes in Hodgkin's disease. *Cancer Treat Rep* 1982;66:639.
50. Thangavelu M, Le BM. Chromosomal abnormalities in Hodgkin's disease. *Hematol Oncol Clin North Am* 1989;3:221.
51. Tilly H, Bastard C, Delastre T, et al. Cytogenetic studies in untreated Hodgkin's disease. *Blood* 1991;77:1298.
52. Steenvoorden AC, Janssen JW, Drexler HD. Ras mutations in Hodgkin's disease. *Leukemia* 1988;2:325.
53. Gravel S, Delsol G, Al ST. Single-cell analysis of the t(14;18)(q32;q21) chromosomal translocation in Hodgkin's disease demonstrates the absence of this translocation in neoplastic Hodgkin and Reed-Sternberg cells. *Blood* 1998;91:2866.
54. Emmerich F, Meiser M, Hummel M, et al. Overexpression of I kappa B alpha without inhibition of NF-kappaB activity and mutations in the I kappa B alpha gene in Reed-Sternberg cells. *Blood* 1999;94:3129.
55. Bargou R, Emmerich F, Krappmann D, et al. Constitutive nuclear factor-kappaB-RelA activation is required for proliferation and survival of Hodgkin's disease tumor cells. *J Clin Invest* 1997;100:2961.
56. Wood K, Roff M, Hay R. Defective IκBα in Hodgkin cell lines with constitutively active NF-κB. *Oncogene* 1998;16:2131.
57. van den Berg A, Visser L, Poppema S. High expression of the CC chemokine TARC in Reed-Sternberg cells. A possible explanation for the characteristic T-cell infiltratein Hodgkin's lymphoma. *Am J Pathol* 1999;154:1685.
58. Bargou R, Leng C, Krappmann D, et al. High-level nuclear NF-kappa B and Oct-2 is a common feature of cultured Hodgkin/Reed-Sternberg cells. *Blood* 1996;87:4340.
59. Kanzler H, Hansmann ML, Kapp U, et al. Molecular single cell analysis demonstrates the derivation of a peripheral blood-derived cell line (L1236) from the Hodgkin/Reed-Sternberg cells of a Hodgkin's lymphoma patient. *Blood* 1996;87:3429.
60. Lee S, Constandinou C, Thomas W, et al. Antigen presenting phenotype of Hodgkin Reed-Sternberg cells:analysis of the HLA class I processing pathway and the effects of interleukin-10 on Epstein-Barr virus-specific cytotoxic T-cell recognition. *Blood* 1998; 92:1020.
61. Diehl V, Kirchner H, Schaadt M, et al. Hodgkin's disease: establishment and characterization of four in vitro cell lies. *J Cancer Res Clin Oncol* 1981;101:111.
62. Gause A, Jung W, Schmits R, et al. Soluble CD8, CD25 and CD30 antigens as prognostic markers in patients with untreated Hodgkin's lymphoma. *Ann Oncol* 1992;3[Suppl 4]:49.
63. Falini B, Bigerna B, Pasqualucci L, et al. Distinctive expression pattern of the BCL-6 protein in nodular lymphocyte predominance Hodgkin's disease. *Blood* 1996;87:465.
64. Carbone A, Gloghini A, Gaidano G, et al. Expression status of BCL-6 and syndecan-1 identifies distinct histogenetic subtypes of Hodgkin's disease. *Blood* 1998;92:2220.
65. Ludewig B, Graf D, Gelderblom HR. Spontaneous apoptosis of dendritic cells is efficiently inhibited by TRAP (CD40-ligand) and TNF-alpha, but strongly enhanced by interleukin-10. *Eur J Immunol* 1995;25:1943.
66. Sarris A, Kliche K, Pethambaram P, et al. Interleukin-10 levels are often elevated in serum of adults with Hodgkin's disease and are associated with inferior failure-free survival. *Ann Oncol* 1999;10:433.
67. Pinkus G, Said J. Hodgkin's disease, lymphocyte predominance type, nodular—further evidence for a B cell derivation. L & H variants of Reed-Sternberg cells express L26, a pan B cell marker. *Am J Pathol* 1988;133:211.
68. Hall P, d'Ardenne A, Stansfeld A. Paraffin section immunohistochemistry. II. Hodgkin's disease and large cell anaplastic (Ki1) lymphoma. *Histopathology* 1988;13:161.
69. Regula DJ, Hoppe R, Weiss L. Nodular and diffuse types of lymphocyte predominance Hodgkin's disease. *N Engl J Med* 1988;318:214.
70. Brauninger A, Kuppers R, Strickler JG. Hodgkin and Reed-Sternberg cells in lymphocyte predominant Hodgkin disease represent clonal populations of germinal center–derived tumor B cells. *Proc Natl Acad Sci U S A* 1997;94:9337.
71. Kanzler H, Kuppers R, Hansmann M, et al. Hodgkin and Reed-Sternberg cells in Hodgkin's disease represent the outgrowth of a dominant tumor clone derived from (crippled) germinal center B cells. *J Exp Med* 1996;184:1495.
72. Mason D, Banks P, Chan J, et al. Nodular lymphocyte predominance Hodgkin's disease. A distinct clinicopathological entity [editorial]. *Am J Surg Pathol* 1994;18:526.
73. Jackson HJ, Parker FJ. *Hodgkin's disease and allied disorders.* New York: Oxford University Press, 1947:312.
74. Lukes R, Butler J, Hicks E. Natural history of Hodgkin's disease as related to its pathlogical picture. *Cancer* 1966;19:317.
75. Harris NL, Jaffe ES, Stein H. A revised European-American classification of lymphoid neoplasms: a proposal from the International Lymphoma Study Group. *Blood* 1994;84:1361.
76. von Wasielewsky R, Werner M, Fischer R, et al. Lymphocyte-predominant Hodgkin's disease. An immunohistochemical analysis of 208 reviewed Hodgkin's disease cases from the German Hodgkin Study Group. *Am J Pathol* 1997;150:793.
77. Burns B, Colby T, Dorfman R. Differential diagnostic features of nodular L & H Hodgkin's disease, including progressive transformation of germinal centers. *Am J Surg Pathol* 1984;8:253.
78. Poppema S, Kaiserling E, Lennert K. Nodular paragranuloma and progressively transformed germinal centers:ultrastructural and immunohistochemical findings. *Virchows Arch [B]* 1979;31:211.

79. Ferry J, Zukerberg L, Harris N. Florid progressive transformation of germinal centers. A syndrome affecting young men, without early progression to nodular lymphocyte predominance Hodgkin's disease. *Am J Surg Pathol* 1992;16:252.
80. Bennett M, MacLennan K, Vaughan HG, et al. Non-Hodgkin's lymphoma arising in patients treated for Hodgkin's disease in the BNLI: a 20-year experience. British National Lymphoma Investigation. *Ann Oncol* 1991;2[Suppl 2]:83.
81. Hansmann M, Wacker H, Radzun H. Paragranuloma is a variant of Hodgkin's disease with predominance of B-cells. *Virchows Arch A Pathol Anat Histopathol* 1986;409:171.
82. Orlandi E, Lazzarino M, Brusamolino E. Nodular lymphocyte predominance Hodgkin's disease (NLPHD): clinical behavior and pattern of progression in 66 patients. In: Proceedings of the Third International Symposium on Hodgkin's Lymphoma, Cologne, Germany, 1995:85.
83. Wickert R, Weisenburger D, Tierens A, et al. Clonal relationship between lymphocytic predominance Hodgkin's disease and concurrent or subsequent large-cell lymphoma of B lineage. *Blood* 1995;86:2312.
84. Sundeen J, Cossman J, Jaffe E. Lymphocyte predominant Hodgkin's disease nodular subtype with coexistent "large cell lymphoma". Histological progression or composite malignancy? *Am J Surg Pathol* 1988;12:599.
85. Stein H, Hansmann M, Lennert K, et al. Reed-Sternberg and Hodgkin cells in lymphocyte-predominant Hodgkin's disease of nodular subtype contain J chain. *Am J Clin Pathol* 1986;86:292.
86. Stoler M, Nichols G, Symbula M, et al. Lymphocyte predominance Hodgkin's disease. Evidence for a kappa light chain-restricted monotypic B-cell neoplasm. *Am J Pathol* 1995;146:812.
87. Carbone A, Gloghini A, Gattei V, et al. Expression of functional CD40 antigen on Reed-Sternberg cells and Hodgkin's disease cell lines. *Blood* 1995;85:780.
88. Timens W, Visser L, Poppema S. Nodular lymphocyte predominance type of Hodgkin's disease is a germinal center lymphoma. *Lab Invest* 1986;54:457.
89. Poppema S. The nature of the lymphocytes surrounding Reed-Sternberg cells in nodular lymphocyte predominance and in other types of Hodgkin's disease. *Am J Pathol* 1989;135:351.
90. Kamel O, Gelb A, Shibuya R, et al. Leu 7 (CD57) reactivity distinguishes nodular lymphocyte predominance Hodgkin's disease from nodular sclerosing Hodgkin's disease, T-cell-rich B-cell lymphoma and follicular lymphoma. *Am J Pathol* 1993;142:541.
91. Hansmann M, Stein H, Dallenbach F, et al. Diffuse lymphocyte-predominant Hodgkin's disease (diffuse paragranuloma). A variant of the B-cell-derived nodular type. *Am J Pathol* 1991;138:29.
92. Krayaldin G, Behm F, Geiser P. Lymphocyte predominant Hodgkin disease: clinicopathologic features and results of treatment—the Pediatric Oncology Group experience. *Med Pediatr Oncol* 1997;29:519.
93. Colby T, Hoppe R, Warnke R. Hodgkin's disease: a clinicopathologic study of 659 cases. *Cancer* 1982;49:1848.
94. Kant J, Hubbard S, Longo D, et al. The pathologic and clinical heterogeneity of lymphocyte-depleted Hodgkin's disease. *J Clin Oncol* 1986;4:284.
95. Bennett M, MacLennan K, Easterling M, et al. The prognostic significance of cellular subtypes in nodular sclerosing Hodgkin's disease: an analysis of 271 non-laparotomised cases (BNLI report no. 22). *Clin Radiol* 1983;34:497.
96. Wijlhuizen T, Vrints L, Jairam R, et al. Grades of nodular sclerosis (NSI-NSII) in Hodgkin's disease. Are they of independent prognostic value? *Cancer* 1989;63:1150.
97. Hess J, Bodis S, Pinkus G, et al. Histopathologic grading of nodular sclerosis Hodgkin's disease. Lack of prognostic significance in 254 surgically staged patients. *Cancer* 1994;74:708.
98. van Spronsen D, Vrints L, Erdkamp F. Disappearance of prognostic value of subclassification of nodular sclerosing Hodgkin's disease in south-east Netherlands since 1972. In: Proceedings of the Third International Symposium on Hodgkin's Lymphoma, Cologne, Germany, 1995:129.
99. Stein H, Herbst H, Anagnostopoulos I, et al. The nature of Hodgkin and Reed-Sternberg cells, their association with EBV, and their relationship to anaplastic large-cell lymphoma. *Ann Oncol* 1991;2[Suppl 2]:33.
100. Neiman R, Rosen P, Lukes R. Lymphocyte depletion Hodgkin's disease. A clinicopathological entity. *N Engl J Med* 1973;288:751.
101. Falini B, Stein H, Pileri S, et al. Expression of lymphoid-associated antigens on Hodgkin's and Reed-Sternberg cells of Hodgkin's disease. An immunocytochemical study on lymph node cytospins using monoclonal antibodies. *Histopathology* 1987;11:1229.
102. Falini B, Bigerna B, Pasqualucci L, et al. Distinctive expression pattern of the BCL-6 protein in nodular lymphocyte predominance Hodgkin's disease. *Blood* 1996;87:465.
103. McBride J, Rodriguez J, Luthra R, et al. T-cell-rich B large-cell lymphoma simulating lymphocyte-rich Hodgkin's disease. *Am J Surg Pathol* 1996;20:193.
104. Ashton-Key M, Thorpe P, Allen J, et al. Follicular Hodgkin's disease. *Am J Surg Pathol* 1995;19:1294.
105. Diehl V, Stein H, Sextro M. Lymphocyte predominant Hodgkin's disease: a European Task Force on Lymphoma project. *Blood* 1996;88:294a.
106. Wasielewski R, Mengel M, Fischer R. Classical Hodgkin's disease: clinical impact of the immunophenotype. *Am J Pathol* 1997;151:1123.
107. Jaffe E, Zarate-Osorno A, Medeiros L. The interrelationship of Hodgkin's disease and non-Hodgkin's lymphomas—lessons learned from composite and sequential malignancies. *Semin Diagn Pathol* 1992;9:297.
108. Travis L, Gonzalez C, Hankey B, et al. Hodgkin's disease following non-Hodgkin's lymphoma. *Cancer* 1992;69:2337.
109. Brauninger A, Hansmann M, Strickler J, et al. Identification of common germinal-center B-cell precursors in two patients with both Hodgkin's disease and non-Hodgkin's lymphoma. *N Engl J Med* 1999;340:1239.
110. Rubin D, Hudnall S, Aisenberg A, et al. Richter's transformation of chronic lymphocytic leukemia with Hodgkin's-like cells is associated with Epstein-Barr virus infection. *Mod Pathol* 1994;7:91.
111. Kuppers R, Rajewsky K. The origin of Hodgkin and Reed/Sternberg cells in Hodgkin's disease. *Annu Rev Immunol* 1998;16:471.
112. Brousset P, Lamant L, Viraben R, et al. Hodgkin's disease following mycosis fungoides: phenotypic and molecular evidence for different tumour cell clones. *J Clin Pathol* 1996;49:504.
113. Stein H, Mason D, Gerdes J, et al. The expression of the Hodgkin's disease associated antigen Ki-1 in reactive and neoplastic lymphoid tissue: evidence that Reed-Sternberg cells and histiocytic malignancies are derived from activated lymphoid cells. *Blood* 1985;66:848.
114. Benharroch D, Meguerian-Bedoyan Z, Lamant L, et al. ALK-positive lymphoma: a single disease with a broad spectrum of morphology. *Blood* 1998;91:2076.
115. Zinzani P, Bendandi M, Martelli M, et al. Anaplastic large-cell lymphoma: clinical and prognostic evaluation of 90 adult patients. *J Clin Oncol* 1996;14:955.
116. Elmberger P, Lozano M, Weisenburger D, et al. Transcripts of the npm-alk fusion gene in anaplastic large cell lymphoma, Hodgkin's disease, and reactive lymphoid lesions. *Blood* 1995;86:3517.
117. Sarris A, Luthra R, Papadimitracopoulou V, et al. Long-range amplification of genomic DNA detects the t(2;5)(p23;q35) in anaplastic large-cell lymphoma, but not in other non-Hodgkin's lymphomas, Hodgkin's disease, or lymphomatoid papulosis. *Ann Oncol* 1997;8[Suppl 2]:59.
118. Pulford K, Lamant L, Morris S, et al. Detection of anaplastic lymphoma kinase (ALK) and nucleolar protein nucleophosmin (NPM)-ALK proteins in normal and neoplastic cells with the monoclonal antibody ALK1. *Blood* 1997;89:1394.
119. Gilbert R. Radiotherapy in Hodgkin's disease (malignant granulomatosis); anatomic and clinical foundations; governing principles, results. *Am J Roentgenol* 1939;41:198.
120. Peters M. A study of survivals in Hodgkin's disease treated radiologically. *AJR Am J Roentgenol* 1950;63:299.
121. Kaplan H. The radical radiotherapy of regionally localized Hodgkin's disease. *Radiology* 1962;78:553.
122. Peters M. Prophylactic treatment of adjacent areas in Hodgkin's disease. *Cancer Res* 1966;26:1232.
123. Lister T, Crowther D, Sutcliffe S, et al. Report of a committee convened to discuss the evaluation and staging of patients with Hodgkin's disease: Cotswolds meeting. *J Clin Oncol* 1989;7:1630.
124. Hughes-Davies L, Tarbell N, Coleman C, et al. Stage IA-IIB Hodgkin's disease: management and outcome of extensive thoracic involvement. *Int J Radiat Oncol Biol Phys* 1997;39:361.
125. Hoppe R, Coleman C, Cox R, et al. The management of stage I–II Hodgkin's disease with irradiation alone or combined modality therapy: the Stanford experience. *Blood* 1982;59:455.
126. Rostock R, Siegelman S, Lenhard R, et al. Thoracic CT scanning for mediastinal Hodgkin's disease: results and therapeutic implications. *Int J Radiat Oncol Biol Phys* 1983;9:1451.
127. Hopper K, Diehl L, Lesar M, et al. Hodgkin disease: clinical utility of CT in initial staging and treatment. *Radiology* 1988;169:17.
128. Castellino RA, Podoloff DA. Diagnostic radiology and nuclear medicine imaging in Hodgkin's disease. In: Mauch PM, Armitage JO, Diehl V, Hoppe RT, Weiss LM, eds. *Hodgkin's disease.* Philadelphia: Lippincott Williams & Wilkins, 1999:241.
129. Webb W, Gatsonis C, Zerhouni E. CT and MRI imaging in staging non-small cell bronchogenic carcinoma: report of the Radiologic Diagnostic Group. *Radiology* 1991;178:705.
130. Mauch P, Larson D, Osteen R, et al. Prognostic factors for positive surgical staging in patients with Hodgkin's disease. *J Clin Oncol* 1990;8:257.
131. Castellino R, Dunnick N, Goffinet D, et al. Predictive value of lymphography for sites of subdiaphragmatic disease encountered at staging laparotomy in newly diagnosed Hodgkin's disease and non-Hodgkin's lymphoma. *J Clin Oncol* 1983;1:532.
132. Gilbert R. La roentgentherapie de la granulomatose maligne. *J Radiol Electrol* 1925;9:509.
133. Sapozink M, Kaplan H. Intracranial Hodgkin's disease. A report of 12 cases and review of the literature. *Cancer* 1983;52:1301.
134. Gobbi P, Cavalli C, Gendarini A, et al. Reevaluation of prognostic significance of symptoms in Hodgkin's disease. *Cancer* 1985;56:2874.
135. Pusey W. Cases of sarcoma and of Hodgkin's disease treated by exposures to X-rays: a preliminary report. *JAMA* 1902;38:166.
136. Senn N. Therapeutical value of roentgen ray in treatment of pseudoleukemia. *N Y Med J* 1903;77:665.
137. Gilbert R. La roentgentherapie de la granulomatose maligne. *J Radiol Electrol* 1925;9:509.
138. Ginzton E, Mallory K, Kaplan H. The Stanford Medical Linear Accelerator: I. Design and development. *Stanford Med Bull* 1957;15:123.
139. Kinzie J, Hanks G, MacLean C, et al. Patterns of care study: Hodgkin's disease relapse rates and adequacy of portals. *Cancer* 1983;52:2223.
140. Lutz W, Larsen R. Technique to match mantle and para-aortic fields. *Int J Radiat Oncol Biol Phys* 1983;9:1753.
141. Horning S, Hoppe R, Kaplan H, et al. Female reproductive potential after treatment for Hodgkin's disease. *N Engl J Med* 1981;304:1377.
141a. Skipper HE, Schabel FM, Wilcox WS. Experimental evaluation of potential anticancer agents. XIII. On the criteria and kinetics associated with "curability" of experimental leukemia. *Cancer Chemother Rep* 1964;35:1.
141b. DeVita VT, Serpick AA. Combination chemotherapy in the treatment of advanced Hodgkin's disease. *Proc Am Assoc Cancer Res* 1967;8:13.
142. Loeffler M, Diehl V, Pfreundschuh M, et al. Dose-response relationship of complementary radiotherapy following four cycles of combination chemotherapy in intermediate-stage Hodgkin's disease. *J Clin Oncol* 1997;15:2275.
143. Bahtia S, Robison LL, Oberlin O. Breast cancer and other second neoplasms after childhood Hodgkin's disease. *N Engl J Med* 1996;334:745.

144. Hancock S, Tucker M, Hoppe R. Factors affecting late mortality from heart disease after treatment of Hodgkin's disease. *JAMA* 1993;270:1949.
145. Horning S, Hoppe R, Mason J, et al. Stanford-Kaiser Permanente G1 study for clinical stage I to IIA Hodgkin's disease: subtotal lymphoid irradiation versus vinblastine, methotrexate, and bleomycin chemotherapy and regional irradiation. *J Clin Oncol* 1997;15:1736.
146. Frei EI. Combined intensive alkylating agents with autologous bone marrow transplantation for metastatic solid tumors. In: Dicke K, Spitzer G, Zander A, eds. *Autologous bone marrow transplantation: proceedings of the first international symposium.* Houston: University of Texas, M.D. Anderson Cancer Center, 1985:509.
147. Reece D, Phillips G. Intensive therapy and autotransplantation in Hodgkin's disease. *Stem Cells* 1994;12:477.
148. Phillips GL, Wolff SN, Herzig RH. Treatment of progressive Hodgkin's disease with intensive chemoradiotherapy and autologous bone marrow transplantation. *Blood* 1989;73:2086.
149. Jagannath S, Dicke K, Armitage J, et al. High-dose cyclophosphamide, carmustine, and etoposide and autologous bone marrow transplantation for relapsed Hodgkin's disease. *Ann Intern Med* 1986;104:163.
150. Josting A, Mapara M, Reiser M. Novel three phase, high-dose sequential chemotherapy with autologous stem cell support for relapsed or refractory Hodgkin's and high-grade Non-Hodgkin's lymphoma. *Ann Oncol* 1999;10:638.
151. Gianni A, Siena S, Bregni M, et al. High-dose sequential chemo-radiotherapy with peripheral blood progenitor cell support for relapsed or refractory Hodgkin's disease—a 6-year update. *Ann Oncol* 1993;4:889.
152. Norton L, Simon R. The Norton-Simon hypothesis revisited. *Cancer Treat Rep* 1986;70:163.
153. Reece D, Connors J, Spinelli J, et al. Intensive therapy with cyclophosphamide, carmustine, etoposide +/− cisplatin, and autologous bone marrow transplantation for Hodgkin's disease in first relapse after combination chemotherapy. *Blood* 1994;83:1193.
154. Yahalom J, Gulati S, Toia M, et al. Accelerated hyperfractionated total-lymphoid irradiation, high-dose chemotherapy, and autologous bone marrow transplantation for refractory and relapsing patients with Hodgkin's disease. *J Clin Oncol* 1993;11:1062.
155. Poen J, Hoppe R, Horning S. High-dose therapy and autologous bone marrow transplantation for relapsed/refractory Hodgkin's disease: the impact of involved field radiotherapy on patterns of failure and survival. *Int J Radiat Oncol Biol Phys* 1996;36:3.
156. Goldstone A. The case for and against high-dose therapy with stem cell rescue for early poor prognosis Hodgkin's disease in first remission. *Ann Oncol* 1998;9[Suppl 5]:83.
157. Mauch P, Tarbell N, Weinstein H. Stage IA and IIA supradiaphragmatic Hodgkin's disease: prognostic factors in surgically staged patients treated with mantle and paraaortic irradiation. *J Clin Oncol* 1988;6:1576.
158. Loeffler M, Pfreundschuh M, Hasenclever D. Prognostic risk factors in advanced Hodgkin's disease. Report of the German Hodgkin Study Group. *Blut* 1988;56:273.
159. Carde P, Burger JM, Henry-Amar M. Clinical stages I and II Hodgkin's disease: a specifically tailored therapy according to prognostic factors. *J Clin Oncol* 1988;6:239.
160. Loeffler M, Pfreundschuh M, Rühl U. Risk factor adapted treatment of Hodgkin's lymphoma: strategies and perspectives. *Recent Results Cancer Res* 1989;117:142.
161. Hasenclever D, Diehl V. A prognostic score for advanced Hodgkin's disease. International Prognostic Factors Project on Advanced Hodgkin's Disease. *N Engl J Med* 1998;339:1506.
162. Lagarde P, Eghbali H, Bonichon F, et al. Brief chemotherapy associated with extended field radiotherapy in Hodgkin's disease. Long-term results in a series of 102 patients with clinical stages I-IIIA. *Eur J Cancer Clin Oncol* 1988;24:1191.
163. Specht LK, Hasenclever D. Prognostic factors of Hodgkin's disease. In: Mauch PM, Armitage JO, Diehl V, Hoppe RT, Weiss LM, eds. *Hodgkin's disease.* Philadelphia: Lippincott Williams & Wilkins, 1999:295.
164. Viviani S, Bonadonna G, Santoro A, et al. Alternating versus hybrid MOPP and ABVD combinations in advanced Hodgkin's disease: ten-year results. *J Clin Oncol* 1996;14:1421.
165. Proctor S, Taylor P, Mackie M, et al. A numerical prognostic index for clinical use in identification of poor-risk patients with Hodgkin's disease at diagnosis. The Scotland and Newcastle Lymphoma Group (SNLG) Therapy Working Party. *Leuk Lymph* 1992;7[Suppl]:17.
166. Hasenclever D, Schmitz N, Diehl V.Is there a rationale for high-dose chemotherapy as first line treatment of advanced Hodgkin's disease? German Hodgkin's Lymphoma Study Group (GHSG). *Leuk Lymph* 1995;15[Suppl 1]:47.
167. Horning SJ, Yahalom J, Tesch H. Treatment of stage III-IV Hodgkin's disease. In: Mauch PM, Armitage JO, Diehl V, Hoppe RT, Weiss LM, eds. *Hodgkin's disease.* Philadelphia: Lippincott Williams & Wilkins, 1999:483.
168. Vijayakumar S, Myrianthopoulos L. An updated dose-response analysis in Hodgkin's disease. *Radiother Oncol* 1992;24:1.
169. Duhmke E, Diehl V, Loeffler M, et al. Randomized trial with early-stage Hodgkin's disease testing 30 Gy vs. 40 Gy extended field radiotherapy alone. *Int J Radiat Oncol Biol Phys* 1996;36:305.
170. Tubiana M, Henry-Amar M, Carde P. Toward comprehensive management tailored to prognostic factors of patients with clinical stages I and II in Hodgkin's disease. The EORTC Lymphoma Group controlled clinical trials: 1964–1987. *Blood* 1989;73:47.
171. Sutcliffe S, Gospodarowicz M, Bergsagel D, et al. Prognostic groups for management of localized Hodgkin's disease. *J Clin Oncol* 1985;3:393.
172. Wirth A, Chao M, Corry J, et al. Mantle irradiation alone for clinical stage I-II Hodgkin's disease: long-term follow-up and analysis of prognostic factors in 261 patients. *J Clin Oncol* 1999;17:230.
173. Noordijk E, Kluin-Nelemans J. Stage I or II Hodgkin's disease: more chemotherapy and less irradiation. *Ned Tijdschr Geneeskd* 1997;141:1281.
174. Ganesan T, Wrigley P, Murray P, et al. Radiotherapy for stage I Hodgkin's disease: 20 years experience at St Bartholomew's Hospital. *Br J Cancer* 1990;62:314.
175. Horning S, Hoppe R, Hancock S. Vinblastine, bleomycin, and methotrexate: an effective adjuvant in favorable Hodgkin's disease. *J Clin Oncol* 1988;6:1822.
176. Bates N, Williams M, Bessell E, et al. Efficacy and toxicity of vinblastine, bleomycin, and methotrexate with involved-field radiotherapy in clinical stage IA and IIA Hodgkin's disease: a British National Lymphoma Investigation pilot study. *J Clin Oncol* 1994;12:288.
177. Gobbi P, Pieresca C, Frassoldati A, et al. Vinblastine, bleomycin, and methotrexate chemotherapy plus extended-field radiotherapy in early, favorably presenting, clinically staged Hodgkin's patients: the Gruppo Italiano per lo Studio dei Linfomi Experience. *J Clin Oncol* 1996;14:527.
178. Noordijk E, Carde P, Hagenbeek A. Combination of radiotherapy and chemotherapy is advisable in all patients with clinical stage I-II Hodgkin's disease. Six-year results of the EORTC-GPMC controlled clinical trials "H7-VF," "H7-F" and "H7-U." *Int J Radiat Oncol Biol Phys* 1997;39:173(abst).
179. Carde P, Noordijk E, Hagenbeek A. Superiority of EBVP chemotherapy in copmbination with involved field irradiation over subtotal nodal irradiation in favorable clinical stage I-II Hodgkin's disease: the EORTC-GPMC H7F randomized trial. *Proc Am Soc Clin Oncol* 1997;16:13.
180. Andrieu J, Montagnon B, Asselain B, et al. Chemotherapy radiotherapy association in Hodgkin's disease, clinical stages IA, II2A: results of a prospective clinical trial with 166 patients. *Cancer* 1980;46:2126.
181. Diehl V, Sieber M, Rüffer U. Treatment of early-stage Hodgkin's disease: considerations in the use of chemotherapy. Presented at the annual meeting of the American Society of Clinical Oncology, Los Angeles, CA, 1998.
182. Radford J, Cowen R, Ryder W. Four weeks of neo-adjuvant chemotherapy significantly reduces the progression rate in patients treated with limited field radiotherapy for clinical stage (CS IA/IIA) Hodgkin's disease. Results of a randomized pilot. *Ann Oncol* 1996;7:66.
183. Bartlett N, Rosenberg S, Hoppe R, et al. Brief chemotherapy, Stanford V, and adjuvant radiotherapy for bulky or advanced-stage Hodgkin's disease: a preliminary report. *J Clin Oncol* 1995;13:1080.
184. Olweny C, Katongole-Mbidde E, Klife C. Childhood Hodgkin's disease in Uganda: a 10-year experience. *Cancer* 1978;42:787.
185. Colonna P, Andrieu J. MOPP chemotherapy alone: a suitable treatment for early stages of Hodgkin's disease? [letter]. *Lancet* 1985;1:1224.
186. Longo D, Glatstein E, Duffey P, et al. Radiation therapy versus combination chemotherapy in the treatment of early-stage Hodgkin's disease: seven-year results of a prospective randomized trial. *J Clin Oncol* 1991;9:906.
187. Biti G, Cimino G, Cartoni C, et al. Extended-field radiotherapy is superior to MOPP chemotherapy for the treatment of pathologic stage I-IIA Hodgkin's disease: eight-year update of an Italian prospective randomized study. *J Clin Oncol* 1992;10:378.
187a. Pavlovsky S, Maschio M, Santarelli MT, et al. Randomized trial of chemotherapy versus chemotherapy plus radiotherapy for stage I/II Hodgkin's disease. *J Natl Cancer Inst* 1989;80:1466.
188. Pavlovsky S, Schvartzman E, Lastiri F, et al. Randomized trial of CVPP for three versus six cycles in favorable-prognosis and CVPP versus AOPE plus radiotherapy in intermediate-prognosis untreated Hodgkin's disease. *J Clin Oncol* 1997;15:2652.
189. Santoro A, Viviani S, Zucali R. Comparative results and toxicity of MOPP vs ABVD combined with radiotherapy (RT) in PS IIB, III (A,B) Hodgkin's disease (HD). Presented at the annual meeting of the American Society of Clinical Oncology, San Diego, CA, 1983.
190. Carde P, Noordijk N, Hagenbeek A. Superiorty of MOPP/ABV over EBVP in combination with involved field irradiation in unfavorable clinical stage I-II Hodgkin's disease: the EORTC H7U randomized trial. *Proc Am Soc Clin Oncol* 1993;12:362.
191. Cosset J, Ferme C, Noordijk E. Combined modality therapy for poor prognosis stages I and II Hodgkin's disease. *Semin Radiat Oncol* 1996;6:185.
192. Hagemeister F, Purugganan R, Fuller L, et al. Treatment of early stages of Hodgkin's disease with novantrone, vincristine, vinblastine, prednisone, and radiotherapy. *Semin Hematol* 1994;31:36.
193. Andre M, Brice P, Cazals D, et al. Results of three courses of Adriamycin, bleomycin, vindesine, and dacarbazine with subtotal nodal irradiation in 189 patients with nodal Hodgkin's disease (stage I, II and IIIA). *Hematol Cell Ther* 1997;39:59.
194. Horning S, Rosenberg S, Hoppe R. Brief chemotherapy (Stanford V) and adjuvant radiotherapy for bulky or advanced Hodgkin's disease: an update. *Ann Oncol* 1996;7[Suppl 4]:105.
195. Brusamolino E, Lazzarino M, Orlandi E, et al. Early-stage Hodgkin's disease: long-term results with radiotherapy alone or combined radiotherapy and chemotherapy. *Ann Oncol* 1994;5[Suppl 2]:101.
196. Colonna P, Jais J, Desablens B, et al. Mediastinal tumor size and response to chemotherapy are the only prognostic factors in supradiaphragmatic Hodgkin's disease treated by ABVD plus radiotherapy: ten-year results of the Paris-Ouest-France 81/12 trial, including 262 patients. *J Clin Oncol* 1996;14:1928.
197. Zittoun R, Audebert A, Hoerni B, et al. Extended versus involved fields irradiation combined with MOPP chemotherapy in early clinical stages of Hodgkin's disease. *J Clin Oncol* 1985;3:207.
197a. Hoppe RT, Cosset JM, Santoro A, et al. Treatment of unfavorable stage I–II Hodgkin's disease. In: Mauch PM, Armitage JO, Diehl V, Hoppe RT, Weiss LM, eds. *Hodgkin's disease.* Philadelphia: Lippincott Williams & Wilkins, 1999:475.
197b. Rüffer U, Sieber M, Pfistner B, et al. Involved field radiation is as effective as extended field radiation following chemotherapy for intermediate stage Hodgkin's disease expecting a reduction of long term side-effects: interim analysis of the HD8 trial (GHSG). *Ann Oncol* 1999;10[Suppl 3]:250.
198. Andrieu J, Bayle-Weisgerber C, Boiron M. The chemotherapy-radiotherapy sequence in the management of Hodgkin's disease. Results of a clinical trial. *Euro J Cancer* 1979;48:153.
199. Preti A, Hagemeister F, McLaughlin P, et al. Hodgkin's disease with a mediastinal mass greater than 10 cm: results of four different treatment approaches. *Ann Oncol* 1994;5[Suppl 2]:97.
200. Pavlovsky S, Maschio M, Santarelli M, et al. Randomized trial of chemotherapy versus chemotherapy plus radiotherapy for stage I-II Hodgkin's disease. *J Natl Cancer Inst* 1988;80:1466.
201. DeVita VJ, Hubbard SM. Hodgkin's disease. *N Engl J Med* 1993;328:560.
202. Longo D, Young R, Wesley M, et al. Twenty years of MOPP therapy for Hodgkin's disease. *J Clin Oncol* 1986;4:1295.

203. Bonadonna G, Valagussa P, Santoro A. Alternating non-cross-resistant combination chemotherapy or MOPP in stage IV Hodgkin's disease. A report of 8-year results. *Ann Intern Med* 1986;104:739.
204. Nissen NI, Pajak TF, Glidewell O. A comparative study of a BCNU containing 4-drug program versus MOPP versus 3-drug combinations in advanced Hodgkin's disease: a cooperative study by the Cancer and Leukemia Group B. *Cancer* 1979;43:31.
205. Bakemeier R, Anderson J, Costello W, et al. BCVPP chemotherapy for advanced Hodgkin's disease: evidence for greater duration of complete remission, greater survival, and less toxicity than with a MOPP regimen. Results of the Eastern Cooperative Oncology Group study. *Ann Intern Med* 1984;101:447.
206. Nicholson WM, Beard ME, Crowther D. Combination chemotherapy in generalized Hodgkin's disease. *Br Med J* 1970;3:7.
207. Sutcliffe SB, Wrigley PF, Peto J. MVPP chemotherapy regimen for advanced Hodgkin's disease. *Br Med J* 1978;1:679.
208. Hancock B. Randomised study of MOPP (mustine, Oncovin, procarbazine, prednisone) against LOPP (Leukeran substituted for mustine) in advanced Hodgkin's disease. British National Lymphoma Investigation. *Radiother Oncol* 1986;7:215.
209. Bonadonna G, Zucali R, Monfardini S, et al. Combination chemotherapy of Hodgkin's disease with adriamycin, bleomycin, vinblastine, and imidazole carboxamide versus MOPP. *Cancer* 1975;36:252.
210. Santoro A, Bonadonna G, Valagussa P. Long-term results of combined chemotherapy-radiotherapy approach in Hodgkin's disease: superiority of ABVD plus radiotherapy versus MOPP plus radiotherapy. *J Clin Oncol* 1987;5:27.
211. Glick J, Young M, Harrington D, et al. MOPP/ABV hybrid chemotherapy for advanced Hodgkin's disease significantly improves failure-free and overall survival: the 8-year results of the intergroup trial. *J Clin Oncol* 1998;16:19.
211a. Canellos GP, Anderson JR, Propert KJ. Chemotherapy of advanced Hodgkin's disease with MOPP, ABVD, or MOPP alternating with ABVD. *N Engl J Med* 1992;327:1478.
212. Somers R, Carde P, Henry-Amar M, et al. A randomized study in stage IIIB and IV Hodgkin's disease comparing eight courses of MOPP versus an alteration of MOPP with ABVD: a European Organization for Research and Treatment of Cancer Lymphoma Cooperative Group and Groupe Pierre-et-Marie-Curie controlled clinical trial. *J Clin Oncol* 1994;12:279.
213. DeVita VJ, Simon RM, Hubbard SM. Curability of advanced Hodgkin's disease with chemotherapy. Long-term follow-up of MOPP-treated patients at the National Cancer Institute. *Ann Intern Med* 1980;92:587.
214. Canellos G, Anderson J, Propert K, et al. Chemotherapy of advanced Hodgkin's disease with MOPP, ABVD, or MOPP alternating with ABVD. *N Engl J Med* 1992;327:1478.
215. Goldie JH, Coldman AJ. A mathematic model for relating the drug sensitivity of tumors to their spontaneous mutation rate. *Cancer Treat Rep* 1979;63:1727.
216. Jones S, Haut A, Weick J, et al. Comparison of Adriamycin-containing chemotherapy (MOP-BAP) with MOPP-bleomycin in the management of advanced Hodgkin's disease. A Southwest Oncology Group Study. *Cancer* 1983;51:1339.
217. Sieber M, Rueffer U, Tesch H. Rapidly alternating COPP+ABV+IMEP (CAI) is equally effective as alternating COPP+ABVD (CA) for Hodgkin's disease: final results of two randomised trials for intermediate (HD5 protocol) and advanced (HD6 protocol) stages. *Leuk Lymph* 1998;29:93.
217a. Duggan D, Petroni G, Johnson J, et al. MOPP/ABV vs ABVD for advanced Hodgkin's disease: a preliminary report of CALGB 8952 (with SWOG, ECOG, NCIC). *Proc Am Soc Clin Oncol* 1997;16:12a.
218. Gregory W, Vaughan-Hudson G, MacLennon K. Alternating ChlVPP/PABlOE versus PABlOE in advanced Hodgkin' s disease. *Leuk Lymph* 1998;29:08a(abst).
219. Schmoll H. Review of etoposide single-agent activity. *Cancer Treat Rev* 1982;9:21.
220. Radford JA, Rohatiner AZS, Dunlop DJ. Preliminary results of a four-centre randomised trial paring weekly VAPEC-B chemotherapy with the ChlVPP/EVA hybrid regimen in previously untreated patients. *Proc Am Soc Clin Oncol* 1997;16:12.
221. Simmonds P, Mead G, Sweetenham J, et al. PACE BOM chemotherapy: a 12-week regimen for advanced Hodgkin's disease. *Ann Oncol* 1997;8:259.
222. Carde P, MacKintosh F, Rosenberg S. A dose and time response analysis of the treatment of Hodgkin's disease with MOPP chemotherapy. *J Clin Oncol* 1983;1:146.
223. Gerhartz HH, Schwencke H, Bazarbashi S. Randomized comparison of COPP/ABVD vs. dose and time-escalated COPP/ABVD with GM-CSF support for advanced Hodgkin's disease. *Blood* 1997;90:389.
224. Hasenclever D, Loeffler M, Diehl V. Rationale for dose escalation of first line conventional chemotherapy in advanced Hodgkin's disease. German Hodgkin's Lymphoma Study Group. *Ann Oncol* 1996;7[Suppl 4]:95.
225. Diehl V. Dose-escalation study for the treatment of Hodgkin's disease. The German Hodgkin Study Group (GHSG). *Ann Hematol* 1993;66:139.
226. Diehl V, Franklin J, Hasenclever D, et al. BEACOPP: a new regimen for advanced Hodgkin's disease. German Hodgkin's Lymphoma Study Group. *Ann Oncol* 1998;9[Suppl 5]:67.
227. Diehl V, Franklin J, Hasenclever D, et al. BEACOPP, a new dose-escalated and accelerated regimen, is at least as effective as COPP/ABVD in patients with advanced-stage Hodgkin's lymphoma: interim report from a trial of the German Hodgkin's Lymphoma Study Group. *J Clin Oncol* 1998;16:3810.
228. Chopra R, McMillan A, Linch D, et al. The place of high-dose BEAM therapy and autologous bone marrow transplantation in poor-risk Hodgkin's disease. A single-center eight-year study of 155 patients. *Blood* 1993;81:1137.
229. Horning S, Chao N, Negrin R, et al. High-dose therapy and autologous hematopoietic progenitor cell transplantation for recurrent or refractory Hodgkin's disease: analysis of the Stanford University results and prognostic indices. *Blood* 1997;89:801.
230. Reece D, Phillips G. Intensive therapy and autologous stem cell transplantation for Hodgkin's disease in first relapse after combination chemotherapy. *Leuk Lymph* 1996;21:245.
231. Carella A, Carlier P, Congiu A, et al. Autologous bone marrow transplantation as adjuvant treatment for high-risk Hodgkin's disease in first complete remission after MOPP/ABVD protocol. *Bone Marrow Transplant* 1991;8:99.
232. Straus D, Gaynor J, Myers J, et al. Prognostic factors among 185 adults with newly diagnosed advanced Hodgkin's disease treated with alternating potentially noncross-resistant chemotherapy and intermediate-dose radiation therapy. *J Clin Oncol* 1990;8:1173.
233. Fabian C, Mansfield C, Dahlberg S, et al. Low-dose involved field radiation after chemotherapy in advanced Hodgkin disease. A Southwest Oncology Group randomized study. *Ann Intern Med* 1994;120:903.
234. Diehl V, Loeffler M, Pfreundschuh M, et al. Further chemotherapy versus low-dose involved-field radiotherapy as consolidation of complete remission after six cycles of alternating chemotherapy in patients with advance Hodgkin's disease. German Hodgkins' Study Group (GHSG). *Ann Oncol* 1995;6:901.
235. Loeffler M, Brosteanu O, Hasenclever D, et al. Meta-analysis of chemotherapy versus combined modality treatment trials in Hodgkin's disease. International Database on Hodgkin's Disease Overview Study Group. *J Clin Oncol* 1998;16:818.
236. Raemaekers J, Burgers M, Henry-Amar M, et al. Patients with stage III/IV Hodgkin's disease in partial remission after MOPP/ABV chemotherapy have excellent prognosis after additional involved-field radiotherapy:interim results from the ongoing EORTC LCG and GPMC phase III trial. The EORTC Lymphoma Cooperative Group and Groupe Pierre-et-Marie-Curie. *Ann Oncol* 1997;8[Suppl 1]:111.
237. Canellos GP, Horvich A. Management of recurrent Hodgkin`s disease. In: Mauch P, Armitage JO, Diehl V, Hoppe RT, Weiss LM, eds. *Hodgkin's disease.* Philadelphia: Lippincott Williams & Wilkins, 1999:507.
238. Van Leeuwen FE, Klokmann WJ, Hagenbeek A. Second cancer risk following Hodgkin's disease: a 20-year follow-up study. *J Clin Oncol* 1994;12:312.
239. Henry-Amar M. Second cancers after treatment of Hodgkin's disease: experience at the International Database on Hodgkin's disease (IDHD). *Bull Cancer* 1992;79:389.
240. Hansmann M, Fellbaum C, Hui P, et al. Morphological and immunohistochemical investigation of non-Hodgkin's lymphoma combined with Hodgkin's disease. *Histopathology* 1989;15:35.
241. Fisher R, De VV, Hubbard S, et al. Prolonged disease-free survival in Hodgkin's disease with MOPP reinduction after first relapse. *Ann Intern Med* 1979;90:761.
242. Longo D, Duffey P, Young R, et al. Conventional-dose salvage combination chemotherapy in patients relapsing with Hodgkin's disease after combination chemotherapy: the low probability for cure. *J Clin Oncol* 1992;10:210.
243. Horwich A, Specht L, Ashley S. Survival analysis of patients with clinical stages I or II Hodgkin's disease who have relapsed after initial treatment with radiotherapy alone. *Eur J Cancer* 1997;33:848.
244. Roach Md, Brophy N, Cox R, et al. Prognostic factors for patients relapsing after radiotherapy for early-stage Hodgkin's disease. *J Clin Oncol* 1990;8:623.
245. Mauch P, Henry-Amar M. International Database on Hodgkin's Disease: a cooperative effort to determine treatment outcome. *Ann Oncol* 1992;3[Suppl 4]:59.
246. Healey EA, Tarbell NJ, Kalish LA. Prognostic factors for patients with Hodgkin`s disease in first relapse. *Cancer* 1993;71:2613.
247. Specht L, Horwich A, Ashley S. Salvage of relapse of patients with Hodgkin's disease in clinical stages I or II who were staged with laparotomy and initially treated with radiotherapy alone. A report from the international database on Hodgkin's disease. *Int J Radiat Oncol Biol Phys* 1994;30:805.
248. Cannellos G, Young RC, De Vita VD. Combination chemotherapy for advanced Hodgkin`s disease in relapse following extensive radiotherapy. *Clin Pharm Ther* 1972;13:750.
249. Santoro A, Viviani S, Villarreal C, et al. Salvage chemotherapy in Hodgkin's disease irradiation failures: superiority of doxorubicin-containing regimens over MOPP. *Cancer Treat Rep* 1986;70:343.
250. Wirth A, Corry J, Laidlaw C, et al. Salvage radiotherapy for Hodgkin's disease following chemotherapy failure. *Int J Radiat Oncol Biol Phys* 1997;39:599.
251. Pfreundschuh M, Rueffer U, Lathan B, et al. Dexa-BEAM in patients with Hodgkin's disease refractory to multidrug chemotherapy regimens: a trial of the German Hodgkin's Disease Study Group. *J Clin Oncol* 1994;12:580.
252. Hagemeister F, Tannir N, McLaughlin P, et al. MIME chemotherapy (methyl-GAG, ifosfamide, methotrexate, etoposide) as treatment for recurrent Hodgkin's disease. *J Clin Oncol* 1987;5:556.
253. Rodriguet MG, Schoppe WD, Fuchs R. Lomustine, etoposide, vindesine, and dexamethasone (CEVD) in Hodgkin's disease refractory to cyclophosphamide, vincristine, procarbacine, and prednisone (COPP) and doxorubicine, bleomycin, vinblastine, and darcarbazine (ABVD): a multi-center trial of the German Hodgkin`s study group. *Cancer Treat Rep* 1987;71:1203.
254. Velasquez WS, Jagannath S, Hagemeister FB. Dexamethasone, high-dose ara-C and cisplatin as salvage treatment for relapsing Hodgkin`s disease. *Proc Am Soc Hematol* 1986;68:242.
255. Ferme C, Bastion Y, Lepage E, et al. The MINE regimen as intensive salvage chemotherapy for relapsed and refractory Hodgkin's disease. *Ann Oncol* 1995;6:543.
256. Bierman P, Bagin R, Jagannath S, et al. High dose chemotherapy followed by autologous hematopoietic rescue in Hodgkin's disease:long-term follow-up in 128 patients. *Ann Oncol* 1993;4:767.
257. Josting A, Katay I, Rueffer U, et al. Favorable outcome of patients with relapsed or refractory Hodgkin's disease treated with high-dose chemotherapy and stem cell rescue at the time of maximal response to conventional salvage therapy (Dex-BEAM). *Ann Oncol* 1998;9:289.
258. Linch D, Winfield D, Goldstone A, et al. Dose intensification with autologous bone-marrow transplantation in relapsed and resistant Hodgkin's disease: results of a BNLI randomised trial. *Lancet* 1993;341:1051.
259. Schmitz N, Sextro M, Pfistner B. HDR-1: high-dose therapy (HDT) followed by hematopoietic stem cell transplantation (HSCT) for relapsed chemosensitive Hodgkin's disease (HD): final results of a randomized GHSG and EBMT trial (HD-R1). *Proc Am Soc Clin Oncol* 1999;18[Suppl 5]:18.

260. Bonfante V, Santoro A, Viviani S, et al. Outcome of patients with Hodgkin's disease failing after primary MOPP-ABVD. *J Clin Oncol* 1997;15:528.
261. Sweetenham JW, Carella AM, Taghipour G. High-dose therapy and autologous stem cell transplantation for adult patients with Hodgkin's disease who fail to enter remission after induction chemotherapy: results in 175 patients reported to the EBMT. *J Clin Oncol* 1999;17:3101.
262. Lazarus H, Rowlings P, Zhang M, et al. Autotransplants for Hodgkin's disease in patients never achieving remission:a report from the Autologous Blood and Marrow Transplant Registry. *J Clin Oncol* 1999;17:534.
263. Reece D, Barnett M, Shepherd J, et al. High-dose cyclophosphamide, carmustine (BCNU), and etoposide (VP16-213) with or without cisplatin (CBV +/- P) and autologous transplantation for patients with Hodgkin's disease who fail to enter a complete remission after combination chemotherapy. *Blood* 1995;86:451.
264. Yuen A, Rosenberg S, Hoppe R, et al. Comparison between conventional salvage therapy and high-dose therapy with autografting for recurrent or refractory Hodgkin's disease. *Blood* 1997;89:814.
265. Andre M, Henry-Amar M, Pico J, et al. Comparison of high-dose therapy and autologous stem-cell transplantation with conventional therapy for Hodgkin's disease induction failure: a case-control study. Societe Francaise de Greffe de Moelle. *J Clin Oncol* 1999;17:222.
266. Josting A, Rüffer U, Franklin J. Prognostic factors and treatment outcome in patients with primary progressive Hodgkin's lymphoma—a report from the German Hodgkin's disease Study Group (GHSG). *Blood* 1999;94(10)[Suppl 1]:2299a.
267. Josting A, Reiser M, Rüffer U. Treatment of primary progressive Hodgkin's and aggressive non Hodgkin's disease—Is there a chance for cure? *J Clin Oncol* 2000;18, 2, 332.
268. Brice P, Bouabdallah R, Moreau P, et al. Prognostic factors for survival after high-dose therapy and autologous stem cell transplantation for patients with relapsing Hodgkin's disease: analysis of 280 patients from the French registry. Societe Francaise de Greffe de Moelle. *Bone Marrow Transplant* 1997;20:21.
269. Sweetenham J, Taghipour G, Milligan D, et al. High-dose therapy and autologous stem cell rescue for patients with Hodgkin's disease in first relapse after chemotherapy: results from the EBMT. Lymphoma Working Party of the European Group for Blood and Marrow Transplantation. *Bone Marrow Transplant* 1997;20:745.
270. Crump M, Smith A, Brandwein J, et al. High-dose etoposide and melphalan, and autologous bone marrow transplantation for patients with advanced Hodgkin's disease: importance of disease status at transplant. *J Clin Oncol* 1993;11:704.
271. Wheeler C, Eickhoff C, Elias A, et al. High-dose cyclophosphamide, carmustine, and etoposide with autologous transplantation in Hodgkin's disease: a prognostic model for treatment outcomes. *Biol Blood Marrow Transplant* 1997;3:98.
272. Milpied N, Fielding A, Pearce R, et al. Allogeneic bone marrow transplant is not better than autologous transplant for patients with relapsed Hodgkin's disease. European Group for Blood and Bone Marrow Transplantation. *J Clin Oncol* 1996;14:1291.
273. Anderson J, Litzow M, Appelbaum F, et al. Allogeneic, syngeneic, and autologous marrow transplantation for Hodgkin's disease: the 21-year Seattle experience. *J Clin Oncol* 1993;11:2342.
274. Gajewski J, Phillips G, Sobocinski K, et al. Bone marrow transplants from HLA-identical siblings in advanced Hodgkin's disease. *J Clin Oncol* 1996;14:572.
275. Rosenthal SR. Significance of tissue lymphocytes in the prognosis of lymphogranulomatosis. *Arch Pathol* 1936;21:628.
276. Westling P. Studies of the prognosis in Hodgkin's disease. *Acta Radiol* 1965;245:5.
277. Peters MV. A study of survivals in Hodgkin's disease treated radiologically. *Am J Roentgenol* 1950;63:299.
278. Culine S, Henry-Amar M, Diebold J, et al. Relationship of histological subtypes to prognosis in early stage Hodgkin's disease: a review of 312 cases in a controlled clinical trial. The Groupe Pierre et Marie Curie. *Eur J Cancer Clin Oncol* 1989;25:551.
279. Diehl V, Sextro M, Franklin J, et al. Clinical presentation, course, and prognostic factors in lymphocyte-predominant Hodgkin's disease and lymphocyte-rich classical Hodgkin's disease: report from the European Task Force on Lymphoma Project on Lymphocyte-Predominant Hodgkin's Disease. *J Clin Oncol* 1999;17:776.
280. Hansmann M, Zwingers T, Boske A, et al. Clinical features of nodular paragranuloma (Hodgkin's disease, lymphocyte predominance type, nodular). *J Cancer Res Clin Oncol* 1984;108:321.
281. Orlandi E, Lazzarino M, Brusamolino E, et al. Nodular lymphocyte predominance Hodgkin's disease: long-term observation reveals a continuous pattern of recurrence. *Leuk Lymph* 1997;26:359.
282. Pappa V, Norton A, Gupta R, et al. Nodular type of lymphocyte predominant Hodgkin's disease. A clinical study of 50 cases. *Ann Oncol* 1995;6:559.
283. Mauch P, Kalish L, Kadin M, et al. Patterns of presentation of Hodgkin disease. Implications for etiology and pathogenesis. *Cancer* 1993;71:2062.
284. Miettinen M, Franssila K, Saxen E. Hodgkin's disease, lymphocytic predominance nodular. Increased risk for subsequent non-Hodgkin's lymphomas. *Cancer* 1983;51:2293.
285. Henry-Amar M. Second cancer after the treatment for Hodgkin's disease: a report from the International Database on Hodgkin's Disease. *Ann Oncol* 1992;3[Suppl 4]:117.
286. Maloney DG, Grillo-Lopez AJ, Bodkin DJ. IDEC-C2B8: results of a phase I multiple-dose trial in patients with relapsed non-Hodgkin's lymphoma. *J Clin Oncol* 1997;15:3266.
287. Lokich L, Pinkus G, Moloney W. Hodgkin's disease in the elderly. *Oncology* 1974;29:484.
288. Specht L, Nissen N. Hodgkin's disease and age. *Eur J Haematol* 1989;43:127.
289. Franklin J, Sieber M, Paulus U. Toxicity and feasibility of the BEACOPP regimen for advanced stage Hodgkin's disease patients older than 65 years. *Ann Oncol* 1999;2:157.
290. Tesch H, Santoro A, Fiedler F. Phase II study of gemcitabine in pretreated Hodgkin's disease. Results of a multicenter study. *Blood* 1997;90:339.
291. Gherlinzoni F, Zinziani PL, Magagnoli M. VBM regimen for Hodgkin's disease in the elderly. *Leuk Lymph* 1998;29:72.
292. Sadural E, Smith LG. Haematological malignancies during pregnancy. *Clin Obstet Gynecol* 38;1995:535.
293. Gelb AB, Van de Rijn M, Warnke RA. Pregnancy-associated lymphomas. A clinicopathologic study. *Cancer* 1996;78:304.
294. Fisher P, Hancock B. Hodgkin's disease in the pregnant patient. *Br J Hosp Med* 1996;56:529.
295. Tirelli U, Errante D, Dolcetti R, et al. Hodgkin's disease and human immunodeficiency virus infection: clinicopathologic and virologic features of 114 patients from the Italian Cooperative Group on AIDS and Tumors. *J Clin Oncol* 1995;13:1758.
296. Carbone A, Dolcetti R, Gloghini A, et al. Immunophenotypic and molecular analyses of acquired immune deficiency syndrome-related and Epstein-Barr virus-associated lymphomas: a comparative study. *Hum Pathol* 1996;27:133.
297. Tirelli U, Vaccher E, Rezza G, et al. Hodgkin disease and infection with the human immunodeficiency virus (HIV) in Italy [letter]. *Ann Intern Med* 1988;108:309.
298. Bellas C, Santon A, Manzanal A, et al. Pathological, immunological, and molecular features of Hodgkin's disease associated with HIV infection. Comparison with ordinary Hodgkin's disease. *Am J Surg Pathol* 1996;20:1520.
299. Andrieu J, Roithmann S, Tourani J, et al. Hodgkin's disease during HIV1 infection: the French registry experience. French Registry of HIV-associated Tumors. *Ann Oncol* 1993;4:635.
300. Tirelli U, Errante D, Vaccher E, et al. Hodgkin's disease in 92 patients with HIV infection: the Italian experience. GICAT (Italian Cooperative Group on AIDS & Tumors). *Ann Oncol* 1992;3[Suppl 4]:69.
301. Rubio R. Hodgkin's disease associated with human immunodeficiency virus infection. A clinical study of 46 cases. Cooperative Study Group of Malignancies Associated with HIV Infection of Madrid. *Cancer* 1994;73:2400.
302. Errante D, Tirelli U, Gastaldi R, et al. Combined antineoplastic and antiretroviral therapy for patients with Hodgkin's disease and human immunodeficiency virus infection. A prospective study of 17 patients. The Italian Cooperative Group on AIDS and Tumors (GICAT). *Cancer* 1994;73:437.
303. Tirelli U, Erranta D, Gisselbrecht C. Epirubicin, bleomycin, vinblastine and prednisone (EBVP) chemotherapy in combination with antiretroviral therapy and primary use of G-CSF for patients with Hodgkin's disease and HIV Infection (HD-HIV). *Proc Am Soc Clin Oncol* 1996;15:304.
304. Levine AM, Cheung T, Tulpule A. Preliminary results of AIDS Clinical Trials Group (ACTG) Study No. 149: phase II trial of ABVD chemotherapy with G-CSF in HIV-infected patients with Hodgkin's disease (HD). *AIDS* 1997;14:12.
305. Tirelli U, Carbone A, Strau DJ. HIV-related Hodgkin's disease. In: Mauch PM, Armitage JO, Diehl V, Hoppe RT, Weiss LM, eds. *Hodgkin's disease.* Philadelphia: Lippincott Williams & Wilkins, 1999:701.
306. Hartmann P, Winkler U, Franzen C. BEACOPP chemotherapeutic regimen for treatment of HIV-infected patients with Hodgkin's lymphoma. *Blood* 1998;92:540.
307. Tarbell N, Thompson L, Mauch P. Thoracic irradiation in Hodgkin's disease: disease control and long-term complications. *Int J Radiat Oncol Biol Phys* 1990;18:275.
308. Hancock S, Hoppe R, Horning S, et al. Intercurrent death after Hodgkin disease therapy in radiotherapy and adjuvant MOPP trials. *Ann Intern Med* 1988;109:183.
309. Boivin J, Hutchison G. Coronary heart disease mortality after irradiation for Hodgkin's disease. *Cancer* 1982;49:2470.
310. Van Leeuwen FE, Swerdlow AJ, Valaguss P. Hodgkin's disease. In: Mauch PM, Armitage JO, Diehl V, Hoppe RT, Weiss LM, eds. *Hodgkin's disease.* Philadelphia: Lippincott Williams & Wilkins, 1999:607.
311. Tucker M. Solid second cancers following Hodgkin's disease. *Hematol Oncol Clin North Am* 1993;7:389.
312. Sandoval C, Pui C, Bowman L, et al. Secondary acute myeloid leukemia in children previously treated with alkylating agents, intercalating topoisomerase II inhibitors, and irradiation. *J Clin Oncol* 1993;11:1039.
313. Valagussa P. Second neoplasms following treatment of Hodgkin's disease. *Curr Opin Oncol* 1993;5:805.
314. Van Leeuwen F, Somers R, Taal B. Increased risk of lung cancer, non-Hodgkin's lymphoma and leukemia following Hodgkin's disease. *J Clin Oncol* 1989;7:1046.
315. Hancock S, Tucker M, Hoppe R. Breast cancer after treatment of Hodgkin's disease. *J Natl Cancer Inst* 1993;85:25.
316. Hancock S, Hoppe R. Long-term complications of treatment and causes of mortality after Hodgkin's disease. *Semin Radiat Oncol* 1996;6:225.
317. Swerdlow A, Douglas A, Hudson G, et al. Risk of second primary cancers after Hodgkin's disease by type of treatment: analysis of 2846 patients in the British National Lymphoma Investigation. *BMJ* 1992;304:1137.
318. Kaldor J, Day N, Bell J, et al. Lung cancer following Hodgkin's disease: a case-control study. *Int J Cancer* 1992;52:677.
319. Bonadonna G. Modern treatment of malignant lymphomas: a multidisciplinary approach? The Kaplan Memorial Lecture. *Ann Oncol* 1994;5[Suppl 2]:5.
320. Chilcote R, Baehner R, Hammond D. Septicemia and meningitis in children splenectomized for Hodgkin's disease. *N Engl J Med* 1976;295:798.
321. Bradlyn A, Harris C, Spieth L. Quality of life assessment in pediatric oncology: a retrospective review of phase III reports. *Soc Sci Med* 1995;41:1463.
322. Kornblith A, Anderson J, Cella D, et al. Hodgkin disease survivors at increased risk for problems in psychosocial adaptation. The Cancer and Leukemia Group B. *Cancer* 1992;70:2214.
323. Joly F, Henry-Amar M, Arveux P, et al. Late psychosocial sequelae in Hodgkin's disease survivors: a French population-based case-control study. *J Clin Oncol* 1996;14:2444.
324. Aaronson NK. Assessing the quality of life of patients in cancer clinical trials: common problems and common sense solution. *Eur J Cancer* 1992;8:1304.
325. Devizzi L, Santoro A, Bonfante V, et al. Vinorelbine: a new promising drug in Hodgkin's disease. *Leuk Lymph* 1996;22:409.

326. Devizzi L, Santoro A, Bonfante V, et al. Vinorelbine: an active drug for the management of patients with heavily pretreated Hodgkin's disease. *Ann Oncol* 1994;5:817.
327. Benchekroun S, Chouffai Z, Harif M. Clinical study of Navelbine activity in Hodgkin's disease. Phase II study. In: Fabre P, ed. *Navelbine (vinorelbine): update and new trends.* Montrouge: Oncologie, Libbey Eurotext, 1991:261.
328. Plunkett W, Huang P, Searcy CE. Gemcitabine: preclinical pharmacology and mechanism of action. *Semin Oncol* 1996;23:3.
329. Kaplan H. Hodgkin's disease: unfolding concepts concerning its nature, management and prognosis. *Cancer* 1980;45:2439.
330. Engert A, Martin G, Amlot P, et al. Immunotoxins constructed with anti-CD25 monoclonal antibodies and deglycosylated ricin A-chain have potent anti-tumour effects against human Hodgkin cells in vitro and solid Hodgkin tumours in mice. *Int J Cancer* 1991;49:450.
331. McLaughlin P, Cabanillas F, Grillo-Lopez AJ. IDEC-C2B8 anti-CD20 antibody: final report on a phase III pivotal trial in patients with relapsed low-grade or follicular lymphoma. *Blood* 1996;88:349.
332. Fitzgerald D, Pastan I. Targeted toxin therapy for the treatment of cancer. *J Natl Cancer Inst* 1989;81:1455.
333. Engert A, Diehl V, Schnell R, et al. A phase-I study of an anti-CD25 ricin A-chain immunotoxin (RFT5-SMPT-dgA) in patients with refractory Hodgkin's lymphoma. *Blood* 1997;89:403.
334. Schnell R, Linnartz C, Katouzi A, et al. Development of new ricin A-chain immunotoxins with potent anti-tumor effects against human Hodgkin cells in vitro and disseminated Hodgkin tumors in SCID mice using high-affinity monoclonal antibodies directed against the CD30 antigen. *Int J Cancer* 1995;63:238.
335. Staak J, Schnell R, Schwartz C. Clinical experience with a novel ricin A-chain immunotoxin (Ki-4.dgA) in patients with refractory CD30+ lymphoma. *Onkologie* 1999;22:132.
336. O'Donoghue JA. The impact of tumor cell proliferation in radioimmunotherapy. *Cancer* 1994;73:974.
337. Winkler U, Stein H, Scheidhauer K. Radioimmunoconjugates for the therapy of Hodgkin's lymphoma: preliminary data of a clinical study using the anti-CD30 antibody 99mTc-BerH2. Fourth International Symposium on Hodgkin's Lymphoma, March 28–April 1, Cologne, Germany. *Leuk Lymph* 1998;29[Suppl.1]:115a.
338. Vriesendorp H, Herpst J, Germack M, et al. Phase I-II studies of yttrium-labeled antiferritin treatment for end-stage Hodgkin's disease, including Radiation Therapy Oncology Group 87-01. *J Clin Oncol* 1991;9:918.
339. Hartmann F, Renner C, Jung W. Treatment of refractory Hodgkin's disease with an anti-CD16/CD30 bispecific antibody. *Blood* 1997;89:2042.
340. Vinciguerra V, Coleman M, Pajak T, et al. MER immunotherapy and combination chemotherapy for advanced, recurrent Hodgkin's disease. Cancer and Leukemia Group B study. *Cancer Clin Trials* 1981;4:99.
341. Margolin K, Aronson F, Sznol M, et al. Phase II trial of high-dose interleukin-2 and lymphokine-activated killer cells in Hodgkin's disease and non-Hodgkin's lymphoma. *J Immunother* 1991;10:214.
342. Bernstein Z, Vaickus L, Friedman N, et al. Interleukin-2 lymphokine-activated killer cell therapy of non-Hodgkin's lymphoma and Hodgkin's disease. *J Immunother* 1991;10:141.
343. Tourani J, Levy V, Briere J, et al. Interleukin-2 therapy for refractory and relapsing lymphomas. *Eur J Cancer* 1991;27:1676.
344. Koziner B. Alpha interferon in patients with progressive and/or recurrent Hodgkin's disease. *Eur J Cancer* 1991;27[Suppl 4]:79.
345. Heslop HE, Brenner MK, Rooney CM. Long-term restoration of immunity against Epstein-Barr virus infection by adoptive transfer of gene-modified virus specific T-lymphocytes. *Nat Med* 1996;2:551.
346. Roskrow M, Suzuki N, Gan Y, et al. Epstein-Barr virus (EBV)-specific cytotoxic T lymphocytes for the treatment of patients with EBV-positive relapsed Hodgkin's disease. *Blood* 1998;91:2925.

CHAPTER 46

Leukemias

SECTION 1

CLARA D. BLOOMFIELD
MICHAEL A. CALIGIURI

Molecular Biology of Leukemias

Leukemia can be broadly defined as a disease whose malignant cell is derived from the hematopoietic system and manifests its expansion in the bone marrow with or without peripheral blood involvement. The cytogenetic study of these malignant cells has revealed that recurrent chromosomal changes occur in over one-half of all cases of leukemia. Most commonly, these are structural changes classified as translocations, inversions, or deletions. Further, it is usually the disruption or deregulation of specific genes at the chromosome breaks that in turn contributes to the process of leukemogenesis.[1,2] In many instances, these genes have also been found to be directly or indirectly involved in the normal development or maintenance of the hematopoietic system. Thus, leukemia results, at least in part, from the disruption or deregulation of genes that normally regulate blood cell development, blood cell homeostasis, or both.[1–5] In this sense, the molecular biology of leukemia is consistent with the paradigm established for cancer in general: Genes that predispose to human cancer (i.e., oncogenes and tumor suppressor genes) are altered or inactivated versions of genes normally involved in the regulation of cell growth, cell development, and cell death.[4,6]

Several generalizations about the molecular biology of leukemia can be made.[7] First, the chromosomal aberrations that result in the disruption or deregulation of genes occur in somatic tissues (i.e., hematopoietic cells) and are not found in nonleukemic cells. The genetic mishap often occurs at a specific point in normal hematopoiesis, giving rise to leukemia of a specific lineage that has arrested at a distinct maturational stage. This strongly suggests that the gene or genes altered in a particular type of leukemia are important in a specific stage of development or homeostasis of its normal cell counterpart. There are, however, some notable exceptions to this, such as the myeloid-lymphoid leukemia (*MLL*) gene that can be involved in leukemia of different or mixed lineages.

The mechanisms by which disrupted or deregulated genes cause leukemia can be broadly classified into two categories. The first is gene fusion, whereby a distinct protein, usually either a transcription factor or receptor tyrosine kinase, fuses with an unrelated gene to create a unique *chimeric* fusion protein that then critically contributes to malignant transformation of the cell. This mechanism predominates in the genesis of myeloid leukemia, but is also found in lymphoid leukemia. The second is gene activation, whereby a gene that normally controls transcription within the cell is inappropriately placed under the control of an active promoter/enhancer from another gene, usually the immunoglobulin (Ig) or T-cell receptor (TCR) promoter/enhancer during the process of antigen receptor gene rearrangement. Chromosomal translocations that result in gene activation usually occur in lymphoid tissue and lead to a deregulation in gene expression.[1,3–5] As discussed in this chapter, more recently it has been appreciated that other genetic and epigenetic events, such as point mutations, gene deletions, and DNA methylation, usually in tumor suppressor genes, can also contribute to the initiation or progression of leukemia.

The improved techniques for the study of chromosomes and the explosive growth in molecular biology are rapidly facilitating the elucidation of genes involved at chromosomal breakpoints in cases of leukemia, and the list of oncogenes is increasing almost daily in the literature. Table 46.1-1 provides the reader with some examples of genes involved in leukemo-

TABLE 46.1-1. Selected Examples of Cytogenetic and Molecular Abnormalities in Leukemia

Cytogenetic Abnormality	*Genes Involved*	*Derivation of Abbreviation*	*Protein Characterization*	*Disease*	*Reference*
FUSIONS INVOLVING THE CORE-BINDING FACTORS (CBFs)					
t(8;21)(q22;q22)	*CBFA2T1/ETO* (8q22)	Eight twenty-one	Zinc finger protein	AML	12
	CBFA2/AML1 (21q22)	Acute myeloid leukemia 1	α subunit of CBF complex		
inv(16)(p13q22)	*MYH11* (16p13)	Myosin heavy chain 11	Smooth muscle myosin heavy chain	AML	18
	CBFB/CBFβ (16q22)	Core binding factor-β	β subunit of CBF complex		
t(3;21)(q26;q22)	*EVI1* (3q26)	Ecotrophic virus integration site 1	Multiple zinc fingers	MDS, AML	24
	CBFA2/AML1 (21q22)	Acute myeloid leukemia 1	α subunit of CBF complex	CML-BC	
FUSIONS INVOLVING THE CBFs AND *TEL* (ETV6)					
t(12;21)(p13;q22)	*TEL* (12p13)	Translocation ETS leukemia	ETS-related transcription factor	ALL	29,30
	CBFA2/AML1 (21q22)	Acute myeloid leukemia 1	α subunit of CBF complex		
FUSIONS INVOLVING *TEL*					
t(5;12)(q33;p13)	*PDGFRβ* (5q33)	Platelet-derived growth factor receptor-β	Tyrosine kinase	Chronic myelomonocytic leukemia	37
	TEL (12p13)	Translocation ETS leukemia	ETS-related transcription factor		
t(9;12)(q34;p13)	*ABL* (9q34)	Abelson	Tyrosine kinase	AML, ALL,	41
	TEL (12p13)	Translocation ETS leukemia	ETS-related transcription factor	atypical CML	
t(12;22)(p13;q11)	*TEL* (12p13)	Translocation ETS leukemia	ETS-related transcription factor	AML	43
	MN1 (22q11)	Meningioma 1	Nuclear protein	MDS	
FUSIONS INVOLVING *MLL*					
t(4;11)(q21;q23)	*AF4* (4q21)	*ALL1* fused chromosome 4	Transactivator	ALL, AML	49,50
	MLL (11q23)	Myeloid lymphoid leukemia	*Drosophila* trithorax homolog		
t(11;19)(q23;p13.3)	*MLL* (11q23)	Myeloid lymphoid leukemia	*Drosophila* trithorax homolog	AML, ALL	176
	ENL (19p13.3)	Eleven nineteen leukemia	Transcription factor		
t(9;11)(p22;q23)	*AF9* (9p22)	*ALL1* fused chromosome 9	Nuclear protein, ENL homology	AML, ALL	177
	MLL (11q23)	Myeloid lymphoid leukemia	*Drosophila* trithorax homolog		
t(11;22)(q23;q13)	*MLL* (11q23)	Myeloid lymphoid leukemia	*Drosophila* trithorax homolog	AML	178
	P300 (22q13)	Protein 300	Adenoviral E1A-associated protein		
t(1;11)(q21;q23)	*AF1q* (1q21)	*ALL1* fused chromosome 1q	No homology to any known protein	AML	60
	MLL (11q23)	Myeloid lymphoid leukemia	*Drosophila* trithorax homolog		
+11 (sole) or normal cytogenetics	*MLL* (11q23)	Myeloid lymphoid leukemia	*Drosophila* trithorax homolog MLL partial tandem duplication	AML	62
FUSIONS INVOLVING *RAR-α*					
t(15;17)(q22;q12-21)	*PML* (15q21)	Promyelocytic leukemia	Zinc finger protein	APL	81,82
	RAR-α (17q21)	Retinoic acid receptor-α	Retinoic acid receptor-α		
t(11;17)(q23;q21)	*PLZF* (11q23)	Promyelocytic leukemia zinc finger	Zinc finger protein	APL	87
	RAR-α (17q21)	Retinoic acid receptor-α	Retinoic acid receptor-α		
FUSIONS INVOLVING *E2A*					
t(1;19)(q23;p13.3)	*PBX1* (1q23)	Pre-B transformation 1	Homeodomain	ALL	95,96
	E2A (19p13.3)	Early region 2A	bHLH transcription factor		
t(17;19)(q22;p13.3)	*HLF* (17q22)	Hepatic leukemia factor	Leucine zipper	ALL	100,101
	E2A (19p13.3)	Early region 2A	bHLH transcription factor		

(continued)

TABLE 46.1-1. *(Continued)*

Cytogenetic Abnormality	*Genes Involved*	*Derivation of Abbreviation*	*Protein Characterization*	*Disease*	*Reference*
FUSION OF *BCR-ABL*					
t(9;22) (q34;q11)	*ABL* (9q34)	Abelson	Tyrosine kinase	ALL, CML	108,109
	BCR (22q11)	Breakpoint cluster region	Serine kinase		
FUSIONS INVOLVING NUCLEOPORIN GENES					
t(6;9) (p23;q34)	*DEK* (6p23)	Not relevant to molecule	Transcription factor	AML	118
	CAN/NUP214 (9q34)	Nuclear pore 214	Nucleoporin		
inv(9) (q34q34)	*SET* (9q34)	Not relevant to molecule	Nuclear protein	AML	118
	CAN/NUP214 (9q34)	Nuclear pore 214	Nucleoporin		
t(7;11) (p15;p15)	*HOXA9* (7p15)	Homeobox A9	Homeobox protein	AML/MDS	122
	NUP98 (11p15)	Nuclear pore 98	Nucleoporin	AML	
GENE ACTIVATION INVOLVING THE IMMUNOGLOBULIN GENES					
t(8;14) (q24;q32)	*MYC* (8q24)	Myelocytomatosis virus	bHLH/bZIP transcription factor	ALL	124,125
	IGH (14q32)	Immunoglobulin heavy chain	Ig heavy chain promoter		
t(2;8) (p12;q24)	*IGK* (2p12)	Immunoglobulin kappa chain	Ig kappa chain promoter	ALL	179
	MYC (8q24)	Myelocytomatosis virus	bHLH/bZIP transcription factor		
t(8;22) (q24;q11)	*MYC* (8q24)	Myelocytomatosis virus	bHLH/bZIP transcription factor	ALL	180
	IGL (22q11)	Immunoglobulin lamda chain	Ig lamda chain promoter		
GENE ACTIVATION INVOLVING THE T CELL RECEPTOR GENES					
t(1;14) (p32;q11)	*TAL1/SCL* (1p33)	T-cell acute leukemia 1/ stem cell leukemia	bHLH transcription factor	ALL	128
	TCRα/δ (14q11)	T-cell receptor-α/δ	T-cell receptor promoter		
t(1;7) (p32;q34)	*TAL1/SCL* (1p32)	T-cell acute leukemia 1/ stem cell leukemia	bHLH transcription factor	ALL	129
	TCRβ (7q34)	T-cell receptor-β	T-cell receptor promoter		
t(7;9) (q34;q34)	*TCRβ* (7q34)	T-cell receptor-β	T-cell receptor promoter	ALL	130
	TAL2/SCL2 (9q34)	T-cell acute leukemia 2/ stem cell leukemia	bHLH transcription factor		
t(7;19) (q34;p13)	*TCRβ* (7q34)	T-cell receptor-β	T-cell receptor promoter	ALL	131
	LYL1 (19p13)	Lymphoid leukemia 1	bHLH transcription factor		
t(8;14) (q24;q11)	*MYC* (8q24)	Myelocytomatosis virus	bHLH/bZIP transcription factor	ALL	132–134
	TCRα/δ (14q11)	T-cell receptor-α/δ	T-cell receptor promoter		
t(11;14) (p15;q11)	*LMO1* (11p15)	LIM only 1	Zinc finger	ALL	136
	TCRα/δ (14q11)	T-cell receptor-α/δ	T-cell receptor promoter		
t(11;14) (p13;q11)	*LMO2* (11p13)	LIM only 2	Zinc finger	ALL	137
	TCRα/δ (14q11)	T-cell receptor-α/δ	T-cell receptor promoter		
t(7;10) (q34;q24)	*TCRβ* (7q34)	T-cell receptor-β	T-cell receptor promoter	ALL	141
	HOX11 (10q24)	Homeobox 11	Homeobox gene		
inv(14) (q11q32.1)	*TCL1* (14q32.1)	T-cell leukemia 1	β-barrel protein family	T-PLL	143
	TCRα/δ (14q11)	T-cell receptor-α/δ	T-cell receptor promoter		
t(14;14) (q11;q32)	*TCL1* (14q32.1)	T-cell leukemia 1	β-barrel protein family	T-PLL	143
	TCRα/δ (14q11)	T-cell receptor-α/δ	T-cell receptor promoter		
t(7;14) (q35;q32.1)	*TCRβ* (7q34)	T-cell receptor-β	T-cell receptor promoter	T-PLL	143
	TCL1 (14q32.1)	T-cell leukemia 1	β-barrel protein family		
t(X;14) (q28;q11)	*TCRα/δ* (14q11)	T-cell receptor-α/δ	T-cell receptor promoter	T-PLL	144
	MTCP1 (Xq28)	Mature T-cell proliferation-1	β-barrel protein family		

ALL, acute lymphoblastic leukemia; AML, acute myeloid leukemia; APL, acute promyelocytic leukemia; bHLH, basic helix-loop-helix; bZIP, basic region/leucine zipper; CML, chronic myeloid leukemia; CMML, chronic myelomonocytic leukemia; ETS, E twenty-six retrovirus; MDS, myelodysplastic syndrome; MLL, myeloid-lymphoid leukemia; T-PLL, T-cell prolymphocytic leukemia.

genesis by either gene fusion or gene activation, their chromosomal location and name derivation, a general description of their function, if known, and the type of leukemia with which they are associated. However, it should be noted that nearly one-half of all cases of leukemia do not have cytogenetic evidence of recurrent structural chromosomal rearrangements, but instead have changes only in chromosome number (e.g., monosomy 7 or trisomy 8), or completely normal cytogenetics. This severely restricts the molecular biologist's ability to focus in on *hot spots* in the genome where evidence of gene fusion or gene activation is likely to be found. Advances in a fraction of such cases have revealed that comparable genetic mechanisms of leukemogenesis are operative even in the absence of structural cytogenetic abnormalities.

In this chapter, we review the most common genetic disruptions that result from the recurrent cytogenetic aberrations in acute and chronic leukemia, and where possible, provide an explanation as to how such alterations contribute to the molecular pathogenesis of the disease. In addition, we review instances in which the molecular basis for leukemia has been determined in the absence of structural cytogenetic abnormalities. Finally, we discuss other genetic alterations, mostly in tumor suppressor genes, that are likely to contribute to the genesis or progression of leukemia. We proceed with a molecular description of leukemia that simply follows the list of the more common molecular defects provided in Table 46.1-1. There is little or no attention to the more traditional revised histologic classification of leukemia to put more emphasis on the genetic basis of leukemia.[8] Derivations of abbreviations used for the genes discussed in the text can be found in Table 46.1-1.

GENE FUSIONS IN LEUKEMIA

GENE FUSIONS INVOLVING CORE-BINDING FACTOR IN LEUKEMIA

Core-binding factor (CBF) is a heterodimeric transcription factor, composed of CBFA2 and CBFB, that is involved in the regulation of hematopoiesis (Fig. 46.1-1*A*). The CBFA2 protein (originally described as AML1) has an amino terminus domain with homology to the *Drosophila* runt protein, which is an early acting factor that regulates the expression of genes involved in segmentation during fly development.[9] The runt homology domain of CBFA2 confers at least two properties to the protein. The first is a DNA-binding domain that recognizes the sequence TGT/cGGT, an enhancer core motif that serves as a regulatory element in several genes important in hematopoiesis, such as *LCK, myeloperoxidase, granulocyte-macrophage colony-stimulating factor, interleukin-3, colony-stimulating factor, neutrophil elastase,* and *TCR*α, β, and γ.[10] The second important function of the runt homology domain of CBFA2 is that it is required for heterodimerization of CBFA2 with its normal partner CBFB. CBFB does not directly bind to DNA, but its binding to CBFA2 is thought to increase the heterodimeric transcription factor's affinity and stability for the target DNA-binding sequence.[9] More recently, the carboxyl terminus of CBFA2 was discovered to contain a transactivation domain that binds the transcriptional coactivator p300, a transcriptional regulator that has been shown to promote transcription via acetylation of histone proteins associated with targeted genes (see Fig. 46.1-1*A*).[11]

The CBF complex is the most frequent target of chromosomal translocations and inversions in human acute leukemia. At the molecular level, the t(8;21)(q22;q22) generates a chimeric gene fusing *CBFA2* with the *CBFA2T1* gene (originally described as *ETO*) at chromosome band 8q22.[12] The reciprocal *CBFA2T1-CBFA2* fusion, on the derivative chromosome 21, is often not expressed and thus does not appear to be essential for leukemogenesis. The CBFA2-CBFA2T1 fusion protein retains the runt homology domain and therefore its protein-protein binding (to CBFB) and its DNA-binding properties. However, the fusion of *CBFA2* with nearly the entire *CBFA2T1* coding sequence does create a protein that lacks the CBFA2 carboxyl terminal transactivation domain and may therefore interfere with CBF-mediated transcriptional activation of hematopoiesis through a dominant-negative mechanism (Fig. 46.1-1*B*).[13]

The CBFA2T1 protein binds to the human homologue of the murine nuclear receptor corepressor (N-COR). N-COR forms a complex with mammalian SIN3A and histone deacetylase 1 (HDAC1) and facilitates repression of transcription by altering chromatin structure via histone deacetylation.[14,15] It is thus possible that in t(8;21) acute myeloid leukemia (AML), the N-COR/SIN3A/HDAC1 complex is recruited to the CBF complex by the CBFA2-CBFA2T1 protein, thereby inducing repression of transcription by deacetylation of CBFA2-targeted genes (see Fig. 46.1-1B). This process may result in the disruption of normal hematopoiesis and may also inactivate tumor suppressor genes and other factors important for neoplastic transformation.[10,16] In support of such a hypothesis, there are data demonstrating that inhibitors of histone deacetylase can reverse CBFA2T1-mediated transcriptional repression and can induce differentiation of *CBFA2-CBFA2T1* leukemia cells.[17]

At the molecular level, inv(16)(p13q22) and t(16;16)(p13;q22) both result in the fusion of the *CBFB* gene, the normal partner of *CBFBA2* shown in Fig. 46.1-1*A* and located at chromosome 16q22, with the *MYH11* gene from chromosome 16p13.[18] The *MYH11* gene encodes a smooth muscle form of the myosin heavy chain, and it is the fusion of its carboxyl terminus with almost the entire *CBFB* gene, including its *CBFA2*-binding domain, that appears important for leukemogenesis. The genomic fusion between these two genes is quite variable, and at least eight different sized fusion transcripts have been described, the biologic and clinical significance of which are unclear.[19] The mechanism whereby the *CBFB-MYH11* fusion gene contributes to malignant transformation remains to be fully elucidated. *In vitro* analyses show that the CBFB-MYH11 chimeric protein can bind to the CBFA2 protein, which in turn can bind its TGT/cGGT core enhancer DNA sequence element, albeit with reduced DNA-binding activity. The carboxyl terminus of MYH11 does contain a functional domain, the myosin long tail, that might mediate homodimerization of the CBFB-MYH11 fusion protein into high-molecular-weight structures. It may therefore be possible that the CBFB-MYH11 homodimers could sequester CBFA2 subunits into a nonfunctional complex, thereby inhibiting the transcriptional activation of genes important for hematopoiesis. Indeed, Adya et al. provided compelling *in vitro* evidence in support of such a hypothesis, demonstrating that the CBFB-MYH11 homodimers could colocalize with the CBFA2 protein in actin filaments outside of the nucleus.[20] These data would therefore support a

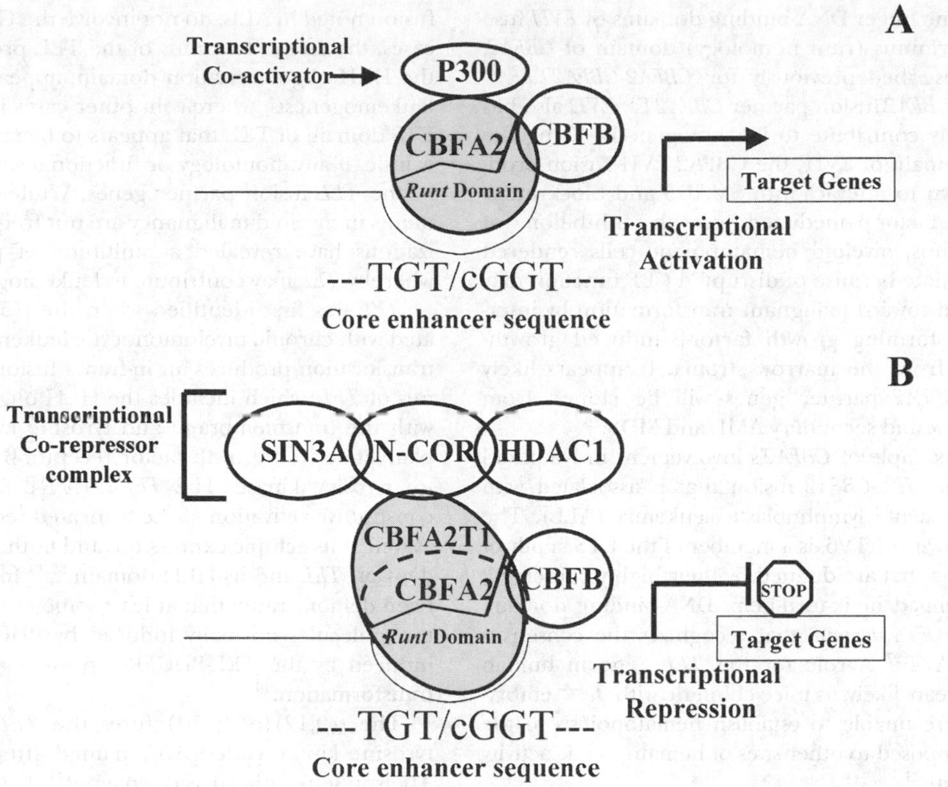

FIGURE 46.1-1. **A:** Schematized representation of the wild-type CBFA2-CBFB transcription factor complex. The DNA-binding domain of CBFA2 (originally described as AML1) recognizes the enhancer core motif of the target gene via its domain that has homology to the *Drosophila* runt protein. The CBFA2 runt domain is also required for heterodimerization with CBFB (originally described as CBFβ), which in turn increases the affinity and stability of CBFA2 binding to the core enhancer sequence, thereby promoting efficient activation of target gene transcription. Additional factors that act as coactivators of transcription participate in this complex formation (e.g., p300), depending on the particular target gene promoter or enhancer involved (e.g., myeloperoxidase, CSF-1 receptor, etc). **B:** Schematized representation of the transcription factor complex that results from the *CBFA2-CBFA2T1* (originally described as *AML1-ETO*) gene fusion in t(8;21)(q22;q22) acute myeloid leukemia. The CBFA2 runt domain is left intact following the fusion, allowing it to (1) recognize and bind to the enhancer core motif of the target gene and (2) heterodimerize with wild-type CBFB. However, its fusion partner, CBFA2T1, forms either a homodimer or a heterodimer (not shown) that then interacts with the nuclear corepressors (N-COR) and SIN3A, which complex with histone deacetylase 1 (HDAC1). This entire complex then facilitates repression of transcription by altering chromatin structure via histone deacetylation. (Adapted from ref. 7.)

dominant negative mechanism of CBFA2 gene inactivation by the CBFB-MYH11 fusion protein, leading to dysregulated hematopoiesis.

Mice have been generated with *Cbfb*$^{+Cbfb\text{-}MYH11}$ embryonic stem cells.[21] The *Cbfb*$^{+Cbfb\text{-}MYH11}$ mice are chimeric, in that they have hematopoietic stem cells with and without the knocked-in *Cbfb-MYH11* gene in the marrow. The mice have defective myeloid and lymphoid differentiation; however, they did not develop any malignancies in their first year of life. To test the hypothesis that additional genetic events might be required, the mice were injected with a single sublethal dose of N-ethyl-N nitrosourea, a potent DNA alkylating mutagen. Within 2 to 6 months after treatment, 84% of the treated *Cbfb*$^{+Cbfb\text{-}MYH11}$ chimeric mice developed acute myelomonocytic leukemia, whereas none of the control populations (*Cbfb*$^{+Cbfb\text{-}MYH11}$ chimeras without injection or wild-type mice with injection) developed leukemia. Leukemic cells expressed the *Cbfb-MYH11* fusion gene and, importantly, the mice did not show evidence of malignancy in other tissues where the *Cbfb-MYH11* fusion gene was not expressed. The data from this elegant experimental model and from others not discussed suggest that alterations in the CBF complex serve to block hematopoietic differentiation, while a *second hit* that targets these particular cells may be necessary to induce frank leukemia. The molecular analysis of human familial platelet disorder (FPD) with predisposition to AML (familial platelet disorder/AML) perhaps reveals the first clinical evidence in support of the mouse model. Patients with familial platelet disorder/AML have haploinsufficiency of *CBFA2,* which causes an autosomal dominant congenital platelet defect and may predispose to the acquisition of additional mutations that cause leukemia.[22]

There are other examples of fusion with *CBFA2* that lead to dysregulation of myeloid hematopoiesis and leukemic transformation. The t(3;21)(q26;q22) noted in myelodysplastic syndromes (MDS), AML, and blast crisis of chronic myeloid leukemia (CML) results in a fusion of *CBFA2* with the *EVI1* gene, where the zinc finger DNA-binding domains of *EVI1* fuse with the amino terminus (runt homology) domain of *CBFA2*, similar to that described previously for *CBFA2-CBFA2T1*.[23,24] However, like the *CBFA2* fusion partner *CBFA2T1*, *EVI1* also has properties that may contribute to leukemogenesis. Using the first zinc finger domain of EVI1, the CBFA2-EVI1 fusion product has been shown to interact with SMAD3 and block transforming growth factor-β–mediated growth inhibition of myeloid cells.[25] Thus, myeloid hematopoietic cells rendered unable to differentiate because of disrupted CBF function may be further induced toward malignant transformation by interference with transforming growth factor-β–induced growth-inhibitory signals from the marrow stroma. It appears likely that additional *CBFA2* partner genes will be cloned from patients with *de novo* and secondary AML and MDS.[26]

An important example of *CBFA2*'s involvement in lymphoid malignancies is the *TEL-CBFA2* fusion that is associated with pediatric B-lineage acute lymphoblastic leukemia (ALL). The *TEL* gene, also known as ETV6, is a member of the ETS family of transcription factors that are defined by their highly conserved, 90–amino acid, winged helix-turn-helix DNA-binding domain, also known as the *ETS domain*, that recognizes the consensus motif C/A GGA A/T.[27] A role for the *TEL* gene in human hematopoiesis appears likely, as mice chimeric with $Tel^{-/-}$ embryonic stem cells were unable to establish hematopoiesis in the bone marrow, as opposed to other sites of hematopoietic activity during development.[28]

The *TEL-CBFA2* fusion of childhood B-lineage ALL results from the t(12;21)(p13;q22). However, it is best identified by fluorescence *in situ* hybridization, because the juxtaposition of bands 12p13 and 21q22 is usually unrecognizable in banded metaphase preparations. The *TEL-CBFA2* fusion occurs in approximately 25% of cases of pediatric ALL and is therefore the most common gene rearrangement in any childhood cancer.[29,30] The fusion product contains the helix-loop-helix (HLH) homooligomerization domain near the amino terminus of *TEL* linked to, essentially, the full-length *CBFA2* gene, including both the runt homology domain as well as the carboxyl terminus transactivation domain. Indeed, this is the only *CBFA2* fusion in human leukemia currently known to incorporate the transactivation domain. It is likely that the *TEL-CBFA2* fusion contributes to a reduction in normal *CBFA2* function via a dominant negative mechanism.[31] However, in addition, this fusion invariably leads to the loss of the remaining wild-type *TEL* allele, suggesting that this might be an important contributor to leukemogenesis as well.[29,32] The mechanism by which such a contribution might occur remains unknown.[33]

The disruption of the CBF complex in t(8;21), inv(16), and t(12;21) confers a favorable prognosis on patients whose leukemic blasts harbor the consequent molecular alterations.[33,34] This does not appear to be the case for the t(3;21). The molecular basis for this clinical observation largely remains obscure, but there is at least preliminary evidence that downstream genes that could confer resistance to standard induction chemotherapy might be dysregulated by disruptions in the CBF complex.[35]

ADDITIONAL GENE FUSIONS WITH TEL

There are several chromosomal translocations in myeloid leukemia that disrupt the *TEL* gene, which, unlike the *TEL-CBFA2* fusion noted in ALL, do not involve the CBF complex. In some cases, the amino terminus of the TEL protein, which includes the HLH oligomerization domain, appears to be required for leukemogenesis, whereas in other cases it is the DNA-binding ETS domain of TEL that appears to be relevant. Further, there is little, if any, homology or functional similarity between most of the *TEL* fusion partner genes. While *TEL* gene rearrangements in myeloid malignancy are not frequent, their characterizations have revealed a multitude of possible mechanisms whereby *TEL* may contribute to leukemogenesis.[36]

TEL was first identified when the t(5;12)(q33;p13) associated with chronic myelomonocytic leukemia was cloned.[37] This translocation produces an in-frame fusion of the amino terminus of *TEL*, which includes the HLH oligomerization domain, with the transmembrane and tyrosine kinase domains of the platelet-derived growth factor receptor-β (PDGFR-β), a receptor tyrosine kinase. The *TEL-PDGFR-β* fusion results in both constitutive activation of the truncated receptor tyrosine kinase as well as its ectopic expression, and both properties are dependent on *TEL* and its HLH domain.[38,39] In model systems it has been demonstrated that at least some of the downstream effector molecules normally induced by PDGF, such as MYC, are induced by the TEL-PDGFR-β protein and are required for transformation.[40]

The t(9;12)(q34;p13) fuses the *TEL* gene with another tyrosine kinase called *ABL*, named after its homologue, the Abelson leukemia virus oncogene.[41] *ABL* is best known as the fusion partner with *BCR* (breakpoint cluster region) in CML (see Philadelphia-Positive Chronic Myeloid Leukemia and Acute Lymphoblastic Leukemia Result from a Fusion of BCR with the Tyrosine Kinase ABL, later in this chapter). The *TEL-ABL* fusion is strikingly similar to the *TEL-PDGFR-β* fusion, in that the in-frame fusion joins the HLH domain of *TEL* with the catalytic (kinase) domain of *ABL*. Once again, the HLH domain serves to oligomerize the ABL kinase, with subsequent constitutive ABL kinase activation. The fusion has been characterized in acute undifferentiated myeloid leukemia, atypical CML, and ALL. The similarities between the roles of *TEL* and *BCR* in their fusion with *ABL* are striking. They both appear to function by primarily inducing ABL oligomerization and consequent activation, i.e., a gain-of-function mechanism. Indeed, comparison of TEL-ABL and BCR-ABL transformation properties and downstream signal transduction events suggests that the fusion proteins are indistinguishable.[42]

The t(12;22)(p13;q11) is found in AML and in MDS. In contrast to the two fusions of *TEL* with tyrosine kinases noted previously, in which the HLH domain of *TEL* functions to oligomerize and activate the kinase, this translocation fuses the carboxyl terminus-containing *ETS* domain of *TEL* with the *MN1* gene that encodes a nuclear protein whose function is unknown. Two types of *MN1-TEL* fusion transcripts have been identified, one that includes the *TEL* HLH domain as well and one that disrupts the *TEL* HLH domain. This suggests that the oligomerization is not likely important in the process of malignant transformation, but rather that the DNA-binding or *ETS* domain is, and that *MN1-TEL*–mediated leukemic transformation occurs via a molecular pathway that normally involves *TEL*. The reciprocal *TEL-MN1* fusion products are not known to contain any functional domains, suggesting little or no contribution of this protein to leukemogenesis.[43]

MLL GENE: FUSIONS WITH MULTIPLE PARTNERS RESULT IN ACUTE LEUKEMIA

In our discussion of the *TEL* gene at chromosome band 12p13, we reviewed how *TEL* can fuse with a variety of partners, in a variety of ways, and participate in the genesis of both lymphoid and myeloid leukemias. However, the best example of a *promiscuous* partner in leukemia is the *MLL* gene located at chromosome band 11q23. This gene fuses with an extraordinary number (over 30) of diverse partner genes, examples of which are shown in Table 46.1-1. The fusions manifest in myeloid, lymphoid, or mixed lineage leukemias (defined by markers of more than one hematopoietic lineage) of infants, children, or adults, the clinical details of which are provided in subsequent chapters. Further, the leukemias involving *MLL* may be *de novo* or primary, but also account for as many as 80% of secondary leukemias that develop in patients who were successfully treated for other tumors at an earlier time with regimens that included topoisomerase II inhibitors.[44–46] Collectively, the clinical and correlative laboratory data support the notion that *MLL* is important for early pluripotent and lineage-specific hematopoiesis, and that disruption of *MLL* at 11q23 can give rise to leukemias of mixed or multiple lineages.

MLL (also known as *ALL1*, *HRX*, and *HTRX1*) was cloned by four independent groups and found to contain at least 36 exons that encode 3968 amino acids with a predicted molecular mass of 431 kD.[47–50] The various names for the single gene at 11q23 are derived from its association with *MLL*, its initial identification in a case of ALL (*ALL1*), and because of its strong homology to the *Drosophila* trithorax protein (*HRX* and *HTRX1*). This trithorax homology includes a highly conserved domain covering the carboxyl terminus known as SET, because it is also found in *s*uvar3-9, *e*nhancer-of-zeste, and *t*rithorax proteins (Fig. 46.1-2*A*).[49–53]

Collectively, the structural and functional data accumulated thus far strongly suggest that wild-type MLL is a maintenance factor for gene expression. For example, in *Drosophila*, trithorax (the MLL fly homologue) maintains homeobox gene expression, critical for normal development of the head, thorax, and abdomen.[52] Gene-targeting studies in mice demonstrated that MLL is a positive regulator of homeobox (*Hox*) gene expression and maintenance.[53,54] Mammalian *Hox* genes encode DNA-binding, homeodomain-containing, helix-turn-helix transcription factors that appear critical in both skeletal and blood cell development.[55] The $Mll^{-/-}$ mouse completely lacks *Hox* gene expression, has defects in yolk sac hematopoiesis, and is lethal to the embryo, while the $Mll^{+/-}$ mouse has a disruption in *Hox* gene expression and various consequent defects in skeletal, neural, craniofacial, and hematopoietic development.[53,56] *In vitro*, $Mll^{-/-}$ embryonic stem cells fail to undergo hematopoietic differentiation.[57] Structure function studies suggest that the SET domain of *MLL* is required for proper regulation of *Hox* gene expression.

Virtually all of the translocations involving *MLL* at 11q23 in human acute leukemia consistently disrupt the gene within an 8.5-kb region located between exons 5 and 11, joining the amino-terminal half of *MLL* to the partner gene. The large *MLL* fusion gene on the derivative 11 chromosome includes the AT hook minor groove DNA-binding motifs, a methyl-CpG binding domain (MCBD), the nuclear localization domain, and all or part of the overlapping transcriptional repression domain. Missing are the two protein-binding zinc finger domains in the mid region and the *trithorax* homology located in the SET domain at the carboxyl terminus of the protein (see Fig. 46.1-2*A*). This derivative chromosome 11 (der 11) thus contains the *MLL* promoter and the amino terminus of *MLL* fused to the carboxyl terminus encoded by the gene at the breakpoint of the partner chromosome and is always the one that is transcribed by the leukemic clone.[58]

In contrast to many of the other common translocations discussed in this chapter, we have thus far learned little about the mechanisms of *MLL*-associated leukemogenesis from the study of its many fusion partners (see Table 46.1-1 and Fig. 46.1-2*A*). There is limited similarity in protein structure between the partner genes currently known to fuse with *MLL* in acute myeloid, lymphoid, or mixed lineage leukemia. To date, 18 *MLL* fusion partner genes have been cloned and sequenced (see Fig. 46.1-2*A*), and there is no one structure-function that can unify their role in the malignant transformation of hematopoietic cells. Most of the cloned partners are novel genes and inference about their functions comes from the study of their homologies or *in vitro* systems. Several partners, such as *AF4*, *ENL*, *AF9*, *CBP*, and *P300* have evidence for transcriptional activation or coactivation domains, suggesting that replacement of the MLL zinc finger and SET domains by these partners could result in uncontrolled expression of MLL target genes, possibly within some lineage-specific, transcriptional context (e.g., *MLL-AF4* in lymphoblasts).[59] However, this alone cannot be the only pathway to malignant transformation, as other partner genes (e.g., *AF1q*) lack homology to any known protein sequence and contribute a minimal portion of its carboxyl terminus to the MLL fusion protein (see Fig. 46.1-2*A*), suggesting this fusion may only contribute through haploinsufficiency or possibly via a dominant negative effect.[60]

The multitude of partners that fuse with *MLL* in acute leukemia led us to hypothesize that the *MLL* gene might be rearranged without structural cytogenetic evidence of translocations, inversions, or deletions at 11q23. We therefore looked for evidence of *MLL* gene rearrangements in cases of AML without cytogenetic abnormalities involving 11q23, including cases with normal cytogenetics. Rearrangement of *MLL* was initially observed in cases of AML with trisomy 11 (+11) as a sole abnormality and in cases of AML with normal cytogenetics.[61] These rearrangements were subsequently not found to result from cryptic fusions with other partner genes, but rather from a partial tandem duplication (PTD) of *MLL* spanning exons 2 through 6 or exons 2 through 8 (see Fig. 46.1-2*B*).[62,63] The putative partially duplicated protein includes duplication of the AT hooks and MCBD, without loss of the carboxyl portion of the protein containing the SET domain. Molecular analysis of the chromosomes in a limited number of cases with +11 or normal cytogenetics and the *MLL* PTD revealed that only one of the alleles carries the rearrangement.[64] Sequence analysis of the genomic fusion in nine cases of *MLL* PTD indicated that the rearrangement is most likely the result of *Alu-Alu*–mediated homologous recombination events within the involved introns.[63,65,66] This is the first demonstration of homologous recombination between *Alu* elements as a consistent mechanism for gene rearrangement in somatic tissue.

The PTD of *MLL* has been found to be present in the majority of AML patients with +11 as a sole cytogenetic abnormality, as well as in some patients with +11 accompanied by

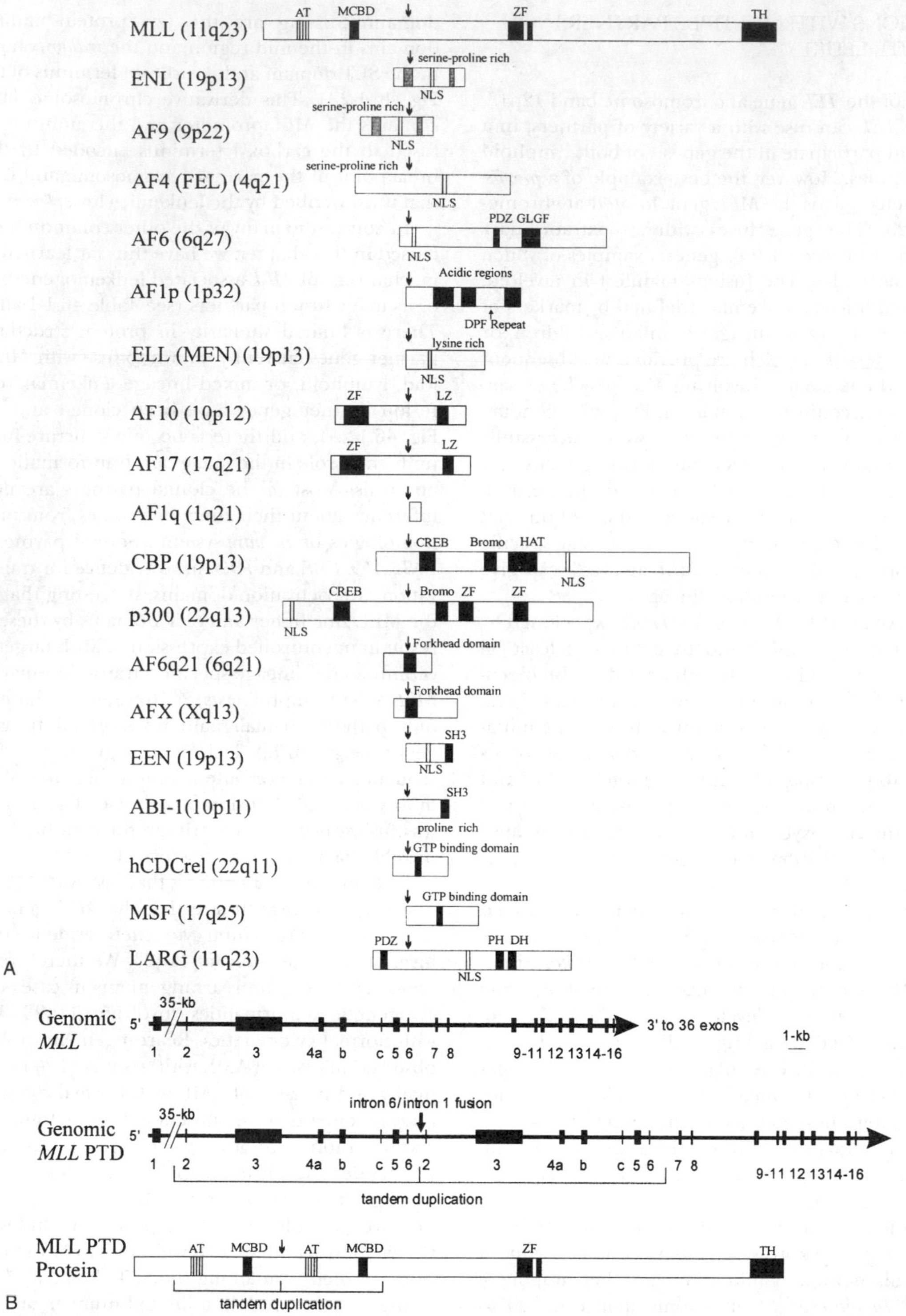

FIGURE 46.1-2. **A:** The MLL protein and its known fusion partners with various motifs identified. Protein motifs are indicated in black. The shaded gray regions in ENL and AF9 indicate known regions of homology. Fusion breakpoints are indicated by *arrows.* AF1q is unique in that its fusion breakpoint occurs six nucleotides upstream of its open reading frame, resulting in a fusion protein without functional domains. Protein motifs are indicated in black. AT, AT hooks; bromo, bromodomain; CREB, cAMP response element-binding protein site; DH, *Dbl* homology domain; DPF, aspartic acid-proline-phenylalanine repeat; GLGF, glycine-leucine-phenylalanine domain; HAT, histone acetyltransferase activity; LZ, leucine zipper; MCBD, methyl-CpG binding domain; NLS, nuclear localization signal; PDZ, PDZ domain; PH, pleckstrin homology domain; SH3, *Src* homology domain; TH, trithorax homology (SET domain); ZF, zinc fingers. **B:** The genomic structures of *MLL* and *MLL* with an exon 6–exon 2 partial tandem duplication (PTD) are shown. Exons are indicated by vertical lines and boxes, and introns are indicated by the horizontal line for each structure. Vertical arrow indicates point of unique self-fusion that results from the PTD. The predicted protein structure for MLL with the 6-2 PTD is illustrated below and can be compared with the wild-type protein at top of the figure (**A**).

additional cytogenetic abnormalities,[67,68] and is the first consistent gene rearrangement associated with recurrent trisomy in human cancer. In a study of 98 AML patients with normal cytogenetics, 11% of patients had rearrangement of *MLL*, and in eight of eight cases in which additional material was available, the *MLL* PTD was documented. In patients with AML and normal cytogenetics, a rearranged *MLL* gene was associated with a poorer prognosis compared with the remaining AML patients with normal cytogenetics.[69] These adverse prognostic data were confirmed in a separate study, but with a lower percentage (6%) of the *MLL* PTD in AML cases with normal cytogenetics.[70] Thus, the *MLL* PTD is an example of a novel gene fusion detectable in a significant fraction of AML patients without structural cytogenetic abnormalities.

MLL gene rearrangements are seen in 80% of infant ALL cases and in approximately 50% of infant AML cases.[71] There have now been several elegant reports of infant twins developing acute leukemia with 11q23 translocations involving *MLL in utero*.[72–74] The concordance rate for the development of 11q23-related acute leukemia in monozygotic twins with shared circulation approaches 100%, with the disease manifesting quickly (i.e., 5 to 24 months of age). The concordance rate for monozygotic twins with shared circulation who develop childhood common ALL, including those with the *TEL-CBFA2* fusion, is estimated to be less than or equal to 5%, with the leukemia often developing 3 to 4 years after birth.[75] These twin studies suggest that proliferating pluripotent progenitor cells in the developing bone marrow are uniquely susceptible to malignant transformation by *MLL*-associated chimeric fusion proteins. Further, the identical *MLL* gene rearrangements found within each pair of twins suggests the leukemic clone arose in one infant and spread via the placental circulation to the other twin infant.

Approximately 80% of leukemias that develop secondarily in patients treated with DNA-topoisomerase II inhibitors such as the epipodophyllotoxins (e.g., etoposide) and the anthracyclines are associated with a chimeric gene fusion involving *MLL*.[44–46] While the *MLL* fusions in secondary AML occur within the 8.5-kb breakpoint cluster region, they are more often distributed in the telomeric region, compared with the more centromeric region in cases of primary AML. Interestingly, the telomeric region has scaffold attachment regions and topoisomerase II consensus binding sites.[76,77] The DNA-topoisomerase II inhibitors stabilize the DNA-topoisomerase II complex after it cleaves double-stranded DNA, allowing for the accumulation of double-strand DNA breaks that are then presumably more susceptible to *MLL* translocations via nonhomologous recombination events. Acute leukemia then develops within 6 to 24 months after diagnosis of the primary malignancy, and typically without antecedent MDS. This is in distinct contrast to the secondary acute leukemias that develop following exposure to alkylating agents, which lack an association with *MLL*, have a chromosome 7q- or 5q- karyotype, have a latency period of 5 to 10 years, and are more often associated with an antecedent MDS.[78]

The short latency noted with *MLL*-associated infant and secondary acute leukemia suggests that the molecular defect itself might be all that is required for malignant transformation, or might predispose the affected hematopoietic stem cells to rapidly undergo additional secondary mutations. For example, if the fusion with an *MLL* partner gene protected against apoptosis or promoted enhanced cell growth, the stimulation from marrow stromal factors in the developing fetus or in the patient recovering from topoisomerase II inhibitor chemotherapy-induced aplasia might lead to the rapid acquisition of additional genetic alterations associated with full transformation of the leukemic clone.[79]

RETINOIC ACID RECEPTOR GENE REARRANGEMENTS IN ACUTE PROMYELOCYTIC LEUKEMIA

Acute promyelocytic leukemia (APL) is one of the best examples of how a molecular characterization of leukemia can provide insights into the pathogenesis and the success of a serendipitous treatment approach. A unique molecular defect, the *PML/RAR-α* fusion, segregates with a single phenotype, FAB M3 AML, and identifies a set of patients who are essentially all initially responsive to differentiation therapy with all-*trans*-retinoic acid (ATRA).[80] *RAR-α* is located on chromosome 17 and encodes a transcriptionally active protein that contains two zinc finger DNA-binding domains and a ligand-binding domain that interacts with retinoic acid derivatives. The promyelocytic leukemia (*PML*) gene is located on chromosome 15 and encodes a protein that also has zinc finger motifs.[81,82] PML proteins are normally localized to macromolecular nuclear organelles called PML oncogenic domains (PODs). With the t(15;17)(q22;q12-21), the resultant PML/RAR-α fusion protein contains each of the functional domains described previously, yet appears to act as a dominant negative inhibitor of wild-type RAR-α function, and disrupts the PODs into a dispersed microparticulate pattern, preventing localization of PML. Both of these effects likely lead to an arrest in myeloid differentiation at the promyelocyte stage, and the subsequent development of APL, but the molecular details of this process are not yet clear.[83] One mechanism for the transcriptional inhibitory effect on myeloid differentiation is the PML/RAR-α fusion protein's ability to bind DNA and form complexes with N-COR and HDAC1, as was shown for the CBFA2-CBFA2T1 fusion protein in Figure 46.1-1*B*. The complex in turn alters chromatin conformation in such a way that transcription of target genes responsible for myeloid differentiation is repressed.[84,85] ATRA appears to overcome the dominant negative actions of the PML/RAR-α fusion protein and allows PML to relocalize to the PODs. It releases the N-COR and HDAC1 complex from the PML/RAR-α DNA-bound protein, allowing RAR-α–mediated transcription and myeloid differentiation to proceed.[86] The serendipitous introduction of ATRA for the treatment of APL turned out to be the first truly effective targeted therapy for the treatment of acute leukemia and has had a profound effect on improving the cure rate for this disease (see Chapter 46.2). Resistance to ATRA likely involves the up-regulation of cellular retinoic acid–binding proteins as well as increased cellular degradation of ATRA.

The disruption of the *RAR-α* locus and its fusion with other nuclear proteins via chromosome translocation is responsible for the APL phenotype (see Table 46.1-1). One of several variant translocations involving *RAR-α* is the t(11;17)(q23;q21), which fuses the *PLZF* (for promyelocytic leukemia zinc finger) gene with *RAR-α* and results in APL that is not responsive to ATRA.[87] When fused with *RAR-α*, PLZF itself is capable of forming complexes with N-COR and HDAC1[88] that in turn inhibit the transcription of target genes responsible for myeloid differentiation. However, unlike PML, PLZF does not disassociate from the complex on exposure to ATRA, thus maintaining a repressed chromatin conformation and consequent inhibition of transcription in the presence of this treatment.[86]

GENE FUSIONS IN B-LINEAGE ACUTE LYMPHOBLASTIC LEUKEMIA INVOLVING THE *E2A* GENE

The *E2A* gene encodes a basic HLH (bHLH) transcription factor that was originally discovered to regulate Ig kappa gene expression,[89] but was subsequently found to have three differentially spliced products involved in multiple regulatory aspects of B-cell development.[90] The amino terminus of the E2A-encoded protein contains two transcriptional activation domains,[91] and the carboxyl terminus contains the bHLH domain. The latter is responsible for both DNA binding and homodimerization or heterodimerization with other bHLH proteins. The various protein partners normally dimerizing with the *E2A* gene products determine its DNA-binding specificity and consequent gene activation during development.[92] The E2A homodimer is itself critically important during normal B-cell development.[93,94] It is the carboxyl end of *E2A* that is disrupted by distinct partner genes in two important gene fusions associated with B-lineage ALL (see Table 46.1-1). Both of the fusion proteins invariably contain the two transcriptional activation domains at the amino terminus of E2A.

The t(1;19)(q23;p13) occurs in childhood pre–B-cell ALL and fuses the amino terminus of *E2A*, including the two transactivation domains, to the homeodomain of *PBX1*, a member of the TALE (three-amino acid extension) family of homeodomain proteins.[95,96] *PBX1* is normally not expressed during B-cell development. The inclusion of the PBX1 homeodomain in the fusion protein is likely critical to leukemogenesis, as it allows complex formation with HOX proteins, substituting for the severed bHLH DNA-binding protein interaction domain of E2A. Thus, although *PBX1*, by itself, has no transactivating ability, its fusion with the strong *E2A* transactivating domains bestows this property on the novel chimeric protein,[97] allowing for activation of genes normally controlled by PBX1-HOX complexes, but with inappropriate expression in the pre-B cell. Indeed, the first of such genes (*WNT-16, EB-1*) have been identified and will likely provide additional insights into the mechanism by which this fusion transcript induces malignant transformation of human pre-B cells.[98,99]

E2A also fuses with the hepatic leukemia factor (*HLF*) gene in the t(17;19)(q22;p13) in a small subset of ALL patients with the pro–B-cell (CD45R+) phenotype and only partial rearrangement of a functional heavy chain gene.[100,101] *HLF* is a basic region/leucine zipper (bZIP) transcription factor whose protein product has structural similarity to the proapoptotic gene product of *Caenorhabditis elegans, CES-2* (for cell-death specification-2).[102] *In vitro* studies demonstrate that the E2A-HLF fusion protein induces strong antiapoptotic gene expression in pro-B cells,[103] and that amino terminus-containing transactivation domains of E2A are critical for this function, while the DNA-binding and protein dimerization motifs of HLF are not.[104] It thus appears that *E2A-HLF* contributes to leukemogenesis by interfering with an evolutionarily conserved lineage-specific suicide pathway in pro-B cells, leading to prolonged survival and subsequent malignant transformation of genetically altered cells normally programmed for cell death.[104]

PHILADELPHIA-POSITIVE CHRONIC MYELOID LEUKEMIA AND ACUTE LYMPHOBLASTIC LEUKEMIA RESULT FROM A FUSION OF *BCR* WITH THE TYROSINE KINASE *ABL*

The Philadelphia chromosome[105] is produced by a t(9;22)(q34;q11)[106] that results in a fusion of the phosphoprotein BCR with the truncated ABL tyrosine kinase protooncogene on chromosome 22.[107–109] The t(9;22) and subsequently the fusion oncoprotein were first noted in patients with CML, and then in 30% to 40% of adults and 3% to 5% of children with ALL.[110] In CML and in ALL, the *ABL* gene consistently fuses within its first intron to *BCR*, thus always contributing its complete tyrosine kinase domain. However, in CML, *BCR* fuses to *ABL* within a 5.8-kb region known as the major breakpoint cluster region that spans exons 12 through 16 to produce a chimeric oncoprotein product known as $p210^{bcr\text{-}abl}$, while in ALL and a minority of patients with CML, *ABL* fuses with *BCR* at various sites within its first intron known as the minor breakpoint cluster region to produce a chimeric oncoprotein product known as $p185^{bcr\text{-}abl}$ or $p190^{bcr\text{-}abl}$. A larger BCR-ABL fusion protein ($p230^{bcr\text{-}abl}$) has been found in a subgroup of CML patients with a more indolent clinical course (reviewed in reference 111).

The ability of the BCR-ABL fusion protein to transform cells has been studied in a host of elegant *in vitro* and *in vivo* systems by numerous investigators and has provided insight into what regions of the fusion protein are required for transformation of cell lines and which signal transduction pathways are likely involved in mediating this transformation. A comprehensive review of this work has been carefully undertaken.[112] The first 63 amino acids of BCR are responsible for the tetramerization of the fusion protein, which is necessary for tyrosine kinase activation and activation of the F-actin binding function within ABL. Tyrosine 177 in the BCR portion of the fusion protein is required for transformation because once phosphorylated by the ABL tyrosine kinase it serves as a docking site for the SH2 domain of Grb-2.[113] The phosphoserine-threonine domain located between amino acids 192 and 413 of BCR may be responsible for activation of the ABL kinase.

The three regions in the ABL portion of the fusion protein that are required for transformation are the SH2 domain, the SH1 tyrosine kinase domain, and the F-actin binding domain.[112] Three properties of the fusion protein appear to contribute critically to its *in vitro* transforming ability: First, BCR-ABL has constitutive and elevated tyrosine kinase activity; second, this dysregulated kinase activity is confined to the cytoplasm, in distinct contrast to the wild-type ABL that moves between the nucleus and the cytoplasm[114,115]; and third, its constitutive activation of the tyrosine kinase domain in the cytoplasm results in the activation of a multitude of both cytoplasmic and nuclear signaling pathways that enhance the cell's growth and survival (Fig. 46.1-3). The substrates activated as a consequence of this signaling include CRKL, CBL, RIN, RAS, RAF, phosphatidylinositol-3-kinase, JUN, MYC, STAT5, PAXILLIN, and FAK (reviewed in references 111 and 112). However, although these studies reveal the complexity by which the BCR-ABL fusion protein can transform *in vitro*, it is unclear how much of this dysregulation is responsible for the clinical disease we know as CML. The use of different promot-

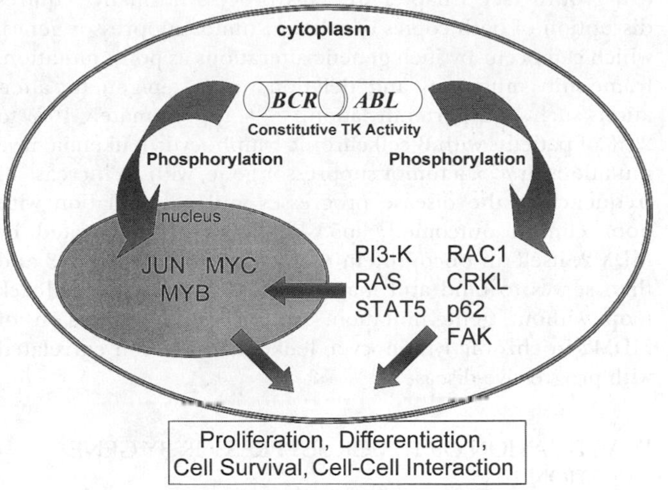

FIGURE 46.1-3. Promiscuous cell signaling by the BCR-ABL oncoprotein. The t(9;22)(q34;q11) results in the fusion of the phosphoprotein BCR with the truncated ABL tyrosine kinase protooncogene. The first 63 amino acids of BCR are responsible for the fusion protein tetramerization and consequent constitutive and elevated tyrosine kinase activity that is restricted to the cytoplasm. This activation results in phosphorylation of a multitude of cellular and nuclear signaling molecules (some of which are shown) whose pathways ultimately affect cell growth, differentiation, and cell survival. PI3-K, phosphatidylinositol-3 kinase; TK, tyrosine kinase.

ers to drive the expression of the oncoprotein, the absence of the *ABL-BCR* gene, and the presence of two wild-type *BCR* and *ABL* alleles may, among other *in vitro* conditions, all serve to sufficiently alter the dose or function of BCR-ABL in the transduced cell lines such that it may bear only some resemblance to what may actually happen *in vivo.* The specific oral ABL kinase inhibitor STI571 was tested in chronic phase CML patients who had failed to respond to interferon therapy, and complete hematologic response (i.e., normalization of counts for greater than or equal to 4 weeks) was obtained in 23 of 24 (96%) patients on treatment for at least 4 weeks, with minimal side effects. A significant fraction of these patients have also achieved a complete cytogenetic response as well, again emphasizing how specific targeting of molecular defects is likely to have a significant effect on treatment outcome (see Chapter 46.3.1).[116]

GENE FUSIONS INVOLVING THE NUCLEOPORIN FAMILY OF PROTEINS

Nucleoporins (NUP) make up the nuclear pore complex (NPC), which promotes the selective transportation of both RNA and protein between the nucleus and the cytoplasm in a bidirectional fashion.[117] In the past several years, a series of gene fusions involving two NUPs have been described in *de novo* AML, treatment-related AML, and in T-cell ALL. The first such fusion to be cloned was *DEK-CAN,* found in children and young adults with t(6;9)(p23;q34) AML (see Table 46.1-1).[118] *CAN,* also called *NUP214,* is an NPC protein that contains multiple NUP-specific Phe-Gly (FG) peptide sequence motifs that mediate protein-protein interaction thought to be required for nuclear-cytoplasmic transport, cell-cycle control, and cell survival.[119,120] *NUP214* fuses with the amino terminus of *DEK,* a putative DNA-binding transcription factor. *NUP214* has also been shown, in a single case of inv(9)(q34q34) AML,[118] to fuse with SET, a nuclear protein that is thought to regulate G_1/S transition by modulating the activity of cyclin E–cyclin-dependent kinase-2 activity via p21^{Cip1}.[121] *SET-NUP214,* like *DEK-NUP214,* is located exclusively in the nucleus, leaves the FG repeat-rich motif intact, and therefore presumably interacts with the same cellular proteins likely to be important in leukemogenesis.[119]

The other important NPC gene involved in leukemogenesis is *NUP98,* located at chromosome 11p15, which, like *NUP214,* lends it amino terminus FG repeat domains to fuse in frame to a variety of partners in acute leukemia. *NUP98* was first identified as part of the t(7;11)(p15;p15), associated primarily with AML.[122] In this instance, *NUP98* fuses with the carboxyl terminus of *HOXA9,* located at chromosome 7p15, a homeobox gene that regulates hematopoietic differentiation. Evidence suggests that this fusion transcript requires the *HOXA9* domains for DNA binding and interaction with PBX proteins, while the FG repeats of NUP98 act as transactivators of gene transcription and recruit cAMP response element (CREB)–binding protein and p300 as requisite transcriptional coactivators. Thus, the properties of the NUP98-HOXA9 fusion protein collectively result in a deregulation of HOX-responsive genes with consequent induction of AML.[123] The other fusion partners of *NUP98* have not yet shed additional light on the mechanism of FG-rich NPC protein-mediated leukemogenesis, but do provide supporting evidence that *NUP98* is a recurrent target primarily in treatment-related AML/MDS.

GENE ACTIVATION IN LEUKEMIA

GENE ACTIVATION INVOLVING IMMUNOGLOBULIN GENES IN B-CELL LEUKEMIA AND LYMPHOMA

In the t(8;14)(q24;q32), the prototypic bHLH/bZIP transcription factor *MYC* is juxtaposed to a region of strong Ig heavy chain enhancer elements. Two variants have also been described in which regulatory portions of the *Igk* gene on chromosome 2 or the *Ig lambda* (λ) gene on chromosome 22 are juxtaposed to the *MYC* locus of chromosome 8 (see Table 46.1-1). In each instance, the B cell experiences a deregulation of *MYC* gene expression because of its inappropriate activation and control by Ig regulatory elements whose expression is B-cell specific. This resultant malignant B-cell transformation takes the form of either Burkitt's lymphoma or ALL. The earliest of these studies were the first to demonstrate that rearrangement of specific genes that resulted from chromosomal translocations were actually at the heart of malignant transformation.[124,125]

MYC is capable of activating gene transcription by forming a heterodimer with MAX, which normally homodimerizes with itself or heterodimerizes with MAD or MXI-1 to repress transcription. Therefore, the overexpression of *MYC* in B lymphocytes, carrying the t(8;14)(q24;q32) or one of its variants, functions to disrupt the normal equilibrium that MAX shares with its partners, ultimately leading to the inappropriate overexpression of a multitude of downstream genes activated by the MYC-MAX heterodimer. How the activation of these downstream events in turn induces the malignant B-cell transformation is still incompletely understood and an area of intense study (reviewed in references 126 and 127).

GENE ACTIVATION INVOLVING T-CELL RECEPTOR GENE IN T-CELL LEUKEMIA AND LYMPHOMA

A comparable group of transcription factors, normally active during early hematopoiesis, but not during more committed T-cell development, are rearranged via chromosome translocation to lie near enhancers within the T-cell receptor *TCRβ* (chromosome 7q34) and *TCRα/δ* (chromosome 14q11) loci. As a consequence, these regulatory genes become inappropriately expressed, and their protein products contribute to T-cell leukemogenesis. They include the bHLH *TAL1/SCL*,[128,129] *TAL2/SCL2*,[130] *LYL1*,[131] as well as *MYC*.[132–134] Each of these specific translocations are listed in Table 46.1-1.

Rearrangements involving *TAL* account for up to 25% of childhood cases of T-cell ALL and T-cell lymphoma, but are seen infrequently in adults. *TAL1* is normally coexpressed with another transcription factor called *LM02*, and both are part of a larger transcriptional complex that includes the zinc finger transcription factors *GATA1* and *E2A*. The complex is likely to be important for normal erythropoiesis.[135] *LM02* and *LM01* are both rearranged near the regulatory elements of *TCR* loci in T-cell ALL (see Table 46.1-1).[136–138] The mouse *Hox11* gene is a homeobox transcription factor that is likely critical for lymphocyte development and survival, in that it prevents apoptosis of splenocytes in the mouse.[139] Further, *Hox11* interacts with a protein serine-threonine phosphatase, PP1C, allowing bypass of the G_2 checkpoint following injury and progression to the M phase.[140] Thus, its juxtaposition within the regulatory regions of the *TCRβ* and *TCRα/δ* loci[141] results in its ectopic expression in T cells, which likely contributes to T-cell ALL via its inhibition of normal programmed cell death and disruption of normal cell cycling, two processes that facilitate tumor progression.

T-cell prolymphocytic leukemia (T-PLL) is a rare form of mature T-cell leukemia characterized by chromosomal inversions and translocations involving chromosome band 14q11, containing the *TCRα/δ* gene. The inv(14)(q11q32.1) and the t(14;14)(q11;q32) each juxtapose the T-cell leukemia-1 (*TCL1*) gene at 14q32.1 to *TCRα/δ*, and the rarely seen t(7;14)(q35;q32.1) juxtaposes *TCL1* to the *TCRβ* gene.[142,143] The t(X;14) (q28;q11) rearranges another gene, *MTCP1*, within the *TCRα/δ* locus as well in T-PLL.[144] While the function of *TCL1* and *MTCP1* remain unknown, they share 40% amino acid identity, and with the elucidation of the three-dimensional structure of *MTCP1* showing a compact eight-stranded β-barrel structure, it appears that these two gene products are the first members of a β-barrel family of proteins.[145]

TUMOR SUPPRESSOR GENES IN LEUKEMIA

INACTIVATION OF TUMOR SUPPRESSOR BY GENE MUTATION

Mutations in tumor suppressor genes that result in functional inactivation likely contribute to the process of malignant transformation by disrupting the signals that normally inhibit cell growth (see Chapter 6). This process normally requires disruption of both copies of relevant tumor suppressor genes, which can occur by such genetic alterations as point mutation, frame-shift mutation, and deletion, or by epigenetic alterations such as hypermethylation.[146,147] Approximately 10% to 20% of patients with B-cell chronic lymphocytic leukemia have mutations in *p53*, a tumor suppressor gene, with an increase in frequency as the disease progresses and a correlation with poor clinical outcome.[148] p53 can also be inactivated by MDM2, itself an oncoprotein that is up-regulated by p53 and then serves to bind and inactivate it in a negative feedback loop without gene mutation. An increased expression of MDM2 in chronic lymphocytic leukemia has been correlated with progressive disease.[149]

INACTIVATION OF TUMOR SUPPRESSOR BY GENE DELETION

The frequent deletion of the human chromosome 9p21 region in leukemia and other cancers led to the search and ultimate discovery of two tumor suppressor genes at this locus, *p16* and *p15*. *p16* blocks cell-cycle progression by inhibiting cyclin-dependent kinase, as does *p15*, whose expression can be induced by transforming growth factor-β.[150–152] A review of the literature on the frequency of *p15* and *p16* deletions ($p15^{del}$ and $p16^{del}$, respectively) in leukemia showed they were frequently deleted in T-lineage ALL, ranging between 47% and 64%, as well as in B-lineage ALL, with a frequency between 20% and 27%. Likewise, in CML lymphoid blast crisis, the frequency of $p15^{del}$ was noted to be 27%, while $p16^{del}$ was 35%. There was little difference in frequency between children and adults with ALL, but $p15^{del}$ and $p16^{del}$ were absent from infants with ALL. The frequency of $p15^{del}$ and $p16^{del}$ was noted to be low in chronic T- and B-cell leukemias and is uncommon in AML, MDS, or CML (i.e., less than or equal to 2%).[153]

ATM is a kinase and putative tumor suppressor gene thought to have a role in cell-cycle checkpoint control. Indeed, patients with the genetic disease ataxia-telangiectasia have a loss of *ATM*, an increased frequency of translocations and inversions involving *TCL1*, and a clonal excess of mature T cells. This develops years before a significant fraction of these patients progress to T-PLL.[154,155] This finding is consistent with a model by which the deregulation of *TCL1* could serve as a tumor initiator, and loss of tumor suppressor genes might function to further promote progression of T-PLL. In strong support of this model and in support of *ATM* as a tumor suppressor gene, a large fraction of sporadic T-PLL cases, many with rearrangements of *TCL1*, have been shown to contain inactivating deletions and missense mutations of *ATM*.[156]

INACTIVATION OF TUMOR SUPPRESSOR BY HYPERMETHYLATION

Methylation of CpG islands located in the 5' regulatory region of genes can lead to the repression of gene transcription and illustrates an epigenetic mechanism for inactivation of tumor suppressor genes.[147] Multiple known tumor suppressor genes have been shown to be inactivated via hypermethylation in leukemia, including *p15* and *p16*. While *p16* is often inactivated by hypermethylation in epithelial tumors, it is *p15* that is frequently inactivated by hypermethylation in hematologic malignancies, most notably in AML and MDS, but also in ALL. Intriguingly, *p16* is not inactivated in these cases by either deletion, methylation, or point mutation.[157–159] In AML, and possibly in MDS, the density of *p15* methylation (i.e., the percent of CpG dinucleotides that are methylated on each allele) appears to correlate best with the degree of gene silencing and may increase as the disease progresses.[157,160] Other candidate tumor suppressor genes, such as *p73* in ALL,[161] have also been shown to be inactivated by hypermethylation.

While most investigations of aberrant CpG island methylation in human cancer have primarily taken a candidate gene approach, we performed a global analysis of the methylation status of 1184 unselected CpG islands in each of 98 primary human tumors including AML using a technique termed *restriction landmark genomic scanning*. This approach showed that an average of 608 CpG islands were aberrantly methylated in these tumors (range, 0 to 4500), and it allowed the identification of patterns of CpG island methylation that were shared within each tumor type, together with a pattern that was specific for acute leukemia. Which tumor suppressor genes are systematically silenced by this process has not yet been determined. However, these data suggest that the methylation of particular subsets of CpG islands has specific consequences for leukemogenesis and is likely an important event in disease progression.[162] One of the exciting avenues being pursued by several laboratories is the reversal of methylation status with pharmacologic agents such as 5-azacytidine, which often results in reexpression of the target gene.

MOLECULAR MONITORING OF LEUKEMIA

ASSESSMENT OF MINIMAL RESIDUAL DISEASE

Molecular analysis can not only play a role in the diagnosis and treatment of leukemia, but may also prove to be useful for monitoring a patient's response to therapy. Both the exponential amplification of small fragments of DNA and RNA by polymerase chain reaction (PCR) and reverse transcription PCR, respectively, and the growing discovery of the unique gene fusions and *Ig* and *TCR* gene rearrangements in leukemia, form the basis for our ability to detect the presence of these genetic alterations while a patient is in complete morphologic and clinical remission. There have been at least two important observations made with the advancement of this technology and the explosion of literature on the subject of minimal residual disease (MRD) in leukemia. First, in some instances (e.g., *MLL* PTD, *BCR-ABL*), the fusion transcripts can be detected in bone marrow, blood samples, or both from normal individuals.[163–167] The reasons for this are not entirely clear, but in some cases the fusions in normal individuals are clearly distinct from the malignant gene fusions and likely occur through entirely different mechanisms.[66,164,165]

Second, the persistence of *PCR-detectable* chimeric or rearranged genes is not at all a guarantee of persistent functional disease or eventual relapse in either CML[168] or some types of AML (e.g., *CBFA2-CBFA2T1*).[169,170] The reasons for this are also not known, but likely involve the presence of the fusion transcript in a normal parental clone, immunologic suppression of MRD by the host, or the absence of additional genetic alterations that were required for tumor initiation, progression, or both.[171] There are some striking examples of how the detection of MRD by PCR can predict relapse in ALL[172] and APL,[173] but most of these studies have yet to be confirmed in large prospective trials with standardized criteria for quantitative methodologies and uniform evaluation intervals. The ability to accurately quantify these genes and gene products using more fully automated technologies[174] might ultimately identify levels of MRD above which relapse is probable and below which relapse is unlikely. However, as we learn more about the evolutionary history of the leukemic clone and the seemingly high likelihood that in many instances, a multitude of genetic alterations are required for leukemogenesis, the simultaneous detection of several such alterations may prove to be more predictive of outcome following the achievement of a clinical complete remission. The incorporation of genetic profiling with cDNA microarray technology is likely to have a significant effect on unraveling the molecular complexity of leukemia for the purposes of diagnosis, classification, treatment, and monitoring clinical outcome.[175]

Acknowledgments

The authors would like to thank Tamra Brooks, John Byrd, Megan Cooper, Todd A. Fehniger, Peter J. Kourlas, Guido Marcucci, Krzysztof Mrózek, Laura Rush, Matthew P. Strout, and Susan P. Whitman for their assistance. This work was supported in part by grants P30 CA16058, U10 CA37027, and T32 CA09338, National Cancer Institute, Bethesda, MD, and the Coleman Leukemia Research Fund.

REFERENCES

1. Croce CM. Role of chromosome translocations in human neoplasia. *Cell* 1987;49:155.
2. Rowley JD. The critical role of chromosome translocations in human leukemias. *Annu Rev Genet* 1998;32:495.
3. Rabbitts TH. Translocations, master genes, and differences between the origins of acute and chronic leukemias. *Cell* 1991;67:641.
4. Rabbitts TH. Chromosomal translocations in human cancer. *Nature* 1994;372:143.
5. Look AT. Oncogenic transcription factors in the human acute leukemias. *Science* 1997;278:1059.
6. Bishop JM. The molecular genetics of cancer. *Science* 1987;235:305.
7. Look AT. Genes altered by chromosomal translocations in leukemias and lymphomas. In: Vogelstein B, Kinzler KW, eds. *The genetic basis of human cancer.* New York: McGraw-Hill, 1998:109.
8. Harris NL, Jaffe ES, Diebold J, et al. World Health Organization classification of neoplastic diseases of the hematopoietic and lymphoid tissues: report of the Clinical Advisory Committee Meeting—Airlie House, November 1997. *J Clin Oncol* 1999;17:3835.
9. Meyers S, Downing JR, Hiebert SW. Identification of AML-1 and the (8;21) translocation protein (AML-1/ETO) as sequence-specific DNA-binding proteins: the runt homology domain is required for DNA binding and protein-protein interactions. *Mol Cell Biol* 1993;13:6336.
10. Downing JR. The AML1-ETO chimaeric transcription factor in acute myeloid leukaemia: biology and clinical significance. *Br J Haematol* 1999;106:296.
11. Kitabayashi I, Yokoyama A, Shimizu K, Ohki M. Interaction and functional cooperation of the leukemia-associated factors AML1 and p300 in myeloid cell differentiation. *EMBO J* 1998;17:2994.
12. Erickson P, Gao J, Chang KS, et al. Identification of breakpoints in t(8;21) acute myelogenous leukemia and isolation of a fusion transcript, AML1/ETO, with similarity to Drosophila segmentation gene, runt. *Blood* 1992;80:1825.
13. Meyers S, Lenny N, Hiebert SW. The t(8;21) fusion protein interferes with AML-1B-dependent transcriptional activation. *Mol Cell Biol* 1995;15:1974.
14. Wang J, Hoshino T, Redner RL, et al. ETO, fusion partner in t(8;21) acute myeloid leukemia, represses transcription by interaction with the human N-CoR/mSin3/HDAC1 complex. *Proc Natl Acad Sci U S A* 1998;95:10860.
15. Gelmetti V, Zhang J, Fanelli M, Minucci S, et al. Aberrant recruitment of the nuclear receptor corepressor-histone deacetylase complex by the acute myeloid leukemia fusion partner ETO. *Mol Cell Biol* 1998;18:7185.
16. Redner RL, Wang J, Liu JM. Chromatin remodeling and leukemia: new therapeutic paradigms. *Blood* 1999;94:417.

17. Wang J, Sauntharajah Y, Redner RL, Liu JM. Inhibitors of histone deacetylase relieve ETO-mediated repression and induce differentiation of AML1-ETO leukemia cells. *Cancer Res* 1999;59:2766.
18. Liu P, Tarle SA, Hajra A, et al. Fusion between transcription factor CBF beta/PEBP2 beta and a myosin heavy chain in acute myeloid leukemia. *Science* 1993;261:1041.
19. Liu PP, Hajra A, Wijmenga C, Collins FS. Molecular pathogenesis of the chromosome 16 inversion in the M4Eo subtype of acute myeloid leukemia [published erratum appears in *Blood* 1997;89:1842]. *Blood* 1995;85:2289.
20. Adya N, Stacy T, Speck NA, Liu PP. The leukemic protein core binding factor beta (CBF-beta)-smooth-muscle myosin heavy chain sequesters CBFalpha2 into cytoskeletal filaments and aggregates. *Mol Cell Biol* 1998;18:7432.
21. Castilla LH, Garrett L, Adya N, et al. The fusion gene Cbfb-MYH11 blocks myeloid differentiation and predisposes mice to acute myelomonocytic leukaemia. *Nat Genet* 1999;23:144.
22. Song WJ, Sullivan MG, Legare RD, et al. Haploinsufficiency of CBFA2 causes familial thrombocytopenia with propensity to develop acute myelogenous leukaemia. *Nat Genet* 1999;23:166.
23. Mitani K, Ogawa S, Tanaka T, et al. Generation of the AML1-EVI-1 fusion gene in the t(3;21)(q26;q22) causes blastic crisis in chronic myelocytic leukemia. *EMBO J* 1994;13:504.
24. Nucifora G, Begy CR, Kobayashi H, et al. Consistent intergenic splicing and production of multiple transcripts between AML1 at 21q22 and unrelated genes at 3q26 in (3;21)(q26;q22) translocations. *Proc Natl Acad Sci U S A* 1994;91:4004.
25. Kurokawa M, Mitani K, Imai Y, et al. The t(3;21) fusion product, AML1/Evi-1, interacts with Smad3 and blocks transforming growth factor-beta-mediated growth inhibition of myeloid cells. *Blood* 1998;92:4003.
26. Roulston D, Espinosa R III, Nucifora G, et al. CBFA2(AML1) translocations with novel partner chromosomes in myeloid leukemias: association with prior therapy. *Blood* 1998;92:2879.
27. Nye JA, Petersen JM, Gunther CV, Jonsen MD, Graves BJ. Interaction of murine ets-1 with GGA-binding sites establishes the ETS domain as a new DNA-binding motif. *Genes Dev* 1992;6:975.
28. Wang LC, Swat W, Fujiwara Y, et al. The TEL/ETV6 gene is required specifically for hematopoiesis in the bone marrow. *Genes Dev* 1998;12:2392.
29. Golub TR, Barker GF, Bohlander SK, et al. Fusion of the TEL gene on 12p13 to the AML1 gene on 21q22 in acute lymphoblastic leukemia. *Proc Natl Acad Sci U S A* 1995;92:4917.
30. Romana SP, Mauchauffe M, Le Coniat M, et al. The t(12;21) of acute lymphoblastic leukemia results in a tel-AML1 gene fusion. *Blood* 1995;85:3662.
31. Hiebert SW, Sun W, Davis JN, et al. The t(12;21) translocation converts AML-1B from an activator to a repressor of transcription. *Mol Cell Biol* 1996;16:1349.
32. Raynaud S, Cave H, Baens M, et al. The 12;21 translocation involving TEL and deletion of the other TEL allele: two frequently associated alterations found in childhood acute lymphoblastic leukemia. *Blood* 1996;87:2891.
33. Rubnitz JE, Pui CH, Downing JR. The role of TEL fusion genes in pediatric leukemias. *Leukemia* 1999;13:6.
34. Bloomfield CD, Lawrence D, Byrd JC, et al. Frequency of prolonged remission duration after high-dose cytarabine intensification in acute myeloid leukemia varies by cytogenetic subtype. *Cancer Res* 1998;58:4173.
35. Lutterbach B, Sun D, Schuetz J, Hiebert SW. The MYND motif is required for repression of basal transcription from the multidrug resistance 1 promoter by the t(8;21) fusion protein. *Mol Cell Biol* 1998;18:3604.
36. Golub TR. TEL gene rearrangements in myeloid malignancy. *Hematol Oncol Clin North Am* 1997;11:1207.
37. Golub TR, Barker GF, Lovett M, Gilliland DG. Fusion of PDGF receptor beta to a novel ets-like gene, tel, in chronic myelomonocytic leukemia with t(5;12) chromosomal translocation. *Cell* 1994;77:307.
38. Carroll M, Tomasson MH, Barker GF, Golub TR, Gilliland DG. The TEL/platelet-derived growth factor beta receptor (PDGF beta R) fusion in chronic myelomonocytic leukemia is a transforming protein that self-associates and activates PDGF beta R kinase-dependent signaling pathways. *Proc Natl Acad Sci U S A* 1996;93:14845.
39. Jousset C, Carron C, Boureux A, et al. A domain of TEL conserved in a subset of ETS proteins defines a specific oligomerization interface essential to the mitogenic properties of the TEL-PDGFR beta oncoprotein. *EMBO J* 1997;16:69.
40. Bourgeade MF, Defachelles AS, Cayre YE. Myc is essential for transformation by TEL/platelet-derived growth factor receptor beta (PDGFRbeta). *Blood* 1998;91:3333.
41. Papadopoulos P, Ridge SA, Boucher CA, Stocking C, Wiedemann LM. The novel activation of ABL by fusion to an ets-related gene, TEL. *Cancer Res* 1995;55:34.
42. Okuda K, Golub TR, Gilliland DG, Griffin JD. p210BCR/ABL, p190BCR/ABL, and TEL/ABL activate similar signal transduction pathways in hematopoietic cell lines. *Oncogene* 1996;13:1147.
43. Buijs A, Sherr S, van Baal S, et al. Translocation (12;22)(p13;q11) in myeloproliferative disorders results in fusion of the ETS-like TEL gene on 12p13 to the MN1 gene on 22q11 [published erratum appears in *Oncogene* 1995;10:809]. *Oncogene* 1995;10:1511.
44. Super HJ, McCabe NR, Thirman MJ, et al. Rearrangements of the MLL gene in therapy-related acute myeloid leukemia in patients previously treated with agents targeting DNA-topoisomerase II. *Blood* 1993;82:3705.
45. Hunger SP, Tkachuk DC, Amylon MD, et al. HRX involvement in de novo and secondary leukemias with diverse chromosome 11q23 abnormalities. *Blood* 1993;81:3197.
46. Pedersen-Bjergaard J, Andersen MK, Johansson B. Balanced chromosome aberrations in leukemias following chemotherapy with DNA-topoisomerase II inhibitors. *J Clin Oncol* 1998;16:1897.
47. Ziemin-van der Poel S, McCabe NR, Gill HJ, et al. Identification of a gene, MLL, that spans the breakpoint in 11q23 translocations associated with human leukemias [published erratum appears in *Proc Natl Acad Sci U S A* 1992;89:4220]. *Proc Natl Acad Sci U S A* 1991;88:10735.
48. Djabali M, Selleri L, Parry P, et al. A trithorax-like gene is interrupted by chromosome 11q23 translocations in acute leukaemias [published erratum appears in *Nat Genet* 1993;4:431]. *Nat Genet* 1992;2:113.
49. Gu Y, Nakamura T, Alder H, et al. The t(4;11) chromosome translocation of human acute leukemias fuses the ALL-1 gene, related to Drosophila trithorax, to the AF-4 gene. *Cell* 1992;71:701.
50. Tkachuk DC, Kohler S, Cleary ML. Involvement of a homolog of Drosophila trithorax by 11q23 chromosomal translocations in acute leukemias. *Cell* 1992;71:691.
51. Jones RS, Gelbart WM. The Drosophila Polycomb-group gene Enhancer of zeste contains a region with sequence similarity to trithorax. *Mol Cell Biol* 1993;13:6357.
52. Simon J. Locking in stable states of gene expression: transcriptional control during Drosophila development. *Curr Opin Cell Biol* 1995;7:376.
53. Yu BD, Hess JL, Horning SE, Brown GA, Korsmeyer SJ. Altered Hox expression and segmental identity in Mll-mutant mice. *Nature* 1995;378:505.
54. Yu BD, Hanson RD, Hess JL, Horning SE, Korsmeyer SJ. MLL, a mammalian trithorax-group gene, functions as a transcriptional maintenance factor in morphogenesis. *Proc Natl Acad Sci U S A* 1998;95:10632.
55. van Oostveen JW, Bijl JJ, Raaphorst FM, Walboomers JJM, Meijer CJLM. The role of Homeobox genes in normal hematopoiesis and hematological malignancies. *Leukemia* 1999;13:1675.
56. Hess JL, Yu BD, Li B, Hanson R, Korsmeyer SJ. Defects in yolk sac hematopoiesis in Mll-null embryos. *Blood* 1997;90:1799.
57. Fidanza V, Melotti P, Yano T, et al. Double knockout of the ALL-1 gene blocks hematopoietic differentiation in vitro. *Cancer Res* 1996;56:1179.
58. Rowley JD. The der(11) chromosome contains the critical breakpoint junction in the 4;11, 9;11, and 11;19 translocations in acute leukemia. *Genes Chromosomes Cancer* 1992;5:264.
59. Dimartino JF, Cleary ML. Mll rearrangements in haematological malignancies: lessons from clinical and biological studies. *Br J Haematol* 1999;106:614.
60. Tse W, Zhu W, Chen HS, Cohen A. A novel gene, AF1q, fused to MLL in t(1;11)(q21;q23), is specifically expressed in leukemic and immature hematopoietic cells. *Blood* 1995;85:650.
61. Caligiuri MA, Schichman SA, Strout MP, et al. Molecular rearrangement of the ALL-1 gene in acute myeloid leukemia without cytogenetic evidence of 11q23 chromosomal translocations. *Cancer Res* 1994;54:370.
62. Schichman SA, Caligiuri MA, Gu Y, et al. ALL-1 partial duplication in acute leukemia. *Proc Natl Acad Sci U S A* 1994;91:6236.
63. Schichman SA, Caligiuri MA, Strout MP, et al. ALL-1 tandem duplication in acute myeloid leukemia with a normal karyotype involves homologous recombination between Alu elements. *Cancer Res* 1994;54:4277.
64. Caligiuri MA, Strout MP, Oberkircher AR, et al. The partial tandem duplication of ALL1 in acute myeloid leukemia with normal cytogenetics or trisomy 11 is restricted to one chromosome. *Proc Natl Acad Sci U S A* 1997;94:3899.
65. So CW, Ma ZG, Price CM, et al. MLL self fusion mediated by Alu repeat homologous recombination and prognosis of AML-M4/M5 subtypes. *Cancer Res* 1997;57:117.
66. Strout MP, Marcucci G, Bloomfield CD, Caligiuri MA. The partial tandem duplication of ALL1 (MLL) is consistently generated by Alu-mediated homologous recombination in acute myeloid leukemia. *Proc Natl Acad Sci U S A* 1998;95:2390.
67. Bernard OA, Romana SP, Schichman SA, et al. Partial duplication of HRX in acute leukemia with trisomy 11. *Leukemia* 1995;9:1487.
68. Caligiuri MA, Strout MP, Schichman SA, et al. Partial tandem duplication of ALL1 as a recurrent molecular defect in acute myeloid leukemia with trisomy 11. *Cancer Res* 1996;56:1418.
69. Caligiuri MA, Strout MP, Lawrence D, et al. Rearrangement of *ALL1 (MLL)* in acute myeloid leukemia with normal cytogenetics. *Cancer Res* 1998;58:55.
70. Dôhner K, Ulrich R, Liebisch C, et al. Prognostic significance of partial tandem duplication of the *MLL* gene in acute myeloid leukemia with normal cytogenetics: a study within a multicenter treatment trial. *Blood* 1999;94(Suppl):499a.
71. Greaves MF. Infant leukaemia biology, aetiology and treatment. *Leukemia* 1996;10:372.
72. Ford AM, Ridge SA, Cabrera ME, et al. In utero rearrangements in the trithorax-related oncogene in infant leukaemias. *Nature* 1993;363:358.
73. Ford AM, Pombo-de-Oliveira MS, McCarthy KP, et al. Monoclonal origin of concordant T-cell malignancy in identical twins. *Blood* 1997;89:281.
74. Gale KB, Ford AM, Repp R, et al. Backtracking leukemia to birth: identification of clonotypic gene fusion sequences in neonatal blood spots. *Proc Natl Acad Sci U S A* 1997;94:13950.
75. Ford AM, Bennett CA, Price CM, et al. Fetal origins of the TEL-AML1 fusion gene in identical twins with leukemia. *Proc Natl Acad Sci U S A* 1998;95:4584.
76. Broeker PL, Super HG, Thirman MJ, et al. Distribution of 11q23 breakpoints within the MLL breakpoint cluster region in de novo acute leukemia and in treatment-related acute myeloid leukemia: correlation with scaffold attachment regions and topoisomerase II consensus binding sites. *Blood* 1996;87:1912.
77. Strissel PL, Strick R, Rowley JD, Zeleznik-Le NJ. An in vivo topoisomerase II cleavage site and a DNase I hypersensitive site colocalize near exon 9 in the MLL breakpoint cluster region. *Blood* 1998;92:3793.
78. Pedersen-Bjergaard J, Rowley JD. The balanced and the unbalanced chromosome aberrations of acute myeloid leukemia may develop in different ways and may contribute differently to malignant transformation. *Blood* 1994;83:2780.
79. Downing JR, Look AT. MLL fusion genes in the 11q23 acute leukemias. In: Freireich EJ, Kantarjian H, eds. *Leukemia: advances in research and treatment.* Boston: Kluwer, 1995.
80. Lo Coco F, Diverio D, Falini B, et al. Genetic diagnosis and molecular monitoring in the management of acute promyelocytic leukemia. *Blood* 1999;94:12.

81. de The H, Lavau C, Marchio A, et al. The PML-RAR alpha fusion mRNA generated by the t(15;17) translocation in acute promyelocytic leukemia encodes a functionally altered RAR. *Cell* 1991;66:675.
82. Kakizuka A, Miller WH Jr, Umesono K, et al. Chromosomal translocation t(15;17) in human acute promyelocytic leukemia fuses RAR alpha with a novel putative transcription factor, PML. *Cell* 1991;66:663.
83. Slack JL. Biology and treatment of acute progranulocytic leukemia. *Curr Opin Hematol* 1999;6:236.
84. Grignani F, De Matteis S, Nervi C, et al. Fusion proteins of the retinoic acid receptor-alpha recruit histone deacetylase in promyelocytic leukaemia. *Nature* 1998;391:815.
85. Lin RJ, Nagy L, Inoue S, et al. Role of the histone deacetylase complex in acute promyelocytic leukaemia. *Nature* 1998;391:811.
86. He LZ, Guidez F, Tribioli C, et al. Distinct interactions of PML-RARalpha and PLZF-RARalpha with co- repressors determine differential responses to RA in APL. *Nat Genet* 1998;18:126.
87. Chen Z, Brand NJ, Chen A, et al. Fusion between a novel Kruppel-like zinc finger gene and the retinoic acid receptor-alpha locus due to a variant t(11;17) translocation associated with acute promyelocytic leukaemia. *EMBO J* 1993;12:1161.
88. Hong SH, David G, Wong CW, Dejean A, Privalsky ML. SMRT corepressor interacts with PLZF and with the PML retinoic acid receptor alpha (RARalpha) and PLZF-RARalpha oncoproteins associated with acute promyelocytic leukemia. *Proc Natl Acad Sci U S A* 1997;94:9028.
89. Murre C, McCaw PS, Baltimore D. A new DNA binding and dimerization motif in immunoglobulin enhancer binding, daughterless, MyoD, and myc proteins. *Cell* 1989;56:777.
90. Reya T, Grosschedl R. Transcriptional regulation of B-cell differentiation. *Curr Opin Immunol* 1998;10:158.
91. Aronheim A, Shiran R, Rosen A, Walker MD. The E2A gene product contains two separable and functionally distinct transcription activation domains. *Proc Natl Acad Sci U S A* 1993;90:8063.
92. Lassar AB, Davis RL, Wright WE, et al. Functional activity of myogenic HLH proteins requires hetero-oligomerization with E12/E47-like proteins in vivo. *Cell* 1991;66:305.
93. Bain G, Maandag EC, Izon DJ, et al. E2A proteins are required for proper B cell development and initiation of immunoglobulin gene rearrangements. *Cell* 1994;79:885.
94. Zhuang Y, Soriano P, Weintraub H. The helix-loop-helix gene E2A is required for B cell formation. *Cell* 1994;79:875.
95. Kamps MP, Murre C, Sun XH, Baltimore D. A new homeobox gene contributes the DNA binding domain of the t(1;19) translocation protein in pre-B ALL. *Cell* 1990;60:547.
96. Nourse J, Mellentin JD, Galili N, et al. Chromosomal translocation t(1;19) results in synthesis of a homeobox fusion mRNA that codes for a potential chimeric transcription factor. *Cell* 1990;60:535.
97. Van Dijk MA, Voorhoeve PM, Murre C. Pbx1 is converted into a transcriptional activator upon acquiring the N-terminal region of E2A in pre-B-cell acute lymphoblastoid leukemia. *Proc Natl Acad Sci U S A* 1993;90:6061.
98. Fu X, McGrath S, Pasillas M, Nakazawa S, Kamps MP. EB-1, a tyrosine kinase signal transduction gene, is transcriptionally activated in the t(1;19) subset of pre-B ALL, which express oncoprotein E2a-Pbx1. *Oncogene* 1999;18:4920.
99. McWhirter JR, Neuteboom ST, Wancewicz EV, et al. Oncogenic homeodomain transcription factor E2A-Pbx1 activates a novel WNT gene in pre-B acute lymphoblastoid leukemia. *Proc Natl Acad Sci U S A* 1999;96:11464.
100. Hunger SP, Ohyashiki K, Toyama K, Cleary ML. Hlf, a novel hepatic bZIP protein, shows altered DNA-binding properties following fusion to E2A in t(17;19) acute lymphoblastic leukemia. *Genes Dev* 1992;6:1608.
101. Inaba T, Roberts WM, Shapiro LH, et al. Fusion of the leucine zipper gene HLF to the E2A gene in human acute B- lineage leukemia. *Science* 1992;257:531.
102. Metzstein MM, Hengartner MO, Tsung N, Ellis RE, Horvitz HR. Transcriptional regulator of programmed cell death encoded by Caenorhabditis elegans gene ces-2. *Nature* 1996;382:545.
103. Inukai T, Inoue A, Kurosawa H, et al. SLUG, a ces-1-related zinc finger transcription factor gene with antiapoptotic activity, is a downstream target of the E2A-HLF oncoprotein. *Mol Cell* 1999;4:343.
104. Inukai T, Inaba T, Ikushima S, Look AT. The AD1 and AD2 transactivation domains of E2A are essential for the antiapoptotic activity of the chimeric oncoprotein E2A-HLF. *Mol Cell Biol* 1998;18:6035.
105. Nowell PC, Hungerford DA. A minute chromosome in human chronic granulocytic leukemia. *Science* 1960;132:1497.
106. Rowley JD. A new consistent chromosomal abnormality in chronic myelogenous leukaemia identified by quinacrine fluorescence and Giemsa staining. *Nature* 1973;243:290.
107. Bartram CR, de Klein A, Hagemeijer A, et al. Translocation of c-abl oncogene correlates with the presence of a Philadelphia chromosome in chronic myelocytic leukaemia. *Nature* 1983;306:277.
108. Shtivelman E, Lifshitz B, Gale RP, Canaani E. Fused transcript of abl and bcr genes in chronic myelogenous leukaemia. *Nature* 1985;315:550.
109. Stam K, Heisterkamp N, Grosveld G, et al. Evidence of a new chimeric bcr/c-abl mRNA in patients with chronic myelocytic leukemia and the Philadelphia chromosome. *N Engl J Med* 1985;313:1429.
110. Bloomfield CD, Peterson LC, Yunis JJ, Brunning RD. The Philadelphia chromosome (Ph1) in adults presenting with acute leukaemia: a comparison of Ph1+ and Ph1- patients. *Br J Haematol* 1977;36:347.
111. Sawyers CL. Chronic myeloid leukemia. *N Engl J Med* 1999;340:1330.
112. Verfaillie CM. Biology of chronic myelogenous leukemia. *Hematol Oncol Clin North Am* 1998;12:1.
113. Pendergast AM, Quilliam LA, Cripe LD, et al. BCR-ABL-induced oncogenesis is mediated by direct interaction with the SH2 domain of the GRB-2 adaptor protein. *Cell* 1993;75:175.
114. Van Etten RA, Jackson P, Baltimore D. The mouse type IV c-abl gene product is a nuclear protein, and activation of transforming ability is associated with cytoplasmic localization. *Cell* 1989;58:669.
115. Lewis JM, Baskaran R, Taagepera S, Schwartz MA, Wang JY. Integrin regulation of c-Abl tyrosine kinase activity and cytoplasmic- nuclear transport. *Proc Natl Acad Sci U S A* 1996;93:15174.
116. Druker BJ, Talpaz M, Resta D, et al. Clinical efficacy and safety of an ABL specific tyrosine kinase inhibitor as targeted therapy for chronic myelogenous leukemia. *Blood* 1999;94(Suppl):368a.
117. Stoffler D, Fahrenkrog B, Aebi U. The nuclear pore complex: from molecular architecture to functional dynamics. *Curr Opin Cell Biol* 1999;11:391.
118. von Lindern M, Breems D, van Baal S, Adriaansen H, Grosveld G. Characterization of the translocation breakpoint sequences of two DEK-CAN fusion genes present in t(6;9) acute myeloid leukemia and a SET-CAN fusion gene found in a case of acute undifferentiated leukemia. *Genes Chromosomes Cancer* 1992;5:227.
119. Fornerod M, Boer J, van Baal S, Morreau H, Grosveld G. Interaction of cellular proteins with the leukemia specific fusion proteins DEK-CAN and SET-CAN and their normal counterpart, the nucleoporin CAN. *Oncogene* 1996;13:1801.
120. Boer J, Bonten-Surtel J, Grosveld G. Overexpression of the nucleoporin CAN/NUP214 induces growth arrest, nucleocytoplasmic transport defects, and apoptosis. *Mol Cell Biol* 1998;18:1236.
121. Estanyol JM, Jaumot M, Casanovas O, et al. The protein SET regulates the inhibitory effect of p21(Cip1) on cyclin E-cyclin-dependent kinase 2 activity. *J Biol Chem* 1999;274:33161.
122. Borrow J, Shearman AM, Stanton VP Jr, et al. The t(7;11)(p15;p15) translocation in acute myeloid leukaemia fuses the genes for nucleoporin NUP98 and class I homeoprotein HOXA9. *Nat Genet* 1996;12:159.
123. Kasper LH, Brindle PK, Schnabel CA, et al. CREB binding protein interacts with nucleoporin-specific FG repeats that activate transcription and mediate NUP98-HOXA9 oncogenicity. *Mol Cell Biol* 1999;19:764.
124. Dalla-Favera R, Bregni M, Erikson J, et al. Human c-myc onc gene is located on the region of chromosome 8 that is translocated in Burkitt lymphoma cells. *Proc Natl Acad Sci U S A* 1982;79:7824.
125. Taub R, Kirsch I, Morton C, et al. Translocation of the c-myc gene into the immunoglobulin heavy chain locus in human Burkitt lymphoma and murine plasmacytoma cells. *Proc Natl Acad Sci U S A* 1982;79:7837.
126. Klein G. Immunoglobulin gene associated chromosomal translocations in B cell derived tumors. *Curr Top Microbiol Immunol* 1999;246:161.
127. Luscher B, Larsson LG. The basic region/helix-loop-helix/leucine zipper domain of Myc proto-oncoproteins: function and regulation. *Oncogene* 1999;18:2955.
128. Begley CG, Aplan PD, Davey MP, et al. Chromosomal translocation in a human leukemic stem-cell line disrupts the T-cell antigen receptor delta-chain diversity region and results in a previously unreported fusion transcript. *Proc Natl Acad Sci U S A* 1989;86:2031.
129. Fitzgerald TJ, Neale GA, Raimondi SC, Goorha RM. c-tal, a helix-loop-helix protein, is juxtaposed to the T-cell receptor- beta chain gene by a reciprocal chromosomal translocation: t(1;7)(p32;q35). *Blood* 1991;78:2686.
130. Xia Y, Brown L, Yang CY, et al. TAL2, a helix-loop-helix gene activated by the (7;9)(q34;q32) translocation in human T-cell leukemia. *Proc Natl Acad Sci U S A* 1991;88:11416.
131. Mellentin JD, Smith SD, Cleary ML. lyl-1, a novel gene altered by chromosomal translocation in T cell leukemia, codes for a protein with a helix-loop-helix DNA binding motif. *Cell* 1989;58:77.
132. Mathieu-Mahul D, Caubet JF, Bernheim A, et al. Molecular cloning of a DNA fragment from human chromosome 14(14q11) involved in T-cell malignancies. *EMBO J* 1985;4:3427.
133. McKeithan TW, Shima EA, Le Beau MM, et al. Molecular cloning of the breakpoint junction of a human chromosomal 8;14 translocation involving the T-cell receptor alpha-chain gene and sequences on the 3' side of MYC. *Proc Natl Acad Sci U S A* 1986;83:6636.
134. Finger LR, Harvey RC, Moore RC, Showe LC, Croce CM. A common mechanism of chromosomal translocation in T- and B-cell neoplasia. *Science* 1986;234:982.
135. Wadman IA, Osada H, Grutz GG, et al. The LIM-only protein Lmo2 is a bridging molecule assembling an erythroid, DNA-binding complex which includes the TAL1, E47, GATA-1 and Ldb1/NLI proteins. *EMBO J* 1997;16:3145.
136. McGuire EA, Hockett RD, Pollock KM, et al. The t(11;14)(p15;q11) in a T-cell acute lymphoblastic leukemia cell line activates multiple transcripts, including Ttg-1, a gene encoding a potential zinc finger protein. *Mol Cell Biol* 1989;9:2124.
137. Royer-Pokora B, Loos U, Ludwig WD. TTG-2, a new gene encoding a cysteine-rich protein with the LIM motif, is overexpressed in acute T-cell leukaemia with the t(11;14)(p13;q11). *Oncogene* 1991;6:1887.
138. Rabbitts TH. LMO T-cell translocation oncogenes typify genes activated by chromosomal translocations that alter transcription and developmental processes. *Genes Dev* 1998;12:2651.
139. Dear TN, Colledge WH, Carlton MB, et al. The Hox11 gene is essential for cell survival during spleen development. *Development* 1995;121:2909.
140. Kawabe T, Muslin AJ, Korsmeyer SJ. HOX11 interacts with protein phosphatases PP2A and PP1 and disrupts a G2/M cell-cycle checkpoint. *Nature* 1997;385:454.
141. Hatano M, Roberts CW, Minden M, Crist WM, Korsmeyer SJ. Deregulation of a homeobox gene, HOX11, by the t(10;14) in T cell leukemia. *Science* 1991;253:79.
142. Russo G, Isobe M, Pegoraro L, et al. Molecular analysis of a t(7;14)(q35;q32) chromosome translocation in a T cell leukemia of a patient with ataxia telangiectasia. *Cell* 1988;53:137.
143. Russo G, Isobe M, Gatti R, et al. Molecular analysis of a t(14;14) translocation in leukemic T-cells of an ataxia telangiectasia patient. *Proc Natl Acad Sci U S A* 1989;86:602.

144. Stern MH, Soulier J, Rosenzwajg M, et al. MTCP-1: a novel gene on the human chromosome Xq28 translocated to the T cell receptor alpha/delta locus in mature T cell proliferations. *Oncogene* 1993;8:2475.
145. Fu ZQ, Du Bois GC, Song SP, et al. Crystal structure of MTCP-1: implications for role of TCL-1 and MTCP-1 in T cell malignancies. *Proc Natl Acad Sci U S A* 1998;95:3413.
146. Levine AJ. Tumor suppressor genes. *Bioessays* 1990;12:60.
147. Baylin SB, Herman JG, Graff JR, Vertino PM, Issa JP. Alterations in DNA methylation: a fundamental aspect of neoplasia. *Adv Cancer Res* 1998;72:141.
148. Cordone I, Masi S, Mauro FR, et al. p53 expression in B-cell chronic lymphocytic leukemia: a marker of disease progression and poor prognosis. *Blood* 1998;91:4342.
149. Shinn CA, Byrd JC, DS N, Flinn IW, Grever MR. Over expression of MDM2 in leukemic cells in previously treated patients with chronic lymphocytic leukemia. *Blood* 1999;94(Suppl):542a.
150. Serrano M, Hannon GJ, Beach D. A new regulatory motif in cell-cycle control causing specific inhibition of cyclin D/CDK4. *Nature* 1993;366:704.
151. Hannon GJ, Beach D. p15INK4B is a potential effector of TGF-beta-induced cell cycle arrest. *Nature* 1994;371:257.
152. Serrano M, Lee H, Chin L, et al. Role of the INK4a locus in tumor suppression and cell mortality. *Cell* 1996;85:27.
153. Drexler HG. Review of alterations of the cyclin-dependent kinase inhibitor INK4 family genes p15, p16, p18 and p19 in human leukemia-lymphoma cells. *Leukemia* 1998;12:845.
154. Stern MH, Theodorou I, Aurias A, et al. T-cell nonmalignant clonal proliferation in ataxia telangiectasia: a cytological, immunological, and molecular characterization. *Blood* 1989;73:1285.
155. Narducci MG, Virgilio L, Isobe M, et al. TCL1 oncogene activation in preleukemic T cells from a case of ataxia- telangiectasia. *Blood* 1995;86:2358.
156. Stilgenbauer S, Schaffner C, Litterst A, et al. Biallelic mutations in the ATM gene in T-prolymphocytic leukemia. *Nat Med* 1997;3:1155.
157. Quesnel B, Guillerm G, Vereecque R, et al. Methylation of the p15(INK4b) gene in myelodysplastic syndromes is frequent and acquired during disease progression. *Blood* 1998;91:2985.
158. Herman JG, Civin CI, Issa JP, et al. Distinct patterns of inactivation of p15INK4B and p16INK4A characterize the major types of hematological malignancies. *Cancer Res* 1997;57:837.
159. Uchida T, Kinoshita T, Nagai H, et al. Hypermethylation of the p15INK4B gene in myelodysplastic syndromes. *Blood* 1997;90:1403.
160. Cameron EE, Baylin SB, Herman JG. p15(INK4B) CpG island methylation in primary acute leukemia is heterogeneous and suggests density as a critical factor for transcriptional silencing. *Blood* 1999;94:2445.
161. Corn PG, Kuerbitz SJ, van Noesel MM, et al. Transcriptional silencing of the p73 gene in acute lymphoblastic leukemia and Burkitt's lymphoma is associated with 5' CpG island methylation. *Cancer Res* 1999;59:3352.
162. Costello JF, Frühwald MC, Smiraglia DJ, et al. Aberrant CpG island methylation has non-random and tumor type-specific patterns. *Nat Genet* 2000;25:132.
163. Schnittger S, Wormann B, Hiddemann W, Griesinger F. Partial tandem duplications of the MLL gene are detectable in peripheral blood and bone marrow of nearly all healthy donors. *Blood* 1998;92:1728.
164. Caldas C, So CW, MacGregor A, et al. Exon scrambling of MLL transcripts occur commonly and mimic partial genomic duplication of the gene. *Gene* 1998;208:167.
165. Marcucci G, Strout MP, Bloomfield CD, Caligiuri MA. Detection of unique ALL1 (MLL) fusion transcripts in normal human bone marrow and blood: distinct origin of normal versus leukemic ALL1 fusion transcripts. *Cancer Res* 1998;58:790.
166. Bose S, Deininger M, Gora-Tybor J, Goldman JM, Melo JV. The presence of typical and atypical BCR-ABL fusion genes in leukocytes of normal individuals: biologic significance and implications for the assessment of minimal residual disease. *Blood* 1998;92:3362.
167. Biernaux C, Loos M, Sels A, Huez G, Stryckmans P. Detection of major bcr-abl gene expression at a very low level in blood cells of some healthy individuals. *Blood* 1995;86:3118.
168. Faderl S, Talpaz M, Kantarjian HM, Estrov Z. Should polymerase chain reaction analysis to detect minimal residual disease in patients with chronic myelogenous leukemia be used in clinical decision making? *Blood* 1999;93:2755.
169. Jurlander J, Caligiuri MA, Ruutu T, et al. Persistence of the AML1/ETO fusion transcript in patients treated with allogeneic bone marrow transplantation for t(8;21) leukemia. *Blood* 1996;88:2183.
170. Nucifora G, Larson RA, Rowley JD. Persistence of the 8;21 translocation in patients with acute myeloid leukemia type M2 in long-term remission. *Blood* 1993;82:712.
171. Greaves M. Silence of the leukemic clone. *N Engl J Med* 1997;336:367.
172. Rubnitz JE, Pui CH. Molecular diagnostics in the treatment of leukemia. *Curr Opin Hematol* 1999;6:229.
173. Diverio D, Rossi V, Avvisati G, et al. Early detection of relapse by prospective reverse transcriptase-polymerase chain reaction analysis of the PML/RARalpha fusion gene in patients with acute promyelocytic leukemia enrolled in the GIMEMA-AIEOP multicenter "AIDA" trial. GIMEMA-AIEOP Multicenter "AIDA" Trial. *Blood* 1998;92:784.
174. Marcucci G, Livak KJ, Bi W, et al. Detection of minimal residual disease in patients with AML1/ETO- associated acute myeloid leukemia using a novel quantitative reverse transcription polymerase chain reaction assay. *Leukemia* 1998;12:1482.
175. Golub TR, Slonim DK, Tamayo P, et al. Molecular classification of cancer: class discovery and class prediction by gene expression monitoring. *Science* 1999;286:531.
176. Rubnitz JE, Morrissey J, Savage PA, Cleary ML. ENL, the gene fused with HRX in t(11;19) leukemias, encodes a nuclear protein with transcriptional activation potential in lymphoid and myeloid cells. *Blood* 1994;84:1747.
177. Nakamura T, Alder H, Gu Y, et al. Genes on chromosomes 4, 9, and 19 involved in 11q23 abnormalities in acute leukemia share sequence homology and/or common motifs. *Proc Natl Acad Sci U S A* 1993;90:4631.
178. Ida K, Kitabayashi I, Taki T, et al. Adenoviral E1A-associated protein p300 is involved in acute myeloid leukemia with t(11;22)(q23;q13). *Blood* 1997;90:4699.
179. Hollis GF, Mitchell KF, Battey J, et al. A variant translocation places the lambda immunoglobulin genes 3' to the c-myc oncogene in Burkitt's lymphoma. *Nature* 1984;307:752.
180. Magrath I, Erikson J, Whang-Peng J, et al. Synthesis of kappa light chains by cell lines containing an 8;22 chromosomal translocation derived from a male homosexual with Burkitt's lymphoma. *Science* 1983;222:1094.

DAVID A. SCHEINBERG
PETER MASLAK
MARK WEISS

SECTION 2

Acute Leukemias

Leukemias are clonal, neoplastic proliferations of immature cells of the hematopoietic system, which are characterized by aberrant or arrested differentiation. Leukemia cells accumulate in the bone marrow cavity, ultimately replacing most of the normal hematopoietic cells, thus resulting in the signs and symptoms of the disease. These include most prominently, bone marrow failure and its consequences of anemia, hemorrhage, and infection. Leukemia cells circulate into the blood and other tissues throughout the body, with patterns characteristic of the particular type of leukemia. The acute leukemias, which can be broadly grouped as either lymphoblastic or myelogenous, can be identified phenotypically and genetically and are characterized by a rapid clinical course usually necessitating immediate treatment. Acute leukemias are derived from, and biologically resemble, primitive hematopoietic progenitor cells; in contrast, chronic leukemias have the phenotype and biologic character of more mature cells. Chronic myeloid leukemia (CML), however, over time may transform to an acute, blastic phase and thereafter more closely resembles an acute leukemia in its biology, clinical course, and need for therapy.

The acute lymphoblastic leukemias (ALLs) are distinguished generally from the lymphomas because the latter resemble more mature lymphoid cells and typically inhabit the lymph nodes, spleen, or other extramedullary sites before spreading to involve the blood or bone marrow. Certain lymphomas, such as lymphoblastic lymphomas and Burkitt's lymphomas, retain features of both the leukemias and lymphomas, but are derived from immature cells and require therapy similar to that used for ALL. Other lymphomas, and sometimes multiple myelomas, however, may spread widely into the blood and bone marrow, and in such a phase, can be described as *leukemic*, but are not true leukemias.

Leukemia (meaning *white blood*) was originally described in 1845 by Virchow.[1] Although acute leukemias are relatively rare cancers, these leukemias are the most carefully studied and best characterized neoplasms. Numerous subtypes have been defined based on morphology, genetics, immunophenotype, and biologic behavior. Oncogenes responsible for leukemogenesis are beginning to be identified, and there is an enlarging body of knowledge regarding the factors regulating leukemia cell growth and function. Multiple drugs capable of killing leukemia cells are now available. Therapeutic strategies that have been developed often result in clinical remissions of adult leukemias and, in a smaller fraction of patients, result in cures. Despite these advances, acute leukemia remains, for most patients, a fulminant and incurable disease, requiring immediate diagnosis and treatment. The course of patients with acute leukemia is often complicated by the severity of the treatments themselves (Fig. 46.2-1).

EPIDEMIOLOGY AND ETIOLOGY

INCIDENCE

The acute leukemias are rare diseases, but have a disproportionately large effect on cancer survival statistics among children and younger adults. Although the acute leukemias account for less than 3% of all cancers, these diseases are the leading cause of death due to cancer in the United States in persons younger than 35 years of age.[2,3] The incidence rate of acute myelogenous leukemias (AMLs) in the United States is approximately 2.5 per 100,000 persons; for ALL, the rate is approximately 1.3 per 100,000 persons. AML has a slight male predominance (1.5:1.0) and accounts for 25% of both acute and chronic leukemias. AML affects approximately 9000 people a year in the United States. ALL affects approximately 4000 people, with a similar predominance of male subjects. The incidences of acute leukemias in the United States have not changed substantially since the 1980s, although there is a slight trend upward among those diagnosed with ALL and a slight decrease in the number of diagnoses of AML in this time period. Incidence rates for acute leukemia are similar worldwide. In ALL, the incidence rates in African Americans are approximately one-half that seen in whites; in AML, rates are similar between these two groups. Age-specific incidences differ dramatically between ALL, which has a median age at diagnosis of 10 years, and AML, which has a median age of 65 years. AML is rare below the age of 40, but the incidence increases progressively with age from approximately 1 per 100,000 at age 40 to more than 15 per 100,000 at age 75 or older. In contrast, ALL has its peak incidence at less than 10 years and has a second smaller increase in persons older than 70 (Fig. 46.2-2).

SECONDARY LEUKEMIAS

For most patients with acute leukemia, the cause of the disease is unknown. Because leukemias are the result of a genetic alteration in a clonogenic cell, which can often be identified by a chromosomal translocation, deletion, or mutation, known and suspected carcinogens have been explored as causative agents in acute leukemia. A clear cause of leukemia can be found in the minority of patients with a history of prior chemotherapy or radiation therapy. Such secondary leukemias, more than 90% of which are myeloid, are notoriously difficult to treat. The chromosomal abnormalities often observed in these secondary leukemias are associated with a poor prognosis, even when observed in patients without a history of prior therapy or toxic exposure.

Secondary myeloid leukemias first became apparent in the early survivors of Hodgkin's disease.[4,5] Studies initially linked the use of alkylating agents such as nitrogen mustard to the increased risk. Among a large cohort of patients treated with chemotherapy and radiotherapy for Hodgkin's disease, 163 cases of secondary leukemia were found.[6] There were dose-related increases in secondary leukemia. More recent studies have not linked radiotherapy, when used alone, to an increased risk.[7] Mechlorethamine (nitrogen mustard), procarbazine, cyclophosphamide, lomustine, teniposide, and chlorambucil were all implicated in the increased risk. The risk for secondary AML was greatest between 2 and 9 years after therapy, with 85% of cases occurring before the tenth year.[6,7]

Curative therapy for childhood ALL has a risk of inducing secondary AML as well.[8–10] The increased risk of AML occurred within 6 years and was originally associated with a T-cell phenotype of the original ALL[8] and use of an epipodophyllotoxin (etoposide or teniposide)[9] or alkylating agent.[10] The risk from epipodophyllotoxins was proportional to the dose intensity of the drug, rather than the cumulative dose, with the highest risks associated with weekly or twice weekly administration.[9] In contrast, secondary AML was not increased in pediatric ALL protocols in which epipodophyllotoxins were not used.[11]

Several additional studies in both adults and children have confirmed the association between treatment with epipodophyllotoxins and secondary AML,[12–14] in particular, monocytic leukemias with abnormalities of chromosome 11q23. Promyelocytic leukemias with t(15;17) have also been associated with etoposide and with other chemotherapeutic agents, such as doxorubicin, that target topoisomerase II.[15]

Dose-dependent risks for secondary AML have also been observed in adults treated with alkylating agents, including platinum-based drugs and radiotherapy for breast cancer[16] and ovarian cancer,[17] and for a variety of neoplasms treated with an autologous bone marrow transplant (BMT) after high-dose radiation and alkylating agent therapy.[18] Among the alkylating agents, cyclophosphamide appears to hold less risk; a study of the incidence of secondary leukemia in patients with breast cancer treated with moderate doses of cyclophosphamide confirms this lower level of risk.[19]

OCCUPATIONAL AND ENVIRONMENTAL EXPOSURES

The clear relationship between the atomic bomb radiation[20] or use of carcinogenic therapies and the development of secondary leukemias has led to the exploration of the possible leukemogenic role of other potential carcinogens in the environment, such as low-dose radiation, chemicals, cigarette smoke, and electromagnetic radiation.[21]

Although electromagnetic fields have received considerable attention as a possible carcinogen, the actual risk of leukemia from exposure to commercial and residential power fields remains controversial.[21–23] There are a large number of conflicting reports, but there is a lack of clear dose-response relationships, and a causal relationship between leukemia and electromagnetic fields, either as a consequence of occupational exposure or residential power use, has little current support.[21–23]

Both ALL and AML risks increased as a result of exposure to the atomic bomb.[20] Risks associated with occupational expo-

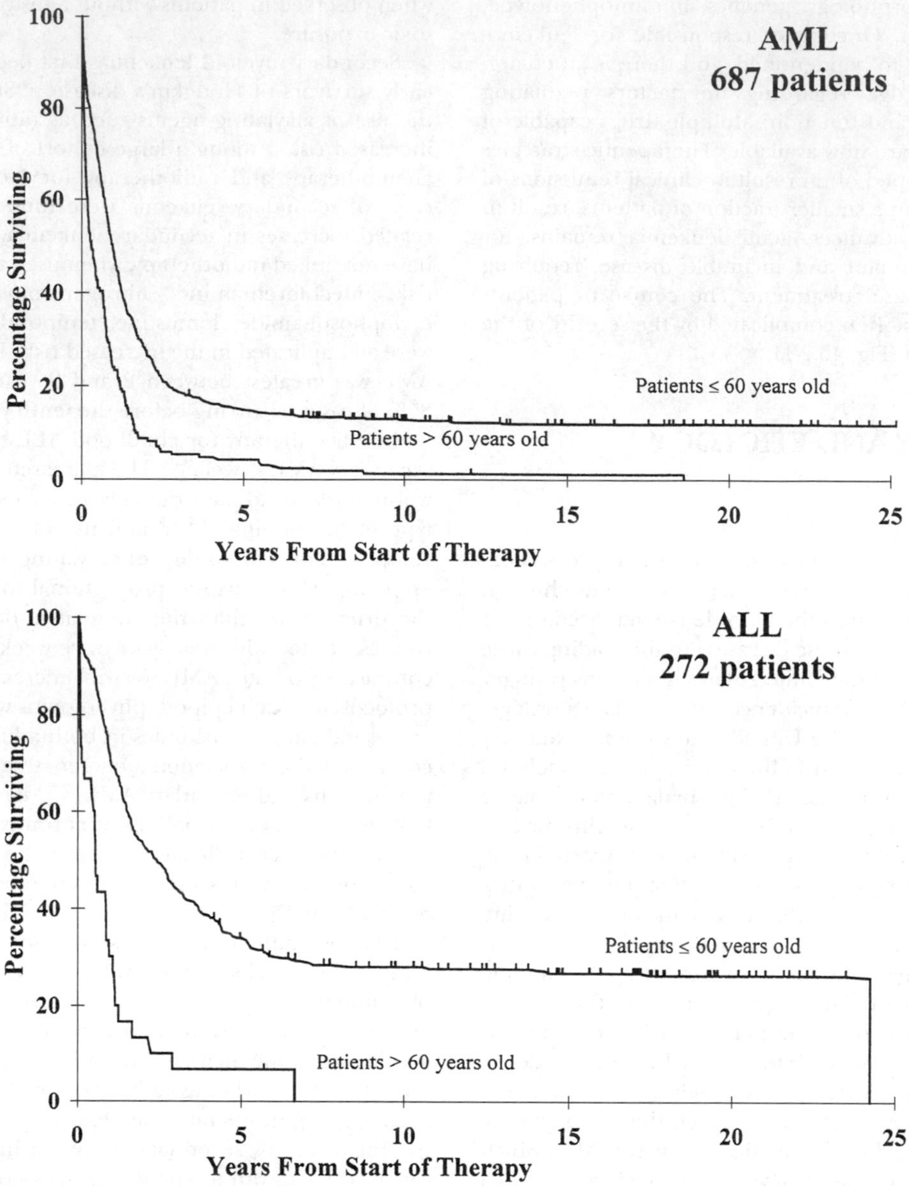

FIGURE 46.2-1. Overall survival for up to 25 years of follow-up in adults treated on protocols at Memorial Hospital, New York City. Patients older than 60 years of age have a substantially worse prognosis for both acute lymphoblastic leukemias (ALL) and acute myelogenous leukemias (AML). Patients treated on more recent protocols have a similar outcome to those on earlier protocols. (Data accrued by B. D. Clarkson, C. Little, D. Tyson, L. Megharian, and D. A. Scheinberg.)

sure to low-dose radiation are controversial. Early suspicions that paternal exposure at power plants resulted in an increased risk for subsequent children of the exposed workers have been disputed.[24,25]

Cigarette smoke contains numerous carcinogens and has been linked in a dose-dependent manner to leukemia,[26–28] particularly in patients older than 60 years and to specific chromosomal alterations known to be associated with chemical mutagens. As much as 20% of AML may be attributable to smoking.[27]

Occupational exposure to benzene has been established as a cause of AML,[29] but low-level exposure in the workplace (e.g., less than 10 parts-per-million) has not been clearly established as a risk. Other occupational exposures to solvents, such as to toluene or butadiene in the shoe and rubber industries, or hair dyes, have not been shown conclusively to increase leukemia risk.[21]

OTHER RISK FACTORS

Viruses, and in particular, RNA retroviruses, have been found to cause many neoplasms in experimental animals, including leukemia of mice[30] and cats; a human retrovirus, human T-cell lymphotropic virus-1, has been identified as the cause of a mature T-cell lymphoma and leukemia in humans.[31] A clear retroviral cause for acute leukemia in humans has not been

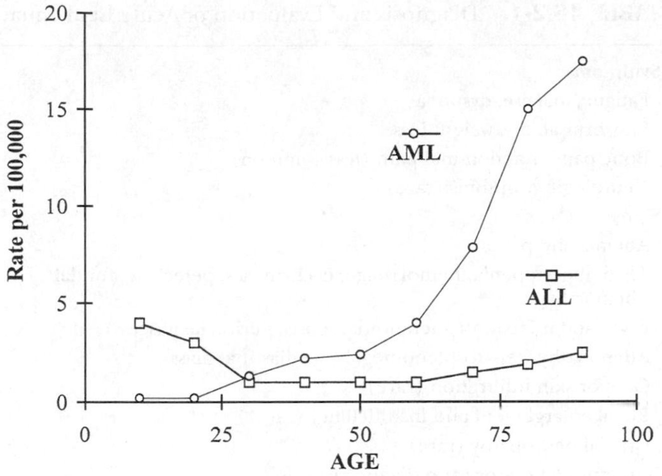

FIGURE 46.2-2. Age-specific incidence of acute myelogenous leukemias (AML) (*circles*) and acute lymphoblastic leukemias (ALL) (*squares*) in the United States. (Adapted from ref. 3.)

identified. Epstein-Barr virus, a DNA virus, has been associated with oncogenesis in acute B-cell leukemias, Burkitt's lymphomas, especially those of endemic origin, and human immunodeficiency virus–associated lymphomas.[31] Epstein-Barr virus may function by increasing lymphoid proliferation in patients; this provides a setting in which a second oncogenic event, possibly *myc* oncogene activation, can result in the clonal, neoplastic proliferation.[32] It has not been demonstrated, however, that simple infection with either an RNA- or DNA-based virus alone is a cause of acute leukemia.

Although leukemias are acquired disorders, there may be significant genetic and immunologic predispositions that allow their occurrence. Several genetic syndromes are associated with increased risk of leukemias, including Down syndrome, Fanconi's anemia, Bloom's syndrome, and ataxia-telangiectasia.[33,34] Down syndrome is associated with 20-fold increased risk of leukemia; this is typically a megakaryoblastic leukemia in children younger than 3 years of age and a pre-B ALL in children who are older.[35] These true leukemias must be differentiated from a transient abnormal myeloproliferative disorder.[36] Patients with transient abnormal myeloproliferative disorder are neonates with hepatosplenomegaly, modest elevations in blasts, and pancytopenia. Although transient abnormal myeloproliferative disorder is a clonal disorder, in two-thirds of cases the disease has a benign course.

An immunologic predisposition for acute leukemia has not been clearly delineated. However, analyses of HLA types with specific cytogenetically defined subgroups of AML have pointed to associations between certain HLA A, B, C, and DR types and common chromosomal translocations or deletions.[37] These correlations may become increasingly important as an understanding of the immune response to these breakpoints becomes clear.[38]

BIOLOGY OF ACUTE LEUKEMIAS

More is known about the pathobiology of the acute leukemia cell than about any other neoplasm. This is the consequence of a confluence of discoveries regarding hematopoietic growth factors, hematopoietic stem cells and progenitor cells, oncogenes, and transcription factors. These discoveries were made possible by the availability of acute leukemia cell lines capable of immortal growth in culture, reliable assays for hematopoietic cell growth, and sensitive tests for specific gene expression and protein expression. The important concepts about leukemia cell growth and function are likely to be useful paradigms that will aid in understanding all cancers.

Cell lines derived from and biologically resembling AML and ALL have been available since the 1980s and have allowed careful study of the growth of leukemia cells under controlled conditions and of the effects of antileukemic agents.[39] Mouse models mimicking human leukemias can be prepared by oncogene transfections.[40] In addition, both cell lines and fresh acute leukemias have been propagated in immunocompromised nude or severe combined immunodeficiency (SCID) mice, thus also allowing controlled study of new therapies under conditions *in vivo* as well.[41] Fresh normal and neoplastic hematopoietic cells can also be grown in intermediate-term cultures or colony-forming assays (over 2 to 8 weeks), in which maturation into specific lineages can be observed and modulated by use of exogenous growth factors, drugs, and differentiating agents.[42–44] This has allowed the elucidation of the sequence and importance of the various growth factors and adhesion molecules during normal and leukemia cell growth and cell death (apoptosis),[45] the identification and isolation of primitive normal stem cells, and the partial reconstitution of normal hematopoiesis *ex vivo*.[42–47] The growth of myeloid leukemia cells *in vitro* appears to be dependent on interleukin (IL)-3, granulocyte-macrophage colony-stimulating factor (GM-CSF), granulocyte colony-stimulating factor (G-CSF), or macrophage colony-stimulating factor (M-CSF) and may be regulated by IL-6 and tumor necrosis factor as well.[43,47,48] Autocrine production of colony-stimulating factors or mutations in their receptors by cells that also express the appropriate receptors on their cell surfaces may allow unregulated proliferation in the absence of exogenous factors.[43,49,50] Comparable assays *in vivo* using immunosuppressed mice that allow spleen colony formation or complete bone marrow reconstitution have demonstrated that viable hematopoiesis for an entire animal may require as few as 30 hematopoietic stem cells.[51,52]

Enzyme marker studies using glucose-6-phosphate dehydrogenase have shown that leukemia cells derive from a single clonogenic cell.[53–55] Depending on the cell of origin, the leukemia clone may involve cells of more than one lineage (e.g., erythroid and myeloid) or only one lineage. Unlike normal hematopoiesis, the clonogenic leukemia cell generally retains only a limited ability to differentiate into different lineages.[56] The cells responsible for leukemia colony growth *in vitro* represent a more primitive subset of the entire leukemia cell population.[57]

There is considerable aberrancy in the differentiation of leukemia cells, as compared with normal cells, when the cell is examined for surface protein phenotype.[58] There may also be abnormalities in apoptosis, or programmed cell death, that leads to persistence of the leukemic clone[45,59] or abnormalities in telomerase, which promotes longevity.[60] Apoptotic death may still be induced with appropriate growth factors *in vitro*, or in the case of promyelocytic leukemia, by clinical use of retinoic acid (see Acute Promyelocytic Leukemia, later in this chapter). It is likely that many leukemogenic translocations or mutations (see Molecular Biology, later in this chapter, and Chapter 45.1) result in dysregulation of the cell cycle.[61]

Heterogeneity of the cells that make up the leukemic population is frequently seen.[53,54,57] Although the leukemic clone may involve multiple lineages, typically leukemia blasts are phenotypically of one lineage; within this lineage, stages of maturation may vary, suggesting incomplete control of differentiation. The phenotypic heterogeneity of the leukemia colony-forming cell also suggests that leukemias may arise at various stages of differentiation. This concept was surmised based on the morphologic and phenotypic characteristics of different leukemias; evidence supporting the concept has been demonstrated in patients with acute promyelocytic leukemia (APL), in which the leukemia clone can be positively identified by use of sensitive polymerase chain reaction (PCR) techniques for the t(15;17). In most cases, the most primitive hematopoietic cells remained normal, whereas more mature progenitors contained the neoplastic translocation.[62]

Despite the achievement of a complete clinical remission after therapy of acute leukemia, normal hematopoiesis derived from cells originally involved with the leukemic clone is sometimes present.[63] Apparently normal granulocytes have exhibited persistence of chromosomal markers of the original leukemia.[64] The continued presence of clonal hematopoiesis may suggest the existence of a preleukemic clone of cells that has a proliferative advantage to other normal cells.[63] In spite of this, hematopoiesis in patients in remission is usually polyclonal or oligoclonal.[65]

TABLE 46.2-1. Diagnosis and Evaluation of Acute Leukemia

Symptoms
Fatigue, malaise, dyspnea
Easy bruisability, weight loss
Bone pain or abdominal pain (less common)
Neurologic symptoms (rare)
Signs
Anemia and pallor
Thrombocytopenia, hemorrhage, ecchymoses, petechiae, fundal hemorrhage
Fever and infection (pneumonia, sepsis, perirectal abscess)
Adenopathy, hepatosplenomegaly, mediastinal mass
Gum or skin infiltration (rare)
Renal enlargement and insufficiency (rare)
Cranial neuropathy (rare)
Important laboratory and diagnostic tests
Complete blood cell count and differential coagulation studies, including fibrinogen
Blood electrolytes and chemistries, including creatinine, uric acid, calcium, phosphorus
Examination of the peripheral blood smear
Examination of the bone marrow aspirate smear and biopsy
Leukemia blast cell surface phenotype, cytogenetics (and molecular genetics if indicated)
Examination of the cerebrospinal fluid (in all patients with acute lymphoblastic leukemias; in patients with acute myelogenous leukemias, only if indicated)
Computed tomography of the chest (in lymphoblastic lymphoma) or of the abdomen (in mature B-cell acute lymphoblastic leukemias)
Human leukocyte antigen typing (for younger patients)

DIAGNOSIS AND CLASSIFICATION OF ACUTE LEUKEMIAS

CLINICAL PRESENTATION

Although the signs and symptoms are relatively nonspecific, the diagnosis of acute leukemia is usually made easily with the history of the illness, the physical examination, and an examination of the blood smear and bone marrow aspirate smear. Additional laboratory examinations (complete blood cell counts, coagulation profile, chemistry profile) or diagnostic imaging (chest radiography, abdominal sonography) are important in the management of the disease, but are not usually necessary for diagnosis. Patients with acute leukemia typically present with a 1- to 3-month history of fatigue or malaise, easy bruisability or frank bleeding, dyspnea, minimal to modest weight loss, fever, bone pain, or abdominal pain (Table 46.2-1). Excessive bleeding after a minor dental procedure or severe epistaxis may bring the patient to the physician's attention. In adults with an antecedent myelodysplastic syndrome, symptoms may date back for up to a year or more.

The physical examination typically shows pallor, consistent with anemia, and hemorrhage (in the gums, as epistaxis, in the stool, in the skin as petechiae or ecchymoses, or as fundal hemorrhage). Less commonly, there is hepatic or splenic enlargement and lymphadenopathy. Fever and infection, usually of respiratory origin are frequent; sepsis may occur. Neurologic signs and symptoms are infrequent at presentation, occur more commonly with ALL, and typically include cranial neuropathies, nausea and vomiting, and headache.

The laboratory evaluation is notable for anemia and thrombocytopenia in most patients, with severe thrombocytopenia (less than 50,000/µL) in more than one-half of patients. The white blood cell (WBC) count can be normal, reduced, or elevated; less than 20% of patients have greater than 100,000 cells per µL, and an equal number of patients have less than 5000 cells per µL. Acute monocytic leukemias and T-cell leukemias may have the highest WBC counts. Examination of the peripheral blood smear shows blasts in almost all cases. Peripheral blood blasts may be absent in some patients with lymphoblastic or Burkitt's lymphoma. Peripheral blood myeloblast levels in excess of 100,000/µL represent a medical emergency requiring prompt reduction in the blast level to prevent leukostasis. The prothrombin time and partial thromboplastin time may be elevated; in APL, this coagulopathy is often associated with reduced fibrinogen and other evidence of disseminated intravascular coagulation (DIC) and is another medical emergency that must be treated urgently (see Principles of Clinical Management of Acute Leukemia, later in this chapter). Subclinical DIC may be present in any form of acute leukemia.

Blood chemistry results are typically normal, but in advanced disease, or in infiltrative cases such as with monocytic leukemias, there may be evidence of renal dysfunction (elevated creatinine). Renal infiltration and enlargement can be documented with ultrasonography. In cases of high cell turnover and cell death, such as in patients with mature B-cell ALL

(ALL-L3), there may be evidence of tumor lysis syndrome at presentation; this syndrome is more commonly seen during the rapid lysis of large numbers of ALL cells, and less often AML cells, during chemotherapy. The laboratory picture of tumor lysis syndrome consists of hypocalcemia, hyperkalemia, hyperphosphatemia, increased lactate dehydrogenase, hyperuricemia and renal insufficiency; if untreated, this syndrome can be fatal (see Principles of Clinical Management of Acute Leukemia, later in this chapter).

The clinical presentation of AML cannot usually be distinguished from ALL without examination of the blasts for immunophenotype and morphology (see Morphology and Cytochemistry, later in this chapter). There are signs and symptoms, however, that are more frequent with certain disease subgroups than with others. Bone pain is more common in ALL, as are signs and symptoms of central nervous system (CNS) infiltration. Lymph node and organ infiltration and enlargement are also more common in ALL and in monocytic subtypes of AML. Gum involvement is seen most frequently in acute monocytic leukemia (AML-M5). Mediastinal masses are found in greater than 50% of patients with T-cell ALL. However, the overlap in symptoms and signs among the leukemia subtypes requires a pathologic diagnosis to be made in all cases. Therefore, a bone marrow aspirate and biopsy, with appropriate cytochemical, immunochemical, and genetic evaluations, must be done in all cases.

The differential diagnosis of acute leukemia includes other neoplastic hematopoietic disorders, such as lymphomas, myelodysplastic syndromes, multiple myeloma, aplastic anemia, severe megaloblastic anemia due to folate or B_{12} deficiency, severe lymphocytosis due to infection, such as with Epstein-Barr virus; severe monocytosis due to tuberculosis; and bone marrow failure with release of early cells, such as in myelophthisis, due to carcinoma. Examination of the bone marrow nearly always excludes the nonhematopoietic conditions because of the presence of increased numbers of blasts. Careful morphologic examination and immunophenotyping of the cells then excludes virtually all the hematopoietic conditions based on lineage and maturational stage; one exception is the myelodysplastic syndromes, which often differ from the acute leukemias only in the percentage of blasts in the marrow. Up to one-third of AMLs in patients older than the age of 60 years have evolved from a prior myelodysplastic syndrome or other hematologic disorder, suggesting that the distinction between refractory anemia with excess blasts or refractory anemia with excess blasts in transformation and true AML after myelodysplasia may be clinically unimportant. These conditions each respond more poorly to chemotherapy than *de novo* AML, and progressive leukemia and bone marrow failure leading to death is the typical outcome.

CLASSIFICATION OF ACUTE LEUKEMIA

Modern classifications of acute leukemia must answer three questions to be diagnostically and prognostically useful: (1) What is the lineage? (2) What is the maturational stage? (3) What is the genotype? Although traditional classifications relied primarily on morphology and cytochemistry,[66–69] these limited characterizations are not always adequate for classifying leukemias into groups that assign the most appropriate therapy or predict outcome. Knowledge of the exact immunophenotype and the genotype, either via cytogenetic analysis or molecular analysis, is critically important before commencing the most appropriate definitive treatment, such as high-dose consolidation chemotherapy, BMT, or prolonged maintenance therapy.

MORPHOLOGY AND CYTOCHEMISTRY

The French-American-British (FAB) group has proposed a widely used classification of eight different types of AMLs (M0 to M7) and three types of ALLs (L1 to L3) based on morphology and cytochemistry[66,67,69]; monoclonal antibody–based immunophenotype is also used in undifferentiated cases in which morphology and cytochemistry are inconclusive[69,70] (Table 46.2-2). Because the treatments of ALL and AML may differ significantly, the most important first step in the diagnostic assignment is to distinguish the lymphoid and myeloid lineages to assign therapy. Among the lymphoid neoplasms, the distinction of FAB L3-ALL (Burkitt's type; mature B cell) is a second important step, as treatment strategies and prognosis differ with this subgroup. Among the myeloid leukemias, identification of FAB M3-AML (APL) is necessary because retinoic acid differentiation therapy is instituted instead of, or concurrently with, chemotherapy. Moreover, there is a significant risk of highly morbid coagulopathy associated with APL. Because current therapies for all subtypes of AML, except APL, are generally similar, and outcomes are typically poor, the advantages of the FAB classification are limited. In addition, morphology and cytochemistry are not diagnostic in 10% to 15% of cases or can be misleading in a small percentage of patients. Moreover, concordance of diagnosis among reviewers may only be 70% to 85%. For these reasons, the FAB classification should always be accompanied by immunophenotypic and genotypic analysis.[70–72]

The FAB classification of AML, as modified by the National Cancer Institute,[71] is based on morphologic examination for lineage, confirmation of lineage by cytochemical stains, quantitation of the number of blasts, and estimation of the degree of differentiation of the cells (see Table 46.2-2). Myeloid leukemia blasts are typically large with round or irregular, smoothly grained nuclei, and with moderate cytoplasm often containing granules or Auer rods; the Auer rods are pathognomonic for myeloblasts. In contrast, lymphoid blasts are typically small with more regular nuclei, clumpier chromatin, and scant, agranular cytoplasm. A cytoplasmic tail, making the cell resemble a hand mirror is sometimes seen. B-lineage leukemia blasts are not distinguishable from T-lineage leukemia blasts based on morphology alone, except if they are mature B-cell type (Burkitt's type, FAB L3) blasts, which have characteristic voluminous, vacuolated, deeply basophilic cytoplasm. Myeloblasts are graded according to the number of and quality of granules (e.g., a type I blast has no granules; a type II blast has up to 15 delicate granules; a type III blast has numerous azurophilic granules). The blasts associated with chronic myelogenous leukemia in blast crisis cannot be distinguished on morphologic or phenotypic grounds alone.

The most important stains for determining lineage initially include myeloperoxidase, which can be positive (golden brown), even in the absence of visible primary azurophilic granules, and Sudan black B, which stains primary and secondary granule lipids black. Myeloid differentiation is inferred if either of these stains are positive in 3% or more blasts. AS-D

TABLE 46.2-2. Classification of Acute Leukemia

Subtype (Incidence)	*Bone Marrow Morphology*	*Typical Immunophenotype*	*Associated Genotype*	*Comments*
AML-M0, undifferentiated AML (5% of AML)	Type 1 blasts >30%; cytochemistry negative	CD13, 33, 34, HLA-DR	N/A	Poorer prognosis
AML-M1, AML with minimal maturation (15% of AML)	Types 1 and II blasts >90%; sudan black or peroxidase positive; occasional Auer rods present	CD13, 14, 15, 33, 34, HLA-DR	Occasionally inv(3)	Inv(3) associated with thrombocytosis
AML-M2, AML with maturation (25% of AML)	Types I, II, and III blasts >30% and <90%; <20% monocytic cells; strong positive Sudan black, peroxidase, or chloroacetate esterase; many Auer rods possible	CD13, 15, 33, 34, HLA-DR	t(8;21) in one-half of cases	t(8;21) has a favorable prognosis; seen in younger adults; associated with extramedullary involvement and splenomegaly
AML-M3, Pronycyclocytic leukemia (APL), (10% of AML)	>30% blasts and abnormal promyelocytes; multiple Auer rods, sometimes in bundles; heavy granulation; strong positive cytochemistry	CD13, 33, 15, less CD34, HLA-DR negative	t(15;17)	Best prognosis of all acute myeloid leukemias; capable of differentiation with retinoic acid therapy; a high risk of disseminated intravascular coagulation; seen in younger adults
AML-M3v (variant)	Abnormal promyelocytes lack granules or Auer rods; weaker cytochemical stains	As for M3, CD2(+)	As for M3	As for M3, may be mistaken for monocytic leukemia
AML-M4, myelomonocytic leukemia (25% of AML)	As for M2, except that monocytic lineage cells are >20% and <80%; peripheral blood has >5000 monocytes/μL; alpha-naphthol stain is positive	CD13, 14, 15, 33, 34, HLA-DR positive	N/A	Evidence of both monocytic and granulocytic differentiation; extramedullary involvement can be seen
AML-M4eo, myelomonocytic leukemia with eosinophilia	Abnormal basophilic eosinophils are seen in the marrow, which is similar to that of M4	As for M4	inv(16); other 16 abnormalities	Good prognosis; extramedullary involvement is often seen
AML-M5 A, monocytic leukemia (5% of AML)	Large blasts with >80% of cells of the monocytic lineage; >80% of cells are monoblasts; alpha-naphthol stain is positive	CD13, 14, 33, 34, HLA-DR	Abnormal 11q23	Poorer prognosis; often seen in older adults; extramedullary disease (skin, gingival, and central nervous system involvement) common
AML-M5 B, monocytic leukemia with differentiation (5% of AML)	As for M5 A except that <80% of monocytic lineage are blasts	As for M5 A, CD34(-)	As for M5 A	As for M5 A; t(8,16) associated with erythrophagocytosis
AML-M6, erythroid leukemia (5% of AML)	>50% of nucleated cells are erythroid; often dysmorphic; >30% of nonerythroid cells are blasts; periodic acid–Schiff is block positive	CD13, 33, 41, 71, HLA-DR, glycophorin A	Deletion 5 and 7 are often seen	Poorer prognosis; often preceded by a myelodysplastic syndrome; seen in older patients
AML-M7, megakaryoblastic leukemia (10% of AML)	>30% blasts of megakaryocytic origin with blebs; micromegakaryoblasts often present; megakaryocytic fragments are seen in the blood; peroxidase is usually negative; alpha-naphthol and periodic acid–Schiff may be positive; platelet peroxidase is positive by electron microscopy	CD41, 61	Occasional inv(3); t(3;3) trisomy 21; t(9;22); t(1;22) in infants	Poor prognosis; often a fibrotic bone marrow makes diagnosis difficult; can be seen in Down syndrome children <3 years old, but must be distinguished from transient abnormal myeloproliferative disorder; is often associated with prior myelodysplastic syndromes, chronic myeloid leukemia blast crisis, or myeloprolif-erative disorders
ALL-L1 (30% of adult ALL)	Small cells with minimal cytoplasm and no granules; rare nucleoli; tdt positive	If B-lineage: CD10, 19, 20, 22, 34, HLA-DR, cytoplasmic Ig; if T-lineage: CD2, 5, 7, 10, 34	t(9;22); t(4;11); t(1:9); hyperdiploid	Most common subtype in children
ALL-L2 (65% of adult ALL)	Larger cells with moderate amounts of cytoplasm and prominent nucleoli; tdt positive	As for ALL-L1	As for ALL-L1	Most common subtype in adults
ALL-L3, B-cell or Burkitt's type leukemia (5% of ALL)	Large round cells with deeply basophilic cytoplasm and vacuoles	CD10, 19, 20, 21, 22, surface Ig	t(8;14); t(2;8); t(8;22)	Poor prognosis with standard ALL treatment regimens

ALL, acute lymphoblastic leukemias; AML, acute myelogenous leukemia; tdt, terminal deoxynucleotidyl transferase.

chloroacetate esterase is another stain (red or blue) for maturing myeloid granules; α-naphthyl butyrate esterase staining (red/brown) is indicative of monocytic differentiation. Acid phosphatase is generally most useful in T-cell ALL, where it stains as a block or patch.

In the small subset of cases in which lineage cannot be indicated by morphology or cytochemistry, immunophenotyping using specific monoclonal antibodies usually determines lineage to be myeloid.[69,70,73] This group is designated AML-M0. The poorer prognosis of this subgroup makes their distinction from L2-ALL and other AML subtypes important.

Another subgroup that is difficult to classify due to its pleomorphic morphology and unhelpful cytochemistry is acute megakaryoblastic leukemia (AML-M7).[67,74] The lineage can sometimes be identified by cytoplasmic blebs; electron microscopy for platelet peroxidase is confirmatory, although this is not a routinely or rapidly available test. Monoclonal antibodies to platelet-specific antigens CD41 and CD61 are usually helpful, but false-positive results are seen often.[67,70,71] This disease is often associated with bone marrow fibrosis and pancytopenia that obscures the percentage of blasts in aspirates and necessitates the use of a bone marrow biopsy for morphologic diagnosis.[67,71]

The FAB classification of ALL into L1 and L2 subtypes is based on an examination of blasts for nuclear cytoplasmic ratio, the number and appearance of nucleoli, the regularity of the nuclear membrane outline, and cell size.[68] In general, L1 has a small size in greater than 50% of cells, a high nuclear cytoplasmic ratio in greater than 75% of cells, up to one small, ill-defined nucleoli in greater than 75% of cells, and a regular nuclear membrane in greater than 75% of cells. L2 generally has the opposite characteristics. L1-type blasts are found more often among children and denote a better prognosis. L2 is more common in adults, but has little prognostic significance in this population. L3-ALL is easily distinguished by its homogeneous large cells and basophilic cytoplasm with prominent vacuolization. L3-ALL cells usually express cell surface immunoglobulin. The ALLs are usually distinguished by the absence of myeloid-specific immunophenotypic markers or cytochemical stains and by the presence of lymphoid immunophenotypic patterns.

Additional diagnostic subgroups not classified by the FAB criteria include mixed lineage (biphenotypic) leukemias, mast cell leukemias, the histiocytoses, juvenile chronic myelogenous leukemia, and eosinophilic leukemias.

IMMUNOPHENOTYPING OF ACUTE LEUKEMIAS

Approximately 160 antigen groups, known as *clusters of differentiation* (CDs), have been identified on the surface of hematopoietic cells by monoclonal antibodies. These antigens are predominantly cell surface glycoproteins, and rarely carbohydrates or glycolipids. Although no leukemia-specific antigens have been identified, the CD antigen characterization of hematopoietic cells using a panel of antibodies can establish lineage with reasonable certainty and may suggest maturational stages of cells. Expression on a cell population of antigens not usually found together can also provide strong evidence for neoplasia. Currently, immunophenotyping plays an important role in the understanding of hematopoietic biology and in the diagnosis of leukemia. The immunophenotype is used (1) to confirm the diagnosis in cases in which the classification is clear; (2) to make a diagnosis when morphology and cytochemistry are equivocal, as in M0-AML; (3) to identify biphenotypic leukemias; (4) to characterize aberrant antigen expression, which can be used to identify a neoplastic clone, even when found as minimal residual disease, as in clinical remission; and (5) to assist in assigning leukemias into prognostic groups.

The lineage and state of maturation of normal hematopoietic cells may be identified by use of a flow cytometer to determine the cell size, granularity, and the presence or absence of a panel of cell surface or cytoplasmic differentiation antigens (designated by their CD numbers). Such analyses, termed *multidimensional* or *multiparameter flow cytometry*, are available at most cancer centers or commercial laboratories. Pathways describing the phenotype of normal B, T, and myeloid cells have been constructed[70,75–78] (Fig. 46.2-3). Acute leukemias can also be characterized by a similar panel of markers, and in general, lineage can be assigned by examination of expression of the same antigens as those found in normal cells.[58,70,79]

Acute lymphoid leukemias of T-cell lineage are characterized by expression of the T-cell markers CD2, CD5, CD7, and sometimes CD1 or dual staining of CD4 and CD8. T-cell ALL or lymphoblastic lymphoma may also express the B-lineage mark-

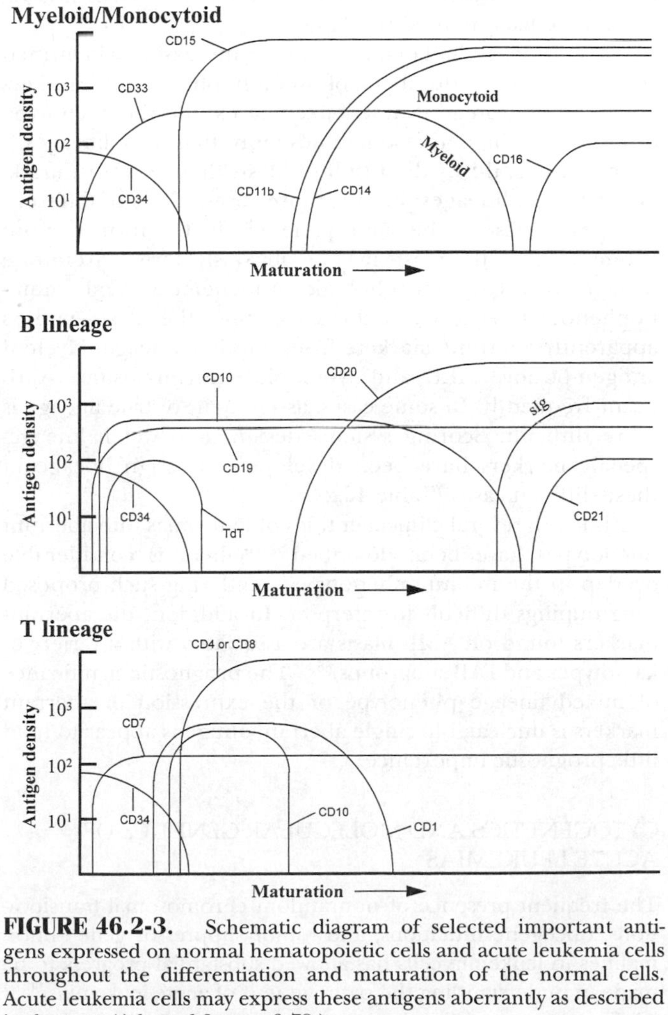

FIGURE 46.2-3. Schematic diagram of selected important antigens expressed on normal hematopoietic cells and acute leukemia cells throughout the differentiation and maturation of the normal cells. Acute leukemia cells may express these antigens aberrantly as described in the text. (Adapted from ref. 78.)

ers CD10 and CD21. Acute lymphoid leukemias of B-cell lineage express CD19, CD10, CD22, and, depending on maturational stage, CD20, and surface immunoglobulin. Acute myeloid leukemias express CD13, CD15, CD33, and, more often if monocytoid, CD14. Terminal deoxyribonucleotidyl transferase is expressed by most lymphoid blasts and approximately 20% of myeloid blasts. CD34 can be expressed by blasts of all lineages, especially if the cells are primitive. HLA-DR is found on virtually all B-lineage leukemias, most myeloid and monocytic leukemias (except FAB M3), and on a rare T-cell ALL.

The pathways of antigen expression, with regard to maturational stage, however, are often aberrant in leukemias.[58,70,78,79] In some cases, there is also abnormal expression of antigens not expected to be found in the lineage.[81–84] Although such infidelity of antigen expression may prevent exact assignment of the maturational stage of the leukemia cell, it may distinguish that cell as neoplastic from within a larger population of normal cells. Thus, aberrant antigen expression, which can be an antigen of the wrong lineage, the simultaneous expression of antigens of different stages of maturation, or the lack of an expected antigen, can provide a useful diagnostic marker for the leukemia cells.[79,81] In addition, such a marker may allow the flow cytometric detection of the leukemia cells at a level of 1 cell in 1000 to 10,000 normal cells, even in patients who have apparently normal bone marrow and blood examination by morphologic criteria.[85] The prognostic significance of this detection is not yet clear, but is likely to predict relapse.[86]

Mixed lineage leukemias are being increasingly identified as use of larger numbers of immunophenotypic markers becomes widespread. These leukemias exhibit the phenotype of more than one, and sometimes more than two, lineages.[83] In most cases, this is the result of blasts that coexpress markers of several lineages; in other rare cases, blasts of different lineages coexist in the same patient.[87] In the former, more common cases, the blasts may be obviously derived from one lineage, based on morphologic, cytochemical, and immunophenotypic criteria; at the same time, the blasts express apparently aberrant markers from another lineage. Myeloid antigen-positive ALL and lymphoid antigen-positive AML occur frequently. In some cases, assignment of true lineage is more difficult. Scoring systems designed to weigh lineage-specific markers have been developed to assign lineage in these difficult cases (Table 46.2-3).[72]

Although several clinical entities of leukemias with aberrant phenotypes have been described,[82,84] there is considerable overlap in the immunophenotypes, rendering such proposed subgroupings difficult to interpret. In addition, the aberrant markers found on AML blasts are associated with a variety of karyotypes and FAB subgroups.[88,89] The prognostic significance of mixed lineage phenotype or the expression of aberrant markers is unclear, but single aberrant antigens appear to hold little prognostic importance.

CYTOGENETICS AND MOLECULAR GENETICS OF ACUTE LEUKEMIAS

The frequent presence of nonrandom chromosomal translocations, oncogene mutations, and tumor suppressor gene abnormalities in leukemia cells has allowed substantial progress to be made in understanding the pathogenesis of acute leukemias,[90–94] in diagnosing and developing prognostic models for subtypes of leukemia,[95–98] and in assessing the effects of therapy or detecting early relapse.[99,100] The molecular genotype or karyotype is rapidly becoming the gold standard for diagnosis and prognosis in many subtypes of acute leukemia. A detailed discussion of the molecular biology of hematopoietic cancer is found in Chapter 45.1.

In ALL, the presence of t(9;22), found in up to 30% of adults, t(4;11), –7 or +8, which are more infrequently seen, are poor prognostic signs. Abnormal karyotypes are seen in approximately 80% of patients with AML.[98] In AML, t(15;17), t(8;21), and inv(16) or t(16;16), have a favorable prognosis, whereas +8, –5, del (5q), –7, del (7q), –20, +11, +13, inv (3), and involvement of 11q23, are unfavorable. Distinct pathologic and clinical syndromes, such as APL, are strongly associated with t(15;17); AML-M2 with t(8;21); AML-M4EO with inv (16) or del 16p and AML-M7 with t(1;22).[98,101] Chemotherapeutic agents that interfere with DNA topoisomerase II, such as epidophyllotoxins or anthracylines, can result in the balanced translocations described previously[102,103] and often appear 1 to 3 years after chemotherapy. In contrast, alkylating agents more typically yield –5, –7, and complex chromosomal abnormalities, 2 to 9 years later, frequently initiate as myelodysplastic syndromes and have a particularly poor prognosis.[104,105]

PRINCIPLES OF THERAPY FOR ACUTE LEUKEMIA

Despite advances, the majority of adult patients with acute leukemia die as a result of the disease (see Fig. 46.2-1).[106] Although most patients initially respond to chemotherapy, relapse is common. The goal of therapy in acute leukemia is the eradication of the leukemic clone with the restoration of normal hematopoiesis. This is usually accomplished by the use of profoundly myelosuppressive chemotherapy, which induces a period of relative bone marrow aplasia with the rapid reduction of leukemia cells. It is during the recovery from aplasia, that a state of clonal competition develops.

Normal stem cells gain a growth advantage and repopulate the bone marrow, establishing the predominance of polyclonal hematopoiesis. Leukemia cells are replaced by normal differentiated progeny, which are capable of providing vital life-sustaining functions. The disease process has been temporarily abated.

The transient nature of the initial clinical response is best understood in the context of the enormous size of the total leukemia burden and the limitations of the effect of modern chemotherapy on this critical mass. Based on data from animal models, it has been estimated that there are approximately 10^{12} leukemia cells in the body at the time of diagnosis. Standard chemotherapy regimens generally result in a 2 to 3 log (99.0% to 99.9%) reduction in the total amount of tumor cells.[107] This places the residual leukemia burden below the level of clinical detection, and based on morphologic criteria, the patient has been placed into a complete remission. Laboratory and clinical evidence, however, would suggest that such a remission is far from complete for the great majority of patients. Although standard morphologic evaluation shows no evidence of residual leukemia, a state of minimal residual disease exists, with estimates for the remaining leukemia burden approaching approximately 10 billion cells. A number of laboratory techniques have been introduced in an effort to increase the resolution of detecting remaining leukemia cells (Table 46.2-4).

TABLE 46.2-3. Assigning Lineage in Mixed Lineage Leukemias[a]

To Assign	*½ Point*	*1 Point*	*2 Points*
Myeloid lineage	CD11b, CD11, CD15	CD33, CD13, CD14, morphology/cytochemistry	Myeloperoxidase
B-lineage	Tdt, IgH rearrangement	CD10, CD19, CD24	cCD22, cμ chain
T-lineage	Tdt, CD7	CD2, CD5, T-cell receptor rearrangement	cCD3

c, cytoplasmic; μ, immunoglobulin M heavy chain; Tdt, terminal deoxyribonucleotidyl transferase.
[a]IgH (heavy chain) rearrangement and T-cell receptor are determined by Southern blot analysis. Any leukemia with two or more points from more than one lineage is scored as a mixed lineage.
(Adapted from ref. 72.)

Although none of the available assays are ideal, current studies of minimal residual disease are attempting to establish the clinical validity of such measures and whether the results from these assays may form the basis for therapeutic decisions in individual patients. The paradigm for this has been provided by the reverse transcriptase-based (RT) PCR assay for the PML/αRAR gene rearrangement used in APL (see Acute Promyelocytic Leukemia, later in this chapter).[71,81,85,97,108–113]

The primary goal of the initial chemotherapy in AML is to achieve a complete response (CR). Despite the limitations of morphologic evaluation, clinical standards have been adopted to define outcomes and establish reference points from which therapies can be compared.[71] CR is defined as less than 5% of blasts in the bone marrow normally regenerated as evidenced by both an acceptable level of cellularity (greater than 20% on bone marrow biopsy) and the restoration of normal hematopoiesis (as reflected by peripheral blood values of at least 1500 neutrophils per μL and 100,000 platelets per μL). Red cell parameters are not usually considered in this definition. The peripheral blood should not contain circulating blasts (in the absence of growth factor use), and there should be no evidence of extramedullary disease. These criteria must be sustained for a period of at least 4 weeks.

CR is the only significant form of clinical response in acute leukemia. The ability to achieve such a response has been directly correlated with survival and is a necessary first step in a curative treatment strategy. Although some research studies have chosen to categorize lesser responses and define partial remission (or response), the inability to morphologically clear leukemia cells from the bone marrow is a treatment failure with grave implications for the patient.

Current treatment strategies divide therapy into two basic parts: induction and postremission therapy. The purpose of remission induction is to achieve a CR. The goal of postremission therapy is to eradicate minimal residual disease, thus preventing relapse and effecting a cure. Different approaches to postremission therapy have been used and defined by a number of studies. Consolidation therapy is used to describe immediate postremission treatment regimens that are similar to induction therapy. The doses of the drugs are either equivalent or slightly attenuated. Intensification is the application of higher doses of active agents while in CR. Maintenance is defined as therapy given in greatly attenuated doses over extended periods.

Relapse is usually heralded by a change in a previously normal complete blood cell count. Reduction in normal cells or the reappearance of blasts in the peripheral blood occur fre-

TABLE 46.2-4. Current Methods Used Frequently for Detection of Minimal Residual Disease

Technique	*Typical No. of Cells Analyzed*	*Materials Analyzed*	*Limits of Sensitivity (%)*	*Example*
Morphology	100–200	Intact cells	5	Standard definition of complete response and relapse[71]
Cytogenetics	20–100	Cells capable of dividing in culture	1–5	Inv(16) in remission bone marrow[108]
Fluorescence *in situ* hybridization	100–1000	DNA	1–2	Trisomy 17 in acute lymphoblastic leukemias[109]
Southern blot	1,000,000	DNA	1–2	TCR gene rearrangements[110]
Multiparameter flow cytometry	50,000–1,000,000	Intact cells	0.001	Aberrant immunophenotype: CD34/56[81]
Polymerase chain reaction	1,000,000	RNA	<.0001	PML/RAR-α in acute promyelocytic leukemia[99]

(Adapted from ref. 35.)

quently; isolated extramedullary relapse is infrequent. Examination of the bone marrow confirms the relapse by demonstrating more than 5% blasts. In situations in which there is only a borderline increase in blasts, it may be necessary to repeat the bone marrow examination in 1 to 2 weeks to confirm relapse.[71]

PRINCIPLES OF CLINICAL MANAGEMENT OF ACUTE LEUKEMIA

The care of the patient with acute leukemia requires the ability to support the individual through the expected complications of myelosuppressive therapy, most notably the period of pancytopenia, which may last for 2 to 5 weeks. Successful clinical management requires a detailed understanding of likely complications accompanied by early therapeutic intervention designed to minimize life-threatening toxicities. With regard to these principles, much of the improvement seen in the care of leukemia patients in the last few years can be directly attributed to advances in supportive care.

Infection and hemorrhage are the primary cause of death in patients with leukemia.[114] Many patients with acute leukemia initially present to the physician with fever and neutropenia. Virtually all patients develop these complications after treatment with chemotherapy. Untreated, infection in the neutropenic host can be rapidly fatal. Therefore, the early institution of antibiotic therapy is necessary.[115,116] Initial antibiotics must provide a broad spectrum of antibacterial coverage, with particular emphasis on gram-negative organisms. The epidemiology of a single center's flora may be instrumental in determining the particular antibiotics used as first-line therapy. Common regimens include an antipseudomonal penicillin or cephalosporin coupled with an aminoglycoside. Monotherapy with a third-generation cephalosporin, such as ceftazidime, or a carbapenem, such as imipenem, is an alternative.

Changes in the initial antibiotic coverage are based either on the sensitivities of the organisms isolated or persistence of fever. Continued fever, despite 4 to 6 days of antibacterial therapy usually requires empiric antifungal therapy with amphotericin B. Additionally, patients with indwelling central venous catheters or other prosthetic devices may require the early institution of vancomycin. Antimicrobial agents should be continued until the absolute neutrophil count has risen above 500/μL. Patients who have a documented bacterial source of infection should complete at least a 10- to 14-day course of therapy, whereas those patients with evidence of infection secondary to invasive mycoses may require a more protracted course of therapy.

Despite the accepted approach to empiric therapy in patients with leukemia and neutropenic fever, there is considerable controversy regarding infection prophylaxis, use of protected environments, reverse isolation, transfusion of granulocytes, or the use of hematopoietic growth factors to accelerate recovery.[117–119] Although the duration of neutropenia has consistently been shortened by the use of G-CSF or GM-CSF in a number of studies, the effect on infectious complications and mortality has been variable.[120–125] Careful attention to oral hygiene with regular use of oral rinsing and cleaning with soft tipped (sponge) devices to prevent gingival trauma may prove useful. Rectal or vaginal manipulations should be avoided.

Immediate access to blood products is critical to sustain the patient; the hemoglobin level should be maintained at 8 g/dL or higher in patients with other medical comorbidities (pulmonary disorders or coronary heart disease). There is a direct relationship between hemorrhage and reductions in the platelet count below 5000 to 10,000/μL. Hence, platelets are not only transfused in response to hemorrhage, but also to prevent hemorrhage. The routine use of platelet transfusions has had a significant effect on the incidence of hemorrhagic death. Patients with uncomplicated thrombocytopenia can be transfused when the platelet count falls below 10,000/μL. Patients who are either febrile or have other complicating medical conditions such as severe mucositis or ongoing coagulopathy, require prophylactic transfusions at higher levels.[126–128]

Some patients become refractory to platelet transfusions. This may result either from alloimmunization in the patients who have received multiple transfusions or may be secondary to other medical conditions such as persistent fever or disseminated intravascular coagulation. This refractoriness poses a particularly difficult management problem for the clinician. Current strategies to overcome alloimmunization include the prevention of sensitization by the use of single, related donor platelets or HLA-matched platelets as well as the use of leukocyte reduction filters.[129] Platelets from a potential bone marrow donor should be avoided in patients who are eligible for allogeneic BMT.

A bleeding diathesis or frank DIC may be present in addition to thrombocytopenia and may result in either hemorrhage or thrombosis. This complication is most frequently associated with APL, but may also be found in other subtypes of acute leukemia either at presentation or after the institution of cytotoxic therapy. The coagulopathy has been attributed to the release of procoagulants from the leukemia cells as they lyse. The contribution of increased fibrinolysis to this hemostatic disorder has come under scrutiny.[130]

The approach to the patient with leukemia-associated coagulopathy remains controversial. Laboratory tests that are useful as indicators of coagulopathy include the platelet count, prothrombin time, activated partial thromboplastin time, thrombin time, fibrinogen, fibrin split products, and D-dimer. Clinical management relies on frequent monitoring of the patient with intervention based on a deteriorating clinical status or worsening trend in a laboratory value such as fibrinogen. The former approach of managing the bleeding diathesis of APL with low-dose heparin (7 to 10 U/kg/h) has largely been replaced by early treatment with retinoids as well as aggressive blood product support.[131,132] Platelets and fresh frozen plasma are transfused multiple times daily to maintain platelet counts above 50,000/μL and fibrinogen levels above 100 mg/dL. The hemostatic abnormalities typically abate after the leukemia burden has been reduced.

Metabolic abnormalities can exist in the leukemia patient at presentation or with the institution of therapy.[133,134] Patients rarely present with disorders of potassium or calcium, but can develop electrolyte problems during treatment with aminoglycosides, amphotericin, or other agents that affect kidney function. Rapid leukemia cell death releases intracellular metabolites, notably uric acid, potassium, and phosphorus, causing a life-threatening metabolic condition known as the *tumor lysis syndrome.* Uric acid, a product of purine metabolism, may then deposit in the joints, causing a gouty arthropathy or, more important, in the renal parenchyma or collecting system, resulting in renal failure. Hyperuricemia may be detected. Prevention of these complications is usually accomplished by instituting vigorous hydration with a brisk urine output (greater than 150 mL/h) and administering allopurinol before beginning cytotoxic therapy. The dose of allopurinol ranges from 300 to 900 mg/d. Alkalinization of the urine by adding sodium bicarbonate to the intravenous fluids, administering a carbonic anhydrase inhibitor (such as acetazolamide), or both are recommended in extreme cases, or in patients allergic to allopurinol, to increase the solubility of the uric acid.

Complications, such as cardiac disturbances with hyperkalemia or the precipitation of calcium phosphate resulting in renal failure due to hyperphosphatemia, can be avoided in most cases with early attention to metabolic disturbances. Correction of these abnormalities is best accomplished by aggressive hydration with concominant diuresis to wash out the toxic by-product of the dying leukemia cells. Additional benefit may be gained by using oral phosphate binders (aluminum hydroxide or calcium acetate) to minimize absorption of additional phosphate from dietary sources. In situations in which hyperkalemia is complicated by renal insufficiency, cation exchange resins (Kayexalate) may be indicated. Extreme circumstances may require renal dialysis to correct multiple abnormalities.

Tumor lysis syndrome most frequently complicates acute lymphoid leukemia (particularly Burkitt's type) and is most problematic in the setting of hyperleukocytosis (peripheral blast counts greater than 100,000/µL). Patients with AML are at a relatively reduced risk of tumor lysis, relative to ALL, but are at an increased risk for sludging of large myeloblasts in the microcirculation (leukostasis), resulting in cerebral or pulmonary compromise often associated with hemorrhage and, in extreme circumstance, leading to death. The ability to rapidly decrease the circulating blast number, however, is an important factor for survival in these patients. Leukapheresis can be used, but, at best, is only a temporizing measure. Instead, immediate treatment with chemotherapy should be undertaken with careful attention to the expected metabolic abnormalities discussed previously.

TREATMENT OF NEWLY DIAGNOSED ACUTE MYELOGENOUS LEUKEMIAS

Untreated, AML is a uniformly fatal disease. Although it is possible to support patients for a period with supportive medical care, they ultimately succumb to the complications associated with bone marrow failure: infection or hemorrhage. Most patients seek medical attention for symptoms related to infection or bleeding, and these patients typically require immediate therapeutic intervention. Other patients are not candidates for cytotoxic therapy because of a poor performance status or other active severe medical comorbidities that complicate their care. In such settings, a supportive strategy may be most appropriate. The risks and potential benefits and alternatives should be carefully considered in each case and discussed with the patient and the family.

Several prognostic factors have been identified in AML (Table 46.2-5).[114,135] The difference in treatment results among various trials using similar chemotherapy may, in part, be explained by the frequency of these negative characteristics within a study population.[136] Age is inversely associated with the ability to achieve remission.[137,138] In patients older than the age of 60 years, standard therapy achieves CR in only 30% to 50% of treated individuals. AML that occurs as a consequence of prior cytotoxic therapy, or that has developed from an antecedent hematologic disorder (e.g., myelodysplastic syndrome) has a particularly poor outcome, with a lower incidence of achieving a CR and shorter duration of survival than for patients with *de novo* AML.[139,140] Multiple studies have demonstrated the prognostic importance of cytogenetic abnormalities in AML, making this the single most important predictor of outcome.[141–143] Patients with a good prognosis are those with t(15;17), t(8;21), or inv(16), whereas poor-risk patients have loss of all or part of chromosome 5 or 7, translocations involving 11q23, or trisomy 8.

TABLE 46.2-5. Prognostic Features in Adult Acute Leukemia

Acute myelogenous leukemias
Age: Older age is associated with a reduced incidence of complete response
Antecedent hematologic disorder or secondary acute myelogenous leukemia: These subgroups have a lower incidence of complete response and a reduced overall survival
Cytogenetics: t(15;17), t(8;21), and inv(16) denote good prognostic subgroups; abnormalities of chromosome 5 or 7, trisomy 8, and t(9;11) denote poor prognostic subgroups
Acute lymphoblastic leukemias
White blood cell count: High count associated with poor prognosis
Leukemic cell immunophenotype: T cell has a favorable prognosis, pre-B cell has an intermediate prognosis, whereas mature B-cell disease has a poor prognosis with standard regimens
Age: Older age associated with worse prognosis
Philadelphia chromosome–positive disease has a worse prognosis
Time to complete response: Patients requiring more than 4 to 5 weeks to achieve a complete response have a lower likelihood of being cured

Historically, the diagnosis of acute leukemia has left the physician with few therapeutic options. During the 1940s, Farber established the modern era of chemotherapy by effectively using antimetabolites in pediatric patients with ALL. Subsequently, a number of other single agents were demonstrated to have antileukemic activity at first in the laboratory and then later in the clinic. Many of the drugs initially used to treat adults with AML had been used in pediatric ALL, but they were not active in AML, and the early clinical results were disappointing. The introduction of cytarabine (Ara-C) dramatically changed the therapy of patients with AML.

Ara-C is the most important drug in use today for the treatment of AML. Much of the clinical investigation done since the 1970s has focused on increasing the efficacy of this drug by either combining it with other agents, escalating the dose, or changing the schedule of administration. Despite some minor modifications made in treatment in the last few years, Ara-C remains the cornerstone of AML therapy.

INDUCTION

Standard induction therapy is based on the combination of Ara-C with an anthracycline or anthracenedione. CR rates in newly diagnosed AML patients younger than the age of 60 years range from 50% to 75%, depending on the patient population studied (Table 46.2-6).[136] In the 1960s, investigators first demonstrated the ability of Ara-C alone to induce responses in approximately 20% to 30% of patients.[144] Ara-C was then tried in combination, at first with 6-thioguanine and later with daunorubicin, and found to increase the incidence of CR to approximately 40% to 50%.[145] When the dose of the Ara-C and daunorubicin used was increased, the response rates improved. Ara-C given for 7 days at 100 mg/m^2/d as a continuous infusion with daunorubicin given at 45 mg/m^2/d for 3 days became the standard regimen and is referred to as the *3 + 7* or *7 + 3* regimen. Patients who do not achieve a CR with one course of induction therapy may still be induced into a CR with a second cycle of this therapy. A randomized trial by the Cancer and Leukemia Group B (CALGB) reported a 59% CR rate using 3 + 7 induction therapy and found this response to be superior to a briefer course of similar therapy.[138,146]

The initial success of increasing response rates through dose intensification prompted studies designed to improve the 3 + 7 combination by either adding agents or further increasing doses. Given the prior results with 6-thioguanine, this agent was added to the daunorubicin and Ara-C to form the DAT or TAD regimens. In a number of nonrandomized, single-arm studies, the CR rates were similar to those obtained with 3 + 7 regimen.[147,148] The CALGB conducted a randomized study between 3 + 7 and DAT and found the addition of 6-thioguanine provided no significant benefit.[149] The extension of the Ara-C infusion to 10 days was also found to be without an advantage. A subsequent study failed to show a statistical advantage to doubling the Ara-C dose during the 7-day infusion, although a greater number of treatment-related deaths were noted in patients younger than 60 years of age.[150]

TABLE 46.2-6. Toronto Leukemia Study Group: Effect of Patient Subsets on Complete Response Rate

Induction therapy
- Ara-C, 100 mg/m^2 IV q12h × 7 days
- 6-thioguanine, 100 mg/m^2 PO q12h × 7 days
- Daunorubicin, 60 m/m^2 IV days 5, 6, and 7

Patient Population	*No. of Patients Achieving Complete Response*	*Percentage Complete Response*
All patients (142)	74	52
Without patients unable to complete therapy (–20 patients)	74	61
Above without patients older than 70 years of age (–44 patients)	64	82
Above without patients with antecedent hematologic disorder (–5 patients)	62	85
Above without patients with secondary acute myelogenous leukemias (–5 patients)	62	91

(Modified from ref. 136.)

As new drugs with antileukemic activity have been introduced into the clinic, trials have been undertaken in an attempt to improve on 3 + 7 induction (Table 46.2-7). The substitution of doxorubicin for daunorubicin produced no significant benefit, but instead resulted in increased gastrointestinal toxicity.[137] In another study, the addition of etoposide to 3 + 7 produced an improved remission duration in a younger cohort of patients.[151] Mitoxantrone, amsacrine, rubidazone, and aclarubicin have all been substituted for daunorubicin in induction, but no clinical trial has demonstrated the unequivocal superiority of any of these second-generation regimens.[152–155]

Three randomized trials have compared idarubicin with daunorubicin and have demonstrated that the idarubicin regimens increased response rates in patients younger than 60 years of age.[156–158] More patients treated with idarubicin were able to achieve CR after only one course. The toxicity profiles between the two regimens were similar. In two of the studies, the idarubicin combination demonstrated a survival advantage. An update of these studies has suggested a survival advantage could still be detected in one trial (but not the other two) with a follow-up of 5 years.[159]

Despite these findings, the anthracycline of choice in the induction regimens remains controversial. Criticism of the idarubicin studies cited previously has centered on the issue of dose equivalency between the idarubicin dose (12 or 13 mg/m^2) and the daunorubicin dose (45 or 50 mg/m^2) used for comparison. The CR rate (58%, 58%, and 59%, respectively) in the daunorubicin arm was lower than other studies that used a standard 3 + 7 induction. Several nonrandomized trials have used higher doses of daunorubicin (70 mg/m^2) and have described response rates similar to those seen with idarubicin, suggesting that the dose of the anthracycline used may be more important than the choice of anthracycline.[147] In addition, preliminary results of a large Eastern Cooperative Oncology Group (ECOG) trial that randomized elderly patients between induction regimens using daunorubicin, idarubicin, or mitoxantrone failed to show an advantage to using the newer agents.[160] Despite conflicting results, idarubicin has been widely adopted as part of current treatment regimens.

The ability of high doses of Ara-C to overcome drug resistance and induce remission has been demonstrated in relapsed disease. Such an approach has been applied to upfront induction therapy in an effort to improve response. Ara-C doses ranging from 0.5 to 6.0 g/m^2/d for 3 to 8 days have been investigated. The effect of these regimens on treatment outcomes has been variable. A University of California, Los Angeles, study randomized patients between a 3 + 7 induction and an intermediate-dose Ara-C regimen and found that both remission rate and actuarial 4-year disease-free survival were similar in the two cohorts.[161] Two other randomized studies, however, have shown a benefit to high-dose Ara-C–based inductions, demonstrating an advantage not in the likelihood of achieving a CR but in producing more durable responses and a superior disease-free survival.[162,163] Toxicity was increased with the high-dose regimens and particularly evident during the postremission period when infections were increased and recovery times delayed.

Hematopoietic growth factors have been tested in clinical trials in an attempt to reduce the toxicities seen with dose-intensive treatments. In older patients, significant toxicity with standard therapy has prevented testing more dose-intensive

TABLE 46.2-7. Representative Treatment Regimens in Acute Myelogenous Leukemias (AML)

Source	*Study Group*	*Induction*	*Postremission*	*Complete Response*	*Outcome*	*Comments*
CALGB[137]	AML: <60 y >60 y	D/A "3 + 7"	Cyclic maintenance with A/D/P/VCR	72% 31%	12-mo median duration complete response	Standard induction
ECOG[173]	*De novo* AML <65 y	DAT	High-dose Ara-C/ AMSA versus T/A versus allogeneic bone marrow transplant	68%	27% event-free survival (4 y) in high-dose Ara-C/AMSA group	Addition of 6-thioguanine; high-dose Ara-C intensification
ALSG[191]	*De novo* AML <70 y	A/D/VP-16 "7-3-7"	A/D/VP-16 "5-2-5"	59%	17-mo median survival	Addition of VP-16 to standard "3 + 7"
MSKCC[156]	*De novo* AML <60 y	IDR/A "3 + 5"	IDR/A "2 + 4" ×2	80%	20-mo median survival	Idarubicin substituted as anthracycline
UCLA[161]	AML	D/IDAC	High-dose Ara-C/Mito → Mito/VP-16 → high-dose Ara-C/ D or allogeneic bone marrow transplant	74%	28% DFS (4 y)	Cytarabine dose increased in induction (intermediate dose)
ALSG[162]	*De novo* AML <60 y	D/high-dose Ara-C/VP-16	A/D/VP-16 "5-2-5" IDR/A	74%	42% actual DFS (4 y)	Cytarabine dose further increased in induction (high dose)
MSKCC[223]	APL (newly diagnosed)	ATRA	"3 + 5" → "2 + 4" ×2	88%	>31-mo median DFS (4 y)	Retinoids as acute promyelocytic leukemia induction with chemotherapy postremission
GIMEMA-AIEOP[230]	APL (newly diagnosed)	ATRA/IDR	IDR/A → Mito/VP-16 → IDR/A followed by maintenance	95%	79% 2-y event-free survival	Combination retinoid/chemotherapy as induction; chemotherapy or retinoid as maintenance
ECOG[121]	*De novo* AML >55 y	D/A + GM-CSF	IDAC + GM-CSF	60%	10-mo median survival	GM-CSF added in induction for poor-risk population

A, cytarabine; ALSG, Australian Leukemia Study Group; AMSA, amsacrine; Ara-C, cytarabine; ATRA, all-*trans*-retinoic acid; CALGB, Cancer and Leukemia Group B; D, daunorubicin; DFS, disease-free survival; ECOG, Eastern Cooperative Oncology Group; GIMEMA-AIEOP, Gruppo Italiano Malattie Ematologiche Maligne dell Adulto-Associazione Italiana di Ematologia ed Oncologia Pediatrica; GM-CSF, granulocyte-macrophage colony-stimulating factor; IDAC, intermediate-dose cytarabine; IDR, idarubicin; Mito, mitoxantrone; MSKCC, Memorial Sloan-Kettering Cancer Center; P, prednisone; T, 6-thioguanine; UCLA, University of California, Los Angeles; VCR, vincristine; VP-16, etoposide.

regimens. Treatment-related mortality in patients older than the age of 60 years is higher compared with younger patients treated with similar therapy and remains a primary cause of treatment failure in this group.[114] As the hematopoietic growth factors had been used successfully to speed granulocyte recovery after chemotherapy in other malignancies, this approach was tested in older patients with AML. Initially, there was concern over using a myeloid growth factor in AML; however, a clinical trial conducted in patients with relapsed disease did not demonstrate stimulation of leukemia cells when growth factor was used in support of chemotherapy.[119] A number of small, nonrandomized studies have investigated the use of either G-CSF or GM-CSF after treatment in poor-risk populations and found an advantage in ameliorating treatment-related toxicity.[164,165] Other studies have explored a novel application of using growth factors to modify drug sensitivity in addition to their potential supportive role. Both G-CSF and GM-CSF have been used before chemotherapy (as priming) in an effort to increase leukemia cell proliferation and increase sensitivity to cell-cycle–specific agents.[160,167,168] None of these trials have demonstrated any benefit to such a strategy.

Given the conflicting data in the early studies, several large randomized trials were conducted in an attempt to clarify the role of growth factors in AML therapy.[120–125] Although these studies have generally demonstrated a decrease in the duration of neutropenia, the significance of this effect has remained controversial. A study from the ECOG was able to show a decrease in treatment-related mortality with GM-CSF, while another large randomized study from CALGB was not able to demonstrate any significant clinical benefit from this growth factor.[120,121] It should be noted that two different forms of the recombinant growth factor were used, which could account for the disparity in outcomes. Moreover, large numbers of patients were removed from treatment in the CALGB study, which may have altered the outcome. Using G-CSF, the French AML Cooperative Study Group demonstrated an increased CR rate but no survival benefit.[122] The Southwest Oncology Group also tested G-CSF in older patients (older than 55 years old) and found a reduction in time of neutrophil recovery and decreased duration of infection, but no difference in either CR rate or overall survival.[124] A separate European and Australian phase III study also showed similar response and survival rates in the G-CSF and control groups, but was able to demonstrate significant reduction in measures of morbidity such as duration of fever, requirements of antimicrobials, and duration of hospitalization.[123] This study was not confined to the older population but included all patients older than the age of 16 years with *de novo* AML seen during the study period. Hence, despite intensive investigation, there is still no consensus regarding growth factor use in AML therapy other than the observation that their use is safe and reduces the neutropenic period. More recently, cost-to-benefit considerations have been introduced into the equation, and future clinical trials may incorporate economic data when dealing with this question.[168]

TABLE 46.2-8. State-of-the-Art Treatment Programs for Adult Acute Leukemia

Acute myelogenous leukemia
Anthracycline- and cytarabine-based induction regimens
Intensive postremission therapy; either bone marrow transplant or high-dose cytarabine is required for prolonged remission
Maintenance therapy is not generally indicated, with the exception of acute promyelocytic leukemia
Acute promyelocytic leukemia
Retinoic acid and anthracycline- and cytarabine-based treatment
Management of disseminated intravascular coagulation
Administration of cryoprecipitate or fresh frozen plasma to maintain fibrinogen >100 mg/dL; platelet transfusions to maintain daily platelet count >50,000/µL
Bone marrow transplant/high-dose cytarabine therapy reserved for relapsed disease
Acute lymphoblastic leukemias
Four or five drug induction regimens using anthracyclines, cyclophosphamide, and/or asparaginase in addition to vincristine and prednisone
Intensive consolidation therapy based on cytarabine combined with anthracyclines, epidophyllotoxins, or antimetabolites
Protracted maintenance therapy (approximately 2 years) based on oral methotrexate combined with mercaptopurine
Prophylactic intrathecal chemotherapy (with or without cranial radiotherapy) for central nervous system prophylaxis

POSTREMISSION THERAPY

Although the exact form of postremission therapy is controversial, the need for such therapy is widely accepted. Induction therapy fails to provide adequate cell kill, and leukemia cells survive the initial treatment. The benefit of postremission therapy was established by two randomized multicenter trials that showed that maintenance therapy was superior to no further treatment in prolonging remission duration.[169,170] This concept of continuing low-dose therapy over a prolonged period was further modified by subsequent clinical trials. The CALGB addressed the question of the duration of maintenance in a randomized study that compared 36 months of therapy versus 8 months of therapy.[149] No benefit was found for the more prolonged duration of treatment. Additional studies have suggested that more intensive therapy delivered within a shorter period appeared to offer clinical benefit.[171,172] One study from ECOG randomized patients younger than than 65 years of age to receive either one course of intensive consolidation versus 2 years of maintenance therapy and found superior survival in patients receiving the more intensive form of therapy.[173] This has led to the concept that state-of-the-art therapy of AML includes induction, intensive consolidations, but no maintenance (Table 46.2-8). However, this concept has been challenged by the experience reported in APL (see Acute Promyelocytic Leukemia, later in this chapter).

The logical progression of the experience that established consolidation was to further intensify the chemotherapy used in postremission treatment. The efficacy of high-dose Ara-C in treating patients with relapsed AML led to regimens for postremission therapy. A number of nonrandomized trials using Ara-C doses ranging from 1 to 3 g/m^2 (typically given every 12 hours for 6 to 12 doses) have reported 4-year disease-free survivals ranging from 30% to 40%.[174,175] These results appear to be superior to the 15% to 20% survival reported with standard consolidation regimens. The most compelling evidence for intensification, however, has been provided by a large randomized study conducted by the CALGB.[80] After achieving remission with a standard 3 + 7 regimen, patients with *de novo* AML were randomized to receive four courses of Ara-C at one of three dose levels: 100 mg/m^2/d for 5 days by continuous infusion (standard-dose arm); 400 mg/m^2/d for 5 days by continuous infusion (intermediate-dose arm); or 3 g/m^2 twice daily via a 3-hour infusion on days 1, 3, and 5 (high-dose arm). A subsequent analysis of this trial according to cytogenetic data underscored the importance of this prognostic factor, with 84% of the patients who had favorable cytogenetics [defined in this study as t(8;21) or inv (16)] able to have prolonged disease-free survival.[176] Although the results from this trial have been used to bolster the argument for single-agent high-dose Ara-C intensification, all patients received four courses of maintenance therapy in the form of attenuated doses Ara-C and daunorubicin in addition to the high-dose Ara-C intensification. The effect of such therapy on outcomes is uncertain, causing some speculation as to whether comparable results can be achieved by administering the high-dose Ara-C intensification alone. Still, the results from this trial compare favorably with studies using allogeneic BMT as postremission therapy and have heightened the debate regarding the standard of care in the postremission setting.

ALLOGENEIC BONE MARROW TRANSPLANTATION

The use of bone marrow or stem cell transplantation as postremission therapy represents dose intensification carried to the extreme of myeloablation. High doses of chemotherapy with or without total body radiation are used in an effort to maximize leukemia cell kill. Hematopoiesis is restored by the infusion of stem cells harvested from an HLA-compatible donor, thereby rescuing the patient from the consequences of bone marrow failure. The donor bone marrow and peripheral blood stem cells (graft) may also have a number of immunologic effects. Because of differences in HLA composition, the graft may reject the host, resulting in graft-versus-host disease (GVHD). This complication may increase the risk of infection and represents a major source of morbidity and mortality in patients who undergo this procedure.[177] This immunologic effect may, however, also translate into antileukemic activity as evidenced by the lower relapse rates observed in patients with GVHD. This graft-versus-leukemia effect is an evolving area of investigation and probably accounts for the lower relapse rates seen in allogeneic BMT as compared with syngeneic (or autologous) transplants in which similar conditioning regimens are used.[178]

Despite treatment-related complications, allogeneic BMT is effective antileukemic therapy. This was first established in a small number of heavily pretreated refractory AML patients who were successfully treated with allogeneic BMT. The concept that the efficacy of this therapy could be improved and its toxicity lessened if transplants were performed earlier in the course of the disease led to a number of nonrandomized trials from large centers or cooperative groups. These trials showed that allogeneic BMTs in first CR using HLA-compatible related donors resulted in 5-year disease-free survival of approximately 45% to 50%, with relapse rates ranging only from 10% to 20%.[179] A significant number of patients, however, succumb to such complications as GVHD, infection, or interstitial pneumonitis, affecting the overall survival of the group as a whole.

Therefore, the major criticism of allogeneic BMT in first CR is that although it is effective therapy with a relatively low incidence of relapse, it is quite toxic, expensive, and not necessarily better than other forms of dose-intensive therapy. The complication rate increases with age, and it is not standard practice to offer allogeneic BMT with a conventional graft to patients older than the age of 50 to 55 years. As the median age of patients with AML is approximately 65 years, it is clear that most patients with this disease are not eligible for this form of therapy. Because of entry criteria, BMT trials report results in younger groups of patients who may do well with other forms of dose-intensive therapy, but are generally not representative of the majority of patients with AML. In addition, only approximately 30% of eligible patients have an HLA-compatible donor. Despite meeting the minimum requirements of age and availability of a donor, a significant number of patients still fail to undergo transplantation.[180] Therefore, it has been estimated that allogeneic BMT is only applicable in 2% to 10% of patients with AML.[106] Strategies using unrelated HLA-matched or haplotype-mismatched individuals as alternative donors or using nonmyeloablative transplant regimens with reduced toxicity as part of a minitransplant for older patients have been introduced and are currently undergoing investigation.[181,182]

AUTOLOGOUS BONE MARROW TRANSPLANTATION

Despite efforts to expand the donor pool for allogeneic BMT, the majority of patients do not have an acceptable HLA-matched donor and cannot undergo allogeneic BMT. In an attempt to allow such patients to undergo high-dose therapy with curative intent, investigators began to explore the use of the patient's own bone marrow, obtained while in CR, as a source of hematopoietic reconstitution.[183] Such an approach was thought to provide the antileukemic benefits associated with high-dose conditioning regimens yet avoid the toxic complications such as GVHD. One major disadvantage, however, is the potential contamination of the autologous graft by residual leukemia cells. The inability of currently available laboratory techniques to reliably detect minimal residual disease and predict outcome based on its presence represents a major problem in leukemia therapy. Hence, there is concern that despite the high-dose conditioning designed to eradicate residual leukemia cells in the body, patients will ultimately relapse because undetectable leukemia cells will be reinfused with the graft. One innovative study from St. Jude Children's Hospital attempted to address this important question.[184] Cells in an autologous bone marrow graft were marked with a neomycin-resistant gene before transplantation into two patients with AML. After clinical relapse of the patients, the neomycin-resistant gene marker was detected in the leukemia blast cells of both patients, implying that the remission marrow that had been reinfused contributed to disease recurrence.

Despite this laboratory evidence and the rationale for attempting to remove minimal residual disease from the stem cell graft, the clinical benefits of purging the graft remain unclear. Clinical trials using unpurged bone marrow as the source for hematopoietic reconstitution in first CR have reported treatment results comparable with studies using a purged graft. Results from these trials have generally reported disease-free survival of approximately 40% to 50%.[183] Relapse rates (50% to 60%) are higher than allogeneic BMT, but, as expected, the toxicities are less. In studies that have used either immunologic or pharmacologic methods to purge bone marrow, there has been a profound suppression of normal bone marrow progenitors, resulting in delayed engraftment and a prolonged period of hematologic recovery.

Given the experience in other malignancies using peripheral blood stem cells as the source of hematopoietic reconstitution after high-dose therapy, this approach has been investigated in patients with AML.[185] One potential advantage to this approach is the hypothesis that there is a difference between the normal stem cell and leukemia cell compartments in recovery rates after a priming stimulus such as chemotherapy. The normal cells are thought to have a temporary competitive growth advantage so that the cells that initially repopulate the peripheral blood are more likely to be normal progenitors instead of clonogenic leukemic stem cells. Therefore, collecting stem cells early in the priming process may be thought to provide the graft with a kinetic purge, making it relatively free from contamination by residual leukemia cells. Some evidence to support this hypothesis has been provided by a study that used standard cytogenetic analysis to assay for contamination of residual leukemia cells and failed to detect them early in the collection process.[186] Further support for the feasibility of this approach as been provided by the experience of harvesting pure populations of progenitor cells after chemotherapy in CML and myelodysplastic syndromes.[187] Studies using newer, more sensitive techniques, such as PCR or multiparameter flow cytometry, will continue to address the issue of graft contamination by minimal residual disease.[188]

The clinical results using peripheral blood stem cells have generally shown a decrease in the duration of neutropenia and thrombocytopenia. The effect on treatment outcomes, however, has been less clear, with some groups reporting relapse rates comparable with trials using unpurged bone marrow grafts.[189] Other studies have shown superior leukemia-free survival using purged bone marrow grafts. Although no studies have appeared, as yet, using purged peripheral stem cells, there has been great interest in intensifying the chemotherapy before collection of these stem cells and, in effect, achieving a form of *in vivo* purging.[190] This approach has been applied in both peripheral stem cell and bone marrow grafts, with the most compelling evidence provided by the results from the Medical Research Council (MRC) AML 10 trial (discussed in the following section).[191]

ASSESSING THE OPTIONS FOR POSTREMISSION THERAPY IN ACUTE MYELOGENOUS LEUKEMIAS

Currently, the options for postremission therapy in younger patients with AML involve three forms of dose-intensive treatments: allogeneic or autologous transplantation and high-dose chemotherapy. These can be applied either alone or in combination. A number of studies have compared the different approaches in an effort to establish the optimal therapy. Although the initial comparisons reported the superiority of allogeneic BMT over chemotherapy, these studies used standard-dose attenuated consolidation regimens.[179] In the modern era, many would consider this suboptimal postremission therapy for patients younger than 60 years of age. More recent studies, however, have compared outcomes in patients who have undergone allogeneic BMT from HLA-compatible donors with those who have received either dose-intensive chemotherapy or autologous BMT.[192–194] The results from several of these studies are summarized in Table 46.2-9. These trials have consistently reported decreased relapse rates with higher treatment-related morbidity and mortality in the BMT groups, but no significant benefit in survival. In fact, a large U.S. intergroup study showed a marginally better overall survival in the cohort treated with a single course of high-dose Ara-C after a standard Ara-C/idarubicin consolidation.[194] In contrast, the MRC 10 trial found a decreased relapse rate with a survival benefit for patients who received autologous BMT after three cycles of intensive postremission chemotherapy.[191] It should be noted that these two studies differed in the amount of therapy patients received before autologous BMT, as well as the conditioning regimen used for the autologous transplant.

The results from these randomized studies have failed to provide a clear answer to the postremission question, but have caused many centers to reevaluate the approach to AML patients in first remission. Although some institutions still recommend allogeneic BMT for suitable candidates with HLA-compatible donors, other centers reserve BMT for relapse. This strategy is based on the relative equivalence of treatment outcomes. Despite a higher risk of relapse with chemotherapy, BMT can salvage some patients who fail chemotherapy-based consolidation, leading to equivalent overall survival while avoiding unnecessary toxicity in those patients who may be cured by chemotherapy alone. Patients should have either a potential donor identified or stem cells (bone marrow or peripheral blood) harvested and cryopreserved during first remission, in the event relapse occurs and a salvage strategy becomes necessary.[194,195] Treatment options are limited in patients who are not candidates for BMT, who are the largest fraction of patients.

TREATMENT OF RELAPSED ACUTE MYELOGENOUS LEUKEMIAS

The majority of patients with AML relapse and ultimately die from the consequences of resistant disease. Chemotherapy is generally not curative in this setting. The data from multiple trials suggest median survivals of only a few months after a second remission is obtained.[196] Both allogeneic and autologous BMT have been reported to provide prolonged disease-free survival in 30% to 40% of patients treated in first relapse or second CR.[197,198] Therefore, suitable patients who have relapsed should undergo BMT as this represents the best chance for cure.

The timing of BMT in relapsed disease is controversial. Previous strategies have relied on the ability of salvage chemotherapy to decrease the leukemia burden and induce a second CR. However, a significant proportion of patients are unable to achieve a second CR, and the ability to proceed to allogeneic BMT may be compromised by the additional morbidity seen with such therapy. This is particularly true as high-dose regimens have been moved up front, limiting the treatments available on relapse. Data from the Fred Hutchinson Cancer Center have suggested that allogeneic BMT performed early in first relapse yields similar results to those transplants performed after a second CR has been obtained.[197] Although a number of centers have adopted this strategy, it requires that patients are able to proceed to allogeneic BMT in a timely manner. The feasibility of this approach, however, is often problematic as the readiness of the transplant facility or the availability of the donor may instead require the patient to receive some form of chemotherapy before allogeneic BMT. Further complicating the application of this relapse strategy has been disagreements over the definition of early relapse and concern regarding the maximal level of leukemia burden that will allow a successful transplantation to take place.

A similar strategy may be used for patients proceeding to autologous BMT.[198] Patients who relapse and previously had stem cells (either peripheral blood or bone marrow) harvested and cryopreserved, may proceed directly to autologous BMT. If no provision has been made for the patient and stem cells have not been collected in first CR, a second remission must be obtained. A number of studies have reported durable disease-free survival of approximately 30% in patients who have received autologous BMT in second CR and approximately 20% in third CR.[199,200] Results were not dependent on whether purged or unpurged marrow was used as the source of hematopoietic reconstitution.

Most patients, however, are not candidates for either type of BMT. For such patients, the goal in treating relapse is to induce a second remission. The ability to achieve a second remission is primarily dependent on the duration of the first remission.[196,201] Several groups have found that the response rates to salvage therapies are lower in patients with first remission durations of 6 to 12 months. Patients with an exceptionally short remission duration (less than 6 months) are unlikely to respond to any of the standard agents now available. In such patients, the use of investigational approaches are appropriate.[202] Alternatively, patients who relapse after 2 years in remission may achieve a second CR by repeating the original induction regimen. Because of the potential cumulative toxicity of the anthracyclines, patients who receive up to three cycles of such chemotherapy require evaluation of cardiac function before additional re-treatment with these agents.

TABLE 46.2-9. Randomized Comparisons of Dose-Intensive Postremission Regimens

Author	*Comparison*	*Outcomes*
Burnett[191]	Autologous BMT (unpurged) versus observation	Superior DFS and OS at 7 y in autologous BMT group
Zittoun[192]	Allogeneic BMT versus autologous BMT (unpurged) versus IC	DFS best with allogeneic BMT versus equivalent OS
Harousseau[193]	Allogeneic BMT versus autologous BMT (unpurged) versus IC	No difference in DFS or OS
Cassileth[194]	Allogeneic BMT versus autologous BMT (purged) versus IC	No difference in DFS, marginal advantage in OS for IC

BMT, bone marrow transplantation; DFS, disease-free survival; IC, intensive chemotherapy; OS, overall survival.

Because most patients with relapsed disease, however, do not respond to repetition of the original induction regimen, research efforts have sought to define the underlying basis for clinical drug resistance with the ultimate goal of identifying new therapeutic approaches. One suspected mechanism of clinical drug resistance that has received much attention is the multidrug-resistant (MDR) phenotype. This laboratory phenomenon describes the observation that cell lines can become cross-resistant to unrelated, structurally diverse chemotherapeutic agents. The mechanism of resistance is linked to a 170- to 180-kD glycoprotein that functions via decreasing the intracellular accumulation of drugs, resulting in decreased cytotoxicity of these agents. The MDR phenotype has been observed in approximately 70% of patients with relapsed or refractory disease but also in 25% to 30% of patients with untreated disease.[203] The variable correlation of clinical response with expression of MDR phenotypes suggests alternative mechanisms may be active in determining resistance of AML cells to current chemotherapy.[204,205] In addition, other potential mediators of drug resistance, such as lung resistance protein, have been described, and the relationship of this resistant phenotype to MDR and outcome remains under investigation.[206] The emphasis on the MDR data may be explained by the potential to use modulators that alter the phenotype and restore chemotherapy sensitivity. Several trials have been undertaken that attempt to use the cyclosporin derivative, PSC-833, in an effort to reverse the MDR phenotype.[207] These studies are ongoing in both relapsed disease and up front as part of a strategy to increase CR rate and improve outcomes. Although such an approach has been shown to be feasible, efficacy remains to be established. A major criticism of this approach is that resistance to the most important antileukemia agent, Ara-C, is not affected by MDR, and that these studies basically ignore a common yet important mechanism of failure. Several investigators, however, have attempted to modify Ara-C efficacy in several different ways: increasing the intracellular concentration of the drug by giving high-dose Ara-C or combining Ara-C with fludarabine or attempting to exploit the cytokinetic properties of hematopoietic growth factors to recruit leukemia cells into cell cycle, thereby increasing the sensitivity to the drug.[167]

Among the drugs tested in the relapsed setting, high-dose Ara-C, either alone or in combination, has consistently been found to have the greatest antileukemic activity.[208,209] Although the dose and schedule of Ara-C has varied somewhat between studies, high-dose Ara-C is usually given at 2 to 3 g/m^2 every 12 hours for eight to 12 doses. Several centers now administer the Ara-C once daily or twice daily on an every other day schedule in an effort to decrease toxicity. Responses to such regimens have ranged from approximately 30% to 50%. Other active agents, such as daunorubicin, mitoxantrone, idarubicin, and etoposide, have been combined with high-dose Ara-C, but the therapeutic advantage of these combinations remain unclear. Substantial differences in treatment results between trials containing similar agents may be explained by patient selection and the small numbers of patients enrolled on these trials.

Patients who fail to achieve CR after receiving two courses of standard dose therapy are considered to have primary refractory disease. The prognosis for such patients is exceptionally poor, and response to salvage regimens is rare. Approximately 20% to 40% of these patients who are able to undergo allogeneic BMT can be rendered free of disease with durable remissions.[210] This ability to salvage primary refractory patients underscores the importance of identifying potential donors early in the therapy of patients who may be eligible for BMT. Patients who are not transplant candidates are best enrolled in investigational studies.

As more patients receive some form of high-dose therapy as their initial treatment, the options at relapse have changed. For some patients relapsing after high-dose Ara-C postremission therapy, studies suggest that either autologous BMT or allogeneic BMT can be curative. Those patients who are not BMT candidates may undergo therapy with alternative salvage regimens. Although the initial reports of potentially non–cross-resistant combinations, such as mitoxantrone/etoposide or carboplatin, were encouraging, subsequent studies have shown that these regimens are relatively ineffective.[211,212] The combination of cyclophosphamide and etoposide, given in near myeloablative doses, has been shown to induce CR in approximately 30% of patients who are refractory to regimens containing high-dose Ara-C.[213] Similar to the experience with other chemotherapy-based salvage regimens, such responses are usually short-lived.

Relapse of AML after allogeneic BMT poses a difficult and frustrating management problem,[214,215] with a median survival of 3 to 4 months. However, results are not significantly improved with current available therapy. Treatment options are determined by the performance status of the patient as well as the interval from transplant to relapse. Although a CR rate of approximately 35% has been reported to standard induction regimens, patients who relapse within the first 100 days after BMT are unlikely to respond and have a high treatment-related mortality. Selected young patients who relapse after 1 year may be candidates for a second allogeneic BMT, but the survival at 3 years has been reported to be approximately 10%. Therapeutic approaches, including the use of G-CSF, modulation of the graft-versus-leukemia effect by discontinuing immunosuppressives such as cyclosporin, or infusing donor leukocytes have been reported to induce remission in this setting.[216] Although donor leukocyte infusions have received much attention, most of the data have been generated in patients with CML and the results of such therapies in AML have been disappointing, although investigations continue.

ACUTE PROMYELOCYTIC LEUKEMIA

APL represents a distinct entity among the myeloid leukemias. The unique biology that characterizes the disease also serves to make it the paradigm for targeted antineoplastic therapy. Historically, the importance of the prompt recognition of this subtype of AML has been stressed because of the coagulopathy associated with the disease and the potential for lethal hemorrhage with the institution of cytotoxic chemotherapy. The incorporation of all-*trans*-retinoic acid (ATRA) into up-front therapy further underscores the importance of rapid and accurate diagnosis.

When treated with standard Ara-C/anthracycline–based chemotherapy, there is a higher rate of periinduction mortality in APL than in the other AML subtypes.[217,218] A variety of supportive interventions have been introduced in an effort to control the hemorrhagic diathesis of the disease, but these complications remain a source of significant morbidity and, even with best available therapy, constitute a major reason for induction failures. Despite the early hazards associated with cytotoxic treatment, the long-term survival in APL with this therapy is far superior to the other subtypes of AML. In groups that have emphasized dose intensity of the anthracycline, long-term disease-free survival as high as 60% has been reported.[219]

The clinical use of ATRA changed the emphasis from cytotoxic therapy and established differentiation therapy as an effective modality in the therapy of human cancer. The initial experience with this agent was reported by Huang et al. and subsequently confirmed by other groups.[220–222] ATRA is not a cytotoxic agent but instead causes a proliferation of the abnormal clone coincident with maturation, eventual terminal differentiation, and ultimately, apoptotic cell death. CR is obtained in 90% to 95% of newly diagnosed cases of APL without inducing aplasia and without the toxic effects associated with standard chemotherapy. Instead of worsening APL-related coagulopathy, there is stabilization and improvement of the condition within days of the institution of ATRA therapy. The biologic effects of ATRA are not restricted to *de novo* disease but are also seen in patients who have relapsed after chemotherapy as demonstrated by CR rates between 85% and 90% in this population.[221,223]

Despite the many advantages of ATRA therapy, it is not without potential complications. Although there is prompt improvement of coagulopathy with ATRA, many trials continue to report a 10% to 15% periinduction mortality due to both thrombosis and hemorrhage as well as the occurrence of a newly recognized toxicity named the *retinoic acid syndrome* (RAS). Approximately 25% of patients develop symptoms consistent with a capillary leak syndrome with features similar to acute respiratory distress syndrome or endotoxic shock.[224] Therefore, RAS is characterized by fever, dyspnea, peripheral edema with resultant weight gain, pleural and pericardial effusions, hypotension, and occasionally renal failure. Untreated, RAS can lead to rapid clinical deterioration and death.

The pathogenesis of RAS and its relationship to the other biologic effects observed with ATRA remain unclear. The description of a similar symptom complex in patients with APL who have not received ATRA has raised the hypothesis that this syndrome is directly related to the underlying disease process.[225] Leukocytosis, which is seen in up to 40% of patients with the institution of ATRA and may be an indicator of a biologic response, has, in some series, been associated with RAS.[226] This observation has lead some investigators to advocate the early institution of cytotoxic chemotherapy with ATRA in patients who initially present with a high WBC count (greater than 5000/μL) or who demonstrate a rapid increase in WBC count during therapy (5000/μL by day 6 ATRA; 10,000/μL by day 10; or 15,000/μL by day 15). Although this strategy has been highly successful in reducing the incidence of RAS, it does expose a significant proportion of these patients to early chemotherapy.[227] Because RAS may occur in as many as one-third of the cases regardless of leukocytosis, alternative strategies have been developed. Early therapy with a short course of high-dose corticosteroids (dexamethasone, 10 mg IV twice a day for 3 or more days) at the first onset of symptoms can effectively halt the progression of RAS and has markedly reduced the mortality from this complication.[223,228] Other investigators have proposed corticosteroid prophylaxis be used with ATRA therapy to avoid the RAS.

Although highly successful in inducing remission, ATRA alone is insufficient therapy for APL.[223] If left on a continuous schedule of ATRA, patients eventually develop resistance to this agent. They are unable to sustain adequate plasma concentrations of the drug and generally relapse within a few months. In addition, most patients have persistent minimal residual disease and remain positive for the PML/RAR-α, the molecular signature of APL, after ATRA monotherapy. These observations have lead to the incorporation of standard chemotherapeutic agents to the treatment of APL.

Initially, ATRA, in conjunction with anthracycline/Ara-C–based postremission regimens, were used as sequential therapy in phase II studies and resulted in improved disease-free survival compared with historical controls treated with similar chemotherapy given without the retinoid. Large randomized studies from both Europe and North America demonstrated the superiority of ATRA-containing regimens over chemotherapy alone.[227,229]

In an effort to exploit the known sensitivity of APL to anthracyclines, extend the durability of remissions obtained with ATRA chemotherapy–based regimens, and reduce ATRA-related toxicity, the Italian cooperative groups, GIMEMA-AIEPO, moved the chemotherapy up to induction by including idarubicin with ATRA (AIDA).[230] Ninety-five percent of patients achieved CR with AIDA induction and, when followed by three courses of postremission chemotherapy, the actuarial event-free survival at 2 years was reported to be 79%. Only 2.5% of patients developed RAS. Sequential ATRA chemotherapy was subsequently compared with simultaneous administration during induction in a large randomized study conducted by the European APL study group.[231] Although the actuarial relapse rates at 2 years were marginally better in the ATRA-plus chemotherapy group, the estimated 2-year survival was statistically similar. In addition, patients who received maintenance in the form of either chemotherapy or intermittent ATRA had superior overall survival. This is in sharp contrast to the other forms of AML in which maintenance therapy after a dose-intensive course of consolidation is generally without benefit.

The unique disruption of the RAR-α locus results in novel fusion proteins that given the current level of sophistication in the laboratory, are readily detectable and provide a useful tool for the clinician. The PML/RAR-α transcript defines sensitivity to ATRA, and the ability of RT-PCR to readily detect the PML/RAR-α fusion product allows for rapid genetic confirmation of the diagnosis, which given the various morphologic variants can be difficult even for the experienced eye.[99,100] In addition to helping in the diagnosis and planning an effective treatment strategy, RT-PCR has facilitated the detection of minimal residual disease and has made APL a paradigm for the use of molecular techniques to monitor therapy.[232]

Despite the spectacular CR rates and the equally impressive survival results, approximately 30% of patients treated in the large randomized studies relapse. Similar to the experience in other AML subtypes, such patients are generally incurable with chemotherapy alone and achieving a second remission may be difficult. Many are resistant to rechallenge with the retinoid, particularly if the disease relapses early (within 6 to 12 months). Arsenic trioxide has been used to achieve CR in heavily pretreated patients.[233] For those patients who are able to obtain a remission, both allogeneic and autologous BMT have been reported to offer a chance for cure. The results with autologous transplantation are dependent on the pretransplant status of minimal residual disease with 75% of patients who were PCR-negative before the autograft in molecular and clinical remission with a median follow-up of 28 months.[234]

The therapy of APL in the modern era is marked by great clinical success accompanied by a new understanding of the fundamental biology of the disease. The promise for future progress in AML may lie in mechanism-based drug design. The observation that arsenic trioxide leads to increased expression of caspases resulting in enhanced apoptosis has prompted investigators to combine this agent with the differentiating effects of ATRA in an attempt to amplify the effect of each agent by exploiting the different mechanisms of action. *In vitro*, this combination has been found to be synergistic, and the investigation of arsenic and ATRA has been undertaken in animal models.[41] The interaction between PML/RAR-α fusion products, corepressor binding proteins, and histone deacetylation have been implicated in the pathogenesis of APL. This has led to interest in a class of drugs, the histone deacetylase inhibitors, that may usher in a new era in the drug therapy of leukemia.

GENERAL PRINCIPLES FOR THE TREATMENT OF ADULT ACUTE LYMPHOBLASTIC LEUKEMIAS

Treatment of adults with ALL has been modeled on therapy developed for childhood ALL. The similarity between the childhood and adult forms of this disease allows for inferences to be drawn from experience in the pediatric population. However, adults with ALL have a far poorer outcome when compared with children. Some of this difference can be attributed to differences in ability to tolerate intensive therapy coupled with an increased incidence of unfavorable cytogenetic subgroups [particularly t(9;22) and t(4;11)] and a decreased incidence of favorable cytogenetic subgroups [such as hyperdiploidy or t(12;21)]. Despite these mitigating features, the distinctly different outcomes of therapy have led to questions regarding how advances in pediatrics can be used in adult ALL. A broad review of the St. Jude experience in pediatric ALL demonstrated a dramatic stepwise improvement in treatment results since the 1970s.[235] However, adults with ALL have not shared in this remarkable success story.[236]

Treatment of adult ALL is typically divided into four broad categories: induction, consolidation, maintenance, and CNS prophylaxis. At presentation, many patients are quite ill with active infection, hemorrhage, or both, and induction regimens for adult ALL have typically emphasized relatively myeloid-sparing cytotoxic agents.

Consolidation therapy is administered at a relatively higher level of intensity to patients already in complete remission. Before beginning this phase of therapy, patients have normal blood counts and generally a good performance status. They are therefore able to tolerate significant myelosuppression with acceptable toxicity.

Maintenance therapy is administered to patients in remission after the more intensive consolidation therapy. It is administered at a low level of intensity, but for a protracted period. Current opinion is that 2 years of maintenance therapy is required for optimal results.

The fourth category of treatment is CNS prophylaxis. This is administered concurrently with systemic chemotherapy. Despite aggressive systemic therapy, the CNS remains a sanctuary site and without specific meningeal-directed therapy approximately 35% of adult patients develop CNS disease.

To understand the natural history of adult ALL and to assign specific therapy, the FAB subclassification (see Morphology and Cytochemistry, earlier in this chapter) is less useful than an immunophenotypic subclassification, which recognizes three major groups: The most common subtype is pre–B-cell ALL, which represents approximately 70% of patients. The term *pre-B* refers to the fact that these cells are committed to the B-cell lineage, as manifested by immunoglobulin gene rearrangement and expression of typical early B-cell markers such as CD19 and terminal deoxyribonucleotidyl transferase, but do not express the hallmark of the mature B cell, surface immunoglobulin. In addition to CD19 and terminal deoxyribonucleotidyl transferase, the lymphoblasts of patients with pre–B-cell ALL typically express CD10, which was previously known as common ALL antigen (CALLA).

The second subtype of ALL is T-cell disease. T-cell ALL and lymphoblastic lymphoma are essentially the same disease. This disease typically affects young adults and has a significant male predominance. The malignant process begins as a rapidly growing mediastinal mass with early dissemination to the bone marrow. Patients present with symptoms related to their mediastinal mass (cough, dyspnea, chest pain) or to bone marrow involvement (infection and bleeding). Patients without evident bone marrow involvement at diagnosis are said to have lymphoblastic lymphoma. Those with scant bone marrow involvement are said to have stage IV lymphoblastic lymphoma and those with significant (greater than 30%) bone marrow involvement are said to have T-cell ALL. These distinctions are largely semantic and are without important clinical implications. All patients with lymphoblastic lymphoma/T-cell ALL require therapy as for ALL.

The third and least common subtype (approximately 5% of adult ALL) is mature B cell ALL. As the name implies, these leukemic cells are slightly more mature than their pre–B-cell counterparts and express surface immunoglobulin. The typical patient is a young man who presents with a rapidly growing abdominal mass (initial sites are typically the appendix and the ileocecal valve) and early dissemination to the bone marrow. The most common presentation is with symptoms related to the abdominal mass (pain, bloating, and small bowel obstruction) or to bone marrow involvement (infection and bleeding). Patients who present to medical attention without evidence of bone marrow involvement are said to have Burkitt's lymphoma. Once significant bone marrow infiltration occurs, this disease is called *mature B-cell ALL.* In contrast to pre–B-cell ALL and T-cell ALL, mature B-cell ALL requires a different treatment regimen for optimal results (see Treatment of Mature B-Cell Acute Lymphoblastic Leukemia, later in this chapter).

PROGNOSTIC FEATURES IN ADULT ACUTE LYMPHOBLASTIC LEUKEMIA

There have been several evaluations of prognostic features in adult ALL. The two most widely accepted multivariate analyses were performed by the German multicenter group and the Memorial Sloan-Kettering group.[237,238] Other analyses have in general supported these two studies and have led to five widely accepted prognostic features: WBC count, age, leukemic cell immunophenotype, Philadelphia chromosome–positive disease, and time to achieve CR (see Table 46.2-5).

Multivariate analyses indicate that a high WBC count at diagnosis is associated with poor prognosis. There is both a reduced likelihood of achieving a CR as well as shorter duration of remission (and overall survival) for those who achieve a CR. An increased WBC count probably has prognostic significance in part on the basis as a measure of tumor burden, but also because of its correlation with adverse cytogenetics [e.g., t(4;11) and t(9;22)]. A high WBC count is probably a continuous variable (the higher the count, the worse the prognosis), and different studies have used different levels of elevated WBC count as their cutoff for an adverse feature. In the Memorial Hospital study, WBC counts greater than 10,000/μL were associated with a lower frequency of achieving a CR, whereas counts greater than 20,000/μL were associated with a shorter duration of CR. The German study indicated that WBC counts greater than 30,000/μL carry an adverse prognosis.

Older age is also associated with a worse prognosis. Age is probably a continuous variable (the older the patient, the worse the prognosis). In pediatric series, adolescent patients typically have the worst prognosis, though in adult series this is almost always the most favorable group. Different studies have defined different ages as having a poor prognosis, the two most important being age 35 years from the German group and age 60 from the Memorial Hospital study.

The immunophenotype of the leukemic cell also carries prognostic implication.[237–239] T-cell disease has a favorable prognosis, pre-B-cell (common) ALL has an intermediate prognosis, whereas mature B-cell disease has a poor prognosis when treated with standard regimens. It should be noted that modern regimens designed specifically for mature B-cell ALL improve the prognosis for this subtype significantly. Previously, null cell ALL was considered to have a poor prognosis. Modern immunophenotyping has essentially eliminated this entity. It is possible that in the past some acute leukemias now classified as AML-M0 would have been considered null cell ALL; not surprisingly these would fare poorly with vincristine/prednisone-based therapy.

Philadelphia chromosome–positive disease carries a poor prognosis. Adult patients with this entity are essentially never cured by chemotherapeutic regimens. A minority of patients with this disease may be cured if they undergo allogeneic transplant in first CR.[240] Other cytogenetic abnormalities also have prognostic implications, but their frequency is not sufficient to be noted in multivariate analysis. Most notable of these is the poor prognosis associated with t(4;11).

Time to achieve a CR during induction therapy carries significant prognostic implications. Patients requiring more than 4 weeks[70,241] or 5 weeks[238] to achieve a CR have a lower likelihood of being cured. It is not clear if this reflects an innate sensitivity to (and curability by) the chemotherapeutic agents used or rather that rapid cytoreduction of the leukemic cell mass minimizes the opportunity for drug resistance to develop and ultimately allows for cure of the patient.

TREATMENT OF NEWLY DIAGNOSED ADULT PATIENTS WITH ACUTE LYMPHOBLASTIC LEUKEMIA

A variety of different treatment regimens for adults with ALL have been developed since the 1970s. These regimens, which borrow heavily from advances made in childhood ALL, have many features in common. Current therapy can induce complete remission in approximately 65% to 85% of adults. However, the majority of these patients subsequently relapse, and overall only 20% to 30% of adults with ALL prove to be cured of their disease (see Fig. 46.2-1).[242–249] The mainstay of induction therapy for ALL has been the combination of vincristine and prednisone. Vincristine and prednisone achieves a CR in approximately 50% of patients. Addition of an anthracycline to induction therapy was demonstrated in a randomized trial to increase the likelihood of achieving a CR (83% vs. 47%).[250] This increased incidence of CR did not translate into improved survival for the patients randomized to receive the anthracycline. Although lacking support from randomized clinical trials, further intensification of induction therapy with cyclophosphamide or L-asparaginase, is widely accepted as improving remission induction, and one or both of these drugs are therefore included in essentially all induction regimens. Current induction regimens are therefore labeled as *four drug* (vincristine, prednisone, anthracycline, and cyclophosphamide or asparaginase) or *five drug* (vincristine, prednisone, anthracycline, cyclophosphamide, and asparaginase) regimens. There are no data currently available to favor one of these induction regimens over another.

Consolidation therapy has evolved over time to include several drugs given in varying sequence. Though there is no standard consolidation therapy, some generalizations can be made. The drug most prominently used in consolidation of adult ALL is Ara-C. Consolidation regimens include Ara-C combined with other drugs, most typically anthracyclines, epidophyllotoxins, or antimetabolites (such as methotrexate or thioguanine). Multiple studies seem to indicate the value of such consolidations. Most of these studies are uncontrolled phase II studies or comparisons with historical controls.[243,246,248,249] The experience at M. D. Anderson is typical in this regard in which implementation of such therapy increased 3-year survival from 15% to 40%.[251] A randomized phase III trial demonstrating the importance of cytarabine-containing consolidations was reported by Fiere et al.[242] In this study, after remission induction, patients were randomized to receive consolidation therapy with cytarabine, doxorubicin, and asparaginase or to immediately receive maintenance therapy. Three-year disease-free survival in the consolidation arm was markedly superior (38%) to the no consolidation arm (0%) (P <.005). Although most authors accept that intensive consolidations are beneficial, there is a report by Ellison et al. of a randomized trial that failed to show significant benefit to cytarabine-based consolidation.[252]

Protracted maintenance therapy is a feature unique to treatment strategies for ALL. All other chemotherapeutically curable human malignancies are typically cured with 3 to 6 months of therapy. In pediatric ALL, maintenance therapy is clearly necessary, and most regimens prescribe 2 to 3 years of such treatment. In adults, the necessity of maintenance therapy has been less clearly addressed. Only a few studies have failed to use maintenance therapy, and the low reported disease-free survival seen in the CALGB study (18% at 3 years) and the ECOG study (13% at 4 years) suggests the importance of maintenance therapy in adult ALL.[253,254] The two most important drugs in maintenance chemotherapy are a combination of oral methotrexate and mercaptopurine. In pediatric ALL, these two drugs alone can be sufficient for maintenance therapy; in adults, however, most maintenance regimens are intensified by incorporating other active agents such as vincristine, prednisone, anthracyclines, and cyclophosphamide.

The CNS, along with the eye and the testis, are viewed as sanctuary sites. These are areas where penetration of systemically administered cytotoxic agents is compromised, leading to the potential of localized relapse. In adults, ocular relapse is extremely rare. Testicular disease occurs occasionally in patients with mature B-cell ALL, less frequently in patients with Philadelphia chromosome–positive ALL, and is extremely uncommon in other adults with ALL. Of the three sanctuary sites, CNS relapse is by far the most common. The incidence of CNS disease at presentation in adult ALL is typically 5% to 10%. Risk factors for developing CNS disease include high WBC count at diagnosis and mature B-cell immunophenotype. Patients who do not receive prophylactic therapy have a cumulative risk of approximately 35% of developing CNS involvement during the course of their disease. Prophylaxis with intrathecal chemotherapy (with or without whole brain irradiation) effectively reduces the cumulative incidence to approximately 10%. Intrathecal chemotherapy can be delivered by lumbar puncture or intraventricularly via Ommaya reservoir. If whole brain irradiation is used, intrathecal chemotherapy can be delivered by lumbar puncture (and requires fewer treatments) to achieve acceptable results. Patients not receiving whole brain irradiation as part of their prophylaxis require a greater number of intrathecal treatments and should have these treatments administered via an Ommaya reservoir. Patients should achieve a complete remission of their systemic disease before having an Ommaya reservoir placed to avoid this surgery in the subset of patients who have primary refractory disease or die during induction therapy. Intrathecal chemotherapy does not require adjustments for body surface area, and a typical adult dose is 12 mg of methotrexate (or 60 mg of cytarabine). A variety of administration schedules have been used, but for patients not receiving brain irradiation, we recommend six doses during the first 2 months of treatment, two doses per month during consolidation therapy, and two doses for every 3 months of maintenance therapy. The addition of whole brain radiotherapy to intrathecal chemotherapy can reduce the amount of intrathecal chemotherapy required for adequate CNS prophylaxis (and obviate the need for an Ommaya reservoir); however, concerns of late toxicity, including loss of cognitive function and leukoencephalopathy,[255] have led many investigators to omit whole brain radiotherapy from prophylactic regimens. CNS prophylaxis, although effective at reducing the incidence of CNS relapse, has no demonstrable effect on systemic relapse or overall survival.[256]

Features common to state-of-the-art treatment programs for adult ALL are summarized in Table 46.2-8. Since the 1970s, treatment regimens that incorporate these features have been developed at many centers. Multiple formulations have been tested that vary the drug dose and schedule during induction, the number and intensity of chemotherapy cycles during consolidation, and the sequencing and duration of maintenance. Despite years of experience with multiple variations of this treatment strategy, no single formulation appears to be superior to the others. The wide variation in reported outcomes of clinical trials would superficially suggest the superiority of certain regimens (Table 46.2-10). Closer inspection, however, does not support this view. Interpretation of the literature is complicated primarily by differences in patient mix and duration of follow-up. It is easy to understand how duration of follow-up affects disease-free survival. Figure 46.2-1 indicates overall survival for the 272 adult patients with ALL treated at Memorial Sloan-Kettering Cancer Center on several sequential treatment protocols. All of these treatment regimens were designed according to the principles listed in Table 46.2-7. Although 2-year survival is almost 50%, the survival curve continues to fall and a plateau is not reached until 6 years out at approximately 24%. There-

TABLE 46.2-10. Clinical Chemotherapy Studies in Adult Acute Lymphoblastic Leukemia

Author	No. of Patients	Median Age	Complete Response (%)	Disease-Free Survival	
				Percentage	At Year
Linker[246]	109	25	88	42	5
Hussein[248]	168	28	68	30	5
Kantarjian[244]	105	30	84	32	5
Cuttner[254]	164	32	63	20	5
Ellison[252]	277	33	64	29	5
Fiere[242]	218	33	77	40	3
Stewart[247]	68	38	76	18	5

fore, studies that report only 2- or 3-year survival markedly overestimate their actual results and can appear superior to regimens that report 5-year survival.

The prognostic features of patients treated on a particular study are as important as duration of follow-up in interpreting the results of clinical trials in adult ALL. Certain patients with adult ALL, such as those with Philadelphia chromosome–positive disease have little likelihood of long-term survival. Because these patients may constitute 15% to 30% of unselected adults with ALL, their inclusion in clinical trials can have a major effect on reported results. Age is another important selection criteria that can vary from study to study with a major effect on reported survival. An analysis by Ohno of the relationship between median age and disease-free survival in 18 published studies of adult ALL reveals a tight correlation between the median age of the patients treated and the long-term disease-free survival.[257] This suggests that the apparent differences in results among published studies likely reflect patient mix rather than differences in treatment regimen.

The uniformity of results seen with vincristine/prednisone-based regimens has led to exploration of new induction approaches in adults. A phase II study at Memorial Sloan-Kettering Cancer Center used an induction regimen of cytarabine combined with a high single dose of mitoxantrone (80 mg/m^2). Vincristine and prednisone were not used during induction therapy. When compared with historical controls, this regimen demonstrated a higher incidence of CR (P = .056), a lower incidence of failure with resistant disease (P = .028), a significantly reduced time to CR (P = .003), and a trend to improved survival.[258] This regimen appeared to have particularly good activity in patients with Philadelphia chromosome–positive disease. A prospective multicenter randomized trial comparing this regimen to a standard four-drug induction regimen is currently ongoing.

TREATMENT OF RELAPSED OR REFRACTORY ADULT PATIENTS WITH ACUTE LYMPHOBLASTIC LEUKEMIA

Most current induction regimens obtain CRs in 65% to 85% of newly diagnosed patients. Early deaths account for some of the induction failures, but in most studies 10% to 25% of patients have disease resistant to vincristine/prednisone-based regimens. In addition to these primary refractory patients, 60% to 70% of patients achieve a CR relapse. Treatment of relapsed and refractory patients is therefore an important and common problem. Numerous regimens have been reported in the setting of relapsed ALL. The most important regimens can be divided into two main groups: those that repeat the regimens used for newly diagnosed patients (this strategy is obviously not used for primary refractory patients) and those that involve high-dose chemotherapy. High-dose regimens appear to obtain a greater incidence of second CRs when compared with reinduction with vincristine/prednisone-based regimens. The high-dose regimens with the greatest likelihood for inducing a second CR are high-dose cytarabine-based regimens.

High-dose cytarabine has been used alone and in combination with a number of different agents. In combination with L-asparaginase,[259–261] doxorubicin,[262] idarubicin,[263,264] or mitoxantrone,[265–268] CRs as high as 72% have been reported in relapsed patients with ALL. Issues of patient mix make it difficult to assess if a specific regimen is superior to others, but in general a combination of high-dose cytarabine and an anthracycline has the greatest likelihood of achieving a second CR in relapsed patients (or a first CR in refractory patients). The toxicity of these regimens should be balanced against the benefits of achieving a CR. However, second CRs are difficult to maintain and typically each succeeding response is briefer than the preceding one. Patients with a suitable allogeneic transplant option should probably be referred for such a transplant in second CR.[269] The role of autologous or matched unrelated transplants in relapsed adult ALL has not been clearly established and should be considered investigational.

CENTRAL NERVOUS SYSTEM RELAPSE IN ADULT ACUTE LYMPHOBLASTIC LEUKEMIA

CNS relapse occurs in approximately 10% of patients who have received appropriate prophylaxis. In the majority of patients, simultaneous bone marrow relapse can be documented. In occasional patients, CNS relapse may occur without demonstrable systemic relapse (so-called isolated CNS relapse); however, this event almost always predicts subsequent bone marrow relapse, and patients with isolated CNS relapse should receive reinduction chemotherapy as well. Treatment of established CNS disease requires a combination of radiotherapy and intrathecal chemotherapy. Radiotherapy should consist of 1800 to 2400 cGy (in 150- to 200-cGy fractions) administered to the whole brain. Higher doses should be avoided because of the risk of late toxicity and the fact that some patients may later require total body irradiation as part of a conditioning regimen for an allogeneic transplant. Despite encouraging results in children, spinal radiotherapy should be avoided in adults because the dose of radiotherapy to marrow-bearing areas subsequently limits the ability to administer necessary systemic chemotherapy. Intrathecal therapy with methotrexate (12 mg) for patients with established CNS disease should be administered intraventricularly via an Ommaya reservoir. Intrathecal chemotherapy can be administered as often as two or three times per week until the CSF is cleared of leukemic blasts, then twice a week for 3 weeks, and twice a month for 2 or 3 additional months. Patients who develop CNS disease despite prophylaxis with intrathecal methotrexate, or those who do not clear the blasts from the CSF promptly (within two treatments) with methotrexate, should receive intraventricular therapy with cytarabine at a dose of 60 mg.

BONE MARROW TRANSPLANT FOR ADULT ACUTE LYMPHOBLASTIC LEUKEMIA

HLA identical sibling BMTs have been used in adults with ALL in a variety of settings. This dose-intense treatment approach has the ability to eradicate leukemia in a subset of patients with disease refractory to conventional chemotherapy. However, the lack of availability of HLA-matched donors and the toxicity and mortality seen with transplant limits the utility of this approach. There is significant controversy over the use and timing of allogeneic transplant in adult ALL. Analysis of patterns of failure highlight a fundamental difference in the use of this modality for ALL compared with AML. Patients with AML (in first or second CR) treated with allogeneic transplant tend to fail therapy because of treatment-related mortality (infectious complications, GVHD, and so forth). Failure because of relapsed AML after allogeneic transplant (for patients in first or second CR) is relatively uncommon. The results for ALL, however, indicate that even for patients who survive the transplant, there is a significant relapse rate, and overall few patients are long-term disease-free survivors. The ability of allogeneic transplants to cure malignant diseases rests in part on the ability of the transplanted (donor) immune system to eliminate residual leukemic cells; this is known as the *graft-versus-leukemia effect.* There is evidence to suggest that this effect may be less important in ALL than in either AML or in CML. Data from the International Bone Marrow Transplant Registry compared identical twin to HLA identical sibling transplants.[270] Presumably, graft-versus-leukemia should be more pronounced in the HLA identical sibling transplants as compared with the identical twin transplants. In this study, there was a significantly higher relapse rate in the identical twin transplants for AML and CML, but not for ALL. This implies that graft-versus-leukemia is less important in ALL. A second indication that graft-versus-leukemia is less active in ALL comes from an analysis of studies of donor T-cell infusions used to treat leukemia that has relapsed after allogeneic BMT. In this study, donor lymphocyte infusions produced CRs in 73% of patients with CML, 29% of patients with AML, and in 0% of patients with ALL.[219] The lack of graft-versus-leukemia in ALL may in part explain the high relapse rate and the relatively low incidence of long-term disease-free survival after allogeneic transplant for adult ALL.

A review of the published experience of allogeneic BMT in adult ALL reveals that only a small fraction of patients are cured by this modality. The results of 192 adults with ALL transplanted at the Fred Hutchinson Cancer Center report a 5-year disease-free survival of only 15% for patients transplanted in second CR or beyond.[269] Another study that suggested more favorable results is difficult to interpret because this study presents combined results for pediatric and adult patients or patients in first CR (who may already be cured) with higher risk patients.[271]

The ability to cure a small subset of relapsed patients with allogeneic transplant has led investigators to test this modality in first CR. However, two large comparisons of allogeneic transplant versus standard chemotherapy for patients in first CR have failed to demonstrate an improved survival for the transplant arm.[272,273] In one of these studies, subset analysis suggests a benefit for certain high-risk patients.[272] This benefit was not confirmed in the other study.[273] Currently, the only group for whom allogeneic transplant in first CR can be routinely recommended is patients with t(9;22) and t(4;11) disease. For other adult patients, allogeneic transplant should be reserved for second CR.

Autologous transplant for adult ALL is even less effective than allogeneic transplant.[274] The extremely poor results for patients in second CR or beyond has led to this modality being tested in first CR. However, both a nonrandomized[244] and randomized trial[275] showed no benefit for autotransplant compared with maintenance chemotherapy. This modality should be considered experimental and not routinely performed in first CR.

TREATMENT OF MATURE B-CELL ACUTE LYMPHOBLASTIC LEUKEMIA

Mature B-cell ALL is an uncommon disorder that accounts for approximately 5% of all patients with ALL. This disease has an extremely poor prognosis when treated with traditional ALL regimens such as those described previously. Studies indicate that a majority of patients with mature B-cell ALL can be cured with certain intensive regimens. The important features of regimens for this disease are rapid cycling of drugs, fractionated cyclophosphamide, high-dose methotrexate, and intensive CNS prophylaxis. Maintenance therapy is not used in these regimens. A retrospective review of the French experience with this form of therapy indicates that 12 of 22 (55%) patients older than the age of 18 years were cured in this poor-risk group of patients.[276]

GRANULOCYTE SARCOMAS, LEUKEMIA CUTIS, AND OTHER EXTRAMEDULLARY LEUKEMIC INVOLVEMENT

Acute leukemia cells may diffusely infiltrate any organ of the body during the course of disease, or may form collections and large masses known as *granulocytic sarcomas* or *chloromas,* due to their green hue from the myeloperoxidase. Diffuse involvement of the skin by acute leukemia cells is referred to as *leukemia cutis* and should be distinguished from Sweet's syndrome, which is an infiltration of the skin by neutrophils. The initial presentation of acute leukemia at a primary extramedullary site with normal marrow and blood findings is extremely rare.[278] However, if extramedullary leukemia is misdiagnosed as carcinoma or lymphoma and treated without leukemia-specific therapy, the prognosis is poor; overt leukemia usually appears within a year, and death occurs at a median of 3 months later. In contrast, granulocytic sarcomas may occur secondarily in approximately 5% of patients, especially in those with (8;21) or (9;11) translocations or inv(16) chromosome abnormalities, and in patients with other monocytic leukemias.[277–279]

The occurrence of extramedullary disease virtually always heralds systemic relapse and should be treated as such.[278] Specific therapy directed at the extramedullary disease, unless it is located in the CNS, is usually not indicated. Treatment of CNS leukemia is discussed earlier in this chapter (see Central Nervous System Relapse in Adult Acute Lymphoblastic Leukemia). The prognostic significance of extramedullary disease is usually negative even when it is associated with other good prognostic signs [e.g., t(8;21)].[279] Extramedullary disease is treated by systemic therapy of the kind used to consolidate or intensify systemic leukemia. Leukemia cutis has been treated by external electron beam therapy, but this has been associated with fatal dermatitis in patients who had also received anthracyclines commonly used to treat AML.[280]

Involvement of the CNS is rare at presentation in AML, in contrast to ALL, in which it occurs more frequently; therefore, in the absence of symptoms of neurologic involvement, examination of the CSF in patients with AML is not indicated at presentation. In patients with ALL, the CSF should be examined routinely during the initiation of treatment and prophylactic intrathecal chemotherapy should be administered; more aggressive therapy should be initiated if the CSF is involved (as described previously). In AML, CNS disease is more common in patients with high blast counts in the blood and with monocytic leukemias, especially the M4EO variant.[281,282] Cranial neuropathies, when present, are most likely to involve the fifth or seventh nerves.[283] Leukemic infiltration of the cranial nerves can occasionally be detected by computed tomography; magnetic resonance imaging is a better choice, but the diagnosis is usually made by demonstration of leukemia blasts in the CSF. Some patients may not display positive CSF findings; emergency treatment with irradiation and intrathecal methotrexate is sometimes indicated even without diagnostic CSF.

Neurologic symptoms, such as headache or confusion, may also be the consequence of leukostasis and microemboli in the cerebral microvasculature; this is a rare occurrence except in myeloid leukemias with blood blast counts in excess of 100,000/μL.[284] In these cases, urgent therapy (either by leukopheresis or chemotherapy) to lower the blast count is indicated.

BIOLOGIC AND IMMUNOLOGIC THERAPIES OF ACUTE LEUKEMIAS

Modern attempts to treat acute leukemias with agents designed to alter the biology and growth of the leukemia cells or to kill the cells via immunologic means have met with variable success.[285–287] Early work focused on nonspecific immunostimulators such as interferon, IL-2, and linomide in the setting of advanced disease; more recently these agents have been proposed for use after induction therapy to eliminate residual leukemia.[288–293] Interferon has demonstrated sporadic and limited success in inducing remissions in ALL of children, but has never achieved the consistent results observed in hairy cell leukemia or chronic myelogenous leukemia.[122,285,288,289] Moreover, the lack of potency and requirement for prolonged use to achieve effects, combined with the marked toxicity of interferons (including fever, malaise, myalgia, neurologic disorders, and cytopenias), make chronic use as a long-term agent for postremission or maintenance therapy difficult. A mechanism of action of interferon in treating acute leukemia has not been demonstrated.

IL-2, which promotes the growth of T cells and natural killer cells and activates natural killer cells to become lymphokine-activated killer cells, has demonstrated potent activity *in vitro* in stimulating autologous effector cells to kill leukemia blasts, and to block leukemia cell growth in culture *in vitro* and in mouse models.[286,287,290–293] Clinical trials of IL-2 have shown significant antileukemia effects in inverse relationship to the leukemic burden[291,293,294]; therefore, studies have focused on the use of IL-2 in patients in remission or posttransplantation. There is some preliminary evidence that relapse rates may be reduced in AML but not in ALL.[274,292,295] IL-2 is also under investigation as a means to enhance specific therapy with monoclonal antibodies directed to AML cells, because of its ability to enhance antibody-dependent cellular cytotoxicity.[296,297]

Specific monoclonal antibody therapy of acute leukemia has been under investigation since 1981 using passively infused murine monoclonal antibodies, radiolabeled monoclonal antibodies, immunotoxins, and, most recently, genetically engineered humanized monoclonal antibodies.[286,287,298–303] Passive serotherapy in relapsed ALL and AML has generally not been effective because of the lack of antibody potency, rapid loss of the target antigen from the leukemia cell surface, and development of human antimurine antibody responses. Attempts to use genetically engineered humanized antibodies, which have greater potency and can be repeatedly infused, have begun to show activity in the setting of residual disease, particularly in APL.[287,297,298,300,301] A new drug-conjugated antibody and an alpha-emitting construct appears to have significant activity in relapsed AML as well.[302,303] Randomized trials to assess the effectiveness of these approaches are in progress. The application of radiolabeled monoclonal antibodies as an ablative agent before BMT in patients with acute leukemia is also under study.[287,304–306] CR rates approaching 100% have been achieved using these combined modalities, without detriment to engraftment or significant worsening of toxicity associated with the transplant; the demonstration of a therapeutic advantage of this approach in survival awaits randomized studies.

Antibody therapy can also be used *ex vivo* to purge bone marrow of residual leukemia before autologous reinfusion.[286,307] Though initial clinical results are encouraging, no randomized studies confirming the efficacy of this approach have been reported.

Active specific immunotherapy (vaccine therapy) has been explored for its potential in the treatment of leukemias. In principle, peptide sequences derived from oncogene products and translocated fusion proteins may serve as leukemia-specific targets for stimulated cytolytic T cells.[38,308] Such approaches are most likely to be effective in the setting of minimal disease or transplantation.

CONCLUSIONS

Two decades of empiric therapy in leukemia have led to long-term cures in a fraction of adult patients with acute leukemia. Advances in the molecular genetics, immunology, and biology of normal and neoplastic hematopoiesis have produced significant progress in understanding the pathogenesis of acute leukemia. This knowledge is leading to an explosion of new, sensitive molecular assays for minimal disease, new diagnostic and prognostic tests, and to more specific, and less toxic therapies. However, there is still a large gap between the patients who initially achieve remission and those who are ultimately cured. The appropriate care of patients with leukemia requires specialized resources and remains a difficult and complicated task with significant morbidity and mortality. Patients with acute leukemias should continue to be referred to cancer centers and enrolled in investigational treatment protocols until a greater fraction of patients achieve long-term survival.

REFERENCES

1. Virchow R. Weisses, Blut and Milztumoren. *Med Z* 1847;16:19.
2. Hernández JA, Land KJ, McKenna RW. Leukemia, myeloma, and other lymphoreticular neoplasms. *Cancer* 1995;75:381.
3. Wingo PA, Tong T, Bolden S. Cancer statistics, 1995. *CA Cancer J Clin* 1995;45:8.
4. Arseneau JC, Sponzo RW, Levin DL, et al. Nonlymphomatous malignant tumors complicating Hodgkin's disease. *N Engl J Med* 1972;287:1119.
5. Aisenberg AC. Acute nonlymphocytic leukemia after treatment for Hodgkin's disease. *Am J Med* 1983;75:449.
6. Kaldor JM, Day NE, Clarke EA, et al. Leukemia following Hodgkin's disease. *N Engl J Med* 1990;322:7.
7. van Leeuwen FE, Chorus AMJ, van den Belt-Dusebout AW, et al. Leukemia risk following Hodgkin's disease: relation to cumulative dose of alkylating agents, treatment with teniposide combinations, number of episodes of chemotherapy, and bone marrow damage. *J Clin Oncol* 1994;12:1063.
8. Pui CH, Behm FG, Raimondi SC, et al. Secondary acute myeloid leukemia in children treated for acute lymphoid leukemia. *N Engl J Med* 1989;321:136.
9. Pui C-H, Ribeiro RC, Hancock ML, et al. Acute myeloid leukemia in children treated with epipodophyllotoxins for acute lymphoblastic leukemia. *N Engl J Med* 1991;325:1682.
10. Tucker MA, Meadows AT, Bioce JD, et al. Leukemia after therapy with alkylating agents for childhood cancer. *J Natl Cancer Inst* 1977;78:459.
11. Neglia JP, Meadows AT, Robison LL, et al. Second neoplasms after acute lymphoblastic leukemia in childhood. *N Engl J Med* 1991;325:1330.

12. Hawkins MM. Secondary leukaemia after epipodophyllotoxins. *Lancet* 1991;338:1408.
13. DeVore R, Whitlock J, Hainsworth JD, Johnson DH. Therapy-related acute nonlymphocytic leukemia with monocytic features and rearrangement of chromosome 11q. *Ann Intern Med* 1989;110:740.
14. Ratain MJ, Kaminer LS, Bitran JD, et al. Acute nonlymphocytic leukemia following etoposide and cisplatin combination chemotherapy for advanced non-small-cell carcinoma of the lung. *Blood* 1987;70:1412.
15. Detourmignies L, Castaigne S, Stoppa AM, et al. Therapy-related acute promyelocytic leukemia: a report on 16 cases. *J Clin Oncol* 1992;10:1430.
16. Curtis RE, Boice JD Jr, Stovall M, et al. Risk of leukemia after chemotherapy and radiation treatment for breast cancer. *N Engl J Med* 1992;326:1745.
17. Travis LB, Holowaty EJ, Bergfeldt K, et al. Rick of leukemia after platinum-based chemotherapy for ovarian cancer. *N Engl J Med* 1999;340:351.
18. Kumar L. Secondary leukaemia after autologous bone marrow transplantation. *Lancet* 1995;345:810.
19. Tallman MS, Gray R, Bennett JM, et al. Leukemogenic potential of adjuvant chemotherapy for early-stage breast cancer: the Eastern Cooperative Oncology Group experience. *J Clin Oncol* 1995;13:1557.
20. Preston DL, Kusumi S, Tomonaga M, et al. Cancer incidence in atomic bomb survivors. Part III: leukemia, lymphoma and multiple myeloma, 1950–1987. *Radiat Res* 1994;137:S68.
21. Sandler DP. Recent studies in leukemia epidemiology. *Curr Opin Oncol* 1995;7:12.
22. Linet MS, Hatch EE, Kleinerman RA, et al. Residential exposure to magnetic fields and acute lymphoblastic leukemia in children. *N Engl J Med* 1997;337:1.
23. Taubes G. Another blow weakens EMF-cancer link. *Science* 1995;269:1816.
24. Doll R, Evans HJ, Darby SC. Paternal exposure not to blame. *Nature* 1994;367:678.
25. Sorahan T, Roberts PJ. Childhood cancer and paternal exposure to ionizing radiation: preliminary findings from the Oxford Survey of Childhood Cancers. *Am J Indust Med* 1993;23:343.
26. Sandler DP, Shore DL, Anderson JR, et al. Cigarette smoking and risk of acute leukemia: associations with morphology and cytogenetic abnormalities in bone marrow. *J Natl Cancer Inst* 1993;85:1994.
27. Siegel M. Smoking and leukemia: evaluation of a causal hypothesis. *Am J Epidemiol* 1993;138:1.
28. Kabat GC, Augustine A, Hebert JR. Smoking and adult leukemia: a case-control study. *J Clin Epidemiol* 1988;41:907.
29. Austin A, Delzell E, Cole P. Benzene and leukemia: a review of the literature and risk assessment. *Am J Epidemiol* 1988;127:419.
30. Ben-David Y, Bernstein A. Friend virus-induced erythroleukemia and the multistage nature of cancer. *Cell* 1991;66:831.
31. Poiesz BJ, Ruscetti FW, Gazdar AF, et al. Detection and isolation of type C retrovirus particles from fresh and cultured lymphocytes of patient with cutaneous T-cell lymphoma. *Proc Natl Acad Sci U S A* 1980;77:7415.
32. Lombardi L, Newcomb EW, Dalla-Favera R. Pathogenesis of Burkitt's lymphoma: expression of an activated *c-myc* oncogene causes the tumorigenic conversion of EBV-infected human B lymphoblasts. *Cell* 1987;49:161.
33. Pui C-H. Childhood leukemias. *N Engl J Med* 1995;332:1618.
34. Taylor AMR, Metcalfe JA, Thick J, Mak Y-F. Leukemia and lymphoma in ataxia telangiectasia. *Blood* 1995;15:423.
35. Pui C-H, Raimondi SC, Borowitz MJ, et al. Immunophenotypes and karyotypes of leukemic cells in children with Down syndrome and acute lymphoblastic leukemia. *J Clin Oncol* 1993;11:1361.
36. Homans A, Verissimo AM, Vlacha V. Transient abnormal myelopoiesis of infancy associated with trisomy 21. *Am J Pediatr Hematol Oncol* 1993;15:392.
37. Joventino LP, Stock W, Lane NJ, et al. Certain HLA antigens are associated with specific morphologic and cytogenetic subsets of acute myeloid leukemia. *Leukemia* 1995;9:433.
38. Bocchia M, Korontsvit T, Xu A, et al. Specific human cellular immunity to bcr-abl oncogene-derived peptides. *Blood* 1996;82:3587.
39. Koeffler HP, Golde DW. Human myeloid leukemia cell lines: a review. *Blood* 1980;56:344.
40. Li S, Ilaria RL Jr, Million RP, Daley GQ, Van Etten RA. The P190, P210 and P230 forms of the bcr/abl oncogene induce a similar chronic myeloid leukemia-like syndrome in mice but have different lymphoid leukemogenic activity. *J Exp Med* 1999;189:1399.
41. Lallemand-Breitenbach V, Guillemin M-C, Janin A, et al. Retinoic acid and arsenic synergize to eradicate leukemic cells in a mouse model of acute promyelocytic leukemia. *J Exp Med* 1999;189:1043.
42. Moore MAS. Hematopoietic reconstruction: new approaches. *Clin Cancer Res* 1995;1:3.
43. Metcalf D. The roles of stem cell self-renewal and autocrine growth factor production in the biology of myeloid leukemia. *Cancer Res* 1989;49:2305.
44. Suda J, Suda T, Ogawa M. Analysis of differentiation of mouse hematopoietic stem cells in culture by sequential replating of paired progenitors. *Blood* 1984;64:393.
45. Wickremasinghe RG, Hoffbrand AV. Biochemical and genetic control of apoptosis: relevance to normal hematopoiesis and hematological malignancies. *Blood* 1999;93:3587.
46. Timens W. Cell adhesion molecule expression and homing of hematologic malignancies. *Crit Rev Oncol Hematol* 1995;19:111.
47. Gabrilove JL. Hematopoietic growth factors. In: Holland JF, et al., eds. *Cancer medicine.* 3rd ed. Philadelphia: Lea & Febiger, 1993:948.
48. Hoang T, Nara N, Wong G, et al. Effects of recombinant GM-CSF on the blast cells of acute myeloblastic leukemia. *Blood* 1986;68:313.
49. Hunter MG, Avalos BR. Deletion of a critical internalization domain in the G-CSFR in acute myelogenous leukemia preceded by severe congenital neutropenia. *Blood* 1999;93:440.
50. Ward AC, van Aesch YM, Schelen AM, Touw IP. Defective internalization and sustained activation of truncated granulocyte-colony stimulating factor receptor found in severe congenital neutropenia/acute myeloid leukemia. *Blood* 1999;93:447.
51. Till JE, McCulloch EA. A direct measurement of the radiation sensitivity of normal mouse bone marrow cells. *Radiat Res* 1961;14:213.
52. Spangrude GJ, Heimfeld S, Weissman IL. Purification and characterization of mouse hematopoietic stem cells. *Science* 1988;241:58.
53. Fialkow PJ, Singer JW, Raskind WH, et al. Clonal development, stem cell differentiation, and clinical remissions in a acute nonlymphocytic leukemia. *N Engl J Med* 1987;317:468.
54. Fialkow PJ, Singer JW, Adamson JW, et al. Acute nonlymphocytic leukemia: heterogeneity of stem cell origin. *Blood* 1981;57:1068.
55. Ferraris AM, Broccia G, Meloni T, et al. Clonal origin of cells restricted to monocytic differentiation in acute nonlymphocytic leukemia. *Blood* 1984;64:817.
56. Griffin JD, Lowenberg B. Clonogeneic cells in acute myeloblastic leukemia. *Blood* 1986;68:1185.
57. Sabbath KD, Ball ED, Larcom P, David RB, Griffin JD. Heterogeneity of clonogenic cells in acute myeloblastic leukemia. *J Clin Invest* 1985;75:746.
58. Terstappen LWMM, Safford M, Unterhalt M, et al. Flow cytometric characterization of acute myeloid leukemia: IV. Comparison to the differentiation pathway of normal hematopoietic progenitor cells. *Leukemia* 1992;6:993.
59. Sachs L, Lotem J. Control of programmed cell death in normal and leukemic cells: new implications for therapy. *Blood* 1993;82:15.
60. Counter CM, Gupta J, Harley CB, Leber B, Bacchetti S. Telomerase activity in normal leukocytes and in hematologic malignancies. *Blood* 1995;85:2315.
61. Hirama T, Koeffler HP. Role of the cyclin-dependent kinase inhibitors in the development of cancer. *Blood* 1995;86:841.
62. Turhan AG, Lemoine FM, Debert C, et al. Highly purified primitive hematopoietic stem cells are PML/RARα negative and generate nonclonal progenitors in acute promyelocytic leukemia. *Blood* 1995;85:2154.
63. Singer JW, Fialkow PJ. Nature of remission in acute myeloid leukemia: more questions than answers. *Leukemia* 1992;6:60.
64. Fearon ER, Burke PJ, Schiffer CA, et al. Differentiation of leukemia cells to polymorphonuclear leukocytes in patients with acute nonlymphocytic leukemia. *N Engl J Med* 1986;315:15.
65. Lo Coco F, Pelicci PG, D'Adamo F, et al. Polyclonal hematopoietic reconstitution in leukemia patients at remission after suppression of specific gene rearrangements. *Blood* 1993;82:606.
66. Bennett JM, Catovsky D, Daniel MT, et al. Proposed revised criteria for the classification of acute myeloid leukemia. *Ann Intern Med* 1985;103:620.
67. Bennett JM, Catovsky D, Daniel MT, et al. Criteria for the diagnosis of acute leukemia of megakaryocytic lineage (M7). *Ann Intern Med* 1985;103:460.
68. Bennett JM, Catovsky D, Daniel MT, et al. The morphological classification of acute lymphoblastic leukaemia: concordance among observers and clinical correlations. *Br J Haematol* 1981;47:553.
69. Jennings CD, Foon KA. Recent advances in flow cytometry: application to the diagnosis of hematologic malignancy. *Blood* 1997;90:2863.
70. Bennett JM, Catovsky D, Daniel MT, et al. Proposed revised criteria for the classification of acute myeloid leukemia. (AML-M0). *Br J Haematol* 1991;78:325.
71. Cheson BD, Cassileth PA, Head DR, et al. Report of the National Cancer Institute-sponsored workshop on definitions of diagnosis and response to acute myeloid leukemia. *J Clin Oncol* 1990;8:813.
72. Catovsky D, Matutes E, Buccheri V, et al. A classification of acute leukaemia for the 1990s. *Ann Hematol* 1991;62:16.
73. Lee EJ, Pollak A, Leavitt RD, Testa JR, Schiffer CA. Minimally differentiated acute nonlymphocytic leukemia: a distinct entity. *Blood* 1987;70:1400.
74. Windebank KP, Tefferi A, Smithson WA, et al. Acute megakaryocytic leukemia (M7) in children. *Mayo Clin Proc* 1989;64:1339.
75. Loken MR, Shah VO, Datilio KL, Civin CI. Flow cytometric analysis of human bone marrow: I. Normal erythroid development. *Blood* 1987;70:1316.
76. Terstappen LWMM, Huang S, Picker LJ. Flow cytometric assessment of human T-cell differentiation in thymus and bone marrow. *Blood* 1992;79:666.
77. Terstappen LWMM, Safford M, Loken MR. Flow cytometric analysis of human bone marrow III. Neutrophil development. *Leukemia* 1990;4:657.
78. Terstappen LWMM. Cell differentiation and maturation in normal bone marrow and acute leukaemia. In: Macey MG, ed. Flow cytometry clinical applications. Oxford: Blackwell, 1995:101.
79. Terstappen LWMM, Safford M, Könemann S, et al. Flow cytometric characterization of acute myeloid leukemia II. Phenotypic heterogeneity at presentation. *Leukemia* 1991;5:757.
80. Mayer RJ, David RB, Schiffer CA, et al. Intensive postremission chemotherapy in adults with acute myeloid leukemia. *N Engl J Med* 1994;331:896.
81. Reading CL, Estey EH, Huh YO, et al. Expression of unusual immunophenotype combinations in acute myelogenous leukemia. *Blood* 1993;81:3083.
82. Cross AH, Goorha RM, Nuss R, et al. Acute myeloid leukemia with T-lymphoid features: a distinct biological and clinical entity. *Blood* 1988;72:579.
83. Greaves MF, Chan LC, Furley AJW, Watt SM, Molgaard HV. Lineage promiscuity in hematopoietic differentiation and leukemia. *Blood* 1986;67:1.
84. Lo Coco F, De Rossi G, Pasqualetti D, et al. CD7 positive acute myeloid leukaemia: a subtype associated with cell immaturity. *Br J Haematol* 1989;73:480.
85. Campana D, Pui C-H. Detection of minimal residual disease in acute leukemia: methodologic advances and clinical significance. *Blood* 1995;85:1416.
86. Syrjälä M, Anttila V-J, Ruutu T, Jansson S-E. Flow cytometric detection of residual disease in acute leukemia by assaying blasts co-expressing myeloid and lymphatic antigens. *Leukemia* 1994;8:1564.
87. Ferrara F, Del Vecchio L. Clinical relevance of acute mixed-lineage leukemias. *Leukemia Lymphoma* 1993;12:11.

88. Ball ED, Davis RB, Griffin JD, et al. Prognostic value of lymphocyte surface markers in acute myeloid leukemia. *Blood* 1991;77:2242.
89. Paietta E, Van Ness B, Bennett J, et al. Lymphoid lineage-associated features in acute myeloid leukaemia: phenotypic and genotypic correlations. *Br J Haematol* 1992;82:324.
90. Rowley JD. Recurring chromosome abnormalities in leukemia and lymphoma. *Semin Hematol* 1990;27:122.
91. Nichols J, Nimer S. Transcription factors, translocations, and acute leukemia. *Blood* 1992;80:2953.
92. Gilliland DG. Molecular genetics of human leukemia. *Leukemia* 1998;12:S7.
93. Look AT. Oncogenic transcription factors in the human acute leukemias. *Science* 1997;278:1059.
94. Korsmeyer SJ. Chromosomal translocations in lymphoid malignancies reveal novel proto-oncogenes. *Annu Rev Immunol* 1992;10:785.
95. Heim S, Mitelman F. Cytogenetic analysis in the diagnosis of acute leukemia. *Cancer* 1992;70:1701.
96. Wetzler M, Dodge RK, Mrózek K, et al. Prospective karyotype analysis in adult acute lymphoblastic leukemia: the cancer and leukemia group B experience. *Blood* 1999;93:3983.
97. Dabaja BS, Faderl S, Thomas D, et al. Deletions and losses in chromosomes 5 or 7 in adult acute lymphocytic leukemia: incidence, associations and implications. *Leukemia* 1999;13:869.
98. Mrózek K, Heinonen K, de la Chapelle A, Bloomfield CD. Clinical significance of cytogenetics in acute myeloid leukemia. *Semin Oncol* 1997;24:17.
99. Miller WH Jr, Levine K, DeBlasio A, et al. Detection of minimal residual disease in acute promyelocytic leukemia by reverse transcription polymerase chain reaction assay for the PML/RAR-α fusion mRNA. *Blood* 1993;82:1689.
100. Miller WH Jr, Kakizuka A, Frankel SR, et al. Reverse transcription polymerase chain reaction for the rearranged retinoic acid receptor α clarifies diagnosis and detects minimal residual disease in acute promyelocytic leukemia. *Proc Natl Acad Sci U S A* 1992;89:2694.
101. Koeffler HP. Syndromes of acute nonlymphocytic leukemia. *Ann Intern Med* 1987;107:748.
102. Levine EG, Bloomfield CD. Leukemias and myelodysplastic syndromes secondary to drug, radiation, and environmental exposure. *Semin Oncol* 1992;19:47.
103. Rubin CM, Arthur DC, Woods WG, et al. Therapy-related myelodysplastic syndrome and acute myeloid leukemia in children: correlation between chromosomal abnormalities and prior therapy. *Blood* 1991;78:2982.
104. Pedersen-Bjergaard J, Philip P. Two different classes of therapy-related and de-novo acute myeloid leukemia. *Cancer Genet Cytogenet* 1991;55:119.
105. Boultwood J, Lewis S, Wainscoat JS. The 5q-Syndrome. *Blood* 1994;84:3253.
106. Brinker H. Estimates of overall treatment results in acute non-lymphocytic leukemia based on age-specific rates of incidence and of complete remission. *Cancer Treat Rep* 1985;69:5.
107. Skipper HE, Schabel FM, Jay R, et al. Experimental evaluation of potential antitumor agents: on the criteria and kinetics associated with curability of experimental leukemia. *Cancer Treat Rep* 1974;4:137.
108. Freireich EJ, Cork A, Stass SA, et al. Cytogenetics for detection of minimal residual disease in acute myeloblastic leukemia. *Leukemia* 1992;6:500.
109. Anastasi J, Vardiman JW, Rudinsky R, et al. Direct correlation of cytogenetic findings with morphology using in situ hybdridization: an analysis of suspicious cells in bone marrow specimens of two patients completing therapy for acute lymphoblastic leukemia. *Blood* 1991;77:2456.
110. Zehnbauer BA, Pardol DM, Burke PJ, Graham ML. Immunoglobulin gene rearrangement in remission bone marrow specimens from patients with acute lymphoblastic leukemia. *Blood* 1986;67:835.
111. San Miguel JF, Martinez A, Macedo A, et al. Immunophenotyping investigation of minimal residual disease is a useful approach for predicting relapse in acute myeloid leukemia patients. *Blood* 1997;90:2465.
112. Bader P, Beck J, Frey A, et al. Serial and quantitative analysis of mixed hematopoietic chimerism by PCR in patients with acute leukemias allows prediction of relapse after allogeneic BMT. *Bone Marrow Transplant* 1998;21:487.
113. Diverio D, Rossi V, Avvisati G, et al. Early detection of relapse by prospective reverse transcriptase-polymerase chain reaction of the PML/RARα fusion gene in patients with acute promyelocytic leukemia enrolled in the GIMEMA-AIOP multicenter "AIDA" trial. *Blood* 1998;92:784.
114. Anderlini P, Luna M, Kantarjian H, et al. Causes of initial remission induction failure in patients with acute myeloid leukemia and myelodysplastic syndrome. *Leukemia* 1996;10:600.
115. Hughes WT, Armstrong D, Bodey GP, et al. Guidelines for the use of antimicrobial agents in neutropenic patients with unexplained fever. A statement by the Infectious Disease Society of America. *J Infect Dis* 1990;161:381.
116. Pizzo P. Fever in immunocompromised patients. *N Engl J Med* 1999;341:893.
117. Uzun O, Anaissie EJ. Antifungal prophylaxis in patients with hematologic malignancies: a reappraisal. *Blood* 1995;86:2063.
118. Straus RG. Therapeutic granulocyte transfusions in 1993. *Blood* 1993;81:1675.
119. Ohno R, Tomonaga M, Kobayashi T, et al. Effect of granulocyte colony-stimulating factor after intensive induction therapy in relapsed or refractory acute leukemia. *N Engl J Med* 1990;323:871.
120. Stone RM, Berg DT, George SL, et al. Granulocyte-macrophage colony-stimulating factor after initial chemotherapy for elderly patients with primary acute myelogenous leukemia. *N Engl J Med* 1995;332:1671.
121. Rowe JW, Andersen JW, Mazza JJ, et al. A randomized placebo-controlled phase III study of granulocyte-macrophage colony-stimulating factor in adult patients (>55 to 70 years of age) with acute myelogenous leukemia: a study of the Eastern Cooperative Oncology Group (E1490). *Blood* 1995;86:457.
122. Dombret H, Chastang C, Fenaux P, et al. A controlled study of recombinant human granulocyte colony-stimulating factor in elderly patients after treatment for acute myelogenous leukemia. *N Engl J Med* 1995;332:1678.
123. Heil G, Hoelzer D, Sanz MA, et al. A randomized, double-blind, placebo-controlled, phase III study of filgrastim in remission induction and consolidation therapy for adults with de novo acute myeloid leukemia. *Blood* 1997;90:4710.
124. Godwin JE, Kopecky KJ, Head DR, et al. A double-blind, placebo controlled trial of granulocyte colony stimulating factor in elderly patients with previously untreated acute myeloid leukemia: a Southwest Oncology Group Study (9031). *Blood* 1998;91:3607.
125. Witz F, Sadoun A, Perrin MC, et al. A placebo-controlled study of recombinant human granulocyte-macrophage colony-stimulating factor administered during and after induction treatment for de novo acute myelogenous leukemia in elderly patients. *Blood* 1998;91:2722.
126. Gmur J, Burger J, Schanz U, Fehr J, Schaffner A. Safety of stringent prophylactic platelet transfusion policy for patients with acute leukemia. *Lancet* 1991;338:1223.
127. Rebulla P, Finazzi G, Marangoni F, et al. The threshold for prophylactic platelet transfusions in adults with acute myeloid leukemia. *N Engl J Med* 1997;337:1870.
128. Wandt H, Frank M, Ehninger G, et al. Safety and cost effectiveness of a 10×10^9/L trigger for prophylactic platelet transfusions compared with traditional 20×10^9/L trigger: a prospective comparative trial in 105 patients with acute myeloid leukemia. *Blood* 1998;91:3601.
129. Trial to Reduce Alloimmunization to Platelets Study Group. Leukocyte reduction and ultraviolet B irradiation of platelets to prevent alloimmunization and refractoriness to platelet transfusions. *N Engl J Med* 1997;337:1861.
130. Tallman MS, Kwaan HC. Reassessing the hemostatic disorder associated with acute promyelocytic leukemia. *Blood* 1992;79:543.
131. Goldberg MA, Ginsburg D, Mayer RJ, et al. Is heparin administration necessary during induction chemotherapy for patients with acute promyelocytic leukemia? *Blood* 1987;69:187.
132. Barbui T, Finazzi G, Falanga A. The impact of all-*trans*-retinoic acid on coagulopathy of acute promyelocytic leukemia. *Blood* 1998;91:3093.
133. O'Regan S, Carson S, Chesney RW, Drummond KN. Electrolyte and acid base disturbances in the management of leukemia. *Blood* 1997;49:345.
134. Mir WA, Delamore IW. Metabolic disorders in acute myeloid leukemia. *Br J Haematol* 1978;40:79.
135. Swirsky DM, DeBastos M, Parish SE, Rees JKH, Hayhoe FGJ. Features affecting outcome during remission induction of acute myeloid leumemia in 619 adult patients. *Br J Hematol* 1986;64:435.
136. Keating A, Baker MA. Effect of exclusion criteria on interpretation of clinical outcome in AML. In: Gale RP, ed. *Acute myelogenous leukemia: progress and controversies.* New York: Wiley-Liss, 1990:235.
137. Yates J, Gildewell O, Wienik P, et al. Cytosine arabinoside with daunorubicin or adriamycin for therapy of acute myelocytic leukemia: A CALGB study. *Blood* 1982;60:454.
138. Rai KR, Holland JF, Glidewell OJ, et al. Treatment of acute myelocytic leukemia: a study by Cancer and Leukemia Group B. *Blood* 1981;58:1203.
139. Neugut AI, Robinson E, Nieves J, Murray T, Tsai WY. Poor survival of treatment-related acute nonlymphocytic leukemia. *JAMA* 1990;264:1006.
140. Gajewski JL, Ho WG, Nimer SD, et al. Efficacy of intensive chemotherapy for acute myelogenous leukemia associated with preleukemic syndrome. *J Clin Oncol* 1989;7:1637.
141. Keating MJ, Smith TL, Kantarjian H, et al. Cytogenetic pattern in acute myelogenous leukemia: a major reproducible determinant of outcome. *Leukemia* 1988;2:403.
142. Schiffer CA, Lee EJ, Tomiyasu T, Wiernik PH, Testa JR. Prognostic impact of cytogenetic abnormalities in patients with de novo acute nonlymphcytic leukemia. *Blood* 1989;73:263.
143. Ferrant A, Lapopin M, Frassoni F, et al. Karyotype in acute myeloblastic leukemia: prognostic significance for bone marrow transplantation in first remission: a European Group for Blood and Marrow Transplantation Study. *Blood* 1997;76:2931.
144. Ellison RR, Holland JF, Weil M, et al. Arabinosyl cytosine: a useful agent in the treatment of acute leukemia in adults. *Blood* 1968;32:507.
145. Carey RW, Ribas-Mundo M, Ellison RR, et al. Comparative study of cytosine arabinoside therapy alone and combined with thioguanine, mercaptopurine, or daunorubicin in acute myelocytic leukemia. *Cancer* 1975;36:1560.
146. Yates JW, Wallace HT Jr, Ellison RR, Holland JF. Cytosine arabinoside (NSC 63878) and daunorubicin (NSC 83142) therapy in acute nonlymphocytic leukemia. *Cancer Chemother Rep* 1973;57:485.
147. Gales RP, Cline MJ. High remission induction rate in acute myeloid leukaemia. *Lancet* 1977;1:49.
148. Amadori S, Papa G, Meloni G, et al. Daunorubicin, cytosine arabinoside and 6-thioguanine (DAT) combination therapy for the treatment of acute nonlymphocytic leukemia. *Leuk Res* 1979;3:147.
149. Preisler H, Davis RB, Kirshner J, et al. Comparison of three remission induction regimens and two post induction strategies for the treatment of acute nonlymphocytic leukemia: a Cancer and Leukemia Group B study. *Blood* 1987;69:1441.
150. Dillman RO, David RB, Green MR, et al. A comparative study of two different doses of cytarabine for acute myeloid leukemia: a phase III trial of cancer and Leukemia Group B. *Blood* 1991;78:2520.
151. Bishop JF, Lowenthal RM, Joshua D, et al. Etoposide in acute nonlymphocytic leukemia. *Blood* 1990;75:27.
152. Arlin Z, Case DC, Moore J, et al. Randomized multicenter trial of cytosine arabinoside with mitoxantrone or daunorubicin in previously untreated adult patients with acute nonlymphocytic leukemia (ANLL). *Leukemia* 1990;4:177.
153. Berman E, Arlin ZA, Gaynor J, et al. Comparative trial of cytarabine and thioguanine in combination with amsacrine or daunorubicin in patients with untreated acute nonlymphocytic leukemia: results of the L-16M protocol. *Leukemia* 1989;3:115.

154. Harousseau JL, Milpied N, Briere J, et al. Double intensive consolidation chemotherapy in adult acute myeloid leukemia. *J Clin Oncol* 1991;8:1432.

155. Hansen OP, Pedersen-Bjergaard J, Ellegaard J, et al. Aclarubicin plus cytosine arabinoside versus daunorubicin plus cytosine arabinoside in previously untreated patients with acute myeloid leukemia: A Danish National Phase III trial. *Leukemia* 1991;5:510.

156. Berman E, Heller G, Santorsa J, et al. Results of a randomized trial comparing idarubicin and cytosine arabinoside with daunorubicin and cytosine arabinoside in adult patients with newly diagnosed acute myelogenous leukemia. *Blood* 1991;77:1666.

157. Vogler WR, Velez-Garcia E, Weiner RS, et al. A phase III trial comparing idarubicine and daunorubicin in combination with cytarabine in acute myelogenous leukemia: a Southeastern cancer study group study. *J Clin Oncol* 1992;10:1103.

158. Wiernik PH, Banks PLC, Case Jr, et al. Cytarabine plus idarubicin or daunorubicin as induction and consolidation therapy for previously untreated adult patients with acute myeloid leukemia. *Blood* 1992;79:313.

159. Berman E, Wiemik P, Vogler R, et al. Long term follow-up of three randomized trial comparing idarubicin and daunorubicin as induction therapies for patients with untreated acute myeloid leukemia. *Cancer* 1997;80(Suppl 2):2181.

160. Rowe JM, Neuberg D, Friedenberg W, et al. A phase III study of daunorubicin vs. idarubicin vs. mitoxantrone for older adult patients (>55yrs) with acute myelogenous leukemia (AML): a study of the Eastern Cooperative Oncology Group (E3993). *Blood* 1998;92(Suppl 1):1284(abst).

161. Schiller G, Gajewski J, Nimer S, et al. A randomized study of intermediate versus conventional-dose cytarabine as intensive induction for acute myelogenous leuaemia. *Br J Haematol* 1992;81:170.

162. Bishop JF, Matthews JP, Young GA, et al. A randomized study of high dose cytarabine in induction in acute myeloid leukemia. *Blood* 1996;87:1710.

163. Weick J, Kopecky K, Appelbaurn F, et al. A randomized investigation of high-dose versus standard dose cytosine arabinoside with daunorubicin in patients with patients with previously untreated acute myeloid leukemia. *Blood* 1996;88:2841.

164. Buchner T, Hiddenman W, Koenigsmann M, et al. Recombinant human granulocyte-macrophage colony-stimulating factor after chemotherapy in patients with acute myeloid leukemia at higher age or after relapse. *Blood* 1991;78:1190.

165. Maslak P, Weiss M, Berman E, et al. Granulocyte colony-stimulating factor following chemotherapy in elderly patients with newly diagnosed acute myelogenous leukemia. *Leukemia* 1996;10:32.

166. Ohno R, Naoe T, Kanamaru T, et al. A double-blind controlled study of granulocyte colony-stimulating factor started two days before induction chemotherapy in refractory acute myeloid leukemia. *Blood* 1994;83:2086.

167. Estey E, Thall P, Andreeff M, et al. Use of granulocyte colony-stimulating factor before, during, and after fludarabine plus cytarabine induction therapy of newly diagnosed acute myelogenous leukemia or myelodysplastic syndromes: comparison with fludarabine plus cytarabine with granulocytes colony-stimulating factor. *J Clin Oncol* 1994;12:671.

168. Bennett CL, Stinson TJ, Tallman MS, et al. Economic analysis of a randomized placebo-controlled phase III study of granulocyte macrophage colony stimulating factor in adult patients (>55 to 70 years of age) with acute myelogenous leukemia. Eastern Cooperative Oncology Group (E1490). *Ann Oncol* 1999;10:177.

169. Buchner T, Urbanitz D, Hiddemann W, et al. Intensified induction and consolidation with and without maintenance chemotherapy for acute myeloid leukemia: two multicenter studies of the German AML Cooperative Group. *J Clin Oncol* 1985;3:1583.

170. Cassileth PA, Harrington DP, Hines JD, et al. Maintenance chemotherapy prolongs remission duration in adult acute nonlymphocytic leukemia. *J Clin Oncol* 1988;6:583.

171. Cassileth PA, Begg CB, Bennett JM, et al. A randomized study of the efficacy of consolidation therapy in adult acute nonlymphocytic leukemia. *Blood* 1984;63:843.

172. Sauter C, Berchtold W, Foop M, et al. Acute myelogenous leukemia: maintenance chemotherapy after early consolidation does not prolong survival. *Lancet* 1984;1:379.

173. Cassileth PA, Lynch E, Hines JD, et al. Varying intensity of postremission therapy in acute myeloid leukemia. *Blood* 1992;79:1924.

174. Bolwell BJ, Cassileth PA, Gale RP. High dose cytarabine: a review. *Leukemia* 1988;2:253.

175. Schiller G, Gajewski J, Territo M, et al. Long-term outcome of high-dose cytarabine consolidation chemotherapy for adults with acute myelogenous leukemia. *Blood* 1992;80:2977.

176. Bloomfield CD, Lawrence D, Arthur DC, et al. Curative impact of intensification with high-dose cytarabine (HiDAC) in acute myeloid leukemia (AML) varies by cytogenetic group. *Blood* 1994;84(Suppl 1):431(abst).

177. Sullivan KM, Weiden PL, Storb R, et al. Influence of acute and chronic graft-versus-host disease on relapse and survival after bone marrow transplantation from HLA-identical siblings as treatment of acute and chronic leukemia. *Blood* 1989;73:1720.

178. Horowitz MM, Gale RP, Sondel PM, et al. Graft-versus-leukemia reactions after bone marrow transplantation. *Blood* 1990;75:555.

179. Stockerl-Goldstein A, Blume K, Allogeneic hematopoietic cell transplantation for adult patients with acute myeloid leukemia. In: Thomas ED, Blume K, Forman S, eds. *Hematopoietic cell transplantation.* 2nd ed. Malden, MA: Blackwell, 1999:823.

180. Berman E, Little C, Gee T, O'Reilly R, Clarkson B. Reasons that patients with acute myelogenous leukemia do not undergo allogeneic bone marrow transplantation. *N Engl J Med* 1992;326:156.

181. Szydlo R, Goldman JM, Klein JP, et al. Results of allogeneic bone marrow transplants for leukemia using donors other than HLA-Identical siblings. *J Clin Oncol* 1997;15:1767.

182. Slavin S, Nagler A, Naparstek E, et al. Nonmyeloablative stem cell transplantation and cell therapy as an alternative to conventional bone marrow transplantation with lethal cytoreduction for the treatment of malignant and nonmalignant hematologic diseases. *Blood* 1998;91:756.

183. Gorin NC. Autlogous stem cell transplantation in acute myelocytic leukemia. *Blood* 1998;92:1073.

184. Brenner MK, Rill DR, Moen RC, et al. Gene-marking to trace origin of relapse after autologous bone-marrow transplantation. *Lancet* 1993;341:85.

185. To LB, Juttner CA. Peripheral blood stem cell autografting: a new therapeutic option for AML? *Br J Hematol* 1987;66:285.

186. To LB, Russell J, Moore S, Juttner CA. Residual leukemia cannot be detected in very early remission peripheral blood stem cell collections in acute non-lymphoblastic leukemia. *Leuk Res* 1987;11:327.

187. Carella AM, Cunningham I, Lerma E, et al. Mobilization and transplantation of Philadelphia-negative peripheral blood progenitor cells early in chronic myelogenous leukemia. *J Clin Oncol* 1997;15:1575.

188. Miyamoto T, Nagafuji K, Harada M, et al. Quantitative analysis of AML 1/ETO transcripts in peripheral blood stem cell harvests from patients with t(8;21) acute myelogenous leukaemia. *Br J Hematol* 1995;91:132.

189. Korbling M, Fliedner TM, Holle R, et al. Autologous blood stem cell (ABSCT) versus purged bone marrow transplantation (pABMT) in standard risk AML: influence of source and cell composition of the autograft on hemopoietic reconstitution and disease-free survival. *Bone Marrow Transplant* 1991;7:343.

190. Stein AS, O'Donnell MR, Chai A, et al. In vivo purging with high-dose cytarabine followed by high dose chemoradiotherapy and reinfusion of unpurged bone marrow for adult acute myelogenous leukemia in first complete remission. *J Clin Oncol* 1996;14:2206.

191. Burnett AK, Goldstone AH, Stevens RM, et al. Randomised comparison of addition of autologous bone-marrow transplantation to intensive chemotherapy for acute myeloid leukaemia in first remission: results of MRC AML 10 trial. *Lancet* 1998;351:700.

192. Zittoun RA, Mandelli F, Willemze R, et al. Autologous or allogeneic bone marrow transplantation compared with intensive chemotherapy in acute myelogenous leukemia. *N Engl J Med* 1995;332:217.

193. Harousseau J-L, Cahn J-Y, Pignon B, et al., Comparison of autologous bone marrow transplantation and intensive chemotherapy as postremission therapy in adult acute myeloid leukemia. *Blood* 1997;90:2978.

194. Cassileth PA, Harrington DP, Appelbaum FR, et al. Chemotherapy compared with autologous or allogeneic bone marrow transplantation in the management of acute myeloid leukemia in first remission. *N Engl J Med* 1998;339:1649.

195. Schiffman K, Clift R, Applebaum FR, et al. Consequences of cryopreserving first remission autologous marrow for use after relapse in patients with acute myeloid leukemia. *Bone Marrow Transplant* 1993;11:227.

196. Keating MJ, Kantarjian H, Smith TL, et al. Response to salvage therapy and survival after relapse in acute myelogenous leukemia. *J Clin Oncol* 1989;7:1071.

197. Clift RA, Buckner CD, Applebaum FR, et al. Allogeneic marrow transplantation during untreated first relapse of acute myeloid leukemia. *J Clin Oncol* 1992;10:1723.

198. Petersen FB, Lynch MHE, Clift RA, et al. Autologous marrow transplantation for patients with acute myeloid leukemia in untreated first relapse or in second complete remission. *J Clin Oncol* 1993;11:1353.

199. Chopra R, Goldstone AH, McMillan AK, et al. Successful treatment of acute myeloid leukemia beyond first remission with autologous bone marrow transplantation using busulfan/cyclophosphamide and unpurged marrow: the British autograft group experience. *J Clin Oncol* 1991;9:1840.

200. Yeager AM, Kaizer H, Santos GW, et al. Autologous bone marrow transplantation in patients with acute nonlymphoblastic leukemia using *ex vivo* in marrow treatment with 4 hydroperocyclophoaphamide. *N Engl J Med* 1986;315:141.

201. Hiddemann W, Martin WR, Sauerland CM, Heinecke A, Bochner T. Definition of refractoriness against conventional chemotherapy in acute myeloid leukemia: a proposal based on the results of retreatment by thiogauanine, cytosine arabinoside, and daunorubicin (TAB 9) in 150 patients with relapse after standardized first line therapy. *Leukemia* 1990;4:184.

202. Vey N, Keating M, Giles F, et al. Effect of complete remission on survival in patients with acute myelogenous leukemia receiving first salvage therapy [letter]. *Blood* 1999;93:3149.

203. Maslak P, Hegewisch-Becker S, Godfrey L, Andreeff M. Flow cytometric determination of the multi-drug resistant phenotype in acute leukemia. *Cytometry* 1994;17:84.

204. Leith CP, Chen I-M, Kopecky KJ, et al. Correlation of multidrug resistance (MDR1) protein expression with functional dye/drug efflux in acute myeloid leukemia by multiparameter flow cytometry: identification of discordant CD34+/MDR1-/efflux+ and MDR1+/efflux- cases. *Blood* 1995;86:2329.

205. Filipits M, Suchomel RW, Zochbauer, et al. Multidrug resistance associated protein in acute myeloid leukemia: no impact on treatment outcome. *Clin Cancer Res* 1997;3:1419.

206. Filipits M, Pohl G, Stranzl T, et al. Expression of the lung resistance protein predicts poor outcome in de novo acute myeloid leukemia *Blood* 1998;91:1508.

207. Advani R, Saba HI, Tallman MS, et al. Treatment of refractory and relapsed acute myelogenous leukemia with combination chemotherapy plus the multidrug resistance modulator PSC 833 (Valspdar). *Blood* 1999;93:787.

208. Herzig RH, Wolff SN, Lazarus HM, et al. High-dose cytosine arabinoside therapy for refractory leukemia. *Blood* 1983;62:361.

209. Bolwell BJ, Cassileth PA, Gale RP. High dose cytarabine: a review. *Leukemia* 1988;2:253.

210. Forman SJ, Schmidt GM, Nademanee AP, et al. Allogeneic bone marrow transplantation as therapy for primary induction failure for patients with acute leukemia. *J Clin Oncol* 1991;9:1570.

211. Ho AD, Lipp T, Ehninger G, et al. Combination of mitoxantrone and etoposide in refractory acute myelogenous leukemia—an active and well-tolerated regimen. *J Clin Oncol* 1988;6:213.

212. Vogler WR, Harrington DP, Winton EF, et al. Phase II clinical trial of carboplatin in relapsed and refractory leukemia. *Leukemia* 1992;6:1072.

213. Brown RA, Herzig RH, Wolff SN, et al. High-dose etoposide and cyclophosphamide without bone marrow transplantation for resistant hematologic malignancy. *Blood* 1990;76:473.

214. Kumar L. Leukemia; management of relapse after allogeneic bone marrow transplantation. *J Clin Oncol* 1994;12:1710.
215. Giralt SA, Champlin RE. Leukemia relapse after allogeneic bone marrow transplantation: a review. *Blood* 1994;84:3603.
216. Kolb H-J, Schattenberg A, Goldman JM, et al. Graft-versus-Leukemia effect of donor lymphocyte transfusions in marrow grafted patients. *Blood* 1995;86:2041.
217. Kantajian HM, Keating MJ, Walters RS, et al. Acute promyelocytic leukemia: M.D. Anderson Hospital experience. *Am J Med* 1986;80:789.
218. Cunningham I, Gee TS, Reich LM, et al. Acute promyelocytic leukemia: treatment results during a decade at Memorial Hospital. *Blood* 1989;73;116.
219. Head D, Kopecky KJ, Weick J, et al. Effect of aggressive daunomycin therapy on survival in acute promyelocytic leukemia. *Blood* 1995;86:1717.
220. Huang ME, Ye YC, Chen SR, et al. Use of all-trans retinoic acid in the treatment of acute promyelocytic leukemia. *Blood* 1988;72:567.
221. Degos L, Dombret H, Chomienne C, et al. All-trans retinoic acid as a differentiating agent in the treatment of acute promyelocytic leukemia. *Blood* 1995;85:2643.
222. Warrell RP Jr, Frankel SR, Miller WH Jr, et al. Differentiation therapy of acute promyelocytic leukemia with tretinoin (all-trans-retinoic acid). *N Engl J Med* 1991;324:1385.
223. Warrell RP, Maslak P, Eardley A, et al. Treatment of acute promyelocytic leukemia with all-trans retinoic acid: an update of the New York experience. *Leukemia* 1994;8:929.
224. Frankel SR, Eardley A, Lauwers G, Weiss M, Warrell RP Jr. The "retinoic acid syndrome" in acute promyelocytic leukemia. *Ann Intern Med* 1992;117:292.
225. Stadler M, Ganser A, Hoelzer D. Acute promyelocytic leukemia. *N Engl J Med* 1994;330:140.
226. Castaigne S, Chomienne C, Daniel MT, et al. All-trans retinoic acid as a differentiation therapy for acute promyelocytic leukemia. I. Clinical results. *Blood* 1990;76:1704.
227. Fenaux P, Le Deley MC, Castaigne S, et al. Effect of all-trans retinoic acid in newly diagnosed acute promyelocytic leukemia: results of a multicenter randomized trial. *Blood* 1993;82:3241.
228. Vahdat L, Maslak P, Miller WH Jr, et al. Early mortality and the retinoic acid syndrome in acute promyelocytic leukemia: impact of leukocytosis, low-dose chemotherapy, PML/RAR-α isoform, and CD13 expression in patients treated with all-trans retinoic acid. *Blood* 1994;8:3843.
229. Tallman MS, Andersen J, Schiffer CA, et al. All-trans retinoic acid in acute promyelocytic leukemia. *N Engl J Med* 1997;337:1021.
230. Mandelli F, Diverio D, Avvisati G, et al. Molecular remission in PML/RARα-positive acute promyelocytic leukemia by combined all-trans retinoic acid and idarubicin (AIDA) therapy. *Blood* 1997;90:1014.
231. Fenaux P, Chastang C, Chevret S, et al. A randomized comparison of all transretinoic acid (ATRA) followed by chemotherapy and ATRA plus chemotherapy and the role of maintenance therapy in newly diagnosed acute promyelocytic leukemia. *Blood* 1999;94:1192.
232. Lo Coco F, Diverio D, Avvisati G, et al. Therapy of molecular relapse in acute promyelocytic leukemia. *Blood* 1999;94:2225.
233. Soignet S, Maslak P, Wang Z-G, et al. Complete remission after treatment of acute promyelocytic leukemia with arsenic trioxide. *N Engl J Med* 1998;339:1341.
234. Meloni G, Diverio D, Vignetti M, et al. Autologous bone marrow transplantation for acute promyelocytic leukemia in second remission: prognostic relevance of pretransplant minimal residual disease by reverse-transcription polymerase chain reaction of the PML/α fusion gene. *Blood* 1997;90:1321.
235. Rivera GK, Pinkel D, Simone JV, Hancock ML, Crist WM. Treatment of acute lymphoblastic leukemia: 30 years' experience at St. Jude Children's Research Hospital. *N Engl J Med* 1993;329:1289.
236. Hoelzer D. Acute lymphoblastic leukemia-progress in children, less in adults. *N Engl J Med* 1993;329:1343.
237. Hoelzer D, Thiel E, Löffler H, et al. Prognostic factors in a multicenter study for treatment of acute lymphoblastic leukemia in adults. *Blood* 1988;71:123.
238. Gaynor J, Chapman D, Little C, et al. A cause-specific hazard rate analysis of prognostic factors among 199 adults with acute lymphoblastic leukemia: the Memorial Hospital experience since 1969. *J Clin Oncol* 1988;6:1014.
239. Boucheix C, David B, Sebban C, et al. Immunophenotype of adult acute lymphoblastic leukemia, clinical parameters and outcome: an analysis of a prospective trial including 562 tested patients (LALA87). *Blood* 1994;84:1603.
240. Barrett AJ, Horowitz MM, Ash RC, et al. Bone marrow transplantation for Philadelphia chromosome-positive acute lymphoblastic leukemia. *Blood* 1992;79:3067.
241. Watkins CH, Hall BE. Monocytic leukemia of the Naegeli and Schilling types. *Am J Clin Pathol* 1940;10:387.
242. Fiere D, Extra JM, David B, et al. Treatment of 218 adult acute lymphoblastic leukemias. *Semin Oncol* 1987;14:64.
243. Hoelzer D, Thiel E, Löffler H, et al. Intensified therapy in acute lymphoblastic and acute undifferentiated leukemia in adults. *Blood* 1984;64:38.
244. Kantarjian HM, Walters RS, Keating MJ, et al. Results of the vincristine, doxorubicin, and dexamethasone regimen in adults with standard-and high-risk acute lymphocytic leukemia. *J Clin Oncol* 1990;8:994.
245. Larson RA, Dodge RK, Burns CP, et al. A five-drug remission induction regimen with intensive consolidation for adults with acute lymphoblastic leukemia: cancer and leukemia group B study 8811. *Blood* 1995;85:2025.
246. Linker CA, Levitt LJ, O'Donnell M, Forman SJ, Ries CA. Treatment of adult acute lymphoblastic leukemia with intensive cyclical chemotherapy: a follow-up report. *Blood* 1991;78:2814.
247. Stewart K, Keating A, Sutton D, et al. Adult acute lymphoblastic leukaemia: the value of therapy intensification. *Leukemia Lymphoma* 1991;4:103.
248. Hussein KK, Dahlberg D, Head D, et al. Treatment of acute ly/mphoblastic leukemia in adults with intensive induction, consolidation, and maintenance chemotherapy. *Blood* 1989;73:57.
249. Schauer P, Arlin ZA, Mertelsmann R, et al. Treatment of acute lymphoblastic leukemia in adults: results of the L-10 and L-10M protocols. *J Clin Oncol* 1983;1:462.
250. Gottlieb AJ, Weinbert V, Ellison RR, et al. Efficacy of daunorubicin in the therapy of adult acute lymphocytic leukemia: a prospective randomized trial by Cancer and Leukemia Group B. *Blood* 1984;64:267.
251. Preti A, Kantarjian HM. Management of adult acute lymphocytic leukemia: present issues and key challenges. *J Clin Oncol* 1994;12:1312.
252. Ellison RR, Mick R, Cuttner J, et al. The effects of postinduction intensification treatment with cytarabine and daunorubicin in adult acute lymphocytic leukemia: a prospective randomized clinical trial by Cancer Leukemia Group B. *J Clin Oncol* 1991;9:2002.
253. Cassileth PA, Anderson JW, Bennett JM, et al. Adult acute lymphocytic leukemia: the Eastern Cooperative Oncology Group experience. *Leukemia* 1992;6:178.
254. Cuttner J, Mick R, Budman DR, et al. Phase III trial of brief intensive treatment of adult acute lymphoblastic leukemia comparing daunorubicin and mitoxantrone-A CALGB study. *Leukemia* 1991;5:425.
255. Inati A, Sallan SE, Cassady JR, et al. Efficacy and morbidity of central nervous system "prophylaxis" in childhood acute lymphoblastic leukemia: eight years' experience with cranial irradiation and intrathecal methotrexate. *Blood* 1983;61:297.
256. Omura GA, Moffitt S, Vogler WR, Salter MM. Combination chemotherapy of adult acute lymphoblastic leukemia with randomized central nervous system prophylaxis. *Blood* 1980;55:199.
257. Ohno R. Current progress in the treatment of adult acute leukemia in Japan. *Jpn J Clin Oncol* 1993;22:85.
258. Weiss M, Maslak P, Feldman E, et al. Cytarabine with high dose mitoxantrone induces rapid complete remissions in adult acute lymphoblastic leukemia (ALL) without the use of vincristine or prednisone. *J Clin Oncol* 1996;148:2480.
259. Capizzi RL, Poole M, Cooper MR, et al. Treatment of poor risk acute leukemia with sequential high-dose Ara-C and asparaginase. *Blood* 1984;63:694.
260. Amadori S, Papa G, Avvisati G, et al. Sequential combination high-dose Ara-C and asparaginase for the treatment of advanced acute leukemia and lymphoma. *Leuk Res* 1984;8:729.
261. Wells RJ, Feusner J, Devney R, et al. Sequential high dose cytosine arabinoside-asparaginase treatment in advance childhood leukemia. *J Clin Oncol* 1985;3:998.
262. Ishii E, Mara T, Ohkubo K, et al. Treatment of childhood acute lymphoblastic leukemia with intermediate-dose cytosine arabinoside and adriamycin. *Med Pediatr Oncol* 1986;14:73.
263. Giona F, Testi A, Amadori G, et al. Idarubicin and high-dose cytarabine in the treatment of refractory and relapsed acute lymphoblastic leukemia. *Ann Oncol* 1990;1:51.
264. Tan C, Steinherz P, Meyers P. Idarubicin in combination with high-dose cytosine arabinoside in patients with acute leukemia in relapse. *Proc Annu Meet Am Assoc Cancer Res* 1990;31:A1133(abst).
265. Hiddemann W, Kreutzman H, Straif K, et al. High-dose cytosine arabinoside in combination with mitoxantrone for the treatment of refractory acute myeloid and lymphoblastic leukemia. *Semin Oncol* 1987;14:73.
266. Leclerc J, Rivard G, Blanch M, et al. The association of once a day high-dose Ara-C followed by mitoxantrone for three days induces a high rate of complete remission in children with poor prognosis acute leukemia. *Blood* 1988;72(Suppl):210(abst).
267. Kantarjian H, Walters R, Keating M, et al. Mitoxantrone and high dose cytosine arabinoside for the treatment of refractory acute lymphocytic leukemia. *Cancer* 1990;65:5.
268. Feldman EJ, Alberts DS, Arlin Z, et al. Phase I clinical and pharmacokinetic evaluation of high-dose mitoxantrone in combination with cytarabine in patients with acute leukemia. *J Clin Oncol* 1993;11:2002.
269. Doney K, Fisher LD, Appelbaum FR, et al. Treatment of adult acute lymphoblastic leukemia with allogeneic bone marrow transplantation. Multivariate analysis of factors affecting acute graft-versus-host disease, relapse, and relapse-free survival. *Bone Marrow Transplant* 1991;7:453.
270. Gale RP, Horowitz MM, Ash RC, et al. Identical-twin bone marrow transplants for leukemia. *Ann Intern Med* 1994;120:646.
271. Weisdorf DJ, Woods WG, Nesbit ME Jr, et al. Allogeneic bone marrow transplantation for acute lymphoblastic leukaemia: risk factors and clinical outcome. *Br J Haematol* 1994;86:62.
272. Sebban C, Lepage E, Vernant J-P, et al. Allogeneic bone marrow transplantation in adult acute lymphoblastic leukemia in first complete remission: a comparative study. *J Clin Oncol* 1994;12:2580.
273. Zhang M-J, Hoelzer D, Horowitz MM, et al. Long-term follow-up of adults with acute lymphoblastic leukemia in first remission treated with chemotherapy or bone marrow transplantation. *Ann Intern Med* 1995;123:428.
274. Attal M, Blaise D, Marit G, et al. Consolidation treatment of adult acute lymphoblastic leukemia: a prospective, randomized trial comparing allogeneic versus autologous bone marrow transplantation and testing the impact of recombinant interleukin-2 after autologous bone marrow transplant. *Blood* 1995;86:1619.
275. Fière D, Lepage E, Sebban C, et al. Adult acute lymphoblastic leukemia: a multicentric randomized trial testing bone marrow transplantation as postremission therapy. *J Clin Oncol* 1993;11:1990.
276. Soussain C, Patte C, Ostronoff M, et al. Small noncleaved cell lymphoma and leukemia in adults. A retrospective study of 65 adults treated with the LMB pediatric protocols. *Blood* 1995;85:664.
277. Tallman MS, Hakimian D, Shaw K, et al. Granulocytic sarcoma is associated with the 8;21 translocation in acute myeloid leukemia. *J Clin Oncol* 1993;11:690.
278. Byrd JC, Edenfield WJ, Shields DJ, Dawson NA. Extramedullary myeloid cell tumors in acute nonlymphocytic leukemia: a clinical review. *J Clin Oncol* 1995;13:1800.
279. Byrd JC, Weiss RB, Arthur DC, et al. Extramedullary leukemia adversely affects hematologic complete remission rate and overall survival in patients with t(8;21) (q22;q22): Results from Cancer and Leukemia Group B 8461. *Blood* 1999;93:2143.

280. Baer MR, Barcos M, Farrell H, et al. Acute myelogenous leukemia with leukemia cutis. *Cancer* 1989;63:2192.
281. Cassileth PA, Sylvester LS, Bennett JM, Begg CB. High peripheral blast counts in adult acute myelogenous leukemia is a primary risk factor for CNS leukemia. *J Clin Oncol* 1988;6:495.
282. Holmes R, Keating MJ, Cork A. A unique pattern of central nervous system leukemia in acute myelomonocytic leukemia associated with inv(16) (p13q22). *Blood* 1985;6:495.
283. Brinch L, Evensen SA, Stavem P. Leukemia in the central nervous system. *J Intern Med* 1988;224:173.
284. McKee LC Jr, Collins RD. Intravascular leucocyte thrombi and aggregates as a course of morbidity and mortality in leukemia. *Medicine* 1974;52:463.
285. Schiffer CA. Interferon studies in the treatment of patients with leukemia. *Semin Oncol* 1995;18:1.
286. Caron PC, Scheinberg DA. Immunotherapy for acute leukemias. *Curr Opin Oncol* 1994;6:14.
287. Jurcic J, Scheinberg DA. Recent developments in the radioimmunotherapy of cancer. *Curr Opin Immunol* 1994;6:715.
288. Meyers JD, Flournoy N, Sanders JE, et al. Prophylactic use of human leukocyte interferon after allogeneic marrow transplantation. *Ann Intern Med* 1987;107:809.
289. Ochs J, Brecher ML, Mahoney D, et al. Recombinant interferon-α given before and in combination with standard chemotherapy in children with acute lymphoblastic leukemia in the first marrow relapse: a Pediatric Oncology Group (POG) pilot study. *J Clin Oncol* 1991;9:777.
290. Lotzová E, Savary CA, Herberman RB. Induction of NK cell activity against fresh human leukemia in culture with interleukin 2. *J Immunol* 1987;138:2718.
291. Foa R. Does interleukin-2 have a role in the management of acute leukemia? *J Clin Oncol* 1993;11:1817.
292. Soiffer RJ, Murray C, Gonin R, Ritz J. Effect of low-dose interleukin-2 on disease relapse after T-cell-depleted allogeneic bone marrow transplantation. *Blood* 1994;84:964.
293. Foa R, Meloni G, Tosti S, et al. Treatment of acute myeloid leukaemia patients with recombinant interleukin 2: a pilot study. *Br J Haematol* 1991;77:491.
294. Meloni G, Foa R, Vignetti M, et al. Interleukin-2 may induce prolonged remissions in advanced acute myelogenous leukemia. *Blood* 1994;84:2158.
295. Benyunes MC, Massumoto AY, Higuchi CM, et al. Interleukin-2 with or without lymphokine-activated killer cells as consolidative immunotherapy after autologous bone marrow transplantation for acute myelogenous leukemia. *Bone Marrow Transplant* 1993;12:159.
296. Caron PC, Lai LT, Scheinberg DA. Interleukin-2 enhancement of cytotoxicity by humanized monoclonal antibody M195 (anti-CD33) in myelogenous leukemia. *Clin Cancer Res* 1995;1:63.
297. Kossman SE, Scheinberg DA, Jurcic JB, Jimenez J, Caron PC. A phase I trial of humanized monoclonal antibody HuM195 (anti-CD33) with low dose Interleukin-2 (IL-2) in acute myelogenous leukemia. *Clin CA Res* 1999;5:2748.
298. Grossbard ML, Press OW, Appelbaum FR, Bernstein ID, Nadler LM. Monoclonal antibody-based therapies of leukemia and lymphoma. *Blood* 1992;80:863.
299. Caron PC, Jurcic JG, Scott AM, et al. A phase IB trial of humanized monoclonal antibody M195 (anti-CD33) in myeloid leukemia: specific targeting without immunogenicity. *Blood* 1994;83:1760.
300. Caron PC, Dumont L, Scheinberg DA. Super-saturating infusional humanized anti-CD33 monoclonal antibody HuM195 in myelogenous leukemia. *Clin CA Res* 1998;4:1421.
301. Jurcic J, DeBlasio T, Dumont L, Yao TJ, Scheinberg DA. Molecular remission induction without relapse and after anti-CD33 antibody in APL. Submitted 1998.
302. Sievers EL, Appelbaum FR, Spielberger RT, et al. Selective ablation of acute myeloid leukemia using antibody-targeted chemotherapy: a phase I study of an anti-CD33 calicheamicin immunoconjugate. *Blood* 1999;93:3678.
303. Jurcic JG, McDevitt MR, Sgouros G, et al. Phase I trial of targeted alpha-particle therapy for myeloid leukemias with bismuth-213-HuM195 (anti CD33). *Proc Am Soc Clin Oncol* 1999;18:7a(abst).
304. Matthews DC, Appelbaum FR, Eary JF, et al. Development of a marrow transplant regimen for acute leukemia using targeted hematopoietic irradiation delivered by ^{131}I-labeled anti-CD45 antibody combined with cyclophosphamide and total body irradiation. *Blood* 1995;85:1122.
305. Schwartz MA, Lovett DR, Redner A, et al. A dose-escalation trial of M195 labeled with iodine 131 for cytoreduction and marrow ablation in relapsed or refractory myeloid leukemias. *J Clin Oncol* 1993;11:294.
306. Jurcic JG, Divgi CR, McDevitt MR, et al. Potential for myeloablation with yttrium-90-labeled HuM195 (anti-CD33): a phase I trial in advance myeloid leukemias. *Blood* 1998;92(Suppl):613a(abst).
307. Selvaggi KJ, Wilson JW, Mills LE, et al. Improved outcome for high-risk acute myeloid leukemia patients using autologous bone marrow transplantation and monoclonal antibody-purged bone marrow. *Blood* 1994;83:1698.
308. Pinilla-Ibarz J, Cathcart K, Korontsvit T, et al. Vaccination of patients with chronic myelogenous leukemia with bcr-abl oncogene breakpoint fusion peptides generates specific immune responses. *Blood* 2000;95:1781.

SECTION **3**

Chronic Leukemias

HAGOP M. KANTARJIAN
STEFAN FADERL
MOSHE TALPAZ

Chronic Myelogenous Leukemia

Chronic myelogenous leukemia (CML) is a clonal myeloproliferative disorder of a pluripotent hematopoietic progenitor cell. It is characterized by excessive proliferation of marrow granulocytes, erythroid precursors, megakaryocytes, and connective tissue–forming cells. Clonal proliferation and transformation of myeloid progenitor cells usually dominate the clinical picture. The CML cells harbor a distinctive cytogenetic abnormality, the Philadelphia chromosome (Ph). It results from a translocation between the long arms of chromosomes 9 and 22. Segments of the *ABL* gene on chromosome 9 are fused to segments of *BCR* on chromosome 22. The *BCR-ABL* fusion genes are translated into chimeric proteins with increased tyrosine kinase activity such as p210. Downstream signaling events, which heavily involve ras pathways, eventually activate genes responsible for the uncontrolled proliferation of the leukemic clone.

CML is divided into three clinical phases. The benign or chronic phase may last for a few years. Transformation through an accelerated phase into a blastic phase typically follows. Whereas outcome in the transformed phases is still unsatisfactory, advances in stem cell transplantation (SCT), interferon-based therapies, and supportive care have had a major effect on prognosis in chronic phase disease. Novel treatments based on immunomodulation and our increasing understanding of signal transduction pathways in the leukemic cells have generated new targets for therapy that are currently being investigated in clinical trials.

Current state-of-the-art therapies result in increasing numbers of patients who achieve complete cytogenetic remissions. However, highly sensitive molecular assays such as fluorescence *in situ* hybridization (FISH) or polymerase chain reaction (PCR) frequently detect *BCR-ABL* rearrangements in these patients. In many cases, these patients stay in remission for many years, raising the question of the significance of *molecular cures* versus *functional cures* and the mechanisms that sustain these remissions. Thus, CML has not only become a paradigm for our understanding of leukemogenesis and targeted drug development, but is also an ideal model for the study of minimal residual disease in hematologic malignancies.

EPIDEMIOLOGY

Some 4000 to 5000 patients are diagnosed with CML in the United States annually. The incidence of CML is 1 to 2 per 100,000 population with a male to female ratio of 1.4 to 2.2:1.0. CML accounts for 7% to 15% of leukemias among adults. The median age at presentation is between 45 and 55 years. One-third of the patients are older than 60 years.[1] This incidence used to be higher in earlier studies and the more recently reported decrease may be a consequence of earlier detection, referral of younger patients to large centers, and exclusion of patients with CML-like conditions such as chronic myelomonocytic leukemia, Ph-negative CML, or other myeloproliferative disorders. Nevertheless, the proportion of patients over age 60 is important when considering therapeutic options such as allogeneic SCT, which is associated with a high treatment-related mortality, or interferon-α (IFN-α), which has more side effects in older patients. CML is uncommon in children and adolescents in whom it accounts for less than 5% of the leukemias.

ETIOLOGY AND PATHOGENESIS

ETIOLOGY

The etiology of CML is unknown. There is little evidence for genetic factors linked to CML. Lack of concordance in monozygotic twins and the demonstration of Ph in hematopoietic progenitor cells only, suggest that CML is an acquired disorder.[2] Offspring of parents with CML do not have a higher incidence of CML than the general population. The incidence of CML is higher among survivors of the atomic bomb explosions in Hiroshima and Nagasaki.[3] Effects of therapeutic doses of radiation on the development of CML are disputed. No association has been established with infectious agents.

MOLECULAR PATHOGENESIS

More than 90% of patients with the clinical picture of CML demonstrate Ph in 95% to 100% of marrow cell metaphases. Through a reciprocal translocation between the long arms of chromosomes 9 and 22, a large 3' segment of the *ABL* gene on chromosome 9q34 is fused to a 5' segment of the *BCR* gene on chromosome 22q11, creating a hybrid *BCR-ABL* gene on 22q11 and, in two-thirds of patients, a reciprocal *ABL-BCR* gene on chromosome 9q+.[4,5] In most cases, *ABL* exons 2 to 11 (also referred to as *a2 to a11*) are transposed into the major breakpoint cluster region (M-bcr) of *BCR* between exons 13 or 14 (also called *b2 or b3*). The *BCR-ABL* fusion mRNA extends over 8.5 kb and contains a b2a2 or b3a2 junction. It is translated into a chimeric protein of 210 kD called p210.[6,7] In most cases, CML cells express either b2a2 or b3a2 transcripts, but in approximately 5% alternative splicing causes expression of both forms. No significant difference exists with respect to response to treatment, prognosis, or clinical features, except for a higher platelet count in patients with b3a2 transcripts.[8,9]

In rare cases of CML, but in 50% of adults and up to 80% of children with Ph-positive acute lymphoblastic leukemia, the breakpoint on chromosome 22 is located centromeric to M-bcr between exons e1 and e2 referred to as the minor breakpoint cluster region (m-bcr). The e1a2 fusion gene is translated into a protein of 190 kD termed p190.[10] A third breakpoint location occurs telomeric from M-bcr, creating a fusion transcript with an e19a2 junction and a protein of 230 kD termed p230 (Fig. 46.3.1-1).[11] Expression of p190 in CML has been associated with monocytosis, and of p230 with the chronic neutrophilic leukemia variant and with thrombocytosis.[12]

In approximately two-thirds of cases, the reciprocal *ABL-BCR* rearrangement can be detected on the derivative chromosome 9q+. The 5' remnant of *ABL* exon 1 is transposed to the 3' tail of *BCR* exons 14 or 15 (b3 or b4). No pathogenetic role in CML has been documented for this rearrangement.[13]

Both *in vitro* and *in vivo* animal experiments using transgenic mice and retrovirus-mediated gene transfer into murine hematopoietic cells have demonstrated that expression of *BCR-ABL* can imitate the clinical manifestations of CML, including the progression from chronic to blastic phase. Thus, the combined data from animal experiments support the role of *BCR-ABL* and its fusion proteins as central mediators of myeloid proliferation and transformation in CML.[14]

Whereas *ABL* encodes a nonreceptor tyrosine kinase (p145) whose activity is rigorously controlled and which is involved in signal transduction and regulation of cell growth, p210 and p190 show increased and uncontrolled kinase activity. Constitu-

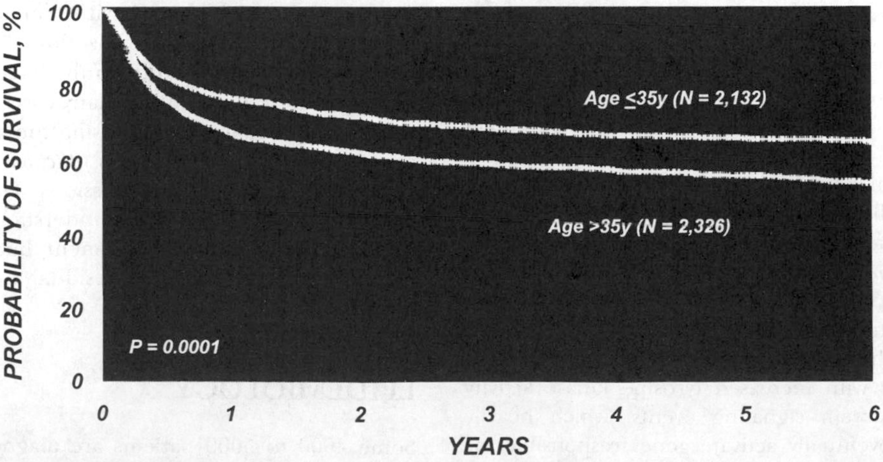

FIGURE 46.3.1-1. Probability of survival after human leukocyte antigen–identical sibling stem cell transplantation for chronic myelogenous leukemia in chronic phase by age, 1991 through 1997. (International Bone Marrow Transplant Registry data, with permission.)

tive activation of the kinases initiates downstream signaling pathways that up-regulate transcription of genes mediating proliferation and transformation of CML hematopoietic progenitor cells. A central element of BCR-ABL signaling is Ras. Activation of Ras is mediated through a series of adapter proteins that in turn also connect p210 to other kinases and signal transduction systems.[7,15]

CELLULAR PATHOGENESIS

CML is dominated by expansion of myeloid progenitor cells at various stages of maturation, their premature release into the circulation, and their tendency to home to extramedullary sites. Clonal expansion may also involve the erythroid, megakaryocytic, and B- as well as occasionally T-lymphoid lineages. The disorderly expansion of leukemic progenitors in chronic phase may reflect both alterations in their proliferative activity and shifts in the balance of self-renewal and differentiation. Although Ph-positive primitive hematopoietic cells (long-term culture-initiating cells) are found in lower frequencies than are colonies of normal progenitor cells and have a longer generation time, they may undergo additional cell divisions.[16] Leukemic progenitor mass is also increased by altered regulation at the stem cell level, shifting the balance between self-renewal and differentiation toward the differentiating cell pool, a process that has been referred to as *discordant maturation.*[17] Stem cells become part of the proliferating compartment, causing the neoplastic population to expand exponentially in later maturational compartments. At this stage, leukemic progenitor cells may also be less responsive to growth regulatory signals from either cytokines or the bone marrow microenvironment.[16–18] Defective adherence of CML progenitors to bone marrow stromal elements further facilitates their premature release into the peripheral blood.[19] Although differentiation remains relatively unaffected during chronic phase disease, transforming events in accelerated and blastic phase substantially deregulate the delicate balance between normal and leukemic progenitor colonies, leading to maturation arrest similar to events observed in acute leukemias.

DIAGNOSIS AND CLINICAL COURSE

CLINICAL MANIFESTATIONS

CML is a triphasic disease (Table 46.3.1-1). At diagnosis, more than 90% of patients are in chronic phase. Symptoms at presentation reflect the increase in mass and turnover of the CML hematopoietic progenitor cells. Patients may complain of lethargy and weakness, night sweats, and weight loss. Increase in abdominal girth and abdominal discomfort may be due to an enlarged spleen. Less frequently, easy bruisability and bleeding are recorded due to platelet dysfunction. Ten percent to 20% of patients from older series and as many as one-half of patients in more recent studies have no symptoms and are diagnosed by routine blood tests. Presentations in accelerated or blastic phases occur in 5% to 10%. Splenomegaly occurs in up to 50% and is the most common finding on physical examination. Generalized lymphadenopathy and fever, rare in chronic phase, may indicate an accelerated disease course.[20,21]

LABORATORY TESTS

Peripheral Blood and Bone Marrow

Myeloid hyperplasia in the marrow associated with neutrophilic leukocytosis, thrombocytosis, and basophilia in the peripheral blood are typical chronic phase CML laboratory features. Peripheral blood leukocytosis exceeding 100×10^9/L occurs in 70% to 90% of patients. Anemia of varying degrees is frequent. The marrow is markedly hypercellular with a myeloid to erythroid ratio between 9:1 to 15:1. Myeloid cells display all stages of maturation, with a preponderance of myelocytes and promyelocytes. Megakaryocytes are frequently increased, especially in accelerated phase. Marrow fibrosis is focal in early dis-

TABLE 46.3.1-1. Phases of Chronic Myelogenous Leukemia

Chronic Phase	*Accelerated Phase*	*Blastic Phase*
No symptoms (if treated) None of the characteristics of accelerated or blastic phase	M. D. Anderson Peripheral blood blasts ≥15% Peripheral blood blasts and promyelocytes ≥30% Peripheral blood basophils ≥20% Platelet count <100 × 10^9/L unrelated to therapy Cytogenetic evolution IBMTR WBC count "difficult to control" with use of busulfan or hydroxyurea Rapid doubling time of WBC (<5 days) ≥10% blasts in peripheral blood/marrow ≥20% blasts and promyelocytes in peripheral blood/bone marrow ≥20% basophils and eosinophils in peripheral blood Anemia or thrombocytopenia unresponsive to busulfan or hydroxyurea Persistent thrombocytosis Clonal evolution Progressive splenomegaly and myelofibrosis	≥30% blasts in blood, marrow, or both Extramedullary infiltrates of leukemic cells Blastic phase is lymphoid in one-third of patients (TdT+, CD10+, CD19+, CD20+, frequent coexpression of myeloid markers), and myeloblastic or undifferentiated in two-thirds of patients

IBMTR, International Bone Marrow Transplant Registry; WBC, white blood cell.

ease stages and may progress to a more diffuse pattern with disease evolution.[22]

Cytogenetic Analysis

Cytogenetic analysis is the gold standard for demonstration of the Ph translocation and other abnormalities that occur frequently with disease progression (clonal evolution).[23] Cytogenetic analysis is tedious and time-consuming, and only 20 to 25 metaphases per sample are examined. In approximately 10% of patients with CML, no t(9;22) is detected by cytogenetic analysis. However, in up to one-third of these patients, molecular studies detect *BCR-ABL* rearrangements. The remaining patients are Ph and *BCR-ABL* negative. These patients carry a worse prognosis and have to be distinguished from typical CML (Table 46.3.1-2).[24]

Molecular Analysis

Molecular assays are used in the diagnosis of CML and the assessment of response to therapeutic modalities. PCR, Southern and Northern blot, and immunoprecipitation can determine the exact breakpoints of the fusion genes, detect *BCR-ABL* transcripts at the RNA level, and demonstrate the p210 protein using antibodies against the N-terminal region of BCR and the C-terminal region of ABL.

Patients on therapy are frequently monitored by PCR and FISH.[25] FISH allows analysis of metaphase and nondividing interphase cells and is easily quantifiable. Interphase FISH can be performed on peripheral blood specimens.[26] However, it overestimates the degree of cytogenetic responses at high Ph-positive percent values and has a false-positive rate of up to 10%. Hypermetaphase FISH is as time efficient as interphase FISH, does not generate false-positive results, but cannot be done on peripheral blood samples.[27] The use of double color probes for FISH is being investigated and may have superior sensitivity and specificity.[28]

PROGRESSION OF CHRONIC MYELOID LEUKEMIA

When treated with chemotherapeutic agents such as hydroxyurea or busulfan, CML invariably progresses into an accelerated phase that is followed after 3 to 18 months by a blastic transformation. Criteria for the definition of accelerated and blastic phase disease have been proposed (see Table 46.3.1-1).[29,30]

Whereas Ph predominates throughout chronic phase, up to 80% of patients develop additional cytogenetic abnormalities when they progress (clonal evolution). Common changes during clonal evolution of CML are trisomy 8, isochromosome i(17q), trisomy 19, and an additional Ph. Trisomy 8 and isochromosome i(17q) are common during myeloid transformation.[23] Alterations of molecular markers during clonal evolution include *p53, RB1, c-MYC, p16, Ras,* and AML/EVI-1, a fusion protein resulting from translocation t(3;21)(q26;q22). Abnormalities of *p53* occur in 20% to 30% of patients and are mainly associated with myeloid transformation.[31,32] Loss of function of *p53* has been associated with suppression of apoptosis and progression into blastic phase. Abnormalities of *RB1* have been associated with lymphoid transformation.

TREATMENT

Criteria for assignment of response to therapies are summarized in Table 46.3.1-3. A number of poor prognostic features

TABLE 46.3.1-2. Differential Diagnosis of Philadelphia Chromosome and *BCR-ABL*–Negative Chronic Myelogenous Leukemia

Condition	*Characteristics*
Leukemoid reaction	Total white blood cell count rarely >100 × 10^9/L Left shift on peripheral blood differential does not usually involve promyelocytes/myelocytes Absence of basophilia Cytoplasmic inclusions (toxic granulation, Döhle bodies) Absence of basophilia Usually elevated leukocyte alkaline phosphatase Usually underlying etiology (infection, shock, hemolysis, chronic inflammation, other underlying malignancy)
Other myeloproliferative disorders (myelofibrosis, polycythemia vera)	Lesser degree of leukocytosis Larger spleen Leukoerythroblastic peripheral blood smear (tear drop cells) Established criteria for diagnosis
Atypical chronic myelogenous leukemia	Dysplastic changes in leukocytes of peripheral blood/bone marrow No basophilia
Chronic neutrophilic leukemia	Leukocytosis usually consisting of mature neutrophils Splenomegaly High leukocyte alkaline phosphatase
Chronic myelomonocytic leukemia, myeloproliferative	Increase in absolute and relative monocyte counts Minimal dysplastic changes in leukocytes No basophilia Immature cells of neutrophil series present
Juvenile chronic myeloid leukemia	Disease of children <4 years old Hepatomegaly and splenomegaly common at presentation Markedly increased fetal hemoglobin levels

TABLE 46.3.1-3. Criteria for Cytogenetic and Hematologic Remissions in Chronic Myelogenous Leukemia

Response	*Parameters*
Complete hematologic response	Complete normalization of peripheral counts (WBC <10 × 10^9/L, platelets <450 × 10^9/L, no immature cells like blasts, promyelocytes, metamyelocytes) No signs and symptoms of disease, disappearance of palpable splenomegaly
Cytogenetic response (in patients in complete hematologic response)	
Complete	No Ph-positive cells (major)
Partial	1–34% Ph-positive cells (major)
Minor	35–90% Ph-positive cells
Partial hematologic response	As for complete hematologic response, except for (1) persistence of immature cells, or (2) platelets <50% pretreatment level but >450 × 10^9/L, or (3) persistent splenomegaly but >50% of pretreatment

Ph, Philadelphia chromosome.
(Adapted from ref. 33.)

have been identified, and prognostic systems have been developed in CML (Table 46.3.1-4). These systems allow patients to be categorized into good-, intermediate-, and poor-risk groups with respective median survivals of 6, 3 to 4, and 2 years in patients receiving conventional therapy. These models are useful in evaluating the effect of new strategies within different risk groups (see Table 46.3.1-4).

HISTORICAL AND CONVENTIONAL TREATMENTS FOR CHRONIC MYELOGENOUS LEUKEMIA

The median survival of patients with CML used to be 3 years, and less than 20% of patients were alive 5 years after diagnosis. Nowadays, patients in chronic phase can expect a median survival time of 5 to 7 years, and up to 9 years in good-prognosis patients. Five and 10-year survival rates are 60% to 70% and 30% to 40%, respectively. Earlier diagnosis, better supportive care, and more effective anti-CML therapies account mostly for this change.[33]

The use of arsenicals (Fowler's solution) was first advocated for the treatment of CML in 1856. In the early 1900s up to approximately 1950, total body or splenic radiation therapy was shown to be effective in controlling the signs and symptoms of CML. Its benefit was, however, short-lived and the overall survival was not affected significantly. It is a rarely used modality today.

In the early 1950s, oral alkylating agents such as busulfan became the new mainstay of treatment.[35] Busulfan is inexpensive and allows long periods of hematologic control, but may be associated with serious side effects such as delayed myelosuppression and pulmonary toxicities (Table 46.3.1-5). Busulfan was replaced by hydroxyurea in the 1970s.[36] Hydroxyurea is a cell-cycle–specific inhibitor of DNA synthesis that allows rapid hematologic control and is well tolerated (see Table 46.3.1-5).

TABLE 46.3.1-4. Prognostic Models in Chronic Myelogenous Leukemia

	Sokal Model	*Synthesis Model*
Characteristics	Age Platelet count Spleen size Percentage blood blasts	Poor-prognosis characteristics Age ≥60 years Spleen ≥10 cm below costal margin Blasts ≥3% in blood or marrow Basophils ≥7% in blood or ≥3% in marrow Platelets ≥700 × 10^9/L Accelerated-phase characteristics Clonal evolution Blood blasts ≥15% Blood blasts and promyelocytes ≥30% Blood basophils ≥20% Platelets <100 × 10^9/L
Risk group[a]	Low risk (<0.8) Intermediate risk (0.8–1.2) High risk (>1.2)	1: 0 to 1 poor-prognosis criteria 2: 2 poor-prognosis criteria 3: ≥3 poor-prognosis criteria 4: ≥1 Accelerated-phase criteria (regardless of number of poor-prognosis criteria)

[a]Risk is based on hazard ratio values in Sokal's model[34] and on summation of poor-prognosis factors in synthesis model.[21]

TABLE 46.3.1-5. Dosage and Side Effects of Hydroxyurea and Busulfan in the Management of Patients with Chronic Myelogenous Leukemia

Drug	*Dosage*		*Side Effects*
Busulfan	0.1 mg/kg PO daily until WBC count decreases by 50%, then reduce dose by 50%; maintain WBC between 20 and 50 × 10^9/L		Severe, prolonged myelosuppression (10%); idiosyncratic pulmonary fibrosis (busulfan lung); fibrosis of the endocardium; Addison's disease–like syndrome
Hydroxyurea	WBC count (×10^9/L)	Hydroxyurea (g)	Nausea and vomiting; skin changes (scaling, atrophy, alopecia, ulcerations)
	>100	5–7	
	80–100	4–5	
	50–80	3–4	
	30–50	2–3	
	20–30	1.5–2.0	
	10–20	1.0–1.5	
	5–10	0.5–1.0	
	Maintain WBC between 2 and 10 × 10^9/L		

WBC, white blood cell.

Both hydroxyurea and busulfan cause complete hematologic remissions in up to 80% of patients. Cytogenetic remissions occur, but are rare, and neither agent has any notable effect on the natural course of the disease. In a large randomized study, both median survival (56 vs. 44 months) and median duration of chronic phase (47 vs. 37 months) were significantly longer in patients treated with hydroxyurea compared with busulfan.[37] Busulfan therapy before allogeneic SCT has also an adverse outcome on posttransplant survival (3-year disease-free survival of 61% for patients treated with hydroxyurea vs. 45% for patients on busulfan).[38]

While other agents (dibromomannitol, melphalan, 6-mercaptopurine, 6-thioguanine, cyclophosphamide, chlorambucil) have also been used in the treatment of CML, they have been associated with worse outcome. Uncontrolled thrombocytosis on therapy with hydroxyurea may respond to anagrelide, the addition of IFN-α, or intermittent therapy with thiotepa (75 mg/m² intravenously every 2 to 4 weeks).

Splenectomy may benefit occasional patients with persistent and symptomatic splenomegaly and refractory cytopenias. Splenectomy pretransplant reduces the time to marrow recovery, but does not influence long-term prognosis.[39]

STEM CELL TRANSPLANTATION

Matched Related Allogeneic Stem Cell Transplantation

SCT has become an effective treatment for CML and can cure a substantial proportion of carefully selected patients with suitable donors. In most studies of chronic phase CML, projected actuarial 3-year to 5-year survival rates range between 50% and 60%, with values up to 80% in large centers. Relapses occur in 15% to 30%, and plateau at 5 to 7 years after transplantation, suggesting a cure for some patients. Late relapses 10 to 12 years posttransplant can occur. Allogeneic SCT is limited by availability of matched siblings and age restrictions. Less than 30% of patients in Europe and North America receive SCT from matched sibling donors.[40]

Transplant-related mortality ranges between 10% and 40%, but can be as high as 68% in subgroups of patients who receive marrows from mismatched or unrelated donors. Several variables influence transplant outcome.[41]

AGE. Younger patients do best (see Fig. 46.3.1-1): Disease-free survival is from 60% to 70%, transplant-related mortality 10%, and probability of relapse 20%. Above age 20, patients appear to have a continuous and inverse relationship between age and survival. Older patients do worse mainly because of an increased treatment-related mortality in this age group; the relapse rates are similar. One center reported favorable outcomes for carefully selected patients above age 50: The 2-year estimated survival rate among 57 such patients was 80%.[42] Results from other transplant centers or registry studies are worse. In the International Bone Marrow Transplant Registry (IBMTR) studies, the 5-year survival rate for patients above age 50 was only 30%. In the European Bone Marrow Transplant Registry (EBMTR), patients over age 45 had a treatment-related mortality of 47% and a 5-year disease-free survival rate of 25%.[43,44]

PHASE OF DISEASE. The largest effect of treatment is achieved in the chronic phase of CML. Disease-free survival rates decrease from 40% to 60% in chronic phase to less than 15% in blastic phase (Fig. 46.3.1-2).[21,38] Transplantation in transformed CML phases is accompanied by increased rates of leukemia relapse and treatment-related mortality. Posttransplant outcome in accelerated phase is better when clonal evolution is the single criterion for disease acceleration: Disease-free survival up to 60% has been reported in these patients.[45] Timing of transplantation in chronic phase is more controversial. Based on earlier data, most centers propose transplantation in early chronic phase CML (i.e., within 1 year of diagnosis) (Fig. 46.3.1-3).[38] However, updates of these data suggest similar rates for 5-year disease-free survival for transplants performed within 12 to 24 months from diagnosis and a critical prognostic cut-off point at around 2 years from diagnosis is suggested.[44,46]

PRETRANSPLANT CHEMOTHERAPY. Anti-CML therapy before transplantation influences posttransplant outcome. Disease-

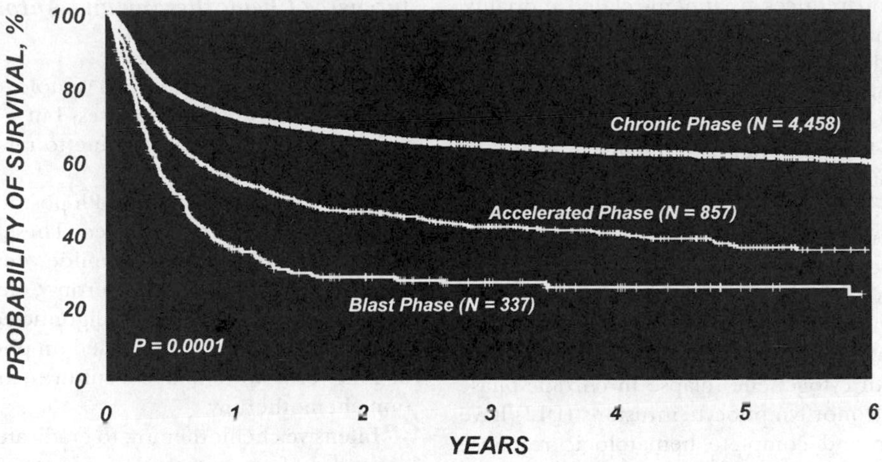

FIGURE 46.3.1-2. Probability of survival after human leukocyte antigen–identical sibling stem cell transplantation for chronic myelogenous leukemia by disease status pretransplant, 1991 through 1997. (International Bone Marrow Transplant Registry data, with permission.)

free survival at 5 years is significantly higher in chronic phase patients pretreated with hydroxyurea than with busulfan (61% vs. 45%). Prior therapy with IFN-α does not appear to affect outcome of matched related SCT. The influence of IFN-α on matched unrelated donor transplantation is more controversial.[47–50]

PREPARATIVE REGIMENS. Results are conflicting regarding the best preparative regimen. Virtually all regimens produce toxic effects, with severe mucositis of the gastrointestinal tract being most common. The combination of busulfan with cyclophosphamide appears as effective as the combination of cyclophosphamide with total body irradiation, except for the more unfavorable toxicity profile of the latter.[51]

GRAFT-VERSUS-HOST DISEASE PROPHYLAXIS. Acute graft-versus-host disease (GVHD) occurs in 8% to 63% of patients and is the cause of death in up to 13%.[38] The rates for chronic GVHD can be as high as 75% with a mortality of up to 10%. The use of methotrexate with cyclosporine has resulted in better outcomes than single methotrexate or methotrexate in other combinations.[52] T-cell depletion pretransplant

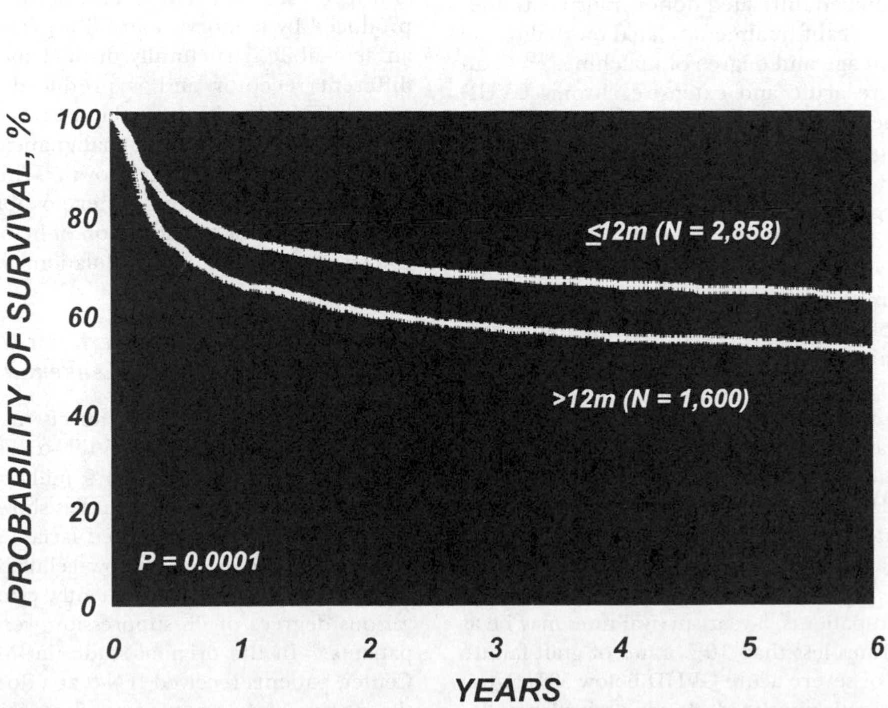

FIGURE 46.3.1-3. Probability of survival after human leukocyte antigen–identical sibling stem cell transplantation for chronic myelogenous leukemia in chronic phase by disease duration, 1991 through 1997. (International Bone Marrow Transplant Registry data, with permission.)

improves tolerance and reduces treatment-related mortality. However, this advantage is offset by increased leukemia relapse, indicating the importance of immune-mediated effects (e.g., graft-versus-leukemia effect) in maintaining remission in CML.[53,54]

The incidence of relapse posttransplant ranges from 10% to 70%. It is lowest in patients transplanted in chronic phase and highest in blastic phase.[55] Second transplants from human leukocyte antigen (HLA)-identical sibling donors can achieve disease-free survival rates up to 30%. Results, however, depend on the time interval between transplant and relapse and are most favorable in the setting of a long first remission duration.[56] IFN-α may induce long-lasting cytogenetic remissions in 20% to 40% of patients with cytogenetic relapse in chronic phase postallogeneic SCT.[57] Donor lymphocyte infusions (DLI) have generated cytogenetic and complete hematologic response rates in 60% to 80% of patients. Disease-free survival at 3 years is between 40% and 85%. Responses are considerably less frequent and short-lived in transformed CML phases. A strong correlation exists between development of GVHD and response to DLI, which supports a role for the graft-versus-leukemia activity generated by infused donor T lymphocytes. DLI toxicity can be substantial and includes myelosuppression and severe GVHD.[58]

Matched Unrelated Donor Transplants

It is possible to identify HLA-compatible unrelated donors for approximately half the patients who lack an HLA-matched sibling through the National Marrow Donor Program in the United States and similar transplant registries throughout the world. The median time from donor search to transplant is approximately 6 months. Although encouraging results have been obtained with matched unrelated donor transplants, they are associated with significant treatment-related morbidity and mortality depending on age and degree of matching.[59,60] Graft failure as well as severe acute and extensive chronic GVHD contribute to a treatment-related mortality above 50% in some groups of patients. Good-risk patients for matched unrelated donor transplants are younger (less than 30 years), in early chronic phase, cytomegalovirus seronegative, and have received non–T-cell–depleted marrow infusions.[60] Molecular matching is emerging as a highly significant parameter of treatment outcome. The EBMTR group analyzed the effect of HLA class II matching on results of matched unrelated donor transplants in 366 patients, two-thirds of whom had been transplanted in chronic phase.[61] Matching at the HLA-DRB1 locus was the most significant factor influencing overall survival, disease-free survival, and treatment-related mortality. Patients transplanted in first chronic phase, with non–T-cell–depleted marrows, and a matched HLA-DRB1 locus had a 2-year survival of 51%, a treatment-related mortality of 47%, and a relapse rate of 2%. Treatment-related mortality was 80% for HLA-DRB1 mismatches.

In carefully selected patients, 5-year survival rates may be as high as 70%, relapse rates less than 10%, rates of graft failure below 10%, and rates of severe acute GVHD below 50%. Until experience with matched unrelated donor transplants has matured, it should be offered preferentially to younger patients in chronic phase who are resistant to IFN-α and who have a fully matched donor available.[60]

Intensive Chemotherapy and Autologous Transplantation

Autografting with unpurged autologous marrow generates transient cytogenetic responses, but a survival advantage has not been proven.[62] Relapse due to reinfused, Ph-positive cells may occur.[63]

To reduce contaminating Ph-positive cells, several purging strategies have been developed. These include *in vitro* manipulations with cyclophosphamide derivatives and biologic response modifiers (interferon-γ, interleukin-2), tyrosine kinase inhibitors, antisense oligonucleotides, ribozymes, positive or negative selections based on phenotype determination or long-term bone marrow cultures, and high-dose combination chemotherapy.

Intensive chemotherapy, to eradicate Ph-positive clones, was patterned after acute leukemia programs. Cytogenetic remissions were induced in 60% to 70% of patients and were complete in 35% to 50%. However, the cytogenetic responses were brief and not improved by maintenance with IFN-α.[64] Intensive chemotherapy has been used preceding autologous SCT as a method for *in vivo* purging that allows collection of Ph-negative marrow and peripheral blood stem cells during early hematopoietic recovery.[65,66]

INTERFERON-α

IFNs are a complex group of naturally occurring proteins produced by eukaryotic cells in response to various stimuli. They have pleiotropic biologic activities including inhibition of cellular proliferation, regulation of cytokine expression, and modulation of the immune system. IFNs consist of three distinct groups of peptides: IFN-α, IFN-β, and IFN-γ. IFN-α and IFN-β are acid stable, bind to the same receptor, and are produced by leukocytes and fibroblasts, respectively. IFN-γ is an acid-labile, structurally distinct molecule that binds to a different receptor and is produced mainly by T lymphocytes.[67] IFN-α has been used most commonly in the treatment of solid and hematologic malignancies. The mechanism of action of IFN-α is not known. While antiproliferation is thought to be important, other possible mechanisms include (1) restoration of cytoadhesion of hematopoietic cells to marrow stroma; (2) immunomodulation; and (3) antiangiogenesis.

Single-Arm Studies of Interferon-α in Chronic Myelogenous Leukemia

The clinical activity of interferons in CML was first demonstrated with partially purified IFN-α (Finnish Red Cross, Helsinki), given at doses of 3 to 9 million U/d to early chronic phase patients. Preliminary studies showed that laboratory indices of disease activity (elevated lactate dehydrogenase and B_{12} levels, increased bone marrow cellularity) normalized among responding patients. Subsequently, cytogenetic responses with various degrees of Ph suppression were found in 41% of the patients.[68] In the original studies at M. D. Anderson Cancer Center, patients received IFN-α at a dose of 5 million U/m^2 or the maximally tolerated lower dose daily.[69] Complete hematologic response rates were 80% and cytogenetic response rates 58%. The estimated median survival was 89 months. Achieving a cytogenetic response after 12 months of therapy conferred a

TABLE 46.3.1-6. Single Arm Studies with Interferon-α

Study	*No. of Patients*	*Complete Hematologic Response (%)*	*Cytogenetic Response (%)*		*Survival (mo)*
			Any	Major	
Alimena et al.[70]	65	46	55	12	—
Ozer et al.[71]	107	59	—	29	66
Mahon et al.[72]	116	80	—	43	60+
Kantarjian et al.[69]	274	80	58	38	89

significant survival benefit by landmark analysis: 5-year survival rates from 12 months into therapy were 90% with a complete cytogenetic response, 88% with a partial cytogenetic response, 76% with a minor cytogenetic response, and 38% in other response categories (P <.001) (Fig. 46.3.1-4). The benefit of cytogenetic response was identified by multivariate analysis, introducing it as a time-dependent variable. It was also observed within each risk group. The 4-year survival dated from the 12-month landmark analysis in good-risk patients was 79% with cytogenetic response versus 62% without cytogenetic response (P <.01); in the intermediate-risk group the rates were 82% versus 35% (P <.01); and in the poor-risk group these rates were 83% versus 39% (P <.01). This study confirmed the independent effect of achieving a cytogenetic response on prolongation of survival, and supported efforts aimed at suppressing Ph-positive clones. Among patients with good-risk disease (50% of patients), the median survival was 102 months, and the major cytogenetic response rate 50%.

Three other trials reported similar results (Table 46.3.1-6). The high hematologic and cytogenetic response rates observed with IFN-α were dose-dependent. Furthermore, survival was significantly influenced by achieving a complete hematologic response at 3 months and a cytogenetic response at 12 months of treatment with IFN-α (see Fig. 46.3.1-4).[70–72a]

Randomized Studies

In four randomized trials from Japan, the United Kingdom, Italy, and Germany patients treated with IFN-α achieved higher rates of major and complete cytogenetic responses than with conventional chemotherapy (Table 46.3.1-7).[73–76] Achievement of cytogenetic response was associated with prolonged survival in the Italian and Japanese trials and in an updated report of the Medical Research Council data from the United Kingdom.[77] An updated report from the Italian Cooperative Study Group on CML with prolonged follow-up (range, 95 to 129 months) demonstrated continued significantly better survival for patients on IFN-α versus chemotherapy.[78] Median and 10-year survival of low-risk patients were 104 months versus 64 months and 47% versus 30% (P = .03), and 69 months versus 46 months and 16% versus 5% for intermediate and high-risk patients (P = .006), respectively. The German trial found a survival benefit with both IFN-α and hydroxyurea therapy compared with busulfan, but no difference between IFN-α and hydroxyurea.[75] When the data were updated for patients who were on IFN-α for more than 3 months and when *intended* versus actually *delivered* therapy was considered, survival was better with IFN-α than with hydroxyurea.[79]

A metaanalysis compared IFN-α with chemotherapy in CML and suggested better survival with IFN-α (57% at 5 years) than

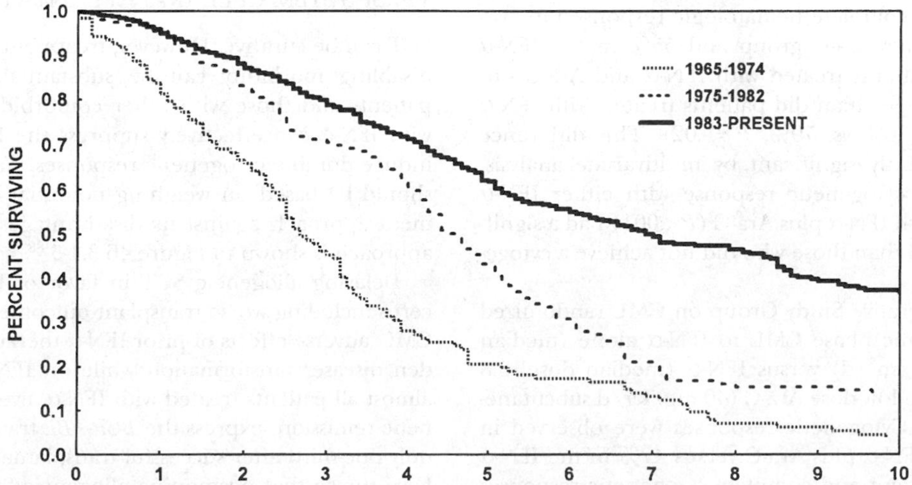

FIGURE 46.3.1-4. Probability of survival of patients in chronic phase chronic myelogenous leukemia on interferon-α (1983 through the present) compared with historical control groups.

TABLE 46.3.1-7. Randomized Studies with Interferon-α

Study	Complete Hematologic Response (%)	Cytogenetic Response (%) Any	Major	Survival Advantage with Interferon-α
Hehlmann et al.[75]	31	18	10	+[a]
Italian Cooperative Study Group[74,78]	62	55	19	+
Allan et al.[77]	68	22	11	+
Ohnishi et al.[76]	39	44	9	+

[a]The study of Hehlmann et al.[75] showed a survival advantage of interferon-α versus busulfan, but not versus hydroxyurea. In a subsequent intent-to-treat analysis, Ansari et al.[79] demonstrated a survival advantage for patients on interferon-α versus both busulfan and hydroxyurea.

with either hydroxyurea (P = .001) or busulfan (P = .00007) (42% at 5 years).[80]

Interferon-α in Combination with Cytosine Arabinoside

IFN-α alone in late chronic and accelerated phases of CML yielded modest results. In a study from M. D. Anderson Cancer Center, 140 patients with Ph-positive early chronic phase CML received IFN-α (5 million U/m^2) in combination with low-dose Ara-C, 10 mg subcutaneously daily, or intermittent Ara-C (7 d/mo).[81] With daily IFN-α and daily Ara-C, complete hematologic responses were seen in 92% of patients and cytogenetic responses in 74% (major 50%, complete 31%). The estimated 4-year survival rate was 70%. The median time to achievement of a major cytogenetic response was also significantly shorter with daily Ara-C (P<.01).

In a French trial, 721 patients in early chronic-phase CML received either hydroxyurea (50 mg/kg), and IFN-α (5 million U/m^2/d) alone, or with monthly courses of Ara-C (20 mg/m^2 for 10 d/mo).[82] The complete hematologic response rate was 66% in the IFN-α plus Ara-C group and 55% in the IFN-α group (P = .003). Patients treated with IFN-α and Ara-C survived significantly longer than did patients treated with IFN-α (3-year survival rate 86% vs. 79%, P = .02). This difference remained independently significant by multivariate analysis. Patients achieving a cytogenetic response with either IFN-α alone (P<.001) or with IFN-α plus Ara-C (P<.001) had a significantly longer survival than those who did not achieve a cytogenetic response.

The Italian Cooperative Study Group on CML randomized 540 patients in chronic phase CML to IFN-α alone (median dose, 3.65 million U/m^2/d) versus IFN-α (median dose, 3.8 million U/m^2/d) with low-dose Ara-C (40 mg/kg/d subcutaneously × 10 d/mo).[83] Cytogenetic responses were observed in 54% of patients on IFN-α plus Ara-C versus 47% in the IFN-α group. The rate of major and complete cytogenetic responses was significantly higher in the combined treatment arm (28% vs. 19%, P= .01). At a median follow-up of 24 months, the study demonstrated a significantly higher survival rate among good-risk patients with IFN-α plus Ara-C versus IFN-α alone (3-year survival rates 85% vs. 80%, P= .03).

Toxicities of Interferon-α and Clinical Management

Toxicities are common with IFN-α. Almost all patients experience some constitutional side effects, up to 50% of patients require dose reductions, and discontinuation of treatment due to toxicity is necessary in up to 18%.[84] Early adverse effects consist of flu-like symptoms and include fever, chills, postnasal dripping, and anorexia. These are usually not dose limiting, can be managed symptomatically (Table 46.3.1-8), and abate once tachyphylaxis develops within 1 to 2 weeks. Common chronic side effects are fatigue, depression, insomnia, weight loss, alopecia, reduced libido, and impotence. Neurotoxicity (lack of concentration, depression, psychosis) is more common in patients with psychiatric problems and those 60 years and older. Autoimmune phenomena occur in less than 5% of patients: hemolytic anemia and thrombocytopenia, Raynaud's phenomenon, collagen vascular disorders, hypothyroidism, and nephrotic syndrome. Cardiac arrhythmias and manifestations of congestive heart failure are rare but mandate discontinuation of therapy as do severe autoimmune phenomena, severe neurotoxicity, and refractory depression.[85]

The use of IFN-α during pregnancy is controversial. IFN-α has antiproliferative and antiangiogenic activities that may affect the placenta and fetal development. Mutagenicity *in vitro* and teratogenicity in animal studies are not documented with IFN-α, but IFN-α caused abortions in rhesus monkeys at dose levels above those used clinically.[86] Case reports of uncomplicated pregnancies with successful delivery of healthy newborns on IFN-α given either at the time of conception or during pregnancy may not be representative, since adverse outcomes may be less frequently reported, and possible damaging consequences for fetal development by IFN-α cannot be excluded.[87] Alternative treatments of pregnant patients with CML are supportive care or pheresis in the first 3 months, then hydroxyurea until delivery, and resumption of IFN-α thereafter.

TREATMENT DECISION ANALYSIS: INTERFERON-α VERSUS STEM CELL TRANSPLANTATION

SCT can be curative. However, treatment-related mortality and disabling morbidity can be substantial, especially in older patients and those with other comorbid conditions. Therapy with IFN-α can effectively suppress the Ph-positive clone and induce durable cytogenetic responses. Any treatment decision should be based on weighing potential benefits of one treatment approach against its disadvantages. An example of this approach is shown in Figure 46.3.1-5.[88,89]

Delaying allogeneic SCT in favor of IFN-α has raised concerns including worse transplant outcome in late chronic phase CML, adverse effects of prior IFN-α therapy on SCT, risk of sudden disease transformation while on IFN-α, and the fact that almost all patients treated with IFN-α, even in complete cytogenetic remission, express the *BCR-ABL* transcript compared with only one-third after successful transplantation. However, studies have shown that postponing allogeneic SCT up to 2 years into chronic phase does not adversely affect outcome. Likewise, prior IFN-α therapy, if discontinued for more than 3 months before transplantation, has no adverse effects on transplantation. The

TABLE 46.3.1-8. Side Effects and Guidelines for Therapy with Interferon-α in Chronic Myelogenous Leukemia

THERAPY

Start cytoreduction with hydroxyurea at dose of 1 to 5 g daily to decrease WBC to between 10 to 20 × 10^9/L before starting IFN-α
Initiate IFN-α at lower dose and increase gradually (3 million U daily for 3 to 7 days, then 5 million U daily for 3 to 7 days, then 5 million U/m^2 or maximally tolerated dose)
Older patients are more sensitive to side effects of IFN-α and may not tolerate full dose
Premedication with acetaminophen may lessen fever and chills
Inject doses at bedtime
Common chronic side effects include a triad of fatigue, depression, and insomnia. Tricyclic antidepressants at low dose (e.g., amitriptyline at bedtime at dose of 12.5 to 50.0 mg) may be of benefit. Neuropsychiatric consultation can be helpful in some cases
Do not reduce the dose of IFN-α if WBC low unless the WBC is below 2 × 10^9/L or platelets are below 50 × 10^9/L
For grade 3 and 4 toxicities, hold dose and restart at 50%; for grade 2 persistent toxicities, reduce dose by 25%
Hold IFN-α for moderate acute intercurrent illness

MONITORING

Monitor complete blood counts weekly until stable, then twice weekly; aim for a WBC between 2 and 4 × 10^9/L and platelets >50 × 10^9/L
Monitor cytogenetic response on bone marrow aspirates every 3 months in the first year, then every 4 to 6 months
Interphase FISH on peripheral blood samples every 3 months until Philadelphia chromosome-positive cells <10%. Hypermetaphase FISH on marrow when Ph-positive cells <10%
Monitor for unusual complications: T_4, thyroid-stimulating hormone

FISH, fluorescence *in situ* hybridization; IFN, interferon; WBC, white blood count.

risk of sudden disease transformation is low during the first 3 years.[90] The significance of persisting *BCR-ABL* transcripts is unknown. Patients in long-term complete cytogenetic remission in whom IFN-α has been discontinued and who are still PCR-positive for *BCR-ABL* have been reported.[91] This observation is consistent with the situation in many other malignant conditions that are considered to be cured despite persistent expression of molecular markers of disease [translocation (14;18), inv(16), translocation (8;21)]. Moreover, long-term cytogenetic responders on IFN-α may become negative.[92]

MANAGEMENT OF ACCELERATED AND BLASTIC PHASE CHRONIC MYELOGENOUS LEUKEMIA

Treatment results in the transformed phases of CML are unsatisfactory.[93] Disease-free survival of selected patients after SCT is less than 15%. IFN-α has no effect on the disease course. Control of elevated white cell counts may be achieved by increasing doses of hydroxyurea and combination with other cytotoxic drugs in the short-term. Symptomatic splenomegaly may be treated with splenectomy. Anemia and thrombocytopenia can be managed with transfusions. New agents and combinations of drugs are being developed and can be offered on investigational protocols.

In one-third of the patients, blastic phase is of lymphoid phenotype with expression of markers such as terminal deoxynucleotidyl transferase (TdT), CD19, CD20, or CD10 common acute lymphoblastic leukemia antigen (CALLA). Most cases with lymphoid blastic phase (80%) coexpress myeloid markers (CD13, CD14, CD33). The remaining two-thirds have an acute myeloblastic or undifferentiated leukemia-like phenotype and form a heterogeneous group. Patients with lymphoid blastic phase respond better to treatment with regimens active against acute lymphoid leukemia. The complete remission rate is 60%, one-half of the patients may have suppression of Ph-positive cells (cytogenetic response), and the remission duration is 9 to 12 months. Patients with myeloid blastic phase have a low objective response rate of 20% to 30%, may respond to high-dose cytosine-arabinoside, other antiacute myeloid leukemia regimens, or to hypomethylating agents such as 5'-deoxyazacitidine (decitabine), and to BCR-ABL tyrosine kinase inhibitors.[94,95]

NEW AGENTS AND APPROACHES

Tyrosine Kinase Inhibitors

Although many molecules along the signaling cascade can be targeted (blockade of SH3, farnesyl transferase, Ras, further downstream targets), inhibition of phosphotyrosine kinase activity has been studied most extensively. Natural inhibitors of tyrosine kinases (herbimycin A, genistein, erbstatin, lavendustin A), extracted from fungal sources, have only broad specificity for a variety of enzyme substrates. To improve target specificity, synthetic compounds have been modeled after the naturally occurring kinase inhibitors. They have been called tyrphostins, and more than 20 of them are known today. Analysis of some of these compounds (AG1112, AG568) showed a growth-inhibitory effect on CML cell lines *in vitro*, inhibition of the tyrosine kinase activity of p210, and induction of differentiation and death in a CML cell blast crisis cell line K562.[96,97] Identification of the crystal structure of several protein kinases allowed the generation of more specific tyrosine kinase inhibitors. In preclinical studies, signal transduction inhibitor 571 (STI571), formerly known as CGP57148B, was found to (1) inhibit the ABL tyrosine kinase at submicromolar concentrations; (2) inhibit the proliferation of BCR-ABL expressing cell lines; (3) inhibit colony formation of BCR-ABL–positive hematopoietic cell lines; and (4) only minimally inhibit the formation of normal bone marrow colonies. Based on these promising results, phase I clinical studies have been conducted in patients with CML in chronic and in transformed phases. Among 54 patients with chronic phase CML who have failed therapy with IFN-α and received STI571 at doses of 300 mg orally daily and more, 96% achieved a complete hematologic remission and 33% a cytogenetic response. After about 3 months of therapy, the cytogenetic response rate is anticipated to exceed 50%, being complete in over 20% to 30%. Responses in de novo patients treated with STI571 may be even higher.[98] In 46

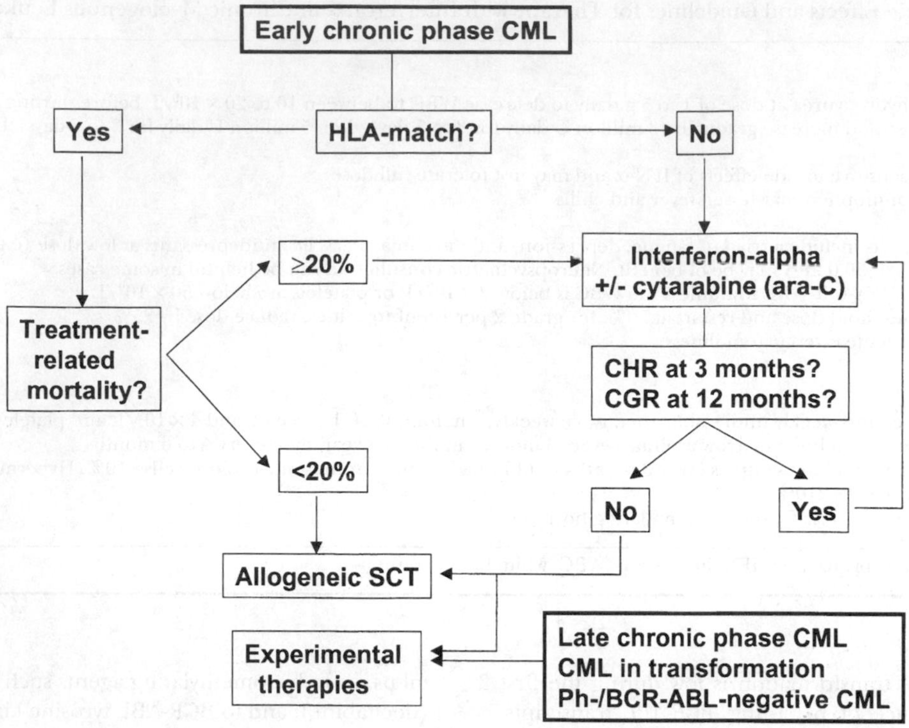

FIGURE 46.3.1-5. Clinical decision making in chronic myelogenous leukemia (CML). For patients in early chronic phase CML, allogeneic stem cell transplantation (SCT) and interferon-α are possible first-line therapies. The decision depends on several factors: (1) availability of a matched sibling; (2) age and performance status of the patient; (3) presence of other comorbid conditions; and (4) socioeconomic situation. For patients who have a matched sibling donor and whose physical condition allows SCT with an acceptable treatment-related morbidity and mortality (less than 20%), allogeneic SCT should be the first choice. For other patients, a trial with interferon-α may be preferable given the manageable side-effect profile with absence of treatment-related mortality. Furthermore, a prospective study on 840 patients below age 56 with chronic phase CML found increased survival with matched sibling allogeneic transplant only in those patients who were younger than 32 years and had intermediate- or high-risk CML. Patients in late chronic phase or accelerated phase should be offered investigational therapies or undergo allogeneic transplantation.[88,89] CGR, cytogenetic response; CHR, complete hematologic response; HLA, human leukocyte antigen.

patients with CML in blastic phase (32 myeloid, 14 acute lymphoid leukemia or lymphoid blast crisis), 18 (39%) patients had a complete clearance of blood and bone marrow leukemic cells. The marrow complete response rate for patients with myeloid blast crisis was 29%, but responses were often transient. In accelerated phase, the hematologic response is about 70%, cytogenetic responses have been noted in 20%, and responses appear durable.[99] STI571 was well tolerated and no dose-limiting toxicity has yet been reached except for myelosuppression at doses of 300 to 800 mg orally daily. Side effects included nausea, vomiting, diarrhea, and muscle cramps, mostly mild in nature.

Antisense Oligonucleotides

Antisense oligonucleotides are short DNA sequences modified to bind target RNA sequences within the cell, preventing translation of the RNA message into functional proteins. Effective targets for antisense approaches are *BCR-ABL* itself, Ras, PI-3-kinase, c-Myb, and c-Myc. *BCR-ABL* antisense oligonucleotides alone or in combination with sequences targeted against additional oncogenes reduce the level of $p210^{bcr\text{-}abl}$ in CML cells and slow the rate of growth and proliferation. Antisense sequences directed against *BCR-ABL* for *ex vivo* purging in autologous SCT are of interest.[100]

Polyethylene Glycol Interferon

Polyethylene glycol interferon is a modified IFN-α molecule that is covalently attached to polyethylene glycol. Polyethylene glycol interferon has a significantly longer half-life than its parent compound and can be given once weekly instead of daily. Early data suggest an improved side-effect profile compared with IFN-α. Complete hematologic remissions and cytogenetic responses have been reported. Results with polyethylene glycol interferon are promising, and further investigations are required to validate its role in the treatment of CML.[101]

Homoharringtonine

Homoharringtonine (HHT) is a plant alkaloid derived from the *Cephalotaxus fortuneii* tree. Used in a low-dose continuous infusion schedule (2.5 mg/m^2 for 14 days for remission induction followed by a 7-day monthly infusion as maintenance), HHT resulted in complete hematologic remission in two-thirds of patients and cytogenetic response in one-third (one-half of which were major).[102] More than one-half of the patients were resistant to prior therapy with IFN-α. In early chronic phase disease, HHT was given for six cycles as remission induction followed by IFN-α maintenance: Complete hematologic remission rate was 92% and cytogenetic response rate was 68%.[103] Combinations of HHT with IFN-α and Ara-C in the clinical setting, including early chronic phase CML, are in progress with promising results.[104]

5-Aza-2'-Deoxycytidine

5-Aza-2'-deoxycytidine (decitabine) is a potent hypomethylating cytidine analogue. Decitabine produced response rates of 25% in blastic phase and 53% in accelerated phase. Further clinical trials are in progress including decitabine in combination with busulfan and cyclophosphamide as part of a preparative regimen for allogeneic SCT, and as salvage therapy together with stem cell rescue after relapse from allogeneic SCT.[105]

Adoptive Immunotherapy

That leukemic cell proliferation is under the control of the immune system is based on several observations: (1) there is an increased frequency of disease recurrence with T-cell depleted SCTs; (2) DLIs in patients who relapse after an allogeneic transplant reestablish cytogenetic remissions in a high percentage of patients; (3) there is a positive correlation between GVHD and reduced risk of relapse after transplant; and (4) cytogenetic response correlates with IFN-associated autoimmune phenomena. Response to DLIs suggests a pivotal role for graft-versus-leukemia activity generated by infused donor T lymphocytes in suppressing Ph-positive clones.

Research is focusing on identification of (1) specific T-cell clones able to eliminate leukemic progenitors and (2) proteins that can serve as targets, even though only a few tumors express structures unique to them. CML is a good model because p210 is uniquely associated with the Ph translocation. Minor histocompatibility antigens, overexpressed normal antigens, and other leukemia-restricted antigens are studied as further immunologic targets.[106] In one study, cultures of CD34-positive CML progenitor cells incubated with granulocyte-macrophage colony-stimulating factor, interleukin-4, and tumor necrosis factor stimulated the formation *in vitro* of dendritic cells, leukemic-antigen-presenting cells that are strong inducers of T-cell responses *in vitro*.[107] Identification of leukemia-specific antigens and stimulation of leukemia-specific T-cell responses may allow us to use immunogenicity of CML cells in approaches such as immune gene therapy and peptide vaccination.

Investigational combined modalities using T-cell–depleted allogeneic SCT upfront (to reduce GVHD and treatment-related mortality), followed by periodic incremental doses of selected T-cell subsets for DLIs (to eradicate minimal residual disease), may render allogeneic SCT safer and more effective and extend its use to older patients and those with unrelated or mismatched donors.

CONCLUSIONS

CML is one of the most extensively studied human malignancies and a prime example of how advances in our understanding of molecular biology can be translated into novel and effective treatment strategies. The most beneficial treatment for the patient in early chronic phase, transplantation versus IFN-α–based therapy, has to be decided on an individual basis. Numerous patient- and treatment-related factors have to be considered, particularly the acceptable threshold of transplant-related mortality, which may be different for different patients. Socioeconomic and logistic factors may play an increasing role in choosing the most appropriate therapy. These recommendations may change drastically as data mature on the efficacy of new investigational treatments, particularly the BCR-ABL tyrosine kinase inhibitor (STI571), and on the safety of new SCT approaches (e.g., mini-SCT). The effect of current treatments in accelerated phases of CML is modest at best, making investigational therapies the best option for these patients.

REFERENCES

1. Kinlen LJ. Leukemia. In: Doll R, Fraumeni JF, Muir DS, eds. *Trend in cancer incidence and mortality. Cancer surveys* 1994, 19/20, 475. Plainview, NY: Cold Spring Harbor Laboratory Press, 1994.
2. Hasle H, Olsen JH. Cancer in relatives of children with myelodysplastic syndrome, acute and chronic myeloid leukaemia. *Br J Haematol* 1997;97:127.
3. Lange R, Moloney W, Yamawaki T. Leukemia in atomic bomb survivors. 1. General observations. *Blood* 1954;9:514.
4. Nowell PC, Hungerford DA. A minute chromosome in human chronic granulocytic leukemia. *Science* 1960;132:1497.
5. Rowley JD. A new consistent chromosomal abnormality in chronic myelogenous leukemia identified by quinacrine, fluorescence and Giemsa staining. *Nature* 1970;243:290.
6. De Klein A, Van Kessel G, Grosveld G, et al. A cellular oncogene is translocated to the Philadelphia chromosome in chronic myelogenous leukemia. *Nature* 1982;300:765.
7. Faderl S, Talpaz M, Estrov Z, Kantarjian HM. The biology of chronic myelogenous leukemia. *N Engl J Med* 1999;341:164.
8. Melo JV. The molecular biology of chronic myeloid leukemia. *Leukemia* 1996;10:751.
9. Shepherd P, Suffolk R, Hasley J, Allan N. Analysis of molecular breakpoint and mRNA transcripts in a prospective randomized trial of interferon in chronic myeloid leukaemia: no correlation with clinical features, cytogenetic response, duration of chronic phase, or survival. *Br J Haematol* 1995;89:546.
10. Kurzrock R, Shtalrid M, Romero P, et al. A novel c-abl protein product in Philadelphia-positive acute lymphoblastic leukemia. *Nature* 1987;325:631.
11. Pane F, Frigeri F, Sindona M, et al. Neutrophilic-chronic myeloid leukemia: a distinct disease with a specific molecular marker. *Blood* 1996;88:2410 [Erratum, *Blood* 1997;89:4244].
12. Melo JV, Myint H, Galton DAG, Goldman JM. P190 BCR-ABL chronic myeloid leukemia: the missing link with chronic myelomonocytic leukaemia? *Leukemia* 1994;8:208.
13. Melo J, Hochhaus A, Yan X-H, Goldman J. Lack of correlation between ABL-BCR expression and response to interferon-α in chronic myeloid leukemia. *Br J Haematol* 1996;92:684.
14. Li S, Ilaria RL Jr, Million RP, Daley GQ, Van Etten RA. The p190, p210, and p230 forms of the BCR/ABL oncogene induce a similar chronic myeloid leukemia-like syndrome in mice but have different leukemogenic activity. *J Exp Med* 1999;189:1399.
15. Verfaillie CM. Biology of chronic myelogenous leukemia. *Hematol Oncol Clin North Am* 1998;12:1.
16. Udomsakdi C, Eaves CJ, Swolin B, et al. Rapid decline of chronic myeloid leukemic cells in long-term culture due to a defect at the leukemic stem cell level. *Proc Natl Acad Sci U S A* 1992;89:6192.
17. Strife A, Lambek C, Wisniewski D, et al. Discordant maturation as the primary biological defect in chronic myelogenous leukemia. *Cancer Res* 1988;48:1035.
18. Eaves CJ, Eaves AC. Cell culture studies in CML. *Baillieres Clin Haematol* 1987;1:931.
19. Verfaillie CM, Hurley R, Zhao RCH, et al. Pathophysiology of CML: do defects in integrin function contribute to the premature circulation and massive expansion of the BCR/ABL positive clone? *J Lab Clin Med* 1997;129:584.
20. Savage DG, Szydlo RM, Goldman JM. Clinical features at diagnosis in 430 patients with chronic myeloid leukemia seen at a referral centre over a 16-year period. *Br J Haematol* 1997;96:111.
21. Kantarjian HM, Deisseroth A, Kurzrock R, Estrov Z, Talpaz M. Chronic myelogenous leukemia: a concise update. *Blood* 1993;82:691.
22. Kamada N, Uchino H. Chronologic sequence in appearance of clinical and laboratory findings characteristic of chronic myelocytic leukemia. *Blood* 1978;51:843.
23. Mitelman F. The cytogenetic scenario of chronic myeloid leukemia. *Leukemia Lymphoma* 1993;11(Suppl 1):11.
24. Cortes J, Talpaz M, O'Brien S, et al. Philadelphia chromosome negative chronic myelogenous leukemia with rearrangement of the breakpoint cluster region: long-term follow-up results. *Cancer* 1995;75:464.
25. Cuneo A, Bigoni R, Emmanuel B, et al. Fluorescence in situ hybridization for the detection and monitoring of the Ph-positive clone in chronic myelogenous leukemia: comparison with metaphase banding analysis. *Leukemia* 1998;12:1718.

26. Muhlmann J, Thaler J, Hilbe W, et al. Fluorescence in situ hybridization (FISH) on peripheral blood smears for monitoring Philadelphia chromosome-positive chronic myeloid leukemia (CML) during interferon treatment: a new strategy for remission assessment. *Genes Chromosomes Cancer* 1998;21:90.
27. Seong D, Kantarjian H, Ro J, et al. Hypermetaphase fluorescence in situ hybridization for quantitative monitoring of Philadelphia chromosome-positive cells in patients with chronic myelogenous leukemia during treatment. *Blood* 1995;86:2343.
28. Grand FH, Chase A, Iqbal S, et al. A two-color BCR-ABL probe that greatly reduces the false positive and false negative rates for fluorescence in situ hybridization in chronic myeloid leukemia. *Genes Chromosomes Cancer* 1998;12:1718.
29. Kantarjian HM, Dixon D, Keating MJ, et al. Characteristics of accelerated disease in chronic myelogenous leukemia. *Cancer* 1988;61:1441.
30. Sokal JE, Baccarani M, Russo D, Tusa S. Staging and prognosis in chronic myelogenous leukemia. *Semin Hematol* 1988;25:49.
31. Ishikura H, Yufu Y, Yamashita S, et al. Biphenotypic blast crisis of chronic myelogenous leukemia: abnormalities of p53 and retinoblastoma genes. *Leukemia Lymphoma* 1997;25:573.
32. Ahuja H, Bar-Eli M, Advani SH, Benchimol S, Cline MJ. Alterations in the p53 gene and the clonal evolution of the blast crisis of chronic myelocytic leukemia. *Proc Natl Acad Sci U S A* 1989;86:6783.
33. Kantarjian HM, Giles FJ, O'Brien SM, Talpaz M. Clinical course and therapy of chronic myelogenous leukemia with interferon-alpha and chemotherapy. *Hematol Oncol Clin North Am* 1998;12:31.
34. Sokal JE, Cox EB, Baccarani M, et al. Prognostic discrimination in "good-risk" chronic granulocytic leukemia. *Blood* 1984;63:789.
35. Galton D. Myleran in chronic myeloid leukemia. *Lancet* 1953;1:208.
36. Kennedy BJ. Hydroxyurea therapy in chronic myelogenous leukemia. *Cancer* 1972;29:1052.
37. Hehlmann R, Heimpel H, Hasford J, et al. Randomized comparison of busulfan and hydroxyurea in chronic myelogenous leukemia: prolongation of survival by hydroxyurea. *Blood* 1993;82:398.
38. Goldman JM, Szydlo R, Horowitz MM, et al. Choice of pretransplant treatment and timing of transplants for chronic myelogenous leukemia in chronoic phase. *Blood* 1993;82:2235.
39. Bouvet M, Babiera GV, Termuhlen PM, et al. Splenectomy in the accelerated or blastic phase of chronic myelogenous leukemia: a single-institution, 25-year experience. *Surgery* 1997;122:20.
40. Horowitz MM, Rowlings PA, Passweg JR. Allogeneic bone marrow transplantation for CML: a report from the International Bone Marrow Transplant Registry. *Bone Marrow Transplant* 1996;17(Suppl 3):S5.
41. Clift RA, Buckner CD, Thomas ED, et al. Marrow transplantation for chronic myelogenous leukemia: a randomized study comparing cyclophosphamide and total body irradiation with busulfan and cyclophosphamide. *Blood* 1994;84:2036.
42. Clift RA, Storb R. Marrow transplantation for CML: the Seattle experience. *Bone Marrow Transplant* 1996;17(Suppl 3):S1.
43. Gratwohl A, Hermanns J, Niederwieser D, et al. Bone marrow transplantation for chronic myeloid leukemia: long-term results. Chronic Leukemia Working Party of the European Group for Bone Marrow Transplantation. *Bone Marrow Transplant* 1993;12:509.
44. Van Rhee F, Szydlo RM, Germans J, et al. Long-term results after allogeneic bone marrow transplantation for chronic myelogenous leukemia in chronic phase: a report from the Chronic Leukemia Working Party of the European Group for Blood and Marrow Transplantation. *Bone Marrow Transplant* 1997;20:553.
45. Cortes J, Talpaz M, O'Brien S, et al. Suppression of cytogenetic clonal evolution with interferon alfa therapy in patients with Philadelphia chromosome-positive chronic myelogenous leukemia. *J Clin Oncol* 1998;16:3279.
46. Clift RA, Anasetti C. Allografting for chronic myeloid leukemia. *Bailleres Clin Haematol* 1997;10:319.
47. Giralt SA, Kantarjian HM, Talpaz M, et al. Effect of prior interferon alfa therapy on the outcome of allogeneic bone marrow transplantation for chronic myelogenous leukemia. *J Clin Oncol* 1993;11:1055.
48. Tomas JF, Lopez-Lorenzo JL, Requena MJ, et al. Absence of influence of prior treatment with interferon on the outcome of allogeneic bone marrow transplantation for chronic myeloid leukemia. *Bone Marrow Transplant* 1998;22:47.
49. Beelen DW, Elmaagacli AH, Schaefer UW. The adverse influence of pretransplant interferon-α (IFN-α) on transplant outcome after marrow transplantation for chronic phase chronic myelogenous leukemia increases with duration of IFN-α exposure [letter]. *Blood* 1999;93:1779.
50. Morton AJ, Gooley T, Hansen JA, et al. Association between pretransplant interferon-alpha and outcome after unrelated donor marrow transplantation for chronic myelogenous leukemia in chronic phase. *Blood* 1998;92:394.
51. Clift RA, Buckner CD, Thomas ED. Marrow transplantation for chronic myeloid leukemia: a randomized study comparing cyclophosphamide and total body irradiation with busulfan and cyclophosphamide. *Blood* 1994;84:2036.
52. Chao NJ, Schmidt GM, Niland JC, et al. Cyclosporine, methotrexate, and prednisone compared with cyclosporine and prednisone for prophylaxis of acute graft-versus-host disease. *N Engl J Med* 1993;329:1225.
53. Horowitz MM, Gage RP, Sondel DM, et al. Graft versus leukemia reactions after bone marrow transplantation. *Blood* 1990;75:555.
54. Goldman JM, Gale RP, Horowitz MM, et al. Bone marrow transplantation for chronic myelogenous leukemia in chronic phase. Increased risk for relapse with T-cell depletion. *Ann Intern Med* 1988;108:806.
55. Arcese W, Goldman JM, D'Arcangelo E, et al. Outcome for patients who relapse after allogeneic bone marrow transplantation for chronic myeloid leukemia. *Blood* 1993;82:3211.
56. Mrsíc M, Horowitz MM, Atkinson K, et al. Second HLA-identical sibling transplants for leukemia recurrence. *Bone Marrow Transplant* 1992;9:269.
57. Higano CS, Raskind WH, Singer JW. Use of α-interferon for the treatment of relapse of chronic myelogenous leukemia in chronic phase after allogeneic bone marrow transplantation. *Blood* 1992;80:1437.
58. Giralt SA, Kolb HJ. Donor lymphocyte infusions. *Curr Opin Oncol* 1996;8:96.
59. McGlave P, Bartsch G, Anasetti C, et al. Unrelated donor marrow transplantation therapy for chronic myelogenous leukemia: initial experience of the National Marrow Donor Program. *Blood* 1993;81:543.
60. Hansen JA, Gooley TA, Martin PJ, et al. Bone marrow transplants from unrelated donors for patients with chronic myeloid leukemia. *N Engl J Med* 1998;338:962.
61. Devergie A, Apperley JF, Labopin M, et al. European results of matched unrelated donor bone marrow transplantation for chronic myeloid leukemia. Impact of HLA class II matching. *Bone Marrow Transplant* 1997;20:11.
62. Khouri IF, Kantarjian HM, Talpaz M, et al. Results with high-dose chemotherapy and unpurged autologous stem cell transplantation in 73 patients with chronic myelogenous leukemia: the MD Anderson experience. *Bone Marrow Transplant* 1996;17:775.
63. Deisseroth AB, Zu Z, Claxton D, et al. Genetic marking shows that Ph^+ cells present in autologous transplants of chronic myelogenous leukemia (CML) contribute to relapse after autologous bone marrow in CML. *Blood* 1994;83:3068.
64. Kantarjian HM, Vellekoop L, McCredie KB, et al. Intensive combination chemotherapy (ROAP) and splenectomy in the management of chronic myelogenous leukemia. *J Clin Oncol* 1985;3:192.
65. Kantarjian HM, Talpaz M, Hester J, et al. Collection of peripheral blood diploid cells from chronic myelogenous leukemia patients early in the recovery phase from myelosuppression induced by intensive-dose chemotherapy. *J Clin Oncol* 1995;13:554.
66. Talpaz M, Kantarjian H, Liang J, et al. Percentage of Philadelphia chromosome (Ph)-negative and Ph-positive cells found after autologous transplantation for chronic myelogenous leukemia depends on percentage of diploid cells induced by conventional-dose chemotherapy before collection of autologous cells. *Blood* 1995;85:3257.
67. Estrov Z, Kurzrock R, Talpaz M. *Interferons. Basic principles and clinical applications.* 1st ed. Austin: R.G. Landes Company, 1993.
68. Talpaz M, Kantarjian HM, McCredie KB, et al. Clinical investigation of human alpha interferon in chronic myelogenous leukemia. *Blood* 1987;69:1280.
69. Kantarjian H, Smith T, O'Brien S, et al. Prolonged survival following achievement of cytogenetic response with alpha interferon therapy in chronic myelogenous leukemia. *Ann Intern Med* 1995;122:254.
70. Alimena G, Morra E, Lazzarino M, et al. Interferon alpha-2b as therapy for Ph^1-positive chronic myelogenous leukemia: a study of 82 patients treated with intermittent or daily administration. *Blood* 1988;72:642.
71. Ozer H, George SL, Schiffer CA, et al. Prolonged subcutaneous administration of recombinant α2b interferon in patients with previously untreated Philadelphia chromosome-positive chronic-phase chronic myelogenous leukemia: effect on remission duration and survival: Cancer and Leukemia Group B Study 8583. *Blood* 1993;82:2975.
72. Mahon FX, Faberes C, Pueyo S, et al. Response at three months is a good predictive factor for newly diagnosed chronic myeloid leukemia patients treated by recombinant interferon-alpha. *Blood* 1998;92:4059.
72a. Ohnishi K, Ohno R, Tomonaga M, et al. A randomized trial comparing interferon-α with busulfan for newly diagnosed chronic myelogenous leukemia in chronic phase. *Blood* 1995;86:916.
73. Allan NC, Richards SM, Shepherd PCA, on behalf of the UK Medical Research Council's Working Parties for Therapeutic Trials in Adult Leukaemia. UK Medical Research Council randomised, multicentre trial of interferon-αn1 for chronic myeloid leukemia: improved survival irrespective of cytogenetic response. *Lancet* 1995;345:1392.
74. The Italian Cooperative Study Group On Chronic Myeloid Leukemia. Interferon alfa-2a as compared with conventional chemotherapy for the treatment of chronic myeloid leukemia. *N Engl J Med* 1994;330:820.
75. Hehlmann R, Heimpel H, Hasford J. Randomized comparison of interferon-α with busulfan and hydroxyurea in chronic myelogenous leukemia. The German CML Study Group. *Blood* 1994;84:4064.
76. Ohnishi K, Ohno R, Tomonaga M, et al. A randomized trial comparing interferon-α with busulfan for newly diagnosed chronic myelogenous leukemia in chronic phase. *Blood* 1995;86:906.
77. Allan NC, Richards SM, Shepherd PCA. Interferon-α therapy with busulfan or hydroxyurea compared with either BU or HU alone in treatment of chronic phase CML. Results from MRC CML III trial. *Int J Hematol* 1996;64(Suppl 1):S68.
78. The Italian Cooperative Study Group on Chronic Myeloid Leukemia. Long-term follow-up of the Italian trial of interferon-alpha versus conventional chemotherapy in chronic myeloid leukemia. *Blood* 1998;92:1541.
79. Ansari H, Hasford J, Hehlmann R, and the German CML Study Group. Fallacies of the intent-to-treat analysis. *J Mol Med* 1997;75:B243.
80. Chronic Myeloid Leukemia Trialists' Collaborative Group. Interferon alfa versus chemotherapy for chronic myeloid leukemia: a meta-analysis of seven randomized trials. *J Natl Cancer Inst* 1997;89:1616.
81. Kantarjian HM, O'Brien S, Smith TL, et al. Treatment of Philadelphia chromosome-positive early chronic phase chronic myelogenous leukemia with daily doses of interferon alpha and low dose cytosine arabinoside. *J Clin Oncol* 1999;17:284.
82. Guilhot F, Chastang C, Michallet M, et al. Interferon alfa-2b combined with cytarabine versus interferon alone in chronic myelogenous leukemia. *N Engl J Med* 1997;337:223.
83. Rosti G, Bonifazi F, De Vivo A, et al. Cytarabine increases karyotypic response in αIFN treated chronic myeloid leukemia patients: results of a national prospective randomized trial of the Italian Cooperative Study Group on CML. *Blood* 1999;94:600a.
84. Quesada JR, Talpaz M, Rios A, Kurzrock R, Gutterman JU. Clinical toxicity of interferons in cancer patients: a review. *J Clin Oncol* 1986;4:234.
85. Sacchi S, Kantarjian H, Cohen P, Pierce S, Talpaz M. Immune-mediated and unusual complications during alpha-interferon therapy in chronic myelogenous leukemia. *J Clin Oncol* 1995;13:2401.

86. Vassiliadis S, Athanassakis I. Type II interferon may be a potential hazardous therapeutic agent during pregnancy. *Br J Haematol* 1992;82:782.
87. Haggstrom J, Adrianson M, Hybbinette T, Harnby E, Thorbert G. Two cases of CML treated with alpha-interferon during second and third trimester of pregnancy with analysis of the drug in the new-born immediately postpartum. *Eur J Haematol* 1996;102
88. Italian Study Group on Chronic Myeloid Leukemia and Italian Group for Bone Marrow Transplantation. Monitoring treatment and survival in chronic myeloid leukemia. *J Clin Oncol* 1999;17:1858.
89. Silver RT, Woolf SH, Hehlmann R, et al. An evidence-based analysis of the effect of busulfan, hydroxyurea, interferon, and allogeneic bone marrow transplantation in treating the chronic phase of chronic myeloid leukemia: developed for the American Society of Hematology. *Blood* 1999;94:1517.
90. Thomas D, Kantarjian H, O'Brien S, et al. "Sudden" blastic phase (SBP) transformation in the first 2 years (YRS) of interferon-α (IFN) therapy (RX) for chronic phase (CP) chronic myelogenous leukemia (CML). *Blood* 1998;92:251a.
91. Talpaz M, Estrov Z, Kantarjian H, et al. Persistence of dormant leukemic progenitors during interferon-induced remission in chronic myelogenous leukemia. *J Clin Invest* 1994;94:1383.
92. Kurzrock R, Estrov Z, Kantarjian H, Talpaz M. Conversion of interferon-induced, long-term cytogenetic remissions in chronic myelogenous leukemia to polymerase chain reaction negativity. *J Clin Oncol* 1998;16:1526.
93. Kantarjian H, Keating M, Talpaz M, et al. Chronic myelogenous leukemia in blast crisis. Analysis of 242 patients. *Am J Med* 1987;83:445.
94. Kantarjian H, O'Brien S, Beran M, et al. Results with decitabine, a hypomethylating agent, in the treatment of chronic myelogenous leukemia in accelerated or blastic phases. *Blood* 1996;88:199b.
95. Walters R, Kantarjian H, Keating M, et al. Therapy of lymphoid and undifferentiated chronic myelogenous leukemia in blast crisis with continuous vincristine and Adriamycin infusions plus high dose decadron. *Cancer* 1987;81:516.
96. Levitzki A, Gazit A. Tyrosine kinase inhibition: an approach to drug development. *Science* 1995;267:1782.
97. Druker BJ, Sawyers CL, Talpaz M, et al. Phase I trial of a specific ABL tyrosine kinase inhibitor, CGP 57148, in interferon refractory chronic myelogenous leukemia patients. *Proc Am Soc Clin Oncol* 1999;18:7a.
98. Druker BJ, Talpaz M, Resta D, et al. Clinical efficacy and safety of an ABL specific tyrosine kinase inhibitor as targeted therapy for chronic myelogenous leukemia. *Blood* 1999;94:368a.
99. Talpaz M, Sawyers CL, Kantarjian H, et al. Activity of an ABL specific tyrosine kinase inhibitor in patients with BCR-ABL-positive acute leukemias, including chronic myelogenous leukemia in blast crisis. *Proc ASCO* 2000;19:4a.
100. Skorski T, Nieborowska-Skorska M, Wlodarski P, et al. Antisense oligodeoxynucleotide combination therapy of primary chronic myelogenous leukemia blast crisis in SCID mice. *Blood* 1996;88:1005.
101. Talpaz M, Cortes J, O'Brien S, et al. Phase I study of polyethylene glycol (PEG) interferon alpha-2b (intron-A) in CML patients. *Blood* 1998;92(Suppl 1):251a.
102. O'Brien SM, Kantarjian H, Keating M, et al. Homoharringtonine therapy induces responses in patients with chronic myelogenous leukemia in late chronic phase. *Blood* 1995;86:3322.
103. Kantarjian HM, Talpaz M, Cortes J, et al. Homoharringtonine and low-dose cytosine (LDara-C) in late chronic phase chronic myelogenous leukemia (CML). *Blood* 1999;94:274b.
104. O'Brien S, Kantarjian H, Koller C, et al. Sequential homoharringtonine and interferon-α in the treatment of early chronic phase chronic myelogenous leukemia. *Blood* 1999;93:4149.
105. Kantarjian HM, O'Brien SM, Estey E, et al. Decitabine studies in chronic and acute myelogenous leukemia. *Leukemia* 1997;11(Suppl 1):S35.
106. Molldrem JJ, Clave E, Jiang YZ, et al. Cytotoxic T lymphocytes specific for a nonpolylmorphic proteinase 3 peptide preferentially inhibit chronic myeloid leukemia colony-forming units. *Blood* 1997;90:2529.
107. Choudhoury A, Gajewski JL, Liang JC, et al. Use of leukemic dendritic cells expressing bcr/abl from CD34 positive chronic myeloid leukemia precursor cells. *Blood* 1997;89:1133.

BRUCE D. CHESON

The Chronic Lymphocytic Leukemias

Chronic lymphocytic leukemia (CLL) is the most common form of leukemia affecting adults in Western countries. The current annual incidence estimates vary from approximately 8100 to 12,500 new cases in the United States.[1,2] An apparent decrease from 3.3 in 100,000 population in 1973 to 2.3 in 100,000 in 1990 may reflect an improved ability to distinguish CLL from other chronic lymphoid leukemias. CLL occurs more often in males, with a relative frequency of 1.3:1 to 2.6:1. The median age at diagnosis of CLL is 62 years; approximately 10% to 15% of patients with CLL present younger than 50 years of age, and 20% are younger than 55 years.[3] A 10-year-old child with CLL has been reported.[4] The increase in younger patients most likely represents the more routine use of automated blood counts and differentials. Although younger patients with stage 0 disease may survive as long as a normal age-matched population, those with more advanced stages of the disease have a median survival comparable to older patients when corrected for non–CLL-related causes of death.[3,5] CLL occurs more commonly in Jewish people of Russian or Eastern European ancestry, and it is infrequent in Japan, China, and Asian countries.[6,7]

No clear etiologic factors exist for CLL, although few carefully conducted studies have been performed.[8] CLL is one of the few leukemias that does not appear to be associated with prior exposure to ionizing radiation, chemicals, or drugs, and it was the only leukemia not associated with atomic bomb explosions.[9–12]

A clear familial incidence of CLL has been established. Approximately 20% of patients with this disease have relatives with CLL or another lymphoid malignancy, although no genetic linkage has yet been identified. Rare sets of twins have been affected.[13,14] A lack of concordance of oncogene expression was reported in monozygous twin sisters who both had CLL.[15] Immigrants from Japan to the United States maintain their low incidence of CLL. The occurrence in spouses has been observed.[16]

CELL OF ORIGIN

The precise origin of the CLL lymphocyte has not been clearly defined. CLL lymphocytes have been assumed to be the malignant counterpart of normal lymphocytes because of their similar morphology. However, whereas B-CLL cells share some immunologic features with normal B cells, marked molecular and immunologic differences distinguish the two cell populations.

CLL cells express pan-B antigens (e.g., HLA class II, CD19, CD20), as well as activation antigens (e.g., CD5, CD23, CD25, CD71), but not terminal differentiation antigens exhibited by plasma cells.[17] This profile supports the hypothesis that the B-CLL cell is an "activated" B lymphocyte, meaning that the cells can be activated without dividing, but it does not suggest that they are in a state of active proliferation. Overexpression of BCL-2 is restricted to the malignant cells. CLL B cells express a restricted repertoire of V_{H1} genes, which is distinct from that of normal B cells.[18]

Two major features that distinguish CLL cells from normal B cells is their expression of CD5 and the barely detectable amount of surface immunoglobulins. Although CD5 was formerly considered to be a restricted T-cell antigen, CD5+ B cells are normally present in the mantle zone of normal lymph nodes, and small numbers can be found in the peripheral blood of normal individuals. CD5+ B cells are found in increased numbers in patients with autoimmune disorders (e.g., rheumatoid arthritis, Sjögren's syndrome, and systemic lupus erythematosus), immune thrombocytopenic purpura, and after allogeneic bone marrow transplantation.[19,20] These observations have led to the current theory that B-CLL is a monoclonal proliferation of mantle zone–based anergic CD5+ self-reactive B cells devoted to the production of polyreactive autoantibodies.[21] A wide variety of growth factors have been implicated in the disordered proliferation and differentiation of B cells in CLL, including tumor necrosis factor,[22] interleukin-2 (IL-2),[23,24] IL-4,[25,26] IL-6,[27] IL-7,[28] IL-8, IL-10, IL-11, IL-12, IL-13, interferon-γ (IFN-γ), granulocyte-macrophage colony-stimulating factor, transforming growth factor-β, and others.[29–34]

IMMUNE FUNCTION AND AUTOIMMUNITY IN CHRONIC LYMPHOCYTIC LEUKEMIA

CLL is characterized by an accumulation of immunologically incompetent B cells. These cells produce reduced amounts of normal immunoglobulins in response to antigenic stimuli.[21] Quantitative and qualitative abnormalities of normal B cells, T cells, and natural killer (NK) cells also have been reported, with a reduction in the number and function of normal T cells and the function of NK cells, and impaired complement activation.[35,36] Elevated levels of circulating IL-2 receptor (IL-2R) may down-regulate helper T-cell function and may play a role in the pathogenesis of the immunodeficiency.[23,24] B-CLL cells express CD40, which down-modulates CD40 ligand (CD154) on CD4+ T cells. Because CD40 ligand allows B cells to respond to T cells, this effect may contribute to the immune incompetence in CLL.[37]

CYTOGENETICS

Conventional banding techniques detect cytogenetic abnormalities in more than 50% of cases of CLL.[38–40] More recently, fluorescent *in situ* hybridization has identified cytogenetic abnormalities in more than 80% of cases.[41–43] The most common cytogenetic abnormality in CLL appears to be deletion of 13q, which is present in 55% of cases. Patients with 13q14 abnormalities tend to experience a more benign course with a normal lifespan. Whether deletion of the breast cancer gene BRCA2 at 13q12 is involved is controversial.[44,45]

Deletions of 11q23 are detected in 18% of cases and are associated with massive lymphadenopathy that is often out of proportion to the increase in peripheral blood lymphocyte count. Trisomy 12 occurs in 16% of cases and is associated with atypical morphology and a poor outcome. Lymphocytes with trisomy 12 tend to have unmutated immunoglobulin variable (V_H) genes, whereas those with 13q14 have evidence of somatic mutations.[46] Mutations or deletions of p53 at 17p13.3 have been reported in approximately 15% of patients. Chromosome 17 abnormalities are found more frequently in cases of atypical CLL and are associated with a higher likelihood of Richter's transformation and a poor prognosis.[47]

BCL-3 translocations, t(14;19)(q32.3;q13.2), are uncommon and, in approximately one-half of cases, occur in association with trisomy 12. These patients tend to be young and have rapidly progressive disease. Of note is the lack of translocations in patients with CLL.

MOLECULAR BIOLOGY AND GENETICS

Lymphocytes from approximately one-half of patients with CLL contain V_H genes that are mutated postgerminal center B cells [immunoglobulin D (IgD)–, CD38+)], whereas the other half are naïve and unmutated (IgD+/IgM+, CD38–).[48–50] These two populations are characterized by markedly different clinical outcomes, with the unmutated group having a significantly shorter survival rate. Studies of gene use in CLL have indicated that there may be nonrandom differential usage of V_H and V_l genes used in the cell of origin, with an apparent increase in the usage of the V_{H1}-69 (51p1) gene from the V_{H1} family.[46,51]

No single oncogene has been implicated in the pathogenesis of CLL. Early reports of cases with the BCL-1 translocation were more likely mantle cell lymphoma (MCL).[52–54] The translocations associated with BCL-2 [t(14;18)(q32;q21)] and BCL-3 [t(14;19)(q32;q13.1)] have been detected in only 5% to 10% of cases.[55,56] However, overexpression of the BCL-2 gene is present in more than 70% of cases, even in the absence of the chromosome rearrangement.[57] The ratio of the antiapoptotic gene BCL2 to the proapoptotic gene BAX is increased in CLL cells, which favors cell survival. Deletions of 13q have been identified using molecular techniques, even in cases without cytogenetic changes. This abnormality was thought to be at the site of the retinoblastoma (RB) suppressor gene but has since been shown to be telomeric to that region with a novel suppressor gene referred to as *DBM* (disrupted in B-cell malignancy).[58] An apparent correlation exists between the antiapoptotic protein Mcl-1 and resistance to chemotherapy.[59]

Considerable interest has focused on the *ATM* gene, which is mutated in patients with ataxia telangiectasia, who are at an increased risk for developing lymphoid neoplasms. The *ATM* gene is located at chromosome 11q22-23 and encodes for a high-molecular-weight protein that is involved in cell-cycle control, DNA repair, and DNA recombination. However, only a subset of patients with deletions at 11q22-23 show mutations in the coding region of the remaining ATM allele,[60] suggesting a pathogenetic role for other genes.

Abnormalities of p53 occur in at least 15% of patients and are associated with a higher percentage of prolymphocytes, advanced stage, chemoresistance, and a poorer outcome.[61–63]

DIAGNOSIS

Most patients with CLL are asymptomatic at presentation, and the diagnosis is often made when lymphocytosis is noted at the

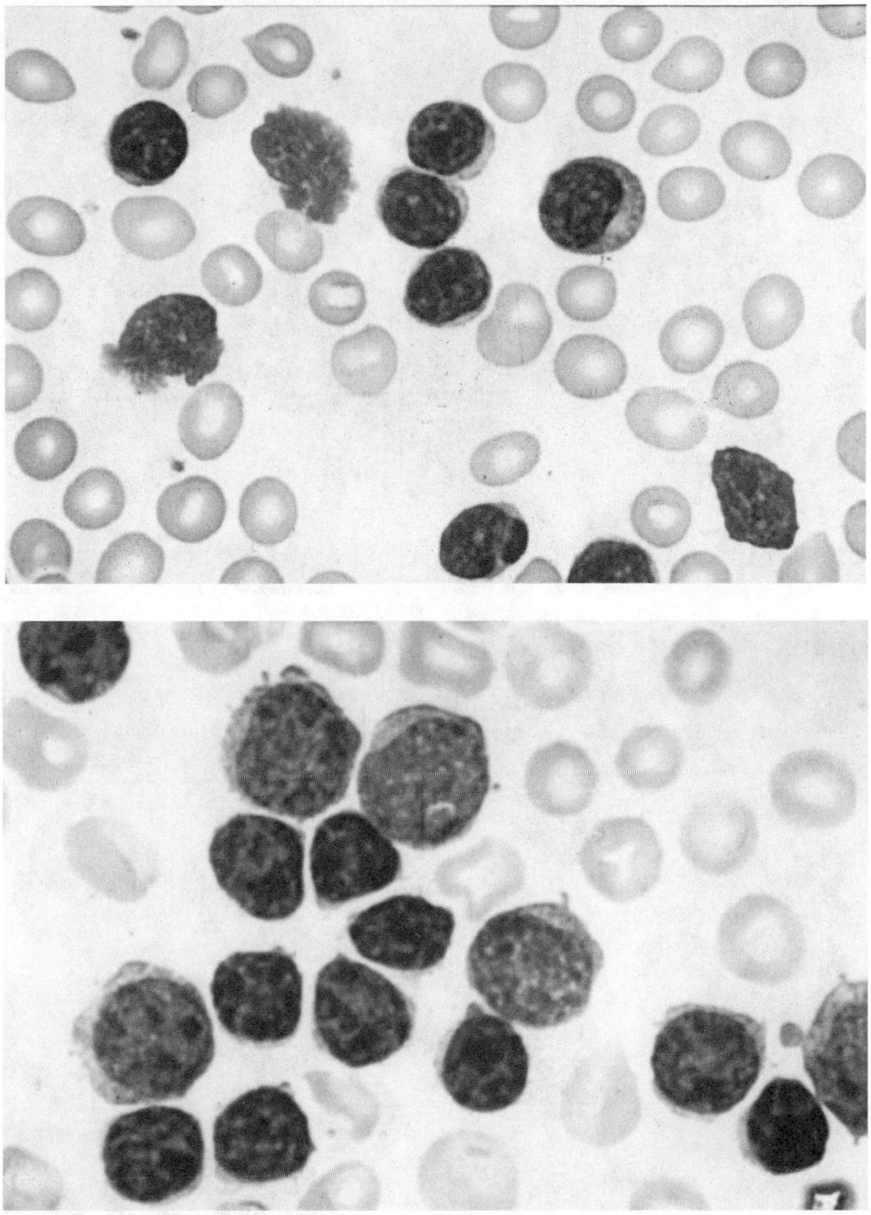

FIGURE 46.3.2-1. Morphologic and immunophenotypic characteristics, respectively, of **(A)** chronic lymphocytic leukemia (small, compact nucleus; no visible nucleoli; homogeneous cells; sIg dim, CD19+, CD20+, CD23+, CD5+, CD103–, CD10–); **(B)** prolymphocytic leukemia (larger, prominent nucleoli; mixed population; sIg+, CD19+, CD20+, CD5+/–, CD23+/–, CD103–, CD10–). (*Figure continues*)

time of a routine complete blood cell count. Physical examination is normal in 20% to 30% of patients at presentation. As the disease progresses, however, generalized adenopathy and splenomegaly are common.

The diagnosis of CLL requires more than 5000 per μL of small, mature-appearing lymphocytes circulating in the peripheral blood that are unexplained by other clinical disorders. The bone marrow aspirate and biopsy are infiltrated by at least 30% lymphocytes. A bone marrow aspirate and biopsy are rarely required to make the diagnosis of CLL, but they may provide prognostic information and are valuable for assessing response to therapy.[64,65]

The immunophenotype of CLL cells readily distinguishes CLL from other disorders associated with increased numbers of circulating atypical lymphoid cells [e.g., prolymphocytic leukemia (PLL), hairy cell leukemia (HCL), and hairy cell variant (HCL_V)], from non-Hodgkin's lymphomas (NHL) in a leukemic phase (e.g., lymphoplasmacytic lymphomas; marginal zone NHL, including splenic lymphoma with villous lymphocytes; mantle cell NHL), and from plasma cell leukemia[66] (Fig. 46.3.2-1). CLL lymphocytes are monoclonal B cells that express CD19, CD20, CD23, and CD5, along with low levels of surface immunoglobulin (sIg). T-cell antigens (e.g., CD2, CD3) are absent.[66] Mouse red blood cell rosettes on peripheral blood lymphocytes are characteristic of CLL, but this test is no longer routinely performed. In an occasional patient, CLL B cells express additional antigens more characteristic of hairy cells, monocytes, or myeloid cells.[17,67] Immunoglobulin heavy-chain gene rearrangements are invariably present but are not required to make the diagnosis.[68] Disorders characterized by CD5– chronic lymphocy-

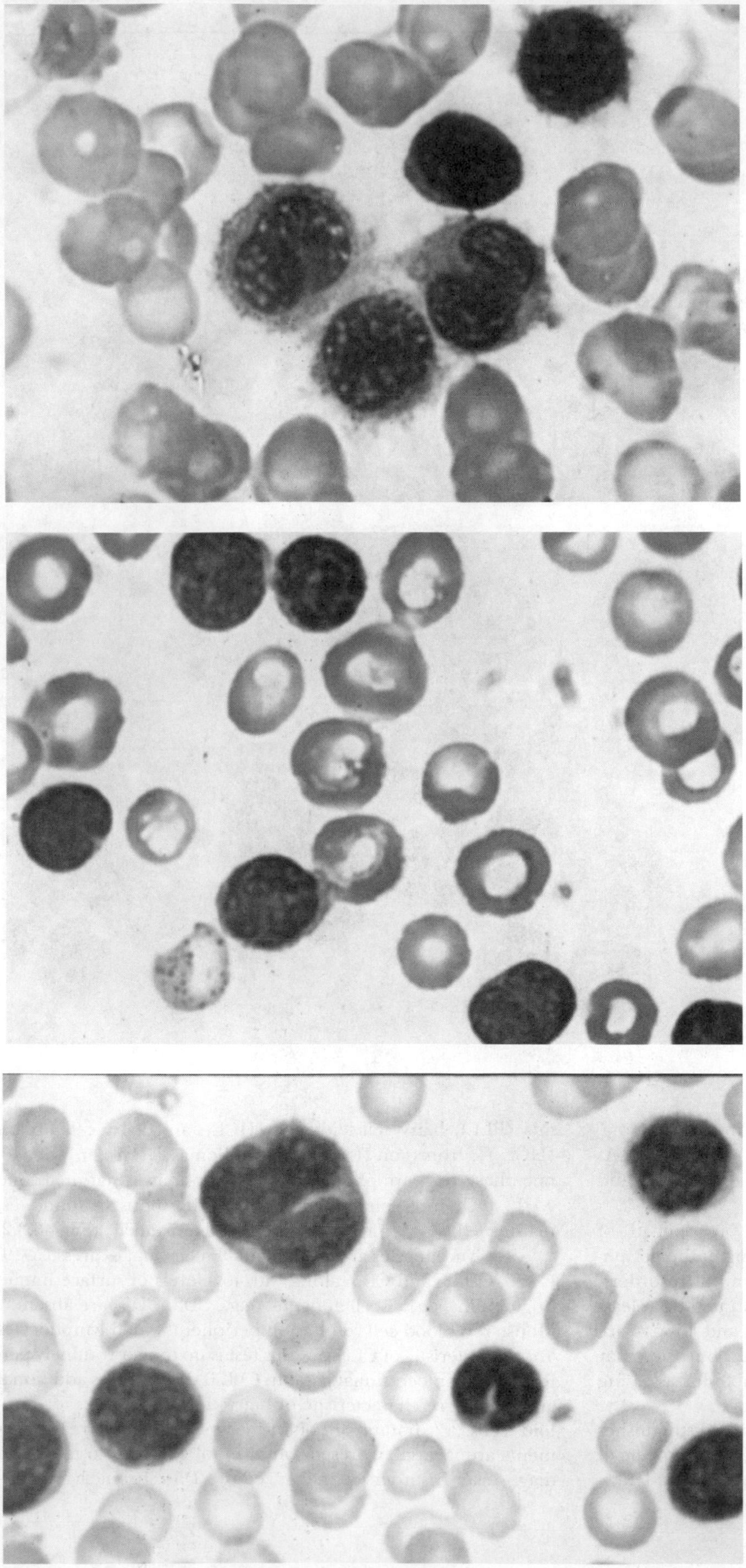

C

D

E

FIGURE 46.3.2-1. *(Continued)* **(C)** hairy cell leukemia (filamentous projections; sIg+, CD19+, CD20+, CD23–, CD5–, CD103+, CD10–); **(D)** follicular small cleaved cell lymphoma (small, cleaved cells; SIg+; CD19+, CD20+, CD5–, CD10+/–, CD23–); and **(E)** mantle cell lymphoma (small to medium cleaved; sIg+, CD19+, CD20+, CD23–, CD5–,CD103–, CD10+). sIg, surface immunoglobulin. (See Color Fig. 46.3.2-1 in the CD-ROM and on the Web at www.LWWoncology.com.)

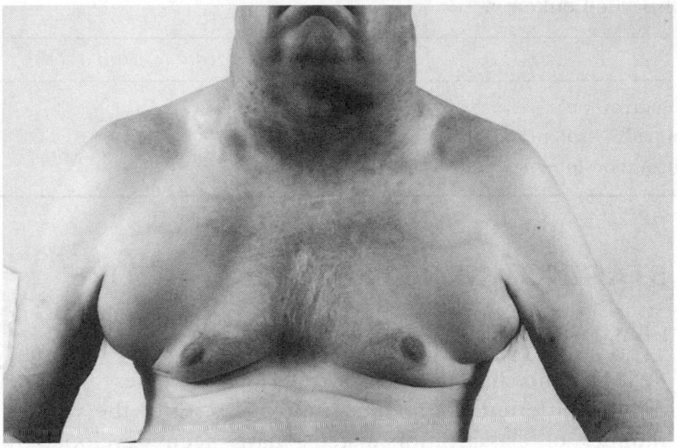

FIGURE 46.3.2-2. Pronounced cervical, supraclavicular, and axillary lymphadenopathy in a patient with chronic lymphocytic leukemia. (See Color Fig. 46.3.2-2 in the CD-ROM and on the Web at www.LWWoncology.com.)

tosis should not be considered CLL because they differ in immunologic, molecular, and functional features.[69]

CLINICAL FEATURES

CLINICAL PRESENTATION

Patients with CLL are generally symptomatic at presentation, and the diagnosis is often made incidentally when a lymphocytosis is noted at the time of a routine evaluation. Physical examination is normal at presentation in 20% to 30% of patients, with lymphadenopathy or hepatosplenomegaly, or both, noted in an additional 40% to 50% of patients. As the disease progresses, however, generalized adenopathy and splenomegaly become common features of this disease (Fig. 46.3.2-2). Pulmonary and central nervous system involvement are uncommon.[70,71]

INFECTIONS

Hypogammaglobulinemia is common in CLL, especially in patients with advanced disease. The increased susceptibility to infections reflects an inability to produce specific antibodies and abnormal activation of the complement system.[36] Historically, the most common pathogens were those that require opsonization for bacterial killing, such as *Streptococcus pneumoniae, Staphylococcus aureus,* and *Haemophilus influenzae.* The increased use of immunosuppressive agents, such as fludarabine, 2-chlorodeoxyadenosine (2-CdA), and 2'-deoxycoformycin (DCF), has markedly altered the spectrum of pathogens encountered in patients with CLL, with an increase in infections seen with opportunistic organisms such as *Candida, Listeria, Pneumocystis carinii, Cytomegalovirus, Aspergillus,* Herpesvirus infections, and others that were rarely encountered before the widespread use of nucleoside analogues.[72–75] A febrile patient with CLL receiving one of the new nucleoside analogues can no longer be assumed to have a common bacterial pathogen, and aggressive diagnostic measures may be required. Prophylactic antimicrobial regimens cannot be routinely recommended for all fludarabine-treated patients because the broad spectrum of potential pathogens would require multiple, potentially toxic drugs. However, such regimens should be considered for patients with extensive prior therapy, who have failed fludarabine, who have a history of recurrent infections, or are on corticosteroids.[75,76]

High-dose intravenous immunoglobulins have been evaluated for their ability to prevent infections in CLL.[77] Although a reduction in the total number of bacterial infections is reported with this treatment, these are primarily of trivial to moderate severity, with no decrease in the total number of major infections, either viral or fungal, or in the number of patients experiencing an infection, and with no improvement in overall survival. The prophylactic use of intravenous immunoglobulins is not cost-effective[78] and should be reserved for select patients with documented, repeated bacterial infections.[79]

Whether myeloid growth factors can protect against chemotherapy-induced myelosuppression has not yet been demonstrated.[80] In one study,[81] the use of granulocyte colony-stimulating factor to support fludarabine therapy reduced the occurrence of pneumonias but not other forms of severe infections.

AGGRESSIVE TRANSFORMATION

Approximately 3% to 15% of CLLs evolve into a more aggressive lymphoid malignancy. The most common of these is Richter's syndrome, which was initially described in 1928 by Maurice Richter.[82] He reported a 46-year-old man with CLL who experienced a rapid clinical deterioration characterized by lymphocytosis, massive and diffuse adenopathy, hepatosplenomegaly, and abdominal discomfort. At autopsy, large abdominal and retroperitoneal lymph nodes were infiltrated not only by small lymphocytes, but with larger cells, which reflected the large cell lymphoma component. Additional cases were subsequently reported by Lortholary et al.,[83] who designated the entity as Richter's syndrome. Richter's syndrome develops in approximately 5% of CLL patients.[84] Patients characteristically present with increasing lymphadenopathy, hepatosplenomegaly, fever, abdominal pain, weight loss, progressive anemia, and thrombocytopenia, with a rapid rise in the peripheral blood lymphocyte count. A lymph node biopsy reveals a large cell lymphoma. This transformation is not clearly related to either the nature or the extent of prior therapy. The large cell lymphoma shares immunologic, cytogenetic, and molecular features with the original CLL clone in one-half of the cases.[85–87] Nucleic acid sequence analysis of the heavy- and light-chain–variable region supports the theory that Richter's syndrome is derived from the same malignant clone in most patients.[88,89] Response of patients with Richter's syndrome to systemic therapy is poor, with a median survival of 4 to 5 months using alkylating agents, but may be longer with nucleoside analogue–based regimens.[84,90]

CLL may also evolve over the years into PLL. This transformation is associated with progressive anemia and thrombocytopenia, with at least 55% prolymphocytes in the peripheral blood.[91] Clinical features include lymphadenopathy, hepatosplenomegaly with a wasting syndrome, and an increasing resistance to therapy.

Anecdotal reports have been published of a transformation to acute lymphoblastic leukemia, plasma cell leukemia, multiple myeloma, or Hodgkin's disease.[91–93]

TABLE 46.3.2-1. Modified Rai Staging System for Chronic Lymphocytic Leukemia

Rai Stage	*Three-Stage System*	*Clinical Features*	*Median Survival (Y)*
0	Low risk	Lymphocytosis in blood and marrow only	>10
I/II	Intermediate risk	Lymphocytosis + lymphadenopathy + splenomegaly ± hepatomegaly	7
III/IV	High risk	Lymphocytosis + anemia + thrombocytopenia	2–4

AUTOIMMUNITY

A positive Coombs' antiglobulin test may be present in 20% to 30% of cases of CLL, with clinical hemolysis in 10% to 25% of patients.[94,95] The frequency of immune thrombocytopenia appears to be approximately 2%.[94,95] The immune hemolysis is more often related to a warm-reactive than a cold antibody. In most cases, these antibodies are polyclonal and, therefore, not produced by the malignant B cells.[21,96] This phenomenon probably reflects impaired interactions among the malignant B cells, normal B cells, and T cells.[21] However, two V_H genes have been shown to be preferentially expressed in cells from CLL patients with warm-reacting antibodies: 51pl/DP-10 gene and a DP-50 gene.[97,98] These observations suggest that, whereas the antibodies that are produced by the CLL are not involved in the red blood cell destruction, they may still be involved in the pathogenesis of the autoimmune hemolytic anemia.

Autoimmune anemia, or thrombocytopenia, generally responds to corticosteroids, such as prednisone, 60 to 100 mg/d, which may be tapered after 1 or 2 weeks after evidence of response. Patients who are unresponsive to corticosteroids may respond to high-dose intravenous immunoglobulins using an initial loading dose daily for 5 days followed by 0.4 g/kg every 3 weeks. Splenectomy may be considered when systemic approaches fail.[99] Splenic irradiation induces only transient responses. Rituximab has been associated with dramatic responses (B. Cheson, unpublished observation).

PURE RED BLOOD CELL APLASIA

Pure red blood cell aplasia has been reported to occur in up to 6% of cases of CLL, although that figure is likely an overestimate.[100] This complication is characterized by severe anemia (hematocrit generally less than 21%) without a reticulocyte response or bone marrow normoblasts and in the absence of neutropenia or thrombocytopenia. Corticosteroids may induce transient responses. Chemotherapy increases the hematocrit in the majority of patients with a response of the CLL. Cyclosporine A, with or without concurrent corticosteroids, may also achieve responses, often within 2 to 3 weeks and without requiring a reduction in tumor mass.[101]

SECOND MALIGNANCIES

Secondary malignancies occur with increased frequency in patients with CLL, related both to the immune defects of the disease as well as the consequences of therapy.[102–108] The most common tumors are lung cancers and melanomas; others include Hodgkin's disease, essential thrombocythemia, multiple myeloma, and acute myeloid leukemia. Coincidence of CLL and chronic myeloid leukemia also has been observed[109,110] (B. Cheson, unpublished observation).

STAGING AND PROGNOSTIC FACTORS

STAGING SYSTEMS

CLL patients have markedly differing outcomes and may require different therapeutic approaches. Over the years, a number of classification systems have been developed to organize CLL patients into risk groups.[111–113] The first widely accepted attempt to identify various prognostic groups of patients was the five-stage Rai classification (Table 46.3.2-1): Stage 0 includes patients with only lymphocytosis (median survival, more than 12.5 years); stage I patients also have lymphadenopathy (median survival, 8.5 years); stage II is characterized by splenomegaly with or without hepatomegaly (median survival, 6 years); stage III includes anemia (not related to hemolysis) (median survival, 2 to 4 years); and stage IV includes thrombocytopenia (median survival, 2 to 4 years).[114] This system was subsequently simplified to three stages: low risk (stage 0), intermediate risk (stages I–II), and high risk (stages III–IV)[115] (Fig. 46.3.2-3). In Europe a few years later, Binet described his three-stage stage system: Stage A patients have fewer than three node-bearing areas (median survival, more than 10 years); stage B patients have three or more node-bearing areas (median survival, 5 years); and stage C patients have anemia and/or thrombocytopenia (median survival, 2 years)[116] (Table 46.3.2-2). The Rai classification is the most commonly used in the United States, whereas the Binet system is often applied in Europe. A major difference between the two systems is the failure of the Binet system to identify Rai stage 0 patients, who have a 10-year survival rate of approximately 60%. Binet stage A patients include all Rai 0, two-thirds of Rai I, and one-third of Rai II. Neither system identifies patients with lymphocytosis and splenomegaly without lymphadenopathy. Nevertheless, the two systems have similar prognostic value. Other staging systems do not appear to provide an advantage over the two already in widespread use.[117,118]

At diagnosis, approximately 20% to 30% of patients are Rai stage 0, and 70% to 80% of patients are in low- or intermediate-risk groups in both the Rai and Binet classifications.[5,106,114,116,118–122]

PROGNOSIS

Clinical features and laboratory studies are used to predict survival in CLL. Montserrat and coworkers[123,124] were the first to use the term *smoldering CLL* to distinguish patients with early-stage disease who were unlikely to progress from those who were more likely to require treatment. The laboratory features included a hemoglobin of 12 g% or higher, a lymphocyte count of less than 30,000 cells per μL, a platelet count of more than 150,000 cells per μL, and a nondiffuse pattern of bone marrow involvement with fewer than 80% lymphocytes.

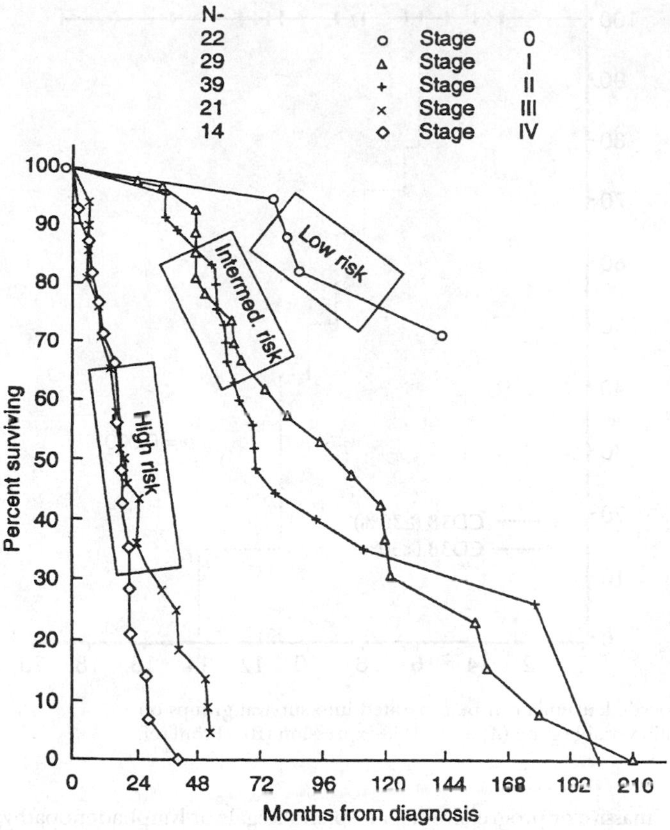

FIGURE 46.3.2-3. Simplification of the five-stage Rai classification into three risk groups based on survival. Stage 0, low risk; stages I and II, intermediate risk; stages III and IV, high risk.

A rapid lymphocyte doubling time appears to be a better predictor of a poor outcome than the absolute number of circulating lymphocytes.[124,125]

In more than one-half of CLL cases, the bone marrow is diffusely infiltrated by small lymphocytes; in the remaining patients, the pattern of infiltration is nodular, interstitial, or a mixture of the two. The diffuse pattern has been suggested to be a strong independent adverse prognostic factor,[121] although this finding does not clearly add to clinical stage.[5,126–129]

Additional features associated with a shorter survival include male gender, black race, poor performance status, abnormal liver chemistries, decreased serum albumin, and vertebral bone marrow involvement detected by magnetic resonance imaging.[106,118,130,131]

Of the numerous immunologic characteristics that have been evaluated, soluble CD23 and serum β_2-microglobulin appear to have a particularly strong predictive value.[132–137] Others include the function of various lymphocyte subpopulations,[138] expression of surface IgM, FMC7, loss of CD23, increased serum levels of soluble CD54,[139–145] and soluble IL-2 receptors.[23,24]

A serum or urine paraprotein can be detected in more than 60% of cases of CLL, including the presence of Bence Jones proteinuria,[146,147] but the level of paraprotein does not appear to have prognostic value. There has been no consistent relationship between hypogammaglobulinemia and survival among series.[118,142,148,149]

Cytogenetic and molecular studies best predict outcome in CLL. Patients with 13q abnormalities experience the longest survival and rarely require therapy, whereas complex abnormalities are associated with the poorest outcome.[43] Deletions of the long arm of chromosome 11 (11q21-25) tend to occur in patients who are younger and have more aggressive disease; peripheral, abdominal, and mediastinal adenopathy; advanced stage; and a shorter survival. Trisomy 12 has a prognosis that is intermediate between the two. Cytogenetic studies are not recommended as part of the routine evaluation of the patient with CLL because they are expensive, difficult to perform, and most important, we do not yet know how to apply the information to treatment decisions.

Although BCL-2 expression has not uniformly correlated with outcome, the ratio of BCL-2 to BAX favors survival in CLL cells with enhanced *in vitro* cell survival and correlates with clinical resistance to chemotherapy and clinical outcome.[150–152] P53 deletions predict for poor response to therapy with fludarabine or pentostatin.[62]

Studies[49,50] have shown a strong independent correlation between V_H gene mutations, CD38 expression, and survival. The V_H mutation status distinguishes more primitive from more mature B cells and appears to separate CLL patients into markedly distinct prognostic groups (Fig. 46.3.2-4).

TABLE 46.3.2-2. Binet Staging System for Chronic Lymphocytic Leukemia

Stage	*Clinical Features*	*Median Survival (Y)*
A	Fewer than three areas of clinical lymphadenopathy; no anemia or thrombocytopenia	12
B	Three or more involved node areas; no anemia or thrombocytopenia	7
C	Hemoglobin ≤10 g/dL and/or <100,000 platelets per μL	2

THERAPY

Patients with low-risk CLL often do not require therapy for many years after diagnosis and eventually die of apparently unrelated causes. Anecdotal reports of transient spontaneous remissions also have been published.[153,154] Many patients with intermediate-risk disease may remain stable for many years as well, whereas others may die from disease-related complications within a few months of diagnosis, despite appropriate therapy. Most patients with high-risk CLL need treatment at diagnosis.

INITIAL APPROACH TO THE PATIENT WITH CHRONIC LYMPHOCYTIC LEUKEMIAS

Currently available therapies do not cure patients with CLL[155] (Fig. 46.3.2-5), yet they may be associated with substantial toxicities. Moreover, early intervention has not been shown to benefit patients with early-stage disease.[107,156–159] The French Cooperative Group on CLL conducted two studies in patients with Binet stage

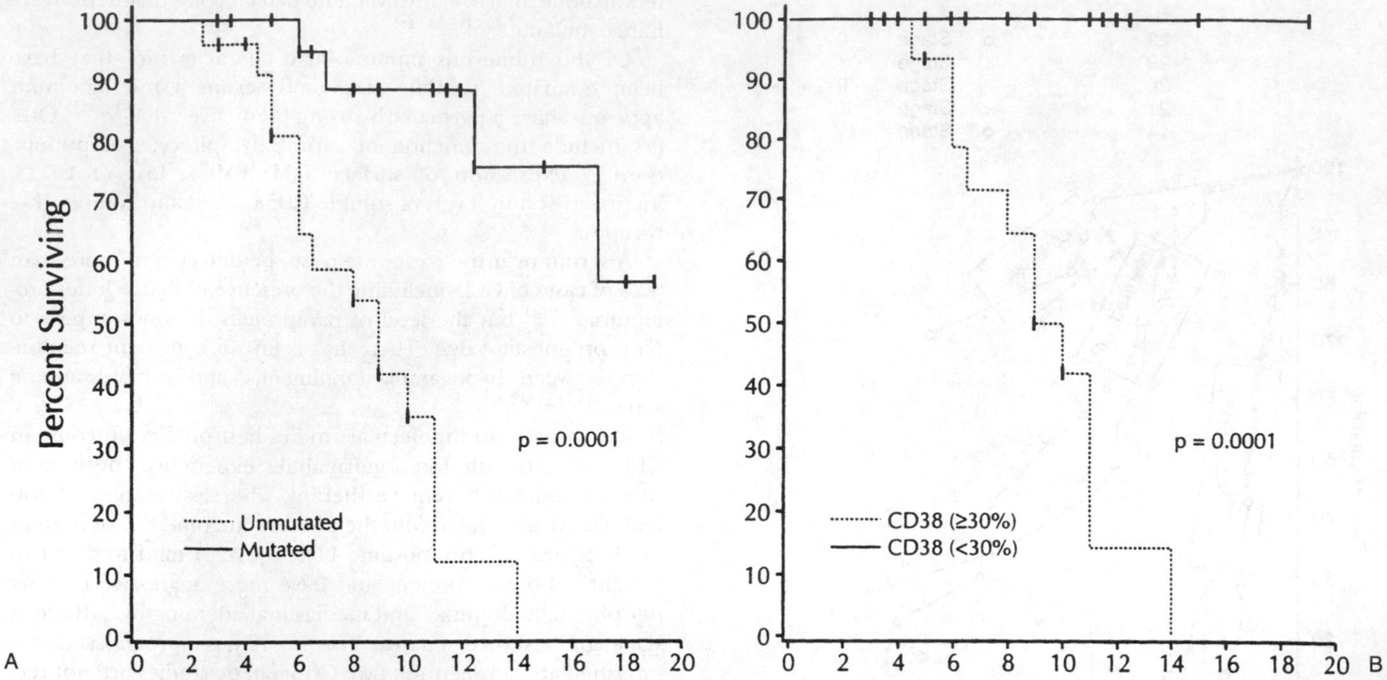

FIGURE 46.3.2-4. Patients with chronic lymphocytic leukemia can be separated into survival groups on the basis of the mutational status of the immunoglobulin variable gene **(A)** and CD38 expression **(B)**. (From ref. 50, with permission.)

A disease.[107,158] In the first study, patients were randomized to daily oral chlorambucil or observation. In the second trial, patients received either intermittent chlorambucil plus prednisone or no initial treatment. Neither study detected an advantage to early intervention. Moreover, a greater number of fatal, secondary solid tumors were reported in the first study, which was not noted in the study using an intermittent drug schedule.[158] Therefore, therapy should not be initiated in patients with early-stage CLL without specific indications, which include disease-related symptoms (e.g., fevers, chills, weight loss, pronounced fatigue); increasing bone marrow failure with anemia and/or thrombocytopenia, autoimmune anemia, or thrombocytopenia; massive or progressive hepatosplenomegaly or lymphadenopathy; and recurrent infections.[65] An elevated lymphocyte count alone is not sufficient to prompt therapy; however, a lymphocyte doubling time of less than 6 months may support the decision to treat.[5,125]

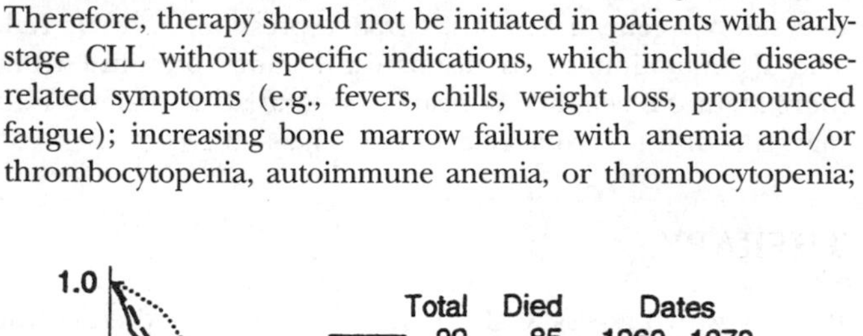

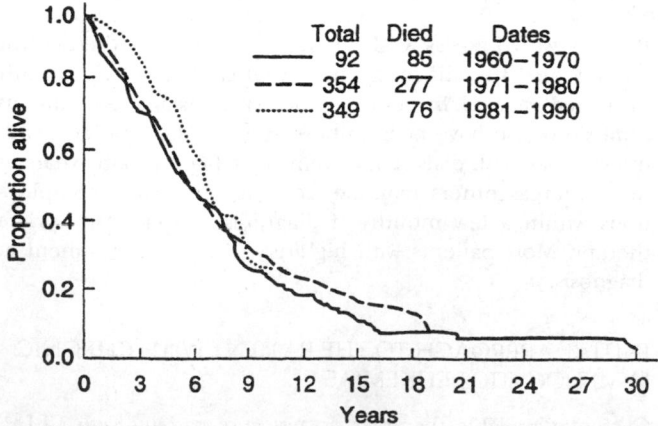

FIGURE 46.3.2-5. Survival of 741 previously untreated patients seen at the M. D. Anderson Cancer Center over three decades, ending in 1990, demonstrating a lack of any incremental improvement in survival with therapies available during that period. (From ref. 155, with permission.)

SINGLE-AGENT CHEMOTHERAPY

The most active classes of chemotherapy drugs in CLL are alkylating agents, such as chlorambucil and cyclophosphamide, and the nucleoside analogues fludarabine, 2-CdA, and DCF (pentostatin).[155,160,161] When chlorambucil is administered orally, either at a dose of 4 to 8 mg/m^2 daily for 4 to 8 weeks, or as pulses of 15 to 30 mg/m^2 every 2 to 4 weeks, responses are attained in approximately 30% to 70% of previously untreated patients, although few of these are complete responses.[157,162,163] The activity of cyclophosphamide appears to be similar to chlorambucil, but it is generally used only when chlorambucil has failed or is poorly tolerated, and in combination regimens.

Corticosteroids are less active than alkylating agents in CLL and should be reserved for patients with autoimmune complications because of the risks of bacterial, viral, and fungal infections; diabetes; and osteoporosis.

PURINE ANALOGUES

Fludarabine (2-fluoro-ara-adenosine monophosphate) is the most active agent for the treatment of CLL (Table 46.3.2-3). The currently recommended schedule of administration of fludarabine is as an intravenous bolus of 25 mg/m^2 daily for 5 consecutive days once a month. Patients failing to respond to two or three courses should be switched to an alternative treatment. Patients who achieve a complete response probably do not warrant additional treatment. For those patients with a par-

TABLE 46.3.2-3. Purine Analogues in Chronic Lymphocytic Leukemia

Study	*Number of Patients*	*Prior Therapy*	*Response Rate (%)* CR	PR
Fludarabine				
Grever et al. 1988[164]	32	+	3	9
Keating et al. 1993[165]	78	+	14 (24)	19
	35	–	37 (37)	6^b
O'Brien et al. 1993[166]	169	+	37	15^b
	95	–	63	16^b
Whelan et al.[a] 1991[167]	15	+	0	20
Hiddemann et al.[a] 1991[100]	20	+	20	35
French Cooperative Group 1996[169]	48	+	18	25
Leporrier et al. 1997[170]	225	–	23	44
Rai et al. 1996[163]	166	–	27	43
Montserrat et al. 1996[171]	68	+	4	28
Sorensen et al. 1997[172]	703	+	3	29
2-CdA				
Saven et al. 1991[160]	90	+	4	40
Juliusson et al. 1993[173]	18	+	39^b	28
Tallman et al. 1995[174]	26	+	0	31
Delannoy et al. 1995[175]	19	–	47	27
Saven et al. 1995[176]	20	–	10	75
Robak et al. 1996[177]	18	–	16	55
	92	+	5	30
Rondelli et al. 1997[178]	19	+	11	57
Robak et al. 1999[179]	46	–	41	50
	67	+	3	22
Robak et al. 1999[180]	43	10	30	40
DCF				
Grever et al. 1985[181]	25	+	4	16
O'Dwyer[182]	29	NS	3	21
Dillman et al. 1989[161]	39	26	3	23
Ho et al. 1990[183]	26	+	0	27
Dearden and Catovsky 1990[184]	17	+	0	35

+, yes; –, no; 2-CdA, 2-chlorodeoxyadenosine; CR, complete response; DCF, 2'-deoxycoformycin; NS, not specified; PR, partial response. Numbers in parentheses indicate "nodular complete remissions" (see section Second-Line Therapy for definition and discussion).
[a]Group C and special exception cases.
[b]Includes nodular CRs.

TABLE 46.3.2-4. Comparisons between Fludarabine and Alkylating Agent Regimens as Initial Therapy of Chronic Lymphocytic Leukemia

Study	*Number of Patients*	*CR/RR*	*DFS*	*OS*
IWCLL[169]	100	–	+	–
Rai et al. 1996[163]	544	+	+	–
Leporrier et al. 1997[170]	695	+	+	±
Spriano et al. 1999[191]	150	+	+	NR

+, significant fludarabine advantage; –, no difference; ±, borderline; CR, complete response; DFS, disease-free survival; IWCLL, International Working Group on Chronic Lymphocytic Leukemia; NR, not reported; OS, overall survival; RR, rate response

tial response, therapy is continued to best response plus two additional courses, not exceeding 1 year of therapy because of concerns of cumulative myelotoxicity. Other schedules have not been as active.[185–187] The oral bioavailability of fludarabine is 50% to 60%, and an oral formulation is in clinical trials.[188]

Fludarabine induces complete remissions in approximately 30% of previously untreated patients, with an overall response rate higher than 70%.[163,165,166,169,170] In a long-term follow-up of a large, single institution series, the median time to progression of responders was 31 months, and the overall median survival was 74 months.[189] Those who achieve an immunophenotypic and molecular complete remission appear to experience a longer survival than those with only a clinical and hematologic remission.[190]

Fludarabine has been compared with an alkylating agent–based regimen in several phase III trials[163,169,170,191] (Table 46.3.2-4).

In a North American Intergroup study, 544 untreated patients with advanced-stage, active disease were randomized to either fludarabine at the standard dose, chlorambucil (40 mg/m^2 single dose), or a combination of the two agents (fludarabine 20 mg/m^2 daily for 5 days; chlorambucil 20 mg/m^2 day 1) every 4 weeks for up to 12 months. Patients who were unsuccessful with one of the single agents were crossed over to receive the alternate drug. The 167 patients in the fludarabine group had an overall response rate of 70%, including 27% complete remissions, which was significantly higher than with chlorambucil (43% responses, 3% complete remissions; $P < .0001$). The duration of response was 32 months with fludarabine versus 18 months with chlorambucil ($P = .0002$), with a median progression-free survival of 27 months with fludarabine and 17 months for chlorambucil ($P < .0001$). However, no apparent prolongation of survival was reported, related in part to the crossover design of the study. The combination arm was prematurely closed because it was more toxic with no likelihood of being more effective than fludarabine alone.

A European collaborative group randomized 196 patients with stage A (2), B (104), or C (89) to either fludarabine or one of two anthracycline-based regimens [cyclophosphamide, doxorubicin, and prednisone (CAP) or cyclophosphamide, doxorubicin, vincristine, and prednisone (CHOP)].[169] A higher response rate was attained with fludarabine in the untreated patients, although the difference was not significant. The advantage for fludarabine was significant for remission duration, with a trend toward a survival advantage ($P = .087$). In a subsequent trial by the International Working Group on CLL, including 486 stage B and 209 stage C patients,[170] a complete hematologic remission was observed in 37% of the fludarabine group, 28% of the CHOP group, and 13% of the CAP-treated patients. The differences were significant between fludarabine and CAP and between CHOP and CAP ($P < .0001$) in response and survival, but not between fludarabine and CHOP ($P = .15$). Nevertheless, fewer deaths were reported in the fludarabine group, resulting in a significant survival advantage ($P = .05$).

These results establish fludarabine as the preferred initial treatment for most patients with CLL. However, for patients who are elderly or those who have a reduced performance status or an active infection, chlorambucil may be a reasonable first-line treatment option. Another alternative is a 3-day schedule of fludarabine, which appears to be almost as active but has fewer associated toxicities.[187]

The major toxicities associated with fludarabine at the currently used schedules are moderate myelosuppression and severe immunosuppression, with occasional neurotoxicity, particularly at higher than recommended doses.[74,192,193] Lymphocyte counts decrease within weeks, particularly CD4 cells, which do not return to normal for 1 year or longer after treatment has been discontinued.[74,166] Fludarabine has not been found to be more myelotoxic but has been associated with more opportunistic infections than alkylating agent regimens.[163,169]

Tumor lysis syndrome is a rare complication of treatment of CLL with alkylating agents, radiation, combination chemotherapy, or fludarabine.[194]

Approximately 55% to 85% of patients who are treated with 2-CdA as their initial therapy respond to this agent, but only 10% to 15% achieve complete remissions, and the duration of response appears to be shorter than reported for fludarabine[176,177,195] (see Table 46.3.2-3). Data with pentostatin as initial therapy are insufficient to assess its level of activity[161] (see Table 46.3.2-3).

COMBINATION REGIMENS

Combination regimens are not clearly superior to single-agent therapy for CLL.[157,169,196–202] The most commonly used multiagent regimens include chlorambucil plus prednisone (CP) or cyclophosphamide, vincristine, and prednisone (CVP). CP and CVP induce responses in fewer than 10% to more than 60% of previously untreated patients, although few of these responses are complete, and the median survival is shorter than 2 years.[157,162,196–198,203] The French Cooperative Group randomized 151 patients with Binet stage B CLL to indefinite daily oral chlorambucil and 140 patients to cyclophosphamide, Oncovin, and prednisone (COP). No difference was noted in response rate, reduction in clinical stage, or overall survival.[204]

More aggressive regimens that include multiple alkylating agents or anthracyclines also have not shown an advantage over less intensive programs.[170,201,202,205,206] One small randomized trial suggested a survival advantage for an attenuated CHOP regimen (including doxorubicin at 25 mg/m^2 every 4 weeks) over COP in a small number of patients with stage C disease.[199] Moreover, data from the same investigators suggest an advantage for CHOP over CAP.[170] However, several other randomized trials and a metaanalysis have not confirmed superiority for anthracycline-containing regimens.[157,159,198,200]

Combinations of fludarabine with chlorambucil, anthracyclines or related compounds, cytarabine, and IFN-α are not clearly better than fludarabine alone.[163,207–214] The addition of prednisone to fludarabine does not increase the response rate but is associated with more frequent opportunistic infections.[72,75,166] Preliminary encouraging data with combinations of fludarabine and cyclophosphamide have led to phase III studies.[215,216]

DCF has been combined with alkylating agents and steroids with high response rates but considerable toxicity.[217]

SECOND-LINE THERAPY

Treatment decisions for relapsed and refractory patients should be based on criteria similar to those used for initial management.[65] Because therapy is palliative in this setting, treatment should not be initiated unless it is clearly needed.

Patients with CLL who relapse after or are refractory to initial treatment should be referred to a clinical trial. For patients who are not eligible for or are unwilling to participate in clinical research, salvage therapy is determined by the initial treatment and response to that treatment. Alkylating agents and fludarabine remain the most widely used drugs in this setting. Most other cytotoxic drugs have failed to show activity.[218,219]

Patients who initially respond to an alkylating agent can often be successfully retreated with that agent; however, the quality of the subsequent response and its duration are usually inferior to the initial treatment.[196,201,205] Response rates with multiple alkylating agents of anthracycline-containing regimens are significantly lower as second-line therapy, with few complete remissions.[169,201,205]

Fludarabine has become the standard agent for treating patients unsuccessful with alkylating agents.[164,166–168,172,185,220,221] Grever et al.[164] were the first to report activity for fludarabine in a series of 32 previously treated patients. Although they achieved only 3% complete responses and 9% partial responses, a large number of other patients experienced major clinical improvement. When current response criteria were applied, the overall response rate was 45%.[65] Keating and coworkers[155,165,220,222] reported 57% complete responses and 36% partial responses of 28 relapsed patients, and 28% complete responses and 10% partial responses of 50 refractory patients (63% of complete responses had residual lymphoid nodules in the bone marrow) (see Table 46.3.2-3). The median time to progression was 18 months for patients who were refractory to alkylating agents and 17 months for patients who had relapsed after prior treatment. Lower response rates and durability of response were noted in patients with advanced-stage disease, extensive prior therapy, and poor performance status.[171,172] When compared with CAP as second-line therapy,[169] fludarabine was associated with a significantly higher response rate as well as a longer remission duration and survival, although these differences were not significant.

Re-treatment with fludarabine is successful in one-half of those patients whose initial response to fludarabine lasted 1 year or longer.[165,189] On the other hand, few effective therapeutic options are available to patients whose disease is refractory to fludarabine.[163,165]

2-Chlorodeoxyadenosine

In general, response rates with 2-CdA for relapsed and refractory patients are in the range of 30% to 40%, but with few complete remissions.[160,174,177] Saven et al.[160] reported 4% complete responses and 40% partial responses of 90 relapsed and refractory patients with CLL, with a median duration of response of 4 months (see Table 46.3.2-3). Variability in response rates among series reflect differences in drug administration schedule, patient selection, response criteria, and other factors.

2-CdA has limited activity in fludarabine failures.[223,224]

2′-Deoxycoformycin (Pentostatin)

Almost one-fourth of alkylating agent failures respond to DCF, although few of these responses are complete or durable[161,181,183,184,193,225–227] (see Table 46.3.2-3).

A few reports of combinations of DCF with other cytotoxic or biologic agents in CLL in relapsed patients have been published.[217,228]

OTHER CHEMOTHERAPY AGENTS

Despite the lack of single-agent data for cisplatin and cytarabine, these drugs have been incorporated into multidrug regimens, although their contribution to those regimens is unclear.[229–231] Theophylline appears to synergize with chlorambucil *in vitro* in inducing apoptosis and has shown clinical activity.[232–234]

Several newer agents are currently under investigation in CLL. Compound GW506U78, a prodrug for ara-G, is a new nucleoside analogue with impressive activity in a variety of hematologic malignancies.[235] Responses have been reported in patients with chronic B-cell and T-cell leukemias, even after failure with fludarabine and alkylating agents.[236,237] Interest in the use of arsenicals in CLL stems from several preclinical studies suggesting that arsenic induces apoptosis of malignant lymphocytes at clinical achievable doses.[238,239] The protein kinase C inhibitors bryostatin and UCN-01, the cyclin inhibitor flavopiridol, and the histone deacetylase inhibitor depsipeptide are being evaluated as single agents and in combinations.[240–244] A variety of *in vitro* observations suggest a potential role for antiangiogenesis agents.[245]

BIOLOGIC THERAPY

Interferon-α

IFN-α has limited activity in CLL, with transient partial responses in patients with limited-stage disease.[246–249] Preliminary data suggesting benefit for IFN maintenance after a response to induction chemotherapy with alkylating agents[246] were not confirmed in studies with fludarabine.[250,251]

Monoclonal Antibodies

Early studies with monoclonal antibodies targeting CD5 did not show adequate activity to pursue in larger trials.[252–254] However, several newer antibodies have shown considerable promise.

The CAMPATH-1H monoclonal antibody recognizes the CD52 antigen, which is present on B cells as well as T cells. This antibody has shown impressive activity against both in CLL and PLL.[255–259] Responses occur in approximately one-third of patients who have been unsuccessful with other treatments, including fludarabine.[260] This agent appears to be more active against peripheral blood and bone marrow involvement than nodal disease.

Rituximab (Rituxan) is an anti-CD20 antibody C2B8 with major activity against follicular lymphomas.[261] However, its activity using the recommended dose and schedule has not been impressive in patients with small lymphocytic leukemia or CLL, with response rates in the range of 10% to 15% and no complete remissions.[261–265] This lack of activity may reflect the dim expression of CD20 on CLL cells. Attempts are being made to improve on this activity by increasing the dose, altering the schedule of administration, or augmenting CD20 expression.[264,266–268] Rituximab may sensitize tumor cells to chemotherapy agents, and combinations of the antibody with fludarabine are in development. Patients with CLL who are treated with this antibody are at risk for potentially life-threatening toxicities characterized by cytokine release syndrome or rapid tumor clearance.[264,269]

The development of antibodies conjugated to radioisotopes, such as iodine 131 or yttrium 90, will be more difficult because of concerns that antibody localization in the bone marrow results in significant myelotoxicity.[270,271]

BONE MARROW TRANSPLANTATION

Allogeneic bone marrow transplantation has been performed to a limited extent in patients with CLL, primarily because these patients tend to be older and it has been difficult to eradicate the disease in the patient.[272–275] Although more than 70% of patients may be induced into a remission with bone marrow transplantation,[272,274,275] only approximately one-half of patients are alive and free of disease after long-term follow-up. The best outcome has been reported for patients with no evidence of minimal residual disease by polymerase chain reaction.[276] However, the treatment-related death rate has been approximately 30% to 50%, related to a high rate of graft-versus-host disease. Whereas some patients with advanced disease clearly benefit from bone marrow transplantation, the occurrence of late relapses raises questions as to how many patients are actually cured.

Submyeloablative preparative regimens, or “mini-transplants,” have been reported to induce successful engraftment without substantial acute graft-versus-host disease. The necessary immunosuppression is provided by a drug such as fludarabine, with a moderately myelosuppressive dose of cyclophosphamide.[277,278] This approach permits eligibility to older patients and those with impaired performance status or organ function. Further refinement of this technology is needed before it becomes a standard approach.

Autologous stem cell transplantation as currently performed has a limited role for patients with CLL, with the possible exception of patients who can be induced into a molecular remission.[272,273,276,279]

OTHER THERAPEUTIC MEASURES

Small, unconfirmed series have suggested a role for such treatments as leukopheresis[285] or photochemotherapy[286] in the management of CLL; however, these approaches have not been widely accepted.

Splenectomy

Splenectomy may play an important role in the palliative management of patients with CLL who have failed systemic treatment for autoimmune hemolytic anemia or thrombocytopenia, who have mechanical complications from splenomegaly that is unresponsive to chemotherapy, or in patients with hypersplenism who are tolerating chemotherapy poorly.[99] Splenectomy may also assist in making the diagnosis of a suspected Richter’s transformation. Thrombocytopenia is the most likely cell type to respond after splenectomy. When performed by an experienced surgeon, the mortality of the procedure is less than 10%.[99]

Radiation Therapy

Radiation therapy has a limited role in the current management of patients with CLL. Older studies suggesting therapeu-

TABLE 46.3.2-5. Revised National Cancer Institute Working Group Guidelines for Chronic Lymphocytic Leukemia

Diagnosis	*Criteria*
Lymphocytes (× 10⁹/L)	>5; ≥B-cell marker (CD19, CD20, CD23) + CD5
"Atypical" cells (%) (e.g., prolymphocytes)	<55
Duration of lymphocytosis	None required
Bone marrow lymphocytes (%)	≥30
Staging	Modified Rai
Eligibility for trials	"Active disease"
Response criteria	
Complete response	
Physical examination	Normal
Symptoms	None
Lymphocytes (× 10⁹/L)	≤4
Neutrophils (× 10⁹/L)	≥1.5
Platelets (× 10⁹/L)	>100
Hemoglobin (g/dL)	>11 (untransfused)
Bone marrow lymphs (%)	<30; no nodules
Partial response	
Physical examination (nodes and/or liver, spleen)	≥50% decrease
Plus one or more of:	
Neutrophils (× 10⁹/L)	≥1.5
Platelets (× 10⁹/L)	>100
Hemoglobin (g/dL)	>11 or 50% improvement
Duration of complete or partial remission	≥2 mo
Progressive disease	
Physical examination (nodes, liver, spleen)	≥50% increase or new
Circulating lymphocytes	≥50% increase
Other	Richter's syndrome
Stable disease	All others

tic benefit have not been substantiated, and it adds little benefit but considerable morbidity when combined with chemotherapy.[280,281] Splenic irradiation to palliate symptoms or in the treatment of autoimmune hemolytic anemia achieves only brief responses.[282–284]

ASSESSMENT OF RESPONSE TO THERAPY IN CHRONIC LYMPHOCYTIC LEUKEMIAS

Several sets of response criteria for CLL have been published.[287–289] The recommendations of the National Cancer Institute Sponsored Working Group on CLL, published first in 1988 and updated in 1996, are the most widely used for clinical research protocols (Table 46.3.2-5).[64,65] These guidelines standardized eligibility, response, and toxicity criteria; provided dose modifications for drug-related myelosuppression; and provided a grading system for infectious complications.

RELATED B-CELL LEUKEMIAS

PROLYMPHOCYTIC LEUKEMIA

PLL can occur either *de novo* or, less often, as a transformation from CLL. In contrast to the small, mature-appearing lymphocytes of CLL, PLL cells are large, with a round nucleus and a prominent nucleolus.[91–93,290] In *de novo* PLL, most of the peripheral blood mononuclear cells tend to be prolymphocytes; in PLL that has transformed from CLL, there is a dimorphic population of lymphocytes in the peripheral blood.[290,291]

Cells from patients with PLL exhibit immunologic differences from B-CLL cells. They may be CD5– and may express CD20 brightly. They lack mouse red blood cell rosettes and more frequently express FMC7.[139,292] In one-fourth of cases, the t(11;14) leads to the BCL-1 rearrangement, suggesting that these cases represent mantle cell lymphoma. A consistent chromosomal abnormality, t(6;12), has been reported in addition to the more common 14q+. A high frequency of somatic mutation in the Vh genes is expressed in PLL.[293] P53 abnormalities are identified in more than 50% of cases, which may confer drug resistance.[62]

Patients with *de novo* PLL tend to be older than those with transformed PLL. They are usually symptomatic and may experience a wasting syndrome. They are generally Rai stage III or IV at presentation, with marked splenomegaly and a higher white blood cell count but less lymphadenopathy. The clinical course tends to be aggressive. Nevertheless, the outcome for those patients who have transformed appears to be even worse. The median survival for *de novo* PLL has been reported to be 3 years, compared with only 9 months for those who have transformed from CLL to PLL. Patients with PLL tend to respond poorly to either single-agent or combination chemotherapy, with overall response rates of less than 25% and rare complete responses. Small series and anecdotal cases suggest impressive activity for fludarabine and pentostatin in refractory PLL[184,294–296] and for cladribine in previously untreated patients.[297]

HAIRY CELL LEUKEMIA

HCL was initially described by Bouroncle et al.[298] in 1958 and called *leukemic reticuloendotheliosis.* This chronic B-cell leukemia is characterized by splenomegaly and pancytopenia and, occasionally, lymphadenopathy.

HCL occurs in approximately 500 new patients each year in the United States, and it makes up 2% of all leukemias. It tends to occur in older persons, with a strong male predominance. Patients generally present with symptoms referable to cytopenias, including infections in 29% and weakness or fatigue in 27%. Less common presentations include left upper quadrant pain related to splenomegaly (5%) or bleeding related to thrombocytopenia (4%). Incidence of second malignancies is increased. The most common findings include palpable splenomegaly (72% to 86%), hepatomegaly (13% to 20%), hairy cells in the peripheral blood (85% to 89%), thrombocytopenia (fewer than 100,000 cells per mm^3, 53%), anemia (hemoglobin less than 12 cells per dL, 71% to 77%), and neutropenia (absolute neutrophil count less than 500 cells per mm^3, 32% to 39%).

The hairy cells generally have an eccentric, spongiform kidney-shaped nucleus, with characteristic filamentous cytoplasmic projections. Bone marrow biopsy is generally required to make the diagnosis, because the aspirate is often not obtainable. The malignant cells are of B-cell origin, expressing CD19, CD20, and the monocyte antigen CD11c. Perhaps the most specific marker is CD103. It is most difficult to distinguish HCL from HCL_v; the latter is often associated with a high circulating white blood cell count, cells containing bilobed nuclei with prominent nucleoli, and a typical bone marrow histology with interstitial infiltration of clumped cells.[299] An important distinguishing, almost diagnostic, feature is the resistance of this disease to treatment with IFN-α, cladribine, and pentostatin.[299]

HCL may be an indolent disorder, and 10% of patients may never require treatment. In most patents, however, treatment is eventually warranted because of massive or progressive splenomegaly, worsening blood counts, recurrent infections, more than 20,000 hairy cells per μL of peripheral blood, or bulky lymphadenopathy. Until the early 1980s, splenectomy was the standard treatment for HCL. In most patients, this procedure improves symptoms related to splenomegaly and peripheral blood counts, often for prolonged periods, but it does not affect the disease itself. Splenectomy now plays a minor role in the management of HCL and is reserved for the rare patient who is refractory to treatment and has splenomegaly that is either symptomatic or is resulting in cytopenias.

The first systemic therapy to demonstrate activity in HCL was IFN. At doses of 2×10^6 $U/m^2/d$ or 3×10^6 U three times per week, IFN produces responses in 80% of patients; however, only 10% of these are complete responses. Although responses generally occur within 3 to 4 months, it may take more than 1 year of therapy to achieve the maximal response. The leukemia invariably recurs after IFN therapy is discontinued, and maintenance therapy is associated with excessive toxicity and expense without any apparent survival benefit. Many patients who recur will again respond when retreated. IFN is associated with flu-like symptoms (fevers, myalgias, malaise) in almost all patients. Other toxicities include rash; application site disorders; and gastrointestinal symptoms, with nausea, vomiting, and anorexia. Reduced doses are associated with less toxicity but lower response rates.

The purine analogues have revolutionized the treatment of patients with HCL.[300,301] In 1984, Spiers et al.[302] first reported complete responses in patients with HCL treated with pentostatin. DCF at doses of 4 mg/m^2 intravenously every other week for 4 to 6 months achieves complete responses in 60% to 89% of previously treated or untreated patients, including those who have been unsuccessful with IFN, with overall response rates of 80% to 90%. Moreover, only 25% of patients have relapsed with more than 5 years of follow-up. In an intergroup trial, 350 previously untreated patients with HCL were randomized to IFN or DCF; the complete response rate was approximately 11% for IFN compared with 76% for DCF, with a significant advantage to DCF in the durability of response.[300]

In 1990, Piro et al.[301] reported 11 complete responses of 12 patients with HCL who had received a single 7-day continuous infusion of 2-CdA. Numerous studies have now confirmed that the original schedule or a 2-hour infusion for 5 to 7 days achieves responses in 80% to more than 90% of patients, including 65% to 80% complete remissions. These responses tend to be durable, with 20% to 30% of patients relapsing with prolonged follow-up. Relapse can be predicted by the demonstration of minimal residual disease using sensitive immunohistochemical methods.[303] In many cases, relapse is characterized only by an increase in bone marrow hairy cells, with no indication for treatment. Most patients who require re-treatment achieve a second durable response.

The results with DCF are equivalent to those with 2-CdA. However, the shorter duration of treatment makes 2-CdA somewhat more attractive, although no advantage exists with regard to toxicity.

New monoclonal antibodies have shown promise for patients with HCL who are unsuccessful with purine analogue therapy or for those with HCL_v.[304,305]

NON-HODGKIN'S LYMPHOMA IN A LEUKEMIC PHASE

Patients with NHL may present with or subsequently develop a leukemic picture,[306,307] most commonly those with a follicular small-cleaved cell histology, MCL, or marginal zone lymphoma. Although morphologic differences exist among these cells, immunophenotyping is necessary to distinguish among these entities.[66] Follicular NHL in a leukemic phase is characterized by cells that are small, with clefts and little or no visible cytoplasm, called *buttock cells.* These cells strongly express sIg, are positive for FMC7, CD22, and CD10, and are negative for CD5 and CD23.[17,66] The leukemic manifestation of MCL is characterized by a mixture of small- to medium-size lymphocytes with nuclei that are generally cleaved but may be nearly round, leading to a misdiagnosis of CLL or PLL and small lymphocytic leukemia. MCL cells also express CD5, but in contrast to CLL cells, they strongly express sIg but not CD23.[66]

Leukemic follicular small-cleaved cell lymphomas and mantle zone lymphomas have a median survival rate of 2.0 to 3.5 years and 2 years, respectively, whereas those derived from a large cell NHL have a median survival of only 1 to 3 months. Patients tend to respond poorly to therapy, including aggressive regimens such as CHOP. Anecdotal reports suggest activity for fludarabine in leukemic forms of low-grade NHL.

Splenic lymphoma with villous lymphocytes is a marginal-zone NHL that generally presents with significant splenomegaly, often with circulating cells exhibiting villous projections.[308,309] The diagnosis may not be apparent until the spleen is examined histologically after splenectomy. The malignant cells are larger than CLL cells and often contain a prominent nucleolus. They tend to stain positively for acid phosphatase, which is not tartrate resistant and which distinguishes them from HCL. The cells express B-cell markers, including CD19, CD20, CD22, SIg, and FMC-7. In contrast to CLL, they are negative for CD5 and CD23. Anemia and thrombocytopenia are common. A small concentration of an IgG or IgM monoclonal gammopathy can be detected in either the serum or urine from most cases. Fludarabine is active in this disorder.[310]

CHRONIC T-CELL LEUKEMIAS

The mature (postthymic) T-cell leukemia disorders consist of large granular lymphocytic leukemia (LGL), T-PLL, adult T-cell leukemia/lymphoma, and the Sézary syndrome. The chronic T-cell leukemias are a heterogeneous group of rare disorders that differ significantly from B-CLL with respect to their immunophenotype, virology, biology, morphology, and response to therapy. The term *T-cell CLL* is no longer used in current classification systems.[66]

Large Granular Lymphocytic Leukemia

LGL is the most common chronic T-cell leukemia.[311] The etiology of this clonal disorder is unknown. It is often diagnosed in the setting of an incidental T-cell lymphocytosis with more than 2000 circulating T cells per μL. The peripheral blood lymphoid cells demonstrate characteristic azurophilic granulation. Monoclonal antibodies directed against the V-gene region of the T-cell receptor gene and the p58 family on NK cells may help make the diagnosis.[312]

Proliferations of LGL may be either CD3+ (T-LGL) or CD3- (NK-LGL). Approximately 95% are CD4–/CD8+, although some cases may be CD4–/CD8–. T-LGL is the most common of these entities and occurs more often in women, with a median age of 57 years. Physical examination is notable for splenomegaly. Neutropenia is common and may be severe, with recurrent infections in 40% of patients. Peripheral blood NK cells are often decreased in numbers. The bone marrow is involved in almost all patients. There is a 30% incidence of rheumatoid arthritis, often with Felty's syndrome. Polyclonal hypergammaglobulinemia, rheumatoid factor, antinuclear antibodies, and circulating immune complexes are often present.[313] Pure red blood cell aplasia also has been reported. More than two-thirds of cases eventually require therapy, primarily because of recurrent infections. Responses may be achieved with alkylating agents, corticosteroids, or cyclosporine A. DCF and 2-CdA have shown activity.[314,315] Splenectomy is generally not associated with long-term benefit.

Disorders associated with an increase in NK cells form a spectrum, from more indolent NK-cell lymphocytosis to an aggressive NK-LGL leukemia/lymphoma. Chronic NK-cell lymphocytosis is a clonal disorder characterized by a sustained increase in cells with a CD3–/CD16+/CD2–/CD8+ phenotype.[316] The bone marrow is usually involved. The median age of patients with NK-LGL is 60 years, and the disease appears to be more common in men. Most patients note constitutional symptoms, but lymphadenopathy or splenomegaly are not common at presentation. Associated diseases include pure red blood cell aplasia and vasculitis syndromes. The outcome is similar to that of T-LGL. However, vasculitis and cytopenias may be life-threatening. Cyclophosphamide may be effective in controlling the vasculitis syndrome.[316] NK-LGL leukemia/lymphoma is an aggressive disease characterized by constitutional symptoms and splenomegaly. Response to therapy is poor, and the median survival rate is only a few months.

T-Cell Prolymphocytic Leukemia

T-PLL is characterized by massive splenomegaly, lymphadenopathy in 40% of patients, and skin infiltration in 20%.[317] The presenting white blood cell count often exceeds 100,000 cells per μL. The malignant cells generally express CD3, CD4, CD5, and CD7, but are negative for CD8– and CD25–, although one-third of cases are CD4+/CD8+ or CD4–/CD8+. There are no apparent clinical differences among these subsets. A consistent abnormality of chromosome 14 has been reported with two breakpoints at 14q11 and 14q32.[317]

The prognosis of T-PLL is poor, with a median survival of 7 months. The purine analogues are active agents; DCF has achieved complete responses in up to 10% of patients, with partial responses in one-third.[296,314] Response rates of more than 70% have been reported in small series with CAMPATH-1H in T-PLL, including almost 60% complete responses.[256]

Adult T-Cell Leukemia/Lymphoma

Adult T-cell leukemia/lymphoma occurs most commonly in patients from the Caribbean and southwestern islands of Japan.[318] This uncommon lymphoid malignancy is associated with infection with human T-cell leukemia virus type 1. The immunophenotype of the malignant cells includes CD2+, CD3+, CD5+, CD4+, CD8–, CD25++, and CD56/57–. The disease exhibits a clinical spectrum ranging from an indolent disease that may not require treatment for several years to an extremely aggressive disease characterized by anemia, hypercalcemia, bone lesions, splenomegaly, skin infiltration, central nervous system involvement, opportunistic infections, circulating leukemia cells, and a very poor outcome.[319,320] DCF has been used with modest success.[321,322]

Sézary Syndrome

One-third of patients with mycosis fungoides will have circulating malignant cells at diagnosis. The peripheral blood of patients with skin patches may reveal circulating cerebriform cells in 0% to 22%, in 9% to 30% of those with plaques, in 27% to 50% with skin tumors, and in 90% to 96% of those with erythroderma. The presence of circulating cells may be an independent negative prognostic factor. Treatment of this disorder is discussed in Chapter 45.4.

REFERENCES

1. Greenlee RT, Murray T, Bolden S, Wingo PA. Cancer statistics, 2000. *CA Cancer J Clin* 2000;50:7.
2. Surveillance Epidemiology and End Results (SEER) Program Report 1998.

3. Mauro FR, Foa R, Gianarelli D, et al. Clinical characteristics and outcome of young chronic lymphocytic leukemia patients: a single institution study of 204 cases. *Blood* 1999;94:448.
4. Sonnier JA, Buchanan GR, Howard-Peebles PN, Rutledge J, Graham Smith R. Chromosomal translocation involving the immunoglobulin kappa-chain and heavy-chain loci in a child with chronic lymphocytic leukemia. *N Engl J Med* 1983;309:590.
5. Montserrat E, Gomis F, Vallespí T, et al. Presenting features and prognosis of chronic lymphocytic leukemia in younger adults. *Blood* 1991;78:1545.
6. Linet MS, Cartwright RA. Chronic lymphocytic leukemia: epidemiology and etiologic findings. *Nouv Rev Fr Hematol* 1988;30(5–6):353.
7. Kwong YL, Wong KF, Chan LC, et al. The spectrum of chronic lymphoproliferative disorders in Chinese people. An analysis of 64 cases. *Cancer* 1994;74:174.
8. Malone KE, Koepsell TD, Daling JR, et al. Chronic lymphocytic leukemia in relation to chemical exposures. *Am J Epidemiol* 1989;130:1152.
9. Bizzozero OJ, Johnson KG, Ciocco A, Kawasaki S, Toyoda S. Radiation-related leukemia in Hiroshima and Nagasaki 1946–1964. *Ann Intern Med* 1967;55:522.
10. Arp JEW, Wolf PH, Checkoway H. Lymphocytic leukemia and exposure to benzene and other solvents in the rubber industry. *J Occup Med* 1983;25:598.
11. Zahm SH, Weisenburger DD, Babbitt PA, et al. Use of hair coloring products and the risk of lymphoma, multiple myeloma, and chronic lymphocytic leukemia. *Am J Public Health* 1992;82:990.
12. Inskip PD, Kleinerman RA, Stovall M, et al. Leukemia, lymphoma, and multiple myeloma after pelvic radiotherapy for benign disease. *Radiat Res* 1993;135:108.
13. Linet MS, Van Natta MI, Brookmeyer R, et al. Familial cancer history and chronic lymphocytic leukemia. *Am J Epidemiol* 1989;130:655.
14. Blattner WA, Strober W, Muchmore AV, et al. Familial chronic lymphocytic leukemia. Immunologic and cellular characterization. *Ann Intern Med* 1976;84:554.
15. Brok-Simoni F, Rechavi G, Katzir N, Ben-Bassat I. Chronic lymphocytic leukaemia in twin sisters: monozygous but not identical. *Lancet* 1987;1:329.
16. Cuttner J. Increased incidence of hematologic malignancies in first-degree relatives of patients with chronic lymphocytic leukemia. *Cancer Invest* 1992;10:103.
17. Freedman AS, Nadler LM. Immunologic markers in B-cell chronic lymphocytic leukemia. In: Cheson BD, ed. *Chronic lymphocytic leukemia: scientific advances and clinical developments.* New York: Marcel Dekker Inc, 1993:1.
18. Johnson TA, Rassenti LZ, Kipps TJ. Ig VH1 genes expressed in B cell chronic lymphocytic leukemia exhibit distinctive molecular features. *J Immunol* 1997;158:235.
19. Plater-Zyberk C, Maini RN, Lam K, Kennedy TD, Janossy G. A rheumatoid arthritis B cell subset expresses a phenotype similar to that in chronic lymphocytic leukemia. *Arthritis Rheum* 1985;28:971.
20. Mizutani H, Furubayashi T, Kashiwagi H, et al. B cells expressing CD5 antigen are markedly increased in peripheral blood and spleen lymphocytes from patients with immune thrombocytopenic purpura. *Br J Haematol* 1991;78:474.
21. Caligaris-Cappio F, Hamblin TJ. B-cell chronic lymphocytic leukemia: a bird of a different feather. *J Clin Oncol* 1999;17:399.
22. Foa R, Massaia M, Cardona S, et al. Production of tumor necrosis factor-alpha by B-cell chronic lymphocytic leukemia cells: a possible regulatory role of TNF in the progression of the disease. *Blood* 1990;76:393.
23. Semenzato G, Foa R, Agostini C, et al. High serum levels of soluble interleukin 2 receptor in patients with B chronic lymphocytic leukemia. *Blood* 1987;70:396.
24. Kay NE, Burton J, Wagner D, Nelson DL. The malignant B cells from B-chronic lymphocytic leukemia patients release TAC-soluble interleukin-2 receptors. *Blood* 1988;72:447.
25. Dancescu M, Rubio-Trujillo M, Biron G, et al. Interleukin 4 protects chronic lymphocytic leukemic B cells from death by apoptosis and upregulates bcl-2 expression. *J Exp Med* 1992;176:1319.
26. Frankfurt OS, Byrnes JJ, Villa L. Protection from apoptotic cell death by interleukin-4 is increased in previously treated chronic lymphocytic leukemia patients. *Leuk Res* 1997;21:9.
27. Aderka D, Maor Y, Novick D, et al. Interleukin-6 inhibits the proliferation of B-chronic lymphocytic leukemia cells that is induced by tumor necrosis factor-α or β. *Blood* 1993;81:2076.
28. Digel W, Schmid M, Heil G, et al. Human interleukin-7 induces proliferation of neoplastic cells from chronic lymphocytic leukemia and acute leukemias. *Blood* 1991;78:753.
29. Kremer JP, Reisbach G, Nerl C, Dormer P. B-cell chronic lymphocytic leukaemia cells express and release transforming growth factor-β. *Br J Haematol* 1992;80:480.
30. Reittie JE, Yong KL, Panayiotidis P, Hoffbrand AV. Interleukin-6 inhibits apoptosis and tumour necrosis factor induced proliferation of B-chronic lymphocytic leukaemia. *Leuk Lymphoma* 1996;22:83.
31. Frishman J, Long B, Knospe W, Gregory S, Plate J. Genes for interleukin 7 are transcribed in leukemic cell subsets of individuals with chronic lymphocytic leukemia. *J Exp Med* 1993;177:955.
32. di Celle PF, Mariani S, Riera L, et al. Interleukin-8 induces the accumulation of B-cell chronic lymphocytic leukemia cells by prolonging survival in an autocrine fashion. *Blood* 1996;87:4382.
33. Jurlander J, Lei CF, Tan J, et al. Characterization of interleukin-10 receptor expression on B-cell chronic lymphocytic leukemia cells. *Blood* 1997;89:4146.
34. Chaouchi N, Wallon C, Goujard C, et al. Interleukin-13 inhibits interleukin-2-induced proliferation and protects chronic lymphocytic leukemia B cells from *in vitro* apoptosis. *Blood* 1996;87:1022.
35. Foa R. Pathogenesis of the immunodeficiency in B-cell chronic lymphocytic leukemia. In: Cheson BD, ed. *Chronic lymphocytic leukemia: scientific advances and clinical developments.* New York: Marcel Dekker Inc, 1993:147.
36. Heath ME, Cheson BD. Defective complement activity in chronic lymphocytic leukemia. *Am J Hematol* 1985;19:63.
37. Cantwell M, Hua T, Pappas J, Kipps TJ. Acquired CD40-ligand deficiency in chronic lymphocytic leukemia. *Nature Med* 1997;3:984.
38. Bird ML, Ueshima Y, Rowley JD, Haren JM, Vardiman JW. Chromosome abnormalities in B cell chronic lymphocytic leukemia and their clinical correlations. *Leukemia* 1989;3:182.
39. Oscier D, Fitchett M, Herbert T, Lambert R. Karyotypic evolution in B-cell chronic lymphocytic leukaemia. *Genes Chromosomes Cancer* 1991;3:16.
40. Juliusson G, Gahrton G. Chromosome abnormalities in B-cell chronic lymphocytic leukemia. In: Cheson BD, ed. *Chronic lymphocytic leukemia: scientific advances and clinical developments.* New York: Marcel Dekker Inc, 1993:83.
41. Anastasi J, Le Beau MM, Vardiman JW, et al. Detection of trisomy 12 in chronic lymphocytic leukemia by fluorescence *in situ* hybridization to interphase cells: a simple and sensitive method. *Blood* 1992;79:1796.
42. Escudier SM, Pereira-Leahy JM, Drach JW, et al. Fluorescent *in situ* hybridization and cytogenetic studies of trisomy 12 in chronic lymphocytic leukemia. *Blood* 1993;81:2702.
43. Stilgenbauer S, Döhner K, Bentz M, Kichter P, Döhner H. Molecular cytogenetic analysis of B-cell chronic lymphocytic leukemia. *Ann Hematol* 1998;76(3–4):101.
44. Garcia-Marco JA, Caldas C, Price CM, et al. Frequent somatic deletion of the 13q12 locus encompassing BRCA2 in chronic lymphocytic leukemia. *Blood* 1996;88:1568.
45. Panayiotidis P, Ganeshaguru K, Rowntree C, et al. Lack of clonal BRCA2 gene deletion on chromosome 13 in chronic lymphocytic leukaemia. *Br J Haematol* 1997;99:708.
46. Oscier D, Thompsett A, Zhu D, Stevenson FK. Differential rates of somatic hypermutation in Vh genes among subsets of chronic lymphocytic leukemia defined by chromosome abnormalities. *Blood* 1997;89:4153.
47. Geisler CH, Philip P, Christensen BE, et al. In B-cell chronic lymphocytic leukaemia chromosome 17 abnormalities and not trisomy 12 are the single most important cytogenetic abnormalities for the prognosis: a cytogenetic and immunophenotypic study of 480 unselected newly diagnosed patients. *Leuk Res* 1997;21:1011.
48. Fais F, Ghiotto F, Hashimoto S, et al. Chronic lymphocytic leukemia B cells express restricted sets of mutated and unmutated antigen receptors. *J Clin Invest* 1998;102:1515.
49. Hamblin T, Davis Z, Gardiner A, Oscier DG, Stevenson FK. Unmutated Ig Vh genes are associated with a more aggressive form of chronic lymphocytic leukemia. *Blood* 1999;94:1848.
50. Damle RN, Wasil T, Fais F, et al. Ig V gene mutation status and CD38 expression as novel prognostic indicators in chronic lymphocytic leukemia. *Blood* 1999;94:1840.
51. Kipps TJ. Immunoglobulin genes in chronic lymphocytic leukemia. *Blood Cells* 1993;19:615.
52. Tsujimoto Y, Yunis JJ, Onorato-Showe L, et al. Molecular cloning of the chromosomal breakpoint of B-cell lymphomas and leukemias with the t(11;14) chromosome translocation. *Science* 1984;224:1403.
53. Madeiros LJ, Van Krieken JH, Jaffe ES, Raffeld M. Association of *bcl*-1 rearrangements with lymphocytic lymphoma of intermediate differentiation. *Blood* 1990;76:2086.
54. Williams ME, Whitefield M, Swerdlow SH. Analysis of the cyclin-dependent kinase inhibitors p18 and p19 in mantle-cell lymphoma and chronic lymphocytic leukemia. *Ann Oncol* 1997;8[Suppl 2]:S71.
55. McKeithan TW, Ohno H, Diaz MO. Identification of a transcriptional unit adjacent to the breakpoint in the 14;19 translocation of chronic lymphocytic leukemia. *Genes Chromosomes Cancer* 1990;1:247.
56. Dyer MJS, Zani VJ, Lu WZ, et al. BCL2 translocations in leukemias of mature B cells. *Blood* 1994;83:3682.
57. Hanada M, Delia D, Aiello A, Stadtmauer E, Reed JC. *bcl-2* gene hypomethylation and high-level expression in B-cell chronic lymphocytic leukemia. *Blood* 1993;82:1820.
58. Bullrich F, Veronese ML, Kitada S, et al. Minimal region of loss at 13q14 in B-cell chronic lymphocytic leukemia. *Blood* 1996;88:3109.
59. Kitada S, Andersen J, Akar S, et al. Expression of apoptosis-regulating proteins in chronic lymphocytic leukemia: correlations with *in vitro* and *in vivo* chemoresponses. *Blood* 1998;91:3379.
60. Stilgenbauer S, Schaffner C, Lichter P, Döhner H. Deletion of bands 11q22-q23 in B-CLL and other lymphoproliferative disorders. *Proceedings of the Eighth International Workshop on CLL.* 1999;17(abst S01).
61. Cordone I, Masi S, Mauro FR, et al. p53 expression in B-cell chronic lymphocytic leukemia: a marker of disease progression and poor prognosis. *Blood* 1998;91:4342.
62. Döhner H, Fischer K, Bentz M, et al. p53 gene deletion predicts for poor survival and non-response to therapy with purine analogs in chronic B-cell leukemias. *Blood* 1995;85:1580.
63. Döhner H. The role of p53 mutations in B-CLL. *Proceedings of the Eighth International Workshop on CLL.* 1999:17(abst S03).
64. Cheson BD, Bennett JM, Rai KR, et al. Guidelines for clinical protocols for chronic lymphocytic leukemia: report of the NCI-sponsored Working Group. *Am J Hematol* 1988;29:152.
65. Cheson BD, Bennett JM, Grever M, et al. National Cancer Institute–sponsored Working Group guidelines for chronic lymphocytic leukemia: revised guidelines for diagnosis and treatment. *Blood* 1996;87:4990.
66. Harris NL, Jaffe ES, Stein H, et al. A revised European-American classification of lymphoid neoplasms: a proposal from the International Lymphoma Study Group. *Blood* 1994;84:1361.
67. Wormsley SB, Baird SM, Gadol N, Rai KR, Sobol RE. Characteristics of CD11c+CD5+ chronic B-cell leukemias and the identification of novel peripheral blood B-cell subsets with chronic lymphoid leukemia immunophenotypes. *Blood* 1990;76:123.
68. Liang R, Chan V, Chan TK, et al. Detection of immunoglobulin gene rearrangement in acute and chronic lymphoid leukemias of B-cell lineage by polymerase chain reaction gene amplification. *Am J Hematol* 1991;38:189.
69. Freedman AS, Freeman G, Whitman J, et al. Studies of *in vitro* activated CD5+ and CD5– B cells. *Blood* 1989;73:202.
70. Berkman N, Polliack A, Breuer R, Okon E, Kramer M. Pulmonary involvement as the major manifestation of chronic lymphocytic leukemia. *Leuk Lymphoma* 1992;8:495.
71. Stagg MP, Gumbart CH. Chronic lymphocytic leukemic meningitis as a cause of the syndrome of inappropriate secretion of antidiuretic hormone. *Cancer* 1987;60:191.
72. Anaissie E, Kontoyiannis DP, Kantarjian H, et al. Listeriosis in patients with chronic lymphocytic leukemia who were treated with fludarabine and prednisone. *Ann Intern Med* 1992;117:466.
73. Spielberger RT, Stock W, Larson RA. Listeriosis after 2-chlorodeoxyadenosine treatment [Letter]. *N Engl J Med* 1993;328:813.

74. Cheson BD. Immunologic and immunosuppressive complications of purine analogue therapy. *J Clin Oncol* 1995;13:2431.
75. Anaissie EJ, Kontoyiannis DP, O'Brien S, et al. Infections in patients with chronic lymphocytic leukemia treated with fludarabine. *Ann Intern Med* 1998;129:559.
76. Byrd JC, Hargis JB, Kester KE, et al. Opportunistic pulmonary infections with fludarabine in previously treated patients with low-grade lymphoid malignancies: a role for *Pneumocystis carinii* pneumonia prophylaxis. *Am J Hematol* 1995;49:135.
77. Cooperative Group for the Study of Immunoglobulin in Chronic Lymphocytic Leukemia. Intravenous immunoglobulin for the prevention of infection in chronic lymphocytic leukemia. A randomized, controlled clinical trial. *N Engl J Med* 1988;319:902.
78. Weeks JC, Tierney MR, Weinstein MC. Cost effectiveness of prophylactic intravenous immune globulin in chronic lymphocytic leukemia. *N Engl J Med* 1991;325:81.
79. Molica S, Musto P, Chiurazzi F, et al. Prophylaxis against infections with low-dose intravenous immunoglobulins (IVIG) in chronic lymphocytic leukemia. Results of a crossover study. *Haematologica* 1996;81:121.
80. Vadhan-Raj S, Velasquez WS, Butler JJ, et al. Stimulation of myelopoiesis in chronic lymphocytic leukemia and in other lymphoproliferative disorders by recombinant human granulocyte-macrophage colony-stimulating factor. *Am J Hematol* 1990;33:189.
81. O'Brien S, Kantarjian H, Beran M, et al. Fludarabine and granulocyte colony-stimulating factor (G-CSF) in patients with chronic lymphocytic leukemia. *Leukemia* 1997;11:1631.
82. Richter MN. Generalized reticular cell sarcoma of lymph nodes associated with lymphocytic leukemia. *Am J Pathol* 1928;4:285.
83. Lortholary P, Boiron M, Ripault P, et al. Leucemie lymphoide chronique secondairemonte associee a une reticulopathie maligne, syndrome de Richter. *Nouv Rev Fr Hematol* 1964;78:621.
84. Robertson LE, Pugh W, O'Brien S, et al. Richter's syndrome: a report on 39 patients. *J Clin Oncol* 1993;11:1985.
85. Michiels JJ, van Dongen JJM, Hagemeijer A, et al. Richter's syndrome with identical immunoglobulin gene rearrangements in the chronic lymphocytic leukemia and the supervening non-Hodgkin lymphoma. *Leukemia* 1989;3:819.
86. Raziuddin S, Assaf HM, Teklu B. T cell malignancy in Richter's syndrome presenting as hyper IgM. Induction and characterization of a novel CD3+, CD4–, CD8+ T cell subset from phytohemagglutinin-stimulated patient's CD3+, CD4+, CD8+ leukemic T cells. *Eur J Immunol* 1989;19:469.
87. Tohda S, Morio T, Suzuki T, et al. Richter syndrome with two B cell clones possessing different surface immunoglobulins and immunoglobulin gene rearrangements. *Am J Hematol* 1990;35:32.
88. Cherepakhin V, Baird SM, Meisenholder GW, Kipps TJ. Common clonal origin of chronic lymphocytic leukemia and high-grade lymphoma of Richter's syndrome. *Blood* 1993;82:3141.
89. Bessudo A, Kipps TJ. Origin of high-grade lymphomas in Richter syndrome. *Leuk Lymphoma* 1995;18(5–6):367.
90. Giles FJ, O'Brien S, Kantarjian HM, et al. Sequential *cis*-platinum, fludarabine, and arabinosyl cytosine (PFA) or cyclophosphamide, fludarabine and arabinosyl cytosine (CFA) in patients with Richter's syndrome. *Blood* 1996;88[Suppl 1]:93a.
91. Melo JV, Catovsky D, Galton DAG. The relationship between chronic lymphocytic leukaemia and prolymphocytic leukaemia. I. Clinical and laboratory features of 300 patients and characterization of an intermediate group. *Br J Haematol* 1986;63:377.
92. Melo JV, Catovsky D, Galton DAG. The relationship between chronic lymphocytic leukaemia and prolymphocytic leukaemia IV. Patterns of evolution of "prolymphocytoid" transformation. *Br J Haematol* 1986;64:77.
93. Melo JV, Catovsky D, Gregory WM, Galton DAG. The relationship between chronic lymphocytic leukaemia and prolymphocytic leukaemia. IV. Analysis of survival and prognostic features. *Br J Haematol* 1987;65:2329.
94. Hamblin TJ, Oscier DJ, Young BJ. Autoimmunity in chronic lymphocytic leukemia. *J Clin Pathol* 1986;39:713.
95. Duhrsen U, Augener W, Zwingers T, Brittinger G. Spectrum and frequency of autoimmune derangements in lymphoproliferative disorders: analysis of 637 cases and comparison with myeloproliferative diseases. *Br J Haematol* 1987;67:235.
96. Kipps TJ, Carson DA. Autoantibodies in chronic lymphocytic leukemia and related systemic autoimmune diseases. *Blood* 1993;81:2475.
97. Efremov DG, Ivanovski M, Siljanovski N, et al. Restricted immunoglobulin VH region repertoire in chronic lymphocytic leukemia patients with autoimmune hemolytic anemia. *Blood* 1996;87:3869.
98. Efremov DG, Ivanovski M, Burrone OR. The pathologic significance of the immunoglobulins expressed by chronic lymphocytic leukemia B-cells in the development of autoimmune hemolytic anemia. *Leuk Lymphoma* 1998;28(3–4):285.
99. Seymour JF, Cusack JD, Lerner SA, Pollock RE, Keating MJ. Case/control study of the role of splenectomy in chronic lymphocytic leukemia. *J Clin Oncol* 1997;15:52.
100. Chikkappa G, Zarrabi MH, Tsan MF. Pure red-cell aplasia in patients with chronic lymphocytic leukemia. *Medicine* 1986;65:339.
101. Chikkappa G, Pasquale D, Zarrabi MH, et al. Cyclosporine and prednisone therapy for pure red cell aplasia in patients with chronic lymphocytic leukemia. *Am J Hematol* 1992;41:5.
102. Travis LB, Curtis RE, Hankey BF, Fraumeni JF Jr. Second cancers in patients with chronic lymphocytic leukemia. *J Natl Cancer Inst* 1992;84:1422.
103. Davis JW, Weiss NS, Armstrong BK. Second cancers in patients with chronic lymphocytic leukemia. *J Natl Cancer Inst* 1987;78:91.
104. Molica S, Alberti A. Second neoplasms in chronic lymphocytic leukemia: analysis of incidence as a function of the length of follow-up. *Haematologica* 1989;74:481.
105. Stern N, Shemesh J, Ramot B. Chronic lymphatic leukemia terminating in acute myeloid leukemia: review of the literature. *Cancer* 1981;47:1849.
106. Catovsky D, Fooks J, Richards S. Prognostic factors in chronic lymphocytic leukaemia: the importance of age, sex and response to treatment in survival. A report from the MRC CLL 1 trial. *Br J Haematol* 1989;72:141.
107. French Cooperative Group on Chronic Lymphocytic Leukemia F. Effects of chlorambucil and therapeutic decision in initial forms of chronic lymphocytic leukemia (stage A): results of a randomized trial on 612 patients. *Blood* 1990;75:1414.
108. Cheson BD, Vena D, Barrett J, Freidlin B. Second malignancies as a consequence of nucleoside analog therapy of chronic lymphoid leukemias. *J Clin Oncol* 1999;17:2454.
109. Maher VE, Gill L, Townes PL, et al. Simultaneous chronic lymphocytic leukemia and chronic myelogenous leukemia. Evidence of a separate stem cell origin. *Cancer* 1993;71:1993.
110. Esteve J, Cervantes F, Rives S, et al. Simultaneous occurrence of B-cell chronic lymphocytic leukemia and chronic myeloid leukemia with further evolution to lymphoid blast crisis. *Haematologica* 1997;82:596.
111. Boggs DR, Sofferman SA, Wintrobe MM, Cartwright GE. Factors influencing the duration of survival of patients with chronic lymphocytic leukemia. *Am J Med* 1966;40:243.
112. Galton DAG. The pathogenesis of chronic lymphocytic leukemia. *Can Med Assoc J* 1966;94:1005.
113. Dameshek W. Chronic lymphocytic leukemia—an accumulative disease of immunologically incompetent lymphocytes. *Blood* 1967;29:566.
114. Rai KR, Sawitsky A, Cronkite EP, et al. Clinical staging of chronic lymphocytic leukemia. *Blood* 1975;46:219.
115. Rai KR. A critical analysis of staging in CLL. In: Gale RP, Rai KR, ed. *Chronic lymphocytic leukemia. Recent progress and future direction.* New York: Alan R Liss, 1987:253.
116. Binet JL, Auquier A, Dighiero G, et al. A new prognostic classification of chronic lymphocytic leukemia derived from a multivariate survival analysis. *Cancer* 1981;48:198.
117. Jaksic B, Vitale B. Total tumour mass score (TTM): a new parameter in chronic lymphocytic leukaemia. *Br J Haematol* 1981;49:405.
118. Mandelli F, De Rossi G, Mancini P, et al. Prognosis in chronic lymphocytic leukemia: a retrospective multicentric study from the GIMEMA group. *J Clin Oncol* 1987;5:398.
119. Skinnider LF, Tan L, Schmidt J, Armitage G. Chronic lymphocytic leukemia. A review of 745 cases and assessment of clinical staging. *Cancer* 1982;50:2951.
120. Baccarani M, Cavo M, Gobbi M, Lauria F, Tura S. Staging of chronic lymphocytic leukemia. *Blood* 1982;59:1191.
121. Rozman C, Montserrat E, Rodríguez-Fernández JM, et al. Bone marrow histologic pattern—the best single prognostic parameter in chronic lymphocytic leukemia: a multivariate survival analysis of 329 cases. *Blood* 1984;64:642.
122. De Rossi G, Mandelli F, Covelli A, et al. Chronic lymphocytic leukemia (CLL) in younger adults: a retrospective study of 133 cases. *Hematol Oncol* 1989;7:127.
123. Montserrat E, Viñolas N, Reverer JC, Rozman C. Natural history of chronic lymphocytic leukemia: on the progression and prognosis of early stages. *Nouv Rev Fr Hematol* 1988;30:359.
124. French Cooperative Group on Chronic Lymphocytic Leukaemia. Natural history of stage A chronic lymphocytic leukaemia untreated patients. *Br J Haematol* 1990;76:45.
125. Montserrat E, Sanchez-Bisono J, Viñolas N, Rozman C. Lymphocyte doubling time in chronic lymphocytic leukaemia: analysis of its prognostic significance. *Br J Haematol* 1986;62:567.
126. Desablens B, Claisse JF, Piprot-Choffat C, Gontier MF. Prognostic value of bone marrow biopsy in chronic lymphoid leukemia. *Nouv Rev Fr Hematol* 1989;31:179.
127. Pangalis GA, Boussiotis VA, Kittas C. B-chronic lymphocytic leukemia. Disease progression in 150 untreated stage A and B patients as predicted by bone marrow pattern. *Nouv Rev Fr Hematol* 1988;30:373.
128. Molica S, Tucci L, Levato D, Docimo C. Clinico-prognostic evaluation of bone marrow infiltration (biopsy versus aspirate) in early chronic lymphocytic leukemia. A single institution study. *Haematologica* 1997;82:286.
129. Zwiebel J, Cheson BD. Prognostic factors in chronic lymphocytic leukemia. *Semin Oncol* 1998;25:42.
130. Lee JS, Dixon DO, Kantarjian HM, Keating MJ, Talpaz M. Prognosis of chronic lymphocytic leukemia: a multivariate regression analysis of 325 untreated patients. *Blood* 1987;69:929.
131. Lecouvet FE, Vande Berg BC, Michaux L, et al. Early chronic lymphocytic leukemia: prognostic value of quantitative bone marrow MR imaging findings and correlations with hematologic variables. *Radiology* 1997;204:813.
132. Reinish W, Willheim M, Hilgarth M, et al. Soluble CD23 reliably reflects disease activity in B-cell chronic lymphocytic leukemia. *J Clin Oncol* 1994;12:2146.
133. Sarfati M, Chevret S, Chastang C, et al. Prognostic importance of serum soluble CD23 level in chronic lymphocytic leukemia. *Blood* 1996;88:4259.
134. Molica S, Levato D, Dell'Olio M, et al. Cellular expression and serum circulating levels of CD23 in B-cell chronic lymphocytic leukemia. Implications for prognosis. *Haematologica* 1996;81:428.
135. Simonsson B, Wibell L, Nilsson K. β_2-microglobulin in chronic lymphocytic leukaemia. *Scand J Haematol* 1980;24:174.
136. Tötterman T, Nilsson K, Simonsson B. Phorbol ester–induced production of beta-2-microglobulin in B-CLL cells: relation to IgM secretory response and disease activity. *Br J Haematol* 1986;62:95.
137. Keating MJ, Lerner S, Kantarjian H, Freireich EJ, O'Brien S. The serum β_2-microglobulin (β_2M) level is more powerful than stage in predicting response and survival in chronic lymphocytic leukemia (CLL). *Blood* 1995;86[Suppl 1]:606(abst 2412).
138. Apostolopoulos A, Symeonidis A, Zoumbos N. Prognostic significance of immune function parameters in patients with chronic lymphocytic leukaemia. *Eur J Haematol* 1990;44:39.
139. Catovsky D, Cherchi M, Brooks D, Bradley J, Zola H. Heterogeneity of B-cell leukemias demonstrated by the monoclonal antibody FMC7. *Blood* 1981;58:406.
140. Caligaris-Cappio F, Gobbi M, Bergui L, et al. B-chronic lymphocytic leukaemia patients with stable benign disease show a distinctive membrane phenotype. *Br J Haematol* 1984;56:655.
141. Dadmarz R, Cawley JC. Heterogeneity of CLL: high CD23 antigen and alpha-IFN receptor expression are features of favourable disease and of cell activation. *Br J Haematol* 1988;68:279.

142. Tefferi A, Phyliky RL. Role of immunophenotyping in chronic lymphocytosis: review of the natural history of the condition in 145 adult patients. *Mayo Clin Proc* 1988;63:806.
143. Hamblin TJ, Oscier DG, Stevens JR, Smith JL. Long survival in B-CLL correlates with surface IgMκ phenotype. *Br J Haematol* 1987;66:21.
144. De Rossi G, Zarcone D, Mauro F, et al. Adhesion molecule expression of B-cell chronic lymphocytic leukemia cells: malignant cell phenotypes define distinct disease subsets. *Blood* 1993;81:2679.
145. Molica S, Levato D, Dell'Olio M, et al. Clinico-prognostic implications of increased levels of soluble CD54 in the serum of B-cell chronic lymphocytic leukemia patients. Results of a multivariate survival analysis. *Haematologica* 1997;82:148.
146. Sinclair D, Dagg JH, Dewar AE, et al. The incidence, clonal origin and secretory nature of serum paraproteins in chronic lymphocytic leukaemia. *Br J Haematol* 1986;64:725.
147. Deegan MJ, Abraham JP, Sawdyk M, Van Slyck EJ. High incidence of monoclonal proteins in the serum and urine of chronic lymphocytic leukemia patients. *Blood* 1984;64:1207.
148. Ultmann JE, Fish W, Osserman E, Gellhorn A. The clinical implications of hypogammaglobulinemia in patients with chronic lymphocytic leukemia and lymphocytic lymphosarcoma. *Ann Intern Med* 1959;51:501.
149. Rozman C, Montserrat E, Viñolas N. Serum immunoglobulins in B-chronic lymphocytic leukemia. Natural history and prognostic significance. *Cancer* 1988;61:279.
150. Robertson LE, Plunkett W, McConnell K, Keating MJ, McDonnell TJ. Bcl-2 expression in chronic lymphocytic leukemia and its correlation with the induction of apoptosis and clinical outcome. *Leukemia* 1996;10:456.
151. Pepper C, Bentley P, Hoy T. Regulation of clinical chemoresistance by bcl-2 and bax oncoproteins in B-cell chronic lymphocytic leukaemia. *Br J Haematol* 1996;95:513.
152. Pepper C, Hoy T, Bentley DP. Bcl-2/Bax ratios in chronic lymphocytic leukaemia and their correlation with *in vitro* apoptosis and clinical resistance. *Br J Cancer* 1997;76:935.
153. Holmes JA, Whittaker JA. Spontaneous remission in chronic lymphocytic leukaemia. *Br J Haematol* 1988;69:97.
154. Ribera J, Vinolas N, Urbano-Ipizua A, et al. "Spontaneous" complete remissions in chronic lymphocytic leukemia: report of three cases and review of the literature. *Blood Cells* 1987;12:481.
155. Keating MJ. Chemotherapy of chronic lymphocytic leukemia. In: Cheson BD, ed. *Chronic lymphocytic leukemia: scientific advances and clinical developments.* New York: Marcel Dekker Inc, 1993:297.
156. Shustik C, Mick R, Silver R, et al. Treatment of early chronic lymphocytic leukemia: intermittent chlorambucil versus observation. *Hematol Oncol* 1988;6:7.
157. Spanish Cooperative Group P. Treatment of chronic lymphocytic leukemia: a preliminary report of Spanish (PETHEMA) trials. *Leuk Lymphoma* 1991;5[Suppl]:89.
158. Dighiero G, Maloum K, Desablens B, et al. Chlorambucil in indolent chronic lymphocytic leukemia. French Cooperative Group on Chronic Lymphocytic Leukemia. *N Engl J Med* 1998;338:1506.
159. CLL Trialists' Collaborative Group. Chemotherapeutic options in chronic lymphocytic leukemia: a meta-analysis of the randomized trials. *J Natl Cancer Inst* 1999;91:861.
160. Saven A, Carrera CJ, Carson DA, Beutler E, Piro LD. 2-Chlorodeoxyadenosine treatment of refractory chronic lymphocytic leukemia. *Leuk Lymphoma* 1991;5[Suppl]:133.
161. Dillman RO, Mick R, McIntyre OR. Pentostatin in chronic lymphocytic leukemia: a phase II trial of Cancer and Leukemia Group B. *J Clin Oncol* 1989;7:433.
162. Sawitsky A, Rai KR, Glidewell O, Silver RT. Comparison of daily versus intermittent chlorambucil and prednisone therapy in the treatment of patients with chronic lymphocytic leukemia. *Blood* 1977;50:1049.
163. Rai KR, Peterson B, Elias L, et al. A randomized comparison of fludarabine and chlorambucil for patients with previously untreated chronic lymphocytic leukemia. A CALGB, SWOG, CTC/NCI-C and ECOG inter-group study. *Blood* 1996;88[Suppl 1]:141a(abst 552).
164. Grever MR, Kopecky KJ, Coltman CA, et al. Fludarabine monophosphate: a potentially useful agent in chronic lymphocytic leukemia. *Nouv Rev Fr Hematol* 1988;30:457.
165. Keating MJ, O'Brien S, Kantarjian H, et al. Long-term follow-up of patients with chronic lymphocytic leukemia treated with fludarabine as a single agent. *Blood* 1993;81:2878.
166. O'Brien S, Kantarjian H, Beran M, et al. Results of fludarabine and prednisone therapy in 264 patients with chronic lymphocytic leukemia with multivariate analysis–derived prognostic model for response to treatment. *Blood* 1993;82:1695.
167. Whelan JS, Davis CL, Rule S, et al. Fludarabine phosphate for the treatment of low grade lymphoid malignancy. *Br J Cancer* 1991;64:120.
168. Hiddemann W, Rottmann R, Wormann B, et al. Treatment of advanced chronic lymphocytic leukemia by fludarabine. Results of a clinical phase-II study. *Ann Hematol* 1991;63:1.
169. French Cooperative Group on CLL, Johnson S, Smith AG, et al. Multicentre prospective randomised trial of fludarabine versus cyclophosphamide, doxorubicin, and prednisone (CAP) for treatment of advanced-stage chronic lymphocytic leukemia. *Lancet* 1996;347:1432.
170. Leporrier S, Chevret B, Cazin B, et al. Randomized comparison of fludarabine, CAP and ChOP, in 695 previously untreated stage B and C chronic lymphocytic leukemia (CLL). Early stopping of the CAP accrual. *Blood* 1997;90[Suppl 1]:529a(abst 2357).
171. Montserrat E, López-Lorenzo JL, Manso F, et al. Fludarabine in resistant or relapsing B-cell chronic lymphocytic leukemia. The Spanish Group experience. *Leuk Lymphoma* 1996;21:467.
172. Sorensen JM, Vena D, Fallavollita A, Chun HG, Cheson BD. Treatment of refractory chronic lymphocytic leukemia with fludarabine phosphate via the Group C mechanism of the National Cancer Institute: 5-year follow-up report. *J Clin Oncol* 1997;15:458.
173. Juliusson G, Liliemark J. High complete remission rate from 2-chloro-2'-deoxyadenosine in previously treated patients with B-cell chronic lymphocytic leukemia: response predicted by rapid decrease in blood lymphocyte count. *J Clin Oncol* 1993;11:679.
174. Tallman MS, Hakimian D, Zonzig C, et al. Cladribine in the treatment of relapsed or refractory chronic lymphocytic leukemia. *J Clin Oncol* 1995;13:983.
175. Delannoy A, Martiat P, Gala JL, et al. 2-Chlorodeoxyadenosine (CdA) for patients with previously untreated chronic lymphocytic leukemia (CLL). *Leukemia* 1995;9:1130.
176. Saven A, Lemon RH, Kosty M, Beutler E, Piro LD. 2-Chlorodeoxyadenosine activity in patients with untreated chronic lymphocytic leukemia. *J Clin Oncol* 1995;13:570.
177. Robak T, Blasinka-Morawiec M, Krykowski E, et al. Intermittent 2-hour intravenous infusions of 2-chlorodeoxyadenosine in the treatment of 110 patients with refractory or previously untreated B-cell chronic lymphocytic leukemia. *Leuk Lymphoma* 1996;22:509.
178. Rondelli D, Lauria F, Zinzani PL, et al. 2-Chlorodeoxyadenosine in the treatment of relapsed/refractory chronic lymphoproliferative disorders. *Eur J Haematol* 1997;58:46.
179. Robak T, Blonski JZ, Urbanska-Rys H, Blasinska-Morawiec M, Skotnicki AB. 2-Chlorodeoxyadenosine (cladribine) in the treatment of patients with chronic lymphocytic leukemia 55 years old and younger. *Leukemia* 1999;13:518.
180. Robak T, Blasinska-Morawiec M, Blonski JZ, Dmoszynska A. 2-Chlorodeoxyadenosine (cladribine) in the treatment of elderly patients with B-cell chronic lymphocytic leukemia. *Leuk Lymphoma* 1999;34:151.
181. Grever MR, Leiby JM, Kraut EH, et al. Low-dose deoxycoformycin in lymphoid malignancy. *J Clin Oncol* 1985;3:1196.
182. O'Dwyer PJ, Wagner B, Leyland-Jones B, et al. 2'-Deoxycoformycin (pentostatin) for lymphoid malignancies. *Ann Intern Med* 1988;108:733.
183. Ho AD, Thaler J, Strykmans P, et al. Pentostatin in refractory chronic lymphocytic leukemia: a phase II trial of the European Organization for Research and Treatment of Cancer. *J Natl Cancer Inst* 1990;82:1416.
184. Dearden C, Catovsky D. Deoxycoformycin in the treatment of mature B-cell malignancies. *Br J Cancer* 1990;62:4.
185. Puccio CA, Mittelman A, Lictman SM, et al. A loading dose/continuous infusion schedule of fludarabine phosphate in chronic lymphocytic leukemia. *J Clin Oncol* 1991;9:1562.
186. Kemena A, O'Brien S, Kantarjian H, et al. A phase II clinical trial of fludarabine in chronic lymphocytic leukemia on a weekly low-dose schedule. *Leuk Lymphoma* 1993;10:187.
187. Robertson LE, O'Brien S, Kantarjian H, et al. A 3-day schedule of fludarabine in previously treated chronic lymphocytic leukemia. *Leukemia* 1995;9:1444.
188. Foran JM, Oscier D, Orchard J, et al. Pharmacokinetic study of single doses of oral fludarabine phosphate in patients with "low-grade" non-Hodgkin's lymphoma and B-cell chronic lymphocyte leukemia. *J Clin Oncol* 1999;17:1574.
189. Keating MJ, O'Brien S, Lerner S, et al. Long-term follow-up of patients with chronic lymphocytic leukemia (CLL) receiving fludarabine regimens as initial therapy. *Blood* 1998;92:1165.
190. Robertson LE, Huh YO, Butler JJ, et al. Response assessment in chronic lymphocytic leukemia after fludarabine plus prednisone: clinical, pathologic, immunophenotypic, and molecular analysis. *Blood* 1992;80:29.
191. Spriano M, Chiurazzi F, Liso V, et al. Multicentre prospective randomized trial of fludarabine versus chlorambucil and prednisone in previously untreated patients with active B-CLL. *Proceedings of the Eighth International Workshop on CLL.* 1999:52(abst P086).
192. Cheson BD, Vena D, Foss F, Sorensen JM. Neurotoxicity of purine analogs: a review. *J Clin Oncol* 1994;12:2216.
193. Cheson BD. Toxicities associated with nucleoside analog therapy. In: Cheson BD, Keating MJ, Plunkett W, ed. *Nucleoside analogs in cancer therapy.* New York: Marcel Dekker Inc, 1997:415.
194. Cheson BD, Frame JN, Vena D, Quashu N, Sorensen JM. Tumor lysis syndrome: an uncommon complication of fludarabine therapy of chronic lymphocytic leukemia. *J Clin Oncol* 1998;16:2313.
195. Juliusson G, Christiansen I, Hansen MM, et al. Oral cladribine as primary therapy for patients with B-cell chronic lymphocytic leukemia. *J Clin Oncol* 1996;14:2160.
196. Montserrat E, Alcala A, Parody R, et al. Treatment of chronic lymphocytic leukemia in advanced stages. A randomized trial comparing chlorambucil plus prednisone versus cyclophosphamide, vincristine, and prednisone. *Cancer* 1985;56:2369.
197. Raphael B, Andersen JW, Silber R, et al. Comparison of chlorambucil and prednisone versus cyclophosphamide, vincristine, and prednisone as initial treatment for chronic lymphocytic leukemia: long-term follow-up of an Eastern Cooperative Oncology Group randomized clinical trial. *J Clin Oncol* 1991;9:770.
198. Hansen MM, Andersen E, Birgens H, et al. CHOP versus chlorambucil + prednisolone in chronic lymphocytic leukemia. *Leuk Lymphoma* 1991;5:97.
199. French Cooperative Group on Chronic Lymphocytic Leukemia. Long-term results of the CHOP regimen in stage C chronic lymphocytic leukaemia. *Br J Haematol* 1989;73:334.
200. Kimby E, Millstedt H. Chlorambucil/prednisone versus CHOP in symptomatic chronic lymphocytic leukemias of B-cell type. A randomized trial. *Leuk Lymphoma* 1991;5[Suppl]:93.
201. Keating MJ, Scouros M, Murphy S, et al. Multiple agent chemotherapy (POACH) in previously treated and untreated patients with chronic lymphocytic leukemia. *Leukemia* 1988;2:157.
202. Keating MJ, Hester JP, McCredie KB, et al. Long-term results of CAP therapy in chronic lymphocytic leukemia. *Leuk Lymphoma* 1990;2:391.
203. Liepman M, Votaw ML. The treatment of chronic lymphocytic leukemia with COP chemotherapy. *Cancer* 1978;41:1664.
204. French Cooperative Group on Chronic Lymphocytic Leukemia. A randomized clinical trial of chlorambucil versus COP in stage B chronic lymphocytic leukemia. *Blood* 1990;75:1422.
205. Kempin S, Lee BJ 3rd, Thaler HT, et al. Combination chemotherapy of advanced chronic lymphocytic leukemia: the M-2 protocol (vincristine, BCNU, cyclophosphamide, melphalan, and prednisone). *Blood* 1982;60:1110.
206. Montserrat E, Alcala A, Alonso C, et al. A randomized trial comparing chlorambucil plus prednisone vs cyclophosphamide, melphalan, and prednisone in the treatment of chronic lymphocytic leukemia stages B and C. *Nouv Rev Fr Hematol* 1988;30:429.
207. Elias L, Stock-Novak D, Grever M, et al. A phase I trial of combination fludarabine and chlorambucil in chronic lymphocytic leukemia. *Proc Am Soc Clin Oncol* 1991;10:221(abst 745).

208. Weiss M, Kempin S, Berman E, Eardley A, Gee T. Results of a phase I study of fludarabine phosphate (FAMP) plus chlorambucil (CLB) in patients with chronic lymphocytic leukemia. *Proc Am Soc Clin Oncol* 1992;11:276(abst 914).
209. Gandhi V, Nowak B, Keating MJ, Plunkett W. Modulation of arabinosylcytosine metabolism by arabinosyl-2-fluoroadenine in lymphocytes from patients with chronic lymphocytic leukemia: implications for combination therapy. *Blood* 1989;74:2070.
210. Gandhi V, Kemena A, Keating MJ, Plunkett W. Fludarabine infusion potentiates arabinosylcytosine metabolism in lymphocytes of patients with chronic lymphocytic leukemia. *Cancer Res* 1992;52:897.
211. O'Brien S, Kantarjian H, Koller C, et al. Fludarabine-prednisone: a highly effective regimen in chronic lymphocytic leukemia (CLL). *Proc Am Soc Clin Oncol* 1992;11:260(abst 850).
212. Foss F, Ihde D, Phelps R, et al. Phase II study of fludarabine and interferon-alfa-2A in advanced mycosis fungoides/Sézary syndrome (MF/SS). *Proc Am Soc Clin Oncol* 1992;11:315(abst 1068).
213. Rummel M, Schenk M, Renner C, et al. Fludarabine and epirubicin in the treatment of CLL as first line therapy or in first relapse—results of a phase-II study. *Blood* 1997;90[Suppl 1]:530a(abst 2359).
214. Bosch F, Perales M, Cobo F, et al. Fludarabine, cyclophosphamide and mitoxantrone (FCM) therapy in resistant or relapsed chronic lymphocytic leukemia (CLL) or follicular lymphoma (FL). *Blood* 1997;90[Suppl 1]:530a(abst 2360).
215. O'Brien S, Kantarjian H, Beran M, et al. Fludarabine (FAMP) and cyclophosphamide (CTX) therapy in chronic lymphocytic leukemia (CLL). *Int J Hematol* 1996;64[Suppl 1]:S56(abst 214).
216. Flinn IW, Byrd JC, Morrison C, et al. Fludarabine and cyclophosphamide: a highly active and well tolerated regimen in patients with previously untreated chronic lymphocytic leukemia. *Blood* 1998;92[Suppl 1]:104a(abst 424).
217. Oken MM, Lee S, Cassileth PA, Krigel RL. Pentostatin, chlorambucil and prednisone for the treatment of chronic lymphocytic leukemia (CLL): Eastern Cooperative Oncology Group (ECOG) protocol E1488. *Proc ASCO* 1998;17:6a(abst 22).
218. Keller JW, Omura GA, Gams RA, Bartolucci AA. Weekly mitoxantrone therapy of Hodgkin's disease, non-Hodgkin's lymphoma, and chronic lymphocytic leukemia. *Am J Clin Oncol* 1987;10:194.
219. O'Brien S, Kantarjian H, Ellis A, et al. Topotecan in chronic lymphocytic leukemia. *Cancer* 1995;75:1104.
220. Keating MJ, Kantarjian H, Talpaz M, et al. Fludarabine: a new agent with major activity against chronic lymphocytic leukemia. *Blood* 1989;74:19.
221. Zinzani PL, Rondelli D, Lauria F, et al. Fludarabine: an effective drug in refractory lymphoproliferative disorders. *Proc Am Soc Clin Oncol* 1992;11:268(abst 881).
222. Keating MJ. Fludarabine monophosphate in the treatment of chronic lymphocytic leukemia. *Semin Oncol* 1990;17[Suppl 8]:49.
223. Saven A, Lemon RH, Piro LD. 2-Chlorodeoxyadenosine for patients with B-cell chronic lymphocytic leukemia resistant to fludarabine [Letter]. *N Engl J Med* 1993;328:812.
224. O'Brien S, Kantarjian H, Estey E, et al. Lack of effect of 2-chlorodeoxyadenosine therapy in patients with chronic lymphocytic leukemia refractory to fludarabine therapy. *N Engl J Med* 1994;330:319.
225. Kefford RF, Fox RM. Deoxycoformycin-induced response in chronic lymphocytic leukaemia: deoxyadenosine toxicity in non-replicating lymphocytes. *Br J Haematol* 1982;50:627.
226. Grever MR, Siaw MFE, Jacob WF, et al. The biochemical and clinical consequences of 2'-deoxycoformycin in refractory lymphoproliferative malignancy. *Blood* 1981;57:406.
227. Ho AD, Ganeshaguru K, Knauf WU, et al. Clinical response to deoxycoformycin in chronic lymphoid neoplasms and biochemical changes in circulating malignant cells *in vivo*. *Blood* 1988;72:1884.
228. Bernard S, Gill P, Rosen P, et al. A phase I trial of alpha-interferon in combination with pentostatin in hematologic malignancies. *Med Pediatr Oncol* 1991;19:276.
229. Velasquez WS, McLaughlin P, Swan F, et al. Dexamethasone, high dose ara-C and cisplatin (DHAP) combination for progressive chronic lymphocytic leukemia. *Blood* 1986;68[Suppl 1]:234a(abst 815).
230. McCroskey RD, Mosher DF, Spencer CD, Prendergast E, Longo WL. Acute tumor lysis syndrome and treatment response in patients treated for refractory chronic lymphocytic leukemia with short-course, high-dose cytosine arabinoside, cisplatin, and etoposide. *Cancer* 1990;66:246.
231. De Rossi G, Mauro FR, Pizzo F, et al. Combination of cytosine-arabinoside (ARA-C), cyclophosphamide and prednisone in the treatment of B-chronic lymphocytic leukemia in advanced stages and progressive disease. *Leuk Lymphoma* 1991;5[Suppl]:101.
232. Binet JL, Mentz F, Leblond V, Merle-Beral H. Synergistic action of alkylating agents and methylxanthine derivatives in the treatment of chronic lymphocytic leukemia. *Leukemia* 1995;9:2159.
233. Makower D, Malik U, Novik Y, Wiernik PH. Therapeutic efficacy of theophylline in chronic lymphocytic leukemia. *Med Oncol* 1999;16:69.
234. Mentz F, Merle-Beral H, Dalloul AH. Theophylline-induced B-CLL apoptosis is partly dependent on cyclic AMP production but independent of CD38 expression and endogenous IL-10 production. *Leukemia* 1999;13:78.
235. Kurtzberg J, Keating MJ, Plunkett W, et al. Compound 506 (2-amino-6-methoxypurine arabinoside) is active against resistant T-cell malignancies: preliminary results of an ongoing phase I trial. *J Clin Oncol* 1996;14:1750(abst 2022).
236. Gandhi V, Keating M, O'Brien S, Plunkett W. Compound GW506U78 in refractory hematologic malignancies: relationship between cellular pharmacokinetics and clinical response. *J Clin Oncol* 1998;16:3607.
237. O'Brien S, Thomas D, Kantarjian H, et al. Compound 506U has activity in mature lymphoid leukemia. *Blood* 1998;92[Suppl 1]:490a(abst 2022).
238. Akao Y, Mizoguchi H, Kojima S, et al. Arsenic induces apoptosis in B-cell leukaemic cell lines *in vitro*: activation of caspases and down-regulation of Bcl-2 protein. *Br J Haematol* 1998;102:1055.
239. Zhu XH, Shen YL, Jing YK, et al. Apoptosis and growth inhibition in malignant lymphocytes after treatment with arsenic trioxide at clinically achievable concentrations. *J Natl Cancer Inst* 1999;91:772.
240. Al-Katib A, Mohammed RM, Dan M, et al. Bryostatin 1–induced hairy cell features on chronic lymphocytic leukemia cells *in vitro*. *Exp Hematol* 1993;21:61.
241. Varterasian ML, Mohammad RM, Eilender DS, et al. Phase I study of bryostatin 1 in patients with relapsed non-Hodgkin's lymphoma and chronic lymphocytic leukemia. *J Clin Oncol* 1998;16:56.
242. Byrd JC, Shinn CA, Bedi A, et al. Flavopiridol has marked *in vitro* activity against B-chronic lymphocytic leukemia (B-CLL) and induces apoptosis independent of p53 status. *Blood* 1997;90[Suppl 1]:531a(abst 2366).
243. Waselenko JK, Przygodzki R, Grever MR, et al. Flavopiridol, UCN-01, FR901228 and gemcitabine have significant *in vitro* activity in *de novo* B-cell prolymphocytic leukemia with aberrant p53 function. *Blood* 1997;90[Suppl 1]:532a(abst 2369).
244. Byrd JC, Shinn C, Ravi R, et al. Depsipeptide (FR901228): a novel therapeutic agent with selective, *in vitro* activity against human B-cell chronic lymphocytic leukemia cells. *Blood* 1999;94:1401.
245. Menzel T, Rahman Z, Calleja E, et al. Elevated intracellular level of basic fibroblast growth factor correlates with stage of chronic lymphocytic leukemia and is associated with resistance to fludarabine. *Blood* 1996;87:1056.
246. Ferrara F, Rametta V, Mele G, et al. Recombinant interferon-alpha2A as maintenance treatment for patients with advanced stage chronic lymphocytic leukemia responding to chemotherapy. *Am J Hematol* 1992;41:45.
247. O'Connell MJ, Colgan JP, Oken MM, et al. Clinical trial of recombinant leukocyte A interferon as initial therapy for favorable histology non-Hodgkin's lymphomas and chronic lymphocytic leukemia. An Eastern Cooperative Oncology Group pilot study. *J Clin Oncol* 1986;4:128.
248. Rozman C, Montserrat E, Viñolas N, et al. Recombinant α2-interferon in the treatment of B chronic lymphocytic leukemia in early stages. *Blood* 1988;71:1295.
249. Molica S, Alberti A. Recombinant alpha-2a interferon in treatment of B-chronic lymphocytic leukemia. A preliminary report with emphasis on previously untreated patients in early stage of disease. *Haematologica* 1990;75:75.
250. O'Brien S, Kantarjian H, Beran M, et al. Interferon maintenance therapy for patients with chronic lymphocytic leukemia in remission after fludarabine. *Blood* 1995;86:1296.
251. Zinzani PL, Bendandi M, Magagnoli M, et al. Results with fludarabine induction and alpha-interferon maintenance protocol in pretreated patients with chronic lymphocytic leukemia and low-grade non-Hodgkin's lymphoma. *Eur J Haematol* 1997;59:82.
252. Dillman RO, Shawler DL, Dillman JB, Royston I. Therapy of chronic lymphocytic leukemia and cutaneous T-cell lymphoma with T101 monoclonal antibody. *J Clin Oncol* 1984;2:881.
253. Hertler AA, Schlossman DM, Borowitz MJ, et al. A phase I study of T101-ricin A chain immunotoxin in refractory chronic lymphocytic leukemia. *J Biol Respir Mod* 1988;7:97.
254. DeNardo GJ, Lewis JP, DeNardo SJ, O'Grady LF. Effect of Lym-1 radioimmunoconjugate on refractory chronic lymphocytic leukemia. *Cancer* 1993;73:1425.
255. Dyer MJS, Hale G, Hayhoe FGJ, Waldmann H. Effects of CAMPATH-1 antibodies *in vivo* in patients with lymphoid malignancies: influence of antibody isotype. *Blood* 1989;73:1431.
256. Pawson R, Dyer MJS, Barge R, et al. Treatment of T-cell prolymphocytic leukemia with human CD52 antibody. *J Clin Oncol* 1997;15:2667.
257. Österborg A, Dyer MJS, Bunjes D, et al. Phase II multicenter study of human CD52 antibody in previously treated chronic lymphocytic leukemia. *J Clin Oncol* 1997;15:1567.
258. Rawstron AC, Davies FE, Evans P, et al. CAMPATH1H therapy for patients with refractory chronic lymphocytic leukemia (CLL). *Blood* 1997;90[Suppl 1]:529a(abst 2356).
259. Dearden C, Matutes E, Dyer MJS, Catovsky D. CAMPATH-1H treatment of T-PLL. *Proceedings of the Eighth International Workshop on CLL.* 1999;:68(abst P131).
260. Bowen AL, Zomas A, Emmett E, et al. Subcutaneous CAMPATH-1H in fludarabine-resistant/relapsed chronic lymphocytic and B-prolymphocytic leukaemia. *Br J Haematol* 1997;96:617.
261. McLaughlin P, Grillo-López AJ, Link BK, et al. Rituximab chimeric anti-CD20 monoclonal antibody therapy of relapsed indolent lymphoma: half of patients respond to a four-dose treatment program. *J Clin Oncol* 1998;16:2825.
262. Maloney DG, Grillo-López AJ, White CA, et al. IDEC-C2B8 (Rituximab) anti-CD20 monoclonal antibody therapy in patients with relapsed low-grade non-Hodgkin's lymphoma. *Blood* 1997;90:2188.
263. Piro LD, White CA, Grillo-Lopez AJ, et al. Extended rituximab (anti-CD20 monoclonal antibody) therapy for relapsed or refractory low-grade or follicular non-Hodgkin's lymphoma. *Ann Oncol* 1999;10:655.
264. Winkler U, Jensen M, Manzke O, et al. Cytokine-release syndrome in patients with B-cell chronic lymphocytic leukemia and high lymphocyte counts after treatment with an anti-CD20 monoclonal antibody (Rituximab, IDEC-C2B8). *Blood* 1999;94:2217.
265. Foran JM, Rohatiner AZ, Cunningham D, et al. European phase II study of rituximab (Chimeric anti-CD20 monoclonal antibody) for patients with newly diagnosed mantle-cell lymphoma and previously treated mantle-cell lymphoma, immunocytoma, and small B-cell lymphocytic lymphoma. *J Clin Oncol* 2000;18:317.
266. O'Brien S, Thomas DA, Freireich EJ, et al. Rituxan has significant activity in patients with CLL. *Blood* 1999;94[Suppl 1]:603a(abst 2684).
267. Venugopal P, Sivaraman S, Huang X, et al. Upregulation of CD20 expression in chronic lymphocytic leukemia (CLL) cells by *in vitro* exposure to cytokines. *Blood* 1998;92[Suppl 1]:247a(abst 1009).
268. Byrd JC, Grever MR, Davis B, et al. Phase I/II study of thrice weekly rituximab in chronic lymphocytic leukemia (CLL)/small lymphocytic lymphoma (SLL): a feasible and active regimen. *Blood* 1999;94[Suppl 1]:704a(abst 3114).
269. Byrd JC, Waselenko JK, Maneatis T, et al. Rituximab therapy in hematologic malignancy patients with circulating tumor cells: association with increased infusion-related side effects and rapid blood tumor clearance. *J Clin Oncol* 1999;17:791.
270. Kaminski MS, Zasadny KR, Francis IR, et al. Iodine-131-anti-B1 radioimmunotherapy for B-cell lymphoma. *J Clin Oncol* 1996;14:1974.

271. Witzig TE, White CA, Wiseman GA, et al. Phase I/II trial of IDEC-Y2B8 radioimmunotherapy for treatment of relapsed or refractory CD20(+) B-cell non-Hodgkin's lymphoma. *J Clin Oncol* 1999;17:3793.
272. Rabinowe SN, Soiffer RJ, Gribben JG, et al. Autologous and allogeneic bone marrow transplantation for poor prognosis patients with B-cell chronic lymphocytic leukemia. *Blood* 1993;82:1366.
273. Khouri IF, Keating MJ, Vriesendorp HM, et al. Autologous and allogeneic bone marrow transplantation for chronic lymphocytic leukaemia: preliminary results. *J Clin Oncol* 1994;12:748.
274. Michallet M, Archimbaud E, Bandini G, et al. HLA-identical sibling bone marrow transplantation in younger patients with chronic lymphocytic leukemia. *Ann Intern Med* 1996;124:311.
275. Khouri IF, Przepiorka D, van Besien K, et al. Allogeneic blood or marrow transplantation for chronic lymphocytic leukaemia: timing of transplantation and potential effect of fludarabine on acute graft-versus-host disease. *Br J Haematol* 1997;97:466.
276. Provan D, Bartlett-Pandite L, Zwicky C, et al. Eradication of polymerase chain reaction–detectable chronic lymphocytic leukemia cells is associated with improved outcome after bone marrow transplantation. *Blood* 1996;88:2228.
277. Slavin S, Nagler A, Naparstek E, et al. Nonmyeloablative stem cell transplantation and cell therapy as an alternative to conventional bone marrow transplantation with lethal cytoreduction for the treatment of malignant and nonmalignant hematologic diseases. *Blood* 1998;91:756.
278. Khouri IF, Keating M, Körbling M, et al. Transplant-lite: induction of graft-versus-malignancy using fludarabine-based nonablative chemotherapy and allogeneic blood progenitor-cell transplantation as treatment for lymphoid malignancies. *J Clin Oncol* 1998;16:2817.
279. Pavletic ZS, Bierman PJ, Vose JM, et al. High incidence of relapse after autologous stem-cell transplantation for B-cell chronic lymphocytic leukemia or small lymphocytic lymphoma. *Ann Oncol* 1998;9:1023.
280. Johnson RE. Treatment of chronic lymphocytic leukemia by total body irradiation alone and combined with chemotherapy. *Int J Radiat Oncol Biol Phys* 1979;5:159.
281. Bennett JM, Raphael B, Moore D, et al. Comparison of chlorambucil and prednisone vs total body irradiation and chlorambucil:prednisone vs cytoxan, vincristine, prednisone for the therapy of active chronic lymphocytic leukemia: a long term follow-up of two ECOG studies. In: Gale RP, Rai KR, ed. *Chronic lymphocytic leukemia: recent progress and future directions.* New York: Alan R Liss, 1987:317.
282. De Rossi G, Biagini C, Lopez M, Tombolini V, Mandelli F. Treatment by splenic irradiation in 22 chronic lymphocytic leukemia patients. *Tumori* 1982;68:511.
283. Chisesi T, Capnist G, Dal Flor S. Splenic irradiation in chronic lymphocytic leukemia. *Eur J Haematol* 1990;46:202.
284. Paule B, Brion N, Brion G. Remission of autoimmune hemolytic anemia associated with chronic lymphocytic leukemia following splenic irradiation. *Nouv Rev Fr Hematol* 1989;31:413.
285. Marti GE, Folks T, Longo DL, Klein H. Therapeutic cytapheresis in chronic lymphocytic leukemia. *J Clin Apheresis* 1983;1:243.
286. Knobler RM, Pirker R, Kokoschka EM, et al. Experimental treatment of chronic lymphocytic leukemia with extracorporeal photochemotherapy. *Blut* 1990;60:215.
287. Committee of the Chronic Leukemia-Myeloma Task Force. Proposed guidelines for protocol studies. *Cancer Chemother Rep* 1973;4:141.
288. Silver RT, Sawitsky A, Rai K, Holland JF, Glidewell O. Guidelines for protocol studies in chronic lymphocytic leukemia. *Am J Hematol* 1978;4:343.
289. International Workshop on Chronic Lymphocytic Leukemia. Chronic lymphocytic leukemia: recommendations for diagnosis, staging, and response criteria. *Ann Intern Med* 1989;110:236.
290. Galton DAG, Goldman JM, Wiltshaw E, et al. Prolymphocytic leukaemia. *Br J Haematol* 1974;27:7.
291. Kjeldsberg CR, Marty J. Prolymphocytic transformation of chronic lymphocytic leukemia. *Cancer* 1981;48:2447.
292. Bennett JM, Catovsky D, Daniel MT, et al. Proposals for the classification of chronic (mature) B and T lymphoid leukaemias. *J Clin Pathol* 1989;42:567.
293. Davi F, Maloum K, Michel A, et al. High frequency of somatic mutations in the VH genes expressed in prolymphocytic leukemia. *Blood* 1996;88:3953.
294. Kantarjian HM, Childs C, O'Brien S, et al. Efficacy of fludarabine, a new adenine nucleoside analogue, in patients with prolymphocytic leukemia and the prolymphocytoid variant of chronic lymphocytic leukemia. *Am J Med* 1991;90:223.
295. Sporn JR. Sustained response of refractory prolymphocytic leukemia to fludarabine. *Acta Haematol* 1991;85:209.
296. Döhner H, Ho AD, Thaler J, et al. Pentostatin in prolymphocytic leukemia: phase II trial of the European Organization for Research and Treatment of Cancer Leukemia Cooperative Study Group. *J Natl Cancer Inst* 1993;85:658.
297. Saven A, Lee T, Schlutz M, et al. Major activity of cladribine in patients with *de novo* B-cell prolymphocytic leukemia. *Blood* 1997;15:37.
298. Bouroncle BA, Wiseman BK, Doan CA. Leukemic reticuloendotheliosis. *Blood* 1958;13:609.
299. Sainati L, Matutes E, Mulligan S, et al. A variant of hairy cell leukemia resistant to alpha-interferon: clinical and phenotypic characteristics of 17 patients. *Blood* 1990;76:157.
300. Grever M, Kopecky K, Foucar MK, et al. A randomized comparison of pentostatin vs alpha-interferon in previously untreated patients with hairy cell leukemia: an intergroup study. *J Clin Oncol* 1995;13:974.
301. Piro LD, Carrera CJ, Carson DA, Beutler E. Lasting remissions in hairy cell leukemia induced by a single infusion of 2-chlorodeoxyadenosine. *N Engl J Med* 1990;322:1117.
302. Spiers ASD, Parekh SJ, Bishop M. Hairy-cell leukemia: induction of complete remission with pentostatin (2'-deoxycoformycin). *J Clin Oncol* 1984;2:1336.
303. Tallman MS, Hakimian D, Rademaker AW, et al. Relapse of hairy cell leukemia after 2-chlorodeoxyadenosine: long-term follow-up of the Northwestern University experience. *Blood* 1996;88:1954.
304. Thomas DA, O'Brien S, Cortes J, et al. Pilot study of rituximab in refractory or relapsed hairy cell leukemia. *Blood* 1999;94[Suppl 1]:705a(abst 3116).
305. Kreitman RJ, Wilson WH, Robbins D, et al. Responses in refractory hairy cell leukemia to a recombinant immunotoxin. *Blood* 1999;94:3340.
306. Come SE, Jaffe ES, Andersen JC, et al. Non-Hodgkin's lymphomas in leukemic phase: clinicopathologic correlations. *Am J Med* 1980;69:667.
307. Mintzer DM, Hauptman SP. Lymphosarcoma cell leukemia and other non-Hodgkin's lymphomas in leukemic phase. *Am J Med* 1983;75:110.
308. Mulligan SP, Matutes E, Dearden C, Catovsky D. Splenic lymphoma with villous lymphocytes: natural history and response to therapy in 50 cases. *Br J Haematol* 1991;78:206.
309. Isaacson PG, Matutes E, Burke M, Catovsky D. The histopathology of splenic lymphoma with villous lymphocytes. *Blood* 1994;84:3828.
310. Lefrère F, Troussard X, Hermine O, et al. Fludarabine for splenic lymphoma with villous lymphocytes (SLVL). *Blood* 1997;90[Suppl 1]:308b(abst 4136).
311. Loughran TP Jr. Clonal diseases of large granular lymphocytes. *Blood* 1993;82:1.
312. Semenzato G, Zambello R, Starkebaum G, Oshimi K, Loughran TP Jr. The lymphoproliferative disease of granular lymphocytes: updated criteria for diagnosis. *Blood* 1997;89:256.
313. McKenna RW, Arthur DC, Gajl-Peczalska J, Flynn P, Brunning RD. Granulated T cell lymphocytosis with neutropenia: malignant or benign chronic lymphoproliferative disorder. *Blood* 1985;66:259.
314. Dearden C, Matutes E, Catovsky D. Deoxycoformycin in the treatment of mature T-cell leukaemias. *Br J Cancer* 1991;64:903.
315. O'Brien S, Kurzrock R, Duvic M, et al. 2-Chlorodeoxyadenosine therapy in patients with T-cell lymphoproliferative disorders. *Blood* 1994;84:733.
316. Tefferi A, Li CY, Witzig TE, et al. Chronic natural killer cell lymphocytosis: a descriptive clinical study. *Blood* 1994;84:2721.
317. Catovsky D. Diagnosis and treatment of CLL variants. In: Cheson BD, ed. *Chronic lymphocytic leukemia: scientific advances and clinical developments.* New York: Marcel Dekker Inc, 1993:369.
318. Uchiyama T, Yodoi J, Sagawa K, Takatsuki K, Uchino H. Adult T-cell leukemia: clinical and hematologic features of 16 cases. *Blood* 1977;50:481.
319. Kinoshita K, Amagasaki T, Ikeda S, et al. Preleukemic state of adult TG cell leukemia: abnormal T lymphocytosis induced by human adult T cell leukemia-lymphoma virus. *Blood* 1985;66:120.
320. Gibbs WN, Lofters WS, Campbell M, et al. Non-Hodgkin lymphoma in Jamaica and its relation to adult T-cell leukemia/lymphoma. *Ann Intern Med* 1987;106:361.
321. Lofters W, Campbell M, Gibbs WN, Cheson BD. 2'-Deoxycoformycin therapy in adult T-cell leukemia/lymphoma. *Cancer* 1987;60:2605.
322. Yamaguchi K, Nishimura H, Kohrogi H, et al. A proposal for smoldering adult T-cell leukemia: a clinicopathologic study of five cases. *Blood* 1983;62:758.

SECTION **4**

NIKHIL C. MUNSHI
GUIDO TRICOT
BART BARLOGIE

Plasma Cell Neoplasms

Plasma cell neoplasms represent a spectrum of diseases characterized by clonal proliferation and accumulation of immunoglobulin-producing cells that are terminally differentiated B cells. The spectrum includes clinically benign conditions, such as monoclonal gammopathy of unknown significance (MGUS) and rare disorders such as Castleman's disease and α heavy-chain disease; indolent conditions such as Waldenström's macroglobulinemia; the more common malignant entity, plasma cell myeloma, a disseminated B-cell malignancy; and a more aggressive form, plasma cell leukemia, with circulating malignant plasma cells in the blood. All of these disorders share common features in the form of plasma cell morphology, production of immunoglobulin molecules, and immune dysfunction. A plasma cell neoplasm is considered to originate from a single B cell, with resultant monoclonal protein secretion that characterizes its type. Occasional oligoclonal or polyclonal protein abnormalities are observed in conditions such as Castleman's disease. Current laboratory data based on complementarity determining region III (CDRIII) confirm the monoclonal origin of this disease.[1]

There are five major classes of immunoglobulin synthesized by normal B cells and plasma cells: IgG, IgA, IgM, IgD, and IgE. The dysfunctional plasma cells secrete one of these molecules or, in some instances, produce only κ or λ light chain molecules.[2–4] Usually, intact immunoglobulin molecules are secreted by the plasma cells; however, there may be a discrepancy in the production of the heavy and light chains leading to an imbalance, with an excess of free light chain that is excreted in the urine (Bence Jones proteinuria). Occasionally, plasma cells do not secrete any paraproteins (nonsecretory type myeloma); however, they usually have cytoplasmic immunoglobulin and produce low levels of immunoglobulins undetectable by current methods. Although myeloma can be associated with any of the immunoglobulin subtypes, the IgM type is predominately associated with other malignant conditions such as Waldenström's macroglobulinemia and chronic lymphocytic leukemia (CLL).

The clinical manifestations of plasma cell dyscrasias range from total absence of any symptoms in subjects with MGUS to formation of tumors, paraproteinemia, hypogammaglobulinemia due to decreased levels of the uninvolved immunoglobulins, bone disease, especially osteolytic lesions, hematopoietic and immune dysfunction, kidney function abnormalities, and infectious problems. These clinical manifestations are the result of a variety of pathogenic mechanisms, including cytokine production by the tumor or by the microenvironment, effect of the tumor mass itself, the deposition of the M protein into various organs, suppression of the T- and B-cell functions, and occasionally autoimmune disorders.

HISTORY

The earliest evidence of myeloma has been reported from the Egyptian mummies; however, the first published clinical description of the disease was reported in 1850 in England. A patient, Thomas Alexander McBean, presented with symptoms of episodes of fatigue, diffuse bone pain, and urinary frequency to Dr. William Macintrye of London in 1845. The urinalysis test results detected a urinary protein with the heat properties often observed for urinary light chains and McIntyre called it "mollities and fragilitas ossium" based on the patient's bony symptoms.[5] Later that year, Dr. Henry Bence Jones also tested urine specimens provided by Macintyre and corroborated the heat properties of urinary light chains. Bence Jones thought that the protein was the "hydrated deuteroxide of albumin" (now called *Bence Jones proteins*) and published his findings several years before Macintyre published his case report.[6] Bence Jones also emphasized the potential importance of looking for this urinary protein in other cases with mollities ossium. After the patient died in 1846, a surgeon, Dr. John Dalrymple, examined several bones and made gross and microscopic observations.[7] His drawings are consistent with morphology of myeloma cells.

The term *multiple myeloma* was coined by Rustizky in 1873 following his independent observation in a similar patient with multiple bone lesions.[8] Kahler in 1889 published a review on this condition and the disease became known, particularly in Europe, as Kahler's disease.[9] Ellinger, in 1899, described the increased serum proteins and sedimentation rate in myeloma.[10] In 1900, Wright described the involvement of plasma cells in this neoplasm instead of original belief of its origin from the red marrow and for the first time he used roentgenographic abnormality in myeloma, which to date remains one of the diagnostic tests.[11]

The development of bone marrow aspiration in 1929,[12] electrophoresis to separate serum proteins in 1937,[13] and a later report of a specific spike in the g globulin region[14] enhanced the diagnosis and understanding of myeloma. Identification of the heavy and light chains in the monoclonal protein by immunoelectrophoresis was described by Grabar in 1953, confirming the monoclonality of immunoglobulin in this disease.[15] Other developments from 1960s to 1980s include a staging system, role of several cytokines such as interleukin-1 (IL-1) and IL-6, and significance of chromosome 13 changes in myeloma.

No effective systemic therapy existed before 1947, when urethan was reported to show initial results in a few patients.[16] However, a subsequent randomized trial indicated that the survival of patients receiving urethan was inferior to that observed with a placebo.[17] The first successful use of chemotherapeutic agent in myeloma was reported in 1958 by Blokhin and colleagues with the use of a racemic mixture of D-and L-phenylalanine mustards (Sarcolysine). Subsequently, the D- and L-isomers of phenylalanine mustard were tested separately, and the antimyeloma activity was found to reside in the L-isomer, melphalan. In 1962, Bergsagel and colleagues of the Southwest Oncology Group reported remissions in approximately one-third of myeloma patients with melphalan.[18] Administration of high doses of the glucocorticoid was first reported to induce remissions in relapsing or refractory myeloma in 1967.[19] The use of melphalan in combination with prednisone was then studied extensively.[20] The role of high-dose therapy was investigated by McElwain and Powles in 1984, and addition of bone marrow transplantation with improved safety and further dose escalation was reported in 1986 by Barlogie et al.[21,22] Since then, numerous developments have taken place including activity of tandem transplant and the role of bisphosphonates and thalidomide.

EPIDEMIOLOGY

According to the most recent data from the Surveillance, Epidemiology, and End Results program, multiple myeloma is a relatively uncommon malignancy in the United States, representing 1.0% of all malignancies in whites and 2.0% in African Americans. Among hematologic malignancies, it constitutes 10% of the tumors and ranks as the second most frequently occurring hematologic cancer in the United States after non-Hodgkin's lymphoma. At any one time, the prevalence of myeloma is around 40,000 and approximately 14,000 new patients are diagnosed each year, with 11,000 people dying each year from myeloma. The disease is more common in men and has average annual age-adjusted (1970 U.S. standard) incidence rates per 100,000 among whites of 4.7 in men and 3.2 in women, whereas for African Americans the incidence is 10.2 in men and 6.7 in women. The increased incidence in African Americans is not explained by factors such as social or economic condition, household size, or family income.[23] The incidence data for other ethnic groups including native Hawaiians, female Hispanics, American Indians from New Mexico, and Alaskan natives also show higher myeloma rates relative to U.S. whites in the same geographic group; however, the Chinese and Japanese populations have a lower incidence than whites.

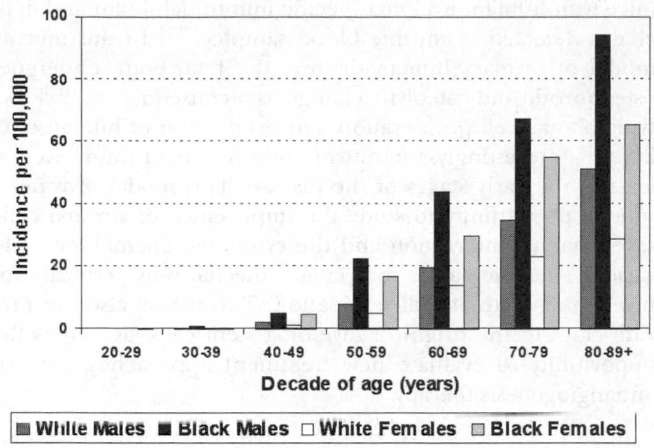

FIGURE 46.4-1. Multiple myeloma average annual age-, sex-, and race-specific incidence per 100,000 in the United States, 1992 to 1996. Increase in incidence is noted with advancing age, and higher incidence is observed in male than female subjects and in African American than white populations.

The incidence of multiple myeloma has slowly increased in the U.S. white population since 1970; however, the incidence among African Americans has increased more prominently during the 1970s, 1980s, and 1990s.

The incidence of myeloma and other plasma cell disorders increases with advancing age. The median age of onset is 68 years. The mortality pattern also closely follows the incidence curves for age distribution with median age at death in men of 70 years and women of 71 years. As seen in Figure 46.4-1, fewer than 2% of patients are younger than 40 years, whereas more than 40% of the patients are older than 70 years.[24] A similar age distribution is also observed in other related plasma cell disorders including MGUS and Waldenström's macroglobulinemia.

ETIOLOGY

ENVIRONMENTAL EXPOSURE

Exposure to ionizing radiation is the strongest single factor linked to an increased risk of multiple myeloma.[25] This has been documented in atomic bomb survivors with a five times greater incidence than the control group and a latent period of approximately 20 years from exposure.[26] People exposed to low levels of radiation also demonstrate an increased incidence of myeloma, including radiologists, people employed in the nuclear industry, or those handling radioactive materials.[27] An increase in myeloma risk with increasing numbers of diagnostic radiographs was demonstrated without an increased risk of leukemia or lymphoma, suggesting that even a low level of radiation may be a risk factor for myeloma. An association between exposure to various chemicals and the risk of multiple myeloma remains ill defined. Exposure to metals, especially nickel; agricultural chemicals; benzene and petroleum products; other aromatic hydrocarbons; and silicon have been considered as potential risk factors.[25,28–33] Alcohol and tobacco consumption has not been clearly linked to myeloma. Among medications, only mineral oil used as a laxative has been reported to be associated with an increased risk of multiple myeloma in some patients.[34,35]

Hereditary and genetic factors may predispose to myeloma development.[36,37] Among 37 families with at least two family members who had myeloma, occurrence among siblings was reported in 25 of the families. However, direct genetic linkage has not been established.[38] Myeloma risk also appears to be enhanced by the presence of HLA-Cw2 in both African American and white populations.

MGUS has been considered a premalignant condition; however, the rate of conversion to myeloma remains extremely small and often associated with additional genetic changes.[39,40] Repeated infections or antigenic stimulation of the plasma cell compartment has also been proposed as a possible predisposing condition for myeloma. In one interesting patient report in the literature, a prior therapy with horse antiserum against tetanus lead to subsequent development of MGUS, which lasted for three decades before conversion to multiple myeloma. At the time of myeloma diagnosis, the serum IgG component was found to react specifically against horse α_2-macroglobulin.[41] This report suggests an initial antigen-driven stimulation of monoclonal protein-producing plasma cells, eventually becoming malignant after acquiring additional genetic alterations.[42]

Epidemiologic studies have not been able to conclusively establish an association between multiple myeloma and infectious or autoimmune diseases. The human herpes virus (HHV-8; Kaposi's sarcoma herpes virus) has been shown to be present in the bone marrow dendritic cells of the majority of patients with multiple myeloma.[43,44] Its association with other lymphoproliferative diseases, such as Castleman's disease,[45] body cavity lymphoma,[46] and Kaposi's sarcoma,[47] has been previously demonstrated. Although this association has been reported by some,[44,48,49] others have failed to identify HHV-8 in dendritic cells from various sources including mobilized peripheral blood stem cells.[50–62] In the initial report, 100% of myeloma patients demonstrated evidence of ORF26 sequences in dendritic cells, compared with zero in normal controls. However, one study reports that 60% of 30 myeloma samples were positive for ORF26, with 44% of 25 normal controls demonstrating positive results. This study also failed to show positivity for the viral genes ORF72 and 75 in both myeloma and control samples.[49] Antibodies against HHV-8 have not been observed in multiple myeloma. Since HHV-8 produces unique gene products, including possible growth-promoting factors for myeloma such as IL-6, insulin-like growth factor-1, and an IL-8-like molecule, the possible linkage of HHV-8 to myeloma is intriguing, with infection of the stromal cell elements, part of the tumor microenvironment, exerting cell survival or antiapoptotic signals on the tumor cells.[63,64]

PATHOGENESIS

Myeloma occurs not only in humans, but also in mice, canines, and hamsters. In fact, genetic susceptibility to plasma cell tumors has been demonstrated in an inbred strain of mice. A common factor in various species has been considered to be the prevalence of endogenous retroviruses.[65,66] Animal models are now providing a basis for understanding the role of various molecular events, including the activation of oncogenes, tumor suppressor genes, and various cytokines, and the role of the microenvironment not only in causing bone destruction but sustaining and promoting growth, survival, drug resistance, and genetic instability.

MURINE MODEL

C57BL/Ka strains of inbred mice spontaneously develop monoclonal gammopathies without tumor formation in 16% of the mice by 2 years.[65,67,68] Other strains, such as BALB/c, have a low spontaneous incidence of monoclonal gammopathies. In BALB/c mouse, however, induction of plasmacytoma or myeloma is easily observed after intraperitoneal injection of mineral oil or its clinically defined component, pristane.[65] Production of such tumors can be blocked by administration of indomethacin and accelerated by subsequent infection of the mice with Abelson's virus. The plasmacytomas develop within the oil or other foreign body–mediated granulomas with lymphoplasmacytic infiltration. Plasmacytoma progression is associated with dysregulated expression of c-MYC as a result of translocation analogous to t(8;14) in humans. These plasmacytomas produce IgA immunoglobulins, and a growth factor present in the peritoneal fluid has been confirmed to be IL-6. Interestingly, however, the C57BL/Ka strain with a high incidence of spontaneous monoclonal gammopathies is relatively resistant to induction of plasmacytoma by mineral oil.

An association between antigenic stimulation of normal B cells and development of plasmacytoma has been demonstrated in the pristine oil–treated BALB/c mouse model. When animals are raised in a germ-free environment, incidence of myeloma after mineral oil stimulation is markedly reduced, whereas that of other lymphoid neoplasms increases.[65] These studies suggest an important role of immune stimulation toward myeloma development.

Human myeloma cell lines can grow and disseminate in a severe combined immunodeficiency (SCID) mouse model, providing a unique opportunity to study this disease in an *in vivo* setting.[69–71] The introduction of fetal human bone in to SCID mice (SCID-Hu) has allowed engraftment and proliferation of primary human myeloma cells in more than 80% of mice with human myeloma-specific immunoglobulin and light chains detected in murine blood samples.[72,73] In this murine model of primary human disease, the fetal bone undergoes osteoporotic and osteolytic change as a consequence of clonotypic plasma cell proliferation and production of human cytokines.[74] Interestingly, the murine bones remain uninvolved at least in the early stages of the disease. This model provides a unique opportunity to study the importance of stromal cell–myeloma cell interaction and the cytokines, chemokines, and various genetic and molecular mechanisms critical for myeloma growth and dissemination. This model also can provide clues to the origin of myeloma stem cells, as well as the opportunity to evaluate new treatment approaches, such as antiangiogenesis therapy.

CYTOGENETIC AND MOLECULAR GENETIC ALTERATIONS

Myeloma karyotypes are complex, with an average of 11 numeric and structural abnormalities per cell.[75–77] The relative incidence of gain or loss of various chromosomes and its p and q arm are shown in Figure 46.4-2. The inherent problem in the low proliferative activity of the tumor cells and possible clonal evolution have been obstacles to identify specific chromosomal and molecular changes in myeloma. However, the newer techniques of multicolor fluorescent *in situ* hybridization (FISH) and spectral karyotyping along with refined G-banding techniques in a large number of patients have identified many nonrandom changes.[78,79]

Partial or complete deletion chromosome 13 q arm confers a poor prognosis, even with high-dose therapy, and suggests a putative tumor suppressor gene.[80] Using the RB1 gene as a probe, FISH analysis reveals RB-1 deletion in more than 40% of these patients.[81] On detailed analysis of the 13q chromosome

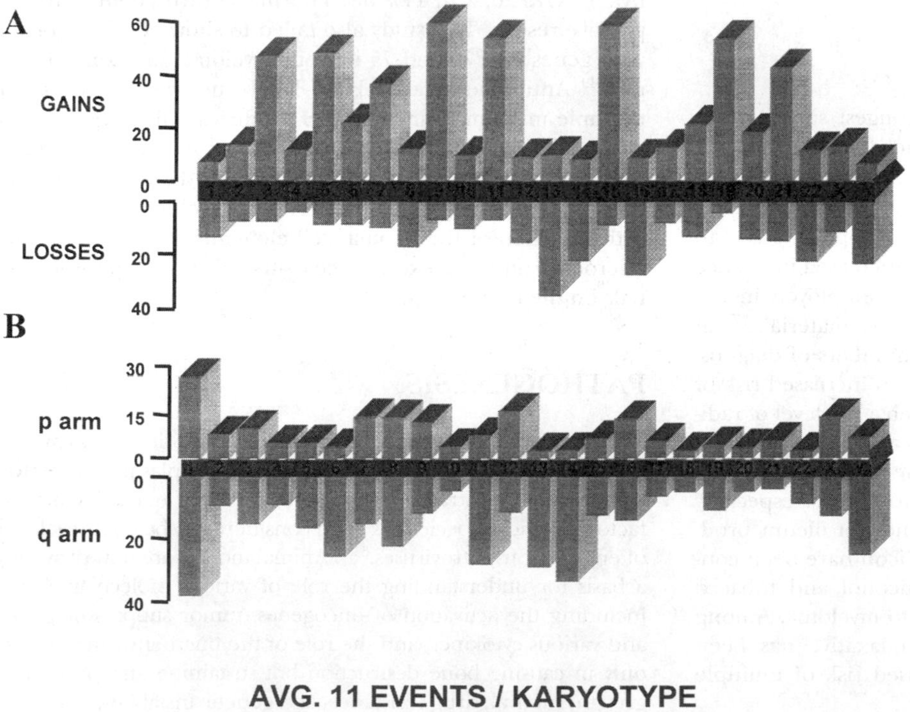

FIGURE 46.4-2. Summary karyotypic abnormalities in 158 patients with evaluable abnormal cytogenetics from study of 492 patients demonstrating *chromosomal chaos.* **A:** Numeric changes with trisomies (gain) and monosomies (loss). **B:** Structural changes involving short (p) and long (q) arms. (Courtesy of Jeffery R. Sawyer.)

with a 11 probe panel of FISH probes, more than 80% of 50 patients showed molecular deletions, with 13q14 representing a critical region most frequently involved.[82] Additionally, constitutive phosphorylation of pRB is reported in myeloma cells, which is further enhanced by IL-6.[83] Cycline D, cycline-dependent kinases (CDK) and CDK inhibitors p15 and p16 (ink), p21 and p27 (cip), and p57 (kip) have also been investigated in myeloma based on their effect on pRB phosphorylation. Abnormalities in p16 in 75% and p15 in 67% of myeloma patients have been reported, suggesting an important defect in the pRB regulatory pathway.[84–87]

The immunoglobulin heavy-chain gene at 14q32 is involved in translocation in 20% to 30% of myeloma by conventional cytogenetics and higher percentage by molecular techniques.[75,76,88] Demonstration of this abnormality in MGUS may suggest its involvement in the initial step of the transformation.[89] The most common translocation involving 14q32 is t(11;14), resulting in overexpression of cycline D.[88,90] Additional interesting partners are 4p, 16q, and chromosome 9. Involved in the 4p16 region are fibroblast growth factor receptor III (FGFR3) and MMSET genes. Mutated FGFR3 has been shown to confer resistance to caspase 3–related apoptosis.[91,92] With the help of spectral karyotyping a nonrandom involvement of t(14:16) (q32:q22-23) has been described. Molecular analysis of the locus at chromosome 16q22 shows fusion of immunoglobulin heavy chain with the sequence near the cMAF oncogene.[93] Additionally, t(9;14) involving PAX5 gene and t(6;14) involving IRF4 genes have been described.[94,95] In the majority of the cases, however, the translocating partner chromosome locus is not identified. Although, 14q32 is one of the common translocation points, its real significance remains unclear in relation to myelomagenesis because of the variety of partner chromosomes involved and lack of prognostic implications.

One of the commonly altered genes in many malignancies is p53. However, in myeloma, abnormalities in p53 in early disease are detected in only 10% of patients.[96–98] However, it represents an important late event associated with progression to an aggressive form of the disease. A study of frequency of p53 gene mutations in a series of 52 patients with myeloma in different clinical phases showed 7 of 52 patients with abnormalities, all with an advanced and clinically aggressive acute leukemic form of multiple myeloma (7 of 16, 43%). Three of these cases with mutated p53 had been evaluated earlier during the indolent form of the disease and were negative for p53 mutations.[96] One study showed poor prognosis in patients with p53 gene deletion, as assessed by FISH when treated with standard-dose therapy.[97] The effect of p53 deletion in relation to high-dose therapy has not yet been evaluated. In contrast to primary patient samples, mutations in p53 are more commonly detected in myeloma cell lines, which are usually derived from patients with aggressive myeloma. MDM2, an important inhibitor of p53 function, is overexpressed in the majority of myeloma cell lines; however, its abnormality is infrequently observed in primary myeloma cells.[99] Changes in another important cell-cycle regulatory gene, c-myc, are also observed in a majority of patients in the form of either abnormal size transcript or high level of expression.[100,101]

An important antiapoptotic gene, BCL-2, is uniformly overexpressed in low-grade non-Hodgkin's lymphoma. In this family of genes, BCL-2 and BCL-XL are antiapoptotic genes, while BAX, BAD, and BCL_{XS} are proapoptotic genes. A balance between these genes determines cell survival. The t(14:18) translocation involving the BCL-2 gene is quite rare (2% to 3%) in myeloma. However, numerous myeloma cell lines as well as primary cells express high levels of BCL-2.[102,103] Its relation with development of drug resistance as well as radiation resistance in myeloma cells is also well described.[104,105,386] The relation of BCL-2 expression and prognosis remains controversial as one small study failed to correlate it with short survival. Another study in 63 patients, however, showed a significant correlation between BCL-2 expression and resistance to therapy with interferon but not melphalan and prednisone.[106] BCL-XL is up-regulated in myeloma cells after exposure to IL-6 through activation of STAT-3.[107,108] It confers a drug-resistant phenotype and in conjunction with BCL-2 leads to increased genetic instability. These and other molecular changes involving gp130, NF-κB, and STATs combined lead to the development and progression of myeloma.[109]

High telomerase activity has also been demonstrated in myeloma cells compared with normal cells, as well as other malignant cell lines.[110] The clinical implication of this activity remains under investigation; however, telomerase activity provides an additional target for therapeutic intervention.

DISEASE EVOLUTION

Multiple myeloma is a germinal center-derived tumor with mainly a post-switch B-cell phenotype characterized by extensive Ig gene hypermutation in the CDRs, which interacts with the antigen. This is reflected in the exceedingly rare occurrence of IgM myeloma. Somatic mutations of other loci, such as BCL-6, have also been reported in the B cells along with the immunoglobulin gene rearrangement.[111] Similar mechanisms may also be affecting other cell-cycle control genes important for cell proliferation and malignant transformation.

As in most malignancies, pathogenesis of multiple myeloma appears to be associated with dysregulated expression and the function of multiple key cellular genes controlling apoptosis, cell growth, and proliferation. Understanding the evolution of myeloma from MGUS has provided a background for a multistep process involving alterations in various oncogenes and tumor suppressor genes. One report suggests the presence of 14q32 abnormalities in patients with MGUS and an additional chromosome 13 change, with a transformation to overt multiple myeloma.[89] This has lead to a theory that a subset of myeloma may originate from prior MGUS with a high incidence of monosomy 13 and a second group of *de novo* myeloma in which other genetic abnormalities may be involved.[89]

CYTOKINES

IL-6 is an important cytokine originally identified as a B-cell differentiation factor that causes proliferation of plasmablastic cells and induces terminal differentiation of B cells into antibody-producing cells. Several studies have confirmed its activity as an autocrine and paracrine growth factor for myeloma cell lines and primary cells.[112–115] Evidence supporting this includes *in vitro* myeloma cell growth in the presence of recombinant IL-6,[83] IL-6 production by some of the myeloma cells themselves,[116] expression of high levels of IL-6 receptors,[112] and suppression of *in vitro* myeloma cell proliferation by anti–IL-6 antibodies.[117]

Close cell–cell contact between myeloma cells and the bone marrow stromal cells triggers a large amount of IL-6 production by stromal cells, which supports the growth of myeloma cells and protects them from apoptosis induced by dexamethasone or other chemotherapeutic agents.[118,119] Correlation has been reported between serum IL-6 levels or C-reactive protein (CRP) levels, an indirect measurement of IL-6 activity, and disease severity as well as extent of bone marrow plasmacytosis[120]; frequent lytic bone lesions; and some tumor-associated symptoms such as fever, fatigue, and weight loss. In addition, indirect evidence of the role of IL-6 in B-cell disorders is provided through IL-6 transgenic mice. These animals have a high incidence of polyclonal plasmacytosis. Transduction of the IL-6 gene in hematopoietic cells in mice leads to a disorder resembling Castleman's disease.[121] IL-6, however, is not an absolute requirement for myeloma cell growth as some of the myeloma cells do not proliferate in response to IL-6, nor do they require IL-6 for their continued growth. Therapy with anti–IL-6 antibody has also not provided significant clinical benefit.[122,123]

Expression by myeloma cells of IL-1β, tumor necrosis factor-β (TNF-β), and hepatocyte growth factor has been described, resulting in development of resistance to therapy, possibly through activation of NF-κB.[124–127] Myeloma cells express a variety of cytokine receptors that play a significant role in cell–cell interactions as well as autocrine and paracrine growth control. A majority of myeloma cell lines and primary cells express IL-6–related receptors gp80 and gp130.[128,129] Additionally, receptors are expressed for TNF-α, IL-11, IL-1, IL-2, IL-7, granulocyte-macrophage colony-stimulating factor (GM-CSF), stem cell factor, leukocyte inhibitory factor, oncostatin-M, and insulin-like growth factor-1 and -2.[130–134] These findings suggest that in addition to IL-6, interferon-γ, IL-1, IL-2, IL-7, GM-CSF, TNF, and insulin growth factor have at least a direct biologic effect on myeloma cells.

The soluble cytokines can be used *in vitro* to expand the pre-B cells to mature plasma cell stage with cytoplasmic immunoglobulin expression. An important combination of cytokines in this regard is IL-6 and IL-3. However, secretion of immunoglobulin requires contact between marrow stromal cells and myeloma cells; this occurs through adhesion molecules on the surface of the myeloma cells and their counterparts on the stromal cell or extracellular matrix in the bone marrow.[135]

The role of angiogenesis in myeloma has been investigated, showing that advanced-stage myeloma is associated with high microvessel density in bone marrow compared with indolent myeloma or MGUS.[136,137] An association between increased bone marrow microvessel density at diagnosis with poor event-free and overall survival has also been reported.[138] Angiogenic factors such as vascular endothelium growth factor-1 (VEGF-1) and fibroblast growth factor are expressed by myeloma cells.[139] This observation has lead to an evaluation of thalidomide as antiangiogenic therapy in myeloma with encouraging results.[140]

ADHESION MOLECULES

Adhesion molecules, especially those expressed by myeloma cells and the bone marrow stromal cells, play an important role in mediating the interaction between the host and tumor cells to regulate tumor growth and migration of these cells *in vivo.* It is believed that after class switching in lymph nodes, myeloma cells home to the bone marrow through acquisition of a variety of adhesion molecules including syndecan-1 (CD138), CD44, very late antigen-4 (VLA-4) (CD49d) and VLA-5 (CD49e), lymphocyte function–associated antigen-1 (LFA-1), intracellular adhesion molecule-1 (CD54), neural cell adhesion molecule (NCAM) (CD56), and MPC-1.[141,142] The homing to the marrow leads to binding of myeloma cells to bone marrow stromal cells, which in turn mediates signal transduction events including IL-6 production by the stromal cells.[72] The adhesion molecules in the bone marrow that myeloma cells bind to, and require for their homing, include heparan sulfate proteoglycan, intracellular adhesion molecule-1, and vascular cellular adhesion molecule-1 (VCAM-1) on the bone marrow stromal cell, as well as fibronectin and type I collagen in the extracellular matrix.[143–146] With further progress of the disease, CD56 (NCAM), syndecan-1 (CD138), and VLA-5 are down-regulated; in the case of syndecan-1, this occurs in response to IL-6. Some of these changes may allow circulation of clonotypic plasma cells in blood. The acquisition of CD11b may also help in invasion and metastatic spread through its interaction with the endothelium. All plasma cells express CD38, which is a receptor for CD31, expressed on endothelial cells with potential implications for trafficking of myeloma cells through blood vessels. Interestingly, the majority of the plasmacytic myeloma cells, but not plasmablastic and plasma cell leukemia cells, have also been reported to express CD31.[147] Other than syndecan-1, matrix metalloproteinase (MMP), especially MMP-2 and MMP-9, have also been implicated in myeloma cell proliferation and spread.[136,148,149] Serum syndecan-1 levels are reflective of tumor burden as is hepatocyte growth factor.[127,150] *In vitro* and *in vivo* studies have documented a role of syndecan-1 in cell–cell and cell–matrix adhesion and in inducing myeloma cell apoptosis.[144] Syndecan-1 expressed by myeloma cell may also serve to trap the growth regulatory molecules such as fibroblast growth factor and insulin-like growth factor as well as angiogenic molecules, such as VEGF and fibroblast growth factor.[149] Expression of different adhesion and surface molecules on normal plasma cells, myeloma cells, and plasma cell leukemia cells are listed in Table 46.4-1.

PHENOTYPE

Myeloma cells display heterogenous phenotypes with differences in the molecules among different patients expressed on the cell surface as well as differences within the same patient at different disease stages.[135] In general, all myeloma cells express high levels of CD38 with immature plasma cell additionally expressing CD45 and the IL-6 receptor.[116,151–153] More mature myeloma cells do not express CD45 and lack the IL-6 receptor expression.[154] A subpopulation of myeloma cells may also express CD10, CD56, or CD49e (VLA-5).[154–157] CD28 expression is associated with more aggressive disease[158,159] and CD20 expression is present in 20% of myeloma patients, which can be further up-regulated with interferon-α.[160] The phenotypic heterogeneity of myeloma cells in fact describes the differentiation process that is an important part of the disease development. The identity of the myeloma stem cell still remains an enigma. B cells expressing CD19 and CD11b can be induced to mature with the help of stromal cells into monotypic plasma cells, suggesting that this cellular compartment may comprise myeloma cell progenitors.[161] Using the allele-specific oligonucleotide PCR and the SCID-hu model, the myeloma stem cell will be better defined in the future.

TABLE 46.4-1. Adhesion Molecule Expression on Normal Plasma Cells and Multiple Myeloma Cells

	Normal Plasma Cell	*Multiple Myeloma Cell*
SURFACE MOLECULES		
CD19	+	±
CD20	+	±
CD28	–	–
CD38	+	+
CD40	+	+[a]
CD45	+	–[b]
ADHESION MOLECULES		
CD11a	+	–
CD11b	–	–[c]
CD44	+	+
CD54	+	+
CD56	–	+[d]
CD58	–	+
LFA-1	–	±
VLA-4	+	+
VLA-5	+	+[d]
MPC-1	+	+[d]
RHAMM	–	+[d]
Syndecan-1	+	+

[a]CD40 expression is enhanced on plasma cell leukemia cells relative to normal plasma cells and multiple myeloma cells.
[b]CD45 on immature myeloma cells.
[c]Expression is gained on plasma cell leukemia cells.
[d]Expression is lost on plasma cell leukemia cells.
(Adapted from ref. 142.)

IMMUNOSUPPRESSION

Myeloma patients present with suppressed immune function from a variety of factors. The most significant observation is suppression of uninvolved immunoglobulins (e.g., in patients with IgG myeloma there is suppression of serum IgA and IgM levels).[162] The factors causing such suppression include the direct role of monoclonal immunoglobulin, increased soluble Fc-receptor or Fc-expressing cells, suppression of helper cell functions through the effect of monoclonal immunoglobulin, and an ill-defined macrophage-related factor that affects B-cell maturation to plasma cell.[163] Recovery of uninvolved immunoglobulin following effective therapy has been associated with improved survival as well as protection from infectious complications. In regard to T-cell function, deficiency of T_4 helper cell is most pronounced.[164] The total T-cell count may be decreased; however, in a substantial number of patients it could be normal with no significant change in CD8 cells.[165–168] There has been demonstration of a stage-dependent suppression of NK cells.[169] Antiidiotypic T-cell response has been demonstrated in the majority of the patients with higher Id-specific T-cell frequency in MGUS and early-stage myeloma compared with advanced disease.[170] This has lead to a provocative hypothesis that in the early stage of the disease immunologic response plays an important role in controlling proliferation of the malignant clone, and at some point the system is overwhelmed or fails, leading to an overt or more aggressive form of the disease. This also provides a scientific basis to develop idiotype-specific T-cell response through vaccination or *in vitro* production of idiotype or myeloma-specific cytotoxic T lymphocytes for therapeutic purpose.[171]

CLINICAL MANIFESTATIONS

Patients with multiple myeloma may be entirely asymptomatic and could be diagnosed on routine blood work or may present with a myriad of symptoms, including hematologic manifestations, bone-related problems, infections, various organ dysfunctions, neurologic complaints, or bleeding tendencies (Table 46.4-2). These signs and symptoms result from direct tumor involvement in the bone marrow or location of various plasmacytomas in the body, the effect of the protein produced by the tumor cells and deposited in various organs, production of cytokines by the tumor cells or by the bone marrow microenvironment, and the effect on the immune system.

ANEMIA

A normochromic normocytic anemia is usually observed in myeloma patients and it may originate from tumor cell involvement in the marrow as well as inadequate erythropoietin responsiveness. Anemia gives rise to fatigue, weakness, and occasionally shortness of breath. In addition to the decreased production of red cells due to marrow infiltration, the effect of various cytokines on erythropoiesis and the effect of renal dysfunction on erythropoietin production may account for some of these effects. High immunoglobulin levels aggravate the anemia due to dilutional effects. In the Durie-Salmon staging system, the level of anemia is considered as one of the criteria to determine the tumor mass load.

RENAL FAILURE

Nephropathy is one of the serious adverse complications that can be observed at the time of clinical presentation. The etiology of renal failure can be multifactorial. However, the most common cause is development of light chain tubular casts leading to interstitial nephritis (myeloma kidney).[172] Another common cause of renal dysfunction is development of hypercalcemia and hypercalciuria leading to osmotic diuresis and vol-

TABLE 46.4-2. Clinical Features of Multiple Myeloma

Symptoms	*Common Cause*
Bone pain	Pathologic fracture
Easy fatigability	Anemia
Polyuria	Hypercalcemia
Nausea and vomiting	Renal failure, hypercalcemia
Recurrent infections	Low uninvolved Ig, low CD4 count
Paraplegia	Cord compression
Confusion, central nervous system symptoms	Hyperviscosity or hypercalcemia
Neurologic symptoms	Nerve compression, amyloidosis, POEMS syndrome

POEMS, polyneuropathy, organomegaly, endocrinopathy, monoclonal gammopathy, and skin changes.

ume depletion and prerenal azotemia. Other modes of kidney involvement in myeloma are light chain deposition disease, which is more commonly associated with κ light chain proteins with impaired glomerular filtration; and AL amyloidosis, which is more frequently associated with λ light chain, especially λ light chain subtype VI, and may have an initial presentation as nephrotic range proteinuria, and renal calcium deposition leading to interstitial nephritis.[173–176] The presence of λ light chain in the urine is also more commonly associated with myeloma kidney when compared with κ light chain. Bence Jones proteins bind to a common peptide segment of Tom-Horsfall glycoprotein to promote heterotypic aggregation.[177–179] Tom-Horsfall protein deposition in the kidney and its measurement in the urine may be a sensitive measure to predict renal dysfunction.[180] Additional factors complicating the renal failure in myeloma patients includes use of nonsteroidal antiinflammatory drugs for pain control, hyperuricemia, nephrotoxic chemotherapeutic agents, intravenous contrast for radiographic studies, and calcium deposition and stones in the kidney.[181] The proteinuria observed in patients with amyloidosis is more often nonspecific, which can help differentiate it from typical myeloma-related kidney problems in which patients have excessive light chain excretion.[182] A demonstration of the development of pathologic renal changes similar to human myeloma-related nephropathy in an IL-6 transgenic mice expressing IL-6 under metallothionein-1 promoter indicates a relationship between constitutive high IL-6 expression in the liver inducing dysproteinemia and long acute-phase response and renal changes.[183]

HYPERCALCEMIA AND BONE DISEASE

The mechanism of bone abnormalities, especially destruction, in myeloma is an unbalanced process of increased osteoclast activity and suppressed osteoblast activity. These changes are exerted by an increase in osteoclast-activating factors produced predominantly by the bone marrow microenvironment but additionally contributed by the myeloma cells.[126,184] These factors include IL-1b, TNF-β (lymphotoxin), and IL-6.[124,125,387] Newly identified factors such as osteoprotegerin and its ligand TRANCE and RANK ligand, which acts as a decoy receptor for TRANCE, have been implicated in the development of bone changes in myeloma.[185,186] TRANCE is a member of the TNF family and was originally discovered to be secreted by T cells to induce maturation of dendritic cells. TRANCE is also secreted by stromal cells and osteoblasts and induces differentiation and maturation of osteoclast progenitors. Its production is elicited by factors such as parathyroid hormone, parathyroid hormone–related protein, and osteoclast-activating factors. Radiographic findings of such destruction are shown in Figure 46.4-3.[184,187] All of these changes lead to the development of osteoporotic changes and subsequent development of lytic bone lesions. These bone changes frequently involve the vertebral column, leading to compression fracture and lytic bone lesions that lead to pain-related complications in this disease. A new onset of back pain or other bone pain is a frequent presenting symptom in myeloma patients. These changes in the cytokine milieu and bone destruction may also lead to development of hypercalcemia, which is observed in approximately 25% of patients at some stage of the disease. It may reflect a high tumor burden and the presence of symptoms related to high calcium, which include mental status changes, lethargy, constipation, and vomiting. High paraprotein levels, low albumin levels, or both, commonly observed in patients with myeloma require measurement of ionized calcium rather than total calcium to reliably diagnose hypercalcemia. Hypercalcemia also contributes to renal failure and should be considered an oncologic emergency requiring prompt intervention.

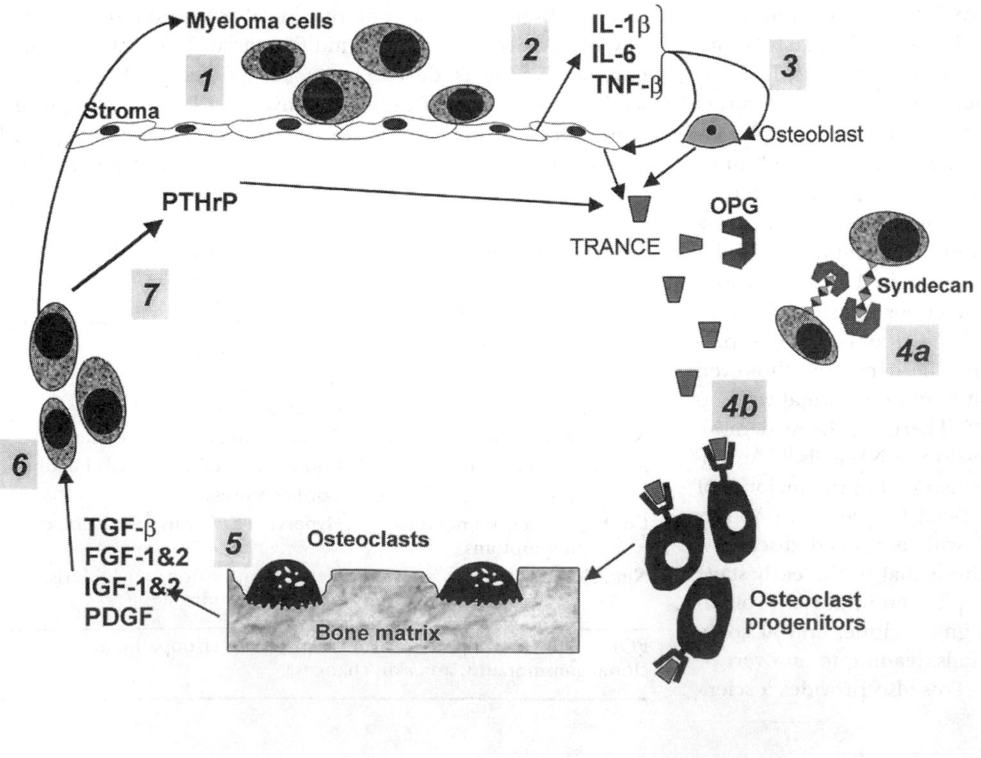

FIGURE 46.4-3. Biology of bone destruction in multiple myeloma (MM): 1. MM cells adhere to stroma. 2. Stromal cells secrete osteoclast-activating factors. 3. Osteoclast-activating factors elicit stroma and osteoblasts to secrete TRANCE. 4a. TRANCE is blocked by osteoprotegerin (OPG); OPG levels are reduced in MM due to syndecan trapping OPG. 4b. Excess TRANCE is available to stimulate osteoclast differentiation and maturation. 5. Increased osteoclastic activity leads to increased cytokine release from the bone matrix. 6. These cytokines stimulate MM cell growth, which increases process 1. 7. These cytokines also cause release of parathyroid hormone–related protein (PTHrP) from MM cells, which activates stromal cells to secrete additional TRANCE. FGF-1 and 2, fibroblast growth factor-1 and 2; IGF-1 and 2, insulin growth factor-1 and 2; IL, interleukin; PDGF, platelet-derived growth factor; TGF-β, transforming growth factor-β; TNF-β, tumor necrosis factor-β. (Adapted from ref. 187.)

INFECTIONS

Myeloma patients are at risk for developing recurrent bacterial infections due to deficiencies in both humoral and cellular immunity.[163,188–190] Various factors including high monoclonal immunoglobulin levels, soluble Fc receptor in serum, and transforming growth factor-β lead to suppression of B-cell function, which in turn leads to depressed uninvolved immunoglobulins.[191–193] This impairment in patients' abilities to mount humoral responses predisposes patients to bacterial infections that are ordinarily opsonized by specific antibodies against the bacterial antigens. Patients also have profound T-cell dysfunction originating from various immunosuppressive cytokines such as transforming growth factor-β secreted by the microenvironment and fas ligand present on the membrane of the myeloma cells. The therapy for myeloma, which frequently includes high-dose corticosteroids, also increases the infection-related risks in these patients.

NEUROLOGIC SYMPTOMS

The most common cause of neurologic abnormalities is related to a tumor mass effect, especially compression of the spinal cord or cranial or spinal nerves. This may present as motor or, less frequently, sensory problems. Depositions of amyloids in the paraneural or *vasa nervorum* may lead to polyneuropathies. An interesting group of symptoms described as POEMS syndrome (*p*olyneuropathy, *o*rganomegaly, *e*ndocrinopathy, *m*onoclonal gammopathy, and *s*kin changes) is observed in osteosclerotic myeloma with prominent sensory neuropathy.[194–198] The biologic and cellular basis of these manifestations is not yet well understood. Leptomeningeal involvement in myeloma has been described, usually in the late phase of the disease and with manifestations involving the CNS.[199,200] Paraneoplastic CNS syndromes have also been described, possibly related to an immune mechanism directed at proteins present in the CNS including the cerebellum. Additionally, neurologic symptoms may occur as a consequence of hypercalcemia or hyperviscosity.

HYPERVISCOSITY

The M components in myeloma can lead to circulatory problems when the serum immunoglobulin levels exceed certain levels. Such effects require sufficient concentration of an M protein; the incidence is highest in Waldenström's macroglobulinemia with IgM, followed by IgA myeloma, and is least common in IgG myeloma.[201–203] It can also be observed when the immunoglobulins have a self-aggregation property leading to increased viscosity. The syndrome is observed usually when serum viscosity exceeds 4.0 centipoule (cp) units relative to normal serum and it usually manifests with circulatory problems involving the CNS, kidneys, and pulmonary function and may also be associated with bleeding complications. Due to varying characteristics of idiotypes, the same level of increased viscosity may produce different severity of symptoms in different patients. Its incidence in IgA myeloma is 25% of the patients, whereas in IgG myeloma it is observed in less than 10% of the patients. In IgG myeloma, the IgG3 subclass is more commonly associated with hyperviscosity.[204] As prompt plasmapheresis can alleviate the symptoms and possibly other irreversible organ damage, a high level of suspicion for this syndrome is important in any patient with paraproteinemia and either mental changes or pulmonary distress.

COAGULOPATHY

Myeloma patients may acquire coagulation abnormalities related to a high level of paraprotein interfering with the normal coagulation cascade or exhibit specific antibody activity leading to a clinical syndrome similar to acquired deficiency of factor VIII.[205–207] Additional factors such as thrombosis in capillary circulation associated with hyperviscosity and anoxia may lead to coagulation-related complications in 15% of patients with IgG myeloma and in more than 33% of the patients with IgA myeloma. Although platelet counts are not suppressed in the early stages of myeloma, functional abnormalities of platelets have been described and may contribute to bleeding-related problems.

Patients may also present in a hypercoagulable state related to acquired deficiencies in protein C, protein S, or lupus anticoagulates, leading to thromboembolic complications.[208]

The fab fragment of the antibody of the myeloma protein binds to fibrin and may prevent its aggregation. This may represent one of the common mechanisms of coagulopathy in myeloma.[209] Additionally, factor X deficiency is reported in patients with systemic AL amyloidosis.[210] However, an inhibitor has not been demonstrated *in vitro* to account for this manifestation.

EXTRAMEDULLARY DISEASE

Extramedullary disease manifestations are uncommon in patients with myeloma at presentation. However, with more aggressive therapy and improved survival an increasing frequency of such manifestations has been observed. Solitary or multiple extramedullary plasmacytomas have been described in the liver, spleen, lymph nodes, kidneys, subcutaneous tissues, and brain parenchyma. Such extramedullary involvement may be suspected in patients who have more aggressive features of myeloma including high lactate dehydrogenase levels, immunoblastic morphology, high tumor cell labeling index, and complex karyotypic features.[211]

DIAGNOSIS

As myeloma patients present with a variety of symptoms not specific to the disease, the diagnosis of myeloma is quite often delayed. An older patient with a new onset of unexplained back pain or bone pain, recurrent infection, anemia, or renal insufficiency should be screened for myeloma. Additional finding such as hyperproteinemia or proteinuria, anemia, hypoalbuminemia, low immunoglobulin levels, or marked elevation of erythrocyte sedimentation rate should prompt a further complete evaluation for diagnosis of plasma cell myeloma.

The initial evaluation includes a hemogram, complete skeletal radiographic survey, serum and urine protein electrophoresis and immunofixation, quantitative immunoglobulin levels, urinary protein excretion in 24 hours, and bone marrow aspiration and biopsy (Table 46.4-3). The diagnostic criteria for MGUS, smoldering and indolent myeloma, and multiple myeloma are shown in Table 46.4-4.

TABLE 46.4-3. Patient Evaluation in Multiple Myeloma

Presence and characterization of monoclonal protein
Serum protein electrophoresis
Quantitative immunoglobulin
24-H urine: total protein and Bence Jones protein immunofixation of urine and serum
Radiologic evaluation
Skeletal survey
Magnetic resonance imaging with short time inversion recovery images
Bone densitometry
Computed tomography to rule out solitary plasmacytoma
Laboratory evaluation
Complete blood cell count with reticulocyte and differential count
Chemistry panel (renal, calcium, albumin, uric acid, lactate dehydrogenase)
β_2-Microglobulin, C-reactive protein
Bone marrow
Aspirate and biopsy
Cytogenetics
Flow cytometry (DNA-cIg)
Plasma cell labeling index
Specialized studies for selected patients
Abdominal fat pad or rectal biopsy for amyloid
Solitary lytic lesion biopsy
Serum viscosity if IgM component or high IgA levels or serum M component >7 g/dL

Ig, immunoglobulin.

STAGING AND RISK ASSESSMENT

Following preliminary investigation, more detailed cellular and molecular studies are required to stage myeloma and evaluate other prognostic variables that determine the patient's probable outcome.

PROTEIN ELECTROPHORESIS

Among patients with myeloma, 70% have IgG, whereas 20% have IgA subtype with an additional 5% to 10% having production of monoclonal light chains only. A small proportion, less than 1%, of patients produce monoclonal IgD, IgE, IgM or have nonsecretory myelomas. Suppression of uninvolved immunoglobulins (e.g., IgM and IgA in IgG myeloma) is present in the majority of the patients at diagnosis. Suppression of all of the three major classes of immunoglobulin should raise the possibility that the patient may have light chain only disease or a nonsecretory disease. When multiple immunoglobulin class suppression is associated with small M peak on serum protein electrophoresis, a less common variety of myeloma involving IgD or IgE may be suspected. Patients producing intact immunoglobulin can also have excess light chain production with excretion in the urine (Fig. 46.4-4). The distribution of κ and λ light chains in the majority of myeloma cases is similar except in IgD myeloma in which λ light chain is more common. Currently, there is no difference in therapeutic approach between the different types of myeloma; however, patients with IgA myeloma, despite a higher initial response rate, have poorer survival outcomes.

Myeloma plasma cells usually produce a single, abnormal, unique, monoclonal antibody with a constant isotype and light chain restriction. Rare occurrences of biclonal and triclonal cases have been reported at the time of diagnosis.[212]

TABLE 46.4-4. Diagnostic Criteria for Multiple Myeloma, Myeloma Variants, and Monoclonal Gammopathy of Unknown Significance

Multiple myeloma
Major criteria
I. Plasmacytoma on tissue biopsy
II. Bone marrow plasmacytosis with >30% plasma cells
III. Monoclonal globulin spike on serum electrophoresis exceeding 3.5 g/dL for IgG or 2 g/dL for IgA, greater than or equal to 1 g/24 h of κ- or λ-light chain excretion on urine electrophoresis in the presence of amyloidosis
Minor criteria
a. Bone marrow plasmacytosis 10% to 30%
b. Monoclonal globulin spike present but less than the level defined above
c. Lytic bone lesions
d. Suppressed uninvolved immunoglobulins; IgM <50 mg/dL, IgA <100 mg/dL, or IgG <600 mg/dL
Diagnosis is confirmed when any of the following features are documented in symptomatic patients with clearly progressive disease. The diagnosis of myeloma requires a minimum of one major and one minor criterion or three minor criteria that must include a + b, that is,
I + b, I + c, I + d (I + a not sufficient)
II + b, II + c, II + d
III + a, III + c, III + d
a + b + c, a + b + d
Indolent myeloma (same as myeloma except)
No bone lesions or only limited bone lesion (less than or equal to three lytic lesions): no compression fractures
M component levels: (a) IgG <7 g/dL; (b) IgA <5/dL
No symptoms or associated disease features, that is,
Performance status >70%
Hemoglobin >10 g/dL
Serum calcium normal
Serum creatinine <2 mg/dL
No infections
Smoldering myeloma (same as indolent myeloma except)
No bone lesions
Bone marrow plasma cells less than or equal to 30%
Monoclonal gammopathy of unknown significance
Monoclonal gammopathy
M component level
IgG less than or equal to 3.5 g/dL
IgA less than or equal to 2 g/dL
Bence Jones protein less than or equal to 1 g/24 h
Bone marrow plasma cells <10%
No bone lesions
No symptoms

Ig, immunoglobulin.
(Adapted from refs. 139, 170, 194, and 195.)

Occurrence of isotype switch and appearance of abnormal protein bands have, however, been reported in myeloma patients after therapy, especially high-dose therapy.[213] This appears to be related to recovery of normal immunoglobulin production rather than alteration in disease biology. This change is also associated with improved survival. Occasionally, patients with initially intact immunoglobulin production relapse with only Bence Jones proteinuria (light chain escape), nonsecretory disease, or high lactate dehydrogenase disease, and this change has been correlated with more aggressive disease.[214]

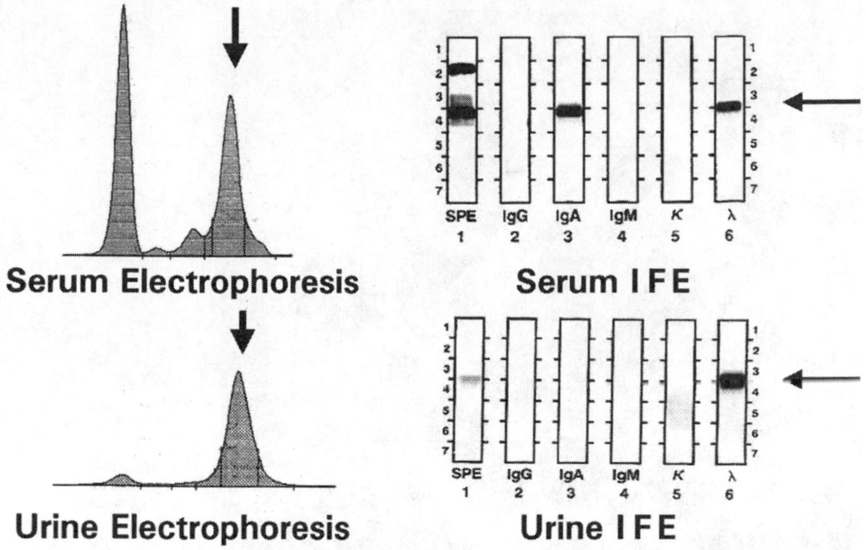

FIGURE 46.4-4. Serum (SPE) and urine protein electrophoresis (*left*) showing abnormal monoclonal protein bands (*arrows*). Quantitation of the M protein is performed by nephelometric measurement of the band. Identification of serum and urine M component by immunofixation electrophoresis (IFE) (*right*). The labels indicate the specificity of the antiserum used in developing the immunofixation pattern. The top is immunoglobulin (IgG) A-γ in serum and bottom is free γ light chain in urine.

Further analysis of a unique variable region in the myeloma-related idiotype (e.g., CDRIII) provides information on the monoclonal nature of the protein and also provides a tool to investigate minimal residual disease by polymerase chain reaction using allele-specific oligonucleotide, thus allowing determination of molecular complete remissions.[215]

BONE MARROW EXAMINATION

Various degrees of bone marrow infiltration are observed in myeloma, with the majority of the patients having an excess number of plasma cells (more than 5%). The pattern of bone marrow involvement (diffuse vs. nodular) is important, as patients with nodular disease seem to have poorer outcomes (in contrast to CLL).[216] The morphology of the plasma cell seems to be an important factor determining severity of the disease. This is based on histologic examination (Bartl grade) in which grade I suggests a slow-growing disease, whereas grade III represents plasmablastic disease with an aggressive course.[217] There is also an increased incidence of cytogenetic abnormalities in patients with Bartl grade III when compared with grade I. As plasma cells contain cytoplasmic immunoglobulins with a constant heavy and light chain, its frequency can be evaluated by flow cytometric analysis using immunohistochemical staining of the plasma cells.[218] When coupled with DNA staining using propidium iodide, two-parameter analysis can detect changes in DNA content in the myeloma cells (Fig. 46.4-5). DNA aneuploidy is observed in the bone marrow of more than 80% of patients, suggesting the existence of chromosomal abnormalities in the majority of patients.[218–220] This also provides an objective marker for evaluation of therapy and to distinguish reactive from clonal plasmacytosis, especially in nonsecretory disease. A hypodiploid tumor cell has also been associated with refractoriness to standard-dose therapy.

CYTOGENETICS

As the myeloma cell represents a mature differentiated cell with low proliferative activity, cytogenetic abnormalities are not frequently found. Abnormalities are detected in only one-third of the patients at the time of diagnosis; however, repeated analysis improves the yield to almost one-half of the patients. The normal karyotypic pattern observed in the remaining half most likely originates from dividing normal hematopoietic cells.[75]

As described previously, a complex karyotypic pattern is frequently observed and its distribution is shown in Figure 46.4-2. Although a predominant constant cytogenetic abnormality has not been identified, certain recurrent changes have been noticed. These include the common B-cell tumor-related changes in the 14q32 region involving the IGH region, chromosome 1q, and chromosome 13–related changes.[221–223] A longitudinal analysis in patients undergoing high-dose chemotherapy has shown clinical evolution including changes involving chromosome 5 and 7, commonly associated with myelodysplastic syndrome.[224] Acquisition of such changes in the myeloma karyotype appears to portend poor prognosis. Detection of chromosome 13 deletion abnormalities at diagnosis as well as after high-dose chemotherapy has now been reported to carry a poor prognosis. The application of FISH technology has improved our ability to detect genetic changes by using interphase cells. The Rb-1 probe detects an abnormality on the 13q14 region, and its deletion has been reported in 40% of patients by interphase FISH, also suggesting a prognostically poor-risk group of patients treated by standard-dose therapy.[225] Interphase FISH analysis for numeric chromosomal aberrations has identified chromosomes 6, 9, and 17 as also carrying favorable outcomes.[79] Plasma cell leukemia has been reported to frequently contain a t(11:14); however, this translocation has also been detected in patients with MGUS without any prognostic relevance.[226]

LABELING INDEX

The proportion of myeloma cells in the cell cycle is small early in the disease. A study of cycling myeloma cells with bromodeoxyuridine or tritiated thymidine methods shows a median of 1% cycling cells at diagnosis. The labeling index has important prognostic significance as patients with more than 1% cells in S phase in bone marrow have worse outcomes.[218,227–230]

RADIOGRAPHIC EVALUATION

The radiographic survey of the bone is a standard diagnostic workup, which shows osteopenia in an early phase of the disease and, with increasing tumor burden, lytic punched out

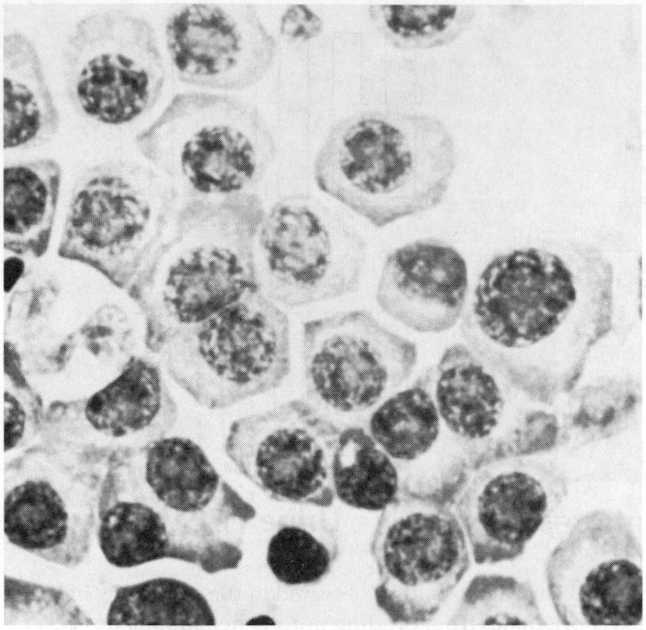

A

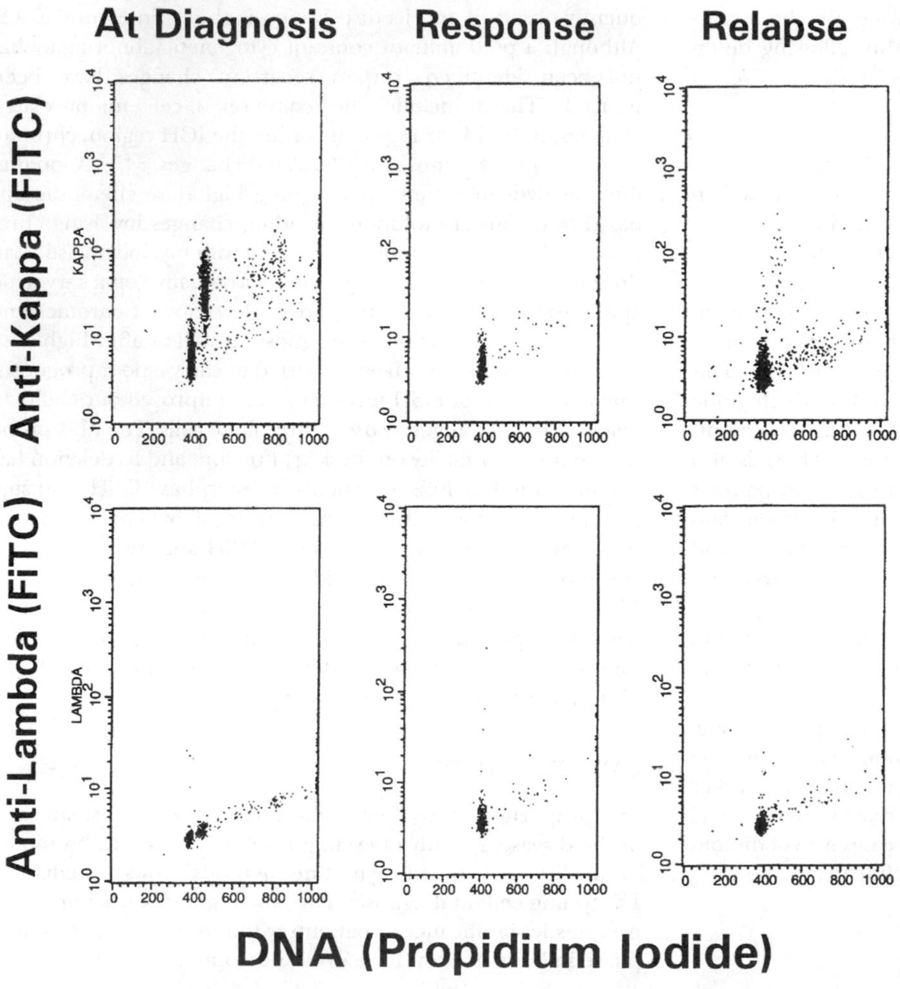

B

FIGURE 46.4-5. **A:** Bone marrow plasma cells in a patient with immunoglobulin G myeloma showing neoplastic plasma cells at various stages of differentiation. **B:** Two-parameter flow cytometry of DNA content of bone marrow cells; abscissa (propidium iodide), and cytoplasmic immunoglobulin (ordinate, anti-κ or γ FiTC). At diagnosis approximately 45% hyperdiploid tumor cells with κ light chain restriction are seen (*left panel*); at the time of maximal response no hyperdiploid light chain restricted cells are seen (*middle panel*); at the time of early relapse reappearance of small hyperdiploid and κ light chain–restricted population (<1%) is indicative of reemergence of a small number of clonal cells that may not yet be apparent on cytologic examination of the bone marrow (*right panel*).

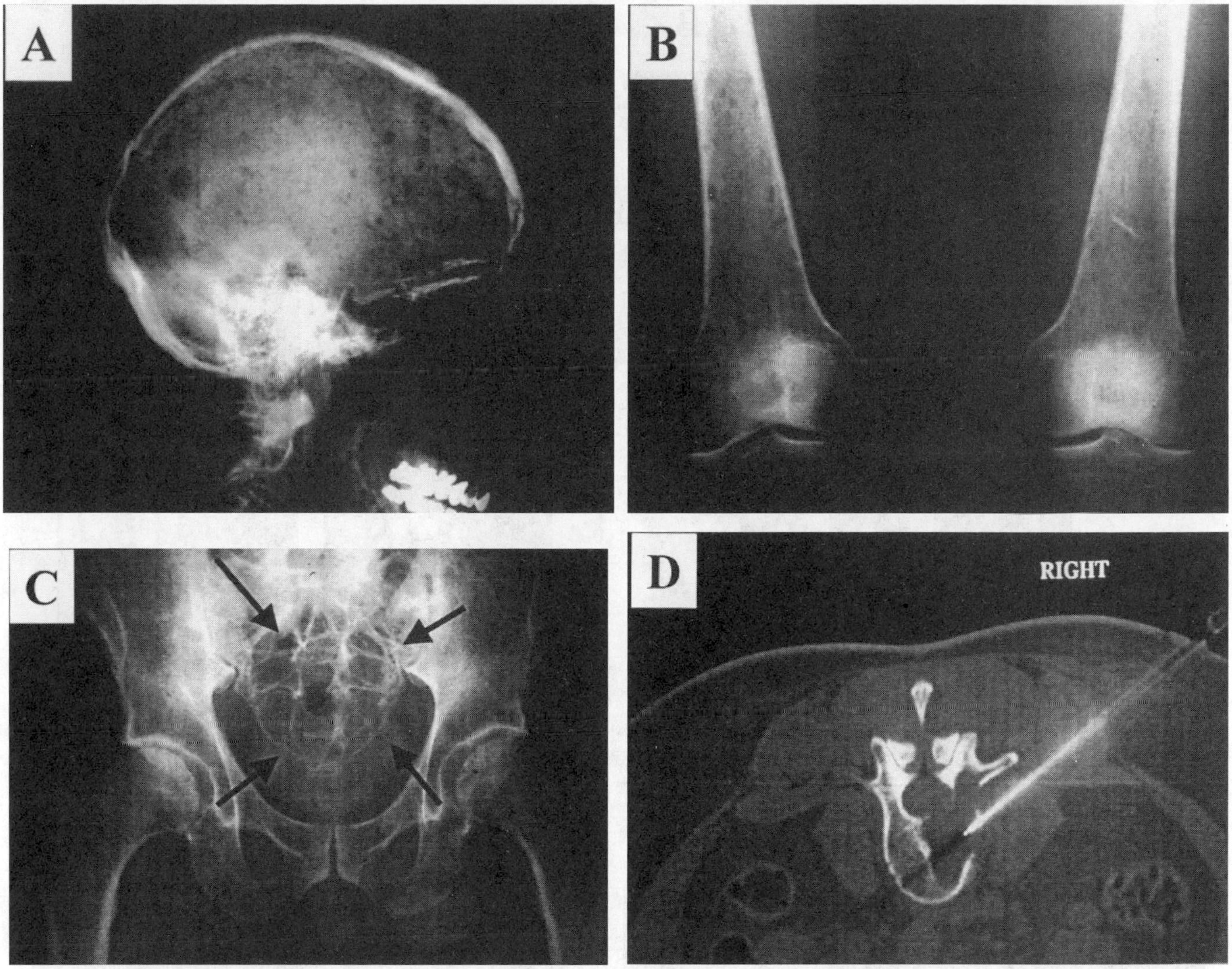

FIGURE 46.4-6. Typical skeletal changes on roentgenogram. **A:** Example of punched-out lytic lesions in skull. **B:** Small lytic lesions in the left femur. **C:** Large lytic lesion in sacrum (*arrows*). **D:** Fine-needle aspiration biopsy of the vertebral lesion. (Courtesy of Hemendra Shah.)

lesions (Fig. 46.4-6). Osteosclerotic lesions are observed in POEMS syndrome.[194–197] Due to the predominant osteolytic activity with osteoblastic inactivity, bone scans are seldom positive unless a recent fracture has occurred and not useful in the diagnosis of multiple myeloma.[231]

As demineralization of bone (osteoporosis) is one of the common manifestations of myeloma, measurement of bone mineral density (BMD) by dual-energy x-ray absorptiometry is an important evaluation at diagnosis.[232] In a study of 66 patients at diagnosis, majority of the patients had decreased BMD: lumbar mean BMD value (Z score) −1.24 ± 1.45. Following standard-dose therapy, lumbar BMD increased 0.7%, while in a group treated with high-dose therapy the improvement was 4.6% ($P = .02$).[233] Similar improvements in BMD have also been noted in patients undergoing high-dose therapy with addition of bisphosphonates[234] and show differential effects of pamidronate on cortical and cancellous bones in patients with myeloma undergoing autotransplants.[233,234]

Magnetic resonance imaging (MRI) of bone marrow provides a better assessment of tumor burden and is essential in the workup of a patient with solitary plasmacytomas of bone.[235] More than 95% of myeloma patients have MRI abnormalities: one-third have diffuse involvement of the bone marrow, one-third have focal lesions, while the other one-third have heterogenous marrow with both focal and diffused involvement. As myeloma is well recognized as a macrofocal disease, random bone marrow sampling may not be entirely diagnostic or predictive of disease status. MRI short tau inversion recovery images (STIR) provide a better assessment of tumor load in myeloma.[236–239] A focal marrow plasmacytoma can be further analyzed through computed tomographically (CT)-guided fine-needle aspiration allowing cytologic diagnosis, which can be combined with further risk assessment through evaluation of cytogenetic and FISH analysis as well as labeling index. As therapies become more effective, the MRI pattern may change as seen in Figures 46.4-7*A*, *B*, and *C*; a diffuse involvement of the marrow may unravel into a focal disease. Normalization of MRI abnormalities may provide a better definition of complete responses as the therapy for this disease with autologous or allogenic transplantations aims toward cure. Positron emission tomography scanning has been evaluated in a small number of studies and may provide a better functional definition of the

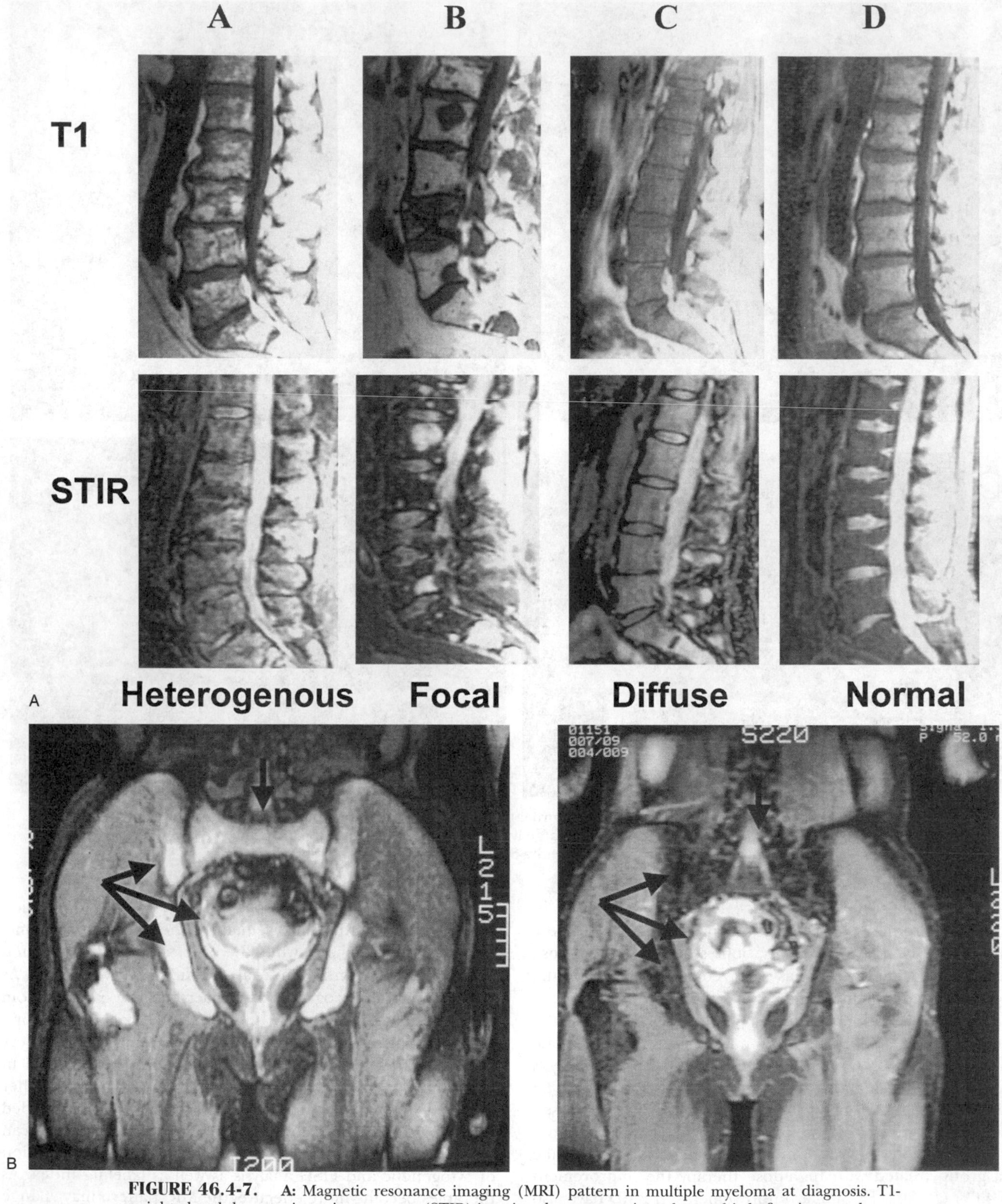

FIGURE 46.4-7. **A:** Magnetic resonance imaging (MRI) pattern in multiple myeloma at diagnosis. T1-weighted and short tau inversion recovery (STIR) imaging shows approximately one-third of patients each presenting with heterogeneous pattern (A), focal plasmacytoma lesions (B), or diffuse homogeneous hyperintense marrow pattern (C). Hyperintensity of marrow on short inversion time inversion recovery image is suggestive of uniform marrow involvement by myeloma. Few patients have a hypointense and homogenous pattern also seen in normal individuals (D). **B:** The hyperintense marrow pattern (*arrows*) suggestive of extensive marrow involvement pretherapy (left) changes to hypointense pattern following complete response and normalization of marrow (right). (*Figure continues*)

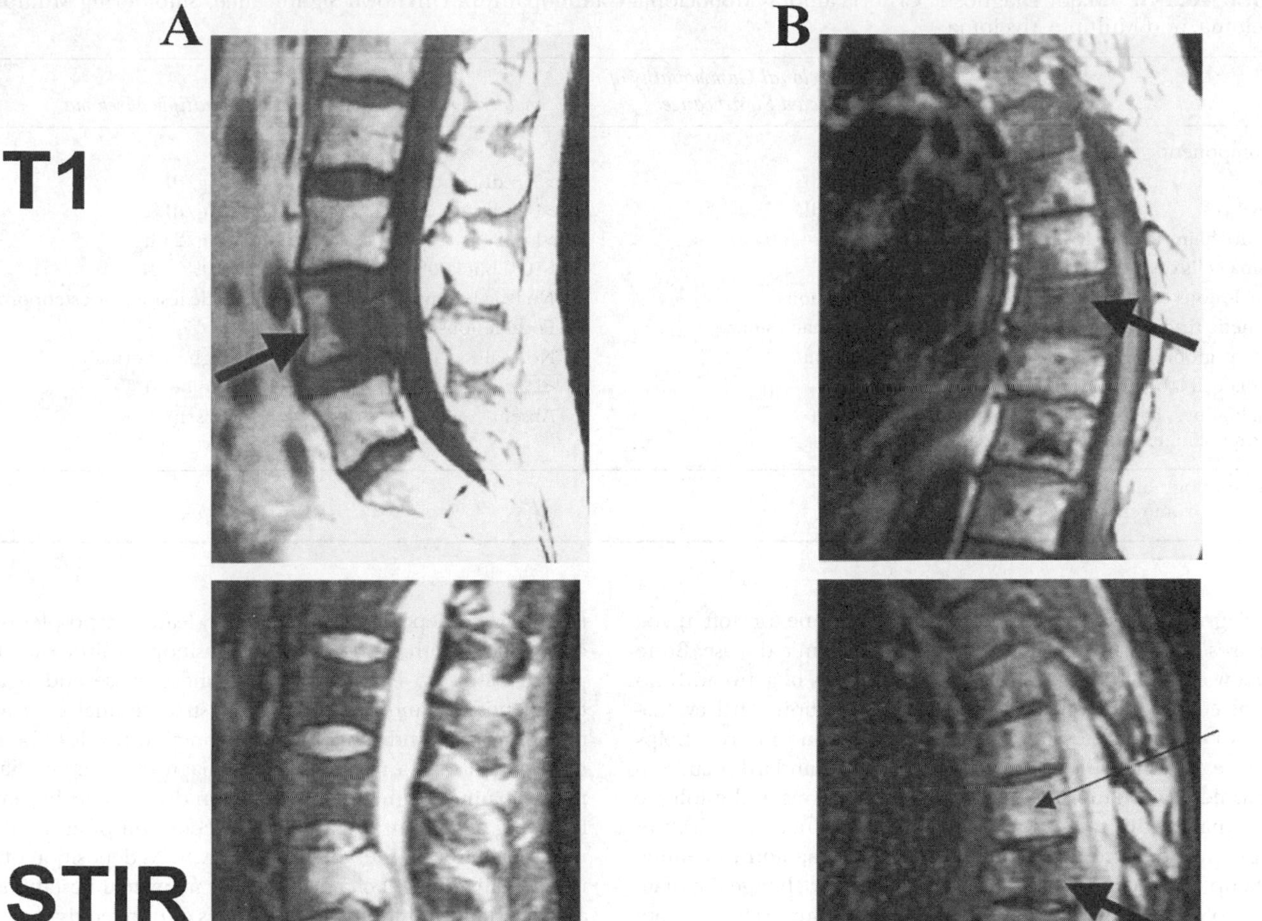

FIGURE 46.4-7. (*Continued*) **C:** MRI is useful in differentiating myelomatous involvement from amyloidosis or infection. The active plasmacytoma appears as bright on a STIR image (A, *arrow*), whereas amyloidosis appears as a dark lesion (B, *thick arrow*). A bright shadow above the amyloid (*thin arrow*) is suggestive of associated small plasmacytoma. Fine-needle aspiration examination in 72 patients with MRI focal disease showed tumor in 92%, indicating that MRI focal lesions in myeloma represent tumor. (Courtesy of Ramesh Avva.)

lesions observed on MRI or CT and allow selection of lesions for biopsy.[240]

DIFFERENTIAL DIAGNOSIS

In the presence of lytic bone lesions and greater than 30% marrow plasmacytosis, the myeloma diagnosis can be readily established. However, in the absence of lytic bone lesions or diffused osteoporosis, other criteria have to be fulfilled to differentiate overt myeloma from MGUS.[39] These include anemia, high levels of monoclonal protein in serum and urine, and marrow plasmacytosis as described in Table 46.4-4.[241,242] Distinguishing smoldering myeloma and monoclonal gammopathy may be difficult as this distinction is essentially based on levels of serum monoclonal proteins and marrow plasmacytosis.[243] The differentiating features are shown in Table 46.4-5, and in the majority of the patients with monoclonal gammopathy, anemia, bone lesions, or MRI abnormalities are absent. Conventional cytogenetic results are usually negative in MGUS; however, monoclonal plasma cells in some cases with MGUS may be aneuploid. Patients with nonsecretory myeloma are diagnosed based on marrow plasmacytosis and bone lesion. MRI abnormalities and CT- or MRI-guided fine-needle aspiration biopsy are important for follow-up of the disease.

TABLE 46.4-5. Major Diagnostic Criteria among Monoclonal Gammopathy of Unknown Significance, Smoldering Multiple Myeloma, and Multiple Myeloma

	Monoclonal Gammopathy of Unknown Significance	*Smoldering Multiple Myeloma*	*Multiple Myeloma*
M component			
IgG	<3 g/dL	>3 g/dL, stable	>3 g/dL
IgA	<1 g/dL	>1 and <2 g/dL, stable	>2 g/dL
Light chain/urine	<1 g/24 h	>1 g/24 h	>1 g/24 h
Plasma cells on marrow biopsy	<10%	>10% but <20%	>10%
Bone lesions on skeletal survey	No lesions	No lytic lesions	Lytic lesions or osteoporosis
Magnetic resonance imaging	No focal lesions	Focal lesions can be present	—
β_2-Microglobulin levels	Normal	Normal	High or normal
Plasma cell labelling index	<1%	<1%	Can be >1%
Renal failure, hypercalcemia, anemia, bone pain, extramedullary disease	Absent	Absent	Present

Ig, immunoglobulin.
(Adapted from refs. 241–243.)

Diagnosis of solitary plasmacytoma of bone or soft tissue requires intense investigation to rule out systemic disease. Bone marrow examination in a true solitary lesion is negative with no clonal cell population on DNA cIg examination. MRI evaluation for myelomatous involvement of the bone marrow helps detect early lesions before their detection by standard roentgenographic examination. Detection of such lesions and cytologic confirmation through CT- or MRI-guided fine-needle aspiration biopsy may help confirm solitary plasmacytoma and its genetic makeup. In case of MGUS, such detection may change the diagnosis to solitary or multiple myeloma. It is important to note that patients with MGUS or solitary plasmacytoma seldom have suppression of uninvolved immunoglobulins.

Besides plasma cell neoplasms, various other conditions can present with monoclonal immunoglobulin secretion. These conditions include other B-cell neoplasms such as CLL and B-cell non-Hodgkin's lymphoma; autoimmune conditions such as cold agglutinin diseases, mixed cryoglobulinemia, hypergammaglobulinemia, and Sjögren's syndrome; inflammatory or storage diseases such as lichen myxedematous, Gaucher's disease, sarcoidosis, and cirrhosis; and rarely other malignancies such as chronic myelogenous leukemia, and colon, breast, or prostate cancer.

Protein deposition disease involving various organs requires additional special diagnostic procedures. Deposition of amyloid protein (amyloidosis) can be clinically suspected based on macroglossia, vascular fragility (*raccoon's eyes,* periorbital subcutaneous hemorrhages), carpal tunnel syndrome, organomegaly, nephropathy, and cardiomegaly with arrhythmia. Detection of Congo red–positive amyloid in perivascular area and in subcutaneous fat, bone marrow, or rectal biopsy and classic apple-green birefringence when visualized under polarized light are diagnostic of AL amyloid. Electrocardiography may reveal a low voltage, and echocardiographic evaluation shows thickening of the interventricular septum or classic spackled pattern in the myocardium. Endomyocardial biopsy may establish the diagnosis of cardiac amyloid. Another manifestation of amyloid deposition includes autonomic dysfunction due to amyloid deposition in the vasa nervorum of the autonomic nerves, leading to orthostatic hypotension. Deposition in adrenal glands leads to hypoadrenalism. Amyloid deposition in spleen may lead to hyposplenism with observation of thrombocytosis. Deposition in liver may be suspected based on elevated alkaline phosphatase and γ-glutamyl transpeptidase, and deposition in gastrointestinal tract leads to malabsorption syndrome. Renal dysfunction needs to be further investigated with a renal biopsy, as diagnosis of light chain cast nephropathy or light chain deposition disease may be reversible following aggressive therapy while deposition of amyloid would require a different therapeutic approach. As deposition of immunoglobulin and light chain can mimic many manifestations of AL amyloid, immunofluorescence analysis of unfixed tissue is important for diagnosis.

PROGNOSTIC VARIABLES

Patients with multiple myeloma have variable disease courses with survival ranging from less than 1 year with aggressive disease to more than 10 years with indolent presentation of sensitive disease. Various characteristics have been identified to predict the possible course of the disease. Evaluation of prognostic factors is important to define therapeutic strategies, permit comparison of clinical trial results, and predict life expectancy after diagnosis. As shown in Table 46.4-6, prognostic factors are related to tumor burden, intrinsic property of the tumor, host and microenvironmental influences, and treatment intervention–related factors.

Studies measuring *in vitro* immunoglobulin production by patients' myeloma cells have lead to the development of clinically applicable methods to estimate tumor mass. A clinical staging system developed by Durie and Salmon for multiple myeloma using standard laboratory measurements has been applied to predict clinical outcomes after standard-dose chemotherapy.[244,245] As shown in Table 46.4-7, this system uses monoclonal protein or immunoglobulin levels in serum, light chain excretion in a 24-hour urine sample, presence of hypercalcemia, anemia, extent of bone lesions, and presence or absence of renal failure. In a study by National Cancer Institute Canada, overall survival with standard-dose therapy in patients with low-disease burden (stage I) was 49 months and with high-tumor burden (stage III) was 25 months. Including the renal failure in

TABLE 46.4-6. Prognostic Variables

TUMOR-RELATED FACTORS
Tumor mass–related factors
β_2-Microglobulin
Serum immunoglobulin
Number of lytic bone lesions
Hemoglobin
Serum calcium
Percentage bone marrow plasmacytosis
Tumor biology-related factors
Monosomy 13 or 13q-
Plasma cell labeling index
Bartl grade
Mitotic activity
Immunoglobulin A myeloma
C-reactive protein
Lactate dehydrogenase
Soluble interleukin-6 receptor
Renal failure
HOST-RELATED FACTORS
Bone marrow microenvironment–related factors
Bone marrow microvessel density
Serum syndecan-1 levels
Matrix metalloptrotease-9 levels
Soluble CD16
Patient-related factors
Albumin
Performance status
Other organ problems not related to myeloma
Treatment-related factors
Less than or equal to 12 mo of prior therapy
Tandem transplant
Second transplant within 6 mo
Achieving complete response

TABLE 46.4-7. Myeloma Staging System

Criteria	*Measured Myeloma Cell Mass (Cells × $10^{12}/m^2$)*
STAGE I	
All of the following	<0.6 (low)
Hemoglobulin >10 g/dL	
Normal serum calcium (<12 mg/dL)	
Skeletal survey normal bone structure (Scale 0) or solitary bone plasmacytoma or osteoporosis only	
Low M component production rates	
IgG value <5 g/dL	
IgA value <3 g/dL	
Urine light chain M component on electrophoresis <4 g/24 h	
STAGE II	
Overall data not as minimally abnormal as shown for stage I and no single value abnormal as defined for stage III	0.6–1.2 (intermediate)
STAGE III	
One or more of the following	>1.2 (high)
Hemoglobin value <8.5 g/dL	
Serum calcium value >12 mg/dL	
Advanced lytic bone lesions, three or more	
High M component production rates	
IgG value >7 g/dL	
IgA value >5 g/dL	
Urine light chain M component on electrophoresis >12 g/24 h	
Subclassification	
A = relatively normal renal function (serum creatinine value >2 mg/dL)	
B = abnormal renal function (serum creatinine value greater than or equal to 2 mg/dL)	

Ig, immunoglobulin.
(From Alexanian R, Balcerzak S, Bonnet JD, et al. Prognostic factors in multiple myeloma. *Cancer* 1975;36:1192, with permission.)

the staging system, patients with stage IIIa disease had a median survival of 30 months and stage IIIb disease, 15 months.[246] The accuracy and predictive value of the Durie-Salmon system is less pronounced in patients undergoing high-dose chemotherapy.[247] The high-dose chemotherapy is probably able to treat the disease burden more successfully, with the patient's outcome depending more on tumor biology factors. As the Durie-Salmon system considers tumor burden variables and depends on subjective interpretation of lytic bone lesions, additional other variables have been investigated to better assess patients' risk.

β_2-microglobulin (β_2m) has been identified as one of the most important predictors of survival in plasma cell myeloma. β_2m is the light chain gene of the class I histocompatibility antigens expressed on the surface of all nucleated cells and shed into the blood. Its renal excretion explains its elevation in renal failure. In multiple myeloma it reflects both tumor burden and renal function.[248,249] High β_2m (greater than 2.5 mg/L) levels carry a poor prognosis with both standard-dose and high-dose therapy.[247] Other independent factors associated with poor prognosis include elevated CRP and less consistently serum IL-6 activity and sIL-6R and IgA isotype.[250] Because CRP levels reflect IL-6 activity and elevated levels can be associated with various acute-phase reactions including inflammation and infections, its predictive value is important only when other possible causes of elevated CRP are ruled out.

The bone marrow plasmacytosis reflects tumor burden and has been considered in prognosticating survival. Peripheral blood monoclonal plasma cell has also been reported as a predictor of survival in myeloma. In a study of 254 patients, blood monoclonal plasma cell count was greater than or equal to 4% in 57% of patients, with median survival of 2.4 years compared with 4.4 years in patients with a count less than 4.[251]

Among the various other disease biology variables, Bartl grading of tumor cells correlates with survival even in patients undergoing high-dose chemotherapy. Flow cytometry of DNA and cytoplasmic immunoglobulin (DNA-cIg) can identify hypodiploid tumor cells, associated with resistance to standard-dose chemotherapy, which can be overcome by high-dose chemotherapy.[252] The plasma cell proliferation rate as measured by the labeling index is a valuable prognostic factor, with an index of greater than 2% predicting inferior survival. One study combining β_2m and labeling index identified a low-risk group with both parameters

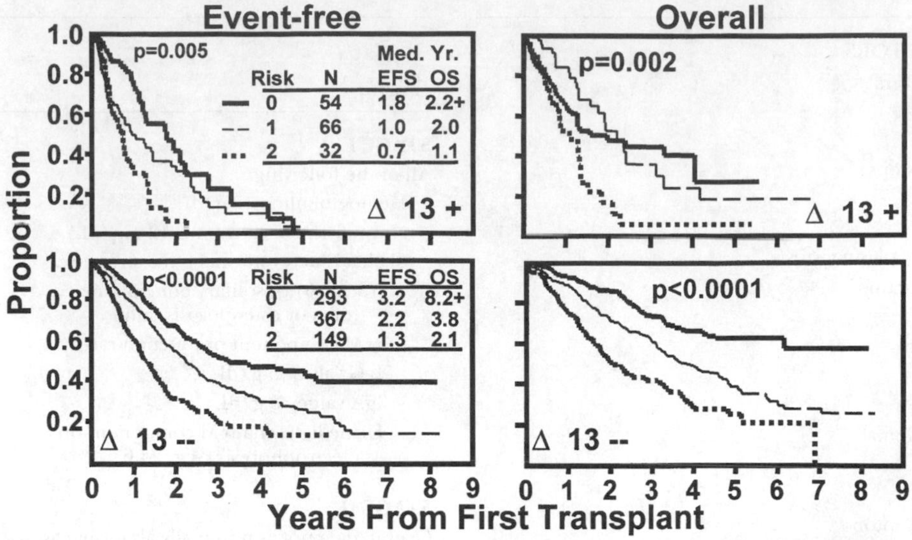

FIGURE 46.4-8. Multivariate analysis of 972 patients undergoing at least one high-dose melphalan with autologous peripheral blood stem cell rescue showed chromosome 13 abnormality, β_2-microglobulin (β_2m) >4.0 mg/L, and C-reactive protein >3 mg/L to be the most significant predictors of poor outcome, followed by >12 months of prior therapy. Patients were divided into three groups based on their β_2m and C-reactive protein values; those with both values normal (risk 0), those with one of the two values abnormal (risk 1), and those with both the values abnormal (risk 2). These patients were evaluated for event-free (EFS) (*left*) and overall survival (OS) (*right*) and divided into those with (*top*) or without (*bottom*) chromosome 13 abnormality. As seen in the figure, patient groups divided based on β_2m and C-reactive protein show significantly superior EFS and OS as the number of risk factors increases (risk 0 to 2). However, within each group the presence of chromosome 13 abnormality (upper panel compared with lower panel) predicts significantly inferior EFS and OS, suggesting adverse effect of chromosome 13 abnormality irrespective of other risk factors.

low, intermediate-risk group with one parameter high, and high-risk group with both parameters high, with median survival of 71 months, 40 months, and 15 months, respectively.[230]

Cytogenetic analysis has now been identified as a major prognosticator in plasma cell myeloma. Abnormalities involving chromosome 13 carry a poor prognosis with short survival as well as inferior response to high-dose chemotherapy. Additional tumor-related factors associated with inferior survival include increased soluble IL-6 receptor level, elevated serum lactate dehydrogenase level usually associated with extramedullary disease, and increased mitotic activity (greater than one per high power field).

Among the microenvironment-related factors, bone marrow microvessel density has been identified as an important prognosticator. High microvessel density in the bone marrow (greater than or equal to four per high power field) at the diagnosis confers shorter event-free (2.7 vs. 4.3 years; $P = .03$) and overall survival (7.9+ vs. 4.3 years; $P = .006$) after high-dose chemotherapy.[138] This may be reflective of increased VEGF expression by myeloma cells or other microenvironmental factors.[139] An increased level of serum syndecan-1 has been described as carrying poor prognosis. Soluble CD16 levels have been correlated with disease activity, with significantly reduced levels of soluble CD16 found in sera from patients with multiple myeloma as compared with MGUS patients and normal controls; a stage-dependent decrease in soluble CD16 was observed in myeloma.[253]

Among therapy- and intervention-related prognostic factors, more than 12 months of prior standard-dose therapy affects survival most significantly in patients undergoing high-dose chemotherapy. Additionally, the tandem transplant and the time between the two transplants are also significantly correlated with superior event-free and overall survival.[247] Age over 65 years has been reported to be associated with inferior survival using standard-dose therapy; however, with high-dose therapy, age does not appear to predict poor survival.[254]

As high-dose therapy is able to overcome the problems related to increased disease burden as well as to some other biologic features associated with drug resistance, some traditional prognostic factors are no longer predictive of survival after high-dose chemotherapy. With this background, in a study of 1000 patients receiving high-dose chemotherapy with melphalan, 200 mg/m^2, the three most significant adverse variables associated with a shorter survival were the presence of chromosome 13 abnormality, β_2m greater than 2.5 mg/L at the time of transplant, and more than 12 months of preceding conventional-dose therapy. When patients are divided into groups with none of the previously mentioned risk factors, presence of one of the risk factors, or presence of both the risk factors, inferior prognosis is associated with an increase in the number of risk factors. As shown in Figure 46.4-8, even among these three groups presence of chromosome 13 abnormality predicts inferior survival, confirming its overriding influence. Additional molecular studies with FISH analysis as well as expression of various proteins such as BCL-family proteins, p53, and activation of STAT and NF-κB pathways in the future may provide new insight into the understanding of predicative factors important for prognostication.

TREATMENT

The diagnosis of a monoclonal protein does not always require immediate treatment of the patient. Although multiple

TABLE 46.4-8. Results of Large Trials for Remission Induction with Combination Chemotherapy Regimens Showing a Statistically Significant Improvement in Survival

Investigation	*Treatment*	*Patients*	*Response Rate (%)*	*Survival Median (mo)*
SWOG 7704[268]	VMCP + VBAP + VCAP	160	54	42
	MP	77	32	23
SWOG 7927	VMCP + VBAP	93	54	48
	VCP	107	28	29
MRC[269]	ABCM	314	61	32
	Melphalan	316	59	24
SWOG[281,a]	VMCP/VBAP	169	36	31
	VMCPP/VBAPP	171	49	40
	VAD	169	50	35

A, doxorubicin (Adriamycin); B, carmustine; C, cyclophosphamide; D, dexamethasone; M, melphalan; MRC, Medical Research Council; P, prednisone; PP, prednisone between cycles; SWOG, Southwest Oncology Group; V, vincristine.
[a]Glucocorticoid dose intensity.

myeloma is generally a disseminated disease, patients can present with solitary plasmacytomas that can be treated with local therapy or they may present with indolent asymptomatic myeloma, which can smolder for a long period of time before becoming symptomatic and requiring treatment.

SOLITARY PLASMACYTOMA

Solitary plasmacytoma requires specialized techniques for more accurate staging including a CT scan and MRI to exclude more disseminated disease. Solitary plasmacytomas of the bone involve vertebral bodies in one-third of the patients and frequently affect men (70%) at a younger age (median, 56 years).[255] A measurable monoclonal protein in the serum is observed in 24% to 54% of the patients and in a large proportion, no detectable monoclonal protein is observed, even on immunofixation. Extramedullary plasmacytomas are diagnosed less frequently and require a complete workup including MRI and positron emission tomography scanning to rule out any additional site or disseminated disease. The optimal therapy for true solitary plasmacytoma is curative-dose radiotherapy with 4000 to 5000 cGy.[256–258] With such a dose, the local tumor recurrence rate has been less than 10%, and 30% of patients with solitary bone lesions compared with more than 70% of patients with solitary extramedullary plasmacytomas have a long disease-free survival.[259,260] The monoclonal protein disappears after radiotherapy in 25% to 50% of the patients, suggesting possible eradication of all detectable disease. Reappearance of monoclonal protein predicts recurrence of disease. It can be anticipated that with better staging with MRI true solitary plasmacytoma of the bone can be cured in a high proportion of patients.[261]

INDOLENT MYELOMA

Myeloma patients with a low tumor mass and slowly progressive disease may present without specific symptoms. These patients generally have less than 20% bone marrow plasmacytosis and low monoclonal protein levels as shown in Table 46.4-5.[243,262] They have no lytic bone lesions, no hypercalcemia or renal disease, and hemoglobin greater than 10 g/dL. In patients with indolent light chain disease, Bence Jones proteinuria does not exceed more than 10 g/d. These patients do not present with cytogenetic abnormalities using conventional karyotyping and do have a low labeling index and low β_2m. Features predictive of early progression to symptomatic myeloma include lytic bone lesions, high serum myeloma protein levels (greater than 3 g/dL IgG or greater than 2 g/dL IgA), and focal MRI abnormalities.[263] Median time to progression is 26 months for all patients, 10 months in patients with bone lesions and high monoclonal protein, and 61 months for those without any of these features. Such indolent myeloma patients are typically not treated with chemotherapy until disease progression, onset of symptoms, or development of new lytic bone lesions. However, pamidronate has been used as *soil-directed* treatment to delay the onset of bone-related complications. Additionally, cytogenetic analysis of bone lesions through CT-guided biopsy provides important prognostic information that may dictate the need for early chemotherapeutic intervention.

SYMPTOMATIC MULTIPLE MYELOMA

Standard-Dose Therapy

Since the observation of induction of remission defined as greater than or equal to 50% decrease in paraprotein levels with melphalan in one-third of the myeloma patients studied, various standard-dose chemotherapeutic combinations have been evaluated. Oral melphalan and prednisone was the first successful combination chemotherapy for myeloma and in subsequent years various other single agents and combinations have been investigated and reported to have significant antimyeloma activity.

MELPHALAN AND PREDNISONE. Treatment with oral melphalan and prednisone was introduced 30 years ago and has remained the standard of therapy, providing symptomatic relief as well as tumor mass reduction.[264] A partial response as defined by greater than 50% reduction in monoclonal protein has been observed in 50% to 60% of the patients and between 3% and 5% of patients achieve a complete response. The absorption of oral melphalan is unpredictable, requiring its ingestion on empty stomach and increase in dose if the patient does not develop cytopenia.[265] With availability of the intravenous formulation, dose and pharmacokinetics are now predictable. In patients receiving melphalan and prednisone, a prompt response was associated with a poor survival, reflecting possibly a highly proliferative tumor. The median response duration was 18 months and overall survival was 24 to 36 months. One of the frequent complications of melphalan and prednisone therapy was the development of cytopenia and eventually myelodysplastic changes in the marrow. With successful treatment with high-dose therapy, melphalan and prednisone are not being used as induction therapy because the ability to mobilize adequate numbers of stem cells decreases with prolonged use of this combination; the incidence of treatment-related myelodysplastic syndrome and acute myeloid leukemia increases and partial resistance even to high-dose chemotherapy develops.

OTHER ALKYLATING AGENT-BASED COMBINATIONS. Various chemotherapeutic combinations have been investigated in myeloma, including vincristine (V), cyclophosphamide (C), carmustine (BCNU; B), melphalan (M), doxorubicin (Adriamycin; A), and prednisone (P). Commonly used combinations include VBMCP or VMCP/VBAP.[266–278] These combinations in randomized studies achieved similar response rates and event-free and overall survival when compared with melphalan and prednisone. Results from large studies evaluating standard-dose chemotherapy regimens are listed in Tables 46.4-8 and 46.4-9. In the majority of the studies, there was no benefit of any of these combinations over melphalan and prednisone, and the toxicity problems, including bone marrow stem cell damage, remained the same. A metaanalysis of 18 published studies with 3814 patients randomized to receive melphalan and prednisone or various other chemotherapeutic combinations showed that melphalan and prednisone and other chemotherapeutic combinations are equivalent.

VINCRISTINE, ADRIAMYCIN, AND DEXAMETHASONE AND HIGH-DOSE DEXAMETHASONE. The role of high-dose corticosteroids was initially investigated in the late 1960s with an observation of therapeutic benefit in small numbers of patients. Glucocorticoids down-regulate IL-6 production and induce apoptosis *in vitro*. The molecular mechanism of corticosteroid-induced apoptosis in myeloma involves a decrease in NF-κB activity through IκB activation. Interestingly, myeloma cells can be rescued from glucocorticoid-mediated killing by addition of IL-6 to *in vitro* cultures or by coculturing them with stromal cells, which are a source of IL-6 *in vivo*. High-dose dexamethasone was evaluated in combination with vincristine and Adriamycin. The dosages of these agents (VAD) were vincristine at 0.25 mg/m^2 and Adriamycin at 9 mg/m^2 given by continuous infusion over 24 hours for 4 days, along with dexamethasone, 40 mg orally on days 1 to 4, 9 to 12, and 17 to 20, with the cycle repeated every 5 weeks.[279,280] More than 50% of refractory myeloma patients showed rapid and marked response, defined as greater than 75% cytoreduction, with better efficacy in patients responsive to prior therapy. Response with VAD was much faster, with the median tumor halving time of 21 days compared with greater than 6 weeks for other combination therapies. The advantages of this combination include quick response, effectiveness in hypercalcemia, quick relief of bone pain, applicability in patients with renal failure, and no cumulative bone marrow stem cell damage, allowing subsequent successful mobilization of stem cells. Studies using high-dose dexamethasone alone given in doses similar to the VAD regimen have shown response rates almost similar to those observed with VAD in primary resistant myeloma but higher in relapsing disease, indicating that dexamethasone is clearly an important agent in VAD. In a study evaluating glucocorticosteroid dose intensity, chemotherapy regimens with higher glucocorticoste-

TABLE 46.4-9. Results of Large Trials for Remission Induction with Multiagent Chemotherapy Compared with Simple Alkylating Agent Therapy That Failed to Show a Survival Advantage

Investigation	*Treatment*	*Patients*	*Response Rate (%)*	*Survival Median (mo)*
Cancer and Leukemia Group B[277]	MCBP	156	56	29
	MCBAP	157	44	26
	MP	146	47	33
Eastern Cooperative Oncology Group[274]	M2	134	74	31
	MP	131	53	30
SECSG[274]	BCP	186	49	36
	MP	187	52	36
Argentine[278]	MeCCMVP	105	46	41
	MP	129	38	39
Canadian[246]	MCBP	116	47	31
	MP	125	31	28
Italian[266]	VMCP-VBAP	158	77	32
	MP	146	64	37
Finnish[273]	MOMeCCA	64	75	41
	MP	66	54	45
Danish[270]	M2	31	45	21
	VMP	32	73	30
	MP	33	58	21
Norwegian[276]	M2	33	74	33
	MP	34	67	33

A, doxorubicin; B, BCNU; C, cyclophosphamide; M, melphalan; MeC, methyl-CCNU; P, prednisone; SECSG, Southeast Cancer Study Group; V or O, vincristine.

roid dose intensity yielded higher response rates and improved survival ($P = .02$).[281] VAD is associated with minimal bone marrow toxicity, and continuous infusion of Adriamycin prevents cardiac toxicity. Randomized comparisons between VAD and other chemotherapeutic combinations have failed to show any survival benefit for VAD; however, lack of stem cell damage provides an advantage in using VAD for initial cytoreduction before stem cell mobilization and transplant. Addition of cyclophosphamide to VAD (CVAD) has been shown to achieve responses in up to 40% of VAD-refractory patients.

INTERFERON. The role and efficacy of interferon in the management of myeloma remains controversial. It has been shown to have up to a 20% response rate in relapsed myeloma patients. Its mode of action remains multifactorial; direct growth inhibitory action as well as its antiangiogenic and immunomodulatory activity may contribute to its overall action. However, in combination with other chemotherapeutic regimens, it has failed to demonstrate beneficial effect.[282] In a metaanalysis of 16 trials involving 2286 patients, response rate was 45.9% in the chemotherapy alone group versus 54.4% for the chemotherapy with interferon group.[283] The difference in overall survival was 5 months. Its role in maintenance therapy after standard-dose therapy has generally been more positive, with demonstration in some of the studies of significant prolongation of survival for groups receiving interferon-α.[282,284] However, other studies have failed to show benefit. A metaanalysis of eight trials involving 929 patients randomized to interferon versus no treatment showed prolongation of relapse-free survival by 7 months and overall survival by 5 months. However, in younger patients and those with lower tumor burden interferon was more effective.[283] Its role, if any, after high-dose therapy is entirely unclear.[285] It is associated with flu-like symptoms, weight loss, impotence, depression, mental status changes, and cytopenia, and its prolonged use has been associated with inability to mobilize stem cells.

Radiation Therapy

Radiation therapy was considered the mainstay of the treatment for myeloma before availability of chemotherapeutic options. However, with more effective chemotherapy, especially high-dose chemotherapy, the role of radiation has now been limited.[286] A definitive role remains in patients with solitary bone and extramedullary plasmacytoma. In this setting, it provides excellent local control, and in a subset of patients it provides long-term disease-free survival when a solitary lesion is confirmed through extensive radiographic workup. Patients with solitary bone plasmacytoma following definitive radiation therapy (4000 to 5000 cGy) have progression-free survival of 30% compared with extramedullary plasmacytoma in which progression-free survival is around 70%.[256–260] The indication for radiation therapy in multiple myeloma remains palliative in cases of impending pathologic fracture and spinal cord compression. In patients with bone pains or symptomatic soft tissue masses, radiation is only considered when patients have failed chemotherapeutic options.[287,288] Radiation to the extensive marrow-containing area, such as the pelvic bone, should be considered carefully in light of the need for collection of stem cells. The dose for palliative radiation therapy has been substantially lower, in the range of 1500 to 2500 cGy. Studies to date have failed to show any benefit of hemibody radiation in multiple myeloma. However, total body radiation has been used in relation with allogeneic transplantation as well as autologous transplantation. More recent studies have demonstrated that total body irradiation does not provide additional cytoreductive potential and it actually increases treatment-related morbidity and mortality and delays immune recovery following high-dose therapy possibly affecting disease control. Total body irradiation as part of conditioning for allogeneic transplantation is especially important in the optimal regimen for achieving engraftment; however, its role in cytoreduction in this setting also remains questionable. Newer studies are evaluating low-dose radiation therapy with or without chemotherapy in nonmyeloablative conditioning regimens that may be associated with lower morbidity and still achieve tumor control through graft versus myeloma effect.

High-Dose Therapy with Peripheral Blood Stem Cell Support

The low incidence of complete response with standard induction chemotherapy, even in newly diagnosed patients, suggests a marked drug resistance that is possibly acquired during a prolonged subclinical course of the disease evidenced by the presence of complex karyotypic aberrations and multiple molecular changes. This observation led to a pilot study by the late Tim McElwain and his colleagues at the Royal Marsden Hospital where they evaluated role of melphalan dose escalation (140 mg/m^2). They reported complete remissions in refractory patients.[21] However, treatment-related mortality was high due to bone marrow toxicity. Bone marrow support in the subsequent studies improved the treatment-related mortality[22] and further dose escalation of melphalan to 200 mg/m^2 and by added total body irradiation provided further improvement in response.[289,290]

HIGH-DOSE THERAPY WITH AUTOLOGOUS HEMATOPOIETIC STEM CELL SUPPORT IN NEWLY DIAGNOSED PATIENTS. Initial demonstration of activity of high-dose melphalan therapy has lead to series of evaluations by various institutions of this treatment with stem cell support to avoid prolonged cytopenia (Table 46.4-10). A large single-institution study from the University of Arkansas for Medical Sciences evaluated intensive remission induction with three non–cross-resistant regimens [VAD, high-dose cyclophosphamide, and etoposide, dexamethasone, Ara-C, and cis-platinum (EDAP)] followed by two cycles of myeloablative therapy with melphalan, 200 mg/m^2, with hematopoietic stem cell support. A total of 231 newly diagnosed multiple myeloma patients aged 70 years or younger were treated on this protocol. The partial remission and complete remission rates after induction therapy were 69% and 14%; after the first high-dose melphalan dose they were 82% and 30%, and after the second transplant, 95% and 48%, respectively. On an intent-to-treat-basis, the true complete remission rate was 37%. With a median follow-up of 37 months, event-free and overall survival were 43 and 62 months, respectively. Treatment-related mortality in the first 12 months on the study was 4%. The median duration of neutropenia less than 500/mL and platelets less than 50,000/mL was 6 and 7 days, respectively.[247]

The superiority of high-dose chemotherapy with autologous bone marrow support was confirmed in a randomized trial conducted by Intergroupe Français du Myelome study. The reported response rate (greater than or equal to 50% reduction in myeloma protein) in 100 patients receiving high-dose therapy

TABLE 46.4-10. Results of High-Dose and Autologous Transplant in Myeloma

Regimen	Therapy	Author	Prior Therapy	Responsive Only	No.	Age	Median Follow-up (y)	Early Death (%)	Complete Response (%)	Median (y) Event-Free Survival	Median (y) Overall Survival
CY 400, MEL 140	—	Cunningham[293]	–	–	63	48	6.1	14	32	1.5	4
MEL 200	ABMT	Cunningham[294]	–	+	53	52	2.6	2	75	2	6.7
MEL-TBI	ABMT purged	Anderson[298]	±	+	52	49	—	2	40	2.6	4.2
BU-CY ± TBI	PBSC, ABMT	Bensinger[295]	+	–	63	51	—	25	30	0.8	2.8
MEL ± TBI	PBSC, ABMT	Bjorkstraud[297]	+	–	207	49	—	4	46	2.4	2.7
TBI-CC	PBSC	Fermand[296]	±	–	63	44	7.5	11	20	3.6	6.4
MEL-TBI	PBSC, ABMT	Harousseau[300]	–	–	133	52	3	4	37	2	3.8
MEL 200 × 2	PBSC	Barlogie[306]	–	–	231	51	4.2	2	41	3.6	5.7

ABMT, autologous bone marrow transplant; BU, busulfan; CC, combination chemotherapy consisting of carmustine, etoposide, melphalan, and cyclophosphamide; CY, cyclophosphamide; MEL, melphalan; PBSC, peripheral blood stem cells; TBI, total body irradiation.

(Mel-140 + total body irradiation) and in a similar number of patients receiving standard-dose VMCP regimen was 81% (22% complete remission) and 57% (5% complete remission), respectively (*P* <.001). Significantly longer event-free (median, 28 vs. 18 months) and overall survival (median, 57 vs. 42 months) were reported with high-dose therapy (Fig. 46.4-9). The projected 5-year event-free survival is 28% and overall survival is 52% with high-dose therapy compared with 10% and 12%, respectively, for the standard therapy arm.[291]

The superiority of high-dose therapy was also confirmed in a pair-mate analysis comparing 116 patients treated on the tandem transplant arm with a similar number of patients selected from 1123 patients treated with standard therapy on various Southwest Oncology Group studies and selected for important prognostic factors. Using an intent-to-treat-approach, compared with standard therapy, patients undergoing tandem transplant as part of the *total therapy* regimen had a superior partial response rate (86% vs. 52%; *P* = .0001) and longer median duration of event-free survival (49 vs. 22 months; *P* = .0001) and overall survival (62+ vs. 48 months; *P* = .01), with a projected 5-year event-free survival of 36% versus 19% and overall survival of 61% versus 39%.[292]

The role of single versus tandem transplants has been evaluated by the French Intergroup. With a short follow-up, no differences in response, complete remission (32% and 33%), or event-free (54% and 57%) and overall survival (71% and 67%) were observed in the whole group. However, a subgroup of patients with low β_2m showed a significant survival benefit with tandem transplant. Longer follow-up will determine if all or a subset of patients may benefit from such an approach.

Other institutions have studied high-dose chemotherapy with stem cell support in myeloma. As seen in Table 46.4-10, complete remissions are obtained in up to 50% of patients and event-free and overall survival are extended to more than 3 years and more than 5 to 6 years, respectively.[293–300]

PREVIOUSLY TREATED PATIENTS. Various investigators have studied high-dose therapy in previously treated patients showing its effectiveness in achieving complete responses. Harousseau et al. report 21% complete response and 66% partial response in 44 refractory or relapsed multiple myeloma patients treated with melphalan, 140 mg/m^2, with peripheral blood stem cell support.[301] The median overall survival was 17 months in this group. Vesole et al. studied 135 patients with advanced refractory myeloma treated with high-dose chemotherapy reporting event-free and overall survival of 21 and 43+ months, respectively.[302] Patients with primary unresponsive disease (not responding to standard induction therapy) had outcomes superior to patients with resistant relapse (relapsing after initial response) with event-free survival of 37 versus 17 months (*P* = .0004) and overall survival of 43+ versus 21 months (*P* = .0003), respectively.

Molecular complete responses have been observed in myeloma after high-dose therapy. Björkstrand et al. have reported sustained molecular complete responses in four of five patients by allele-specific oligonucleotide polymerase chain reaction for CDRIII up to 33 months from high-dose therapy.[303]

Various factors need special consideration in the management of myeloma with high-dose chemotherapy. These factors include source of stem cell, conditioning regimen, timing of transplant, and tumor-cell purging.

TIMING OF HIGH-DOSE THERAPY. To obtain high-quality hematopoietic stem cells, ideal timing for stem cell collection is early in the course of the induction treatment. Ability to collect adequate stem cells (greater than or equal to 2×10^6 CD34+ cells/kg) in patients with less than 12 months of prior therapy is 86% compared with 48% in patients with more than 24 months of prior therapy.[304] The role of early high-dose therapy (n = 91) compared with initial standard-dose therapy followed by high-dose therapy at the time of relapse (n = 94) has been investigated by Fermand et al. in a randomized trial. Overall survival was similar in both arms after early and late transplant (median, 64.6 and 64 months, respectively). Median event-free survival was 39 months after high-dose therapy, whereas median time to transplant after randomization to conventional chemotherapy was only 13 months (Fig. 46.4-9). However, patients randomized to early high-dose therapy had a longer time without symptoms, treatment, and

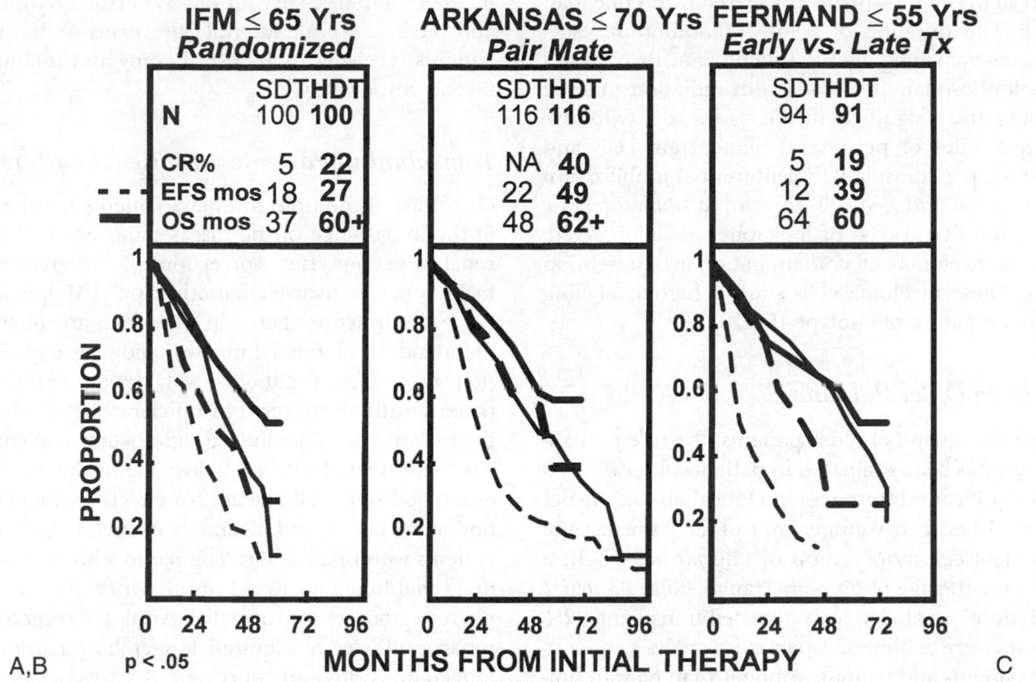

FIGURE 46.4-9. Comparative trials of high-dose therapy (HDT) versus standard dose chemotherapy (SDT). **A:** IFM-90 (Intergroupe Français de Myelome) randomized trial with 100 patients accrued to each arm comparing SDT with vincristine, melphalan, cyclophosphamide, prednisone/vincristine, carmustine, Adriamycin, and prednisone and HDT with melphalan, 140 mg/m^2, plus total body irradiation (800 cGy). Higher complete response rates and significantly longer event-free and overall survival were noted with HDT. **B:** Pair-mate comparison of 116 patients receiving HDT with total therapy as opposed to mainly vincristine, Adriamycin, dexamethasone (VAD)-based chemotherapy according to Southwest Oncology Group trials, matched for β_2m, creatinine, and age. With total therapy, complete response was obtained in 40% and both event-free and overall survivals were markedly extended. **C:** Randomized study of early high-dose therapy with melphalan, 140 mg/m^2, plus total body irradiation (800 cGy) versus initial standard dose therapy followed by high-dose therapy at relapse. With early high-dose therapy a superior complete response rate and event-free survival was observed with superior quality of life; however, overall survival was similar between the two arms. CR, complete response; EFS, event-free survival; OS, overall survival.

treatment-related toxicity, thus providing a rationale for early high-dose therapy.[305] A delay in high-dose chemotherapy and transplantation may lead to increased drug resistance, as well as further genetic changes resulting in more aggressive disease. An ongoing Intergroup trial in the United States randomizing patients to up-front high-dose therapy or standard therapy with high-dose therapy as a salvage treatment should also further define the role of high-dose therapy.

HIGH-DOSE REGIMEN. High-dose melphalan (140 to 200 mg/m^2) with or without total body irradiation is the most common conditioning regimen used in myeloma.[250,289,302,306–309] Melphalan's predominant myelotoxicity and metabolism independent of renal function is ideal for multiple myeloma patients who commonly have renal function abnormalities. Melphalan seems to be superior to thiotepa when given with total body irradiation, with patients achieving longer relapse-free and overall survival duration.[310] A combination regimen containing high-dose carboplatin with etoposide and Cytoxan (cyclophosphamide) or a combination with CBV has also been investigated in resistant patients with only occasional responses.[311–313] However, no regimen has shown marked superiority over others. The addition of total body irradiation has not been shown to improve cytoreduction, and in fact it increases morbidity and treatment-related mortality. A poor outcome in one study using total body irradiation was considered to be related to delayed immune recovery.

STEM CELL PURGING. Myeloma cell contamination as evaluated by polymerase chain reaction or sensitive immunofluorescence is universally observed in stem cell products. Purging of tumor cells by positive selection of CD34+ cells leads to a 3- to 5-log reduction in contamination.[314–316] Negative selection by the monoclonal antibody cocktail containing CD10 (common acute lymphoblastic leukemia antigen); CD20 (a pan B-cell antigen); and PCA-1, (plasma cell-associated antigen) or peanut agglutinin (PNA) and anti-CD19 antibodies results in undetectable myeloma cells by conventional flow cytometry.[298] The early follow-up results from these studies have not revealed any significant advantage in responses or survival, but they consistently show a delay in engraftment posttransplantation. Even when cells were purged using fluorescence-activated cell sorting of early hematopoietic stem cells (CD34+, Thy1+, Lin-) devoid of any clonal B cells, relapses were frequent and patients had delayed hematopoietic engraftment and suppressed immune status for prolonged periods of time.[317,318] These effects lead to infectious complications. As complete responses are observed in 30% to 50% of patients, greater emphasis needs to be placed on achieving better tumor cytoreduction in the patient.

HEMATOPOIETIC STEM CELL SOURCE. Mobilized peripheral blood stem cells provide faster engraftment compared with bone marrow. Myeloma patients with less than 1 year of prior therapy had faster granulocyte and platelet recovery after peripheral blood stem cell transplants compared with bone marrow autografts.[319] The duration of prior chemotherapy, especially with stem cell–damaging agents (melphalan, BCNU, and high-doses of cyclophosphamide) along with radiation to bone marrow–containing areas, significantly affects the ability to procure adequate quantities of peripheral blood stem cells and engraftment kinetics posttransplant.[320] Differential mobilization with cyclophosphamide and GM-CSF of normal hematopoietic stem cells during the first 3 days of leukapheresis is observed, while peak levels of myeloma cell contamination are present on subsequent days. These myeloma cells show a higher labeling index and a more immature phenotype (CD19+).[321]

Transplantation in Older Patients

Because myeloma is a disease of older patients, the role of high-dose chemotherapy has been evaluated in patients older than 65 years of age. No significant differences in clinical characteristics have been observed between younger and older patients. Age does not impair stem cell mobilization or engraftment.[254] In a study of patients over the age of 65 years (range, 65 to 83 years) undergoing high-dose melphalan with stem cell transplant, 22% complete responses were achieved. A pair-mate analysis was conducted for these patients and patients younger than 65 with similar high-dose therapy who were matched for relevant prognostic features. Results showed no significant difference in event-free survival (2.1 vs. 1.5 years; $P = .2$) and overall survival (3.9 vs. 3.7 years; $P = .4$) for younger versus older patients, respectively (Fig. 46.4-10). In a study involving 71 older patients (age greater than 60 years) receiving intermediate-dose melphalan at 100 mg/m^2 with stem cell support applied two to three times, the older patients were compared with 71 pair-mates matched for age and β2M and treated with oral melphalan and prednisone. Complete response rates were observed in 47% versus 5% ($P <.001$), median event-free survival was 34 versus 17.7 months ($P <.001$), and median overall survival 56+ versus 48 months ($P <.01$) in patients receiving high-dose therapy and melphalan and prednisone, respectively.[322]

Transplant in Patients with Renal Failure

One-third of multiple myeloma patients have renal dysfunction in the initial stage of the disease, and one-half of them recover renal function after correction of hypercalcemia, improved hydration, or effective chemotherapy.[323] Melphalan[324] and busulfan,[325] both active agents in myeloma, are pharmacokinetically independent of renal function, allowing high-dose administration in myeloma patients with renal dysfunction. Thirty-six patients with severe renal insufficiency (creatinine clearance less than 40 mL/min), including eight patients on chronic hemodialysis, were treated with high-dose melphalan followed by peripheral blood stem cell rescue. No effects on median half-life, area under the curve, and clearance of melphalan were observed in patients with renal failure compared with patients who had normal renal function. Renal insufficiency did not affect posttransplant engraftment or overall survival. However, the patients with renal insufficiency required longer hospitalization due to prolonged mucositis and anorexia.

Myelodysplastic Syndrome after High-Dose Therapy in Myeloma

Treatment-related myelodysplastic syndrome and acute myeloid leukemia are well-recognized complications following alkylating agent therapy. Myeloma patients with their advanced age may have coexisting myelodysplastic syndrome at a preclinical stage detected by cytogenetic changes that may be exacerbated by alkylating agent therapy[224] and may be further affected by high-

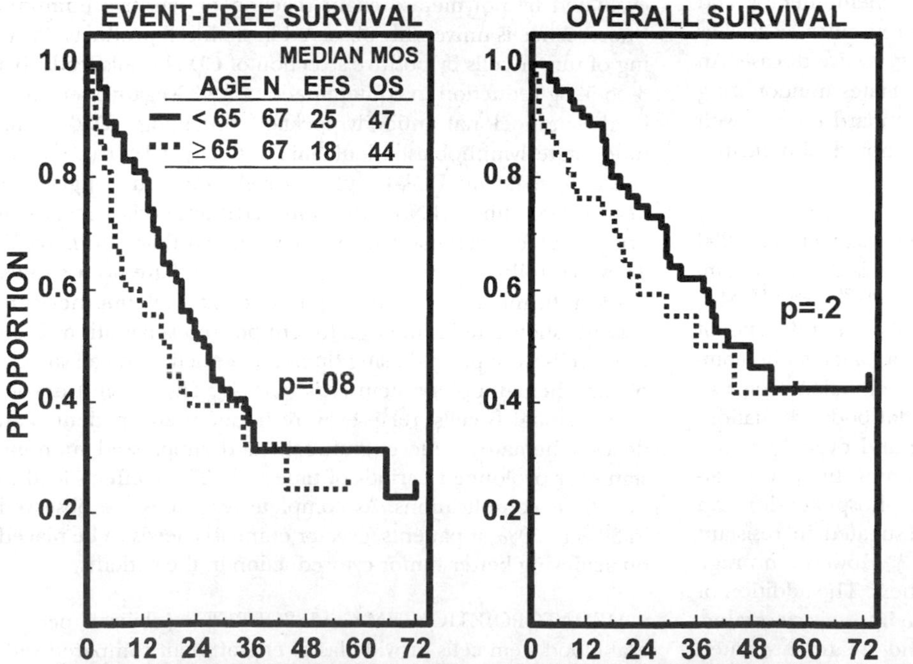

FIGURE 46.4-10. Outcome of 67 patients over the age of 65 and undergoing high-dose chemotherapy with autologous stem cell rescue were compared with a matched pair of patients with age less than 65 and similar prognostic features including chromosome 13 abnormality, C-reactive protein, β_2m, and months of prior therapy and treated with similar high-dose chemotherapy. There is no difference in overall (OS) and event-free survival (EFS) between the two groups, suggesting that when myeloma patients are treated with high-dose therapy older age does not predict for poor outcome.

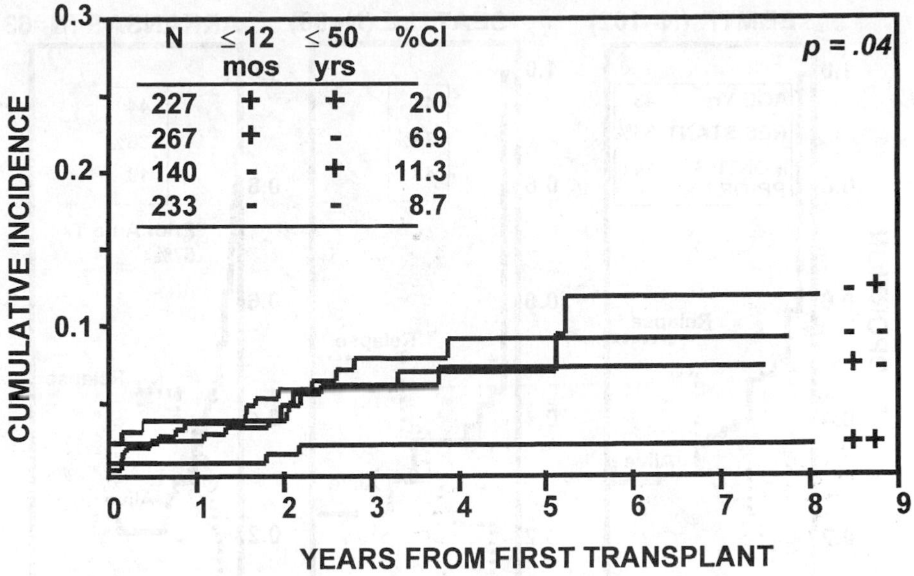

FIGURE 46.4-11. Development of myelodysplasia using cytogenetic criteria (-5 or del 5q, -7 or del 7q, trisomy 8, del 20q11) following autologous hematopoietic stem cell–supported high-dose therapy with melphalan, 200 mg/m^2 (one or two cycles). Cumulative incidence of cytogenetic myelodysplastic syndrome in relationship to months of prior therapy (≤12 vs. >12 months) and age (≤50 vs. >50 years). Patients with no more than 12 months of prior therapy and aged 50 years or younger had the lowest risk of myelodysplastic syndrome compared with the three other groups.

dose melphalan and stem cell transplant. In myeloma following high-dose therapy and stem cell support increased incidence of cytogenetically detected myelodysplastic syndrome is observed. The increase observed after 2 years was lowest in patients less than 50 years age and with less than 12 months of prior standard-dose therapy (1% to 2%); and it increased to 7% to 10% in older patients (>50 years) with more than 12 months of prior therapy, especially when CD34 mobilization was impaired (Fig. 46.4-11). Thus, in the background of older age and cumulative DNA damage caused by standard-dose alkylating agent therapy, the hematopoietic reconstitution following high-dose therapy may lead to excess telomeric shortening with genomic instability and an increased chance of myelodysplastic syndrome and acute myeloid leukemia.[326,327]

Allogeneic Transplantation

Patients with identical siblings have an option of syngeneic transplantation with true tumor-free graft.[328] In the setting of maximal cytoreductive therapy data from the European Bone Marrow Registry involving 16 patients undergoing syngeneic transplant, a complete response rate of 50% and median event-free and overall survival of 32 and 60 months were seen.

HLA-matched sibling donor transplantation enables myeloma patients to achieve 15% to 30% long-term disease-free survival, as shown by various large groups and summarized in Table 46.4-11.[298,329–332] In this study, between 30% and 50% of patients achieved a complete remission; however, an extremely high 1-year mortality (up to 50%) has been reported (Fig. 46.4-12). This unusually high treatment-related mortality compared with other diseases, including chronic myelogenous leukemia and acute leukemia, might be related to the older patient population, an immunosuppressed state due to the disease, corticosteroid treatment leading to higher bacterial and fungal infections, and the prior long duration of chemotherapy.[333] Definitive evidence of graft-versus-myeloma effect has been demonstrated and is considered responsible for the reduced probability of disease progression.[334,335] However, outcome after allografts are poor compared with autografts both as primary and salvage therapy. European Bone Marrow Transplant Registry retrospective analysis in a matched pair setting showed superior overall survival after autotransplants (34 vs. 18 months).[336] Surprisingly, even autograft performed as salvage in patients with resistant or relapsed disease resulted in superior overall survival (32 vs. 20 months), compared with allotransplant.[337] This is mainly due to excessive treatment-related mortality associated with allografts. Newer approaches are now being investigated with nonmyeloablative transplants, TK gene–transduced donor lymphocyte infusion, and CD6-depleted transplants and CD4+ donor lymphocyte infusion to reduce treatment-related mortality and improve overall survival.[298]

Salvage Therapies

Patients unresponsive or relapsing after standard alkylating agent therapies such as melphalan and prednisone are responsive to

TABLE 46.4-11. Allogeneic Transplant Results

Source	*No.*	*Early Death (%)*	*Complete Response (%)*	*Survival*
EBMT Registry	162	25	44	34% 5-y RFS in complete response patients
IBMT Registry	264	50	—	—
Seattle	80	56	35	33% 5-y RFS in complete response patients
Arkansas	63	52	31	28% 5-y RFS

EBMT, European Bone Marrow Transplant; IBMT, International Bone Marrow Transplant; RFS, relapse-free survival.

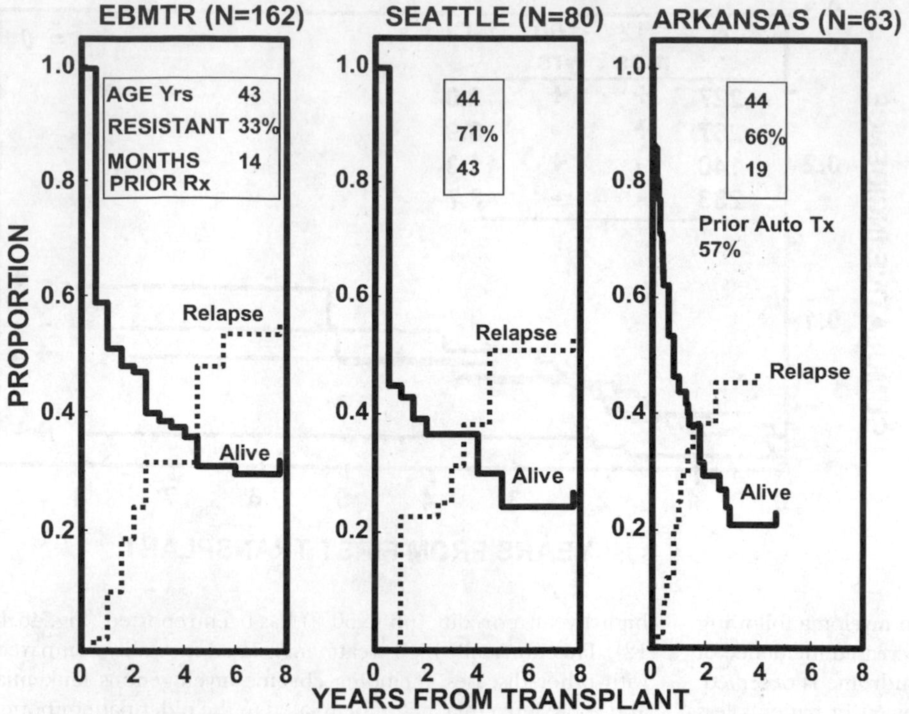

FIGURE 46.4-12. Results of allogeneic transplantation from three large groups show high early mortality with relapse-free survival around 25% to 30%. However, later relapses are observed. EBMTR, European Bone Marrow Transplant Registry; Rx, treatment; Tx, transplant.

high-dose dexamethasone pulsing alone or in combination with drugs such as VAD or CVAD.[306,338–340] Such patients still remain candidates for high-dose melphalan with peripheral blood stem cell rescue if adequate quantities of stem cells can be procured after salvage therapies. Patients relapsing after prior VAD and autotransplant have been treated with combination chemotherapy consisting of dexamethasone in a pulsing fashion and cyclophosphamide, 400 mg/m^2/d, etoposide, 40 mg/m^2/d, and cisplatin, 15 mg/m^2/d by continuous infusion for 4 days (DCEP). In a study of 57 patients relapsing after tandem transplant, more than 40% achieved greater than or equal to 75% tumor mass reduction, including true complete remission in 13% patients.[341] The responses were seen in high-risk disease settings, including chromosome 13 abnormalities and high labeling index. The efficacy of thalidomide in this setting (see Thalidomide, later in this chapter) has led to the evaluation of a combination of DCEP with thalidomide and Adriamycin (DTPACE) followed by G-CSF administration as induction therapy before transplantation. The preliminary results of this combination appear to be extremely promising, with more than 75% of previously treated patients achieving partial response after two cycles. These combinations, with success in the salvage setting, are now being evaluated as induction therapy and posttransplant consolidation. In fact, superior overall and event-free survival have been reported in high-risk patients (chromosome 13 abnormalities) receiving posttransplant DCEP consolidation.[342]

Newer Phase I Agents

BISPHOSPHONATES. The second- and third-generation bisphosphonates, pamidronate and zoledronate, reduce skeletal complications and bone pain in myeloma (Table 46.4-12).[343,344] The mechanism of action includes down-regulation of osteoclast activity, decreased IL-6 production, and induction of apoptosis of osteoclasts through inhibition of farnesyl and geranyl-geranyl transferase activity.[345,346] Besides reducing bone-related problems,

TABLE 46.4-12. Summary of Published Placebo-Controlled Trials of Bisphosphonates in Patients with Multiple Myeloma

	Belch et al.[384]	*Lahtinen et al.*[385]	*Berenson et al.*[343]
Number of evaluable patients	166	336	377
Bisphosphonate therapy	Etidronate, 5 mg/kg daily (oral)	Clodronate, 2.4 g/d (oral) for 24 mo	Pamidronate, 90 mg (IV q4wk × 9 cycles)
Lytic bone lesions	0	+	0
Pathologic fractures	0	0	+
Radiation therapy	NA	NA	+
Bone pain	0	0	+
Hypercalcemia	0	0	+
Survival	—	0	+

0, no effect; +, beneficial effect; –, harmful effect; NA, not assessed.

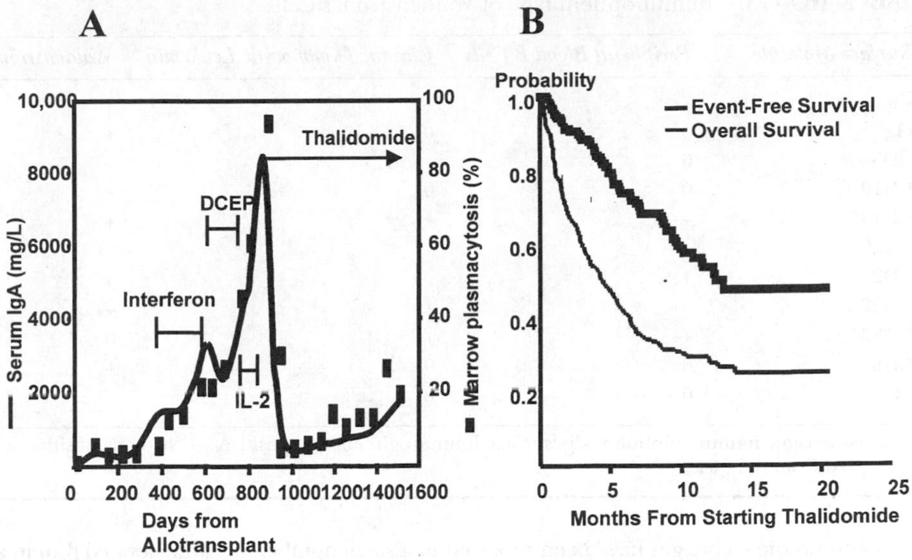

FIGURE 46.4-13. **A:** A patient initially undergoing allogeneic transplantation followed by interleukin-2 treatment and salvage therapy with DCEP (dexamethasone, cyclophosphamide, etoposide, cis-platinum) at relapse without response was treated with escalating doses of thalidomide starting at 200 mg and increasing to 800 mg daily. Within 12 weeks the patient had achieved a complete response, with normalization of bone marrow plasmacytosis from 95% involvement before thalidomide and reduction of immunoglobulin A from over 8 g/dL to normal range. The patient was maintained at a 400 mg daily dose. Following sustained response for over 16 months, the patient showed signs of relapse and is being treated with a higher thalidomide dose now. **B:** Event-free and overall survival of 89 relapsed or refractory myeloma patients treated with single-agent thalidomide.

continued administration over 21 months showed some survival advantage (21 vs. 14 months; $P = .041$) in a subgroup of patients receiving salvage chemotherapy and pamidronate versus same chemotherapy alone.[343,347] *In vitro* cytotoxic effects have been observed in myeloma cell lines,[348,349] tumor specimens, and the SCID-hu system. Preliminary reports of pamidronate alone administered frequently, every 2 weeks, have shown response or delay in disease progression in occasional patients.[350]

THALIDOMIDE. In 180 patients, thalidomide was investigated using incremental doses of 200 to 800 mg. Thalidomide may act in many different ways including through antiangiogenic activity, down-regulation of anti–TNF-α activity, immunomodulation, and changes in adhesion molecules.[351,352] In this group of patients with advanced posttransplant relapsed myeloma, a partial response was attained in 26% and an overall response was observed in 34% of patients with single-agent thalidomide.[140] As the major toxicities are somnolence, constipation, neurologic symptoms, and fatigue, it may be an ideal drug to combine with other traditional chemotherapeutic regimens (Fig. 46.4-13).

OTHER POTENTIAL AGENTS. With the success of thalidomide, newer potent antiangiogenic agents and thalidomide analogues are of interest in myeloma. Other potential agents under investigation include TNF-α inhibitors, oral tamoxifen, arsenic trioxide, and a newer generation of bisphosphonates.[131,353–355] Additionally, with altered ras activity and high telomerase levels in myeloma, approaches directed at these molecular targets are being investigated. The SCID-hu model provides a perfect setting for such evaluation before human studies.

WALDENSTRÖM'S MACROGLOBULINEMIA

Dr Jan Waldenström first described a condition in two patients characterized by bleeding tendencies from mucosa, anemia, lymphadenopathy, and high serum viscosity with high molecular mass M component.[356] This disease subsequently was recognized to have lymphoplasmacytic differentiation that differed from myeloma in various aspects including absence of lytic bone disease and presence of hepatosplenomegaly, lymphadenopathy, or both.

Macroglobulinemia is less frequent than myeloma, affecting approximately 1500 people a year in the United States, with a higher incidence in men and in whites than in African Americans and a median age at diagnosis of 63 years.[357,388] The pathogenetic mechanisms are not well understood. However, mechanisms similar to those in myeloma can be considered. Familial occurrence and a case report of occurrence in monozygotic twins have been reported.[358,359] A patient working as a canary breeder developed macroglobulinemia and showed reactivity of monoclonal IgM to an antigen in the canary droppings, suggesting a role of constant antigenic stimulation in the pathogenesis of the disease.[360] Infrequency of the disease, however, has limited detailed epidemiologic and pathogenetic studies. Like myeloma the tumor cells are postantigen selection memory B cells with somatic hypermutation and rearrangement in the variable region and unique CDR. The normal B cells produce IgM as primary immune response and with further antigenic stimulation and selection undergo class switching and produce IgG. Waldenström's macroglobulinemia cells, with production of IgM, are arrested before class switching. However, no clonal diversity is observed and no isotype switching is reported.

Viral infections with hepatitis C virus appear to be a significant risk for cryoglobulinemia, which is often associated with Waldenström's macroglobulinemia. The role of Kaposi's sarcoma herpes virus, which has been reported to be present in dendritic cells derived from bone marrow from patients with Waldenström's macroglobulinemia, and hepatitis G virus are unclear in pathogenesis of this disease.[361–363] Phenotypically the malignant cells are surface and cytoplasmic Ig+ cells expressing various pan B-cell markers such as CD19, CD20, and CD22. CD5 and CD23 are observed in a small number of patients. The immunophenotypic differences between cells in multiple myeloma, Waldenström's macroglobulinemia, CLL, and normal B cells are shown in Table 46.4-13.[364] Bone marrow examination shows various subtypes from small lymphocytes to lymphocytes with varying levels of plasmacytoid differentiation to presence of mature plasma cells along with mast cells and Dutcher bodies.

TABLE 46.4-13. Immunophenotype of Waldenström's Cells

Surface Molecule	*Peripheral Blood B Cells*	*Chronic Lymphocytic Leukemia*	*Waldenström's Macroglobulinemia*	*Multiple Myeloma*
sIg	++	+	+	0
cIg	0	0	+	++
CD5	0	++	±	0
CD10	0	0	±	+
CD19	++	++	+	0/+
CD20	++	+	++	0/+
CD21	++	++	+	0
CD22	++	+	++	0
CD23	++	++	0	0
CD38	0	0	+	++
PCA1	0	0	+	++

cIg, cytoplasmic immunoglobulin; sIg, surface immunoglobulin; +, positive; ++, strongly positive; ±, variable; 0, negative.
(Adapted from ref. 364.)

Chromosomal changes have been reported in a small number of patients with Waldenström's macroglobulinemia, mainly due to low proliferative potential of this disease. Complex karyotypic changes include trisomies, deletions, and structural abnormalities of various chromosomes.[365] As with myeloma and other B-cell tumors, translocations involving 14q32 are reported with various partners.[366,367] These includes chromosome 18 (BCL-2), 8 (c-myc), 11 (PRAD-1), and importantly, chromosome 9 involving PAX5 gene, which is expressed at a higher level in normal pre-B cells, and its expression decreases as the cells become plasma cells.[368]

The clinical presentation is variable and is related to high IgM levels and lymphoplasmacytic cell infiltration of various organs.[369] The usual manifestations related to tissue infiltration include pulmonic symptoms with cough and dyspnea, gastrointestinal infiltration with diarrhea and bleeding, skin plaques, and periorbital exophthalmos and nerve palsies. The large molecular size of IgM leads to higher serum viscosity than seen with comparable levels of IgG or IgA. Hyperviscosity is seldom seen with IgG or IgA levels less than 5 g/dL, whereas IgM levels of greater than 3 g/dL may lead to clinical manifestations. Relative plasma viscosity above 5 cp is usually associated with symptoms. Hyperviscosity may present with fatigue, blurred vision, headache, shortness of breath, mucosal bleeding, and mental status changes or coma. Type I cryoglobulinemia, which is caused by physicochemical interactions with the paraprotein and observed in small numbers of patients, may present with purpura, urticaria, Raynaud's phenomenon, acrocyanosis, malleolar ulcers, or necrosis.[370] Cryoglobulinemia type II, which is due to antibody reactivity, may present with arthralgia, proteinuria, renal failure, polyneuropathy, and mononeuritis.[364,371] Additional special presentation may be related to the presence of cold agglutinins leading to a mild hemolytic anemia or exacerbation of Raynaud's phenomenon. Severe demyelinating sensorimotor neuropathies is observed in 10% of the patients. One-half of these patients have detectable antibodies against myelin-associated glycoprotein (anti-MAG antibodies).[372,373,389] Sensory or ataxic neuropathy is observed more commonly in patients with anti-MAG antibodies. The frequency of common presenting features is listed in Table 46.4-14.

Laboratory evaluation usually shows anemia; however, early leukopenia and thrombocytopenia in untreated patients is uncommon. Elevated erythrocyte sedimentation rate, monoclonal IgM protein in serum with occasional light chains in the urine, and elevated β_2m in a subset of patients is observed. Bone marrow shows typical lymphoplasmacytic infiltration with the presence of mast cells. CT scan evaluation of chest, abdomen, and pelvis may show the presence of lymphadenopathy with enlargement of liver, spleen, or both. Skeletal survey is done to rule out IgM myeloma as bone lesions are not seen in Waldenström's macroglobulinemia. Depending on clinical findings of immunologic effects or involvement of other organs, specialized test are required. Tissue infiltration may require confirmation with biopsies.

Asymptomatic presentation of Waldenström's macroglobulinemia does not require immediate cytoreductive therapy as it does not alter the outcome and delays chemotherapy-related bone marrow suppression. Patients with preserved hemoglobin and low β_2m are ideal candidates for observation. Patients with high IgM-related symptoms, such as hyperviscosity, hemolytic anemia, neuropathy, and cryoglobulinemia, benefit from plasmapheresis without conventional chemotherapy.[374–376]

Patients who are symptomatic from the disease or have marked hepatosplenomegaly, cytopenia, or progressive disease have been treated with alkylating agents. Chlorambucil alone or with corticosteroids produces response rates as defined by greater than 50% drop in paraproteins and tumor mass in 60% to 75% of previously untreated patients, and complete responses observed in less than 5% of the patients.[377] Responses are slow and may take up to 12 to 18 months from the beginning of treat-

TABLE 46.4-14. Clinical Manifestations in 260 Patients with Waldenström's Macroglobulinemia

Clinical Findings	*Frequency (%)*
SYMPTOMS	
Severe fatigue	85
Bleeding	60
Neurologic	17
Bone pain	10
SIGNS	
Lymphadenopathy	40
Hepatomegaly	30
Splenomegaly	30
Hepatosplenomegaly	25

ment. Treatment is continued until maximal reduction is observed. Median survival from diagnosis is more than 10 years. More aggressive combination therapy with multiple agents has achieved more than 80% response rate. However, there is no improvement in overall survival. Prolonged alkylating agent therapy has led to development of myelodysplastic syndrome or acute myeloid leukemia in up to 10% of the patients.

Purine analogues fludarabine at a dose of 25 mg/m^2 intravenously for 5 days every 4 weeks and cladribine at a dose of 0.1 mg/kg by continuous infusion for 7 days have produced responses in up to 80% of previously untreated patient populations and complete responses in 10% of patients. Effectiveness of purine analogues in previously treated patients has been in the range of 30%, with higher responses in patients relapsing after cessation of prior therapy and less frequent responses in patients with resistant relapse.[263,390–394] Patients relapsing after receiving one purine analogue do not usually respond to another purine analogue. In a large prospective multicenter study by the Southwest Oncology Group in newly diagnosed patients, however, fludarabine showed only 39% response rate.[378] Younger patients are shown to respond better than older patient populations. Anemia, β_2m greater than 2.5 mg/dL, and IgM greater than 4 g/dL were predicative of poor outcome in that study. The major side effects with purine analogues are prolonged cumulative cytopenia and immunosuppression leading to opportunistic infections. Nonchemotherapeutic treatment options include Rituxan (anti-CD20 mo-ab) with 20% to 30% responses in small studies,[364] and interferon-α with a 30% response rate.[395–398] High-dose dexamethasone pulsing has produced some responses in refractory patients.[379,380] There have been reports of occasional responses following splenectomy.[381,382] The role of high-dose chemotherapy has been evaluated in six patients with extensive prior therapy showing five patients achieving a partial response and one patient achieving a complete response.[383] However, as prolonged prior therapy affects stem cell mobilization, especially after purine analogues and chlorambucil, mobilization, at an earlier stage of the treatment, is necessary. The role of thalidomide in this disease remains under investigation.

PERSPECTIVE

New discoveries in molecular biology, better understanding of B-cell development and immune regulation, and improved imaging techniques have advanced our understanding of the biology of multiple myeloma and related plasma cell neoplasms in the last decade. A new entity of multiple myeloma with chromosome 13 abnormalities has been recognized, carrying an extremely adverse prognosis even with high-dose chemotherapy. A putative tumor suppressor molecule is under investigation and a risk-based therapeutic approach is applied with more aggressive treatment in this subgroup of patients, including up-front allogeneic transplantation. High-dose chemotherapy has been clearly shown to be effective in improving complete response rates and event-free and overall survival in comparison with standard-dose therapy. It has been successfully applied in older patients or in the presence of renal dysfunction. Over 40% of patients now achieve complete remission compared with 5% with standard-dose therapy a decade ago, and for the first time durable complete responses have been reported in patients without standard risk factors and absence of chromosome 13 abnormalities. MRI with inversion recovery images provides better assessment of bone marrow involvement with myeloma cells and CT- and MRI-guided fine-needle aspiration biopsies provide cytologic and molecular diagnosis of the residual bone lesions. Progress is being made in better defining complete responses and now includes normalization of MRI (MRI complete response). Preliminary investigations appear to predict superior survival in such patients. Allogeneic transplants continue to remain difficult, with up to 50% 1-year morality. However, nonmyeloablative allogeneic transplant regimens are being evaluated to decrease treatment-related morality while at the same time using graft-versus-myeloma effect to achieve disease control, especially in patients with chromosome 13 changes. The demonstration of the role of neoangiogenesis in myeloma has led to identification of an effective new agent, thalidomide, in refractory myeloma patients. With its different spectrum of adverse effects, it may be an ideal drug to be combined with chemotherapeutic agents. Soil-directed therapy with the use of bisphosphonates has shown antitumor effects along with improvement in bone density and a decrease in skeletal events.

Future directions include investigation of thalidomide in induction as well as maintenance therapy, evaluation of post–high-dose chemotherapy consolidation with chemotherapeutic agents, development of tumor cell–specific cytotoxic T lymphocytes, and safe administration of allogeneic transplantation. Better understanding of the molecular mechanism of the disease, especially of factors that prevent apoptosis with the help of subtractive libraries and micro array chips, should provide newer tools to effectively and specifically treat this disease.

REFERENCES

1. Bakkus MH. Ig gene sequences in the study of clonality. *Pathol Biol (Paris)* 1999;47:128.
2. Macro M, Andre I, Comby E, et al. IgE multiple myeloma. *Leuk Lymphoma* 1999;32:597.
3. Blade J, Kyle RA. Nonsecretory myeloma, immunoglobulin D myeloma, and plasma cell leukemia. *Hematol Oncol Clin North Am* 1999;13:1259.
4. Poncet JC, Toussirot E, Wendling D. Specific features of immunoglobulin D multiple myeloma. *Revue Du Rhumatisme* [English Edition] 1997;64:410.
5. Macintyre W. Case of mollities and fragilitas ossium, accompanied with urine strongly charged with animal matter. *Med Chir Trans Lond* 1859;33:211.
6. Bence J. On a new substance occurring in the urine of a patient with mollities and fragilits ossium. *Phil Trans R Soc Lond* 1848;55:673.
7. Dalrymple J. On the microscopical character of mollities ossium. *Dublin Q J Med Sci* 1846;2:85.
8. Rustizky J. Multiple myeloma. *Deutsch Z Chir* 1873;3:162.
9. Kahler O. Zur Symptomatologie des multiplen Myeloma: beobachtung von Albumosurie. *Prog Med Wochnschr* 1889;14:33.
10. Ellinger A. Das Vorkommen des Bence Jones' schen Korpes in Harn bei Tumoren des Knochenmarks und seine diagnostische Bedeutung. *Deutsch Arch Klin Med* 1899;62:266.
11. Wright J. A case of multiple myeloma. *Bull Johns Hopkins Hosp* 1933;52:156.
12. Arinkin M. Die intravitale Untersuchungs-Methodik des Knochenmarks. *Folia Haematol (Lepiz)* 1929;38:233.
13. Tiselius A. Electrophoresis of serum globulin. II Electrophoretic analysis of normal and immune sera. *Biochem J* 1937;31:1464.
14. Longsworth L. Electrophoretic patterns of normal and pathological human blood serum and plasma. *J Exp Med* 1939;70:399.
15. Grabar P. Methode permettant l'etude conjugee des proprietes electrphoretiques et immunochimiques d'un melange de proteines. Application au serum sanguin. *Biochim Biophys Acta* 1953;10:193.
16. Alwall N. Urethane and stilbamidine in multiple myeloma: report on 2 cases. *Lancet* 1947;2:388.
17. Holland JR, Hosley H, Scharlau C, et al. A controlled trial of urethane treatment in multiple myeloma. *Blood* 1966;27:328.
18. Bergsagel D. Evaluation of new chemotherapeutic agents in the treatment of multiple myeloma. IV. L-Phenylalanine mustard (NSC-8806). *Cancer Chemother Rep* 1962;21:87.
19. Salmon SE, Shadduck RK, Schilling A. Intermittent high-dose prednisone (NSC-10023) therapy for multiple myeloma. *Cancer Chemother Rep* 1967;51:179.
20. Alexanian R, Bonnet J, Gehan E, et al. Combination chemotherapy for multiple myeloma. *Cancer* 1972;30:382.

21. McElwain T, Powles R. High-dose intravenous melphalan for plasma-cell leukemia and myeloma. *Lancet* 1983;1:822.
22. Barlogie B, Hall R, Zander A, Dicke K, Alexanian R. High-dose melphalan with autologous bone marrow transplantation for multiple myeloma. *Blood* 1986;67:1298.
23. Cohen HJ, Crawford J, Rao MK, Pieper CF, Currie MS. Racial differences in the prevalence of monoclonal gammopathy in a community-based sample of the elderly [published erratum appears in *Am J Med* 1998;105:362]. *Am J Med* 1998;104:439.
24. Devesa SS, Silverman DT, Young JL Jr, et al. Cancer incidence and mortality trends among whites in the United States, 1947–84. *J Natl Cancer Inst* 1987;79:701.
25. Riedel DA, Pottern LM. The epidemiology of multiple myeloma. *Hematol Oncol Clin North Am* 1992;6:225.
26. Ichimaru M, Ishimaru T, Mikami M, Matsunaga M. Multiple myeloma among atomic bomb survivors in Hiroshima and Nagasaki, 1950–76: relationship to radiation dose absorbed by marrow. *J Natl Cancer Inst* 1982;69:323.
27. Omar RZ, Barber JA, Smith PG. Cancer mortality and morbidity among plutonium workers at the Sellafield plant of British Nuclear Fuels. *Br J Cancer* 1999;79:1288.
28. Bergsagel DE, Wong O, Bergsagel PL, et al. Benzene and multiple myeloma: appraisal of the scientific evidence. *Blood* 1999;94:1174.
29. Lundberg I, Milatou-Smith R. Mortality and cancer incidence among Swedish paint industry workers with long-term exposure to organic solvents. *Scand J Work Environ Health* 1998;24:270.
30. Salmon SE, Kyle RA. Silicone gels, induction of plasma cell tumors, and genetic susceptibility in mice: a call for epidemiologic investigation of women with silicone breast implants [editorial]. *J Natl Cancer Inst* 1994;86:1040.
31. Tricot GJ, Naucke S, Vaught L, et al. Is the risk of multiple myeloma increased in patients with silicone implants? *Curr Top Microbiol Immunol* 1996;210:357.
32. Cuzick J, De Stavola B. Multiple myeloma—a case-control study. *Br J Cancer* 1988;57:516.
33. Fritschi L, Siemiatycki J. Lymphoma, myeloma and occupation: results of a case-control study. *Int J Cancer* 1996;67:498.
34. Doody MM, Linet MS, Glass AG, et al. Risks of non-Hodgkin's lymphoma, multiple myeloma, and leukemia associated with common medications. *Epidemiology* 1996;7:131.
35. Linet MS, Harlow SD, McLaughlin JK. A case-control study of multiple myeloma in whites: chronic antigenic stimulation, occupation, and drug use. *Cancer Res* 1987;47:2978.
36. Brown LM, Linet MS, Greenberg RS, et al. Multiple myeloma and family history of cancer among blacks and whites in the U.S. *Cancer* 1999;85:2385.
37. Grosbois B, Jego P, Attal M, et al. Familial multiple myeloma: report of fifteen families. *Br J Haematol* 1999;105:768.
38. Watanabe T, Suzuki Y, Murakami S, Komatsu M. [Multiple myeloma in siblings]. *Rinsho Ketsueki* 1999;40:135.
39. Kyle RA. Monoclonal gammopathy of undetermined significance. *Am J Med* 1978;64:814.
40. Avet-Loiseau H, Facon T, Daviet A, et al. 14q32 translocations and monosomy 13 observed in monoclonal gammopathy of undetermined significance delineate a multistep process for the oncogenesis of multiple myeloma. Intergroupe Francophone du Myelome. *Cancer Res* 1999;59:4546.
41. Seligmann M, Sassy C, Chevalier A. A human IgG myeloma protein with anti- 2 macroglobulin antibody activity. *J Immunol* 1973;110:85.
42. Salmon SE, Seligmann M. B-cell neoplasia in man. *Lancet* 1974;2:1230.
43. Rettig MB, Ma HJ, Vescio RA, et al. Kaposi's sarcoma-associated herpesvirus infection of bone marrow dendritic cells from multiple myeloma patients [see comments]. *Science* 1997;276:1851.
44. Said JW, Rettig MR, Heppner K, et al. Localization of Kaposi's sarcoma-associated herpesvirus in bone marrow biopsy samples from patients with multiple myeloma [see comments]. *Blood* 1997;90:4278.
45. Soulier J, Grollet L, Oksenhendler E, et al. Kaposi's sarcoma-associated herpesvirus-like DNA sequences in multicentric Castleman's disease [see comments]. *Blood* 1995;86:1276.
46. Said W, Chien K, Takeuchi S, et al. Kaposi's sarcoma-associated herpesvirus (KSHV or HHV8) in primary effusion lymphoma: ultrastructural demonstration of herpesvirus in lymphoma cells. *Blood* 1996;87:4937.
47. Schalling M, Ekman M, Kaaya EE, Linde A, Biberfeld P. A role for a new herpes virus (KSHV) in different forms of Kaposi's sarcoma. *Nat Med* 1995;1:707.
48. Chauhan D, Bharti A, Raje N, et al. Detection of Kaposi's sarcoma herpesvirus DNA sequences in multiple myeloma bone marrow stromal cells. *Blood* 1999;93:1482.
49. Tisdale JF, Stewart AK, Dickstein B, et al. Molecular and serological examination of the relationship of human herpesvirus 8 to multiple myeloma: orf 26 sequences in bone marrow stroma are not restricted to myeloma patients and other regions of the genome are not detected. *Blood* 1998;92:2681.
50. Cull GM, Carter GI, Timms JM, et al. Low incidence of human herpesvirus 8 in stem cell collections from myeloma patients. *Bone Marrow Transplant* 1999;23:759.
51. Tarte K, Chang Y, Klein B. Kaposi's sarcoma-associated herpesvirus and multiple myeloma: lack of criteria for causality. *Blood* 1999;93:3159.
52. De Greef C, Van De Voorde W, Bakkus M, et al. Kaposi's sarcoma-associated herpesvirus (KSHV/HHV-8) DNA sequences are absent in leukapheresis products and ex vivo expanded CD34+ cells from multiple myeloma patients. *Br J Haematol* 1999;106:1033.
53. Harada N, Hata H, Matsuno F, et al. Absence of Kaposi's sarcoma-associated herpesvirus (KSHV) in bone marrow cells from Japanese myeloma patients [letter]. *Leukemia* 1999; 13:1465.
54. Bellos F, Goldschmidt H, Dorner M, Ho AD, Moos M. Bone marrow derived dendritic cells from patients with multiple myeloma cultured with three distinct protocols do not bear Kaposi's sarcoma associated herpesvirus DNA. *Ann Oncol* 1999;10:323.
55. Olsen SJ, Tarte K, Sherman W, et al. Evidence against KSHV infection in the pathogenesis of multiple myeloma. *Virus Res* 1998;57:197.
56. Yi Q, Ekman M, Anton D, et al. *Blood* dendritic cells from myeloma patients are not infected with Kaposi's sarcoma-associated herpesvirus (KSHV/HHV-8). *Blood* 1998; 92:402.
57. Tarte K, Olsen SJ, Yang Lu Z, et al. Clinical-grade functional dendritic cells from patients with multiple myeloma are not infected with Kaposi's sarcoma-associated herpesvirus. *Blood* 1998;91:1852.
58. Parravicini C, Lauri E, Baldini L, et al. Kaposi's sarcoma-associated herpesvirus infection and multiple myeloma [letter; comment]. *Science* 1997;278:1969.
59. Cottoni F, Uccini S. Kaposi's sarcoma-associated herpesvirus infection and multiple myeloma [letter; comment]. *Science* 1997;278:1972; discussion 1972.
60. Masood R, Zheng T, Tupule A, et al. Kaposi's sarcoma-associated herpesvirus infection and multiple myeloma [letter; comment]. *Science* 1997;278:1970.
61. Whitby D, Boshoff C, Luppi M, Torelli G. Kaposi's sarcoma-associated herpesvirus infection and multiple myeloma [letter; comment]. *Science* 1997;278:1971.
62. Brousset P, Meggetto F, Attal M, Delsol G. Kaposi's sarcoma-associated herpesvirus infection and multiple myeloma [letter; comment]. *Science* 1997;278:1972; discussion 1972.
63. Berenson JR, Vescio RA. HHV-8 and multiple myeloma. *Pathol Biol (Paris)* 1999;47:115.
64. Berenson JR, Bergsagel PL, Munshi N. Initiation and maintenance of multiple myeloma. *Semin Hematol* 1999;36:9.
65. Potter M. Experimental plasmacytomagenesis in mice. *Hematol Oncol Clin North Am* 1997;11:323.
66. Radl J. Multiple myeloma and related disorders. Lessons from an animal model. *Pathol Biol (Paris)* 1999;47:109.
67. Radl J. Animal model of human disease. Benign monoclonal gammopathy (idiopathic paraproteinemia). *Am J Pathol* 1981;105:91.
68. Radl J, Croese JW, Zurcher C, Van den Enden-Vieveen MH, de Leeuw AM. Animal model of human disease. Multiple myeloma. *Am J Pathol* 1988;132:593.
69. Huang YW, Richardson JA, Vitetta ES. Anti-CD54 (ICAM-1) has antitumor activity in SCID mice with human myeloma cells. *Cancer Res* 1995;55:610.
70. Feo-Zuppardi FJ, Taylor CW, Iwato K, et al. Long-term engraftment of fresh human myeloma cells in SCID mice. *Blood* 1992;80:2843.
71. Ahsmann EJ, van Tol MJ, Oudeman-Gruber J, et al. The SCID mouse as a model for multiple myeloma. *Br J Haematol* 1995;89:319.
72. Urashima M, Chen BP, Chen S, et al. The development of a model for the homing of multiple myeloma cells to human bone marrow. *Blood* 1997;90:754.
73. Yaccoby S, Barlogie B, Epstein J. Primary myeloma cells growing in SCID-hu mice: a model for studying the biology and treatment of myeloma and its manifestations. *Blood* 1998;92:2908.
74. Yaccoby S, Barlogie B, Epstein J. Primary myeloma cells growing in SCID-hu mice: a model for studying the biology and treatment of myeloma and its manifestations. *Blood* 1998;92:2908.
75. Sawyer J, Waldron J, Jagannath S, Barlogie B. Cytogenetics findings in 200 patients with multiple myeloma. *Cancer Genet Cytogenet* 1995;82:41.
76. Dewald GW, Kyle RA, Hicks GA, Greipp PR. The clinical significance of cytogenetic studies in 100 patients with multiple myeloma, plasma cell leukemia, or amyloidosis. *Blood* 1985;66:380.
77. Gould J, Alexanian R, Goodacre A, et al. Plasma cell karyotype in multiple myeloma. *Blood* 1988;71:453.
78. Sawyer JR, Lukacs JL, Munshi N, et al. Identification of new nonrandom translocations in multiple myeloma with multicolor spectral karyotyping. *Blood* 1998;92:4269.
79. Perez-Simon JA, Garcia-Sanz R, Tabernero MD, et al. Prognostic value of numerical chromosome aberrations in multiple myeloma: a FISH analysis of 15 different chromosomes. *Blood* 1998;91:3366.
80. Tricot G, Sawyer J, Jagannath S, et al. Poor prognosis in multiple myeloma is associated only with partial or complete deletion of chromosome 13 or abnormalities involving 11q and not with other karyotype abnormalities. *Blood* 1995;86:4250.
81. Dao DD, Sawyer JR, Epstein J, et al. Deletion on of the retinoblastoma gene on multiple myeloma. *Leukemia* 1994;8:1280.
82. Shaughnessy J, Barlogie B. Chromosome 13 deletion in myeloma. *Curr Top Microbiol Immunol* 1999;246:199.
83. Urashima M, Ogata A, Chauhan D, et al. Interleukin-6 promotes multiple myeloma cell growth via phosphorylation of retinoblastoma protein. *Blood* 1996;88:2219.
84. Ng MH, Chung YF, Lo KW, et al. Frequent hypermethylation of p16 and p15 genes in multiple myeloma. *Blood* 1997;89:2500.
85. Tasaka T, Berenson J, Vescio R, et al. Analysis of the p16INK4A, p15INK4B and p18INK4C genes in multiple myeloma. *Br J Haematol* 1997;96:98.
86. Urashima M, Teoh G, Ogata A, et al. Characterization of p16(INK4A) expression in multiple myeloma and plasma cell leukemia. *Clin Cancer Res* 1997;3:2173.
87. Kawano MM, Mahmoud MS, Ishikawa H. Cyclin D1 and p16INK4A are preferentially expressed in immature and mature myeloma cells, respectively. *Br J Haematol* 1997;99:131.
88. Hallek M, Bergsagel LP, Anderson KD. Multiple myeloma: increasing evidence for a multistep transformation process. *Blood* 1998;91:3.
89. Avet-Loiseau H, Li JY, Morineau N, et al. Monosomy 13 is associated with the transition of monoclonal gammopathy of undetermined significance to multiple myeloma. Intergroupe Francophone du Myelome. *Blood* 1999;94:2583.
90. Chesi M, Bergsagel PL, Brents LA, et al. Dysregulation of cyclin D1 by translocation into an IgH gamma switch region in two multiple myeloma cell lines [see comments]. *Blood* 1996;88:674.
91. Chesi M, Nardini E, Brents LA, et al. Frequent translocation t(4;14)(p16.3;q32.3) in multiple myeloma is associated with increased expression and activating mutations of fibroblast growth factor receptor 3. *Nat Genet* 1997;16:260.
92. Chesi M, Nardini E, Lim RS, et al. The t(4;14) translocation in myeloma dysregulates both FGFR3 and a novel gene, MMSET, resulting in IgH/MMSET hybrid transcripts. *Blood* 1998;92:3025.
93. Chesi M, Bergsagel PL, Shonukan OO, et al. Frequent dysregulation of the c-maf proto-oncogene at 16q23 by translocation to an Ig locus in multiple myeloma. *Blood* 1998;91:4457.

94. Iida S, Rao PH, Butler M, et al. Deregulation of MUM1/IRF4 by chromosomal translocation in multiple myeloma. *Nat Genet* 1997;17:226.
95. Mahmoud MS, Huang N, Nobuyoshi M, et al. Altered expression of Pax-5 gene in human myeloma cells. *Blood* 1996;87:4311.
96. Neri A, Baldini L, Trecca D, et al. p53 gene mutations in multiple myeloma are associated with advanced forms of malignancy. *Blood* 1993;81:128.
97. Drach J, Ackermann J, Fritz E, et al. Presence of a p53 gene deletion in patients with multiple myeloma predicts for short survival after conventional-dose chemotherapy. *Blood* 1998;92:802.
98. Portier M, Moles JP, Mazars GR, et al. p53 and RAS gene mutations in multiple myeloma. *Oncogene* 1992;7:2539.
99. Teoh G, Urashima M, Ogata A, et al. MDM2 protein overexpression promotes proliferation and survival of multiple myeloma cells. *Blood* 1997;90:1982.
100. Selvanayagam P, Blick M, Narni F, et al. Alteration and abnormal expression of the *c-myc* oncogene in human multiple myeloma. *Blood* 1988;71:30.
101. Greil R, Fasching B, Loidl P, Huber H. Expression of the c-Myc proto-oncogene in multiple myeloma and chronic lymphocytic leukemia: an in situ analysis. *Blood* 1991;78:180.
102. Pettersson M, Jernberg-Wiklund H, Larsson LG, et al. Expression of the Bcl-2 gene in human multiple myeloma cell lines and normal plasma cells. *Blood* 1992;79:495.
103. Puthier D, Pellat-Deceunynck C, Barille S, et al. Differential expression of Bcl-2 in human plasma cell disorders according to proliferation status and malignancy. *Leukemia* 1999;13:289.
104. Tu Y, Xu FH, Liu J, et al. Upregulated expression of BCL-2 in multiple myeloma cells induced by exposure to doxorubicin, etoposide, and hydrogen peroxide. *Blood* 1996;88:1805.
105. Tu Y, Renner S, Xu F, et al. BCL-X expression in multiple myeloma: possible indicator of chemoresistance. *Cancer Res* 1998;58:256.
106. Sangfelt O, Osterborg A, Grander D, et al. Response to interferon therapy in patients with multiple myeloma correlates with expression of the Bcl-2 oncoprotein. *Int J Cancer* 1995;63:190.
107. Ogata A, Chauhan D, Urashima M, et al. Blockade of mitogen-activated protein kinase cascade signaling in interleukin 6-independent multiple myeloma cells. *Clin Cancer Res* 1997;3:1017.
108. Catlett-Falcone R, Landowski TH, Oshiro MM, et al. Constitutive activation of Stat3 signaling confers resistance to apoptosis in human U266 myeloma cells. *Immunity* 1999;10:105.
109. Feinman R, Koury J, Thames M, et al. Role of NF-kappaB in the rescue of multiple myeloma cells from glucocorticoid-induced apoptosis by bcl-2. *Blood* 1999;93:3044.
110. Shammas M, Batchu RB, Hurley LH, et al. Inhibitors of telomerase can reduce the proliferative potential of myeloma cells. *Blood* 1999;94:311a.
111. Sahota SS, Davis Z, Hamblin TFS. Discordant somatic mutation of immunoglobulin variable region genes and bcl-6 genes in chronic lymphocytic leukemia. *Blood* 1999;94:662.
112. Klein B, Zhang XG, Lu ZY, Bataille R. Interleukin-6 in human multiple myeloma. *Blood* 1995;85:863.
113. Klein B, Zhang X, Jourdan M, et al. Paracrine rather than autocrine regulation of myeloma-cell growth and differentiation by interleukin-6. *Blood* 1989;73:517.
114. Anderson KC, Lust JA. Role of cytokines in multiple myeloma. *Semin Hematol* 1999;36:14.
115. Treon SP, Anderson KC. Interleukin-6 in multiple myeloma and related plasma cell dyscrasias. *Curr Opin Hematol* 1998;5:42.
116. Hata H, Xiao HQ, Petrucci MT, et al. Interleukin-6 gene expression in multiple myeloma: a characteristic of immature myeloma cells. *Blood* 1993;81:3357.
117. Villunger A, Egle A, Kos M, et al. Constituents of autocrine IL-6 loops in myeloma cell lines and their targeting for suppression of neoplastic growth by antibody strategies. *Int J Cancer* 1996;65:498.
118. Grigorieva I, Thomas X, Epstein J. The bone marrow stromal environment is a major factor in myeloma cell resistance to dexamethasone. *Exp Hematol* 1998;26:597.
119. Hardin J, MacLeod S, Grigorieva I, et al. Interleukin-6 prevents dexamethasone-induced myeloma cell death. *Blood* 1994;84:3063.
120. Papadaki H, Kyriakou D, Foudoulakis A, et al. Serum levels of soluble IL-6 receptor in multiple myeloma as indicator of disease activity. *Acta Haematol* 1997;97:191.
121. Brandt SJ, Bodine DM, Dunbar CE, Nienhuis AW. Dysregulated interleukin 6 expression produces a syndrome resembling Castleman's disease in mice. *J Clin Invest* 1990;86:592.
122. Bataille R, Barlogie B, Lu ZY, et al. Biologic effects of anti-interleukin-6 murine monoclonal antibody in advanced multiple myeloma. *Blood* 1995;86:685.
123. Legouffe E, Liautard J, Gaillard JP, et al. Human anti-mouse antibody response to the injection of murine monoclonal antibodies against IL-6. *Clin Exp Immunol* 1994;98:323.
124. Cozzolino F, Torcia M, Aldinucci D, et al. Production of interleukin-1 by bone marrow myeloma cells. *Blood* 1989;74:380.
125. Garrett R, Durie B, Nedwin G, et al. Production of lymphotoxin, a bone resorbing cytokine, by cultured human myeloma cells. *N Engl J Med* 1987;317:526.
126. Mundy GR, Raisz LG, Cooper RA, Schechter GP, Salmon SE. Evidence for the secretion of an osteoclast stimulating factor in myeloma. *N Engl J Med* 1974;291:1041.
127. Borset M, Hjorth-Hansen H, Seidel C, Sundan A, Waage A. Hepatocyte growth factor and its receptor c-met in multiple myeloma. *Blood* 1996;88:3998.
128. Klein B. Update of gp130 cytokines in multiple myeloma. *Curr Opin Hematol* 1998;5:186.
129. Tupitsyn N, Kadagidze Z, Gaillard JP, et al. Functional interaction of the gp80 and gp130 IL-6 receptors in human B cell malignancies. *Clin Lab Haematol* 1998;20:345.
130. Nishimoto N, Ogata A, Shima Y, et al. Oncostatin M, leukemia inhibitory factor, and interleukin 6 induce the proliferation of human plasmacytoma cells via the common signal transducer, gp130. *J Exp Med* 1994;179:1343.
131. Jourdan M, Tarte K, Legouffe E, et al. Tumor necrosis factor is a survival and proliferation factor for human myeloma cells. *Eur Cytokine Network* 1999;10:65.
132. Georgii-Hemming P, Wiklund HJ, Ljunggren O, Nilsson K. Insulin-like growth factor I is a growth and survival factor in human multiple myeloma cell lines. *Blood* 1996; 88:2250.
133. Hjorth-Hansen H, Waage A, Borset M. Interleukin-15 blocks apoptosis and induces proliferation of the human myeloma cell line OH-2 and freshly isolated myeloma cells. *Br J Haematol* 1999;106:28.
134. Jelinek DF, Witzig TE, Arendt BK. A role for insulin-like growth factor in the regulation of IL-6-responsive human myeloma cell line growth. *J Immunol* 1997;159:487.
135. Epstein J. Myeloma stem cell phenotype. Implications for treatment. *Hematol Oncol Clin North Am* 1997;11:43.
136. Vacca A, Ribatti D, Presta M, et al. Bone marrow neovascularization, plasma cell angiogenic potential, and matrix metalloproteinase-2 secretion parallel progression of human multiple myeloma. *Blood* 1999;93:3064.
137. Vacca A, Ribatti D, Roncali L, et al. Bone marrow angiogenesis and progression in multiple myeloma. *Br J Haematol* 1994;87:503.
138. Munshi N, Wilson C, Penn J, et al. Angiogenesis in newly diagnosed multiple myeloma (MM): poor prognosis with increased microvessel density (MVD) in bone marrow biopsies (BMBX). *Blood* 1998;92:98a.
139. Bellamy WT, Richter L, Frutiger Y, Grogan TM. Expression of vascular endothelial growth factor and its receptors in hematopoietic malignancies. *Cancer Res* 1999; 59:728.
140. Singhal S, Mehta J, Desikan R, et al. Antitumor activity of thalidomide in refractory multiple myeloma [see comments]. *N Engl J Med* 1999;341:1565.
141. Ridley RC, Xiao H, Hata H, et al. Expression of syndecan regulates human myeloma plasma cell adhesion to type I collagen. *Blood* 1993;81:767.
142. Teoh G, Anderson KC. Interaction of tumor and host cells with adhesion and extracellular matrix molecules in the development of multiple myeloma. *Hematol Oncol Clin North Am* 1997;11:27.
143. Dhodapkar MV, Sanderson RD. Syndecan-1 (CD 138) in myeloma and lymphoid malignancies: a multifunctional regulator of cell behavior within the tumor microenvironment. *Leuk Lymphoma* 1999;34:35.
144. Dhodapkar MV, Abe E, Theus A, et al: Syndecan-1 is a multifunctional regulator of myeloma pathobiology: control of tumor cell survival, growth, and bone cell differentiation. *Blood* 1998;91:2679.
145. Wijdenes J, Vooijs WC, Clement C, et al. A plasmocyte selective monoclonal antibody (B-B4) recognizes syndecan-1. *Br J Haematol* 1996;94:318.
146. Vacca A, Di Loreto M, Ribatti D, et al. Bone marrow of patients with active multiple myeloma: angiogenesis and plasma cell adhesion molecules LFA-1, VLA-4, LAM-1, and CD44. *Am J Hematol* 1995;50:9.
147. Vallario A, Chilosi M, Adami F, et al. Human myeloma cells express the CD38 ligand CD31. *Br J Haematol* 1999;105:441.
148. Barille S, Akhoundi C, Collette M, et al. Metalloproteinases in multiple myeloma: production of matrix metalloproteinase-9 (MMP-9), activation of proMMP-2, and induction of MMP-1 by myeloma cells. *Blood* 1997;90:1649.
149. Kaushal GP, Xiong X, Athota AB, et al. Syndecan-1 expression suppresses the level of myeloma matrix metalloproteinase-9. *Br J Haematol* 1999;104:365.
150. Dhodapkar MV, Kelly T, Theus A, et al. Elevated levels of shed syndecan-1 correlate with tumour mass and decreased matrix metalloproteinase-9 activity in the serum of patients with multiple myeloma [published erratum appears in *Br J Haematol* 1998 May;101:398]. *Br J Haematol* 1997;99:368.
151. Jensen GS, Mant MJ, Pilarski LM. Sequential maturation stages of monoclonal B lineage cells from blood, spleen, lymph node, and bone marrow from a terminal myeloma patient. *Am J Hematol* 1992;41:199.
152. Pilarski LM, Jensen GS. Monoclonal circulating B cells in multiple myeloma. A continuously differentiating, possibly invasive, population as defined by expression of CD45 isoforms and adhesion molecules. *Hematol Oncol Clin North Am* 1992;6:297.
153. Jensen GS, Mant MJ, Belch AJ, et al. Selective expression of CD45 isoforms defines CALLA+ monoclonal B-lineage cells in peripheral blood from myeloma patients as late stage B cells. *Blood* 1991;78:711.
154. Kawano MM, Huang N, Harada H, et al. Identification of immature and mature myeloma cells in the bone marrow of human myelomas. *Blood* 1993;82:564.
155. Epstein J, Barlogie B, Katzmann J, Alexanian R. Phenotypic heterogeneity in aneuploid multiple myeloma indicates pre-B cell involvement. *Blood* 1988;71:861.
156. Omede P, Boccadoro M, Fusaro A, Gallone G, Pileri A. Multiple myeloma: 'early' plasma cell phenotype identifies patients with aggressive biological and clinical characteristics. *Br J Haematol* 1993;85:504.
157. Kawano MM, Mahmoud MS, Huang N, et al. High proportions of VLA-5- immature myeloma cells correlated well with poor response to treatment in multiple myeloma. *Br J Haematol* 1995;91:860.
158. Zhang XG, Olive D, Devos J, et al. Malignant plasma cell lines express a functional CD28 molecule. *Leukemia* 1998;12:610.
159. Robillard N, Jego G, Pellat-Deceunynck C, et al. CD28, a marker associated with tumoral expansion in multiple myeloma. *Clin Cancer Res* 1998;4:1521.
160. Treon SP, Shima Y, Preffer FI, et al. Treatment of plasma cell dyscrasias by antibody-mediated immunotherapy. *Semin Oncology* 1999;26:97.
161. Thomas X, Xiao HQ, Chang R, Epstein J. Circulating B lymphocytes in multiple myeloma patients contain an autocrine IL-6 driven pre-myeloma cell population. *Curr Top Microbiol Immunol* 1992;182:201.
162. Pilarski LM, Andrews EJ, Mant MJ, Ruether BA. Humoral immune deficiency in multiple myeloma patients due to compromised B-cell function. *J Clin Immunol* 1986;6:491.
163. Munshi NC. Immunoregulatory mechanisms in multiple myeloma. *Hematol Oncol Clin North Am* 1997;11:51.
164. Pilarski LM, Mant MJ, Ruether BA, et al. Abnormal clonogenic potential of T cells from multiple myeloma patients. *Blood* 1985;66:1266.
165. Herrmann F, Lochner A, Jauer B, Sieber G, Ruhl H. Lymphocyte subsets in the peripheral blood of patients with multiple myeloma and benign monoclonal gammopathy. *Klin Wochensch* 1983;61:819.
166. Ludwig H, Fritz E. [Lymphocyte subpopulations in multiple myeloma. Shift in the helper/suppressor cell relation]. *Acta Medica Austriaca* 1982;9:215.

167. Mellstedt H, Holm G, Pettersson D, et al. T cells in monoclonal gammopathies. *Scand J Haematol* 1982;29:57.
168. Mills KH, Cawley JC. Abnormal monoclonal antibody-defined helper/suppressor T-cell subpopulations in multiple myeloma: relationship to treatment and clinical stage. *Br J Haematol* 1983;53:271.
169. Osterborg A, Nilsson B, Bjorkholm M, Holm G, Mellstedt H. Natural killer cell activity in monoclonal gammopathies: relation to disease activity. *Eur J Haematol* 1990;45:153.
170. Yi Q, Osterborg A, Bergenbrant S, et al. Idiotype-reactive T-cell subsets and tumor load in monoclonal gammopathies. *Blood* 1995;86:3043.
171. Yi Q, Osterborg A. Idiotype-specific T cells in multiple myeloma: targets for an immunotherapeutic intervention? *Med Oncol* 1996;13:1.
172. Solomon A, Weiss DT, Kattine AA. Nephrotoxic potential of Bence Jones proteins [see comments]. *N Engl J Med* 1991;324:1845.
173. Khamlichi AA, Rocca A, Touchard G, et al. Role of light chain variable region in myeloma with light chain deposition disease: evidence from an experimental model. *Blood* 1995;86:3655.
174. Pozzi C, Fogazzi GB, Banfi G, et al. Renal disease and patient survival in light chain deposition disease. *Clin Nephrol* 1995;43:281.
175. Kyle RA. Monoclonal proteins and renal disease. *Annu Rev Med* 1994;45:71.
176. Clark AD, Shetty A, Soutar R. Renal failure and multiple myeloma: pathogenesis and treatment of renal failure and management of underlying myeloma. *Blood Rev* 1999;13:79.
177. Huang ZQ, Sanders PW. Localization of a single binding site for immunoglobulin light chains on human Tamm-Horsfall glycoprotein. *J Clin Invest* 1997;99:732.
178. Huang ZQ, Sanders PW. Biochemical interaction between Tamm-Horsfall glycoprotein and Ig light chains in the pathogenesis of cast nephropathy. *Lab Invest* 1995;73:810.
179. Sanders PW. Pathogenesis and treatment of myeloma kidney. *J Lab Clin Med* 1994;124:484.
180. Huang ZQ, Kirk KA, Connelly KG, Sanders PW. Bence Jones proteins bind to a common peptide segment of Tamm-Horsfall glycoprotein to promote heterotypic aggregation. *J Clin Invest* 1993;92:2975.
181. Reeves WB, Foley RJ, Weinman EJ. Nephrotoxicity from nonsteroidal anti-inflammatory drugs. *South Med J* 1985;78:318.
182. Kyle RA, Greipp PR. Amyloidosis (AL): clinical and laboratory features in 229 cases. *Mayo Clin Proc* 1983;58:665.
183. Fattori E, Della Rocca C, Costa P, et al. Development of progressive kidney damage and myeloma kidney in interleukin-6 transgenic mice. *Blood* 1994;83:2570.
184. Roodman GD. Mechanisms of bone lesions in multiple myeloma and lymphoma. *Cancer* 1997;80:1557.
185. Lacey DL, Timms E, Tan HL, et al. Osteoprotegerin ligand is a cytokine that regulates osteoclast differentiation and activation. *Cell* 1998;93:165.
186. Simonet WS, Lacey DL, Dunstan CR, et al. Osteoprotegerin: a novel secreted protein involved in the regulation of bone density [see comments]. *Cell* 1997;89:309.
187. Tricot G. New Insights into role of microenvironment in multiple myeloma. *Lancet* 2000;355:248.
188. Ullrich S, Zolla-Pazner S. Immunoregulatory circuits in myeloma. *Clin Haematol* 1982;11:87.
189. Broder S, Humphrey R, Durm M, et al. Impaired synthesis of polyclonal (non-paraprotein) immunoglobulins by circulating lymphocytes from patients with multiple myeloma Role of suppressor cells. *N Engl J Med* 1975;293:887.
190. Jacobson DR, Zolla-Pazner S. Immunosuppression and infection in multiple myeloma. *Semin Oncol* 1986;13:282.
191. Cook G, Campbell JD, Carr CE, Boyd KS, Franklin IM. Transforming growth factor beta from multiple myeloma cells inhibits proliferation and IL-2 responsiveness in T lymphocytes. *J Leukocyte Biol* 1999;66:981.
192. Kyrtsonis MC, Repa C, Dedoussis GV, et al. Serum transforming growth factor-beta 1 is related to the degree of immunoparesis in patients with multiple myeloma. *Med Oncol* 1998;15:124.
193. Urashima M, Ogata A, Chauhan D, et al. Transforming growth factor-beta1: differential effects on multiple myeloma versus normal B cells. *Blood* 1996;87:1928.
194. Soubrier MJ, Dubost JJ, Sauvezie BJM. Syndrome at FSGoP. POEMS syndrome: a study of 25 cases and a review of the literature. *Am J Med* 1994;97:543.
195. Schey S. Osteosclerotic myeloma and 'POEMS' syndrome. *Blood Rev* 1996;10:75.
196. Lacy MQ, Gertz MA, Hanson CA, Inwards DJ, Kyle RA. Multiple myeloma associated with diffuse osteosclerotic bone lesions: a clinical entity distinct from osteosclerotic myeloma (POEMS syndrome). *Am J Hematol* 1997;56:288.
197. Miralles GD, O'Fallon JR, Talley NJ. Plasma-cell dyscrasia with polyneuropathy. The spectrum of POEMS syndrome. *N Engl J Med* 1992;327:1919.
198. Waldenstrom JG, Adner A, Gydell K, Zettervall O. Osteosclerotic "plasmocytoma" with polyneuropathy, hypertrichosis and diabetes. *Acta Med Scand* 1978;203:297.
199. Leifer D, Grabowski T, Simonian N, Demirjian ZN. Leptomeningeal myelomatosis presenting with mental status changes and other neurologic findings. *Cancer* 1992;70:1899.
200. Truong LD, Kim HS, Estrada R. Meningeal myeloma. *Am J Clin Pathol* 1982;78:532.
201. Pruzanski W, Watt JG. Serum viscosity and hyperviscosity syndrome in IgG multiple myeloma. Report on 10 patients and a review of the literature. *Ann Intern Med* 1972;77:853.
202. Preston FE, Cooke KB, Foster ME, Winfield DA, Lee D. Myelomatosis and the hyperviscosity syndrome. *Br J Haematol* 1978;38:517.
203. Chandy KG, Stockley RA, Leonard RC, et al. Relationship between serum viscosity and intravascular IgA polymer concentration in IgA myeloma. *Clin Exp Immunol* 1981;46:653.
204. Capra JD, Kunkel HG. Aggregation of gamma-G3 proteins: relevance to the hyperviscosity syndrome. *J Clin Invest* 1970;49:610.
205. Perkins HA, MacKenzie MR, Fudenberg HH. Hemostatic defects in dysproteinemias. *Blood* 1970;35:695.
206. Lackner H. Hemostatic abnormalities associated with dysproteinemias. *Semin Hematol* 1973;10:125.
207. Kelsey PR, Leyland MJ. Acquired inhibitor to human factor VIII associated with paraproteinaemia and subsequent development of chronic lymphatic leukaemia. *Br Med J Clin Res Ed* 1982;285:174.
208. Deitcher SR, Erban JK, Limentani SA. Acquired free protein S deficiency associated with multiple myeloma: a case report. *Am J Hematol* 1996;51:319.
209. Coleman M, Vigliano EM, Weksler ME, Nachman RL. Inhibition of fibrin monomer polymerization by lambda myeloma globulins. *Blood* 1972;39:210.
210. Furie B, Greene E, Furie BC. Syndrome of acquired factor X deficiency and systemic amyloidosis in vivo studies of the metabolic fate of factor X. *N Engl J Med* 1977;297:81.
211. Barlogie B, Smallwood L, Smith T, Alexanian R. High serum levels of lactic dehydrogenase identify a high-grade lymphoma-like myeloma. *Ann Intern Med* 1989;110:521.
212. Pizzolato M, Bragantini G, Bresciani P, et al. IgG1-kappa biclonal gammopathy associated with multiple myeloma suggests a regulatory mechanism. *Br J Haematol* 1998;102:503.
213. Zent CS, Wilson CS, Tricot G, et al. Oligoclonal protein bands and Ig isotype switching in multiple myeloma treated with high-dose therapy and hematopoietic cell transplantation. *Blood* 1998;91:3518.
214. Kozuru M, Uike N, Takahira H, et al. Immunoglobulin class switch from IgA1 to IgG2 and simultaneous association with Bence Jones proteinuria in the escape phase in a myeloma patient treated with interferon alpha. *Br J Haematol* 1997;98:114.
215. Billadeau D, Quam L, Thomas W, et al. Detection and quantitation of malignant cells in the peripheral blood of multiple myeloma patients. *Blood* 1992;80:1818.
216. Barlogie B, Gale RP. Multiple myeloma and chronic lymphocytic leukemia: commonalities and differences in biology and therapy. *Leuk Lymphoma* 1991;26:27.
217. Bartl R, Frisch B. Clinical significance of bone marrow biopsy and plasma cell morphology in MM and MGUS. *Pathol Biol (Paris)* 1999;47:158.
218. Barlogie B, Alexanian R, Pershouse M, Smallwood L, Smith L. Cytoplasmic immunoglobulin content in multiple myeloma. *J Clin Invest* 1985;76:765.
219. Latreille J, Barlogie B, Dosik G, et al. Cellular DNA content as a marker of human multiple myeloma. *Blood* 1980;55:403.
220. Latreille J, Barlogie B, Johnston D, Drewinko B, Alexanian R. Ploidy and proliferative characteristics in monoclonal gammopathies. *Blood* 1982;59:43.
221. Bergsagel PL, Nardini E, Brents L, Chesi M, Kuehl WM. IgH translocations in multiple myeloma: a nearly universal event that rarely involves c-myc. *Curr Top Microbiol Immunol* 1997;224:283.
222. Tricot G, Sawyer JR, Jagannath S, et al. Unique role of cytogenetics in the prognosis of patients with myeloma receiving high-dose therapy and autotransplants. *J Clin Oncol* 1997;15:2659.
223. Sawyer JR, Tricot G, Mattox S, Jagannath S, Barlogie B. Jumping translocations of chromosome 1q in multiple myeloma: evidence for a mechanism involving decondensation of pericentromeric heterochromatin. *Blood* 1998;91:1732.
224. Govindarajan R, Jagannath S, Flick J, et al. Preceeding standard therapy is the likely cause of MDS after autotransplants for multiple myeloma. *Br J Haematol* 1996;95:349.
225. Dao DD, Sawyer JR, Epstein J, et al. Deletion of the retinoblastoma gene in multiple myeloma. *Leukemia* 1994;8:1280.
226. Avet-Loiseau H, Li JY, Facon T, et al. High incidence of translocations t(11;14)(q13;q32) and t(4;14)(p16;q32) in patients with plasma cell malignancies. *Cancer Res* 1998;58:5640.
227. Greipp PR, Katzmann JA, O'Fallon WM, Kyle RA. Value of β2-microglobulin level and plasma cell labeling indices as prognotic factors in patients with newly diagnosed myeloma. *Blood* 1988;72:219.
228. Durie BG, Salmon SE, Moon TE. Pretreatment tumor mass, cell kinetics, and prognosis in multiple myeloma. *Blood* 1980;55:364.
229. Witzig TE, Gonchoroff NJ, Katzmann JA, et al. Peripheral blood B-cell labeling indices are a measure of disease activity in patients with monoclonal gammopathies. *J Clin Oncol* 1988;6:1041.
230. Greipp PR, Lust JA, O'Fallon WM, et al. Plasma cell labeling index and beta 2-microglobulin predict survival independent of thymidine kinase and C-reactive protein in multiple myeloma [see comments]. *Blood* 1993;81:3382.
231. Agren B, Lonnqvist B, Björkstrand B, Rudberg U, Aspelin P. Radiography and bone scintigraphy in bone marrow transplant multiple myeloma patients. *Acta Radiol* 1997;38:144.
232. Mariette X, Khalifa P, Ravaud P, et al. Bone densitometry in patients with multiple myeloma [see comments]. *Am J Med* 1992;93:595.
233. Mariette X, Bergot C, Ravaud P, et al. Evolution of bone densitometry in patients with myeloma treated with conventional or intensive therapy. *Cancer* 1995;76:1559.
234. Chodimella U, Dhodapkar M, Weinstein R, et al. Differential effects of pamidronate (PAM) on cortical and cancellous bone in patients with myeloma (MM) undergoing autotransplants (AT). *Proc Am Soc Clin Oncol* 1998:10.
235. Moulopoulos LA, Dimopoulos MA, Weber D, et al. Magnetic resonance imaging in the staging of solitary plasmacytoma of bone. *J Clin Oncol* 1993;11:1311.
236. Moulopoulos LA, Dimopoulos MA, Smith T, et al. Prognostic significance of magnetic resonance imaging in patients with asymptomatic multiple myeloma. *J Clin Oncol* 1995;13:251.
237. Moulopoulos LA, Dimopoulos MA. Magnetic resonance imaging of the bone marrow in hematologic malignancies. *Blood* 1997;90:2127.
238. Vande Berg BC, Lecouvet FE, Michaux L, et al. Magnetic resonance imaging of the bone marrow in hematological malignancies. *Eur Radiol* 1998;8:1335.
239. Kusumoto S, Jinnai I, Itoh K, et al. Magnetic resonance imaging patterns in patients with multiple myeloma. *Br J Haematol* 1997;99:649.
240. el-Shirbiny AM, Yeung H, Imbriaco M, et al. Technetium-99m-MIBI versus fluorine-18-FDG in diffuse multiple myeloma. *J Nucl Med* 1997;38:1208.
241. Merlini G, Waldenstrom JG, Jayakar SD. A new improved clinical staging system for multiple myeloma based on analysis of 123 treated patients. *Blood* 1980;55:1011.
242. Woodruff RK, Wadsworth J, Malpas JS, Tobias JS. Clinical staging in multiple myeloma. *Br J Haematol* 1979;42:199.
243. Kyle RA, Greipp PR. Smoldering multiple myeloma. *N Engl J Med* 1980;302:1347.
244. Salmon SE, Smith BA. Immunoglobulin synthesis and total body tumor cell number in IgG multiple myeloma. *J Clin Invest* 1970;49:1114.

245. Durie B, Salmon S. Clinical staging system for myeloma: correlation of measured myeloma cell mass with presenting clinical features, response to treatment, and survival. *Cancer* 1975;36:842.
246. Bergsagel DE, Bailey AJ, Langley GR, et al. The chemotherapy on plasma-cell myeloma and the incidence of acute leukemia. *N Engl J Med* 1979;301:743.
247. Barlogie B, Jagannath S, Desikan KR, et al. Total therapy with tandem transplants for newly diagnosed multiple myeloma. *Blood* 1999;93:55.
248. Child JA, Norfolk DR, Cooper EH. Serum beta 2-microglobulin in myelomatosis [letter]. *Br J Haematol* 1986;63:406.
249. Garewal H, Durie BG, Kyle RA, et al. Serum beta 2-microglobulin in the initial staging and subsequent monitoring of monoclonal plasma cell disorders. *J Clin Oncol* 1984;2:51.
250. Vesole DH, Tricot G, Jagannath S, et al. Autotransplants in multiple myeloma: what have we learned? *Blood* 1996;88:838.
251. Witzig TE, Gertz MA, Lust JA, et al. Peripheral blood monoclonal plasma cells as a predictor of survival in patients with multiple myeloma [see comments]. *Blood* 1996;88:1780.
252. Barlogie B, Alexanian R, Dicke KA, et al. High-dose chemoradiotherapy and autologous bone marrow transplantation for resistant multiple myeloma. *Blood* 1987;70:869.
253. Mathiot C, Galon J, Tartour E, et al. Soluble CD16 in plasma cell dyscrasias. *Leuk Lymphoma* 1999;32:467.
254. Siegel DS, Desikan KR, Mehta J, et al. Age is not a prognostic variable with autotransplants for multiple myeloma. *Blood* 1999;93:51.
255. Dimopoulos MA, Moulopoulos A, Delasalle K, Alexanian R. Solitary plasmacytoma of bone and asymptomatic multiple myeloma. *Hematol Oncol Clin North Am* 1992;6:359.
256. Woodruff RK, Whittle JM, Malpas JS. Solitary plasmacytoma. I: extramedullary soft tissue plasmacytoma. *Cancer* 1979;43:2340.
257. Mill WB, Griffith R. The role of radiation therapy in the management of plasma cell tumors. *Cancer* 1980;45:647.
258. Liebross RH, Ha CS, Cox JD, et al. Solitary bone plasmacytoma: outcome and prognostic factors following radiotherapy. *Int J Radiat Oncol Biol Phys* 1998;41:1063.
259. Corwin J, Lindberg RD. Solitary plasmacytoma of bone vs. extramedullary plasmacytoma. *Cancer* 1979;43:1007.
260. Woodruff RK, Malpas JS, White FE. Solitary plasmacytoma. II: solitary plasmacytoma of bone. *Cancer* 1979;43:2344.
261. Fruehwald FX, Tscholakoff D, Schwaighofer B, et al. Magnetic resonance imaging of the lower vertebral column in patients with multiple myeloma. *Invest Radiol* 1988;23:193.
262. Alexanian R. Localized and indolent myeloma. *Blood* 1980;56:521.
263. Dimopoulos MA, Moulopoulos A, Smith T, Delasalle KB, Alexanian R. Risk of disease progression in asymptomatic multiple myeloma. *Am J Med* 1993;94:57.
264. Bergsagel DE, Sprague CC, Austin C, Griffith KM. Evaluation of new chemotherapeutic agents in the treatment of myeloma IV: phenylalaine mustard. *Cancer Chemother Rep* 1962;21:87.
265. Alexanian R, Haut A, Khan AU, et al. Treatment for multiple myeloma. Combination chemotherapy with different melphalan dose regimens. *JAMA* 1969;208:1680.
266. Boccadoro M, Marmont F, Tribalto M, et al. Multiple myeloma: VMCP/VBAP alternating combination chemotherapy is not superior to melphalan and prednisone even in high-risk patients. *J Clin Oncol* 1991;9:444.
267. Gregory WM, Richards MA, Malpas JS. Combination chemotherapy versus melphalan and prednisolone in the treatment of multiple myeloma: an overview of published trials [see comments]. *J Clin Oncol* 1992;10:334.
268. Salmon SE, Haut A, Bonnet JD, et al. Alternating combination chemotherapy and levamisole improves survival in multiple myeloma: a Southwest Oncology Group Study. *J Clin Oncol* 1983;1:453.
269. MacLennan IC, Chapman C, Dunn J, Kelly K. Combined chemotherapy with ABCM versus melphalan for treatment of myelomatosis. The Medical Research Council Working Party for Leukaemia in Adults [see comments]. *Lancet* 1992;339:200.
270. Hansen OP, Clausen NA, Drivsholm A, Laursen B. Phase III study of intermittent 5-drug regimen (VBCMP) versus intermittent 3-drug regimen (VMP) versus intermittent melphalan and prednisone (MP) in myelomatosis. *Scand J Haematol* 1985;35:518.
271. Birgens HS, Hansen OP, Clausen NT. A methodological evaluation of 14 controlled clinical trials in myelomatosis. *Scand J Haematol* 1985;35:26.
272. Palva IP, Ahrenberg P, Ala-Harja K, et al. Treatment of multiple myeloma with an intensive 5-drug combination or intermittent melphalan and prednisone; a randomised multicentre trial. Finnish Leukaemia Group. *Eur J Haematol* 1987;38:50.
273. Palva IP, Ahrenberg P, Ala-Harja K, et al. Treatment of multiple myeloma in old patients. Finnish Leukaemia Group. *Eur J Haematol* 1989;43:328.
274. Palva IP, Ahrenberg P, Ala Harja K, et al. Intensive chemotherapy with combinations containing anthracyclines for refractory and relapsing multiple myeloma. Finnish Leukaemia Group. *Eur J Haematol* 1990;44:121.
275. Cohen HJ, Silberman HR, Tornyos K, Bartolucci AA. Comparison of two long-term chemotherapy regimens, with or without agents to modify skeletal repair, in multiple myeloma. *Blood* 1984;63:639.
276. Kildahl-Andersen O, Bjark P, Bondevik A, et al. Multiple myeloma in central and northern Norway 1981–1982: a follow-up study of a randomized clinical trial of 5-drug combination therapy versus standard therapy. *Eur J Haematol* 1988;41:47.
277. Cooper MR, McIntyre OR, Propert KJ, et al. Single, sequential, and multiple alkylating agent therapy for multiple myeloma: a CALGB Study. *J Clin Oncol* 1986;4:1331.
278. Pavlovsky S, Saslavsky J, Tezanos Pinto M, et al. A randomized trial of melphalan and prednisone versus melphalan, prednisone, cyclophosphamide, MeCCNU, and vincristine in untreated multiple myeloma. *J Clin Oncol* 1984;2:836.
279. Barlogie B, Smith L, Alexanian R. Effective treatment of advanced multiple myeloma refractory to alkylating agents. *N Engl J Med* 1984;310:1353.
280. Alexanian R, Barlogie B, Dixon D. High-dose glucocorticoid treatment of resistant myeloma. *Ann Intern Med* 1986;105:8.
281. Salmon SE, Crowley JJ, Grogan TM, et al. Combination chemotherapy, glucocorticoids, and interferon alfa in the treatment of multiple myeloma: a Southwest Oncology Group study [see comments]. *J Clin Oncol* 1994;12:2405.
282. Mandelli F, Avvisati F, Amadori S, et al. Maintenance treatment with recombinant interferon alfa-2b in patients with multiple myeloma responding to conventional induction chemotherapy. *N Engl J Med* 1990;322:1430.
283. Gisslinger H. Interferon alpha in the therapy of multiple myeloma. *Leukemia* 1997;11(Suppl 5):S52.
284. Ludwig H, Cohen AM, Polliack A, et al. Interferon-alpha for induction and maintenance in multiple myeloma: results of two multicenter randomized trials and summary of other studies. *Ann Oncol* 1995;6:467.
285. Ludwig H, Fritz E, Zulian GB, Browman GP. Should-alpha-interferon be included as standard treatment in multiple myeloma? *Eur J Cancer* 1998;34:12.
286. Hu K, Yahalom J. Radiotherapy in the management of plasma cell tumors. *Oncology* 2000;14:101.
287. Wallington M, Mendis S, Premawardhana U, et al. Local control and survival in spinal cord compression from lymphoma and myeloma. *Radiother Oncol* 1997;42:43.
288. Rowell NP, Tobias JS. The role of radiotherapy in the management of multiple myeloma. *Blood Rev* 1991;5:84.
289. Barlogie B, Dicke KA, Alexanian R. High dose melphalan for refractory myeloma—the M.D. Anderson experience. *Hematol Oncol* 1988;6:167.
290. McElwain TJ, Selby PJ, Gore ME, et al. High-dose chemotherapy and autologous bone marrow transplantation for myeloma. *Eur J Haematol* 1989;51(Suppl):152.
291. Attal M, Harousseau JL, Stoppa AM, et al. A prospective, randomized trial of autologous bone marrow transplantation and chemotherapy in multiple myeloma. Intergroupe Francais du Myelome. *N Engl J Med* 1996;335:91.
292. Barlogie B, Jagannath S, Vesole D, et al. Superiority of tandem autologous transplantation over standard therapy for previously untreated multiple myeloma. *Blood* 1996;89:789.
293. Cunningham D, Paz-Ares L, Milan S, et al. High-dose melphalan and autologous bone marrow transplantation as consolidation in previously untreated myeloma. *J Clin Oncol* 1994;12:759.
294. Cunningham D, Paz-Ares L, Gore ME, et al. High-dose melphalan for multiple myeloma: long-term follow-up data. *J Clin Oncol* 1994;12:764.
295. Bensinger WI, Rowley SD, Demirer T, et al. High-dose therapy followed by autologous hematopoietic stem-cell infusion for patients with multiple myeloma. *J Clin Oncol* 1996;14:1447.
296. Fermand JP, Ravaud P, Chevret S, et al. High-dose therapy and autologous blood stem cell transplantation in multiple myeloma: preliminary results of a randomized trial involving 167 patients. *Stem Cells* 1995;13:156.
297. Björkstrand B, Ljungman P, Bird JM, et al. Autologous stem cell transplantation in multiple myeloma: results of the European Group for Bone Marrow Transplantation. *Stem Cells* 1995;13:140.
298. Anderson KC, Andersen J, Soiffer R, et al. Monoclonal antibody-purged bone marrow transplantation therapy for multiple myeloma. *Blood* 1993;82:2568.
299. Reiffers J, Marit G, Boiron JM. Autologous blood stem cell transplantation in high-risk multiple myeloma [letter]. *Br J Haematol* 1989;72:296.
300. Harousseau JL, Attal M, Divine M, et al. Autologous stem cell transplantation after first remission induction treatment in multiple myeloma. A report of the French Registry on autologous transplantation in multiple myeloma. *Stem Cells* 1995;13:132.
301. Harousseau JL, Milpied N, Laporte JP, et al. Double-intensive therapy in high-risk multiple myeloma. *Blood* 1992;79:2827.
302. Vesole DH, Barlogie B, Jagannath S, et al. High-dose therapy for refractory multiple myeloma: improved prognosis with better supportive care and double transplants. *Blood* 1994;84:950.
303. Björkstrand B, Ljungman P, Bird JM, Samson D, Gahrton G. Double high-dose chemoradiotherapy with autologous stem cell transplantation can induce molecular remissions in multiple myeloma. *Bone Marrow Transplant* 1995;15:367.
304. Tricot G, Jagannath S, Vesole D, et al. Peripheral blood stem cell transplant for multiple myeloma: identification of favorable variables for rapid engraftment in 225 patients. *Blood* 1995;85:588.
305. Fermand JP, Ravaud P, Chevret S, et al. Early versus late high dose therapy and autologous peripheral blood stem cell transplantation in multiple myeloma. *Blood* 1996;88:685a.
306. Barlogie B, Alexanian R. Therapy of primary resistant and relapsed multiple myeloma. *Onkologie* 1986;9:210.
307. Desikan KR, Fassas A, Siegel D, et al. Superior outcome with melphalan 200 mg/m^2 (MEL 200) for scheduled second autotransplant compared with MEL+TBI or CTX for myeloma (MM) in pre-tx-2 PR. *Blood* 1997;90:231a.
308. Schey SA, Kazmi M, Ireland R, Lakhani A. The use of intravenous intermediate dose melphalan and dexamethasone as induction treatment in the management of de novo multiple myeloma. *Eur J Haematol* 1998;61:306.
309. Selby P, Zulian G, Forgeson G, et al. The development of high dose melphalan and of autologous bone marrow transplantation in the treatment of multiple myeloma: Royal Marsden and St Bartholomew's Hospital studies. *Hematol Oncol* 1988;6:173.
310. Jagannath S, Barlogie B. Autologous bone marrow transplantation for multiple myeloma. *Hematol Oncol Clin North Am* 1992;6:437.
311. Fermand JP, Levy Y, Gerota J, et al. Treatment of aggressive multiple myeloma by high-dose chemotherapy and total body irradiation followed by blood stem cells autologous graft. *Blood* 1989;73:20.
312. Ventura GJ, Barlogie B, Hester JP, et al. High dose cyclophosphamide, BCNU and VP-16 with autologous blood stem cell support for refractory multiple myeloma. *Bone Marrow Transplant* 1990;5:265.
313. Adkins DR, Salzman D, Boldt D, et al. Phase I trial of dacarbazine with cyclophosphamide, carmustine, etoposide, and autologous stem-cell transplantation in patients with lymphoma and multiple myeloma. *J Clin Oncol* 1994;12:1890.

314. Lemoli RM, Fortuna A, Motta MR, et al. Concomitant mobilization of plasma cells and hematopoietic progenitors into peripheral blood of multiple myeloma patients: positive selection and transplantation of enriched CD34+ cells to remove circulating tumor cells. *Blood* 1996;87:1625.
315. Vescio RA, Hong CH, Cao J, et al. The hematopoietic stem cell antigen, CD34, is not expressed on the malignant cells in multiple myeloma. *Blood* 1994;84:3283.
316. Schiller G, Vescio R, Freytes C, et al. Transplantation of CD34+ peripheral blood progenitor cells after high-dose chemotherapy for patients with advanced multiple myeloma. *Blood* 1995;86:390.
317. Gazitt Y, Reading CC, Hoffman R, et al. Purified CD34+Lin-Thy+ stem cells do not contain clonal myeloma cells. *Blood* 1995;86:381.
318. Tricot G, Gazitt Y, Leemhuis T, et al. Collection, tumor contamination, and engraftment kinetics of highly purified hematopoietic progenitor cells to support high dose therapy in multiple myeloma. *Blood* 1998;91:4489.
319. Harousseau JL, Attal M, Divine M, et al. Comparison of autologous bone marrow transplantation and peripheral blood stem cell transplantation after first remission induction treatment in multiple myeloma. *Bone Marrow Transplant* 1995;15:963.
320. Tricot G, Jagannath S, Vesole D, et al. Peripheral blood stem cell transplants for multiple myeloma: identification of favorable variables for rapid engraftment in 225 patients. *Blood* 1995;85:588.
321. Gazitt Y, Tian E, Barlogie B, et al. Differential mobilization of myeloma cells and normal hematopoietic stem cells in multiple myeloma after treatment with cyclophosphamide and granulocyte-macrophage colony-stimulating factor. *Blood* 1996;87:805.
322. Palumbo A, Triolo S, Argentino C, et al. Dose-intensive melphalan with stem cell support (MEL100) is superior to standard treatment in elderly myeloma patients. *Blood* 1999;94:1248.
323. Barlogie B, Alexanian R, Jagannath S. Plasma cell dyscrasias. *JAMA* 1992;268:2946.
324. Tricot G, Alberts DS, Johnson C, et al. Safety of autotransplants with high-dose melphalan in renal failure: a pharmacokinetic and toxicity study. *Clin Cancer Res* 1996;2:947.
325. Mansi J, da Costa F, Viner C, et al. High-dose busulfan in patients with myeloma. *J Clin Oncol* 1992;10:1569.
326. Shapiro F, Engelhardt M, Ngok D, Han W, Moore MAS. Telomere length shortening and recovery following high-dose chemotherapy with autologous peripheral stem cell rescue. *Blood* 1997;88:601a.
327. Boultwood J, Fidler C, Kusec R, et al. Telomere length in myelodysplastic syndromes. *Am J Hematol* 1997;56:266.
328. Bensinger WI, Demirer T, Buckner CD, et al. Syngeneic marrow transplantation in patients with multiple myeloma. *Bone Marrow Transplant* 1996;18:527.
329. Gahrton G. Allogeneic bone marrow transplantation in multiple myeloma. *Pathol Biol (Paris)* 1999;47:188.
330. Gahrton G, Tura S, Ljungman P, et al. An update of prognostic factors for allogeneic bone marrow transplantation in multiple myeloma using matched sibling donors. European Group for Blood and Marrow Transplantation. *Stem Cells* 1995;13:122.
331. Gahrton G, Tura S, Ljungman P, et al. Allogeneic bone marrow transplantation in multiple myeloma. European Group for bone marrow transplantation [see comments]. *N Engl J Med* 1991;325:1267.
332. Bensinger W, Buckner C, Anasetti C, et al. Allogeneic marrow transplantation for multiple myeloma: an analysis of risk factors on outcome. *Blood* 1996;88:2787.
333. Kulkarni S, Powles RL, Treleaven JG, et al. Impact of previous high-dose therapy on outcome after allografting for multiple myeloma. *Bone Marrow Transplant* 1999;23:675.
334. Tricot G, Vesole DH, Jagannath S, et al. Graft-versus-myeloma effect: proof of principle. *Blood* 1996;87:1196.
335. Mehta J, Singhal S. Graft-versus-myeloma. *Bone Marrow Transplant* 1998;22:835.
336. Björkstrand B, Ljungman P, Svensson H, et al. Allogenic bone marrow transplantation versus autologous stem cell transplantation in multiple myeloma: a retrospective case-matched study from the european group for blood and marrow transplantation. *Blood* 1996;88:4711.
337. Mehta J, Tricot G, Jagannath S, et al. Salvage autologous or allogeneic transplantation for multiple myeloma refractory to or relapsing after a first-line autograft? *Bone Marrow Transplant* 1998;21:887.
338. Mineur P, Menard JF, Le Loet X, et al. VAD or VMBCP in multiple myeloma refractory to or relapsing after cyclophosphamide-prednisone therapy (protocol MY 85). *Br J Haematol* 1998;103:512.
339. Gertz MA, Kalish LA, Kyle RA, et al. Phase III study comparing vincristine, doxorubicin (Adriamycin), and dexamethasone (VAD) chemotherapy with VAD plus recombinant interferon alfa-2 in refractory or relapsed multiple myeloma. An Eastern Cooperative Oncology Group study. *Am J Clin Oncol* 1995;18:475.
340. Dimopoulos MA, Weber D, Kantarjian H, Delasalle KB, Alexanian R. HyperCVAD for VAD-resistant multiple myeloma. *Am J Hematol* 1996;52:77.
341. Munshi NC, Desikan KR, Jagannath S, et al. Dexamethasone, cyclophosphamide, etoposide, and cis-platinum (DCEP): an effective regimen for relapse after high-dose chemotherapy and autologous transplantation. *Blood* 1996;88:586a.
342. Desikan R, Siegel D, Fassas A, et al. DCEP consolidation after tandem autotransplants (AT) in high risk multiple myeloma (MM)—improved prognosis compared with matched historical controls. *ASH Abstract*, 1998.
343. Berenson JR, Lichtenstein A, Porter L, et al. Efficacy of pamidronate in reducing skeletal events in patients with advanced multiple myeloma. *N Engl J Med* 1996;334:488.
344. Apperley JF, Croucher PI. Bisphosphonates in multiple myeloma. *Pathol Biol (Paris)* 1999;47:178.
345. Berenson JR, Lipton A. Bisphosphonates in the treatment of malignant bone disease. *Annu Rev Med* 1999;510:237.
346. Shipman CM, Croucher PI, Russell RG, Helfrich MH, Rogers MJ. The bisphosphonate incadronate (YM175) causes apoptosis of human myeloma cells in vitro by inhibiting the mevalonate pathway. *Cancer Res* 1998;58:5294.
347. Berenson JR, Lichtenstein A, Porter L, et al. Long-term pamidronate treatment of advanced multiple myeloma patients reduces skeletal events. Myeloma Aredia Study Group. *J Clin Oncol* 1998;16:593.
348. Aparicio A, Gardner A, Tu Y, et al. In vitro cytoreductive effects on multiple myeloma cells induced by bisphosphonates. *Leukemia* 1998;12:220.
349. Shipman CM, Rogers MJ, Apperley JF, et al. Anti-tumour activity of bisphosphonates in human myeloma cells. *Leuk Lymphoma* 1998;32:129.
350. Dhodapkar MV, Singh J, Mehta J, et al. Anti-myeloma activity of pamidronate in vivo. *Br J Haematol* 1998;103:530.
351. Kruse FE, Joussen AM, Rohrschneider K, Becker MD, Volcker HE. Thalidomide inhibits corneal angiogenesis induced by vascular endothelial growth factor. *Graefes Archive for Clinical and Experimental Opthalmology* 1998;236:461.
352. Raje N, Anderson K. Thalidomide—a revival story [editorial; comment]. *N Engl J Med* 1999;341:1606.
353. Barlogie B, Epstein J, Selvanayagam P, Alexanian R. Plasma cell myeloma—new biological insights and advances in therapy. *Blood* 1989;73:865.
354. Rousselot P, Labaume S, Marolleau JP, et al. Arsenic trioxide and melarsoprol induce apoptosis in plasma cell lines and in plasma cells from myeloma patients. *Cancer Res* 1999;59:1041.
355. Munshi NC, Barlogie B, Desikan KR, Wilson C. Novel approaches in myeloma therapy. *Semin Oncol* 1999;26:28.
356. Waldenstrom J. Incipient myelomatosis or "essential hyperglobulinemia with fibrinogenopenia: a new syndrome? *Acta Med Scand* 1944;117:216.
357. Groves FD, Travis LB, Devesa SS, Ries LA, Fraumeni JF Jr. Waldenstrom's macroglobulinemia: incidence patterns in the United States, 1988–1994. *Cancer* 1998;82:1078.
358. Fine JM, Muller JY, Rochu D, et al. Waldenstrom's macroglobulinemia in monozygotic twins. *Acta Med Scand* 1986;220:369.
359. Renier G, Ifrah N, Chevailler A, et al. Four brothers with Waldenstrom's macroglobulinemia. *Cancer* 1989;64:1554.
360. James JM, Brouet JC, Orvoenfrija E, et al. Waldenstrom's macroglobulinaemia in a bird breeder: a case history with pulmonary involvement and antibody activity of the monoclonal IgM to canary's droppings. *Clin Exp Immunol* 1987;68:397.
361. Izumi T, Sasaki R, Shimizu R, et al. Hepatitis C virus infection in Waldenstrom's macroglobulinemia [letter]. *Am J Hematol* 1996;52:238.
362. Izumi T, Sasaki R, Tsunoda S, et al. B cell malignancy and hepatitis C virus infection. *Leukemia* 1997;11:516.
363. Silvestri F, Barillari G, Fanin R, et al. Risk of hepatitis C virus infection, Waldenstrom's macroglobulinemia, and monoclonal gammopathies [letter; comment]. *Blood* 1996;88:1125.
364. Dimopoulos MA, Panayiotidis P, Moulopoulos LA, Sfikakis P, Dalakas M. Waldenstrom's macroglobulinemia: clinical features, complications, and management. *J Clin Oncol* 2000;18:214.
365. Calasanz MJ, Cigudosa JC, Odero MD, et al. Cytogenetic analysis of 280 patients with multiple myeloma and related disorders: primary breakpoints and clinical correlations. *Genes Chromosomes Cancer* 1997;18:84.
366. van den Akker TW, Radl J, Franken-Postma E, Hagemeijer A. Cytogenetic findings in mouse multiple myeloma and Waldenstrom's macroglobulinemia. *Cancer Genet Cytogenet* 1996;86:156.
367. Nishida K, Taniwaki M, Misawa S, Abe T. Nonrandom rearrangement of chromosome 14 at band q32.33 in human lymphoid malignancies with mature B-cell phenotype. *Cancer Res* 1989;49:1275.
368. Iida S, Rao PH, Nallasivam P, et al. The t(9;14)(p13;q32) chromosomal translocation associated with lymphoplasmacytoid lymphoma involves the PAX-5 gene. *Blood* 1996;88:4110.
369. Waldenstrom JG. Macroglobulinemia—a review. *Haematologica* 1986;71:437.
370. Andriko JA, Aguilera NS, Chu WS, Nandedkar MA, Cotelingam JD. Waldenstrom's macroglobulinemia: a clinicopathologic study of 22 cases. *Cancer* 1997;80:1926.
371. Pruzanski W, Chu R, Damji NF, Galler S, Norman CS. Anemia, splenomegaly and hyperviscosity syndrome. *Can Med Assoc J* 1980;123:731.
372. Meier C, Roberts K, Steck A, et al. Polyneuropathy in Waldenstrom's macroglobulinaemia: reduction of endoneurial IgM-deposits after treatment with chlorambucil and plasmapheresis. *Acta Neuropathol* 1984;64:297.
373. Virella G, Lopes-Virella MF. Effects of therapeutically useful thiols (DL-penicillamine and alpha-mercaptopropionylglycine) on immunoglobulins. *Clin Exp Immunol* 1970;7:85.
374. Waldenstrom JG. Plasmapheresis—bloodletting revived and refined. *Acta Med Scand* 1980;208:1.
375. Waldenstrom JG. Plasmapheresis and cold sensitivity of immunoglobulin molecules. II. A study of macroglobulinemia polyclonalis spuria and immune complex disease. *Acta Med Scand* 1984;216:467.
376. Buskard NA, Galton DA, Goldman JM, et al. Plasma exchange in the long-term management of Waldenstrom's macroglobulinemia. *Can Med Assoc J* 1977;117:135.
377. Petrucci MT, Avvisati G, Tribalto M, Giovangrossi P, Mandelli F. Waldenstrom's macroglobulinaemia: results of a combined oral treatment in 34 newly diagnosed patients. *J Intern Med* 1989;226:443.
378. Dhodapkar M, Jacobson J, Gertz M, et al. Phase II intergroup trial of fludarabine in Waldenstrom's macroglobulinemia: results of Southwest Oncology Group trial (SWOG 9003) in 220 patients. *Blood* 1997;90:577a.
379. Clamon GH, Corder MP, Burns CP. Successful doxorubicin therapy of primary macroglobulinemia resistant to alkylating agents. *Am J Hematol* 1980;9:221.
380. Jane SM, Salem HH. Treatment of resistant Waldenstrom's macroglobulinemia with high dose glucocorticosteroids. *Aust NZ J Med* 1988;18:77.
381. Humphrey JS, Conley CL. Durable complete remission of macroglobulinemia after splenectomy: a report of two cases and review of the literature. *Am J Hematol* 1995;48:262.
382. Takemori N, Hirai K, Onodera R, Kimura S, Katagiri M. Durable remission after splenectomy for Waldenstrom's macroglobulinemia with massive splenomegaly in leukemic phase. *Leuk Lymphoma* 1997;26:387.

383. Desikan KR, Dhodapkar M, Siegel D, et al. High-dose therapy with autologous peripheral blood stem cell support for Waldenstrom's macroglobulinemia: a pilot study. *Br J Hematol* 1999;105:993.
384. Belch A, Shelley W, Bergsagel D, et al. A randomized trial of maintenance versus no maintenance melphalan and prednisone in responding multiple myeloma patients. *Br J Cancer* 1988;57:94.
385. Lahtinen R, Laakso M, Palva I, Virkkunen P, Elomaa I. Randomised, placebo-controlled multicentre trial of clodronate in multiple myeloma. Finnish Leukaemia Group [published erratum appears in *Lancet* 1992;340:1420; see comments]. *Lancet* 1992;340:1049.
386. Gazitt Y, Fey V, Thomas C, Alvarez R. Bcl-2 overexpression is associated with resistance to dexamethasone, but not melphalan, in multiple myeloma cells. *Int J Oncol* 1998;13:397.
387. Bataille R, Manolagas SC, Berenson JR. Pathogenesis and management of bone lesions in multiple myeloma. *Hematol Oncol Clin North Am* 1997;11:349.
388. Herrinton LJ, Weiss NS. Incidence of Waldenström's macroglobulinemia. *Blood* 1993; 82:3148.
389. Dalakas MC, Flaum MA, Rick M, Engel WK, Gralnick HR. Treatment of polyneuropathy in Waldenström's macroglobulinemia: role of paraproteinemia and immunologic studies. *Neurology* 1983;33:1406.
390. Dimopoulos MA, Weber DM, Kantarjian H, et al. 2-Chlorodeoxyadenosine therapy of patients with Waldenstrom macroglobulinemia previously treated with fludarabine. *Ann Oncol* 1994;5:288.
391. Dimopoulos MA, Kantarjian H, Weber D, et al. Primary therapy of Waldenström's macroglobulinemia with 2-chlorodeoxyadenosine. *J Clin Oncol* 1994;12:2694.
392. Kantarjian HM, Alexanian R, Koller CA, et al. Fludarabine therapy in macroglobulinemic lymphoma. *Blood* 1990;75:1928.
393. Zinzani PL, Gherlinzoni F, Bendandi M, et al. Fludarabine treatment in resistant Waldenström's macroglobulinemia. *Eur J Haematol* 1995;54:120.
394. Betticher DC, Hsu Schmitz SF, Ratschiller D, et al. Cladribine (2-CDA) given as subcutaneous bolus injections is active in pretreated Waldenström's macroglobulinaemia. Swiss Group for Clinical Cancer Research (SAKK). *Br J Haematol* 1997;99:358.
395. Quesada JR, Alexanian R, Kurzrock R, et al. Recombinant interferon gamma in hairy cell leukemia, multiple myeloma, and Waldenström's macroglobulinemia. *Am J Hematol* 1988;29:1.
396. Ohno R, Kodera Y, Ogura M, et al. Treatment of plasma cell neoplasm with recombinant leukocyte A interferon and human lymphoblastoid interferon. *Cancer Chemother Pharmacol* 1985;14:34.
397. Rotoli B, De Renzo A, Frigeri F, et al. A phase II trial on alpha-interferon (alpha IFN) effect in patients with monoclonal IgM gammopathy. *Leuk Lymphoma* 1994;13:463.
398. Legouffe E, Rossi JF, Laporte JP, et al. Treatment of Waldenström's macroglobulinemia with very low doses of alpha interferon. *Leuk Lymphoma* 1995;19:337.
399. Durie BGM, Dixon D, Carter S, et al. Improved survival duration with combination chemotherapy induction for multiple myeloma: a Southwest Oncology Group study. *J Clin Oncol* 1986;4:1127

SECTION 5

HAGOP M. KANTARJIAN
ELIHU ESTEY

Myelodysplastic Syndromes

The myelodysplastic syndromes (MDS) are heterogeneous clonal hematopoietic stem cell disorders grouped together because of the presence of dysplastic changes in one or more of the hematopoietic lineages.[1,2] Dysplasia signifies abnormal or discordant nuclear cytoplasmic maturation and is the morphologic hallmark of apoptosis. Indeed, MDS is associated with apoptosis[3–6] and excessive proliferation, resulting in the paradoxic picture of peripheral cytopenias and cellular marrows. The common findings in MDS include anemia-associated problems, infections and bleeding, generally in elderly patients, frequent exposure to carcinogens or leukemogenic agents, a wide range of transformation rates (10% to 80%) to acute leukemia, and a high incidence of cytogenetic abnormalities associated with poor prognoses.[7] The MDS were previously referred to as *smoldering leukemia* or *preleukemia, oligoblastic leukemia,* or *hematopoietic dysplasia,*[8] implying an indolent course. More recent studies have emphasized the aggressive nature and poor prognosis of some subsets of *high-risk* MDS, defined by excess marrow or peripheral blasts, cytogenetic abnormalities, or both.[9,10]

INCIDENCE

The estimated incidence of MDS is 7000 to 12,000 new cases in the United States annually.[11] With a median survival of 1 to 3 years, the estimated prevalence is 10,000 to 25,000 cases. The true incidence of MDS is probably underestimated, because the diagnosis is often overlooked or not reported. Those cases often receive no specific therapy because of older age, complicating medical illnesses, and unavailability of effective low-risk treatment modalities. Some MDS may be misdiagnosed as other entities such as hypoplastic or aplastic anemia (hypoplastic MDS), acute myelogenous leukemia (AML) (high blast percent), or myeloproliferative disorders (high white blood cell counts).

ETIOLOGY

The etiology of most MDS cases is unknown. Smoking and exposures to ionizing irradiation, organic chemicals, heavy metals, herbicides, pesticides, fertilizers, stone and cereal dusts, exhaust gases, nitroorganic explosives, petroleum and diesel derivatives, alkylating agents, benzene, solvents other than benzene (e.g., toluene, xylene), chloramphenicol, and marrow-damaging agents including chemotherapeutic agents may increase the risk of developing MDS.[12–16] Patients with clear exposure to such agents are referred to as having *secondary MDS* or *treatment-related MDS* and constitute approximately 20% to 30% of MDS cases. Their proportion is increasing as more patients with other cancers are exposed to and cured with such treatments. Secondary MDS accounts for 30% of MDS cases referred to M. D. Anderson Cancer Center since 1990, compared with 15% before 1990. Alkylating agents (melphalan, chlorambucil, cyclophosphamide, procarbazine) and radiation therapy are associated with the highest risk of development of MDS.[17] Their effects are synergistic, particularly in older patients. Patients with Hodgkin's disease and other lymphomas, myeloma, breast and ovarian cancers, and those undergoing stem cell transplantation (SCT) are often exposed to such treatments.[17,18] Among patients with Hodgkin's disease or lymphoma undergoing autologous SCT with high-dose cyclophosphamide and total body irradiation, the estimated cumulative risk of developing MDS at 5 to 6 years is 11% to 18%, the risk being higher with use of total body irradiation, with increasing age, with longer time from first treatment to transplant, and with low platelet counts at time of SCT.[18] X-chromosome inactivation analysis has shown replacement of polyclonal hematopoiesis with clonal hematopoiesis preceding the development of MDS in some patients. Patients with MDS

TABLE 46.5-1. French-American-British Classification of Myelodysplastic Syndromes

Myelodysplastic Syndrome Category	*Percentage Marrow Blasts*	*Percentage Peripheral Blasts*	*Others*	*Percentage of Myelodysplastic Syndromes*	*Percentage Acute Myeloid Leukemia Transformation*
Refractory anemia	<5	≤1	—	10–40	10–20
Refractory anemia with ringed sideroblasts	<5	≤1	>15% ringed sideroblasts	10–20	10–35
Refractory anemia with excessive blasts	5–20	<5	—	25–30	50+
Refractory anemia with excessive blasts in transformation	21–29	≥5	Auer rods	10–30	60–100
Chronic myelomonocytic leukemia	≤20	<5	Monocytosis >10^9/L	10–20	40+

(From ref. 20, with permission.)

are older than those with AML and have a higher incidence of unfavorable chromosomal abnormalities, including losses of parts or all of chromosome 5 or 7.

There is no known association between viral or other infections and development of MDS. There may be an increased risk of MDS in families of patients with MDS. Rare familial forms of MDS or AML and monosomy 7 have been described.[19] Studies of the frequency of specific polymorphism in enzymes activating, detoxifying, or both activating and detoxifying carcinogens in MDS patients versus normal controls may help in understanding the disease pathophysiology and identifying individuals at risk for developing MDS.

CLASSIFICATION AND RISK GROUPS

The French-American-British (FAB) classification categorizes patients with MDS based on the percentage of marrow and peripheral blasts and the presence of monocytosis and Auer rods. Categories include refractory anemia (RA), RA with ringed sideroblasts (RARS), RA with excess blasts (RAEB), and RAEB in transformation (RAEBT). Chronic myelomonocytic leukemia (CMML), a hybrid disorder of excessive myeloid proliferation, monocytosis, and dysplastic changes in the erythroid and megakaryocytic series, is sometimes considered as a fifth MDS category or as a separate disorder[20,21] (Table 46.5-1).

The FAB classification of MDS has shortcomings.[22] For example, Auer rods, which characterize RAEBT, have been associated with favorable rather than poor prognosis.[23] Confusion arises when monocytosis is present with 5% to 29% blasts as to whether such cases should be referred to as *RAEBT* (if blasts more than 20%) or as a separate category of accelerated-phase CMML. Finally, there is great variability in prognosis within a single FAB subtype, indicating the need to incorporate further information into the FAB system.[24] Investigators have attempted to improve on the classification by including prognostically relevant variables such as the percentage of marrow blasts, chromosomal abnormalities, and cytopenias (anemia or thrombocytopenia).[25,26]

An International Prognostic Scoring System (IPSS) was developed that assigns points to each of several prognostic factors[27] (Table 46.5-2). It divides patients into low, intermediate-1, intermediate-2, and high-risk groups with median survivals of 5.7, 3.5, 1.2, and 0.4 years, respectively. Although it is an improvement

TABLE 46.5-2. International Prognostic Scoring System and Model

	Score Value				
Prognostic Variable	0	0.5	1.0	1.5	2.0
Marrow blasts (%)	<5	5–10	—	11–20	21–30
Karyotype[a]	Good	Intermediate	Poor		
Cytopenias[b]	0–1	2–3			

International Prognostic Scoring System Risk Group	*Score Value*	*Survival Median/ 5-Y Percentage*	*Percentage 5-Y Acute Myeloid Leukemia Transformation*
Low	0	5.7/55	15
Intermediate-1	0.5–1.0	3.5/35	30
Intermediate-2	1.5–2.0	1.2/7	65
High	≥2.5	0.4/0	100

[a]Good, normal, -Y, del (5q), del (20q); poor, complex (≥3 abnormalities), chromosome 7 anomalies; intermediate, others.
[b]Cytopenias: hemoglobin <10 g/dL, granulocytes <1.5 × 10^9/L, platelets <100 × 10^9/L.
(From ref. 27, with permission.)

TABLE 46.5-3. Prognosis in Myelodysplastic Syndrome According to the International Prognostic Scoring System (IPSS)

	International Prognostic Scoring System (n = 816)		*M. D. Anderson (n = 219)*	
IPSS Risk	Percentage of Total	Median Survival (y)	Percentage of Total	Median Survival (y)
Low	33	5.7	13	2.1
Intermediate-1	38	3.5	41	1.2
Intermediate-2	22	1.2	30	0.7
High	7	0.4	16	0.4

(Data from refs. 24 and 27.)

over the FAB system, the IPSS also suffers from variability within single risk groups. For example, the median survivals of patients with IPSS low and intermediate-1 groups referred to M. D. Anderson were only 2.1 and 1.2 years, respectively, significantly different from those reported in the IPSS study (5.7 and 3.5 years, respectively), despite similar therapeutic measures (Table 46.5-3).[24,27] The IPSS was derived from newly diagnosed untreated patients, and survival was calculated from diagnosis. However, patients referred to tertiary centers have often had prior therapy, the patients were referred because of some need for therapy, and their survival was measured from the referral date. Thus, latent variables, unrecognized by the prognostic models and related to the referral, might account for differences in prognosis of different study groups categorized in the same IPSS risk groups. Investigations of aberrant cellular or molecular events in MDS (e.g., RAS mutations, apoptosis, clonality, loss of suppressor genes, methylation, and others) may yield new clinically relevant biologic prognostic factors.

BIOLOGY AND PATHOPHYSIOLOGY

Preclinical studies have provided insight into different pathophysiologic processes in MDS, and several models of MDS evolution have been proposed.[28,29]

The clonal nature of MDS appears restricted to hematopoietic population subsets.[30,31] Primitive progenitors (CD34+, Thy 1+) and T cells, perhaps in the earlier MDS phases, appear nonclonal. Late-stage hematopoietic cells of myeloid and erythroid lineage, as well as B-cell lymphocytes, were often clonal.[30–35] Hematopoietic recovery in remission marrows is frequently nonclonal.[35,36]

In some patients, nonclonal CD8+ T cells directed against HLA class I–restricted antigens may suppress normal hematopoiesis, as evidenced by enhanced *in vitro* growth of granulocyte-macrophage colony-forming units following T-cell depletion (cyclosporin, anti-CD8).[37] This provides the rationale for the use of immunosuppressive therapy in MDS.

In vitro colony formation is generally reduced in MDS and correlates with survival.[8,38] Addition of growth factors [erythropoietin, granulocyte colony-stimulating factor (G-CSF), granulocyte-macrophage colony-stimulating factor (GM-CSF), interleukin-3 (IL-3)] increases colony formation. This provided hope that at least some patients in early MDS phases or with mild lineage involvement may benefit from such therapy. Serum levels of growth factors (e.g., erythropoietin) were inversely correlated with the degree of cytopenia, indicating appropriate host compensatory mechanisms. Cytopenias may be improved with pharmacologic doses of growth factors.

Dysplasia appears to signify high apoptotic rates, explaining the unilineage or multilineage peripheral cytopenias.[3–6] According to one hypothesis, the primary lesion in MDS is the high cell death rate, which is counterbalanced by a compensatory early phase of excessive hematopoiesis. This is supported by studies demonstrating both increased apoptosis and proliferation[3–6] and may explain the apparent paradox of peripheral cytopenia and hypercellular marrows. Increased apoptosis has also been observed in the marrow microenvironment cells, suggesting that the primitive stem cell involved is a progenitor to both hematopoietic and stromal cells.[5]

What might contribute to increased apoptosis? High levels of tumor necrosis factor-α (TNF-α) or other proapoptotic cytokines, and the effect of TNF-α on induction of Fas expression on CD34+ cells, may be pathophysiologic.[39,40] Elevated TNF-α levels in MDS may be restricted to the earlier phases (RA, RARS) and were not found in normal control subjects or in patients with AML.[41,42] The source of TNF-α production may be the increased marrow macrophages in MDS, which may be stimulated by elevated macrophage colony-stimulating factor (M-CSF) levels, through point mutations in c-fms, which encodes the M-CSF receptor.[43–45] That TNF-α production in MDS is relevant is suggested by (1) enhanced *in vitro* colony growth in MDS by incubation with TNF-α neutralizing antibodies[46]; and (2) the correlation of TNF-α levels with severity of anemia, poor response to erythropoietin, and increased apoptosis.[5,41,47] Strategies to suppress TNF-α levels may help therapeutically.

Other proapoptotic cytokines of interest include interferon-γ and IL-1β. Interferon-γ production appears to be important in aplastic anemia but less so in MDS.[42] IL-1β levels are highest in RA, tend to correlate with apoptosis but not proliferation, and may be due to deficient production of the receptor antagonist in MDS stromal cells, which increase IL-1β levels and thus apoptosis.[48]

Involvement of the Fas/Fas ligand system in MDS apoptosis has also been proposed,[4,5] as well as a role for other molecular events including Ras mutations or aberrations in the RAS pathways that may be dysfunctional without Ras mutations.[49] Understanding the pathophysiology of RAS in MDS and CMML (10% to 25% with Ras mutations) may result in rational intervention approaches with RAS inhibitors (antisense, farnesyl-transferase inhibitors). Antiapoptotic signaling pathways, including bcl-2 overexpression, and shortening of telomeres may be important in advanced MDS states.[4,5,50]

Chromosomal abnormalities may serve as *fingerprints* for the molecular abnormalities. Chromosome 5 abnormalities (losses in the long arm, 5q-) are common. Many hematopoietic growth regulatory genes have been mapped to this region.[51] These include M-CSF, GM-CSF, IL-4 and IL-5, CD-14, interferon regulatory factor-1, the receptors for platelet-derived growth factor and M-CSF (Fms), and others. Fms is a tyrosine kinase protooncogene, and the viral form of Fms (v-Fms) has transforming properties. Fms point mutations have been described in patients with MDS and AML and those receiving chemotherapy, suggesting its possible role in MDS pathogenesis.[45,52] Other abnormalities include mutations in p53, overexpression of bcl-2 and c-mpl, deletions of IRF-1, methylation of p15^{INK4b} and others.[53–57] C-mpl expression was low in low-risk MDS and high in RAEB, RAEBT, and CMML (40% to 45%). In RAEB and RAEBT, c-mpl expression correlated with other adverse features and with poor survival ($P = .02$).[54]

How do these observations fit into a general multistep pathophysiologic process in MDS? It is possible that an initial injury results in suppression of normal hematopoietic stem cell growth and differentiation, directly or through stimulation of an immunologic response of polyclonal T cells. The cytotoxic suppressor T cells induce hematopoietic suppression through production of proapoptotic cytokines including TNF-α and the Fas/Fas ligand system. The roles of increased M-CSF, c-fms mutation, increased macrophages and contribution to TNF-α production, and interferon-γ and IL-1β need further elucidation. These processes are more prominent in the early phase of MDS (RA, RARS), producing excessive apoptosis and cytopenias, and are more amenable to therapeutic approaches including growth factors, antiapoptotic strategies (e.g., against TNF-α), and immunomodulation (e.g., cyclosporin A, antithymocyte globulins [ATG], corticosteroids). As compensatory proliferation continues, and perhaps mediated by the process of telomeric shortening and genomic instability, the hematopoietic progenitor cells allow the escape and growth advantage of clonal malignant hematopoiesis. This process may predominate in MDS advanced phases (RAEB, RAEBT, CMML), in which proliferation and maturation arrest (rather than apoptosis) are frequent, and in which a new set of molecular events dictate the pathophysiology, including enhanced Bcl-2 and p53 mutations, RAS mutations and dysfunction, and hypermethylation of p15^{INK4b} (leading to suppression of tumor suppressor genes). In these stages, more appropriate investigations include AML-like strategies to suppress the abnormal clone, or ones directed against specific molecular targets including hypomethylating agents or RAS inhibitors.

Thus, MDS might appropriately be divided into two distinct entities, early and late MDS, which are governed by different sets of pathophysiologic processes and in which different directed strategies should be investigated.

CLINICAL MANIFESTATIONS

The median age in MDS is 65 to 75 years, with a clear-cut age-related incidence. Younger patients who develop MDS have generally had exposure to leukemogenic agents. There is a male preponderance with a male to female ratio of 1.3:1.0. Presenting manifestations are due to cytopenia-associated problems including fatigue, pallor, infections, and bleeding (Table 46.5-4). Lymphadenopathy and hepatosplenomegaly are uncommon, occurring in less than 10% to 20% of patients. Central nervous system involvement is rare.

LABORATORY FEATURES

Anemia is the most common finding; neutropenia and thrombocytopenia are frequent. Monocytosis greater than 10^9/L in

TABLE 46.5-4. Presentation of Myelodysplastic Syndrome (M. D. Anderson, 1980–1999, 1358 Patients)

Characteristic	*Category*	*Percentage*
Age (y)	≥60 [median]	64 [64.5]
Splenomegaly	Any	11
Hepatomegaly	Any	8
Hemoglobin (g/dL)	<10	58
Platelets (× 10^9/L)	<50	43
	50–100	24
Granulocytes (× 10^9/L)	<0.5	23
French-American-British category	Refractory anemia	24
	Refractory anemia with ringed sideroblasts	4
	Refractory anemia with excessive blasts	28
	Refractory anemia with excessive blasts in transformation	30
	Chronic myelomonocytic leukemia	13
Karyotype	Diploid, -Y	41
	inv 16,t(8;21)	1.5
	Chromosome 5 or 7 abnormalities	30
	Trisomy 8	7
	20q-	2
	Other abnormalities	12
	Insufficient metaphases	7
Fatigue	Yes	61
Infections	Yes	21
Bleeding	Yes	6

the peripheral blood, in the setting of other MDS features, leads to a diagnosis of CMML. Smears of the bone marrow and blood show various degrees of dysplasia (mild, moderate, severe) in one or more lineages (myeloid, erythroid, megakaryocytic). While the degree and lineage involvement by dysplasia have been correlated with prognosis, assessment of dysplasia may be subjective. Blasts in MDS are myeloid in origin as determined by histochemistry (myeloperoxidase-positive, positive monocytic stain results) and by immunophenotyping (CD13, CD14, CD33 positivity); some cases exhibit B-lineage lymphoid (CD19 or CD10) or mixed-lineage morphologies.

Bone marrow biopsies or aspirates are usually hypercellular, but may be normocellular or hypocellular. Twenty percent of cases may have a cellularity below 20%, which may be important in the context of immune-mediated mechanisms and of immunomodulatory strategies. Other abnormalities include hypogranulation or hyposegmentation (Pelger-Huët–like) of granulocytes; anisocytosis, poikilocytosis, and macrocytosis of peripheral red cells; and marrow dyserythropoiesis including ringed sideroblasts, asynchronous maturation, abnormal nuclear shapes, and chromatin clumping. Peripheral platelet dysplasia may be noted with large abnormally granular platelets or hypogranular platelets. Marrow micromegakaryocytes are also frequent.

Cytochemical stains of importance in the workup of MDS include stains for (1) iron to identify ringed sideroblasts, (2) myeloperoxidase to identify abnormal granulation of myeloblasts, (3) periodic acid–Schiff to identify abnormal erythroblasts, (4) reticulin to define the degree of fibrosis, and (5) platelet antibodies to mark micromegakaryocytes.[58]

Blood chemistries should include B_{12} and folic acid levels to exclude vitamin deficiency–induced MDS-like changes. Serum and urinary lysozymes may be increased in CMML. Hypokalemia (lysozyme-induced renal tubular loss), renal dysfunction (leukemic involvement), and hyperuricemia may be present. Testing for the human immunodeficiency virus excludes MDS-like changes associated with human immunodeficiency virus–positive disease.[59]

Additional abnormalities observed in MDS include polyclonal gammopathies in up to one-third of patients, monoclonal gammopathies or hypogammaglobulinemia, the presence of autoimmune antibodies, and B- or T-cell abnormalities.

Cytogenetic studies demonstrate karyotypic abnormalities in 40% to 75% of patients. These are more common in higher risk MDS and secondary MDS and often involve chromosome 5 or 7 abnormalities, trisomy 8, 20q-, and complex abnormalities (see Table 46.5-4).[7,51,60] A characteristic chromosomal abnormality involving 5q23, or the 5q- syndrome, is often associated with an indolent form of RA.[51] Patients with MDS may infrequently demonstrate *favorable* chromosomal abnormalities such as t(8;21) or inversion 16.[61]

DIFFERENTIAL DIAGNOSIS

Dysplastic changes in the bone marrow are not pathognomonic for MDS, and the first concern is to exclude more treatable conditions associated with cytopenias. These include B_{12} or folic acid deficiencies; exposure to antibiotics, chemotherapy, ethanol, benzene or lead; or a regenerating bone marrow following hypoplasia induced by drugs or infections. Patients with human immunodeficiency virus–positive disease, chronic inflammation, tuberculosis, liver disorders, hypersplenism, Hodgkin's disease, lymphomas, and metastatic disease to the marrow may present with cytopenias and marrow dysplastic changes. In these situations, appropriate tests and an observation period clarify the diagnosis.

Hypoplastic MDS with a marrow cellularity of less than 10% to 20% may be confused with aplastic or hypoplastic anemia.[62] Cytogenetic studies may help in the differential diagnosis, but some aplastic conditions may also be clonal or associated with cytogenetic abnormalities.[63] MDS with maturation arrest at the promyelocytic stage may be confused with acute promyelocytic leukemia; this is clarified by the characteristic promyelocytic blastic morphology and appropriate cytogenetic and molecular studies. Predominance of myelofibrosis in MDS may confuse it with myelofibrosis[64] or occasionally with hairy cell leukemia, because of the constellation of cytopenia, dry marrow aspiration, fibrosis, and splenomegaly in an elderly man. A high blast percentage may result in difficulty classifying MDS-RAEBT versus AML, but this distinction may not be critical for therapeutic choices or prognosis.

SIGNIFICANCE OF THE 30% BLAST CUTOFF TO DISTINGUISH HIGH-RISK MYELODYSPLASTIC SYNDROMES FROM ACUTE MYELOID LEUKEMIA

The 30% blast cutoff has been traditionally proposed by the FAB classification to distinguish MDS from AML. The original intent was to avoid misdiagnosis and treatment of benign conditions as AML. This was supported by the view that MDS are indolent disorders often observed or treated with supportive care.

More recent studies have shown that high-risk MDS has as poor a prognosis as AML, and that other factors, some known, such as cytogenetic abnormalities, and others yet to be discovered (apoptotic, proliferative, angiogenesis, and methylation patterns, molecular abnormalities), may provide more rational methods to classify AML and MDS. In multivariate analysis, when account was taken of cytogenetics, patients with AML and high-risk MDS had similar outcomes following the use of anti-AML chemotherapy, independent of the blast percent.[9,65] Thus, the use of 30% marrow blasts to distinguish and to assign different treatments to AML versus high-risk MDS may not be relevant. A committee of the World Health Organization has recommended that patients with 20% or more marrow blasts be treated as they would for AML.[66]

SPECIFIC SUBTYPES OF MYELODYSPLASTIC SYNDROMES

5Q SYNDROME

This syndrome is often found in elderly women who present with isolated anemia.[51] The median age is 65 years; the female to male ratio is 3:1. The disease presents as RA or RARS, has an indolent course, rarely transforms to AML, and is associated with a median survival longer than 5 years. The peripheral blood shows macrocytic anemia and normal or slightly elevated white blood cell and platelet counts. The bone marrow may show characteristic monolobulated megakaryocytes. Cytogenetic studies usually demonstrate 5q23 as the single abnormality. Additional chromosome abnormalities, when present, are associated with a worse prognosis. Since repeated transfusions are a major component of supportive care, iron-chelating therapy (desferioxamine) is important in these patients, particularly if they have received more than 20 units of packed red cells, or when serum ferritin levels exceed 400 to 800 mg/L.

OTHER MYELODYSPLASTIC SYNDROME SUBTYPES

Hypoplastic MDS,[62] like aplastic anemia, may respond to immunomodulatory therapy such as corticosteroids, cyclosporin A, or ATG. Some cases may have disease induced by T-cell suppression of normal hematopoiesis. Myelofibrosis may predominate in some MDS cases[64] and raises the differential diagnosis of acute or chronic myelofibrosis, AML-M7 (megakaryocytic leukemia), and occasionally hairy cell leukemia.

Rarely, MDS may present with prominent eosinophilia or monocytosis without fulfilling the criterion of 10^9/L peripheral monocytes. These are referred to as *MDS with eosinophilia* or *with monocytosis.* The latter is probably a variant of CMML without excessive myeloproliferation.

CHRONIC MYELOMONOCYTIC LEUKEMIA

Originally categorized as MDS, CMML is now recognized as a hybrid disorder characterized by increased myeloid proliferation with monocytosis and erythroid and megakaryocytic dysplasia.[67,68] Thus, it shares characteristics of both MDS and myeloproliferative disorders in different lineages. The median age of patients is 65 to 75 years; there is a male predominance with a ratio of 2:1. Anemia and thrombocytopenia are common; hepatosplenomegaly is present in 25% to 50%; extramedullary disease involves the skin and subcutaneous tissues. Gingival or central nervous system involvement is rare. Patients with CMML and significant leukocytosis may present with organ infiltration and dysfunction including pulmonary insufficiency, cardiac decompensation, and renal failure. This may be exacerbated once treatment has started, and patients may develop bilateral lung infiltrates (leukemic cell necrosis and inflammation) and a picture resembling adult respiratory distress syndrome. Subtle renal dysfunction at the start may worsen transiently on therapy as tumor lysis complications develop. Patients presenting with severe leukocytosis, monocytosis, and organ dysfunction may benefit from leukapheresis, measures to prevent tumor lysis (allopurinol, alkalinization, hydration, oral aluminum hydroxide to bind calcium), corticosteroids, and, at times, early hemodialysis for renal failure. Cytogenetic abnormalities are less frequent than in MDS. When present, they involve monosomy 7, trisomy 8, or other structural changes including 12p. Ras mutations are more common in CMML than in MDS (30% to 40%). The median survival of patients with CMML is approximately 18 months. Characteristics associated with shorter survival include increased marrow blasts, anemia, thrombocytopenia, cytogenetic abnormalities, and perhaps older age and excessive monocytosis.

THERAPY

BACKGROUND

The standard of care in MDS is generally accepted to be supportive care. This practice reflects (1) the older age and concomitant medical problems of MDS patients, making AML-like combination regimens risky; (2) the lack of effective nontoxic modalities; and (3) the prevailing notion that MDS is an indolent disorder. However, as discussed, the 30% blast cutoff is arbitrary, and survival of patients with high-risk MDS is similar to that of patients with AML. Hence, the same treatment considerations in elderly AML patients also apply to MDS. The belief that MDS is incurable except with allogeneic SCT is now contradicted by studies using AML-type therapy and intensive supportive care for patients with MDS. In such studies, the overall 3-year complete response duration rates of 25% were similar, among comparable age groups, to patients undergoing allogeneic SCT.[9,69]

There is marked heterogeneity in MDS. An indolent course is generally seen only in patients with RA or RARS, or low- and intermediate-1 IPSS risk groups. Other patients, making up the majority of referrals to specialized centers, have a poor prognosis and estimated median survivals of 1 year or less, similar to patients with AML. Low-risk MDS generally refers to RA and RARS in the FAB classification and to the low-risk IPSS group. High-risk patients include RAEB and RAEBT in the FAB classification and the high- and intermediate-2 IPSS risk groups. The intermediate-1 IPSS categorization depends on the population under study, being *lower* risk in community-based studies, and *higher* risk in studies from specialized centers (see Table 46.5-3).

GENERAL TREATMENT PRINCIPLES

Treatment strategies should be individualized to the patient's condition and disease manifestations. MDS may be appropriately divided into two generally distinct entities pathophysiologically and for therapeutic purposes: low-risk and high-risk MDS. Patients with low-risk MDS and minimal findings should be observed. If they develop significant cytopenias and complications, growth factor support, as single agents or in combinations, may be indicated depending on patient's symptoms and frequency of transfusions and infections. For patients with low-risk MDS, trials of high doses of vitamins (e.g., B_6) or androgens could benefit occasional patients. Immunomodulatory therapy with corticosteroids, cyclosporin A, and ATG may benefit 30% to 50% of selected patients. Low-risk patients may also be offered investigational single-agent chemotherapy, cytokines, antiapoptotic, or targeted modalities. Because of the poor prognosis of high-risk MDS, efforts should be made to involve patients in investigational studies including novel single chemotherapeutic agents, cytokines, gene or other targeted approaches (e.g., RAS-inhibitors, monoclonal antibodies), or AML-type combination regimens.

SUPPORTIVE CARE

Most patients succumb to complications of marrow failure and cytopenias before transformation has occurred. Patients with anemia may be transfused with packed red cells when symptoms develop. If the frequency of transfusions increases (e.g., more than 1 to 2 per month), trials of vitamins, androgens, erythropoietin alone or in combinations, and immunomodulatory strategies may be indicated. With granulocytopenia and repeated infectious episodes (e.g., two or more) antibiotic prophylaxis with or without G-CSF appears reasonable, although not established in randomized studies or in high-risk patient subsets.

Thrombocytopenia may be managed with platelet transfusions when platelets are reduced below 10×10^9/L or if bleeding

TABLE 46.5-5. Combination Chemotherapy in Myelodysplastic Syndromes

Study	*Treatment*	*No. Treated*	*Percentage Complete Response*	*Percentage Mortality*	*Median Survival (mo)*
De Witte[92]	Ida Ara-C	50	52	8	15
Ruutu[96]	Ida Ara-C	40	53	10	12
Invenizzi[97]	Ida Ara-C	25	48	8	12
Economopoulos[98]	Ida Ara-C	22	54	9	18
Wattel[99]	Zorubicin, mitoxantrone, Ara-C	99	41	16	11
Bernstein[100]	Daunorubicin or mitoxantrone, Ara-C	33	79	6	13
Parker[94]	Fludarabine, Ara-C, granulocyte colony-stimulating factor, Ida	19	63	0	NA
Estey[93]	Ida, HDAra-C, fludarabine + Ara-C	168	60	—	—

Ara-C, cytarabine; HDAra-C, high-dose Ara-C; Ida, idarubicin.

occurs. Patients may become refractory to platelet transfusions; investigational strategies with cytokines, immunomodulation, new agents, or chemotherapy combinations should then be considered.

VITAMINS, ANDROGENS, DIFFERENTIATING AGENTS, AND INTERFERON

Although occasional patients may benefit from vitamin B_6, androgens, and corticosteroids, the approaches have had a low success rate. Differentiating agents have been investigated including vitamin D, vitamin A, retinoids, hexamethylene bisacetamide, and sodium phenylbutyrate. These were associated with low response rates,[70–75] as did interferon alone or with chemotherapy and vitamins.[76]

HEMATOPOIETIC GROWTH FACTORS

Erythropoietin has improved anemia and reduced transfusion requirements in 16% to 25% of selected patients, despite elevated endogenous erythropoietin levels in 85% of patients.[77] Better responses are noted in RA and RAEB compared with RARS (22% vs. 7%), in patients without transfusion requirements, in the absence of ringed sideroblasts, or with low to normal serum levels of endogenous erythropoietin (below 2000 U/L). Erythropoietin, 10,000 U, 3 times weekly, or 40,000 U weekly, may show benefit within 8 weeks of therapy.

G-CSF and GM-CSF improve neutropenia in 70% to 80% of patients and occasionally in other lineage cytopenias. Randomized studies comparing supportive care with G-CSF or GM-CSF have not shown them to reduce infectious episodes, prolong survival, or influence the rate of transformation to acute leukemia.[78,79] Combinations of G-CSF and erythropoietin may synergize in improving cytopenias.[80,81] Other cytokines investigated include IL-3 alone and in combinations, IL-6, and IL-11, and thrombopoietins for thrombocytopenia.[82–85] Growth factors with low-dose cytarabine were not better than chemotherapy alone.[86]

LOW-DOSE CYTARABINE

Large-scale analyses of cytarabine, 10 to 20 mg/m^2 daily for up to 3 weeks, in MDS showed response rates of 10% to 15%.[87] Cytotoxicity, rather than differentiation, was the anti-MDS mechanism. Morbidity and mortality were substantial, and survival was not improved. Randomized studies of low-dose cytarabine, one with GM-CSF, versus supportive care did not show a survival benefit with cytarabine.[88,89]

ACUTE MYELOID LEUKEMIA–TYPE COMBINATION REGIMENS

In the early 1980s, two retrospective studies showed that regimens used to treat AML could induce complete response in patients with MDS.[90,91] Since then, several studies reported on the use of intensive chemotherapy in MDS[92–101] (Table 46.5-5). Remission rates have ranged from 40% to 60% and mortality from 20% to 40%. Appropriate supportive care measures and prophylactic antibiotics have reduced this mortality to 6% to 20%. Complete response rates were 70% to 80% with favorable or normal karyotypes, and 40% to 50% with unfavorable karyotypes. Cytogenetic remissions generally accompanied complete responses.[35,36] Factors influencing outcome were age, karyotype, and FAB diagnosis. Patients most likely to benefit were younger than 50 years, had normal karyotypes, and had RAEBT[95] (Table 46.5-6). Long-term event-free survival was possible with intensive chemotherapy: Among age-comparable groups, the 3-year complete response and survival rates were similar with intensive chemotherapy versus allogeneic SCT[69] (see Table 46.5-6).

ALLOGENEIC STEM CELL TRANSPLANTATION

Allogeneic SCT is applicable to a small subset of MDS patients because of age restrictions, concomitant medical conditions, and donor availability. Disease-free survival rates of 30% to 50% have been reported.[102–104] Results were better in younger patients, with low-risk MDS, and if transplant was applied within 1 year from diagnosis.[102] Failure was primarily due to transplant-associated mortality in low-risk MDS and to disease recurrence in high-risk MDS. In the latter disorders, the long-term follow-up to studies showed 3-year survival rates of 23%, similar to those with intensive chemotherapy.[69,102] Allogeneic SCT after tumor reduction to less than 5% blasts in high-risk MDS produced better results, but may have selected inherently better patients.[103] In an update of the Seattle experience, patients were evaluated by the IPSS.[104] The disease-free survival rates were 60% in low-risk, 36% in intermediate-1, and 28% in intermediate-2 risk groups. This is compared with 5-year survival rates of 55%, 35%, and 7%, respectively, for unselected patients not receiving SCT. Consider-

TABLE 46.5-6. Outcome of Myelodysplastic Syndrome with Acute Myeloid Leukemia–Type Chemotherapy by Different Characteristics and Therapy

Therapy	*Study Group*	*Number*	*Percentage Complete Response*	*Percentage Survival at 3 Y*	*Complete Response Duration*
Intensive chemotherapy	Myelodysplastic syndrome total (M. D. Anderson Cancer Center 1992 to present)	403	53	11	17
	CG favorable	146	58	17	32
	CG unfavorable	241	50	5	6
	Myelodysplastic syndrome, age ≤60 years	151	56	25	30
	CG favorable	46	65	32	47
	CG unfavorable	100	51	6	3
Allogeneic stem cell transplantation	Anderson et al.[102]		NA	23	23

CG, cytogenetics.

ing the risk to benefit ratios (early transplant mortality but potential event-free survival) and the comparison of disease-free survival versus survival rates, it appears that SCT may benefit high-risk MDS patients.

While autologous SCT has been advocated as a treatment for MDS, this applies to patients who have achieved complete response, could be harvested, and were candidates for the procedure. The 2-year survival rate was only 39%, despite the highly selected nature of the patients.[105]

Improvement in results of SCT may occur through (1) targeted marrow ablative approaches (e.g., radiolabeled monoclonal antibodies against CD33 or CD45); (2) reductions in SCT-related mortality (e.g., mini-SCT); (3) preallogeneic and postallogeneic SCT-effective chemotherapy or immunomodulation; and (4) broader application of safer procedures in the setting of matched unrelated donor transplant.[106]

NOVEL AGENTS AND STRATEGIES

Topotecan

Topotecan, a topoisomerase I inhibitor, given as a single agent at 2 mg/m^2 by continuous infusion daily for 5 days every 4 to 6 weeks, produced complete response in 31% of patients.[107] Side effects were severe mucositis and diarrhea (23% and 17%, respectively).

Combinations of topotecan, 1.25 mg/m^2 daily × 5 and Ara-C 1 g/m^2 over 2 hours daily × 5, every 4 to 6 weeks, were given with intensive supportive care, prophylactic antibiotics, and the use of the protected environment among patients 50 years or older. Eighty-six patients have been treated (59 MDS, 27 CMML). Their median age was 64 years; 35% had prior therapy and 50% had unfavorable chromosomal abnormalities. Complete response was observed in 56% and induction mortality in 7%.[35] Complete response rates were higher with RAEB than with RAEBT and CMML (complete response rate of 80% vs. 47% vs. 44%; $P = .01$), but were similar by different age groups and cytogenetic abnormalities. Median complete response duration was 8 months, and median survival was 14 months. Severe mucositis or diarrhea occurred in only 3%. This suggested a possible role for topotecan in patients with poor prognoses (older, poor cytogenetics), who have a high incidence of expression of the multidrug resistance phenotype and may benefit from agents that are not multidrug resistance–dependent, such as topoisomerase I inhibitors. Investigations to improve prognosis include (1) addition of cyclophosphamide to topotecan and Ara-C; (2) consolidation strategies in complete response (targeted therapies, immunomodulation, anticytokines); (3) newer topoisomerase I inhibitors[108,109]; and (4) different dose schedules (e.g., oral topotecan in lower dose, longer exposure schedules).

Hypomethylating Agents

DNA site-specific methylation may be associated with tumor resistance and progression in many solid and hematologic cancers including MDS.[110] In MDS, frequent hypermethylation of p15^{INK4b} has been reported.[56,57,111] Agents shown to induce general and selective hypomethylation include 5-azacitidine, decitabine, and the newer methyl transferase antisense inhibitors.

Following pilot studies of continuous intravenous and subcutaneous 5-azacitidine in MDS, Silverman et al. conducted a large-scale randomized trial of subcutaneous 5-azacitidine, 75 mg/m^2 daily × 7 every 4 weeks (n = 99), versus observation (n = 92) in 191 patients with high-risk MDS.[112,113] Cross-over to 5-azacitidine was allowed if there was progression on the observation arm. Responses occurred in 61% of 5-azacitidine–treated MDS patients (9% complete response, 15% partial response, 35% hematologic improvement) versus 5% in the observation arm ($P < .01$). The median time to leukemia transformation (21 vs. 13 months; $P < .01$) and the median survival (24 vs. 14 months; P = .10) were longer among 5-azacitidine–treated patients.[112] Quality of life was also improved.[113] Thus, 5-azacitidine therapy effectively modified the natural history of MDS.

Wijermans et al. treated elderly patients with high-risk MDS with decitabine, 40 to 50 mg/m^2 over 24 hours daily × 3 every 6 weeks (120 to 150 mg/m^2/course), and later at 15 mg/m^2 over 4 hours every 8 hours for 3 days (135 mg/m^2/course) every 6 weeks.[114] In an update of 125 patients in three studies (median age, 70 years; IPSS risk intermediate-1 in 35, intermediate-2 in 38, and high-risk in 52) 49% responded: complete response in 24 (20%), partial response in 12 (10%), and hematologic improvement in 23 (19%).[114] Response rates were 58% in IPSS high-risk and 39% and 45% in IPSS intermediate-1 and -2 risk groups, respectively. Ten patients (8%) died during therapy. In 15 patients with chromosomal abnormalities who obtained complete response, disappearance of the cytogenetic abnormalities was noted. The median response duration was 9 months. The median survival was 15 months: 19 months in intermediate -1, 13 months in intermediate -2, and 14 months in high-risk patients. Hypermethylation at three cytosine residues in the 5' region of the p15 gene was detected in 59% of patients. Efficient reduction of methylation with decitabine therapy either accompanied or preceded suppression of bone marrow blasts and improvement of cytopenias. However, responses to decitabine also occurred in the absence of p15 hypermethylation, suggesting that p15 is one but not the only molecular target of pharmacologic demethylation in MDS, or that decitabine may induce anti-MDS activity through mechanisms other than hypomethylation.[111]

Other Chemotherapeutic Agents

Homoharringtonine, a semisynthetic plant alkaloid, showed activity in chronic myelogenous leukemia and AML.[115] Feldman et al. treated 15 patients with MDS with homoharringtonine, 5 mg/m^2 by continuous infusion daily for 9 days every month, and observed four responses (27%).[116] Significant myelosuppression and high induction mortality discouraged further studies. Lower dose schedules of homoharringtonine, 2.5 mg/m^2 daily × 7, alone or in combinations, may prove effective and less toxic.[115]

Amifostine

Amifostine, an organic thiophosphonate, increases normal hematopoiesis *in vitro*, suppresses apoptosis, and inhibits production of TNF-α and other inflammatory cytokines. In a multiinstitutional study, patients with MDS received amifostine, 200 or 400 mg/m^2 intravenously 3 times weekly for 3 weeks every 5 weeks. Among 75 evaluable patients, single or multilineage hematologic response was observed in 27 (36%). A 50% decrease in blasts was noted in ten patients (13%) and a 50% decrease in ringed sideroblasts in nine patients (total 16 patients). Ten of the 16 also had peripheral blood responses.[117] Other studies reported lower response rates.[118]

Immunotherapy

Immunosuppression may be pathophysiologic in some MDS cases, and immune therapy may be beneficial.[119] Patients with hypoplastic MDS have had complete and durable remissions with therapies similar to those used in aplastic anemia. ATG resulted in responses in 44% of patients.[120] Cyclosporin A resulted in clinical improvements in 14 of 17 patients treated for low-risk MDS.[121] Studies of combinations of ATG, cyclosporine A, growth factors, and corticosteroids are in progress.

Other Strategies

Monoclonal antibodies targeted against surface antigens expressed in MDS (e.g., CD33 and CD45) may be useful.[122] Anti-TNF strategies using pentoxifylline-based combinations were not beneficial.[123] Other anti-TNF strategies may incorporate amifostine and pentoxifylline or use soluble TNF receptors alone or in combination with amifostine, pentoxifylline, and anti-Fas ligand. Antiangiogenesis therapy with thalidomide, 200 to 800 mg orally daily, produced complete response in only one of nine patients in one study[124]; another study reported clinical benefits in 10 of 20 evaluable patients (50%).[125] Based on the association of p53 mutations with MDS,[53,126] Bishop et al. investigated whether inactivation of p53 RNA by antisense and rebound in p53 expression through the use of OL(1)p53 would be effective. Only one of ten high-risk MDS patients treated had a transient response.[127] Approaches attempting to enhance immunologic response in MDS, using linomide or IL-2, have not been successful.[128,129] Investigations of the new RAS inhibitors and antitelomeric strategies will be of interest in MDS.[130,131]

Agents with interesting differentiation properties include hexamethylene bisacetamid and sodium phenylbutyrate. In two studies in MDS, hexamethylene bisacetamid given by continuous infusion induced complete response in three patients and partial response in six patients among a total of 57 patients treated (objective response rate, 17%).[74,132] Sodium phenylbutyrate, a histone deacetylase inhibitor, was given to 27 patients at doses up to 440 mg/kg daily × 7 every 4 weeks: 17 had improvements in granulocyte counts and 3 had improvements in platelet counts.[71]

Correlative Studies and Mechanism of Actions

While each of these new approaches has provided encouraging results, little is known about how they influence specifically the pathophysiology of MDS. Understanding how these agents affect methylation, cytokines, and genes involved in apoptosis or proliferation cascades may refine treatments to be more selective and less toxic and help combine them in more appropriate simultaneous and sequential schedules.

SUMMARY

While several strategies were initially thought to be hopeful in MDS (e.g., low-dose Ara-C, growth factors), progress has been modest. Better understanding of the pathophysiology of MDS (e.g., apoptosis, clonality, cytokines) may produce tailored strategies. The improved classification of MDS may allow more appropriate therapies for low- versus high-risk groups. Growth factors and immunosuppressive strategies may improve results in low-risk MDS, while the combination of more selective anti-MDS agents (topoisomerase I inhibitors, hypomethylating agents) may improve outcome in high-risk MDS. Progress in SCT (graft-versus-MDS, mini-SCT, preparative regimens) could result in its broader applications. Finally, it is hoped that new targets and targeted therapies will emerge that will add to our knowledge and better treatment of MDS.

REFERENCES

1. Heaney M, Golde D. Myelodysplasia. *N Engl J Med* 1999;340:1649.
2. Hofman W-K, Hoelzer D. Current therapeutic options in myelodysplastic syndromes. *Hematology* 1999;4:91.
3. Raza A, Mundle S, Shetty V, et al. Novel insights into the biology of myelodysplastic syndromes: excessive apoptosis and the role of cytokines. *Int J Hematol* 1996;63:265.
4. Rajapaksa R, Ginzton N, Rott LS, Greenberg PL. Altered oncoprotein expression and apoptosis in myelodysplastic syndrome marrow cells. *Blood* 1996;88:4275.
5. Raza A, Gezer S, Mundle S, et al. Apoptosis in bone marrow biopsy samples involving stromal and hematopoietic cells in 50 patients with myelodysplastic syndromes. *Blood* 1995;6:268.

6. Clark DM, Lampert IA. Apoptosis is a common histopathological finding in myelodysplasia: the correlate of ineffective haematopoiesis. *Leuk Lymphoma* 1990;2:415.
7. Noel P, Tefferi A, Pierre RV, Jenkins RB, Dewald GW. Karyotypic analysis in primary myelodysplastic syndromes. *Blood Rev* 1993;7:10.
8. Greenberg PL, Mara B. The preleukemic syndrome: correlation in vitro parameters of granulopoiesis with clinical features. *Am J Med* 1979;66:951.
9. Estey E, Thall P, Beran M, et al. Effect of diagnosis (refractory anemia with excess blasts, refractory anemia with excess blast in transformation, or acute myeloid leukemia [AML]) on outcome of AML-type chemotherapy. *Blood* 1997;90:2969.
10. Morel P, Declercq C, Hebbar M, Bauters F, Fenaux P. Prognostic factors in myelodysplastic syndromes: critical analysis of the impact of age and gender and failure to identify a very-low-risk group using standard mortality ratio techniques. *Br J Haematol* 1996;94:116.
11. Cartwright RA. Incidence and epidemiology of the myelodysplastic syndromes. In: Multi GJ, Galton DAG, eds. *The myelodysplastic syndromes.* London: Churchill Livingstone, 1992:23.
12. West RR, Stafford DA, Farrow A, Jacobs A. Occupational and environmental exposures and myelodysplasia: a case-control study. *Leuk Res* 1995;19:127.
13. Nisse C, Lorthois C, Dorp V, et al. Exposure to occupational and environmental factors in myelodysplastic syndromes: preliminary results of a case-control study. *Leukemia* 1995;9:693.
14. Rigolin GM, Cuneo A, Roberti MG, et al. Esposure to myelotoxic agents and myelodysplasia: case-control study and correlation with clinicobiologic findings. *Br J Haematol* 1998;103:189.
15. Brown LM, Blair A, Gibson R, et al. Pesticide exposures and other risk factors for leukemia among men in Iowa and Minnesota. *Cancer Res* 1990;50:6585.
16. Garfinkel L, Boffeta P. Association between smoking and leukemia in two American cancer society prospective studies. *Cancer* 1990;65:2356.
17. Kantarjian HM, Keating MJ. Therapy-related leukemia and myelodysplastic syndrome. *Semin Oncol* 1987;14:435.
18. Stone RM, Neuberg D, Soiffer R, et al. Myelodysplastic syndrome as a late complication following autologous bone marrow transplantation for non-Hodgkin's lymphoma. *J Clin Oncol* 1994;12:2535.
19. Paul B, Reid MM, Davison EV, Abela M, Hamilton PJ. Familial myelodysplasia: progressive disease associated with emergence of monosomy 7. *Br J Haematol* 1987;65:321.
20. Bennett JM, Catovsky D, Daniel MT, et al. Proposals for the classification of the myelodysplastic syndromes. *Br J Haematol* 1982;51:189.
21. Michaux JL, Martiat P. Chronic myelomonocytic leukemia (CMML) a myelodysplastic or myeloproliferative syndrome? *Leuk Lymphoma* 1993;9:35.
22. Verhoef GEG, Pittaluga S, Wolfe-Peters CDE, Boogaerts MA. FAB classification of myelodysplastic syndromes: merits and controversies. *Ann Hematol* 1995;71:3.
23. Seymour J, Estey E. The contribution of Auer rods to the classification and prognosis of myelodysplastic syndromes. *Leuk Lymphoma* 1995;17:79.
24. Estey E, Keating M, Pierce S, Beran M. Application of the international scoring system for myelodysplasia to M. D. Anderson patients. *Blood* 1997;90:2843.
25. Sanz GF, Sanz MA, Vallespi T, Canizo M. Two regression models and a scoring system for predicting survival and planning treatment in myelodysplastic syndromes: a multivariate analysis of prognostic factors in 370 patients. *Blood* 1989;74:395.
26. Morel P, Hebbar M, Lai JL, Duhamel A. Cytogenetic analysis has strong independent prognostic value in de novo myelodysplastic syndromes and can be incorporated in a new scoring system: a report on 408 cases. *Leukemia* 1993;7:1315.
27. Greenberg P, Cox C, LeBeau M, et al. International scoring system for evaluating prognosis in myelodysplastic syndromes. *Blood* 1997;89:2079.
28. Gallagher A, Darley RL, Padua R. The molecular basis of myelodysplastic syndromes. *Haematologica* 1997;82:191.
29. Rosenfeld CS, List A. A hypothesis for the pathogenesis of myelodysplastic syndrome: implications for new therapies. *Leukemia* 2000;14:2.
30. Janssen JWG, Buschle M, Layton M, et al. Clonal analysis of myelodysplastic syndromes: evidence of multipotent stem cell origin. *Blood* 1989;73:248.
31. Tefferi A, Thibodeau SN, Solberg LA Jr. Clonal studies in the myelodysplastic syndrome using X-linked restriction fragment length polymorphisms. *Blood* 1990;75:1770.
32. Saitoh K, Miura I, Takahashi N, Miura AB. Fluorescence in situ hybridization of progenitor cells obtained by fluorescence-activated cell sorting for the detection of cells affected by chromosome abnormality trisomy 8 in patients with myelodysplastic syndromes. *Blood* 1998;92:2886.
33. Van Kamp H, Fibbe WE, Jansen RPM, et al. Clonal involvement of granulocytes and monocytes, but not of T and B lymphocytes and natural killer cells in patients with myelodysplasia: analysis by X-linked restriction fragment length polymorphisms and polymerase chain reaction of the phosphoglycerate kinase gene. *Blood* 1992;80:1774.
34. Kroef MJPL, Fibbe WE, Mout R, et al. Myeloid but not lymphoid cells carry the 5q deletion: polymerase chain reaction analysis of loss of heterozygosity using mini-repeat sequences on highly purified cell fractions. *Blood* 1993;81:1849.
35. Beran M, Kantarjian H, O'Brien S, et al. Topotecan, a topoisomerase I inhibitor, is active in the treatment of myelodysplastic syndromes and chronic myelomonocytic leukemia. *Blood* 1996;88:2473.
36. Beran M, Estey EH, O'Brien S, et al. Topotecan and cytarabine is an active combination regimen in myelodysplastic syndromes and chronic myelomonocytic leukemia. *J Clin Oncol* 1999;17:2819.
37. Molldrem JJ, Jiang YZ, Stetler-Stevenson M, et al. Hematological response of patients with myelodysplastic syndrome to anti-thymocyte globulin is associated with a loss of lymphocyte-mediated inhibition of CFU-GM and alterations in T-cell receptor Vb profiles. *Br J Haematol* 1998;102:1314.
38. Greenberg P. In vitro hemopoietic cell culture studies in MDS. *Semin Oncol* 1992;19:34.
39. Selleri C, Sato T, Anderson S, Young NS, Maciejewski JP. Interferon-gamma and tumor necrosis factor-alpha suppress both early and late stages of hematopoiesis and induce programmed cell death. *J Cell Physiol* 1995;165:538.
40. Maciejewski J, Selleri C, Anderson S, Young NS. Fas antigen expression on CD34+ human marrow cells is induced by interferon γ and tumor necrosis factor α and potentiates cytokine-mediated hematopoietic suppression in vitro. *Blood* 1995;85:3183.
41. Verhoef GEG, De Schouwer P, Ceuppens JL, et al. Measurement of serum cytokine levels in patients with myelodysplastic syndromes. *Leukemia* 1992;12:1268.
42. Kitagawa M, Saito I, Kuwata T, et al. Overexpression of tumor necrosis factor (TNF)-α and interferon (IFN)-γ bone marrow cells from patients with myelodysplastic syndromes. *Leukemia* 1997;11:2049.
43. Kitagawa M, Kamiyama R, Kasuga T. Increase in number of bone marrow macrophages in patients with myelodysplastic syndromes. *Eur J Haematol* 1993;51:56.
44. Janowska-Wieczorek A, Belch AR, Jacobs A, et al. Increased circulating colony-stimulating factor-1 in patients with preleukemia, leukemia, and lymphoid malignancies. *Blood* 1991;77:1796.
45. Tobal K, Pagliuca A, Bhatt B. Mutation of the human FMS gene (M-CSF receptor) in myelodysplastic syndromes and acute myeloid leukemia. *Leukemia* 1990;4:486.
46. Gersuk GM, Yamaguchi M, Beckham C, et al. A role for FAS, FAS-ligand and TNF-α in the dysregulation of hematopoiesis in myelodysplastic syndrome (MDS). *Blood* 1996;88(Suppl 1):639a.
47. Stasi R, Brunetti M, Bussa S, et al. Serum levels of tumour necrosis factor-α predict response to recombinant human erythropoietin in patients with myelodysplastic syndrome. *Clin Lab Haematol* 1997;19:197.
48. Mundle SD, Venugopal P, Cartlidge JD, et al. Indication of an involvement of interleukin-1β converting enzyme-like protease in intramedullary apoptotic cell death in the bone marrow of patients with myelodysplastic syndromes. *Blood* 1996;88:2640.
49. Paquette RL, Landaw EM, Pierre RV, et al. N-ras mutations are associated with poor prognosis and increased risk of leukemia in myelodysplastic syndrome. *Blood* 1993;82:590.
50. Ohyashiki JH, Ohyashiki K, Fujimura T, et al. Telomere shortening associated with disease evolution patterns in myelodysplastic syndromes. *Cancer Res* 1994;54:3557.
51. Boultwood J, Lewis S, Waincoar JS. The 5q-syndrome. *Blood* 1994;84:3253.
52. Ridge SA, Worwood M, Oscier D, Jacobs A, Padua RA. Fms mutations in myelodysplastic, leukemic, and normal subjects. *Proc Natl Acad Sci U S A* 1990;87:1377.
53. Mori N, Hidai H, Yokota J, et al. Mutations of the p53 gene in myelodysplastic syndrome and overt leukemia. *Leukemia Res* 1995;19:869.
54. Bouscary D, Preudhomme C, Ribrag V, et al. Prognostic value of c-mpl expression in myelodysplastic syndromes. *Leukemia* 1995;9:783.
55. Willman CL, Sever CE, Pallavicini MG, et al. Deletion of *IRF-1*, mapping to chromosome 5q31.1, in human leukemia and preleukemic myelodysplasia. *Science* 1993;259:968.
56. Uchida T, Kinoshita T, Nagai H, et al. Hypermethylation of the $p15^{INK4b}$ gene in myelodysplastic syndromes. *Blood* 1997;90:1403.
57. Quensel B, Guillerm G, Vereecque R, et al. Methylation of the $p15^{INK4b}$ gene in myelodysplastic syndromes is frequent and acquired during disease progression. *Blood* 1998;91:2985.
58. Seo IS, Li C-Y, Yam LT. Myelodysplastic syndrome: diagnostic implications of cytochemical and immunocytochemical studies. *Mayo Clin Proc* 1993;68:47.
59. Schneider DR, Picker LJ. Myelodysplasia in the acquired immune deficiency syndrome. *Am J Clin Pathol* 1985;84:144.
60. Wattel E, Lai JL, Hebbar M, Preudhomme C. De novo myelodysplastic syndrome with deletion of long arm of chromosome 20: a subtype of MDS with distinct hematological and prognostic features? *Leuk Res* 1993;17:921.
61. Estey E, Trujillo J, Cork A, O'Brien S, et al. AML-associated cytogenetic abnormalities (inv(16), del(16), t(8;21)) in patients with myelodysplastic syndromes. *Hematol Pathol* 1992;6:43.
62. Nand S, Godwin JE. Hypoplastic myelodysplastic syndromes. *Cancer* 1988;62:958.
63. Appelbaum FR, Barrall J, Storb R, et al. Clonal cytogenetic abnormalities in patients with otherwise typical aplastic anemia. *Exp Hematol* 1987;15:1134.
64. Lambertenghi-Deliliers G, Orazi A, Luksch R, Annaloro C, Soligo D. Myelodysplastic syndrome with increased marrow fibrosis: a distinct clinicopathological entity. *Br J Haematol* 1991;78:161.
65. Estey EH, Keating MJ, Dixon DO, et al. Karyotype is prognostically more important than FAB system's distinction between myelodysplastic syndrome and acute myelogenous leukemia. *Hematol Pathol* 1987;7:203.
66. Harris NL, Jaffe ES, Diebold J, et al. World Health Organization Classification of neoplastic diseases of the hematopoietic and lymphoid tissues: report of the Clinical Advisory Committee Meeting. *J Clin Oncol* 1999;17:3835.
67. Fenaux P, Benscart R, Lai JL, Jouet JP, Bauters F. Prognostic factors in adult chronic myelomonocytic leukemia: analysis of 107 cases. *J Clin Oncol* 1988;6:1417.
68. Bennett JM, Catovsy D, Daniel MT, et al. The chronic myeloid leukemias: guidelines for distinguishing chronic granulocytic, atypical chronic myeloid and chronic myelomonocytic leukemia. *Br J Haematol* 1994;87:746.
69. Anderlini P, Pierce S, Kantarjian H, Estey E. AML-type chemotherapy for myelodysplasia. *J Clin Oncol* 1996;14:1404.
70. Doll DC, Ringenberg QS, Yarbro JW. Danazol therapy in acquired idiopathic sideroblastic anemia. *Acta Haematol* 1987;77:170.
71. Gore SD, Miller CB, Weng LJ, et al. Clinical development of sodium phenylbutyrate as a putative differentiating agent in myeloid malignancies. *Anticancer Res* 1997;17:3938a.
72. Kurzrock R, Estey E, Talpaz M. All-trans retinoic acid: tolerance and biologic effects in myelodysplastic syndrome. *J Clin Oncol* 1993;11:1489.
73. Koeffler HP, Heitjan D, Mertelsmann R, et al. Randomized study of 13-cis retinoic acid v placebo in the myelodysplastic disorders. *Blood* 1988;71:703.
74. Andreeff M, Stone R, Michaeli J, et al. Hexamethylene bisacetamide in myelodysplastic syndrome and acute myelogenous leukemia: a phase II clinical trial with a differentiation-inducing agent. *Blood* 1992;80:2604.
75. Morosetti R, Koeffler HP. Differentiation therapy in myelodysplastic syndromes. *Semin Hematol* 1996;33:236.

76. Hellstrom E, Robert KH, Gahrton G, et al. Therapeutic effects of low-dose cytosine arabinoside, alpha-interferon, 1 alpha-hydroxyvitamin D_3 and retinoic acid in acute leukemia and myelodysplastic syndromes. *Eur J Haematol* 1988;40:449.
77. Hellstrom-Lindberg E. Efficacy of erythropoietin in the myelodysplastic syndromes: a meta-analysis of 205 patients from 17 studies. *Br J Haematol* 1995;89:67.
78. Willemze R, van der Lely N, Zwierzina H, et al. A randomized phase I/II multicenter study of recombinant human granulocyte-macrophage colony-stimulating factor (GM-CSF) therapy for patients with myelodysplastic syndromes and a relatively low risk of acute leukemia. *Ann Hematol* 1992;64:173.
79. Greenberg P, Taylor K, Larson R, et al. Phase III randomized multicenter trial of G-CSF vs. observation for myelodysplastic syndromes. *Blood* 1993;82(Suppl 1):196a(abst).
80. Negrin RS, Stein R, Doherty K, et al. Maintenance treatment of the anemia of myelodysplastic syndromes with recombinant human granulocyte colony-stimulating factor and erythropolietin: evidence for in vivo synergy. *Blood* 1996;87:4076.
81. Hellstrom-Lindberg E, Ahlgren T, Beguin Y, et al. Treatment of anemia in myelodysplastic syndromes with granulocyte colony-stimulating factor plus erythropoietin: results from a randomized phase II study and long-term follow-up of 71 patients. *Blood* 1998;92:68.
82. Nand S, Sosman J, Godwin JE. A phase I/II study of sequential interleukin 3 and granulocyte-macrophage colony-stimulating factor in myelodysplastic syndromes. *Blood* 1994;83:357.
83. Gordon MS, Nemunaitis J, Hoffman R, et al. A phase I trial of recombinant human interleukin-6 in patients with myelodysplastic syndromes and thrombocytopenia. *Blood* 1995;85:3066.
84. Tepler I, Elias L, Smith JW II, et al. A randomized placebo-controlled trial of recombinant human interleukin-11 in cancer patients with severe thrombocytopenia due to chemotherapy. *Blood* 1996;87:3615.
85. Fanucchi M, Glapsy J, Crawford J, et al. Effects of polyethylene glycol-conjugated recombinant human megakaryocyte growth and development factor in platelet counts after chemotherapy for lung cancer. *N Engl J Med* 1997;336:404.
86. Gerhartz HH, Marcus R, Delmer A. A randomized phase II study of low-dose cytosine arabinoside plus GM-CSF in MDS with a high risk of developing leukemia. *Leukemia* 1994;8:16.
87. Cheson BD, Jasperese DM, Simon R, Friedman MA. A critical appraisal of low-dose cytosine arabinoside in patients with acute non-lymphocytic leukemia and myelodysplastic syndromes. *J Clin Oncol* 1986;4:1857.
88. Miller KB, Kim K, Morrison FS, et al. The evaluation of low-dose ara-C in the treatment of myelodysplastic syndromes—a phase III intergroup study. *Ann Hematol* 1992;65:162.
89. Gerhartz H, Marcus R, Delmer A, et al. A randomized phase II study of low-dose cytosine arabinoside (LD-ara-C) plus granulocyte-macrophage colony-stimulating factor (rhGM-CSF) in myelodysplastic syndromes (MDS) with a high risk of developing leukemia. *Leukemia* 1994;8:16.
90. Mertelsmann R, Thaler HT, To L, et al. Morphological classification, response to therapy, and survival in 263 adult patients with acute nonlymphoblastic leukemia. *Blood* 1980;56:773.
91. Armitage JO, Dick FR, Needleman SW, et al. Effect of chemotherapy for the dysmyelopoietic syndrome. *Cancer Treat Rep* 1981;65:601.
92. De Witte T, Suciu S, Peetermans M, et al. Intensive chemotherapy for poor prognosis myelodysplasia (MDS) and secondary acute myeloid leukemia (sAML) following MDS of more than 6 months duration: a pilot study by the Leukemia Cooperative Group of the European Organization for Research and Treatment in Cancer (EORTC-LCG). *Leukemia* 1995;9:1805.
93. Estey E. Treatment of acute myelogenous leukemia and myelodysplastic syndromes. *Semin Hematol* 1995;32:132.
94. Parker JE, Pagliuga A, Mijovic A, et al. Fludarabine, cytarabine, G-CSF and idarubicin (FLAG-IDA) for the treatment of poor-risk myelodysplastic syndromes and acute myeloid leukemia. *Br J Haematol* 1997;99:939.
95. Fenaux P, Morel P, Rose C, et al. Prognostic factors in adult de novo myelodysplastic syndromes treated by intensive chemotherapy. *Br J Haematol* 1991;77:497.
96. Ruutu T, Hanninen A, Jarventie G, et al. Intensive chemotherapy of poor prognosis myelodysplastic syndromes and acute myeloid leukemia following MDS with idarubicin and cytarabine. *Leuk Lymphoma* 1997;21:133.
97. Invernizzi R, Pecci A, Rossi G, et al. Idarubicin and cytosine arabinoside in the induction and maintenance therapy of high-risk myelodysplastic syndromes. *Haematologica* 1997;82:9.
98. Economopoulos T, Papageorgiou E, Stathakis N, et al. Treatment of high-risk myelodysplastic syndromes with idarubicin and cytosine arabinoside supported by granulocyte-macrophage colony-stimulating factor. *Leuk Lymphoma* 1995;20:385.
99. Wattel E, de Botton S, Lai J, et al. Long-term follow-up of de novo myelodysplastic syndromes treated with intensive chemotherapy: incidence of long-term survivors and outcome of partial responders. *Br J Haematol* 1997;98:983.
100. Bernstein SH, Brunetto VL, Davey FR, et al. Acute myeloid leukemia-type chemotherapy for newly diagnosed patients without antecedent cytopenias having myelodysplastic syndrome as defined by French-American-British criteria: a Cancer and Leukemia Group B study. *J Clin Oncol* 1996;14:2486.
101. Loffler H, Schmitz N, Gassmann W. Intensive chemotherapy and bone marrow transplantation for myelodysplastic syndromes. *Hematol Oncol Clin North Am* 1992;6:619.
102. Anderson JE, Appelbaum FR, Schoch G, et al. Allogeneic marrow transplantation for myelodysplastic syndrome with advanced disease morphology: a phase II study of busulfan, cyclophosphamide, and total-body irradiation and analysis of prognostic factors. *J Clin Oncol* 1996;14:220.
103. Casto-Malaspina H, Childs B, Gillio A, et al. Improved disease-free survival in patients with low risk (<5% marrow blasts) myelodysplastic syndromes treated with HLA-identical sibling-derived T-cell depleted (SBA-E) marrow transplants. *Blood* 1994;34:518A(abst).
104. Appelbaum F, Anderson J. Allogeneic bone marrow transplantation for myelodysplastic syndrome-outcomes analysis according to IPSS score. *Leukemia* 1998;12(Suppl 1):S25.
105. de Witte T, van Biezen A, Hermans J, et al. Autologous bone marrow transplantation for patients with myelodysplastic syndrome (MDS) or acute myeloid leukemia following MDS. *Blood* 1997;90:3863.
106. Anderson J, Anasetti C, Appelbaum F, et al. Unrelated donor marrow transplantation for myelodysplasia (MDS) and MDS-related acute myeloid leukemia. *Br J Haematol* 1996; 93:59.
107. Beran M, Estey E, O'Brien S, et al. Results of topotecan single-agent therapy in patients with myelodysplastic syndromes and chronic myelomonocytic leukemia. *Leuk Lymphoma* 1998;31:521.
108. Vey N, Kantarjian H, Tran H, et al. Phase I and pharmacologic study of 9-aminocamptothecin colloidal dispersion formulation in patients with refractory or relapsed acute leukemia. *Ann Oncol* 1999;10:577.
109. Kantarjian H, Cortes J, O'Brien S, et al. 9-nitro-20-(S)-camptothecin (9-NC, RFS2000): an effective agent for treatment of chronic myelogenous leukemia (CML). *Am Soc Clin Oncol* 1999:83.
110. Baylin SB, Herman JG, Graff JR, et al. Alterations in DNA methylation—a fundamental aspect of neoplasia. *Adv Cancer Res* 1998;72:141.
111. Daskalakis MNTT, Wijermans P, Jomes PA, Lubbert M. Frequent hypermethylation of p15/INK4B in patients with myelodysplastic syndromes is decreased following treatment with 5-aza-2'-deoxycytidine (decitabine). *Blood* 1998;92(Suppl 1):715a.
112. Silverman LR, Demakos EP, Peterson B, et al. A randomized controlled trial of subcutaneous azacytidine (AZA C) in patients with myelodysplastic syndromes (MDS): a study of the Cancer and Leukemia Group B. *Am Soc Clin Oncol* 1998;34:12a.
113. Kornblith AB, Silverman LR. The impact of 5-azacytidine on the quality of life of patients with myelodysplastic syndrome (MDS) treated in a randomized phase III trial of the Cancer and Leukemia Group B. *Am Soc Clin Oncol* 1998;34:189.
114. Wijermans P, Luebbert M, Verhoef G, et al. DNA demethylating therapy in MDS—the experience with 5-aza-2'-deoxycytidine (decitabine). *Blood* 1999;94(Suppl 1):306a.
115. Kantarjian H, Keating M, McCredie K, Freireich E. Phase II study of homoharringtonine in refractory acute myelogenous leukemia. *Cancer* 1989;63:813.
116. Feldman EJ, Seiter KP, Ahmed T, Baskind P, Arlin ZA. Homoharringtonine in patients with myelodysplastic syndrome (MDS) and MDS evolving to acute myeloid leukemia. *Leukemia* 1996;10:40.
117. List A, Holmes H, Greenberg P, Bennett J, Oster W. Phase II study of amifostine in patients with myelodysplastic syndromes. *Blood* 1999;94(Suppl 1):305a.
118. Bowen DT, Denzlinger C, Brugger W, et al. Poor response rate to a continuous schedule of amifostine therapy for "low/intermediate risk" myelodysplastic patients. *Br J Haematol* 1998;103:785.
119. Biesma DH, van den Tweel JG, Vendonck LF. Immunosuppressive therapy for hypoplastic myelodysplastic syndrome. *Cancer* 1997;70:1548.
120. Molldrem JJ, Caples M, Mavroudis D, et al. Antithymocyte globulin for patients with myelodysplastic syndrome. *Br J Haematol* 1997;99:699.
121. Jonasova A, Neuwirtova R, Cermak J, et al. Cyclosporin A therapy in hypoplastic MDS patients and certain refractory anemias without hypoplastic bone marrow. *Br J Haematol* 1998;100:304.
122. Caron PC, Dumont L, Scheinberg DA. Supersaturating infusional humanized anti-CD33 monoclonal antibody HuM195 in myelogenous leukemia. *Clin Cancer Res* 1998;4:1421.
123. Nemunaitis J, Rosenfield C, Getty L, et al. Pentoxifylline and ciprofloxacin in patients with myelodysplastic syndrome. *Am J Clin Oncol* 1995;18:189.
124. Thomas DA, Aguayo A, Estey E, et al. Thalidomide as anti-angiogenesis therapy in refractory or relapsed leukemias. *Blood* 1999;94(Suppl 1):507a(abstr).
125. Raza A, Lisak L, Andrews C, et al. Thalidomide produces transfusion independence in patients with long-standing refractory anemias and myelodysplastic syndromes. *Blood* 1999;94(Suppl 1):661a(abst).
126. Wattel E, Preudhomme C, Hecquet B, et al. p53 mutations are associated with resistance to chemotherapy and short survival in hematologic malignancies. *Blood* 1994;84:3148.
127. Bishop MR, Iversen PL, Bayever E, et al. Phase I trial of an antisense oligonucleotide OL(1)p53 in hematologic malignancies. *J Clin Oncol* 1996;14:1320.
128. Nand S, Stock W, Stiff P, et al. A phase II trial of interleukin-2 in myelodysplastic syndromes. *Br J Haematol* 1998;101:205.
129. Rosenfeld CS, Zeigler ZR, Shadduck RK, Nilsson B. Phase II study of roquinimex in myelodysplastic syndrome. *Am J Clin Oncol* 1997;20:189.
130. Sharma S, Raymond E, Soda H, et al. Preclinical and clinical strategies for development of telomerase and telomere inhibitors. *Ann Oncol* 1997;8:1063.
131. Rowinsky EK, Windle JJ, Von Hoff DD. Ras protein farnesyltransferase: a strategic target for anticancer therapeutic development. *J Clin Oncol* 1999;17:3631.
132. Rowinsky EK, Conley BA, Jones RJ, et al. Hexamethylene bisacetamide in myelodysplastic syndrome: effect of five-day exposure to maximal therapeutic concentrations. *Leukemia* 1992;6:526.

Susanne M. Arnold Andrew M. Lowy
Roy Patchell Kenneth A. Foon

CHAPTER 47

Paraneoplastic Syndromes

Tumors may produce signs and symptoms at sites distant from the primary tumor or its metastases and these are referred to as *paraneoplastic syndromes.* The syndromes may be due to (1) tumor production of substances that directly or indirectly cause distant symptoms, (2) depletion of normal substances that leads to a paraneoplastic manifestation, or (3) host response to the tumor that results in the syndrome. The evidence for the existence of a paraneoplastic syndrome may range from the mere association of the syndrome with the presence of an actively growing tumor to the cloning of the gene responsible for the syndrome. Among the best characterized of the paraneoplastic syndromes are those producing polypeptide hormones, such as adrenocorticotropin (ACTH) or parathyroid hormone, that affect organ function at remote sites. In such situations, the paraneoplastic syndrome parallels the underlying malignancy, and treatment of the underlying tumor leads to disappearance of the hormone. Additional tumor-derived proteins responsible for paraneoplastic syndromes have been identified, including various growth factors and cytokines such as interleukin-1 (IL-1) and tumor necrosis factor (TNF). Antibodies produced by certain malignancies may lead to neurologic paraneoplastic syndromes such as the Eaton-Lambert syndrome. Many paraneoplastic syndromes, especially those of an immune etiology, do not respond to treatment of the underlying malignancy.

The paraneoplastic syndrome may be the first sign of a malignancy, and its recognition may be critical for early cancer detection. Certain paraneoplastic syndromes that secrete proteins can be used as tumor markers in monitoring patients before and after therapy. In some situations, the underlying disease cannot be treated, but the symptoms and complications of the paraneoplastic syndrome must be treated. This chapter reviews the wide range of paraneoplastic syndromes including the endocrinologic, hematologic, gastrointestinal (GI), renal, cutaneous, and neurologic paraneoplastic syndromes.

ENDOCRINOLOGIC MANIFESTATIONS OF CANCER

Endocrine syndromes of cancer are caused by the tumor's direct production of hormones, hormone-precursors, or cytokines, as well as cancer metabolism of steroids to active forms.[1]

ECTOPIC ADRENOCORTICOTROPIC HORMONE SYNDROME

In 1928, Brown first described the syndrome of ectopic ACTH overproduction, when he reported a patient with small cell lung carcinoma and associated hirsutism, diabetes mellitus, hypertension, and adrenal hyperplasia.[2] The syndrome was further characterized in 1965 when 88 patients with Cushing's syndrome and cancer were described.[3] This report was the first to suggest that tumors produced ACTH or an ACTH-like substance, which led to adrenal hyperplasia and hypercortisolism, coining the term *ectopic ACTH production.* Subsequently, propiomelanocortin (POMC), the precursor hormone of ACTH, was described, containing not only ACTH, but melanocyte stimulating hormone, β-lipotropin, endorphins, and enkephalins.[4–6]

Many normal tissues produce minute amounts of POMC, while carcinomas produce higher quantities, and in some instances can convert these to active ACTH, producing the Cushing's syndrome. Patients with ectopic ACTH syndrome have a much higher ratio of ACTH precursors to endogenous ACTH, when compared with patients with Cushing's disease (hypercortisolism secondary to a pituitary adenoma).[7] The molecular con-

TABLE 47-1. Tumors Associated with Ectopic Adrenocorticotropic Hormone

Tumor type	*Liddle, Island, Ney, et al. (3)*	*Crapo (10)*	*Howlett, Drury, Perry, et al. (22)*	*Wajchenberg, Mendonca, Liberman, et al. (11)*	*Odell (1)*
Small cell lung carcinoma	50	49	19	8	50
Bronchial carcinoid	8	8	37	17	2
Thymic carcinomas	10	12	12	25	10
Pancreas	10	6	12	25	10
Pheochromocytoma	3	2	6	25	5
Medullary cancer of the thyroid	2	6			5
Gastrointestinal carcinoid	6				
Adenocarcinoma	7	2			
Miscellaneous	10	10	12		18

trol of this process lies in the fact that three promoter regions control transcription of the POMC gene. In normal pituitary glands the P_2 promoter is active, while in cancer-associated ACTH production, the P_1 promoter predominates.[8] It is postulated that loss of tumor suppressor genes leads to overproduction of the C-fos oncogene, which leads to increased POMC gene expression, along with many other proteins in the oncogenic cascade.[9] Some neoplasms then convert pro-ACTH to active ACTH, resulting in the ectopic ACTH syndrome.[1]

Ectopic ACTH is commonly associated with small cell carcinoma of the lung, but can also be found in a variety of neoplasms (Table 47-1). While 3% to 7% of patients with small cell carcinoma of the lung develop Cushing's syndrome, many patients with small cell carcinoma of the lung secrete ACTH precursors without the development of the syndrome.[10]

Clinical Presentation

Cushing's initial description of the peripheral effects of a hyperfunctioning pituitary adenoma included truncal obesity, purple striae, hypertension, fatigue, moon facies, buffalo hump, weakness, depression, amenorrhea, hirsutism, and edema. The differential diagnosis of a patient with hypercortisolism includes Cushing's disease, adrenal dysfunction, ectopic ACTH production, and corticotropin-releasing hormone (CRH) overproduction. Pituitary overproduction (Cushing's disease) is the most common etiology, occurring in 55% to 82% of patients, while adrenal dysfunction occurs in 5% to 32%, ectopic ACTH production in 11% to 25%, and CRH overproduction in less than 1% to 2%.[11–14] Although signs and symptoms of hypercortisolism are not specific, several features of ectopic ACTH production are distinguishing: Myopathy with weakness, muscle wasting, hyperpigmentation, and hypokalemia are more common in ectopic ACTH production. Cushing's disease is more common in young women (3 to 1), whereas older men (at higher risk for lung cancer) typically have ectopic ACTH production.[10] Commonly, hirsutism, severe hypertension, and hyperpigmentation are noted on physical evaluation, while glucose intolerance, hypokalemia, and metabolic alkalosis make up the usual biochemical profile. The hypokalemia can be severe and life threatening.

Diagnosis

Distinguishing between pituitary adenoma, ectopic ACTH production, and primary adrenal disorders is the primary focus of the diagnostic workup (Fig. 47-1). The two most common screening tests for cortisol overproduction are the 24-hour urinary free cortisol and the low-dose dexamethasone suppression test. In normal subjects cortisol production should be suppressed by a relatively low dose of dexamethasone, whereas patients with Cushing's disease or ectopic ACTH production are not affected.

With reliable radioassays of ACTH, plasma levels can be determined early in the diagnostic workup. In primary adrenal disease, ACTH levels are low, while in ACTH-dependent Cushing's syndrome the ACTH level is elevated.[14] Classically, plasma ACTH and ACTH precursor levels in ectopic ACTH production are much higher than in Cushing's disease (pituitary adenoma);

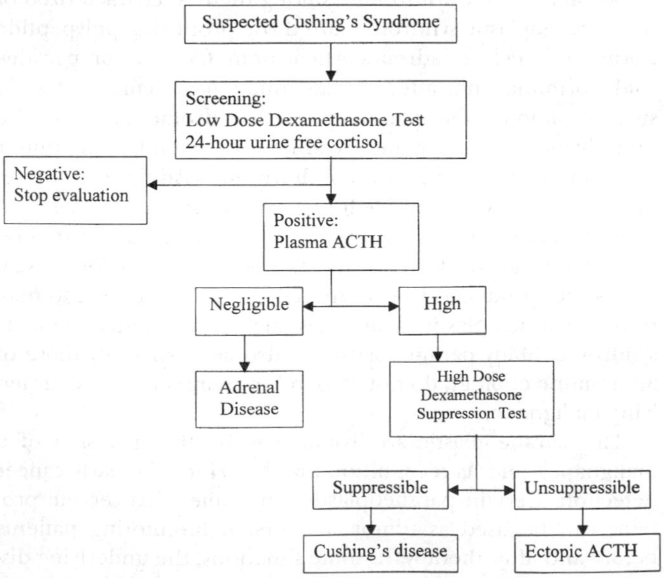

FIGURE 47-1. Diagnostic algorithm for the evaluation of patients with suspected Cushing's syndrome. See text for details of various tests. ACTH, adrenocorticotropic hormone.

however, there is a great deal of overlap, particularly in the case of slow-growing malignancies such as bronchial carcinoids. Once primary adrenal disease is eliminated, with normal or elevated ACTH levels, a high-dose dexamethasone suppression test is indicated. High-dose dexamethasone suppresses cortisol production (and thus the urinary study results) in patients with Cushing's disease but not ectopic ACTH production or primary adrenal disorders.[10] False-positive dexamethasone suppression test results are seen when dexamethasone is metabolized more rapidly than normal. Drugs such as diphenylhydantoin, phenobarbital, and primidone, as well as disease states such as thyrotoxicosis cause rapid dexamethasone metabolism. Furthermore, bronchial carcinoids can have ACTH and cortisol suppression with high-dose dexamethasone testing in 40% to 50% of cases.[15]

While the reliability of the dexamethasone suppression test is good, the test is cumbersome and its performance characteristics (sensitivity and specificity) are not perfect. For these reasons, the metyrapone and CRH stimulation tests have been developed. In both tests the sensitivity of pituitary adenoma to stimulation by either cortisol deprivation (metyrapone) or directly (CRH) is exploited. Metyrapone blocks the production of cortisol in the adrenal by inhibiting the conversion of 11-deoxycortisol to cortisol, leading to an increased ACTH secretion in normal patients, thus testing the integrity of the adrenal-cortisol-pituitary feedback loop. Patients with Cushing's disease show stimulated ACTH production, whereas ectopic ACTH production is unaffected. In the largest reported study, the metyrapone test correctly predicted Cushing's in 71% of patients with ACTH-dependent Cushing's syndrome. The combination of the dexamethasone suppression test and the metyrapone test predicted 82% of the cases (significantly better than either test alone).[16] Similarly, pituitary adenomas are generally responsive to ovine CRH stimulation, while ectopic ACTH-producing tumors are not. In one report of 41 patients with ACTH-dependent hypercortisolism, 29 of 33 patients with pituitary adenoma were stimulated with ovine CRH, whereas none of the 8 patients with ectopic ACTH production were stimulated.[17] This led to a sensitivity of 88%, a specificity of 100%, and a diagnostic accuracy of 90%, which compared favorably with the standard dexamethasone suppression test. Again, the combination of CRH stimulation and dexamethasone suppression led to a superior diagnostic accuracy of 98%.

Other evaluations that are more invasive or less well established in diagnosing Cushing's syndrome include inferior petrosal blood sampling with or without CRH stimulation,[18] continuous dexamethasone infusion,[19] and serum chromogranin A.[20] Inferior petrosal venous samples show a marked gradient with peripheral samples in pituitary adenoma. The diagnostic accuracy is high, but the test is expensive and invasive. One hundred twenty-one patients were evaluated with 7-hour continuous infusion dexamethasone at 1 mg/h. The sensitivity for pituitary disease was 100%, the specificity was 90%, and the diagnostic accuracy was 98%. This evaluation was thought to be more convenient and accurate, but these results have not been confirmed. Serum chromogranin A has been shown to be a potential marker of ectopic production. The results, at this point, are preliminary, however.

Treatment

Localization is the most important aspect of therapy. Since a major portion of patients with ectopic ACTH have lung cancer, chest evaluation is initially in order. Plain radiographs followed by computed tomography (CT) detect more than 90% of the lung tumors associated with ACTH production.[11,21,22] The exception is bronchial carcinoid tumors, which are visualized on 36% of initial radiographs, but are localized by CT scan in approximately 85% of cases.[23] Octreotide receptor scintigraphy has been promoted for localizing ACTH-producing tumors, because many such tumors have octreotide receptors.[24] An additional advantage of localizing tumors with octreotide receptor scintigraphy is the suggestion of possible therapy with either somatostatin analogues or radiolabeled octreotide.

TABLE 47-2. Drugs Used for Treating Ectopic Adrenocorticotropic Hormone Production

Drug	*Dose*
Ketoconazole	400–1200 mg/d
Metyrapone	500–4000 mg/d
Aminoglutethimide	500–2000 mg/d
Mitotane	4–12 g/d
Sandostatin	300–1500 μg/d

Surgery is the treatment of choice in patients with early-stage tumors producing Cushing's syndrome because it can completely alleviate symptoms. In one series of 41 patients with ectopic ACTH and absence of small cell cancer of the lung, 16 of 21 (76%) patients with localized tumors were cured of Cushing's syndrome with surgery. Specifically, 81% of bronchial carcinoid tumors were cured with resection, and 9 of 12 (75%) patients with occult ACTH production were palliated with bilateral adrenalectomy.[25] While bilateral adrenal removal is effective in treating Cushing's syndrome, the patient must have lifelong glucocorticoid and mineralocorticoid replacement. Patients with severe muscle weakness and uncontrolled hypertension are candidates for this approach. The use of laparoscopic adrenalectomy has been reported to effectively palliate patients with Cushing's with minimal morbidity and no mortality reported.[26]

The majority of patients do not have surgically resectable disease and may have ongoing symptoms related to Cushing's syndrome. Medical therapy for ectopic ACTH production centers on inhibiting cortisol production with mitotane, aminoglutethimide, metyrapone, or ketoconazole (Table 47-2).[27–29] Mitotane is effective in lowering cortisol levels; however, it is rarely used because of its severe toxicity and slow onset of action. Aminoglutethimide is used in only limited situations, because of incomplete responses. Metyrapone is an effective treatment, particularly in combination with aminoglutethimide. Because of its rapid onset of action and favorable toxicity profile, ketoconazole has evolved as the therapy of choice for ectopic ACTH. In one small study, 66% of patients with ectopic ACTH production had a hormonal response and symptomatic improvement with ketoconazole at a dose of 400 to 1200 mg/d. A minority developed symptomatic hypoadrenalism.

Suppression of primary ACTH production can be accomplished by two means: cytotoxic chemotherapy, for the primary problem, and octreotide suppression of ACTH release. In general, chemotherapy alone is not associated with control of Cushing's syndrome, but is combined with adrenal suppression in most cases. As well, if patients show significant localization with octreotide receptor scintigraphy, a trial of octreotide may be in order. In one small study of ten patients treated with octreotide, four had significant rapid responses.[30] The combination of ketoconazole and octreotide has also been reported.[31]

SYNDROME OF INAPPROPRIATE ANTIDIURETIC HORMONE

The syndrome of inappropriate antidiuretic hormone production (SIADH) was first reported in two patients with lung cancer and hyponatremia.[32] The proposed etiology was an abnormal production of ADH or an ADH-like substance by the cancer. In 1968, arginine vasopressin (ADH) was extracted from cancers associated with this syndrome, confirming the original hypothesis.[33] While the majority of small cell lung tumors positively stain for arginine vasopressin by radioimmune assay,[34–36] only 3% to 15% of patients with small cell lung carcinoma have this syndrome.[37,38] Clearly, as with ectopic ACTH production, the vast majority of tumors that contain these substances does not produce the clinical syndrome.

The pathophysiology of SIADH is well described. After vasopressin is released, it binds to specific receptors in the renal collecting ducts and ascending limb of the loop of Henle. Excess water is reabsorbed and increased sodium is delivered to the distal nephron. This increases intravascular volume, which in turn increases renal perfusion and decreases proximal tubular resorption of sodium. ADH secretion continues in SIADH despite the decrease in plasma osmolality, causing eventual hyponatremia.[39,40]

Clinical Features and Diagnosis

The cardinal features of SIADH are water intoxication and hyponatremia, including the following principal findings: decreased serum osmolarity, inappropriate elevation of urine osmolarity with urine sodium levels greater than 20 mEq/L, euvolemia (absence of hypovolemia), normal renal function, normal adrenal function, and normal thyroid function. Most patients are asymptomatic, but when symptoms develop they generally reflect central nervous system toxicity. In its early stages, patients complain of fatigue, anorexia, headaches, and mild altered mental status. As the syndrome progresses, patients may experience continued delirium, confusion, fatigue, and seizures. Ultimately, patients develop refractory seizures, coma, and rarely death. Most patients, however, experience minimal symptoms and are discovered on routine laboratory evaluation when they have hyponatremia.

In evaluating a patient with hyponatremia and cancer, other causes of hyponatremia need to be considered. In general, the first step in evaluating patients with hyponatremia is to assess volume status. SIADH is one of the so-called euvolemic hyponatremic states. Therefore, it is necessary to eliminate states associated with volume overload such as congestive heart failure, nephrotic syndrome, malignant ascites, and significant liver disease. It is also essential to exclude extrarenal volume depletion and renal sodium wasting. Once the patient is determined to be euvolemic, other causes of euvolemic hyponatremia must be ruled out, including hypothyroidism, renal dysfunction, and Addison's disease. A careful review of medications is also essential.

Once the diagnosis of SIADH is made, a wide variety of etiologies must be considered, including central nervous system diseases, pulmonary diseases, and drugs. Tumor-associated SIADH is a diagnosis of exclusion. For the purposes of treatment, however, differentiating tumor-related SIADH from other causes of SIADH is not necessary. Of note, it is rarely necessary to perform a water-loading test in order to make the diagnosis of SIADH. Because these patients are often unable to excrete free water, they can develop significant water intoxication, leading to serious morbidity in this setting.

The principal malignancy associated with SIADH is small cell lung carcinoma, although others have been described (non–small cell lung cancer, head and neck cancers, and others). Seventy-five percent of all SIADH associated with malignancy is secondary to small cell lung carcinoma. Previously it was proposed that SIADH was a marker of tumor burden as well as a negative prognostic factor.[41] However, more recent reports have indicated that SIADH is neither an indicator of poor outcome nor disease burden.[42] Indeed, many patients with small cell lung carcinoma only develop SIADH after treatment.[43] Of interest, several chemotherapeutic agents commonly used in oncology cause transient SIADH including vincristine, vinblastine, vinorelbine, ifosfamide, cyclophosphamide, and cisplatin.[44–46]

Treatment

As with any syndrome associated with ectopic hormone production, treating the underlying disease is the most effective means of controlling SIADH. Chemotherapy treatment of the associated small cell lung cancer is generally associated with improvement in the syndrome. SIADH has not been shown to be a negative prognostic factor in terms of response to chemotherapy. In situations in which brain metastases are present, the addition of radiation therapy is important. Because surgery is not generally thought to be an effective modality in patients with small cell lung cancer, surgery is rarely undertaken in patients with malignancy-associated SIADH. In chemotherapy-related SIADH, the offending drug should be stopped.

Supportive measures such as fluid restriction and pharmacologic therapy can be undertaken to treat SIADH. Patients with sodium levels under 130 mmol/L are placed on a free water restriction (500 mL/d), in addition to treatment of the primary malignancy.[47] In the event that this measure does not bring the serum sodium above 130 mmol/L, pharmacologic agents such as demeclocycline can be instituted. Demeclocycline inhibits the effect of arginine vasopressin on the kidneys.[48] The recommended dose of demeclocycline is 600 to 1200 mg/d in divided doses. Other less common medications that have reported efficacy include fludrocortisone, urea, and lithium. Finally, in severe cases in which patients have life-threatening convulsions or coma, patients can be treated with hypertonic saline solution with intravenous furosemide. It is important not to raise the serum sodium too rapidly (the recommendation is 1 mEq/L/h) due to the risk of central pontine myelinolysis.[49] It is generally thought that hypertonic saline and Lasix treatment should be carried out in the intensive care unit setting.

HYPOCALCEMIA

Although most of the discussion regarding disturbance of calcium balance and malignancy revolves around hypercalcemia, hypocalcemia is actually more common in patients with bone metastases.[50,51] Tumors associated with lytic bone metastases such as breast, prostate, and lung cancers, can lead to hypocalcemia.[52,53] Also, rarely, hypocalcemia can occur in patients whose tumors secrete calcitonin (i.e., medullary carcinoma of the thyroid). More common than hypercalcemia, hypocalcemia is rarely symptomatic. Patients occasionally develop the features of hypocalcemia such as tetany and neuromuscular irritability, but can show mild neuromuscular dysfunction by electromyography. Therapy, consisting of calcium infusion, is reserved for those patients with findings of neuromuscular irritability or symptoms such as tetany and seizures. Signs of neuromuscular irritability including Chvostek's sign and Trousseau's sign (carpal spasm with decreased blood flow) indicate the need for calcium infusion. For a discussion of hypercalcemia, please refer to the chapter on Metabolic Emergencies (see Chapter 51.3).

ONCOGENOUS OSTEOMALACIA

Rickets is a well-recognized inborn error of metabolism, while the adult counterpart, osteomalacia, is usually secondary to intestinal malabsorption syndrome, renal tubular acidosis, and chronic renal insufficiency. Oncogenous osteomalacia is a rare syndrome characterized by osteomalacia, hypophosphatemia, hyperphosphaturia, and decreased vitamin D levels. Mean age at diagnosis is approximately 35 years. Patients typically present with bone pain, phosphaturia, renal glycosuria, hypophosphatemia, normocalcemia with normal parathyroid hormone function, low 1,25-$(OH)_2$-D_3, and increased alkaline phosphatase. The proposed mechanisms include inhibition of the conversion of 1,25-dihydroxyvitamin D and a tumor-secreted *phosphaturic substance.* It is usually associated with benign mesenchymal tumors including hemangiomas and hemangiopericytomas, but rarely is seen with multiple myeloma and prostate cancer.[54–58] The typical tumor involves prominent giant cells, spindle cells, and a high degree of vascularity. Approximately one-half of the tumors are in the lower extremities, and the remaining tumors are divided between the head and upper extremities with some patients having tumors at multiple sites. The definitive therapy is removal of the tumor, if possible. Otherwise, treatment requires large doses of vitamin D and phosphate.

CALCITONIN PRODUCTION BY TUMORS

Calcitonin is a polypeptide hormone that is produced by C cells of the thyroid. Calcitonin prevents calcium release from bone and causes increased renal excretion of calcium, sodium, and phosphate.[59] Because medullary thyroid carcinoma produces calcitonin, calcitonin serum levels are a sensitive tumor marker to monitor this disease. They are also useful in identifying patients with multiple endocrine neoplasia type 2, a familial disorder involving an association of medullary carcinoma of the thyroid, pheochromocytoma, and parathyroid adenomas.

A variety of tumors, including small cell lung cancer, carcinoids, breast cancer, and GI cancer also may secrete calcitonin.[60–62] While calcitonin levels may reflect clinical tumor status in these diseases, they are not used as tumor markers. Furthermore, there is no known paraneoplastic syndrome associated with calcitonin.

CHROMOGRANIN A

Chromogranin A is a 68-kD glycoprotein found in the neurosecretory granules of normal and malignant amine precursor uptake and decarboxylation cells.[63,64] Chromogranin A is released into the circulation via exocytosis from neuroendocrine storage vesicles. It may act in neuroendocrine secretion by binding intravesicular calcium. Its sequence is nearly identical to pancreastatin, which inhibits insulin and somatostatin secretion from the pancreas.[65] As with calcitonin, it is unknown whether chromogranin A is associated with a paraneoplastic syndrome. Chromogranin A secretion is most commonly associated with small cell lung cancer and neuroendocrine tumors.[66–68]

GONADOTROPINS

The human hormones with gonadotropic properties are follicle-stimulating hormone (FSH), luteinizing hormone (LH), and human chorionic gonadotropin (HCG).[69] These three hormones are composed of two polypeptide chains; α and β subunits. The α subunit is common to all of the hormones and the β subunit determines biologic and immunologic specificity. Both subunits are required for bioactivity. In normal individuals, the pituitary produces FSH and LH. Biologically active HCG is produced by the placenta and is therefore normally found only in pregnant women. Because the levels of FSH and LH vary under normal physiologic conditions, the β-HCG hormone is typically used for following paraneoplastic syndromes.

Gonadotropin secretion may occur in pituitary tumors, gestational trophoblastic tumors, germ cell tumors, hepatoblastomas in children, bronchogenic carcinomas, and GI cancers.[70–73] Gonadotropins measured in tumors arising in gestational tissue, testes, ovaries, and endocrine organs are valuable tumor markers and are discussed in the following chapters: Cancers of the Endocrine System, Gynecologic Tumors, Cancer of the Ovary, and Cancer of the Testes.

Although many studies have suggested elevations in HCG in a number of common tumors, it may also be elevated in nonmalignant chronic diseases. Values for the α and β subunits of HCG are significantly higher in cancer patients than in patients with nonmalignant disease.[69,74] Elevations of β-FSH, thyroid-stimulating hormone-β, and β-LH have not been observed. With rare exceptions, however, these markers are not routinely used to follow common cancers.

The frequency of symptoms associated with tumor-produced gonadotropin is unknown. The most common problem is a male patient presenting with unexplained gynecomastia. In this situation, a β-HCG determination should be performed as well as a careful examination of the testes and radiographic examination of the chest and mediastinum. Germ cell tumors of the testes or extragonadal sites and lung cancers are the most frequent causes of the combination of gynecomastia and HCG elevation.[75] Other extragonadal tumors that produce HCG include lung cancer, adrenal carcinoma, hepatoma, GI tract tumors, and tumors of the genitourinary tract.[76–82] Histologic specimens have revealed that all of these tumors contain syncytial giant cells or choriocarcinomatous elements similar to trophoblastic germ cell tumors. Conversely, 40% of patients with extragonadal germ cell tumors *masquerading* as poorly differentiated carcinomas had immunohistochemical staining for β-HCG and α-fetoprotein without serum elevation of these markers.[83] Many of these patients responded to chemotherapy, as would be expected of germ cell tumors.

TUMOR-PRODUCED HUMAN PLACENTAL LACTOGEN, GROWTH HORMONE–RELEASING HORMONE, PROLACTIN, AND THYROTROPIC SUBSTANCE

Human placental lactogen (hPL) has been detected in a small percentage of patients with nontrophoblastic nongonadal tumors.[84,85] This may be associated with elevated levels of estrogen, HCG, and gynecomastia. hPL in nonpregnant women is diagnostic of malignancy.[85]

Elevated growth hormone levels have been reported in rare patients with gastric and lung cancer.[86] Whether this is due to ectopic production or overproduction by cells that retain the ability to secrete growth hormone from primordial origin remains controversial.

Growth hormone–releasing hormone production has been reported in nonpituitary tumors and, like pituitary tumors, results in acromegaly.[87–89] This 44 amino acid peptide has been isolated from pancreatic tumors as well as bronchial and foregut carcinoids. Secretion of growth hormone–releasing hormone can be controlled by administration of long-acting somatostatin analogues. The definitive therapy is removal of the tumor, whenever possible.

Patients with cancers of the lung, colon, breast, ovary, and cervix, as well as hypernephroma have been reported with elevated prolactin levels, and one case was associated with galactorrhea.[90–92] Symptoms can be subtle; male subjects may only exhibit decreased libido, whereas postmenopausal women may have no symptoms. Treatment of the tumor decreases prolactin levels. Because these cases are extremely rare, it is important to exclude the presence of a pituitary lesion in patients with elevated prolactin levels.

Tumor-associated thyroid-stimulating hormone production without thyrotoxicosis has been reported.[93] An association has been reported between hyperthyroidism and gestational trophoblastic disease with biochemical hyperthyroidism.[94] This may also be seen in testicular tumors. In some cases, the excess HCG produced by trophoblastic tumors appears to be the thyroid-stimulating substance.[95]

HYPOGLYCEMIA

Insulinomas frequently produce hypoglycemia; however, hypoglycemia associated with non–islet cell tumors is an unusual paraneoplastic syndrome. Mesenchymal tumors including a variety of sarcomas and mesotheliomas are the most common cause of non–islet cell–induced hypoglycemia. Rarely, adrenal carcinomas, GI cancers, and varied other tumors have been associated.[90,96] These tumors are typically large, often invade the liver, and have a protracted course. The patient may present with typical signs and symptoms of hypoglycemia, including generalized neurologic abnormalities.

These tumors may cause hypoglycemia by a variety of mechanisms including production of nonsuppressible insulin-like growth factors-1 and -2 (IGF-1 and -2), hypermetabolism of glucose, production of substances stimulating ectopic insulin release, massive liver infiltration, production of hepatic glucose inhibitor, insulin binding by an M protein in myeloma, insulin receptor proliferation, or rarely ectopic insulin production.[97–102] The most likely mechanism is tumor production of IGFs (also called *somatomedins*), a family of peptide hormones normally produced by the liver under growth hormone regulation.[103–106] Several reports have specifically identified excess production of PRO-IGF-2, which binds to insulin and IGF receptors in malignancy. This in turn down-regulates growth hormone secretion and decreases hepatic production of IGF-binding proteins with eventual hypoglycemia.[107,108]

The treatment of paraneoplastic hypoglycemia initially involves glucose infusion. Following this, tumor debulking should be carried out, although the long-term effect of debulking is poorly understood. If treatment of the tumor is not possible, then the use of subcutaneous and long-acting intramuscular glucagon or high-dose corticosteroids might be considered.

HEMATOLOGIC MANIFESTATIONS OF CANCER

Paraneoplastic syndromes that involve hematopoietic cells and clotting factors are extremely common. While the etiologies of most of these paraneoplastic abnormalities remain unexplained, advances in the understanding of hormones and growth factors that regulate hematopoiesis has led to a better understanding of some of these disorders.[109,110]

ERYTHROCYTOSIS

Erythrocytosis secondary to a wide variety of tumors is well described in the literature. The most common solid tumor leading to erythrocytosis is renal cell carcinoma, which is often associated with elevated serum erythropoietin levels. Benign renal lesions such as cystic kidneys may also cause erythrocytosis, and other tumors of the kidneys such as Wilms' tumor and hemangiomas rarely cause erythrocytosis. The next most common malignancy leading to erythrocytosis is hepatoma, also likely secondary to erythropoietin production. Cerebellar hemangioblastomas are also known to produce erythrocytosis. Other tumors leading to erythrocytosis include uterine fibroids, adrenal tumors, and pheochromocytomas.[111,112] Adrenal cortical tumors and virilizing ovarian tumors can produce androgenic hormones that may lead to erythrocytosis.[113] Prostaglandins produced from tumors can enhance the effect of erythropoietin and lead to erythrocytosis.

It is still important to rule out other causes of erythrocytosis even in the presence of a tumor. Polycythemia rubra vera is typically associated with elevated white count and platelets as well as splenomegaly. There are obvious causes of polycythemia secondary to arterial desaturation associated with hemoglobulinopathies, carboxyhemoglobin, and so forth. Erythropoietin can be measured from the blood when it is suspected that it is overproduced secondary to a tumor. Erythrocytosis secondary to tumors is usually not high enough to require treatment, but if the hematocrit is extremely high (i.e., greater than 55% for a man or greater than 50% for a woman) phlebotomy can be used. Control of the tumor usually controls the erythrocytosis, as well.

ANEMIA

The most common anemias in cancer patients are the normocytic normochromic anemia of chronic disease, anemia secondary to bone marrow invasion, which may be associated with leukoerythroblastosis, and anemia secondary to chemotherapy and radiation therapy. Normochromic, normocytic anemia, or anemia of cancer, is a common paraneoplastic syndrome, characterized by low serum iron, normal or increased ferritin, normal iron stores, and a low serum erythropoietin level. It is thought that IL-1, TNF, and transforming growth factor-β are produced by tumors and effect a decreased erythropoietin response.[114]

A rare cause of anemia in cancer patients is pure red cell aplasia. The relationship of thymoma and pure red cell aplasia often associated with hypogammaglobulinemia is well described in the literature.[115,116] Pure red cell aplasia may also be associated with a variety of lymphoid malignancies including chronic lymphocytic leukemia (CLL) and large granular lymphocytic lymphoma and leukemia.[117] Rarely, pure red cell aplasia is associated with solid tumor malignancies.

Autoimmune hemolytic anemias are typically associated with B-cell malignancies including CLL and lymphomas,[118,119] and arise secondary to immunoregulatory abnormalities in these diseases, rather than a direct secretion of tumor-derived substances. Hallmarks of the disease are a positive direct antiglobulin test result, elevated reticulocyte count, decreased haptoglobin, and elevated lactate dehydrogenase. Warm antibody hemolytic anemia is most commonly associated with lymphomas, CLL, and mucin-producing adenocarcinomas. Cold agglutinin disease is most common in Waldenström's macroglobulinemia and lymphomas.[120] Autoimmune hemolytic anemia is rarely associated with solid tumor malignancies; however, an association with ovarian, GI, lung, breast, and renal cell cancers has been reported.[121] Corticosteroid treatment appears to be less effective in autoimmune hemolytic anemia associated with carcinomas than in those that are idiopathic or associated with lymphoid malignancies. The Coombs' test result may revert to negative with control of the tumor.

Microangiopathic hemolytic anemia is characterized by fragmentation of red cells and is observed in diseases associated with lesions in small blood vessels such as thrombotic thrombocytopenic purpura, congenital vascular abnormalities, and the hemolytic uremic syndrome. Microangiopathic hemolytic anemia has also been reported in association with malignancy.[122,123] Such patients may have intimal proliferation of arterioles, intravascular tumor growth, or intravascular fibrin precipitation. Thrombocytopenias may also be associated. Disseminated intravascular coagulation (DIC) may contribute to microangiopathic hemolytic anemia in metastatic carcinomas by inducing the red cell fragmentation from fibrin strands. Patients typically have pronounced schistocytosis with *microspherocytes*, which are spherocyte-shaped erythrocytes less than 5 μm in diameter. The reticulocyte count is typically increased and a leukoerythroblastic blood picture may predominate. The mechanism remains unknown. The microangiopathic hemolytic anemia syndrome may respond to effective anticancer therapy. It is typically associated with adenocarcinoma of the GI tract, heart, lung, and prostate, as well as after mitomycin C chemotherapy.

GRANULOCYTOSIS

Granulocytosis with elevation of the white blood cell count above $15 \times 10^9/l$ without infection or leukemia is common in neoplasms.[124–127] Isolated or associated monocytosis is also described.[128] Neoplasms most commonly associated with granulocytosis include Hodgkin's disease, lymphoma, and a variety of solid tumors including gastric, lung, pancreatic, and brain, as well as malignant melanoma. The granulocytosis associated with a paraneoplastic leukemoid reaction consists of mature neutrophils with some band forms seen. This differs significantly from chronic myelogenous leukemia in which there are many more immature cells, basophils, and eosinophils; a decreased leukocyte alkaline phosphatase; elevated vitamin B_{12} and vitamin B_{12}–binding capacity; and the presence of the Philadelphia chromosome. The common mechanism associated with tumor-associated granulocytosis is tumor production of growth factors including granulocyte colony-stimulating factor, granulocyte-macrophage colony-stimulating factor, IL-3, IL-1, and a variety of others.[129,130]

GRANULOCYTOPENIA

Granulocytopenia is typically secondary to chemotherapy, radiation therapy, or tumor infiltration of bone marrow. It is possible in some cases that the tumors may produce a factor that suppresses granulopoiesis by interfering with any number of growth factors. As well, there are rare reports of antibodies against granulocytes in patients with Hodgkin's disease and nonchemotherapy-induced neutropenia.[131] Neutropenia associated with large granular lymphocytic leukemia and lymphoma may be caused by immune dysregulation of T cells. The preferred therapy for severe granulocytopenia is direct stimulation with growth factors including granulocyte colony-stimulating factor, granulocyte-macrophage colony-stimulating factor, or both.

EOSINOPHILIA AND BASOPHILIA

Eosinophilia is commonly associated with Hodgkin's disease and mycosis fungoides and is rarely associated with other lymphomas and solid tumors.[132] The tumor cells may be producing a factor that specifically stimulates eosinophil production. In one study, a tumor-associated eosinophil-stimulating factor was found to be a glycoprotein of 45 kD.[133] Other candidate cytokines include granulocyte-macrophage colony-stimulating factor, IL-3, and IL-5, which are involved in the development and differentiation of eosinophils.[134] Eosinophilia is rarely of sufficiently high counts to lead to symptoms of Löffler's-like syndrome, which is associated with nodular pulmonary infiltrates with cough and fever. Basophilia is associated with chronic myelogenous leukemia and a variety of other myeloproliferative disorders, but is not typically associated with symptoms.[135]

THROMBOCYTOSIS

Thrombocytosis is quite common in cancer patients and may be associated with Hodgkin's disease, lymphomas, and a variety of carcinomas and leukemias.[136] Thrombocytosis is expected early in the course of a variety of myeloproliferative diseases including polycythemia rubra vera and chronic myelogenous leukemia. It is, of course, the hallmark of primary thrombocytosis. Thrombocytosis may also be associated with inflammatory disorders, hemorrhage, iron deficiency, hemolytic anemia, and postsplenectomy. The thrombocytosis secondary to malignancies may be secondary to overproduction of thrombopoietin.[137] Thrombosis and hemorrhage are rarely associated with this paraneoplastic syndrome and treatment is not generally indicated.

THROMBOCYTOPENIA

Thrombocytopenia in cancer patients is typically secondary to chemotherapy, radiation therapy, DIC, or tumor infiltration of bone marrow. A syndrome similar to idiopathic thrombocytopenia purpura is commonly seen in lymphoid malignancies including CLL and lymphomas, as well as Hodgkin's disease. Rarely, solid tumors such as lung, breast, and GI cancers have been associated with a similar syndrome.[138–143] These patients may have bleeding, petechia, and purpura and may respond to high-dose prednisone, splenectomy, or both. Other common causes of thrombocytopenia, such as heparin-induced thrombocytopenia, thiazide diuretics, and a variety of other drugs, should be ruled out. Typical of any other idiopathic thrombocytopenia purpura, the patients have adequate or increased megakaryocytes in the bone marrow associated with the thrombocytopenia and do not respond to transfused platelets.

THROMBOPHLEBITIS

The association of cancer and thrombophlebitis was first observed by Trousseau and this association still bears his name.[144] The incidence of thrombophlebitis in cancer patients is quite common and migratory thrombophlebitis is well documented. Recurrent deep venous thrombosis, warfarin resistance, and thrombosis at unusual sites should increase suspicion of occult malignancy in a patient without a known diagnosis of cancer. The greatest risk of migratory thrombophlebitis is with pancreatic cancer; however, it may be seen in a variety of adenocarcinomas, including breast, ovarian, and prostate cancer.[123] The activation of coagulation by tissue factor is clearly implicated in the patients with solid tumors when compared with normal controls.[145] As well, mucinous adenocarcinomas produce a sialic acid moiety that can activate factor X, causing a hypercoagulable state.[146] It is likely that cancer-related thrombosis represents a complex imbalance of coagulation and fibrinolysis: Increased fibrinogen and platelet catabolism; decreased protein C, S, and antithrombin; direct generation of thrombin; and thrombocytosis all represent abnormalities associated with malignancy.[147]

The treatment, although difficult, must be initiated with heparin; however, it is often unsuccessful and long-term therapy with either warfarin or heparin is typically not satisfactory. Initial reports of the beneficial effects of low-molecular-weight heparin in cancer patients with thrombosis[148] are supported by a retrospective metaanalysis. In this study, a significant reduction in mortality was reported in cancer patients treated with low-molecular-weight heparin compared with those treated with unfractionated heparin for deep venous thrombosis. The cause of reduced mortality appeared to be an indirect effect that persisted well beyond discontinuation of the drug.[149] Treatment of the underlying malignancy is the most definitive therapy, but usually in these particular diseases is also unsuccessful.

COAGULOPATHIES AND DISSEMINATED INTRAVASCULAR COAGULATION

The most common coagulation abnormalities in cancer patients are elevated levels of fibrin or fibrinogen degradation products, thrombocytosis, and hyperfibrinogenemia, representing overcompensated DIC with fibrinolysis. This may be accompanied by an increased synthesis of fibrinogen and various clotting factors and platelets. Overt DIC with consumption of platelets and clotting factors and bleeding is rare and is most commonly associated with acute promyelocytic leukemia and adenocarcinomas.[150] DIC is detected by a combination of abnormal prothrombin time, thrombocytopenia, and hypofibrinogenemia.[151,152] The platelet count is abnormal in more than 90% of cases of DIC. The most useful confirmation test for DIC is the measurement of fibrin degradation products. Identification and treatment of precipitating factors is critical in the management of DIC. Some investigators have advocated replacement of coagulation factors and platelets in combination with heparin. The use of heparin alone is controversial and is more commonly used with thromboembolic or necrotizing complications typically seen in the chronic DIC of malignancy. A variety of other therapies including antiplatelet drugs and fibrinolytic inhibitors and activators have been suggested, but have no proven efficacy. Epsilon amino caproic acid is contraindicated. Treatment of the underlying malignancy is essential.

NONBACTERIAL THROMBOTIC ENDOCARDITIS

Nonbacterial thrombotic endocarditis may lead to thrombotic or hemorrhagic complications and may occur with or without DIC.[153–155] It is characterized by sterile verrucous fibrin platelet lesions in the left-sided heart valves. A typical presentation is emboli to the brain and other organs associated with focal or diffuse neurologic abnormalities. Typical diffuse abnormalities include confusion, seizures, and disorientation. The definitive diagnostic test is cerebral angiography showing multiple arterial occlusions. While some patients may have heart murmurs, the majority do not. Echocardiography picks up vegetations larger than 2 mm. The association of nonbacterial thrombotic endocarditis is most common with adenocarcinoma of the lung. Other adenocarcinomas are less frequently associated, and rarely nonadenocarcinomas, lymphomas, and leukemias are associated.[156] Bleeding may be found in the skin, central nervous system, genitourinary tract, upper respiratory tract, GI tract, and lower respiratory tract. Treatment of the underlying malignancy is the primary therapy. Anticoagulants are not indicated.

GASTROINTESTINAL MANIFESTATIONS OF CANCER

PROTEIN-LOSING ENTEROPATHY

Protein-losing enteropathy is a disorder defined by an excessive loss of serum proteins into the GI tract, which generally leads to hypoproteinemia. It was postulated that the hypoproteinemia associated with protein-losing enteropathy was due to impaired protein synthesis. However, it has been shown that synthesis of proteins in these patients is normal or slightly increased, while the serum half-life of protein such as albumin is dramatically decreased.[157] It has also been shown that enteric loss of proteins contributes to, but is not the sole etiology of, the hypoproteinemia seen in patients with this disorder.[158]

Normally, the GI tract plays a small role in the catabolism of serum proteins.[159] Approximately 10% of all normal protein loss of albumin and globulin loss is through the GI tract.[160] It is thought that malignancy-related protein-losing enteropathy results from the increased mucosal permeability to serum proteins due to abnormal cellular structure, mucosal erosion or ulceration or lymphatic obstruction.[161] Hypoalbuminemia can be seen in virtually any cancer of the GI tract including esophageal, gastric, colonic, and carcinoid syndrome.[162] It has also been described in acquired immunodeficiency syndrome (AIDS) patients with Kaposi's sarcoma.[163] Intestinal involvement of lymphoma including Waldenström's macroglobulinemia, Hodgkin's disease, and non-Hodgkin's lymphoma can lead to protein-losing enteropathy.[164,165]

In contrast to renal protein loss, the protein loss in GI disorders is independent of the size of the protein. Therefore, proteins of various sizes such as albumin, immunoglobulins, and ceruloplasmin all are lost equivalently in contrast to patients with nephrotic syndrome. Once the protein loss becomes greater than the body's ability to synthesize proteins, decreased protein levels in the serum result. Usually, this decline in serum proteins progresses until a new set point is reached. At that point, the protein level stabilizes and a new homeostasis is achieved. Also, of note, in both GI as well as non-GI sources of hypoproteinemia, proteins of long serum half-life (i.e., albumin) tend to be more affected than proteins of shorter serum half-life (i.e., retinol-binding protein). Other serum constituents associated with these proteins may be affected by the hypoproteinemia. Specifically, constituents that depend on carrier proteins, such as iron, copper, and calcium, may be depressed when patients develop hypoproteinemic states.

Clinically, patients with protein-losing enteropathy develop hypoproteinemia. This may or may not be associated with peripheral edema, but is rarely associated with severe edema or anasarca. Despite the fact that globulin levels are depressed, the patients rarely develop opportunistic infections and rarely develop coagulopathy even though clotting factors are also lost. Patients may or may not have other GI symptoms, such as diarrhea.

The diagnosis of protein-losing enteropathy is generally not difficult. Patients are noted to be hypoproteinemic on routine chemistry evaluation. Other sources of hypoproteinemia such as malnutrition and liver disease must be excluded. In the past, cumbersome nuclear studies were performed looking for protein loss in the stool. These have largely been replaced by new techniques using α_1-antitrypsin, a protein, which is not degraded in the lower GI tract. Therefore, if it is lost in excessive amounts it is excreted unchanged in the stool. Clearance of this protein is used to confirm the diagnosis of protein-losing enteropathy.[166] It should be noted that the presence of diarrhea could abnormally influence the interpretation of this study.[166] Also, fecal occult blood can falsely elevate this study result.

Once the diagnosis of protein-losing enteropathy has been made in association with cancer, the treatment consists of treatment of the primary malignancy. In situations with lymphatic obstruction, a low-fat diet should be instituted. Patients frequently require the use of medium-chain triglycerides, which do not require intestinal lymphatic transport. With appropriate treatment of the cancer and dietary therapy, approximately 50% of the patients improve with treatment.[157]

ANOREXIA AND CACHEXIA IN THE CANCER PATIENT

Cancer anorexia-cachexia syndromes (CACS), as it is now referred, is the most common paraneoplastic syndrome, consisting of anorexia, nausea, and weight loss. While it afflicts patients with solid tumors most commonly, more than 50% of all cancer patients have some demonstrable weight loss, and 15% experience loss of greater than 10% of their normal body weight.[167] Survival is negatively affected if a patient has greater than 10% weight loss,[167] in part due to problems with infection and wound healing.[168] Problems associated with weight loss may be exacerbated by treatment with surgery, chemotherapy, or radiation. As well, cancer therapy can lead to new difficulties with food intake such as postoperative ileus, esophagitis, and stomatitis.

Multifactorial derangements in biochemical pathways lead to cancer-related decreased food intake.[162] Tumors produce factors that change the patient's perception of food, particularly taste and smell, which leads to a lack of enjoyment. The central nervous system's control of appetite can be altered by tumor factors,[163] such as serotonin. Local obstruction and abnormal swallowing interfere with food intake when tumors involve these portions of the alimentary tract. Maldigestion and malabsorption may result from obstruction of biliary or pancreatic secretions. When patients become nauseated due to either anatomic factors related to their tumor or as a result of chemotherapy or radiation treatment, they may develop a psychological aversion for food, which is difficult to control.

Cancer patients possess abnormally high serum levels of IL-1β, TNF-α, IL-6, IFN-γ, and serotonin,[169,170] produced as a response to the tumor, rather than by the tumor itself. Administration of these cytokines is capable of reproducing CACS, thus further supporting their role in its etiology.[171] The physiologic changes induced by the tumor through these cytokines are numerous and result in progressive weight loss through a variety of mechanisms (i.e., serotonin changing the taste and smell of food). As well, in cancer patients, there is an increased basal energy expenditure with alterations in carbohydrate, protein, and lipid metabolism. In cases of starvation, weight loss arises primarily from fat stores, whereas in cancer patients there is equal loss of fat and skeletal muscle.[172] Skeletal proteins are frequently sacrificed in accelerated gluconeogenesis with the loss of amino acids and subsequent loss of lean body mass.[173] However, CACS is not solely a state of starvation; the tumor continues to grow while the host is depleted with an increase in total body protein conversion and destruction of peripheral muscle stores.[173] Even when sufficient calories are supplied to patients through various means, the patients are unable to incorporate amino acids into lean body proteins.[173] A cancer-driven inflammatory response can divert resources used for production of normal serum proteins to other organ sites (i.e., liver).[174] Malnourished cancer patients also lose a great deal of their lipid reserve; a decrease in lipoprotein lipase, responsible for moving triglycerides into fat cells, results in weight loss.[175] Treatment with individual anticytokine antibodies reverses specific features of CACS, but no single antibody eradicates all aspects of the syndrome.[176]

When clinically evaluating a cancer patient for CACS, appetite, intake over prior weeks, weight, and weight loss are all critical. In one study, a weight less than 90% of ideal body weight, 10% weight loss over the last 6 months, or both were associated with a poor prognosis.[177] Plasma proteins such as albumin have limited value in evaluating CACS, because they are affected by factors other than nutrient status. Immune responsiveness assessed by delayed type hypersensitivity skin tests, as well as total lymphocyte count, correlate not only with the patient's nutrient status, but also the ability to fight off various infections. In summary, the best means of determining a patient's nutrient status is a history and physical examination by an experienced clinician.

Treating patients with malnutrition and cancer is similar to treating other forms of severe stress such as burns, trauma, and sepsis; the primary objective is adequate caloric intake excluding calories from protein sources. Often the most difficult decision facing the clinician is choosing the route of administration. The widespread availability of total parenteral nutrition has made this an attractive option, particularly when patients are severely anorexic. However, numerous studies have found no survival benefit using total parenteral nutrition in cancer patients, with an increase in infectious and mechanical complications.[178] It has become axiomatic to use the GI tract for nutritional support whenever possible, because it has the benefit of being less expensive and more physiologic, and it maintains gut barrier function. The Harris-Benedict equation is useful for determining basal caloric needs. Generally, stress factors of cancer (estimated at 20% to 30% of the basal metabolic rate) are added to the patient's caloric needs. If other forms of stress are present, such as infection, these factors should be added. In addition to the caloric needs, 1.0 to 1.5 g of protein per kilogram of body weight is also given, and 25% to 40% of nonprotein calories should be in the form of lipid. The enteral formulations have been developed to balance these factors. When total parenteral nutrition is necessary, these same formulas are used for determining calorie protein and lipid intake. Once nutritional support is initiated, a 24-hour urine collection for nitrogen loss should be undertaken. If the patient has no diarrhea, 2 g of nitrogen should be added for insensible losses of nitrogen in the stool. Using these values, a nitrogen balance can be calculated; this balance should be positive, meaning that the patient receives more nitrogen than he or she excretes. This is critical in determining whether the patient is receiving adequate caloric intake.

Pharmacologic approaches to improving nutritional status in the cancer patient include appetite stimulants, corticosteroids and progestational agents, anabolic steroids, antidepressants, analgesics, and antiemetics. Unfortunately, most of these medications are of marginal benefit. Several studies have examined the utility of corticosteroids and found that in the short-term, they can increase appetite and elevate mood, but are limited because of progressive muscle weakness. Progestational agents including megestrol acetate and medroxyprogesterone acetate are appetite stimulants. Eight prospective randomized studies have now revealed that although these agents do stimulate appetite and weight gain, no survival benefit is associated with their use.[179] One study found that 12 weeks of megestrol acetate (480 mg daily) produced an average weight gain of 5.41 kg, but no gain in performance status or quality of life.[180] The major risk of progestational agents is an increased risk of thromboembolic events. Cannabinoids such as dronabinol have been used, but most of these studies related to their use are in patients with AIDS-related anorexia, and definitive data in cancer patients are pending.

Unfortunately, the current therapy for CACS remains largely ineffective. Nutritional support, counseling, and the use of progestational agents continue to play the predominant role in management. Novel agents such as cytokine inhibitors have yet to be tested in randomized controlled trials.

RENAL MANIFESTATIONS OF NONRENAL CANCER

Patients with nonrenal carcinoma develop many important renal complications. Treatment-related nephropathies, tubular interstitial defects, glomerular abnormalities, and fluid and electrolyte disorders are seen in many patients with cancer. Radiation nephritis and drug-induced toxicities from antineoplastic drugs (e.g., cisplatin), antibiotics, analgesics, and radiographic contrast agents all induce various forms of renal failure. Infiltrative disorders from leukemias and lymphomas, tubular precipitation abnormalities such as protein cast nephropathy, uric acid nephropathy, hypercalcemic nephropathy, and obstructive nephropathy lead to tubular interstitial diseases. Membranous glomerulopathy, minimal change disease, amyloidosis, and consumptive coagulopathy all lead to glomerular abnormalities. Finally, hypercalcemia, hypocalcemia, hyponatremia, and tumor lysis syndrome, covered in other areas of this book, lead to fluid and electrolyte disorders. While renal manifestations of systemic cancer and its therapy are common, several classes of renal insult are specifically paraneoplastic in nature.

GLOMERULAR DISORDERS

Most cases of membranous nephropathy are idiopathic, but a reasonable number have been associated with cancers, especially in the elderly. In an early report of 101 patients with idiopathic nephrotic syndrome, 11% had cancer with 8% having membranous nephropathy.[181] In 80% of cases the diagnosis of nephrotic syndrome is made concurrently or after the malignant disease, lending credence to the idea that it is a paraneoplastic process. Nephrotic range proteinuria, hypertension, and microscopic hematuria characterize the syndrome. Sixty percent of cancers of the stomach, lung, and colon have membranous nephropathy,[182] while other cancers such as rectal, pancreas, head and neck, ovary, bile duct, prostate, breast, kidney, and skin rarely produce glomerulonephritis.[183,184] Immunofluorescence studies reveal granular deposits of immunoglobulin and complement, whereas electron microscopy shows evidence of subepithelial deposits, which are the pathologic hallmarks of this process. Immune complexes are thought to play a role in malignancy-associated glomerular disease.[182] The responsible antigens include fetal antigens, autologous nontumor antigens, tumor-associated antigens, and viral antigens.[185]

Nephrotic syndrome has been reported to resolve with successful treatment of the underlying malignancy.[186] Other standard therapies include loop diuretics to symptomatically treat the peripheral edema associated with the syndrome. As well, careful monitoring for the development of thrombosis is warranted in severe protein wasting, especially renal vein thrombosis.

Other glomerular diseases include membranoproliferative glomerulonephritis[187] and minimal change disease.[183] Hodgkin's disease is the cause of most cases of minimal change disease, while other lymphoproliferative disorders, pancreatic carcinoma, and mesothelioma are also seen.[188,189] There is a parallel relationship between the activity of the lymphoma and the degree of proteinuria. Other cancer-associated glomerulopathies include focal and segmental glomerulosclerosis with CLL, T-cell lymphomas, and acute myelogenous leukemia; IgA nephropathy with lung, head and neck, and pancreatic cancers, mycosis fungoides, and liposarcoma; and membranoproliferative glomerulonephritis with CLL, Burkitt's, and other lymphomas, hairy cell leukemia, and malignant melanoma. Rarely rapidly progressive glomerulonephritis has been associated with lymphoma and monoclonal gammopathies.[190]

MICROVASCULAR LESIONS

Hemolytic uremic syndrome is most often seen after chemotherapeutic agents such as mitomycin C, but has also been reported in malignancy. Giant hemangiomas and hemangioendotheliomas[191] and specific malignancies such as acute promyelocytic leukemia, prostate, gastric, and pancreatic cancers are the most common culprits. A renal vasculitis secondary to Henoch-Schönlein purpura has also been reported in a patient with lung cancer, but this is an extremely rare complication of malignancy. More frequent is the association of renal vasculitis secondary to a process such as cryoglobulinemia, a known complication of hepatocellular carcinoma and concomitant hepatitis C disease.[190]

TUMOR INFILTRATION

Autopsy series show the kidney is commonly affected by infiltrative and metastatic processes[192]; 40% to 60% of patients with leukemia have tumor infiltration of the kidney. Non-Hodgkin's lymphoma more commonly invades the kidney than Hodgkin's disease,[193] although not all series support this distinction.[194] There is a strong association between bone marrow involvement by tumor and renal infiltration. In both non-Hodgkin's lymphoma as well as Hodgkin's disease the involvement tends to be nodular and bilateral, whereas in leukemia the involvement is infiltrative.[195] Treatment of the underlying malignancy often results in resolution of the renal lesions. Other tubular abnormalities, such as protein cast precipitation syndrome, paraprotein disease, uric acid nephropathy, hypercalcemia, and obstructive uropathy, are discussed in Metabolic Emergencies, Chapter 51.3, and Plasma Cell Neoplasms, Chapter 46.4.

CUTANEOUS PARANEOPLASTIC SYNDROMES

A wide variety of cutaneous syndromes are associated with malignancies and may precede, be concurrent with, or follow the discovery of the underlying malignancy. It is critical that once a potential cutaneous paraneoplastic syndrome has been diagnosed, an appropriate systemic evaluation for a neoplasm is undertaken. The initial workup includes detailed medical history, complete physical examination, and routine screening laboratory tests. This is followed by studies directed by the abnormalities discovered during the preliminary evaluation, emphasizing those malignancies most strongly associated with the particular skin lesion. Some cutaneous syndromes are uncommon and usually are associated with cancer, whereas other cutaneous lesions are extremely common and associated with benign disorders or cancers. Certain cutaneous lesions are always associated with a particular tumor, whereas others are associated with a variety of malignancies. In general, the cause of the cutaneous lesions is typically unknown.

PIGMENTED LESIONS AND KERATOSES

Acanthosis nigricans (Table 47-3) is characterized by a gray-brown hyperpigmented, symmetric, velvety plaque that often affects the neck, axilla, and flexor areas and anogenital region. There are four groups: the malignant, inherited, endocrine, and idiopathic. The malignant form appears the same as the benign form, but may progress rapidly; pruritus is common. The malignant variety may precede the tumor, occur simultaneously, or even follow the appearance of the tumor. It affects men and women equally and is typically associated with adenocarcinomas of the GI tract, predominantly gastric cancer, but has also been associated with a variety of other adenocarcinomas including lung, breast, ovarian, and even hematologic malignancies.[196–198] The pathogenesis remains uncertain.

Tripe palms is associated with thickened palms and characterized by exaggerated ridges with a velvety texture and brown hyperpigmentation.[199,200] Virtually, all of these cases are associated with cancer, and, in most patients, occur in association with acanthosis nigricans. The condition is usually associated with lung and gastric cancer.

Melanosis is caused by abnormal deposition of melanin, causing diffuse gray-brown pigmentation in the skin.[201–203] Melanosis may appear before or after the primary melanoma is detected, and it is often accentuated in light-exposed areas of the upper body. Histopathology demonstrates melanin granules in perivascular or interstitial melanophages; free granules may be seen in the dermis. Melanosis can also be caused by ACTH-producing tumors.[204] Hemochromatosis from iron deposition may appear similar to melanosis.

The sign of Leser-Trélat is characterized by the sudden appearance of seborrheic keratoses. Such keratoses may occur in elderly patients, and one could argue reports of cutaneous lesions regressing after the cancer is treated are only coincidental.[205,206] Adenocarcinoma of the stomach is the most common malignancy; lymphoma, breast cancer, and squamous cell carcinoma are also reported.[207]

Acrokeratosis paraneoplastica or Bazex's syndrome is characterized by symmetric psoriasiform acral hyperkeratosis. It is almost always associated with cancer, typically squamous cell carcinoma of the esophagus, head and neck, or lungs.[208,209] The skin lesions may precede the detection of the tumor or parallel the growth of the malignancy. Antigenic cross-reaction of basement membrane and tumor antigens, as well as secretion of growth factors such as insulin-like growth factor-1 (ILGF-1) or transforming growth factor-α are postulated to cause this syndrome.[210]

Paget's disease of the breast is characterized by erythematous keratotic patches over the areola, nipple, or accessory breast tissue and is associated with breast cancer.[211] Extramammary Paget's disease is an erythematous exudative dermatitis located on the vulva in women, the genitals in men, and the perianal area in both sexes. Histopathologically, Paget's disease demonstrates large pale cells within the epidermis, and often in the cutaneous appendages. Extramammary Paget's disease is associated with an internal malignancy in 50% of cases. Most of these cancers are usually related to the site of the dermatosis. The most common sites of Paget's disease are in decreasing order: breast, uterus, rectum, bladder, vagina, and prostate gland.

NEUTROPHILIC DERMATOSES

Sweet's syndrome is associated with fever, neutrophilia, and the appearance of erythematous painful raised cutaneous plaques. The distribution is typically on the face, neck, and upper extremities. Histopathology demonstrates a dermal infiltration of well-differentiated neutrophils, as opposed to leukemia cutis, which contains immature myeloid blasts. This syndrome may be associated with an underlying malignancy (approximately 20%), most frequently, acute myelogenous leukemia. Some cases have been associated with myeloproliferative and lymphoproliferative disorders, myelodysplastic syndromes, and carcinomas.[212–214] Sweet's syndrome may precede the detection of malignancy by many years or occur concomitantly. The etiol-

TABLE 47-3. Pigmented Lesions and Keratoses

Disease	*Description*	*Malignancy*	*Cause*	*Comments*
Acanthosis nigricans[a]	Gray-brown symmetric velvety plaques on the neck, axilla, flexor areas, and anogenital region	Adenocarcinomas; predominantly gastric	Unknown	Benign form present from birth and associated with various syndromes
Tripe palms[a]	Hyperpigmented velvety thickened palms with exaggerated ridges	Gastric; lung	Unknown	Often associated with acanthosis nigricans
Generalized melanosis	A diffuse gray-brown skin pigmentation	Melanoma; adrenocorticotropic hormone producers	Melanin deposits in dermis	May be seen in benign conditions
Sign of Leser-Trélat	Sudden appearance of seborrheic (wart-like) keratoses	Gastric; lymphoma; breast	Unknown	Differentiate from noncancerous seborrheic keratoses
Acrokeratosis paraneoplastica or Bazex's disease[a]	Symmetric, psoriasiform acral hyperkeratosis; pruritus of nose, toes, ears, and nail dystrophy	Squamous cell carcinoma of the esophagus; head and neck; lung	Unknown	Males older than 40 years
Paget's disease	Erythematous keratotic patch over areola, nipple, or accessory breast tissue	Breast	Paget cells are either migrants (cancerous) or Langerhans cells	Occurs in fewer than 3% of breast cancers; extramammary Paget's seen in the anogenital region and commonly associated with cancer
Sweet's syndrome[a]	Erythematous painful raised cutaneous plaques	Hematologic malignancies, various carcinomas	Unknown	May respond to steroids; 10% to 15% associated with cancer
Pyoderma gangrenosum[a]	Painful papules, ulcers, violaceous borders and purulent exudates	Basal, squamous skin cancers; cutaneous T-cell non-Hodgkin's lymphoma	Unknown	Neutrophilic infiltrate

[a]True paraneoplastic syndrome.

ogy is thought to be hypersensitivity, and response to corticosteroids is usually prompt.

The lesions of pyoderma gangrenosum appear as painful papules that subsequently ulcerate with violaceous irregular borders and a purulent, hemorrhagic exudate with a necrotic base. Histopathology demonstrates a lymphocytic vasculitis or neutrophilic infiltrate. It is associated with basal and squamous cell carcinomas as well as cutaneous T-cell lymphomas.[215]

ERYTHEMAS

Erythema gyratum repens (Table 47-4) is an unusual progressive scaling erythema with prorates and a wood grain appearance.[216–218] It is almost always associated with internal malignancies, most commonly lung, breast, uterus, and GI tract.

Necrolytic migratory erythema is a rare disorder characterized by circinate and gyrate areas of blistering and erosive erythema on the face, abdomen, and limbs.[219,220] It is the hallmark of a glucagonoma. The eruption clears following resection of the tumor.

Flushing is an episodic reddening of the face and neck, lasting a few minutes, typically associated with the carcinoid syndrome but also seen with leukemia, medullary carcinoma of the thyroid, renal cell carcinoma, and other forms.[221–223] Vasoactive peptides such as serotonin are thought to mediate this syndrome.[224,225]

Erythema annulare centrifugum is characterized by slowly migrating annular and configurate erythematous lesions; rarely, it is associated with cancer, but this association remains unproven.[226,227]

Exfoliative dermatitis is a progressive erythema followed by scaling, which is classically associated with cutaneous T-cell lymphoma but may be seen in other lymphomas.[228,229]

ENDOCRINE AND METABOLIC LESIONS

Systemic nodular panniculitis or subcutaneous fat necrosis (Table 47-5) is characterized by violaceous nodules associated with adenocarcinoma of the pancreas and may be accompanied by polyarthralgia, fever, and eosinophilia.[230] Similar lesions are seen with pancreatitis, due to the release of pancreatic enzymes such as lipase, amylase, and trypsin into the serum.[231]

Cushing's syndrome is associated with broad purple striae, hyperpigmentation, telangiectasia, atrophy of the skin, and mild hirsutism. Cushing's syndrome is caused by increased ACTH, typically from small cell lung cancer, thyroid cancer, testicular cancer, ovarian cancer, adrenal tumors, and a variety of other tumors.[6,11]

Addison's syndrome is characterized by generalized hyperpigmentation, especially in scars, pressure points, and points of friction. This syndrome is caused by decreased glucocorti-

TABLE 47-4. Erythemas

Disease	*Description*	*Malignancy*	*Cause*	*Comments*
Erythema gyratum repens[a]	Progressive scaling erythema with pruritus appearance	Lung, breast, uterus, gastrointestinal	Unknown	Almost always associated with malignancies
Necrolytic migratory erythema[a]	Circinate and gyrate blistering, and erosive erythema on face, abdomen, limbs	Glucagonoma	Glucagon or metabolic product	
Flushing[a]	Episodic reddening of face and neck	Carcinoids, medullary thyroid carcinoma	Serotonin or other vasoactive peptides	
Erythema annulare centrifugum	Slowly migrating annular and configurate erythematous lesions	Prostate, myeloma, other	Unknown	Occurs also with infections and other disorders
Exfoliative dermatitis	Progressive erythema followed by scaling	Cutaneous T-cell and other lymphomas, Hodgkin's disease	Unknown	Accounts for 10% to 20% of all exfoliative dermatitis

[a]True paraneoplastic syndromes.

coids and may be seen with malignant replacement of the adrenal gland.

Hirsutism is associated with virilism and is caused by increased glucocorticoids and testosterone, typically from adrenal and ovarian tumors.

BULLOUS AND URTICARIAL LESIONS

Paraneoplastic pemphigus is most frequently seen in B-cell lymphoproliferative disorders including lymphomas and CLL, as well as Castleman's disease, thymoma, Waldenström's macroglobulinemia, and spindle cell neoplasms.[232–234] Patients develop painful bullous ulcers and intraepidermal and lichenoid skin lesions. Internal organ involvement is common and respiratory failure causes death in 30% of patients with this disorder.[235] Patients with paraneoplastic pemphigus demonstrate autoantibodies to desmogleins 1 and 3, which cause acantholytic blistering.[236] Antibodies to other cytoskeletal elements such as plakins have also been described.[235] The course of the disease is progressive and independent of the underlying malignancy. Corticosteroids and cyclosporin have been advocated and high-dose cyclophosphamide without stem cell rescue has been successful in one patient.[237] Table 47-6 describes the bullous and urticarial lesions.

Bullous pemphigoid is characterized by large tense bullae. Histopathology demonstrates absent acantholysis. It is reported to be associated with lymphomas, but this remains controversial.

TABLE 47-5. Endocrine and Metabolic Lesions

Disease	*Description*	*Malignancy*	*Cause*	*Comments*
Systemic nodular panniculitis[a] (nodular relapsing fat necrosis; Weber-Christian disease)	Recurrent crops of tender violaceous subcutaneous nodules; may be accompanied by abdominal pain, fat necrosis in bone marrow, lungs, and other organs	Adenocarcinoma of pancreas	Due to release of pancreatic enzymes into circulation on fatty tissues	May be associated with pancreatitis
Cushing's syndrome	Broad purple striae, atrophy, hirsutism hyperpigmentation (uncommon), plethora, telangiectasia, mild hirsutism	Small cell lung cancer, thyroid, testes, ovary, adrenal tumors; pancreatic islet cell, pituitary	Increased adrenocorticotropic hormone	
Addison's syndrome	Hyperpigmentation, especially scars, pressure points, points of friction; increased amounts of hair	Adrenal gland invasion, lymphomas or carcinomas	Decreased glucocorticoids	Usually related to nonmalignant diseases
Hirsutism	Increased hair in male distribution	Adrenal tumors, ovarian tumors	Increased glucocorticoid and testosterone	Associated with virilism

[a]True paraneoplastic syndrome.

TABLE 47-6. Bullous and Urticarial Lesions

Disease	*Description*	*Malignancy*	*Cause*	*Comments*
Paraneoplastic pemphigus[a]	Bullae of the skin, oral blisters	Lymphomas, Kaposi's sarcoma, breast cancer	Autoantibodies react to desmogleins 1 and 3 and other cytoskeletal elements	
Bullous pemphigoid	Large tense bullae with histologically absent acantholysis	Rarely lymphomas, miscellaneous	Unknown	Questionable association with malignancy
Dermatitis herpetiformis	Pleomorphic symmetric subepidermal bullae particularly with scarring	Lymphomas, miscellaneous	Related to autoantibodies	
Muir-Torre syndrome	Sebaceous gland neoplasm	Colon cancer, lymphoma	Unknown	

[a]True paraneoplastic syndrome.

Muir-Torre syndrome is a sebaceous gland neoplasm that may precede, follow, or coexist with visceral cancers.[238–240] It is most often associated with GI tract adenocarcinoma of the colon, genitourinary tract, or lymphoma.

MISCELLANEOUS LESIONS

Acquired ichthyosis (Table 47-7) is characterized by generalized dry, crackling skin, hyperkeratotic palms and soles, and rhomboidal scales. It is most commonly associated with Hodgkin's disease, but may be seen with lymphomas, multiple myeloma, and other malignancies.[241,242] It has also been associated with Kaposi's sarcoma and AIDS-related Kaposi's sarcoma.[243,244] Remission of the cancers may be accompanied by disappearance of the ichthyosis.

Dermatomyositis is a rare severe inflammatory myelopathy with erythema or telangiectasias of the knuckles, upper chest, or periorbital regions.[245–248] Dermatomyositis has been linked to malignancies, especially in adults after the age of 40. Frequency of cancer in adults is reported to vary from 10% to 50%, increasing with age. Malignancy can precede, follow, or occur with dermatomyositis; the most frequent pattern is onset of cancer within 1 year of the diagnosis of dermatomyositis.

Pachydermoperiostosis is characterized by thickening of the skin and creation of new folds; thickened lips, ears, and lids; macroglossia; clubbing; thickening of the forehead and scalp; and

TABLE 47-7. Miscellaneous Lesions

Disease	*Description*	*Malignancy*	*Cause*	*Comments*
Acquired ichthyosis[a]	Generalized dry, crackling skin, hyperkeratotic palms and soles, rhomboidal scales	Hodgkin's disease, other lymphomas, multiple myeloma, other	Unknown	Should be differentiated from hereditary, which occurs before age 20
Dermatomyositis[a]	Erythema or telangiectasias of the knuckles, chest, periorbital region	Miscellaneous	Unknown	Malignant disease reported in up to 50%, precedes carcinoma by days to years
Pachydermoperiostosis[a]	Thickening of skin and creation of new folds; thickened lips, ears, lids; thick forehead, scalp; clubbing; excessive sweating	Lung	Unknown	May be seen in lung abscess and benign tumors
Hypertrichosis lanuginosa (malignant down)[a]	Rapid development of fine, long, silky hair, especially on ears and forehead	Lung, colon, bladder, uterus, gallbladder	Unknown	High association with cancer
Pruritus[a]		Lymphomas, leukemias, multiple myelomas, central nervous system tumors, abdominal tumors	Unknown	Failure to determine a cutaneous cause of generalized pruritus necessitates an evaluation for an underlying systemic disease

[a]True paraneoplastic syndrome.

excessive sweating.[249] The cause of this syndrome is unknown, but it is most often associated with bronchogenic carcinoma.

Hypertrichosis lanuginosa (malignant down) is the development of long, silky hair on the ears, forehead, and possibly the entire body, associated with lung, colon, bladder, and a variety of other cancers.[250,251]

Pruritus may be the initial feature of an occult malignancy or the clinical manifestations of a previously diagnosed tumor. It is most frequently associated with Hodgkin's disease, but may be seen with polycythemia vera, cutaneous T-cell lymphomas, and a variety of other diseases.[252–254] Severe pruritus localized in the nostrils has been reported in some patients with advanced brain tumors.

Amyloid deposits, which may manifest as macroglossia, superficial waxy yellow and pink elevated nodules on the skin, may be associated with multiple myeloma or Waldenström's macroglobulinemia. They may also be associated with benign disorders such as primary systemic amyloid.

Herpes zoster is a vesicular eruption in a dermatomal pattern typically associated with the immunosuppression associated with Hodgkin's disease, lymphomas, and leukemias.[255–257]

HEREDITARY DISORDERS

Cowden's disease (Table 47-8) is characterized by multiple hamartomas and is a rare autosomal dominant condition characterized by both benign and malignant tumors.[258–261] The main features are fibromas of the oral mucosa characterized by *cobblestoning* of the tongue and acral palmoplantar keratoses. Multiple facial trichilemmomas appear to be pathognomonic. There is an increased prevalence of malignancy, most often in women, typically breast and thyroid cancer.

Gardener's syndrome is an autosomal dominant condition with a high malignant transformation rate. The syndrome includes multiple osteomas, fibromas, lipomas, desmoid tumors, fibrosarcomas, epidermoid cysts, and leiomyoma, as well as dental abnormalities.[262,263] The hallmark is intestinal polyposis of the colon and rectum, with development of colon carcinoma before the age of 30 in at least one-half of the patients. If untreated, death occurs before the age of 50; therefore, total colectomy is recommended for prevention.

Peutz-Jeghers syndrome is autosomal dominant characterized by hamartomatous polyps of the GI tract and mucocutaneous pigmentation of the lips, face, and oral mucosa and is commonly associated with both benign and malignant neoplasms.[264–268] There is a risk of approximately 2% to 3% of adenocarcinomas of the GI tract, and the carcinomas may arise in the hamartomatous polyps. Non-GI carcinomas affect mainly the breast, genitals, and pancreas. Cancers develop more frequently at younger ages.

Keratosis palmaris et plantaris or tylosis is an autosomal dominant disease associated with esophageal carcinoma. The disease consists of discreet hyperkeratotic papules on the palms and soles.[269–271]

Neurofibromatosis or von Recklinghausen is an autosomal dominant syndrome and is characterized by neurofibromas and café au lait spots. Malignancies develop in a minority of patients and are most often pheochromocytoma.[272]

The nevoid basal cell carcinoma syndrome is an autosomal dominant syndrome with early onset of multiple basal cell carcinomas, multiple jaw cysts, and anomalies of the skeletal system, specifically rib abnormalities such as ectopic calcification in the pits of the hands and feet.[273–275] The pits are pathognomonic of the syndrome, occurring in approximately two-thirds of adults with the syndrome. Medulloblastoma is the most common tumor. Leiomyomas and fibromas of the ovary can also occur. Central nervous system tumors have also been reported in early childhood. There are numerous additional hereditary disorders associated with malignancy described in Table 47-8.[276–281]

NEUROLOGIC MANIFESTATIONS OF CANCER

Remote effects of cancer on the central nervous system are neurologic disorders of unknown cause that occur exclusively, or with increased frequency, in patients with cancer.[282] Technically, the phrase *neurologic paraneoplastic syndrome* is a more general description that refers to any neurologic dysfunction that occurs in cancer patients that is not caused by metastasis or direct invasion of the nervous system by cancer. However, both phrases (*neurologic paraneoplastic syndromes* and *remote effects of cancer on the nervous system*) are often used interchangeably in the more restrictive sense and are used that way in this review.

The neurologic paraneoplastic disorders can logically be separated into anatomic categories, although there is often overlap. This is particularly true of the dementias, which are often lumped together with brain stem, cerebellar, and spinal cord lesions under the rubric of *carcinomatous encephalomyelitis.* The older term *carcinomatous neuromyopathy* has been used to describe all the remote effects of cancer on the nervous system as well as the disorders of peripheral nerves and muscle associated with cancer.

FREQUENCY

Even though most patients with cancer can be demonstrated to have some mild degree of neuromuscular dysfunction (usually in the form of myopathy or peripheral neuropathy), the frequency of clearly defined, symptomatic neurologic paraneoplastic syndromes is extremely low. Recognized neurologic paraneoplastic syndromes occur in less than 1% of patients with cancer.[282]

However, the situation is complicated by the fact that not all patients with neurologic syndromes that appear to be paraneoplastic actually have an underlying cancer. In approximately 50% of patients with known cancer, the nervous system symptoms precede the discovery of the underlying malignancy.[282,283] The probability that a given paraneoplastic syndrome is associated with an underlying cancer in patients who have not had a tumor identified varies with the specific type of paraneoplastic syndrome (Table 47-9).

PATHOGENESIS

The cause and pathogenesis of the neurologic paraneoplastic syndromes are not known. However, a variety of causative mechanisms have been proposed to explain the individual syndromes.[282] In 1888, Oppenheim was the first to suggest that the tumors themselves released substances that were directly neurotoxic.[284] No known paraneoplastic syndromes have been shown to be caused by this mechanism, although the nervous system can be secondarily affected when tumors release hormones [e.g., adrenocorti-

TABLE 47-8. Hereditary Disorders

Disease	*Description*	*Malignancy*	*Heredity*	*Comments*
Cowden's disease (multiple hamartoma syndrome)	Fibromas of oral mucosa with "cobblestoning" of the tongue, facial trichilemmomas	Thyroid, breast carcinomas	Autosomal dominant	Associated with multiple hamartomas, lipomas, neuromas, hemangiomas, thyroid adenomas
Gardner's syndrome	Bony exostoses, epidermal cysts, sebaceous cysts, dermoid tumors, lipomas, fibromas	Adenocarcinoma of large or small bowel	Autosomal dominant	Hallmark is polyposis of the colon
Peutz-Jeghers syndrome	Hamartomatous polyps of the GI tract and mucocutaneous pigmentation of the lips, face, and oral mucosa	GI adenocarcinomas	Autosomal dominant	Associated with benign or malignant neoplasm
Keratosis palmaris et plantaris (Tylosis)	Hyperkeratosis of palms and soles after age 10	Esophageal carcinoma	Autosomal dominant	95% incidence of carcinoma by age 65
Neurofibromatosis (von Recklinghausen)	Neurofibromas, café au lait spots	Pheochromocytoma	Autosomal dominant	Malignancies develop in a minority of patients
Nevoid basal cell carcinoma syndrome	Multiple basal cell carcinomas, pits on soles and palms, jaw cysts, skeletal abnormalities	Medulloblastoma, fibrosarcoma (jaw)	Autosomal dominant	Infrequent association with internal malignancy
Tuberous sclerosis (Bourneville)	Pigmented macules, adenomas, fibromas	Neurologic malignancies	Autosomal dominant	Malignancies develop in a minority of patients
Cerebelloretinal hemangioblastoma (von Hippel-Lindau)	Retinal malformation, papilledema	Neurologic malignancies	Autosomal dominant	Malignancies develop in a minority of patients
Encephalotrigeminal syndrome (Sturge-Weber)	Capillary or cavernous hemangiomas within the cutaneous distribution of the trigeminal nerve	Neurologic malignancies	Autosomal dominant	Malignancies develop in a minority of patients
Ataxia-telangiectasia	Telangiectasias	Lymphomas, leukemias	Autosomal recessive	IgA ± IgE deficiency; sinopulmonary infections, tumors in <10%
Bloom's syndrome	Photosensitivity, telangiectasias, erythema of face	Leukemias	Autosomal recessive	Stunted growth, high incidence
Fanconi's anemia	Patchy hyperpigmentation	Leukemias	Autosomal recessive	High incidence
Chediak-Higashi syndrome	Recurrent pyoderma, giant melanosomes, dilution of skin and hair color	Lymphomas	Autosomal recessive	High incidence
Werner's syndrome (adult progeria)	Scleroderma-like changes, premature aging, leg ulcers, short stature	Sarcomas, meningiomas, others	Autosomal recessive	Cancers in approximately 10%
Wiskott-Aldrich syndrome	Eczematous dermatitis, pyoderma	Lymphomas	Sex linked (male)	>10% incidence
Bruton's sex-linked agammaglobulinemia	Recurrent infections	Lymphomas, leukemias	Sex linked	>5% incidence

GI, gastrointestinal.

cotropin hormone (ACTH) and parathyroid hormone related peptide (PTHRP)] and cytokines [e.g., tumor necrosis factors (TNF) and the interleukins (ILs)].

Opportunistic infections have also been invoked as a possible cause of paraneoplastic syndromes. Progressive multifocal encephalitis, formerly classified as a paraneoplastic syndrome, has been shown to arise from the JC virus[285]; it is possible that other infections may be responsible for other paraneoplastic syndromes. Detection of 14-3-3 protein, commonly found in the CSF of patients with Creutzfeldt-Jakob disease, has also been found in the CSF of 12.5% of patients with paraneoplastic neurologic syndromes (including paraneoplastic cerebellar degeneration and limbic encephalitis). Although this etiologic link to slow viruses is intriguing, it is not clear how the 14-3-3 protein is involved in the development of paraneoplastic syndromes,[286] and further research in this area is warranted.

Another possible mechanism involves competition by the tumor for a biochemical nutrient or substrate. In this way, large metastatic carcinoid tumors produce an encephalopathy by depletion of tryptophan and niacin.[287] However, no evidence has been found of competition for a vital nutrient in any of the known paraneoplastic syndromes. Furthermore, it is unlikely that the small tumors frequently associated with paraneoplastic

TABLE 47-9. Estimated Incidence of Neurologic Disorders That Are Paraneoplastic Syndromes

Syndrome	*Percent Paraneoplastic*
Lambert-Eaton myasthenic syndrome	60
Subacute cerebellar degeneration	50
Subacute sensory neuronopathy	20
Opsoclonus-myoclonus (children)	50
Opsoclonus-myoclonus (adults)	20
Sensory motor peripheral neuropathy	10
Encephalomyelitis	10
Dermatomyositis	10

(From ref. 283, with permission.)

syndromes could consume enough of any substrate to produce a deficiency syndrome, and paraneoplastic syndromes usually run a course independent of that of the tumor.

There is increasing evidence that many of these syndromes are mediated by a T-lymphocyte mechanism. Pathologic study of the central nervous system of patients with paraneoplastic syndromes shows an intense inflammatory infiltrate (including T cells),[288,289] while T-cell receptor studies show that tumor-infiltrating T lymphocytes are specifically targeted to neuronal antigens.[290] Peripheral blood lymphocytes show an increase in memory helper T cells in seropositive patients with paraneoplastic syndromes versus seronegative controls.[291] Further, a report of cytotoxic T-cell activity in a patient with paraneoplastic sensory neuronopathy and anti-Hu antibodies provides provocative data regarding the relationship of T cells to the paraneoplastic process.[292] Further study in this area is ongoing.

The most widely accepted cause of many neurologic paraneoplastic syndromes appears to involve an autoimmune reaction. It is likely that certain antigenic molecules normally produced only in the central nervous system are produced ectopically by specific tumors. When the immune system reacts to these antigens, the neural tissues that share the same or similar antigens are also attacked. Subacute cerebellar degeneration, optic neuritis, opsoclonus-myoclonus, subacute sensory neuropathy, myasthenia gravis, and the Lambert-Eaton myasthenic syndrome (LEMS) have all been associated with the production of autoantibodies.[293] The most compelling evidence resides in the well-described LEMS in which autoantibodies against voltage-gated calcium channels are expressed by small cell lung cancer,[294] although no paraneoplastic syndrome has yet been proven conclusively to be caused by an autoimmune reaction.

DIAGNOSIS

Because most neurologic paraneoplastic syndromes occur in patients who do not have cancer or have not had a diagnosis of cancer made before the neurologic syndrome develops, diagnosis is often difficult. The clinical problem is twofold: (1) Either the patient is known to have cancer, and the question is whether the neurologic symptoms are due to a remote effect or to metastatic disease, or (2) the patient is not known to have cancer and the questions are whether there is a paraneoplastic syndrome present and does the patient need to be carefully evaluated for an occult cancer.

In the first instance, remote effects are so rare and metastatic disease so common that in the patients with known cancer the physician is obligated to consider and rule out all of the other neurologic complications of systemic cancer before diagnosing a paraneoplastic syndrome. Neurologic symptoms that may cause diagnostic difficulty include dementia, cerebellar dysfunction, and weakness of the extremities. Dementia is one of the well-described remote effects of cancer on the nervous system. However, similar symptoms may occur in patients with multiple cerebral metastases, leptomeningeal involvement, or in older patients with low brain reserve and systemic metabolic alterations or early neurodegenerative disorders such as Alzheimer's disease. Cerebral metastases are usually visible on MRI and CT scans, while with neurodegenerative disorders, one usually sees hydrocephalus on neuroimaging and CSF abnormalities. Also, if the patient has become acutely demented, metabolic brain disease is a possible diagnosis, as are the late effects of radiation therapy to the brain for previous metastasis. In patients with lymphoma, infections of the central nervous system including progressive multifocal leukoencephalopathy, toxoplasmosis, and fungal meningitis must also be considered.

If cerebellar dysfunction develops in a patient with a known cancer, it is much more likely that the patient is suffering from a metastasis in the cerebellum than from a remote effect. Clinically, subacute cerebellar degeneration as a remote effect is characterized by bilateral appendicular signs (point to point test difficulties in both upper and lower extremities) and by dysarthria, usually without nystagmus. Dementia is common as well. Metastatic disease of the cerebellum usually causes difficulties with gait without involvement of the upper extremities or speech (midline lesion), or it causes unilateral ataxia without gross dysarthria (hemispheral lesion). An MRI or CT scan usually clarifies the diagnosis.

The most serious diagnostic problems arise in patients developing weakness of the lower extremities with absent reflexes and with or without bladder or bowel dysfunction. The physician may suspect a paraneoplastic peripheral neuropathy, but invasion of the cauda equina by leptomeningeal tumor is more likely. The diagnosis can usually be established by careful examination of the CSF and spinal imaging studies.

Most paraneoplastic neurologic diseases, such as sensomotor peripheral neuropathy, dementia, and acute transverse myelopathy, occur only slightly more commonly in patients with cancer than in the general population. In such patients, a careful search for an underlying neoplasm is unlikely to be fruitful and is probably not warranted. However, several neurologic syndromes occur exclusively or with a much higher frequency in patients with cancer. These syndromes include dermatomyositis in middle-aged and elderly men, subacute cerebellar degeneration, subacute sensory neuropathy, and a subacute motor neuropathy. Any patient presenting with one of the previously mentioned neurologic syndromes deserves a careful search for an occult cancer. If the initial search result is negative, a tumor should still be suspected until a definitive diagnosis is established.

AUTOANTIBODIES

Some patients with paraneoplastic syndromes develop detectable autoantibodies and these are outlined in Table 47-10. When

TABLE 47-10. Antineuronal Antibodies and Associated Paraneoplastic Syndromes and Cancers

Antibody	*Site of Activity*	*Genes*	*Cellular Function*	*Clinical Syndrome*	*Cancers*
Anti-Hu (ANNA-1)	Panneuronal	HuD, HuC, Hel-N1/N2	RNA binding	Paraneoplastic encephalomyelitis, paraneoplastic sensory neuronopathy, PCD, autonomic	SCLC, sarcoma, neuroblastoma
Anti-Ri (ANNA-2)	Central nervous system neurons	Nova-1	RNA binding	Paraneoplastic opsoclonus-myoclonus, PCD	Breast, gynecologic, SCLC, bladder
Anti-Yo (APCA)	Purkinje cell	CDR34/62/3, PCD-17	Leucine zipper	PCD	Ovary, uterus, breast, SCLC
Anti-Tr	Purkinje cell	?	?	PCD	Hodgkin's, non-Hodgkin's lymphoma
Anti-VGCC	Presynaptic neuromuscular junction	MysB, Synaptotagmin	Ach release	Lambert-Eaton myasthenic syndrome	SCLC, Hodgkin's disease
Anti-CAR	Photoreceptors	Recoverin	Calcium binding	Cancer-associated retinopathy	SCLC, melanoma
Antiamphiphysin	Synapse; central nervous system neurons	Amphiphysin	Synaptic vesicle protein	Stiff-person syndrome, encephalitis	Breast, SCLC
Anti-AchR	Postsynaptic neuromuscular junction	?MHC	Ach receptor	Myasthenia	Thymoma
Anti-Ta	Nucleus	Ma1, Ma2	?	Limbic encephalitis	Testis

Ach, acetylcholine; MHC, major histocompatibility complex; PCD, paraneoplastic cerebellar degeneration; SCLC, small cell carcinoma of the lung; VGCC, voltage-gated calcium channel.

found in the patient without a history of cancer, a search for an underlying malignancy should be undertaken. While several of these are most commonly associated with one specific syndrome (as in anti–voltage-gated calcium channel and LEMS), they are not absolutely specific to a particular syndrome. For example, anti-Hu autoantibodies are seen in paraneoplastic encephalomyelitis, sensory neuronopathy, cerebellar degeneration, and opsoclonus-myoclonus.[295] Specific cancers are often associated with various paraneoplastic syndromes: 90% of anti-Yo autoantibodies indicates an underlying breast or gynecologic cancer.[293] However, autoantibodies are not required for the diagnosis of a paraneoplastic disorder to be made. Conversely, the presence of an autoantibody does not always herald the development of a paraneoplastic syndrome. Individual autoantibodies are discussed under the specific paraneoplastic syndromes with which they are associated.

TREATMENT

Treatment for most neurologic paraneoplastic syndromes is generally ineffective. The major exceptions are LEMS in which plasmapheresis and 3,4-diaminopyridine therapy are effective, and opsoclonus-myoclonus, which often responds to corticosteroid therapy. As well, treatment of the underlying malignancy has been successful in LEMS and opsoclonus-myoclonus.[296] A report of the successful use of protein A immunoadsorption in a wide variety of neurologic paraneoplastic syndromes is encouraging,[297] but waits confirmation in larger randomized studies before it can be recommended as a standard of care. A possible reason for the general failure of treatment in these disorders is that most of the syndromes have a rapid onset, and there is usually insufficient time to make a diagnosis and start treatment before irreversible damage is done. It is also postulated that immunosuppression may promote tumor growth, thus resulting in more rapid cancer-related deaths in these patients.

SPECIFIC SYNDROMES

Encephalomyelitis

Encephalomyelitis is a global term for paraneoplastic syndromes with an intense inflammatory response, perivascular lymphocyte cuffing, and lymphocyte accumulation in brain or spinal cord.[298] The manifestation of the paraneoplastic inflammatory process can be quite varied, depending on the affected area of the central nervous system. For example, spinal cord involvement can lead to transverse myelitis or motor neuropathy, while sympathetic autonomic effects can lead to orthostatic hypotension.[293] It is unclear why specific areas of the central nervous system are affected in individual patients. There is no known treatment and thc disorder runs a subacute course ending in severe debilitation.

Paraneoplastic Cerebellar Degeneration

Paraneoplastic cerebellar degeneration is a disorder that is characterized clinically by cerebellar signs and symptoms (ataxia, dysarthria, dysphagia) and pathologically by the diffuse loss of Purkinje cells in the cerebellum.[299] It is the most common paraneoplastic syndrome that affects the central nervous system, yet affects less than 1% of patients with cancer. Although the syndrome is sometimes present in patients without cancer, it is most often associated with cancers of the lung (especially small cell carcinoma), ovary, breast, and lymphomas (especially Hodgkin's disease).[300–302]

Evidence of diffuse cerebellar dysfunction is the most common clinical presentation of the disorder. In the majority of cases, the neurologic signs and symptoms antedate the discovery of underlying cancer by months to years.[282] The onset of symptoms is usually abrupt, with symmetric ataxia of the arms and legs progressing over weeks to months, usually associated with dysarthria and sometimes nystagmus. The seropositive patients appear to progress more rapidly.[303] In addition, a mild to moderate degree of dementia is often present. MRI and CT initially show no abnormalities; however, as the disease progresses, some degree of cerebellar atrophy is usually found on imaging studies. CSF may be normal, but there is usually a mild pleocytosis and increased protein.[304] There is frequently an increase in the CSF IgG, and oligoclonal bands may also be present.[282,283,302] The clinical course is one of subacute worsening and then stabilization at a severe level of neurologic dysfunction, with improvement highly unlikely.

Several autoantibodies have been found in association with paraneoplastic cerebellar degeneration.[303–305] When present, the titers of these antibodies are usually much higher in the CSF than in the serum, suggesting synthesis within the central nervous system. The most commonly found autoantibodies are high-titer polyclonal IgG anti-Purkinje cell antibodies (anti-Yo antibodies). These antibodies are found almost exclusively in female patients with paraneoplastic cerebellar degeneration and underlying cancers of the breast, ovary, or female genital tract.[306]

Other patients do not have anti-Yo antibodies but instead have other, less specific, autoantibodies including type 1 antineuronal nuclear autoantibodies (anti-Hu antibodies)[295] and anti-Ri antibodies.[304] Anti-Hu antibodies are more commonly associated with paraneoplastic encephalomyelitis and sensory neuronopathy; however, some patients with small cell lung carcinoma may develop a cerebellar syndrome that is clinically indistinguishable from the anti-Yo associated form, even though these patients lack anti-Yo and have only anti-Hu antibodies. A separate group of patients have been identified who have breast cancer, anti-Ri antibodies, and cerebellar degeneration (often with opsoclonus-myoclonus) in the absence of either anti-Yo or anti-Hu antibodies. In addition, some patients with Hodgkin's disease and a number of other neoplasms may have paraneoplastic cerebellar degeneration in the complete absence of any antineuronal antibodies.

In most instances, patients with paraneoplastic cerebellar degeneration have similar clinical presentations and clinical courses.[292] However, spontaneous remissions do occur, predominantly in patients with Hodgkin's disease and without anti-Purkinje cell autoantibodies.[300]

Limbic Encephalitis

Paraneoplastic limbic encephalitis is a rare complication of testicular neoplasms, small cell lung carcinoma, and other cancers; it can also occur in the absence of cancer.[282] Pathologically, the syndrome is characterized by loss of neurons in the amygdala, hippocampus, and insular cortex, occasionally with additional involvement of other deep gray matter structures.[302,307] There is usually gliosis, lymphocyte cuffing of blood vessels, and microglial nodules. The clinical manifestations include subacute development of personality changes and loss of short-term memory occurring over days to weeks. Less commonly there can be seizures, hallucinations, and disorientation. Autoantibodies have been described in patients with limbic encephalitis and testicular cancer. These anti-Ta antibodies recognize proteins (Ma1 and Ma2) present in the nucleus and cytoplasm of neurons. The function of these proteins is unknown.[308] There is no proven treatment, although there have been anecdotal reports of improvement when the underlying primary tumor responded to treatment.

Paraneoplastic Opsoclonus-Myoclonus

Opsoclonus is a problem of saccadic instability and consists of high-amplitude, involuntary, chaotic, conjugate, saccadic eye movements. These are often associated with focal myoclonus and ataxia. Opsoclonus is seen in two settings. In children, opsoclonus can be a self-limited condition that is probably due to a viral infection that involves the brain stem and is not related to cancer. More rarely, opsoclonus (with or without myoclonus) can also be a paraneoplastic syndrome. In children, the paraneoplastic syndrome is most often associated with neuroblastoma and occurs in approximately 2% of patients with neuroblastoma.[309] Approximately 50% of children who present with opsoclonus have an underlying neuroblastoma.[310] In one-half the cases, the opsoclonus predates the diagnosis of cancer. Paraneoplastic opsoclonus-myoclonus in children responds to corticosteroids; however, in a review 69% of these patients had long-term residual neurologic damage.[311]

In adults, opsoclonus-myoclonus is much less common than in children and less likely to be associated with an underlying neoplasm. Only approximately 20% of adults who present with opsoclonus have tumors,[282] and unlike children, the most commonly associated tumor is lung cancer.[312] As with many paraneoplastic syndromes, the neurologic abnormalities usually precede the diagnosis of an underlying neoplasm. The clinical picture is one of progressive eye movement abnormalities and myoclonus. The CSF usually shows a mild pleocytosis with slightly increased protein. Neuroimaging study results are usually normal. Treatment is rarely effective, but spontaneous remissions and remissions after treatment of the primary tumor occur infrequently. Neuropathologic findings run the spectrum from normal to a picture similar to paraneoplastic cerebellar degeneration with loss of Purkinje cells. Anti-Hu and anti-Ri antibodies have been found in a small number of cases, but no consistent pattern or presence of antibodies has been identified.[282]

Cancer-Associated Retinopathy

Degeneration of the photoreceptors in the retina is a rare paraneoplastic syndrome. In more than 90% of the described cases, small cell carcinoma of the lung is the primary tumor; malignant melanoma is the second most common primary tumor associated with the condition. The major pathologic findings are widespread degeneration of the rods, cones, and ganglion cells of the retina.[313] There is also usually degeneration of the outer neuronal layer of the retina with lymphocytic infiltration. Clinical findings consist of photosensitivity, scotomatous visual loss, and attenuation of the caliber of retinal arterioles. Frequently, decreased color vision, night blindness, and decreased visual acuity are also present. The CSF is usually normal. Electroretinography is abnormal; however, visual-evoked responses are normal. Serum autoantibodies that react with retinal cells have been identified in some, but not all cases. Antineuronal antibodies recognizing the photoreceptor recoverin are the best described.[314] Corticosteroids have sometimes resulted in improved visual symptoms.

Subacute Sensory Neuronopathy

Subacute sensory neuronopathy is a rare paraneoplastic disorder that presents with sensory loss in the extremities. The disorder occurs in patients with cancer but more commonly is found in patients without cancer and in association with primary Sjögren's syndrome.[302,315,316] In most patients, the sensory symptoms precede the diagnosis of cancer, and only approximately 20% of patients with the syndrome are ever demonstrated to have an underlying neoplasm.[282] When present, the most common underlying cancer is small cell carcinoma of the lung in 90% of cases.[316] Women are affected more often than men.

Pathologic findings consist of severe neuronal loss of primary sensory neurons in the dorsal root ganglia and gasserian ganglia. The cell loss is often patchy and sensory large fibers (e.g., proprioceptive nerves) are preferentially involved. There is often variable lymphocytic infiltration of the ganglia and secondary loss of white matter tracts in the posterior columns. The initial clinical symptoms are numbness, tingling, and dysesthetic pain in the distal extremities. The sensory loss progresses over days to weeks to involve all four extremities and ascends to involve the trunk and face. Deep tendon reflexes are lost; however, motor power is usually normal. The disease tends to stabilize after several months at a severe level of disability; most patients are unable to walk. Treatment with corticosteroids and plasmapheresis has not been successful. Occasionally, the syndrome remits spontaneously or improves after the primary tumor is treated.

Subacute Motor Neuronopathy

Subacute motor neuronopathy is a condition associated primarily with Hodgkin's disease and other lymphomas (although there have been rare occurrences with other tumors).[317] The syndrome is characterized by subacute, progressive lower extremity weakness without significant sensory loss. The weakness is of the lower motor neuron type. Nerve conduction velocities are normal, and electromyography shows evidence of denervation. There is usually a mild elevation of protein in the CSF without pleocytosis. Pathologic findings include anterior horn cell degeneration, demyelination of the anterior (motor) nerve roots, and variable demyelination of spinal cord white matter. A specific motor neuropathy, Guillain-Barré syndrome, is increased in frequency in patients with Hodgkin's disease and is therefore labeled a paraneoplastic syndrome.[203]

Unlike most other neurologic paraneoplastic syndromes, subacute motor neuronopathy usually develops *after* the diagnosis of the underlying neoplasm has been made, and the disorder frequently develops while the cancer is in remission (e.g., following *curative* mantle radiotherapy). The weakness usually does not produce profound debilitation and runs a course independent of the underlying malignancy. Typically, the weakness stabilizes or improves after several months. Presently, there is no effective treatment.

Paraneoplastic Sensomotor Peripheral Neuropathy

Mixed motor and sensory peripheral neuropathies are extremely common in cancer patients. In most cases the neuropathies are caused by neurotoxic chemotherapy, malnutrition, or metabolic problems that are not per se paraneoplastic. However, a rare subacute or chronic sensomotor neuropathy has been described,[315] and is most frequently associated with lung cancer. The neuropathy involves the distal extremities in a characteristic glove and stocking distribution; bulbar structures are usually not involved. The CSF is usually normal or shows only a mild increase in protein. Nerve conduction study results are usually consistent with an axonal neuropathy, and electromyography demonstrates denervation. Pathologic study of nerves shows axonal degeneration, segmental demyelination, or a combination of the two. The neuropathy tends to stabilize and remain chronic. However, the condition can also remit and recur. No specific treatment is available.

Lambert-Eaton Myasthenic Syndrome

LEMS is a disorder of the myoneural junction that results in proximal muscle weakness. Approximately 40% of patients do not have an underlying cancer; women make up the majority of patients in this group.[318] Of the 60% of patients with an underlying neoplasm, approximately two-thirds have small cell lung carcinoma.[203]

LEMS is caused by an antibody attack on the presynaptic nerve terminal, specifically on the voltage-dependent calcium channels.[319] The antibodies block the entry of calcium into the terminal in response to an action potential and this decreases acetylcholine release. LEMS has been induced in animals by passive transfer experiments in which animals were injected with IgG from patients with the disorder.[294,320]

The clinical findings include muscle weakness and fatigability that is usually worse in the proximal muscles. Unlike classic myasthenia gravis, the weakness usually does not involve the bulbar musculature, although approximately 30% of patients experience dysphagia. Approximately one-half of patients have symptoms of cholinergic dysautonomia (e.g., dry mouth and impotence).[293]

Nerve conduction velocities show a characteristic pattern with normal conduction velocities and initially low amplitude compound muscle action potential. After exercise, the CMAPs increase to near normal levels. Repetitive nerve stimulation studies show a decrement of the compound muscle action potentials at low stimulation rates and an increase in the compound muscle action potentials at high stimulation rates.

In contrast to most paraneoplastic syndromes, the LEMS has been reported to respond to plasmapheresis, intravenous immune globulin, and immunosuppression.[282] Drugs that increase transmitter release (e.g., 3,4-diaminopyridine) relieve symptoms and may be beneficial in maintenance therapy. Pyridostigmine propagates the effect of 3,4-diaminopyridine, but is usually ineffective when given alone.[293] Treatment of the underlying cancer also results in clinical improvement.

Dermatomyositis and Polymyositis

Dermatomyositis and polymyositis are inflammatory myopathies characterized by the subacute development of proximal muscle weakness, with or without pain and muscle tenderness.[321] Dermatomyositis has the classic heliotrope rash over the face, elbows, knees, and knuckles, in addition to the muscle weakness. Both conditions are usually idiopathic and are associated with cancer in only approximately 10% of cases.[322] The muscle syndrome usually precedes the diagnosis of the underlying cancer. When the characteristic findings are present in men older than 40 years, there is a higher incidence of underlying cancer, especially carcinoma of the lung, and a search for cancer is warranted. The most commonly associated cancers are breast and lung tumors.

In addition to proximal symmetric muscle weakness and skin changes, there is usually an elevation in muscle creatinine kinase. Electromyography is consistent with a myopathic process, and muscle biopsy usually shows inflammatory infiltrates, necrotic fibers, and atrophic fibers, sometimes in a perifascicular pattern. Treatment with immunosuppressive agents, including corticosteroids, is the standard therapy. The syndrome follows an inconsistent course and often is independent of that of the tumor.

Miscellaneous Syndromes

The following syndromes have been described that have less concrete supporting data and are so rare that an in-depth review is not warranted. Stiff-person syndrome has been reported rarely in women with breast cancer, often preceding the oncologic diagnosis. Symptoms include painful muscle cramps and stiffness. Antiamphiphysin autoantibodies are associated with this syndrome.[323] Acute necrotizing myopathy has been described in several patients with rapid progression of symmetric, proximal muscle weakness, with pathologic evidence of muscle fiber necrosis without inflammation.[324] Paraneoplastic vasculitic neuropathy is a syndrome characterized by nonsystemic subacute vasculitic neuropathy, usually due to small cell lung and lymphoma. Neuropathy varies from mononeurotherapy multiplex to polyneuropathy. Axonal neuropathy is the characteristic finding in electrophysiologic studies, while the microscopic evaluation reveals a vasculitis. Unlike most other paraneoplastic syndromes, treatment of the underlying cancer or immunotherapy for vasculitis is helpful.[325] Myasthenia gravis, a classic paraneoplastic syndrome associated with thymoma, is discussed in depth in Neoplasms of the Mediastinum, Chapter 32, and is not discussed here.

MISCELLANEOUS PARANEOPLASTIC SYNDROMES

HYPERTROPHIC OSTEOARTHROPATHY

A clinical syndrome, presumably hypertrophic osteoarthropathy (HOA), has been in the medical literature since antiquity. Hippocrates described the syndrome, which was most certainly digital clubbing, 25 centuries ago, and this syndrome was called *hippocratic fingers.* In the past, the problem was termed *pulmonary HOA,*[326] but because other nonpulmonary diseases can cause the syndrome, the term was simplified to HOA. In 1992, an international workshop on HOA met in Florence, Italy, and established a consensus for the diagnosis classification and assessment of this syndrome.[327]

To fulfill diagnostic criteria of this disease, both digital clubbing and periostosis must be present. Digital clubbing can be defined as paronychial soft tissue expansion associated with the loss of the curved linear lucency normally present at the junction between the nail and the skin. This may progress to a prominent bulbus enlargement of the distal end of the digit, representing an underlying increase in vascular and connective tissues. Periostosis is represented by periosteal proliferation in tubular bones, particularly the tibia and femurs. Incomplete forms of HOA have been recognized including clubbing alone, isolated periostosis, and pachydermia associated with any of the minor manifestations of the syndrome (synovial effusions, seborrhea, folliculitis, hyperhidrosis, hypertrophic gastropathy, and acroosteolysis).[328] Some investigators have also used a response to nonsteroidal antiinflammatory agents to confirm the diagnosis of HOA.[329]

HOA can be characterized as either primary or secondary. The secondary forms are either generalized or localized. The localized forms are seen in patients with hemiplegia, aneurism, infectious arthritis, and patent ductus arteriosis. The generalized syndromes are more common and are associated with six major disease categories including pulmonary diseases, cardiac diseases, liver disease, intestinal disease, mediastinal disease, and miscellaneous problems. By far the most common are the pulmonary syndromes including non–small cell lung cancer, metastatic malignancy, cystic fibrosis, pulmonary fibrosis, chronic infections such as abscess or bronchiectasis, and arteriovenous fistula. Cyanotic congenital heart disease is the most likely etiology of cardiac-associated HOA. Cirrhosis is the most common liver problem associated with HOA, but the syndrome can also be seen with hepatic carcinoma. Inflammatory bowel disease including Crohn's disease and ulcerative colitis, as well as other chronic infections and bowel malignancies, are rarely associated with HOA. The mediastinal diseases associated with HOA are esophageal carcinoma, thymoma, and achalasia, while the miscellaneous category is headed by Grave's disease and thalassemia.

The treatment of HOA is somewhat disappointing. As with virtually all paraneoplastic syndromes, successful treatment of the underlying disease is associated with a rapid resolution of the problem. However, in most cases of lung cancer the disease is generally in an advanced state and, therefore, successful treatment is difficult. Patients with severe pain have been successfully treated with nonsteroidal antiinflammatory drugs.[330] Surgery and other arthritic treatments such as colchicine have been less successful.[331] Liver transplantation in patients with liver diseases associated with HOA has been related to dramatic improvement in symptoms,[332] as has lung transplantation in patients with underlying lung disease.[333] Many times, however, the symptoms can be quite debilitating and do not respond to therapy.

FEVER

Fever occurs in many patients with cancer. The causes of fever in cancer patients include infection, tumor, drug fever, reaction to blood products, and autoimmune diseases. Thirty percent of patients with cancer develop fever at some point during the course of their malignancy,[334] with the majority having an underlying infection.[335] The major differential point in determining whether the fever is due to infection is the presence or absence of neutropenia. In patients with low white blood cell count, infection causes more than two-thirds of all fevers,[336] while patients with normal white blood cell counts are infected far less frequently. Twenty percent of fevers in nonneutropenic patients are secondary to infection, whereas 45% remain unexplained after complete evaluation.[337]

In the absence of infection, it is thought that cancer cells can produce cytokines, which cause fever. Renal cell carcinoma is the most common cancer associated with fever in up to one-half of patients,[338] while hepatoma patients develop fever one-third of the time.[339] Pel-Ebstein fever is seen in patients with Hodgkin's disease and is an important prognostic feature of this disease. Fever is also seen in patients with non-Hodgkin's lymphoma.[340] Acute leukemia, osteosarcoma, atrial myxoma, adrenal carcinoma, pheochromocytoma, and hypothalamic tumors are also rarely associated with the development of fever.[341]

The endogenous pyrogens have been well described over the past 20 years. IL-1 replaces the term *endogenous pyrogen*, which was initially used to describe this cytokine associated with Hodgkin's disease.[342] Subsequently, IL-1 has been shown to increase circulating neutrophils and cortisol and be intimately involved in the acute phase response. TNF (α and β subtypes) has also been shown to cause fever, although it does not use the same receptors as IL-1 and appears to induce IL-1.[343] As well, interferon and IL-6 have been shown to produce fever, and it is expected that several more cytokines will eventually be added to the class of endogenous pyrogens.[344]

The most important point in the management of fever in patients with cancer is evaluating for infection. In patients with neutropenia this could be life threatening, but it is also important in nonneutropenic patients. If infection is excluded, nonsteroidal antiinflammatory drugs are a reasonable means to manage patients with fever. Nonsteroidal drugs effect a decrease in fever by inhibiting cyclooxygenase, reducing prostaglandin E_2 synthesis. Some investigators use the response to nonsteroidal antiinflammatory drugs to differentiate fever caused by infection from that caused by a tumor. In two separate studies, response to indomethacin and naproxen was associated with a high incidence of tumor-related fever compared with infectious etiologies.[345,346] Corticosteroids are also effective antipyretics, both through inhibition of prostaglandin E_2 and blocking transcription of mRNA for pyrogenic cytokines.[344]

REFERENCES

1. Odell W. Endocrine/metabolic syndromes of cancer. *Semin Oncol* 1997;214:299.
2. Brown WH. A case of pluriglandular syndrome: diabetes of bearded women. *Lancet* 1928,2.1022.
3. Liddle GW, Island DP, Ney RL, et al. Non-pituitary neoplasms and Cushing's syndrome. *Arch Intern Med* 1963;11:471.
4. Odell WD, Wolfsen AR, Yoshimoto Y, et al. Ectopic peptide synthesis—a universal concomitant of neoplasia. *Trans Assoc Am Physicians* 1977;90:204.
5. Baylin SB, Mendelsohn G. Ectopic (inappropriate) hormone production by tumors: mechanism involved and the biological and clinical implications. *Endocr Rev* 1980;1:45.
6. Wajchenberg BL, Mendonca BB, Liberman B, et al. Ectopic adrenal corticotropic hormone syndrome. *Endocr Rev* 1994;15:752.
7. Stewart PM, Gibson S, Crosby SR, et al. ACTH precursors characterize the ectopic ACTH syndrome. *Clin Endocrinol* 1994;40:199.
8. Kraus J, Buchfelder M, Holt V. Regulatory elements of the human proopiomelanocortin gene promoter. *DNA Cell Biol* 1993;12:527.
9. Amsler U, Pasi A, Qu B. A novel hypothesis: specific oncogenes and tumor suppression genes are involved in the expression of the proopiomelanocortin gene by small cell lung cancer. *Med Hypotheses* 1994;42:397.
10. Crapo L. Cushing's syndrome: a review of diagnostic tests. *Metabolism* 1979;28:955.
11. Wajchenberg BL, Mendonca BB, Liberman B, et al. Ectopic ACTH syndrome. *J Steroid Biochem Mol Biol* 1995;53:139.
12. Carpenter PC. Diagnostic evaluation of Cushing's syndrome. *Endocrinol Metab Clin North Am* 1988;17:455.
13. Oldfield EH, Doppman JL, Nieman LK, et al. Petrosal's sign is sampling with and without corticotropin-releasing hormone for the differential diagnosis of Cushing's syndrome. *N Engl J Med* 1991;325:897.
14. Odell WD, Appleton WS. Hormonal manifestations of cancer. In: Wilson JD, Foiter DW, eds. *Williams endocrinology*. 8th ed. Philadelphia: WB Saunders, 1990.
15. Pass HI, Doppman J, Nieman L, et al. Management of the ectopic ACTH-syndrome due to thoracic carcinoids: the HIH experience and review of the world literature. *Ann Thorac Surg* 1990;50:52.
16. Avgerinos PC, Wanovski JA, Oldfield EH, et al. The metyrapone and dexamethasone suppression tests for the differential diagnosis of the adrenocorticotropin-dependent Cushing syndrome: a comparison. *Ann Intern Med* 1994;121:318.
17. Nieman LK, Chrousos GP, Oldfield EH, et al. The ovine corticotropin-releasing hormone stimulation test and the dexamethasone suppression test in the differential diagnosis of Cushing's syndrome. *Ann Intern Med* 1986;105:862.
18. Midgette AS, Aron DC. High dose dexamethasone suppression testing versus inferior petrosal sign and sampling and the differential diagnosis of adrenocorticotropin-dependent Cushing's syndrome: a decision analysis. *Am J Med Sci* 1995;309:162.
19. Biemond P, de Jong FH, Lamberts SW. Continuous dexamethasone infusion for seven hours in patient with Cushing's syndrome. A superior differential diagnostic test. *Ann Intern Med* 1990;112:738.
20. Nobels FR, de Herder WW, Kwekkeboom DJ, et al. Serum chromatin A in a differential diagnosis of Cushing's syndrome. *Eur J Endocrinol* 1994;131:589.
21. Jex RK, Little van Heerden JA, Carpenter PC, et al. Ectopic ACTH syndrome diagnostic and therapeutic aspects. *Am J Surg* 1985;149:276.
22. Howlett TA, Drury PL, Perry L, et al. Diagnosis and management of ACTH-dependent Cushing's syndrome: comparison of the features in ectopic and pituitary ACTH production. *Clin Endocrinol* 1986;24:699.
23. Leinung MC, Young WF Jr, Whitaker MD, et al. Diagnosis of corticotropin-producing bronchial carcinoid tumors causing Cushing's syndrome. *Mayo Clin Proc* 1990;65:1315.
24. de Herder WW, Krenning EP, Malchoff CD, et al. Somatostatin receptor scintigraphy: its value in tumor localization in patients with Cushing's syndrome caused by ectopic corticotropin or corticotropin-releasing hormone secretion. *Am J Med* 1994;96:305.
25. Zeiger MA, Pass HI, Doppman JD, et al. Surgical strategy in the management of non-small cell ectopic adrenal corticotropic hormone syndrome. *Surgery* 1992;112:994.
26. Pujol J, Viladrich M, Rafecas A, et al. Laparoscopic adrenalectomy. A review of 30 initial cases. *Surg Endosc* 1999;13:488.
27. Misbin RI, Canary J, Willard D. Amino glutethimide in the treatment of Cushing's syndrome. *J Clin Pharmacol* 1976;16:645.
28. Jeffcoate WJ, Rees LH, Tomlin S, et al. Metyrapone in the long-term management of Cushing's disease. *BMJ* 1977;2:215.
29. Winquist EW, Laskey J, Crump M, et al. Ketoconazole in the management of paraneoplastic Cushing's syndrome secondary to ectopic adrenal corticotropin production. *J Clin Oncol* 1995;13:157.
30. Woodhouse NJ, Dagogo-Jack S, Ahmed M, et al. Acute and long-term effects of octreotide in patients with ACTH-dependent Cushing's syndrome. *Am J Med* 1993;95:305.
31. Vignati F, Loli P. Additive effect of ketoconazole and octreotide in the treatment of severe adrenocorticotropin-dependent hypercortisolism. *J Clin Endocrinol Metab* 1996;81:2885.
32. Schwartz WB, Bennet W, Curelop S, Bartter FC. A syndrome of renal sodium loss in hyponatremia probably resulting from inappropriate secretion of anti-diuretic hormone. *Am J Med* 1957;23:529.
33. Vorherr H, Massry S, Utiger R, et al. Anti-diuretic principle in malignant tumor extracts from patients with inappropriate ADH syndrome. *J Clin Endocrinol Metab* 1968;28:162.
34. Hamilton BPM. Presence of neurophysin proteins in tumors associated with the syndrome of inappropriate ADH secretion. *NY Acad Sci* 1975;248:153.
35. Legros JJ. The radioimmunoassay of human neurophysins: contribution to the understanding of the physiopathology of neurohypophyseal. *NY Acad Sci* 1975;248:281.
36. Legros JJ, Geenen V, Carvelli T, et al. Neurophysins as markers of vasopressin and oxytocin release. *Horm Res* 1990;34:151.
37. Rasham JW, Anderson G. Incidence of paramalignant disorders in bronchogenic carcinoma. *Thorax* 1975;30:86.
38. Lokich JJ. The frequency in clinical biology of ectopic hormone syndromes of small cell carcinoma. *Cancer* 1982;50:2111.
39. Hays R. Alteration in luminal membrane structure by antidiuretic hormone. *Am J Physiol* 1983;245:289.
40. Barri Y, Knochel J. Hypercalcemia and electrolyte disturbances in malignancy. *Hematol Oncol Clin North Am* 1996;10:775.
41. Comis RL, Miller N, Ginsberg SJ. Abnormalities in water homeostasis in small cell anaplastic lung cancer. *Cancer* 1980;45:2414.
42. Bondy PK, Gilby ED. Endocrine function in small cell and differential carcinoma of the lung. *Cancer* 1982;50:2147.
43. List AF, Hainsworth JD, Davis BW, et al. A syndrome of inappropriate secretion of anti-diuretic hormone (SIADH) in small cell lung cancer. *J Clin Oncol* 1986;4:1191.
44. Steele TH, Serpick AA, Block JB. Anti-diuretic response to cyclophosphamide in man. *J Pharmacol Exp Ther* 1973;185:245.
45. Cutting H. Inappropriate secretion of anti-diuretic hormone secondary to vincristine therapy. *Am J Med* 1971;51:269.
46. Goldberg M. Hyponatremia. *Med Clin North Am* 1981;65:251.
47. Glover D, Glick J. Metabolic oncologic emergencies. *CA Cancer J Clin* 1987;37:302.

48. Cerrill D, State R, Birge J, et al. Demeclocycline treatment in the syndrome of inappropriate anti-diuretic hormone secretion. *Ann Intern Med* 1975;83:654.
49. Ayus J, Krothapali R, Arieff A. Treatment of symptomatic hyponatremia and its relation to brain damage. *N Engl J Med* 1987;317:1190.
50. Raskin P, McClain CJ, Medsger TA. Hypocalcemia associated with metastatic bone disease. *Arch Intern Med* 1973;132:539.
51. Hall TC, Griffiths CT, Petranek JR. Hypocalcemia: an unusual metabolic complication of breast cancer. *N Engl J Med* 1966;275:1474.
52. Sackner MA, Spivak AP, Balian LJ. Hypocalcemia in the presence of osteoblastic metastases. *N Engl J Med* 1960;262:173.
53. Ehrlich M, Goldsten M, Heinemann HO. Hypocalcemia, hypoparathyroidism and osteoblastic metastases. *Metabolism* 1963;12:516.
54. Ryan EA, Reiss E. Oncogenous osteomalacia. Review of the world literature of 42 cases and report of two new cases. *Am J Med* 1984;77:501.
55. Salassa RM, Jowsey J, Arnaud C. Hypophosphatemia osteomalacia associated with "nonendocrine" tumors. *N Engl J Med* 1970;283:65.
56. Stanbury W. Tumor-associated hypophosphatemia, osteomalacia and rickets. *Clin Endocrinol Metab* 1972;1:256.
57. Daniels RA, Weisenfeld I. Tumorous phosphaturic osteomalacia. Report of a case associated with multiple hemangiomas of bone. *Am J Med* 1979;67:155.
58. Siris ES, Clemens TL, Dempster DW, et al. Tumor-induced osteomalacia. Kinetics of calcium, phosphorus, and vitamin D metabolism and characteristics of bone histomorphometry. *Am J Med* 1987;82:307.
59. Tashjian AH, Wolfe HJ, Voelkel EF. Human calcitonin: immunologic assay, cytologic localization and studies of medullary thyroid carcinoma. *Am J Med* 1974;56:840.
60. Silva OL, Broder LE, Doppman JL, et al. Calcitonin as a marker for bronchogenic cancer: a prospective study. *Cancer* 1979;44:680.
61. Bertagna XY, Nicholson WE, Pettengill OS, et al. Ectopic production of high molecular weight calcitonin and corticotropin by human small cell carcinoma cells in tissue culture: evidence for separate precursors. *J Clin Endocrinol Metab* 1978;47:1390.
62. Hillyard V, Coombes RC, Greenberg PB, et al. Calcitonin in breast and lung cancer. *Clin Endocrinol* 1976;5:1.
63. O'Connor DT, Bernstein KN. Radioimmunoassay of chromogranin A in plasma as a measure of exocytotic sympathoadrenal activity in normal subjects and patients with pheochromocytoma. *N Engl J Med* 1984;311:764.
64. Wilson BS, Lloyd RV. Detection of chromogranin in neuroendocrine cells with a monoclonal antibody. *Am J Pathol* 1984;115:458.
65. Huttner WB, Benedum UM. Chromogranin A and pancreastatin. *Nature* 1987;325:305.
66. Sobol RE, O'Connor DT, Addison J, et al. Elevated serum chromogranin A concentrations in small cell lung carcinoma. *Ann Intern Med* 1986;105:698.
67. O'Connor DT, Frigon RP, Sokoloff RI. Human chromogranin A: purification and characterization from catecholamine storage vesicles of human pheochromocytoma. *Hypertension* 1984;6:2.
68. O'Connor DT, Deftos LJ. Secretion of chromogranin A by peptide-producing endocrine neoplasms. *N Engl J Med* 1986;314:1145.
69. Blackman MR, Weintraub BD, Rosen SW, et al. Human placental and pituitary glycoprotein hormones and their subunits as tumor markers: a quantitative assessment. *J Natl Cancer Inst* 1980;65:81.
70. Kenimer JG, Hershman JM, Higgins HP. The thyrotropin in hydatidiform moles is human chorionic gonadotropin. *J Clin Endocrinol Metab* 1975;40:481.
71. Faiman C, Colwell JA, Ryan RJ, et al. Gonadotropin secretion from a bronchogenic carcinoma. *N Engl J Med* 1967;277:1395.
72. Fusco FD, Rosen SW. Gonadotropin-producing anaplastic large-cell carcinomas of the lung. *N Engl J Med* 1966;275:507.
73. Anderson T, Waldmann TA, Javadpour N, Glatstein E. Testicular germ-cell neoplasms: recent advances in diagnosis and therapy. *Ann Intern Med* 1979;90:373.
74. Vaitukaitis JL, Ross GT, Braunstein GD, Rayford PL. Gonadotropins and their subunits: basic and clinical studies. *Recent Prog Horm Res* 1976;32:289.
75. Rudnick P, Odell WD. In search of a cancer. *N Engl J Med* 1971;284:405.
76. Muggia FM, Rosen SW, Weintraub BD, Hansen HH. Ectopic placental proteins in nontrophoblastic tumors: serial measurements following chemotherapy. *Cancer* 1975;36:1327.
77. Kahn CR, Rosen SW, Weintraub BD, et al. Ectopic production of chorionic gonadotropin and its subunits by islet cell tumors: a specific marker for malignancy. *N Engl J Med* 1977;197:565.
78. Bender RA, Weintraub BD, Rosen SW. Prospective evaluation of two tumor-associated proteins in pancreatic adenocarcinoma. *Cancer* 1979;45:591.
79. Broder LE, Weintraub BD, Rosen SW, et al. Placental proteins and their subunits as tumor markers in prostatic carcinoma. *Cancer* 1977;40:211.
80. Metz SA, Weintraub B, Rosen SW, et al. Ectopic secretion of chorionic gonadotropin by a lung carcinoma. Pituitary gonadotropin and subunit secretion and prolonged chemotherapeutic remission. *Am J Med* 1978;65:325.
81. Tashjian AH Jr, Weintraub BD, Barowksy NJ, et al. Subunits of human chorionic gonadotropin: unbalanced synthesis and secretion by clonal cell strains derived from a bronchogenic carcinoma. *Proc Natl Acad Sci U S A* 1973;70:1419.
82. Skrabanek P, Kirrane J, Powell D. A unifying concept of chorionic gonadotropin production in malignancy. *Invest Cell Pathol* 1979;2:75.
83. Greco FA, Fer MF, Oldham RD, et al. Intracytoplasmic localization of ectopic β-human chorionic gonadotropin and α-fetoprotein in suspected extragonadal germ cell cancers by immunohistochemical methods. *Clin Res* 1980;28:415A.
84. Weintraub BD, Rosen SW. Ectopic production of human chorionic somatomammotrophin by nontrophoblastic cancers. *J Clin Endocrinol Metab* 1971;32:94.
85. Rosen SW, Weintraub BD, Vaitukaitis JL, et al. Placental proteins and their subunits as tumor markers. *Ann Intern Med* 1975;82:71.
86. Steiner H, Dahlback O, Waldenstrom J. Ectopic growth-hormone production and osteoarthropathy in carcinoma of the bronchus. *Lancet* 1968;1:783.
87. Sonksen PH, Ayres AB, Braimbridge M, et al. Acromegaly caused by pulmonary carcinoid tumors. *Clin Endocrinol* 1976;5:505.
88. Scheithauer BW, Bloch B, Carpenter PC, Brazeau P. Ectopic secretion of a growth hormone-releasing factor. Report of a case of acromegaly with bronchial carcinoid tumor. *Am J Med* 1984;76:605.
89. Boizel R, Labat F, Bachelot I, et al. Acromegaly due to a growth hormone releasing hormone secreting bronchial carcinoid tumor. Further information on the abnormal responsiveness of the somatotroph cells and their recovery after successful treatment. *J Clin Endocrinol Metab* 1987;64:304.
90. Blackman MR, Rosen SW, Weintraub BD. Ectopic hormones. *Adv Intern Med* 1978;23:85.
91. Lees LH. The biosynthesis of hormones by nonendocrine tumors—a review. *J Endocrinol* 1975;67:143.
92. Ilan Y, Sibirsky O, Livni N, et al. Plasma and tumor prolactin in colorectal cancer. *Dig Dis Sci* 1995;40:2010.
93. Hennen G. Characterization of a thyroid-stimulating factor in human cancer tissue. *J Clin Endocrinol Metab* 1967;27:610.
94. Odell WD, Bates RW, Rivlin RS, et al. Increased thyroid function without clinical hyperthyroidism in patients with choriocarcinoma. *J Clin Endocrinol Metab* 1963;23:658.
95. Cave WT Jr, Dunn JT. Choriocarcinoma with hyperthyroidism: probable identity of the thyrotropin with human chorionic gonadotropin. *Ann Intern Med* 1976;85:60.
96. Odell WD, Wolfsen AR. Humoral syndromes associated with cancer. *Ann Rev Med* 1978;29:379.
97. Sluiter WJ, Marrink J, Houwen B. Monoclonal gammopathy with an insulin binding IgG(k) M-component associated with severe hypoglycemia. *Br J Haematol* 1986;62:679.
98. Stuart CA, Prince MJ, Peters EJ, et al. Insulin receptor proliferation: a mechanism for tumor-associated hypoglycemia. *J Clin Endocrinol Metab* 1986;63:879.
99. Younus S, Soterakis J, Sossi AJ, et al. Hypoglycemia secondary to metastases to the liver. A case report and review of the literature. *Gastroenterology* 1977;72:334.
100. Kiang DT, Bauer GE, Kennedy BJ. Immunoassayable insulin in carcinoma of the cervix associated with hypoglycemia. *Cancer* 1973;31:801.
101. Silvert CK, Rossini AA, Ghazvinian S, et al. Tumor hypoglycemia: deficient splanchnic glucose output and deficient glucagon secretion. *Diabetes* 1976;25:202.
102. Solomon J. Case report: spurious hypoglycemia and hyperkalemia in myelomonocytic leukemia. *Am J Med Sci* 1974;267:359.
103. Zapf J, Walter H, Froesch ER. Radioimmunological determination of insulin-like growth factors I and II in normal subjects and in patients with growth disorders and extrapancreatic tumor hypoglycemia. *J Clin Invest* 1981;68:3121.
104. Gorden P, Hendricks CM, Kahn CR, et al. Hypoglycemia associated with non-islet cell tumor and insulin like growth factors. *N Engl J Med* 1981;305:1452.
105. Li TCM, Reed C, Stubenbard WT, et al. Surgical cure of hypoglycemia associated with cystosarcoma phylloides and elevated NSILP. *Am J Med* 1983;74:1080.
106. Van Wyk JJ, Underwood LE, Hintz RL, et al. The somatomedins: a family of insulin-like hormones under growth hormone control. *Recent Prog Horm Res* 1974;30:259.
107. Daughaday W, Emanuele M, Brooks M, et al. Synthesis and secretion of IGF-II by leiomyosarcoma with associated hypoglycemia. *N Engl J Med* 1988;319:1434.
108. Ron D, Powers A, Pandian M, et al. Increased IGF-II production and consequent suppression of GH secretion: a dual mechanism for tumor-induced hypoglycemia. *J Clin Endocrinol Metab* 1989;68:701.
109. Hocking W, Goodman J, Golde D. Granulocytosis associated with tumor cell production of colony stimulating activity. *Blood* 1983;61:600.
110. Clark SC, Kamen R. The human hematopoietic colony stimulating factors. *Science* 1987;236:1229.
111. Hammond D, Winnick S. Paraneoplastic erythrocytosis and ectopic erythropoietins. *Ann N Y Acad Sci* 1974;230:219.
112. Valentine WN, Hennessy TG, Lang E, et al. Polycythemia: erythrocytosis and erythema. *Ann Intern Med* 1968;69:587.
113. Lees LH. The biosynthesis of hormones by nonendocrine tumors—a review. *J Endocrinol* 1975;67:143.
114. Spivak J. Cancer-related anemia: its cause and characteristics. *Semin Oncol* 1994;21(Suppl 3):3.
115. Jacobs EM, Hutter RVP, Pool JL, Ley AB. Benign thymoma and selective erythroid aplasia of the bone marrow. *Cancer* 1959;12:47.
116. Vasavada PJ, Bournigal LJ, Reynolds RW. Thymoma associated with pure red cell aplasia and hypogammaglobulinemias. *Postgrad Med* 1973;54:93.
117. Akard LP, Brandt J, Lee L, et al. Chronic T cell lymphoproliferative disorder and pure red cell aplasia. *Am J Med* 1987;83:1069.
118. Barry KG, Crosby WH. Autoimmune hemolytic anemia arrested by removal of an ovarian teratoma: review of the literature and report of a case. *Ann Intern Med* 1957;47:1002.
119. Packman CH, Leddy JP. Acquired hemolytic anemia due to warm-reacting autoantibodies. In: Beutler I, Lichtman MA, Coller BS, Kipps TJ, eds. *Williams hematology.* New York: McGraw-Hill, 1995:677.
120. Frenkel E, Bick R, Rutherford C. Anemia of malignancy. *Hematol Oncol Clin North Am* 1997;10:861.
121. Spira MA, Lynch EC. Autoimmune hemolytic anemia and carcinoma: an unusual association. *Am J Med* 1979;67:753.
122. Antman KH, Skarin AT, Mayer RJ, et al. Microangiopathic hemolytic anemia and cancer: a review. *Medicine (Baltimore)* 1979;58:377.
123. Sack GH, Levin J, Bell WR. Trousseau's syndrome and other manifestations of chronic disseminated coagulopathy in patients with neoplasms. *Medicine (Baltimore)* 1977;56:1.
124. Robinson WA. Granulocytosis in neoplasia. *Ann N Y Acad Sci* 1974;230:212.

125. Meyer LM, Rotter SD. Leukemoid reaction (hyperleukocytosis) in malignancy. *Am J Clin Pathol* 1942;12:218.
126. Fahey RJ. Unusual leukocyte response in primary carcinoma of the lung. *Cancer* 1952;4:930.
127. Hughes WF, Highley CS. Marked leukocytosis resulting from carcinomatosis. *Ann Intern Med* 1952;37:1095.
128. Barrett O Jr. Monocytosis in malignant disease. *Ann Intern Med* 1970;73:991.
129. Hocking W, Goodman J, Golde E. Granulocytosis associated with tumor production of colony stimulating factor. *Blood* 1983;61:600.
130. Sato K, Fujii Y, Kakiuchi T, et al. Paraneoplastic syndrome of hypercalcemia and leukocytosis caused by squamous carcinoma cells (T3M-1) producing parathyroid hormone-related protein, interleukin 2, and granulocyte colony stimulating factor. *Cancer Res* 1989;49:4740.
131. Heyman M, Walsh T. Autoimmune neutropenia and Hodgkin's disease. *Cancer* 1987;59:1903.
132. Wardlaw AJ, Kay AB. Eosinopenia and eosinophilia. In: Beutler E, Lichtman MA, Coller BS, Kipps TJ, eds. *Williams hematology*. New York: McGraw-Hill, 1995:844.
133. Slungaard A, Ascensao J, Zanjani E, Jacob HS. Pulmonary carcinoma with eosinophilia: demonstration of a tumor-derived eosinophilopoietic factor. *N Engl J Med* 1983;309:778.
134. Weller P. The immunobiology of eosinophils. *N Engl J Med* 1991;324:1110.
135. Lichtman MA. Basophilopenia, basophilia, and mastocytosis. In: Beutler E, Lichtman MA, Coller BS, Kipps TJ, eds. *Williams hematology*. New York: McGraw-Hill, 1995:852.
136. Levin J, Conley CL. Thrombocytosis associated with malignant disease. *Arch Intern Med* 1964;114:497.
137. Estrov Z, Talpaz M, Maligit G, et al. Elevated plasma thrombopoietin activity in patients with cancer related thrombocytosis. *Am J Med* 1995;98:551.
138. Kim HD, Boggs DR. A syndrome resembling idiopathic thrombocytopenic purpura in 10 patients with diverse forms of cancer. *Am J Med* 1979;67:371.
139. Doan C, Bouroncle BA, Wiseman BK. Idiopathic and secondary thrombocytopenic purpura. Clinical study and evaluation of 381 cases over a period of 28 years. *Ann Intern Med* 1960;53:861.
140. Bellone JD, Kunicki TS, Aster RH. Immune thrombocytopenia associated with carcinoma. *Ann Intern Med* 1983;99:470.
141. Kaden BR, Rosse WF, Hauch TW. Immune thrombocytopenia in lymphoproliferative diseases. *Blood* 1979;53:545.
142. Khilanani P, Al-Sarraf M. The association of autoimmune thrombocytopenia and Hodgkin's disease. *Oncology* 1973;28:238.
143. Jones SE. Autoimmune disorders and malignant lymphoma. *Cancer* 1973;31:1092.
144. Trousseau A. Phlegmasia alba dolens. Clinique medicale de l'Hotel-Dieu de Paris, London. *N Sydenham Soc* 1865;3:94.
145. Kakkar A, DeRuvo N, Chinswangwatanakul V, et al. Extrinsic-pathway activation in cancer with high factor VIIa and tissue factor. *Lancet* 1995;346:1004.
146. Pineo G, Brain M, Gallus A. Tumors, mucus production and hypercoagulability. *Ann NY Acad Sci* 1974;230:262.
147. Bick R, Struass J, Frenkel E. Thrombosis and hemorrhage in oncology patients. *Hematol Oncol Clin North Am* 1997;10:875.
148. Green D, Hull RD, Brant R, Pineo GF. Lower mortality in cancer patients treated with low-molecular weight heparin versus standard heparin. *Lancet* 1992;339:1476.
149. Siragusa S, Cosmi B, Piovella F, et al. Low-molecular-weight heparins and unfractionated heparin in the treatment of patients with acute venous thromboembolism: results of a meta-analysis. *Am J Med* 1996;100:269.
150. Grainick HR, Abrell E. Studies of the procoagulant and fibrinolytic activity of promyelocytes in acute promyelocytic leukemia. *Br J Hematol* 1973;24:59.
151. Goodnight SH Jr. Bleeding and intravascular clotting in malignancy: a review. *Ann NY Acad Sci* 1974;230:271.
152. Siegal T, Seligsohn U, Aghai E, Modan M. Clinical and laboratory aspects of disseminated intravascular coagulation (DIC): a study of 118 cases. *Thromb Haemost* 1978;39:122.
153. MacDonald RA, Robbins SL. The significance of nonbacterial thrombotic endocarditis: autopsy and clinical study of 78 patients. *Ann Intern Med* 1957;46:255.
154. Studdy P, Wiloughby JMT. Non-bacterial thrombotic endocarditis in early cancer. *Br J Med* 1976;1:752.
155. Rosen P, Armstrong D. Nonbacterial thrombotic endocarditis in patients with malignant neoplastic disease. *Am J Med* 1973;54:23.
156. Gonzales Quintela A, Candela M, Vidal C, et al. Non-bacterial thrombotic endocarditis in cancer patients. *Acta Cardiol* 1991;46:1.
157. Waldmann TA. Protein losing enteropathy. *Gastroenterology* 1966;50:422.
158. Waldmann TA. Protein losing enteropathies. In: Haubrich WS, Kalser MA, Roth JL, Schaffner F, eds. *Bockus gastroenterology*. 4th ed. Philadelphia, WB Saunders, 1985:1814.
159. Florent C, L'Hirondel C, Dexmazures C, et al. Intestinal clearance of alpha1-anti-trypsin. A sensitive method for the detection of protein losing enteropathy. *Gastroenterology* 1981;81:777.
160. Thomas DW, Sinatra FR, Merritt RJ. Random fecal alpha1-anti-trypsin concentration in children with gastrointestinal disease. *Gastroenterology* 1981;80:776.
161. Jeffries GH. Protein losing enteropathy. In: Sleisenger MH, Fortrand JS, eds. *Gastrointestinal disease: pathophysiology, diagnosis, management*. 4th ed. Philadelphia, WB Saunders, 1989:283.
162. Schwartz M, Jarnum S. Protein losing gastroenteropathy: hypoproteinemia due to gastrointestinal protein loss of varying aetiology, diagnosed by means of 131I-albumin. *Dan Med Bull* 1961;8:1.
163. Laine L, Politoske EJ, Gill P. Protein losing enteropathy in acquired immune deficiency syndrome due to intestinal Kaposi's sarcoma. *Arch Intern Med* 1987;147:1174.
164. Bedine MS, Yeardley JH, Elliot HL, et al. Intestinal involvement in Waldenström's macroglobulinemia. *Gastroenterology* 1973;65:308.
165. Sum PT, Hoffman MM, Webster DR. Protein losing gastroenteropathy in patients with gastrointestinal cancer. *Can J Surg* 1964;7:1.
166. Strygler B, Nicor MJ, Santangelo WC, et al. Alpha1-anti-trypsin excretion in stool in normal subjects and in patients with gastrointestinal disorders. *Gastroenterology* 1990;99:1380.
167. DeWys WD, Begg D, Lavin PT, et al. Prognostic effect of weight loss prior to chemotherapy in cancer patients. *Am J Med* 1980;69:491.
168. Hickman DM, Miller RA, Rambeau JL, et al. Serum albumin and body weight as predictors of post-operative course in colorectal cancer. *JPEN J Parenter Enteral Nutr* 1980;4:314.
169. Langstein HN, Norton JA. Mechanisms of cancer cachexia. *Hematol Oncol Clin North Am* 1991;5:103.
170. Mantovani G, Maccio A, Lai P, et al. Cytokine involvement in cancer anorexia/cachexia: role of megestrol acetate and medroxyprogesterone acetate on cytokine downregulation and improvement of clinical symptoms. *Crit Rev Oncol* 1998;9:99.
171. Oliff A, Defeo-Jones D, Boyer M. Tumors secreting human TNF/cachectin induce cachexia in mice. *Cell* 1987;50:555.
172. Tisdale MJ. Cancer cachexia: metabolic alterations and clinical manifestations. *Nutrition* 1997;13:1.
173. Lundholm K, Byland AC, Holm J, et al. Skeletal muscle metabolism in patients with malignant tumors. *Eur J Cancer* 1976;12:465.
174. Warren RS, Jeevanandam M, Brennan MF. Protein synthesis in tumor-influenced hepatocyte. *Surgery* 1985;98:275.
175. Kralovic RC, Zepp A, Canedella RJ. Studies of the mechanism of fat depletion in experimental cancer. *Eur J Cancer* 1977;13:1071.
176. Moldawer LL, Copeland EM. Proinflammatory cytokines, nutritional support, and the cachexia syndrome: interactions and therapeutic options. *Cancer* 1997;79:1828.
177. Seltzer MH, Slocum BA, Cataldi-Betcher EL, et al. Instant nutritional assessment: absolute weight loss and surgical mortality. *JPEN J Parenter Enteral Nutr* 1982;6:218.
178. Body JJ. The syndrome of anorexia-cachexia. *Curr Opin Oncol* 1999;11:255.
179. Ottery FD, Walsh D, Strawford A. Pharmacologic management of anorexia/cachexia. *Semin Oncol* 1998;25(Suppl 6):35.
180. Vadell C, Segui MA, Giminez-Arnau JM, et al. Anticachectic efficacy of megestrol acetate at different doses and versus placebo in patients with neoplastic cachexia. *Am J Clin Oncol* 1998;4:347.
181. Lee JC, Yamauchi H, Hopper J. The association of cancer and nephrotic syndrome. *Ann Intern Med* 1966;64:41.
182. Dinh BL, Brassard A. Renal lesion associated with the Walker 256 adenocarcinoma in the rat. *Br J Exp Pathol* 1968;49:145.
183. Zimmerman SW, Vishnu-Moorthy A, Burkholder PM, et al. Glomerulopathies associated with neoplastic disease. In: Rieselbach RE, Garnick NB, eds. *Cancer in the kidney*. 1st ed. Philadelphia: Lea & Febiger, 1982.
184. Stuart K, Faloon BG, Cardi NA. Development of nephrotic syndrome in a patient with prostatic carcinoma. *Am J Med* 1986;80:295-298.
185. Eagen JW, Lewis EJ. Glomerulopathies of neoplasia. *Kidney Int* 1977;11:297.
186. Coltharp W, Lee S, Miller R, et al. Nephrotic syndrome complicating adenocarcinoma of the lung with resolution after resection. *Ann Thorac Surg* 1991;51:308.
187. Heaton JM, Menzin MA, Carney DN. Extrarenal malignancy and the nephrotic syndrome. *J Clin Pathol* 1975;28:944.
188. Whelan TV, Hirszel P. Minimal-change nephropathy associated with pancreatic carcinoma. *Arch Intern Med* 1988;148:975.
189. Schroeter NJ, Rushing DA, Parker JP, et al. Minimal-change in nephrotic syndrome associated with malignant mesothelioma. *Arch Intern Med* 1986;148:1834.
190. Maesaka J, Mittel S, Fishbane S. Paraneoplastic syndromes of the kidney. *Semin Oncol* 1997;24:373.
191. Lesesne J, Rothschild N, Erickson B. Cancer-associated hemolytic-uremic syndrome: analysis of 85 cases from a national registry. *J Clin Oncol* 1989;7:781.
192. Martinez-Maldonado M, Ramirez de Arellano JA. Renal involvement in malignant lymphomas: a survey of 49 cases. *J Urol* 1966;95:485.
193. Richmond J, Sherman RS, Diamond HD, et al. Renal lesions associated with malignant lymphoma. *Am J Med* 1962;32:184.
194. Weimar G, Culp DA, Loening S, et al. Urogenital involvement by malignant lymphomas. *J Urol* 1981;125:230.
195. Shapiro JH, Ramsay CG, Jacobson HG, et al. Renal involvement in lymphomas and leukemias in adults. *AJR Am J Roentgenol* 1962;88:928.
196. Brown J, Winkelmann RK. Acanthosis nigricans, a study of 90 cases. *Medicine* 1968;47:33.
197. Curth HO, Hilberg AW, Machacek GF. The site and histology of the cancer associated with malignant acanthosis nigricans. *Cancer* 1962;15:364.
198. Ackerman AB, Lantis LR. Acanthosis nigricans associated with Hodgkin's disease: concurrent remission and exacerbation. *Arch Dermatol* 1967;95:202.
199. Cohen RP, Grossman ME, Almeida L, Kurzrock R. Tripe palms and cancer. *Clin Dermatol* 1993;11:165.
200. Cohen PR, Kurzrock R. Malignancy-associated tripe palms. *J Am Acad Dermatol* 1992;27(2 Pt 1):271.
201. Fitzpatrick TB, Montgomery H, Lerner AB. Pathogenesis of generalized dermal pigmentation secondary to malignant melanoma and melanuria. *J Invest Dermatol* 1954;22:163.
202. Eldar M, Weinberger A, Ben Bassat M, et al. Diffuse melanosis secondary to disseminated malignant melanoma. *Cutis* 1980;25:416.
203. Sexton M, Snyder CR. Generalized melanosis in occult primary melanoma. *J Am Acad Dermatol* 1989;20:261.
204. Nelson DH, Meakin JW, Thorn GW, et al. ACTH-producing pituitary tumors following adrenalectomy for Cushing's syndrome. *Ann Intern Med* 1960;52:560.
205. Venencie PY, Perry HO. Sign of Leser-Trélat: report of two cases and review of the literature. *J Am Acad Dermatol* 1984;10:83.
206. Sperry K, Wall J. Adenocarcinoma of the stomach with eruptive seborrheic keratoses: the sign of Leser-Trélat. *Cancer* 1980;45:2434.

207. Holdiness MR. The sign of Leser-Trélat. *Int J Dermatol* 1986;25:564.
208. Richard M, Giroux JM. Acrokeratosis paraneoplastica (Bazex's syndrome). *J Am Acad Dermatol* 1987;16:178.
209. Boudoulas O, Camisa C. Paraneoplastic acrokeratosis: Bazex's syndrome. *Cutis* 1986;37:449.
210. Bolognia JL. Bazex's syndrome. *Clin Dermatol* 1993;11:37.
211. Ashikari R, Park K, Huvos AG, Urban JA. Paget's disease of the breast. *Cancer* 1970;26:680.
212. Cohen PR, Kurzrock R. Sweet's syndrome and malignancy. *Am J Med* 1987;82:1220.
213. Cooper PH, Innes DJ, Greer KE. Acute febrile neutrophilic dermatosis (Sweet's syndrome) and myeloproliferative disorders. *Cancer* 1983;51:1518.
214. Cohen PR, Talpaz M, Kurzrock R. Malignancy-associated Sweet's syndrome. *J Clin Oncol* 1988;6:1887.
215. Cohen P, Kurzrock R. Mucocutaneous paraneoplastic syndromes. *Semin Oncol* 1997;24:334.
216. Langolis JC, Shaw JM, Odland GF. Erythema gyratum repens unassociated with internal malignancy. *J Am Acad Dermatol* 1985;12:911.
217. Solomon H. Erythema gyratum repens. *Arch Dermatol* 1969;100:639.
218. Thomson J, Stankler J. Erythema gyratum repens. *Br J Dermatol* 1970;82:406.
219. Hashizume T, Kiryu H, Noda K, et al. Glucagonoma syndrome. *J Am Acad Dermatol* 1988;19:377.
220. Mallinson CN, Bloom SR, Warin AP, et al. A glucagonoma syndrome. *Lancet* 1974;2:1.
221. Murray JS, Paton RR, Pope CE. Pancreatic tumor associated with flushing and diarrhea. *N Engl J Med* 1961;264:436.
222. Cunliffe WJ, Black MM, Hall R, et al. A calcitonin secreting thyroid carcinoma. *Lancet* 1968;2:63.
223. Plaskin J, Landau Z, Coslovsky R. A carcinoid-like syndrome caused by a prostaglandin secreting renal cell carcinoma. *Arch Intern Med* 1980;140:1095.
224. Wilkin JK. Flushing reactions: consequences and mechanisms. *Ann Intern Med* 1981;95:468.
225. Resnick RH, Gray SJ. Serotonin metabolism and the carcinoid syndrome: a review. *Med Clin North Am* 1960;44:1323.
226. Shelley WB. Erythema annulare centrifugum. *Arch Dermatol* 1964;90:54.
227. Mahood JM. Erythema annulare centrifugum: a review of 24 cases with special reference to its associations with underlying disease. *Clin Exp Dermatol* 1983;8:383.
228. Abrahams F, McCarthy JT, Sanders SL. 101 cases of exfoliative dermatitis. *Arch Dermatol* 1963;87:96.
229. Nicolis GD, Helwig EB. Exfoliative dermatitis: a clinicopathologic study of 135 cases. *Arch Dermatol* 1973;108:788.
230. MacMahon HE, Brown PA, Shen EM. Acinar cell carcinoma of the pancreas with subcutaneous fat necrosis. *Gastroenterology* 1965;49:555.
231. Hughes PSH, Apisarnthanarax P, Mullins F. Subcutaneous fat necrosis associated with pancreatic disease. *Arch Dermatol* 1975;111:506.
232. Anhalt GJ, Kim SC, Stanley JR, et al. Paraneoplastic pemphigus. An autoimmune mucocutaneous disease associated with neoplasia. *N Engl J Med* 1990;323:1729.
233. Krain LS, Bierman SM. Pemphigus vulgaris and internal malignancy. *Cancer* 1974;33:1091.
234. Armin A, Nadimi H, Robinson J. Pemphigus vulgaris and malignancy. *Int J Oral Surg* 1985;14:376.
235. Nousari H, Anhalt G. Pemphigus and bullous pemphigoid. *Lancet* 1999;354:667.
236. Amagai M, Nishikawa T, Nousari HC, et al. Antibodies against desmoglein 3 (pemphigus vulgaris antigen) are present in sera from patients with paraneoplastic pemphigus and cause acantholysis in vivo in neonatal mice. *J Clin Invest* 1998;102:775.
237. Nousari H, Brodsky R, Jones R, et al. Immunoablative high-dose cyclophosphamide without stem cell rescue in paraneoplastic pemphigus: report of a case and review of this new therapy for severe autoimmune disease. *J Am Acad Dermatol* 1999;40:750.
238. Finan MC, Connolly SM. Sebaceous gland tumors and systemic disease: a clinicopathologic analysis. *Medicine* 1984;63:232.
239. Housholder MS, Zeligman I. Sebaceous neoplasms associated with visceral carcinomas. *Arch Dermatol* 1980;116:61.
240. Burgdorf WHC, Pitha J, Fahmy A. Muir-Torre syndrome. Histologic spectrum of sebaceous proliferations. *Am J Dermatopathol* 1986;8:202.
241. Aram H. Acquired ichthyosis in mycosis fungoides. *J Assoc Milit Dermatol* 1984;10:32.
242. Polisky RB, Bronson DM. Acquired ichthyosis in a patient with adenocarcinoma of the breast. *Cutis* 1986;38:359.
243. Krakowski A, Brenner S, Covo J, et al. Acquired ichthyosis in Kaposi's sarcoma. *Dermatologica* 1973;147:348.
244. Young L, Steinman HK. Acquired ichthyosis in a patient with acquired immunodeficiency syndrome and Kaposi's sarcoma. *J Am Acad Dermatol* 1987;16:395.
245. Cox NH, Lawrence CM, Langtry JAA, et al. Dermatomyositis. Disease associations and an evaluation of screening investigations for malignancy. *Arch Dermatol* 1990;126:61.
246. Basset-Seguin M, Roujeau JC, Gherardi R, et al. Prognostic factors and predictive signs of malignancy in adult dermatomyositis. *Arch Dermatol* 1990;126:633.
247. Barnes BE. Dermatomyositis and malignancy: a review of the literature. *Ann Intern Med* 1976;84:68.
248. Sigurgeirsson B, Lindelöf B, Edhag O, et al. Risk of cancer in patients with dermatomyositis or polymyositis. *N Engl J Med* 1992;326:363.
249. Vogl A, Goldfischer S. Pachydermoperiostosis. Primary or idiopathic hypertrophic osteoarthropathy. *Am J Med* 1962;33:166.
250. Lyell A, Whittle CH. Hypertrichosis lanuginosa acquired type. *Br J Dermatol* 1951;63:411.
251. Hegedus SI, Schorr WF. Acquired hypertrichosis lanuginosa and malignancy. *Arch Dermatol* 1972;106:84.
252. Lober CW. Should the patient with generalized pruritus be evaluated for malignancy? *J Am Acad Dermatol* 1988;19(2 Pt 1):350.
253. Rajka G. Investigation of patients suffering from generalized pruritus, with special references to systemic diseases. *Acta Derm Venereol* 1966;46:190.
254. Cormia FE. Pruritus, an uncommon but important symptom of systemic cancer. *Arch Dermatol* 1965;92:36.
255. Schimpff S, Serpick A, Stoler B, et al. Varicella-zoster infection in patients with cancer. *Ann Intern Med* 1972;76:241.
256. Dolin R, Reichman RC, Mazur MH, Whitley RJ. Herpes zoster-varicella infections in immunosuppressed patients. *Ann Intern Med* 1978;89:375.
257. Huberman M, Fossieck BE Jr, Bunn PA Jr, et al. Herpes zoster and small cell bronchogenic carcinoma. *Am J Med* 1980;68:214.
258. Lloyd KM II, Denis M. Cowden disease: a possible new symptom complex with multiple system involvement. *Ann Intern Med* 1963;58:136.
259. Salem OS, Steck WD. Cowden's disease (multiple hamartoma and neoplasia syndrome). A case report and review of the English literature. *J Am Acad Dermatol* 1983;8:686.
260. Elston DM, James WD, Rodman OG, et al. Multiple hamartoma syndrome (Cowden's disease) associated with non-Hodgkin's lymphoma. *Arch Dermatol* 1986;122:572.
261. Starink TM, Van der Veen JPW, Arwert F, et al. The Cowden syndrome: a clinical and genetic study in 21 patients. *Clin Genet* 1986;29:222.
262. Leppard B, Bussey HJR. Epidermoid cysts, polyposis coli and Gardner's syndrome. *Br J Surg* 1975;62:387.
263. Thomas KE, Watne AL, Johnson JE, et al. Natural history of Gardner's syndrome. *Am J Surg* 1968;115:218.
264. Reid JD. Intestinal carcinoma in the Peutz-Jeghers syndrome. *JAMA* 1974;229:833.
265. Perzin KH, Bridge MF. Adenomatous and carcinomatous changes in hamartomatous polyps of the small intestine (Peutz-Jeghers syndrome): report of a case and review of the literature. *Cancer* 1982;49:971.
266. Ryo UY, Roh SK, Balkin RB, et al. Extensive metastases in Peutz-Jeghers syndrome. *JAMA* 1978;239:2268.
267. Giardiello FM, Welsh SB, Hamilton SR, et al. Increased risk of cancer in the Peutz-Jeghers syndrome. *N Engl J Med* 1987;316:1511.
268. Trau H, Schewach-Millet M, Fisher BK, et al. Peutz-Jeghers syndrome and bilateral breast carcinoma. *Cancer* 1982;50:788.
269. Howel-Evans W, McConnell RB, Clarke CA, et al. Carcinoma of the oesophagus with keratosis palmaris et plantaris (tylosis). A study of two families. *Q J Med* 1958;107:413.
270. Bennion SD, Patterson JW. Keratosis punctata palmaris et plantaris and adenocarcinoma of the colon: a possible familial association of punctate keratoderma and gastrointestinal malignancy. *J Am Acad Dermatol* 1984;10:587.
271. Murata Y, Kumano K, Tani M. Acquired diffuse keratoderma of the palms and soles with bronchial carcinoma: report of a case and review of the literature. *Arch Dermatol* 1988;124:497.
272. Crowe FW. Axillary freckling as a diagnostic aid in neurofibromatosis. *Ann Intern Med* 1964;61:1142.
273. Howell JB. Nevoid basal cell carcinoma syndrome. Profile of genetic and environmental factors in oncogenesis. *J Am Acad Dermatol* 1984;11:98.
274. Howell JB, Freeman RG. Structure and significance of the pits with their tumors in the nevoid basal cell carcinoma syndrome. *J Am Acad Dermatol* 1980;2:224.
275. Gorlin RJ. Nevoid basal-cell carcinoma syndrome. *Medicine* 1987;66:98.
276. Butterworth T, Wilson M Jr. Dermatologic aspects of tuberous sclerosis. *Arch Dermatol Syph* 1941;43:1.
277. Christoferson LA, Gustafson MB, Petersen AG. Von Hippel-Lindau's disease. *JAMA* 1961;178:280.
278. Doll R, Kinlen L. Immunosurveillance and cancer: epidemiologic evidence. *BMJ* 1970;4:420.
279. Frizzera G, Rosai J, Dehner LP, et al. Lymphoreticular disorders in primary immunodeficiencies: new findings based on an up-to-date histologic classification of 35 cases. *Cancer* 1980;46:692.
280. Helm F, Helm J. Cutaneous markers of internal malignancies. In: Helm F, ed. *Cancer dermatology*. Philadelphia: Lea & Febiger, 1979:247.
281. Epstein CJ, Martin GM, Schultz AL, Motulsky AG. Werner's syndrome: a review of the symptomatology, natural history, pathologic features, genetics, and relationship to the natural aging process. *Medicine (Baltimore)* 1966;45:177.
282. Posner JB. Paraneoplastic syndromes. In: Posner JB, ed. *Neurologic complications of cancer*. Philadelphia: F.A. Davis, 1995:353.
283. Posner JB. Paraneoplastic syndromes. *Neurol Clin* 1991;9:919.
284. Oppenheim H. Uber Hirnsymptome bei Carcinomatose ohne nachweisbare. Veranderungen im Gehirn. *Charite-Annalen (Berlin)* 1888;13:335.
285. Houff S, Major E, Katz D, et al. Involvement of the JC virus-infected mononuclear cells from the bone marrow and spleen in the pathogenesis of progressive multifocal leukoencephalopathy. *N Engl J Med* 1998;318:301.
286. Saiz A, Graus F, Dalmau J, et al. Detection of 14-3-3 brain protein in the cerebrospinal fluid of patients with paraneoplastic neurologic disorders. *Ann Neurol* 1999;46:774.
287. Patchell RA, Posner JB. Neurologic complications of carcinoid. *Neurology* 1986;36:745.
288. Dalmau J, Furneaux HM, Rosenblum MK, Graus F, Posner JB. Detection of the anti-Hu antibody in specific regions of the nervous system and tumor from patients with paraneoplastic encephalomyelitis/sensory neuronopathy. *Neurology* 1991;41:1757.
289. Jean WC, Dalmau J, Ho A, Posner JB. Analysis of the IgG subclass distribution and inflammatory infiltrates in patients with anti-Hu-associated paraneoplastic encephalomyelitis. *Neurology* 1994;44:140.
290. Voltz R, Dalmau J, Posner JB, Rosenfeld MR. T-cell receptor analysis in anti-Hu associated paraneoplastic encephalomyelitis. *Neurology* 1998;51:1146
291. Benyahia B, Liblau R, Merle-Beral H, et al. Cell mediated auto-immunity in paraneoplastic neurologic syndromes with anti-Hu antibodies. *Ann Neurol* 1999;45:162.
292. Tanaka K, Tanaka M, Inuzuka T, et al. Cytotoxic T lymphocyte-mediated cell death in paraneoplastic sensory neuronopathy with anti-Hu antibody. *J Neurol Sci* 1999;163:159.
293. Dalmau J, Posner J. Paraneoplastic syndromes affecting the nervous system. *Semin Oncol* 1997;24:318.

294. Lang B, Newsom-Davis J, Wray D. Autoimmune aetiology for myasthenic (Eaton-Lambert) syndrome. *Lancet* 1981;1:224.
295. Dalmau J, Graus F, Rosenblum MK, et al. Anti-Hu-associated paraneoplastic encephalomyelitis/sensory neuronopathy. A clinical study of 71 patients. *Medicine (Baltimore)* 1992;71:59.
296. Grisold W, Drlicek M, Liszka-Setinek U, et al. Anti-tumour therapy in paraneoplastic disease. *Clin Neurol Neurosurg* 1995;97:106.
297. Batchelor T, Platten M, Hochberg F. Immunoadsorption therapy for paraneoplastic syndromes. *J Neurooncol* 1999;40:131.
298. Henson RA, Urich H. Encephalomyelitis with carcinoma. In: Henson R, Urich H, eds. *Cancer and the nervous system.* 1st ed. London: Blackwell Scientific, 1992:314.
299. Verschuuren J, Chuang L, Rosemblum MK, et al. Inflammatory infiltrates and complete absence of Purkinje cells in anti-Yo associated paraneoplastic cerebellar degeneration. *Acta Neuropathol (Berl)* 1996;91:519.
300. Hammack JE, Kotanides H, Rosenblum MK, Posner JB. Paraneoplastic cerebellar degeneration: clinical and immunologic findings in 21 patients with Hodgkin's disease. *Neurology* 1992;42:1938.
301. Peterson K, Rosenblum M, Kotenides H, et al. Paraneoplastic cerebellar degeneration I: a clinical analysis of 55 anti-Yo antibody positive patients. *Neurology* 1992;42:1931.
302. Henson RA, Urich H. Remote effects of malignant disease: certain intracranial disorders. In: Vinken PJ, Bruyn GW, Klawans HL, eds. *Handbook of clinical neurology.* Amsterdam: North-Holland, 1979:625.
303. Anderson NE, Rosenblum MK, Posner JB. Paraneoplastic cerebellar degeneration: clinical-immunological correlations. *Ann Neurol* 1988;24:559.
304. Dropcho EJ, Kline LB, Riser J. Antineuronal (anti-Ri) antibodies in a patient with steroid-responsive opsoclonus-myoclonus. *Neurology* 1993;43:207.
305. Tsukamoto T, Yamamoto H, Iwasaki Y, et al. Antineural autoantibodies in patients with paraneoplastic cerebellar degeneration. *Arch Neurol* 1989;46:1225.
306. Hinton R. Paraneoplastic neurologic syndromes. *Hematol Oncol Clin North Am* 1996;10:909.
307. Brain WR, Norris FH, eds. *The remote effects of cancer on the nervous system.* New York: Grune & Stratton, 1965.
308. Voltz R, Gultekin S, Rosenfeld M, et al. A serologic marker of paraneoplastic limbic and brain-stem encephalitis in patients with testicular cancer. *N Engl J Med* 1999;340:1788.
309. Altman AJ, Baehner RL. Favorable prognosis for survival in children with coincident opso-myoclonus and neuroblastoma. *Cancer* 1976;37:846.
310. Telander RL, Smithson WA, Groover RV. Clinical outcome in children with acute cerebellar encephalopathy and neuroblastoma. *J Pediatr Surg* 1989;24:11.
311. Russo C, Cohn S, Petruzzi M, et al. Long-term neurologic outcome in children with opsoclonus-myoclonus associated with neuroblastoma: a report from the Pediatric Oncology Group. *Med Pediatr Oncol* 1997;28:284.
312. Digre KB. Opsoclonus in adults. *Arch Neurol* 1986;43:1165.
313. Jacobson DM, Thirkill CE, Tipping SJ. A clinical triad to diagnose paraneoplastic retinopathy. *Ann Neurol* 1990;28:162.
314. Adamus G, Guy J, Schmiel J, et al. Role of anti-recoverin autoantibody in cancer associated retinopathy. *Invest Ophthalmol US Sci* 1993;34:2626.
315. Croft PB, Urich H, Wilkinson M. Peripheral neuropathy of sensorimotor type associated with malignant disease. *Brain* 1967;90:31.
316. Chalk CH, Windebank AJ, Kimmel DW, McManis PG. The distinctive clinical features of paraneoplastic sensory neuronopathy. *Can J Neurol Sci* 1992;19:346.
317. Schold SC, Cho ES, Somasundaram M, et al. Subacute motor neuronopathy: a remote effect of lymphoma. *Ann Neurol* 1979;5:271.
318. O'Neill JH, Murray NMF, Newsom-Davis J. The Lambert-Eaton myasthenic syndrome. A review of 50 cases. *Brain* 1988;111:577.
319. Leys K, Lang B, Johnston I, et al. Calcium channel autoantibodies in the Lambert-Eaton myasthenic syndrome. *Ann Neurol* 1991;29:307.
320. Fukunaga H, Engel AG, Lang B, et al. Passive transfer of Lambert-Eaton myasthenic syndrome with IgG from man to mouse depletes the presynaptic membrane active zones. *Proc Natl Acad Sci U S A* 1983;80:7636.
321. Plotz PH, Dalakas M, Leff RL, et al. Current concepts in the idiopathic inflammatory myopathies: polymyositis, dermatomyositis, and related disorders. *Ann Intern Med* 1989;111:143.
322. Dalakas MC, ed. *Polymyositis and dermatomyositis.* Boston: Butterworths, 1988.
323. Folli F, Solimena M, Cofiell R, et al. Autoantibodies to a 128-kd synaptic protein in three women with stiff-man syndrome and breast cancer. *N Engl J Med* 1993;328:546.
324. Levin M, Mazaffar T, Al-Lozi M, et al. Paraneoplastic necrotizing myopathy: clinical and pathologic features. *Neurology* 1998;50:764.
325. Oh S. Paraneoplastic vasculitis of the peripheral nervous system. *Neurol Clin* 1997;15:849.
326. Altman RD, Gray RG. Bone disease. In: Katzwa WA, ed. *Diagnosis and management of rheumatic diseases.* 2nd ed. Philadelphia: Lippincott, 1988:620.
327. Martinez-Lavin M, Matucci-Cerinic M, Jajic I, Pineda C. Hypertrophic osteoarthropathy: consensus on its definition, classification, assessment and diagnostic criteria. *J Rheumatol* 1993;20:1386.
328. Matucci-Cerinic M, Lotti T, Jajic I, et al. The clinical spectrum of pachydermoperiostosis (primary hypertrophic osteoarthropathy). *Medicine* 1991;70:208.
329. Caldwell DS, McCallum RM. Rheumatic manifestations of cancer. *Med Clin North Am* 1986;70:385.
330. Martinez-Lavin M, Weisman MH, Pineda CJ. Hypertrophic osteoarthropathy. In: Schumacher HR Jr, ed. *Primer on rheumatic diseases.* 9th ed. Atlanta: Arthritis Foundation, 1988:240.
331. Matucci-Cerinic M, Ceruso M, Lotti T, et al. The medical and surgical treatment of finger clubbing and hypertrophic osteoarthropathy. A blind study with coltrosine and a surgical approach to finger clubbing resection. *Clin Exp Rheumatol* 1992;10(Suppl 7):67.
332. Pitt P, Mowat A, Williams R, Hamilton E. Hepatic hypertrophic osteoarthropathy in liver transplantation. *Ann Rheumatol Dis* 1994;53:338.
333. Sansores RH, Villalba-Caloca J, Romerez-Venegas A, et al. Reversal of digital clubbing after lung transplantation. *Chest* 1995;107:283.
334. Greenberg SB, Taber L. Fever of unknown origin. In: Mackowiak PA, ed. *Fever: basic mechanisms in management.* New York: Raven Press, 1991:183.
335. Bodey GP. Overview of the problem of infections in the immunocompromised host. *Am J Med* 1985;79(Suppl 5B):56.
336. Wade JC. Management of infection in patients with acute leukemia. *Hematol Oncol Clin North Am* 1993;7:293.
337. Pizzo PA, Robichaud KJ, Wesley R, Commers JR. Fever in the pediatric and young adult patient with cancer. *Medicine* 1982;61:153.
338. Friocourt L, Jouquan J, Khoury S, et al. Fever in adult renal cancer. In: *Renal tumors: proceedings of the first international symposium on kidney tumors.* New York: Alan R. Liss, 1982:283.
339. Ashraf SJ, Arya SC, El-Sayed M, et al. A profile of primary hepatocellular carcinoma patients in the gizan area of Saudi Arabia. *Cancer* 1986;58:2163.
340. Larson EB, Featherstone HJ, Petersdorf RG. Fever of undetermined origin: diagnosis and follow-up of 105 cases, 1970–1980. *Medicine* 1982;61:269.
341. Dominguez EA, Rupp ME, Preagim LC. Fever without neutropenia. In: Abeloff MD, Armitage JO, Lichter AS, Niederhuber JE, eds. *Clinical oncology.* New York: Churchill Livingstone, 1995.
342. Bodel P, Ralph P, Wenc K, et al. Endogenous pyrogen production by Hodgkin's disease and human histiocytic lymphoma cell lines in vivo. *J Clin Invest* 1980;65:514.
343. Dinarello C, Cannon J, Wolff S, et al. Tumor necrosis factor (cachectin) is an endogenous pyrogen and induces production of interleukin 1. *J Exp Med* 1986;163:1433.
344. Dinarello C, Bunn P. Fever. *Semin Oncol* 1997;24:288.
345. Warshaw AL, Carey RW, Robinson DR. Control of fever associated with visceral cancers by indomethacin. *Surgery* 1981;89:414.
346. Chang JC, Gross HM. Utility of naproxen in the differential diagnosis of fever of undetermined origin in patients with cancer. *Am J Med* 1983;76:597.

Frank A. Greco
John D. Hainsworth

CHAPTER **48**

Cancer of Unknown Primary Site

Cancers of unknown primary site are common. Their exact incidence is unknown, because many of such patients are "assigned" other diagnoses (an issue discussed later in Carcinoma of Unknown Primary Site As a Distinct Clinicopathologic Entity) and are, therefore, not represented accurately in tumor registries. Nonetheless, unknown primary cancers accounted for 2% of all cancer diagnoses reported by Surveillance, Epidemiology and End Results registries between 1973 and 1987.[1] We believe that a more realistic estimate of the incidence of these patients is 6% of all invasive cancers in the United States per year (approximately 80,000 to 90,000 patients). Within this heterogeneous patient group are found several clinical presentations and histologic tumor types. The largest group of patients has metastatic carcinoma of unknown primary site. Others have equivocal histologic diagnoses and tumors that create difficulty in classification using the time-honored method of light-microscopical examination. Specialized pathologic studies are essential in delineating the type of neoplasm present in many of these patients and, at times, may suggest the site of origin. Extreme heterogeneity in clinical presentations, histologic appearances, and natural histories has rendered systematic evaluation of such patients difficult, and an established base of knowledge has developed slowly. Only a few investigators have been interested in detailed studies of these patients. Therefore, past information suffers from many generalizations and is not representative of the entire patient population. These data are derived from grouping all patients and deal primarily with results of various chemotherapeutic regimens.

Over the last few decades, several important oncologic issues have changed. Combination chemotherapy, often used with surgery or radiation therapy, has proved to be potentially curative for selected patients with several metastatic tumors. In addition, palliation and prolongation of survival have been demonstrated after systemic therapy for patients with many other tumor types. Furthermore, treatment continues to evolve and improve. Such therapeutic improvements have relevance for patients with cancers of unknown primary site, because some have these responsive neoplasms (i.e., with occult primaries or atypical histologies).

Diagnostic pathology has improved remarkably. More routine use of electron microscopy and the emerging fields of immunohistochemistry and molecular genetics are contributing to more precise diagnosis of neoplasms. Now possible is defining more reliably the histology and, at least in selected patients, the origin and biology of neoplasms. In concert with evolving diagnostic techniques, several clinical syndromes and features are being recognized and are helping physicians to understand and better manage patients with unknown primary cancer. Oncologists are rethinking issues involving patients with cancers of unknown primary site.

Appropriate patient management requires an understanding of several clinicopathologic features that help to identify patients with more responsive tumors. Typically, patients with cancer of unknown primary site develop symptoms or signs at a metastatic site, and the diagnosis is made by biopsy of a metastatic lesion. History, physical examination, and other appropriate evaluation of such patients fail to identify the primary site. The initial biopsy should be generous, because many studies may be required. Routine light-microscopical histology establishes the neoplastic process and provides a practical classification system by which the patient subsequently can be evaluated and managed. The broad category of cancers of unknown primary site offers four major light-microscopical diagnoses: (1) poorly differentiated neoplasm, (2) well-differentiated and moderately well-differentiated adenocarcinoma, (3) squamous cell carcinoma, and (4) poorly differentiated carcinoma (with or without

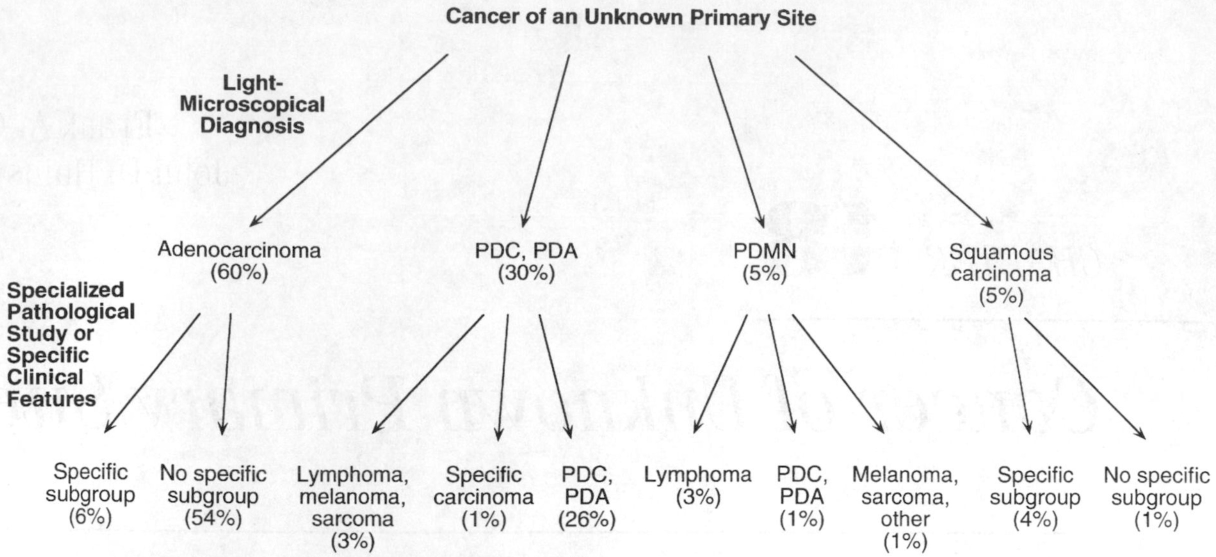

FIGURE 48-1. Relative size of various clinical and histologic subgroups of patients as determined by optimal clinical and pathologic evaluation. PDA, poorly differentiated adenocarcinoma; PDC, poorly differentiated carcinoma; PDMN, poorly differentiated malignant neoplasm. (From Hainsworth JD, Greco FA. Treatment of patients with cancer of an unknown primary site. *N Engl J Med* 1995;329:257, with permission.)

features of adenocarcinoma). These diagnoses vary with respect to clinical characteristics, recommended diagnostic evaluation, treatment, and prognosis. The approximate size of the various groups and subsets of patients are illustrated according to clinicopathologic evaluation in Figure 48-1.

POORLY DIFFERENTIATED NEOPLASMS OF UNKNOWN PRIMARY SITE

If pathologists are confident of a cancer but cannot differentiate a general category of neoplasm (e.g., carcinoma, lymphoma, melanoma, sarcoma), it is designated as a poorly differentiated neoplasm of unknown primary site. A more precise diagnosis is essential in patients having this type of cancer, because many have responsive tumors. Approximately 5% of all patients with cancers of unknown primary site (nearly 4000 U.S. patients annually) present with this diagnosis on initial light-microscopical appearance, but few remain without a defined lineage after specialized pathologic study. The most frequent tumor for which effective therapy is available is non-Hodgkin's lymphoma. In reported series, 35% to 65% of poorly differentiated neoplasms were found to be lymphomas after further pathologic study.[2–5] Most of the remaining tumors in this group are carcinomas. Melanoma and sarcoma together account for fewer than 15% of all tumors in such patients.

The evaluation of poorly differentiated tumors requires specialized pathologic studies. Immunoperoxidase tumor staining, electron microscopy, and genetic analysis can be helpful in the differential diagnosis. The most common cause of a nonspecific light-microscopical diagnosis is an inadequate or poorly handled biopsy specimen. If possible, fine-needle aspiration biopsy should not be performed in affected patients as an *initial* diagnostic procedure, because the histologic pattern is not preserved and the ability to perform special studies is limited. We have documented several instances in which a fine-needle aspiration has suggested a specific diagnosis, which was proved later to be incorrect by an incisional biopsy. Frequently, a more definitive diagnosis can be made by obtaining a larger biopsy. Communication with pathologists is important, as special tissue processing may be necessary for some pathologic studies. In addition, all clinical information also may help pathologists to narrow down, or become more certain of, diagnoses. Some neoplasms remain unclassifiable by light microscopy, even with an adequate biopsy specimen. Additional pathologic study always is indicated in such cases.

IMMUNOPEROXIDASE TUMOR STAINING

Immunoperoxidase staining is the specialized technique most widely available for the classification of neoplasms. Often, immunoperoxidase staining can be done on formalin-fixed, paraffin-embedded tissue, which broadens its applicability, rendering repeat biopsy unnecessary in some patients. Immunoperoxidase antibodies are either monoclonal or polyclonal and are directed at cell components or products, which can include enzymes [e.g., prostatic acid phosphate, neuron-specific enolase (NSE)]; normal tissue components [e.g., keratin, desmin, vimentin, neurofilaments, common leukocyte antigen (CLA)]; hormones and hormone receptors (e.g., estrogen receptor); oncofetal antigens [e.g., α-fetoprotein (AFP)]; carcinoembryonic antigen (CEA); and other substances (e.g., S-100 protein, chromogranin). Many new antibodies are being developed, and this area of diagnostic pathology is a dynamic and evolving field. Usually, specific diagnoses cannot be made on the basis of immunoperoxidase staining alone, because none of these reagents is directed at tumor-specific antigens. Staining also can be extremely variable, and a particular stain may be negative; yet, other data may nonetheless support a particular tumor type. For example, a neuroendocrine carcinoma does not stain invariably with all neuroendocrine reagents. Therefore, results must be interpreted in conjunction with the light-microscopical appearance and the clinical picture. Some immunoperoxidase staining patterns that are useful in the differential diagnosis of neoplasms are outlined in Table 48-1.

Usually, several important questions can be answered by immunoperoxidase staining. The CLA stain usually can be used to make the important distinction between lymphoma and carcinoma.[6,7] Staining for NSE, chromogranin, and synaptophysin can suggest a neuroendocrine carcinoma (e.g., small cell lung cancer, carcinoid, islet cell tumor, etc.).[8–10] Staining for prostate-specific antigen (PSA) strongly suggests prostate carcinoma in a man with metastatic adenocarcinoma.[10,11] Certain staining characteristics can suggest breast carcinoma (e.g., estrogen or progesterone receptors, gross cystic fluid protein 15), amelanotic melanoma (e.g., positive staining for S-100 protein, vimentin, HMB-45), or sarcoma (e.g., positive staining for desmin, vimentin, factor VIII antigen).[12–16] Staining for human chorionic gonadotropin (HCG) or AFP can suggest the diagnosis of a germ cell tumor in an appropriate clinical situation.[17,18]

Several problems are associated with immunoperoxidase stains. Technical expertise is required to perform these tests accurately and reproducibly, and proper interpretation requires an experienced pathologist. Appropriate control slides are stained and examined concurrently, because nonspecific staining occasionally is a problem. Care must be taken to avoid overinterpretation, because no staining pattern is entirely specific. Certain stains, particularly CLA and PSA, are relatively specific; however, false-positive and false-negative results can occur with any of these stains. For example, some carcinomas stain with vimentin, some sarcomas stain with keratin, and a wide variety of carcinomas (other than neuroendocrine and germ cell tumors) stain with NSE and HCG, respectively.

In some circumstances, diagnoses based on immunoperoxidase staining in patients with poorly differentiated neoplasms of unknown primary site can be used to plan therapy and to predict outcome. Undifferentiated neoplasms identified as lymphoma on the basis of positive CLA staining respond well to the combination chemotherapy used for non-Hodgkin's lymphoma.[2] In 35 patients with equivocal routine light-microscopical histology and positive CLA staining, treatment with a variety of standard lymphoma regimens results in an actuarial disease-free survival of 45% at 30 months. These patients' outcome was similar to that of a group of concurrently treated patients who had non-Hodgkin's lymphomas with typical light-microscopical histology. In patients whose diagnoses were based on immunoperoxidase staining with tumors other than lymphoma, only limited data exist concerning treatment outcome.

TABLE 48-1. Immunoperoxidase Tumor-Staining Patterns Useful in the Differential Diagnosis of Poorly Differentiated Neoplasms

Tumor Type	*Immunoperoxidase Staining*
Carcinoma	Epithelial stains (e.g., cytokeratin, EMA) (+)
	CLA, S-100, vimentin (–)
Lymphoma	CLA (+), rare false (–)
	EMA occasionally (+)
	All other stains (–)
Sarcoma	
Mesenchymal	Vimentin (+)
	Epithelial stains usually (–)
Rhabdomyosarcoma	Desmin (+)
Angiosarcoma	Factor VIII antigen (+)
Melanoma	S-100, vimentin, HMB-45 (+)
	NSE often (+)
	Synaptophysin (–)
	Epithelial stains (–)
Neuroendocrine tumor	NSE, chromogranin, synaptophysin (+)
	Epithelial stains (+)
Germ cell tumor	HCG, AFP (+)
	Placental alkaline phosphatase (+)
	Epithelial stains (+)
Prostate cancer	PSA (+), rare false (–) and (+)
	Epithelial stains (+)
Breast cancer	ER, PR (+)
	Gross cystic fluid protein 15 (+)
	Epithelial stains (+)
Thyroid	
Follicular	Thyroglobulin (+)
Medullary	Calcitonin (+)

+, positive result; –, negative result; AFP, α-fetoprotein; CLA, common leukocyte antigen; EMA, epithelial membrane antigen; ER, estrogen receptor; HCG, human chorionic gonadotropin; NSE, neuron-specific enolase; PR, progesterone receptor; PSA, prostate-specific antigen.

ELECTRON MICROSCOPY

A diagnosis can be made by electron microscopy in some poorly differentiated neoplasms. Electron microscopy is not widely available, requires special tissue fixation, is relatively expensive, and should be reserved for the study of neoplasms with unclear lineage after routine light microscopy and immunoperoxidase staining. Like immunoperoxidase staining, electron microscopy is reliable in differentiating lymphoma from carcinoma. It may be superior to immunoperoxidase staining for the identification of poorly differentiated sarcoma. Other structures, such as neurosecretory granules (neuroendocrine tumors) or premelanosomes (melanoma), can suggest a particular tumor. Often, undifferentiated tumors have nonspecific ultrastructural features; therefore, the absence of a particular ultrastructural finding cannot be used to rule out a specific diagnosis. Some neoplasms defy further classification despite specialized pathologic study.

In some instances, electron microscopy provides evidence for adenocarcinoma or squamous cell carcinoma. Features of adenocarcinoma include intercellular and intracellular lumina and surface microvilli. Squamous carcinomas are characterized by frequent and prominent desmosomes and by prominent bundles of prekeratin filaments in the adjacent cytoplasm. Usually, determining the origin of poorly differentiated adenocarcinoma or squamous carcinoma is not possible by electron-microscopical features. Treatment implications are unclear for adenocarcinoma and squamous carcinoma recognized only by ultrastructural features.

GENETIC ANALYSIS

The identification of chromosomal abnormalities and genetic changes associated with neoplasms is becoming increasingly important. The use of tumor-specific chromosomal abnormalities in diagnosis still is limited, but future research likely will identify many additional specific genetic abnormalities.

The biology of the primary tumor in patients with unknown primary neoplasms remains an enigma. Certainly, these tumors possess a metastatic phenotype. Some of these primary tumors may regress or involute or grow very slowly. Possibly some arise from embryonic epithelial "rest cells" that did not complete their appropriate migration. Often, karyotypic analysis of metastatic carcinomas demonstrates diverse multiple complex abnormalities, and is not yet helpful (in most instances) for diagnosis or classification, but is more representative of advanced neoplasms of many types (e.g., various chromosome 1p abnormalities).[19] Overexpression of p53, bcl-2, C-myc, Ras, and Her-2-neu has been observed in unknown primary carcinomas[20–22]; however, controversy continues regarding the frequency of expression and the clinical relevance. Tumors that strongly express p53 and bcl-2 may be more responsive to platinum-based chemotherapy.[21] Recently, we showed that 10% of the poorly differentiated carcinomas are strongly positive for Her-2-neu staining (F. A. Greco and J. D. Hainsworth, unpublished data). Patients affected by these tumors will be reasonable candidates for an anti-Her-2-neu antibody therapeutic trial. Recently, DNA microarrays have been studied in acute leukemias,[23] and this technique holds promise as a method of classifying neoplasms on the basis of gene expression monitoring, perhaps identifying specific genetic patterns or fingerprints independent of previous histologic and biologic knowledge. In the future, this and other techniques may identify more specific tumor lineages or primary tumor types subject to specific therapies in patients with unknown primary cancers. On the other hand, the pathogenesis of some carcinomas of unknown primary site may arise from specific genetic lesions. Possibly, many such tumors have similar gene expression distinct from specific carcinomas of recognized primary sites. This possibility is suggested by the unusual occurrence of metastatic adenocarcinoma of unknown primary site in monozygotic twin brothers with a primary immunodeficiency disorder (X-linked hyper-IgM syndrome).[24] The technology is now available to classify unknown primary carcinoma by gene expression, a technique that also has the potential to identify their primary origin and to provide more specific therapy by pharmacogenomic evaluation. As more precise and specific genetic lesions are identified in primary neoplasms and their metastases (e.g., lung, breast, ovary, germ cell), we can expect these data to provide more useful diagnostic and therapeutic information for unknown primary cancers. The identification of germ cell tumors already has met this expectation.

Chromosomal abnormalities have been well characterized in several hematopoietic neoplasms. Most B-cell non-Hodgkin's lymphomas are associated with tumor-specific immunoglobulin gene rearrangements, and typical chromosomal changes have been identified in some B-cell and T-cell lymphomas and in Hodgkin's disease.[25,26] In the rare instance when the diagnosis of lymphoma cannot be established definitively with either immunoperoxidase staining or electron microscopy, detection of chromosomal translocations t(14:18); t(8:14); or t(11:14) or the presence of an immunoglobulin gene rearrangement provides definitive diagnostic information.

A few other nonrandom chromosomal rearrangements associated with nonlymphoid tumors have been identified. A chromosomal translocation, t(11:22), has been found in peripheral neuroepitheliomas and frequently in Ewing's tumor.[27,28] An isochromosome of the short arm of chromosome 12 (i12p) and other chromosome 12 abnormalities are found in a large percentage of germ cell tumors.[29,30] A recently developed genomic hybridization technique can detect extra 12p material in paraffin-embedded tissue specimens.[31] This technique likely will improve the applicability of testing, as tissue culture is not necessary. Several other nonrandom cytogenetic abnormalities found in other tumors include t(2:13) in alveolar rhabdomyosarcoma; 3p deletion in small cell lung cancer; 1p deletion in neuroblastoma; t(X:18) in synovial sarcoma; and 11p deletion in Wilms' tumor. Polymerase chain reaction has been used to identify Epstein-Barr viral genomes in the tumor cells of patients with cervical lymph node metastases of unknown primary site, suggesting nasopharyngeal primaries.[32] Among head and neck tumors, Epstein-Barr virus has been associated only with nasopharyngeal carcinoma. Because some of these tumor types discussed are poorly differentiated and often are metastatic at the time of diagnosis, identification of these genetic changes may provide a specific diagnosis. Genetic diagnosis has been applied successfully to a subset of patients with carcinoma of unknown primary site (see Poorly Differentiated Carcinoma, later in this chapter).

ADENOCARCINOMA OF UNKNOWN PRIMARY SITE

CLINICAL CHARACTERISTICS

Well-differentiated and moderately well-differentiated adenocarcinoma are the most frequent light-microscopical diagnoses in patients with carcinoma of unknown primary site, accounting for approximately 60% of patients (some 50,000 U.S. patients annually). Typically, patients with this diagnosis are elderly and have metastatic tumors at multiple sites. Frequently, the sites of tumor involvement determine the clinical presentation; common metastatic sites include lymph nodes, liver, lung, and bone.

Often, the clinical course is dominated by symptoms and signs related to the metastases. The primary site becomes obvious in only 15% to 20% of patients during life.[33] At autopsy, however, a primary site is detected in 70% to 80% of patients. The most common primary sites identified at autopsy are the lung and pancreas, accounting for approximately 40%.[34] Other gastrointestinal sites (e.g., stomach, colon, liver) are frequent, although adenocarcinomas from a wide variety of other primary sites occasionally are encountered. Adenocarcinomas of the breast, prostate, and ovary are rare in patients in this group.[34] Also, an unexpected metastatic pattern seems to be observed; for example, occult pancreatic primaries more frequently involve bone rather than liver.

Historically, as a group, patients with metastatic adenocarcinoma of unknown primary site have a very poor prognosis, with inexorable progression and a median survival of only 3 to 4 months. This finding is not surprising, considering the fact that many such patients harbor lung or gastrointestinal neoplasms. Many patients in this group have widespread metastases and poor performance status at the time of diagnosis. However, stereotyping *all* patients with adenocarcinoma of unknown primary site would be an error, because within this large group are subsets of patients with more favorable prognoses. In addition, chemotherapy has improved considerably in the last 5 years, and many patients now candidates for chemotherapy have a reasonable expectation of clinical benefit and improved survival.

PATHOLOGY

The diagnosis of well-differentiated or moderately well-differentiated adenocarcinoma is based on light-microscopical features, particularly the formation of glandular structures by neoplastic cells. We have considered patients with well-differentiated or moderately well-differentiated adenocarcinoma as one group. These histologic features are shared by adenocarcinomas, and the site of the primary tumor usually cannot be determined by histologic examination. Typically, certain histologic features are associated with a particular tumor type (e.g., papillary features with ovarian cancer and signet-ring cells with gastric cancer). However, these characteristics are not specific enough to be used as definitive evidence of the primary site. Immunoperoxidase stains and electron microscopy are of limited value in identifying the site of origin of most well-differentiated or moderately well-differentiated adenocarcinomas. The stain for PSA is an exception because it is relatively specific for prostate cancer, and it should be used in men with suggestive clinical findings. Positive immunoperoxidase staining for estrogen or progesterone receptors and gross cystic fluid protein 15 suggests metastatic breast cancer in women with metastatic adenocarcinoma. Occasionally, neuroendocrine stains (e.g., NSE, chromogranin, synaptophysin) can identify an unsuspected neuroendocrine neoplasm. Several other stains or batteries of stains have been evaluated,[35–38] but none are truly tumor-specific and, if used, should be used in connection with all other clinical data.

The diagnosis of poorly differentiated adenocarcinoma should be viewed differently, because some affected patients are distinctive in tumor biology and responsiveness to systemic therapy (see Poorly Differentiated Carcinoma, later in this chapter). Usually, this diagnosis is made when only minimal or questionable glandular formation is seen on histologic examination or, on occasion, when tumors exhibit positive staining for mucin but have no "glandular features." Well-differentiated adenocarcinoma, poorly differentiated adenocarcinoma, and poorly differentiated carcinoma are diagnoses that probably represent parts of a spectrum of tumor differentiation rather than specific, sharply demarcated entities. These histologies represent a heterogeneous group of tumors with various biologic and clinical properties. Different pathologists may use slightly different criteria for making each of these three diagnoses. Therefore, an appropriate approach is to perform additional study with immunoperoxidase staining or electron microscopy in all poorly differentiated adenocarcinomas.

DIAGNOSTIC EVALUATION

An exhaustive search for the primary site is not indicated because it rarely can be found. Therefore, the clinical evaluation should be performed to evaluate any suspicious clinical symptoms or signs and to determine the extent of metastatic disease. Initial evaluation should include a thorough history and physical examination, standard laboratory screening tests (i.e., complete blood cell count, liver function tests, serum creatinine, urinalysis), and chest radiography. All men should have a serum PSA determination, and all women should undergo mammography. Computed tomography (CT) scans of the abdomen can identify a primary site in 10% to 35% of affected patients and frequently are useful in identifying additional sites of metastatic disease.[39,40] Additional symptoms, signs, or abnormal physical and laboratory findings should be evaluated with appropriate diagnostic studies. Extensive imaging evaluation of asymptomatic areas rarely is useful in identifying a primary site, is expensive, and often results in confusing or false-positive results.

Positron emission tomography (PET) may be an important addition for the evaluation of potential primary sites. These data are very limited now, but one small series identified likely primary sites in 7 of 29 patients (24%).[41] The availability of various tumor markers (CEA; CA-15-3; CA-19-9; CA-125, B-HCG, α-fetoprotein) has not proved, in general, to be useful for diagnosis or prognosis but can be used to follow the response to therapy.[42,43]

TREATMENT

The group of patients with adenocarcinoma of unknown primary site contains several clinically defined subgroups for which useful, rather specific therapy can be given. Therapy can be useful also for some patients who are not a part of one of these subgroups, as empiric chemotherapy recently has improved.

Peritoneal Carcinomatosis in Women

Adenocarcinoma causing diffuse peritoneal involvement is typical of ovarian carcinoma, although carcinomas from the gastrointestinal tract, lung, or breast occasionally can produce this clinical picture. In several women described with diffuse peritoneal carcinomatosis, no primary site was found in the ovaries or elsewhere in the abdomen at the time of laparotomy.[44–49] These patients frequently had histologic features typical of ovarian carcinoma, such as papillary configuration or psammoma bodies. This syndrome has been termed *multifocal extraovarian serous carcinoma* or *peritoneal papillary serous carcinoma.* These patients have a primary peritoneal carcinoma. In the early 1980s, several anecdotal case reports documented excellent responses to cisplatin-based chemotherapy in women with this syndrome.[44–47] This tumor is more common in women with a family history of ovarian cancer, and preventive oophorectomy, as expected, does not protect them from this disease.[48] As for ovarian carcinoma, the incidence of primary peritoneal carcinoma is increased in women with *BRCA1* mutations.[49]

Table 48-2 summarizes the results of seven series including a total of 258 women with this syndrome.[50–56] The clinical features are similar to ovarian carcinoma or abdominal carcinomatosis. Many patients have elevated serum levels of CA-125 antigen. An occasional patient will present with pleural effusion only. Metastases outside the peritoneal cavity are unusual, and their histologic features are similar to those of ovarian carcinoma (usually papillary configurations but also other histologies, including poorly differentiated carcinoma). The initial treatment plan for most patients included laparotomy with surgical cytoreduction, and the majority of these patients was treated with cisplatin-based combination chemotherapy. A few

TABLE 48-2. Therapy for Women with Peritoneal Adenocarcinomatosis of Unknown Primary Site

Study	*Number of Patients*	*Therapy*	*Complete Response Rate (%)*	*Long-Term Survival (%)*	*Median Survival (mo)*
Lele et al., 1988[50]	23	Surgical cytoreduction and cisplatin-based chemotherapy	22	26	19
Strnad et al., 1989[52]	18	Surgical cytoreduction and cisplatin-based chemotherapy	39	17	23
Dalrymple et al., 1989[51]	31	Surgical cytoreduction and cisplatin-based or chlorambucil chemotherapy	10	6	11
Ransom et al., 1990[53]	33	Surgical cytoreduction and cisplatin-based chemotherapy	13	9	17
Fromm et al., 1990[54]	74	Surgical cytoreduction, cisplatin alone, or in combination or melphalan alone	20	25	24
Bloss et al., 1993[55]	33	Surgical cytoreduction, cisplatin-based chemotherapy	35	15	20
Piver et al., 1997[56]	46	Surgical cytoreduction, cisplatin-based chemotherapy: paclitaxel-based chemotherapy	40	Too early	19
Totals	258		22	16	18

patients received cisplatin, chlorambucil, or melphalan alone. Recent series have documented the activity of paclitaxel.[56] A summary of the results in 258 women are as follows: Twenty-two percent (range, 10% to 40%) of all patients had a complete response to chemotherapy, median survival was 18 months (range, 11 to 24 months), and long-term survival (more than 2 years) was 16% (range, 6% to 26%).

Frequently, women with metastatic adenocarcinoma involving the peritoneal surface and no obvious primary site have biologically distinct tumors and often are responsive to chemotherapy. The site of origin of these carcinomas likely is the peritoneal surface (primary peritoneal carcinoma). Because ovarian epithelium is in part an extension of the mesothelial surface, some carcinomas arising from the peritoneal (mesothelial) surface may share a similar lineage (Müllerian derivation) and biology with ovarian carcinoma. Certainly, this possibility should be considered and would not be surprising (e.g., papillary mesothelioma). Optimal management of these patients includes aggressive surgical cytoreduction followed by postoperative chemotherapy. Cisplatin or carboplatin plus paclitaxel considered optimal for the treatment of advanced ovarian cancer would seem a reasonable choice for initial chemotherapy, and the results are likely to be similar to ovarian carcinoma.[57,58] Approximately 20% of the patients in this group have complete responses to therapy, and some 16% have prolonged disease-free survival.

We have encountered a few men with this syndrome (papillary adenocarcinoma), but confirming the precise biology is difficult, and the lesions may be metastatic from an occult primary tumor arising elsewhere. A trial of chemotherapy also should be considered.

Women with Axillary Lymph Node Metastases

Breast cancer should be suspected in women who have axillary lymph node involvement with adenocarcinoma. Occasionally, the histologic finding is poorly differentiated carcinoma. Men with occult breast cancer can present in this fashion but are rare. The initial lymph node biopsy should include measurement of estrogen and progesterone receptors. Elevated levels provide strong evidence for the diagnosis of breast cancer.[59] If no other metastases are identified, these patients may have stage II breast cancer with an occult primary, which is potentially curable with appropriate therapy. A few reports using PET and magnetic resonance imaging scans have identified occult breast cancer even with normal mammography results.[60,61] Additional study is necessary before these procedures are recommended routinely in this setting. Modified radical mastectomy has been recommended in affected patients, even when physical examination and mammography results are normal. An occult breast primary has been identified after mastectomy in 44% to 80% of patients.[62–64] Usually, primary tumors are less than 2 cm in diameter; in occasional patients, only noninvasive tumor is identified in the breast.[65] Prognosis after primary therapy is similar to that of other patients with stage II breast cancer.[62–66] Radiation therapy to the breast after axillary lymph node dissection is an effective alternative primary therapy. Adjuvant systemic chemotherapy is indicated in this setting and is similar to standard therapy for stage II breast cancer.

Women with metastatic sites in addition to the axillary lymph nodes may have metastatic breast cancer with an occult primary tumor. Such women should be managed as if they have metastatic breast cancer. Elevated serum levels of CA-15-3 or CA-27-29 suggest the possibility of breast cancer. Estrogen and progesterone receptor status is of particular importance because those with positive hormone receptors may derive major palliative benefit from hormonal therapy, chemotherapy, or both.

Men with Possible Prostate Carcinoma

PSA concentrations should be measured in men with adenocarcinoma of unknown primary site. These tumors also can be stained for PSA. Even when clinical features (i.e., metastatic patterns) do not suggest prostate cancer, a positive PSA (serum or tumor stain) is reason for a trial of hormonal therapy.[67,68] Osteoblastic bone metastases also are an indication for an empiric hormone trial, regardless of the PSA findings.

Chemotherapy for Metastatic Adenocarcinoma of Unknown Primary Site

Approximately 90% of patients with well-differentiated or moderately differentiated adenocarcinoma of unknown primary site are not listed in one of the several foregoing clinical subgroups. In the past, chemotherapy of various types has produced low response rates, very few complete responses, and no long-term survivals.[69]

The results of chemotherapy in reported series of 10 or more patients from 1964 to 1991 have been reviewed. A total of 1102 patients were reported in 33 trials.[33,70–93] The only single agent studied adequately was 5-fluorouracil (5-FU), with response rates ranging from 0% to 16%.[33,70,71] Cisplatin has been reported as a single drug in only one series,[72] with a response rate of 19%. Other single agents (including methotrexate, doxorubicin, mitomycin C, vincristine, and semustine) that have been reported produced response rates from 6% to 16%.[73] The FAM regimen (5-FU, doxorubicin, and mitomycin C) and various modifications have been used often, their use based on the demonstrated activity of these combination regimens in some gastrointestinal cancers.[71 85] Response rates varied from 8% to 39% (mean, 20%); complete responders registered fewer than 1%; median survival was 4 to 15 months (mean, 6 months); survival beyond 2 years was rare; and disease-free survival beyond 3 years was nonexistent.

These data should be viewed with several factors in mind. Some of the series are small, and large randomized comparisons are lacking. In addition to those with adenocarcinomas, some patients with poorly differentiated carcinoma of unknown primary site were included in many of these series. The patients did not undergo standard evaluation or comparison in regard to sites of metastasis (nodal vs. visceral), performance status, gender, or age.

Cisplatin-based combination chemotherapy has not been evaluated adequately. However, two small randomized comparisons of doxorubicin with or without cisplatin[74,77] (subject to the many confounding factors previously mentioned) demonstrated no difference in median survival but more toxicity in the cisplatin-containing arm. A third, more recent, small randomized trial[94] did show the superiority of cisplatin, epirubicin, and mitomycin C as compared to mitomycin C alone (median survival, 9.4 months vs. 5.4 months). We also have seen some useful clinical responses to cisplatin or carboplatin-based chemotherapy and to 5-FU plus leucovorin. The combination of 5-FU and leucovorin has not been evaluated adequately but does not appear active in patients with liver metastasis arising from an unknown primary site,[95] a group most likely to have gastrointestinal primaries.

Several retrospective analyses have identified clinical and pathologic features associated with a more favorable response to empiric chemotherapy.[96–99] Some of these features include tumor location in lymph nodes, female gender, and poorly differentiated histology. Patients with liver or bone involvement have a relatively poor prognosis.[96]

Recent chemotherapy has improved considerably for patients who have adenocarcinoma and poorly differentiated carcinoma but do not fit into a specific "treatable" subset. The introduction of several new drugs with rather broad-spectrum antineoplastic activity is changing the standard treatment for patients having any of several common epithelial cancers. These drugs include the taxanes, gemcitabine, vinorelbine, and the topoisomerase I inhibitors. We have completed several phase II trials incorporating paclitaxel and docetaxel into first-line therapy for patients with carcinoma of unknown primary site. The initial trial included 71 patients, and the preliminary results of the first 55 patients were published.[100] The chemotherapy regimen, patients' characteristics, and treatment results are summarized in Table 48-3, and the survival curve is shown in Figure 48-2 for all 71 patients (F. A. Greco and J. D. Hainsworth, unpublished data). With a minimum follow up of 34 months, the median survival was 11 months, and the 1-, 2-, and 3-year survivals were 48%, 20%, and 14%, respectively. This paclitaxel-based regimen delivered in a multicenter community-based setting (Minnie Pearl Research Network) was well tolerated and easily administered in the outpatient area. Only patients who had carcinoma of unknown primary site (any histology) and were not in a previously defined treatable subset, with the exception of poorly differentiated neuroendocrine carcinoma, were eligible for this trial. The response rate of 66 evaluable patients was 48%, with ten complete responses (15%). The toxicity was moderate, primarily myelosuppression, but with only 12 hospitalizations for fever-neutropenia and no treatment-related deaths. Long-term follow-up for these 71 patients (minimum follow-up, 34 months) is of interest; the median survival was 11 months, and the median 1-, 2-, and 3-year actual survivals of patients with complete response (20 months, 80%, 40%, 20%, respectively) was significantly longer ($P = .025$) than those with partial response or stable disease (11 months, 50%, 15%, 10%, respectively). This latter group survived significantly longer ($P = .033$) than did patients who progressed on therapy (Fig. 48-3).

Subsequently, we turned our attention to docetaxel and have performed two sequential phase II trials in the same patient population with either docetaxel (75 mg/m^2) and cisplatin (75 mg/m^2) given every 3 weeks in 26 patients or docetaxel (65 mg/m^2) and carboplatin [area under the curve (AUC) = 5] every 3 weeks in 47 patients (F. A. Greco and J. D.

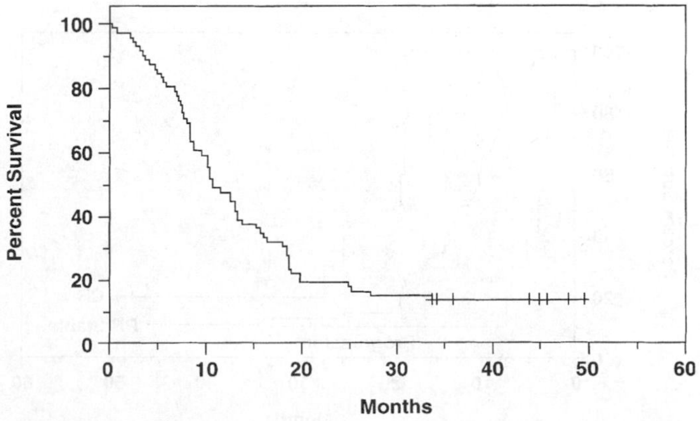

FIGURE 48-2. Survival curve for 71 patients with adenocarcinomas or poorly differentiated carcinoma. Patients with poor prognostic features were selected. The minimum follow-up is 34 months; median survival is 11 months; 1-, 2-, and 3-year survivals are 48%, 20%, and 14%, respectively.

TABLE 48-3. Summary of Phase II Trial of Paclitaxel, Carboplatin, and Extended-Schedule Oral Etoposide

REGIMEN

Repeat the following regimen at 21-day intervals for four to six courses:

Paclitaxel	200 mg/m^2, 1-hour IV infusion, day 1
Carboplatin	AUC = 6.0 IV, day 1
Etoposide	Alternating doses of 50 mg and 100 mg daily PO, days 1–10

PATIENT CHARACTERISTICS

Characteristic (N = 71)	*Number of Patients*
Age (y)	
Median	71
Range	31–82
Gender (male-female)	35:36
Histology	
Adenocarcinoma (well-differentiated)	34 (48%)
PDC or PDA	30 (42%)
Neuroendocrine carcinoma (poorly differentiated)	6 (9%)
Squamous carcinoma	1 (1%)

RESULTS

		Survival (%)		
Results	*Response Rate*	1 y	2 y	3 y
Entire group	48% (15% complete)	48	20	14
Adenocarcinoma	46%	47	21	13
PDC and PDA	50%	49	20	14

PDA, poorly differentiated adenocarcinoma; PDC, poorly differentiated carcinoma.

Hainsworth, unpublished data January 1999). These combinations also were active, but the docetaxel-plus-cisplatin regimen was associated with substantial gastrointestinal toxicity, and the carboplatin regimen was associated with more myelosuppression. More than 20% of all patients responded to these regimens, with no differences for those with well-differentiated adenocarcinoma or poorly differentiated carcinoma. Although the follow-up is shorter than that of the paclitaxel-based trial, the 1 and 2 year survivals are similar. By combining these taxane-based chemotherapy trials, a total of 144 patients (71 on paclitaxel regimen, 73 on docetaxel regimens) have been treated and followed up (Fig. 48-4). Some preliminary analysis of these patients is of interest. The median follow-up is 25 months, and median survival is 10 months, with actuarial sur-

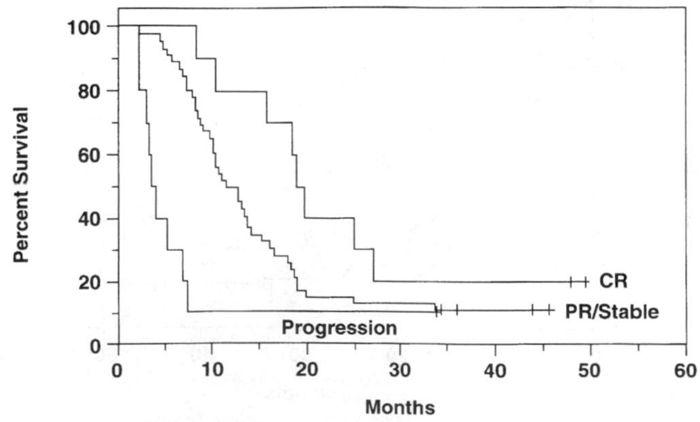

FIGURE 48-3. Survival curve for patients with complete response (CR) was significantly better (0.025) than for those with partial response (PR) or stable tumor, which in turn was better (0.033) than for those with progressive tumor.

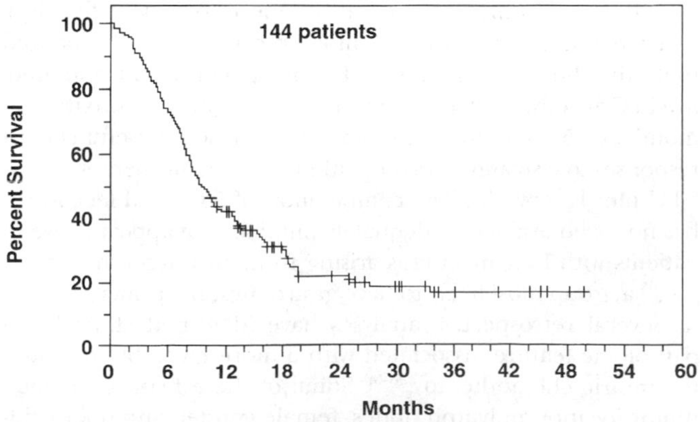

FIGURE 48-4. Survival curve for 144 patients who received taxane-based combination chemotherapy. With a median follow-up of 25 months, the median survival is 10 months, and the 1-, 2-, 3-, and 4-year survivals are 42%, 22%, 17%, and 17%, respectively.

vival at 1, 2, 3, and 4 years of 42%, 22%, 17%, and 17%, respectively. Complete responders, partial responders, and stable disease patients survive significantly longer than do those with progressive disease, and the study revealed a major trend for improvement in survival for poorly differentiated neuroendocrine carcinomas (too few in number to reach statistical significance). No difference was seen in survival for adenocarcinoma versus the poorly differentiated carcinomas. However, patients with known favorable subsets were not included in these trials. Women survived significantly longer than did men, and those with performance status 0, 1 (Eastern Cooperative Oncology Group scale) lived longer than did those with performance status 2. The progression-free survival of these 144 patients reveals that a small number of patients remain alive without progressive cancer: 1 year, 16%; 2 years, 9%; and 3 years, 9%. A subsequent, recently reported trial by others of 72 patients confirmed the activity of paclitaxel and carboplatin with a 41% response rate.[101] The median survival had not been reached but was greater than 8 months.

These data are encouraging. The patients who have more common unknown primary adenocarcinoma or poorly differentiated carcinoma but do not fit into any previously defined "treatable" subset now can attain substantial clinical benefits from taxane-based combination chemotherapy. Despite the fact that randomized trials still are lacking, both the median survival and 1-, 2-, and 3-year survival results are superior to the results seen in the past and are now comparable to the survivals of several other groups of advanced carcinoma patients receiving various types of chemotherapy (e.g., extensive-stage small cell lung cancer and advanced non–small cell lung cancer). Certainly, vast room for improvement exists, and basic and clinical research remain a priority for further enhancing the therapy for such patients.

We have continued to study empiric chemotherapy. Recently, gemcitabine was tested as secondary therapy in previously treated patients, and a response rate of only approximately 10% was observed, but several other patients had minor response or subjective improvement (or both). Topotecan given orally is being evaluated in previously treated patients. For previously untreated patients, the combination of paclitaxel, carboplatin, gemcitabine (followed by weekly paclitaxel consolidation) is ongoing.

SQUAMOUS CARCINOMA OF UNKNOWN PRIMARY SITE

Squamous carcinoma at a metastatic site represents approximately 5% of all patients with unknown primary carcinomas (nearly 4000 U.S. patients annually). Effective treatment is available for patients with certain clinical syndromes, and appropriate evaluation of these patients is important.

SQUAMOUS CARCINOMA INVOLVING CERVICAL AND SUPRACLAVICULAR LYMPH NODES

The cervical lymph nodes are the most common metastatic site. Usually, patients are middle-aged or elderly, and frequently they have abused tobacco or alcohol. When the upper or middle cervical lymph nodes are involved, a primary tumor in the head and neck region should be suspected. Clinical evaluation should include an examination of the oropharynx, hypopharynx, nasopharynx, larynx, and upper esophagus by direct endoscopy, with biopsy of any suspicious areas. CT of the neck better defines the disease in the neck and occasionally identifies a primary site. PET scanning also may identify primary sites but remains controversial.[102,103] Detection of Epstein-Barr virus genome in the tumor tissue is highly suggestive of a nasopharyngeal primary site[31] (see Genetic Analysis, earlier in this chapter), particularly in poorly differentiated carcinomas. Other genetic studies of squamous cell carcinoma of the head and neck region have shown genetic alterations in "normal tissue" as a precursor of invasive carcinoma.[104] Further study is indicated, as these findings do not yet have a practical application. When the lower cervical or supraclavicular lymph nodes are involved, a primary lung cancer should be suspected. Fiberoptic bronchoscopy should be performed if the chest radiograph and head and neck examination results are normal, as this has a high yield, frequently identifying a lung primary.[105]

When no primary site is identified, local treatment should be given to the involved neck. The reported results in more than 1400 patients are primarily retrospective, single-institution experiences, often using a variety of treatment modalities.[106–129] In many of these series, a large minority of patients had poorly differentiated carcinoma and adenocarcinoma (see Special Issues, Single Site of Neoplasm, later in this chapter). A substantial percentage (usually 30% to 40%) of patients achieved long-term disease-free survival after local treatment modalities. The results obtained using radical neck dissection, high-dose radiation therapy, or a combination of these modalities have been similar. The volume of tumor in the involved neck influences outcome, with N1 or N2 disease having a significantly higher cure rate than N3 disease or massive neck involvement.[126,128] Poorly differentiated carcinoma also represents a poor prognostic factor in such patients. When resection alone is used as the primary treatment modality, a primary tumor in the head and neck subsequently becomes apparent in 20% to 40% of patients. Primary tumors surface less commonly when radiation therapy is used, presumably owing to the eradication of occult head and neck primary sites within the irradiation field. Radiation therapy dosages and techniques should be similar to those used in patients with primary head and neck cancer,[117] and the nasopharynx, oropharynx, and hypopharynx may be included in the irradiated field.

Patients with low cervical and supraclavicular nodes do not do as well, because lung cancer is a frequent site of occult primary tumors. Patients with no detectable disease below the clavicle should be treated with aggressive local therapy, because 10% to 15% of these patients will have long-term disease-free survival. Chemotherapy also should be considered for such patients.

The role of chemotherapy for metastatic squamous carcinoma in cervical lymph nodes is controversial. One small nonrandomized comparison of patients treated with local modalities alone or with local modalities combined with chemotherapy (cisplatin and 5-FU) showed a higher complete response rate (81% vs. 60%) and longer median survival time (>37 months vs. 24 months) in patients also receiving chemotherapy.[120] Paclitaxel-based chemotherapy may be more effective. Neoadjuvant chemotherapy and radiation therapy in locally advanced head and neck carcinoma is gaining acceptance, and consideration of chemotherapy for these unknown primary tumor patients now would also seem reasonable. In those who receive local therapy first, adjuvant platinum-based or paclitaxel-based chemotherapy should be considered.

SQUAMOUS CARCINOMA INVOLVING INGUINAL LYMPH NODES

Most patients with a tumor in inguinal lymph nodes have a detectable primary site in the genital or anorectal areas. Careful examination of vulva, vagina, cervix, penis, and scrotum is important and should include biopsy of any suspicious areas. Digital examination and anoscopy should be performed to exclude lesions in the anorectal area. Identification of a primary site in such patients is important, because curative therapy is available for carcinomas of the vulva, vagina, cervix, and anus, even after spread to regional lymph nodes. Nearly 50% of patients with inguinal presentations have poorly differentiated carcinoma. For patients in whom no primary site is identified, surgical resection with or without radiation therapy to the inguinal area sometimes results in long-term survival.[73,124] Such patients should be considered also for neoadjuvant or adjuvant chemotherapy.

SQUAMOUS CARCINOMA METASTATIC TO OTHER SITES

Usually, metastatic tumor in areas other than the cervical or inguinal lymph nodes represents metastasis from an occult primary lung cancer. CT scans of the chest and fiber-optic bronchoscopy should be considered. Chemotherapy with regimens employed in the treatment of non–small cell lung cancer may be considered in patients with good performance status. Other rare presentations include primary tumors from the head and neck, esophagus, anus, and skin.

Patients with the diagnosis of poorly differentiated squamous carcinoma should be evaluated carefully, particularly if other clinical features are atypical for lung cancer (i.e., young patients, nonsmokers, unusual metastatic sites). Occasionally, adenocarcinomas, particularly in the breast, undergo squamous differentiation at metastatic sites. As with the diagnosis of poorly differentiated adenocarcinoma, this histologic diagnosis (squamous cell) sometimes is based on minimal histologic findings. Additional pathologic evaluation with immunoperoxidase stains or electron microscopy should be considered. When the diagnosis remains unclear, such patients should be considered for a trial of therapy for poorly differentiated carcinoma.

POORLY DIFFERENTIATED CARCINOMA (WITH OR WITHOUT FEATURES OF ADENOCARCINOMA) OF UNKNOWN PRIMARY SITE

Patients with poorly differentiated carcinoma or adenocarcinoma of unknown primary site appear to represent distinctive subgroups with specific therapeutic implications. They account for approximately 30% of all patients with carcinoma of unknown primary site (nearly 25,000 U.S. patients annually); approximately two-thirds have poorly differentiated carcinoma, and one-third has poorly differentiated adenocarcinoma. Often, chemotherapy trials in the past included such patients and the more common patients with well-differentiated adenocarcinoma of unknown primary. All such patients were assumed to be similar, and they experienced both a poor response to 5-FU-based chemotherapy and a short survival. These chemotherapy trials included drugs likely to be useful in a palliative sense for a minority of patients with gastrointestinal, lung, and breast carcinomas. Some patients with poorly differentiated carcinomas have responsive neoplasms, and some are curable with cisplatin-based combination chemotherapy.[99,130–138] Clinical and pathologic evaluation is, therefore, crucial in patients with poorly differentiated carcinoma.

CLINICAL CHARACTERISTICS

The clinical characteristics in this diverse group of patients appear to differ—albeit with considerable overlap—from the characteristics of patients with well-differentiated adenocarcinoma. The median age of this patient group is younger, although both groups have a wide age range. Often, patients with poorly differentiated carcinoma reveal a history of rapid progression of symptoms (often <30 days) and have objective evidence of rapid tumor growth.[34,99,130] Most important, the location of metastases often differs, and the predominant sites of involvement frequently are lymph nodes, mediastinum, and retroperitoneum, occurring much more commonly than in well-differentiated adenocarcinoma. Some of these relatively distinctive clinical features are useful in identifying chemotherapy-responsive subsets of patients (see following Pathologic Evaluation section).

PATHOLOGIC EVALUATION

Light-microscopical features that can differentiate chemotherapy-responsive tumors from nonresponsive tumors have not been identified.[131] Even with careful retrospective review of these tumors, responsive tumors of well-defined types (e.g., germ cell tumor, lymphoma) only rarely are identified.

These tumors should undergo routine additional pathologic study with immunoperoxidase staining; in selected tumors, electron microscopy and genetic analysis also are appropriate. The use of routine light microscopy alone is not adequate to assess such tumors. The information provided by these additional pathologic studies has been summarized previously (see Poorly Differentiated Neoplasms, earlier in this chapter). The frequency of more specific diagnoses, particularly lymphoma, is much lower in the carcinoma group than in the group initially diagnosed by routine light microscopy as poorly differentiated neoplasm. This is not surprising, because carcinoma is a more specific diagnosis. Other diagnoses still may be suggested.

To assess the clinical utility of immunoperoxidase tumor cell staining in patients with poorly differentiated carcinoma of unknown primary site, we retrospectively performed a battery of stains on archival tumors from patients treated prospectively.[132] Poorly differentiated carcinoma or poorly differentiated adenocarcinoma was diagnosed on the basis of routine light-microscopical examination, and all patients were treated before the technology of immunoperoxidase staining was used routinely (1978 to 1983). Therefore, results of immunoperoxidase staining could be correlated with clinical outcome in this group of similarly treated patients with a long median follow-up. Immunoperoxidase staining confirmed the diagnoses of poorly differentiated carcinoma in 49 patients (56%) and yielded other diagnoses in 16 patients (18%): melanoma in eight patients, lymphoma in four, prostatic carcinoma in one, and neuroendocrine tumor in three (see Neuroendocrine Carcinoma of Unknown Primary Site, later in this chapter). In 24 patients (28%), the immunoperoxidase staining pattern was inconclusive; electron microscopy occasionally was helpful in clarifying the diagnosis in affected patients. Seventy-five patients (86%) received combination chemotherapy with a cisplatin-based regimen, and 24 patients (28%) had a complete response. Nine of these patients later were given specific diagnoses by immunoperoxidase staining; lymphoma was diagnosed in four patients, melanoma in four patients, and yolk sac tumor in one patient. All patients with an immunoperoxidase diagnosis of lymphoma had clinical features compatible with lymphoma and are long-term survivors. Patients with immunoperoxidase features suggesting melanoma were surprisingly responsive to chemotherapy, with three of seven complete responses and two long-term survivors. Patients with melanoma diagnosed by immunoperoxidase staining alone should not be excluded from a trial of cisplatin-based therapy. Immunoperoxidase staining is useful in the routine evaluation of metastatic poorly differentiated carcinoma of unknown primary site, as occasionally it can suggest the lineage of the tumor and can have specific therapeutic implications. Others have reported similar findings in patients treated with cisplatin-containing chemotherapy.[139]

Immunoperoxidase staining should be used in the evaluation of poorly differentiated carcinomas to do the following: (1) confirm the diagnosis of carcinoma; (2) identify a primary site of a recognized carcinoma (e.g., prostate); (3) identify patients who may have other neoplasms, such as lymphoma or melanoma (although therapeutic recommendations for neoplasms other than lymphoma identified in this manner remain to be established); and (4) identify a group of patients in whom electron microscopy may provide important additional information.

Electron microscopy can be useful for a small minority of these carcinomas. In general, electron microscopy should be reserved for those tumors not diagnosed by immunoperoxidase stains. Lymphoma can be diagnosed reliably (in most instances) in those tumors mistakenly believed to be carcinoma. In addition, sarcoma, melanoma, mesothelioma, and neuroendocrine tumors occasionally are defined by subcellular features. Neuroendocrine differentiation is particularly important.

Chromosomal or genetic analysis is becoming an increasingly important method of diagnosis. Specific abnormalities have been identified in several neoplasms. Evaluation for these abnormalities may be useful in patients with poorly differentiated carcinoma of unknown primary site. In reference to germ cell tumors, Motzer et al.[140] performed genetic analysis on tumors in 40 patients with primarily midline carcinomas of uncertain histology. In 12 of the 40 patients with poorly differentiated carcinoma, abnormalities of chromosome 12 (e.g., i[12p]; del[12p]; multiple copies of 12p) were diagnostic of germ cell tumor. Other specific abnormalities were diagnostic of melanoma (two patients), lymphoma (one patient), peripheral neuroepithelioma (one patient), and desmoplastic small cell tumor (one patient). Of the germ cell tumors diagnosed on the basis of genetic analysis, five achieved a complete response to cisplatin-based chemotherapy. This outcome confirms our previously formulated hypothesis that some of these patients have histologically atypical germ cell tumors.[130,134] These genetic findings can be diagnostic in these patients. Additional specific genetic abnormalities or gene expression monitoring in solid tumors likely will improve our ability further to establish tumor lineage or biology and, it is hoped, also will improve therapy. Preliminary results using polymerase chain reaction to identify Epstein-Barr viral genomes in neck nodes have established an occult nasopharyngeal primary in some patients.

Autopsy data looking specifically at patients with poorly differentiated carcinoma of unknown primary site are limited. Additionally, the number of postmortem examinations in medicine in general is declining. On the basis of limited necropsy data we have accumulated, primary sites appear to be found in only a minority of such patients (40%). These findings are contrary to those for well-differentiated adenocarcinoma of unknown primary site, in which the primary site is found in most patients (>75%) at autopsy.[34]

DIAGNOSTIC EVALUATION

The clinical evaluation of patients with poorly differentiated carcinoma of unknown primary site is similar to that described for patients with well-differentiated adenocarcinoma of unknown primary site. A medical history, physical examination, routine laboratory testing, and chest radiograph should be obtained for each patient. Any clues are followed with appropriate diagnostic testing. CT scans of the chest and abdomen should be performed in all patients in this group, owing to the frequency of mediastinal and retroperitoneal involvement. Serum levels of HCG and AFP should be measured because substantial elevations of these markers suggest the diagnosis of germ cell tumor. Serum tumor markers, such as CEA, CA-125, CA-19-9, and CA-15-3, can be helpful in monitoring response to chemotherapy. PET scanning may have a role in diagnosis and after therapy, but further data are necessary before recommending PET scanning as standard.

TREATMENT

When additional pathologic studies identify a specific neoplasm (e.g., lymphoma, sarcoma), appropriate therapy can be administered. Patients with elevated serum levels of HCG or AFP and clinical features suggestive of extragonadal germ cell tumor (e.g., mediastinal or retroperitoneal mass) should be treated with chemotherapy that is effective for germ cell tumors, even when pathologic examination results are not diagnostic.

Most affected patients have multiple metastases and only the nonspecific diagnoses of poorly differentiated carcinoma or poorly differentiated adenocarcinoma despite additional pathologic study. The first reports showing that some of these patients (a small subset) have highly responsive tumors appeared in the late 1970s.[133–136] Most such patients were young men with mediastinal tumors; serum levels of HCG or AFP frequently were elevated. Most of these patients were thought to have histologically atypical extragonadal germ cell tumors. Although several other tumor lineages subsequently have been identified in these patients (i.e., thymoma, neuroendocrine tumors, sarcomas, lymphomas), most still defy precise classification.

Further evidence for the responsiveness of many other tumors in patients with poorly differentiated carcinoma of unknown primary site has accumulated during the last 20 years. On the basis of encouraging results in a few patients treated from 1976 to 1978, we prospectively studied the role of cisplatin-based therapy for patients with poorly differentiated carcinoma of unknown primary site. In a series of reports, we have documented a high overall response rate and long-term disease-free survival in a minority of such patients.[130–138] Our experience in the treatment of 220 such patients, accumulated between 1978 and 1989, is summarized in Table 48-4. Most of the patients in this group did not have clinical characteristics strongly suggestive of extragonadal germ cell tumor. However, involvement of the mediastinum, retroperitoneum, and peripheral lymph node groups was relatively common. In the early years of this study, most patients received treatment with cisplatin, vinblastine, and bleomycin (PVB) with or without doxorubicin, then the most commonly used regimen for the treatment of advanced testicular cancer. Later, as etoposide replaced vinblastine, these patients received cisplatin and etoposide with or without bleomycin. All patients received an initial treatment trial of two courses of therapy, and responding patients received a total of four treatment courses. Major tumor responses were seen in 138 of 220 patients (62%), and 58 patients (26%) had complete response to treatment.

Our most recent update of this initial group of patients shows the following: 12% (26 patients) of the entire group has remained alive and free of tumor at a minimum follow-up of 6 years, with a range of 6 to 17 years (median, 11 years). Fourteen patients who were relapse-free at a minimum of 11 months at the time of our original report[141] cannot be documented now as alive and free of the original tumor. Six patients are lost to follow-up, though each was known to be alive and relapse-free at 1, 2.5, 3, 3.5, 4, and 7 years, respectively. Four patients died with progressive carcinoma of unknown primary site (two at 1 year and two at 7 years after initial chemotherapy). Three patients developed new cancers: one brain tumor, one pancreatic carcinoma, one lymphoma (two at 9 years and one at 17 years, respectively, after the initial therapy). One patient died of an unrelated cause 4 years after therapy.

The survival curves for the entire group of 220 patients and for the subset of 58 (26%) who had a complete response to chemotherapy are shown in Figures 48-5 and 48-6. The median survival of complete responders was approximately 3 years. Median survival for all patients was 20 months. Of the 58 complete responders, 22 patients remain alive and relapse-free (38%), representing 10% of the entire group of 220. Four additional patients were treated in an "adjuvant setting" after resection of all gross tumor and all remain alive, bringing the total to 12% of all patients relapse-free. These long-term survival statistics are not censored. Patients who are lost to follow-up (six), died of second unrelated cancers (three), or died of other causes (one) are included as deaths on the curves. It is of note that 50 of the 220 patients were treated by oncologists outside our center, and their long-term results are equivalent. These results in a large series of patients support the notion that these poorly differentiated histologic types, as a whole, represent more sensitive tumors than well-differentiated adenocarcinoma, and substantial prolongation of life is possible for some of these patients, with the expectation of cure for a small minority.

In only 32 of the 220 patients (14%) was the primary site or specific tumor type eventually identified (Table 48-5). In 19 of these 32 patients, the definitive diagnosis was made at repeat biopsy later during the course of the disease or at autopsy. In the remainder, retrospective specialized pathology studies provided the basis for diagnosis. All six lymphomas were identified

TABLE 48-4. Clinical Characteristics of 220 Patients with Poorly Differentiated Carcinoma of Unknown Primary Site

Characteristics	*Number of Patients (%)*
GENDER	
Female	54
Male	166
RACE	
White	209
African American	9
Asian American	2
PERFORMANCE STATUS	
ECOG 0, 1	188
ECOG 2, 3	32
DOMINANT METASTATIC SITE	
Mediastinum	43 (20)
Retroperitoneum	42 (19)
Lung	29 (13)
Lymph nodes (cervical, axillary, inguinal)	20 (9)
Liver	11 (5)
Pleura-peritoneum	6
Bone	5
Pelvic mass	4
Pancreas	3
Soft tissue	2
Brain	2
Other (one each)	3
Multiple sites (no dominant site)	50 (23)
SERUM TUMOR MARKERS	
HCG (N = 206)	
Normal	174
Elevated	32 (16)
AFP (N = 201)	
Normal	190
Elevated	11 (5)
LDH (N = 199)[a]	
Normal	103
Elevated	96 (48)
CEA (N = 127)	
Normal	80
Elevated	47 (37)
NUMBER OF METASTATIC SITES	
1	57 (26)
2	67 (31)
3	60 (27)
>3	36 (16)

AFP, α-fetoprotein; CEA, carcinoembryonic antigen; ECOG, Eastern Cooperative Oncology Group; HCG, human chorionic gonadotropin; LDH, lactate dehydrogenase.
[a]Thirty-two of 96 patients had liver metastases as possible source for elevated LDH.

retrospectively: four by immunoperoxidase staining, one by repeat biopsy at the time of tumor relapse, and one by genetic analysis (detection of an immunoglobulin gene rearrange-

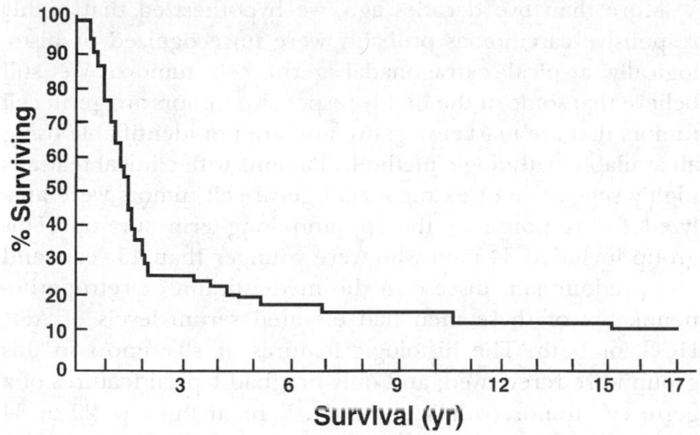

FIGURE 48-5. Survival curve for all 220 patients with poorly differentiated carcinoma (12% at 17 years).

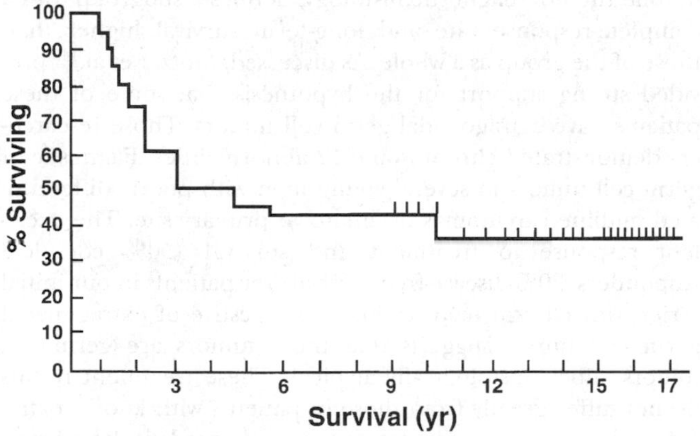

FIGURE 48-6. Survival curve of complete responders (38% at 17 years).

ment). However, only 30 autopsies were performed, and in only 11 (37%) was a primary site identified. In the remainder, metastatic, poorly differentiated carcinoma or poorly differentiated adenocarcinoma with no primary site was found. This observation is nearly opposite for those patients with well-differentiated adenocarcinoma; in nearly 80% of them, a primary tumor was found at autopsy. In addition, nine patients were thought to have melanoma on the basis of pathologic review or special pathologic studies; however, none of these patients had a known primary site, and none had typical light-microscopical findings of melanoma.

Since 1989, we have either seen or collected clinical and pathologic data from 700 additional patients with carcinomas of unknown primary site. Before 1997, the majority of these patients with poorly differentiated carcinomas received cisplatin plus etoposide with or without bleomycin, and the results are similar to those of the 220 previously reported patients. We are reviewing all these data.

In the last 5 years, we have treated most patients with carboplatin and etoposide, with or without a taxane (paclitaxel or docetaxel), either as initial therapy or after first relapse. The response rate appears similar to those of cisplatin-based regimens. Furthermore, we have explored the paclitaxel-based[100] and docetaxel-based chemotherapy (unpublished data) in this group, in addition to the well-differentiated adenocarcinoma group, and found these regimens useful. We are attempting to confirm that taxane-based chemotherapy is superior to other chemotherapy regimens.

At present, the treatment for most patients with poorly differentiated carcinoma (with or without features of adenocarcinoma) is controversial, but we think that they should be treated initially with a regimen containing paclitaxel, carboplatin, and oral etoposide. Follow-up with docetaxel-based therapy is less, but early results support a similar survival rate. The optimal regimen has not been defined. Treatment after

TABLE 48-5. Specific Pathologic Diagnoses Confirmed

	Method of Diagnosis						
Diagnosis	Autopsy	Rebiopsy (After Initial Therapy)	Review of Light Microscopy	Electron Microscopy	Immunoperoxidase Staining	Genetic Analysis	*Total*
Lymphoma		1			4	1	6
Sarcoma (no primary site)		1		5			6
Lung							
Adenocarcinoma	6						6
Mixed adenocarcinoma, small cell carcinoma		1					1
Germ cell tumor							
Extragonadal		2	1				3
Testis		1					1
Carcinoid tumor[a]	2	1					3
Peripheral neuroepithelioma						1	1
Kidney carcinoma	1						1
Pancreatic carcinoma	2						2
Prostate carcinoma					1		1
Breast carcinoma		1					1
Total	11	8	1	5	5	2	32

[a]Primary sites identified in two of three patients (rectum, one; lung, one).

relapse from primary therapy is difficult, but some new drugs, including gemcitabine, occasionally produce clinical benefit. For those patients with features highly suggestive of an extragonadal germ cell tumor, we continue to recommend the classic regimen of cisplatin and etoposide with or without bleomycin. We do not use bleomycin now, as it does not appear to improve the therapy of known germ cell tumors when four courses of chemotherapy are administered, and occasionally it produces severe pulmonary toxicity, particularly if thoracic irradiation is administered later.

Other investigators also have demonstrated the responsiveness of these poorly differentiated tumors.[94,101,142–145] Complete remissions are seen in a minority (10% to 20%) of these patients, as is a small cohort (5% to 10%) of long-term disease-free survivors. Usually, these results were seen with combination chemotherapy, cisplatin-based or carboplatin-based. Results with carboplatin-based combinations are at least as good as previous results using cisplatin, vinblastine, and bleomycin and are achieved with less toxicity. More recently, taxane-based combination chemotherapy has broadened the usefulness of therapy for many affected patients. A therapeutic trial of two courses should be given. Responders should complete a total of at least four treatment courses. No evidence substantiates that more prolonged treatment will improve results, and nearly all long-term survivors have received only four to six treatment courses. In patients with residual palpable or radiographic abnormalities, surgical resection or radiation therapy should be contemplated.

Although the foregoing results represent marked improvement as compared with the dismal historical results (response rate <30%, no complete responders, no long-term survivors), this group of patients is heterogeneous, and many patients have relatively unresponsive tumors. Many such patients should be considered for either taxane-based chemotherapy (as discussed) or investigational trials of newer approaches.

Favorable Prognostic Factors

As only a minority of patients have excellent treatment responses, we have analyzed patients for clinical features predictive of treatment responsiveness and long-term survival.[141] Prognostic features evaluated in a multivariate analysis included age, gender, smoking history, serum tumor marker status (HCG, AFP), serum chemistries, number of metastatic sites, predominant site of tumor involvement, and light-microscopical histology (poorly differentiated carcinoma vs. poorly differentiated adenocarcinoma). The probability of complete response to therapy and various features is illustrated in Table 48-6. Several features were independently predictive of favorable treatment outcome, including tumor location in the retroperitoneum or peripheral lymph nodes, tumor limited to one or two metastatic sites, younger age, and negative smoking history.

Because most of the highly responsive tumors cannot be identified despite extensive pathologic evaluation, a variety of clinical features have been found to be useful as prognostic indicators (Table 48-6). Although evaluation of these clinical features allows the identification of patients with a higher chance of complete response, none of these indicators is specific enough to be able to exclude a patient reliably from a therapeutic trial. However, these features can better define relatively poor prognostic subsets and more favorable subsets of patients.

More than two decades ago, we hypothesized that highly responsive carcinomas probably were unrecognized or histologically atypical extragonadal germ cell tumors. We still believe that some of the highly responsive tumors are germ cell tumors that are marker-negative and are not identifiable using all available pathologic methods. Patients with clinical features highly suggestive of extragonadal germ cell tumors were analyzed for response to therapy and long-term survival. This group included 34 men who were younger than 45 years and had predominant disease in the mediastinum or retroperitoneum. Six of these men had elevated serum levels of AFP, HCG, or both. The histologic features of all tumors in this group were rereviewed, and only one had typical features of a germ cell tumor (yolk sac tumor).[131] In this group, 29 of 34 patients (85%) responded to therapy, with 17 patients (50%) having complete response. Seven patients in this group (20%) remain disease-free. Therefore, selection of patients with *clinical features* highly suggestive of extragonadal germ cell tumor, despite the nondiagnostic histology, defines a subgroup with a complete-response rate and long-term survival higher than those of the group as a whole. As discussed, Motzer et al.[140] provided strong support for the hypothesis that some of these patients have extragonadal germ cell tumors. Those researchers demonstrated chromosome 12 abnormalities diagnostic of germ cell tumors in several young men with poorly differentiated midline carcinomas of unknown primary site. The excellent response to treatment and survival (50% complete responders, 20% disease-free survival) for patients in our initial series with clinical features highly suggestive of extragonadal germ cell tumor suggests that these tumors are germ cell tumors, albeit histologically atypical. These treatment results do not differ greatly from those in patients with known extragonadal germ cell tumors treated with standard cisplatin-based therapy.[146,147] If feasible, genetic analysis on tumor tissue should be performed as a diagnostic test for selected patients with carcinoma of unknown primary site.

Responsive tumors are heterogeneous in their origin, and only a small subset of patients have histologically atypical germ cell tumors. A few of the patients have non-Hodgkin's lymphoma. Certain lymphomas may be confused with anaplastic carcinomas; some lymphomas, notably the Ki-1 lymphomas, also can stain positively with epithelial membrane antigen, further complicating their differentiation from carcinoma.[148] It is hoped that this confusion will be minimized or eliminated with the routine use of immunoperoxidase staining for CLA. A second group of highly responsive tumors are poorly differentiated neuroendocrine carcinomas. The origin of such tumors remains speculative, but they may be an anaplastic variant of occult primary carcinoid.

The nature of the other responsive tumors in this heterogeneous group of patients remains even more speculative. Malignant thymoma is a tumor recently recognized to be responsive to cisplatin-based therapy, with some patients experiencing long-term complete remissions.[149] Some patients with poorly differentiated carcinoma located predominantly in the mediastinum may have thymoma. In our original series, a few patients who were long-term survivors were identified as having "melanoma" on the basis of immunoperoxidase stains. This diagnosis seems unusual because melanoma is a tumor that normally is unresponsive to chemotherapy. Possibly, melanomas identifiable only by immunoperoxidase staining or electron

TABLE 48-6. Clinical and Pathologic Characteristics Predictive of Chemotherapy Responsiveness

Clinical and Pathologic Characteristics	*Number of Patients*	*Number of Complete Responders (%)*	*P Value*
AGE			
≤35 y	81	28 (35)	.01
>35 y	139	34 (24)	
GENDER			
Male	166	48 (29)	NS
Female	54	14 (26)	
DOMINANT TUMOR LOCATION			
Retroperitoneum-peripheral nodes	62	32 (52)	<.001
All others	158	30 (19)	
SMOKING HISTORY			
>10 pack-years	117	24 (21)	.007
≤10 pack-years	103	38 (37)	
LIGHT-MICROSCOPICAL HISTOLOGY			
PDC	142	43 (30)	NS
PDA	51	9 (18)	
NUMBER OF METASTATIC SITES			
1 or 2	124	46 (37)	<.001
>2	96	16 (17)	
CHEMOTHERAPY			
PVB ± A	116	29 (25)	NS
Cisplatin/etoposide	104	33 (32)	
SERUM MARKERS			
LDH			
Normal	103	36 (35)	.01
Elevated	96	18 (18)	
CEA			
Normal	80	26 (33)	<.001
Elevated	47	2 (4)	

A, doxorubicin (Adriamycin); CEA, carcinoembryonic antigen; LDH, lactate dehydrogenase; NS, not significant; PDA, poorly differentiated adenocarcinoma; PDC, poorly differentiated carcinoma; PVB, cisplatin (platinum), vinblastine, and bleomycin.

microscopy represent a uniquely chemotherapy-sensitive subset. Finally, some responsive tumors possibly represent a heretofore undefined tumor type. Alternatively, some may represent highly undifferentiated—and therefore perhaps chemotherapy-sensitive—epithelial tumors from occult primary sites, which usually are much less responsive to systemic therapy. Future knowledge and refinements in genetic diagnosis may establish the identity of many of these tumors.

Table 48-7 shows the relation of response and long-term survival (>6 years) to the site of dominant tumor involvement. Regardless of other factors, dominant tumor in the retroperitoneum, peripheral lymph nodes, or mediastinum is fairly favorable. Forty-five of 105 patients in these categories had a complete response, and 20 patients remain alive and relapse-free (19%).

Prognostic factors also have been evaluated in a large series of patients reported from the M. D. Anderson Hospital.[96,150] This large group was heterogeneous, containing patients with all histologic subtypes. Those with clinical features of extragonadal germ cell tumors were excluded, and only a minority of patients with poorly differentiated carcinoma received cisplatin-based treatment as used in the treatment of germ cell tumors. Some of the same clinical features that we identified were found to be important prognostic features, including limited number of organ sites involved, tumor location in lymph nodes (including mediastinum and retroperitoneum) other than the supraclavicular lymph nodes, and female gender (seen also in our recent series). In addition, the relatively poor outcome of patients with adenocarcinoma as compared to other histologies was confirmed. However, they could not identify a subset of patients with poorly differentiated carcinoma and long-term survival after chemotherapy.[150] Although these prognostic features are useful, occasional excellent responses

TABLE 48-7. Chemotherapy Response, Survival, and Predominant Site of Tumor

Dominant Tumor Site	*Number of Patients*	*Overall Response Rate (CR+PR) (%)*	*Number of Complete Responders (%)*	*Number of Relapse-Free Survivors >6 y (%)*
Retroperitoneum	42	35 (83)	21 (50)	10 (28)
Peripheral lymph nodes[a] (cervical, axillary, inguinal)	20	14 (70)	11 (55)	6 (40)
Mediastinum	43	29 (67)	13 (30)	4 (14)
Bone	5	3 (60)	1 (20)	1 (20)
Pelvic mass	4	4 (100)	1 (25)	1 (25)
Lung	29	21 (72)	6 (21)	1 (4)
Liver	11	5 (45)	1 (9)	1 (9)
Pleura-peritoneum	6	2 (33)	1 (17)	0
Multiple sites (no dominant site)	50	25 (50)	5 (10)	1 (4)
Other sites[b]	10	4 (40)	2 (20)	1 (10)
Total	220	142 (65)	58 (28)	26 (12)

CR, complete response; PR, partial response.
[a]Includes four patients treated in adjuvant setting.
[b]Sites include pancreas (three patients); brain (two); subcutaneous tissue (two); stomach (one); parotid (one); and nasopharynx (one).

are seen even in patient groups with "unfavorable" clinical features. At present, even these patients should be considered for a trial of chemotherapy.

NEUROENDOCRINE CARCINOMA OF UNKNOWN PRIMARY SITE

Improved pathologic methods for diagnosing neuroendocrine tumors has resulted in the recent recognition of a wider spectrum of these neoplasms. The incidence of unknown primary neuroendocrine tumors is not known, but an estimate suggests approximately 4000 U.S. patients annually. Most of the well-described adult neuroendocrine tumors have distinctive histology and a known primary site of origin (Table 48-8). The well-differentiated or low-grade neuroendocrine tumors (typical carcinoid, islet cell tumors, and others) occasionally present without a recognizable primary site and usually possess an indolent biologic behavior. Carcinoid tumors of unknown primary site appear to be increasing.[1] A second group of neuroendocrine tumors are poorly differentiated by light microscopy but have "neuroendocrine features (typical small cell, atypical carcinoid, or poorly differentiated neuroendocrine carcinoma) and act aggressively. A third group of neuroendocrine tumors, recently recognized, has high-grade biology and no distinctive neuroendocrine features by light microscopy. The initial diagnosis in this group usually is poorly differentiated carcinoma, and neuroendocrine features are recognized only when immunoperoxidase staining (or, more definitively, if electron microscopy) is performed. Neuroendocrine carcinomas of unknown primary site occur in each of these three categories.

LOW-GRADE NEUROENDOCRINE CARCINOMA

Occasionally, metastatic neuroendocrine tumors with histologic features typical of low-grade well-differentiated carcinoid or islet cell tumor are found without obvious primary site. In this situation, metastatic tumor usually involves the liver or bone (or both) and sometimes is associated with clinical syndromes produced by the secretion of bioactive substances (e.g., carcinoid syndrome, glucogonoma syndrome, vipomas, Zollinger-Ellison syndrome). In some affected patients, further evaluation reveals primary sites in the small intestine, rectum, pancreas, or bronchus.

As predicted by the histologic appearance, these neuroendocrine tumors usually exhibit an indolent biology, and slow progression over years is likely. Management should follow guidelines established for metastatic carcinoid or islet cell tumors from obvious primary sites. Often, these neoplasms are refractory to systemic chemotherapy, and cisplatin-based chemotherapy produces low response rates.[151] Depending on the clinical situation, appropriate management may include local therapy (resection of isolated metastasis, hepatic artery ligation-embolization), treatment of associated syndromes with somatostatin analogs, streptozocin, doxorubicin, 5-FU-based systemic therapy, or symptomatic management.

SMALL CELL CARCINOMA

Patients with a history of cigarette smoking and small cell undifferentiated carcinoma at a metastatic site usually have a lung primary tumor. CT of the chest and fiber-optic bronchoscopy should be performed. Perhaps PET scanning may be useful in this setting, but data are limited. If a pulmonary lesion is identified, affected patients should be treated according to recommendations for small cell lung cancer. Small cell carcinoma

TABLE 48-8. Adult Neuroendocrine Tumors with Known Primary Sites

Indolent Biology	*Aggressive Biology*
Carcinoid tumor (many primary sites)	Small cell lung cancer, atypical or poorly differentiated carcinoids (many primary sites)
Islet cell tumor, pancreas	Extrapulmonary small cell carcinoma (many primary sites)
Pheochromocytoma, adrenal	Peripheral neuroepithelioma (usually in adolescents)
Medullary carcinoma, thyroid	Merkel cell tumor, skin
Paraganglioma-neurons	Neuroblastoma, adrenal

can arise also from a variety of extrapulmonary primary sites. Patients with localizing symptoms should undergo appropriate diagnostic studies.

When no primary site is identified, patients with small cell carcinoma should be treated with combination chemotherapy as recommended for small cell lung cancer. We have found that paclitaxel, carboplatin, and oral etoposide is a very active therapy for these patients and have continued to evaluate this regimen. Initially, these tumors are chemotherapy-sensitive, and major palliative benefit can be derived from treatment. An occasional patient will enjoy long-term benefit. In the rare instance in which the tumor appears at a single metastatic site, the addition of radiation therapy or resection (or both) to combination chemotherapy should be considered.

POORLY DIFFERENTIATED NEUROENDOCRINE CARCINOMA

In approximately 10% of poorly differentiated carcinomas, electron microscopy reveals neurosecretory granules, a finding diagnostic of neuroendocrine carcinoma. These tumors have been called *poorly differentiated neuroendocrine tumors, atypical carcinoids,* or *primitive neuroectodermal tumors.* In some of these tumors, neuroendocrine features are recognizable by light microscopy; in others, the light-microscopical diagnosis is "poorly differentiated carcinoma." Though electron microscopy is the most accurate means of pathologic diagnosis, most of the tumors also have typical immunoperoxidase staining patterns with positive staining for neuron specific enolase, chromogranin, and synaptophysin.

Previously, we reported on a group of 29 patients with poorly differentiated neuroendocrine tumors[137] and later updated our experience to include 51 patients, 46 treated with combination chemotherapy (Table 48-9). Most of these patients had clinical evidence of high-grade tumor, and most had metastases in multiple sites. Thirty-three of 43 evaluable patients (77%) responded to chemotherapy with a cisplatin-based combination regimen. Thirteen patients (26%) had complete responses, and eight remain continuously disease-free more than 2 years after completion of therapy. Our more recent experience would favor the use of paclitaxel, carboplatin, and oral etoposide in such patients.

The origin of these poorly differentiated neuroendocrine carcinomas remains unclear. In four of our patients, specific diagnoses were made either subsequently in their clinical course or at autopsy. Two patients had carcinoid tumors with "undifferentiated" growth pattern (both presented with abdominal carcinomatosis); one had small cell lung cancer; and one had extragonadal germ cell tumor with predominant neuroendocrine differentiation. Likely some additional patients with small cell histology had small cell lung cancer with occult primary tumor, but more than one-half of these patients had no smoking history, and the absence of overt pulmonary involvement renders this diagnosis unlikely in most patients. Probably, some of these tumors are undifferentiated variants of well-recognized neuroendocrine tumors (e.g., carcinoid tumor), without a recognizable primary site. In the undifferentiated form, the clinical and pathologic characteristics no longer resemble the characteristics of the more differentiated counterpart. Anaplastic or

TABLE 48-9. Poorly Differentiated Neuroendocrine Tumors of Unknown Primary Site in 51 Patients

Features	*Number of Patients*
CLINICAL CHARACTERISTICS	
Male	34
Female	17
Smoking (>10 pack-years)	25
DOMINANT TUMOR SITE	
Retroperitoneum	13
Peripheral lymph nodes	7
Mediastinum	6
Bone	6
Liver	6
Other	8
Multiple sites (no dominant site)	6
TREATMENT	
Cisplatin-based combinations	38
Cyclophosphamide, doxorubicin, vincristine with or without etoposide	8
Surgical excision only	3
Radiation therapy only	2
RESPONSE TO CHEMOTHERAPY	
Complete response	13 (26%)
Partial response	20
No response or nonevaluable	10
Continuously disease-free	8 (15%)

atypical carcinoid tumors arising in the gastrointestinal tract are responsive to cisplatin-based chemotherapy, whereas carcinoid tumors with typical histology usually are resistant.[151] A few reports of patients with "extrapulmonary small cell carcinoma of unknown primary site" also have documented chemotherapy responsiveness and occasional long-term survival after systemic therapy.[152,153] However, the term *extrapulmonary small cell carcinoma* implies the existence of a known primary site (e.g., head and neck, salivary gland, prostate, cervix, esophagus, bladder, etc.); therefore, these tumors are more aptly described as *neuroendocrine carcinoma of unknown primary site.*

Although the origins of these poorly differentiated neuroendocrine tumors remain undefined, the presence of neurosecretory granules in the tumors of patients with poorly differentiated carcinoma identifies a highly treatable subgroup. Molecular genetic studies may be helpful if an 11:22 translocation (peripheral neuroepithelioma or soft tissue Ewing's sarcoma) or i(12p) abnormality (germ cell tumor) is identified. All patients with disease not otherwise specifically diagnosed should be treated with a trial of combination chemotherapy. As are small cell neuroendocrine carcinomas, these tumors are very sensitive to the combination of paclitaxel, carboplatin, and oral etoposide. Some patients with a single site of tumor involvement may be curable with local treatment modalities alone; however, a course of adjuvant chemotherapy also should be considered in such patients if clinically feasible.

SPECIAL ISSUES

CARCINOMA OF UNKNOWN PRIMARY SITE AS A DISTINCT CLINICOPATHOLOGIC ENTITY

We have been struck over the last two decades by the number of times patients and their referring physicians (often oncologists) are very frustrated by unknown primary cancer. Often, they are somewhat obsessed with finding the primary site or at least giving their patients a more specific diagnosis. Many reasons underlie these feelings. Some patients think that their oncologists are not clever enough as diagnosticians and seek the advice of others. Some oncologists feel relatively inadequate and wonder what other tests they might order; some have been relatively tentative, not feeling confident in recommending any therapy. Certainly, a reasonable clinical and pathologic evaluation of these patients and their tumors is indicated, with oncologists being aware of possible primary sites and the relevance in particular patients. However, once these considerations and evaluation are complete and no additional helpful information is forthcoming (as often is the case), physicians should stop, discuss the issue with their patients and their families, and accept the clinicopathologic diagnosis as an unknown primary tumor. Indeed, most patients at this point have unknown primary cancer; such tumors only occasionally surface during life and often cannot even be found at autopsy. Patients will be better served, and physicians will eventually feel more comfortable—and therefore manage these patients more effectively—once their patients accept and understand this diagnosis as a distinct clinicopathologic entity. They have a diagnosis.

A second very practical issue in the United States is the determination of Medicare reimbursement for chemotherapy for cancer diagnoses. Most typically, these reimbursements are determined by Medicare (and several other third-party insurers) by consulting two compendia: the *American Hospital Formulary Drug Information* (AHFS) and the *United States Pharmacopeia Drug Information* (USPDI). Their entries are listed by an indication index or by tumor types [ICD-9(*International Classification of Diseases*-9) codes] and a generic drug index. Tumor types and drugs used for a particular tumor type are listed. The list is based on published literature showing "effectiveness" or clinical benefit in a specific tumor type. This system is particularly arbitrary. The diagnosis code for unknown primary cancer is not listed at all in AHFS or USPDI. Therefore, no drugs are listed as "useful" for patients with unknown primary cancer. Usually, Medicare will not pay for any drug not listed as an indication.

Many patients with unknown primary cancer are coded with another diagnosis by oncologists. At times, this is a "good guess" of the possible primary tumor (e.g., non–small cell lung cancer in patients with lung lesions or mediastinal node involvement; hepatoma, pancreatic, or colon cancer for patients with liver involvement, etc.). Furthermore, patients at times are assigned a diagnosis based on the pathology report alone (e.g., adenocarcinoma consistent with pancreatic or colon primary tumor). Certainly, this practice allows for reimbursement for some drug costs by a system that otherwise has not even recognized unknown primary cancer. This activity, in turn, causes the true incidence of unknown primary cancer to be underestimated. Recently, we and others provided the editors of AHFS and USPDI with considerable data concerning unknown primary cancer, and we hope that the diagnosis code and specific drugs useful for this entity will appear in their pages soon.

Currently, more than enough clinical and pathologic data allow classification of patients confidently as having an unknown primary cancer, and the more global acceptance of this entity will help these patients to establish an identity, will stimulate more interest by physician investigators, and eventually will improve general understanding of such patients and their tumors.

EXTRAGONADAL GERM CELL CANCER SYNDROME

Selected patients with poorly differentiated carcinoma almost certainly have germ cell tumors, although the histologic features are atypical even when generous pathologic specimens are available for study. Chromosomal analysis (as discussed) may provide a definitive diagnosis in some of these patients, particularly if their tumor cells contain specific chromosome 12 abnormalities. Even if they are not found or in the absence of a genetic study, young people who have mediastinal or retroperitoneal masses or multiple lung nodules (with or without elevated serum levels of HCG or AFP) should be suspected of harboring a germ cell tumor. Lymphomas should be ruled out by immunoperoxidase stains, electron microscopy, or (if necessary) cytogenetic studies. The "extragonadal germ cell cancer syndrome" was described in 1979.[133,134] The full syndrome displays the following features: (1) It occurs in young men (<50 years); (2) tumors are predominantly located in the midline (mediastinum, retroperitoneum) or multiple pulmonary nodules; (3) the symptom interval is short (<3 months) and history is of rapid tumor growth; (4) serum levels of HCG, AFP, or both are elevated; and (5) a good response to previously administered radiation therapy or chemotherapy is demonstrated.

Few patients have all elements of this syndrome. These clinical features are those of extragonadal germ cell tumors but, without definitive histology, the diagnosis is not unequivocal. In rare cases, women can develop these tumors, and the other features also are not absolute. Any one feature suggests the possibility of a germ cell tumor. Treatment with cisplatin-based therapy is prudent in affected patients who may have atypical germ cell tumors.

SINGLE SITE OF NEOPLASM

In situations in which only one site of neoplasm is identified (e.g., one node group or one large mass), the possibility of an unusual primary tumor mimicking metastatic disease should be considered. Several unusual tumors could present in this fashion, including Merkel-cell tumors, skin adnexal tumors (e.g., apocrine, eccrine, and sebaceous carcinomas), and even sarcomas, melanomas, or lymphomas that are interpreted mistakenly as metastatic carcinoma (pathologically and clinically). Usually, patients with one site of involvement have metastatic carcinoma, and many other sites are present but are not detectable. In the absence of any other documented metastatic disease, such patients should be treated with aggressive local therapy (i.e., resection, radiation therapy, or both) because a minority will enjoy long-term disease-free survival. Patients who present with isolated cervical, supraclavicular, and inguinal adenopathy often have squamous cell carcinoma, but a minority harbor poorly differentiated carcinoma and adenocarcinoma. In addition to receiving definitive local therapy, these patients also should receive either neoadjuvant or adjuvant platinum-based or paclitaxel-based chemotherapy, but knowing whether this treatment is superior to local therapy alone is difficult.

On occasion, patients will present with apparent solitary metastasis of adenocarcinoma or poorly differentiated carcinoma in the brain, liver, subcutaneous tissue, intestine, or other areas. In most instances, other metastases will become clinically apparent with time. Certainly, some examples highlight resection or irradiation of these single areas and illustrate patients doing well with no evidence of recurrence. At times, the resection may be planned as palliative, particularly with a brain metastasis. The method of choice in managing these patients is to resect the single lesion. After resection, and depending on the other clinical circumstances, patients may be candidates for chemotherapy, particularly if their histology is poorly differentiated carcinoma. In those patients with single metastases (i.e., brain), radiation therapy is a prudent consideration after surgical resection. Often, isolated axillary carcinoma in women arises from an occult breast cancer and has important therapeutic implications (see Adenocarcinoma of Unknown Primary Site, earlier in this chapter).

UNSUSPECTED GESTATIONAL CHORIOCARCINOMA

In young women with poorly differentiated carcinoma or anaplastic neoplasms, particularly with lung nodules, oncologists must be aware of the possibility of metastatic gestational choriocarcinoma. The history of recent pregnancy, spontaneous abortion, or missed menstrual periods should suggest this possibility. In this group of patients, serum HCG levels invariably are elevated. On occasion, biopsy specimens do not show the classic appearance of choriocarcinoma but simply that of metastatic carcinoma, usually poorly differentiated. Ultrasonography or CT scan of the abdomen may show an enlarged uterus, and a dilation and curettage may be indicated in such patients. Most affected patients are curable with single-agent methotrexate.

ISOLATED PLEURAL EFFUSION

Occasionally, an isolated pleural effusion containing carcinoma in women will represent metastatic disease from occult ovarian carcinoma or primary peritoneal carcinomatosis. Even when affected patients have no symptoms or signs and an abdominopelvic CT scan result is normal, the primary tumor may reside in the abdomen or pelvis. Such occult abdominal neoplasms may arise from the ovary or the peritoneal surface (see Adenocarcinoma of Unknown Primary Site, Peritoneal Carcinomatosis in Women, earlier in this chapter) and most characteristically cause a pleural effusion. In the absence of clues of neoplasm in the abdomen, an elevated plasma CA-125 level suggests the possibility of this phenomenon. In the absence of clinical findings in the abdomen, laparoscopy or exploratory laparotomy might be diagnostic, but these procedures are not therapeutic in this setting. Some of these tumors are particularly responsive to chemotherapy with paclitaxel and a platinum agent.

An isolated pleural effusion can be a manifestation of a peripheral lung carcinoma (usually adenocarcinoma), a mesothelioma or, rarely, a lesion from other sites. Diagnosis may be difficult; at times the primary tumor is not apparent even after thorocostomy and chest tube drainage. Usually, cytology shows adenocarcinoma. Electron microscopy may reveal ultrastructural features diagnostic of mesothelioma. The therapy for such patients is difficult. In those with poor performance status or advanced age, a trial of tamoxifen or megestrol acetate is reasonable. In fit patients, a trial of chemotherapy (as discussed) for unknown primary carcinoma should be considered.

GERM CELL TUMORS WITH METASTASES OF OTHER HISTOLOGIES

On occasion, patients with germ cell tumors, particularly extragonadal primaries, may have a metastatic lesion that consists of only somatic tumor cells. This is particularly true for neuroendocrine or sarcomatous differentiation. Patients, therefore, may be diagnosed as having a neuroendocrine tumor or sarcoma. In these rare instances, a primary germ cell tumor (usually extragonadal) is present elsewhere and subsequently will be clinically apparent. Making the diagnosis initially is difficult. An elevated plasma AFP or HCG level is suggestive. The presence of a mediastinal, retroperitoneal, or testicular mass supports this possibility. Chromosomal analysis of tumor tissue may be diagnostic if a specific chromosome 12 abnormality is found. If affected patients have metastatic germ cell tumor with metastases of other histologies, the treatment of choice is cisplatin-based chemotherapy. Such patients appear to have a worse prognosis than do those with typical germ cell tumors, probably because the somatic cell tumors are less sensitive to chemotherapy.

MELANOMA AND "AMELANOTIC" MELANOMA

Approximately 10% to 15% of all melanomas presenting with an unknown primary site are believed to be "amelanotic." We have viewed this diagnosis with considerable skepticism. At times, the only reason for the pathologic diagnosis is the histologic pattern's similarity to melanoma, even though no pigment is demonstrated. In our experience, detailed pathologic and molecular study occasionally has revealed a group of other specific diagnoses, including lymphomas, neuroendocrine tumors, germ cell tumors, sarcomas, and poorly differentiated carcinoma (otherwise not specified).

Melanosomes or premelanosomes seen on electron micrographs have been considered diagnostic of melanoma but, on rare occasion, these structures are seen in other tumors. Some believe amelanotic melanomas do not always form premelanosomes, opening the question as to whether they really are melanomas. Immunoperoxidase panels also are useful in suggesting the diagnosis of melanoma (see Table 48-1). Of considerable interest is that in our original series of 220 patients with poorly differentiated carcinoma, 9 later were thought possibly to harbor amelanotic melanoma on the basis of immunoperoxidase stains or electron microscopy (or both). Generally, these patients responded well to cisplatin-based chemotherapy, and several had long-term survival, an unexpected result for "melanoma."

Certainly, the history of a resected, abraded, or frozen pigmented skin lesion would favor a metastatic melanoma in affected individuals. In addition, the rare primary visceral melanoma should be considered (eye, adrenal, bowel, etc.) as the source of the disease in questionable cases. Except in those patients who are discovered not to have melanoma but a specific tumor lineage requiring relatively specific therapy, the therapy for a questionable amelanotic melanoma is the same as that for carcinoma of unknown primary site presenting in a single site (local resection with or without radiation therapy). Such patients may have stage II melanoma and are potentially curable with resection. For patients with poorly differentiated tumor, including amelanotic melanoma, we also favor chemotherapy after local treatment.

EVOLVING ROLE OF PROGNOSTIC FACTORS: THERAPEUTIC IMPLICATIONS

The prognoses of those small groups of patients with squamous cell carcinoma and poorly differentiated neoplasm (otherwise not classified) are relatively good. Many patients with poorly differentiated carcinoma have chemotherapy-responsive tumors, and complete responses and long-term survival have been documented for a minority of patients. Conversely, in the past, the even larger group of patients with well-differentiated adenocarcinoma has had relatively resistant tumors, with virtually no complete responses to chemotherapy and no long-term survivals. In the last several years, patients with other "favorable" factors have been recognized. Such patients, many managed with specific therapies, have a better prognosis than do those in the group as a whole. We have stressed that both pathologic and clinical factors now can define several patients with a better prognosis (Table 48-10). Although other unrecognized favorable features undoubtedly exist, apparently the prognosis of patients who do not fit into a favorable subset have a particularly poor prognosis, regardless of their initial light-microscopical diagnosis (well-differentiated adenocarcinoma or poorly differentiated carcinoma). Patients in this group recently have been treated with taxane-based chemotherapy, and the treatment does appear to improve the response rate (with some complete responses) and survival of these groups of patients with historically very poor prognoses. The degree of response seen in poorly differentiated neuroendocrine carcinoma also is noteworthy. Furthermore, the taxane-based chemotherapy appears as effective, with less toxicity, as cisplatin-based chemotherapy, even for those patients within favorable prognostic subsets who otherwise require chemotherapy. The one exception is patients with the extragonadal germ cell syndrome, for whom cisplatin-based therapy remains the treatment of choice. Further study of such patients with poor prognoses is necessary to continue to build on the progress seen with taxane-based combination chemotherapy.

"SHRINKING POPULATION" OF PATIENTS WITH CANCER OF UNKNOWN PRIMARY SITE

As our ability to identify specific tumor lineages (lymphoma, germ cell tumors, sarcoma, melanoma, etc.) improves, the total population of patients with cancer of unknown primary site is becoming smaller. In the future, advances in molecular genetics may enable the diagnosis of most neoplasms with a specific genetic fingerprint. In addition, subsets of patients with more favorable prognostic features (neuroendocrine tumors, peripheral lymph node sites, retroperitoneum, etc.) now are apparent. Many affected patients are likely to be labeled or more specifically identified, at least into a treatable or responsive clinicopathologic subset. This evolution is likely to continue, as improved chemotherapy now is developing for patients with many advanced neoplasms (including non–small cell lung, ovarian, urothelial, head and neck, colorectal, esophageal, thymic, and pancreatic cancers). The remaining patients who do not fit a "responsive subset" will be the true unknown primary patients in the future. Paradoxically effective treatment for them will remain very difficult.

TABLE 48-10. Favorable Prognostic Factors in Cancer of Unknown Primary Site

DEFINITE
Poorly differentiated malignant neoplasm (otherwise not classified): 60% lymphomas
Extragonadal germ cell syndrome (PDA or PDC)
Retroperitoneal or peripheral lymph node involvement (PDA, PDC, WDA)
Squamous cell carcinomas (head and neck or inguinal area)
Isolated axillary adenopathy—women, very rare in men (WDA, PDC, PDA)
Peritoneal carcinoma—women, rare in men (WDA, PDC, PDA)
Blastic bone metastases or increased PSA in serum or tumor: men (WDA, PDA, PDC)
Neuroendocrine carcinoma, high-grade or poorly differentiated (small cell and others)
Neuroendocrine carcinoma, low-grade or well-differentiated (carcinoid and islet cell type)
Single site of metastasis (WDA, PDC, PDA)
PROBABLE
Women
Performance status 0, 1
Nonsmoker
Two sites of metastasis
Estrogen receptor–positive or progesterone receptor–positive tumor
Normal LDH, CEA

CEA, carcinoembryonic antigen; LDH, lactate dehydrogenase; PDA, poorly differentiated adenocarcinoma; PDC, poorly differentiated carcinoma; PSA, prostate-specific antigen; WDA, well-differentiated adenocarcinoma.

CONCLUSION: FUTURE TRENDS

The recognition of subsets of responsive tumors in patients within the large heterogeneous population of cancers of unknown primary site represents an improvement in the management of such patients. Approximately 40% of all patients fall within a defined subset with important treatment implications (see Fig. 48-1). Often, such patients with more responsive tumors can be defined with appropriate clinical and pathologic evaluation. A summary of several subsets and an outline of the evaluation necessary for their identification is given in Table 48-11. As the therapy for various neoplasms improves, the outcomes for more patients with cancers of unknown primary site also improves. Recently, taxane-based combination chemotherapy has been shown to be useful for many of these patients. A therapeutic trial is the only absolute method to determine whether a patient has a responsive tumor. Even for most responsive carcinomas, the tumor origin, biology, and precise lineage often continue to be an enigma. Consequently, groups of patients with insensitive tumors remain. Improved therapy for such patients

TABLE 48-11. Carcinoma of Unknown Primary Site: Summary of Evaluation and Therapy for Responsive Subsets

Type	*Clinical Evaluation*[a]	*Special Pathologic Studies*	*Subsets*	*Therapy*	*Prognosis*
Adenocarcinoma (well-differentiated or moderately differentiated)	Abdominal CT scan	Men: PSA stain	1. Women: axillary node involvement	Treat as primary breast cancer	Poor for entire group but improving
	Men: serum PSA	Women: ER, PR	2. Women: peritoneal carcinomatosis	Surgical cytoreduction + chemotherapy (as in ovarian cancer)	Better for subsets
	Women: mammogram, serum CA-15-3, serum CA-125		3. Men: blastic bone metastases, high serum PSA, or PSA tumor staining	Hormonal therapy for prostate cancer	
	Additional studies to evaluate symptoms, signs		4. Single metastatic site	Lymph node dissection ± radiation therapy	
Squamous carcinoma	Cervical node presentation[b]: panendoscopy	Genetic analysis	1. Cervical adenopathy: nasopharyngeal cancer (identified by PCR for Epstein-Barr viral genes)	Radiation therapy ± neck dissection ± chemotherapy	25%–50% 5-y survival
	Supraclavicular presentation[b]: bronchoscopy		2. Supraclavicular	Radiation therapy ± chemotherapy	5%–15% 5-y survival
	Inguinal presentation[b]: pelvic and rectal examinations, anoscopy		3. Inguinal adenopathy	Inguinal node dissection ± radiation therapy ± chemotherapy	15%–20% 5-y survival
Poorly differentiated carcinoma, poorly differentiated adenocarcinoma	Chest, abdominal CT scans, serum HCG, AFP; Additional studies to evaluate symptoms, signs	Immunoperoxidase staining	1. Atypical germ cell tumors (identified by chromosomal abnormalities only)	Treatment for germ cell tumor	40%–50% cure rate
		Electron microscopy	2. Predominant tumor location in retroperitoneum, peripheral nodes	Cisplatin/etoposide	Prolongation of survival; 10%–20% cured
		Genetic analysis			
Neuroendocrine carcinoma	CT abdomen, chest	Immunoperoxidase staining	1. Low-grade	Treat as advanced carcinoid	Indolent biology
		Electron microscopy	2. Small cell carcinoma	Paclitaxel-carboplatin-etoposide or platinum-etoposide	High response rate
			3. Poorly differentiated		Prolongation of survival; rarely cured

AFP, α-fetoprotein; CT, computed tomography; ER, estrogen receptor; HCG, human chorionic gonadotropin; PCR, polymerase chain reaction; PR, progesterone receptor; PSA, prostate-specific antigen.
[a]In addition to history, physical examination, routine laboratory tests, and chest x-ray films.
[b]May also present with poorly differentiated carcinoma, and management and outcome is similar.

probably will follow advances in the treatment of non–small cell lung cancer, pancreatic cancer, and the other gastrointestinal cancers, because most insensitive carcinomas probably arise from these occult primary sites.

We have established a registry—a repository for pathologic material—and are collecting and cataloging patients' data from other physicians around the country. Pathologic material, clinical summaries, and follow-up data from all such patients are being requested. A bank of unstained slides is maintained, and special stains developed in the future may be evaluated rapidly. We are establishing a frozen-tissue bank for genetic studies. Eventually, further studies may provide a better assessment of the frequency and spectrum of these neoplasms and could improve our knowledge of their biology and, subsequently, the therapy for affected patients.

REFERENCES

1. Muir C. Cancer of unknown primary site. *Cancer* 1995;75:353.
2. Horning SJ, Carrier EK, Rouse RV, et al. Lymphomas presenting as histologically unclassified neoplasms: characteristics and response to treatment. *J Clin Oncol* 1989;7:1281.
3. Hales SA, Gatter KC, Heryet A, Mason DY. The value of immunocytochemistry in differentiating high-grade lymphoma from other anaplastic tumours: a study of anaplastic tumours from 1940 to 1960. *Leuk Lymphoma* 1989;1:59.

4. Gatter KC, Alcock C, Heryet A, Mason DY. Clinical importance of analysing malignant tumours of uncertain origin with immunohistochemical techniques. *Lancet* 1985;1:1302.
5. Azar HA, Espinoza CG, Richman AV, et al. "Undifferentiated" large cell malignancies: an ultrastructural and immunocytochemical study. *Hum Pathol* 1982;13:323.
6. Warnke RA, Gatter KC, Falini B, et al. Diagnosis of human lymphoma with monoclonal antileukocyte antibodies. *N Engl J Med* 1983;109:1275.
7. Battifora H, Trowbridge IS. A monoclonal antibody useful for the differential diagnosis between malignant lymphoma and nonhematopoietic neoplasms. *Cancer* 1983;51:816.
8. Tapra FJ, Polak JM, Barbosa AJA, et al. Neuron-specific enolase is produced by neuroendocrine tumors. *Lancet* 1981;1:808.
9. O'Connor DT, Burton D, Deftos LJ. Immunoreactive human chromogranin A in diverse polypeptide hormone producing human tumors and normal endocrine tissues. *J Clin Endocrinol Metab* 1983;57:1084.
10. Mackey B, Ordonez NG. Pathological evaluation of neoplasms with unknown primary tumor site. *Semin Oncol* 1993;20:206.
11. Allhof EP, Proppe KH, Chapman CM. Evaluation of prostate-specific acid phosphatase and prostate-specific antigen. *J Urol* 1983;57:1084.
12. Denk H, Knepler R, Artlieb U, et al. Proteins of intermediate filaments: an immunohistochemical and biochemical approach to the classification of soft tissue tumors. *Am J Pathol* 1983;110:193.
13. Osborn M, Weber K. Biology of disease: tumor diagnosis by intermediate filament type—a novel tool for surgical pathology. *Lab Invest* 1983;48:372.
14. Kahn HJ, Marks A, Thom H, et al. Role of antibody to S-100 protein in diagnostic pathology. *Am J Clin Pathol* 1983;79:341.
15. Gown AM, Vogel AM, Hoak D, et al. Monoclonal antibodies specific for melanocytic tumors distinguish subpopulations of melanocytes. *Am J Pathol* 1986;123:195.
16. Kaufmann O, Deidesteimer T, Muehlenberg M, et al. Immunohistochemical differentiation of metastatic breast carcinomas from metastatic adenocarcinomas of other primary sites. *Histopathology* 1996;29:233.
17. Bosman FT, Giard RWM, Nieuwenhuijen-Kruseman AC, et al. Human chorionic gonadotrophin and alpha fetoprotein in testicular germ cell tumors: a retrospective immunohistochemical study. *Histopathology* 1980;4:673.
18. Kurman KJ, Scardino PT, McIntire KR, et al. Cellular localization of alpha fetoprotein and human chorionic gonadotropin in germ cell tumors of the testis using an indirect immunoperoxidase technique: a new approach to classification utilizing tumor markers. *Cancer* 1977;40:2136.
19. Abbruzzese JL, Lenzi R, Raber MN, et al. The biology of unknown primary tumors. *Semin Oncol* 1993;20:238.
20. Bar-Eli M, Abbruzzese JL, Lee-Jackson D, et al. P53 gene mutation spectrum in human unknown primary tumors. *Anticancer Res* 1993;13:1619.
21. Briasoulis E, Tsakos M, Fountzilas G, et al. Bcl2 and p53 protein expression in metastatic carcinoma of unknown primary origin: biological and clinical implications. A Hellenic Cooperative Oncology Group study. *Anticancer Res* 1998;18:1907.
22. Pavlidis N, Briasoulis E, Baj M, et al. Overexpression of C-myc, Ras and C-erb-2 oncoproteins in carcinoma of unknown primary origin. *Anticancer Res* 1995;15:2563.
23. Golub TR, Slovim DK, Tamayo P, et al. Molecular classification of cancer: class discovery and class prediction by gene expression monitoring. *Science* 1999;286:531.
24. Wood LA, Venner PM, Pabst HF. Monozygotic twin brothers with primary immunodeficiency presenting with metastatic adenocarcinoma of unknown primary. *Acta Oncologica* 1998;37:771.
25. Arnold A, Cossman J, Bakhshi A, et al. Immunoglobulin-gene rearrangements as unique clonal markers in human lymphoid neoplasms. *N Engl J Med* 1983;309:1593.
26. Rowley JD. Recurring chromosome abnormalities in leukemia and lymphoma. *Semin Hematol* 1990;27:122.
27. Turc-Carel C, Philip I, Berger MP, et al. Chromosomal translocation in Ewing's sarcoma. *N Engl J Med* 1983;309:497.
28. Whang-Peng J, Triche TJ, Knutsen T, et al. Chromosome translocation in peripheral neuroepithelioma. *N Engl J Med* 1984;311:584.
29. Atkin NB, Baker MC. Specific chromosome change, i(12p), in testicular tumors. *Lancet* 1982;2:1349.
30. Ilson DH, Motzer RJ, Rodriguez E, et al. Genetic analysis in the diagnosis of neoplasms of unknown primary tumor site. *Semin Oncol* 1993;20:229.
31. Summersgill B, Goker H, Osin P, et al. Establishing germ cell origin of undifferentiated tumors by identifying gain of 12p material using comparative genomic hybridization analysis of paraffin-embedded samples. *Diagn Mol Pathol* 1998;7:260.
32. Feinmesser R, Miyazaki I, Chenng R, et al. Diagnosis of nasopharyngeal carcinoma by DNA amplification of tissue obtained by fine-needle aspiration. *N Engl J Med* 1992;326:17.
33. Schildt RA, Kennedy PS, Chen TT, et al. Management of patients with metastatic adenocarcinoma of unknown origin: a Southwest Oncology Group study. *Cancer Treat Rep* 1983; 67:77.
34. Nystrom JS, Weiner JM, et al. Metastatic and histologic presentations in unknown primary cancer. *Semin Oncol* 1977;4:53.
35. Brown RW, Campagna LB, Dunn JK, Cagle PT. Immunohistochemical identification of tumor markers in metastatic adenocarcinoma. A diagnostic adjunct in the determination of primary site. *Am J Clin Pathol* 1997;107:12.
36. Kaufman O, Deidesheimer T, Muehlenberg M, Deicke P, Dietel M. Immunohistochemical differentiation of metastatic breast carcinomas from metastatic adenocarcinomas of other common primary sites. *Histopathology* 1996;29:233.
37. Lagendijk JH, Mullink H, VanDiest PJ, Meijer GA, Meijer CJ. Tracing the origin of adenocarcinomas with unknown primary using immunohistochemistry: differential diagnosis between colonic and ovarian carcinomas as primary sites. *Hum Pathol* 1998;29:491.
38. Tot T. Adenocarcinomas metastatic to the liver: the value of cytokeratins 20 and 7 in the search for unknown primary tumors. *Cancer* 1999;85:171.
39. McMillan JH, Levine E, Stephens RH. Computed tomography in the evaluation of metastatic adenocarcinoma from an unknown primary site. *Radiology* 1982;143:143.
40. Karsell PR, Sheedy PF, O'Connell MJ. Computerized tomography in search of cancer of unknown origin. *JAMA* 1982;248:340.
41. Kole AC, Nieweg OE, Prium J, et al. Detection of unknown occult primary tumors using positron emission tomography. *Cancer* 1998;82:1160.
42. Currow DC, Findlay M, Cox K, Harnett PR. Elevated germ cell markers in carcinoma of unknown primary site do not predict response to platinum-based chemotherapy. *Eur J Cancer* 1996;32A:2357.
43. Pavlidis N, Kalef-Ezra J, Briasoulis E, et al. Evaluation of six tumor markers in patients with carcinoma of unknown primary. *Med Pediatr Oncol* 1994;22:162.
44. Hochstere H, Wernz JC, Muggia FM. Intra-abdominal carcinomatosis with histologically normal ovaries [Letter]. *Cancer Treat Rep* 1984;68:931.
45. Gooneratne S, Sassone M, Blaustein A, Talerman A. Serous surface papillary carcinoma of the ovary: a clinicopathologic study of 26 cases. *Int J Gynecol Pathol* 1982;1:258.
46. Chen KT, Flam MS. Peritoneal papillary serous carcinoma with long-term survival. *Cancer* 1986;58:1371.
47. August CZ, Murad TM, Newton M. Multiple focal extraovarian serous carcinoma. *Int J Gynecol Pathol* 1985;4:11.
48. Tobacman JK, Greene MH, Tucker MA, et al. Intra-abdominal carcinomatosis after prophylactic oophorectomy in ovarian cancer-prone families. *Lancet* 1982;2:795.
49. Schorge JO, Muto MG, Welch WR, et al. Molecular evidence for multifocal papillary serous carcinoma of the peritoneum in patients with germ-line BRCA1 mutations. *J Natl Cancer Inst* 1998;90:841.
50. Lele SB, Piver MJ, Mathara J, et al. Peritoneal papillary carcinoma. *Gynecol Oncol* 1988;31:315.
51. Dalrymple JC, Bannatyne P, Russell P, et al. Extraovarian peritoneal serous papillary carcinoma: a clinicopathologic study of 31 cases. *Cancer* 1989;64:110.
52. Strnad CM, Grosh WW, Baxter J, et al. Peritoneal carcinomatosis of unknown primary site in women. *Ann Intern Med* 1989;111:213.
53. Ransom DT, Patel SR, Keeney GL, et al. Papillary serous carcinoma of the peritoneum: a review of 33 cases treated with cisplatin-based chemotherapy. *Cancer* 1990;66:1091.
54. Fromm GL, Gershenson DM, Silva EG. Papillary serous carcinoma of the peritoneum. *Obstet Gynecol* 1990;75:89-95.
55. Bloss JD, Liao SY, Buller RE, et al. Extraovarian peritoneal serous papillary carcinoma: a case-control retrospective comparison to papillary adenocarcinoma of the ovary. *Gynecol Oncol* 1993;50:347.
56. Piver MS, Eltabbakh GH, Hempling RE, et al. Two sequential studies for primary peritoneal carcinoma: induction with weekly cisplatin followed by either cisplatin/doxorubicin/cyclophosphamide or paclitaxel/cisplatin. *Gynecol Oncol* 1997;67:141.
57. Muggia FM, Baranda J. Management of peritoneal carcinomatosis of unknown primary tumor site. *Semin Oncol* 1993;20:268.
58. McGuire WP, Hoskins WJ, Brady MF, et al. A phase III trial comparing cisplatin/cytoxan and cisplatin/taxol in advanced ovarian cancer. *Proc Am Soc Clin Oncol* 1993;12:255.
59. Bhatia SK, Saclarides TJ, Witt TR, et al. Hormone receptor studies in axillary metastases from occult breast cancer. *Cancer* 1987;59:1170.
60. Block EF, Meyer MA. Positron emission tomography in diagnosis of occult adenocarcinoma of the breast. *Am Surg* 1998;64:906.
61. Schorn C, Fischer U, Luftner-Nagel S, Westerhof JP, Grabbe E. MRI of the breast in patients with metastatic disease of unknown primary. *Eur Radiol* 1999;9:470.
62. Ashikari R, Rosen PP, Urban JA, Senoo T. Breast cancer presenting as an axillary mass. *Ann Surg* 1976;183:415.
63. Patel J, Nemoto T, Rosner D, et al. Axillary lymph node metastases from an occult breast cancer. *Cancer* 1981;47:2923.
64. Merson M, Andreola S, Galimberti V, et al. Breast carcinoma presenting as axillary metastases without evidence of a primary tumor. *Cancer* 1992;70:504.
65. Rosen PP. Axillary lymph node metastases in patients with occult noninvasive breast carcinoma. *Cancer* 1980;46:1298.
66. Ellerbroek N, Holmes F, Singletary E, et al. Treatment of patients with isolated axillary nodal metastases from an occult primary carcinoma consistent with breast origin. *Cancer* 1990;66:1461.
67. Tell DT, Khoury JM, Taylor HG, et al. Atypical metastasis from prostate cancer: clinical utility of the immunoperoxidase technique for prostate-specific antigen. *JAMA* 1985;253:3574.
68. Gentile PS, Carloss HW, Huang T-Y, et al. Disseminated prostate carcinoma simulating primary lung cancer. *Cancer* 1988;62:711.
69. Sporn JR, Greenberg BR. Empirical chemotherapy for adenocarcinoma of unknown primary tumor site. *Semin Oncol* 1993;20:261.
70. Johnson RO, Castro R, Ansfield FJ. Response of primary unknown cancers to treatment with 5-fluorouracil. *Cancer Chemother Rep* 1964;38:63.
71. Moertel CG, Reitemeier RJ, Schutt AJ, Hahn RG. Treatment of the patient with adenocarcinoma of unknown origin. *Cancer* 1972;30:1469.
72. Wagener DJT, de Muelder PHM, Burghouts JT, et al. Phase II trial of cisplatin for adenocarcinoma of unknown primary site. *Eur J Cancer* 1991;27:755.
73. Casciato DA. Metastasis of unknown origin. In: Haskell CM, ed. *Cancer treatment*, 4th ed. Philadelphia: WB Saunders, 1995:1128.
74. Milliken ST, Tattersall MHN, Woods RL, et al. Metastatic adenocarcinoma of unknown primary site: a randomized study of two combination chemotherapy regimens. *Eur J Cancer Clin Oncol* 1987;23:1645.
75. McKeen E, Smith F, Haidak D, et al. Fluorouracil, Adriamycin and mitomycin-C for adenocarcinoma of unknown origin. *Proc Am Assoc Cancer Res* 1980;21:358(abst).
76. Woods RL, Fox RM, Tattersall MHN, et al. Metastatic adenocarcinoma of unknown primary: a randomized study of two combination-chemotherapy regimens. *N Engl J Med* 1980;303:87.

77. Eagan RT, Thermean TM, Rubin J, et al. Lack of value for cisplatin added to mitomycin-doxorubicin combination chemotherapy for carcinoma of unknown primary site. *Am Clin Oncol* 1987;10:82.
78. Goldberg RM, Smith FP, Ueno W, et al. Fluorouracil, adriamycin and mitomycin in the treatment of adenocarcinoma of unknown primary. *J Clin Oncol* 1986;4:395.
79. Kambhu I, Kelsen D, Niedzwiecki D, et al. Phase II trial of mitomycin-C, vindesine, and adriamycin and predictive variables in the treatment of patients with adenocarcinoma of unknown primary site. *Proc Am Assoc Cancer Res* 1986;27:734(abst).
80. Flore JJ, Kelsen DP, Gralla RJ, et al. Adenocarcinoma of unknown primary origin. Treatment with vindesine and doxorubicin. *Cancer Treat Rep* 1985;69:591.
81. Valentine J, Rosenthal S, Arseneau JC. Combination chemotherapy for adenocarcinoma of unknown primary origin. *Cancer Clin Trials* 1979;2:265.
82. Rudnick S, Tremont S, Staab E, et al. Evaluation and therapy of adenocarcinoma of unknown primary. *Proc Am Soc Clin Oncol* 1981;1:379(abst).
83. Sulkes A, Uziely B, Isacson R, et al. Combination chemotherapy in metastatic tumors of unknown origin. *Isr J Med Sci* 1988;24:604.
84. Van der Gaast A, Verweij J, Planting AST, et al. 5-Fluorouracil, doxorubicin, and mitomycin C (FAM) combination chemotherapy for metastatic adenocarcinoma of unknown primary. *Eur J Cancer Clin Oncol* 1988;24:765.
85. Treat J, Falchuk SC, Tremblay C, et al. Phase II trial of methotrexate-FAM in adenocarcinoma of unknown primary. *Eur J Cancer Clin Oncol* 1989;25:1053.
86. Alberts AS, Falkson G, Falkson HC, et al. Treatment and prognosis of metastatic carcinoma of unknown primary: analysis of 100 patients. *Med Pediatr Oncol* 1989;17:188.
87. Walach N, Horn Y. Combination chemotherapy in the treatment of adenocarcinoma of unknown primary origin. *Cancer Treat Rep* 1987;71:605.
88. Anderson H, Thatcher N, Rankin E, et al. VAC (vincristine, Adriamycin and cyclophosphamide) chemotherapy for metastatic carcinoma from an unknown primary site. *Eur J Cancer Clin Oncol* 1983;19:49.
89. Bedikian AY, Valdivieso M, Bodey GP, et al. Sequential chemotherapy for adenocarcinoma of unknown primary. *Am J Clin Oncol* 1983;6:219.
90. Jadeja J, Legha S, Burgess M, et al. Combination chemotherapy with 5-FU, Adriamycin, cyclophosphamide, and *cis*-platinum in the treatment of adenocarcinoma of unknown primary and undifferentiated carcinomas. *Proc Am Soc Clin Oncol* 1983;2:926(abst).
91. Pasterz R, Savoraj N, Burgess M. Prognostic factors in metastatic carcinoma of unknown primary. *J Clin Oncol* 1986;4:1652.
92. Becouarn Y, Brunet R, Barbe-Gaston C. Fluorouracil, doxorubicin, cisplatin and altretamine in the treatment of metastatic carcinoma of unknown primary. *Eur J Cancer Clin Oncol* 1989;25:861.
93. Lenzi R, Abbruzzese J, Amato R, et al. Cisplatin, 5-FU, and folinic acid for the treatment of carcinoma of unknown primary. A phase II study. *Proc Am Soc Clin Oncol* 1991;10:1055(abst).
94. Falkson CI, Cohen GL. Mitomycin C, epirubicin and cisplatin versus mitomycin C alone as therapy for carcinoma of unknown primary origin. *Oncology* 1998;55:116.
95. Nole F, Colleoni M, Buzzoni R, et al. Fluorouracil plus folinic acid in metastatic adenocarcinoma of unknown primary site suggestive of a gastrointestinal primary. *Tumori* 1993;79:116.
96. Abbreuzese JL, Abbruzzese MC, Hess KR, et al. Unknown primary carcinoma: natural history and prognostic factors in 657 consecutive patients. *J Clin Oncol* 1994;12:1272.
97. Hainsworth JD, Johnson DH, Greco FA. Cisplatin-based combination chemotherapy in the treatment of poorly differentiated carcinoma and poorly differentiated adenocarcinoma of unknown primary site: results of a 12-year experience. *J Clin Oncol* 1992;10:912.
98. Theodore C, Fizazi K, Borol C, et al. Carcinoma of an unknown primary site (CUP): results of a chemotherapy strategy based on histologic differentiation. *Proc Am Soc Clin Oncol* 1997;15:308a(abst).
99. van der Gaast A, Verweij J, Henzen-Logmans SC, Rodenburg CJ, Stoter G. Carcinoma of unknown primary: identification of a treatable subset. *Ann Oncol* 1990;1:119.
100. Hainsworth JD, Erland JB, Kalman LA, et al. Carcinoma of unknown primary: treatment with 1-hour paclitaxel, carboplatin, and extended schedule etoposide. *J Clin Oncol* 1997;15:2385.
101. Pavlidis N, Kalofonos H, Bafaloukos D, et al. Cisplatin/Taxol combination chemotherapy in 72 patients with metastatic cancer of unknown primary site: a phase II trial of the Hellenic Cooperative Oncology Group. *Proc Am Soc Clin Oncol* 1999;18:195a(abst).
102. Assar OS, Fischbein NG, Caputo GR, et al. Metastatic head and neck cancer: role and usefulness of FDG PET in locating occult primary tumors. *Radiology* 1999;210:177.
103. Braams JW, Pruim J, Kole AC, et al. Detection of unknown primary head and neck tumor by positron emission tomograph. *Int J Oral Maxillofac Surg* 1997;26:112.
104. Califano J, Westra WH, Koch W, et al. Unknown primary head and neck squamous carcinoma: molecular indemnification of the site of origin. *J Natl Cancer Inst* 1999;91:599.
105. Jones AS, Cook JA, Phillips DE, et al. Squamous carcinoma presenting as an enlarged cervical lymph node. *Cancer* 1993;72:1756.
106. Barrie JR, Knapper WH, Strong EW. Cervical nodal metatases of unknown origin. *Am J Surg* 1970;120:466.
107. Jesse RH, Perez CA, Fletcher GH. Cervical lymph node metastasis: unknown primary cancer. *Cancer* 1973;31:854.
108. Coker DD, Casterline PF, Chambers RG, Jacques DA. Metastases to lymph nodes of the head and neck from an unknown primary site. *Am J Surg* 1977;134:517.
109. Jose B, Bosch A, Caldwell WL, Frias Z. Metastasis to neck from unknown primary tumor. *Acta Radiol Oncol* 1979;18:161.
110. Nordstrom DG, Tewfik HH, Latourette HB. Cervical lymph node metastases from an unknown primary. *Int J Radiat Oncol Biol Phys* 1979;5:73.
111. Fermont AC. Malignant cervical lymphadenopathy due to an unknown primary. *Clin Radiol* 1980;31:355.
112. Leipzig B, Winter ML, Hokanson JA. Cervical nodal metastases of unknown origin. *Laryngoscope* 1981;91:593.
113. Pacini P, Olmi P, Cellai E, Chiavacci A. Cervical lymph node metastases from an unknown primary tumour. *Acta Radiol Oncol* 1981;20:311.
114. Spiro RH, DeRose G, Strong EW. Cervical node metastasis of occult origin. *Am J Surg* 1983;146:441.
115. Mobit-Tabatabasi MA, Dasmaphapatra KS, Rush BF Jr, Ohanian M. Management of squamous cell carcinoma of unknown origin in cervical lymph nodes. *Am Surg* 1986; 52:152.
116. Yang ZY, Hu YH, Yan JH, et al. Lymph node metastases in the neck from an unknown primary: report on 113 patients. *Acta Radiol Oncol* 1983;22:17.
117. Carlson LS, Fletcher GH, Oswald MJ. Guidelines for the radiotherapeutic techniques for cervical metastases from an unknown primary. *Int J Radiat Oncol Biol Phys* 1986;12:2101.
118. McCunniff AJ, Raber M. Metastatic carcinoma of the neck from an unknown primary. *Int J Radiat Oncol Biol Phys* 1986;12:1849.
119. Bataini JP, Rodriguez J, Jaulerry C, et al. Treatment of metastatic neck nodes secondary to an occult epidermoid carcinoma of the head and neck. *Laryngoscope* 1987;97:1080.
120. De Braud F, Heilbrun LK, Ahmed K, et al. Metastatic squamous cell carcinoma of an unknown primary localized to the neck: advantages of an aggressive treatment. *Cancer* 1989;64:510.
121. Marcial-Vega VA, Cardenes H, Perez CA, et al. Cervical metastasis from unknown primaries: radiotherapeutic management and appearance of subsequent primaries. *Int J Radiat Oncol Biol Phys* 1990;19:919.
122. LeFevre JL, Coche-Dequeant D, Ton Van J, et al. Cervical lymph nodes from unknown primary tumor in 190 patients. *Am J Surg* 1990;160:443.
123. Weir L, Keane T, Cummings B, et al. Radiation treatment of cervical lymph node metastasis from an unknown primary: an analysis of outcome by treatment volume and other prognostic factors. *Radiother Oncol* 1995;35:206.
124. Brizel DM, Albers MF, Fisher SR, et al. Hyperfractionated irradiation with or without concurrent chemotherapy for locally advanced head and neck cancer. *N Engl J Med* 1998;338:1798.
125. Wendt TG, Grabenbauer GG, Rodel CM, et al. Simultaneous radiochemotherapy versus radiotherapy alone in advanced head and neck cancer: a randomized multicenter study. *J Clin Oncol* 1998;16:1318.
126. Coletier PJ, Garden AS, Morrison WH, et al. Postoperative radiation for squamous cell carcinoma metastatic to cervical lymph nodes from an unknown primary site: outcomes and patterns of failure. *Head Neck* 1998;20:674.
127. Fernandez JA, Suarez C, Martinez JA, et al. Metastatic squamous cell carcinoma in cervical lymph nodes from an unknown primary tumor: prognostic factors. *Clin Otolaryngol* 1998;23:158.
128. Medini E, Medini AM, Lee CK, Gapany M, Levitt SR. The management of metastatic squamous cell carcinoma in cervical lymph nodes from an unknown primary. *Am J Clin Oncol* 1998;21:121.
129. Guarischi A, Keane TJ, Elhakim T. Metastatic inguinal nodes from an unknown primary neoplasm: a review of 56 cases. *Cancer* 1987;59:572.
130. Greco FA, Vaughn WK, Hainsworth JD. Advanced poorly differentiated carcinoma of unknown primary site: recognition of a treatable syndrome. *Ann Intern Med* 1986; 104:547.
131. Hainsworth JD, Wright EP, Gray GF Jr, Greco FA. Poorly differentiated carcinoma of unknown primary site: correlation of light microscopic findings with response to cisplatin-based combination chemotherapy. *J Clin Oncol* 1987;5:1272.
132. Hainsworth JD, Wright EP, Johnson DH, Davis BW, Greco FA. Poorly differentiated carcinoma of unknown primary site: clinical usefulness of immunoperoxidase staining. *J Clin Oncol* 1991;9:1931.
133. Richardson RL, Greco FA, Wolff S, et al. Extragonadal germ cell malignancy: value of tumor markers in metastatic carcinoma of young males. *Proc Am Assoc Cancer Res* 1979;20:204(abst).
134. Richardson RL, Schoumacher RA, Fer MF, et al. The unrecognized extragonadal germ cell cancer syndrome. *Ann Intern Med* 1981;94:181.
135. Hainsworth JD, Greco FA. Poorly differentiated carcinoma of unknown primary site. In: Fer MF, Greco FA, Oldham R, eds. *Poorly differentiated neoplasms and tumors of unknown origin*. Orlando: Grune & Stratton, 1986:189.
136. Fox RM, Woods RL, Tattersall MHN. Undifferentiated carcinoma in young men: the atypical teratoma syndrome. *Lancet* 1979;1:1316.
137. Hainsworth JD, Johnson DH, Greco FA. Poorly differentiated neuroendocrine carcinoma of unknown primary site: a newly recognized clinicopathologic entity. *Ann Intern Med* 1988;109:364.
138. Hainsworth JD, Greco FA. Treatment of patients with cancer of an unknown primary site. *N Engl J Med* 1995;329:257.
139. van der Gaast A, Verweij J, Planting AS, et al. The value of immunohistochemistry in patients with poorly differentiated adenocarcinoma and undifferentiated carcinoma of unknown primary site. *J Cancer Res Clin Oncol* 1996;122:181.
140. Motzer RJ, Rodriguez E, Reuter VE, et al. Molecular and cytogenic studies in the diagnosis of patients with midline carcinomas of unknown primary site. *J Clin Oncol* 1995;13:274.
141. Hainsworth JD, Johnson DH, Greco FA. Cisplatin-based combination chemotherapy in the treatment of poorly differentiated carcinoma and poorly differentiated adenocarcinoma of unknown primary site: results of a 12 year experience at a single institution. *J Clin Oncol* 1992;10:912.
142. Raber MN, Faintuch J, Abbruzzese J, et al. Continuous infusion 5-fluorouracil, etoposide and *cis*-diamminedichloroplatinum in patients with metastatic carcinoma of unknown primary site. *Ann Oncol* 1991;2:519.
143. Pavlidis N, Kosmidis P, Skaros D, et al. Subsets of tumors responsive to cisplatin or combinations in patients with carcinoma of unknown primary site. *Ann Oncol* 1992:236.
144. Zarba J, Izzo J, Hahjoubi R, et al. Treatment of unknown primary adenocarcinoma with fluorouracil, mitomycin, epirubicin and platinum. *Eur J Cancer* 1991;27[Suppl 2]:1350(abst).
145. Briasoulis E, Txavaris N, Fountzilas G, et al. Combination regimen with carboplatin, epi-

rubicin and etoposide in metastatic carcinomas of unknown primary site: a Hellenic Cooperative Oncology Group phase II trial. *Oncology* 1998;55:426.
146. Hainsworth JD, Einhorn LH, Williams SD, et al. Advanced extragonadal germ cell tumors: successful treatment with combination chemotherapy. *Ann Intern Med* 1982;97:7.
147. Israel A, Bosl GJ, Golbey RB, et al. The results of chemotherapy for extragonadal germ cell tumors in the cisplatin era: the Memorial Sloan Kettering Cancer Center experience (1975–1982). *J Clin Oncol* 1985;3:1073.
148. Agnarsson BA, Kadin ME. Ki-1 positive large cell lymphoma: a morphologic and immunologic study of 19 cases. *Am J Surg Pathol* 1988;12: 264.
149. Loehrer PJ, Perez CA, Roth LM, et al. Chemotherapy for advanced thymoma: preliminary results of an intergroup study. *Ann Intern Med* 1990;113:520.
150. Lenzi R, Hess KR, Abbruzzese MC, et al. Poorly differentiated carcinoma and poorly differentiated adenocarcinoma of unknown primary origin: favorable subsets of patients with unknown primary cancer? *J Clin Oncol* 1997;15:2056.
151. Moertel CG, Kovals LK, O'Connell MJ, et al. Treatment of neuroendocrine carcinomas with combined etoposide and cisplatin: evidence of major therapeutic activity in the anaplastic variants of these neoplasms. *Cancer* 1991;68:227.
152. van der Gaast A, Verwey J, Prins E, Splinter TAW. Chemotherapy as treatment of choice in extrapulmonary undifferentiated small cell carcinoma. *Cancer* 1990;65:422.
153. Kasimis BS, Wuerker RB, Malefatto JP, Moran EM. Prolonged survival of patients with extrapulmonary small cell carcinoma arising in the neck. *Med Pediatr Oncol* 1983;11:27.

David L. Bartlett

CHAPTER 49

Peritoneal Carcinomatosis

Peritoneal carcinomatosis is defined as the spread and implantation of tumor cells throughout the peritoneal cavity, and it is considered an incurable disease state leading to significant patient suffering. However, oncologists should recognize peritoneal carcinomatosis not as a terminal event for the patient but as a regional disease entity that requires special attention and as a therapeutic challenge for consideration of novel management strategies. Although the primary histology dictates the clinical course, important concepts of diagnosis and treatment are common among all forms. Also, the palliative management of complications, such as bowel obstruction and ascites, warrants special consideration. The purpose of this chapter is to provide a general overview of peritoneal carcinomatosis as a regional stage of metastatic disease. This includes a discussion of the biology of tumor spread and implantation and techniques for early recognition of peritoneal tumors. General concepts regarding regional treatment approaches are reviewed.

PATHOPHYSIOLOGY

The peritoneum is a serous lining of mesothelial cells with a rich vascular and lymphatic capillary network.[1] The flow of abdominal fluid provides clues to the development and pattern of peritoneal carcinomatosis. Gravity, diaphragmatic and intestinal movement, and diaphragmatic and omental absorption via lymphatics leads to a characteristic peritoneal fluid circulation (Fig. 49-1).[2] Lymphatic endothelial cells have been shown to form channels extending from the peritoneal cavity directly into lymphatics,[3] most notably in the diaphragm. Flessner et al.[4] demonstrated that the absorption of ^{125}I-labeled albumin from the peritoneal cavity concentrated in the diaphragm and abdominal wall peritoneum but not in the visceral peritoneum. The most dependent recess is the pouch between the rectum and uterus or bladder. Hagiwara et al.[5] demonstrated a site-specific correlation between the number of milky spots at specific peritoneal locations and the number of infiltrating tumor cells. Milky spots represent an immunologic filter similar to the lymphatic drainage of solid organs and seem to represent sites where peritoneal fluid drains into lymphatic channels. If fluid is actively absorbed into these spots, it is easy to hypothesize that free clumps of tumor cells could become trapped at these spots and develop into tumors. Milky-spot tissues are found in the hepatoduodenal ligament, base of mesentery, appendiceal epiploicae, gonadal fat (corresponding to the pouch of Douglas), and the greater omentum. The omentum contains the highest concentration of milky spots. The constant flux of fluid, the sites of absorption and filtration, and gravity all play a role in the pattern of peritoneal tumors. It has been proposed that more aggressive, invasive tumors have a "stickier" phenotype and are more likely not to follow the experimental observations of peritoneal spread but have a more random distribution close to the initial site of peritoneal contamination.[6] In addition, more aggressive, invasive tumors are better at forming tumors on moving surfaces, such as the serosal surface of the small bowel.

Tumor cells reach the peritoneal cavity by direct invasion of aggressive gastrointestinal (GI) tumors through the serosal lining of the organ or through a pressure-burst effect of less invasive tumors that push through the serosal surface without tissue invasion. This is characteristic of appendiceal and ovarian tumors, in which even a benign tumor can grow large enough to break through the wall of the organ and contaminate the peritoneal cavity with neoplastic cells.[7] It is possible for hematogenous metastases from extraperitoneal tumors to invade secondarily or burst into the abdominal cavity, leading to peritoneal carcinomatosis. A final source for peritoneal contamination of tumor cells is iatrogenic spillage of neoplastic

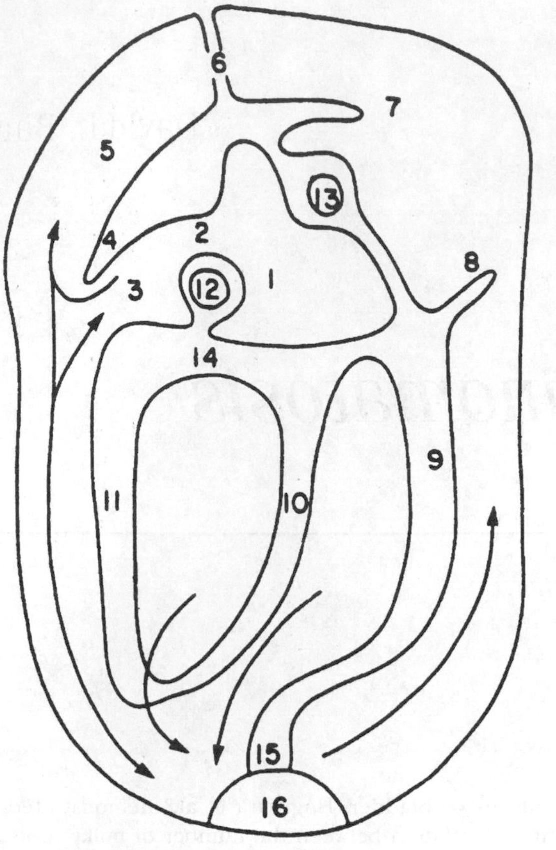

FIGURE 49-1. Circulation of fluid in the peritoneal cavity. Flow is generated by diaphragmatic movement, absorption of material from the diaphragmatic lymphatic channel, and gravity. 1, Lesser sac; 2, foramen of Winslow; 3, Morison's pouch; 4, right triangular ligament; 5, right subphrenic space; 6, falciform ligament; 7, left subphrenic space; 8, phrenocolic ligament; 9, bare area of the descending colon; 10, root of the small bowel mesentery; 11, bare area of ascending colon; 12, duodenum; 13, esophagus; 14, root of the transverse mesocolon; 15, bare area of the rectum; 16, bladder. (From ref. 2, with permission.)

cells. A classic example is during cholecystectomy in the setting of unrecognized gallbladder cancer, in which the subserosal plane of tumor cell invasion is dissected during the resection, spilling tumor cells throughout the region.[8] It is also possible to contaminate the peritoneal cavity during a needle biopsy for diagnosis.

Seeding of the peritoneal cavity with tumor cells does not necessarily lead to implantation, proliferation, and formation of carcinomatosis.[9] Different tumors and heterogeneous cell populations within a single tumor will lead to different efficiencies with regard to tumor formation after peritoneal seeding.[10] The requirements for peritoneal tumor seeding are different from the requirements for hematogenous metastases. The tumor cells must make their way into the cavity, then stick to the peritoneal surface via adhesion molecules.[11] They must avoid immunologic destruction and, once implanted, be able to stimulate angiogenesis for continued growth. In general, this can be accomplished with a less aggressive tumor cell than that required for hematogenous spread. Also, it may be possible for tumors to grow to a limited extent within the peritoneal cavity without implantation and vascularization but relying on nutrients within peritoneal exudate for survival.

DIAGNOSIS

Although the follow-up and early detection of metastatic cancers in general is in debate in the absence of effective therapy,[12] the early diagnosis of peritoneal spread of cancer would be preferable in the setting of experimental protocols for regional therapy. In other cases, the early detection of peritoneal spread might alter the management of the primary tumor or avoid surgical exploration for hepatic or pulmonary metastasectomy. However, peritoneal spread is diagnosed in most patients after surgical exploration for bowel complications or after clinical ascites develops. At this stage in the setting of invasive tumors, a regional therapy approach is probably beyond any chance of success.

Standard imaging tests, including ultrasonography and helical computed tomography (CT) scans, are notably insensitive for the detection of peritoneal tumor. The sensitivity of CT scan for peritoneal nodules measuring smaller than 1 cm is on the order of 15% to 30%.[13] Ultrasonography is similarly insensitive. It is important to consider findings other than solid-tumor detection that may suggest the presence of peritoneal carcinomatosis. These include the presence of ascites, fixing together of bowel loops, thickening of mesentery, and omental matting.

Advances in magnetic resonance imaging (MRI) have been demonstrated to improve significantly detection of peritoneal tumor nodules.[14] Low et al.[15] have demonstrated that abdominal MRI is superior to helical CT for the detection of peritoneal and bowel wall abnormalities. It may be that MRI of the peritoneal cavity is improved with dilute oral barium contrast materials. In general, CT scans are easier to interpret for the general oncologist and are cheaper to obtain and, therefore, are still more widely used than MRI. For patients on clinical protocol, however, improved imaging should be a goal for the oncologist, to aid in follow-up of peritoneal disease. Nelson et al.[16] studied intraperitoneal infusion of contrast material before CT scanning, but this did not significantly improve the sensitivity for detection of peritoneal metastases.

Positron emission tomography (PET) imaging for metastatic GI tumors is under investigation at numerous institutions and may improve the sensitivity for detecting small nodules. In general, PET has not been shown to be sensitive for lesions measuring smaller than 1 cm in the abdominal cavity. Extrahepatic peritoneal nodules of smaller than 1 cm were not detected by [^{18}F]fluorodeoxyglucose (FDG) PET scanning as a preoperative screen for patients undergoing hepatic metastasectomy for colorectal cancer.[17]

Another mechanism for screening for peritoneal spread of tumor involves peritoneal lavage cytology. This can be performed as a percutaneous closed technique or at the time of laparoscopy or laparotomy for resection of primary disease. The sensitivity of this test depends on the ability to lavage completely all regions of the peritoneal cavity and the ability to detect cancer cells accurately. Sensitivity may be improved using polymerase chain reaction techniques or immunohistochemistry.[18,19] The sensitivity also depends on the number of cells being shed into the peritoneal cavity by the tumor. Even in cases with advanced, grossly evident peritoneal metastases, the ascites can be negative for tumor cells. A study by Fujiwara et al.[20] compared closed abdominal lavage cytology to second-look laparotomy. In this study, 14 patients who had positive cytology results also had positive disease on second-look laparotomy. Three patients with negative cytology had positive disease on second-look laparotomy. The other 23 patients had negative cytology and negative second-look laparotomy. This illustrates the fact that cytology can be helpful in predicting the presence of carcinomatosis, but it is not as sensitive as direct inspection and palpation of the peritoneal surfaces.

Much has been studied regarding the prognostic utility of lavage cytology for patients at high risk of peritoneal spread, as in the case of gastric cancer, colon cancer, and pancreatic cancer.[21,22] Positive cytology correlates with full-thickness invasion through the bowel wall, as would be expected.[23] Positive cytology also seems to correlate with a poor prognosis for peritoneal recurrence.[24,25] It is not clear, however, whether cytology has any added prognostic value over the stage of the primary tumor. It should be noted also that cells shed into the peritoneal cavity may not be viable or may not be able to establish new tumor sites; therefore, the presence of tumor cells may not predict the development of carcinomatosis.

By far the most sensitive modality for detecting the spread of tumor is direct visualization of the peritoneal surfaces along with palpation of the abdominal contents. Visualization of the peritoneal surfaces can be accomplished with a minimally invasive approach. Laparoscopy is now used routinely in most cancer centers as a staging modality for patients with resectable pancreatic and gastric cancers. Its greatest utility is in diagnosing small peritoneal metastases and small surface liver metastases that are not detected on imaging tests.[26] The minimally invasive laparoscopy allows for safe, directed peritoneal lavage for cytology as well. Laparoscopy should be considered for the detection of peritoneal surface tumors in patients in whom therapy would be altered or investigational therapy considered for tumor spread in this fashion. This includes patients who are considered for preoperative neoadjuvant regional therapy before surgical resection for resectable pancreatic and gastric cancer. Laparoscopy may also be of utility in patients with carcinomatosis who should be followed up for response to therapy to determine whether to change therapies or continue the current treatment strategy.[27,28] Repeat laparoscopy for following up disease status at intervals during therapy is feasible. The adhesions after multiple tumor debulkings and laparoscopies may ultimately limit the sensitivity of detection and increase the risk of laparoscopy. Open abdominal exploration and palpation of the peritoneal surfaces is extremely sensitive for even small 1- to 2-mm peritoneal surface nodules. Palpation of the areas at high risk should be performed during any cancer surgery for intraperitoneal malignancies. This includes the greater omentum, the deepest recess of the pelvic peritoneum, the base of the small bowel mesentery and transverse mesocolon, the falciform ligament, and the diaphragm.

HISTOLOGIC SUBTYPES

PSEUDOMYXOMA PERITONEI

Classically, the diagnosis of *Pseudomyxoma peritonei* includes any low-grade or benign tumor within the abdominal cavity that produces copious amounts of mucinous ascites. The term was first coined in 1884 by Werth[29] as a description of the gelatinous material filling the peritoneal cavity of a patient with a ruptured cystadenoma of the ovary. In 1901, Fraenkel[30] first associated *P peritonei* with a ruptured mucocele of the appendix. Because of the relative rarity of this clinical entity, it is generally poorly understood by oncologists. The spectrum of conditions that are considered to fall under the general diagnosis of *P peritonei* is quite large.[7] This leads to confusion in determining the expected clinical outcome and treatment approaches for this condition.

The condition of diffuse mucinous ascites can be caused by any tumor that has spread into the peritoneal cavity and produces significant amounts of mucin. This includes well-differentiated adenocarcinomas of the GI tract and benign mucin-secreting adenomas of the appendix.[7] A benign tumor of the appendix can grow to a size that ruptures the wall of the appendix and leads to spillage of benign cells into the peritoneal cavity. These cells can then continue to proliferate and produce copious amounts of mucin despite a completely benign histology, with the inability to invade into tissues and metastasize hematogenously or via lymphatics. The most important prognosticator for patients with mucinous ascites is, therefore, whether the primary tumor is benign or malignant.

Clinical evidence of malignancy includes the presence of lymph node metastases and gross evidence of an invasive phenotype. Histologically, malignant tumors will have moderate to abundant cellularity, show evidence of invasion, and demonstrate cellular atypia and nuclear pleomorphism consistent with malignancy. Benign tumors have scant cellularity with no evidence of invasion into tissues and no cellular atypia. In difficult cases, it is helpful to examine the primary tumor carefully to determine whether the primary tumor represents invasion of tumor cells through the wall of the organ or a benign process that has ruptured the wall without invasion.

The site of origin of cells producing mucinous ascites often is difficult to define. This is especially the case when, in women, both the appendix and the ovaries are obliterated by tumor. Although the ovary can be a site for mucinous borderline tumors of low malignant potential or mucinous carcinomas, these are almost never associated with diffuse copious mucinous ascites.[7] Therefore, all cases of *P peritonei* with benign-appearing mucinous epithelial cells emanate from an appendiceal mucinous adenoma. These tumors often involve the ovaries at early stages but should not be confused with a primary ovarian cancer. Ruptured ovarian follicles may allow for a rich soil and sticky surface on which benign tumor cells can stick and proliferate. In surgical debulking procedures, appendectomy and bilateral oophorectomy should be performed.

Ronett et al.[31] have extensive experience in *P peritonei*, and they have classified cases of *P peritonei* into three pathologically and prognostically distinct groups: (1) disseminated peritoneal adenomucinosis; (2) peritoneal mucinous carcinomatosis; and (3) peritoneal mucinous carcinomatosis with intermediate or discordant features (Table 49-1). They have shown distinct difference in survival and prognosis in patients with disseminated peritoneal adenomucinosis as compared to those with carcinomatosis or discordant features (Fig. 49-2). This work verifies the importance of differentiating a malignant from a benign diagnosis. In their study, the median survival for patients with disseminated peritoneal adenomucinosis had not been reached with a median follow-up of approximately 6 years, whereas the median survival for patients with a malignant tumor producing mucinous ascites was approximately 16 months.

TABLE 49-1. Distinguishing Pathologic Features of Disseminated Peritoneal Adenomucinosis and Peritoneal Mucinous Carcinomatosis

Feature	*DPAM*	*PMCA*
Primary site	Appendix	Appendix, colon, small intestine
Primary diagnosis	Mucinous adenoma	Mucinous adenocarcinoma
Surgical appearance	Mucinous ascites with redistribution	Carcinomatosis with invasive implants
Peritoneal tumor		
Cellularity	Scant	Moderate to abundant
Morphology	Abundant extracellular mucin containing simple to focally proliferative mucinous epithelium	Moderate to abundant extracellular mucin containing extensively proliferative mucinous epithelium or mucinous glands, clusters of cells, or individual cells consistent with carcinoma
Cytologic atypia	Minimal	Moderate to marked
Mitotic activity	Rare	Infrequent to frequent
Lymph node involvement	Rare	Frequent
Parenchymal organ invasion	Rare (except for ovary)	Frequent

DPAM, disseminated peritoneal adenomucinosis; PMCA, peritoneal mucinous carcinomatosis.
(Reproduced from ref. 7, with permission.)

Despite this dramatic difference in prognosis, most studies include all forms of *P peritonei* together, and this confuses outcome determinants for therapy in this condition. It would be best not to use the term *P peritonei* without further classification into mucinous adenocarcinoma or benign mucinous tumors. The treatment approach should be different for patients with benign mucin-producing tumors as compared to those with mucinous carcinomatosis. Patients with benign tumors should be treated with aggressive surgical debulking to limit the symptoms of compression and abdominal distention caused by extensive mucinous ascites within the abdominal cavity. It has been reported that long-term disease-free survival can be accomplished with repeated tumor debulking.[32] The extent of required surgery and the indication for chemotherapy are controversial.[33] The complication rate of the procedure should be seriously considered in recommending treatment for a condition with such an indolent course. It may be that aggressive regional chemotherapy approaches should not be offered until their efficacy has been better defined in carcinomas. In the case of low-grade mucinous carcinomatosis, the uniformly poor prognosis encourages innovative and aggressive approaches. This includes intensive regional chemotherapy in combination with cytoreduction (as discussed in the Intraperitoneal Chemotherapy section).

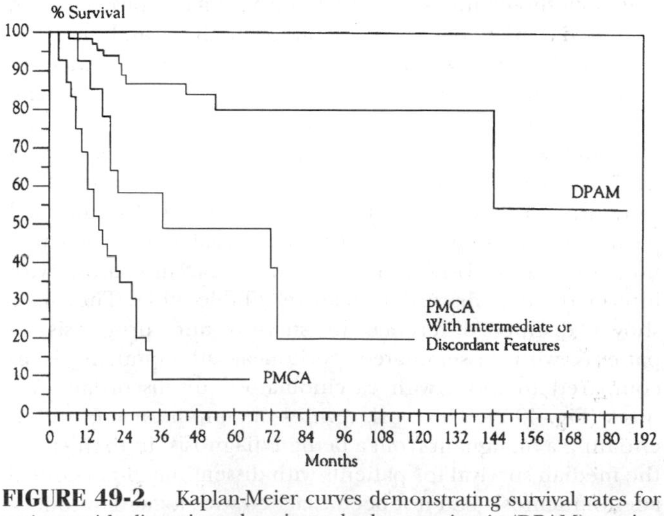

FIGURE 49-2. Kaplan-Meier curves demonstrating survival rates for patients with disseminated peritoneal adenomucinosis (DPAM), peritoneal mucinous carcinomatosis (PMCA), and PMCA with intermediate or discordant features. There is a statistically significant difference in survival between the three groups ($P<.0001$). (From ref. 7, with permission.)

Because of inconsistencies in pathologic diagnosis as well as different philosophies with regard to aggressiveness of surgery, it is difficult to define the prognosis and the best treatment strategies. The largest series of mucinous appendiceal tumors with peritoneal spread has been reported by Sugarbaker and Chang.[34] A total of 385 patients were reviewed. Patients with benign adenomucinosis had a 5-year survival of 80%, as compared to those with low-grade mucinous carcinomas, who had a 5-year survival of approximately 25%. The 5-year survival for those patients undergoing a complete resection was approximately 80%, as compared to those undergoing an incomplete resection, in which it was approximately 25%. It is probably not a coincidence that characteristics of surgical debulking and pathology lead to similar survival rates: Complete resection is more likely in patients with benign mucinous neoplasms as compared to those with more infiltrative mucinous carcinomas. As discussed later in the Surgery section, the fact that complete cytoreduction has an improved prognosis over incomplete cytoreduction does nothing to support aggressive surgery for this disease. Of note, the mortality rate for extensive cytoreduction and early postoperative intraperitoneal chemotherapy in the Sugarbaker and Chang[34] series is 2%, with major morbidity of 27%.

Gough et al.[35] (from the Mayo Clinic) reviewed 56 patients with the malignant form of *P peritonei*. Only 20% of their patients had complete cytoreduction, and they reported a 10-year survival rate of 32%. Smith et al.[36] (from the Memorial Sloan-Kettering Cancer Center) reviewed 17 patients undergoing surgical debulking for *P peritonei* without histologic classification. They reported a 10-year survival rate of 60%.

In summary, the entity of *P peritonei* is becoming better defined. Classification of the benign and malignant subtypes is essential and should be used to define and compare therapeutic approaches for this disease. The use of aggressive surgery and regional chemotherapy approaches remains experimental and requires investigation in a multiinstitutional randomized format to make standard treatment recommendations.

PERITONEAL MESOTHELIOMA

Peritoneal mesothelioma is a primary tumor of the mesothelial lining of the peritoneum. It is a rare tumor of approximately two cases per million population per year, but the incidence appears to be increasing. Tumors can be classified into benign lesions, borderline malignant lesions, and malignant tumors.[37] Benign lesions include adenomatoid mesothelioma and localized fibrous mesothelioma, which are rare tumors treated by surgical excision alone, with a good prognosis. Borderline tumors include multicystic peritoneal mesothelioma and well-differentiated papillary mesothelioma of the peritoneum.[38–40] Both of these tumors carry an indolent course, which can be treated with surgical debulking. These borderline tumors are characterized by local recurrences that can ultimately lead to complications within the abdominal cavity. It is not clear whether the tumors themselves will ultimately lead to the death of the patient. In a review of 22 patients, none died directly because of their disease, but several died as a result of complications of therapy.[41] One patient who died 29 years after he received a diagnosis of well-differentiated papillary mesothelioma had residual disease but died of unrelated causes. Microscopically, well-differentiated papillary mesothelioma consists of mesothelial cells in a well-developed papillary pattern with bland mesothelial appearance and cuboidal epithelium. It can be difficult to differentiate histologically the well-differentiated papillary mesothelioma from diffuse malignant mesothelioma, so multiple sections of tumor should be examined.

The malignant peritoneal mesotheliomas are less common than pleural mesotheliomas and have been associated with asbestos exposure and abdominal therapeutic radiation.[42] The association of malignant peritoneal mesothelioma and asbestos exposure has been reported to be as high as 83%; however, in our experience, it is much lower. These tumors often present with nonspecific abdominal pain and increasing abdominal girth secondary either to tumor mass or to the development of ascites. The diagnosis can be suggested by cytologic examination of ascites and verified by percutaneous biopsy of the omentum. These tumors tend to present with diffuse involvement of the peritoneal cavity, including an omental "cake" and diaphragmatic and pelvic tumor deposits (Fig. 49-3).

The epithelial type of malignant peritoneal mesothelioma is the most common type and has the best prognosis. The sarcomatoid and mixed (elements of both epithelial and sarcomatoid) forms are more aggressive, leading to fixed abdominal contents and an inability to successfully debulk these tumors surgically. Even among the primary epithelial form, there may be a spectrum of phenotypic aggressiveness and a variable clinical course. Some patients primarily experience ascites with no significant invasiveness to the tumors themselves, allowing for easy debulking and management of ascites. Other patients have more aggressive forms that can invade through the diaphragm to involve the chest, through the wall of the intestine (leading to complications of intestinal obstruction and bleeding), and into lymph nodes. The more invasive forms are difficult to debulk and have a worse prognosis. The sarcomatoid

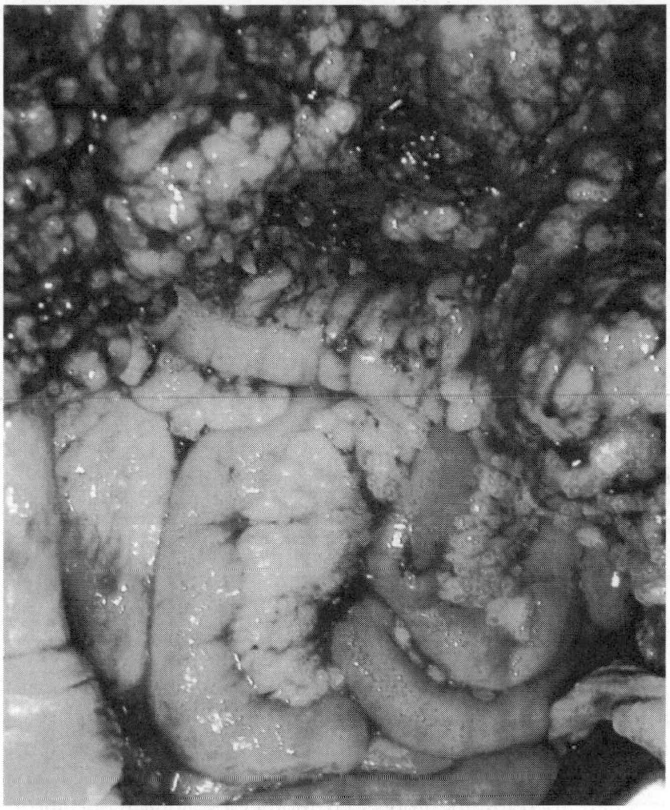

FIGURE 49-3. Diffuse malignant peritoneal mesothelioma of the papillary form. A thick omental "cake" is evident here, as is disease involving the mesentery of the small bowel. Notice the general sparing of the mobile surfaces of the small intestine. This disease was successfully debulked and treated with continuous hyperthermic peritoneal perfusion.

and mixed forms are rapidly growing tumors leading to intraabdominal complications and death within a year.[43]

Death from malignant mesothelioma is usually caused by complications from intraperitoneal progression. Hematogenous metastases are extremely rare, and secondary involvement of the chest occurs at a late stage and is usually not a life-threatening feature of this disease. Lymphatic metastases can be identified within the abdominal cavity with the more aggressive forms of epithelial mesothelioma and the sarcomatoid mesothelioma.[44] Patients with peritoneal mesothelioma in general have a better prognosis than those with pleural mesothelioma. CA-125 levels may be increased in patients with diffuse mesothelioma and can be followed up for response to therapy.

The natural history of diffuse mesothelioma is difficult to define. Reported series are small, owing to the rarity of this disease. Original reports suggested that the median survival was less than 1 year from the time of diagnosis.[45] However, multiple varied treatment approaches, usually combining surgical debulking with chemotherapy or total abdominal radiation (or both), may result in long-term survival.[46] Langer et al.[47] demonstrated a median survival of 22 months using surgical debulking and intraperitoneal chemotherapy with cisplatin and etoposide. No control, untreated arm is included in these trials to prove that the natural history is not sometimes indolent. It is also difficult to know whether adjuvant therapies improve the results of surgical debulking alone, as no series exists of aggressive surgical debulking alone for this disease. It is suggested, however, that the package of treatment strate-

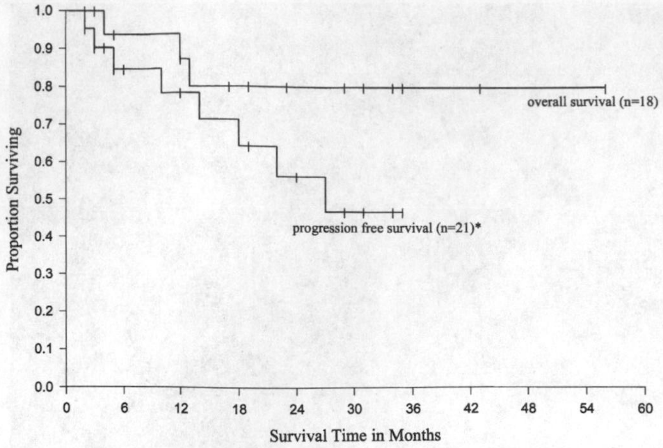

FIGURE 49-4. Kaplan-Meier survival curve for 18 patients treated with continuous hyperthermic peritoneal perfusion with cisplatin at the National Cancer Institute for peritoneal mesothelioma. *The progressive free survival analysis includes three patients who have been treated twice. (Adapted from ref. 50.)

gies that have been used can successfully alter the natural history of this disease. Lederman et al.[48] reported that six of ten patients remain free of disease up to 6 years after diagnosis after treatment with surgical debulking, combination chemotherapy, and whole abdomen radiation. Whole abdomen radiation is not well tolerated and has not gained widespread acceptance. Other investigators have used intraperitoneal chemotherapy alone (cisplatin or cisplatin plus mitomycin C) with modest clinical responses and improvement in ascites but have failed to demonstrate a survival benefit. Markman and Kelsen[49] reported 47% palliation of ascites and a median survival of 9 months in 19 patients who were treated with intraperitoneal cisplatin and mitomycin C.

We have explored the combination of extensive surgical debulking followed by intraoperative, intraperitoneal chemotherapy in the form of continuous hyperthermic peritoneal perfusion with cisplatin combined with early postoperative intraperitoneal dwell chemotherapy with 5-fluorouracil (5-FU) and paclitaxel.[50] Patients who presented with incapacitating ascites have complete resolution of their ascites and long-term disease-free survival. The median time to progression after treatment in 18 patients was approximately 27 months, with a median overall survival not being reached after a median potential follow-up of 19 months (Fig. 49-4). Ninety percent of patients had complete resolution of their ascites after therapy. Three patients were treated after recurrence of ascites approximately 2 years after their primary treatment, and all had resolution of their ascites again after retreatment. Other investigators have demonstrated similar success using the hyperthermic peritoneal treatment with mitomycin C for mesothelioma.[51]

PRIMARY PERITONEAL CARCINOMA

Primary peritoneal carcinoma has been called by many names, including *papillary carcinoma of the peritoneum, extraovarian papillary serous carcinoma, serous surface papillary carcinoma,* and *psammocarcinoma.*[52–54] The cell of origin for primary peritoneal carcinoma is not clear. Both the germinal epithelium of the ovary and the mesothelium of the peritoneum arise from the same embryologic origin; therefore, the peritoneum may retain the multipotentiality of the Müllerian system, allowing for the development of a primary carcinoma. Hereditary predisposition may play a role in this disease, as patients have an increased risk with the BRCA1 mutation.[55]

Primary peritoneal carcinoma diffusely involves the peritoneal surface while sparing or only minimally involving the ovaries. It is histologically indistinguishable from primary epithelial ovarian carcinoma, and its diagnosis requires differentiation from mesothelioma and ovarian cancer. Immunohistochemistry differentiates this from peritoneal mesothelioma.[56] Primary ovarian cancer is ruled out by the following criteria[57]: (1) Both ovaries must be normal in size; (2) the extraovarian involvement must be greater than the involvement on the surface of the ovary; (3) the ovarian component must be less than 5 × 5 mm within the ovary or confined to the ovarian surface; and (4) the cytologic characteristics must be of the serous type. This is a tumor described almost exclusively in women. Patients are older than those with epithelial ovarian cancers. The presentation of primary peritoneal carcinoma is abdominal distention and diffuse nonspecific abdominal pain secondary to ascites.

In general, these tumors are treated as ovarian cancers with cytoreduction and adjuvant therapy with platinum-based chemotherapeutic regimens. The median survival for women with primary peritoneal carcinoma has been reported to range from 12 to 25 months. This is similar or slightly worse than for epithelial ovarian cancer. Carboplatin or cisplatin in combination with paclitaxel leads to a high response rate and a reported median survival of 40 months.[52,58]

DESMOPLASTIC SMALL ROUND CELL TUMORS

The rare desmoplastic small round cell tumors typically occur in adolescents and young men and present with extensive involvement of the peritoneal surfaces. Rapid multifocal growth and hematogenous metastases to the liver, lungs, and lymph nodes are common. Reported median survival is 17 months, and long-term survival is uncommon. A combination of aggressive surgical debulking and systemic chemotherapy with cyclophosphamide, doxorubicin, and vincristine interspersed with ifosfamide, etoposide, and mesna (P6 protocol) appears to lead to an improved outcome.[59] The genetics of this tumor are interesting in that a consistent chromosomal translocation has been identified, which results in fusion of the Ewing's sarcoma gene with the Wilms' tumor gene.[60] This tumor can sometimes be difficult to differentiate from malignant peritoneal mesothelioma.

GASTROINTESTINAL PRIMARY TUMORS

GI primary tumors are the most common source of peritoneal carcinomatosis in male patients. This includes colon cancer, gastric cancer, pancreatic cancer, gallbladder cancer, and primary small bowel adenocarcinomas. The range of aggressiveness of these cancers is quite broad. However, as opposed to appendiceal tumors, the majority of other GI primary tumors are aggressive, invasive forms. The most important risk factor for developing peritoneal carcinomatosis is the depth of invasion of the primary tumor. If the tumor has invaded through the serosa (T3), the entire peritoneal surface is at risk for the development of carcinomatosis. These patients should be considered for adjuvant regional chemotherapy.

Patients with peritoneal carcinomatosis from these types of aggressive GI cancers usually present with symptoms of partial small bowel obstruction, as opposed to diffuse ascites, as is seen with the less invasive malignancies. Successful management of these patients with a regional approach is unlikely by the time they develop symptoms and complications of intraperitoneal spread. Because of their invasive nature, these tumors often invade the retroperitoneum and bowel wall and extensively involve lymphatics, where intraperitoneal chemotherapy may not reach. Adequate surgical debulking becomes less feasible for these aggressive GI malignancies. The treatment goal should be prophylaxis against the development of carcinomatosis or treatment of those patients who are incidentally found, at the time of primary resection, to have minimal peritoneal spread that can be managed with complete surgical excision. Because of the uniformly poor prognosis with peritoneal spread, an aggressive, prophylactic regional chemotherapy approach seems warranted.

GYNECOLOGIC PRIMARY TUMORS

Ovarian, endometrial, and cervical cancer can all invade into the peritoneal cavity and have a clinical course dominated by intraperitoneal spread of the tumor. Ovarian tumors (similar to appendiceal primary tumors) can lead to peritoneal contamination even in the setting of relatively low-grade, minimally aggressive tumors.[61] As compared to GI tumors (other than appendiceal), the ovarian carcinomatosis is less aggressive and, therefore, more amenable to surgical cytoreduction and regional intraperitoneal chemotherapy. Because of the sensitivity of ovarian tumors to systemic chemotherapy, carcinomatosis from an ovarian primary tumor represents a rare instance in which systemic chemotherapy can provide a long-term disease-free interval and potential cure.[62] It has been demonstrated that surgical debulking can improve the response and results of systemic chemotherapy.[63] The systematic staging of the peritoneal surface in patients with primary ovarian cancer is required to document microscopic metastases to the peritoneum, which would alter the treatment paradigm. Ascites is a common complication of peritoneal carcinomatosis from ovarian cancer, and palliation of ascites can play a significant role in the management of this disease.

OTHER FORMS

Other forms of peritoneal carcinomatosis are less common, and peritoneal spread does not normally dominate the clinical course of these tumors. Among these lesions are tumors from the genitourinary tract, such as testicular cancer, transitional cell cancer of the bladder, and renal cancer.[64] We have seen hemangiopericytoma, adrenal cancer, and pediatric solid tumors contaminate the peritoneal cavity. Peritoneal sarcomatosis is discussed in Chapter 39. Breast cancer can also lead to peritoneal carcinomatosis and ascites, which can be the only site of progressive disease in some patients. Palliation of ascites in these patients may improve their overall prognosis.

TREATMENT

SURGERY

Surgical debulking for peritoneal carcinomatosis is standard for the management of benign and low-grade malignant processes, such as *P peritonei*, mesothelioma, and ovarian cancer. In these settings, the goal of debulking is to "reset the clock" for development of symptoms. The more tumor that is removed, the longer the interval until the tumor grows to a symptomatic stage. Investigational strategies combine surgical cytoreduction with regional therapy. The goal of cytoreduction in this case is to leave behind only tumors smaller than 5.0 mm in diameter so as to allow for topical chemotherapy to penetrate and treat all cells within the tumor.[65] The best scenario is complete cytoreduction, wherein only microscopic disease is left behind. This is similar to bathing cells with chemotherapy in a Petri dish, ensuring delivery of chemotherapy to the cells.

Common sites for tumor spread should be closely examined, and resection of tumors is indicated where possible. This includes complete resection of the greater omentum, lesser omentum, falciform ligament, and peritoneum overlying the diaphragm; the base of the small bowel and transverse colon mesentery; and the pelvis. The splenic hilum is often involved with tumor, necessitating a splenectomy. Appendices epiploicae commonly are involved and may require limited bowel resections. The most difficult sites in which to achieve complete clearance are the hepatoduodenal ligament and pelvis. Oophorectomy, hysterectomy, partial bladder resection, and sigmoid colon resection may be required in the pelvis. Care must be taken to preserve blood supply to the stomach when dissecting the lesser omentum. The extent of resection should be dictated by the realistic treatment goal. Complete removal of all microscopic disease in the peritoneal cavity is not realistic, so the goal is to remove macroscopic disease in the hopes that chemotherapy or other adjuvant therapy will be more effective. An extensive procedure to remove pelvic peritoneal drop metastases in the setting of unresectable hepatic hilar disease does not make sense. Incidental extensive stripping of the peritoneum to address microscopic disease is not generally accepted, as all surfaces and all microscopic disease cannot be addressed.

Except in ovarian cancer, extensive cytoreduction for peritoneal carcinomatosis has not been objectively studied. Numerous trials demonstrate improved prognosis in patients who undergo complete debulking as compared to those whose tumors cannot be debulked,[52,66,67] but this is only a mirror of the aggressiveness of the tumor or late presentation. The ability to debulk completely correlates with an improved prognosis, but this should not be accepted as an indication to perform the procedure. Nevertheless, well-controlled trials are extremely difficult to perform in this disease state, and many definitive answers will not be obtained for some time. It is generally accepted in the setting of indolent, benign, or low-grade tumors, in which survival is dictated by complications of regional growth, that tumor debulking can extend survival. It is also accepted that intraperitoneal approaches that require direct absorption of chemotherapy into tumors will be more successful in the setting of minimal to microscopic residual disease. Complications of the procedure and quality of life must be considered in the decision for aggressive surgery. Enterotomies can lead to fistulas, bowel anastomoses can dehisce (leading to peritonitis), and a permanent colostomy may not be a reasonable outcome for a disease with an expected indolent course.

Sugarbaker[68] has been a proponent of aggressive peritoneal resection for carcinomatosis in selected circumstances. He has described "peritonectomy" procedures, which have been widely quoted in the literature, by which the peritoneum and associated expendable structures are removed. The six procedures are (1) omentectomy-splenectomy; (2) left upper quadrant stripping; (3) right upper quadrant stripping; (4) lesser omentectomy and cholecystectomy; (5) pelvic peritoneal stripping, including hysterectomy and sigmoid colectomy; and (6) antrectomy. The procedures were undertaken only where gross tumor was present. The morbidity of such procedures in the context of intraperitoneal chemotherapy has been reported by the same group for 200 patients undergoing aggressive cytoreductive surgery and hyperthermic, intraoperative, intraperitoneal chemotherapy. The mortality rate was 1.5%, and grade III and grade IV morbidity were seen in 27% of patients.[69]

INTRAPERITONEAL CHEMOTHERAPY

Systemic chemotherapy has been notoriously poor for the treatment of peritoneal carcinomatosis. This is mostly due to the fact that most GI solid tumors are not sensitive to chemotherapy, but other theoretic concerns exist regarding the successful penetration of chemotherapy into the peritoneal cavity (and into solid tumors in general). It should be noted that ovarian cancer patients with peritoneal carcinomatosis can be cured with systemic chemotherapy in rare cases.[63] The concept of delivering chemotherapy directly into the peritoneal cavity is appealing, theoretically allowing higher concentrations to be delivered to the tumor while minimizing systemic side effects. The mesothelial lining acts as a barrier to absorption of chemotherapy agents. Casper et al.[70] demonstrated 30-fold higher peritoneal concentration of cisplatin when delivered into the peritoneal cavity as compared to intravenous delivery. High concentrations of chemotherapy topically applied to tumor cells should be more effective than what can be achieved with intravascular delivery.

The pharmacokinetic rationale for intraperitoneal chemotherapy has been recognized for many years,[71] and intraperitoneal chemotherapy trials blossomed in the early 1980s.[72–75] Larger, water-soluble and ionized compounds exit the peritoneal compartment more slowly than smaller lipid-soluble and un-ionized molecules. Pharmacokinetic models of peritoneal delivery have been developed.[76,77] Patients with peritoneal carcinomatosis may have decreased clearance of all drugs from the peritoneal cavity due to obstruction of lymphatic channels. In addition, the majority of compounds delivered into the peritoneal cavity are cleared by the portal circulation and, therefore, may be metabolized by the liver. Compounds that have a delayed clearance from the peritoneal cavity may allow for prolonged exposure of slowly dividing cells to the chemotherapy agent. If the agent requires mitosis for efficacy, this improves the chance of it being effective, compared to the relatively brief exposure provided by systemic delivery. Finally, by confining the treatment to direct absorption, systemic binding agents can be delivered and bind and inactivate systemically absorbed drug to minimize systemic toxicity.[78]

The main pitfalls for intraperitoneal chemotherapy include the difficulty in obtaining even distribution throughout the peritoneal cavity and the limited absorption of agents into tumor nodules.[79] Prior abdominal surgery leads to numerous loculations within the peritoneal cavity and prevents even distribution of intraperitoneal agents. Prolonged intraperitoneal dwell chemotherapy can be hampered by scarring around the delivery catheter, allowing for escape of tumor cells within protected areas of the abdomen. Large treatment volumes (>2 liters) have been shown to improve distribution.[80] Intraoperative and early postoperative intraperitoneal chemotherapy may allow for treatment of all peritoneal surfaces before dense, loculated scarred areas develop, but this may increase the morbidity associated with the procedure.[81] A randomized trial of adjuvant intraperitoneal chemotherapy with carbon-absorbed mitomycin in gastric cancer was prematurely terminated due to a statistically significant increase in major postoperative morbidity in the patients receiving chemotherapy.[82]

The ideal setting for ensuring complete distribution of chemotherapy to the peritoneal cavity is intraoperative treatment at the time of surgical debulking. Recirculating circuits and physical manipulation of abdominal contents during therapy may enhance distribution. Studies suggest, and logic concludes, that the best means for ensuring complete distribution during intraperitoneal therapy is to manipulate the contents of the peritoneal cavity by hand during treatment. This can be accomplished by a variety of techniques with the patient under general anesthesia, allowing a hand to be inserted into the abdominal cavity without spilling the chemotherapy solution.

Tumor penetration of drugs delivered into the peritoneal cavity has been studied. Los et al.[83] demonstrated that the tumor concentration of cisplatin was significantly elevated after intraperitoneal delivery, as compared to systemic delivery, at a depth of 1.0 mm but not at 1.5 mm. Increasing pressure within the peritoneal cavity may improve penetration, and vasoactive agents that decrease capillary uptake of drugs in the tumor may allow for deeper penetration of drugs. Larger molecules may penetrate more deeply into some tissues than low-molecular-weight agents because of decreased capillary permeability and vascular washout of the compounds. On the other hand, if increased interstitial pressure occurs within tumors, as has been described, this may be an advantage to low-molecular-weight agents. Although it is easy to determine clearance from the peritoneal cavity and easy to assume that decreased clearance leads to increased exposure of intraperitoneal tumor to chemotherapy, it is not clear how decreased clearance correlates with absorption into tumor tissue. Decreased clearance may correlate with decreased tumor absorption, which may be counterproductive. On the other hand, for the treatment of microscopic cells that have not developed into tumor nodules, prolonged exposure in the peritoneal cavity should be advantageous.

A variety of agents have been delivered into the peritoneal cavity, and these are summarized in Table 49-2. The mean peritoneal cavity peak concentrations over peak plasma concentra-

TABLE 49-2. Pharmacokinetic Advantages Associated with Intraperitoneal Antineoplastic Drug Delivery

Agent	*Peak Peritoneal Cavity to Plasma Concentration Ratio*
Carboplatin	18
Cisplatin	20
Mitomycin C	72
Methotrexate	92
5-Fluorouracil	298
Doxorubicin	474
Mitoxantrone	620
Paclitaxel	>1000

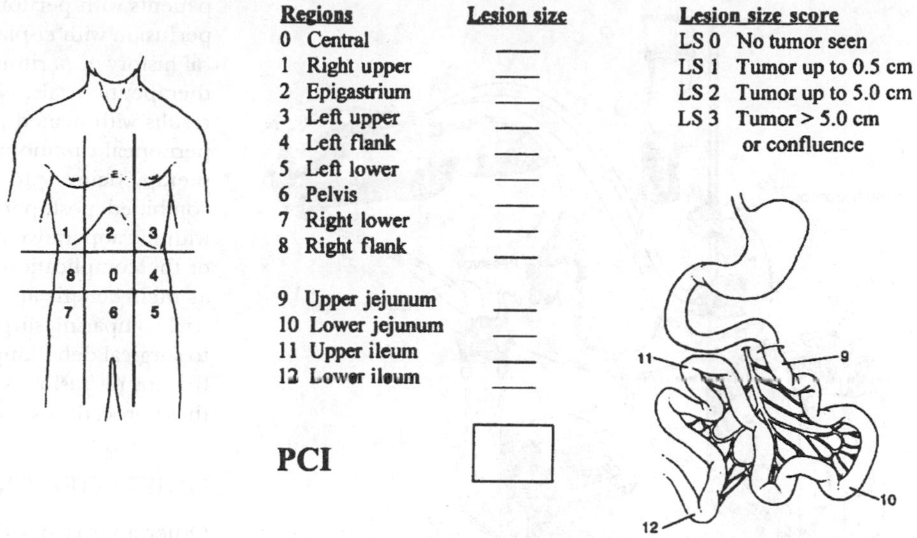

FIGURE 49-5. Proposed standardized scheme for assessing extensive peritoneal disease. The peritoneal cancer index (PCI) represents the sum of the lesion size scores for the different regions. (Reproduced from ref. 85, with permission.)

tions range from 20 in the case of cisplatin to more than 600 for cytarabine and mitoxantrone and more than 1000 for paclitaxel. Regional toxicity has not been a major problem with most of these agents. Even mitomycin C, which is considered a very caustic agent to tissues when infiltrated, has been delivered into the peritoneal cavity safely. The most common agents that have been used in intraperitoneal trials include cisplatin, mitomycin C, 5-FU, and, recently, paclitaxel. Gemcitabine currently is being studied with intraperitoneal delivery.

In general, trials of intraperitoneal chemotherapy have been poorly controlled, with numerous treatment regimens for different histologies of varying prognosis at different stages of peritoneal involvement, making interpretation of results difficult.[81,84] In addition, the combination of aggressive surgical debulking and intraoperative or early postoperative chemotherapy make the interpretation of morbidity difficult. Sugarbaker[85] has used a complex scheme for assessing the extent of peritoneal disease and completeness of resection (Fig. 49-5). Adoption of this or similar standardized criteria should help in the standardization and interpretation of clinical trials. Histologic grade and clinical invasive phenotyping should also improve trial interpretation.

The utility and advantages of intraperitoneal chemotherapy have been demonstrated in randomized trials. Sugarbaker et al.[86] performed a small randomized trial comparing postoperative adjuvant 5-FU delivered intravenously (n = 30) to intraperitoneal delivery (n = 36) for patients with high-risk primary colorectal cancers. Although there was no difference in survival between the groups, the patients with intraperitoneal delivery had a significantly lower incidence of intraperitoneal recurrences and less hematologic and hepatic toxicity. More recently, the combined Southwest Oncology Group, Gynecologic Oncology Group, and Eastern Cooperative Oncology Group Intergroup Study examined intravenous versus intraperitoneal cisplatin with intravenous cyclophosphamide for stage III ovarian cancer.[87] This large, randomized, prospective, phase III trial demonstrated a significant survival advantage for patients receiving intraperitoneal cisplatin (49 vs. 41 months). In addition, this group experienced significantly less clinical hearing loss, neutropenia, and neuromuscular toxicity. Yu et al.[88] examined early postoperative intraperitoneal chemotherapy as compared to no treatment after resection of gastric cancer (n = 248). This group demonstrated no overall survival benefit, but subset analysis suggested improved survival for stage III disease, as might be expected (49% 5-year survival vs. 18%). Follow-up trials should be focused on stage III disease. These results should stimulate continued interest in the peritoneal delivery of chemotherapy for peritoneal carcinomatosis and emphasize the need for randomized trials for GI malignancies to define better the advantages of intraperitoneal delivery.

One procedure that is becoming increasingly popular across the world for the treatment of peritoneal carcinomatosis is the intraoperative combination of hyperthermia and chemotherapy delivered as a recirculating perfusion.[89–95] Temperatures of 41°C to 42°C are maintained in the tissues over a period of 90 minutes by recirculating fluid that passes through a roller pump and heat exchanger delivering high concentrations of chemotherapy to the peritoneal cavity (Fig. 49-6). The most common drugs used in this fashion have been cisplatin and mitomycin C.[96] The theoretic advantages of this technique include the improved mixing and surface exposure associated with the increased pressure and high flow rates of the perfusate along with intraoperative manipulation of the abdominal contents. The hyperthermia has been demonstrated to have selective cytotoxicity against cancer cells while the normal cells recover.[97] In addition, hyperthermia has been shown to enhance chemotherapy penetration into tumors,[98] improve intraperitoneal pharmacokinetics,[99] and work synergistically with chemotherapy to kill cancer cells.[100]

This therapy has been demonstrated to be successful in randomized trials in Japan for completely resected advanced gastric cancer (Table 49-3). These trials include mitomycin C as the active agent or mitomycin C and cisplatin in combination. Fujimoto et al.[101] reported an 8-year survival of 88% in patients receiving hyperthermic perfusion with mitomycin C for high-risk (serosal invasion) gastric cancers, as compared to 49% for surgery alone. Peritoneal recurrence was 23% in the control group, as compared to 1% in the treatment group.

We have reported our results with continuous hyperthermic peritoneal perfusion in a phase I study with tumor necrosis fac-

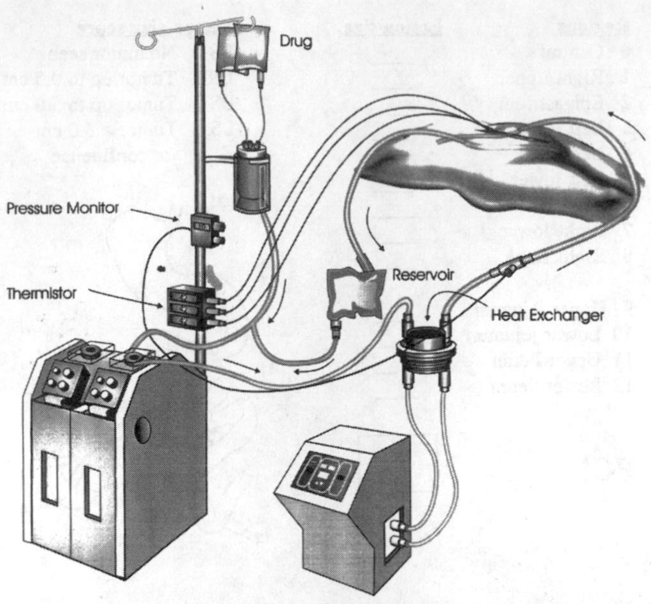

FIGURE 49-6. Peritoneal perfusion technique used at the National Cancer Institute. Chemotherapy solution is circulated through the roller pump, then through a heat exchanger and into the abdominal cavity. The outflow is collected from the pelvis and passes to a small reservoir and then back through the roller pump. Peritoneal temperatures are monitored via three probes inserted in different places in the peritoneal cavity, and intraabdominal pressures are monitored during the procedure.

tor and cisplatin against all forms of peritoneal carcinomatosis.[102] In that trial and subsequent trials, the response of patients with peritoneal mesothelioma stands out as being notable. We have demonstrated a median progression-free survival of 26 months and overall 2-year survival rate of 80% in patients with peritoneal mesothelioma treated with peritoneal perfusion with cisplatin.[50] This compares favorably to the natural history of peritoneal mesothelioma and the results of other therapeutic trials. Numerous centers are now reporting their results with heated peritoneal perfusion for different forms of peritoneal carcinomatosis. In an attempt to maximize chemotherapy delivery to these tumors, we (and others) have now combined postoperative intraperitoneal dwell chemotherapy with intraoperative heated peritoneal perfusion. Close scrutiny of the complication rates with these procedures is important, as their benefit at this point is only theoretic. A randomized trial comparing surgical debulking and systemic chemotherapy to surgical debulking plus intraoperative hyperthermic chemotherapy perfusion is necessary to demonstrate the true utility of these procedures.

OTHER INTRAPERITONEAL THERAPIES

Other approaches for regional therapy for peritoneal carcinomatosis have been investigated. Total abdominal irradiation, in combination with surgical debulking and chemotherapy, has been shown to be effective in peritoneal mesothelioma and has been studied in other malignancies.[103] In general, the toxicity of total abdominal irradiation is unsatisfactory; therefore, this treatment approach has not become standard. Photodynamic therapy of the peritoneal cavity is under active investigation for all forms of peritoneal carcinomatosis. Patients receive an intravenous photosensitizing dose of dihematoporphyrin ethers followed by exposure of the peritoneal surfaces to laser light.[104] The approach has undergone phase I studies, but its efficacy has not been reported in phase II studies. Intraperitoneal immunotherapy approaches are under investigation, including the intraperitoneal delivery of adoptively transferred lymphocytes.[105] Gene therapy approaches are also being investigated, as intraperitoneal tumor cells may be ideally exposed

TABLE 49-3. Clinical Results of Multiarm Studies Evaluating the Efficacy of Prophylactic or Therapeutic Continuous Hyperthermic Peritoneal Perfusion Immediately after Resection for Gastric Cancer

Study	*No. of Subjects*	*Treatment Arm*	*Agent and Dose*	*Duration (min.)*	*Temperature (ºC)*	*Follow-Up (y)*	*Survival (%)*	*P-value*
Koga et al.[110]	26	CHPP	Mitomycin C, 8–10 mg/L	60	44–45	2.5	83	*NS*
	21	Control	—	—	—	2.5	67	—
Koga et al.[111]	38	CHPP	Mitomycin C, 8–10 mg/L	60	44–45	5	72	*<.04*
	55	Control[a]	—	—	—	5	60	
Fujimoto et al.[112]	30	CHPP	Mitomycin C, 10 mg/L	120	45–47	1	80	*<.001*
	29	Control	—	—	—	1	34	—
Fujimura et al.[96]	22	CHPP	Mitomycin C, 30 mg/kg, and cisplatin, 300 mg/kg	60	41–42	3	68	*<.01*[b]
	18	CNPP	Mitomycin C, 30 mg/kg, and cisplatin, 300 mg/kg	60	37–38	3	51	—
	18	Control	—	—	—	3	23	—
Hamazoe et al.[113]	42	CHPP	Mitomycin C, 10 mg/L	60	48–50	5	64	*NS*
	40	Control	—	—	—	—	53	—

CHPP, continuous hyperthermic peritoneal perfusion; CNPP, continuous normothermic peritoneal perfusion; NS, not significant.
[a]Historical control group.
[b]CHPP or CNPP versus control.
[Adapted from Alexander HR, Buell JF, Fraker DL. Rationale and clinical status of continuous hyperthermic peritoneal perfusion (CHPP) for the treatment of peritoneal carcinomatosis. In: DeVita V, Hellman S, Rosenberg S (eds.), *Principles and practice of oncology updates.* Philadelphia: JB Lippincott, 1995:1–9.]

to intraperitoneal delivered vectors, leading to a high transduction efficiency.[106]

PALLIATION

Major complications of peritoneal carcinomatosis include partial and complete obstruction of the GI tract, leading to crampy abdominal pain, nausea, and vomiting. The other significant complication is the development of ascites, which can become incapacitating and the direct cause of death. The palliative management of these entities by the oncologist is required. Patients with crampy, abdominal pain suggesting partial small bowel obstruction should be worked up with a CT scan and upper GI series. A determination should be made about whether a simple bypass or resection of an obstructed region can be performed, in which case the appropriate operation is undertaken. In the setting of diffuse disease that cannot be bypassed, a percutaneous endoscopic gastrostomy tube should be inserted for palliation.[107] This is a simple procedure that can be performed with minimal complications, yet provides lasting palliation. Signs of peritonitis or systemic sepsis should raise concerns of a closed loop obstruction that may require emergent surgical resection. It is often helpful to ensure patency of the rectum in patients being explored for bypass of a small bowel obstruction in the setting of peritoneal carcinomatosis. A shelf of tumor in the pelvic peritoneal recess may lead to obstruction, placing a proximal bowel anastomosis at risk. Rarely, patients may require a colostomy or ileostomy for palliation. The nutritional management of patients who require a palliative gastrostomy in the setting of peritoneal carcinomatosis and bowel obstruction is controversial. In general, it is accepted that total parenteral nutrition does nothing to improve the quality of life or prolong survival in patients having peritoneal carcinomatosis secondary to aggressive GI malignancies. However, in the case of low-grade malignancies, these patients can survive for a very long time after palliative gastrostomy; therefore, parenteral nutrition should be considered. We have had the experience of managing a patient on total parenteral nutrition for more than a year with a good quality of life after palliative gastrostomy in the setting of a low-grade, mucinous adenocarcinoma causing compressive bowel obstruction.

Management of malignant ascites is a challenge for the oncologist. In cases of malignant mesothelioma and ovarian cancer, the best therapy may involve aggressive surgical debulking and intraperitoneal chemotherapy. Numerous patients who have been considered terminal because of incapacitating ascites have been treated successfully in this manner. Schilsky et al.[84] demonstrated successful resolution of ascites with intraperitoneal dwell chemotherapy with 5-FU and cisplatin. Diuretics are ineffective in the management of malignant ascites, and intermittent paracentesis may be effective in the short term but invariably leads to electrolyte imbalance, hypoproteinemia, hypovolemia, and, ultimately, renal failure and death. Peritoneovenous shunts can be effective and should be considered. Straus et al.[108] reported that 89% of their shunts relieved symptoms of nausea, distention, loss of appetite, and dyspnea and that 79% of the shunts functioned for longer than 3 months or until death. Qazi and Savlov[109] reported 70% effective palliation with peritoneovenous shunt. As these shunts are rather easy to insert (under local anesthesia in most cases) with at least temporary palliation, they should be considered in patients with reasonable performance status and incapacitating ascites.

REFERENCES

1. Henriksen JH, Winkler K. Peritoneum and ascites formation. In: Bengmark S, ed. *The peritoneum and peritoneal access.* London: Wright Publishers, 1989:94.
2. Levison ME, Pontzer RE. Peritonitis and other intra-abdominal infections In: Mandell GL, Douglas RG Jr, Bennett JE, eds. *Principles and practice of infectious diseases.* New York: John Wiley and Sons, 1979:476.
3. Watters WB, Buck RC. Scanning electron microscopy of mesothelial regeneration in the rat. *Lab Invest* 1972; 26(5):604.
4. Flessner MF, Fenstermacher JD, Blasberg RG, Dedrick RL. Peritoneal absorption of macromolecules studied by quantitative autoradiography. *Am J Physiol* 1985;248:H26.
5. Hagiwara A, Rakahashi T, Sawai K, et al. Milky spots at the implantation site for malignant cells in peritoneal dissemination in mice. *Cancer Res* 1993;53:687.
6. Sugarbaker P. Observations concerning cancer spread within the peritoneal cavity and concepts supporting an ordered pathophysiology. In: Sugarbaker P, ed. *Peritoneal carcinomatosis: principles of management.* Boston: Kluwer Academic Publishers, 1996:79.
7. Ronnett BM, Shmookler BM, Sugarbaker PH, Kurman RJ. *Pseudomyxoma peritonei*: new concepts in diagnosis, origin, nomenclature, and relationship to mucinous borderline (low malignant potential) tumors of the ovary. *Anat Pathol* 1997;2:197.
8. Bartlett DL. Tumors of the gallbladder. In: Blumgart L, Fong Y, eds. *Surgery of the liver and biliary tract.* London: Harcourt, Brace, 2000 *(in press).*
9. Weiss L. Metastatic inefficiency: intravascular and intraperitoneal implantation of cancer cells. *Cancer Treat Res* 1996;82:1.
10. Veatch AL, Carson LF, Ramakrishnan S. Phenotypic variations and differential migration of NIH:OVCA R-3 ovarian carcinoma cells isolated from athymic mice. *Clin Exp Metastasis* 1995;13:165.
11. Liebman JM, Burbelo PD, Yamada Y, Feldman R, Kleinman HK. Altered expression of basement-membrane components and collagenases in ascitic xenografis of OVCA R-3 ovarian cancer cells. *Int J Cancer* 1993;55:102.
12. Graham RA, Wang S, Catalano PJ, Haller DG. Postsurgical surveillance of colon cancer: preliminary cost analysis of physician examination, carcinoembryonic antigen testing, chest x-ray, and colonoscopy. *Ann Surg* 1998;228:59.
13. Archer AG, Sugarbaker PH, Jelinek JS. Radiology of peritoneal carcinomatosis. *Cancer Treat Res* 1996;82:263.
14. Chou CK, Liu GC, Su JH, et al. MRI demonstration of peritoneal implants. *Abdom Imaging* 1994;19:95.
15. Low RN, Semelka RC, Worawattarakul S, Alzate GD, Sigeti JS. Extrahepatic abdominal imaging in patients with malignancy: comparison of MR imaging and helical CT, with subsequent surgical correlation. *Radiology* 1999;21:625.
16. Nelson RC, Chezmar JL, Hoel MJ, Buck DR, Sugarbaker PH. Peritoneal carcinomatosis: preoperative CT with intraperitoneal contrast material. *Radiology* 1992;182:133.
17. Fong Y, Waldinger PF, Akhurst T, et al. Utility of 18F-FDG positron emission tomography scanning on selection of patients for resection of hepatic colorectal metastases. *Am J Surg* 1999;178:282.
18. Nakao A, Oshima K, Takeda S, et al. Peritoneal washings cytology combined with immunocytochemical staining in pancreatic cancer. *Hepatogastroenterology* 1999;46:2974.
19. Vogel P, Ruschoff J, Kummel S, et al. Immunocytology improves prognostic impact of peritoneal tumour cell detection compared to conventional cytology in gastric cancer. *Eur J Surg Oncol* 1999;25:515.
20. Fujiwara K, Yamauchi H, Yoshida T, et al. Relationship between peritoneal washing cytology through implantable port system (IPS-cytology) and second-look laparotomy in ovarian cancer patients with unmeasurable residual diseases. *Gynecol Oncol* 1998;70:231.
21. Kodera Y, Yamamura Y, Shimizu Y, et al. Peritoneal washing cytology: prognostic value of positive findings in patients with gastric carcinoma undergoing a potentially curative resection. *J Surg Oncol* 1999;72:60.
22. Makary MA, Warshaw AL, Centeno BA, et al. Implications of peritoneal cytology for pancreatic cancer management. *Arch Surg* 1998;133:361.
23. Funami Y, Tokumoto N, Miyauchi H, Ochiai T, Kuga K. Prognostic value of peritoneal lavage cytology and chemotherapy during surgery for advanced gastric cancer. *Int Surg* 1999;84: 220.
24. Bando E, Yonemura Y, Takeshita Y, et al. Intraoperative lavage for cytological examination in 1,297 patients with gastric carcinoma. *Am J Surg* 1999;178:256.
25. Hayes N, Wayman J, Wadehra V, et al. Peritoneal cytology in the surgical evaluation of gastric carcinoma. *Br J Cancer* 1999;79:520.
26. Jerby BL, Milsom JW. Role of laparoscopy in the staging of gastrointestinal cancer. *Oncology* (Huntingt) 1998;12:1353.
27. Huizing MT, van Warmerdam LJ, Rosing H, et al. Phase I and pharmacologic study of the combination paclitaxel and carboplatin as first-line chemotherapy in stage III and IV ovarian cancer. *J Clin Oncol* 1997;15:1953.
28. Abu-Rustum NR, Barakat RR, Siegel PL, et al. Second-look operation for epithelial ovarian cancer: laparoscopy or laparotomy? *Obstet Gynecol* 1996;88:549.
29. Werth H. Klinische und anatomische untersuchungen zue lehre von den bauchgeschwuelsten und der laparotomie. *Arch Gynaekol* 1884;24:100.
30. Fraenkel E. Ueber das sogennante pseudomyxoma peritonei. *Muench Med Wochenschr* 1901;48:965.
31. Ronnett BM, Zahn CM, Kurman RJ, et al. Disseminated peritoneal adenomucinosis and peritoneal mucinous carcinomatosis: a clinicopathologic analysis of 109 cases with emphasis on distinguishing pathologic features, site of origin, prognosis, and relationship to *Pseudomyxoma peritonei. Am J Surg Pathol* 1995;19:1390.
32. Little JM, Halliday JP, Glenn DC. *Pseudomyxoma peritonei. Lancet* 1969;27:659.
33. Sugarbaker PH, Kern K, Lack E. Malignant *Pseudomyxoma peritonei* of colonic origin. Natural history and presentation of a curative approach to treatment. *Dis Colon Rectum* 1987;30:772.

34. Sugarbaker PH, Chang D. Results of treatment of 385 patients with peritoneal surface spread of appendiceal malignancy. *Ann Surg Oncol* 1999;6:727.
35. Gough DB, Donohue JH, Schutt AJ, et al. *Pseudomyxoma peritonei:* long-term patient survival with an aggressive regional approach. *Ann Surg* 1994;219:112.
36. Smith JW, Kemeny N, Caldwell C, et al. *Pseudomyxoma peritonei* of appendiceal origin. The Memorial Sloan-Kettering Cancer Center experience. *Cancer* 1992;70:396.
37. Kass ME. Pathology of peritoneal mesothelioma. In: Sugarbaker P, ed. *Peritoneal carcinomatosis: drugs and diseases.* Boston: Kluwer Academic Publishers, 1996:213.
38. Hutchinson R, Sokhi GS. Multicystic peritoneal mesothelioma: not a benign condition. *Eur J Surg* 1992;158:451.
39. Miles JM, Hart WR, McMahon JT. Cystic mesothelioma of the peritoneum. *Cleve Clin Q* 1986;53:109.
40. Hoekman K, Tognon G, Risse EKJ, Bloemsma CA, Vermorken JB. Well-differentiated papillary mesothelioma of the peritoneum: a separate entity. *Eur J Cancer* 1996;43A:255.
41. Daya D, McCaughey W. Well-differentiated papillary mesothelioma of the peritoneum: a clinicopathologic study of 22 cases. *Cancer* 1990;65:292.
42. Manavoglu O, Orhan B, Evrensel T, et al. Malignant peritoneal mesothelioma following asbestos exposure. *J Environ Pathol Toxicol Oncol* 1996;15:191.
43. Averbach AM, Sugarbaker PH. Peritoneal mesothelioma: treatment approach based on natural history. *Cancer Treat Res* 1996;81:193.
44. Kannerstein M, Churg J. Peritoneal mesothelioma. *Hum Pathol* 1977;8:83.
45. van Gelder T, Hoogsteden HC, Versnel MA, et al. Malignant peritoneal mesothelioma: a series of 19 cases. *Digestion* 1989;43:222.
46. Antman K, Osteen R, Klegar K, et al. Early peritoneal mesothelioma: a treatable malignancy. *Lancet* 1985;2:977.
47. Langer CJ, Rosenblum N, Hogan M, et al. Intraperitoneal cisplatin and etoposide in peritoneal mesothelioma: favorable outcome with a multimodality approach. *Cancer Chemother Pharmacol* 1993;32:204.
48. Lederman GS, Recht A, Herman T, et al. Long-term survival in peritoneal mesothelioma. *Cancer* 1987;59:1882.
49. Markman M, Kelsen D. Efficacy of cisplatin-based intraperitoneal chemotherapy as treatment of malignant peritoneal mesothelioma. *J Cancer Res Clin Oncol* 1992;118:547.
50. Park BJ, Alexander HR, Libutti SK, et al. Treatment of primary peritoneal mesothelioma by continuous hyperthermic peritoneal perfusion (CHPP). *Ann Surg Oncol* 1999;6:582.
51. Loggie BW, Fleming RA, Geisinger KR. Cytologic assessment before and after intraperitoneal hyperthermic chemotherapy for peritoneal carcinomatosis. *Acta Cytol* 1996;40:1154.
52. Kennedy AW, Markman M, Webster KD, et al. Experience with platinum-paclitaxel chemotherapy in the initial management of papillary serous carcinoma of the peritoneum. *Gynecol Oncol* 1998;71:288.
53. Whitcomb BP, Kost ER, Hines JF, Zahn CM, Hall KL. Primary peritoneal psammocarcinoma: a case presenting with an upper abdominal mass and elevated CA-125. *Gynecol Oncol* 1999;73:331.
54. Chu CS, Menzin AW, Leonard DG, Rubin SC, Wheeler JE. Primary peritoneal carcinoma: a review of the literature. *Obstet Gynecol Surv* 1999;54:323.
55. Bandera CA, Muto MM, Schorge J. BRCA1 gene mutations in women with papillary serous carcinoma of the peritoneum. *Obstet Gynecol* 1998;92:596.
56. Ordonez NG. Role of immunohistochemistry in distinguishing epithelial peritoneal mesotheliomas from peritoneal and ovarian serous carcinomas. *Am J Surg Pathol* 1998;22:1203.
57. Chu CS, Menzin AW, Leonard DGB, Rubin SC, Wheeler JE. Primary peritoneal carcinoma: a review of the literature. *Obstet Gynecol Surv* 1999;54:323.
58. Menzin AW, Aikins JK Jr, Wheeler JE, Rubin SC. Surgically documented responses to paclitaxel and cisplatin in patients with primary peritoneal carcinoma. *Gynecol Oncol* 1996;62:55.
59. Schwarz RE, Gerald WL, Kushner BH, et al. Desmoplastic small round cell tumors: prognostic indicators and results of surgical management. *Ann Surg Oncol* 1998;5:416.
60. Benjamin LE, Fredericks WJ, Barr FG, Rauscher FR. Fusion of the EWS1 and WT1 genes as a result of the t(11;22)(p13;q12) translocation in desmoplastic small round cell tumors. *Med Pediatr Oncol* 1996;27:434.
61. Gershenson DM, Silva EG, Tortolero-Luna G, et al. Serous borderline tumors of the ovary with noninvasive peritoneal implants. *Cancer* 1998;83:2157.
62. Benedetti-Panici P, Greggi S, Scambia G, et al. Very high-dose chemotherapy with autologous peripheral stem cell support in advanced ovarian cancer. *Eur J Cancer* 1995;31A:1987.
63. Munkarah AR, Hallum AV, Morris M, et al. Prognostic significance of residual disease in patients with stage IV epithelial ovarian cancer. *Gynecol Oncol* 1997;64:13.
64. Chrysikopoulos H, Manlatis V, Roussakis A, Pappas J, Andreou J. Peritoneal metastases from transitional cell carcinoma of the urinary tract: CT and MR imaging. *Abdom Imaging* 1998;23:91.
65. Alexander HR, Bartlett DL, Libutti SK. National Cancer Institute experience with regional therapy for unresectable primary and metastatic cancer of the liver or peritoneal cavity. In: Markman M, ed. *Regional chemotherapy: clinical research and practice (current clinical oncology).* Totowa, NJ: Humana Press, 2000:127.
66. Bristow RE, Montz FJ, Lagasse LD, Leuchter RS, Karlan BY. Survival impact of surgical cytoreduction in stage IV epithelial ovarian cancer. *Gynecol Oncol* 1999;72:278.
67. Portilla AG, Sugarbaker PH, Chang D. Second-look surgery after cytoreduction and intraperitoneal chemotherapy for peritoneal carcinomatosis from colorectal cancer: analysis of prognostic features. *World J Surg* 1999;23:23.
68. Sugarbaker PH. Peritonectomy procedures. *Ann Surg* 1995;221:29.
69. Stephens AD, Alderman R, Chang D, et al. Morbidity and mortality analysis of 200 treatments with cytoreductive surgery and hyperthermic intraoperative intraperitoneal chemotherapy using the coliseum technique. *Ann Surg Oncol* 1999;6:790.
70. Casper ES, Kelsen DP, Alcock NW, Lewis JL Jr. IP cisplatin in patients with malignant ascites: pharmacokinetic evaluation and comparison with the IV route. *Cancer Treat Rep* 1983;67:235.
71. Dedrick RL, Myers CE, Bungay PM, DeVita VT Jr. Pharmacokinetic rationale for peritoneal drug administration in the treatment of ovarian cancer. *Cancer Treat Rep* 1978;62:1.
72. Howell SB, Pfeifle CE, Olshen RA. Intraperitoneal chemotherapy with melphalan. *Ann Intern Med* 1984;101:14.
73. Howell SB, Pfeifle CE, Wung WE. Intraperitoneal cisplatin with sodium thiosulfate protection. *Ann Intern Med* 1982;97:845.
74. Speyer JL, Collins JM, Dedrick R. Phase I pharmacological studies of 5-fluorouracil administered intraperitoneally. *Cancer Res* 1980;40:567.
75. Markman M, Howell SB, Lucas WE. Combination intraperitoneal chemotherapy with cisplatin, cytarabine, and doxorubicin for refractory ovarian carcinoma and other malignancies principally confined to the peritoneal cavity. *J Clin Oncol* 1984;1:1321.
76. Dedrick RL. Interspecies scaling of regional drug delivery. *J Pharm Sci* 1986;75:1047.
77. Cho H-K, Lush RM, Bartlett DL, et al. Pharmacokinetics of cisplatin administered by continuous hyperthermic peritoneal perfusion (CHPP) to patients with peritoneal carcinomatosis. *J Clin Pharmacol* 1999;39:1.
78. Howell SB, Pfeifle CG, Wung WE, et al. Intraperitoneal cisplatin with systemic thiosulfate protection. *Ann Intern Med* 1982;97:845.
79. Dedrick RL, Flessner MF. Pharmacokinetic problems in peritoneal drug administration: tissue penetration and surface exposure. *J Natl Cancer Inst* 1997;89:480.
80. Dunnick NR, Jones RB, Doppman JL, Speyer J, Myers CE. Intraperitoneal contrast infusion for assessment of intraperitoneal fluid dynamics. *AJR Am J Roentgenol* 1979;133:221.
81. Dlias D, Dubé P, Blot F, et al. Peritoneal carcinomatosis treatment with curative intent: the Institut Gustave-Roussy experience. *Eur J Surg Oncol* 1997;23:317.
82. Rosen HR, Jatzko G, Repse S, et al. Adjuvant intraperitoneal chemotherapy with carbon-adsorbed mitomycin in patients with gastric cancer: results of a randomized multicenter trial of the Austrian Working Group for Surgical Oncology. *J Clin Oncol* 1998;16:2733.
83. Los G, Mutsaers PHA, van der Vijgh WJF, et al. Direct diffusion of *cis*-diamminedichloroplatinum(II) in intraperitoneal tumors after intraperitoneal chemotherapy: a comparison with systemic chemotherapy. *Cancer Res* 1989;49:33.
84. Schilsky RL, Choi KE, Grayhack J, et al. Phase I clinical and pharmacologic study of intraperitoneal cisplatin and fluorouracil in patients with advanced intraabdominal cancer. *J Clin Oncol* 1990;8:2054.
85. Sugarbaker PH. Successful management of microscopic residual disease in large bowel cancer. *Cancer Chemother Pharmacol* 1999;43:S15.
86. Sugarbaker PH, Gianola FJ, Speyer JC, et al. Prospective, randomized trial of intravenous versus intraperitoneal 5-fluorouracil in patients with advanced primary colon or rectal cancer. *Surgery* 1985;98:414.
87. Alberts DS, Liu PY, Hannigan EV, et al. Intraperitoneal cisplatin plus intravenous cyclophosphamide versus intravenous cisplatin plus intravenous cyclophosphamide for stage III ovarian cancer. *N Engl J Med* 1996;335:1950.
88. Yu W, Whang I, Suh I, et al. Prospective randomized trial of early postoperative intraperitoneal chemotherapy as an adjuvant to resectable gastric cancer. *Ann Surg* 1998;228:347.
89. Elias D, Antoun S, Raynard B, et al. Treatment of peritoneal carcinomatosis using complete excision and intraperitoneal chemohyperthermia: a phase I–II study defining the best technical procedures. *Chirurgie* 1999;124:380.
90. Zoetmulder FA, van der Vange N, Witkamp AJ, et al. Hyperthermic intraperitoneal chemotherapy (HIPEC) in patients with peritoneal *Pseudomyxoma* or peritoneal metastases of colorectal carcinoma; good preliminary results from the Netherlands Cancer Institute. *Ned Tijdschr Geneeskd* 1999;143:1863.
91. Gilly FN, Beaujard A, Glehen O, et al. Peritonectomy combined with intraperitoneal chemohyperthermia in abdominal cancer with peritoneal carcinomatosis: phase I–II study. *Anticancer Res* 1999;19:2317.
92. Cavaliere F, di Filippo F, Cosimelli M, et al. The integrated treatment of peritoneal carcinomatosis: a preliminary experience. *J Exp Clin Cancer Res* 1999;18:151.
93. Sugarbaker PH. Successful management of microscopic residual disease in large bowel cancer. *Cancer Chemother Pharmacol* 1999;43:S15.
94. Fujimoto S, Takahashi M, Mutou T, Kobayashi K, Toyosawa T. Successful intraperitoneal hyperthermic chemoperfusion for the prevention of postoperative peritoneal recurrence in patients with advanced gastric carcinoma. *Cancer* 1999;85:529.
95. Huff T, Brand E. *Pseudomyxoma peritonei*: treatment with the argon beam coagulator. *Obstet Gynecol* 1992;80:569.
96. Fujimura T, Yonemura Y, Muraoka K, et al. Continuous hyperthermic peritoneal perfusion for the prevention of peritoneal recurrence of gastric cancer: randomized controlled study. *World J Surg* 1994;18:150.
97. Giovanella BC, Stehlin JS Jr, Morgan AC. Selective lethal effect of supranormal temperatures on human neoplastic cells. *Cancer Res* 1976;36:3944.
98. Benoit L, Duvillard C, Rat P, Chauffert B The effect of intra-abdominal temperature on the tissue and tumor diffusion of intraperitoneal cisplatin in a model of peritoneal carcinomatosis in rats. *Chirurgie* 1999;124:375.
99. Zakris EL, Dewhirst MW, Riviere JE, et al. Pharmacokinetics and toxicity of intraperitoneal cisplatin combined with regional hyperthermia. *J Clin Oncol* 1987;5:1613.
100. Miller RC, Richards M, Baird C, Martin S, Hall EJ. Interaction of hyperthermia and chemotherapy agents; cell lethality and oncogenic potential. *Int J Hyperthermia* 1994;10:89.
101. Fujimoto S, Takahashi M, Mutou T, Kobayashi K, Toyosawa T. Successful intraperitoneal hyperthermic chemoperfusion for the prevention of postoperative peritoneal recurrence in patients with advanced gastric carcinoma. *Cancer* 1999;85:529.
102. Bartlett DL, Buell JF, Libutti SK, et al. A Phase I trial of continuous hyperthermic peritoneal perfusion with tumor necrosis factor and cisplatin in the treatment of peritoneal carcinomatosis. *Cancer* 1998;83:1251.
103. Wong CS, Harwood AR, Cummings BJ, et al. Total abdominal irradiation for cancer of the colon. *Radiother Oncol* 1984;2:209.
104. Sindelar WF, DeLaney TF, Tochner Z, et al. Technique of photodynamic therapy for disseminated intraperitoneal malignant neoplasms: phase I study. *Arch Surg* 1991;126:318.

105. Freedman RS, Lenzi R, Kudelka AP, et al. Intraperitoneal immunotherapy of peritoneal carcinomatosis. *Cytokines Cell Mol Ther* 1998;4:121.
106. Lechanteur C, Princen F, Lo Bue S, et al. HSV-1 thymidine kinase gene therapy for peritoneal carcinomatosis. *Adv Exp Med Biol* 1998;451:119.
107. Scheidbach H, Horbach T, Groitl H, Hohengerger W. Percutaneous endoscopic gastrostomy/jejunostomy (PEG/PEJ) for decompression in the upper gastrointestinal tract. Initial experience with palliative treatment of gastrointestinal obstruction in terminally ill patients with advanced carcinomas. *Surg Endosc* 1999;13:1103.
108. Straus AK, Roseman DL, Shapiro TM. Peritoneovenous shunting in the management of malignant ascites. *Arch Surg* 1979;114:489.
109. Qazi R, Savlov ED. Peritoneovenous shunt for palliation of malignant ascites. *Cancer* 1982;49:600.
110. Koga S, Hamazoe R, Maeta M, et al. Prophylactic therapy for peritoneal recurrence of gastric cancer by continuous hyperthermic peritoneal perfusion with mitomycin C. *Cancer* 1988;61:232.
111. Kaibara N, Hamazoe R, Iitsuka Y, Maeta M, Koga S. Hyperthermic peritoneal perfusion combined with anticancer chemotherapy as prophylactic treatment of peritoneal recurrence of gastric cancer. *Hepatogastroenterology* 1989;36:75.
112. Fujimoto S, Shrestha RD, Kokuban M, et al. Positive results of combined therapy of surgery and intraperitoneal hyperthermic perfusion for far-advanced gastric cancer. *Ann Surg* 1990;212:592.
113. Hamazoe R, Maeta M, Kaibara N. Intraperitoneal thermochemotherapy for prevention of peritoneal recurrence of gastric cancer. *Cancer* 1994;73:2048.

CHAPTER 50

Immunosuppression-Related Malignancies

SECTION 1 AIDS-Related Malignancies

ROBERT YARCHOAN
RICHARD F. LITTLE

Individuals with human immunodeficiency virus (HIV) infection are at substantially increased risk of developing a number of neoplasms (Table 50.1-1).[1,2] Three malignant conditions are now considered as defining acquired immunodeficiency syndrome (AIDS) when they occur in HIV-infected individuals: Kaposi's sarcoma (KS), certain aggressive non-Hodgkin's lymphomas (NHLs), and invasive cervical cancer.[3] The risk of KS among gay and bisexual men with AIDS is greater than 100,000-fold that of the background population.[4] Also, NHLs occur overall with approximately 60-fold greater frequency than expected based on rates of NHL in HIV-negative populations.[5] There are conflicting data regarding the excess frequency of cervical cancer in HIV-infected women,[6,7] but cervical intraepithelial neoplasia appears to be more difficult to control and invasive cancer appears to be more aggressive in HIV infection.[8]

In addition, a number of other cancers that do not confer a diagnosis of AIDS occur with increased incidence among HIV-infected persons. In one study, a probabilistic matching algorithm comparing over 1 million people with AIDS, cancer, or both, the occurrence of several non–AIDS-defining cancers was found to be significantly increased in HIV infection (see Table 50.1-1); these include angiosarcoma (36.7-fold), Hodgkin's disease (7.6-fold), multiple myeloma (4.5-fold), brain cancer (3.5-fold), and seminoma (2.9-fold).[1] Age-, sex-, and period-adjusted standardized incidence ratios (SIR) in New South Wales, Australia, identified an increased incidence of Hodgkin's disease (SIR 18.3), multiple myeloma (SIR 12.1), leukemia (SIR 5.76), lip cancer (SIR 5.94), and lung cancer (SIR 3.80).[2] Thus, oncologists can expect to see a variety of malignant conditions with increased frequency in HIV-infected patients. One pattern that is emerging is that many tumors highly associated with HIV [such as KS or primary central nervous system lymphoma (PCNSL)] appear to be caused by oncogenic viruses. It will be important to understand the mechanisms by which HIV and these viruses interact, and this understanding should in turn lead to an increased appreciation for the pathogenesis of other tumors. On the other hand, certain tumor associations with HIV may have arisen because cohorts at risk for HIV may also have risk factors for other tumors (e.g., from increased exposure to other oncogenic viruses, increased cigarette smoking, and so forth) rather than because of HIV itself or HIV-induced alterations in immune function. Also, it should be pointed out that the relative risk of a large number of tumors is not increased in HIV disease, and this must be considered in evaluating the potential role of immunosurveillance in the pathogenesis of such tumors.

This chapter focuses primarily on those tumors that are considered as AIDS defining, but in general, certain principles common to the treatment of HIV-infected patients with cancer apply to various malignant conditions. The treatment of such patients can be

TABLE 50.1-1. Post–Acquired Immunodeficiency Syndrome Relative Risks of Various Malignant Conditions in Patients with Acquired Immunodeficiency Syndrome

Tumor	*Relative Risk*[a]	*95% Confidence Interval*
Kaposi's sarcoma	310.2	291.6–329.5
Non-Hodgkin's lymphoma	112.9	103.6–123.4
Invasive cervical cancer	2.9	0.7–16.0
Anal cancer	31.7	11.6–69.2
Non–acquired immunodeficiency syndrome cancers	1.9	1.5–2.3
Angiosarcoma	36.7	4.4–132.5
Soft tissue sarcoma	7.2	1.5–21.0
Hodgkin's disease	7.6	4.1–13.1
Leukemia	11.0	3.0–28.3
Multiple myeloma	4.5	0.9–13.2
Brain	3.5	1.4–7.2
Seminoma or germinoma	2.9	1.1–6.3
Squamous cell carcinoma, unusual sites	6.8	1.4–19.8
Lung, adenocarcinoma	2.5	1.0–5.0

[a]Relative risk calculations based on comparisons of the cancer experiences of people with acquired immunodeficiency syndrome and those of the general population under 70 years of age by matching population-based cancer and acquired immunodeficiency syndrome registries in the United States and Puerto Rico.
(Data from ref. 1.)

quite complex and requires expertise in both the tumor and HIV infection. The goals of cancer therapy (i.e., curative versus palliative), and the relationship of these goals to the status of the underlying HIV infection should be evaluated in each case.

KAPOSI'S SARCOMA

A cluster of cases of KS among young homosexual men in 1982 was one of the first epidemiologic signs of the AIDS epidemic.[9] One hundred sixty-two cases of KS were reported over an 11-month period that year, with most cases indexed to New York City. This was a striking epidemiologic finding given that only three cases had been reported in the period 1961 to 1979 for the same age group in New York City.[9] KS is now the most common tumor seen in HIV-infected patients.[10–12]

AIDS-associated KS well illustrates the interactions of basic, clinical, and applied sciences in unraveling the determinants of disease, resulting in both disease prevention and improved therapy. For many years, a relatively indolent form of KS had been sporadically reported in elderly men in Eastern Europe and countries bordering the Mediterranean (classic KS).[13] More recently, KS has been observed with increased frequency in Africa and in transplantation recipients. It was suggested from the initial pattern of the AIDS epidemic, even before the identification of HIV as the cause of AIDS, that sexual transmission of an infectious agent was likely to be involved in the etiology of KS. Specifically, those at highest risk for developing KS were those with evidence of cellular immune deficiency and whose sexual partners had sex with other men.[10,14,15] After the 1984 joint discovery of HIV as the causative agent of AIDS by Gallo[16] and Montagnier,[17] studies showed that the epidemiologic pattern of KS was not satisfactorily explained by HIV epidemiology alone, and the search for a KS cofactor intensified. During this period, institution of educational and preventive strategies resulted in changes in sexual practices,[18] and lower rates of sexually transmitted diseases in groups at high risk for KS.[19] Since then, there has been a decreasing incidence and prevalence of HIV infection as well as of KS among homosexuals in the United States and other western industrialized countries.[3,19] Before 1985, KS was reported as the initial manifestation of AIDS in approximately 30% of cases,[20] but in the period 1992 through 1997, it was the initial manifestation in 12.5%.[3] The decrease in KS as the index disease for AIDS has occurred in part because the Centers for Disease Control (CDC) revised its definition of AIDS in 1992 to include a CD4 cell count under 200/μL,[21] and thus cases of KS that occur at lower CD4 cell counts are excluded from the index-case count. However, there has been a further decline in incident cases from 60 to 20 per 1000 person-years between 1992 and 1997,[21] invoking cause beyond a simple change in case definition. It should be noted, however, that KS is much more frequent in other areas of the world, particularly sub-Saharan Africa. In parts of Uganda, for example, KS represents almost one-half of all cases of cancers in male subjects and is the second most frequent tumor in female subjects.[22,23]

In 1994, Drs. Chang, Moore, and their colleagues discovered a new herpesvirus, called KS-associated herpesvirus (KSHV) or human herpesvirus-8 (HHV-8), and subsequent studies showed that this was an essential causative agent for all forms of KS.[24,25] This discovery has in turn enabled seroepidemiologic analyses of its pattern of infection indicating that populations with a high incidence of KS also had a high incidence of KSHV infection and that the epidemic of KSHV infection in gay men in the United States emerged almost simultaneously with that of HIV.[26] The seroincidence of KSHV then appeared to taper beginning after 1983, in concert with efforts to encourage safer sex practices among gay men at risk for HIV infection. Also, as discussed later (see Treatment), improved treatments for the underlying HIV infection may have contributed to the decline in KS incidence.[27,28]

KSHV transmission correlates with a history of sexually transmitted disease and the number of male sexual partners: Strictly heterosexual men appear to have a relatively lower risk.[29,30] Coinfection with both KSHV and HIV increases the risk of developing KS by as much as 10,000-fold as compared with KSHV infection alone, and disease manifestation occurs at a younger age. Individuals infected with KSHV but not HIV can develop KS, but it is rare and usually occurs after their fifth decade of life. The risk of developing AIDS-KS appears to be related to the CD4 cell count. The majority of cases occur when the CD4 cell count is below 200/μL, and the risk increases substantially as the CD4 cell count falls below 100/μL.[4,31] The 10-year probability of developing KS after coinfection with both HIV and KSHV approaches 50%.[30] Also, there is evidence that the risk of KS appears to be higher for those who acquire KSHV subsequent to HIV infection,[32] suggesting there is an important role for immune surveillance of KSHV and the risk of KS.

PATHOGENESIS

KS is a multicentric tumor that arises simultaneously in multiple nonmetastatic sites (Fig. 50.1-1). The lesions are highly vascular,

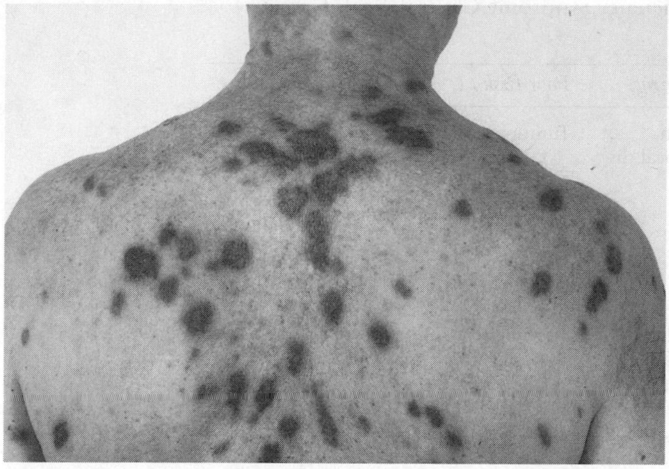

FIGURE 50.1-1. Cutaneous manifestation of Kaposi's sarcoma. (See Color Fig. 50.1-1 in the CD-ROM and on the Web at www.LWWoncology.com.)

accounting for their purplish hue. Microscopically, the tumors are characterized by a predominance of spindle-shaped cells.[33] There is heterogeneity of the cells that make up the lesions, but vascular endothelial cell histogenesis of both the vascular and spindle cell components of KS is suggested by the cellular expression of endothelial cell-associated antigens such as factor VIII–related antigen, HLA DR antigens, E92, and OKM5.[33] However, there remains some uncertainty as to the cell of origin of this tumor. Cells in KS lesions also stain for coexpression of macrophage markers (PAM-1, CD68, and CD14).[34,35] Although advanced KS may involve monoclonal proliferation,[36] there is evidence that proangiogenic factor-driven hyperproliferation of endothelial-derived spindle cells is important at all stages of the disease.[37,38] Spindle cells produce and respond to proangiogenic factors such as basic fibroblast growth factor and vascular endothelial growth factor (VEGF).[37,39]

The angiogenic polypeptide cytokine oncostatin M, which is produced by activated lymphoid cells, shares functional similarity and structural homology to leukemia inhibitory factor and interleukin-6 (IL-6),[40–42] and has autocrine growth properties for cells derived from AIDS-KS.[43,44] Cells exposed to oncostatin M develop spindle morphology, increase proliferation in soft agar, and increase secretion of IL-6,[44] and induction of basic fibroblast growth factor.[45] The soluble form of IL-6 receptor-α (sIL-6α) makes cells expressing gp 130 (the oncostatin M receptor) responsive to IL-6.[46] Since AIDS-KS cells express high levels of IL-6, it is likely that, in the presence of soluble IL-6 receptor-α, cells with the oncostatin M receptor acquire an IL-6 autocrine growth loop.[46,47]

The discovery in 1994 of a novel herpesvirus called KSHV or HHV-8 has introduced some clarity regarding this complex array of cellular markers and cytokine pathways.[25] Essentially all patients with KS are infected with this virus and KSHV/HHV-8 appears to represent an essential factor in the pathogenesis of KS.[48–53] KSHV/HHV-8 is present in the flat endothelial cells lining vascular spaces of KS lesions as well as in typical KS spindle cells.[50] KSHV/HHV-8 can induce the production of a number of virally encoded mimics of human cytokines and other factors involved in KS pathogenesis.[54,55] KSHV encodes for viral homologues to human IL-6, macrophage inhibitory protein, and interferon regulatory factor. It alters other cellular angiogenic factors, which, also, with viral IL-6 and the viral macrophage inhibitory proteins, have the potential for stimulating spindle cells as well as angiogenesis.[54,55] Also, the constitutively active KSHV/HHV-8–encoded G-protein coupled receptor (KSHV GPCR), expressed on infected cells,[56] up-regulates production of VEGF and other angiogenic factors.[57] In addition, there is some evidence that the kinase domain region (KDR) receptor for VEGF is up-regulated in cells infected with KSHV, providing a basis for the paracrine effects of this angiogenic factor in KS.[58] The KSHV GPCR can also cause oncogenic transformation in transfected cells.[59] Moreover, chemokines, such as IL-8 and growth-related protein-α can activate KSHV GPCR over constitutive levels *in vitro*, suggesting that endogenous chemokines may be evolved in KS pathogenesis, in part through KSHV-related pathways.[60]

Although HIV can markedly increase the incidence of KS in KSHV/HHV-8–infected individuals, the precise role of HIV in KS pathogenesis is somewhat unclear. A number of observations invoke the role of HIV Tat protein as a coregulator of KS development. *In vitro*, HIV Tat protein can stimulate endothelial and KS-derived spindle cell growth and proliferation.[61] Normal vascular cells acquire spindle morphology and become responsive to the mitogenic effect of Tat after culture with inflammatory cytokines. Tat promotes adhesion of AIDS-KS and normal vascular cells through a specific interaction with the integrin receptors α_5, β_1, and $\alpha_v\beta_3$, whose expression is increased by inflammatory cytokines.[62,63] However, the degree of extracellular Tat released in HIV-infected patients is unclear. Other mechanisms by which HIV may potentiate the development of KS include increased levels of IL-6 and decreased cellular immunity (perhaps permitting increased KSHV/HHV-8 replication). These mechanisms may explain why in some cases, KS appears to improve with effective treatment of HIV.[64,65]

STAGING AND PROGNOSIS

The unique clinical presentation of KS requires a departure from the standard oncologic staging approach. The widely used tumor, node, metastasis system (TNM), or other staging systems that incorporate histologic grade and biologic indices as the primary prognostic variables,[66] are not satisfactory in KS for a number of reasons. One is the multicentric nature of the disease. Lesions arise simultaneously at multiple sites without an obvious primary site (see Fig. 50.1-1). Almost all KS patients would be classified as having metastatic disease using the TNM system, but multiple areas of skin involvement may not necessarily imply a worse prognosis relative to more focal involvement. Indeed, it is not at all clear how to use the term *metastatic* in relation to KS. Also, assessment of tumor bulk is extremely difficult in KS. Consequently, staging has been relatively nonstandardized, relative to other cancers.

Uniform staging is central to response assessment and is necessary to help compare results among trials and with historic controls. The most widely used staging system for KS, devised by the AIDS Clinical Trials Group Oncology Committee, is the TIS staging system (Table 50.1-2). This system scores patients based on the extent of tumor involvement (T), the immune status of the patient (I), and other AIDS-related systemic illness (S) in an attempt to stratify risk of poor prognosis.[67,68] The TIS system stages patients as being overall either good risk or poor risk, depending on the presence or absence of localized tumor versus more extensive tumor with associated edema, ulceration, vis-

TABLE 50.1-2. Revised Acquired Immunodeficiency Syndrome Clinical Trials Group Staging Classification for Kaposi's Sarcoma[a]

	Good Risk (0; All of the Following)	*Poor Risk (1; Any of the Following)*
Tumor (T)	Confined to skin and/or lymph nodes and/or nonnodular oral disease confined to the palate	Tumor-associated edema or ulceration; extensive oral KS; gastrointestinal KS; KS in other nonnodal viscera
Immune system (I)	CD4 cells ≥150/μL	CD4 cells <150/μL
Systemic illness (S)	No history of opportunistic infection or thrush; no B symptoms (unexplained fever, night sweats, >10% involuntary weight loss, or diarrhea) persisting more than 2 wk; performance status ≥70 (Karnofsky)	History of opportunistic infections, thrush, or both; B symptoms present; performance status <70; other HIV-related illness (e.g., neurologic disease, lymphoma)

HIV, human immunodeficiency virus; KS, Kaposi's sarcoma.
[a]The revised CD4 cutoff of 150 cells/μL[68] is lower than the original proposal of 200 cells/μL. Example of staging: A patient with KS restricted to the skin, CD4 count of 10 cells/μL, and a history of *Pneumocystis carinii* pneumonia would be $T_0I_1S_1$.
(Data from refs. 67 and 68.)

ceral disease, or extensive oral KS; CD4 cells over or below 150/μL; and the presence or absence of antecedent opportunistic infections, thrush, constitutional symptoms, other HIV-related illness, and Karnofsky's performance status. Good risk is designated with a subscript 0, and poor risk by the subscript 1, the summary taking the form T_0 or $_1$, I_0 or $_1$, S_0 or $_1$. A patient who is poor risk in any single category is considered poor risk overall.

Although this staging system is subject to observer bias, it is nevertheless predictive of survival. One of the most important prognostic factors is the CD4 count. A CD4 cell count greater than 150 to 200 cells/μL implies a better prognosis,[68–70] regardless of visceral involvement by KS.[68]

The extent of KS lesions as a prognostic factor has not uniformly been validated,[69,70] but the potentially confounding role of immunosuppression degree was not adequately controlled for in certain analyses. The degree of immunosuppression predicts life expectancy after the diagnosis of KS.[71] The clinical course of KS is quite variable, from remarkably indolent to rapidly fulminant, but there are no clear criteria on which to assess the risk of aggressive versus indolent disease. KS behavior can be affected by the degree of immunosuppression or alternatively by the degree of HIV replication.[61–63,72] There is evidence that KS may become more indolent with good control of HIV, but the long-term course of KS in patients with highly active antiretroviral regimens is not known. The role of other factors, such as the activity of KSHV/HHV-8, are not well understood at present, but could potentially contribute to risk assessment.

TREATMENT

During the 1980s, KS was a frequent cause of death in AIDS patients.[73,74] In the late 1990s, however, a number of advances in the therapy of this disease have been seen. While KS is still a cause of considerable morbidity and mortality in HIV-infected individuals, better tumor control is now attainable in most patients than was possible several years ago. In addition, there is evidence that the development of highly effective antiretroviral regimens has contributed to a decline in the incidence of KS in HIV-infected individuals.[75,76] Finally, advances in understanding the pathogenesis of KS offer the possibility of developing new pathogenesis-based therapies that may be less toxic than the current agents.

In order to best understand the effect of more recent advances in the therapy of KS, it is useful to recount the standard therapy for this condition as of approximately 1993 to 1994. Overall, the initial therapies identified as being active against KS during the first few years of the AIDS epidemic can be divided into three groups: local measures, immunotherapy (interferon-α), and cytotoxic chemotherapeutic agents.

Local Therapy

Local therapies include surgical excision of the lesions, cryotherapy, photodynamic therapy, intralesional injections, radiation therapy, and topical application of various drugs and are most useful for patients with limited cutaneous disease that is cosmetically disturbing to the patient.[77] Intralesional injection or iontophoresis of low-dose vinblastine (0.1 mL of 0.1 mg/mL) or 3% sodium tetradecyl sulfate injection (0.1 to 0.3 mL) causes a nonspecific necrosis or sclerosis of mucocutaneous tissue with sometimes reasonable cosmetic outcome for small lesions.[78–81] Cryotherapy is easy to administer and unlike surgical excision, it can be accomplished without local anesthesia.[82] However, cryotherapy can cause permanent destruction of melanocytes, particularly in dark-skinned individuals. Topical 9-*cis* retinoic acid (Panretin Gel), approved by the U.S. Food and Drug Administration (FDA) for use in KS, may result in responses in over 45% of lesions but can cause local inflammation and lightening of the skin, yielding inadequate cosmesis in some cases.[83,84]

Radiotherapy is useful for localized disease, but as with other nonsystemic therapies, does not control disease outside of the treatment area. In addition, there are reports of a decreased tolerance to radiation among AIDS-KS patients, particularly on the mucosal surfaces where severe mucositis can occur.[85,86] Reappearance of KS in the area of previous irradiation can occur. Radiotherapy is useful as adjunctive therapy in severe disease to treat areas of painful involvement that may respond only slowly to systemic therapy. The use of carbon dioxide laser therapy to remove tumors of the mouth, oropharynx, and larynx has been reported to result in immediate improved oral intake and with less toxicity than is sometimes seen with radiation to the oral cavity.[87] Radiotherapy is also useful for cosmetic purposes, such as involvement of the eyelid or conjunctiva, when other local therapies are not practical. Applied doses vary between 800 rad given over one fraction to 3000 rad given over ten fractions, depending on the site of involvement, and disease status entering into the dosing algorithm. Complete responses can be seen in over 90% of lesions, but sometimes residual radiation-induced pigmentation or telangiectasia, which can at times be severe, limits the cosmetic outcome.[85,88] Doses of 1500 rad for oral lesions and doses of 2000 rad for lesions involving eyelids, conjunctiva, and genitals have been shown to be sufficient to produce shrinkage of the tumor and good palliation of the symptoms. Short-course radiotherapy may be useful and effective in some settings. Treatment comparisons of either 1600 rad over four fractions over 4 days or 800 rad as a single fraction yielded similar response rates of 78% to 81%. The toxicity was somewhat site dependent, and thus single-fraction therapy may not be appropriate in all cases.[89] Radiation therapy can be used for palliation of visceral disease, including pulmonary involvement, and may be reasonably well tolerated in some circumstances.[90]

Photodynamic therapy has been reported to be effective in KS, yielding high response rates, and has the advantage over other local therapies in that 40 to 50 lesions can be treated during a single session.[91,92] It is frequently associated with moderate pain and then photosensitivity for a number of weeks following the treatment.

Immunotherapy

Immunotherapy with interferon-α was identified as being active in KS in the early 1980s, particularly in patients with over 200 CD4 cells/μL and disease limited to the skin.[93,94] Interferon-α appears to be more effective when used in combination with zidovudine monotherapy than when used alone,[95] and as will be discussed below, studies are underway to test this agent in combination with potent combination anti-HIV therapy (see Antiangiogenesis Approches, later in this chapter). The use of interferon-α is associated with a decreased white blood count, flu-like symptoms, and sometimes depression.

Cytotoxic Chemotherapy

Early in the AIDS-KS epidemic, several cytotoxic chemotherapeutic agents were found to yield tumor responses with acceptable toxicity.[96] Vinca alkaloids (either vincristine, vinblastine, or an alternating regimen of the two) were among the first to be studied. Other active single-agent drugs included etoposide, bleomycin, and doxorubicin. Subsequently, several studies showed that the combination of doxorubicin, bleomycin, and vinca alkaloids (ABV) was effective, even in patients with extensive KS or disease that was refractory to other therapies.[97,98] The initial clinical studies of ABV in KS generally used relatively high doses of doxorubicin, either 40 mg/m^2 every 4 weeks or 20 mg/m^2 every 2 to 3 weeks.[97,98] Impressive response rates of 84% and 88%, respectively, were seen. However, the therapy was frequently limited by neutropenia and concomitant non-KS opportunistic infections. Also, although many patients derived benefit from such agents and regimens, as late as 1999 it was not infrequent to see patients die with severe, progressive KS in spite of optimal therapy.

This situation has improved somewhat with the development of two new chemotherapeutic approaches for KS: liposomal anthracyclines and paclitaxel.[99] Liposomal formulations of anthracyclines were considered in part because they were predicted to have a smaller volume of distribution than unencapsulated drug and thus remain in the circulation for longer periods of time.[100,101] Two such formulations, liposomal daunorubicin (DaunoXome) and pegylated liposomal doxorubicin (Doxil) have now been developed and found to be active in patients with KS and have prolonged half-lives as compared with unencapsulated forms. Moreover, there is some evidence that encapsulation of the drugs in liposomes helps target them to KS lesions, in part because of the sequestering of blood that occurs because of the leaky blood vessels in the lesions.[102] In early clinical studies, both preparations were found to induce major tumor responses, even in patients who had failed standard chemotherapy.[100,103]

With this background, liposomal anthracyclines as single agents were tested against active combination regimens in several randomized trials. In one study, liposomal daunorubicin (40 mg/m^2 every 2 weeks) was found to have a response rate comparable with ABV, although with somewhat less neutropenia.[104] It is noteworthy that the 28% major response rate of ABV in this study was substantially less than that found on previous studies. One likely reason for this is that the dose of doxorubicin used (10 mg/m^2 every 2 weeks) was less than that used in the earlier ABV studies. Another likely reason is that the patients in this randomized trial had advanced HIV disease with a median CD4 count of 29 cells/μL. The substantial difference in response rates to ABV in these two trials highlights the sensitivity of KS response rates to disease status and other parameters.

In two separate trials, pegylated liposomal doxorubicin was found to have better response rates against KS than either bleomycin plus vincristine (BV) or an ABV regimen with either less or roughly comparable toxicities.[105,106] In the study comparing it with BV, the major response rate to pegylated liposomal doxorubicin alone was 58%. Both of these liposomal preparations have now been approved by the FDA for the therapy of KS.

To address whether the liposomal anthracyclines were better used alone or in place of doxorubicin in combination regimens, a study of liposomal doxorubicin alone compared with liposomal doxorubicin, bleomycin, and vincristine (DBV) in patients with advanced KS was initiated.[107] At a protocol-mandated interim analysis on 126 evaluable patients (62 on liposomal doxorubicin and 64 on DBV), the major tumor responses (partial and complete responses) were similar in the two treatment arms (79% on liposomal doxorubicin vs. 80% on the combination regimen). However, more patients receiving DBV had toxicities requiring cessation of treatment than did patients receiving liposomal doxorubicin alone, and there was a trend toward better survival in favor of liposomal doxorubicin alone (11 vs. 18 deaths, $P = .079$). The study concluded that single-agent liposomal doxorubicin had equivalent activity but lower toxicity than DBV, and all patients were switched to liposomal doxorubicin alone.

Paclitaxel was also developed for use in KS during this period based on observations that it targets cellular microtubules (such as vinca alkaloids shown to be active in KS, albeit causing the opposite effect) and its *in vitro* inhibition of a KS-derived spindle cell line.[108] An initial trial of paclitaxel at the National Cancer Institute (NCI) using a dose of 135 to 175

TABLE 50.1-3. Therapies for Patients with Advanced Kaposi's Sarcoma

Therapy	*Response Rates*
COMMONLY USED STANDARD THERAPIES	
Liposomal anthracyclines	
Doxorubicin	59%[106]
Daunorubicin	25% [104]
Paclitaxel	59–71%[109,110]
ALTERNATIVE THERAPIES	
Adriamycin/bleomycin/ vinca alkaloids	24–88% (higher response rates with higher doxorubicin doses, but greater toxicity)[97,104,105,379,380]
Vincristine/vinblastine	45%[381]
Bleomycin/vinca alkaloids	23%[106]

mg/m^2 administered over 3 hours every 3 weeks showed substantial activity in patients with advanced KS; 20 of 28 assessable patients had complete or partial responses for a major response rate of 71.4%.[108,109] It was noteworthy that five of six patients with pulmonary KS responded, as did four patients who had previously received anthracycline therapy.

Gill, Scadden, and their colleagues at the University of Southern California and Harvard University conducted a second trial of paclitaxel in 56 mostly previously treated patients with advanced KS.[110] This trial used a somewhat different regimen: 100 mg/m^2 of paclitaxel administered over 3 hours every 2 weeks. Overall, the major response rate in this trial was 59%. It was noteworthy that of the 32 patients who had received prior anthracycline therapy, 55% responded. In both trials, neutropenia was the dose-limiting toxicity, and a number of patients had improvement in KS-related symptoms. Largely based on the results of these two studies, the FDA approved paclitaxel as second-line therapy for KS in 1997. Also, it is important to emphasize that corticosteroids can result in dramatic acceleration of KS growth. Premedication with 10 mg of dexamethasone is adequate for premedication in taxane-based therapy, but corticosteroids should otherwise be avoided when possible.

The development of the liposomal anthracyclines and paclitaxel for KS appears to have enabled better palliation of symptoms with less toxicity than was possible with previous regimens, and at the present time, most oncologists treating KS patients consider these to be the two most valuable modalities for the treatment of advanced KS (Table 50.1-3). For most such patients, the liposomal anthracyclines (and especially liposomal doxorubicin) are generally considered the preferred first-line therapy. Paclitaxel is generally considered as a valuable second-line therapy, although for patients with particularly severe KS, some oncologists use it as initial therapy (this is a deviation from the current FDA labeling of the drug). Other therapies that are considered useful in some patients include ABV, weekly alternating vincristine and vinblastine, or BV.

In an attempt to explore the relative merits of these agents as first-line therapy for KS, von Roenn and colleagues in the Eastern Cooperative Oncology Group and the AIDS Malignancy Consortium of the NCI have initiated a phase III trial comparing liposomal doxorubicin (Doxil), 20 mg/m^2 every 3 weeks, with paclitaxel, 100 mg/m^2 every 2 weeks in patients with advanced, untreated KS. This study should provide valuable guidance for therapy in advanced KS.

Experimental Approaches to the Treatment of Kaposi's Sarcoma

Although the development of liposomal anthracyclines and paclitaxel has improved the therapeutic armamentarium for advanced KS, these agents have the potential for substantial toxicity. In particular, both cause bone marrow and immunologic suppression, although there is evidence that paclitaxel is relatively sparing of CD4 cells as compared with other cytotoxic agents.[111] Moreover, even in the absence of HIV infection, the regeneration of CD4 cells after cytotoxic therapy can take many months, especially in adults or older children.[112] For these reasons, there is a substantial interest in developing effective less toxic pathogenesis-based therapies.

ANTIANGIOGENESIS APPROACHES. One active area of research in this regard is the inhibition of new blood vessel growth, a field that has been pioneered by Folkman and colleagues.[113–115] KS is a highly vascular tumor, and for this reason, there is currently an interest in exploring the use of angiogenesis inhibitors in patients with KS. Compounds of interest that have been in phase I or II testing include pentosan polysulfate,[116] TNP-470 (an analogue of the fungal product fumagillin),[117,118] IL-12,[119] IM-862,[120] SU5416, and thalidomide.[121,122] Preliminary results from two initial phase II trials of thalidomide both showed that this agent had activity in a subset of patients with KS.[121,122]

IL-12 possesses a number of interesting immunologic and antiangiogenic characteristics that make it a potentially attractive agent for HIV-associated KS. There is evidence that HIV-infected patients have a specific defect in T-cell help for cellular response (Th1 cells), and that IL-12 selectively stimulates such responses.[123,124] In addition, IL-12 has been shown to be a potent inhibitor of angiogenesis,[115,125] possibly through induction of inducible protein 10, a potent inhibitor of angiogenesis.[125–127] Interestingly, the constitutively active KSHV GPCR expressed on KS cells is inhibited by inducible protein 10,[128] leading to potentially decreased production of VEGF and other angiogenic factors by KSHV/HHV-8–infected cells.[59,129] A potential concern in the use of IL-12 is that it has been shown to slightly increase HIV replication *in vitro*.[130] However, this can easily be controlled by anti-HIV drugs.[130] Preliminary results from a phase I trial of IL-12 in patients with KS show that it has some activity.[119] In the future, it may also be of interest to explore the possible clinical utility of inducible protein 10 in this disease.

The results seen with thalidomide and IL-12, plus advances in angiogenesis research, have led to further interest in this approach to the treatment of KS. The AIDS Malignancy Consortium is conducting studies of novel antiangiogenic agents, including a phase I trial of the metalloproteinase inhibitor col-3 and of IM-862 versus placebo for evidence of therapeutic effect. There has been substantial interest in two biologic anti-angiogenesis agents, endostatin and angiostatin,[131,132] and as development proceeds, they may be studied in KS.

Finally, it should be noted that interferon-α can inhibit angiogenesis,[133] and that this may be one mechanism for its anti-KS activity. Initial studies suggested that this agent was principally active in patients with disease limited to the skin and with over

200 CD4 cells/μL.[93,94,134] However, subsequent trials suggested that this agent also manifested anti-KS activity in patients with lower CD4 counts if given with nucleoside anti-HIV therapy.[95] To extend these observations, the AIDS Malignancy Consortium is now studying the effectiveness of interferon-α in combination with highly active antiretroviral therapy (AIDS Malignancy Consortium Trial 004) in patients with HIV-associated KS.

RETINOIC ACIDS. KS-derived spindle cells have been shown to proliferate in response to IL-6 and certain retinoids have been shown to down-regulate IL-6 receptors, at least on myeloma lines, and to have an antiproliferative effect on KS-derived cell lines.[135–137] Much of the initial interest in the retinoids centered on all-*trans*-retinoic acid. However, the results with this agent were inconclusive.[138–140] Also, a problem with the use of all-*trans*-retinoic acid is that it rapidly induces enzymes that significantly increase its metabolism, resulting in a substantially diminished area under the time concentration curve.[141] In part because of this and in part because it has a different pattern of receptor binding, more recent clinical work has focused on 9-*cis* retinoic acid. Preliminary reports from two clinical trials have provided evidence that this agent is active when administered orally to patients with KS.[142,143] The response rates in these studies were 46% and 37%. The most frequent side effects were headache and skin changes. Additional studies will be needed to further define the role of this agent in KS. As noted previously, topical 9-*cis* retinoic acid has been approved by the FDA for use in KS.

HORMONAL APPROACHES. One of the interesting epidemiologic features of AIDS-KS is that the vast majority of patients are male.[10] This male predominance is more than can be explained by patterns of KSHV/HHV-8 infection,[51,144] and it suggests that there may be some hormonal effect on the disease pathogenesis. Several years ago, Lundardi-Iskandar, Gallo, and coworkers found that a factor in the urine of pregnant women blocked the growth of a KS-derived cell line.[145] This factor was initially thought to be human chorionic gonadotropin, but subsequent investigation has suggested that it is a related urinary protein that is found in certain preparations of human chorionic gonadotropin.[146] Early clinical trials have shown that preparations of human chorionic gonadotropin containing this factor could induce regressions in KS.[147,148] Ongoing studies are now focused on better defining this active factor.

KAPOSI'S SARCOMA–ASSOCIATED HERPESVIRUS, HUMAN HERPESVIRUS-8, AND HUMAN IMMUNODEFICIENCY VIRUS–RELATED APPROACHES. The discovery of KSHV/HHV-8 has opened up many avenues of research in KS.[24,25] Most of the cells in KS lesions are infected with KSHV/HHV-8 in a latent state.[52] However, a small percentage of cells in KS lesions appear to contain KSHV/HHV-8 in a lytic state of replication, and if these few cells are important in ongoing tumor pathogenesis, then antiherpes drugs might have anti-KS activity. Although preliminary evidence suggests that antiherpes drugs such as acyclovir, foscarnet, or ganciclovir do not substantially decrease the population of KSHV/HHV-8–infected cells in the circulation, there is some anecdotal evidence of KS remissions being associated with the use of foscarnet.[49,149,150] Perhaps more noteworthy is the finding from a randomized clinical trial of oral ganciclovir that administration of this agent was associated with a lower rate of KS.[151] This result indicates that an antiherpes drug can reduce the incidence of KS, although it still remains unclear as to how it can affect established lesions.

While the role of ongoing KSHV/HHV-8 replication in the growth of KS lesions is still unclear, there is somewhat better evidence of a linkage between KS growth and HIV replication. The incidence of KS is much higher among patients coinfected with HIV and KSHV/HHV-8 than in those with just KSHV/HHV-8 infection, and there are reports of KS regression during highly active anti-HIV therapy.[152] Also, there is evidence that the incidence of KS has declined in HIV-infected patients since the introduction of potent combination anti-HIV therapy.[153] Possible mechanisms for this association include interaction of HIV Tat protein with KS-derived spindle cells,[154] HIV-induced immunosuppression, HIV-related cytokine dysregulation, and the possible role of other HIV-encoded proteins. These epidemiologic findings provide a paradigm for the prevention of a tumor by antiviral control of the underlying viral and immunosuppressive disease.

ACQUIRED IMMUNODEFICIENCY SYNDROME–ASSOCIATED LYMPHOMAS

EPIDEMIOLOGY AND OVERVIEW

Beginning in 1973, before recognition of the AIDS epidemic, there was a clear increase in reported cases of lymphoma.[176–178] This trend overlapped with the early years of the epidemic, and from 1973 to 1988, there was a 50% increase in the incidence of NHL based on analysis of the NCI's Surveillance, Epidemiology, and End Results program data.[155] The incidence rates for primary brain lymphomas increased during the same period.[156] The increased incidence rates for large cell immunoblastic and small noncleaved cell NHL observed during the 1980s has been attributed largely, although not entirely, to the AIDS epidemic.[155]

Immune dysfunction had previously been associated with the development of lymphoproliferative disease and lymphomas, and with this background, investigators were alerted early in the AIDS epidemic to the possibility that this new disease might be associated with lymphomagenesis.[157] Indeed, as early as 1982, only 1 year after AIDS was recognized as a new epidemic disease, four cases of aggressive lymphoma in young men ranging in age from 24 to 35 years were reported within a 10-month period in the San Francisco area.[158,159] This was seen as remarkable because only one case of aggressive lymphoma had been reported in the age group 20 to 39 years for the period 1977 to 1980. It was thus recognized that the then-termed *KS and opportunistic infection syndrome* may predispose affected persons to more than one kind of tumor.[14,15,158]

Additional significance to the emerging problem of NHL was highlighted in 1985 with publication of the Surveillance, Epidemiology, and End Results program database, which suggested a ninefold increase of the morbidity odds ratio for aggressive lymphomas among *never-married men* (a term used to approximate homosexual men for epidemiologic purposes) in the San Francisco area 1981 to 1982 as compared with 1973 to 1980.[160] Ultimately, it was found that there was an overall 60-fold increase in the ratio of observed cases of NHL in HIV-infected persons compared with that expected in the HIV-negative population.[5] Because of these epidemiologic and immunologic considerations, NHL of high-grade pathologic type (diffuse, undifferentiated) and of B-cell or unknown immunologic phenotype, diagnosed by biopsy, was included in the case definition of AIDS in 1985.[161]

NHL is now the second most common AIDS-associated malignancy and is the AIDS-defining diagnosis in roughly 3% of HIV-positive patients.[3,162] It is not clear what percentage of HIV-infected patients ultimately develop NHL, since the occurrence of a second AIDS-defining event is not reportable. Estimates of incidence up to 10% per year with a prevalence of 4.5% to 25.0% have been documented in certain patient populations.[163–166] In addition to an increased risk of NHL in HIV-infected persons, the pattern of presentation differs from the HIV-negative population. Over 80% of lymphomas in HIV-infected patients are high-grade B-cell lymphomas,[5,167,168] whereas only 10% to 15% of lymphomas among HIV-negative patients are of this type.[169]

Data collected by the NCI suggest that between 8% and 27% of the approximately 40,000 annual cases of NHL are HIV-related.[11] In a long-term follow-up of patients participating in phase I trials of zidovudine, the predicted occurrence of NHL by Kaplan-Meier statistics was 8% after 24 months and 29% after 36 months of zidovudine.[163] A high risk of lymphoma development was also observed in patients followed for a long time on a phase I trial of didanosine.[166] Lymphoma risk appeared to be increased with the degree and duration of immunosuppression. These reports suggested that anti-HIV therapy might possibly increase the cumulative risk of HIV-infected individuals developing lymphoma by extending overall survival.[163,166] However, when these reports were published, concern arose that nucleoside reverse transcriptase inhibitors might directly contribute to development of lymphoma. The finding that that lifetime exposure in rodents was associated with vaginal tumors and the subsequent finding that administration of high-dose zidovudine to pregnant mice was associated with increased cancer rates among the offspring, further raised concern that these drugs were potentially carcinogenic in humans.[170–172] Clinical studies have not supported these concerns, however. First, some studies have reported relatively low overall rates of the development of lymphoma. In one study, only 24 (2.3%) of 1030 AIDS patients receiving zidovudine developed NHL.[162] With 1463 person-years of follow-up, the rate was 1.6 per 100 person-years of therapy. Also, data from a case-control study provided no evidence that the use of zidovudine increased the risk of lymphoma in HIV infection.[173]

Another piece of evidence arguing against a role of zidovudine increasing the risk of B-cell lymphoma is that zidovudine is not implicated in lymphomagenesis or in inducing B-cell activation.[174] Also, it is worth remembering that an increased incidence of lymphoma in HIV-infected patients was found even before the introduction of zidovudine.[161]

The excess risk of developing AIDS-NHL appears to be independent of the particular risk group for HIV acquisition[5,165,175] or lifestyle factors such as drug use,[175] although one autopsy series suggested that patients with a prior history of KS had a 5.3-fold higher risk of NHL compared with HIV-infected patients with other AIDS-defining illnesses.[164] The risk, however, does vary with age. It has been reported that the excess risk of NHL in HIV is approximately 360-fold for the age group under 19 years, and 20-fold for the age group over 60 years of age.[5] However, NHL is a rare disease in western children (0.1 to 0.3 per 100,00),[176] such that a small number of excess cases translate into higher ratios of observed versus expected cases.[5] It has also been reported that male subjects and whites are at higher risk than other groups,[177] but this feature does not distinguish AIDS-NHL from the epidemiology of non–AIDS-NHL.[178,179] NHL is the most frequent AIDS-related malignancy among hemophiliacs,[161] primarily because KS appears so rarely in this group.

There may be innate biologic characteristics that predispose certain HIV-infected persons to develop NHL. In a study of 746 HIV-infected persons, the 3'A variant of stromal cell-derived factor-1 chemokine was associated with an approximate doubling of the NHL risk in heterozygotes and a fourfold increase in homozygotes.[180] The stromal cell-derived factor-1 3'A chemokine variant is carried by 37% of whites and 11% of blacks and may contribute to the lower risk of AIDS-NHL in blacks compared with whites.

A deletion in the CCR5 chemokine receptor gene has been reported to alter the risk for HIV infection and progression to AIDS.[181] In a matched case-control study, the CCR5 deletion variant CCR5-Δ32 offered approximately a threefold protection against NHL.[182] By contrast, the AIDS-protective variant CCR2-64I had no significant effect on the risk of lymphoma. The CCR5 gene was not associated with a difference in risk for Kaposi's sarcoma, or development of opportunistic infections.[183] Costimulation of normal B cells with the CCR5 ligand RANTES (regulated on activation, normally T-cell expressed and secreted) induces a proliferative response, indicating that RANTES is a mitogen for B cells.[184,185] Perhaps the CCR5-Δ32 mutation is protective through a mechanism involving a decreased response of B cells to the mitogenic activity of RANTES.[183] It is possible that such factors may provide a means of assessing the risk of NHL in HIV-infected persons and provide insights for preventive and treatment approaches for this disease.

It is conceivable that potent antiretroviral therapy (PAT) for HIV infection will have an effect on the incidence of AIDS-NHL. In the Australian AIDS registration data, NHL has decreased by 37.5% as an AIDS-defining diagnosis since 1994, coincident with the introduction of PAT as common anti-HIV therapy.[186] The French database has also suggested a decrease in NHL: Of 66,202 HIV-seropositive subjects, the incidence of lymphoma (peripheral and primary CNS) per 1000 patient-years in the first half of 1997 decreased 44% compared with the incidence in the first half of 1996.[28] The effect of PAT on PCNSL may be clearer. This effect is not surprising as PCNSL most commonly develops in patients with fewer that 50 CD4 cells/μL[163,166,187] and as PAT can profoundly increase the CD4 counts. In a prospective study, the probabilities of developing focal brain lesions were analyzed for linear trend comparing 1991 through 1996, a period before PAT, with 1997 through 1998, when PAT became commonly available. The odds ratio of developing PCNSL was 0.46 in the PAT era compared with pre-PAT.[188] Others studies have found less evidence of a substantial effect on the incidence of lymphoma. An analysis of data from the Multicenter AIDS Cohort Study showed that the incidence of NHL as the AIDS-defining condition has remained fairly constant over time.[27] Among a total of 6587 patients enrolled in AIDS Clinical Trials Group trials between November 1987 and February 1997, incidence rates of both KS and NHL per 100 person-years declined in concert with decreases in mortality, but the decreases in NHL were somewhat inconsistent, suggesting that current therapies have not appreciably ameliorated the incidence of NHL.[76] It is hard to predict the ultimate effect PAT will have on the development of NHL. On the one hand, it may reduce the immediate incidence through its beneficial effect on the viral load and CD4 count. On the other hand, as patients live longer with PAT, there may be a cumulative increase in the risk of patients developing NHL.

PATHOLOGY AND CLASSIFICATION

Efforts to understand disease mechanisms for AIDS-NHL have involved consideration of NHL occurring in other conditions of disordered immunity. Immune-suppressive therapy in solid organ transplantation is associated with a 30- to 300-fold increase in the risk of lymphomas and has been used as a model of AIDS-associated lymphomagenesis.[168,189] These lymphoproliferations can sometimes respond to reduction in immunosuppressive therapy, but in other instances can also be aggressive and poorly responsive to treatment.[190–193] The congenital immunodeficiency syndromes also confer a predisposition to malignancy, providing yet another model in which to consider lymphomagenesis.[194,195] For example, in ataxia-telangiectasia, there are specific immune defects that have been identified and linked to chromosome breakpoints in genes involved in both the immune system and in certain malignancies such as Burkitt's lymphoma.[196,197] Further illustrating the role of immune dysfunction is the increased frequency of lymphoproliferative disease and lymphomas occurring in patients with autoimmune disease.[198,199] Autoimmune factors in HIV infection are suggested by the finding that antibodies to the HIV-1 gp41 protein cross-react with self MHC class II antigens, triggering chronic antigenic stimulation of B cells.[200] Further, immunoglobulin somatic hypermutation with the preferential use of the V_H4 family of immunoglobulin-variable genes (molecular events that are produced under chronic lymphoproliferative conditions) has been seen in AIDS-associated lymphomas.[201–203] Elevated serum IL-6 levels in HIV-infected patients have also been associated with a higher risk of certain forms of NHL.[166,204] Thus, chronic antigen stimulation from HIV, concomitant infections, or autoimmune phenomena can potentially lead to B-cell proliferation and oligoclonal expansion in a multistep process rapidly progressing from clinically undetectable hyperplastic adenopathy[205,206] to malignant monoclonal lymphoma in the setting of immunosuppression or other host factors such as deregulated cytokine production (i.e., IL-6, IL-10, tumor necrosis factor-β).[166,204,207,208]

HISTOLOGY

AIDS-NHLs are histologically heterogeneous and are almost invariably derived from monoclonal B-cell populations,[209–212] although there are sporadic reports of T-cell lymphomas associated with HIV.[213,214] There are three major categories of HIV-associated B-cell lymphomas: (1) Burkitt's and Burkitt-like lymphomas; (2) B-cell immunoblastic lymphomas; and (3) the rarely occurring primary effusion lymphomas (PEL), also termed *body cavity lymphomas*.[5,167,209,212,215–220] The Revised European-American Classification of Lymphoid Neoplasms classifies all these lymphomas as either (1) Burkitt's and Burkitt-like, which includes small non–cleaved cell lymphomas (SNCCL) and account for approximately 20% of the cases; and (2) diffuse large B-cell lymphoma, which include the large non–cleaved cell and large cell-immunoblastic plasmacytoid types and account for approximately 60% of cases.[221,222] HIV-associated PCNSLs are almost always of this latter morphologic type.[223] The World Health Organization proposes a unique classification for PEL.[224]

Occasional lymphomas arising in HIV-infected individuals have been reported to be polyclonal.[225] These tumors are most often Epstein-Barr virus (EBV)-negative tumors with no evidence of c-myc rearrangement. Less frequently, these polyclonal tumors are found to be EBV-positive with similarities to lymphoproliferations seen in transplant patients. Polyclonality is said to confer a favorable prognosis.[226] However, most authorities agree that the majority of AIDS-lymphomas are monoclonal.[217] Other lymphomas that are seen in the setting of HIV but are not AIDS-defining conditions, include classical Hodgkin's disease,[227,228] polymorphic lymphoproliferative disorders resembling post-transplant-associated lymphoproliferative disease,[229] and lymphomatoid granulomatosis.[230] Multicentric Castleman's disease is sporadically reported in patients with AIDS-NHL and KS and is of interest because of its association with KSHV/HHV-8 and other similarities with lymphomagenesis.[231]

SYSTEMIC LYMPHOMAS

As noted previously, the vast majority of systemic lymphomas developing in HIV-infected individuals are either diffuse large cell lymphomas or SNCCL. The presence of distinct genetic pathways for AIDS-SNCCL and AIDS-diffuse large cell lymphomas correlates with a number of clinical features that distinguish these two groups of tumors, including differences in the age of onset, CD4 counts at the time of presentation, time elapsed since HIV infection, and clinical presentation (Table 50.1-4).[209] EBV expression patterns are distinct from posttransplant lymphoproliferative disorders related to iatrogenic immunosuppression and are heterogeneous among AIDS-NHLs.[232] These patterns appear to correlate with histiogenic origin of the malignant clone.[233]

Large B-cell lymphomas in HIV-infected patients are associated with EBV infection in 70% to 90% of cases and are more likely to occur later in the course of HIV infection in older patients with relatively low CD4 cell counts.[209,234] Cells tend to exhibit EBV-latency type 3 expression and in particular express Epstein-Barr nuclear antigen-2 (EBNA-2) and latent membrane protein-1 (LMP-1), which are EBV-specific antigenic targets.[235–237] It has been hypothesized that HIV-infected patients have a defect in these EBV-specific cytotoxic T-cell responses, thus allowing immune escape of the emerging lymphomatous clone. The viral oncogene LMP-1 may be involved in lymphomagenesis by increasing the threshold for cells to undergo programmed cell death[238] through up-regulation of the cellular antiapoptotic oncogene, bcl-2.[239,240] Unlike HIV-negative lymphomas of similar histology in which translocations of bcl-2 are often found,[221,241,242] rearrangements of bcl-2 are not generally found in peripheral AIDS-NHLs.[212] However, bcl-2 may be densely expressed in some cases.[243] EBNA-2 expression has been reported to be associated with extranodal disease,[244] which is a prominent feature of the large cell AIDS-NHLs.

SNCCL is more likely to occur earlier in the course of HIV infection in younger patients with relatively preserved CD4 cell counts. Only a minority of cases (25% to 40%) express EBV.[209,245] If EBV is found in SNCCL, EBNA-2 and LMP-1 are not typically expressed, as is also observed in EBV-positive cases of (sporadic) Burkitt's lymphoma in the general population. The lack of EBV protein expression could contribute to the ability of tumor cells to escape the relatively intact immune surveillance in these patients.

The different patterns of EBV expression found in these lymphomas may relate in part to the observation that the synthesis of

TABLE 50.1-4. Comparison of Human Immunodeficiency Virus–Associated Lymphomas

	Lymphoma Subtypes			
Feature	Burkitt	Burkitt-like	Immunoblastic	Primary Effusion Lymphoma
Presentation	++CNS +Systemic ++Bone marrow	++Systemic +Bone marrow	+++CNS +++Gastrointestinal/extra-nodal ±Bone marrow	Effusions
Prior acquired immuno-deficiency syndrome	<30%	Variable	>75%	>75%
CD4 cells	Normal (or decreased)	Decreased	Decreased	Decreased
Epstein-Barr virus	30–50% –LMP-1, –EBNA-2	80% –LMP-1, –EBNA-2	>90% +LMP-1, +EBNA	>90%
Human herpesvirus-8	Negative	Negative	Negative	100%
C-myc	>65%	>65%	20%	Negative
BCL-6	Negative	Negative	20%	Negative
BCL-2	Negative	Negative	Occasional	Negative
p53	60%	60%	Negative	Negative
RAS	15%	15%	15%	Negative

BCL, B-cell lymphoma; CNS, central nervous system; EBNA, Epstein-Barr nuclear antigen; LMP, low-molecular weight protein.
(Adapted from refs. 209, 216, 382, and 383.)

various EBV transformation-associated proteins is regulated by different cellular factors depending on the differentiation stage of the host cell.[233] A number of these tumors express BCL-6, a protein selectively expressed by germinal center (GC) B cells, and it has been suggested that these lymphomas may originate from the GC.[246] Deregulated BCL-6 expression may contribute to lymphomagenesis by preventing post-GC differentiation.[247,248] Syndecan-1 (syn-1) is a proteoglycan that is not expressed in GC B cells, but it is expressed in specific subsets of post-GC B cells, including immunoblasts and plasma cells. It is absent on circulating and peripheral B lymphocytes, but is reexpressed on their differentiation into immobilized plasma cells.[249] BCL-6 and syn-1 appear to segregate into two major phenotypic subsets, suggesting that tumors displaying the BCL-6+/syn-1– phenotype originate from GC-related B cells, whereas tumors displaying the BCL-6–/syn-1+ phenotype derive from post-GC B cells. The differential expression of BCL-6 and syn-1 appears to be related to expression of LMP-1. Among EBV-infected AIDS-NHL, expression of the LMP-1 antigen can be found only in BCL-6–/syn-1+ tumors, suggesting that the GC stage is not permissive for LMP-1 expression, and that tumors expressing LMP-1 derive from more mature post-GC B cells. Cases with immunoblastic plasmacytoid features and LMP-1 expression thus appear to be BCL-6–/syn-1+ with post-GC histiogenic origin, whereas most SNCCL and large non–cleaved cell lymphomas appear to originate from more immature GC B cells expressing BCL-6+/syn-1– and LMP-1–. Such considerations may provide insight into the complicated pattern of EBV expression in NHL.

Clustering of the protooncogenes c-myc, BCL-6, and the tumor suppressor gene product p53 is also predictable according to histologic subtype: C-myc activation is seen among 65% to 100% of SNCCL cases, but rarely in large cell lymphomas.[245] Inappropriately regulated expression of c-myc, which can be independent of EBV infection in AIDS-NHL,[245] may contribute to lymphomagenesis by causing the down-regulation of lymphocyte function-associated antigen-1 adhesion molecules and loss of B-cell adhesion to cytotoxic T cells and natural killer cells.[250] This may provide another mechanism for malignant cells to escape immune surveillance. BCL-6 rearrangements occur in approximately 20% of large cell lymphomas, but are not found in SNCCL. p53 overexpression is restricted to SNCCL, possibly resulting in disruptions in programmed cell death.[245] A small number of cases of both large cell and SNCCL have been observed to express activated RAS, potentially distinguishing these tumors from those found in the immunocompetent host.[245]

The Burkitt-like AIDS-NHL may be a distinct clinical entity from the HIV-negative morphologic counterpart. Most AIDS–Burkitt-like lymphomas appear to have a molecular pattern similar to that of typical Burkitt's lymphoma: The c-myc oncogene appears to be rearranged in the majority of cases but not the bcl-2 gene,[216] whereas in HIV-negative Burkitt-like lymphomas, rearrangement of c-myc is uncommon, and the bcl-2 gene is rearranged in 30% of cases.[251] However, some features clearly differentiate AIDS–Burkitt-like lymphomas from AIDS-Burkitt's lymphomas. The frequency of EBV infection in AIDS–Burkitt-like lymphomas (80%) is similar to that in diffuse large cell lymphoma, but the pattern of viral latency is similar to that seen in Burkitt's lymphoma (i.e., no LMP-1 or EBNA-2 expression) in approximately 60% of the cases. Also, patients with AIDS–Burkitt-like lymphomas usually have a relatively low CD4 count, similar to that seen in the diffuse large cell immunoblastic lymphomas. However, Burkitt-like lymphomas do not seem to share the predilection for CNS involvement associated with Burkitt's lymphoma. Burkitt-like lymphomas may be a morphologic variant in a continuum from Burkitt's lymphoma to diffuse large cell lymphomas in the context of the range of immunodepletion that occurs in HIV-infected patients.

PRIMARY EFFUSION LYMPHOMA

PEL, also termed *body cavity lymphoma*, is a rare entity, and as the name implies, these tumors typically grow mainly in the pleural, pericardial, and abdominal cavities as lymphomatous effu-

TABLE 50.1-5. Selected Regimens and Outcomes for Acquired Immunodeficiency Syndrome–Associated Non-Hodgkin's Lymphoma

Regimen	*Evaluable Patients*	*Median Baseline CD4 Cells/μL*	*Complete Response Rate (%)*	*Median Overall/Disease-Free Survival (mo)*	*Author*
Low or standard dose m-BACOD	175	100 (low) 107 (standard)	41 (low) 52 (standard)	8/8	Kaplan et al.[283]
ACVB/LNH84	141	227	63	9/16	Gisselbrecht et al.[289]
Low or standard dose CHOP plus HAART	53	119	35 (low) 37 (standard)	Not available	Ratner et al.[288]
Infusional CDE	21	87	62	18/not available	Sparano et al.[384]
Dose-adjusted EPOCH	23	255	79	72%/83% at 23 mo (median, not yet reached)	Little et al.[294]

ACVB, doxorubicin, cyclophosphamide, vindesine, bleomycin, and prednisolone; CDE, cyclophosphamide, doxorubicin, and etoposide; CHOP, cyclophosphamide, hydroxydaunorubicin (Adriamycin),vincristine (Oncovin), and prednisone; EPOCH, etoposide, prednisone, vincristine, cyclophosphamide, and doxorubicin; HAART, highly active antiretroviral treatment; m-BACOD, methotrexate, bleomycin, doxorubicin (Adriamycin), cyclophosphamide, vincristine (Oncovin), dexamethasone.

sions.[217,252–255] Sometimes, however, the initial presentation can be nodal, and in some cases the tumor can involve soft tissue or the gastrointestinal tract. PELs exhibit distinctive clinical and biologic features, including immunoblastic morphology and indeterminate immunophenotype. Monoclonality can be established by the finding of clonal immunoglobulin gene rearrangements indicating late B-cell genotype derivation that may have undergone antigenic selection.[203,256] These tumors are universally associated with KSHV/HHV-8 and appear to follow the same epidemiologic pattern as KS (i.e., the greatest frequency of occurrence is among those who acquire HIV infection from an individual who has sex with other men).[253] The majority of PELs are also EBV positive, although some PEL cell lines are EBV negative, and these usually lack rearrangements in c-myc.[253,257–260] There is evidence that VEGF is involved in the pathogenesis of this tumor.[261] KSHV/HHV-8 up-regulates production of VEGF, and SCID/beige mice inoculated intraperitoneally with BCBL-1 cells (an KSHV/HHV-8 infected PEL cell line) develop effusion lymphoma. Treatment with neutralizing anti-VEGF antibody inhibits formation of the lymphoma.[262] While the role of KSHV/HHV-8 is unclear, this virus may have a direct transforming role in PEL. In particular, viral BCL-2, IL-6, and cyclin D homologues may serve to delay apoptotic cell death or stimulate lymphomatous cell proliferation.[54,59,259] These observations may provide insights toward developing novel therapeutic strategies for this rare tumor. These tumors are often quite resistant to cytotoxic chemotherapy.

CLINICAL PRESENTATION AND STAGING OF PERIPHERAL LYMPHOMAS

HIV-related NHLs frequently present as advanced stage 3 or 4 disease and behave aggressively with unusual patterns of organ involvement.[163,167,263,264] The majority of patients present with either a rapidly growing mass lesion or the development of systemic *B* symptoms (unexplained fever, drenching night sweats, or unexplained weight loss in excess of 10% of the normal body weight).[265] Extranodal involvement is common, including the bone marrow (25% to 40%), gastrointestinal tract (26%), and the CNS (17% to 32%).[167,168,211]

In addition to the standard NHL staging for HIV-negative patients, CD4 cell count, HIV viral load, and CNS assessment should be performed on all HIV-infected patients with lymphoma. Computed tomography of the brain with contrast is adequate to assess for parenchymal brain lesions, but magnetic resonance imaging with gadolinium has the potential advantage of revealing evidence of leptomeningeal involvement by lymphoma.[266] Cytologic examination of the cerebrospinal fluid should be performed in all cases.

NHL is significantly associated with a worse prognosis than many other complications of AIDS.[267] For systemic lymphomas, the factor most correlated with prognosis is the CD4 cell count. With standard therapy, patients with fewer than 100 CD4 cells/μL have a median survival of approximately 4 months, whereas those with 100 or greater CD4 cells/μL have a median survival of 11 months.[263,268] Other factors associated with poor outcome are age over 35 to 40 years, high serum lactate dehydrogenase levels, presence of extranodal sites, intravenous drug use, and preexisting AIDS diagnosis.[269,270] The international prognostic index for lymphoma is thus of some utility in AIDS-lymphomas, although its use is not widely reported.[271] In a multivariate analysis of 192 patients, patients who had none or one of such factors had a median survival of 46 weeks, and 30% were alive at 144 weeks, suggesting longer term survival can be achieved in the subset of patients without unfavorable characteristics.[272] With the advent of PAT, it is quite possible that overall prognosis in AIDS-NHL will improve.

TREATMENT OF PERIPHERAL ACQUIRED IMMUNODEFICIENCY SYNDROME LYMPHOMAS

Nearly two decades into the AIDS epidemic, optimal therapy for AIDS-NHL remains incompletely defined (Table 50.1-5). As noted previously, patients who develop AIDS-NHL continue to have a poor prognosis in spite of efforts to sort out the role of dose-intensive chemotherapy regimens for the immunocompromised host. The rapid improvements in therapy for the underlying HIV infection complicate the ability to compare clinical trials conducted at different times. To put this in perspective, it is instructive to consider some of the issues that have motivated the different treatment strategies for AIDS-NHL.

At the beginning of the AIDS epidemic, oncologists who treated AIDS-NHL recognized that patients frequently tolerated multiagent chemotherapy poorly, and that responses occurred in only a low percentage of patients and were often of short duration.[211,273,274] Importantly, in the early 1980s, prophylaxis against opportunistic infections had not yet been defined as standard practice,[275] and PAT was not available. At that point in time, second- and third-generation lymphoma regimens such as m-BACOD, ProMACE-CytaBOM, and MACOP-B were being explored in AIDS-NHL based on preliminary evidence that they may have been more efficacious in the treatment of lymphoma.[276–279] However, these regimens themselves were observed to sometimes cause opportunistic infections such as *Pneumocystis carinii* pneumonia in HIV-negative patients.[279,280] In 1993, an intergroup randomized trial failed to show that these regimens were more effective than cyclophosphamide, hydroxydaunorubicin (Adriamycin), Oncovin, and prednisone (CHOP) in HIV-negative patients and were perhaps associated with greater toxicity.[281] Before that report, based on early observations that these lymphoma regimens were toxic in AIDS patients, investigators began to consider lower dose modifications of the second- and third-generation lymphoma regimens in an attempt to reduce the toxicity and immunodeficiency caused by these regimens.[282] A large randomized trial comparing standard- with low-dose m-BACOD was completed in 1997, showing equivalent results in both groups, with complete responses ranging from 41% to 52%, but with a lower incidence of febrile neutropenia in the low-dose group.[283] However, the incidence of opportunistic infections was equivalent in both groups, and the low-dose arm was not shown to yield an improved survival outcome. Also, this study was not designed or adequately powered to determine if the subset of patients with more favorable HIV prognostic characteristics might have benefited from the higher dose intensity of the standard dose m-BACOD.[284] This issue is potentially important, as some studies of aggressive lymphomas in HIV-negative patients have suggested that chemotherapy dose intensity is associated with curative potential.[285] However, the strategy of low-dose chemotherapy clearly resulted in better quality of life with fewer treatment-related hospitalizations for a substantial proportion of the patients treated. In addition, several small studies using dose-reduced CHOP in AIDS-NHL have generally shown equivalent efficacy to standard dose CHOP, although the numbers are relatively small for assessment.[286–288]

At least one study suggests that more intensive chemotherapy may benefit the subset of patients with favorable prognostic factors. In a prospective multicenter study, 141 patients, with a median CD4 cell count of 227/µL, were treated with three cycles of doxorubicin, 75 mg/m^2; cyclophosphamide, 1200 mg/m^2; vindesine, 2 mg/m^2 for 2 days; bleomycin, 10 mg for 2 days; and prednisolone, 60 mg/m^2 for 5 days, followed by a consolidation phase of high-dose methotrexate plus leucovorin, ifosfamide, etoposide, asparaginase, and cytarabine (LNH84) and CNS prophylaxis with intrathecal methotrexate.[289] Zidovudine was started after chemotherapy. Eighty-nine patients (63%) achieved complete remission and 19 (13%) partial remission. With a median follow-up of 28 months, median survival and disease-free survival were 9 and 16 months, respectively. Twenty-three patients subsequently died of opportunistic infections while in complete remission. This study, conducted in the era before PAT, demonstrates that a subset of patients with AIDS-NHL were able to tolerate aggressive antilymphoma therapy and appeared to do reasonably well in terms of lymphoma-free survival. This study also highlights the potential importance of improved anti-HIV therapy in patients free of lymphoma.

A greater understanding of HIV disease has resulted in the standard prophylaxis against opportunistic infections and more effective treatment of the underlying HIV infection. These therapies have translated into improved survival and quality of life for patients with HIV disease. Prophylaxis for opportunistic infections clearly plays a major role during cytotoxic chemotherapy in such patients, but it is as yet unclear how advances in antiretroviral therapy will affect the treatment outcome of AIDS-NHL. To explore this issue, investigators have begun to administer newer antiretroviral regimens along with the chemotherapy regimens.[204,290] This is a complicated issue and as yet only scant data exist to guide best use of these drugs during chemotherapy. Preliminary results were recently reported from an NCI-sponsored trial conducted by the AIDS Malignancy Consortium. This trial involved 63 patients with a median CD4 cell count of 136/µL who received either modified or full-dose CHOP while receiving PAT with stavudine, lamivudine, and indinavir.[288] Sixty percent of patients had stage 3 or 4 lymphoma. HIV viral loads were stable, with many remaining below the level of detection for the test throughout the course of chemotherapy. The overall complete response rate for the trial was equivalent between the two dose groups: 33% for the modified and 32% for the full-dose group. These rates are similar to those previously reported without PAT,[274,283,286] although such comparisons may be of limited value. Pharmacokinetic data were collected and compared with historic controls. Elimination of cyclophosphamide was decreased from 70 mL/min/m^2 in historic controls to 39 mL/min/m^2 in the study patients, but without apparent effect on toxicity of the regimen. Doxorubicin elimination and the area under the time concentration curve of indinavir were similar to that in previous studies of these agents. These results highlight the feasibility of administering antineoplastic and antiretroviral drugs concomitantly, in spite of the potential complicated pharmacokinetics involved in this approach. At the same time, they show that there may be pharmacokinetic interactions and that there is room for improvement in the therapy of this disease.

In a study of 12 patients with AIDS-NHL treated with 96-hour continuous intravenous infusion of cyclophosphamide, doxorubicin, and etoposide (CDE) plus filgrastim, patients also received saquinavir and one or two nucleoside analogue anti-HIV drugs. Severe mucositis occurred in 8 of 12 patients (67%) treated with CDE plus saquinavir, which is more than the 3 in 25 (12%) rate of this toxicity in a previous trial of CDE without saquinavir.[291] This raises the possibility that pharmacokinetic interactions may have contributed to these different rates of toxicity. In addition, such approaches may affect the consistency of antiretroviral dosing.[287,291] In another trial of CDE, plasma etoposide levels were reported to be decreased by 11% to 38% on chemotherapy cycles given with didanosine compared with cycles without didanosine administration.[292] These results serve as a reminder that there may be complex and unexpected drug interactions when one attempts to combine complex chemotherapy regiments with complex anti-HIV regimens and that these interactions may affect the outcome of either therapy.

Preliminary results from a study at the NCI showed that 19 of 24 patients (79%) with HIV-associated NHL had a complete response using a modification of chemotherapy with etoposide, prednisone, vincristine, cyclophosphamide, and doxorubicin (EPOCH).[293,294] Cyclophosphamide was initially dosed according to CD4 count (187 mg/m^2 for CD4 cells less than 100/µL; 375 mg/m^2 if CD4 cells 100/µL or greater), and then adjusted up or down each cycle (by 187 mg/m^2 to a maximum of 750 mg/m^2)

depending on the neutrophil nadir. Antiretroviral therapy was suspended until completion of chemotherapy (maximum of six cycles), and then restarted. The median progression-free survival and overall survival had not been reached, but were 83% and 79%, respectively, at 22.5 months. Over 90% of the planned maximum dose intensity of doxorubicin [10 mg/m^2/24 hours continuous intravenous infusion (CIV) for 4 days], etoposide (50 mg/m^2/24 hours CIV × 4 days), and vincristine (0.4 mg/m^2/24 hours CIV × 4 days), and 56% of the cyclophosphamide was administered with relatively little associated toxicity. Febrile neutropenia occurred in only 12% of the cycles administered. No new opportunistic infections developed in these patients despite the withdrawal of antiretroviral treatment on initiation of chemotherapy (*Pneumocystis carinii* pneumonia prophylaxis was administered to all patients, and *Mycobacterium avium-complex* prophylaxis to at-risk patients). All patients who had responded to antiretroviral therapy before development of AIDS-NHL responded again to PAT when it was subsequently started postchemotherapy. CD4 counts recovered to baseline within 12 months after PAT reinstitution.[294] While this strategy may have the advantage of optimizing dose intensity and protecting patients against development of resistant HIV, some physicians may feel uncomfortable withdrawing antiretroviral therapy (even for a relatively short period of time), and the results require further study.

A high percentage (15% to 20%) of HIV-associated lymphomas have involvement of the CNS at presentation.[263] CNS progression is a potentially important cause of mortality in this setting,[274] and as patients potentially live longer with better antiretroviral treatment after chemotherapy, CNS relapse may become a relatively more important issue. Therefore, in HIV-associated lymphomas, routine CNS prophylaxis with intrathecal methotrexate or cytosine arabinoside should be considered standard practice.[187,295]

Novel approaches to AIDS-NHL are clearly needed. Infusional chemotherapy regimens appear to have a favorable toxicity profile and may be useful in AIDS-NHL, but comparative trials with conventional intravenous bolus regimens have not been conducted. Until such data are available, it is unclear whether the encouraging data from small phase II trials of CDE and etoposide, prednisone, vincristine, cyclophosphamide, and doxorubicin truly represent an advance in the treatment of this condition. There is current interest in the potential role of the anti-CD20 monoclonal antibody, rituximab (Rituxan) in AIDS-NHL, and trials are currently planned to test this approach. Interest has also evolved in the use of stem cell transplantation in AIDS-NHL. Both autologous and allogeneic transplantation, with transfer of HIV-resistant genes into the marrow infusate are areas of interest being studied in clinical trials. In a collaborative trial being conducted by investigators at the National Institutes of Health, nonmyeloablative matched-sibling donor allogeneic transplantation is being studied with encouraging initial results.[296]

PRIMARY CENTRAL NERVOUS SYSTEM LYMPHOMA IN ACQUIRED IMMUNODEFICIENCY SYNDROME

OVERVIEW AND PATHOLOGY

PCNSL makes up approximately 19% of AIDS-NHLs, which is substantially higher than that in non–AIDS-NHL (approximately 1%).[165,222,297] The frequency of PCNSL is more than 3000-fold higher in patients with AIDS than in the general population, occurring in up to 12% of HIV-infected individuals.[298] From 20% to 30% of CNS lesions in patients with AIDS are ultimately found to have PCNSL.[5,299,300] PCNSL is the second most common mass lesion found in patients with AIDS, and the most common brain tumor in this population.[301,302] The survival of patients with HIV-associated PCNSL is 2 to 5 months, which is substantially shorter than that in the non–HIV-infected population with PCNSL.[298,303] PCNSL occurs most frequently in patients with a CD4 cell count less than 50/µL and can occur in the setting of other CNS pathology such as toxoplasmosis.[163,303,304]

Definitive diagnosis of focal brain lesions in AIDS patients requires biopsy and yields a greater than 92% diagnostic rate.[305] However, there is often some reluctance to do this procedure. While stereotactic biopsy is generally safe, the location of some lesions poses technical challenge and can introduce potential morbidity to the patient as well as risk to the surgical team.[306] Therefore, in many medical centers it has become standard practice to treat AIDS patients who have focal brain lesions and antitoxoplasmosis antibodies empirically with antitoxoplasmosis therapy, reserving biopsy for those patients who are seronegative for antitoxoplasma antibodies or fail to respond to treatment.[307] However, delay in diagnosis can adversely affect survival in AIDS-PCNSL.[308] Such factors necessitate consideration of alternative, less invasive diagnostic modalities.

Computed tomography or magnetic resonance imaging scans usually demonstrate single or multiple contrast-enhancing masses that are not reliably distinguishable from toxoplasmosis or other CNS processes. Preliminary studies suggest that ^{18}F-fluoro-2-deoxyglucose and positron emission tomography may have some utility in distinguishing malignant and nonmalignant conditions, since high FDG uptake most likely represents a malignant process.[309] Also, there is some evidence that thallium 201 single photon emission computed tomography might be a useful, noninvasive method for differentiating intracranial lymphoma from nonneoplastic lesions in patients with AIDS.[310,311] However, these modalities have not been confirmed in large studies, and a high degree of intercenter variability in procedure may reduce the reliability of these techniques.

It has been shown that detection of CSF EBV DNA by polymerase chain reaction (PCR) in HIV-infected patients is reliably associated with PCNSLs,[312] lending support for the use of this assay as a diagnostic test for this condition. The basis for this approach is the observation that nearly all HIV-associated PCNSLs are associated with EBV infection.[313] In a series of 95 patients, including 40 patients with AIDS-PCNSL, the sensitivity and specificity of PCR for EBV DNA detection in lumbar CSF were 80% and 100%, respectively.[312] Lumbar puncture and subsequent assessment of EBV DNA would have allowed a correct diagnosis in 63.2% of patients with AIDS-PCNSL and excluded this diagnosis in 76.3% of patients without lymphoma (because EBV DNA was not detected).[312] Another group reported an even higher diagnostic confidence of AIDS-related focal brain lesions using minimally invasive procedures.[314] By combining CSF EBV DNA detection by PCR with ^{201}Tl single photon emission computed tomography, the presence of increased uptake, positive EBV DNA, or both had 100% sensitivity and 100% negative predictive value. Because PCNSL likelihood is extremely high in patients with hyperactive lesions and positive EBV DNA, brain biopsy may be avoided, and patients could promptly undergo definitive therapy.[314]

Most cases of PCNSL are of immunoblastic morphology with plasmacytic differentiation, large cell lymphomas with immunoblastic features, or are centroblastic polymorphic lymphomas.[223] SNCCL are rare. EBV is consistently detected by

PCR. The bcl-2 oncoprotein and LMP-1 of EBV are frequently strongly expressed. In a study of 11 AIDS-related primary brain lymphomas, LMP-1 and bcl-2 were expressed in all cases but one,[315] potentially implicating their involvement in CNS lymphomagenesis. Expression of mutated p53, or rearrangement of bcl-2 or the c-myc oncogene is not reported.[316,317] The precise histogenetic derivation and the molecular pathogenesis of PCNSL is poorly understood. Evidence suggests that these tumors may be segregated into two major biologic categories based on the expression pattern of BCL-6, LMP-1, and BCL-2.[318] In an analysis of 26 AIDS-related and 23 AIDS-unrelated PCNSL cases, expression of BCL-6 protein, which is restricted to GC B cells throughout physiologic B-cell maturation, was detected in all of the AIDS-unrelated PCNSL. However, only 56% of the AIDS-related cases expressed BCL-6. Expression of BCL-6 was mutually exclusive with expression of EBV-encoded LMP-1, and with few exceptions, of BCL-2. All but one PCNSL expressed hMSH2, which among mature B cells selectively stains GC B cells. Thus, a proportion of AIDS-PCNSLs may represent a divergent biologic spectrum from their non-AIDS counterparts.

TREATMENT

Treatment modalities for immunocompetent patients are applied to patients with AIDS-PCNL, but generally with substantially more toxicity and poorer results. PCNSL is highly responsive to whole brain irradiation, and a substantial proportion of patients can be expected to have complete tumor eradication; however, they have a high likelihood of subsequently succumbing to opportunistic infection[319] or recurrent lymphoma.[320] In a study of 55 AIDS patients with biopsy-proven primary CNS lymphomas, all tumors responded both clinically and radiologically to whole brain radiation therapy consisting of 4000 rad in 267-rad fractions over 3 weeks or an equivalent dose.[319] The mean duration of survival from the appearance of symptoms consistent with the mass lesion was significantly greater in patients who received radiation therapy than in those who did not (134 vs. 42 days). Autopsy findings showed that patients who did not receive radiation therapy generally died from tumor progression, whereas those who completed radiation therapy often died of opportunistic infections. Such observations emphasize the need for early diagnosis and treatment, and for treatment of opportunistic infections and the underlying HIV infection.[319] Relapse can occur remote from the primary site, but also within the radiation port.

Experience combining chemotherapy with radiotherapy suggests that a subgroup of patients can benefit from this approach, with survival reaching over 1 year.[320,321] However, this is still shorter than survival in non-AIDS patients, and still only a minority of patients so treated have survival greater than 1 year.[322]

Surgery has no therapeutic role in PCNSL since microscopic tumor infiltration into brain parenchyma extends from the site of primary involvement.[323]

EFFECT OF ANTIRETROVIRAL THERAPY ON PRIMARY CENTRAL NERVOUS SYSTEM LYMPHOMA INCIDENCE

Since AIDS-PCNSL appears to be an opportunistic illness associated with profound CD4 depletion (usually occurring in patients with less than 50 CD4 cells), it might be expected that better therapy for HIV would result in a decrease in the incidence of PCNSL. A large medical records analysis showed a decrease in the incidence of PCNSL from 8.5 cases per 1000 person-years in early 1994 to 0.9 cases per 1000 person-years in late 1996 ($P = .04$). This change was coincident with changes in antiretroviral treatment patterns and an increase in the use of two or more drugs from 20% to 46% of patients.[75] Other data support these findings.[28,188] However, many patients are now developing resistance to available therapies, and it is possible that the incidence may increase in the near future. Also, it is possible that the cumulative incidence of AIDS-related lymphomas may rise as patients live longer with HIV infection.[163]

HODGKIN'S DISEASE

EPIDEMIOLOGY

Although Hodgkin's disease is not an AIDS-defining condition, its association with HIV is apparent for several reasons: it presents in HIV-infected patients with distinct clinical and biologic characteristics that distinguish it from its HIV-negative counterpart (*primary* Hodgkin's disease); and it occurs with somewhat increased frequency among HIV-infected patients.[1,324,325] By contrast, many registries have indicated a slight decrease in primary Hodgkin's disease incidence in recent decades.[326] An eightfold excess of Hodgkin's disease in HIV-infected patients has been found by linking AIDS and cancer registry data.[12] However, there is some controversy over the epidemiology, as some studies have not found an increased incidence of Hodgkin's disease in areas of high prevalence for HIV infection.[327,328]

Overall, Hodgkin's disease of the nodular sclerosis subtype (the most frequent subtype in HIV-negative patients) has increased over time, whereas Hodgkin's disease of mixed cellularity has declined.[326] However, among HIV-infected patients, the most common histologic subtype is mixed cellularity, followed by lymphocyte depleted.[228,329–334]

PATHOGENESIS

EBV infection appears to be more predominant among cases of HIV-associated Hodgkin's disease than in cases of primary Hodgkin's disease.[334] Monoclonal expansions of EBV-infected cells have been found in from 78% to 100% of HIV-related Hodgkin's disease, but in only 15% to 48% of primary Hodgkin's disease cases.[227,333,335] EBV-encoded LMP-1 has been demonstrated in the tumor cells in from 25% to 50% of primary Hodgkin's disease cases, but in up to 100% of both the nodular sclerosing and mixed cellularity subtypes of Hodgkin's disease in HIV-positive patients.[335] The pattern of EBV gene expression may favor immune escape in HIV-related Hodgkin's disease. The EBV latency C promoter drives expression of the immunodominant EBNAs that are targeted by cytotoxic T lymphocytes. In EBV-associated Hodgkin's disease, the C promoter is inactive and the immunodominant EBNAs are thus not expressed.[336] This finding may be relevant to the frequent occurrence of Hodgkin's disease in relatively immunocompetent HIV-infected patients.[228,331,333]

CLINICAL PRESENTATION, TREATMENT, AND PROGNOSIS

Patients with HIV-associated Hodgkin's disease generally present at a younger age, with higher stage disease, less fre-

TABLE 50.1-6. Comparison of Human Immunodeficiency Virus–Associated Hodgkin's Disease and Primary Hodgkin's Disease

Feature	*Reference 333*		*Reference 331*		*Reference 228*
	HIV+ (n = 114)	HIV– (n = 104)	HIV+ (n = 45)	HIV– (n = 407)	HIV+ (n = 46)
Age (median)	29	38	30	31	27
CD4 (median)	275	N/A	306	N/A	—
Histology (%)					
MC	45	29	49	20	41
LD	21	—	4	—	22
NS	30	59	40	—	22
Mediastinal disease (%)					
NS	27	80	10	71	—
MC	23	21	3	—	—
Stage III–IV (%)	81	44	75	—	89
Extranodal disease (%)	63	29	33	—	>41
Epstein-Barr virus–positive tumor (%)	78	25			
B symptoms (%)	77	35	80	—	83
Prior acquired immunodeficiency syndrome diagnosis (%)	17	N/A	11	N/A	6

HIV, human immunodeficiency virus; LD, lymphocyte depleted; MC, mixed cellularity; NS, nodular sclerosing.

quent mediastinal involvement, more frequent involvement of extranodal sites of disease, and more frequent occurrence of B symptoms compared with their HIV-negative counterparts (Table 50.1-6).[333] These differences are more than can be accounted for by the overrepresentation of the mixed cellularity histologic subtype in HIV-associated Hodgkin's disease,[331] a histologic subtype that involves the mediastinal less often compared with nodular sclerosing Hodgkin's disease. Compared with AIDS-associated NHL, in which the CD4 cell count is frequently less than 100/µL, the median CD4 cell count in HIV-associated Hodgkin's disease has been reported to be over 275 cells/µL in large patient series.[228,331,333]

Prognosis is generally poorer for HIV-Hodgkin's disease than for primary Hodgkin's disease. HIV-Hodgkin's disease patients frequently have a number of features that have been associated with poor prognosis in primary non–HIV-associated Hodgkin's disease, including male sex, large number of sites involved, and mixed cellularity or lymphocyte-depleted histology.[337] Because of this, the precise contribution of HIV infection per se to the poor prognosis is uncertain. In general, complete response rates are relatively high with systemic chemotherapy (50% to over 80%),[333,338,339] although rates as low as 14% have also been reported.[340] Relapse of Hodgkin's disease and progression of AIDS are common, contributing to poor overall survival. The CD4 cell count at the time of diagnosis is a prognostic factor. Patients with a CD4 cell count less than 250 to 200 CD4 cells/µL have a median survival of less than 11 months,[331,333] whereas higher CD4 cell counts are associated with somewhat better outcome. Although most patients do not have an AIDS diagnosis when they develop HIV-Hodgkin's disease, 48% to 71% develop AIDS within 3 years after treatment for HIV-Hodgkin's disease,[331,333] compared with development of AIDS in 22% for most other HIV-infected patients with similar CD4 cell counts.[341] These findings underscore the need for skilled management of the underlying HIV.

Most patients with HIV-Hodgkin's disease are treated with conventional chemotherapy regimens (i.e., radiotherapy, mechlorethamine, vincristine, procarbazine, and prednisone; doxorubicin, bleomycin, vinblastine, and dacarbazine; or alternating the two regimens; epirubicin, bleomycin, vinblastine, and prednisone; or combined modality therapy).[329,338,342] Because of the occurrence of multiple poor prognostic factors in HIV-Hodgkin's disease, most oncologists advocate use of systemic chemotherapy in all clinically staged patients. The CNS is rarely involved, so CNS prophylaxis is not commonly used. Strategies to improve outcome have included the use of antiretrovirals and colony-stimulating factors, but before the use of protease inhibitor anti-HIV therapy, outcomes were essentially equivalent among trials.[338,339,343] It is hoped that treatment outcomes with PAT may change these grim statistics.

ANOGENITAL CANCERS IN HUMAN IMMUNODEFICIENCY VIRUS INFECTION

Cervical cancer was added to the CDC list of AIDS-defining conditions in 1993.[21] Anal cancer, though not an AIDS-defining condition, is also relatively prevalent among HIV-infected women and homosexual and bisexual men with HIV infection.[344] These cancers are associated with human papillomavirus (HPV) infection[345] and appear to be more aggressive in HIV-infected than in non–HIV-infected individuals. It is thus recommended that HIV-infected women undergo regular periodic cervical Papanicolaou (Pap) testing. The CDC has recommended cytologic screening as part of the initial evaluation when HIV seropositivity is diagnosed. The CDC recommends that if the initial Pap smear is normal, at least one additional evaluation should be repeated within 6 months.[346] If the repeat result is normal, then reevaluation should be done at least annually. If the initial or follow-up Pap smear shows severe inflammation with reactive squamous cellular changes, another Pap smear should be collected within 3 months. If the initial or follow-up Pap smear shows squamous intraepithelial lesions or atypical squamous cells of undetermined significance, the woman should be referred for a colposcopic examination of the lower genital tract and, if indicated, undergo colposcopically directed biopsies. HIV infection is not an indication for colposcopy among women with normal Pap smear results. Because of the common occurrence of HPV-associated cytologic abnormalities in the anal mucosa of both HIV-infected women and homosexual men, some experts have suggested that routine periodic cytologic examination of the anal mucosa should also be considered in high-risk individuals.[6,347–349] A model to estimate the clinical benefits and cost-effectiveness of screening HIV-positive homosexual and bisexual men for anal squamous intraepithelial lesions and anal squamous cell cancer indicates that Pap screening every 1 to 2 years beginning in early HIV disease would result in an incremental cost-effectiveness ratio of $13,000 to $16,000 per quality-adjusted life year saved, and thus offers quality-adjusted life expectancy benefits at a cost comparable with other accepted clinical preventive interventions.[350]

CERVICAL CANCER

Epidemiology

Squamous intraepithelial lesions, vulvovaginal condyloma acuminata, and anal intraepithelial neoplasia are seen with approximately fivefold increase in HIV-infected women compared with women not infected with HIV.[6,351,352] The prevalence of cervical intraepithelial neoplasia has been reported to range from 11% to 29% overall for HIV-infected women,[6,353] which may be higher than the 4% to 13% prevalence in HIV-negative women.[354,355] Among sexually active women, HIV-infected women have a substantially higher rate of persistent HPV infections of the types most strongly associated with intraepithelial lesions and invasive cervical cancer (i.e., HPV-16 or HPV-18).[356,357] HPV infection is associated with development of squamous intraepithelial lesions[358] and increased prevalence of HPV infection among HIV-infected women may explain the increased incidence of squamous intraepithelial lesions in this population.[359] Greater immune suppression is associated with increased incidence of high-grade cervical intraepithelial neoplasia in HIV-infected women, who may also present with invasive cervical cancer at a younger age and with more aggressive advanced stage disease compared with HIV-seronegative women.[8,360] This suggests that progression of HPV-associated dysplasia to frank invasive anogenital cancers may be more rapid in this population. Women with a CD4 cell count less than 500/μL appear to be at greater risk for poor outcome.[360] The incidence of invasive cervical cancer appears unchanged since the advent of PAT,[75] but it is unclear whether this is due to reduce usage of these medications among the women at highest risk for both HIV and HPV, or some other factor. Likewise, the effect of PAT on the incidence of anal squamous intraepithelial lesions is as yet unclear, but the data suggest that PAT may not result in regression of these lesions.[361]

Progressive immune deficiency may increase the risk of persistent oncogenic HPV infection,[347,362] but the association between HIV infection and HPV-associated anogenital disease could also be related to molecular mechanisms of HIV modulation of HPV expression.[363] For example, HIV Tat increases HPV-16 upstream regulatory region-directed chloramphenicol acetyltransferase expression driven by the native HPV-16 promoter (P97). Tat also reverses E2-mediated repression of P97-directed chloramphenicol acetyltransferase expression. Treatment of cells with HIV, Tat, or IL-6 modulates the expression of naturally integrated HPV-18 genes at the transcriptional level. However, in cell lines, the translation of HPV-18 proteins seems to occur only during HIV coinfection.[364,365] HIV Rev and Rev-responsive elements appear to modulate expression of the HPV type 16 L1 protein in epithelial cells.[366,367]

Among women infected with HPV-16 who have not developed cervical intraepithelial neoplasia, the amount of HPV-16 DNA in cervicovaginal lavage is significantly increased in those who are infected with HIV.[368] Consistent with this thesis is the observation that women with HIV viral loads over 10,000 copies per milliliter are at relatively higher risk of HPV infection-related abnormal PAP smear results.[369] Also, HPV appears to be more persistent in the anal mucosa of HIV-infected individuals.[370] Thus, it appears that HIV may be a cofactor for the oncogenic effects of HPV.

Therapy

Standard therapy for preinvasive cervical neoplasia, including cryotherapy, laser therapy, cone biopsy, and loop excision, appears to be somewhat less effective in women with HIV infection due to the twofold higher frequency of recurrence even among those with high CD4 cell count.[371] The lower the CD4 count, the higher the risk for recurrence. Preliminary data suggest that early preinvasive lesions can regress with effective antiretroviral therapy,[372] and that PAT reduces recurrence and progression following standard excisional therapy.[373]

Invasive cervical cancer should be approached with the same principles of oncologic management that guide treatment of cervical cancer in HIV-negative patients. Patients with well-controlled HIV infection and relative immune preservation can be expected to have outcomes similar to that of HIV-negative women. Patients with advanced HIV disease may be more intolerant of the myelosuppressive effects of radiation therapy and combination chemotherapy. When such therapy is administered concomitantly with antiretroviral therapy, potential for overlapping toxicity of the various agents should be considered in the therapeutic plan. Following surgery, recurrence is common.[374]

ANAL CANCER

Evidence of HPV infection of the anal canal and anal cancer and the immediate precursor lesions, high-grade anal intraepithelial neoplasia, are common among HIV-infected women[6] and among men who have sex with men, especially those with HIV or immunosuppression.[347,375] HPV infection of the anal epithelium has been reported to be double that of cervical and the prevalence of anal cytologic abnormalities in HIV-infected women have been reported to be 14% to 27%[6,352] compared with 7% in HIV-negative women.[352] Among men, a longitudinal study conducted of 287 HIV-seronegative and 322 HIV-seropositive men attending a community-based clinic revealed anal HPV DNA at entry among 91.6% of men with HIV and 65.9% of men without HIV.[370] History of recent anal warts predicted for HPV DNA in all men. Anal squamous intraepithelial lesions do not appear to regress in patients receiving PAT, but among those with high CD4 cell counts the effect appears to be variable.[376]

For invasive anal cancer, standard combined chemotherapy and radiation appears to effectively control disease in most patients.[377,378] Patients with CD4 counts less than 200/µL appear more likely to suffer treatment-related toxicity including cytopenias, intractable diarrhea, or moist desquamation requiring hospitalization or a colostomy either for a therapy-related complication or for salvage. Patients with CD4 of 200/µL or greater appear to have better disease control with acceptable morbidity.

FUTURE DIRECTIONS

Most AIDS-associated cancers are virally mediated neoplastic processes. In this regard, HIV can play a varied role. It can induce an immunosuppressed host in which oncogenic viral infection and opportunistic neoplasia can develop relatively unchecked, and it can serve to stimulate the immune system to secrete cytokines that promote cellular proliferation and oligoclonal expansions of cells infected with a variety of known oncogenic viruses. Molecular interactions between HIV-related proteins (or factors induced by HIV) and genomic sequences in some of these viruses may modulate their oncogenic potential. Many AIDS-associated cancers thus appear to be preventable. However, as with other cancers, it is unlikely that behavioral prevention alone will eliminate these epidemic neoplasms. Great strides in the treatment of HIV infection have been made, although it is too soon to determine the ultimate effect of these advances on opportunistic neoplastic disease. The greater understanding of the virologic and molecular basis of these cancers may provide opportunities for advancement in prevention and treatment through antiangiogenesis approaches, antiviral-, vaccine-, and immune-based therapies. Research in AIDS malignancies has the potential to affect a number of other important fields in oncology, including general tumor angiogenesis, viral oncogenesis, immunologic control of tumors, and molecular pathogenesis of tumors. This should prove to be a fruitful area of research over the next decade.

REFERENCES

1. Goedert JJ, Cote TR, Virgo P, et al. Spectrum of AIDS-associated malignant disorders. *Lancet* 1998;351:1833.
2. Grulich AE, Wan X, Law MG, Coates M, Kaldor JM. Risk of cancer in people with AIDS. *AIDS* 1999;13:839.
3. MMWR. Surveillance for AIDS-defining opportunistic illnesses, 1992–1997. Atlanta: Centers for Disease Control and Prevention, 1999:SS2.
4. Biggar RJ, Rosenberg PS, Cote T. Kaposi's sarcoma and non-Hodgkin's lymphoma following the diagnosis of AIDS. Multistate AIDS/Cancer Match Study Group. *Int J Cancer* 1996;68:754.
5. Beral V, Peterman T, Berkelman R, Jaffe H. AIDS-associated non-Hodgkin lymphoma. *Lancet* 1991;337:805.
6. Williams AB, Darragh TM, Vranizan K, et al. Anal and cervical human papillomavirus infection and risk of anal and cervical epithelial abnormalities in human immunodeficiency virus-infected women. *Obstet Gynecol* 1994;83:205.
7. Chiasson MA, Ellerbrock TV, Bush TJ, Sun XW, Wright TC Jr. Increased prevalence of vulvovaginal condyloma and vulvar intraepithelial neoplasia in women infected with the human immunodeficiency virus. *Obstet Gynecol* 1997;89:690.
8. Northfelt DW. Cervical and anal neoplasia and HPV infection in persons with HIV infection. *Oncology (Huntingt)* 1994;8:33;discussion 38.
9. MMWR. Kaposi's sarcoma and pneumocystis pneumonia among homosexual men—New York City and California. Atlanta: Centers for Disease Control, 1981.
10. Beral V, Peterman TA, Berkelman RL, Jaffe HW. Kaposi's sarcoma among persons with AIDS: a sexually transmitted infection? *Lancet* 1990;335:123.
11. Rabkin CS, Biggar RJ, Horm JW. Increasing incidence of cancers associated with the human immunodeficiency virus epidemic. *Int J Cancer* 1991;47:692.
12. Biggar RJ, Rabkin CS. The epidemiology of AIDS-related neoplasms. *Hematol Oncol Clin North Am* 1996;10:997.
13. Kaposi M. Idiopathisches multiples Pigmensarkom der Haut. *Arch Derm Syph* 1872;4:265.
14. Gottlieb MS, Schroff R, Schanker HM, et al. *Pneumocystis carinii* pneumonia and mucosal candidiasis in previously healthy homosexual men: evidence of a new acquired cellular immunodeficiency. *N Engl J Med* 1981;305:1425.
15. Masur H, Michelis MA, Greene JB, et al. An outbreak of community-acquired *Pneumocystis carinii* pneumonia: initial manifestation of cellular immune dysfunction. *N Engl J Med* 1981;305:1431.
16. Gallo RC, Salahuddin SZ, Popovic M, et al. Frequent detection and isolation of cytopathic retroviruses (HTLV-III) from patients with AIDS and at risk for AIDS. *Science* 1984;224:500.
17. Laurence J, Brun-Vezinet F, Schutzer SE, et al. Lymphadenopathy-associated viral antibody in AIDS. Immune correlations and definition of a carrier state. *N Engl J Med* 1984; 311:1269.
18. deFrancesco S, Austin D, Bordowitz G, Carlomusto J, Hoskins V. The design and development of AIDS educational materials. *Int Conf AIDS* 1990;6:306(abst F.D.898).
19. MMWR. US HIV and AIDS cases reported through December 1994. HIV/AIDS Surveillance Report. Vol. 6. Atlanta: Centers for Disease Control and Prevention, 1995:1.
20. Safai B, Johnson KG, Myskowski PL, et al. The natural history of Kaposi's sarcoma in the acquired immunodeficiency syndrome. *Ann Intern Med* 1985;103:744.
21. MMWR. 1993 Revised classification system for HIV infection and expanded surveillance case definition for AIDS among adolescents and adults. *MMWR* 1992;41(RR-17).
22. Wabinga HR, Parkin DM, Wabwire-Mangen F, Mugerwa JW. Cancer in Kampala, Uganda, in 1989-91: changes in incidence in the era of AIDS. *Int J Cancer* 1993;54:26.
23. Parkin DM, Wabinga H, Nambooze S, Wabwire-Mangen F. AIDS-related cancers in Africa: maturation of the epidemic in Uganda. *AIDS* 1999;13:2563.
24. Moore PS, Chang Y. Detection of herpesvirus-like DNA sequences in Kaposi's sarcoma in patients with and without HIV infection. *N Engl J Med* 1995;332:1181.
25. Chang Y, Cesarman E, Pessin M, et al. Identification of herpesvirus-like DNA sequences in AIDS-associated Kaposi's sarcoma. *Science* 1994;266:1865.
26. O'Brien TR, Kedes D, Ganem D, et al. Evidence for concurrent epidemics of human herpesvirus 8 and human immunodeficiency virus type 1 in US homosexual men: rates, risk factors, and relationship to Kaposi's sarcoma. *J Infect Dis* 1999;180:1010.
27. Jacobson LP. *Impact of highly effective antiretroviral therapy on the incidence of malignancies among HIV-infected individuals.* Second National AIDS Malignancy Conference, Bethesda, MD, April 6–8, 1998.
28. Costagliola D. Clinical manifestations of HIV infections in the era of highly active antiretroviral treatment (HAART) in France. *Int Conf AIDS* Vol. 12, Geneva, 1998.
29. Kedes DH, Operskalski E, Busch M, et al. The seroepidemiology of human herpesvirus 8 (Kaposi's sarcoma-associated herpesvirus): distribution of infection in KS risk groups and evidence for sexual transmission. *Nat Med* 1996;2:918.
30. Martin JN, Ganem DE, Osmond DH, et al. Sexual transmission and the natural history of human herpesvirus 8 infection. *N Engl J Med* 1998;338:948.
31. Melbye M, Cook P, Hjalgrim H, et al. *Risk factors for HHV-8 seropositivity and progression to Kaposi's sarcoma in a cohort of homosexual men, 1981–96.* 1st National AIDS Malignancy Conference, Bethesda, MD, April 1, 1997, Vol. 14. Lippincott-Raven.
32. Renwick N, Halaby T, Weverling GJ, et al. Seroconversion for human herpesvirus 8 during HIV infection is highly predictive of Kaposi's sarcoma. *AIDS* 1998;12:2481.
33. Rutgers JL, Wieczorek R, Bonetti F, et al. The expression of endothelial cell surface antigens by AIDS-associated Kaposi's sarcoma. Evidence for a vascular endothelial cell origin. *Am J Pathol* 1986;122:493.
34. Uccini S, Ruco LP, Monardo F, et al. Co-expression of endothelial cell and macrophage antigens in Kaposi's sarcoma cells. *J Pathol* 1994;173:23.
35. Russell Jones R, Orchard G, Zelger B, Wilson Jones E. Immunostaining for CD31 and CD34 in Kaposi sarcoma. *J Clin Pathol* 1995;48:1011.
36. Rabkin CS, Janz S, Lash A, et al. Monoclonal origin of multicentric Kaposi's sarcoma lesions. *N Engl J Med* 1997;336:988.
37. Ensoli B, Nakamura S, Salahuddin SZ, et al. AIDS-Kaposi's sarcoma-derived cells express cytokines with autocrine and paracrine growth effects. *Science* 1989;243:223.
38. Miles SA, Rezai AR, Salazar-Gonzalez JF, et al. AIDS Kaposi sarcoma-derived cells produce and respond to interleukin 6. *Proc Natl Acad Sci U S A* 1990;87:4068.
39. Friedlander M, Brooks PC, Shaffer RW, et al. Definition of two angiogenic pathways by distinct alpha v integrins. *Science* 1995;270:1500.
40. Zarling JM, Shoyab M, Marquardt H, et al. a growth regulator produced by differentiated histiocytic lymphoma cells. *Proc Natl Acad Sci U S A* 1986;83:9739.
41. Vasse M, Pourtau J, Trochon V, et al. Oncostatin M induces angiogenesis in vitro and in vivo. *Arterioscler Thromb Vasc Biol* 1999;19:1835.
42. Modur V, Feldhaus MJ, Weyrich AS, et al. Oncostatin M is a proinflammatory mediator. In vivo effects correlate with endothelial cell expression of inflammatory cytokines and adhesion molecules. *J Clin Invest* 1997;100:158.
43. Nair BC, DeVico AL, Nakamura S, et al. Identification of a major growth factor for AIDS-Kaposi's sarcoma cells as oncostatin M. *Science* 1992;255:1430.
44. Miles SA, Martinez-Maza O, Rezai A, et al. Oncostatin M as a potent mitogen for AIDS-Kaposi's sarcoma-derived cells. *Science* 1992;255:1432.
45. Wijelath ES, Carlsen B, Cole T, et al. Oncostatin M induces basic fibroblast growth factor expression in endothelial cells and promotes endothelial cell proliferation, migration and spindle morphology. *J Cell Sci* 1997;110:871.
46. Murakami-Mori K, Taga T, Kishimoto T, Nakamura S. The soluble form of the IL-6 receptor (sIL-6R alpha) is a potent growth factor for AIDS-associated Kaposi's sarcoma (KS) cells; the soluble form of gp130 is antagonistic for sIL-6R alpha-induced AIDS-KS cell growth. *Int Immunol* 1996;8:595.
47. Murakami-Mori K, Taga T, Kishimoto T, Nakamura S. AIDS-associated Kaposi's sarcoma (KS) cells express oncostatin M (OM)- specific receptor but not leukemia inhibitory factor/OM receptor or interleukin-6 receptor. Complete block of OM-induced KS cell growth and OM binding by anti-gp130 antibodies. *J Clin Invest* 1995;96:1319.
48. Whitby D, Howard MR, Tenant-Flowers M, et al. Detection of Kaposi sarcoma associated her-

pesvirus in peripheral blood of HIV-infected individuals and progression to Kaposi's sarcoma. *Lancet* 1995;346:799.
49. Humphrey RW, O'Brien TR, Newcomb FM, et al. Kaposi's sarcoma (KS)-associated herpesvirus-like DNA sequences in peripheral blood mononuclear cells (PBMCs): association with KS and persistence in patients receiving anti-herpes drugs. *Blood* 1996;88:297.
50. Boshoff C, Schulz TF, Kennedy MM, et al. Kaposi's sarcoma-associated herpesvirus infects endothelial and spindle cells. *Nat Med* 1995;1:1274.
51. Gao SJ, Kingsley L, Li M, et al. KSHV antibodies among Americans, Italians and Ugandans with and without Kaposi's sarcoma. *Nat Med* 1996;2:925.
52. Staskus KA, Zhong W, Gebhard K, et al. Kaposi's sarcoma-associated herpesvirus gene expression in endothelial (spindle) tumor cells. *J Virol* 1997;71:715.
53. Davis DA, Humphrey RW, Newcomb FM, et al. Detection of serum antibodies to a Kaposi's sarcoma-associated herpesvirus-specific peptide. *J Infect Dis* 1997;175:1071.
54. Moore PS, Boshoff C, Weiss RA, Chang Y. Molecular mimicry of human cytokine and cytokine response pathway genes by KSHV. *Science* 1996;274:1739.
55. Boshoff C, Endo Y, Collins PD, et al. Angiogenic and HIV-inhibitory functions of KSHV-encoded chemokines. *Science* 1997;278:290.
56. Arvanitakis L, Geras-Raaka E, Varma A, Gershengorn MC, Cesarman E. Human herpesvirus KSHV encodes a constitutively active G-protein-coupled receptor linked to cell proliferation. *Nature* 1997;385:347.
57. Bais C, Santomasso B, Coso O, et al. G-protein-coupled receptor of Kaposi's sarcoma-associated herpesvirus is a viral oncogene and angiogenesis activator. *Nature* 1998;391:86.
58. Flore O, Rafii S, Ely S, et al. Transformation of primary human endothelial cells by Kaposi's sarcoma-associated herpesvirus. *Nature* 1998;394:588.
59. Cesarman E, Nador RG, Bai F, et al. Kaposi's sarcoma-associated herpesvirus contains G protein-coupled receptor and cyclin D homologs which are expressed in Kaposi's sarcoma and malignant lymphoma. *J Virol* 1996;70:8218.
60. Gershengorn MC, Geras-Raaka E, Varma A, Clark-Lewis I. Chemokines activate Kaposi's sarcoma-associated herpesvirus G protein-coupled receptor in mammalian cells in culture. *J Clin Invest* 1998;102:1469.
61. Ensoli B, Barillari G, Salahuddin SZ, Gallo RC, Wong-Staal F. Tat protein of HIV-1 stimulates growth of cells derived from Kaposi's sarcoma lesions of AIDS patients. *Nature* 1990;345:84.
62. Barillari G, Gendelman R, Gallo RC, Ensoli B. The Tat protein of human immunodeficiency virus type 1, a growth factor for AIDS Kaposi sarcoma and cytokine-activated vascular cells, induces adhesion of the same cell types by using integrin receptors recognizing the RGD amino acid sequence. *Proc Natl Acad Sci U S A* 1993;90:7941.
63. Albini A, Barillari G, Benelli R, Gallo RC, Ensoli B. Angiogenic properties of human immunodeficiency virus type 1 Tat protein. *Proc Natl Acad Sci U S A* 1995;92:4838.
64. Du Clary F, Bendenoun M, Eliaszewicz M, Treilhou M, Dupont B. Prolonged recovery of visceral Kaposi sarcoma in two AIDS patients treated with HAART including antiprotease 6 months after the end of chemotherapy: first report. *Int Conf AIDS* Vol. 12, Geneva, 1998.
65. Santambrogio S, Ridolfo AL, Tosca N, et al. *Effect of highly active antiretroviral treatment (HAART) in patients with AIDS-associated Kaposi's sarcoma (KS).* 12th World AIDS Conference, Geneva, June 28 to July 3, 1998.
66. Ohori M, Wheeler TM, Scardino PT. The New American Joint Committee on Cancer and International Union Against Cancer TNM classification of prostate cancer. Clinicopathologic correlations. *Cancer* 1994;74:104.
67. Krown SE, Metroka C, Wernz JC. Kaposi's sarcoma in the acquired immunodeficiency syndrome: a proposal for uniform evaluation, response, and staging criteria. *J Clin Oncol* 1989; 7:1201.
68. Krown SE, Testa MA, Huang J. AIDS-related Kaposi's sarcoma: prospective validation of the AIDS Clinical Trials Group staging classification. AIDS Clinical Trials Group Oncology Committee. *J Clin Oncol* 1997;15:3085.
69. Tambussi G, Repetto L, Torri V, et al. Epidemic HIV-related Kaposi's sarcoma: a retrospective analysis and validation of TIS staging. GICAT. Gruppo Italiano Collaborativo AIDS e Tumori. *Ann Oncol* 1995;6:383.
70. Antinori A, Izzi I, Ammassari A, et al. Evaluation of different staging systems for Kaposi's sarcoma in HIV-infected patients. *J Cancer Res Clin Oncol* 1992;118:635.
71. Jacobson LP, Kirby AJ, Polk S, et al. Changes in survival after acquired immunodeficiency syndrome (AIDS): 1984–1991. *Am J Epidemiol* 1993;138:952.
72. Mellors JW, Munoz A, Giorgi JV, et al. Plasma viral load and CD4+ lymphocytes as prognostic markers of HIV-1 infection. *Ann Intern Med* 1997;126:946.
73. Mitsuyasu RT, Taylor JMG, Glaspy J, Fahey JL. Heterogeneity of epidemic Kaposi's sarcoma. Implications for therapy. *Cancer* 1986;57:1657.
74. Yarchoan R, Venzon DJ, Pluda JM, et al. CD4 count and the risk for death in patients infected with HIV receiving antiretroviral therapy. *Ann Intern Med* 1991;115:184.
75. Jones J, Hanson D, Ward J. *Effect of antiretroviral therapy on recent trends in cancers among HIV-infected persons.* Second National AIDS Malignancy Conference, Bethesda, MD, April 6–8, 1998.
76. Rabkin CS, Testa MA, Huang J, Von Roenn JH. Kaposi's sarcoma and non-Hodgkin's lymphoma incidence trends in AIDS Clinical Trial Group study participants. *J Acquir Immune Defic Syndr* 1999;21(Suppl 1):S31.
77. Northfelt DW. Treatment of Kaposi's sarcoma. Current guidelines and future perspectives. *Drugs* 1994;48:569.
78. Serfling U, Hood AF. Local therapies for cutaneous Kaposi's sarcoma in patients with acquired immunodeficiency syndrome. *Arch Dermatol* 1991;127:1479.
79. Konzelman JL, Smith K, Swango P, et al. Vinblastine iontophoresis of Kaposi's sarcoma (KS). *Int Conf AIDS*, Vol. 8, Amsterdam, 1992.
80. Smith KJ, Konzelman JL, Lombardo FA, et al. Iontophoresis of vinblastine into normal skin and for treatment of Kaposi's sarcoma in human immunodeficiency virus-positive patients. The Military Medical Consortium for Applied Retroviral Research. *Arch Dermatol* 1992;128:1365.
81. Lucatorto FM, Sapp JP. Treatment of oral Kaposi's sarcoma with a sclerosing agent in AIDS patients. A preliminary study. *Oral Surg Oral Med Oral Pathol* 1993;75:192.
82. Kaliebe T, Schmitz T, Schroder U, Maciejewski W, Breit R. Cryotherapy of AIDS-related Kaposi's sarcoma. *Int Conf AIDS*, Vol. 9, 1993.
83. Dman-Kien AF, Conant M. North American phase 3 study (protocol L1057T-31) of Panretin gel (LGD1057, ALRT1057) for cutaneous AIDS-related Kaposi's sarcoma. *Int Conf AIDS* 1998;12:319.
84. Bodsworth N. Topical 9-cis-retinoic acid (Panretin) gel as treatment of cutaneous AIDS-related Kaposi's sarcoma: interim results of an international, placebo-controlled trial (ALRT 1057-503). International Panretin KS Study Group, *Int Conf AIDS*, Vol. 12, Geneva, 1998.
85. Kirova YM, Belembaogo E, Frikha H, et al. Radiotherapy in the management of epidemic Kaposi's sarcoma: a retrospective study of 643 cases. *Radiother Oncol* 1998;46:19.
86. Hughes-Davies L, Young T, Spittle M. Radiosensitivity in AIDS patients [letter]. *Lancet* 1991;337:1616.
87. Hadderingh RJ, van der Meulen FW. Carbon dioxide laser treatment of oral Kaposi's sarcoma. *Int Conf AIDS*, Vol. 5, 1989.
88. Conill C, Alsina M, Verger E, Henriquez I. Radiation therapy in AIDS-related cutaneous Kaposi's sarcoma. *Dermatology* 1997;195:40.
89. Harrison M, Harrington KJ, Tomlinson DR, Stewart JS. Response and cosmetic outcome of two fractionation regimens for AIDS-related Kaposi's sarcoma. *Radiother Oncol* 1998;46:23.
90. Nobler MP. Pulmonary irradiation for Kaposi's sarcoma in AIDS. *Am J Clin Oncol* 1985;8:441.
91. Schweitzer VG, Visscher D. Photodynamic therapy for treatment of AIDS-related oral Kaposi's sarcoma. *Otolaryngol Head Neck Surg* 1990;102:639.
92. Bernstein ZP, Wilson BD, Oseroff AR, et al. Photofrin photodynamic therapy for treatment of AIDS-related cutaneous Kaposi's sarcoma. *AIDS* 1999;13:1697.
93. Krown SE, Real FX, Cunningham-Rundles S, et al. Preliminary observations on the effect of recombinant leukocyte A interferon in homosexual men with Kaposi's sarcoma. *N Engl J Med* 1983;308:1071.
94. Groopman JE, Gottlieb MS, Goodman J, et al. Recombinant alpha-2 interferon therapy for Kaposi's sarcoma associated with the acquired immunodeficiency syndrome. *Ann Intern Med* 1984;100:671.
95. Fischl MA, Finkelstein DM, He W, et al. A phase II study of recombinant human interferon-alpha 2a and zidovudine in patients with AIDS-related Kaposi's sarcoma. AIDS Clinical Trials Group. *J Acquir Immune Defic Syndr Hum Retrovirol* 1996;11:379.
96. Volberding PA, Abrams DI, Conant M, et al. Vinblastine therapy for Kaposi's sarcoma in the acquired immunodeficiency syndrome. *Ann Intern Med* 1985;103:335.
97. Laubenstein LJ, Krigel RL, Odajnyk CM, et al. Treatment of epidemic Kaposi's sarcoma with etoposide or a combination of doxorubicin, bleomycin, and vinblastine. *J Clin Oncol* 1984;2:1115.
98. Gill PS, Rarick M, McCutchan JA, et al. Systemic treatment of AIDS-related Kaposi's sarcoma: results of a randomized trial. *Am J Med* 1991;90:427.
99. Yarchoan R. Therapy for Kaposi's sarcoma: recent advances and experimental approaches. *J Acquir Immune Defic Syndr* 1999;21(Suppl 1):S66.
100. Presant CA, Scolaro M, Kennedy P, et al. Liposomal daunorubicin treatment of HIV-associated Kaposi's sarcoma. *Lancet* 1993;341:1242.
101. Gill PS, Espina BM, Muggia F, et al. Phase I/II clinical and pharmacokinetic evaluation of liposomal daunorubicin. *J Clin Oncol* 1995;13:996.
102. Harrison M, Tomlinson D, Stewart S. Liposomal-entrapped doxorubicin: an active agent in AIDS-related Kaposi's sarcoma. *J Clin Oncol* 1995;13:914.
103. Northfelt DW, Dezube BJ, Thommes JA, et al. Efficacy of pegylated-liposomal doxorubicin in the treatment of AIDS-related Kaposi's sarcoma after failure of standard chemotherapy. *J Clin Oncol* 1997;15:653.
104. Gill PS, Wernz J, Scadden DT, et al. Randomized phase III trial of liposomal daunorubicin versus doxorubicin, bleomycin, and vincristine in AIDS-related Kaposi's sarcoma. *J Clin Oncol* 1996;14:2353.
105. Northfelt DW, Dezube B, Thommes J, et al. Randomized comparative trial of Doxil vs. adriamycin, bleomycin, and vincristine (ABV) in the treatment of severe AIDS-related Kaposi's sarcoma (AIDS-KS). *3rd Conf Retro Opportun Infect* 1996:123.
106. Stewart S, Jablonowski H, Goebel FD, et al. Randomized comparative trial of pegylated liposomal doxorubicin versus bleomycin and vincristine in the treatment of AIDS-related Kaposi's sarcoma. International Pegylated Liposomal Doxorubicin Study Group. *J Clin Oncol* 1998;16:683.
107. Mitsuyas R, Roenn JY, Krown S, et al. *Comparison study of liposomal doxorubicin (DOX) alone or with bleomycin and vincristine (DBV) for treatment of advanced AIDS-associated Kaposi's sarcoma (AIDS-KS): AIDS Clinical Trial Group (ACTG) protocol 286.* American Society of Clinical Oncology, Denver, May 17–20, 1997.
108. Saville MW, Lietzau J, Pluda JM, et al. Treatment of HIV-associated Kaposi's sarcoma with paclitaxel. *Lancet* 1995;346:26.
109. Welles L, Saville MW, Lietzau J, et al. Phase II trial with dose titration of paclitaxel for the therapy of human immunodeficiency virus-associated Kaposi's sarcoma. *J Clin Oncol* 1998;16:1112.
110. Gill P, Scadden D, Groopman J, et al. Low dose paclitaxel (Taxol) is highly effective in the treatment of patients with advanced AIDS-related Kaposi's sarcoma. In: *J AIDS & HR, 1st National AIDS Malignancy Conference*, Bethesda, MD, April 1, 1997, Vol. 14, Lipppincott-Raven.
111. Hakim FT, Cepeda R, Kaimei S, et al. Constraints on CD4 recovery postchemotherapy in adults: thymic insufficiency and apoptotic decline of expanded peripheral CD4 cells. *Blood* 1997;90:3789.
112. Mackall CL, Fleisher TA, Brown MR, et al. Age, thymopoiesis, and CD4+ T-lymphocyte regeneration after intensive chemotherapy. *N Engl J Med* 1995;332:143.
113. Ingber D, Fujita T, Kishimoto S, et al. Synthetic analogues of fumagillin that inhibit angiogenesis and suppress tumour growth. *Nature* 1990;348:555.
114. D'Amato RJ, Loughnan MS, Flynn E, Folkman J. Thalidomide is an inhibitor of angiogenesis. *Proc Natl Acad Sci U S A* 1994;91:4082.
115. Voest EE, Kenyon BM, O'Reilly MS, et al. Inhibition of angiogenesis *in vivo* by interleukin 12. *J Natl Cancer Inst* 1995;87:581.

116. Pluda JM, Shay LE, Foli A, et al. Administration of pentosan polysulfate to patients with human immunodeficiency virus-associated Kaposi's sarcoma. *J Natl Cancer Inst* 1993;85:1585.
117. Pluda JM, Wyvill K, Lietzau J, et al. *A phase I trial of TNP-470 (AGM-1470) administered to patients with HIV-associated Kaposi's sarcoma (KS).* The First National Conference on Human Retroviruses and Related Infections, Washington, DC, December 12–16, 1993.
118. Dezube BJ, Von Roenn JH, Holden-Wiltse J, et al. Fumagillin analog in the treatment of Kaposi's sarcoma: a phase I AIDS Clinical Trial Group study. AIDS Clinical Trial Group No. 215 Team. *J Clin Oncol* 1998;16:1444.
119. Little R, Pluda J, Wyvill K, et al. *Interleukin 12 (IL-12) appears to be active in AIDS-associated Kaposi's sarcoma (KS): early results of a pilot study.* 7th Conference on Retroviruses and Opportunistic Infections, San Francisco, January 30 to February 2, 2000.
120. Tulpule A, Espina BM, Cabriales S, et al. *IM862 nasal solution is an active anti-angiogenic agent in the treatment of AIDS-related Kaposi's sarcoma.* American Society of Clinical Oncology 35th Anual Meeting, Atlanta, May 15–18, 1999.
121. Welles L, Little R, Wyvill K, et al. *Preliminary results of a phase II study of oral thalidomide in patients with HIV infections and Kaposi's sarcoma (KS).* 1st National AIDS Malignancy Conference, Bethesda, MD, April 1, 1997, Vol. 14, Lippincott-Raven.
122. Bower M, Howard M, Gracie F, Phillips R, Fife K. *A Phase II study of thalidomide for Kaposi's sarcoma: activity and correlation with KSHV DNA load.* 1st National AIDS Malignancy Conference, Bethesda, MD, April 1, 1997, Vol. 14, Lippincott-Raven.
123. Clerici M, Lucey DR, Berzofsky JA, et al. Restoration of HIV-specific cell-mediated immune responses by interleukin-12 in vitro. *Science* 1993;262:1721.
124. Chougnet C, Wynn TA, Clerici M, et al. Molecular analysis of decreased interleukin-12 production in persons infected with human immunodeficiency virus. *J Infect Dis* 1996;174:46.
125. Sgadari C, Angiolillo AL, Tosato G. Inhibition of angiogenesis by interleukin-12 is mediated by the interferon-inducible protein 10. *Blood* 1996;87:3877.
126. Angiolillo AL, Sgadari C, Taub DD, et al. Human interferon-inducible protein 10 is a potent inhibitor of angiogenesis in vivo. *J Exp Med* 1995;182:155.
127. Sgadari C, Angiolillo AL, Cherney BW, et al. Interferon-inducible protein-10 identified as a mediator of tumor necrosis in vivo. *Proc Natl Acad Sci U S A* 1996;93:13791.
128. Geras-Raaka E, Varma A, Ho H, Clark-Lewis I, Gershengorn MC. Human interferon-gamma-inducible protein 10 (IP-10) inhibits constitutive signaling of Kaposi's sarcoma-associated herpesvirus G protein-coupled receptor. *J Exp Med* 1998;188:405.
129. Russo JJ, Bohenzky RA, Chien MC, et al. Nucleotide sequence of the Kaposi sarcoma-associated herpesvirus (HHV8). *Proc Natl Acad Sci U S A* 1996;93:14862.
130. Foli A, Saville MW, Baseler MW, Yarchoan R. Effects of the Th1 and Th2 stimulatory cytokines interleukin-12 and interleukin-4 on human immunodeficiency virus replication. *Blood* 1995;85:2114.
131. O'Reilly MS, Holmgren L, Shing Y, et al. Angiostatin: a novel angiogenesis inhibitor that mediates the suppression of metastases by a Lewis lung carcinoma. *Cell* 1994;79:315.
132. O'Reilly MS, Boehm T, Shing Y, et al. Endostatin: an endogenous inhibitor of angiogenesis and tumor growth. *Cell* 1997;88:277.
133. Chang E, Boyd A, Nelson CC, et al. Successful treatment of infantile hemangiomas with interferon-alpha-2b. *J Pediatr Hematol Oncol* 1997;19:237.
134. Gelmann EP, Preble OT, Steis R, et al. Human immunoblastoid interferon treatment of Kaposi's sarcoma in the acquired immunodeficiency syndrome. *Am J Med* 1985;78:737.
135. Miles SA, Rezai AR, Salazar-Gonzalez JF, et al. AIDS Kaposi sarcoma-derived cells produce and respond to interleukin 6. *Proc Natl Acad Sci U S A* 1990;87:4068.
136. Corbeil J, Rapaport E, Richman DD, Looney DJ. Antiproliferative effect of retinoid compounds on Kaposi's sarcoma cells. *J Clin Invest* 1994;93:1981.
137. Sidell N, Taga T, Hirano T, Kishimoto T, Saxon A. Retinoic acid-induced growth inhibition of a human myeloma cell line via down-regulation of IL-6 receptors. *J Immunol* 1991;146:3809.
138. Gill PS, Espina BM, Moudgil T, et al. All-*trans* retinoic acid for the treatment of AIDS-related Kaposi's sarcoma: results of a pilot phase II study. *Leukemia* 1994;8:S26.
139. Bailey J, Pluda JM, Foli A, et al. Phase I/II study of intermittent all-trans-retinoic acid, alone and in combination with interferon alfa-2a, in patients with epidemic Kaposi's sarcoma. *J Clin Oncol* 1995;13:1966.
140. Von Roenn J, von Gunten C, Mullane M, et al. All-transretinoic acid (TRA) in the treatment of AIDS-related Kaposi's sarcoma. *Abstracts of the IXth International Conference on AIDS IVth STD World Congress* 1993;I:397(abst PO-B12-1571).
141. Adamson PC, Boylan JF, Balis FM, et al. Time course of induction of metabolism of all-*trans*-retinoic acid and the up-regulation of cellular retinoic acid-binding protein. *Cancer Res* 1993;53:472.
142. Aboulafia D, Norris D, Grossman RJ, et al. Interim analysis of phase ii study (protocol L1057-28) of Panretin Capsules (LGD1057, ARLT1057) for AIDS-related Kaposi's sarcoma. 2nd National AIDS Malignancy Meeting, Bethesda, MD, April 6–8, 1998. *J Acquir Immune Defic Syndr Hum Retrovirol* Vol 17, Lippincott, Williams & Wilkins.
143. Friedman-Kien A, Dezube B, Lee J, et al. *Oral 9-cis-retinoic acid is active in AIDS related Kaposi's sarcoma: AIDS Associated Malignancy Consortium Study 002.* 2nd National AIDS Malignancy Meeting, Bethesda, MD, April 6–8, 1998, Vol. 17, Lippincott, Williams & Wilkins.
144. Lennette ET, Blackbourn DJ, Levy JA. Antibodies to human herpesvirus type 8 in the general population and in Kaposi's sarcoma patients. *Lancet* 1996;348:858.
145. Lundardi-Iskandar Y, Bryant JL, Zeman RA, et al. Tumorigenesis and metastasis of neoplastic Kaposi's sarcoma cell line in immunodeficient mice blocked by a human pregnancy hormone. *Nature* 1995;375:64.
146. Lunardi-Iskandar Y, Bryant JL, Blattner WA, et al. Effects of a urinary factor from women in early pregnancy on HIV-1, SIV and associated disease. *Nat Med* 1998;4:428.
147. Gill PS, Lunardi-Ishkandar Y, Louie S, et al. The effects of preparations of human chorionic gonadotropin on AIDS-related Kaposi's sarcoma. *N Engl J Med* 1996;335:1261.
148. Gill PS, McLaughlin T, Espina BM, et al. Phase I study of human chorionic gonadotropin given subcutaneously to patients with acquired immunodeficiency syndrome-related mucocutaneous Kaposi's sarcoma. *J Natl Cancer Inst* 1997;89:1797.
149. Morfeldt L, Torssander J. Long-term remission of Kaposi's sarcoma following foscarnet treatment in HIV-infected patients. *Scand J Infect Dis* 1994;26:749.
150. Humphrey RW, Davis DA, Newcomb FM, Yarchoan R. Human herpesvirus 8 (HHV-8) in the pathogenesis of Kaposi's sarcoma and other diseases. *Leuk Lymphoma* 1998;28:25564.
151. Martin DF, Kuppermann BD, Wolitz RA, et al. Oral ganciclovir for patients with cytomegalovirus retinitis treated with a ganciclovir implant. Roche Ganciclovir Study Group. *N Engl J Med* 1999;340:1063.
152. Chieco-Bianchi L. *HAART Treatment for AIDS-Related KS.* 1999 International Meeting of the Institute of Human Virology, August 28 to September 2, 1999.
153. Jones J. *Effect of antiretroviral therapy on recent trends in cancers among HIV infected persons.* 2nd National AIDS Malignancy Conference, Bethesda, MD, April 6, 1998.
154. Ensoli B, Barillari G, Gallo RC. Cytokines and growth factors in the pathogenesis of AIDS-associated Kaposi's sarcoma. *Immunol Rev* 1992;127:147.
155. Greiner TC, Medeiros LJ, Jaffe ES. Non-Hodgkin's lymphoma. *Cancer* 1995;75:370.
156. Eby NL, Grufferman S, Flannelly CM, et al. Increasing incidence of primary brain lymphoma in the US. *Cancer* 1988;62:2461.
157. Gail MH, Pluda JM, Rabkin CS, et al. Projections of the incidence of non-Hodgkin's lymphoma related to acquired immunodeficiency syndrome. *J Natl Cancer Inst* 1991;83:695.
158. MMWR. Diffuse, undifferentiated non-Hodgkin's lymphoma among homosexual males—United States. *MMWR* 1982;31:277.
159. Ziegler JL, Miner RC, Rosenbaum E, et al. Outbreak of Burkitt's-like lymphoma in homosexual men. *Lancet* 1982;2:631.
160. Biggar RJ, Horm J, Lubin JH, et al. Cancer trends in a population at risk of acquired immunodeficiency syndrome. *J Natl Cancer Inst* 1985;74:793.
161. MMWR. Current trends revision of the case definition of acquired immunodeficiency syndrome for national reporting—United States. *MMWR* 1985;34:373.
162. Moore RD, Kessler H, Richman DD, Flexner C, Chaisson RE. Non-Hodgkin's lymphoma in patients with advanced HIV infection treated with zidovudine. *JAMA* 1991;265:2208.
163. Pluda JM, Yarchoan R, Jaffe ES, et al. Development of non-Hodgkin lymphoma in a cohort of patients with severe HIV infection on long-term antiretroviral therapy. *Ann Intern Med* 1990;113:276.
164. Ridolfo AL, Santambrogio S, Mainini F, et al. High frequency of non-Hodgkin's lymphoma in patients with HIV-associated Kaposi's sarcoma. *AIDS* 1996;10:181.
165. Cote TR, Biggar RJ, Rosenberg PS, et al. Non-Hodgkin's lymphoma among people with AIDS: incidence, presentation and public health burden. AIDS/Cancer Study Group. *Int J Cancer* 1997;73:645.
166. Pluda JM, Venzon DJ, Tosato G, et al. Parameters affecting the development of non-Hodgkin's lymphoma in patients with severe human immunodeficiency virus infection receiving antiretroviral therapy. *J Clin Oncol* 1993;11:1099.
167. Tirelli U, Spina M, Vaccher E, et al. Clinical evaluation of 451 patients with HIV related non-Hodgkin's lymphoma: experience on the Italian cooperative group on AIDS and tumors (GICAT). *Leuk Lymphoma* 1995;20:91.
168. Levine AM. Lymphoma complicating immunodeficiency disorders. *Ann Oncol* 1994; 5(Suppl 2):29.
169. National Cancer Institute sponsored study of classifications of non-Hodgkin's lymphomas: summary and description of a working formulation for clinical usage. The Non-Hodgkin's Lymphoma Pathologic Classification Project. *Cancer* 1982;49:2112.
170. Zhang Z, Diwan BA, Anderson LM, et al. Skin tumorigenesis and Ki-ras and Ha-ras mutations in tumors from adult mice exposed in utero to 3'-azido-2',3'-dideoxythymidine. *Mol Carcinogen* 1998;23:45.
171. Olivero OA, Beland FA, Fullerton NF, Poirier MC. Vaginal epithelial DNA damage and expression of preneoplastic markers in mice during chronic dosing with tumorigenic levels of 3'-azido-2',3'-dideoxythymidine. *Cancer Res* 1994;54:6235.
172. Olivero OA, Anderson LM, Diwan BA, et al. Transplacental effects of 3'-azido-2',3'-dideoxythymidine (AZT): tumorigenicity in mice and genotoxicity in mice and monkeys. *J Natl Cancer Inst* 1997;89:1602.
173. Levine AM, Bernstein L, Sullivan-Halley J, et al. Role of zidovudine antiretroviral therapy in the pathogenesis of acquired immunodeficiency syndrome-related lymphoma. *Blood* 1995;86:4612.
174. Widney D, Yawetz S, van der Meyden M, et al. Effects of zidovudine on B lymphocyte activation. *Cell Immunol* 1994;158:140.
175. Armenian HK, Hoover DR, Rubb S, et al. Risk factors for non-Hodgkin's lymphomas in acquired immunodeficiency syndrome (AIDS). *Am J Epidemiol* 1996;143:374.
176. Philip T. Burkitt's lymphoma in Europe. In: Lenoir G, O'Connor G, Olweny C, eds. *Burkitt's lymphoma: a human cancer model.* Lyon: IARC, 1985:107.
177. Obrams GI, Grufferman S. Epidemiology of HIV associated non-Hodgkin lymphoma. *Cancer Surv* 1991;10:91.
178. Cantor KP, Fraumeni JF Jr. Distribution of non-Hodgkin's lymphoma in the United States between 1950 and 1975. *Cancer Res* 1980;40:2645.
179. Ries L, Hankey B, Miller B, et al. *Cancer statistics review, 1973–1988.* Bethesda, MD: NIH, 1991:2789.
180. Rabkin CS, Yang Q, Goedert JJ, et al. Chemokine and chemokine receptor gene variants and risk of non-Hodgkin's lymphoma in human immunodeficiency virus-1-infected individuals. *Blood* 1999;93:1838.
181. Michael NL, Chang G, Louie LG, et al. The role of viral phenotype and CCR-5 gene defects in HIV-1 transmission and disease progression. *Nat Med* 1997;3:338.
182. Dean M, Carrington M, Winkler C, et al. Genetic restriction of HIV-1 infection and progression to AIDS by a deletion allele of the CKR5 structural gene. Hemophilia Growth and Development Study, Multicenter AIDS Cohort Study, Multicenter Hemophilia Cohort Study, San Francisco City Cohort, ALIVE Study. *Science* 1996;273:1856.
183. Dean M, Jacobson LP, McFarlane G, et al. Reduced risk of AIDS lymphoma in individuals heterozygous for the CCR5-delta32 mutation. *Cancer Res* 1999;59:3561.
184. Bacon KB, Premack BA, Gardner P, Schall TJ. Activation of dual T cell signaling pathways by the chemokine RANTES. *Science* 1995;269:1727.
185. Taub DD, Turcovski-Corrales SM, Key ML, Longo DL, Murphy WJ. Chemokines and T lymphocyte activation: I. Beta chemokines costimulate human T lymphocyte activation in vitro. *J Immunol* 1996;156:2095.

186. Grulich AE. AIDS-associated non-Hodgkin's lymphoma in the era of highly active antiretroviral therapy. *J Acquir Immune Defic Syndr* 1999;21(Suppl 1:)S27.
187. Levine AM. Epidemiology, clinical characteristics, and management of AIDS-related lymphoma. *Hematol Oncol Clin North Am* 1991;5:331.
188. Antinori A, Cingolani A, Ammassari A, et al. *AIDS-related focal brain lesions in the era of HAART.* 6th Conference on Retroviruses and Opportunistic Infections, Chicago, January 31 to February 4, 1999.
189. Hoover R, Fraumeni JF Jr. Risk of cancer in renal-transplant recipients. *Lancet* 1973;2:55.
190. Nalesnik MA, Jaffe R, Starzl TE, et al. The pathology of posttransplant lymphoproliferative disorders occurring in the setting of cyclosporine A-prednisone immunosuppression. *Am J Pathol* 1988;133:173.
191. Sokal EM, Antunes H, Beguin C, et al. Early signs and risk factors for the increased incidence of Epstein-Barr virus-related posttransplant lymphoproliferative diseases in pediatric liver transplant recipients treated with tacrolimus. *Transplantation* 1997;64:1438.
192. Natkunam Y, Elenitoba-Johnson KS, Kingma DW, Kamel OW. Epstein-Barr virus strain type and latent membrane protein 1 gene deletions in lymphomas in patients with rheumatic diseases. *Arthritis Rheum* 1997;40:1152.
193. Cheung AN, Chan AC, Chung LP, et al. Post-transplantation lymphoproliferative disorder of donor origin in a sex-mismatched renal allograft as proven by chromosome in situ hybridization. *Mod Pathol* 1998;11:99.
194. Gatti RA, Good RA. The immunological deficiency diseases. *Med Clin North Am* 1970;54:281.
195. Henley WL. Immunodeficiency disorders. *Pediatr Ann* 1976;5:418.
196. Hecht F, Hecht BK. Chromosome changes connect immunodeficiency and cancer in ataxia- telangiectasia. *Am J Pediatr Hematol Oncol* 1987;9:185.
197. Xu Y, Ashley T, Brainerd EE, et al. Targeted disruption of ATM leads to growth retardation, chromosomal fragmentation during meiosis, immune defects, and thymic lymphoma. *Genes Dev* 1996;10:2411.
198. Santana V, Rose NR. Neoplastic lymphoproliferation in autoimmune disease: an updated review. *Clin Immunol Immunopathol* 1992;63:205.
199. Jaffe ES. *An increased risk of B-cell lymphomas in autoimmune lyphoproliferative syndrome.* 3rd National AIDS Malignancy Meeting, Bethesda, MD, May 26–27, 1999, National Cancer Institute.
200. Golding H, Robey FA, Gates FT, et al. Identification of homologous regions in human immunodeficiency virus virus I gp41 and human MHC class II beta 1 domain. *J Exp Med* 1988;167:914.
201. Ng VL, Hurt MH, Herndier BG, Fry KE, McGrath MS. VH gene use by HIV type 1-associated lymphoproliferations. *AIDS Res Hum Retroviruses* 1997;13:135.
202. Riboldi P, Gaidano G, Schettino EW, et al. Two acquired immunodeficiency syndrome-associated Burkitt's lymphomas produce specific anti-i IgM cold agglutinins using somatically mutated VH4-21 segments. *Blood* 1994;83:2952.
203. Bessudo A, Cherepakhin V, Johnson TA, et al. Favored use of immunoglobulin V(H)4 Genes in AIDS-associated B-cell lymphoma. *Blood* 1996;88:252.
204. Levine AM, Tulpule A, Espina B, et al. Low dose methotrexate, bleomycin, doxorubicin, cyclophosphamide, vincristine, and dexamethasone with zalcitabine in patients with acquired immunodeficiency syndrome-related lymphoma. Effect on human immunodeficiency virus and serum interleukin-6 levels over time. *Cancer* 1996;78:517.
205. Przybylski GK, Goldman J, Ng VL, et al. Evidence for early B-cell activation preceding the development of Epstein-Barr virus-negative acquired immunodeficiency syndrome-related lymphoma. *Blood* 1996;88:4620.
206. Joshi VV, Kauffman S, Oleske JM, et al. Polyclonal polymorphic B-cell lymphoproliferative disorder with prominent pulmonary involvement in children with acquired immune deficiency syndrome. *Cancer* 1987;59:1455.
207. Amadori A, Gallo P, Zamarchi R, et al. IgG oligoclonal bands in sera of HIV-1 infected patients are mainly directed against HIV-1 determinants. *AIDS Res Hum Retroviruses* 1990;6:581.
208. Silvestris F, Williams RC Jr, Dammacco F. Autoreactivity in HIV-1 infection: the role of molecular mimicry. *Clin Immunol Immunopathol* 1995;75:197.
209. Gaidano G, Pastore C, Lanza C, Mazza U, Saglio G. Molecular pathology of AIDS-related lymphomas. Biologic aspects and clinicopathologic heterogeneity. *Ann Hematol* 1994;69:281.
210. Carbone A, Tirelli U, Gloghini A, Volpe R, Boiocchi M. Human immunodeficiency virus-associated systemic lymphomas may be subdivided into two main groups according to Epstein-Barr viral latent gene expression. *J Clin Oncol* 1993;11:1674.
211. Ziegler JL, Beckstead JA, Volberding PA, et al. Non-Hodgkin's lymphoma in 90 homosexual men. Relation to generalized lymphadenopathy and the acquired immunodeficiency syndrome. *N Engl J Med* 1984;311:565.
212. Knowles DM. Etiology and pathogenesis of AIDS-related non–Hodgkin's lymphoma. *Hematol Oncol Clin North Am* 1996;10:1081.
213. Chadburn A, Cesarman E, Jagirdar J, et al. CD30 (Ki-1) positive anaplastic large cell lymphomas in individuals infected with the human immunodeficiency virus. *Cancer* 1993;72:3078.
214. Hollingsworth HC, Stetler-Stevenson M, Gagneten D, et al. Immunodeficiency-associated malignant lymphoma. Three cases showing genotypic evidence of both T- and B-cell lineages. *Am J Surg Pathol* 1994;18:1092.
215. Levine AM. Acquired immunodeficiency syndrome-related lymphoma. *Blood* 1992;80:8.
216. Davi F, Delecluse HJ, Guiet P, et al. Burkitt-like lymphomas in AIDS patients: characterization within a series of 103 human immunodeficiency virus-associated non-Hodgkin's lymphomas. Burkitt's Lymphoma Study Group. *J Clin Oncol* 1998;16:3788.
217. Knowles DM. Immunodeficiency-associated lymphoproliferative disorders. *Mod Pathol* 1999;12:200.
218. Raphael MM, Audouin J, Lamine M, et al. Immunophenotypic and genotypic analysis of acquired immunodeficiency syndrome-related non-Hodgkin's lymphomas. Correlation with histologic features in 36 cases. French Study Group of Pathology for HIV-Associated Tumors. *Am J Clin Pathol* 1994;101:773.
219. Cesarman E, Chang Y, Moore PS, Said JW, Knowles DM. Kaposi's sarcoma-associated herpesvirus-like DNA sequences in AIDS- related body-cavity-based lymphomas. *N Engl J Med* 1995;332:1186.
220. Carbone A, Gloghini A, Gaidano G, et al. AIDS-related Burkitt's lymphoma. Morphologic and immunophenotypic study of biopsy specimens. *Am J Clin Pathol* 1995;103:561.
221. Harris NL, Jaffe ES, Stein H, et al. A revised European-American classification of lymphoid neoplasms: a proposal from the International Lymphoma Study Group. *Blood* 1994;84:1361.
222. Biggar RJ, Rabkin CS. The epidemiology of acquired immunodeficiency syndrome-related lymphomas. *Curr Opin Oncol* 1992;4:883.
223. Morgello S. Epstein-Barr and human immunodeficiency viruses in acquired immunodeficiency syndrome-related primary central nervous system lymphoma. *Am J Pathol* 1992;141:441.
224. Harris NL, Jaffe ES, Diebold J, et al. World Health Organization classification of neoplastic diseases of the hematopoietic and lymphoid tissues: report of the Clinical Advisory Committee meeting-Airlie House, Virginia, November 1997. *J Clin Oncol* 1999;17:3835.
225. Shiramizu B, Herndier B, Meeker T, Kaplan L, McGrath M. Molecular and immunophenotypic characterization of AIDS-associated, Epstein-Barr virus-negative, polyclonal lymphoma. *J Clin Oncol* 1992;10:383.
226. Kaplan LD, Shiramizu B, Herndier B, et al. Influence of molecular characteristics on clinical outcome in human immunodeficiency virus-associated non-Hodgkin's lymphoma: identification of a subgroup with favorable clinical outcome. *Blood* 1995;85:1727.
227. Moran CA, Tuur S, Angritt P, Reid AH, O'Leary TJ. Epstein-Barr virus in Hodgkin's disease from patients with human immunodeficiency virus infection. *Mod Pathol* 1992;5:85.
228. Rubio R. Hodgkin's disease associated with human immunodeficiency virus infection. A clinical study of 46 cases. Cooperative Study Group of Malignancies Associated with HIV Infection of Madrid. *Cancer* 1994;73:2400.
229. Kingma DW, Mueller BU, Frekko K, et al. Low-grade monoclonal Epstein-Barr virus-associated lymphoproliferative disorder of the brain presenting as human immunodeficiency virus- associated encephalopathy in a child with acquired immunodeficiency syndrome. *Arch Pathol Lab Med* 1999;123:83.
230. Jaffe ES, Wilson WH. Lymphomatoid granulomatosis: pathogenesis, pathology and clinical implications. *Cancer Surv* 1997;30:233.
231. Cesarman E, Knowles DM. The role of Kaposi's sarcoma-associated herpesvirus (KSHV/HHV-8) in lymphoproliferative diseases. *Semin Cancer Biol* 1999;9:165.
232. Shibata D, Weiss LM, Hernandez AM, et al. Epstein-Barr virus-associated non-Hodgkin's lymphoma in patients infected with the human immunodeficiency virus. *Blood* 1993;81:2102.
233. Contreras-Brodin BA, Anvret M, Imreh S, et al. B cell phenotype-dependent expression of the Epstein-Barr virus nuclear antigens EBNA-2 to EBNA-6: studies with somatic cell hybrids. *J Gen Virol* 1991;72:3025.
234. Hamilton-Dutoit SJ, Pallesen G, Franzmann MB, et al. AIDS-related lymphoma: histopathology, immunophenotype, and association with Epstein-Barr virus as demonstrated by *in situ* nucleic acid hybridization. *Am J Pathol* 1991;138:149.
235. Murray RJ, Kurilla MG, Brooks JM, et al. Identification of target antigens for the human cytotoxic T cell response to Epstein-Barr virus (EBV): implications for the immune control of EBV-positive malignancies. *J Exp Med* 1992;176:157.
236. Khanna R, Burrows SR, Nicholls J, Poulsen LM. Identification of cytotoxic T cell epitopes within Epstein-Barr virus (EBV) oncogene latent membrane protein 1 (LMP1): evidence for HLA A2 supertype-restricted immune recognition of EBV-infected cells by LMP1-specific cytotoxic T lymphocytes. *Eur J Immunol* 1998;28:451.
237. Redchenko IV, Rickinson AB. Accessing Epstein-Barr virus-specific T-cell memory with peptide-loaded dendritic cells. *J Virol* 1999;73:334.
238. Wang D, Liebowitz D, Kieff E. An EBV membrane protein expressed in immortalized lymphocytes transforms established rodent cells. *Cell* 1985;43:831.
239. Finke J, Lange W, Mertelsmann R, Dolken G. BCL 2 induction is part of the strategy of Epstein-Barr virus. *Leuk Lymphoma* 1994;12:413.
240. Henderson S, Rowe M, Gregory C, et al. Induction of bcl-2 expression by Epstein-Barr virus latent membrane protein 1 protects infected B cells from programmed cell death. *Cell* 1991;65:1107.
241. Gaidano G, Pastore C, Volpe G. Molecular pathogenesis of non-Hodgkin lymphoma: a clinical perspective. *Haematologica* 1995;80:454.
242. Lai R, Arber DA, Chang KL, Wilson CS, Weiss LM. Frequency of bcl-2 expression in non-Hodgkin's lymphoma: a study of 778 cases with comparison of marginal zone lymphoma and monocytoid B-cell hyperplasia. *Mod Pathol* 1998;11:864.
243. Schlaifer D, Brousset P, Attal M, et al. bcl-2 proto-oncogene and Epstein-Barr virus latent membrane protein-1 expression in AIDS-related lymphoma. *Histopathology* 1994;25:77.
244. Hamilton-Dutoit SJ, Rea D, Raphael M, et al. Epstein-Barr virus-latent gene expression and tumor cell phenotype in acquired immunodeficiency syndrome-related non-Hodgkin's lymphoma. Correlation of lymphoma phenotype with three distinct patterns of viral latency. *Am J Pathol* 1993;143:1072.
245. Ballerini P, Gaidano G, Gong JZ, et al. Multiple genetic lesions in acquired immunodeficiency syndrome-related non-Hodgkin's lymphoma. *Blood* 1993;81:166.
246. Carbone A, Gaidano G, Gloghini A, et al. BCL-6 protein expression in AIDS-related non-Hodgkin's lymphomas: inverse relationship with Epstein-Barr virus-encoded latent membrane protein-1 expression. *Am J Pathol* 1997;150:155.
247. Flenghi L, Ye BH, Fizzotti M, et al. A specific monoclonal antibody (PG-B6) detects expression of the BCL-6 protein in germinal center B cells. *Am J Pathol* 1995;147:405.
248. Cattoretti G, Chang CC, Cechova K, et al. BCL-6 protein is expressed in germinal-center B cells. *Blood* 1995;86:45.
249. Sanderson RD, Lalor P, Bernfield M. B lymphocytes express and lose syndecan at specific stages of differentiation. *Cell Regulation* 1989;1:27.
250. Inghirami G, Grignani F, Sternas L, et al. Down-regulation of LFA-1 adhesion receptors by C-myc oncogene in human B lymphoblastoid cells. *Science* 1990;250:682.
251. Yano T, van Krieken JH, Magrath IT, et al. Histogenetic correlations between subcategories of small noncleaved cell lymphomas. *Blood* 1992;79:1282.
252. Knowles DM, Inghirami G, Ubriaco A, Dalla-Favera R. Molecular genetic analysis of three

AIDS-associated neoplasms of uncertain lineage demonstrates their B-cell derivation and the possible pathogenetic role of the Epstein-Barr virus. *Blood* 1989;73:792.
253. Nador RG, Cesarman E, Chadburn A, et al. Primary effusion lymphoma: a distinct clinicopathologic entity associated with the Kaposi's sarcoma-associated herpes virus. *Blood* 1996;88:645.
254. Arvanitakis L, Mesri EA, Nador RG, et al. Establishment and characterization of a primary effusion (body cavity-based) lymphoma cell line (BC-3) harboring Kaposi's sarcoma-associated herpesvirus (KSHV/HHV-8) in the absence of Epstein-Barr virus. *Blood* 1996;88:2648.
255. Green I, Espiritu E, Ladanyi M, et al. Primary lymphomatous effusions in AIDS: a morphological, immunophenotypic, and molecular study. *Mod Pathol* 1995;8:39.
256. Stamatopoulos K, Kosmas C, Stavroyianni N, Belessi C, Papadaki T. Selection of immunoglobulin diversity gene reading frames in B cell lymphoproliferative disorders. *Leukemia* 1999;13:601.
257. Jaffe ES. Primary body cavity-based AIDS-related lymphomas. Evolution of a new disease entity [editorial; comment]. *Am J Clin Pathol* 1996;105:141.
258. Karcher DS, Alkan S. Human herpesvirus-8-associated body cavity-based lymphoma in human immunodeficiency virus-infected patients: a unique B-cell neoplasm. *Hum Pathol* 1997;28:801.
259. Friborg J Jr, Kong WP, Flowers CC, et al. Distinct biology of Kaposi's sarcoma-associated herpesvirus from primary lesions and body cavity lymphomas. *J Virol* 1998;72:10073.
260. Carbone A, Cilia AM, Gloghini A, et al. Establishment and characterization of EBV-positive and EBV-negative primary effusion lymphoma cell lines harbouring human herpesvirus type-8. *Br J Haematol* 1998;102:1081.
261. Aoki Y, Jaffe ES, Chang Y, et al. Angiogenesis and hematopoiesis induced by Kaposi's sarcoma-associated herpesvirus-encoded interleukin-6. *Blood* 1999;93:4034.
262. Aoki Y, Tosato G. *Pathophysiological role of vascular endothelial growth factory/vascular permeability factor (VEGF/VPF) in primary effusion lymphomas.* 3rd National AIDS Malignancy Meeting, Bethesda, MD, May 26–27, 1999. National Cancer Institute.
263. Levine AM. AIDS-associated malignant lymphoma. *Med Clin North Am* 1992;76:253.
264. Levine AM, Gill PS, Muggia F. Malignancies in the acquired immunodeficiency syndrome. *Curr Probl Cancer* 1987;11:209.
265. Carbone PP, Kaplan HS, Musshoff K, Smithers DW, Tubiana M. Report of the Committee on Hodgkin's Disease Staging Classification. *Cancer Res* 1971;31:1860.
266. Yousem DM, Patrone PM, Grossman RI. Leptomeningeal metastases: MR evaluation. *J Comput Assist Tomogr* 1990;14:255.
267. Luo K, Law M, Kaldor JM, McDonald AM, Cooper DA. The role of initial AIDS-defining illness in survival following AIDS. *AIDS* 1995;9:57.
268. Tirelli U, Errante D, Spina M, et al. Long-term survival of patients with HIV-related systemic non-Hodgkin's lymphomas. *Hematol Oncol* 1996;14:7.
269. Hagemeister FB, Khetan R, Allen P, et al. Stage, serum LDH, and performance status predict disease progression and survival in HIV-associated lymphomas. *Ann Oncol* 1994; 5(Suppl 2):41.
270. Vaccher E, Tirelli U, Spina M, et al. Age and serum lactate dehydrogenase level are independent prognostic factors in human immunodeficiency virus-related non-Hodgkin's lymphomas: a single-institute study of 96 patients. *J Clin Oncol* 1996;14:2217.
271. Navarro JT, Ribera JM, Oriol A, et al. International prognostic index is the best prognostic factor for survival in patients with AIDS-related non-Hodgkin's lymphoma treated with CHOP. A multivariate study of 46 patients. *Haematologica* 1998;83:508.
272. Straus DJ, Huang J, Testa MA, Levine AM, Kaplan LD. Prognostic factors in the treatment of human immunodeficiency virus-associated non-Hodgkin's lymphoma: analysis of AIDS Clinical Trials Group protocol 142—low-dose versus standard-dose m-BACOD plus granulocyte-macrophage colony-stimulating factor. National Institute of Allergy and Infectious Diseases. *J Clin Oncol* 1998;16:3601.
273. Levine AM, Gill PS, Meyer PR, et al. Retrovirus and malignant lymphoma in homosexual men. *JAMA* 1985;254:1921.
274. Gill PS, Levine AM, Krailo M, et al. AIDS-related malignant lymphoma: results of prospective treatment trials. *J Clin Oncol* 1987;5:1322.
275. MMWR. Guidelines for prophylaxis against *Pneumocystis carinii* pneumonia for persons infected with human immunodeficiency virus type 1. *MMWR* 1989;38(Suppl S-5):1.
276. Shipp MA, Yeap BY, Harrington DP, et al. The m-BACOD combination chemotherapy regimen in large-cell lymphoma: analysis of the completed trial and comparison with the M-BACOD regimen. *J Clin Oncol* 1990;8:84.
277. Skarin AT, Canellos GP, Rosenthal DS, et al. Improved prognosis of diffuse histiocytic and undifferentiated lymphoma by use of high dose methotrexate alternating with standard agents (M- BACOD). *J Clin Oncol* 1983;1:91.
278. Klimo P, Connors JM. MACOP-B chemotherapy for the treatment of diffuse large-cell lymphoma. *Ann Intern Med* 1985;102:596.
279. Longo DL, DeVita VT Jr, Duffey PL, et al. Superiority of ProMACE-CytaBOM over ProMACE-MOPP in the treatment of advanced diffuse aggressive lymphoma: results of a prospective randomized trial. *J Clin Oncol* 1991;9:25.
280. Browne MJ, Hubbard SM, Longo DL, et al. Excess prevalence of *Pneumocystis carinii* pneumonia in patients treated for lymphoma with combination chemotherapy. *Ann Intern Med* 1986;104:338.
281. Fisher RI, Gaynor ER, Dahlberg S, et al. Comparison of a standard regimen (CHOP) with three intensive chemotherapy regimens for advanced non-Hodgkin's lymphoma. *N Engl J Med* 1993;328:1002.
282. Levine AM, Wernz JC, Kaplan L, et al. Low-dose chemotherapy with central nervous system prophylaxis and zidovudine maintenance in AIDS-related lymphoma. A prospective multi-institutional trial. *JAMA* 1991;266:84.
283. Kaplan LD, Straus DJ, Testa MA, et al. Low-dose compared with standard-dose m-BACOD chemotherapy for non-Hodgkin's lymphoma associated with human immunodeficiency virus infection. National Institute of Allergy and Infectious Diseases AIDS Clinical Trials Group. *N Engl J Med* 1997;336:1641.
284. Wilson WH. Chemotherapy for AIDS-related lymphomas [letter; comment]. *N Engl J Med* 1997;337:1172; discussion, 1173.
285. Kwak LW, Halpern J, Olshen RA, Horning SJ. Prognostic significance of actual dose intensity in diffuse large-cell lymphoma: results of a tree-structured survival analysis. *J Clin Oncol* 1990;8:963.
286. Kaplan LD, Kahn JO, Crowe S, et al. Clinical and virologic effects of recombinant human granulocyte-macrophage colony-stimulating factor in patients receiving chcmotherapy for human immunodeficiency virus-associated non-Hodgkin's lymphoma. *J Clin Oncol* 1991;9:929.
287. Vaccner E, Spina M, Santarossa S, et al. Concomitant CHOP chemotherapy (CT) and highly active antiretroviral therapy (HAART) in patients with HIV-related non-Hodgkin's lymphoma (HIV-NHL). *Int Conf AIDS*, Vol. 12, Geneva, 1998.
288. Ratner L, Redden D, Hamzeh F, et al. *Chemotherapy for HIV-NHL in combination with HAART.* 3rd National AIDS Malignancy Meeting, Bethesda, MD, May 26–28, 1999.
289. Gisselbrecht C, Oksenhendler E, Tirelli U, et al. Human immunodeficiency virus-related lymphoma treatment with intensive combination chemotherapy. French-Italian Cooperative Group. *Am J Med* 1993;95:188.
290. Gabarre J, Lepage E, Thyss A, et al. Chemotherapy combined with zidovudine and GM-CSF in human immunodeficiency virus-related non-Hodgkin's lymphoma. *Ann Oncol* 1995;6:1025.
291. Sparano JA, Wiernik PH, Hu X, et al. Saquinavir enhances the mucosal toxicity of infusional cyclophosphamide, doxorubicin, and etoposide in patients with HIV- associated non-Hodgkin's lymphoma. *Med Oncol* 1998;15:50.
292. Sparano J, Wiernik P, Hu X, Sarta C, Schwartz E. Pilot Trial of infusional cyclophosphamide, doxorubicin, and etoposide plus didanosine and filgrastim in patients with human immunodeficiency virus-associated non-Hodgkin's lymphoma. *J Clin Oncol* 1996;14:3026.
293. Wilson WH, Bryant G, Bates S, et al. EPOCH chemotherapy: toxicity and efficacy in relapsed and refractory non-Hodgkin's lymphoma. *J Clin Oncol* 1993;11:1573.
294. Little RF, Pearson D, Steinberg S, et al. *Dose-Adjusted EPOCH Chemotherapy (CT) in previously untreated HIV-associated non-Hodgkin's lymphoma (HIV-NHL).* American Society of Clinical Oncology35th Annual Meeting, Atlanta, May 15–18, 1999.
295. Schurmann D, Grunewald T, Weiss R, et al. Intensive treatment of AIDS-related non-Hodgkin's lymphomas with the MACOP-B protocol. *Eur J Haematol* 1995;54:73.
296. Tisdale J, Little RF, Childs R, Barret J. Unpublished observation, 1999.
297. von Gunten CF, Von Roenn JH. Clinical aspects of human immunodeficiency virus-related lymphoma. *Curr Opin Oncol* 1992;4:894.
298. Goplen AK, Dunlop O, Liestol K, et al. The impact of primary central nervous system lymphoma in AIDS patients: a population-based autopsy study from Oslo. *J Acquir Immune Defic Syndr Hum Retrovirol* 1997;14:351.
299. Biggar RJ, Burnett W, Mikl J, Nasca P. Cancer among New York men at risk of acquired immunodeficiency syndrome. *Int J Cancer* 1989;43:979.
300. Cote TR, Manns A, Hardy CR, Yellin FJ, Hartge P. Epidemiology of brain lymphoma among people with or without acquired immunodeficiency syndrome. AIDS/Cancer Study Group. *J Natl Cancer Inst* 1996;88:675.
301. DeAngelis LM. Primary brain tumors in the acquired immunodeficiency syndrome. *Curr Opin Neurol* 1995;8:419.
302. Ruiz A, Post MJ, Bundschu C, Ganz WI, Georgiou M. Primary central nervous system lymphoma in patients with AIDS. *Neuroimaging Clin North Am* 1997;7:281.
303. Levine AM, Sullivan-Halley J, Pike MC, et al. Human immunodeficiency virus-related lymphoma. Prognostic factors predictive of survival. *Cancer* 1991;68:2466.
304. Camilleri-Broet S, Davi F, Feuillard J, et al. AIDS-related primary brain lymphomas: histopathologic and immunohistochemical study of 51 cases. The French Study Group for HIV- Associated Tumors. *Hum Pathol* 1997;28:367.
305. Iacoangeli M, Roselli R, Antinori A, et al. Experience with brain biopsy in acquired immune deficiency syndrome-related focal lesions of the central nervous system. *Br J Surg* 1994;81:1508.
306. Yarchoan R, Jaffe ES, Little R. Diagnosing central nervous system lymphoma in the setting of AIDS: a step forward [editorial; comment]. *J Natl Cancer Inst* 1998;90:346.
307. Mathews C, Barba D, Fullerton SC. Early biopsy versus empiric treatment with delayed biopsy of non-responders in suspected HIV-associated cerebral toxoplasmosis: a decision analysis. *AIDS* 1995;9:1243.
308. Holloway RG, Mushlin AI. Intracranial mass lesions in acquired immunodeficiency syndrome: using decision analysis to determine the effectiveness of stereotactic brain biopsy. *Neurology* 1996;46:1010.
309. Hoffman JM, Waskin HA, Schifter T, et al. FDG-PET in differentiating lymphoma from nonmalignant central nervous system lesions in patients with AIDS. *J Nucl Med* 1993;34:567.
310. Ruiz A, Ganz WI, Post MJ, et al. Use of thallium-201 brain SPECT to differentiate cerebral lymphoma from toxoplasma encephalitis in AIDS patients. *AJNR Am J Neuroradiol* 1994;15:1885.
311. O'Malley JP, Ziessman HA, Kumar PN, et al. Diagnosis of intracranial lymphoma in patients with AIDS: value of 201TI single-photon emission computed tomography. *AJR Am J Roentgenol* 1994;163:417.
312. Cingolani A, De Luca A, Larocca LM, et al. Minimally invasive diagnosis of acquired immunodeficiency syndrome-related primary central nervous system lymphoma. *J Natl Cancer Inst* 1998;90:364.
313. MacMahon EM, Glass JD, Hayward SD, et al. Epstein-Barr virus in AIDS-related primary central nervous system lymphoma. *Lancet* 1991;338:969.
314. Antinori A, De Rossi G, Ammassari A, et al. Value of combined approach with thallium-201 single-photon emission computed tomography and Epstein-Barr virus DNA polymerase chain reaction in CSF for the diagnosis of AIDS-related primary CNS lymphoma. *J Clin Oncol* 1999;17:554.
315. Camilleri-Broet S, Davi F, Feuillard J, et al. High expression of latent membrane protein 1 of Epstein-Barr virus and BCL-2 oncoprotein in acquired immunodeficiency syndrome-related primary brain lymphomas. *Blood* 1995;86:432.

316. Bergmann M, Blasius S, Bankfalvi A, Mellin W. Primary non-Hodgkin lymphomas of the CNS-proliferation, oncoproteins and Epstein-Barr-virus. *Gen Diagn Pathol* 1996;141:235.
317. Jellinger KA, Paulus W. Primary central nervous system lymphomas—new pathological developments. *J Neurooncol* 1995;24:33.
318. Larocca LM, Capello D, Rinelli A, et al. The molecular and phenotypic profile of primary central nervous system lymphoma identifies distinct categories of the disease and is consistent with histogenetic derivation from germinal center-related B cells. *Blood* 1998;92:1011.
319. Baumgartner JE, Rachlin JR, Beckstead JH, et al. Primary central nervous system lymphomas: natural history and response to radiation therapy in 55 patients with acquired immunodeficiency syndrome. *J Neurosurg* 1990;73:206.
320. Deangelis LM. Current management of primary central nervous system lymphoma. *Oncology* 1995;9:63; discussion 71.
321. Chamberlain MC. Long survival in patients with acquired immune deficiency syndrome-related primary central nervous system lymphoma. *Cancer* 1994;73:1728.
322. Forsyth PA, Yahalom J, DeAngelis LM. Combined-modality therapy in the treatment of primary central nervous system lymphoma in AIDS. *Neurology* 1994;44:1473.
323. Deangelis LM, Yahalom J, Rosenblum M, Posner JB. Primary CNS lymphoma: managing patients with spontaneous and AIDS- related disease. *Oncology* 1987;1:52.
324. Reynolds P, Saunders LD, Layefsky ME, Lemp GF. The spectrum of acquired immunodeficiency syndrome (AIDS)-associated malignancies in San Francisco, 1980–1987. *Am J Epidemiol* 1993;137:19.
325. Hessol NA, Katz MH, Liu JY, et al. Increased incidence of Hodgkin disease in homosexual men with HIV infection. *Ann Intern Med* 1992;117:309.
326. Hartge P, Devesa SS, Fraumeni JF Jr. Hodgkin's and non-Hodgkin's lymphomas. *Cancer Surv* 1994;19:423.
327. Harnly ME, Swan SH, Holly EA, Kelter A, Padian N. Temporal trends in the incidence of non-Hodgkin's lymphoma and selected malignancies in a population with a high incidence of acquired immunodeficiency syndrome (AIDS). *Am J Epidemiol* 1988;128:261.
328. Bernstein L, Levin D, Menck H, Ross RK. AIDS-related secular trends in cancer in Los Angeles County men: a comparison by marital status. *Cancer Res* 1989;49:466.
329. Monfardini S, Tirelli U, Vaccher E, Foa R, Gavosto F. Hodgkin's disease in 63 intravenous drug users infected with human immunodeficiency virus. Gruppo Italiano Cooperativo AIDS & Tumori (GICAT). *Ann Oncol* 1991;2(Suppl 2):201.
330. Serraino D, Carbone A, Franceschi S, Tirelli U. Increased frequency of lymphocyte depletion and mixed cellularity subtypes of Hodgkin's disease in HIV-infected patients. Italian Cooperative Group on AIDS and Tumours. *Eur J Cancer* 1993;14:1948.
331. Levy R, Colonna P, Tourani JM, et al. Human immunodeficiency virus associated Hodgkin's disease: report of 45 cases from the French Registry of HIV-Associated Tumors. *Leuk Lymphoma* 1995;16:451.
332. Bouabdallah R, Quiles N, Bonnet E, et al. Hodgkin's disease (HD) in HIV infected patients: clinical, histologic and therapeutic aspects. *Int Conf AIDS*, Vol. 9, 1993.
333. Tirelli U, Errante D, Dolcetti R, et al. Hodgkin's disease and human immunodeficiency virus infection: clinicopathologic and virologic features of 114 patients from the Italian Cooperative Group on AIDS and Tumors. *J Clin Oncol* 1995;13:1758.
334. Bellas C, Santon A, Manzanal A, et al. Pathological, immunological, and molecular features of Hodgkin's disease associated with HIV infection. Comparison with ordinary Hodgkin's disease. *Am J Surg Pathol* 1996;20:1520.
335. Audouin J, Diebold J, Pallesen G. Frequent expression of Epstein-Barr virus latent membrane protein-l in tumour cells of Hodgkin's disease in HIV-positive patients. *J Pathol* 1992;167:381.
336. Deacon EM, Pallesen G, Niedobitek G, et al. Epstein-Barr virus and Hodgkin's disease: transcriptional analysis of virus latency in the malignant cells. *J Exp Med* 1993;177:339.
337. Tubiana M, Henry-Amar M, Hayat M, et al. Prognostic significance of the number of involved areas in the early stages of Hodgkin's disease. *Cancer* 1984;54:885.
338. Levine AM, Cheung T, Huang J, Testa M. Prospective, multicenter phase II trial of ABVD chemotherapy with G-CSF in HIV-infected patients with Hodgkin's disease (HD): AIDS Clinical Trials Group (ACTG) study 149. *Proc Annu Meet Am Soc Clin Oncol* 1997;16 (abst).
339. Errante D, Gabarre J, Ridolfo AL, et al. Hodgkin's disease in 35 patients with HIV infection: an experience with epirubicin, bleomycin, vinblastine and prednisone chemotherapy in combination with antiretroviral therapy and primary use of G-CSF. *Ann Oncol* 1999;10:189.
340. Tirelli U, Errante D, Oksenhendler E, et al. Prospective study with combined low-dose chemotherapy and zidovudine in 37 patients with poor-prognosis AIDS-related non-Hodgkin's lymphoma. French-Italian Cooperative Study Group. *Ann Oncol* 1992;3:843.
341. Venet A, Tourani JM, Beldjord K, et al. Actuarial rate of clinical and biological progression in a cohort of 250 HIV-1-seropositive subjects. Laennec HIV Study Group. *Clin Exp Immunol* 1990;80:151.
342. Andrieu JM, Roithmann S, Tourani JM, et al. Hodgkin's disease during HIV1 infection: the French registry experience. French Registry of HIV associated Tumors. *Ann Oncol* 1993;4:635.
343. Errante D, Tirelli U, Gastaldi R, et al. Combined antineoplastic and antiretroviral therapy for patients with Hodgkin's disease and human immunodeficiency virus infection. A prospective study of 17 patients. The Italian Cooperative Group on AIDS and Tumors (GICAT). *Cancer* 1994;73:437.
344. Palefsky JM. Human papillomavirus infection and anogenital neoplasia in human immunodeficiency virus-positive men and women. *J Natl Cancer Inst* Monogr 1998;23:15.
345. Frisch M, Glimelius B, van den Brule AJ, et al. Sexually transmitted infection as a cause of anal cancer. *N Engl J Med* 1997;337:1350.
346. MMWR. *1993 sexually transmitted diseases treatment guidelines.* Atlanta: Centers for Disease Control and Prevention, 1993.
347. Palefsky JM, Holly EA, Ralston ML, Jay N. Prevalence and risk factors for human papillomavirus infection of the anal canal in human immunodeficiency virus (HIV)-positive and HIV-negative homosexual men. *J Infect Dis* 1998;177:361.
348. Northfelt DW, Swift PS, Palefsky JM. Anal neoplasia. Pathogenesis, diagnosis, and management. *Hematol Oncol Clin North Am* 1996;10:1177.
349. Palefsky JM, Holly EA, Ralston ML, et al. Anal cytological abnormalities and anal HPV infection in men with Centers for Disease Control group IV HIV disease. *Genitour Med* 1997;73:174.
350. Goldie SJ, Kuntz KM, Weinstein MC, et al. The clinical effectiveness and cost-effectiveness of screening for anal squamous intraepithelial lesions in homosexual and bisexual HIV-positive men. *JAMA* 1999;281:1822.
351. Wright TC Jr, Ellerbrock TV, Chiasson MA, Van Devanter N, Sun XW. Cervical intraepithelial neoplasia in women infected with human immunodeficiency virus: prevalence, risk factors, and validity of Papanicolaou smears. New York Cervical Disease Study. *Obstet Gynecol* 1994;84:591.
352. Hillemanns P, Ellerbrock TV, McPhillips S, et al. Prevalence of anal human papillomavirus infection and anal cytologic abnormalities in HIV-seropositive women. *AIDS* 1996;10:1641.
353. Spinillo A, Tenti P, Zappatore R, et al. Prevalence, diagnosis and treatment of lower genital neoplasia in women with human immunodeficiency virus infection. *Eur J Obstet Gynecol Reprod Biol* 1992;43:235.
354. Wright TC, Ellerbrock TV, Chiasson MA, Dole P. Cervical disease in HIV-infected women: prevalence, incidence, risk factors, detection and use of loop electrosurgical excision for treatment. *HIV Infect Women Conf* 1995:S59.
355. Edelman M, Fox AS, Alderman EM, et al. Cervical Papanicolaou smear abnormalities in inner city Bronx adolescents: prevalence, progression, and immune modifiers. *Cancer* 1999;87:184.
356. Motti PG, Dallabetta GA, Daniel RW, et al. Cervical abnormalities, human papillomavirus, and human immunodeficiency virus infections in women in Malawi. *J Infect Dis* 1996;173:714.
357. Sun XW, Kuhn L, Ellerbrock TV, et al. Human papillomavirus infection in women infected with the human immunodeficiency virus. *N Engl J Med* 1997;337:1343.
358. Carter JJ, Koutsky LA, Wipf GC, et al. The natural history of human papillomavirus type 16 capsid antibodies among a cohort of university women. *J Infect Dis* 1996; 174:927.
359. Klein RS, Ho GY, Vermund SH, Fleming I, Burk RD. Risk factors for squamous intraepithelial lesions on Pap smear in women at risk for human immunodeficiency virus infection. *J Infect Dis* 1994;170:1404.
360. Maiman M, Fruchter RG, Guy L, et al. Human immunodeficiency virus infection and invasive cervical carcinoma. *Cancer* 1993;71:402.
361. Palefsky JM. Anal squamous intraepithelial lesions: relation to HIV and human papillomavirus infection. *J Acquir Immune Defic Syndr* 1999;21(Suppl 1):S42.
362. Petry KU, Scheffel D, Bode U, et al. Cellular immunodeficiency enhances the progression of human papillomavirus-associated cervical lesions. *Int J Cancer* 1994;57:836.
363. Vernon SD, Hart CE, Reeves WC, Icenogle JP. The HIV-1 tat protein enhances E2-dependent human papillomavirus 16 transcription. *Virus Res* 1993;27:133.
364. Tornesello ML, Buonaguro FM, Beth-Giraldo E, Giraldo G. Human immunodeficiency virus type 1 tat gene enhances human papillomavirus early gene expression. *Intervirology* 1993;36:57.
365. Dolei A, Curreli S, Pierangeli A, et al. HIV induces the expression of naturally integrated HPV18 both at the transcriptional and the translational level. *Int Conf AIDS*, Vol. 11, 1996.
366. Tan W, Schwartz S. The Rev protein of human immunodeficiency virus type 1 counteracts the effect of an AU-rich negative element in the human papillomavirus type 1 late 3' untranslated region. *J Virol* 1995;69:2932.
367. Tan W, Felber BK, Zolotukhin AS, Pavlakis GN, Schwartz S. Efficient expression of the human papillomavirus type 16 L1 protein in epithelial cells by using Rev and the Rev-responsive element of human immunodeficiency virus or the cis-acting transactivation element of simian retrovirus type 1. *J Virol* 1995;69:5607.
368. Wright T, Sun XW, Ellerbrock TV, Chiasson MA. Comparison of the amount of HPV 16 DNA in cervicovaginal secretions of HIV-infected and -uninfected women, using quantitative competitive-polymerase chain reaction (QC-PCR). *Int Conf AIDS*, Geneva, Vol. 12, 1998.
369. Luque AE, Demeter LM, Reichman RC. Association of human papillomavirus infection and disease with magnitude of human immunodeficiency virus type 1 (HIV-1) RNA plasma level among women with HIV-1 infection. *J Infect Dis* 1999;179:1405.
370. Chlow CC, Hawes SE, Kuypers JM, et al. Effect of HIV infection on the natural history of anal human papillomavirus infection. *Int Conf AIDS*, Geneva, Vol. 12, 1998.
371. Maiman M, Fruchter RG, Serur E, et al. Recurrent cervical intraepithelial neoplasia in human immunodeficiency virus-seropositive women. *Obstet Gynecol* 1993;82:170.
372. Heard I, Schmitz V, Costagloila D, Orth G, Kazatchkine MD. Early regression of cervical lesions in HIV-seropositive women receiving highly active antiretroviral treatments (HAART). *Int Conf AIDS*, Geneva, Vol. 12, 1998.
373. Robinson W, Hamilton C, Michaels S, Kissinger P. *The effect of excisional therapy and highly active antiretroviral therapy on cervical intraepithelial neoplasis HIV-infected women.* 3rd National AIDS Malignancy Meeting, Bethesda, MD, May 26–27, 1999.
374. Leyria C, Flichman JC, Wainstein C, Blumtritt CC. Human papilloma virus (HPV) lesions in HIV+ and AIDS patients. *Int Conf AIDS*, Geneva, Vol. 12, 1998.
375. Friedman HB, Saah AJ, Sherman ME, et al. Human papillomavirus, anal squamous intraepithelial lesions, and human immunodeficiency virus in a cohort of gay men. *J Infect Dis* 1998;178:45.
376. Palefsky JM, Holly EA, Ralston ML, et al. *The effect of HAART on the natural history of anal squamous intraepithelial lesions in HIV+ men.* 3rd National AIDS Malignancy Meeting, Bethesda, MD, May 26–27, 1999.
377. Hocht S, Wiegel T, Kroesen AJ, et al. Low acute toxicity of radiotherapy and radiochemotherapy in patients with cancer of the anal canal and HIV-infection. *Acta Oncol* 1997;36:799.
378. Hoffman R, Welton ML, Klencke B, Weinberg V, Krieg R. The significance of pretreatment CD4 count on the outcome and treatment tolerance of HIV-positive patients with anal cancer. *Int J Radiat Oncol Biol Phys* 1999;44:127.

379. Tavio M, Vaccher E, Antinori A, et al. Combination chemotherapy with doxorubicin, bleomycin, and vindesine for AIDS-related Kaposi's sarcoma. *Cancer* 1996;77:2117.
380. Gill P, Mitsuyasu R, Montgomery T, et al. AIDS Clinical Trials Group Study 094: a phase I/II trial of ABV chemotherapy with zidovudine and recombinant human GM-CSF in AIDS-related Kaposi's sarcoma. *Cancer J Sci Am* 1997;3:278.
381. Kaplan L, Abrams D, Volberding P. Treatment of Kaposi's sarcoma in acquired immunodeficiency syndrome with an alternating vincristine-vinblastine regimen. *Cancer Treat Rep* 1986;70:1121.
382. Gaidano G, Carbone A, Dalla-Favera R. Pathogenesis of AIDS-related lymphomas: molecular and histogenetic heterogeneity. *Am J Pathol* 1998;152:623.
383. Knowles DM, Chamulak GA, Subar M, et al. Lymphoid neoplasia associated with the acquired immunodeficiency syndrome (AIDS): the New York University Medical Center experience with 105 patients (1981–1986). *Ann Intern Med* 1988;108:744.
384. Sparano JA, Wiernik PH, Strack M, et al. Infusional cyclophosphamide, doxorubicin and etoposide in HIV-related non-Hodgkin's lymphoma: a follow-up report of a highly active regimen. *Leuk Lymphoma* 1994;14:263.

***SECTION* 2**

STANLEY R. RIDDELL

Transplantation-Related Malignancies

The transplantation of hematopoietic stem cells to restore bone marrow function after high-dose cytotoxic therapy for malignant and nonmalignant diseases and the surgical implantation of an allogeneic solid organ to restore organ function have become increasingly effective therapeutic modalities. The survival of patients undergoing hematopoietic stem cell and solid organ transplantation has improved as a result of more effective prophylaxis and treatment of infections in the early posttransplant period and the introduction of refined immunosuppressive regimens for preventing or treating graft-versus-host disease (GVHD) and graft rejection, respectively.[1–7] As larger numbers of patients are being cured of their underlying disease with transplantation, late complications, including the development of a malignancy, have assumed greater importance in the medical management of transplant patients.

The development of registries that collect data on large numbers of patients who have received hematopoietic stem cell or solid organ transplants has provided a mechanism to identify the late development of malignancies in transplant recipients.[8,9] The method most commonly used for analysis of the risk of a new malignancy is the standardized incidence ratio, which refers to the incidence of the malignancy observed in patients who have undergone transplantation compared with the expected incidence in the general population of the same age and gender. In the 1980s and 1990s, large numbers of patients undergoing hematopoietic stem cell transplantation (HSCT) and solid organ allografting have been followed, and several malignancies that occur with increased frequency compared with the general population have been identified.

IMMUNE SURVEILLANCE AND TUMOR DEVELOPMENT

It has been hypothesized that the host has a natural immunologic resistance against the development of cancer and that the prolonged or intense immunosuppression that is administered to transplant recipients would result in the frequent development of tumors. Class I and II major histocompatibility complex (MHC) molecules expressed on the surface of cells bind cellular peptides for presentation to CD8+ and CD4+ T cells, respectively, and this provides a mechanism whereby T cells, which are essential for protecting the host from virus infection, could also recognize and eliminate cells that have developed mutations that induce malignant transformation. Studies have shown that many common tumors in humans do present antigens to T cells, but there has been little direct evidence to support a role for immune surveillance in the development of these cancers.

Although immune surveillance does not appear to limit the development of common malignancies in normal hosts, the observation that many cancers that develop in chronically immunosuppressed transplant recipients are associated with oncogenic viruses such as Epstein-Barr virus (EBV) and human herpesvirus-8 (HHV-8), or with exposure to ultraviolet light suggests that immune surveillance mechanisms may function against these highly antigenic tumors. Virus-associated malignancies often undergo complete regression with withdrawal of immunosuppressive drugs or after restoration of functional T-cell responses to viral antigens by adoptive immunotherapy, and these observations provide direct evidence of a role for host immunity in containing the outgrowth of these tumors. Thus, immunodeficient transplant recipients provide a unique opportunity to reexamine the role of the immune system in tumor development and to determine the principles for effectively treating tumors in humans with immunotherapy.

HEMATOPOIETIC STEM CELL TRANSPLANT RECIPIENTS

Approximately 12,000 allogeneic and 18,000 autologous stem cell transplants are performed worldwide each year.[10] Several studies have demonstrated that patients who have received either an allogeneic or autologous HSCT are at an increased risk for the development of a new malignancy compared with the general population. Allogeneic HSCT recipients are at increased risk for the development of lymphoproliferative disorders and solid tumors, and autologous HSCT recipients are at increased risk for developing acute myeloid leukemia (AML) or myelodysplastic syndrome (MDS) and solid tumors. The peak time for the occurrence of these malignancies after transplant suggests distinct factors are involved in their pathogenesis. Solid tumors show a steady increase in incidence with time, lymphoproliferative disorders typically occur during the first year at the height of the immunodeficiency, and AML and MDS primarily occur in the first 3 years after transplant (Fig. 50.2-1).

SOLID TUMORS AFTER HEMATOPOIETIC STEM CELL TRANSPLANTATION

Epidemiology

Early studies in rhesus monkeys and in dogs given gamma irradiation and either autologous or allogeneic HSCT revealed a strik-

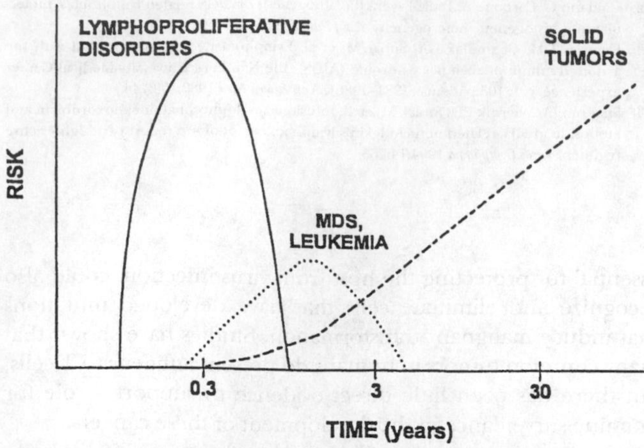

FIGURE 50.2-1. Time course and relative risk of the major categories of malignancies that develop after hematopietic stem cell transplantation. MDS, myelodysplastic syndrome. (Reproduced with permission from Deeg HJ, Socie G. Malignancies after hematopietic stem cell transplantation: many questions, some answers. *Blood* 1998;91:1833.)

ing increase in the development of solid tumors when compared with control unirradiated animals.[11–13] Tumors developed in these animal models a median of 8 years after transplantation, and it was anticipated that long-term follow-up of humans who received cytotoxic conditioning and HSCT might similarly reveal an increase in the incidence of solid tumors. The first large study to address the development of solid tumors in HSCT recipients evaluated 2145 patients who underwent allogeneic or syngeneic HSCT between 1970 and 1987 as treatment for leukemia or aplastic anemia. In this study, 13 solid tumors developed a median of 56 months (range, 2.5 to 163.0 months) after transplantation.[14] The histology of these malignancies was varied and included glioblastoma, melanoma, squamous cell carcinoma of the skin or oral cavity, basal cell carcinoma of the skin, adenocarcinoma of the gastrointestinal tract and lung, and hepatoma. Subsequent studies at other centers confirmed the late development of solid tumors in HSCT recipients.[15–17] These early studies validated the concern raised by animal models of stem cell transplantation and identified a need to evaluate larger numbers of patients to define the risk of individual tumors and to elucidate the pathogenesis of tumor development in these patients.

A multicenter study analyzed the occurrence of solid tumors in 19,220 patients who received allogeneic or syngeneic HSCT between 1964 and 1992.[18] Overall, the ratio of observed to expected (O/E) cases of new solid tumors was 2.7, with a cumulative incidence rate of 2.2% at 10 years and 6.7% at 15 years.[18] The rapid increase in the incidence of solid tumors between 10 and 15 years suggests that the risk will be even greater with longer follow-up. Cancers that occur with significantly increased frequency in HSCT recipients include melanoma (O/E = 5.0), cancers of the buccal cavity or oropharynx (O/E = 11.1), liver (O/E = 7.5), brain (O/E = 7.6), thyroid (O/E = 6.6), bone (O/E = 13.4), and connective tissues (O/E = 8.0) (Table 50.2-1). Breast, lung, gastrointestinal, and genitourinary tumors, which represent the most common malignancies in the general population, are not increased in HSCT recipients (Table 50.2-2).

The factors associated with a significantly increased risk of solid tumor development in HSCT recipients are younger age at

TABLE 50.2-1. Ratio of Observed to Expected Cases of Solid Tumors in Hematopoietic Stem Cell Transplant Recipients: Tumors That Occur with Increased Frequency Compared with the General Population[a]

Site of Tumor Development	*Ratio of Observed to Expected Cases*	*95% Confidence Interval*
Melanoma	5.0	2.5–8.9
Buccal cavity or oropharynx	11.1	6.5–17.8
Liver	7.5	1.5–22.0
Brain or other central nervous system	7.6	3.8–13.5
Thyroid	6.6	2.8–12.9
Connective tissue	8.0	2.2–20.5
Bone	13.4	4.3–31.3

[a] The *P* value for the ratio of observed to expected cases for all tumors is <.05.
(Adapted from ref. 18.)

the time of transplant and the use of total body irradiation in the pretransplant conditioning regimen.[18] The risk of developing a tumor posttransplant is 36 times higher than expected for children who are younger than the age of 10 years at the time of transplant, 4.6 times higher for patients aged 10 to 29, and nearly normal for those patients who are aged 30 and older. The excess risk in children younger than age 10 years is primarily due to the development of brain and thyroid tumors in patients who have received pretransplant cranial irradiation. Total body irradiation in doses of greater than 10 Gy in a single dose or greater than 13 Gy in fractionated doses is associated with an increased risk for squamous cell carcinoma of the oral cavity (relative risk = 3.0), melanoma (relative risk = 8.2), thyroid (relative risk = 5.8), and central nervous system (CNS) tumors (relative risk = 4.3).[18]

The analysis of risk factors does not support a role for defective immune surveillance in the development of most solid tumors after HSCT because T-cell depletion of the stem cell graft; acute, chronic, or both acute and chronic GVHD; or transplantation from MHC-mismatched donors are not associated with an increased risk. However, there may be a potential role for immune deficiency or dysregulation in the development of melanoma and squamous cell carcinoma of the oral cavity in HSCT recipients. Transplantation of stem cells that are depleted

TABLE 50.2-2. Ratio of Observed to Expected Cases of Solid Tumors in Hematopoietic Stem Cell Transplant Recipients: Tumors That Occur with the Same Frequency as in the General Population

Site of Tumor Development	*Ratio of Observed to Expected Cases*	*95% Confidence Interval*
Breast	1.1	0.4–2.2
Lung	0.7	0.1–2.6
Colon	0.7	0.0–3.8
Rectum	2.2	0.3–7.9
Cervix	0.7	0.0–3.9
Uterus	1.4	0.0–7.9

(Adapted from ref. 18.)

of donor T cells to prevent GVHD confers an increased risk for melanoma (relative risk = 4.5).[18] Additionally, patients who develop chronic GVHD and require longer than 1 year of immunosuppressive therapy exhibit a significantly increased risk of squamous cell carcinoma of the buccal cavity (relative risk = 6.0) and skin (relative risk = 22.6).[18]

Solid tumors also develop with increased frequency in recipients of autologous HSCT, although the available data are derived from analysis of smaller numbers of patients and are not sufficient to accurately define the risk for specific tumors.[15,19] However, the types of solid tumors reported after autologous HSCT are similar to those seen in allogeneic HSCT recipients and include squamous and basal cell carcinoma of the skin, melanoma, CNS tumors, and thyroid carcinoma. The major risk factor for the development of solid tumors after autologous HSCT is the use of total body irradiation in the conditioning regimen. Studies assessing larger numbers of autologous HSCT recipients will be helpful in further defining the epidemiology of tumors in these patients. Because autologous HSCT recipients do not develop GVHD or receive immunosuppressive drug therapy, comparison of the incidence and types of malignancies that develop in these patients with allogeneic HSCT recipients may assist in elucidating the contributions of GVHD and immunosuppressive drug therapy to the pathogenesis of tumor development.

Pathogenesis

The mechanisms operative in the genesis of solid tumors developing after HSCT have not been fully elucidated.[20] The use of total body irradiation is associated with a higher risk of solid tumor development, suggesting that DNA damage induced by ionizing radiation is an important contributor to tumorigenesis. Chronic GVHD is a risk factor for squamous cell cancer of the oral cavity, suggesting that chronic inflammation induced by alloreactivity at the local site, prolonged treatment with immunosuppressive drugs, decreased immune surveillance, or all of these factors may be involved in the development of tumors at this site.[18,21] DNA from viruses with known oncogenic potential, such as human papilloma virus and EBV, have occasionally been detected in squamous cell carcinomas developing in the skin or at mucosal sites in immunosuppressed patients, and additional studies are necessary to determine if these viruses contribute significantly to tumor development in HSCT recipients.[22–25]

The association of T-cell depleted transplantation with an increased risk of melanoma suggests a potential role for defective T-cell function in the pathogenesis of melanoma. T cells reactive with melanocyte differentiation antigens such as Melan A, gp100, and tyrosinase, which are expressed in both normal melanocytes and melanomas, have been identified in normal individuals.[26] A role in immune surveillance has not been proven, but such T cells are expanded in the blood and tumor infiltrates of some patients with melanoma, recognize and kill tumor cells *in vitro*, and can mediate tumor regression after *in vitro* expansion and adoptive transfer to tumor-bearing hosts.[27,28]

Clinical Features, Diagnosis, and Management

The clinical features of solid tumors developing in HSCT recipients have not been distinguishable from tumors of the same histology developing in normal individuals, and diagnosis and management should be performed in accordance with standard practice for tumors of the same stage in nontransplant patients.

The increase in the incidence of second malignancies after HSCT does have an effect on long-term survival of these patients. A study that examined the causes of late deaths in patients free of their original disease 2 years after allogeneic HSCT found that new cancers accounted for 6% of the late deaths.[29] The median follow-up of patients in this study was only 80 months, and tumors that exhibit a longer latency may yet emerge. Thus, longer follow-up of HSCT recipients will be essential to fully evaluate the risk of solid tumor development and the effect on long-term survival. The current data would suggest that all HSCT recipients should be counseled pretransplant as to their risk of solid tumor development and that symptoms or signs that may be indicative of a malignancy be promptly evaluated to ensure early diagnosis and institution of therapy.

Newer approaches to allogeneic HSCT are being developed that use less intensive conditioning regimens either not containing total body irradiation or using lower doses of irradiation.[30,31] These approaches are not myeloablative and rely on the allogeneic graft-versus-tumor effect to eradicate the underlying malignancy. If such less intensive conditioning regimens prove to be equally efficacious as conventional myeloablative regimens and are widely adopted, the risk of secondary malignancies in allogeneic HSCT recipients may be reduced.

LYMPHOPROLIFERATIVE DISORDERS ASSOCIATED WITH EPSTEIN-BARR VIRUS IN HEMATOPOIETIC STEM CELL TRANSPLANT RECIPIENTS

Epidemiology

Posttransplant lymphoproliferative disorders (PTLDs), the overwhelming majority of which are of donor B cell origin and associated with EBV infection, are a life-threatening complication of allogeneic HSCT.[32–35] In contrast to solid tumors, which typically develop after an interval of several years, PTLDs most commonly develop during the first 6 months after HSCT and represent the most frequent new malignancy in the first 5 years after transplant.[20,36] In a large multicenter study of 18,014 patients who received allogeneic HSCT between 1969 and 1992, the cumulative incidence of PTLD was 1.0% at 10 years.[36] More than 80% of the cases occurred in the first year after transplant with the peak incidence in the third month posttransplant.

The risk of developing a PTLD differs dramatically in subsets of patients, depending on factors that interfere with the reconstitution of T-cell immunity. The use of MHC-mismatched donors, the administration of anti–T-cell antibodies in the preparative regimen or as GVHD prophylaxis or therapy, and depletion of T cells from the stem cell inoculum are all associated with an increased risk of PTLD.[15,33–36] Recipients of transplants from unrelated donors or donors mismatched at two or more MHC alleles with the recipient have a 3.7-fold greater risk of PTLD than recipients of transplants from matched related donors.[36] The use of antithymocyte globulin or anti-CD3 monoclonal antibodies as prophylaxis or therapy for GVHD is also associated with a markedly increased risk of PTLD.[14,36]

Patients who receive a stem cell transplant that is depleted of T cells to prevent GVHD are at higher risk (relative risk = 9.1) for developing PTLD than those who receive unmodified bone marrow or peripheral blood stem cells.[36] However, the method used to deplete T cells from the stem cell inoculum influences the risk of PTLD. A high risk of PTLD is seen when T-cell depletion is performed using monoclonal antibodies directed against surface markers expressed only by T cells or by both T cells and natural killer cells (relative risk = 12.8), or using sheep red blood cell E-rosetting techniques (relative risk = 15.6).[36] In contrast, depletion of T cells using techniques that eliminate both T and B cells, such as with the CAMPATH-1 antibody, which recognizes the CD52 surface molecule; elutriation, which removes lymphocytes based on size and density; or agglutination with soybean lectin, does not increase the risk of PTLD compared with unmodified HSCT.[36–40] The lower incidence of PTLD with these methods of T-cell depletion is presumably due to the removal of EBV-infected B cells from the stem cell inoculum.[37,39,41]

Pathogenesis

EBV is a ubiquitous human gamma herpesvirus that establishes a persistent infection in more than 90% of adults, and the near universal association of this virus with PTLD implies a direct role in tumor development. During primary EBV infection in normal hosts, the virus enters B lymphocytes by an interaction between the viral envelope glycoprotein gp350/220 and the B-cell surface molecule CD21, which serves as the receptor for the C3d complement fragment.[42] Some infected B cells may express the entire array of viral genes and undergo lytic infection and cell death, but a characteristic of primary EBV infection is expression of a limited set of viral proteins that include EBNA-1, EBNA-2, EBNA-3A, EBNA-3B, EBNA-3C, EBNA-LP, LMP-1, LMP-2A, and LMP-2B.[43] This pattern of EBV gene expression, termed the *latency III program*, is responsible for the proliferation of B cells observed in the early stages of primary EBV infection and in PTLD developing in immunosuppressed patients.

How EBV induces B-cell proliferation continues to be the subject of intense investigation. The consensus is that immortalization of B cells requires the coordinated action of several EBV proteins. EBNA-1 is required for maintenance of the viral episome, and EBNA-2 functions as a transcriptional activator that induces the expression of viral and cellular genes that regulate cell growth.[44–46] LMP-1 acts as an analogue of a constitutively active form of the CD40 signaling molecule in B cells and activates NF-κB.[47–49] The expression of LMP-1 as a transgene in mice resulted in the development of oligoclonal or monoclonal B-cell lymphomas, suggesting that this molecule is critically involved in B-cell transformation.[50]

In response to primary infection with EBV, immunocompetent hosts mount both a humoral and cellular immune response that limits the spread of replicating virus and eliminates the proliferating EBV-infected B cells that express the latency III program of viral genes. The T-cell response is characterized by major expansions of CD3+ CD8+ cytotoxic T cells (CTLs) that recognize both EBV lytic phase viral antigens and, with the notable exception of EBNA-1, antigens that are expressed in the proliferating EBV-infected B cells.[51–53] The elimination of proliferating EBV-infected B cells by CTLs assists in terminating the acute infection. However, residual virus remains in resting memory B cells in which the viral DNA persists as an episome and EBNA-1 is the only viral gene that is expressed.[44,54–56] The presence of glycine/alanine repeat sequences in the EBNA-1 protein precludes its efficient processing and presentation to CTLs, thus latently infected B cells are able to evade immune elimination and serve as a reservoir for reactivation.[57] Reactivation of EBV in latently infected B cells may be characterized by expression of the lytic program of gene expression and production of new virions, or the latency III program that induces B-cell proliferation. Because of this persistent reservoir of virus, memory CTL responses to EBV must be maintained for the life of the host to prevent the outgrowth of EBV-infected B cells.

The balance that is established between host T-cell immunity and persistent EBV in immunocompetent hosts is acutely and dramatically perturbed in the setting of allogeneic HSCT. The administration of cytotoxic therapy before HSCT destroys the host T cells, which are required to maintain EBV in a latent state, and also eliminates the reservoir of host EBV-infected B cells. The infusion of unmanipulated allogeneic stem cells from an EBV-seropositive donor provides a new source of EBV-infected B cells and replaces the host EBV strain with the EBV strain of the donor.[58] Reconstitution of EBV-specific T-cell immunity is essential to reestablish control of EBV infection. However, a quantitative deficiency of EBV-specific CTLs is common in the first 6 months after allogeneic transplant.[59,60] T-cell depletion of the stem cell graft, which reduces the number of EBV-specific T cells administered to the recipient, or the use of monoclonal anti T-cell antibodies for GVHD prophylaxis or therapy, which eliminates EBV-specific T cells *in vivo*, further impairs T-cell recovery. In the setting of a severe deficiency of EBV-specific CTLs, EBV may reactivate, induce polyclonal proliferation of B cells, and result in the emergence of rapidly growing oligoclonal or monoclonal populations.

Clinical Features and Diagnosis

PTLD in HSCT recipients commonly presents with fever and progressive lymphadenopathy. Involvement of pharyngeal lymphoid tissue with an exudative pharyngitis is observed in one-third of patients.[38] The lesions may be extranodal and involve the spleen, liver, lungs, gastrointestinal tract, kidneys, and CNS. Thus, PTLD should be included in the differential diagnosis of symptoms or signs related to these organs in a patient at high risk.

The diagnosis is usually established by biopsy and demonstration of the presence of EBV in involved tissue. Tumors developing after HSCT almost always consist of oligoclonal or monoclonal populations of donor B cells and most commonly exhibit a monomorphic diffuse large cell morphology, although plasmacytoid or polymorphic morphology are also seen.[38,61] The presence of EBV in the tumor is established by Southern blot of DNA extracted from tumor tissue or by analysis of EBV gene expression in tissue sections. Two EBV-encoded RNAs (EBERs) are abundantly expressed in PTLD and can be detected in tissue sections by *in situ* hybridization.[62] Immunohistochemical staining with antibodies against EBV proteins can also be used to confirm the presence of EBV in thc tumor.[63] Analysis of Ig gene rearrangements or characterization of repeat sequences at EBV DNA episomal joints is used to determine the clonality of tumor cells. Detection of high EBV DNA levels by polymerase chain reaction analysis of DNA in peripheral blood has been associated with PTLD and may be useful for early diagnosis and monitoring response to therapy.[64]

Therapy and Prophylaxis of Posttransplant Lymphoproliferative Disorders

The development of PTLD in HSCT recipients is an ominous sign due to the propensity for these tumors to grow rapidly, and urgent therapy is usually necessary. Reduction in the intensity of immunosuppression is indicated, although this may not be possible in patients with severe GVHD. Surgical resection or irradiation may be appropriate as a temporary measure to control anatomically localized disease, but recurrences at other sites are common. Efforts to treat PTLD with chemotherapy regimens similar to those used to treat non-Hodgkin's lymphoma are only occasionally successful in HSCT recipients in part due to the toxicity of administering systemic chemotherapy to these patients.

Anecdotal reports and studies in small numbers of patients have examined systemic therapy with antiviral drugs and interferon-α. Although the administration of acyclovir or ganciclovir is often used as a component of therapy for PTLD, these drugs target the viral thymidine kinase, which is expressed in the replicative phase of EBV infection but not in proliferating EBV-infected B cells. These agents do not inhibit the growth of EBV-transformed B cells *in vitro* and would not be expected to be beneficial for PTLD. Pharmacologic induction of the viral thymidine kinase gene in EBV-infected cells by administration of arginine butyrate has been reported to render EBV-associated PTLD susceptible to ganciclovir and induce a complete regression in four of six patients.[65] The administration of interferon-α and immunoglobulin was reported to induce regression of PTLD in a small number of patients in an early study, but this approach has not been widely adopted.[32]

The infusion of anti–B-cell monoclonal antibodies directed at the CD21 and CD24 surface molecules has induced regression of PTLD in approximately 50% of patients. However, this approach is less effective in patients with oligoclonal or monoclonal disease and, at the present time, these antibodies are not commercially available.[66–68] The use of anti-CD20 monoclonal antibody (Rituxan) has been reported to induce remission of PTLD after HSCT in some patients, and the results of additional studies of this agent are eagerly awaited.[69,70]

The association of deficient EBV-specific T-cell immunity with the development of PTLD has led to efforts to restore T-cell responses to EBV by the adoptive transfer of T cells obtained from the stem cell donor. Support for this approach was provided by a study of five patients who developed PTLD after T-cell–depleted allogeneic HSCT and received infusions of unirradiated donor peripheral blood mononuclear cells containing 1×10^6 CD3+ T cells per kilogram of recipient body weight.[71] Clinical and pathologic regression of the PTLD was observed in all five patients, and three of these patients became long-term survivors. Two patients with pulmonary involvement developed fatal respiratory failure after the lymphocyte infusions, and two of the three surviving patients developed chronic GVHD.[71] In a subsequent report, 19 patients with PTLD were treated with donor lymphocytes, and 16 achieved complete pathologic and clinical resolution of their disease.[38] Studies analyzing the frequency of EBV-specific CTLs in the blood before and after therapy demonstrated a rapid amplification of EBV-specific CTLs to levels equivalent to normal donors. However, due to the presence of alloreactive T cells in the donor cells used for therapy, GVHD developed in 50% of the patients treated with this approach.[38]

An approach to cellular therapy of PTLD that alleviates the problem of GVHD uses donor T cells that are enriched for EBV-specific reactivity and depleted of alloreactivity by *in vitro* culture. The infusion of such cultured EBV-specific T cell lines is effective in treatment of established PTLD in HSCT recipients. Transferred T cells can be identified in the regressing tumor and persist in the blood for longer than 18 months after infusion.[72,73] The prophylactic administration of EBV-specific T cell lines to patients who have received a T-cell–depleted HSCT has been effective in preventing PTLD in these high-risk patients.[74] At the present time, the major impediment to the broader application of cellular therapy for EBV-associated PTLD is the technical expertise and resources required to isolate EBV-reactive T cells.

HODGKIN'S DISEASE AND LATE-ONSET NON-HODGKIN'S LYMPHOMAS IN HEMATOPOIETIC STEM CELL TRANSPLANT RECIPIENTS

Epidemiology

Hodgkin's disease has been reported to occur with increased frequency in immunosuppressed patients, including solid organ transplant recipients and human immunodeficiency virus (HIV)-infected patients.[75,76] The incidence of Hodgkin's disease has been evaluated in 18,531 allogeneic HSCT recipients and compared with the incidence in the general population.[77] Eight cases of Hodgkin's disease were observed in the HSCT patients, which was significantly more than expected in the age- and sex-matched general population (O/E = 6.2). There was a trend toward a significantly increased risk in patients who developed grade 3 or 4 GVHD. The majority of cases were of mixed cellularity histology and contained the EBV genome; however, in contrast to EBV-associated PTLD, which typically occurs in the first 6 months after transplant, the onset of Hodgkin's disease occurred at a median of 4.2 years after transplant.[77] Cases of late-onset non-Hodgkin's lymphoma have also been reported in HSCT recipients, but the majority of these are T cell in origin and an association with lymphotropic viruses, such as EBV or human T-cell lymphotropic virus, has not been demonstrated.[78]

Clinical Manifestations and Management

The cases of Hodgkin's disease reported in HSCT recipients were characterized by an aggressive histology, with 75% being mixed cellularity or lymphocyte depleted. Therapy with conventional chemotherapy or radiotherapy is usually effective, however, with six of the eight patients in the largest series alive 2.7 to 9.6 years after the diagnosis of Hodgkin's disease.[77]

ACUTE LEUKEMIA AND MYELODYSPLASTIC SYNDROME AFTER HEMATOPOIETIC STEM CELL TRANSPLANTATION

Epidemiology

AML and MDS are well-recognized complications of conventional chemotherapy and radiotherapy for Hodgkin's disease, non-Hodgkin's lymphoma, breast cancer, and other malignancies.[79–82] Patients who receive high-dose chemotherapy and autologous HSCT for non-Hodgkin's lymphoma and Hodgkin's disease have also been reported to have an increased risk of secondary AML or MDS compared with the general population. In three large series, the cumulative incidence of AML/MDS in recipients of autologous HSCT for non-Hodgkin's lymphoma or Hodgkin's disease was 5% at 5 years,[83] 18% at 6 years,[84] and 14.5% at 5 years,[85] respectively. Risk factors for the development of AML/MDS were age older than 40 years at the time of transplant, pretransplant irradiation, pretransplant therapy with alkylating agents, mobilization of stem cells with VP-16, and a low pretransplant platelet count.[83–86] In one study, the use of total body irradiation in the conditioning regimen was a risk factor for the development of AML/MDS after transplant.[83]

Rare cases of leukemia developing in donor cells after allogeneic HSCT have also been reported.[87–90] In these cases, the donor reportedly remained healthy and the mechanism of leukemogenesis in the recipient remained unexplained. Inadvertent transplantation of marrow from a donor with AML has also been reported.[91]

Pathogenesis

The pathogenesis of secondary AML/MDS in patients who receive conventional chemotherapy or combined chemoradiotherapy is related to DNA damage in hematopoietic stem cells induced by alkylating agents, epidophyllotoxins, or ionizing radiation. It is unclear whether the risk of AML/MDS is entirely due to damage to stem cells from prior chemotherapy or if the conditioning regimen administered immediately before transplant further adds to the risk. A study of patients with multiple myeloma who underwent autologous HSCT found that the risk of developing AML/MDS correlated with the intensity and duration of pretransplant conventional chemotherapy.[92] However, the increased risk of AML/MDS when total body irradiation was a component of the conditioning regimen suggests that there may be additional contributions from regimen-related damage to residual stem cells in the patient or to the marrow stroma.[83]

Cytogenetic abnormalities are occasionally found in the marrow of patients being evaluated for autologous HSCT. In a few cases in which the marrow was morphologically normal and was used for transplant despite the presence of cytogenetic alterations, the patients developed MDS or AML in the first 12 months after transplant.[93] Thus, cytogenetic analysis of the bone marrow should be considered in patients with extensive prior therapy who are being evaluated for HSCT.

Clinical Features and Management

The clinical features of AML/MDS after autologous HSCT are the same as those seen in cases of secondary AML/MDS that develop after conventional chemotherapy or low-dose radiation. These include frequent abnormalities of chromosomes 5 and 7 and a poor response to therapy. A small number of patients who have developed AML/MDS after autologous HSCT have subsequently been treated with a second high-dose cytotoxic regimen followed by allogeneic HSCT.[94] This approach is complicated by a high risk of regimen-related toxicity but can be curative.

ORGAN TRANSPLANT RECIPIENTS

The transplantation of allogeneic solid organs has become a widely used and often life-saving therapy, with more than 20,000 procedures performed in 1997 in the United States.[95] However, recipients of organ allografts generally require life-long therapy with immunosuppressive drugs to prevent or treat episodes of graft rejection and are at increased risk for the development of a malignancy. The overwhelming majority of tumors arising in solid organ transplant recipients are *de novo* malignancies of recipient origin,[9,96,97] or recurrence of a malignancy existing in the recipient before transplant.[98–100] However, a malignancy of donor origin may occasionally arise in the transplanted organ *de novo* or be inadvertently transmitted to the recipient via the transplanted organ.[101–106] Polymorphic molecular markers that differ between donor and recipient can be used to determine the origin of the malignancy, and these studies should be considered in suspicious cases because withdrawal of immunosuppression can sometimes result in regression of donor-derived malignancies.[102,103]

Data from single institutions and large international registries have shown that the incidence of cancer in organ allograft recipients is increased three- to fourfold compared with the general population.[9,97,107–109] The incidence of tumor development increases with the length of observation after transplant. In two studies of renal allograft recipients, the risk of developing cancer at 20 years after transplant was 40% to 50% compared with a 6% cumulative risk in the general population of age-matched individuals.[97,108] Similar to the findings in HSCT recipients, malignancies that develop frequently in the general population, such as those occurring in breast, lung, prostate, colon, and cervix, are not increased in solid organ transplant recipients.[110,111] The incidence of cancers of the skin and lip, and B-cell lymphoproliferative diseases are increased in both solid organ transplant and HSCT recipients.[9,97,108,112] Kaposi's sarcoma (KS), which is rarely seen in HSCT recipients, is significantly increased in organ allograft recipients.[113,114]

CANCER OF THE SKIN AND LIP

Epidemiology

Cancer of the skin or lip is the most common neoplasm developing in organ allograft recipients, and the risk of a cutaneous neoplasm is increased 3.2- to 24.0-fold compared with the general population.[115] The most dramatic increase is in squamous cell carcinoma, but the risk of developing basal cell carcinoma, melanoma, and Merkel's cell carcinoma is also significantly increased. The cumulative incidence of skin cancer increases with time after transplantation (Table 50.2-3). The incidence of skin cancer in renal transplant recipients was 70% at 20 years in a study from Australia where sun exposure is high,[116] and 40% in a study from the Netherlands.[115] In two studies of heart transplant recipients, the incidence of skin cancer was 44% and 35% at 7 and 10 years, respectively.[117,118] In the general population, basal cell carcinoma of the skin occurs five times more frequently than squamous cell carcinoma, whereas in organ transplant recipients, squamous cell carcinoma occurs one to three times more frequently than basal cell carcinoma.[114]

Cumulative sun exposure, the length of time after transplant, and mismatching between donor and recipient at the HLA-B locus or homozygosity at the HLA-DR locus have been identified as risk factors for the development of skin cancer in organ transplant recipients.[117,119,120] Features prevalent in patients with skin cancer in the general population, including light skin and blonde or red hair, are also prevalent in transplant recipients.

The length of time from transplant is an important risk factor and presumably reflects the contributions of immunosuppressive drug therapy to tumorigenesis. Insufficient data are available to conclude whether specific immunosuppressive drugs or the intensity of the regimen influences the risk of skin cancer. Patients who receive cyclosporine in addition to azathioprine and prednisolone[121] or who receive OKT3[117] have been reported to be

TABLE 50.2-3. Cumulative Incidence of Skin Cancer in Organ Transplant Recipients

Study	*Transplant Type*	*Follow-Up (y)*	*Cumulative Incidence (%)* Squamous Cell Carcinoma	Basal Cell Carcinoma	Squamous Cell Carcinoma + Basal Cell Carcinoma
Bouwes Bavnick et al.[116]	Renal	11	35	32	45
		20	58	54	70
Hartevelt et al.[115]	Renal	10	9	8	10
		20	35	10	40
Lampros et al.[117]	Heart	10	32	10	34
Espana et al.[118]	Heart	7	28	16	44

at higher risk for the development of skin cancer. However, other studies have not found an association between the type of immunosuppressive drug regimen used and the risk of skin cancer.[116]

Sun exposure and cigarette smoking are risk factors for the development of cancer of the lip in organ transplant recipients. In addition to an increased incidence of malignant lesions, transplant recipients have a higher incidence of leukoplakia and dysplastic lesions of the lip when compared with age- and sex-matched controls.[122]

Pathogenesis

Multiple factors may be involved in the pathogenesis of cancers of the skin and lip in organ allograft recipients, including underlying genetic predisposition, environmental factors, immunologic alterations induced by the transplant, immunosuppressive drugs, and viral infection. The mechanism by which transplantation and immunosuppressive drug therapy potentiates the development of skin cancer remains elusive. In murine models, tumors induced by ultraviolet light are often highly antigenic when transplanted into syngeneic mice, suggesting defects in the host immune response are required for tumor formation.[123] There is evidence that ultraviolet light induces local immunosuppressive effects that facilitate the establishment of tumors, and immunosuppressive drugs may potentiate this local impairment in host immunity.[124,125] Consistent with this hypothesis, the skin of renal allograft recipients exhibits a decrease in the density of CD4+ and CD8+ T lymphocytes, and CD1a+ dermal Langerhans' cells when compared with normal controls.[126] Moreover, melanomas that occur in solid organ transplant recipients lack the mononuclear cell infiltrates that are frequently seen in tumors in immunocompetent hosts and are associated with a good prognosis.[127] A potential role for cyclosporine in tumorigenesis that is distinct from its immunosuppressive properties has been identified. Exposure of tumor cells to cyclosporine increases the production of transforming growth factor-β, which results in increased tumor cell motility and invasiveness *in vitro* and enhanced tumor growth and metastasis *in vivo*.[128]

The association of viral infections with the development of malignancies in immunosuppressed patients has prompted a search for viruses in skin cancers in organ allograft recipients. There have been reports of the detection of human papillomavirus DNA in a significant fraction of skin cancers in organ transplant recipients.[22,24,129–133] However, other studies have failed to detect human papilloma-virus, and the role of this agent in the development of skin cancer in transplant recipients remains controversial.[25,134] EBV DNA and gene expression has been detected in tumors from 10 of 15 cardiac allograft recipients with squamous cell carcinoma, suggesting a potential role for EBV as a cofactor in tumor development.[25]

Clinical Features, Management, and Prevention

Skin disorders that resemble malignancies, such as warts, hyperkeratoses, and keratoacanthomas, are frequently observed in transplant patients, and a biopsy should be performed for suspicious lesions for accurate diagnosis. Premalignant lesions have been successfully treated with topical tretinoin[135] or a combination of low-dose etretinate and topical tretinoin.[136]

Skin cancers in organ transplant recipients are generally considered to be more aggressive than tumors that develop in the general population. Fifty percent to 80% of patients have multiple lesions, and individual lesions characteristically exhibit greater local invasiveness.[108,137] Squamous cell carcinomas in organ transplant patients are also more likely to metastasize to lymph nodes and distant sites.[137] Treatment of skin cancers in these patients is performed with the same modalities used for tumors in the general population, including surgical excision, cryosurgery, or radiotherapy.

Given the aggressive nature of skin cancers in organ allograft recipients, it is essential to educate patients about the hazards associated with sun exposure, provide strategies for protecting the skin from sunlight, and promote awareness of the importance of early detection and treatment.[138,139] Chemoprophylaxis of skin cancer with systemic retinoids may also be appropriate in high-risk patients. Acitretin has been suggested to reduce the number of new tumors in renal transplant recipients and to prevent keratotic skin lesions and skin cancer in a placebo-controlled trial.[140,141] The most effective preventive measure for skin cancer may come from the development of novel approaches to induce specific tolerance to the donor organ that do not require long-term administration of drugs that cause global immunosuppression.[142]

EPSTEIN-BARR VIRUS–ASSOCIATED LYMPHOPROLIFERATIVE DISORDERS IN ORGAN TRANSPLANT RECIPIENTS

Epidemiology

PTLDs associated with EBV infection are the second most frequent malignancy in solid organ transplant recipients.[114] In a study of 45,141 kidney transplant recipients and 7634 heart transplant recipients, the incidence of PTLD during the first year after transplant was 0.2% for kidney transplant recipients and 1.2% for heart transplant recipients.[143] These rates are 20 and 120 times higher, respectively, than the incidence of non-Hodgkin's lymphoma in the general population.[143] The incidence of PTLD is highest in the first year after transplant, but these tumors may develop with increased frequency for more than 6 years after transplant. PTLD in organ allograft recipients develop in host B cells, although the EBV strain may be derived from reactivation of latent virus in the host or virus transmitted with the donor organ.[144,145] Transplant recipients who are EBV seronegative and receive an organ from an EBV-seropositive donor are up to 76 times more likely to develop a PTLD than EBV-seropositive recipients.[146–148]

The drug regimen used to prevent or treat graft rejection influences the risk of PTLD, with the highest risk of PTLD observed in patients who receive cyclosporine, FK-506, or anti-CD3 monoclonal antibodies.[143] Heart, lung, or heart and lung transplants have a higher incidence of PTLD than patients receiving kidney or liver transplants because intensive immunosuppression must be maintained in these patients to prevent life-threatening graft rejection.[143] The administration of anti-CD3 monoclonal antibodies confers a particularly high risk of PTLD related both to the suppression of T-cell function and the release of T-cell cytokines that activate B cells.[149]

Pathogenesis

The pathogenesis of PTLD occurring in solid organ transplant recipients is similar to that in HSCT recipients and reflects defective control of EBV by the host immune response. The immunosuppressive drugs administered to organ transplant patients potently suppress EBV-specific CTL activity *in vitro* and *in vivo*.[150] A study of 30 cardiothoracic transplant recipients who received cyclosporin A and azathioprine as rejection prophylaxis showed that EBV-specific CTL activity in the peripheral blood was suppressed or undetectable in all patients during the first 6 months after transplant.[151] Recovery of EBV-specific T-cell responses is further impaired in patients who require additional immunosuppressive therapy with prednisone or azathioprine to treat rejection episodes.[151] These studies support a deficiency of EBV-specific CTLs as the critical factor in pathogenesis, but the clinical presentation of PTLD in organ allograft recipients suggests that local factors at the tumor site also play a role. Tumors frequently involve the transplanted organ, the CNS, and the gastrointestinal tract, suggesting that immunoregulatory factors in the microenvironment may act in concert with a deficiency of EBV-specific CTLs to predispose to the development of PTLD. The organ allograft is a site of chronic antigenic stimulation, and local cytokines produced by alloreactive T cells have been suggested to promote the activation and growth of EBV-infected B cells.[152]

Clinical Features, Diagnosis, and Management

Patients developing PTLD may present with an infectious mononucleosis syndrome, including fever, peripheral lymphadenopathy, and tonsillar enlargement. Occasionally, the disease presents with a fulminant course characterized by rapidly progressive diffuse multiorgan involvement and severe systemic symptoms. More commonly, PTLD presents with localized lesions in lymph nodes, extranodal sites, such as the gastrointestinal tract, CNS, lung, and the transplanted organ, or both nodes and extranodal sites.[153–155]

The diagnosis of PTLD is made by biopsy of involved tissue as described earlier for HSCT recipients. Three morphologic variants of PTLD are recognized in solid organ transplant recipients. These include plasmacytic hyperplasia, which is typically polyclonal, polymorphic B cell hyperplasia, which is typically monoclonal, and monomorphic lymphoma or multiple myeloma, which is monoclonal and contains alterations in oncogenes, tumor suppressor genes, or both, in addition to the EBV genome.[61,156] Studies suggest that patients with the monomorphic/myeloma morphology or with bcl-6 mutations have a poor response to therapy.[157,158]

A standard approach to the management of PTLD in organ allograft recipients has not been established. The therapeutic approach may depend on the site of tumor involvement, the rate of tumor growth, and the necessity to maintain intense immunosuppression. Initial therapy frequently consists of a reduction or withdrawal of immunosuppressive drug therapy, which can result in expansion of endogenous EBV-specific T cells and complete regression of the tumor.[159,160] However, this strategy may lead to rejection of the organ allograft, which, with the exception of renal transplant recipients who can return to dialysis therapy, can have disastrous consequences. Anatomically localized lesions may be amenable to surgical resection or limited field irradiation, but tumor recurrence is common.

Systemic therapy is usually necessary to control PTLD that fails to regress after a reduction in immunosuppressive therapy. The use of a combination of anti-B cell monoclonal antibodies targeting CD21 and CD24 for PTLD in organ transplant recipients resulted in a 55% survival at a median of 61 months, although the subset of patients with visceral disease, CNS involvement, or onset longer than 1 year after transplant responded poorly to therapy.[68] Early results with the anti-CD20 antibody (Rituxan) suggest a comparable response rate, although the follow-up on these patients is short.[161]

Chemotherapy has been used in patients who fail to respond to a reduction in immunosuppression or who have rapidly progressive disease. In small studies, standard regimens used for non-Hodgkin's lymphoma, such as cyclophosphamide, hydroxydaunorubicin (Adriamycin), Oncovin, and prednisone or ProMACE-CytaBOM have induced durable complete remissions in the majority of patients.[162,163] However, other studies have reported significantly less promising results due both to a high incidence of infectious complications related to neutropenia and refractory disease.[155,164]

Based on the encouraging results in allogeneic HSCT recipients, the use of cellular immunotherapy to restore EBV-specific T-cell immunity is being explored as therapy for PTLD occurring in solid organ transplant recipients. In contrast to the allogeneic HSCT recipients who have an immunocompetent stem cell donor that can be used as a source of T cells for therapy, EBV-specific T cells must be generated from the organ transplant recipient's blood before transplant and cryopreserved for later use. The feasibility of isolating and adoptively transferring EBV-reactive T cells from both EBV-seropositive and EBV-seronegative organ transplant recipients has been demonstrated.[165,166] The transfer of EBV-specific T cells resulted in an increase in the frequency of EBV-specific CTLs in the blood, and in a single patient with an established PTLD was associated with tumor regression.[166]

LATE-ONSET LYMPHOMAS AND HODGKIN'S DISEASE IN ORGAN TRANSPLANT RECIPIENTS

The overwhelming majority of PTLD are EBV-associated and of B cell origin, but well-documented cases of T-cell lymphoproliferative disorders have been described in organ transplant recipients. The T-cell lymphoproliferations typically occur several years after transplant, involve the bone marrow and peripheral blood at presentation, and are not related to EBV, human T-cell lymphotropic virus, or HHV-8 infection.[167] The prognosis for these patients is poor despite the administration of chemotherapy and reduction of immunosuppression.[167]

Hodgkin's disease has also been reported in organ allograft recipients, and the tumors are usually EBV positive.[76] The clinical presentation is typical of Hodgkin's disease in the general population, and these patients respond to conventional therapy.

KAPOSI'S SARCOMA

Epidemiology

The incidence of Kaposi's sarcoma is up to 500 times greater in organ transplant recipients than in the general population.[168–170] An analysis of patients reported to the Cincinnati Transplant Tumor Registry revealed that more transplant patients are diagnosed with KS than with colorectal, breast, or prostate cancer.[114] The major risk factors for the development of KS in organ transplant recipients include African or Middle Eastern origin and the use of antilymphocyte serum for immunosuppression.[171]

A human gamma herpesvirus termed *HHV-8* has been detected in KS lesions but not in uninvolved tissues from the same individual, leading to speculation that it plays either a direct causative role or is a critical cofactor in the pathogenesis of this tumor.[172–175] The role of HHV-8 in KS in organ transplant recipients has been examined by analysis of the serostatus of recipients and donors. The presence of HHV-8 antibodies before or after transplantation is highly predictive of the development of posttransplant KS, supporting a role for reactivation of endogenous HHV-8 or transmission of HHV-8 in the pathogenesis of KS.[171] The direct transmission of HHV-8 by the organ allograft has been demonstrated and, in conjunction with intensive immunosuppression, associated with the development of posttransplant KS.[176,177]

Pathogenesis

The finding of HHV-8 DNA in KS lesions suggests that this herpes virus is central to the pathogenesis of the tumor. HHV-8 has been shown to reactivate soon after transplantation, and increasing levels of virus in the blood are associated with the development of KS.[178] Despite tantalizing leads from molecular studies of HHV-8 reviewed in the preceding chapter, the mechanisms by which HHV-8 induces tumor formation have not been elucidated. The role played by immunosuppressive drug therapy in the development of KS is also unresolved. *In vitro*, corticosteroids activate the lytic cycle of HHV-8 gene expression, suggesting that immunosuppression may increase viral load *in vivo*.[179] The spontaneous regression in KS lesions observed with withdrawal of immunosuppression in organ transplant recipients or with the resolution of immunodeficiency in HIV infection suggests that cellular immune responses have a crucial role in control of HHV-8 infection and preventing the development of KS. CD8+ CTLs specific for antigens expressed in latent and lytic infection have been identified in HHV-8 seropositive individuals,[180] and it anticipated that future studies will address the role of deficient T-cell responses to HHV-8 in the pathogenesis of KS.

Clinical Features and Management

Sixty percent of organ allograft recipients with KS present with localized skin or mucosal lesions, and the remainder present with visceral disease involving the gastrointestinal tract, lungs, and lymph nodes.[114,181] The diagnosis of KS, which can be difficult in cases of visceral disease, is made by biopsy and histologic analysis. The mainstay of therapy for KS developing after solid organ transplant is reduction in immunosuppressive therapy. This intervention alone induces a complete response in approximately 25% of patients.[114,181] However, reintroduction of intensive immunosuppression to treat episodes of graft rejection has been associated with recurrence of the tumor. Due to the inability to maintain reduced levels of immunosuppression in many organ allograft recipients, chemotherapy using regimens described for KS in HIV infection is frequently required to control KS.[181,182] Novel less toxic approaches to treat KS are likely to emerge as the biology of these tumors is better understood. Cellular therapy with HHV-8–specific T cells may have a role in future therapeutic strategies. Additionally, KS cells have been shown to express the interleukin-4 receptor, and administration of interleukin-4 linked to a toxin molecule was highly effective in mediating tumor regression in a mouse xenograft model of established subcutaneous KS.[183]

OTHER HUMAN HERPESVIRUS-8–ASSOCIATED MALIGNANCIES IN ORGAN TRANSPLANT RECIPIENTS

HHV-8 has also been associated with other malignancies, including primary effusion lymphoma in HIV-infected patients and multicentric Castleman's diseases in both HIV-positive and -negative patients.[184,185] Primary effusion lymphoma with integrated HHV-8 DNA has been reported to occur rarely in solid organ transplant recipients and can be distinguished from the more common PTLD by the presence of malignant pleural, peritoneal, or pericardial effusions without tumor mass, or adenopathy.[186,187]

REFERENCES

1. Goodman JL, Winston DJ, Greenfield RA, et al. A controlled trial of fluconazole to prevent fungal infections in patients undergoing bone marrow transplantation. *N Engl J Med* 1992;326:845.
2. Goodrich JM, Bowden RA, Fisher L, et al. Ganciclovir prophylaxis to prevent cytomegalovirus disease after allogeneic marrow transplant. *Ann Intern Med* 1993;118:173.
3. Winston DJ, Ho WG, Bartoni K, et al. Ganciclovir prophylaxis of cytomegalovirus infection and disease in allogeneic bone marrow transplant recipients. *Ann Intern Med* 1993;118:179.
4. Gane E, Saliba F, Valdecasas GJ, et al. Randomised trial of efficacy and safety of oral ganciclovir in the prevention of cytomegalovirus disease in liver-transplant recipients. *Lancet* 1997;350:1729.
5. Merigan TC, Renlund DG, Keay S, et al. A controlled trial of ganciclovir to prevent cytomegalovirus disease after heart transplantation. *N Engl J Med* 1992;326:1182.
6. Fraund S, Pethig K, Franke U, et al. Ten year survival after heart transplantation: palliative procedure or successful long term treatment? *Heart* 1999;82:47.
7. McGiffin DC, Kirklin JK, Naftel DC, Bourge RC. Competing outcomes after heart transplantation: a comparison of eras and outcomes. *J Heart Lung Transplant* 1997;16:190.
8. Horowitz MM, Rowlings PA. An update from the International Bone Marrow Transplant Registry and the Autologous Blood and Marrow Transplant Registry on current activity in hematopoietic stem cell transplantation. *Curr Opin Hematol* 1997;4:395.

9. Penn I. Occurrence of cancers in immunosuppressed organ transplant recipients. *Clin Transplant* 1998;147.
10. Horowitz M. Uses and growth of hematopoietic cell transplantation. In: Thomas ED, Blume KG, Forman SJ, eds.. *Hematopoietic cell transplantation.* Malden, MA: Blackwell, 1999:12.
11. Broerse JJ, Hollander CF, van Zwieten MJ. Tumour induction in Rhesus monkeys after total body irradiation with X-rays and fission neutrons. *Int J Radiat Biol* 1981;40:671.
12. Deeg HJ, Prentice R, Fritz TE, et al. Increased incidence of malignant tumors in dogs after total body irradiation and marrow transplantation. *Int J Radiat Oncol Biol Phys* 1983;9:1505.
13. Deeg HJ, Storb R, Prentice R, et al. Increased cancer risk in canine radiation chimeras. *Blood* 1980;55:233.
14. Witherspoon RP, Fisher LD, Schoch G, et al. Secondary cancers after bone marrow transplantation for leukemia or aplastic anemia. *N Engl J Med* 1989;321:784.
15. Bhatia S, Ramsay NK, Steinbuch M, et al. Malignant neoplasms following bone marrow transplantation. *Blood* 1996;87:3633.
16. Kolb HJ, Guenther W, Duell T, et al. Cancer after bone marrow transplantation. *Bone Marrow Transplant* 1992;10:135.
17. Socie G, Henry-Amar M, Cosset JM, et al. Increased incidence of solid malignant tumors after bone marrow transplantation for severe aplastic anemia. *Blood* 1991;78:277.
18. Curtis RE, Rowlings PA, Deeg HJ, et al. Solid cancers after bone marrow transplantation. *N Engl J Med* 1997;336:897.
19. Andre M, Henry-Amar M, Blaise D, et al. Incidence of second cancers (SC) and causes of death after autologous stem cell transplantation (ASCT) for Hodgkin's disease. *Blood* 1995;(Suppl 1)86:460a.
20. Deeg HJ, Socie G. Malignancies after hematopoietic stem cell transplantation: many questions, some answers. *Blood* 1998;91:1833.
21. Kolb HJ, Duell T, Socie G, et al. New malignancies in patients surviving more than 5 years after marrow transplantation. *Blood* 1995;(Suppl 1)86:460a.
22. Lutzner MA, Orth G, Dutronquay V, et al. Detection of human papillomavirus type 5 DNA in skin cancers of an immunosuppressed renal allograft recipient. *Lancet* 1983;2:422.
23. Orozco-Topete R, Archer-Dubon C, Valadez-Huerta N, et al. Cutaneous neoplasms and human papillomavirus in renal transplant patients: experience of one center in Mexico. *Transplant Proc* 1996;28:3314.
24. Shamanin V, zur Hausen H, Lavergne D, et al. Human papillomavirus infections in nonmelanoma skin cancers from renal transplant recipients and nonimmunosuppressed patients. *J Natl Cancer Inst* 1996;88:802.
25. Ternesten-Bratel A, Kjellstrom C, Ricksten A. Specific expression of Epstein-Barr virus in cutaneous squamous cell carcinomas from heart transplant recipients. *Transplantation* 1998;66:1524.
26. Pittet MJ, Valmori D, Dunbar PR, et al. High frequencies of naive Melan-A/MART-1-specific CD8(+) T cells in a large proportion of human histocompatibility leukocyte antigen (HLA)-A2 individuals. *J Exp Med* 1999;190:705.
27. Rosenberg SA. A new era for cancer immunotherapy based on the genes that encode cancer antigens. *Immunity* 1999;10:281.
28. Van Pel A, van der Bruggen P, Coulie PG, et al. Genes coding for tumor antigens recognized by cytolytic T lymphocytes. *Immunol Rev* 1995;145:229.
29. Socie G, Stone JV, Wingard JR, et al. Long-term survival and late deaths after allogeneic bone marrow transplantation. *N Engl J Med* 1999;341:14.
30. McSweeney PA, Storb R. Mixed chimerism: preclinical studies and clinical applications. *Biol Blood Marrow Transplant* 1999;5:192.
31. Giralt S, Estey E, Albitar M, et al. Engraftment of allogeneic hematopoietic progenitor cells with purine analog-containing chemotherapy: harnessing graft-versus-leukemia without myeloablative therapy. *Blood* 1997;89:4531.
32. Shapiro RS, Chauvenet A, McGuire W, et al. Treatment of B-cell lymphoproliferative disorders with interferon alfa and intravenous gamma globulin. *N Engl J Med* 1988;318:1334.
33. Antin JH, Bierer BE, Smith BR, et al. Selective depletion of bone marrow T lymphocytes with anti-CD5 monoclonal antibodies: effective prophylaxis for graft-versus-host disease in patients with hematologic malignancies. *Blood* 1991;78:2139.
34. Gerritsen EJ, Stam ED, Hermans J, et al. Risk factors for developing EBV-related B cell lymphoproliferative disorders (BLPD) after non-HLA-identical BMT in children. *Bone Marrow Transplant* 1996;18:377.
35. Zutter MM, Martin PJ, Sale GE, et al. Epstein-Barr virus lymphoproliferation after bone marrow transplantation. *Blood* 1988;72:520.
36. Curtis RE, Travis LB, Rowlings PA, et al. Risk of lymphoproliferative disorders after bone marrow transplantation: a multi-institutional study. *Blood* 1999;94:2208.
37. Hale G, Waldmann H. Risks of developing Epstein-Barr virus-related lymphoproliferative disorders after T-cell-depleted marrow transplants. *Blood* 1998;91:3079.
38. O'Reilly RJ, Small TN, Papadopoulos E, et al. Biology and adoptive cell therapy of Epstein-Barr virus-associated lymphoproliferative disorders in recipients of marrow allografts. *Immunol Rev* 1997;157:195.
39. Flinn I, Orentas R, Noga SJ, et al. Low risk of Epstein-Barr virus (EBV)-associated posttransplant lymphoproliferative disease (PTLD) in patients receiving elutriated allogeneic marrow transplants may reflect depletion of EBV infected lymphocytes from the graft. *Blood* 1995;(Suppl 1)85:626a.
40. Gross TG, Steinbuch M, DeFor T, et al. B cell lymphoproliferative disorders following hematopoietic stem cell transplantation: risk factors, treatment and outcome. *Bone Marrow Transplant* 1999;23:251.
41. Gross TG, Hinrichs SH, Davis JR, et al. Depletion of EBV-infected cells in donor marrow by counterflow elutriation. *Exp Hematol* 1998;26:395.
42. Nemerow GR, Moore MD, Cooper NR. Structure and function of the B-lymphocyte Epstein-Barr virus/C3d receptor. *Adv Cancer Res* 1990;54:273.
43. Kieff E. Epstein-Barr virus and its replication. In: Fields BN, Knipe DM, Howley PM, eds. *Fields virology.* Philadelphia: Raven Press, 1996:2343.
44. Kempkes B, Pich D, Zeidler R, Sugden B, Hammerschmidt W. Immortalization of human B lymphocytes by a plasmid containing 71 kilobase pairs of Epstein-Barr virus DNA. *J Virol* 1995;69:231.
45. Grossman SR, Johannsen E, Tong X, Yalamanchili R, Kieff E. The Epstein-Barr virus nuclear antigen 2 transactivator is directed to response elements by the J kappa recombination signal binding protein. *Proc Natl Acad Sci U S A* 1994;91:7568.
46. Hsieh JJ, Hayward SD. Masking of the CBF1/RBPJ kappa transcriptional repression domain by Epstein-Barr virus EBNA2. *Science* 1995;268:560.
47. Kilger E, Kieser A, Baumann M, Hammerschmidt W. Epstein-Barr virus-mediated B-cell proliferation is dependent upon latent membrane protein 1, which simulates an activated CD40 receptor. *EMBO J* 1998;17:1700.
48. Busch LK, Bishop GA. The EBV transforming protein, latent membrane protein 1, mimics and cooperates with CD40 signaling in B lymphocytes. *J Immunol* 1999;162:2555.
49. Liebowitz D. Epstein-Barr virus and a cellular signaling pathway in lymphomas from immunosuppressed patients. *N Engl J Med* 1998;338:1413.
50. Kulwichit W, Edwards RH, Davenport EM, et al. Expression of the Epstein-Barr virus latent membrane protein 1 induces B cell lymphoma in transgenic mice. *Proc Natl Acad Sci U S A* 1998;95:11963.
51. Callan MF, Tan L, Annels N, et al. Direct visualization of antigen-specific CD8+ T cells during the primary immune response to Epstein-Barr virus in vivo. *J Exp Med* 1998;187:1395.
52. Callan MF, Steven N, Krausa P, et al. Large clonal expansions of CD8+ T cells in acute infectious mononucleosis. *Nat Med* 1996;2:906.
53. Cohen JI. The biology of Epstein-Barr virus: lessons learned from the virus and the host. *Curr Opin Immunol* 1999;11:365.
54. Miyashita EM, Yang B, Babcock GJ, Thorley-Lawson DA. Identification of the site of Epstein-Barr virus persistence in vivo as a resting B cell. *J Virol* 1997;71:4882.
55. Decker LL, Klaman LD, Thorley-Lawson DA. Detection of the latent form of Epstein-Barr virus DNA in the peripheral blood of healthy individuals. *J Virol* 1996;70:3286.
56. Chen F, Zou JZ, di Renzo L, et al. A subpopulation of normal B cells latently infected with Epstein-Barr virus resembles Burkitt lymphoma cells in expressing EBNA-1 but not EBNA-2 or LMP1. *J Virol* 1995;69:3752.
57. Levitskaya J, Coram M, Levitsky V, et al. Inhibition of antigen processing by the internal repeat region of the Epstein-Barr virus nuclear antigen-1. *Nature* 1995;375:685.
58. Gratama JW, Oosterveer MA, Zwaan FE, et al. Eradication of Epstein-Barr virus by allogeneic bone marrow transplantation: implications for sites of viral latency. *Proc Natl Acad Sci U S A* 1988;85:8693.
59. Lucas KG, Small TN, Heller G, Dupont B, O'Reilly RJ. The development of cellular immunity to Epstein-Barr virus after allogeneic bone marrow transplantation. *Blood* 1996;87:2594.
60. Crawford DH, Mulholland N, Iliescu V, Hawkins R, Powles R. Epstein-Barr virus infection and immunity in bone marrow transplant recipients. *Transplantation* 1986;42:50.
61. Knowles DM, Cesarman E, Chadburn A, et al. Correlative morphologic and molecular genetic analysis demonstrates three distinct categories of posttransplantation lymphoproliferative disorders. *Blood* 1995;85:552.
62. Ambinder RF, Mann RB. Detection and characterization of Epstein-Barr virus in clinical specimens. *Am J Pathol* 1994;145:239.
63. Young L, Alfieri C, Hennessy K, et al. Expression of Epstein-Barr virus transformation-associated genes in tissues of patients with EBV lymphoproliferative disease. *N Engl J Med* 1989;321:1080.
64. Rooney CM, Loftin SK, Holladay MS, et al. Early identification of Epstein-Barr virus-associated post-transplantation lymphoproliferative disease. *Br J Haematol* 1995;89:98.
65. Faller DV, Hermine O, Small T, et al. Treatment of Epstein-Barr virus (EBV)-associated lymphomas and PTLD using arginine butyrate to induce viral TK gene expression: initial findings of a phase I/II trial. *Blood* 1999;94(Suppl 1):523a.
66. Fischer A, Blanche S, Le Bidois J, et al. Anti-B-cell monoclonal antibodies in the treatment of severe B-cell lymphoproliferative syndrome following bone marrow and organ transplantation. *N Engl J Med* 1991;324:1451.
67. Blanche S, Le Deist F, Veber F, et al. Treatment of severe Epstein-Barr virus-induced polyclonal B-lymphocyte proliferation by anti-B-cell monoclonal antibodies. *Ann Intern Med* 1988;108:199.
68. Benkerrou M, Jais JP, Leblond V, et al. Anti-B-cell monoclonal antibody treatment of severe posttransplant B-lymphoproliferative disorder: prognostic factors and long-term outcome. *Blood* 1998;92:3137.
69. Faye A, Van Den Abeele T, Peuchmaur M, Mathieu-Boue A, Vilmer E. Anti-CD20 monoclonal antibody for post-transplant lymphoproliferative disorders. *Lancet* 1998;352:1285.
70. Kuehnle I, Huls HH, Liu Z, et al. CD20 monoclonal antibody (rituximab) for therapy of epstein-barr virus lymphoma after hemopoietic stem-cell transplantation. *Blood* 2000;95:1502.
71. Papadopoulos EB, Ladanyi M, Emanuel D, et al. Infusions of donor leukocytes to treat Epstein-Barr virus-associated lymphoproliferative disorders after allogeneic bone marrow transplantation. *N Engl J Med* 1994;330:1185.
72. Rooney CM, Smith CA, Ng CY, et al. Use of gene-modified virus-specific T lymphocytes to control Epstein-Barr-virus-related lymphoproliferation. *Lancet* 1995;345:9.
73. Heslop HE, Ng CY, Li C, et al. Long-term restoration of immunity against Epstein-Barr virus infection by adoptive transfer of gene-modified virus-specific T lymphocytes. *Nat Med* 1996;2:551.
74. Rooney CM, Smith CA, Ng CY, et al. Infusion of cytotoxic T cells for the prevention and treatment of Epstein-Barr virus-induced lymphoma in allogeneic transplant recipients. *Blood* 1998;92:1549.
75. Tirelli U, Errante D, Dolcetti R, et al. Hodgkin's disease and human immunodeficiency virus infection: clinicopathologic and virologic features of 114 patients from the Italian Cooperative Group on AIDS and Tumors. *J Clin Oncol* 1995;13:1758.
76. Garnier JL, Lebranchu Y, Dantal J, et al. Hodgkin's disease after transplantation. *Transplantation* 1996;61:71.

77. Rowlings PA, Curtis RE, Passweg JR, et al. Increased incidence of Hodgkin's disease after allogeneic bone marrow transplantation. *J Clin Oncol* 1999;10:3122.
78. Zutter MM, Durnam DM, Hackman RC, et al. Secondary T-cell lymphoproliferation after marrow transplantation. *Am J Clin Pathol* 1990;94:714.
79. Abrahamsen JF, Andersen A, Hannisdal E, et al. Second malignancies after treatment of Hodgkin's disease: the influence of treatment, follow-up time, and age. *J Clin Oncol* 1993;11:255.
80. Travis LB, Curtis RE, Boice JD Jr, Hankey BF, Fraumeni JF Jr. Second cancers following non-Hodgkin's lymphoma. *Cancer* 1991;67:2002.
81. Curtis RE, Boice JD Jr, Stovall M, et al. Risk of leukemia after chemotherapy and radiation treatment for breast cancer. *N Engl J Med* 1992;326:1745.
82. Levine EG, Bloomfield CD. Leukemias and myelodysplastic syndromes secondary to drug, radiation, and environmental exposure. *Semin Oncol* 1992;19:47.
83. Darrington DL, Vose JM, Anderson JR, et al. Incidence and characterization of secondary myelodysplastic syndrome and acute myelogenous leukemia following high-dose chemoradiotherapy and autologous stem-cell transplantation for lymphoid malignancies. *J Clin Oncol* 1994;12:2527.
84. Stone RM, Neuberg D, Soiffer R, et al. Myelodysplastic syndrome as a late complication following autologous bone marrow transplantation for non-Hodgkin's lymphoma. *J Clin Oncol* 1994;12:2535.
85. Miller JS, Arthur DC, Litz CE, et al. Myelodysplastic syndrome after autologous bone marrow transplantation: an additional late complication of curative cancer therapy. *Blood* 1994;83:3780.
86. Krishnan A, Bhatia S, Slovak ML, et al. Predictors of therapy-related leukemia and myelodysplasia following autologous transplantation for lymphoma: an assessment of risk factors. *Blood* 2000;95:1588.
87. Fialkow PJ, Thomas ED, Bryant JI, Neiman PE. Leukaemic transformation of engrafted human marrow cells in vivo. *Lancet* 1971;1:251.
88. Thomas ED, Bryant JI, Buckner CD, et al. Leukaemic transformation of engrafted human marrow cells in vivo. *Lancet* 1972;1:1310.
89. Newburger PE, Latt SA, Pesando JM, et al. Leukemia relapse in donor cells after allogeneic bone-marrow transplantation. *N Engl J Med* 1981;304:712.
90. Deeg HJ, Sanders J, Martin P, et al. Secondary malignancies after marrow transplantation. *Exp Hematol* 1984;12:660.
91. Niederwieser DW, Appelbaum FR, Gastl G, et al. Inadvertent transmission of a donor's acute myeloid leukemia in bone marrow transplantation for chronic myelocytic leukemia. *N Engl J Med* 1990;322:1794.
92. Govindarajan R, Jagannath S, Flick JT, et al. Preceding standard therapy is the likely cause of MDS after autotransplants for multiple myeloma. *Br J Haematol* 1996;95:349.
93. Chao NJ, Nademanee AP, Long GD, et al. Importance of bone marrow cytogenetic evaluation before autologous bone marrow transplantation for Hodgkin's disease. *J Clin Oncol* 1991;9:1575.
94. Anderson J. Allogeneic hematopoietic cell transplantation for myelodysplastic and myeloproliferative disorders. In: Thomas ED, Blume KG, Forman SJ, eds. *Hematopoietic cell transplantation.* Malden, MA: Blackwell, 1999:872.
95. United Network for Organ Sharing Web Site. Available at http://www.unos.org.
96. Penn I. Tumors after renal and cardiac transplantation. *Hematol Oncol Clin North Am* 1993;7:431.
97. Birkeland SA, Storm HH, Lamm LU, et al. Cancer risk after renal transplantation in the Nordic countries, 1964–1986. *Int J Cancer* 1995;60:183.
98. Penn I. Effect of immunosuppression on preexisting cancers. *Transplant Proc* 1993;25:1380.
99. Doutrelepont JM, De Pauw L, Gruber SA, et al. Renal transplantation exposes patients with previous Kaposi's sarcoma to a high risk of recurrence. *Transplantation* 1996;62:463.
100. Gazdar AF. Tumors arising after organ transplantation. *JAMA* 1997;277:154.
101. Hoppner W, Grosse K, Dreikorn K. Renal cell carcinoma in a transplanted kidney: successful organ-preserving procedure. *Urol Int* 1996;56:110.
102. Conlon PJ, Smith SR. Transmission of cancer with cadaveric donor organs. *J Am Soc Nephrol* 1995;6:54.
103. Loh E, Couch FJ, Hendricksen C, et al. Development of donor-derived prostate cancer in a recipient following orthotopic heart transplantation. *JAMA* 1997;277:133.
104. Detry O, Bonnet P, Honore P, Meurisse M, Jacquet N. What is the risk of transferral of an undetected neoplasm during organ transplantation? *Transplant Proc* 1997;29:2410.
105. Healey PJ, Davis CL. Transmission of tumours by transplantation. *Lancet* 1998;352:2.
106. Suranyi MG, Hogan PG, Falk MC, et al. Advanced donor-origin melanoma in a renal transplant recipient: immunotherapy, cure, and retransplantation. *Transplantation* 1998;66:655.
107. First MR, Peddi VR. Malignancies complicating organ transplantation. *Transplant Proc* 1998;30:2768.
108. London NJ, Farmery SM, Will EJ, Davison AM, Lodge JP. Risk of neoplasia in renal transplant patients [published erratum appears in *Lancet* 1995;9(8976):714]. *Lancet* 1995;346:403.
109. Sheil AG. Cancer in immune-suppressed organ transplant recipients: aetiology and evolution. *Transplant Proc* 1998;30:2055.
110. Kelly DM, Emre S, Guy SR, et al. Liver transplant recipients are not at increased risk for nonlymphoid solid organ tumors. *Cancer* 1998;83:1237.
111. Stewart T, Tsai SC, Grayson H, Henderson R, Opelz G. Incidence of de-novo breast cancer in women chronically immunosuppressed after organ transplantation. *Lancet* 1995;346:796.
112. Gupta AK, Cardella CJ, Haberman HF. Cutaneous malignant neoplasms in patients with renal transplants. *Arch Dermatol* 1986;122:1288.
113. Erer B, Angelucci E, Muretto P, et al. Kaposi's sarcoma after allogeneic bone marrow transplantation. *Bone Marrow Transplant* 1997;19:629.
114. Penn I. Neoplastic complications of organ transplantation. In: Ginns LC, Cosimi AB, Morris PJ, eds. *Transplantation.* Malden, MA: Blackwell, 1999:770.
115. Hartevelt MM, Bavinck JN, Kootte AM, Vermeer BJ, Vandenbroucke JP. Incidence of skin cancer after renal transplantation in The Netherlands. *Transplantation* 1990;49:506.
116. Bouwes Bavinck JN, Hardie DR, et al. The risk of skin cancer in renal transplant recipients in Queensland, Australia. *Transplantation* 1996;61:715.
117. Lampros TD, Cobanoglu A, Parker F, et al. Squamous and basal cell carcinoma in heart transplant recipients. *J Heart Lung Transplant* 1998;17:586.
118. Espana A, Redondo P, Fernandez AL, et al. Skin cancer in heart transplant recipients. *J Am Acad Dermatol* 1995;32:458.
119. Sheil AG. Skin cancer in renal transplant recipients. *Transplant Sci* 1994;4:42.
120. Bouwes Bavinck JN, Vermeer BJ, van der Woude FJ, et al. Relation between skin cancer and HLA antigens in renal-transplant recipients. *N Engl J Med* 1991;325:843.
121. Jensen P, Hansen S, Moller B, et al. Skin cancer in kidney and heart transplant recipients and different long-term immunosuppressive therapy regimens. *J Am Acad Dermatol* 1999;40:177.
122. King GN, Healy CM, Glover MT, et al. Increased prevalence of dysplastic and malignant lip lesions in renal-transplant recipients. *N Engl J Med* 1995;332:1052.
123. Kripke ML. Immunoregulation of carcinogenesis: past, present, and future. *J Natl Cancer Inst* 1988;80:722.
124. Hill LL, Shreedhar VK, Kripke ML, Owen-Schaub LB. A critical role for Fas ligand in the active suppression of systemic immune responses by ultraviolet radiation. *J Exp Med* 1999;189:1285.
125. Shreedhar VK, Pride MW, Sun Y, Kripke ML, Strickland FM. Origin and characteristics of ultraviolet-B radiation-induced suppressor T lymphocytes. *J Immunol* 1998;161:1327.
126. Galvao MM, Sotto MN, Kihara SM, Rivitti EA, Sabbaga E. Lymphocyte subsets and Langerhans cells in sun-protected and sun-exposed skin of immunosuppressed renal allograft recipients. *J Am Acad Dermatol* 1998;38:38.
127. Penn I. Malignant melanoma in organ allograft recipients. *Transplantation* 1996;61:274.
128. Hojo M, Morimoto T, Maluccio M, et al. Cyclosporine induces cancer progression by a cell-autonomous mechanism. *Nature* 1999;397:530.
129. Barr BB, Benton EC, McLaren K, et al. Human papilloma virus infection and skin cancer in renal allograft recipients. *Lancet* 1989;1:124.
130. Mansat-Krzyzanowska E, Dantal J, Hourmant M, et al. Frequency of mucosal HPV DNA detection (types 6/11, 16/18, 31/35/51) in skin lesions of renal transplant patients. *Transplant Int* 1997;10:137.
131. Arends MJ, Benton EC, McLaren KM, et al. Renal allograft recipients with high susceptibility to cutaneous malignancy have an increased prevalence of human papillomavirus DNA in skin tumours and a greater risk of anogenital malignancy. *Br J Cancer* 1997;75:722.
132. Euvrard S, Chardonnet Y, Pouteil-Noble C, et al. Association of skin malignancies with various and multiple carcinogenic and noncarcinogenic human papillomaviruses in renal transplant recipients. *Cancer* 1993;72:2198.
133. Stark LA, Arends MJ, McLaren KM, et al. Prevalence of human papillomavirus DNA in cutaneous neoplasms from renal allograft recipients supports a possible viral role in tumour promotion. *Br J Cancer* 1994;69:222.
134. McGregor JM, Farthing A, Crook T, et al. Posttransplant skin cancer: a possible role for p53 gene mutation but not for oncogenic human papillomaviruses. *J Am Acad Dermatol* 1994;30:701.
135. Euvrard S, Verschoore M, Touraine JL, et al. Topical retinoids for warts and keratoses in transplant recipients. *Lancet* 1992;340:48.
136. Rook AH, Jaworsky C, Nguyen T, et al. Beneficial effect of low-dose systemic retinoid in combination with topical tretinoin for the treatment and prophylaxis of premalignant and malignant skin lesions in renal transplant recipients. *Transplantation* 1995;59:714.
137. Barrett WL, First MR, Aron BS, Penn I. Clinical course of malignancies in renal transplant recipients. *Cancer* 1993;72:2186.
138. Cowen EW, Billingsley EM. Awareness of skin cancer by kidney transplant patients. *J Am Acad Dermatol* 1999;40:697.
139. Seukeran DC, Newstead CG, Cunliffe WJ. The compliance of renal transplant recipients with advice about sun protection measures. *Br J Dermatol* 1998;138:301.
140. McKenna DB, Murphy GM. Skin cancer chemoprophylaxis in renal transplant recipients: 5 years of experience using low-dose acitretin. *Br J Dermatol* 1999;4:656.
141. Bavinck JN, Tieben LM, Van der Woude FJ, et al. Prevention of skin cancer and reduction of keratotic skin lesions during acitretin therapy in renal transplant recipients: a double-blind, placebo-controlled study. *J Clin Oncol* 1995;13:1933.
142. Harlan DM, Kirk AD. The future of organ and tissue transplantation: can T-cell costimulatory pathway modifiers revolutionize the prevention of graft rejection? *JAMA* 1999;282:1076.
143. Opelz G, Henderson R. Incidence of non-Hodgkin lymphoma in kidney and heart transplant recipients. *Lancet* 1993;342:1514.
144. Haque T, Thomas JA, Falk KI, et al. Transmission of donor Epstein-Barr virus (EBV) in transplanted organs causes lymphoproliferative disease in EBV-seronegative recipients. *J Gen Virol* 1996;77:1169.
145. Cen H, Breinig MC, Atchison RW, Ho M, McKnight JL. Epstein-Barr virus transmission via the donor organs in solid organ transplantation: polymerase chain reaction and restriction fragment length polymorphism analysis of IR2, IR3, and IR4. *J Virol* 1991;65:976.
146. Walker RC, Paya CV, Marshall WF, et al. Pretransplantation seronegative Epstein-Barr virus status is the primary risk factor for posttransplantation lymphoproliferative disorder in adult heart, lung, and other solid organ transplantations. *J Heart Lung Transplant* 1995;14:214.
147. Sokal EM, Antunes H, Beguin C, et al. Early signs and risk factors for the increased incidence of Epstein-Barr virus-related posttransplant lymphoproliferative diseases in pediatric liver transplant recipients treated with tacrolimus. *Transplantation* 1997;64:1438.
148. Swinnen LJ. Treatment of organ transplant-related lymphoma. *Hematol Oncol Clin North Am* 1997;11:963.
149. Swinnen LJ, Costanzo-Nordin MR, Fisher SG, et al. Increased incidence of lymphoproliferative disorder after immunosuppression with the monoclonal antibody OKT3 in cardiac-transplant recipients. *N Engl J Med* 1990;323:1723.

150. Burman K, Crawford DH. Effect of FK 506 on Epstein-Barr virus specific cytotoxic T cells. *Lancet* 1991;337:297.
151. Haque T, Thomas JA, Parratt R, et al. A prospective study in heart and lung transplant recipients correlating persistent Epstein-Barr virus infection with clinical events. *Transplantation* 1997;64:1028.
152. Haque T, Crawford DH. The role of adoptive immunotherapy in the prevention and treatment of lymphoproliferative disease following transplantation. *Br J Haematol* 1999;106:309.
153. DeMario MD, Liebowitz DN. Lymphomas in the immunocompromised patient. *Semin Oncol* 1998;25:492.
154. Swinnen LJ. Overview of posttransplant B-cell lymphoproliferative disorders. *Semin Oncol* 1999;(Suppl 14) 5:21.
155. Leblond V, Sutton L, Dorent R, et al. Lymphoproliferative disorders after organ transplantation: a report of 24 cases observed in a single center. *J Clin Oncol* 1995;13:961.
156. Frizzera G, Hanto DW, Gajl-Peczalska KJ, et al. Polymorphic diffuse B-cell hyperplasias and lymphomas in renal transplant recipients. *Cancer Res* 1981;41:4262.
157. Chadburn A, Chen JM, Hsu DT, et al. The morphologic and molecular genetic categories of posttransplantation lymphoproliferative disorders are clinically relevant. *Cancer* 1998;82:1978.
158. Cesarman E, Chadburn A, Liu YF, et al. BCL-6 gene mutations in posttransplantation lymphoproliferative disorders predict response to therapy and clinical outcome. *Blood* 1998;92:2294.
159. Khatri VP, Baiocchi RA, Peng R, et al. Endogenous CD8+ T cell expansion during regression of monoclonal EBV-associated posttransplant lymphoproliferative disorder. *J Immunol* 1999;163:500.
160. Starzl TE, Nalesnik MA, Porter KA, et al. Reversibility of lymphomas and lymphoproliferative lesions developing under cyclosporin-steroid therapy. *Lancet* 1984;1:583.
161. Milpied N, Antoine C, Garnier JL, et al. Humanized anti-CD20 monoclonal antibody (rituximab) in B post-transplant lymphoproliferative disorders: a retrospective analysis of 32 patients. *Ann Oncol* 1999;10:5(abst).
162. Garrett TJ, Chadburn A, Barr ML, et al. Posttransplantation lymphoproliferative disorders treated with cyclophosphamide-doxorubicin-vincristine-prednisone chemotherapy. *Cancer* 1993;72:2782.
163. Swinnen LJ, Mullen GM, Carr TJ, Costanzo MR, Fisher RI. Aggressive treatment for post-cardiac transplant lymphoproliferation. *Blood* 1995;86:3333.
164. Morrison VA, Dunn DL, Manivel JC, et al. Clinical characteristics of post-transplant lymphoproliferative disorders. *Am J Med* 1994;97:14.
165. Haque T, Amlot PL, Helling N, et al. Reconstitution of EBV-specific T cell immunity in solid organ transplant recipients. *J Immunol* 1998;160:6204.
166. Khanna R, Bell S, Sherritt M, et al. Activation and adoptive transfer of Epstein-Barr virus-specific cytotoxic T cells in solid organ transplant patients with posttransplant lymphoproliferative disease. *Proc Natl Acad Sci U S A* 1999;96:10391.
167. Hanson MN, Morrison VA, Peterson BA, et al. Posttransplant T-cell lymphoproliferative disorders—an aggressive, late complication of solid-organ transplantation [see comments]. *Blood* 1996;88:3626.
168. Ziegler JL, Templeton AC, Vogel CL. Kaposi's sarcoma: a comparison of classical, endemic, and epidemic forms. *Semin Oncol* 1984;11:47.
169. Biggar RJ, Rabkin CS. The epidemiology of AIDS-related neoplasms. *Hematol Oncol Clin North Am* 1996;10:997.
170. Stribling J, Weitzner S, Smith GV. Kaposi's sarcoma in renal allograft recipients. *Cancer* 1978;42:442.
171. Farge D, Lebbe C, Marjanovic Z, et al. Human herpes virus-8 and other risk factors for Kaposi's sarcoma in kidney transplant recipients. *Transplantation* 1999;67:1236.
172. Chang Y, Cesarman E, Pessin MS, et al. Identification of herpesvirus-like DNA sequences in AIDS-associated Kaposi's sarcoma. *Science* 1994;266:1865.
173. Moore PS, Chang Y. Detection of herpesvirus-like DNA sequences in Kaposi's sarcoma in patients with and without HIV infection. *N Engl J Med* 1995;332:1181.
174. Weiss RA, Whitby D, Talbot S, Kellam P, Boshoff C. Human herpesvirus type 8 and Kaposi's sarcoma. *Monogr Natl Cancer Inst* 1998;51.
175. Alkan S, Karcher DS, Ortiz A, et al. Human herpesvirus-8/Kaposi's sarcoma-associated herpesvirus in organ transplant patients with immunosuppression. *Br J Haematol* 1997; 96:412.
176. Regamey N, Tamm M, Wernli M, et al. Transmission of human herpesvirus 8 infection from renal-transplant donors to recipients. *N Engl J Med* 1998;339:1358.
177. Parravicini C, Olsen SJ, Capra M, et al. Risk of Kaposi's sarcoma-associated herpes virus transmission from donor allografts among Italian posttransplant Kaposi's sarcoma patients. *Blood* 1997;90:2826.
178. Mendez JC, Procop GW, Espy MJ, et al. Relationship of HHV8 replication and Kaposi's sarcoma after solid organ transplantation. *Transplantation* 1999;67:1200.
179. Hudnall SD, Rady PL, Tyring SK, Fish JC. Hydrocortisone activation of human herpesvirus 8 viral DNA replication and gene expression in vitro. *Transplantation* 1999;67:648.
180. Osman M, Kubo T, Gill J, et al. Identification of human herpesvirus 8-specific cytotoxic T-cell responses. *J Virol* 1999;73:6136.
181. Shepherd FA, Maher E, Cardella C, et al. Treatment of Kaposi's sarcoma after solid organ transplantation. *J Clin Oncol* 1997;15:2371.
182. Gill PS, Rarick M, McCutchan JA, et al. Systemic treatment of AIDS-related Kaposi's sarcoma: results of a randomized trial. *Am J Med* 1991;90:427.
183. Husain SR, Kreitman RJ, Pastan I, Puri RK. Interleukin-4 receptor-directed cytotoxin therapy of AIDS-associated Kaposi's sarcoma tumors in xenograft model. *Nat Med* 1999;5:817.
184. Cesarman E, Chang Y, Moore PS, Said JW, Knowles DM. Kaposi's sarcoma-associated herpesvirus-like DNA sequences in AIDS-related body-cavity-based lymphomas. *N Engl J Med* 1995;332:1186.
185. Soulier J, Grollet L, Oksenhendler E, et al. Kaposi's sarcoma-associated herpesvirus-like DNA sequences in multicentric Castleman's disease. *Blood* 1995;86:1276.
186. Dotti G, Fiocchi R, Motta T, et al. Primary effusion lymphoma after heart transplantation: a new entity associated with human herpesvirus-8. *Leukemia* 1999;13:664.
187. Jones D, Ballestas ME, Kaye KM, et al. Primary-effusion lymphoma and Kaposi's sarcoma in a cardiac-transplant recipient. *N Engl J Med* 1998;339:444.

CHAPTER **51**

Oncologic Emergencies

SECTION **1** JOACHIM YAHALOM

Superior Vena Cava Syndrome

Superior vena cava syndrome (SVCS) is the clinical expression of obstruction of blood flow through the SVC. Characteristic symptoms and signs may develop quickly or gradually when this thin-walled vessel is compressed, invaded, or thrombosed by processes in the superior mediastinum. The first pathologic description of SVC obstruction, in a patient with syphilitic aortic aneurysm, appeared in 1757.[1] In 1954, Schechter[2] reviewed 274 well-documented cases of SVCS reported in the literature; 40% of them were due to syphilitic aneurysms or tuberculosis mediastinitis. These entities have since virtually disappeared, and cancer of the lung is now the underlying process in approximately 70% of patients with SVCS. It is estimated that, in the United States, 15,000 people develop SVCS each year.[3]

ANATOMY AND PATHOPHYSIOLOGY

The SVC is the major vessel for drainage of venous blood from the head, neck, upper extremities, and upper thorax. It is located in the middle mediastinum and is surrounded by relatively rigid structures, such as the sternum, trachea, right bronchus, aorta, pulmonary artery, and the perihilar and paratracheal lymph nodes. The SVC extends from the junction of the right and left innominate veins to the right atrium, for a distance of 6 to 8 cm. The distal 2 cm of the SVC is within the pericardial sac, with a point of relative fixation of the vena cava at the pericardial reflection. The azygos vein, the main auxiliary vessel, enters the SVC posteriorly, just above the pericardial reflection. The width of the SVC is 1.5 to 2.0 cm and it maintains blood at a low pressure. The SVC is thin-walled, compliant, and easily compressible, and is vulnerable to any space-occupying process in its vicinity. The SVC is completely encircled by chains of lymph nodes that drain all the structures of the right thoracic cavity and the lower part of the left thorax. The auxiliary azygos vein is also threatened by enlargement of paratracheal nodes. Other critical structures in the mediastinum, such as the main bronchi, esophagus, and the spinal cord, may be involved by the same process that led to obstruction of the SVC.[4–6]

When the SVC is fully or partially obstructed, an extensive venous collateral circulation may develop. The azygos venous system is the most important alternative pathway. Carlson[7] found that dogs could not survive sudden ligation of the SVC below the level of the azygos vein, but they tolerated well ligation of the SVC above it. He could, however, successfully obstruct the SVC and the azygos vein in operations performed in two stages, presumably by allowing time for collaterals to form. Other collateral systems are the internal mammary veins, lateral thoracic veins, paraspinous veins, and the esophageal venous network. The subcutaneous veins are important pathways, and their engorgement in the neck and thorax is a typical physical finding in SVCS. Despite these collateral pathways, venous pressure is almost always elevated in the upper compartment if there is obstruction of the SVC. Venous pressures have been recorded as high as 200 to 500 cm H_2O in severe SVCS.[8]

ETIOLOGY AND NATURAL HISTORY

SVCS usually has an insidious onset and progresses to typical symptoms and signs. Review of the data from three series (Table 51.1-1) shows dyspnea to be the most common symptom.[9–11]

TABLE 51.1-1. Common Symptoms and Physical Findings of Superior Vena Cava Syndrome

Symptoms	*Patients Affected*[a] *(%)*	*Physical Findings*	*Patients Affected*[a] *(%)*
Dyspnea	63	Venous distention of neck	66
Facial swelling and head fullness	50	Venous distention of chest wall	54
Cough	24	Facial edema	46
Arm swelling	18	Cyanosis	20
Chest pain	15	Plethora of face	19
Dysphagia	9	Edema of arms	14

[a]Analysis based on data from 370 patients.[9–11]

Dyspnea occurred in 63% of patients with SVCS. A sensation of fullness in the head and facial swelling was reported by 50% of the patients. Other complaints were cough (24%), arm swelling (18%), chest pain (15%), and dysphagia (9%). The characteristic physical findings were venous distention of the neck (66%) and chest wall (54%), facial edema (46%), plethora (19%), and cyanosis (19%). These symptoms and signs may be aggravated by bending forward, stooping, or by lying down.

Malignant disease is the most common cause of SVCS. The percentage of patients in different series with a confirmed diagnosis of malignancy varies from 78% to 86% (Table 51.1-2). Lung cancer was diagnosed in 65% of 415 patients analyzed in these series.[4,10–12] Armstrong et al.[9] did a retrospective review of 4100 cases treated for bronchogenic carcinoma between 1965 and 1984, and they identified 99 patients (2.4%) with SVCS. Salsali and Cliffton[13] observed SVCS in 4.2% of 4960 patients with lung cancer; 80% of the tumors inducing SVCS were of the right lung. Small cell lung cancer (SCLC) is the most common histologic subtype (Table 51.1-3), and it was found in 38% of the patients who had lung cancer and SVCS. In six large series of SCLC, 9% to 19% of patients demonstrated SVCS.[14–19] The second most common histologic subtype is squamous cell carcinoma, found in 26% of lung cancer patients with SVCS.

Lymphoma involving the mediastinum was the cause of SVCS in 8% of patients reported in the series (see Table 51.1-2). Armstrong et al.[9] found SVCS in 1.9% of 952 lymphoma patients. Perez-Soler et al.[20] identified 36 cases (4%) of SVCS among 915 patients with non-Hodgkin's lymphoma (NHL) treated at the M. D. Anderson Cancer Center. Twenty-three patients (64%) had diffuse large cell lymphoma, 12 (33%) had lymphoblastic lymphoma, and one patient had follicular large cell lymphoma. Of their patients with diffuse large cell lymphoma and lymphoblastic lymphoma, 7% and 21% had SVCS, respectively. In a series of patients with primary mediastinal B-cell lymphoma with sclerosis, SVCS was present in 57% of patients.[21] Hodgkin's lymphoma commonly involves the mediastinum, but it rarely causes SVCS. Other primary mediastinal malignancies that cause SVCS are thymoma and germ cell tumors. Breast cancer is the most common metastatic disease that causes SVCS.[4,10,12] In one report, breast cancer was the cause of SVCS in 11% of cases.[22]

Nonmalignant conditions causing SVCS are not as rare as previously reported.[9,23] When the data were collected from general hospitals, as many as 22% of patients had noncancerous causes of SVCS.[4,10,12] Parish et al.[10] reported 19 patients with benign causes of SVCS, and Schraufnagel et al.[4] included 16 such patients in his series. Fifty percent of the patients in both reports had a diagnosis of mediastinal fibrosis, which was probably due to histoplasmosis. Parish et al.[10] reported six patients with thrombosis of SVC, and in five, the thrombosis developed in the presence of central vein catheters or pacemakers. Sculier and Field[24] reviewed 24 cases of central venous catheter–induced SVC. Of these, 18 were caused by pacemaker catheters. LeVeen peritoneovenous shunts, Swan-Ganz catheters, and hyperalimentation catheters were also involved. The increasing use of these devices for the delivery of chemotherapy agents or for hyperalimentation contributes to the development of SVCS in the cancer patient.[25]

Obstruction of SVC in the pediatric age group is rare and has a different etiologic spectrum. The causative factors are mainly iatrogenic[26] secondary to cardiovascular surgery for congenital heart disease, ventriculoatrial shunt for hydrocephalus, and SVC catheterization for parenteral nutrition. In a report of

TABLE 51.1-2. Primary Pathologic Diagnoses for Superior Vena Cava Syndrome

Histologic Diagnosis	*Bell et al.,*[11] *159 Patients (%)*	*Schraufnagel et al.,*[4] *107 Patients (%)*	*Parish et al.,*[10] *86 Patients (%)*	*Yellin et al.,*[12] *63 Patients (%)*	*Total, 415 Patients (%)*
Lung cancer	129 (81)	67 (63)	45 (52)	30 (48)	271 (65)
Lymphoma	3 (2)	10 (9)	8 (9)	13 (21)	34 (8)
Other malignancies (primary or metastatic)	4 (3)	14 (13)	14 (16)	8 (13)	40 (10)
Nonneoplastic	2 (1)	16 (15)	19 (22)	11 (18)	50 (12)
Undiagnosed	21 (13)	—	—	—	21 (5)

TABLE 51.1-3. Lung Cancer Subtypes Associated with Superior Vena Cava Syndrome

Histology	*Number of Patients*	*Percentage of Patients*
Small cell	142	38
Squamous cell	97	26
Adenocarcinoma	52	14
Large cell	43	12
Unclassified	34	9
Total	**370**	**100**

175 children with SVCS, 70% were iatrogenic. Of the remaining 53 cases, 37 (70%) were caused by mediastinal tumors, eight (15%) were caused by benign granuloma, and four (7.5%) by congenital anomalies of the cardiovascular system. Two-thirds of the tumors causing SVCS in childhood are lymphomas.[26,27] Of 16 children reported from St. Jude Children's Research Hospital with SVCS at presentation, eight were diagnosed with NHL, four had acute lymphoblastic leukemia, two had Hodgkin's disease, one had neuroblastoma, and one had a yolk sac tumor.[22] Most children who developed SVCS late in the course of their malignancy had recurrent solid tumors.[28] Issa et al.[27] reported that mediastinal fibrosis secondary to histoplasmosis caused SVCS in 7 (5%) of the 150 patients reviewed.

DIAGNOSTIC PROCEDURES

SVCS has long been considered to be a potentially life-threatening medical emergency.[5,23,29] It was common practice to immediately apply radiation therapy with initial high-dose fractions, sometimes even before the histologic diagnosis of the primary lesion was established.[23,29,30] Diagnostic procedures, such as bronchoscopy, mediastinoscopy, thoracotomy, or supraclavicular lymph node biopsy, were often avoided because they were considered to be hazardous in the presence of SVCS.[5,23] However, the safety of these invasive procedures in patients with SVCS has markedly improved, and the modern treatment of SVCS has become disease-specific from the outset.[4,31,32] Temporizing emergency mediastinal irradiation before biopsy is rarely used because it may preclude proper interpretation of the specimen in almost one-half of patients.[33]

The clinical identification of SVCS is simple because the symptoms and signs are typical and unmistakable. The chest film shows a mass in most patients. Only 16% of the patients studied by Parish had normal chest films.[10] The most common radiographic abnormalities are superior mediastinal widening and pleural effusion (Table 51.1-4). Computed tomography (CT) provides more detailed information about the SVC, its tributaries, and other critical structures, such as the bronchi and the cord.[34] The additional information is necessary because the involvement of these structures requires prompt action for relief of pressure. CT phlebography provides excellent imaging information on the site and extent of obstruction and the status of collaterals.[35] Helical CT phlebography replaced the combination of CT and digital phlebography that was advocated in the past.[36] The role of magnetic resonance imaging has been insufficiently investigated but appears promising, especially because this modality is noninvasive.[37]

TABLE 51.1-4. Chest Radiographic Findings for 86 Patients with Superior Vena Cava Syndrome

Finding	*Number of Patients*	*Percentage of Patients*
Superior mediastinal widening	55	64
Pleural effusion	22	26
Right hilar mass	10	12
Bilateral diffuse infiltrates	6	7
Cardiomegaly	5	6
Calcified paratracheal nodes	4	5
Mediastinal (anterior) mass	3	3
Normal	14	16

(From ref. 10, with permission.)

Contrast venography provides important information for determining if the vena cava is completely obstructed or remains patent and extrinsically compressed.[31,38] Dyet and Moghissi[39] demonstrated by venography that 41% of patients with SVCS have a patent SVC that is displaced or involved but not obstructed by a tumor. Another 19% have SVC obstruction below the azygos vein, for which collateral venous compression should be adequate. Venography is valuable if surgical bypass is considered for the obstructed vena cava.[40] Lokich and Goodman[23] stated that venograms are relatively contraindicated because the interruption of the integrity of the vessel wall, in the presence of increased intraluminal pressures, may result in excessive bleeding from the puncture site. However, no evidence of this complication has been reported. Although a venography can confirm the clinical diagnosis and outline the anatomy, priority should still be given to procedures that help establish the histologic diagnosis. Radionuclide technetium (Tc) 99m venography is an alternative, minimally invasive method of imaging the venous system.[41–43] Although images that are obtained by this method are not as well defined as those achieved with contrast venography, they demonstrate patency and flow patterns. Collateral circulation can be evaluated in a general manner and quantified to some degree by radionuclide venography. Gallium single photon emission CT may be of value in selected cases.[44]

In 58% of 107 patients reported by Schraufnagel et al.,[4] the SVCS developed before the primary diagnosis was established. The diagnostic procedures used in different studies are summarized in Table 51.1-5. Sputum cytology established the diagnosis for almost one-half of patients. Cytologic diagnosis is as accurate as tissue diagnosis in small cell carcinoma.[45] Bronchoscopy supplies the malignant cells for cytologic evaluation in most cases of small cell disease.[46] In the presence of pleural effusion, thoracocentesis established the diagnosis of malignancy in 71% of patients. Biopsy of a supraclavicular node, especially if there was a suspicious palpatory finding, was rewarding in two-thirds of the reported attempts. SCLC and NHL often involve the bone marrow. A biopsy of the bone marrow may provide the diagnosis and stage for these patients. Mediastinoscopy has a very high success rate for providing a diagnosis, and a complication rate of approximately 5%.[47] Reports by Jahangiri and Goldstraw[48] (34 patients) and Mineo

TABLE 51.1-5. Positive Yield of Diagnostic Procedures for Patients with Superior Vena Cava Syndrome

	Number of Procedures	*Number Positive*	*Percentage Positive*
Sputum cytology	59	29	49
Thoracocentesis	14	10	71
Bone marrow biopsy	13	3	23
Lymph node biopsy	95	64	67
Bronchoscopy	124	65	52
Mediastinoscopy	105	95	90
Thoracotomy	49	48	98

et al.[47] (80 patients), on using mediastinoscopy for patients with SVCS whose histologic diagnosis could not be established with less invasive techniques, confirmed the safety and high diagnostic yield of mediastinoscopy. No perioperative mortality was recorded and the diagnosis yield was excellent.

Percutaneous transthoracic CT-guided fine-needle biopsy is emerging as an effective and safe alternative to an open biopsy or mediastinoscopy.[49,50] Successful diagnostic transluminal atherectomy also has been reported.[51] A thoracotomy is diagnostic if all other procedures have failed.

Ahmann[31] examined the traditional opinion that diagnostic procedures carry with them significant hazard, primarily excessive bleeding.[23,29] He reviewed 843 invasive and semiinvasive diagnostic procedures and found that only ten reported complications, none of them fatal. Ahmann[31] and others[12,32] found minimal evidence to suggest that diagnostic procedures such as venographies, thoracotomies, bronchoscopies, mediastinoscopies, and lymph node biopsies carry an excessive risk in patients with SVCS. In 163 patients treated at Memorial Sloan-Kettering Cancer Center for anterior mediastinal mass, 44 underwent general anesthesia. There were no deaths and only four patients had prolonged intubation, demonstrating the low risk of modern anesthesia in thoracic patients.[52]

MANAGEMENT

The goals of treatment of SVCS are to relieve symptoms and to attempt the cure of the primary malignant process. SCLC, NHL, and germ cell tumors constitute almost one-half of the malignant causes of SVCS. These disorders are potentially curable, even in the presence of SVCS. The treatment of SVCS should be selected according to the histologic disorder and stage of the primary process. The prognosis of patients with SVCS strongly correlates with the prognosis of the underlying disease.

When the therapeutic goal is only palliation of SVCS, or when urgent treatment of the venous obstruction is required, direct opening of the occlusion should be considered. The newer techniques of endovascular stenting and angioplasty with possible thrombolysis should provide prompt relief of symptoms before more specific cancer therapy.[3]

SMALL CELL LUNG CANCER

Chemotherapy alone or in combination with thoracic irradiation therapy is the standard treatment for SCLC.[53] Both chemotherapy and radiotherapy as initial treatments are effective in rapidly improving the symptoms of SVCS.[19] In an analysis of 50 patients with SCLC who presented with SVCS, investigators from Ontario, Canada recorded a response rate to chemotherapy of 93% and a similar response to mediastinal irradiation of 94%.[19] In this series, 70% of patients remained SVCS-free before death. It is of interest that, when the total treatment of SCLC included both chemotherapy and radiation, the risk of SVCS recurrence was significantly lower than when the treatment was chemotherapy alone.[19] A small randomized trial, however, could not show that the addition of mediastinal radiation after chemotherapy in patients with SCLC and SVCS increased the protection from local recurrence or improved the survival rate.[16]

Among 643 patients with SCLC, Sculier et al.[15] identified 55 patients (8.5%) with SVCS. One-half of patients developed the manifestations of SVCS before the histologic diagnosis was established. In the other patients, the syndrome developed after the pathologic diagnosis of SCLC was made, but before a specific treatment was started. Symptomatic relief of SVCS was obtained in 35 of 48 patients (73%) initially treated with chemotherapy and in three of seven patients (43%) who were initially treated with radiation. Relief of SVCS occurred within 7 to 10 days after initiation of therapy. In SCLC patients with recurrent or persistent SVCS after initial chemotherapy, the obstruction responded in five of seven patients (71%) who received additional chemotherapy and in 25 of 32 patients (78%) who received radiotherapy.[19] These data support retreatment of SVCS for palliation of symptoms.

In some series of SCLC, SVCS was a favorable prognostic sign,[15,16,18] whereas its presence did not affect survival in other reports.[14,17] A study of 408 patients with SCLC by Wurschmidt et al.[18] showed that the presence of SVCS independently predicted for better survival. Other independent predictors for better survival were stage and performance status.[18] The reason for the possible association of SVCS with better prognosis remains obscure. It is of interest to note that some researchers found a higher incidence of brain metastases at the time of diagnosis in SCLC patients with SVCS compared to patients without SVCS.[17,18,53]

Although randomized trials of the contribution of thoracic irradiation to chemotherapy have not consistently demonstrated an advantage to the combined modality approach, metaanalysis of these studies showed a small but significant improvement in local control and survival of patients with limited disease with the addition of radiotherapy.[54,55] The optimal sequence of the two modalities, and the dose and fractionation of radiotherapy, have not been fully established yet.[56] However, the use of combination chemotherapy as the initial modality, with subsequent rapid shrinkage of the tumor, may eliminate the necessity of irradiating a large volume of lung tissue. When chemotherapy is administered, the arm veins should be avoided. Veins of the lower extremities provide an alternative simple venous access.

NON-HODGKIN'S LYMPHOMA

The most extensive experience in treating SVCS secondary to NHL is reported from the M. D. Anderson Cancer Center.[20] Twenty-two patients with diffuse large cell lymphoma and eight patients with lymphoblastic lymphoma were evaluated for results of treatment. The patients were treated with chemotherapy alone, chemotherapy combined with irradiation, or radiotherapy alone. All patients achieved complete relief of SVCS symptoms within 2 weeks of the onset of any type of treatment. No treatment modality appeared to be superior in achieving clinical improvement. The presence of dysphagia, hoarseness, or stridor was a major adverse prognostic factor for patients with lymphoma presenting with SVCS. Eighteen of 22 patients (81%) with large cell lymphoma achieved complete response. Relapse occurred in all six patients treated with irradiation alone, in four of seven patients treated with chemotherapy alone, and in five of nine patients treated with chemotherapy and radiotherapy. The median survival rate was 21 months. All eight patients with lymphoblastic lymphoma achieved complete response. Six relapses occurred in this group, and all were in sites not initially involved. Median survival was 19 months.

From these results, the researchers concluded that SVCS secondary to lymphoma is rarely an emergency that requires treatment before a histologic diagnosis is made. They recommended that the choice of treatment should be based on the histologic diagnosis and that the patients should undergo, if possible, a complete staging workup before therapy. However, lymphangiography should be avoided to prevent embolization of contrast material that could result in respiratory failure. They advocated chemotherapy as the treatment of choice, because it provides both local and systemic therapeutic activity. They suggested that local consolidation with radiation therapy may be beneficial in patients with large cell lymphoma with mediastinal masses larger than 10 cm.

A similarly favorable experience in children with T-cell lymphoma or leukemia (nine patients) and Hodgkin's disease (two patients) presenting with SVCS was reported from Israel.[57] Tissue diagnosis was obtained before specific therapy in all children; SVCS responded to chemotherapy within 2 to 10 days, and the overall 3-year disease-free survival rate was 78%.

NONMALIGNANT CAUSES

Patients with nonmalignant causes of SVCS differ significantly from patients with malignant disease. If the cause is not malignant, the patients often have symptoms long before they seek medical advice; it takes more time to establish the diagnosis; and their survival is markedly longer.[4] Schraufnagel et al.[4] reported that the average survival rate was 9 years if the primary process was benign, compared with an average survival of 5 months for patients with lung cancer. Mahajan et al.[58] reviewed the literature of benign SVCS and reported 16 new cases. Twelve (75%) of these 16 patients had a mediastinal granuloma that was attributed to histoplasmosis. Most patients had an insidious onset of SVCS and were relatively young. Ten patients who were available for a follow-up of 1 to 11 years were all doing well at the time of the report. It was suggested that the good prognosis of patients with benign SVCS caused by fibrosing mediastinitis does not provide a role for SVC bypass surgery.[58,59] However, Nieto and Doty[38] advocated surgery for SVCS caused by benign disorders if the syndrome develops suddenly, progresses, or persists after 6 to 12 months of observation for possible collateral development.[38] In patients whose histoplasmosis complement fixation titers suggest active disease, ketoconazole treatment may prevent recurrent SVCS.[60]

CATHETER-INDUCED OBSTRUCTION

In catheter-induced SVCS, the mechanism of obstruction is usually thrombosis. Streptokinase, urokinase, or recombinant tissue-type plasminogen activator may cause lysis of the thrombus early in its formation.[24,61–64] Heparin and oral anticoagulants may reduce the extent of the thrombus and prevent its progression. Removal of the catheter, if possible, is another option and should be combined with anticoagulation to avoid embolization. In patients for whom electrodes of a pacemaker must be changed, the broken wire should be removed to prevent the risk of developing SVCS.[24,61,65] Percutaneous transluminal angioplasty, with or without thrombolytic therapy, and stent insertion have been successfully used to open catheter-induced SVC obstructions.[62,66–69]

TREATMENT

RADIATION THERAPY

In patients with SVCS as a result of non-SCLC, radiotherapy has long been the primary treatment. The likelihood of relieving the symptoms and signs of SVCS is high,[5,9] but the overall prognosis for these patients is poor.[4,5,9,25] In the series of Armstrong et al.,[9] the 1-year survival for these patients was 17%, and the survival at 2 years declined to 2%. More recently, the use of percutaneous metal stent insertion to improve blood flow through the SVC has been introduced as an alternative to palliative radiation therapy in malignant SVCS.[3,70]

Radiotherapy is an optional treatment for most patients with SVCS.[23,29,30] It is also used as an effective initial treatment if a histologic diagnosis cannot be established and the clinical status of the patient is deteriorating. However, some reviews suggest that SVC obstruction alone rarely represents an absolute emergency that requires radiotherapy without a specific diagnosis, and endovascular stenting may be used as an alternative to radiotherapy for obtaining immediate relief of the obstruction.[3,12,31,32,70] Yet, SVCS may be the earliest manifestation of invasive involvement of additional critical structures in the thorax (Table 51.1-6), such as the bronchi. Under such circumstances, prompt treatment with irradiation may be required without any delay.

The fractionation schedule of radiation that has been recommended includes two to four large initial fractions of 3 to 4 cGy, followed by conventional fractionation to a total dose of 30 to 50 cGy.[5,23,29] However, no data clearly support a particular fractionation scheme.[19] In one study, patients treated with initial high-dose fractions showed a slightly faster symptomatic improvement than patients receiving conventional-dose radiation.[9] Improvement within 2 weeks or less was observed in 70% of those treated with initial high-dose fractions and in 56% of patients receiving conventional-dose therapy. This difference was not statistically significant.

A radiotherapy study evaluated the efficacy of treating patients with SVCS with a short course of hypofractionated irradiation.[71] The study compared a regimen of 8 Gy per fraction once a week to a total dose of 24 Gy to a program of delivering

TABLE 51.1-6. Complications of Malignant Invasion Associated with Superior Vena Cava Syndrome

Complication	*Number of Patients[a] (%)*
ESOPHAGUS	
Symptoms of dysphagia or esophageal dysfunction	26 (24)
Anatomic evidence of esophageal invasion	6 (6)
TRACHEA	
Displaced on examination or roentgenogram	7 (7)
Compressed or invaded by lesion	14 (13)
VOCAL CORD PARALYSIS	
Unilateral	6 (6)
Bilateral	3 (3)
PERICARDIUM	
Tamponade	3 (3)
Neoplastic invasion at necropsy	6 (6)

[a]Some patients may have had more than one complication.
(From ref. 4, with permission.)

only two fractions of 8 Gy (total of 16 Gy) within 1 week. Transient dysphagia was the main side effect in almost one-half of patients in both programs. The 24-Gy regimen resulted in a complete resolution of symptoms in 56% of patients and a partial response in another 40%. The 16-Gy regimen yielded a complete response in only 28% of patients. The mean time for SVCS recurrence and the median overall survival rate were longer in the higher-dose regimen (6 months and 9 months, respectively) compared to the low-dose regimen (3 months and 3 months, respectively).

Serial venograms and autopsies[31] suggest that the symptomatic improvement achieved by radiotherapy is not always due to improvement of flow through the SVC, but it is probably also a result of the development of collaterals after the pressure in the mediastinum is eased.

The field of radiation for SVCS induced by lung cancer should encompass the gross tumors with appropriate margins, and mediastinal, hilar, and supraclavicular lymph nodes. In Armstrong et al.'s series,[9] supraclavicular failures occurred in 8 of 91 patients (9%) receiving radiation therapy to the supraclavicular fossae and in two of six patients (33%) not receiving therapy to these lymph nodes.[9]

ENDOVASCULAR STENTING AND ANGIOPLASTY

Percutaneous transluminal angioplasty using the balloon technique, insertion of expandable wire stents, or both, has been successfully used to open and maintain the patency of SVC obstruction resulting from malignant and benign causes.[3,69,70,72]

Thrombolysis is often an integral part of the endovascular management of SVCS because thrombosis is often a critical component of the obstruction and lysis is necessary to allow the passage of the wire. Balloon dilatation (angioplasty) may also be used before stenting. Most reports have emphasized the use of combination endovascular therapy—thrombolysis, angioplasty, and stent therapy.[3]

The experience with stenting has been growing rapidly. Most experience has been with three stents: the Gianturco Z-stent, the Wallstent, and the Palmaz stent. The Wallstent is the most commonly used device.[3] It is self-expanding and built of woven stainless steel wire. Its tight weave deters tumor ingrowth.

Total occlusion of the SVC is not a contraindication to stent therapy, and a success rate of 85% in total occlusion situations has been reported.[73] The largest experience in using stents to open malignant obstruction of the SVC was reported by Nicholson et al. in Great Britian.[70] The British team used Wallstents in 75 patients and obtained improvement of obstruction in all patients; 90% remained free of symptoms until death. This study retrospectively compared stent therapy with radiation therapy and found that only 12% of patients treated with radiation remained free of SVCS until death. However, long-term experience in maintaining patency after stent therapy in patients with SVCS from benign causes who are expected to have long survival, is still limited.[69]

Complication rates for endovascular therapy have ranged from 0% to 50% and include bleeding, stent migration, stent occlusion, and pulmonary embolus.[3] Most complications can be successfully treated with percutaneous methods.

SURGERY

The experience with successful direct bypass graft for SVC obstruction is limited. It was recommended that autologous grafts of almost the same size as the SVC should be used.[74] Doty et al.[75] used a composite spiral graft, which was constructed from the patient's saphenous vein. They reported 23 years of experience with this procedure in 16 patients with benign obstruction of SVC; 14 patients maintained patency and 15 were relieved of symptoms of SVCS. Avashti and Moghissi[76] reported successful bypasses of obstructed SVCs using Dacron protheses. Magnan and associates[77] used an expanded polytetrafluoroethylene prosthesis to reconstruct the SVC in nine patients with malignancy-induced SVCS and in one patient with chronic mediastinitis. In all, patients' symptoms disappeared promptly after the operation, the grafts remained open, and survival rates at 1, 2, and 5 years were 70%, 25%, and 12.5%, respectively.[77]

The preferred bypass route is between an innominate or jugular vein on the left side and the right atrial appendage, using an end-to-end anastomosis.[45] Piccione et al.[78] used the autologous pericardium to reconstruct the SVC after resection for malignant obstruction. In patients with malignancy-induced SVCS, surgical intervention should be considered only after other therapeutic maneuvers with irradiation and chemotherapy have been exhausted. Most patients with SVCS of benign origin have long survivals without surgical intervention.[58,59] However, if the process progresses rapidly or if there is arterosternal goiter or aortic aneurysm, surgical intervention may relieve the obstruction.

THROMBOLYTIC THERAPY

Thrombolysis is an important component of comprehensive endovascular therapy.[3] Successful experience with thrombolytic agents was also obtained in the treatment of catheter-induced SVCS.[24,64,79] A review of the response of SVCS to thrombolytic therapy from the Cleveland Clinic[64,80] showed that in 8 of 11 patients (73%) with a central venous catheter, lysed after thrombolytic therapy compared with only one of five patients who responded to thrombolytic therapy in the absence of a central catheter. The higher yield of thrombolytic therapy in patients with catheters is probably related to the mechanism of obstruction, the ability to deliver the agent directly to the thrombus, and to earlier recognition of SVCS in patients with malfunctioning catheters. In the Cleveland Clinic experience,[64] urokinase was more effective than streptokinase, and a delay administering therapy beyond 5 days of symptom onset was associated with a treatment failure. Favorable experience with recombinant tissue-type plasminogen activator as a thrombolytic agent for catheter-induced SVCS has been reported.[62,63]

GENERAL MEASURES

Medical measures other than specific chemotherapy may be beneficial in temporarily relieving the symptoms of SVCS. Bed rest with the head elevated and oxygen administration can reduce the cardiac output and venous pressure. Diuretic therapy and a reduced-salt diet to reduce edema may have an immediate palliative effect, but the risk of thrombosis enhanced by dehydration should not be ignored. Steroids are commonly used, but their effectiveness has never been properly evaluated. They may improve obstruction by decreasing a possible inflammatory reaction associated with tumor or with irradiation. However, Green and colleagues[81] demonstrated the lack of inflammatory reaction and edema after radiotherapy for experimental SVCS, but documentation in a controlled fashion is lacking. Thrombolytic therapy with urokinase, streptokinase, and recombinant tissue-type plasminogen activator was effective in SVCS induced by indwelling catheters.[62,64,79,80]

RECOMMENDATIONS

In patients without a clear cause of SVCS, an efficient diagnostic effort should be attempted before any oncologic treatment. However, percutaneous endovascular intervention should be considered, because it relieves symptoms without masking the diagnosis.

Three deep-cough sputum specimens should be obtained for cytologic analysis. A positive cytologic evaluation provides reliable pathologic information, particularly in the diagnosis of SCLC.[45] If there is pleural effusion, thoracocentesis should be performed and the centrifuge-prepared specimen examined for the presence of malignant cells. If a suspicious lymph node is palpable, particularly in the supraclavicular area, a needle or open biopsy should be the next diagnostic step. In the absence of positive sputum results, pleural effusion, or accessible suspicious lymph node analysis, a bronchoscopy should be performed, and brushing, washing, and biopsy samples should be obtained for cytologic and histologic analysis. If these efforts do not provide the histologic diagnosis of the primary process, percutaneous transthoracic fine-needle biopsy under CT or fluoroscopic guidance is safe and highly effective.[49,51] In the rare patient for whom less-invasive procedures have failed to establish the diagnosis, the location of the suspicious lesion in the chest and the experience of the surgical team should determine whether mediastinoscopy or thoracotomy is performed.

During the diagnostic process, the patient can benefit from bed rest with the head elevated and with oxygen administration. Some clinicians advocate the use of diuretics and steroids (6 to 10 mg of dexamethasone given orally or intravenously every 6 hours) as a temporary palliative measure if the patient is uncomfortably symptomatic. Anticoagulation is of no proven benefit and may interfere with diagnostic procedures. After the cause of SVCS has been established, treatment of the primary process should promptly follow. Combination chemotherapy with an appropriate regimen is the treatment of choice for SCLC and NHL. Radiation therapy of the lesion and adjacent nodal areas may enhance control after initial response to chemotherapy. Non-SCLC causing SVCS is best treated with radiation therapy or endovascular stent insertion or both. The incorporation of CT scan information into a carefully designed treatment plan may enable the administration of a total radiation dose of more than 5000 cGy, which may provide long-term local control for some patients. Most patients with nonmalignant causes for SVCS have an indolent course and a good prognosis. Percutaneous transluminal angioplasty or stent insertion should be considered an effective alternative to surgery. However, the long-term maintenance of patency with stent insertion is still unknown. Surgery is indicated only when the process is rapidly progressing or caused by a retrosternal goiter or an aortic aneurysm. If SVCS is induced by a catheter, the catheter should be removed if possible. Heparin should be administered during the removal of the catheter to prevent embolization. In catheter-induced SVCS, urokinase, streptokinase, or recombinant tissue-type plasminogen activator are of value if used early in the thrombotic process.[60–62,80]

The clinical course of SVCS rarely represents an absolute emergency. In these situations, the bronchus is likely to be obstructed by the same basic process, and irradiation may have to be started immediately, even before the histologic diagnosis is established.

REFERENCES

1. Hunter W. The history of an aneurysm of the aorta, with some remarks on aneurysms in general. *Med Observ Inq* 1757;1:323.
2. Schechter MM. The superior vena cava syndrome. *Am J Med Sci* 1954;227:46.
3. Schindler N, Vogelzang RL. Superior vena cava syndrome. Experience with endovascular stents and surgical therapy. *Surg Clin North Am* 1999;79:683.
4. Schraufnagel DE, Hill R, Leech JA, Pare JAP. Superior vena caval obstruction. Is it an emergency? *Am J Med* 1981;70:1169.
5. Davenport D, Ferree C, Blake D, Raben M. Radiation therapy in the treatment of superior vena caval obstruction. *Cancer* 1978;42:2600.
6. Rubin P, Hicks GL. Biassociation of superior vena caval obstruction and spinal-cord compression. *N Y State J Med* 1973;73:2176.
7. Carlson HA. Obstruction of the superior vena cava: an experimental study. *Arch Surg* 1934;29:669.
8. Roswit B, Kaplan G, Jacobson HG. The superior vena cava syndrome in bronchogenic carcinoma. *Radiology* 1953;61:722.
9. Armstrong BA, Perez CA, Simpson JR, Hederman MA. Role of irradiation in the management of superior vena cava syndrome. *Int J Radiat Oncol Biol Phys* 1987;13:531.
10. Parish JM, Marschke RF, Dines DE, Lee RE. Etiologic considerations in superior vena cava syndrome. *Mayo Clin Proc* 1981;56:407.
11. Bell DR, Woods RL, Levi JA. Superior vena caval obstruction: a 10-year experience. *Med J Aust* 1986;145:566.
12. Yellin A, Rosen A, Reichert N, Lieberman Y. Superior vena cava syndrome. The myth—the facts. *Am Rev Respir Dis* 1990;141:1114.
13. Salsali M, Cliffton EE. Superior vena caval obstruction in carcinoma of lung. *N Y State J Med* 1969;69:2875.
14. Dombernowsky P, Hansen HH. Combination chemotherapy in the management of superior vena caval obstruction in small-cell anaplastic of the lung. *Acta Med Scand* 1978;204:513.

15. Sculier JP, Evans WK, Feld R, et al. Superior vena caval obstruction in small cell lung cancer. *Cancer* 1986;57:847.
16. Spiro SG, Shah S, Harper PG, et al. Treatment of obstruction of the superior vena cava by combination chemotherapy with and without irradiation in small-cell carcinoma of the bronchus. *Thorax* 1983;38:501.
17. Urban T, Lebeau B, Chastang C, et al. Superior vena cava syndrome in small-cell lung cancer. *Arch Intern Med* 1993;153:384.
18. Wurschmidt F, Bunemann H, Heilmann HP. Small cell lung cancer with and without superior vena cava syndrome: a multivariate analysis of prognostic factors in 408 cases. *Int J Rad Oncol Biol Phys* 1995;33:77.
19. Chan RH, Dar AR, Yu E, et al. Superior vena cava obstruction in small-cell lung cancer. *Int J Radiat Oncol Biol Phys* 1997;38:513.
20. Perez-Soler R, McLaughlin P, Velasquez WS, et al. Clinical features and results of management of superior vena cava syndrome secondary to lymphoma. *J Clin Oncol* 1984;2:260.
21. Lazzarino M, Orlandi E, Paulli M, et al. Primary mediastinal B-cell lymphoma with sclerosis: an aggressive tumor with distinctive clinical and pathologic features. *J Clin Oncol* 1993;11:2306.
22. Chen JC, Bongard F, Klein SR. A contemporary perspective on superior vena cava syndrome. *Am J Surg* 1990;97:1005.
23. Lokich JJ, Goodman R. Superior vena cava syndrome: clinical management. *JAMA* 1975;231:58.
24. Sculier JP, Feld R. Superior vena cava obstruction system: recommendation for management. *Cancer Treat Rev* 1985;12:209.
25. Bertrand M, Presant CA, Klein L, Scott E. Iatrogenic superior vena cava syndrome. A new entity. *Cancer* 1984;54:376.
26. Janin Y, Becker J, Wise L, et al. Superior vena cava syndrome in childhood and adolescence: a review of the literature and report of three cases. *J Pediatr Surg* 1982;17:290.
27. Issa PY, Brihi ER, Janin Y, Slim MS. Superior vena cava syndrome in childhood: report of ten cases and review of the literature. *Pediatrics* 1983;71:337.
28. Ingram L, Rivera GK, Shapiro DN. Superior vena cava syndrome associated with childhood malignancy: analysis of 24 cases. *Med Pediatr Oncol* 1990;18:476.
29. Perez CA, Presant CA, Van Amburg AL III. Management of superior vena cava syndrome. *Semin Oncol* 1978;5:123.
30. Scarantino C, Salazar OM, Rubin R, et al. The optimum radiation schedule in the treatment of superior vena caval obstruction: importance of ^{99m}Tc scintinangiograms. *Int J Radiat Oncol Biol Phys* 1979;5:1987.
31. Ahmann FR. A reassessment of the clinical implications of the superior vena cava syndrome. *J Clin Oncol* 1984;2:961.
32. Shimm DS, Lugue GL, Tigsby LC. Evaluating the superior vena cava syndrome. *JAMA* 1981;245:951.
33. Loeffler JS, Leopold KA, Recht A, et al. Emergency prebiopsy radiation for mediastinal masses: impact on subsequent pathologic diagnosis and outcome. *J Clin Oncol* 1986;4:716.
34. Yedlicka JW, Schultz K, Moncada R, Flisak M. CT findings in superior vena cava obstruction. *Semin Roentgenol* 1989;24:84.
35. Qanadli SD, El Hajjam M, Bruckert F, et al. Helical CT phlebography of the superior vena cava: diagnosis and evaluation of venous obstruction. *AJR Am J Roentgenol* 1999;172:1327.
36. Moncada R, Cardella R, Demos TC, et al. Evaluation of superior vena cava syndrome by axial CT and CT phlebography. *AJR Am J Roentgenol* 1984;143:731.
37. Hansen ME, Spritzer CE, Sostman HD. Assessing the patency of mediastinal and thoracic inlet veins: value of MR imaging. *AJR Am J Roentgenol* 1990;155:1177.
38. Nieto AF, Doty DB. Superior vena cava obstruction: clinical syndrome, etiology and treatment. *Curr Prob Cancer* 1986;10:442.
39. Dyet JF, Moghissi K. Role of venography in assessing patients with superior vena cava obstruction caused by bronchial carcinoma for bypass operations. *Thorax* 1980;35:628.
40. Stanford W, Jolles H, Ell S, Chiu LC. Superior vena cava obstruction: a venographic classification. *AJR Am J Roentgenol* 1987;148:259.
41. Son YH, Wetzel RA, Wilson WA. ^{99m}Tc pertechnetate scintiphotography as diagnostic and followup aids in major vascular obstruction due to malignant neoplasm. *Radiology* 1968;91:349.
42. Van Houtte P, Fruhling J. Radionuclide venography in the evaluation of superior vena cava syndrome. *Clin Nucl Med* 1981;6:177.
43. Conte FA, Orzel JA. Superior vena cava syndrome and bilateral subclavian vein thrombosis: CT and radionuclide venography correlation. *Clin Nucl Med* 1986;11:698.
44. Swayne LC, Kaplan IL. Gallium SPECT detection of neoplastic intravascular obstruction of superior vena cava. *Clin Nucl Med* 1989;14:823.
45. Yesner R, Gerstl B, Auerbach O. Application of the World Health Organization classification of lung carcinoma to biopsy material. *Ann Thorac Surg* 1965;1:33.
46. Ihde DC, Cohen MH, Bernath AM, et al. Serial fiberoptic bronchoscopy during chemotherapy of small cell carcinoma of the lung. *Chest* 1978;74:531.
47. Mineo TC, Ambrogi V, Nofroni I, et al. Mediastinoscopy in superior vena cava obstruction: analysis of 80 consecutive patients. *Ann Thorac Surg* 1999;68:223.
48. Jahangiri M, Goldstraw P. The role of mediastinoscopy in superior vena caval obstruction. *Ann Thorac Surg* 1995;59:453.
49. Cosmos L, Haponik EF, Dariak JJ, Summer WR. Neoplastic superior vena caval obstruction: diagnosis with percutaneous needle aspiration. *Am J Med Sci* 1987;293:99.
50. Reyes CV, Thompson KS, Massarani-Wafai R, et al. Utilization of fine-needle aspiration cytology in the diagnosis of neoplastic superior vena caval syndrome. *Diagn Cytopathol* 1998;19:84.
51. Dake MD, Zemel G, Dolmatch BL, Katzen BT. The cause of superior vena cava syndrome diagnosis with percutaneous atherectomy. *Radiology* 1990;174:957.
52. Ferrari LR, Bedford RF. General anesthesia prior to the treatment of anterior mediastinal masses in pediatric cancer patients. *Anesthesiology* 1990;72:991.
53. Seifter EJ, Ihde DC. Therapy of small cell lung cancer: a perspective on two decades of clinical research. *Semin Oncol* 1988;15:278.
54. Warde P, Payne D. Does thoracic irradiation improve survival and local control in limited stage small cell carcinoma of the lung? A meta-analysis. *J Clin Oncol* 1992;10:890.
55. Pignon JP, Arriagada R, Ihde DC, et al. A meta-analysis of thoracic radiotherapy for small-cell lung cancer. *N Engl J Med* 1992;327:1618.
56. Murray N, Coy P, Pater JL, et al. Importance of timing for thoracic irradiation in the combined modality treatment of limited-stage small-cell lung cancer. *J Clin Oncol* 1993;11:336.
57. Yellin A, Mandel M, Rechavi G, et al. Superior vena cava syndrome associated with lymphoma. *Am J Dis Child* 1992;146:1060.
58. Mahajan V, Strimlan V, Van Ordstrand HS, Loop FD. Benign superior cava syndrome. *Chest* 1975;68:32.
59. Effler DB, Groves LK. Superior vena caval obstruction. *J Thorac Cardiovasc Surg* 1962;43:574.
60. Urshel HC Jr, Razzuk MA, Netto GJ, Disiere J, Chung SY. Sclerosing mediastinitis: improved management with histoplasmosis titer and ketoconazole. *Ann Thorac Surg* 1990;50:215.
61. Goudevonos JA, Reid PG, Adams PC, Holden MP, Williams DO. Pacemaker-induced superior vena cava syndrome: report of four cases and review of the literature. *PACE* 1989;12:1890.
62. Fine DG, Shepherd RF, Welch TJ. Thrombolytic therapy for superior vena cava syndrome [Letter]. *Lancet* 1989;1:1200.
63. Greenberg S, Kosinski R, Daniels J. Treatment of superior vena cava thrombosis with recombinant tissue type plasminogen activator. *Chest* 1991;99:1298.
64. Gray BH, Olin JW, Grador RA, et al. Safety and efficacy of thrombolytic therapy for superior vena cava syndrome. *Chest* 1991;99:54.
65. Blackburn T, Dunn M. Pacemaker-induced superior vena cava syndrome: consideration of management. *Am Heart J* 1988;116:893.
66. Grace AA, Sutters M, Schofield PM. Balloon dilation of pacemaker-induced stenosis of the superior vena cava. *Br Heart J* 1991;65:225.
67. Montgomery JH, D'Souza VJ, Dyer RB, et al. Non-surgical treatment of the superior vena cava syndrome. *Am J Cardiol* 1985;56:829.
68. Sunder SK, Ekong EA, Sivalingam K, Kumar A. Superior vena cava thrombosis due to pacing electrodes: successful treatment with combined thrombolysis and angioplasty. *Am Heart J* 1992;123:790.
69. Kee ST, Kinoshita L, Razavi MK, et al. Superior vena cava syndrome: treatment with catheter-directed thrombolysis and endovascular stent placement. *Radiology* 1998;206:187.
70. Nicholson AA, Ettles DF, Arnold A, et al. Treatment of malignant superior vena cava obstruction: metal stents or radiation therapy. *J Vasc Interv Radiol* 1997;8:781.
71. Rodrigues CI, Njo KH, Karim ABMF. Hypofractionated radiation therapy in the treatment of superior vena cava syndrome. *Lung Cancer* 1993;10:221.
72. Shah R, Sabanathan S, Lowe RA, et al. Stenting in malignant obstruction of superior vena cava. *J Thorac Cardiovasc Surg* 1996;112:335.
73. Crowe MT, Davies CH, Gaines PA, et al. Percutaneous management of superior vena cava occlusions. *Cardiovasc Intervent Radiol* 1995;18:367.
74. Scherck JP, Kerstein MD, Stansel HC. The current status of vena caval replacement. *Surgery* 1974;76:209.
75. Doty JR, Flores JH, Doty DB. Superior vena cava obstruction: bypass using spiral vein graft. *Ann Thorac Surg* 1999;67:1111.
76. Avashti RB, Moghissi K. Malignant obstruction of the superior vena cava and its palliation. *J Thorac Cardiovasc Surg* 1977;74:244.
77. Magnan PE, Thomas P, Giudicelli R, Fuentes P, Branchereau A. Surgical reconstruction of the superior vena cava. *Cardiovasc Surg* 1994;2:598.
78. Piccione W Jr, Faber LP, Warren WH. Superior vena caval reconstruction using autologous pericardium. *Ann Thorac Surg* 1990;50:417.
79. Meister FL, McLaughlin TF, Tenney RD, Sholkoff SD. Urokinase. A cost-effective alternative treatment of superior vena cava thrombosis and obstruction. *Arch Intern Med* 1989;149:1209.
80. Comerota AJ. Safety and efficacy of thrombolytic therapy for superior vena caval syndrome. *Chest* 1991;99:3.
81. Green J, Rubin P, Holzwasser G. The experimental production of superior vena cava obstruction. *Radiology* 1963;81:406.

SECTION **2**

BRIAN G. FULLER
JOHN D. HEISS
EDWARD H. OLDFIELD

Spinal Cord Compression

Spinal cord compression from metastatic cancer remains an important source of morbidity despite the fact that with early diagnosis, treatment is effective in 90% of patients.[1] Technical improvements in spinal imaging, radiation therapy, and surgery have allowed treatment of spinal cord compression to be dispensed with greater precision. However, the most important weapon against the devastation of paraplegia or sphincter dysfunction is a heightened awareness of possible spinal cord compression in the cancer patient and early intervention.

Despite its common occurrence, there have been few prospective studies[1–4] and randomized trials have been exceedingly rare.[5–7] At the dawn of the new millennium, treatment recommendations are based largely on empiric experiences described in retrospective reports. However, the pathophysiology of cord compression and the factors that predict treatment outcome are well known.

Malignant spinal cord compression is defined as the compressive indentation, displacement, or encasement of the spinal cord's thecal sac by metastatic or locally advanced cancer. Compression can occur via posterior extension of a vertebral body mass, resulting in compression of the anterior aspect of the spinal cord, or through anterior or anterolateral extension of a mass arising from the dorsal elements or invading the vertebral foramen, respectively. Intramedullary spinal cord metastases produce edema, distortion, and compression of the spinal cord parenchyma, resulting in symptoms and signs that are similar to epidural spinal cord compression. Virtually any neoplasm capable of metastasis or local invasion can produce malignant spinal cord compression. The response to nonsurgical therapy and the duration of survival following treatment can vary considerably among the different histologic tumor types. Therapy for the individual patient can be optimized once the tumor's histologic type is known and the extent, severity, and mechanism of spinal compression are established.

The degree of pretreatment neurologic dysfunction is the strongest predictor of treatment outcome. Ambulation can be preserved in greater than 80% of patients who are ambulatory at presentation.[1,2,8–10] Paraplegia, quadriplegia, and loss of bowel or bladder function are potential consequences of cord compression if it is diagnosed late or left untreated. Once lost, neurologic function cannot be regained in the majority of patients. The diagnosis of cord compression is easy to establish with contemporary diagnostic evaluations, and with early intervention the results of treatment are good to excellent. Therefore, the key to successful management is a heightened awareness of signs and symptoms, specifically newly developed back pain or motor dysfunction, leading to early diagnosis and treatment.

EPIDEMIOLOGY

In adults, metastatic spinal cord compression occurs in roughly 3.0% to 7.4% of patients with lung, prostate, and breast cancer,[8] and the overall frequency of malignant spinal cord compression has been reported to be approximately 5%.[11,12] Spinal cord compression is the second most frequent neurologic complication of metastatic cancer.[13] It can be identified at autopsy in 5% to 10% of patients dying of cancer.[14,15] Ten percent of adult patients with malignant spinal cord compression present without a known primary tumor or with cord compression as the initial presentation of a malignancy.[13] Cord compression at initial presentation is more commonly seen at general hospitals than at regional cancer centers.[16] Tertiary referral centers specializing in cancer may see 50 to 100 cases per annum, although the true incidence of malignant spinal cord compression is not known.[17] Intramedullary lesions make up only 0.8% to 3.8% of all cases of metastatic spinal cord compression.[18] Second episodes of malignant spinal cord compression occur in 7% to 16% of cases.[19,20]

In children, the frequency of metastatic spinal cord compression is approximately 4.0% to 5.5%.[21–23] In one report roughly 50% of cases presented with cord compression at the time of initial diagnosis, and 50% developed compression from secondary spinal metastases.[23] The most frequent tumor types producing pediatric cord compression are neuroblastoma (7.9% to 50%), Ewing's sarcoma (15% to 28.5%), rhabdomyosarcoma (15% to 28%), osteosarcoma (6% to 9%), lymphoma (6.0% to 7.5%), and leukemia (6%).[21–24] Cord compression has been reported to be more frequent in male than in female children, reflecting the epidemiology of childhood cancer.[21,23,24]

PATHOPHYSIOLOGY

In the majority of cases, vertebral body metastases result from the hematogenous dissemination of tumor clonogens that express tropism for the vertebral column bone marrow. More frequently growing in the well-vascularized marrow space of the posterior vertebral body, spinal metastases can produce cord compression in two ways. The first results from continued growth and obliteration of the marrow space with expansion into the epidural space, producing impingement on the anterior thecal sac and its surrounding venous plexus (Fig. 51.2-1). Alternatively, destruction of cortical bone by tumor can result in vertebral body collapse with anterior angulation and posterior displacement of bony fragments into the epidural space against the thecal sac and epidural venous plexus. Compression of the cord, its blood vessels, and nerve roots can also occur from the posterolateral direction via invasion of tumor through the neural foramen. Paraspinous tumors or expanding paraaortic nodal metastases use this mechanism of compression. Posterior thecal sac compression from metastatic involvement of the neural arch does occur but with less frequency. Finally, intramedullary metastases that result from hematogenous dissemination produce internal compression of the spinal cord structures and parenchymal vasculature. The signs and symptoms of intramedullary cord compression are similar to those of external cord compression. However, myelography is less reliable for detection of intramedullary compression. Patterns of metastatic involvement of the spine are illustrated in Figure 51.2-2 and displayed in Figures 51.2-3, 51.2-4, 51.2-5, and 51.2-6.

In an early study of spinal cord compression employing Murphy-Sturm lymphoma in Sprague-Dawley rats, Rubin demonstrated the ability of radiation to produce neurologic recovery and the absence of significant radiation-induced edema in the treated spinal cord.[25] Usio et al., using a Walker 256 carci-

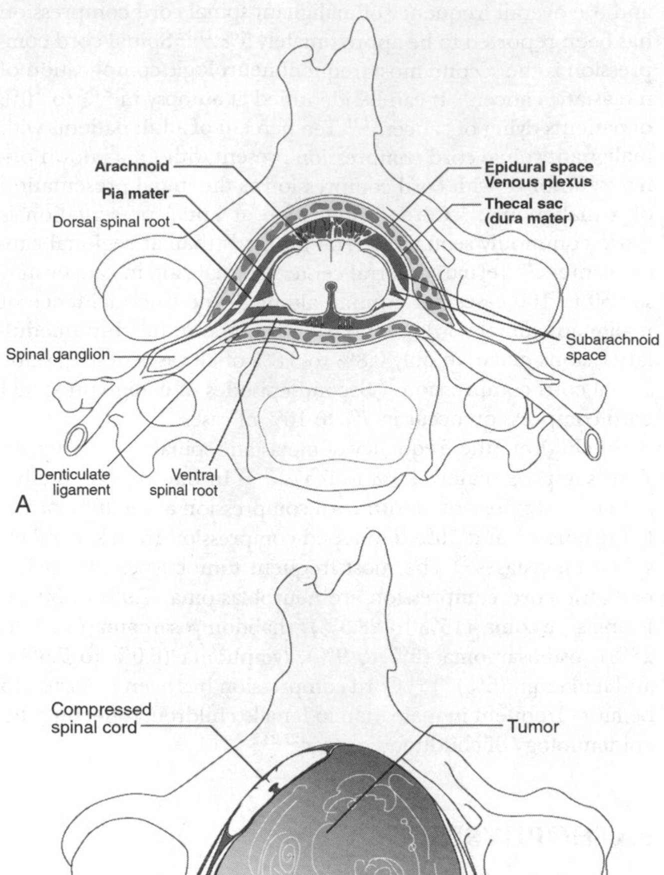

FIGURE 51.2-1. An appreciation of the anatomic relationships within the spinal canal is important in understanding the pathophysiology of spinal cord compression. **A:** The normal spinal cord structures are shown. Note the relationship of the epidural venous plexus to the vertebral body and bony canal. **B:** The change in these relationships produced by a metastatic tumor arising from the vertebral body is illustrated. Note the obliteration of the epidural venous plexus and the compressive displacement of the spinal cord and its nerve roots. (Courtesy of Howard Bartner and Martha Blalock.)

noma cord compression model in rats, were able to document the early development of white matter necrosis and gliosis with preservation of large blood vessels.[26] Similar findings were reported by Ikeda et al. using a rabbit model of malignant epidural cord compression. Early pathologic changes included axonal swelling and white matter edema. Later changes consisted of white matter necrosis with relative sparing of gray matter. Microangiography of the compressed spinal cords revealed preservation of the anterior and posterior spinal arteries, while the central arteries were deformed and decreased in number. Stenosis and obstruction of the epidural venous plexus was observed in the earliest stages of neurologic dysfunction.[27]

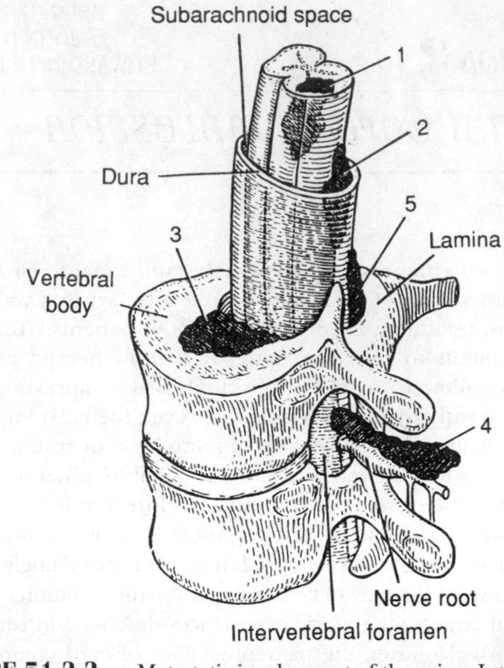

FIGURE 51.2-2. Metastatic involvement of the spine. Intramedullary metastases reach the cord through hematogenous dissemination and grow within the cord parenchyma (1). Leptomeningeal metastases involve the meningeal membranes of the subarachnoid space, which are extramedullary and intradural (2). Epidural metastases usually arise from the highly vascular posterior aspect of the vertebral body and produce compression of the anterior aspect of the spinal cord (3). Epidural compression can also result from paravertebral tumors that invade the vertebral foramina (4) and, less often, from metastases arising in the epidural space itself (5). (Adapted from ref. 103.)

An analysis of spinal cord blood flow in rats with cord compression by Kato et al. revealed three distinct phases in the development of spinal cord compression: (1) initial circulatory disturbance resulting in white matter edema and neurologic dysfunction secondary to venous outflow obstruction; (2) decreased spinal cord blood flow resulting from vasogenic edema and mechanical compression of the cord; and (3) rapid loss of spinal cord blood flow in small arterioles and capillaries resulting in infarction with preservation of large extramedullary nutritional vessels.[28] The validity of this sequence of events was further confirmed by Arbit et al., who found loss of medullary centrifugal blood vessels at the level of compression, with preservation of radicular and subcommissural vessels. Spongy vacuolization and pallor of the white matter as well as spinal cord edema were also described.[29]

Within the spinal cord itself, existing evidence suggests that the pathophysiology of spinal cord compression is vascular in nature.[26,28–34] This has been shown repeatedly in animal models and has been corroborated by autopsy findings.[35] Initial extension of tumor into the epidural space results in compression of the epidural venous plexus, which normally drains blood from the spinal cord. Compression of the venous plexus leads to venous stasis. Relative hypoxia, increased vascular permeability, and interstitial edema appear to selectively involve the white matter,[27–29] although increased vascular permeability was observed involving gray matter in one model.[26] Edema in the spinal cord caused by increased vascular permeability impairs spinal cord function, resulting in weakness and sensory impairment. Interstitial edema increases the pressure within

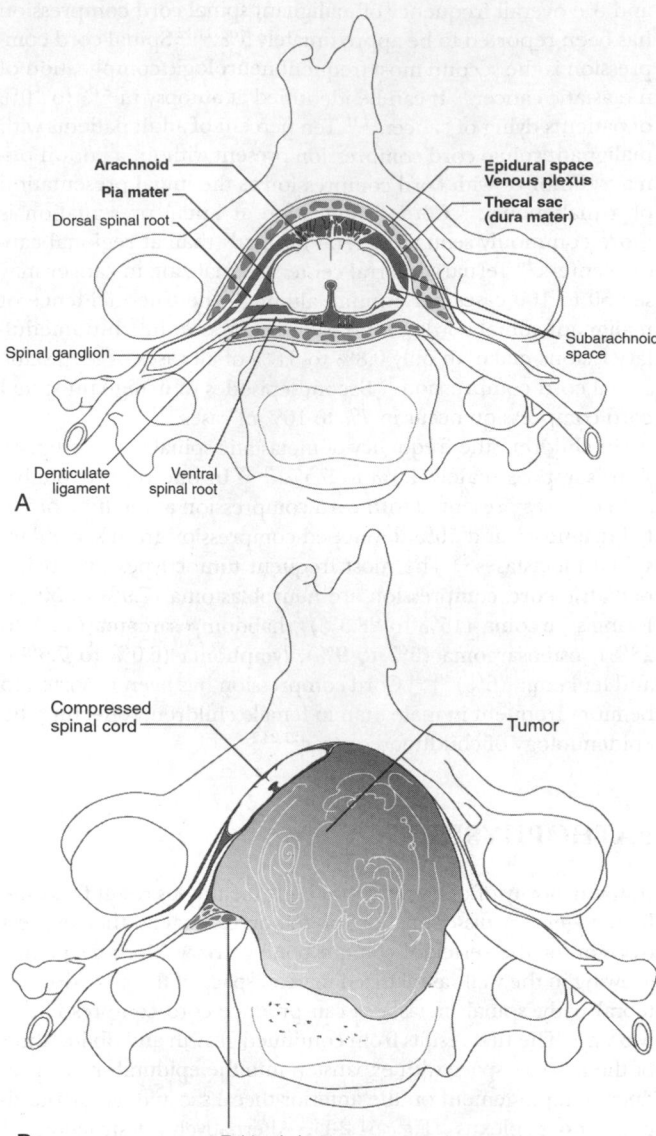

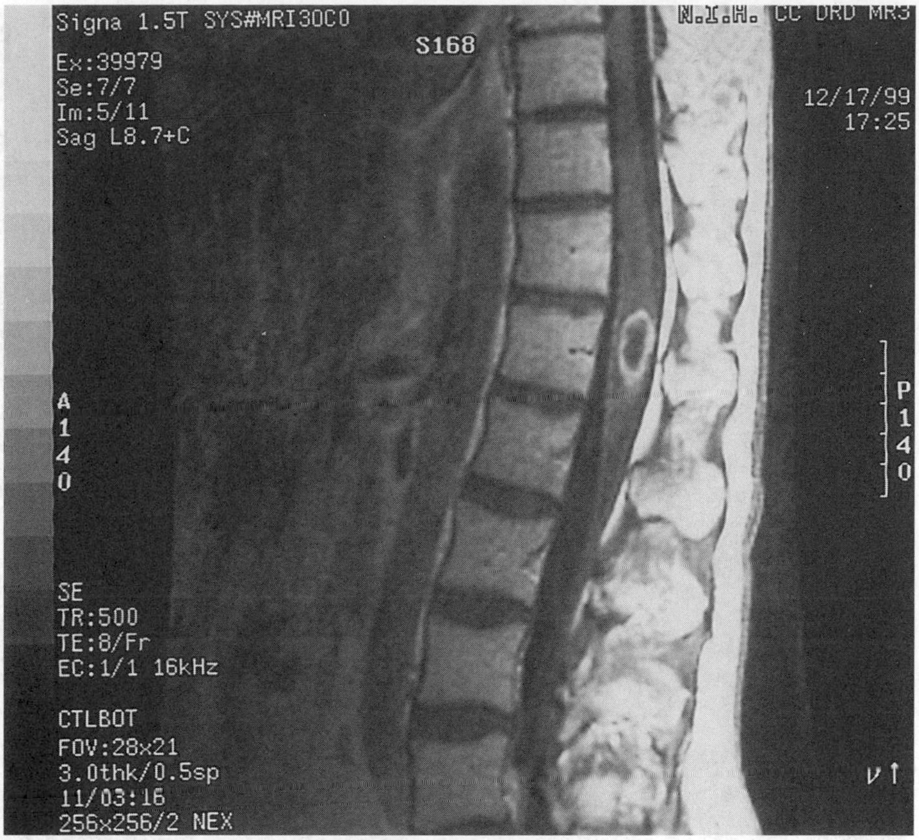

FIGURE 51.2-3. This sagittal view of a magnetic resonance image demonstrates an intramedullary metastasis in the lumbar spine from renal cell carcinoma.

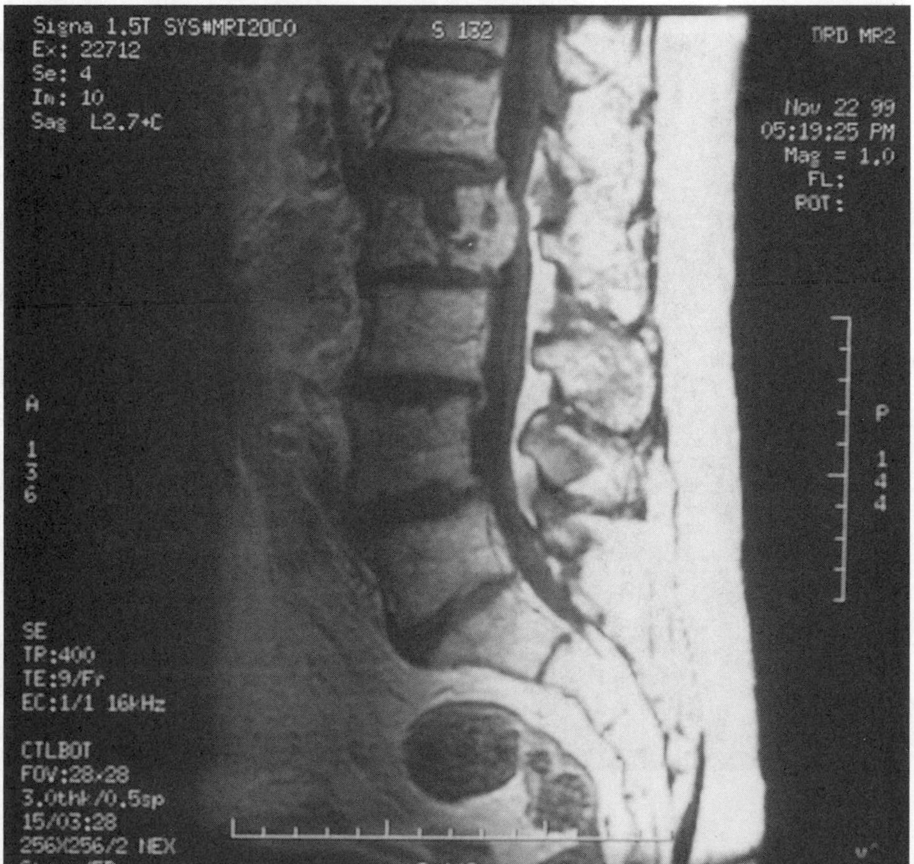

FIGURE 51.2-4. This sagittal magnetic resonance image of the lumbar spine demonstrates anterior compression of the cauda equina below the conus medullaris. Note the pathologic fracture of the L-2 vertebral body and the retropulsed bone fragments compressing the thecal sac.

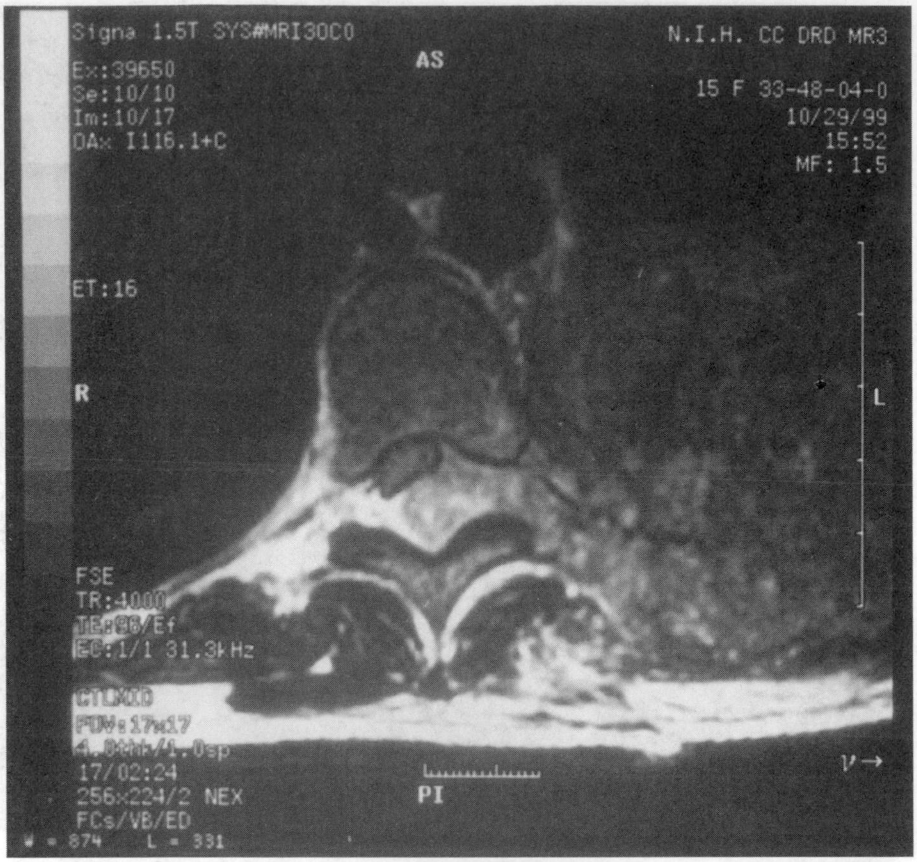

FIGURE 51.2-5. This axial view from a magnetic resonance image of the thoracic spine demonstrates posterolateral compression of the spinal cord resulting from invasion of the left neuroforamen.

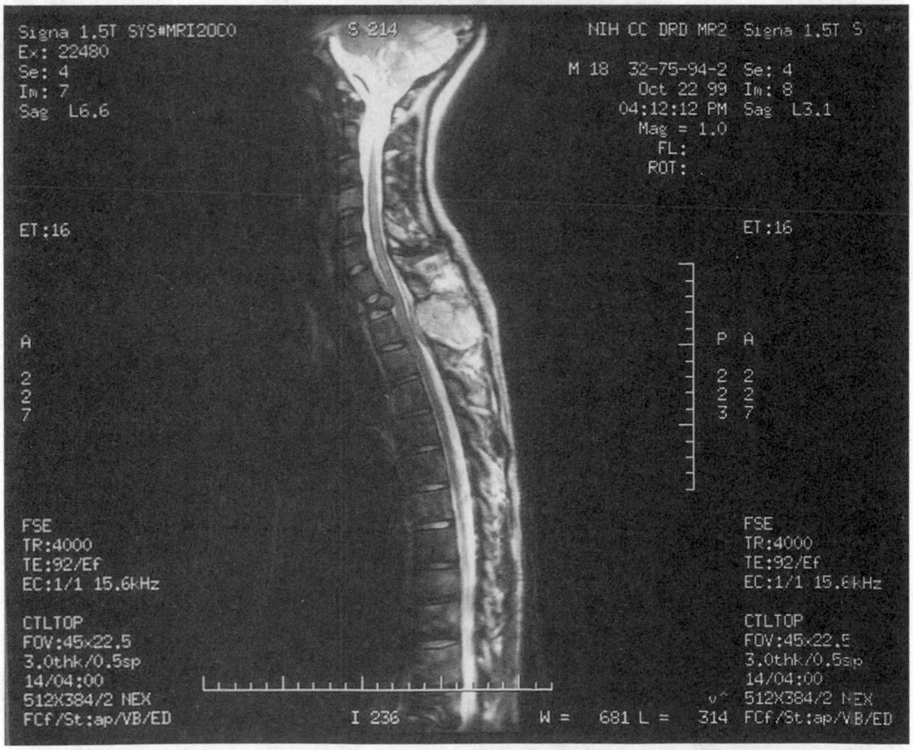

FIGURE 51.2-6. A sagittal magnetic resonance image of the spine demonstrating posterior compression of the spinal cord from a metastasis arising in the spinous process. Laminectomy is the most useful approach for tumors arising posterior to the cord.

small arterioles early in the evolution of spinal cord compression and therefore retards blood flow. In the more advanced stages, pressure on small intramedullary arterioles produced by increasing interstitial edema combined with progressive direct physical pressure on the spinal cord by the expanding mass ultimately leads to arrest of capillary blood flow, resulting in ischemia of white matter. If left untreated, there is infarction of ischemic white matter and permanent neurologic loss.

Siegal and colleagues have evaluated the roles of cytokines, inflammatory mediators, and neurotransmitters in the pathophysiology of cord compression in a series of reports.[45–50] Spinal cord injury from compression was associated with increased water content, increased vascular permeability, and increased specific gravity in the compressed spinal cord as well as increased extravasation of blood cells into the cord parenchyma.[45] Treatment with dexamethasone phosphate was shown to reduce tissue-specific gravity in the compressed cord and to delay the onset of paralysis.[46,47] Similar results were obtained with indomethacin, which also decreased the elevated water content and reduced prostaglandin E_2 (PGE_2) levels in the compressed segments of the spinal cord.[46,47]

Later experiments demonstrated the ability of free dexamethasone to decrease free water content and PGE_2 levels in compressed segments of the spinal cord.[48] The potential role of glutamate in the production of cytotoxic edema was suggested when it was shown that N-methyl-D-aspartate receptor antagonists reduced the spinal cord free water.[49] This group also demonstrated that inhibitors of serotonin synthesis could reduce the elevated serotonin levels associated with spinal cord injury. Serotonin receptor antagonists reduced PGE_2 synthesis, reduced spinal cord vascular permeability, and delayed the onset of paraplegia.[50] These studies form the basis for development of new pharmacologic approaches to the treatment of cord compression.

The role of vascular endothelial growth factor (VEGF) in the pathophysiology of malignant spinal cord compression is being increasingly recognized. In the early stages of malignant spinal cord compression, venous stasis and relative hypoxia stimulate VEGF production.[44] VEGF increases vascular permeability and vasogenic edema in the spinal cord in response to transient ischemia[36] and trauma.[37,38] The progressive hypoxia, resulting from interstitial edema and decreased microcapillary perfusion, continues to drive VEGF production. Several observations suggest that the beneficial effects of dexamethasone are at least in part meditated by its effect on VEGF activity. Dexamethasone down-regulates VEGF gene expression,[39–41] inhibits VEGF activity,[42] and prevents the VEGF-induced cytoskeletal changes associated with vascular permeability (i.e., plasmalemmal ruffling and widening of intracellular spaces) in rat brain endothelial cells.[43] A model of the pathophysiology of malignant spinal cord compression is presented in Figure 51.2-7.

The importance of the magnitude, rate, and duration of compression in regard to the neurologic outcome was studied in dogs with an epidural inflatable balloon by Tarlov et al. Paraparesis resulting from rapid compression of the cord could be reversed if decompression occurred within 9 hours. Paraparesis resulting from more gradual compression over 20 to 48 hours could be successfully reversed by decompression within the next 7 days, emphasizing that neurologic deficits are more likely to be reversed if compression occurs gradually rather than rapidly.[30–32] This has also been observed in humans. Rades et al. reported 96 patients treated with radiotherapy for spinal cord compression who were compared based on the duration of motor symptoms before treatment. Improvement of neurologic function 2 weeks after radiotherapy occurred in a higher percentage (89%) of patient with deficits that developed greater than 14 days before treatment, compared with patients who developed symptoms less than 14 days before treatment (12%). A separate cohort of patients with severe deterioration of motor function occurring within 48 hours before treatment experienced improvement in only 6% of cases.[51]

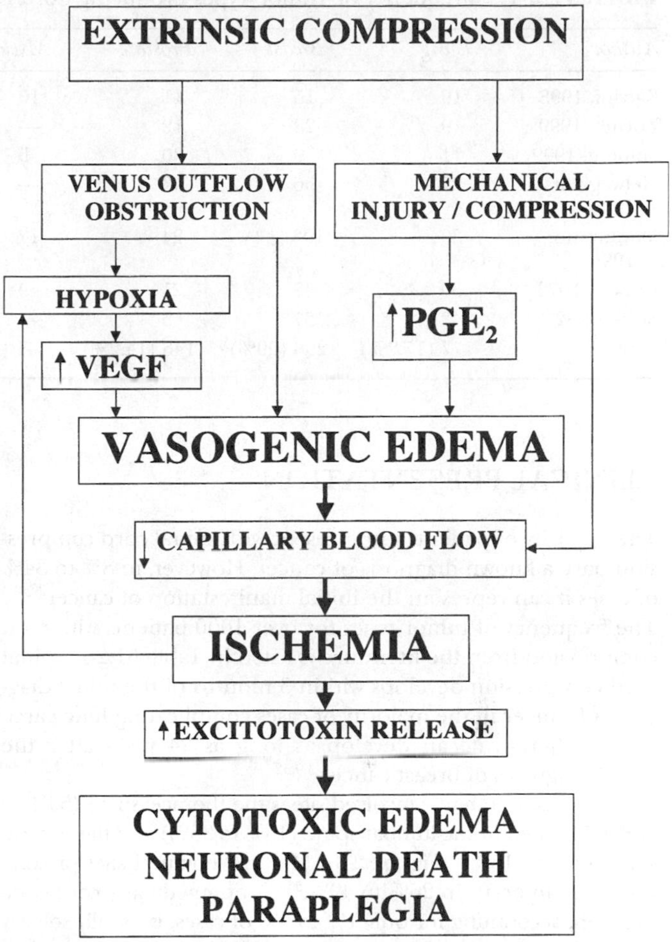

FIGURE 51.2-7. A simplified schematic representation of the pathophysiologic changes leading to neuronal damage from cord compression. Several histologic studies suggest that the initial pathophysiologic changes resulting in vasogenic edema are confined principally to white matter.[27–29] PGE_2, prostaglandin E_2; VEGF, vascular endothelial growth factor.

In summary, spinal cord damage and loss of neurologic function result from venous stasis, spinal cord edema, reduced capillary blood flow, ischemia, and mechanical compression culminating in infarction. Prostaglandins, cytokines, excitatory neurotransmitters, and inflammatory mediators regulate the sweeping pathophysiologic changes associated with hypoxia, edema, ischemia, and injury resulting from malignant compression. The rapidity of progression of neurologic symptoms indicates the severity of spinal cord injury and the likelihood of permanent neurologic loss. Dexamethasone and other antiinflammatory agents can delay the onset of paralysis and improve symptoms until decompressive measures intervene.

TABLE 51.2-1. Frequency of Tumor Types Producing Cord Compression

Author	*Lung*	*Breast*	*Prostate*	*Myeloma*	*Renal*	*Lymphoma*	*Other*	*Sarcoma*	*Total*
Katrini, 1998	19	15	11	10	3	7	33	3	101
Kovner, 1999	9	28	12	—	—	9	21	—	79
Solberg, 1999	11	9	30	5	6		25	—	86
Helweg-Larson, 1996	27	56	43	—	6	—	17	4	153
Maranzano, 1995	38	103	24	17	7	9	45	—	243
Gilbert, 1978	30	48	21	9	17	26	62	22	235
Stark, 1982	43	37	5	—	4	—	42	1	132
Total	177 (17.2%)	296 (29%)	146 (14.2%)	41 (4%)	43 (4.2%)	51 (5%)	245 (23.8%)	30 (2.9%)	1029 (100%)

CLINICAL PRESENTATION

The majority of patients who present with spinal cord compression have a known diagnosis of cancer. However, in 8% to 34% of cases it can represent the initial manifestation of cancer.[52–54] The frequency of tumor types for over 1000 patients with cord compression from the literature is listed in Table 51.2-1. Spinal cord compression develops within 3 months of the initial diagnosis of cancer in the majority of cases complicating lung carcinoma, whereas it can develop as long as 24 years after the initial diagnosis of breast cancer.[3,9,52]

The most frequently involved site is the thoracic spine (59% to 78%), followed by the lumbar spine (16% to 33%) and the cervical spine (4% to 15%) (Fig. 51.2-8). Multiple epidural sites of compression can occur in 26% to 49%.[55–59] Intramedullary cord compression, accounting for only 1% to 4% of cases, is usually solitary and is often associated with parenchymal brain metastases.[18,55,60,146]

Pain accompanies malignant spinal cord compression in 70% to 96% of cases.[7,52,53,61,62] It usually precedes the diagnosis of spinal cord compression by days to months.[52,63] The pain may be local, radicular, or both. Local pain is present in the vast majority of cases and is caused by expansion, destruction, or fracture of the involved vertebral elements. The site of compression can usually be localized to the site of back or neck pain. Local back or neck pain is usually dull, aching, constant, and progressive. Back pain from vertebral destruction resulting in retropulsion of bone fragment is often worse in the supine position, a feature distinguishing cord compression from a herniated disc. Local back or neck pain can be exacerbated by movement, sneezing, straining, or neck flexion. The location of the involved vertebral body can usually be established by gentle spinal percussion. Radicular pain, which is usually, but not always, associated with local back or neck pain, is caused by compression of the nerve roots or cauda equina. Radicular pain is often shooting in quality and localizes to within one to two vertebral segments of the compression. Bilateral band-like girdle pain is characteristic of thoracic cord lesions, and unilateral radicular pain is more characteristic of lumbar or cervical lesions. Radicular pain from a cervical or lumbar lesion may involve the shoulder, hip, groin, perineum, or extremity.

Weakness, the second most common symptom at presentation, is usually what prompts the patient to seek medical intervention. Weakness, which usually follows the development of local or radicular pain, can develop gradually in association with progressive balance disturbance and numbness. Initial unilateral weakness is common when paresis develops gradually. Complete loss of motor and sensory function below the affected level (cord shock) can occur abruptly as vascular insufficiency progresses to frank ischemia. Neurologic examination of the patient with cord shock reveals absent motor, sensory, reflex, and autonomic function below the level of the lesion, and the affected extremities demonstrate flaccidity and absence of tone. Absence of perineal and anal reflexes and painless overflow incontinence complete the neurologic presentation. Flaccidity and areflexia are gradually replaced by paraplegia in flexion. Compression of the upper

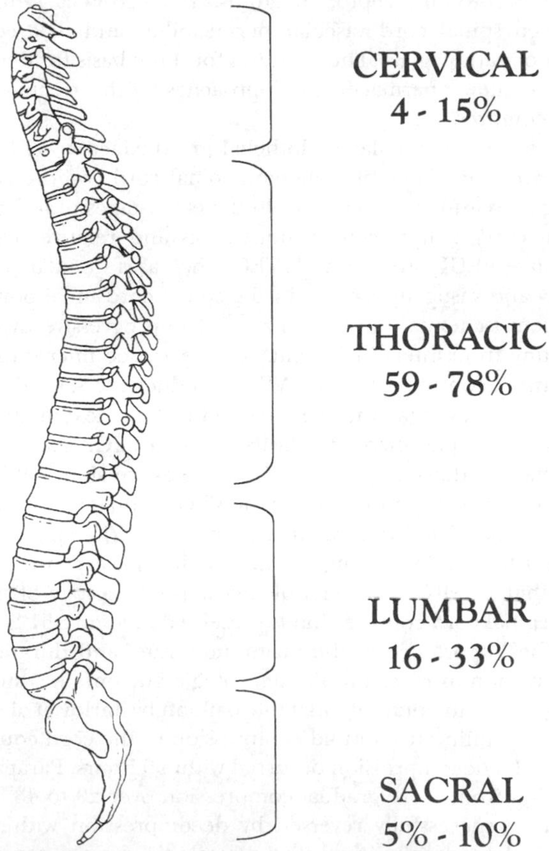

FIGURE 51.2-8. The frequency of involvement in the different regions of the spine is shown.

TABLE 51.2-2. Frequency of Symptoms and Signs Accompanying Cord Compression

Author	*Pain (%)*	*Weakness (%)*	*Sensory Dysfunction (%)*	*Autonomic Dysfunction (%)*	*No. of Patients*
Törmä, 1957	96	86	80	64	250
Gilbert, 1978	96	76	51	57	130
Martenson, 1985	94	85	57	52	77
Helweg, 1996	88	61	78	40	153
Kovner, 1999	70	91	46	44	79

cervical spinal cord can produce paralysis of the upper extremities and respiratory failure, if acute. Chronic injuries of the cervical spine can produce wasting of the intrinsic muscles of the hand, forearm, or arm as well as progressive weakness of the intercostal muscles and diaphragm, leading ultimately to respiratory arrest. Lesions involving the conus medullaris or cauda equina produce flaccid paralysis of the lower extremities, absent or flexor plantar responses, saddle anesthesia, urinary retention leading to incontinence, and male impotence. The frequency of symptoms and signs of cord compression is presented in Table 51.2-2.

DIAGNOSTIC EVALUATION

The diagnostic evaluation of suspected cord compression should include a careful history, physical and neurologic examination, radiologic evaluation including a sagittal magnetic resonance imaging (MRI) survey of the spine, and, if indicated, urgent consultation by physicians in neurology, neurosurgery, radiation oncology, and medical oncology, when compression is caused by a chemosensitive neoplasm. Clear indications of epidural cord compression such as focal weakness, ataxia, and unexplained bowel or bladder dysfunction accompanied by back pain in the cancer patient demand urgent evaluation.

The medical history obtained from the cancer patient suspected of spinal cord compression should emphasize the onset, quality, location, and temporal pattern of back or neck pain. Back pain associated with spinal cord compression may be exacerbated by movement, lying flat, neck flexion, straight leg raising, straining, coughing, or sneezing. Symptoms of motor dysfunction are often described as stiffness or weakness that usually begins in one extremity and remains unilateral in nerve root compression but becomes bilateral with compression of the spinal cord or conus medullaris. Paresthesias due to involvement of the spinothalamic tract begin distally, usually in the foot, and ascend to the level of involvement. Numbness and paresthesias are typically noticed later in the history than motor dysfunction.

Physical examination should emphasize localization of the level of suspected compression. This is often best initialized by asking the patient to point out the site of the back pain. Gentle percussion over the spine can confirm the site of involvement and help elucidate other sites of vertebral metastases. Flexor and extensor motor testing, deep tendon and plantar reflex assessment, sensory level identification via pin prick, and anal sphincter tone assessment are required components of any diagnostic evaluation for cord compression.

There are several radiologic and tumor imaging techniques that are potentially useful in the diagnosis and treatment of cord compression. Plain radiographic films continue to be quite useful in evaluation of cord compression associated with bony involvement of the spine or due to compression fracture. However, they are relatively insensitive for detecting bone involvement and soft tissue masses, and they cannot demonstrate the actual spinal cord itself.

Despite these limitations, plain films can be useful in diagnosing cord compression and in planning therapy. Plain radiographs detect bony abnormalities in 72% of patients with epidural cord compression.[5] Plain film radiographs detect the presence and location of epidural metastases in 83% of patients complaining of back pain. Vertebral body collapse, destruction of the pedicle, and blastic or sclerotic changes are characteristic findings observable with plain film radiography. However, paraspinous masses or vertebral body involvement resulting in less than 50% destruction of the cortex cannot be appreciated with plain film techniques. In addition, in up to 60% of patients with epidural compression by lymphoma and pediatric malignancies, plain films may be normal. Posterior or posterolateral compression resulting from a paraspinous mass invading the vertebral foramen is most common with these tumor types. Computed tomography (CT) and MRI are able to detect posterior or posterolateral cord compression secondary to neuroforamina invasion and are superior to plain films, bone scintigraphy, or myelography in that regard.

Myelography has the advantage over plain films of visualizing the level of the compression as indicated by a blockage of myelographic contrast. However, multiple sites of compression, which may be present in greater than 30% of cases, may require more than one subarachnoid puncture. For these reasons, CT, and to a much greater extent MRI, have emerged as the most useful techniques for imaging cord compression.

Bone scintigraphy is more sensitive than plain films in detecting metastatic involvement and provides information about the entire skeleton in a single examination. This facilitates screening the skeletal system for potential sources of referred pain, and it is useful in planning radiation therapy to multiple sites. However, bone scintigraphy is not as sensitive and specific in detecting spinal metastases as MRI[64–66] and is incapable of describing the soft tissue and spinal cord anatomy required for the proper diagnosis and treatment of cord compression. Furthermore, primarily osteolytic metastases produced by multiple myeloma, lymphoma, and other malignancies may not be detected by bone scan.[67,68]

In the pre-MRI era, myelography and CT were the imaging modalities of choice for the diagnosis of cord compression, and either or both of these tests are mandatory when MRI is not available or is nondiagnostic. When a complete myelographic block is detected following routine lumbar injection, an additional injection from above through a C-1 to C-2 puncture is

TABLE 51.2-3. Patterns of Radiographic Impingement, Compression, or Both

Author	*No. of Patients*	*More Than One Site of Impingement or Compression*	*Impingement or Compression in More Than One Region*	*Cervical Spine Impingement or Compression*
Pigott, 1994	62	13/62 (20%)	N/A	5/62 (8%)
Heldmann, 1996	65	32/65 (49%)	N/A	N/A
Cook, 1998	85	33/85 (39%)	24/85 (28%)	11/85 (13%)
Shiff, 1998	65	26/65 (40%)	68/337 (20%)[a]	33/337 (10%)
Khaw, 1999	100	43/100 (43%)	N/A	11/100 (11%)
Total	337	147/377 (39%)	92/422 (22%)	60/587 (10%)

[a]Estimated based on percentage of cases with imaging of the entire spine.

required to evaluate possible additional sites of compression. CT following metrizamide myelography is an alternative to a C-1 to C-2 puncture in patients with a complete myelographic bloc. However, MRI is superior to both CT and myelography in convenience, anatomic detail, and cost.[69] Yet CT exceeds MRI in the evaluation of vertebral stability and bone destruction. Therefore, CT should be obtained before vertebral body resection or surgical stabilization of the vertebral column.

Positron emission tomography has been used to evaluate metabolic changes in the cervical spinal cord following mechanical spinal cord compression[70,71] and to identify intramedullary spinal cord metastases.[72] Although positron emission tomography is increasingly being studied in the setting of malignant spinal cord compression,[61,72] its current role is not completely defined.

MRI has replaced myelography and CT scanning as the diagnostic procedure of choice for evaluating cord compression.[61,64,73–80] MRI has a sensitivity of 93%, a specificity of 97%, and an overall diagnostic accuracy of 95% in detecting cord compression.[75] It is superior to bone scintigraphy in sensitivity and specificity for spinal metastases[64–66] and can distinguish between benign and metastatic causes of vertebral body collapse with a sensitivity of 97.6%, a specificity of 100%, and an overall accuracy of 98.2%.[75] The advantages of MRI over myelography for evaluating cord compression include its noninvasive ability to image soft tissue anatomy in great detail (tumors, spinal cord) and its ability to image multiple levels of cord impingement in one examination. Paraspinous and neuroforaminal tumors are not as easily identified with myelography as with MRI.[80] In addition, MRI allows avoidance of the 16% to 24% chance of neurologic deterioration following lumbar puncture for myelography.[81] MRI excels in demonstrating intramedullary metastases that can be missed completely by myelography.

The advantages of MRI over CT include its ability to distinguish the spinal cord proper from other soft tissue masses in the spinal canal, and its ability to assess thecal sac impingement in the presence of disrupted cortical bone as is frequently encountered with myeloma and blastic lesions from prostate cancer. MRI is safer, more convenient, better tolerated, more informative, and less expensive than other techniques used to diagnose cord compression. Jordan et al. compared the cost of evaluation of spinal cord compression with and without MRI. Establishing the diagnosis of cord compression was 65% more expensive when MRI was not used.[69]

Because of its diagnostic accuracy and ability to image multiple levels of involvement, MRI is extremely useful in planning local treatment. Identification of paravertebral tumor, neuroforamina invasion, and additional sites of vertebral metastases is important for designing radiotherapy portals and for planning surgical resection. Multiple sites of cord and nerve root impingement or compression are frequent. Myelography detects multiple sites of impingement in approximately 30% of cases, and MRI detects multiple sites in approximately 40% to 50% of cases[55–59] (Table 51.2-3). The frequency of multiple sites of impingement and compression decreases by approximately 50% when imaging is limited to only one spinal region (i.e., thoracic or lumbar).[58] It is therefore imperative that the entire spine be evaluated radiologically. A sagittal T1 nonenhanced survey of the entire spine quickly and easily identifies multiple sites of compression and should guide the acquisition of axial views through areas of involvement. Bone metastases appear as dark botches relative to normal bone marrow in unenhanced T1 images. CSF and edematous tumor appear bright on T2 sequences. T2 sequences display CSF brightly, producing images that are similar to a myelogram. Axial T2 sequences can be useful in identifying small tumor nodules on nerve roots. Focal blastic lesions may produce decreased intensity on T2 images. In most cases of suspected epidural cord compression, MRI can be performed without contrast. However, gadolinium contrast images may complement noncontrast images in demonstrating paravertebral tumor and intramedullary metastases (see Fig. 51.2-3). Visualization of leptomeningeal involvement requires MRI contrast.[82] Myelography with or without CT is mandatory when MRI is nondiagnostic, when it is not available, or in cases of claustrophobia or severe scoliosis.

TREATMENT

The diagnosis of cord compression requires emergent treatment. Delays in initiating treatment have been associated with deterioration in motor and autonomic function.[54] Animal models and clinical results have documented better functional outcome when pretreatment motor loss has been gradual and worse functional outcome when the onset of motor loss has been rapid.[30–32,51]

Rades et al. reported significantly better motor function and ambulation in patients with gradual rather than rapid onset of pretreatment paresis.[51] Despite these differences in expected outcome based on the rate of neurologic progression, there is no justification for delaying therapy once the diagnosis of cord compression has been made. Although untreated epidural cord compression is not fatal, the consequences of paralysis are devastating and loss of ambulation has been associated with shortened survival in a number of reports.[1,2,9,10,83–87]

TABLE 51.2-4. Effect of Motor Function on Treatment Outcome

	Laminectomy and Radiation[88]		*Radiation Alone*[2]	
Pretreatment Condition	No. Ambulatory/ No. Treated	Percentage Ambulatory	No. Ambulatory/ No. Treated	Percentage Ambulatory
Ambulatory	67/68	99	107/109	98
Paretic	41/50	82	49/82	60
Paraplegic	5/9	55	2/18	11

(Adapted from refs. 2 and 88.)

Treatment of cord compression should be individualized, but started immediately. Ambulatory patients with radiographic evidence of early cord compression and no motor or sensory dysfunction can be treated safely without dexamethasone.[1,8] All other patients should be administered corticosteroids as soon as the diagnosis of cord compression is reached, regardless of whether diagnostic workup is complete. Surgical indications include spinal instability, retropulsion of bone fragments producing compression, previous radiotherapy at the site of compression, and lack of tissue diagnosis in the setting of rapid neurologic deterioration. Patients without an initial diagnosis of cancer can be biopsied using CT or MRI guidance if neurologic dysfunction is absent or is evolving slowly. Radiotherapy should follow surgical resection if the site has not been previously irradiated. All other patients should be considered for primary radiotherapy alone. Chemotherapy can be used as initial therapy for the highly chemosensitive adult or pediatric tumors in patients who are not candidates for surgery or radiation therapy.

The results of treatment of cord compression have improved in recent years as a result of earlier diagnosis with the greater availability of MRI and due to a heightened awareness of cord compression as a potential oncologic emergency.[2,57,58,61,84,88–90] The pretreatment degree of neurologic dysfunction is the strongest predicator of therapeutic outcome. Eighty percent to 100% of patients with minimal or no ambulatory dysfunction retain ambulation posttreatment.[2,4,5,7–10,52,53,83,87,90–93] Paraparesis improves with treatment in 34% to 63% of cases,[2,8,10,88,92] whereas paraplegia improves in up to 10% to 55% of cases.[2,8,9,88,92] The influence of pretreatment motor function is summarized in Table 51.2-4.

Surgical techniques used to resect epidural tumors have become increasingly specialized. Laminectomy, the classic surgical approach for the treatment of cord compression is primarily reserved for resection of posterior or posterolateral tumors, despite the favorable results reported by Landmann et al.[88] When used for treatment of anterior epidural compression, the goal of laminectomy is to relieve pressure on the spinal cord via removal of the spinous processes and laminae from one vertebra above to one vertebra below the level of compression. While this approach does not readily allow debulking of tumor anterior to the spinal cord, it does allow relaxation of the spinal cord away from the impinging mass. However, the results of a laminectomy for tumors anterior to the spinal cord have been disappointing.[7,14,94,95] This is in part due to the inability to resect tumor anterior to the spinal cord, but more importantly due to the decreased spinal instability that can develop when posterior supporting elements are removed from an often eroded or collapsed vertebral body.

The development of alternatives to laminectomy, including techniques for anterior decompression[34,96–98] and newer techniques such as endoscopically assisted anterior decompression,[99] coupled with the limitations of laminectomy, have resulted in laminectomy being no longer regarded as the standard neurosurgical procedure for treatment of anterior epidural cord compression. As a general principle, the location of involvement within the vertebral column should determine the neurosurgical approach. Anterior decompression with spinal stabilization should be considered for tumors in the vertebral body producing anterior epidural compression, and laminectomy should be used for the minority of cases in which tumor involves the posterior vertebral elements or invades the neuroforamina.

Recommendations regarding the use of surgery or radiotherapy alone or in combination should be individualized. Despite the common occurrences of cord compression, there have been no randomized trials containing more than 30 patients in each arm.[5–7] Thus, the guidelines for treatment of cord compression are largely empiric. Appropriate treatment recommendation can only be made after assessing the patient's expected survival; the location, number, and mechanism of spinal cord compression(s); the tumor histology; the rapidity of neurologic progression; and any history of previous radiotherapy administered to the site under current consideration.

CORTICOSTEROIDS

Corticosteroids (dexamethasone, methylprednisolone) are among the most effective treatments of neurologic dysfunction resulting from cord compression. Dexamethasone reduces edema, inhibits PGE_2 synthesis, and decreases the specific gravity of the compressed spinal cord.[48] It also was shown to delay the onset of paraplegia in experimental cord compression.[45,48] Although the mechanisms of dexamethasone action are not completely understood, dexamethasone has been shown to down-regulate VEGF expression in smooth muscle cells[100,101] and to prevent cytoskeletal changes associated with increased vascular permeability.[43] Despite the established role of dexamethasone in treatment of cord compression, the optimal dose and schedule have never been proven.[8]

There have been several prospective evaluations of dexamethasone in the treatment of cord compression, yet the superiority of high- versus low-dose dexamethasone has never been proven. Greenberg et al. reported the results of a prospective trial of high-dose dexamethasone and radiation for epidural cord compression. Eighty-three patients with epidural cord compression received 100 mg of intravenous dexamethasone at the time of diagnosis, followed by 96 mg for 3 days, and a subsequent taper of dexamethasone dose during the course of radiotherapy. Fifty-seven percent of patients were ambulatory following treatment. This result was no better than those previously reported for lower dose corticosteroid regimens. However, 64% of patients reported substantial pain reduction the first day of therapy.[4] Sørensen et al. conducted a prospective randomized trial of high-dose dexamethasone versus no corticosteroid therapy. In 57 patients treated with radiation for cord compression, 81% of the dexamethasone group and 65% of the radiation alone group were ambulatory at 3 months.[5] A prospective randomized study comparing a single high dose of intravenous dexamethasone (100 mg) with conventional dose intravenous dexamethasone (10 mg), both followed by 4 mg orally every 6 hours, demonstrated no significant benefit for the initial high-dose bolus.[6] While a prolonged administration of high-dose corticosteroids may have been a more worthy trial regimen, serious toxicities from high-dose dexamethasone have been reported in up to 14% of patients.[4,5,102]

Thus, the results of clinical trials support a role for corticosteroids in the treatment of cord compression, but they have not indicated an advantage for higher versus lower doses. Currently, there is no clear benefit, other than pain relief, from the routine use of high-dose corticosteroids in patients who can otherwise be treated with conventional doses. We recommend an initial 10-mg dose of intravenous dexamethasone. The dose can be increased incrementally if no improvement is detected in the first 4 to 8 hours. After 2 days on a stable dose of intravenous dexamethasone, therapy can be switched to 4 to 8 mg of oral dexamethasone given every 6 hours. Corticosteroid doses are tapered every 4 days in a manner described by Byrne.[103] If neurologic decline results from dose reduction, the dose is maintained at effective levels until dose reduction is possible. Patients without neurologic dysfunction other than back or neck pain should be managed without corticosteroids whenever possible. Maranzano demonstrated that the use of steroids can be safely avoided in selected patients with no evidence of neurologic dysfunction, or with radiculopathy only. Twenty patients were reviewed who had tumors invading less than 50% of the *spinal cord diameter* and involving not more than two vertebral levels, or greater than two vertebral levels in patients with radiculopathy. All patients received 30 Gy in ten fractions. The results were equivalent or superior to those achieved with the use of dexamethasone.[2,4] Sixteen patients were ambulatory before treatment, and all 20 patients were ambulatory posttreatment. Palliation of pain was achieved in 85% of patients.[1]

SURGERY

Although radiation therapy is currently the treatment of choice for most spinal metastases, radioresistant and recurrent neoplasms remain therapeutic dilemmas.[34] Accepted indications for surgery are (1) unknown diagnosis, (2) spinal instability or compression by bone, (3) failure to respond to radiotherapy, and (4) maximal allowable radiation dose already administered to the spinal cord.[14] Patients who may require surgery should also have chest radiography, electrocardiography, and blood tests, including complete blood count, electrolytes, glucose, creatinine, blood urea nitrogen, hepatic enzymes, prothrombin and partial thromboplastin times, platelet count, and type and crossmatch.

When the diagnosis is in doubt and open surgery is not indicated, fluoroscopic or CT-guided percutaneous vertebral biopsy may diagnose metastatic carcinoma with less incisional pain and a shorter recuperative period than open surgery.[104,105] A paraspinal or a transpedicular approach can be used to place the needle, depending on the position and size of the tumor. CT guidance facilitates precise needle placement and avoidance of neurologic injury. Local anesthesia and mild sedation allow neurologic monitoring during the procedure, which can be performed in less than 1 hour.

Surgical decompression of the spinal cord should be approached from the side of the impinging mass.[106] Since typically the site of metastatic tumor involvement is the vertebral body rather than the neural arch, tumor or pathologic fracture usually compresses the anterior surface of the spinal cord. Anterior tumors are not exposed by laminectomy, which has little therapeutic benefit and causes spinal instability in such cases.[35] Findlay noted that 51% of patients with cord compression had vertebral collapse, defined as over 50% loss of vertebral height, and that 25% of patients treated with laminectomy sustained major neurologic deterioration related to their surgery.[94,95] In keeping with the premise that decompression should occur from the side of the spinal cord compression, laminectomy should be reserved for the removal of posterior lesions.

Anterior decompression with mechanical stabilization has supplanted laminectomy as the principal surgical treatment for epidural metastases arising from the vertebral body. This approach allows total removal of the pathologic vertebral body via thoracotomy or a retroperitoneal approach.[29] The vertebral body is replaced with methylmethacrylate, which is supplemented with a metal prosthesis that attaches to the adjacent vertebral bodies.[29,107] Moore and Uttley reported their results with anterior decompression and stabilization in 26 patients with anterior vertebral collapse who suffered from spinal cord compression or intractable pain.[108] Of 16 patients who were unable to walk preoperatively, 10 were ambulatory after surgery, 3 were not, and 3 died. Of seven patients who were operated on for intractable pain, five were pain free and two died. Morbidity included wound infection, CSF discharge, and the need for posterior stabilization later. During the period of the study (1982 to 1987) 20 additional patients were considered unsuitable for surgery because of "multiple levels of disease, complete paraplegia, or a parlous general condition."[109] Even though anterior spinal decompression and fusion is more effective than laminectomy, its effectiveness appears to be limited to patients in good medical condition who have myelopathy from anteriorly placed tumors. In addition, metastatic disease must be focal since spinal stabilization devices require a foundation of solid, rather than tumor-infiltrated, bone at adjacent spinal levels. Surgical decompression entails considerable mortality, morbidity, and convalescence, even in selected patients. To reduce operative blood loss, intravascular[109] or intravertebral[110] embolization of the vasculature of vertebral metastases may be performed preoperatively.

The indiscriminate use of laminectomy in candidates for radiation has been challenged. While some reports have suggested a more favorable outcome with combined laminectomy and radiation, selection bias prevents the assessment of differences in outcome in those studies.[5,12,88] Indeed, several retrospective studies and one small prospective study failed to demonstrate significant differences in outcome for radiation alone as compared with laminectomy and radiation.[2,7,52,53,85]

In a retrospective study from Memorial Sloan-Kettering Cancer Center, Gilbert et al. found no advantage for the addition of laminectomy to radiation in the treatment of cord compression.[52] Two hundred thirty-five patients with greater than 80% extradural block on myelography were reviewed. Sixty-five underwent surgical decompression followed by radiation, and 170 were treated with radiation alone. Patients with lymphoma or paraplegia usually received radiotherapy alone. Those with uncertain diagnosis, prior radiotherapy, or rapid progression of symptoms underwent surgery. Of the 235 patients, 34% were ambulatory, 41% paraparetic, and 17% paraplegic. Forty-six percent of the laminectomy group were ambulatory after treatment, as compared with 49% in the radiation alone group. Tumors considered radiosensitive (lymphoma, seminoma, myeloma, and neuroblastoma) responded better to either treatment than tumors not considered radiosensitive (carcinoma, sarcoma, melanoma). Patients with rapid development of weakness (over 48 hours) responded more frequently to radiation (7 of 13) compared with those treated with laminectomy (0 of 9; $P < .002$). The duration of neurologic improvement was greater for patients with radiosensitive tumors; however, the duration of improvement was similar for laminectomy and for radiation alone. Fifty eight percent of patients who were ambulatory before treatment remained so after treatment.[52] Although superior results have been reported in more contemporary series, others have also reported that laminectomy adds little to the efficacy of radiotherapy.[2,7,53,85,111]

A small prospective study of laminectomy plus radiotherapy was reported by Young et al.[7] Twenty-nine patients were randomized to laminectomy plus radiation (16 patients) or radiation alone (13 patients). One-half (three of six) of the surgically treated patients who were ambulatory before treatment remained so after treatment, whereas all (five of five) retained ambulation following radiotherapy. Forty-four percent of nonambulatory patients were ambulatory after laminectomy, as compared with 33% after radiation. By 4 months the rate of ambulation for patients in both groups was 33%. Sphincter function and pain relief were likewise similar in each treatment group. There were no significant differences in outcome.[7] Although this series has been criticized for its small numbers, it is the only prospective randomized trial comparing laminectomy and radiation with radiation alone. The results, which suggest that laminectomy does not contribute to the efficacy of radiotherapy, are corroborated by several retrospective analyses.[2,52,53]

In contrast to the experience in adults, laminectomy in children with spinal cord compression often improves neurologic outcome over radiation, radiation and chemotherapy, or chemotherapy alone.[22,24] Because pediatric sarcomas are often located in a posterolateral location in the epidural space, they are amenable to removal via laminectomy, which relieves spinal cord compression more rapidly than chemotherapy and radiotherapy and prevents permanent spinal cord injury from developing.

RADIATION THERAPY

Radiation plays a central role in the treatment of newly diagnosed epidural cord compression. The goals of treatment are decompression of the spinal cord and nerve roots through cytoreduction of tumor, prevention of progressive neurologic symptoms, relief of pain, prevention of further structural damage to the vertebral column, and the establishment of durable local control. Radiation reduces pain in approximately 70% of patients, improves motor function in 45% to 60%, and reverses paraplegia in up to 11% to 21%.[2,52,83,89] While most patients with previously untreated metastatic cord compression are candidates for emergent radiation, patients with compression from retropulsed bone, those with spinal instability, or those without a clinical or pathologic diagnosis of cancer and a rapidly progressing loss of neurologic function should be considered for surgery. Children, and in certain circumstances adults with highly chemosensitive tumors, should be considered for initial chemotherapy. Immediate surgical decompression should be considered for any patient with neurologic progression during radiotherapy. The results of several radiotherapy series are listed in Table 51.2-5.

TABLE 51.2-5. Results of Radiotherapy for Malignant Spinal Cord Compression

No. of Patients	*Dose per Fraction (cGy)*	*Total Dose (cGy)*	*Pain Palliated (%)*	*Ambulation Preserved (%)*	*Paresis Improved (%)*	*Plegia Improved (%)*	*Ambulatory Pretreatment (%)*	*Ambulatory Posttreatment (%)*	*Reference*
170	400 × 3 then 200 × 10–14	2000–4000	—	79	45	3	43	49	Gilbert, 1978
83	500 × 3 then 300 × 5	3000	82	89	35	0	46	57	Greenberg, 1980
66	300 (median)	3000 (median)	—	100	25	0	53	62	Martenson, 1985
59	300 × 10; 400 × 3–5[a]	2000–4000	—	100	35	7	22	42	Kim, 1990
70	400–500; 300 × 10[a]	3000–4500	—	66	30	16	34	39	Leviov, 1993
209	500 × 3 then 300 × 5; 300 × 10[a]	3000	82	98	60	11	52	76	Maranzano, 1995
153	400 × 7	2800	83	97	39	21	52	58	Helweg-Larsen, 1996
20	300 × 10	3000	85	100	100	—	80	100	Maranzano, 1996
49	800 × 2	1600	67	91	50	0	47	63	Maranzano, 1997
79	500 × 3 then 300 × 5	3000	60–62	90	50	20	29	51	Kovner, 1999

[a]The semicolon indicates that more than one fractionation scheme was used.

There has been and continues to be interest in hypofractionated regimens for palliation of cord compression. A seminal experience in this regard was reported by Greenberg et al.,[4] who treated patients with hypofractionated radiotherapy and initial high-dose dexamethasone. Patients received 100 mg of intravenous dexamethasone and 500 cGy per fraction daily for the first 3 days of treatment. Following a 4-day rest, radiation was continued in 300-cGy fractions to a total dose of 3000 cGy. Fifty-seven percent of patients were ambulatory after treatment. No patients with total paraplegia regained ambulation. Ambulation was preserved in 62% of patients with radiosensitive tumors and 55% of those with less radiosensitive tumors. Patients with renal and prostate tumors had the highest rate of ambulation following treatment, and patients with lung cancer had the least favorable outcome. Although these results are no better than those reported for conventional regimens, the achievement of pain relief in 64% of patients after the first day of treatment was impressive.[4]

Maranzano et al. have addressed several issues regarding the radiotherapy of cord compression including hypofractionation in a series of reports from 1989 to 2000. A prospective study of radiotherapy and corticosteroids without surgical resection was reported in 1995.[2] Of the 209 evaluable patients, 52% had minimal or no neurologic impairment, 39% were paraparetic and unable to walk, and 9% were paraplegic at presentation. Ambulation was maintained in 94% of those with minimal or no neurologic impairment. Treatment consisted of 3000 cGy in ten fractions (used primarily for radioresponsive tumors, i.e., seminoma, lymphoma, myeloma) or the fractionation scheme of Greenberg et al. (500 cGy × 3, 4-day rest, 300 cGy × 5). High-dose intravenous corticosteroid (1 g of methylprednisolone) was used for paraparetic or paraplegic patients, and standard-dose dexamethasone (16 mg/d) was used in all other patients. Sixty percent of paraparetic, nonambulant patients regained their ability to walk. Only 11% of paraplegic patients became ambulatory. Overall, 76% of patients were ambulant after treatment. Sphincter dysfunction improved in 44% of patients. Those with favorable histologies (breast, prostate, lymphoma, myeloma, seminoma, small cell carcinoma) more frequently enjoyed restoration of gait and recovery of bladder function. The median survival for the group was 6 months, and 28% were alive at 1 year. Ambulation before treatment was associated with a median survival of 8 months, versus 4 months for those nonambulant before treatment ($P = .02$). Ambulation after treatment was associated with a median survival of 9 months versus 1 month for nonambulant patients after treatment ($P < .01$). Survival for favorable tumor types was 10 months versus 3 months for unfavorable histologies ($P < .01$). Clearly, early diagnosis of cord compression was the factor that most significantly influenced the outcome in this study. Tumor histology had the greatest influence on outcome in patients with loss of ambulation, bladder dysfunction, or paraplegia. This study also demonstrated that the results of radiotherapy plus corticosteroids compared favorably with the results of laminectomy.[2]

In a subsequent report, Maranzano et al. demonstrated that corticosteroids could be omitted from the treatment of cord compression in selected patients. Twenty patients with cord compression and no neurologic dysfunction, or dysfunction limited to radiculopathy, were evaluated. This group included patients with intact motor and sensory function and tumors involving less than 50% of the spinal cord diameter or fewer than two vertebrae longitudinally. Patients with radiculopathy or greater than two vertebral levels involved were included. Six patients presented with radiculopathy, and 14 patients presented with cord impingement. Radiotherapy consisted of 3000 cGy in ten fractions. Back pain responded in 85% of cases. All patients were ambulatory without support following treatment, including four patients who had required support for ambulation before therapy. These excellent results suggest that routine administration of corticosteroids in patients with asymptomatic early cord compression is not necessary.[1]

More recently, the same authors explored the use of hypofractionated regimens for treatment of cord compression. Fifty-three patients with radiographic evidence of cord compression and unfavorable histology with or without neurologic defects, or patients with favorable histology (breast, prostate, myeloma, lymphoma) who presented with plegias, paresis, or low performance status (Eastern Cooperative Oncology Group performance score of less than or equal to 2) and short life expectancy were treated with a single 800-cGy fraction generally delivered via a posterior port. This treatment was repeated after 1 week in responding or stable patients. Of 49 evaluable patients, 4 also received laminectomy, and 4 patients did not receive the second fraction due to systemic disease progression. Pain relief was achieved in 67% of patients, motor function remained intact or improved in 63%. None of the paraplegic patients regained ambulation. The authors claimed that the results were not substantially different from previously published results in similar patients.[2] However, the results were numerically inferior to those achieved with 3000 cGy in ten fractions.[86]

In another publication from this group, two hypofractionated regimens were compared in patients with cord compression from prostate cancer. There was no difference in palliation of pain, neurologic outcome, or survival based on the treatment regimen.[87] These studies have demonstrated that hypofractionated regimens, despite producing more acute toxicity, are reasonably well tolerated and relatively effective. However, split courses and large fraction sizes are fundamentally radiobiologically unfavorable due to the likely presence of tumor hypoxia and the proliferation of tumor during splits in treatment.[125] These considerations combined with the lack of radiographic response data to evaluate the success of these regimens, and the complete absence of data describing late toxicities, prevents the routine recommendation of these schedules. The 800 cGy × 2 regimen may be appropriate for the bedridden paraplegic hospice patient requiring palliation of back pain caused by a cord compression.

In a report from Hanover, Germany, 96 patients with motoric deficits were divided into two subgroups based on the duration of development of motoric deficits: 1 to 13 days (49 patients), group A; and greater than or equal to 14 days (47 patients), group B. The two groups were comparable in pretreatment ambulatory function (33% and 32%, respectively). At 2 weeks and 3 months, more patients were ambulatory in group B (77% and 81%) than in group A (31% and 30%). A separate group of patients (31) with rapid loss of motor function within 48 hours of presentation was evaluated. At 2 weeks and 3 months, only 13% and 15% of patients were ambulatory. In this third group of patients with rapid loss of motor function, 65% had experienced further deterioration by 2 weeks posttreatment.[51] Thus, the success of radiotherapy in reversing paralysis correlates with the rapidity of loss of motor function. Recovery of ambulation occurs more frequently in patients with gradual rather than abrupt loss of ambulation.[51,112] Delays in the recovery of ambulation can last as long as

15 months.[112] These findings are consistent with the results of experimental mechanical cord injury in dogs.[30–32]

The role of corticosteroids during radiotherapy has not been adequately studied. Although corticosteroids are universally prescribed and subsequently tapered during or after radiotherapy, corticosteroids do not appear to be necessary in patients who present with no neurologic dysfunction.[1] Radiation produces no clinically significant spinal cord edema itself,[25] and the benefit of corticosteroids is temporary.[26] Maintaining corticosteroids during radiation is clearly indicated if symptoms progress on withdrawal; however, routine maintenance of corticosteroids throughout the course of radiotherapy is unnecessary. High-dose corticosteroids have no proven greater efficacy than low-dose corticosteroids and remain controversial. High-dose corticosteroid therapy and radiation was significantly superior to radiation alone in one study, but whether similar results could have been achieved with low-dose corticosteroids was not determined.[5] A prospective study of high- versus low-dose corticosteroids revealed no difference in the rate of ambulatory patients after treatment.[6] Despite this, the routine use of high-dose corticosteroids has been advocated by some investigators.[4,8,103,113]

An analysis of prognostic factors in 153 patients treated with radiotherapy and/or laminectomy for cord compression was reported by Helweg-Larsen et al. As has been shown repeatedly in numerous studies, ambulation pretreatment predicted ambulation posttreatment. Tumor type was shown to influence the interval from initial diagnosis to development of cord compression. Shorter intervals were observed in patients with lung cancer, and the longest intervals were observed in patients with breast cancer ($P < .0005$). Lung cancer patients also had more severe gait dysfunction at diagnosis than did patients with other tumor types ($P = .003$). Likewise, the interval between initial diagnosis of cancer and the development of cord compression was predictive of the severity of gait dysfunction. Shorter intervals were associated with more severe gait disturbance ($P = .016$). Survival posttreatment was dependent on the interval from diagnosis to cord compression, the pretreatment gait function, and most importantly, ambulation posttreatment. The median survival for ambulatory patients posttreatment was 7.9 months compared with 1.2 months for nonambulatory patients posttreatment.[114]

Radiotherapy Technique

The size and configuration of radiotherapy portals should be designed using all relevant data from the history and physical examination, plain films, bone scans, myelograms, CT, and spinal MRI. An MRI with sagittal views of the entire length of the spine should be carefully studied to identify any additional sites of cord compression before completing the radiotherapy treatment plan. Additional sites of epidural compression can be detected in 10% to 50% of patients depending on the imaging modality and the length of spine evaluated (see Table 51.2-3).[55–59,64,73,115,116] Although MRI is superior to CT myelography, either study is capable of defining vertebral and paravertebral involvement, and either is adequate for treatment planning.

Radiation portals should be centered on the site of epidural compression. Of the 16% to 25% of patients who develop recurrent cord compression after radiation, 64% of early recurrences (within the first 3 months) are within two vertebral bodies of the site of initial compression.[20] Accordingly, radiation portals customarily extend two vertebral bodies above and two vertebral bodies below the site of compression. Adjacent sites of bony involvement and paravertebral masses should also be encompassed in the treatment port. Lesions in the cervical spine, a common site for myeloma, should be treated with opposed lateral fields to reduce radiation exposure of the pharyngeal mucosa. Thoracic spine lesions are generally treated with a simple posterior field. Although the majority of compressing metastases develop in the posterior aspect of the vertebral body, the radiation dose should be prescribed to a depth corresponding to the anterior aspect of the involved vertebral body. This ensures full-dose delivery to the tumor and adequate treatment of the entire bone. The anterior edge of the affected vertebral body can be determined with a lateral spine simulator film. If this depth equals or exceeds the midplane of the patient, or if beam energies sufficient to prevent greater than a 110% hot spot on the spinal cord are not available, opposed anteroposterior fields should be used. Ad hoc prescription of a depth for posterior fields without measurement of the prescription depth should be discouraged. The lumbar spine is usually treated with opposed anteroposterior fields, since the lumbar vertebrae are generally at midplane.

An important goal of radiotherapy for epidural compression is to deliver an effective palliative dose of radiation expeditiously without exceeding the spinal cord tolerance. To this end, an optimal dose and fractionation scheme has not been established. Radioresponsive tumors, such as neuroblastoma, can be treated with 2000 to 3000 cGy.[117] Epidural cord compression caused by lymphoma more often responds completely when total doses greater than 2500 cGy are employed.[118] Patients with cord compression by malignant melanoma are more likely to respond to total doses greater than 3000 cGy. Complete recovery is more often associated with higher total doses, rather than with the use of large doses per fraction.[119,120]

Initial large daily fractions (400 to 500 cGy) produce more rapid neurologic recovery in animal models with cord compression.[25,113] In contrast, larger doses per fraction provided less durable pain relief from bone metastases[121] and neurologic recovery from cord compression is not superior to that achieved by conventional dose regimens.[4,91,119,122] Nevertheless, some authors continue to recommend delivery of large doses per fraction (400 to 500 cGy) on the first 3 days of treatment to achieve rapid lysis of tumor, followed by smaller doses (200 to 300 cGy) for the remainder of the treatment.[4,9,123] By convention, patients usually receive 200 to 300 cGy per fraction to a total dose not exceeding 3000 to 4000 cGy to the spinal cord in 2 to 4 weeks.[124] The results of several radiotherapy series are summarized in Table 51.2-5.

CHEMOTHERAPY

Neurologic recovery from spinal cord compression in response to chemotherapy has been reported in adults and children.[126–142] In adults, cytotoxic chemotherapy and hormonal therapy have been used to successfully alleviate spinal cord compression from prostate cancer,[130,135,138,139] Hodgkin's disease,[133,140] myeloma,[127,141] germ cell tumors,[131,137] lymphoma,[128,136,141] and breast cancer.[129] The use of chemotherapy combined with radiation was associated with a prolonged survival in patients presenting with epidural cord compression from non-Hodgkin's lymphoma.[142] These studies suggest that in certain cases, chemotherapy should be considered more frequently than is currently accepted. Chemotherapy can be used in combination with radiotherapy for treatment of spinal cord compression,[141] or alone in adults who are not surgical or radiation candidates, but who have chemosensitive tumors such as lymphoma, small cell carcinoma, myeloma, breast, prostate, or germ cell tumors.[127–142]

PEDIATRIC SPINAL CORD COMPRESSION

Malignant spinal cord compression in children differs from that in adults in several respects including the tumor types that most frequently produce compression, the mechanisms of impingement, and most importantly the approach to treatment. Unlike in adults, motor weakness can be as frequent a symptom as local pain, being present in 82% to 100% of cases.[24,117,143] Neuroblastoma, Ewing's sarcoma, Wilms' tumor, lymphoma, and soft tissue and bone sarcomas are the most frequent tumor types producing compression in children,[22–24] yet they are infrequently encountered in adults (see Table 51.2-1). The majority of tumors causing cord compression in children do so via neuroforaminal invasion producing the so-called dumbbell tumors.[22,24,144,145] Unlike treatment of adult malignant spinal cord compression, there is a greater emphasis on the use of chemotherapy in pediatric patients. This is due to the greater chemosensitivity of most pediatric cancers and the profound interest in avoiding iatrogenic spinal deformities and second cancers in children, which can result from radiotherapy.

The most impressive results of pediatric cord compression treatment with chemotherapy were reported by Hayes et al. Fourteen patients with spinal cord compression from neuroblastoma or Ewing's sarcoma received combination chemotherapy alone. All patients with neurologic signs or symptoms (10 of 14) experienced complete or near complete recovery following chemotherapy.[126] Sanderson et al. had similar results. Four of four patients presenting with paraparesis or paraplegias from cord compression by neuroblastoma had complete neurologic recovery following treatment with chemotherapy alone.[134]

When chemotherapy is used for treatment of spinal cord compression, the response to treatment should be monitored closely by a multidisciplinary team including a neurosurgeon, pediatric oncologist, radiation oncologist, and neuroradiologist so that alternate interventions can be instituted quickly to alleviate neurologic progression.

Klein et al. reviewed 112 cases of pediatric cord compression from St. Jude Children's Hospital. Patients with soft tissue sarcomas treated with laminectomy as a component of their overall treatment had statistically superior ambulation following treatment compared with those who received chemotherapy or radiation alone.[22] Raffel et al. studied children with severe cord compression as evidenced by greater than 50% replacement of the spinal canal by tumor on MRI or CT.[24] Twenty-five of 26 children treated with laminectomy improved compared with four of seven treated nonsurgically. Since posterior cord compression resulting from vertebral foramen invasion occurs in a larger percentage of pediatric cases, laminectomy may be of greater benefit than in adults.

However, in a retrospective analysis of pediatric neuroblastoma with cord compression, there was no significant difference based on whether or not laminectomy was used. There were, however, numerically more ambulatory patients following surgical treatment.[145] Thus, pediatric patients with soft tissue or bone sarcomas and severe neurologic dysfunction from compression should be considered for osteoplastic laminotomy or laminectomy followed by adjuvant chemotherapy or radiation. In other circumstances, treatment with initial chemotherapy alone may be appropriate.

TABLE 51.2-6. Recommendations for Management of Patients with Metastatic Cord Compression[a]

RADIATION THERAPY ONLY
Known radiosensitive tumor with no spinal instability or bony compression of the spinal cord (with or without a rapidly progressing neurologic deficit)
Spinal involvement without a rapidly progressing neurologic deficit, spinal instability, or bony compression of the spinal cord (regardless of radiosensitivity)
SURGERY FOLLOWED BY RADIATION
Pathologic fracture with spinal instability or compression of the spinal cord by bone
Unradioresponsive tumor with rapidly progressive neurologic deficit
Unknown tissue diagnosis (if radiosensitive tumor is suspected, needle biopsy can provide the diagnosis)
SURGERY ONLY[b]
Initial or recurrent cord compression in a previously radiated site
Failure to respond to radiation
CHEMOTHERAPY
Pediatric patients with chemoresponsive tumors
Adjuvant treatment in adults with chemosensitive tumors
Initial or recurrent cord compression by a chemosensitive tumor in a site of previous radiation or surgery
PEDIATRIC CORD COMPRESSION
Chemotherapy as primary treatment for chemoresponsive tumors
Laminectomy for sarcomas, severe compression, or progressive symptoms during treatment
Radiotherapy in patients with radioresponsive tumors that have failed chemotherapy
Radiotherapy or chemotherapy as adjuvant to laminectomy

[a]Corticosteroids should be used in the early phases of therapy in all cases with neurologic dysfunction.
[b]The surgical approach should be determined by the tumor site (anterior vs. posterior).

CONCLUSION

Paraplegia from epidural cord compression is preventable if diagnosis and treatment are instituted before severe neurologic deficits develop. A heightened awareness of the significance of new or progressive back pain is the most important factor in the successful treatment of cord compression. Plain films, myelography, MRI, or CT should be obtained when the history and neurologic examination suggest spinal involvement with tumor or cord compression. Corticosteroids should be administered in symptomatic patients when the diagnosis has been established, and oncology, neurology, neurosurgery, and radiation oncology consultants should provide urgent evaluations.

Fortunately, management recommendations can be made despite the lack of definitive randomized trials evaluating contemporary treatments. Treatment recommendations are outlined in Table 51.2-6. Radiotherapy is indicated in all patients with minimal or no neurologic deficits. Radiation should also be administered following surgery in patients who have not previously received radiation. Spinal instability, compression from bone fragments, previous radiotherapy, and neurologic progression during radiotherapy are indications for surgery in appropriate candidates. Surgery should be considered in patients with a life expectancy of greater than 2 months. The surgical approach should be determined by the location of vertebral involvement and direction of compression.

Chemotherapy should be the initial treatment for children with chemosensitive tumors. Patients treated with chemotherapy should be monitored closely so that immediate intervention can proceed if there is an inadequate response or neurologic progression. Children with severe neurologic deficits from cord compression should be considered for primary laminectomy. Adults with chemotherapy-sensitive or hormone-sensitive tumors should receive chemotherapy as an adjuvant or as the primary treatment if radiation or surgery are contraindicated. Corticosteroid therapy remains one of the most effective treatments for acute spinal cord compression.

REFERENCES

1. Maranzano E, Latini P, Beneventi S, et al. Radiotherapy without steroids in selected metastatic spinal cord compression patients. A phase II trial. *Am J Clin Oncol* 1996;19:179.
2. Maranzano E, Latini P. Effectiveness of radiation therapy without surgery in metastatic spinal cord compression: final results from a prospective trial. *Int J Radiat Oncol Biol Phys* 1995;15:959.
3. Helweg-Larsen S. Clinical outcome in metastatic spinal cord compression. A prospective study of 153 patients. *Acta Neurol Scand* 1996;94:269.
4. Greenberg HS, Kim JH, Posner JB. Epidural spinal cord compression from metastatic tumor: results with a new treatment protocol. *Ann Neurol* 1980;8:361.
5. Sorenson S, Helweg-Larsen S, Mouridsen H, Hansen HH. Effect of high-dose dexamethasone in carcinomatous metastatic spinal cord compression treated with radiotherapy: a randomised trial. *Eur J Cancer* 1994;30A:22.
6. Vecht CJ, Haaxima-Reiche H, Van Putten WLT, et al. Initial bolus of conventional versus high dose dexamethasone in metastatic spinal cord compression. *Neurology* 1989;39:1255.
7. Young RF, Post EM, King GA. Treatment of spinal epidural metastases. Randomized prospective comparison of laminectomy and radiotherapy. *J Neurosurg* 1980;53:741.
8. Loblaw DA, Laperriere NJ. Emergency treatment of malignant extradural spinal cord compression: an evidence-based guideline. *J Clin Oncol* 1998;16:1613.
9. Kovner F, Spigel S, Rider I, et al. Radiation therapy of metastatic spinal cord compression. Multidisciplinary team diagnosis and treatment. *J Neurooncol* 1999;42:85.
10. Solberg A, Bremnes RM. Metastatic spinal cord compression: diagnostic delay, treatment, and outcome. *Anticancer Res* 1999;19:677.
11. Barron KD, Hirano A, Araki S, Terry RD. Experiences with metastatic neoplasms involving the spinal cord. *Neurology* 1959;9:91.
12. Bach F, Agerlin N, Sorensen JB, et al. Metastatic spinal cord compression secondary to lung cancer. *J Clin Oncol* 1992;10:1781.
13. Boogerd W, van der Sande JJ. Treatment of complications: diagnosis and treatment of spinal cord compression in malignant disease. *Cancer Treat Rep* 1993;19;129.
14. Black P. Spinal epidural tumors. In Wilkins RH, Rengachary SS, eds. *Neurosurgery*. New York: McGraw-Hill, 1985:1062.
15. Walsh GL, Gokaslan ZL, McCutcheon IE, et al. Anterior approaches to the thoracic spine in patients with cancer: indications and results. *Ann Thorac Surg* 1997;64:1611.
16. Grant R, Papadopoulos SM, Sandler HM, Greenberg HS. Metastatic epidural spinal cord compression: current concepts and treatment. *J Neurooncol* 1994;19:79.
17. Posner JB. Management of central nervous system metastases. *Semin Oncol* 1977;4:81.
18. Grosh W, Greco FA. Spinal cord compression: comparison of extradural and intramedullary metastases. *J Tenn Med Assoc* 1981;74:821.
19. Helweg-Larsen S, Hansen SW, Sorensen PS. Second occurrence of symptomatic metastatic spinal cord compression and findings of multiple spinal epidural metastases. *Int J Radiat Oncol Biol Phys* 1995;33:595.
20. Kaminski HJ, Diwan VG, Ruff RL. Second occurrence of spinal epidural metastases. *Neurology* 1991;41:744.
21. Lewis DW, Packer RJ, Raney B, et al. Incidence, presentation and outcome of spinal cord disease in children with systemic cancer. *Pediatrics* 1986;78:438.
22. Klein SL, Sanford RA, Muhlbauer MS. Pediatric spinal epidural metastases. *J Neurosurg* 1991;74:70.
23. Bouffet E, Marec-Berard P, Thiesse P, et al. Spinal cord compression by secondary epi- and intradural metastases in childhood. *Childs Nerv Syst* 1997;13:383.
24. Raffel C, Neave VCD, Lavine S, McComb JG. Treatment of spinal cord compression by epidural malignancy in childhood. *Neurosurgery* 1991;28:349.
25. Rubin P. Extradural spinal cord compression by tumor. Part I: experimental production and treatment trials. *Radiology* 1993;263:1243.
26. Ushio Y, Posner R, Posner JB, Shapiro WR. Experimental spinal cord compression by epidural neoplasms. *Neurology* 1977;27:422.
27. Ikeda H, Ushio Y, Hayakawa T, Mogami H. Edema and circulatory disturbance in the spinal cord compressed by epidural neoplasms in rabbits. *J Neurosurg* 1980;52:203.
28. Kato A, Ushio Y, Hayakawa T, et al. Circulatory disturbance of the spinal cord with epidural neoplasm in rats. *J Neurosurg* 1985;63:260.
29. Arbit E, Galicich JH. Vertebral body reconstruction with a modified Harrington rod distraction system for stabilization of the spine affected with metastatic disease. *J Neurosurg* 1995;83:617.
30. Tarlov IM, Klinger H, Vitale S. Spinal cord compression studies. I Experimental techniques to produce acute and gradual compression. *Arch Neurol Psychiatry* 1957;70:813.
31. Tarlov IM, Klinger H. Spinal cord compression studies. II. Time limits for recovery after acute compression in dogs. *Arch Neurol Psychiatry* 1954;71:271.
32. Tarlov IM. Spinal cord compression studies. III. Time limits for recovery after gradual compression in dogs. *Arch Neurol Psychiatry* 1954;71:588.
33. Doppman JL, Girton M. Angiographic study of the effect of laminectomy in the presence of acute anterior epidural masses. *J Neurosurg* 1976;45:19.
34. Siegal T, Siegal T. Current considerations in the management of neoplastic spinal cord compression. *Spine* 1989;14:223.
35. Kakulas BA, Harper CG, Shibasaki K, Bedbrook GM. Vertebral metastases and spinal cord compression. *Clin Exp Neurol* 1978;15:98.
36. Hayashi T, Sakurai M, Abe K, et al. Expression of angiogenic factors in rabbit spinal cord after transient ischaemia. *Neuropathol Appl Neurobiol* 1999;25:63.
37. Vaquero J, Zurita M, de Oya S, Coca S. Vascular endothelial growth/permeability factor in spinal cord injury. *J Neurosurg* 1999;90(Suppl 4):220.
38. Bartholdi D, Rubin BP, Schwab ME. VEGF mRNA induction correlates with changes in the vascular architecture upon spinal cord damage in the rat. *Eur J Neurosci* 1997;9:2549.
39. Steinbrech DS, Mehrara BJ, Saadeh PB, et al. VEGF expression in an osteoblast-like cell line is regulated by a hypoxia response mechanism. *Am J Physiol Cell Physiol* 2000;278:C853.
40. Klekamp JG, Jarzecka K, Hoover RL, et al. Vascular endothelial growth factor is expressed in ovine pulmonary vascular smooth muscle cells in vitro and regulated by hypoxia and dexamethasone. *Pediatr Res* 1997;42:744.
41. Heiss JD, Papavassiliou E, Merrill MJ, et al. Mechanism of dexamethasone suppression of brain tumor-associated vascular permeability in rats. Involvement of the glucocorticoid receptor and vascular permeability factor. *J Clin Invest* 1996;98:1400.
42. Gonzalez MV, Gonzalez-Sancho JM, Caelles C, Munoz A, Jimenez B. Hormone-activated nuclear receptors inhibit the stimulation of the JNK and ERK signalling pathways in endothelial cells. *FEBS Lett* 1999;459:272.
43. Criscuolo GR, Balledux JP. Clinical neurosciences in the decade of the brain: hypotheses in neuro-oncology. VEG/PF acts upon the actin cytoskeleton and is inhibited by dexamethasone: relevance to tumor angiogenesis and vasogenic edema. *Yale J Biol Med* 1996;69:337.
44. Dang CV, Semenza GL. Oncogenic alterations of metabolism. *Trends Biochem Sci* 1999;24:68.
45. Siegal T, Siegal TZ, Shapira Y, et al. Experimental neoplastic spinal cord compression. Evoked potentials, edema, prostaglandins, and light and electron microscopy. *Spine* 1987;12:440.
46. Siegal T, Shohami E, Siegal TZ. Indomethacin and dexamethasone treatment in experimental spinal cord compression. Part I. Effect on water content and specific gravity. *Neurosurgery* 1988;22:328.
47. Siegal T, Shoshami E, Shapira Y, Siegal TZ. Indomethacin and dexamethasone treatment in experimental spinal cord compression. Part II. Effect on edema and prostaglandin synthesis. *Neurosurgery* 1988;22:334.
48. Siegal T, Siegal T, Shohami E, Shapira Y. Comparison of soluble dexamethasone sodium phosphate with free dexamethasone and indomethacin in treatment of experimental neoplastic spinal cord compression. *Spine* 1988;13:1171.
49. Siegal T, Siegal T, Shohami E, Lossos F. Experimental neoplastic spinal cord compression: effect of ketamine and MK-801 on edema and prostaglandins. *Neurosurgery* 1990;26:963.
50. Siegal T. Spinal cord compression: from laboratory to clinic. *Eur J Cancer* 1995;31A:1748.
51. Rades D, Blach M, Nerreter V, Bremer M, Karstens JH. Metastatic spinal cord compression. Influence of time between onset of motoric deficits and start of irradiation on therapeutic effect. *Strahlenther Onkol* 1999;175:378.
52. Gilbert RW, Kim J-H, Posner JB. Epidural spinal cord compression from metastatic tumor: diagnosis and treatment. *Ann Neurol* 1978;3:40.
53. Stark RJ, Henson RA, Evans SJW. Spinal metastases. A retrospective survey from a general hospital. *Brain* 1982;105:189.
54. Husband DJ. Malignant spinal cord compression: prospective study of delays in referral and treatment. *BMJ* 1998;317:18.
55. Pigott KH, Baddeley H, Maher EJ. Pattern of disease in spinal cord compression on MRI scan and implications for treatment. *Clin Oncol (R Coll Radiol)* 1994;6:7.
56. Heldmann U, Myschetzky PS, Thomsen HS. Frequency of unexpected multifocal metastasis in patients with acute spinal cord compression. Evaluation by low-field MR imaging in cancer patients. *Acta Radiol* 1997;38:372.
57. Cook AM, Lau TN, Tomlinson MJ, et al. Magnetic resonance imaging of the whole spine in suspected malignant spinal cord compression: impact on management. *Clin Oncol (R Coll Radiol)* 1998;10:39.
58. Schiff D, O'Neill BP, Wang CH, O'Fallon J. Neuroimaging and treatment implications of patients with multiple epidural spinal metastases. *Cancer* 1998;83:1593.
59. Khaw FM, Worthy SA, Gibson MJ, Gholkar A. The appearance on MRI of vertebrae in acute compression of the spinal cord due to metastases. *J Bone Joint Surg Br* 1999;81:830.
60. Crasto S, Duca S, Davini O, et al. MRI diagnosis of intramedullary metastases from extra-CNS tumors. *Eur Radiol* 1997;7:732.
61. Bilsky MH, Lis E, Raizer J, Lee H, Boland P. The diagnosis and treatment of metastatic spinal tumor. *Oncologist* 1999;4:459.
62. Helweg-Larsen S, Sorensen PS. Symptoms and signs in metastatic spinal cord compres-

sion: a study of progression from first symptom until diagnosis in 153 patients. *Eur J Cancer* 1994;30A:396.
63. Portenoy RK, Lipton RB, Foley KM. Back pain in the cancer patient: an algorithm for evaluation and management. *Neurology* 1987;37:134.
64. St. Amour TE, Hodges SC, Laakman RW, Tamas DE, eds. *MRI of the spine*. New York: Raven, 1994:435.
65. Frank JA, Ling A, Patronas NJ, et al. Detection of malignant bone tumors: MRI vs. scintigraphy. *AJR Am J Roentgenol* 1990;155:1043.
66. Algra PR, Bloem JL, Tissing H, et al. Detection of vertebral body metastases: comparison between MR imaging and bone scintigraphy. *Radiographics* 1991;11:219.
67. Avrahami E, Tadmor R, Dally O, Hadar H. Early MR demonstration of spinal metastases in patients with normal radiographs and CT and radionuclide bone scans. *J Comput Assist Tomogr* 1989;13:598.
68. Gjorup T, Hartling OJ, Munck-Hansen J, Munck O. Bone-scan "cold" lesion caused by an osteolytic metastasis from an adenocarcinoma of the thyroid. *Eur J Nucl Med* 1985;10:470.
69. Jordan JE, Donaldson SS, Enzmann DR. Cost effectiveness and outcome assessment of magnetic resonance imaging in diagnosing cord compression. *Cancer* 1995;75:2579.
70. Kamoto Y, Sadato N, Yonekura Y, et al. Visualization of the cervical spinal cord with FDG and high-resolution PET. *J Comput Assist Tomogr* 1998;22:487.
71. Baba H, Uchida K, Sadato N, et al. Potential usefulness of ^{18}F-2-fluoro-deoxy-D-glucose positron emission tomography in cervical compressive myelopathy. *Spine* 1999;24:1449.
72. Poggi M, Fuller B, et al. Intramedullary spinal cord metastasis from renal cell carcinoma: confirmation by positron emission tomography (*submitted*).
73. Smoker WRK, Goderski JC, Knutzon RK, et al. The role of MR imaging in evaluating metastatic spinal disease. *AJR Am J Roentgenol* 1987;149:1241.
74. Godersky JC, Smoker WR, Knutzon R. Use of magnetic resonance imaging in the evaluation of metastatic spinal disease. *Neurosurgery* 1987;21:676.
75. Li KC, Poon PY. Sensitivity and specificity of MRI in detecting malignant spinal cord compression and in distinguishing malignant from benign compression fractures of vertebrae. *Magn Reson Imaging* 1988;6:547.
76. Lien HH, Blomlie V, Heimdal K. Magnetic resonance imaging of malignant extradural tumors with acute spinal cord compression. *Acta Radiol* 1990;31:187.
77. Carmody RF, Yang PJ, Seeley GW, et al. Spinal cord compression due to metastatic disease: diagnosis with MR imaging versus myelography. *Radiology* 1989;173:225.
78. Quint DJ. Indications for emergent MRI of the central nervous system. *JAMA* 2000;283:853.
79. Ratanatharathorn V, Powers WE. Epidural spinal cord compression from metastatic tumor: diagnosis and guidelines for management. *Cancer Treat Rev* 1991;18:55.
80. Sze G. Magnetic resonance imaging in the evaluation of spinal tumors. *Cancer* 199115;67(Suppl 4):1229.
81. Hollis PH, Malis LI, Zappulla RA. Neurological deterioration after lumbar puncture below complete spinal subarachnoid block. *J Neurosurg* 1986;64:253.
82. Gomori JM, Heching N, Siegal T. Leptomeningeal metastases: evaluation by gadolinium enhanced spinal magnetic resonance imaging. *J Neurooncol* 1998;36:55.
83. Leviov M, Dale J, Stein M, et al. The management of metastatic spinal cord compression: a radiotherapeutic success ceiling. *Int J Radiat Oncol Biol Phys* 1993;27:231.
84. Hicks F, Thom V, Alison D, Corcoran G. Spinal cord compression: the hospice perspective. *J Palliat Care* 1993;3:9.
85. Martenson JA, Evans RG, Lie MR, et al. Treatment outcome and complications in patients treated for malignant epidural spinal cord compression (SCC). *J Neuro-Oncol* 1985;3:77.
86. Maranzano E, Latini P, Perrucci E, et al. Short-course radiotherapy (8 Gy × 2) in metastatic spinal cord compression: an effective and feasible treatment. *Int J Radiat Oncol Biol Phys* 1997;38:1037.
87. Maranzano E, Latini P, Beneventi S, et al. Comparison of two different radiotherapy schedules for spinal cord compression in prostate cancer. *Tumori* 1998;84:472.
88. Landmann C, Hunig R, Gratzl O. The role of laminectomy in the combined treatment of metastatic spinal cord compression. *Int J Radiat Oncol Biol Phys* 1992;24:627.
89. Turner S, Marosszeky B, Timms I, Boyages J. Malignant spinal cord compression: a prospective evaluation. *Int J Radiat Oncol Biol Phys* 1993;26:141.
90. Sorensen PS, Borgesen SE, Rohde K, et al. Metastatic epidural spinal cord compression. *Cancer* 1990;65:1502.
91. Kim RY, Spencer SA, Meredith RF, et al. Extradural spinal cord compression: analysis of factors determining functional prognosis—a prospective study. *Radiology* 1990;176:279.
92. Sundaresan N, Sachdev VP, Holland JF, et al. Surgical treatment of spinal cord compression from epidural metastasis. *Clin Oncol* 1995;13:2330.
93. Katagiri H, Takahashi M, Inagaki J, et al. Clinical results of nonsurgical treatment for spinal metastases. *Int J Radiat Oncol Biol Phys* 1998;42:1127.
94. Findlay GFG. The role of vertebral body collapse in the management of malignant spinal cord compression. *J Neurol Neurosurg Psychiatry* 1987;50:151.
95. Findlay GFG. Adverse effects of the management of malignant spinal cord compression. *J Neurol Neurosurg Psychiatry* 1984;47:761.
96. Harrington KD. Anterior cord compression and spinal stabilization for patients with metastatic lesions of the spine. *J Neurosurg* 1984;61:107.
97. Sundaresan N, DiGiacinto GV, Krol G, Hughes JEO. Spondylectomy for malignant tumors of the spine. *J Clin Oncol* 1989;7:1485.
98. Moore AJ, Uttley D. Anterior decompression and stabilization of the spine in malignant disease. *Neurosurgery* 1989;24:713.
99. McLain RF. Endoscopically assisted decompression for metastatic thoracic neoplasms. *Spine* 1998;23:1130.
100. Nauck M, Karakiulakis G, Perruchoud AP, Papakonstantinou E, Roth M. Corticosteroids inhibit the expression of the vascular endothelial growth factor gene in human vascular smooth muscle cells. *Eur J Pharmacol* 1998;341:309.
101. Nauck M, Roth M, Tamm M, et al. Induction of vascular endothelial growth factor by platelet-activating factor and platelet-derived growth factor is downregulated by corticosteroids. *Am J Respir Cell Mol Biol* 1997;16:398.
102. Heimdal K, Hirschberg H, Slettebo H, Watne K, Nome O. High incidence of serious side effects of high-dose dexamethasone treatment in patients with epidural spinal cord compression. *J Neuro-Oncol* 1992;12:141.
103. Byrne TN. Current concepts. Spinal cord compression from epidural metastases. *N Engl J Med* 1992;327:614.
104. Ottolenghi CE. Aspiration biopsy of the spine: technique for the thoracic spine and results of twenty-eight biopsies in this region and over-all results of 1050 biopsies of other spinal segments. *J Bone Joint Surg Am* 1969;51:1531.
105. Adapon BD, Legada BD, Lim EVA, et al. CT-guided closed biopsy of the spine. *J Comput Assist Tomogr* 1981;5:73.
106. Bell GR. Surgical treatment of spinal tumors. *Clin Orthop* 1997;335:54.
107. Pennin RG, McBroom RJ. Spinal fixation after anterior decompression for symptomatic spinal metastasis. *Neurosurgery* 1988;22:324.
108. Moore AJ, Uttley D. Anterior decompression and stabilization of the spine in malignant disease. *Neurosurgery* 1989;24:713.
109. Choi IS, Berenstein A, Scott J. The use of ethyl alcohol in the treatment of malignant tumors. *AJNR Am J Neuroradiol* 1985;6:462.
110. Chiras J, Cognard C, Rose M, et al. Percutaneous injection of an alcoholic embolizing emulsion as an alternative preoperative embolization for spine tumor. *AJNR Am J Neuroradiol* 1993;14:1113.
111. Cobb CA, Leavens ME, Eckles N. Indications for nonoperative treatment of spinal cord compression due to breast cancer. *J Neurosurg* 1977;47:653.
112. Helwig-Larsen S, Rasmusson B, Sorensen PS. Recovery of gait after radiotherapy in paralytic patients with metastatic epidural spinal cord compression. *Neurology* 1990;40:1234.
113. Henson JW, Posner JB. Neurologic complications. In: Holland JF, Frei E, Bast RC, et al., eds. *Cancer medicine*. Philadelphia: Lea & Febiger, 1993:2268.
114. Helweg-Larsen S, Sorensen PS, Kreiner S. Prognostic factors in metastatic spinal cord compression: a prospective study using multivariate analysis of variables influencing survival and gait function in 153 patients. *Int J Radiat Oncol Biol Phys* 2000;46:1163.
115. Van der Sande JJ, Kroger R, Boogerd W. Multiple spinal epidural metastases; an unexpectedly frequent finding. *J Neurol Neurosurg Psychiatry* 1990;53:1001.
116. Calkins AR, Olson MA, Ellis JH. Impact of myelography on the radiotherapeutic management of malignant spinal cord compression. *Neurosurgery* 1986;19:614.
117. Punt J, Pritchard J, Pincott J, Till K. Neuroblastoma: a review of 21 cases presenting with spinal cord compression. *Cancer* 1980;45:3095.
118. Friedman M, Kim TH, Panahon AM. Spinal cord compression in malignant lymphoma. *Cancer* 1976;37:1485.
119. Rate WR, Solin LJ, Turrisi AT. Palliative radiotherapy for metastatic malignant melanoma: brain metastases, bone metastases, and spinal cord compression. *Int J Radiat Oncol Biol Phys* 1988;15:859.
120. Herbert SH, Solin LJ, Rate WR, Schultz DJ, Hanks GE. The effect of palliative radiation therapy on epidural compression due to metastatic malignant melanoma. *Cancer* 1991;67:2472.
121. Bates T. A review of local radiotherapy in the treatment of bone metastases and cord compression. *Int J Radiat Oncol Biol Phys* 1991;23:217.
122. Podd TJ, Carpenter DS, Baughan CA, Percival D, Dyson P. Spinal cord compression: prognosis and implications for treatment fractionation. *Clin Oncol* 1992;4:341.
123. Faul CM, Flickinger JC. The use of radiation in the management of spinal metastases. *J Neuro-Oncol* 1995;23:149.
124. Leibel SA. ACR appropriateness criteria. Expert Panel on Radiation Oncology, American College of Radiology. *Int J Radiat Oncol Biol Phys* 1999;43:125.
125. Hall E. *Radiobiology for the radiologist*, 4th ed. Philadelphia: Lippincott Williams & Wilkins, 1993.
126. Hayes FA, Thompson EI, Hvizdala E, O'Conor D, Green AA. Chemotherapy as an alternative to laminectomy and radiation in the management of epidural tumor. *J Pediatr* 1984;104:221.
127. Sinoff CL, Blumsohn A. Spinal cord compression in myelomatosis: response to chemotherapy alone. *Eur J Cancer Clin Oncol* 1989;25:197.
128. Posner JB, Howieson J, Cvitkovic E. "Disappearing" spinal cord compression: oncolytic effect of glucocorticoids (and other chemotherapeutic agents) on epidural metastases. *Ann Neurol* 1977;2:409.
129. Boogerd W, van der Sande JJ, Kroger R, Bruning PF, Somers R. Effective systemic therapy for spinal epidural metastases from breast carcinoma. *Eur J Cancer Clin Oncol* 1989;25:149.
130. Edelman IS. Paraplegia secondary to metastatic prostate cancer treated with stilbestrol: report of a case. *Ann Intern Med* 1949;31:1098.
131. Friedman HM, Sheetz S, Levine HL, Everett JR, Hong WK. Combination chemotherapy and radiation therapy. The medical management of epidural spinal cord compression from testicular cancer. *Arch Intern Med* 1986;146:509.
132. Marshall LF, Langfitt TW. Combined therapy for metastatic extradural tumors of the spine. *Cancer* 1977;40:2067.
133. Burch PA, Grossman SA. Treatment of epidural cord compression from Hodgkin's disease with chemotherapy. *Am J Med* 1988;84:555.
134. Sanderson IR, Pritchard J, Marsh MT. Chemotherapy as the initial treatment of spinal cord compression due to disseminated neuoblastoma. *J Neurosurg* 1989;70:688.
135. Sasagawa J, Guton H, Miyabayashi H, Yamaquchi O, Shiraiara Y. Hormonal treatment of symptomatic spinal cord compression in advanced prostate cancer. *Int Urol Nephrol* 1991;21:351.
136. Clarke PRR, Saunders M. Steroid-induced remission in spinal canal reticulum cell sarcoma. *J Neurosurg* 1975;42:346.
137. Cooper K, Bajorin D, Shapiro W, et al. Decompression of epidural metastases from germ cell tumors with chemotherapy. *J Neurooncol* 1990;8:275.
138. Gonzalez-Barcena D, Vadillo-Buenfil M, Cortez-Morales A, et al. Luteinizing hormone-releasing hormone antagonist cetrorelix as primary single therapy in patients with advanced prostatic cancer and paraplegia due to metastatic invasion of spinal cord. *Urology* 1995;45:275.

139. Wakisaka M, Takagishi Y. Paraparesis due to metastatic prostatic cancer effectively treated with a high dose of diethylstilbestrol diphosphate: a case report. *Hinyokika Kiyo* 1993;39:1055.
140. Gershanovich ML, Arkhipov AI, Vilensky BS. Nitrosourea derivatives for the treatment of Hodgkin's disease involving the central nervous system: a study of 23 cases. *Bull Cancer (Paris)* 1990;77:821.
141. Wallington M, Mendis S, Premawardhana U, Sanders P, Shahsavar-Haghighi K. Local control and survival in spinal cord compression from lymphoma and myeloma. *Radiother Oncol* 1997;42:43.
142. Rathmell AJ, Gospodarowicz MK, Sutcliffe SB, Clark RM. Localized extradural lymphoma: survival, relapse pattern and functional outcome. *Radiother Oncol* 1992;24:14.
143. Conrad EU 3d, Olszewski AD, Berger M, Powell E, Bruckner J. Pediatric spine tumors with spinal cord compromise. *J Pediatr Orthop* 1992;12:454.
144. King D, Goodman J, Hawk T, Boles ET Jr, Sayers MP. Dumbbell neuroblastomas in children. *Arch Surg* 1975;110:888.
145. Hoover M, Bowman LC, Crawford SE, et al. Long-term outcome of patients with intraspinal neuroblastoma. *Med Pediatr Oncol* 1999;32:353.
146. Schiff D, O'Neill BP. Intramedullary spinal cord metastases: clinical features and treatment outcome. *Neurology* 1996;47:906.
147. Törmä T. Malignant tumors of the spine and spinal epidural space: a study based on 250 histologically verified cases. *Acta Chir Scand* 1957;225:1.

SECTION **3**

RAYMOND P. WARRELL, JR.

Metabolic Emergencies

Patients with cancer may develop a number of metabolic and endocrinologic problems, frequently to an exaggerated degree. This section reviews metabolic complications of cancer that require urgent therapy for treatment or prevention.

HYPERCALCEMIA

EPIDEMIOLOGY

Hypercalcemia is the most common life-threatening metabolic disorder in patients with cancer. The prevalence of this disorder approximates 15 to 20 cases per 100,000 persons.[1,2] The incidence varies depending on the underlying cancer diagnosis, being highest in myeloma and breast cancer (approximately 40%), intermediate in non–small cell lung cancer, and uncommon in colon, prostate, and small cell lung carcinomas.[3–5]

DIFFERENTIAL DIAGNOSIS

Hypercalcemia is associated with a wide variety of pathologic states (Table 51.3-1). Primary hyperparathyroidism and cancer are the two most common causes of hypercalcemia, and both diseases are prevalent.[6,7] Patients who present with a recent onset of symptomatic hypercalcemia and weight loss are more likely to have a malignant disorder. In hypercalcemic patients who require hospitalization, cancer has been previously diagnosed or becomes apparent after minimal diagnostic evaluation in most cases. By contrast, asymptomatic hypercalcemia and chronic symptoms are the most common presentations of primary hyperparathyroidism. The diagnostic evaluation and differential diagnosis of patients with hypercalcemia have been reviewed.[8–10] Generally, an elevation in serum calcium with a low or normal serum immunoreactive parathyroid hormone (PTH) level, especially when combined with an increase in serum PTH-related protein (see Parathyroid Hormone and the Parathyroid Hormone–Related Protein, later in this chapter) can exclude the diagnosis of primary hyperparathyroidism with high confidence.[11]

Serum calcium is highly bound to albumin, and measurements of total serum calcium fluctuate with changes in serum protein concentrations. Occasional patients with myeloma present with striking elevations of total serum calcium due solely to an increase in serum calcium-binding proteins.[12] Measurements of ionized calcium by ion-specific electrode are essential in such cases. However, for most patients an approximate estimate of the severity of hypercalcemia can be made by using one of several formulas that adjust serum calcium levels for serum albumin concentration, as follows:

$$\text{Corrected [calcium] (mg/dL)}^* = \text{measured [calcium] (mg/dL)} - \text{[albumin] (g/dL)} + 4.0$$ [13]

CLINICAL MANIFESTATIONS

Patients with hypercalcemia can present with a wide variety of symptoms affecting multiple organ symptoms (Table 51.3-2). The severity of the presentation is not exclusively related to the degree of elevation in serum calcium. Patients with a slight-to-moderate elevation (12 to 13 mg/dL) may be obtunded if the increase has occurred acutely. Conversely, patients with long-standing hypercalcemia (such as those with parathyroid carcinoma) may tolerate a serum calcium greater than 14 mg/dL with few symptoms. Other factors (especially age, performance status, sites of metastases, and hepatic or renal dysfunction) also contribute to the severity of symptoms.

In patients with evolving hypercalcemia, fatigue, lethargy, constipation, nausea, and polyuria are the most common initial complaints. It is important to evaluate the serum calcium in patients who have these relatively nonspecific complaints because the combination of polyuria and nausea can lead to rapid dehydration and substantial worsening of the hypercalcemic state. Patients in late stages may present in stupor or coma, and the condition is easily mistaken for diabetic ketoacidosis or drug overdose.

PATHOPHYSIOLOGY

In the past, cancer-related hypercalcemia was conveniently categorized according to the presence or absence of bone involvement. Hypercalcemia in the former group was believed to be associated with direct bone destruction by cancer cells (so-called local osteolytic hypercalcemia), and the second group was characterized by various humorally mediated mechanisms.[14] However, it is now evident that hypercalcemia, even in patients with extensive osteolysis, is mediated by factors released by malignant cells that ultimately act to resorb calcium from bone. Some of these factors also stimulate calcium

*Concentrations in milligrams per deciliter can be converted to SI units after multiplication by 0.2495, which yields a concentration expressed in millimoles per liter.

TABLE 51.3-1. Diseases Associated with Hypercalcemia

Endocrine and metabolic diseases	
	Primary hyperparathyroidism
	Hyperthyroidism
	Pheochromocytoma
	Osteopetrosis
	Infantile hyperphosphatasia
	Familial hypercalcemia with hypercalciuria
Cancer	
Infectious diseases	
	Tuberculosis
	Coccidioidomycosis
	Human immunodeficiency virus infection
Renal insufficiency	
Granulomatous diseases	
	Sarcoidosis
	Berylliosis
Dietary and drug-related	
	Vitamin D intoxication
	Vitamin A intoxication, retinoids
	Calcium supplements
	Lithium
	Milk-alkali syndrome

reabsorption from the renal tubule, but this effect is secondary in importance to accelerated osteoclastic bone resorption.

Parathyroid Hormone and the Parathyroid Hormone–Related Protein

Many patients with cancer-related hypercalcemia have biochemical characteristics suggestive of PTH stimulation, including increased tubular reabsorption of calcium, hypophosphatemia with phosphaturia, and elevated levels of *nephrogenous* cyclic adenosine monophosphate. However, most studies of *ectopic hyperparathyroidism* were based on bioassays or measurements of immunoreactive material.[15] Studies examining PTH-specific mRNA in tumors have confirmed that ectopic PTH production is not a common cause of cancer-related hypercalcemia.[16] Other than cases of parathyroid carcinoma,[17] tumor secretion of authentic PTH by malignant tumors is exceptionally rare.[18,19] Nonetheless, primary hyperparathyroidism caused by parathyroid adenomas is a common feature of the heritable multiple endocrine neoplasia syndromes 1 and 2a.

A PTH-related protein (PTH-RP), which is elaborated by cancer cells and binds to the PTH receptor, has now been fully characterized.[20–23] Genes encoding PTH-RP and authentic

TABLE 51.3-2. Clinical Manifestations of Cancer-Related Hypercalcemia

General:	dehydration, weight loss, anorexia, pruritus, polydipsia
Neuromuscular:	fatigue, lethargy, muscle weakness, hyporeflexia, confusion, psychosis, seizure, obtundation, coma
Gastrointestinal:	nausea, vomiting, constipation, obstipation, ileus
Genitorenal:	polyuria, renal insufficiency
Cardiac:	bradycardia, prolonged P-R interval, shortened Q-T interval, wide T wave, atrial or ventricular arrhythmias

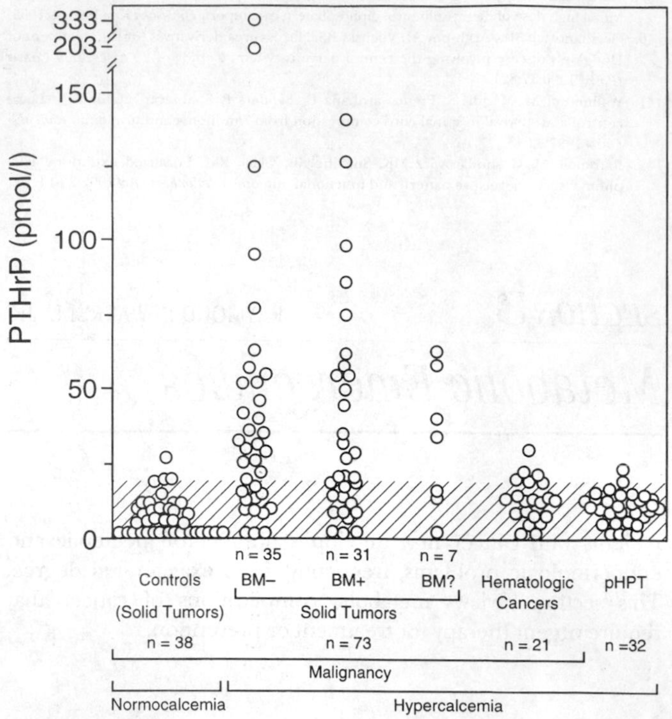

FIGURE 51.3-1. Plasma levels of parathyroid-related protein (PTHrP) in normocalcemic control patients with solid tumors, patients with solid tumors with (BM+) or without (BM–) bone metastases or in whom the presence or absence of bone metastases was not determined (BM?), patients with various hematologic cancers, and patients with primary hyperparathyroidism (pHPT). (From ref. 34, with permission.)

human PTH have been mapped to the short arms of chromosomes 12 and 11, respectively. The proteins are homologous for only 8 of the first 13 amino acids in the amino-terminal portion, which contains the receptor-binding domain. PTH-RP is widely distributed in normal tissues such as brain, kidney, parathyroid, skin, atrium, uterus, and breast.[24–27] PTH-RP mediates the effects of a protein known as *Indian hedgehog* that is a negative regulator of chondrocyte differentiation.[28,29] The protein seems to be involved only in local signaling and under normal conditions is not released into the general circulation.

Although at least one case of elevated PTH-RP has been reported in association with a benign tumor (called *humoral hypercalcemia of benignancy*),[30] this phenomenon is extremely rare. PTH-RP appears to be the most common mediator of cancer-related hypercalcemia.[31–37] Increased blood levels of PTH-RP are commonly found in patients with solid tumors (Fig. 51.3-1), particularly patients with squamous (epidermoid) carcinomas.[32–34] Elevated serum PTH-RP levels have been found in 30% to 50% of hypercalcemic patients with breast cancer,[33–35] even though this disease was formerly thought to characterize the bone metastasis form of hypercalcemia. The factor does not appear to be associated with most hematologic cancers such as myeloma or lymphoma.[32–34,36] However, the viral *tax* protein transactivates the PTH-RP gene promoter,[38,39] and high levels of PTH-RP have been reported in patients with human T-cell lymphotropic virus 1–associated leukemia and lymphoma.[40] The factor is elaborated at sites of bone metastases in breast[41] and prostate[42] cancer, and women with high basal levels of immunoreactive PTH-RP in the primary tumor appear more likely to develop metastases in bone than in soft tissues.[43] The absolute serum level of PTH-RP is not affected by hypocalcemic treatment.[44,45] Several studies have shown that patients with high levels tend to have an inferior response when treated with bisphosphonates[46,47] and a poorer life expectancy.[48]

Vitamin D_3

Elevated serum 1,25 $(OH)_2$-vitamin D_3 levels have been reported in patients with Hodgkin's disease, non-Hodgkin's lymphoma, myeloma,[49–52] and occasional patients with solid tumors.[53] This effect probably results from increased enzymatic conversion of 25-OH-vitamin D_3 by 1_α-vitamin D-hydroxylase, similar to well-documented processes that occur in patients with granulomatous disease. However, these observations do not necessarily establish an etiologic association. The measured elevations in serum vitamin D_3 concentrations in such patients have generally been well below levels that are known to cause hypercalcemia in patients with sarcoidosis.[54] The levels are also below serum levels in subjects who have ingested oral calcitriol and who remain normocalcemic.[55] Moreover, serum vitamin D_3 levels may not be appropriately suppressed in hypercalcemic patients with elevated PTH-RP levels.[56] Whether vitamin D_3 plays a critical pathophysiologic role, acting alone or in concert with other factors, or acts merely as a marker of tumor burden is still unclear. Nonetheless, normalization of serum vitamin D_3 levels and resolution of hypercalcemia occur with control of the underlying disease.

Prostaglandins

Prostaglandins have long been implicated as circulating mediators of cancer-related hypercalcemia, and certain prostaglandins (notably of the E series) have potent bone-resorptive activity *in vitro*.[57] Although occasional hormonally induced flares of hypercalcemia in breast cancer have been linked to prostaglandin release,[58] cancer-related hypercalcemia rarely responds clinically to treatment with classic cyclooxygenase inhibitors (such as aspirin or nonsteroidal antiinflammatory drugs).[57,59] Furthermore, circulating levels of prostaglandin E in hypercalcemic patients are far too low to account for the observed degree of accelerated bone resorption.[60] Thus, prostaglandins may have an important (but time-dependent and highly focal) role in cancer-related osteolysis.[61]

Cytokines

A number of soluble osteoclast-activating factors have been isolated that are potent inducers of bone resorption *in vitro*. The transforming growth factors (TGFs) are released in an autocrine manner by many cancer cells and regulate both resorption and formation of normal bone. TGF-α shares partial amino acid homology with epidermal growth factor, binds to the epidermal growth factor receptor, and is a potent inducer of bone resorption *in vitro*, both alone and in combination with PTH-RP.[62,63] Conversely, TGF-β is secreted by osteoblasts and may regulate osteoblast growth and differentiation. Thus, dysregulated TGF secretion might lead to uncoupling of the normal processes of bone resorption and formation and could partly account for the mixed lytic and blastic appearance of skeletal metastases in diseases such as breast and prostate cancer.

Interleukin-6 increases bone resorption *in vitro*,[64] acts as an autocrine growth factor in myeloma,[65] and may be associated with hypercalcemia in kidney cancer.[66] Hypercalcemia induced *in vivo* by interleukin-6 administration is blocked by treatment with specific neutralizing antibodies.[67] Other cytokines, including interleukin-1,[68] tumor-derived hematopoietic colony-stimulating factors,[69] and tumor necrosis factor [particularly tumor necrosis factor-β (lymphotoxin)],[70] are also potent inducers of bone resorption *in vitro*. However, clinical therapy with supra-pharmacologic amounts of therapeutic recombinant cytokines is not associated with hypercalcemia. Thus, although the focal interaction of these factors at sites of bone involvement may be complex, there is little evidence that circulating cytokines are important mediators of cancer-related hypercalcemia.

SUMMARY

With the discovery of the PTH-RP and its high prevalence in patients with cancer-related hypercalcemia, a unifying hypothesis for the etiology of this syndrome has become more apparent. PTH-RP, not normally released to the general circulation, is a potent mediator of hypercalcemia. In general, patients who elaborate this factor, particularly patients with epidermoid carcinomas, are more resistant to treatment with antihypercalcemic drugs. Osteotropic tumors, such as breast and prostate cancer, appear to require proximity to bone in order to effect bone resorption, possibly via release of TGFs, PTH-RP, prostaglandins, or all three. The extensive osteolysis observed in multiple myeloma may be due to focally increased production of interleukin-6 and tumor necrosis factor-β that accelerates bone resorption by normal osteoclasts. A large number of patients with cancer have lytic bone disease, but only a small proportion develop hypercalcemia; thus, interaction of these factors and amplification of the pathophysiology by the kidney must also occur.

TREATMENT OF CANCER-RELATED HYPERCALCEMIA

GENERAL MEASURES

Although the best treatment for cancer-related hypercalcemia is therapy directed at the underlying disease, hypercalcemia most commonly occurs in patients with advanced disease who have failed prior cytotoxic therapy. The usual therapies for hypercalcemia are directed at decreasing serum calcium by increasing urinary calcium excretion or decreasing bone resorption by inhibition of osteoclast function.[71,72] For practical purposes, increased intestinal absorption of calcium does not make an important contribution to hypercalcemia in patients with cancer. Low-calcium diets are generally unpalatable and distinctly ineffective; their use is strongly discouraged.

Where possible, immobilization should be minimized because inactivity tends to aggravate hypercalcemia. Drugs that inhibit urinary calcium excretion (e.g., thiazides) or agents that may decrease renal blood flow (nonsteroidal antiinflammatory drugs and H_2-receptor antagonists) should be discontinued if possible. Patients should be carefully interviewed with respect to dietary aberrations, and medications containing calcium, vitamin D, vitamin A, or other retinoids should be stopped.

Formerly, hypercalcemic patients were commonly treated with vigorous intravenous hydration and diuretics for several

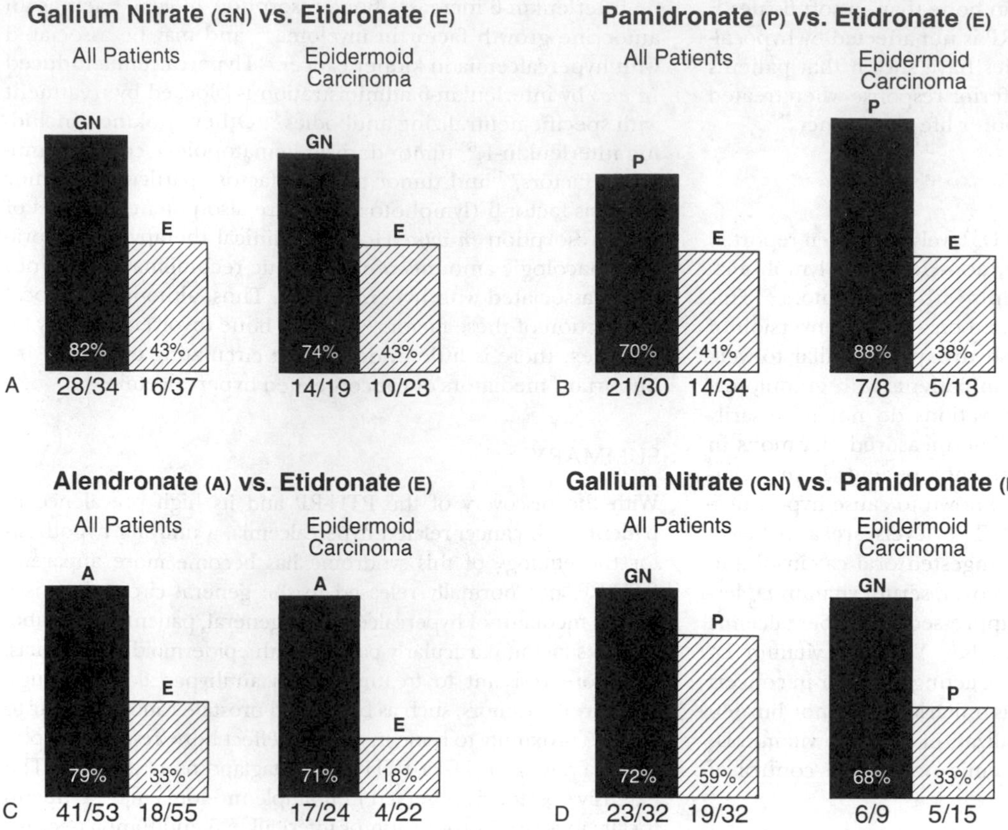

FIGURE 51.3-2. Results from four randomized double-blind comparisons of the major drugs used for acute treatment of cancer-related hypercalcemia. Bars depict proportion of patients who achieved a normal serum calcium value subsequent to treatment with the assigned agent. All analyses are based on *intent to treat.* Numbers at bottom indicate number of patients responding over number of patients treated per group. The test drugs were administered on the following dose-schedules: **(A)** gallium nitrate (200 mg/m^2) as a continuous IV infusion daily for 5 days, and etidronate (7.5 mg/kg) as a 4-hour infusion daily for 5 days[131]; **(B)** pamidronate (60 mg) as a single 24-hour infusion, and etidronate (7.5 mg/kg) as a 4-hour infusion daily for 3 days[90]; **(C)** alendronate (10 or 15 mg) as a single 2-hour infusion, and etidronate (7.5 mg/kg) as a 4-hour infusion daily for 3 days[105]; **(D)** gallium nitrate (200 mg/m^2) as a continuous IV infusion daily for 5 days, and pamidronate (60 or 90 mg) as a single 24-hour infusion.[95]

days, and specific hypocalcemic drugs were reserved for patients who did not respond to hydration. As noted in Intravenous Fluids and Diuretics, later in this chapter, this approach is outdated. Most patients benefit substantially from the early introduction of specific antihypercalcemic therapy, and this approach leads to more rapid clinical improvement, lower overall toxicity, and decreased cost.

SPECIFIC MEASURES

Until recently, the literature on the treatment of cancer-related hypercalcemia contained few controlled studies. Interpretation of older clinical trial results is therefore confounded by enormous variability in patient selection, underlying diagnoses, severity of hypercalcemia, and unique methods of reporting results.[73] Figure 51.3-2 depicts results from four major clinical studies, all of which were well-designed, randomized, double-blinded, and which generally employed similar entry and response criteria. Table 51.3-3 summarizes current therapies with an estimate of their relative clinical efficacy in acutely restoring normocalcemia.

Intravenous Fluids and Diuretics

Hypercalcemic patients frequently present with dehydration owing to vomiting and obligate water losses associated with calciuresis. Fluid repletion, usually with isotonic saline, has been a mainstay of acute therapy, because volume expansion and natriuresis can increase renal blood flow and enhance calcium excretion.[74] The rate of fluid administration depends on a clinical estimate of the extent of dehydration, cardiovascular function, and renal excretory capacity. Assuming renal and cardiac functions are adequate, saline infusion at a rate of 300 to 400 or more mL/h can be used for 3 to 4 hours in severely dehydrated patients. Slower hydration is indicated for less severe disturbances or in patients with congestive heart failure or oliguria. Serum calcium, creatinine, potassium, and magnesium should be reassessed frequently during this period.

The heroic degrees of saline hydration and forced diuresis that made up past therapy for cancer-related hypercalcemia[75] are no longer indicated. Such treatment is excessively toxic since it frequently causes fluid overload and occasionally life-threatening pulmonary edema. The resulting weight gain and lower extremity edema that occurs in hypoproteinemic patients with advanced cancer may not resolve during the life of that individual and can be severely disabling. Moreover, hydration (with or without diuretics) is not very effective. In a prospective study of 16 patients with serum calcium greater than or equal to 13.0 mg/dL (3.25 mmol/L), only five patients (31%) achieved normocalcemia with normal saline (4000 cc/d × 2 days).[76] Although furosemide-induced natriuresis theoretically enhances urinary calcium excretion, no controlled studies were ever conducted to indicate that hypercalcemic patients benefit from routine furosemide treatment. Furosemide also increases the risk for developing hypovolemia; the resultant decrease in glomerular filtration may actually stimulate renal calcium reabsorption, inadvertently reinduce dehydration, and worsen the clinical condition. Therefore, the use of furosemide should be restricted to balancing fluid intake and urinary output in patients who have been fully rehydrated. In most hospitalized patients, fluid administration should not be employed alone, and treatment with antiresorptive drugs

TABLE 51.3-3. Therapy for the Treatment of Cancer-Related Hypercalcemia

	Pamidronate	*Gallium Nitrate*	*Calcitonin*	*Plicamycin*	*Normal Saline*	*Oral Phosphorus*	*Corticosteroids*
Dose	60–90 mg IV over 24 h	100–200 mg/m²/d by continuous IV infusion, up to 5 d	2–8 U/kg SC or IM every 6–12 h	10–50 (usually 25) μg/kg IV by brief infusion	200–400 (+) mL/h	1–3 g/d orally, divided doses	40–100 mg/d prednisone (or equivalent)
Indications	Moderate to severe hypercalcemia	Moderate to severe hypercalcemia	Mild to moderate hypercalcemia; acute control	Moderate to severe hypercalcemia	Hypovolemia, dehydration	Mild to moderate hypercalcemia, hypophosphatemia	Hypercalcemia from myeloma, lymphoma, hormonal *flare*
Onset of action	24–48 h	24–48 h	1–4 h	24–48 h	12–24 h	24–48 h	3–5 d
Relative potency (%)[a]	60–75	75–80	30	5	20	30	0–40 (depending on disease)
Advantages	Highly effective, decreases bone resorption	Highly effective, decreases bone resorption	Minimal toxicity	Moderately effective	Corrects dehydration	Orally available; minimal toxicity	Orally available
Disadvantages and toxicity	Fever, venous irritation	Prolonged infusion, nephrotoxicity, hypophosphatemia	Nausea, hypersensitivity	Nausea, nephrotoxicity, hepatotoxicity, thrombocytopenia, coagulopathy	Pulmonary edema hypernatremia, fluid overload	Nausea, diarrhea extraosseous calcification	Hyperglycemia, gastritis, osteopenia

[a]Potency is defined as the expected proportion of patients with a serum calcium greater than or equal to 12.0 mg/dL who achieve normocalcemia after a single course of therapy.

should be initiated promptly following rehydration for control of hypercalcemia.

Bisphosphonates

Bisphosphonates (formerly diphosphonates), chemical analogues of pyrophosphate that are resistant to hydrolysis by pyrophosphatase, have become the most commonly used drugs for the treatment of hypercalcemia. Bisphosphonates adsorb to the surface of crystalline hydroxyapatite and inhibit calcium release from bone by interfering with the metabolic activity of osteoclasts.[77] There are numerous bisphosphonates available or undergoing clinical investigation, including etidronate, clodronate, pamidronate, zoledronate, alendronate, tiludronate, ibandronate, and risedronate. As a class, bisphosphonates have low oral bioavailability (less than 1%), and none of these agents is currently recommended as an oral therapy for hypercalcemia.

Intravenous pamidronate has become the most widely prescribed drug for treatment of hypercalcemia. This drug is well-tolerated and its side effects are usually limited to infusion-site irritation, fever, and flu-like symptoms that occur after the first infusion in approximately 20% of patients. Although multiple doses and schedules have been tested,[78,79] pamidronate is most commonly given at doses of 60 or 90 mg infused over 2 hours. Although the higher dose has been suggested for patients with more sever hypercalcemia (e.g., a total serum calcium greater than 13.0 mg/dL), there are conflicting data whether any substantial dose-response relationship exists above 60 mg.[80–83] Similar doses have been widely used to reduce skeletal morbidity from bone metastases.[84]

Considerable data indicate that the response to pamidronate is inferior in patients whose hypercalcemia is mediated by PTH-RP.[85–88] The hypocalcemic effect also appears to decrease with repeated dosing.[88] This reduced activity is clinically important because PTH-RP is the most common cause of cancer-related hypercalcemia.

Alendronate has also been studied by the intravenous route in hypercalcemia,[89,90] but this formulation is not widely available. The usual doses are 10 or 15 mg administered over 2 hours. Oral alendronate is widely used for treatment of postmenopausal osteoporosis; however, there are no data available supporting oral alendronate as a treatment for hypercalcemia. Based on similarly designed randomized studies compared with etidronate (see Fig. 51.3-2),[78,89] pamidronate and alendronate appear to have comparable degrees of clinical efficacy.

Among other bisphosphonates, etidronate has been compared with pamidronate, alendronate, and gallium nitrate in randomized double-blind studies. The response to etidronate in all three studies was similar: 42%, 33%, and 43%, respectively[78,83,89] (see Fig. 51.3-2). This result was significantly inferior relative to each of the other agents tested, and these data have largely accounted for its diminished use. Clodronate is available in Europe, but current data suggest that it is not as effective as pamidronate.[91,92] Ibandronate[93] and zoledronate[94,95] are other bisphosphonates undergoing clinical testing that are more potent (on a milligram per milligram basis) than earlier bisphosphonates. However, it is unclear if increased potency will translate to improved clinical efficacy, and early results suggest comparable clinical activity.

Gallium Nitrate

Gallium nitrate is a potent inhibitor of bone resorption.[96–98] Elemental gallium is incorporated into bone[99,100] and renders hydroxyapatite less soluble and more resistant to cell-mediated resorption.[126] However, the drug's principal mechanism of action is inhibition of an ATPase-dependent proton pump that is located in the ruffled membrane of the osteoclast.[101] This effect impairs osteoclast acidification and consequent dissolution of the underlying bone matrix. Randomized double-blind studies have demonstrated superiority of gallium nitrate compared with calcitonin[102] and etidronate[103] for acute treatment of resistant hypercalcemia, and preliminary data from one study also suggested superiority compared with pamidronate (see Fig. 51.3-2).[83]

Following administration as a continuous intravenous infusion (200 mg/m^2/d over 24 hours for up to 5 days), gallium nitrate induces normocalcemia in 70% to 90% of patients.[83,96,102,103] The maximal hypocalcemic effect occurs several days after the drug has been discontinued; therefore, the drug infusion should be discontinued once the patient has achieved normocalcemia. In earlier studies that used high-dose gallium nitrate as primary cancer treatment, nephrotoxicity was dose-limiting; however, the incidence of renal insufficiency in controlled hypercalcemia studies has been similar to calcitonin, etidronate, and pamidronate.[83,102,103] Like the bisphosphonates, gallium nitrate should be started after the patient has been rehydrated and urinary output ensured. A daily urinary output of 2000 mL should be maintained during the infusion. Concurrent use of highly nephrotoxic drugs, such as aminoglycosides, amphotericin B, and cisplatin, should be avoided.

Calcitonin

Pharmacologic doses of calcitonin reduce serum calcium by increasing renal calcium excretion and inhibiting bone resorption.[104] Calcitonin is especially advantageous due to its rapid onset of action (2 to 4 hours)[102,105] and its lack of serious toxicity (other than rare hypersensitivity reactions). Notwithstanding these desirable features, the hypocalcemic effect of calcitonin is relatively weak; the acute response peaks at 48 hours and diminishes thereafter despite continued treatment.[102] Less than 30% of hypercalcemic patients treated with calcitonin as a single agent achieve a normal serum calcium value. High doses of calcitonin (6 to 8 IU/kg every 6 hours) should be employed for acute treatment of hypercalcemia. Absent thrombocytopenia, the drug should be administered intramuscularly rather than subcutaneously to ensure complete absorption. Corticosteroids probably do not enhance the hypocalcemic effects of calcitonin in patients whose underlying disease is not steroid-responsive.[102] The drug does not appear to be effective when administered by nasal insufflation.[106] Because of its rapid action, calcitonin has been increasingly used in combination with more potent antiresorptive drugs such as gallium nitrate and pamidronate, and this combination, in addition to vigorous intravenous hydration, is excellent therapy for critically ill patients with acute severe hypercalcemia.[107]

Corticosteroids

Corticosteroids acutely inhibit osteoclast-mediated bone resorption *in vitro*[108] and decrease gastrointestinal calcium resorption.[109] Corticosteroids are most useful in patients whose underlying tumor is responsive to the cytostatic action of these drugs. These diseases include myeloma, lymphoma, leukemia, and occasional patients with carcinoma of the breast (particularly those who have a hypercalcemic *flare* during hormonal therapy). Corticosteroids do not have consistent hypocalcemic activity in other diseases[110,111] and should not be used in these conditions due to adverse effects. Prednisone (40 to 100 mg/d or its equivalent) is usually effective in controlling hypercalcemia caused by hematologic cancers; lower doses (15 to 30 mg/d) may suffice for patients with hypercalcemic flares caused by breast cancer. However, most patients who require therapy should be treated with a specific antiresorptive drug.

Phosphates

An increase in serum phosphorus concentration decreases osteoclastic activity, inhibits calcium resorption from bone, and causes a significant reduction in urinary calcium excretion.[112] However, administration of exogenous phosphate to hypercalcemic patients also shifts calcium from blood to other tissues that can result in severe toxicity. Oral phosphate (0.5 to 3.0 g/d) may be highly effective, particularly in mild forms of hypercalcemia[113]; principal side effects are diarrhea and nausea, which may lead to noncompliance. Serum phosphorus concentrations should be monitored in all patients who receive phosphates, especially patients with decreased renal function or preexisting hyperphosphatemia.[114] Serum creatinine should be regularly monitored to avoid renal insufficiency. When the [calcium × phosphorus product] (expressed in milligrams per deciliter) exceeds 55, phosphate should be discontinued.

Intravenous phosphate is highly effective and the onset of hypocalcemic action occurs more rapidly than with any other hypocalcemic therapy. However, renal failure, hypotension, extraskeletal calcification, and severe hypocalcemia are common sequelae of parenteral phosphate therapy,[115] and the use of intravenous phosphate has largely been abandoned. Although uncommon, these effects have occasionally been seen with oral phosphates.[114,116]

Plicamycin

Plicamycin (formerly mithramycin) induces hypocalcemia by a direct cytotoxic effect on osteoclasts,[117] thereby decreasing cell-mediated bone resorption. Plicamycin is administered at doses ranging from 10 to 50 μg/kg of body weight. The usual dose is 25 μg/kg or a total dose of 1.5 to 2.0 mg given as a brief infusion. Since the onset of action occurs after 24 to 48 hours,[118,119] doses should not be repeated more frequently than every 2 days. Except for nausea, single injections are generally well tolerated; the incidence of adverse effects (renal insufficiency, hepatotoxicity, thrombocytopenia, and a hemorrhagic diathesis) increases with multiple injections.[120]

GENERAL APPROACH TO TREATMENT OF HYPERCALCEMIA

Patients with hypercalcemia can be divided according to those who require urgent in-hospital therapy and those for whom outpatient therapy can be considered. Table 51.3-4 presents a list of considerations that influence this level of care decision. Hospitalization should be considered for any patient with a serum calcium greater than 12.0 mg/dL or for any patient with significant signs and symptoms, particularly nausea, dehydration, or confusion. Hypercalcemia that has evolved slowly may

TABLE 51.3-4. Approach to the Management of Patients with Cancer-Related Hypercalcemia: Criteria to Ascertain Level of Care

Outpatient	*Inpatient*
Serum calcium <12.0 mg/dL	Serum calcium ≥12.0 mg/dL
No significant nausea	Nausea or vomiting
Able to ingest fluids	Dehydration
Fatigue	Altered mental status
Normal renal function	Renal insufficiency
Stable cardiac rhythm	Cardiac arrhythmia
Mild constipation	Obstipation, ileus
Companion for supervision	Lives alone
Access to emergency care	Limited access to medical care

rapidly progress after a patient begins vomiting or if mentation is impaired.

EMERGENCY TREATMENT OF HOSPITALIZED PATIENTS

Intravenous hydration should be initiated immediately in patients who require hospitalization. Furosemide should be given only if diuresis is inadequate or to treat problems related to fluid retention. Most patients with significant hypercalcemia (total calcium greater than or equal to 12.0 mg/dL) do not respond satisfactorily to intravenous fluids, and pamidronate, which is now first-line therapy, should be administered shortly after hydration has been started and satisfactory urinary output established. Patients who do not respond to two pamidronate infusions (administered 48 to 72 hours apart) should be considered for additional therapy, such as gallium nitrate. For patients with a serum calcium greater than or equal to 15.0 mg/dL or severe symptoms (e.g., coma, cardiac irritability), calcitonin (8 U/kg as an intramuscular injection every 6 hours for 2 to 3 days) can be added immediately to provide an acute hypocalcemic effect.[107,121] Corticosteroids should also be given, but only if the underlying disease is steroid-responsive. Mithramycin should generally be reserved for patients without thrombocytopenia or significant renal or hepatic dysfunction who do not respond to pamidronate or gallium nitrate. Hypercalcemic patients with marked renal insufficiency (especially those with myeloma) should be considered candidates for immediate dialysis.[122]

AMBULATORY MANAGEMENT OF HYPERCALCEMIC PATIENTS

One of the major goals of outpatient therapy is to reduce the need for hospitalization. Ambulatory patients must receive clear instructions regarding increased oral fluid intake. The amount of fluid should be stated in terms that the patient and family understand. It is imperative that a family member or companion attend the patient to ensure that nausea caused by worsening hypercalcemia does not lead to further dehydration. Diuretics such as furosemide should not be added since the risk of dehydration outweighs any theoretical benefits in ambulatory patients who are not edematous.

The most commonly used therapy is pamidronate (60 to 90 mg intravenously over 2 to 4 hours). The schedule can be titrated according to the patients needs, but the drug is usually given every 7 to 14 days. Oral bisphosphonates are not useful. In patients with PTH-RP–mediated hypercalcemia, neutral phosphorus (1 to 3 g/d in divided doses) can be quite useful in the setting of hypophosphatemia, so long as renal function is maintained. Oral corticosteroids are helpful if the underlying disease is steroid-responsive. The use of calcitonin has largely been supplanted by the bisphosphonates. Plicamycin can also be administered in doses of 10 to 25 μg/kg once or twice per week with close monitoring for evidence of myelosuppression or changes in renal or hepatic function.[123]

MANAGEMENT OF CHRONIC RECURRENT HYPERCALCEMIA

The management of acute hypercalcemic episodes is relatively straightforward. However, an increasing problem is the patient whose underlying disease is poorly or incompletely responsive to primary antitumor therapy, and who continues to develop multiple episodes of hypercalcemia. In this setting, the primary goal of treatment is to prevent exacerbations that require repeated hospitalization. Several principles underlie the management of such patients. First, hypocalcemic treatment must be given on a chronic schedule and must not reserved for treatment of acute recurrent episodes, even if the patient is relatively normocalcemic. Second, the dosing schedule of pamidronate, once initiated, can be progressively intensified up to a maximum of 90 mg IV twice per week. Third, hypocalcemic drugs should be continued indefinitely unless the patient has sustained a major antitumor response. Patients should not be declared *pamidronate-resistant.* Rather, the bisphosphonate should be continued on a maximally intensive schedule and additional drugs, including gallium nitrate, calcitonin, oral phosphate, and plicamycin, should be added to the regimen until the serum calcium can be consistently maintained below 12.0 mg/dL.

HYPERURICEMIA

Uric acid is formed as a result of the sequential catalysis of hypoxanthine and xanthine by xanthine oxidase. Renal insufficiency develops when urine becomes supersaturated with urate and crystals of uric acid form in the renal tubules and distal collecting system.[124] Uric acid stones may also develop, although this presentation is more commonly associated with chronic hyperuricemia.

Renal complications and arthritis are the most important consequences of acute or chronic hyperuricemia. The disorder occurs most commonly in hematologic neoplasms, particularly the leukemias, high-grade lymphomas, and myeloproliferative diseases.[125–127] Acute urate nephropathy has also been reported after chemotherapy for solid tumors. Patients at highest risk include those with bulky high-grade lymphomas, patients with high leukocyte counts undergoing remission-induction chemotherapy for acute or chronic leukemia, and individuals with preexisting renal impairment (especially those with ureteral obstruction). Hyperuricemia is also a side effect of certain agents, notably diuretics (thiazides and furosemide), and antituberculosis drugs (pyrazinamide, ethambutol, and nicotinic acid).

TREATMENT

Recognition of patients at risk is essential for proper therapy. It is essential that prophylactic measures be undertaken *before* cytotoxic therapy is initiated. Drugs that tend to elevate serum urate or that produce an acidic urine (thiazides and salicylates) should be withdrawn. All patients should receive intravenous hydration to correct preexisting deficits of intravascular volume and to ensure continued urinary output. Increased urinary volume decreases the concentration of urate in urine and thus minimizes problems with respect to urate solubility.[128] Although furosemide theoretically promotes increased tubular urate reabsorption, this effect is outweighed by its acute diuretic action; thus, the drug can be safely used to maintain satisfactory urine output so long as fluid status and serum electrolytes are monitored and replaced. Alkalinization of the urine should be initiated to maintain a urine pH greater than or equal to 7.0. Although oral sodium bicarbonate can be used, it is usually simpler to add sodium bicarbonate solution (50 to 100 mmol/L) to intravenous fluids and then to adjust the admixture so that an alkaline urine pH is maintained. Acetazolamide (an inhibitor of carbonic anhydrase) may be used to increase the effects of alkalinization. However, it must be emphasized that alkalinization is secondary to the overall goal of decreasing urinary uric acid concentration by increasing urinary volume.

The mainstay of current drug therapy is allopurinol, which inhibits xanthine oxidase and consequently increases plasma and urinary concentrations of xanthine and hypoxanthine. Although xanthine is somewhat more soluble than uric acid, allopurinol has occasionally been associated with renal failure due to xanthine nephropathy.[129] The drug is generally well tolerated. The most common adverse reaction is a blanching, erythematous skin rash that indicates hypersensitivity. The onset of this reaction is usually delayed for several days after initial administration, and the drug can usually be continued throughout periods of greatest risk in patients who have not had prior exposure. In acute situations, the drug is administered orally once or twice per day in daily doses ranging from 300 to 900 mg. The dose of certain drugs that are metabolized by xanthine oxidase (e.g., 6-mercaptopurine) must be substantially reduced during treatment with allopurinol.

Patients in renal failure and allopurinol-sensitive individuals represent uncommon but difficult management problems.[130] Intravenous administration of uricase has also been useful in certain circumstances.[131,132] In the face of acute oliguria, ultrasonography or computed tomographic (CT) scanning should be used to evaluate possible ureteral obstruction by urate calculi. Administration of intravenous contrast agents for pyelography should be avoided due to an increased risk of acute tubular necrosis.[133] Peritoneal or hemodialysis has been quite effective in reversing renal failure due to urate deposition.

TUMOR LYSIS SYNDROME

The tumor lysis syndrome occurs as a result of the rapid release of intracellular contents into the blood stream, which then increase to life-threatening concentrations. The syndrome is characterized by hyperuricemia, hyperkalemia, hyperphosphatemia, and hypocalcemia.[127,134,135] Lethal cardiac arrhythmias are the most serious consequences of hyperkalemia. Hyperphosphatemia may result in acute renal failure.[136,137] Elevated serum phosphorus may also decrease renal function, which can lead to further reductions in urinary potassium and phosphate excretion. Hypocalcemia, a result of hyperphosphatemia, may cause muscle cramps, cardiac arrhythmias, and tetany.[138]

The tumor lysis syndrome occurs most commonly in diseases with large tumor burdens and high proliferative fractions that are exquisitely sensitive to cytotoxic treatment. These disorders include high-grade lymphomas,[139] leukemias with high leukocyte counts,[140] and (much less commonly) solid tumors.[141,142] The syndrome has been observed not only with agents that have potent myelosuppressive activity, but also with drugs such as interferon-α,[143] tamoxifen,[144] cladribine,[145] and intrathecal methotrexate.[146] Although not related to tumor lysis, severe hypocalcemia has been associated with estrogenic treatment of prostate cancer[147] and with accelerated bone formation in patients with leukemia.[148]

TREATMENT

Recognition of risk and prevention are essential to management. Patients at risk should be identified before the initiation of chemotherapy. If possible, intravenous hydration should be started 24 to 48 hours before administration of chemotherapy. Any acid–base or electrolyte disorders should be corrected (although intravenous administration of sodium bicarbonate may aggravate symptoms of hypocalcemia). Treatment with allopurinol should be undertaken along with other measures to minimize hyperuricemia as described previously. Serum electrolytes, uric acid, phosphorus, calcium, and creatinine should be checked every few hours for 3 to 4 days after initiating cytotoxic treatment. The frequency of monitoring should depend on the clinical condition of the patient. If significant hyperkalemia or hypocalcemia become evident, an electrocardiogram should be obtained and the cardiac rhythm should be monitored while these abnormalities are corrected. In most patients, hypocalcemia can be corrected with intravenous administration of calcium gluconate; however, patients who have persistent hypocalcemia should be treated with calcitriol until the syndrome resolves.[149] Hyperkalemia (serum $[K^+]$ greater than or equal to 5.0 mg/dL) should be treated with an oral sodium-potassium exchange resin (e.g., Kayexalate, 15 g orally every 6 hours) or with combined insulin and glucose therapy.

In the face of acutely worsening renal function after administration of chemotherapy, consideration should be given to the *early* initiation of renal dialysis in order to rapidly control serum concentrations of potassium, calcium, phosphate, and uric acid, as well as other problems related to uremia. The dose of many drugs, especially antineoplastics, requires substantial modification in the presence of renal insufficiency.

LACTIC ACIDOSIS

Lactic acidosis is a rare but potentially severe metabolic complication in patients with cancer. Type A lactic acidosis results from impaired delivery of oxygen to peripheral tissue and is commonly seen with shock and septicemia. Type B lactic acidosis is associated with a variety of diseases (including diabetes, renal failure, liver disease, infection, and cancer) as well as drugs (such as metformin), toxins, and hereditary diseases.[150–152] Lactic acidosis is characterized by decreased arterial pH (less than 7.37) secondary to accumulation of blood lactate (greater than 2 mEq/L). The disorder is a consequence of both increased lactate production and impaired use. Lactate is a metabolite of pyruvate and is produced in a cytosolic reaction catalyzed by lactic dehydrogenase, an enzyme with an absolute requirement for nicotinamide adenine dinucleotide (NAD). Consequently, the concentrations of pyruvate, hydrogen ion, and NAD regulate lactate metabolism. Accelerated glycogenolysis increases pyruvate production and decreases tissue oxygen, which in turn decreases levels of NAD. As NAD is depleted, gluconeogenesis is halted and pyruvate increases. Anaerobic metabolism of pyruvate to lactate is increased, which also leads to accumulation of NADH and hydrogen ion.[153]

In a review of 25 cases of lactic acidosis in which the underlying tumor was believed to represent the primary etiologic factor, more than two-thirds were associated with leukemia or lymphoma.[154] The development of lactic acidosis coincided with the onset of progressive disease in the hematologic cancers, whereas most patients with solid tumors had extensive liver metastases. Antiviral drugs, such as azidothymidine and fialuridine, have produced hepatic failure and severe lactic acidosis.[155,156] Typically, the patient with lactic acidosis presents with hyperventilation and hypotension. Nonspecific clinical symptoms such as tachycardia, weakness, nausea, and stupor may proceed to frank shock as the acidosis worsens. Laboratory studies show decreased blood pH, a widened anion gap (greater than 18), and low serum bicarbonate.[151] It must be noted that primary cancer-induced lactic acidosis is a rare event, and the diagnostic workup should always search for other, potentially more treatable causes.

The prognosis for patients with a serum lactate concentration greater than 4 mEq/L is exceedingly poor; however, the outcome is largely determined by the underlying disease and not the acidosis per se. Several reports have suggested that administration of sodium bicarbonate may actually increase lactate and CO_2 production and impair oxygen delivery.[155–157] Although some deleterious effects of severe acidemia on cardiovascular function could theoretically be ameliorated by sodium bicarbonate,[158] no study has shown a convincing survival advantage for alkali therapy in this condition.[159] Despite ongoing controversy, bicarbonate administration remains a reasonably safe and conservative therapy.[152,160–162]

HYPOGLYCEMIA

Insulin-producing islet cell tumors are the most frequent cause of hypoglycemia in patients with cancer; however, more than 250 cases of hypoglycemia associated with non–islet cell tumors have also been reported.[163] Non–islet cell tumors associated with hypoglycemia tend to be large. In such patients, mesenchymal tumors (fibrosarcomas, leiomyomas, rhabdomyosarcomas, liposarcomas, and mesotheliomas) account for approximately 50% of cases; another 25% are hepatomas.[163–166] Classic symptoms of hypoglycemia (e.g., weakness, dizziness, diaphoresis, and nausea) are nonspecific and may develop slowly. In the initial phases, symptoms tend to be worse in the early morning (due to overnight fasting) and improve after ingestion of food. However, patients may also present acutely with seizures, coma, and focal or diffuse neurologic deficits.

PATHOPHYSIOLOGY

Several etiologic mechanisms for cancer-related hypoglycemia have been proposed: (1) secretion of insulin-like substances; (2) excessive glucose use by the tumor that exceeds hepatic production; and (3) failure of counterregulatory mechanisms that usually prevent hypoglycemia (e.g., reduction in levels of growth hormone). Various substances with nonsuppressible insulin-like activities have been detected in serum from patients with hypoglycemia. These factors are composed of two general classes: one of relatively low-molecular-weight substances that are soluble in acid ethanol, and the other of high molecular weight that are acid-ethanol precipitable. The low-molecular-weight compounds consist of four peptides, the insulin-like growth factors (IGF-1, IGF-2, somatomedin A, and somatomedin C).[167,168] The IGFs share a high degree of amino acid similarity with proinsulin, are bound by circulating proteins that inactivate them, and mediate their biologic activities after binding to specific cell surface receptors.[167,168] They do not react with antiinsulin antibodies and they have only 1% to 2% of the specific metabolic activity of insulin. Insulin itself has a weak affinity for the IGF-1 receptor but not for IGF-2R. IGFs appear to act as growth factors for various tumors and have been proposed as targets for anticancer therapy.

In most patients with non–islet cell tumors that have been associated with hypoglycemia, serum levels of IGF-1 have been appropriately suppressed, whereas levels of IGF-2 have been relatively normal (as measured by radioimmunoassay).[168] However, it now appears that the high-molecular-weight, nonsuppressible-insulin-like-activities molecule is actually a propeptide of IGF-2, so-called big IGF-2, secreted by tumor cells that are incompletely cleaved.[169] The large size either prevents formation of an acid-labile subunit from binding or impairs binding of a critical molecule (IGF-binding protein 3), which inactivates the protein; thus, the bound molecule retains its biologic activity.[170–171]

Accelerated glucose use by large tumors may also account for cancer-related hypoglycemia in some patients. It has been estimated that a 1-kg tumor may use from 50 to 200 g of glucose per day.[172] Since the liver can produce approximately 700 g of glucose per day, hepatic production should theoretically be sufficient to prevent hypoglycemia. However, many patients with hypoglycemia have tumors that weigh several kilograms along with extensive hepatic metastases; thus, the combination of accelerated glucose use with impaired production may lead to hypoglycemia.

Finally, a failure of the usual counterregulatory mechanisms in patients with large tumors may also induce hypoglycemia.[173] Impaired liver function can decrease glycogenolysis and gluconeogenesis. Certain patients with cancer have a depressed hyperglycemic response to the administration of glucagon[174]; depressed secretion of counterregulatory hormones such as glucagon, adrenocorticotropic hormone (ACTH), glucocorticoids, and growth hormone has also been reported. However, there remains little direct evidence to support this hypothesis as an important clinical mechanism of tumor-induced hypoglycemia.

THERAPY

Therapy of hypoglycemia should match the severity of the condition. As with most paraneoplastic syndromes, specific antitumor therapy is the preferred treatment. To date, chemotherapeutic agents that are cytotoxic for islet cells or that block insulin release or activity have had little effect on production, release, or activity of IGFs. Mild hypoglycemia can usually be managed by increasing the frequency of meals. In patients with more severe or unpredictable symptoms, the administration of corticosteroids and glucagon may afford symptomatic relief. Intravenous infusions of glucose provide temporary support while other specific treatment is administered (i.e., surgery, chemotherapy, or radiation). Under certain circumstances, continuous infusions of glucagon using portable pumps have been used with some success.[173]

ADRENAL FAILURE

Symptomatic adrenocortical insufficiency due to destruction of cortical tissue by metastatic carcinoma is uncommon. More common are iatrogenic causes such as surgical adrenalectomy, treatment with mitotane (o-p'-DDD) and inhibitors of steroid synthesis such as aminoglutethimide, chronic corticosteroid therapy, and occasionally adrenal hemorrhage.[174–179] Nonetheless, technical improvements in CT and magnetic resonance imaging have increased the likelihood of making an antemortem diagnosis of adrenal metastases. In one study, 19% of patients with metastatic cancer and enlargement of the adrenal glands by CT scans developed symptoms of adrenal insufficiency.[174] In a separate study wherein 15 patients with metastatic cancer and adrenal enlargement on CT scan were evaluated by ACTH stimulation, one-third were judged to have adrenal insufficiency. Further clinical study revealed symptoms of nausea, anorexia, and orthostatic hypotension in all of these patients.[175] Adrenal insufficiency may thus develop insidiously in patients with adrenal metastasis, and CT scans and ACTH testing may be useful diagnostic tools.

CLINICAL MANIFESTATIONS

Classic signs and symptoms of adrenal insufficiency include weakness, weight loss, anorexia, hyperpigmentation, and postural hypotension. One or more of these symptoms are evident in almost all patients, but the onset of symptoms is frequently insidious. Circulatory collapse and shock are uncommon but may develop with the onset of infection. Biochemical evaluation frequently reveals a mild acidosis (without an anion gap), hyponatremia, and hypokalemia.

EVALUATION AND TREATMENT

Because an ACTH-stimulation test is a benign procedure, this test is recommended when symptoms suggestive of adrenal insufficiency are evident. Typically, patients receive Cosyntropin, 0.25 mg intravenously, and serum cortisol is monitored at baseline, 30 minutes, and 1 hour. An increase in serum cortisol of 5 to 7 μg/dL over baseline levels (to a minimum of 15 μg/mL) is considered normal. If adrenal insufficiency is strongly suspected on clinical grounds, steroid replacement (or stress doses of steroids) should be started immediately, and subsequent therapy can be reevaluated when results of the ACTH test become available.

Physiologic glucocorticoid replacement is attained by administration of cortisone acetate (25 mg in the morning and 12.5 mg in the early evening). During periods of stress (e.g., operative procedures or infection), these doses may need to be doubled or tripled. Occasionally, mineralocorticoid replacement (0.05 to 0.1 mg of fludrocortisone) is required in addition to cortisone acetate. In patients with no adrenocortical function whatsoever, maintenance doses of dexamethasone or prednisone do not provide adequate mineralocorticoid coverage and fludrocortisone must be given. Pharmacologic doses of parenteral glucocorticoids are required in the setting of acute adrenal failure and circulatory collapse. Typically, aqueous-soluble forms of hydrocortisone (e.g., sodium succinate salt) at doses of 100 mg intravenously every 8 hours are required. Thereafter, the patient should be monitored for evidence of hyperglycemia, hypokalemia, or hypernatremia.

REFERENCES

1. Raue F. Epidemiological aspects of hypercalcemia of malignancy. *Rec Res Cancer Res* 1994;137:99.
2. Vassilopoulou-Sellin R, Newman B, Taylor SH, et al. Incidence of hypercalcemia in patients with malignancy referred to a comprehensive cancer center. *Cancer* 1993;71:1309.
3. Brada M, Rowley M, Grant DJ, et al. Hypercalcemia in patients with disseminated breast cancer. *Acta Oncol* 1990;29:577.
4. Coggeshall J, Merrill W, Hande K, et al. Implications of hypercalcemia with respect to diagnosis and treatment of lung cancer. *Am J Med* 1986;80:325.
5. Van Dijk JM. Hypercalcemia in prostatic carcinoma: case report and review of the literature. *Am J Clin Oncol* 1993;16:329.
6. Axelrod DM, Bockman RS, Wong GY, et al. Distinguishing features of primary hyperparathyroidism in patients with breast cancer. *Cancer* 1987;60:1620.
7. Hutchesson ACJ, Bundred NJ, Ratcliffe WA. Survival in hypercalcemic patients with cancer and co-existing primary hyperparathyroidism. *Postgrad Med J* 1995;71:28.
8. Lafferty FW. Differential diagnosis of hypercalcemia. *J Bone Miner Res* 1991;6(Suppl 2):S51.
9. Schmidt-Gayk H, Haerdt H. Differential diagnosis of hypercalcemia: laboratory assessment. *Rec Res Cancer Res* 1994;137:122.
10. Nussbaum SR, Potts JT Jr. Immunoassays for parathyroid hormone 1–84 in the diagnosis of hyperparathyroidism. *J Bone Miner Res* 1991;6(Suppl 2):S43.
11. Ratcliffe WA, Hutcheson ACJ, Bundred NJ, et al. Role of assays for parathyroid hormone-related protein in investigation of hypercalcemia. *Lancet* 1992;339:164.
12. Annesley TM, Burritt MF, Kyle RA. Artifactual hypercalcemia in multiple myeloma. *Mayo Clin Proc* 1982;57:572.
13. Payne RB, Carver ME, Morgan DB. Interpretation of serum total calcium: effects of adjustment for albumin concentration on frequency of abnormal values and on detection of change in the individual. *J Clin Pathol* 1979;32:56.
14. Stewart AF, Horst R, Deftos LJ, et al. Biochemical evaluation of patients with cancer-associated hypercalcemia: evidence for humoral and non-humoral groups. *N Engl J Med* 1980;303:1377.
15. Skrabanek P, McPartlin J, Powell D. Tumor hypercalcemia and "ectopic hyperparathyroidism." *Medicine* 1980;59:262.
16. Simpson EL, Mundy GR, D'Souza SM, et al. Absence of parathyroid messenger RNA in nonparathyroid tumors associated with hypercalcemia. *N Engl J Med* 1983;309:325.
17. Wynne AG, Van Heerden J, Carney JA, et al. Parathyroid carcinoma: clinical and pathological features in 43 patients. *Medicine* 1992;71:197.
18. Nussbaum SR, Gaz RD, Arnold A. Hypercalcemia and ectopic secretion of parathyroid hormone by an ovarian carcinoma with rearrangement of the gene for parathyroid hormone. *N Engl J Med* 1990;323:1324.
19. Strewler GJ, Budayr AA, Clark OH, et al. Production of parathyroid hormone by a malignant nonparathyroid tumor in a hypercalcemic patient. *J Clin Endocrinol Metab* 1993;76:1373.
20. Moseley JM, Kubota M, Dieffenbach-Jagger H, et al. Parathyroid hormone-related protein purified from a human lung cancer cell line. *Proc Natl Acad Sci U S A* 1987;84:5048.
21. Suva LJ, Winslow GA, Wettenhall REH, et al. A parathyroid hormone-related protein implicated in malignant hypercalcemia: cloning and expression. *Science* 1987;237:894.
22. Mangin M, Webb AC, Dreyer BE, et al. Identification of a cDNA encoding a parathyroid hormone-like peptide from a human tumor associated with humoral hypercalcemia of malignancy. *Proc Natl Acad Sci U S A* 1988;85:597.
23. Abol-Samra A-B, Juppner H, Force T, et al. Expression cloning of a common receptor for parathyroid hormone and parathyroid hormone-related peptide from rat osteoblast-like cells: a single receptor stimulates intracellular accumulation of both cAMP and inositol triphosphates and increases intracellular free calcium. *Proc Natl Acad Sci U S A* 1992;89:2732.
24. Weir EC, Brines ML, Ikeda K, et al. Parathyroid hormone-related peptide gene is expressed in the mammalian central nervous system. *Proc Natl Acad Sci U S A* 1990;87:108.
25. Thiede MA, Daifotis AG, Weir EC, et al. Intrauterine occupancy controls expression of the parathyroid hormone-related peptide gene in preterm rat myometrium. *Proc Natl Acad Sci U S A* 1990;87:6969.
26. Yamamoto M, Harm SC, Grasser WA, et al. Parathyroid hormone-related protein in the rat urinary bladder: a smooth muscle relaxant produced locally in response to mechanical stretch. *Proc Natl Acad Sci U S A* 1992;89:5326.
27. Deftos LJ, Burton DW, Brandt DW. Parathyroid hormone-like protein is a secretory product of atrial myocytes. *J Clin Invest* 1993;92:727.
28. Vortkamp A, Lee K, Lanske B, et al. Regulation of cartilage differentiation by Indian Hedgehog and PTH-related protein. *Science* 1996;273:613.

29. Lanske B, Karaplis AC, Kaechong L, et al. PTH/PTHrP receptor in early development and Indian hedgehog-regulated bone growth. *Science* 1996;273:663.
30. Knecht TP, Behling CA, Burton DW, et al. The humoral hypercalcemia of benignancy: a newly appreciated syndrome. *Am J Clin Pathol* 1996;105:487.
31. Burtis WJ, Brady TG, Orloff JJ, et al. Immunochemical characterization of circulating parathyroid hormone-related protein in patients with humoral hypercalcemia of cancer. *N Engl J Med* 1990;322:1106.
32. Rankin W, Grill V, Martin TJ. Parathyroid hormone-related protein and hypercalcemia. *Cancer* 1997;80:1564.
33. Wysolmerski JJ, Broadus AE. Hypercalcemia of malignancy: the central role of parathyroid hormone related protein. *Annu Rev Med* 1994;45:189.
34. Blind E. Humoral hypercalcemia of malignancy: role of parathyroid hormone-related protein. *Rec Res Cancer Res* 1994;137:20.
35. Bucht E, Rong H, Pernow Y, et al. Parathyroid hormone-related protein in patients with primary breast cancer and eucalcemia. *Cancer Res* 1998;58:4113.
36. Firkin F, Schneider H, Grill V. Parathyroid hormone-related protein in hypercalemia associated with hematological malignancy. *Leuk Lymphoma* 1998;29:499.
37. Dunbar ME, Wysolmerski JJ, Broadus AE. Parathyroid hormone-related protein: from hypercalcemia of malignancy to developmental regulatory molecule. *Am J Med Sci* 1996;312:287.
38. Watanabe T, Yamaguchi K, Takasuki K, et al. Constitutive expression of parathyroid hormone-related protein gene in human T-cell leukemia virus type 1 (HTLV-1) carriers and adult T-cell leukemia patients that can be transactivated by HTLV-1 tax gene. *J Exp Med* 1990;172:759.
39. Prager D, Rosenblatt JD, Ejima E. Hypercalcemia, parathyroid hormone-related protein expression and human T-cell leukemia virus infection. *Leuk Lymphoma* 1994;14:395.
40. Motokura T, Fukumoto S, Matsumoto T, et al. Parathyroid hormone-related protein in adult T-cell leukemia-lymphoma. *Ann Intern Med* 1989;111:484.
41. Powell GJ, Southby J, Danks JA, et al. Localization of parathyroid hormone-related protein in breast cancer metastases: increased incidence in bone compared with other sites. *Cancer Res* 1991;51:3059.
42. Iwamura M, Sant'Agnese PA, Wu G, et al. Immunohistochemical localization of parathyroid hormone-related protein in human prostate cancer. *Cancer Res* 1993;53:1724.
43. Bouizar Z, Spyratos F, Deytieux S, et al. Polymerase chain reaction analysis of parathyroid hormone-related protein gene expression in breast cancer patients and occurrence of bone metastases. *Cancer Res* 1993;53:5076.
44. Budayr AA, Zysset E, Jenzer A, et al. Effects of treatment of malignancy-associated hypercalcemia on serum parathyroid hormone-related protein. *J Bone Miner Res* 1994;9:521.
45. Body JJ, Dumon JC, Thirion M, et al. Circulating PTH-RP concentration in tumor-induced hypercalcemia: influence on the response to bisphosphonate and changes after therapy. *J Bone Miner Res* 1993;8:701.
46. Wimalawansa SJ. Significance of plasma PTH-rp in patients with hypercalcemia of malignancy treated with bisphosphonate. *Cancer* 1994;73:2223.
47. Gurney H, Grill V, Martin TJ. Parathyroid hormone-related protein and response to pamidronate in tumour-induced hypercalcaemia. *Lancet* 1993;341:1611.
48. Pecherstorfer M, Schilling T, Blind E, et al. Parathyroid hormone-related protein and life expectancy in hypercalcemic cancer patients. *J Clin Endocrinol Metab* 1994;78:1268.
49. Seymour JF, Gagel RF. Calcitriol: the major humoral mediator of hypercalcemia in Hodgkin's disease and non-Hodgkin's lymphoma. *Blood* 1993;82:1383.
50. Seymour JF, Gagel RF, Hagemeister FB, et al. Calcitriol production in hypercalcemic and normocalcemic patients with non-Hodgkin lymphoma. *Ann Intern Med* 1994;121:633.
51. Cox M, Haddad JG. Lymphoma, hypercalcemia, and the sunshine vitamin [Editorial]. *Ann Intern Med* 1994;121:709.
52. Adams JS, Fernandez M, Gacad MA, et al. Vitamin D metabolite-mediated hypercalcemia and hypercalciuria in patients with AIDS and non-AIDS-related lymphoma. *Blood* 1989;73:235.
53. Shigeno H, Yamamoto I, Dokoh S, et al. Identification of 1,24 (R)-dihydroxyvitamin D_3-like bone-resorbing lipid in a patient with cancer-associated hypercalcemia. *J Clin Endocrinol Metab* 1985;61:761.
54. Sandler LM, Winearls CG, Fraher LJ, et al. Studies of the hypercalcemia of sarcoidosis: effects of steroids and exogenous vitamin D_3 on the circulating concentrations of 1,25-dihydroxy vitamin D_3. *Q J Med* 1984;53:165.
55. Broadus AE, Erickson SB, Gertner JM, et al. An experimental model of 1,25-dihydroxyvitamin D-mediated hypercalciuria. *J Clin Endocrinol Metab* 1984;59:202.
56. Schweitzer DH, Hamdy NAT, Frolich M, et al. Malignancy-associated hypercalcemia: resolution of controversies over vitamin D metabolism by a pathophysiological approach to the syndrome. *Clin Endocrinol* 1994;41:251.
57. Brenner BE, Harvey HA, Lipton A, et al. A study of prostaglandin E2, parathormone, and response to indomethacin in patients with hypercalcemia of malignancy. *Cancer* 1982;49:556.
58. Valentin-Opran A, Eilon G, Saez S, et al. Estrogens and antiestrogens stimulate release of bone-resorbing activity by cultured human breast cancer cells. *J Clin Invest* 1985;75:726.
59. Metz SA, McRae JR, Robertson RP. Prostaglandins as mediators of paraneoplastic syndromes: review and update. *Metabolism* 1981;30:299.
60. Robertson RB, Baylink DJ, Metz SA, et al. Plasma prostaglandin E in patients with cancer with and without hypercalcemia. *J Clin Endocrinol Metab* 1976;43:1330.
61. Bringhurst FR, Bierer BE, Godeau F, et al. Humoral hypercalcemia of malignancy: release of a prostaglandin-stimulating bone-resorbing factor *in vitro* by human transitional-cell carcinoma cells. *J Clin Invest* 1986;77:456.
62. Ibbotson KJ, Twardzik DR, D'Souza SM, et al. Stimulation of bone resorption in vitro by synthetic transforming growth factor-α. *Science* 1985;228:1007.
63. Guise TA, Yoneda T, Yates AJ, et al. The combined effect of tumor-produced parathyroid hormone-related protein and transforming growth factor-α enhance hypercalcemia in vivo and bone resorption in vitro. *J Clin Endocrinol Metab* 1993;77:40.
64. Ishimi Y, Miyaura C, Jin CH, et al. IL-6 is produced by osteoblasts and induces bone resorption. *J Immunol* 1990;145:3297.
65. Bataille R, Jourdan M, Zhang X-G, et al. Serum levels of interleukin-6, a potent myeloma cell growth factor, as a reflection of disease severity in plasma cell dyscrasias. *J Clin Invest* 1989;84:604.
66. Weissglas MG, Schamhart DH, Lowik CW, et al. The role of interleukin-6 in the induction of hypercalcemia in renal cell carcinoma transplanted into nude mice. *Endocrinology* 1997;138:1879.
67. Yoneda T, Nakai M, Moriyama K, et al. Neutralizing antibodies to human interleukin 6 reverse hypercalcemia associated with a human squamous carcinoma. *Cancer Res* 1993;53:737.
68. Stashenko P, Dewhirst FE, Peros WJ, et al. Synergistic interactions between interleukin-1, tumor necrosis factor, and lymphotoxin in bone resorption. *J Immunol* 1987;138:1464.
69. Sato K, Mimura H, Han DC, et al. Production of bone-resorbing activity and colony-stimulating activity in vivo and in vitro by a human squamous cell carcinoma associated with hypercalcemia and leukocytosis. *J Clin Invest* 1986;78:145.
70. Garrett IR, Durie BGM, Nedwin GE, et al. Production of lymphotoxin, a bone-resorbing cytokine, by cultured human myeloma cells. *N Engl J Med* 1987;317:526.
71. Chisholm MA, Mulloy AL, Taylor AT. Acute management of cancer-related hypercalcemia. *Ann Pharmacother* 1996;30:507.
72. Barri YM, Knochel JP. Hypercalcemia and electrolyte disturbances in malignancy. *Hematol Oncol Clin North Am* 1996;10:775.
73. Warrell RP Jr. Questions about clinical trials in hypercalcemia [Editorial]. *J Clin Oncol* 1988;6:759.
74. Massry SG, Friedler RM, Coburn JW. Excretion of phosphate and calcium: physiology of their renal handling and relation to clinical medicine. *Arch Intern Med* 1973;131:828.
75. Suki WN, Yium JJ, Von Minden M, et al. Acute treatment of hypercalcemia with furosemide. *N Engl J Med* 1970;283:836.
76. Hosking DJ, Cowley A, Bucknall CA. Rehydration in the treatment of severe hypercalcemia. *Q J Med* 1981;200:473.
77. Carano A, Teitelbaum SL, Konsek JD, et al. Bisphosphonates directly inhibit the bone resorption activity of isolated avian osteoclasts in vitro. *J Clin Invest* 1990;85:456.
78. Gucalp R, Ritch P, Wiernik PH, et al. Comparative study of pamidronate disodium and etidronate disodium in the treatment of cancer-related hypercalcemia. *J Clin Oncol* 1992;10:134.
79. Gucalp R, Theriault R, Gill I, et al. Treatment of cancer-associated hypercalcemia: double-blind comparison of rapid and slow intravenous infusion regimens of pamidronate disodium and saline alone. *Arch Intern Med* 1994;154:1935.
80. Nussbaum SR, Younger J, VandePol CJ, et al. Single-dose intravenous therapy with pamidronate for the treatment of hypercalcemia of malignancy: comparison of 30-, 60-, and 90-mg dosages. *Am J Med* 1993;95:297.
81. Body JJ, Dumon JC. Treatment of tumour-induced hypercalcaemia with the bisphosphonate pamidronate: dose-response relationship and influence of tumour type. *Ann Oncol* 1994;5:359.
82. Gallacher SJ, Ralston SH, Fraser WD, et al. A comparison of low versus high dose pamidronate in cancer-associated hypercalcemia. *Bone Miner* 1991;15:249.
83. Bertheault-Cvitkovic F, Armand J-P, Tubiana-Hulin M, et al. Randomized, double blind comparison of pamidronate vs. gallium nitrate for acute control of cancer-related hypercalcemia. *Proceedings of the 9th EORTC/NCI Symposium on New Drugs in Cancer Therapy* 1996;140.
84. Hortobagyi GN, Theriault RL, Lipton A, et al. Long-term prevention of skeletal complications of metastatic breast cancer with pamidronate. *J Clin Oncol* 1998;16:2038.
85. Gallacher SJ, Fraser WD, Logue FC, et al. Factors predicting the acute effect of pamidronate on serum calcium in hypercalcemia of malignancy. *Calcif Tissue Int* 1992;51:419.
86. Walls J, Ratcliffe WA, Howell A, et al. Response to intravenous bisphosphonate therapy in hypercalcemic patients with and without bone metastases: the role of parathyroid hormone-related protein. *Br J Cancer* 1994;70:169.
87. Dodwell DJ, Abbas SK, Morton AR, et al. Parathyroid hormone-related protein (50–69) and response to pamidronate therapy for tumour-induced hypercalcemia. *Eur J Cancer* 1991;27:1629.
88. Body JJ, Louviaux I, Dumon JC. Decreased efficacy of bisphosphonates for recurrences of tumor-induced hypercalcemia-mechanisms and influence of the tumor type. *Proc Am Soc Clin Oncol* 1998;17:169.
89. Warrell RP Jr, Mullane M, Bilezikian J, et al. Treatment of cancer-associated hypercalcemia with alendronate: a randomized double-blind comparison with etidronate. *Proc Am Soc Clin Oncol* 1993;12:438.
90. Nussbaum SR, Warrell RP Jr, Rude R, et al. A dose-response study of alendronate for the treatment of malignancy-associated hypercalcemia. *J Clin Oncol* 1993;11:1618.
91. O'Rourke NP, McCloskey EV, Vasikaran S, et al. Effective treatment of malignant hypercalcemia with a single intravenous infusion of clodronate. *Br J Cancer* 1993;67:560.
92. Kanis JA, McCloskey EV. Clodronate. *Cancer* 1997;80(Suppl):1691.
93. Pecherstorfer M, Herrmann Z, Body JJ, et al. Randomized phase II trial comparing different doses of the bisphosphonate ibandronate in the treatment of hypercalcemia of malignancy. *J Clin Oncol* 1996;14:268.
94. Body JJ, Ford JM, Vigneron AM, et al. A dose finding study of zoledronate intravenous infusion in patients with tumour induced hypercalcemia. *J Bone Miner Res* 1996;11(Suppl):S485
95. Body JJ. Clinical research update: zoledronate. *Cancer* 1997;80(Suppl 1):1699.
96. Warrell RP Jr, Bockman RS, Coonley CJ, et al. Gallium nitrate inhibits calcium resorption from bone and is effective treatment for cancer-related hypercalcemia. *J Clin Invest* 1984;73:1487.
97. Hall TJ, Chambers TJ. Gallium inhibits bone resorption by a direct effect on osteoclasts. *Bone Miner* 1990;8:211.

98. Warrell RP Jr, Alcock NW, Skelos A, et al. Gallium nitrate inhibits accelerated bone turnover in patients with bone metastases. *J Clin Oncol* 1987;5:292.
99. Bockman RS, Repo MA, Warrell RP, et al. Distribution of trace levels of therapeutic gallium in bone as mapped by synchrotron x-ray microscopy. *Proc Natl Acad Sci U S A* 1990;87:4149.
100. Bockman RS, Bosley A, Blumenthal NC, et al. Gallium increases bone calcium and crystallite perfection of hydroxyapatite. *Calcif Tissue Int* 1986;39:376.
101. Blair HC, Teitelbaum SL, Tan H-L, et al. Reversible inhibition of osteoclastic activity by bone-bound gallium (III). *J Cell Biochem* 1992;48:401.
102. Warrell RP Jr, Israel R, Frisone M, et al. A randomized double-blind study of gallium nitrate versus calcitonin for acute treatment of cancer-related hypercalcemia. *Ann Intern Med* 1988;108:669.
103. Warrell RP Jr, Heller G, Murphy WP, et al. A randomized double-blind study of gallium nitrate compared to etidronate for acute control of cancer-related hypercalcemia. *J Clin Oncol* 1991;9:1467.
104. Austin LA, Heath H III. Calcitonin: physiology and pathophysiology. *N Engl J Med* 1981;304:269.
105. Wisneski LA. Salmon calcitonin in the acute management of hypercalcemia. *Calcif Tissue Int* 1990;46:S26.
106. Dumon JC, Magritte A, Body JJ. Nasal human calcitonin for tumour-induced hypercalcemia. *Calcif Tissue Int* 1992;51:18.
107. Warrell RP Jr, Crown JP. Recovery from extreme hypercalcemia [Letter]. *Lancet* 1993;342:375.
108. Raisz LG, Trummel CL, Wener JA, et al. Effect of glucocorticoids on bone resorption in tissue culture. *Endocrinology* 1972;90:961.
109. Kimberg DB, Baerg RD, Gershon E, et al. Effect of cortisone treatment on the active transport of calcium by the small intestine. *J Clin Invest* 1971;50:1309.
110. Percival RC, Yates AJP, Grey RES, et al. Role of glucocorticoids in the management of malignant hypercalcemia. *BMJ* 1984;289:287.
111. Kristensen B, Ejlertsen B, Holmegaard SN, et al. Prednisolone in the treatment of severe malignant hypercalcemia in metastatic breast cancer: a randomized study. *J Intern Med* 1992;232:237.
112. Yates AJ, Oreffo ROC, Mayor K, et al. Inhibition of bone resorption by inorganic phosphate is mediated by both reduced osteoclast formation and decreased activity of mature osteoclasts. *J Bone Miner Res* 1991;6:473.
113. Heath DA. The use of inorganic phosphate in the management of hypercalcemia. *Metab Bone Dis Rel Res* 1980;2:213.
114. Ayala G, Chertow BS, Shah JH, et al. Acute hyperphosphatemia and acute persistent renal insufficiency induced by oral phosphate therapy. *Ann Intern Med* 1975;83:520.
115. Carey RW, Schmott GW, Kopald HH, et al. Massive extraskeletal calcification during phosphate treatment of hypercalcemia. *Arch Intern Med* 1968;122:150.
116. Laflamme GH, Jowsey J. Bone and soft tissue changes with oral phosphate supplements. *J Clin Invest* 1972;51:2834.
117. Kiang DT, Loken MK, Kennedy BJ. Mechanism of the hypocalcemic effect of mithramycin. *J Clin Endocrinol Metab* 1979;48:341.
118. Ralston SH, Gardner MD, Dryburgh FJ, et al. Comparison of aminohydroxypropylidene diphosphonate, mithramycin, and corticosteroids/calcitonin in treatment of cancer-associated hypercalcemia. *Lancet* 1985;2:907.
119. Thurlimann B, Waldburger R, Semm HJ, et al. Plicamycin and pamidronate in symptomatic tumor-related hypercalcemia: a prospective randomized crossover trial. *Ann Oncol* 1992;3:619.
120. Green L, Donehower RC. Hepatic toxicity of low doses of mithramycin in hypercalcemia. *Cancer Treat Rep* 1984;68:1379.
121. Thiebaud D, Jacquet AF, Burckhardt P. Fast and effective treatment of malignant hypercalcemia: combination of suppositories of calcitonin and a single infusion of 3-amino 1-hydroxypropylidene-1-bisphosphonate. *Arch Intern Med* 1990;150:2125.
122. Miach PJ, Dawborn JK, Martin TJ, et al. Management of the hypercalcemia of malignancy by peritoneal dialysis. *Med J Aust* 1975;1:782.
123. Bilezkian JP. Management of acute hypercalcemia. *N Engl J Med* 1992;326:1196.
124. Klinenberg JR, Kippen I, Bluestone R. Hyperuricemic nephropathy: pathophysiologic features and factors influencing urate deposition. *Nephron* 1975;14:88.
125. Cohen LF, Balow JE, Magrath IT, et al. Acute tumor lysis syndrome. A review of 37 patients with Burkitt's lymphoma. *Am J Med* 1980;68:486.
126. Garnick MB, Mayer RB. Acute renal failure associated with neoplastic disease and its treatment. *Semin Oncol* 1978;5:155.
127. Kalemkerian GP, Darwish B, Varterasian ML. Tumor lysis syndrome in small cell carcinoma and other solid tumors. *Am J Med* 1997;103:363.
128. Conger JD, Falk SA. Intrarenal dynamics in the pathogenesis and prevention of acute urate nephropathy. *J Clin Invest* 1977;59:786.
129. Hande KR, Hixson CV, Chabner BA. Postchemotherapy purine excretion in lymphoma patients receiving allopurinol. *Cancer Res* 1981;41:2273.
130. Simmonds HA, Cameron JS, Morris GS, et al. Allopurinol in renal failure and the tumor lysis syndrome. *Clin Chim Acta* 1986;160:189.
131. Jankovic M, Zurlo MG, Rossi E, et al. Urate-oxidase as hypouricemic agent in a case of acute tumor lysis syndrome. *Am J Pediatr Hematol Oncol* 1985;7:202.
132. Wolf G, Hegewisch-Becker S, Hossfeld DK, Stahl RA. Hyperuricemia and renal insufficiency associated with malignant disease: urate oxidase as an efficient therapy? *Am J Kidney Dis* 1999;34:E20.
133. Mandell GA, Swacus JR, Rosenstock J, et al. Danger of urography in hyperuricemic children with Burkitt's lymphoma. *J Can Assoc Radiol* 1983;34:273.
134. Arrambide K, Toto RD. Tumor lysis syndrome. *Semin Nephrol* 1993;13:273.
135. Castro MP, VanAuken J, Spencer-Cisek P, et al. Acute tumor lysis syndrome associated with concurrent biochemotherapy of metastatic melanoma—a case report and review of the literature. *Cancer* 1999;85:1055.
136. Vachvanichsanong P, Maipang M, Dissaneewate P, et al. Severe hyperphosphatemia following acute tumor lysis syndrome. *Med Pediatr Oncol* 1995;24:63.
137. Thatte L, Oster JR, Singer I, et al. Review of the literature: severe hyperphosphatemia. *Am J Med Sci* 1995;310:167.
138. Abramson EC, Gajardo H, Kukreja SC. Hypocalcemia in cancer. *Bone Miner* 1990;10:161.
139. Fleming DR, Doukas MA. Acute tumor lysis syndrome in hematologic malignancies. *Leuk Lymphoma* 1992;8:315.
140. Razis E, Arlin ZA, Ahmed T, et al. Incidence and treatment of tumor lysis syndrome in patients with acute leukemia. *Acta Haematol* 1994;91:171.
141. Drakos P, Bar-Ziv J, Catane R. Tumor lysis syndrome in nonhematologic malignancies. *Am J Clin Oncol* 1994;17:502.
142. Persons DA, Garst J, Vollmer R, et al. Tumor lysis syndrome and acute renal failure after treatment of non-small-cell lung carcinoma with combination irinotecan and cisplatin. *Am J Clin Oncol-Cancer Clin Trials* 1998;21:426.
143. Fer MF, Bottino GC, Sherwin SA, et al. Atypical tumor lysis syndrome in a patients with T-cell lymphoma treated with recombinant leukocyte interferon. *Am J Med* 1984;77:953.
144. Cech P, Block JB, Cone IA, et al. Tumor lysis syndrome after tamoxifen flare. *N Engl J Med* 1986;315:263.
145. Dann EJ, Gillis S, Polliack A, et al. Brief report: tumor lysis syndrome following treatment with 2-chlorodeoxyadenosine for refractory chronic lymphocytic leukemia. *N Engl J Med* 1993;329:1547.
146. Simmons ED, Somberg KA. Acute tumor lysis syndrome after intrathecal methotrexate administration. *Cancer* 1991;67:2062.
147. Harley HA, Mason R, Phillips PJ. Profound hypocalcemia associated with oestrogen treatment of carcinoma of the prostate. *Med J Aust* 1983;2:41.
148. Schenkein DP, O'Neill WC, Shapiro J, et al. Accelerated bone formation causing profound hypocalcemia in acute leukemia. *Ann Intern Med* 1986;105:375.
149. Dunlay RW, Camp MA, Allon M, et al. Calcitriol in prolonged hypocalcemia due to the tumor lysis syndrome. *Ann Intern Med* 1989;110:162.
150. Uribarri J, Oh MS, Carroll HJ. D-Lactic acidosis: a review of clinical presentation, biochemical features, and pathophysiologic mechanisms. *Medicine* 1998;77:73.
151. Ishihara K, Szerlip H. Anion gap acidosis. *Semin Nephrol* 1998;18:83.
152. Adrogué HJ, Madias NE. Management of life-threatening acid-base disorders. *N Engl J Med* 1998;338:26.
153. Gore DC, Jahoor F, Hibbert JM, et al. Lactic acidosis during sepsis is related to increased pyruvate production, not deficits in tissue oxygen availability. *Ann Surg* 1996;224:97.
154. Sculier JP, Nicaise C, Klastersky J. Lactic acidosis: a metabolic complication of extensive metastatic cancer. *Eur J Clin Oncol* 1983;19:597.
155. Sundar K, Suarez M, Banogon PE, et al. Zidovudine-induced fatal lactic acidosis and hepatic failure in patients with acquired immunodeficiency syndrome: report of two patients and review of the literature. *Crit Care Med* 1997;25:1425.
156. McKenzie R, Fried MW, Sallie R, et al. Hepatic failure and lactic acidosis due to fialuridine (FIAU), an investigational nucleoside analogue for chronic hepatitis B. *N Engl J Med* 1995;333:1099.
157. Narins RG, Cohen JJ. Bicarbonate therapy for organic acidosis: the case for its continued use. *Ann Intern Med* 1987;106:615.
158. Cooper DJ, Walley KR, Wiggs BR, et al. Bicarbonate does not improve hemodynamics in critically ill patients who have lactic acidosis. A prospective controlled clinical study. *Ann Intern Med* 1990;112:492.
159. Stacpoole PW. Lactic acidosis: the case against bicarbonate therapy [Editorial]. *Ann Intern Med* 1986;105:276.
160. Ritter JM, Doktor HS, Benjamin N. Paradoxical effect of bicarbonate on cytoplasmic pH. *Lancet* 1990;335:1243.
161. Stacpoole PW, Wright EC, Baumgartner TG, et al. A controlled clinical trial of dichloroacetate for treatment of lactic acidosis in adults. *N Engl J Med* 1992;327:1564.
162. Gutierrez G, Wulf ME. Lactic acidosis in sepsis: a commentary. *Intensive Care Med* 1996;22:6.
163. Daughaday WH. Hypoglycemia in patients with non-islet cell tumors. *Endocrinol Metab Clin North Am* 1988;18:91.
164. LeRoith D, Clemmons D, Nissley P, et al. Insulin-like growth factors in health and disease. *Ann Intern Med* 1992;116:854.
165. Macaulay VM. Insulin-like growth factors and cancer. *Br J Cancer* 1992;65:311.
166. Daughaday WH, Emanuele MA, Brooks MH, et al. Synthesis and secretion of insulin-like growth factor II by a leiomyosarcoma with associated hypoglycemia. *N Engl J Med* 1988;319:1434.
167. Ishida S, Noda M, Kuzuya N, et al. Big insulin-like growth factor II-producing hepatocellular carcinoma associated with hypoglycemia. *Intern Med* 1995;34:1201.
168. Shapiro ET, Bell GI, Polonsky KS, et al. Tumor hypoglycemia: relationship to high molecular weight insulin-like growth factor-II. *J Clin Invest* 1990;85:1672.
169. Zapf J, Futo E, Peter M, et al. Can "big" insulin-like growth factor II in serum of tumor patients account for the development of extrapancreatic tumor hypoglycemia? *J Clin Invest* 1992;90:2574.
170. Daughaday WH, Trivedi B, Baxter RC. Serum "big insulin-like growth factor II from patients with tumor hypoglycemia lacks normal E-domain O-linked glycosylation, a possible determinant of normal propeptide processing. *Proc Natl Acad Sci U S A* 1993;90:5823.
171. Zapf J. IGFs: function and clinical importance: role of insulin-like growth factor (IGF) II and IGF binding proteins in extrapancreatic tumour hypoglycaemia. *J Intern Med* 1993;234:543.
172. Tisdale MJ, Brennan RA. Metabolic substrate utilization by a tumour cell line which induces cachexia *in vivo*. *Br J Cancer* 1986;54:601.
173. Davis MR, Shamoon H. Deficient counterregulatory hormone responses during hypoglycemia in a patient with insulinoma. *J Clin Endocrinol Metab* 1991;72:788.
174. Hoff AO, Vassilopoulou-Sellin R. The role of glucagon administration in the diagnosis and treatment of patients with tumor hypoglycemia. *Cancer* 1998;82:1585.

175. Samaan NA, Pham FK, Sellin RV, et al. Successful treatment of hypoglycemia using glucagon in a patient with an extrapancreatic tumor. *Ann Intern Med* 1990;113:404.
176. Subramanian S, Goker H, Kanji A, et al. Clinical adrenal insufficiency in patients receiving megestrol therapy. *Arch Intern Med* 1997;157:1008.
177. Redman DG, Pazdur R, Zingas AP, et al. Prospective evaluation of adrenal insufficiency in patients with adrenal metastasis. *Cancer* 1987;60:103.
178. Gamelin E, Beldent V, Rousselet M-C, et al. Non-Hodgkin's lymphoma presenting with primary adrenal insufficiency: a disease with an underestimated frequency? *Cancer* 1992;69:2333.
179. Hug V, Kau S, Hortobagyi GN, et al. Adrenal failure in patients with breast carcinoma after long-term treatment of cyclic alternating oestrogen progesterone. *Br J Cancer* 1991;63:454.
180. Dahlberg PJ, Goellner MH, Pehling GB. Adrenal insufficiency secondary to adrenal hemorrhage: two case reports and a review of cases confirmed by computed tomography. *Arch Intern Med* 1990;150:905.
181. Siu SCB, Kitzman DW, Sheedy PF II, et al. Adrenal insufficiency from bilateral adrenal hemorrhage. *Mayo Clin Proc* 1990;65:664.

SECTION **4**

MCCLELLAN M. WALTHER

Urologic Emergencies

Urologic oncologic emergencies may arise secondary to the underlying malignancy, treatment, or unrelated medical conditions. Initial evaluation of symptoms of sepsis, hematuria, urinary obstruction, priapism, and other urologic emergencies leads to diagnosis and initial management. Urologic consultation may be necessary for definitive treatment.

URINARY TRACT INFECTION

URINARY SEPSIS

Neutropenic sepsis occurs after 1.1% to 14.0% of cycles of chemotherapy, most frequently associated with malignancies that impair granulocyte function or with more intensive bone marrow suppression, such as CHOP-M (cyclophosphamide, doxorubicin, vincristine, prednisone, with methotrexate) or similar regimens.[1,2] Of the sepsis episodes, as many as 8.9% are urosepsis.[1] Urinary tract infections are most frequently associated with urethral catheterization and require surveillance in immunocompromised patients.[3,4]

Treatment includes broad-spectrum antibiotic coverage until sensitivity results are available (Chapter 54). Broad-spectrum antibiotic coverage resulting in appropriate empiric antibiotic treatment has been associated with improved survival and shorter hospital stay, compared to inappropriate empiric antibiotic coverage.[5,6] Use of antibiotics before hospital admission, advanced patient age, and male gender have been predictive of a resistant uropathogen.[7]

Altered renal function, flank pain, urinary retention, or other signs or symptoms of urinary obstruction requires immediate evaluation to provide relief. Percutaneous nephrostomy gives direct drainage of an obstructed infected ureter and allows manual irrigation of viscous purulent fluid if drainage is not adequate.

PERIURETHRAL ABSCESS

Periurethral abscess is a life-threatening infection of the male urethra and periurethral tissues.[8] Patients present with sepsis and perineal or scrotal abscess or phlegmon. Urethral strictures, found in 60% to 85% of these patients, cause a high urethral voiding pressure, and lead to periurethral extravasation of infected urine, particularly after urethral instrumentation.[8,9] The infection can range from a small abscess confined by Buck's fascia, to an extensive necrotizing fasciitis of the penis, scrotum, and perineum.

The differential diagnosis includes tissue edema, follicular abscess, perirectal abscess, Fournier's gangrene, and penile or urethral cancer.[10,11] Physical examination will identify urethral involvement, extent of phlegmon, and crepitance caused by gas-forming organisms. Urinalysis and culture usually isolate gram-negative and anaerobic bacteria. Retrograde urethrogram will demonstrate diagnostic extravasation of contrast into the periurethral tissues.[12,13]

Treatment of periurethral abscess consists of emergent débridement and suprapubic drainage of urine. In the presulfonamide era, mortality was at least 50%.[9] Broad-spectrum antibiotic coverage for gram-negative organisms and anaerobes, using aminoglycoside and cephalosporins, have been associated with a 1.6% mortality.[8] Additional débridement and skin grafts or secondary wound closure can be required with extensive tissue necrosis.

As many as 20% of patients develop recurrent periurethral abscess during follow-up, apparently due to extensive urethral stricture disease. Evaluation after resolution of sepsis should exclude contributory factors, such as an unstable bladder, urethral diverticula, or watering-pot perineum. Construction of a perineal urethrostomy may prevent abscess recurrence and should be considered if significant urethral disease is present.[8,9,14]

CYSTITIS

Cystitis, defined symptomatically as an irritation of the bladder, presents with suprapubic discomfort, frequency, dysuria, and urgency. Severe manifestations include urge incontinence and hematuria. Patients may present with acute exsanguinating hematuria but more commonly develop milder symptoms and pathologic disease. The etiology may be related to a toxic chemical agent, radiation, thrombocytopenia with subsequent bleeding, or myelosuppression with associated infection.

General measures taken in the initial evaluation of patients with cystitis should exclude urinary infection and the presence of malignancy. Symptomatic relief of discomfort on voiding can be obtained with urinary analgesics, such as phenazopyridine hydrochloride (Pyridium). Suprapubic discomfort, frequency, urgency, and urge incontinence require antispasmodics to obtain relief; oxybutynin chloride (Ditropan), propantheline bromide (Pro-Banthine), hyoscyamine sulfate (Cystospaz, Levsin), and flavoxate hydrochloride (Urispas) are used for this purpose. Combinations of drugs, sometimes including antiseptics, are often helpful. These include Urised (methenamine, methylene blue, phenyl salicylate, benzoic acid, atropine sulfate, and hyoscyamine), Pyridium Plus (phenazopyridine, hyoscyamine, and butabarbital), and Azogantrisin (sulfisoxazole and phenazopyridine). Severe symptoms may require belladonna and opium rectal suppositories. Patients with mild voiding dysfunction associated with chronic bladder pain may benefit from a trial of tricyclic antidepressants.[15] Many treatment measures are unique to each etiology.

CHEMICAL CYSTITIS

Oxazaphosphorines

Cyclophosphamide (Cytoxan), the most commonly used oxazaphosphorine, is an alkylating agent first used in the treatment of malignant tumors in Europe in 1957. Currently, Cytoxan has a role in the treatment of solid tumors and lymphomas, as well as benign inflammatory states, Wegener's granulomatosis and rheumatoid arthritis being the most common. Other oxazaphosphorines—ifosfamide, trophosphamide, and sufosfamide—have been used since the 1970s for the treatment of solid malignancies and lymphomas. Dose-limiting toxicity with these compounds is usually urinary tract toxicity.

Urinary symptoms, including frequency, urgency, dysuria, and nocturia, develop in as many as 24% of patients treated with oral Cytoxan.[16] Microhematuria occurs in 7% to 53% of patients and gross hematuria in 0.6% to 15.0%.[16–19] Gross hematuria can range from lightly stained urine to exsanguinating hemorrhage. Symptoms usually occur soon after Cytoxan is given but may occur years later.[17] Malignant lesions, usually transitional cell carcinoma, occur in 2% to 5.5% of patients who receive oral Cytoxan for nonmalignant disease.[16,19,20] The entire urothelium can be affected, but the bladder is the most frequently involved area.

Bladder pathology has been attributed to toxic metabolites of these compounds. Hepatic microsomal cells break down cyclophosphamide to hydroxycyclophosphamide, then by target cells to aldophosphamide, and then to phosphoramide mustard, the active antineoplastic metabolite, and acrolein, which has no significant antitumor activity.[21–23] Similarly, ifosfamide is metabolized to iphosphoramide mustard and acrolein.[22] Urinary excretion of acrolein is believed to be the major source of urothelial toxicity.[22] Most normal cells are able to break down the toxic metabolites and diminish their effect. Glutathione is a naturally occurring thiol that can confer such protection in most cells but is present in low levels in urine.[21] Oxazaphosphorine toxicity has been demonstrated in several animal models with their systemic administration and by instillation of their normal metabolic products directly into the bladder.[24–26]

Bladder damage from these compounds is cumulative and generally dose-related. "Cytoxan cystitis" occurs frequently and early after intravenous therapy, especially dose-intensive regimens. Fibrosis has been found in as many as 25% of children receiving high-dose cyclophosphamide.[27] Severe hematuria and telangiectasia are more common in these patients.[27] Cystitis usually takes weeks to develop after oral treatment but has been seen after as little as one dose.[28] Oxazaphosphorine cystitis is potentiated by prior pelvic radiation.[17,29]

Laboratory values reveal normal coagulation profiles, a normal platelet count, and negative urine culture. Because these patients are at risk for developing urothelial malignancies, episodes of cystitis and hematuria must be evaluated, including urinalysis and urine cytology. Patients receiving cyclophosphamide develop markedly abnormal cytologies, including marked atypia, increased nuclear size, and bizarrely shaped cytoplasm, which frequently resolves with cessation of the drug.[30] These findings can be suggestive of malignancy and need to be interpreted with caution.[31] Patients with abnormal cytologies that have not been investigated previously should undergo a thorough urologic evaluation. Cystoscopy may reveal a tumor or changes compatible with Cytoxan cystitis (Fig. 51.4-1). Acutely diffuse inflammation is seen. Chronic changes include a pale bladder mucosa with telangiectasia. Areas of edema can be present with patchy hemorrhagic areas that stain with methylene blue, an indicator of mucosal injury.[24] Biopsies reveal hyperemia, hemorrhage, edema, mucosal thinning, and ulceration of the urothelium. Necrosis of mucosa, muscle, and small arterioles and telangiectasia can be present.[24,26,32] Atypia can be prominent, and abundant mitoses often occur.[26,30,32] These findings are similar to those seen after radiation therapy. Mucosal lesions of cyclophosphamide-induced cystitis may be identified early, before the appearance of microscopic hematuria.[33]

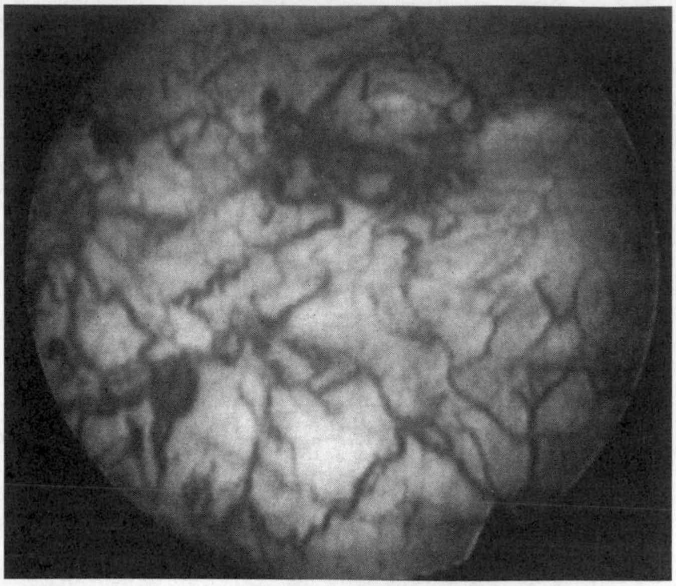

FIGURE 51.4-1. Cytoxan cystitis. Microscopic hematuria is found in approximately one-half of patients receiving oral Cytoxan. Increased vascularity with fragile "corkscrew" vessels are seen at cystoscopy here. Submucosal hemorrhage adjacent to larger vessels occurred after bladder distention. Fulgaration of these small vessels will temporarily alleviate bleeding. Radiation cystitis appears similar at cystoscopy. (See Color Fig. 51.4-1 in the CD-ROM and on the Web at www.LWWoncology.com.)

Hemorrhagic cystitis is managed by stopping or reducing the drug. Replacing the drug, usually with azathioprine, is necessary in as many as one-third of patients who develop severe cystitis after chronic oral administration.[34] Hydration and diuresis are routinely used to dilute the metabolites in the urine and minimize their toxicity after intravenous administration.[23] The cystitis usually improves within several days after cessation of the drug but can occasionally persist for months. Patients receiving high doses of oxazaphosphorines require additional measures to counter their effects.[35] Bladder irrigation is helpful in many of these patients taking cyclophosphamide.[36]

Sodium 2-mercaptoethane sulfonate (mesna) was designed to function in the urinary tract to detoxify azophosphorine metabolites with urothelial toxicity. Mesna is a sulfhydryl compound that is administered intravenously and rapidly excreted by the urinary tract. After intravenous administration, mesna undergoes oxidation, forming disulfide bonds and making an unreactive dimer (dimesna). One concern regarding such a class of drugs is that they might affect the antineoplastic properties of oxazaphosphorines. Mesna and dimesna are very hydrophilic and do not normally penetrate cells, explaining its antineoplastic sparing effect.[23] This unreactive form—dimesna—is filtered by the kidneys and undergoes tubular reabsorption, where one-third of it is reduced to its active form, mesna, by glutathione reductase.[23] In the urinary tract, the sulfhydryl group of mesna complexes with the terminal methyl group of acrolein, joining the compound to the double bond of acrolein and forming a nontoxic thioether.[23] The presence of mesna also inhibits spontaneous breakdown of cyclophosphamide to acrolein in the urine.[37] In addition to decreasing chemical cystitis, the risk of bladder cancer is significantly reduced when mesna is used in the Sprague-Dawley rat model.[38]

Oral mesna is well absorbed but slow to achieve adequate urinary concentrations. It has an unpleasant taste, which makes patient compliance poor, particularly when there is concomitant administration of a chemotherapy that induces nausea.[21] Mesna is best given intravenously, and the manufacturer recommends three doses. A loading dose equivalent to 20% (wt/wt) of the ifosfamide dose, given 15 minutes before the ifosfamide, is followed by two similar doses 4 and 8 hours after the ifosfamide.[23] Doses as high as 60% to 120% (wt/wt) have been used with cyclophosphamide, given at a similar schedule. The timing of dosages of mesna is important, as the half-life of mesna is 35 minutes, while that of cyclophosphamide is 4 hours.[23,39] Mesna toxicity is minimal, the major side effects being diarrhea, headaches, and limb pain.[21]

Another thiol compound, N-acetyl-L-cysteine, has been used less extensively to ameliorate the effects of oxazaphosphorines. Animal data demonstrate that the bladder is protected when it is given at a dose of 1:1 (wt/wt) with cyclophosphamide in a similar schedule as mesna.[40] Problems with N-acetyl-L-cysteine include a wide distribution in the body with low urinary levels. High intravenous doses or intravesical administration is required to reach effective concentrations.[41] Conflicting data concerning impairment of antitumor activity have not been resolved.

Bone Marrow Transplantation

Hemorrhagic cystitis occurs in approximately 2% of conditioning regimens not containing Cytoxan and is frequently related to thrombocytopenia.[29] The incidence of hemorrhagic cystitis in regimens with cyclophosphamide is 5% to 15%.[29,42–44] Allogeneic bone marrow and unrelated transplantation appear to have a higher risk than autologous bone marrow transplantation.[42,43] Prior cyclophosphamide, radiation, urethral catheterization, infection (bacterial or previous viral), concurrent medication, or coagulation disorders (thrombocytopenia) can all contribute to the development of hemorrhagic cystitis in these patients. Prior administration of busulfan, an alkyl sulfonate, increases the risk of hemorrhagic cystitis to as high as 36%, compared to 4% in patients receiving the same regimen without prior exposure.[45] Concomitant use of these agents is associated with hemorrhagic cystitis in 0.5% to 50.0% of patients.[29,44,46,47] Patients with acute bleeding have decreased survival compared to patients without bleeding.[43]

Several viruses have been implicated in the etiology of hemorrhagic cystitis in patients undergoing bone marrow transplantation, either as viral reactivation or a new infection. These include polyoma (BK) virus,[29,48] adenovirus,[42] especially adenovirus 11,[48,49] papovavirus, influenza A, and cytomegalovirus.[47,48] Patients in whom viral particles were recovered developed hematuria later after transplantation (55 days)[48] than patients with so-called idiopathic hemorrhagic cystitis (25 to 27 days).[29] The viral type also had a longer duration than idiopathic cystitis.[48,49] Diagnosis of viral cystitis is improving with polymerase chain reaction technology.[50]

It has been recommended that patients receiving the combination of Cytoxan and busulfan should receive continuous bladder irrigation during treatment.[47] Prophylactic treatment with mesna seems equally efficacious[51–53] and does not appear to affect engraftment.[54] Mesna 60% (wt/wt) has been an adequate dose in children, but adults appear to require a higher dose [120% to 160% (wt/wt)].[54] Treatment in these patients is symptomatic.

Intravesical Chemotherapy

Intravesical treatment of superficial bladder tumors with chemotherapeutic agents or biologic modifiers may cause a chemical cystitis or inflammatory response with marked symptoms. Several agents are commonly used. Thiotepa is well tolerated, although 2% to 49% of patients experience cystitis[55,56] and approximately one-third develop hematuria.[55] One-third of patients receiving epodyl[56] and 26% to 50% of patients receiving doxorubicin (Adriamycin) develop cystitis.[56,57] Mitomycin C is best tolerated, with 6% to 33% of patients developing cystitis, and one-third developing hematuria.[55–57] Most hematuria is microscopic. Significant hemorrhagic cystitis is uncommon with any of these agents. Bladder contractures have rarely been reported in patients receiving thiotepa or mitomycin.

Most patients receiving bacille Calmette-Guérin develop irritative voiding symptoms, which can be the most severe of all intravesical treatments. Biopsies in these patients reveal acute and chronic inflammatory changes and granuloma formation. Urinary analgesics and antispasmodics are particularly helpful in this group. If symptoms are prolonged, isoniazid and acetaminophen or ibuprofen are given until symptoms resolve. It is uncommon for treatment regimens to be stopped because of toxicity.[58]

Other

Oral 9-nitrocamptothecin, a water-insoluble topoisomerase I inhibitor, and other camptothecins are associated with dose-related hematuria in up to 25% of patients.[59] Hematuria may be a chemical cystitis related to the significant urinary elimination of the drug, although it can also be associated with profound thrombocytopenia. Increasing fluid intake to 3 liters/d has been associated with decreased cystitis and ability to finish treatment.

Busulfan, an alkyl sulfonate used in the treatment of chronic granulocytic leukemia, has also been reported as a cause of hemorrhagic cystitis.[45,60,61] As many as 16% of patients in regimens with intravenous busulfan and without cyclophosphamide develop hemorrhagic cystitis.[29] Cystoscopy in these patients reveals generalized inflammation and edema. Biopsies demonstrate metaplastic changes in the urothelium, submucosal inflammation, and telangiectasia.[60] Both cystoscopic and histologic findings are similar to radiation or oxazaphosphorine cystitis. Bladder malignancies have not been associated with its use. Given orally, a cumulative dose of 2 to 5 kg appears necessary to induce these changes.[60,62] Stopping the drug and alleviation of irritative symptoms are the primary treatment.

Other chemotherapeutic regimens that do not include agents with known bladder toxicity appear to be able to induce a cystitis and hematuria without associated thrombocytopenia.[63] The mechanism in these patients is not clear, although bleomycin has been suggested to be the culprit.[63,64]

INTRAVESICAL PHOTOTHERAPY

Kelly and Snell first performed treatment of superficial bladder tumors with "phototherapy" in 1975. Treatment involves administration of an intravenous photosensitizer (usually a hematoporphyrin derivative), waiting 2 days, and then activation of the compound with light. The time lag allows preferential uptake of sensitizer by tumor, with normal tissue levels decreasing, thus increasing the therapeutic index. An optical fiber placed in the bladder through a cystoscope transmits light to activate the sensitizer. Patients whose entire bladder mucosa is illuminated develop marked bladder irritation with suprapubic discomfort, urgency, and urge incontinence. Symptoms can be surprisingly mild the first day after activation but peak in the second and third day. Symptoms improve quickly and usually resolve by 4 to 6 weeks. Cystoscopy initially reveals exuberant local reaction and edema.[65] Biopsies initially reveal coagulative necrosis and hemorrhage.[65] Later, acute and chronic inflammation and atypia are present.[66] The acute response can resolve with little residual effect visually apparent. Bladder fibrosis and reflux are unpredictable side effects of this therapy. Treatment of the acute symptoms includes Foley drainage to put the bladder to rest and B&O suppositories for control of bladder discomfort.

RADIATION

Patients undergoing primary radiotherapy of malignant pelvic tumors, most commonly uterine, bladder, and prostate neoplasms, can suffer direct or incidental damage to the bladder. The risk is increased when urinary infection is present, repeated or high-dose radiation is given, or when surgery has been performed in the area. Cyclophosphamide, given systemically in combination with pelvic radiotherapy, greatly increases the risk of radiation cystitis.[67]

In the first 4 to 6 weeks after treatment, an acute inflammatory response with resultant irritative symptoms or hematuria (or both) develops. Mild symptoms occur in as many as 50% to 82% of patients and generally do not require medication.[68,69]

Hemorrhagic cystitis can occur later, even years after successful treatment,[69] and frequently is associated with tumor recurrence.[70] The time between treatment and development of delayed symptoms (frequency, dysuria, and hematuria) is proportional to the dose received.[69] Patients with late cystitis develop bladder ulcers, bladder fibrosis, and ureteral strictures. They require thorough evaluation, as these patients are at increased risk for transitional cell carcinoma of the bladder. Bladder biopsies should be performed sparingly, as the bladder mucosa heals poorly.

Approximately 3.7% of patients receiving intravaginal intracavitary radiation alone (3200 cGy) for stage I endometrial carcinoma after radical hysterectomy have been reported to develop cystitis.[71] When external-beam radiation (4000 to 5400 cGy) is added, 4.0% to 6.5% of patients develop cystitis.[71,72] Patients undergoing definitive radiation treatment of cervical carcinoma have a risk of cystitis that is dose-related.[70,73] At doses of less than 6000 cGy, the development of cystitis has been strongly linked to recurrent tumor.[70] The incidence of cystitis in this group is 2.8% to 8.0%.[69,74,75] Between 1.2% and 18.0% of patients receiving external-beam radiation (3000 to 8500 cGy) for bladder cancer developed cystitis,[70,76,77] 8% hematuria,[70] and 5% a contracted bladder.[77] Chronic cystitis developed in 15% of patients.

Radiation to the prostate (5000 to 7200 cGy) and draining lymph nodes (5000 cGy) for cure of prostate cancer elicits dysuria and mild to moderate hematuria in 18% to 40% of patients.[78,79] Between 0.8% and 8.3% develop severe dysuria or hematuria, and 3.4% to 9.0% develop strictures or urethral obstruction as a delayed presentation.[78–80]

During the acute phase, cystoscopy reveals edema, erythema, and increased vascularity, which can be associated with a mild decrease in bladder capacity. Later, the bladder is pale, and telangiectasia is present. Focal areas of hyperemia and bullous edema may be present. Often there is no focal area of bleeding. With extensive damage, necrosis and calcification can occur. Biopsy findings are dose- and time-dependent. In the first 24 hours, there is erythema due to hyperemia. This develops into a diffuse inflammatory response with hyperemia, edema, lymphocytic infiltration, and degeneration of the urothelium with atypia.[68,69,81] Shallow ulcers are occasionally seen but usually occur as a late response. This response lasts up to 4 months after therapy.[82] Later, sclerosing endarteritis, fibrosis, and atrophy occur. There may be edema and an inflammatory infiltrate. There can be ulceration, and healing is poor.[77,82,83] Treatment is symptomatic.

ANTIBIOTICS

While most cystitis seen in the setting of oncologic care is related to antineoplastic agents, penicillins used in the treatment of chemotherapy related infections represent another source. Methicillin, nafcillin, ticarcillin, piperacillin, carbenicillin, and penicillin G have all been implicated. The incidence of cystitis associated with the use of these agents is small, occurring in 4% to 8% of patients.[84] Symptoms are typical of cystitis. Laboratory investigation reveals eosinophilia, pyuria, hematuria, proteinuria, and negative urine cultures. The submucosal deposition of C3, immunoglobulins G and M, and dimethoxyphenylpenicilloyl, a methicillin antigen, supports a hypersensitivity etiology.[84–86] A diffuse hemorrhagic cystitis is seen at cystoscopy.[85] Biopsies show an intense inflammatory reaction with erosion.[87] With repeated use, the time to development of symptoms shortens. Symptoms usually resolve promptly on cessation of the drug or substitution with an unrelated drug.[85,86]

BLADDER HEMORRHAGE

Severe cystitis can result in hemorrhage resulting in clot retention and requiring transfusion. If bedside bladder clot evacua-

TABLE 51.4-1. Management of Bladder Hemorrhage

Medical management	
	Maintain platelet count >50,000/mm^3.
	Correct prothrombin time, partial thromboplastin time with necessary factors, fresh-frozen plasma.
	Stop medications that adversely affect clotting.
	Minimize constipation, straining to eliminate.
	Transfuse with blood as needed.
	Sedate as needed.
Bedside management	
	Place large-bore Foley and evacuate clots with piston syringe.
	If irrigation is clear and bladder is emptied, replace Foley with three-way catheter for continuous irrigation.
Operative management	
	Conservative measures
	Perform cystoscopic evacuation of clots and fulgaration after bleeding parameters are normalized.
	Use three-way continuous bladder irrigation after cystoscopy.
	Intravesical instillation for hematuria
	Perform cystoscopic evacuation of clots and fulgaration after bleeding parameters are normalized.
	Obtain cystogram; if no reflux, start continuous bladder irrigation in operating room, choosing less toxic agent (silver nitrate, alum, etc.) first.
	If life-threatening bleeding persists, reevaluate medical management, cystoscopy, fulgarate, exclude reflux, and consider formalin instillation in operating room. Irrigate bladder with saline afterward to remove residual formalin.

tion and continuous irrigation are not successful, cystoscopic evacuation of clots with fulguration of bleeding sites will cure most patients (Table 51.4-1). Correction of thrombocytopenia before cystoscopy will frequently stop bleeding and is necessary to prevent further bleeding episodes. Patients resistant to conservative therapy have been treated with intravesical instillation of chemical astringents or fixatives started immediately after cystoscopic treatment and cystogram to exclude vesicoureteral reflux.[88] Bladder instillation is performed using gravity drainage with minimal hydrostatic head required for filling.

Silver nitrate is a cauterizing agent that results in cellular protein coagulation and eschar formation. A 0.5% to 1.0% water solution as continuous bladder irrigation has been used in the management of radiation and chemical cystitis.[89] Chloride salts in solution or from ulcerated mucosal lesions are avoided as they can result in precipitation of silver chloride.[90] When effective, bleeding usually stops within 24 to 72 hours.

Continuous irrigation with 1% alum is used in a similar manner as silver nitrate.[91,92] Specific toxicities are related to aluminum absorption and include renal dysfunction, altered mental status, and encephalopathy.[93,94]

Formalin is a tissue fixative and embalming agent. Because of its potential toxicity, formalin is used only in the management of patients with life-threatening hematuria unresponsive to other measures. After cystoscopic examination, a 1% to 5% solution of formalin is instilled for 3 to 10 minutes in the operating room.[95–97] Complications and response are directly related to concentration and duration of exposure. Complications include bladder rupture, vesicorectal or vesicovaginal fistula, renal failure, acidosis, altered mental status, and chemical skin burns.[96,98–100] Formalin toxicity may be abrogated by dialysis to decrease blood levels and correct the metabolic acidosis.

Formaldehyde exists as a gas and has a maximum solubility of 37% in aqueous solution. A 37% aqueous solution of formaldehyde is equivalent to a 100% solution of formalin. Dilution of formaldehyde to formalin in treatment concentrations is best performed in the pharmacy.

Bladder irrigation with any chemical agent can be irritating, with local pain and bladder spasms requiring medical treatment. Complications related to intravesical instillation of chemical agents include ureteral stricture, bladder fibrosis with loss of volume, and death.[90,91,95,101] With signs of toxicity, the bladder irrigation is changed to water or saline to wash out any residual drug. As bladder healing occurs, hematuria can frequently recur if the underlying pathology still exists.

Other less-tried regimens have been shown to have activity in the treatment of radiation- or cyclophosphamide-induced hemorrhagic cystitis. These include intravesical installation of prostaglandins,[102,103] oral pentosanpolysulphate,[104] conjugated estrogens,[102,103] or hyperbaric oxygen.[105–107] Open cystotomy with bladder packing has rarely been used.[108]

URINARY OBSTRUCTION

Urinary obstruction associated with loss of renal function can lead to accumulation of water, urea, and electrolytes as well as loss of renal concentrating ability. Immediately after release of obstruction, these can lead to brisk diuresis, hypovolemia, and shock. Patients are monitored hourly for elevated urine output and if not able to match with oral intake, require intravenous supplementation.[109,110] Rarely, patients with severe fluid and electrolyte disturbances may require dialysis.[111]

UPPER TRACTS

Malignant ureteral obstruction occurs in as many as 4.4% of patients with advanced cancer.[112] The most common associated malignancies are prostate, bladder, cervical, colon, or lymphoid cancers.[113,114] Definitive radiation treatment of cervical cancer has been reported to have a continuous increasing of risk of 0.15% per year over 25 years.[115] Ureteral obstruction may be an incidental finding on computed tomography imaging and associated with altered renal function. Radionuclide imaging may be helpful if the clinical picture is not diagnostic of obstruction.[116]

Cystoscopic placement of ureteral stents maintains quality of life better than percutaneous nephrostomy.[117] Stent placement may be difficult when the ureteral orifices are obscured by local tumor invasion. Ureteral stents placed for obstruction at the bladder level are more predisposed to bleeding and obstruction than are those placed for retroperitoneal metastases causing extrinsic ureteral obstruction. As many as 49% to 63% of patients with bladder malignancies may end up with percutaneous nephrostomy.[111,113]

Patients undergoing percutaneous nephrostomy placement can usually undergo antegrade placement of a ureteral stent.[118] These stents can be changed cystoscopically, taking care not to lose access to the ureteral orifice. Ureteral stents are generally changed every 3 months to prevent encrustation and obstruction.[119] Minor hematuria and bladder spasms are often associated with ureteral stent placement and treated symptomatically. As many as 5% of patients have significant bleeding, usually associated with tumor invasion in the bladder.[113]

Patients with ureteral obstruction and urinary conduits may require initial percutaneous nephrostomy followed by internalization of the ureteral stent.[120] Percutaneous management with ureteroscopic incision of a benign stricture has been affective in up to 57% of patients.[121] Residual ureteral stricture requiring definitive surgical treatment is uncommon, as most responses to treatment are short-lived. Late strictures after radiation therapy have had limited success with excision and ureteral reimplantation.[115]

Untreated patients with bilateral ureteral obstruction succumb to renal failure within a month.[114] Recovery of renal function after relief of obstruction depends on duration of obstruction and initial renal function.[122] Preservation of renal parenchyma and renal function has been reported as long as 5 months after complete unilateral ureteral obstruction.[123] When there is partial ureteral obstruction, return to normal function has been reported in 68% of patients, with marked improvement in 24%.[114] Patients with ureteral obstruction from hormone-sensitive prostate cancer have had longer survival[111–113] than those with gastric, pancreatic, or colon cancer.[111,124]

LOWER TRACT

Prostate

Urinary voiding symptoms may occur in debilitated patients after surgery, chemotherapy, or significant medical events. Symptoms may range from urinary frequency with decreased force of stream and nocturia to urinary retention.

Urinary retention may be obstructive, pharmacologic, neurogenic, or psychogenic in nature.[125] Patient medical and voiding history is examined with these factors in mind. Urinary tract infection or prostatitis should be detected early and treated appropriately. Manipulation of the urinary tract or prostate in these patients is kept to a minimum to prevent sepsis.

Relief of urinary obstruction with catheter drainage offers immediate relief. Patients with urethral stricture disease, benign prostatic hypertrophy, prostate cancer, meatal stenosis, or phimosis can be challenging to catheterize. Urethral dilation or use of a specialized angulated (Coudé) catheter to pass an enlarged prostate median lobe may be necessary. Placement of suprapubic trochar drainage is performed when urethral catheterization is not possible or there are concerns about promoting sepsis. Individuals especially trained in their use best perform these procedures. Minor surgical procedures can be performed to relieve phimosis or meatal stenosis.

Permanent affects on ability to void can occur after abdominoperineal resection, radical hysterectomy, or extensive pelvic operations that interrupt normal pelvic parasympathetic innervation to the bladder. Temporary loss of voiding may occur secondary to anticholinergic agents that block detrusor activity, pain that results in increased sympathetic bladder neck tone, and narcotics that inhibit the urge to void. Of patients with urinary retention as a presenting complaint, as many as 18% to 23% will reestablish normal voiding if given a voiding trial.[126,127] Of patients with urinary retention after nonurologic surgery, as many as 69% reestablish normal voiding patterns if placed on intermittent self-catheterization, generally within 3 months.[128]

Evaluation of urinary retention associated with nonsurgical medical disorders is less well defined. Assessment of prehospital admission American Urological Association voiding symptom score in all these patients is helpful in identifying patients who may require treatment of prostate obstruction.[129–133] Urodynamics may be indicated to distinguish bladder outlet obstruction from impaired detrusor contractility.[134] Transurethral resection of the prostate remains the standard against which other treatment regimens for urinary retention due to benign prostate hypertrophy are measured.[135] Use of alternative methods, such as holmium laser resection, urethral stent, or chronic indwelling catheter drainage, may be dictated by available technology or patient health.

Patients with urinary retention due to prostate cancer had good relief of obstruction 1 month after bilateral orchiectomy.[136] Similar results have been observed using luteinizing hormone–releasing hormone antagonists, although improvement may take longer.[137] Urethral stents have been used to hasten spontaneous voiding.

Urethra

Patients in whom a catheter cannot be passed may have benign prostatic hypertrophy or urethral stricture disease. A Coudé catheter more easily follows the natural angulation of the urethra into the bladder. A small catheter may pass through a stricture that is not severe.[138] Urethral dilation by trained personnel may be required. Forceful advancement of the catheter is to be avoided, as the integrity of the urethra can be violated, contributing to bleeding, urinary extravasation, local cellulitis, and stricture formation.[139] Cystoscopic placement of a Foley catheter may be required if this occurs. Urethral bleeding after traumatic catheter placement or inflation of a balloon in the urethra will stop when the Foley is in place if coagulation parameters are normal. Urine should be checked for infection and treated appropriately.

A Foley catheter balloon may not deflate, preventing its removal. Scissors removal of the valve will allow drainage if that is the location of the obstruction. Obstruction at a distal level can be relieved by balloon rupture with a spinal needle under ultrasound guidance.[138] Suprapubic or transvaginal routes are preferred, although the transrectal route is technically feasible.

PRIAPISM

Priapism is the emergent condition defined as sustained painful erection of the corpora cavernosal tissue not associated with sexual stimulation. Two types of priapism have been described, ischemic (low-flow) and nonischemic (high-flow), with different treatment and prognosis.

Ischemic priapism is associated with decreased penile venous outflow and stasis of blood resulting in intracavernosal blood acidosis and low oxygen tension. Ischemic priapism is treated emergently, as irreversible cellular damage and corporal fibrosis, which can result in erectile dysfunction, occur within 24 to 48 hours. Ischemic priapism may be caused by sickle cell disorders, oral or injected medications, or tumor infiltrate.[140–142] Nonischemic priapism usually results from perineal trauma with injury to the internal pudendal artery with arteriovenous fistula formation.[143–145] Nonischemic priapism is painless, can increase in tumescence after sexual stimuli, and can be managed electively.

Patient history may reveal drug use, sickle cell anemia, perineal trauma, or malignancy. Priapism is usually found in men but has been reported rarely in women.[146] On physical examination, the corpora cavernosa are rigid. The glans, an extension of the corpora spongiosa, is usually soft. Voiding symptoms may occur in as many as 25% of patients when tumor involves the corpora spongiosa or urethra.[147] Pseudopriapism is characterized by rigidity and edema associated with metastases rather than venous stasis. Pain is thought to be due to tissue anoxia. In malignant priapism, tumor infiltration of the cavernosa or invasion of venous drainage is thought to lead to stasis and thrombosis.

As many as 10% of patients develop priapism related to malignancy.[148,149] Penile metastases are most often symptom-free, with associated priapism in 20% to 53% of patients.[150] Prostate, bladder, and kidney cancer are most commonly involved in adults.[150,151] Leukemia is the most common malignant cause in children.[149,152] Needle biopsy or aspiration of the firm corpora cavernosa can confirm the diagnosis. The management of priapism varies according to cause.[153-157]

Treatment of malignant priapism is initially aimed at relief of pain and anxiety with hydration, analgesia, and rest.[153] Treatment of the underlying malignancy can be associated with relief.[150] Hormonal therapy of prostate cancer and chemotherapy of leukemia[156,158] would have higher expectations of response. Radiation is palliative if more emergent relief is needed or therapeutic options are limited. Intracavernosal injection of pharmacologic agents has had anecdotal success.[159,160] Without systemic treatment, survival in malignant priapism is poor, as most patients have metastatic disease at presentation.[150,161,162] Sixty percent of patients died at a median of 4 months (range, 0.2 to 60 months) after developing priapism.[150]

Surgical treatment of priapism involves creation of a shunt between the glans penis and the corpora cavernosa.[163] Under anesthesia, a tru-cut needle placed through the glans into each corpora cavernosum will achieve this. Anoxia occurring during priapism or shunting performed as treatment can result in impotence. A penile prosthesis may be required if the corpora cavernosa become fibrosed and unable to distend in normal fashion.

PARAPHIMOSIS

Paraphimosis is the pathologic state occurring after retraction of the foreskin proximal to the glans penis, characterized by local swelling and difficulty in returning the foreskin to its normal position. Retention of the preputial ring proximal to the coronal sulcus is associated with tissue tension greater than lymphatic pressure and results in edema of the prepuce and glans. If not reduced, the edema can become massive, associated with pain and skin breakdown. Manual reduction is usually performed, using anesthetic jelly and pressure to remove edema. The penis is grasped with both hands, placing the last three fingers along the shaft. The index fingers are used to pull the foreskin over the glans, while the thumbs push the glans back through the constricting ring of the prepuce.[139] When this is not possible, a local anesthetic block may be required to release the trapped foreskin.[138] A dorsal slit procedure will allow relief of an acute constricting paraphimosis or phimosis if conservative measures fail.

REFERENCES

1. Wilkinson TJ, Robinson BA. Neutropenic sepsis complicating treatment of solid tumours, lymphoma and myeloma. *Clin Oncol (R Coll Radiol)* 1992;4:355.
2. Rotstein C, Cummings KM, Nicolaou AL, Lucey J, Fitzpatrick J. Nosocomial infection rates at an oncology center. *Infect Control* 1988;9:13.
3. Bryan CS, Reynolds KL. Hospital-acquired bacteremic urinary tract infection: epidemiology and outcome. *J Urol* 1984;132:494.
4. Rosser CJ, Bare RL, Meredith JW. Urinary tract infections in the critically ill patient with a urinary catheter. *Am J Surg* 1999;177:287.
5. Leibovici L, Shraga I, Drucker M, et al. The benefit of appropriate empirical antibiotic treatment in patients with bloodstream infection. *J Intern Med* 1998;244:379.
6. Leibovici L, Drucker M, Konigsberger H, et al. Septic shock in bacteremic patients: risk factors, features and prognosis. *Scand J Infect Dis* 1997;29:71.
7. Leibovici L, Greenshtain S, Cohen O, Wysenbeek AJ. Toward improved empiric management of moderate to severe urinary tract infections. *Arch Intern Med* 1992;152:2481.
8. Walther MM, Mann BB, Finnerty DP. Periurethral abscess. *J Urol* 1987;138:1167.
9. Baker WJ, Wilkey JL, Barson LJ. An evaluation of the management of peri-urethral phlegmon in 272 consecutive cases at the Cook County Hospital. *J Urol* 1949;61:943.
10. Tashiro S, Hinman F. Periurethral and perirectal infections: pathologic and clinical differentiation. *J Urol* 1947;57:338.
11. Paty R, Smith AD. Gangrene and Fournier's gangrene. *Urol Clin North Am* 1992;19:149.
12. Veiga-Pires JA, Elebute EA. Urethrocystography in the male. *Br J Urol* 1967;39:194.
13. Finestone EO. Urinary extravasation (periurethral phlegmon) pathogenesis and experimental study. *Surg Obstet Gynecol* 1941:73:918
14. Wilkey JL, Barson LJ, Portney FR. Urinary extravasation and periurethral phlegmon: clinical analysis of 100 cases. *J Urol* 1959;82:657.
15. Pranikoff K, Constantino G. The use of amitriptyline in patients with urinary frequency and pain. *Urology* 1998;51:179.
16. Stillwell TJ, Benson RC Jr, DeRemee RA, McDonald TJ, Weiland LH. Cyclophosphamide-induced bladder toxicity in Wegener's granulomatosis. *Arthritis Rheum* 1988;31:465.
17. Stillwell TJ, Benson RC Jr, Burgert EO Jr. Cyclophosphamide-induced hemorrhagic cystitis in Ewing's sarcoma. *J Clin Oncol* 1988;6:76.
18. Lawrence HJ, Simone J, Aur RJ. Cyclophosphamide-induced hemorrhagic cystitis in children with leukemia. *Cancer* 1975;36:1572.
19. Talar-Williams C, Hijazi YM, Walther MM, et al. Cyclophosphamide-induced cystitis and bladder cancer in patients with Wegener's granulomatosis. *Ann Intern Med* 1996;124:477.
20. Fairchild WV, Spence CR, Solomon HD, Gangai MP. The incidence of bladder cancer after cyclophosphamide therapy. *J Urol* 1979;122:163.
21. Shaw IC, Graham MI. Mesna—a short review. *Cancer Treat Rev* 1987;14:67.
22. Cox PJ. Cyclophosphamide cystitis—identification of acrolein as the causative agent. *Biochem Pharmacol* 1979;28:2045.
23. Schoenike SF, Dana WJ. Ifosfamide and mesna. *Clin Pharm* 1990;9:179.
24. Chaviano AH, Gill WB, Ruggiero KJ, Vermeulen CW. Experimental Cytoxan cystitis and prevention by acetylcysteine. *J Urol* 1985;134:598.
25. Brock N, Pohl J, Stekar J. Detoxification of urotoxic oxazaphosphorines by sulfhydryl compounds. *J Cancer Res Clin Oncol* 1981;100:311.
26. Philips FS, Sternberg SS, Cronin AP, Vidal PM. Cyclophosphamide and urinary bladder toxicity. *Cancer Res* 1961;21:1577.
27. Johnson WW, Meadows DC. Urinary-bladder fibrosis and telangiectasia associated with long-term cyclophosphamide therapy. *N Engl J Med* 1971;284:290.
28. Host H, Nissen-Meyer R. A preliminary clinical study of cyclophosphamide. *Cancer Chemother Rep* 1960;9:47.
29. Brugieres L, Hartmann O, Travagli JP, et al. Hemorrhagic cystitis following high-dose chemotherapy and bone marrow transplantation in children with malignancies: incidence, clinical course, and outcome. *J Clin Oncol* 1989;7:194.
30. Forni AM, Koss LG, Geller W. Cytological study of the effect of cyclophosphamide on the epithelium of the urinary bladder in man. *Cancer* 1964;17:1348.
31. Liedberg CF, Rausing A, Langeland P. Cyclophosphamide hemorrhagic cystitis. *Scand J Urol Nephrol* 1970;4:183.
32. Koss LG. A light and electron microscopic study of the effects of a single dose of cyclophosphamide on various organs in the rat: I. The urinary bladder. *Lab Invest* 1967;16:44.
33. Kimura M, Tomita Y, Morishita H, Takahashi K. Presence of mucosal change in the urinary bladder in nonhematuric patients with long-term exposure and/or accumulating high-dose cyclophosphamide. Possible significance of follow-up cystoscopy on preventing development of cyclophosphamide-induced hemorrhagic cystitis. *Urol Int* 1998;61:8.
34. Fauci AS, Haynes BF, Katz P, Wolff SM. Wegener's granulomatosis: prospective clinical and therapeutic experience with 85 patients for 21 years. *Ann Intern Med* 1983;98:76.
35. Droller MJ, Saral R, Santos G. Prevention of cyclophosphamide-induced hemorrhagic cystitis. *Urology* 1982;20:256.
36. Blume KG, Beutler E, Bross KJ, et al. Bone-marrow ablation and allogeneic marrow transplantation in acute leukemia. *N Engl J Med* 1980;302:1041.
37. Brock N, Stekar J, Pohl J, Niemeyer U, Scheffler G. Acrolein, the causative factor of urotoxic side-effects of cyclophosphamide, ifosfamide, trofosfamide and sufosfamide. *Arzneimittelforschung* 1979;29:659.
38. Petru E, Schmahl D. Anticancer drugs: second malignancies—risk reduction. *Cancer Treat Rev* 1987;14:337.
39. Cytoxan. In: Schumacher MM, Dowd AL, eds, *Physician's Desk Reference.* Montvale, NJ: Medical Economics Company, 1991:723.
40. Tolley DA. The effect of N-acetyl cysteine on cyclophosphamide cystitis. *Br J Urol* 1977; 49:659.
41. Ormstad K, Ohno Y. N-acetylcysteine and sodium 2-mercaptoethane sulfonate as sources of urinary thiol groups in the rat. *Cancer Res* 1984;44:3797.
42. Sencer SF, Haak, RJ, Weisdorf DJ. Hemorrhagic cystitis after bone marrow transplantation. Risk factors and complications. *Transplantation* 1993;56:875.
43. Nevo S, Swan V, Enger C, et al. Acute bleeding after bone marrow transplantation (BMT)—incidence and effect on survival. A quantitative analysis in 1,402 patients. *Blood* 1998;91:1469.
44. Seber A, Shu XO, Defor T, Sencer S, Ramsay N. Risk factors for severe hemorrhagic cystitis following BMT. *Bone Marrow Transplant* 1999;23:35.

45. Thomas AE, Patterson J, Prentice HG, et al. Haemorrhagic cystitis in bone marrow transplantation patients: possible increased risk associated with prior busulfan therapy. *Bone Marrow Transplant* 1987;1:347.
46. Nevill TJ, Barnett MJ, Klingemann HG, et al. Regimen-related toxicity of a busulfan-cyclophosphamide conditioning regimen in 70 patients undergoing allogeneic bone marrow transplantation. *J Clin Oncol* 1991;9:1224.
47. Atkinson K, Biggs J, Noble G, et al. Preparative regimens for marrow transplantation containing busulfan are associated with haemorrhagic cystitis and hepatic veno-occlusive disease but a short duration of leucopenia and little oro-pharyngeal mucositis. *Bone Marrow Transplant* 1987;2:385.
48. Arthur RR, Shah KV, Baust SJ, Santos GW, Saral R. Association of BK viruria with hemorrhagic cystitis in recipients of bone marrow transplants. *N Engl J Med* 1986;315:230.
49. Miyamura K, Takeyama K, Kojima S, et al. Hemorrhagic cystitis associated with urinary excretion of adenovirus type 11 following allogeneic bone marrow transplantation. *Bone Marrow Transplant* 1989;4:533.
50. Echavarria MS, Ray SC, Ambinder R, Dumler JS, Charache P. PCR detection of adenovirus in a bone marrow transplant recipient: hemorrhagic cystitis as a presenting manifestation of disseminated disease. *J Clin Microbiol* 1999;37:686.
51. Turkeri LN, Lum LG, Uberti JP, et al. Prevention of hemorrhagic cystitis following allogeneic bone marrow transplant preparative regimens with cyclophosphamide and busulfan: role of continuous bladder irrigation. *J Urol* 1995;153:637.
52. Meisenberg B, Lassiter M, Hussein A, et al. Prevention of hemorrhagic cystitis after high-dose alkylating agent chemotherapy and autologous bone marrow support. *Bone Marrow Transplant* 1994;14:287.
53. Vose JM, Reed EC, Pippert GC, et al. Mesna compared with continuous bladder irrigation as uroprotection during high-dose chemotherapy and transplantation: a randomized trial. *J Clin Oncol* 1993;11:1306.
54. Blacklock H, Ball L, Knight C, Schey S, Prentice G. Experience with mesna in patients receiving allogeneic bone marrow transplants for poor prognostic leukaemia. *Cancer Treat Rev* 1983;10:45.
55. Heney NM, Koontz WW, Barton B, et al. Intravesical thiotepa versus mitomycin C in patients with Ta, T1 and TIS transitional cell carcinoma of the bladder: a phase III prospective randomized study. *J Urol* 1988;140:1390.
56. Lamm D. Intravesical therapy of superficial bladder cancer. *AUA Update Series* 1983;2:2.
57. Herr H, Laudone V. Intravesical therapy for superficial bladder cancer. *AUA Update Series* 1989;8:90.
58. Lamm DL, Stogdill VD, Stogdill BJ, Crispen RG. Complications of bacillus Calmette-Guérin immunotherapy in 1,278 patients with bladder cancer. *J Urol* 1986;135:272.
59. Verschraegen CF, Natelson EA, Giovanella BC, et al. A phase I clinical and pharmacological study of oral 9-nitrocamptothecin, a novel water-insoluble topoisomerase I inhibitor. *Anticancer Drugs* 1998;9:36.
60. Pode D, Perlberg S, Steiner D. Busulfan-induced hemorrhagic cystitis. *J Urol* 1983;130:347.
61. Bandini G, Belardinelli A, Rosti G, et al. Toxicity of high-dose busulfan and cyclophosphamide as conditioning therapy for allogeneic bone marrow transplantation in adults with haematological malignancies. *Bone Marrow Transplant* 1994;13:577.
62. Millard RJ. Busulfan-induced hemorrhagic cystitis. *Urology* 1981;18:143.
63. Cantwell BM, Harris AL, Patrick D, Hall RR. Hemorrhagic cystitis after IV bleomycin, vinblastine, cisplatin, and etoposide for testicular cancer. *Cancer Treat Rep* 1985;70:548.
64. Creagan ET, Ahmann DL, Schutt AJ, Green SJ. Phase II study of the combination of vinblastine, bleomycin, and cisplatin in advanced malignant melanoma. *Cancer Treat Rep* 1982;66:567.
65. Benson RC, Kinsey JH, Cortese DA, Farrow GM, Utz DC. Treatment of transitional cell carcinoma of the bladder with hematoporphyrin derivative phototherapy. *J Urol* 1983;130:1090.
66. Prout GR, Lin CW, Benson R, et al. Photodynamic therapy with hematoporphyrin derivative in the treatment of superficial transitional cell carcinoma of the bladder. *N Engl J Med* 1987;317:1251.
67. Jayalakshmamma B, Pinkel D. Urinary-bladder toxicity following pelvic irradiation and simultaneous cyclophosphamide therapy. *Cancer* 1976;38:701.
68. Fajardo LF, Berthrong M. Radiation injury in surgical pathology. *Am J Surg Pathol* 1978;2:159.
69. Oration JP. Complications following radiation therapy in carcinoma of the cervix and their treatment. *Am J Obstet Gynecol* 1964;88:854.
70. Dean RJ, Lytton B. Urologic complications of pelvic irradiation. *J Urol* 1978;119:64.
71. Kucera H, Vavra N, Weghaupt K. Benefit of external irradiation in pathologic stage I endometrial carcinoma: a prospective clinical trial of 605 patients who received postoperative vaginal irradiation and additional pelvic irradiation in the presence of unfavorable prognostic factors. *Gynecol Oncol* 1990;38:99.
72. Jampolis S, Martin P, Schroder P, Horiot JC. Treatment tolerance and early complications with extended field irradiation in gynaecological cancer. *Br J Radiol* 1977;50:195.
73. Montana GS, Fowler WC. Carcinoma of the cervix: analysis of bladder and rectal radiation dose and complications. *Int J Radiat Oncol Biol Phys* 1989;16:95.
74. Montana GS, Fowler WC, Varia MA, Walton LA, Mack Y. Analysis of results of radiation therapy for Stage II carcinoma of the cervix. *Cancer* 1985;55:956.
75. Buchler DA, Kline JC, Peckham BM, Boone ML, Carr WF. Radiation reactions in cervical cancer therapy. *Am J Obstet Gynecol* 1971;111:745.
76. Shiels RA, Nissenbaum MM, Mark SR, Browde S. Late radiation cystitis after treatment for carcinoma of the bladder. *S Afr Med J* 1986;70:727.
77. Ram MD. Visceral complications of supervoltage radiotherapy for carcinoma of the bladder. *Br J Surg* 1970;57:409.
78. Ray GR, Cassady JR, Bagshaw MA. Definitive radiation therapy of carcinoma of the prostate. A report on 15 years of experience. *Radiology* 1973;106:407.
79. Taylor WJ, Richardson RG, Hafermann MD. Radiation therapy for localized prostate cancer. *Cancer* 1979;43:1123.
80. Harisiadis L, Veenema RJ, Senyszyn JJ, et al. Carcinoma of the prostate: treatment with external radiotherapy. *Cancer* 1978;41:2131.
81. Warren S VII. Effects of radiation on the urinary system. *Arch Pathol* 1942;34:1079.
82. Haemorrhagic cystitis after radiotherapy. *Lancet* 1987;1:304.
83. Gowing NF III. Pathological changes in the bladder following irradiation. *Br J Radiol* 1960;33:484.
84. Relling MV, Schunk JE. Drug-induced hemorrhagic cystitis [clinical conference]. *Clin Pharm* 1986;5:590.
85. Bracis R, Sanders CV, Gilbert DN. Methicillin hemorrhagic cystitis. *Antimicrob Agents Chemother* 1977;12:438.
86. Marx CM, Alpert SE. Ticarcillin-induced cystitis cross-reactivity with related penicillins. *Am J Dis Child* 1984;138:670.
87. Cook FV, Farrar WE Jr, Kreutner A. Hemorrhagic cystitis and ureteritis, and interstitial nephritis associated with administration of penicillin G. *J Urol* 1979;122:110.
88. West NJ. Prevention and treatment of hemorrhagic cystitis. *Pharmacotherapy* 1997;17:696.
89. Kumar AP, Wrenn ELJ, Jayalakshmamma B, et al. Silver nitrate irrigation to control bladder hemorrhage in children receiving cancer therapy. *J Urol* 1976;116:85.
90. Raghavaiah NV, Soloway MS. Anuria following silver nitrate irrigation for intractable bladder hemorrhage. *J Urol* 1977;118:681.
91. Arrizabalaga M, Extramiana J, Parra JL, et al. Treatment of massive haematuria with aluminous salts. *Br J Urol* 1987;60:223.
92. Goel AK, Rao MS, Bhagwat AG, et al. Intravesical irrigation with alum for the control of massive bladder hemorrhage. *J Urol* 1985;133:956.
93. Sherrard DJ. Aluminum toxicity. *Kidney* 1988;20:31.
94. Murphy CP, Cox RL, Harden EA, et al. Encephalopathy and seizures induced by intravesical alum irrigations. *Bone Marrow Transplant* 1992;10:383.
95. Donahue LA, Frank IN. Intravesical formalin for hemorrhagic cystitis: analysis of therapy. *J Urol* 1989;141:809.
96. Godec CJ, Gleich P. Intractable hematuria and formalin. *J Urol* 1983;130:688.
97. Dewan AK, Mohan GM, Ravi R. Intravesical formalin for hemorrhagic cystitis following irradiation of cancer of the cervix. *Int J Gynecol Obstet* 1993;42:131.
98. Vicente J, Rios G, Caffaratti J. Intravesical formalin for the treatment of massive hemorrhagic cystitis: retrospective review of 25 cases. *Eur Urol* 1990;18:204.
99. Sarnak MJ, Long J, King AJ. Intravesicular formaldehyde instillation and renal complications. *Clin Nephrol* 1999;51:122.
100. Axelsen RA, Leditschke JF, Burke JR. Renal and urinary tract complications following the intravesical instillation of formalin. *Pathology* 1986;18:453.
101. Jerkins GR, Noe HN, Hill DE. An unusual complication of silver nitrate treatment of hemorrhagic cystitis: case report. *J Urol* 1986;136:456.
102. Yamamoto M, Hibi H, Ohmura M, Miyake K. Successful treatment of hemorrhagic cystitis secondary to cyclophosphamide chemotherapy with intravesical instillation of prostaglandin F2 alpha. *Hinyokika Kiyo* 1994;40:833.
103. Miller LJ, Chandler SW, Ippoliti CM. Treatment of cyclophosphamide-induced hemorrhagic cystitis with prostaglandins. *Ann Pharmacother* 1994;28:590.
104. Hampson SJ, Woodhouse CR. Sodium pentosanpolysulphate in the management of haemorrhagic cystitis: experience with 14 patients. *Eur Urol* 1994;25:40.
105. Lee HC, Liu CS, Chiao C, Lin SN. Hyperbaric oxygen therapy in hemorrhagic radiation cystitis: a report of 20 cases. *Undersea Hyperb Med* 1994;21:321.
106. Weiss JP, Mattei DM, Neville EC, Hanno PM. Primary treatment of radiation-induced hemorrhagic cystitis with hyperbaric oxygen: 10-year experience. *J Urol* 1994;151:1514.
107. Mathews R, Rajan N, Josefson L, Camporesi E, Makhuli Z. Hyperbaric oxygen therapy for radiation induced hemorrhagic cystitis. *J Urol* 1999;161:435.
108. Andriole GL, Yuan JJ, Catalona WJ. Cystotomy, temporary urinary diversion and bladder packing in the management of severe cyclophosphamide-induced hemorrhagic cystitis. *J Urol* 1990;143:1006.
109. O'Reilly PH, Brooman PJ, Farah NB, Mason GC. High pressure chronic retention. Incidence, aetiology and sinister implications. *Br J Urol* 1986;58:644.
110. Howards SS. Post-obstructive diuresis: a misunderstood phenomenon. *J Urol* 1973;110:537.
111. Norman RW, Mack FG, Awad SA, et al. Acute renal failure secondary to bilateral ureteric obstruction: review of 50 cases. *Can Med Assoc J* 1982;127:601.
112. Paul AB, Love C, Chisholm GD. The management of bilateral ureteric obstruction and renal failure in advanced prostate cancer. *Br J Urol* 1994;74:642.
113. Shekarriz B, Shekarriz H, Upadhyay J, et al. Outcome of palliative urinary diversion in the treatment of advanced malignancies. *Cancer* 1999;85:998.
114. Zadra JA, Jewett MA, Keresteci AG, et al. Nonoperative urinary diversion for malignant ureteral obstruction. *Cancer* 1987;60:1353.
115. McIntyre JF, Eifel PJ, Levenback C, Oswald MJ. Ureteral stricture as a late complication of radiotherapy for stage IB carcinoma of the uterine cervix. *Cancer* 1995;75:836.
116. Dubovsky EV, Russell CD. Advances in radionuclide evaluation of urinary tract obstruction. *Abdom Imaging* 1998;23:17.
117. Yachia D. Overview: role of stents in urology. *J Endourol* 1997;11:379.
118. Harding JR. Percutaneous antegrade ureteric stent insertion in malignant disease. *J R Soc Med* 1993;86:511.
119. Watson G. Problems with double-J stents and nephrostomy tubes. *J Endourol* 1997;11:413.
120. Soper JT, Blaszczyk TM, Oke E, Clarke-Pearson D, Creasman WT. Percutaneous nephrostomy in gynecologic oncology patients. *Am J Obstet Gynecol* 1988;158:1126.
121. Meretyk S, Clayman RV, Kavoussi LR, Kramolowsky EV, Picus DD. Endourological treatment of ureteroenteric anastomotic strictures: long- term follow-up. *J Urol* 1991;145:723.
122. Shokeir AA, Provoost AP, Nijman RJ. Recoverability of renal function after relief of chronic partial upper urinary tract obstruction. *B J U Int* 1999;83:11.
123. Okubo K, Suzuki Y, Ishitoya S, Arai Y. Recovery of renal function after 153 days of complete unilateral ureteral obstruction. *J Urol* 1998;160:1422.

124. Donat SM, Russo P. Ureteral decompression in advanced nonurologic malignancies. *Ann Surg Oncol* 1996;3:393.
125. Bakht FR, Guerriero WG. Genitourinary emergencies. *Prim Care* 1989;16:905.
126. Taube M, Gajraj H. Trial without catheter following acute retention of urine. *Br J Urol* 1989;63:180.
127. Murray K, Massey A, Feneley RC. Acute urinary retention—a urodynamic assessment. *Br J Urol* 1984;56:468.
128. Anderson JB, Grant JB. Postoperative retention of urine: a prospective urodynamic study. *BMJ* 1991;302:894.
129. Barry MJ, Fowler FJJ, O'Leary MP, et al. The American Urological Association symptom index for benign prostatic hyperplasia. The Measurement Committee of the American Urological Association. *J Urol* 1992;148:1549.
130. Kaplan SA, Olsson CA, Te AE. The American Urological Association symptom score in the evaluation of men with lower urinary tract symptoms: at 2 years of follow-up, does it work? *J Urol* 1996;155:1971.
131. Lawrence K. Measurement properties of the AUA symptom score: a methodological clarification. *Br J Urol* 1996;77:175.
132. Guess HA. Epidemiology and natural history of benign prostatic hyperplasia. *Urol Clin North Am* 1995;22:247.
133. Meigs JB, Barry MJ, Giovannucci E, et al. Incidence rates and risk factors for acute urinary retention: the health professionals follow-up study. *J Urol* 1999;162:376.
134. Chancellor MB, Blaivas JG, Kaplan SA, Axelrod S. Bladder outlet obstruction versus impaired detrusor contractility: the role of outflow. *J Urol* 1991;145:810.
135. Holtgrewe HL. Transurethral prostatectomy. *Urol Clin North Am* 1995;22:357.
136. Thomas DJ, Balaji VJ, Coptcoat MJ, Abercrombie GF. Acute urinary retention secondary to carcinoma of the prostate. Is initial channel TURP beneficial? *J R Soc Med* 1992;85:318.
137. Hampson SJ, Davies JH, Charig CR, Shearer RJ. LHRH analogues as primary treatment for urinary retention in patients with prostatic carcinoma. *Br J Urol* 1993;71:583.
138. Stine RJ, Avila JA, Lemons MF, Sickorez GJ. Diagnostic and therapeutic urologic procedures. *Emerg Med Clin North Am* 1988;6:547.
139. Neuwirth H, Frasier B, Cochran ST. Genitourinary imaging and procedures by the emergency physician. *Emerg Med Clin North Am* 1989;7:1.
140. Fowler JEJ, Koshy M, Strub M, Chinn SK. Priapism associated with the sickle cell hemoglobinopathies: prevalence, natural history and sequelae. *J Urol* 1991;145:65.
141. Hamre MR, Harmon EP, Kirkpatrick DV, Stern MJ, Humbert JR. Priapism as a complication of sickle cell disease. *J Urol* 1991;145:1.
142. Banos JE, Bosch F, Farre M. Drug-induced priapism. Its aetiology, incidence and treatment. *Med Toxicol Adverse Drug Exp* 1989;4:46.
143. Ilkay AK, Levine LA. Conservative management of high-flow priapism. *Urology* 1995;46:419.
144. Bastuba MD, Saenz DT, Dinlenc CZ, et al. Arterial priapism: diagnosis, treatment and long-term follow-up. *J Urol* 1994;151:1231.
145. Hakim LS, Kulaksizoglu H, Mulligan R, Greenfield A, Goldstein I. Evolving concepts in the diagnosis and treatment of arterial high flow priapism. *J Urol* 1996;155:541.
146. Monllor J, Tano F, Arteaga PR, Galbis F. Priapism of the clitoris. *Eur Urol* 1996;30:521.
147. Belville WD, Cohen JA. Secondary penile malignancies: the spectrum of presentation. *J Surg Oncol* 1992;51:134.
148. Kulmala RV, Lehtonen TA, Tammela TL. Preservation of potency after treatment for priapism. *Scand J Urol Nephrol* 1996;30:313.
149. Winter CC, McDowell G. Experience with 105 patients with priapism: update review of all aspects. *J Urol* 1988;140:980.
150. Chan PT, Begin LR, Arnold D, et al. Priapism secondary to penile metastasis: a report of two cases and a review of the literature. *J Surg Oncol* 1998;68:51.
151. Perez LM, Shumway RA, Carson CC, Fisher SR, Hudson WR. Penile metastasis secondary to supraglottic squamous cell carcinoma: review of the literature *J Urol* 1992;147:157.
152. Nelson JH, Winter CC. Priapism: evolution of management in 48 patients in a 22-year series. *J Urol* 1977;117:455.
153. Powars DR, Johnson CS. Priapism. *Hematol Oncol Clin North Am* 1996;10:1363.
154. Mulhall JP, Honig SC. Priapism: etiology and management. *Acad Emerg Med* 1996;3:810.
155. Lee M, Cannon B, Sharifi R. Chart for preparation of dilutions of alpha-adrenergic agonists for intracavernous use in treatment of priapism. *J Urol* 1995;153:1182.
156. Becker HC, Pralle H, Weidner W. Therapy of priapism in high counting myeloid leukemia—a combined oncological-urological approach. Two case reports. *Urol Int* 1985;40:284.
157. Altebarmakian VK, Rabinowitz R, Rana SR, Ettinger LJ. Transglandular cavernosum-spongiosum shunt for leukemic priapism in childhood. *J Urol* 1980;123:287.
158. Schreibman SM, Gee TS, Grabstald H. Management of priapism in patients with chronic granulocytic leukemia. *J Urol* 1974;111:786.
159. van Driel MF, Mooibroek JJ, Mensink HJ. Treatment of priapism by injection of adrenaline into the corpora cavernosa penis. *Scand J Urol Nephrol* 1991;25:251.
160. Shantha TR, Finnerty DP, Rodriquez AP. Treatment of persistent penile erection and priapism using terbutaline. *J Urol* 1989;141:1427.
161. Yokoi K, Miyazawa N, Muraki J, et al. Penile metastasis from lung cancer. *Jpn J Clin Oncol* 1992;22:297.
162. Daniels GFJ, Schaeffer AJ. Renal cell carcinoma involving penis and testis: unusual initial presentations of metastatic disease. *Urology* 199137:369.
163. Kulmala R. Treatment of priapism: primary results and complications in 207 patients. *Ann Chir Gynaecol* 1994;83:309.

CHAPTER **52**

Treatment of Metastatic Cancer

PATRICK Y. WEN
PETER MCLAREN BLACK
JAY S. LOEFFLER

SECTION **1**

Metastatic Brain Cancer

Brain metastases are a common complication in cancer patients[1] and an increasingly important cause of morbidity and mortality. In adults, brain metastascs are the most common cause of brain tumors, occurring five to ten times more frequently than primary tumors.[2,3] In recent years, there have been important advances in the diagnosis and management of this condition.[2–4] As a result, most patients receive effective palliation, and the majority do not die from their brain metastases. Further studies defining the optimal role of conventional treatments and future advances in the use of chemotherapy, radiosurgery, and more novel cancer therapies may lead to further increases in the effectiveness of treatments for brain metastases.

Brain metastases develop when tumor cells originating in tissues outside the nervous system spread secondarily to directly involve the brain. Intracranial metastases may involve the brain parenchyma, the cranial nerves, the blood vessels (including the dural sinuses), the dura, the leptomeninges, and the inner table of the skull. Of the intracranial metastases, the most common are intraparenchymal metastases, and these are the main focus of this chapter.

INCIDENCE AND EPIDEMIOLOGY

Brain metastases develop in approximately 10% to 30% of adults and 6% to 10% of children with cancer.[2–9] It is estimated that each year in the United States, there are between 97,800 and 170,000 new cases of brain metastases.[2,3,5,9] This number may be increasing as a result of the increased ability of magnetic resonance imaging (MRI) to detect small metastases and prolonged survival due to improvement in systemic therapy.[2,3,9–11]

In adults, the most common primary tumors responsible for brain metastases are lung (50%), breast (15% to 20%), unknown primary (10% to 15%), melanoma (10%), and colon (5%) (Table 52.1-1).[2,3,5,6,12] In children, the most common sources of brain metastases are sarcomas, neuroblastoma, and germ cell tumors.[2,3,7,13,14] Certain tumors almost never metastasize to the brain parenchyma. These include carcinomas of the esophagus, oropharynx, and prostate and nonmelanoma skin cancers.

METHOD OF SPREAD AND DISTRIBUTION

The most common mechanism of metastasis to the brain is by hematogenous spread.[2] These metastases are usually located directly beneath the gray-white junction.[14] Brain metastases tend to occur at this site because the blood vessels decrease in size at this point and act as a trap for clumps of tumor cells. Brain metastases also tend to be more common at the terminal "watershed areas" of arterial circulation.[2,14] The distribution of metastases roughly follows the relative weight of (and blood flow to) each area. Approximately 80% of brain metastases are located in the cerebral hemispheres, 15% in the cerebellum,

TABLE 52.1-1. Frequency of Brain Metastases by Primary Tumor Type

Primary Tumor	*No. of Patients*	*Percentage*
Lung	270	48
Breast	82	15
Melanoma	50	9
Colon	26	5
Other known primary	72	13
Unknown primary	61	11
Total	561	100

(Pooled data from ref. 178, ref. 16, and ref. 12.)

and 5% in the brain stem.[14] For unclear reasons, pelvic (prostate and uterus) and gastrointestinal tumors have a predilection to metastasize to the posterior fossa.[14]

Metastases from breast, colon, and renal cell carcinoma are often single, while melanoma and lung cancer have a greater tendency to produce multiple metastases.[2,3,14] Studies using MRI suggest that the percentage of single metastases is lower than was previously believed, accounting for only one-third to one-fourth of patients with cerebral metastases.[3,15] With the widespread use of MRI and new improvements in MRI contrast agents and resolution, the proportion of multiple metastases probably will be even higher in the future.

CLINICAL MANIFESTATIONS

It is estimated that more than two-thirds of patients with cerebral metastases experience neurologic symptoms during the course of their illness.[2,3] The clinical features due to brain metastases are extremely variable, and the presence of brain metastases should be suspected in any cancer patient who develops new neurologic symptoms. The majority of patients present with progressive neurologic dysfunction resulting from a gradually expanding tumor mass and the associated edema or, rarely, to the development of obstructive hydrocephalus. Approximately 10% to 20% of patients present acutely with seizures, while another 5% to 10% present acutely as a result of strokes caused by embolization of tumor cells or invasion or compression of an artery by tumor or as a result of hemorrhage into a metastases.[10,16,17] Melanoma, choriocarcinoma, thyroid, and renal carcinoma have a particular propensity to bleed.[10]

The clinical presentation of brain metastases is similar to that of other brain tumors and includes headaches, focal neurologic dysfunction, cognitive dysfunction, and seizures. Headaches occur in approximately 40% to 50% of patients with brain metastases. These headaches are usually dull and nonthrobbing and often are indistinguishable from tension headaches.[18] The headaches are usually on the same side as the tumor, although they can be diffuse. Headaches characteristic of increased intracranial pressure, such as early morning headaches or headaches exacerbated by coughing, bending, and straining, are present in fewer than one-half of patients with brain metastases. These headaches may be associated with nausea, vomiting, and transient visual obscurations. Patients with multiple metastases and posterior fossa metastases have a higher frequency of headaches.[2] Papilledema is present in fewer than 10% of patients at the time of presentation. Focal neurologic dysfunction is the presenting symptom of 20% to 40% of patients. Hemiparesis is the most common complaint, but the precise symptom varies depending on the location of the metastases.[2] Cognitive dysfunction, including memory problems and mood or personality changes, are the presenting symptoms in one-third of patients, while seizures are the presenting symptom in another 10% to 20%.[19–22]

DIAGNOSIS

Brain metastases must be distinguished from primary brain tumors, abscesses, demyelination, cerebral infarctions or hemorrhages, progressive multifocal leukoencephalopathy, and effects of treatment, including irradiation necrosis. In a study by Patchell et al.,[23] 11% of patients who were initially thought to have a single brain metastasis eventually turned out to have a different diagnosis after the lesion was subjected to biopsy. One-half of the nonmetastatic lesions were primary brain tumors, while the other one-half were infections. The false-positive rate for diagnosis of multiple metastases is undoubtedly significantly less than the 11% for single metastases. Nonetheless, in any patient where the diagnosis of brain metastases is in doubt, a biopsy should be performed, since this is the only reliable method of establishing the diagnosis.

Breast cancer patients with a single dura-based lesion pose a particular diagnostic dilemma. The incidence of meningiomas is increased in patients with breast cancer so that it is important to differentiate a dura-based metastasis from a meningioma.[24,25] Frequently, imaging studies will be inconclusive, and these patients will require a biopsy or surgical resection of the lesion to establish the diagnosis.

In addition to diagnosing the brain metastases, it is also important to differentiate those patients with single or solitary metastases from patients with multiple brain metastases, since their subsequent treatment will be different. The term *single brain metastasis* refers to an single cerebral lesion, and no implication is made regarding the extent of extracranial disease. In contrast, the term *solitary brain metastasis* describes the relatively rare occurrence of a single brain metastasis that is the only known site of metastatic cancer in the body.[2,14]

IMAGING STUDIES

Although computed tomographic (CT) scans detect the majority of brain metastases, the best diagnostic test for brain metastases is contrast-enhanced MRI.[15,26,27] This test is more sensitive than enhanced CT scanning or nonenhanced MRI in detecting lesions in patients suspected of having cerebral metastases and in differentiating these metastases from other central nervous system (CNS) lesions.[26,27] Radiographic features that help to differentiate brain metastases from other CNS lesions include the presence of multiple lesions (which helps to distinguish metastases from gliomas or other primary tumors), localization of the lesion at the gray-white junction, more circumscribed margins, and relatively large amounts of vasogenic edema compared to the size of the lesion.[3] Triple-dose contrast administration may help to clarify the presence of metastases in selected patients with equivocal lesions or to detect additional lesions in patients with a single lesion on conventional single-dose contrast MRI.[28,29] Magnetization-transfer MRI, a technique that increases the contrast between enhancing and nonenhancing lesions by suppressing background signal, [27,30,31] may also increase the sensitivity of MRI. However, the usefulness of these approaches is limited by their availability and cost. In general, they may have a limited role in selected patients with a single or a small number of metastases on standard MRI and who are being considered for aggressive local therapy. In these patients, the detection of additional lesions may change the usefulness of surgery or radiosurgery. Functional imaging techniques, such as single-photon emission computed tomography, positron emission tomography, magnetic resonance spectroscopy, and perfusion and diffusion MRI, do not have a role in the diagnosis of brain metastases but may help in differentiating tumor from radiation necrosis.[27]

BRAIN METASTASES WITHOUT A KNOWN PRIMARY TUMOR

In the majority of patients (80%), brain metastases develop after the diagnosis of systemic cancer (metachronous presentation).[2] However, in some patients, brain metastases may be diagnosed before the primary tumor is found (precocious presentation) or at the same time (synchronous presentation). For patients who present with brain metastases without a known primary tumor, the lung should be the focus of the evaluation. More than 60% of these patients will have a lung primary or pulmonary metastases from a primary tumor located elsewhere.[2,32–34] Other frequent causes include malignant melanoma and colon cancer, while the primary remains unknown in approximately 25% to 30% of cases.[32–34] Breast cancer is an uncommon cause of brain metastases without a known primary tumor, possibly due to its earlier detection on physical examination and its tendency to produce brain metastases in the setting of widely disseminated disease.[33] The history and physical examination will demonstrate the site of origin in one-third to one-fourth of patients. In others, the chest radiograph is the most useful test. If it is nondiagnostic, a chest CT scan should be performed, as this significantly increases the likelihood of detecting a lung tumor.[32] These patients should also have a CT scan of the abdomen and pelvis and a bone scan to determine the extent of metastatic disease.

MANAGEMENT

The management of patients with brain metastases can be divided into symptomatic therapy and definitive therapy. Symptomatic therapy includes the use of corticosteroids for the treatment of peritumoral edema, anticonvulsants for control of seizures, and anticoagulants or inferior vena cava (IVC) filters for the management of venous thromboembolic disease.[3,10] Definitive therapy includes such treatments as surgery, radiotherapy, chemotherapy, and hormonal therapy directed at eradicating the tumor itself.

SYMPTOMATIC THERAPY

Corticosteroids

Corticosteroids were first used for treating peritumoral edema by Kofman et al.[35] in 1957 in patients with breast cancer. Subsequently, Galicich et al.[36] introduced the use of dexamethasone in 1961, and this has remained the standard treatment for peritumoral edema ever since. Corticosteroids produce their antiedema effect by reducing the permeability of tumor capillaries[37] and are indicated in any patient with symptomatic edema. Most patients are usually started on dexamethasone, which has the advantage over other corticosteroids of having relatively little mineral corticoid activity, reducing the potential for fluid retention. In addition, dexamethasone may be associated with a lower risk of infection and cognitive impairment.[37] The usual starting dose is a 10-mg load, followed by 4 mg four times daily, although there is some evidence that lower doses (4 to 8 mg/d) may be as effective.[38] While most patients improve symptomatically within 24 to 72 hours, neuroimaging studies may not show a decrease in the amount of edema for up to 1 week.[39] In general, headaches tend to respond better than focal deficits. If 16 mg of dexamethasone is insufficient, the dose may be increased up to 100 mg/d. Steroids are usually tapered after irradiation, although the taper may begin earlier in patients with little peritumoral edema.

Despite their usefulness, corticosteroids are associated with a large number of well-known side effects, including myopathy, weight gain, fluid retention, hyperglycemia, insomnia, gastritis, acne, and immunosuppression.[40] The frequency of these complications can be reduced by using the lowest possible dose of corticosteroids. There is increasing evidence that brain tumor patients on corticosteroids are at increased risk of developing *Pneumocystis carinii* pneumonitis.[41,42] This complication can be prevented by treating patients, especially those older than the age of 50, who are on prolonged courses of corticosteroid with trimethoprim-sulfamethoxazole prophylaxis.[3]

Anticonvulsants

Seizures are the presenting symptom in approximately 10% to 20% of patients with brain metastases and are present at some stage of the illness in another 10% to 20% of patients.[19–22] Patients with brain metastases who present with seizures should be treated with standard anticonvulsants. To minimize toxicity, the lowest effective dose of medication should be used and polytherapy avoided whenever possible. Electroencephalography may be useful if the diagnosis of seizures is in doubt but is not routinely needed for patients who give a clear history of seizures or do not have symptoms suggestive of seizures.

In addition to the usual complications of anticonvulsants, brain tumor patients experience an increased incidence of particular side effects, especially drug rashes. Approximately 20% of brain tumor patients treated with phenytoin and carbamazepine develop a morbilliform rash, and a small percentage develop Stevens-Johnson syndrome,[43–45] while patients receiving phenobarbital have an increased incidence of shoulder-hand syndrome.[46]

In addition to producing adverse effects, anticonvulsants also have clinically significant interactions with other drugs commonly used in patients with brain metastases. Phenytoin induces the hepatic metabolism of dexamethasone and significantly reduces its half-life and bioavailability.[47] Conversely, dexamethasone may also reduce phenytoin levels.[48] A number of chemotherapeutic agents commonly used in cancer patients interact with phenytoin, causing the levels to fall and potentially leading to breakthrough seizures,[49] while hepatic enzyme–inducing anticonvulsants, such as phenobarbital and phenytoin, may interfere with chemotherapeutic agents, such as taxol.[50]

Because the risk of seizures in patients with infratentorial metastases is very small, anticonvulsant therapy is usually not indicated. The role of anticonvulsant therapy in patients with supratentorial brain metastases who have not had a seizure is controversial. Cohen et al.[20] retrospectively reviewed 160 patients with brain metastases and who have not had a seizure and found that those patients receiving prophylactic anticonvulsant therapy with phenytoin had the same frequency of late seizures (10%) as patients receiving no treatment.[20] However, two-thirds of patients who developed seizure while on phenytoin had a subtherapeutic serum phenytoin concentration. Glantz et al.[21] conducted a prospective, placebo-controlled, randomized study involving 74 patients and evaluated the efficacy of valproic acid in protecting patients with newly diagnosed brain metastases from seizures. There was no significant difference in the incidence of seizures between patients receiving valproic acid (35%) or placebo (24%), suggesting that prophylactic anticonvulsants were not effective in these patients. Weaver et al.[51] conducted a prospective randomized study of prophylactic anticonvulsants in 100 brain tumor patients, including 60 with metastases who have not had seizures.[22] Overall, 26% of patients had seizures. There was no difference in the seizure rate between patients taking anticonvulsants and those who were on no medications. Recently, Glantz et al.[51] reviewed the evidence concerning the efficacy of prophylactic anticonvulsants. Because the number of patients in these studies was small, they also performed a metaanalysis of the randomized clinical trials addressing this issue. They concluded that there was no statistical evidence showing a significant benefit of prophylactic anticonvulsant.

Because of the increased incidence of allergic reactions in patients with brain metastases receiving anticonvulsant therapy and of the lack of clear evidence that anticonvulsant therapy reduces the incidence of seizures, routine anticonvulsant therapy is probably unnecessary in patients with brain metastases who have not experienced a seizure. Possible exceptions to this are patients with brain metastases in areas of high epileptogenicity (e.g., motor cortex), patients with multiple melanoma metastases,[52] and patients with both brain metastases and leptomeningeal metastases.[10] These patients have a higher incidence of seizures and may benefit from prophylactic anticonvulsant therapy.

Venous Thromboembolic Disease

Venous thromboembolic disease is common in patients with brain metastases, occurring in approximately 20% of patients.[53] The optimal therapy is unknown. These patients are often perceived to be at increased risk of intracranial hemorrhage with anticoagulation because of the vascularity of the tumors and anecdotal case reports of hemorrhage. As a result, the majority of brain metastases patients with venous thromboembolic disease are managed with IVC filters rather than anticoagulation. However, this may not be the optimum approach, since there is a high rate of complications with filtration devices in these patients. In a retrospective study of 42 patients with intracranial malignancy and venous thromboembolic disease treated with IVC filters, the complication rate was 62%. Fifty-seven percent developed IVC or filter thrombosis, recurrent deep venous thrombosis, or postphlebitic syndrome, and 12% developed recurrent pulmonary embolism.[54] In addition to the high complication rate with IVC filters, there is increasing evidence that the risk of intracranial hemorrhage in patients with primary brain tumors who are anticoagulated outside the immediate postoperative period may not be significantly increased.[55] More recently, Schiff and DeAngelis[56] reviewed the experience at the Memorial Sloan-Kettering Cancer Center with anticoagulation in patients with brain metastases who developed venous thromboembolic disease.[56] Of the 42 patients who received anticoagulation at some stage of their treatment, only 3 (7%) experienced cerebral hemorrhage, 2 in the setting of supratherapeutic anticoagulation. These studies suggest that anticoagulation may be more effective than IVC filter placement and is acceptably safe when the prothrombin time is maintained in the therapeutic range, especially in patients with brain metastases that generally do not hemorrhage, such as breast cancer.

DEFINITIVE TREATMENT

The management of brain metastases is directed at relieving neurologic symptoms and achieving long-term control of the tumors. The therapeutic modalities available include surgery, radiotherapy, chemotherapy, and hormonal therapy. The optimal combination of therapies for each patient depends on careful evaluation of numerous factors, including the location, size, and number of brain metastases; patient age, general condition, and neurologic status; extent of systemic cancer; as well as the tumor's response to past therapy and its potential response to future treatments.[3]

Surgery

The role of surgery in patients with brain metastases is to provide immediate relief of symptoms resulting from the mass effect of the tumor, to establish a histologic diagnosis, and to improve local control of the tumor. Recent advances in neuroanesthesia and neurosurgery, including the use of computer-assisted stereotaxy, intraoperative functional mapping, intraoperative ultrasonography, and functional and intraoperative MRI, have significantly improved the safety of surgical resection of brain metastases.[3,57,58]

For surgical candidates, the most important factor to consider is the extent of the extracranial disease. Patients with extensive systemic disease generally have a very limited prognosis and only rarely benefit from surgery. Other important factors influencing the decision concerning surgery include the presence of single or multiple metastases, the location of the tumor, the neurologic status of the patient, and the interval between diagnosis of the primary neoplasm and the brain metastasis.[3,59–61]

SINGLE BRAIN METASTASES. Until relatively recently, the optimal treatment for patients with a single brain metastasis was controversial. A number of uncontrolled retrospective studies suggested that patients with a single brain metastasis who underwent surgical resection in addition to radiotherapy generally had better outcomes than patients treated with radiotherapy alone. However, these studies were limited by the inevitable selection bias resulting from the inclusion of patients in better condition in surgical series.[10,59–65] There are now three randomized prospective studies that have evaluated the role of surgery as an adjunct to whole brain radiotherapy (WBRT) for patients with a single brain metastasis.[23,66–68]

Patchell et al.[23] were the first to address this issue in a prospective randomized study. Fifty-four patients with or without active systemic cancer and a single brain metastasis were randomly assigned to receive either biopsy of the metastases followed by WBRT (36 Gy in 12 fractions) or surgical resection followed by radiotherapy. Six of the 54 patients (11%) did not have a metastasis and were excluded from the study, leaving 48 patients. The patients treated with surgery and WBRT had fewer local recurrences (20% vs. 52%), improved survival (40 weeks vs. 15 weeks), and a better quality of life as measured by the Karnofsky performance status than did patients receiving WBRT alone. The median time to recurrence for patients receiving surgery and radiotherapy was more than 59 weeks, compared to 21 weeks for patients receiving WBRT alone. A multivariate analysis showed that the factors that correlated significantly with increased survival were surgical treatment of the metastasis, the absence of extracranial disease, longer time to the development of the brain metastasis, and younger age.

A second prospective randomized trial evaluating the role of surgery for patients with single brain metastasis was conducted by Vecht et al.[66,67] In this study, 63 patients with a single brain metastasis documented by CT scanning were randomly chosen to receive either surgery and WBRT or WBRT alone. The radiotherapy dose was an unconventional scheme of two fractions a day of 2 Gy each, for a total of 40 Gy given over 2 weeks. Unlike Patchell's study, patients randomly selected to receive radiotherapy alone did not undergo a stereotactic biopsy to confirm the diagnosis of metastases, and MRI was not performed to exclude multiple small metastases that may have been missed by CT imaging. The overall survival of patients treated with surgery and radiotherapy was significantly longer than that of patients treated with radiotherapy alone (10 months vs. 6 months; $P = .04$). In addition, combined treatment also resulted in significantly increased functionally independent survival (FIS) (7.5 months vs. 3.5 months; $P = .06$). The greatest benefit was seen in patients with stable extracranial disease (median survival, 12 vs. 7 months; median FIS, 9 vs. 4 months). Patients with active extracranial disease had a median survival of only 5 months and a FIS of 2.5 months and did not appear to benefit from the addition of surgery. This is consistent with the concept that the extent of systemic disease largely determines the survival of the patient and overcomes any potential advantage the addition of surgery may have provided in controlling the brain metastasis.[9] Patients older than 60 years had decreased survival rates as compared to younger patients (hazard ratio of dying, 2.74; $P = .001$), consistent with the general importance of age as an adverse prognostic factor for brain tumors.

In contrast to these two studies, a more recent multicenter randomized study conducted by Mintz et al.[68] failed to detect a difference in survival or quality of life between patients who underwent surgery plus radiotherapy and those having radiotherapy alone. In this study, the 43 patients randomly assigned to radiotherapy alone had a median survival of 6.3 months, while the 41 patients randomly assigned to surgery and radiotherapy had a median survival of only 5.6 months. The failure of this study to demonstrate that the addition of surgery to radiotherapy improved the outcome of patients may be due to the fact that it included patients with a lower baseline median Karnofsky performance score (KPS) and a higher proportion of extracranial disease.[68,69]

A fourth study, conducted by the Radiation Therapy Oncology Group (RTOG) and the Southwest Oncology Group, was initially intended to be a randomized study comparing surgery and radiotherapy to radiotherapy alone. However, because of poor patient accrual, its design was changed to a prospective physician preference trial. Ultimately, 80 of the 97 registered patients were evaluable. Patients treated with surgery and radiotherapy showed greater neurologic improvement (79% vs. 59%), decreased recurrence (22% vs. 45%), and improved survival, when corrected for other prognostic factors, compared to patients receiving radiotherapy alone.[70] Overall, these studies provide support for the use of surgery in addition to WBRT for patients with a single brain metastasis and stable extracranial disease.

MULTIPLE BRAIN METASTASES. The role of surgery in patients with multiple brain metastases is usually limited to resection of a large, symptomatic, or life-threatening lesion, to obtain tissue for diagnosis in patients without a known primary tumor, or to differentiate a brain metastasis from other cerebral lesions, such as a meningioma.[3] However, as surgical techniques have improved, the ability to resect multiple lesions is becoming more feasible. In one study, Bindal et al.[71] evaluated the efficacy of surgery in 56 patients with multiple brain metastases. These patients were divided into those who had one or more lesions remaining after surgery (group A; n = 30) and those who had all lesions removed (group B; n = 26). In addition, the patients in group B were matched by tumor type, presence or absence of extracranial disease, and time from diagnosis of primary tumor to diagnosis of brain metastases to a group of patients undergoing surgery for a single metastasis (group C; n = 26). The median survivals for patients in groups A, B, and C were 6, 14, and 14 months, respectively. These results suggest that if all the lesions can be removed surgically in patients with multiple brain metastases, the outcome is significantly improved, and comparable to the outcome of patients who underwent surgery for a single lesion. In a second study, Hernandez-Avila et al.[72] evaluated the outcome of 34 patients with multiple metastases treated with surgery. The median survival of patients with controlled systemic disease was 17 months, compared to only 3.1 months for those with active systemic disease, suggesting that surgery for patients with multiple metastases may be feasible in patients with limited systemic disease. However, in contrast to these studies, Hazuka et al.[73] found that surgery was of little benefit in patients with multiple brain metastases. They reported a series consisting of 28 patients with a single metastasis and 18 patients with multiple metastases. The patients with multiple metastases who underwent surgery and radiotherapy had a median survival of only 5 months, compared to 12 months for those with single brain metastases. In these studies, the surgical morbidity and mortality for patients with multiple brain metastases were low and comparable to those reported for patients with a single metastasis undergoing surgery. However, these conflicting results render it difficult to draw firm conclusions regarding the value of surgical resection in patients with multiple brain metastases.

RECURRENT METASTATIC BRAIN TUMORS. Surgery may have a role in patients who develop recurrent disease after standard treatment for brain metastases, especially if there is a single, symptomatic lesion. In an early study, Sundaresan et al.[74] reported the results of reoperation in 21 patients with brain metastasis. Two-thirds of the patients experienced neurologic improvement, and the median duration of the improvement was 6 months. There was no mortality, and only one patient developed increased neurologic deficits after surgery.

Bindal et al.[75] reviewed the experience from M. D. Anderson Cancer Center of 48 patients who underwent reoperation for recurrent brain metastasis.[75] The median interval between the first craniotomy and the diagnosis of recurrence was 6.7 months and the median survival after reoperation was 11.5 months. After surgery, 75% of patients improved symptomatically. Multivariate analysis revealed that survival was negatively affected by the presence of systemic disease ($P = .008$); KPS exceeded 70 ($P = .008$); time to recurrence was less than 4 months ($P = .008$); age exceeded 40 years ($P = .051$); and the primary tumor type was breast or melanoma ($P = .028$). There was no operative mortality. Five patients (10.4%) developed new or increased neurologic deficits after surgery.

Arbit et al.[76] reported the results from Memorial Sloan-Kettering Cancer Center of 109 patients with recurrent brain metastases from non–small cell lung cancer (NSCLC). Thirty-two of these patients (30%) underwent a reoperation. The median interval between the first and second operation was 5 months. The median survival after the second operation was 10 months. The group of patients who underwent reoperation survived significantly longer (median survival, 15 months from the time of the first operation) than a group of 77 patients who did not undergo a second procedure (median survival, 10 months; $P < .001$).

These results provide support for surgical resection of recurrent brain metastases in selected patients with symptomatic lesions. Factors that should be considered include the length of time since the initial operation, location of the recurrent tumor, age and performance status of the patient, extent of extracranial disease, and radiosensitivity of the tumor.[9,77] In general, the sooner the metastasis recurs after initial resection, the less likely reoperation will provide a significant period of palliation.[3,77]

Radiotherapy

PRIMARY RADIOTHERAPY. Radiotherapy has been the mainstay of treatment for patients with brain metastases for more than 40 years. The median survival of patients with brain metastases who are not treated or are treated with corticosteroids alone is 1 to 2 months. Conventional WBRT increases the median survival to 3 to 6 months.[2,3,12] Irradiation is effective in the palliation of neurologic symptoms and also significantly decreases the likelihood of death due to neurologic causes (Fig. 52.1-1). However, for most patients, overall survival is more likely to be determined by the activity and extent of extracranial disease rather than the success or failure of radiotherapy or surgery in controlling brain metastases.

The main goal of radiotherapy for the treatment of brain metastases is to improve neurologic deficits cause by the tumor deposit. The overall response rate is symptom-dependent but ranges from 50% to 85%.[19,78,79] In one study, 74% of patients had improvement of neurologic symptoms, such as headaches, and 65% maintained this for the duration of their lives or for at least 9 months.[80] Cranial nerve deficits improve in approximately 40% of patients. However, the potential for improvement is directly related to the time from diagnosis to radiotherapy.[2,3] Early treatment is generally associated with a better outcome. The majority of patients with significant neurologic dysfunction improve with the use of steroids and radiotherapy, while fewer than 50% of patients with moderate neurologic dysfunction will improve after therapy.[78]

The optimal dose fractionation schedules for patients with brain metastases have been evaluated with randomized trials conducted by the RTOG.[78,81,82] The RTOG completed two trials of several dose-fraction schedules that were subsequently reported together.[78] In the first trial, patients were randomly assigned to 40 Gy in 4 weeks, 40 Gy in 3 weeks, 30 Gy in 3 weeks, or 30 Gy in 2 weeks. The second trial randomly assigned patients to 40 Gy in 3 weeks, 30 Gy in 2 weeks, or 20 Gy in 1 week. The overall response rate and median survival were equivalent in all arms of these studies. The median survival was 18 weeks in the first trial and 15 weeks in the second trial. Brain metastases was the cause of death in 40% of patients in both trials. Patients treated in the shortest time, with larger fractions, responded more quickly, but the duration of the clinical response and the time to progression were similar in each treatment arm. Symptoms were palliated in 75% to 80% of the patients in all treatment arms of these protocols.[82]

To explore the efficacy and toxicity of ultrarapid treatment schedules, the RTOG treated 26 patients with 10 Gy in one fraction and 36 patients with 12 Gy in two fractions.[83] While the promptness of response, percentage of patients demonstrating neurologic improvement, and overall survival were similar to the more protracted schedules described, the median duration of improvement was only 4 weeks compared to 10 weeks in the protracted radiotherapy trials.

While the studies of the RTOG failed to identify the best dose and fractionation schedule for the treatment of brain metastasis, they allowed the identification of clinical factors associated with better survival.[84,85] Patients with breast cancer and no soft tissue metastases, ambulatory lung cancer patients with no extracranial disease, or other ambulatory patients with no extracranial metastases had a median survival of 28 weeks versus 11 weeks for the remaining patients. There was no survival advantage to any fractionation scheme, even among this selected group of patients.

To examine the role of irradiation dose escalation in this prognostically favorable subset of patients with brain metastases, the RTOG randomly assigned 309 of these patients to either 30 Gy in 10 fractions or 50 Gy in 20 fractions.[86] The median survival of the 30-Gy arm was 18 weeks, and that of the 50-Gy arm was 17 weeks. The 1-year survival rate, response rate, time to achieving response, duration of response, and time to progression were the same for both arms, suggesting that there was no therapeutic benefit to dose escalation.

Another approach that has been explored to improve the results of WBRT for patients with brain metastases is the use of

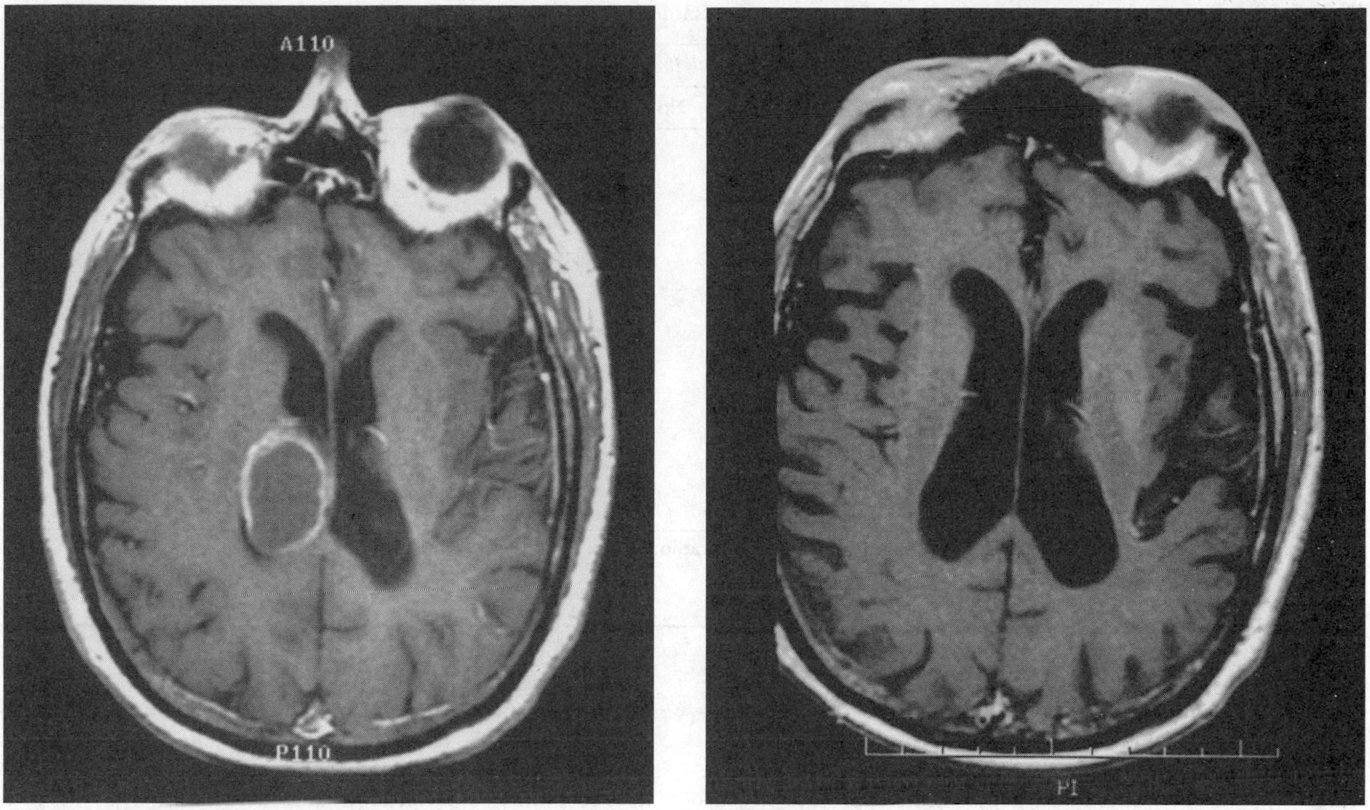

A B

FIGURE 52.1-1 Axial T1-weighted magnetic resonance imaging with gadolinium of 66-year-old man with a single metastasis from colon cancer. **A:** Before whole brain radiotherapy. **B:** After whole brain radiotherapy showing almost complete resolution of the metastasis.

accelerated fractionation. Accelerated fractionation is a technique that uses multiple fractions of radiotherapy per day with the goal to decrease overall treatment time and reduce the risk of tumor cell repopulation. The RTOG performed a phase I and phase II trial of accelerated fractionation for patients with single or multiple brain metastases with controlled, stable, or absent primary disease or in patients with uncontrolled primary disease but no evidence of extracranial metastases.[87] The entire brain was treated twice daily with 1.6-Gy fractions to a total dose of 32 Gy and then a twice-daily boost to encompass all of the disease. The boost dose was increased in successive groups from 16 Gy to 22.4 Gy to 32 Gy to 42.4 Gy. The median survival increased from 4.2 months at a 48-Gy total dose to 5.3 months at a 54.4-Gy total dose to 4.8 months at 60 Gy to 6.4 months at 70.4 Gy. The 1-year survival for 48 Gy was 15%, and the other arms had a 30% 1-year survival. Based on these encouraging results, the RTOG conducted a randomized phase III study comparing accelerated hyperfractionated radiotherapy (1.6 Gy b.i.d.) to a total dose of 54.4 Gy versus standard therapy consisting of 30 Gy in 10 daily fractions in patients with unresected brain metastases, limited systemic disease, and good KPS (≥70). There were 429 evaluable patients, two-thirds of whom had lung primaries. However, the median survival in both groups was 4.5 months, suggesting that there was no benefit of accelerated hyperfractionation over conventional therapy.[88]

The use of biochemical modification (irradiation sensitizers) of irradiation effect has also been explored in patients with brain metastases. However, the results to date have been generally disappointing. Studies using radiosensitizers, such as misonidazole[89] and bromodeoxyuridine,[90] failed to show any additional benefit over radiotherapy alone. Nonetheless, there continues to be interest in irradiation sensitizers and agents, such as gadolinium texaphyrin,[91,92] RSR 13,[93] and pentoxifylline,[94] are currently being evaluated in clinical trials. There is also interest in the concurrent use of radiotherapy with chemotherapeutic agents, such as the topoisomerase II inhibitor lucanthone.[95]

There is currently no consensus on the optimal irradiation schedule for patients with brain metastases. The standard treatment regimen for brain metastasis now includes all of the dose ranges evaluated in the early RTOG studies[78] and is dependent on such issues as the severity of CNS symptomatology, extent of systemic disease, and physician preference. Typical irradiation treatment schedules consist of total doses of 30 to 50 Gy in 1.5- to 4-Gy daily fractions. The most common treatment schedule employed consists of 30 Gy in 10 fractions over 2 weeks.[96] For patients with good prognosis who are likely to survive more than 1 year, more prolonged fractionation (e.g., 40 Gy in 2-Gy fractions) may reduce the long-term morbidity from irradiation.

POSTOPERATIVE RADIOTHERAPY. The goal of postoperative WBRT in patients with solitary brain metastasis is to destroy microscopic residual cancer cells at the site of resection and at other locations within the brain. Theoretically, this should reduce the recurrence rate and prolong survival. Although it is standard practice for patients to receive postoperative radiotherapy as adjuvant therapy to surgery, until

TABLE 52.1-2. Studies Evaluating the Role of Postoperative Radiotherapy

	No. of Patients		*Patients with Brain Recurrence (%)*			*Median Survival (mo)*		
Study	XRT	No XRT	XRT	No XRT	P	XRT	No XRT	P
Dosoretz et al., 1980[97]	12	21	50	52	NS	8	10	NS
Smalley et al., 1987[98]	34	51	21	85	NA	21	12	.02
DeAngelis et al., 1989[99]	79	19	45	65	.03	21	4	NS
Hagen et al., 1990[100]	12	21	50	52	NS	8	10	NS
Armstrong et al., 1994[101]	32	32	47	38	NS	10	14	NS
Skibber et al., 1996[102]	22	12	32	72	NA	18	6	.002
Patchell et al., 1998[103a]	49	46	18	70	.001	11	10	NS

NA, not available; NS, not significant; XRT, postoperative whole brain radiotherapy.
[a]Only prospective randomized study.
(Modified from ref. 103.)

recently the value of this approach was based only on retrospective studies (Table 52.1-2).[97–102] Some of these studies demonstrated that adjuvant WBRT reduced the recurrence rate,[98,99,102] and two studies demonstrated prolonged survival.[98,102] Recently, Patchell et al.[103] published the results of a randomized trial that examined the role of postoperative WBRT in patients with single metastasis.[103] In this study, 95 patients underwent surgical resection of the metastasis and were then randomly assigned to treatment with WBRT (50.4 Gy in 28 fractions) or no further treatment. Patients who received irradiation were significantly less likely to fail in the brain (18% vs. 70%; $P<.001$), and this was true both at the original site of disease (10% vs. 46%; $P<.001$) and other areas of the brain (14% vs. 37%; $P<.01$). Treated patients were also less likely to die of neurologic causes (14% vs. 44%; $P=.003$), but there was no difference in overall survival (48 vs. 43 weeks; $P=.39$) or duration of functional independence (37 vs. 35 weeks; $P=.61$) between the treated and untreated groups. The results of this study suggest that postoperative WBRT in patients with a resected solitary metastasis significantly reduces the incidence of neurologic death but has little impact on the overall survival of the patient, who is mainly dependent on the extent of systemic disease. The authors of this study concluded that the reduction of neurologic death justifies the routine use of postoperative radiotherapy. However, the relatively small size of this study precluded any subgroup analysis. As a result, it remains unclear whether all patients who undergo surgical resection should also receive adjuvant radiotherapy. There may be certain groups of patients, such as those with radio-resistant tumors, such as melanoma or renal cell cancer, for whom WBRT may not be useful after complete surgical resection of the metastases. In addition, the long-term neurocognitive complications of WBRT and its effects on quality of life have not been fully evaluated.

LATE TOXICITY. An important benefit of aggressive treatment for brain metastases is the likelihood that some patients will become long-term survivors. In these patients, late complications of WBRT can be debilitating. These complications include leukoencephalopathy and brain atrophy leading to neurocognitive deterioration and dementia; brain necrosis resulting in more specific neurologic sequelae, depending on the site of necrosis; and communicating hydrocephalus, causing cognitive, gait, and bladder dysfunction.[10,40,104] Neuroendocrine dysfunction, such as hypothyroidism, may also occur.[40,105] The risk for late complications from WBRT is related to total dose, fraction size, patient age, extent of disease, and neurologic impairment at presentation.[106] Prior or concurrent chemotherapy may also effect the occurrence of late CNS toxicity. If WBRT is to be given, a dose-fraction schedule should be used, which takes into account the overall clinical status of the patient while maximizing the palliation of symptoms and, if appropriate, minimizing the risk of long-term complications. In a retrospective review by DeAngelis et al.[104] of 70 patients treated with postoperative radiotherapy using no less than 300-cGy fractions, 11% showed evidence of dementia.[104] Therefore, patients with good prognosis, such as those with single brain metastasis with no or controlled systemic disease, are best treated with daily fractions of 200 cGy or less to decrease the likelihood of long-term CNS toxicity (e.g., 40 to 45 Gy in 1.8- to 2.0-Gy daily fractions).

REIRRADIATION. Occasionally, patients are reirradiated with whole brain or partial brain radiotherapy at the time of brain recurrence. The percentage of patients who undergo reirradiation is quite small, since most patients who recur within the CNS also have progressive extracranial disease and are treated with supportive measures only. However, there are times when recurrence of brain metastasis develops in a patient with controlled systemic disease. Patients with a solitary or a few (≤3) metastases are candidates for treatment with radiosurgery, as this will have less toxicity than repeating WBRT (discussed later in Stereotactic Radiosurgery) and is more likely to be effective than systemic therapy. Other

TABLE 52.1-3. Radiosurgery for Brain Metastases: Results of Representative Series

Study	Technique	Patients/Lesions Treated	Dose (Gy)	Local Control (%)	Median Survival (mo)	Necrosis (%)
Mehta et al., 1992[115]	Linac	40/58	18	82	6.6	0
Kilhstrom et al., 1993[123]	GK	160/235	30	94	NA	NA
Engenhart et al., 1993[120]	Linac	69/102	17	94	6–12[a]	3
Flickinger et al., 1994[116]	GK	157/229	16	89	10	0
Alexander et al., 1995[114]	Linac	248/421	15	89 (65)[b]	9 (7)[b]	3
Valentino, 1995[124]	Linac	139/>139	20–30	86	12.5	NA
Auchter et al., 1996[117]	Linac, GK	122/122	17	86	12	0
Flickinger et al., 1996[121]	GK	116/116	16	85	11	4
Joseph et al., 1996[122]	Linac	120/189	25	94	8	4
Fukuoka et al., 1996[125]	GK	130/>215	14–30	93	8	4.6
Gerosa et al., 1996[126]	GK	225/343	21.1	88	9.3	3.9
Shirato et al., 1997[141]	Linac	39/39	25	92	8.7	0
Breneman et al., 1997[128]	Linac	84/145	16	25	11	2
Shiau et al., 1997[129]	GK	100/219	18.5	77	12	4
Cho et al., 1998[119]	Linac	73/136	17.5	80[b]	7.8	8
Weltman et al., 1998[197]	Linac	34/69	18	NA	6.4	NA
Schoeggl et al., 1999[130]	GK	97/>200	20	94	6	1

GK, gamma knife; Linac, linear accelerator; NA, not available.
[a]Six months with disseminated disease and 12 months with no extracranial disease.
[b]Actuarial.

patients should be considered for treatment with systemic chemotherapy or hormonal therapy. For patients not eligible for radiosurgery or systemic therapy, treatment with whole or partial brain radiation may be indicated. Several retrospective studies have addressed this issue.[107–110] A recent review evaluated 189 patients from three separate studies who were reirradiated.[109] The overall clinical response rate was 42% to 75%, and the median survival from the time of reirradiation was between 3.5 and 5 months. The published techniques of reirradiation include doses from 8 Gy in 2 weeks to 30.6 Gy in 3 weeks, with the median of approximately 20 Gy in 2 weeks, but there is no consensus on which dose fractionation schedule is appropriate or how long after the initial course of radiotherapy it is appropriate to reirradiate.[110] Some investigators have argued that reirradiation should be considered for patients who remain in good general condition but experience neurologic deterioration 4 or more months after a satisfactory response to the initial course of WBRT.[110] The tolerance of the brain is more than likely to be exceeded by reirradiation but, with the limited survival of these patients, there are inadequate data to evaluate the consequences of this treatment.

Stereotactic Radiosurgery

Stereotactic radiosurgery is a technique of external irradiation that uses multiple convergent beams to deliver a high single dose of radiation to a radiographically discrete treatment volume.[111] Radiosurgery can be performed with high-energy roentgenograms produced by linear accelerators, with gamma rays from the gamma knife and, less frequently, with charged particles, such as protons produced by cyclotrons.[112] All the stereotactic irradiation techniques result in rapid fall-off of dose at the edge of the target volume, resulting in a clinically insignificant radiation dose to normal nontarget tissue. Metastases are usually small (<3 cm) radiographically discrete lesions that are noninvasive, rendering them ideal targets for radiosurgery.[113]

An increasing number of uncontrolled studies confirm the effectiveness of stereotactic radiosurgery in treating brain metastases (Table 52.1-3). To date, more than 1780 patients with more than 2700 lesions have been reported in the literature.[111,113] Radiosurgery produces local control rates of 73% to 94% and is associated with a 5% to 10% risk of irradiation necrosis. The median survival from these series ranges from 6 to 15 months, with an average of 9.4 months.[3,111–131] In a multiinstitutional trial involving 116 patients treated with radiosurgery for single brain metastasis using a mean dose of 17.5 Gy, local tumor control was obtained in 99 patients (85%).[116] The 2-year actuarial tumor control rates for the entire group was 67% ± 8%, with a plateau in the curve at 18 months. In a multivariate analysis, better local control was obtained in patients who received WBRT in addition to radiosurgery and in those patients with "radioresistant" histologies (melanoma and renal cell carcinoma). In the largest series to date, Alexander et al.[114] reported the results of radiosurgery using a linear accelerator for the treatment of 248 patients with 421 metastatic lesions. At the time of radiosurgery, 77 patients had no evidence of systemic disease, while 171 patients had stable systemic disease. Of the lesions treated, 126 were classified as radioresistant (melanoma, renal cell carcinoma, and sarcoma), with the remaining 295 lesions representing all other histologies. With a median observation period of 26 months, 48 of 421 lesions (11%) progressed within the radiosurgery volume. The actuarial 1-, 2-, and 3-year local control rates were 85%, 65%, and 65%, respectively. Radioresistant histologies had statistically equal control rates as other lesions. The median survival for the entire group was 9.4 months, measured from the radiosurgery treatment. In a multivariate analysis, the absence of systemic disease (relative risk, 4.4; $P = .0001$) and age younger than 60 years (relative risk, 1.6; $P = .002$) were factors associated with improved survival. The development of symptomatic irradiation necrosis requiring reoperation for increasing mass effect and steroid dependency occurred in 7% of patients in this series.

The optimal role for radiosurgery in patients with brain metastases and its effectiveness in prolonging patient survival remains unclear. However, a recent study by Kondziolka et al. [132] comparing WBRT to WBRT with radiosurgery for patients with multiple metastases (two to four) was stopped at interim analysis because of the significantly better tumor control seen in the group receiving both treatments. In this study, 27 patients with two to four brain metastases (all ≤25 mm in diameter) and a known primary tumor were randomly assigned to WBRT alone or with radiosurgery. Combination therapy was associated with a much lower rate of local failure at 1 year (8% vs. 100%) and a longer median time to local failure (36 vs. 6 months). However, there was no significant improvement in median survival (11 vs. 7.5 months; $P = .22$), which was related to the extent of extracranial disease. An RTOG trial (95-08) is currently under way in which patients with one to three untreated brain metastases will be randomly assigned to WBRT or WBRT and radiosurgery. The study will provide further data on the usefulness of adding radiosurgery to WBRT.

The studies by Patchell et al.,[23] Vecht et al.,[66] and Noordijk et al.[67] indicate that there is a survival advantage for patients with a single brain metastasis treated with surgery and radiotherapy as compared to radiotherapy alone. Many clinical investigators believe that radiosurgery can act as an alternative to surgical resection.[111,113,115,117,121,131] Moreover, radiosurgery has several potential advantages over surgery. It can be used to treat metastases in surgically inaccessible areas of the brain, such as the brain stem. Since it is a noninvasive procedure that can be performed on an outpatient basis, it is associated with less morbidity than surgery. In addition, there is increasing evidence that radiosurgery may also be more cost-effective than surgery.[131,133] In the study by Mehta et al.,[133] the average cost per week of survival was $310 for radiotherapy, $524 for resection plus irradiation, and $270 for radiosurgery plus irradiation.[133]

While there are no completed randomized trials comparing radiosurgery to surgery, Auchter et al.[117] identified 122 patients who met the selection criteria used by Patchell et al.[23] and were treated with WBRT (median, 37.5 Gy) followed by a radiosurgery boost (median, 17 Gy). The overall local control rate was 86%, with an actuarial median survival of 56 weeks and a neurologic median survival of KPS greater than 70 of 44 weeks. These results are comparable to the surgery and irradiation therapy arms of the studies by Patchell et al.,[23] Vecht et al.,[66] and Noordijk et al.[67] and better than the arms of the whole brain treatment alone. In a second retrospective study, Muacevic et al.[134] compared 52 patients with single brain metastasis treated with surgery and WBRT with 56 patients treated with radiosurgery alone. The 1-year local tumor control rates after surgery and radiosurgery were 75% and 83%, respectively, and the 1-year neurologic death rates were 37% and 39%, respectively, suggesting that the local tumor control rates are similar in the two groups. The 1-year survival rate and median survival were 53% and 68 weeks, respectively, in the surgical group and 43% and 35 weeks, respectively, in the radiosurgical group. The shorter overall survival time in the radiosurgery group was related to higher rate of death from systemic disease. Brandt et al.[135] also compared surgery and radiosurgery in a series of 56 patients. In this study, the median survival of the radiosurgically treated patients was 11.4 months, comparable to the 10.4 months for the surgically treated patients. In a fourth study, by Shu et al.,[136] patients with single brain metastases treated with radiosurgery had a median survival of 16 months. In contrast, Bindal et al.[137] conducted a retrospective study comparing 34 consecutive patients treated with radiosurgery with 62 clinically matched patients treated surgically. The median survival for patients treated surgically was 16.4 months, compared to 7.5 months for those treated with radiosurgery ($P = .0009$). Based on these results, the authors concluded that surgery was superior to radiosurgery for the treatment of a single brain metastasis. However, the low local control rate in the radiosurgically treated patients in this study (61%) and differences in the extent of systemic disease between the surgery and radiosurgery groups may have accounted for the poor results of radiosurgery. Ideally, a prospective randomized study comparing surgery to radiosurgery in the treatment of single brain metastases would resolve the issue of the relative efficacy of these two treatments. However, previous attempts at such a study have been unsuccessful due to poor patient accrual as a result of patient or physician preference (or both) for either surgery or radiosurgery.

The role of WBRT in patients treated with radiosurgery is controversial, especially for patients with relatively radioresistant tumors, such as melanoma.[121,131] In the study by Patchell et al.,[103] 37% of patients failed in other sites within the brain if they did not receive whole brain irradiation. While some studies have shown improved local control in patients who received whole brain radiotherapy in addition to radiosurgery,[116] overall patient survival is generally not increased.[114,123,131] Currently, most centers treat patients with brain metastases with both radiosurgery and whole brain radiotherapy (Fig. 52.1-2) and limit the use of up-front radiosurgery alone to cases for which there are no alternatives, such as prior high-dose irradiation to the head and neck area or when the patient refuses whole brain radiation therapy. However, there are several retrospec-

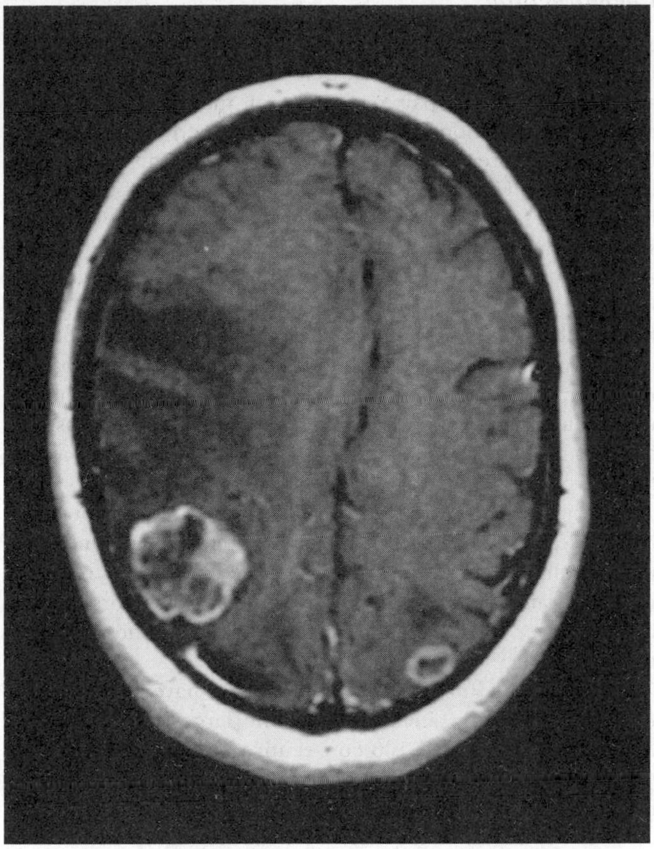
A

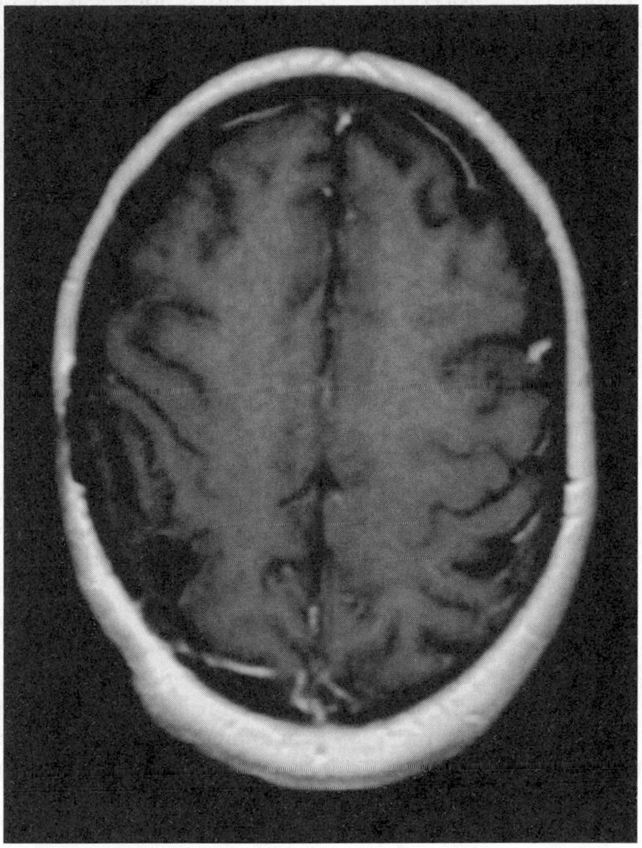
B

FIGURE 52.1-2 A 48-year-old woman with non–small cell lung cancer presenting with lethargy and left-sided weakness. **A:** Axial T1-weighted magnetic resonance imaging shows a 3-cm enhancing metastasis in the right anterior parietal lobe and a smaller 1-cm metastasis in the left parietal lobe. The right parietal lesion was resected, and the left parietal lesion was treated with stereotactic radiosurgery (1800 cGy), followed by whole brain radiation therapy. **B:** Follow-up magnetic resonance imaging 6 months later showing no residual tumor at either site. Twenty months after her surgery, the patient remains well neurologically, with no evidence of recurrent metastases in her brain. However, she has developed recurrent disease in her lung.

tive studies suggesting that for selected patients, radiosurgery alone may be as effective as the combination of radiosurgery and WBRT, with potentially less morbidity.[138–141] In a study by Sneed et al.,[138] the outcome of 62 patients with up to four newly diagnosed brain metastases treated with radiosurgery alone were compared with 43 patients with newly diagnosed metastases treated with the combination of radiosurgery and WBRT. The median survival and the 1-year local freedom from progression (FFP) were the same for radiosurgery alone and for radiosurgery and WBRT (median survival, 11.3 vs. 11.1 months; 1-year local FFP, 71% vs. 79%, respectively). More patients treated with radiosurgery failed in the brain (new metastases or local failure or both) than those receiving the combination of radiosurgery and WBRT (brain FFP at 1 year, 28% for radiosurgery compared to 69% for the combination of radiosugery and WBRT). However, brain control, allowing for successful salvage of a first failure, was not significantly different between the two groups. This study suggests that omission of WBRT in the initial management of patients treated with radiosurgery for up to four brain metastases does not appear to compromise survival or intracranial control and allows for salvage therapy as indicated. A second small retrospective study of 35 patients with melanoma brain metastases found no difference in survival between the patients treated with radiosurgery and the combination of radiosurgery and WBRT.[139] A third study by Pirzkall et al.[140] comparing the outcome of 158 patients with one to three brain metastases treated by radiosurgery with 78 patients treated with radiosurgery and WBRT also found no statistical difference in survival and local control between the two groups, although there was a trend toward improved local control and increased survival in the group that received WBRT. Randomized studies comparing radiosurgery and the combination of radiosurgery and WBRT are currently under way to assess survival, quality of life, and cost-effectiveness in patients with newly diagnosed brain metastases.

COMPLICATIONS OF RADIOSURGERY. Acute complications within the first week of treatment are uncommon, occurring in fewer than 10% of patients.[114,128,129,142] These include seizures (2.3% to 6.1%), headaches, exacerbation of preexisting neurologic deficits (2% to 6%), nausea (especially in patients receiving more than 375 cGy to the area postrema) and, rarely, hemorrhage.[125] The risk of seizures can be reduced by treating patients with anticonvulsants before the radiosurgery procedure.[114] Patients with lesions near the posterior fossa may benefit from premedication with antiemetics. Acute neurologic deficits can be reduced by using doses of less than 30 Gy.[113]

Subacute complications occurring within 6 months of treatment consists of alopecia in patients whose scalp received more than 4.4 Gy of irradiation[114] and neurologic deterioration due to necrosis and peritumoral edema.[113]

Chronic complications due to irradiation necrosis occur in approximately 8% to 16% of patients. These patients present with increased seizures, headaches, or worsening neurologic deficits.[113,114,120] These side effects can usually be treated with corticosteroids. However, 5% to 10% of patients develop severe symptomatic necrosis and may require surgical resection.[113,114] Cranial nerve palsies are rare and develop in fewer than 1% of patients.[142]

PROGNOSTIC FACTORS. Young patients with good performance status, limited extracranial disease, and one or two small lesions are particularly suited to treatment by radiosurgery.[113,114,131] Poor prognostic factors include poor performance status (<70), progressive systemic disease, large tumor size, infratentorial location, and multiple metastases (more than two lesions).[113,119,122] The efficacy of radiosurgery appears to be independent of the histology of the lesion. Radioresistant tumors, such as renal cell carcinoma,[143] malignant melanoma,[144,145] and NSCLC[146] have statistically the same control rate as other tumors.[111,113]

SUMMARY. The introduction of radiosurgery over the last decade represents one of the major advances in the treatment of brain metastases. For patients with a single small asymptomatic or mildly symptomatic lesion, radiosurgery can probably be used as a substitute for surgery with comparable outcomes.[113,117] Radiosurgery also has an important role in patients with recurrence of brain metastasis after whole brain radiotherapy and, perhaps, in the initial treatment of patients with several metastases and limited systemic disease.

Interstitial Brachytherapy

Interstitial brachytherapy involves the implantation of radioactive nuclides into the wall of the surgical cavity to deliver an additional dose of radiation to the residual tumor while limiting the irradiation to the surrounding brain. The relatively sharp border between metastases and the surrounding brain renders them ideal lesions for brachytherapy. Brachytherapy for metastases has been evaluated in several small uncontrolled studies using iodine 125 sources, and median survivals have ranged from 9 to 18.3 months.[147–149] Although brachytherapy is rarely performed for small lesions suitable for radiosurgery, it may have a limited role for metastases that are too large for radiosurgery.

A more recent brachytherapy strategy involves using a photon radiosurgery system. This is a battery-powered miniature x-ray generator with an attached probe that can be placed stereotactically into metastases at the time of craniotomy to deliver a single fraction of high-dose radiation (12.5 Gy) in less than an hour.[149,150] Preliminary results suggest that this procedure is well tolerated and produces effective local tumor control.[149,150]

Chemotherapy

The role of chemotherapy for the treatment of patients with brain metastases has not been defined. At present, chemotherapy is rarely used as part of the overall management of brain metastases. Traditionally, it had been assumed that the blood–brain barrier prevented chemotherapeutic agents from entering the CNS. However, there is evidence that the blood–brain barrier is in fact partially disrupted within brain tumors.[151] This suggests that other factors may also contribute to the generally disappointing results of chemotherapy for brain metastases, such as the intrinsic resistance to chemotherapy of many tumors that metastasize to the brain; the use of chemotherapeutic agents designed to penetrate the blood–brain barrier rather than agents known to be most effective against the primary malignancy; and the tendency for brain metastases to develop after the failure of primary chemotherapeutic agents to control systemic disease.[151,152]

Although the overall results of chemotherapy for brain metastases have been generally disappointing, a number of uncontrolled studies have demonstrated favorable response rates in brain metastases from chemosensitive tumors, such as breast cancer, small cell lung cancer (SCLC), and germ cell tumors.[2,3,151,152]

Patients with metastatic breast cancer have been treated with chemotherapy since 1970. In the largest series to date, Rosner et al.[153] treated 100 consecutive breast cancer patients with brain metastases with several chemotherapy regimens, including cyclophosphamide, 5-fluorouracil, and prednisone, or with this regimen together with methotrexate and vincristine. These patients had not received prior chemotherapy for their systemic disease. Overall, 50% of patients had an objective response (10% had a complete response, and 40% had a partial response). In addition, 9% had stable disease. The median duration of remission for complete responders was 10 months and, for partial responders, it was 7 months. Rosner et al.[154] subsequently treated an additional 26 patients with progressive brain metastases from breast cancer with four different chemotherapeutic regimens: cyclophosphamide, 5-fluorouracil, and prednisone; cyclophosphamide, 5-fluorouracil, and prednisone together with methotrexate and vincristine; cyclophosphamide and doxorubicin (Adriamycin); and mitomycin and vinblastine (Velban).[154] Objective responses were seen in 61% of patients, while another 15% had stable disease. The median survival for responders was 12 months, compared to 2.4 months for nonresponders. Interestingly, prior systemic chemotherapy did not affect the response of the brain metastases, arguing against the concept of the brain as a pharmacologic sanctuary.

Franciosi et al.[155] treated 56 patients with brain metastases from breast cancer with the combination of cisplatin and etoposide for a maximum of six cycles and observed complete responses in 13%, partial responses in 26%, and stable disease in 21% of patients. The median survival was approximately 8 months. Boogerd et al.[156] treated 20 patients with cyclophosphamide, methotrexate, and 5-fluorouracil, or cyclophosphamide, doxorubicin, and 5-fluorouracil. Seven patients had recurrent disease after WBRT. Objective tumor regression occurred in 76% of patients after two cycles of chemotherapy. The median duration of neurologic remission was 30 weeks, and the median survival was 25 weeks. When the results of these chemotherapy patients were compared to 29 historic controls treated with WBRT, the neurologic response rate, duration of response, and median survival were better in those patients treated with chemotherapy.

Several other small series have reported responses to a variety of regimens, including a combination of drugs combining thioguanine, procarbazine, dibromodulcitol, lomustine (CCNU), 5-fluorouracil, and hydroxyurea designed to improve the efficacy of CCNU.[157] Recently, there has also been a report of patients with brain metastases from breast cancer responding to high-dose chemotherapy.[158]

There have also been many studies evaluating the response of brain metastases from SCLC to chemotherapy.[151,159] Kristensen et al.[159] reviewed 12 patient series with a total of 116 patients published between 1981 and 1990. Eleven of these studies contained an epipodophyllotoxin and, in five, this was combined with either cisplatin or carboplatin. The overall response rate to chemotherapy without irradiation in patients with intracranial metastases at diagnosis was 76%, while the response rate at relapse was 43%. These results suggest that intracranial metastases from SCLC respond to chemotherapy as readily as other metastatic locations of SCLC.

Favorable responses have also been seen with chemotherapy for metastases from choriocarcinoma, germ cell tumors, and ovarian cancer.[151,160–162] The results of chemotherapy for brain metastases from less chemosensitive tumors, such as NSCLC and melanoma, have been generally disappointing. However, newer regimens, such as thioguanine, procarbazine, dibromodulcitol, CCNU, 5-fluorouracil, and hydroxyurea[157]; carboplatin and etoposide[155]; cisplatin and etoposide[163]; cisplatin and tenoposide[164]; and tenoposide alone[165] for NSCLC[166] and temozolamide for melanoma have produced slightly higher response rates. In a study by Franciosi et al.,[155] 43 patients with NSCLC were treated with cisplatin and etoposide. The combined complete and partial response rates were 30%, and median survival was 8 months.

Overall, these studies suggest that chemotherapy has some activity against brain metastases, especially from chemosensitive tumors, such as breast cancer, SCLC, and choriocarcinoma. In these patients, chemotherapy may have a role as palliative therapy in patients with recurrent disease after radiotherapy or possibly as initial treatment in patients with small asymptomatic tumors. As newer drugs are introduced, the effectiveness of chemotherapy for brain metastases may improve.

Hormonal Therapy

In patients with hormone-responsive tumors, such as breast cancer, there are anecdotal reports of patients responding to hormonal agents, such as tamoxifen[167] and megestrol acetate.[168]

PROGNOSIS

The median survival of patients with untreated brain metastases is approximately 1 month.[169] The addition of steroids increases survival to 2 months,[14,79] while whole brain radiotherapy further improves survival to 3 to 6 months.[12,78,79,85,170,171] Patients with single brain metastases and limited extracranial disease who are treated with surgery and WBRT have a median survival of approximately 10 to 16 months.[23,64,66,67] Favorable prognostic factors include the absence of systemic disease, young age (<60 years), good performance status (KPS ≥70), long time to development of metastasis, surgical resection, less than three lesions, and possibly response to steroids.[2,3,64,78,85,172–175] Patients with brain metastases as the only manifestation of an undetected primary tumor also have a favorable prognosis, with an overall median survival of 13.4 months.[176] Breast cancer patients with brain metastases generally have a more favorable prognosis than brain metastases from other types of primary tumor.[82,84,85] On the other hand, patients with colorectal carcinoma tend to have a poorer prognosis.[177] This may be due to the tendency of these patients to have a higher frequency of cerebellar metastases, which are associated with an adverse prognosis.

Recently, Gaspar et al.[173] performed a recursive partitioning analysis of prognostic factors from three RTOG brain metastases trials and identified three prognostic classes. Class 1 patients had a KPS of 70 or higher, were younger than 65 years of age, had a controlled primary and no extracranial metastases, and had a median survival of 7.1 months. Class 3 patients had a KPS of less than 70 and a median survival of 2.3 months. Class 2 patients included all remaining patients and had a median survival of 4.2 months. Agboola et al.[174] evaluated the validity of this classification system in 125 patients with brain metastases treated with surgical resection and WBRT. The median survival in classes 1, 2, and 3 were 14.8 months, 9.9 months, and 6 months, respectively. Use of this classification may identify patients most likely to benefit from treatment and potentially allows new therapies to be evaluated on homogeneous patient groups.[174,175]

REFERENCES

1. Clouston PD, DeAngelis LM, Posner JB. The spectrum of neurological disease in patients with systemic cancer. *Ann Neurol* 1992;31:268.
2. Patchell R. Brain metastases. *Handbook Neurol* 1997;25:135.
3. Wen PY, Loeffler JS. Management of brain metastases. *Oncology* 1999;13:941.
4. Davey P. Brain metastases. *Curr Probl Cancer* 1999;23:59.
5. Posner JB. Management of brain metastases. *Rev Neurol* 1992;148:477.
6. Sawaya R, Bindal RK. Metastatic brain tumors. In: Kaye AH, Laws ER, eds. *Brain tumors.* Edinburgh: Churchill Livingstone, 1995:923.
7. Graus F, Walker RW, Allen JC. Brain metastases in children. *J Pediatr* 1983;103:558.
8. Takakura K, Sano K, Hojo S, et al. *Metastatic tumors of the central nervous system.* Tokyo: Igaku-Shoin, Ltd, 1982.
9. Johnson JD, Young B. Demographics of brain metastasis. *Neurosurg Clin North Am* 1996;7:337.
10. Posner JB. *Neurologic complications of cancer.* Philadelphia: FA Davis Co, 1995.
11. Paterson AH, Agarwal M, Lees A, et al. Brain metastases in breast cancer patients receiving adjuvant chemotherapy. *Cancer* 1982;49:651.
12. Zimm S, Wampler GL, Stablein D, et al. Intracerebral metastases in solid tumor patients: natural history and results of treatment. *Cancer* 1981;48:384.
13. Bouffet E, Doumi N, Thiesse P, et al. Brain metastases in children with solid tumors. *Cancer* 1997;79:403.
14. Delattre JY, Krol G, Thaler HT, Posner JB. Distribution of brain metastases. *Arch Neurol* 1988;45:741.
15. Sze G, Milano E, Johnson C, et al. Detection of brain metastases: comparison of contrast-enhanced MR with unenhanced MR and contrast CT. *Am J Neuroradiol* 1990;11:785.
16. Cairncross JG, Posner JB. The management of brain metastases. In: Walker MD, eds. *Oncology of the nervous system.* Boston: Nijhoff, 1983:341.
17. Nutt SH, Patchell RA. Intracranial hemorrhage associated with primary and secondary tumors. *Neurosurg Clin North Am* 1992;3:591.
18. Forsyth PA, Posner JB. Headaches in patients with brain tumors: a study of 111 patients. *Neurology* 1993;43:1678.
19. Coia LR, Aaronson N, Linggood R, et al. A report of the consensus workshop panel on the treatment of brain metastases. *Int J Radiat Oncol Biol Phys* 1992;23:223.
20. Cohen N, Strauss G, Lew R, et al. Should prophylactic anticonvulsants be administered to patients with newly diagnosed cerebral metastases? A retrospective analysis. *J Clin Oncol* 1988;6:1621.
21. Glantz M, Cole B, Friedberg M, et al. A randomized, blinded, placebo-controlled trial of divalproex sodium prophylaxis in adults with newly diagnosed brain tumors. *Neurology* 1996;46:985.

22. Weaver S, DeAngelis LM, Fulton D, et al. A prospective randomized study of prophylactic anticonvulsants in patients with primary or metastatic brain tumors and without seizures. *Ann Neurol* 1997;42:430.
23. Patchell RA, Tibbs PA, Walsh JW, et al. A randomized trial of surgery in the treatment of single metastases to the brain. *N Engl J Med* 1990;322:494.
24. Schoenberg BS, Christine BW, Whisnant JO. Nervous system neoplasms and primary malignancy of other sites: the unique association between meningiomas and breast cancer. *Neurology* 1975;25:705.
25. Rubinstein AB, Schein M, Reichenthal E. The association of carcinoma of the breast with meningioma. *Surg Gynecol Obstet* 1989;169:334.
26. Davis PC, Hudgins PA, Peterman SB, et al. Diagnosis of cerebral metastases: double-dose delayed CT vs contrast-enhanced MR imaging. *AJNR Am J Neuroradiol* 1991;12:293.
27. Schaefer PW, Budzik RF, Gonzalez RG. Imaging of cerebral metastases. *Neurosurg Clin North Am* 1996;7:393.
28. Sze G, Johnson C, Kawamura Y, et al. Comparison of single- and triple-dose contrast material in the MR screening of brain metastases. *AJNR Am J Neuroradiol* 1988;19:821.
29. Yuh WT, Fisher DJ, Runge VM, et al. Phase III multicenter trial of high-dose gadoteridol in MR evaluation of brain metastases. *AJNR Am J Neuroradiol* 1994;15:1037.
30. Finelli DA, Hurst GC, Gullapali RP, et al. Improved contrast of enhancing brain lesions of postgadolinium, T_1-weighted spin-echo images with the use of magnetization transfer. *Radiology* 1994;190:553.
31. Peretti-Viton P, Taieb D, Viton JM, et al. Contrast-enhanced magnetization transfer MRI in metastatic lesions of the brain. *Neuroradiology* 1998;40:783.
32. Latief KH, White CS, Protopapas Z, et al. Search for a primary lung neoplasm in patients with brain metastasis: is the chest radiograph sufficient? *AJR Am J Roentgenol* 1997;168:1339.
33. Merchut MP. Brain metastases from undiagnosed systemic neoplasms. *Arch Intern Med* 1989;149:1076.
34. Van de Pol M, van Aalst VC, Wilmink JT, Twijnstra A. Brain metastases from an unknown primary tumor: which diagnostic procedures are indicated? *J Neurol Neurosurg Psychiatry* 1996;61:321.
35. Kofman S, Garvin JS, Nagamani D, et al. Treatment of cerebral metastases from breast cancer with prednisone. *JAMA* 1957;163:1473.
36. Galicich JH, French LA, Melby JC. Use of dexamethasone in the treatment of cerebral edema associated with brain tumors. *Lancet* 1961:81:46.
37. Batchelor T, DeAngelis LM. Medical management of cerebral metastases. *Neurosurg Clin North Am* 1996;7:435.
38. Vecht CJ, Hovestadt A, Verbiest HBC, et al. Dose-effect relationship of dexamethasone on Karnofsky performance in metastatic brain tumors: a randomized study of doses of 4, 8, and 16 milligrams per day. *Neurology* 1994;44:675.
39. Vecht CJ, Verbiest HBC. Use of glucocorticoids in neuro-oncology. In: Wiley RG, ed. *Neurological complications of cancer.* New York: Marcel Dekker Inc, 1995:199.
40. Delattre JY, Posner JB. Neurological complications of chemotherapy and radiation therapy. In: Aminoff MJ, ed. *Neurology and general medicine.* New York: Churchill Livingstone, 1994:421.
41. Henson JW, Jalaj JK, Walker RW, et al. *Pneumocystis carinii* pneumonia in patients with primary brain tumors. *Arch Neurol* 1991;48:406.
42. Slivka A, Wen PY, Shea WM, Loeffler JS. Pneumocystis pneumonia during steroid taper in patients with primary brain tumors. *Am J Med* 1993;94:216.
43. Delattre JY, Safai B, Posner JB. Erythema multiforme and Stevens-Johnson syndrome in patients receiving cranial irradiation and phenytoin. *Neurology* 1988;38:194.
44. Mamon H, Wen PY, Loeffler JS. Allergic skin reactions to anticonvulsant medications in patients receiving cranial radiation. *Epilepsia* 1999;40:341.
45. Khe HX, Delattre J-Y, Poisson M. Stevens-Johnson syndrome in a patient receiving cranial irradiation and carbamazepine. *Neurology* 1990;40:1144.
46. Taylor LP, Posner JB. Phenobarbital rheumatism in patients with brain tumor. *Ann Neurol* 1989;25:92.
47. Werk EE, Choi Y, Sholiton Z, et al. Interference in the effect of dexamethasone by diphenylhydantoin. *N Engl J Med* 1969;281:32.
48. Lawson LA, Blouin RA, Smith RB, et al. Phenytoin-dexamethasone interaction: a previously unreported observation. *Surg Neurol* 1981;16:23.
49. Grossman SA, Sheidler VR, Gilbert MR. Decreased phenytoin levels in patients receiving chemotherapy. *Am J Med* 1989;87:505.
50. Fetell MR, Grossman SA, Fisher JD, et al. Preirradiation paclitaxel in glioblastoma multiforme: efficacy, pharmacology, and drug interactions. New Approaches to Brain Tumor Therapy Central Nervous System Consortium. *J Clin Oncol* 1997;15:3121.
51. Glantz MJ, Cole BF, Forsyth PA, et al. Anticonvulsant prophylaxis in patients with brain tumors: a systematic review of the evidence (*in press*).
52. Byrne TN, Cascino TL, Posner JB. Brain metastasis from melanoma. *J Neurooncol* 1983;1:313.
53. Sawaya R, Zuccarello M, Elkalliny M, et al. Postoperative venous thromboembolism and brain tumors: I. Clinical profile. *J Neurooncol* 1992;14:119.
54. Levin JM, Schiff, Loeffler JS, et al. Complications of therapy for venous thromboembolic disease in patients with brain tumors. *Neurology* 1993;43:1111.
55. Ruff RL, Posner JB. The incidence and treatment of peripheral venous thombosis in patients with glioma. *Ann Neurol* 1983;13:334.
56. Schiff D, DeAngelis LM. Therapy of venous thromboembolism in patients with brain metastases. *Cancer* 1994;73:493.
57. Kelly PJ, Abe H, Aida T, et al. Results of computed tomography-based computer-assisted stereotactic resection of metastatic intracranial tumors. *Neurosurgery* 1988;22:7.
58. Lang FF, Sawaya R. Surgical treatment of metastatic brain tumors. *Semin Surg Oncol* 1998;14:53.
59. Sundaresan N, Galicich J. Surgical treatment of brain metastases: clinical and computerized tomography evaluation of the results of treatment. *Cancer* 1985;55:1382.
60. Galicich JH, Sundaresan N, Arbit E, et al. Surgical treatment of single brain metastasis: factors associated with survival. *Cancer* 1980;45:381.
61. Winston KR, Walsh JW, Fischer EG. Results of operative treatment of intracranial metastatic tumors. *Cancer* 1980;45:2639.
62. White K, Fleming T, Laws E. Single metastasis to the brain. Surgical treatment in 122 consecutive patients. *Mayo Clin Proc* 1981;56:424.
63. Pieper DR, Hess KR, Sawaya RE. Role of surgery in the treatment of brain metatases in patients with breast cancer. *Ann Surg Oncol* 1997;4:484.
64. Wronski M, Arbit E, McCormick B, Wronski M. Surgical treatment of 70 patients with brain metastases from breast carcinoma. *Cancer* 1997;80:1746.
65. Mandell L, Harris B, Sullivan M, et al. The treatment of single brain metastasis from non-oat cell lung carcinoma. Surgery and radiation vs. radiation alone. *Cancer* 1986;58:641.
66. Vecht CJ, Haaxma-Reiche EM, Noordijk GW, et al. Treatment of single brain metastasis: radiotherapy alone or combined with neurosurgery? *Ann Neurol* 1993;583.
67. Noordijk EM, Vecht CJ, Haaxma-Reiche H, et al. The choice of treatment of single brain metastasis should be based on extracranial tumor activity and age. *Int J Radiat Oncol Biol Phys* 1994;29:711.
68. Mintz AP, Kestle J, Rathbone MP, et al. A randomized trial to assess the efficacy of surgery in addition to radiotherapy in patients with a single brain metastasis. *Cancer* 1996;78:1470.
69. Mintz AP, Cairncross JG. Treatment of a single brain metastasis. The role of radiation following surgical resection. *JAMA* 1998;280:1527.
70. Sause W, Crowley J, Morantz R, et al. Solitary brain metastasis: results of an RTOG/SWOG protocol evaluating surgery + RT versus RT alone. *Am J Clin Oncol* 1990;3:427.
71. Bindal RK, Sawaya R, Leavens ME, et al. Surgical treatment of multiple brain metastases. *J Neurosurg* 1993;79:210.
72. Hernandez-Avila G, Black PMcL, Loeffler JS, et al. Is it worth operating on a patient with more than one intracranial metastasis? (Abstract 32) Congress of Neurological Surgeons, forty-ninth annual meeting, 1999.
73. Hazuka MB, Burleson W, Stroud DN, et al. Multiple brain metastases are associated with poor survival in patients treated with surgery and radiotherapy. *J Clin Oncol* 1993;11:369.
74. Sundaresan N, Sachdev V, DiGiacinto G. Reoperation for brain metastases. *J Clin Oncol* 1988;6:1625.
75. Bindal RK, Sawaya R, Leavens ME, et al. Reoperation for recurrent metastatic brain tumors. *J Neurosurg* 1995;83:600.
76. Arbit E, Wronski M, Burt M, Galicich JH. The treatment of patients with recurrent brain metastases. *Cancer* 1995;76:765.
77. Kaye A. Malignant brain tumors: late reoperation for metastatic tumors. In: Little J, Awad I, eds. *Reoperative neurosurgery.* Baltimore: Williams & Wilkins, 1992:72.
78. Borgelt B, Gelber R, Kramer S, et al. The palliation of brain metastases. Final results of the first two studies by the Radiation Therapy Oncology Group. *Int J Radiat Oncol Biol Phys* 1980;6:1.
79. Sneed PK, Larson DA, Wara WM. Radiotherapy for cerebral metastases. *Neurosurg Clin North Am* 1996;7:505.
80. Cairncross JG, Kim JH, Posner JB. Radiation therapy for brain metastasis. *Ann Neurol* 1980;7:529.
81. Vermeulen SS. Whole brain radiotherapy in the treatment of metastatic brain tumors. *Semin Surg Oncol* 1998;14:64.
82. Berk L. An overview of radiotherapy trials for the treatment of brain metastases. *Oncology* 1995;9:1205.
83. Borgelt B, Gelber R, Larson M, et al. Ultra-rapid high dose irradiation for the palliation of brain metastases: final results of the first two studies by the Radiation Therapy Oncology Group. *Int J Radiat Oncol Biol Phys* 1981;7:1633.
84. Gelber R, Larson M, Borgelt B, et al. Equivalence of radiation schedules for the palliative treatment of brain metastases in patients with favorable prognosis. *Cancer* 1981;48:1749.
85. Diener-West M, Dobbins TW, Phillips TL, et al. Identification of an optimal subgroup for treatment evaluation of patients with brain metastases using RTOG study 7916. *Int J Radiat Oncol Biol Phys* 1989;16:669.
86. Kurtz JM, Gelber R, Brady LW, et al. The palliation of brain metastases in a favorable patient population. A randomized clinical trial by the Radiation Therapy Oncology Group. *Int J Radiat Oncol Biol Phys* 1981;7:891.
87. Sause W, Scott C, Krisch R, et al. Phase I/II trial of accelerated fractionation in brain metastases RTOG 85-28. *Int J Radiat Oncol Biol Phys* 1993;26:653.
88. Murray KJ, Scott C, Greenberg HM, et al. A randomized phase III study of accelerated hyperfractionation versus standard in patients with unresected brain metastases: a report of the Radiation Therapy Oncology Group (RTOG) 9104. *Int J Radiat Oncol Biol Phys* 1997;39:571.
89. Kamarnicky LT, Phillips TL, Martz K, et al. A randomized phase III protocol for the evaluation of misonidazole combined with radiation in the treatment of patients with brain metastases (RTOG-7916). *Int J Radiat Oncol Biol Phys* 1991;20:53.
90. Phillips TL, Scott CB, Leibel SA, et al. Results of a randomized comparison of radiotherapy and bromodeoxyuridine with radiotherapy alone for brain metastases: report of RTOG trial 89-05. *Int J Radiat Oncol Biol Phys* 1995;33:339.
91. Carde P, Timmerman D, Koprowski C, et al. Gadolinium-texaphyrin (GD-TEX) radiation sensitizer: improved survival in a phase IB/II trial in patients with brain metastases. *Proc Am Soc Clin Oncol* 1998;17:379a(abst 1463).
92. Viala J, Vanel D, Meingan P, et al. Phases IB and II multidose trial of gadolinium texaphyrin, a radiation sensitizer detectable at MR imaging: preliminary results in brain metastases. *Radiology* 1999;212:755.
93. Kleinberg L, Grossman SA, Piantadosi S, et al. Phase I trial to determine the safety, pharmacodynamics, and pharmacokinetics of RSR 13, a novel radioenhancer, in newly diagnosed glioblastoma multiforme. *J Clin Oncol* 1999;17:2593.
94. Johnson FE, Harrison BR, McKirgan LW, et al. A phase II evaluation of pentoxifylline combined with radiation in the treatment of brain metastases. *Int J Oncol* 1998;13:801.

95. Del Rowe JD, Bello J, Mitnick R, et al. Accelerated regression of brain metastases in patients receiving whole brain radiation and the topoisomerase II inhibitor, lucanthone. *Int J Radiat Oncol Biol Phys* 1999;43:89.
96. Coia LR, Hanks GE, Martz K, et al. Practice patterns of palliative care for the United States 1984–1985. *Int J Radiat Oncol Biol Phys* 1993;25:209.
97. Dosoretz DE, Blitzer PH, Russell AH, et al. Management of solitary metastasis to the brain: the role of elective brain irradiation following complete surgical resection. *Int J Radiat Oncol Biol Phys* 1980;6:1727.
98. Smalley S, Schray M, Laws E, et al. Adjuvant radiation therapy after surgical resection of solitary brain metastasis: association with pattern of failure and survival. *Int J Radiat Oncol Biol Phys* 1987;13:1611.
99. DeAngelis LM, Mandell LR, Thaler HT, et al. The role of postoperative radiotherapy after resection of single brain metastases. *Neurosurgery* 1989;24:798.
100. Hagen N, Cirrincione C, Thaler H, et al. The role of radiation therapy following resection of single brain metastasis from melanoma. *Neurology* 1990;40:158.
101. Armstrong JG, Wronski M, Galicich J, et al. Postoperative radiation for lung cancer metastatic to the brain. *J Clin Oncol* 1994;12:2340.
102. Skibber JM, Soong S, Austin L, et al. Cranial irradiation after surgical excision of brain metastases in melanoma patients. *Ann Surg Oncol* 1996;3:118.
103. Patchell RA, Tibbs PA, Regine WF, et al. Postoperative radiotherapy in the treatment of single brain metastases to the brain. *JAMA* 1998;280:1485.
104. DeAngelis L, Delattre J-Y, Posner JB. Radiation-induced dementia in patients cured of brain metastases. *Neurology* 1989;39:789.
105. Heikens J, Michiels EM, Behrendt H, et al. Long-term neuro-endocrine sequelae after treatment for childhood medulloblastoma. *Eur J Cancer* 1998;34:1592.
106. Schultheiss TE, Kun LE, Ang KK, et al. Radiation response of the central nervous system. *Int J Radiat Oncol Biol Phys* 1995;31:1093.
107. Kurup P, Reddy S, Hendrikson FR. Results of re-irradiation for cerebral metastases. *Cancer* 1980;46:2587.
108. Hazuka MB, Kinzie JJ. Brain metastases: results and effects of re-irradiation. *Int J Radiat Oncol Biol Phys* 1988;15:433.
109. Wong WW, Schild SE, Sawyer TE, Shaw EG. Analysis of outcome in patients reirradiated for brain metastases. *Int J Radiat Oncol Biol Phys* 1996;34:585.
110. Cooper JS, Steinfield A, Lerch IA. Cerebral metastases: value of reirradiation in selected patients. *Radiology* 1990;174:883.
111. Loeffler JS, Barker FG, Chapman PH. Role of radiosurgery in the management of central nervous system metastases. *Cancer Chemother Pharmacol* 1999;43:S11.
112. Phillips MH, Stelzer KJ, Griffin TW, et al. Stereotactic radiosurgery: a review and comparisons of methods. *J Clin Oncol* 1994;12:1085.
113. Boyd TS, Mehta MP. Stereotactic radiosurgery for brain metastases. *Oncology* 1999;13:1397.
114. Alexander E III, Moriarty TM, Davis RB, et al. Stereotactic radiosurgery for the definitive, noninvasive treatment of brain metastases. *J Natl Cancer Inst* 1995;87:34.
115. Mehta MP, Rozental JM, Levin AB, et al. Defining the role of radiosurgery in the management of brain metastases. *Int J Radiat Oncol Biol Phys* 1992;24:619.
116. Flickinger JC, Kondziolka D, Lunsford LD, et al. A multi-institutional experience with stereotactic radiosurgery for solitary brain metastasis. *Int J Radiat Oncol Biol Phys* 1994;28:797.
117. Auchter RM, Lamond JP, Alexander E III, et al. A multi-institutional outcome and prognostic factor analysis of radiosurgery for resectable single brain metastasis. *Int J Radiat Oncol Biol Phys* 1996;35:27.
118. Alexander E, Moriarty TM, Loeffler JS. Radiosurgery for metastases. *J Neurooncol* 1996;27:279.
119. Cho KH, Hall WA, Gerbi BJ, et al. Patient selection criteria for the treatment of brain metastases with stereotactic radiosurgery. *J Neurooncol* 1998;40:73.
120. Engenhart R, Kimmig B, Hover K, et al. Long term follow-up for brain metastases treated with percutaneous single high dose radiation. *Cancer* 1993;71:1353.
121. Flickinger JC, Lunsford LD, Somaza S, Kondziolka D. Radiosurgery: its role in brain metastasis management. *Neurosurg Clin North Am* 1996;7:497.
122. Joseph J, Adler JR, Cox RS, Hancock SL. Linear accelerator-based stereotaxic radiosurgery for brain metastases: the influence of number of lesions on survival. *J Clin Oncol* 1996;14:1085.
123. Kihlstrom L, Karlson B, Lindquist C. Gamma knife surgery for brain metastasis: implications for survival based on 16 years experience. *Stereotact Funct Neurosurg* 1993;61:45.
124. Valentino V. The results of radiosurgical management of 139 single cerebral metastases. *Acta Neurochir* 1995;63:95.
125. Fukuoka S, Seo Y, Takanashi S, et al. Radiosurgery of brain metastases with the gamma knife. *Stereotact Funct Neurosurg* 1996;66:193.
126. Gerosa M, Nicolato A, Severi F, et al. Gamma knife radiosurgery for intracranial metastases: from local tumor control to increased survival. *Stereotact Funct Neurosurg* 1996;66:184.
127. Weltman E, Salvajoli JV, Oliveira VC, et al. Score index for stereotactic radiosurgery of brain metastases. *J Radiosurg* 1998;1:89.
128. Breneman JC, Warnick RE, Albright RE, et al. Stereotactic radiosurgery for the treatment of brain metastases: results of a single institution series. *Cancer* 1997;79:551.
129. Shiau CY, Sneed PK, Shu HK, et al. Radiosurgery for brain metastases: relationship of dose and pattern of enhancement to local control. *Int J Radiat Oncol Biol Phys* 1997;37:375.
130. Schoeggl A, Kitz K, Ertl A, et al. Prognostic factor analysis of multiple brain metastases after gamma knife radiosurgery: results of 97 patients. *J Neurooncol* 1999;42:169.
131. Young RF. Radiosurgery for the treatment of brain metastases. *Semin Surg Oncol* 1998;14:70.
132. Kondziolka D, Patel A, Lunsford LD, et al. Stereotactic radiosurgery plus whole brain radiotherapy versus radiotherapy alone for patients with multiple brain metastases. *Int J Radiat Oncol Biol Phys* 1999;45:427.
133. Mehta M, Noyes W, Craig B, et al. A cost-effectiveness and cost-utility analysis of radiosurgery vs. resection for single-brain metastases. *Int J Radiat Oncol Biol Phys* 1997;39:445.
134. Muacevic A, Kreth FW, Horstmann GA, et al. Surgery and radiotherapy compared with gamma knife radiosurgery in the treatment of solitary cerebral metastases of small diameter. *J Neurosurg* 1999;91:35.
135. Brandt RA, Cruz J, Sciuajolitz J, et al. Neurosurgical treatment of brain metastases: microsurgery or radiosurgery. From the American Association of Neurological Surgeons Annual Meeting. 1996:328(abst).
136. Shu HK, Sneed PK, Shiau CY, et al. Factors influencing survival after gamma knife radiosurgery for patients with single and multiple brain metastases. *Cancer J Sci Am* 1996;2:335.
137. Bindal AK, Bindal RK, Hess KR, et al. Surgery versus radiosurgery in the treatment of brain metastases. *J Neurosurg* 1996;84:748.
138. Sneed PK, Lamborn KR, Forstner JM, et al. Radiosurgery for brain metastases: is whole brain radiotherapy necessary? *Int J Radiat Oncol Biol Phys* 1999;43:549.
139. Grob JJ, Regis J, Laurans R, et al. Radiosurgery without whole brain radiotherapy in melanoma brain metastases. Club de Cancerologie Cutanee. *Eur J Cancer* 1998;34:1187.
140. Pirzkall A, Debus J, Lohr F, et al. Radiosurgery alone or in combination with whole-brain radiotherapy for brain metastases. *J Clin Oncol* 1998;16:3563.
141. Shirato H, Takamura A, Tomita M, et al. Stereotactic irradiation without whole brain irradiation for single brain metastases. *Int J Radiat Oncol Biol Phys* 1997;37:385.
142. Loeffler JS, Alexander E. Radiosurgery for the treatment of intracranial metastases. In: Alexander E, Loeffler JS, Lunsford D, eds. *Stereotactic radiosurgery*. New York: McGraw-Hill, 1993.
143. Becker G, Duffner F, Kortmann R, et al. Radiosurgery for the treatment of brain metastases in renal cell carcinoma. *Anticancer Res* 1999;19:1611.
144. Mori Y, Kondziolka D, Flickinger JC, et al. Stereotactic radiosurgery for cerebral metastatic melanoma: factors affecting local disease control and survival. *Int J Radiat Oncol Biol Phys* 1998;42:581.
145. Lavine SD, Petrovitch Z, Cohen-Gadol AA, et al. Gamma knife radiosurgery for metastatic melanoma: an analysis of survival, outcome, and complications. *Neurosurgery* 1999;44:59.
146. Williams J, Enger C, Wharam M, et al. Stereotactic radiosurgery for brain metastases: comparison of lung carcinoma vs. non-lung tumors. *J Neurooncol* 1998;37:79.
147. Bernstein M, Cabantog A, Laperriere N, et al. Brachytherapy for recurrent single brain metastases. *Can J Neurol Sci* 1995;22:13.
148. Schulder M, Black PM, Shrieve DC, et al. Permanent low-activity iodine-125 implants for cerebral metastases. *J Neurooncol* 1997;33:213.
149. McDermott MW, Cosgrove GR, Larson DA, et al. Interstitial brachytherapy for intracranial metastases. *Neurosurg Clin North Am* 1996;7:485.
150. Cosgrove GR, Hochberg FH, Zervas NT, et al. Interstitial irradiation of brain tumors using a miniature radiosurgery device: initial experience. *Neurosurgery* 1997;40:518.
151. Lesser GJ. Chemotherapy of cerebral metastases from solid tumors. *Neurosurg Clin North Am* 1996;7527.
152. Buckner JC. The role of chemotherapy in the treatment of patients with brain metastases from solid tumors. *Cancer Metastasis Rev* 1991;10:335.
153. Rosner D, Nemoto T, Lane WW. Chemotherapy induces regression of brain metastases in breast carcinoma. *Cancer* 1986;58:832.
154. Rosner D, Flowers A, Lane WW. Chemotherapy induces regression of brain metastases in breast carcinoma patients: update study. *Proc Annu Meet Am Soc Clin Oncol* 1993; A508(abst).
155. Franciosi V, Cocconi G, Michiara M, et al. Front-line chemotherapy with cisplatin and etoposide for patients with brain metastases from breast carcinoma, nonsmall cell lung carcinoma, or malignant melanoma: a prospective study. *Cancer* 1999;85:1599.
156. Boogerd W, Dalesio O, Bais EM, et al. Response of brain metastases from breast cancer to systemic chemotherapy. *Cancer* 1992;69:972.
157. Kaba SE, Kyritsis AP, Hess K, et al. TPDC-FuHu chemotherapy for the treatment of recurrent metastatic brain tumors. *J Clin Oncol* 1997;15:1063.
158. Fleming DR, Goldsmith GC, Stevens DA, Herzig RH. Dose-intensive chemotherapy for breast cancer with brain metastases: a case series. *Am J Clin Oncol* 1999;22:371.
159. Kristensen CA, Kristjansen PEG, Hansen HH. Systemic chemotherapy of brain metastases from small-cell lung cancer: a review. *J Clin Oncol* 1992;10:1498.
160. Rustin GJ, Newlands ES, Begent RH, et al. Weekly alternating etoposide, methotrexate, and actinomycin/vincristine and cyclophosphamide chemotherapy for the treatment of CNS metastases of choriocarcinoma. *J Clin Oncol* 1989;7:900.
161. Cooper KG, Kitchener HC, Parkin DE. Cerebral metastases from epithelial ovarian carcinoma treated with carboplatin. *Gynecol Oncol* 1994;55:318.
162. Cormio G, Gabriele A, Maneo A, et al. Complete remission of brain metastases from ovarian carcinoma with carboplatin. *Eur J Obstet Gynecol Reprod Biol* 1998;78:91.
163. Malacarne P, Santini A, Maestri A. Response of brain metastases from lung cancer to systemic chemotherapy with carboplatin and etoposide. *Oncology* 1996;53:210.
164. Minotti V, Crino L, Meacci ML, et al. Chemotherapy with cisplatin and tenoposide for cerebral metastases in non-small cell lung cancer. *Lung Cancer* 1998;20:93.
165. Boogerd W, van der Sande JJ, van Zandwijk N. Tenoposide sometimes effective in brain metastases from non-small cell lung cancer. *J Neurooncol* 1999;41:285.
166. Kelly K, Bunn PA Jr. Is it time to reevaluate our approach to the treatment of brain metastases in patients with non-small cell lung cancer? *Lung Cancer* 1998;20:85.
167. Pors H, Edler von Eyben F, Sorensen OS, et al. Long-term remission of multiple brain metastases with tamoxifen. *J Neurooncol* 1991;10:173.
168. Van der Gaast A, Alexieva-Figusch J, Vecht C, et al. Complete remission of a brain metastasis to third line hormonal treatment with megestrol acetate. *Am J Clin Oncol* 1990;13:507.
169. Markesbery WR, Brooks WH, Gupta GD, et al. Treatment for patients with cerebral metastases. *Arch Neurol* 1978;35:754.

170. Lagerwaard FJ, Levendag PC, Nowak PJ, et al. Identification of prognostic factors in patients with brain metastases: a review of 1292 patients. *Int J Radiat Oncol Biol Phys* 1999;43:795.
171. Hsiung CY, Leung SW, Wang CJ, et al. The prognostic factors of lung cancer patients with brain metastases treated with radiotherapy. *J Neurooncol* 1998;36:71.
172. Swift P, Phillips T, Martz K, et al. CT characteristics of patients with brain metastases treated in RTOG study 79-16. *Int J Radiat Oncol Biol Phys* 1993;25:209.
173. Gaspar L, Scott C, Rotman M, et al. Recursive partitioning analysis (RPA) of prognostic factors in three Radiation Therapy Oncology Group (RTOG) brain metastases trials. *Int J Radiat Oncol Biol Phys* 1997;37:745.
174. Agboola O, Benoit B, Cross P, et al. Prognostic factors derived from recursive partition analysis (RPA) of Radiation Therapy Oncology Group (RTOG) brain metastases trials applied to surgically resected and irradiated brain metastatic cases. *Int J Radiat Oncol Biol Phys* 1998;42:155.
175. Lagerwald FJ, Levendag PC, Nowak PJ, et al. Identification of prognostic factors in patients with brain metastases: a review of 1292 patients. *Int J Radiat Oncol Biol Phys* 1999;43:795.
176. Nguyen LN, Maor MH, Oswald MJ. Brain metastases as the only manifestation of an undetected primary tumor. *Cancer* 1998;83:2181.
177. Wronski M, Arbit E. Resection of brain metastases from colorectal carcinoma in 73 patients. *Cancer* 1999;85:12677.
178. Markesbery WR, Brooks WH, Gupta GD, Young AB. Treatment for patients with cerebral metastases. *Arch Neurol* 1978;35:754.

SECTION 2

JOE B. PUTNAM, JR.

Metastatic Cancer to the Lung

Metastases often represent diffuse systemic or untreatable spread of a primary neoplasm. However, selected patients with metastases isolated to the lung may be resected safely and achieve prolonged survival compared to patients with unresectable metastases. In general, patients with complete resection of pulmonary metastases have associated prolonged survival (regardless of histology) compared to patients with unresectable metastases. This observation is surprising because surgery alone cannot control micrometastases. After complete resection of pulmonary metastases (including multiple and bilateral metastases), the long-term survival rate (more than 5 years) may be expected in approximately one-third of patients.

HISTORICAL PERSPECTIVE

The history of resection of pulmonary metastases has been reviewed.[1,2] One of the earliest resections for pulmonary metastases was performed after resection of a chest wall sarcoma in 1882 by Weinlechner.[1] In 1883, Kronlein[3] resected a recurrent chest wall sarcoma in a young woman. The patient lived for several years after the surgery and died of recurrent disease. The first resections of a pulmonary metastasis as a separate procedure were described in 1926 by Divis[4] and in 1930 by Torek.[5] One of the first long-term survivors of any pulmonary metastasectomy was reported by Barney and Churchill[6] after resection of a metastasis from a patient with renal cell carcinoma. Local control of the primary tumor was achieved, and the patient survived for 23 years after resection of the metastasis and died from unrelated causes. Alexander and Haight[7] reported the first large series (25 patients) of metastasectomy in 1947. Multiple metastases from osteochondroma of the tibia were resected in 1953 by Mannix, with the patient surviving more than 2 years.[1] Other authors[8–10] have noted that certain clinical characteristics may enable clinicians to identify patients with more favorable disease-free and overall survival rate prognoses. Since the late 1970s, resection of solitary and multiple pulmonary metastases from sarcomas and various other primary neoplasms have been performed with long-term survival in up to 40% of patients so treated.[11]

IDENTIFICATION OF PULMONARY METASTASES

Routinely, clinicians may evaluate patients for pulmonary metastases based on screening chest roentgenograms (Fig. 52.2-1) obtained at various intervals after resection of the primary. Although their specificity exceeds 95% when nodules consistent with metastases are identified, their sensitivity [compared to computed tomography (CT) of the chest] is low, and this deficiency has prompted some clinicians to screen patients at high risk of recurrent metastases with CT chest scans (Fig. 52.2-2). Duda et al.[12] examined 130 patients with soft tissue and bone sarcomas. Sixty-six patients had no evidence of pulmonary metastases on chest x-ray (CXR) and subsequently had linear tomography or CT of the chest performed. Only 1 of 53 patients with a normal CXR and no local recurrence had an abnormal tomogram. Two patients of 13 with locally recurrent sarcoma and a normal CXR had an abnormal tomogram. The authors concluded that a screening CXR in the absence of local recurrence is the most cost-effective test. However, tomograms should be performed for evaluation of the extent of disease (e.g., pulmonary metastases) in patients with locally recurrent sarcomas.[12]

CT has replaced linear tomograms as the examination of choice in patients with suspected pulmonary metastases[13] (see Fig. 52.2-2). CT scans of the chest provide a sensitive and specific noninvasive examination for patients with pulmonary metastases.[14–16] CT scans of the chest are sensitive and identify smaller nodules (3 to 7 mm) earlier than conventional linear tomography, although these nodules may not necessarily be metastases. Theoretically, earlier detection and treatment of metastases can improve survival. However, in one study that detected occult metastases during median sternotomy with bilateral lung exploration, survival was not improved over patients having a single thoracotomy, even though a significant percentage of patients would be expected to have occult metastases.[17]

Magnetic resonance imaging (MRI) is routinely performed to evaluate the local site of resection for recurrence. MRI is not routinely helpful for the radiographic diagnosis of pulmonary metastases; rather, CT of the chest is preferred.[18] MRI is helpful when the pulmonary metastases are of great size and may abut or invade the mediastinum.[19] Pulmonary metastases from sarcomas "push" tissue rather than invade, and exploration is often required to determine the extent of host-tumor interactions. The MRI may assist the surgeon in planning the approach needed for resection of these complex intrathoracic neoplasms.

Lucas et al.[20] examined the role of whole body [^{18}F]fluorodeoxyglucose positron emission tomography (FDG PET) in the

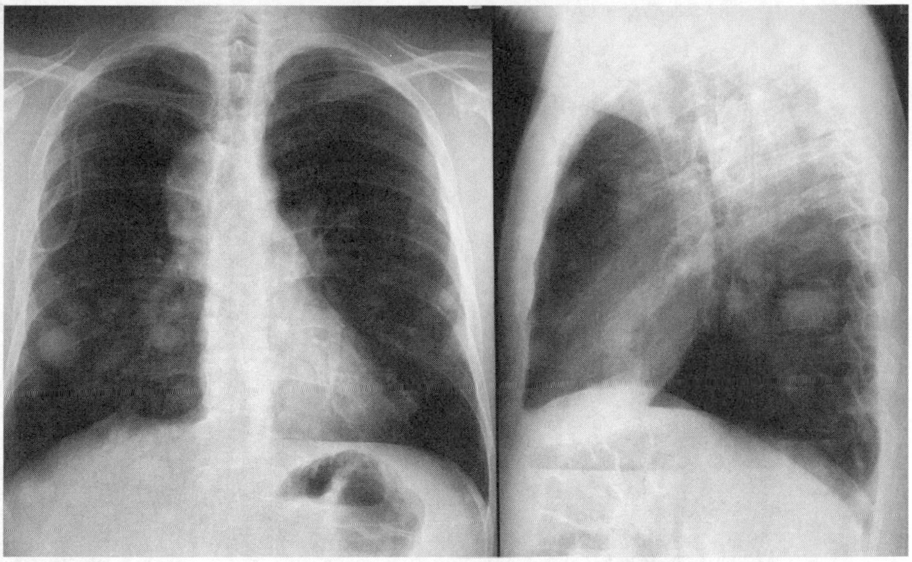

FIGURE 52.2-1. Chest x-ray (posteroanterior and lateral views) of patient with multiple metastases from malignant fibrous histiocytoma. The number and location of these metastases preclude resection.

diagnosis of pulmonary metastases from soft tissue tumors. The authors made 70 comparisons between FDG PET and chest CT for the identification of lung metastases. The sensitivity of FDG PET was 86.7% and the specificity was 100% (13 true-positive, two false-negative). CT of the chest had a sensitivity of 100% and a specificity of 96.4%. However, FDG PET identified 13 other sites of metastases. The authors suggested that FDG PET might be used for evaluation of local recurrence as well as pulmonary and extrathoracic metastases. The use of all three modalities (CT of the chest, MRI, and FDG PET) may most

A

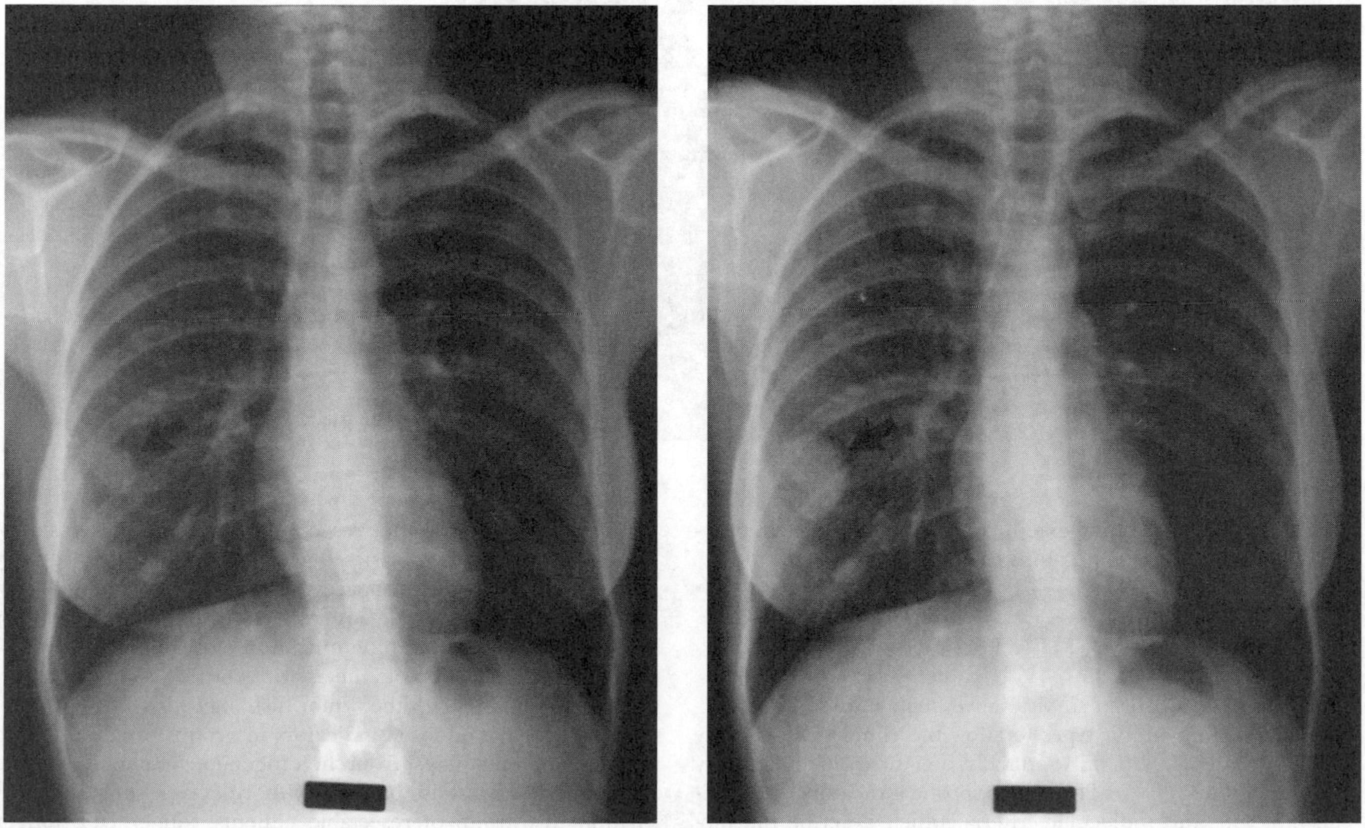

B

FIGURE 52.2-2. Correlation of chest x-ray and computed tomography in a patient with pulmonary metastases from soft tissue sarcoma. Serial chest x-rays **(A,B)** and corresponding computed tomography of the chest **(C,D)** were taken 4 months apart. The patient subsequently underwent median sternotomy and complete resection of bilateral pulmonary metastases. (*continued*)

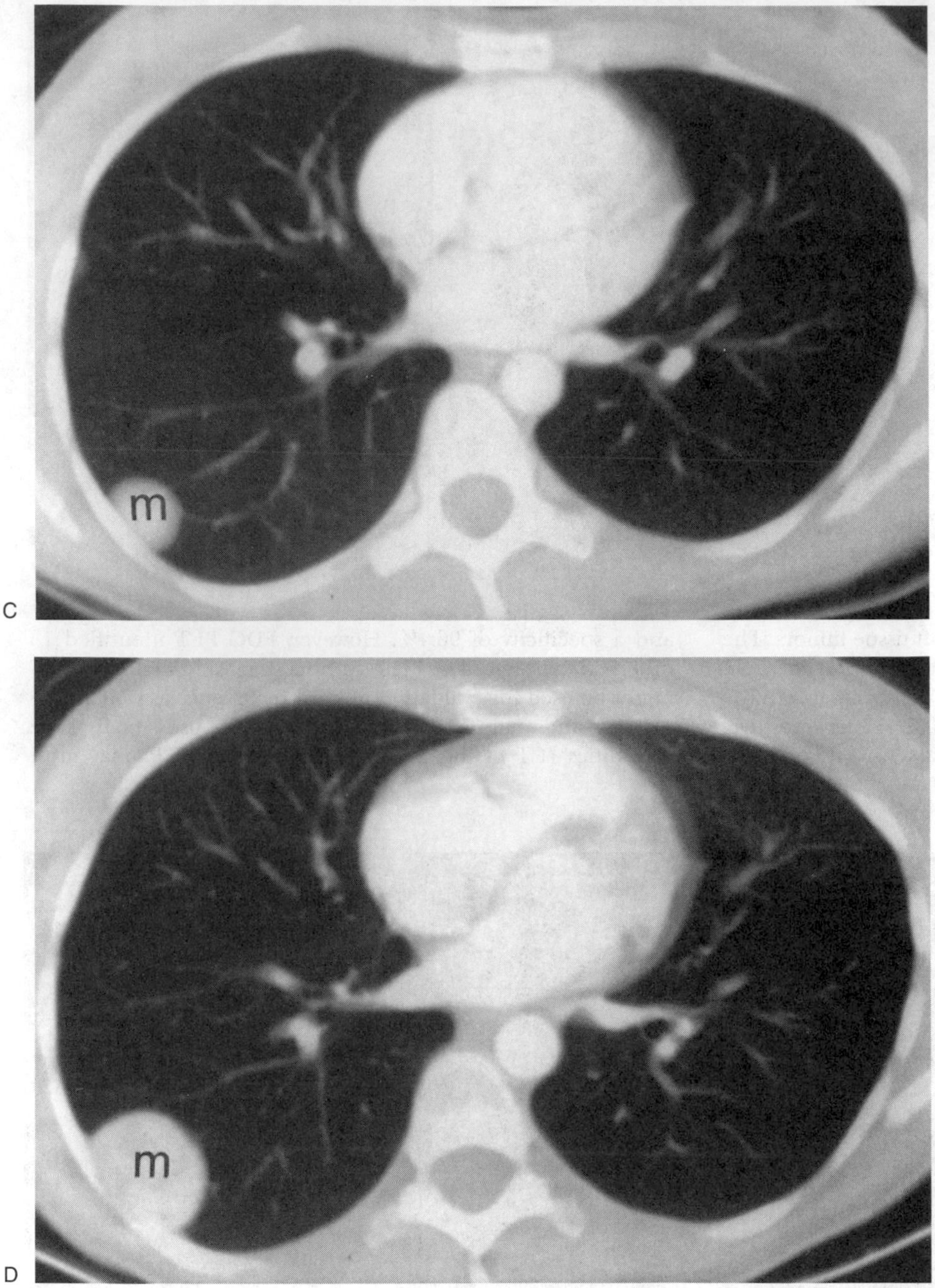

FIGURE 52.2-2. *(Continued)*

accurately define the total extent of disease. The cost effectiveness of these three examinations has not been studied.[20]

SELECTION OF PATIENTS FOR SURGERY

Predictors for improved survival have been studied retrospectively for various tumor types to allow the clinician to identify selected patients who will optimally benefit from pulmonary metastasectomy.[8,11,21–25] These "prognostic indicators" are clinical, biologic, and molecular criteria, which describe the biologic interaction between the metastases and the patient, and the association of the two with prolonged survival. These prognostic indicators may be used to identify those patients who are most likely to benefit after resection of pulmonary metastases. Many patients with metastases will not benefit from surgery because of a biologically aggressive tumor [e.g., extensive disease, a short disease-free interval (DFI) between control of their primary tumor and identification of unresectable pulmonary metastases, and rapid metastatic growth]. Biologic characteristics also differ with the tumor histology.

Analysis of prognostic indicators in groups of patients with pulmonary metastases from heterogeneous tumors describe prolonged survival in patients with resectable metastases.[8,23] Within this group of resectable patients, longer DFI, longer tumor-doubling time (TDT), fewer numbers of metastases, and specific primary histology may be favorably associated with improved survival.[8,21,22,24] A disadvantage of studying prognostic indicators in heterogeneous groups of neoplasms is the wide variability in biologic characteristics of metastases, particularly among different primary neoplasms. The study of pulmonary metastases from patients with the same tumor histology will provide better information on prognostic indicators that may influence survival after resection of these metastases.

Pastorino and colleagues[26] retrospectively reviewed more than 5000 patients with metastases treated with resection. Overall, actuarial 5-year survival was 36%, 10-year survival was 26%, and 15-year survival was 22%. Patients could generally be staged by the presence of favorable clinical indicators. These indicators included a DFI of more than 3 years, a solitary pulmonary nodule, and germ cell histology.[26]

Kandioler and colleagues[27] confirmed the biologically favorable characteristics of patients with pulmonary metastases who could be completely resected of their disease. Overall median survival for a heterogeneous population of patients with pulmonary metastases was 60 months.

PREPARATION OF THE PATIENT FOR METASTASECTOMY

The patient's overall medical condition and prior treatment must be considered in planning resection of pulmonary metastases. As with any patient undergoing thoracotomy, the patient must have sufficient physiologic reserves to withstand the anesthesia and the surgical procedure. Routine blood chemistries, chest roentgenogram, and CT of the chest and abdomen are routinely performed. CT of the area of primary neoplasm and other studies may be obtained to evaluate the site for local recurrence.[28] Only if appropriate system-related symptoms were identified, such as headaches or neurologic deficits, or bone pain, would a brain CT or bone scan, respectively, be obtained. The evaluation of pulmonary function includes arterial blood gas measurement, xenon ventilation-perfusion lung scans, DLCO (carbon monoxide diffusing capacity of the lungs), and maximal oxygen consumption (MVO_2). These studies are obtained to evaluate the patient's suitability for general anesthesia and one-lung anesthesia and to estimate the potential for sufficient postoperative pulmonary reserve. Cardiac assessment (e.g., electrocardiogram, stress test) may be necessary for older patients. For patients previously treated with Adriamycin chemotherapy, an echocardiogram should be obtained to evaluate ejection fraction as a measure of extent of cardiomyopathy.

If preoperative chemotherapy has been given, surgery should be delayed a minimum of 4 weeks or longer to allow for sufficient bone marrow recovery [for low absolute leukocyte count (fewer than 5000 cells per mm^3) or low platelet count (fewer than 50,000 per mm^3)]. If marrow suppression precludes recovery of platelets, then perioperative support with platelet transfusions may be required. Absolutely no smoking is permitted for a minimum of 2 weeks before surgery to enhance pulmonary hygiene. Patients are encouraged to use an incentive spirometer several times daily. The patient is routinely admitted to the hospital the morning of surgery.

In the operating room, two large-bore intravenous lines, a radial arterial line, and oxygen saturation monitors are placed. A central line is not routinely used for wedge resections of the lung. A Foley catheter is placed routinely if the operation is expected to exceed 3 hours or if a thoracic epidural catheter is placed for perioperative analgesia. The pertinent radiographic examinations (chest roentgenograms and CT scans of the chest) are displayed prominently in the operating room. After intubation with a single-lumen endotracheal tube, a bronchoscopy is performed to evaluate the distal trachea and tracheobronchial tree. A double-lumen endotracheal tube is used to facilitate sequential exposure and palpation of the lungs.

TABLE 52.2-1. Advantages and Disadvantages of Various Surgical Resections

Medial sternotomy	
Advantages	Bilateral thoracic explorations with one incision.
	Less patient discomfort.
Disadvantages	Resection may be difficult for lesions posterior and medial (near the hilum).
	Difficult exposure to the left lower lobe in patients with obesity, congestive heart failure, or chronic obstructive pulmonary disease (increased thoracic anterior-posterior diameter).
Posterolateral thoracotomy	
Advantages	"Standard" approach.
	Excellent exposure of the hemithorax.
Disadvantages	Patient discomfort (although minimized with thoracic epidural anesthesia).
	Only one hemithorax may be explored at one operation.
	A second operation is needed for bilateral metastases.
Video-assisted thoracic surgery	
Advantages	Lobectomy potentially less immunosuppressive.
	Excellent visualization.
	Minimal morbidity and discomfort.
	Excellent exposure for visceral pleural metastases.
	May identify unresectable metastases, pleural studding, etc.
Disadvantages	Unable to fully evaluate metastases in the lung parenchyma.
	Learning curve.
	Length of procedure.
	Potential for increased costs.
	Potential for higher costs (staplers, disposable instruments).

SURGICAL INCISIONS

Surgical procedures for resection include single thoracotomy, staged bilateral thoracotomy, or median sternotomy. These procedures have almost no mortality and minimal morbidity.[11,17,29–34] The procedure chosen does not influence survival in patients resected of all disease; however, various advantages and disadvantages are inherent to each approach (Table 52.2-1). Patients with pulmonary metastases may also undergo multiple procedures for re-resection of metastases, with prolonged survival after complete resection.[35–37]

For median sternotomy, the patient is positioned supine with the entire anterior thorax exposed from the neck to the umbilicus and laterally to the anterior axillary line. The sternum is divided and the lungs sequentially deflated. The pulmonary ligament is divided to mobilize the lung completely. The deflated lung is palpated to identify metastases, and these are resected with a surgical stapling device or other means (laser or Bovie electrocautery). The deflated right lung may be brought completely into the field by placing folded sponges behind the hilum (for elevation). Metastases may be resected with the lung inflated, but the metastases must be marked with a suture, and metastases deep within the parenchyma may be difficult to resect with wedge excision alone. The lung is reinflated.

Exposure of the left lower lobe through a median sternotomy may be more difficult than exposure of the other lobes because of the overlying heart. With appropriate gentle traction on the pericardium, the left lower lobe can be exposed readily and brought into the operative field. Technical aids, such as an internal mammary artery retractor, may provide for better exposure, particularly for basilar (left lower lobe) tumors or posterior hilar left lower lobe masses.

The posterolateral thoracotomy is a familiar and "standard" approach to pulmonary resection for carcinoma of the lung, although several authors encourage median sternotomy for both resection of lung carcinoma[38] and for pulmonary metastases.[17] In contrast to median sternotomy, posterolateral thoracotomy (either with division of the latissimus dorsi or "muscle sparing") may be more uncomfortable for the patient during the postoperative convalescence. Improvements in postoperative pain management with intercostal nerve analgesia, thoracic epidural analgesia, and patient-controlled analgesia can control or even eliminate postoperative pain. The posterior or posterolateral thoracotomy does provide better exposure for metastases located posterior and near the hilum, particularly on the left side, and limits the surgeon to one hemithorax. In only rare circumstances would bilateral thoracotomies be performed in the same patient during the same operation.

RESECTION OF PULMONARY METASTASES

Patients with bilateral metastases may be explored with a median sternotomy, staged bilateral thoracotomies, or posterolateral thoracotomy. Prior evaluation of patients with sarcomas and unilateral nodules demonstrated bilateral metastases in 38% to 60% of patients.[17,33] Postresection survival from median sternotomy and from bilateral staged thoracotomies is similar.[17] Numbers of nodules, presence of unilateral or bilateral nodules, location of nodules, and the size of various nodules can be identified and, if required, resected through a median sternotomy. A median sternotomy is recommended for the initial exploration and resection in patients with unilateral or bilateral nodules, and in patients with pulmonary metastases from osteogenic sarcoma (OST) or soft tissue sarcoma (STS), and should be considered the procedure of choice in patients with suspected bilateral metastases.[32,34] Multiple authors have advocated median sternotomy for lobectomy for resection of primary carcinoma of the lung,[38–40] particularly in patients with impaired pulmonary function. A posterolateral thoracotomy approach may be required for left lower lobectomy in patients with obesity, cardiomegaly, or an elevated left hemidiaphragm.[38]

All nodules are resected with a margin of normal tissue. Nodules should not be "shelled out," because viable tumor cells remain on the periphery of the resected area. Often the decision of margin adequacy is the surgeon's alone, because lung parenchyma may become distorted around the nodule after resection, giving the illusion of a "positive" or "close" margin. Mediastinal lymph nodes can also be examined for potentially rare involvement from pulmonary metastases.[10,41]

Laser-assisted pulmonary resection using the neodymium:yttrium aluminum garnet laser may provide a better means of resecting pulmonary metastases than with the surgical stapler.[29] Disadvantages of laser resection may include longer operating time and the potential for prolonged postoperative air leaks; however, use of the laser may enhance preservation of lung parenchyma with less distortion.[42] Bovie electrocautery may also spare lung parenchyma by removing the metastases with minimal distortion of remaining lung. Air leaks can be sealed by the use of fibrin glue.[43]

Thoracoscopic resection or video-assisted thoracic surgery (VATS) using high-resolution video cameras may be helpful for diagnosis of metastases[44,45]; however, its usefulness is limited to metastases identified on the surface or outer one-third of the lung. Metastases within the lung parenchyma may be undetectable with this technique.[46] Landreneau and associates[47] have described minimal morbidity and no mortality in 41 patients who underwent 52 thoracoscopic pulmonary resections for small lesions (less than 3 cm) in the outer one-third of the lung parenchyma.

At this time, wedge resection of pulmonary metastases using VATS techniques has no proven advantage over resection using standard "open" techniques. Even patients at increased physiologic risk from thoracotomy may tolerate a simple wedge resection of the lung without difficulty. VATS may be inadequate to detect all metastases. McCormack and colleagues[48] demonstrated that a combination of chest CT and VATS had a 56% failure rate to detect and resect all lesions. The frequency of bilateral and occult metastases, particularly in sarcoma, precludes the use of thoracoscopy. Thoracoscopy *may* play a role in highly selected patients with a solitary metastasis of nonsarcomatous origin with a long DFI.

Complications specific to thoracoscopic resection of pulmonary metastases have been described. The subjective risks of an incomplete, inadequate, or inconsistent operation must be compared to the benefits of the VATS approach. The surgeon must consider the technical skills required, the desired objectives for the patient, the instrumentation available for manipulation of the lung and other thoracic organs, and an assessment of the risk of a "closed" versus "open" procedure. An inadequate resection of pulmonary metastases may cause more morbidity than the benefits achieved by VATS. The obvious chest wall implant from tumor seeding has devastating effects on the patient.[49] Postoperative pain from periosteal injury affects some patients. Patient selection remains a critical step in the appropriate use of VATS in thoracic surgical oncology.[50] VATS is considered appropriate for diagnosis or intrathoracic staging (Fig. 52.2-3).

SURVIVAL ANALYSIS

Survival may be absolute or actuarial and is usually calculated from the time the surgical procedure is performed until death

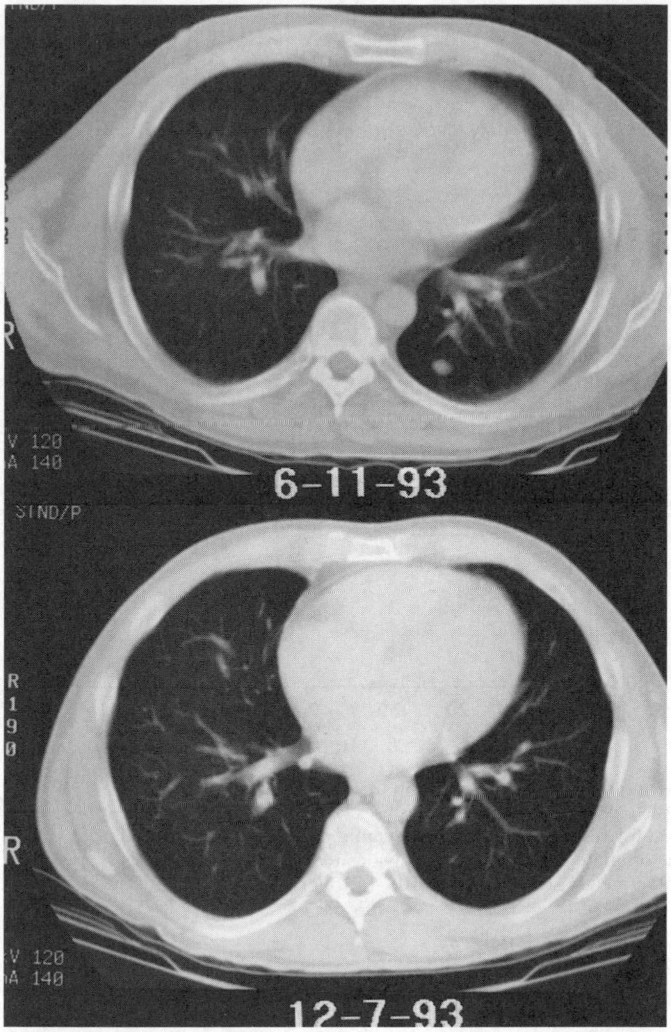

A

B

FIGURE 52.2-3. **A:** Computed tomography with a peripheral nodule in a 45-year-old man with a prior history of a superficial melanoma (Clark's level 2) removed from his forearm 2 years previously. **B:** Video-assisted thoracic surgery resection was performed for complete resection of a granuloma. No other intrathoracic lesions were noted. The patient has remained free of disease from his melanoma. An open procedure, thoracotomy, was avoided. Minimal scarring is present.

or the date of last follow-up. For example, patients followed for a minimum of 5 years (survivors) or until death provide an absolute 5-year survival rate (number patients alive of all patients studied); patients followed for varying periods (i.e., 2 to 7 years) may be evaluated using an actuarial survival curve. Actuarial survival and disease-free survival may be estimated using the method of Kaplan and Meier.[51] Patients, grouped into two or more populations, are defined as meeting or not meeting an objective criteria and compared so that differences in survival can be evaluated. Univariate analysis (or comparisons between groups) may be made using the generalized Wilcoxon test of Gehan[52] or log-rank test; if sample sizes are small, the Thomas exact test[53] may be used. Cox's proportional hazards model[54] would be used to determine the relative effect of various prognostic indicators on survival. Univariate analysis identifies the most important prognostic indicators. Multivariate analysis evaluates the predictive ability of two or more prognostic indicators to provide additional prognostic value.

RESULTS OF RESECTION OF SARCOMATOUS PULMONARY METASTASES

An evaluation of prognostic indicators and results of resection of pulmonary metastasectomy is difficult, because numerous primary histologies are often combined to discuss the value of pulmonary metastasectomy. Although identification of trends is helpful, analysis of factors that are associated with improved survival depend on a single histology and a group of patients sufficiently large from which to draw conclusions. Prognostic indicators have been reviewed to assess their association, singularly and in combination, with postresection survival in patients with pulmonary metastases and to assist clinically in better selecting appropriate patients for resection of pulmonary metastases. Age and gender of the patient; histology, stage, grade, and location of the primary tumor; disease-free survival; number of nodules on preoperative radiologic studies; whether the metastases are unilateral or bilateral, or synchronous or metachronous; and TDT all may be evaluated preoperatively. In addition, resectability, technique of resection, nodal spread, the number of metastases and their location, and re-resection may be examined postoperatively.

OSTEOGENIC SARCOMA

Pulmonary metastases from OST occur in up to 80% of patients who relapse after treatment for their primary neoplasm, whether or not they receive adjuvant chemotherapy.[55–57] Ninety percent of all recurrences occur within 3 years.[58] Because these metastases are often isolated to the lungs, surgical resection may render a significant number of patients disease-free and enhance long-term survival.[44,55,56,59–61] The 5-year survival rate may range up to 50%.[62]

Various groups have evaluated survival and prognostic factors in patients with pulmonary metastases from OST. Series from the National Cancer Institute in the early 1980s evaluated 80 patients with primary OST of the extremity. Forty-three patients developed pulmonary metastases. Thirty-nine patients were deemed resectable and underwent one or more thoracic explorations for resection of their metastases. The 5-year survival rate was 38%. Various prognostic factors were analyzed. Fewer number of nodules (three or less), longer DFI, resectable metastases, and fewer metastases identified and resected were associated with longer postthoracotomy survival. A multivariate analysis did not find any combination of factors to be more predictive than the number of nodules identified on preoperative tomograms.[9] Surgical resectability was the only predictive factor associated with prolonged survival for recurrent OST.[55]

Chemotherapy has been effective in prolonging the DFI between the surgical treatment of the primary tumor and the appearance of pulmonary metastases. Chemotherapy offers no survival advantage in treating bulk metastases from OST; however, chemotherapy may prevent or cure micrometastatic disease not amenable to surgery.[60] Goorin et al.[55] reported on 113 patients treated with adjuvant therapy for primary OST. Adjuvant chemotherapy improved event-free survival over surgery alone (P = .00) for primary OST. Relapses occurred in the lungs in more than 80% of patients. Survival after relapse was not influenced by chemotherapy. The only factor associated with improved survival after relapse (in the lungs) was complete resection of all metastases, rendering the patient disease-free (P = .03).[55]

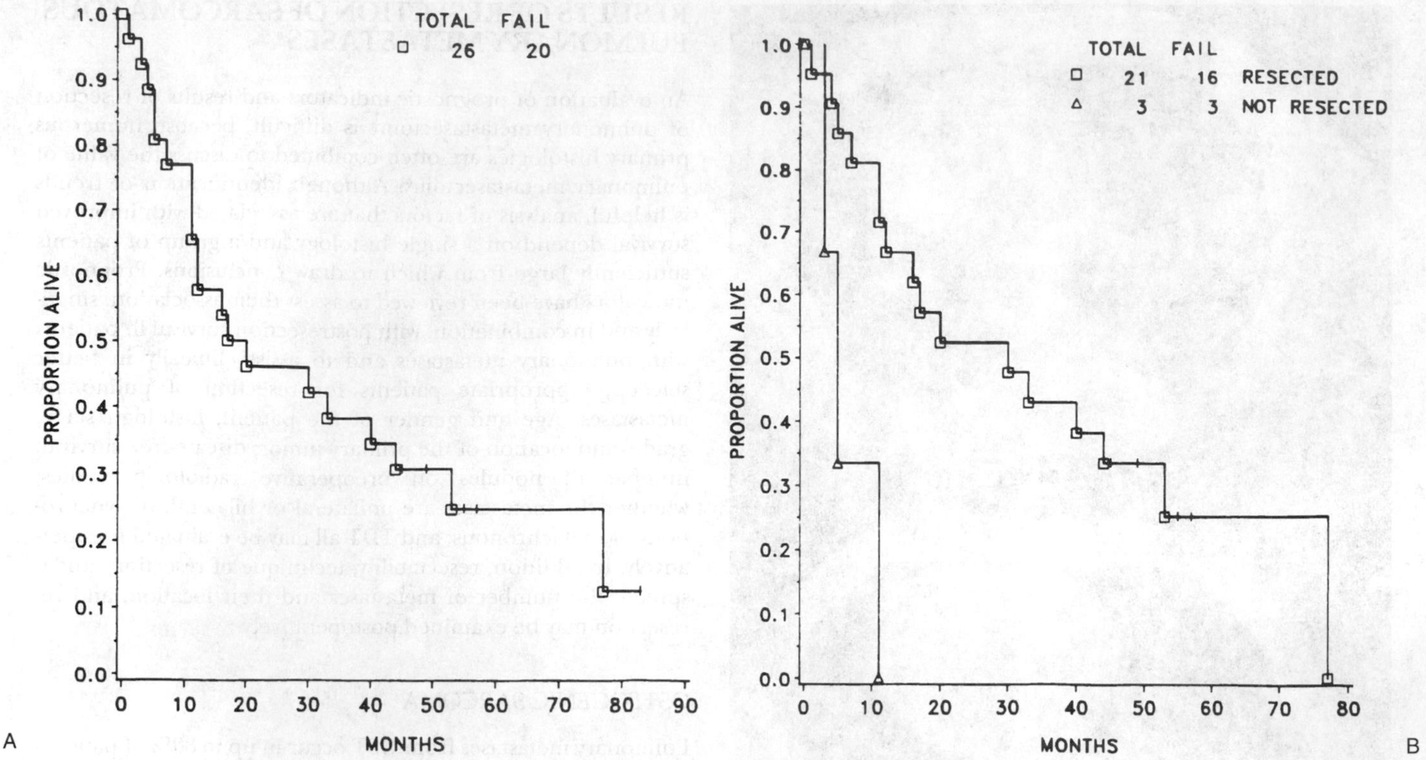

FIGURE 52.2-4. **A:** Overall survival for patients with pulmonary metastases from soft tissue sarcoma. Patients were selected for surgery based on the potential for complete resection of their metastases. The 5-year survival rate was 25%. (From ref. 103, with permission.) **B:** Survival for resectable and nonresectable patients with pulmonary metastases from soft tissue sarcoma. Patients with complete resection have an associated survival advantage over patients with incomplete resection or unresectable metastases. (From ref. 103, with permission.)

More recently, the value of chemotherapy for treatment of patients with pulmonary metastases from OST was examined by Antunes and colleagues[63] in a review of 198 patients operated on for OST of the limbs. The patients were treated with a combination of chemotherapy and surgery. The patients received three cycles of preoperative chemotherapy with methotrexate, Adriamycin, and cisplatin. Patients underwent surgery approximately 1 month later and received chemotherapy postoperatively (Adriamycin and ifosfamide). With chemotherapy and surgery for pulmonary metastases, the 3-year survival rate was 61%, compared to 79% in patients without metastases. Of all patients with pulmonary metastases who died, they died of progressive pulmonary metastases. Chemotherapy to achieve a biologic response, followed by surgery for "salvage" and local control, followed by more chemotherapy for micrometastatic disease, is a reasonable and effective means of treatment of pulmonary metastases from OST. Patients with synchronous pulmonary metastases with their primary tumor have a worse survival rate, even with chemotherapy and complete resection.[64,65]

SOFT TISSUE SARCOMAS

STSs comprise a family of nonossifying malignant neoplasms arising from mesenchymal connective tissues. As with OST, local recurrence is common (20%), and metastases are predominantly to the lungs[66] (Fig. 52.2-4). Casson et al.[67] evaluated determinants of 5-year survival in 58 patients who had complete resection and who were followed until death or for a minimum of 5 years. Absolute 5-year survival was 25% (15 of 58 patients). Favorable prognostic factors included TDT of more than 40 days, unilateral disease, three or fewer nodules identified on preoperative tomograms, two or fewer metastases resected, and tumor histology (median survival of 33 months for malignant fibrous histiocytoma vs. 17 months for all others). Using multivariate analysis, the number of nodules (four or more) was the most significant prognostic indicator. The addition of tumor histology (malignant fibrous histiocytoma) improved the predictive ability of this model.[67]

One study[10] evaluated 67 patients with histologically documented pulmonary metastases from STS treated at the National Cancer Institute. Significant preoperative predictors of enhanced survival included TDT (more than 20 days), number of metastases on preoperative tomograms (four or fewer nodules), and the DFI (more than 12 months). Predictive ability was improved when all three prognostic factors were combined. These patients represent the patients who have the best response (i.e., prolonged postresection survival) to pulmonary metastasectomy.[10,68]

Patients with recurrent pulmonary metastases and complete resection also have improved postresection survival.[35–37] Increased age and female gender were associated with an increased risk of death from disease in resected patients with recurrent pulmonary metastases in contrast to initial isolated pulmonary metastases.[36] Resectable patients and those with one metastasis have the best postresection survival.[35]

Chemotherapy given before resection of pulmonary metastases has variable impact on postresection survival. In a study of patients with pulmonary metastases from STS,[69] chemotherapy (doxorubicin, cyclophosphamide, and dacarbazine) was given before metastasectomy. Time from treatment initiation to thoracotomy ranged from 1 to 57 months. Patients were grouped according to response. Five patients had a complete response (not surgically confirmed) and recurred 5 to 57 months later. Seven patients had a partial response. Twelve patients had either no change or progression. Thirty-eight procedures were performed. Resectable patients had a median survival of 30 months and an actuarial 5-year survival rate of 25% (see Fig. 52.2-4*A*). Complete resection was associated with an improved survival compared to unresectable patients (see Fig. 52.2-4*B*). No differences were found in postresection survival between any groups. Postthoracotomy survival cannot be predicted from initial response to this chemotherapy regimen.[69]

Adriamycin and ifosfamide have activity in more than 20% of patients with metastatic sarcoma. In addition, the combination of both chemotherapeutic agents may be greater than either single agent. The value of chemotherapy as an adjuvant is unknown, but several studies suggest a modest relapse-free and survival benefit. The authors[70] correctly note that patients with STSs should be studied in prospective clinical trials. Newer and more active chemotherapeutic agents are needed.[70]

CHILDHOOD SARCOMAS

Primary sarcomas of childhood, such as Ewing's sarcoma and rhabdomyosarcoma, commonly spread to the lungs[71,72]; however, other sites of metastasis are frequent, with the exception of metastases associated with OST. Chemotherapy remains the major treatment modality for metastases in multiple sites. Pulmonary resection for metastases may be required to document metastases in the lungs or to assess the tumor's response to chemotherapy or the viability of the remaining tumor. Resection of all disease in the lung may enhance postresection survival in these children with resectable metastases. Children undergoing median sternotomy for resection of pulmonary metastases from OST have almost a complete recovery of preoperative pulmonary function.[73]

Ewing's sarcoma and OST metastasize preferentially to the lungs in children and may be resected. Patients with resectable pulmonary metastases from Ewing's sarcoma have prolonged survival (actuarial 5-year survival rate, 15%; median, 28 months) compared to those patients explored but found to have unresectable metastases (no survivors beyond 22 months; median survival, 12 months; $P = .0047$). Patients with four or fewer nodules have better survival than patients with four or more nodules.[74] Other studies[71,72,75] support these findings.

OST metastasizes preferentially to the lungs.[61] Resection of pulmonary metastases from OST also results in prolonged postresection survival.[44,55,59,76,77] Adjuvant therapy, such as chemotherapy[55,59,60,78] or lung irradiation,[79,80] may also be valuable, particularly for micrometastases. Post resection survival may be as high as 40% at 5 years.[44]

NONPULMONARY METASTASES FROM SARCOMAS

Location of sarcomatous recurrence or metastases may vary by the original location or histology of the primary tumor. Biopsy of suspicious lesions is needed to confirm the presence of local recurrence or distant metastases. A needle biopsy, or a core biopsy, may be considered.[81]

Metastases from OST and STSs occur most commonly in the lungs but may also occur in other organs. Potter et al.[66] noted that only 53% of recurrences in those patients completely resected of primary sarcoma recurred in the lung. In another early study[82] of 255 patients with STS treated with preoperative chemotherapy and radiation followed by limb-sparing surgery, 85 patients developed metastatic disease (isolated local recurrence, 13; isolated pulmonary metastases, 43; lung and other, 11; and multiple sites, 18). Poor 2-year survival rate (less than 10%) occurred in those patients with multiple recurrence sites. Resection of isolated metastases appears to benefit a portion of patients with metastatic disease.[82] More recently, Billingsley et al.[83] noted that, in patients with primary extremity sarcoma, 23% of all patients develop metastases. Of these patients, 73% develop pulmonary metastases. Other sites of metastasis include the skin and soft tissues of the head and neck, trunk, and extremities.[83]

In contrast to the expected pulmonary site for metastases, myxoid liposarcomas may metastasize preferentially to extrathoracic sites. In one study from the University of Texas M. D. Anderson Cancer Center in Houston,[84] 102 patients with myxoid tumors had 33 distant recurrences. Extrapulmonary soft tissue sites were the most common (e.g., the retroperitoneum, chest wall, pleura, pericardium, pelvic sidewall, and soft tissue of the back; n = 31), whereas pulmonary metastases were rare (n = 2). In this study, pleomorphic tumors more frequently recurred in the lung (10 of 18 patients recurred: three of ten extrapulmonary, seven of ten pulmonary) than did the myxoid tumors ($P < .05$; myxoid vs. pleomorphic).[84]

Angiosarcoma is a high-grade aggressive sarcoma with local recurrences likely in 20% of patients and distant metastases in 49%. The location of metastases is commonly the lungs, lymph nodes, soft tissues, bone, liver, and other sites.[85]

In another study,[86] of 981 patients with sarcoma, 65 were noted as having developed hepatic metastases. Most patients (n = 61) had an intraabdominal primary site of high-grade leiomyosarcoma. Even with resection in 14 patients, all recurred; however, a median survival of 30 months was achieved. The opportunity for complete resection of hepatic metastases is rare, but complete resection of hepatic metastases must be considered to obtain a survival advantage.[87]

In patients with brain metastases from STSs, complete resection may also provide a survival advantage (14 months vs. 6 months) compared to patients with incomplete resection. The authors concluded that complete resection of brain metastases from STS patients with a good performance status (Karnofsky performance score greater than 70) is associated with a good prognosis. Even if synchronous lung metastases were present, complete resection of all metastases provided the patient with a survival of 11.8 months (median).[88]

COLORECTAL NEOPLASMS

Colorectal metastases commonly spread to local or regional nodes or are trapped in the liver through the portal venous drainage. Patients with prior colorectal neoplasms have had pulmonary metastases resected with prolonged postresection survival. An absolute distinction cannot be made between a single carcinomatous metastasis and a primary bronchogenic carcinoma except by direct visual comparison between the two neoplasms. As with other isolated pulmonary metastases, patients with pulmonary metastases from colorectal carcinoma may be resected safely with low morbidity and mortality and long-term survival (see Fig. 52.2-4). Reports[89–94] describe 5-year survival rates ranging from 21% up to 50% after resection of pulmonary metastases from colon carcinoma. Differences in age and gender of the patient and location, grade, and stage of the primary colorectal cancer are not associated with either improved or worsened survival after resection of these metastases. Patients with metachronous liver lesions excised for cure may also be candidates for resection of pulmonary metastases. Sauter et al.[95] evaluated 49 patients with isolated pulmonary metastases (n = 18) and hepatic metastases (n = 31). Patients with pulmonary metastases had a 47% 5-year survival rate compared to patients with hepatic metastases (5-year survival, 19%). Of 1578 patients treated for colon and rectal cancer, 117 of 1013 patients with rectal carcinoma (11.5%) and 20 of 565 patients with colon cancer (3.5%) recurred in the lungs.[96] In 66 patients who underwent resection of pulmonary metastases from colorectal adenocarcinoma, patients with a solitary metastasis had a longer postresection survival than others.[94] The 5-year survival rate was 38% in both studies. In another study of 62 patients,[93] metastases less than 3 cm in diameter were associated with improved survival.

In a series from the Mayo Clinic, McAfee et al.[97] reported 139 patients who underwent resection of pulmonary metastases from colorectal carcinoma. Operative mortality was 1.4%. Overall, the 5-year survival rate was 30.5%, and the median follow-up was 7 years. Patients with a solitary pulmonary metastasis and those with a preoperative carcinoembryonic antigen (CEA) level of less than 4.0 ng/mL had a better postthoracotomy than others. A longer DFI and metastases smaller than 3 cm in diameter were not associated with improved survival.

Patients with resection of colon metastases from the lung and the liver have a survival advantage with complete resection.[98,99] Forty-eight patients had both liver and lung metastases. Twenty-five patients underwent resection of these metastases, and the remaining 23 patients did not. Median survival was longer after resection of the last metastasis than in those individuals who did not undergo resection (16 months vs. 6 months; $P < .001$). The authors also noted that patients with metachronous resections survived longer than patients with synchronous resections (median of 70 months vs. 22 months; $P < .001$). Robinson et al.[100] noted that the ideal candidate for resection is a patient younger than 50 years old with a solitary liver metastasis and a 4-year interval between the colorectal cancer resection and the occurrence of the pulmonary metastasis. The patient least suited for resection is one older than 70 years with multiple liver metastases and synchronous disease.[100] In addition, a French study[101] examined 43 patients who previously had undergone complete resection of hepatic metastasis and then developed pulmonary metastases. The median survival was 19 months, and the 5-year survival was estimated to be 11%. Patients with a CEA of more than 0.5 ng/mL had a significantly lower probability of survival than those with lower levels (less than 0.5 ng/mL; $P = .0018$).[101]

In patients with colorectal metastases to both liver and lung, complete resection is generally associated with improved survival. Whether the liver metastases occur first and then the lung metastases, or whether lung metastases occur first followed by liver metastases, complete surgical resection tends to be associated with longer survival. Poorer survival was noted in those patients who cannot be completely resected or who are deemed unresectable without operation. Of the total population of patients with colorectal metastases, those individuals with completely resectable lung or hepatic metastases represent a small percentage and one with the most favorable "biology" of the tumor. The surgeon can take advantage of this biologically favorable subset of patients. With complete resection of both lung and hepatic metastases, survival may be enhanced.

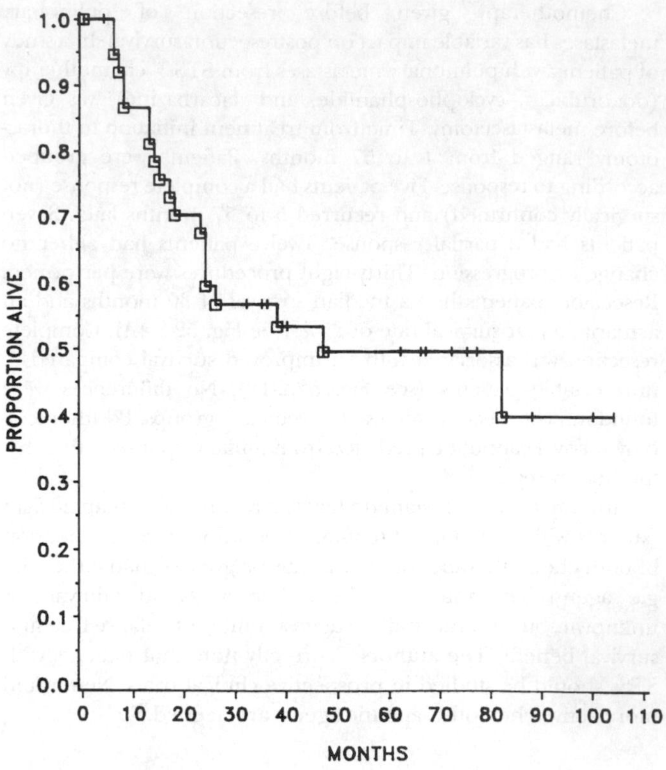

FIGURE 52.2-5. Overall survival for patients after resection of pulmonary metastases from breast carcinoma. The 5-year survival rate was 50%.

BREAST CARCINOMA

Patients with metastases from breast carcinoma usually do poorly because metastases occur in multiple sites. Patanaphan and colleagues[102] described 145 patients with metastatic breast carcinoma (145 of 558; 26%) in whom bone (51%), lung (17%), brain (16%), and liver (6%) metastases occurred. Overall median survival was 12 months for patients with lung metastases, most of whom were treated with palliative chemotherapy, irradiation, or both.[102] Lanza and associates[103] reviewed 44 women with a prior history of breast cancer who underwent pulmonary resection for new pulmonary lesions. Seven patients were excluded who had benign nodules (n = 3) or unresectable metastases (n = 4). In 37 resectable patients, actuarial 5-year survival was 50% (Fig. 52.2-5). A DFI of more than 12 months was associated with a longer median survival (82 months) and 5-year survival rate (57%) compared with patients with a DFI of less than 12 months (15 months median; 0% 5-year survival; P = .004). Estrogen receptor–positive status tended to be associated with a longer postthoracotomy survival (P = .098). Another favorable prognostic factor included positive receptor status of the primary tumor that was associated with improved 3-year survival (61%) compared to negative receptor status (38%). Resection of solitary metastasis resulted in a 35% 5-year survival rate compared to 0% for resection of five or more metastases.[104] More recently, favorable selection of patients has enabled survival to increase up to 62% at 5 years in one series.[105]

Staren et al.[174] evaluated 33 patients treated with surgical resection of pulmonary metastases from breast carcinoma and compared the results to that of 30 patients treated primarily with systemic chemotherapy and hormonal therapy. Patients having complete resection of metastases had a better median survival than patients with medical therapy, particularly when single nodules were compared (58 months median survival vs. 34 months, respectively). The 5-year survival rate in patients treated with some surgical resection was 36%, compared to 11% in those patients treated with other than surgical treatment.

TESTICULAR NEOPLASMS

Nonseminomatous testicular tumors can be diagnosed by the occurrence of new pulmonary nodules identified on CXR or by CT scan.[106,107] Metastatic testicular seminoma most commonly is identified as mediastinal nodal enlargement. CT scan, therefore, is more accurate in diagnosis of seminomatous metastases than plain chest roentgenograms.[108]

Cytoreductive surgery for disseminated nonseminomatous germ cell tumors of the testis may be performed after chemotherapy for removal of residual metastatic disease. The response to chemotherapy may be assessed when no further reduction in size of the nodules is noted. The majority of patients require retroperitoneal lymph node dissections (69%), although thoracotomies may be required in 18% of patients. Several authors[109–111] evaluated 80 patients with germ cell tumors and lung metastases treated with chemotherapy and subsequent surgery. Thirty-five percent (n = 28) achieved complete response after chemotherapy. Thirty-six patients with partial response underwent surgery for resection of metastases in the abdomen (n = 17), the lungs (n = 15), or both (n = 4). Twenty-seven of 36 patients achieved complete response after both chemotherapy and surgery. Carter et al.[112] noted that extensive pulmonary metastases (unresectable metastases) are a predictor of ultimate treatment failure.

Liu and colleagues[113] evaluated the role of pulmonary metastasectomy for testicular germ cell tumors over a 28-year period. The typical patient was young (median age, 27 years) and complete resection generally could be accomplished. Most of these patients had already undergone chemotherapy. Viable metastasis was present in 44% of the patients; 25% had metastasis to other sites after resection of their pulmonary metastasis. Overall, the 5-year survival rate was 68%, and for the patients diagnosed after 1985, the survival rate was 82%. The authors of the study noted that extrathoracic metastasis (nonpulmonary visceral sites) as well as the presence of viable tumor in the resected specimens were adverse prognostic indicators. Of interest was the observation that preoperative tumor markers were normal in the majority of patients and that patients with multiple metastases predominated. Approximately one-half of the patients had synchronous presentation of their metastasis, and 66% of patients had no viable tumor; mature teratoma and fibrosis/necrosis were equally represented. Patients with metastases outside the pulmonary parenchyma and elevated tumor markers from viable tumor had a worse prognosis. Parenchymal resection not only removed all identifiable disease but also provided a measure as to the effectiveness of their chemotherapy treatment.[113] More recently, 28 patients with pulmonary metastases from germ cell/testicular neoplasms were treated with bleomycin, etoposide, and cisplatin. Complete response was achieved in 21 patients (75%), and a complete response was achieved in 11 patients. Resection of residual mass was necessary in 12 patients with normalized serum markers. Overall, the cure rate was 89.3%. Resection of the residual mass was recommended for histology and may modify subsequent treatment.[114]

The value of repeat surgical resection of pulmonary metastasis has not been as well studied as individuals having only one resection. In one report of 396 operations in 330 patients,[27] the authors identified a subgroup of 35 patients who had undergone reoperation for pulmonary metastasis. In this group, the 5- and 10-year survival rates were 48% and 28%, respectively. The favorable prognostic factors included a DFI of more than 1 year. No survival advantage was associated with histology (epithelial carcinoma, osteosarcoma, or STS). In this patient population, successful repeat surgical resections of pulmonary metastasis and survival advantage are probably related to a favorable biologic behavior. The specific criteria for this favorable behavior are not yet known.[27]

GYNECOLOGIC NEOPLASMS

Fuller and colleagues[115] from the Massachusetts General Hospital reviewed a 40-year experience of treating 15 patients with pulmonary metastases from gynecologic cancer, which included primary tumors involving the cervix (6), endometrium (3), and ovary (2), as well as two uterine sarcomas and two choriocarcinomas. The 5-year survival rate was 36%. Lesions less than 4 cm in diameter and a DFI of more than 36 months were associated with prolonged survival.

Levenback et al.[116] reviewed 45 patients with pulmonary metastases from uterine sarcomas. Most patients (71%) had unilateral lesions, and 51% had only one lesion. The 5-year survival rate was 43%. Unilateral metastases or fewer numbers of metastases were not significantly associated with prolonged survival.

Kumar[181] reviewed 97 patients with metastatic gestational trophoblastic disease; chemotherapy was the treatment of choice. Selective thoracotomy in patients with solitary lung metastases reduced the treatment time and need for further aggressive chemotherapy. Overall, 2-year survival after diagnosis was 65%. A DFI of less than 1 year was associated with poorer survival.

Barter et al.[117] studied 2116 patients with primary cervical malignancy between 1969 and 1984 and found 88 patients (4.16%) with pulmonary lesions consistent with metastases. Prognosis was poor with chemotherapy only (median survival, 8 months; only 2 of 88 long-term survivors). Imachi et al.[118] identified 50 of 817 patients (6.1%) treated for carcinoma of the uterine cervix who developed pulmonary metastases. Eighty-one percent of patients had local recurrence or other metastases, and chemotherapy was given. The authors suggest that surgery may be considered for patients with pulmonary metastases without extrathoracic metastases. Resection of pulmonary metastases from squamous cell carcinoma (SCC) of the uterine cervix also has been described.[119]

RENAL CELL CARCINOMA

Various series have examined the value of resection of pulmonary metastases from renal cell carcinoma. Five-year survival rates have ranged from 21%[120] to 60%.[121] Schott et al.[122] reported 39 of 938 patients (4.1%) with pulmonary metastases after nephrectomy for renal carcinoma. Patients with pulmonary metastases less than 2 cm in diameter and limited to one site had prolonged survival and DFI compared to other patients. Dernevik and colleagues[120] resected 33 patients for pulmonary metastases and evaluated them with a minimum follow-up period of 5 years or until death. Longer DFI (more than 1 year) was better than a shorter DFI (less than 1 year). Pogrebniak and associates[121] from the National Cancer Institute reported 23 patients who underwent resection of pulmonary metastases from renal cell carcinoma, 18 of which had previous interleukin-2–based immunotherapy. Resectable patients (15 of 23; 65%) had a longer survival (mean, 49 months; median not yet reached) compared to unresectable patients (median, 16 months, P = .02). Postresection survival did not depend on tomogram nodules, resected nodules, or the DFI.[123]

The 5-year survival rate after complete resection was 44% in one study of 50 patients undergoing resection of metastases from renal cell carcinoma.[123] Twelve patients had repeat resection (42% 5-year survival after second resection). Complete resection was the most important factor associated with 5-year survival.

MELANOMA

The overall biologic behavior of melanoma cannot be predicted. Most commonly, pulmonary metastases occur in addition to other visceral sites, and overall long-term survival is poor. Immunotherapy has been used with some favorable results. In the rare patients who present with isolated pulmonary metastases, resection may be associated with long-term survival.[124] Current 5-year survival ranges from 4.5% to 25%. In a large series of 1521 patients with American Joint Committee on Cancer stage IV melanoma, 5-year survival was only 4% (median survival, 8.3 months).[125,126]

Gorenstein and colleagues[127] evaluated 56 patients with histologically proven pulmonary metastases from melanoma. The overall postresection survival was 25% at 5 years. Patients with earlier primary-stage melanoma, or patients with metastases to the lungs as the first site of metastasis, had longer postresection survival than other patients. Location of the primary tumor, histology, thickness, Clark level, nodal metastases, TDT, or type of resection of the primary tumor was not associated with improved postresection survival.

Harpole et al.[128] evaluated pulmonary metastases in 945 patients with melanoma out of a population of 7564 melanoma patients. Bilateral and multiple metastases were present in the majority of these patients. Multivariate predictors of survival included complete resection, DFI, chemotherapy, two or fewer metastases, negative lymph nodes, and histologic type. The 5-year survival rate for all patients (n = 7564) was 4%, in contrast to 20% 5-year survival in patients with resection of pulmonary metastases.

SQUAMOUS CELL CARCINOMA

Patients with primary SCC outside the lungs frequently have disease metastasize to the lungs. These secondary lung neoplasms may be resected with subsequent survival benefit.[129] With solitary pulmonary lesions after treatment of primary SCC elsewhere in the body, the origin of the lesion is uncertain. The lesion may represent a solitary metastasis, a primary bronchogenic carcinoma, or a benign process. The recommended treatment for such a solitary lesion is bronchoscopy thoracic exploration and excisional biopsy. If a SCC is identified, a lobectomy and mediastinal lymph node dissection should be performed in the same manner as if the lesion were a second primary neoplasm. Less desirable is a generous wedge excision and mediastinal lymph node dissection, because local control may be limited.

Finley et al.[130] described factors associated with improved survival in patients with SCC metastases from head and neck cancers. These included complete resection, control of primary tumor, early stage of the head and neck primary, one nodule on CXR, and longer DFI (more than 2 years) from primary resection. Complete resection of all malignant disease was associated with a 5-year survival rate of 29%. The number of nodules was not significantly associated with survival. In eight patients with more than one nodule, median survival was 2 years, and no 5-year survivors were reported. Therefore, the benefits of resection of multiple pulmonary metastases from head and neck primary SCC are not completely clear. In another study of 44 patients,[131] 5-year survival after pulmonary resection was 43%. Mazer et al.[131] noted that single nodules, primary tumor stage, or absence of locoregional recurrence were not associated with enhanced survival. The presence of mediastinal disease was associated with the worst outcome.

Lefor and colleagues[132] attempted to correlate primary carcinomas of the head and neck with subsequent development of pulmonary metastases or second primary lung carcinomas. An algorithm was used that considered the DFI, histology, radiographic findings, and characteristics of the lung lesion, as well as the identification of mediastinal lymphadenopathy. The authors recommended that treatment of indeterminate lesions be treated as primary lung carcinomas (e.g., with lobectomy and mediastinal lymph node dissection) because this strategy provides the best local control of the disease and potential for cure.

WILMS' TUMOR

Patients with Wilms' tumor may present with pulmonary metastases at diagnosis or relapse after initial treatment.[133] Early diagnosis using CT may identify metastases in up to 36% of patients.[134] Pulmonary metastases may be resected safely from children with Wilms' tumor.[71,135] In contrast,[136] 211 patients entered on the National Wilms' Tumor Study whose initial relapse was in the lungs did not show any survival advantage to resection of pulmonary metastases compared to treatment with chemotherapy and whole lung irradiation.

METASTASIS OR PRIMARY BRONCHOGENIC CARCINOMA?

Pulmonary metastases from sarcomas or other distinctive nonpulmonary neoplasms are usually easy to diagnose. However, solitary carcinomatous metastasis from breast or colon, or SCC metastasis from head and neck primary tumors, are difficult to distinguish from primary lung carcinoma. Patients with two or more pulmonary nodules can be considered to have metastases. In tumors without a propensity for bilaterality (e.g., nonsarcomatous histology), a solitary pulmonary nodule may be approached through a lateral thoracotomy incision. A generous wedge excision or lobectomy and mediastinal lymph node dissection should be performed. The final pathology may suggest histology amenable to adjuvant therapy.

Traditionally, a comparison of the primary neoplasm and the lung nodule using light microscopy has been the only method for determining origin of the lung nodule or neoplasm. Electron microscopy[137] or specific molecular or genetic characteristics may identify more precisely the origin of such neoplasms. Monoclonal antibodies can assist in discriminating between primary bronchogenic adenocarcinoma and colon carcinoma metastatic to the lung.[138] Characteristics of amplified K-ras oncogene expression present in the primary tumor can be used to identify pulmonary metastases.[139] Monoclonal antibodies can identify colorectal carcinoma metastases.[140] The monoclonal antibody was not sufficient to discriminate primary lung from metastatic adenocarcinoma. Flow cytometry and DNA analysis have been used[95,141,142] to describe primary carcinomas of the lung and to distinguish them from metastases.

Algorithms have been developed[132] for patients with SCCs of the head and neck who develop pulmonary nodules after treatment. Characteristics of metastases and of primary lung carcinoma were examined in an attempt to better direct subsequent therapy.

RECURRENT PULMONARY METASTASES

If pulmonary metastases recur in the lungs, resection can again be accomplished safely with prolonged postthoracotomy survival.[143] Patients are screened by the criteria in Table 52.2-2. Patients with pulmonary metastases may undergo multiple procedures for re-resection of metastases, with prolonged survival after complete resection. Several studies have reviewed results of multiple resections for recurrent pulmonary metastases. Rizzoni and associates[37] described 29 patients with recurrent pulmonary metastases from STSs who underwent two or more resections of pulmonary metastases. Patients with favorable tumor biology [resectable metastases, longer TDT, three or fewer nodules, longer DFI (more than 6 months)] had longer survival. No operative mortality occurred, and the complication rate was 7.5%. Median survival was 14.5 months and overall 5-year survival was 22%. Resectable patients had a median survival of 24 months. These findings were confirmed by Casson and colleagues,[35] who described 39 patients with adult

TABLE 52.2-2. Criteria for Resection of Pulmonary Metastases

Pulmonary parenchymal nodules or changes consistent with metastases
Absence of uncontrolled extrathoracic metastases
Control of the patient's primary tumor
Potential for complete resection
Sufficient pulmonary parenchymal reserve after resection
Additional criteria for partial or complete resection of pulmonary metastases:
Provide a diagnosis
Evaluate the effects of chemotherapy on residual disease
Obtain tumor for markers, immunohistochemical studies, vaccine, etc.
Palliate symptoms
Decrease tumor burden

STSs. Thirty-four patients were resectable (median survival, 28 months; 5-year survival, approximately 32%). Unresectable patients had a median survival of 7 months. Survival after resection of a solitary recurrent metastasis was 65 months (median) compared to patients with two or more nodules (median, 14 months; $P = .01$).

Repeat resection of pulmonary metastasis may salvage a subset of pediatric patients with sarcomatous histologies, including OST, nonrhabdomyosarcoma STS, and Ewing's sarcoma. At the National Cancer Institute, 70 patients underwent at least one reoperation between 1965 and 1995.[144] Osteosarcoma predominated (36 patients), and single-wedge resection was the most common operation performed (84%). The authors noted that complete resection was the most important and favorable prognostic factor. Patients with complete resection had improved survival compared with those who were incompletely resected. Median survival was 2.25 years; in resectable patients, median survival was 5.6 years, compared to 0.7 year in unresectable patients ($P < .0001$). The authors concluded that an aggressive surgical approach in patients with small numbers of nodules, a longer DFI, and the ability to obtain a complete resection is warranted and associated with prolonged survival.[144]

EXTENDED RESECTION OF PULMONARY METASTASES

Pneumonectomy or other extended resection of pulmonary metastases may be performed safely in selected patients with associated long-term disease-free survival. Fewer than 3% of all patients undergoing resection of pulmonary metastases will require an extended resection. Pneumonectomy or *en bloc* resection of pulmonary metastases with chest wall or other thoracic structures, such as diaphragm, pericardium, and superior vena cava, have been performed in a small number of patients with good results.[145] In this series of pneumonectomy (n = 19) and other extended resection (n = 19), the 5-year actuarial survival rate was 25%. Mortality was 5% and occurred in those patients having pneumonectomy often after multiple prior wedge resections for metastases.

Pneumonectomy is performed infrequently for resection of pulmonary metastases. The need for pneumonectomy may be evident in the large metastases that involve the majority of one lung and that compress the heart and shift the mediastinum

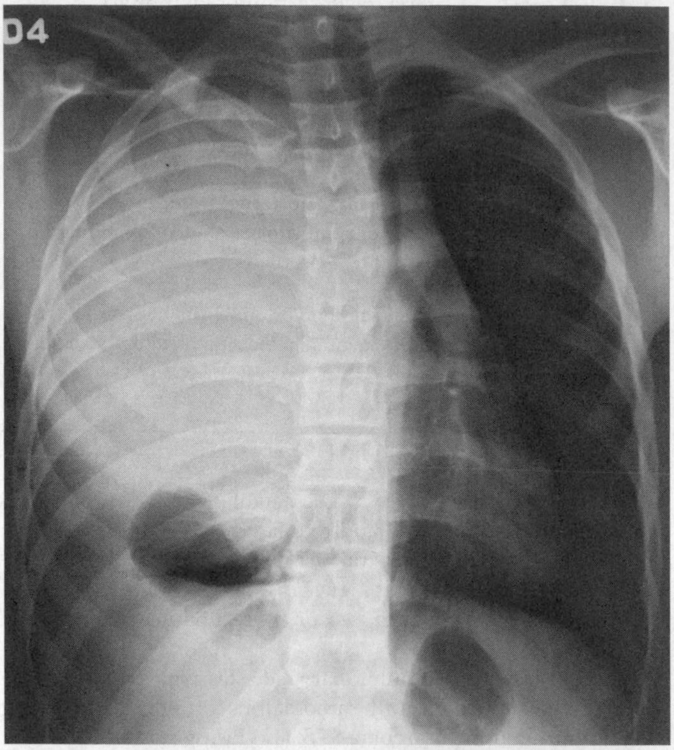
A

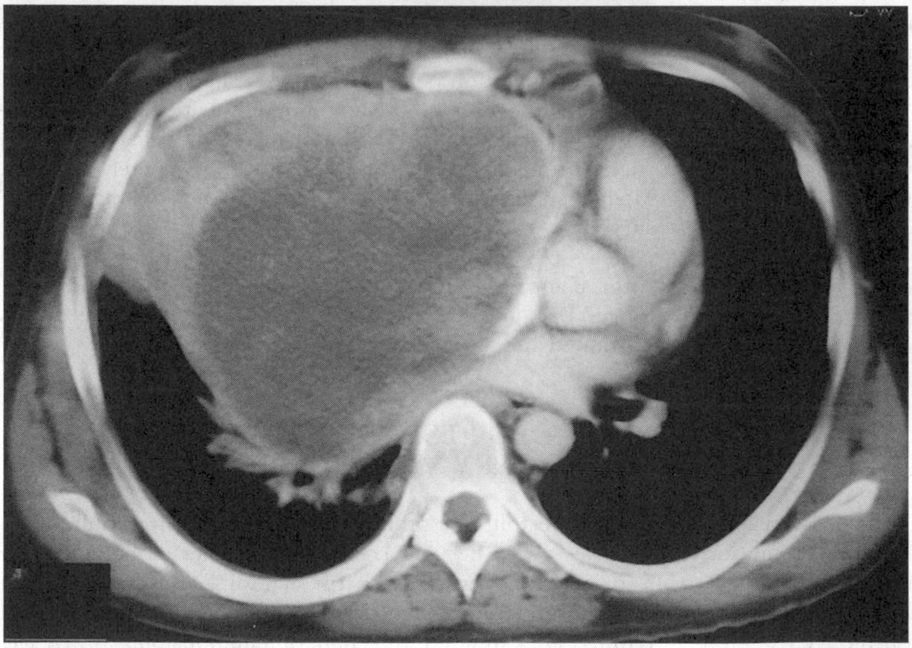
B

FIGURE 52.2-6. **A:** Chest roentgenogram with a massive pulmonary metastasis from malignant fibrous histiocytoma compressing and shifting the mediastinum into the contralateral hemithorax. Compression of the heart and airway is noted. Impairment of ventilation to the involved hemithorax and secondary compression of the contralateral hemithorax further impairs ventilation. **B:** Chest computed tomography with a massive pulmonary metastasis from osteogenic sarcoma compressing the superior vena cava, right heart, and right lung, and shifting the mediastinum into the left chest. Resection often requires extracorporeal support to allow decompression and manipulation of the heart and pulmonary veins. An approach to the right pulmonary artery and veins and the right mainstem bronchus via a median sternotomy allows for control of the pulmonary vasculature and airway before removal of the tumor.

(Fig. 52.2-6). In a French study of 42 patients treated over 10 years,[146] 29 patients underwent pneumonectomy for sarcoma; 12 for carcinoma; and one for a lipoma. Most metastases were centrally located. Two postoperative deaths occurred, and four patients had major complications; five patients (12%) had recurrences in the residual lung. The median survival was only 6.25 months, and the 5-year survival rate was 16%. The standard surgical mortality for operations for pulmonary metastases is less than 1%. Patients with large centrally located metastases may require pneumonectomy for complete resection. Although mortality for pneumonectomy for pulmonary metastases corresponds to mortality for other histologies, the 5-year survival rate of only 16% demands careful selection of patients before resection. The authors suggest that young patients, those with a long DFI, and those with normal CEA levels (e.g., patients with metastases from colorectal carcinoma) be considered as potential candidates for pneumonectomy for pulmonary metastases.[146]

The value of pneumonectomy was also examined by retrospective review of the International Registry of Lung Metastases.[147] Of the 5206 patients who were enrolled, 133 patients (2.6%) had undergone pneumonectomy for pulmonary

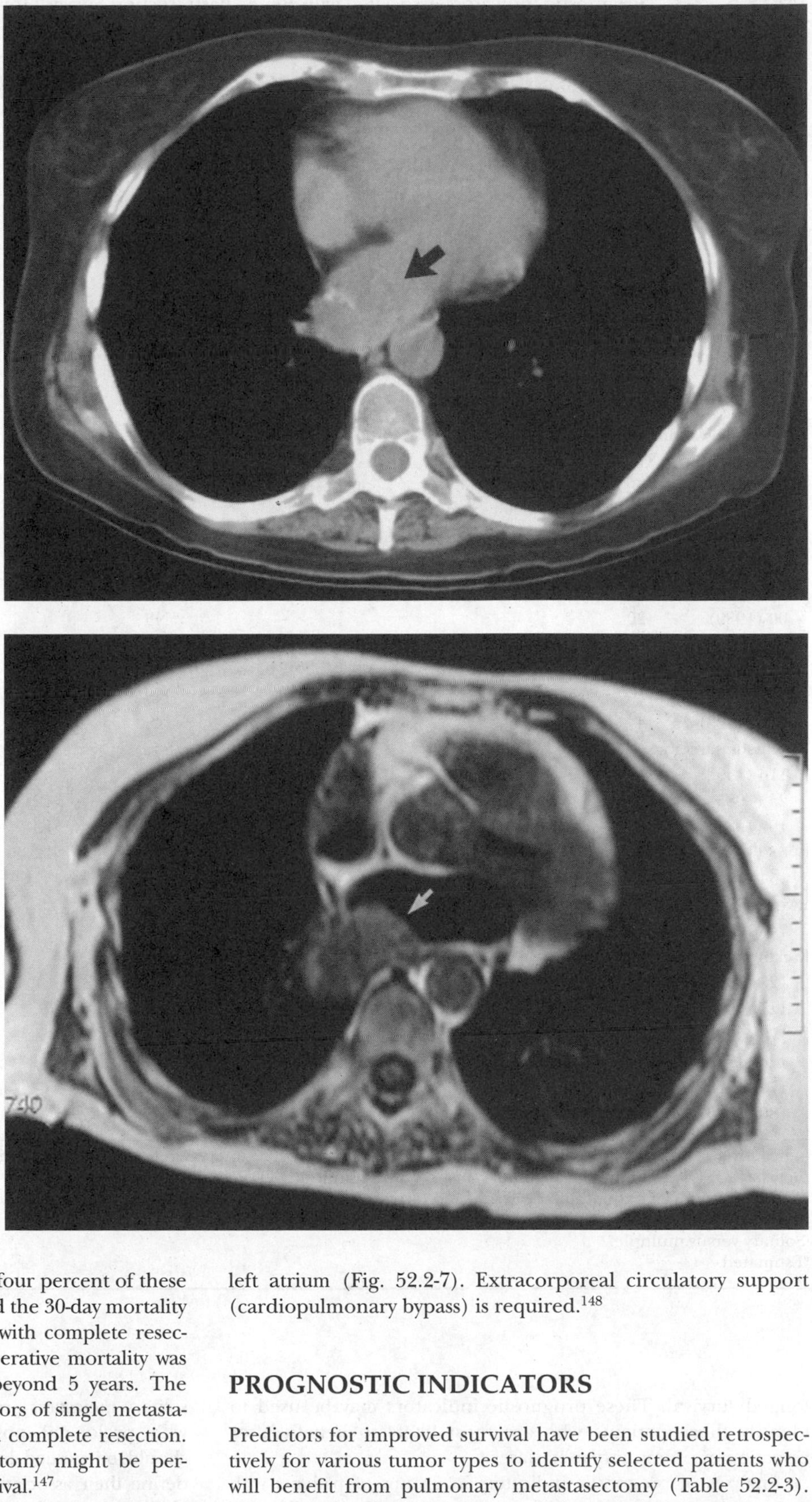

A

B

FIGURE 52.2-7. Metastatic synovial cell sarcoma. The patient has an azygoesophageal mass abutting the left atrium and esophagus without direct invasion. The mass is confirmed by chest computed tomography **(A)** and magnetic resonance imaging **(B)**. Pulmonary metastases were resected. Using hypothermic circulatory arrest, the patient also underwent complete resection of the posterior wall of the left atrium *en bloc* with the metastasis. Patch reconstruction of the posterior wall of the left atrium was required.

metastases between 1962 and 1994. Eighty-four percent of these patients underwent complete resection, and the 30-day mortality rate was 3.6%. Five-year survival was 20% with complete resection. For incomplete resection, the perioperative mortality was 19%, and the majority did not survive beyond 5 years. The authors identified favorable prognostic factors of single metastasis, negative mediastinal lymph nodes, and complete resection. The authors concluded that pneumonectomy might be performed safely with adequate long-term survival.[147]

Intraatrial extension of sarcoma through the pulmonary vein is rare but may also be safely treated with pulmonary resection and pneumonectomy, and resection of the tumor from the left atrium (Fig. 52.2-7). Extracorporeal circulatory support (cardiopulmonary bypass) is required.[148]

PROGNOSTIC INDICATORS

Predictors for improved survival have been studied retrospectively for various tumor types to identify selected patients who will benefit from pulmonary metastasectomy (Table 52.2-3). These prognostic indicators are clinical, biologic, and molecular criteria that describe the biologic interaction between the metastases and the patient and their association with pro-

TABLE 52.2-3. Prognostic Indicators Associated with Better Postresection Survival for Patients with Pulmonary Metastases from Various Tumor Types[a]

Reference	*N*	*Stage of Primary*	*Number of Nodules* CT	*Number of Nodules* *FLT*	*Metastases Resected*	*TDT (mo)*	*Resectability DFI (mo)*	*Median Survival (mo)*	*Percentage of 5-Y Survival*
Breast									
174 (1992)	33	–						58	36
103 (1992)	44	NS	NS		+	>12		47[b]	50
149 (1988)	50	–		NS		>18		13	12
Colorectal									
97 (1992)	139	NS		1[c]	+	NS		36	30.5
90 (1988)	66	NS		1[c]			>24	42	38
153 (1979)	35	+		NS[c]		NS			22
93 (1989)	27	NS		NS[c]			27		9
94 (1986)	27	NS		NS[c]	+		>24	35	21
175 (1985)	62	NS		1[c]		NS		24	42
Osteogenic sarcoma									
176 (1992)	102				+				58
25 (1985)	38			≤4	NS	+	NS		
61 (1987)	39		<4	<6	+	NS		20	38
9 (1983)	38		≤3	≤4	NS	+	>6	26	40
150 (1988)	27			1		>12		28	47 (at 3 y)
152 (1984)	32			NS	+	NS		24	32
60 (1989)	20				+	NS			37
Renal									
121 (1992)	23		NS	NS	+	NS		>49[b]	60
177 (1988)	39			NS[c]	+	NS		36	32.7
151 (1983)	44			NS		NS	>24	33	27
Soft tissue sarcomas									
116 (1992)	45			NS	+	NS			43
25 (1985)	67		≤4	>20 d	+		>12		
10 (1984)	67		≤4	<16	>20 d	+	>12	8	10
68 (1989)	63	NS	≤5	≤3	NS	NS	>12	20.3	27
154 (1989)	28				NS	NS			35[d]
Ewing's sarcoma									
74 (1987)	19			≤4	+	NS		28[b]	15
Melanoma									
128 (1992)	98			+	+	+		22[b]	20
127 (1991)	56	NS	NS	NS	NS	+	NS	18	25
178 (1990)	29	NS		NS	+	NS		11[b]	4.5
126 (1988)	31	NS	NS	NS	NS	NS		13	7[d]
179 (1988)	47				+	NS		19	25
180 (1985)	17			NS		NS		16.5	11.1

–, negative; +, positive; CT, computed tomography; DFI, disease-free interval between control of primary tumor and identification of pulmonary metastases; FLT, full lung linear tomograms; NS, not significant; TDT, tumor-doubling time.
[a]Age and gender of patient, tumor grade, and location of primary tumor are rarely prognostic indicators for either improved or poorer survival.
[b]Resectable patients only.
[c]Solitary versus multiple.
[d]Estimated.

longed survival. These prognostic indicators may be used to identify those patients who are most likely to benefit after resection of pulmonary metastases.

Analyses of prognostic indicators in groups of patients with pulmonary metastases from heterogeneous tumors describe prolonged survival in patients with resectable metastases. Resectable patients, longer DFI, longer TDT, fewer numbers of metastases, or solitary metastasis are prognostic indicators generally associated with prolonged postresection survival. Prognostic indicators should be studied in patients with the same primary tumor to define their association with postresection survival. A wide variability exists in the characteristics of pulmonary metastases from different primary neoplasms and the subsequent survival of patients with these metastases. The study of prognostic indicators from the same primary neoplasm yields the most precise information on association with postresection survival. Age or gender does not usually influence postthoracotomy survival. Neither age nor gender should be considered as prognostic factors.

DISEASE-FREE INTERVAL

The DFI extends from resection of the primary tumor until pulmonary metastases are detected. A short DFI may indicate a poor prognosis because metastases may be multiple and growing rapidly. A longer DFI may represent a less biologically aggressive tumor and correlate with a longer postresection survival.

The DFI may also be defined as the time between resection of the pulmonary metastases and recurrence of metastases in the lungs or elsewhere. DFIs of more than 12 months are usually associated with improved survival in patients with breast carcinoma,[149] colorectal carcinoma,[90,94] OST,[150] STS,[10,25] and renal cell carcinoma.[151] Patients with pulmonary metastases from OST and a DFI of more than 6 to 12 months demonstrated a survival advantage[9,150] in contrast to others who demonstrated no such advantage.[25,60,61,152] In STS, a DFI of more than 12 months[10,25,68] was usually associated with a better postresection survival. Evaluation of patients with Ewing's sarcoma[74] did not reveal differences in survival based on DFI.

LOCATION AND STAGE OF PRIMARY TUMOR

Postresection survival is not usually influenced by the specific anatomic location of the primary tumor. Postresection survival in patients with more advanced stage primary neoplasms does not usually differ from patients with earlier stage disease. Still, initial or primary stage may suggest the biologic aggressiveness of the tumor. Schlappack et al.[149] found that a negative nodal status predicted improved postresection survival for patients with breast cancer. McCormack et al.[153] found better postthoracotomy survival in patients with Duke's class A colorectal carcinoma (5-year survival, 37.5%) compared to Duke's class C patients (5-year survival, 15%), although this was not confirmed by the study by McAfee et al.[97]

NUMBER OF NODULES ON PREOPERATIVE IMAGING STUDIES

CT has replaced linear tomograms as the examination of choice in patients with suspected pulmonary metastases. CT of the chest provides a sensitive and specific study for patients with pulmonary metastases. CT of the chest is sensitive but less specific than conventional linear tomography or CXR. Nodules may or may not represent metastases. Theoretically, earlier detection and treatment of metastases can improve survival. Laterality (unilateral or bilateral) of pulmonary metastases does not directly influence postresection survival; the number of nodules is a more precise prognostic indicator.

In patients with OST or STS, better postresection survival was found in patients with fewer number of nodules identified on preoperative full lung linear tomograms or CT scans of the chest. CT scans are more sensitive than other studies, and better survival was noted in those patients with OST with fewer than four nodules[61] and those with STS with five or fewer nodules.[68] Full lung tomograms were performed in several older studies. Patients with OST with fewer than four metastases identified on full lung tomography,[9,25] or four or fewer nodules in STS,[10,25,68] had better postresection survival than those individuals with more nodules. Unilateral or bilateral pulmonary metastases do not influence postresection survival; the number of nodules is a more precise prognostic indicator.

NUMBER OF METASTASES RESECTED

Nodules on preoperative roentgenograms usually correspond to the number of metastases present; however, not all nodules are malignant.[126] Usually, the fewer the number of pulmonary metastases at the time of resection, the better the postresection survival. Postresection survival after complete resection of pulmonary metastases has been examined in patients with pulmonary metastases from multiple histologies to evaluate the influence of number of metastases resected. Patients with OST and with fewer than six[150] or four or fewer[9] metastases resected, or patients with STS and fewer than 16 metastases,[10] had a better postresection survival than patients with more metastases resected. Postresection survival for number of metastases resected after complete resection has been examined in patients with pulmonary metastases from OST[152] or STS.[68,154]

TUMOR-DOUBLING TIME

TDT is calculated[155–157] by measuring the same metastasis on similar studies (e.g., serial chest roentgenograms) separated by a minimum of 10 to 14 days. The most rapidly growing nodule is selected, and changing diameters of the metastasis is plotted on semilogarithmic paper. A formula may be used to precisely calculate TDT:

$$TDT = T[\ln {}^{2}\!/_{3} \times \ln(M2/M1)] = 0.231 \times T/\ln(M2/M1)$$

where ln is the natural logarithm, M1 is the first measurement, M2 is the second measurement, and T is the number of days between measurements.

Metastases from the same primary may or may not grow at similar rates, because differing growth rates between tumor nodules reflect heterogeneity of metastases from the primary. The TDT indirectly reveals the biologic nature or aggressiveness of the metastases, which influences the patient's postresection survival. The TDT may vary based on the size of the metastasis itself or the effect of chemotherapy.

Pulmonary metastases initially grow exponentially, and the growth rate slows with increased size. Growth may also be expressed by "Gompertzian" kinetics,[158,159] which considers a gradual diminution in TDT with time and increased size of the metastasis. TDT only reflects the growth rate during the interval measured.

TDT is not a significant predictor of postresection survival in patients with pulmonary metastases from OST.[9,25] TDT of more than 20 days in patients with STS resulted in a better postthoracotomy survival than those patients with rapid TDTs (less than 20 days). One study of patients with STS[68] found no correlation between TDT and postresection survival.

RESECTABILITY

Complete resection consistently correlates with improved postthoracotomy survival for patients with pulmonary metastases. If pulmonary metastases cannot be completely removed, the postthoracotomy survival is shortened for patients with most tumors in comparison to those individuals completely resected.

ENDOBRONCHIAL OR NODAL METASTASES

Involvement of mediastinal lymph nodes from pulmonary metastases is rare. Udelsman et al.[41] noted that patients with endobronchial metastases from adult STSs have a short postresection survival rate. Seven of 11 patients with endobronchial metastases lived 6 months or less. Jablons et al.[68] found that survival is poor (5 months) in patients with mediastinal lymph node involvement from STSs compared to patients without nodal metastases (31 months).

MULTIVARIATE ANALYSIS OF PROGNOSTIC INDICATORS

Multivariate analysis of prognostic factors may define which patients are most likely to achieve long-term survival. Separate prognostic variables may be combined to enhance the predictive value for survival. Jablons et al.[68] noted the DFI, gender, resectability, and truncal location in patients with pulmonary metastases from STSs to be the best predictors of postthoracotomy survival. Putnam et al.[10] noted that a DFI of more than 12 months, a TDT of more than 20 days, and four or fewer nodules on preoperative full lung tomograms as a single prognostic indicator was the best predictor of postthoracotomy survival in patients with pulmonary metastases from STSs. Roth et al.[25] compared prognostic indicators in patients with OST and STS. TDT, number of metastases on preoperative full lung tomograms, and DFI, when combined, improved predictive ability over any single indicator or pair of indicators.

NOVEL TREATMENT STRATEGIES

MOLECULAR AND GENETIC STRATEGIES

Molecular events associated with pulmonary metastases have been identified in patients with OST. Amplification of the MDM2 gene (the human homologue of a murine p53 binding protein) may regulate p53 protein function by inactivating the protein and deregulating or enhancing tumor growth. In one small study,[160] no detectable MDM2 gene amplification in primary OST was found compared to 14% of metastases (three pulmonary metastases, one local metastasis). Amplification of MDM2 may be associated with metastases and tumor progression in OST.

In STS, alterations (mutations) of the p53 gene (a tumor suppressor gene) may provide for uncontrolled cell growth. Restoration of normal p53 (wild-type) in STS may provide for more controlled cell growth or even programmed cell death (apoptosis). In one *in vitro* study,[161] transduction of wild-type p53 into STSs bearing mutated p53 genes altered the malignant potential of the tumor. After transduction, transfected cells expressed wild-type p53, decreased cell proliferation, decreased colony formation in soft agar, and demonstrated decreased tumor formation in severe combined immunodeficient (SCID) mice *in vivo.* The ability to restore wild-type p53 function in STS *in vitro* and in SCID mice may ultimately be considered as future therapy for patients with STS.[161] Other investigations have shown that pulmonary metastases from STS can develop from clonal expansion of primary tumor cells bearing p53 mutations.[162] Examination of tissue specimens from OST and STS demonstrated p53 mutations in 25% of OSTs, yet in only 1 of 16 metastases.[163] Use of specific molecular markers may provide better selection of patients who will optimally benefit from surgery, chemotherapy, or other treatment modalities.

Other targets of gene therapy may include those chemotherapy-resistant tumors or those tumors with greater propensity for metastatic spread. Overexpression of the MDR1 gene product P glycoprotein is an important predictor of poor prognosis in osteosarcoma patients treated with chemotherapy. In these patients, the MDR phenotype is not *de novo* more aggressive (e.g., more metastatic); however, the poor outcome of patients with the MDR phenotype related to P glycoprotein overexpression is related to the cells' failure to respond to cytotoxic drugs.[164]

In another study,[165] 42% of patients with OSTs had metastases that expressed ErbB-2 and correlated with early development of pulmonary metastasis and poor survival. ErbB-2, therefore, may enhance tumor growth and promote metastases. These authors recommended that ErbB-2 might be considered as a prognostic factor for patients with osteosarcoma.

ErbB-2 protein is expressed in approximately 42% of osteosarcomas. It has been strongly correlated with early pulmonary metastasis and poor survival. ErbB-2 may enhance tumor aggressiveness and metastasis in osteosarcoma. As a marker, ErbB-2 may be useful as a prognostic indicator.[165]

A rodent model of OST has been developed with high propensity for pulmonary metastases. In this metastatic tumor model, matrix metalloproteinase 2 activity is increased as well as expression of vascular endothelial growth factor messenger RNA.[166]

Gene therapy strategies are being studied also. Systematic delivery of recombinant adenovirus (Ad) vector containing herpes simplex virus thymidine kinase (TK) gene [with an Osteocalcin (OC) promoter (Ad-OC-TK)] supplemented with the prodrug acyclovir (ACV) may be an effective strategy for osteosarcoma metastases to the lungs.[167]

Preclinical studies noted that, after Ad-OC-beta-gal administration, specific beta-gal expression was found in tumor cells deposited in the lung. Induced rat osteogenic lung metastases in nude rats were followed by systemic Ad-OC-TK and intraperitoneal ACV treatment, resulting in decreased numbers of tumor nodules and increased survival in treated animals compared to controls. Ad-OC-TK/ACV may be a future treatment for pulmonary metastases from osteosarcoma. Other preclinical treatment methods may include nebulized interleukin-2 liposomes.[168]

REGIONAL DRUG DELIVERY TO THE LUNG

Novel drug delivery systems may enhance chemotherapy treatment effects by increasing drug concentration in lung tissues and minimizing systemic effects of such treatment. In many patients, surgery has been used as salvage treatment after maximal chemotherapy response has been achieved. Systemic toxicity may limit the amount of chemotherapy given to an individual patient. Regional drug delivery to the lungs minimizes systemic drug delivery, preventing systemic toxicity; however, this technique dramatically increases the drug delivered to the lung over a short period. This isolated lung perfusion technique may be done unilaterally, with the contralateral lung serving as an "oxygenator" while the ipsilateral lung is perfused. Bilateral pulmonary perfusion may be performed, although extracorporeal circulatory support (cardiopulmonary bypass) is required.

Preclinical studies in rodents with experimental pulmonary metastases from a methylcholanthrene-induced syngeneic sarcoma[169–171] have shown that chemotherapy may be delivered to pulmonary tissue in significantly higher concentrations than with systemic delivery. Minimal to no systemic toxicity was noted. In this model, isolated single-lung perfusion with Adriamycin (doxorubicin) was safe and effective.[169] This simple microsurgical technique was performed in rats. After left thoracotomy, the pulmonary artery and pulmonary vein were isolated and clamped. The lung was flushed before infusing doxorubicin. The infusion occurred over 10 minutes. Then the drug was flushed out before removing the cannulas and restoring circulation. A perfusion concentration of 255 mg/L caused less general toxicity than a systemic dose equivalent to 75 mg/m^2, the extraction ratio was 58%, and the pulmonary tissue concentration of Adriamycin was 25-fold higher than with the systemic dose. The technique was also effective: Nine of ten animals treated at 320 mg/L had complete eradication of metastases from an implanted methylcholanthrene-induced sarcoma.[169]

Previous clinical studies of lung perfusion[172,173] have shown higher drug concentrations in pulmonary tissue, although clinical tumor response has been mixed. Johnston and colleagues[173] described a continuous perfusion of the lungs with Adriamycin (single lung, continuous perfusion) as a safe technique and subsequently applied their technique clinically. Drug concentrations in normal lung and tumor generally increased with higher drug dosages. Two of eight patients had major complications: One patient developed pneumonia and sternal dehiscence; one patient developed respiratory failure 4 days after lung perfusion. No objective responses occurred (none of four patients with sarcomas). Although continuous perfusion with a pump circuit offers some theoretical advantages, the technique is cumbersome, equipment-intensive, and time-consuming, and it has the inherent problem of the incompatibility of Adriamycin and heparin. Pass et al.[172] examined isolated single-lung perfusion with tumor necrosis factor-α, interferon-γ, and moderate hyperthermia for patients with unresectable pulmonary metastases. No hospital deaths occurred, and a short-term (less than 6 months) decrease in nodule size was noted in 3 of 15 patients.

Phase I studies in patients with unresectable pulmonary metastases from STS are currently under way at the University of Texas M. D. Anderson Cancer Center. A paucity of effective treatment and the potential for high drug concentrations for pulmonary metastases by regional lung perfusion warrants further clinical study.

REFERENCES

1. Meade RH. *A history of thoracic surgery.* Springfield, IL: Charles C Thomas Publisher, 1961.
2. Martini N, McCormack PM. Evolution of the surgical management of pulmonary metastases. *Chest Surg Clin North Am* 1998;8:13.
3. Kronlein RU. Ueber Lungenchirirugie. *Berlin Klin Wschr* 1884;9:129.
4. Divis G. Ein Beitrag zur operativen Behandlung der Lungengeschwultse. *Acta Chir Scand* 1927;62:329.
5. Torek F. Removal of metastatic carcinoma of the lung and mediastinum: suggestions as to technic. *Arch Surg* 1930;21:1416.
6. Barney JD, Churchill EJ. Adenocarcinoma of the kidney with metastasis to the lung cured by nephrectomy and lobectomy. *J Urol* 1939;42:269.
7. Alexander J, Haight C. Pulmonary resection for solitary metastatic sarcoma and carcinoma. *Surg Gynecol Obstet* 1947;85:129.
8. Takita H, Edgerton F, Karakousis C, et al. Surgical management of metastases to the lung. *Surg Gynecol Obstet* 1981;194:191.
9. Putnam JB, Roth JA, Wesley MN, Johnston MR, Rosenberg SA. Survival following aggressive resection of pulmonary metastases from osteogenic sarcoma: analysis of prognostic factors. *Ann Thorac Surg* 1983;38:516.
10. Putnam JB, Roth JA, Wesley MN, Johnston MR, Rosenberg SA. Analysis of prognostic factors in patients undergoing resection of pulmonary metastases from soft tissue sarcomas. *J Thorac Cardiovasc Surg* 1984;87:260.
11. Pastorino U, Buyse M, Friedel G, et al. Long-term results of lung metastasectomy: prognostic analyses based on 5206 cases. *J Thorac Cardiovasc Surg* 1997;113:37.
12. Duda RB, Beatty JD, Kokal WA, Riihimaki DU, Terz JJ. Radiographic evaluation for pulmonary metastases in sarcoma patients. *J Surg Oncol* 1988;38:271.
13. Davis SD. CT evaluation for pulmonary metastases in patients with extrathoracic malignancy. *Radiology* 1991;180:1.
14. Chang AE, Schaner EG, Conkle DM, et al. Evaluation of computed tomography in the detection of pulmonary metastases: a prospective study. *Cancer* 1979;43:913.
15. Schaner EG, Chang AE, Doppman JL, et al. Comparison of computed and conventional whole lung tomography in detecting pulmonary nodules: a prospective radiologic-pathologic study. *AJR Am J Roentgenol* 1978;131:51.
16. Pass HI, Dwyer A, Makuch R, Roth JA. Detection of pulmonary metastases in patients with osteogenic and soft-tissue sarcomas: the superiority of CT scans compared with conventional linear tomograms using dynamic analysis. *J Clin Oncol* 1985;3:1261.
17. Roth JA, Pass HI, Wesley MN, et al. Comparison of median sternotomy and thoracotomy for resection of pulmonary metastases in patients with adult soft-tissue sarcomas. *Ann Thorac Surg* 1986;42:134.
18. Lise M, Rossi CR, Alessio S, Foletto M. Multimodality treatment of extra-visceral soft tissue sarcomas M0: state of the art and trends. *Eur J Surg Oncol* 1995;21:125.
19. Wyttenbach R, Vock P, Tschappeler H. Cross-sectional imaging with CT and/or MRI of pediatric chest tumors. *Eur Radiol* 1998;8:1040.
20. Lucas JD, O'Doherty MJ, Wong JC, et al. Evaluation of fluorodeoxyglucose positron emission tomography in the management of soft-tissue sarcomas. *J Bone Joint Surg Br* 1998;80:441.
21. Takita H, Merrin C, Didolkar MS, et al. The surgical management of multiple lung metastases. *Ann Thorac Surg* 1992;24:359.
22. Morrow CE, Vassilopoulos PP, Grage TB. Surgical resection for metastatic neoplasms of the lung: experience at the University of Minnesota Hospitals. *Cancer* 1980;45:2981.
23. Wright JO III, Brandt B III, Ehrenhaft JL. Results of pulmonary resection for metastatic lesions. *J Thorac Cardiovasc Surg* 1982;83:94.
24. Mountain CF, McMurtrey MJ, Hermes KE. Surgery for pulmonary metastasis: a 20-year experience. *Ann Thorac Surg* 1984;38:323.
25. Roth JA, Putnam JB, Wesley MN, Rosenberg SA. Differing determinants of prognosis following resection of pulmonary metastases from osteogenic and soft tissue sarcoma patients. *Cancer* 1985;55:1361.
26. Long-term results of lung metastasectomy: prognostic analyses based on 5206 cases. The International Registry of Lung Metastases. *J Thorac Cardiovasc Surg* 1997;113:37.
27. Kandioler D, Kromer E, Tuchler H, et al. Long-term results after repeated surgical removal of pulmonary metastases. *Ann Thorac Surg* 1998;65:909.
28. Sauter ER, Hoffman JP, Eisenberg BL. Diagnosis and surgical management of locally recurrent soft-tissue sarcomas of the extremity. *Semin Oncol* 1993;20:451.
29. Kodama K, Doi O, Higashiyama M, Tatsuta M, Iwanaga T. Surgical management of lung metastases. Usefulness of resection with the neodymium:yttrium-aluminum-garnet laser with median sternotomy. *J Thorac Cardiovasc Surg* 1991;101:901.
30. Pastorino U, Valente M, Gasparini M, et al. Median sternotomy and multiple lung resections for metastatic sarcomas. *Eur J Cardiothorac Surg* 1990;4:477.
31. Kelm C, Achatzy R, Ritscher R, et al. Surgery of lung metastases. *Thorac Cardiovasc Surg* 1988;36:118.
32. Vogt-Moykopf I, Meyer G. Surgical technique in operations on pulmonary metastases. *Thorac Cardiovasc Surg* 1986;34(2):125.
33. Johnston MR. Median sternotomy for resection of pulmonary metastases. *J Thorac Cardiovasc Surg* 1983;85:516.
34. Meng RL, Jensik RL, Kittle CF, Faber LP. Median sternotomy for synchronous bilateral pulmonary operations. *J Thorac Cardiovasc Surg* 1980;80:7.
35. Casson AG, Putnam JB, Natarajan G, et al. Efficacy of pulmonary metastasectomy for recurrent soft tissue sarcoma. *J Surg Oncol* 1991;47:1.
36. Pogrebniak HW, Roth JA, Steinberg SM, Rosenberg SA, Pass HI. Reoperative pulmonary resection in patients with metastatic soft tissue sarcoma [see comments]. *Ann Thorac Surg* 1991;52:197.
37. Rizzoni WE, Pass HI, Wesley MN, Rosenberg SA, Roth JA. Resection of recurrent pulmonary metastases in patients with soft-tissue sarcomas. *Arch Surg* 1986;121:1248.
38. Urschel HC Jr, Razzuk MA. Median sternotomy as a standard approach for pulmonary resection. *Ann Thorac Surg* 1986;41:130.
39. Watanabe Y, Ichihashi T, Iwa T. Median sternotomy as an approach for pulmonary surgery. *Thorac Cardiovasc Surg* 1988;36:227.
40. Asaph JW, Keppel JF. Midline sternotomy for the treatment of primary pulmonary neoplasms. *Am J Surg* 1984;147:589.
41. Udelsman R, Roth JA, Lees D, Jelenich SE, Pass HI. Endobronchial metastases from soft tissue sarcoma. *J Surg Oncol* 1986;32:145.

42. Landreneau RJ, Haxelrigg SR, Johnson JA, et al. Neodymium:yttrium-aluminum garnet laser–assisted pulmonary resections. *Ann Thorac Surg* 1991;51:973.
43. Vincent JG, van de Wal HJ, Meijer JM, van Herwaarden C, Lacquet LK. Postponing the limits. Multiple and repeated pulmonary metastasectomy by parenchyma sparing electrocautery excision. *Helv Chir Acta* 1990;57:295.
44. Snyder CL, Saltzman DA, Ferrell KL, Thompson RC, Leonard AS. A new approach to the resection of pulmonary osteosarcoma metastases. Results of aggressive metastasectomy. *Clin Orthop* 1991;Sept:247.
45. LoCicero J III, Frederiksen JW, Hartz RS, Michaelis LL. Laser-assisted parenchyma-sparing pulmonary resection. *J Thorac Cardiovasc Surg* 1989;97:732.
46. Landreneau RJ, Herlan DB, Johnson JA, et al. Thorascopic neodymium:yttrium-aluminum garnet laser–assisted pulmonary resection. *Ann Thorac Surg* 1991;52:1176.
47. Landreneau RJ, Hazelrigg SR, Ferson PF, et al. Thoracoscopic resection of 85 pulmonary lesions. *Ann Thorac Surg* 1992;54:415.
48. McCormack PM, Bains MS, Begg CB, et al. Role of video-assisted thoracic surgery in the treatment of pulmonary metastases: results of a prospective trial. *Ann Thorac Surg* 1996;62:213.
49. Walsh GL, Nesbitt JC. Tumor implants after thoracoscopic resection of a metastatic sarcoma. *Ann Thorac Surg* 1995;59:215.
50. Celik M, Halezeroglu S, Senol C, et al. Video-assisted thoracoscopic surgery: experience with 341 cases. *Eur J Cardiothorac Surg* 1998;14:113.
51. Kaplan EL, Meier P. Nonparametric estimation from incomplete observations. *J Am Stat Assoc* 1958;53:457.
52. Gehan EA. A generalized Wilcoxon test for comparing arbitrarily singly censored samples. *Biometrika* 1965;522:203.
53. Thomas DG. Exact and asymptotic methods for the combination of 2 × 2 tables. *Comput Biomed Res* 1975;8:423.
54. Cox DR. Regression models and life-tables. *J R Stat Soc B* 1972;34:187.
55. Goorin AM, Shuster JJ, Baker A, et al. Changing pattern of pulmonary metastases with adjuvant chemotherapy in patients with osteosarcoma: results from the multiinstitutional osteosarcoma study. *J Clin Oncol* 1991;9:600.
56. Al Jilaihawi AN, Bullimore J, Mott M, Wisheart JD. Combined chemotherapy and surgery for pulmonary metastases from osteogenic sarcoma. Results of 10 years experience. *Eur J Cardiothorac Surg* 1988;2:37.
57. Huth JF, Eilber FR. Patterns of recurrence after resection of osteosarcoma of the extremity. *Arch Surg* 1989;124:122.
58. Korholz D, Verheyen J, Kemperdick HF, Gobel U. Evaluation of follow-up investigations in osteosarcoma patients: suggestions for an effective follow-up program. *Med Pediatr Oncol* 1998;30:52.
59. Pastorino U, Gasparini M, Tavecchio L, et al. The contribution of salvage surgery to the management of childhood osteosarcoma. *J Clin Oncol* 1991;9:1357.
60. Belli L, Scholl S, Livartowski A, et al. Resection of pulmonary metastases in osteosarcoma. A retrospective analysis of 44 patients. *Cancer* 1989;63:2546.
61. Meyer WH, Schell MJ, Kumar AP, et al. Thoracotomy for pulmonary metastatic osteosarcoma. An analysis of prognostic indicators of survival. *Cancer* 1987;59:374.
62. Saeter G, Hoie J, Stenwig AE, et al. Systemic relapse of patients with osteogenic sarcoma. Prognostic factors for long term survival. *Cancer* 1995;75:1084.
63. Antunes M, Bernardo J, Salete M, et al. Excision of pulmonary metastases of osteogenic sarcoma of the limbs. *Eur J Cardiothorac Surg* 1999;15:592.
64. Bacci G, Briccoli A, Mercuri M, et al. Osteosarcoma of the extremities with synchronous lung metastases: long-term results in 44 patients treated with neoadjuvant chemotherapy. *J Chemother* 1998;10:69.
65. Harris MB, Gieser P, Goorin AM, et al. Treatment of metastatic osteosarcoma at diagnosis: a Pediatric Oncology Group study. *J Clin Oncol* 1998;16:3641.
66. Potter DA, Glenn J, Kinsella T, et al. Patterns of recurrence in patients with high-grade soft-tissue sarcomas. *J Clin Oncol* 1985;3:353.
67. Casson AG, Putnam JB, Natarajan G, et al. Five-year survival after pulmonary metastasectomy for adult soft tissue sarcoma. *Cancer* 1992;69:662.
68. Jablons D, Steinberg SM, Roth J, et al. Metastasectomy for soft tissue sarcoma. Further evidence for efficacy and prognostic indicators. *J Thorac Cardiovasc Surg* 1989;97:695.
69. Lanza LA, Putnam JB Jr, Benjamin RS, Roth JA. Response to chemotherapy does not predict survival after resection of sarcomatous pulmonary metastases. *Ann Thorac Surg* 1991;51:219.
70. O'Byrne K, Steward WP. The role of chemotherapy in the treatment of adult soft tissue sarcomas. *Oncology (Huntingt)* 1999;56:13.
71. Di Lorenzo M, Collin PP. Pulmonary metastases in children: results of surgical treatment. *J Pediatr Surg* 1988;23:762.
72. Lembke J, Havers W, Doetsch N, Rohm N, Sadony V. Long-term results following surgical removal of pulmonary metastases in children with malignomas. *Thorac Cardiovasc Surg* 1986;34:137.
73. Paul KP, Toomes H, Vogt Moykopf I. Lung volumes following resection of pulmonary metastases in paediatric patients—a retrospective study. *Eur J Pediatr* 1990;149:862.
74. Lanza LA, Miser JS, Pass HI, Roth JA. The role of resection in the treatment of pulmonary metastases from Ewing's sarcoma. *J Thorac Cardiovasc Surg* 1987;94:181.
75. Winkler K. Surgical treatment of pulmonary metastases in childhood. *Thorac Cardiovasc Surg* 1986;34:133.
76. Ellis PM, Tattersall MH, McCaughan B, Stalley P. Osteosarcoma and pulmonary metastases: 15-year experience from a single institution. *Aust N Z J Surg* 1997;67:625.
77. Beattie EJ, Harvey JC, Marcove R, Martini N. Results of multiple pulmonary resections for metastatic osteogenic sarcoma after two decades. *J Surg Oncol* 1991;46:154.
78. Yamaguchi H, Nojima T, Yagi T, et al. The alteration in the pattern of pulmonary metastasis with adjuvant chemotherapy in osteosarcoma. *Int Orthop* 1988;12:305.
79. Burgers JM, van Glabbeke M, Busson A, et al. Osteosarcoma of the limbs. Report of the EORTC-SIOP 03 trial 20781 investigating the value of adjuvant treatment with chemotherapy and/or prophylactic lung irradiation. *Cancer* 1988;61:1024.
80. Zaharia M, Caceres E, Valdivia S, Moran M, Tejada F. Postoperative whole lung irradiation with or without Adriamycin in osteogenic sarcoma. *Int J Radiat Oncol Biol Phys* 1986;12:907.
81. Dodd LG, Chai C, McAdams HP, Layfield LJ. Fine needle aspiration of osteogenic sarcoma metastatic to the lung. A report of four cases. *Acta Cytologica* 1998;42:754.
82. Huth JF, Elber FR. Patterns of metastatic spread following resection of extremity soft-tissue sarcomas and strategies for treatment. *Semin Surg Oncol* 1988;4:20.
83. Billingsley KG, Lewis JJ, Leung DH, et al. Multifactorial analysis of the survival of patients with distant metastasis arising from primary extremity sarcoma. *Cancer* 1999;85:389.
84. Pearlstone DB, Pisters PW, Bold RJ, et al. Patterns of recurrence in extremity liposarcoma: implications for staging and follow-up. *Cancer* 1999;85:85.
85. Meis-Kindblom JM, Kindblom LG. Angiosarcoma of soft tissue: a study of 80 cases. *Am J Surg Pathol* 1998;22:683.
86. Jaques DP, Coit DG, Casper ES, Brennan MF. Hepatic metastases from soft-tissue sarcoma. *Ann Surg* 1995;221:392.
87. Hafner GH, Rao U, Karakousis CP. Liver metastases from soft tissue sarcomas. *J Surg Oncol* 1995;58:12.
88. Bindal RK, Sawaya RE, Leavens ME, Taylor SH, Guinee VF. Sarcoma metastatic to the brain: results of surgical treatment. *Neurosurgery* 1994;35:185; discussion, 190.
89. Murray KD. Excision of pulmonary metastasis of colorectal cancer. *Semin Surg Oncol* 1991;7:157.
90. Brister SJ, de Varennes B, Gordon PH, Sheiner NM, Pym J. Contemporary operative management of pulmonary metastases of colorectal origin. *Dis Colon Rectum* 1988;31:786.
91. Roberts DG, Lepore V, Cardillo G, et al. Long-term follow-up of operative treatment for pulmonary metastases. *Eur J Cardiothorac Surg* 1989;3:292.
92. Scheele J, Altendorf Hofmann A, Stangl R, Gall FP. Pulmonary resection for metastatic colon and upper rectum cancer. Is it useful? *Dis Colon Rectum* 1990;33:745.
93. Goya T, Miyazawa N, Kondo H, et al. Surgical resection of pulmonary metastases from colorectal cancer: 10-year follow-up. *Cancer* 1989;64:1418.
94. Mansel JK, Zinsmeister AR, Pairolero PC, Jett JR. Pulmonary resection of metastatic colorectal adenocarcinoma. A ten year experience. *Chest* 1986;89:109.
95. Sauter ER, Bolton JS, Willis GW, Farr GH, Sardi A. Improved survival after pulmonary resection of metastatic colorectal carcinoma. *J Surg Oncol* 1990;43:135.
96. Pihl E, Hughes ES, McDermott FT, Johnson WR, Katrivessis H. Lung recurrence after curative surgery for colorectal cancer. *Dis Colon Rectum* 1987;30:417.
97. McAfee MK, Allen MS, Trastek VF, et al. Colorectal lung metastases: results of surgical excision. *Ann Thorac Surg* 1992;53:780.
98. Murata S, Moriya Y, Akasu T, Fujita S, Sugihara K. Resection of both hepatic and pulmonary metastases in patients with colorectal carcinoma. *Cancer* 1998;83:1086.
99. McCormack PM, Burt ME, Bains MS, et al. Lung resection for colorectal metastases. 10-year results. *Arch Surg* 1992;127:1403.
100. Robinson BJ, Rice TW, Strong SA, Rybicki LA, Blackstone EH. Is resection of pulmonary and hepatic metastases warranted in patients with colorectal cancer? *J Thorac Cardiovasc Surg* 1999;117:66.
101. Regnard JF, Grunenwald D, Spaggiari L, et al. Surgical treatment of hepatic and pulmonary metastases from colorectal cancers. *Ann Thorac Surg* 1998;66:214.
102. Patanaphan V, Salazar OM, Risco R. Breast cancer: metastatic patterns and their prognosis. *South Med J* 1988;81:1109.
103. Lanza LA, Natarajan G, Roth JA, Putnam JB Jr. Long-term survival after resection of pulmonary metastases from carcinoma of the breast. *Ann Thorac Surg* 1992;54:244; discussion, 248.
104. Friedel G, Linder A, Toomes H. The significance of prognostic factors for the resection of pulmonary metastases of breast cancer. *Thorac Cardiovasc Surg* 1994;42:71.
105. Simpson R, Kennedy C, Carmalt H, McCaughan B, Gillett D. Pulmonary resection for metastatic breast cancer. *Aust N Z J Surg* 1997;67:717.
106. Lien HH, Lindskold L, Fossa SD, Aass N. Computed tomography and conventional radiography in intrathoracic metastases from non-seminomatous testicular tumor. *Acta Radiol* 1988;29:547.
107. Tesoro-Tess JD, Pizzocaro G, Zanoni F, et al. Reliability of diagnostic imaging after orchiectomy alone in follow-up of clinical stage I testicular carcinoma: excessive cost with potential risk. *Lymphology* 1987;20:161.
108. Williams MP, Husband JE, Heron CW. Intrathoracic manifestations of metastatic testicular seminoma: a comparison of chest radiographic and CT findings. *AJR Am J Roentgenol* 1987;149:473.
109. Kulkarni RP, Reynolds KW, Newlands ES, et al. Cytoreductive surgery in disseminated non-seminomatous germ cell tumours of testis. *Br J Surg* 1991;78:226.
110. Van Schil P, Vaneerdeweg W, Schoofs E, Van Oosterom A, Bourgeois N. Surgical excision of pulmonary metastases from primary testicular cancer—case reports. *Acta Chir Belg* 1989;89:175.
111. Carsky S, Ondrus D, Schnorrer M, Majek M. Germ cell testicular tumours with lung metastases: chemotherapy and surgical treatment. *Int Urol Nephrol* 1992;24:305.
112. Carter GE, Lieskovsky G, Skinner DG, Daniels JR. Reassessment of the role of adjunctive surgical therapy in the treatment of advanced germ cell tumors. *J Urol* 1987;138:1397.
113. Liu D, Abolhoda A, Burt ME, et al. Pulmonary metastasectomy for testicular germ cell tumors: a 28-year experience. *Ann Thorac Surg* 1998;66:1709.
114. Schnorrer M, Ondrus D, Carsky S, et al. Management of germ cell testicular cancer with pulmonary metastases. *Neoplasma* 1996;43:47.
115. Fuller AF Jr, Scannell JG, Wilkins EW Jr. Pulmonary resection for metastases from gynecologic cancers: Massachusetts General Hospital experience, 1943–1982. *Gynecol Oncol* 1985;22:174.
116. Levenback C, Rubin SC, McCormack PM, et al. Resection of pulmonary metastases from uterine sarcomas. *Gynecol Oncol* 1992;45:202.
117. Barter JF, Soong SJ, Hatch KD, Orr JW, Shingleton HM. Diagnosis and treatment of pulmonary metastases from cervical carcinoma. *Gynecol Oncol* 1990;38:347.
118. Imachi M, Tsukamoto N, Matsuyama T, Nakano H. Pulmonary metastasis from carcinoma of the uterine cervix. *Gynecol Oncol* 1989;33:189.

119. Seki M, Nakagawa K, Tsuchiya S, et al. Surgical treatment of pulmonary metastases from uterine cervical cancer. Operation method by lung tumor size. *J Thorac Cardiovasc Surg* 1992;104:876.
120. Dernevik L, Berggren H, Larsson S, Roberts D. Surgical removal of pulmonary metastases from renal cell carcinoma. *Scand J Urol Nephrol* 1985;19:133.
121. Pogrebniak HW, Haas G, Linehan WM, Rosenberg SA, Pass HI. Renal cell carcinoma: resection of solitary and multiple metastases. *Ann Thorac Surg* 1992;54:33.
122. Schott G, Weissmuller J, Vecera E. Methods and prognosis of the extirpation of pulmonary metastases following tumor nephrectomy. *Urol Int* 1988;43:272.
123. Fourquier P, Regnard JF, Rea S, Levi JF, Levasseur P. Lung metastases of renal cell carcinoma: results of surgical resection. *Eur J Cardiothorac Surg* 1997;11:17.
124. Ollila DW, Morton DL. Surgical resection as the treatment of choice for melanoma metastatic to the lung. *Chest Surg Clin North Am* 1998;8:183.
125. Barth A, Wanek LA, Morton DL. Prognostic factors in 1,521 melanoma patients with distant metastases. *J Am Coll Surg* 1995;181:193.
126. Pogrebniak HW, Stovroff M, Roth JA, Pass HI. Resection of pulmonary metastases from malignant melanoma: results of a 16-year experience. *Ann Thorac Surg* 1988;46:20.
127. Gorenstein LA, Putnam JB, Natarajan G, Balch CA, Roth JA. Improved survival after resection of pulmonary metastases from malignant melanoma [see comments]. *Ann Thorac Surg* 1991;52:204.
128. Harpole DH Jr, Johnson CM, Wolfe WG, George SL, Seigler HF. Analysis of 945 cases of pulmonary metastatic melanoma. *J Thorac Cardiovasc Surg* 1992;103:743.
129. Nibu K, Nakagawa K, Kamata S, et al. Surgical treatment for pulmonary metastases of squamous cell carcinoma of the head and neck. *Am J Otolaryngol* 1997;18:391.
130. Finley RK, Verazin GT, Driscoll DL, et al. Results of surgical resection of pulmonary metastases of squamous cell carcinoma of the head and neck. *Am J Surg* 1992;164:594.
131. Mazer TM, Robbins KT, McMurtrey MJ, Byers RM. Resection of pulmonary metastases from squamous carcinoma of the head and neck. *Am J Surg* 1988;156:238.
132. Lefor AT, Bredenberg CE, Kellman RM, Aust JC. Multiple malignancies of the lung and head and neck. Second primary tumor or metastasis? *Arch Surg* 1986;121:265.
133. Macklis RM, Oltikar A, Sallan SE. Wilms' tumor patients with pulmonary metastases. *Int J Radiat Oncol Biol Phys* 1991;21:1187.
134. Wilimas JA, Douglass EC, Magill HL, Fitch S, Hustu HO. Significance of pulmonary computed tomography at diagnosis in Wilms' tumor. *J Clin Oncol* 1988;6:1144.
135. de Kraker J, Lemerle J, Voute PA, et al. Wilm's tumor with pulmonary metastases at diagnosis: the significance of primary chemotherapy. International Society of Pediatric Oncology Nephroblastoma Trial and Study Committee. *J Clin Oncol* 1990;8:1187.
136. Green DM, Breslow NE, Ii Y, et al. The role of surgical excision in the management of relapsed Wilms' tumor patients with pulmonary metastases: a report from the National Wilms' Tumor Study. *J Pediatr Surg* 1991;26:728.
137. Herrera GA, Alexander CB, Jones JM. Ultrastructural characterization of pulmonary neoplasms. II. The role of electron microscopy in characterization of uncommon epithelial pulmonary neoplasms, metastatic neoplasms to and from lung, and other tumors, including mesenchymal neoplasms. *Surv Synth Pathol Res* 1985;4:163.
138. Ghoneim AH, Brisson ML, Fuks A, Mobasher AA, Kreisman H. Monoclonal anti-CEA antibodies in the discrimination between primary pulmonary adenocarcinoma and colon carcinoma metastatic to the lung. *Mod Pathol* 1990;3:613.
139. Slebos RJ, Habets GG, Evers SG, Mooi WJ, Rodenhuis S. Allele-specific detection of K-ras oncogene expression in human non-small-cell lung carcinomas. *Int J Cancer* 1991;48:51.
140. Flint A, Lloyd RV. Pulmonary metastases of colonic carcinoma. Distinction from pulmonary adenocarcinoma. *Arch Pathol Lab Med* 1992;116:39.
141. Nomori H, Hirohashi S, Noguchi M, Matsuno Y, Shimosato Y. Tumor cell heterogeneity and subpopulations with metastatic ability in differentiated adenocarcinoma of the lung. Histologic and cytofluorometric DNA analyses. *Chest* 1991;99:934.
142. Salvati F, Teodori L, Gagliardi L, et al. DNA flow cytometric studies of 66 human lung tumors analyzed before treatment. Prognostic implications. *Chest* 1989;96:1092.
143. Groeger AM, Kandioler D, Mueller MR, et al. Survival after surgical treatment of recurrent pulmonary metastases. *Eur J Cardiothorac Surg* 1997;12:703.
144. Temeck BK, Wexler LH, Steinberg SM, et al. Reoperative pulmonary metastasectomy for sarcomatous pediatric histologies. *Ann Thorac Surg* 1998;66:908.
145. Putnam JB Jr, Suell DM, Natarajan G, Roth JA. Extended resection of pulmonary metastases: is the risk justified? *Ann Thorac Surg* 1993;55:1440.
146. Spaggiari L, Grunenwald DH, Girard P, Solli P, Le Chevalier T. Pneumonectomy for lung metastases: indications, risks, and outcome. *Ann Thorac Surg* 1998;66:1930.
147. Koong HN, Pastorino U, Ginsberg RJ. Is there a role of pneumonectomy in pulmonary metastases? *Ann Thorac Surg* 1999;68:2039.
148. Heslin MJ, Casper ES, Boland P, Gold JP, Burt ME. Preoperative identification and operative management of intraatrial extension of lung tumors. *Ann Thorac Surg* 1998;65:544.
149. Schlappack OK, Baur M, Steger G, Dittrich C, Moser K. The clinical course of lung metastases from breast cancer. *Klin Wochenschr* 1988;66:790.
150. Pastorino U, Valente M, Gasparini M, et al. Lung resection as salvage treatment for metastatic osteosarcoma. *Tumori* 1988;74:201.
151. Jett JR, Hollinger CG, Zinsmeister AR, Pairolero PC. Pulmonary resection of metastatic renal cell carcinoma. *Chest* 1983;84:442.
152. Goorin AM, Delorey MJ, Lack EE, et al. Prognostic significance of complete surgical resection of pulmonary metastases in patients with osteogenic sarcoma: analysis of 32 patients. *J Clin Oncol* 1984;2:425.
153. McCormack PM, Attiyeh FF. Resected pulmonary metastases from colorectal cancer. *Dis Colon Rectum* 1979;22:553.
154. Pastorino U, Valente M, Gasparini M, et al. Lung resection for metastatic sarcomas: total survival from primary treatment. *J Surg Oncol* 1989;40:275.
155. Collins VP, Loeffler RK, Tivey H. Observations on growth rates of human tumors. *AJR Am J Roentgenol* 1956;76:988.
156. Joseph WL, Morton DL, Adkins PC. Prognostic significance of tumor doubling time in evaluating operability in pulmonary metastatic disease. *J Thorac Cardiovasc Surg* 1971;61:23.
157. Joseph WL, Morton DL, Adkins PC. Variation in tumor doubling time in patients with pulmonary metastatic disease. *J Surg Oncol* 1971;3:143.
158. Gompertz B. On the nature of the function expressive of the law of human mortality, and on a new mode of determining the value of life contingencies. *Philos Trans* 1825;513.
159. Laird AK. Dynamics of tumor growth. *Br J Cancer* 1960;18:490.
160. Ladanyi M, Cha C, Lewis R, et al. MDM2 gene amplification in metastatic osteosarcoma. *Cancer Res* 1993;53:16.
161. Pollock R, Lang A, Ge T, et al. Wild-type p53 and a p53 temperature-sensitive mutant suppress human soft tissue sarcoma by enhancing cell cycle control. *Clin Cancer Res* 1998;4:1985.
162. Pollock RE, Lang A, Luo J, el-Naggar AK, Yu D. Soft tissue sarcoma metastasis from clonal expansion of p53 mutated tumor cells. *Oncogene* 1997;12:2035.
163. Mousses S, McAuley L, Bell RS, Kandel R, Andrulis IL. Molecular and immunohistochemical identification of p53 alterations in bone and soft tissue sarcomas. *Mod Pathol* 1996;9:1.
164. Scotlandi K, Serra M, Nicoletti G, et al. Multidrug resistance and malignancy in human osteosarcoma. *Cancer Res* 1996;56:2434.
165. Onda M, Matsuda S, Higaki S, et al. ErbB-2 expression is correlated with poor prognosis for patients with osteosarcoma. *Cancer* 1996;77:71.
166. Asai T, Ueda T, Itoh K, et al. Establishment and characterization of a murine osteosarcoma cell line (LM8) with high metastatic potential to the lung. *Int J Cancer* 1998;76:418.
167. Shirakawa T, Ko SC, Gardner TA, et al. *In vivo* suppression of osteosarcoma pulmonary metastasis with intravenous osteocalcin promoter-based toxic gene therapy. *Cancer Gene Ther* 1998;5:274.
168. Khanna C, Anderson PM, Hasz DE, et al. Interleukin-2 liposome inhalation therapy is safe and effective for dogs with spontaneous pulmonary metastases. *Cancer* 1997;79:1409.
169. Weksler B, Lenert J, Ng B, Burt M. Isolated single lung perfusion with doxorubicin is effective in eradicating soft tissue sarcoma lung metastases in a rat model. *J Thorac Cardiovasc Surg* 1994;107:50.
170. Weksler B, Ng B, Lenert JT, Burt ME. Isolated single-lung perfusion with doxorubicin is pharmacokinetically superior to intravenous injection. *Ann Thorac Surg* 1993;56:209.
171. Weksler B, Schneider A, Ng B, Burt M. Isolated single lung perfusion in the rat: an experimental model. *J Appl Physiol* 1993;74:2736.
172. Pass HI, Mew DJ, Kranda KC, et al. Isolated lung perfusion with tumor necrosis factor for pulmonary metastases. *Ann Thorac Surg* 1996;61:1609.
173. Johnston MR, Minchen RF, Dawson CA. Lung perfusion with chemotherapy in patients with unresectable metastatic sarcoma to the lung or diffuse bronchioloalveolar carcinoma. *J Thorac Cardiovasc Surg* 1995;110:368.
174. Staren ED, Salerno C, Rongione A, Witt TR, Faber LP. Pulmonary resection for metastatic breast cancer. *Arch Surg* 1992;127:1282.
175. Wilking N, Petrelli NJ, Herrera L, Regal AM, Mittelman A. Surgical resection of pulmonary metastases from colorectal adenocarcinoma. *Dis Colon Rectum* 1985;28:562.
176. Pastorino U, Gasparini M, Valente M, et al. Primary childhood osteosarcoma: the role of salvage surgery. *Ann Oncol* 1992;3[Suppl 2]:S43.
177. Schott G, Weissmuller J, Vecera E. Methods and prognosis of the extirpation of pulmonary metastases following tumor nephrectomy. *Urol Int* 1988;43:272.
178. Karp NS, Boyd A, DePan HJ, Harris MN, Roses DF. Thoracotomy for metastatic malignant melanoma of the lung. *Surgery* 1990;107:256.
179. Wong JH, Euhus DM, Morton DL. Surgical resection for metastatic melanoma to the lung. *Arch Surg* 1988;123:1091.
180. Thayer JO Jr, Overholt RH. Metastatic melanoma to the lung: long-term results of surgical excision. *Am J Surg* 1985;149:558.
181. Kumar J, Ilancheran A, Ratnam SS. Pulmonary metastases in gestational trophoblastic disease: a review of 97 cases. *Br J Obstet Gynaecol* 1988;95:70.

SECTION **3**

H. RICHARD ALEXANDER
CARMEN J. ALLEGRA
THEODORE S. LAWRENCE

Metastatic Cancer to the Liver

Metastatic cancer in the liver can represent the sole or life-limiting component of disease for many patients with a variety of tumor histologies, including colorectal cancer, ocular melanoma, neuroendocrine tumors, and, less commonly, other histologies. The liver is a common site of hematogenous metastases for tumors arising in the gastrointestinal tract, presumably because of the unique venous drainage through the portal venous system to the liver. On the other hand, factors that predispose ocular melanoma to metastasize almost exclusively to liver are unknown; liver metastases must occur through hematogenous spread via the arterial system. Once metastases to the liver are diagnosed, the prognosis is generally poor. Even with aggressive therapy, the median survival for patients with ocular melanoma in the liver is between 2 and 7 months[1,2] and 12 to 24 months for patients with colorectal cancer.[3] Because of the unique vascular anatomy of the liver, a number of regional therapies designed to maximize efficacy while minimizing systemic toxicity have been under clinical evaluation. For patients with colorectal cancer the ability to resect disease is associated with 5-year disease-free survival in 20% to 50% of patients,[4–8] and patients with liver metastases from functional neuroendocrine tumor can derive substantial palliative benefit from resection.[9,10] Infusional therapy is administered into the hepatic artery using intermittent percutaneous catheterization with or without particle embolization of the tumor neovasculature or via continuous hepatic artery infusional (HAI) therapy with indwelling implantable pumps. Local ablative therapy is administered via laparotomy or percutaneously placed probes or needles to deliver cryotherapy or radiofrequency ablation of tumors or direct injection of cytotoxic agents such as ethanol. Combined approaches have been used, such as adjuvant HAI after resection or local ablation, in an attempt to prolong disease control in the liver. Newer regional therapies, such as isolated hepatic perfusion (IHP) or intraarterial delivery of gene-modified viral vectors are being evaluated.

Much of the data regarding regional therapy for hepatic metastases relate to colorectal cancer because of its high incidence. It is estimated that 150,000 new cases of colorectal carcinoma occur annually in the United States and approximately 75,000 deaths occur.[11] Synchronous hepatic metastases are identified in 10% to 20% of patients with colorectal cancer[12] and are the sole or life-limiting component of disease in up to 60% of patients.[13] Only a small proportion of patients have resectable disease[14] and therefore the vast majority of patients are best suited for a regional therapy as mentioned previously. This section reviews the natural history of patients with hepatic metastases and the advances in imaging modalities. The results of resection alone or with adjuvant therapy for patients with resectable disease are presented as well as results with other regional therapies such as local ablative techniques, HAI therapies, and newer approaches such as IHP (Table 52.3-1).

NATURAL HISTORY OF LIVER METASTASES

The natural history of hepatic metastases from various histologies has been largely derived from retrospective studies and without the benefit of routine imaging modalities currently available. For patients who are staged using computed tomography (CT), magnetic resonance imaging (MRI), or, for patients with neuroendocrine tumors, somatostatin receptor scintigraphy, survival may appear better than historic controls for whom the number and extent of hepatic metastases were not easily quantified (Fig. 52.3-1). In addition, it has become increasingly apparent that there is considerable variability in the rate of progression of disease in the liver. This is reflected by the fact that in patients with colorectal cancer metastatic to liver, there are occasional long-term survivors, and there is a considerable disparity between median and mean survival (see Fig. 52.3-1). In one series from Roswell Park Cancer Institute of 30 patients with untreated colorectal cancer metastatic to liver, the mean survival was 16 months, with a range of 2 to 58 months.[15] A classification system for staging of hepatic metastases has been proposed based on the number and distribution of lesions in the liver.[16] Heterogeneity in tumor progression has also been demonstrated in patients with neuroendocrine tumors metastatic to liver.[17]

In an older series of 125 patients with colorectal metastases to liver staged primarily with technetium 99 sulfur colloid scans, the overall median survival was 12.5 months.[3] Extent of disease and histologic grade of the tumor were the two most important factors influencing survival. Those with four or more nodules, hepatomegaly, or abnormal liver test results had a median survival of less than 12 months. The immediate cause of death was liver failure in almost 90% of patients despite the coexistence of metastases to other sites in 40% of patients. In another series of 175 patients with hepatic metastases from colorectal cancer, factors potentially influencing survival were subjected to a multifactorial analysis.[18] Although median survival in the group was only 6.1 months, one patient survived for 67 months. Extent of disease as reflected by the number of hepatic nodules, bilobar disease, or abnormal liver test results was independently correlated with survival. Stage of the primary tumor and number of positive lymph nodes also correlated with outcome. In a series from the United Kingdom of 90 patients with colorectal cancer metastatic to liver there was a median survival of 10.3 months.[19]

In a more recent series of 544 patients with unresectable colorectal liver metastases documented by laparotomy, CT, or ultrasound, the factors that independently predicted outcome on multivariate analysis were performance status, extent of liver disease (number of involved segments), abnormal liver test results (prothrombin time and alkaline phosphatase), and site of primary.[14] Those with no adverse factors (i.e., normal performance status and liver test results) had a 1-year survival of 46%. The apparent beneficial effect from chemotherapy in retrospective studies of patients with liver metastases from colorectal cancer and other histologies[3,14,18,20] probably reflects selection bias rather than true treatment effect. In general, patient factors such as gender or age do not influence survival, whereas performance status, which reflects tumor burden, does.[3,14,18,19]

In patients with treated primary ocular melanoma the overall 5-year survival is approximately 70%, but once metastases occur the liver is the sole or life-limiting component of disease in 70% to 80% of patients.[2,21] Age older than 50 years and male gender are

TABLE 52.3-1. Various Regional Treatments under Clinical Evaluation for Cancers Confined to the Liver

Treatment	*Advantages*	*Disadvantages*
Resection	5-y survival: 20–50% for colorectal cancer patients	Disease-free survival is low; limited number of patients suitable
Infusional therapy		
Chemoembolization	Can palliate large symptomatic tumor deposits	May require repeated percutaneous catheterizations
	Effects are prompt	Staged treatments are usually necessary
Hepatic artery infusion	Allows significant dose escalation, has high response rates	Implantable pump is expensive, requires laparotomy
	Fluorodeoxyuridine has high hepatic extraction, minimizing systemic toxicity	
Local ablative therapy (cryotherapy, radiofrequency ablation, local injection)	Can obliterate established hepatic metastases	Requires operative procedure to apply treatment (cryotherapy)
	Minimal injury to normal hepatic tissue	Does not treat microscopic disease
		Limitations on size and number of lesions that can be treated

associated with a shorter survival after recurrence,[2] but the most important factor influencing outcome is the presence of liver metastases[22] (see Fig. 52.3-1). In one study, median survival in patients with recurrence was 19 months, but only 7 months when the liver was involved.[22] Although survival is longer in patients with liver metastases diagnosed by screening (5 vs. 3 months) and in those receiving treatment (5 vs. 2 months), the differences in terms of individual patient benefit are negligible and highlight the grave prognosis associated with liver metastases.[1]

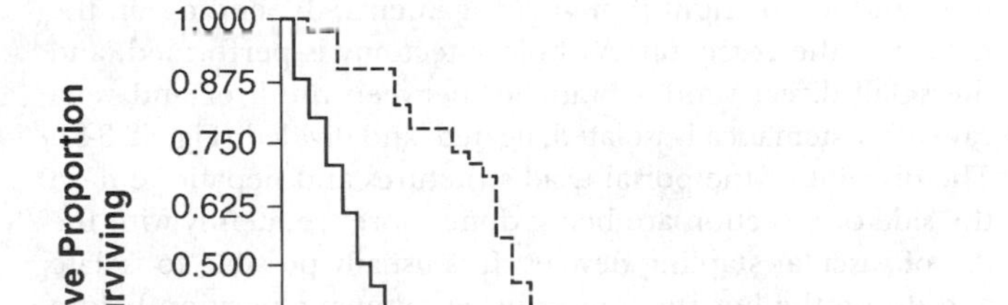

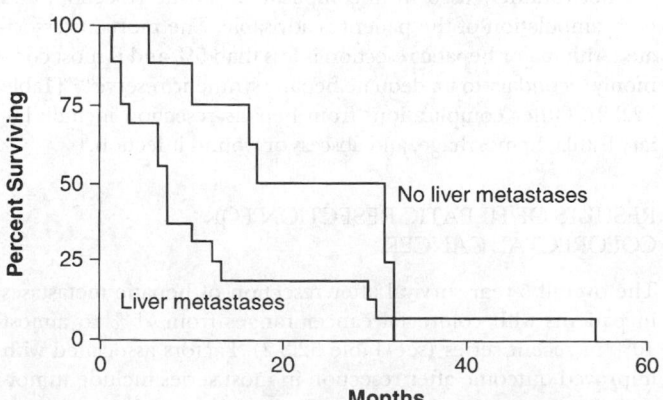

FIGURE 52.3-1. **A:** Survival in patients with untreated colorectal cancer with metastases confined to the liver based on percent hepatic replacement of less than or equal to 20 (*dotted line*) or greater than 20 (*solid line*). **B:** Survival in patients with metastatic ocular melanoma with or without hepatic metastases. (Modified from refs. 19 and 22.)

Ayoub and coworkers reported outcome in more than 1500 patients with metastases from unknown primary tumors.[20] Five hundred patients had metastases to liver, of whom 27% (135 patients) eventually had primary tumors diagnosed arising from lung, colon or rectum, or pancreas. The presence of liver metastases was associated with a significantly shorter survival, but was most favorable in those with neuroendocrine histology. Sutliff and coworkers have shown that the pattern of progression in patients with metastatic gastrinoma to liver is highly variable.[17] Over a follow-up interval of 29 months, 5 of 19 (26%) demonstrated no growth of tumor, whereas 42% had rapid growth in less than 1 year. Tumor progression, most commonly in liver, is the main determinant of survival in patients with gastrinoma.[23,24] For patients with other functional neuroendocrine tumors, liver metastases and the development of the uncontrolled sequelae from excess hormone production are the main causes of death.[25]

IMAGING OF HEPATIC METASTASES

Currently there are several imaging options available for assessment of liver metastases. Considerable advancement in imaging technology has made it possible to accurately detect the number, size, and distribution of hepatic lesions and frequently distinguish between malignant or benign lesions. The most commonly used tests include CT scan, MRI, ultrasound, and, more recently, positron emission tomography using the glucose analogue, [^{18}F]fluorodeoxyglucose. Ultrasound is commonly used for screening because of its availability and relative inexpensiveness, but has its most important application as an intraoperative modality to assess suitably for resection and to gauge the adequacy of treatment when using cryotherapy. In general, intraoperative ultrasound identifies 20% more occult lesions in the liver compared with CT scan[26] and therefore should be used before any contemplated resection.

CT scan is used most commonly to assess a patient with possible hepatic metastases. It has the advantages of being widely available and, by using new generation rapid acquisition scanners, the entire chest, abdomen, and pelvis can be evaluated in a single study.[5] Moreover, the use of rapid helical or spiral CT allows for a scan of the entire abdomen in a single breath hold, eliminating the problem of respiratory misregistration. Because liver tumors have a variable degree of vascularity and derive their perfusion from the arterial tree, CT arterioportography has been used to enhance the sensitivity of the test, particularly for hypovascular lesions, but involves placement of a catheter and injection of contrast into the superior mesenteric artery with capture of images during both the arterial and portal venous phase of hepatic perfusion.[27] Dual arterial and venous phase CT scans after intravenous injection of contrast agent using high-speed helical CT scanners are now commonly used in place of CT arterioportography,[28] but may have limited additional sensitivity for detection of hypovascular tumors compared with portal phase CT alone.[29] On the other hand, because hypervascular lesions are frequently isoattenuating in relation to normal liver parenchyma, arterial phase helical CT detects more liver metastases than conventional portal venous phase CT in this setting.[30]

MRI scanning is also used routinely and has particular advantages for imaging of focal liver lesions. Two contrast agents with liver specificity are currently being used; one is manganese pyridoxal disphosphate, a paramagnetic agent taken up by hepatocytes, and the other is superparamagnetic iron oxide particles, which are taken up by the reticuloendothelial system.[31–33] The optimal MRI protocols for evaluation of liver lesions vary depending on the available equipment and contrast agents being used. Although there are disadvantages with MRI because of motion artifact from the heart or aorta, it can distinguish benign cysts or hemangiomas from malignant lesions based on characteristic findings on T1 versus T2 spin-weighted sequences.[31]

Positron emission tomography scanning uses the glucose analogue [^{18}F]fluorodeoxyglucose, which is selectively retained in malignant tissue because of increased glucose metabolism compared with nonneoplastic tissue. It has been shown to have sensitivity comparable with CT scan and can often distinguish benign and malignant lesions, but has potential for false-positive findings in abscesses and false-negative findings in hepatocellular carcinoma.[34] Somatostatin receptor scintigraphy has been used with increasing regularity and is extremely accurate in imaging neuroendocrine tumors,[35–37] with the exception of insulinoma, and may be superior to MRI in detecting islet cell tumors in liver.[35] In addition, because hemangiomas are not visible on somatostatin receptor scintigraphy, the study can be used to distinguish benign versus malignant lesions when there are equivocal findings on CT or MRI.[38]

RESECTION OF HEPATIC METASTASES

RESECTION OF METASTATIC DISEASE: TECHNICAL CONSIDERATIONS

The benefit of resection in selected patients with hepatic metastases from colorectal cancer and potentially other histologies, such as neuroendocrine tumors, has been fairly well established in the literature. Several advances in hepatic surgery have made hepatic resection a more routine procedure with minimal patient morbidity. Initial evaluation of the abdominal cavity at exploration should be carefully done to exclude the presence of extrahepatic disease. Intraoperative ultrasound should be routinely used to screen for the presence of deep-seated or occult metastases, and resection should be based when possible on functional anatomic considerations, including segmental resection, to preserve unaffected hepatic parenchyma and minimize blood loss during resection (Fig. 52.3-2). The liver is mobilized, including division of the falciform and left or right triangular ligaments, depending on the nature of the resection. A cholecystectomy is performed, and the small direct venous branches between the liver and vena cava are systematically isolated, ligated, and divided (Fig. 52.3-3). The division of the portal triad structures and hepatic vein on the side of resection are being done more frequently with the use of vascular stapling devices. It is usually possible to isolate and divide the hepatic vein in its extrahepatic position before commencing parenchymal dissection. Vascular inflow occlusion via the Pringle's maneuver and maintenance of a low central venous pressure minimizes blood loss during dissection of the hepatic parenchyma.[39,40] Extensive resection involving contiguous vena caval resection or reimplantation of the hepatic veins are rarely indicated but have been reported.[41,42] Argon beam coagulation helps with hemostasis after resection. Drains are not routinely used in uncomplicated hepatic resection, and early ambulation of the patient is advisable. The mortality associated with major hepatic resection is less than 5% and is most commonly secondary to inadequate hepatic synthetic reserve[5–8] (Table 52.3-2). Other complications from hepatic resection include biliary fistula, hemorrhage, and abscess or wound infection.[6]

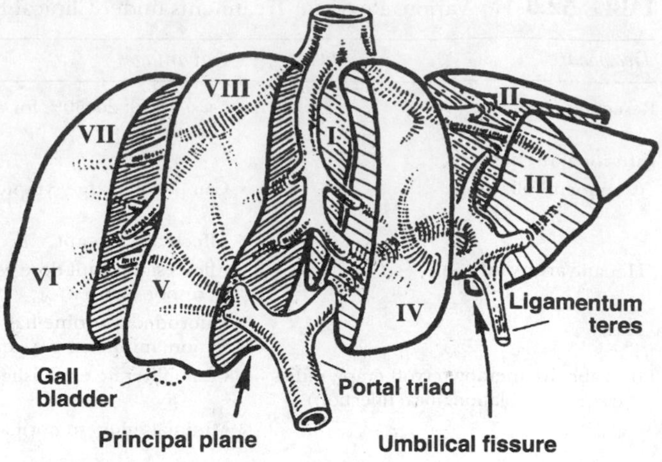

FIGURE 52.3-2. Segments of the liver used in planning hepatic resection. The principal plane divides the right and left lobes of the liver. Extent of hepatic resection planned on the basis of an understanding of the segmental anatomy of the liver has resulted in minimal morbidity and mortality associated with the procedure. (Modified from ref. 6.)

RESULTS OF HEPATIC RESECTION FOR COLORECTAL CANCER

The overall 5-year survival after resection of hepatic metastases in patients with colorectal cancer ranges from 25% to almost 40% in recent series (see Table 52.3-2). Factors associated with improved outcome after resection in most series include tumor- and treatment-related variables. Patient characteristics, such as age or gender, have not been identified as significant prognostic variables, but elevation in preoperative serum carcinoembryonic antigen levels is associated with poorer outcome in most series.[43–45] Tumor-related factors associated with poor outcome

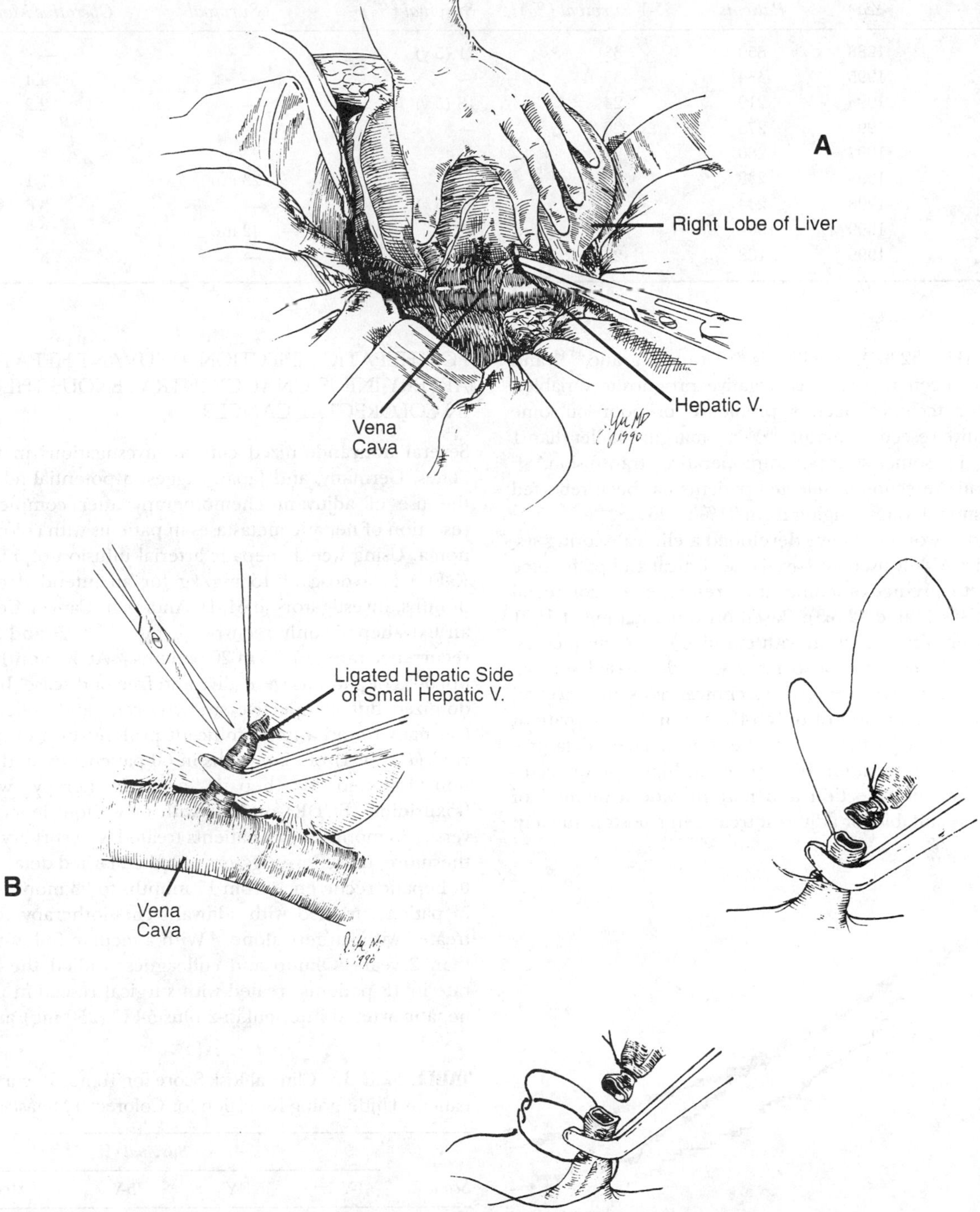

FIGURE 52.3-3. **A:** Technique of isolation and **B:** division of the direct venous tributaries between the inferior vena cava and the liver that are routinely divided before a right or left hepatic lobectomy. V, vein. (From ref. 4, with permission.)

after resection include positive lymph node status of the primary tumor, a disease-free interval between resection of the primary tumor and liver metastases less than 1 year, and the presence of extrahepatic disease, including regional periportal lymph nodes. With respect to the liver metastases, factors that generally reflect advanced tumor burden, such as increasing number of lesions,[43,46,47] size of largest lesion larger than 5 or 10 cm,[47,48] bilobar distribution of disease,[49,50] percent hepatic replacement,[51] or weight of resected specimen,[43] have been shown to predict shorter survival compared with those without these

TABLE 52.3-2. Results of Resection of Colorectal Liver Metastases from Selected Series

Author	*Year*	*No. of Patients*	*5-Y Survival (%)*	*Disease-Free Survival (%)*	*Median Survival*	*Operative Mortality*
Hughes[55]	1988	859	33	21 (5 y)	—	—
Scheele[48]	1995	434	33	—	—	4.4
Doci[51]	1995	219	24	18 (5 y)	—	2.2
Nadig[49]	1997	275	26	—	—	4
Jamison[52]	1997	280	27	—	2.7 y	4
Bekalakos[50]	1998	238	29	—	23 mo	1.1
Cady[43]	1998	244	—	30 (5 y)	—	3.6
Fong[45]	1999	1001	37	—	42 mo	2.8
Ambiru[54]	1999	168	26	11 mo (median)	—	3.5

parameters (Fig. 52.3-4). Satellitosis,[48,52] tumor grade,[43,44] and ploidy[53] have been reported as negative prognostic variables. Treatment or technical factors predictive of poor outcome include positive resection margin,[46,48,50,54] margin smaller than 1 cm,[55] and, in some studies, intraoperative transfusion.[44,52] Repeat hepatic resection in selected patients has been reported with 5-year survival rates ranging from 21% to 26%.[56–60]

Fong and coworkers[45] have developed a clinical scoring system using five widely used and available clinical and pathologic parameters to predict outcome after resection of colorectal liver metastases (Table 52.3-3). Based on the outcome of 1001 patients undergoing resection with curative intent, an increasing clinical risk score was associated with decreased survival (Fig. 52.3-5). Of note, patients with a clinical risk score of 5 had an actuarial 5-year survival of only 14% and in fact no patient had survived 5 years at the time of the report. These data provide a basis for stratification of patients at high risk of recurrence after hepatic resection and may provide a method of selecting those suitable for adjuvant treatments postoperatively.

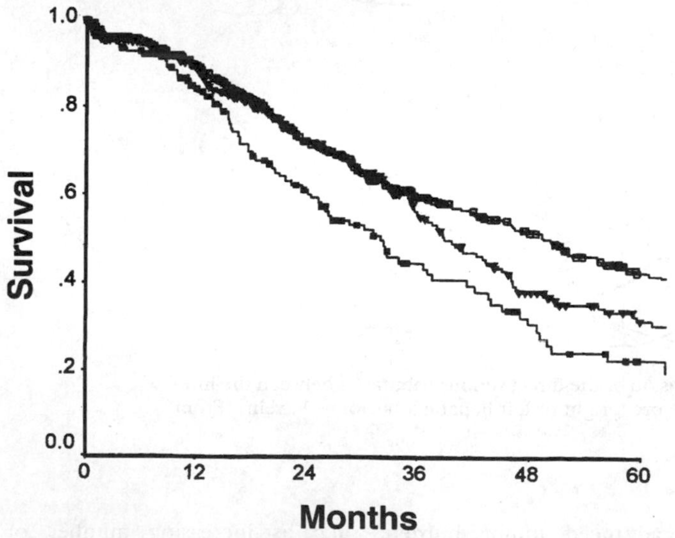

FIGURE 52.3-4. Five-year overall survival in patients undergoing resection of hepatic metastases from colorectal cancer based on number of lesions. Survival is better in patients with one lesion (*open square*) compared with those with two or three (*filled triangles*) or four or more lesions (*filled boxes*). (From ref. 45, with permission.)

POSTHEPATIC RESECTION ADJUVANT HEPATIC ARTERY INFUSIONAL OR INTRAVENOUS THERAPY IN COLORECTAL CANCER

Several nonrandomized clinical investigations in the United States, Germany, and Japan suggest a potential advantage for the use of adjuvant chemotherapy after complete surgical resection of hepatic metastases in patients with colorectal carcinoma. Using weekly hepatic arterial infusion of 5-fluorouracil (5-FU) at a dose of 15 mg/kg for an intended course of 6 months, investigators at M. D. Anderson Cancer Center noted an extrahepatic-only recurrence rate of 33% and a liver-only recurrence rate of 17% in 20 patients.[61] At 39 months of follow-up, 50% of patients were alive and free of disease. In a nonrandomized but prospective study, Lorenz and colleagues from Germany found a nonsignificant prolongation in median survival ($P = .064$) of 52 months in 60 patients treated with resection followed by hepatic arterial therapy with either floxuridine (FUDR) or 5-FU with or without leucovorin (LV) versus 33 months in 21 patients treated with surgery alone. Furthermore, these investigators noted a marked delay in the time to hepatic recurrence from 17 months to 63 months ($P = .015$) in patients treated with adjuvant chemotherapy versus those treated with surgery alone.[62] With a median follow-up of more than 2 years, Okuno and colleagues studied the recurrence rate in 18 patients treated with surgical resection followed by hepatic arterial interleukin-2 plus 5-FU (250 mg) and mitomy-

TABLE 52.3-3. Clinical Risk Score for Tumor Recurrence in Patients Undergoing Resection for Colorectal Metastases to Liver[a]

	Survival (%)			
Score	1-Y	3-Y	5-Y	Median (mo)
0	93	72	60	74
1	91	66	44	51
2	89	60	40	47
3	86	42	20	33
4	70	38	25	20
5	71	27	14	22

[a]Each risk factor is one point: node-positive primary, disease-free interval less than 12 months, greater than one tumor, size greater than 5 cm, carcinoembryonic antigen greater than 200 ng/mL. (Modified from ref. 45.)

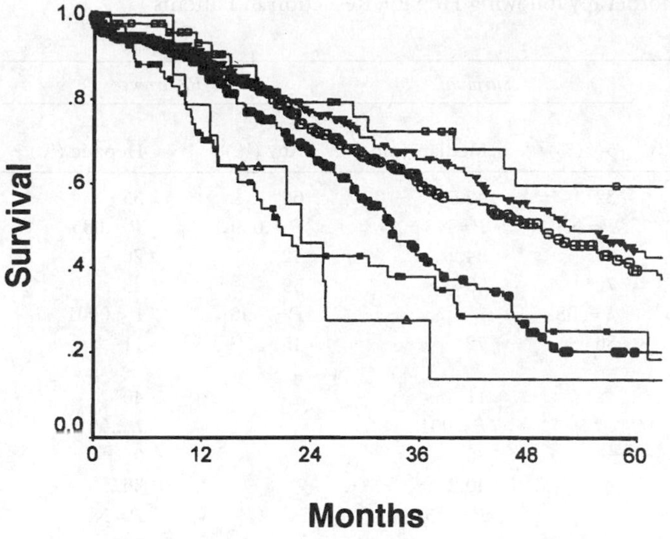

FIGURE 52.3-5. Five-year overall survival in 1001 patients with metastatic colorectal cancer to the liver undergoing resection with curative intent. Outcome was analyzed based on the absence or presence of various prognostic factors as outlined in Table 52.3-3. Patients with 0 or 1 prognostic factor had improved survival compared with those with increasing numbers of adverse prognostic variables (P <.0001). *Open box* score = 0; *filled triangle* score = 1; *open circle* score = 2; *filled circle* score = 3; *filled box* score= 4; and *open triangle* score = 5. (From ref. 45, with permission.)

cin C (4 mg) given weekly for 6 months and found an overall recurrence rate of 22% with no recurrences in the liver (17% lung; 6% pelvis).[63] More recently, investigators in Japan performed a retrospective investigation of 174 patients who had been treated with hepatic resection for metastases resulting from colorectal carcinoma and identified three separate groups, including those treated with surgery alone (66 patients), surgery plus hepatic artery infusion (78 patients), and surgery plus peripheral venous infusion (30 patients).[64] The hepatic arterial therapy consisted of 5-FU, 50 $mg/m^2/d \times$ 14 days, plus bolus injections of an anthracycline analogue, aclarubicin (40 mg), suspended in a lipid contrast medium given every 3 to 6 months for up to 3 years. These investigators noted that the patients treated with surgery followed by hepatic artery infusion had a significantly decreased hepatic recurrence rate and a more prolonged disease-free and overall survival compared with either of the other groups and had a 5-year survival rate of 35% compared with 13% for those treated with surgery plus peripheral venous infusion therapy and 9% for those treated with surgery alone. Investigators from Tokyo retrospectively analyzed 115 patients with hepatic-only metastatic colorectal carcinoma treated with potentially curative therapy with resection alone (40 patients) versus surgery followed by either hepatic arterial (28 patients) or intraportal vein (ten patients) 5-FU/LV, with or without mitomycin C, versus surgery followed by either oral or systemic intravenous mitomycin C, or 5-FU, or oral tegafur with or without uracil (37 patients).[65] These investigators found an overall 5-year survival for all patients of 42.2%. Estimates of median survivals from the published graphs show survivals of 35, 43, and 60 months for those patients treated with surgery alone versus surgery plus HAI versus surgery plus systemic therapy, respectively. Although these differences did not reach statistical significance, the disease-free survival appeared to be statistically worse in patients treated with surgery alone compared with those who received systemic adjuvant therapy. Nonami and colleagues from Japan, in a nonrandomized trial, treated patients with metastatic colorectal carcinoma using surgery alone (26 patients) or surgery followed by hepatic arterial 5-FU (250 mg/kg/d × 14 days) plus an anthracycline (20 to 40 mg/kg days 1 and 8), plus mitomycin C (4 to 8 mg/kg days 1 and 8) (31 patients) every 3 months for 1 year.[66] These investigators noted an approximately 12% 5-year survival rate for patients treated with surgery alone versus 57% for those treated with surgery followed by hepatic artery chemotherapy.

Based on relatively promising results from nonrandomized studies, several groups have conducted prospective randomized studies with the goal of defining the role of adjuvant chemotherapy in patients with metastatic colorectal carcinoma treated with complete surgical resection of hepatic metastases. As shown in Table 52.3-4, an intergroup trial randomized 109 patients with isolated hepatic metastases from colorectal carcinoma to treatment with either surgery alone (56 patients) or surgery followed by continuous hepatic artery infusion of FUDR for four cycles plus systemically administered 5-FU for 12 cycles (53 patients).[67] Although none of the survival differences reached a statistically significant level, those patients treated with surgery followed by chemotherapy enjoyed a 63% 5-year survival versus 32% for those treated with surgery alone. The median survival for those treated with surgery plus chemotherapy of 34.2 months was less, albeit not significantly less, than those treated with surgery (47.5 months). A significant decrease in overall recurrence rate was noted for the group treated with surgery plus chemotherapy (42% vs. 66%) as well as a decrease in hepatic-only recurrences (26% vs. 55%) compared with those treated with resection alone. Investigators from Memorial Sloan-Kettering Cancer Center randomized 74 patients with hepatic-only disease to surgery followed by hepatic arterial FUDR and dexamethasone plus systemic therapy with 5-FU plus LV for 6 months and 82 patients to surgery followed by systemic therapy with 5-FU/LV alone for 6 months.[68] These investigators found a statistically significant improvement in 2-year survival rate of 86% for those treated with both HAI and systemic chemotherapy versus those treated with surgery followed by systemic chemotherapy alone (72%) ($P = .023$) (see Table 52.3-4). Furthermore, although the overall recurrence rates were not different between the two groups, there was a marked decrease in hepatic recurrence in the group treated with the addition of HAI chemotherapy (10% vs. 40%, $P = .000012$). Toxicities were similar for the two groups of patients, with the exception of a greater incidence of grade 3 to 4 diarrhea and an 18% incidence of hyperbilirubinemia (greater than 3) in those patients treated with the addition of the hepatic artery therapy. In all but one patient, the bilirubin returned to normal.

Lygidakis and colleagues from Greece found an almost threefold increase in median survival from 11 to 30 months and a decrease in hepatic recurrence rates from 40% to 0% in patients treated with surgery followed by chemoimmunotherapy.[69] Chemoimmunotherapy consisted of splenic and gastroduodenal artery infusion of interferon-γ and interleukin-2 emulsified in radiographic contrast medium. In addition, patients received bolus transarterial infusion of mitomycin C, carboplatin, 5-FU, LV, and an anthracycline analogue every 3 to 6 months for 3 years. In contrast to these studies, Lorenz and colleagues from Germany prospectively randomized a total of 226 patients to treatment with

TABLE 52.3-4. Prospective Randomized Trials of Adjuvant Chemotherapy following Hepatic Resection in Patients with Metastatic Colorectal Cancer

			Survival		*Recurrence*	
Group	*Regimen*	*No. of Patients*	5-Y (%)	Median (mo)	Any (%)	Hepatic (%)
Intergroup[67]	Surgery	56	32	47.5	66	55
	vs.		P = NS	P = NS	P = .039	P = .035
	Surgery → FUDR HAI × 4 + 5-FU IV × 12	53	63	34.2	42	26
Memorial Sloan-Kettering Cancer Center[68]	Surgery → 5-FU/LV IV × 6 mo	82	72[a]	59	59	43
	vs.		P = .03		P = .096	P<.0001
	Surgery→ 5-FU/LV + FUDR/DEX HAI × 6 mo	74	86	72	45	11
Greece[69]	Surgery	20		11		40
	vs.			P<.001		P<.001
	Surgery → Immunochemotherapy HAI	20		30		0
Germany[70]	Surgery	113		40.8		36.7
	vs.			P = .15		P = NS
	Surgery → 5-FU/LV HAI	113		34.5		33.3

DEX, dexamethasone; 5-FU, 5-fluorouracil; FUDR, floxuridine; HAI, hepatic artery infusion; LV, leucovorin.
[a]Two-year survival.

surgery alone (113 patients) versus surgery followed by hepatic arterial 5-FU (1000 mg/m²/d) plus LV (200 mg/m²/d) given for 5 days each month for 6 months (see Table 52.3-4). The investigators found no difference in overall median survival or time to disease progression and concluded that it was highly unlikely that the addition of chemotherapy to surgical resection would improve survival by more than 15%.[70] However, the power of this study to detect differences was markedly reduced by a substantial decrease in the number of patients completing the chemotherapy (only 34 of 113 randomized to the adjuvant arm). These studies generally support the use of adjuvant chemotherapy after surgical resection of hepatic metastases in high-risk patients with colorectal carcinoma.

NEOADJUVANT THERAPY FOR INITIALLY UNRESECTABLE COLORECTAL HEPATIC METASTASES

Chemotherapy has also been used in a neoadjuvant setting for those patients initially deemed inoperable with the goal of enabling resection. Bismuth and coworkers treated 53 patients with initially unresectable disease with systemic chemotherapy, which included 5-FU/LV and oxaliplatin, for an average of 8 months before resection and for at least 6 months after surgery. Major hepatectomy was performed in 37 patients and minor resections in the balance of patients. Although surgical complications occurred in 14 patients, there was no operative mortality. Although hepatic recurrence was observed in 66% of patients, the overall 5-year survival was found to be 40%, suggesting a potential role for neoadjuvant chemotherapy in patients initially considered unresectable.[71]

RESULTS OF RESECTION FOR NONCOLORECTAL CANCERS

Series of hepatic resection for tumor histologies other than colorectal cancer have been reported, but the benefit of this approach has not been conclusively demonstrated. Table 52.3-5 summarizes

TABLE 52.3-5. Results of Resection of Noncolorectal Cancers from Selected Series

Author	*Histology*	*No. of Patients*	*Actuarial 5-Y Survival (%)*	*Median Survival (mo)*
Chen et al.[77]	Neuroendocrine	15	73	NR
Que et al.[10]	Neuroendocrine	74	73[a]	NR
Harrison et al.[84]	Genitourinary[b]	34	60	NR
Jaques et al.[81]	Sarcoma	14	0	30
Harrison et al.[84]	Breast/melanoma sarcoma	41	26	32
Elias et al.[80]	Breast	21	9	26
Raab et al.[79]	Breast	34	18	27

NR, not reached.
[a]Four-year actuarial survival.
[b]Includes renal (five), testicular (nine), adrenal (seven), ovary (seven), uterine (four), and cervix (two).
(Modified from ref. 225.)

outcomes of selected series of patients with different histologies. There are anecdotal reports of long-term survivors after hepatic resection for noncolorectal gastrointestinal primary tumors such as gastric or pancreatic cancer[72,73]; however, this is not considered standard treatment as most patients with advanced upper intestinal adenocarcinomas have recurrences at multiple sites in addition to liver such as lymph nodes and peritoneum. Five-year survival in patients undergoing resection of neuroendocrine hepatic metastases ranges from 10% to 54%.[10,74–78] Chen and coworkers reported that outcome was significantly improved in patients undergoing resection compared with a retrospectively matched cohort who did not undergo resection.[77] Actuarial 5-year survival after resection of clinically isolated hepatic metastases in breast cancer patients is reported between 9% and 18%.[79,80] Based on the typical systemic pattern of recurrence in patients with advanced breast cancer, this approach must be considered palliative in nature with little expectation of long-term disease control. Other histologies for which hepatic resection has been reported include metastatic soft tissue sarcoma[81] and cutaneous[82] or ocular[83] melanoma. Actuarial 5-year survival of 60% has been reported for patients undergoing resection for tumors arising from the genitourinary tract, including testicular, adrenal, ovarian, renal, uterine, and cervix.[84,85] Presumably, patients with noncolorectal cancers and hepatic metastases were selected for operation based on factors thought to be favorable such as a long interval of radiographically isolated and resectable liver metastases and good operative risk.

INFUSIONAL THERAPY FOR HEPATIC METASTASES

HEPATIC ARTERY INFUSIONAL THERAPY: TECHNICAL CONSIDERATIONS

HAI therapy has had substantial clinical application based on the development of an implantable pump (or port) that can deliver a continuous infusion of therapeutic agents via the hepatic artery and the availability of agents that have an established pharmacokinetic advantage for HAI delivery because of a high first-pass extraction in liver and a concentration-dependent therapeutic effect. The implantable pump is a low-profile dual-chamber device that is placed in a subcutaneous pocket over the lower abdominal wall connected to a catheter that is positioned in the gastroduodenal artery for infusion of agents into the liver via the hepatic artery.[86] The pump is activated by filling the inner chamber with saline or therapeutic agent and as the inner reservoir expands it compresses a hydrofluorocarbon gas contained in the outer chamber from a gas to a liquid (see Chapter 29.2). The body temperature then expands the gas, thereby compressing the inner chamber's contents through a resistor to maintain constant flow into the arterial catheter.

The two most important technical considerations in placing the device are to ensure that the entire liver is perfused with the therapeutic agent and that no extrahepatic visceral perfusion occurs. Typically patients undergo preoperative angiography to define the arterial anatomy of the liver. All accessory or aberrant arterial vessels should be ligated. In addition, careful dissection of the gastroduodenal artery and hepatic artery should be performed to ensure that no collateral flow to the viscera occurs. Distribution of the infusate is assessed with fluorescein intraoperatively and postoperatively using technetium 99–labeled albumin scintigraphy before commencing therapy. Interestingly, a positive arterial nuclide scan using technetium 99–labeled macroaggregated albumin has been shown to predict tumor response to subsequent intraarterial therapy.[87]

As an alternative, an arterial catheter connected to a subcutaneously placed port can be used that is accessed with a noncoring Huber's needle and the infusate delivered by an external programmable infusion pump.[88] This device has been used because of the considerably higher cost of the implanted pump although maintenance costs are higher with the port. Fordy and coworkers evaluated the frequency of treatment interruptions and complication rates associated with the use of either device in 95 patients undergoing a total of 959 treatment cycles.[88] The port was associated with a significantly higher incidence of catheter blockages requiring nurse intervention, and in ten cases the needle dislodged during infusion. Because of the higher complication rate with ports, there were treatment interruptions in 5.7% of treatments compared with only 1.7% for pumps. Curley and coworkers reviewed the technical aspects of arterial port or pump placement in 180 patients[89] and found aberrant hepatic arterial anatomy in 37% of patients. Ligation of the variant vessel is normally all that is required except in rare circumstances in which temporary occlusion of the variant vessel results in severe ischemia of one hepatic lobe. In this case, a two-cannulae system may be necessary. Although the early complication rate (within 30 days of the procedure) is 5% for both ports and pumps, the late complication rate is twofold greater for ports (49%) versus pumps (28%). Operative mortality from placement of any device is less than 1%.[90]

Treatment responses have been reported to be the same after HAI therapy in colorectal cancer patients with aberrant arterial anatomy compared with those with normal anatomy by some[89] but not by others.[91] Burke and coworkers found that aberrant arterial anatomy occurred in 18% of patients and was associated with reduced effectiveness after 4 months of therapy.[91] Complete perfusion of the liver is essential for adequate delivery of drug to tumor[92] and if incomplete or misperfusion is demonstrated after catheter placement, it can usually be corrected by selective angiography and coil embolization of the necessary artery.[93] It also appears that surgeon experience is an important factor in minimizing complications during device placement.[94] Because of the desire to minimize complications and treatment interruptions in patients with a potentially limited life expectancy, the implanted pump is most commonly used.

It has long been known that established tumor metastases derive their blood supply from the arterial anatomy.[95] FUDR is a 5-FU derivative[96] that has a high first-pass extraction in liver, 94% to 99% compared with 20% to 55% for 5-FU.[97,98] After injection of FUDR into the hepatic artery or portal vein, the mean concentration of FUDR in liver is similar, but tumor concentrations of FUDR are significantly higher after intraarterial injection.[99] Furthermore, FUDR is rapidly cleared from the systemic circulation and has a short (less than 10-minute) serum half-life. Other drugs with a short serum half-life and for which there is a pharmacokinetic advantage for intraarterial therapy include cisplatin, doxorubicin, mitomycin C, and bischlorethylnitroureas.[4]

HEPATIC ARTERY INFUSIONAL THERAPY FOR COLORECTAL CANCER

A number of phase II studies have evaluated continuous HAI of FUDR administered over a 14-day interval repeated every 28

TABLE 52.3-6. Hepatic Arterial Infusion Therapy Toxicity

Reference	Regimen	No. of Patients	Chemical Hepatitis (%)	Biliary Sclerosis (%)	Ulcer (%)	Gastritis (%)
Kemeny[106]	0.3 mg/kg/d FUDR	48	42	19	17	8
Chang[107]	0.2–0.3 mg/kg/d FUDR	24	79	21	17	21
Kemeny[104]	0.3 mg/kg/d FUDR, leucovorin, 15 mg/m²/d, and 20 mg dexamethasone	62	49	3	—	8
Stagg[102]	0.1 mg/kg/d FUDR × 7 days, 15 mg/kg bolus 5-fluorouracil days 15, 22, 29 with 5-week cycle	64	14	0	—	—

FUDR, floxuridine.

days in patients with colorectal cancer metastatic to liver, many of whom had failed prior systemic therapy with 5-FU.[90,100] These studies documented that HAI with FUDR or 5-FU consistently resulted in overall response rates substantially greater than that seen with systemic therapy. In ten reported trials, the mean response rate was 42% (range, 15% to 83%) and median survival ranged from 12 to 26 months.[101] However, the initial results with FUDR administered via HAI were associated with an unacceptable incidence of biliary toxicity manifested by ischemic cholangiopathy and increased serum bilirubin (Table 52.3-6). Several modifications have been made to the initial regimens to optimize efficacy and minimize toxicity, including alternating FUDR and 5-FU,[102] reducing the dose of FUDR, and adding LV[103] and dexamethasone.[104]

Kemeny and coworkers reported that 0.3 mg/kg/d of FUDR, 15 $mg/m^2/d$ of LV, and 20 mg of dexamethasone administered as a 14-day infusion to 33 previously untreated patients with metastatic colorectal cancer to liver resulted in an overall response rate of 78% and a median duration of survival of almost 25 months.[104] In 29 previously treated patients, the regimen resulted in an overall response rate of 52% and a median survival of 13.5 months. The addition of dexamethasone was associated with a significantly lower incidence of biliary sclerosis compared with the same regimen without dexamethasone (3% vs. 21%, respectively) without adversely affecting response rates (75% vs. 69%, respectively).

A number of prospective random assignment trials were reported in the 1980s and 1990s comparing FUDR administered via HAI to either systemic therapy or best supportive care (Table 52.3-7). In general, all studies demonstrated a significantly superior response rate for HAI compared with systemic therapy, but this did not consistently translate into a survival advantage due to several possible explanations. Three of the five studies conducted in the United States, including the two largest, allowed patient crossover, thereby obscuring any potential survival advantage for HAI therapy. The dose of FUDR used in these trials, 0.3 mg/kg/d, was associated with significant toxicity, resulting in treatment interruptions for many patients. In addition, technical difficulties with pump placement or function prevented some patients from receiving HAI therapy. For example, in the Northern California Oncology Group trial, 9 of 67 patients randomized to HAI therapy did not receive therapy because of technical difficulties with pump placement or function, and of 50 evaluable patients receiving HAI therapy, one-half of the patients terminated therapy because of toxicity rather than disease progression.[105] Twenty-eight of 65 patients receiving intravenous therapy crossed over to HAI therapy, and although median survival was longer in those treated with HAI versus intravenous only, these differences may be due largely to a favorable selection bias in those able to undergo crossover treatment. Another prospective random assignment trial from the Memorial Sloan-Kettering Cancer Center evaluated response and survival for patients with laparotomy-confirmed unresectable disease confined to liver treated with HAI or intravenous therapy.[106] Although there was a significantly higher response rate with HAI therapy compared with intravenous therapy (50% vs. 20%, respectively), no overall survival differences were observed. Of note, in both studies in which crossover was allowed, the responses to those previously treated with intravenous therapy were lower than those treated initially with HAI. In the study from the National Cancer Institute, significant biliary sclerosis was observed in 21% of patients.[107] In an unplanned subgroup analysis, there was a significant survival advantage in the group with histologically negative periportal lymph nodes who received HAI therapy. Because patients in the intravenous therapy arm did not have the benefit of surgical staging, improved outcome in the HAI node-negative group was presumably due to more accurate surgical staging and exclusion of those with occult extrahepatic disease. The other United States trial that did not allow crossover to HAI therapy was from the Mayo Clinic, and no difference in overall survival was observed between groups.[108]

Two European studies did show a survival advantage, but patients were randomized to HAI therapy or best supportive care, which included cytotoxic therapy in only one-third of patients, a control treatment arm not commonly used in the United States. The study from the United Kingdom treated patients with 0.2 mg/kg/d of FUDR, which was well tolerated.[109] Overall survival and improved quality of life were observed in the treated versus best supportive care group in whom intravenous chemotherapy was administered for palliation of symptoms only. The French study also demonstrated a survival benefit with HAI therapy; only one-half of the patients in the control arm received systemic therapy.[110]

Two metaanalyses of the published prospective random assignment trials have concluded there is a modest survival advantage to HAI therapy[111,112] (Fig. 52.3-6). Currently, there is another ongoing prospective random assignment trial in the United States (cancer and leukemia group B 9841). This is a noncrossover design trial with stratification parameters for extent of hepatic involvement, prior chemotherapy, and the presence or absence of synchronous primary disease. The HAI treatment arm will receive a 14-day infusion of 0.18 mg/kg/d of

TABLE 52.3-7. Hepatic Arterial Infusion Therapy: Randomized Trials in Colorectal Cancer

			Response Rate			*Survival Progression*		*Trial Design*	
Reference	*Regimen*	No. of Patients	Complete Response (%)	Partial Response (%)	Total (%)	Free	Overall	Crossover	Extrahepatic Disease
Kemeny[106]	HAI, 0.3 mg/kg/d FUDR	48	2	48	50	9	17	Yes	No
	IV 0.15 mg/kg/d FUDR	51	0	20	20	5	12		
Chang[107]	HAI, 0.2–0.3 mg/kg/d FUDR	32	5	57	62	7	17	No	Yes
	IV 0.1125 mg/kg/d FUDR	32	3	14	17	9	12		
Hohn[105]	HAI, 0.2–0.3 mg/kg/d FUDR	50	8	34	42	13	17	Yes	Yes
	IV ≥ 0.075 mg/kg/d FUDR	65	5	5	10	7	16		
Martin[108]	HAI, 0.3 mg/kg/d FUDR	33	—	—	48	15.7	12.6	No	Yes
	IV 5-FU + 500 mg/m²/d × q5wk	36	—	—	21	6	10.5		
Rougier[110]	HAI, 0.3 mg/kg/d FUDR	81	6	37	43	14.5	15	No	Yes
	IV 5-FU[a]	82	2	7	9	5.5	11		
Wagman[226]	HAI 0.3–0.5 mg/kg/d FUDR	31	—	—	56	—	19.8	Yes	Yes
	IV 5-FU 10–15 mg/kg weekly	10	—	—	0	—	11.6		
Allen-Mersh[109]	HAI 0.2 mg/kg/d FUDR	51	—	—	5	—	13	No	No
	Supportive care[a]	49	—	—	0	—	6.3		

5-FU, 5-fluorouracil; FUDR, floxuridine; HAI, hepatic artery infusion.
[a]One-third to one-half of patients received cytotoxic therapy.

FUDR, 10 mg/m² of LV, and 20 mg of dexamethasone, a combination previously associated with a 78% response rate and a low incidence of biliary toxicity.[104] The systemic therapy arm will receive 425 mg/m²/d of 5-FU and 20 mg/m²/d of LV for 5 days.

OTHER APPLICATIONS OF HEPATIC ARTERY INFUSIONAL THERAPY

HAI therapy has been used with other agents for patients with various histologies, including interleukin-2 and chemotherapy for colorectal cancer patients,[113] doxorubicin for hepatocellular cancer patients,[114] and carboplatin[115] or fotemustine[116] for patients with metastatic ocular melanoma to liver. Leyvraz and coworkers treated 31 patents with ocular melanoma metastatic to liver with 100 mg/m² as a 4-hour infusion weekly for 3 weeks followed by a repeat cycle every 21 days via an implanted intraarterial port.[116] Objective radiographic responses were observed in 12 of 30 assessable patients (40%), and the median duration of response was 11 months. These data are similar to those reported with chemoebolization[117] and show encouraging activity in a disease for which there are no good options.

INTERMITTENT HEPATIC ARTERY INFUSION THERAPY

The use of HAI therapy requires a surgical procedure coupled with the risk of infection and bleeding associated with the

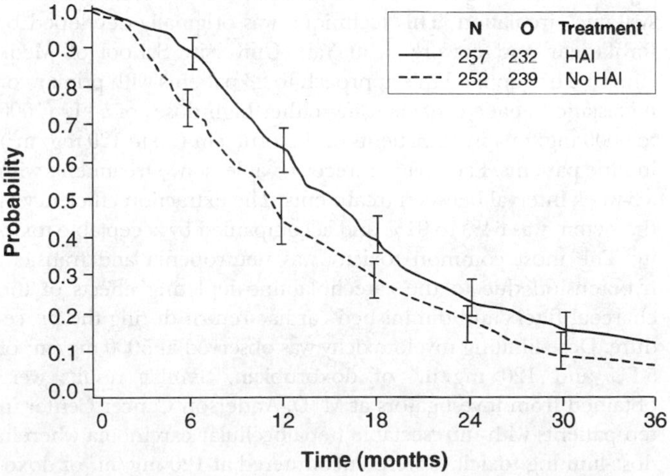

FIGURE 52.3-6. Five-year overall survival in patients with metastatic colorectal cancer to the liver treated with hepatic artery infusional (HAI) therapy using a floxuridine-based regimen compared with systemic therapy (No HAI). Survival curves based on a metaanalysis of the published literature of phase III random assignment trials comparing these two treatment strategies. HAI therapy has a significantly improved survival compared with those treated with no HAI therapy (Log rank test, $P = .0009$). (From ref. 112, with permission.)

requirement for the placement of a semipermanent catheter and port. One approach to circumvent the cost and toxicities associated with chronic indwelling devices is the use of an intermittently placed percutaneous hepatic arterial catheter. The feasibility of this approach has been demonstrated by several groups.[118,119] Jung and colleagues demonstrated the safety and feasibility of the approach in 21 patients with primary or metastatic cancer in the liver. Major complications requiring catheter removal and reimplantation occurred in 19% of patients. Patients with metastatic breast cancer to the liver were treated with percutaneous hepatic artery infusion of cisplatin, 120 mg/m^2 (31 patients), or vinblastine, 2 mg/m^2 (26 patients), daily for 5 days each month via percutaneous hepatic artery catheters.[71,120] Partial responses were noted in 19% of patients treated with platinum and 36% of those treated with vinblastine, and toxicities were found to be acceptable with both regimens. Experience using this approach in 36 patients treated at the University of Nebraska has been published.[121] Patients entered onto this trial had unresectable hepatic metastases from colorectal carcinoma and were treated with FUDR plus LV continuously for 4 days via hepatic arterial infusion followed in 1 week by intravenous continuous infusion 5-FU and oral LV for 21 days each month for six cycles followed by maintenance systemic 5-FU and oral LV. The overall response rate was 45%, with a median survival of 1 year.

HEPATIC ARTERY INFUSION WITH VENOUS FILTRATION

An interesting approach to enable the use of high doses of chemotherapy while limiting systemic toxicities involves the use of venous filtration wherein high doses of cytotoxins may be administered into the arterial supply while the liver and hepatic venous blood is collected via a catheter positioned in the retrohepatic vena cava and in which balloons are inflated above and below the hepatic veins to isolate and collect hepatic venous effluent. The collected blood is passed through a charcoal-containing device capable of filtering the cytotoxic compounds and returned to the systemic circulation. This technique was originally developed by Ravikumar and coworkers at Yale University School of Medicine.[122] They applied this approach to 23 patients with primary or metastatic hepatic cancers using either high doses of 5-FU (1000 to 5000 mg/m^2) in 12 patients or doxorubicin (50 to 120 mg/m^2) in nine patients. Each patient received at least two treatments with a 3-week interval between treatments. The extraction efficiency of the system was 64% to 91% and accompanied by acceptable toxicity. The most common toxicity was neutropenia and transient hypotension due to the catecholamine-depleting effects of the charcoal filters and diminished cardiac return during the procedure. Dose-limiting myelotoxicity was observed at 5000 mg/m^2 of 5-FU and 120 mg/m^2 of doxorubicin. Similar results were obtained from investigators at M. D. Anderson Cancer Center in ten patients with unresectable hepatocellular carcinoma wherein dose-limiting toxicities were encountered at 120 mg/m^2 of doxorubicin. This approach holds promise for the delivery of relatively high doses of chemotherapy into an isolated organ; however, because the isolation is not complete, systemic toxicities limit drug exposure; thus, the value of this approach clearly requires further investigation.

In an attempt to simplify the technique, Ku and colleagues from Japan have developed a single-catheter technique of hepatic isolation and charcoal hemoperfusion that required only a single cutdown rather than the three needed for the double-balloon technique described previously.[123] They compared their single-catheter technique with the original technique as developed by Ravikumar in 16 patients, with either primary or metastatic cancer to the liver. Nine of these patients were treated using the new technique and seven using the original double-balloon technique. Although this group found either technique feasible and relatively safe, their study suggests that the single-catheter technique may result in a significant decrease in systemic exposure, presumably due to greater efficiency of removal of the cytotoxin from the venous effluent. The hemofiltration concept was further tested in 23 patients with hepatic metastases from colorectal cancer (seven previously treated with 5-FU/LV) who were treated with hepatic arterial chemotherapy using a combination of mitomycin (30 to 50 mg/m^2) and epirubicin (60 to 90 mg/m^2) combined with intraperitoneal cisplatin (60 mg/m^2) coupled with a venous filtration catheter placed in the retrohepatic inferior vena cava.[124] This high-dose regimen was supplemented with four subsequent cycles of the same agents given at more standard doses. The investigators found this regimen to be feasible and associated with acceptable toxicities that included grade 3 to 4 hematologic (12%), gastrointestinal (19%), and hepatic effects (9%) and pain (9%). They identified an overall response rate of 59%, with a median duration of response of 10 months and an overall median survival of 14 months. In a subsequent study from investigators in Belgium, hemofiltration was used in eight patients with unresectable hepatic metastases from colorectal carcinoma. This group used hepatic arterial infusion of 5-FU, mitomycin C, and doxorubicin. They noted a 46% overall response rate with essentially negligible major gastrointestinal or renal toxicities.[125]

ISOLATED HEPATIC PERFUSION

IHP is a regional treatment that has been used at a limited number of centers since its original clinical application in the 1950s[126] and is similar to isolated limb perfusion used for extremity melanoma or sarcoma in which the cancer-bearing region is perfused with a recirculating closed circuit containing a reservoir, heat exchanger for delivery of hyperthermia, and roller pump (see Chapter 29.3).[127] IHP is administered via a major operative procedure during which the liver is extensively mobilized to prevent leak of systemic perfusate during treatment. Venous outflow is from a cannula positioned in an isolated segment of the retrohepatic inferior vena cava and arterial inflow is through a cannula or cannulae placed in the gastroduodenal artery and sometimes in the portal vein. During perfusion the splanchnic portal venous and inferior vena caval blood flow is temporarily occluded and must be shunted to the systemic circulation using a venovenous bypass circuit similar to that used in hepatic transplantation procedures.[128]

Because of its technical complexity, the morbidity associated with the procedure reported in older series, and the lack of documented efficacy using chemotherapeutics alone,[127] it has not gained widespread or consistent clinical evaluation. However, in the early 1990s, several centers initiated trials of IHP using tumor necrosis factor (TNF) and melphalan with the benefit of continuous intraoperative leak monitoring using radiolabeled erythrocytes or albumin to ensure minimal or no

TABLE 52.3-8. Summary of Isolated Hepatic Perfusion Trial Using Tumor Necrosis Factor and Chemotherapeutics

Authors	*No. of Patients*	*Agent(s)*	*Dose*	*Duration (h)*	*Temperature (°C)*	*Results*
De Vries, 1998[130,131]	8	Melphalan	1 mg/kg	1	>41	Mortality 33%
		TNF	0.4 mg			5/6 PR
	1	TNF alone	0.8 mg			
Hafström, 1998[133,136]	11	Melphalan	0.5 mg/kg	1	39	Mortality 18%
		TNF	30–200 μg			Morbidity 45%
						3/11 PR
Oldhafer, 1999[132]	6	Melphalan	60–140 mg	1	40–41	Mortality 0%
		TNF	200–300 μg			1 CR, 2 PR (50%)
Alexander, 1998[134]	34	Melphalan	1.5 mg/kg	1	39.5–40.0	Mortality 3%
		TNF	1.0 mg			1 CR, 25 PR (75%)

CR, complete response; PR, partial response; TNF, tumor necrosis factor.

leak of perfusate during treatment.[129] There are data from three centers in Europe and the National Cancer Institute in Bethesda, Maryland, reporting results with IHP using TNF and melphalan (Table 52.3-8). De Vries and coworkers treated nine patients with advanced unresectable metastatic cancer confined to liver and reported a considerable treatment mortality of 33% but did observe significant antitumor activity.[130,131] However, the median duration of response was only 18 weeks, and median survival was 10 months. Oldhafer and coworkers reported a series of 12 patients of whom six received TNF and melphalan.[132] Tumor biopsies obtained on posttreatment day 1 showed tumor necrosis in most patients and there was an overall radiographic response rate of 50% and a median survival of 11 months. A Swedish group treated 11 patients and had an operative mortality of 18%. Antitumor activity was observed in three of six patients with ocular melanoma to liver and in zero of five patients with colorectal cancer. The modest antitumor activity may be secondary to the low doses of agents used, only 0.2 to 0.3 mg of TNF and 0.5 mg/kg of melphalan, which are considerably lower than the maximum safe tolerated doses determined in phase I trials at the National Cancer Institute.[127,133]

Alexander and coworkers from the National Cancer Institute reported results in 34 patents with metastatic unresectable cancers confined to liver using 1 mg of TNF and 1.5 mg/kg of melphalan.[134] Treatment mortality was 3% and despite the fact that most had received previous therapy and many had advanced tumor burden in liver, there was an overall radiographic response rate of 75%. Responses were consistent across all histologies treated, including ocular melanoma and colorectal cancer and observed in those with advanced disease (Table 52.3-9). More recently, results in 51 patents with isolated unresectable colorectal cancer confined to liver treated with IHP using TNF and melphalan or melphalan alone followed by HAI therapy using FUDR and LV have been presented by the group.[135] Seventy-three percent of patents had failed previous systemic therapy with a 5-FU–based regimen. There was one treatment-related mortality (2%). Of note, the overall responses remained

TABLE 52.3-9. Response to Isolated Hepatic Perfusion Based on Number of Lesions, Diameter of Largest Tumor, or Percent Hepatic Replacement in Patients Treated with Tumor Necrosis Factor and Melphalan

	No. of Patients	*Partial Response or Complete Response*	*Percentage*
Overall	33	25	75
Number of radiographically imageable lesions			
1–4	9	7	78
5–19	13	9	69
≥20	11	9	81
Diameter largest lesion (cm)			
<5	4	2	50
5.0–9.9	12	9	75
≥10	17	14	82
Hepatic replacement (%)			
<20	6	5	83
20–49	15	10	66
≥50	12	10	83

(From ref. 134, with permission.)

TABLE 52.3-10. Outcome in Patients with Neuroendocrine Tumors Metastatic to the Liver after Chemoembolization

Reference	Histology	Treatment	No. of Patients	Response Rate: Objective	Response Rate: Hormonal[a]	Median Survival (mo)
Ruszniewski[227]	Carcinoid, islet cell	Embolization only	24	6/18	8/14	ND
Therasse[228]	Carcinoid	Doxorubicin (60 mg mean)	23	6/17	10/11	24 (mean)
Marlink[229]	Carcinoid, islet cell	Embolization only	10	9/10	7/10	ND
Kim[136]	Carcinoid	Carcinoid, cisplatin (150 mg), doxorubicin (50 mg)	30	11/30	21/16	15
	Islet cell	Islet cell, 5-fluorouracil (350 mg), streptozotocin (150–200 mg)				
Perry[230]	Carcinoid, gastrinoma	Doxorubicin (30–60 mg)	30	14/18	11/16	24
Ajani[231]	Islet cell	Embolization only	22	12/20	9/11	34

ND, not determined.
[a]Defined as 50% decrease; expressed as fraction of patients evaluable.

similar to their initial report, 77% for patents treated with TNF and melphalan IHP and 74% for patents treated with IHP using melphalan alone, but median time to progression in liver was significantly prolonged with the addition of HAI therapy (10 months vs. 14.5 months, respectively). These data suggest that continued clinical evaluation of IHP for patients with advanced refractory metastatic cancers confined to liver is warranted.

Chemoembolization

Chemoembolization involves the administration of chemotherapy followed by vascular occlusion using a variety of agents such as degradable starch microspheres, gelatin powders, polyvinyl chloride, or pledgets. Responding patients usually undergo multiple procedures over time as tumors and vasculature regrow. This approach has been widely applied in the treatment of primary hepatocellular carcinoma (see Chapter 33.5). For patients with metastatic cancer, the most common application is in patients with unresectable metastases from carcinoid or islet cell tumors. Because most tumors are highly vascular and have an indolent course in many patients, a partial response can provide long-term palliation. Furthermore, many patients who do not achieve an objective response have improvements in symptoms resulting from hormonal secretion. The overall objective response rate tends to be in the range of 30% to 50%, and the great majority of patients show reduced hormone secretion and improvement of symptoms (Table 52.3-10). Although there has been a shift in practice from embolization alone to chemoembolization with a variety of agents, there is no clear evidence that the use of chemotherapy improves response or patient outcome.[136]

Chemoembolization has also been attempted for patients with colorectal cancer metastatic to the liver. In contrast to neuroendocrine tumors, most patients with metastatic colorectal cancer demonstrate a more aggressive course both within the liver and systemically. Two small randomized trials showed no statistically significant benefit of chemoembolization over embolization only (Table 52.3-11).

Embolization procedures cause significant pain (requiring narcotic analgesics), fever, nausea, and malaise lasting 2 to 7 days in nearly all patients. Portal venous thrombosis, while rarely seen (in contrast to hepatocellular carcinoma), is an absolute contraindication to hepatic arterial embolization.

Chemoembolization Plus Adjuvant Chemotherapy

Chemoembolization appears to have value as a local therapy for patients with liver-only or liver-predominant unresectable carcinoma. Given the potential value of adjuvant chemotherapy after hepatic resection, at least two groups have sought to investigate the potential value of adjuvant chemotherapy after chemoembolization in patients with gastrointestinal malignancies metastatic to the liver. The Puget Sound Oncology Consortium performed an investigation of alternating systemic continuous infusion 5-FU (250 $mg/m^2/d$ for 28 days) interspersed with two or three transcatheter arterial chemoembolization treatments using foam particles with cisplatin in 32 patients. Although this group believed that toxicity was acceptable with this regimen, they did have grade 3 toxicities occur in 81% of patients and grade 4 in 31%. Furthermore, the overall 40% response rate, median duration of response of 4.2 months and overall median survival of 14.3 months are similar to what one might anticipate with systemic chemotherapy alone.[137] A similar experience was published by the Southwest Oncology Group, who combined chemoembolization (collagen mixed with cisplatin, mitomycin C, and doxorubicin) with systemic continuous infusion 5-FU/LV in 31 patients. This group found an overall response rate of 29% with a median survival of 14 months.[138] These outcomes are similar to what one might have anticipated with the use of systemic chemotherapy alone. Thus, the value of combining hepatic chemoembolization with adjuvant chemotherapy using agents currently available does not appear promising.

LOCAL ABLATIVE THERAPY

Several techniques are being used for local ablation of hepatic metastases, including cryotherapy, percutaneous injection of toxic agents, hyperthermic coagulative necrosis, and newer experimental techniques (Table 52.3-12).[139] The goal of local ablative therapy is to achieve complete necrosis of the tumor

TABLE 52.3-11. Outcome in Patients with Colorectal Cancer Metastatic to the Liver after Chemoembolization

Reference	*Treatment*	*Previously Treated*	*No. of Patients*	*Response Rate* Objective	Carcinoembryonic Antigen[a]	*Median Survival (mo)*
Sanz-Altamira[232]	1000 mg 5-FU 10 mg MMC	Yes	40	8/35	18/29	10
Tellez[233]	Cisplatin, MMC, doxorubicin	Yes	30	17/27	19/20	8.6
McGinn[234]	Radiation, floxuridine, MMC	Yes	26	3/25		5
Martinelli[235]	Embolization only[b]	Yes	11	6/24	9/14	9.3
	Embolization with 5-FU (750 mg/m^2) Interferon-α (9 × 10^6 U)		13			
Goldberg[236]	Angiotensin II 5-FU (1 g)	No	21	2/21		9
Hunt[237]	No treatment	No	20	ND	ND	7.9
	Embolization only		22			7.0
	Embolization + 500 mg 5-FU[b]		19			10.7
Civalleri[238]	MMC (10 mg/m^2)	No	39	10/39	ND	14

5-FU, 5-fluorouracil; MMC, mitomycin C; ND, not determined.
[a]Defined as 50% decrease; expressed as fraction of patients evaluable.
[b]Randomized trial.

with minimal injury to surrounding normal hepatic parenchyma. Currently, their use is indicated in patients who are not surgical candidates, for those whose tumors are not amenable to resection because of multiple tumors involving both lobes, tumors arising in cirrhotic livers in which preservation of parenchyma is imperative, tumors straddling the interlobar plane that would otherwise require an extended resection, recurrent tumors after previous resection in which reresection may be unsafe or anatomically impossible, and as an adjunct to surgical resection by treating microscopically positive margins.

Limitations of local ablation therapies include the inability to treat subclinical or occult tumor deposits, inability to treat tumors larger than several centimeters in diameter, inability to treat tumors abutting major vascular structures, and difficulty in assessing the adequacy of tissue destruction during therapy. Real-time ultrasound and MRI scanning are routinely used during treatment, but further refinement in technique and imaging is required.

CRYOTHERAPY

Cryotherapy is a term representing the *in situ* destruction of tissue by the freeze and thaw process. James Arnott first used freezing to decrease the size of breast and cervical cancers in England in 1845.[140] The most widespread application has been in the field of dermatology in which the cure rate for skin tumors has been reported at 97% to 98%. Subsequently, encouraging results have been reported with deep tumors of

TABLE 52.3-12. Techniques for Local Ablation

Mechanism	*Technique*	*Needle or Probe Size*	*Zone of Necrosis*	*Advantages*	*Disadvantages*
Freezing	Cryotherapy	6–12 mm	3–5 cm	Large zone of necrosis Easily followed by ultrasound	Requires laparotomy Large probe size
Hyperthermic coagulative necrosis	Radiofrequency or microwave ablation	14–20 gauge	2 cm	Percutaneous technique	Small zone of necrosis
Local injection therapy	Ethanol Acetic acid Chemotherapy Hot saline	20–22 gauge	3 cm	Simple, inexpensive	Inhomogeneous distribution
Experimental	Gene transfer Intralesional TIL Focused ultrasound	Variable	Variable	Variable	Efficacy unknown

TIL, tumor infiltrating lymphocytes.
(Modified from ref. 239.)

the liver, lung, breast, prostate, and brain. The process of freezing tissue can cause direct cellular destruction that is dependent on the rate of tissue cooling, and this can be variable during cryosurgery. Microcirculatory failure secondary to freezing within the vasculature and subsequent vascular damage may be an additional tumoricidal mechanism.[141]

Two main technical advances have made cryotherapy applicable to liver tumors on a broad scale. The first is the development of vacuum-insulated cryoprobes that allow controlled freezing of tumors deep within the liver, and the second is the use of intraoperative ultrasound to allow precise probe placement into the center of tumors and to monitor the progression of the freeze margin in real time.[142] The most commonly used probes range from 6 to 12 mm in diameter and a disk-shaped probe can be used for freezing thin surface lesions or for freezing a positive or close resection margin. Liquid nitrogen is circulated through the tip of the probes at a temperature of –196°C, which results in a probe-tip temperature between –160°C and –180°C. The probe is placed into the center of the lesion under ultrasound guidance to ensure that uniform freezing will extend symmetrically in all directions from the tip of the probe. Repeated freeze and thaw cycles can improve tumor cell killing[143] and vascular inflow occlusion to the liver (Pringle's maneuver) can improve the cooling rate and may allow successful freezing of larger tumors with smaller probes.

The 8-mm probe can reliably create a spheric ice ball of 3 cm, and the 12-mm probe can create an ice ball of 5 cm in nonischemic liver. Newer cryosurgical systems are designed to allow simultaneous circulation of liquid nitrogen through multiple probes.[144] Smaller 2- to 3-mm needle tip probes have been used in combination to freeze large tumors and minimize bleeding from the probe tract in the liver. Smaller probes can be inserted through laparoscopic ports. The advancing interface between frozen tissue and normal tissue can be monitored by ultrasound as a distinct hyperechoic ring.[145] The advancement of this ring is monitored until it extends at least 1 cm beyond the tumor in all directions. The ice ball creates an acoustic shadow, making it impossible to monitor the advancement of all edges simultaneously. The ultrasound transducer should be moved as necessary to visualize the entire circumference and ensure complete freezing to 1 cm beyond the tumor.

A number of studies were published in the early 1990s from centers reporting their initial experience with the technique. Zhou et al. from the Shanghai Medical University in China reported a series of 107 patients with primary liver cancer treated with cryotherapy[146] and observed a 5-year survival of 15% for 49 patients treated with cryotherapy. Onik and coworkers reported a series of 59 patients with unresectable hepatic metastases treated with cryosurgery.[147] At a median follow-up of 21 months the disease-free survival rate was 27% and overall survival was 52.5%. The number of tumors treated ranged from one to 16, and 73% of patients treated had bilobar disease and many had tumors directly abutting major vessels. Ravikumar and coworkers reported an initial series of 32 patients treated with cryosurgery resulting in a 2-year disease-free survival of 28% and overall survival of 62%.[148] A second series from the same investigator[26] reported results in 21 patients undergoing cryosurgery and at a median follow-up of 16 months. In both series, the liver recurrence rate was approximately 25% to 30%, and one-half of patients failed systemically. Preketes and coworkers have reported their results of cryosurgery in 38 patients with unresectable multiple liver metastases from colorectal carcinoma.[149] They report a 12.5% 2-year survival rate for the 11 patients receiving cryotherapy alone.

TABLE 52.3-13. Factors with Independent Prognostic Significance in Colorectal Patients Undergoing Cryotherapy of Hepatic Metastases

Low pretreatment carcinoembryonic antigen value
Diameter largest lesion <3 cm
No extrahepatic disease
Node-negative involvement of primary tumor
Metachronous (vs. synchronous) liver metastases
Successful cryotherapy of all hepatic lesions

(Data from ref. 154.)

Currently, the world literature reports results in more than 900 patients treated with the technique,[150] with more recent reports detailing patient, treatment, and tumor parameters associated with successful outcome.[151–155] Seifert and Morris reported that 116 patients with colorectal cancer treated with cryotherapy had an overall morbidity of 28%.[154] There was a single mortality secondary to treatment (0.9%). Factors found to be independently correlated with favorable outcome after therapy are listed in Table 52.3-13. In a second report of 85 patients presumably also included in the first series, the mean disease-free interval at the cryosite was 42 months and was 60% at 3 years.[155] The median hepatic disease-free interval was 15 months and 17% at 3 years. Weaver and coworkers reported a median survival of 34 months and an 82% hepatic recurrence rate in 136 patients undergoing 158 cryotherapy procedures.[153] Repeat[156] and laparoscopic treatments[157,158] have been reported.

A single prospective random assignment trial evaluating cryosurgery versus conventional resection in patients with liver metastases from a variety of histologies has been reported.[159] Liver recurrences and overall survival were similar in both groups, and the authors concluded that cryotherapy is as effective as surgical resection for liver metastases. However, the heterogeneous nature of the patients treated and the unconventional treatment administered routinely to patients postoperatively make the interpretation of the data difficult. Others have reported results in patients with neuroendocrine[160] or other tumors[161,162] of the liver and have reported good palliation and a greater than 90% reduction in circulating tumor-related functional proteins (i.e., gastrin or 5-hydroxyindoleacetic acid) in more than 90% of patients for a median of 10 to 13 months after cryotherapy.[160,163]

In general, cryotherapy is considered a safe and effective means for treating hepatic tumors of all histologies with low morbidity. Cryotherapy has also been used in conjunction with hepatic resection to assist in resection of a deep-seated lesion,[164,165] treat an inadequate margin after resection,[166] and in addition to resection to preserve hepatic tissue.[167] The main advantage of cryotherapy over surgery is the minimal damage suffered by the normal hepatic parenchyma and the avoidance of the risk of hemorrhage and damage to bile ducts that occurs during parenchymal dissection. Most patients experience an increase in liver enzymes to approximately twice normal, with normalization by postoperative day 5. Leukocytosis and low-grade fevers are common. Hemorrhage from the probe tract is generally easily controlled with pressure, packing with absorbable gelatin sponge or absorbable knitted fabric, or both. Complications related specifically to cryotherapy include pleural effusions in 6%, hepatic cracking with associated intraoperative hemorrhage in 4%, biliary fistula in 3%, abscess in 1.7%, and myoglobinuria with renal failure in 1.4%.[150,168]

CRYOTHERAPY PLUS ADJUVANT CHEMOTHERAPY

Given the potential value of adjuvant chemotherapy in the setting of hepatic resection, it may be reasonable to expect a similar improvement in outcome with the addition of adjuvant chemotherapy to other local ablative therapies, including cryotherapy. A study from Australia (38 patients) and one from New Zealand (30 patients) investigated the value of adjuvant chemotherapy after cryotherapy in patients who had hepatic colorectal metastases that were deemed inoperable.[149,169] Each of these groups of investigators found the regimen of hepatic cryotherapy followed by hepatic arterial chemotherapy using 5-FU plus LV to be relatively safe and well tolerated, and each found a similar median survival of approximately 18 months in patients treated with the combined approach. In a small group of 11 patients nonrandomly treated with cryotherapy alone in the Australian trial, the investigators noted a median survival of only 8 months, suggesting that adjuvant chemotherapy may well be a useful adjunct to hepatic cryotherapy. Using systemic 5-FU plus LV, a group of investigators from Roswell Park Cancer Institute found that the use of this adjuvant systemic chemotherapy in four patients treated with prior cryotherapy was highly toxic and recommended caution when combining systemic adjuvant chemotherapy with cryotherapy.[170]

MICROWAVE TISSUE COAGULATION AND RADIOFREQUENCY ABLATION

Another form of local ablative therapy for liver tumors is percutaneous microwave or hyperthermic coagulation. A probe inserted into the middle of a tumor emits microwaves or radiowaves from its tip, which heats the surrounding tissue. Energy penetrates a few centimeters into the surrounding tissue, causes molecular vibration of dipoles (particularly of water), and is converted to heat, resulting in tissue coagulative necrosis. A single electrode emitting 2450 MHz for 60 seconds produces coagulation necrosis of a spindle-shaped region approximately 2 cm in diameter.[171] Evaluation of the zone of necrosis in real time can be achieved with ultrasound, which shows strong hyperechogenic foci representing cellular destruction. Percutaneous microwave coagulation has efficacy in ablating hepatocellular tumors up to 6.5 cm in diameter.[172] Microwave therapy has advantages over laser photocoagulation as a larger zone of necrosis can be obtained with a shorter treatment.[173] In contrast to other forms of local ablation, the zone of cellular destruction does not extend beyond the tip of the electrode. This allows precise treatment at the deep edge of the tumor where ultrasound visualization is often limited.[171]

A number of studies have been reported outlining results in patients treated with percutaneous or open radiofrequency thermal ablation (RFA) (Table 52.3-14). The success of RFA in successful ablation of primary or metastatic tumor deposits within the liver is influenced by the expertise and diligence of the treating physician to ensure that an adequate zone of thermal necrosis has been delivered to the entire tumor. For large tumors, this requires multiple consecutive propregnant placements and, because the zone of thermal necrosis cannot be definitively imaged with intraoperative ultrasound, it is somewhat difficult to determine which areas within a large tumor have or have not been adequately treated. Solbiati and coworkers reported results in 29 patients with 44 hepatic metastases ranging in size from 1.3 to 5.1 cm in diameter.[174] The authors report successful ablation of all identifiable tumor in 91% of treated metastases, but a local progression rate of 34%. Liviaghi and coworkers subsequently reported a series of 14 patients with liver metastases and one patient with a primary cholangiocarcinoma treated with RFA.[175] Fourteen of 25 lesions were completely obliterated and ranged in size from 1.2 to 3.9 cm. Partial necrosis in 12 additional lesions was noted, with diameters ranging from 1.5 to 4.5 cm. Nagata and coworkers reported results of RFA treatment in 173 patients with primary or hepatic cancers.[176] Additional therapy, including arterial embolization, radiotherapy, immunotherapy, and systemic chemotherapy, were also combined with RFA treatment in this series. Treatments were administered percutaneously, and more than 80% of patients underwent more than four sessions of RFA. In 45 patients treated with metastatic tumor deposits, there was no response or disease progression in 53%. Cuschieri and coworkers reported results of microscopically administered ultrasound-guided RFA of hepatic tumors and successfully achieved total ablation in seven of eight patients with metastatic colorectal cancer to the liver.[177] At the time of publication, follow-up ranged from 6 to 20 months, and eight of ten patients remained free of tumor. The largest series of patients treated with RFA was reported by Curley and coworkers from the M. D. Anderson Cancer Center.[178] The investigators treated 123 patients with RFA either using the percutaneous or open operative technique with ultrasound guidance. A total of 169 tumors ranging in size from 0.5 to 12 cm (median diameter, 3.4 cm) were ablated. Three-fourths of patients underwent open operative RFA, and there were no treatment-related deaths in the study. The authors report three tumor recurrences in 169 treated lesions (1.8%) at a median follow-up of 15 months (see Table 52.3-14). The low recurrence rate may be due to the fact that many patients were treated operatively to facilitate probe placement and more reliably assess adequacy of therapy. In addition, the authors used inflow occlusion via the Pringle's maneuver, which may have enhanced the effectiveness of the thermal ablation. However, it should be noted the intraoperative use of RFA does not take full advantage of its technology. For example,

TABLE 52.3-14. Local Recurrence after Radiofrequency Ablation of Hepatic Neoplasms

Author	*No. of Patients*	*Local Recurrence Rate*
Rossi, 1995[240]	24	54% mean follow-up 24 mo
Solbiati, 1997[174]	29	34% at 1 y
Nagata, 1997[176]	45[a]	29%
Allgaier, 1999[241]	10	0% mean 145 d
Cuschieri, 1999[177]	10	0% with follow-up 6–26 mo
Curley, 1999[178]	123	1.8% with median follow-up 15 mo

[a]Metastatic colorectal cancers only.

the small probe size and the fact that the tissue is cauterized along the track eliminates the risk of bleeding from the probe track or cracking of the liver on removal of the probe. For patients undergoing operative local ablative therapy, the use of cryotherapy allows one to use real-time intraoperative ultrasound to accurately assess the adequacy of the zone of destruction, which is more difficult to assess using RFA. In practice, the technology behind the various local ablative therapies is evolving, and, as smaller probe sizes are developed and techniques for monitoring adequacy of tissue destruction are refined, the advantages of one form of ablative therapy over another may become increasingly obscure.

RADIOFREQUENCY ABLATION PLUS ADJUVANT CHEMOTHERAPY

A group of investigators from Japan investigated the feasibility of combining intrahepatic artery 5-FU (750 to 1250 mg) administered as a weekly 5-hour infusion with RFA therapy in nine patients with hepatic metastases from colorectal carcinoma.[179] These investigators found the combination to be feasible and safe with three of nine patients surviving for more than 2 years. Clearly, the potential value of adjuvant chemotherapy in the setting of local therapy using radiofrequency should be further investigated.

INTERSTITIAL LASER PHOTOCOAGULATION

Interstitial laser photocoagulation is a minimally invasive technique for local ablation of tumors first developed in 1983.[180] A thin optical fiber is inserted percutaneously into the center of a liver tumor and a laser light is delivered to the tip of the fiber. The laser light emitted from the fiber tip is absorbed as heat by the surrounding tumor. The laser light penetrates the surrounding tissue in an isotropic fashion around the fiber tip. In general, 1 to 2 W of continuous near-infrared laser energy is delivered for durations of 300 to 1000 seconds. Most of the work has been performed with a neodymium:yttrium aluminum garnet laser. Cells in the target volume undergo coagulative necrosis resulting from protein denaturation at temperatures greater than 60°C.[181] Special diffusion fiber tips have been developed to allow even scatter and penetration of the laser light throughout the tumor, avoiding a local charring effect that subsequently blocks laser penetration.[182]

As with cryotherapy, the zone of tissue necrosis can be followed in real time by ultrasound and MRI.[183] The accuracy of ultrasound during the treatment of large tumors is inferior to the results with cryotherapy.[184] Tumors up to 9 cm have been treated with this technique using multiple probes and multiple treatment sessions. In general, a single probe is adequate for a tumor 0.5 cm in diameter. If multiple probes are necessary, they are spaced 1.0 to 1.5 cm apart. This is adequate to achieve complete homogeneous necrosis between the fiber tips.[184] As with cryotherapy, this treatment is less effective in tumors close to large vessels, as the blood flow cools the adjacent tissue, preventing thermal necrosis. The advantage over cryotherapy is the small size of the delivery fibers, allowing accurate and safe percutaneous insertion.

Clinical reports of interstitial laser photocoagulation are limited. Amin and coworkers reported results in a total of 55 tumors with interstitial laser photocoagulation.[185] Eighty-two percent of tumors had a partial response (greater than 50% necrosis identified on CT imaging), and 38% underwent complete necrosis. Metastases smaller than 4 cm responded better than larger tumors. Complications were minimal, but included pain, subcapsular hematoma, and pleural effusion. Nolsoe and coworkers reported a pilot study of 11 patients with 16 colorectal liver metastases.[186] Twelve of 16 tumors were considered completely destroyed by the procedure, including a 3.7-cm tumor. No serious complications were encountered. Amin and coworkers compared interstitial laser photocoagulation in 54 colorectal liver metastases with percutaneous alcohol injection in 22 tumors.[184] They report that 52% of tumors treated with photocoagulation had complete necrosis of the tumor on dynamic CT scan compared with zero patients receiving alcohol injection. There were no major complications in either group, but pain was more significant in the alcohol-injected group.

In summary, interstitial laser photocoagulation is a safe and simple technique for treating small localized liver tumors. The zone of necrosis is smaller than with cryotherapy, thereby requiring multiple probes per tumor. This makes following the progression of cellular destruction with ultrasound more difficult and increases the chance of leaving viable cells. Further refinements in imaging may make this treatment more successful.

PERCUTANEOUS ETHANOL INJECTION

Percutaneous ethanol injections into malignant deposits in the liver have most broadly been applied to the treatment of patients with hepatocellular carcinomas. The density of tumors associated with hepatocellular carcinoma and the common occurrence of this malignancy in the setting of severe underlying hepatic disease lends itself to this form of local therapy as opposed to surgical resection, which is often not possible in patients with severe underlying hepatic cirrhosis. Currently, there are no randomized studies comparing the value of percutaneous ethanol injection with any of the other local modalities for the treatment of patients with hepatic malignancy. Thus, its value relative to other local techniques is uncertain. However, there have been several series of patients with hepatocellular carcinoma treated by percutaneous ethanol injection reported in the literature, primarily from investigators in Japan and Italy. In patients with hepatocellular carcinoma with either single or multiple hepatic tumors treated with curative intent, the investigators from Japan found 3- and 5-year overall survival rates of 62% to 65% and 28% to 52%, respectively.[187,188] The 3-year recurrence rate for these patients was approximately 60% to 65%, with the vast majority of new recurrences occurring in portions of the liver not previously treated with ethanol injections. The 3- and 5-year overall survival rates were slightly better in the studies from Italy (approximately 70% and 40%, respectively); however, these differences may well be attributed to the differences in the underlying hepatic disease, which is an important prognostic factor.[189,190] Patients classified as Child's A have a 2-year survival, approximately twofold greater than those patients classified as Child's C (approximately 90% vs. less than 40%, respectively). In addition to Child's classification, the prognosis of patients with hepatocellular carcinoma is negatively influenced by a greater number of deposits of carcinoma as well as increasing size of the deposits and elevated pretreatment α-fetoprotein levels.[191] Although generally restricted to patients with tumors smaller than approximately 3 to 5 cm in size, Livraghi and colleagues published their experience with percutaneous ethanol injection in 108 patients with hepatocellular carcinoma with tumors larger than 5 cm and performed in a single session under general anesthesia. Despite the size of the lesions treated, this group found a 3-year survival of 57% for those in patients with single lesions measuring 5.0 to 8.5 cm and 42% for those with multiple lesions measuring 5 to 10 cm.[192] The overall rate of major complications in this study was less than 5%, thus suggesting that percutaneous ethanol injections may be a useful modality even in the setting of lesions up to 10 cm in size.

Although no randomized comparisons between percutaneous ethanol injection and hepatectomy have been performed, several studies address this issue through retrospective comparisons of the use of contemporary patient cohorts. In a cohort study from Spain,[193] patients with solitary hepatocellular carcinomas smaller than or equal to 4 cm were treated with surgical resection (n = 33) or percutaneous ethanol injection (n = 30). Despite a significant increased proportion of Child's A patients in the surgically treated group (91% vs. 33%) and a decreased proportion of patients with ascites (6% vs. 47%), these authors found that the overall survival rates in the two groups were not different. Similar results were obtained in a study of 40 patients with solitary hepatocellular carcinomas smaller than 2 cm in diameter treated by Kotoh and colleagues wherein 17 were treated with hepatectomy, 12 with percutaneous ethanol injection, and 11 with a combination of percutaneous ethanol injections and arterial embolization with gel-containing mitomycin C and Adriamycin. These authors found no difference in median survival (3.5 to 4.0 years) or recurrence rates (70% to 80%) between patients undergoing hepatectomy versus those treated with ethanol injection with or without arterial embolization despite a greater proportion of patients with Child's class A disease in the surgically treated group (73% vs. 36%).[194] In a large retrospective analysis of 391 patients, Livraghi and colleagues found no difference in 3-year survival for 120 patients treated by surgical resection (79% Child's A; 40% Child's B) versus 155 treated by percutaneous ethanol injection (71% Child's A; 41% Child's B); however, they noted a significantly inferior (threefold lower) survival for those patients who were not treated with either percutaneous ethanol injection or hepatectomy.[195] Similarly, Orlando and colleagues used a matched historic comparison group to compare the outcome of this untreated group (65 patients) with small hepatocellular carcinomas (smaller than 4 cm) with 35 patients treated by percutaneous ethanol injection and found that the 3-year survival of patients treated with percutaneous ethanol injections was superior to the historic comparison group (33% vs. 14%, respectively), but that the primary difference in survival outcome was restricted to those patients with Child's A disease (71% vs. 21%, respectively) whereas those with Child's B had a similar, but poor, 3-year survival outcome regardless of whether they were treated with percutaneous ethanol injections or left untreated (9% for both groups).[196] These results suggest that percutaneous ethanol injections may be associated with a more favorable outcome compared with those patients who are treated with best supportive care only and that clinical outcome with this form of local therapy may be similar to that of hepatectomy.

Given the potential value of percutaneous ethanol injections and transcatheter arterial embolization, several groups have combined these two approaches. In 86 patients with Child's class A or B cirrhosis and large hepatocellular carcinomas (3.1 to 8.0 cm), Lencioni and colleagues found 69% and 47% 3- and 5-year survivals, with 56% and 82% recurrence rates at 3 and 5 years in patients treated with transcatheter arterial chemoembolization (gelatin sponge with epirubicin emulsified in iodized oil) followed by percutaneous ethanol injection.[197] Investigators in Germany compared the survival of 132 patients with inoperable hepatocellular carcinoma nonrandomly treated with best supportive care (45 patients) or percutaneous ethanol infusion (15 patients), or transcatheter arterial chemoembolization (33 patients), or the combination of both local therapies (39 patients).[198] These investigators found that patients treated with a combination of percutaneous ethanol infusion and transarterial chemoembolization had an improved survival when compared with those patients treated with either chemoembolization alone or with best supportive care only. However, patients treated with chemoembolization alone had larger and more advanced hepatic disease compared with those treated with ethanol alone or the combination of local therapies, as ethanol injections (either alone or combined with chemoembolization) were reserved for those patients with fewer than three lesions with none larger than 5 cm in size. Those assigned to supportive care had disease too advanced to be treated by either chemoembolization or alcohol injections. Given these caveats, the supportive care group had the worst median survival compared with any of the treatment groups (2 months vs. 25 months in the combination group). Although these data support the use and feasibility of combining transarterial chemoembolization with percutaneous ethanol injection, the true value of this combined approach versus either approach used individually requires further investigations using a randomized prospective trial design.

RESULTS OF WHOLE LIVER IRRADIATION WITH OR WITHOUT CHEMOTHERAPY

Early studies demonstrated that whole liver radiation produces temporary palliation of pain for patients with cancer metastatic for the liver.[199] However, it was soon discovered that doses greater than 30 to 35 Gy could produce a condition that has become known as *radiation hepatitis*.[200–202] Radiation hepatitis is better described as radiation-induced liver disease (RILD), as the pathologic evaluation shows no evidence of hepatitis. Patients who develop RILD present 2 weeks to 3 months after the completion of radiation therapy with weight gain and bloating, and, in severe cases, confusion. Jaundice as a presenting symptom is uncommon (and suggests that the patient has already developed impending liver failure). Physical examination reveals anicteric ascites and painful hepatomegaly. Laboratory evaluation shows a marked elevation of alkaline phosphatase out of proportion to the typically modest increases in alanine aminotransferase, aspartate aminotransferase, and bilirubin (which tends to be unconjugated), elevations in prothrombin time and partial thromboplastin time, and thrombocytopenia. Paracentesis and radiologic studies (CT, MRI, or both) fail to show progressive disease. Liver biopsy reveals venoocclusive disease pathologically identical to that resulting from a variety of insults. Although most patients recover in 1 to 2 months, 10% to 20% develop overt liver failure and death.[203,204]

A tolerable whole liver dose produces only short-term palliation and patient survival (Table 52.3-15). This is true regardless

TABLE 52.3-15. Results of Treatment of Metastatic Cancer to the Liver Treated with Whole Liver Irradiation Alone

Reference	*Histology[a]*	*Dose (Gy/Fractions)*	*No. of Patients*	*Decrease in Pain (% Total)*	*Median Survival (mo)*	*Radiation-Induced Liver Disease[b]*
Borgelt,[242] RTOG 76-05	38% colorectal	21–30/7–19	103	55	3	0
Leibel,[243] RTOG 80-03	48% colorectal	21/7 (± misonidazole)	187	80/7[c]	4	0
Prasad[244]	33% colorectal	25/16	27	70	4	0
Russell,[245] RTOG 84-05	60% colorectal	27/15	53		4	0
		30/20	69	Not determined	4	0
		33/22	51		4	2

RTOG, Radiation Therapy Oncology Group.
[a]Predominant histology.
[b]Number of patients with grade 3 radiation-induced liver disease.
[c]Objective response (computed tomographic scan).

of whether the radiation is given daily or twice daily in 1.5-Gy fractions. To attempt to improve on these results, whole liver radiation has been combined with systemic and hepatic arterial chemotherapy. The most widely used drugs have been 5-FU[205] and FUDR,[206,207] as both are cytotoxic and radiosensitizing agents. The objective response rates and survival after combination chemoradiotherapy appears to be somewhat superior to that obtained by radiation alone (Table 52.3-16). Whole liver radiation tolerance does not seem to be affected by the concurrent use of fluoropyrimidines in contrast with other chemotherapeutic agents such as alkylating agents or mitomycin C,[208–210] which appear to increase RILD risk. Tolerable courses (5% chance of RILD) for whole liver radiation in patients who have not received alkylator therapy appear to be 21 Gy in 3-Gy fractions, 25 Gy in 2.5-Gy fractions, and 30 Gy in 2-Gy fractions.

Three techniques have been explored to increase focal radiation dose: yttrium 90 microspheres, interstitial implantation of radioactive sources, and three-dimensional conformal external-beam radiation. The theory behind the use of ^{90}Y microspheres is described in the chapter on hepatocellular carcinoma (see Chapter 33.5). A number of phase I trials have been conducted in patients with metastatic disease to the liver (chiefly colorectal cancer) demonstrating that an estimated whole liver absorbed dose of 100 to 150 Gy is tolerable. Fur-

TABLE 52.3-16. Results of Treatment of Metastatic Cancer to the Liver Treated with Whole Liver Irradiation with Chemotherapy

Reference	*Dose (Gy/Fractions)*	*Chemotherapy*	*Route*	*No. of Patients*	*Response (% Total)*	*Median Survival (mo)*	*Hepatic Toxicity[a]*
Byfield[246]	15–30/12[c]	FUDR	HA	28	ND	9	1
Friedman[247]	1354–21/5–7	5-FU, doxorubicin	HA	22	48[b]	>3	1
Herbsman[248]	25–30/15	FUDR	HA	13	70[d]	16	0
Lawrence[221]	33/22	FUDR	HA	19	39[b]	7	0
	36/24			13	ND	ND	3
Lokich[249]	19.5–30/10–12	5-FU or FUDR	HA	12	63[d]	ND	0
McCracken[208]	19.5/13	5-FU, mitomycin C	HA	13	(Adjuvant)	ND	1
Raju[250]	21/1.5	FUDR or 5-FU	HA or IV[e]	12	83[d]	14	0
Rotman[251]	22.5–32.3/15	5-FU	IV	27	83[d]	6	0
Sherman[252]	15–30/7–10	5-FU or procarbazine + hydroxyurea ± cyclophosphamide ± 5-FU	IV	50[f]	90[d]	4	0
Webber[253]	25/10	FUDR	HA	25	72[d]	12	0
Wiley[254]	25.5/17	5-FU	HA	19	37[b]	6	0
Woldberding[255]	21/17	5-FU, doxorubicin, methotrexate	HA	27	33	7	0

5-FU, 5-fluorouracil; FUDR, fluorodeoxyuridine; HA, intraarterial hepatic infusion; ND, not determined.
[a]Number of patients with grade 3 radiation hepatitis.
[b]Objective response (computed tomography or radionuclide scan documenting 50% decrease in bidimensional product).
[c]Split-course therapy.
[d]Subjective response (e.g., decrease in pain).
[e]FUDR (HA) in four patients; 5-FU IV in eight patients.
[f]Includes 19 patients who received radiation therapy only.

thermore, in the range of 20% to 25% of patients have shown objective responses.[211–214] Should ^{90}Y microspheres become available for clinical use in the United States, it will be important to administer them with careful attention to technical details such as avoiding pulmonary shunting and perfusion of other organs (such as the stomach) by aberrant blood vessels.

A second method of delivering high doses of radiation to parts of the liver is to use interstitial brachytherapy (placement of radioactive sources inside the tumor). In one series, 22 patients were treated with a single high dose-rate application of ^{192}iridium placed in catheters implanted at the time of laparotomy. The time of irradiation ranged from 10 minutes to 4.5 hours as a function of the size and number of lesions.[215] In another approach, permanent ^{125}I seeds have been implanted at the time of laparotomy or under ultrasound guidance.[216] The maximum tumor size in this latter series was smaller than 5 cm. Additional phase II experience is required to assess the efficacy of these approaches.

External-beam irradiation can be used to treat patients with localized unresectable metastatic cancer to the liver. These efforts have been based on the hypothesis that, just as substantial fractions of the liver can be resected if the remaining fraction can support liver function, focal high-dose liver radiation can be safely administered if sufficient normal liver is spared. As summarized in the chapter on hepatobiliary cancer (see Chapter 33.5), conformal planning can use beams not confined to the axial plane to reduce normal liver irradiation.[217,218] Furthermore, three-dimensional planned treatment has allowed the development of a quantitative understanding of the relationships among dose, volume, and risk of complication.[218,219]

A phase I and II trial for patients with unresectable hepatic cancer using either standard two-dimensional techniques[220] or three-dimensional conformal external-beam irradiation combined with hepatic arterial FUDR have demonstrated that high-dose focal radiation can produce up to a 50% response rate in previously treated patients.[221,222] However, the freedom from hepatic progression in one study was only 29% at 1 year, suggesting that higher doses will be required to produce long-term control.[222] More recent results support the hypothesis that the dose delivered is an important prognostic factor in both local control and survival for patients with metastatic colorectal cancer. In this study, dose is prescribed (to a maximum of 90 Gy) according to the fraction of normal liver that is spared based on a normal tissue complication probability model (see Chapter 33.5). Patients who could receive greater than or less than 70 Gy have a median survival in excess of 17 months, which approaches that achieved by surgical resection. Dose was an independent prognostic factor, and was not correlated with tumor size.[223]

CONCLUSIONS

Despite the fact that isolated hepatic metastases are a significant clinical problem frequently associated with a poor prognosis, there are evolving regional treatment strategies that increasingly expand the options available for patients afflicted with this condition. For patients with resectable hepatic deposits primarily of colorectal, neuroendocrine, or genitourinary origin, the benefit in terms of overall survival or palliation appears to be well established. For patients undergoing resection for colorectal cancer, various patient, tumor, and treatment variables have been identified as important prognostic factors and can be used to select patients for adjuvant therapy. For those with unresectable colorectal cancers confined to the liver, HAI therapy using FUDR-based regimens have high response rates, but the influence on overall survival has not been conclusively demonstrated. Local ablative therapies have the advantage of being able to ablate local tumor deposits, but their influence on overall survival has not been demonstrated. As the technology behind local ablative treatments advances, they will no doubt become more widely used alone or in combination with postablation HAI, systemic therapy, or both. Chemoembolization has been used in patients with advanced cancers of the liver and can result in palliation in a significant percentage of those treated. Newer therapies, including IHP and gene therapy, are under active clinical evaluation and may gain more widespread acceptance with further refinement of treatment in the future. HAI of a recombinant adenoviral construct containing the wild-type p53 gene is being evaluated in patients with metastatic colorectal cancer to the liver.[224] The range of regional therapies highlight the acknowledged importance and difficulty in treating hepatic metastases and provide an expectation that durable complete disease control within the liver with an associated improvement in quality of life and overall survival may be routinely achieved.

REFERENCES

1. Gragoudas ES, Egan KM, Seddon JM, et al. Survival of patients with metastases from uveal melanoma. *Ophthalmology* 1991;98:383.
2. Rajpal S, Moore R, Karakousis CP. Survival in metastatic ocular melanoma. *Cancer* 1983;52:334.
3. Goslin R, Steele G Jr, Zamcheck N. Factors influencing survival in patients with hepatic metastases from adenocarcinoma of the colon or rectum. *Dis Colon Rectum* 1982;25:749.
4. Daly JM, Kemeny NE. Metastatic cancer to the liver. In: DeVita VT, Hellman S, Rosenberg SA, eds. *Cancer: principles & practice of oncology* (5th ed). Philadelphia: Lippincott–Raven, 1997:2551.
5. Fong Y, Salo J. Surgical therapy of hepatic colorectal metastasis. *Semin Oncol* 1999;26:514.
6. Yoon SS, Tanabe KK. Surgical treatment and other regional treatments for colorectal cancer liver metastases. *Oncologist* 1999;4:197.
7. Choti MA, Bulkley GB. Management of hepatic metastases. *Liver Transplant Surg* 1999;5:65.
8. Curley SA, Vecchio R. New trends in the surgical treatment of colorectal cancer liver metastases. *Tumori* 1998;84:281.
9. Chen H, Pruitt A, Nicol TL, Gorgulu S, Choti MA. Complete hepatic resection of metastases from leiomyosarcoma prolongs survival. *J Gastrointest Surg* 1998;2:151.
10. Que FG, Nagorney DM, Batts KP, Linz LJ, Kvols LK. Hepatic resection for metastatic neuroendocrine carcinomas. *Am J Surg* 1995;169:36.
11. Landis SH, Murray T, Bolden S, Wingo PA. Cancer statistics, 1999. *CA Cancer J Clin* 1999;49:8.
12. Görög D, Toth A, Weltner J. Prognosis of untreated liver metastasis from rectal cancer. *Acta Chir Hung* 1997;36:106.
13. Burke D, Allen-Mersh TG. Colorectal liver metastases. *Postgrad Med J* 1996;72:464.
14. Rougier P, Milan C, Lazorthes F, et al. Prospective study of prognostic factors in patients with unresected hepatic metastases from colorectal cancer. *Br J Surg* 1995;82:1397.
15. Palmer M, Petrelli NJ, Herrera L. No treatment option for liver metastases from colorectal adenocarcinoma. *Dis Colon Rectum* 1989;32:698.
16. Petrelli NJ, Bonnheim DC, Herrera LO. A proposed classification system for liver metastases from colorectal carcinoma. *Dis Colon Rectum* 1984;27:249.
17. Sutliff VE, Doppman JL, Gibril F, et al. Growth of newly diagnosed, untreated metastatic gastrinomas and predictors of growth patterns. *J Clin Oncol* 1997;15:2420.
18. Lahr CJ, Soong S-J, Cloud G, et al. A multifactorial analysis of prognostic factors in patients with liver metastases from colorectal carcinoma. *J Clin Oncol* 1983;1:720.
19. Finan PJ, Marshall RJ, Cooper EH, Giles GR. Factors affecting survival in patients presenting with synchronous hepatic metastases from colorectal cancer: a clinical and computer analysis. *Br J Surg* 1985;72:373.
20. Ayoub J-P, Hess KR, Abbruzzese MC, et al. Unknown primary tumors metastatic to liver. *J Clin Oncol* 1998;16:2105.
21. Seregard S, Kock E. Prognostic indicators following enucleation for posterior uveal melanoma. *Acta Ophthalmol Scand* 1995;73:340.
22. Kath R, Hayungs J, Bornfeld N, et al. Prognosis and treatment of disseminated uveal melanoma. *Cancer* 1993;72:2219.
23. Weber HC, Venzon DJ, Fishbein VA, et al. Determinants of metastatic rate and survival in patients with Zollinger-Ellison syndrome (ZES): a prospective long-term study. *Gastroenterology* 1995;108:1637.

24. Yu F, Venzon DJ, Serrano J, et al. Prospective study of the clinical course, prognostic factors, causes of death, and survival in patients with long-standing Zollinger-Ellison syndrome. *J Clin Oncol* 1999;17:615.
25. Fraker DL, Jensen RT. Cancer of the endocrine system. In: DeVita VT Jr, Hellman S, Rosenberg SA, eds. *Cancer: principles and practice of oncology.* Philadelphia: Lipincott–Raven, 1997:1678.
26. Ravikumar TS, Buenaventura S, Salem RR, D'Andrea B. Intraoperative ultrasonography of liver: detection of occult liver tumors and treatment by cryosurgery. *Cancer Detect Prev* 1994;18:131.
27. Inoue E, Fujita M, Hosomi N, et al. Double phase CT arteriography of the whole liver in the evaluation of hepatic tumors. *J Comput Assist Tomogr* 1998;22:64.
28. Johnson DBS, Francis IR, Eckhauser FE, Knol JA, Chang AE. Dual-phase helical CT of nonfunctioning islet cell tumors. *J Comput Assist Tomogr* 1998;22:59.
29. Ch'en IY, Katz DS, Jeffrey B Jr, et al. Do arterial phase helical CT images improve detection or characterization of colorectal liver metastases? *J Comput Assist Tomogr* 1997;21:391.
30. Oliver JH III, Baron RL, Federle MP, Jones BC, Sheng R. Hypervascular liver metastases: do unenhanced and hepatic arterial phase CT images affect tumor detection? *Radiology* 1997;205:709.
31. Paley MR, Ros PR. Hepatic metastases: computed tomography versus magnetic resonance imaging in 1997. *Endoscopy* 1997;29:524.
32. Reimer P, Tombach B. Hepatic MRI with SPIO: detection and characterization of focal liver lesions. *Eur Radiol* 1998;8:1198.
33. Awaya H, Ito K, Jonjo K, et al. Differential diagnosis of hepatic tumors with delayed enhancement at gadolinium-enhanced MRI: a pictorial essay. *Clin Imaging* 1998;22:180.
34. Delbeke D, Martin WH, Sandler MP, et al. Evaluation of benign vs malignant hepatic lesions with positron emission tomography. *Arch Surg* 1998;133:510.
35. Gibril F, Reynolds JC, Doppman JL, et al. Somatostatin receptor scintigraphy: its sensitivity compared with that of other imaging methods in detecting primary and metastatic gastrinomas. A prospective study. *Ann Intern Med* 1996;125:26.
36. Termanini B, Gibril F, Reynbolds JC, et al. Value of somatostatin receptor scintigraphy: a prospective study in gastrinoma of its effect on clinical management. *Gastroenterology* 1997;112:335.
37. Lamberts SWJ, Bakker WH, Reubi JC, Krenning EP. Somatostatin receptor imaging in the localization of endocrine tumors. *N Engl J Med* 1990;323:1246.
38. Termanini B, Gibril F, Doppman JL, et al. Distinguishing small hepatic hemangiomas from vascular liver metastases in gastrinoma: use of a somatostatin-receptor scintigraphic agent. *Radiology* 1997;202:151.
39. Emond JC, Kelley SC, Heffron TG, et al. Surgical and anesthetic management of patients undergoing major hepatectomy using total vascular exclusion. *Liver Transplant Surg* 1996;2:91.
40. Melendez JA, Arslan V, Fischer ME, et al. Perioperative outcomes of major hepatic resections under low central venous pressure anesthesia: blood less, blood transfusion, and the risk of postoperative renal dysfunction. *J Am Coll Surg* 1998;187:620(abst).
41. Nakamura S, Suzuki S, Konno H, Baba S. Resection of metastatic liver tumors with special reference to hepatic venous system. *Hepato-gastroenterology* 1998;45:24.
42. Miyazaki M, Ito H, Nakagawa K, et al. Aggressive surgical resection for hepatic metastases involving the inferior vena cava. *Am J Surg* 1999;177:294.
43. Cady B, Jenkins RL, Steele GD Jr, et al. Surgical margin in hepatic resection for colorectal metastasis. A critical and improvable determinant of outcome. *Ann Surg* 1998;227:566.
44. Ohlsson B, Stenram U, Tranberg K-G. Resection of colorectal liver metastases: 25-year experience. *World J Surg* 1998;22:268.
45. Fong Y, Fortner J, Sun RL, Brennan MF, Blumgart LH. Clinical score for predicting recurrence after hepatic resection for metastatic colorectal cancer. *Ann Surg* 1999;230:309.
46. Fuhrman GM, Curley SA, Hohn DC, Roh MS. Improved survival after resection of colorectal liver metastases. *Ann Surg Oncol* 1995;2:537.
47. Fong Y, Cohen AM, Fortner JG, et al. Liver resection for colorectal metastases. *J Clin Oncol* 1997;15:938.
48. Scheele J, Stang R, Altendorf-Hofmann A, Paul M. Resection of colorectal liver metastases. *World J Surg* 1995;19:59.
49. Nadig DE, Wade TP, Fairchild RB, Virgo KS, Johnson FE. Major hepatic resection. Indications and results in a National Hospital System from 1988 to 1992. *Arch Surg* 1997;132:115.
50. Bakalakos EA, Kim JA, Young DC, Martin EW Jr. Determinants of survival following hepatic resection for metastatic colorectal cancer. *World J Surg* 1998;22:399.
51. Doci R, Bignami P, Montalto F, Gennari L. Prognostic factors for survival and disease-free survival in hepatic metastases from colorectal cancer treated by resection. *Tumori* 1995;81:143(abst).
52. Jamison RL, Donohue JH, Nagorney DM, et al. Hepatic resection for metastatic colorectal cancer results in cure for some patients. *Arch Surg* 1997;132:505.
53. Cady B, Stone MD, McDermott WV Jr, et al. Technical and biological factors in disease-free survival after hepatic resection for colorectal cancer metastases. *Arch Surg* 1992;127:561.
54. Ambiru S, Miyazaki M, Isono T, et al. Hepatic resection for colorectal metastases. *Dis Colon Rectum* 1999;42:632.
55. Hughes KS, Simon R, Songhorabodi S. Resection of the liver for colorectal carcinoma metastases: a multi-institutional study of indications for resection. *Surgery* 1988;103:278.
56. Kin T, Nakajima Y, Kanehiro H, et al. Repeat hepatectomy for recurrent colorectal metastases. *World J Surg* 1998;22:1087.
57. Fernandez-Trigo V, Shamsa F, Sugarbaker PH. Repeat liver resections from colorectal metastasis. *Surgery* 1995;117:296.
58. Bines SD, Doolas A, Jenkins L, Millikan K, Roseman DL. Survival after repeat hepatic resection for recurrent colorectal hepatic metastases. *Surgery* 1996;120:591.
59. Adam R, Bismuth H, Castaing D, et al. Repeat hepatectomy for colorectal liver metastases. *Ann Surg* 1997;225:51.
60. Chiappa A, Zbar AP, Biella F, Staudacher C. Survival after repeat hepatic resection for recurrent colorectal metastases. *Hepato-gastroenterology* 1999;46:1065.
61. Curley SA, Roh MS, Chase JL. Adjuvant hepatic arterial infusion chemotherapy after curative resection of colorectal liver metastases. *Am J Surg* 1993;66:746.
62. Lorenz M, Staib-Sebler E, Loch B. The value of postoperative hepatic arterial infusion following curative liver resection. *Anticancer Res* 1997;17:3825.
63. Okuno K, Shigeoka H, Lee YS. Adjuvant hepatic arterial IL-2 and MMC, 5-FU after curative resection of colorectal liver metastases. *Hepato-gastroenterology* 1996;43:688.
64. Ambiru S, Miyazaki H, Ito H. Adjuvant regional chemotherapy after hepatic resection for colorectal metastases. *Br J Surg* 1999;86:1025.
65. Kokudo N, Seki M, Ohta H, et al. Effects of systemic and regional chemotherapy after hepatic resection for colorectal metastases. *Ann Surg Oncol* 1998;5:706.
66. Nonami T, Takeuchi Y, Yasui M. Regional adjuvant chemotherapy after partial hepatectomy for metastatic colorectal carcinoma. *Semin Oncol* 1997;24:S6-130.
67. Kemeny MM, Adak S, Lipsitz S. Results of the intergroup [Eastern Cooperative Oncology Group (ECOG) and Southwest Oncology Group (SWOG)] prospective randomized study of surgery alone versus continuous hepatic artery infusion of FuDR and continuous systemic infusion of 5FU after hepatic resection for colorectal liver metastases. *Proc Am Soc Clin Oncol* 1999;18:1012.
68. Kemeny N, Huang Y, Cohen A, et al. Hepatic arterial infusion of chemotherapy after resection of hepatic metastases from colorectal cancer. *N Engl J Med* 1999;341:2039.
69. Lygidakis NJ, Ziras N, Parissis J. Resection versus resection combined with adjuvant pre- and post-operative chemotherapy—immunotherapy for metastatic colorectal liver cancer. A new look at an old problem. *Hepato-gastroenterology* 1995;42:155.
70. Lorenz M, Müller H-H, Schramm H, et al. Randomized trial of surgery versus surgery followed by adjuvant hepatic arterial infusion with 5-fluorouracil and folinic acid for liver metastases of colorectal cancer. *Ann Surg* 1998;228:756.
71. Fraschini G, Fleishman G, Charnsangavej C. Continuous 5-day infusion of vinblastine for percutaneous hepatic arterial chemotherapy for metastatic breast cancer. Cancer Treat Rep 1987;11:1005.
72. Ochiai T, Sasako M, Mizuno S. Hepatic resection for metastatic tumours from gastric cancer: analysis of prognostic factors. *Br J Surg* 1994;81:1175.
73. Bines SD, England G, Deziel DJ, et al. Synchronous, metachronous and multiple hepatic resections of liver tumors originating from primary gastric tumors. *Surgery* 1993;114:799.
74. Thompson GB, van Heerden JA, Grant CS, Carney JA, Ilstrup DM. Islet cell carcinomas of the pancreas: a twenty-year experience. *Surgery* 1988;104:1011.
75. Declore R, Friesen SR. Gastrointestinal neuroendocrine tumors. *J Am Coll Surg* 1994;178:188.
76. Godwin JD. Carcinoid tumors: an analysis of 2837 cases. *Cancer* 1975;36:560.
77. Chen H, Hardacre JM, Uzra A, Cameron JL, Choti MA. Isolated liver metastases from neuroendocrine tumors: does resection prolong survival? *J Am Coll Surg* 1998;187:88.
78. Ihse I, Persson B, Tibblin S. Neuroendocrine metastases of the liver. *World J Surg* 1995;19:76.
79. Raab R, Nussbaum KT, Behrend M, Weimann A. Liver metastases of breast cancer: results of liver resection. *Anticancer Res* 1998;18:2231.
80. Elias D, Lasser PH, Montrucolli D, Bonvallot S, Spielmann M. Hepatectomy for liver metastases from breast cancer. *Eur J Surg Oncol* 1995;21:510.
81. Jaques DP, Coit DG, Casper ES, Brennan MF. Hepatic metastases from soft-tissue sarcoma. *Ann Surg* 1995;221:392.
82. Schwartz SI. Hepatic resection for noncolorectal nonneuroendocrine metastases. *World J Surg* 1995;19:72.
83. Salmon RJ, Levy C, Plancher C, et al. Treatment of liver metastases from uveal melanoma by combined surgery-chemotherapy. *Eur J Surg Oncol* 1998;24:127.
84. Harrison LE, Brennan MF, Newman E, et al. Hepatic resection for noncolorectal, nonneuroendocrine metastases: a fifteen-year experience with ninety-six patients. *Surgery* 1997;121:625.
85. Fujisaki S, Takayama T, Shimada K, et al. Hepatectomy for metastatic renal cell carcinoma. *Hepato-gastroenterology* 1997;44:817.
86. Niederhuber JE, Ensminger W, Gyves J, et al. Regional chemotherapy of colorectal cancer metastatic to the liver. *Cancer* 1984;53:1336.
87. Daly JM, Butler J, Kemeny N, et al. Predicting tumor response in patients with colorectal hepatic metastases. *Ann Surg* 1985;202:384.
88. Fordy C, Burke D, Earlam S, Twort P, Allen-Mersh TG. Treatment interruptions and complications with two continuous hepatic artery floxuridine infusion systems in colorectal liver metastases. *Br J Surg* 1995;82:1023.
89. Curley SA, Chase JL, Roh MS, Hohn DC. Technical considerations and complications associated with the placement of 180 implantable hepatic arterial infusion devices. *Surgery* 1993;114:928.
90. Kemeny NE, Ron IG. Hepatic arterial chemotherapy in metastatic colorectal patients. *Semin Oncol* 1999;26:524.
91. Burke D, Earlan S, Fordy C, Allen-Mersh TG. Effect of aberrant hepatic arterial anatomy on tumour response to hepatic artery infusion of floxuridine for colorectal liver metastases. *Br J Surg* 1995;82:1098.
92. Sigurdson ER, Ridge JA, Daly JM. Fluorodeoxyuridine uptake by human colorectal hepatic metastases after hepatic artery infusion. *Surgery* 1986;100:285.
93. Bloom AI, Gordon RL, Ahl KH, et al. Transcatheter embolization for the treatment of misperfusion after hepatic artery chemoinfusion pump implantation. *Ann Surg Oncol* 1999;6:350.
94. Campbell KA, Burns RC, Sitzmann JV, et al. Regional chemotherapy devices: effect of experience and anatomy on complications. *J Clin Oncol* 1993;11:822.
95. Breedis C, Young G. Blood supply of neoplasms of the liver. *Am J Pathol* 1954;30:969.
96. Dorr RT, Von Hoff DD. Floxuridine. In: Anonymous, *Cancer chemotherapy handbook.* Norwalk, CT: Appleton & Lange, 1994:489.
97. Ensminger WD, Rosowsky A, Raso V, et al. A clinical-pharmacologic evaluation of hepatic arterial infusions of 5-fluoro-2'-deoxyuridine and 5-fluorouracil. *Cancer Res* 1978;38:3784.
98. Ensminger WD, Walker SC, Stetson PL, et al. Clinical pharmacology of hepatic arterial infusions of 5-bromo-2'-deoxyuridine. *Cancer Res* 1996;54:2121.

99. Sigurdson ER, Ridge JA, Kemeny N, Daly JM. Tumor and liver drug uptake following hepatic artery and portal vein infusion in man. *J Clin Oncol* 1987;5:1836.
100. Venook AP. Update on hepatic intra-arterial chemotherapy. *Oncology* 1997;11:947.
101. Kemeny NE. Regional chemotherapy of colorectal cancer. *Eur J Cancer* 1995;31A:1271.
102. Stagg RJ, Venook AP, Chase JL, et al. Alternating hepatic intra-arterial floxuridine and fluorouracil: a less toxic regimen for treatment of liver metastases from colorectal cancer. *J Natl Cancer Inst* 1991;83:423.
103. Kemeny N, Seiter K, Conti JA, et al. Hepatic arterial floxuridine and leucovorin for unresectable liver metastases from colorectal carcinoma. New dose schedules and survival update. *Cancer* 1994;73:1134.
104. Kemeny N, Conti JA, Cohen A, et al. Phase II study of hepatic arterial floxuridine, leucovorin, and dexamethasone for unresectable liver metastases from colorectal carcinoma. *J Clin Oncol* 1994;12:2288.
105. Hohn DC, Stagg RJ, Friedman MA, et al. A randomized trial of continuous intravenous versus hepatic intraarterial floxuridine in patients with colorectal cancer metastatic to the liver: the Northern California oncology group trial. *J Clin Oncol* 1989;7:1646.
106. Kemeny N, Daly J, Reichman B, et al. Intrahepatic or systemic infusion of fluorodeoxyuridine in patients with liver metastases from colorectal carcinoma. *Ann Intern Med* 1987;107:459.
107. Chang AE, Schneider PD, Sugarbaker PH, et al. A prospective randomized trial of regional versus systemic continuous 5-fluorodeoxyuridine chemotherapy in the treatment of colorectal liver metastases. *Ann Surg* 1987;206:685.
108. Martin JK, O'Connel MJ, Wieand HS, et al. Intra-arterial floxuridine vs systemic fluorouracil for hepatic metastases from colorectal cancer. *Arch Surg* 1990;125:1022.
109. Allen-Mersh TG, Earlam S, Fordy C, Abrams K, Houghton J. Quality of life and survival with continuous hepatic-artery floxuridine infusion for colorectal liver metastases. *Lancet* 1994;344:1255.
110. Rougier P, LaPlanche A, Huguier M, et al. Hepatic arterial infusion of floxuridine in patients with liver metastases from colorectal carcinoma: long-term results of a prospective randomized trial. *J Clin Oncol* 1992;10:1112.
111. Harmantas A, Rothstein LE, Langer B. Regional versus systemic chemotherapy in the treatment of colorectal carcinoma metastatic to the liver. Is there a survival difference? Meta-analysis of the published literature. *Cancer* 1996;78:1639.
112. Anonymous. Reappraisal of hepatic arterial infusion in the treatment of nonresectable liver metastases from colorectal cancer. *J Natl Cancer Inst* 1999;88:252.
113. Okuno K, Yasutomi M, Kon M, et al. Intrahepatic interleukin-2 with chemotherapy for unresectable liver metastases: a randomized multicenter trial. *Hepato-gastroenterology* 1999;46:1116.
114. Minoyama A, Yoshikwa M, Ebara M, et al. Study of repeated arterial infusion chemotherapy with a subcutaneously implanted reservoir for advanced hepatocellular carcinoma. *J Gastroenterol* 1995;30:356.
115. Cantore M, Fiorentini G, Aitini E, et al. Intra-arterial hepatic carboplatin-based chemotherapy for ocular melanoma metastatic to the liver. Report of a phase II study. *Tumori* 1994;80:37.
116. Leyvraz S, Spataro V, Bauer J, et al. Treatment of ocular melanoma metastatic to the liver by hepatic arterial chemotherapy. *J Clin Oncol* 1997;15:2589.
117. Mavligit GM, Charnsangavej C, Carrasco CH, et al. Regression of ocular melanoma metastatic to the liver after hepatic arterial chemoembolization with cisplatin and polyvinyl sponge. *JAMA* 1988;260:974.
118. Jung HY, Shim HJ, Kwak BK. Percutaneously implantable catheter-port system for chemotherapeutic infusion through the hepatic artery. *AJR Am J Roentgenol* 1999;172:641.
119. Maruyama M, Takamatsu S, Nagahama T. Adjuvant hepatic arterial infusion chemotherapy for gastrointestinal malignancies with removable hepatoarterial catheter. *J Surg Oncol* 1999;71:246.
120. Fraschini G, Fleishman G, Yap HY. Percutaneous hepatic arterial infusion of cisplatin for metastatic breast cancer. *Cancer Treat Rep* 1987;71:313.
121. Copur MS, Matamoros A, Capadano M. Alternating hepatic arterial infusion and systemic chemotherapy for liver metastases from colorectal cancer: a phase II trial using intermittent percutaneous hepatic arterial access. *Proc Am Soc Clin Oncol* 1999;18:955.
122. Ravikumar TS, Pizzorno G, Bodden W, et al. Percutaneous hepatic vein isolation and high-dose hepatic arterial infusion chemotherapy for unresectable liver tumors. *J Clin Oncol* 1994;12:2723.
123. Ku Y, Tominaga M, Iwasaki T, et al. Percutaneous hepatic venous isolation and extracorporeal charcoal hemoperfusion for high-dose intraarterial chemotherapy in patients with colorectal hepatic metastases. *Surg Today* 1996;26:305.
124. Dazzi C, Fiorentini G, Davitti B. High-dose intra-arterial plus intraperitoneal chemotherapy combined with hemofiltration in liver metastases from colorectal cancer. *Tumori* 1994;80:204.
125. Taton G, Ghanem G, Pandin P. First results of a clinical pilot study on intraarterial chemotherapy with haemofiltration of locally advanced gastrointestinal cancers. *Acta Chir Belg* 1996;96:206.
126. Ausman RK. Development of a technic for isolated perfusion of the liver. *N Y State J Med* 1961;61:3393.
127. Alexander HR, Bartlett DL, Libutti SK. Isolated hepatic perfusion: a potentially effective treatment for patients with metastatic or primary cancers confined to the liver. *Cancer J Sci Am* 1998;4:2.
128. Diebel LN, Wilson RF, Bender J, Paules B. A comparison of passive and active shunting for bypass of the retrohepatic IVC. *J Trauma* 1991;31:987.
129. Barker WC, Andrich MP, Alexander HR, Fraker DL. Continuous intraoperative external monitoring of perfusate leak using I-131 human serum albumin during isolated perfusion of the liver and limbs. *Eur J Nucl Med* 1995;22:1242.
130. de Vries MR, Rinkes IH, van de Velde CJ, et al. Isolated hepatic perfusion with tumor necrosis factor alpha and melphalan: experimental studies in pigs and phase I data from humans. *Recent Results Cancer Res* 1998;147:107.
131. de Vries MR, Rinkes IH, van de Velde CJ, et al. Isolated hepatic perfusion with tumor necrosis factor alpha and melphalan: experimental studies in pigs and phase I data from humans. *Recent Results Cancer Res* 1998;147:107.
132. Oldhafer KJ, Lang H, Frerker M, et al. First experience and technical aspects of isolated liver perfusion for extensive liver metastasis. *Surgery* 1998;123:622.
133. Hafström L, Naredi P. Isolated hepatic perfusion with extracorporeal oxygenation using hyperthermia TNFα and melphalan: Swedish experience. *Rec Res Cancer Res* 1998;147:120.
134. Alexander HR Jr, Bartlett DL, Libutti SK, et al. Isolated hepatic perfusion with tumor necrosis factor and melphalan for unresectable cancers confined to the liver. *J Clin Oncol* 1998;16:1479.
135. Bartlett DL, Libutti SK, Alexander HR. Results of isolated hepatic perfusion (IHP) in patients with regionally advanced unresectable colorectal cancer. *Soc Surg Oncol* 1999;14(abst).
136. Kim YH, Ajani JA, Carrasco CH. Selective hepatic arterial chemoembolization for liver metastases in patients with carcinoid tumor or islet cell carcinoma. *Cancer Invest* 1999;17:474.
137. Bavisotto LM, Patel NH, Althaus SJ, et al. Hepatic transcatheter arterial chemoembolization alternating with systemic protracted continuous infusion 5-fluorouracil for gastrointestinal malignancies metastatic to liver: a phase II trial of the Puget Sound Oncology Consortium (PSOC 1104). *Clin Cancer Res* 1999;5:95.
138. Leichman CG, Jacobson JR, Modiano M. Hepatic chemoembolization combined with systemic infusion of 5-fluorouracil and bolus leucovorin for patients with metastatic colorectal carcinoma: a Southwest Oncology Group pilot trial. *Cancer* 1999;86:775.
139. D'Agostino HB, Solinas A. Percutaneous ablation therapy for hepatocellular carcinomas [comment]. *AJR Am J Roentgenol* 1995;164:1165.
140. Arnott J. *On the treatment of cancer by the regulated application of an anaesthetic temperature.* London: J. Churchill, 1851:32.
141. Rubinsky B, Lee CY, Bastacky J, Onik G. The process of freezing and the mechanism of damage during hepatic cryosurgery. *Cryobiology* 1990;27:85.
142. Ravikumar TS, Steele GD. Hepatic cryosurgery. *Surg Clin North Am* 1989;69:433.
143. Stewart GJ, Preketes A, Horton M, Ross WB, Morris DL. Hepatic cryotherapy: double-freeze cycles achieve greater hepatocellular injury in man. *Cryobiology* 1995;69:215.
144. Cuschieri A, Crosthwaite G, Shimi S, et al. Hepatic cryotherapy for liver tumors. Development and clinical evaluation of a high-efficiency insulated multineedle probe system for open and laparoscopic use. *Surg Endosc* 1995;9:483.
145. Onik G, Kane R, Steele G, et al. Monitoring hepatic cryosurgery with sonography. *AJR Am J Roentgenol* 1986;147:665.
146. Zhou XD, Tang ZY, Yu YQ, et al. The role of cryosurgery in the treatment of hepatic cancer: a report of 113 cases. *J Cancer Res Clin Oncol* 1993;120:100.
147. Onik GM, Atkinson D, Zemel R, Weaver ML. Cryosurgery of liver cancer. *Semin Surg Oncol* 1993;9:309.
148. Ravikumar TS, Kane R, Cady B, et al. A 5-year study of cryosurgery in the treatment of liver tumors. *Arch Surg* 1991;126:1520.
149. Preketes AP, Caplehorn JR, King J, et al. Effect of hepatic artery chemotherapy on survival of patients with hepatic metastases from colorectal carcinoma treated with cryotherapy. *World J Surg* 1995;19:768.
150. Seifert JK, Junginger T, Morris DL. A collective review of the world literature on hepatic cryotherapy. *J R Coll Surg Edinburg* 1998;43:141.
151. Dale PS, Souza JW, Brewer DA. Cryosurgical ablation of unresectable hepatic metastases. *J Surg Oncol* 1998;68:242.
152. Yeh KA, Fortunato L, Hoffman JP, Eisenberg BL. Cryosurgical ablation of hepatic metastases from colorectal carcinomas. *Am Surg* 1997;63:63.
153. Weaver ML, Ashton JG, Zemel R. Treatment of colorectal liver metastases by cryotherapy. *Semin Surg Oncol* 1998;14:163.
154. Seifert JK, Morris DL. Prognostic factors after cryotherapy for hepatic metastases from colorectal cancer. *Ann Surg* 1998;228:201.
155. Seifert JK, Morris DL. Indicators of recurrence following cryotherapy for hepatic metastases from colorectal cancer. *Br J Surg* 1999;86:234.
156. Seifert JK, Morris DL. Repeat hepatic cryotherapy for recurrent metastases from colorectal cancer. *Surgery* 1999;125:233.
157. Iannitti DA, Heniford T, Hale J, Grundfest-Broniatowski S, Gagner M. Laparoscopic cryoablation of hepatic metastases. *Arch Surg* 1998;133:1011.
158. Heniford BT, Arca MJ, Jannitti DA, Walsh RM, Gagner M. Laparoscopic cryoablation of hepatic metastases. *Semin Surg Oncol* 1998;15:194.
159. Korpan NN. Hepatic cryosurgery for liver metastases. Long-term follow-up. *Ann Surg* 1997;225:193.
160. Bilchik AJ, Sarantou T, Foshag LJ, Giuliano AE, Ramming KP. Cryosurgical palliation of metastatic neuroendocrine tumors resistant to conventional therapy. *Surgery* 1997;122:1040.
161. Bilchik AJ, Sarantou T, Wardlaw JC, Ramming KP. Cryosurgery causes a profound reduction in tumor markers in hepatoma and noncolorectal hepatic metastases. *Am Surg* 1997;63:796.
162. Crews KA, Kuhn JA, McCarty TM, et al. Cryosurgical ablation of hepatic tumors. *Am J Surg* 1997;174:614.
163. Seifert JK, Cozzi PJ, Morris DL. Cryotherapy for neuroendocrine liver metastases. *Semin Surg Oncol* 1998;14:175.
164. Polk W, Fong Y, Karpeh M, Blumgart LH. A technique for the use of cryosurgery to assist hepatic resection. *J Am Coll Surg* 1995;180:171.
165. Johnson LB, Krebs TL, Van Echo D, et al. Cytoablative therapy with combined resection and cryosurgery for limited bilobar hepatic colorectal metastases. *Am J Surg* 1997;174:610.
166. Dwerryhouse SJ, Seifert JK, McCall JL, et al. Hepatic resection with cryotherapy to involved or inadequate resection margin (edge freeze) for metastases from colorectal cancer. *Br J Surg* 1998;85:185.
167. Wallace JR, Christians KK, Pitt HA, Quebbeman EJ. Cryotherapy extends the indications for treatment of colorectal liver metastases. *Surgery* 1999;126:766.
168. Ross WB, Horton M, Bertolino P, Morris DL. Cryotherapy of liver tumours—a practical guide. *HPB Surg* 1995;8:167.
169. Stubbs RS, Alwan MH, Booth MWC. Hepatic cryotherapy and subsequent hepatic arterial chemotherapy for colorectal metastases to the liver. *HPB Surg* 1998;11:97.
170. Rodriguez-Bigas MA, Klippenstein D, Meropol NJ. A pilot study of cryochemotherapy for hepatic metastases from colorectal cancer. *Cryobiology* 1996;33:600.

171. Murakami R, Yoshimatsu S, Yamashita Y, et al. Treatment of hepatocellular carcinoma: value of percutaneous microwave coagulation. *AJR Am J Roentgenol* 1995;164:1159.
172. Hamazoe R, Hirooka Y, Ohtani S, Katoh T, Kaibara N. Intraoperative microwave tissue coagulation as treatment for patients with nonresectable hepatocellular carcinoma. *Cancer* 1995;75:794.
173. Seki T, Wakabayashi M, Nakagawa T, et al. Ultrasonically guided percutaneous microwave coagulation therapy for small hepatocellular carcinoma. *Cancer* 1994;74:817.
174. Solbiati L, Goldberg SN, Ierace T, et al. Hepatic metastases: percutaneous radio-frequency ablation with cooler-tip electrodes. *Radiology* 1997;205:367.
175. Livraghi T, Goldberg SN, Monti F, et al. Saline-enhanced radio-frequency tissue ablation in the treatment of liver metastases. *Radiology* 1997;202:205.
176. Nagata Y, Hiraoka M, Nishimura Y, et al. Clinical results of radiofrequency hyperthermia for malignant liver tumors. *Int J Radiat Oncol Biol Phys* 1997;38:359.
177. Cuschieri A, Bracken J, Boni L. Initial experience with laparoscopic ultrasound-guided radiofrequency thermal ablation of hepatic tumours. *Endoscopy* 1999;31:318.
178. Curley SA, Izzo F, Delrio P, et al. Radiofrequency ablation of unresectable primary and metastatic hepatic malignancies: results in 123 patients. *Ann Surg* 1999;230:9.
179. Kainuma O, Asano T, Aoyama H. Combined therapy with radiofrequency thermal ablation and intra-arterial infusion chemotherapy for hepatic metastases from colorectal cancer. *Hepato-gastroenterology* 1999;46:1071.
180. Bown SG. Phototherapy of tumours. *World J Surg* 1983;7:700.
181. Amin Z, Harries SA, Lees WR, Bown SG. Interstitial tumour photocoagulation. *Endosc Surg Allied Technol* 1993;1:224.
182. van Hillegersberg R, van Staveren HJ, Kort WJ, Zondervan PE, Terpstra OT. Interstitial Nd:YAG laser coagulation with a cylindrical diffusing fiber tip in experimental liver metastases. *Lasers Surg Med* 1994;14:124.
183. Gewiese B, Beuthan J, Fobbe F, et al. Magnetic resonance imaging-controlled laser-induced interstitial thermotherapy. *Invest Radiol* 1994;29:345.
184. Amin Z, Bown SG, Lees WR. Local treatment of colorectal liver metastases: a comparison of interstitial laser photocoagulation (ILP) and percutaneous alcohol injection (PAI). *Clin Radiol* 1993;48:166.
185. Amin Z, Donald JJ, Masters A, et al. Hepatic metastases: interstitial laser photocoagulation with real-time US monitoring and dynamic CT evaluation of treatment. *Radiology* 1993;187:339.
186. Nolsoe CP, Torp-Pedersen S, Burcharth F, et al. Interstitial hyperthermia of colorectal liver metastases with a US-guided Nd-YAG laser with a diffuser tip: a pilot clinical study. *Radiology* 1993;187:333.
187. Ebara M, Ohto M, Sugiura N. Percutaneous ethanol injection for the treatment of small hepatocellular carcinoma. Study of 95 patients. *J Gastroenterol Hepatol* 1990;5:616.
188. Shiina S, Tagawa K, Niwa Y. Percutaneous ethanol injection therapy for hepatocellular carcinoma: results in 146 patients. *AJR Am J Roentgenol* 1993;160:1023.
189. Lencioni R, Pinto F, Armillotta N. Long-term results of percutaneous ethanol injection therapy for hepatocellular carcinoma in cirrhosis: a European experience. *Eur Radiol* 1997;7:514.
190. Giorgio A, Tarantino L, Mariniello N. Percutaneous ethanol injection under general anesthesia for hepatocellular carcinoma: 3 year suvival in 112 patients. *Eur J Ultrasound* 1998;8:201.
191. Castellano L, Calandra M, Del Vecchio Blanco C. Predictive factors of survival and intrahepatic recurrence of hepatocellular carcinoma in cirrhosis after percutaneous ethanol injection: analysis of 71 patients. *J Hepatol* 1997;27:862.
192. Livraghi T, Benedini V, Lazzaroni S. Long term results of single session percutaneous ethanol injection in patients with large hepatocellular carcinoma. *Cancer* 1998;83:48.
193. Castells A, Bruix J, Bru C. Treatment of small hepatocellular carcinoma in cirrhotic patients: a cohort study comparing surgical resection and percutaneous ethanol injection. *Hepatology* 1993;18:1121.
194. Kotoh K, Sakai H, Sakamoto S. The effect of percutaneous ethanol injection therapy on small solitary hepatocellular carcinoma is comparable to that of hepatectomy. *Am J Gastroenterol* 1994;89:194.
195. Livraghi T, Bolondi L, Buscarini L. No treatment, resection and ethanol injection in hepatocellular carcinoma: a retrospective analysis of survival in 391 patients with cirrhosis. *J Hepatol* 1995;22:522.
196. Orlando A, Cottone M, Virdone R. Treatment of small hepatocellular carcinoma associated with cirrhosis by percutaneous ethanol injection. A trial with a comparison group. *Scand J Gastroenterol* 1997;32:598.
197. Lencioni R, Paolicchi A, Moretti M. Combined transcatheter arterial chemoembolization and percutaneous ethanol injection for the treatment of large hepatocellular carcinoma: local therapeutic effect and long-term survival rate. *Eur Radiol* 1998;8:439.
198. Allgaier HP, Deibert P, Olschewski M. Survival benefit of patients with inoperable hepatocellular carcinoma treated by a combination of transarterial chemoembolization and percutaneous ethanol injection—a single-center analysis including 132 patients. *Int J Cancer* 1998;79:601.
199. Phillips R, Karnofsky DA, Hamilton LD, Nickson JJ. Roentgen therapy of hepatic metastases. *AJR Am J Roentgenol* 1954;71:826.
200. Ingold DK, Reed GB, Kaplan HS, Bagshaw MA. Radiation hepatitis. *AJR Am J Roentgenol* 1965;93:200.
201. Ogata K, Hizawa A, Yoshida M. Hepatic injury following irradiation—a morphologic study. *Tukushima J Exp Med* 1963;9:240.
202. Reed GB, Cos AJ. The human liver after radiation injury. A form of veno-occlusive disease. *Am J Pathol* 1966;48:597.
203. Lawrence TS, Robertson JM, Anscher MS, et al. Hepatic toxicity resulting from cancer treatment. *Int J Radiat Oncol Biol Phys* 1995;31:1237.
204. Jirtle RL, Anscher MS, Alati T. Radiation sensitivity of the liver. *Adv Radiat Biol* 1990;14:269.
205. Byfield JE, Calabro-Jones P, Klisak LL, Kulhanian F. Pharmacologic requirements for obtaining sensitization of human tumor cells in vitro to combined 5-fluorouracil or forafur and x rays. *Int J Radiat Oncol Biol Phys* 1982;8:1923.
206. Bruso CE, Shewach DS, Lawrence TS. Fluorodeoxyuridine-induced radiosensitization and inhibition of DNA double strand break repair in human colon cancer cells. *Int J Radiat Oncol Biol Phys* 1990;19:1411.
207. Heimburger DK, Shewach DS, Lawrence TS. The effect of fluorodeoxyuridine on sublethal damage repair in human colon cancer cells. *Int J Radiat Oncol Biol Phys* 1991;21:983.
208. McCracken JD, Weatherall TJ, Oishi N, Janaki L, Boyer C. Adjuvant intrahepatic chemotherapy with mitomycin and 5-FU combined with hepatic irradiation in high-risk patients with carcinoma of the colon: a Southwest Oncology Group phase II pilot study. *Cancer Treat Rep* 1985;69:129.
209. Hadda E, Le Bourgeois JP, Kuentz M, Lobo P. Liver complications in lymphomas treated with a combination of chemotherapy and radiotherapy: preliminary results. *Int J Radiat Oncol Biol Phys* 1983;9:1313.
210. Schacter L, Crum E, Spitzer T, et al. Fatal radiation hepatitis: a case report and review of the literature. *Gynecol Oncol* 1986;24:373.
211. Andrews JD, Walker SC, Ackermann RJ, et al. Hepatic radioembolization with Yttrium-90 containing glass microspheres: preliminary results and clinical follow-up. *J Nucl Med* 1993;35:1637.
212. Anderson JH, Goldberg JA, Bessent RG. Glass yttrium-90 microspheres for patients with colorectal liver metastases. *Radiother Oncol* 1988;25:137.
213. Herba MJ, Ilescas FF, Thirlwell MP. Hepatic malignancies: improved treatment with intraarterial Y-90. *Radiology* 1988;169:311.
214. Gray BN, Anderson JE, Burton MA. Regression of liver metastases following treatment with yttrium-90 microspheres. *Aust N Z J Surg* 1992;62:105.
215. Thomas DS, Nauta RJ, Rodgers JE. Intraoperative high-dose rate interstitial irradiation of hepatic metastases from colorectal carcinoma. Results of a phase I–II trial. *Cancer* 1993;71:1977.
216. Donath D, Nori D, Turnbull A, Kaufman N, Fortner JG. Brachytherapy in the treatment of solitary colorectal metastases to the liver. *J Surg Oncol* 1990;44:55.
217. Ten Haken RK, Lawrence TS, McShan DL, et al. Technical considerations in the use of 3-D beam arrangements in the abdomen. *Radiother Oncol* 1991;22:19.
218. Lawrence TS, Tesser RJ, Ten Haken RK. An application of dose volume histograms to the treatment of intrahepatic malignancies with radiation therapy. *Int J Radiat Oncol Biol Phys* 1990;19:1041.
219. McGinn CJ, Ten Haken RK, Ensminger WD, et al. Treatment of intrahepatic cancers with radiation doses based on a normal tissue complication probability model. *J Clin Oncol* 1998;16:2246.
220. Mohuiddin M, Chen E, Ahmad N. Combined liver radiation and chemotherapy for palliation of hepatic metastases from colorectal cancer. *J Clin Oncol* 1996;14:722.
221. Lawrence TS, Dworzanin LM, Walker-Andrews SC. Treatment of cancers involving the liver and porta hepatis with external beam irradiation and intraarterial hepatic fluorodeoxyuridine. *Int J Radiat Oncol Biol Phys* 1990;20:555.
222. Robertson JM, Lawrence TS, Walker S, et al. The treatment of colorectal liver metastases with conformal radiation therapy and regional chemotherapy. *Int J Radiat Oncol Biol Phys* 1995;32:445.
223. Dawson LA, McGinn NJ, Ensminger W, Walker SC, Lawrence TS. Preliminary results of escalated focal liver radiation and hepatic artery floxuridine for unresectable liver malignancies. *Proc Am Soc Clin Oncol* 1999;18:86a.
224. Habib NA, Hodgson HJF, Lemoine N, Pignatelli M. A phase I/II study of hepatic artery infusion with twp53-CMV-Ad in metastatic malignant liver tumours. *Human Gene Ther* 1999;10:2019.
225. Bartlett DL, Fong Y. Solitary small hepatic metastases: when and how? In: Blumgart L, Poston G, eds. *Clinical challenges in hepatobiliary and pancreatic surgery.* Oxford: Isis Medical Media Limited, 1999.
226. Wagman LD, Kemeny MM, Leong L, et al. A prospective, randomized evaluation of the treatment of colorectal cancer metastatic to the liver. *J Clin Oncol* 1990;8:1885.
227. Ruszniewski P, Rougier P, Legmann P. Hepatic arterial chemoembolization in patients with liver metastases of endocrine tumors. *Cancer* 1993;71:2624.
228. Therasse E, Briettmayer F, Roche A. Transcatheter chemoembolization of progressive carcinoid liver metastasis. *Radiology* 1993;189:541.
229. Marlink RG, Lokich JJ, Robins JR, Clouse ME. Hepatic arterial embolization for metastatic hormone-secreting tumors. *Cancer* 1990;65:2227.
230. Perry LJ, Stuart K, Stokes KR, Clouse ME. Hepatic arterial chemoembolization for metastatic neuroendocrine tumors. *Surgery* 1994;116:1111.
231. Ajani JA, Carrasco CH, Charnsagavej C, et al. Islet cell tumors metastatic to the liver: effective palliation by sequential hepatic artery embolization. *Ann Intern Med* 1988;108:340.
232. San-Altamira PM, Spence LD, Huberman MS. Selective chemoembolization in the management of hepatic metastases in refractory colorectal carcinoma. *Dis Colon Rectum* 1997;40:770.
233. Tellez C, Benson IAB, Lyster MT. Phase II trial of chemoembolization for the treatment of metastatic colorectal carcinoma to the liver and review of the literature. *Cancer* 1998;82:1250.
234. McGinn CJ, Robertson JM, Lawrence TS, et al. A phase I/II trial of chemoembolization with mitomycin C following hepatic arterial fluorodeoxyuridine/leucovorin and whole liver radiotherapy for patients with intrahepatic malignancies. *Cancer Ther* 1998;1:88.
235. Martinelli DJ, Wadler S, Bakal CW. Utility of embolization or chemoembolization as second line treatment in patients with advanced or recurrent colorectal carcinoma. *Cancer* 1994;74:1706.
236. Goldberg JA, Kerr DJ, Wilmott N, McKillop JH, McArdle CS. Regional chemotherapy for colorectal liver metastases: a phase II evaluation of targeted hepatic arterial 5-fluorouracil for colorectal liver metastases. *Br J Surg* 1990;77:1238.
237. Hunt TM, Flowerdew ADS, Birch SJ, et al. Prospective randomized controlled trial of hepatic arterial embolization or infusion chemotherapy with 5-fluorouracil and degradable starch microspheres for colorectal liver metastases. *Br J Surg* 1990;77:779.
238. Civalleri D, Pector C, Hakansson L, et al. Treatment of patients with irresectable liver metastases from colorectal cancer by chemo-occlusion and degradable starch microspheres. *Br J Surg* 1994;81:1338.

239. Alexander HR, Bartlett DL, Fraker DL, Libutti SK. Regional treatment strategies for unresectable primary or metastatic cancer confined to the liver. In: DeVita VT Jr, Hellman S, Rosenberg SA, eds. *Cancer: principles and practice of oncology.* Philadelphia: Lippincott, 1996:1.
240. Rossi S, di Stasi M, Buscarini E, et al. Percutaneous radiofrequency interstitial thermal ablation in the treatment of small hepatocellular carcinoma: report of 24 patients. *Cancer J Sci Am* 1995;1:73.
241. Allgaier HP, Diebert P, Zuber I, Olschewski M, Blum HE. Percutaneous radiofrequency interstitial thermal ablation of small hepatocellular carcinoma. *Lancet* 1999;353:1676.
242. Borgelt BB, Gelber R, Brady LW, Griffin T, Hendrickson FR. The palliation of hepatic metastases: results of the Radiation Therapy Oncology Group pilot study. *Int J Radiat Oncol Biol Phys* 1981;7:587.
243. Liebel SA, Pajak TF, Massullo V. A comparison of misonidazole sensitized radiation therapy to radiation therapy alone for the palliation of hepatic metastases: results of a Radiation Therapy Oncology Group randomized prospective trial. *Int J Radiat Oncol Biol Phys* 1987;7:105.
244. Prasad B, Lee M-S, Henderson FR. Irradiation of hepatic metastases. *Int J Radiat Oncol Biol Phys* 1977;2:129.
245. Russell AH, Clyde C, Wasserman TH, Turner SS, Rotman M. Accelerated hyperfractionated hepatic irradiation in the management of patients with liver metastases: results of the RTOG dose escalating protocol. *Int J Radiat Oncol Biol Phys* 1993;27:117.
246. Friedman M, Cassidy M, Levine M, et al. Combined modality therapy of hepatic metastasis. Northern California Oncology Group Pilot Study. *Cancer* 1979;44:906.
247. Friedman M, Cassidy M, Levine M, et al. Combined modality therapy of hepatic metastasis. Northern California Oncology Group Pilot Study. *Cancer* 1979;44:906.
248. Herbsman H, Hassan A, Gardner B. Treatment of hepatic metastases with a combination of hepatic artery infusion chemotherapy and external radiotherapy. *Surg Gynecol Obstet* 1978;127:13.
249. Lokich J, Kinsella T, Perri J, Malcomb A, Clouse M. Concomitant hepatic radiation and intraarterial fluorinated pyrimidines therapy: correlation of liver scan, liver function tests, and plasma CEA with tumor response. *Cancer* 1981;48:2569.
250. Raju PL, Maruyama Y, DeSimone P, MacDonald J. Treatment of liver metastases with a combination of chemotherapy and hyperfractionated external radiation therapy. *Am J Clin Oncol* 1987;10:41.
251. Rotman M, Kuruvilla AM, Choi K. Response of colo-rectal hepatic metastases to concomitant radiotherapy and hyperfractionated external radiation therapy. *Int J Radiat Oncol Biol Phys* 1986;12:2179.
252. Sherman DM, Weichselbaum R, Order SE, et al. Palliation of hepatic metastasis. *Cancer* 1978;41:2013.
253. Webber BM, Soderberg CH, Leone LA, Rege VB, Glicksman AS. A combined treatment approach to management of hepatic metastases. *Cancer* 1978;42:1087.
254. Wiley AL, Wirtanen GW, Stephenson JA, et al. Combined hepatic artery 5-fluorouracil and irradiation of liver metastases. A randomized study. *Cancer* 1989;64:1783.
255. Wolberding P, Friedman MA, Resser KJ, Phillip TL. Therapy of liver tumors metastatic from colorectal cancer with whole-liver radiation combined with 5-FU, adriamycin, and methotrexate. *Cancer Chemother Pharmacol* 1982;9:17.

SECTION 4

HOLLY K. BROWN
JOHN H. HEALEY

Metastatic Cancer to the Bone

Most of the more than 560,000 people in the United States who die of cancer each year have tumor metastasis.[1] Bone is the third most common organ involved by metastasis, behind lung and liver.[2] In breast cancer, bone is the second most common site of metastatic spread, and 90% of patients dying of breast cancer have bone metastasis.[2,3] Breast and prostate cancers metastasize to bone most frequently, which reflects the high incidence of both of these tumors, as well as their prolonged clinical courses.[2] Other tumors that commonly cause symptomatic bone metastases include kidney and thyroid cancer and multiple myeloma. The increasing age and size of the population leads to an increased number of cases of cancer. This, coupled with longer patient survival, increases the incidence of metastatic lesions to bone. Patients with bone metastasis from breast cancer have an average 2-year survival from the time of presentation with their first bone lesion. As more patients are living with bone metastases, the challenge is to improve their quality of life.

Current management of skeletal cancer involves a multimodality approach, including systemic therapies (chemotherapy, hormone and immune therapies, and other drugs such as bisphosphonates), radiation (external-beam and targeted radioisotopes), and surgery. Medical, radiation, surgical, and orthopedic oncologists, with diagnostic assistance from radiologists and pathologists, form a multidisciplinary team to manage these complex and often very ill patients. Early detection and aggressive management of metastases should be the goal, to maintain and maximize patients' quality of life and functional level. Nihilism is no longer appropriate. However, due to economic considerations and a dearth of data to support intensive surveillance for metastases, physicians may be lulled into a sense of complacency. Currently, care is optimized in only a fraction of patients with bone metastases.

PRESENTATION

Patients with metastatic disease to the skeleton most often present with pain as the principal symptom. The pain associated with bone metastasis comprises two components: biologic and mechanical. *Biologic pain* is related to the local release of cytokines and chemical mediators by the tumor cells, periosteal irritation, stimulation of intraosseous nerves by these mediators, and the pressure or mass effect of the tumor tissue within the bone. *Mechanical pain* is related to the loss of bone strength and stiffness caused by the metastatic lesion, which leads to activity-related pain. Mechanical pain is seen most often with osteolytic lesions but can also occur in osteoblastic lesions, because the disorganized pattern of tumor-related bone lacks structural integrity.

The initial pain pattern of a metastasis mimics that of primary bone tumors and osteonecrosis. The symptoms are intermittent but may be sharp and severe. Pain tends to be worst at night and may be partially relieved by activity. As the lesion progresses, symptoms become more constant and take on a more mechanical character.

Patients with metastatic disease can present with a pathologic fracture. Pathologic fractures most often occur with osteolytic lesions. The majority of pathologic fractures are seen in patients with metastatic breast cancer. In one study, the incidence of pathologic fracture was 8% in 1800 cancer patients, with 53% of those fractures occurring secondary to breast cancer metastases.[4] Other malignant culprits for pathologic fracture in this series were kidney in 11%, lung in 8%, thyroid in 5%, lymphoma in 5%, and prostate in 3%.[4]

Hypercalcemia of malignancy occurs in 5% to 10% of patients with bone metastasis and is seen predominantly in breast cancer, multiple myeloma, and squamous carcinomas of the lung. Thirty percent of patients with breast cancer will develop hypercalcemia during the course of their disease.[5] Hypercalcemia is mediated by multiple factors: local osteolysis caused by the skeletal metastasis, parathyroid-like hormone released by the tumor cells and having both a local (paracrine) and systemic (endocrine) effect, and disuse osteolysis related to the immobility of these patients.

Neurologic abnormality related to spinal cord compression can occur with spinal metastasis. Knowledge of the course and character of neurologic symptoms is important in directing the radiographic evaluation and treatment plan. Neurologic compromise secondary to spinal involvement with metastasis has a major impact on quality of life and function.

Systemic issues include generalized debilitation, leading to immobility. Bed rest exacerbates hypercalcemia and can lead to atelectasis, thromboembolic disease, and skin pressure necrosis. In addition, patients with systemic malignancy who are immobilized are prone to developing disseminated intravascular coagulation. Careful screening for these conditions is imperative in the management of these patients. Doppler ultrasound tests are a convenient and sensitive way of identifying deep venous thrombosis. Loss of ambulatory ability is a poor prognostic factor in metastatic disease, particularly spine disease. Performance status should be specifically quantified as part of the preoperative evaluation.[6,7]

PATHOGENESIS

The pattern of metastatic involvement of bone is related to blood flow. Metastases most commonly occur in the more heavily vascularized parts of the skeleton, particularly the axial skeleton, including the ribs and the vertebral column, as well as the proximal ends of the long bones.[8] Batson's plexus is a low-pressure, high-volume, valveless system of vertebral veins that communicates with the pelvic venous plexus. The high number of vertebral metastases in prostate cancer is attributed to Batson's plexus. Arterial spread may also be important. The patterns of metastatic distribution to bone seen after intracardiac injection of tumor cells in animal models are similar to those seen clinically.[9] Histopathologic evaluation of metastatic development and distribution in these animal models confirms that the metastatic lesions originate at the terminal end of the major arteries supplying the bone.[10] Specific radiographic evaluation of metastatic disease in the spine indicates a role for arterial spread as well.[11]

A great deal of research has been conducted recently into the mechanisms of tumor metastasis. Tumor metastasis is believed to be related to several factors: angiogenesis, which allows for primary tumor growth and subsequent access to the systemic circulation to colonize secondary sites[9]; adhesion via cell surface molecules, which allow tumor cells to attach to other cells and to extracellular matrix components; invasion, mediated by proteolytic enzymes such as matrix metalloproteinases,[12,13] which allow tumor cells to pass across extracellular matrix barriers; and proliferation, which is mediated by growth factors and the uncoupling of the normal mechanisms of cell growth and suppression. Of particular interest in bone metastases is the ability of tumor-released factors to cause osteolysis. There is evidence that this osteolysis is mediated by stimulation of osteoclastic bone resorption by tumor cytokines and direct bone degradation by tumor cells.[8] Matrix metalloproteinases appear not only to mediate the ability of tumor cells to invade via basement membrane hydrolysis but also directly to degrade bone matrix.[12,13] Better understanding of the molecular mechanisms of metastatic tumor spread allows for the development of new therapies to target these areas, as well as more effective use of existing techniques.

DIAGNOSTIC EVALUATION

A careful history and physical examination, including careful breast or prostate evaluations and thyroid palpation, remain the cornerstone for identification of the site of primary disease in patients who present with a bone lesion without a known primary tumor. In those patients with a history of cancer and a new bone lesion, the coexistence of disease other than metastasis must be ruled out.

Plain radiographs remain the most specific test for diagnosing bone diseases. Scintigraphy is extremely sensitive and practical for use in metastatic evaluation, because it can screen the entire body at one time. Certainly, any abnormality found on bone scan should be correlated with plain radiographs.

Metastatic disease is characterized by the presence of multiple bone lesions. Single metastases occur rarely and must be differentiated from primary bone tumors. Typically, the so-called solitary metastasis is merely the first of many lesions to be identified. Thyroid and renal cancers and myeloma (plasmacytoma) are the most likely to present with an isolated metastasis. Even patients with these favorable cancers typically develop widespread disease, suggesting that there is unrecognized dissemination of cancer at the time that the first bone metastasis is identified.[14,15]

Diagnostic workup entails the use of several laboratory tests to help narrow the differential diagnosis and identify the primary site of disease. A basic screening panel includes a complete blood cell count with platelets, to evaluate for anemia and myelosuppression; serum calcium, phosphorus, and alkaline phosphatase levels to identify markers of bone turnover and evaluate for hypercalcemia; and assessment of serum electrolytes, liver function tests, and an erythrocyte sedimentation rate for systemic evaluation. If clinically indicated, such additional specific tests as the following can be ordered: parathyroid hormone level, to evaluate for metabolic bone disease; serum or urine protein electrophoresis or b_2-microglobulin if multiple myeloma or lymphoma is suspected; or specific markers such as cancer antigen 125 for breast cancer or prostate-specific antigen for prostate cancer. Biochemical markers of bone turnover, such as urine N-telopeptide and urine deoxypyridinoline, also are noted to have a significant association with the probability of bone metastasis.[16]

The technique of screening blood and marrow with polymerase chain reaction (PCR) or reverse transcriptase–PCR (RT-PCR) for specific tumor cell DNA is being investigated as a tool for diagnosing metastatic disease and following the response to systemic therapy. The attraction of PCR technology is that it can detect a very small number of tumor cells (1 tumor cell in 10 to 100 million normal cells), potentially identifying patients with marrow or circulating cancer cells who are at risk for the development of clinical metastases. As technology improves, the genetics of tumors are being better defined and the PCR technique is becoming more standardized, such that it is likely to prove a useful adjuvant in the diagnosis of, and monitoring of therapeutic response in, bone metastases patients.[17]

Chest radiography and computed tomographic (CT) scans of the chest, abdomen, and pelvis also are used in the diagnostic workup of bone lesions without a known primary lesion. These studies can help to identify the primary tumor in 85% of patients, as well as identifying additional sites of metastatic disease.[18] They are particularly useful because the predominant lesions causing metastases of unknown origin are lung and renal carcinomas.

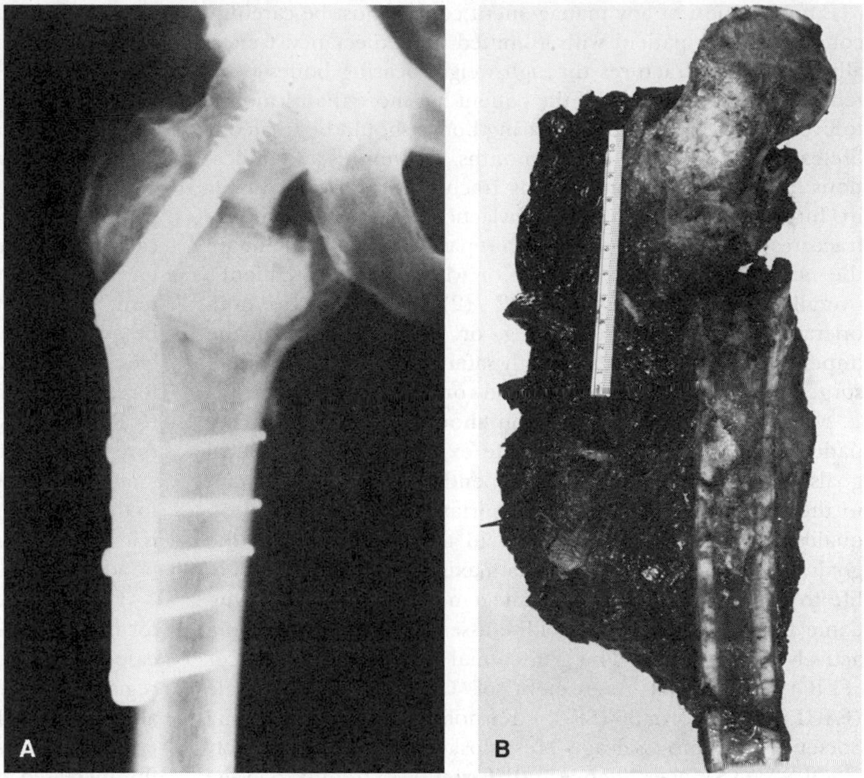

FIGURE 52.4-1. Dedifferentiated chondrosarcoma presents as a predominantly lytic, destructive lesion in an older patient, mimicking a metastatic lesion. Internal fixation in this case is inappropriate, and a biopsy is needed to exclude the presence of a primary bone tumor, particularly with a solitary bone lesion such as this. **A:** Compression hip screw and cement used for internal fixation of a fractured chondrosarcoma. **B:** Gross appearance of the resected bone after removing the screw. White-gray cartilage percolates across the fracture site and down the intramedullary canal.

A firm diagnosis must be obtained before a fracture involving a solitary bone lesion is fixed internally. Magnetic resonance imaging (MRI) can be helpful in differentiating pathologic fracture due to osteoporosis from that due to metastatic disease, particularly in the spine. MRI is also helpful in delineating the soft tissue extension and component of tumors involving bone. When the diagnosis cannot be discerned from clinical information and the baseline tests of plain films and bone scan, MRI can be a helpful diagnostic adjuvant.[19,20]

Solitary bone lesions warrant a biopsy before treatment. Primary bone sarcomas occur in the same population under consideration for metastatic disease. Lytic phases of dedifferentiated chondrosarcoma and Paget's sarcoma can also produce pathologic fractures (Fig. 52.4-1). In addition, metabolic bone disease is in the differential diagnosis of skeletal abnormalities in this older age group (older than 40 years). Brown tumor of hyperparathyroidism can produce multiple lytic bone lesions, and osteoporosis can lead to pathologic fracture, particularly in the spine. Osteomalacia can mimic metastatic disease by producing multiple fractures throughout the skeleton, resulting in a bone scan indistinguishable from that seen with multiple metastatic foci. All of these entities must be distinguished from metastatic disease, as the management of such conditions is very different from that for metastases.

Bone scan can be of further assistance in planning a biopsy. When the symptomatic lesion involves a weight-bearing bone, biopsy worsens the fracture risk by creating a new hole in the bone cortex. Bone scan can identify other bone lesions and possibly locate one that can be subjected to biopsy with greater ease and less morbidity.

CT-guided needle biopsy is usually satisfactory when the lesion is osteolytic, offering diagnostic accuracy of 80%. When the lesion is osteoblastic or exhibits a thick overlying cortical rim, inserting a needle and obtaining an adequate tissue sample is extremely difficult. Such cases necessitate open surgical biopsy. Regardless of whether the biopsy of a weight-bearing bone is performed by closed or open technique, there is a genuine fracture risk. Weight bearing must be protected until bone healing occurs, which experimentally has been shown to require at least 6 weeks. Sufficient tissue for immunohistochemical studies should always be obtained to improve the ability of the biopsy to yield a definitive tissue diagnosis.

TREATMENT GOALS

There are four main goals in managing patients with metastatic disease to the skeleton: pain relief, preservation and restoration of function, skeletal stabilization, and local tumor control (e.g., relief of tumor impingement on normal structures, prevention of release of chemical mediators that have local and systemic effects).

Symptomatic relief is usually satisfactory from a combination of radiation and medical therapy. Most patients without a fracture do not require surgery for the bone metastasis; however, fractures are best treated by operative internal fixation. Even when fractures can heal by nonoperative therapy, the protracted treatment time required for closed management is inappropriate, as this period generally is increased by the presence of tumor negatively affecting the ability of the fracture to heal. The goals of surgical intervention vary in metastatic tumor patients. Primary goals are to allow immediate weight bearing and return to activity, not necessarily to promote fracture healing. Prosthetic replacement and stabilization with polymethyl methacrylate are frequently selected, whereas such techniques would be avoided in the treatment of nonneoplastic fractures.

The duration of any management course must be carefully considered in a patient with a limited life expectancy. Generally, pathologic fractures through weight-bearing bones (e.g., femur) should be treated if the patient has more than 1 month to live, whereas non–weight-bearing bones should be treated if life expectancy is more than 3 months. Definitions and indications for treatment of impending fractures are discussed later in Impending Fractures: Prophylactic Fixation. Impending fractures warrant fixing if (1) such repair will help to eliminate the need for narcotic analgesics or will reduce the patient's overall pain by approximately 50%, (2) equally effective nonoperative treatments are lacking, or (3) treatment for the impending fracture is significantly safer or more effective than surgery once the bone has fractured completely.

Management and intervention should be tailored to the patient's overall prognosis and life expectancy. The medical goals of patient comfort and independence are predominant in these situations. Increasing importance is being placed on quality-of-life issues and measures in these patients, and the goals of therapy have shifted from maximization of duration of life to maximization of pain management and function. Outcome measures and quality-of-life assessment tools are being actively investigated. The Functional Living Index–Cancer (FLIC); Functional Assessment of Cancer Therapy Scale (FACT), Short Form 36 (SF-36); Karnofsky Scale; International Society of Limb Salvage–Musculoskeletal Tumor Society (ISOLS-MSTS) assessment; and Toronto Extremity Salvage Score (TESS) are tools currently in use. The Memorial Sloan-Kettering Cancer Center (MSKCC) is moving toward use of the FACT and away from the FLIC.[21–24] Other tools are being developed and validated that pertain not only to patients with cancer but also to those with musculoskeletal issues. These new functional assessments strive to combine the recently developed American Academy of Orthopaedic Surgeons Modems with oncologic assessments such as the Health-Related Quality of Life (HR-QOL) and the FACT. These tools will become increasingly important in evaluating the efficacy and value of new therapies for patients with metastatic bone disease.

IMAGING OF BONE LESIONS

PLAIN RADIOGRAPHY

Plain radiographs are the foundation of evaluation, surgical planning, and monitoring of metastatic lesions of bone. Radiographs are a fast, inexpensive, and readily available technique for evaluating bone metastases. Other techniques may be more sensitive, but radiographs give the best integration of overall bone structure and alignment and correlate best with clinical features. Therefore, plain radiography should be the first test ordered in the evaluation of bone pain.

Three radiographic patterns of metastatic disease typically are seen: osteolytic, osteoblastic, and mixed.[25] Because of variations in the bone microenvironment and clonal differentiation of tumors, different patterns may exist throughout the skeleton or within a single bone. Prostate cancer metastases are classically osteoblastic, breast cancer bone lesions usually show a lytic or mixed pattern, and lung cancer metastases are predominantly lytic. Radiographic variability can also be seen during the course of therapy, as the radiographic appearance of a lesion changes during treatment. Osteoblastic areas seen radiographically correspond to the reaction of the host bone to the metastases, not to the tumor itself. Fast-growing tumors tend to have a lytic or mixed pattern, and the bone reaction cannot keep pace with the rate of tumor growth. Reactive bone often lacks mechanical strength, as it forms in a random pattern lacking normal Haversian structure.

Periosteal changes can also occur with metastatic disease to the bone. Rapidly growing tumor can elevate the periosteum, causing an irregular periosteal reaction. Lung cancer and prostate cancer with cortical involvement commonly display this pattern. Stress fracture through the underlying bone lesion can also be associated with periosteal reaction. Nevertheless, periosteal elevation is usually a hallmark of primary bone neoplasm; therefore, sarcoma should be excluded when periostitis is present.

Radiographs assist greatly in surgical planning. Disease spreads diffusely within long bones. In patients with proximal femoral metastases in whom radiographic evaluation is confined to the hip, potential lesions distal in the femur are overlooked. It is important that the entire bone be imaged, so that all lesions can be addressed and stabilized during the same operative procedure.

Finally, sequential radiographs of involved areas are important for monitoring response to treatment, local recurrence, and disease progression. X-ray films of subsequently symptomatic regions are important for identifying further metastatic foci, allowing for early intervention and management. In addition, certain tumors (most notably multiple myeloma) do not stimulate the increased bone turnover required for positive readings on bone scan. Patients with such tumors are best evaluated for other foci of skeletal disease by a plain radiographic skeletal survey.

BONE SCINTIGRAPHY

Technetium diphosphonate bone scans are extremely valuable in identifying occult bone lesions and diagnosing metastatic disease. Whereas 30% to 50% of bone mineral must be lost for a lesion to appear on plain radiograph, bone scans show skeletal involvement much earlier. Bone scintigraphy is an essential part of cancer staging for skeletal metastases, identifies sites of both symptomatic and asymptomatic lesions, and locates potential sources of referred pain. In 85% of patients with metastatic cancer to bone and a single symptomatic focus, multiple additional foci will be seen on bone scan. Certain tumors, such as lung cancer and melanoma, grow rapidly and evoke little reactive bone formation, leading to false-negative scans. In addition, multiple myeloma is notorious for resulting in false-negative bone scans. Bone scans lack anatomic detail and, although they can localize the site of involvement, the specific characteristics of the lesion are not visualized. Bone scan results should be correlated with additional imaging modalities such as plain-film radiographs or CT scans.

Bone scintigraphy can be used to evaluate the response to chemotherapy, hormone therapy, or radiation therapy, by reflecting the biology of the lesion and the extent of the host response. The method has been most useful in evaluating treatment in breast cancer patients. Up to 15% of patients will experience an initial increase in radioisotope uptake on bone scan with treatment, called the *flare phenomenon*.[26] This reflects new bone formation as a healing response around the quiescent lesion. Over time, the surrounding bone heals, and osteoblast activity, which is estimated by the uptake on bone scan, will diminish. Development of additional scintigraphic lesions early in treatment does not necessarily reflect disease progression. Instead, this can reflect healing and ossification of areas where the tumor did not evoke a response initially.

A limitation of the bone scan technique is that it measures solely the metabolic activity of the bone and not its structural integrity. Biologic control of the tumor does not necessarily translate into mechanical restoration of the skeleton. Therefore, close correlation of follow-up bone scan information with plain radiographs or CT scanning is necessary.

COMPUTED TOMOGRAPHY

CT scanning is very effective in evaluating the three-dimensional integrity of bone and the characteristics of lesions identified on bone scan.[27] It helps to confirm the presence of metastatic disease, particularly when evaluating lesions localized to the pelvic and shoulder girdles. Spine lesions can also be imaged by CT scans but are better evaluated by MRI in most circumstances.[28] CT scanning is superior to MRI in demonstrating bone mineral content and cortical integrity and is therefore more useful in evaluating the structure of the involved bone. MRI will often show extensive marrow involvement in a bone, even though the structural integrity is preserved. CT scans help to discriminate between the presence of cellular and structurally significant disease.

MAGNETIC RESONANCE IMAGING

MRI is an excellent technique for evaluating bone marrow, which is the first site of metastatic involvement of bone.[19,28–30] Though it is very sensitive for this indication, it is nonspecific. However, MRI is particularly useful in round cell lesions such as leukemia, lymphoma, and multiple myeloma, which replace the marrow space. The high fat content of bone marrow translates to high signal intensity or brightness on T1-weighted and low signal intensity on T2-weighted images. This essentially provides a contrast medium juxtaposed to the tumor, which, because of its high water content, has high signal intensity on T2-weighted and low signal intensity on T1-weighted images.

MRI provides good three-dimensional anatomic information throughout the skeleton and is excellent in defining soft tissues and delineating soft tissue involvement by tumor. In the spine, MRI is especially useful because it is sensitive for tumor involvement, shows sagittal and cross-sectional alignment, and details tumor present in the spinal canal, dural impingement, and spinal cord compression. MRI is particularly helpful in distinguishing between pathologic fracture due to osteoporosis and that due to tumor. This is particularly important for postmenopausal women, who may experience both metastatic disease and osteoporosis.[30] MRI is useful in the evaluation of skeletal metastatic disease but is an imperfect discriminator and therefore requires close correlation with additional studies and the clinical situation.

POSITRON EMISSION TOMOGRAPHY

Positron emission tomographic (PET) scanning is a newly used tool in the evaluation of metastatic bone disease. Though nonspecific, PET scans identify metabolically active areas by their differential uptake of radiolabeled glucose ([^{18}F]fluorodeoxyglucose), similar to the technetium labeling of areas of bone turnover in bone scan. PET scanning was used in a study of 29 patients with bone metastases and an unknown primary tumor in whom conventional diagnostic workup had failed.[31] In these 29 patients, all but one known metastatic site was visualized by PET scan, and additional metastatic sites were identified in 5 patients. PET was able to identify the primary tumor in only 7 of these 29 patients (24%).[31] Data regarding the current clinical relevance of PET scanning are limited. The technique is used predominantly in an investigational role. However, PET scanning does show utility in selected instances for diagnosis of bone and soft tissue metastases.

THERAPEUTIC MODALITIES

Multiple therapeutic modalities are available in the armamentarium for management of metastatic disease to bone. These modalities comprise three broad categories: systemic therapy, radiation therapy, and surgery.

SYSTEMIC THERAPY

Systemic therapies include chemotherapy, bone marrow transplantation, hormone therapy, immunotherapy, and medications. The medical oncologist directs the majority of systemic management. Systemic chemotherapy with antineoplastic agents is primary tumor–specific. Until the development of bisphosphonates, no specific drugs were directed to the general entity of bone metastases. Bisphosphonates have shown great utility in the management of patients with metastatic bone lesions, most notably in cases of breast cancer and multiple myeloma.

Bisphosphonates

Bisphosphonates are stable analogs of naturally occurring inorganic pyrophosphate. They inhibit the precipitation of calcium phosphate *in vitro* and biologic calcification *in vivo*. They also inhibit bone resorption, particularly that occurring in certain metastatic lesions of bone. The mechanism by which bisphosphonates inhibit bone resorption is inhibition of osteoclasts by interruption of the †mevalonate metabolic pathway and, possibly, by causing osteoclast apoptosis as well.

First-generation bisphosphonates such as clodronate and etidronate, second-generation drugs such as tiludronate and pamidronate, and third-generation medications such as ibandronate and zoledronate, have differing potencies and effects. The bisphosphonates are generally safe compounds with few side effects. The drugs are not metabolized in the human body, with 50% to 60% of each dose rapidly absorbed by bone, followed by slow renal elimination; the other 40% to 50% is rapidly excreted by the kidneys.

Bisphosphonates have proven efficacy in the treatment of hypercalcemia of malignancy, Paget's disease of bone, osteoporosis, and bone metastasis in breast cancer and multiple myeloma. Pamidronate is approved for use in hypercalcemia of malignancy, Paget's disease, and bone metastasis, whereas therapeutic approval for other bisphosphonates varies: Etidronate is approved for use in hypercalcemia of malignancy, alendronate for the treatment of osteoporosis, and tiludronate for the treatment of Paget's disease. Pamidronate, 90 mg by IV infusion every 3 to 4 weeks, is the dosing regimen that has been shown to provide the most rapid onset of pain reduction and increased mobility, with minimal side effects.[32] Several large randomized trials have been performed to analyze the efficacy of pamidronate in the management of metastatic bone lesions.[33]

Theriault et al.[33] reported on their randomized, double-blind trial involving 372 patients with breast cancer and at least one lytic bone lesion who received standard hormone therapy. The skeletal morbidity was significantly reduced in the patients receiving pamidronate; however, there was no significant difference in survival or objective bone response rate. Not until 6 months was a difference observed between the two groups, at which point the curves diverged, with an upward shift of the placebo group's skeletal event rate curve, though the curves for both treatment groups maintained the same slope.[34]

Hortobagyi et al.[35] reported on their randomized, double-blind trial involving 382 patients with metastatic breast cancer and lytic bone lesions who were receiving standard chemotherapy. Again, a significantly decreased risk of bone lesion complications was seen in the pamidronate group as compared to the placebo group.[35]

Berenson et al.[36] reported on their randomized, double-blind trial of 392 patients with stage III myeloma and at least one lytic bone lesion who were receiving either first-line or second-line antimyeloma chemotherapy. There was a significant reduction in skeletal events in the pamidronate group, although survival was not different between the pamidronate and placebo patients. Again, the skeletal event curves of the pamidronate and placebo groups diverged, in this instance from the initiation of the study. The placebo group's curve was shifted upward, but the two curves continued to have similar slopes, as was seen in the breast cancer trials.[36]

In light of the outcomes from these large randomized trials, bisphosphonates have been added to the therapeutic armamentarium in the treatment of bone metastasis due to breast cancer or multiple myeloma. Although bisphosphonates have not been proven to be efficacious in managing bone metastasis due to other tumors, theoretically these compounds should be of value in all cancers causing lytic bone lesions. There is also evidence that bisphosphonates may actually prevent the development of bony metastases. In several animal models, injected tumor cells failed to establish colonies in bone that had been pretreated with bisphosphonate.[37,38] The magnitude of benefit of bisphosphonates in other cancers, its possible early use in the management of patients with metastatic disease, and the details of the mechanism of action of this drug class all warrant further investigation. Despite their benefits, bisphosphonates act over the course of several months. When a more rapid response is needed, radiation therapy or surgery (or both) still are required.

Chemotherapy and Hormone Therapy

Because of the significant percentage of patients with breast cancer who develop metastatic bone lesions, the effects of chemotherapy and hormone therapy on these lesions have been investigated. The goals of chemotherapy and hormone therapy in patients with metastatic disease involving bone are pain control, disease stabilization, and reduction of the risk of morbid skeletal events (e.g., pathologic fracture). In a series of patients from the M. D. Anderson Cancer Center who were treated with 5-fluorouracil, doxorubicin, and cyclophosphamide, bone lesions showed an 18% complete and a 65% partial response to the regimen. Hormone-sensitive breast carcinoma has a predilection to metastasize to bone; therefore, hormone therapy can be effective in these cases. As with other therapies, a peritreatment lesion "flare" may occur that makes the evaluation of overall response difficult. However, the use of chemotherapy and hormone therapy in metastatic breast cancer has been shown to prolong survival and can render patients better able to respond to bone lesion–specific therapy such as bisphosphonates or systemic radionuclides, reducing overall skeletal morbidity.[39]

RADIATION THERAPY

External-Beam Radiation Therapy

Radiation is an important technique for treatment of tumor that has metastasized to the bone. The indications for radiation therapy are pain relief and suppression of local tumor growth. Suppression of local tumor growth is important in the treatment of impending fractures, after surgical fixation of metastatic lesions, and in the treatment of neural compression. This is exemplified by irradiation of tumor for spinal cord compression. Tumor reduction and pain relief can begin immediately, particularly for very radiosensitive round cell tumors. Thoughtfully planned treatment with high-energy radiation causes minimal morbidity, and the benefits far exceed the risks in most situations. Radiation is of therapeutic value in patients with localized symptomatic lesions and should be considered in all but the few cases in whihc either the disease is very responsive to systemic treatment (e.g., germ cell tumor, lymphoma) or the lesions are resectable for cure.

Despite its efficacy, radiation therapy should not be used indiscriminately. Marrow fibrosis can be a late complication that precludes chemotherapy. The radiation oncologist must collaborate with the medical oncologist and surgical personnel to optimize treatment. This interdisciplinary cooperation is critical in the management of an impending fracture. Occasionally, a lesion will heal with radiation therapy, especially if it is mechanically protected.[40] Treating an isolated lesion may allow the radiation oncologist to use a narrower radiation field. However, fracture and subsequent intramedullary fixation necessitate treatment of the entire bone, which can be difficult to implement if a radiation treatment protocol has already been applied within the new field.

More than 80% of patients with a limited number of well-localized bony metastases can be treated effectively by external-beam irradiation.[41–43] High-dose radiation, coupled with careful subsequent observation, is suitable, cost-effective oncologic management for most cancer patients, especially if the available chemotherapeutic regimens are not well established. Radiation may render the patient asymptomatic and control the disease for an extended period.

Patients with numerous areas of skeletal involvement require systemic therapy. Chemotherapy or endocrine therapy is the most appropriate. If symptoms persist over the course of several months, alternative management for localized disease should be considered. External-beam irradiation to the most symptomatic or potentially troublesome areas should be used to supplement systemic therapy. Hemibody radiation or systemic radionuclide therapy should be considered for widely disseminated bone disease.[44–46]

Metastases involving the spine are best treated early in the course of disease because progression can produce grave morbidity.[47,48] The spine should be braced until the lesions can heal. Irradiation of a weight-bearing bone such as the femur should be undertaken only after careful evaluation of the potential fracture risk produced by the underlying lesion (as discussed later in Impending Fractures: Prophylactic Fixation). There is an increased risk of pathologic fracture in the peri-irradiation period due to an induced hyperemic response at the periphery of the tumor. This weakens the adjacent bone and increases the risk of spontaneous fracture. Mechanical protection is important until the bone's structural integrity has been restored. Identification of disease progression and management of associated morbidity by the treatment team is very important during the course of irradiation, because other treatments often are suspended during this time. The interdisciplinary communication essential for high-quality treatment often is best provided through a medical practice environment in which all the specialists are in geographic proximity. This minimizes the need for excessive travel by the patient who is experiencing a limitation in mobility and is at risk for fracture.

TREATMENT PLANNING. Data from a patient's medical history, physical examination, bone radiographs, and three-dimensional imaging help to direct radiation fields. The radiation fields should include all soft tissue masses as identified by the aforementioned studies. The margin of normal tissue treated around the lesion is variable. The goal, as in surgery, is to avoid having to treat the same bone on multiple occasions. MRI is used to image proximal and distal lesions in the spine. Appropriate radiation portals can then be defined to avoid repetitive irradiation of the spinal cord. Careful planning in this fashion avoids overtreatment and complications such as transverse myelitis, bowel toxicity, and peripheral edema.

Radiation suppresses hematopoiesis in the bones within the treatment portal. Marrow suppression is a more significant concern in patients receiving chemotherapy, as combined myelosuppression can be severe. Aggressive chemotherapy regimens that depress stem cell populations are the most dangerous in this regard. Complete blood cell counts must be closely monitored, often on a daily basis.

PAIN RELIEF. Irradiation achieves at least partial relief of pain in 80% to 90% of patients.[49] The speed of response varies. When the cause of pain is neurologic, tumor regression can be prompt and relief rapid. Spinal cord compression from lymphoma is a classic example of this phenomenon.[50,51] Most symptomatic bony metastases begin to respond over the course of 10 to 14 days. Seventy percent of patients experience some pain relief within 2 weeks of starting therapy and, within 3 months, 90% of patients achieve pain relief.[52] Tong et al.,[53] from the Radiation Treatment Oncology Group (RTOG), found that approximately 55% to 70% of patients who responded initially did not develop recurrent pain in the treatment field. These data support other studies that note sustained pain relief for 1 year or more in 55% to 65% of patients.[54] There is no convincing evidence that different histologic cancers respond differently to irradiation. Although undoubtedly there are some variations, they seem to be as great among cancers of the same histologic type as they are between primary cancer types.[55]

Evaluation of pain relief and tumor responsiveness has failed to account properly for the mechanical contribution to pain. Even when cancer cells respond well to therapy, lytic tumors may lack matrix, and thus the underlying bone may require more time to restore its mechanical strength. This may explain the clinical observation that radiation is less successful in palliating lung and kidney cancer lesions, which tend to be predominantly lytic. The RTOG reported that patients with breast and prostate metastases, cancers that have a significant amount of associated matrix, derived better pain relief from irradiation than did patients with long bone lesions from other primary tumors.[53] Patients with more severe and frequent pain as well as those in whom other treatments have failed are in a poor prognostic category.

When patients do not achieve relief on a therapeutic schedule consistent with that already described, a separate etiology should be considered for the pain. The clinician should have a high index of suspicion for comorbid conditions. A sudden increase in pain after the start of treatment may indicate that a pathologic fracture has occurred. Radiographic and orthopedic evaluation should be obtained before the radiation course is continued.

RADIATION DOSE AND FRACTIONATION. The optimal dose and fractionation regimen for palliative therapy of metastatic bone lesions is debated.[42,49,56] Dose, duration, and fractionation of treatment are interrelated concerns. Metastatic cancer patients with limited life expectancies should receive effective treatment over as short a time course as possible. Short-term toxicity is the major concern in patients with pathologic fractures because of their reduced life expectancies. Short-course irradiation minimizes the number of treatments and necessary travel time while producing high response rates.

The RTOG's randomized study of differing dose fractionation schedules in 759 patients reported no significant difference in pain relief among five different schedules of fractionation (270 cGy × 15, 300 cGy × 10, 300 cGy × 5, 400 cGy × 5, and 500 cGy × 5).[43,53] Complete pain relief and the elimination of the need for narcotic analgesics occurred more frequently with protracted fractionation. According to Blitzner's reanalysis of the RTOG data,[43] the 270 × 15 or 300 × 10 regimens were most effective. At the Royal Marsden Hospital, 288 patients were treated for painful bony metastases with either 800 cGy × 1 or 300 cGy × 10.[42,57] The response rate in each arm of the trial was 80%. Retrospective analysis of single low-dose (400- to 1500-cGy) versus multiple moderate-dose (2000- to 4000-cGy) programs have shown remarkably little difference.[58,59] These studies indicate that there is no consistent dose-response relationship governing pain relief after the irradiation of bone metastases. The heterogeneous nature of patients studied, however, and differences in posttreatment survival times may mask such a relationship.

Some authorities continue to recommend higher doses and longer courses of irradiation to palliate bone metastases. The effectiveness of high-dose therapy is supported by Arcangeli and Micheli,[60] who reported that doses of more than 4000 cGy effected a higher complete response rate. Therefore, patients with a projected long survival and good performance status may be best treated by a full dose (more than 4000 cGy) with conventional fractionation.

Patients with disseminated bone metastases are candidates for hemibody radiation.[59] This method is an alternative for patients for whom localized treatment would be inadequate and effective systemic therapy is lacking. The usual protocol is the administration of 6 to 10 Gy in one fraction to the upper, middle, or lower body. Premedication with antiemetics and corticosteroids and hydration are necessary to treat the acute radiation effects. Response rates are consistently in excess of 70%, with more than

20% of patients experiencing complete pain relief and fewer than 50% requiring additional irradiation for recurrent bone pain. Toxicity occurs in fewer than 10% of patients, and severe toxicity is less common in treatment of the middle or lower body. Prostate cancer appears to be particularly well suited for this form of therapy: Persistent palliation of pain until death has been noted in 82% of patients receiving upper body irradiation and in 67% of those receiving lower body irradiation. However, concerns regarding the permanent impact on bone marrow reserve, with the possible future need for chemotherapy in these patients, has made hemibody radiation less popular, particularly in the setting of available systemic radiopharmaceuticals that target metastatic foci and do not carry similar systemic risks.

Systemic Radionuclides

The systemic administration of radionuclides can be very effective in treating symptomatic bone metastases. This approach is appealing as compared with any other local or systemic therapy in that it treats all involved sites rapidly and selectively, thereby reducing toxicity and enhancing the therapeutic ratio.[49] Strategies include using a carrier that seeks the tumor or a vehicle that localizes in bone matrix. The antineoplastic effect both relieves pain and allows for healing of the underlying bone lesion. Iodine 131 is the prototype, localizing within well-differentiated thyroid carcinoma cells.

Strontium 89 is the most commonly used radioisotope in bony metastatic disease and is advocated for a variety of primary cancer histologic types.[61,62] It localizes in the mineral of bone by combining with the calcium component of hydroxyapatite. Actively calcifying areas concentrate most of the isotope, just as with radionuclide scintigraphy. Therefore, it has particular efficacy in osteoblastic lesions, such as those occurring with metastatic prostate or breast cancer. Degradation of the isotope in the host bone administers local short-acting radiation to the adjacent tumor cells. ^{89}Sr has very good response rates ranging from 51% to 91%. Patients with prostate cancer showed more than 80% symptomatic improvement after ^{89}Sr therapy. The only significant toxic effect of ^{89}Sr is myelotoxicity, with a 25% reduction in platelets and leukocytes, and it is usually temporary.

The low-energy β-emission of ^{89}Sr is safer and better tolerated than are high-energy isotopes such as orthophosphate 32. Other radiopharmaceuticals are also available, including such isotopes as ^{186}Rh, tin-11m-diethylenetriaminepentaacetic acid, ^{153}Sm, and gallium nitrate. The mechanism of action relates to the half-life of the isotope in the lesion, the penetrance and mean energy of emitted radioactive particle, and the delivered dose. Isotopes with short half-lives, such as ^{186}Rh, emit both γ rays, permitting imaging of lesions, and β-particles, which confer therapeutic value. All agents cause bone marrow suppression, which is worse in heavily pretreated patients undergoing chemotherapy. However, premedication, as is required with hemibody radiation, is not necessary with the use of systemic radionuclides.

Radiopharmaceuticals can cause an initial exacerbation of pain (the flare response) in 10% to 15% of patients. A flare response can indicate good overall analgesic value.[63] In addition, it has been shown that ^{89}Sr can be safely used in conjunction with external-beam irradiation, either in patients who have previously received wide-field radiation and present with symptomatic bony lesions or in patients who have not received previous external-beam irradiation and so can receive external-beam irradiation subsequent to treatment with ^{89}Sr.[64,65]

SURGERY

General Considerations

BONE MECHANICS. Bone strength depends on a combination of material and structural properties.[66] Material properties are of greatest importance when overall bone geometry remains unchanged. Alterations in bone mineral content influence strength and stiffness exponentially.[67] Alterations in bone proteins after chemotherapy or radiation therapy may influence the ability of bone to reconstitute. Bone structural properties reflect the underlying geometry and distribution of material in space, integrating the contribution of medullary trabecular bone and cortical compact bone. Both lytic and blastic lesions dramatically alter the bone modulus of elasticity and reduce bone strength. Lytic disease reduces bone strength more so than blastic metastases.[68,69] However, blastic metastases also reduce bone strength secondary to the disorganized nature of this tumor-related bone.

Most of the compressive strength of bone is due to its mineral component, whereas it is the combination of mineral and protein that lends strength in tension.[70] During normal activity, most forces are either of compression or tension. Torsional or rotational forces, which come into play when the lower extremity is planted and the patient pivots, are also important.[71] These forces typically occur during transfers such as getting into and out of a chair. Bone is weakest in torsion. A single 6-mm drill hole, the size used for bone biopsy, reduces torsional strength 50%.[71–73] Larger defects create even greater stress risers, decreasing torsional strength by 70% and more.[68] Defects larger than the diameter of the bone are termed *open segment defects* and can reduce both bending and torsional strength as much as 90%. Weak bone tends to fracture in a transverse configuration, as compared with normal bone, which fractures in an oblique or spiral pattern. Overall bone alignment usually is good in pathologic fractures as long as a large destructive lesion is not present.

BONE BIOLOGY. The local presence of cancer precludes bone healing in most pathologic fracture situations. The rapid growth of metastatic lesions overwhelms the healing response. Gainor and Buchert[40] evaluated 123 patients with pathologic long bone fractures. Healing occurred in 45 of the 129 fractures (35%). Healing rates were related to tumor type: In this series, 67% of fractures due to multiple myeloma, 44% of fractures due to renal cancer, and 37% of fractures due to breast cancer healed. No pathologic fractures due to lung cancer healed.

The length of patient survival correlated best with fracture healing rates, although healing was considered multifactorial. The five factors that related to the healing of pathologic fractures included diagnosis, survival, internal fixation, postoperative irradiation, and chemotherapy.[40] Melanoma and lung and colorectal cancers failed to heal. Lesions due to multiple myeloma and breast and renal cancers tended to heal most frequently; however, they also occurred earlier in the course of these diseases, while other therapeutic options still remained. Survival was directly related to diagnosis, and this correlated with improved healing rates for patients living longer than 6 months. Rigid internal fixation supplemented with bone cement was found to increase the probability of bone union. Bone cement not only contributes to stability but also may present a mechanical obstacle to tumor growth in the fracture region. High doses of postoperative radiation (>3000 cGy) were associated with poor healing. Because of the variety of agents and therapeutic courses of chemotherapy, this series could not extrapolate the influence of chemotherapy on fracture healing. However, other studies suggest that healing is reduced 50% by such common agents as methotrexate and doxorubicin.[74]

Other systemic factors may make a contribution to fracture healing in patients with metastatic bony lesions, including osteoporosis, hormone manipulation, and cachexia.

Fracture Treatment

Management of pathologic fractures with internal fixation or prosthetic replacement is the most effective and expedient means by which to control pain and restore function. Effective orthopedic procedures for metastatic disease convert open segment to closed segment defects, restore bone strength in bending and torsion, and allow immediate weight bearing. Stabilization of a fracture requires control of the proximal and distal fracture fragments. In this respect, fracture location is an important consideration, and management strategies are different for epiphyseal, metaphyseal, and diaphyseal locations.

EPIPHYSEAL FRACTURES. Epiphyseal fractures present the easiest problem. Fracture healing is not a consideration, even with nondisplaced fractures, because it almost never occurs. Resection of the fracture and associated diseased tissue is appropriate, and arthroplasty should be performed, usually involving a cemented implant. Stem length should be chosen to treat existing or potential lesions within the same bone. Widespread use of bisphosphonate therapy may reduce the need for long-stemmed prostheses in the future.

METAPHYSEAL FRACTURES. Metaphyseal fractures are more complex. The fracture geometry, quality and quantity of residual bone, and histologic subtype must be considered. It is especially important to judge the fracture healing potential using the Gainor criteria discussed in the previous Bone Biology section. If a patient is early in the course of treatment, effective systemic therapies are available, and the tumor is sensitive to irradiation, internal fixation can support the bone while healing occurs. Lymphoma, occasionally myeloma, and breast cancer are the tumor types for which a long-term, bone-healing strategy has merit.

Internal fixation methods are familiar to orthopedists who treat nonpathologic fractures. Techniques can be classified according to their use of load-bearing devices (plates and screws) or load-sharing devices (intramedullary rods). A good indication for plate and screw fixation in metaphyseal fractures is densely sclerotic bone, for which intramedullary fixation or the insertion of a prosthetic device with a long intramedullary stem would be very difficult. One drawback of plate and screw fixation is that the entire bone is not stabilized in the same procedure. This leaves the patient susceptible to a future fracture proximal or distal to the fixation. Plating techniques also are more prone to failure than are intramedullary fixation methods. Dijstra,[75] citing a series of 167 fractures, reported that plate fixation is associated with an 11% failure rate within 7 weeks and a 40% cumulative 5-year failure rate. However, intramedullary fixation of metaphyseal fractures often is impractical because of inadequate control of the epiphyseal fracture fragment by the device.

Prosthetic replacement of metaphyseal lesions can be very difficult. Generally, the bone in the surrounding apophyseal areas should be saved because it helps to retain soft tissue attachments. Examples of these areas are the greater and lesser trochanters of the hip and the greater and lesser tuberosities of the humerus. Securing these attachments to a hemiarthroplasty device in a dependable fashion is difficult. When necessary, supplemental fixation methods with mesh, tension bands, wires, or cable systems can be used, but the constructs are usually unsatisfactory and result in persistent muscle weakness and pain. In addition, it is difficult to assess bone alignment and length accurately when treating metaphyseal fractures with prosthetic replacement. In these instances, the significant bone loss resulting from the metastatic lesion that indicates prosthetic replacement also eliminates or distorts the typical bony landmarks needed to orient the reconstruction. Problems with limb length inequality, joint instability, and limb weakness typically follow such surgical attempts.

DIAPHYSEAL FRACTURES. Diaphyseal lesions are treated successfully by intramedullary fixation. The method requires the establishment of excellent fixation proximal and distal to the fracture. This often is possible even when there is total destruction of the affected area. Fixation is achieved by combining interlock screw fixation with cementing of the bony defect. Flexion and bending strength are well restored with intramedullary rods.[76] Compression strength depends on the magnitude and extent of the bone deficiency. Methyl methacrylate cement used to fill bone gaps restores strength in compression. Torsional strength and stiffness are restored poorly by intramedullary devices; therefore, successful use of such devices requires the limitation of torsional forces and the use of appropriate interlocking technique and cement to control the proximal and distal bone fragments.[77,78] If such control is lacking, plate fixation should be considered.

When diaphyseal lesions are combined with a metaphyseal tumor deposit, prosthetic replacement with a long-stemmed device removes the metaphyseal disease and stabilizes the diaphyseal shaft fracture with strong intramedullary fixation.[79,80] The secondary tumor deposit should be treated, in most instances, even if this necessitates opening of the fracture site. Closed intramedullary fracture treatment should be reserved only for those fractures that will heal with stabilization and supplemental radiation or in patients with rapidly advancing preterminal disease in whom the fixation alone will outlast the patient's projected survival. Long-term success of the technique requires good apposition of bone fragments and removal of local tumor so that healing occurs.

OTHER MANAGEMENT OPTIONS. Although most surgeons and patients choose internal fixation or prosthetic replacement as the most effective treatment of pathologic fractures, other management options are available. These include external fixation, cast or brace immobilization, and amputation.

External fixation and cast or brace immobilization can be considered in patients (1) with extensive localized disease that cannot be immobilized by internal means; (2) who are preterminal and in whom analgesic modalities such as narcotics or rhizotomy can control symptoms; or (3) in whom infection, nadir sepsis, pneumonia, or other temporary medical problems prevent surgery. These measures can be used in the hospital and translate well to outpatient, home, or hospice care situations.

Amputation continues to play a role in the management of metastatic cancer, with complications of disease and therapy triggering the need for amputation.[81,82] The indications for amputation fall into three categories: (1) extremity lesions that cannot be reconstructed or are inappropriately reconstructed; (2) complications of the tumor or treatment, such as a fungating infected lesion; and (3) intractable pain.

Acrometastases (metastases that occur in the distal extremity) present at variable times during the progression of metastatic disease. They are rare, occurring in 0.007% to 0.3% of patients with osseous metastasis, and usually represent a preterminal event. Lung, renal, and esophageal cancer accounted for 48% of the primary lesions causing the 31 cases of acrometastases reviewed by Healey et al.[83] In this review, seven of the cases were the first presentation of cancer, and another seven cases constituted the first presentation of metastatic disease.

Amputation is quite suitable for a distal extremity lesion, particularly in the foot. Depending on the primary diagnosis, amputation may provide an opportunity for extended disease control of early or solitary metastases. Because rehabilitation of distal sites can be difficult and time-consuming, amputation presents the best way to relieve symptoms and resume function.[83,84] More proximal amputations are considered in the lower extremity, particularly when complex reconstruction would be required. The aggressive treatment methods developed for limb salvage in primary bone tumors are an inappropriate use of time and resources in skeletal metastases. Intractable pain is sometimes an indication for amputation, but rhizotomy and chordotomy can accomplish the same goal while retaining the extremity.

Recent interest has been demonstrated in a technique that uses radiographically guided percutaneous injection of polymethyl methacrylate into certain metastatic bony lesions. The basic goal of this technique is to address mechanical symptoms by improving the mechanical stability, particularly in compression, of bones involved by lytic lesions. In vertebroplasty, under radiographic guidance, liquid methyl methacrylate is injected directly into vertebral body lesions. One of the major complications of the injection technique is the extravasation of cement from within the contained bony space, with impingement on adjacent structures. This is particularly important in the spine, where spinal cord compression by cement can cause catastrophic neurologic compromise and requires immediate surgical decompression.[85,86] With use of this technique for pelvic lesions, reported complications include intraarticular extension of cement into the hip joint and extravasation around the sciatic nerve.[87] One of the contraindications of the technique is associated fracture, which allows for extravasation of the injected cement outside the bone. Because of the complications associated with percutaneous injection of polymethyl methacrylate, it is important to coordinate the procedure to allow for emergent surgical backup to address acute extravasation issues.[85]

Tumor Excision

The metastatic tumor deposit should be excised under most fracture circumstances and in selected instances of bone biopsy, treatment of impending fracture, and solitary bone metastasis. Treatment options consist of intralesional excision, wide excision, or excision plus a surgical adjuvant.

Intralesional therapy occurs either at the time of biopsy or as a planned intervention. Once the biopsy confirms metastatic disease, a decision must be made as to whether to remove all gross disease, debulking the tumor, or to rely on external irradiation and systemic therapy for local control of the lesion. It is helpful if the members of the oncology team discuss the treatment options before beginning a course of therapy. Judgment, sensitivity, and skill are needed to integrate the biopsy process with overall tumor management and to prepare the patient and his or her family appropriately before surgery. Combining biopsy with tumor removal and bone stabilization best meets the goals of diagnosis, pain relief, and functional restoration. This is particularly important because biopsy further disrupts the already weakened bone.

Intralesional curettage of tumor in and around the fracture site is the principal strategy in addressing metastatic lesions involving bone. Eliminating gross tumor achieves an immediate "partial response" that could take weeks to be achieved by other methods, improving local tumor control. Furthermore, the remaining structural bone is identified. The resultant defect can be filled much more effectively with methyl methacrylate cement, giving better long-term stability to the fractured bone.[88]

Extralesional excision can be accomplished by either marginal or wide excision. The appeal of complete local excision is obvious. It is the most effective way to eliminate the biologic contribution to pain while correcting the structural deficiency. Isolated solitary metastases should be evaluated for potential resectability.[7,89] Occasional cures are reported after resection of bone metastases, but these are infrequent. Radical ablative surgery usually is not appropriate. A long interval between primary tumor presentation and the development of a metastatic focus argues well for cancer resectability. Patients with a projected long survival, such as those with renal or thyroid cancers, are best suited to undergo extralesional excision of metastases. The sacroiliac region and spine are common sites of a solitary metastasis. Tumors in these areas are large and bulky, and the surgery is dangerous. Plasmacytomas should also be considered for resection. Even if systemic disease later develops, some clinicians contend that survival may be prolonged in surgically resected cases.[14,90]

Surgical adjuvants are helpful, whether intralesional or excisional procedures are considered, and include angiography, cryosurgery, chemotherapy, and radiation therapy. Preoperative angiography and tumor embolization greatly reduce blood flow and intraoperative hemorrhage, particularly in vascular tumors such as thyroid and renal cell carcinoma.[91–94] Cryosurgery can be used in the local management of bone lesions[95]; Marcove[96] pioneered its use in metastatic disease. It is particularly suited for cancers that have failed to respond to systemic treatment or local radiation therapy and in which local tumor progression is expected.

The addition of chemotherapeutic agents to the methyl methacrylate bone cement used in implant and fixation constructs is under investigation as a method of local delivery of antineoplastic drugs for enhanced local, and potentially systemic, disease con-

TABLE 52.4-1. Mirels' Scoring System to Predict Pathologic Fracture[105]

Variable	*Points* 1	2	3
Site	Upper extremity	Lower extremity	Pertrochanteric
Pain	Mild	Moderate	Mechanical
Radiograph	Blastic	Mixed	Lytic
Size (% of shaft)	0–33	34–67	68–100
Score	*No. of Patients*	*Fracture Rate (%)*	
0–6	11	0	
7	19	5	
8	12	33	
9	7	57	
10–12	18	100	

trol. Preliminary studies show promising results, but further clinical investigation is required before this method can be entered into the therapeutic armamentarium.[97,98]

Radiation therapy remains the principal surgical adjuvant. It should be delivered to the entire surgical field and extend the length of any prosthesis or internal fixation device.[41,52] This addresses tumor cells that have been spread by the surgical procedure along the intramedullary canal and soft tissues. Local tumor control helps to prevent destabilization of the implant construct by preventing local tumor progression from affecting the structural integrity of the bone in which the implant is fixed.

Impending Fractures: Prophylactic Fixation

There is no specific definition of an impending fracture, and the indications for operative treatment of impending fractures continue to be controversial. This controversy remains extant in part because of the evidence in the literature. Snell and Beals,[99] in their review of 19 pathologic femur fractures due to metastatic breast cancer, found that a lesion of 2.5-cm diameter involving the femoral cortex with pain, irrespective of location, was a positive predictor of pathologic fracture. Parrish and Murray[100] reported on their experience with 104 pathologic fractures due to metastatic disease and identified increasing pain, more than 33% cortical destruction, and lack of radiographic improvement after radiation therapy as indicators of impending fracture. Fidler,[101] in his retrospective study of 19 long bone fractures, showed that with 50% or more cortical involvement in a long bone, there is at least a 50% incidence of spontaneous fracture. Zickel and Mouradian,[102] in their retrospective review of 34 patients, found that size did not correlate with risk of fracture and that, instead, pure lysis on radiography, medial cortical involvement at the hip, and increasing pain were indicative of a high risk of fracture. Harrington,[103] in his review of the literature, summarized the positive predictors of pathologic fracture through a metastatic lesion as (1) a lesion of 2.5-cm or larger diameter involving the femur, (2) lytic destruction of at least 50% of the cortex of a long bone, and (3) continued pain with weight bearing after radiation therapy.

Keene et al.[104] evaluated clinical and radiographic risk factors in an attempt to predict pathologic fracture of the femur. This study involved 2673 breast cancer patients who had undergone skeletal surveys. Of these, 203 patients had evaluable proximal femoral metastases. The authors found no criteria to identify the bone at risk for fracture. They concluded that plain radiographic measurements are insufficient to identify high-risk lesions. This study, however, was limited to the single anteroposterior radiographic evaluation present in the skeletal survey.

Mirels[105] proposed a graduated scoring system that further refined the risk-factor criteria. Included are clinical and radiographic factors, which generate a composite score from 0 to 12 that correlates with fracture risk. Four factors—anatomic site, pain pattern, radiographic nature, and lesion size—were each evaluated on a 0 to 3 scale. Table 52.4-1 depicts this scoring system and its ability to predict pathologic fracture. Mirels investigated 78 lesions followed up over the course of 6 months. Fifty-one lesions resulted in fracture, and 27 did not. The mean score for the nonfracture patients was 7, versus a mean score of 10 for the fracture patients; however, there was significant overlap between the two groups. The author concluded that lesions with scores of less than 7 could be irradiated, whereas those with a higher score should be managed with internal fixation followed by postoperative irradiation.

Equally valuable is the ability of this scoring system to predict which lesions would not fracture.[105] The fracture rate was small (5%) when the lesion was less than two-thirds of the bone diameter, but it increased to 81% for lesions larger than two-thirds of the shaft diameter. It was stressed that standard radiographs are inadequate to grade many lesions, and CT scanning was recommended to improve diagnostic accuracy. Mirels[105] also made an important distinction between pain and "functional" pain, the latter being pain that worsens with weight bearing. Thus, functional pain reflects the structural insufficiency of bone and was found to be the most significant indicator of bone failure, enjoying an almost universal success in predicting fracture. Lesions measuring larger than twice the bone diameter were closely associated with functional pain. Fracture probability in patients with smaller lesions was only 10%.

The scientific foundation for predicting fracture risk has been improved and summarized by Callaway and Healey.[106] Computer modeling of the proximal femur in *in vitro* testing has allowed some investigators to predict femoral strength more accurately.[107–109] Evaluating intertrochanteric and subtrochanteric lesions subject to bending forces, these researchers found that endosteal reabsorption of one-half the cortical width weakens the bone by 70% and leaves the patient at high fracture risk. Similar analysis is not available for other anatomic sites.

At the MSKCC, a functional system has been used that has practical implications.[30,110,111] In each of the following four circumstances, major bone loss has usually been encountered surgically, and the bone was found to be essentially fractured:

- A painful medullary lytic lesion resulting in endosteal reabsorption of at least 50% of the cortical thickness
- A painful lytic lesion involving the cortex that is larger than the cross-sectional diameter of the bone
- A painful cortical lesion more than 2.5-cm long
- A lesion producing functional pain after radiation therapy

Prophylactic fixation should be performed as described earlier in Fracture Treatment.

SPECIFIC ANATOMIC SITES

For each site, unique patterns of metastases and functional and prognostic implications exist. The spine, proximal femur, and pelvis cause the most problems and will be dealt with individually.

SPINE

Metastatic disease most often affects the vertebral bodies. The lumbar spine is the site of the greatest number of metastases.[112] However, any site within the spine can develop symptomatic metastases. The primary cancers responsible for spinal metastases are breast, lung, and prostate. Among reports regarding the prevalence of spine metastases, most emanate from referral centers. However, Stark et al.[48] note that from a general hospital, lung cancer was responsible in 33%, breast cancer in 28%, other identifiable sites in 25%, and unknown primary lesions in 14% of cases. Remarkably, in 47% of the 131 patients with neurologic symptoms reported by Stark et al.,[48] the spinal metastases were the initial presentation of malignant disease. In an autopsy study of 832 patients dying of metastatic cancer, 36% were found to have spinal metastases, and 26% of these patients had negative plain radiographs of the spine despite the gross evidence of tumor.[113]

Pain is the most common presenting symptom. It may be caused by intraosseous disease, motion segment instability, vertebral fracture, epidural compression, or nerve root impingement. Vascular insufficiency of the spine can also occur due to tumor or to associated spinal instability, surgery, radiation therapy, or embolization of the spinal arteries.[114] Neurologic deficit is seen commonly in symptomatic patients. Myelopathy, radiculopathy, or cauda equina syndromes are recorded. Of particular importance is loss of proprioception and sphincter function. These are harbingers of serious neurologic damage and are much less likely to return after any form of treatment.

Various staging systems for vertebral involvement have been advanced.[115,116] The Tomita system is the most logical and offers the greatest clinical applicability.[117] It identifies disease involving the vertebral body, pedicle, posterior spinous elements, epidural space, and paraspinal region as distinct components. Clinical staging has also been identified as an important prognostic factor. Tokuhashi et al.[118] have identified six parameters for staging, each of which is assigned 0 to 2 points: (1) general condition, (2) number of extraspinal bone metastases, (3) number of vertebral metastases, (4) visceral metastases, (5) primary cancer site, and (6) severity of spinal cord palsy. Outcome was correlated to total score. These authors recommended that an excisional operation be performed in patients with 9 or more points, whereas palliative surgery is indicated for the more seriously ill, those patients scoring fewer than 5 points.[118]

The natural history of metastases is variable. Influential factors are anatomic location of metastases, functional status, treatment, and primary tumor histology. Tomita et al.[119] reported on a group of 78 patients with epidural metastases who were treated with irradiation and high-dose steroids. Among the patients, 2 improved and 11 became paraplegic, whereas in 65, symptoms stabilized. There was a major difference in outcome based on the ability to restore ambulation. Ambulators had a 53-week survival in contrast to nonambulators, who survived less than 5 weeks.

Radiation is the first line of treatment for most patients with spinal metastases and pain. Rao et al.[120] reported on 19 patients with cervical metastases without neurologic deficits. All patients received radiation therapy or chemotherapy. Symptomatic control lasted for 6 months, with subsequent deterioration that necessitated another treatment. Median survival was less than 15 months. The authors concluded that nonoperative treatment is appropriate for most patients without neurologic signs, particularly if the expected survival is in the 6- to 12-month range.[120] Similarly, Young et al.[47] performed a randomized trial of radiation therapy versus laminectomy and posterior decompression of the spinal cord. They found no benefit from this form of surgery and therefore favored nonoperative treatment. However, the series was small, was not stratified for tumor location, and preceded the application of modern spine instrumentation methods.

Surgery may be important to improve the quality of life of these patients.[121] The goals of surgery in metastatic spine disease are to decompress the spinal cord and neural elements and to stabilize the spine. Laminectomy alone rarely accomplishes these goals and may further destabilize the spine.[47] It is indicated for rare posterior element disease or peripheral root compression only.

The debate continues as to whether an anterior, posterior, or combined anterior-posterior approach is better. Proponents of anterior decompression contend that it is often preferable because it addresses the primary site of the disease.[122,123] Harrington,[122] in his original report of 14 patients, found that 9 of 12 patients with major neurologic dysfunction recovered completely, 2 recovered partially, and 1 was unchanged. Vertebral body resection and cement and rod vertebral body reconstruction achieved excellent pain relief in 13 of 14 patients. Sundaresan et al.[124] reported on 101 vertebral body resections. Patients were stabilized anteriorly or posteriorly as required; pins and cement usually were inserted to replace the vertebral body. Seventy-eight percent regained ambulatory ability, and 85% experienced pain relief. Morbidity was the least in patients who were treated *de novo* and underwent subsequent radiation therapy. In a follow-up study of 54 patients with *de novo* surgery, Sundaresan et al.[115] noted that 25 patients survived 2 years or more, with 92% maintaining ambulatory ability. The overall complication rate in this series was a low 15%.

Rosenthal et al.[125] reviewed a 3-year experience at the MSKCC, where anterior corpectomy and reconstruction with pins and cement were used for metastatic disease. Deterioration in function or pain control occurred in 7 months for cervical lesions, in 11 months for lumbar lesions, and in 22 months for thoracic lesions. Junctional sites were more unstable, leading to early deterioration. Anterior surgery alone was satisfactory for

A 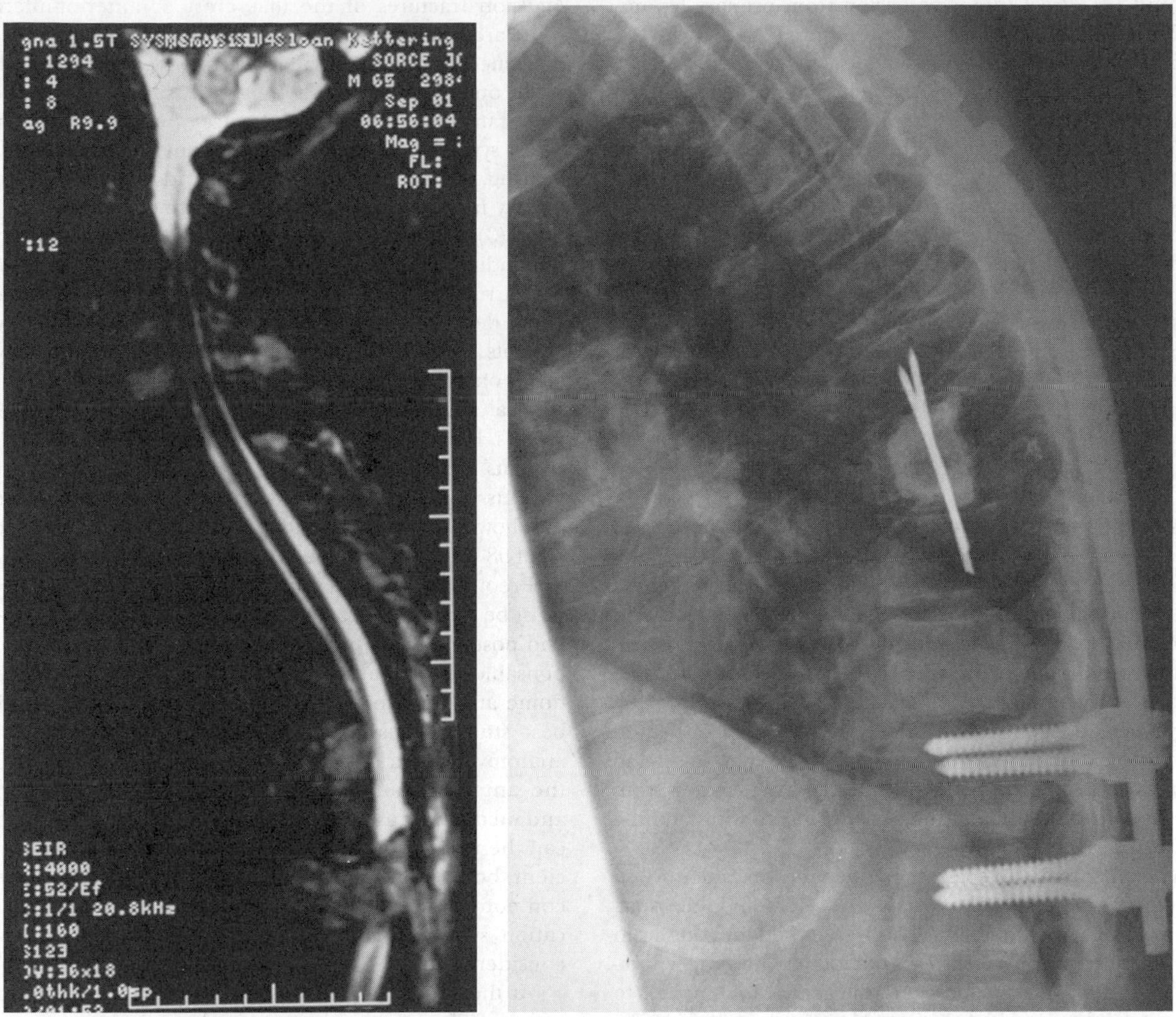 B

FIGURE 52.4-2. Metastatic disease involving the spine with fracture and spinal cord compression at T9. **A:** T2 stir, fat-suppressed magnetic resonance imaging scan demonstrating multiple-level vertebral involvement with extension of tumor involving the T9 vertebral body into the spinal canal with cord impingement. **B:** Postoperative radiograph after decompression and stabilization using the single-stage posterolateral, transpedicular approach with anterior reconstruction with pins and cement and long posterior fusion with pedicle screw fixation.

patients with short survival times. If survival was expected to exceed the durability of the anterior reconstruction, then staged, posterior stabilization was recommended. Currently, the group at MSKCC is advocating a posterolateral, transpedicular approach that permits circumferential neural decompression, corpectomy, anterior pin and cement fixation, and segmental posterior fixation (Fig. 52.4-2).[126] This strategy has achieved excellent tumor control, pain relief, and neurologic preservation in a preliminary series of 25 patients. It is particularly suitable for patients with extensive epidural disease and those who have had a previous thoracotomy or thoracic irradiation or who have significant pulmonary disease, which is a relative contraindication for thoracotomy.

Segmental spine fixation, including pedicle fixation, has greatly improved the ability to stabilize the spine posteriorly.[127] Anterior devices, including plates or multiple rod fixation, have greatly expanded the options for vertebral body reconstruction.[128–131] Each anterior construct can be combined with bone or synthetic replacements for the vertebra. The choice here depends on the expected survival of the patient. In most situations, survival is insufficient for bone healing to occur and is well within the limits of synthetic durability. This is in distinction to the case for curative resection of solitary metastases or primary tumors.

Finally, Tomita et al.[132] have described total *en bloc* spondylectomy for metastatic and primary disease in a selected series of 24 patients. This is the most oncologically sound procedure described to date, removing the posterior elements as a single segment and resecting the vertebral body as a single segment. Careful spine stabilization and meticulous technique have prevented neurologic damage. Eighteen patients had substantial neurologic improvement. Among the 12 patients who were alive at 14-month review, no local recurrence was found. These results are in contrast to the high local recurrence rates (up to 49%) that have been reported by King et al.[133] and other experienced spine surgeons.

Current surgical indications agreed on by most authors are (1) cord compression with myelopathy, (2) bone impinging into the spinal canal and producing thecal compression, (3) spinal instability with unremitting mechanical pain, (4) fracture-dislocation of the spine, (5) radiculopathy with progressive or uncontrolled symptoms, (6) tumor growth unresponsive to radiation therapy, and (7) direct tumor extension from primary lesions, such as Pancoast tumor invading the vertebra.

Embolization of spinal metastases from renal carcinoma has been recommended as the sole treatment for patients with late-stage disease. O'Reilly et al.[93] described this treatment in four patients who achieved progressive neurologic improvement that lasted for 12 weeks or more. Preoperative tumor embolization is warranted in renal carcinoma and, possibly, in other hypervascular lytic tumors. Olerud et al.[92] noted that the average blood loss was cut by two-thirds after embolization in 11 cases of renal cancer, as compared with 18 similar procedures in which embolization was not performed. The value of embolization in the treatment of other tumors has not been as well documented, but it is often useful in the treatment of metastases to difficult sites such as the acetabulum.

PROXIMAL FEMUR

Fractures of the proximal femur are the most common surgical problem in bony metastatic disease. Sixty-six percent of pathologic long bone fractures involve the femur, and 80% of these occur in the proximal portion. The femoral neck is the location for approximately 52% of these fractures, with the intertrochanteric region responsible for another 15% and the subtrochanteric region for the remaining 33%.[134] Walking, rising from a chair, climbing stairs, and even lifting the leg to swing out of bed all apply forces in excess of three times one's body weight on the hip joint and proximal femur. Underlying mechanical weakness from even a treated metastasis leaves the bone unable to withstand the forces of normal activity.

It is a tragic mistake to spare the patient an operation when the procedure can make an important improvement in the quality of the patient's remaining life. This is true even for patients in whom anticancer therapy and resuscitation are no longer indicated. As in other anatomic locations, the goal of treatment is to reduce pain and maintain function. Maintenance of function usually means preservation of walking ability but, in severely disabled patients, functional restoration means regaining transfer ability, which facilitates nursing care. General indications for surgery are a life expectancy of at least 1 month, a general physical condition adequate to tolerate surgery, a result from surgery that will expedite patient mobilization and facilitate general care, and bone adequate to support fixation or a prosthesis proximal or distal to the fracture.[134] Conversely, patients with major neurologic impairment or potential large persistent narcotic requirement are unlikely to benefit greatly from surgery.

Generally, all fractures require supplemental radiation therapy to treat underlying tumor. Treatment of the fracture frequently exposes new areas to tumor spread. Tumor can be seeded down the femoral canal during intramedullary reaming, insertion of an intramedullary device, or injection of cement down the canal. This newly contaminated region must be treated with radiation to avoid tumor proliferation and a new fracture distal to the implant.

Surgical treatment is largely dependent on fracture location and anatomy, which is discussed earlier, in Fracture Treatment.

PELVIS AND ACETABULUM

Most patients with pelvic and acetabular metastases have pain; however, it does not always arise directly from the hip joint. Avulsion fractures of the iliac crest or anterior-inferior iliac spine are common and should be treated nonoperatively. However, mechanical insufficiency of the acetabulum can be managed only surgically. The general surgical indications for metastatic disease involving the acetabulum are (1) continued acute symptoms despite management with protected weight bearing, antineoplastic treatment, and analgesics; (2) unsatisfactory function and pain control 1 to 3 months after irradiation; (3) a pathologic fracture of the acetabulum; or (4) an impending fracture in the ipsilateral femur requiring surgery.

Harrington and Rock[135,136] described four types of acetabular bone deficiency and their surgical management among 58 patients with pelvic metastases. Their classification system is based on the extent of bony involvement by tumor and reflects surgical treatment. Overall results were good for most patient groups. Pain relief was effective for at least 6 months in 67% of patients and for more than 2 years in 43%. Eighty percent of patients remained ambulatory for 6 months or more. Harrington did, however, treat a generally favorable group of patients, with 30 of 58 (51%) surviving 2 years or more after surgery.

Preoperative evaluation, including Judet radiographs, must be performed carefully, to define disease in the anterior and posterior acetabular columns.[137,138] CT scanning is indispensable to evaluate the medial acetabulum and acetabular dome and to define any associated soft tissue mass. It is the best study for assessing overall bone integrity. Pathologic anatomy is better described by a four-part system that assesses the anterior column, posterior column, acetabular dome, and medial wall as separate components. Bone in each region can then be graded as sufficient or insufficient, whereby sufficient bone provides adequate support for the acetabular component and insufficient bone does not. Thus, the classification system combines both anatomic and reconstructive considerations.

At the MSKCC, this four-part system was used to analyze a series of 55 patients who required surgical reconstruction of the acetabulum for metastatic disease.[139] In this series, ten patients (18%) had insufficiency of both anterior and posterior columns, whereas 36 patients (65%) had single column insufficiency. Forty-two of 55 patients (76%) had an insufficient medial wall combined with either an insufficient column or dome, and 47 patients (85%) had an acetabular fracture. In all 55 patients, the reconstruction was reinforced with pins or cannulated screws incorporated into cement, using a modified Harrington technique. This allows for bypass of major acetabular defects with proximal fixation of the socket into the remaining iliac bone. Insertion of pins or screws can be performed in an antegrade fashion from the iliac crest, using a vector guide, or retrograde from the bone defect. A protrusio ring "revision" hip socket can be used to transfer load to the remaining intact cortical bone when medial wall defects are present (Fig. 52.4-3). Of the 41 out of the 55 patients (75%) in this series that were evaluable at 3 months, 34 (83%) experienced significant pain relief, 9 of 18 nonambulatory patients had regained walking ability, and 14 of 17 patients maintained their ability to ambulate in the community. Fourteen of 55 patients (25%) developed significant local disease progression, but only 5 patients (9%) experienced fixation failure. Early complications developed in 12 patients (22%). Of the 21 patients (38%) who had more than 1 year of follow-up, 14 (67%) continued to experience improved pain relief and 12 (57%) remained com-

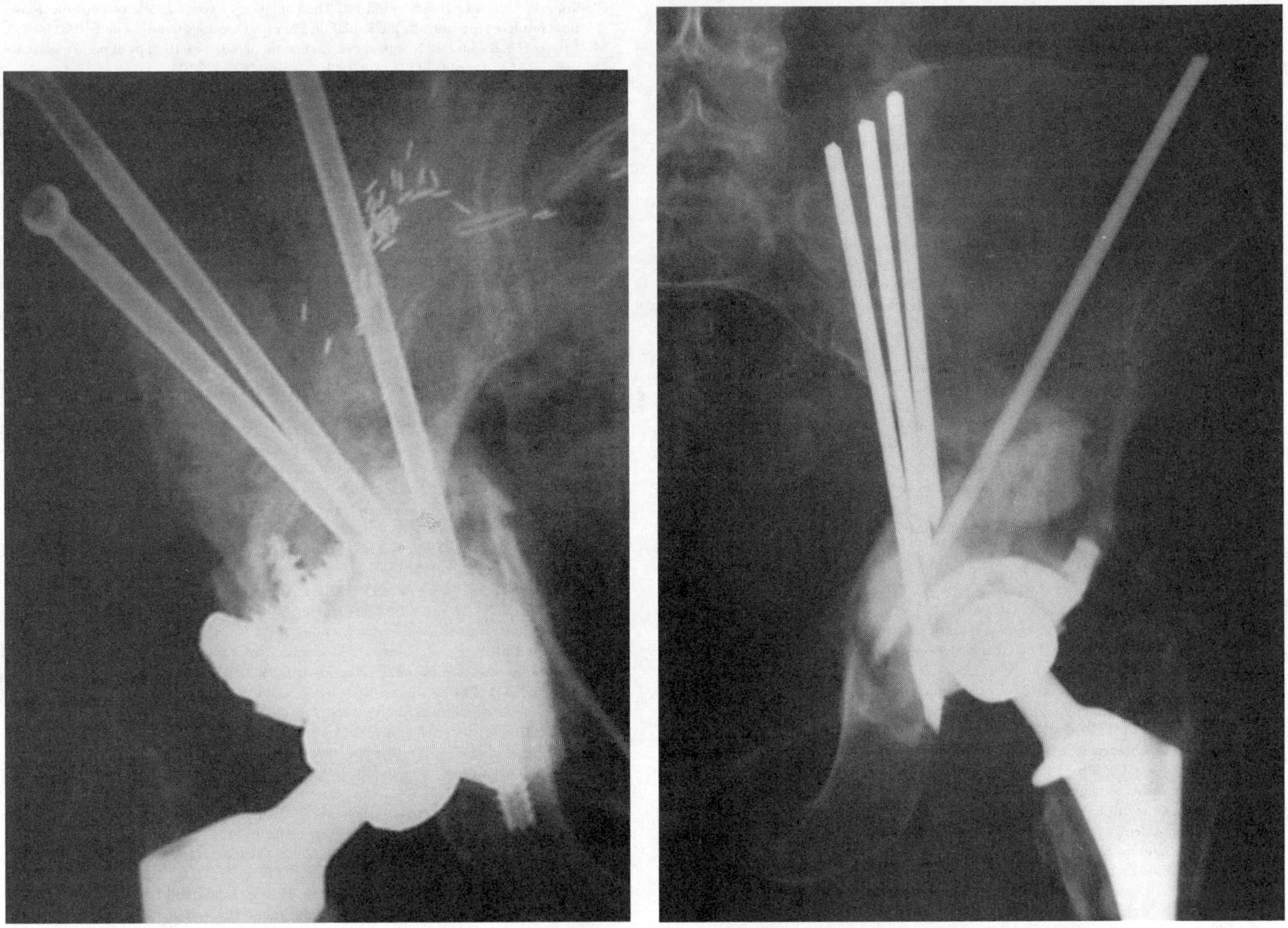

A B

FIGURE 52.4-3. Reconstructions using the techniques outlined for metastatic cancer to the pelvis and acetabulum. **A:** Plain radiograph shows the use of antegrade cannulated screws, a protrusio ring acetabular component (Healey Cup, Biomet, Warsaw, IN) with fixation screws, and cement to reconstruct a large acetabular defect with medial wall deficiency. **B:** Reconstruction of a large lesion involving the posterior column, medial wall, and acetabular dome using antegrade pins, a protrusio ring acetabular component, and cement. The prominent lateral iliac pin demonstrates pin back-out. The protrusio ring acetabular component lateralizes the socket and helps to bypass the central defect.

munity or household ambulators. In this series, despite the fact that patients with significant acetabular metastasis had a short life expectancy, the positive effect on both pain relief and functional improvement validated the role of surgery in managing this group. Acetabular reconstruction using the outlined techniques showed a low incidence of fixation failure, supporting the biomechanical stability of the construct and providing sufficient durability in these patients.

Finally, massive pelvic involvement can be treated by acetabular resection and reconstruction using a saddle prosthesis (Waldemar Link, Hamburg, Germany), as reported by Aboulafia et al.,[140] or with a pelvic endoprosthesis. Such aggressive surgical approaches may help selected patients with intermediate-term life expectancies.

When coupled with systemic measures to control bony metastases, local care with radiation therapy and/or judicious surgery can achieve the goals of pain relief and functional preservation in patients surviving with metastatic cancer that involves bone.

REFERENCES

1. Landis SH, Murray T, Bolden S, Wingo PA. Cancer statistics, 1999. *CA Cancer J Clin* 1999;49(1):8.
2. Walther HE. *Krebsmetastasen.* Basel: Bens Schwabe Verlag, 1948.
3. Mundy GR, Yoneda T. Facilitation and suppression of bone metastasis. *Clin Orthop* 1995;312:34.
4. Higinbotham NL, Marcove RC. The management of pathological fractures. *J Trauma* 1965;5:792.
5. Galasko CSB, Burn JI. Hypercalcemia in patients with advanced mammary cancer. *Br Med J* 1971;3:573.
6. Roila F, Lupattelli M, Sassi M, et al. Intra- and interobserver variability in cancer patients' performance status assessed according to Karnofsky and ECOG scales. *Ann Oncol* 1991;2:437.
7. Takashi M, Takagi Y, Sakata T, Shimoji T, Miyake K. Surgical treatment of renal cell carcinoma metastases: prognostic significance. *Int Urol Nephrol* 1995;27:1.
8. Mundy GR. Mechanisms of bone metastasis. *Cancer* 1997;80[Suppl 8]:1546.
9. Sasaki A, Alcalde RE, Nishiyama A, et al. Angiogenesis inhibitor TNP-470 inhibits human breast cancer osteolytic bone metastasis in nude mice through the reduction of bone resorption. *Cancer Res* 1998;58(3):462.
10. Yoneda T. Arterial microvascularization and breast cancer colonization in bone. *Histol Histopathol* 1997;12(4):1145.
11. Sugiyama A. Study of vertebral metastasis by MR imaging: significance of T2* weighted image (gradient field echo) and metastatic pattern. *Nippon Igaku Hoshasen Gakkai Zasshi* 1994;54(8):767.
12. Cockett MI, Murphy G, Birch ML, et al. Matrix metalloproteinases and metastatic cancer. *Biochem Soc Symp* 1998;63:295.

13. Sanchez-Sweatman OH, Lee J, Orr FW, Singh G. Direct osteolysis induced by metastatic murine melanoma cells: role of matrix metalloproteinases. *Eur J Cancer* 1997;33(6):918.
14. Holland J, Trenkner DA, Wasserman TH, Fineberg B. Plasmacytoma treatment results and conversion to myeloma. *Cancer* 1992;69:1513.
15. Tongaonkar HB, Kulkarni JN, Kamat MR. Solitary metastases from renal cell carcinoma: a review. *J Surg Oncol* 1992;49:45.
16. Demers LM, Costa L, Chinchilli VM, et al. Biochemical markers of bone turnover in patients with metastatic bone disease. *Clin Chem* 1995;41(10):1489.
17. Raj GV, Moreno JG, Gomella LG. Utilization of polymerase chain reaction technology in the detection of solid tumors. *Cancer* 1998;82(8):1419.
18. Rougraff BT, Kneisl JS, Simon MA. Skeletal metastases of unknown origin. *J Bone Joint Surg Am* 1993;75(9):1276.
19. Gosfield E, Alavi A, Kneeland B. Comparison of radionuclide bone scans and magnetic resonance imaging in detecting spinal metastases. *J Nucl Med* 1993;34:2191.
20. Pomeranz SJ, Pretorius HT, Ramsingh PS. Bone scintigraphy and multimodality imaging in bone neoplasia: strategies for imaging in the new health care climate. *Semin Nucl Med* 1994;24:188.
21. Cella DF, Tulsky DS, Gray G, et al. The Functional Assessment of Cancer Therapy scale: development and validation of the general measure. *J Clin Oncol* 1993;11(3):570.
22. Clohisy DR, Le CT, Umen AJ. Measuring health status in patients with skeletal metastases. *Am J Clin Oncol* 1997;20(4):424.
23. Davis AM, Bell RS, Badley EM, Yoshida K, Williams JI. Evaluating functional outcome in patients with lower extremity sarcomas. *Clin Orthop* 1999;358:90.
24. Verger E, Salamero M, Conill C. Can Karnofsky Performance Status be transformed to the Eastern Cooperative Oncology Group Scoring Scale and vice versa? *Eur J Cancer* 1992;28A(8–9):1328.
25. Wilner D, ed. Cancer metastasis to bone. In: Wilner D, ed. *Radiology of bone tumors.* Philadelphia: WB Saunders, 1982:3641.
26. Pollne JJ, Witztum KF, Ashburn WL. The flare phenomenon of radionuclide bone scan in metastatic prostate cancer. *Am J Radiol* 1984;142:773.
27. Weissman RB, Gilbert M, Wang H, Grossman SA. The use of computed tomography of the spine to identify patients at high risk for epidural metastases. *J Clin Oncol* 1985;3:1541.
28. Zimmer WD, Berquist TH, McLeod RA, et al. Bone tumors: magnetic resonance imaging versus computed tomography. *Radiology* 1985;155:709.
29. Colletti PM, Dang HT, Deseran MW, et al. Spinal MR imaging in suspected metastases: correlation with skeletal scintigraphy. *Magn Reson Imaging* 1991;9:349.
30. Tan SB, Kozak JA, Mawad ME. The limitations of magnetic resonance imaging in the diagnosis of pathologic vertebral fractures. *Spine* 1991;16:919.
31. Kole AC, Nieweg OE, Pruim J, et al. Detection of unknown occult primary tumors using positron emission tomography. *Cancer* 1998;82(6):1160.
32. Cascinu S, Graziano F, Alessandroni P, et al. Different doses of pamidronate in patients with painful osteolytic bone metastases. *Support Care Cancer* 1998;6:139.
33. Fulfaro F, Casuccio A, Ticozzi C, Ripamonti C. The role of bisphosphonates in the treatment of painful metastatic bone disease: a review of phase III trials. *Pain* 1998;78:157.
34. Theriault RL, Lipton A, Horrobaggi ON, et al. Pamidronate reduces skeletal morbidity in women with advanced breast cancer and lytic bone lesions: a randomized placebo-controlled trial. *J Clin Oncol* 1999;17(3):846.
35. Hortobaggi ON, Theriault RL, Lipton A, et al. Long-term prevention of skeletal complications of metastatic breast cancer with pamidronate. *J Clin Oncol* 1998;16(6):2038.
36. Berenson JR, Lichtenstein A, Porter L, et al. Long-term pamidronate treatment of advanced multiple myeloma patients reduces skeletal events. *J Clin Oncol* 1998;16(2):593.
37. Tamura H, Ishii S, Enomoto K, et al. Evaluation of the therapeutic efficacy of bisphosphonate (BP) to bone metastasis of breast cancer in a rat model. *Proc Annu Meet Am Assoc Cancer Res* 1994;35:A2787(abst).
38. Goodship AE, Walker PC, McNally D, Chambers T, Green JR. Use of a bisphosphonate (pamidronate) to modulate fracture repair in ovine bone. *Ann Oncol* 1994;5[Suppl 7]:S53.
39. Harvey HA. Issues concerning the role of chemotherapy and hormonal therapy of bone metastases from breast carcinoma. *Cancer* 1997;80[8 Suppl]:1646.
40. Gainor BJ, Buchert P. Fracture healing in metastatic bone disease. *Clin Orthop* 1983;178:297.
41. Takahashi I, Niibe H, Mitsuhashi N, et al. Palliative radiotherapy of bone metastasis. *Adv Exp Med Biol* 1992;324:227.
42. Bates T, Yarnold JR, Blitzer P, et al. Bone metastasis consensus statement. *Int J Radiat Oncol Biol Phys* 1992;23:215.
43. Blitzer P. Reanalysis of the RTOG study of the palliation of symptomatic osseous metastasis. *Cancer* 1985;55:1468.
44. Ahmed M, Bjurholm A, Kreicbergs A, Schultzberg M. Sensory and autonomic innervation of the facet joint in the rat lumbar spine. *Spine* 1993;18:2121.
45. Algara M, Valls A, Ruiz V, et al. Half-body irradiation: palliative efficacy and predictive factors of response in 78 procedures. *Med Clin (Barc)* 1994;103:85.
46. Zelefsky MJ, Scher HI, Forman JD, et al. Palliative hemiskeletal irradiation for widespread metastatic prostate cancer: a comparison of single dose and fractionated regimens. *Int J Radiat Oncol Biol Phys* 1989;17:1281.
47. Young RF, Post EM, King GA. Treatment of spinal epidural metastases: randomized prospective comparison of laminectomy and radiotherapy. *J Neurosurg* 1980;53:741.
48. Stark RJ, Henson RA, Evans SJ. Spinal metastases: a retrospective survey from a general hospital. *Brain* 1982;105:189.
49. Porter AT, Fontanesi J. Palliative irradiation for bone metastasis: a new paradigm [Editorial]. *Int J Radiat Oncol Biol Phys* 1994;29:1199.
50. Lucraft HH. Primary lymphoma of bone: a review of 13 cases emphasizing orthopedic problems. *Clin Oncol (R Coll Radiol)* 1991;3:265.
51. Lewis SJ, Bell RS, Fernandes BJ, Burkes RL. Malignant lymphoma of bone. *Can J Surg* 1994;37:43.

Allen KL, Johnson TW, Hibbs GG. Effective bone palliation as related to various treatment regimens. *Cancer* 1976;37(2):984.

53. Tong D, Gillick L, Hendrickson FR. The palliation of symptomatic osseous metastases: final results of the study by the Radiation Therapy Oncology Group. *Cancer* 1982;50:893.
54. Gilbert HA, Kagan HR, Nussbaum H. Evaluation of radiation therapy of bone metastases: pain relief and qualify of life. *AJR Am J Roentgenol* 1977;129:1095.
55. Bauer HC, Wedin R. Survival after surgery for spinal and extremity metastases: prognostication in 241 patients. *Acta Orthop Scand* 1995;66:143.
56. Cole DJ. A randomized trial of a single treatment versus conventional fractionation in the palliative radiotherapy of painful bone metastases. *Clin Orthop* 1989;1:59.
57. Price P, Hoskin PJ, Easton E. Low dose single fraction radiotherapy in the treatment of metastatic bone pain: a pilot study. *Radiother Oncol* 1988;12:297.
58. Garmatis CJ, Chu FCH. The effectiveness of radiation therapy in the treatment of bone metastases from breast cancer. *Radiology* 1978;126:235.
59. Varga O, Glicksman AS, Boland J. Single-dose radiation therapy in the palliation of metastatic disease. *Radiology* 1969;93:1180.
60. Arcangeli G, Micheli A. The responsiveness of bone metastases to radiotherapy: the effect of site histology and radiation dose on pain relief. *Radiother Oncol* 1989;14:95.
61. Perez CA, Cosmatos D, Garcia DM, Eisbruch A, Poulter CA. Irradiation in relapsing carcinoma of the prostate. *Cancer* 1993;71:1110.
62. Porter AT, McEwan AJB, Powe JE. Results of a randomized phase-III trial to evaluate the efficacy of strontium-89 adjuvant to local field external beam irradiation in the management of endocrine resistant metastatic prostate cancer. *Int J Radiat Oncol Biol Phys* 1993;25:805.
63. Houston SJ, Rubens RD. The systemic treatment of bone metastases. *Clin Orthop* 1995;312:95.
64. Robinson RG, Preston DF, Scheifelbein M, Baxter KG. Strontium 89 therapy for the palliation of pain due to osseous metastases. *JAMA* 1995;274(5):420.
65. McEwan AJB, Porter AT, Venner PM, Amyotte G. An evaluation of the safety and efficacy of treatment with Strontium-89 in patients who have previously received wide field radiotherapy. *Antibody Immunoconj Radiopharm* 1990;3:9.
66. Reilly DT, Burstein AH. Review article: the mechanical properties of cortical bone. *J Bone Joint Surg Am* 1974;56:1001.
67. Reilly DT, Burstein AH, Frankel VH. The elastic modulus for bone. *J Biomech* 1974;7:271.
68. Hipp JA, Katz G, Hayes WC. Local demineralization as a model for bone strength reductions in lytic transcortical metastatic lesions. *Invest Radiol* 1991;26:934.
69. Hipp JA, Rosenberg AE, Hayes WC. Mechanical properties of trabecular bone within and adjacent to osseous metastases. *J Bone Miner Res* 1992;7:1165.
70. Burnstein AH, Zika JM, Heiple KG, Klein L. Contribution of collagen and mineral to the elastic-plastic properties of bone. *J Bone Joint Surg Am* 1975;57:956.
71. Brooks DB, Burstein AH, Frankel VH. The biomechanics of torsional fractures: the stress concentration effect of a drill hole. *J Bone Joint Surg Am* 1970;52:507.
72. Burnstein AH, Currey J, Frankel VH, et al. Bone strength: the effect of screw holes. *J Bone Joint Surg Am* 1972;54:1143.
73. Hipp JA, Edgerton BC, An KN, Hayes WC. Structural consequences of transcortical holes in long bones loaded in torsion. *J Biomech* 1990;23:1261.
74. Pelker RR, Friedlaender GE, Panjabi MM, et al. Chemotherapy-induced alterations in the biomechanics of rat bone. *J Orthop Res* 1985;3:91.
75. Dijstra S, Wiggers T, Van Geel BN, Boxma H. Impending and actual pathological fractures in patients with bone metastases of the long bones: a retrospective study of 233 surgically treated fractures. *Eur J Surg* 1994;160:535.
76. Martens M, Frankel VH, Burstein AH. Ultimate properties of intramedullary nails. *Injury* 1972;4:18.
77. Van Der Hulst RR, Van Den Wildenberg FA, Vroemen JP, Greve JW. Intramedullary nailing of (impending) pathologic fractures. *J Trauma* 1994;36:211.
78. Williams WW, Hudson I, Hall AJ, et al. Nailing of impending and pathological fractures of the proximal femur. *Int Orthop* 1992;169:93.
79. Keating JF, Burke T, Macauley P. Proximal femoral replacement for pathological fracture. *Injury* 1990;21:231.
80. Chan D, Carter SR, Grimer RJ, Sneath RS. Endoprosthetic replacement for bony metastases. *Ann R Coll Surg Engl* 1992;74:13.
81. Malawer MM, Buch RG, Thompson WE, Sugarbaker PH. Major amputations done with palliative intent in the treatment of local bony complications associated with advanced cancer. *J Surg Oncol* 1991;47:121.
82. Leiger JF, Tauber LN. Solitary metastasis of occult prostatic carcinoma simulating osteogenic sarcoma. *Cancer* 1968;22:168.
83. Healey JH, Turnbull AD, Miedema B, Lane JM. Acrometastases: a study of twenty-nine patients with osseous involvement of the hands and feet. *J Bone Joint Surg Am* 1986;68(5):743.
84. Morris DM, House HC. The significance of metastasis to the bones and soft tissues of the hand. *J Surg Oncol* 1985;28:146.
85. Cotten A, Boutry N, Cortet B, et al. Percutaneous vertebroplasty: state of the art. *Radiographics* 1998;18(2): 311.
86. Cotten A, Dewatre F, Cortet B, et al. Percutaneous vertebroplasty for osteolytic metastases and myeloma: effects of the percentage lesion filling and the leakage of methylmethacrylate at clinical follow-up. *Radiology* 1996;200(2):525.
87. Weill AH, Kobaiter H, Chiras J. Acetabulum malignancies: technique and impact on pain of percutaneous injection of acrylic surgical cement. *Eur Radiol* 1998;8(1):123.
88. Harrington KD, Johnston JO, Turner RA, Green DL. The use of methylmethacrylate as an adjunct in the internal fixation of malignant neoplastic fractures. *J Bone Joint Surg Am* 1972;54:1665.
89. Althausen P, Althausen A, Jennings LC, Mankin HJ. Prognostic factors and surgical treatment of osseous metastases secondary to renal cell carcinoma. *Cancer* 1997;80(6):1103.
90. Loftus CM, Michelsen CB, Rapoport F, Antunes JL. Management of plasmacytomas of the spine. *Neurosurgery* 1983;13:30.
91. Sundaresan N, Choi IS, Huges JE, Sachder VP, Berenstein A. Treatment of spinal metastases from kidney cancer by presurgical embolization and resection. *J Neurosurg* 1990;73:548.
92. Olerud C, Jonsson H Jr, Lofberg AM, Lovelius LE, Sjostrom L. Embolization of spinal metastases reduces preoperative blood loss: 21 patients operated on for renal cell carcinoma. *Acta Orthop Scand* 1993;64:9.

93. O'Rielly GV, Kleefield J, Klein LA, et al. Embolization of solitary spinal metastases from renal cell carcinoma: alternative therapy for spinal cord or nerve root compression. *Surg Neurol* 1989;31:268.
94. Roscoe MW, McBroom RJ, St. Louis E, Grossman H, Perrin R. Preoperative embolization in the treatment of osseous metastases from renal cell carcinoma. *Clin Orthop* 1989;238:302.
95. Malawar MM, Marks MR, McChecney D. The effect of cryosurgery and polymethylmethacrylate (PMMA) in dogs with experimental bone defects comparable to tumor defects. *Clin Orthop* 1988;226:229.
96. Marcove RC. A 17-year review of cryosurgery in the treatment of bone tumors. *Clin Orthop* 1982;163:231.
97. Wang HM, Galasko CSB, Crank S, Oliver G, Ward CA. Methotrexate loaded acrylic cement in the management of skeletal metastases: biomechanical biological and systemic effect. *Clin Orthop* 1995;312:173.
98. Karagiri H, Saro K, Takahashi M, et al. Use of Adriamycin-impregnated methylmethacrylate in the treatment of tumor metastasis in the long bones. *Arch Orthop Trauma Surg* 1997;116(6–7):329.
99. Snell WE, Beals RK. Femoral metastases and fractures from breast cancer. *Surg Gynecol Obstet* 1964;119:22.
100. Parrish FF, Murray JA. Surgical treatment for secondary neoplastic fractures. *J Bone Joint Surg Am* 1970;52:665.
101. Fidler M. Prophylactic internal fixation of secondary neoplastic deposits in long bones. *Br Med J* 1973;1:341.
102. Zickel RE, Mouradian WH. Intramedullary fixation of pathological fractures and lesions of the subtrochanteric region of the femur. *J Bone Joint Surg Am* 1976;58:1061.
103. Harrington KD. New trends in the management of lower extremity metastases. *Clin Orthop* 1982;169:53.
104. Keene JS, Sellinger DS, McBeath AA, Engber WD. Metastatic breast cancer in the femur: a search for the lesion at risk of fracture. *Clin Orthop* 1986;203:282.
105. Mirels H. Metastatic disease in long bones: a proposed scoring system for diagnosing impending pathologic fractures. *Clin Orthop* 1989;249:256.
106. Callaway GH, Healey JH. Surgical management of metastatic carcinoma. *Curr Opin Orthop* 1990;1:416.
107. McBroom RJ, Cheal EJ, Hayes WC. Strength reductions from metastatic cortical defects in long bones. *J Orthop Res* 1988;6:369.
108. Hipp JA, McBroom RJ, Cheal EJ, Hayes WC. Structural consequences of endosteal metastatic lesions in long bones. *J Orthop Res* 1989;7:828.
109. Beaupre GS, Carter DR, Dueland RT, Caler WE, Spengler DM. A biomechanical assessment of plate fixation with insufficient bony support. *J Orthop Res* 1988;6:721.
110. Robbins SG, Lane JM, Healey JH, Cornell CN. Metastatic bone disease: epidemiology, biology, diagnosis, and treatment. In: Lane JM, Healey JH, eds. *Diagnosis and management of pathologic fractures.* New York: Raven Press, 1993:99.
111. Lane JM, Sculco TP, Zolan S. Treatment of pathological fractures of the hip by endoprosthetic replacement. *J Bone Joint Surg Am* 1980;62:954.
112. Schaberg J, Gainor BJ. A profile of metastatic carcinoma of the spine. *Spine* 1985;10:19.
113. Wong DA, Fornasier VL, MacNab I. Spinal metastases: the obvious, the occult, and the impostors. *Spine* 1990;15:1.
114. Smith MD, Emery SE, Dudley A, Murray KJ, Leventhal M. Vertebral artery injury during anterior decompression of the cervical spine: a retrospective review of ten patients. *J Bone Joint Surg Br* 1993;75:410.
115. Sundaresan N, Digriacinto GV, Huges JE, Cafferty M, Vallejo A. Treatment of neoplastic spinal cord compression: results of a prospective study. *Neurosurgery* 1991;29:645.
116. Weinstein JN, Differential diagnosis and surgical treatment of pathologic spine fractures. In: Eilert RE, ed. *Instructional Course Lectures.* Illinois: American Academy of Orthopaedic Surgeons; 1992:301.
117. Tomita K, Toribatake Y, Kawahara N, Ohnari H, Kose H. Total en bloc spondylectomy and circumspinal decompression for solitary spinal metastasis. *Paraplegia* 1994;32:36.
118. Tokuhashi Y, Matsuzaki H, Toriyama S, Kawano H, Ohsaka S. Scoring system for the preoperative evaluation of metastatic spine tumor prognosis. *Spine* 1990;15:1110.
119. Tomita T, Galicich JH, Sundaresan N. Radiation therapy for spinal epidural metastases with complete block. *Acta Radiol Oncol* 1983;22:135.
120. Rao S, Badani K, Schildhauer T, Borges M. Metastatic malignancy of the cervical spine: a nonoperative history. *Spine* 1992;17[Suppl 10]:S407.
121. Solini A, Paschero B, Orsini G, Guercio N. The surgical treatment of metastatic tumors of the lumbar spine. *Ital J Orthop Traumatol* 1985;11:427.
122. Harrington KD. The use of methylmethacrylate for vertebral-body replacement and anterior stabilization of pathological fracture-dislocations of the spine due to metastatic malignant disease. *J Bone Joint Surg Am* 1981;63(1):36.
123. Harrington KD. Metastatic tumors of the spine: diagnosis and treatment. *J Am Acad Orthop Surg* 1993;1(2):76.
124. Sundaresan N, Galicich JH, Lane JM, Bains MS, McCormack P. Treatment of neoplastic epidural cord compression by vertebral body resection and stabilization. *J Neurosurg* 1985;63:676.
125. Rosenthal HG, Healey JH, Peterson M, et al. Outcome analysis of corpectomy without posterior instrumentation. In: Brown KLB, ed. *Complications of limb salvage: prevention, management, and outcome.* Montreal: International Society of Limb-Sparing Surgery, 1991.
126. Bilsky MH, Boland PJ, Lis E, Raizer JJ, Healey JH. Single stage posterolateral transpedicle approach (PTA) for spondylectomy, epidural decompression, and circumferential fusion of spinal metastases. *Spine* 1999.
127. Roy-Camille R, Saillant G, Mazel C. Internal fixation of the lumbar spine with pedicle screw plating. *Clin Orthop* 1986;203:7.
128. Zdeblick TA, Shirado O, McAfee PC, deGroot H, Warden KE. Anterior spinal fixation after lumbar corpectomy: a study in dogs. *J Bone Joint Surg Am* 1991;73:527.
129. McAfee PC, Zdeblick TA. Tumors of the thoracic and lumbar spine: surgical treatment via the anterior approach. *J Spinal Disord* 1989;2:145.
130. Kaneda K, Asano S, Hashimoto T, Satoh S, Fujiya M. The treatment of osteoporotic-post-traumatic vertebral collapse using the Kaneda device and a bioactive ceramic vertebral prosthesis. *Spine* 1992;17:S295.
131. Bohm H, Harms J, Donk R, Zielke K. Correction and stabilization of angular kyphosis. *Clin Orthop* 1990;258:56.
132. Tomita K, Kawahara N, Baba H, et al. Total en bloc spondylectomy: a new surgical technique for primary malignant vertebral tumors. *Spine* 1997;22(3):324.
133. King GJ, Kostuik JP, McBroom RJ, Richardson W. Surgical management of metastatic renal carcinoma of the spine. *Spine* 1991;16:265.
134. Sim FH. Instructional Course Lectures—metastatic bone diseases: management of lesions of hip and acetabulum. In: *American Academy of Orthopaedic Surgeons 66th Annual Meeting.* Anaheim, CA; 1999.
135. Harrington KD. Pathological fractures of the pelvis and acetabulum. In: Harrington KD, ed. *Orthopaedic management of metastatic bone disease.* St Louis: Mosby, 1988:215.
136. Rock MG, Harrington KD. Pathologic fractures of the acetabulum and the pelvis. *Orthopedics* 1992;15:569.
137. Sarolaine ER, Ebraheim NA, Jackson WT, Conover SR. Modified Judet radiographic projection in evaluation of acetabular insufficiency secondary to metastatic disease. *Orthopedics* 1990;13:1154.
138. Sim FH. Metastatic bone disease of the pelvis and femur. In: Eilert RE, ed. *Instructional Course Lectures.* Illinois: American Academy of Orthopaedic Surgeons: 317.
139. Marco RAW, Sheth DS, Boland PJ, et al. Functional and oncological outcome of acetabular reconstruction for the treatment of metastatic disease. *Journal of Bone and Joint Surgery* 2000;82A(5):642.
140. Aboulafia AJ, Faulks W, Li W, et al. Reconstruction using the Saddle prosthesis following excision of malignant periacetabular tumors. In: Brown KLB, ed. *Complications of limb salvage: prevention, man†agement, and outcome.* Montreal: International Society of Limb-Sparing Surgery, 1991.

DAVID S. SCHRUMP
DAO M. NGUYEN

SECTION 5

Malignant Pleural and Pericardial Effusions

MALIGNANT PLEURAL EFFUSION

Forty percent of all pleural effusions are due to malignancy,[1] and cancer is the second leading cause of pleural effusion in patients older than 50 years of age. Approximately 100,000 cases of malignant pleural effusion (MPE) occur annually in the United States, and MPE is the initial manifestation in 10% to 50% of cancer patients.[2] Two-thirds of MPEs are attributable to lung carcinoma (35%) or breast carcinoma (23%) and lymphoma (10%). Carcinomas of unknown primary origin account for an additional 12% of MPEs.[3] Presence of MPE frequently indicates advanced and incurable disease. Although the overall prognosis of patients with MPE depends on the histology and extent of their primary disease, significant palliation can be achieved in these individuals by accurate and timely diagnosis and interventions associated with minimal morbidity.

PATHOGENESIS OF MALIGNANT PLEURAL EFFUSION

The pleural space functions as a mechanical coupling system between the lung and the chest wall. The normal pleural space is between 7 and 27 μm in width and is filled with 10 to 40 mL of hypoproteinemic plasma.[4,5] Most of the pleural fluid originates from the capillary bed of the parietal pleura. The major route of pleural fluid efflux is through the parietal pleural lymphatics, which have a clearance capacity 28 times greater than the rate of fluid formation.[6] Under normal conditions, a dynamic equilibrium exists between the osmotic and hydrostatic pressures that control the secretion and absorption of the pleural fluid. Accumulation of fluid within the pleural space may be the consequence of any of the following[7]:

- Increased hydrostatic pressure in the microvascular circulation
- Decreased oncotic pressure in the microvascular circulation
- Decreased pressure in the pleural space
- Increased permeability of the microvascular circulation
- Impaired lymphatic drainage from the pleural space
- Transudation of fluid from the peritoneum via lymphatics or anatomic defects in the diaphragm

MPEs typically arise as the result of altered microvascular permeability, as well as diffuse metastatic involvement of mediastinal or subpleural lymphatics. Pulmonary parenchymal tumors (primary or metastatic) may erode the visceral pleura, spilling cells and disrupting the normal resorption of fluid by the visceral pleura. Alternatively, the parietal and visceral pleura themselves are common sites of deposits, resulting in increased capillary permeability due to inflammation, overt endothelial disruption, or obstruction of efferent flow with elevated lymphatic hydrostatic pressure. Primary or metastatic involvement of hilar or mediastinal lymph nodes obstructs normal visceral and parietal lymphatic drainage, resulting in pleural effusion.[8] In an autopsy study of 29 patients with lung cancer, Meyer[9] observed that the development of pleural effusion was closely related to malignant infiltration of mediastinal lymph nodes but not the extent of pleural metastases. Typically, involvement of the mesothelial surface results in exfoliation of tumor cells into the pleural fluid; however, few malignant cells will be found in the pleural fluid in the setting of submesothelial involvement.

Occasionally, pleural effusions in cancer patients are negative for malignancy despite exhaustive diagnostic efforts. Although related to the underlying cancer, these paramalignant effusions are not due to metastatic disease involving the pleura but rather are caused by obstruction of the hilar-mediastinal lymph nodes or bronchial obstruction, resulting in pneumonitis or atelectasis. Such paramalignant effusions, if associated with non–small cell lung cancer, should not preclude patients from undergoing potentially curative resection if otherwise indicated. However, in most lung cancer patients, cytologically negative pleural effusions eventually are found to be inoperable.[10,11] Decker et al.[11] observed that only 4 of 73 patients (5.5%) with lung cancer and cytologically negative pleural effusions had resectable disease,[11] demonstrating that pleural effusions of any kind in lung cancer patients typically are indicative of locally advanced, incurable disease. Furthermore, occult malignant cells have been detected by pleural washing in nearly 15% of patients undergoing resection of presumed stage I non–small cell lung cancer[12]; survival of these individuals is as poor as that reported for patients with stage III disease, indicating the ominous nature of pleural space metastases of any kind in lung cancer patients.

CLINICAL PRESENTATION

MPE is often an initial manifestation of cancer; nearly 50% of individuals presenting with MPE have no history of malignancy.[13,14] Most patients with MPE are symptomatic, with dyspnea of varying severity being the predominant symptom; cough and chest discomfort ranging from dull ache (often characterized as heaviness or pressure) to sharp pleuritic pain may also be present.[13] Physical examination usually reveals decreased breath sounds, with dullness to percussion and diminished tactile fremitus. Tracheal deviation and low cardiac output related to mediastinal compression occasionally may be seen with large effusions.

DIAGNOSIS AND EVALUATION

Radiographic Examinations

As little as 200 mL of pleural fluid, evidenced by blunting of the costophrenic angle, can be detected by standard posterolateral and lateral chest radiographs. Upright posteroanterior, lateral, and lateral decubitus chest radiographs that allow assessment of "free-flowing" pleural effusion should be performed as initial investigations. Particularly in the setting of a newly diagnosed effusion, computed tomographic (CT) scan of the chest should be performed to define fluid loculations or hilar lymphadenopathy, pleural masses, and parenchymal disease. Complete opacification of the hemithorax occurs in approximately 15% of MPE; an opacified hemithorax with mediastinal shift toward the contralateral side indicates massive effusion, whereas opacification without a shift may be due to a combination of pleural fluid and lung collapse resulting from proximal airway obstruction, effusion with mediastinal fixation by malignant lymphadenopathy, or malignant mesothelioma.[15]

Invasive Diagnostic Maneuvers

After appropriate radiographic assessment, thoracentesis should be performed to obtain fluid for biochemical and cytopathologic analysis, to relieve symptoms, and to determine the extent of lung expansion after pleural fluid drainage. In the presence of free-flowing effusion, thoracentesis can be safely performed at the level of the posterior sixth or seventh intercostal space, removing 500 to 1000 mL of fluid. In the presence of a large pleural effusion occupying more than 50% of the pleural cavity, gradual drainage of the fluid is prudent to avoid postexpansion pulmonary edema.[16–18] If the pleural collection is loculated, ultrasound- or CT-guided drainage is recommended. A small sample of pleural fluid should be sent for biochemical analysis; the remaining fluid should be processed for cytopathologic examination.

After thoracentesis, patients frequently experience less dyspnea and chest heaviness, even in situations in which the lung fails to expand after evacuation of the effusion due to encasement with malignant or inflammatory "peel." Possible complications of thoracentesis include bleeding, pneumothorax requiring tube thoracostomy (in approximately 5%), vagovagal reaction, pain from reexpansion of the lung and apposition of pleural surfaces, and reexpansion pulmonary edema.[19,20]

The initial cytology result is positive in approximately one-half of patients who are ultimately found to have MPE. If initial cytology results are negative, repeat thoracentesis should be performed, since malignant cells will be identified in an additional 20% of patients. Closed pleural biopsy performed either by random sampling of the pleura just before thoracentesis (to minimize lung injury) or using CT guidance may be considered to expedite diagnosis of patients with presumed MPE. However, recent data indicate that closed pleural biopsy is complementary to pleural fluid cytology and only slightly increases the yield in diagnosing malignancy.[21] In a direct comparison of closed pleural biopsy with cytologic examination, Nance et al.[22] observed that pleural biopsy was diagnostic in 45% of patients with MPE, 75% of whom had positive cytology results; pleural biopsy was informative in only 3% of patients whose cytology results were negative.[22] The low yield of closed pleural biopsy is related to the focal nature of metastatic disease in the pleural space. In contrast, thoracoscopy performed either by direct pleuroscopy under local anesthesia with intravenous sedation or with video assistance under general anesthesia has a diagnostic yield of nearly 100% for malignant disease involving the pleura.[23–25] Therefore, patients whose effusions remain undiagnosed after two thoracentesis procedures should be referred for thoracoscopy.

Biochemical and Pathologic Analysis

Pleural fluid obtained by diagnostic thoracentesis should be routinely sent for protein, glucose, and lactate dehydrogenase (LDH) analysis and for cell counts, cultures, and pathologic examinations. MPE is most commonly exudative (LDH >200 U/mL; fluid-serum LDH ratio >0.6; fluid-serum protein ratio >0.5).[26] Frequently, fluid is blood-tinged or grossly hemorrhagic, owing to disruption of capillaries or venules by direct tumor invasion or cytokine-mediated vasodilation.[15] Typically, the pleural fluid is hypercellular, with leukocytes (1000 to 10,000 cells/mm^3, predominantly lymphocytes and monocytes), reactive mesothelial cells, and exfoliated tumor cells. Approximately one-third of MPEs are acidic (pH <7.3), with glucose-serum ratios of less than 0.5. These biochemical parameters correlate with advanced disease, poor response to palliative pleurodesis maneuvers, and diminished survival in patients with MPE.[27,28]

The diagnosis of MPE is confirmed in approximately 50% of patients after initial cytopathologic evaluation. Second and third thoracentesis procedures may increase the diagnostic yield to 65% and 70%, respectively[3,29]; analysis of carcinoembryonic antigen has not proven to be specific enough to discriminate benign from malignant epithelial effusions.[30] Pleural fluid cytology is positive in fewer than 33% of patients with lymphomas and leukemias; cytogenetic studies can confirm the malignant nature of pleural effusions in 80% of these individuals.[3]

Almost all patients with malignant pleural mesothelioma present with effusions. Atypical mesothelial cells are nearly always present in all pleural effusions irrespective of the underlying malignancy, and differentiating malignant mesothelioma from metastatic adenocarcinoma can be difficult. Analysis of hyaluronidase levels (which frequently are elevated in malignant pleural mesothelioma) has not proven to be sufficiently sensitive to be diagnostic[31]; as such, immunohistochemistry techniques must be used to distinguish epithelial pleural mesotheliomas from pulmonary adenocarcinomas. In general, pulmonary adenocarcinomas tend to express carcinoembryonic antigen, LeuM1, B72.3, and BerEP4; in contrast, the majority of epithelial mesotheliomas do not express these antigens.[32] Histopathologic diagnosis of malignant mesothelioma frequently requires relatively large tissue samples obtained by thoracoscopy techniques.

TREATMENT

The treatment of MPE should focus on palliation of symptoms and must be tailored to the patient's physical condition and prognosis. Overall, 54% and 84% of patients with MPE succumb within 1 month and 3 months, respectively, after diagnosis. However, survival is related to the histology of the underlying disease. Patients with malignant effusions secondary to breast cancer may live 1 year or more, whereas individuals with ovarian cancer have an average survival of 9 months. In contrast, patients with lung or gastric carcinomas typically do not survive more than 3 months after detection of MPE.[2]

Thoracentesis

Thoracentesis may be an appropriate treatment for MPE in patients with limited life expectancy who cannot tolerate any surgical procedure. Recurrent effusions are observed in 97% of individuals within 30 days after thoracentesis. In general, pleurodesis immediately after thoracentesis is not effective, since residual pleural fluid dilutes the sclerosing agent, thus diminishing its irritant effects on the pleura. Loculations may form after such treatment, rendering definitive therapy of the pleural effusion more complicated. In patients presenting with MPE as the initial manifestation of breast cancer, small cell lung cancer, germ cell tumors, or lymphoma, thoracentesis followed by systemic chemotherapy may successfully treat disease in the pleural space. However, most patients with MPE require more aggressive intervention to prevent recurrence.

Tube Thoracostomy with or without Pleurodesis

After thoracentesis and reexpansion of the lung, pleural fluid should be completely evacuated with a tube thoracostomy to allow apposition of the visceral and parietal pleura. Recurrent effusions are noted in 60% to 100% of patients after tube thoracostomy drainage alone; in general, obliteration of the pleural space, either by parietal pleurectomy or instillation of sclerosants causing inflammation and subsequent pleural symphysis, is required to ensure durable relief. Chemical pleurodesis is the preferred treatment for patients with MPE, and the efficacy of this intervention depends on (1) complete drainage of the pleural space and reexpansion of the lung to ensure apposition of the pleural surfaces and (2) instillation of an effective sclerosing agent into the pleural space and retention of this agent in the chest for several hours to induce an inflammatory fibrosis.

The chest tube (28 Fr. to 32 Fr.) is routinely inserted at the level of the sixth or seventh intercostal space laterally and directed posteriorly to the most dependent portion of the pleural cavity. Once complete drainage is achieved (as confirmed by chest radiograph and daily drainage of <150 mL), the sclerosing agent (suspended or dissolved in 100 to 150 mL of normal saline) is instilled into the pleural space via the chest tube. The tube is then clamped for 1 to 2 hours, during which time the patient changes position periodically to enhance distribution of the sclerosant; subsequently the tube is unclamped and connected to suction. The tube is removed when the daily drainage is again less than 150 mL.

Traditionally, this method of treatment requires hospitalization for 4 to 6 days and placement of a large-bore chest tube for complete evacuation of the exudative effusion prior to chemical pleurodesis. However, several studies have indicated that pigtail catheter drainage and sclerosis may be as successful as more traditional chest tube pleurodesis procedures.[33,34] Recently, outpatient management of MPE with a small-bore all-purpose drainage catheter (10.3 Fr.) and bleomycin pleurodesis has been described.[35] Pleural fluid was drained by a catheter connected to a collection bag until drainage was less than 100 mL/day. Bleomycin (60 U in 50 mL of 5% dextrose in water) was then instilled to the chest via the drainage catheter, and the tube was removed 24 hours after pleurodesis. Fifty-three percent of patients treated in this manner experienced complete responses, and an additional 25% had partial responses. In another study, MPE was drained by a 12-Fr. van Sonnenberg pigtail catheter inserted under ultrasound guidance in 15 patients, 11 of whom had loculated pleural effusion (which necessitated this method of drainage).[36] Talc (5 g suspended in 100 mL of injectable normal saline) was instilled into the pleural cavity once pleural fluid drainage was less than 100 mL/day. Control of MPE was achieved in 80% of these cases; additional talc instillation was required in two patients to treat residual pockets of effusion with good results. These data suggest that outpatient management of MPE may be appropriate in patients with MPE who typically have limited life expectancies.

Pleurodesis Agents

Various agents have been used in the last 50 years to induce adhesive obliteration of the pleural space. Nitrogen mustard was one of the first agents used to treat MPE. The overall response rate was 52%.[37,38] The main complications related to its use were bone marrow suppression, pain, fever, nausea, and vomiting. Thiotepa, 5-fluorouracil, and bacille Calmette-Guérin[39,40] were also used but were found to have limited efficacy and unacceptable toxicity. Radioactive zinc, gold, chromium, or phosphorus were used in the 1940s to treat MPE, with a cumulative response rate of approximately 53%.[41,42] The main disadvantages of radioactive colloids were cost, short half-lives, and potential hazards to treatment personnel; these agents are no longer used clinically.

Certain chemicals have been extensively evaluated in both randomized and nonrandomized clinical studies for their efficacy as pleurodesis agents. None of them except bleomycin are known to possess antitumor activity. They induce intense pleural inflammation and, subsequently, adhesive fibrosis of the parietal and visceral pleurae.

TETRACYCLINE-DOXYCYCLINE. Tetracycline was extensively used as a sclerosing agent to treat pleural effusions of benign and malignant etiologies because of its efficacy, low cost, and safety. The overall efficacy of tetracycline in controlling MPE was 70%.[43,44] The usual dose was 500 to 1000 mg diluted in 100 mL of normal saline. The main side effects were pleuritic pain (20% to 70%) at the time of drug instillation and low-grade fever (33%). Lidocaine (20 mL of 1% or 2% solution) could be mixed with tetracycline prior to administration to decrease pleuritic pain. Injectable tetracycline is no longer available in the United States since 1991, because the drug preparations did not meet the U.S. Food and Drug Administration purity standards; as such, the tetracycline derivatives doxycycline and minocycline have been used for pleurodesis. Three small, uncontrolled clinical trials have reported response rates of 67% to 88% after doxycycline pleurodesis.[45–47] The side effects are similar to those observed with tetracycline. Most patients require repeated doxycycline instillation for successful pleurodesis. In these reported series, only 15% of patients responded to a single treatment, and 9% required more than four instillations. Intrapleural minocycline (300 mg with 1% lidocaine) was given to seven patients with MPE, of whom six responded (86%).[48] The small number of patients studied, unspecified criteria for success, and duration of treatment response make for difficult comparisons of minocycline with other agents.

BLEOMYCIN. Intrapleural administration of bleomycin (60 to 120 U) achieves pleurodesis in 65% of patients with MPE (range, 62% to 81%).[49–52] Intrapleural bleomycin is well tolerated and associated with few side effects.[53] In a multicenter, randomized trial,[43] bleomycin was superior to tetracycline for pleurodesis; 70% of patients treated with bleomycin had successful control of their MPE, as compared to only 47% of patients treated with tetracycline. However, bleomycin is expensive; typically, each treatment dose ranges from US $1100 to $1300. Bleomycin has been compared with less expensive talc pleurodesis in a prospective randomized study of 29 women with MPE secondary to breast cancer. Of 22 evaluable patients (with 3 patients having had bilateral pleurodesis), all 10 patients (100%) treated with talc had complete control of their MPE, as compared to 10 of 15 patients (67%) receiving bleomycin.[51]

TALC. Chambers[54] was the first to use talc to treat MPE.[54] Talc produces an intense chemical pleuritis that effectively obliterates the pleural space.[55] Asbestos-free, gas-sterilized, or heat-sterilized talc USP may be administered via chest tube as a slurry (5 g in 100 mL of normal saline) or insufflated as a powder during thoracoscopy or thoracotomy. Talc pleurodesis is highly effective, with the overall response rates ranging from 80% to 100%.[54,56–67] The most commonly reported adverse effects of talc pleurodesis are fever (16%) and pain (7%). Less common complications include empyema, pneumonitis (similar to acute respiratory distress syndrome), and respiratory failure.[65,68,69] Pulmonary complications noted in earlier series have not been observed as frequently in more recent trials and tend to occur in patients who receive 10 to 12 g of talc or undergo either bilateral pleurodesis or unilateral pleurodesis in conjunction with pleural biopsy (raising the possibility of talc emboli). Viallat et al.[64] reviewed their experience with thoracoscopic talc poudrage pleurodesis for MPE in 360 cases, including 88 mesothelioma patients and 272 individuals with effusions secondary to a variety of malignancies. Approximately 3 to 4.5 g of heat-sterilized asbestos-free talc was insufflated via atomizer during thoracoscopy. Pleurodesis was successful in 90% of 327 evaluable patients at 1 month, and 82% of individuals had lifelong pleurodesis. Complications included fever (10%), empyema (2.5%), pulmonary infection (0.8%), and malignant invasion of the thoracoscopy trocar site in a mesothelioma patient. Aelony et al.[67] reported effective talc pleurodesis using thoracoscopy in patients whose pleural

TABLE 52.5-1. Efficiency of Sclerosing Agents Used in Treating Patients with Malignant Pleural Effusion

Agents	*Response (%)* Mean	Range
Talc	98	72–100
Bleomycin	64	31–85
Tetracycline	72	25–100
Doxycycline	73	68–88
Quinacrine	86	64–100
Nitrogen mustard	44	27–95

(Adapted from ref. 71.)

fluid was acidic (<7.2), with a response rate of 88%. This high success rate compares favorably with the low response (57%) previously reported by Rodriguez-Panadero and Mejias.[28] Failure of talc thoracoscopic pleurodesis in these two studies was more closely correlated with the presence of trapped lung than with low pleural fluid pH.

Talc has consistently been shown to be superior to other commonly used sclerosing agents, such as tetracycline-doxycycline and bleomycin. The efficacy of past and currently used pleurodesis agents is summarized in Table 52.5-1. In a randomized controlled trial, Fentiman et al.[56] compared the efficacy of talc poudrage and tetracycline in 33 breast cancer patients with MPE. Ninety-two percent of patients receiving talc had successful pleurodesis, as compared to only 42% of patients receiving tetracycline. In another study, successful pleurodesis was observed in 97% of patients undergoing intrapleural talc insufflation by thoracoscopy, as compared to 70% and 47% of patients receiving bleomycin and tetracycline, respectively.[63] Thoracoscopic talc poudrage was also very effective in producing durable pleurodesis in patients with recalcitrant MPE who failed prior treatment with tetracycline.[67] Zimmer et al.[70] prospectively evaluated the efficacy of either bleomycin (60 U; 14 patients) or talc slurry (5 g; 19 patients) administered at the bedside via tube thoracostomy in 33 patients. Permanent control of MPE was noted in 79% of patients receiving bleomycin and 90% of patients treated with talc pleurodesis. The difference, however, did not reach statistical significance ($P = .34$). Due to the high cost of bleomycin, the authors recommended talc as the agent of choice for bedside chest tube pleurodesis. Talc poudrage has traditionally been performed by insufflating dry sterilized talc powder into the pleural cavity via the thoracoscope to ensure proper distribution and coating of the pleural surfaces. This technique incurs high costs due to operating room charges and specialized equipment. Pleurodesis achieved via talc slurry administered by thoracostomy tube appears to be more cost-effective than thoracoscopic talc poudrage (Table 52.5-2). A phase III randomized clinical trial comparing talc slurry via chest tube and talc insufflation by thoracoscopy is being conducted in North America with the participation of the Cancer and Leukemia Group B, the Eastern Cooperative Oncology Group, the Southwest Oncology Group, and the North Central Cancer Treatment Group[71]; the primary end points are evaluation of efficacy and cost-effectiveness of these two pleurodesis techniques.

QUINACRINE. Quinacrine (mepacrine), an antimalarial agent, has been a popular drug for pleurodesis of pleural effusion in Scandinavian countries. As with other aforementioned

TABLE 52.5-2. Efficacy of Talc Pleurodesis by Thoracoscopic Talc Poudrage or Talc Slurry by Tube Thoracostomy for Malignant Pleural Effusion

Study	*No. of Patients*	*Successful Pleurodesis[a] (%)*
THORACOSCOPIC TALC POUDRAGE		
Fentiman et al.[56]	12	92
Boniface et al.[58]	270	93
Marchandise et al.[57]	33	87
Hartman et al.[63]	33	90
Viallat et al.[64]	360	90
Yim et al.[154]	28	96
Ladjimi et al.[59]	218	78
Weissberg et al.[60]	169	92
Canto et al.[61]	128	86
Sanchez-Armengol[62]	119	87
Aelony et al.[67]	42	92
Total	1412	90 (average)
TALC SLURRY		
Yim et al.[154]	29	90
Webb et al.[66]	28	100
Kennedy et al.[155]	40	78
Chambers et al.[54]	22	86
Zimmer et al.[70]	19	90
Total	138	89 (average)

[a]As defined by parameters delineated in each study.

sclerosing agents, intrapleural instillation of quinacrine produces significant chemical pleuritis that promotes intrapleural adhesion formation.[72] The response rates to intrapleural quinacrine range from 75% to 100% and 70% to 90% after thoracentesis or chest tube drainage, respectively, in controlled clinical series.[72] Toxicities associated with quinacrine include fever, hypotension, and hallucination.[73]

CORYNEBACTERIUM PARVUM. Injection of the lipopolysaccharide extracts of *C parvum* (an anaerobic gram-positive bacterium) into the pleural space induces a strong, nonspecific inflammatory reaction.[74] Clinical experience with this agent was described in reports from nine studies performed in Europe, but *C parvum* is not available in the United States. Intrapleural injection of 3.5 to 14.0 g of *C parvum* (commercially available as Copravax, Wellcome Research, Beckenham, Kent, UK) has resulted in a cumulative response rate of 76% (129 of 169 evaluable patients), although significant variability has been noted in these studies (response rates ranging from 32% to 90%). The main untoward side effects include pain (43%), nausea (39%), and fever (5%). *C parvum* has been reported to be as effective as bleomycin or tetracycline[75–77] for chemical pleurodesis.

BIOLOGIC RESPONSE MODIFIERS. Chemical agents used for pleurodesis induce inflammatory adhesion of the pleurae, thus obliterating the pleural space and preventing reaccumulation of pleural effusion. Biologic response modifiers, such as interferons and interleukins, have been used to treat MPE primarily on the basis of their antitumor activity. Adequate drug levels can be achieved only by high systemic doses that are associated with severe side effects. Regional intrapleural administration of these agents yields biologically relevant drug concentrations with fewer systemic side effects. None of these agents, however, are routinely used to treat MPE. (They are briefly discussed here for academic interest.)

Interferons. Goldman et al.[78] studied the toxicity and efficacy of intrapleural administration of interferon-2b (50 million to 75 millions units) for MPE associated with cancers of different histologies in 23 patients. The pleural fluid was completely evacuated, and interferon was instilled via the chest tube for a maximum of three treatments per patient. Complete and partial resolution of MPE was documented in 14 of 20 evaluable patients (70%). The most common side effect was the flu-like syndrome followed by grade 3 hematologic toxicity in three patients who received high doses of 75 million units. Other studies also indicated somewhat lower response rates and similar toxicity profiles.[79,80]

Interleukin-2. Intrapleural administration of recombinant interleukin-2 (rIL-2) as a means to treat MPE has been evaluated in numerous small phase I trials.[81–84] Yasumoto and Ogura[82] treated 43 patients with MPE due to non–small cell lung cancer with daily intrapleural administrations of rIL-2 for an average of 14 days (5 to 33 days) after pleural effusion had been completely evacuated. Control of MPE was achieved in 21 of 35 evaluable patients (60%), with 13 experiencing complete disappearance of MPE. More impressive was the observation of disappearance of malignant cells in the pleural fluid samples sequentially obtained during treatment for cytologic analysis. This was noted in 26 of 35 evaluable patients (74%) and the effect lasted for more than 4 weeks in 19 patients (54%). This observation had also been reported by other investigators.[84] Viallat et al.[81] studied the effects and toxicity profiles of intrapleural injections of rIL-2 in 23 patients with MPE associated with cancers of various histologies. Objective responses were observed in 5 of 21 evaluable patients (24%). Side effects included fever, transient increase in pleural effusion, skin rash, and pruritus. Staphylococcus empyema attributed to prolonged chest tube drainage was noted in two patients.[81]

OK432. OK432 is a heat- and penicillin-treated lyophilized powder of the SU substrain of *Streptococcus pyogenes* A3. This immune modulator has recently been found to be useful in treating malignant ascites. Malignant ascites may decrease in volume and even disappear. The OK432 therapy increases neutrophils, macrophages, and lymphocyte[85] counts and augments autologous tumoricidal activity of large granular lymphocytes in ascites fluid.[86] Luh et al.[87] conducted a randomized trial to compare the efficacy of OK432 and mitomycin C in controlling MPE caused by lung cancer. Twenty-six patients received weekly injections of OK432 for 4 weeks. The overall response rate was 88%: 73% (19 of 26 patients) had complete response, and 15% (4 of 26 patients) experienced partial response. Fever, chills, and local pleuritic chest pain were the most common side effects and were observed in 80% of cases.

Intrapleural Chemotherapy

Few clinical studies were conducted to investigate the efficacy of intrapleural chemotherapy for MPE. Regional chemotherapy in the form of intrapleural chemotherapy for malignant mesothelioma is discussed in Chapter 40.2. The overall response rates of intrapleural chemotherapy are low, and the treatments, even though regional, are associated with significant systemic side effects. Unless studied within a context of a clinical trial, intrapleural chemotherapy has no role in the management of MPE.

Intrapleural combinations of cisplatin (100 mg/m^2) and cytosine arabinoside (600 to 1200 mg/m^2) have been used to treat MPE in two studies.[88,89] This combination produced a complete response in only 27% of the patients, and adverse effects including pain (66%), cardiopulmonary symptoms (54%), bone marrow suppression (52%), and renal toxicity (34%) were noted in 76% of the patients, suggesting that significant systemic absorption of the chemotherapeutic agents occurred in these individuals. Intrapleural doxorubicin at doses ranging from 10 to 40 mg has produced complete responses in 12 of 55 (22%) evaluable patients.[90–92] Adverse effects included pain (29%), fever (15%), nausea and vomiting (29%), and anorexia (24%). Repeated, escalating doses of etoposide (100 to 225 mg/m^2) have been administered intrapleurally to nine patients with MPE,[93] of whom none experienced clinical responses.

Cost-Effectiveness of Pleurodesis for Malignant Pleural Effusions

The most effective and economic method for the treatment of MPE is still a matter of debate. It is important for physicians who manage patients with MPE to be knowledgeable regarding the efficacy, toxicities, and costs of available treatment modalities. Even though the sclerosant is not expensive ($0.15 to $0.50 for a 2.5- to 10-g dose), the cost of talc pleurodesis performed by thoracoscopy is high because of operating room and professional fees. The total cost of treatment has been determined to be $20,996 (1992 U.S. dollars). The high success rate may justify the expense of talc pleurodesis. The 6-month cost of talc pleurodesis, estimated to be $149 per symptom-free day, should drop significantly if the procedure is performed by pleuroscopy under intravenous sedation and local anesthesia or by instillation of talc slurry via chest tube. Both these techniques are as effective as talc poudrage performed by video-assisted thoracoscopic surgery under general anesthesia. Bleomycin is the most expensive pleurodesis agent, the cost per dose averaging $1104; however, the total cost of treatment is relatively low, owing to the high efficiency of pleurodesis achieved with a single administration of this drug. The 6-month cost per symptom-free day was approximately $132 in an analysis reported by Belani et al.[71] Tetracycline and its currently available substitute, doxycycline, are costly ($159 and $218 per symptom-free day, respectively), given the fact that repeated administrations of these agents are required to achieve successful pleurodesis, thus prolonging hospitalization and increasing the risk of treatment-related complications.

Pleurectomy

Stripping of the parietal pleura is 100% effective in controlling MPE. Although it may have a role in the treatment of malignant pleural mesothelioma,[94] pleurectomy via thoracotomy is not routinely performed because the morbidity (23%) and mortality (10%)[95,96] cannot be justified in debilitated patients for whom less invasive and equally successful treatment options may be available. However, several recent studies have indicated that parietal pleurectomy can be performed via video-assisted thoracoscopic surgery (VATS) with acceptable risk in patients. Waller et al.[97] performed VATS parietal pleurectomy in 19 patients with MPE secondary to mesothelioma or metastatic adenocarcinoma. Symptomatic recurrent effusion occurred in three patients (15.7%). Tumor seeding at the thoracoscopic trocar sites occurred in 5 of 13 mesothelioma patients. More recently, Harvey et al.[98] performed VATS pleurectomy in 11 (5 non–small cell lung cancer, 4 breast cancer, 1 mesothelioma, 1 cancer of unknown primary) patients, with no recurrence and one death (1 of 11; 9%) due to sepsis from a necrotic tumor involving the liver. Other complications included prolonged air leak (one patient) and bleeding requiring reoperation and transfusion (one patient). The results of these two small series should not be viewed as justifications for more liberal application of VATS parietal pleurectomy as the first line of treatment for MPE. Instead, parietal pleurectomy should be reserved for malignant effusions that are refractory to less invasive and less expensive interventions.[96]

Pleuroperitoneal Shunt

The pleuroperitoneal shunt, introduced in 1982, has been evaluated as a therapeutic option for the treatment of MPE.[97] It may be used for recurrent effusions that are refractory to tube thoracostomy and pleurodesis or for MPE associated with trapped lung.[99–101] The most commonly used device is the Denver pleuroperitoneal shunt (Denver Biomaterials, Inc., Golden, CO). The shunt is a silicone rubber conduit consisting of a unidirectional valved pump chamber connecting to pleural and peritoneal catheters. The pumping chamber can be implanted into a subcutaneous pocket or exteriorized as an external pumping chamber. Because of the negative pressure differential between the pleural and peritoneal cavities, manual compression of the pumping chamber is required for fluid drainage from the chest. Each compression transports 1.5 mL of fluid, and patients are frequently asked to compress the pump for 5 to 10 minutes four times daily. Implantation of the shunt can be performed under local or general anesthesia. Petrou et al.[100] used pleuroperitoneal shunt in 63 patients with recurrent MPE and trapped lung. There were no operative deaths, and complications were noted in 5 patients (8%). Effective palliation was achieved in more than 95% of cases. Catheter occlusion was noted in eight patients (12%) at 1 week to 4 months after insertion, with five patients requiring replacement or revision of the shunt and three patients requiring shunt removal and treatment of empyema. Contraindications include pleural infection, multiple loculations, inability of the patient to press the chamber, short life expectancy, and obliterated peritoneal space.[102] The need for active pumping of the chamber a minimum of 400 times per day limits its usefulness to patients with excellent performance status. In addition, the shunt may malfunction over time, further limiting its usefulness. As such, the pleuroperitoneal shunt should be considered as one of the last alternatives for patients with refractory effusions.[71]

Indwelling Pleural Catheter

Malignant pleural fluid can be drained for prolonged periods by a small-caliber biocompatible silicone rubber indwelling catheter. The Tenckoff (Quinton Instrument, Seattle, WA) and Denver (Denver Biomaterials) catheters have similar design, consisting of a 15-Fr. translucent silicone rubber tube with a radiopaque stripe, a felt or polyester cuff, and a plastic occluding device that may be opened to drain the fluid. The catheter is inserted in the operating room under local anesthesia. Two small skin incisions are made in the anterolateral chest. The catheter is brought through a 15-cm subcutaneous tunnel between these two incisions. The pleural cavity is accessed with a needle and, using the Seldinger technique and a Tear Apart Introducer kit (Quinton Instrument), the catheter is introduced into the pleural cavity and positioned so that the felt cuff on the catheter lies just within the exit wound. The advantages of pleural catheter placement are the ease of insertion and minimal discomfort due to the catheter, rapid drainage of recurrent symptomatic effusion, and minimal or no hospitalization required for catheter insertion and care. Robinson et al.[103] used the Tenckoff catheter to manage MPE in nine patients, with three patients having bilateral catheter placement for a total of 12 catheters inserted. Four of the nine patients had recurrent pleural effusion after failed tube thoracostomy and chemical pleurodesis. None of the patients had trapped lung. The authors reported excellent palliation of symptoms in all patients. Complications were minor, with insertion-site cellulitis that was easily managed with oral antibiotic in 3 of 12 catheter sites (25%).

A phase III trial comparing the efficacy of the Denver pleural catheter versus chest tube and doxycycline sclerotherapy for recurrent symptomatic MPE in 144 patients was recently completed (99 patients had Denver catheter, and 45 patients had doxycycline pleurodesis).[104] The Denver pleural catheter was as effective as doxycycline pleurodesis in relieving symptoms related to MPE and improving quality of life. At 90 days, pleurodesis was achieved in 69% of patients treated with Denver pleural catheter alone, as compared to 50% of patients treated with doxycycline. No patient in the catheter group experienced fluid reaccumulation. Moreover, patients treated with pleural catheter had shorter hospital stay (mean, 1.83 days) than those treated with chest tube and doxycycline pleurodesis (mean, 6.83 days). Pleural catheter, either a Tenckoff or a Denver catheter, is indicated for recurrent MPEs refractory to pleurodesis or those associated with trapped lung. The pleural catheter is particularly useful in debilitated patients in whom a reliable and painless method of fluid drainage is required or in patients with effusions secondary to chemosensitive malignancies.

External-Beam Irradiation

Only lymphomatous pleural effusions seem to respond favorably to external-beam irradiation. Close to 90% of malignant lymphoma effusions have been controlled by mediastinal and hemithorax irradiation in a small series of patients (1.4 to 2.3 Gy).[105]

SUMMARY

The prognosis of patients with MPE varies with the histologic type of the primary tumor. In general, 65% of patients with MPE are dead within 3 months and 80% within 6 months. As such, treatment of MPE should focus on expeditious and cost-efficient palliation. Our approach to patients with MPE having good performance status is talc pleurodesis. Indwelling pleural catheters have been frequently used for intermittent drainage of effusions

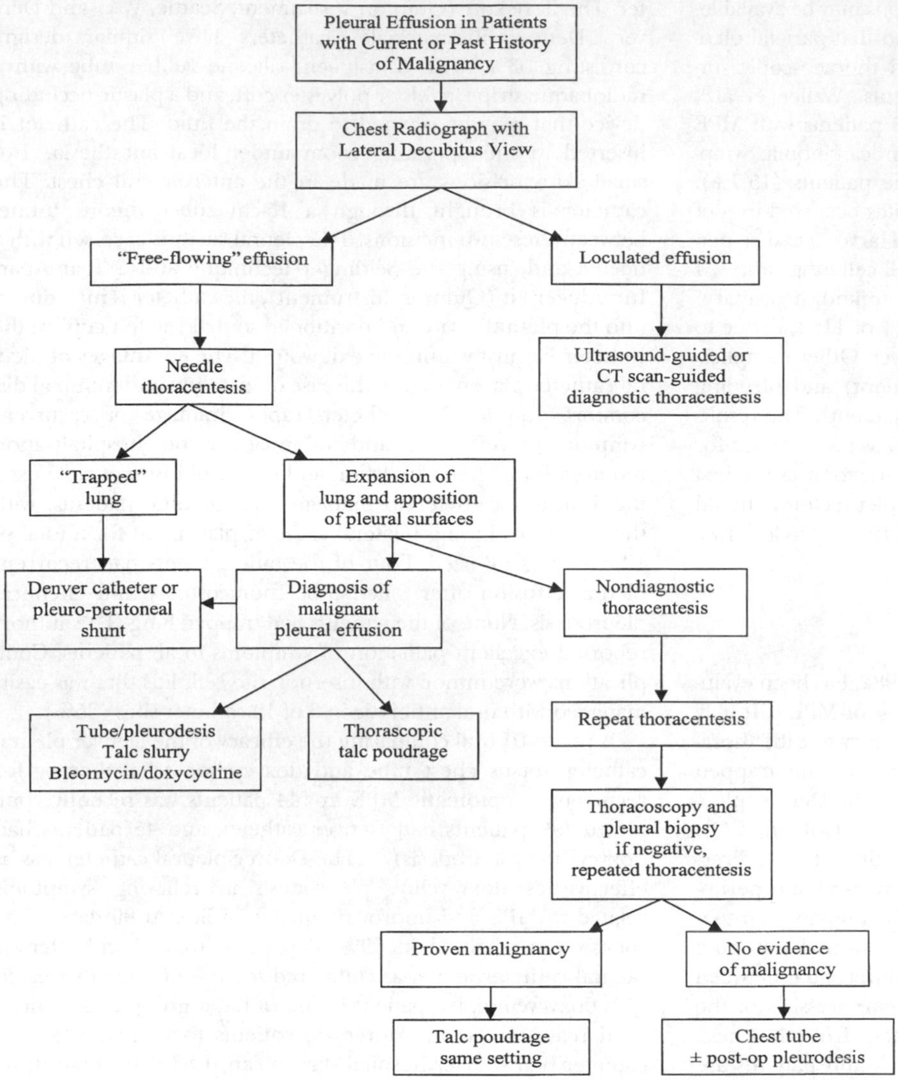

FIGURE 52.5-1. Treatment algorithm for malignant pleural effusion. CT, computed tomography.

in patients with trapped lung or limited life expectancies, as well as individuals on protocols requiring sequential analysis of molecular end points in tumor cells readily obtained from malignant effusions. The algorithm for the diagnosis and treatment of malignant pleural effusion is outlined in Figure 52.5-1.

MALIGNANT PERICARDIAL EFFUSION

Patients with malignant pericardial disease may be asymptomatic or may present with a number of manifestations, with pericardial effusion being the most common. Pericardial tamponade due to malignant pericardial effusion (MPCE) accounts for at least 50% of all reported cases of pericardial fluid collection that require intervention. Similar to cancerous pleural effusions, MPCEs are frequently indicative of advanced incurable malignancy; overall median survival of patients with MPCE is less than 6 months.

PATHOGENESIS AND ETIOLOGY

Malignant cells gain access to the pericardium either via direct invasion from an adjacent tumor or by hematogenous or lymphatic routes.[106–108] Many cardiac and pericardial metastases as well as pericardial effusions result from retrograde progression of disease through lymphatic channels draining the heart and pericardium.[106,108] The normal lymphatic circulation of the heart and pericardium consists of an extensive subendocardial plexus that drains via an intercommunicating system of myocardial channels into a subepicardial plexus. Efferent branches form from this subepicardial plexus and unite into larger trunks that initially follow, then subsequently diverge from, the coronary artery vessels near the aortic root and drain either directly into a cardiac node between the innominate artery and superior vena cava or into a pretracheal node and then into the cardiac node.[108] The cardiac node, in turn, drains into the mediastinal system. In addition, the subepicardial plexus interconnects with a superficial adventitial plexus of lymphatics surrounding the aorta.[109] The latter plexus drains through the paraaortic node and enters directly into the thoracic duct or the paratracheal system.[110] The parietal pericardium contains a relatively unimportant lymphatic system.[110] Thus, pericardial fluid drains primarily via the subepicardial plexus through a few large trunks to the cardiac node and then into the mediastinal nodal system; a secondary pathway involves communication with the lymphatic plexus of the aortic adventitia. Thus, lymphatics from the heart and pericardium appear to have a vulnerable isthmus-like section near the base of the heart. Consequently, impairment of cardiac lymphatic drainage with retrograde epicardial invasion may occur with limited mediastinal metastases.[108] Obstruction of epicardial venous and lymphatic drainage by neoplastic invasion alters the equilibrium between hydrostatic and osmotic forces and capillary filtration favoring fluid accumulation in the pericardial space. The rate of fluid accumulation (which can be rapid if accompanied by intrapericardial hemorrhage) and the degrees of pericardial compliance (which can be low from prior inflammation, irradiation, or tumor infiltration) determine the severity of clinical manifestations of MPCE.

Metastases involving the heart or pericardium (or both) occur relatively frequently in cancer patients.[111–113] Several autopsy series,[114–116] including one by Klatt and Heitz,[114] have indicated that cardiac metastases occur in approximately 10% of patients dying from cancer; the epicardium is involved in 75% of metastatic lesions, and pericardial effusions are present in one-third of these cases.[115,116] Metastasis from the lung (all histologies) and breast and hematologic malignancies account for three-fourths of MPCEs, with lung cancer being the most common etiology; virtually all malignancies (except primary brain tumors) may cause MPCE.

Neoplasms that invade the mediastinal lymphatics and obstruct pericardial lymphatic flow are commonly associated with pericardial effusion. Kline[117] observed cardiac metastases in 61 of 716 cancer patients; all the patients with cardiac involvement had metastases in mediastinal lymph nodes and lymphatics of the epicardium and pericardium. Metastases to the pericardium or heart have been noted in approximately 30% of patients dying from lung cancer,[118] 65% of whom have pericardial effusion; the predominant metastatic pathway involves the hilar lymphatics in these individuals.

CLINICAL PRESENTATION

In most cases, MPCE is observed in patients with a previous diagnosis of cancer, typically at late stages of their disease. MPCE is rarely seen as the initial manifestation of extracardiac malignancy; only 90 cases were reported in the English-language literature over a 55-year period.[119] The most common symptoms attributed to pericardial effusion are dyspnea, cough, chest pain, fever, and edema. Nonspecific complaints are also frequent; as such, pericardial effusion may remain unsuspected in patients in whom nonspecific symptoms are attributed to disease progression. The frequency of cardiac tamponade as the initial manifestation of malignant effusion is highly variable and depends on the rate of fluid accumulation, volume of the fluid, and underlying cardiac function. The pericardium may distend over a period to accommodate a large volume of fluid prior to the clinical appearance of tamponade. Impedance of right atrial and ventricular filling by pericardial fluid results in cardiac tamponade. Signs and symptoms of cardiac tamponade include dyspnea, orthopnea, low output (peripheral vasoconstriction, cold clammy extremities, poor capillary refill, and diaphoresis), jugular venous distention, distant heart sounds, pulsus paradoxus, and narrowed pulse pressure. Electrocardiography may show low voltage complexes in all leads and electrical alternans.

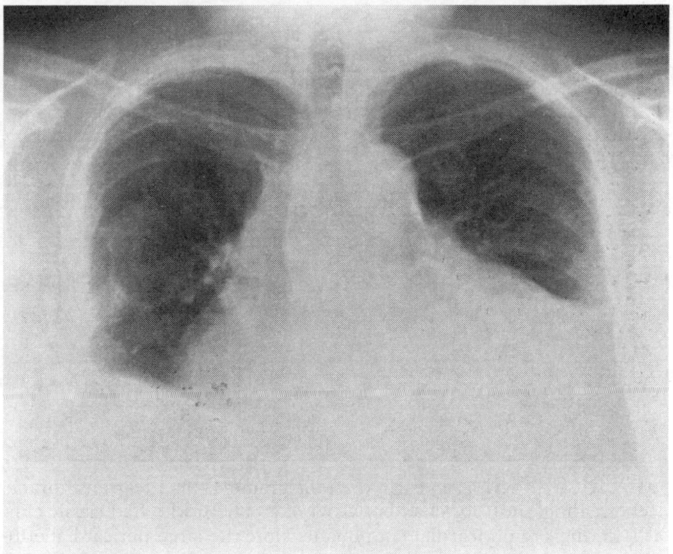

FIGURE 52.5-2. Posteroanterior chest radiograph of a patient with significant pericardial effusion as indicated by an enlarged cardiac silhouette.

DIAGNOSTIC MODALITIES

Radiographic and Echocardiographic Studies

Pericardial effusion in asymptomatic patients is most frequently detected by plain posteroanterior and lateral chest radiographs. The typical finding on chest radiograph is an enlarged globular water-bottle pericardial silhouette (Fig. 52.5-2). Moreover, when pericardial effusion and tamponade are caused by malignancy, concomitant parenchymal involvement or pleural effusion (or both) are observed in 30% to 50% of cases, respectively.[120] Once disease is suspected, echocardiography should be performed to confirm the presence and hemodynamic significance of pericardial effusion. Two-dimensional echocardiography can define the location and amount of effusion, as well as the presence of pericardial or intracardiac masses. Right atrial and ventricular collapse are the most common echocardiographic signs of cardiac tamponade, with sensitivity ranging from 38% to 60% and specificity ranging from 50% to 100% (Fig. 52.5-3).[121] Echocardiography is frequently used to provide guidance for safe and accurate pericardiocentesis.[122,123]

Pericardial effusion can also be diagnosed by CT scan, which can detect as little as 50 mL of pericardial fluid (Fig. 52.5-4). This is not the diagnostic method of choice for pericardial effusion, since it is time-consuming to perform and is no more accurate than echocardiography. CT scan may be helpful in evaluating intrapericardial masses as well as defining the nature of the pericardial fluid, as the attenuation coefficients for exudates, chyle, serous fluid, or blood may differ.[121,124,125]

Cytopathology and Histopathology

The foregoing imaging techniques provide information regarding the amount and hemodynamic significance of pericardial effusion but not its benign or malignant nature. Only 50% to 60% of pericardial effusions in cancer patients are confirmed by cytologic examination to be malignant.[126–128] Posner

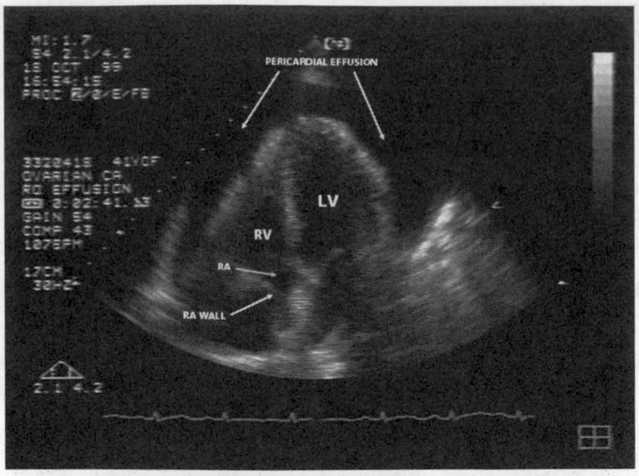

FIGURE 52.5-3. An early diastolic frame from the transthoracic echocardiogram (four-chamber view) of a patient who had classic clinical findings of pericardial tamponade. Note the large pericardial effusion (2-cm dark "echo-free" space) circumferentially around the heart. Early diastolic collapse of the right atrium—a useful, characteristic echo finding of tamponade physiology—is clearly seen where the right atrial cavity (RA) wall (*arrow*) is deviated inward, into the RA chamber. LV, left ventricle; RV, right ventricle. (Courtesy of Eben E. Tucker, M.D., NHLBI, National Institutes of Health, Bethesda, MD.)

et al.[129] studied 31 patients with pericardial disease associated with various malignancies. Fifty-eight percent of the patients had MPCE, 32% had idiopathic pericarditis, and 10% had radiotherapy-induced pericarditis. Pericardiocentesis and cytologic examination of the fluid identified malignancy in 85% of positive cases; open biopsy was required for diagnosis in the remaining 15%. Weiner et al.[116] reviewed 95 cases of pericardial effusion treated initially by pericardiocentesis. Malignant

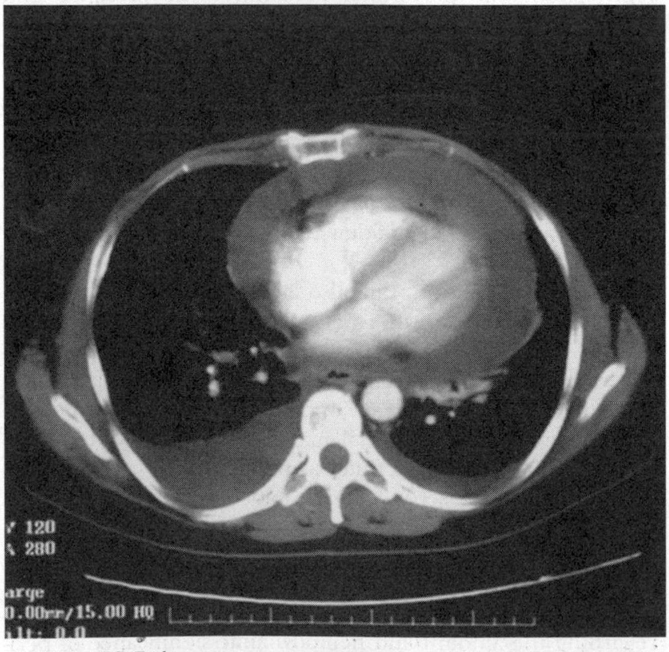

FIGURE 52.5-4. The chest computed tomographic scan of this patient with metastatic ovarian carcinoma shows a large malignant pericardial effusion and bilateral malignant pleural effusions (right more than left).

cells were identified in pericardial fluid from two-thirds of cancer patients; cytology correlated with histologic diagnosis of the underlying malignancy in 100% of these individuals. Press and Livingston[130] reviewed 190 cases of MPCE diagnosed by pericardiocentesis. Pericardial fluid was positive for malignant cells in 151 patients with documented neoplastic pericarditis (specificity, 79%); hence, cytologic examination of pericardial fluid remains valuable in the diagnosis of MPCE, especially when positive for malignant cells. In contrast, parietal pericardial biopsy is frequently nondiagnostic, since the principal site of malignant infiltration is the visceral pericardium and its subepicardial lymphatics. Clarke and Cosgrove[131] performed a prospective study to determine the diagnostic value of pericardial biopsy in 25 patients with malignancy and pericardial effusions. Fluid cytology revealed malignant cells in 11 patients (44%), of whom only 5 had histologic evidence of malignancy in pericardial biopsy specimens.

TREATMENT

The goals of treatment for MPCE include relief of immediate symptoms, confirmation of the malignant nature of the fluid, and prevention of recurrence. Although simple pericardiocentesis may be life-saving in cases of cardiac tamponade, this procedure alone is rarely adequate therapy for MPCE because of the high rate of fluid reaccumulation[120]; thus, if initially performed, pericardiocentesis should be followed by a more definitive medical or surgical procedure to prevent recurrence. Therapy for MPCE should be tailored to the performance status and prognosis of each patient; options include surgical procedures, such as subxiphoid pericardiostomy (pericardial window), transthoracic pericardial window or pericardiectomy (either by video-assisted thoracoscopy or thoracotomy), and medical interventions, such as percutaneous tube pericardiostomy with or without intrapericardial instillation of sclerosing agents.

Subxiphoid Pericardiostomy (Subxiphoid Pericardial Window)

The subxiphoid pericardiostomy approach is now the most commonly performed surgical procedure for benign as well as MPCEs. This procedure can be performed under local anesthesia with intravenous sedation or general anesthesia (Fig. 52.5-5). It can be performed as the initial procedure for MPCE in medically stable patients or after needle pericardiocentesis in patients with signs and symptoms of significant cardiac tamponade. A small vertical skin incision is made from the xyphoid process caudally for 4 to 6 cm. The upper linear alba is divided in the midline, and the xyphoid is either bisected or resected. The peritoneum is not open. The preperitoneal fat is dissected cephalad by blunt finger dissection. The plane between the posterior sternum and the anterior pericardium is then developed to allow insertion of a retractor to elevate the lower end of the sternum. The pericardium is identified as the bulging, grayish white, fibrous membrane. The anterior pericardium is then incised, fluid is drained, and samples are collected for cytologic and microbiologic analyses. The pericardium then is explored digitally to identify adhesions and tumor masses. A piece of pericardium (2 to 4 cm^2) is excised and submitted for microbiologic as well as pathologic studies. Through a separate stab wound in the

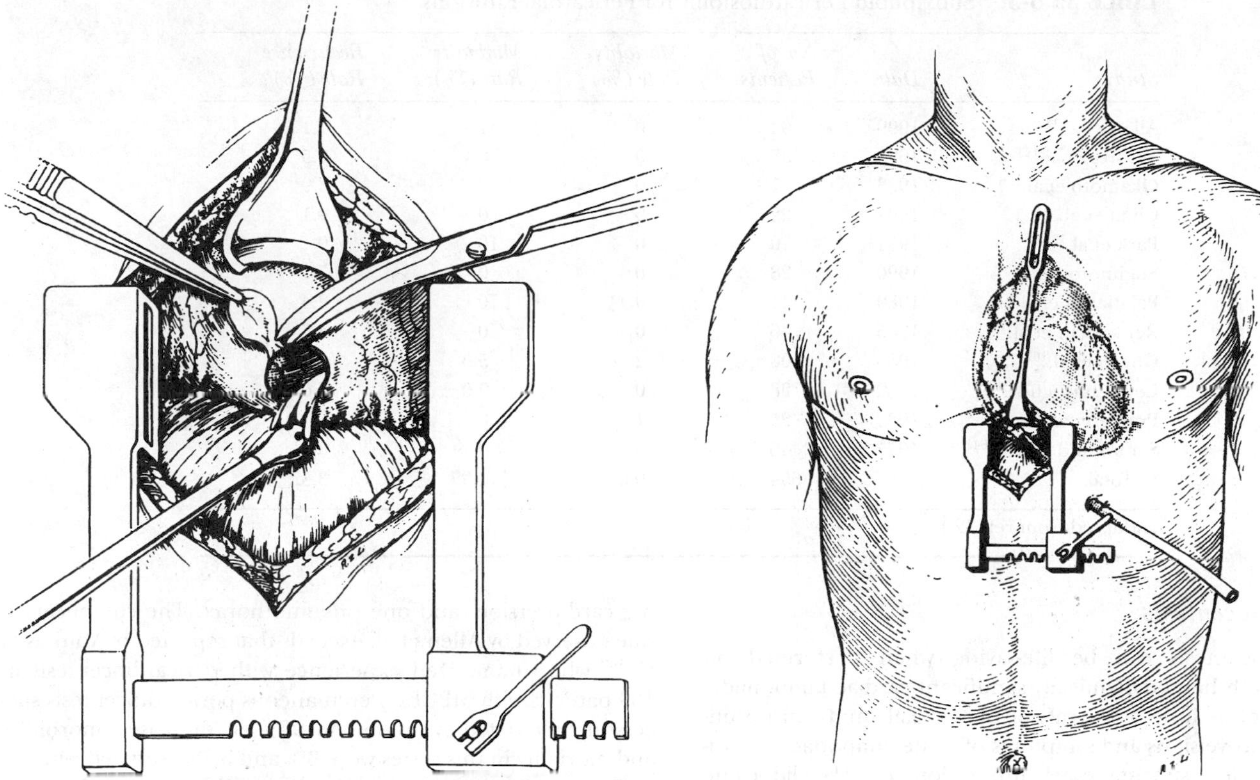

A B

FIGURE 52.5-5. Subxiphoid pericardial window (pericardiostomy). Resection of a small pericardial segment and evacuation of the effusion **(A)** and insertion of a pericardial tube via a separate stab wound in the upper abdominal wall **(B)**. (From ref. 126, with permission.)

upper abdomen, a 28-Fr. curved chest tube is placed in the pericardial space through the pericardial window for postoperative drainage. Some authors advocate leaving the tube in place for 4 to 5 days, regardless of the drainage amount, to promote local inflammation and fusion of the visceral and parietal pericardium. No attempts are made to create a communication between the pericardial space and either the pleural or peritoneal space. Allen et al.[132] noted that autopsies of six patients who had undergone the subxiphoid procedure revealed complete pericardial symphysis with extensive adhesions. A comprehensive review of the clinical experience pertaining to 654 patients with effusion of different etiologies who underwent subxiphoid pericardiostomy has indicated an overall mortality rate of approximately 0.46% (range, 0% to 5%), an overall morbidity rate of approximately 1.53% (range, 0% to 10%), and a recurrence rate of approximately 3.5% (range, 0% to 9.1%). These low mortality, morbidity, and recurrence rates compare very favorably with those attributable to percutaneous pericardiocentesis and pericardiostomy with or without sclerosis (0.7% mortality, 3% morbidity, and 13% recurrence; Tables 52.5-3, 52.5-4).

Partial Pericardiectomy or Pericardial Window via Thoracotomy

Before the recent resurrection of subxiphoid pericardial window as the preferred surgical treatment for pericardial effusion, pericardial window or even pericardiectomy via a thoracotomy incision were advocated. Piehler et al.[133] reviewed their experience with surgical management of pericardial effusions in 145 patients and suggested that the extent of pericardial resection influenced incidence of recurrent effusions. However, several recent series indicate no difference in recurrence rates of patients treated by subxiphoid pericardiostomy as compared to those undergoing transthoracic drainage.[134,135] More importantly, postoperative complications (pneumonia, pleural effusion, respiratory failure, cardiac arrhythmia, deep vein thrombosis, and pulmonary embolism) are much less frequent after subxiphoid pericardial drainage as compared to transthoracic pericardial resection (10% vs. 50%, respectively). Thus, transthoracic pericardial resection is not a suitable initial procedure for drainage of MPCE.

If possible, VATS[136–138] should be used if transthoracic pericardial resection is required for recurrent effusion after subxiphoid pericardiostomy or for diagnosis and treatment of simultaneous pleural-parenchymal pathology. Compared to thoracotomy, minimally invasive approaches are more suitable interventions in debilitated cancer patients. The potential limitation of VATS pericardiectomy is the need for general anesthesia and single-lung ventilation. Pericardial resection via laparoscopy or video-assisted subxiphoid pericardial window have been reported[139]; however, there is no added benefit of these expensive minimally invasive techniques compared to standard subxiphoid pericardiostomy. Pericardial-peritoneal shunt, using a Denver pleuroperitoneal catheter with pumping chamber, has been used to treat MPCE in a limited number of patients[140]; experience with this technique is too limited to allow adequate assessment of its clinical utility, although it may be suitable for pericardial effusions that are refractory to repeated pericardiostomy procedures.

TABLE 52.5-3. Subxiphoid Pericardiostomy for Pericardial Effusions

Study	*Date*	*No. of Patients*	*Mortality Rate (%)*	*Morbidity Rate (%)*	*Recurrence Rate (%)*
Allen et al.[132]	1999	94	0	1.1	1.1
Moores et al.[126]	1995	155	0	0	2.5
Okamoto et al.[156]	1993	51	0	0	3.9
Chan et al.[157]	1991	22	5	0	9.1
Park et al.[135]	1991	10	0	10	0
Sugimoto et al.[158]	1990	28	0	0	7.1
Palatianos et al.[159]	1989	41	0	0	2.4
Reitknecht et al.[160]	1985	46	0	0	4.5
Ghosh et al.[161]	1985	108	2	5.5	4.6
Levin and Aaron[162]	1982	28	0	7.0	7.0
Prager et al.[163]	1982	25	1	0	0
Santos and Frater[164]	1977	46	0	0	0
Total		654	0.67	1.97	3.52

(Adapted from ref. 32.)

Pericardiocentesis

Pericardiocentesis can be life-saving when performed on patients with hemodynamically significant cardiac tamponade. Removal of as little as 50 mL of pericardial fluid can significantly improve signs and symptoms of acute tamponade. Traditionally, after subcutaneous infiltration of 1% lidocaine (Xylocaine) local anesthetic solution, the needle is inserted at the right side of the xyphoid process and directed 45 degrees dorsally, aiming toward the tip of the left scapula (Fig. 52.5-6). In cancer patients with symptomatic pericardial effusion, pericardiocentesis may be performed to stabilize patients prior to more definitive drainage procedures, such as percutaneous tube pericardiostomy or subxiphoid pericardial window.

As the sole treatment for MPCE, pericardiocentesis is associated with recurrence requiring further treatment in up to 70% of cases.[141] This procedure has been associated with a significant incidence of complications, some of which are fatal even when performed by experienced physicians. Allen et al.[132] observed clinically significant complications in 5 of 23 patients (22%) undergoing percutaneous pericardiocentesis, including three right ventricular perforations (with one fatality) requiring surgical interventions, one ventricular arrhythmia requiring cardioversion, and one pneumothorax. The complication rate observed by Allen et al. exceeds that reported by Vaitkus et al.,[142] who summarized experience with pericardiocentesis in 139 patients with MPCEs. Percutaneous pericardiocentesis successfully alleviated symptoms in 97% of the cases; morbidity and mortality in this series were 3% and 0.7%, respectively.

Echocardiography may reduce complications and improve the success of the pericardiocentesis by delineating the size and location of the effusion relative to cardiac structures. Overall rates of complication and success are approximately 2.4% and 100%, respectively, after ultrasound-guided pericardial drainage[144,145] as compared to 4.8% and 90%, respectively, after unassisted pericardiocentesis.[131,146]

Percutaneous Tube Pericardiostomy and Pericardial Sclerotherapy

The rates of fluid reaccumulation have been reported to range from as low as 44% to as high as 70% after pericardiocentesis.[147] It is now a common practice to place a 9-Fr. pigtail draining catheter into the pericardial space after successful needle pericardiocentesis using the Seldinger technique to enable more complete

TABLE 52.5-4. Percutaneous Catheter Drainage for Pericardial Effusions

Study	*Technique*	*Date*	*No. of Patients*	*Mortality Rate (%)*	*Morbidity Rate (%)*	*Recurrence Rate (%)*
Allen[132]	Catheter	Present series	23	4.3	17.4	33.3
Celermajer et al.[143]	Catheter	1991	36	3.0	5.6	19.4
Kopecky et al.[165]	Catheter	1986	42	0	2.4	24.0
Shepherd[120]	Catheter-sclerosis	1987	58	0	10.3	17.0
Davis[166]	Catheter-sclerosis	1984	33	0	0	0
Ziskind et al.[151]	Balloon-pericardiostomy	1993	50	2.0	20.0	4.0
Lemmon and Ziskind[167]	Balloon-pericardiostomy	1993	81	0	14.0	11.0
Di Segni et al.[153]	Balloon-pericardiostomy	1995	8	0	12.5	0
Total			331	1.16	10.28	13.59

(Adapted from ref. 32.)

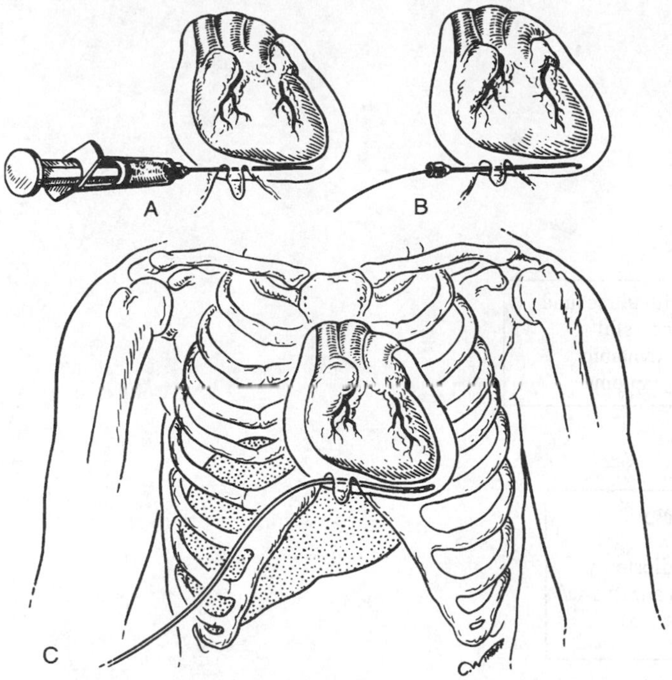

FIGURE 52.5-6. Percutaneous pericardiocentesis and placement of an indwelling catheter for pericardial effusion. (From DWO Moores, SW Dziuban. Pericardial drainage procedures. *Chest Surg Clin North Am* 1995;5:359, with permission.)

evacuation of the effusion and provide access for sclerotherapy. Although several agents have been used in the past, tetracycline and its currently available derivative, doxycycline, have been most extensively evaluated as sclerosing agents for pericardial effusion. Maher et al.[147] reported their experience with 93 patients with MPCE treated by percutaneous pericardial drainage followed by tetracycline or doxycycline sclerosis. Successful placement of the pericardiostomy tube was achieved in 85 patients (91.4%). Pericardial effusion was controlled in 75 of the 85 patients (88%); 10 of the 85 patients (12%) did not respond to sclerosis, of whom 8 subsequently underwent surgical pericardiostomy. Sclerotherapy necessitated one to eight instillations of tetracycline or doxycycline (median, 3); 50 patients required three or more instillations to control their effusions. Treatment-related complications (in decreasing order of frequency) included pain, catheter occlusion, fever, and atrial arrhythmias. The apparently favorable results of this minimally invasive treatment strategy are offset by the need for repeated instillations of the sclerosing agent to achieve pericardial symphysis. Liu et al.[148] recently conducted a prospective study to evaluate the efficacy and toxicity of bleomycin versus doxycycline as the sclerosing agents for MPCE. Bleomycin was found to be as effective as doxycycline in achieving satisfactory control of MPCE, yet with much less retrosternal pain. As a result, these authors recommended that bleomycin be considered the first-line chemical sclerosing agent for treating MPCE. In addition to bleomycin or doxycycline, other sclerosing agents used for treating MPCE include OK-432 (a penicillin-treated and heat-treated lyophilized powder of the *Staphylococcus aureus* substrain A3),[148] cisplatin,[149] vinblastine,[150] and sterile talc. The clinical utility of these adjunctive sclerosing agents is not known, and their use cannot be considered standard of care at this time.

Percutaneous Balloon Tube Pericardiostomy

Percutaneous balloon tube pericardiostomy, initially advocated by Ziskind et al.[151] and subsequently studied by others,[152,153] appears to be an extension of the more commonly performed percutaneous tube pericardiostomy. After successful pericardiocentesis, dilatation of the needle tract is performed under fluoroscopy using a balloon catheter. Ziskind et al.[151] reported that this technique was effective in relieving pericardial effusion in 46 of 50 patients (92%). Procedure-related complications included fever (six patients), pleural effusion requiring chest tube placement or thoracentesis (eight patients), small pneumothorax (two patients), and right ventricular injury requiring surgery (one patient), for an overall clinically significant complication rate of 18%. Even though this is an effective minimally invasive technique of pericardial drainage, its widespread application may be limited by the need for specialized equipment as well as for interventional cardiologists or radiologists. The high incidence of inadvertent pleural effusions requiring drainage renders this technique less attractive compared with others discussed.

Local or Systemic Therapies for Malignant Pericardial Effusion

Radiotherapy is generally reserved for MPCE associated with lymphoma or breast carcinoma. Vaitkus et al.[142] reviewed the experience of 54 patients treated with radiotherapy as the primary mode of therapy for MPCE. Of these patients, 39 (72%) underwent initial pericardiocentesis. The majority received neither systemic nor other direct pericardial intervention. Radiation therapy was successful in controlling MPCE in 36 patients (66.7%). The highest success rates were noted in leukemia-lymphoma and breast cancer patients (93% and 71%, respectively). Surprisingly, 45% of patients with other solid tumors had adequate control of their effusions. Although noninvasive, radiotherapy requires repeated visits or even prolonged hospitalization and may theoretically cause acute pericarditis or myocarditis. These potential complications may not be relevant in many patients, owing to their limited survival.

Patients with MPCE secondary to lymphoma or breast carcinoma may have effusions controlled with systemic chemotherapy. Vaitkus et al.[142] reported their experience with 46 patients with breast tumor (n = 38), lymphoma (n = 2), or other solid tumors (n = 6) treated with systemic chemotherapy. Thirty-six patients (78%) underwent initial therapeutic pericardiocentesis. Systemic chemotherapy prevented recurrence of effusion in 31 patients (67%); successful control of effusion was achieved in more than two-thirds of these individuals irrespective of whether pericardiocentesis preceded systemic therapy.

SUMMARY

MPCE is frequently an indication of advanced, incurable malignancy. Hence, the goals of intervention include relief of symptoms and prevention of recurrence. The treatment of MPCE should proceed in a stepwise fashion (Fig. 52.5-7). Surgical interventions (subxiphoid pericardiostomy) or medical interventions (ultrasound-guided percutaneous tube pericardiostomy and sclerotherapy) have acceptable risks and provide excellent results. We favor surgical drainage as the primary

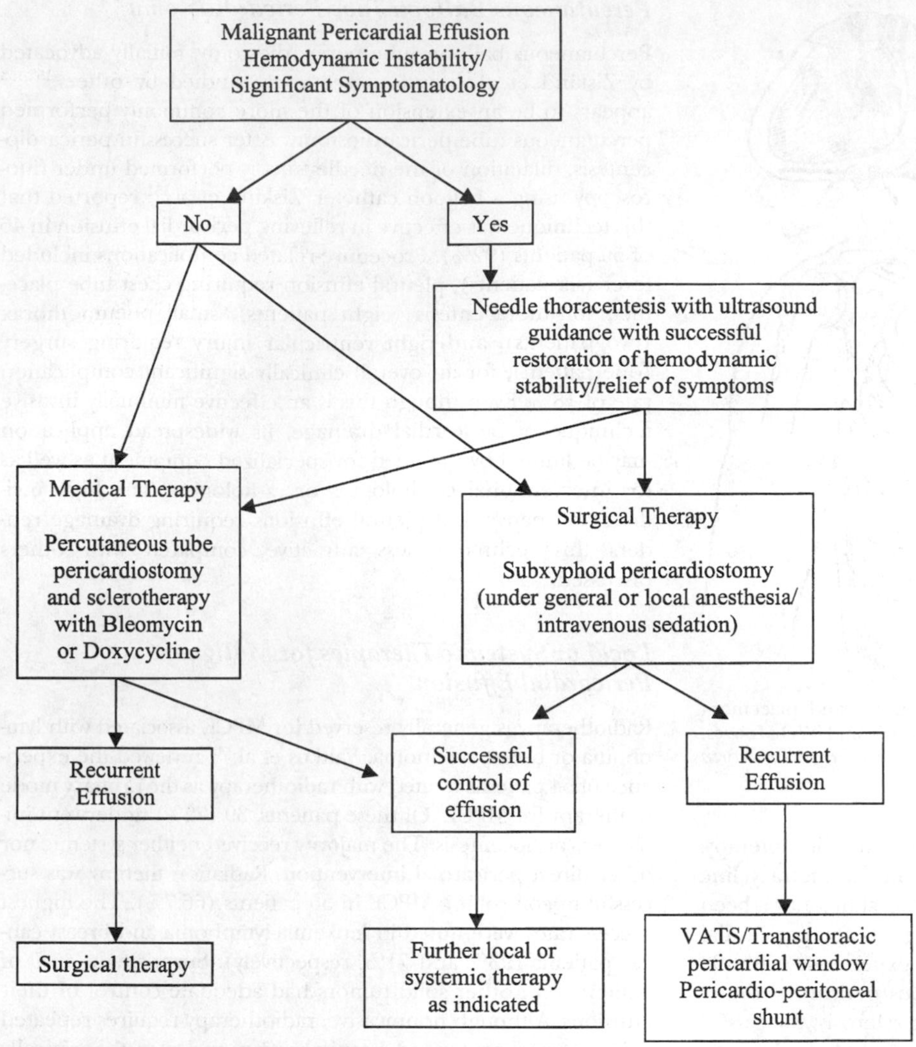

FIGURE 52.5-7. Treatment algorithm for malignant pericardial effusion. VATS, video-assisted thoracoscopic surgery.

approach for patients with MPCE because of its simplicity and extremely high success rate without the need for intrapericardial instillation of sclerosing agents and tube manipulations that may be associated with patient discomfort. Recurrent MPCE can be managed either by repeat pericardiostomy or insertion of a shunt. Patients responding to treatment with complete control of the effusion should have a meaningful survival with life expectancy (average, 9 months) contingent on the histology of the underlying malignancy.

REFERENCES

1. Matthew RA, Coppage L, Shaw C, Filderman AE. Malignancies metastatic to the pleura. *Invest Radiol* 1990;25:601.
2. Fenton KN, Richardson JD. Diagnosis and management of malignant pleural effusion. *Am J Surg* 1995;170:69.
3. Hausheer FH, Yarbro JW. Diagnosis and treatment of malignant pleural effusion: an overview. *Semin Oncol* 1985;12:54.
4. Agostini E, Miserocchi G, Bonanni MV. Thickness and pressure of the pleural liquid in some mammals. *Respir Physiol* 1969;6:245.
5. Wang NS. Morphological data of pleura—normal conditions. In: Chretien J, Hirsh A, eds. *Disease of the pleura.* New York: Masson, 1982:10.
6. Lee FK, Olak J. Anatomy and physiology of the pleural space. *Chest Surg Clin North Am* 1994;4:391.
7. Moores DWO. Management of malignant pleural effusion. *Chest Surg Clin North Am* 1994;4:481.
8. DeCamp MM, Mentzer SJ, Swanson SJ, Sugarbaker DJ. Malignant effusive disease of the pleura and pericardium. *Chest* 1997;112:291S.
9. Meyer PC. Metastatic carcinoma of the pleura. *Thorax* 1966;21:473.
10. Canto A, Ferrer G, Romangosa V. Lung cancer and pleural effusion. *Chest* 1985;87:649.
11. Decker DR, Dines DE, Payne WS. The significance of a cytologically negative pleural effusion in bronchogenic carcinoma. *Chest* 1978;74:640.
12. Dresler CM, Fratelli C, Babb J. Prognostic value of positive pleural lavage in patients with lung cancer resection. *Ann Thorac Surg* 1999;67:1435.
13. Chernow B, Sahn SA. Carcinomatous involvement of the pleura: an analysis of 96 patients. *Am J Med* 1977;63:695.
14. Martini N, Bain MS, Beattie EJ Jr. Indications for pleurectomy in malignant pleural effusion. *Cancer* 1975;35:734.
15. Sahn SA. Pleural effusion in lung cancer. *Clin Chest Med* 1993;14:189.
16. Ratliff JL, Chavez CM, Hamchuk A. Reexpansion pulmonary edema. *Chest* 1973;64:654.
17. Trapnell DH, Thurston JGB. Lateral pulmonary edema after pleural aspiration. *Lancet* 1970;1:1376.
18. Yamazaki S, Ogawa J, Shohyu A. Pulmonary blood flow to rapidly re-expanded lung on spontaneous pneumothorax. *Chest* 1982;81:118.
19. Collins TR, Sahn SA. Thoracentesis: clinical value, complications, technical problem and patient experience. *Chest* 1987;91:817.
20. Seneff MG, Corwin RW, Gold LH. Complications associated with thoracentesis. *Chest* 1986;90:97.
21. Kennedy L, Sahn SA. Noninvasive evaluation of the patient with pleural effusion. *Chest Surg Clin North Am* 1994;4:451.
22. Nance KV, Shermer RW, Askin FB. Diagnostic efficacy of pleural biopsy as compared with that of pleural fluid examination. *Mod Pathol* 1991;4:320.
23. Boutin C, Vaalat JR, Cargnino P. Thoracoscopy in malignant pleural effusions. *Am Rev Respir Dis* 1981;124:58.
24. Menzies R, Charboneau M. Thoracoscopy for the diagnosis of pleural disease. *Ann Intern Med* 1991;114:271.

25. DeCamp MM, Jaklitsch MT, Mentzer SJ, Harpole DH. The safety and versatility of video-thoracoscopy: a prospective analysis of 895 cases. *J Am Coll Surg* 1995;181:113.
26. Assi Z, Caruso JL, Herndon J, Patz EF. Cytologically proved malignant pleural effusion. *Chest* 1998;113:1302.
27. Sahn SA, Good TJ. Pleural fluid in malignant pleural effusion. *Ann Intern Med* 1988;108:345.
28. Rodriguez-Panadero F, Mejias IL. Low glucose and pH levels in malignant pleural effusions. *Am Rev Respir Dis* 1989;139:663.
29. Salyer WR, Eggleston JC, Erozan YS. Efficacy of pleural needle biopsy and pleural fluid cytopathology in the diagnosis of malignant neoplasms involving the pleura. *Chest* 1975;67:536.
30. Pavesi F, Lotzniker M, Cremaschi P. Detection of malignant pleural effusions by tumor marker evaluation. *Eur J Cancer Clin Oncol* 1988;24:1005.
31. Rasmussen KN, Faher V. Hyaluronic acid in 247 pleural fluid. *Scand J Respir Dis* 1967;48:366.
32. Hammar SP. The pathology of benign and malignant pleural disease. *Chest Surg Clin North Am* 1994;4:405.
33. Morrison MC, Muller PR, Lee MJ. Sclerotherapy of malignant pleural effusion through sonographically placed small-bore catheter. *AJR Am J Roentgenol* 1992;158:41.
34. Parker LA, Charnock GC, Delany DJ. Small-bore catheter drainage and sclerotherapy for malignant pleural effusion. *Cancer* 1989;64:1218.
35. Patz EF. Malignant pleural effusions. Recent advances and ambulatory sclerotherapy. *Chest* 1998;113:74S.
36. Thompson RL, Yau JC, Donnelly RF, Gowan DJ, Matzinger FRK. Pleurodesis with iodized talc for malignant effusions using pigtail catheters. *Ann Pharmacother* 1998;32:739.
37. Austin EH, Flye MW. The treatment of recurrent malignant pleural effusion. *Ann Thorac Surg* 1979;28:190.
38. Greenwald DW, Phillips C, Bennett JM. Management of malignant pleural effusion. *J Surg Oncol* 1978;10:361.
39. Richman SP, Hersh EM, Gutterman JU, et al. Administration of BCG cell wall skeleton into malignant effusions: toxic and therapeutic effects. *Cancer Treat Rep* 1981;65:383.
40. Anderson AP, Brinker H. Intracavitary thiotepa in malignant pleural and peritoneal effusion. *Acta Radiol Ther Phys Biol* 1968;7:369.
41. Kent EM, Moses C. Radioactive isotopes in the palliative management of carcinomatosis of the pleura. *J Thorac Surg* 1951;22:503.
42. Card RY, Cold DR, Hensche UK. Summary of 10 years of the use of radioactive colloids in intracavitary therapy. *J Nucl Med* 1960;1:195.
43. Ruckdeschel JC, Moores D, Lee JY, et al. Intrapleural therapy for malignant pleural effusions. A randomized comparison of bleomycin and tetracycline [published erratum appears in *Chest* 1993 May;103(5):1640]. *Chest* 1991;100:1528.
44. Gravelyn TR, Michelson MK, Gross BH, Sitrin RG. Tetracycline pleurodesis for malignant pleural effusions. A 10-year retrospective study. *Cancer* 1987;59:1973.
45. Heffner JE, Standerfer RJ, Torstveit J, Unruh L. Clinical efficacy of doxycycline for pleurodesis. *Chest* 1994;105:1743.
46. Mansson T. Treatment of malignant pleural effusion with doxycycline. *Scand J Infect Dis Suppl* 1988;53:29.
47. Kitamura S, Sugiyama Y, Izumi T. Intrapleural doxycycline for control of malignant pleural effusion. *Curr Ther Res* 1981;30:515.
48. Hatta T, Tsubota N, Yoshimura M, Yanagawa M. Intrapleural minocycline for postoperative air leakage and control of malignant pleural effusion. *Kyobu Geka* 1990;43:283.
49. Ostrowski MJ. An assessment of the long-term results of controlling the reaccumulation of malignant effusions using intracavitary bleomycin. *Cancer* 1986;57:721.
50. Kessinger A, Wigton RS. Intracavitary bleomycin and tetracycline in the management of malignant pleural effusions: a randomized study. *J Surg Oncol* 1987;36:81.
51. Hamed H, Fentiman IS, Chaudary MA, Rubens RD. Comparison of intracavitary bleomycin and talc for control of pleural effusions secondary to carcinoma of the breast. *Br J Surg* 1989;76:1266.
52. Moores DW. Malignant pleural effusion. *Semin Oncol* 1991;18:59.
53. Ostrowski MJ, Halsall GM. Intracavitary bleomycin in the management of malignant effusions: a multicenter study. *Cancer Treat Rep* 1982;66:1903.
54. Chambers JS. Palliative treatment of neoplastic pleural effusion with intercostal intubation and talc installation. *West J Surg Obstet Gynecol* 1958;66:26.
55. Colt HG, Russack V, Chiu Y, et al. A comparison of thoracoscopic talc insufflation, slurry, and mechanical abrasion pleurodesis. *Chest* 1997;111:442.
56. Fentiman IS, Rubens RD, Hayward JL. A comparison of intracavitary talc and tetracycline for the control of pleural effusions secondary to breast cancer. *Eur J Cancer Clin Oncol* 1986;22:1079.
57. Marchandise FX, Vandenplas O, Wallon J, Francis C. Thoracoscopy in the diagnosis and management of chronic pleural effusions. *Acta Clin Belg* 1993;48:5.
58. Boniface E, Guerin JC. Value of talc administration using thoracoscopy in the symptomatic treatment of recurrent pleurisy. Apropos of 302 cases. *Rev Mal Respir* 1989;6:133.
59. Ladjimi S, M'Raihi L, Djemel A, et al. Results of talc administration using thoracoscopy in neoplastic pleurisies. Apropos of 218 cases. *Rev Mal Respir* 1989;6:147.
60. Weissberg D, Ben-Zeev I. Talc pleurodesis. Experience with 360 patients. *J Thorac Cardiovasc Surg* 1993;106:689.
61. Canto A, Rivas J, Moya J, et al. Pleural effusion of malignant etiology. Thoracoscopic use of talc as an effective method of pleurodesis. *Med Clin (Barc)* 1985;84:806.
62. Sanchez-Armengol A, Rodriguez-Panadero F. Survival and talc pleurodesis in metastatic pleural carcinoma, revisited. Report of 125 cases. *Chest* 1993;104:1482.
63. Hartman DL, Gaither JM, Kesler KA, et al. Comparison of insufflated talc under thoracoscopic guidance with standard tetracycline and bleomycin pleurodesis for control of malignant pleural effusions. *J Thorac Cardiovasc Surg* 1993;105:743.
64. Viallat JR, Rey F, Astoul P, Boutin C. Thoracoscopic talc poudrage pleurodesis for malignant effusions. A review of 360 cases. *Chest* 1996;110:1387.
65. Kennedy L, Rusch VW, Strange C, Ginsberg RJ, Sahn SA. Pleurodesis using talc slurry. *Chest* 1994;106:342.
66. Webb WR, Ozmen V, Moulder PV, Shabahang B, Breaux J. Iodized talc pleurodesis for the treatment of pleural effusions. *J Thorac Cardiovasc Surg* 1992;103:881.
67. Aelony Y, King RR, Boutin C. Thoracoscopic talc poudrage in malignant pleural effusions: effective pleurodesis despite low pleural pH. *Chest* 1998;113:1007.
68. Rinaldo JE, Owens GR, Rogers RM. Adult respiratory distress syndrome following intrapleural instillation of talc. *J Thorac Cardiovasc Surg* 1983;85:523.
69. Bouchama A, Chastre J, Gaudichet A, Soler P, Gibert C. Acute pneumonitis with bilateral pleural effusion after talc pleurodesis. *Chest* 1984;86:795.
70. Zimmer PW, Hill M, Casey K, Harvey E, Low DE. Prospective randomized trial of talc slurry vs bleomycin in pleurodesis for symptomatic malignant pleural effusions. *Chest* 1997;112:430.
71. Belani CP, Pajeau TS, Bennett CL. Treating malignant pleural effusion cost consciously. *Chest* 1998;113:78S.
72. Stiksa G, Korsgaard R, Simonsson BG. Treatment of recurrent pleural effusion by pleurodesis with quinacrine. Comparison between instillation by repeated thoracenteses and by tube drainage. *Scand J Respir Dis* 1979;60:197.
73. Borja ER, Pugh RP. Single-dose quinacrine (atabrine) and thoracostomy in the control of pleural effusions in patients with neoplastic disease. *Cancer* 1973;31:899.
74. Rossi GA, Felletti R, Balbi B, et al. Symptomatic treatment of recurrent malignant pleural effusions with intrapleurally administered *Corynebacterium parvum*. Clinical response is not associated with evidence of enhancement of local cellular-mediated immunity. *Am Rev Respir Dis* 1987;135:885.
75. Walker-Renard PB, Vaughan LM, Sahn SA. Chemical pleurodesis for malignant pleural effusions. *Ann Intern Med* 1994;120:56.
76. Hillerdal G, Kiviloog J, Nou E, Steinholtz L. *Corynebacterium parvum* in malignant pleural effusion. A randomized prospective study. *Eur J Respir Dis* 1986;69:204.
77. Ostrowski MJ, Priestman TJ, Houston RF, Martin WM. A randomized trial of intracavitary bleomycin and *Corynebacterium parvum* in the control of malignant pleural effusions. *Radiother Oncol* 1989;14:19.
78. Goldman CA, Skinnider LF, Maksymiuk AW. Interferon instillation for malignant pleural effusions. *Ann Oncol* 1993;4:141.
79. Davis M, Williford S, Muss HB, et al. A phase I-II study of recombinant intrapleural alpha interferon in malignant pleural effusions. *Am J Clin Oncol* 1992;15:328.
80. Rosso R, Rimoldi R, Salvati F, et al. Intrapleural natural beta interferon in the treatment of malignant pleural effusions. *Oncology* 1988;45:253.
81. Viallat JR, Boutin C, Rey F, et al. Intrapleural immunotherapy with escalating doses of interleukin-2 in metastatic pleural effusions. *Cancer* 1993;71:4067.
82. Yasumoto K, Ogura T. Intrapleural application of recombinant interleukin-2 in patients with malignant pleurisy due to lung cancer. A multi-institutional cooperative study. *Biotherapy* 1991;3:345.
83. Suzuki H, Abo S, Kitamura M, Hashimoto M, Izumi K. The intrapleural administration of recombinant interleukin-2 (rIL-2) to patients with malignant pleural effusion: clinical trials. *Surg Today* 1993;23:1053.
84. Astoul P, Viallat JR, Laurent JC, Brandely M, Boutin C. Intrapleural recombinant IL-2 in passive immunotherapy for malignant pleural effusion. *Chest* 1993;103:209.
85. Kanato M, Torisu M. New approach to the management of malignant ascites with a streptococcal preparation OK432: II. Intraperitoneal inflammatory cell mediated tumor cell destruction. *Surgery* 1983;93:365.
86. Uchida A, Micksche M, Hoshino T. Intrapleural administration of OK432 in cancer patients: augmentation of autologous tumor killing activity of tumor-associated large granular lymphocytes. *Cancer Immunol Immunother* 1984;18:5.
87. Luh KT, Yang PC, Kuo SH, et al. Comparison of OK-432 and mitomycin C pleurodesis for malignant pleural effusion caused by lung cancer. A randomized trial. *Cancer* 1992;69:674.
88. Markman M, Cleary S, King ME, Howell SB. Cisplatin and cytarabine administered intrapleurally as treatment of malignant pleural effusions. *Med Pediatr Oncol* 1985;13:191.
89. Rusch VW, Figlin R, Godwin D, Piantadosi S. Intrapleural cisplatin and cytarabine in the management of malignant pleural effusions: a Lung Cancer Study Group trial. *J Clin Oncol* 1991;9:313.
90. Kefford RF, Woods RL, Fox RM, Tatterall MH. Intracavitary Adriamycin nitrogen mustard and tetracycline in the control of malignant effusions: a randomized study. *Med J Aust* 1980;2:447.
91. Desai SD, Figueredo A. Intracavitary doxorubicin in malignant effusions [Letter]. *Lancet* 1979;1:872.
92. Masuno T, Kishimoto S, Ogura T, et al. A comparative trial of LC9018 plus doxorubicin and doxorubicin alone for the treatment of malignant pleural effusion secondary to lung cancer. *Cancer* 1991;68:1495.
93. Holoye PY, Jeffries DG, Dhingra HM, et al. Intrapleural etoposide for malignant effusion. *Cancer Chemother Pharmacol* 1990;26:147.
94. Soysal O, Karaoglanoglu N, Demiracan S, et al. Pleurectomy/decortication for palliation in malignant pleural mesothelioma: results of surgery. *Eur J Cardiothorac Surg* 1997;11:210.
95. Martini N, Bains MS, Beattie EJJ. Indications for pleurectomy in malignant effusion. *Cancer* 1975;35:734.
96. Fry WA, Khandekar JD. Parietal pleurectomy for malignant pleural effusion. *Ann Surg Oncol* 1995;2:160.
97. Waller DA, Morritt GN, Forty J. Video-assisted thoracoscopic pleurectomy in the management of malignant pleural effusion. *Chest* 1995;107:1454.
98. Harvey JC, Erdman CB, Beattie EJ. Early experience with videothoracoscopic hydrodissection pleurectomy in the treatment of malignant pleural effusion. *J Surg Oncol* 1995;59:243.
99. Tsang V, Fernando HC, Goldstraw P. Pleuroperitoneal shunt for recurrent malignant pleural effusions. *Thorax* 1990;45:369.
100. Petrou M, Kaplan D, Goldstraw P. Management of recurrent malignant pleural effusions. The complementary role talc pleurodesis and pleuroperitoneal shunting. *Cancer* 1995;75:801.

101. Reich H, Beattie EJ, Harvey JC. Pleuroperitoneal shunt for malignant pleural effusions: a one-year experience. *Semin Surg Oncol* 1993;9:160.
102. Ponn RB, Blancaflor J, D'Agostino RS, et al. Pleuroperitoneal shunting for intractable pleural effusions. *Ann Thorac Surg* 1991;51:605.
103. Robinson RD, Fullertyon DA, Albert JD, Sorensen J, Johnston MR. Use of pleural Tenckoff catheter to palliate malignant pleural effusion. *Ann Thorac Surg* 1994;57:286.
104. Putnam JB, Ponn R, Olak J, et al. A phase III trial of treatment for malignant pleural effusions: PLEURX pleural catheter (PC) versus chest tube + doxycycline sclerosis (CT-S). *Chest* 1997;112:26S.
105. Weick JK, Kiely JM, Harrison EGJ, Carr DT, Scanlon PW. Pleural effusion in lymphoma. *Cancer* 1973;31:848.
106. Hancock EW. Neoplastic pericardial disease. *Cardiol Clin* 1990;8:673.
107. Olopade OI, Ultmann JE. Malignant effusion. *CA Cancer Clin J* 1991;41:166.
108. Fraser RS, Viloria JB, Wang N-S. Cardiac tamponade as a presentation of extracardiac malignancy. *Cancer* 1980;45:1679.
109. Johnson RA. Lymphatics of blood vessels. *Lymphology* 1969;2:44.
110. Haagensen CD, Feind CR, Herter FP, Slanetz CA, Weinberg JA. *The lymphatics in cancer.* Philadelphia: WB Saunders, 1972:245.
111. Roberts WC, Glancy DL, DeVita VT Jr. Heart in malignant lymphoma (Hodgkin's disease, lymphosarcoma, reticulum cell sarcoma and mycosis fungoides). A study of 196 autopsy cases. *Am J Cardiol* 1968;22:85.
112. Hanfling SM. Metastatic cancer to the heart: review of the literature and report of 127 cases. *Circulation* 1960;22:474.
113. Nelson BE, Rose PG. Malignant pericardial effusion from squamous cell cancer of the cervix. *J Surg Oncol* 1993;52:203.
114. Klatt EC, Heitz DR. Cardiac metastases. *Cancer* 1990;65:1456.
115. Abraham KP, Reddy V, Gattuso P. Neoplasms metastatic to the heart: review of 3314 consecutive autopsies. *Am J Cardiovasc Pathol* 1990;3:195.
116. Weiner HG, Kristensen IB, Haubeck A. The diagnostic value of pericardial cytology: an analysis of 95 cases. *Acta Cytol* 1991;35:149.
117. Kline IK. Cardiac lymphatic involvement by metastatic tumor. *Cancer* 1972;29:799.
118. Tamura A, Mashubara O, Yoshimura N. Cardiac metastasis of lung cancer. A study of metastatic pathways and clinical manifestations. *Cancer* 1992;70:437.
119. Fincher R-ME. Case report: malignant pericardial effusion as the initial manifestation of malignancy. *Am J Med Sci* 1993;305:106.
120. Shepherd F, Morgan C, Evans W, et al. Medical management of pericardial effusion by tetracycline sclerosis. *Am J Cardiol* 1987;60:1161.
121. Chong HH, Plotnick GD. Pericardial effusion and tamponade: evaluation, imaging modalities, and management. *Compr Ther* 1995;21:378.
122. Goldberg BB, Pollack HM. Ultrasonically guided pericardiocentesis. *Am J Cardiol* 1973;31:490.
123. Callahan JA, Sewart JB, Tajik AJ. Pericardiocentesis assisted by two-dimensional echocardiography. *J Thorac Cardiovasc Surg* 1983;85:877.
124. Johnson FE, Wolverson MK, Sundaram M, Heiberg E. Unsuspect malignant pericardial effusion causing cardiac tamponade: rapid diagnosis by computed tomography. *Chest* 1998;82:501.
125. Copland NL, Kennish AJ, Burgess NL. Pericardial mesothelioma masquerading as a benign pericardial effusion. *J Am Coll Cardiol* 1984;4:1307.
126. Moores DW, Allen KB, Faber LP, et al. Subxiphoid pericardial drainage for pericardial tamponade. *J Thorac Cardiovasc Surg* 1995;109:546.
127. Iles R, Lininger L. Subxiphoid pericardial drainage for pericardial tamponade. *J Thorac Cardiovasc Surg* 1995;109:546.
128. Hsu FI, Keef D, Desiderio D, Downey RJ. Echocardiographic and surgical correlation of pericardial effusions in patients with malignant disease. *J Thorac Cardiovasc Surg* 1998;115:1215.
129. Posner MR, Cohen GI, Skarin AT. Pericardial disease in patients with cancer. The differentiation of malignant from idiopathic and radiation-induced pericarditis. *Am J Med* 1981;71:407.
130. Press OW, Livingston R. Management of malignant pericardial effusion and tamponade. *JAMA* 1987;257:1088.
131. Clarke DP, Cosgrove DO. Real-time ultrasound scanning in the planning and guidance of pericardiocentesis. *Clin Radiol* 1987;38:119.
132. Allen KB, Faber LP, Warren WH, Shaar CJ. Pericardial effusion: subxiphoid pericardiostomy versus percutaneous catheter drainage. *Ann Thorac Surg* 1999;67:437.
133. Piehler JM, Pluth JR, Schaff HV, et al. Surgical management of effusive pericardial disease. Influence of extent of pericardial resection on clinical course. *J Thorac Cardiovasc Surg* 1985;90:506.
134. Naunheim KS, Kesler KA, Fiore AC, et al. Pericardial drainage: subxiphoid vs. transthoracic approach. *Eur J Cardiothorac Surg* 1991;5:99.
135. Park JS. Surgical management of pericardial effusion in patients with malignancies. Comparison of subxiphoid window versus pericardiectomy. *Cancer* 1991;67:76.
136. Liu HP, Chang C-H, Lin PJ, et al. Thoracoscopic management of effusive pericardial disease: indications and technique. *Ann Thorac Surg* 1994;58:1695.
137. Mack MJ, Landreneau RJ, Hazelrigg SR, Acuff TE. Videothoracoscopic management of benign and malignant pericardial effusion. *Chest* 1993;103:390.
138. Hazelrigg SR, Mack MJ, Landreneau RJ, et al. Thoracoscopic pericardiectomy for effusive pericardial disease. *Ann Thorac Surg* 1993;56:792.
139. Yim AP, Ho JKS. Video-assisted subxiphoid pericardiectomy. *J Laparoendosc Surg* 1995;5:193.
140. Wang N, Feikes JR, Mogensen T, Vhymeister EE, Bailey LLM. Pericardioperitoneal shunt: an alternative treatment for malignant pericardial effusion. *Ann Thorac Surg* 1994;57:289.
141. Akagi Y, Hirokawa Y, Kagemoto M, et al. Optimum fractionation for high-dose-rate endoesophageal brachytherapy following external irradiation of early stage esophageal cancer. *Int J Radiat Oncol Biol Phys* 1999;43:525.
142. Vaitkus PT, Herrmann HC, LeWinter MM. Treatment of malignant pericardial effusion. *JAMA* 1994;272:59.
143. Celermajer DS, Boyer MJ, Bailey BP, Tattersall MH. Pericardiocentesis for symptomatic malignant pericardial effusion: a study of 36 patients. *Med J Aust* 1991;154:19.
144. Callahan JA, Seward JB, Nishimura RA, et al. Two-dimensional echocardiographically guided pericardiocentesis: experience in 117 consecutive patients. *Am J Cardiol* 1985;55:476.
145. Gatenby RA, Hartz WH, Kessler HB. Percutaneous catheter drainage for malignant pericardial effusion. *J Vasc Interv Radiol* 1991;2:151.
146. Wong B, Murphy J, Chang CJ, Haaenein K, Dunn M. The risk of pericardiocentesis. *Am J Cardiol* 1979;44:1110.
147. Maher EA, Shepherd FA, Todd TJR. Pericardial sclerosis as the primary management of malignant pericardial effusion and cardiac tamponade. *J Thorac Cardiovasc Surg* 1996;112:637.
148. Liu G, Crump M, Goss PE, Dancey J, Shepherd FA. Prospective comparison of the sclerosing agents doxycycline and bleomycin for the primary management of malignant pericardial effusion and cardiac tamponade. *J Clin Oncol* 1996;14:3141.
149. Fiorentino MV, Daniele O, Morandi P. Intrapericardial instillation of platin in malignant pericardial effusion. *Cancer* 1988;62:1904.
150. Primrose WR, Clee MD, Johnston RN. Malignant pericardial effusion managed with vinblastine. *Clin Oncol* 1983;9:76.
151. Ziskind AA, Pearce AC, Lemmon CC, et al. Percutaneous balloon pericardiotomy for the treatment of cardiac tamponade and large pericardial effusions: description of technique and report of the first 50 cases. *J Am Coll Cardiol* 1993;21:1.
152. Palacios IF, Tuzcu ME, Ziskind AA, Younger J, Block PC. Percutaneous balloon pericardial window for patients with malignant pericardial effusion and tamponade. *Cathet Cardiovasc Diagn* 1991;22:244.
153. Di Segni E, Lavee J, Kaplinsky E, Vered Z. Percutaneous balloon pericardiostomy for treatment of cardiac tamponade. *Eur Heart J* 1995;16:184.
154. Yim AP, Chan AT, Lee TW, Wan IY, Ho JK. Thoracoscopic talc insufflation versus talc slurry for symptomatic malignant pleural effusion. *Ann Thorac Surg* 1996;62:1655.
155. Kennedy L, Rusch VW, Strange C, Ginsberg RJ, Sahn SA. Pleurodesis using talc slurry. *Chest* 1994;106:342.
156. Okamato H, Shinkae T, Yamakido M, Saijo N. Cardiac tamponade caused by primary lung cancer and the management of pericardial effusion. *Cancer* 1993;71:93.
157. Chan A, Rishchin D, Clerk CP, Woodruff RK. Subxiphoid partial pericardiostomy with or without sclerosant instillation in the treatment of symptomatic pericardial effusions in patients with malignancy. *Cancer* 1991;68:1021.
158. Sugimoto JT, Little AG, Ferguson MK. Pericardial window: mechanism of efficacy. *Ann Thorac Surg* 1990;50:442.
159. Palatianos GM, Thurer RJ, Pompeo MQ, Kaiser GA. Clinical experience with subxiphoid drainage of pericardial effusion. *Ann Thorac Surg* 1989;48:381.
160. Reitknecht F, Regal AM, Antkowiak JG, Takita H. Management of cardiac tamponade in patients with malignancy. *J Surg Oncol* 1985;30:19.
161. Ghosh SC, Larrieu AJ, Ablaza SGG, Grana VP. Clinical experience with subxiphoid pericardial decompression. *Int Surg* 1985;70:5.
162. Levin BH, Aaron BL. The subxiphoid pericardial window. *Surg Gynecol Obstet* 1982;155:804.
163. Prager RL, Wilson CH, Bender HW. The subxiphoid approach to pericardial disease. *Ann Thorac Surg* 1982;34:6.
164. Santos GH, Frater RWN. The subxiphoid approach in the treatment of pericardial effusion. *Ann Thorac Surg* 1977;23:477.
165. Kopecky SL, Callahan JA, Tajik J, Seward JB. Percutaneous pericardial catheter drainage: report of 42 consecutive cases. *Ann J Cardiol* 1986;58:633.
166. Davis S, Rambotti P, Grignani F. Interpericardial tetracycline sclerosis in the management of malignant pericardial effusion: an analysis of thirty-three cases. *J Clin Oncol* 1984;2:631.
167. Lemmon CC, Ziskind AA. Percutaneous balloon pericardiotomy: nonsurgical alternative for treating malignancy-related pericardial effusions. *Cardiol B Rev* 1993;10:53.

FRANCESCO M. MARINCOLA
DOUGLAS J. SCHWARTZENTRUBER

SECTION **6**

Malignant Ascites

The collection of intraperitoneal fluid in a patient with known intraabdominal cancer is most likely due to intraperitoneal spread of disease and if neoplastic cells are identified, the term *malignant ascites* is used. This finding has multiple implications: (1) the recognition of small quantities of intraperitoneal fluid may have staging and prognostic significance and alter a planned surgical intervention; (2) symptomatic large collections are a sign of disseminated carcinomatosis and may reflect end-stage disease. Although the expected survival in this case is on the order of months,[1] several palliative options can be considered; (3) the presence of malignant ascites may be part of a clinical picture amenable to curative efforts. In such cases, as lymphoma and ovarian cancer, strategies aimed at obtaining regression of tumor and prolongation of survival should be considered.

The therapeutic approaches used to treat patients with malignant ascites may include extensive surgical debulking in preparation for local or systemic chemotherapy,[2–4] intracavitary chemotherapy with or without hyperthermia,[3–9] phototherapy,[10] instillation of biologic response modifiers,[11–15] and intracavitary particle radiation.[16] Although prolongation of survival has been attributed to some of these therapies, no definitive study has ever demonstrated effectiveness or superiority of one strategy over the other.[17] It is possible that the lack of randomized clinical trials reflects the skepticism of many investigators about the therapeutic effectiveness of available options and the desire to explore new treatment modalities in the context of phase I or phase II studies.

DIAGNOSIS AND WORKUP

Abdominal distension and changes in abdominal girth are classic symptoms of ascites (Table 52.6-1). Signs of ascites include dullness to percussion, shifting dullness, and fluid wave. These may be totally absent in smaller effusions (100 mL or less) diagnosed incidentally during the workup of malignancy by ultrasonography,[18] magnetic resonance imaging, or computed tomography.[19] In these cases, radiologic techniques are useful to guide probes for diagnostic purpose into effusions that are not clinically evident.[20] Delayed enhancement of ascitic fluid after intravenous administration of contrast agents has been associated with bloody effusion and malignant characteristics. However, a prospective study failed to show sufficient specificity of this technique.[21]

Nonneoplastic causes of ascites include congestive heart failure, cirrhosis, renal or pancreatic disease, hypoproteinemia, infectious processes, and benign gynecologic conditions such as endometriosis. Although malignant ascites represents approximately 10% of all cases of ascites,[22] in a patient with advanced cancer it is the most likely diagnosis. As a rule of thumb, a small amount of ascitic fluid along the gutter or in the pelvis of an asymptomatic patient with known intraperitoneal malignancy undergoing systemic therapy should not be aspirated since it can be assumed to be secondary to the malignancy itself. A peritoneal tap is indicated when a definitive diagnosis of malignant ascites is necessary for staging purposes or when planning surgical resection. Other indications may include malignant ascites in cancer patients with no known intraperitoneal disease or in cryptogenic ascites. This is particularly true for female patients because of the high likelihood of a gynecologic primary that may benefit from tumor debulking followed by systemic or locoregional therapy.[23]

TABLE 52.6-1. Assessment of the Patient with Ascites: Diagnosis/Workup

HISTORY
Increasing abdominal girth: "clothes don't fit"
Ingestion and early satiety
Ankle swelling
Easy fatigability
Shortness of breath
PHYSICAL EXAMINATION
Fluid wave
Shifting dullness
RADIOGRAPHIC STUDIES
Abdominal flat plate: generalized ground-glass appearance; air-filled small bowel loops occupy central position and are separated by fluid between loops; psoas shadows obscured
Ultrasound, abdominal computed tomography: both are sensitive tests that definitively diagnose small amounts of ascites
PARACENTESIS
Gross character on inspection: bloody, serous, milky, and turbid
Cell count and differential
Chemistries: total protein, lactic dehydrogenase, carcinoembryonic antigen, CA-125, amylase, bilirubin
Cytology
Microbiology: Gram's stain and culture

The ascitic fluid should be evaluated for various chemistry, tumor, and cytologic markers (Tables 52.6-1 and 52.6-2). Five hundred milliliters of fluid are generally sufficient to collect enough cells for cytologic evaluation; if no cancer cells are found with this amount, additional fluid will not be more informative. A serous (rather than bloody) character of the fluid suggests a hydraulic cause such as portal hypertension, cardiac failure, nephrotic syndrome, reduced oncotic pressure, or pancreatic ascites. Infection is generally associated with other systemic symptoms, whereas tubercular and malignant ascites may be particularly difficult to differentiate as several markers, except cholesterol,[24] express a similar pattern. The presence of chylous fluid can be related to obstruction or injury of large retroperitoneal lymphatic channels seen with extensive intraabdominal lymphomas or after external beam radiation.[25]

Only a minority of all causes of ascitic fluid collections is malignancy, particularly in children,[22] and approximately one-third of patients with known malignancy have nonmalignant causes of ascites.[26] Thus, assays have been described that help determine the neoplastic origin of the ascites.[27–29] A prognostic significance has been attributed to biochemical or immuno-

TABLE 52.6-2. Tools for the Evaluation of Malignant Serous Effusions

	References
Standard biochemical and cytologic determinations	
Ascites/serum ratio for protein, lactic dehydrogenase, fibronectin, cholesterol, erythrocyte and leukocyte count, cultures, Papanicolaou's stain of pelleted ascites	24,33,99–101
Immunochemical stains	
Carcinoembryonic antigen, CA-125, urokinase receptor, human chorionic gonadotropin, vascular endothelial growth factor	34,35,102–106
Immunochemical combinations	
Anti–carcinoembryonic antigen/B72.3/PASd, anti-p53/B72.3/c-erbB-2	27,36,107
Cytogenetic analysis	
Benign versus malignant mesothelial cells	28
Computerized interactive morphometry	
Benign versus malignant lymphocytosis	42
In situ hybridization	
For detection of oncogene expression	108
Detection of cytokines, cytokine receptors, adhesion molecules, etc.	
Interleukin-6, tumor necrosis factor, tumor necrosis factor or interleukin-2 receptor, intracellular adhesion molecule-1, and so forth	32,104,109–113
Endoscopic ultrasound guided fine-needle aspiration of ascitic fluid	
Small effusions noted during endoscopy	20,114
Laparoscopic evaluation and biopsy	
Most sensitive test for ascites of unknown origin	38

logic markers.[30–32] Peritoneal fluid cytology yields a diagnosis in a large proportion of patients.[26] The presence of elevated ascitic/serum ratios of protein or lactic dehydrogenase, carcinoembryonic antigen, CA-125, fibronectin, or cholesterol favor neoplasm.[24,33] Others proposed the measurement of human chorionic gonadotropin in serum and ascitic fluid for the identification of gynecologic malignancies.[34] Vascular endothelial growth factor levels have been noted to be significantly elevated in malignant ascites compared with ascites from benign causes.[35] Immunochemical combinations have been described for the diagnosis of adenocarcinomas and other malignancies.[27,36] El-Habashi et al.[36] reported the use of a battery of monoclonal antibodies against p53, B72.3, and c-erbB-2 as complement to conventional cytology to enhance diagnostic sensitivity and accuracy.

Approximately 20% of patients with malignant ascites present without an identified primary cause.[37] In these patients, particularly women,[23] attempts to identify the tumor of origin should be undertaken because the identification of the primary histology may influence the treatment strategy. Laparoscopy in 129 patients with unknown primary identified carcinomatosis in 60%[38] and laparoscopy with peritoneal biopsy was able to establish the cause of ascites in 86% of these cases. Although laparoscopy in patients with ascites has been rarely associated with prolonged leak from the port site[38,39] or port site recurrence,[40] it can be considered a safe tool for the evaluation of ascites. Approximately 75% of women presenting with malignant ascites of unknown origin have a gynecologic cause (ovary, uterus, or cervix) and another 10% a gastrointestinal cause, while in men the gastrointestinal etiology predominates.[23,37,41,42] Other histologies should be considered, particularly when a primary tumor deposit is not recognized after routine studies of the abdominal cavity. These unusual causes of malignant ascites may create a difficult diagnostic challenge such as the differentiation of mesothelioma cells from normal mesothelial cells[28,29] or the analysis of lymphoid-rich effusions in the case of lymphoma.[42] Unusually, ascites can be the result of cancer treatment.[43]

TREATMENT OF MALIGNANT ASCITES

As the pathogenesis of malignant ascites differs from the pathogenesis of most ascitic fluid collections secondary to benign processes, the treatment is often different in many respects.[23] Excess fluid formation[44] as well as obstruction of lymphatic channels[45,46] are believed to be the most relevant factors inducing malignant ascites. Since most of the time there is no underlying venous obstruction, portal hypertension is unusual and vascular shunting procedures are not indicated. Several strategies have been used with the primary goal of achieving palliation, as the presence of malignant ascites is perceived as a sign of end-stage disease. A survey of practicing physicians suggested that the most common mean of managing malignant ascites is paracentesis, which is also believed to be the most effective.[17] After paracentesis, diuretics and peritoneovenous shunting were most commonly used. In particular cases, radical surgical procedures or aggressive intracavitary therapies have been advocated, however, to date no well-controlled prospective randomized trial has been performed to compare alternative treatments. The encouraging results reported by many pilot phase I or II studies involving intracavitary instillation of chemotherapeutic agents have not matured, with few exceptions, into randomized phase III trials. The median survival of patients with symptomatic malignant ascites is approximately 2 months (Table 52.6-3).[23] In general for nonovarian malignant ascites, the focus is on palliation of symptoms. Patients with malignant ascites secondary to ovarian cancer represent an exception because they have a significantly better survival expectation.[47] Thus, investigation of female patients presenting with ascites of unknown origin should be particularly thorough. Patients with large volume nonovarian

TABLE 52.6-3. Patient Survival after Peritoneovenous Shunting

	Underlying Malignancy			*Patient Survival*	
	Ovary	Gastrointestinal (Colon, Stomach, Pancreas, Hepatobiliary)	Other	Median (wk)	Percentage Alive at 1 Y
Summary of studies published before 1985	85	52	99	5–16	0–12
More recent investigations (published since 1985)					
Kostroff, 1985[79]	11	8	12	8	0
Campioni, 1986[115]	8	14	20	7	7
Sonnenfeld, 1986[80]	—	16	11	8	0
Roussel, 1986[116]	12	10	14	13	0
Soderlund, 1986[81]	7	15	2	7	4
Shepherd, 1988[117]	2	8	4	6	7
Edney, 1989[118]	8	24	13	33	13
Smith, 1989[119]	3	23	24	22	4
Holm, 1989[86]	1	7	5	Not available	0
Gough, 1993[50]	9	13	20	20	Not available
Schumacher, 1994[82]	17	34	38	10	Not available
Faught, 1995[120]	21	—	4	11	Not available
Wickremesekera, 1997[121]	—	21	—	22	Not available
Total	184	224	266	5–33	0–13

ascites have a high mortality (41%) following major abdominal surgery. For these patients, Yazdi et al.[48] have suggested intraperitoneal chemotherapy or peritoneovenous shunt placement at the time of the abdominal operation.

DIURESIS AND RESTRICTION OF SALT AND FLUID INTAKE

Loop diuretics, salt restriction, and aldosterone-inhibiting diuretics are generally not beneficial since sodium retention is not a cause of malignant ascites, although spironolactone is seldom used. Pockros et al.[49] noted that cancer patients with portal hypertension-related ascites caused by massive hepatic metastases were most likely to experience palliation when treated with diuretics. The administration of albumin was never proven beneficial in delaying fluid reaccumulation nor more effective than crystalloid solutions in restoring intravascular volume depletion after drainage of large quantities of peritoneal fluid.

REPEATED PARACENTESIS AND EXTERNAL DRAINS

Symptoms of malignant ascites may be relieved by repeated abdominal taps as needed. Gough et al.[50] reported no difference in survival and quality of life between patients treated with repeated abdominal paracentesis and patients treated with peritoneovenous shunts. However, several concerns are raised by this approach, including the risk of infection, electrolyte and fluid imbalances secondary to the sudden depletion of body fluids, and the risk of causing intraperitoneal visceral injury. For this reason multiple methodologies describing the implantation of permanent drains in the peritoneal cavity have been described.[51] Although good palliation can be achieved in this fashion, the life span of these drains is limited by the need for removal because of malfunction or infection. Lorentzen et al.[52] have reported the use of ultrasonically guided insertion of peritoneogastric shunts in patients with malignant ascites using a Denver shunt connected to a gastrostomy tube. This technique allows intermittent removal of fluid that, on pumping, is shunted to the stomach lumen. Others have advocated peritoneal-urinary drainage for the treatment of refractory ascites.[53] These methods have potential benefits compared with the external drain (in which the ascitic fluid is totally removed from the body) and peritoneovenous shunts (returning the drained fluid from the peritoneal cavity directly to the intravascular space).

INTRACAVITARY THERAPY

Instillation of radioactive isotopes, including colloidal suspensions of $^{32}CrPO_4$, was originally reported with minimal side effects.[16] Weisberger et al. performed intraperitoneal administration of nitrogen mustard in seven patients with advanced ovarian cancer with effective reduction of the amount of ascites in all patients.[54] The rationale for this therapeutic approach is based on the intuition that, due to limited peritoneal absorption, some drugs could be administered in high concentrations in the peritoneum with relatively few systemic effects.[55] Cisplatin and mitoxantrone used alone or in combination with other agents have become first-line chemotherapeutic agents for the treatment of peritoneal carcinomatosis.[5,56,57] Cisplatin is mostly used for the intraperitoneal treatment of ovarian carcinoma because of its high effectiveness against this cancer when given systemically. To enhance the local effectiveness of intraperitoneally administered cisplatin while diminishing the side effects related to its systemic absorption, intravenous administration of thiosulfate has been recommended.[56] Kirmani et al. reported a 30% complete response rate in patients who underwent intraperitoneal cisplatin and etoposide administration after failure of first-line platin-containing systemic treatments.[58]

This study was performed on patients with small bulk of disease (less than 2 cm) and suggested that, as for systemic therapy, the load of tumor may play a role in the response rate. Several authors have investigated the use of intraperitoneal treatment in combination with debulking surgery[8] or after first-line systemic therapy.[59] As previously discussed, Howell et al. reported a 49-month median survival with intraperitoneal instillation of cisplatin in 25 patients with microscopic disease (less than 0.5 cm) after first-line chemotherapy. The dose intensity of cisplatin administration has been increased without added toxicity. Bonetti et al. administered high-dose intraperitoneal cisplatin twice a week.[60] Hagiwara et al. reported a 92% response rate with the intraperitoneal administration of cisplatin lactic acid oligomer microspheres in patients with malignant ascites.[61] Park et al. reported their experience in treating 18 patients with primary peritoneal mesothelioma with continuous hyperthermic peritoneal perfusion and cisplatinum.[3] Thirteen of the 18 patients had associated malignant ascites. Continuous hyperthermic peritoneal perfusion with cisplatinum was successful in 12 of the 13 cases. The median progression-free survival in this study was 26 months and the overall 2-year survival was 80%, superior to the survival reported in historical controls. The same group has evaluated the feasibility of a combination continuous hyperthermic peritoneal perfusion, cisplatinum, and tumor necrosis factor.[15] This combination was evaluated in 27 patients with peritoneal carcinomatosis of multiple etiologies. There was no mortality, the complication rate was minimal, and the clinical outcome of this modality of treatment is presently under investigation. Gilly et al. reported resolution of malignant ascites in 11 of 12 patients treated with intraperitoneal chemotherapy and hyperthermia consisting of either cisplatin or mitomycin C after surgical resection of bulk disease. Intraperitoneal instillation of the chemotherapeutic agent was done after closure of the abdominal cavity and heated at the inflow temperature of 46° to 49°C.[7] Patients had ascites secondary to digestive or ovarian primary; the median survival was 11.2 months, and the 1-year survival rate was 46.9%. Similarly, Loggie et al. reported a median survival of 10.1 months in patients with nonovarian malignant ascites treated with cytoreductive surgery and intraperitoneal hyperthermic chemotherapy with mitomycin C.[47] Interestingly, in the same trial, 12 additional patients who did not present with ascites but had positive cytologic evaluations at the time of operation were treated with the same treatment protocol. None of these patients developed ascites subsequent to this treatment and their median survival was 32.7 months, suggesting that intraperitoneal hyperthermic chemotherapy may have a role in preventing the formation of malignant ascites. Several other authors have addressed the use of hyperthermia in combination with local chemotherapy for the treatment of gastrointestinal malignancies with similar results.[8,9]

To evaluate the relative effectiveness of intraperitoneal versus systemic administration of cisplatin in patients with ovarian cancer, Kirmani et al. completed a phase III randomized trial.[62] This is the only randomized trial addressing the efficacy of intracavitary versus systemic therapy for peritoneal carcinomatosis. In this study, patients (29) were randomized to receive six cycles of intraperitoneal cisplatin (22 mg/m^2) and etoposide (350 mg/m^2). As an example of the importance of prospective randomized trials, in spite of the anecdotally derived enthusiasm for intracavitary therapy, no difference was noted in response rate (48% intraperitoneally vs. 52% intravenously). The rate of complete response at second-look laparotomy was 31% and 33%, respectively, and at a median follow-up of 46 months there was no difference in response duration and survival. Furthermore, there was no difference in response rate in relation to the bulk of tumor present at the time of chemotherapy (less than or equal to or greater than 1 cm). The authors concluded that the small number of patients tested did not allow a definitive dismissal of the usefulness of the intraperitoneal approach. To our knowledge, no follow-up evaluation of a larger cohort of patients has been published since, and the same group has turned its interest toward the evaluation of new agents such as the intraperitoneal instillation topotecan.[63] Other alternatives to cisplatin have been suggested including the intraperitoneal administration of carboplatin, etoposide, and granulocyte-macrophage colony-stimulating factor,[64] with a partial response rate of 69%. Steller et al. reported the treatment of small-volume residual ovarian cancer with continuous hyperthermic peritoneal perfusion and carboplatin in the context of a phase I trial.[4] This well-tolerated modality of treatment may have important applications for novel therapies given intraperitoneally.

Biologic response modifiers have been used as an alternative to chemotherapeutic agents for the treatment of intraperitoneal carcinomatosis. Single-agent interferon-α,[11,14] or interferon-β,[65] tumor necrosis factor,[66] and interleukin-2, with or without adoptive administration of lymphokine-activated killer cells,[12,13,65,67] have been reported with variable success. A randomized trial has compared the effectiveness of interleukin-2, interferon-α or interferon-β for the control of malignant effusions, suggesting a higher efficacy of interleukin-2, particularly in patients with mesothelioma.[65] Others have reported effectiveness of the combined intraperitoneal administration of interleukin-2 and OK-423 in patients with ascites secondary to gastric malignancy.[68] The authors reported an incidence of cytologic disappearance of cancer and decrease of ascites in 81% of 22 evaluable patients. The role of interferon-γ has also been explored in patients with malignant ascites because of the ability of this cytokine to induce up-regulation of tumor-associated antigens,[69] major histocompatibility complex molecules, or both in tumor cells.[70] This property suggested possible therapeutic usefulness combining this cytokine with the administration of major histocompatibility complex–restricted T cells in view of the enhanced lysability of tumor cells expressing higher amounts of major histocompatibility complex molecules.[71] Phase I studies of adoptive cellular immunotherapy with intraperitoneal injection of activated human blood monocytes have shown the feasibility of this approach.[72] Radioiodinated monoclonal antibodies directed against tumor markers have also been used.[73]

RADICAL SURGERY

Peritonectomy has been advocated by Sugarbaker[2]: this is an extensive debulking procedure using a ball-type electrocautery device. It includes six possible steps: (1) greater omentectomy-splenectomy; (2) left upper quadrant peritonectomy; (3) right upper quadrant peritonectomy; (4) lesser omentectomy-cholecystectomy with stripping of the omental bursa; (5) pelvic peritonectomy with sleeve resection of the sigmoid colon; and (6) antrectomy. The purpose of the procedure is cytoreduction in preparation for intraperitoneal chemotherapy. The authors reported good long-term results in selected patients affected with peritoneal carcinomatosis, sarcomatosis, and mesothelioma.[2,74,75] Intraperitoneal chemotherapy included mitomycin C and 5-fluorouracil for patients with adenocarcinoma and cisplatin and doxorubicin for patients with sarcoma.[75] Among patients with enteric carcinomatosis, favorable prognostic characteristics were identified that include low-grade histopathology, absence of lymph nodal metastases, and completeness of the cytoreductive procedure (survival at 3 years was 99%).[74] A follow-up report from the same group identified a significant difference in 5-year survival between patients with stage III gastric cancer who had undergone surgery alone (18.4%) versus patients who underwent additional intraperitoneal chemotherapy (49.1%; $P = .011$).[63] In this series patients had resectable gastric cancer and no ascites. This randomized study demonstrates, in principle, that intraperitoneal chemotherapy may have a role in the treatment of aggressive, nonovarian, intraabdominal cancers likely to lead to malignant ascites. A pilot study describing the use of photodynamic therapy as adjuvant therapy after aggressive debulking of disseminated intraperitoneal malignancies by Sindelar et al.[10] has shown a 26% disease-free survival rate at 18 months. These results in selected patients, however, still await confirmation by a randomized trial.

PERITONEOVENOUS SHUNTING

An extensive discussion about the application of shunting procedures for the treatment of malignant ascites has been reviewed by Alexander and Fraker.[76] In patients with symptomatic malignant ascites, internal peritoneovenous shunting represents the standard modality of care. The devices consist of (1) a length of multiply perforated tubing to be inserted in the free peritoneal cavity, (2) a length of tubing to be inserted into the superior vena cava (or other large venous vessel), and (3) a unidirectional flow valve connecting the two limbs (Fig. 52.6-1). The two most popular devices are the LeVeen shunt and the Denver shunt. The latter shunt has a one-way pump that can be manually pumped by the patient or physician to clear debris. Originally, the shunts were used for the treatment of ascites secondary to nonmalignant causes, but this technique was eventually applied to malignant ascites as well.[77–82] Briefly, the principle underlying the function of the shunt takes advantage of the pressure gradient (5 to 15 cm H_2O) existing between the abdominal and the thoracic cavities. On inspiration, the further increase in pressure gradient (due to increased negative pressure within the thorax) drains fluid from the abdominal cavity by allowing the unidirectional valve to open. The surgical procedure for the placement of the shunt can be done under local or general anesthesia. Prophylactic antibiotic coverage is recommended, as with the placement of any prosthetic material. In the traditional approach, a muscle-splitting subcostal incision is performed and the intraperitoneal portion of the shunt is placed using a nonabsorbable pursestring suture to secure the limb in a watertight fashion. Current product guidelines recommend the percutaneous insertion of the peritoneal catheter using a peel-away introducer if allowed by the patient's anatomy. A second incision is performed in the neck to expose the internal jugular vein in which the venous portion of the shunt will be introduced. Alternatively, the venous catheter may be inserted percutaneously into the subclavian vein. A subcutaneous pocket is fashioned for the pump over the lower rib cage (in the case of a Denver shunt) and a subcutaneous tunnel is developed linking the abdominal and neck or chest incision. The venous limb is passed through the tunnel and introduced in

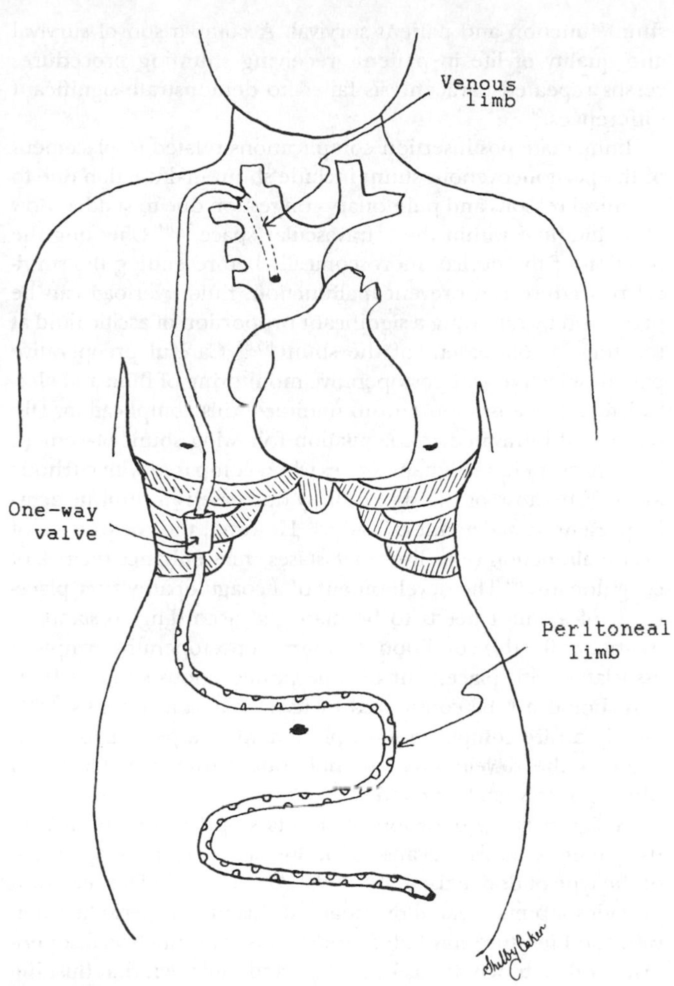

FIGURE 52.6-1. The peritoneovenous shunt *in situ*.

the central venous system according to the chosen technique. Before placement of the intravenous portion of the shunt, the flow of ascitic fluid through the device needs to be demonstrated to exclude malpositioning or kinking within the abdominal cavity. Before terminating the procedure, shunt placement needs to be checked either fluoroscopically or with a portable chest and abdominal radiograph as malposition or kinking of the catheter may be responsible for immediate malfunction.

The indication for the placement of a peritoneovenous shunt has traditionally been the relief of symptoms caused by malignant ascites refractory to medical management. It is, therefore, reasonable to expect that, with the development of more effective systemic or intraperitoneal therapy the need for this procedure will decline. The median survival of 674 patients with refractory malignant ascites (gastrointestinal primary in 33%, ovarian primary in 27%, and other malignancies in 39%) undergoing placement of a peritoneovenous shunt is 5 to 33 weeks with 0% to 13% of patients alive at 1 year (Table 52.6-3). Therefore, the goal of the peritoneovenous shunt placement is to minimize the side effects caused by the procedure and the presence of a foreign body and provide significant palliation. The wide variation in the range of patient survival after placement of a peritoneovenous shunt is most likely due to differences in patient selection criteria. Other variables such as protein content[83] or number of neoplastic cells in the ascitic fluid[83] have accounted for differences in shunt function and patient survival. A comparison of survival and quality of life in patients receiving shunting procedures versus repeated paracentesis failed to demonstrate significant differences.[50]

Immediate postinsertion complications related to placement of the peritoneovenous shunt include shunt malfunction due to technical reasons and pulmonary congestion due to sudden flow of ascitic fluid within the intravascular space.[79,84] Checking the position of the device fluoroscopically before ending the surgical procedure can prevent malfunction; fluid overload can be prevented by removing a significant proportion of ascitic fluid at the time of placement of the shunt.[85,86] Careful preoperative patient selection and postoperative monitoring of fluid and electrolyte balance is important to minimize this complication. Disseminated intravascular coagulation following shunt placement is a rare event in malignant ascites when compared with cirrhotic ascites[87] because of the significantly decreased fibrinolytic activity present in malignant effusion.[88] However, the coexistence of liver malfunction (e.g., liver metastases) may enhance the risk of coagulopathy.[89] The development of a coagulopathy after placement of a shunt needs to be managed according to standard treatment for this condition. A common postoperative symptom associated with placement of a peritoneovenous shunt is fever and should not be considered by itself as a sign of sepsis.[77,79,90] Finally, a rare complication of placement of a peritoneovenous shunt is the development of pulmonary tumor embolization with a possibly fatal outcome.[91]

A significant proportion of shunts stop functioning before the patient's demise because of occlusion, which is independent of the type of device used.[50,78–80,84,86] Although the Denver shunt provides a pump that allows manual flushing at periodic intervals, the literature has failed to demonstrate functional superiority of this device. It has been reported, however, that flushing of the Denver shunt combined with the administration of thrombolytic agents can occasionally restore shunt function.[84] Relocation of the catheter is usually necessary to establish patency since thrombolytic agents are infrequently successful in this situation. The goal in reestablishing flow in the system is correction of the source, avoiding replacement of the entire shunt. Shunt malfunction is usually manifested by recurrence of ascites and can be demonstrated by visualization of nucleotide in the lungs after intraperitoneal injection of 99mTc macroaggregate albumin.[92] A shuntogram performed by percutaneous injection of radiographic contrast agents into the venous limb of the shunt (into the pump reservoir if a Denver shunt) helps determine the site of obstruction. We previously described shunt occlusion by thrombofibrinous encasement of the venous limb, manifesting as a characteristic contrast outline of the tubing during shuntogram.[93]

Another complication of peritoneovenous shunt placement is infection in the peritoneal cavity. This can be associated with postoperative leakage of peritoneal fluid around the insertion site and is prevented by placing watertight double-pursestring sutures. The development of spontaneous bacterial peritonitis, unrelated to operative infection or to perforation of a viscous due to the malignant process, is, for unknown reasons, less likely in patients with malignant ascites than in cirrhotic patients. It has been noted that malignant peritoneal fluid has significantly higher concentrations of transferrin than cirrhotic ascites. As transferrin concentration in peritoneal fluid is inversely correlated with bacterial growth, it is possible that patients with malignant ascites are somewhat more protected against peritonitis than cirrhotic patients.[94] Evidence of hematologic dissemination of tumor cells from the ascitic fluid and tumor growth along the shunt tract has been reported and it is likely to occur relatively often.[78,91,95,96] However, this theoretical risk has not been a problem, most likely because of the limited survival of these patients.

The decision to place a peritoneovenous shunt should be made after consideration of the various risks and potential benefits. According to Souter et al.,[97] a patient with malignant ascites whose only considered therapeutic goal is palliation, should first undergo repeated paracentesis and medical management with diuretics. If the rate of reaccumulation of the fluid is rapid, fluid consistency is not viscous or bloody, there is no evidence of intracavitary loculation,[83] and the expected survival is more than 3 months, shunting should be considered. Contraindications for placement of the shunt are presence of intraperitoneal infection and cardiac or renal insufficiency. To avoid the massive fluid shifts associated with drainage of refractory ascites, Daimon et al. proposed the use of extracorporeal ultrafiltration of the ascites followed by intravenous reinjection of the ultrafiltered fluid.[98] Among the various patients treated in this fashion, two had malignant ascites. This approach was well tolerated and both patients died of their primary disease free of symptoms related to ascites.

In summary, malignant ascites represents in most instances a debilitating symptom of end-stage cancer. Purely palliative measures on one extreme and aggressive therapeutic intervention on the other represent the wide range of treatment options. Reported survival of patients treated with curative intent, in general, is better than that of patients receiving palliative procedures, but clearly reflects differences in patient selection (differences in stage, histology, extent of disease, and so forth). No randomized studies have been performed to evaluate the treatment of malignant ascites. Several questions remain unanswered, such as the value of a peritoneovenous shunt insertion compared with medical management or intermittent drainage; the role of external versus internal drains; and the effectiveness of locoregional curative efforts. Scant information is available regarding the effectiveness of intracavitary versus systemic therapy.

REFERENCES

1. van de Molengraft FJ, Vooijs GP. Survival of patients with malignancy-associated effusions. *Acta Cytol* 1989;33:911.
2. Sugarbaker PH. Peritonectomy procedures. *Ann Surg* 1995;221:29.
3. Park BJ, Alexander HR, Libutti SK, et al. Treatment of primary peritoneal mesothelioma by continuous hyperthermic peritoneal perfusion (CHPP). *Ann Surg Oncol* 1999;6:582.
4. Steller MA, Egorin MJ, Trimble EL, et al. A pilot phase I trial of continuous hypethermic peritoneal perfusion with high-dose carboplatin as primary treatment of patients with small-volume residual ovarian cancer. *Cancer Chemother Pharmacol* 1999;43:106.
5. Markman M, Howell SB, Lucas WE, Pfeifle CE, Green MR. Combination intraperitoneal chemotherapy with cisplatin, cytarabine, and doxorubicin for refractory ovarian carcinoma and other malignancies principally confined to the peritoneal cavity. *J Clin Oncol* 1984;2:1321.
6. McClay EF, Howell SB. Intraperitoneal therapy in the management of patients with ovarian cancer. *Hematol Oncol Clin North Am* 1992;6:915.
7. Gilly FN, Carry PY, Brachet A, et al. Treatment of malignant peritoneal effusion in digestive and ovarian cancer. *Med Oncol Tumor Pharmacother* 1992;9:177.
8. Sayag AC, Gilly FN, Carry PY, et al. Intraoperative chemohyperthermia in the management of digestive cancers. A general review of literature. *Oncology* 1993;50:333.
9. Fujimoto S, Shrestha RD, Kokubun M, et al. Positive results of combined therapy of surgery and intraperitoneal hyperthermic perfusion for far-advanced gastric cancer. *Ann Surg* 1990;212:592.
10. Sindelar WF, DeLaney TF, Tochner Z, et al. Technique of photodynamic therapy for disseminated intraperitoneal malignant neoplasms. Phase I study. *Arch Surg* 1991;126:318.

11. Bezwoda WR, Seymour L, Dansey R. Intraperitoneal recombinant interferon-alpha 2b for recurrent malignant ascites due to ovarian cancer. *Cancer* 1989;64:1029.
12. Steis RG, Urba WJ, VanderMolen LA, et al. Intraperitoneal lymphokine-activated killer-cell and interleukin-2 therapy for malignancies limited to the peritoneal cavity. *J Clin Oncol* 1990;8:1618.
13. Eggermont AM, Sugarbaker PH. Efficacy of intracavitary administration of cyclophosphamide, interleukin-2 and lymphokine activated killer cells against established intraperitoneal tumor. *Acta Med Austriaca* 1989;16:47.
14. Stuart GC, Nation JG, Snider DD, Thunberg P. Intraperitoneal interferon in the management of malignant ascites. *Cancer* 1993;71:2027.
15. Bartlett DL, Buell JF, Libutti SK, et al. A phase I trial of continuous hypethermic peritoneal perfusion with tumor necrosis factor and cisplatin in the treatment of peritoneal carcinomatosis. *Cancer* 1998;83:1251.
16. Jackson GL, Blosser NM. Intracavitary chromic phosphate (32-P) colloidal suspension therapy. *Cancer* 1981;48:2596.
17. Lee CW, Bociek G, Faught W. A survey of practice in management of malignant ascites. *J Pain Symptom Manag* 1998;16:96.
18. Goldberg BB, Goodman GA, Clearfield HR. Evaluation of ascites by ultrasound. *Radiology* 1970;96:15.
19. Wall SD, Hricak H, Bailey GD, et al. MR imaging of pathologic abdominal fluid collections. *J Comput Assist Tomogr* 1986;10:746.
20. Chang KJ, Albers CG, Nguyen P. Endoscopic ultrasound-guided fine needle aspiration of pleural and ascitic fluid. *Am J Gastroenterol* 1995;90:148.
21. Cooper C, Silverman PM, Davros WJ, Zeman RK. Delayed contrast enhancement of ascitic fluid on CT: frequency and significance [see comments]. *AJR Am J Roentgenol* 1993;161:787.
22. Runyon BA. Care of patients with ascites. *N Engl J Med* 1994;330:337.
23. Parsons SL, Watson SA, Steele RJC. Malignant ascites. *Br J Surg* 1996;83:6.
24. Sood A, Garg R, Kumar R, et al. Ascitic fluid cholesterol in malignant and tubercular ascites. *JAPI* 1995;43:745.
25. Lentz SS, Schray MF, Wilson TO. Chylous ascites after whole-abdomen irradiation for gynecologic malignancy. *Int J Radiat Oncol Biol Phys* 1990;19:435.
26. Runyon BA. Malignancy-related ascites and ascitic fluid humoral tests of malignancy [editorial]. *J Clin Gastroenterol* 1994;18:94.
27. Shield PW, Callan JJ, Devine PL. Markers for metastatic adenocarcinoma in serous effusion specimens. *Diagn Cytopathol* 1994;11:237.
28. Granados R, Cibas ES, Fletcher JA. Cytogenetic analysis of effusions from malignant mesothelioma. A diagnostic adjunct to cytology. *Acta Cytol* 1994;30.711.
29. Ferrandez-Izquierdo A, Navarro-Fos S, Gonzalez-Devesa M, Gil-Benso R, Llombart-Bosch A. Immunocytochemical typification of mesothelial cells in effusions: in vivo and in vitro models. *Diagn Cytopathol* 1994;10:256.
30. Nishiyama M, Takashima I, Tanaka T, et al. Carcinoembryonic antigen levels in the peritoneal cavity: useful guide to peritoneal recurrence and prognosis for gastric cancer. *World J Surg* 1995;19:133.
31. Rubin SC, Finstad CL, Wong GY, et al. Prognostic significance of HER-2/neu expression in advanced epithelial ovarian cancer: a multivariate analysis. *Am J Obstet Gynecol* 1993;168:162.
32. Plante M, Rubin SC, Wong GY, et al. Interleukin-6 level in serum and ascites as a prognostic factor in patients with epithelial ovarian cancer. *Cancer* 1994;73:1882.
33. Bansai S, Kaur K, Bansai AK. Diagnosing ascitic ethiology on a biochemical basis. *Hepatogastroenterology* 1998;45:1673.
34. Grossmann M, Hoermann R, Gocze PM, et al. Measurement of human chorionic gonadotropin-related immunoreactivity in serum, ascites and tumour cysts of patients with gynaecologic malignancies. *Eur J Clin Invest* 1995;25:867.
35. Zebrowski BK, Liu W, Ramirez K, et al. Markedly elevated levels of vascular endothelial growth factor in malignant ascites. *Ann Surg Oncol* 1999;6:373.
36. el-Habashi A, el-Morsi B, Freeman SM, el-Didi M, Marrogi AJ. Tumor oncogenic expression in malignant effusions as a possible method to enhance cytologic diagnostic sensitivity. An immunocytochemical study of 87 cases. *Am J Clin Pathol* 1995;103:206.
37. Ringenberg QS, Doll DC, Loy TS, Yarbro JW. Malignant ascites of unknown origin. *Cancer* 1989;64:753.
38. Chu CM, Lin SM, Peng SM, Wu CS, Liaw YF. The role of laparoscopy in the evaluation of ascites of unknown origin. *Gastrointest Endosc* 1994;40:285.
39. Menzies RI, Fitzgerald JM, Mulpeter K. Laparoscopic diagnosis of ascites in Lesotho. *BMJ* 1985;291:473.
40. Wexner SD, Cohen SM. Port site metastases after laparoscopic colorectal surgery for cure of malignancy. *Br J Surg* 1995;82:295.
41. Wilailak S, Linasmita V, Srivannaboon S. Malignant ascites in female patients: a seven year review. *J Med Assoc Thai* 1999;82:15.
42. Walts AE, Svidler R, Tolmachoff T, Marchevsky AM. Lymphoid-rich effusions. Diagnosis by morphometry using the CAS 200 System. *Am J Clin Pathol* 1994;101:526.
43. Kemeny N, Seiter K, Martin D, et al. A new syndrome: ascites, hyperbilirubinemia, and hypoalbuminemia after biochemical modulation of fluorouracil with N-phosphonacetyl-L-aspartate (PALA) [see comments]. *Ann Intern Med* 1991;115:946.
44. Hirabayashi K, Graham J. Genesis of ascites in ovarian cancer. *Am J Obstet Gynecol* 1970;106:492.
45. Feldman GB, Knapp RC. Lymphatic drainage of the peritoneal cavity and its significance in ovarian cancer. *Am J Obstet Gynecol* 1974;119:991.
46. Coates G, Bush RS, Aspin N. A study of ascites using lymphoscintigraphy with 99m Tc-sulfur colloid. *Radiology* 1973;107:577.
47. Loggie BW, Perini M, Fleming RA, Russell GB, Geisenger K. Treatment and prevention of malignant ascites associated with disseminated intraperitoneal malignancies by aggressive combined-modality therapy. *Am Surg* 1997;63:137.
48. Yazdi GP, Miedema BW, Humphrey LJ. High mortality after abdominal operaton in patients with large-volume malignant ascites. *J Surg Oncol* 1996;62:93.
49. Pockros PJ, Esrason KT, Nguyen C, Duque J, Woods S. Mobilization of malignant ascites with diuretics is dependent on ascitic fluid characteristics. *Gastroenterology* 1992;103:1302.
50. Gough IR, Balderson GA. Malignant ascites. A comparison of peritoneovenous shunting and nonoperative management. *Cancer* 1993;71:2377.
51. Lomas DA, Wallis PJ, Stockley RA. Palliation of malignant ascites with a Tenckhoff catheter. *Thorax* 1989;44:828.
52. Lorentzen T, Sengelov L, Nolsoe CP, et al. Ultrasonically guided insertion of a peritoneogastric shunt in patients with malignant ascites. *Acta Radiol* 1995;36:481.
53. Rozenblit GN, Del Guercio LR, Rundback JH, Poplausky MR, Lebovics E. Peritoneal-urinary drainage for treatment of refractory ascites: a pilot study. *J Vasc Intervent Radiol* 1998;9:998.
54. Weisberger AS, Levine B, Storasli JP. Use of nitrogen mustard in the treatment of serous effusions of neoplastic origin. *JAMA* 1955;159:1704.
55. Dedrick RL, Myers CE, Bungay PM, DeVita VT Jr. Pharmacokinetic rationale for peritoneal drug administration in the treatment of ovarian cancer. *Cancer Treat Rep* 1978;62:1.
56. Howell SB, Pfeifle CL, Wung WE, et al. Intraperitoneal cisplatin with systemic thiosulfate protection. *Ann Intern Med* 1982;97:845.
57. Lorusso V, Catino A, Gargano G, et al. Mitoxantrone in the treatment of recurrent ascites of pretreated ovarian carcinoma. *Eur J Gynaecol Oncol* 1994;15:75.
58. Kirmani S, Lucas WE, Kim S, et al. A phase II trial of intraperitoneal cisplatin and etoposide as salvage treatment for minimal residual ovarian carcinoma. *J Clin Oncol* 1991;9:649.
59. Howell SB, Zimm S, Markman M, et al. Long-term survival of advanced refractory ovarian carcinoma patients with small-volume disease treated with intraperitoneal chemotherapy. *J Clin Oncol* 1987;5:1607.
60. Bonetti A, Howell SB, McClay E, et al. High-dose biweekly intraperitoneal cisplatin: an effective way to increase cisplatin dose intensity. *Gynecol Oncol* 1993;49:318.
61. Hagiwara A, Takahashi T, Sawai K, et al. Clinical trials with intraperitoneal cisplatin microspheres for malignant ascites—a pilot study. *Anticancer Drug Des* 1993;8:463.
62. Kirmani S, Braly PS, McClay EF, et al. A comparison of intravenous versus intraperitoneal chemotherapy for the initial treatment of ovarian cancer. *Gynecol Oncol* 1994;54:338.
63. Plaxe SC, Christen RD, O'Quigley J, et al. Phase I and pharmacokinetic study of intraperitoneal topotecan. *Invest New Drugs* 1998;16:147.
64. McClay EF, Braly PD, Kirmani S, et al. A phase II trial of intraperitoneal high-dose carboplatin and etoposide with granulocyte macrophage-colony stimulating factor support in patients with ovarian carcinoma. *Am J Clin Oncol* 1995;18:23.
65. Lissoni P, Barni S, Tancini G, et al. Intracavitary therapy of neoplastic effusions with cytokines: comparison among interferon alpha, beta and interleukin-2. *Support Care Cancer* 1995;3:78.
66. del Mastro L, Venturini M, Giannessi PG, et al. Intraperitoneal infusion of recombinant human tumor necrosis factor and mitoxantrone in neoplastic ascites: a feasibility study. *Anticancer Res* 1995;15:2207.
67. Ottow RT, Eggermont AM, Steller EP, Sugarbaker PH. The requirements for successful immunotherapy of intraperitoneal cancer using interleukin-2 and lymphokine-activated killer cells. *Cancer* 1987;60:1465.
68. Yamaguchi Y, Satoh Y, Miyahara E, et al. Locoregional immunotherapy of malignant ascites by intraperitoneal administration of OK-423 plus IL-2 in gastric cancer patients. *Anticancer Res* 1995;15:2201.
69. Guadagni F, Roselli M, Schlom J, Greiner JW. In vitro and in vivo regulation of human tumor antigen expression by human recombinant interferons: a review. *Int J Biol Markers* 1994;9:53.
70. D'Acquisto R, Markman M, Hakes T, et al. A phase I trial of intraperitoneal recombinant gamma-interferon in advanced ovarian carcinoma. *J Clin Oncol* 1988;6:689.
71. Rivoltini L, Baracchini KC, Viggiano V, et al. Quantitative correlation between HLA class I allele expression and recognition of melanoma cells by antigen specific cytotoxic T lymphocytes. *Cancer Res* 1995;55:3149.
72. Wiesel ML, Faradji A, Grunebaum L, et al. Hemostatic changes in human adoptive immunotherapy with activated blood monocytes or derived macrophages. *Ann Hematol* 1992;65:75.
73. Buckman R, De Angelis C, Shaw P, et al. Intraperitoneal therapy of malignant ascites associated with carcinoma of ovary and breast using radioiodinated monoclonal antibody 2G3. *Gynecol Oncol* 1992;47:102.
74. Sugarbaker PH, Jablonski KA. Prognostic features of 51 colorectal and 130 appendiceal cancer patients with peritoneal carcinomatosis treated by cytoreductive surgery and intraperitoneal chemotherapy. *Ann Surg* 1995;221:124.
75. Sugarbaker PH. Intraperitoneal chemotherapy for treatment and prevention of peritoneal carcinomatosis and sarcomatosis. *Dis Colon Rectum* 1994;37:S115.
76. Alexander HR, Fraker DL. Shunting procedures for malignant ascites and pleural effusions. In: Lotze MT, Rubin JB, eds. *Regional therapy for malignant ascites and pleural effusions.* Philadelphia: Lippincott–Raven, 1997:271.
77. Holman JM Jr, Albo D Jr. Peritoneovenous shunting in patients with malignant ascites. *Am J Surg* 1981;142:774.
78. Souter RG, Wells C, Tarin D, Kettlewell MG. Surgical and pathologic complications associated with peritoneovenous shunts in management of malignant ascites. *Cancer* 1985;55:1973.
79. Kostroff KM, Ross DW, Davis JM. Peritoneovenous shunting for cirrhotic versus malignant ascites. *Surg Gynecol Obstet* 1985;161:204.
80. Sonnenfeld T, Tyden G. Peritoneovenous shunts for malignant ascites. *Acta Chir Scand* 1986;152:117.
81. Soderlund C. Denver peritoneovenous shunting for malignant or cirrhotic ascites. A prospective consecutive series. *Scand J Gastroenterol* 1986;21:1161.
82. Schumacher DL, Saclarides TJ, Staren ED. Peritoneovenous shunts for palliation of the patient with malignant ascites. *Ann Surg Oncol* 1994;1:378.
83. Qazi R, Savlov ED. Peritoneovenous shunt for palliation of malignant ascites. *Cancer* 1982;49:600.
84. Lund RH, Moritz MW. Complications of Denver peritoneovenous shunting. *Arch Surg* 1982;117:924.

85. Reinhold RB, Lokich JJ, Tomashefski J, Costello P. Management of malignant ascites with peritoneovenous shunting. *Am J Surg* 1983;145:455.
86. Holm A, Halpern NB, Aldrete JS. Peritoneovenous shunt for intractable ascites of hepatic, nephrogenic, and malignant causes. *Am J Surg* 1989;158:162.
87. Ragni MV, Lewis JH, Spero JA. Ascites-induced LeVeen shunt coagulopathy. *Ann Surg* 1983;198:91.
88. Scott-Coombes DM, Whawell SA, Vipond MN, Crnojevic L, Thompson JN. Fibrinolytic activity of ascites caused by alcoholic cirrhosis and peritoneal malignancy. *Gut* 1993; 34:1120.
89. Tempero MA, Davis RB, Reed E, Edney J. Thrombocytopenia and laboratory evidence of disseminated intravascular coagulation after shunts for ascites in malignant disease. *Cancer* 1985;55:2718.
90. Greig PD, Langer B, Blendis LM, Taylor BR, Glynn MF. Complications after peritoneovenous shunting for ascites. *Am J Surg* 1980;139:125.
91. Smith RR, Sternberg SS, Paglia MA, Golbey RB. Fatal pulmonary tumor embolization following peritoneovenous shunting for malignant ascites. *J Surg Oncol* 1981;16:27.
92. Singh A, McAfee JG, Thomas FD, Grossman ZD. Radionuclide assessment of peritoneovenous shunt patency. *Clin Nucl Med* 1979;4:447.
93. Schwartzentruber DJ, Leapman SB, Filo RS, Madura JA. Thrombofibrinous sheath occlusion of peritoneovenous shunts. *Surgery* 1987;102:534.
94. Romero A, Perez-Arellano JL, Gonzalez-Villaron L, et al. Effect of transferrin concentration on bacterial growth in human ascitic fluid from cirrhotic and neoplastic patients. *Eur J Clin Invest* 1993;23:699.
95. Maat B, Oosterlee J, Spaas JA, White H, Lammes FB. Dissemination of tumour cells via LeVeen shunt [letter]. *Lancet* 1979;1:988.
96. Tarin D, Price JE, Kettlewell MG, et al. Mechanisms of human tumor metastasis studied in patients with peritoneovenous shunts. *Cancer Res* 1984;44:3584.
97. Souter RG, Tarin D, Kettlewell MG. Peritoneovenous shunts in the management of malignant ascites. *Br J Surg* 1983;70:478.
98. Daimon S, Yasuhara S, Saga T, et al. Efficacy of extracorporeal ultrafiltration of ascitic fluid as a treatment of refractory ascites. *Nephrol Dial Transplant* 1998;13:2617.
99. Chen SJ, Wang SS, Lu CW, et al. Clinical value of tumour markers and serum-ascites albumin gradient in the diagnosis of malignancy-related ascites. *J Gastroenterol Hepatol* 1994;9:396.
100. Lee CM, Changchien CS, Shyu WC, Liaw YF. Serum-ascites albumin concentration gradient and ascites fibronectin in the diagnosis of malignant ascites. *Cancer* 1992;70:2057.
101. Scholmerich J, Volk BA, Kottgen E, Ehlers S, Gerok W. Fibronecting concentration in ascites differentiates between malignant and cirrhotic ascites. *Gastroenterology* 1984;87:1160.
102. Nystrom JS, Dyce B, Wada J, Bateman JR, Haverback B. Carcinoembryonic antigen titers on effusion fluid. A diagnostic tool? *Arch Intern Med* 1977;137:875.
103. Pedersen N, Schmitt M, Ronne E, et al. A ligand-free, soluble urokinase receptor is present in the ascitic fluid from patients with ovarian cancer. *J Clin Invest* 1993; 92:2160.
104. Onsrud M, Shabana A, Austgulen R, Nustad K. Comparison between soluble tumor necrosis factor receptors and CA125 in peritoneal fluids as a marker for epithelial ovarian cancer. *Gynecol Oncol* 1995;57:183.
105. Vergote IB, Onsrud M, Bormer OP, Sert BM, Moen M. CA125 in peritoneal fluid of ovarian cancer patients. *Gynecol Oncol* 1992;44:161.
106. Kraft A, Weindel K, Ochs A, et al. Vascular endothelial growth factor in the sera and effusions of patients with malignant ascites. *Cancer* 1999;85:178.
107. Robinson RJ, Royston D. Comparison of monoclonal antibodies AUA1 and BER EP4 with anti- CEA for detecting carcinoma cells in serous effusions and distinguishing them from mesothelial cells. *Cytopathology* 1993;4:267.
108. Athanassiadou PP, Veneti SZ, Kyrkou KA, Athanassiades PH. Detection of c-Ha-ras oncogene expression in pleural and peritoneal smear effusions by in situ hybridization. *Cancer Detect Prev* 1993;17:585.
109. Giavazzi R, Nicoletti MI, Chirivi RG, et al. Soluble intercellular adhesion molecule-1 (ICAM-1) is released into the serum and ascites of human ovarian carcinoma patients and in nude mice bearing tumour xenografts. *Eur J Cancer* 1994;30A:1865.
110. Moradi MM, Carson LF, Weinberg B, et al. Serum and ascitic fluid levels of interleukin-1, interleukin-6, and tumor necrosis factor-alpha in patients with ovarian epithelial cancer. *Cancer* 1993;72:2433.
111. Andus T, Gross V, Holstege A, et al. High concentrations of soluble tumor necrosis factor receptors in ascites. *Hepatology* 1992;16:749.
112. Andus T, Gross V, Holstege A, et al. Evidence for the production of high amounts of interleukin-6 in the peritoneal cavity of patients with ascites. *J Hepatol* 1992;15:378.
113. Hurteau JA, Simon HU, Kurman C, Rubin L, Mills GB. Levels of soluble interleukin-2 receptor-alpha are elevated in serum and ascitic fluid from epithelial ovarian cancer patients [see comments]. *Am J Obstet Gynecol* 1994;170:918.
114. Gerdes B, Tobollik S, Lausen M. [Rectal endosonography for detection of free fluid in the abdomen]. *Chirurg* 1994;65:709.
115. Campioni N, Pasquali Lasagni R, Vitucci C, et al. Peritoneovenous shunt and neoplastic ascites: a 5-year experience report. *J Surg Oncol* 1986;33:31.
116. Roussel JG, Kroon BB, Hart GA. The Denver type for peritoneovenous shunting of malignant ascites. *Surg Gynecol Obstet* 1986;162:235.
117. Shepherd KE, Miller BJ. Peritoneovenous shunts–devices of last resort. *Can J Surg* 1988;31:444.
118. Edney JA, Hill A, Armstrong D. Peritoneovenous shunts palliate malignant ascites. *Am J Surg* 1989;158:598.
119. Smith DA, Weaver DW, Bouwman DL. Peritoneovenous shunt (PVS) for malignant ascites. An analysis of outcome. *Am Surg* 1989;55:445.
120. Faught W, Kirkpatrick JR, Krepart GV, Heywood MS, Lotocki RJ. Peritoneovenous shunt for palliation of gynecologic malignant ascites. *J Am Coll Surg* 1995;180:472.
121. Wickremesekera SK, Stubbs RS. Peritoneovenous shunting for malignant ascites. *NZ Med J* 1997;110:33.

CHAPTER 53

Hematopoietic Therapy

SECTION 1

PETER L. PERROTTA
EDWARD L. SNYDER

Transfusion Therapy

Despite the increasing use of hematopoietic growth factors, transfusion therapy continues to play an important role in the care of oncology patients. In fact, transfusion therapy has become increasingly critical as improved therapeutic regimens prolong the survival of patients with malignant disease. These patients often require frequent blood transfusions when they develop severe anemia, hemorrhage, thrombocytopenia, and coagulation disorders caused by their disease, treatment, or both.

The development of sterile, disposable, and flexible plastic containers has resulted in the concept of *blood component therapy*.[1] Whole blood is first separated into cellular and noncellular components including red blood cells, platelets, and plasma. Individual blood components are then stored under optimal conditions and only that portion of blood required by the patient is transfused (Table 53.1-1). Thus, blood resources that often reach critically low inventory levels in the blood bank are more efficiently used.[2] Anticoagulants and additives currently used in blood collection containers allow storage of liquid red cells for up to 42 days. These advances have essentially eliminated the use of whole blood for allogeneic blood transfusion. Cancer patients may also require coagulation factor concentrates, albumin, or immune globulin, all of which are prepared by fractionating human plasma. Cell separators capable of collecting platelets, plasma, granulocytes, peripheral blood stem cells, and more recently, red blood cells,[3] are playing an increasingly important role in transfusion medicine.

Routine blood bank procedures including ABO typing, antibody screening, and compatibility testing identify most patients at risk for serious immune-mediated red cell transfusion reactions. Furthermore, a better understanding of red cell, platelet, and leukocyte antigen structure, as well as the immune responses to these antigens, has vastly improved transfusion therapy. Changes in recruiting and screening blood donors, as well as advances in the testing of donor blood, have drastically reduced the risk of viral transmission in the United States and Europe. All units of blood collected in the United States are tested for hepatitis B, hepatitis C, human immunodeficiency virus 1 and 2 (HIV), human T-cell lymphotropic virus-I and II (HTLV-I/II), and syphilis. Nucleotide amplification testing for hepatitis C and HIV is now performed in most European countries and the United States. Nevertheless, there remain significant risks of transfusion therapy. Complications that are not unique to oncology patients include acute and delayed hemolytic, febrile nonhemolytic, allergic, and septic reactions. Of particular concern in patients who receive large numbers of allogeneic transfusions is the development of HLA alloimmunization and graft-versus-host disease (GVHD). The presence of numerous recipient red cell alloantibodies can also severely limit the number of compatible units that will be available for a patient. Development of platelet alloantibodies can result in a refractory state to platelet transfusions. Fortunately, routine precautions taken in oncology patients including leukoreduction and irradiation of all cellular blood products have reduced the incidence of alloimmunization and GVHD.

Although the hazards of blood transfusion are relatively small, the expected benefit of a transfusion must still outweigh any risk to the patient. Therefore, practitioners of hematology and oncology need to clearly understand the indications and complications of blood transfusion therapy to minimize the

TABLE 53.1-1. Use of Blood Transfusion Components in Oncology Patients

Component	*Typical Indications for Oncology Patients*
Red blood cells	Symptomatic acute and chronic anemias
Red blood cells frozen and deglycerolized	Symptomatic anemia in patient who has developed alloantibodies to common red cell antigens
Leukocyte reduced components	Symptomatic anemia, reduce febrile reactions from leukocyte antibodies, alternative to cytomegalovirus-seronegative components, prevent HLA alloimmunization
Washed components	Remove potentially harmful plasma antibodies, may decrease severe febrile reactions if leukoreduction is not effective
Platelet components	Thrombocytopenia with bleeding or as a prophylactic measure
HLA matched/selected platelets and cross-match–compatible platelets	HLA-alloimmunized thrombocytopenic patients with decreased platelet survival by immune mechanisms
Fresh frozen plasma	Replacement of labile and stable plasma coagulation factors for which specific factor concentrates are not available, liver dysfunction, disseminated intravascular coagulation, hypofibrinogenemia
Cryoprecipitate	Fibrinogen replacement
Granulocytes by apheresis	Neutropenic patient with documented infection unresponsive to antibiotics

exposure of patients to unnecessary allogeneic blood products and to prevent wasting of limited blood resources.

BLOOD COMPONENT THERAPY

RED BLOOD CELLS

Preparation and Storage

Red blood cells, formerly called *packed cells*, are prepared by first centrifuging whole blood and then by removing most of the plasma. A standard whole blood collection involves removing 450 ± 45 mL of whole blood[4] into sterile containers containing an anticoagulant and preservative solution. Solutions composed of citrate, phosphate buffers, and dextrose (CPD) originally allowed storage of red cells for 21 days at 1 to 6°C. It was later found that red cell shelf life could be increased to 35 days by adding adenine to the preservative solution (CPDA-1). Adenine improves cell viability by increasing intracellular adenosine triphosphate (ATP) levels, whereas dextrose provides a substrate for red cell metabolism. Shelf life is further extended to 42 days by using an additive solution that contains a higher concentration of adenine than is present in CPDA-1 units.[5] The hematocrit of red cell units varies from 70% (CPDA-1) to 55% to 60% (additive solution). Citrate contained in blood preservatives inhibits clotting by binding calcium. Symptomatic hypocalcemia and alkalosis related to citrate toxicity are rare complications of red cell therapy limited to massively transfused patients. Red blood cells with rare antigen profiles can be frozen within 6 days of collection and stored for up to 10 years. They are frozen in approximately 40% glycerol to avoid cell dehydration and damage during the freezing process. Frozen red cells are indicated for oncology patients who have an alloantibody to a high-incidence antigen or have multiple alloantibodies.

Indications for Red Cell Transfusion

The decision to transfuse red cells is no longer based solely on a patient's hematocrit.[6] The patient's overall clinical status and laboratory parameters are both considered when deciding to transfuse a patient. Symptoms and signs of anemia include excessive fatigue, malaise, headache, tachycardia, and hypotension. Acute blood loss of greater than 30% total blood volume leads to hypotensive shock. Oncology patients typically have more slowly developing chronic anemias that are tolerated better than rapid onset anemias due to the ability of the body's fluid compensatory mechanisms. Red cell transfusion is rarely indicated when the hemoglobin is greater than 10 g/dL and is often not considered until the hemoglobin is less than 7 g/dL.[7] Younger patients usually tolerate a given degree of anemia better than older patients who may have underlying coronary, myocardial, or pulmonary disease. Patients with unstable angina or acute myocardial infarction may benefit from red cells when their hemoglobin is less than 10 g/dL.[8] Thus, red cell transfusion should be based on clinical criteria rather than broadly applied threshold hemoglobin values. Transfusing a single red cell unit typically increases the hemoglobin by 1 g/dL (hematocrit by 3%) in the absence of active red cell destruction.

Antibody Screening, Antibody Identification, and Cross-Matching

Even in emergency situations, a properly labeled sample must be sent to the blood bank before a red cell unit is issued. This sample is used to type a patients' red cells for ABO and Rh status. *Front typing* involves reacting patient red cells with commercial antibodies directed against the A, B, and D antigens. Blood grouping is confirmed during *back typing* in which patient serum is tested for anti-A and anti-B antibodies using commercial type A and B cells. Following blood grouping, recipient serum or plasma is screened for atypical red cell antibodies. Antibody screening is performed by incubating a patient's serum with two to four commercial group O red screening cells that together express most clinically significant red cell antigens on their membrane surface. If an antibody is present in the patient sample, it reacts with the screening cell(s) and causes red cell agglutination. Antibody screening is often referred to as the *indirect antiglobulin test*. Antigen-antibody reactions can be enhanced by adding various substances such as polyethylene glycol, low-ionic strength saline, and albumin. Most blood banks perform *tube testing* in which red cell agglutinates are identified in standard test tubes, but there are a number of newer techniques that are being used to detect antigen-antibody reactions. These include gel systems based on the differential mobility of red cell agglutinates through gel columns, and capture systems in which test red cells are immobilized on microtiter plates. Newer automated and semiautomated systems will likely replace tube testing for the majority of ABO grouping, Rh typing, and antibody screening in the future.

Antibody identification is performed by testing a patient's serum against a *panel* of 8 to 12 commercial group O red cells of known antigen phenotype. The antibody can usually be identified based on the reactivity pattern. A number of techniques are used to facilitate red cell antibody identification. Most use substances that either enhance or suppress the reactivity of a specific antibody. Some patient's serum reacts with all panel cells, a situation termed *panreactivity* or *panagglutinins.* Panagglutinins can be caused by (1) a single antibody directed against a high-incidence antigen present on all panel test red cells, (2) multiple antibodies that in total react with all test cells, or (3) an autoantibody. Autoantibodies are often found in warm autoimmune hemolytic anemias, in which case the patient's serum also reacts with his or her own red cells (positive auto control).

The direct antiglobulin test (DAT), or direct Coombs, is performed to identify *in vivo* coating of red cells with globulins, IgG and C3d in particular. It is performed by incubating a suspension of patient red cells with antihuman antibodies directed against IgG, IgA, IgM, C3, or C4. A positive DAT result implies that the patient's red cells are coated with the corresponding globulin. DATs are no longer performed on volunteer blood donors because they are positive in up to 1 per 7000 blood donors, and more importantly, have no clinical significance.[9] In addition, DATs are not routinely performed at most large medical centers as part of routine pretransfusion testing; the test must be specifically requested. Positive DAT results are also seen in patients with delayed hemolytic transfusion reactions (DHTRs), autoimmune hemolytic anemias, autoimmune disorders (systemic lupus erythematosus), and malignancy (especially B-cell malignancies such as chronic lymphocytic leukemia).

Cross-matching is performed by reacting patient serum with donor red cells from the unit selected for transfusion. If no reaction is observed, the unit is released as *compatible.* Cross-matching is only omitted in emergency life-threatening situations in which there is truly insufficient time to perform compatibility testing. Many hospitals supply group O Rh negative red cells in the emergency or operating rooms until a patient sample is received in the blood bank. Type-specific uncross-matched blood (e.g., A positive unit transfused to A positive recipient) is permitted only when the recipient's ABO Rh status is known with certainty. Use of type-specific blood is particularly helpful when supplies of O negative red cells are severely limited during blood shortages. More recently, *computer cross-matches* have been instituted at several hospitals in North America.[10] Patients of known ABO and Rh types and who have a negative antibody screen are provided computer-selected ABO compatible blood while omitting the cross-match step described previously. Although a true serologic cross-match is not performed, the computer cross-match is safe in the vast majority of transfusions if appropriate safeguards are in place to prevent typing errors and to ensure proper patient identification.

Red Cell Autoantibodies

Oncology patients may develop autoimmune hemolytic anemias as a direct result of their disease or from treatment of that disease. In particular, patients with chronic lymphocytic leukemia, non-Hodgkin's and Hodgkin's lymphoma, and plasma cell disorders frequently develop warm autoimmune hemolytic anemia. Autoantibodies consist of immunoglobulins (IgG, IgM) that react with a wide range of self-antigens including membrane and intracellular components, adsorbed plasma proteins, and nuclear antigens. The DAT result is positive in most cases. Patients with warm autoimmune hemolytic anemia often require transfusion. The blood bank may have difficulty identifying compatible red cell units because the patient's serum not only reacts with his or her own red cells, but also with those of all donor red cells. Therefore, additional time may be required to exclude the presence of a significant underlying alloantibody that is obscured by the autoantibody. Upward of 25% of previously transfused autoimmune hemolytic anemia patients may have an underlying alloantibody.[11] An underlying alloantibody, if undetected, may result in accelerated red cell destruction of a transfused red cell unit that carries the corresponding antigen. Therefore, transfusion therapy must be carefully planned and used in these patients. Autoimmune antibodies often appear to have specificity for Rh antigens (e.g., anti-E), but transfusing antigen-negative red cells (e.g., E negative) is not indicated as *in vivo* red cell survival of antigen-negative cells is usually no better than with antigen-positive cells.

BLOOD DONATIONS

Blood donations can be divided into several categories as follows: (1) *autologous* is donation of one's blood for one's own use, (2) *allogeneic* or homologous is donation of one's blood for use by others, and (3) *directed* is donation of one's blood for use by a specific recipient. Directed donations are important to some cancer patients. A friend or family member of a potential recipient typically donates a directed donor unit. In fact, blood supplies can be greatly supplemented by relatives and friends of oncology patients during critical periods of their treatment. Depending on institutional guidelines directed units not needed by the intended recipient may be *crossed over* to the general blood bank stock and distributed to other patients provided the donor meets all requirements for allogeneic donation.

Autologous Transfusions

The most commonly used forms of autologous transfusion include preoperative blood donation, acute normovolemic hemodilution, and autologous blood salvage. Each type of autologous transfusion may be useful in certain oncology patients.[12] Many blood centers provide autologous preoperative blood donation services in which a patient's blood is drawn and stored for later use, usually during a surgical procedure.[13] Although the criteria for autologous donations are less stringent than those for allogeneic donors, oncology patients are often too anemic to donate their own blood. Patients must feel well on the day of donation and cannot be hypotensive, febrile, or septic because of the risk of bacterial contamination. Thus, the donor cannot have open wounds, such as from a recent biopsy, or have indwelling vascular or urinary catheters. Platelets and granulocytes contained in an autologous blood unit rapidly degrade with storage and are essentially nonfunctional by the time the unit is transfused. If the autologous unit is stored as whole blood, the plasma contained in this unit has low levels of labile coagulation factors. Plasma can be separated from autologous whole blood and frozen to maintain the activity of all coagulation factors. Although autologous blood is intended for the patient–donor, most blood centers test autologous units for the same transfusion disease markers required for allogeneic blood. Preoperative blood donation can be used in older oncology patients, although there is a higher risk of anemia and more serious cardiovascular complications associated with the donation.[14] The use of autologous blood decreases the risk of viral infection, but the risk of bacterial contamination remains. Autologous preoperative blood donation is not crossed over because most of these patients do not meet all requirements for allogeneic blood donation.

Acute normovolemic hemodilution is performed by removing blood from a patient immediately before surgery and replacing the blood volume with crystalloid or colloid solutions to maintain hemodynamic stability.[15] The withdrawn blood is then later reinfused. Autologous blood salvage is performed by collecting and then returning blood lost during or shortly following operative procedures using intraoperative salvage devices.[16] This technique is primarily employed in cardiac and orthopedic surgery. Autologous blood salvage is generally contraindicated in cancer surgery because of the risk of returning contaminating tumor cells to the systemic circulation. There is some evidence that irradiating salvaged blood with 50 Gy can destroy the proliferative ability of malignant cells, but more studies are needed before this technique can be safely applied to cancer surgery.[17]

Autologous Platelet Donation

Although oncology patients can *bank* their own red cells through autologous donation, it is not usually feasible for these patients to donate autologous platelets. Platelets stored in the liquid phase at room temperature have a shelf life of only 5 days. Platelets collected by apheresis and frozen preserved in dimethyl sulfoxide can be stored at –80°C.[18] They are then thawed, washed, and resuspended in autologous plasma or other solutions before transfusion. Platelets prepared by this technique do undergo a number of structural and metabolic changes that decreases their recovery and survival as compared with liquid-stored platelet concentrates.[19] Furthermore, most patients cannot donate enough platelets to support a full course of induction chemotherapy. It is possible, however, to store significant numbers of frozen autologous platelets for patients who are refractory to platelet transfusion provided the blood bank is technically capable of preparing and storing these specialized products.[20]

Directed Blood Donation and Dedicated Donor Units

Directed blood donations are those donations made for a specific patient. These units, most frequently obtained from family members or friends, can greatly augment the blood supply. Donors wishing to make directed donations must meet the same criteria for blood donation as other allogeneic donors. These units undergo all required testing for transmissible diseases. Therefore, due to the possibility of unexpected test results, it is important that the donor understand his or her blood will be tested for viral diseases such as HIV and hepatitis C. In fact, directed blood donors are more likely to be positive for some infectious disease markers than other allogeneic blood donors.[2] This increased frequency of positive infectious disease markers most likely reflects in part the higher percentage of first-time donors in the directed donor group who were not previously screened.

The cytomegalovirus (CMV) status of the blood donor and the needs of the oncology patient also affect the use of directed blood donation. CMV-seronegative blood products are often required by oncology patients, in particular, those patients who are marrow transplant candidates or recipients. As in the allogeneic donor pool, many directed donor units are seropositive for CMV. Thus, units from some directed donors may not be appropriate for the intended recipient. In this situation, the patient's oncologist must decide if a CMV-seropositive directed unit can be transfused to that patient. CMV status of directed units may be less of a concern as prestorage leukodepleted blood products prepared using cyclic good manufacturing practices gain further acceptance as an alternative to CMV-seronegative products.

Dedicated donor blood units are primarily used by pediatric oncology patients to reduce their exposure to blood from different donors. A dedicated unit is simply a unit of allogeneic red cells that is specifically set aside by the blood bank for use by a single patient. The unit is obtained from the general blood bank stock or from a directed donor. When necessary, small aliquots are removed from the units for transfusion. This approach is not feasible in adult oncology patients because of the larger blood volume requirements. However, a single dedicated unit could supply as many as ten separate transfusions in a pediatric patient, thus dramatically reducing multiple donor exposures.

PLATELET TRANSFUSION THERAPY

Preparation and Storage

Plastic primary collection bags with attached satellite containers allow harvesting of platelets as a by-product of red cell separation. In the United States, platelets are usually prepared by the platelet-rich plasma method, whereas the buffy coat method is used in Europe.[21] Each *random donor* platelet unit (RDP) prepared by differential centrifugation of a single whole blood collection contains at least 5.5×10^{10} platelets suspended in 50 mL of plasma. The shelf life of all platelet preparations is 5 days when stored at 20 to 24°C under constant agitation in plastic containers that allow oxygen diffusion. Storage longer than 5 days is precluded by the increased risk of bacterial growth and the development of platelet function abnormalities. RDP are typically administered in four to six unit *pools*. In the absence of conditions associated with decreased platelet survival, each RDP unit should increase a recipient's platelet count by 5000 to 10,000/μL. Single donor platelets (SDPs) prepared by apheresis are often transfused to oncology patients in order to minimize their exposure to multiple donors. SDPs contain more than 3×10^{11} platelets suspended in approximately 200 mL of plasma. Thus, one SDP is equivalent to five to six average RDP units.

ABO type-specific platelets are provided whenever possible. This is because transfusing out-of-type platelets may result in a postplatelet increment 10% to 20% less than that expected for ABO type-specific platelets. In addition, Rh antigens found on the small number of contaminating red cells present in platelet concentrates are sufficient to immunize a small number of Rh-negative recipients. If Rh-negative platelet concentrates are not available for an Rh-negative patient, Rh-positive platelets can be transfused followed by administration of Rh immune globulin within 72 hours of transfusion. Until relatively recently, only intramuscular Rh immune globulin was available to prevent Rh immunization. These injections could be dangerous in oncology patients who have low platelet numbers and coagulation disorders. Fortunately, an intravenous preparation has been licensed for preventing Rh alloimmunization (WinRho, NABI, Boca Raton, FL).[22] This therapy has been proven effective, and is clearly more convenient and less painful to the patient.

Indications for Platelet Transfusion

Platelets are transfused to thrombocytopenic patients who are actively bleeding or to severely thrombocytopenic patients as a prophylactic precautionary measure.[23] Spontaneous bleeding is rarely encountered when a patient's platelet count is more than 20,000/μL. In fact, studies suggest that oncology patients receiving chemotherapy can tolerate platelet counts as low as 5,000 to 10,000/μL.[24–26] Postsurgical patients with platelet counts more than 50,000/μL may require platelet transfusions to control or prevent postoperative bleeding. Overall coagulation status should also be considered because patients with plasma coagulation factor disorders are more likely to bleed at marginal platelet counts. Actively bleeding patients on aspirin, an irreversible inhibitor of platelet function, may require transfusions at higher platelet counts. Obviously, transfused platelets are similarly inhibited if the patient remains on aspirin.

Platelet Refractory State

Platelet refractoriness is a major problem for cancer patients who are dependent on platelet transfusions. There are many causes of an apparent lack of response to platelet transfusions, either through immune or nonimmune mechanisms (Table 53.1-2). In most cases, platelet refractoriness is attributed to nonimmune causes including sepsis, splenomegaly, and disseminated intravascular coagulation.[27] The corrected count increment (CCI) is used to identify patients who are refractory to platelet transfusions through either HLA or platelet alloimmunization. The CCI is calculated as follows:

$$\text{CCI} = \frac{\text{Post}(\ /\mu\text{L}) - \text{Pre}(\ /\mu\text{L})}{\text{Number of platelets} \times 10^{-11}} \times \text{BSA}(\text{m}^2)$$

where Pre is pretransfusion platelet count, Post is posttransfusion platelet count drawn 1 to 4 hours after completion of the transfusion, number of platelets transfused (1 RDP unit approximately 0.5×10^{11} platelets; 1 SDP unit approximates 3.0×10^{11} platelets), and BSA is body surface area in square meters. Patients with a low CCI (less than 5000) may benefit from cross-match–compatible platelets or HLA-matched single donor platelets.

Platelet cross-matching is performed by adding recipient serum to wells coated with donor platelets. After appropriate antibodies and an indicator reagent are added, the compatibility of the patient's serum and the donor's platelets is determined based on reactivity patterns. An incompatible cross-match predicts a poor CCI more than 90% of the time, whereas a negative cross-match is only 50% predictive of a successful transfusion.[28] Depending on a particular hospital's blood supplier, cross-match–compatible platelets or HLA-selected platelets may be more readily available.[29] Some centers use a combination of the two techniques: Platelet units are selected for cross-matching based on the HLA type of the donor and recipient.

TABLE 53.1-2. Potential Causes of Platelet Refractoriness in Cancer Patients

Nonimmune	*Immune*
Hypersplenism	HLA antibodies
Disseminated intravascular coagulation	Platelet-specific antibodies
Sepsis	Circulating immune complexes
Drugs (amphotericin, and so forth)	Autoantibodies (autoimmune thrombocytopenia)
Viremia	
Bleeding	
Radiotherapy, chemotherapy, or both	
Vasculitis	

Cross-match–compatible and HLA-selected platelets are not readily available in all blood banks. Increasing the dose of standard platelet concentrates can be considered until these products are obtained. For example, a dose of eight to ten RDPs is transfused instead of the more typical four to six unit pools. In fact, investigators have suggested that higher platelet doses (approximately 4 to 6×10^{11} platelets per dose) given prophylactically to patients with hematologic malignancies reduce the number of platelet transfusions and thus, the number of donor exposures.[30] Ideally, the platelets are ABO identical because ABO incompatibility may decrease posttransfusion platelet increments by 10% to 20%.[31] Some medical centers provide *platelet drips* to bleeding refractory patients. Three-unit RDP pools are continuously infused through an electromechanical pump every 4 hours, providing a total of 18 RDP units over 24 hours. Electromechanical pumps do not appear to harm platelets.[32] Platelet drips could theoretically maintain a lower platelet count, but this has not been proven. There are no studies that have fully compared the efficacy of intermittent platelet boluses and platelet drips in refractory patients. Corticosteroids, chemotherapy, splenectomy, and intravenous immunoglobulin, effective treatments for many autoimmune thrombocytopenias, are not useful in platelet refractory patients.

Leukocyte reduction filters, as well as ultraviolet B irradiation, decrease the rate of HLA alloimmunization to platelets.[33,34] Therefore, leukocyte reduced filtered blood products should be provided to oncology patients who require many platelet transfusions (see Leukoreduction, later in this chapter). Presumably, leukoreduction removes donor antigen-presenting cells, which may play a key role in initiating HLA alloimmunization.

GRANULOCYTES

Granulocytes continue to play a small role in the supportive care of neutropenic oncology patients with serious infections, including allogeneic and autologous marrow transplant recipients. Improvements in apheresis collection technique now allow collection of larger numbers of granulocytes (6 to 8 × 10^{10}) from volunteer donors than was previously possible.[35] These changes include the administration of corticosteroids or growth factors to white cell donors before apheresis.[36] Granulocytes are typically transfused to neutropenic oncology patients who have developed gram-positive or gram-negative bacterial sepsis unresponsive to antibiotic therapy for a minimum of 24 to 48 hours (Table 53.1-3).[37] Granulocytes collected from nonstimulated (no corticosteroids or growth factors) healthy donors contain at least 1 × 10^{10} neutrophils per unit. These units can be stored for only 24 hours at 20° to 24°C without agitation. Granulocyte units contain 20 to 25 mL of red cells and thus must be cross-matched with the recipient's serum. Donated granulocytes are rarely HLA matched for the recipient, even for those patients with known HLA antibodies because there are little data suggesting that HLA-matched granulocytes have improved survival and recovery. Granulocytes should be irradiated (2500 cGy) to inactivate the large number of lymphocytes found in the product. They are considered for patients who have an absolute neutrophil count less than 500/μL and a reasonable chance of marrow recovery.

Because of their short half-life, granulocytes are typically provided daily until the patient can maintain an absolute neutrophil count greater than 500/μL without transfusion or until the infection resolves. Infusion of larger numbers of granulocytes (on the order of 6 to 8 × 10^{10} granulocytes) produces measurable increases in adult recipient neutrophil counts, but the optimal dose and frequency remain undefined. Febrile reactions to granulocytes are common, the reactions seem to be more severe when amphotericin is infused near the time of granulocyte transfusions. Overall, the additional benefit of granulocyte transfusions for these neutropenic patients as compared with antibiotic treatment alone is unclear as there are no well-controlled clinical trials. In addition, the clinical benefit of transfusing larger numbers of granulocytes collected from donors stimulated by corticosteroids or growth factors has not been proven. The collection of granulocytes, or any blood component, by apheresis is not an entirely innocuous process. The donor is at risk for uncommon, but potentially serious adverse reactions including hydroxyethyl starch–related hypotension and anaphylaxis and citrate-induced hypocalcemia. Hydroxyethyl starch is used as a sedimenting agent to maximize granulocyte yields. Minor, but typically tolerable, side effects of pretreating granulocyte donors with dexamethasone (insomnia, flushing), granulocyte colony-stimulating factor, or both (bone pain, headaches, insomnia) occur in a substantial number of donors.[38] The long-term effects of granulocyte colony-stimulating factor on volunteer donors are unknown.

Adverse recipient reactions to granulocytes are common because of the activity of transfused white cells, as well as their degradation products. These reactions are typical of febrile nonhemolytic transfusion reactions (FNTRs) following other blood product administration. Granulocytes should be transfused slowly, 1 to 2 mL/min through a standard microaggregate filter. Obviously, a leukocyte reduction filter should *never* be used to administer granulocytes. In addition, the recipient should be premedicated with acetaminophen or some other antiinflammatory agent before the granulocyte transfusion.

TABLE 53.1-3. General Guidelines for Granulocyte Transfusions

Absolute neutrophil count <500/μL
Reversible myeloid hypoplasia caused by chemotherapy or disease
Documented infection that has not responded to appropriate antibiotics for a minimum of 24 to 48 hours
Fever of unknown origin unresponsive to broad-spectrum antibiotics

PLASMA

Plasma is prepared by centrifuging whole blood and then freezing the removed plasma within 8 hours of collection. Rapid freezing maintains the activity of labile coagulation factors such as factors V and VIII. The most commonly available form of plasma, fresh frozen plasma (FFP), contains all coagulation factors, other plasma proteins, and complement. FFP should not be used for volume expansion because there is a risk of transfusion-transmitted disease (TTD); other safer non-plasma substitutes are available. A unit of FFP contains from 180 to 270 mL of plasma. The primary indications for FFP transfusion in oncology patients include deficiencies of multiple coagulation factors as seen in liver disease, disseminated intravascular coagulation, and hypofibrinogenemia.[39] It is often used for urgent reversal of warfarin therapy in bleeding patients and before procedures. FFP is not the treatment of choice for replacing most individual clotting factors because of the large volumes that would be required to obtain adequate factor levels. The patient's cardiovascular and fluid status may preclude the use of large amounts of plasma. In fact, large transfusions of FFP can produce fluid overload and subsequent heart failure in some patients. FFP is not the treatment of choice for coagulopathies in cases in which virally inactivated or recombinant products exist such as for deficiencies of factor VIII (hemophilia A) or factor IX (hemophilia B).

CRYOPRECIPITATE

Cryoprecipitate is prepared by thawing FFP between 1°C and 6°C. A single 10- to 15-mL unit of cryoprecipitate contains fibrinogen (100 to 350 mg/U), Factor VIII (at least 80 IU/U), and some von Willebrand factor. Thus, a similar dose of fibrinogen can be provided in a much smaller volume as compared with FFP. Use of cryoprecipitate is generally limited to patients with severe hypofibrinogenemia (less than 100 mg/dL) and von Willebrand's disease. It should *not* be used alone in disseminated intravascular coagulation because it contains no factor V. Cryoprecipitate, thrombin, and calcium are combined to make *fibrin glue.*[40] This biologic sealant is most often used to limit surgical bleeding. Since cryoprecipitate is used, the recipient is exposed to the risks of TTD. A fibrin sealant that contains solvent and detergent-treated plasma has been approved by the Food and Drug Administration.

PLASMA DERIVATIVES

Albumin

Solutions containing 5% human albumin in saline are primarily used to replace intravascular volume and more rarely, to treat hypoalbuminemia. Its use as a volume expander has decreased because other nonplasma colloidal solutions such as dextran and hydroxyethyl starch are readily available. Albumin is also used to replace plasma removed during apheresis. Albumin prepared in the United States is virally inactivated by heat treatment. Properly prepared albumin has not been reported to transmit viral disease including hepatitis B virus, hepatitis C virus (HCV), and HIV types 1 and 2. Albumin is not a viable nutritional source for patients with chronic protein deficiency states seen in oncology patients.[41]

Immunoglobulins

Immune globulin products include intravenously administered immune globulin, intramuscularly administered immune globulin, and several specialized products such as Rh(D) immune globulin and hepatitis B immune globulin. In the United States, immune globulin products are prepared from donor plasma screened for TTDs. Individual plasma units are then pooled and separated by alcohol fractionation or by anion exchange chromatography that results in a product that is considered safe from virus transmission.[42] Polyspecific intravenous immune globulin is used to treat immune-mediated thrombocytopenias, autoimmune hemolytic anemias, and demyelinating polyneuropathies such as Guillain-Barré syndrome. It is also provided to patients with primary and secondary immune deficiencies. Patients who are IgA-deficient are at risk of anaphylaxis due to production of IgG anti-IgA immunoglobulin. For these patients, IgA-deficient preparations should be used. Some immunoglobulin preparations use a chemical inactivation step employing solvent and detergent processing to reduce infectivity for lipid enveloped viruses including HIV and hepatitis C. Specific immune globulin preparations are made from donors with hyperimmune serum and can be used prophylactically or after exposure to prevent infections from viruses such as hepatitis B.

TABLE 53.1-4. Complications of Blood Transfusion Therapy in Cancer Patients

Immune Mediated	*Nonimmune Mediated*
Acute hemolytic transfusion reaction	Transfusion-associated bacterial sepsis
Delayed extravascular hemolytic reaction	Circulatory overload and cardiac failure
Febrile transfusion reaction	Viral transmission
Allergic transfusion reactions	Iron overload
Alloimmunization	Hypocalcemia
Transfusion-associated graft-versus-host disease	Hypothermia
Transfusion-associated acute lung injury	Factor depletion and thrombocytopenia by dilution

Clotting Factors

Antihemophilic factor (factor VIII) and factor IX are commercially available derivatives prepared from large pools of human plasma. These products were originally high risk for transmitting viruses until virus-inactivation methods were developed that did not damage the product's coagulant activity. These methods include heat inactivation and solvent and detergent exposure. Individual coagulation factors of extremely high purity are produced using antibody-affinity purification procedures. Recombinant factors VIII, IX, and VIIa are currently available and should be considered as an alternative to pooled products in specific situations. The use of these products in cancer patients is generally limited to replacement of individual clotting factors or to the treatment of specific factor inhibitors.

TRANSFUSION REACTIONS AND COMPLICATIONS

Oncology patients, like other transfusion recipients, experience adverse reactions to blood component therapy. Although cancer patients per se are not at an increased risk for the more common febrile and allergic transfusion reactions, they are likely to experience one of these reactions if they are or have been multiply transfused during their treatment. Most reactions occur during or shortly after a blood transfusion, but may present several hours to days later. In general, transfusion reactions are broadly categorized as immune or nonimmune based on their presumed mechanism (Table 53.1-4). Of particular concern to cancer patients is (1) the development of alloimmunization, or antibodies to red cell or platelet membranes components, through repeated allogeneic blood exposure, and (2) posttransfusion associated GVHD, a potentially fatal, but uncommon complication. Chronic iron overload and secondary hemochromatosis, long-term complications of red cell transfusion therapy, also occur in patients with hematologic malignancies who experience long-term survival.[43]

ACUTE INTRAVASCULAR HEMOLYTIC REACTIONS

Acute intravascular hemolytic transfusion reactions (AIHTRs) are serious complications that are usually avoided by carefully adhering to standard protocols for administering blood products. These reactions occur in blood recipients who have preexisting antibodies directed against antigens present on the transfused red cells. ABO incompatibility remains the most common cause of immediate intravascular hemolytic reactions, but they are also caused by incompatibility within other blood group systems such as Duffy (Fy^a, Fy^b) and Kidd (Jk^a, Jk^b). Transfusion of ABO incompatible blood is typically due to clerical errors involving misidentification of the patient.[44] Proper labeling of clots used by the blood bank for compatibility testing and careful identification of patients are the best ways to prevent potentially fatal ABO incompatible reactions. Donor erythrocytes carrying either A, B, or both antigens avidly bind to the recipient's naturally occurring anti-A, anti-B, or both antibodies. This binding results in complement fixation, formation of the C5b-9 membrane attack complex, and finally, hemolysis. It is now clear that biologic response modifiers such as proinflammatory cytokines [interleukin-1 (IL-1), tumor necrosis factor-α], chemokines (IL-8), and complement fragments (C3a, C5a) play a major role in the pathophysiology of AIHTRs.[45]

AIHTRs present as fever, chills, the sudden onset of back pain, hypotension, tachycardia, diaphoresis, and dyspnea. The symptoms are usually evident in recipients shortly after beginning the transfusion. Laboratory studies reveal an increase in unconjugated bilirubin up to 2 to 3 mg/dL and marked elevation of lactate dehydrogenase. The classic signs of intravascular hemolysis include acute onset hemoglobinuria and hemoglobinemia. The DAT or direct Coombs' test, becomes reactive due to the coating of *donor* red cells with the *recipient's* antibodies. AIHTRs are medical emergencies. Treatment consists of immediately stopping the transfusion, close monitoring of vital signs, and use of intravenous fluids to maintain urine output greater than 100 mL/h with or without a loop diuretic (Table 53.1-5). Blood pressure and airway support, pressors, and mechanical ventilation may be necessary. Dialysis should be considered in patients who develop renal failure as result of acute red cell hemolysis and subsequent acute tubular necrosis.

DELAYED EXTRAVASCULAR HEMOLYTIC REACTIONS

DHTRs typically occur in patients who initially have a negative antibody screen on pretransfusion testing, but who then experience accelerated destruction of transfused red cells 7 to 14 days posttransfusion. In most cases, red cell destruction is caused by an antibody that is of low titer, below the detection limits of most routine screening techniques. On reexposure to the offending antigen, the antibody rapidly forms and binds to the transfused red cells. DHTRs are also caused by primary sensitization in which a patient synthesizes a new antibody. Antibodies implicated in DHTRs usually fix complement only to the C3 level and thus, cause extravascular as opposed to intravascular hemolysis. Antibodies most commonly identified in DHTRs include those directed against Rh (E, c), Duffy, Kidd, and Kell blood group antigens. DHTRs are often diagnosed following an unexpected posttransfusion drop in hematocrit, an elevation of unconjugated bilirubin, and the appearance of a newly positive DAT. There is usually a delay of 3 days to 2 weeks between transfusion and the onset of extravascular hemolysis. Only rarely do delayed reactions cause intravascular hemolysis with associated hemoglobinemia and hemoglobinuria, but in any case, these patients should be followed until the hemolysis resolves. DHTRs should also be recognized to avoid unnecessary diagnostic procedures that are considered to evaluate an unexpected decrease in hematocrit. These patients typically do not develop cytokine storm and are for the most part asymptomatic.

FEBRILE NONHEMOLYTIC REACTIONS

FNTRs following red cell and platelet transfusions are common in cancer patients. They are presumably caused by antibodies (leukoagglutinins) in the recipient that are directed against HLA-, leukocyte-specific, or both antigens on donor white blood cells and platelets. Reactions between leukoagglutinins present in the transfused product and recipient leukocyte antigens may also play a role. Formation of leukocyte antigen-antibody complexes then results in complement binding and release of endogenous pyrogens such as IL-1, IL-6, and tumor necrosis factor-α. Cytokines generated by leukocytes during platelet and red cell storage may also contribute to FNTRs.[46] Symptoms typically occur during or several hours after the transfusion and include low-grade (greater than 1°C increase) and high-grade fevers accompanied by shaking chills. Rarely vomiting, dyspnea, hypotension, and decreased oxygen saturation ensue. The severity of symptoms is often directly related to the number of leukocytes contained in the product or the rate of transfusion. Leukoreduction of blood components decreases, but does not eliminate, the frequency of FNTRs and therefore, white cell–reduced products should be considered in patients who have experienced febrile reactions. Premedication with an antipyretic such as acetaminophen may minimize mild FNTRs, but is not entirely effective. Antihistamines do not prevent or treat FNTRs. Corticosteroids can minimize FNTRs if they are administered several hours before the transfusion and should be considered for patients who have had several severe reactions. Intravenous or intramuscular meperidine can resolve severe rigors in a matter of minutes.[47] If symptoms do not resolve in less than 4 hours or are especially severe, other complications such as sepsis caused by contaminated blood

TABLE 53.1-5. Identification and Initial Management of Transfusion Reactions in Oncology Patients

Reaction	*Symptoms and Signs*	*Management*
Acute intravascular hemolytic reaction	Back pain, fever, hypotension, shock, dyspnea, hemoglobinuria, hemoglobinemia, positive direct Coombs' test result	Stop transfusion, IV fluids, vasopressor support, maintain diuresis, corticosteroids, dialysis if indicated
Delayed extravascular hemolytic reaction	Anemia, jaundice, fever, positive direct Coombs' test result	Stop transfusion, fluid support, follow laboratory results (hematocrit, lactate dehydrogenase, bilirubin)
Febrile reaction	Fever, chills, rigors, mild dyspnea	Stop transfusion, antipyretics, consider leukoreduced product for subsequent transfusions
Allergic (mild)	Pruritus and urticaria *only*	Antihistamines, may continue transfusion if symptoms improve in <30 minutes, otherwise stop transfusion
Allergic (anaphylactic)	Urticaria, bronchospasm, dyspnea, nausea, hypotension	Stop transfusion, antihistamines, vasopressor support, corticosteroids, consider premedication or washed red blood cells for subsequent transfusions
Septic reaction	Rapid onset of chills, fever, hypotension	Stop transfusion, culture product and patient, vasopressor support, IV fluids, broad-spectrum antibiotics

products, or a hemolytic reaction should be seriously considered. Under some circumstances, it may be difficult to distinguish between FNTRs from other causes of fever in immunocompromised cancer patients. Specific conditions that can mimic benign FNTRs include preexisting or impending patient sepsis, infusion of a contaminated unit of blood or platelets, and a hemolytic transfusion reaction.

ALLERGIC REACTIONS

Allergic reactions to plasma, platelets, and red cells are relatively common in cancer patients. They present as pruritus, urticaria, or both, usually in the absence of fever. Allergic reactions are classically IgE mediated and most symptoms are attributed to histamine release. At times it is difficult to distinguish between allergic and febrile transfusion reactions when urticarial symptoms are accompanied by low-grade fever. Other common symptoms and signs include pruritus, erythema, papular rashes, and wheals. Severe anaphylaxis resulting in bronchospasm and hypotension rarely occur, but can be life threatening. As in other allergic processes, symptoms are not dose related and severe manifestations can occur following small exposures. Treatment of mild allergic reactions consists of stopping the transfusion and administering diphenhydramine or other antihistamines. For mild allergic reactions (e.g., pruritus and hives only without fever or vasomotor instability), it is reasonable to resume transfusing the same unit provided the symptoms promptly resolve. If the symptoms recur after the transfusion is restarted, a new unit should then be obtained. Severe anaphylactic reactions with bronchospasm and cardiovascular collapse are fortunately rare and should be treated like any other anaphylactic reaction with corticosteroids, vasopressors, and airway support. Washed red cells in which the residual donor plasma has been removed and replaced by saline may benefit patients with repeated or severe allergic reactions.[48] Leukocyte reduction filters are not helpful because they do not remove the implicated soluble mediators.

SEPTIC REACTIONS

Blood products are rarely contaminated by bacteria during the collection process. This may occur if the donor is transiently bacteremic at the time of collection or if the arm is improperly cleansed before venipuncture.[49] Transfusing blood products that are contaminated by bacteria is potentially dangerous and can result in profound hypotension, shock, and death. Currently, there are no laboratory tests to screen for bacterial contamination and contaminated units cannot be easily identified on pretransfusion inspection. The risk of septic transfusion reactions (STRs) is higher for platelet transfusions than for other blood components because platelets are stored at room temperature.[50] Refrigeration of red cells markedly diminishes the growth of most bacteria. Common organisms that cause STRs include gram-positive (*Staphylococcus* sp.) and gram-negative (*Enterobacter, Yersinia, Pseudomonas* sp.) bacteria.[51] *Yersinia enterocolitica* is a more common cause of red cell STRs because this organism grows at cold temperature and multiplies during refrigerated storage of red blood cell products.[52] Blood cultures should be obtained from patients who develop high fevers during or shortly after transfusion, especially if they become hypotensive. A Gram's stain or acridine orange stain of the suspected contaminated product is helpful when organisms are seen, but this test is not highly sensitive. Both the patient and the implicated blood unit should be cultured whenever a STR is suspected. Other symptoms associated with STRs are attributed to preformed endotoxin and cytokines and include skin flushing, severe rigors, and cardiovascular collapse. These symptoms may occur during or minutes to hours after completing the transfusion. Treatment includes fluids and cardiovascular support. Broad-spectrum antibiotics should be started immediately, even before culture results can guide further therapy. Severe febrile reactions can mimic STRs, but febrile reactions are self-limited in nature and are generally not associated with profound hypotension.

TRANSFUSION-RELATED ACUTE LUNG INJURY

Transfusion-related acute lung injury (TRALI) is a rare but serious complication of blood transfusion that presents as noncardiogenic pulmonary edema. It typically occurs within 6 hours of transfusion and is clinically identical to the adult respiratory distress syndrome. The most common clinical findings include the rapid onset of dyspnea, tachypnea, cyanosis, fever, and hypotension.[53] Lung auscultation reveals diffuse crackling and decreased breath sounds. Invasive cardiac monitoring shows normal cardiac pressures and function with hypoxemia and decreased pulmonary compliance. Radiographic findings include diffuse, fluffy infiltrates consistent with pulmonary edema. The presumed etiology involves immune-mediated reaction of HLA antibodies or other leukoagglutinins with white cells, which subsequently leads to leukocyte activation.[54] Granulocytes are first activated in the peripheral circulation by HLA or other Ag-Ab complexes. The activated leukocytes then migrate to the lungs where they bind to the pulmonary capillary bed via integrins and other cell adhesion molecules. Proteolytic enzymes are then released that destroy tissue, resulting in a capillary leak syndrome and pulmonary edema. More recently, reactive lipid products released from donor cell membranes have been associated with the development of TRALI.[55] TRALI should be suspected in patients with rapid onset respiratory distress following transfusion therapy or pulmonary edema without hypervolemia and congestive heart failure. Definitive diagnosis requires identifying HLA, granulocyte antibodies, or both in either the donor's or recipient's serum. The corresponding antigens should also be found on the recipient's or donor's leukocytes. This specialized testing is performed in few specialized laboratories. Approximately 80% to 90% of patients with TRALI survive with supportive care consisting of aggressive respiratory support, supplemental oxygen, and mechanical ventilation when necessary. Based on the presumed pathogenesis of TRALI, leukoreduced blood products could potentially decrease the incidence of TRALI. Drugs used to treat TRALI have included corticosteroids and diuretics, but there are no controlled studies demonstrating the efficacy of these agents because of the low incidence of TRALI.

TRANSFUSION-ASSOCIATED GRAFT-VERSUS-HOST DISEASE

Transfusion-associated GVHD is a rare complication of blood transfusion that is fatal in approximately 90% of patients. Transfusion-associated GVHD occurs when donor immunocompetent T and natural killer cells attack recipient cells because these recipient cells appear foreign due to differences in major or minor histocompatibility antigens.[56] GVHD is commonly seen following allogeneic bone marrow transplant, but may also rarely occur in immunodeficient or immunosuppressed patients following blood transfusion. Removing T cells from donor grafts can minimize acute GVHD in oncology patients, but is associated with increased graft failure and a decrease in a beneficial graft-versus-leukemia or graft-versus-tumor effect. The risk of transfusion-associated GVHD is related to the number of viable T lymphocytes transfused, the recipient's immune status, and the HLA disparity between donor and recipient. Therefore, multiply transfused patients who receive cells from donors who share HLA haplotypes (haploidentical) with the recipient are at greatest risk. Clinically, transfusion-associated GVHD is characterized by the acute onset of rash, abdominal pain, diarrhea, liver function abnormalities, and bone marrow suppression beginning 2 to 30 days following transfusion. The maculopapular rash seen is similar to that observed in acute GVHD following bone marrow transplant. Biopsy of the skin can confirm the diagnosis. Pancytopenia in transfusion-associated GVHD may be severe and is attributed to destruction of recipient marrow stem cells by donor lymphocytes. Immunosuppressive therapy with prednisone and cyclosporine has not been reported effective in transfusion-associated GVHD. There is no known effective treatment for transfusion-associated GVHD, but therapeutic strategies have been proposed based on the presumed mechanism of its onset.[57] Fortunately, transfusion-associated GVHD can be prevented by irradiating products before transfusion. Specifically, irradiating cellular blood products with 2500 cGy inactivates donor lymphocytes and is the most effective method for preventing transfusion-associated GVHD.[58]

TRANSFUSION-TRANSMITTED DISEASE

The risk of TTD, primarily viral transmission, has dramatically decreased over the past 25 years. Bacterial contamination of units is not usually considered a TTD, but actually is far more common than viral or fungal transmission. The use of volunteer donors and predonation screening questionnaires were the earliest effective steps taken to reduce the risk of transfusion-related hepatitis and HIV. These risks continue to drive government-mandated pretransfusion testing requirements.[59] The development of enzyme immunoassays in the 1970s and nucleotide testing in the late 1990s have further decreased the risk of TTD[60] (Table 53.1-6). Transfusion-associated HIV and hepatitis are a persistent problem in parts of the world that do not have access to screening tests.

Pretransfusion TTD testing in the United States includes screening for syphilis, hepatitis B (HBsAg, anti-Hbc), hepatitis C (anti-HCV), HIV (anti-HIV-1/2, HIV-1 p24 antigen), and HTLV (anti-HTLV-I/II). Serum alanine aminotransferase, measured in most European countries as a nonspecific surrogate marker of hepatitis, is no longer required by American Association of Blood Bank standards.[61] Positive screening test results are confirmed by supplemental or confirmatory testing. Current estimates for the risk of transfusion-related HIV range from 1:500,000 to 1:750,000 units transfused.[62] Despite improvements in tests used to detect HIV antibodies in donors, the *window period* in which HIV could be transmitted by an infected, but HIV seronegative, donor remained in 1996 at approximately 25 days. The introduction of screening for HIV-1 p24 antigen in 1997 decreased the window period to approximately 15 days. The implementation of HIV nucleotide testing will further decrease the window period to an estimated 10 days.

Routine vaccination of infants and young children with hepatitis B vaccine should also decrease the risk of transfusion-transmitted hepatitis B as these children enter the blood donor pool. Chronic carriers of hepatitis B (HBsAg positive, anti-Hbc IgG positive, HBeAg positive or negative, anti-HBe positive or negative) can transmit the disease through blood donation or by other blood-borne exposures. Those carriers with measurable HBeAg are probably more infectious and accordingly, more likely to transmit disease through blood exposure or by vertical transmission. The chances of a health care worker contracting hepatitis B from a single contaminated needle stick is estimated to be between 2% and 40%. By contrast, the chances of acquiring HIV from a single contaminated needle stick is less than 1%. These differences may be at least in part related to the higher number of viral particles present in the blood of carriers of hepatitis B. The rate of transmitting hepatitis C through needle stick is probably on the order of 5%.[63] Nevertheless, health care workers must strictly adhere to universal precautions to protect themselves and their patients.

Genomic testing for HCV RNA was implemented in the United States and Europe to detect seronegative, yet infectious units. Nucleotide testing for hepatitis C and HIV is typically performed on samples pooled from multiple donors.[64] The importance of hepatitis C transmission in blood therapy has been confirmed in many countries by retrospective review. During these reviews, recipients of blood components from donors later found to be positive by anti-HCV screening (instituted in 1991) are examined. A large percentage of these recipients, up to 75%, are found to be anti-HCV positive.[65,66] Unlike hepatitis B, the majority of those recipients who become HCV seropositive develop chronic liver disease. Therefore, these patients must be offered counseling that addresses the complications of hepatitis C, as well as the risk to close contacts and family members.[67] Nucleotide amplification testing will decrease the incidence of transfusion-related hepatitis C by narrowing the window period from approximately 60 to 80 to 10 to 20 days. Hepatitis G virus has been transferred by blood transfusion, but its significance is unclear in that transfusion-acquired infection has not been associated with acute or chronic hepatitis.[68]

Several techniques have been developed to inactivate viruses in plasma including solvent and detergent treatment and photochemical inactivation using psoralens and long wavelength ultraviolet A light.[69] Methods used to inactivate infectious pathogens in cellular blood components such as platelets and red cells are not currently available but are under clinical development. Due to the low risk of viral infection by transfusion and the fact that most patients who receive plasma also receive cellular blood components, the cost-effectiveness of virally inactivated plasma is low.[70] Albumin, immune globulin, factor concentrates, and other plasma derivatives are also virally attenuated by standard treatment protocols.

TABLE 53.1-6. Risks of Transfusion-Transmitted Disease

Organism	*Estimated Risk Per Unit Transfused in the United States Per Transfusion*	*Pretransfusion Testing*
Hepatitis B virus	1:65,000	HBsAg, anti-Hbc, serum alanine aminotransferase
Hepatitis C virus	1:100,000 (prenucleotide testing); 1:500,000[a] (postnucleotide testing)	Anti-HCV, nucleotide testing
Human immunodeficiency virus 1 and 2	1:500,000 to 1:750,000 (prenucleotide testing); 1:1,000,000[a] (postnucleotide testing)	Anti-HIV-1/2, p24 antigen, nucleotide testing
Human T-cell lymphotropic virus (HTVL) I and II	1:650,000	Anti-HTLV-I/II
Cytomegalovirus (CMV)	1:10 to 1:20 (see text)	Some units tested for anti-CMV antibodies
Parvovirus B19	Unknown	None
Bacterial contamination	1:1500 to 1:2500	None
Treponema pallidum	Rare	Rapid plasma reagin
Parasites (*Plasmodium* sp., *Ehrlichia* sp., *Babesia microti*)	Rare	None
New variant Creutzfeldt-Jacob disease	Theoretically possible	Deferral based on history

[a]Estimated (tests too recently introduced).
HBsAg, hepatitis B surface antigen; Hbc, hepatitis B core.

Other pathogens such as CMV and parvovirus B19 are common in the general donor population and may pose a serious threat in immunocompromised and splenectomized patients.[71] Approximately 40% to 60% of blood donors have been exposed to CMV during their lifetime and thus, have developed antibodies directed against CMV. However, only approximately 2% of CMV-seropositive donors are actively infected, in which case transfusion of their blood to an immunocompromised recipient could cause potentially serious disease. The actual risk of posttransfusion seroconversion of a CMV-negative recipient who receives CMV-untested blood depends on the prevalence of CMV seropositivity in the donor population. This prevalence varies widely in different parts of the United States and other countries.

A number of other infectious diseases are known or are suspected to be transmitted by blood transfusion. These include malaria, Chagas' disease, leishmaniasis, and toxoplasmosis.[72] Parvovirus B19, malaria, and babesiosis are of particular risk to immunocompromised patients. The risk of acquiring babesiosis by blood transfusion is unknown because it is endemic in many areas and often results in asymptomatic infection. Small clusters of blood transfusion–associated babesiosis have been described attributed to single asymptomatic blood donors.[73] Thus, oncologists should recognize that babesiosis can cause febrile hemolytic disorders after diagnosis because it is a potentially fatal, yet treatable disease. Transmission of *Borrelia burgdorferi* by transfusion has not yet been documented. The risk of new variant Creutzfeldt-Jakob disease, first described in 1996, is unknown. It is unclear whether new variant Creutzfeldt-Jakob disease is transmissible by blood transfusion, and this route of transmission has not been reported.[74] Fears of transmitting new variant Creutzfeldt-Jakob disease, however, have resulted in implementation of a universal white blood cell reduction policy in the United Kingdom.[75] In the United States, donors are now deferred *indefinitely* if they have spent 6 months or more, cumulatively, in the United Kingdom from 1980 through 1996. This policy will have a negative effect on blood supplies.

USE OF SPECIAL BLOOD PRODUCTS IN ONCOLOGY PATIENTS

Cancer patients are often immunosuppressed as a result of their disease, treatment, or both. Accordingly, they are prone to a wide variety of viral and bacterial infections and to harmful cellular-mediated immune responses. By virtue of their frequent exposure to transfusions, they are highly susceptible to developing HLA alloantibodies that can adversely effect their therapy if appropriate precautions are not taken. Specifically, HLA antibodies are implicated in common febrile transfusion reactions and the development of refractoriness to platelet transfusions. Thus, oncology patients should receive blood products that have been specially processed to prevent these and other complications. Currently available special blood products include those that are leukoreduced, irradiated blood products, and CMV seronegative or CMV *safe.* Patients should be individually considered for each of these products, and the patient's needs must be periodically reevaluated.

LEUKOREDUCTION

Leukocytes contained in blood components can provoke febrile nonhemolytic reactions, induce HLA alloimmunization, and transmit CMV to both immunocompetent and immunosuppressed recipients. Leukocytes are effectively removed from red cell and platelet concentrates by leukocyte reduction filters. Currently used third-generation leukocyte reduction filters remove 3 to 4 $\log_{10}$ of the total intact leukocytes found in red cell and platelet concentrates. American Association of Blood Bank standards require that units labeled leukoreduced contain less than 5×10^6 residual white cells. Red cells are leukoreduced shortly after blood collection (pre-storage leukodepletion), following refrigerated storage (poststorage leukodepletion), or at the bedside during transfusion. Filters are similarly used to leukoreduce platelet concentrates. Platelets collected by modern apheresis devices are designed to directly collect leukoreduced platelets. Many physicians believe that these products do not require further leukoreduction. White cell reduction by each of these techniques requires quality control measures (using cyclic good manufacturing practices) that verify adequate leukoreduction of cellular blood products.

Leukoreduction reduces the incidence and severity of febrile transfusion reactions and decreases the risk of HLA alloimmunization. Specifically, leukoreduced products are less likely to stimulate the HLA alloantibodies implicated in both febrile transfusion reactions and antibody-mediated platelet reactions. Other generally accepted benefits of white cell reduction include delaying platelet refractoriness and decreasing the risk of transmitting white cell–related infectious agents including CMV and HTLV-I/II.[76] Thus, leukodepleted products are recommended for all autologous and allogeneic bone marrow and peripheral blood stem cell transplant recipients and candidates. They are also indicated for patients with leukemia, lymphoma, and aplastic anemia. Patients with solid tumors who are not transplant patients but who have large anticipated cellular blood product needs should also receive leukoreduced products, as should any patient with chronic transfusion needs (thalassemia, sickle cell disease).

Prestorage leukoreduced products are preferable because they are also devoid of cytokines and other biologic response modifiers that play a role in transfusion complications. Many of these proteins are not efficiently removed by leukocyte reduction filters.[77] This is particularly true in platelet concentrates stored at room temperature because there is continued elaboration of biologically active substances such as tumor necrosis factor, IL-1 and IL-6.[78] With the dramatic decrease in the risk of viral transmission, investigators are focusing on the immunomodulatory effects of blood transfusion.[79] These effects involve associations between allogeneic transfusion and bacterial infection, tumor progression, and tumor recurrence.[80,81] Universal leukoreduction of both red cells and platelets is required in a number of countries including the United Kingdom and will be implemented shortly in the United States.

IRRADIATION

Blood components are irradiated to prevent potentially lethal transfusion-associated GVHD by interfering with the ability of lymphocytes to proliferate. Irradiation of supportive blood components is indicated in bone marrow or peripheral blood stem cell transplant recipients, patients with congenital immunodeficiency states, neonates, premature infants, and during intrauterine exchange transfusion.[82] Directed blood donations made by relatives should also be irradiated. Patients with acquired immunodeficiency syndrome commonly receive irradiated components, although there is no clear increased risk of transfusion-associated GVHD in this population. Standard guidelines recommend irradiating red blood cells, platelets, and granulocytes with a minimum dose of 2500 cGy.[83] Platelets and red cells are not adversely affected by this exposure. It is not believed necessary to irradiate FFP or cryoprecipitate because they do not contain viable leukocytes. Leukoreduction is *not* a substitute for irradiation as transfusion-associated GVHD has been described following transfusion of leukoreduced, nonirradiated blood.[84] Bone marrow or peripheral blood stem cells must never be irradiated before transplant for obvious reasons.

There is preliminary evidence from a murine transfusion model that photochemical treatment with psoralen S-59 and long wavelength ultraviolet light can prevent transfusion-associated GVHD.[85] Using a murine transfusion model, clinical and histologic evidence of GVHD could be prevented by both gamma irradiating or photochemically treating splenic leukocytes. Photochemical treatment was originally developed to inactivate contaminating viruses, bacteria, and leukocytes in blood components. This technology is currently under investigation in the United States and Europe.

CYTOMEGALOVIRUS-SERONEGATIVE AND CYTOMEGALOVIRUS SAFE

CMV infection is a leading cause of morbidity and mortality in marrow and solid organ transplant patients. Most serious CMV infections develop in these populations as a result of latent reactivation of recipient CMV, but nevertheless, CMV can be transmitted by blood transfusion. Therefore, blood banks supply products that have a low potential of transmitting CMV. These products include CMV-seronegative units prepared from donors who are CMV IgG antibody negative and leukodepleted components. The latter refers to blood components leukoreduced in a blood center or laboratory using good manufacturing techniques and strict quality control measures. Depending on the donor population, as many as 80% to 90% of blood donors may be CMV seropositive. In this situation, the demand for CMV-seronegative products can easily exceed supply. In addition, CMV-seronegative products are capable of transmitting CMV disease; CMV seronegativity does not guarantee the product is incapable of causing acute CMV disease. Studies suggest that CMV seronegative and leukodepleted filtered products are equivalent in preventing CMV transmission.[76] In this study, however, all five deaths attributed to CMV pneumonitis occurred in patients who received leukoreduced products.

Many transfusion specialists consider quality-assured leukodepleted units as CMV "safe" in that they are unlikely to transmit CMV disease. In addition to CMV-seronegative marrow and solid organ transplant recipients, CMV-seronegative or -safe components are generally indicated for premature infants, during intrauterine transfusions, for patients with congenital immunodeficiencies, CMV-seronegative pregnant women, and seronegative patients with HIV. The British Committee for Standards in Hematology concluded that leukoreduced components are an "effective alternative" to seronegative products for preventing transfusion-related CMV transmission.[86]

APHERESIS

Apheresis, derived from the Greek word meaning to take away, is the process of selectively removing one component of whole blood and returning the remainder to the donor or patient. Today, sophisticated and highly automated blood cell separators are available for processing large volumes of donor or patient blood to remove the desired blood component. There are two broad applications of apheresis: apheresis for blood component collection and therapeutic apheresis. Apheresis is currently used in blood centers to collect plasma, platelets, granulocytes, and peripheral blood stem cells. In the United

States, most plasma used by the fractionation industry to produce coagulation factor concentrates, albumin, and immune globulin is obtained by *plasmapheresis. Plateletpheresis* provides many of the single donor platelets used by oncology patients. Collecting large numbers of platelets from specific donors is important to many patients who poorly respond to platelet transfusion as a result of alloimmunization to HLA or platelet-specific antibodies. *Leukapheresis* is used to describe the removal of granulocytes (used for granulocytes transfusions in neutropenic cancer patients), peripheral blood stem cells (autologous or allogeneic), and other mononuclear cells. Red cell units are being collected using automated cell separators.

Therapeutic apheresis is a procedure commonly performed for a variety of conditions.[87] Generally recognized indications for *plasma* exchange include thrombotic thrombocytopenic purpura, Waldenström's macroglobulinemia, myasthenia gravis, chronic inflammatory demyelinating polyneuropathy, the Guillain-Barré syndrome, and rheumatoid arthritis. Plasma exchange may help prevent the initiation or continuation of dialysis in patients with rapidly progressive renal failure secondary to multiple myeloma.[88] Therapeutic plasmapheresis has been used in cancer patients who develop a wide array of paraneoplastic syndromes, but its efficacy has not been confirmed by clinical trials.[89] Simple removal of red cells from patients with polycythemia is performed by simple phlebotomy and does not require a cell separator. On the other hand, automated separators very efficiently exchange red cells in patients in sickle cell crisis and patients with *Babesia* infection. Oncology patients with myeloid leukemias may require cellular apheresis to reduce tumor burden before receiving chemotherapy.[90]

Leukapheresis is typically performed in acute or chronic myeloid leukemia in blast crisis when the blast count exceeds 100,000/μL. Patients may or may not have symptoms of leukostasis or hyperviscosity at these levels. Lymphoid leukemias are less likely to produce leukostatic symptoms, but are also treated by leukopheresis in certain situations, or when the blast count is rapidly increasing. As blood viscosity increases, flow in cerebral and myocardial circulations slows, resulting in tissue hypoperfusion and organ hypoxia. The presence of central nervous system or pulmonary symptoms may be an indication for more urgent care. A single leukapheresis can reduce the leukocyte count by 20% to 50% and reduce hyperviscosity symptoms. On occasion, the cell count may actually rise postleukapheresis as malignant cells are released from the spleen and lymphoid organs. Leukapheresis is rarely needed for chronic myelogenous leukemia in chronic phase. *Thrombocytapheresis* is used for patients with myeloproliferative disease who have platelet counts over 1,000,000/μL. These patients with significant thrombocytosis may be actively hemorrhaging or show signs of thrombosis. The platelet count invariably rebounds postprocedure unless chemotherapy is initiated. Prophylactic plateletpheresis is rarely indicated for such patients.

CONCLUSIONS

EFFECT OF GROWTH FACTORS ON TRANSFUSION MEDICINE

Hematopoietic growth factors as applied to oncologic transfusion therapy are designed to limit the exposure of patients to allogeneic blood.[43,91] The isolation, characterization, and subsequent synthesis of erythropoietin by recombinant technology (rHuEPO) was one of the most important advances in decreasing red cell transfusions. Use of rHuEPO has dramatically reduced the transfusion needs of patients with a various anemias.[92] rHuEPO has also been employed to increase the yield of autologous donations and to stimulate erythropoiesis after surgery. Granulocyte colony-stimulating factor has been shown to decrease infection rates in neutropenic patients undergoing chemotherapy, replacing marginally effective granulocyte transfusions. The limitations and risks of platelet transfusion therapy continue to drive the development of agents that stimulate platelet production in oncology patients.[93] There is rapid growth in the use of growth factors including FLT-3 ligand, c MPL ligand (thrombopoietin),[94] and various combinations of growth factors. IL-11, in particular, has been approved by the U.S. Food and Drug Administration for preventing severe thrombocytopenia in patients receiving myelosuppressive chemotherapy. Thrombopoietic growth factors also have the potential to stimulate platelet apheresis donors, increase stem cell harvest yields, and expand progenitor cells *ex vivo*.[95] Development of neutralizing antibodies against endogenous thrombopoietin has plagued clinical testing of thrombopoietic growth factors.

BLOOD SUBSTITUTES

Red cell substitutes currently in development include hemoglobin-based oxygen carriers (HBOCs), perfluorocarbon emulsions, and liposome-encapsulated hemoglobin.[78] The two major types of blood substitutes, HBOCs and perfluorocarbon emulsions, are in phase II and III clinical trials. None are currently approved for clinical use in the United States.[96] HBOCs are artificially derived products with oxygen-carrying properties. They are structurally similar to hemoglobin but do not contain red cell stroma, which is toxic and leads to renal damage. Development of HBOCs has been hampered by the relatively short half-life of these oxygen carriers in the circulation. Perfluorocarbon s are synthetic hydrocarbons that have the ability to carry dissolved oxygen. The particles circulate for only a few hours until they are removed by the reticuloendothelial system. Research efforts to modify or remove red blood cell antigens from donor units is proceeding slowly, but a truly universal compatible red cell unit may one day be within reach.

REFERENCES

1. Rossi EC. *Principles of transfusion medicine.* 2nd ed. Baltimore, MD: Williams & Wilkins, 1996.
2. Wallace EL, Churchill WH, Surgenor DM, et al. Collection and transfusion of blood and blood components in the United States, 1992. *Transfusion* 1995;35:802.
3. Knutson F, Rider J, Franck V, et al. A new apheresis procedure for the preparation of high-quality red cells and plasma. *Transfusion* 1999;39:565.
4. Vengelen-Tyler V, American Association of Blood Banks. *Technical manual.* 13th ed. Bethesda, MD: American Association of Blood Banks, 1999.
5. Klein H. *Standards for blood banks and transfusion services.* 17th ed. Bethesda, MD: American Association of Blood Banks, 1996.
6. Welch HG, Meehan KR, Goodnough LT. Prudent strategies for elective red blood cell transfusion. *Ann Intern Med* 1992;116:393.
7. Hasley PB, Lave JR, Kapoor WN. The necessary and the unnecessary transfusion: a critical review of reported appropriateness rates and criteria for red cell transfusions. *Transfusion* 1994;34:110.
8. Hebert PC, Wells G, Blajchman MA, et al. A multicenter, randomized, controlled clinical trial of transfusion requirements in critical care. Transfusion Requirements in Critical Care Investigators, Canadian Critical Care Trials Group. *N Engl J Med* 1999;340:409.
9. McCullough JJ. *Transfusion medicine.* New York: McGraw-Hill, 1998.

10. Judd WJ. Requirements for the electronic crossmatch. *Vox Sang* 1998;74:409.
11. Leger R, Garratty G. Evaluation of methods for detecting alloantibodies underlying warm autoantibodies. *Transfusion* 1999;39:11.
12. Toy PT, Menozzi D, Strauss RG, et al. Efficacy of preoperative donation of blood for autologous use in radical prostatectomy. *Transfusion* 1993;33:721.
13. Goodnough LT, Brecher ME, Kanter MH, et al. Transfusion medicine. Second of two parts—blood conservation. *N Engl J Med* 1999;340:525.
14. Gandini G, Franchini M, Bertuzzo D, et al. Preoperative autologous blood donation by 1073 elderly patients undergoing elective surgery: a safe and effective practice. *Transfusion* 1999;39:174.
15. Kreimeier U, Messmer K. Hemodilution in clinical surgery: state of the art 1996. *World J Surg* 1996;20:1208.
16. Ereth MH, Oliver WC Jr., Santrach PJ. Perioperative interventions to decrease transfusion of allogeneic blood products. *Mayo Clin Proc* 1994;69:575.
17. Hansen E, Knuechel R, Altmeppen J, et al. Blood irradiation for intraoperative autotransfusion in cancer surgery: demonstration of efficient elimination of contaminating tumor cells. *Transfusion* 1999;39:608.
18. Bock M, Schleuning M, Heim MU, et al. Cryopreservation of human platelets with dimethyl sulfoxide: changes in biochemistry and cell function. *Transfusion* 1995;35:921.
19. Funke I, Wiesneth M, Koerner K, et al. Autologous platelet transfusion in alloimmunized patients with acute leukemia. *Ann Hematol* 1995;71:169.
20. Torretta L, Perotti C, Pedrazzoli P, et al. Autologous platelet collection and storage to support thrombocytopenia in patients undergoing high-dose chemotherapy and circulating progenitor cell transplantation for high-risk breast cancer. *Vox Sang* 1998;75:224.
21. Murphy S, Heaton WA, Rebulla P. Platelet production in the Old World—and the New. *Transfusion* 1996;36:751.
22. Anderson B, Shad AT, Gootenberg JE, et al. Successful prevention of post-transfusion Rh alloimmunization by intravenous Rho (D) immune globulin (WinRho SD). *Am J Hematol* 1999;60:245.
23. Contreras M. Consensus conference on platelet transfusion. Final statement. *Blood Rev* 1998;12:239.
24. Rebulla P, Finazzi G, Marangoni F, et al. The threshold for prophylactic platelet transfusions in adults with acute myeloid leukemia. Gruppo Italiano Malattie Ematologiche Maligne dell'Adulto. *N Engl J Med* 1997;337:1870.
25. Navarro JT, Hernandez JA, Ribera JM, et al. Prophylactic platelet transfusion threshold during therapy for adult acute myeloid leukemia: 10,000/microL versus 20,000/microL. *Haematologica* 1998;83:998.
26. Wandt H, Frank M, Ehninger G, et al. Safety and cost effectiveness of a 10 × 10(9)/L trigger for prophylactic platelet transfusions compared with the traditional 20 × 10(9)/L trigger: a prospective comparative trial in 105 patients with acute myeloid leukemia. *Blood* 1998;91:3601.
27. Contreras M. Diagnosis and treatment of patients refractory to platelet transfusions. *Blood Rev* 1998;12:215.
28. Friedberg RC, Donnelly SF, Mintz PD. Independent roles for platelet crossmatching and HLA in the selection of platelets for alloimmunized patients. *Transfusion* 1994;34:215.
29. Kekomaki S, Volin L, Koistinen P, et al. Successful treatment of platelet transfusion refractoriness: the use of platelet transfusions matched for both human leucocyte antigens (HLA) and human platelet alloantigens (HPA) in alloimmunized patients with leukaemia. *Eur J Haematol* 1998;60:112.
30. Norol F, Bierling P, Roudot-Thoraval F, et al. Platelet transfusion: a dose-response study. *Blood* 1998;92:1448.
31. Duquesnoy RJ, Anderson AJ, Tomasulo PA, et al. ABO compatibility and platelet transfusions of alloimmunized thrombocytopenic patients. *Blood* 1979;54:595.
32. Snyder EL, Rinder HM, Napychank P. In vitro and in vivo evaluation of platelet transfusions administered through an electromechanical infusion pump. *Am J Clin Pathol* 1990;94:77.
33. Leukocyte reduction and ultraviolet B irradiation of platelets to prevent alloimmunization and refractoriness to platelet transfusions. The Trial to Reduce Alloimmunization to Platelets Study Group. *N Engl J Med* 1997;337:1861.
34. Novotny VM. Prevention and management of platelet transfusion refractoriness. *Vox Sang* 1999;76:1.
35. Stroncek DF, Jaszcz W, Herr GP, et al. Expression of neutrophil antigens after 10 days of granulocyte-colony-stimulating factor. *Transfusion* 1998;38:663.
36. Liles WC, Huang JE, Llewellyn C, et al. A comparative trial of granulocyte-colony-stimulating factor and dexamethasone, separately and in combination, for the mobilization of neutrophils in the peripheral blood of normal volunteers. *Transfusion* 1997;37:182.
37. Klein HG, Strauss RG, Schiffer CA. Granulocyte transfusion therapy. *Semin Hematol* 1996;33:359.
38. McCullough J, Clay M, Herr G, et al. Effects of granulocyte-colony-stimulating factor on potential normal granulocyte donors. *Transfusion* 1999;39:1136.
39. Lundberg G. Practice parameter for the use of fresh-frozen plasma, cryoprecipitate, and platelets. Fresh-Frozen Plasma, Cryoprecipitate, and Platelets Administration Practice Guidelines Development Task Force of the College of American Pathologists. *JAMA* 1994;271:777.
40. Jackson MR, MacPhee MJ, Drohan WN, et al. Fibrin sealant: current and potential clinical applications. *Blood Coagul Fibrinolysis* 1996;7:737.
41. Erstad BL, Gales BJ, Rappaport WD. The use of albumin in clinical practice. *Arch Intern Med* 1991;151:901.
42. Tabor E. The epidemiology of virus transmission by plasma derivatives: clinical studies verifying the lack of transmission of hepatitis B and C viruses and HIV type 1. *Transfusion* 1999;39:1160.
43. Dunphy FR, Harrison BR, Dunleavy TL, et al. Erythropoietin reduces anemia and transfusions: a randomized trial with or without erythropoietin during chemotherapy. *Cancer* 1999;86:1362.
44. Linden JV, Paul B, Dressler KP. A report of 104 transfusion errors in New York State. *Transfusion* 1992;32:601.
45. Capon SM, Goldfinger D. Acute hemolytic transfusion reaction, a paradigm of the systemic inflammatory response: new insights into pathophysiology and treatment. *Transfusion* 1995;35:513.
46. Snyder EL. The role of cytokines and adhesive molecules in febrile non-hemolytic transfusion reactions. *Immunol Invest* 1995;24:333.
47. Burks LC, Aisner J, Fortner CL, et al. Meperidine for the treatment of shaking chills and fever. *Arch Intern Med* 1980;140:483.
48. Heddle NM, Klama L, Meyer R, et al. A randomized controlled trial comparing plasma removal with white cell reduction to prevent reactions to platelets. *Transfusion* 1999;39:231.
49. Goldman M, Blajchman MA. Blood product-associated bacterial sepsis. *Transfusion Med Rev* 1991;5:73.
50. Morrow JF, Braine HG, Kickler TS, et al. Septic reactions to platelet transfusions. A persistent problem. *JAMA* 1991;266:555.
51. Krishnan LA, Brecher ME. Transfusion-transmitted bacterial infection. *Hematol Oncol Clin North Am* 1995;9:167.
52. Stubbs JR, Reddy RL, Elg SA, et al. Fatal *Yersinia enterocolitica* (serotype 0:5,27) sepsis after blood transfusion. *Vox Sang* 1991;61:18.
53. Popovsky MA, Moore SB. Diagnostic and pathogenetic considerations in transfusion-related acute lung injury. *Transfusion* 1985;25:573.
54. Silliman CC. Transfusion-related acute lung injury. *Transfusion Med Rev* 1999;13:177.
55. Silliman CC, Voelkel NF, Allard JD, et al. Plasma and lipids from stored packed red blood cells cause acute lung injury in an animal model. *J Clin Invest* 1998;101:1458.
56. Vogelsang GB, Hess AD. Graft-versus-host disease: new directions for a persistent problem. *Blood* 1994;84:2061.
57. Saigo K, Ryo R. Therapeutic strategy for post-transfusion graft-vs.-host disease. *Int J Hematol* 1999;69:147.
58. Williamson LM, Warwick RM. Transfusion-associated graft-versus-host disease and its prevention. *Blood Rev* 1995;9:251.
59. Dodd RY. The risk of transfusion-transmitted infection. *N Engl J Med* 1992;327:419.
60. Schreiber GB, Busch MP, Kleinman SH, et al. The risk of transfusion-transmitted viral infections. The Retrovirus Epidemiology Donor Study. *N Engl J Med* 1996;334:1685.
61. Menitove J. *Standards for blood banks and transfusion services.* 19th ed. Bethesda, MD: American Association of Blood Banks, 1999.
62. Lackritz EM, Satten GA, Aberle-Grasse J, et al. Estimated risk of transmission of the human immunodeficiency virus by screened blood in the United States. *N Engl J Med* 1995;333:1721.
63. Hamid SS, Farooqui B, Rizvi Q, et al. Risk of transmission and features of hepatitis C after needlestick injuries. *Infect Control Hosp Epidemiol* 1999;20:63.
64. Cardoso MS, Koerner K, Kubanek B. Mini-pool screening by nucleic acid testing for hepatitis B virus, hepatitis C virus, and HIV: preliminary results. *Transfusion* 1998;38:905.
65. Long A, Spurll G, Demers H, et al. Targeted hepatitis C lookback: Quebec, Canada. *Transfusion* 1999;39:194.
66. Dike AE, Christie JM, Kurtz JB, et al. Hepatitis C in blood transfusion recipients identified at the Oxford Blood Centre in the national HCV look-back programme. *Transfusion Med* 1998;8:87.
67. Zarski JP, Leroy V. Counselling patients with hepatitis C. *J Hepatol* 1999;31:136.
68. Heuft HG, Berg T, Schreier E, et al. Epidemiological and clinical aspects of hepatitis G virus infection in blood donors and immunocompromised recipients of HGV-contaminated blood. *Vox Sang* 1998;74:161.
69. Corash L. Inactivation of viruses, bacteria, protozoa, and leukocytes in platelet concentrates: current research perspectives. *Transfusion Med Rev* 1999;13:18.
70. Pereira A. Cost-effectiveness of transfusing virus-inactivated plasma instead of standard plasma. *Transfusion* 1999;39:479.
71. Moor AC, Dubbelman TM, VanSteveninck J, et al. Transfusion-transmitted diseases: risks, prevention and perspectives. *Eur J Haematol* 1999;62:1.
72. Dodd RY. Transmission of parasites by blood transfusion. *Vox Sang* 1998;74:161.
73. Dobroszycki J, Herwaldt BL, Boctor F, et al. A cluster of transfusion-associated babesiosis cases traced to a single asymptomatic donor. *JAMA* 1999;281:927.
74. Turner ML, Ironside JW. New-variant Creutzfeldt-Jakob disease: the risk of transmission by blood transfusion. *Blood Rev* 1998;12:255.
75. Murphy MF. New variant Creutzfeldt-Jakob disease (nvCJD): the risk of transmission by blood transfusion and the potential benefit of leukocyte-reduction of blood components. *Transfusion Med Rev* 1999;13:75.
76. Bowden RA, Slichter SJ, Sayers M, et al. A comparison of filtered leukocyte-reduced and cytomegalovirus (CMV) seronegative blood products for the prevention of transfusion-associated CMV infection after marrow transplant. *Blood* 1995;86:3598.
77. Geiger TL, Perrotta PL, Davenport R, et al. Removal of anaphylatoxins C3a and C5a and chemokines interleukin 8 and RANTES by polyester white cell-reduction and plasma filters. *Transfusion* 1997;37:1156.
78. Muylle L, Wouters E, Peetermans ME. Febrile reactions to platelet transfusion: the effect of increased interleukin 6 levels in concentrates prepared by the platelet-rich plasma method. *Transfusion* 1996;36:886.
79. Blajchman MA. Transfusion-associated immunomodulation and universal white cell reduction: are we putting the cart before the horse? *Transfusion* 1999;39:665.
80. McAlister FA, Clark HD, Wells PS, et al. Perioperative allogeneic blood transfusion does not cause adverse sequelae in patients with cancer: a meta-analysis of unconfounded studies. *Br J Surg* 1998;85:171.
81. Amato AC, Pescatori M. Effect of perioperative blood transfusions on recurrence of colorectal cancer: meta-analysis stratified on risk factors. *Dis Colon Rectum* 1998;41:570.
82. Przepiorka D, LeParc GF, Stovall MA, et al. Use of irradiated blood components: practice parameter. *Am J Clin Pathol* 1996;106:6.

83. Guidelines on gamma irradiation of blood components for the prevention of transfusion-associated graft-versus-host disease. BCSH Blood Transfusion Task Force. *Transfusion Med* 1996;6:261.
84. Akahoshi M, Takanashi M, Masuda M, et al. A case of transfusion-associated graft-versus-host disease not prevented by white cell-reduction filters. *Transfusion* 1992;32:169.
85. Grass JA, Wafa T, Reames A, et al. Prevention of transfusion-associated graft-versus-host disease by photochemical treatment. *Blood* 1999;93:3140.
86. Chapman J, Forman K, Kelsey P, et al. Guidelines on the clinical use of leucocyte-depleted blood components. *Transfusion Med* 1998;8:59.
87. Rock G, Herbert C. The Canadian Apheresis Group and therapeutic plasma exchange. *Transfusion Sci* 1999;20:145.
88. Moist L, Nesrallah G, Kortas C, et al. Plasma exchange in rapidly progressive renal failure due to multiple myeloma. A retrospective case series. *Am J Nephrol* 1999;19:45.
89. Graus F, Vega F, Delattre JY, et al. Plasmapheresis and antineoplastic treatment in CNS paraneoplastic syndromes with antineuronal autoantibodies. *Neurology* 1992;42:536.
90. Strauss RG, Ciavarella D, Gilcher RO, et al. An overview of current management. *J Clin Apheresis* 1993;8:189.
91. Thatcher N, De Campos ES, Bell DR, et al. Epoetin alpha prevents anaemia and reduces transfusion requirements in patients undergoing primarily platinum-based chemotherapy for small cell lung cancer. *Br J Cancer* 1999;80:396.
92. Goldberg MA. Erythropoiesis, erythropoietin, and iron metabolism in elective surgery: preoperative strategies for avoiding allogeneic blood exposure. *Am J Surg* 1995;170:37S.
93. Webb IJ, Anderson KC. Risks, costs, and alternatives to platelet transfusions. *Leuk Lymphoma* 1999;34:71.
94. Kaushansky K. Thrombopoietin: the primary regulator of platelet production. *Blood* 1995;86:419.
95. Kuter DJ. Thrombopoietins and thrombopoiesis: a clinical perspective. *Vox Sang* 1998;74:75.
96. Winslow RM. New transfusion strategies: red cell substitutes. *Annu Rev Med* 1999;50:337.

SECTION **2**

DENNIS L. COOPER
STUART SEROPIAN

Autologous Stem Cell Transplantation

High-dose chemotherapy and autologous proximal stem cell rescue is now considered standard therapy for relapsed Hodgkin's disease[1] and intermediate-grade lymphomas,[2] and it is currently being tested as part of initial therapy for patients with adverse risk features and one of the following diagnoses: Hodgkin's disease, non-Hodgkin's lymphoma (NHL), multiple myeloma, breast cancer, and germ cell tumors. The movement of high-dose therapy from a treatment of last resort to a more proximal position is due in large part to improvements in supportive care that have nearly eliminated treatment-related mortality and have, at the same time, facilitated the transfer of much of the care from the hospital to the outpatient setting.[3–5] Perhaps the most important advance in the ability to support patients receiving high-dose therapy has been the use of peripheral blood stem cells (PBSCs). The duration of neutropenia and thrombocytopenia after marrow "ablative" therapy and PBSC rescue is now only moderately longer than that expected after aggressive standard therapy. In most centers, advanced age has become much less important than comorbidity as an important barrier to treatment, and the improved therapeutic index of high-dose therapy has resulted in exploratory studies for the treatment of refractory autoimmune disorders, including systemic lupus erythematosus, rheumatoid arthritis, and multiple sclerosis.[6]

In many respects, because of the availability of PBSC and growth factors, treatment-induced myelosuppression is no longer considered an obstacle to treatment. However, several issues remain unresolved with the use of PBSCs, including the growing recognition that a substantial percentage of collections are contaminated with tumor cells. In fact, strategies for PBSC mobilization have focused on increasing the collections of progenitor cells with much less attention given to the impact on tumor cell mobilization. In addition, a small percentage of patients can still not achieve acceptable PBSC collections, a finding that highlights our ignorance of the biology of stem cell mobilization and the fact that only modest progress has been made in the ability to successfully expand progenitor cells *in vitro.*

Finally, as the general ease of collection and use of PBSCs compared with bone marrow has changed the focus from the procedure ("transplantation") to the treatment, it is clear that high-dose therapy has not been able to overcome significant drug resistance. These results suggest that newer drugs for preparative regimens (including monoclonal antibodies) and novel treatment strategies to eliminate minimal residual disease are needed to further substantially improve cure rates.

HISTORY

In the aftermath of the destruction caused by the atomic bomb at the end of World War II and the subsequent nuclear arms race, a dramatic increase in research was directed at reducing or avoiding bone marrow injury from radiation. In a landmark paper published in 1949, Jacobson et al.[7] reported that lead shielding of the spleen prevented death from bone marrow aplasia in mice after a lethal dose of total body irradiation. Protected mice developed only transient leukopenia and thrombocytopenia and had histologic evidence of bone marrow regeneration 8 days after radiation. In contrast, control mice died without evidence of residual hematopoiesis. Although the authors recognized that a "cellular factor" from the spleen could be responsible for bone marrow recovery in the experimental group, they favored a humoral mechanism because survival in spleen-shielded mice was significantly increased even if the spleen was removed shortly after radiation.[8] Indeed, it was another 7 years before the humoral theory of bone marrow recovery was finally laid to rest.

In retrospect, survival in Jacobson's mice proved that stem cells circulate in the blood and restore hematopoiesis. Thus, bone marrow recovery in the mice that had a splenectomy soon after irradiation must have been due to migration of protected (by lead shielding) stem cells from the spleen to the blood and then to the bone marrow. However, investigators of several studies in mice,[9] guinea pigs,[10] and dogs[11] are generally given credit for confirming the normal presence of circulating hematopoietic progenitor cells in mammals, and in 1975, the presence of pluripotential stem cells in the blood of humans was unequivocally demonstrated.[12]

Although the presence of circulating progenitor cells was established, it was unknown whether enough cells could be collected to reconstitute hematopoiesis in a patient who had received marrow ablative therapy. Indeed, *in vitro* assays showed that an equivalent number of nucleated cells from the bone marrow produced substantially more granulocyte colonies than did the same number of cells from the blood.[13] An important exception to the latter finding was observed in patients in the chronic phase of chronic myelogenous leukemia (CML).[14] In affected patients, the percentage of colony-forming cells collected from the buffy coat layer was higher than in the bone marrow and was approximately fivefold higher than in bone marrow cells from healthy volunteers.[14] These data provided a rationale for rescuing aggressively treated patients in blast crisis with autologous cells harvested at the time of diagnosis,[15] but the data also clearly indicated that the results in CML patients could not be generalized to patients with other diseases.

In fact, the first clinical trials of PBSC rescue in the late 1970s and early 1980s appeared to establish important differences between the engraftment potential of blood stem cells of CML patients and normal donors. Goldman et al.[15] reported complete engraftment in 19 of 20 patients with CML in transformation who were given myeloablative therapy and then rescued with autologous chronic phase, buffy coat cells. In contrast, two patients, one with Ewing's sarcoma[16] and one with paroxysmal nocturnal hemoglobinuria,[17] did not engraft with blood stem cells from healthy identical twin siblings. In both patients, normal hematopoiesis was restored after bone marrow infusions from the same healthy donors. The effectiveness of syngeneic bone marrow but not PBSCs from normal donors used to restore hematopoiesis was in agreement with laboratory experiments that showed important differences in the capacity for self-renewal between blood and bone marrow cells.[18] Because no further reports of PBSC rescue in patients with diseases other than CML were published for the next 5 years, the results of these early clinical studies must have been particularly discouraging.

The first semi-successful PBSC transplantations were reported in 1985 by Juttner et al.[19] in two patients with acute nonlymphocytic leukemia (ANLL). These were also the first "mobilized" stem cell transplantations, as leukapheresis was timed to coincide with the period of hematopoietic recovery after induction chemotherapy. Previous work from the same group had shown that, after aggressive chemotherapy, granulocyte-macrophage colony-forming units (GM-CFUs) were increased 25-fold higher than the mean level in normal subjects and were also higher than the GM-CFU yield from 1 L of bone marrow.[20] In the clinical trial, both patients had rapid evidence of trilineage recovery after being given mobilized stem cells after high-dose therapy. In one patient, however, transient recovery was followed by significant neutropenia and thrombocytopenia before leukemia recurred; in the other patient, disease recurrence precluded assessment of the long-term viability of the graft.

Subsequently, five centers described PBSC transplantations in a total of eight patients.[21–25] In four of the studies, PBSCs were collected after chemotherapy, and in one report of two patients,[24] stem cells were collected during steady-state myelopoiesis. Although these studies showed the feasibility of PBSC rescue, important reservations remained about the broader use of PBSCs. For example, because four of the six patients with mobilized PBSC transplantations had acute leukemia, the mobilizing chemotherapy was intensively myelosuppressive and was associated with a prolonged period of aplasia. As a result, the applicability of chemotherapy mobilization for patients with other diseases was unclear. Similarly, in the patients who had nonmobilized collections, the long period (28 days in one patient) that was required to collect enough progenitor cells was impractical for patients with aggressive disease. Finally, these studies did not establish the number of progenitor cells necessary for engraftment, nor did they establish the durability of PBSC autografts. Thus, in view of the known effectiveness of autologous bone marrow rescue, most centers reserved PBSC transplantation for patients who were not eligible for autologous bone marrow transplantation. Potential candidates included patients with marrow tumor involvement, previous pelvic irradiation, or bone marrow hypocellularity.

The transition toward the use of PBSCs, now complete for autologous rescue and moving in that direction for allogeneic transplantations,[26] has been made possible because of the tremendous number of progenitor cells that can be collected relatively easily and noninvasively.

STEM CELL MOBILIZATION

In 1976, Richman et al.[27] reported that, as blood counts recovered after chemotherapy, a significant increase in circulating neutrophil progenitor cells was seen, and these authors speculated that large-volume apheresis could be used to collect enough stem cells to avert the myelosuppressive effects of chemotherapy. Twelve years later, hematopoietic growth factors were shown to mimic[28] as well as to potentiate the effect of chemotherapy[29] in mobilizing progenitor cells. In addition to neutrophil precursors, megakaryocyte progenitors also were increased[28]; however, in the absence of assays that measured self-renewal and pluripotential capacity, the ability of circulating "mobilized" progenitor cells to establish permanent trilineage engraftment remained speculative. Accordingly, in most early clinical trials, blood progenitor cells were used in addition to autologous bone marrow. These studies confirmed that neutrophil recovery was more rapid in patients given the blood progenitor cells, but the studies also showed an improvement in platelet and red blood cell recovery.[30–34] The latter findings provided the rationale for mobilized progenitor cells to be used alone with bone marrow held in reserve and, more recently, without the need to harvest "backup" bone marrow. In 1994, rescue with PBSCs surpassed the use of bone marrow after high-dose therapy.

The discovery of the CD34 antigen as a stem cell marker significantly facilitated the development of strategies to maximize the mobilization and collection of blood progenitor cells. The CD34 antigen was initially described in 1984 on tissue culture cells derived from a patient with ANLL and was subsequently found to be present on nearly all colony-forming progenitor cells detected by *in vitro* assays.[35] The "stemness" of CD34+ cells was established by successfully engrafting lethally irradiated baboons and, later, humans with CD34+-selected cells.[36,37] These studies suggested that both pluripotential and more committed progenitor cells are contained within the small fraction of bone marrow (1% to 2%) and peripheral blood mononuclear cells that are CD34+.

The presence of the semi-unique CD34 antigen on the surface of stem cells enabled the development of a flow cytometry assay that provides a rapid quantitative analysis of stem (CD34+) cell number.[38] Enumeration of stem cells by flow cytometry has virtually replaced more intensive and time-consuming *in vitro* assays in which the adequacy of stem cell collection is inferred from the number of progenitor colonies that are formed in agar after 2 weeks of growth. With the availability of same-day results

TABLE 53.2-1. Mobilization Strategies

Strategy	*Method*	*Advantage*	*Disadvantage*
G-CSF[a]	G-CSF, 10–20 μg/kg/d,[b] beginning on Friday. Begin 10 L collection on Monday,[c] and continue daily until >2.5 × 10^6 CD34+ cells/kg are collected. G-CSF continued until last day of pheresis.	Avoid weekend pheresis; hospitalization unnecessary; no neutropenia	2–4 d of pheresis usually required; yields generally not high enough to do CD34 selection
Chemotherapy plus G-CSF[a]	Disease-specific chemotherapy followed by G-CSF, 10 μg/kg/d. Begin pheresis when CD34 count is >10 cells/μL or when WBC and platelets increase after nadir (usually 10–14 days after chemotherapy)	Additional treatment against malignancy; higher yields	May require hospitalization; difficult to predict time of pheresis; longer period of G-CSF use; possibly greater expense

G-CSF, granulocyte colony-stimulating factor; WBC, white blood cell.
[a]Some investigators have used granulocyte-macrophage colony-stimulating factor, but available data do not support that it is as effective a mobilizing agent as G-CSF.
[b]Higher yields may be obtained with twice daily injections, but this therapy is less convenient for patient.
[c]Some investigators begin pheresis when the CD34+ count is more than 10 cells/μL.

of the CD34+ blood cell count permitted by flow cytometry, apheresis can be optimally timed to coincide with rising CD34+ cell counts rather than with a surrogate marker, such as neutrophil recovery. Similarly, because the collected number of CD34+ cells also can be counted quickly, apheresis procedures can be limited to the number required to reach the target number of CD34+ cells. In fact, well-mobilized patients often require only one procedure to achieve an adequate collection.

The CD34 count of the infused product is generally considered the most reliable factor for predicting the speed and durability of engraftment after high-dose therapy. After myeloablative therapy, the infusion of more than 5 × 10^6 CD34+ cells per kilogram results in neutrophil and platelet recovery within 14 days in nearly 85% of patients, and 95% have recovery within 20 days.[39] With an intermediate dose (between 2.5 and 5.0 × 10^6 CD34+ cells per kilogram), neutrophil recovery appears to be as rapid as at higher CD34+ cell numbers, but a detectable incidence of delayed platelet recovery is reported, particularly in more heavily pretreated patients and in those given posttransplantation myeloid growth factors.[40,41] A minimum number of CD34+ cells per kilogram that is required for engraftment has not been defined, in part because many regimens are not truly myeloablative. In a study of 48 patients who received 1.0 to 2.5 × 10^6 CD34+ cells per kilogram, all patients achieved neutrophil engraftment at a median of day 11, but 19% had delayed platelet recovery beyond 21 days and 9% had a delay longer than 100 days.[42] The clinical significance of lower CD34 cell doses is longer duration of hospitalization, longer use of antibiotics, and an increased and more prolonged need for transfusions.[43] Taken together, these results suggest that the use of 5 × 10^6 CD34+ cells per kilogram or more is optimal; 2.5 × 10^6 CD34+ cells per kilogram or more is acceptable; and in patients who only achieve between 1.0 and 2.4 × 10^6 CD34+ cells per kilogram, the decision to proceed to transplantation must be individualized.

At present, blood progenitor cells are mobilized in most patients with the use of chemotherapy followed by growth factors or with growth factors alone (Table 53.2-1). The combination of myelosuppressive chemotherapy plus growth factors generally is considered the most productive strategy for mobilizing stem cells and, in comparison with the use of growth factors alone, offers the advantage of providing additional treatment against the underlying disorder. In fact, with the tremendous number of CD34+ cells that are often mobilized into the blood by chemotherapy plus growth factors, often only a single apheresis is required, and the costs and toxicities associated with multiple aphereses can be reduced. On the other hand, the apparent advantages resulting from a reduction in the number of aphereses may be more than offset by the costs and toxicity associated with the use of more myelosuppressive chemotherapy, including the prolonged use of growth factors as well the potential need for hospitalization, intravenous antibiotics, and transfusions. In addition, because no advantage may exist for giving more stem cells than the number necessary to ensure rapid neutrophil and platelet engraftment (between 2.5 and 5.0 × 10^6 CD34+ cells per kilogram), a strong argument can be made for using a less toxic mobilization program.

Although much of the earlier stem cell mobilizing literature was dominated by the use of intensively myelosuppressive regimens, it is clear that, in most patients, standard disease-specific chemotherapy followed by granulocyte colony-stimulating factor (G-CSF) is generally sufficient to collect an adequate number of stem cells. For example, in a group of patients with NHL in whom high-dose therapy and stem cell rescue was planned as part of initial therapy, Pettengell et al.[44] required only a single pheresis to collect more than 2.5 × 10^6 CD34+ cells per kilogram after treatment with vincristine, doxorubicin, prednisone, VP-16, and bleomycin (VAPEC-B) and G-CSF. Even in more heavily pretreated relapsed NHL patients, the well-tolerated combination of ifosfamide, carboplatin, and etoposide followed by G-CSF resulted in successful mobilization (2.0 × 10^6 CD34+ cells per kilogram or more) in 86% of patients, and 61% of patients had 6.0 × 10^6 CD34+ cells per kilogram or more collected.[45] Similarly, the outpatient regimen of cyclophosphamide, 1.5 g/m^2, followed by G-CSF, 10 μg/kg, is a reliable and safe mobilizing program that can be timed to avoid the need for weekend pheresis.[46] In breast cancer patients, Taxol[47] or Taxol-based combinations[48] have been particularly potent in mobilizing stem cells. For example, compared with cyclophosphamide plus G-CSF, the addition of Taxol was associated with a greater than tenfold increase in CD34+ cells per kilogram per collection.[48]

An alternative to the use of chemotherapy plus growth factors for stem cell mobilization is the use of growth factors alone. Mobilization with growth factors, although generally not as productive as the combination of chemotherapy plus growth factors, offers several practical advantages. First, the potential morbidity and need for hospitalization secondary to myelosuppressive chemotherapy can be avoided. Second, the timing of pheresis can be scheduled, making weekend pheresis unnecessary. Finally, the lack of significant acute or known long-term toxicity with growth factors makes them acceptable for stem cell mobilization when normal donors are used for stem cell mobilization. G-CSF is the most commonly used cytokine when growth factors are used alone. GM-CSF is inferior to G-CSF as a mobilizing agent, but the combination of GM-CSF plus G-CSF may mobilize a higher number of early progenitor cells (CD34+, CD38–) than either cytokine used alone.[49] Because it is not clear that the increase in earlier progenitor cells resulting from the combination of cytokines offers any significant advantage, G-CSF is currently most often used alone.

INADEQUATE MOBILIZATION OF STEM CELLS

The failure to mobilize stem cells (less than 1.0×10^6 CD34+ cells per kilogram) is associated with the type and number of previous treatments. Thus, in a population of patients with Hodgkin's disease and NHL who received mobilizing chemotherapy and growth factors, an average decrease of 0.2×10^6 CD34+ cells per kilogram was noted for every cycle of previous chemotherapy.[50] Although this study did not specifically correlate the type of chemotherapy and its impact on stem cell mobilization, it is known that some drugs are more toxic to stem cells than others. Because of their association with myelodysplasia (MDS) and leukemia, it is not surprising that melphalan, nitrosourea agents, nitrogen mustard, and procarbazine are potent stem cell toxins. Less well known for causing stem cell toxicity are fludarabine[51,52] and high cumulative doses (7.5 g/m^2 or more) of cytosine arabinoside.[53] The use of prior wide-field radiation also has been correlated with a reduction in stem cell mobilization. Mediastinal radiation appears to be as toxic as pelvic radiation.[50]

When stem cell collections are inadequate after treatment with growth factors or chemotherapy plus growth factors, inconsistent results have been achieved with alternative strategies. In patients who do not have effective mobilization with G-CSF alone, the use of myelosuppressive chemotherapy plus G-CSF may be worthwhile, but it is unproven as an effective strategy. In patients who do not have adequate mobilization after chemotherapy plus G-CSF, no data are available to suggest that the benefits of more myelosuppressive regimens outweigh the risks associated with more prolonged neutropenia.

The use of autologous bone marrow in poorly mobilized patients also has been disappointing and suggests that the inability to collect adequate stem cells should be considered a marker for an injured bone marrow. For example, Watts et al.[54] described 12 patients in whom fewer than 1.0×10^6 CD34+ cells per kilogram and fewer than 1×10^5 granulocyte-monocyte colony-forming cells per kilogram were mobilized. When a subsequent bone marrow harvest was given in addition to collected stem cells, 5 of the 12 patients experienced transplantation-related mortality; 4 of 11 assessable patients had neutrophil recovery delayed beyond 21 days, and eight patients had delayed platelet recovery.[54]

In patients who experience a poor mobilization either with G-CSF alone or with chemotherapy plus G-CSF, it appears that a variable number can achieve an acceptable (but rarely optimal) number of stem cells after higher doses of G-CSF alone. In a preliminary report, Fraipont et al.[55] studied 27 patients, 25 of whom had collections of less than 2.0×10^6 CD34+ cells per kilogram after chemotherapy plus G-CSF. Seven patients remobilized with chemotherapy plus G-CSF achieved similar stem cell collections to the first mobilization. In patients remobilized with 10 μg/kg G-CSF alone, the peripheral CD34 count, as well as the number of CFU-GM and CD34+ cells collected per apheresis, was statistically increased in the group treated with G-CSF only.[55] Similarly, Jennis et al.[56] studied 20 patients who had unsuccessful initial mobilization (median total collection of 0.57×10^6 CD34+ cells per kilogram), 16 of whom previously had been treated with chemotherapy plus G-CSF, 5 μg/kg twice daily, and four of whom had been treated with G-CSF alone. After a 7-day period of G-CSF withdrawal, G-CSF was given at a dose of 16 μg/kg twice daily. The median total collection for the second collection was 1.53×10^6 CD34+ cells per kilogram, and only two patients did not achieve a cumulative stem cell collection considered adequate to undergo high-dose therapy.[56] Using a slightly different strategy, Gazitt et al.[57] immediately treated mobilization failures (fewer than 0.2×10^6 CD34+ cells per kilogram after 2 to 3 days of pheresis) with G-CSF, 32 μg/kg/d, with apheresis beginning approximately 5 days later. An adequate number of CD34+ cells was collected in 15 of 17 patients.[57] In all three of the studies just described, patients who went on to receive high-dose therapy and stem cell rescue recovered neutrophil and platelets at a median time that was only slightly prolonged compared to more optimally mobilized patients.

Weaver et al.[58] showed that, in patients who obtained fewer than 2.5×10^6 CD34+ cells per kilogram after first mobilization, the yield of second stem cell collections was significantly increased, regardless of whether chemotherapy plus G-CSF or G-CSF alone was used.[58] These results suggested that the first mobilization attempt had a priming effect on the second or that other factors may have compromised the first attempt. Chemotherapy plus G-CSF and G-CSF alone proved equally but only mildly effective, because fewer than one-half of the patients had enough (more than 2.5×10^6 CD34+ cells per kilogram) collected to proceed to transplantation. A relationship appears to exist between G-CSF dose and the yield of CD34+ cells collected, but it did not reach statistical significance.

The sum of the studies discussed suggest that, in patients who achieve suboptimal first collections (1.0 to 2.4×10^6 CD34+ cells per kilogram), approximately one-half or more may achieve a safe (2.5×10^6 CD34+ cells per kilogram or fewer) cumulative stem cell collection after a second mobilization with high-dose (32 μg/kg) G-CSF alone. However, a significant qualitative difference may exist between "hard-to-mobilize" patients who achieve marginal yields (1.0 to 2.4×10^6 CD34+ cells per kilogram) and "nonmobilizable" patients (fewer than 1.0×10^6 CD34+ cells per kilogram).[59] Indeed, more recent engraftment data suggest that the former group may not really need or significantly benefit from the second collection,[42] whereas the latter group has a high incidence of transplantation-related mortality, despite the use of backup bone marrow in addition to blood stem cells.[54] Further studies clearly are required to determine whether high-dose G-CSF is effective in nonmobilizing patients.

Combinations of GM-CSF and G-CSF also have been tested in patients who did not achieve a blood CD34 level considered appropriate (10 cells per microliter) for collection or in whom an institutionally acceptable number of CD34 cells could not be collected with the first collection. In one preliminary report, 10 of 11 patients treated with 10 μg/kg GM-CSF for 2 days followed by G-CSF, 10 to 16 μg/kg, for 4 days achieved CD34+ cell collections of more than 1×10^6 cells per kilogram, including four patients who obtained more than 4×10^6 per kilogram.[60] Nine patients who went on to receive high-dose therapy achieved neutrophil engraftment at a median of 11 days. The median time to platelet engraftment was delayed at 27 days. In a second study, GM-CSF (10 μg/kg) and G-CSF (10 μg/kg) were used concurrently, and a statistically significant increase in the collected number of CD34 cells was seen in the second mobilization, including 13 of 23 patients who achieved an "acceptable" cumulative CD34+ cell dose of more than 3×10^6 CD34+ cells per kilogram.[61] After high-dose therapy, neutrophil and platelet engraftment were said to be rapid. However, in neither study just described was the cytokine combination compared with high-dose G-CSF alone. In addition, it would appear that many of the patients in the second study would not be considered nonmobilizable. Thus, successful results in this group cannot necessarily be extrapolated to those who have previously shown very little or no evidence of progenitor mobilization.

Although the optimal cytokine cocktail for mobilization is unknown, promising results have been achieved with the combination of stem cell factor (SCF) and G-CSF. In a phase I/II randomized trial, patients with NHL in chemosensitive first relapse were randomized to either G-CSF alone (10 μg/kg/d) or the same dose of G-CSF with escalating doses of SCF (5 to 20 μg/kg/d).[62] Leukapheresis was performed on days 5 to 7. Although no significant differences were observed in the yield of CD34+ cells between the two groups, a second analysis limited to the cohort that had been extensively pretreated showed a sixfold increase in the median number of CD34+ cells per kilogram that were collected in the group receiving G-CSF plus any dose of SCF. A second randomized study in patients with multiple myeloma compared cyclophosphamide (Cytoxan), 4 g/m^2, followed by G-CSF, 5 μg/kg/d, with or without the addition of SCF, 20 μg/kg/d.[63] The median number of CD34+ cells per kilogram collected was nearly three times higher in the group receiving SCF, and 65% of the patients had more than 5×10^6 CD34+ cells per kilogram collected in a single leukapheresis, compared with 40% in the group given G-CSF alone. Like the studies of GM-CSF already discussed, it is possible that, in these two cohorts, similar results could have been achieved with higher doses of G-CSF. The apparent dramatic impact of the addition of SCF to the heavily pretreated patients in the first study, however, suggests more than a simple dose-response effect.

To date, only one preliminary report of the combination of SCF and G-CSF in previously nonmobilizable (fewer than 1×10^6 CD34+ cells per kilogram) patients has been published.[64] Ten patients were treated with SCF, 20 μg/kg/d, and G-CSF, 10 μg/kg/d. Pheresis was timed to a blood CD34 count of 10 cells per microliter and continued until a minimum "engraftable dose" of 1×10^6 CD34 cells per kilogram was achieved. If the CD34 count did not reach 10 cells per microliter by day 8, patients were removed from study. All ten patients achieved an engraftable dose after a median of 2.5 collections. These results, although exciting, are incomplete, because no information was presented on subsequent engraftment after high-dose therapy. If a defective bone marrow microenvironment plays a role in poor mobilization, then it is at least theoretically possible that such patients might require more rather than fewer stem cells.

The conflicting and somewhat disappointing results in nonmobilizing patients underscores how little is known about the biology of stem cell mobilization. In fact, the mechanism(s) of progenitor cell mobilization is unknown, including whether cytokines and chemotherapy act through the same or different pathways. Similarly, it is not known whether alternative mobilization strategies differentially impact on tumor cell mobilization, a variable that ultimately may prove to be more important than optimizing the number of stem cells harvested.

TUMOR CONTAMINATION

One of the early indications for the use of PBSCs was pathologic evidence of bone marrow tumor involvement. Implicit in this recommendation was the probability that the blood was likely to be less contaminated with tumor cells than bone marrow. In fact, several studies in breast cancer and neuroblastoma patients show that the concentration of tumor cells is significantly less in blood stem cell collections.[65–69] This advantage may be reduced or eliminated because of the larger number of cells in the PBSC graft and because of the effects of mobilization.[70] In a study of lymphoma patients, for example, less than 1 log fewer tumor cells was found in the bone marrow than in the blood under baseline conditions.[71] However, the advantage of blood over marrow disappeared and in some cases was reversed after mobilization.[71] In six of seven patients followed closely during mobilization, tumor cells increased and, in two cases, tripled compared to baseline levels. Similarly, in patients with multiple myeloma, neoplastic plasma cells appear to be concomitantly mobilized with progenitor cells after treatment with high-dose cyclophosphamide and G-CSF.[72] In six patients who underwent CD34+ cell selection, tumor cells were decreased by 2 to 3 logs, but were still detectable in five of six patients.

Chemotherapy can also result in tumor cell mobilization in patients with solid tumors. In 42 previously untreated patients with solid tumors and no evidence of blood involvement, circulating tumor cells were detected in nine patients (21%) after mobilization with chemotherapy and G-CSF, including 100% of patients with breast cancer and 50% of patients with small cell lung cancer.[73] The peripheralization of tumor cells with stem cell mobilization is related to stage of disease and appears to be substantially reduced by prior effective chemotherapy. In a study of breast cancer patients in whom leukapheresis was performed after each of three planned cycles of chemotherapy plus G-CSF, tumor cell contamination was significantly lower, albeit not eliminated, after the second and third courses of treatment.[74] In addition, the use of effective chemotherapy in the mobilization regimen may have the additional benefit of inhibiting tumor clonogenic growth.[75] Nevertheless, the effect of different mobilization strategies on tumor cell contamination has not been well studied.

The clinical significance of administering tumor-contaminated stem cells is unclear. Gene marking studies in three different malignancies show that infused tumor cells contribute to relapse,[76–78] but no data suggest that they are the sole or even principal cause of recurrence. In patients with breast cancer, two studies have shown comparable outcomes in patients who did and did not have occult tumor in their stem cell product.[79,80] In patients with multiple myeloma, higher numbers of circulating tumor cells were associated with a shorter time to recurrence and a decrease in overall survival, but the presence of circulating tumor cells was not significant in a multivariate analysis that included plasma cell labeling index and β_2 microglobulin.[81] These latter results suggest that the presence of circulating tumor cells was a sign of more aggressive disease rather than a direct cause of failure.

To date, studies in which occult tumor cells are reduced by purging or CD34 selection have shown the most impressive results in patients with low-grade lymphoma. Investigators from the Dana Farber Cancer Institute have updated their experience with patients with follicular lymphoma treated with total body irradiation (TBI)/cyclophosphamide and a purged bone marrow product.[82] Of 113 patients who were evaluable by polymerase chain reaction (PCR) technology, 48 patients had PCR-negative marrows after purging, only six of whom relapsed. In contrast, 49 of 65 patients with a persistently positive PCR relapsed after transplantation. Importantly, no obvious differences were noted between the two populations of patients with respect to stage, B symptoms, gender, bulky disease, remission status at harvest, or histologic evidence of marrow involvement. Although it can be argued that the pattern of relapse in previous sites of disease is evidence against the importance of infused tumor cells, it is also possible that infused tumor cells homed to sites of prior disease because of a favorable microenvironment.[83] In another study of patients with lymphoma, a potential positive impact of purging was inferred from the observation that patients who received lower doses of GM-CFU after purging had a lower relapse rate.[84] A similar correlation between the effectiveness of *ex vivo* purging as reflected by a more profound reduction in postpurging GM-CFU colony formation was previously established in patients with leukemia.[85] A case-matched comparison of purged versus unpurged marrow in lymphoma patients by the European Blood and Marrow Transplant Registry showed a benefit for purging in overall survival but not in progression-free survival.[86] However, the use of different purging protocols and imbalances in the use of conditioning regimens make it difficult to interpret these data.

In patients with multiple myeloma, a randomized study showed that CD34 selection reduced tumor cell contamination of stem cells by a mean of 3.1 logs, but a preliminary analysis showed no benefit in terms of disease-free or overall survival rates.[87,88] As noted earlier in this section, the failure of CD34 selection to improve the clinical outcome in this group of patients likely represents incomplete tumor cell purging[72] as well as the inability to eradicate disease with the conditioning regimen.[81] Importantly, CD34 selection may not be benign. Because of the concomitant T-cell, natural killer cell, and monocyte depletion, there may be an increased risk of opportunistic infections that are otherwise rare in the autologous setting. In a study from Seattle, 7 of 31 patients (22.6%) seropositive for cytomegalovirus developed cytomegalovirus disease, and four patients (12.9%) died. In patients given unselected cells at the same institution, the risk of infection and disease were only 4.2% and 2.1%, respectively.[89]

Prospects for further improvement in tumor purging appear strongest for patients with CD20+ B-cell lymphoma; Rituximab (Rituxan) alone or in combination with chemotherapy results in profound B-cell depletion and achievement of a PCR-negative status in some patients with low-grade lymphomas.[90] Rituxan, perhaps in combination with other B-cell depletion strategies, will be intensively tested over the next several years. For patients with aggressive lymphomas, myeloma, and breast cancer, however, it seems clear that even substantial improvement in tumor purging will have little clinical benefit in the absence of better conditioning programs and more effective posttransplantation therapy.

PRACTICAL CONSIDERATIONS FOR THE POTENTIAL HIGH-DOSE THERAPY AND AUTOLOGOUS STEM CELL RESCUE PATIENT

Because of the potential deleterious effect of prior therapy on stem cell mobilization, the possibility that a patient may be a candidate for high-dose therapy should be considered from the time of diagnosis. For example, given the current importance of high-dose therapy in multiple myeloma[91] and the stem cell toxicity of melphalan and prednisone combination therapy, induction with VAD (vincristine, doxorubicin, dexamethasone) or dexamethasone alone should be considered for initial treatment.[41] Similarly, MOPP (Mustargen, Oncovin, procarbazine, and prednisone)-like regimens, which are already considered second-line for most patients with Hodgkin's disease, should probably not be used until stem cells are collected. More recently, fludarabine, which is playing an increasingly important role in the treatment of low-grade B-cell lymphomas, has been identified as a stem cell toxin in some studies,[51,52,92] but not in others.[93] These results suggest that potential high-dose therapy candidates should have stem cells collected before fludarabine therapy, or at least before extensive treatment.

Stem cell mobilization can be accomplished with chemotherapy plus G-CSF or with G-CSF alone. In general, chemotherapy plus G-CSF is favored by most clinicians because of the additional antineoplastic effect afforded by chemotherapy.[94] If CD34+ cell selection also is being considered, the higher yields achieved with chemotherapy plus G-CSF may be important because of the obligatory loss of CD34+ cells that occurs during selection.

Despite evidence of a dose-response effect when G-CSF is used alone for mobilization,[95] the data are conflicting regarding the efficacy of higher doses of G-CSF when used in conjunction with chemotherapy. Demirer et al.[96] have presented unpublished data showing that, after treatment with three different cyclophosphamide-based regimens, G-CSF, 16 μg/kg/d, resulted in higher yields than 10 μg/kg/d. On the other hand, a preliminary report of a randomized study did not show a greater effect for higher doses of G-CSF when combined with chemotherapy.[97] Currently, in most patients, G-CSF, 10 μg/kg/d, is started 1 to 4 days after chemotherapy to hasten hematopoietic recovery and to increase the yield of stem cells.[98] However, in nonheavily pretreated patients (i.e., those in first remission) who are treated with highly myelosuppressive mobilizing regimens, the brisk myeloid rebound that occurs with higher doses of G-CSF can be associated with symptoms of hyperleukocytosis.[99] Lower doses of G-CSF can be considered in such patients.

The timing of stem cell collection after chemotherapy plus G-CSF can be optimized (lower number of procedures) by measuring the blood CD34+ cell count during the period of brisk neutrophil recovery. If collection is started when the CD34 count exceeds 20 cells per microliter, the majority of patients can collect more than 2×10^6 CD34+ cells per kilogram in one or two procedures.[100–103] However, because patients who show less evidence of mobilization (5 to 15 cells per microliter) may also obtain a potentially engraftable number of CD34+ cells (more than 1×10^6 cells per kilogram) with three or more leukaphereses,[104] the use of the 20 cells per microliter value should be limited to patients who can be anticipated to be good mobilizers (nonheavily pretreated). In settings in which the blood CD34 count is unavailable, it would appear that the best time to begin collection is when the white blood cell (WBC) count has increased to more than 3,000 to 10,000 per microliter[44,48,105,106] and the patient has a rising platelet count.[96,107]

The target number of stem cells is generally at least 2.5×10^6 CD34+ cells per kilogram, but at more than 5.0×10^6 CD34+ cells per kilogram, most patients have WBC and platelet recovery within 2 weeks.[39] Particularly if CD34+ cell selection or tandem transplantations are possible, higher doses are clearly desirable. Although, as noted earlier in this section, more than 1×10^6 CD34+ cells per kilogram is considered sufficient to establish engraftment in most patients, 10% to 20% have slowed or incomplete platelet recovery.[42] In addition, because a substantial percentage of patients who are transplanted relapse and require additional treatment, it is unclear whether marrow reserve in such patients is adequate to sustain treatment.

After stem cell infusion, considerable controversy exists regarding the utility of hematopoietic growth factors.[108–115] Although most studies show a favorable impact of G-CSF on shortening the period of neutropenia, it is much less certain that G-CSF is of significant clinical benefit. For example, it is possible that shorter reported periods of hospitalization with the use of posttransplantation G-CSF may simply reflect clinicians' tendency to discharge patients once they reach a certain WBC count.[109,116] It also seems possible that patients who are most likely to benefit from the addition of G-CSF are those who have received fewer progenitor cells[110]; however, the administration of posttransplantation G-CSF in this group is also associated with delays in platelet engraftment, suggesting that G-CSF may drive a limited number of progenitor cells toward neutrophil differentiation.[40,114,117]

If G-CSF is used after transplantation, most but not all[118] studies suggest that there is no benefit to beginning G-CSF immediately versus delaying 5 to 7 days after stem cell infusion.[119–122] In addition, in patients who were treated with G-CSF beginning on day 0, the use of G-CSF at a dose of 16 µg/kg/d was no more effective than at a dose of 5 µg/kg/d for accelerating neutrophil engraftment.[123] Larger randomized trials clearly are necessary to define the value, if any, for the use of posttransplantation G-CSF.

HIGH-DOSE THERAPY REGIMENS: NEW DIRECTIONS

In contrast to allogeneic transplantation, for which increasing evidence indicates that cure can, and perhaps most often is, achieved by an immunologic effect of the graft, cure after autologous rescue requires complete tumor eradication by the high-dose regimen. As a result, it seems likely that preparative programs for the two procedures eventually may radically diverge. Allogeneic conditioning programs have moved toward less acutely toxic, more intentionally immunosuppressive programs to facilitate donor engraftment.[124,125] In contrast, further improvement in autologously rescued patients will require the development of programs with greater antineoplastic activity. However, little evidence of progress in the construction of more effective autologous high-dose regimens has been seen over a period of 15 years, and it seems likely that the better outcomes reported more recently are more likely due to improvements in patient selection and supportive care.

Alkylating agents have been the nucleus of most preparative programs, primarily because they demonstrate a disproportionate ratio of marrow to nonmarrow toxicity that is uniquely amenable to dose escalation followed by stem cell replacement. In addition, *in vitro* studies show a steep dose-response curve against tumor cell lines and minimal cross-resistance with other alkylating agents.[126,127] Indeed, in contrast to drugs such as anthracyclines, vinca alkaloids, and topoisomerase inhibitors, it is extremely difficult, even under tissue culture conditions, to make tumor cells more than a few-fold resistant to alkylating agents. As a result, minor degrees of drug resistance can theoretically be overcome by dose escalation or by the addition of other alkylating agents. Finally, analogous to other curative regimens, the combination of alkylating agents with nonoverlapping extramyeloid toxicity is theoretically possible with maintenance of near-maximum tolerated doses of each agent.[128] Thus, most high-dose drug regimens, particularly exemplified by the different generations of STAMP (solid tumor autologous marrow program), have used two or more alkylating agents.[129] External-beam radiation, which shares many of the same advantageous biologic features of alkylating agents, cannot be dose-escalated, except to very limited fields; thus, the use of TBI has been limited to highly radiation-sensitive neoplasms, such as leukemia and lymphoma. It is not certain that radiation is superior to chemotherapy, however, even in the latter two diseases.

In clinical practice, dose escalation of alkylating agent–based regimens has been limited by excessive nonmarrow toxicity, including mucositis, pneumonitis, and veno-occlusive disease.[128,129] In fact, new toxicities not predicted by single-agent studies have emerged when high doses of alkylating agents have been used in combination. As a result, the initial promise of all of the currently used programs has not been realized: Significant drug resistance has not been overcome by the modest dose escalation permitted by stem cells and growth factors. In fact, with the exception of a small percentage of patients with refractory Hodgkin's disease, the vast majority of cures after high-dose therapy and autologous stem cell rescue have been observed in patients with chemosensitive lymphoid malignancies.[130–132]

Currently, several strategies are being explored to improve the results of high-dose therapy (Table 53.2-2). First, as morbidity, mortality, and cost are reduced, high-dose therapy will increasingly be explored earlier in treatment, when there is less likelihood of significant drug resistance. Promising results with early high-dose therapy have already been achieved in randomized studies of patients with multiple myeloma[91] and NHL[133] and is being further tested in ongoing trials.

A second approach has been to increase the intensity of preparative regimens. Based on favorable reports from single-institution studies,[134–137] the Southwest Oncology Group tested the addition of high-dose etoposide to Cytoxan and TBI in patients with either relapsed or refractory NHL.[138] Patients who were not candidates for TBI received BCNU (bischloroethylnitrosourea), along with the same doses of Cytoxan plus etoposide used in the

TABLE 53.2-2. Improving the Results of High-Dose Therapy (HDT): New Approaches and Limitations

Strategy	*Advantage*	*Disadvantage*	*Comments*	*References*
Early HDT	Treatment before established drug resistance	Treatment given to patients who may not need it	Positive study in NHL, multiple myeloma; suggestive studies in germ cell tumors	31, 133, 144, 172
"Intensified" HDT	Possibly overcome moderate drug resistance	Increased toxicity of adding additional agent	Suggestive results in patients with high-risk lymphoma; promising early results with addition of radiolabeled monoclonal antibody in lymphoma, leukemia	138, 140, 141
Tandem transplantations	Substantial increase in dose intensity	Possible increase in toxicity	Suggestive evidence in myeloma, germ cell tumors, Hodgkin's disease	143–146, 172
POSTTRANSPLANTATION THERAPY IN PATIENTS WITH MRD				
Induction of GVH-like disease	Thought to play major role in allogeneic transplantation	Toxicity of agents used to induce autoaggression syndrome	Suggestive evidence in myeloma, lymphoma	147, 150
Dendritic cell vaccines with tumor proteins	Minimal toxicity	None	Suggestive evidence in myeloma, lymphoma	152, 173
Posttransplantation monoclonal antibody (e.g., Rituxan, Herceptin)	Evidence of activity after chemotherapy relapse; minimal toxicity	None	Evidence of response in lymphoma patients after autologous and allogeneic transplantations	153, 174
Posttransplantation chemotherapy	Use of non–cross-resistant chemotherapy at time of MRD	Limited bone marrow reserve in some patients, unlikely that chemotherapy will overcome significant drug resistance	Aggressive posttransplantation therapy feasible in patients with multiple myeloma	155

GVH, graft-versus-host; HDT, high-dose therapy; MRD, minimum residual disease; NHL, non-Hodgkin's lymphoma.

TBI regimen. The authors reported that, in primary induction and salvage therapy failures, the results with the more aggressive regimens appeared to be superior than their previous results with cyclophosphamide and TBI but without etoposide. In patients with chemosensitive disease, the more intensive regimen was not better than the group's previous experience. Patients treated with this regimen had a high incidence of grade III–IV mucosal (63%) and grade II or lower skin toxicity (30%) and a 10.6% treatment-related mortality. As a result, further increments in treatment are unlikely. A preliminary report of a study in which amifostine was added to decrease mucosal and skin toxicity did not show any obvious benefit.[139]

Another method of intensifying high-dose therapy in patients with NHL or leukemia is to deliver all or part of the TBI in the form of targeted radioactive monoclonal antibody. Theoretically, radiation delivered in the form of tagged monoclonal antibodies could allow higher doses of radiation to be delivered to tumor-bearing areas without a similar increase in radiation to the lungs and liver. The Seattle group has shown the feasibility of such an approach in patients with lymphoma[140] and leukemia.[141]

In view of the difficulties inherent in increasing the doses or the number of drugs included in high-dose regimens, an alternative approach is to give "conventional" high-dose therapy for two or more cycles. At modestly escalated doses, this strategy can be safely accomplished with growth factors alone, but at higher doses of therapy, stem cells with or without growth factors can be used to accelerate myeloid recovery. At the Dana Farber Cancer Institute, four courses of high-dose CHOP [cyclophosphamide (Cytoxan), doxorubicin, vincristine, prednisone], in which the Cytoxan dose was increased more than fivefold and doxorubicin was increased by 50%, were used in patients with poor-prognosis lymphoma. The study showed that 70% of patients achieved a durable complete response.[142] This regimen is currently being compared with CHOP in a randomized study. Gianni et al.[133] randomized patients with intermediate-grade lymphoma to standard MACOP-B (methotrexate-leucovorin, Adriamycin, cyclophosphamide, Oncovin, prednisone, bleomycin) versus sequential courses of high-dose therapy in which stem cell rescue is given after a final course of marrow ablative therapy. A highly statistically significant benefit was found in disease-free survival, and borderline significant improvement was noted in overall survival favoring the high-dose arm. Patients who relapsed after MACOP-B and then were treated with high-dose therapy did poorly. The latter finding suggests either that drug resistance is more easily overcome earlier in treatment or, alternatively, that several cycles of standard therapy induces a level of drug resistance that makes later dose intensification less effective. Tandem cycles of high-dose therapy also have shown promising results in patients with refractory Hodgkin's disease,[143] recurrent germ cell tumors,[144] and as consolidation therapy for patients with multiple myeloma.[145,146] The use of tandem versus single courses of high-dose therapy is being tested in ongoing clinical trials.

Finally, although high-dose therapy alone may not be curative in most patients, interest is increasing in using the achievement of minimal residual disease as a platform for additional posttransplantation therapy. Several approaches are being explored, including the induction of an autologous graft-versus-host reaction[147–151]; posttransplantation vaccination with tumor-specific proteins[152]; subsequent therapy with monoclonal antibodies, such as Rituxan[153,154] and trastuzumab (Herceptin); and, finally, the use of additional non–cross-resistant chemotherapy.[155]

LATE TOXICITY: MYELODYSPLASIA

A review of published studies suggests that extensive prior alkylating-agent chemotherapy and TBI-containing preparative regimens are the most important risk factors for the development of MDS and ANLL after high-dose therapy and autologous stem cell rescue.[156–166] In individuals with neither risk factor (e.g., breast cancer patients), the risk of MDS and ANLL does not appear to be substantially increased above that expected after conventional treatment.[161,166] Similarly, in patients with Hodgkin's disease and multiple myeloma who are conditioned with high-dose chemotherapy alone, most of the risk of MDS and ANLL appears to be due to prior cumulative stem cell injury from agents such as mechlorethamine, chlorambucil, melphalan, and nitrosourea agents.[162,165]

On the other hand, there appears to be an increased risk of MDS after treatment with TBI-based regimens that is independent of prior therapy. In a study from Nebraska, late MDS in NHL patients was limited to those who received TBI.[158] Of even greater concern is the observed risk of MDS and ANLL in follicular lymphoma patients transplanted in first remission. In one series of patients conditioned with TBI/cyclophosphamide, 5 of 75 patients (6.6%) at risk developed MDS.[167] Before transplantation, these patients had only received 6 to 8 cycles of CHOP, suggesting that the preparative regimen of TBI/cyclophosphamide was the major cause of the subsequent MDS.

The mechanism(s) by which TBI in the preparative regimen contributes to the development of MDS is unclear, because the infused stem cells are not exposed to the radiation and the remaining *in situ* marrow is theoretically destroyed. Although damage to the bone marrow stroma leading to late marrow injury is possible, the rarity of MDS after allogeneic transplantation despite identical conditioning regimens is evidence against a toxic microenvironment. A more likely probability is that most, if not all, preparative regimens are not completely myeloablative[168,169] and that marrow that is genetically damaged but not destroyed eventually achieves a growth advantage, leading to MDS and leukemia. This sequence of events presumably does not occur after allogeneic stem cell transplantation because host hematopoiesis is destroyed or suppressed by a graft-versus–endogenous marrow effect.[170] MDS may be more common after TBI-based regimens either because radiation is a more potent mutagen or because it is less myeloablative than high-dose chemotherapy regimens.

Some studies have implicated blood stem cells as a risk factor for the development of MDS and ANLL. Traweek et al.[157] and, more recently, Andre et al.[164] reported a trend toward an increased incidence of MDS and AML in patients who received PBSC alone or in combination with bone marrow compared with bone marrow alone. Similarly, in an update of an earlier series from the University of Minnesota,[156] Bhatia et al.[160] reported a significantly higher actuarial incidence of MDS in patients who received PBSC (35.8%) than bone marrow (4.1%) in patients transplanted for Hodgkin's disease and NHL. These data are difficult to interpret because the use of PBSC versus marrow was not random, and in some patients, PBSC may have been used because of a prior marrow injury (e.g., hypocellular marrow or previous pelvic radiotherapy) more likely to be associated with late MDS and ANLL. In contrast to these results, investigators from the University of Nebraska have not found an increased incidence of MDS and ANLL in patients who received PBSC.[170] The uncertain susceptibility of stem cells to the damaging effects of prior therapy provides a further rationale for the early collection of stem cells in potential candidates for high-dose therapy.

It seems likely that the risk of MDS and ANLL should be lower in the future, given the trend away from the use of high cumulative doses of agents toxic to stem cells in potential high-dose therapy candidates. For example, in a study from Arkansas[162] no cases of MDS and ANLL were reported in 71 patients with multiple myeloma treated with a brief course of VAD followed by tandem transplantations. In contrast, cytogenetic abnormalities suggestive of MDS and ANLL were observed in 7 of 111 patients who had received an average of 2 years of chemotherapy before receiving tandem courses of high-dose therapy and stem cell rescue.

It should also be emphasized that bone marrow cytogenetic abnormalities after transplantation do not indicate that MDS or ANLL is inevitable. In a preliminary report, only 28% of patients with clonal cytogenetic abnormalities developed MDS and ANLL.[171] Even in patients with notoriously ominous abnormalities, such as partial or complete deletions of chromosome 5, 5 of 17 patients did not develop MDS. Similarly, 16 of 37 patients with deletions of chromosome 7 did not develop MDS, and deletions of chromosome 20 were not predictive of MDS. These results show that clonal cytogenetic abnormalities (estimated to be present sporadically in as many as 50% of patients transplanted at the Dana Farber Cancer Institute[159]) are far more common than the true incidence of bone marrow morphologic dysplasia or late ANLL. This fact would also suggest that the reported 15% to 20% incidence of posttransplantation MDS is much higher than the true incidence of clinical MDS.

FUTURE DIRECTIONS

During the first decade of the twenty-first century, clinical trials in patients with unfavorable prognostic factors should provide substantial insight into the effectiveness of early high-dose therapy. Even for patients who are not cured, quality-of-life studies may provide a further rationale for treating patients briefly but intensively. In patients with drug-sensitive, potentially curable disease, strategies to measure and eliminate tumor cell contamination from stem cell products may incrementally improve cure rates. However, a theoretically perfect purging program will appear ineffective in the absence of more effective antineoplastic therapy. In this regard, the incorporation of monoclonal antibodies into conditioning regimens may allow more intensive therapy to be delivered without proportional toxicity. Posttransplantation immune modulation will likely assume a more important role in overall treatment, especially for patients with a high likelihood of microscopic disease.

REFERENCES

1. Marshall NA, DeVita VT Jr. Hodgkin's disease and transplantation: a room with a (non-transplanter's) view. *Semin Oncol* 1999;26:67.
2. Philip T, Guglielmi C, Hagenbeek A, et al. Autologous bone marrow transplantation as compared with salvage chemotherapy in relapses of chemotherapy-sensitive non-Hodgkin's lymphoma. *N Engl J Med* 1995;333:1540.

3. Schwartzberg LS, Birch R, West WH, et al. Sequential treatment including high-dose chemotherapy with peripheral blood stem cell support in patients with high-risk stage II–III breast cancer: outpatient administration in community cancer centers. *Am J Clin Oncol* 1998;21:523.
4. Weaver CH, Schwartzberg L, Zhen B, et al. High-dose chemotherapy and peripheral blood stem cell infusion in patients with non-Hodgkin's lymphoma: results of outpatient treatment in community cancer centers. *Bone Marrow Transplant* 1997;20:753.
5. Seropian S, Nadkarni R, Jillella AP, et al. Neutropenic infections in 100 patients with non-Hodgkin's lymphoma or Hodgkin's disease treated with high-dose BEAM chemotherapy and peripheral blood progenitor cell transplant: outpatient treatment is a viable option. *Bone Marrow Transplant* 1999;23:599.
6. Burt RK, Traynor AE, Pope R, et al. Treatment of autoimmune disease by intense immunosuppressive conditioning and autologous hematopoietic stem cell transplantation. *Blood* 1998;92:3505.
7. Jacobson LO, Marks EK, Robson MJ, Gaston E, Zirkle RE. The effect of spleen protection on mortality following X-irradiation. *J Lab Clin Med* 1949;34:1538.
8. Jacobson LO. Evidence for a humoral factor (or factors) concerned in recovery from radiation injury: a review. *Cancer Res* 1952;12:315.
9. Goodman JW, Hodgson GS. Evidence for stem cells in the peripheral blood of mice. *Blood* 1962;19:702.
10. Malinin TI, Perry VP, Kerby CC, Dolon MF. Peripheral leukocyte infusion into lethally irradiated guinea pigs. *Blood* 1965;25:693.
11. Cavins JA, Scheer SC, Thomas ED, Feerebee JW. The recovery of lethally irradiated dogs given infusions of autologous leukocytes preserved at –80°C. *Blood* 1964;23:38.
12. Barr RD, Whang-Peng J, Perry S. Hematopoietic stem cells in human peripheral blood. *Science* 1975;190:284.
13. McCarthy DM, Goldman JM. Transfusion of circulating stem cells. *Crit Rev Clin Lab Sci* 1984;20:1.
14. Goldman JM, Th'ng KH, Lowenthal RM. *In vitro* colony forming cells and colony stimulating factor in chronic granulocytic leukaemia. *Br J Cancer* 1974;30:1.
15. Goldman JM, Catovsky D, Goolden AWG, Johnson SA, Galton DAG. Buffy coat autografts for patients with chronic granulocytic leukaemia in transformation. *Blut* 1981;42:149.
16. Abrams RA, Glaubiger D, Appelbaum FR, Deisseroth AB. Result of attempted reconstitution using isologous peripheral blood mononuclear cells: a case report. *Blood* 1980;56:516.
17. Hershko C, Gale RP, Ho WG, Cline MJ. Cure of aplastic anaemia in paroxysmal nocturnal haemoglobinuria by marrow transfusion from identical twin: failure of peripheral-leucocyte transfusion to correct marrow aplasia. *Lancet* 1979;1:945.
18. Micklem HS, Anderson N, Ross E. Limited potential of circulating haemopoietic stem cells. *Nature* 1975;256:41.
19. Juttner CA, To LB, Haylock DN, Branford A, Kimber RJ. Circulating autologous stem cells collected in very early remission from acute nonlymphoblastic leukaemia produce prompt but incomplete haemopoietic reconstitution after high dose melphalan or supralethal chemoradiotherapy. *Br J Haematology* 1985;61:739.
20. To LB, Haylock DN, Kimber RJ, Juttner CA. High levels of circulating haemopoietic stem cells in very early remission from acute non-lymphoblastic leukaemia and their collection and cryopreservation. *Br J Hematol* 1984;58:399.
21. Reiffers J, Bernard P, David B, et al. Successful autologous transplantation with peripheral blood hemopoietic cells in a patient with acute leukemia. *Exp Hematol* 1986;14:312.
22. Korbling M, Dorken B, Ho AD, et al. Autologous transplantation of blood-derived hemopoietic stem cells after myeloablative therapy in a patient with Burkitt's lymphoma. *Blood* 1986;67:529.
23. Bell AJ, Figes A, Oscier DG, Hamblin TJ. Peripheral blood stem cell autografting. *Lancet* 1986;1:1027.
24. Kessinger A, Armitage JO, Landmark JD, Weisenburger D. Reconstitution of human hematopoietic function with autologous cryopreserved circulating stem cells. *Exp Hematol* 1986;14:192.
25. Tilly H, Bastit D, Lucet JC, et al. Haemopoietic reconstitution after autologous peripheral blood stem cell transplantation in acute leukaemia. *Lancet* 1986;154:154.
26. Bensinger W, Martin P, Clift R, et al. A prospective, randomized trial of peripheral blood stem cells or marrow for patients undergoing allogeneic transplantation for hematologic malignancies. *Blood* 1999;94[Suppl 1]:368(abst).
27. Richman CM, Weiner RS, Yankee RA. Increase in circulating stem cells following chemotherapy in man. *Blood* 1976;47:1031.
28. Duhrsen U, Villeval JL, Boyd J, et al. Effects of recombinant human granulocyte colony-stimulating factor on hematopoietic progenitor cells in cancer patients. *Blood* 1988;72:2074.
29. Socinski MA, Cannistra SA, Elias A, et al. Granulocyte-macrophage colony stimulating factor expands the circulating haemopoietic progenitor cell compartment in man. *Lancet* 1988;1:1194.
30. Gianni AM, Bregni M, Siena S, et al. Rapid and complete hemopoietic reconstitution following combined transplantation of autologous blood and bone marrow cells. A changing role for high dose chemo-radiotherapy? *Hematol Oncol* 1989;7:139.
31. Sheridan WP, Begley CG, Juttner CA, et al. Effect of peripheral-blood progenitor cells mobilised by filgrastim (G-CSF) on platelet recovery after high-dose chemotherapy. *Lancet* 1992;339:640.
32. Peters WP, Rosner G, Ross M, et al. Comparative effects of granulocyte-macrophage colony-stimulating factor (GM-CSF) and granulocyte colony-stimulating factor (G-CSF) on priming peripheral blood progenitor cells for use with autologous bone marrow after high-dose chemotherapy. *Blood* 1993;81:1709.
33. Bolwell BJ, Fishleder A, Andresen SW, et al. G-CSF primed peripheral blood progenitor cells in autologous bone marrow transplantation: parameters affecting bone marrow engraftment. *Bone Marrow Transplant* 1993;12:609.
34. Chao NJ, Schriber JR, Grimes K, et al. Granulocyte colony-stimulating factor "mobilized" peripheral blood progenitor cells accelerate granulocyte and platelet recovery after high-dose chemotherapy. *Blood* 1993;81:2031.
35. Civin CI, Strauss LC, Brovall C, et al. Antigenic analysis of hematopoiesis III. A hematopoietic progenitor cell surface antigen defined by a monoclonal antibody raised against KG-1a cells. *J Immunol* 1984;133:157.
36. Berenson RJ, Andrews RG, Bensinger WI, et al. Antigen CD34+ marrow cells engraft lethally irradiated baboons. *J Clin Invest* 1988;81:951.
37. Berenson RJ, Bensinger WI, Hill RS, et al. Engraftment after infusion of CD34+ marrow cells in patients with breast cancer or neuroblastoma. *Blood* 1991;77:1717.
38. Siena S, Bregni M, Brando B, et al. Flow cytometry for clinical estimation of circulating hematopoietic progenitors for autologous transplantation in cancer patients. *Blood* 1991;77:400.
39. Weaver CH, Hazelton B, Birch R, et al. An analysis of engraftment kinetics as a function of the *CD34* content of peripheral blood progenitor cell collections in 692 patients after the administration of myeloablative chemotherapy. *Blood* 1995;86:3961.
40. Bensinger W, Appelbaum F, Rowley S, et al. Factors that influence collection and engraftment of autologous peripheral-blood stem cells. *J Clin Oncol* 1995;13:2547.
41. Tricot G, Jagannath S, Vesole D, et al. Peripheral blood stem cell transplants for multiple myeloma: identification of favorable variables for rapid engraftment in 225 patients. *Blood* 1995;85:588.
42. Weaver CH, Potz J, Redmond J, et al. Engraftment and outcomes of patients receiving myeloablative therapy followed by autologous peripheral blood stem cells with a low CD34+ cell content. *Bone Marrow Transplant* 1997;19:1103.
43. Ketterer N, Salles G, Raba M, et al. High CD34(+) cell counts decrease hematologic toxicity of autologous peripheral blood progenitor cell transplantation. *Blood* 1998;91:3148.
44. Pettengell R, Morgenstern GR, Woll PJ, et al. Peripheral blood progenitor cell transplantation in lymphoma and leukemia using a single apheresis. *Blood* 1993;82:3770.
45. Moskowitz CH, Bertino JR, Glassman JR, et al. Ifosfamide, carboplatin, and etoposide: a highly effective cytoreduction and peripheral blood progenitor cell mobilization regimen for transplant-eligible patients with non-Hodgkin's lymphoma. *J Clin Oncol* 1999;17:3776.
46. Jones HM, Jones SA, Watts MJ, et al. Development of a simplified single apheresis approach for peripheral-blood progenitor-cell transplantation in previously treated patients with lymphoma. *J Clin Oncol* 1994;12:1693.
47. Burtness BA, Psyrri A, Rose M, et al. A phase I study of paclitaxel for mobilization of peripheral blood progenitor cells. *Bone Marrow Transplant* 1999;23:311.
48. Demirer T, Buckner CD, Storer B, et al. Effect of different chemotherapy regimens on peripheral-blood stem-cell collections in patients with breast cancer receiving granulocyte colony-stimulating factor. *J Clin Oncol* 1997;15:684.
49. Lane TA, Law P, Maruyama M, et al. Harvesting and enrichment of hematopoietic progenitor cells mobilized into the peripheral blood of normal donors by granulocyte-macrophage colony-stimulating factor (GM-CSF) or G-CSF: potential role in allogeneic marrow transplantation. *Blood* 1995;85:275.
50. Haas R, Mohle R, Fruhauf S, et al. Patient characteristics associated with successful mobilizing and autografting of peripheral blood progenitor cells in malignant lymphoma. *Blood* 1994;83:3787.
51. O'Donnell P, Loper K, Flinn I, et al. Effect of fludarabine chemotherapy on peripheral blood stem cell transplantation. *Blood* 1998;92[Suppl 1]:120(abst).
52. Laszlo D, Galieni P, Scalia G, et al. Fludarabine containing–regimens may adversely affect peripheral blood stem cell harvesting in low-grade non-Hodgkin lymphoma patients. *Blood* 1998;92[Suppl 1]:273.
53. Moskowitz CH, Glassman JR, Wuest D, et al. Factors affecting mobilization of peripheral blood progenitor cells in patients with lymphoma. *Clin Cancer Res* 1998;4:311.
54. Watts MJ, Sullivan AM, Leverett D, et al. Back-up bone marrow is frequently ineffective in patients with poor peripheral-blood stem-cell mobilization. *J Clin Oncol* 1998;16:1554.
55. Fraipont V, Sautois B, Baudoux E, et al. Failure of adequate mobilization of peripheral blood progenitor cell with chemotherapy and G-CSF: G-CSF alone is superior to chemotherapy + G-CSF for second mobilization. *Blood* 1998;92[Suppl 1]:268(abst).
56. Jennis A, Pecora A, Preti R, et al. High-dose G-CSF stem cell mobilization after initial stem cell mobilization failure. *Blood* 1998;92[Suppl 1]:271(abst).
57. Gazitt Y, Freytes CO, Callander N, et al. Successful PBSC mobilization with high-dose G-CSF for patients failing a first round of mobilization. *J Hematother* 1999;8:173.
58. Weaver CH, Tauer K, Zhen B, et al. Second attempts at mobilization of peripheral blood stem cells in patients with initial low CD34+ cell yields. *J Hematother* 1998;7:241.
59. Stiff PJ. Management strategies for the hard-to-mobilize patient. *Bone Marrow Transplant* 1999;23:S29.
60. Buddharaju LN, Tricot G, Rapoport AP, et al. Successful mobilization of CD34+ cells using GM-CSF plus G-CSF in patients with mobilization failure after initial chemotherapy and cytokine combinations. *Blood* 1999;94[Suppl 1]:1467.
61. Bashey A, Corringham S, Fields KK, et al. Use of concurrent GM-CSF and G-CSF administration to re-mobilize patients who fail initial mobilization: results on twenty-three patients from two centers. *Blood* 1999;94[Suppl 1]:327.
62. Moskowitz CH, Stiff P, Gordon MS, et al. Recombinant methionyl human stem cell factor and filgrastim for peripheral blood progenitor cell mobilization and transplantation in non-Hodgkin's lymphoma patients—results of a phase I/II trial. *Blood* 1997;89:3136.
63. Facon T, Harousseau JL, Maloisel F, et al. Stem cell factor in combination with filgrastim after chemotherapy improves peripheral blood progenitor cell yield and reduces apheresis requirements in multiple myeloma patients: a randomized, controlled trial. *Blood* 1999;94:1218.
64. Powles R, Cunningham D, Kulkarni S, et al. Combination of Ancestin (r-metHu stem cell factor) and filgrastim for peripheral blood stem cell collection in patients who have previously failed to mobilize with G-CSF alone. *Blood* 1999;94[Suppl 1]:606(abst).
65. Ross AA, Cooper BW, Lazarus HM, et al. Detection and viability of tumor cells in peripheral blood stem cell collections from breast cancer patients using immunocytochemical and clonogenic assay techniques. *Blood* 1993;82:2605.
66. Datta YH, Adams PT, Drobyski WR, et al. Sensitive detection of occult breast cancer by the reverse-transcriptase polymerase chain reaction. *J Clin Oncol* 1994;12:475.

67. Franklin WA, Shpall EJ, Archer P, et al. Immunocytochemical detection of breast cancer cells in marrow and peripheral blood of patients undergoing high dose chemotherapy with autologous stem cell support. *Breast Cancer Res Treat* 1996;41:1.
68. Miyajima Y, Horibe K, Fukuda M, et al. Sequential detection of tumor cells in the peripheral blood and bone marrow of patients with stage IV neuroblastoma by the reverse transcription-polymerase chain reaction for tyrosine hydroxylase mRNA. *Cancer* 1996; 77:1214.
69. Vredenburgh JJ, Silva O, Broadwater G, et al. The significance of tumor contamination in the bone marrow from high-risk primary breast cancer patients treated with high-dose chemotherapy and hematopoietic support. *Biol Blood Marrow Transplant* 1997;3:91.
70. Ross AA. Minimal residual disease in solid tumor malignancies: a review. *J Hematother* 1998;7:9.
71. Leonard BM, Hetu F, Busque L, et al. Lymphoma cell burden in progenitor cell grafts measured by competitive polymerase chain reaction: less than one log difference between bone marrow and peripheral blood sources. *Blood* 1998;91:331.
72. Lemoli RM, Cavo M, Fortuna A. Concomitant mobilization of plasma cells and hematopoietic progenitors into peripheral blood of patients with multiple myeloma. *J Hematother* 1996;5:339.
73. Brugger W, Bross KJ, Glatt M, et al. Mobilization of tumor cells and hematopoietic progenitor cells into peripheral blood of patients with solid tumors. *Blood* 1994;83:636.
74. Gluck S, Ross AA, Layton TJ, et al. Decrease in tumor cell contamination and progenitor cell yield in leukapheresis products after consecutive cycles of chemotherapy for breast cancer treatment. *Biol Blood Marrow Transplant* 1997;3:316.
75. Passos-Coelho JL, Ross AA, Kahn DJ, et al. Similar breast cancer cell contamination of single-day peripheral-blood progenitor-cell collections obtained after priming with hematopoietic growth factor alone or after cyclophosphamide followed by growth factor. *J Clin Oncol* 1996;14:2569.
76. Brenner MK, Rill DR, Moen RC, et al. Gene-marking to trace origin of relapse after autologous bone-marrow transplantation. *Lancet* 1993;341:85.
77. Deisseroth AB, Zu Z, Claxton D, et al. Genetic marking shows that Ph+ cells present in autologous transplants of chronic myelogenous leukemia (CML) contribute to relapse after autologous bone marrow in CML. *Blood* 1994;83:3068.
78. Rill DR, Santana VM, Roberts M, et al. Direct demonstration that autologous bone marrow transplantation for solid tumors can return a multiplicity of tumorigenic cells. *Blood* 1994;84:380.
79. Cooper BW, Moss TJ, Ross AA, Ybanez J, Lazarus HM. Occult tumor contamination of hematopoietic stem-cell products does not affect clinical outcome of autologous transplantation in patients with metastatic breast cancer. *J Clin Oncol* 1998;16:3509.
80. Weaver CH, Moss T, Schwartzberg LS, et al. High-dose chemotherapy in patients with breast cancer: evaluation of infusing peripheral blood stem cells containing occult tumor cells. *Bone Marrow Transplant* 1998;21:1117.
81. Gertz MA, Witzig TE, Pineda AA, et al. Monoclonal plasma cells in the blood stem cell harvest from patients with multiple myeloma are associated with shortened relapse-free survival after transplantation. *Bone Marrow Transplant* 1997;19:337.
82. Freedman AS, Neuberg D, Mauch P, et al. Long-term follow-up of autologous bone marrow transplantation in patients with relapsed follicular lymphoma. *Blood* 1999;94:3325.
83. Freedman AS, Gribben JG, Nadler LM. High dose therapy and autologous stem cell transplantation in follicular non-Hodgkin's lymphoma. *Leuk Lymphoma* 1998;28:219.
84. Fouillard L, Laporte JP, Labopin M, et al. Autologous stem-cell transplantation for non-Hodgkin's lymphomas: the role of graft purging and radiotherapy posttransplantation—results of a retrospective analysis on 120 patients autografted in a single institution. *J Clin Oncol* 1998;16:2803.
85. Rowley SD, Jones RJ, Piantadosi S, et al. Efficacy of *ex vivo* purging for autologous bone marrow transplantation in the treatment of acute nonlymphoblastic leukemia. *Blood* 1989;74:501.
86. Williams CD, Goldstone AH, Pearce RM, et al. Purging of bone marrow in autologous bone marrow transplantation for non-Hodgkin's lymphoma: a case-matched comparison with unpurged cases by the European Blood and Marrow Transplant Lymphoma Registry. *J Clin Oncol* 1996;14:2454.
87. Vescio R, Schiller G, Stewart AK, et al. Multicenter phase III trial to evaluate CD34(+) selected versus unselected autologous peripheral blood progenitor cell transplantation in multiple myeloma. *Blood* 1999;93:1858.
88. Stewart AK, Schiller G, Vescio R, et al. CD34 selection does not prolong disease free or overall survival in myeloma patients undergoing autologous stem cell transplant: results of a phase III study. *Blood* 1999;94[Suppl 1]:714.
89. Holmberg LA, Boeckh M, Hooper H, et al. Increased incidence of cytomegalovirus disease after autologous CD34-selected peripheral blood stem cell transplantation. *Blood* 1999;94:4029.
90. Czuczman MS, Grillo-Lopez AJ, White CA, et al. Treatment of patients with low-grade B-cell lymphoma with the combination of chimeric anti-CD20 monoclonal antibody and CHOP chemotherapy. *J Clin Oncol* 1999;17:268.
91. Attal M, Harousseau JL, Stoppa AM, et al. A prospective, randomized trial of autologous bone marrow transplantation and chemotherapy in multiple myeloma. Intergroupe Francais du Myelome. *N Engl J Med* 1996;335:91.
92. Perales M, Marin P, Alfaro J, et al. Impact of fludarabine on peripheral blood progenitor cells mobilization in patients with indolent lymphoproliferative disorders. *Blood* 1999; 94[Suppl 1]:139.
93. Itala M, Pelliniemi TT, Rajamaki A, Remes K. Autologous blood cell transplantation in B-CLL: response to chemotherapy prior to mobilization predicts the stem cell yield. *Bone Marrow Transplant* 1997;19:647.
94. Gajewski JL, Donato M, Anderlini P, et al. Intensive chemotherapy with G-CSF mobilization yields improved peripheral blood progenitor cell collection, quicker recovery after high-dose chemotherapy and reduces progression risk compared to G-CSF alone. *Blood* 1999;94[Suppl 1]:665(abst).
95. Weaver CH, Birch R, Greco FA, et al. Mobilization and harvesting of peripheral blood stem cells: randomized evaluations of different doses of filgrastim. *Br J Haematol* 1998;100:338.
96. Demirer T, Buckner CD, Bensinger WI. Optimization of peripheral blood stem cell mobilization. *Stem Cells* 1996;14:106.
97. Ings SJ, Schey S, Hancock B, et al. Results of a BNLI randomized trial of G-CSF dose after cyclophosphamide 1.5 gm/m^2 for progenitor cell mobilization. *Blood* 1999;94[Suppl 1]:666(abst).
98. Schwartzberg L, Heffernan M, Birch R, West W. Comparison of different G-CSF schedules in conjunction with cyclophosphamide, etoposide, and cisplatin for peripheral blood stem cell (PBSC) mobilization. *Blood* 1994;82[Suppl 1]:641(abst).
99. Salloum E, Stoessel KM, Cooper DL. Hyperleukocytosis and retinal hemorrhages after chemotherapy and filgrastim administration for peripheral blood progenitor cell mobilization. *Bone Marrow Transplant* 1998;21:835.
100. Meldgaard Knudsen L, Gaarsdal E, Jensen L, Nikolaisen K, Johnsen HE. Evaluation of mobilized CD34+ cell counts to guide timing and yield of large-scale collection by leukapheresis. *J Hematother* 1998;7:45.
101. de Fabritiis P, Gonzalez M, Meloni G, et al. Monitoring of CD34+ cells during leukapheresis allows a single, successful collection of hemopoietic progenitors in patients with low numbers of circulating stem cells. *Bone Marrow Transplant* 1999;23:1229.
102. Birhiray R, Plank D, Rushing D, et al. Peripheral blood CD34 count as a predictive tool for collection of stem cells for autologous transplantation. *Blood* 1999;94[Suppl 1]:3356.
103. Fontao-Wendel R, Lazar A, Melges S, Altobeli C, Wendel S. The absolute number of circulating CD34+ cells as the best predictor of peripheral hematopoietic stem cell yield. *J Hematother* 1999;8:255.
104. Ballester OF, Wilcox P, Hill C, et al. Peripheral blood CD34+ count predicts the adequacy of stem cell collection for autologous transplants. *Blood* 1998;92[Suppl 1]:296(abst).
105. Ho AD, Gluck S, Germond C, et al. Optimal timing for collections of blood progenitor cells following induction chemotherapy and granulocyte-macrophage colony-stimulating factor for autologous transplantation in advanced breast cancer. *Leukemia* 1993;7:1738.
106. Dreger P, Marquardt P, Haferlach T, et al. Effective mobilisation of peripheral blood progenitor cells with "Dexa-BEAM" and G-CSF: timing of harvesting and composition of the leukapheresis product. *Br J Cancer* 1993;68:950.
107. Krieger MS, Schiller G, Berenson JR, et al. Collection of peripheral blood progenitor cells (PBPC) based on a rising WBC and platelet count significantly increases the number of CD34+ cells. *Bone Marrow Transplant* 1999;24:25.
108. Dunlop DJ, Fitzsimons EJ, McMurray A, et al. Filgrastim fails to improve haemopoietic reconstitution following myeloablative chemotherapy and peripheral blood stem cell rescue. *Br J Cancer* 1994;70:943.
109. Spitzer G, Adkins DR, Spencer V, et al. Randomized study of growth factors post-peripheral-blood stem-cell transplant: neutrophil recovery is improved with modest clinical benefit. *J Clin Oncol* 1994;12:661.
110. Klumpp TR, Mangan KF, Goldberg SL, Pearlman ES, Macdonald JS. Granulocyte colony-stimulating factor accelerates neutrophil engraftment following peripheral-blood stem-cell transplantation: a prospective, randomized trial. *J Clin Oncol* 1995;13:1323.
111. Tarella C, Castellino C, Locatelli F, et al. G-CSF administration following peripheral blood progenitor cell (PBPC) autograft in lymphoid malignancies: evidence for clinical benefits and reduction of treatment costs. *Bone Marrow Transplant* 1998;21:401.
112. McQuaker IG, Hunter AE, Pacey S, Haynes AP, Iqbal A, Russell NH. Low dose filgrastim significantly enhances neutrophil recovery following autologous peripheral-blood stem-cell transplantation in patients with lymphoproliferative disorders: evidence for clinical and economic benefit. *J Clin Oncol* 1997;15:451.
113. Linch DC, Milligan DW, Winfield DA, et al. G-CSF after peripheral blood stem cell transplantation in lymphoma patients significantly accelerated neutrophil recovery and shortened time in hospital: results of a randomized BNLI trial. *Br J Haematol* 1997;99:933.
114. Kawano Y, Takaue Y, Mimaya J, et al. Marginal benefit/disadvantage of granulocyte colony-stimulating factor therapy after autologous blood stem cell transplantation in children: results of a prospective randomized trial. The Japanese Cooperative Study Group of PBSCT. *Blood* 1998;92:4040.
115. Ojeda E, Garcia-Bustos J, Aguado M, et al. A prospective randomized trial of granulocyte colony-stimulating factor therapy after autologous blood stem cell transplantation in adults. *Bone Marrow Transplant* 1999;24:601.
116. Ojeda E, Garcia-Bustos J, Aguado MJ, et al. G-CSF after PBSC transplantation [Letter]. *Br J Haematol* 1998;101:594.
117. Shpall EJ, Jones RB, Bearman SI, et al. Transplantation of enriched CD34-positive autologous marrow into breast cancer patients following high-dose chemotherapy: influence of CD34-positive peripheral-blood progenitors and growth factors on engraftment. *J Clin Oncol* 1994;12:28.
118. Colby C, McAfee SL, Finkelstein DM, Spitzer TR. Early vs delayed administration of G-CSF following autologous peripheral blood stem cell transplantation [see comments]. *Bone Marrow Transplant* 1998;21:1005.
119. Faucher C, Le Corroller AG, Chabannon C, et al. Administration of G-CSF can be delayed after transplantation of autologous G-CSF-primed blood stem cells: a randomized study. *Bone Marrow Transplant* 1996;17:533.
120. Bolwell BJ, Pohlman B, Andresen S, et al. Delayed G-CSF after autologous progenitor cell transplantation: a prospective randomized trial. *Bone Marrow Transplant* 1998;21:369.
121. Maiolino A, Biasoli I, Nucci M, Spector N, Pulcheri W. Delayed G-CSF after autologous bone marrow transplantation [Letter]. *Bone Marrow Transplant* 1998;22:832.
122. Bence-Bruckler I, Bredeson C, Atkins H, et al. A randomized trial of granulocyte colony-stimulating factor (Neupogen) starting day 1 vs day 7 postautologous stem cell transplantation. *Bone Marrow Transplant* 1998;22:965.
123. Bolwell B, Goormastic M, Dannley R, et al. G-CSF post-autologous progenitor cell transplantation: a randomized study of 5, 10, and 16 micrograms/kg/day. *Bone Marrow Transplant* 1997;19:215.
124. Khouri IF, Keating M, Korbling M, et al. Transplant-lite: induction of graft versus malignancy

using fludarabine-based nonablative chemotherapy and allogeneic blood progenitor-cell transplantation as treatment for lymphoid malignancies. *J Clin Oncol* 1998;16:2817.

125. Slavin S, Nagler A, Naparstek E, et al. Nonmyeloablative stem cell transplantation and cell therapy as an alternative to conventional bone marrow transplantation with lethal cytoreduction for the treatment of malignant and nonmalignant hematologic diseases. *Blood* 1998;91:756.
126. Frei ED, Canellos GP. Dose: a critical factor in cancer chemotherapy. *Am J Med* 1980;69:585.
127. Frei ED, Cucchi CA, Rosowsky A, et al. Alkylating agent resistance: *in vitro* studies with human cell lines. *Proc Natl Acad Sci U S A* 1985;82:2158.
128. Peters WP, Eder JP, Henner WD, et al. High-dose combination alkylating agents with autologous bone marrow support: a phase 1 trial. *J Clin Oncol* 1986;4:646.
129. Eder JP, Antman K, Peters W, et al. High-dose combination alkylating agent chemotherapy with autologous bone marrow support for metastatic breast cancer. *J Clin Oncol* 1986;4:1592.
130. Philip T, Armitage JO, Spitzer G, et al. High-dose therapy and autologous bone marrow transplantation after failure of conventional chemotherapy in adults with intermediate-grade or high-grade non-Hodgkin's lymphoma. *N Engl J Med* 1987;316:1493.
131. Lazarus HM, Rowlings PA, Zhang MJ, et al. Autotransplants for Hodgkin's disease in patients never achieving remission: a report from the Autologous Blood and Marrow Transplant Registry. *J Clin Oncol* 1999;17:534.
132. Josting A, Reiser M, Rueffer U, et al. Treatment of primary progressive Hodgkin's and aggressive non-Hodgkin's lymphoma: is there a chance for cure? *J Clin Oncol* 2000;18:332.
133. Gianni AM, Bregni M, Siena S, et al. High-dose chemotherapy and autologous bone marrow transplantation compared with MACOP-B in aggressive B-cell lymphoma. *N Engl J Med* 1997;336:1290.
134. Gulati S, Yahalom J, Acaba L, et al. Treatment of patients with relapsed and resistant non-Hodgkin's lymphoma using total body irradiation, etoposide, and cyclophosphamide and autologous bone marrow transplantation. *J Clin Oncol* 1992;10:936.
135. Blume KG, Forman SJ. High-dose etoposide (VP-16)-containing preparatory regimens in allogeneic and autologous bone marrow transplantation for hematologic malignancies. *Semin Oncol* 1992;19:63.
136. Horning SJ, Negrin RS, Chao JC, et al. Fractionated total-body irradiation, etoposide, and cyclophosphamide plus autografting in Hodgkin's disease and non-Hodgkin's lymphoma. *J Clin Oncol* 1994;12:2552.
137. Weaver CH, Petersen FB, Appelbaum FR, et al. High-dose fractionated total-body irradiation, etoposide, and cyclophosphamide followed by autologous stem-cell support in patients with malignant lymphoma. *J Clin Oncol* 1994;12:2559.
138. Stiff PJ, Dahlberg S, Forman SJ, et al. Autologous bone marrow transplantation for patients with relapsed or refractory diffuse aggressive non-Hodgkin's lymphoma: value of augmented preparative regimens—a Southwest Oncology Group trial. *J Clin Oncol* 1998;16:48.
139. Rodriguez R, Nademanee A, Ivers B, et al. Amifostine before fractionated total body irradiation, followed by VP-16, Cytoxan and autologous PBSCT for patients with relapsed NHL, HD and acute leukemia: toxicity analysis. *Blood* 1999;94[Suppl 1]:145(abst).
140. Liu SY, Eary JF, Petersdorf SH, et al. Follow-up of relapsed B-cell lymphoma patients treated with iodine-131-labeled anti-CD20 antibody and autologous stem-cell rescue. *J Clin Oncol* 1998;16:3270.
141. Matthews DC, Appelbaum FR, Eary JF, et al. Phase I study of (131)I-anti-CD45 antibody plus cyclophosphamide and total body irradiation for advanced acute leukemia and myelodysplastic syndrome. *Blood* 1999;94:1237.
142. Janicek M, Kaplan W, Neuberg D, et al. Early restaging gallium scans predict outcome in poor-prognosis patients with aggressive non-Hodgkin's lymphoma treated with high-dose CHOP chemotherapy. *J Clin Oncol* 1997;15:1631.
143. Ahmed T, Lake DE, Beer M, et al. Single and double autotransplants for relapsing/refractory Hodgkin's disease: results of two consecutive trials. *Bone Marrow Transplant* 1997;19:449.
144. Margolin BK, Doroshow JH, Ahn C, et al. Treatment of germ cell cancer with two cycles of high-dose ifosfamide, carboplatin, and etoposide with autologous stem-cell support [see comments]. *J Clin Oncol* 1996;14:2631.
145. Barlogie B, Jagannath S, Desikan KR, et al. Total therapy with tandem transplants for newly diagnosed multiple myeloma. *Blood* 1999;93:55.
146. Barlogie B, Jagannath S, Vesole DH, et al. Superiority of tandem autologous transplantation over standard therapy for previously untreated multiple myeloma. *Blood* 1997;89:789.
147. Giralt S, Weber D, Colome M, et al. Phase I trial of cyclosporine-induced autologous graft-versus-host disease in patients with multiple myeloma undergoing high-dose chemotherapy with autologous stem-cell rescue. *J Clin Oncol* 1997;15:667.
148. Hess AD, Thoburn CJ. Immunobiology and immunotherapeutic implications of syngeneic/autologous graft-versus-host disease. *Immunol Rev* 1997;157:111.
149. Meehan KR, Arun B, Gehan EA, et al. Immunotherapy with interleukin-2 and alpha-interferon after IL-2-activated hematopoietic stem cell transplantation for breast cancer. *Bone Marrow Transplant* 1999;23:667.
150. Vogelsang G, Bitton R, Piantadosi S, et al. Immune modulation in autologous bone marrow transplantation: cyclosporine and gamma-interferon trial. *Bone Marrow Transplant* 1999;24:637.
151. Wu DY, Goldschneider I. Cyclosporin A–induced autologous graft-versus-host disease: a prototypical model of autoimmunity and active (dominant) tolerance coordinately induced by recent thymic emigrants. *J Immunol* 1999;162:6926.
152. Reichardt VL, Okada CY, Liso A, et al. Idiotype vaccination using dendritic cells after autologous peripheral blood stem cell transplantation for multiple myeloma—a feasibility study. *Blood* 1999;93:2411.
153. Tsai DE, Moore HCF, Hardy CL, et al. Rituximab (anti-CD20 monoclonal antibody) therapy for progressive intermediate-grade non-Hodgkin's lymphoma after high-dose therapy and autologous peripheral stem cell transplantation. *Bone Marrow Transplant* 1999;24:521.
154. Rapoport AP, Jaberi P, Fassas A, et al. Autotransplantation for refractory aggressive B-cell lymphoma followed by post-transplant Rituxan plus GM-CSF and consolidative chemotherapy. *Blood* 1999;94[Suppl 1]:404 (abst).
155. Desikan R, Munshi N, Zangari M, et al. DCEP consolidation chemotherapy after two cycles of melphalan-based high dose therapy—high incidence of complete response and superior outcome in comparison with matched historical controls. *Blood* 1999;94[Suppl 1]:316(abst).
156. Miller JS, Arthur DC, Litz CE, et al. Myelodysplastic syndrome after autologous bone marrow transplantation: an additional late complication of curative cancer therapy. *Blood* 1994;83:3780.
157. Traweek ST, Slovak ML, Nademanee AP, et al. Clonal karyotypic hematopoietic cell abnormalities occurring after autologous bone marrow transplantation for Hodgkin's disease and non-Hodgkin's lymphoma. *Blood* 1994;84:957.
158. Darrington DL, Vose JM, Anderson JR, et al. Incidence and characterization of secondary myelodysplastic syndrome and acute myelogenous leukemia following high-dose chemoradiotherapy and autologous stem-cell transplantation for lymphoid malignancies. *J Clin Oncol* 1994;12:2527.
159. Stone RM, Neuberg D, Soiffer R, et al. Myelodysplastic syndrome as a late complication following autologous bone marrow transplantation for non-Hodgkin's lymphoma. *J Clin Oncol* 1994;12:2535.
160. Bhatia S, Ramsay NK, Steinbuch M, et al. Malignant neoplasms following bone marrow transplantation. *Blood* 1996;87:3633.
161. Laughlin MJ, McGaughey DS, Crews JR, et al. Secondary myelodysplasia and acute leukemia in breast cancer patients after autologous bone marrow transplant. *J Clin Oncol* 1998;16:1008.
162. Govindarajan R, Jagannath S, Flick JT, et al. Preceding standard therapy is the likely cause of MDS after autotransplants for multiple myeloma. *Br J Haematol* 1996;95:349.
163. Deeg HJ, Socie G. Malignancies after hematopoietic stem cell transplantation: many questions, some answers. *Blood* 1998;91:1833.
164. Andre M, Henry-Amar M, Blaise D, et al. Treatment-related deaths and second cancer risk after autologous stem-cell transplantation for Hodgkin's disease. *Blood* 1998;92:1933.
165. Harrison CN, Gregory W, Hudson GV, et al. High-dose BEAM chemotherapy with autologous haemopoietic stem cell transplantation for Hodgkin's disease is unlikely to be associated with a major increased risk of secondary MDS/AML. *Br J Cancer* 1999;81:476.
166. Sobecks RM, Le Beau MM, Anastasi J, Williams SF. Myelodysplasia and acute leukemia following high-dose chemotherapy and autologous bone marrow or peripheral blood stem cell transplantation. *Bone Marrow Transplant* 1999;23:1161.
167. Freedman AS, Gribben JG, Neuberg D, et al. High-dose therapy and autologous bone marrow transplantation in patients with follicular lymphoma during first remission. *Blood* 1996;88:2780.
168. Laporte JP, Fouillard L, Douay L, et al. GM-CSF instead of autologous bone-marrow transplantation after the BEAM regimen. *Lancet* 1991;338:601.
169. Baranov AE, Selidovkin GD, Butturini A, Gale RP. Hematopoietic recovery after 10-Gy acute total body radiation. *Blood* 1994;83:596.
170. Anderson JR, Vose J, Kessinger A. Myelodysplastic syndrome after autologous transplant for lymphoma [Letter]. *Blood* 1994;84:3988.
171. LaCasce A, Neuberg D, Janosova A, et al. Clonal karyotypic abnormalities after autologous bone marrow transplantation for non-Hodgkin's lymphoma are common and not always associated with myelodysplastic syndrome. *Blood* 1999;94:344.
172. Bokemeyer C, Kollmannsberger C, Meisner C, et al. First-line high-dose chemotherapy compared with standard-dose PEB/VIP chemotherapy in patients with advanced germ cell tumors: a multivariate and matched pair analysis. *J Clin Oncol* 1999;17:3450.
173. Kwak LW. Tumor vaccination strategies combined with autologous peripheral stem cell transplantation. *Ann Oncol* 1998;9:S41.
174. Cuellar-Ambrosi F, Seropian S, McGuirk J, et al. Allogeneic peripheral blood stem cell transplant for patients with high risk aggressive non-Hodgkin's lymphoma. *Blood* 1999;94[Suppl 1]:381b (abst).

SECTION 3

RICHARD W. CHILDS

Allogeneic Stem Cell Transplantation

HISTORICAL PERSPECTIVE

The concept that allogeneic hematopoietic progenitor cells could be used to rescue marrow function in humans after myeloablative doses of whole body irradiation or high-dose chemotherapy arose predominantly from research in mouse models. Mice, after exposure to lethal doses of irradiation, could be reproducibly rescued from marrow aplasia after intravenous infusion of splenocytes or bone marrow cells.[1,2] These observations were followed by mostly unsuccessful clinical applications of bone marrow transplantation (BMT) in humans in the late 1950s, predominantly owing to a limited knowledge of the methods required for the safe application of dose-intensive chemotherapy or total body irradiation (TBI).[3] However, through the dedicated persistence of researchers such as Thomas et al.,[4] who pioneered in the field, the biology and mechanisms required to optimize the procedure were gradually defined. Identification of the HLA system as the major determinant of transplantation outcome was the breakthrough required to establish the field of allogeneic BMT as a successful clinical discipline.[5]

By the 1970s, BMT began to gain acceptance in the medical community as its application expanded from the treatment of patients with hematologic malignancies, such as acute leukemia and chronic myelogenous leukemia (CML), to the treatment of patients with nonmalignant hematologic conditions, such as congenital immunodeficiency syndromes and aplastic anemia. The improved safety and efficacy of dose-intensive treatment regimens, as well as the development of better supportive care measures, laid the foundation for successful allogeneic BMT during this period.

The potential of allogeneic BMT to cure otherwise fatal hematologic malignancies rapidly became established. However, the numerous toxicities associated with the procedure—namely, severe organ toxicity from dose-intensive conditioning, graft rejection, opportunistic infections, and graft-versus-host disease (GVHD)—were quickly defined as well.[4] Although a number of effective drugs became available to prevent or manage many of these complications, such as cyclosporin A (CSA) for the prevention of acute GVHD and ganciclovir for the treatment of cytomegalovirus (CMV) infection, transplant-related mortality remained high, in the range of 30% to 40%.[6] Furthermore, attempts to improve transplantation outcome by preventing disease relapse through intensification of the conditioning regimen proved to be largely unsuccessful, mostly owing to an increase in toxicities associated with these intensified regimens.

Great strides were made in the field of allogeneic hematopoietic stem cell transplantation (SCT) in the 1990s, in improving both transplantation safety and efficacy. The association of an increased risk of leukemic relapse after T-cell depletion of the allograft, as well as the observation that relapse was less likely in patients with a history of acute or chronic GVHD, lent credence to the concept that a donor immune-mediated antimalignancy effect, called *graft-versus-leukemia* (GVL), occurred after such procedures.[7,8] The most compelling evidence for the GVL effect is seen in patients with relapsed CML after transplantation who are successfully induced back into a complete and durable remission following the infusion of donor lymphocytes. Similar GVL effects after donor lymphocyte infusion (DLI) have been observed in other malignancies, including acute leukemias, chronic lymphocytic leukemia (CLL), Hodgkin's and non-Hodgkin's lymphoma, and multiple myeloma.

The success of DLI, particularly in relapsed CML, has generated intense interest in exploring the nature of this powerful immune effect and has raised the question of whether GVL alone, without toxic high-dose chemotherapy or radiotherapy, could be sufficient to eradicate some hematologic malignancies. To answer this question, a number of investigators have explored the concept of using low-intensity, immunosuppressive but nonmyeloablative conditioning regimens to permit engraftment of the donor immune system for the generation of GVL effects while sparing patients the toxicities associated with myeloablative therapy. Early results have been encouraging, demonstrating that such transplantation regimens are well tolerated, with a decreased incidence of transplant-related morbidity and mortality, even in high-risk patients.[278–285] More important, they have demonstrated that GVL alone, without toxic myeloablative conditioning, is sufficient to cure some hematologic malignancies.[279,282,286] These findings highlight the unique and potentially curative immune aspects that are intrinsic to this form of therapy.

ALLOGENEIC HEMATOPOIETIC STEM CELL TRANSPLANTATION FOR HEMATOLOGIC MALIGNANCIES

The relationship between the intensity of chemo/radiotherapy and the antitumor effect led to the development of most high-intensity BMT strategies. Myeloablative doses of chemo/radiotherapy, which are intended to eradicate the malignancy completely, are followed by the infusion of compatible donor hematopoietic progenitor cells to rescue the patient from conditioning-induced bone marrow aplasia. This concept is applied most appropriately to malignancies such as leukemia that originate from the bone marrow itself. However, increasing evidence reveals that even the most intense of conditioning regimens often does not completely eradicate leukemic clones. Rather, a powerful immune reaction generated from donor cells against residual leukemia (GVL) ensues in the majority of responding patients, rendering them leukemia-free.[9–15] It is through the combination of these two components—dose-intensive tumor killing followed by the GVL effect—that allogeneic hematopoietic SCT has its curative potential.

ALLOGENEIC HEMATOPOIETIC STEM CELL TRANSPLANTATION FOR NONMALIGNANT DISORDERS

Allogeneic hematopoietic SCT can be used to successfully treat nonmalignant diseases associated with defective bone marrow function or metabolic disorders associated with lysosomal enzyme defects. These disorders, although nonmalignant, often result in an extremely poor quality of life and may have long-term life-threatening sequelae, thus justifying the risks of morbidity and mortality associated with the procedure. The list of nonmalignant diseases curable by allogeneic hematopoietic SCT is long and includes severe aplastic anemia, Fanconi's anemia, thalassemia major, chronic granulomatous disease, sickle cell anemia, and a number of immunodeficiency syndromes, such as the severe combined immunodeficiency syndrome, Chédiak-Higashi disease, and the Wiskott-Aldrich syndrome.[16–20] Because the eradication of malignant cells is not a concern, the preparative regimens used in these diseases usually are of lower intensity or do not include irradiation, serving primarily to provide sufficient immunosuppression to allow for the engraftment of normal donor bone marrow cells. In some diseases, particularly sickle cell anemia and thalassemia major in children, excellent results have been achieved with disease-free survivals greater then 95%.[21–23]

PREPARATIVE REGIMENS

In the treatment of malignant diseases, the primary purpose of the preparative regimen is to eradicate malignant cells and to induce immunosuppression in the recipient so that rejection is prevented and engraftment of the donor hematopoietic system is permitted. The decision to use a particular preparative regimen often is guided by the sensitivity of the underlying malignancy to the agents contained within that regimen. Although a number of different agents have been used for their antitumor effects in hematologic malignancies, in general, they can be divided into two categories: TBI-based and chemotherapy-based.

Most regimens based on TBI are composed of high-dose cyclophosphamide given as 60 mg/kg IV on 2 consecutive days, followed by varying doses of fractionated TBI to a cumulative dose of 1200 to 1500 cGy.[24–26] Although there is some evidence that the higher doses of TBI may be more effective in terms of preventing disease relapse, toxicity appears to increase concomitantly, thus negating any overall benefit.[27–29] Results, in terms of toxicity and disease-free survival, appear similar between regimens composed of TBI and etoposide (60 mg/kg) and those composed of TBI and cyclophosphamide.[30]

Although a number of chemotherapy-based regimens that do not include irradiation have been used,[31–34] the combination of cyclophosphamide (60 mg/kg IV on 2 consecutive days) and busulfan (4 mg/kg PO on 4 consecutive days) has gained increasing popularity and use since its conception in the early 1980s.[35] Similar to the experience with TBI, dose intensification of chemotherapy-based regimens usually results in increased toxicity, thus negating any potential survival benefit that might occur as a result of less disease relapse.

The decision guiding which preparative regimen to use often is based on the predicted tumor-specific activity of that regimen. In general, radiation- and chemotherapy-based regimens are associated with an equal probability of achieving long-term disease-free survival. Two randomized trials evaluating cyclophosphamide (60 mg/kg × 2) and busulfan versus TBI and cyclophosphamide (60 mg/kg × 2) in patients with chronic-phase CML revealed equal efficacy between both regimens.[36,37] However, in acute lymphocytic leukemia (ALL), TBI-based regimens may be the treatment of choice, as a randomized trial reported a significantly increased risk of relapse in patients with ALL who received conditioning with chemotherapy alone (busulfan and etoposide).[38]

The toxicity profile of preparative regimens varies considerably, a factor that often determines the choice of which regimen to use for an individual patient. In general, TBI-based regimens are associated with a higher risk of secondary malignancies and growth retardation, while chemotherapy-based regimens, particularly those containing busulfan, are associated with a higher risk of severe mucositis and venoocclusive disease (VOD), with minimal effects on growth and development.[39–44]

TABLE 53.3-1. Toxicity Profiles of Conditioning Regimens

	TBI	*Chemotherapy Alone*	*NST*
Sterility	++	+	–
Mucositis	+	++	–
Venocclusive disease	±	++	–
Growth retardation	++	±	–
Secondary malignancies	++	±	?
Cataracts	++	±	–

NST, nonmyeloablative stem cell transplantation; TBI, total body irradiation; +, moderately associated with; ++, highly associated with; –, not associated with; ±, occasionally to rarely associated with; ?, unknown but anticipated to be low.

A number of investigators have explored the concept of using low-intensity preparative regimens (either low-dose chemotherapy, low-dose TBI, or both) in attempts to decrease the risk of toxicity and mortality associated with myeloablative conditioning.[45–48] The preparative regimen in such nonmyeloablative stem cell transplantations (NSTs; discussed later in Nonmyeloablative Allogeneic Stem Cell Transplantation) does not eradicate host hematopoiesis and is used primarily to induce immunosuppression in the recipient to allow for engraftment of donor cells for the subsequent generation of GVL effects. Such low-intensity transplantations rely completely on the GVL effect to eradicate malignancy. Although these regimens vary considerably between institutions, preliminary results are promising, showing high degrees of donor engraftment with considerably less conditioning-related toxicity than is seen with conventional high-dose myeloablative regimens, even in older (older than 55 years) and debilitated patients. Most of the severe and life-threatening complications associated with conventional preparative regimens, such as VOD, pneumonitis, and severe mucositis, have rarely been observed with NST. More important, sufficient engraftment of donor immune cells has been achieved to induce complete remission in a number of different hematologic malignancies.[278–283] The improved safety profile of NST, in both the short and long term, will likely make this transplantation approach the procedure of choice for patients at high risk for complications with conventional dose-intensive regimens (i.e., older or debilitated patients). Furthermore, NST may have its greatest benefit among younger patients in whom growth retardation, sterility, and the risk of secondary malignancy may be completely avoided. The toxicity profiles of TBI-based, chemotherapy-based, and nonmyeloablative transplantation regimens are shown in Table 53.3-1.

GRAFT-VERSUS-LEUKEMIA EFFECT

CLINICAL SIGNIFICANCE

The concept that donor immune cells might make an important contribution to the antileukemic effect of allogeneic BMT was first suggested in the 1950s on the basis of observations in animal

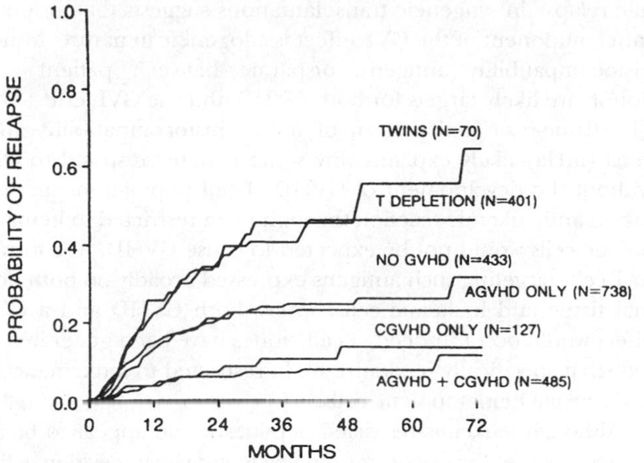

FIGURE 53.3-1. Actuarial probability of relapse after bone marrow transplantation for early leukemia according to type of graft and development of graft-versus-host disease (GVHD). AGVHD, acute GVHD; CGVHD, chronic GVHD. (From ref. 9, with permission.)

models. Mice with leukemia given syngeneic BMTs died of leukemia, whereas mice given allogeneic cells were rescued from leukemia but died from acute GVHD.[50] Subsequently, a large body of evidence began to point toward similar antileukemic effects in humans, mediated through donor cells after allotransplantation. Observations supporting this donor-mediated antileukemic (GVL) effect initially were based on the observation that relapse of leukemia was less likely in patients who developed GVHD after BMT than in those who never developed GVHD.[51] Additional support for the GVL effect included the observation that leukemic relapse occurred more frequently in identical twin transplants and in transplantations in which recipients received T-lymphocyte–depleted marrow for the prevention of GVHD.[52,53] Furthermore, recipients of T-cell–depleted transplants have an increased risk of relapse even after adjusting for GVHD, further supporting an antileukemic effect of donor immune cells separate from acute GVHD. Patients with a history of both acute and chronic GVHD were observed to have the lowest risk of relapse.[9] Data from the International Bone Marrow Transplant Registry showing the relationship of GVHD, T-cell depletion, and the type of allograft to the probability of relapse are shown in Figure 53.3-1.[54] Data from this registry suggest that these effects vary according to the type of leukemia but are most evident in patients with chronic-phase CML undergoing transplantation. Further indirect evidence for the GVL effect includes the observation that up to 50% of patients with CML have small numbers of cells that are Philadelphia-chromosome positive or remain positive for the bcr/abl transcript for months after allogeneic BMT. In the majority of cases, these abnormal cells and bcr/abl transcripts become undetectable over time.[55–58] Additionally, abrupt discontinuation of CSA after detection of disease relapse in CML has been associated with reinduction of cytogenetic remission.[59,60]

Finally, the most compelling evidence supporting the powerful and potentially curative nature of the GVL effect is the observation that complete and durable remissions can be induced by the transfusion of lymphocytes from the marrow donor, without chemotherapy or radiotherapy, in patients with CML who have relapsed after marrow transplantation.[61–66] The efficacy of DLI for the treatment of relapsed leukemia is disease-dependent, with remission induction occurring in a substantially higher percentage of patients with chronic-phase CML than in patients with advanced CML or other acute leukemias.[49] In general, 70% to 80% of patients with cytogenetic or hematologic relapse of CML can be expected to achieve a molecular remission after DLI, with 87% of these patients remaining disease-free at 3 years.[67,68] Remissions usually are not observed until months after DLI, consistent with the time required to expand antileukemic clones (Fig. 53.3-2).

In contrast to the relatively high efficacy of DLI in relapsed chronic-phase CML, only a minority of patients with relapsed acute leukemia achieve remission after this approach. In a report from the European Group for Blood and Marrow Transplant, only 29% of patients with relapsed acute myelogenous leukemia (AML) and none with relapsed ALL (0 of 11) achieved remission after DLI.[67,68] Unlike chronic-phase CML, remission after DLI for advanced-phase CML and acute leukemia appears to be of limited duration, with the majority of responders experiencing relapse within 1 year of treatment. The poor response of accelerated or blast crisis CML to DLI is perhaps due to clonal evolution of the leukemia leading to selective expansion of malignant cells capable of escaping immune recognition.[69]

Disease regression after DLI has also been described in patients with multiple myeloma, CLL, and non-Hodgkin's lymphoma who experience relapse after allotransplantation, although too few have been treated to define the efficacy of this approach in these diseases.[70,71]

The major complication associated with DLI is acute and chronic GVHD. Acute GVHD, which may be severe or life-threatening (grade III or IV) in 15% to 20% of cases, may develop after DLI in up to 70% to 80% of patients.[64–68,72] The propensity for GVHD after DLI is likely affected by the relatively large dose of T lymphocytes that traditionally have been infused (1 to 10 × 10^7 CD3 cells/kg), as well as the fact that these cells are usually given without GVHD prophylaxis. Two approaches to reduce the incidence of GVHD after DLI have been developed. One approach is to selectively infuse lymphocytes depleted of CD8+ T cells: This approach was investigated based on the experience that allografts depleted of CD8+ cells were associated with a low incidence of GVHD without an increased risk of relapse.[73–75] Several nonrandomized trials have shown that DLI depleted of CD8+ cells can reinduce remission, with a rate of GVHD that is lower than that observed with unmanipu-

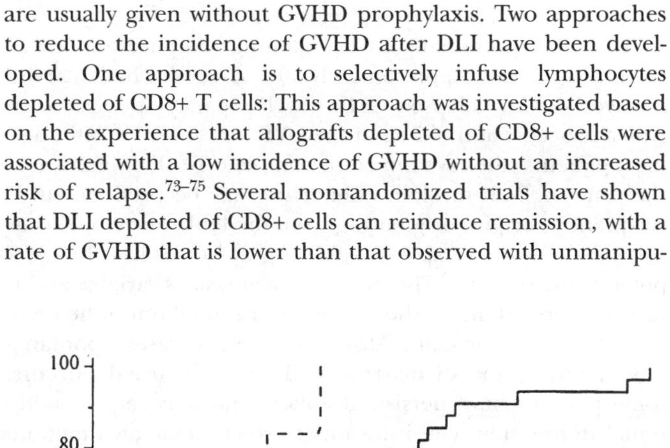

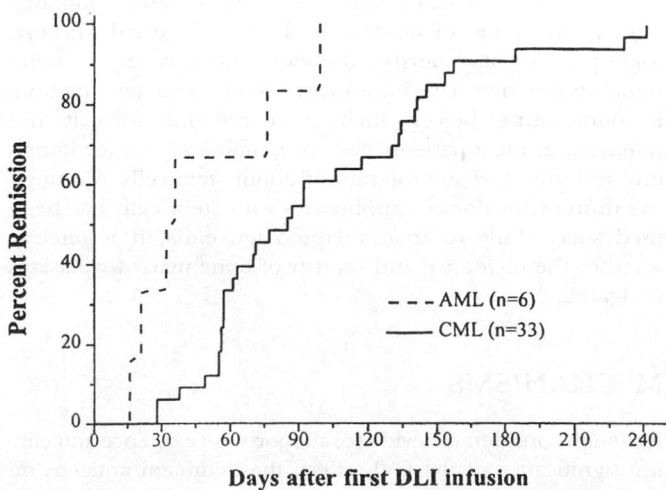

FIGURE 53.3-2. Time to complete remission in acute (AML) and chronic myelogenous leukemia (CML) patients treated with donor lymphocyte infusion (DLI). (From ref. 49, with permission.)

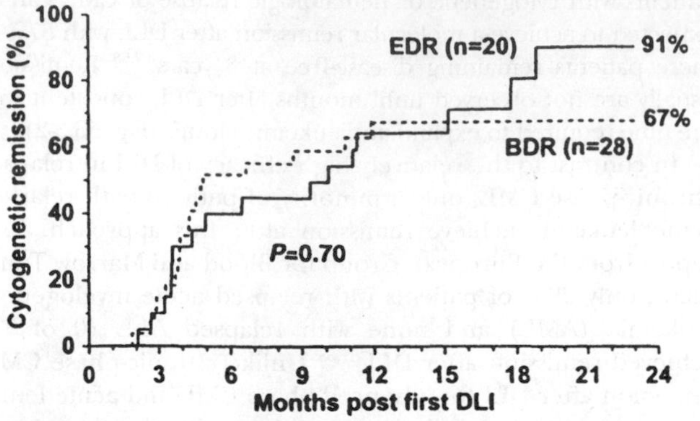

FIGURE 53.3-3. Probability of achieving cytogenetic remission for 48 patients who received escalating-dose (EDR) or bulk-dose infusion regimens (BDR) dated from the first (or only) infusion of donor lymphocytes (DLI). (From ref. 79, with permission.)

lated DLI.[76,77] The other strategy involves the infusion of donor lymphocytes in multiple aliquots, starting at low cell numbers and escalating the dosage at variable intervals until a GVL effect is achieved.[78] This approach is based on the premise that lower T-cell numbers might induce remission while decreasing the risk of GVHD. One trial comparing these two different lymphocyte infusion approaches in patients with relapsed chronic-phase CML revealed a significantly lower incidence of GVHD in the group that received dose-escalating lymphocyte infusions than in the group receiving traditional single "bulk-dose" regimens (10% vs. 44%). Importantly, although the incidence of acute GVHD was extremely low in the escalating-dose group, the GVL effect was preserved, with 91% of these patients achieving a complete remission by 2 years (Fig. 53.3-3).[79]

The other potentially life-threatening complication of DLI is marrow aplasia. Approximately 30% to 40% of patients who receive DLI for relapsed CML develop pancytopenia, which typically occurs at the time of the GVL response.[67,68] Although most patients still have mixed or complete T-cell chimerism at the time of DLI, myeloid chimerism may be predominantly recipient in origin, originating from the leukemic clone, thus leaving the marrow aplastic after a graft-versus-host hematopoietic effect occurs. The duration of aplasia is variable and is directly dependent on the number of residual donor hematopoietic progenitor cells. Although, in most cases, spontaneous reconstitution of marrow by donor cells usually occurs, some patients have persistent aplasia and may require additional donor stem cell infusions to rescue marrow function. Reconditioning before such stem cell infusions is not required, as most patients have predominantly donor immunity and therefore are tolerant of donor stem cells. Although the infusion of donor lymphocytes with stem cells has been used successfully to treat relapsed leukemia, it is unclear whether the incidence and severity of bone marrow aplasia is mitigated.[80]

MECHANISMS

Although considerable evidence supports the existence and clinical significance of the GVL effect, the dominant antigens on leukemic cells and the effector cells mediating the antileukemic effect are not well characterized. The high incidence of leukemic relapse in syngeneic transplantations suggests that a significant component of the GVL effect is allogeneic in nature. Minor histocompatibility antigens, disparate between patient and donor, are likely targets for both GVHD and the GVL effect.[81–87] The tissue-restricted pattern of minor histocompatibility antigens (mHa) likely explains why some patients respond to DLI without the development of GVHD: T-cell populations mediating an antileukemic reaction through mHa restricted to hematopoietic cells would not be expected to cause GVHD, in contrast to T cells targeting such antigens expressed broadly on both normal tissue and leukemic cells, where both GVHD and a GVL effect would occur. Indeed, T-cell clones have been generated *in vitro* that specifically recognize mHa restricted to leukemic cells and normal hematopoietic cells.[81,86]

Although leukemia-restricted peptides would appear to be an attractive target for donor immune cells, convincing evidence has not yet been found to implicate a specific antileukemic effect in GVL. However, the observation that some patients with relapsed leukemia achieve remission after DLI without GVHD lends credence to the notion that GVL may occasionally be a targeted antileukemic process. *In vitro*, it is possible to generate T-cell clones against leukemia cells as well as leukemia-specific peptides. Peptides corresponding to the binding region of P210 BCR/ABL in CML, and the fusion region of the hybrid protein PML/RAR in acute promyelocytic leukemia, can be used to generate T-cell populations with leukemia-specific cytolytic activity.[88–93] Although potentially attractive for targeted immunotherapeutic approaches, no clear evidence supports the hypothesis that these leukemia-specific peptides are a target for GVL.[94]

The nature of the effector cells mediating the GVL effect is not entirely known. In animal models, these effectors often are leukemia- and mouse strain–specific, thus limiting insight into the GVL process in humans. Both CD4+ T helper cells and CD8+ cytotoxic T cells with direct antileukemic activity have been isolated from patients after allogeneic BMT, therefore implicating both as having a role in GVL.[95–100] CD4+ T cells appear to play a particularly important role in the GVL effect in CML. Indeed CD4+ T cells have been generated that are cytolytic to CML cells *in vitro* and can be used successfully to treat relapsed leukemia in patients after BMT.[76,77] Although other cell populations such as natural killer cells, lymphokine-activated killer cells, and $\gamma\delta$ T cells may have antileukemic activity, it is not clear what their overall contribution is to the GVL effect.[101,102] The ability to separate GVL from GVHD will depend on the future delineation of these effector populations and their target antigens.

COMPLICATIONS OF ALLOGENEIC HEMATOPOIETIC STEM CELL TRANSPLANTATION

Allogeneic hematopoietic SCT is associated with a number of complications, many unique to this type of therapy, which can be divided into two general categories: toxicities related to conditioning and toxicities related to the transplantation of an allogeneic immune system into the patient—specifically, graft rejection, GVHD, and infectious complications associated with immunosuppression.

The complications associated with myeloablative doses of chemo/radiotherapy vary in terms of incidence and severity, depending on the intensity and type of agents used in conditioning. These complications may occur as an immediate side effect, at or shortly after administration of the preparative regimen, or in a delayed fashion, years after transplantation. Commonly observed immediate toxicities include nausea and vomiting, mucositis, parotid gland inflammation related to TBI, and neutropenia with associated fever or opportunistic bacterial or invasive fungal infection.

High-dose cyclophosphamide may be associated with hemorrhagic cystitis or, more rarely, rapidly progressive heart failure.[103,104] The routine use of mesna, hydration, and forced diuresis has largely eliminated early hemorrhagic cystitis.[105] In contrast, late hemorrhagic cystitis, occurring beyond 72 hours after cyclophosphamide infusion, remains a continuing problem in allogeneic BMT and usually is viral in origin (polyoma virus BK or adenovirus).[106] High-dose busulfan is associated with grand mal seizures; many busulfan-containing regimens use seizure prophylaxis with phenytoin (Dilantin) or phenobarbital.[107]

Opportunistic infections as a consequence of preparative regimen–induced neutropenia remain a significant complication associated with allogeneic BMT. Most fungal and bacterial infections originate from microorganisms colonizing the skin, oral cavity, perianal area, or gastrointestinal or respiratory tract. The most common life-threatening infections occur during the neutropenic period and involve gram-negative and aerobic gram-positive bacteria. These pathogens gain entry into the host through indwelling vascular catheters or as a consequence of the breakdown of gastrointestinal mucosa related to high-dose chemo/radiotherapy. Decontamination of the gastrointestinal tract with nonabsorbable antibiotics such as neomycin or vancomycin have met with mixed success, with poor patient compliance being a major drawback to this approach.[108,109] Such prophylactic oral quinolones as ciprofloxacin and norfloxacin appear to decrease the incidence of febrile neutropenia and gram-negative infections, although possibly at the expense of more episodes of gram-positive bacteremia.[110,111]

Candida and *Aspergillus* species are the most common fungal pathogens, frequently causing infection during periods of neutropenia or systemic corticosteroid use for GVHD. Oral triazoles, such as fluconazole, have been shown in randomized trials to decrease the incidence of opportunistic candidal infections but have no impact on the incidence of infections with resistant species such as *Aspergillus* or *Candida krusei*.[112,113] It is unclear whether the shortened duration of absolute neutropenia associated with the use of recombinant hematopoietic growth factors [i.e., granulocyte colony-stimulating factor (G-CSF)] will lead to a decrease in the incidence of infections by these opportunistic pathogens.

VENOOCCLUSIVE DISEASE

One of the most serious life-threatening complications of dose-intensive chemo/radiotherapy is hepatic VOD. VOD produces a clinical syndrome of jaundice, tender hepatomegaly, and unexplained weight gain or ascites.[114,115] Clinically evident VOD occurs in approximately 30% of allogeneic BMT patients conditioned with busulfan-containing regimens, with approximately 25% of those affected having severe life-threatening disease leading to progressive liver failure, hepatic encephalopathy, or hepatorenal syndrome. The exact pathogenesis of VOD is unknown, although the earliest event is believed to be endothelial damage due to BMT conditioning, leading to fibrinogen and collagen deposition in vessel walls at the interface of hepatic sinusoids and terminal venules, which ultimately become obstructed. Damage to zone three hepatocytes also is present. Predisposing factors for VOD include a history of liver disease, advanced age, elevated liver enzymes before transplantation, dose intensity of the conditioning regimen, presence of acute GVHD, and transplants from alternative donors such as matched, unrelated donors or haploidentical donors.[116–118] The diagnosis of VOD is based on the presence of clinical criteria (jaundice, tender hepatomegaly, and unexplained weight gain or ascites); there is a 90% correlation between the presence of all three criteria and a histologic confirmation by liver biopsy.[119]

Therapy for established VOD is unsatisfactory and consists mostly of measures to support renal function, fluid balance, and coagulation status. Recombinant tissue plasminogen activator (tPA) and prostaglandin E_1 have had mixed success, making it unclear what, if any, role these agents should play in the treatment of established disease.[120–123] In a single-institution trial, defibrotide, a polydeoxyribonucleotide with activity in several vascular disorders, was used to treat patients with severe VOD after SCT. The drug was well tolerated and showed promising efficacy, with 42% of patients having complete resolution of VOD, warranting further investigation of this agent.[124] The therapeutic drug monitoring of busulfan, with appropriate dose adjustments, appears to be useful in reducing the incidence of VOD in patients receiving this agent. Data regarding pharmacologic prophylaxis against VOD have been contradictory. One double-blind, randomized trial showed a significant reduction in the incidence of VOD in patients taking ursodiol prophylaxis as compared to those taking placebo (50% vs. 15%). Ursodiol was well tolerated and may prove particularly useful as prophylaxis in patients defined to be at high risk for VOD.[125]

PULMONARY COMPLICATIONS

Pulmonary complications occur frequently after allogeneic BMT and may be related to infectious agents, diffuse alveolar hemorrhage, or pulmonary edema, or may have an idiopathic origin. Common infectious etiologies include *Aspergillus* species or other fungi, respiratory syncytial virus, and CMV. Late pneumonia from *Pneumocystis carinii* may occur up to 1 year after transplantation and usually is related to prolonged CD4+ lymphopenia associated with T-cell depletion of the allograft or GVHD. Interstitial pneumonitis (IP), characterized by fever, hypoxia, and diffuse pulmonary infiltrates, occurs in 20% to 40% of patients, usually within the first 3 months of transplantation, and may be lethal in up to one-half of cases.[126–130] Nearly 90% of the cases of IP either are related to CMV infection or have an idiopathic origin [idiopathic interstitial pneumonitis (IIP)].[131] The incidence of early CMV pneumonitis appears to have decreased significantly in the 1990s through the use of both effective prophylactic regimens (intravenous immunoglobulin and ganciclovir) and better methods for early detection of CMV reactivation. Patient-specific risk factors for IP include older age, prior history of exposure to pulmonary toxic drugs such as bleomycin, history of acute or chronic GVHD, dose intensity of the conditioning regimen, or use of TBI.[126–130,132,133] Regimens that use a lower dose rate or total dose of TBI, as well as hyperfractionated TBI, may be associated with a lower risk of IP.

Bronchoscopy with bronchoalveolar lavage should be used in all patients with IP to differentiate IIP from infectious causes or diffuse alveolar hemorrhage. Empiric use of anti-CMV agents such as ganciclovir or foscarnet should be considered when bronchoalveolar lavage is not feasible. Although evidence exists supporting the efficacy of high-dose steroids in patients with diffuse alveolar hemorrhage, their effectiveness in the treatment of IIP remains equivocal.[134,135]

LATE COMPLICATIONS

The delayed complications associated with allogeneic SCT depend on patient age at transplantation and are a consequence of the effects of long-term damage to normal tissues by either the preparative regimen or chronic GVHD. These effects include growth retardation, infertility, endocrine failure, cataracts, renal insufficiency, restrictive pulmonary defects, neurocognitive defects, and secondary malignancies.[136,137] The use of TBI in the conditioning regimen seems to be the major factor associated with secondary malignancies.[138–140] On long-term follow-up of 1036 patients undergoing BMT for a wide range of malignant and nonmalignant conditions, a 12.6% incidence of secondary neoplasms was reported at 15 years, a rate that was 3.8 times higher than that for an age-matched control population.[141] The most frequently observed secondary neoplasms were of the skin and oral cavity, with older patient age and use of CSA for chronic GVHD being significant risk factors for new malignant disease.

EPSTEIN-BARR VIRUS LYMPHOPROLIFERATIVE DISORDER

Posttransplantation Epstein-Barr virus (EBV)–associated lymphoproliferative disorder (LPD) represents an aggressive and potentially fatal B-cell lymphoid proliferation that occurs after 5% to 30% of allogeneic transplantations. This lymphoma originates from B cells infected with EBV, typically of donor origin, and usually stems from a deficiency of EBV-specific cytotoxic T cells associated with the use of immunosuppressive drugs or T-cell depletion of the allograft.[142–144] EBV LPD can be successfully treated by infusing unmanipulated donor leukocytes that contain cytotoxic T cells presensitized to EBV.[145] One trial in children receiving T-cell-depleted transplants from HLA-mismatched donors demonstrated that the prophylactic infusion of *ex vivo*–generated EBV-specific T cells can successfully prevent EBV LPD without causing acute GVHD.[146] Others have shown that B-cell depletion of the allograft can also be used to prevent this disorder.[147] The use of Rituximab (Rituxan), a monoclonal antibody to the B-cell antigen CD20, has recently been shown to be an alternative strategy that can successfully treat established LPD.[148]

GRAFT-VERSUS-HOST DISEASE

GVHD is the consequence of immunocompetent donor T cells targeting recipient tissues that possess antigens absent from the donor.[149–151] The major target tissues of GVHD are the skin, liver, and gastrointestinal tract, although other tissues may be involved. The diagnosis of acute GVHD may be based on one or a myriad of characteristic clinical and laboratory findings.[152–155] Skin manifestations include an erythematous maculopapular rash often involving the palms and soles and, under severe circumstances, may be associated with desquamation. Hepatic involvement is characterized by a rise in alkaline phosphatase and total bilirubin, often in association with a mild to moderate increase in hepatic transaminases. Gastrointestinal GVHD predominantly involves the distal small bowel and colon and clinically is associated with cramping abdominal pain and watery diarrhea, which may be voluminous and bloody under severe circumstances. Endoscopic findings are variable and may range from mild bowel edema to total denuding of intestinal mucosa; colonic biopsy usually reveals classic pathologic features showing crypt cell necrosis with apoptotic bodies and lymphocytic infiltrates, although disease involvement can be patchy and missed on random biopsy. Upper gastrointestinal involvement, although more rare, may be associated with recurrent nausea, vomiting, and dyspepsia.[156] Traditionally, acute GVHD has been divided into severity grades I through IV, depending on the extent of skin involvement, volume of diarrhea, or level of bilirubin elevation (Table 53.3-2).[157]

Donor T cells are the principle mediators of GVHD. In an HLA-mismatched setting, CD8+ T cells may target major histocompatibility complex (MHC) class I mismatched antigens,

TABLE 53.3-2. Glucksberg Clinical Stage and Grade of Acute Graft-Versus-Host Disease

Stage	*Skin*	*Liver*	*Intestinal Tract*
1	Maculopapular rash <25% of body surface	Bilirubin 34–50 μmol/L	>500 mL diarrhea/d
2	Maculopapular rash 25–50% of body surface	Bilirubin 51–102 μmol/L	>1000 mL diarrhea/d
3	Generalized erythroderma	Bilirubin 103–225 μmol/L	>1500 mL diarrhea/d
4	Generalized erythroderma with bullous formation and desquamation	Bilirubin >255 μmol/L	Severe abdominal pain with or without ileus

Grade	*Degree of Organ Involvement*
I	Stage 1–2 skin rash; no gastrointestinal tract involvement; no liver involvement; no decrease in clinical performance
II	Stage 1–3 skin rash; stage 1 gastrointestinal tract involvement or stage 1 liver involvement (or both); mild decrease in clinical performance
III	Stage 2–3 skin rash; stage 2–3 gastrointestinal tract involvement or stage 2–4 liver involvement (or both); marked decrease in clinical performance
IV	Similar to grade III with stage 2–4 organ involvement; extreme decrease in clinical performance

(From refs. 152 and 157, with permission.)

while CD4+ T cells are responsible for the recognition and targeting of MHC class II mismatched antigens.[158–162] The antigens that are disparate between patient and donor and serve as a target for GVHD in HLA-identical sibling transplants are referred to as *minor histocompatibility antigens* (mHa). Relatively few mHa have been characterized to date, although there is increasing evidence to suggest that the degree of disparity between recipient and donor mHa is a major determinant for the development of both acute and chronic GVHD.[163–166] The development of GVHD is a multistep process in which recipient tissues are recognized as foreign by the donor immune system, followed by the activation and expansion of GVHD effector populations, ultimately leading to T-cell–mediated direct cytotoxic damage of target tissues.

GVHD remains a significant contributor to transplant-related morbidity and mortality. The incidence and severity of GVHD is determined by a number of variables, including degrees of HLA disparity between patient and donor, use of a T-cell–replete versus T-cell–depleted allograft, patient age, and the agents used in GVHD prophylaxis.[167–169] Furthermore, acute GVHD after T-cell–replete allogeneic BMT often is most severe within the first month after transplantation and appears to be exacerbated by conditioning-induced cytokine release from damaged recipient tissues. In general, the incidence of clinically significant acute GVHD (grades II through IV) in patients undergoing a T-cell–replete allogeneic SCT (from an HLA-identical sibling) in which conventional GVHD prophylaxis is used (CSA and methotrexate) is on the order of 30% to 40%, with approximately 15% of patients developing severe grade III or IV disease.[167] In recipients of partially matched related donor or partially matched unrelated donor transplants, acute GVHD occurs more frequently, affecting more than 70% of patients.[170]

The two most common methods for preventing acute GVHD include the use of prophylactic immunosuppressive agents and the use of allografts from which donor T cells have been depleted. Although the combined use of CSA and methotrexate has been found to be superior to either agent alone in the prevention of GVHD, the addition of prednisone to these agents does not appear to offer any additional benefit.[171–173] In both HLA-identical sibling and unrelated transplantations, T-cell depletion is the most effective method for preventing GVHD but is associated with an increased risk of graft rejection, opportunistic viral infection, and leukemic relapse. Although the risk of disease relapse is leukemia-specific, a large retrospective analysis from the International Bone Marrow Transplant Registry showed clear evidence that T-cell depletion was associated with a lower disease-free survival in CML.[174] Novel methods of T-cell depletion that appear to decrease this risk of acute GVHD without increasing the risk of disease relapse include the use of allografts that have been selectively depleted of CD8+ T cells and the use of T-cell–depleted transplants followed by a delayed infusion of donor lymphocytes months after the original transplantation to preserve the GVL effect.[74,75,175]

The mainstay of therapy for the treatment of acute GVHD is corticosteroid therapy, usually in association with CSA or FK506. Approximately 40% to 60% of patients with grade II to IV GVHD can be expected to respond to these agents.[176–178] One randomized trial of low-dose (2 mg/kg) versus high-dose (10 mg/kg) methylprednisolone for acute GVHD showed no difference in response rates with either regimen.[179] Response to steroids appears to predict survival, with steroid-refractory patients being at a significantly higher risk of transplant-related mortality than steroid-responsive patients. Antithymocyte globulin (ATG) has been used with minimal success in patients with steroid-refractory disease, and it appears to be inferior to steroids or CSA as an initial therapy for acute GVHD.[180] Other approaches that have shown early promise for the treatment of steroid-resistant disease include the use of the immunosuppressive drug mycophenolate mofetil, monoclonal antibodies that target a number of different T-cell antigens, and extracorporeal photopheresis.[181–187]

Chronic GVHD occurs in 15% to 50% of long-term survivors of allogeneic BMT and typically manifests with symptoms 3 months to 2 years after transplantation. The etiology of chronic GVHD appears to be related to alloreactive T cells that infiltrate and damage tissues and cause abnormalities in immune regulation.[188–190] The greatest risk factor for chronic GVHD is a prior history of acute GVHD, although older patient age, use of mismatched or unrelated donors, a history of DLI for relapsed malignancy, and use of peripheral blood stem transplants also appear to increase the risk.[191,192] Patients with chronic GVHD often are severely immunocompromised, either as a consequence of the immunosuppressive therapy used to treat the disorder or from the underlying immune dysregulation associated with the disease process. Chronic GVHD is lethal in approximately 20% to 30% of cases, with death being predominantly related to infectious causes.[193] Patients with a particularly poor prognosis include those with hepatic involvement or thrombocytopenia.

Chronic GVHD is traditionally classified as either limited or extensive, limited disease being defined as localized skin involvement with or without mild hepatic involvement and extensive disease being generalized skin involvement with or without other target organ involvement. The characteristic clinical manifestations are numerous and include lichenoid or sclerodermatous skin involvement, hepatic cholestasis, friable nails, dry eyes (Sjögren's syndrome), fasciitis, xerostomia, lichenoid buccal changes, bronchiolitis obliterans, vaginal dryness, serositis, malabsorption, diarrhea, gastrointestinal dysmotility, and pancytopenia. Treatment depends on the extent of disease. Systemic disease typically is treated with alternate-day CSA or FK506 and low-dose corticosteroids.[194] Patients not responding to standard therapy often benefit from alternative therapies, including mycophenolate mofetil, psoralen and ultraviolet A for skin involvement, thalidomide, total lymphoid irradiation and, more recently, extracorporeal photopheresis.[186,195–197] As infections are the main cause of death, prophylaxis for organisms such as *P carinii* and encapsulated bacteria usually is warranted, particularly in those patients receiving systemic immunosuppressive therapy.

GRAFT FAILURE

Failure to achieve or maintain sustained donor hematopoietic engraftment after allogeneic transplantation is referred to as *graft failure.* Graft failure may manifest as persistent neutropenia, without evidence of engraftment (primary graft failure) or as initial engraftment followed by a delayed fall in blood counts (late or secondary graft failure). *Graft rejection* is the term used to describe graft failure that occurs as a consequence of the active rejection of donor hematopoietic cells by residual immunocompetent host cells. Clinically, graft rejection manifests as transient donor engraftment followed by a lymphocytosis of recipient origin, which ultimately leads to the rejection of donor hematopoietic cells and pancytopenia or, in some cases, autologous hematopoietic recovery. The mediators of graft rejection include natural killer cells or residual recipient T cells recognizing donor-mismatched MHC molecules or, in an HLA-matched setting, mHa.[198–200]

Primary graft failure should be suspected in all transplant patients who remain pancytopenic for longer than 3 to 4 weeks. It is associated with a significant risk of death from hemorrhage or infection. Although graft failure occurs in fewer than 2% of patients undergoing allogeneic SCT from an HLA-identical sibling, the incidence increases for recipients of T-cell–depleted transplants, particularly those from HLA-mismatched or unrelated donors.[201–203] Other risk factors for graft rejection include the infusion of low stem cell numbers (i.e., $<1 \times 10^6$ CD34+ cells/kg), history of multiple blood transfusions, HLA disparity between the patient and donor, use of low-intensity or dose-reduced conditioning regimens, and transplantation for severe aplastic anemia.[204,205] Although graft rejection is more common after BMT for aplastic anemia, the addition of TBI or ATG to the conditioning regimen (usually high-dose cyclophosphamide) has decreased the incidence from 30% to less than 10%.[206]

Differentiating graft failure from pancytopenia related to other causes, including marrow suppression from infection, medications, or chronic GVHD, is important. Furthermore, it is important to give early consideration for a second donor stem cell infusion, given the difficult logistics of collecting more donor cells. Non–immunologically mediated graft failure has been successfully treated with hematopoietic growth factors such as granulocyte-macrophage colony-stimulating factor or G-CSF, followed by a second infusion of donor stem cells in those who fail to experience hematopoietic recovery.[207–209] Graft rejection, in which donor hematopoietic cells are no longer detectable by cytogenetic or molecular methods, requires repeat conditioning to eradicate these host "rejection" cells, followed by the infusion of a second donor allograft. Although the outcome in patients requiring a second donor marrow infusion for graft failure often is poor, successful and sustained donor engraftment has been reported in 57% of primary and 37% of secondary graft failure patients.[210]

CYTOMEGALOVIRUS INFECTION

CMV is a member of the herpesvirus family and may be associated with serious and life-threatening pathology after allogeneic BMT.[211,212] Most patients who develop CMV disease do so as a consequence of viral reactivation from a previous primary infection. The cellular immune system plays an important role in the suppression of viral reactivation. Disruption of cellular immunity associated with T-cell depletion, GVHD, or immunosuppressive therapy can lead to CMV reactivation and subsequent disease. The clinical features of CMV disease include pneumonitis, hepatitis, upper gastrointestinal involvement, and colitis. Reactivation tends to occur 3 weeks to 100 days after transplantation and is most strongly associated with acute GVHD and pretransplantation seropositivity of the recipient to CMV. Prior to the development of reactivation screening techniques and prophylactic drug regimens, CMV pneumonitis was observed in 10% to 30% of patients and was fatal in 50% to 90% of cases.[213]

Effective prevention can be achieved through the use of CMV-negative or leukocyte-filtered blood products (in seronegative patient-donor pairs) and prophylactic intravenous immunoglobulin and ganciclovir.[214–218] As CMV will never reactivate in 40% to 50% of patients, an alternative and effective approach is to reserve ganciclovir use for patients with detectable viral reactivation, either by polymerase chain reaction methods or by immunofluorescent techniques designed to detect viral antigen on the surface of neutrophils (CMV antigenemia).[219] Both techniques allow for early detection and treatment of CMV reactivation long before symptoms develop. Indeed, these early detection methods have dramatically decreased the incidence and mortality associated with CMV disease.

A recently investigated alternative to CMV drug prophylaxis is to infuse CMV-specific cytotoxic lymphocytes generated from donor cells *in vitro*, early after T-cell–depleted transplantation.[220] This cell-based approach for the prevention of CMV reactivation has shown early success and may serve as a paradigm for future protocols that use tumor-specific T cells to prevent disease relapse.

SOURCES OF ALLOGENEIC HEMATOPOIETIC STEM CELLS

ALLOGENEIC PERIPHERAL BLOOD STEM CELL TRANSPLANTS

Based on the success of autologous peripheral blood stem cell (PBSC) transplants, allogeneic transplantation regimens, which use peripheral blood–derived stem cells as apposed to marrow cells, have been used with increasing frequency since the mid-1990s, with early favorable clinical outcome.[221–227] The recombinant growth factor G-CSF usually is given to donors for 4 to 6 consecutive days (10 μg/kg/d) to mobilize hematopoietic progenitors into the circulation, followed by one or two leukapheresis procedures. G-CSF-mobilized PBSC transplants contain higher numbers of progenitor cells than do marrow grafts, usually in the range of 5 to 10×10^6 CD34+ cells/kg. Although the use of lower doses of G-CSF is associated with a decreased incidence of cytokine-related side effects, the number of CD34+ cells mobilized into circulation may be lower, necessitating additional leukapheresis procedures.[228]

PBSC transplants have potential advantages for both the donor and the patient. Donors do not require hospitalization and are spared the pain and potential risks of general anesthesia associated with marrow harvesting, although the long-term consequences of G-CSF administration remain unknown. Also, PBSC grafts contain higher numbers of hematopoietic progenitor cells, natural killer cells, and T cells, as compared with bone marrow.[229] Engraftment, therefore, usually is faster, and the GVL effect may be enhanced.[230] Initial concerns that the 10- to 20-fold higher T-cell dose in peripheral blood allografts might be associated with a greater risk of acute GVHD have been dispelled. Indeed, two trials comparing allogeneic bone marrow to PBSC transplantation have shown that PBSCs are associated with a shorter period of neutropenia and red blood cell and platelet transfusion dependence, with an equal probability of acute and chronic GVHD.[231,232] The failure to observe a correlation between the number of T lymphocytes in the allograft and GVHD might be related to the polarizing of donor T cells by G-CSF to a type 2 (suppressor) cytokine profile.

A phase III trial of allogeneic transplantation in 138 patients with hematologic malignancies found that PBSC grafts were associated with more rapid engraftment and better disease-free and overall survival than marrow grafts, without a greater risk of acute GVHD.[233] Neutrophil engraftment occurred 6 days earlier (day 15 vs. day 21), and platelet recovery occurred 8 days earlier (day 13 vs. day 21) among those receiving PBSC transplants. The incidence of acute grade III or IV GVHD was equal between groups, occurring in 16% of PBSC graft and 13% of bone marrow graft recipients. The cumulative incidence of chronic GVHD was also similar, occurring in 38% of PBSC and 28% of marrow recipients. This study provided the first evidence that PBSC transplantation may be associated with a survival advantage over conventional marrow transplantation. Two-year survival in the PBSC group was 71%, as compared to 51% in the marrow group, a statistically significant difference that led to the early termination of this trial. These, as well as the previously mentioned benefits, make it likely that PBSC transplantation will replace BMT in the allogeneic setting.

UMBILICAL CORD BLOOD TRANSPLANTATION

Umbilical cord blood is a new and promising source of hematopoietic progenitor cells for transplantation in both malignant and nonmalignant disorders. The realization that cord blood, obtained from the placenta after delivery, contained long-term repopulating progenitor cells led to its investigational use as a source of stem cells for allogeneic transplantation.[234–237] Cord blood has been shown to contain primitive hematopoietic stem cells with remarkable proliferative potential, which may overcome the limitation of relatively low absolute cell numbers.[238–240] Also, the immature lymphocytes in cord blood appear to decrease the risk and severity of acute and chronic GVHD, potentially permitting greater HLA disparity and expanding donor availability.

In a trial evaluating umbilical cord transplants in 44 children with malignant and nonmalignant hematologic diseases receiving grafts from an HLA-identical or single-antigen-mismatched donor, 85% engrafted and only 3% developed grade II or worse acute GVHD.[235] A subsequent multiinstitutional study from Europe reported similar engraftment rates in 78 recipients of cord blood from related donors, with acute GVHD occurring in 9% of the recipients of HLA-matched cord blood and in 50% of the recipients of HLA-mismatched cord blood.[241] Neutrophil engraftment was favorably associated with a younger patient age (younger than 6 years) and weight (<20 kg) and occurred in 85% of patients receiving 37 million or more mononuclear cells per kilogram of recipient body weight. In the recipients of unrelated cord blood, neutrophil engraftment occurred in 94% of those who received 37 million or more mononuclear cells per kilogram, with only 32% of patients developing grade II or worse GVHD.

These early successes have led to the creation of an increasing number of umbilical cord blood banks worldwide. However, graft failure, which is most closely associated with patient size, age, and low cord stem cell doses, remains a significant problem that will likely limit the applicability of this approach in adults.

UNRELATED DONORS

Although allogeneic hematopoietic SCT is a potentially curative modality for a number of otherwise fatal malignancies, only one-third or so of patients have access to an HLA-identical sibling. The growing demand for donors has led to research in the development of techniques for the use of alternative sources of stem cells. The knowledge that the HLA system played a critical role in transplantation outcomes led to the successful use of HLA-matched unrelated donors (MUDs) and subsequent establishment of volunteer donor registries.[242–245] More than 5 million typed volunteer donors have been registered worldwide, and it is estimated that nearly 70% of white patients will have an HLA-A, -B and -DR-matched unrelated donor.[246] Because of the increasing availability of volunteer unrelated donors, it is anticipated that more than 2000 MUD transplantations will be performed in the year 2000.[247] Nonetheless, finding a suitable unrelated donor remains a significant problem for many patients, particularly ethnic and racial minority individuals.

Early MUD transplantations involved donors who were chosen on the basis of serologic HLA typing. The subsequent development of high-resolution molecular HLA typing revealed that many of these serologically typed donors often were mismatched, likely contributing to the increased risk of graft rejection and severe GVHD observed in these trials.[248] The results of extensive published data on unrelated donor transplantations reveal engraftment rates of 85% to 100%, grade II or worse acute GVHD in 21% to 98%, chronic GVHD in 50% to 74%, and disease-free survival rates of between 1% and 74%.[247,249–252] This wide range in outcome is explained mostly by variations in patient populations, transplantation methods, and HLA typing techniques. The use of molecular-based typing has been associated with a significant improvement in transplantation outcome, including a decrease in life-threatening acute and chronic GVHD.[253,254] Furthermore, typing beyond HLA-A, -B, and -DR loci may be of further benefit, as other MHC antigens appear to have a significant impact on transplantation outcome.[256,257]

More precise HLA typing has also increased the difficulty of finding a completely matched donor. T-cell depletion of MUD allografts is associated with a decrease in severe acute and chronic GVHD, although there appears to be no beneficial impact on overall survival.[258] There is some evidence, however, that survival may be better in the recipients of MUD transplants containing higher stem cell doses.[259] This observation has stimulated interest in the development of transplants that use higher total CD34+ cell doses—for instance, through the use of G-CSF-mobilized PBSC allografting. Whether this approach will improve the outcome of unrelated transplantations, particularly in terms of prolonging patient survival, remains to be determined.[255] Future trials that optimize donor selection, conditioning regimens, and GVHD prophylaxis will be required to improve the outcome of MUD transplantations.

MISMATCHED RELATED DONORS

The availability of haploidentical ("half-matched") related donors has led to the use of mismatched family members as an alternative source of stem cells for those patients who lack an HLA-identical sibling.[259–261] The majority of patients with living family members would be expected to have a relative who could serve as a partially mismatched donor. These donors may actually have a closer histocompatibility profile than MUDs, as the shared donor haplotype is genetically identical to that of the patient, which may be associated with better matching of mHa. Furthermore, potential family donors can usually be identified quickly and usually are more readily available than are MUDs. The number of mismatched MHC antigens in the patient is conventionally used to define the degree of mismatch and may range from three (haploidentical) to zero antigens, depending on the number of phenotypically shared antigens coming from the mismatched haplotype.[247]

Graft rejection, GVHD, and ineffective immunity leading to fatal opportunistic infection are the major immune-mediated complications associated with HLA disparity; the greater the HLA disparity, the higher these risks.[262,263] Early as well as recent trials comparing outcome in patients receiving partially mismatched related versus matched sibling donor allografts showed that engraftment, GVHD, and survival were inferior in the recipients of partially mismatched transplants.[264,265] More intensified conditioning regimens have resulted in better engraftment at the expense of more regimen-related organ toxicity.

Severe GVHD exceeded 50% in early trials using unmanipulated allografts, with T-cell doses in the allograft correlating with the probability of developing severe GVHD.[266,267] T-cell depletion, as in matched unrelated transplants, is associated with a significant decrease in the incidence of severe GVHD, although the incidence of graft rejection is increased.[268–270] Through the use of modified conditioning regimens and more effective T-cell depletion methods, several groups have begun to report improved outcome using mismatched family donors. Henslee-Downey et al.[271,272] were the first to report similar 3-year disease-free survivals in patients with lymphoblastic leukemia using partially matched related donors versus matched sibling donors (39% vs. 37%). Subsequently, other investigators have reported regimens with modified conditioning and T-cell depletion techniques associated with a high rate of donor engraftment and a low risk of GVHD, with long-term disease-free survivals in the range of 20% to 40%.[273,274] These results are significant, as most patients treated in these trials had advanced, high-risk hematologic malignancies associated with poor transplantation outcome, even in a matched sibling setting.

Another recently explored approach involves the induction of donor T-cell anergy to recipient alloantigens. This technique involves *ex vivo* culturing of haploidentical donor marrow with recipient lymphocytes in the presence of CTLA-4 immunoglobulin to inhibit the "second signal" required for T-cell activation. Donor T cells in this environment do not receive costimulation and are therefore rendered "tolerant" to recipient alloantigens. Although only a small number of haploidentical transplantations have been performed using this approach, early results have been encouraging, without the occurrence of graft rejection or death from acute GVHD.[275]

Although opportunistic infections and disease relapse remain problematic, modifications in this procedure have demonstrated that the use of full haplotype mismatched donors can be tolerated and is a viable transplantation alternative in patients lacking matched sibling donors. The improvement in haploidentical transplants will likely lead to randomized trials comparing partially mismatched related donors to MUDs to discern which alternative stem cell source is preferable.

NONMYELOABLATIVE ALLOGENEIC STEM CELL TRANSPLANTATION

Allogeneic hematopoietic SCT using high-dose, myeloablative chemo/radiotherapy is associated with a high incidence of treatment-related complications and a 20% to 35% risk of transplant-related mortality. Debilitated or older patients with hematologic malignancies are at particularly high risk, thus limiting the applicability of this potentially curative treatment modality to relatively younger patients with a good performance status.[276,277] The desirable antitumor effects of dose-intensive conditioning often are offset by their substantial and potentially life-threatening toxicities. A greater understanding and appreciation of the powerful and potentially curative nature of the GVL effect led to the notion that GVL alone, without intensive cytoreductive therapy, might be sufficient to obtain long-term control of hematologic malignancies. Patients with relapsed leukemia after allogeneic transplantation whose disease is induced into remission after DLI lend the greatest credence to this concept.

Subsequent to these observations, a number of investigators began to explore the concept of using low-intensity conditioning regimens, immunosuppressive enough to permit engraftment of the donor immune system for the generation of GVL effects while sparing patients the toxicities associated with myeloablative therapy.[278–280] Although NST is still in its infancy, a number of institutions investigating a variety of nonmyeloablative approaches have reported remarkable early success.[281–284] Despite the use of low-intensity conditioning, engraftment rates have been high, and long-term remissions, induced purely through a donor immune-mediated antitumor effect, have been observed in a variety of different hematologic and nonhematologic malignancies.[285] Importantly, regimen-related toxicity and mortality appear to be low, thus expanding eligibility for allogeneic transplantation to include older or debilitated patients, as well as allowing for exploration of graft-versus-tumor (GVT) effects in other treatment-refractory or incurable malignancies. Furthermore, the majority of late side effects attributed to myeloablative conditioning, including growth retardation, sterility, endocrinopathies, cataracts, and secondary malignancies, will likely be avoided using nonmyeloablative transplants.

NONMYELOABLATIVE CONDITIONING REGIMENS

Although a variety of low-intensity conditioning regimens have been explored, they are all, by definition, nonmyeloablative, as recipient hematopoietic stem cells are not eradicated, allowing for the possibility of autologous hematopoietic recovery. Two features are common to all these regimens: First, they avoid acute and chronic toxicities of dose-intensive chemo/radiotherapy by using a relatively low-intensity nontoxic preparative regimen and, second, they attempt to induce sufficient host immunosuppression to allow for engraftment of the donor immune system.

The minimum amount of immunosuppression required to allow for donor engraftment is unlikely to be defined, as it depends on multiple variables, including the competence of the patient's immune system (related to the amount and intensity of prior therapy), degree of patient-donor HLA and mHa disparity, donor immunocompetence, and the dose of T cells in the allograft. Nonetheless, a number of different conditioning regimens with variable degrees of intensity have been used successfully to establish donor engraftment with minimum toxicity, including regimens consisting of purine analogs in combination with alkylating agents, low-dose TBI alone, or thymic irradiation in combination with cyclophosphamide with or without ATG.

Based on results from canine preclinical trials, Storb et al.[286,287] pioneered a novel NST approach that uses low-dose TBI (200 cGy) as well as pre- and posttransplantation immunosuppression with CSA and mycophenolate mofetil to prevent both graft rejection and GVHD. This regimen usually achieves a state of recipient-donor mixed chimerism, which can serve as a platform for the subsequent infusion of donor lymphocytes to enhance GVL effects. Although a heterogeneous population of patients has been treated with a variety of different regimens, conditioning associated toxicity and mortality appear to be significantly lower than with conventional myeloablative approaches. Because host hematopoietic elements are not ablated, recovering myeloid cells are usually of both recipient and donor origin (mixed chimerism). This state of mixed chimerism has both beneficial and negative effects on transplantation outcome. Mixed chimerism is capable of inducing donor and recipient tolerance, thus preventing the development of acute GVHD.[288,289] However, mixed chimerism also is associated with an increased risk of graft failure, and the tolerance that it induces may inhibit beneficial GVL effects. These negative aspects of mixed chimerism can be overcome by infusing donor lymphocytes, which can shift chimerism from a mixed to a complete donor type, thus avoiding tolerance and enhancing the GVL effect.

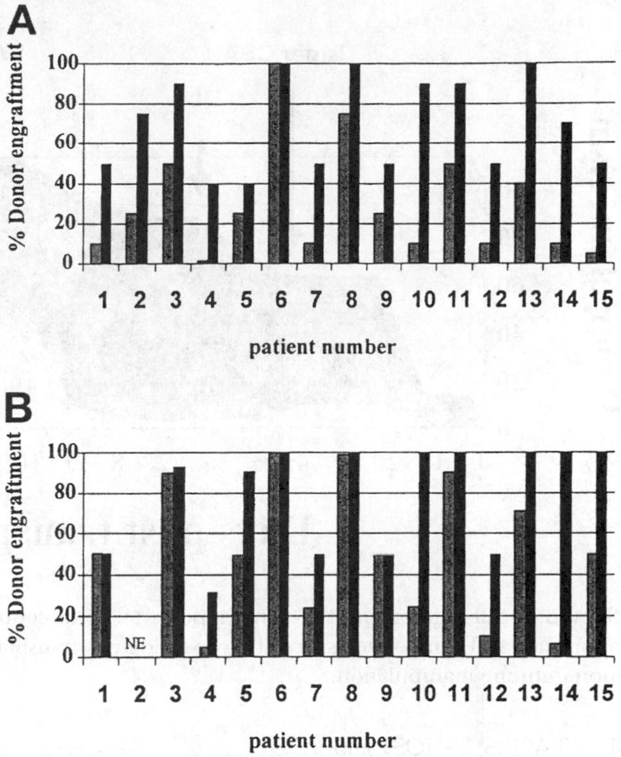

FIGURE 53.3-4. Percentage of donor T (CD3+) cells (*black bars*) and myeloid (CD14+ and CD15+) cells (*gray bars*) in 15 individual patients on days 14 **(A)** and 30 **(B)** after transplantation. NE, nonevaluable. (From ref. 289, with permission.)

NONMYELOABLATIVE TRANSPLANTATION TOXICITY

Conditioning-induced toxicity is relatively mild with nonmyeloablative regimens as compared to myeloablative approaches (see Table 53.3-1). Most patients tolerate the preparative regimen well, without the occurrence of mucositis or requirement for total parenteral nutrition. VOD occurs infrequently, is usually mild, and is observed predominantly with the use of regimens that contain busulfan.[279] Although most patients become pancytopenic, the occurrence of partial autologous hematopoietic recovery appears to shorten the overall depth and duration of neutropenia while reducing platelet and red blood cell transfusion requirements. Most trials have reported transplantation-related mortality rates in the range of 10% to 15%, which is remarkably low given the advanced age and poor performance status of the majority of these patients. Some low-intensity protocols, particularly those that use low-dose TBI alone, appear ideally suited for outpatient use.[286] NST is too new to make any conclusions regarding long-term complications, although it is reasonable to assume that growth retardation, sterility, and secondary malignancies will be observed with reduced frequency as compared to conventional myeloablative transplantation.

ENGRAFTMENT AFTER NONMYELOABLATIVE STEM CELL TRANSPLANTATION

The ability to establish engraftment of donor hematopoietic and lymphoid cells is directly related to the degree of host immunosuppression induced by the preparative regimen. Most, if not all, NST regimens result in some degree of early donor-recipient mixed chimerism. Although graft rejection occurs with a higher frequency than with myeloablative approaches, in general, more than 80% of patients can be expected to have long-term stable donor engraftment. Regimens that use low-dose TBI alone are associated with a higher incidence of graft rejection, although the addition of fludarabine appears to overcome this problem.[290,291]

We evaluated the engraftment kinetics in 50 patients with hematologic and nonhematologic malignancies receiving an NST from an HLA-identical or single-locus mismatched sibling donor using a preparative regimen of cyclophosphamide (60 mg/kg × 2) and fludarabine (25 mg/m^2 × 5).[292] Lineage-specific chimerism analysis using the polymerase chain reaction of minisatellite regions was performed on myeloid (CD14+ and CD15+) and T cells (CD3+) obtained weekly from peripheral blood. A unique pattern of engraftment was observed in which myeloid cells at the time of neutrophil recovery were mixed chimeric (both donor and patient), although predominantly recipient in origin, in contrast to T cells, which were also mixed chimeric but predominantly donor in origin (Fig. 53.3-4*A*). By day 30, half of the patients had made the transition to full-donor T-cell chimerism, while myeloid chimerism often remained mixed (Fig. 53.3-4*B*). After the withdrawal of CSA and, in some patients, after DLI, chimerism changed to a complete donor type in all cellular lineages in the majority of cases. The establishment of full-donor T-cell chimerism consistently preceded full-donor myeloid chimerism, compatible with a graft-versus-host hematopoietic effect.[289] Forty-eight of 50 patients (96%) ultimately achieved stable donor engraftment, with only 2 (4%) experiencing graft rejection, which was followed by complete autologous hematopoietic recovery. Of note, acute GVHD and GVL effects were usually not observed until full-donor T-cell chimerism was

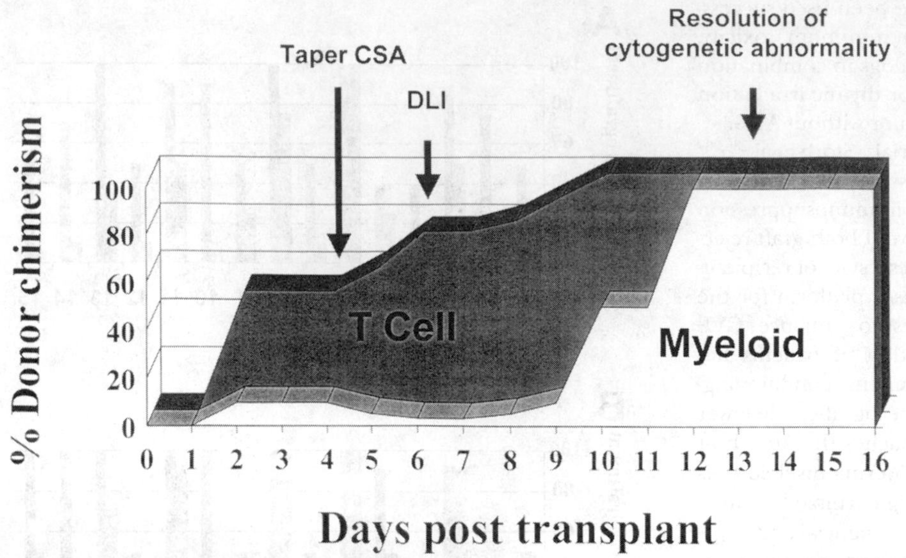

FIGURE 53.3-5. Typical pattern of donor engraftment in myeloid and T-cell lineages in a 56-year-old man undergoing nonmyeloablative stem cell transplantation for chronic myelomonocytic leukemia (CMML). CSA, cyclosporin A; DLI, donor lymphocyte infusion.

achieved. T-cell chimerism, therefore, appears to be of central importance and can be used successfully to guide posttransplantation immune manipulation.

GRAFT-VERSUS-HOST DISEASE

Although mixed T-cell chimerism is associated with GVHD tolerance, withdrawal of CSA and giving DLI, usually to enhance a GVL effect, often results in a rapid transition to full-donor T-cell chimerism and may be associated with the onset of acute GVHD. Acute GVHD appears to be the major nonrelapse life-threatening complication associated with NST. Several trials have reported grade II through IV acute GVHD rates of 30% to 50%, this outcome being lethal in up to 15% of treated patients.[278–280,290,292] Older patient age, prior history of autologous transplantation, and rapid T-cell engraftment appear to be associated with an increased risk of GVHD. We observed a six-fold increase in acute GVHD in those patients who had 90% or more donor T-cell chimerism by day 14 after transplantation. The majority of NST regimens have used CSA or FK506 alone for prophylaxis of GVHD. Future strategies to decrease the incidence and severity of acute GVHD, which include the additional use of prophylactic drugs such as methotrexate or mycophenolate mofetil, or methods to deplete alloreactive T cells selectively, will likely improve the safety of these novel regimens.

GRAFT-VERSUS-LEUKEMIA EFFECT AFTER NONMYELOABLATIVE STEM CELL TRANSPLANTATION

GVL effects after NST have been observed in a heterogeneous group of hematologic malignancies, with some patients achieving durable remissions.[278–283,286,289,293–295] To date, too few patients have been treated in any one disease category to make any generalizations regarding the antileukemic potential of this approach. However, the induction of molecular remissions in CML, CLL, and low-grade non-Hodgkin's lymphoma suggest that the GVL reactions induced after NST are at least as powerful as those after conventional BMT and will likely be of curative potential. Furthermore, complete remissions in advanced and chemotherapy-refractory diseases have been achieved in debilitated and older patients (i.e., older than 60 years) who normally would have been ineligible for a standard myeloablative transplantation due to an unacceptably high risk of treatment-related mortality.[296]

As autologous hematopoietic recovery usually occurs, recurrent and sometimes progressive disease may be observed during the first 3 to 6 months after transplantation. The onset of the GVL effect typically is delayed from the time of transplant conditioning and usually follows the establishment of full-donor T-cell chimerism and the withdrawal of GVHD prophylaxis or DLI.[289] Figure 53.3-5 shows the typical pattern of donor engraftment in myeloid and T-cell lineages in a 56-year-old man undergoing NST for CMML using this approach. Mixed T-cell chimerism on day 30 improved in the direction of the donor after withdrawal of CSA and a DLI of 2×10^6 CD3+ cells/kg. Myeloid recovery was mixed but predominantly autologous in origin. After 100% donor T-cell chimerism was established, a brief period of leukopenia was followed by a rapid increase in the percentage of donor myeloid cells, consistent with a graft-versus-host hematopoietic effect. A 20q- cytogenetic abnormality, which was observed in all bone marrow metaphases on day 60, was no longer detectable by the day 100 analysis, and the patient remains in remission more than 24 months after transplantation without ever having developed GVHD. Similar patterns of delayed disease regression have been observed in patients with CML, CLL, and Hodgkin's and non-Hodgkin's lymphomas.

GRAFT-VERSUS-TUMOR EFFECTS

The low risk of transplant-related mortality with NST renders this approach appealing for the investigation of GVT effects in patients with metastatic and treatment-refractory solid tumors. In 1997, my colleagues and I initiated a pilot trial to investigate for GVT effects in patients with metastatic renal cell carcinoma and melanoma in whom conventional therapy had failed and who had an HLA-compatible sibling.[284,289,297,298] We chose to investigate for GVT effects in these two malignancies owing to their highly immunogenic profiles and known sensitivity to immunomodulation-based therapy (interleukin-2 and interferon-α), in which T cells are believed to be the principle mediators of an antitumor response. None of the first eight patients with melanoma had a sustained disease response. However, several patients with advanced, treatment-refractory metastatic renal cell carcinoma have had a disease response, including three with a complete response, two of whom remain in remission longer than 2 years after transplantation. The disease regressions we observed were typically delayed in onset, occurring at a median of 4 months after transplantation, and followed the withdrawal of CSA, establishment of 100% donor T-cell chimerism and, in one patient, following a DLI, all compatible with a donor-mediated GVT effect. These results illustrate that antitumor effects induced through an allogeneic immune system may be as or more potent than strategies designed to enhance autologous antitumor immunity. They also provide the first evidence that a GVT effect alone can induce complete and clinically meaningful regression of a metastatic solid tumor. Similar trials have been initiated to investigate for GVT effects in patients with other treatment-refractory tumors.

FUTURE DIRECTIONS FOR NONMYELOABLATIVE STEM CELL TRANSPLANTATION

The results of these early trials have been encouraging, showing that low-intensity transplantation regimens are well tolerated with a low risk of transplant-related toxicity and mortality, even in high-risk patients. More important, the trials have shown that adequate engraftment of the donor immune system can be achieved for the generation of powerful antitumor effects, without the use of toxic myeloablative conditioning regimens. Indeed, they provide strong evidence that the GVL effect may be the primary modality, contributing to the curative potential of allogeneic hematopoietic SCT in some malignancies. Because toxicity is decreased, patient eligibility for allogeneic transplantation will likely be expanded to include older or debilitated patients who were historically ineligible for standard BMT. Furthermore, the ability to generate GVL effects resulting in complete remissions of hematologic malignancies will likely lead to prospective randomized trials comparing NST to more conventional myeloablative transplantations. Finally, NST appears to be the ideal platform from which to investigate safely for more targeted adoptive allogeneic immunotherapeutic approaches that use tumor-specific T cells to enhance the antimalignancy effect of allogeneic lymphocytes.

RESULTS OF CONVENTIONAL ALLOGENEIC TRANSPLANTATION FOR HEMATOLOGIC MALIGNANCIES

Allogeneic hematopoietic SCT is potentially curative for a number of different hematologic malignancies, including acute and chronic leukemias, myelodysplastic syndromes, Hodgkin's and non-Hodgkin's lymphoma, and multiple myeloma. The indications for allogeneic SCT vary according to disease categories and are influenced by factors such as cytogenetic abnormalities, response to prior therapy, patient age and performance status, disease status (remission vs. relapsed), disease-specific prognostic factors and, most important, availability of a suitable allogeneic stem cell donor. The decision of whether to proceed with allogeneic transplantation often is difficult and controversial and ultimately is guided by the potential benefits and risks of such therapy. Diseases such as CML, curable only by allograft transplantation, are associated with an excellent posttransplantation outcome and high probability of long-term disease-free survival, justifying the risks of regimen-related toxicity. Conversely, diseases such as multiple myeloma are associated with a high risk of treatment-related mortality and disease relapse, making the decision to proceed with transplantation more difficult.[298] Nevertheless, for the majority of patients who undergo this approach, allogeneic SCT remains the only chance of cure.

CHRONIC MYELOGENOUS LEUKEMIA

CML is a clonal myeloproliferative disease of hematopoietic stem cell origin, characterized by an early chronic phase of 3 to 5 years' duration followed by an accelerated phase of 3 to 6 months, which ultimately terminates in a fatal blastic phase. Although a minority of patients have sustained cytogenetic remission of the Philadelphia chromosome [t(9;22)] after treatment with interferon-α, allogeneic SCT remains the only treatment approach with definitive curative potential. Patient age, disease status (chronic phase vs. accelerated or blastic phase), and the time interval from diagnosis to transplant (i.e., <1 year vs. >1 year) are the most powerful predictors of long-term survival following allogeneic transplantation.[299–303] In general, 65% to 80% of patients with chronic-phase CML who receive a transplant can expect to be cured, in contrast to a minority (10% to 15%) who undergo transplantation in the accelerated or blastic phase. Patients with chronic-phase CML who receive a transplant within 1 year of diagnosis have the best outcome, with long-term disease-free survivals of 75% to 80%. A study from the Fred Hutchinson Cancer Center involving 196 patients undergoing allogeneic SCT from a matched unrelated donor reported a 5-year survival of 75%, a rate that compared favorably to that institution's results using HLA-matched sibling donors.[304]

Among hematologic malignancies, CML appears most susceptible to the GVL effect.[54] The majority of CML patients who experience disease relapse after allogeneic SCT can expect to be induced back into remission with DLI.[61–66] This sensitivity to GVL has led to a number of trials investigating NST as a less toxic approach for patients with chronic-phase CML. Early results using NST have been promising, with several molecular remissions having been reported.[279,282] Notably, patients older than 60 years have been successfully treated with minimal conditioning-associated toxicity, an important finding given the median age at diagnosis of 65 years.[296] These favorable results will expand patient eligibility for this curative modality to include the majority of older patients who are diagnosed with CML and who have a suitable donor, and will likely lead to randomized trials comparing NST with conventional myeloablative approaches.

ACUTE MYELOGENOUS LEUKEMIA

With the exception of those with favorable or low-risk karyotypic abnormalities [i.e., t(8;21), t(15;17), inv or del(16)], most patients with AML are at high risk for disease relapse after chemotherapy-induced remission.[305,306] Allogeneic SCT after first complete remission (CR1) is associated with a lower risk of relapse, with studies demonstrating 5-year disease-free survivals of 46% to 62%.[306–310] Patients in CR2 or with untreated relapsed AML usually are curable only by allogeneic SCT, although they are less likely to achieve long-term survival (22% to 30%).[311,312] Therefore, the decision to perform transplantation after CR1 is influenced by the predicted increase in disease-free survival versus the risk of regimen-related mortality. Based on these observations, it is reasonable to proceed to transplantation in CR1 in patients who are at intermediate or high risk of relapse (i.e., normal karyotype, abnormal chromosome 5 or 7, complex karyotype abnormalities), withholding the procedure until first relapse or CR2 in lower-risk patients. Primary chemotherapy-refractory AML, although associated with a significantly worse prognosis than AML in remission, is salvageable by allogeneic SCT in 10% to 20% of cases.

ACUTE LYMPHOBLASTIC LEUKEMIA

Although 65% to 85% of adults with ALL achieve remission with primary chemotherapy, 60% to 70% eventually experience relapse, which is rarely curable with salvage chemotherapy. Factors associated with a poor outcome (high risk) include age older than 60 years, leukocyte count greater than 30,000 on presentation, and chromosomal translocations involving t(4;11), t(1;19), t(8;14), or the Philadelphia chromosome t(9;22), which can be found in 15% to 30% of adult ALL cases.[313–316] In adults, allogeneic SCT performed during CR1 usually is reserved for patients with high-risk features, for whom cure with chemotherapy is unlikely.[317,318] Several studies of allogeneic SCT in high-risk patients who received a transplant during CR1 have reported long-term disease-free survivals of 41% to 61%, rates considerably higher than those observed with chemotherapy alone.[319,320] Allogeneic SCT usually is recommended in CR2 for patients lacking high-risk factors, as disease will be cured in some with chemotherapy alone. Furthermore, the long-term disease-free survival rate (35% to 40%) is comparable in these patients, regardless of whether they undergo transplantation in CR1 or CR2.[321] As chemotherapy is considerably more effective in achieving durable remissions in children, allogeneic SCT usually is reserved for those who fail to be cured with primary therapy or who have Philadelphia chromosome–positive ALL.[322]

MYELODYSPLASTIC SYNDROME

Allogeneic SCT is the only curative therapy available for patients with myelodysplastic syndrome (MDS). In general, 30% to 50% of patients with MDS can be expected to achieve long-term disease-free survival.[323] Factors associated with improved outcome include younger age, lower pretransplantation marrow blast percentage, shorter disease duration, and favorable cytogenetics. A retrospective trial of 131 patients with MDS undergoing allogeneic BMT reported disease-free and overall survival rates of 34% and 41%, respectively.[324] Disease-free survival depended on pretransplantation bone marrow blast percentages, with refractory anemia/refractory anemia with ringed sideroblasts (RA/RARS), refractory anemia with excess blasts (RAEB), refractory anemia with excess blasts in transformation (RAEB-T), and secondary AML patients having disease-free survivals of 52%, 34%, 19%, and 26%, respectively.

A retrospective analysis of transplantation events in relation to the International Prognostic Scoring System cytogenetic categories showed that cytogenetic abnormalities alone were highly predictive of posttransplantation outcome.[325] The event-free survival for good-, intermediate-, and poor-risk cytogenetic subgroups were 51%, 40%, and 6%, respectively, with corresponding relapse rates of 19%, 12%, and 82%. International Prognostic Scoring System cytogenetic categories were defined as good-risk if patients had normal karyotype, -Y alone, del(5q) alone, or del(20q) alone: poor-risk if patients had anomalies of chromosome 7 or complex cytogenetics (three or more anomalies); and intermediate-risk if other karyotypic anomalies were present that did not meet the criteria for good- or poor-risk. The identification of an extremely high incidence of relapse in the poor-risk group (82%) is important, as new and more effective treatment strategies should be directed specifically toward these patients.

OTHER HEMATOLOGIC MALIGNANCIES

The role of allogeneic SCT in multiple myeloma, CLL, and Hodgkin's and non-Hodgkin's lymphoma is less well defined than in the acute leukemias or chronic-phase CML.[326–331] Most studies published to date have consisted of small retrospective analyses or anecdotal case reports. Nevertheless, reports of durable remissions in patients with relapsed or chemotherapy-refractory disease, often in association with GVHD or after DLI, provide strong evidence that these diseases are susceptible to a potentially curative GVL effect.

The largest series to date of patients with CLL undergoing allogeneic BMT reported a 49% disease-free survival at 27 months, with an extraordinarily high treatment-related mortality of 46%.[326] Although a number of patients with multiple myeloma have achieved long-term disease-free survival after allogeneic SCT, transplant-related mortality may be as high as 50%, thus limiting the full therapeutic potential of this approach.[327] Regimens with reduced transplant-related toxicities, such as NST, may avoid these complications and improve disease-free survival. Indeed several studies exploring NST in diseases such as low-grade non-Hodgkin's lymphoma, CLL, and multiple myeloma have shown early promising results, with durable complete responses being achieved in all disease categories.[278,280,283,284,294] Although CLL and low-grade non-Hodgkin's lymphoma are notorious for delayed relapses, the observation of molecular remissions raises the prospect that NST may have curative potential in these diseases.

FUTURE PROSPECTS

Allogeneic SCT remains the only curative treatment modality for a large number of patients with hematologic malignancies. Exciting advances in the field have made this approach an essential component in the treatment of an increasing number of malignant diseases. Furthermore, an expanded understanding of the requirements for the engraftment of donor cells and of the basic immunologic mechanisms involved in GVHD and GVL reactions have greatly improved both the safety and efficacy of the procedure. The eventual identification of leukemia- and tumor-specific antigens will likely lead to more targeted allogeneic immunotherapy approaches that avoid the morbidity associated with GVHD. The discovery that GVL effects alone have curative potential for a number of different malignancies already has led to new transplantation approaches that appear destined to reduce transplant-related mortality and improve long-term outcome for patients undergoing this procedure.

REFERENCES

1. Jacobson LO, Simmons EL, Marks EK, et al. The risk of the spleen in radiation injury and recovery. *J Lab Clin Med* 1956;35:746.
2. Lorenz E, Congdon CC, Uphoff D. Modification of acute irradiation injury in mice and guinea pigs by bone marrow injections. *Radiology* 1952;58:863.
3. Thomas ED, Lochte HL, Waa Ching Lu, Ferrebee JU. Intravenous infusion of bone marrow in patients receiving radiation and chemotherapy. *N Engl J Med* 1957;257:491.
4. Thomas ED, Storb R, Clift RA, et al. Bone marrow transplantation. *N Engl J Med* 1975;292:832.
5. Daussett J, Rapapert FT, Ivany IP, Colongani J. Tissue alloantigens and transplantation. In: Bainer H, Cleton FJ, Eernisse JC, eds. *Histocompatibility Testing.* Copenhagen: Munksgaad, 1965:63.
6. Bortin MM, Horowitz MM, Barrett AJ, et al. Changing trends in allogeneic bone marrow transplantation for leukemia in the 1980's. *JAMA* 1992;262:607.
7. Sullivan K, Storb R, Buckner C, et al. Graft versus host disease as adoptive immunotherapy in patients with advanced hematological malignancies. *N Engl J Med* 1989;320:828.
8. Kolb HJ, Mittermuller J, Clemm CH, et al. Donor leukocyte transfusions for treatment of recurrent CML in marrow transplant patients. *Blood* 1990;76;2462.
9. Horowitz MM, Gale RP, Sondel PM, et al. Graft vs. leukemia reactions after bone marrow transplantation. *Blood* 1990;75:555.
10. Weiden PL, Flourney N, Thomas ED, et al. Antileukemia effect of graft-versus-host disease in human recipients of allogeneic grafts. *N Engl J Med* 1979;300:1068.
11. O'Kunewick JP, Meredith RF, eds. *Graft-versus-leukemia in man and animal models.* Boca Raton, FL: CRC Press, 1981.
12. Sosman JA, Sondel PM. The graft versus leukemia effect following bone marrow transplantation: a review of laboratory and clinical data. *Hematol Rev* 1987;2:77.
13. Weiden Pl, Sullivan KM, Flourney N, Storb R, Thomas ED. Antileukemia effect of chronic graft versus-host-disease: contribution to improved survival after allogeneic marrow transplantation. *N Engl J Med* 1981;304:1529.
14. Butturini A, Bortin MM, Gale RP. Graft-vs-leukemia following bone marrow transplantation. *Bone Marrow Transplant* 1987;2:233.
15. Butturini A, Gale RP. The role of T-cells in preventing relapse in chronic myelogenous leukemia. *Bone Marrow Transplant* 1987;2:351.
16. Fischer A, Landais P, Friedrich FW, et al. Bone marrow transplantation (BMT) in Europe for primary immunodeficiency disease: a report from the European Group for Immunodeficiency Disease. *Blood* 1994;83:1149.
17. Filipovitch AH, Shapiro RS, Ramsay NKC, et al. Unrelated donor bone marrow transplantation for correction of lethal congenital immunodeficiencies. *Blood* 1992;80:270.
18. Lenarsky C, Weinberg K, Kohn DB, Parkman R. Unrelated donor BMT for Wiskott-Aldrich syndrome. *Bone Marrow Transplant* 1993;12:145.
19. Barrett AJ, McCarthy DM. Bone marrow transplantation for genetic disorders. *Blood Rev* 1990;4:116.
20. Lucarelli G, Galimberti M, Polchi P, et al. Bone marrow transplantation in patients with thalassemia. *N Engl J Med* 1990;322:417.
21. Lucarelli G, Polchi P, Izzi T, et al. Marrow transplantation for thalassemia following treatment with busulfan and cyclophosphamide. *Lancet* 1985;1:1355.
22. Blazar DR, Ramsay NKC, Kersey JH. Pretransplant conditioning with busulfan and cyclophosphamide for nonmalignant diseases. *Transplantation* 1985;39:597.
23. Walters MC, Patience M, Leisenring W, et al. Bone marrow transplantation for sickle cell disease. *N Engl J Med* 1996;335:369.
24. Deeg HJ, Sullivan KM, Buckner CD, et al. Marrow transplantation for acute non-lymphoblastic leukemia in first remission; toxicity and long-term follow up of patients conditioned with single dose or fractionated total body irradiation. *Bone Marrow Transplant* 1986;1:151.
25. Thomas ED, Clift RA, Hersman J, et al. Marrow transplantation for acute nonlymphoblastic leukemia in first remission using fractionated or single dose irradiation. *Int Radiat Oncol Biol Phys* 1982;8:817.
26. Brockstein JA, Kernan NA, Groshen S, et al. Allogeneic bone marrow transplantation after hyperfractionated total body irradiation and cyclophosphamide in children with acute leukemia. *N Engl J Med* 1987;317:1618.
27. Clift RA, Buckner CD, Applebaum FA, et al. Allogeneic marrow transplants for patients with chronic myelogenous leukemia in the chronic phase: a randomized trial of two irradiation regimens. *Blood* 1991;77:1660.
28. Clift RA, Buckner CD, Applebaum FA, et al. Allogeneic marrow transplants for patients with acute myelogenous leukemia in first remission: a randomized trial of two irradiation regimens. *Blood* 1988;76:1867.
29. Kim TH, Khan FM, Galvin JM. A report of the working party: comparison of total body irradiation techniques for bone marrow transplantation. *Int J Radiat Oncol Biol Phys* 1980;6:779.
30. Snyder DS, Negrin RS, O'Donnell MR, et al. Fractionated total-body irradiation and high-dose etoposide as a preparatory regimen for bone marrow transplantation for 94 patients with chronic myelogenous leukemia in chronic phase. *Blood* 1994;84:1672.
31. Locatelli E, Pession A, Bonetti F, et al. Busulfan, cyclophosphamide and melphalan as conditioning regimen for bone marrow transplantation in children with myelodysplastic syndrome. *Leukemia* 1994;8:844.
32. Emminger W, Emminger-Schmidmeier W, Haas OA, et al. Treatment of infant leukemia with busulfan cyclophosphamide + etoposide and bone marrow transplantation. *Bone Marrow Transplant* 1992;10:313.
33. Ratanatharathorn V, Karanes C, Lum LG, et al. Allogeneic bone marrow transplantation in high risk myeloid disorders using busulfan, cytosine arabinoside and cyclophosphamide (BAC). *Bone Marrow Transplant* 1992;9:49.
34. Zander AR, Culbert S, Jaggenath S, et al. High dose cyclophosphamide BCNU, and VP-1 (CBV) as a conditioning regimen for allogeneic bone marrow transplantation for patients with acute leukemia. *Cancer* 1987;59:1083.
35. Santos GW, Tutschka PJ, Brookmeyer R, et al. Marrow transplantation for acute nonlymphocytic leukemia after treatment with busulfan and cyclophosphamide. *N Engl J Med* 1983;309:1347.
36. Clift RA, Buckner CD, Thomas ED, et al. Marrow transplantation for chronic myeloid leukemia: a randomized study comparing cyclophosphamide and total body irradiation with busulfan and cyclophosphamide. *Blood* 1994;84:2036.
37. Devergie A, Blaise D, Attal M, et al. Allogeneic bone marrow transplantation for chronic myeloid leukemia in first chronic phase: a randomized trial of busulfan-cytoxan versus cytoxan–total body irradiation as preparative regimen: a report from the French Society of Bone Marrow Graft. *Blood* 1995;85:2263.
38. Blume KG, Kopecky KJ, Henslee-Downey JP, et al. A prospective randomized comparison of total body irradiation–etoposide versus busulfan-cyclophosphamide as preparatory regimens for bone marrow transplantation in patients with leukemia who were not in first remission: a Southwest Oncology Group Study. *Blood* 1993;81:2187.
39. Baglin TP. Veno-occlusive disease of the liver complicating bone marrow transplantation. *Bone Marrow Transplant* 1994;13:1.
40. Ozkaynak M, Weinberg K, Kohn D, et al. Hepatic veno-occlusive disease post–bone marrow transplantation in children conditioned with busulfan and cyclophosphamide: incidence, risk factors, and clinical outcome. *Bone Marrow Transplant* 1991;7:467.
41. Weiner RS, Bortin MM, Gale RP, et al. Risk factors associated with interstitial pneumonia following allogeneic bone marrow transplantation for leukemia. *Transplant Proc* 1985;17:470.
42. Kolb HJ, Bender-Gotze CH. Late complications after allogeneic bone marrow transplantation. *Bone Marrow Transplant* 1990;4:61.
43. Sanders JE, Pritchard S, Mahoney P et al. Growth and development following marrow transplantation for leukemia. *Blood* 1986;68:1129.
44. Leiper AD, Stanhorpe R, Lou T, et al. The effect of total body irradiation and bone marrow transplantation during childhood and adolescence on growth and endocrine function. *Br J Haematol* 1987;67:419.
45. Giralt S, Estey E, Albitar M, et al. Engraftment of allogeneic hematopoietic progenitor cells with purine analog–containing chemotherapy: harnessing graft-versus-leukemia without myeloablative therapy. *Blood* 1997;89:4531.
46. Slavin S, Nagler A, Naparastak E, et al. Nonmyeloablative stem cell transplantation and cell therapy as an alternative to conventional bone marrow transplantation with lethal cytoreduction for the treatment of malignant and nonmalignant hematologic diseases. *Blood* 1998;91:756.
47. Khouri I, Keating MJ, Korbling M, et al. Transplant-lite: induction of graft-versus-malignancy using fludarabine-based nonablative chemotherapy and allogeneic progenitor-cell transplantation as treatment for lymphoid malignancies. *J Clin Oncol* 1998;16:2817.
48. Childs R, Clave E, Contentin N, et al. Engraftment kinetics after nonmyeloablative allogeneic peripheral blood stem cell transplantation: full donor T-cell chimerism preceded alloimmune responses. *Blood* 1999;94(9):3234.
49. Collins RH Jr, Shpilberg O, Drobyski WR et al. Donor leukocyte transfusions in 140 patients with relapsed malignancy after allogeneic transplantation. *J Clin Oncol* 1997;15:433.
50. Barnes DHW, Loutit JF. Treatment of murine leukemia with x-rays and homologous bone marrow. *Br J Haematol* 1957;3:241.
51. Weiden PL, Sullivan KM, Flournoy N, et al. Antileukemic effect of chronic graft-versus-leukemia disease. Contribution to improved survival after allogeneic marrow transplantation. *N Engl J Med* 1981;304:1529.
52. Gale RP, Horowitz MM, Ash RC, et al. Identical twin bone marrow transplants for leukemia. *Ann Intern Med* 1994;120:646.
53. Goldman JM, Gale RP, Horowitz MM, et al. Bone marrow transplantation for chronic myelogenous leukemia in chronic phase. Increased relapse associated with T-cell depletion. *Ann Intern Med* 1988;108:806.
54. Horowitz MM, Gale RP, Sondel PM, et al. Graft-versus-leukemia reactions after bone marrow transplantation. *Blood* 1991;75:555.
55. Offit K, Burns JP, Cunningham L, et al. Cytogenetic analysis of chimerism and leukemia relapse in chronic myelogenous leukemia patients after T-cell depleted bone marrow transplantation. *Blood* 1990;75:1346.
56. Lee M, Khouri I, Champlin R, et al. Detection of minimal residual disease by polymerase chain reaction of bcr/abl transcripts in chronic myelogenous leukemia following allogeneic bone marrow transplantation. *Br J Haematol* 1992;82:708.
57. DeLage R, Soiffer RJ, Dear K, Ritz J. Clinical significance of bcr/abl gene rearrangement detected by polymerase chain reaction after allogeneic bone marrow transplantation in chronic myelogenous leukemia. *Blood* 1991;78:2759.
58. Pignon JM, Henni T, Amselem S, et al. Frequent detection of minimal residual disease by use of the polymerase chain reaction in long-term survivors after bone marrow transplantation for chronic myeloid leukemia. *Leukemia* 1990;4:83.
59. Higano C, Brixey M, Bryant E, et al. Durable complete remission of acute nonlymphocytic leukemia associated with discontinuation of immunosuppression following relapse after allogeneic bone marrow transplantation: a case report of a probable graft-versus-leukemia effect. *Transplantation* 1990;50:175.
60. Collins R, Rogers Z, Bennett M, et al. Hematologic relapse of chronic myelogenous leukemia following allogeneic bone marrow transplantation: apparent graft-versus-leukemia effect following abrupt discontinuation of immunosuppression. *Bone Marrow Transplant* 1992;10:391.
61. Kolb HJ, Beisser K, Holler E, et al. Donor buffy coat transfusions for adoptive immunotherapy in human and canine chimeras. *Periodicum Biologorum* 1991;93:81.
62. Kolb HJ, Mittermuller J, Clemm C, et al. Donor leukocyte transfusions for treatment of

recurrent chronic myelogenous leukemia in marrow transplant patients. *Blood* 1990; 76:2462.

63. Porter DL, Roth MS, McGarigle C, Ferrara JIM, Antin JH. Induction of graft versus-host disease as immunotherapy for relapsed chronic myeloid leukemia. *N Engl J Med* 1994;330:100.
64. Bar BMAM, Schattenberg A, Mensink EJBM, et al. Donor leukocyte infusions for chronic myeloid leukemia relapsed after allogeneic bone marrow transplantation. *J Clin Oncol* 1993;11:513.
65. Helg C, Roux E, Beris P, et al. Adoptive immunotherapy for recurrent CML after BMT. *Bone Marrow Transplant* 1993;12:125.
66. Drobyski WR, Keever CA, Roth MS, et al. Salvage immunotherapy using donor leukocyte infusions as treatment for relapsed chronic myelogenous leukemia after bone marrow transplantation: efficacy and toxicity of a defined T-cell dose. *Blood* 1993;82:2310.
67. Kolb HJ, Schattenberg A, Goldman J, et al. Graft vs leukemia effect of donor lymphocyte transfusions in marrow grafted patients. *Blood* 1995;86(5):2041.
68. van Rhee F, Kolb HJ. Donor leukocyte transfusions for leukemic relapse. *Curr Opin Hematol* 1995;2:423.
69. Dermime S, Mavroudis D, Jiang YZ, et al. Immune escape from a graft-versus-leukemia effect may play a role in the relapse of myeloid leukemias following allogeneic bone marrow transplantation. *Bone Marrow Transplant* 1997;19:989.
70. Verdonck L, Lokhorst H, Dekker A, et al. Graft-versus-myeloma effect in two cases. *Lancet* 1996;347:800.
71. VanBesien KW, de Lima M, Giralt SA, et al. Management of lymphoma recurrence after allogeneic transplantation: the relevance of graft-versus lymphoma effect. *Bone Marrow Transplant* 1997;19:977.
72. Dazzi F, Szydio RM, Goldman JM. Donor lymphocyte infusions for relapse of chronic myeloid leukemia after allogeneic stem cell transplantation: Where do we now stand? *Exp Hematol* 1999;27:1477.
73. Nimer S, Giorgi J, Gajewski J, et al. Selective depletion of CD8-positive cells for prevention of graft-versus-host disease following bone marrow transplantation: a randomized control trial. *Transplantation* 1994;57:82.
74. Champlin RE, Jansen J, Ho W, et al. Retention of graft-versus-leukemia using selective depletion of CD8-positive T lymphocytes for prevention of graft versus host disease following bone marrow transplantation for chronic myelogenous leukemia. *Tranplant Proc* 1991;23:1695.
75. Champlin R, Giralt S, Przepiorka D, et al. Selective depletion of CD8-positive T lymphocytes for allogeneic bone marrow transplantation: engraftment, graft-versus-host disease and graft-versus-leukemia. *Prog Clin Biol Res* 1992;377:385.
76. Giralt SA, Hetser J, Huh Y, et al. CD8-depleted donor lymphocyte infusion as treatment for relapsed chronic myelogenous leukemia after allogeneic bone marrow transplantation. *Blood* 1995;86:4337.
77. Alyea E, Soiffer RJ, Canning C, et al. Toxicity and efficacy of defined doses of CD4+ donor lymphocytes for treatment of relapse after allogeneic bone marrow transplantation. *Blood* 1998;91:3671.
78. Mackinnon S, Papadoupoulos EB, Carabasi MH, et al. Adoptive immunotherapy evaluating escalating doses of donor leukocytes for relapse of chronic myeloid leukemia after bone marrow transplantation: separation of graft-versus-leukemia responses from graft-versus-host disease. *Blood* 1995;86:1261.
79. Dazzi F, Szydlo RM, Craddock C, et al. Comparison of single-dose and escalating-dose regimens of donor lymphocyte infusions for relapse after allografting for chronic myeloid leukemia. *Blood* 2000;95:67.
80. Siegert W, Bever J, Kingreen D, et al. Treatment of relapse after allogeneic bone marrow transplantation with unmanipulated G-CSF mobilized peripheral blood stem cell preparation. *Bone Marrow Transplant* 1998;22(6):579.
81. Falkenburg JHF, Goselink HM, van der Harst D, et al. Growth inhibition of clonogenic leukemic precursor cells by minor histocompatibility antigen specific cytotoxic T-lymphocytes. *J Exp Med* 1991;174:27.
82. Wang W, Meadowa LR, den Haan JMM, et al. A male-specific histocompatibility antigen derived from the SMCY protein. *Science* 1995;269:1588.
83. Den Haan JMM, Sherman NE, Blokland E, et al. Identification of a graft-versus-host disease–associated minor histocompatibility antigen. *Science* 1995;268:1476.
84. De Bueger M, Bakker A, van Rood JJ, van der Woude F, Goulmy E. Tissue distribution of minor histocompatibility antigens. *J Immunol* 1992;149:1788.
85. Marijt WAF, Kernan NA, Diaz-Barrientos TH, et al. Multiple minor histocompatibility antigen– specific cytotoxic T lymphocyte clones can be generated during graft rejection after HLA identical bone marrow transplantation. *Bone Marrow Transplant* 1995;16:125.
86. Van der Harst D, Gdulmy E, Falkenberg JHF, et al. Recognition of minor histocompatibility antigens on lymphocytic and myeloid leukemic cell lines by cytotoxic T-cell clones. *Blood* 1994;83:1060.
87. Barrett AJ, Jiang YZ. Immune responses to chronic myeloid leukemia: review. *Bone Marrow Transplant* 1992;9:305.
88. Oettel K, Wesly O, Albertini M, et al. Allogeneic T-cell clones able to selectively destroy Philadelphia chromosome–bearing (Ph^{1+}) can also recognize Ph^{1-} cells from the same patient. *Blood* 1994;83:3390.
89. Sosman JA, Oettel KR, Smith SD, et al. Specific recognition of human leukemic cells by allogeneic T cells: II. Evidence for HLA-D restricted determinants on leukemic cells that are cross reactive with determinants present on unrelated nonleukemic cells. *Blood* 1990;75:2005.
90. Faber L, van Luxemberg-Heijs S, Willemze R, et al. Generation of leukemia reactive cytotoxic T lymphocyte clones from the HLA-identical bone marrow donor of a patient with leukemia. *J Exp Med* 1992;176:1283.
91. Chen W, Peace BJ, Rovira DK, et al. T-cell immunity to the joining region of p210 BCR-ABL protein. *Proc Natl Acad Sci U S A* 1992;89:1469.
92. Ten Bosch GJA, Toornvliet AC, Melief CJM, et al. Specific recognition of peptides corresponding to the joining region of p210 BCR-ABL by human T cells. *Blood* 1994;82:521(abst).
93. Cullis J, Barrett AJ, Lechler R, et al. Binding of pcr/abl junctional peptides to MHC class I molecules: studies in antigen processing defective cell lines. *Leukemia* 1994;8:165.
94. Hoffman T, Theobald M, Bunjes D, et al. Frequency of bone marrow T-cells responding to HLA-identical non-leukemic and leukemic stimulator cells. *Bone Marrow Transplant* 1993;12:1.
95. Faber LM, van Luxemberg-Heijs SAP, Veenhof WFJ, et al. Generation of CD4+ cytotoxic T-lymphocyte clones from a patient with severe graft-versus-host disease after allogeneic bone marrow transplantation: implications for graft-versus-leukemia reactivity. *Blood* 1995;86:2821.
96. Delain M, Tiberghien P, Racadot E, et al. Variability of the alloreactive T-cell response to human leukemic blasts. *Leukemia* 1994;8:642.
97. Jiang Y, Kanfer E, MacDonald D. Graft versus leukemia following allogeneic bone marrow transplantation: emergence of cytotoxic T lymphocytes reacting to host leukemic cells. *Bone Marrow Transplant* 1991;8:253.
98. Truitt RL, Atasoylu AA. Contribution of CD4+ and CD8+ T cells to graft-versus-host disease and graft-versus-leukemia reactivity after transplantation of MHC-compatible bone marrow. *Bone Marrow Transplant* 1991;8:51.
99. Weiss L, Weigensberg M, Morecki S, et al. Characterization of effector cells of graft versus leukemia following allogeneic bone marrow transplantation in mice inoculated with murine B-cell leukemia. *Cancer Immunol Immunother* 1990;31:236.
100. Okunewick JP, Kociban DL, Machen LL, et al. The role of CD4 and CD8 T cells in the graft versus leukemia response in Rauscher murine leukemia. *Bone Marrow Transplant* 991;8:445.
101. Hercend T, Takvorian T, Nowill A, et al. Characterization of natural killer cells with anti-leukemia activity following allogeneic bone marrow transplantation. *Blood* 1986;67:301.
102. Morecki S, Gelfand Y, Levi S, et al. Activated long-term peripheral blood cultures as preparation for adoptive alloreactive therapy in cancer patients. *J Hematother* 1997;6:115.
103. Lamb LS Jr, Henslee-Downey PJ, Parrish RS, et al. Increased frequency of TCR gamma delta + T cells in disease-free survivors following T-cell depleted, partially mismatched, related donor bone marrow transplantation for leukemia. *J Hematother* 1996;5:530.
104. Appelbaum FR, Strauchen JA, Graw RG. Acute lethal carditis caused by high dose combination chemotherapy. A unique clinical and pathological entity. *Lancet* 1976;1:58.
105. Haselberger MB, Schwinghammer TL. Efficacy of Mesna for prevention of hemorrhagic cystitis after high-dose cyclophosphamide therapy. *Ann Pharmacother* 1995;29:918.
106. Arthur RR, Shahk V, Baust SJ, et al. Association of BK viruria with hemorrhagic cystitis in recipients of bone marrow transplants. *N Engl J Med* 1986;315:230.
107. De la Camara R, Thomas JF, Figuera-Randa J, et al. High-dose Busulfan and seizures. *Bone Marrow Transplant* 1991;5:363.
108. Guiot HF, van den Broek PJ, van der Meer JW, et al. Selective antimicrobial modulation of the intestinal flora of patients with acute nonlymphocytic leukemia: a double-blind placebo controlled study. *J Infect Dis* 1983;147:615.
109. Pizzo PA. Considerations for the prevention of infectious complications in immunocompromised patients with cancer. *Rev Infect Dis* 1989;11:1551.
110. Schmeisser T, Kurrie E, Arnold R, et al. Norfloxacin for the prevention of bacterial infection during severe granulocytopenia after bone marrow transplantation. *Scand J Infect Dis* 1988;20:625.
111. Menichetti F, Felicini R, Bucaneve G, et al. Norfloxacin prophylaxis for neutropenic patients undergoing bone marrow transplantation. *Bone Marrow Transplant* 1989;4:489.
112. Goodman JL, Winston DJ, Greenfield RA, et al. A controlled trial of fluconazole to prevent fungal infections in patients undergoing bone marrow transplantation. *N Engl J Med* 1992;326:845.
113. Winston DJ, Chandrasekar PH, Lazarus HM, et al. Fluconazole prophylaxis of fungal infections in patients with acute leukemia. Results of a randomized placebo-controlled, double-blind, multicenter trial. *Ann Intern Med* 1993;118:495.
114. Bearman SI. The syndrome of hepatic veno-occlusive disease after bone marrow transplantation. *Blood* 1995;5:363.
115. Bearman SI, Appelbaum FR, Buckner CD, et al. Regimen-related toxicity in patients undergoing bone marrow transplantation. *J Clin Oncol* 1988;6:15628.
116. Rollins BJ. Hepatic veno-occlusive disease. *Am J Med* 1986;81:297.
117. McDonald GB, Sharma P, Matthews DE, et al. Veno-occlusive disease of the liver after bone marrow transplantation: diagnosis, incidence, and predisposing factors. *Hepatology* 1984;4:116.
118. Atkinson K, Biggs J, Noble G, et al. Preparative regimens for marrow transplantation containing Busulfan are associated with hemorrhagic cystitis and hepatic veno-occlusive disease but a short duration of leucopenia and little oro-pharyngeal mucositis. *Bone Marrow Transplant* 1987;2:385.
119. Carreras E, Granena A, Navasa M, et al. On the reliability of clinical criteria for the diagnosis of hepatic veno-occlusive disease. *Ann Hematol* 1993;66:7780.
120. Ibraham A, Pico JL, Ostronoff M, et al. Use of prostaglandin E1 for the treatment of veno-occlusive disease of the liver following autologous bone marrow transplantation. *Bone Marrow Transplant* 1990;5[Suppl 2]:82.
121. Baglin TP, Harper P, Marcus RE. Veno-occlusive disease of the liver complicating ABMT successfully treated with recombinant tissue plasminogen activator. *Bone Marrow Transplant* 1990;5:439.
122. Patton DF, Harper JL, Woolbridge TN, et al. Treatment of VOD of the liver with bolus tissue plasminogen activator and continuous infusion antithrombin III concentrate. *Bone Marrow Transplant* 1996;17:443.
123. Bearman SI, Lee JL, Baron AE, et al. Treatment of hepatic venoocclusive disease with recombinant human tissue plasminogen activator and heparin in 42 marrow transplant patients. *Blood* 1997;89(5):1501.
124. Richardson PG, Elias AD, Krishnan A, et al. Treatment of severe veno-occlusive disease with defibrotide: compassionate use results in response without significant toxicity in a high-risk population. *Blood* 1998;92(3):737.
125. Essel J, Schroeder M, Harman G, et al. Ursodiol prophylaxis against hepatic complications of allogeneic BMT: a randomized, double-blind placebo-controlled trial. *Ann Intern Med* 1988;128:975.
126. Weiner RS, Bortin MM, Gale RP. Risk factors associated with interstitial pneumonitis following allogeneic bone marrow transplantation for leukemia. *Transplant Proc* 1985;17: 470.

127. Piedbois P, Cordonnier C, Levy C, et al. Diffuse interstitial pneumonitis following BMT—incidence and relationship with parameters of single fraction TBI. *Bone Marrow Transplant* 1988;3:273.
128. Granena A, Carreras E, Rozman C, et al. Interstitial pneumonitis after BMT: 15 years experience in a single institution. *Bone Marrow Transplant* 1993;11:453.
129. Meyers JD, Flournoy N, Thomas ED. Non-bacterial pneumonitis after allogeneic bone marrow transplantation: a review of ten years' experience. *Rev Infect Dis* 1982;4:1119.
130. Appelbaum FR, Meyers JD, Fefer A, et al. Nonbacterial nonfungal pneumonia following marrow transplantation in 100 identical twins. *Transplantation* 1982;33:265.
131. Wingard JR, Mellits ED, Sostrin MB, et al. Interstitial pneumonitis after allogeneic bone marrow transplantation. Nine-year experience at a single institution. *Medicine (Baltimore)* 1988;67(3):175.
132. Hartsell F, Czyzewski EA, Ghalie R, et al. Pulmonary complications of bone marrow transplantation: a comparison of total body irradiation and cyclophosphamide to Busulfan and cyclophosphamide. *Int J Radiat Oncol Biol Phys* 1995;32(1):69.
133. Shanker G, Scott Bryson J, Jennings D, et al. Idiopathic pneumonia syndrome after allogeneic bone marrow transplantation in mice. Role of pretransplant radiation conditioning. *Am J Respir Cell Mol Biol* 1999;20(6):1116.
134. Haselton DJ, Klekamp JG, Christman BW. Use of high-dose corticosteroids and high-frequency oscillatory ventilation for treatment of a child with diffuse alveolar hemorrhage after bone marrow transplantation: case report and review of the literature. *Crit Care Med* 200;28(1):245.
135. Chao NJ, Duncan SR, Long GD, at al. Corticosteroid therapy for diffuse alveolar hemorrhage in autologous BMT recipients. *Ann Int Med* 1991;114:145.
136. Kolb HJ, Poetscher C. Late effects after allogeneic bone marrow transplantation. *Curr Opin Hematol* 1997;4(6):401.
137. Deeg HJ, Flournoy N, Sullivan KM, et al. Cataracts after total body irradiation and marrow transplantation: a sparing effect of dose fractionation. *Int J Radiat Oncol Biol Phys* 1984;10:957.
138. Fraunfelder FT, Meyer SM. Ocular toxicity of antineoplastic agents. *Ophthalmology* 1983;90:1.
139. Witherspoon RP, Fisher LD, Schoch G, et al. Secondary cancers after bone marrow transplantation for leukemia or aplastic anemia. *N Engl J Med* 1989;321:784.
140. Bhatia S, Ramsay N, Steinbuch M, et al. Malignant neoplasms following bone marrow transplantation. *Blood* 1996;87:3633.
141. Kolb HJ, Socie G, Duell T, et al. Malignant neoplasms in long-term survivors of bone marrow transplantation: late effects. Working Party of the European Cooperative Group for Blood and Marrow Transplantation and the European Late Effect Project Group. *Ann Intern Med* 1999;131(10):738.
142. Lones MA, Lopez-Terrada D, Shintaku IP. Posttransplant lymphoproliferative disorder in pediatric bone marrow transplant recipients: disseminated disease of donor origin demonstrated by fluorescence in situ hybridization. *Arch Pathol Lab Med* 1998;122(8):708.
143. Gerritsen EJ, Stam ED, Hermans J. Risk factors for developing EBV-related B cell lymphoproliferative disorders (BLPD) after non-HLA-identical BMT in children. *Bone Marrow Transplant* 1996;18(2):377.
144. Orazi A, Hromas RA, Neiman RS, et al. Posttransplantation lymphoproliferative disorders in bone marrow recipients are aggressive diseases with a high incidence of adverse histologic and immunobiologic features. *Am J Clin Pathol* 1997;107:419.
145. Papadopoulos EB, Ladanyi M, Emanuel D. Infusion of donor leukocytes to treat Epstein-Barr virus–associated lymphoproliferative disorders after allogeneic bone marrow transplantation. *N Engl J Med* 1994;330:1185.
146. Rooney CM, Smith CA, Ng CY, et al. Infusion of cytotoxic T cells for the prevention and treatment of Epstein-Barr virus–induced lymphoma in allogeneic transplant recipients. *Blood* 1998;92:1549.
147. Cavazzana-Calvo M, Bensoussan D, Jabado N, et al. Prevention of EBV-induced B-lymphoproliferative disorder by ex vivo marrow B-cell depletion in HLA-phenoidentical or nonidentical T-depleted bone marrow transplantation. *Br J Haematol* 1998;103:543.
148. Kuehnle I, Huls MH, Liu Z, et al. CD20 monoclonal antibody (rituximab) for therapy of Epstein-Barr virus lymphoma after hemopoietic stem-cell transplantation. *Blood* 2000; 95:1502.
149. Magriko K, Karo S, Hagihara M. Stable clonal expansion of T-cells induced by bone marrow transplantation. *Blood* 1996;87:789.
150. Dietrich PY, Caignard A, Diu A, et al. Analysis of T-cell receptor variability in transplanted patients with acute graft-versus-host disease. *Blood* 1992;80:2419.
151. Dietrich PY, Caignard A, et al. In vivo T-cell clonal amplification at time of acute graft-versus-host disease. *Blood* 1994;84:2815.
152. Glucksberg H, Storb R, Fefer A, et al. Clinical manifestations of graft-vs-host disease in human recipients of marrow from HLA-matched sibling donors. *Transplantation* 1974;18:295.
153. Bertheau P, Hadengue A, Cazalshatem D, et al. Chronic cholestasis in patients after allogeneic bone marrow transplantation: several diseases are often associated. *Bone Marrow Transplant* 1995;16:261.
154. Vogelsang GB, Hess AD, Santos GW. Acute graft-vs-host disease: clinical characteristics in the cyclosporine era. *Medicine* 1988;67:163.
155. Deeg HJ, Cottler-Fox M. Clinical spectrum and pathophysiology of acute graft-vs-host disease. In: Burakoff SJ, Deeg HJ, Ferrara J, Atkinson K, eds. *Graft-vs-host disease.* New York: Marcel Dekker Inc, 1990:311.
156. Weisdorf DJ, Snover DC, Haake R, et al. Acute gastrointestinal graft-vs-host disease: clinical significance and response to immunosuppressive therapy. *Blood* 1990;76:624.
157. Thomas ED, Storb R, Clift RA, et al. Bone marrow transplantation. *N Engl J Med* 1975;292:895.
158. Roosnek E, Hogendijk S, Zawadynski S, et al. The frequency of pretransplant donor cytotoxic T-cell precursors with anti-host specificity predicts survival of patients transplanted with bone marrow donors other than HLA-identical siblings. *Transplantation* 1993;56:691.
159. Schwarer AP, Jiang YZ, Brookes PA, et al. Frequency of anti-recipient alloreactive helper T-cell precursors in donor blood and graft-versus-host disease after HLA-identical sibling bone marrow transplantation. *Lancet* 1993;341:203.
160. Theobald M, Nierle T, Bunjes D, et al. Host-specific interleukin-2-secreting donor T-cell precursors as predictors of acute graft-versus-host disease in bone marrow transplantation between HLA-identical siblings. *N Engl J Med* 1992;327:1613.
161. Nierle T, Bunjes D, Arnold R, et al. Quantitative assessment of posttransplant host-specific interleukin-2-secreting T-helper cell precursors in patients with and without graft-versus-host disease after allogeneic HLA-identical sibling bone marrow transplantation. *Blood* 1993;81:841.
162. Theobald M, Bunjes D. Pretransplant detection of human minor histocompatibility antigen-specific naive and memory interleukin-2 secreting T-cells within class-I major histocompatibility complex (MHC)–restricted CD8+ and class-II MHC-restricted CD4+ T-cell subsets. *Blood* 1993;82:298.
163. Den Haan JMM, Sherman NE, Blokland E, et al. Identification of a graft versus host disease–associated human minor histocompatibility antigen. *Science* 1995;268:1476.
164. Perreault C, Decary F, Brochu S, et al. Minor histocompatibility antigens. *Blood* 1990;76:1269.
165. Goulmy E, Voogt P, van Els C, et al. The role of minor histocompatibility antigens in GVHD and rejection: a mini-review [Review]. *Bone Marrow Transplant* 1001;7[Suppl 1]:10.
166. Goulmy E, Schipper R, Pool J, et al. Mismatches of minor histocompatibility antigens between HLA-identical donors and recipients and the development of graft-versus-host disease after bone marrow transplantation. *N Engl J Med* 1996;334:281.
167. Nash RA, Pepe MS, Storb R, et al. Acute graft-versus-host disease: analysis of risk factors after allogeneic marrow transplantation and prophylaxis with cyclosporin and methotrexate [see comments]. *Blood* 1992;80:1838.
168. Hagglund H, Bostrom L, Remberger M, et al. Risk factors for acute graft-versus-host disease in 291 consecutive HLA identical bone marrow transplant recipients. *Bone Marrow Transplant* 1995;16:747.
169. Gale RP, Bortin MM, Van Bekkum DW, et al. Risk factors for acute graft-versus-host disease. *Br J Haematol* 1987;67:397.
170. Henslee-Downey PJ. Mismatched bone marrow transplantation. *Curr Opin Oncol* 1995;7:115.
171. Storb R, Deeg HJ, Pepe M, et al. Graft-versus-host disease prevention by methotrexate combined with cyclosporine compared to methotrexate alone in patients given marrow grafts for severe aplastic anemia: long-term follow-up of a controlled trial. *Br J Haematol* 1989;72:567.
172. Storb R, Leisenring W, Deeg HJ, et al. Long-term follow-up of a randomized trial of graft-versus-host disease prevention by methotrexate/cyclosporine versus methotrexate alone in patients given marrow grafts for severe aplastic anemia. *Blood* 1994;83:2749.
173. Storb E, Pepe M, Anasetti C, et al. What role for prednisone in prevention of acute graft-versus-host disease in patients undergoing marrow transplantation? *Blood* 1990;76:1037.
174. Marmount A, Horowitz MM, Gale RP, et al. T-cell depletion of HLA-identical transplants in leukemia. *Blood* 1991;78:2120.
175. Barrett AJ, Mavroudis D, Tisdale J, et al. T cell depleted bone marrow transplantation and delayed T cell add-back to control acute GVHD and conserve a graft-versus-leukemia effect. *Bone Marrow Transplant* 1998;21(6):543.
176. Neudorf S, Filipovich A, Ramsay N, et al. Prevention and treatment of acute GVHD. *Semin Hematol* 1984;21:91.
177. Bacigalupo A, Van Lint MT, Frassoni F, et al. High dose methylprednisolone for the treatment of acute GVHD. *Blut* 1983;46:125.
178. Kanojia MD, Anagnostou AA, Zander AR, et al. High dose methylprednisolone treatment for acute GVHD after bone marrow transplantation in adults. *Transplantation* 1984;37:246.
179. Van Lint MT, Uderzo C, Losasciulli A, et al. Early treatment of acute GVHD with high or low dose methylprednisolone. A multicenter randomized trial from the Italian Group for Bone Marrow Transplantation. *Blood* 1998;92:2288.
180. Martin PJ, Schoch G, Fisher L, et al. A retrospective analysis of therapy for acute graft-versus-host disease: secondary treatment. *Blood* 1991;77:1821.
181. Hebart H, Ehninger G, Schmidt H, et al. Treatment of steroid-resistant graft-versus-host disease after allogeneic bone marrow transplantation with antiCD3/TCR monoclonal antibodies. *Bone Marrow Transplant* 1995;15:891.
182. Anasetti C, Martin PJ, Hansen JA, et al. A phase I–II study evaluating the murine anti-IL-2 receptor antibody 2A3 for treatment of acute graft-versus-host disease. *Transplantation* 1990;50:49.
183. Anasetti C, Hansen JA, Waldmann TA, et al. Treatment of acute graft-versus-host disease with humanized anti-Tac: an antibody that binds to the interleukin-2 receptor. *Blood* 1994;84:1320.
184. Antin JH, Weinstein HJ, Guinan EC, et al. Recombinant human interleukin-1 receptor antagonist in the treatment of steroid-resistant graft-versus-host disease. *Blood* 1994;84:1342.
185. Lipsky JJ. Mycophenolate mofetil (drug profile). *Lancet* 1996;348:1357.
186. Greinix HT, Volc-Platzer B, Rabitsch W, et al. Successful use of extracorporeal photochemotherapy in the treatment of severe acute and chronic graft-versus-host disease. *Blood* 1998;92:3098.
187. Ringden O. Management of graft-versus-host disease. *Eur J Haematol* 1993;51:1.
188. Sullivan KM, Shulman HM, Storb R, et al. Chronic graft-versus-host disease in 52 patients: adverse natural course and successful treatment with combination immunosuppression. *Blood* 1981;57:267.
189. Shulman HM, Sullivan KM, Weiden PL, et al. Chronic graft-versus-host disease syndrome in man. A long-term clinico-pathologic study of 20 Seattle patients. *Am J Med* 1980;69:204.
190. Ferrara JLM, Deeg HJ. Graft-versus-host disease. *N Engl J Med* 1991;324:667.
191. Loughran TP Jr, Sullivan K, Morton T, et al. Value of day 100 screening studies for predicting the development of chronic graft-versus-host disease after allogeneic bone marrow transplantation. *Blood* 1990;76:228.
192. Wingard JR, Piantadosi S, Vogelsang GB, et al. Predictors of death from chronic graft-versus-host disease after bone marrow transplantation. *Blood* 1989;74:1428.

193. Atkinson K. Chronic graft-versus-host disease. *Bone Marrow Transplant* 1990;5:69.
194. Sullivan KM, Witherspoon RP, Storb R, et al. Alternating-day cyclosporine and prednisone for treatment of high-risk chronic graft-versus-host disease. *Blood* 1988;72:555.
195. Volc-Platzer B, Honigsmann H, Hinterberger W, et al. Photo-chemotherapy improves chronic cutaneous graft-versus-host disease. *J Am Acad Dermatol* 1990;23:220.
196. Vogelsang GB, Farmer ER, Hess AD, et al. Thalidomide for the treatment of chronic GVHD. *N Engl J Med* 1992;325:1055.
197. Mookerjee B, Altomonte V, Vogelsang G. Salvage therapy for refractory chronic graft-versus-host disease with mycophenolate mofetil and tacrolimus. *Bone Marrow Transplant* 1999; 24:517.
198. Voogt PJ, Fibbe WE, Marijt WA, et al. Rejection of bone marrow graft by recipient-derived cytotoxic T lymphocytes against minor histocompatibility antigens. *Lancet* 1990;335:131.
199. Goss GD, Wittwer MA, Bezwoda WR, et al. Effects of natural killer cells on syngeneic bone marrow: in vitro and in vivo studies demonstrating graft failure due to NK cells in an identical twin treated by bone marrow transplantation. *Blood* 1985;66:1043.
200. Bosserman LD, Murray C, Takvorian T, et al. Mechanism of graft failure in HLA-matched and HLA-mismatched bone marrow transplant recipients. *Bone Marrow Transplant* 1989;4:239.
201. Champlin RE, Horowitz MM, Van Bekkum DW, et al. Graft failure following bone marrow transplantation for severe aplastic anemia: risk factors and treatment results. *Blood* 1989;73:606.
202. Kernan NA, Bordignon C, Heller G, et al. Graft failure after T-cell depleted human leukocyte antigen identical marrow transplants for leukemia: I. Analysis of risk factors and results of secondary transplants. *Blood* 1989;74:2227.
203. Martin PJ, Hansen JA, Torok-Storb B, et al. Graft failure in patients receiving T-cell depleted HLA-identical allogeneic marrow transplants. *Bone Marrow Transplant* 1988;3:445.
204. Niederwieser D, Pepe M, Storb R, et al. Improvement in rejection, engraftment rate and survival without increase in graft-versus-host disease by high marrow cell dose in patients transplanted for aplastic anemia. *Br J Haematol* 1988;69:23.
205. Anasetti C, Amos D, Beatty PG, et al. Effect of HLA compatibility on engraftment of bone marrow transplants in patients with leukemia or lymphoma. *N Engl J Med* 1989;320:197.
206. Deeg Hj, Self S, Storb R, et al. Decreased incidence of marrow graft rejection in patients with severe aplastic anemia: changing impact of risk factors. *Blood* 1986;68:1363.
207. Nemunaitis J, Singer JW, Buckner CD, et al. Use of recombinant human granulocyte-macrophage colony-stimulating factor in graft failure after bone marrow transplantation. *Blood* 1990;76:245.
208. Weisdorf DJ, Verfaillie CM, Davies SM, et al. Hematopoietic growth factors for graft failure after bone marrow transplantation: a randomized trial of granulocyte-macrophage colony-stimulating factor (GM-CSF) versus sequential GM-CSF plus granulocyte-CSF. *Blood* 1995;85:3452.
209. Bolger GB, Sullivan KM, Storb R, et al. Second marrow infusion for poor graft function after allogeneic marrow transplantation. *Bone Marrow Transplant* 1986;1:21.
210. Davies SM, Weisdorf DJ, Haake RJ, et al. Second infusion of bone marrow for treatment of graft failure after allogeneic bone marrow transplantation. *Bone Marrow Transplant* 1994;14:73.
211. Emanuel D, Cunningham I, Jules-Elysee K, et al. Cytomegalovirus pneumonia after bone marrow transplantation successfully treated with the combination of ganciclovir and high-dose intravenous immunoglobulin. *Ann Intern Med* 1988;109:777.
212. Paulin T, Ringdén O, Ljungman P, et al. Symptomatic cytomegalovirus infection after bone marrow transplantation. *Clin Transplant* 1989;3:279.
213. Weiner RS, Bortin MM, Gale RP, et al. Interstitial pneumonitis after bone marrow transplantation. *Ann Intern Med* 1986;104:168.
214. Bowden RA, Slichter SJ, Sayers MH, et al. Use of leukocyte-depleted platelets and cytomegalovirus-seronegative red blood cells for prevention of primary cytomegalovirus infection after marrow transplant. *Blood* 1981;78:246.
215. Winston DJ, Ho WG, Lin C-H, et al. Intravenous immunoglobulin for prevention of cytomegalovirus infection anti-interstitial pneumonia after bone marrow transplantation. *Ann Intern Med* 1987;106:12.
216. Bowden RA, Sayers M, Flournoy N, et al. Cytomegalovirus immune globulin and seronegative blood products to prevent primary cytomegalovirus infection after marrow transplantation. *N Engl J Med* 1986;314:1006.
217. Atkinson K, Downs K, Golenia M, et al. Prophylactic use of ganciclovir in allogeneic bone marrow transplantation: absence of clinical cytomegalovirus infection. *Br J Haematol* 1991;79:57.
218. Goodrich J, Bowden R, Fisher L, et al. Ganciclovir prophylaxis to prevent cytomegalovirus disease after allogeneic marrow transplant. *Ann Intern Med* 1993;118:173.
219. Ljungman P, Lore K, Aschan J, et al. Use of a semi-quantitative PCR for cytomegalovirus DNA as a basis for preemptive antiviral therapy in allogeneic bone marrow transplant patients. *Bone Marrow Transplant* 1996;17:583.
220. Walther EA, Greenberg PD, Gilbert MJ, et al. Reconstitution of cellular immunity against cytomegalovirus in recipients of allogeneic bone marrow by transfer of T-cell clones from donor. *N Engl J Med* 1995;333:1038.
221. Kessinger A, Smith DM, Strandjord SE, et al. Allogeneic transplantation of blood-derived T-cell-depleted haemopoietic stem cells after myeloablative treatment in a patient with acute lymphoblastic leukaemia. *Bone Marrow Transplant* 1989;4:643.
222. Russell NH, Hunter A, Rogers S., et al. Peripheral-blood stem-cells as an alternative to marrow for allogeneic transplantation [Letter]. *Lancet* 1993;341:1482.
223. Bensinger WI, Weaver C, Appelbaum F, et al. Transplantation of allogeneic peripheral blood stem cells mobilized by recombinant human granulocyte colony-stimulating factor. *Blood* 1995;85:1655.
224. Korbling M, Przepiorka D, Huh Y, et al. Allogeneic blood stem cell transplantation for refractory leukaemia and lymphoma: potential advantages of blood over marrow allograft. *Blood* 1995;85:1659.
225. Russell JA, Kuider J, Weaver M, et al. Collection of progenitor cells for allogeneic transplantation from peripheral blood of normal donors. *Bone Marrow Transplant* 1995;15:111.
226. Schmitz N, Dreger P, Suttorp M, et al. Primary transplantation of allogeneic peripheral-blood progenitor cells mobilized by filgrastim (granulocyte-colony-stimulating factor). *Blood* 1995;85:1666.
227. Russell JA, Brown C, Bowen T, et al. Allogeneic blood cell transplants for haematological malignancy: preliminary comparison of outcomes with bone marrow transplantation. *Bone Marrow Transplant* 1996;17:703.
228. Grigg AP, Roberts AW, Raunow H, et al. Optimizing dose and scheduling of filgrastim (GCSF) for mobilization and collection of peripheral blood progenitor cells in normal volunteers. *Blood* 1995;86:4437.
229. Dreger P, Haferlach T, Eckstein V, et al. G-CSF-mobilized peripheral blood progenitor cells for allogeneic transplantation: safety, kinetics of mobilization, and composition of the graft. *Br J Haematol* 1994;87:609.
230. Ottinger HD, Beelen DW, Scheulen B, et al. Improved immune reconstitution after allotransplantation of peripheral blood stem cells instead of bone marrow. *Blood* 1997;88:2775.
231. Schmitz N, Bacigalupo A, Hasenclever D, et al. Allogeneic bone marrow transplantation vs filgrastim-mobilised peripheral blood progenitor cell transplantation in patients with early leukemia: first results of a randomised multicentre trial of the European Group for Blood and Marrow Transplantation. *Bone Marrow Transplant* 1998;21:995.
232. Bensinger WI, Clift R, Martin P, et al. Allogeneic peripheral blood stem cell transplantation in patients with advanced hematologic malignancies: a retrospective comparison with marrow transplantation. *Blood* 1996;88:2794.
233. Bensinger W, Martin P, Clift R, et al. A prospective randomized trial of peripheral blood stem cells (PBSC) or marrow (BM) for patients undergoing allogeneic transplantation for hematologic malignancy. *Blood* 1999;94[Suppl 1]:368a(abst).
234. Gluckman E, Broxmeyer HE, Auerbach AD, et al. Hematopoietic reconstitution in a patient with Fanconi's anemia by means of umbilical cord blood from an HLA-identical sibling. *N Engl J Med* 1989;321:1174.
235. Wagner JE, Kernan NA, Steinbuch M, et al. Allogeneic sibling umbilical-cord blood transplantation in children with malignant and non-malignant disease. *Lancet* 1995;346:214.
236. Kurezberg J, Laughlin M, Graham ML, et al. Placental blood as a source of hematopoietic stem cells for transplantation into unrelated recipients. *N Engl J Med* 1996;335:157.
237. Wagner JE, Rosenthal J, Sweerman R, et al. Successful transplantation of HLA-matched and HLA-mismatched umbilical cord blood from unrelated donors; analysis of engraftment and acute graft-versus-host disease. *Blood* 1996;88:795.
238. Mayani H, Lansdorp PM. Thy-1 expression is linked to functional properties of primitive hematopoietic progenitor cells from human umbilical cord blood. *Blood* 1994;83:2410.
239. Morrison SJ, Wandycz AM, Akashi K, et al. The aging of hematopoietic stem cells. *Nat Med* 1996;2:1011.
240. Vaziri H, Dragowska W, Allsop RC, et al. Evidence for a mitotic clock in human hematopoietic stem cells: loss of telomeric DNA with age. *Proc Natl Acad Sci U S A* 1994;91:9857.
241. Gluckman E, Rocha V, Boyer-Chammard B, et al. Outcome of cord blood transplantation from related and unrelated donor. *N Engl J Med* 1997;337:373.
242. Anasetti C, Amos D, Beatty PG, et al. Effect of HLA compatibility on engraftment of bone marrow transplants in patients with leukemia or lymphoma. *N Engl J Med* 1989;320:197.
243. Ash RC, Casper JT, Chitambar CR, et al. Successful allogeneic transplantation of T-cell-depleted bone marrow from closely HLA-matched unrelated donors. *N Engl J Med* 1990;322:485.
244. Beatty PG, Hansen JA, Longton GM, et al. Marrow transplantation from HLA-matched unrelated donors for treatment of hematologic malignancies. *Transplantation* 1991;51:443.
245. Balduzzi A, Gooley T, Anasetti C, et al. Unrelated donor marrow transplantation in children. *Blood* 1995;86:3247.
246. Oudshoorn M, Cornelissen JJ, Fibbe WE, et al. Problems and possible solutions in finding an unrelated bone marrow donor: results of consecutive searches for 240 Dutch patients. *Bone Marrow Transplant* 1997;20:1011.
247. Henslee-Downey PJ, Gluckman E. Allogeneic transplantation from donors other than HLA-identical sibling. *Hematol Oncol Clin North Am* 1999;13:1017.
248. Clay TM, Bidwell JL, Howard MR, et al. PCR-fingerprinting for selection of HLA-matched unrelated marrow donors. *Lancet* 1991;337:1049.
249. Hansen JA, Gooley TA, Martin PJ, et al. Bone marrow transplants from unrelated donors for patients with chronic myeloid leukemia. *N Engl J Med* 1998;338:962.
250. Davies SM, Wagner JE, Shu X-O, et al. Unrelated donor bone marrow transplantation for children with acute leukemia. *J Clin Oncol* 1997;15:557.
251. Kernan NA, Bartsch G, Ash RC, et al. Analysis of 462 transplantations from unrelated donors facilitated by the National Marrow Donor Program. *N Engl J Med* 1993;328:593.
252. Hongeng S, Krance RW, Bowman LC, et al. Outcomes of transplantation with matched-sibling and unrelated donor bone marrow in children with leukemia. *Lancet* 1997;350:767.
253. Speiser DE, Tiercy JM, Rufer N, et al. High resolution HLA matching associated with decreased mortality after unrelated bone marrow transplantation. *Blood* 1996;10:4455.
254. Nademanee A, Schmidt GM, Parker P, et al. The outcome of matched unrelated donor bone marrow transplantation in patients with haematologic malignancies using molecular typing for donor selection and graft-versus-host disease prophylaxis regimen of cyclosporin, methotrexate, and prednisone. *Blood* 1995;86:1228.
255. Ringdén O, Remberger M, Bornhauser M, et al. Peripheral blood stem cell transplantation from unrelated donors: a comparison with marrow transplantation. *Blood* 1999;94:455.
256. Petersdorf EW, Longton GM, Anasetti C, et al. Definition of HLA-DQ as a transplantation antigen. *Proc Natl Acad Sci U S A* 1996;93:15358.
257. Petersdorf EW, Longton GM, Anasetti C, et al. Association of HLA-C disparity with graft failure after marrow transplantation from unrelated donors. *Blood* 1997;89:1818.
258. Wagner JE, King R, Kollman C, et al. Unrelated donor bone marrow transplantation (UBMT) in 5075 patients with malignant and non-malignant disorders: impact of marrow T cell depletion. *Blood* 1998;92[Suppl 1]:686a(abst).

259. Sierra J, Storer B, Hansen JA, et al. Transplantation of marrow cells from unrelated donors for treatment of high-risk acute leukemia: the effect of leukemic burden, donor HLA-matching, and marrow cell dose. *Blood* 1997;89:4226.
260. Powles RL, Morgenstern GR, Kay HEM, et al. Mismatched family donors for bone marrow transplantation as treatment for acute leukemia. *Lancet* 1983;1:612.
261. Beatty PG, Clift RA, Mickelson EM, et al. Marrow transplantation from related donors other than HLA-identical siblings. *N Engl J Med* 1985;313:765.
262. Anasetti C, Amos D, Beatty PG, et al. Effect of HLA compatibility on engraftment of bone marrow transplants in patients with leukemia or lymphoma. *N Engl J Med* 1989; 320:197.
263. Ash RC, Horowitz MM, Gale RP, et al. Bone marrow transplantation from related donors other than HLA-identical siblings: effect of T-cell depletion. *Bone Marrow Transplant* 1991;7:443.
264. Ash RC, Horowitz MM, Gale RP, et al. Bone marrow transplantation from related donors other than HLA-identical siblings: effect of T-cell depletion. *Bone Marrow Transplant* 1991;7:443.
265. Szydlo R, Goldman JM, Klein JP, et al. Results of allogeneic bone marrow transplants for leukemia using donors other than HLA-identical siblings. *J Clin Oncol* 1997;15:1767.
266. Beatty PG, Clift RA, Mickelson EM, et al. Marrow transplantation from related donors other than HLA-identical siblings. *N Engl J Med* 1985;313:765.
267. Beatty PG, Hansen JA, Longton GM, et al. Marrow transplantation from HLA-matched unrelated donors for treatment of hematologic malignancies. *Transplantation* 1991;51:443.
268. Henslee PJ, Thompson JS, Romond EH, et al. T-cell depletion of HLA and haploidentical marrow reduces graft-versus-host disease but it may impair a graft-versus-leukemia effect. *Transplant Proc* 1987;19:2701.
269. Trigg ME, Sondel PM, Billing R, et al. Mismatched bone marrow transplantation in children with hematologic malignancy using T-lymphocyte depleted bone marrow. *J Biol Response Mod* 1985;4:602.
270. O'Reilly RJ, Collins NH, Kernan N, et al. Transplantation of marrow-depleted T-cells by soybean lectin agglutination and E-rosette depletion: major histocompatibility complex–related graft resistance in leukemic transplant patients. *Transplant Proc* 1985;17:455.
271. Fleeting DR, Henslee-Downey PJ, Romond EH, et al. Allogeneic bone marrow transplantation with T cell–depleted partially matched related donors for advanced acute lymphoblastic leukemia in children and adults: a comparative matched cohort study. *Bone Marrow Transplant* 1996;17:917.
272. Henslee-Downey PJ, Abhyankar SH, Parrish RS, et al. Use of partially mismatched related donors extends access to allogeneic marrow transplant. *Blood* 1997;89:3804.
273. Aversa F, Tabilio A, Terenzi A, et al. Successful engraftment of T-cell-depleted haploidentical "three-loci" incompatible transplants in leukemia patients by addition of recombinant human granulocyte colony-stimulating factor–mobilized peripheral blood progenitor cells to bone marrow inoculum. *Blood* 1994;84:3948.
274. Aversa F, Tabilio A, Velardi A, et al. Treatment of high-risk acute leukemia with T-cell depleted stem cells from related donors with one fully mismatched I-ILA haplotype. *N Engl J Med* 1998;339:1186.
275. Guinan EC, Boussiotis VA, Neuberg D, et al. Transplantation of anergic histocompatible bone marrow allografts. *N Engl J Med* 1999;340:1704.
276. Ringdén O, Nilsson B. Death by graft-versus-host disease associated with HLA mismatch, high recipient age, low marrow cell dose, and splenectomy. *Transplantation* 1985;40:39.
277. Barrett AJ, Horowitz MM, Gale RP, et al. Marrow transplantation for acute lymphoblastic leukemia: factors affecting relapse and survival. *Blood* 1989;74:862.
278. Giralt S, Estey E, Albitar M, et al. Engraftment of allogeneic hemapoietic progenitor cells with purine analog–containing chemotherapy: harnessing graft-versus-leukaemia without myeloablative therapy. *Blood* 1997;89:4531.
279. Slavin S, Nagler A, Naparstak E, et al. Nonmyeloablative stem cell transplantation and cell therapy as an alternative to conventional bone marrow transplantation with lethal cytoreduction for the treatment of malignant and non malignant hematologic diseases. *Blood* 1988;91:756.
280. Khouri I, Keating MJ, Korbling M, et al. Transplant-lite: induction of graft-versus-malignancy using fludarabine-based nonablative chemotherapy and allogeneic progenitor cell transplantation as treatment for lymphoid malignancies. *J Clin Oncol* 1998;16:2817.
281. Sykes M, Preffer F, McAfee S, et al. Mixed lymphohaemopoietic chimerism and graft-versus-lymphoma effects after non-myeloablative therapy and HLA mismatched bone marrow transplantation. *Lancet* 1999;353:1755.
282. Childs R, Epperson D, Bahceci E, et al. Molecular remission of chronic myeloid leukaemia following a non-myeloablative allogeneic peripheral blood stem cell transplant: in vivo and in vitro evidence for a graft-versus-leukaemia effect. *Br J Haematol* 1999;107:396.
283. Grigg A, Bardy P, Byron K, et al. Fludarabine-based non-myeloablative chemotherapy followed by infusion of HLA-identical stem cells for relapsed leukaemia and lymphoma. *Bone Marrow Transplant* 1999;23:107.
284. Childs R, Clave E, Tisdale J, et al. Successful treatment of metastatic renal cell carcinoma with a nonmyeloablative allogeneic peripheral blood progenitor cell transplant: evidence for a graft-versus-tumor effect. *J Clin Oncol* 1999;17:2044.
285. Craddock C. Nonmyeloablative stem cell transplants. *Curr Opin Hematol* 1999;6:383.
286. Storb R, Yu C, Sandmaier BM, et al. Mixed hematopoietic chimerism after marrow allografts: transplantation in the ambulatory care setting. *Ann NY Acad Sci* 1999;872:372.
287. Storb R, Yu C, Wagner J, et al. Stable mixed hematopoietic chimerism in DLA-identical littermate dogs given sublethal total body irradiation before and pharmacological immunosuppression after marrow transplantation. *Blood* 1997;89:3048.
288. Sykes M, Sheard MA, Sachs DH. Graft-versus-host-related immunosuppression is induced in mixed chimeras by alloresponses against either host or donor lymphohematopoietic cells. *J Exp Med* 1988;168:2391.
289. Childs R, Clave E, Contenin N, et al. Engraftment kinetics after nonmyeloablative allogeneic peripheral blood stem cell transplantation: full donor T-cell chimerism recedes alloimmune responses. *Blood* 1999;94:3234.
290. Sandmaier BM, McSweeny P, Yu C, et al. Nonmyeloablative transplants: Preclinical and clinical results. *Semin Oncol* 2000;2(Suppl5):78.
291. Niederwieser D, Wolff D, Hegenbart U, et al. Hematopoietic stem cell transplants (HSCT) from HLA matched and 1 allele mismatched unrelated donors using a nonmyeloablative regimen. *Blood* 1999;94[Suppl 1]:561a(abst).
292. Childs R, Contenin N, Clave E, et al. Reduced toxicity and transplant related mortality (TRM) following non-myeloablative allogeneic peripheral blood stem cell transplantation for malignant disease. *Blood* 1999;94[Suppl 1]:393a(abst).
293. Kottaridis P, Chakravarty R, Milligan D, et al. A non-myeloablative regimen for allografting high-risk patients: low toxicity, stable engraftment without GVHD, disease control and potential for GVL with adoptive immunotherapy. *Blood* 1999;94[Suppl 1]:348a(abst).
294. Khouri I, Lee M, Palmer L, et al. Transplant-lite using fludarabine-cyclophosphamide (FC) and allogeneic stem cell transplant (AlloSCT) for low grade lymphoma (LGL). *Blood* 1999;94[Suppl 1]:348a(abst).
295. Michallet M, Bilger K, Garban F, et al. Allogeneic hematopoietic stem cell transplants after immune-ablative preparative regimen: a report of 92 cases. *Blood* 1999;94[Suppl 1]:348a(abst).
296. Shimoni A, Anderlini P, Andersson B, et al. Allogeneic transplantation for leukaemia in patients older than 60 years of age should not exclude treatment with non-myeloablative regimens. *Blood* 1999;94[Suppl 1]:710a(abst).
297. Childs R, Contentin N, Clave E, et al. Sustained regression of metastatic renal cell carcinoma following non-myeloablative allogeneic peripheral blood stem cell transplantation: a new applicant of allogeneic immunology. *Blood* 1999;94[Suppl 1]:710a(abst).
298. Bensinger WI, Buckner CD, Anasetti C, et al. Allogeneic bone marrow transplantation for multiple myeloid: an analysis of risk factors on outcome. *Blood* 1996;88:2787.
299. Biggs JC, Szer J, Grilley P, et al. Treatment of chronic myeloid leukemia with allogeneic bone marrow transplantation after preparation with BuCy 2. *Blood* 1992;80:1353.
300. Clift RA, Buckner CD, Thomas ED, et al. Marrow transplantation for patients in accelerated phase of chronic myeloid leukemia. *Blood* 1994;84:4368.
301. Goldman J, Apperley JF, Jones L, et al. Bone marrow transplantation for patients with chronic myeloid leukemia. *N Engl J Med* 1986;314:202.
302. McGlave P, Arthur D, Haake R, et al. Therapy of chronic myelogenous leukemia with allogeneic bone marrow transplantation. *J Clin Oncol* 1987;5:1033.
303. Wagner JE, Zahurak M, Piantadosi S, et al. Bone marrow transplantation of chronic myelogenous leukemia in chronic phase: evaluation of risks and benefits. *J Clin Oncol* 1992;10:779.
304. Hansen JA, Gooley TA, Martin PJ, et al. Bone marrow transplants from unrelated donors for patients with chronic myeloid leukemia. *N Engl J Med* 1998;338:962.
305. Keating MJ, Smith TL, Kantarjian H, et al. Cytogenetic patterns in acute myelogenous leukemia: a major reproducible determinant of outcome. *Leukemia* 1988;2:403.
306. Grimwade D, Walker H, Oliver F, et al. The importance of diagnostic cytogenetics on outcome in AML: analysis of 1,612 patients entered into the MRC AML 10 trial. *Blood* 1998;92:2322.
307. Bostrom B, Brunning RD, McGlave P, et al. Bone marrow transplantation for acute nonlymphocytic leukemia in first remission: analysis of prognostic factors. *Blood* 1985;65:1191.
308. Forman SJ, Spruce WE, Farbstein MJ, et al. Bone marrow ablation followed by allogeneic marrow grafting during first complete remission of acute nonlymphocytic leukemia. *Blood* 1983;61:439.
309. Helenglass G, Powles RL, McElwain TJ, et al. Melphalan and total body irradiation (TBI) versus cyclophosphamide and TBI as conditioning for allogeneic matched sibling bone marrow transplants for acute myeloblastic leukemia in first remission. *Bone Marrow Transplant* 1988;3:21.
310. McGlave PB, Haake RJ, Bostrom BC, et al. Allogeneic bone marrow transplantation for acute nonlymphocytic leukemia in first remission. *Blood* 1988;72:1512.
311. Buckner CD, Clift RA, Thomas ED, et al. Allogeneic marrow transplantation for patients with acute non-lymphoblastic leukemia in second remission. *Leuk Res* 1982;6:395.
312. Appelbaum FR, Clift RA, Buckner CD, et al. Allogeneic marrow transplantation for acute nonlymphoblastic leukemia after first complete relapse. *Blood* 1983;61:949.
313. Hoelzer D, Ludwig WD, Thiel D, et al. Improved outcome in adult B-cell acute lymphoblastic leukemia. *Blood* 1996;87:495.
314. Hoelzer D, Thiel E, Loffler T, et al. Prognostic factors in a multicentric study for treatment of active lymphoblastic leukemia in adults. *Blood* 1988;71:123.
315. Laport GE, Larson R. Treatment of adult acute lymphoblastic leukemia. *Semin Oncol* 1997;24:70.
316. Faderl S, Kantarjian M, Talpaz M, et al. Clinical significance of cytogenetic abnormalities in adult acute lymphoblastic leukemia. *Blood* 1998;91:3996.
317. Barrett AJ, Horowitz MM, Ash RC, et al. Bone marrow transplantation for Philadelphia chromosome–positive acute lymphoblastic leukemia. *Blood* 1992;79:3067.
318. Chao NJ, Forman SJ, Schmidt GM, et al. Allogeneic bone marrow transplantation for high-risk acute lymphoblastic leukemia during first complete remission. *Blood* 1991;78:1923.
319. Forman SJ. The role of allogeneic bone marrow transplantation in the treatment of high-risk acute lymphocytic leukemia in adults. *Leukemia* 1997;11[Suppl 4]:S18.
320. Chao NJ, Forman SJ, Schmidt GM, et al. Allogeneic bone marrow transplantation for high-risk acute lymphoblastic leukemia during first complete remission. *Blood* 1991;78:1923.
321. Sanders JE, Thomas ED, Buckner CD, et al. Marrow transplantation for children with acute lymphoblastic leukemia in second remission. *Blood* 1987;70:324.
322. Barrett AJ, Horowitz MM, Pollock BH, et al. Bone marrow transplants from HLA-identical siblings as compared with chemotherapy for children with acute lymphoblastic leukemia in a second remission. *N Engl J Med* 1994;331:1253.
323. Anderson JE, Appelbaum FR, Fisher LD, et al. Allogeneic bone marrow transplantation for 93 patients with myelodysplastic syndrome. *Blood* 1993;82:677.
324. Runde V, de Witte T, Arnold R, et al. Bone marrow transplantation from HLA-identical siblings as first-line treatment in patients with myelodysplastic syndromes: early trans-

plantation is associated with improved outcome. Chronic Leukemia Working Party of the European Group for Blood and Marrow Transplantation. *Bone Marrow Transplant* 1998;21:255.

325. Nevill T, Fung H, Shepard J, et al. Cytogenetic abnormalities in primary myelodysplastic syndrome are highly predictive of outcome after allogeneic bone marrow transplantation. *Blood* 1998;92:1910.
326. Michallet M, Archimbaud E, Bandini G, et al. HLA-identical sibling bone marrow transplantation in younger patients with chronic lymphocytic leukemia. European Group for Blood and Marrow Transplantation and the International Bone Marrow Transplant Registry. *Ann Intern Med* 1996;124:311.
327. Gahrton G, Tura S, Ljungman P, et al. Prognostic factors in allogeneic bone marrow transplantation for multiple myeloma. *J Clin Oncol* 1995;13:1312.
328. Chopra R, Goldstone AH, Pearce R, et al. Autologous versus allogeneic bone marrow transplantation for non-Hodgkin's lymphoma: a case-controlled analysis of the European Bone Marrow Transplant Group Registry data. *J Clin Oncol* 1992;10:1690.
329. Ratanatharathorn V, Uberti J, Karanes C, et al. Prospective comparative trial of autologous versus allogeneic bone marrow transplantation in patients with non-Hodgkin's lymphoma. *Blood* 1994;84:1050.
330. Anderson JE, Litzow MR, Appelbaum FR, et al. Allogeneic, syngeneic, and autologous marrow transplantation for Hodgkin's disease: the 21-year Seattle experience. *J Clin Oncol* 1993;11:2342.
331. Dann EJ, Daugherty CK, Larson RA. Allogeneic bone marrow transplantation for relapsed and refractory Hodgkin's disease and non-Hodgkin's lymphoma. *Bone Marrow Transplant* 1997;20:369.

SECTION **4**

JAMES D. GRIFFIN

Hematopoietic Growth Factors

The hematopoietic growth factors (HGFs) are a family of cytokines that regulate the proliferation, differentiation, and viability of hematopoietic progenitor cells and mature blood elements. More than 20 different cytokines have been discovered, all of which are believed to have effects on blood cell development or function, and many of these have been tested in preclinical or clinical trials in cancer patients over the last 15 years. Four HGFs—erythropoietin (EPO), granulocyte colony-stimulating factor (G-CSF), granulocyte-macrophage colony-stimulating factor (GM-CSF), and interleukin-11 (IL-11)—have been approved by the U.S. Food and Drug Administration for specific uses (Table 53.4-1), and other approvals are likely in the future. Early phase I and II trials indicated that G-CSF or GM-CSF had the potential to ameliorate myelosuppression in many circumstances, and now there is abundant evidence from randomized, phase III trials that this is the case. Similarly, EPO has been shown to be an effective treatment for the anemia of cancer in some patients, and IL-11 has been shown to reduce chemotherapy-associated thrombocytopenia in some circumstances. In addition, G-CSF, GM-CSF, and other growth factors are now commonly used to induce transient mobilization of hematopoietic stem and progenitor cells into the blood to allow collection for both autologous and allogeneic stem cell transplantation. Finally, other new cytokines [such as thrombopoietin (TPO)] with well-defined effects on thrombopoiesis are being investigated in on-going clinical trials. Overall, the ability to use HGFs therapeutically to enhance hematopoiesis has now become an important and widely used part of the treatment of certain cancers and has led to improved safety of high-dose chemotherapy and bone marrow transplantation in particular. This is still a field with many questions, however, and the cost-effectiveness of cytokine use in many areas of cancer treatment is still unknown. This chapter focuses on the four HGFs currently approved by the U.S. Food and Drug Administration for one or more applications in cancer and then summarizes the current state of clinical development of other cytokines of potential interest in cancer medicine.

OVERVIEW OF HEMATOPOIETIC GROWTH FACTORS

All the formed elements of the blood—leukocytes, erythrocytes, and platelets—are derived from multipotent stem cells found primarily in the marrow. Because the life span of blood cells is relatively short, large numbers of cells need to be replenished daily, and this daily requirement may be further increased by bleeding or acute infection. Most of the stem cells are not actively cycling, and it is thought that hematopoiesis is maintained by the activity of only a small fraction of the total stem cell pool at any given point in time. As these cells mature, however, they become progressively more committed to a single lineage, creating a series of "progenitor" cells that are actively proliferating and very sensitive to regulation by HGFs. Interestingly, recent studies have identified stem cells with hematopoietic potential in other tissues, including brain and muscle.[1] The significance of these cells and their potential for clinical development is of considerable interest.

There has been a dramatic increase in the knowledge of the regulation of hematopoiesis as the genes for individual HGFs have been cloned and recombinant proteins produced (Table 53.4-2). The existence of HGFs has been recognized for more than 35 years but, before cloning of HGF genes, they could be studied only as partially purified "activities" secreted by activated normal cells or certain cancer cell lines. The large number of cytokines now believed to be involved in potentially regulating hematopoiesis and the complexity of that regulation were unanticipated, and the remarkable history of the development of this field has been extensively reviewed.[2–9] Some factors, such as Steel factor and Flt3 ligand, appear to have effects predominantly on stem and progenitor cells and minimal effects on more mature cells. In contrast, more lineage-restricted factors, such as EPO and G-CSF, have prominent effects on progenitor cells and mature cells and minimal effects on stem cells.

It is likely that a baseline production of growth factors maintains hematopoiesis in a steady state. Many HGFs are secreted by cells in the marrow microenvironment and may be concentrated either on the cell surface of stromal cells or on extracellular matrix proteins in the marrow. One exception to this is the apparently exclusive production of EPO outside the marrow, in the kidney and liver. In emergency situations, HGFs can be produced in many tissues. For example, keratinocytes, fibroblasts, and endothelial cells can produce large amounts of G-CSF, GM-CSF, IL-1,

TABLE 53.4-1. Major Hematopoietic Growth Factors in Clinical Use for Cancer Treatment

Hematopoietic Growth Factor	*Generic Name*	*Molecular Weight*	*Amino Acids*	*Hematopoietic Effects*	*Applications in Cancer*
EPO	Epoetin alpha	30 kD	165	Red cell lineage	Chemotherapy- or cancer-associated anemia
G-CSF	Filgrastim	18 kD	175	Neutrophil lineage	Reduce febrile neutropenia in patients receiving myelosuppressive chemotherapy
GM-CSF	Sargramostim, Molgramostim	15–20 kD	127	Neutrophils, eosinophils, monocytes	Accelerate hematopoietic reconstitution after bone marrow transplantation; marrow failure after bone marrow transplantation
Interleukin-11	Oprelvekin	23 kD	199	Megakaryocyte	Chemotherapy-associated thrombocytopenia

EPO, erythropoietin; G-CSF, granulocyte colony-stimulating factor; GM-CSF, granulocyte-macrophage colony-stimulating factor.
Note: Includes hematopoietic growth factors approved by the U.S. Food and Drug Administration for one or more clinical applications in cancer patients.

and others in response to inflammation or other types of activation. Interestingly, some HGFs circulate in detectable levels in the blood, while many others do not. The serum concentrations of EPO, G-CSF, and TPO vary inversely with red cell oxygen-carrying capacity, neutrophil count, and platelet count, respectively. However, except for EPO, the mechanisms to "sense" the need for increased synthesis of a specific cytokine *in vivo* are not well understood. In the case of bacterial infections, certain bacterial cell wall products, such as lipopolysaccharides, are potent inducers of G-CSF synthesis by macrophages and other cells. In addi-

TABLE 53.4-2. Selected Hematopoietic Growth Factors and Other Cytokines in Clinical Development for Applications in Cancer Therapy

Factor	*Other Names*	*Hematopoietic Activities*	*Gene Location*	*Potential Cancer Applications*[a]
Erythropoietin	EPO	Red cell lineage	7q11-q22	Treatment of chemotherapy- and cancer-associated anemia
Granulocyte CSF	G-CSF	Neutrophil lineage	17q11-21	Accelerate neutrophil recovery after chemotherapy or BMT
				Reduce incidence of febrile neutropenia and infections
				Mobilize progenitor cells
Granulocyte-macrophage CSF	GM-CSF	Granulocyte-macrophage	5q31.1	Accelerate neutrophil recovery after chemotherapy or BMT
				Reduce incidence of febrile neutropenia and infections
				Mobilize progenitor cells
				Gene therapy of tumors
Thrombopoietin	TPO	Megakaryocytes	3q26-27	Reduce chemotherapy-associated thrombocytopenia
	MGDF	Platelets		Generation of megakaryocytes and platelets *in vitro*
Macrophage CSF	M-CSF	Macrophage	1p13-21	Activate tumoricidal functions of macrophages
	CSF-1	Osteoclast		Reduce incidence of severe fungal infections
Interleukin-1	IL-1	Multilineage[b]	α. 2q12-21	Accelerate reconstitution of hematopoiesis
		Immune cells	β. 2q12-21	Expand progenitor cells *ex vivo*
Interleukin-2	IL-2	T cells	4q26-28	Activate tumoricidal T and NK cells; generate lymphokine-activated killer cells
Interleukin-3	IL-3	Multilineage	5q31.1	Accelerate reconstitution of hematopoiesis
	Multi-CSF			Mobilize progenitor cells
				Expand progenitor cells *ex vivo*
Interleukin-4	IL-4	Immune cells[c]	5q31.1	Modulate immune response to tumor cells
				Gene therapy of tumors
Interleukin-6	IL-6	Multilineage	7p21	Accelerate reconstitution of hematopoiesis
		Immune cells		Expand progenitor cells *ex vivo*
Interleukin-11	IL-11	Megakaryocyte	19q13-3-13.4	Reduce chemotherapy-associated thrombocytopenia
				Reduce treatment-associated gastrointestinal toxicity
Interleukin-12	IL-12	NK cells	p35, 3p12-13.2	Activate tumoricidal T cells and NK cells
		T cells	p40, 5q31-33	
Steel factor	c-kit ligand	Multilineage	12q14.3-qter	Accelerate reconstitution of hematopoiesis
				Mobilize progenitor cells
				Expand progenitor cells *ex vivo*

BMT, bone marrow transplant; CSF, colony-stimulating factor; MGDF, megakaryocyte growth and development factor; NK, natural killer.
[a]The applications listed include those based on preclinical or *in vitro* studies, as well as those based on clinical trials in humans.
[b]Multilineage includes red cell, neutrophil, monocyte, and megakaryocyte lineages.
[c]Immune cells include T lymphocytes, NK cells, and B lymphocytes.

tion, a number of cytokines associated with an acute immune response, such as interferon-γ and tumor necrosis factor, will induce secretion of G-CSF and GM-CSF by a variety of other cells. Other factors, such as GM-CSF and IL-3, rarely circulate in detectable levels even during severe neutropenia.

New insights into cytokine biology have been recently obtained by studying mice engineered to lack one or more cytokines. These knockout mice have provided information in some cases that challenges hypotheses of cytokine function based on many years of tissue culture studies.[8,10,11] For example, mice deficient in GM-CSF production are not leukopenic and, in fact, have so far been found to have only a pulmonary defect that resembles pulmonary alveolar proteinosis.[12] Similarly, mice deficient in IL-3 have normal production of granulocytes, red cells, and platelets but have defects in mast cells and certain immune responses.[13,14] Mice with natural mutations in the macrophage colony-stimulating factor or colony-stimulating factor-1 (CSF-1) gene have reduced macrophage number and severe osteopetrosis. Other cytokine-deficient mice also have significant hematopoietic defects. Mice that are deficient in G-CSF,[15] EPO,[16] and TPO[17] are selectively neutropenic, anemic, and thrombocytopenic, respectively. Steel factor–deficient mice may be severely anemic, depending on the exact mutation.[18,19] Overall, these emerging results further suggest that the cytokine network that regulates hematopoiesis is complex, with overlapping and redundant functions for some factors and unclear functions for other factors. To investigate these possibilities, mice deficient in multiple factors are now being studied. These mice will likely provide further insights into the critical events of hematopoietic regulation.[20]

BIOLOGIC FEATURES OF THE MAJOR HEMATOPOIETIC GROWTH FACTORS IN CLINICAL USE

ERYTHROPOIETIN

EPO is the primary regulator of the late stages of red cell production, and both humans and mice deficient in EPO production develop severe anemia. The biology and pharmacology of EPO have been reviewed extensively.[21–25] The EPO gene is located on human chromosome 7q11-22, and the cDNA was cloned in 1984.[26–28] The mature protein contains 165 amino acids and has a molecular weight of 30,400 daltons. EPO is produced in the kidney in response to hypoxia or decreased oxygen-carrying capacity of the blood. The mechanism is still not completely understood, but it is clear that transcription of the EPO gene is regulated in part by a pathway that involves an oxygen-binding heme protein.[29] Occasional patients present with erythrocytosis secondary to either a renal tumor causing local hypoxia related to compression or, more rarely, secondary to secretion of EPO by the tumor.

EPO binds to bone marrow cells expressing the EPO receptor and stimulates proliferation of erythroid colony-forming cells and a subset of less mature burst-forming units. Cloning of the EPO receptor was reported in 1989,[30] and it was shown to be a single-chain transmembrane protein that is believed to function as either a monomer or homodimer. The receptor is a member of the HGF receptor superfamily and shares homology with the receptors for G-CSF, GM-CSF, IL-2, TPO, and other cytokines.[31,32] Interestingly, the receptor interacts with the gp55 protein of the Friend erythroleukemia virus, and the resulting activation of the EPO receptor is involved in causing erythroleukemias of mice.[33–35] In addition, other recent studies with the Friend erythroleukemia virus suggest that the EPO receptor may also interact with a transmembrane tyrosine kinase termed *Ron/stk*. Mutations in the distal end of the EPO receptor are associated with familial erythrocytosis[36–38] but have not yet been associated with human erythroleukemias.

The serum concentration of EPO in normal individuals is approximately 4 to 30 U/L, and the half-life of recombinant EPO administered intravenously in humans is 9 to 13 hours. Serum EPO levels reproducibly start to rise as the hematocrit drops below approximately 35% and can increase 100- to 1000-fold with severe anemia. In cancer patients with chronic anemias, the EPO level is often inappropriately low.[39,40] The clinical indications for EPO treatment are described in detail later in the section Treatment of Anemia in Cancer Patients. In cancer patients, EPO treatment is indicated for chemotherapy-associated anemia not due to other causes (iron deficiency, marrow involvement with tumor, etc.) and is most likely to have benefit if the serum EPO level is abnormally low.

Toxic effects of EPO in cancer patients are generally minimal. The hypertension and thrombotic events seen in patients with chronic renal failure treated with EPO are rarely seen in cancer patients with normal renal function. Monitoring of hematocrit is required to avoid erythrocytosis.

GRANULOCYTE COLONY-STIMULATING FACTOR

G-CSF (filgrastim, lenograstim) regulates the production, maturation, and function of cells of the neutrophil lineage.[8,41–43] G-CSF was initially investigated in the mouse as a factor with potent capacity to differentiate myeloid leukemia cell lines and was later purified from mouse lung–conditioned medium.[44] Human G-CSF was purified from medium conditioned by bladder and head and neck cancer cell lines, and the gene was then cloned.[45,46] The human gene is located on chromosome 17q11-21 and encodes a mature polypeptide of 175 amino acids with a molecular weight of 18,800 daltons. In tissue culture studies, G-CSF induces proliferation and differentiation of cells of the neutrophil lineage. In the mouse, knockout of the G-CSF gene produces severe neutropenia but has minimal effect on other lineages.[15] Hammond et al.[47] have also shown that dogs induced to form neutralizing antiantibodies to G-CSF become profoundly neutropenic.[47] G-CSF may also enhance several functions of neutrophils, but the significance of this observation is unknown. Overall, it is clear that G-CSF is critically involved in regulating neutrophil production.

G-CSF is produced by many different cell types, and expression of G-CSF can be rapidly induced by exposure of epithelial cells, macrophages, endothelial cells, and marrow stromal cells to inflammatory stimuli, particularly endotoxin. Unlike many other hemopoietins, there is readily detectable G-CSF in the serum of normal individuals, with a typical range of 20 to 100 pg/mL. The serum level varies inversely with neutrophil concentration in the blood, and in bacteremic, neutropenic patients, serum levels can exceed 2000 pg/mL.

The receptor for G-CSF is widely expressed, not only on myeloid lineage cells but on endothelial cells and epithelial cancer cell lines. The function of nonhematopoietic G-CSF receptors is not clear, however. The receptor for G-CSF is a member of the cytokine receptor superfamily[48,49] and is composed of a single known transmembrane protein of approximately 100 kD molecular weight. Mutations in the cytoplasmic domain of the receptor have recently been demonstrated in a small number of patients with congenital neutropenia and acute myeloblastic leukemia.[50] The mutations truncate the receptor, possibly removing a domain involved in the differentiation-inducing function of G-CSF.[50] Function of the truncated receptor in murine models suggests that the receptor may be activated to an excessive level by G-CSF.[51]

Administration of G-CSF to humans results in a dose-dependent increase in circulating neutrophils accompanied by expansion of the myeloid components in the marrow and accelerated production of neutrophils due to reduced transit time from stem cell to mature neutrophil. The fraction of myeloid progenitor cells in S-phase in the marrow is increased, and there is some suggestion that G-CSF enhances entry of quiescent stem and progenitor cells into the cell cycle. Neutrophils produced in response to G-CSF therapy have been shown to be functionally normal in terms of standard assays for phagocytosis and activation of the respiratory burst and further appear to have normal function *in vivo.* Marrow aspirates performed on patients receiving G-CSF or other myeloid growth factors may show a striking left shift, and circulating neutrophils have interesting morphologic changes consistent with activation, including Döhle's inclusion bodies, toxic granulation, and an increase in band forms. The elimination half-life of G-CSF in the serum is in the range of 1.3 to 4.2 hours but appears to vary with neutrophil mass, suggesting that neutrophils may contribute to metabolizing the cytokine.[52]

Toxic side effects of G-CSF in humans have been generally mild. Some patients experience bone pain during administration, but fever and weight gain are rare. Chronic administration of G-CSF has been associated with benign splenomegaly,[53] presumably due to extramedullary hematopoiesis. Bone scan abnormalities have also been reported, including an apparent "flare" of metastatic bone lesions and increased uptake in the axial skeleton or juxtaarticular regions.[54] In many patients, there is an acute response to intravenous injections of G-CSF characterized by abrupt, but transient, neutropenia.[55] Occasionally, patients will have transient dyspnea and pulmonary infiltrates on chest radiography. In patients with underlying severe pulmonary disease, these effects can be clinically significant.[56] The acute neutropenia is believed to be due to up-regulation of neutrophil adhesion receptors followed by either intravascular aggregation or margination, and is generally not seen with subcutaneous administration.[55,57] In patients with normal marrow function, prolonged administration of G-CSF can lead to very high neutrophil counts, and it is recommended that in most cases, G-CSF should be discontinued or dose-reduced when the neutrophil count exceeds 10,000 cells/μL. Once G-CSF is discontinued, the absolute neutrophil count typically falls by approximately 50% per day and will return to baseline in 4 to 6 days. Careful studies in normal volunteers have also shown that some alterations of blood chemistries are common but of no apparent clinical consequence.[58]

GRANULOCYTE-MACROPHAGE COLONY-STIMULATING FACTOR

GM-CSF (sargramostim, molgramostim) is a potent growth factor for the myeloid lineage in tissue culture and was cloned by Wong et al.[59] GM-CSF is a glycoprotein with an approximate molecular weight of 22,000 daltons, and the gene has been localized to chromosome 5q31 in close proximity to the gene for IL-3.[60] GM-CSF can be produced by many cells in the body, particularly by activated T cells. Recombinant or purified natural GM-CSF stimulates granulocyte-macrophage and eosinophil colony formation and cooperates with EPO to stimulate growth of erythroid bursts. GM-CSF also stimulates the activity of multiple neutrophil functions and primes these cells to respond more vigorously to other stimuli.[61,62] Changes in expression of neutrophil adhesion molecules are particularly prominent, including up-regulation of the beta-2 integrin CD11/CD18 both *in vitro* and *in vivo*.[63]

A mouse in which the GM-CSF gene has been knocked out does not have demonstrable defects in hematopoiesis but develops a severe lung disorder similar to pulmonary alveolar proteinosis.[12,64] Interestingly, patients with this disorder have been shown to have defects in expression, function, or mutations in the beta chain of the receptor for GM-CSF.[65,66] Receptors for GM-CSF are normally found on both hematopoietic and nonhematopoietic cells, including endothelial cells and some tumor cell lines, such as melanoma and lung cancer cells. The function of these receptors, if any, on nonhematopoietic cells is unclear. The receptor is a heterodimer, composed of a ligand-binding alpha chain and a beta chain necessary for high-affinity binding and signal transduction. The alpha chain uniquely binds GM-CSF, but the same beta chain is also used by the receptors for IL-3 and -5.

Administration of GM-CSF to humans results in a dose-dependent increase in blood neutrophils, eosinophils and, to a lesser extent, macrophages and sometimes lymphocytes. This is accompanied by a dramatic left shift in the myeloid series in the marrow. There is no significant effect on the red cell or platelet lineages. The toxic effects of GM-CSF have been evaluated extensively. If given intravenously in particular, the first dose of GM-CSF may be accompanied by acute but self-limited neutropenia thought to be due to up-regulation of adhesion receptors on neutrophils.[55] Occasional patients may experience brief dyspnea. Many patients experience a low-grade fever, myalgias, and fatigue. At high doses, weight gain, pericarditis, pleuritis, and a capillary leak syndrome may develop,[67] but this is rare at doses in current use. The activities and toxicities of GM-CSF and G-CSF have been directly compared in very few studies. In a randomized study after autologous stem cell transplantation for breast cancer, the efficacy and toxicities of the two factors were equivalent.[68]

There are several formulations of recombinant GM-CSF available, including yeast-derived (sargramostim) and *Escherichia coli*–derived (molgramostim) versions. At present, various formulations of GM-CSF seem to have similar biologic effects. Sargramostim is glycosylated and therefore has a lower specific activity than Molgramostim (because of its higher molecular weight). Manufacturer's directions should be read carefully when changing between formulations of GM-CSF. The recommended dosing for sargramostim is 250 $\mu g/m^2/d$ in patients receiving chemotherapy. Subcutaneous administration is generally preferred over short-term intravenous administration, due to reduced toxicity and equivalent efficacy. However, if clinically indicated, intravenous administration of GM-CSF is acceptable.

CLINICAL APPLICATIONS OF HEMATOPOIETIC GROWTH FACTORS IN CANCER THERAPY

TREATMENT OF ANEMIA IN CANCER PATIENTS

Pathophysiology

Anemia in cancer patients is common and may contribute significantly to quality of life. Anemia can be multifactorial in the cancer patient and can be caused by blood loss, iron or vitamin deficiency, chemotherapy, radiation to the marrow, stem cell damage, hemolysis, hypersplenism, drug toxicity, or tumor involvement of the marrow. An entity known as *anemia of cancer* has been described but may be multifactorial and is likely related to anemia of chronic disease. In both anemias, EPO production is inadequate for the degree of anemia.[69] There may also be an impaired response to EPO by marrow progenitor cells. Stem cell depletion may be more common than generally appreciated because of increasing use of higher doses and repeated courses of chemotherapy and radiation. Radiation involving the pelvis or spine is particularly problematic because of the large volume of marrow in those bones.

Clinical Trials with Erythropoietin

Use of EPO in anemia associated with cancer has been extensively investigated.[70–72] Trials have been conducted in patients with anemia due to marrow involvement with lymphoproliferative disorders[73]; in those with myelodysplastic syndromes (MDSs) or solid tumors; in those developing anemia after chemotherapy,[74–76] autologous transplantation,[77] allogeneic transplantation,[78] or radiation therapy[79]; and in those with anemia of cancer. The rates of response, generally defined as an increase in hemoglobin or a decrease in transfusion requirements (or both), are fairly high in most groups of patients, typically in the range of 50%.[76,80–83] Lack of response correlates with high pretreatment serum level of endogenous EPO. Patients who have an increase in hemoglobin of more than 0.5 g/dL within 2 weeks have a high likelihood of a sustained response.[84] The benefit of EPO treatment with cyclical chemotherapy has been confirmed in several randomized, placebo-controlled multicenter trials, and response has been associated with improved performance status and quality of life.[85] However, despite the high response rate and the apparent reduction in transfusions, EPO therapy is expensive, and careful selection of patients most likely to benefit is warranted.[86]

Subcutaneous EPO administration three times weekly appears to be at least as effective as daily intravenous administration. Higher doses are not clearly better than lower doses, but there is a threshold effect, and intravenous doses less than 100 U/kg and subcutaneous doses less than 50 U/kg may be associated with lower response rates. A reasonable approach would be 50 to 150 U/kg three times weekly by subcutaneous injection, which could be increased to 300 U/kg after 6 weeks without response. Interestingly, late responses are fairly common, and nine weeks of therapy or more may be required in some responding patients. Since many patients fail to respond even to higher levels of EPO, there has been considerable interest in predicting early in the course of treatment which patients are not likely to respond. Several algorithms have been generated and suggest that failure to increase hemoglobin by more than 0.5 g/dL or serum ferritin by more than 400 ng/mL after 2 weeks of treatment predicts for failure.[84,87] Iron deficiency will prevent response to EPO and should be considered in selected nonresponsive patients.[88] Finally, most studies so far have involved concurrent administration of EPO with chemotherapy. Other schedules in which EPO is given before or at the end of chemotherapy are being investigated.

CISPLATIN-ASSOCIATED ANEMIA. Approximately 40% of patients receiving cisplatin chemotherapy develop anemia, and many will require transfusion. Studies of EPO administration to treat cisplatin-induced anemia have generally been positive, even in elderly patients.[81,82,89] Henry and Abels[76] performed three randomized double-blind, placebo-controlled trials of EPO for anemic cancer patients not receiving concomitant chemotherapy, patients receiving chemotherapy that did not include cisplatin, and patients receiving cisplatin-containing chemotherapy. Patients not receiving chemotherapy received 100 U/kg three times weekly, while those on chemotherapy received 150 U/kg three times weekly. Overall, the trials involved 413 patients. Patients receiving EPO in all three trials had a statistically significant increase in hematocrit as compared to placebo-treated patients.[76] Quality of life improved significantly for EPO-treated patients, with an overall response rate of approximately 50% in all three groups. Similar results were reported by Cascinu et al.,[74] who performed a randomized, double-blind trial with EPO versus placebo in 100 patients with cisplatin-associated anemia (hemoglobin <90 g/L), administering EPO at 100 U/kg subcutaneously thrice weekly. After 9 weeks of therapy, the mean hemoglobin levels of the EPO-treated group were statistically different from placebo patients: EPO patients went from a baseline of 86.3 ± 6.2 g/dL to 105.1 ± 9.4 g/dL at 9 weeks, while placebo patients went from a baseline of 87.3 ± 5.2 g/dL to 81.2 ± 11 g/dL at 9 weeks. Also, only 20% of EPO-treated patients required blood transfusion versus 56% of placebo-treated patients. No significant side effects of EPO treatment were encountered. Another multicenter, double-blind, placebo-controlled trial was conducted by Case et al.,[75] who randomly assigned 153 anemic cancer patients receiving cyclic chemotherapy to EPO, 150 U/kg three times weekly, or placebo. EPO-treated patients had a statistically significant increase in hematocrit and a trend toward lower transfusion requirements. Again, no significant side effects were encountered. Also, ten Bokkel Huinink et al.[90] randomly chose 122 ovarian cancer patients receiving platinum-based chemotherapy to EPO or control arms, and demonstrated a significant reduction in transfusion requirement. Overall, these multiple, randomized, controlled trials indicate that EPO is safe and effective for therapy of both chemotherapy-associated and non–chemotherapy-associated chronic anemias in patients with solid tumors. Treatment reduces need for transfusion and improves quality of life for many patients.[91] Recently, EPO therapy in children receiving cisplatin-based therapy has also been shown to reduce the need for transfusions.[92]

ANEMIAS ASSOCIATED WITH MYELODYSPLASTIC SYNDROMES. The role of EPO in treating anemia associated with hematologic malignancies is somewhat less clear, particularly for the anemia of MDS. Most studies reported to date are uncontrolled and have included only small numbers of patients.[93–100] The response rates tend to be more than 25%, although a few patients will respond to higher doses of EPO.[101] A metaanalysis of 205 patients with an MDS from 17 different studies found an overall response rate of only 16%, with a particularly low response rate—7.5%—in patients with refractory anemia with ringed sideroblasts. Factors that predicted for a low response rate were transfusion dependence, high serum EPO, and refractory anemia with ringed sideroblasts. Several studies have looked at sequential or combined use of a myeloid growth factor with EPO,[101–104] but responses are not clearly higher with the doses and schedules studied so far. As is the case for the anemia of cancer, late EPO responses may be observed,[105] necessitating long courses of therapy in clinical trials. At present, EPO appears to benefit only a small number of patients with MDS, primarily patients with low serum EPO levels and minimal transfusion requirement. In recent studies, the combined use of EPO with G-CSF has been encouraging, with a higher fraction of patients responding to the combination.[106,107]

BONE MARROW TRANSPLANTATION. The available data suggest that EPO treatment may be useful for treatment of anemia associated with allogeneic bone marrow transplantation, but is not clearly useful as an adjunct for autologous transplantation.[108] Several randomized, controlled studies have compared EPO versus placebo after autologous or allogeneic transplantation.[78,109,110] Biggs et al.[78] gave EPO (300 U/kg intravenously three times weekly) or placebo to 91 patients undergoing allotransplantation. There was no reduction in red blood cell or platelet transfusion requirement and no reduction in hospital stay.[78] Link et al.[109] randomly selected 107 patients undergoing allotransplantation to EPO (150 U/kg/d by continuous intravenous infusion) or placebo until patients reached 7 days of transfusion independence or day 41.[109] The time to transfusion independence was reduced by EPO from 27 days to 19 days, but the number of transfusions required in the peritransplantation period was similar. EPO-treated patients had a somewhat smaller transfusion requirement from days 42 to 100. The same authors conducted a randomized trial of identical design with 57 patients undergoing autologous transplantation.[109] No difference in transfusion requirement was observed. Chao et al.[110] conducted a placebo-controlled trial of EPO (600 U/kg three times weekly) starting 3 weeks before autologous bone marrow transplantation in 35 patients with lymphoma.[110] All patients also received G-CSF after marrow reinfusion. No differences were observed in transfusion requirement or hematopoietic recovery. Similar results were reported when EPO was combined with GM-CSF in a nonrandomized study of autologous marrow transplantation with historical controls.[111] However, other recent studies have suggested a benefit in combining EPO with G-CSF after transplantation.[112] Another potential use of EPO is in the treatment of late-onset anemia after transplantation, concerning which encouraging pilot studies have been presented.[113] Overall, EPO has been of modest benefit in the allogeneic marrow transplantation setting.

Overall, EPO has an important role in the therapy of anemia in some cancer patients. In the individual cancer patient, the clinician needs to look carefully for treatable causes of anemia, such as iron deficiency or blood loss and to consider the underlying illness and other factors, such as the serum EPO level, to determine whether a course of EPO treatment is warranted.

REDUCTION OF CHEMOTHERAPY-ASSOCIATED NEUTROPENIA

Myelosuppression Associated with Standard-Dose Chemotherapy

Neutropenia and infection are major causes of morbidity and mortality in cancer patients and are dose-limiting for many types of chemotherapy. It is standard practice to treat all neutropenic, febrile patients with broad-spectrum antibiotics, even though many patients do not have documented infections. This adversely affects quality of life, increases hospital costs, and often results in reduction of chemotherapy doses for subsequent cycles. Reducing the incidence of febrile neutropenia and infection are major goals of CSF therapy in this setting.

GRANULOCYTE COLONY-STIMULATING FACTOR. G-CSF has been extensively investigated in clinical trials as an adjunct to cancer chemotherapy, and its use in this setting has been extensively reviewed.[114–117] The initial phase I and phase II studies in bladder cancer and small cell lung cancer patients established that G-CSF administration by either subcutaneous or intravenous routes caused a dramatic, dose-dependent increase in blood neutrophil counts. Data from numerous phase I and phase II studies predicted that administration of G-CSF after standard-dose, myelosuppressive chemotherapy would shorten the duration of neutropenia, but it was not clear from these early trials whether this would translate into clinical benefit. The efficacy of G-CSF has now been established in a series of randomized, controlled clinical trials in which the chemotherapy was sufficient to cause febrile neutropenia in more than 40% of the control group. A pivotal trial was conducted by Crawford et al.,[118] who randomly chose patients with small cell lung cancer to receive G-CSF or placebo after a myelosuppressive regimen containing cyclophosphamide, doxorubicin, and etoposide (CAE). The incidence of febrile neutropenia was significantly reduced in patients receiving G-CSF. Further, length of hospital stay, incidence of confirmed infections, and days of antibiotic use were reduced by approximately 50%.[118] The results of this study have been confirmed by several additional randomized, controlled phase III studies (small cell lung cancer patients receiving CAE chemotherapy[119]; non-Hodgkin's lymphoma patients receiving vincristine, doxorubicin, prednisolone, etoposide, cyclophosphamide, and bleomycin[120]; and patients with various types of cancer receiving several different chemotherapy regimens[121]). In none of these randomized studies was there a clear difference in mortality, tumor response rate, or survival. Thus, despite the fact that some epithelial tumor cells express G-CSF receptors, there does not appear to be any adverse effect of G-CSF on tumor growth when given with chemotherapy. In these randomized studies, the toxicity of G-CSF has been minimal and was generally limited to medullary bone pain that can usually be relieved with analgesics.

The timing of G-CSF after chemotherapy has been investigated in patients receiving melphalan (25 mg/m^2).[57] Delaying administration to 8 days after completion of chemotherapy appeared to be somewhat less effective than immediate administration, and it is now general practice to start G-CSF 24 to 48 hours after completing chemotherapy administration, typically continuing until the neutrophil count has recovered to 10,000/μL. However, administration of G-CSF for a defined period of only 7 days had benefit.[57] Also, there is considerable interest in evaluating G-CSF schedules with lower doses than the standard 5 μg/kg/d. In a randomized trial, Toner et al.[122] found that 2 μg/kg/d was as effective as 5 μg/kg/d in reducing the duration and severity of chemotherapy-related neutropenia. Also, shorter courses of G-CSF therapy are being investigated.[123]

GRANULOCYTE-MACROPHAGE COLONY-STIMULATING FACTOR. Administration of GM-CSF after standard-dose chemotherapy has also been extensively evaluated. In phase I and phase II studies where GM-CSF was administered in alternate cycles, shortening of the duration of neutropenia has been observed.[67] In larger, randomized, placebo-controlled studies, however, benefit has in some cases been limited to subsets of patients.[124–126] In one randomized study in patients with small cell lung cancer receiving CAE chemotherapy, GM-CSF reduced the duration of neutropenia but not the incidence of febrile neutropenia, days in hospital, or antibiotic use. Similarly, in a randomized trial of GM-CSF in patients with germ cell cancer receiving vinblastine, ifosfamide, and platinum, no significant beneficial effects were seen.[124] When given with 21 days of oral etoposide, GM-CSF did not significantly reduce neutropenia or neutropenic complications in a randomized study in patients with advanced cancers.[127] However, in a randomized study of fluorouracil, doxorubicin, and cyclophosphamide therapy in 142 patients with breast cancer, GM-CSF reduced the median duration of severe neutropenia (absolute neutrophil count <500/μL) to 2.8 days as compared to 6.8 days with placebo ($P<.001$) and reduced the duration of an absolute neutrophil count less than 1000/μL to 6.0 versus 9.1 days, respectively.[128] In children with solid tumors, GM-CSF reduced the duration of neutropenia but not the rate of febrile neutropenia.

There are very few studies in which the activities of GM-CSF and G-CSF have been directly compared. In one randomized study comparing these two growth factors after cyclophosphamide (7 g/m^2), patients treated with G-CSF recovered neutrophils slightly more rapidly, but patients treated with GM-CSF recovered platelets more rapidly; overall, both GM-CSF and G-CSF were thought to be effective.[129]

Concurrent Administration of Growth Factors with Chemotherapy or Radiation Therapy

Although the number of relevant studies is small, there is concern that simultaneous administration of GM-CSF or G-CSF with chemotherapy or radiation may lead to serious toxicity.[130] In a randomized trial in limited-stage small cell lung cancer patients receiving platinum, etoposide, and chest radiation, patients receiving GM-CSF had more thrombocytopenia, more toxic deaths, more antibiotic use, and longer hospital stays.[131] Similarly, patients with non–small cell lung cancer given G-CSF with cisplatin, etoposide, and radiation therapy had worse thrombocytopenia than controls.[132] Concern has also been raised about continuing G-CSF up to less than 48 hours before the next cycle of chemotherapy.[133] In contrast, concurrent administration of G-CSF with weekly cycles of dose-intensive vinorelbine did not lead to an apparent increase in myelosuppression.[134] However, until more information is available, concurrent administration of myelosuppressive chemotherapy with growth factors should remain investigational, and the special situation where both chemotherapy and radiation therapy are given concurrently with a growth factor should be avoided.

Treatment of Febrile Neutropenia

Although CSFs have been shown to reduce the incidence of febrile neutropenia in patients receiving myelosuppressive chemotherapy, it is clear that most patients receiving *standard* types of chemotherapy regimens will not develop febrile neutropenia or infection and would, therefore, not benefit from CSF administration. Since CSFs are expensive, are inconvenient for patients, and may have some toxic effects, there is increasing interest in better defining who is most likely to benefit so as to restrict use to appropriate patients. The American Society of Clinical Oncology (ASCO) generated a set of guidelines based on a thorough evidence-based analysis of published literature through 1997[135–137] and concluded that use of CSFs in chemotherapy sessions where the incidence of febrile neutropenia was expected to be less than 40% was not likely to be cost-effective. When less myelosuppressive chemotherapy was planned, CSF administration was recommended only for individual patients with high-risk factors, such as decreased marrow reserve, or those who have had a previous episode of febrile neutropenia with the same chemotherapy regimen. In many institutions, it is now common practice to withhold CSFs until a patient has had an episode of febrile neutropenia or infection and then to initiate CSF prophylaxis with the next cycle. The alternative to this approach is to dose-reduce or delay chemotherapy. For many situations where there is no firm evidence that dose or dose intensity are valuable, this is a very reasonable alternative to CSFs. Enthusiasm for use of a CSF should be highest for those tumors where it is clear that there is value in maintaining maximum scheduled chemotherapy dose with respect to tumor response rate, quality of life, or survival. The ASCO guideline authors did conclude that some "high-risk" patients could be reasonable candidates for CSF therapy before occurrence of an episode of febrile neutropenia. Such patients would include those with reduced marrow function (due to prior pelvic radiation therapy, prior extensive chemotherapy, or marrow involvement with tumor); those with preexisting neutropenia for any reason; those with any other preexisting immune dysfunction; those with active infection; and those with a documented previous episode of chemotherapy-induced febrile neutropenia or infection. A summary of the ASCO guidelines is shown in Table 53.4-3.

One of the inevitable problems faced by authors of guidelines is in defining what constitutes a benefit. GM-CSF and G-CSF can reduce the incidence of febrile neutropenia in aggressive regimens. When viewed as supportive therapy, the benefits of GM-CSF or G-CSF in this situation are clear. However, the larger question of whether the entire treatment program of aggressive chemotherapy with growth factor (or stem cell) support has led to a clinically significant benefit for the patient as compared to standard treatment has often not been addressed. Ultimately, the clinical indications for use of HGFs will need to be linked to treatment plans where high-dose therapy results in improved quality of life or prolonged survival.

An alternative to prophylactic use of G-CSF or GM-CSF after chemotherapy is administration of a CSF to patients who develop febrile neutropenia in an effort to shorten hospitalization, reduce antibiotic use, and improve outcome. In the largest randomized study so far, 218 patients with febrile neutropenia were randomly assigned to receive G-CSF or placebo along with antibiotics. G-CSF–treated patients had 1 day less neutropenia, but duration of fever and hospital stay was not reduced. Similarly, GM-CSF failed to reduce significantly median duration of fever

TABLE 53.4-3. Summary of American Society of Clinical Oncology Guidelines for Administration of Granulocyte Colony-Stimulating Factor and Granulocyte-Macrophage Colony-Stimulating Factor

Indication	*Recommendation*	*Comments and Alternative Approaches*
Primary CSF administration (administration of a CSF with all courses of a treatment regimen)	Use in adults treated with chemotherapy for which the incidence of febrile neutropenia is anticipated to be >40%	May be indicated in "high-risk" patients (marrow compromise, immunocompromised, active infection, etc.); alternative strategy: less myelosuppressive chemotherapy
Secondary CSF administration (administration of a CSF in all subsequent cycles after an episode of febrile neutropenia)	Use in situations in which maintaining dose intensity is essential	Alternative is dose reduction
Afebrile, neutropenic patients	Not indicated	
Febrile neutropenia	Use with antibiotics in patients predicted to have a poor outcome (pneumonia, hypotension, sepsis syndrome, fungal infection)	Available data suggest benefits for CSF administration, but studies not definitive
Increasing dose intensity	Not indicated	Data needed to establish the value of higher dose intensity
Adjuncts to progenitor cell transplantation	CSF use reasonable in autologous setting	Useful for mobilization of PBPCs; possible benefit after allogeneic-BMT
Delayed engraftment–graft failure	Use of a CSF is warranted	
Acute myeloid leukemia	Can be used in patients older than 55 y to shorten neutropenia; not recommended for "priming"	No consistent effect on CR rate or survival
Myelodysplastic syndromes	Use intermittently only in subset of patients who have severe neutropenia and recurrent infections	
Concurrent administration of CSFs with chemotherapy and radiation therapy	Avoid	Available data, although limited, suggest increased toxicity
Use of CSFs in the pediatric patient	Guidelines for adults generally applicable	

BMT, bone marrow transplantation; CR, complete response; CSF, colony-stimulating factor; PBPCs, peripheral blood progenitor cells.
(From refs. 135–137, with permission.)
(http://www.asco.org/prof/pp/html/guide/csf/m_csf.htm)

or hospital stay in patients with febrile neutropenia in two trials.[138,139] However, in patients with tissue infections, the addition of GM-CSF to antibiotics significantly improved outcome. Of 121 patients randomly chosen to receive G-CSF, GM-CSF, or placebo, CSF-treated patients had significantly shorter neutropenia, fever, hospital stay, and overall hospital costs.[140] Similarly, in a placebo-controlled study in children, both GM-CSF[141] and G-CSF[142] significantly reduced hospital stay, antibiotic use, and duration of neutropenia. In 134 adult cancer patients with febrile neutropenia, GM-CSF treatment reduced duration of neutropenia but not days of hospital stay or cost.[143] It may be possible to identify groups of patients in whom GM-CSF is most likely to have benefit.[123] Overall, with both positive and negative studies, the indications for CSFs in febrile neutropenia remain unknown, and additional studies are warranted, particularly emphasizing both cost and quality-of-life issues.[135] At present, the benefits of a CSF to low-risk patients are unclear. In contrast, some high-risk neutropenic patients with documented infections are candidates for CSF treatment, particularly those with pneumonia, prolonged neutropenia, or fungal infections.[139] There is no current indication for CSF administration to afebrile neutropenic patients.[144]

INCREASE OF CHEMOTHERAPY DOSE INTENSITY

Dose Escalation

There is experimental evidence for a steep dose-response curve for many chemotherapy agents, and this has generated considerable interest in using CSFs to facilitate administration of higher doses of chemotherapy drugs where dose is limited primarily by myelosuppression. A variety of phase I trials have been reported in which the possibility that use of GM-CSF[145] or G-CSF would allow escalation of doses of single chemotherapy drugs or multiagent chemotherapy, but placebo-controlled, randomized studies are lacking. The reported phase I studies suggest that escalation of chemotherapy drug dose to levels higher than "standard" has often been possible. However, this approach overall has had limited success, in part due to the fact that thrombocytopenia and nonhematologic side effects often emerge quickly as dose-limiting toxicities. For example, G-CSF was used to investigate accelerated delivery of doxorubicin, 50 mg/m^2 × 2; etoposide, 120 mg/m^2 × 3; and ifosfamide, 2 g/m^2 given every 14 days.[146] Optimal on-time administration was feasible in 66% of 48 patients for three courses but feasible for only 23% for six courses. Twenty-two of 48 patients were withdrawn from the study, including 12 patients with sepsis (4 fatal) or grade 4 thrombocytopenia. Overall, dose-intensity was 1.8 times higher than when the same regimen was used at a 3-week interval.[146] In a randomized study in extensive small cell carcinoma of the lung, it was not possible to increase dose significantly with the addition of GM-CSF.[147] However, in a study of breast cancer patients receiving docetaxel and mitoxantrone, G-CSF allowed a significant increase in maximum tolerated dose of both drugs.[148]

Maintenance of Dose Intensity

There have been a number of studies indicating that either G-CSF or GM-CSF can improve the ability to maintain dose intensity in multicycle regimens. In a randomized study, Pettengell et al.[120] compared G-CSF to placebo in patients with lymphoma receiving vincristine, doxorubicin (Adriamycin), prednisone, VP-16, and bleomycin chemotherapy and found a significant reduction of treatment delays related to myelosuppression and an overall increase in dose intensity of 13%. Similarly, G-CSF treatment led to an 8% increase in dose intensity of CAE chemotherapy as compared to placebo in patients with small cell lung cancer.[119] However, it has been difficult to demonstrate so far that use of a CSF for maintenance of dose intensity in most standard chemotherapy regimens provides a significant advantage in terms of response or disease-free survival.[149] Overall, despite the attractiveness of the concept, use of CSFs to permit dose escalation of chemotherapy (without stem cell rescue) remains a research question. For standard regimens in which the expected incidence of treatment delay or dose reduction is high (i.e., >40%) and in which it is thought that dose intensity is critical, use of G-CSF or GM-CSF is likely to improve on-time, full-dose delivery. The value of dose maintenance will need to be established, however, by prospective, randomized trials in each tumor type.

ADJUNCTS TO AUTOLOGOUS OR ALLOGENEIC TRANSPLANTATION

Acceleration of Hematopoietic Reconstitution after Autologous or Allogeneic Transplantation

GM-CSF and G-CSF have been extensively investigated as adjuncts to autologous and allogeneic stem cell transplantation. Both GM-CSF[150–155] and G-CSF[110,156–159] have been shown in randomized, placebo-controlled trials to reduce the period of neutropenia after autologous bone marrow transplantation. In some, but not all, of these studies, hospital stay, antibiotic use, infections, or platelet transfusions were also reduced. There has been no evidence of reduced mortality or increase in tumor response rates. In studies with autologous, mobilized blood stem cells, G-CSF also reduces the duration of neutropenia, but the overall impact on the transplant procedure may be less than when marrow stem cells are used for the transplantation.[160,161] Interestingly, administration of G-CSF after blood stem cell autologous transplant can be delayed for several days without loss of efficacy.[162] In children, the use of G-CSF after autologous blood transplantation is controversial.[163] In studies with allogeneic marrow transplantation, addition of a CSF tended to reduce neutropenia, but infection rate and hospital stay have not been consistently reduced.[117,164–171] The use of GM-CSF after blood stem cell transplantation has shown only marginal benefit.[172]

The potential use of growth factors for treatment of graft failure or delayed engraftment after either autologous or allogeneic transplantation has been explored to a limited extent, and results are encouraging for both GM-CSF and G-CSF.[173–179] It is clear that while not all patients will respond, neutrophil counts can be rapidly increased in many cases. Combining GM-CSF and G-CSF in a sequential manner did not improve results over GM-CSF alone.[174] In many cases, retransplantation with growth factor–mobilized blood stem cells has been of great value.[180]

Mobilization of Peripheral Blood Progenitor Cells by Hematopoietic Growth Factors

One of the most remarkable effects of G-CSF and GM-CSF is transient mobilization of hematopoietic progenitor and stem cells into the peripheral blood. This unexpected phenomenon was first noted during early phase I studies with GM-CSF[181] and G-CSF[182] and has now been observed with several other cytokines, such as IL-3[183] and even EPO.[184] The effects of either GM-CSF or G-CSF appear to be independent and additive to the effects of myelosuppressive chemotherapy[181] and, in some circumstances, mobilization with growth factor is as good as with a combination of growth factor and cyclophosphamide.[185] The concentration of progenitor cells in the blood of normal individuals is too low to render harvesting of these cells practical. GM-CSF or G-CSF increases progenitor cell concentration approximately tenfold and, when administered after some types of chemotherapy, such as high-dose cyclophosphamide,[186] the increase in blood progenitor cell concentration can be 100-fold or more. However, interpatient variability is substantial, and mobilization is generally reduced in patients with extensive prior exposure to chemotherapy or radiation, particularly to the pelvis. Nonetheless, GM-CSF-mobilized or G-CSF-mobilized progenitor cells can be collected from most cancer patients by leukapheresis in sufficient quantity to replace marrow harvests for autologous transplantation protocols. The mobilized cells may be more immature than the progenitor cells that are resident in the blood of untreated individuals.[187] Patients receiving peripheral blood progenitor cells tend to reconstitute earlier and to require fewer platelet transfusions than patients receiving autologous marrow.[188] As a result, using GM-CSF or G-CSF to assist in mobilizing progenitor cells has become used in autologous transplantation protocols for many different tumors.[186,189–193] G-CSF–mobilized or GM-CSF–mobilized peripheral blood progenitor cells also offer advantages in allogeneic transplantation.[194] In this situation, no chemotherapy is administered, but collection of adequate amounts of progenitor cells with several episodes of leukapheresis is well tolerated by normal donors.[195] Reconstitution is prompt and durable,[196–198] and preliminary results of a randomized trial comparing allogeneic marrow with blood stem cells favors the blood source.[199] Recent studies suggest that combinations of cytokines may be more effective than single cytokines. Winter et al.[200] compared the mobilizing effects of GM-CSF and G-CSF, either alone or in various combinations, including adding G-CSF for 5 days after 7 days of GM-CSF and adding GM-CSF after 7 days of G-CSF. When used individually, GM-CSF and G-CSF administration resulted in mobilization of approximately the same number of progenitor cells, approximately a 35-fold increase over pretreatment values.[200] Administration of G-CSF to patients already receiving GM-CSF resulted in an increase to approximately 80-fold over baseline. Interestingly, the combination of G-CSF and stem cell factor may have particularly good ability to mobilize stem cells, and a number of studies are ongoing with this combination.[201,202] Thus, cytokine combinations may be more efficacious than single cytokines for mobilization, and other combinations and schedules should be tested.

Most studies using cytokine-mobilized peripheral blood progenitor cells have also given G-CSF or GM-CSF after transplant to accelerate reconstitution. This approach seems reasonable at present in autologous transplantation, but additional studies are needed in allogeneic transplants of blood stem cells. The hematopoietic reconstitution observed after peripheral blood progenitor cell transplantations may be sufficiently fast so that the cost-effectiveness of G-CSF or GM-CSF will need to be carefully evaluated.

Tumor cell contamination of progenitor cells collected from the blood could limit the success of these products for autologous transplantation, as is the case for autologous marrow transplantation.[203–206] Recent efforts to reduce tumor cell contamination have focused on either immunologic purging of contaminating tumor cells or positive selection of progenitor cells using the CD34 cell surface marker.[205,207,208] In general, mobilized stem cell products have a high likelihood of containing tumor cells.[209]

Ex Vivo *Expansion of Hematopoietic Progenitor Cells*

One area of active research is the potential use of growth factors to permit *ex vivo* expansion of either marrow or blood stem cells. When partially purified stem cells are cultured with mixtures of growth factors, typically containing Steel factor and a variety of HGFs, substantial expansion of progenitor cells has been observed. However, currently only limited expansion of hematopoietic stem cells has been achieved, and there is the potential that there will not be enough true hematopoietic stem cells to effect long-term permanent reconstitution if these expanded populations are used in transplantation settings. It is possible that there are yet unknown cytokines that will induce stem cell proliferation while inhibiting differentiation, and such cytokines might be ideal for this process. Alternatively, expanded progenitor cells may have some uses, even if the stem cell content is decreased. For example, progenitor cells may be useful to accelerate hematopoietic recovery after myelosuppressive, but not myeloablative, chemotherapy regimens.

TREATMENT OF LEUKEMIAS

Acute Myelogenous Leukemia

Infection related to neutropenia remains a major cause of morbidity and mortality during all phases of the treatment of acute myelogenous leukemia (AML), and any reduction of chemotherapy- or disease-associated neutropenia could be beneficial. The use of GM-CSF and G-CSF in AML therapy has been approached with justifiable caution, however, since both of these cytokines are excellent growth factors for leukemia cells *in vitro,* and there remains concern that these factors could either accelerate leukemic cell growth, reduce chemotherapy response, or enhance toxicity. AML cells from most patients have receptors for both GM-CSF and G-CSF,[210–212] and both factors induce rapid proliferation of leukemic cells without any evidence of terminal differentiation. Thus, administration of either factor carries the risk of promoting leukemic cell proliferation. In the small number of clinical trials conducted so far, however, administration of G-CSF or GM-CSF immediately after standard chemotherapy has not been associated with leukemic cell regrowth or early relapse. Ohno et al.[213] randomly assigned a heterogeneous group of patients with acute leukemia to G-CSF or no treatment during induction therapy. There was a 1-week reduction in the duration of severe neutropenia but no decrease in antibiotic use or hospital stay. The complete remission rate was not decreased by G-CSF, and long-term outcome was unchanged.[213] The results of this study were confirmed in a large study conducted in 31 centers in Europe and Australia in which 521 adult patients with AML were randomly chosen to receive G-CSF or placebo after induction and consolidation therapy.[214] Patients in the G-CSF arm had a statistically significant improvement in duration of neutropenia, a 5-day reduction in the median duration of hospital stay, and a reduction in duration of antibiotic use. There was no significant difference reported in rate of complete remission or overall survival.[214] The Southwest Oncology Group randomly selected 234 patients older than age 55 and having *de novo* or secondary AML to receive G-CSF or placebo.[215] Patients on the G-CSF arm had a 3- to 4-day reduction in the duration of severe neutropenia after induction therapy and also reduced antibiotic use and days of fever. However, there was no reduction in the incidence of severe infections or any difference in complete remission rate or overall survival.[215]

ACUTE MYELOID LEUKEMIA IN THE ELDERLY. GM-CSF has been investigated in two large randomized group trials in induction therapy of AML in older patients.[216,217] An Eastern Cooperative Group Study randomly chose 124 AML patients ages 55 to 70 to receive GM-CSF or placebo after induction therapy.[217] The study drug was started on day 11 if a day-10 marrow was hypoplastic, and patients who entered complete remission received the study drug after consolidation therapy as well. Patients receiving GM-CSF experienced a significant reduction of infectious toxicity and a marginal improvement in median survival. Ten percent of GM-CSF–treated patients experienced severe infections, as compared to 36% of placebo patients. Mortality of patients who developed fungal infections was also lower with GM-CSF treatment, and overall early mortality (within 30 days) was significantly reduced in the GM-CSF arm. However, the beneficial effects of GM-CSF in an elderly population with AML were not confirmed in a larger Cancer and Leukemia Group B study reported by Stone et al.[216] In that study, 388 patients older than age 60 were randomly assigned to GM-CSF or placebo. There was no difference in remission rate, incidence of severe infections, or early deaths. There was a significant decrease in median duration of neutropenia for patients receiving GM-CSF, but the absolute difference was small (15 vs. 17 days).

Considering all the studies in which patients with AML have been randomly chosen to receive growth factor (G-CSF or GM-CSF) or placebo, it appears that although there may be some reduction in duration of neutropenia during induction therapy, this has not resulted in any significant reduction of severe infections or improvement in remission rate and survival.[218,219] At this time, the use of growth factors in myeloid leukemias, particularly in the elderly, requires additional study.

"PRIMING" OF ACUTE MYELOID LEUKEMIA CELLS AND DIFFERENTIATION THERAPY WITH GROWTH FACTORS. Several investigators have tried to take advantage of the fact that GM-CSF or G-CSF induces proliferation of myeloid leukemic cells[212] by using these cytokines to induce leukemic cells to initiate or increase DNA synthesis, followed immediately by administration of chemotherapy with drugs such as cytosine arabinoside, which are most effective against cells actively synthesizing DNA. This approach, termed *priming,* is remarkably effective in the laboratory.[220] However, although pilot studies suggested that GM-CSF and cytosine arabinoside could be coadministered without undue toxicity,[221] larger studies did not suggest that this approach had any benefit in terms of increased complete remission rate or increased survival.[222,223] One explanation is that the CSFs promote viability as well as proliferation of leukemic cells, and they may be paradoxically reducing cell death due to cytotoxic chemotherapy. At present, there is no indication for using CSFs as priming agents outside of a clinical trial.

Acute Lymphoblastic Leukemia

The use of cytokines during induction therapy of adult acute lymphoblastic leukemia (ALL) has not been extensively investigated. A prospective, multicenter trial reported by Ottmann et al.[224] randomly chose 76 patients to receive G-CSF or no growth factor during induction therapy. Patients in the G-CSF arm had a statistically significant reduction in the duration of severe neutropenia (8 days vs. 12.5 days), a lower incidence of nonviral infections, and fewer interruptions of scheduled chemotherapy.[224] The complete remission rates in the G-CSF and control groups were the same (95%), and the probability of disease-free survival at 20 months was also identical. A randomized Cancer and Leukemia Group B trial arrived at similar conclusions.[225] Adults who received intensive chemotherapy for ALL benefited from G-CSF treatment in terms of more rapid recovery of neutrophils, but overall outcome was unchanged. Thus, as is the case for adults with AML, adults with ALL treated with G-CSF have less neutropenia and probably fewer infections but no real improvement in disease outcome.

Myelodysplastic Syndromes

Anemia, neutropenia, and thrombocytopenia are common and chronic problems for patients with MDSs and, as a result, MDS patients have been among the first groups to receive HGFs.[226–228] The use of EPO to treat anemias of MDS patients was described earlier in the section Treatment of Anemia in Cancer Patients. In phase I and phase II trials, both GM-CSF[229–232] and G-CSF[229–232] have been shown to increase the neutrophil count by at least twofold in a variable number of patients (but generally less than 50%) and inevitably for only as long as the cytokine was administered. Even minimal red cell and platelet responses have been uncommon with both GM-CSF and G-CSF. A randomized trial of GM-CSF or observation was conducted in which 133 neutropenic patients with MDS were entered and followed up for 90 days.[233] Patients treated with GM-CSF had a statistically significant increase in neutrophils after 30, 60, and 90 days of treatment[233] and a significant reduction in major infections during the treatment period (15%, GM-CSF; 33%, observation). However, GM-CSF did not increase in hemoglobin or platelets, change transfusion requirement, or reduce the incidence of conversion to AML. The increase in neutrophil counts has been confirmed in other large studies of MDS patients treated with GM-CSF by Willemze et al.,[231] who treated 101 cases with two different daily doses of GM-CSF for 8 weeks. Of 82 evaluable patients, 66% had an increase in neutrophil count of twofold or more during the study, but sustained neutrophil responses, red cell responses, and platelet responses were rare. Interestingly, neutrophil responses in MDS patients may require only very low doses of GM-CSF.[234] There is no evidence so far that GM-CSF preferentially stimulates proliferation of normal progenitor cells rather than MDS progenitor cells. Serial karyotype analysis in one study showed that karyotypes of patients on GM-CSF remained abnormal or became increasingly abnormal over the study duration.[235] There is no clear evidence that GM-CSF administration accelerates development of acute leukemia, although some patients with advanced MDS may have an increase in blood or marrow blasts that may decrease after withdrawal of cytokine. Combinations of GM-CSF and EPO may have increased activity as compared to either agent alone.[106]

G-CSF is also effective at increasing neutrophil counts of patients with MDS.[236,237] In a randomized phase III trial of G-CSF versus observation, the G-CSF–treated arm had a statistically significant increase in neutrophil count.[238] However, the survival for patients with refractory anemia with excess blasts was significantly shorter in the G-CSF arm at the time of the initial analysis of the study.[238] It is not clear whether this is possibly due to an increased number of poor prognosis patients having been randomly assigned to the G-CSF arm or whether this is an effect of G-CSF. The combination of G-CSF with EPO may have significant advantages and deserves further study.[107,112,239]

Both GM-CSF[232,240] and G-CSF[241] have been used as adjuncts to chemotherapy in patients with MDS to reduce myelosuppression. Both factors appear to reduce myelosuppression, but there is no clear effect on response rates or rates of infection.[232,241] The beneficial effects of G-CSF on recovery from neutropenia have been confirmed in recent randomized trials.[242,243]

Overall, the use of GM-CSF and G-CSF remains experimental in MDS, with no clear demonstration of benefit in large patient populations. However, in the individual neutropenic patient with repeated infections, a trial of G-CSF or GM-CSF is reasonable.

REDUCTION OF CHEMOTHERAPY-RELATED THROMBOCYTOPENIA

Interleukin-11

IL-11 (Neumega) is a growth factor produced by stromal cells and has activity on progenitor cells, B cells, intestinal crypt cells, and osteoclasts, but not on stem cells.[244–249] Preliminary studies in both animals and humans suggested that IL-11 increased platelet counts, presumably through an effect on megakaryocytes.[250,251] Side effects in a phase I clinical study in breast cancer patients included fatigue, myalgia, and arthralgia and a grade 3 central nervous system event in one patient but no fever or capillary leak syndrome.[251] The incidence of severe thrombocytopenia after cyclophosphamide and doxorubicin appeared to be reduced.[251] Several randomized placebo controlled clinical trials have shown a reduction in the need for platelet transfusions in the settin g of intensive chemotherapy.[252,253] In autologous transplantation, IL-11 did not reduce platelet transfusion requirement.[254] *In vitro*, IL-11 acts synergistically with several other HGFs to support proliferation of hematopoietic progenitor cells,[245,246] suggesting that combinations of IL-11 with other growth factors will be worth exploring in clinical trials. Interestingly, IL-11 reduces chemotherapy- or radiation therapy–induced damage to the intestine in animal models,[255,256] and it is possible that this factor will reduce therapy-associated gastrointestinal toxicity in humans.[257] IL-11 is currently approved for use in treating chemotherapy-associated thrombocytopenia.

Thrombopoietin (Megakaryocyte Growth and Development Factor)

TPO was cloned by several groups after either purification of the protein from plasma of thrombocytopenic animals, by using the receptor for ligand affinity purification, or by clever expression cloning strategies.[258–261] The receptor for TPO has been identified as c-MPL, the cellular homologue of a viral oncogene that causes a myeloproliferative syndrome in mice. TPO levels vary inversely with the platelet count,[262] suggesting that TPO secretion can be directly induced by thrombocytopenia. TPO induces proliferation of megakaryocyte progenitor cells,[263] expansion of megakaryocytes *in vivo,* and production and release of platelets.[264] Further, TPO acts synergistically with several other growth factors to enhance megakaryocyte differentiation and proliferation.[265] Randomized, placebo-controlled clinical trials in cancer patients have shown a benefit for TPO administration,[266,267] but development has been slowed by rare instances of thrombocytopenia. This cytokine has not yet been approved for use in cancer patients, and its final role in cancer chemotherapy is still to be determined.

LONG-TERM EFFECTS OF GROWTH FACTOR ADMINISTRATION

The long-term consequences of administration of HGFs are not yet known. In children with congenital neutropenias responsive to G-CSF, some have now received this cytokine for several years. Although splenomegaly, apparently related to extramedullary hematopoiesis, has been observed, few serious side effects have been reported.[53] One interesting case has been described in which G-CSF–related extramedullary hematopoiesis was confused with recurrent lymphoma.[208] However, there is no evidence to date that CSF administration by itself predisposes patients to develop leukemia or myelodysplasia. Concern has been raised that administration of CSFs with chemotherapy may increase the cumulative stem cell damage that can occur with some types of chemotherapy drugs or radiation. In fact, in a mouse model, repeated sequential administration of cyclophosphamide and G-CSF was more toxic to stem cells than cyclophosphamide alone.[269] It is possible that CSFs will induce more stem cells to enter the cell cycle and, therefore, potentially become more sensitive to chemotherapy-induced DNA damage. Careful follow-up of patients receiving aggressive chemotherapy with growth factor support is warranted, particularly if these patients later undergo autologous progenitor cell transplantation, or during other situations in which the marrow is stressed, such as during serious bacterial or viral infections.

CONCLUSIONS

There is little doubt that the use of HGFs represents a significant advance in the supportive care available to cancer patients. At present, there are a number of clinical situations wherein administration of a growth factor is warranted, such as after myelosuppressive chemotherapy where there is a high likelihood of febrile neutropenia and after autologous progenitor cell transplantation. Patients who have already had an episode of febrile neutropenia should receive a growth factor if there are good reasons to maintain dose intensity. Ultimately, however, the utility of high-dose chemotherapy needs to be established in each tumor in terms of survival or improved quality of life. Finally, cytokines are expensive, and further efforts to define cost-effectiveness in useful terms are needed. However, despite these cautions, the remarkable ability to manipulate hematopoiesis with growth factors is likely to be beneficial to cancer patients in many different situations.

REFERENCES

1. Bjornson CR, Rietze RL, Reynolds BA, Magli MC, Vescovi AL. Turning brain into blood: a hematopoietic fate adopted by adult neural stem cells in vivo. *Science* 1999;283:534.
2. Metcalf D. The molecular control of cell division, differentiation commitment and maturation in haematopoietic cells. *Nature* 1989;339:27.
3. Uchida N, Fleming WH, Alpern EJ, Weissman IL. Heterogeneity of hematopoietic stem cells. *Curr Opin Immunol* 1993;5:177.
4. Sachs L. The molecular control of hematopoiesis: from clonal development in culture to therapy in the clinic. *Int J Cell Cloning* 1992;10:196.
5. Dexter TM, Heyworth CM. Growth factors and the molecular control of haematopoiesis. *Eur J Clin Microbiol Infect Dis* 1994;13:S3.
6. Ogawa M. Differentiation and proliferation of hematopoietic stem cells. *Blood* 1993;81:2844.
7. Metcalf D. The molecular control of granulocytes and macrophages. *Ciba Found Symp* 1997;204:40.
8. Metcalf D. The molecular control of hematopoiesis: progress and problems with gene manipulation. *Stem Cells* 1998;16:314.
9. Metcalf D. The Charlotte Friend Memorial Lecture. The role of hematopoietic growth factors in the development and suppression of myeloid leukemias. *Leukemia* 1997;11:1599.
10. Metcalf D. Hematopoietic regulators: redundancy or subtlety? *Blood* 1993;82:3515.
11. Lieschke GJ. CSF-deficient mice—what have they taught us? *Ciba Found Symp* 1997;204:60.
12. Dranoff G, Crawford AD, Sadelain M, et al. Involvement of granulocyte-macrophage colony-stimulating factor in pulmonary homeostasis. *Science* 1994;264:713.
13. Mach N, Lantz CS, Galli SJ, et al. Involvement of interleukin-3 in delayed-type hypersensitivity. *Blood* 1998;91:778.
14. Lantz CS, Boesiger J, Song CH, et al. Role for interleukin-3 in mast-cell and basophil development and in immunity to parasites. *Nature* 1998;392:90.
15. Lieschke GJ, Grail D, Hodgson G, et al. Mice lacking granulocyte colony-stimulating factor have chronic neutropenia, granulocyte and macrophage progenitor cell deficiency, and impaired neutrophil mobilization. *Blood* 1994;84:1737.
16. Wu H, Liu X, Jaenisch R, Lodish HF. Generation of committed erythroid BFU-E and CFU-E progenitors does not require erythropoietin or the erythropoietin receptor. *Cell* 1995;83:59.
17. de Sauvage FJ, Shiuh-Ming L, Carver-Moore K, et al. Deficiencies in early and late stages of megakaryocytopoiesis in TPO-KO mice. *Blood* 1995;86:1007a.
18. Lev S, Blechman JM, Givol D, Yarden Y. Steel factor and c-kit protooncogene: genetic lessons in signal transduction. *Crit Rev Oncog* 1994;5:141.
19. Besmer P, Manova K, Duttlinger R, et al. The kit-ligand (Steel factor) and its receptor c-kit/W: pleiotropic roles in gametogenesis and melanogenesis. *Dev Suppl* 1993;125.
20. Zhan Y, Lieschke GJ, Grail D, Dunn AR, Cheers C. Essential roles for granulocyte-macrophage colony-stimulating factor (GM-CSF) and G-CSF in the sustained hematopoietic response of *Listeria monocytogenes*–infected mice. *Blood* 1998;91:863.
21. Petersdorf SH, Dale DC. The biology and clinical applications of erythropoietin and the colony-stimulating factors. *Adv Intern Med* 1995;40:395.
22. Alter BP. Biology of erythropoiesis. *Ann NY Acad Sci* 1994;731:36.
23. Sawyer ST, Penta K. Erythropoietin cell biology. *Hematol Oncol Clin North Am* 1994;8:895.
24. Lok S, Foster DC. The structure, biology and potential therapeutic applications of recombinant thrombopoietin. *Stem Cells* 1994;12:586.
25. Markham A, Bryson HM. Epoetin alfa. A review of its pharmacodynamic and pharmacokinetic properties and therapeutic use in nonrenal applications. *Drugs* 1995;49:232.
26. Lee-Huang S. Cloning and expression of human erythropoietin cDNA in *Escherichia coli*. *Proc Natl Acad Sci U S A* 1984;81:2708.
27. Lin FK, Suggs S, Lin CH, et al. Cloning and expression of the human erythropoietin gene. *Proc Natl Acad Sci U S A* 1985;82:7580.
28. Jacobs K, Shoemaker C, Rudersdorf R, et al. Isolation and characterization of genomic and cDNA clones of human erythropoietin. *Nature* 1985;313:806.
29. Ebert BL, Bunn HF. Regulation of the erythropoietin gene. *Blood* 1999;94:1864.
30. D'Andrea AD, Lodish HF, Wong GG. Expression cloning of the murine erythropoietin receptor. *Cell* 1989;57:277.
31. D'Andrea AD, Fasman GD, Lodish HF. A new hematopoietic growth factor receptor superfamily: structural features and implications for signal transduction. *Curr Opin Cell Biol* 1990;2:648.
32. D'Andrea AD, Fasman GD, Lodish HF. Erythropoietin receptor and interleukin-2 receptor beta chain: a new receptor family. *Cell* 1989;58:1023.
33. Li JP, D'Andrea AD, Lodish HF, Baltimore D. Activation of cell growth by binding of Friend spleen focus-forming virus gp55 glycoprotein to the erythropoietin receptor. *Nature* 1990;343:762.
34. D'Andrea AD, Moreau JF, Showers MO. Molecular mimicry of erythropoietin by the spleen focus-forming virus gp55 glycoprotein: the first stage of Friend virus–induced erythroleukemia. *Biochim Biophys Acta* 1992;1114:31.
35. Zon LI, Moreau JF, Koo JW, Mathey-Prevot B, D'Andrea AD. The erythropoietin receptor transmembrane region is necessary for activation by the Friend spleen focus-forming virus gp55 glycoprotein. *Mol Cell Biol* 1992;12:2949.
36. Sokol L, Luhovy M, Guan Y, et al. Primary familial polycythemia: a frameshift mutation in the erythropoietin receptor gene and increased sensitivity of erythroid progenitors to erythropoietin. *Blood* 1995;86:15.
37. de la Chapelle A, Sistonen P, Lehvaslaiho H, Ikkala E, Juvonen E. Familial erythrocytosis genetically linked to erythropoietin receptor gene. *Lancet* 1993;341:82.

38. de la Chapelle A, Traskelin AL, Juvonen E. Truncated erythropoietin receptor causes dominantly inherited benign human erythrocytosis. *Proc Natl Acad Sci U S A* 1993;90:4495.
39. Spivak JL. Cancer-related anemia: its causes and characteristics. *Semin Oncol* 1994;21:3.
40. Spivak JL. The biology and clinical applications of recombinant erythropoietin. *Semin Oncol* 1998;25:7.
41. Morstyn G, Foote M, Perkins D, Vincent M. The clinical utility of granulocyte colony-stimulating factor: early achievements and future promise. *Stem Cells* 1994;1:213.
42. Dale DC, Liles WC, Summer WR, Nelson S. Review: granulocyte colony-stimulating factor—role and relationships in infectious diseases. *J Infect Dis* 1995;172:1061.
43. Marty M. The optimal dose of glycosylated recombinant human granulocyte colony stimulating factor for use in clinical practice: a review. *Eur J Cancer* 1994;3:S20.
44. Metcalf D, Nicola NA. Proliferative effects of purified granulocyte colony-stimulating factor (G-CSF) on normal mouse hemopoietic cells. *J Cell Physiol* 1983;116:198.
45. Nagata S, Tsuchiya M, Asano S, et al. Molecular cloning and expression of cDNA for human granulocyte colony-stimulating factor. *Nature* 1986;319:415.
46. Souza LM, Boone TC, Gabrilove J, et al. Recombinant human granulocyte colony-stimulating factor: effects on normal and leukemic myeloid cells. *Science* 1986;232:61.
47. Hammond WP, Csiba E, Canin A, et al. Chronic neutropenia. A new canine model induced by human granulocyte colony-stimulating factor. *J Clin Invest* 1991;87:704.
48. Fukunaga R, Seto Y, Mizushima S, Nagata S. Three different mRNAs encoding human granulocyte colony-stimulating factor receptor. *Proc Natl Acad Sci U S A* 1990;87:8702.
49. Larsen A, Davis T, Curtis BM, et al. Expression cloning of a human granulocyte colony-stimulating factor receptor: a structural mosaic of hematopoietin receptor, immunoglobulin, and fibronectin domains. *J Exp Med* 1990;172:1559.
50. Dong F, Brynes RK, Tidow N, et al. Mutations in the gene for the granulocyte colony-stimulating factor receptor in patients with acute myeloid leukemia preceded by severe congenital neutropenia. *N Engl J Med* 1995;333:487.
51. Hermans MH, Antonissen C, Ward AC, et al. Sustained receptor activation and hyperproliferation in response to granulocyte colony-stimulating factor (G-CSF) in mice with a severe congenital neutropenia/acute myeloid leukemia–derived mutation in the G-CSF receptor gene. *J Exp Med* 1999;189:683.
52. Layton JE, Hockman H, Sheridan WP, Mortsyn G. Evidence for a novel in vivo control mechanism of granulopoiesis: mature cell-related control of a regulatory growth factor. *Blood* 1989;74:1303.
53. Bonilla MA, Dale D, Zeidler C, et al. Long-term safety of treatment with recombinant human granulocyte colony-stimulating factor (r-metHuG-CSF) in patients with severe congenital neutropenias. *Br J Haematol* 1994;88:723.
54. Stokkel MP, Valdes Olmos RA, Hoefnagel CA, Richel DJ. Tumor and therapy associated abnormal changes on bone scintigraphy. Old and new phenomena. *Clin Nucl Med* 1993;18:821.
55. Lieschke GJ, Cebon J, Morstyn G. Characterization of the clinical effects after the first dose of bacterially synthesized recombinant human granulocyte-macrophage colony-stimulating factor. *Blood* 1989;74:2634.
56. Schilero GJ, Oropello J, Benjamin E. Impairment in gas exchange after granulocyte colony stimulating factor (G-CSF) in a patient with the adult respiratory distress syndrome. *Chest* 1995;107:276.
57. Morstyn G, Campbell L, Lieschke G, et al. Treatment of chemotherapy-induced neutropenia by subcutaneously administered granulocyte colony-stimulating factor with optimization of dose and duration of therapy. *J Clin Oncol* 1989;7:1554.
58. Stroncek DF, Clay ME, Petzoldt ML, et al. Treatment of normal individuals with granulocyte-colony-stimulating factor: donor experiences and the effects on peripheral blood CD34+ cell counts and on the collection of peripheral blood stem cells. *Transfusion* 1996;36:601.
59. Wong GG, Witek JS, Temple PA, et al. Human GM-CSF: molecular cloning of the complementary DNA and purification of the natural and recombinant proteins. *Science* 1985;228:810.
60. Yang YC, Kovacic S, Kriz R, et al. The human genes for GM-CSF and IL 3 are closely linked in tandem on chromosome 5. *Blood* 1988;71:958.
61. Gasson JC, Weisbart RH, Kaufman SE, et al. Purified human granulocyte-macrophage colony-stimulating factor: direct action on neutrophils. *Science* 1984;226:1339.
62. Lopez AF, Williamson DJ, Gamble JR, et al. Recombinant human granulocyte-macrophage colony-stimulating factor stimulates in vitro mature human neutrophil and eosinophil function, surface receptor expression, and survival. *J Clin Invest* 1986;78:1220.
63. Socinski MA, Cannistra SA, Sullivan R, et al. Human granulocyte-macrophage colony-stimulating factor induces the expression of the CD11b surface adhesion molecule on granulocyte in vivo. *Blood* 1988;72:691.
64. Stanley E, Lieschke GJ, Grail D, et al. Granulocyte/macrophage colony-stimulating-factor-deficient mice show no major perturbation of hematopoiesis but develop a characteristic pulmonary pathology. *Proc Natl Acad Sci U S A* 1994;91:5592.
65. Dirksen U, Nishinakamura R, Groneck P, et al. Human pulmonary alveolar proteinosis associated with a defect in GM-CSF/IL-3/IL-5 receptor common beta chain expression. *J Clin Invest* 1997;100:2211.
66. Seymour JF, Begley CG, Dirksen U, et al. Attenuated hematopoietic response to granulocyte-macrophage colony-stimulating factor in patients with acquired pulmonary alveolar proteinosis. *Blood* 1998;92:2657.
67. Antman KS, Griffin JD, Elias A, et al. The effect of recombinant human granulocyte-macrophage colony-stimulating factor (rhGM-CSF) on chemotherapy-induced myelosuppression. *N Engl J Med* 1988;319:593.
68. Caballero MD, Vazquez L, Barragan JM, et al. Randomized study of filgrastim versus molgramostim after peripheral stem cell transplant in breast cancer. *Haematologica* 1998;83:514.
69. Miller CB, Jones RJ, Piantadosi S, Abeloff MD, Spivak JL. Decreased erythropoietin response in patients with the anemia of cancer. *N Engl J Med* 1990;322:1689.
70. Adamson JW, Spivak JL. Physiologic basis for the pharmacologic use of recombinant human erythropoietin in surgery and cancer treatment. *Surgery* 1994;115:7.
71. Henry DH. Recombinant human erythropoietin for the treatment of anemia in patients with advanced cancer. *Semin Hematol* 1993;30:12.
72. Spivak JL. Recombinant human erythropoietin and the anemia of cancer [Editorial]. *Blood* 1994;84:997.
73. Oster W, Herrmann F, Gamm H, et al. Erythropoietin for the treatment of anemia of malignancy associated with neoplastic bone marrow infiltration. *J Clin Oncol* 1990;8:956.
74. Cascinu S, Fedeli A, Del Ferro A, Luzi Fedeli S, Catalano G. Recombinant human erythropoietin treatment in cisplatin-associated anemia: a randomized, double-blind trial with placebo. *J Clin Oncol* 1994;12:1058.
75. Case D Jr, Bukowski RM, Carey RW, et al. Recombinant human erythropoietin therapy for anemic cancer patients on combination chemotherapy. *J Natl Cancer Inst* 1993;85:801.
76. Henry DH, Abels RI. Recombinant human erythropoietin in the treatment of cancer and chemotherapy-induced anemia: results of double-blind and open-label follow-up studies. *Semin Oncol* 1994;21:21.
77. Ayash LJ, Elias A, Hunt M, et al. Recombinant human erythropoietin for the treatment of the anaemia associated with autologous bone marrow transplantation. *Br J Haematol* 1994;87:153.
78. Biggs JC, Atkinson KA, Booker V, et al. Prospective randomised double-blind trial of the in vivo use of recombinant human erythropoietin in bone marrow transplantation from HLA-identical sibling donors. The Australian Bone Marrow Transplant Study Group. *Bone Marrow Transplant* 1995;15:129.
79. Lavey RS, Dempsey WH. Erythropoietin increases hemoglobin in cancer patients during radiation therapy. *Int J Radiat Oncol Biol Phys* 1993;27:1147.
80. Falkson CI, Keren-Rosenberg S, Uys A, et al. Recombinant human erythropoietin in the treatment of cancer-related anaemia. *Oncology* 1994;51:497.
81. Cascinu S, Del Ferro E, Fedeli A, et al. Recombinant human erythropoietin treatment in elderly cancer patients with cisplatin-associated anemia. *Oncology* 1995;52:422.
82. Gamucci T, Thorel MF, Frasca AM, Giannarell D, Calabresi F. Erythropoietin for the prevention of anaemia in neoplastic patients treated with cisplatin. *Eur J Cancer* 1993;2:S13.
83. Abels RI. Use of recombinant human erythropoietin in the treatment of anemia in patients who have cancer. *Semin Oncol* 1992;19:29.
84. Adamson JW, Ludwig H. Predicting the hematopoietic response to recombinant human erythropoietin (Epoetin alfa) in the treatment of the anemia of cancer. *Oncology* 1999;56:46.
85. Thatcher N. Management of chemotherapy-induced anemia in solid tumors. *Semin Oncol* 1998;25:23.
86. Jilani SM, Glaspy JA. Impact of epoetin alfa in chemotherapy-associated anemia. *Semin Oncol* 1998;25:571.
87. Ludwig H, Fritz E, Leitgeb C, et al. Prediction of response to erythropoietin treatment in chronic anemia of cancer. *Blood* 1994;84:1056.
88. Cazzola M, Ponchio L, Beguin Y, et al. Subcutaneous erythropoietin for treatment of refractory anemia in hematologic disorders. Results of a phase I/II clinical trial. *Blood* 1992;79:29.
89. Onat H, Inanc SE, Dalay N, et al. Effect of cisplatin on erythropoietin and iron changes [Letter]. *Eur J Cancer* 1993;5:777.
90. ten Bokkel Huinink WW, de Swart CA, van Toorn DW, et al. Controlled multicentre study of the influence of subcutaneous recombinant human erythropoietin on anaemia and transfusion dependency in patients with ovarian carcinoma treated with platinum-based chemotherapy. *Med Oncol* 1998;15:174.
91. Barosi G, Marchetti M, Liberato NL. Cost-effectiveness of recombinant human erythropoietin in the prevention of chemotherapy-induced anaemia. *Br J Cancer* 1998;78:781.
92. Varan A, Buyukpamukcu M, Kutluk T, Akyuz C. Recombinant human erythropoietin treatment for chemotherapy-related anemia in children. *Pediatrics* 1999;103:E16.
93. Bowen D, Culligan D, Jacobs A. The treatment of anaemia in the myelodysplastic syndromes with recombinant human erythropoietin. *Br J Haematol* 1991;77:419.
94. van Kamp H, Prinsze-Postema TC, Kluin PM, et al. Effect of subcutaneously administered human recombinant erythropoietin on erythropoiesis in patients with myelodysplasia. *Br J Haematol* 1991;78:488.
95. Stein RS, Abels RI, Krantz SB. Pharmacologic doses of recombinant human erythropoietin in the treatment of myelodysplastic syndromes. *Blood* 1991;78:1658.
96. Kurzrock R, Talpaz M, Estey E, et al. Erythropoietin treatment in patients with myelodysplastic syndrome and anemia. *Leukemia* 1991;5:985.
97. Ghio R, Balleari E, Ballestrero A, et al. Subcutaneous recombinant human erythropoietin for the treatment of anemia in myelodysplastic syndromes. *Acta Haematol* 1993;90:58.
98. Stone RM, Bernstein SH, Demetri G, et al. Therapy with recombinant human erythropoietin in patients with myelodysplastic syndromes. *Leuk Res* 1994;18:769.
99. Isnard F, Najman A, Jaar B, et al. Efficacy of recombinant human erythropoietin in the treatment of refractory anemias without excess of blasts in myelodysplastic syndromes. *Leuk Lymphoma* 1994;12:307.
100. Rose EH, Abels RI, Nelson RA, McCullough DM, Lessin L. The use of r-HuEpo in the treatment of anaemia related to myelodysplasia (MDS). *Br J Haematol* 1995;89:831.
101. Runde V, Aul C, Ebert A, Grabenhorst U, Schneider W. Sequential administration of recombinant human granulocyte-macrophage colony-stimulating factor and human erythropoietin for treatment of myelodysplastic syndromes. *Eur J Haematol* 1995;54:39.
102. Negrin RS, Stein R, Vardiman J, et al. Treatment of the anemia of myelodysplastic syndromes using recombinant human granulocyte colony-stimulating factor in combination with erythropoietin. *Blood* 1993;82:737.
103. Imamura M, Kobayashi M, Kobayashi S, et al. Failure of combination therapy with recombinant granulocyte colony-stimulating factor and erythropoietin in myelodysplastic syndromes. *Ann Hematol* 1994;68:163.
104. Hansen PB, Johnsen HE, Hippe E, Hellstrom-Lindberg E, Ralfkiaer E. Recombinant human granulocyte-macrophage colony-stimulating factor plus recombinant human erythropoietin may improve anemia in selected patients with myelodysplastic syndromes. *Am J Hematol* 1993;44:229.
105. Lewinski UH, Floru S, Cohen AM, Mittelmann M. Recombinant human erythropoietin in the treatment of myelodysplastic syndromes—response patterns. *Leuk Lymphoma* 1994;15:149.

106. Stasi R, Pagano A, Terzoli E, Amadori S. Recombinant human granulocyte-macrophage colony-stimulating factor plus erythropoietin for the treatment of cytopenias in patients with myelodysplastic syndromes. *Br J Haematol* 1999;105:141.
107. Hellstrom-Lindberg E, Negrin R, Stein R, et al. Erythroid response to treatment with G-CSF plus erythropoietin for the anaemia of patients with myelodysplastic syndromes: proposal for a predictive model. *Br J Haematol* 1997;99:344.
108. Klaesson S. Clinical use of rHuEPO in bone marrow transplantation. *Med Oncol* 1999;16:2.
109. Link H, Boogaerts MA, Fauser AA, et al. A controlled trial of recombinant human erythropoietin after bone marrow transplantation. *Blood* 1994;84:3327.
110. Chao NJ, Schriber JR, Long GD, et al. A randomized study of erythropoietin and granulocyte colony-stimulating factor (G-CSF) versus placebo and G-CSF for patients with Hodgkin's and non-Hodgkin's lymphoma undergoing autologous bone marrow transplantation. *Blood* 1994;83:2823.
111. Pene R, Appelbaum FR, Fisher L, et al. Use of granulocyte-macrophage colony-stimulating factor and erythropoietin in combination after autologous marrow transplantation. *Bone Marrow Transplant* 1993;11:219.
112. Vannucchi AM, Bosi A, Ieri A, et al. Combination therapy with G-CSF and erythropoietin after autologous bone marrow transplantation for lymphoid malignancies: a randomized trial. *Bone Marrow Transplant* 1996;17:527.
113. Fujimori Y, Kanamaru A, Saheki K, et al. Recombinant human erythropoietin for late-onset anemia after allogeneic bone marrow transplantation. *Int J Hematol* 1998;67:131.
114. Ganser A, Karthaus M. Clinical use of hematopoietic growth factors. *Curr Opin Oncol* 1996;8:265.
115. Fisher DC, Peters WP. Advances in the clinical use of granulocyte colony-stimulating factor and granulocyte-macrophage colony-stimulating factor to intensify cancer chemotherapy. *Curr Opin Hematol* 1994;1:221.
116. Le Corroller AG, Moatti JP. The economic evaluation of hematopoietic growth factors in high-dose chemotherapy. *Anticancer Drugs* 1998;9:917.
117. Lifton R, Bennett JM. Clinical use of granulocyte-macrophage colony-stimulating factor and granulocyte colony-stimulating factor in neutropenia associated with malignancy. *Hematol Oncol Clin North Am* 1996;10:825.
118. Crawford J, Ozer H, Stoller R, et al. Reduction by granulocyte colony-stimulating factor of fever and neutropenia induced by chemotherapy in patients with small-cell lung cancer. *N Engl J Med* 1991;325:164.
119. Trillet-Lenoir V, Green J, Manegold C, et al. Recombinant granulocyte colony stimulating factor reduces the infectious complications of cytotoxic chemotherapy. *Eur J Cancer* 1993;3:319.
120. Pettengell R, Gurney H, Radford JA, et al. Granulocyte colony-stimulating factor to prevent dose-limiting neutropenia in non-Hodgkin's lymphoma: a randomized controlled trial. *Blood* 1992;80:1430.
121. Gebbia V, Testa A, Valenza R, et al. A prospective evaluation of the activity of human granulocyte-colony stimulating factor on the prevention of chemotherapy-related neutropenia in patients with advanced carcinoma. *J Chemother* 1993;5:186.
122. Toner GC, Shapiro JD, Laidlaw CR, et al. Low-dose versus standard-dose lenograstim prophylaxis after chemotherapy: a randomized, crossover comparison. *J Clin Oncol* 1998;16:3874.
123. Ribas A, Albanell J, Bellmunt J, et al. Five-day course of granulocyte colony-stimulating factor in patients with prolonged neutropenia after adjuvant chemotherapy for breast cancer is a safe and cost-effective schedule to maintain dose-intensity. *J Clin Oncol* 1996;14:1573.
124. Bajorin DF, Nichols CR, Schmoll HJ, et al. Recombinant human granulocyte-macrophage colony-stimulating factor as an adjunct to conventional-dose ifosfamide-based chemotherapy for patients with advanced or relapsed germ cell tumors: a randomized trial. *J Clin Oncol* 1995;13:79.
125. Gerhartz HH, Engelhard M, Meusers P, et al. Randomized, double-blind, placebo-controlled, phase III study of recombinant human granulocyte-macrophage colony-stimulating factor as adjunct to induction treatment of high-grade malignant non-Hodgkin's lymphomas. *Blood* 1993;82:2329.
126. Kaplan LD, Kahn JO, Crowe S, et al. Clinical and virologic effects of recombinant human granulocyte-macrophage colony-stimulating factor in patients receiving chemotherapy for human immunodeficiency virus–associated non-Hodgkin's lymphoma: results of a randomized trial. *J Clin Oncol* 1991;9:929.
127. Weiss GR, Shaffer DW, DeMoor C, et al. A randomized phase I study of oral etoposide with or without granulocyte-macrophage colony-stimulating factor for the treatment of patients with advanced cancer. *Anticancer Drugs* 1996;7:402.
128. Jones SE, Schottstaedt MW, Duncan LA, et al. Randomized double-blind prospective trial to evaluate the effects of sargramostim versus placebo in a moderate-dose fluorouracil, doxorubicin, and cyclophosphamide adjuvant chemotherapy program for stage II and III breast cancer. *J Clin Oncol* 1996;14:2976.
129. Bregni M, Siena S, Di Nicola M, et al. Comparative effects of granulocyte-macrophage colony-stimulating factor and granulocyte colony-stimulating factor after high-dose cyclophosphamide cancer therapy. *J Clin Oncol* 1996;14:628.
130. Petros WP, Crawford J. Safety of concomitant use of granulocyte colony-stimulating factor or granulocyte-macrophage colony-stimulating factor with cytotoxic chemotherapy agents. *Curr Opin Hematol* 1997;4:213.
131. Bunn P Jr, Crowley J, Kelly K, et al. Chemoradiotherapy with or without granulocyte-macrophage colony-stimulating factor in the treatment of limited-stage small-cell lung cancer: a prospective phase III randomized study of the Southwest Oncology Group. *J Clin Oncol* 1995;13:1632.
132. Momin F, Kraut M, Lattin P, Valdivieso M. Thrombocytopenia in patients receiving chemoradiotherapy and g-csf for locally advanced non-small cell lung cancer (nsclc). *Proc Annu Meet Am Soc Clin Oncol* 1992;11:983a.
133. Tjan-Heijnen VC, Biesma B, Festen J, et al. Enhanced myelotoxicity due to granulocyte colony-stimulating factor administration until 48 hours before the next chemotherapy course in patients with small-cell lung carcinoma *J Clin Oncol* 1998;16:2708.
134. Livingston RB, Ellis GK, Gralow JR, et al. Dose-intensive vinorelbine with concurrent granulocyte colony-stimulating factor support in paclitaxel-refractory metastatic breast cancer. *J Clin Oncol* 1997;15:1395.
135. American Society of Clinical Oncology. Recommendations for the use of hematopoietic colony-stimulating factors: evidence-based, clinical practice guidelines. *J Clin Oncol* 1994;12:2471.
136. American Society of Clinical Oncology. Update of recommendations for the use of hematopoietic colony-stimulating factors: evidence-based clinical practice guidelines. *J Clin Oncol* 1996;14:1957.
137. American Society of Clinical Oncology. 1997 update of recommendations for the use of hematopoietic colony-stimulating factors: evidence-based, clinical practice guidelines. *J Clin Oncol* 1997;15:3288.
138. Biesma B, de Vries EG, Willemse PH, et al. Efficacy and tolerability of recombinant human granulocyte-macrophage colony-stimulating factor in patients with chemotherapy-related leukopenia and fever. *Eur J Cancer* 1990;26:932.
139. Bodey GP, Anaissie E, Gutterman J, Vadhan-Raj S. Role of granulocyte-macrophage colony-stimulating factor as adjuvant treatment in neutropenic patients with bacterial and fungal infection. *Eur J Clin Microbiol Infect Dis* 1994;13:S18.
140. Mayordomo JI, Rivera F, Diaz-Puente MT, et al. Improving treatment of chemotherapy-induced neutropenic fever by administration of colony-stimulating factors. *J Natl Cancer Inst* 1995;87:803.
141. Riikonen P, Saarinen UM, Makipernaa A, et al. Recombinant human granulocyte-macrophage colony-stimulating factor in the treatment of febrile neutropenia: a double blind placebo-controlled study in children. *Pediatr Infect Dis J* 1994;13:197.
142. Mitchell PL, Morland B, Stevens MC, et al. Granulocyte colony-stimulating factor in established febrile neutropenia: a randomized study of pediatric patients. *J Clin Oncol* 1997;15:1163.
143. Vellenga E, Uyl-de Groot CA, de Wit R, et al. Randomized placebo-controlled trial of granulocyte-macrophage colony-stimulating factor in patients with chemotherapy-related febrile neutropenia. *J Clin Oncol* 1996;14:619.
144. Hartmann LC, Tschetter LK, Habermann TM, et al. Granulocyte colony-stimulating factor in severe chemotherapy-induced afebrile neutropenia. *N Engl J Med* 1997;336:1776.
145. Clark DA, Neidhart JA. Granulocyte-macrophage colony-stimulating factor with dose-intensified treatment of cancer. *Semin Hematol* 1992;29:27.
146. Trillet-Lenoir V, Soler-Michel C. Granulocyte colony stimulating factor (G-CSF) enables dose intensification of chemotherapy in small cell lung cancer (SCLC). *Proc Annu Meet Am Soc Clin Oncol* 1994;13:1141a.
147. Pujol JL, Douillard JY, Riviere A, et al. Dose-intensity of a four-drug chemotherapy regimen with or without recombinant human granulocyte-macrophage colony-stimulating factor in extensive-stage small-cell lung cancer: a multicenter randomized phase III study. *J Clin Oncol* 1997;15:2082.
148. Kouroussis C, Androulakis N, Kakolyris S, et al. Dose-escalation study of docetaxel in combination with mitoxantrone as first-line treatment in patients with metastatic breast cancer. *J Clin Oncol* 1999;17:862.
149. Johnston EM, Crawford J. Hematopoietic growth factors in the reduction of chemotherapeutic toxicity. *Semin Oncol* 1998;25:552.
150. Gulati SC, Bennett CL. Granulocyte-macrophage colony-stimulating factor (GM-CSF) as adjunct therapy in relapsed Hodgkin disease. *Ann Intern Med* 1992;116:177.
151. Rabinowe SN, Neuberg D, Bierman PJ, et al. Long-term follow-up of a phase III study of recombinant human granulocyte-macrophage colony-stimulating factor after autologous bone marrow transplantation for lymphoid malignancies. *Blood* 1993;81:1903.
152. Link H, Boogaerts MA, Carella AM, et al. A controlled trial of recombinant human granulocyte-macrophage colony-stimulating factor after total body irradiation, high-dose chemotherapy, and autologous bone marrow transplantation for acute lymphoblastic leukemia or malignant lymphoma. *Blood* 1992;80:2188.
153. Gorin NC, Coiffier B, Hayat M, et al. Recombinant human granulocyte-macrophage colony-stimulating factor after high-dose chemotherapy and autologous bone marrow transplantation with unpurged and purged marrow in non-Hodgkin's lymphoma: a double-blind placebo-controlled trial. *Blood* 1992;80:1149.
154. Nemunaitis J, Rabinowe SN, Singer JW, et al. Recombinant granulocyte-macrophage colony-stimulating factor after autologous bone marrow transplantation for lymphoid cancer. *N Engl J Med* 1991;324:1773.
155. Advani R, Chao NJ, Horning SJ, et al. Granulocyte-macrophage colony-stimulating factor (GM-CSF) as an adjunct to autologous hemopoietic stem cell transplantation for lymphoma. *Ann Intern Med* 1992;116:183.
156. Gisselbrecht C, Prentice HG, Bacigalupo A, et al. Placebo-controlled phase III trial of lenograstim in bone-marrow transplantation. *Lancet* 1994;343:696.
157. Klumpp TR, Mangan KF, Goldberg SL, Pearlman ES, Macdonald JS. Granulocyte colony-stimulating factor accelerates neutrophil engraftment following peripheral-blood stem-cell transplantation: a prospective, randomized trial. *J Clin Oncol* 1995;13:1323.
158. Stahel R, Jost L, Pichert G, et al. Controlled study of filgrastim after high-dose chemotherapy and ABMT for high risk lymphoma [Abstract]. Presented at the Molecular Biology of Hematopoiesis Eighth Symposium. Basel, Switzerland: July 1993.
159. Stahel RA, Jost LM, Cerny T, et al. Randomized study of recombinant human granulocyte colony-stimulating factor after high-dose chemotherapy and autologous bone marrow transplantation for high-risk lymphoid malignancies. *J Clin Oncol* 1994;12:1931.
160. Linch DC, Milligan DW, Winfield DA, et al. G-CSF after peripheral blood stem cell transplantation in lymphoma patients significantly accelerated neutrophil recovery and shortened time in hospital: results of a randomized BNLI trial. *Br J Haematol* 1997;99:933.
161. Ojeda E, Garcia-Bustos J, Aguado M, et al. A prospective randomized trial of granulocyte colony-stimulating factor therapy after autologous blood stem cell transplantation in adults. *Bone Marrow Transplant* 1999;24:601.
162. Bolwell BJ, Pohlman B, Andresen S, et al. Delayed G-CSF after autologous progenitor cell transplantation: a prospective randomized trial. *Bone Marrow Transplant* 1998;21:369.

163. Kawano Y, Takaue Y, Mimaya J, et al. Marginal benefit/disadvantage of granulocyte colony-stimulating factor therapy after autologous blood stem cell transplantation in children: results of a prospective randomized trial. The Japanese Cooperative Study Group of PBSCT. *Blood* 1990;892:4040.
164. De Witte T, Gratwohl A, Van Der Lely N, et al. Recombinant human granulocyte-macrophage colony-stimulating factor accelerates neutrophil and monocyte recovery after allogeneic T-cell-depleted bone marrow transplantation. *Blood* 1992;79:1359.
165. Lazarus HM, Rowe JM. Clinical use of hematopoietic growth factors in allogeneic bone marrow transplantation. *Blood Rev* 1994;8:169.
166. Powles R, Smith C, Milan S, et al. Human recombinant GM-CSF in allogeneic bone-marrow transplantation for leukaemia: double-blind, placebo-controlled trial. *Lancet* 1990;336:1417.
167. Asano S, Masaoka T, Takabu F. Beneficial effect of recombinant human glycosylated granulocyte colony-stimulating factor in marrow-transplanted patients: results of multicenter phase II-III studies. *Transplantation Proc* 1991;23:1701.
168. Hiraoka A, Masaoka T, Mizoguchi H, et al. Recombinant human non-glycosylated granulocyte-macrophage colony-stimulating factor in allogeneic bone marrow transplantation: double-blind placebo-controlled phase III clinical trial. Japanese *J Clin Oncol* 1994;24:205.
169. Nemunaitis J, Anasetti C, Storb R, et al. Phase II trial of recombinant human granulocyte-macrophage colony-stimulating factor in patients undergoing allogeneic bone marrow transplantation from unrelated donors. *Blood* 1992;79:2572.
170. Nemunaitis J, Buckner CD, Appelbaum FR, et al. Phase I/II trial of recombinant human granulocyte-macrophage colony-stimulating factor following allogeneic bone marrow transplantation. *Blood* 1991;77:2065.
171. Schriber JR, Chao NJ, Long GD, et al. Granulocyte colony-stimulating factor after allogeneic bone marrow transplantation. *Blood* 1994;84:1680.
172. Legros M, Fleury J, Bay JO, et al. rhGM-CSF vs placebo following rhGM-CSF-mobilized PBPC transplantation: a phase III double-blind randomized trial. *Bone Marrow Transplant* 1997;19:209.
173. Vadhan-Raj S, Buescher S, LeMaistre A, et al. Stimulation of hematopoiesis in patients with bone marrow failure and in patients with malignancy by recombinant human granulocyte-macrophage colony-stimulating factor. *Blood* 1988;72:134.
174. Weisdorf DJ, Verfaillie CM, Davies SM, et al. Hematopoietic growth factors for graft failure after bone marrow transplantation: a randomized trial of granulocyte-macrophage colony-stimulating factor (GM-CSF) versus sequential GM-CSF plus granulocyte-CSF. *Blood* 1995;85:3452.
175. Ippoliti C, Przepiorka D, Giralt S, et al. Low-dose non-glycosylated rhGM-CSF is effective for the treatment of delayed hematopoietic recovery after autologous marrow or peripheral blood stem cell transplantation. *Bone Marrow Transplant* 1993;11:55.
176. Vose JM, Bierman PJ, Kessinger A, et al. The use of recombinant human granulocyte-macrophage colony stimulating factor for the treatment of delayed engraftment following high dose therapy and autologous hematopoietic stem cell transplantation for lymphoid malignancies. *Bone Marrow Transplant* 1991;7:139.
177. Nemunaitis J, Singer JW, Buckner CD, et al. Use of recombinant human granulocyte-macrophage colony-stimulating factor in graft failure after bone marrow transplantation. *Blood* 1990;76:245.
178. Nemunaitis J. The role of hematopoietic growth factor in the treatment of graft failure. *Bone Marrow Transplant* 1993;12:S50.
179. Sierra J, Terol MJ, Urbano-Ispizua A, et al. Different response to recombinant human granulocyte-macrophage colony-stimulating factor in primary and secondary graft failure after bone marrow transplantation. *Exp Hematol* 1994;22:566.
180. Zecca M, Perotti C, Marradi P, et al. Recombinant human G-CSF-mobilized peripheral blood stem cells for second allogeneic transplant after bone marrow graft rejection in children. *Br J Haematol* 1996;92:432.
181. Socinski MA, Cannistra SA, Elias A, et al. Granulocyte-macrophage colony stimulating factor expands the circulating hematopoietic progenitor cell compartment in humans. *Lancet* 1988;1:1194.
182. Duhrsen U, Villeval JL, Boyd J, et al. Effects of recombinant human granulocyte colony-stimulating factor on hematopoietic progenitor cells in cancer patients. *Blood* 1988;72:2074.
183. Brugger W, Bross K, Frisch J, et al. Mobilization of peripheral blood progenitor cells by sequential administration of interleukin-3 and granulocyte-macrophage colony-stimulating factor following polychemotherapy with etoposide, ifosfamide, and cisplatin. *Blood* 1992;79:1193.
184. Kessinger A, Bishop MR, Jackson JD, et al. Erythropoietin for mobilization of circulating progenitor cells in patients with previously treated relapsed malignancies. *Exp Hematol* 1995;23:609.
185. Desikan KR, Barlogie B, Jagannath S, et al. Comparable engraftment kinetics following peripheral-blood stem-cell infusion mobilized with granulocyte colony-stimulating factor with or without cyclophosphamide in multiple myeloma. *J Clin Oncol* 1998;16:1547.
186. Gianni AM, Tarella C, Siena S, et al. Durable and complete hematopoietic reconstitution after autografting of rhGM-CSF exposed peripheral blood progenitor cells. *Bone Marrow Transplant* 1990;6:143.
187. Pettengell R, Testa NG, Swindell R, Crowther D, Dexter TM. Transplantation potential of hematopoietic cells released into the circulation during routine chemotherapy for non-Hodgkin's lymphoma. *Blood* 1993;82:2239.
188. Beyer J, Schwella N, Zingsem J, et al. Hematopoietic rescue after high-dose chemotherapy using autologous peripheral-blood progenitor cells or bone marrow: a randomized comparison. *J Clin Oncol* 1995;13:1328.
189. Negrin RS, Kusnierz-Glaz CR, Still BJ, et al. Transplantation of enriched and purged peripheral blood progenitor cells from a single apheresis product in patients with non-Hodgkin's lymphoma. *Blood* 1995;85:3334.
190. Bensinger W, Singer J, Appelbaum F, et al. Autologous transplantation with peripheral blood mononuclear cells collected after administration of recombinant granulocyte stimulating factor. *Blood* 1993;81:3158.
191. Abboud CN, Liesveld JL, Belanger TJ, et al. Prospective randomized trial of four peripheral blood stem cell (PBSC) mobilization regimens in cancer patients undergoing autologous marrow transplantation (ABMT). *Proc Annu Meet Am Soc Clin Oncol* 1995;14:706a.
192. Pileri A, Tarella C, Bregni M, et al. GM-CSF-exposed peripheral blood progenitors as sole source of stem cells for autologous transplantation in two patients with multiple myeloma. *Haematologica* 1990;1:79.
193. Juttner CA, Fibbe WE, Nemunaitis J, Kanz L, Gianni AM. Blood cell transplantation: report from an International Consensus Meeting. *Bone Marrow Transplant* 1994;14:689.
194. Bishop MR, Tarantolo SR, Jackson JD, et al. Allogeneic-blood stem-cell collection following mobilization with low-dose granulocyte colony-stimulating factor. *J Clin Oncol* 1997;15:1601.
195. Lane TA, Law P, Maruyama M, et al. Harvesting and enrichment of hematopoietic progenitor cells mobilized into the peripheral blood of normal donors by granulocyte-macrophage colony-stimulating factor (GM-CSF) or G-CSF: potential role in allogeneic marrow transplantation. *Blood* 1995;85:275.
196. Weaver CH, Buckner CD, Longin K, et al. Syngeneic transplantation with peripheral blood mononuclear cells collected after the administration of recombinant human granulocyte colony-stimulating factor. *Blood* 1993;82:1981.
197. Molina L, Chabannon C, Viret F, et al. Granulocyte colony-stimulating factor-mobilized allogeneic peripheral blood stem cells for rescue graft failure after allogeneic bone marrow transplantation in two patients with acute myeloblastic leukemia in first complete remission [Letter]. *Blood* 1995;85:1678.
198. Korbling M, Przepiorka D, Huh YO, et al. Allogeneic blood stem cell transplantation for refractory leukemia and lymphoma: potential advantage of blood over marrow allografts. *Blood* 1995;85:1659.
199. Bensinger W, Martin P, Clift R, et al. A prospective, randomised trial of peripheral blood stem cells (pbsc) or marrow (bm) for patients undergoing allogeneic transplantation for hematologic malignancies. *Blood* 1999;94:1637a.
200. Winter JN, Lazarus HM, Rademaker A, et al. Phase I/II study of combined granulocyte colony-stimulating factor and granulocyte-macrophage colony-stimulating factor administration for the mobilization of hematopoietic progenitor cells. *J Clin Oncol* 1996;14:277.
201. Facon T, Harousseau JL, Maloisel F, et al. Stem cell factor in combination with filgrastim after chemotherapy improves peripheral blood progenitor cell yield and reduces apheresis requirements in multiple myeloma patients: a randomized, controlled trial. *Blood* 1999;94:1218.
202. Glaspy JA, Shpall EJ, LeMaistre CF, et al. Peripheral blood progenitor cell mobilization using stem cell factor in combination with filgrastim in breast cancer patients. *Blood* 1997;90:2939.
203. Ross AA, Cooper BW, Lazarus HM, et al. Incidence of tumor cell contamination in peripheral blood stem cell (PBSC) collections from breast cancer patients [Abstract]. *Proc Annu Meet Am Soc Clin Oncol* 1993;12:77a.
204. Craig JI, Langlands K, Parker AC, Anthony RS. Molecular detection of tumor contamination in peripheral blood stem cell harvests. *Exp Hematol* 1994;22:898.
205. Shpall EJ, Jones RB, Bearman SI, et al. Transplantation of enriched CD34-positive autologous marrow into breast cancer patients following high-dose chemotherapy: influence of CD34-positive peripheral-blood progenitors and growth factors on engraftment. *J Clin Oncol* 1994;12:28.
206. Vora AJ, Toh CH, Peel J, Greaves M. Use of granulocyte colony-stimulating factor (G-CSF) for mobilizing peripheral blood stem cells: risk of mobilizing clonal myeloma cells in patients with bone marrow infiltration. *Br J Haematol* 1994;86:180.
207. Schiller G, Vescio R, Freytes C, et al. Transplantation of CD34+ peripheral blood progenitor cells after high-dose chemotherapy for patients with advanced multiple myeloma. *Blood* 1995;86:390.
208. Gazitt Y, Reading CC, Hoffman R, et al. Purified CD34+ Lin− Thy+ stem cells do not contain clonal myeloma cells. *Blood* 1995;86:381.
209. Franklin WA, Glaspy J, Pflaumer SM, et al. Incidence of tumor-cell contamination in leukapheresis products of breast cancer patients mobilized with stem cell factor and granulocyte colony-stimulating factor (G-CSF) or with G-CSF alone. *Blood* 1999;94:340.
210. Griffin JD, Young D, Herrmann F, et al. Effects of recombinant human GM-CSF on proliferation of clonogenic cells in acute myeloblastic leukemia. *Blood* 1986;67:1448.
211. Kelleher C, Miyauchi J, Wong G, et al. Synergism between recombinant growth factors. GM-CSF and G-CSF, acting on the blast cells of acute myeloblastic leukemia. *Blood* 1987;69:1498.
212. Vellenga E, Young DC, Wagner K, et al. The effects of GM-CSF and G-CSF in promoting growth of clonogenic cells in acute myeloblastic leukemia. *Blood* 1987;69:1771.
213. Ohno R, Hiraoka A, Tanimoto M, et al. No increase of leukemia relapse in newly diagnosed acute myeloid leukemia (AML) who received granulocyte-colony stimulating factor (G-CSF) for life-threatening infection during induction and consolidation therapy [Abstract]. *Blood* 1993;81:561.
214. Heil G, Hoelzer D, Sanz MA, et al. Results of a randomized, double-blind placebo controlled phase III study of filgrastim in remission induction and early consolidation therapy for adults with de novo acute myeloid leukemia. *Blood* 1995;86:1053a.
215. Godwin JE, Kopecky KJ, Head DR, et al. A double blind placebo controlled trial of G-CSF in elderly patients with previously untreated acute myeloid leukemia, a Southwest Oncology Group Study. *Blood* 1995;86:1723a.
216. Stone RM, Berg DT, George SL, et al. Granulocyte-macrophage colony-stimulating factor after initial chemotherapy for elderly patients with primary acute myelogenous leukemia. Cancer and Leukemia Group B. *N Engl J Med* 1995;332:1671.
217. Rowe JM, Andersen JW, Mazza JJ, et al. A randomized placebo-controlled phase III study of granulocyte-macrophage colony-stimulating factor in adult patients (>55 to 70 years of age) with acute myelogenous leukemia: a study of the Eastern Cooperative Oncology Group (E1490). *Blood* 1995;86:457.
218. Estey E. Hematopoietic growth factors in the treatment of acute leukemia. *Curr Opin Oncol* 1998;10:23.
219. Ganser A, Heil G. Use of hematopoietic growth factors in the treatment of acute myelogenous leukemia. *Curr Opin Hematol* 1997;4:191.

220. Cannistra SA, Groshek P, Griffin JD. Granulocyte-macrophage colony-stimulating factor enhances the cytotoxic effects of cytosine arabinoside in acute myeloblastic leukemia and in the myeloid blast crisis phase of chronic myeloid leukemia. *Leukemia* 1989;3:328.
221. Cannistra SA, DiCarlo J, Groshek P, et al. Simultaneous administration of granulocyte-macrophage colony-stimulating factor and cytosine arabinoside for the treatment of relapsed acute myeloid leukemia. *Leukemia* 1991;5:230.
222. Estey E, Thall PF, Kantarjian H, et al. Treatment of newly diagnosed acute myelogenous leukemia with granulocyte-macrophage colony-stimulating factor (GM-CSF) before and during continuous-infusion high-dose ara-C + daunorubicin: comparison to patients treated without GM-CSF. *Blood* 1992;79:2246.
223. Lowenberg B, Boogaerts MA, Daenen SM, et al. Value of different modalities of granulocyte-macrophage colony-stimulating factor applied during or after induction therapy of acute myeloid leukemia. *J Clin Oncol* 1997;15:3496.
224. Ottmann OG, Hoelzer D, Gracien E, et al. Concomitant granulocyte colony-stimulating factor and induction chemoradiotherapy in adult acute lymphoblastic leukemia: a randomized phase III trial. *Blood* 1995;86:444.
225. Larson RA, Dodge RK, Linker CA, et al. A randomized controlled trial of filgrastim during remission induction and consolidation chemotherapy for adults with acute lymphoblastic leukemia: CALGB study 9111. *Blood* 1998;92:1556.
226. Greenberg PL. Treatment of myelodysplastic syndromes with hemopoietic growth factors. *Semin Oncol* 1992;19:106.
227. Schuster MW. Will cytokines alter the treatment of myelodysplastic syndrome? *Am J Med Sci* 1993;305:72.
228. Ganser A, Seipelt G, Eder M, et al. Treatment of myelodysplastic syndromes with cytokines and cytotoxic drugs. *Semin Oncol* 1992;19:95.
229. Vadhan-Raj S, Keating M, LeMaistre A, et al. Effects of recombinant human granulocyte-macrophage colony-stimulating factor in patients with myelodysplastic syndromes. *N Engl J Med* 1987;317:1545.
230. Ganser A, Volkers B, Greher J, et al. Recombinant human granulocyte-macrophage colony-stimulating factor in patients with myelodysplastic syndromes—a phase I/II trial. *Blood* 1989;73:31.
231. Willemze R, van der Lely N, Zwierzina H, et al. A randomized phase-i/ii multicenter study of recombinant human granulocyte-macrophage colony-stimulating factor (gm-csf) therapy for patients with myelodysplastic syndromes and a relatively low risk of acute leukemia. EORTC leukemia cooperative group *Ann Hematol* 1992;64:173.
232. Economopoulos T, Papageorgiou E, Stathakis N, et al. Treatment of myelodysplastic syndromes with human granulocytic-macrophage colony stimulating factor (GM-CSF) or GM-CSF combined with low-dose cytosine arabinoside. *Eur J Haematol* 1992;49:138.
233. Schuster MW, Larson RA, Thompson JA, et al. Granulocyte-macrophage colony-stimulating factor (GM-CSF) for myelodysplastic syndrome (MDS): results of a multi-center randomized controlled trial. *Blood* 1990;76:318a.
234. Rose C, Wattel E, Bastion Y, et al. Treatment with very low-dose GM-CSF in myelodysplastic syndromes with neutropenia. A report on 28 cases. *Leukemia* 1994;8:1458.
235. Gradishar WJ, Le Beau MM, O'Laughlin R, Vardiman JW, Larson RA. Clinical and cytogenetic responses to granulocyte-macrophage colony-stimulating factor in therapy-related myelodysplasia. *Blood* 1992;80:2463.
236. Negrin RS, Haeuber DH, Nagler A, et al. Treatment of myelodysplastic syndromes with recombinant human granulocyte colony-stimulating factor. a phase I-II trial. *Ann Intern Med* 1989;110:976.
237. Negrin RS, Haeuber DH, Nagler A, et al. Maintenance treatment of patients with myelodysplastic syndromes using recombinant human granulocyte colony-stimulating factor. *Blood* 1990;76:36.
238. Greenberg P, Taylor K, Larson R, et al. Phase III randomized multicenter trial of G-CSF vs. observation for myelodysplastic syndromes (MDS). *Blood* 1993;82:196a.
239. Ganser A, Maurer A, Contzen C, et al. Improved multilineage response of hematopoiesis in patients with myelodysplastic syndromes to a combination therapy with all-*trans*-retinoic acid, granulocyte colony-stimulating factor, erythropoietin and alpha-tocopherol. *Ann Hematol* 1996;72:237.
240. Gerhartz HH, Marcus R, Delmer A, et al. A randomized phase II study of low-dose cytosine arabinoside (LD-AraC) plus granulocyte-macrophage colony-stimulating factor (rhGM-CSF) in myelodysplastic syndromes (MDS) with a high risk of developing leukemia. EORTC Leukemia Cooperative Group. *Leukemia* 1994;8:16.
241. Estey E, Thall P, Andreeff M, et al. Use of granulocyte colony-stimulating factor before, during, and after fludarabine plus cytarabine induction therapy of newly diagnosed acute myelogenous leukemia or myelodysplastic syndromes: comparison with fludarabine plus cytarabine without granulocyte colony-stimulating factor. *J Clin Oncol* 1994;12:671.
242. Bernasconi C, Alessandrino EP, Bernasconi P, et al. Randomized clinical study comparing aggressive chemotherapy with or without G-CSF support for high-risk myelodysplastic syndromes or secondary acute myeloid leukaemia evolving from MDS. *Br J Haematol* 1998;102:678.
243. Ossenkoppele GJ, van der Holt B, Verhoef GE, et al. A randomized study of granulocyte colony-stimulating factor applied during and after chemotherapy in patients with poor risk myelodysplastic syndromes: a report from the HOVON Cooperative Group. Dutch-Belgian Hemato-Oncology Cooperative Group. *Leukemia* 1999;13:1207.
244. Du XX, Williams DA. Interleukin-11: a multifunctional growth factor derived from the hematopoietic microenvironment. *Blood* 1994;83:2023.
245. Du XX, Scott D, Yang ZX, et al. Interleukin-11 stimulates multilineage progenitors, but not stem cells, in murine and human long-term marrow cultures. *Blood* 1995;86:128.
246. Lemoli RM, Fogli M, Fortuna A, et al. Interleukin-11 stimulates the proliferation of human hematopoietic CD34+ and CD34+CD33–DR– cells and synergizes with stem cell factor, interleukin-3, and granulocyte-macrophage colony-stimulating factor. *Exp Hematol* 1993;21:1668.
247. Du XX, Neben T, Goldman S, Williams DA. Effects of recombinant human interleukin-11 on hematopoietic reconstitution in transplant mice: acceleration of recovery of peripheral blood neutrophils and platelets. *Blood* 1993;81:27.
248. Anderson KC, Morimoto C, Paul SR, et al. Interleukin-11 promotes accessory cell-dependent B-cell differentiation in humans. *Blood* 1992;80:2797
249. Yang YC, Yin T. Interleukin-11 and its receptor. *Biofactors* 1992;4:15.
250. Nash RA, Seidel K, Storb R, et al. Effects of rhIL-11 on normal dogs and after sublethal radiation. *Exp Hematol* 1995;23:389.
251. Gordon MS, Hoffman R, Battiato L, et al. Recombinant human interleukin eleven (Neumega rhIL-11 growth factor; rhIL-11) prevents severe thrombocytopenia in breast cancer patients receiving multiple cycles of cyclophosphamide (C) and doxorubicin (A) chemotherapy [Abstract]. *Proc Annu Meet Am Soc Clin Oncol* 1994;13:326a.
252. Isaacs C, Robert NJ, Bailey FA, et al. Randomized placebo-controlled study of recombinant human interleukin-11 to prevent chemotherapy-induced thrombocytopenia in patients with breast cancer receiving dose-intensive cyclophosphamide and doxorubicin. *J Clin Oncol* 1997;15:3368.
253. Tepler I, Elias L, Smith JW 2nd, et al. A randomized placebo-controlled trial of recombinant human interleukin-11 in cancer patients with severe thrombocytopenia due to chemotherapy. *Blood* 1996;87:3607.
254. Vredenburgh JJ, Hussein A, Fisher D, et al. A randomized trial of recombinant human interleukin-11 following autologous bone marrow transplantation with peripheral blood progenitor cell support in patients with breast cancer. *Biol Blood Marrow Transplant* 1998;4:134.
255. Du XX, Doerschuk CM, Orazi A, Williams DA. A bone marrow stromal-derived growth factor, interleukin-11, stimulates recovery of small intestinal mucosal cells after cytoablative therapy. *Blood* 1994;83:33.
256. Potten CS. Interleukin-11 protects the clonogenic stem cells in murine small-intestinal crypts from impairment of their reproductive capacity by radiation. *Int J Cancer* 1995; 62:356.
257. Schwertschlag US, Trepicchio WL, Dykstra KH, et al. Hematopoietic, immunomodulatory and epithelial effects of interleukin-11. *Leukemia* 1999;13:1307.
258. Chang MS, McNinch J, Basu R, et al. Cloning and characterization of the human megakaryocyte growth and development factor (MGDF) gene. *J Biol Chem* 1995;270:511.
259. Sohma Y, Akahori H, Seki N, et al. Molecular cloning and chromosomal localization of the human thrombopoietin gene. *Febs Lett* 1994;353:57.
260. Lok S, Kaushansky K, Holly RD, et al. Cloning and expression of murine thrombopoietin cDNA and stimulation of platelet production in vivo. *Nature* 1994;369:565.
261. Gurney AL, Kuang WJ, Xie MH, et al. Genomic structure, chromosomal localization, and conserved alternative splice forms of thrombopoietin. *Blood* 1995;85:981.
262. Kuter DJ, Rosenberg RD. The reciprocal relationship of thrombopoietin (c-Mpl ligand) to changes in the platelet mass during busulfan-induced thrombocytopenia in the rabbit. *Blood* 1995;85:2720.
263. Banu N, Wang JF, Deng B, Groopman JE, Avraham H. Modulation of megakaryocytopoiesis by thrombopoietin: the c-Mpl ligand. *Blood* 1995;86:1331.
264. Kaushansky K. Thrombopoietin: the primary regulator of platelet production. *Blood* 1995;86:419.
265. Broudy VC, Lin NL, Kaushansky K. Thrombopoietin (c-mpl ligand) acts synergistically with erythropoietin, stem cell factor, and interleukin-11 to enhance murine megakaryocyte colony growth and increases megakaryocyte ploidy in vitro. *Blood* 1995;85:1719.
266. Basser RL, Rasko JE, Clarke K, et al. Randomized, blinded, placebo-controlled phase I trial of pegylated recombinant human megakaryocyte growth and development factor with filgrastim after dose-intensive chemotherapy in patients with advanced cancer. *Blood* 1997;89:3118.
267. Fanucchi M, Glaspy J, Crawford J, et al. Effects of polyethylene glycol-conjugated recombinant human megakaryocyte growth and development factor on platelet counts after chemotherapy for lung cancer. *N Engl J Med* 1997;336:404.
268. Friedman HD, Sanderson SO, Stein CK, et al. Extramedullary granulopoiesis mimicking recurrent lymphoma after prolonged administration of human recombinant granulocyte colony-stimulating factor. *Ann Hematol* 1998;77:79.
269. Hornung RL, Longo DL. Hematopoietic stem cell depletion by restorative growth factor regimens during repeated high-dose cyclophosphamide therapy. *Blood* 1992;80:77.

Brahm H. Segal
Thomas J. Walsh
Steven M. Holland

CHAPTER 54

Infections in the Cancer Patient

Infections are major causes of morbidity and mortality in patients with cancer. The risk of infection is principally related to the intensity and duration of immunosuppressive chemotherapy. It is essential to know the patient's quantitative and qualitative immune defects and to stratify the risk for specific pathogens in the context of the history, physical examination, and radiologic and laboratory data.

In the 1980s, there was a shift in the relative prevalence of specific pathogens afflicting patients with cancer. Whereas in the 1960s and 1970s, gram-negative bacterial pathogens (Enterobacteriaceae and *Pseudomonas aeruginosa*) were the principal causes of bacteremia, in the 1990s and 1980s, gram-positive bacterial pathogens became predominant.[1] Today, filamentous fungi are a major cause of mortality in allogeneic bone marrow transplant (BMT) recipients and in patients with prolonged neutropenia. The spectrum of invasive fungal infections has dramatically increased. Examples of such emerging pathogens include *Fusarium, Acremonium, Scedosporium,* and dematiaceous (dark-walled fungi) species, and the yeast *Trichosporon beigelii.* This population is also at risk for a broad spectrum of viral and protozoal infections.

We describe the clinical manifestations and treatment of the major pathogens encountered in an oncology population. Specific infectious syndromes, such as fever without a documented source, pneumonia, skin infection, gastrointestinal infection, and sepsis, are reviewed. We also discuss novel approaches aimed at prevention and early diagnosis of infections and immune augmentation strategies.

FACTORS PREDISPOSING TO INFECTION IN PATIENTS WITH CANCER

Patients with cancer are a highly varied population, both in terms of the underlying malignancy and the level of immunosuppression. We describe specific categories of immunosuppression and the pathogens to which these patients are most susceptible. Multiple predisposing factors may exist in a single patient, thus increasing the spectrum of likely pathogens. The major categories of immunologic deficits in persons with cancer and the pathogens to which they are susceptible are summarized in Table 54-1.

ABSOLUTE NEUTROPHIL COUNT GREATER THAN 500/μL AND NO IMMUNOSUPPRESSIVE THERAPY

The group with absolute neutrophil count greater than 500/μl and no immunosuppressive therapy represents the least immunosuppressed patients with cancer, but some level of risk of infection may still exist. The malignancy itself may be associated with an immune defect. Malignancies associated with defective immunoglobulin production lead to increased susceptibility to encapsulated bacteria, principally *Streptococcus pneumoniae.* Such patients may have recurrent sinopulmonary infections, septicemia, and disseminated infection. Patients with chronic lymphocytic leukemia frequently have hypogammaglobulinemia or dysglobulinemia.[2] Low levels of both total immunoglobulin G (IgG) and specific antibodies to pneumococcal polysaccharide capsule are associated with an increased rate of infections in these patients.[2] A decision analysis suggested that routine administration of immunoglobulin to patients with chronic lymphocytic leukemia and hypogammaglobulinemia reduces the frequency of bacterial infections, but is not cost-effective.[3]

Patients with multiple myeloma and other related gammaglobulinopathies also are often functionally hypogammaglobulinemic; the total level of immunoglobulin production is elevated, but the repertoire of antibody production is restricted. Savage et al.[4] noted a biphasic pattern of infection among patients with multiple myeloma. Infections by *S pneumoniae* and

TABLE 54-1. Predominant Immunologic Defects and Associated Pathogens in Patients with Cancer

Abnormality	*Bacterial*	*Fungal*	*Protozoal*	*Viral*
Qualitative defect of phagocytic function or neutropenia	Gram positive	*Candida* sp.		
	Staphylococcus aureus	*Aspergillus* sp.		
	Streptococcus sp.	*Fusarium* sp.		
	Nocardia sp.	Dematiaceous molds		
	Gram negative	*Trichosporon* sp.		
	Escherichia coli	Zygomycetes		
	Klebsiella sp.	Other filamentous fungi		
	Enterobacter sp.			
	Proteus sp.			
	Pseudomonas aeruginosa			
	Stenotrophomonas maltophilia			
	Acinetobacter sp.	*Candida* sp.		
Defective cell-mediated immunity	*Mycobacterium* sp.	*Cryptococcus neoformans*	*Pneumocystis carinii*[a]	Cytomegalovirus
	Nocardia sp.	*Histoplasma capsulatum*	*Toxoplasma gondii*	Epstein-Barr virus
	Listeria monocytogenes	*Coccidioides immitis*	*Strongyloides stercoralis*	Varicella zoster virus
	Salmonella sp.			
Defective humoral immunity	Encapsulated bacteria	*Cryptococcus neoformans*		Community respiratory viruses
Splenectomy	Encapsulated bacteria			
	Salmonella sp.			
	Babesia microti			
	Malaria			
	Capnocytophaga canimorsus			

[a]*Pneumocystis carinii* is more accurately classified as a fungus, but has historically been classified as a protozoan.

Haemophilus influenzae occurred early in the disease and in patients responding to chemotherapy, whereas infections by *Staphylococcus aureus* and gram-negative pathogens occurred more commonly in advanced disease and during neutropenia. Serum from patients with multiple myeloma may be defective in the activation of C3, the major opsonin of the complement system, which likely further contributes to susceptibility to pneumococcal infection.[5] One randomized study showed that prophylactic intravenous immunoglobulin protected against life-threatening and recurrent infections in patients with multiple myeloma.[6] The patients who benefited most from immunoglobulin therapy were those with poor IgG antibody responses to pneumococcal vaccination.

Patients with hairy cell leukemia appear to have a defect in cell-mediated immunity, leaving them prone to develop an unusually high frequency of opportunistic atypical mycobacterial infections.[7] Patients with untreated Hodgkin's disease have significant abnormalities in T-cell number and function, which persist in the majority of long-term survivors.[8] Such patients are at increased risk for toxoplasmosis, nocardiosis, pneumocystosis, cryptococcosis, mycobacterial infections, and herpes zoster. Most opportunistic infections occurred during poorly controlled malignancy when patients were receiving corticosteroids, myeloablative chemotherapy, or both.[9]

Adrenal tumors and ectopic adrenocorticotropic hormone–secreting tumors resulting in high levels of cortisol[10,11] and T-cell leukemias[12] are associated with defects in cellular immunity resulting in an increased risk of mucosal candidiasis, *Pneumocystis carinii* pneumonia (PCP), and invasive aspergillosis.

Solid tumors may predispose patients to infection because of anatomic factors. Tumors that overgrow their blood supply become necrotic, thus forming a nidus for infection. Head and neck tumors may cause erosion through the fascial planes of the neck and floor of the mouth, predisposing patients to serious infections caused by mouth flora. Lemierre's syndrome, a septic thrombophlebitis of the neck with possible embolization to the tricuspid valve and lung and dissemination to other organs, is usually caused by *Fusobacterium* species, which are anaerobic oral commensal organisms.[13] This infection may develop during the course of uncontrolled head and neck cancer. Head and neck cancers may also increase the risk of aspiration pneumonia. Endobronchial lung tumors are associated with recurrent postobstructive pneumonias. Abdominal tumors may obstruct hollow viscera, such as the genitourinary or hepatobiliary tracts, predisposing to pyelonephritis and cholangitis, respectively. Direct invasion through the colonic mucosa is associated with local abscess formation and sepsis by enteric flora. *Streptococcus bovis* bacteremia is highly associated with colon cancer. Breast tumors increase the risk of mastitis and abscess formation, usually by *Staphylococcus aureus.*

Therapy for the underlying malignancy, independent of the immunosuppression, may be associated with an increased risk of infection. Local radiation therapy is associated with loss of epithelial integrity, necrosis, loss of blood supply, and consequent poor ability to repair wounds. Visceral complications include radiation pneumonitis, esophagitis, and enteritis. Implantable hardware necessary for administration of chemotherapy, such as cuffed intravenous catheters and Ommaya reservoirs, are potential niduses of infection.

Patients with malignancy commonly experience malnutrition, which increases the risk of infection. Weight loss frequently precedes the diagnosis of cancer, and the nausea, mucositis, and enteritis that follow antineoplastic chemotherapy worsen malnutrition.

NEUTROPENIA

Neutropenia may develop independently of chemotherapy in certain patients with cancer. In acute leukemia, the marrow may be replaced with malignant cells so that virtually no normal circulating neutrophils exist. Similarly, patients with premalignant hematologic disease, such as myelodysplastic syndrome, may have associated bone marrow failure. Patients also may develop neutropenia due to tumor-related autoimmune neutrophil destruction.[14] Persons rendered neutropenic by myeloablative chemotherapy are likely to be at greater risk for life-threatening infections due to the concomitant disruption of epithelial mucosal barriers by such agents.

The relationship between circulating leukocytes and risk of infection was established by Bodey et al.[15] in a classic early study of 52 patients with acute lymphocytic leukemia or acute myelogenous leukemia. The frequency of severe infections was highest when the absolute neutrophil count (ANC) was less than 100/μL and proportionately less frequent at 100 to 500/μL and 500 to 1000/μL, respectively. This relationship was sustained whether the patient was in relapse or remission, although the overall risk of infection was greater during relapse. Ninety percent of disseminated fungal infections and 78% of septicemias occurred when the ANC was less than 500/μL. No further reduction in the rate of serious infections occurred at ANC greater than 1000 to 1500/μL. In addition to the depth of neutropenia, the risk of infection was strongly related to the duration of neutropenia. A neutrophil count of less than 100/μL resulted in infections in all patients within 3 weeks and in severe infections within 6 weeks. The likelihood of survival from severe infections was related to both the initial granulocyte level and whether an increase in the neutrophil count occurred within the first week. With an initial ANC of less than 100/μL and no increase within the first week, mortality was 80%.

The risk of invasive aspergillosis is also directly related to the period of neutropenia. In patients with leukemia, Gerson et al.[16] showed that aspergillosis was uncommon when neutropenia lasted for less than 14 days. However, after 14 days, the risk of aspergillosis increased in direct proportion to the length of neutropenia. Invasive aspergillosis is also a major cause of mortality in patients with persistent neutropenia secondary to aplastic anemia.[17] Since the mid-1980s, an increasing spectrum of fungal pathogens has been encountered in patients with prolonged neutropenia, including *Fusarium* species, dark-walled molds, and *Trichosporon* species.[18,19]

Diagnosis of infection in granulocytopenic patients may be hampered by the lack of typical symptoms and signs. Sickles et al.[20] compared the clinical manifestations of infections in neutropenic and nonneutropenic patients with cancer. Fever was present in virtually all patients with an ANC less than 100/μL and in 90% of patients with 101 to 1000/μL. However, physical findings of infection, including fluctuance, exudate, local heat and swelling, ulceration, and local adenopathy, were less frequent in neutropenic than in nonneutropenic patients with similar infections. Local erythema and tenderness were sensitive indicators of infection in neutropenic patients. In neutropenic patients with pneumonia, sputum and physical examination signs of consolidation were less frequent than in nonneutropenic patients as were localizing symptoms and pyuria in cases of urinary tract infection. Local infections more commonly led to bacteremia with an ANC less than 100/μL. Thus, fever is a relatively sensitive sign of infection in the neutropenic patient, whereas other findings of infection are often lacking. The high likelihood of systemic infection and mortality in febrile neutropenic patients constitutes the rationale for initiating empiric antibacterial therapy before a documented source of infection or culture data are available.

MUCOSAL IMMUNITY

The mucosal linings in the gastrointestinal, sinopulmonary, and genitourinary tracts constitute the first line of host defense against a variety of pathogens. Chemotherapy and radiation therapy cause defects in mucosal immunity at several different levels. The physical protective barrier conferred by the epithelial lining is compromised, thus allowing access to colonizing microflora. In BMT patients, chronic graft-versus-host disease (GVHD) further compromises mucosal immunity. These patients have defective salivary immunoglobulin secretion,[21] and corticosteroids profoundly compromise mucosa–associated lymphoid tissue by inducing apoptosis of M cells and depleting lymphoid follicles of T and B cells.[22]

Mucosal epithelial cells secrete a variety of antimicrobial peptides, including lactoferrin (iron sequestration), lysozyme (hydrolysis of peptidoglycan of gram-positive bacteria), and phospholipase A2 (cleavage of structural phospholipids of bacteria).[23] Defensins are a group of small cysteine-rich antibacterial peptides (molecular weight, approximately 4 kD) located abundantly in the primary (azurophilic) granules of neutrophils and in a variety of mucosal epithelial cells, including bronchial epithelium and Paneth's cells within small intestinal crypts.[23] Neutropenia and loss of the epithelial cell anatomic barrier and local production of antimicrobial proteins likely predispose to typhlitis (neutropenic enterocolitis). Synthetically produced antimicrobial peptides are potential therapeutic candidates for augmenting mucosal immunity.[24]

IMMUNOSUPPRESSIVE AGENTS NOT RELATED TO NEUTROPENIA

Corticosteroids

Corticosteroids have profound effects on the distribution and function of neutrophils, monocytes, and lymphocytes. They induce a neutrophilic leukocytosis by accelerating the release of neutrophils from the bone marrow and by inhibiting the egress of neutrophils from the circulation. Corticosteroids reduce adherence of neutrophils to the endothelium, thus inhibiting migration to inflammatory sites, and inhibit neutrophil fungicidal activity.[25]

Corticosteroids elicit a peripheral blood monocytopenia that lasts for 24 hours. In addition, a number of monocyte functions are impaired, including chemotaxis, bactericidal activity, and production of interleukin-1 (IL-1) and tumor necrosis factor-α (TNF-α).[26]

Corticosteroids inhibit T-cell activation, leading to reduced proliferative responses and cytokine production, and also induce a redistribution of lymphocytes out of the circulation, leading to peripheral lymphocytopenia. This redistribution predominantly involves T cells.[27] At high doses, corticosteroids also inhibit immunoglobulin generation by B cells.[28]

In patients with cancer, corticosteroids are seldom the only immunosuppressive agents being administered, and it is therefore difficult to delineate the degree of impairment in host defense elicited by the corticosteroid regimen alone. Infections that occur in patients with collagen vascular diseases treated with corticosteroids are associated with both impaired phagocytic function (such as *S aureus* and Enterobacteriaceae) and cell-mediated immunity (such as herpes zoster, and *P carinii*).[26] In this population, the incidence of infectious complications increases when the adult equivalent of prednisone, 20 to 40 mg/d, is administered for longer than 4 to 6 weeks.[27,29] In patients with cancer, the most intensive corticosteroid regimens (usually the equivalent of prednisone, 1 g daily) are used to treat BMT recipients with GVHD, leading to a global suppression of phagocytic and cell-mediated activity and rendering these patients highly susceptible to a broad spectrum of bacterial, fungal, viral, and protozoal pathogens. In addition to immunosuppression, corticosteroids directly stimulate the growth of *Aspergillus fumigatus in vitro*,[30] possibly via sterol-binding proteins in the fungus.

Methotrexate

Methotrexate inhibits dihydrofolate reductase, an enzyme required for the synthesis of DNA and certain amino acids. At the high doses used in antineoplastic chemotherapy, methotrexate is highly immunosuppressive. As with other cytotoxic agents, methotrexate causes bone marrow suppression and mucositis. Trimethoprim-sulfamethoxazole, an antifolate drug commonly used as prophylaxis against *P carinii* infection in this population, may aggravate the hematologic toxicity of methotrexate.[31]

In patients with collagen vascular disease treated with low-dose methotrexate, the infection rate was low. The most common opportunistic pathogens were *P carinii* and herpes zoster.[26] Other reported infections included aspergillosis, histoplasmosis, nocardiosis, mycobacterial infections, and *Listeria monocytogenes* meningitis.[26] Epstein-Barr virus (EBV)–associated B-cell lymphoproliferative disease has been identified in a few patients with collagen vascular diseases treated with methotrexate.[32] Thus, long-term use of low-dose methotrexate can lead to significant depression of cell-mediated immunity, independent of its myeloid toxicity.

Cyclosporin A

Cyclosporin A (CSA) is a potent inhibitor of T-cell activation that is commonly used in the postengraftment period after BMT. CSA is a prodrug that binds to the intracellular protein, cyclophilin. The resulting complex in turn inhibits the calcium-regulated protein phosphatase, calcineurin, a protein required for signal transduction after activation of the T-cell receptor. Calcium-dependent production of the potent neutrophil chemoattractant, IL-8, is inhibited by CSA.[33] Compared with methotrexate, CSA is associated with less mucositis, and in some studies, more rapid myeloid recovery in BMT recipients.[34,35]

Fludarabine

Fludarabine is a fluorinated analog of adenine that has been used in a variety of hematologic malignancies, including chronic lymphocytic leukemia, hairy cell leukemia, and low-grade lymphomas. Fludarabine is a lymphotoxic compound, primarily affecting CD4+ lymphocytes. The combination of fludarabine and corticosteroids is more immunosuppressive than either agent alone.[36] Fludarabine plus prednisone results in a uniform depression of CD4+ cells that may persist for several months after completion of therapy.[37] In one series, 14 of 264 patients (5%) with chronic lymphocytic leukemia developed either PCP or listeriosis, and three cases occurred more than 1 year after therapy in patients who were in remission. Other opportunistic pathogens reflecting T-cell depression include disseminated varicella, mycobacteria, and fungi.[38] Prophylaxis with trimethoprim-sulfamethoxazole (which has activity against both *P carinii* and *L monocytogenes*) appears to be warranted.

Interleukin-2

Patients receiving high-dose IL-2 for malignancy have an increased risk of bacterial infections. Among 345 patients with cancer enrolled in a multicenter study of IL-2, 88 (26%) had bacteremia.[39] *S aureus* followed by coagulase-negative staphylococci were the most common pathogens. The frequency of sepsis in IL-2 recipients was several-fold greater than in nonneutropenic patients with indwelling central catheters. IL-2 causes a profound but reversible defect in neutrophil chemotaxis that may account for the increased frequency of infections.[39]

SPLENECTOMY

The spleen is a reservoir in which rapid antigen presentation occurs, leading to the production of opsonizing antibodies by B cells. Splenic macrophages remove both opsonized and nonopsonized particles from the blood stream. The removal of nonopsonized bacteria is a particularly important function to protect against encapsulated bacteria to which the patient is not immune.

Asplenic patients are principally at risk for overwhelming sepsis by encapsulated bacteria. The most common pathogen is *S pneumoniae*, but other pathogens include *Haemophilus influenzae* and *Neisseria meningitidis*. It is best to immunize individuals against encapsulated bacteria in advance of splenectomy. If this is not feasible, immunization is still advisable after splenectomy, because such patients are still capable of mounting a protective antibody response. In a study of asplenic patients, IgG responses to immunization with pneumococcal, *H influenzae* type b, and meningococcal vaccines were normal by day 28.[40] Patients with Hodgkin's disease, most of whom were asplenic, had normal IgG responses to pneumococcal polysaccharide vaccine. Molrine et al.[40] suggest reimmunization of asplenic persons every 5 years with the pneumococcal polysaccharide vaccine based on a potential increased risk for disease as protective antibody levels wane over time.

Asplenic patients should be advised to seek medical attention when fever occurs. Prophylaxis with penicillin has been traditionally used after splenectomy. However, the growing frequency of antimicrobial resistance among *S pneumoniae* isolates raises a note of caution. In a surveillance study, the overall percentages of respiratory pneumococcal isolates from the United States with intermediate and high-level resistance to penicillin were 28% and 16%, respectively.[41] A significant minority of penicillin-resistant isolates are cross-resistant to cephalosporins, macrolides, and trimethoprim-sulfamethox-

TABLE 54-2. Time Line of Principal Immune Defects and Infectious Complications in Bone Marrow Transplant Recipients

	Months after Transplantation		
	<1	1–6	>6
Principal immune defect	Neutropenia	T-cell, humoral Phagocytic (qualitative)	Humoral
Pathogens	Bacteria *Staphylococcus* sp. *Streptococcus* sp. Enterobacteriaceae *Pseudomonas aeruginosa* Fungi *Candida* sp. *Aspergillus* sp. Herpes simplex virus	Fungi *Aspergillus* sp. *Candida* sp. *Cryptococcus neoformans* Dimorphic fungi *Pneumocystis carinii* Viruses Cytomegalovirus Epstein-Barr virus Varicella zoster virus Respiratory viruses	Respiratory viruses Varicella zoster virus Encapsulated bacteria

[a]Note that graft-versus-host disease necessitating intensive immunosuppressive therapy leads to lack of reconstitution of phagocytic (qualitative) and cell-mediated immunity, thus prolonging the period of risk for both common bacterial and opportunistic infections.

azole.[41] Newer generation quinolones have reliable activity against penicillin-resistant pneumococci, though a Canadian study documented an increased frequency of quinolone-resistant pneumococcal isolates in association with increased use of these agents.[42] Physicians should be aware of local patterns of resistance to guide prophylactic and empiric antibiotic therapy.

Other pathogens associated with a more fulminant course in asplenic individuals include *Capnocytophaga* species,[43,44] babesiosis,[45] malaria, and *Salmonella* species. *Capnocytophaga canimorsus* infection is typically associated with dog bites and can lead to sepsis with or without evidence of cellulitis. *Babesia microti* is transmitted by the *Ixodes* tick, which is also the vector for Lyme disease. When in Lyme-endemic regions in the spring to autumn periods, patients should follow basic precautions to avoid tick bites (long sleeves, tick repellants) and be vigilant about fever. The diagnosis of babesiosis is confirmed by a peripheral blood smear showing characteristic intraerythrocytic inclusions.

BONE MARROW TRANSPLANTATION

The spectrum of pathogens to which BMT recipients are most susceptible follows a time line corresponding to the predominant immune defects observed at different periods (Table 54-2). In the early stage of BMT, neutropenia is the principal host defense defect. These patients are at risk for the same spectrum of bacterial and fungal infections that afflict nontransplant patients who have been treated with potent myeloablative therapy (see Neutropenia, earlier in this chapter). Severe mucocutaneous herpes simplex virus (HSV) infection is also commonly observed in the first month of transplantation in association with chemotherapy-induced mucositis. After myeloid engraftment, fever and mucositis typically resolve, and the risk of serious bacterial and fungal infections decreases.

After myeloid engraftment, a qualitative dysfunction of phagocytes persists due to corticosteroid therapy and other immunosuppressive agents (see Immunosuppressive Agents Not Related to Neutropenia, earlier in this chapter). The risk of infection by filamentous fungi during this period is strongly associated with the severity of GVHD and requirement for potent immunosuppressive regimens. Impairment in neutrophil chemotaxis has been noted in some patients and may increase the risk of infection.[46,47] Alveolar macrophage function in patients studied within 4 months of allogeneic BMT was impaired based on chemotaxis, phagocytosis, and killing of bacterial and candidal species.[48] These observations may, in part, account for the increased risk of pneumonia during this period.

Defects in cell-mediated immunity persist for several months even in uncomplicated allogeneic transplant recipients, thus predisposing these patients to a variety of opportunistic infections, such as candidiasis, *P carinii*, cytomegalovirus (CMV), and herpes zoster (see Table 54-2). Repopulation of specific T-cell subsets occurs at different rates, resulting in a lower than normal CD4+ (helper T cell) to CD8+ (suppressor-cytotoxic T cell) ratio for the first 6 months after engraftment.[49] In addition to quantitative T-cell deficiencies, loss of T-cell receptor diversity is observed.[50] During the first 100 days of transplantation, delayed hypersensitivity responses, proliferative responses to mitogens and antigens, and T-cell–mediated activation of B cells to produce immunoglobulin are impaired.[51] By 1 year after engraftment, BMT recipients without chronic GVHD have normalized CD4+/CD8+ ratios, and in general, have normal *in vivo* and *in vitro* T-cell responses.

Defective reconstitution of humoral immunity is a major factor contributing to increased infection susceptibility in the late transplant period. Winston et al.[52] noted an unusually high frequency of pneumococcal infections between 7 and 36 months after transplantation. All infections occurred after trimethoprim-sulfamethoxazole prophylaxis for *P carinii* was halted. The risk of pneumococcal infection was associated with serum opsonic deficiency for *S pneumoniae.* Kalhs et al.[53,54] showed that functional asplenia, as determined by the presence of Howell-Jolly bodies in peripheral blood smears, was a late complication of allogeneic BMT only in patients with severe GVHD. Thus, even in BMT recipients who have had an uncomplicated course, fever in the late transplant period must be evaluated promptly (similar to patients with asplenia) because of the risk of overwhelming infection by one of these pathogens (see Table 54-2).

During periods of severe GVHD, the immunosuppressive regimen is intensified to include high-dose corticosteroids in combination with CSA and possibly an antilymphocyte globulin preparation. CD4+ lymphocytopenia may, in part, result from GVHD-induced injury of thymic epithelial cells.[55] Whereas mature and cooperative T- and B-cell functions are generally reconstituted by 1 year after engraftment in uncomplicated allogeneic BMT, chronic GVHD is associated with persistently depressed cell-mediated and humoral immunity.

Autologous transplants are associated with less infectious complications than allogeneic transplants due to reduced severity of GVHD and earlier reconstitution of T-cell immunity. Allogeneic transplantation using alternative donors (such as HLA-matched unrelated donors, partially mismatched related donors, and mismatched cord blood) has a higher risk of GVHD and usually requires depletion of mature donor T cells, leading to delayed immune reconstitution and, consequently, a greater risk of infectious complications.

ALTERATIONS IN MICROFLORA COLONIZATION

A shift in the normal respiratory flora toward colonization with aerobic gram-negative bacilli occurs in sick hospitalized patients.[56] This may be due to changes in the fibronectin content of cell surfaces in debilitated persons, leading to reduced adherence by the normal anaerobic flora, thus favoring colonization by aerobic gram-negative bacilli.[57] In immunocompromised patients with cancer, alterations in bowel flora leading to acquisition of more virulent bacteria are well documented. This change is exacerbated by the use of broad-spectrum antibiotics that may suppress the normal anaerobic bowel flora. Patients with acute leukemia are frequent stool carriers of *P aeruginosa*, and nosocomial infections are often preceded by enteric colonization by the infecting strain.

In a classic study, Schimpff et al.[58] collected surveillance cultures from the nose, gingiva, axilla, and rectum of hospitalized patients with acute nonlymphocytic leukemia. Infection nearly always occurred during neutropenia, and in approximately 85% of cases, the infecting organism had been isolated in surveillance cultures before the onset of disease. In almost one-half of the cases, the pathogen was acquired after hospital admission.

BACTERIAL PATHOGENS IN CANCER PATIENTS

STAPHYLOCOCCUS SPECIES

Since the 1980s, there has been a marked increase in the proportion of bacterial infections and bacteremia caused by *Staphylococcus* species. The frequency of *S aureus* infections has remained stable, whereas the incidence of infections caused by coagulase-negative staphylococci has increased, almost certainly due to widespread use of broad-spectrum antibiotics and surgically implantable central venous catheters. Coagulase-negative staphylococci are considered to be low pathogens of low virulence, and their isolation from blood is frequently dismissed as a skin contaminant. In patients with cancer, coagulase-negative staphylococci may produce a localized catheter-associated infection, bacteremia, or, less frequently, metastatic infection. The majority of nosocomial coagulase-negative staphylococci are resistant to antistaphylococcal penicillins, making vancomycin the initial drug of choice for such infections. However, given the increased prevalence of serious infections due to vancomycin-resistant enterococci (VRE), an antistaphylococcal penicillin should be used for staphylococci sensitive to one of these agents.

S aureus is the most common cause of surgical wound infections and can cause both local and systemic disease. In some instances a toxic shock syndrome occurs, manifesting as fever, hypotension, gastrointestinal toxicity, rash, and skin exfoliation. Prompt initiation of antibiotics, fluid resuscitation, removal of surgical packing, and wound débridement are required. In patients with cancer, disruptions of the skin barrier from indwelling intravenous catheters or biopsy sites are additional portals of entry.

The incidence of methicillin-resistant *S aureus* (MRSA) isolates causing nosocomial blood stream infections in the United States is increasing. In a 3-year surveillance study of more than 10,000 cases of nosocomial bacteremia, almost 30% of *S aureus* isolates were methicillin resistant.[59] Among hematology and oncology patients, the rate was 25%. These observations highlight the need to be familiar with the resistance patterns of bacterial pathogens at one's institution to guide empiric antibiotic therapy before the availability of culture results (see Evaluation and Management of Febrile Neutropenia without an Apparent Source, later in this chapter).

MRSA isolates are typically broadly resistant to all antibiotics, except vancomycin. Clinical *S aureus* isolates have been isolated with intermediate resistance to vancomycin.[60,61] Preventing emergence and spread of these organisms requires careful attention to infection control guidelines and judicious use of antibiotics.

Patients with MRSA infection should be kept in private rooms, under contact precautions. Gown and gloves should be worn by hospital staff in cases of a draining wound or other situations in which spread to hands and clothing is likely to occur. Attempts at eradication of nasal carriage of *S aureus* with topical mupirocin and other agents have produced mixed results, and MRSA may develop resistance to mupirocin.[62]

ENTEROCOCCUS SPECIES

An increased incidence of nosocomial infections caused by multidrug-resistant enterococcal species has been observed. Approximately 50% of *Enterococcus faecium* and the minority of *Enterococcus faecalis* isolates are resistant to vancomycin[59] and are typically multiply resistant to penicillin, ampicillin, and aminoglycosides. Patients with cancer who spend a significant time in the hospital are at high risk for being colonized by drug-resistant *Enterococcus* species. The portal of entry for enterococcal bacteremia may be an indwelling central catheter or defects in the gut mucosa from chemotherapy or radiation toxicity. Tumor invasion of the gut may predispose to bacteremia by *Enterococcus* species, as well as *Streptococcus bovis*.

Ampicillin is the drug of choice for sensitive *Enterococcus* isolates. For serious infections (e.g., bacteremia), addition of an aminoglycoside for synergy is reasonable because even sensitive strains are intrinsically tolerant to the bactericidal activity of penicillins and vancomycin. The newly licensed streptogramin antibiotic, quinupristin/dalfopristin (Synercid), is active against most strains of *E faecium* but not *E faecalis*.[63] Linezolid, a prototype of the oxazolidinone group of antimicrobial agents, has broad activity against gram-positive pathogens, including MRSA and VRE, and is being evaluated in clinical trials.[64]

Chloramphenicol, fluoroquinolones, tetracyclines, and rifampin may also have activity against VRE. Prevention and infection control methods, including prudent use of antibiotics (restriction of vancomycin usage), isolation of colonized and infected patients, surveillance, hand washing, and use of appropriate barrier protections, are critical for reducing rates of VRE infection.

VIRIDANS STREPTOCOCCI

Viridans streptococci, also called *α-hemolytic streptococci*, are oral commensal organisms. In the nonimmunocompromised population, they are the most common cause of native valve endocarditis, which usually has a subacute course. In neutropenic patients, viridans streptococci are more virulent. Cytosine arabinoside (Ara-C), a highly mucotoxic agent, and prophylaxis with ciprofloxacin or trimethoprim-sulfamethoxazole (presumably, by selecting for resistant streptococci) are the major risk factors for bacteremia by viridans streptococci.[65–67]

Neutropenic patients with viridans streptococcal bacteremia may have a 24- to 48-hour prodrome of low-grade fever and facial flushing, followed by a high fever and chills. In approximately 25% of patients, bacteremia is complicated by a shock syndrome, characterized by hypotension, respiratory distress syndrome, renal failure, and a maculopapular rash usually starting at the trunk and spreading centrifugally to the face and extremities.[65] Desquamation of the palms and soles may subsequently occur. Endocarditis is observed in a minority of patients. Septic shock may be more common in children than in adults.[68,69]

In a secondary analysis of 909 bacteremias in patients previously enrolled in trials of neutropenic fever, 13% were caused by viridans streptococci.[70] All 52 patients with viridans streptococcal bacteremia who received initial vancomycin survived, compared with an 86% survival rate in patients whose vancomycin therapy was delayed 2 to 3 days ($P = .004$). Of the empiric monotherapy regimens used for febrile neutropenia, ceftazidime has the poorest activity against viridans streptococci, thus prompting some investigators to add vancomycin empirically in patients with neutropenic fever and significant chemotherapy-induced mucositis (see Evaluation and Management of Febrile Neutropenia without an Apparent Source, later in this chapter).[71]

MISCELLANEOUS GRAM-POSITIVE BACTERIA

In the 1990s, there has been an emerging spectrum of gram-positive bacterial infections in patients with cancer. The widespread use of surgically implanted central venous catheters and fluoroquinolone prophylaxis may be contributing to the more frequent isolation of these bacteria. They include *Corynebacterium jeikeium, Bacillus cereus, Stomatococcus mucilaginosus,* and *Leuconostoc* species.[1] These bacteria are associated with localized catheter and wound infections, bacteremia, and disseminated infection.

C jeikeium is a common cutaneous commensal organism that has been associated with infection of prosthetic devices, such as vascular catheters, peritoneal dialysis catheters, prosthetic valves, and ventricular shunts. *C jeikeium* is highly resistant to antibiotics, except vancomycin.

In a review of *C jeikeium* infections in patients with hematologic malignancies, skin lesions were present in one-half of the cases, pulmonary lesions occurred in approximately one-third of cases, and one-third of the patients died.[72] In neutropenic patients, survival was strongly associated with resolution of neutropenia. Virtually all of these patients had an indwelling central venous catheter, which was likely to be the principal portal of entry. In a series of BMT recipients with *C jeikeium* bacteremia, all eight patients who received appropriate antibiotic therapy and who had their central intravenous catheters removed survived regardless of persistent neutropenia.[73] Mortality was greater than 50% in those patients who received no antibiotics and in those who received antibiotics without removal of the central venous catheter. Current treatment consists of prompt initiation of vancomycin and consideration of removal of the infected intravenous catheters.

In neutropenic children, *Bacillus cereus* was associated with a primary cutaneous infection involving vesicular and pustular lesions.[74] *Stomatococcus mucilaginosus* appears to be particularly virulent in neutropenic patients and has been associated with septic shock, respiratory distress syndrome, and meningitis.[75] *Leuconostoc, Lactobacillus,* and *Pediococcus* species are often resistant to vancomycin,[76] but most isolates are susceptible to penicillin.

ENTEROBACTERIACEAE

The Enterobacteriaceae include several pathogenic species, including *Escherichia coli, Klebsiella, Proteus, Enterobacter, Serratia,* and *Citrobacter* species. Patients with neutropenia are at highest risk for bacteremia and life-threatening infections by these pathogens. The principal portal of entry appears to be translocation of bacteria from the alimentary tract.

There has been an increasing frequency of infection due to Enterobacteriaceae and other gram-negative bacteria (such as *Stenotrophomonas maltophilia* and *Acinetobacter* species), which are highly resistant to β-lactam antibiotics. Bush et al.[77] presented an updated classification of β-lactamases, which include three groups of enzymes: (1) group 1 cephalosporinases (also referred to as *Bush group 1 β-lactamases*) are not well inhibited by clavulanic acid; (2) group 2 penicillinases, cephalosporinases, and extended spectrum β-lactamases are generally inhibited by β-lactamase inhibitors; and (3) group 3 metallo-β-lactamases that hydrolyze penicillins, cephalosporins, and carbapenems and confer broad resistance to almost all β-lactam antibiotics. Table 54-3 summarizes commonly used antibacterial agents in patients with cancer.

Extended spectrum β-lactamase–producing pathogens (most common in *E coli* and *Klebsiella* species) may not be detected with standard susceptibility testing because of different susceptibility patterns among third-generation cephalosporins. In one study of a nosocomial outbreak of extended spectrum β-lactamases producing *Klebsiella* strain (as indicated by ceftazidime resistance), use of other third-generation cephalosporins was associated with a poorer outcome.[78] Carbapenems (imipenem and meropenem) have consistent bactericidal activity against extended spectrum β-lactamase–producing strains and should be considered drugs of choice in serious infections by these pathogens.

The Bush group 1 β-lactamases may not be initially expressed (repressed), but are induced (de-repressed) after exposure to broad-spectrum cephalosporins, and confer resistance to virtually all β-lactam antibiotics with the exception of the carbapenems and cefepime. This group of β-lactamases is characteristic of *Enterobacter* species, but is also observed in *P aeruginosa, Citrobacter, Serratia,* and indole-positive *Proteus* species. Thus, if an

TABLE 54-3. Commonly Used Antibacterial Agents in Patients with Cancer

Antibiotic	*Spectrum*	*Usual Daily Dose[a]*	*Comments*
Ceftazidime	Enterobacteriaceae, *Pseudomonas aeruginosa,* less reliable activity against gram-positive bacteria, poor anaerobic activity	2 g q8h	Inactivated by extended spectrum β-lactamases and Bush group 1 β-lactamases
Cefepime	Enterobacteriaceae, *P aeruginosa,* most gram-positive bacteria, poor anaerobic activity	2 g q8–12h	Active against extended spectrum β-lactamases and Bush group 1 producing gram-negative bacteria; active against most gram-positive bacteria, except *Enterococcus* sp.
Extended-spectrum penicillins (e.g., ticarcillin, piperacillin, azlocillin)	Enterobacteriaceae, *P aeruginosa,* most gram-positive bacteria, anaerobes	3–4 g q4–6h	Should be paired with an aminoglycoside or ciprofloxacin for treatment of neutropenic fever; combination with β-lactamase inhibitors (e.g., piperacillin/tazobactam, ticarcillin/clavulanate); confers broader activity against Enterobacteriaceae and enteric anaerobes
Carbapenems (imipenem, Meropenem)	Enterobacteriaceae, *P aeruginosa,* most gram-positive bacteria, anaerobes	Imipenem, 500 mg q6h; Meropenem, 1 g q8h	Broadest spectrum of activity; some *P aeruginosa* isolates are resistant (see text); inactive against *Stenotrophomonas maltophilia*
Aztreonam	Enterobacteriaceae, *P aeruginosa*	2 g q6–8h	Requires pairing with vancomycin for neutropenic fever in patients with β-lactam allergies; often inactive against extended spectrum β-lactamases and cephalosporinase-producing gram-negative bacteria
Vancomycin	Exclusively gram-positive bacteria	1 g q12h	Growing frequency of resistance among *Enterococcus* sp.; *Leuconostoc* sp., *Pediococcus* sp. are intrinsically resistant
Quinolones	Enterobacteriaceae, *P aeruginosa,* newer generation agents have increased activity against gram-positive bacteria		Prophylaxis against aerobic gram-negative rods in neutropenic patients; resistant *P aeruginosa* and Enterobacteriaceae infections reported (see text)
Trimethoprim-sulfamethoxazole	Enterobacteriaceae (growing resistance); active against *Stenotrophomonas maltophilia, Burkholderia cepacia, Listeria monocytogenes, Pneumocystis carinii, Nocardia* sp.; no activity against *P aeruginosa*		Effective prophylaxis against *P carinii;* potential hypersensitivity and bone marrow toxicity
Aminoglycosides	Enterobacteriaceae, *P aeruginosa,* synergistic activity against sensitive *Enterococcus* sp.		Should be paired with an antipseudomonal β-lactam agent if used for neutropenic fever or gram-negative bacteremia
Metronidazole	Exclusive anaerobic activity	500–750 mg q6–8h	First choice agent for *Clostridium difficile* (oral); add to ceftazidime or cefepime for suspected abdominal or perirectal infection

[a]Doses apply to adults with normal renal function.

Enterobacter species is isolated from a blood culture, it is reasonable to change the initial antibiotic regimen to a carbapenem, knowing the potential for induction of a cephalosporinase if third-generation cephalosporin therapy is continued.

PSEUDOMONAS AERUGINOSA

Infections caused by *P aeruginosa* in patients with cancer have diminished since the 1960s and 1970s. Currently, approximately 5% to 10% of bacteremias are caused by this organism in patients with neutropenia. This reduction may reflect the widespread use of fluoroquinolones as prophylaxis as well as the availability of agents with potent antipseudomonal activity, such as ceftazidime, that are used as initial empiric therapy for febrile neutropenia.

Bodey et al.[79] retrospectively analyzed 410 cases of *P aeruginosa* bacteremia in patients with cancer. The overall rate was 4.7 cases per 1000 admissions and was most common among patients with leukemia. Neutropenia was the dominant risk factor. The infections were highly virulent, with 33% of patients developing septic shock and 32% having pneumonia. Other sites of infection included soft tissue, urinary tract, perirectal region, and central venous catheters. Patients who received an antipseudomonal β-lactam antibiotic, with or without an aminoglycoside, had survival

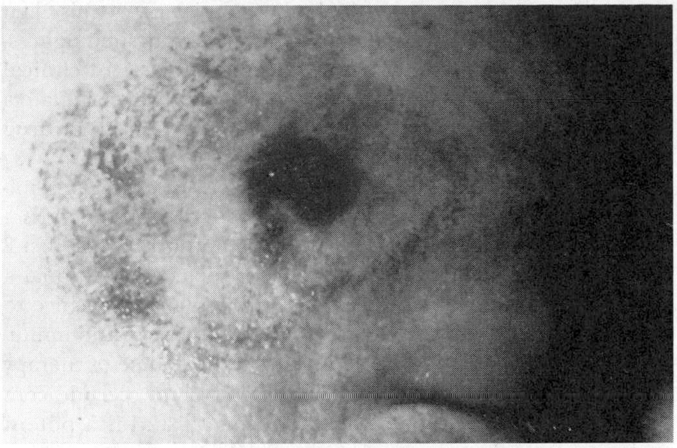

FIGURE 54-1. Lesions of ecthyma gangrenosum in a neutropenic patient with bacteremia due to *Pseudomonas aeruginosa.* The ecthyma lesions are in the necrotic ulcerative edge.

rates of 72% and 71%, respectively, compared with 29% survival in patients who received only an aminoglycoside.

The site of disease often reflects where colonization has occurred.[58] Colonization of the upper airway may lead to pneumonia after aspiration of infected droplets. Typhlitis (neutropenic enterocolitis) and perineal cellulitis may follow colonization of the gut by *P aeruginosa.* Pathologically, *P aeruginosa* invades small arteries and veins, leading to thrombosis, hemorrhage, and infarction. This angioinvasion is most evident in cases of ecthyma gangrenosum in which *P aeruginosa* invades cutaneous blood vessels and perivascular connective tissue, leading to coagulative necrosis of the dermis (Fig. 54-1). The lesions of ecthyma gangrenosum usually evolve from erythematous macules to papules, and ultimately necrotic nodules and bullae. The lesions may present in any stage with minimal or absent inflammatory infiltrate.

Initial optimal antibiotic therapy for *P aeruginosa* bacteremia consists of an antipseudomonal β-lactam antibiotic and an aminoglycoside. It is reasonable to continue aminoglycoside therapy until clinical stability and sterilization of blood have been achieved. Emergence of resistance to cephalosporins and carbapenems during monotherapy for *P aeruginosa* infections may occur. Carbapenem resistance results from an alteration of a porin protein on the outer membrane of the bacteria, preventing penetration of the antibiotic and β-lactamase production.[80] Emergence of resistance to carbapenems during therapy for *P aeruginosa* is well documented and may result in treatment failure. Quinolone-resistant *P aeruginosa* isolates are being observed with increasing frequency. See sections on Neutropenic Fever and Manifestations and Therapy of Infections, later in this chapter.

STENOTROPHOMONAS (XANTHOMONAS) MALTOPHILIA

Stenotrophomonas maltophilia colonizes hospital environments and establishes carriage generally in patients who have been treated with broad-spectrum antimicrobial agents. This organism has become an increasingly important cause of nosocomial infections in patients with cancer.[81] Clinical manifestations include bacteremia, pneumonia, endocarditis, mastoiditis, and meningitis. Vartivarian et al.[82] reviewed 17 cases of mucocutaneous and soft tissue infections caused by *S maltophilia* in patients with cancer. These infections manifested as mucocutaneous ulcerations, primary cellulitis (usually catheter related), and metastatic cellulitis consisting of multiple hard, tender nodules with surrounding or distant cellulitic areas resembling disseminated fungal infection, and one case of ecthyma gangrenosum, resembling *P aeruginosa.* Disseminated cellulitic lesions were most common in patients with refractory leukemia and were frequently associated with septic shock, multiorgan failure, and pneumonia.

Stenotrophomonas maltophilia is resistant to imipenem, and isolates are often broadly resistant to other agents. The organism elaborates a metallo-β-lactamase, which hydrolyzes carbapenems. The majority of strains are susceptible to trimethoprim-sulfamethoxazole, which is the preferred initial antibiotic for this organism, pending susceptibility data.

ACINETOBACTER SPECIES

Acinetobacter calcoaceticus and *Acinetobacter baumannii* are the principal pathogenic species within this genus. These gram-negative coccobacilli are ubiquitous, easily colonize hospital environments, and have been associated with nosocomial outbreaks. *Acinetobacter* species are frequently multidrug resistant, and the risk of infection in one nosocomial outbreak was associated with quinolones.[83] In the largest series of *Acinetobacter* septicemia in patients with cancer (95 cases), 80% of cases were thought to be catheter related and responded to catheter removal and antimicrobial therapy.[84] Infection was polymicrobial in 25% of cases.[84]

CLOSTRIDIUM SPECIES

Clostridium species include highly virulent toxin-producing species as well as relatively avirulent saprophytes. Toxin-producing species can cause invasive disease such as myonecrosis (gas gangrene), emphysematous cholecystitis and pyelonephritis, necrotizing enterocolitis (typhlitis), and septic shock (see Intraabdominal Infections, later in this chapter). *Clostridium perfringens* and *Clostridium septicum* are the most common clostridial species to cause bacteremia in patients with cancer. *Clostridium tertium* sepsis is less commonly observed, but is highly virulent.[85] Cases of infection due to clostridial species other than *C perfringens, C septicum,* and *C tertium* are usually only associated with fever, without evidence of organ involvement, and a low mortality.

Extraintestinal clostridial infections can be devastating. The morbidity and mortality associated with clostridial bacteremia depends on the virulence of the species and the immune status of the host. Clostridial bacteremia after septic abortion is usually self-limited, but clostridial bacteremia with septic shock and myonecrosis requires emergent surgical débridement.

Bodey et al.[86] evaluated 136 episodes of bacteremia due to clostridial species in patients with cancer. Most cases were associated with leukemia, gastrointestinal, and genitourinary malignancies. Eighty-three cases were monomicrobial and 53 were polymicrobial. In 45% of cases of polymicrobial bacteremia, three or more organisms were isolated from the blood. Isolates associated with clostridial sepsis consisted predominantly of enteric flora: *E coli, Klebsiella* species, and *Bacteroides* species. Polymicrobial bacteremias were more likely to result in septic shock and death. The overall survival rate from clostridial bacteremia was 58%, a dramatically poorer prognosis than monomicrobial bacteremias caused by aerobic gram-positive and gram-negative species.

Local and systemic clostridial infections are associated with gastrointestinal and genitourinary neoplasms. They are normally commensals, but proliferate in tissues with a low redox potential, such as necrotic tumors. Damage to the mucosa by chemotherapy or radiation therapy likely further predisposes to local invasion and dissemination. Local bowel invasion by clostridial species can result in necrotizing colitis (typhlitis), which typically involves the cecum but can extend to other regions of the bowel.

Clostridial infections often have a fulminant course. Acute hemolysis, myonecrosis, diffuse spreading cellulitis, and septic shock have a high mortality. Clostridial myonecrosis may respond to rapid surgical débridement. A needle aspiration or biopsy of the infected tissue showing large, thick gram-positive rods is highly suggestive of the diagnosis. However, staining of the organism in clinical material may be variable or appear to be gram negative. In patients with leukemia, clostridial soft tissue infection and septic shock may be particularly rapid, precluding surgical intervention.

Clindamycin and metronidazole are both active against *Clostridia*. Clindamycin, in addition to its antianaerobic activity, may have a theoretical value of reducing toxin production. In a mouse model of myonecrosis by *C perfringens*, clindamycin and metronidazole were each more effective than penicillin.[87] The initial antibiotic regimen should also include an agent active against aerobic enteric flora, such as ceftriaxone, since deep soft tissue infections are often polymicrobial. In neutropenic patients, metronidazole or clindamycin plus an antipseudomonal β-lactam (such as ceftazidime or cefepime), with or without an aminoglycoside, are reasonable regimens.

MYCOBACTERIA

Host defense against *Mycobacterium* species relies principally on functional T lymphocytes. It is therefore surprising that the incidence of *Mycobacterium tuberculosis* (MTB) infection in BMT recipients is relatively low. In two large BMT centers in the United States, MTB infection occurred in approximately 1 per 1000 patients.[88,89] In a Saudi Arabian study, the incidence of tuberculosis was 0.6% among BMT recipients.[90] In contrast, a study in Hong Kong, a highly endemic area for MTB, reported a 5.5% incidence of MTB in BMT recipients.[91] Therefore, an extra level of vigilance for MTB is necessary among patients who have resided in endemic countries.

In patients with compromised T-cell immunity, the clinical manifestations of infection due to MTB may be atypical, and disseminated disease is more common than in immunocompetent patients.[92] The chest radiographic appearance is highly variable and may include an isolated nodule, an infiltrate, or a diffuse reticulonodular pattern indicative of hematogenous dissemination. The chest radiographic result may be negative in patients with disseminated extrapulmonary tuberculosis. Cavitary lung disease is less commonly observed in immunocompromised hosts. Extrapulmonary manifestations may include meningitis, brain abscess, vertebral or paravertebral abscess, septic joint, hepatic and splenic disease, and bone marrow involvement. Patients who consume unpasteurized dairy products are at increased risk of gastrointestinal tuberculosis caused by *Mycobacterium bovis*. In addition, systemic iatrogenic *M bovis* infection may rarely occur after intravesicular therapy with bacille Calmette-Guérin for bladder cancer.[93]

Because of the varied manifestations of MTB, a high index of suspicion may be required to make the diagnosis. For example, a new pulmonary nodule or infiltrate may be mistaken for aspergillosis, and gastrointestinal tuberculosis may be mistaken for GVHD. A definitive diagnosis should be pursued aggressively and early. Detection of mycobacterial DNA in clinical specimens by polymerase chain reaction (PCR) may facilitate a more rapid diagnosis, although cultures are required for drug susceptibility testing.

Due to the increased frequency of drug-resistant isolates, initial therapy for tuberculosis consists of a four-drug regimen (isoniazid, rifampin, pyrazinamide, and ethambutol) for the first 2 months. If a positive clinical response is seen, an additional 4 months of isoniazid and rifampin (if the isolate is sensitive to these agents) is administered. In patients with profound immunosuppression, it is reasonable to extend the course of therapy to 9 months, given the potential increased risk for recrudescent infection. Rifampin is both metabolized by, and is a potent inducer of, the hepatic cytochrome P-4503A isozyme, creating the potential for adverse drug–drug interactions with other drugs (such as CSA and antifungal azoles) used in this patient group that are also metabolized through this pathway. Consultation with MTB specialists is advised for suspected or confirmed multidrug-resistant tuberculosis.

Prevention of infection relies on compliance with established infection control measures, including respiratory isolation of persons with presumed or known active tuberculosis in negative pressure rooms. Given the low prevalence of tuberculosis in cancer centers in the United States, we suggest that skin testing be reserved for patients with some additional risk factor for tuberculosis (such as residence in an endemic country or human immunodeficiency virus infection).

Infection with nontuberculous mycobacteria (atypical mycobacteria) is well described among patients with cancer. Pathogenic species include *Mycobacterium avium* complex, *Mycobacterium kansasii*, *Mycobacterium haemophilum*, and the *Mycobacterium fortuitum-chelonae* complex. Clinical manifestations include pneumonia, soft tissue or wound infections, and central catheter infections that may require surgical excision of the infected tunnel site[94] (see Implanted Vascular Catheters, later in this chapter). Patients with hairy cell leukemia appear to be particularly susceptible to *M kansasii* infection.[95] Sites of involvement include the lungs, lymph nodes, liver, and spleen, and disseminated disease. *M haemophilum* may cause fatal pneumonia and disseminated cutaneous lesions.[96] This organism has a unique requirement for iron supplementation for growth, and therefore the microbiology laboratory should be alerted that this diagnosis is being considered. Speciation of mycobacterial isolates is essential because atypical mycobacteria are typically resistant to regimens for MTB. DNA probes are used to rapidly identify isolates at the species level.

NOCARDIA

Nocardia infections are most frequent in patients with impaired T-cell immunity. Patients with Hodgkin's and non-Hodgkin's lymphoma receiving immunosuppressive therapy appear to be at particularly high risk for nocardiosis.[97–99] Nocardiosis is relatively uncommon in BMT recipients, with an incidence of 0.3% to 0.7%.[100,101] In the largest series, nocardiosis occurred exclusively in allogeneic transplant recipients and developed in both the early and late transplant period (median time, 210 days).[100]

The lungs are the most common site of infection for bronchopneumonia, lobar pneumonia, nodules, and necrotizing abscesses with cavitation observed. Empyema and extension to the chest wall occur. The lesion may be mistaken for a tumor. Extrapulmonary nocardiosis may occur in the presence or absence of pulmonary disease. Brain abscess, meningitis, osteomyelitis, soft tissue mass, cutaneous abscess, catheter exit site infection, liver abscess, bacteremia, and disseminated disease are seen.

Nocardia species are slender, filamentous, beaded, branching gram-positive rods. When nocardiosis is considered, a modified acid fast smear should be ordered because *Nocardia* species stain variably when the conventional acid fast smear is used. Visualization of *Nocardia* species in histologic specimens may also be variable due to weak uptake of stains. A combination of Gram's staining and staining using the Ziehl-Neelsen (acid alcohol decolorizing agent) and Fite (sulfuric acid used instead of alcohol) methods may increase the diagnostic yield.[100] Although *Nocardia* species grow on a variety of media, it is important to alert the microbiology laboratory so that appropriate culture conditions are used.

Therapy consists of high-dose trimethoprim-sulfamethoxazole (15 to 20 mg of trimethoprin/kg daily in three to four divided doses). Combination therapy consisting of a sulfonamide plus an agent with presumed synergy, such as amikacin, imipenem, minocycline, or ceftriaxone, also is frequently used.[100] Surgical drainage or resection should be considered in cases refractory to medical therapy. However, the time course of resolution is slow, and the therapy must be continued for months.

FUNGAL INFECTIONS

CANDIDIASIS

Oropharyngeal and Esophageal Candidiasis

Oral mucosal candidiasis, also called *thrush*, indicates T-cell immunodeficiency. In patients with cancer, conditions that predispose to oral candidiasis include cytotoxic chemotherapy causing mucosal disruption, high-dose corticosteroids, and use of broad-spectrum antibiotics.

The diagnosis of oral candidiasis is usually made visually. White adherent plaques develop on the palate, buccal mucosa, tongue, or gingiva. The differential diagnosis includes chemotherapy-induced mucositis, bacterial infections, and HSV infection. A wet mount or Gram's stain showing pseudohyphae establishes the diagnosis. A culture of the oral mucosa that grows *Candida* species is not by itself diagnostic as these species commonly colonize the mouth. Therapy for oropharyngeal candidiasis includes local treatments such as nystatin or clotrimazole troches or oral fluconazole.

Esophageal candidiasis is a more severe mucosal disease that typically manifests with odynophagia. The differential diagnosis includes esophageal infection by HSV, CMV (in BMT recipients), and bacterial infections (see Esophagitis, later in this chapter). Systemic antifungal therapy (fluconazole or amphotericin B) is required.

Candidemia

Candida species are the fourth most common nosocomial blood culture isolates in the United States.[102] In some series, the attributable mortality to candidemia was 40% to 60%.[103] This high mortality may reflect the fact that these patients often have serious comorbidities, such as malignancy, neutropenia, and illness requiring prolonged periods in the intensive care unit. In a European surveillance study of candidemia in cancer patients, the overall 30-day mortality was 39%, with increased mortality occurring in older patients, in those with poorly controlled malignancy, and in cases in which *Candida* (*Torulopsis*) *glabrata* was isolated.[104] In a retrospective study of 476 cases of candidemia at M. D. Anderson Cancer Center, the mortality was 52%. Neutropenia, a high APACHE (Acute Physiology and Chronic Health Education) score, and disseminated disease were associated with poorer outcomes.[105]

Candida albicans is the most common species isolated from the blood. The proportion of non-*albicans Candida* species varies among different centers. Among patients with cancer, non-*albicans Candida* species account for approximately 45% of cases of systemic candidiasis.[106] Among non-*albicans Candida* species, *Candida tropicalis* was the most common isolate followed by *C glabrata, C parapsilosis,* and *C krusei.*[106] The proportion of non-*albicans Candida* isolates has direct clinical significance. *C krusei* is always resistant to fluconazole, and *C glabrata* is variably resistant. When either of these two species are isolated from the blood, amphotericin B therapy is necessary. *C tropicalis* is more virulent than *C albicans* in immunocompromised animal models[107] and often has a more severe clinical course in patients.[108] Cutaneous dissemination, arthralgias, myalgias, and renal failure appear to be more common in *C tropicalis* infection.[108] *C parapsilosis* is mostly associated with vascular catheters and lipid formulations used for total parenteral nutrition. Some *C guilliermondi* and *C lusitaniae* isolates are resistant to amphotericin B.

Antifungal susceptibility testing is becoming more common and gaining acceptance. Standard guidelines and interpretive breakpoints for susceptibility testing of fluconazole, itraconazole, and 5-flucytosine against yeasts have been proposed by the National Committee for Clinical Laboratory Standards. These may be useful in select cases in which resistance is suspected and in epidemiologic studies.

Isolation of *Candida* species from blood remains unreliable even with modern blood culture isolation systems.[18] The sensitivity for detecting candidemia has been significantly improved by the lysis centrifugation system (Isolator, Wampole Laboratories, Cranbury, NJ) and the BacTAlert system (Organon Teknika, Durham, NC), which detect candidemia earlier and more reliably than conventional broth systems.[18] However, in single organ infection and in early disseminated candidiasis, even lysis centrifugation culture has limited sensitivity.[109] Nonculture methods, such as amplification by PCR, antigen detection, and detection of metabolites, are investigational and may prove useful in complementing culture methods.[110]

All candidemic patients, both neutropenic and nonneutropenic, should be treated with fluconazole or amphotericin B. Isolation of a *Candida* species from only a single blood culture (whether drawn from a catheter or peripheral vein), should be considered indicative of hematogenously disseminated disease. The rationale for early antifungal therapy is to avoid sequelae, such as endophthalmitis and hepatosplenic candidiasis. In a retrospective study of 155 cases of catheter-associated fungemia in patients with cancer, a significant proportion of patients who did not receive antifungal therapy after isolation of a *Candida* species from the blood (possibly because the isolate was considered to be a contaminant or candidemia was considered to be transient) subsequently developed disseminated candidiasis.[111]

TABLE 54-4. Antifungal Agents Commonly Used in Patients with Cancer

Agent	*Dose*	*Indications*
Amphotericin B (conventional)	0.5–0.6 mg/kg/d	Empirical antifungal therapy for neutropenic fever; candidemia; esophageal candidiasis
	0.7–1.0 mg/kg/d	Acute disseminated candidiasis; infections due to *Candida tropicalis, Candida parapsilosis, Cryptococcus neoformans,* dimorphic fungi (e.g., *Histoplasma capsulatum, Coccidioides immitis*)
	1.0–1.5 mg/kg/d	*Aspergillus* sp., other invasive filamentous fungi
Lipid formulations of amphotericin B		All three lipid formulations licensed for presumed or proven invasive fungal infections refractory to conventional amphotericin B or in patients intolerant of amphotericin B
Amphotericin B colloidal dispersion	5 mg/kg/d	
Amphotericin B lipid complex	5 mg/kg/d	
Liposomal amphotericin B	3–5 mg/kg/d	Empirical therapy for neutropenic fever (3 mg/kg/d)
5-flucytosine[a]	25 mg/kg q6h	May be used in combination with amphotericin B for disseminated candidiasis and cryptococcosis
Itraconazole[b]	400–800 mg/d	Stable patients with non–life-threatening fungal infection; maintenance therapy after control of infection achieved; highly active against dematiaceous molds (see text)
Fluconazole	400–800 mg/d	Prophylaxis in bone marrow transplantation; candidemia and invasive candidiasis (in stable patients); maintenance therapy for cryptococcal infections; *Trichosporon species* infection (combine with amphotericin B in neutropenic patients)
Third-generation triazoles		Broad-spectrum activity against yeasts and filamentous fungi; oral and intravenous formulations (currently investigational)
Voriconazole		
Posaconazole (SCH 56592)		
Ravuconazole (BMS 207147)		
Echinocandins		Broad-spectrum activity against yeasts and filamentous fungi; intravenous form available; currently investigational
Caspofungin (MK-0991)		
FK-463		

[a]Monitoring of serum levels required given potential of myelotoxicity (peak target, 40–60 μg/mL). Dose adjustment with reduced renal function.
[b]Monitoring of serum levels recommended [peak greater than 1 μg/mL (high-pressure liquid chromatography) or greater than 4.0 μg/mL (bioassay)].

The site of blood collection, either from a central catheter or peripheral site, had no predictive value in defining the risk of subsequent disseminated disease.[111]

A large randomized study comparing intravenous fluconazole (400 mg daily) with amphotericin B (0.5 mg/kg daily) as therapy for candidemia in nonneutropenic patients found both regimens equally effective.[112] In uncomplicated candidemia, at least 2 weeks of antifungal therapy after the last positive culture result should be administered. Due to the increased frequency of *Candida* isolates with intermediate or complete resistance to fluconazole, a National Institute of Allergy and Infectious Disease Mycosis Study Group trial is underway to compare fluconazole plus amphotericin B versus fluconazole alone in nonneutropenic patients with candidemia.

Management of candidemia in neutropenic patients is more controversial. Amphotericin B has been the standard therapy, but use of fluconazole in this population has increased. In a consensus conference dealing with the management of candidal infections, 17 of 20 investigators chose fluconazole for treatment of uncomplicated candidemia in stable neutropenic patients if no prior azole prophylaxis was administered and no evidence of hematogenous seeding or deep organ involvement existed.[103] A randomized multicenter study[113] and a matched cohort study[114] showed that fluconazole and amphotericin B had comparable efficacy in invasive candidiasis in neutropenic and nonneutropenic patients. In centers in which non-*albicans Candida* species (most notably, *C krusei* and *C glabrata*) are frequently isolated, we believe that it is prudent to use amphotericin B initially. Candiduria in the neutropenic patient should be treated with systemic antifungal therapy because of the risk of systemic infection in this population.

In unstable patients with candidemia such as those with hypotension or hematogenously seeded deep organ infections, amphotericin B (1.0 mg/kg daily) should be initiated. Acute disseminated candidiasis may occur during neutropenia and is characterized by hypotension, skeletal muscle involvement (typically causing severe pain), multiorgan failure, and cutaneous lesions. We suggest adding 5-flucytosine in these settings for synergy (Table 54-4). 5-flucytosine is also likely to be advantageous in central nervous system (CNS) candidiasis because of its excellent cerebrospinal fluid penetration. Inotropic support and hemodynamic monitoring may be necessary.

The requirement for intravenous catheter removal in candidemia has never been evaluated in a randomized study. Early catheter removal may reduce the likelihood of late complications by eliminating a potential nidus of ongoing candidemia. Removal of intravenous catheters in candidemic patients has been shown to reduce the time to sterilization of the blood in nonneutropenic patients.[115] The opposing argument is that in patients who have received cytotoxic chemotherapy, candidemia is likely to arise from defects in the gut mucosa rather than the catheter.[116] Most investigators in the consensus panel would remove nonsurgically implanted catheters, but would attempt to sterilize surgically implanted catheters with antifungal treatment.[103] If the catheter is not immediately removed, we advise rotating antifungal infusions through all ports to increase the likelihood of catheter sterilization. Clinical instability, lack of resolution of fever, and persistent candidemia after 1 to 2 days of antifungal therapy are each indications to replace all catheter devices.

Chronic Disseminated Candidiasis

Chronic disseminated candidiasis typically affects the liver and spleen. During neutropenia, these organs, as well as kidneys, lungs, skin, bone, and other sites, become seeded by *Candida* species in the blood stream (which may be undetected by blood culture).[117] The only symptom may be persistent fever. After resolution of neutropenia, numerous target lesions in the liver and spleen become apparent by radiologic imaging, such as computed tomography (CT), ultrasonography, or magnetic resonance imaging. A liver biopsy is required for a definitive diagnosis, but because the lesions are discrete, the biopsy result may be falsely negative. An open or laparoscopic-guided liver biopsy is recommended if a percutaneous biopsy is nondiagnostic. Various acceptable therapeutic approaches exist. In stable patients, fluconazole (400 to 800 mg daily) may be used.[113,114] Alternatively, amphotericin B (0.7 to 1.0 mg/kg daily) may be initially administered, followed by a prolonged course of fluconazole once fever has resolved and the lesions are improved. Because lipid formulations of amphotericin B preferentially accumulate in the reticuloendothelial system, a pharmacodynamic rationale exists for their use in refractory cases. Amphotericin B lipid complex (ABLC) has been used successfully in the treatment of hepatosplenic candidiasis in children.[118]

Hepatosplenic candidiasis per se is not a contraindication for subsequent antineoplastic myeloablative chemotherapy.[119] Patients in whom fever and lesions have resolved with antifungal therapy can undergo further episodes of neutropenia without progression of the fungal infection if antifungal therapy is reinitiated during the neutropenic periods.[119]

ASPERGILLOSIS

Prolonged and persistent neutropenia is a critical risk factor for aspergillosis.[16] The more frequent use of allogeneic BMT for malignancy has expanded the risk factors for aspergillosis. Wald et al.[120] conduced a case-control analysis of 158 cases of proven or probable cases of aspergillosis among BMT recipients. The onset of infection was bimodal, with the first peak occurring at a mean of 16 days after transplant (before or shortly after engraftment) and the second peak occurring at a mean of 96 days after transplant. Risk factors for late aspergillosis (after day 40 of transplantation) included age older than 18 years, diagnosis other than chronic myelogenous leukemia in chronic phase, an unrelated donor, acute GVHD (grade 2 to 4), neutropenia, and corticosteroid use. Among autologous BMT recipients, aspergillosis was most likely to occur during neutropenia and was rare after engraftment. In contrast, aspergillosis was more likely to occur after the first 40 days in allogeneic transplant recipients. Other series from Europe[121] and Asia[122] have also

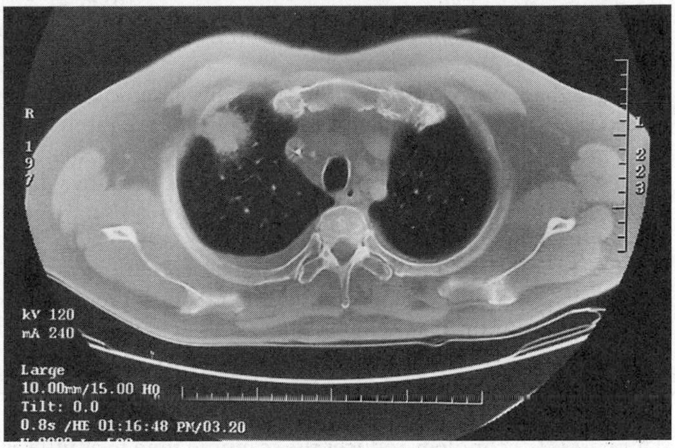

FIGURE 54-2. Computed tomographic scan of the chest in a neutropenic patient with invasive pulmonary infection by *Aspergillus fumigatus.* The lesion in the right upper lobe consist of a hazy infiltrate surrounding a denser nodular lesion. This *halo sign* is most commonly associated with angioinvasive infection by *Aspergillus* species. Other filamentous fungi and *Pseudomonas aeruginosa* may have a similar appearance.

the postengraftment period in BMT recipients, with GVHD being an important risk factor. The reasons for the increased proportion of aspergillosis in the postengraftment period are likely twofold: (1) a reduction in the neutropenic period as a result of myelopoietic growth factors and infusion of larger numbers of myeloid progenitors and (2) increased proportion of unrelated donors and HLA-mismatched transplants, which predispose to GVHD.

Aspergillosis can involve virtually any organ in the immunocompromised host, but sinopulmonary disease is the most common. Alveolar macrophages constitute the first line of host defense against aerosolized conidia. After germination, neutrophils are the dominant host defense arm against the hyphal stage. Invasive aspergillosis in the neutropenic host may present as fever, sinus pain or congestion, cough, pleuritic chest pain, and hemoptysis. Erosion through a large central blood vessel wall can lead to massive pulmonary hemorrhage and exsanguination. The radiographic appearance of pulmonary aspergillosis includes bronchopneumonia, lobar consolidation, segmental pneumonia, nodular lesions resembling septic emboli, and cavitary lesions (Fig. 54-2).

The CNS is a common target site for hematogenously disseminated aspergillosis (see Central Nervous System Infection, later in this chapter). Gastrointestinal aspergillosis usually coexists with pulmonary disease, but in rare instances it is the sole organ involved.[123] In an early study, involvement of the gastrointestinal tract was documented at autopsy in approximately 50% of cases of disseminated aspergillosis.[123] The manifestations include abdominal pain, gastrointestinal infarction with hemorrhage, perforation, and polymicrobial sepsis. Early diagnosis of isolated gastrointestinal aspergillosis followed by resection of the involved bowel and systemic antifungal therapy may be life saving. Other sites of disseminated aspergillosis include the skin, heart, eye, bone, kidney, liver, and thyroid.

Isolation of an *Aspergillus* species from a sputum or bronchoalveolar lavage specimen should be presumed to represent invasive disease in neutropenic patients.[124] In the study by Wald et al.[120] a mucosal isolate of an *Aspergillus* species had a positive predictive value of 60% for invasive disease among BMT recipients; during the neutropenic period, the positive predictive value was 94%.

Early diagnosis of aspergillosis in highly immunocompromised patients remains difficult. Blood cultures are rarely positive, sputum and bronchoalveolar cultures have approximately 50% sensitivity in focal pulmonary lesions, and definitive diagnosis often requires an invasive procedure and is usually only made when the disease is advanced.

CT scanning of the chest may facilitate early detection of aspergillosis. A CT scan may show peripheral or subpleural nodules inapparent on plain chest radiographs. The *halo sign* is a characteristic chest CT feature of angioinvasive organisms.[125] The hazy alveolar infiltrates appear to correspond to regions of ischemia and are highly suggestive of invasive aspergillosis.[125] Ultrafast CT technology reduces the scanning time to as little as 5 minutes, thus permitting wider application to seriously ill patients. Early recognition of pulmonary aspergillosis followed by intensive antifungal therapy and surgical resection of localized disease (see discussion later in this section) has led to improved survival.[126]

PCR-based detection of subclinical aspergillosis is a promising tool for early diagnosis. In a European study, 134 patients underwent at least two bronchoalveolar lavages at the time of BMT, and PCR for *Aspergillus* species was performed.[127] Of seven patients whose bronchoalveolar lavage was PCR positive and culture and cytology were negative, five developed invasive pulmonary aspergillosis within the first 100 days of transplant. A larger study to prospectively evaluate the predictive value of PCR screening of whole blood for *Aspergillus* species DNA among allogeneic BMT recipients is underway. A sensitive double-sandwich enzyme-linked immunosorbent assay for detection of the fungal cell wall constituent galactomannan has been developed.[128] Clinical trials are now essential to delineate which of these diagnostic methods, or which combination, provides the optimal positive and negative predictive value for invasive disease among high-risk patients, and how this information should be translated into a rational therapeutic algorithm.

Aspergillus fumigatus followed by *Aspergillus flavus* are the most common species causing invasive disease in neutropenic patients and after BMT. Therapy for invasive aspergillosis in neutropenic patients and in BMT recipients involves high-dose conventional amphotericin B (1.0 to 1.5 mg/kg daily) or a lipid formulation of amphotericin B. *Aspergillus terreus* is an emerging pathogen in this population that is notable for being resistant to amphotericin B.[129] In cases of invasive *A terreus* infection, the third-generation triazole, voriconazole, may be of value based on *in vitro* sensitivity data.[129]

Surgical excision of locally invasive disease, such as sinusitis, primary cutaneous lesions, intravitreal disease, or bone lesions should be performed. Removal of infected intravenous and peritoneal dialysis catheters and silk sutures in bronchial stumps are also necessary components of therapy. In neutropenic patients and in allogeneic BMT recipients, combined surgery and systemic antifungal therapy should be used in cases of apparent localized disease because of the risk of subclinical dissemination.

The indications for and timing of thoracic surgery for aspergillosis are controversial. In postpneumonectomy patients, infection of the bronchial stump should be débrided and sutures removed. Invasive pleural and pericardial aspergillosis should be treated with decortication and stripping. When possible, pulmonary aspergillosis adjacent to major vessels should be surgically removed to avoid exsanguinating hemoptysis. In a retrospective series of patients with acute leukemia and pulmonary filamentous mycosis (mostly caused by *Aspergillus* species), hemoptysis most commonly occurred shortly after resolution of neutropenia.[130]

Patients who recover from an episode of invasive aspergillosis are at risk for relapse during a subsequent course of myeloablative chemotherapy. In the largest series, a retrospective analysis was performed on 48 patients with definite or probable aspergillosis who subsequently were treated with BMT (77% allogeneic).[131] All patients received systemic antifungal therapy, and approximately 40% underwent surgical resection as initial therapy. Forty-one of 48 (85%) patients received secondary prophylaxis at the time of BMT; the regimens included itraconazole, amphotericin B (conventional and lipid formulations), and combinations of agents with wide variability in dosage and duration. The overall incidence of relapse was 29% among patients receiving secondary prophylaxis and 57% among those who did not. Fourteen of 16 (88%) patients who had relapses died. Other smaller series have also shown that systemic antifungal therapy (with and without surgical resection) of primary fungal infection followed by secondary prophylaxis can suppress reactivation in the majority of patients subsequently undergoing additional myeloablative chemotherapy or BMT.[132,133]

We advise using high-dose amphotericin B (1.0 to 1.5 mg/kg daily) or a lipid formulation of amphotericin B for secondary prophylaxis of invasive aspergillosis during neutropenia after intensive chemotherapy for leukemia or preparative regimens for BMT. Oral itraconazole is more suitable as a maintenance regimen after resolution of neutropenia and mucositis. Antifungal prophylaxis should be reinitiated preemptively during GVHD. Surgical resection does not obviate the need for secondary antifungal prophylaxis during subsequent chemotherapy given the likelihood of residual foci of disease not apparent on diagnostic imaging.

An additional component in treating aspergillosis is reversal or amelioration of immunosuppression. In patients with neutropenia and disseminated aspergillosis, resolution of neutropenia is critical for survival. Granulocyte colony-stimulating factor (G-CSF) and granulocyte-macrophage colony-stimulating factor (GM-CSF) may accelerate myelopoiesis and reduce the neutropenic period as well as augment neutrophil activity. Use of these agents for treatment of serious fungal infections is limited so far to case reports. Corticosteroid therapy should be reduced or discontinued if at all feasible. Granulocyte transfusions may stabilize progressive invasive aspergillosis refractory to antifungal chemotherapy and allow more time until recovery from neutropenia (see Granulocyte Transfusions, later in this chapter).

ZYGOMYCOSIS

Risk factors for zygomycosis (also termed *mucormycosis*) include diabetic ketoacidosis, protein-calorie malnutrition, iron overload, and prolonged neutropenia.[134] Patients receiving potent myeloablative chemotherapy for leukemia are at risk for locally invasive as well as disseminated disease.

Zygomycosis typically manifests as rhinocerebral or pulmonary disease after inhalation of spores. In rhinocerebral disease, fever, facial pain, and headache are common findings. Contiguous extension may lead to orbital involvement with proptosis and extraocular muscle paresis, involvement of hard palate, and spread to the brain. An eschar over the palate is suggestive of zygomycosis, but other filamentous fungi can produce similar findings in highly immunocompromised persons. Occasionally, isolated primary cutaneous disease may follow minor trauma. Injection drug users may inject contaminating spores directly into the blood stream and may present with isolated space-occupying lesions of the brain or other organs. Therapy for zygomycosis involves high-dose amphotericin B (conventional or lipid formulations) plus early and aggressive surgical débridement. Itraconazole is not active against *Zygomycetes* species.

CRYPTOCOCCUS NEOFORMANS

Among patients with cancer, lymphoreticular malignancy and corticosteroid therapy appear to be major risk factors.[135] Host defense against cryptococcal infection is dependent on T-cell immunity. Isolated neutropenia is rarely associated with cryptococcal infection. Immunoglobulins directed against capsular epitopes and complement facilitate phagocytosis of the organism and likely play a role in host defense.[136,137] The principal portal of entry of this organism is via inhalation. Spread to the blood and then to the CNS is a prerequisite for subsequent development of cryptococcal meningitis.

Although meningitis is the most common presentation of cryptococcal infection, other manifestations include primary pneumonia, fungemia, and cutaneous and visceral dissemination. In the pre–acquired immunodeficiency syndrome (AIDS) era, patients who died early during therapy were more likely to have rapidly progressive infection, cerebrospinal fluid with high opening pressure, a low glucose level, less than 20 leukocytes/μL, a positive india ink preparation, culture of cryptococci from extraneural sites, and high titers of cryptococcal antigen in serum and cerebrospinal fluid.[135] A more recent study of non-AIDS–associated cryptococcal disease showed that mortality was highest among persons with malignancy.[138] Additional CNS complications include development of a mass lesion, obstructive hydrocephalus requiring shunting,[139] and vision loss. Vision loss may be a consequence of endophthalmitis, a space-occupying lesion in the visual pathway, direct invasion of the optic nerve (which may cause vision loss over several hours), and as a consequence of elevated intracranial pressure.[140]

Optimal therapy for non-AIDS–associated cryptococcal disease is not well defined. In a classic study, Bennett et al.[141] showed that the combination of amphotericin B plus 5-flucytosine for 6 weeks was superior to amphotericin B alone administered for 10 weeks in non-AIDS–associated cryptococcal meningitis. In AIDS-associated cryptococcal meningitis, the optimal regimen currently is amphotericin B (0.7 mg/kg daily) plus 5-flucytosine (100 mg/kg daily) for the first 2 weeks, followed by life-long maintenance fluconazole therapy (400 mg daily).[142,143] This is an appropriate regimen to use in non-AIDS–associated cryptococcal infection in the absence of modern randomized trials. In neutropenic patients, reduction of the dosage of 5-flucytosine may be considered to avoid delay in myeloid recovery. Because fluconazole is well tolerated, continuing therapy with this agent for several months (or longer if intensive immunosuppressive therapy is continued) is reasonable. In a retrospective series, fluconazole was as efficacious as amphotericin B as initial therapy for non-AIDS–associated cryptococcal disease.[138] Further studies are required to evaluate initial therapy with fluconazole in different populations with cryptococcal disease.

EMERGING OPPORTUNISTIC FUNGAL PATHOGENS

Trichosporon Species

Trichosporon species typically infect profoundly neutropenic patients and those receiving corticosteroid therapy. Acute disseminated trichosporonosis typically manifests with refractory fungemia, funguria, cutaneous lesions, renal failure, pulmonary lesions, and chorioretinitis.[144,145] Disseminated trichosporonosis may yield a false-positive cryptococcal latex antigen test result because of cross-reactivity with the polysaccharide capsule of *C neoformans*.[146] This cross-reactivity may be clinically important because patients treated with high-dose corticosteroid therapy are at risk for both infections, and *C neoformans* typically responds to amphotericin B therapy, whereas *Trichosporon* species are usually resistant.

In vitro and experimental infections indicate that most *Trichosporon* species are inhibited, but not killed, by achievable serum levels of conventional amphotericin B.[147] Fluconazole has superior activity in experimental infections and is recommended as the preferred antifungal agent.[148,149] Combination therapy with high-dose amphotericin B (1.0 to 1.5 mg/kg daily) and fluconazole (800 mg daily or 12 mg/kg daily in children) may have synergy against some strains based on murine models of trichosporonosis.[148]

Blastoschizomyces capitatus (formerly *Trichosporon capitatus*) usually presents as a chronic disseminated infection, resembling chronic candidiasis.[150] A CT scan may show lesions suggestive of hepatosplenic candidiasis, and definitive diagnosis requires either a positive blood culture result or biopsy. CNS involvement is also observed. *B capitatus* does not cross-react with the cryptococcal latex agglutination test.

Malassezia Species

Malassezia furfur is often associated with lipid parenteral nutrition administered through a central venous catheter in immunocompromised patients or premature infants.[151] Clinical manifestations, including persistent fungemia, pulmonary infiltrates, and thrombocytopenia, occur in premature infants but not in adults. Blood culture recovery is enhanced by addition of olive oil or other long-chain fatty acids to the culture plates.

M furfur is often refractory to amphotericin B therapy. Fluconazole therapy is probably the drug of choice, but discontinuation of lipid infusions and removal of the central catheter are important for successful resolution of fungemia. In neutropenic patients and patients treated with corticosteroids, a folliculitis resembling disseminated candidiasis may occur. This infection is a localized process and does not imply disseminated infection. *Malassezia pachydermatis* is a less common cause of infection than *M furfur* and has similar clinical manifestations.

Dematiaceous (Dark-Walled) Molds

Dark-walled molds contain melanin in their cell walls that imparts a brown or olive-green pigment in culture. In immunocompromised patients, soft tissue infection, sinusitis, CNS infection, pneumonia, fungemia, and disseminated disease are observed. Subcutaneous infection is most frequently caused by *Alternaria* species.[152] *Bipolaris, Cladophialophora* (*Xylohypha* or *Cladosporium*) *bantiana, Wangiella,* and *Dactylaria* species have strong predispositions to cause CNS disease.[153]

Definitive diagnosis of phaeohyphomycosis requires documentation of fungal invasion and recovery of the mold from culture of tissue specimens. Positive results of Fontana-Masson staining of tissue specimens, which detects phenolic compounds, including melanin, are suggestive, but not diagnostic, of phaeohyphomycosis.[154] Disseminated infection by *Bipolaris* species may yield a positive blood culture result.

Therapy in immunocompromised patients involves surgical excision of localized disease when feasible and systemic antifungal therapy. Amphotericin B (1.0 to 1.5 mg/kg daily) is standard initial therapy. Sensitivity to amphotericin B is variable, and clinical failures have been reported. Itraconazole has been shown to be effective in cases of phaeohyphomycosis refractory to amphotericin B.[249] Our practice has been to use amphotericin B plus itraconazole as initial therapy for phaeohyphomycosis in severely immunosuppressed patients, followed by prolonged itraconazole maintenance therapy once stabilization has been achieved. Monitoring of serum itraconazole levels is necessary to document oral absorption.

Fusarium Species

Fusarium species are soil saprophytes that have been associated with soft tissue infection, onychomycosis, and keratitis in immunocompetent hosts. With the widespread use of intensive antineoplastic therapy and BMT, more than 150 cases of invasive and disseminated fusariosis have been reported, most within the 1990s.[155] The clinical findings and histologic appearance may be indistinguishable from aspergillosis. In the absence of a definitive culture diagnosis, the likelihood of infection by a *Fusarium* species is substantially increased by the presence of disseminated cutaneous lesions and isolation of a mold from blood culture.

Boutati and Anaissie[155] made important observations about invasive and disseminated fusariosis in a retrospective review of 43 cases occurring in patients with hematologic malignancies at M. D. Anderson Cancer Center. Most cases of disseminated fusariosis were diagnosed during neutropenia, and a high risk of relapse was associated with subsequent myelosuppression. Similar to aspergillosis, a bimodal distribution of fusariosis occurred in BMT recipients (before and after myeloid engraftment). The skin was identified as an important portal of entry. Initial localized manifestations included onychomycosis, paronychia, and cellulitis. Early identification of localized skin disease and surgical débridement may be life saving. Inhalation of spores is another major portal of entry, leading to fungal sinusitis and pneumonia.

Survival from disseminated fusariosis is critically dependent on resolution of neutropenia. Despite the poor response, amphotericin B (1.0 to 1.5 mg/kg daily) or a lipid formulation (greater than or equal to 5 mg/kg/d) is standard therapy. We use G-CSF and granulocyte transfusions in combination with antifungal therapy to try to control the infection until myeloid recovery occurs.

Scedosporium Species

Scedosporium apiospermum (*Pseudallescheria boydii*) and *Scedosporium prolificans* are the principal pathogenic species in the genus *Scedosporium.* In neutropenic patients, *P boydii* is a virulent pathogen, which clinically and histologically resembles aspergillosis. Invasion of blood vessels leading to infarction is common. *P boydii* causes sinopulmonary disease, endophthalmitis, and dissemination to the CNS. The infection can also spread directly from the skin to bone and joint. Establishing a culture diagnosis of *P boydii* is important because of its frequent resistance to amphotericin B. *P boydii* is usually susceptible to azoles, and *in vitro* studies and some clinical experience suggest that the combination of amphotericin B plus an azole (e.g., fluconazole, itraconazole, or miconazole) may provide enhanced activity.[156] Surgical resection of localized lesions is strongly advised. *S prolificans* causes a similar spectrum of disease as *P boydii* and is generally resistant to all antifungal agents.

ENDEMIC DIMORPHIC FUNGI

Endemic dimorphic fungi are so named because of their characteristic geographic distribution. These organisms include *Histoplasma capsulatum, Coccidioides immitis, Blastomyces dermatitidis,* and *Penicillium marneffei* (*P marneffei* is endemic in Southeast Asia). These fungi are dimorphic, existing in nature in the mycelial stage, and convert to yeast stage at body temperature. Because some of these pathogens may be quiescent during the initial infection and only manifest clinically during a subsequent period of severe depression or cell-mediated immunity, a detailed travel history is essential.

Endemic mycoses in the central United States include histoplasmosis and blastomycosis. In the immunocompetent host, inhalation of *Histoplasma* microconidia is typically asymptomatic, but may manifest with acute fever, pulmonary infiltrates, and hypoxia. Immunocompromised patients have a higher risk of disseminated histoplasmosis involving the liver, spleen, lymph nodes, bone marrow, adrenal glands, mucocutaneous tissues, gastrointestinal tract, and CNS. The chest radiograph may show a miliary reticulonodular appearance, suggestive of tuberculosis. An acute sepsis syndrome with hypotension and disseminated intravascular coagulation, adrenal crisis, and meningitis are additional potentially lethal complications.

A rapid diagnosis of histoplasmosis can be made by Giemsa staining of a peripheral blood smear of bone marrow aspirate demonstrating characteristic intracellular yeast forms. Lysis centrifugation is the preferred blood culture system. Antigen detection from blood and urine is a sensitive and specific method in disseminated disease.[157] Antibody detection may also be useful, but false-negative results may occur in immunocompromised patients. Biopsy of specimens may show intracellular or narrow budding yeasts suggestive of the diagnosis, which should be confirmed by culture. In the immunocompromised patient, histoplasmosis should be treated with high-dose amphotericin B (1.0 to 1.5 mg/kg of body weight daily). Prolonged therapy with itraconazole may be initiated after stabilization of disease and should probably be continued for the duration of immunosuppression.

Blastomyces dermatitides may present as an acute pulmonary infection resembling bacterial pneumonia, or as a chronic infection resembling tuberculosis or lung cancer. Extrapulmonary manifestations include involvement of bone, prostate, and CNS. Skin disease resulting from direct inoculation includes large ulcerative and verrucous lesions.

Coccidioides immitis is endemic in the southwestern United States. In normal persons, infection is usually symptomatic or self-limited. In patients with compromised cell-mediated immunity, *C immitis* is likely to be more virulent. In an early review of *C immitis* infection in immunocompromised patients, disseminated disease occurred in almost one-half of the cases and was associated with a high mortality.[158] Progression of infection was often fulminant, and evidence of pulmonary disease frequently occurred after signs of dissemination manifested.[158] Diagnosis is most easily established by serology (in systemic disease) or demonstration of pathognomonic spherules in sputum or tissue samples. Coccidioidomycosis can involve virtually any organ in disseminated disease, but has a particular trophism for bone and the CNS. Therapy for disseminated disease generally requires amphotericin B followed by maintenance fluconazole. Intracisternal amphotericin B should be added in cases of meningitis.

ANTIFUNGAL AGENTS

Azoles

The antifungal activity of azoles principally results from inhibition of the enzyme, lanosterol 14-α-demethylase, which converts lanosterol to ergosterol, a critical component of the fungal cell membrane. These agents also inhibit the cytochrome P-450–dependent enzymes of the fungal respiratory chain. One of the potential toxicities of these compounds is that, to varying degrees, they inhibit mammalian hepatic cytochrome P-450 mixed function oxidases (e.g., 3A4, 3C9, and 3C19), which are involved in the metabolism of numerous drugs. Thus, the potential exists for serious and even life-threatening drug–drug interactions resulting from toxic levels of drugs metabolized by cytochrome P-450 system when they are administered concurrently with the antifungal azoles. The triazoles fluconazole and itraconazole are the most commonly used azoles in patients with cancer (see Table 54-4).

Fluconazole

Fluconazole has activity against yeasts, dermatophytes, and dimorphic fungi, but not against *Aspergillus* species and other filamentous fungi. It has a favorable pharmacokinetic profile. The oral bioavailability of fluconazole exceeds 90%, and absorption is not affected by food or gastric pH. Fluconazole effectively penetrates the CNS, making it a valuable drug for maintenance therapy for cryptococcal and coccidioidal meningitis. The elimination half-life is approximately 30 hours. Drug–drug interactions with fluconazole appear to be less severe than with itraconazole and ketoconazole.

The minimum dose of fluconazole for candidemia or invasive candidiasis is 400 mg daily in adults or 8 to 10 mg/kg/d in children. Dosage reduction is required in patients with renal impairment (creatinine clearance less than 50 mL/min). Clinical experience has been gained using dosages of 800 mg or greater,[159] and several investigators recommend using such a dosage in patients with invasive candidiasis until control of infection is achieved.[103]

One of the major uses of fluconazole in patients with cancer is as a prophylactic agent. In BMT recipients, two double-blind, placebo-controlled trials have shown that prophylactic fluconazole controlled yeast colonization and reduced the rate of mucosal candidiasis and invasive *Candida* infections.[160,161] The use of empiric amphotericin B for prolonged neutropenic fever also was delayed. A reduction in mortality was noted in one of the studies.[161] In an autopsy series of BMT recipients performed at the Fred Hutchinson Cancer Research Center, fluconazole prophylaxis was associated with a reduction in candidal infections, most notably in hepatic candidiasis, but infections by *Aspergillus* species were increased.[162]

Fluconazole prophylaxis has produced mixed results in patients with leukemia receiving chemotherapy. In one randomized study, fluconazole prophylaxis was associated with a reduction in skin and mucosal infection and delay in empiric amphotericin B, but with no significant difference in invasive candidiasis or mortality in comparison with the placebo arm.[163] In another study, fluconazole prophylaxis reduced fungal colonization, invasive infection, and fungal infection-related mortality in patients with leukemia receiving intensive cytotoxic chemotherapy.[164] The major concern with prophylactic fluconazole is the emergence of resistant *Candida* species[165] (see Candidemia, earlier in this chapter).

Itraconazole

Itraconazole has antifungal activity against yeasts, dermatophytes, and dimorphic fungi, and in contrast to fluconazole, is also active against *Aspergillus* species and dark-walled molds. Itraconazole is not active against *Fusarium* species or the agents of zygomycosis.

Itraconazole is available in oral form (capsules and solution) but its oral bioavailability can be erratic. The parenteral solution of itraconazole has been made available in the United States. However, little is known about its use in neutropenic hosts or BMT recipients. Itraconazole is soluble only at an acidic pH, and thus absorption is compromised in patients with achlorhydria and in those patients taking antacids or H_2-receptor antagonists. Absorption is enhanced when itraconazole is taken with food or an acidic beverage. The cyclodextrin preparation of itraconazole is in solution form and has approximately a twofold increased bioavailability compared with that of itraconazole capsules. Because of the inconsistent absorption, plasma itraconazole levels should be monitored. There is no established target plasma itraconazole level that has been clearly associated with clinical response. In a cyclosporin-methylprednisolone animal model, plasma itraconazole levels were shown to correlate with microbiologic clearance of experimental aspergillosis.[166] Based on such studies, we recommend that the plasma itraconazole level should be at least 4 μg/mL by bioassay or 1 μg/mL by high-pressure liquid chromatography in the setting of invasive fungal infection.

Itraconazole is approved as a second-line agent for treatment of aspergillosis in patients intolerant of amphotericin B. In a nonrandomized, compassionate use protocol, itraconazole had comparable efficacy compared with amphotericin B in the treatment of invasive aspergillosis in a variety of patient populations.[167,168] We advise that amphotericin B (conventional or lipid formulation) be the initial agent of choice for invasive mold infections in neutropenic or otherwise severely immunosuppressed patients with cancer. The bioavailability of the oral preparation of itraconazole is unreliable, making it more suitable as a maintenance regimen after control of infection has been achieved. Randomized, prospective studies are required to delineate the optimal role of parenteral itraconazole in neutropenic patients and BMT recipients.

Third-Generation Azoles

In view of the lack of antifungal activity of fluconazole against filamentous fungi, the increasing frequency of fluconazole-resistant *Candida* species, and the inconsistent oral absorption of itraconazole, newer azoles have been developed to overcome some of these limitations. Voriconazole, posaconazole (SCH 56592), and ravuconazole (BMS 207147) are third-generation triazoles that are currently being evaluated in clinical trials.

These agents can be administered orally or intravenously and have activity against *Candida* species (including species that are resistant to fluconazole), *Aspergillus* species, dematiaceous molds, *Fusarium* species, and dimorphic fungi.[169]

AMPHOTERICIN B. Amphotericin B is a member of the polyene group of antifungal agents whose principal mechanism of action is binding to ergosterol, a sterol present in fungal cell membranes. Amphotericin B is active against the majority of fungal pathogens. However, *in vitro* and clinical resistance to amphotericin B has been encountered in a variety of pathogenic fungi afflicting patients with cancer, including isolates of *Candida lusitaniae, Trichosporon beigelii, Pseudallescheria boydii, Fusarium* species, and *Aspergillus terreus.* High dosages (1.0 to 1.5 mg/kg daily) of conventional amphotericin B are required for invasive filamentous fungal infections.

Multiple toxicities are observed with conventional amphotericin B. Acute infusion-related events include fever, rigors, myalgias, nausea, and, less commonly, hypotension, flushing, and bronchospasm. Fever and rigors may result from release of IL-1 and TNF-α from monocytes[170,171] and tend to be most severe during the initial infusions and abate with subsequent administrations. Infusion-related reactions can be lessened with slowing the infusion rate and premedication with acetaminophen, antiemetics, low-dose hydrocortisone (25 to 50 mg in adults), and meperidine (reduces rigors).

The principal long-term adverse effect of amphotericin B is nephrotoxicity. Azotemia occurs in a large proportion of patients receiving amphotericin B, and nephrotoxicity may be compounded by concomitant administration of other nephrotoxic agents such as CSA and aminoglycosides. The azotemia in part results from an increase in tubular glomerular feedback leading to a reduction in glomerular filtration. Administration of normal saline (2 to 4 mEq/kg) before amphotericin can prevent or ameliorate this physiologic azotemia. Long-term administration of amphotericin B is almost invariably associated with renal potassium and magnesium wasting, requiring aggressive electrolyte replacement, often for weeks after the drug has been stopped. Renal tubular acidosis is also observed. Normochromic normocytic anemia likely mediated by suppression of erythropoietin synthesis is another common toxicity.[172]

The toxicity of amphotericin B not only contributes to patient morbidity, but also limits the maximum dosages that can be administered. Lipid formulations of amphotericin B have significantly less nephrotoxicity and, in the case of liposomal amphotericin B, reduced infusion-related toxicity. These lipid formulations (in addition to the newer broad-spectrum azoles and antifungal peptides) are therefore highly promising drugs that are evolving as important alternatives to conventional amphotericin B. Three lipid preparations of amphotericin B have been licensed: liposomal amphotericin B (LAMB or AmBisome), ABLC, and amphotericin B colloidal dispersion (ABCD). These lipid preparations have different biochemical and pharmacokinetic properties, which have been discussed in detail elsewhere.[169,173] All have reduced nephrotoxicity compared with that of conventional amphotericin B.

LIPOSOMAL AMPHOTERICIN B. LAMB is the only true liposomal preparation of amphotericin B, consisting of unilamellar spheric vesicles. Walsh et al.[174] compared LAMB (343 patients) with conventional amphotericin B (344 patients) in neutropenic cancer patients with fever persisting for 5 days or more in a prospective randomized double-blind multicenter study of empiric antifungal therapy. Standard dosages of the two regimens were used (LAMB at 3 mg/kg daily and conventional amphotericin B at 0.6 mg/kg daily), and dose reductions were allowed in cases of renal insufficiency. The liposomal preparation was associated with a reduced incidence of nephrotoxicity, and infusion-related side effects, including fever, chills, hypotension, hypertension, and hypoxia. Fewer proven breakthrough invasive fungal infections (11 proven, six probable) occurred in the LAMB arm in comparison with 30 (27 proven, three probable) in the conventional amphotericin B arm ($P = .009$). A significantly lower incidence of breakthrough candidemia occurred in the LAMB versus the conventional amphotericin B arm 93 versus 12 patients, respectively ($P = .03$). Survival at 7 days after study drug initiation was approximately 90% in both groups. A European study of LAMB versus conventional amphotericin B found reduced nephrotoxicity in the LAMB arm.[174a] In a prospective, randomized trial comparing LAMB (3 or 5 mg/kg daily) with ABLC (5 mg/kg daily) as empiric therapy for persistent febrile neutropenia, patients receiving LAMB had significantly reduced infusion-related toxicity and nephrotoxicity.[175]

AMPHOTERICIN B LIPID COMPLEX. ABLC derives its name from being a complex of two phospholipids arranged in a ribbon-like structure. In the largest series, ABLC (5 mg/kg/d) was evaluated on an emergency use basis in 556 patients with definite or probable invasive mycosis in which the infection was refractory or the patient was intolerant to standard antifungal agents.[176] Among patients with significant azotemia at baseline, the mean serum creatinine improved over the course of ABLC therapy. Among 291 confirmed cases of fungal infection, response to ABLC occurred in 55 of 130 (42%) cases of aspergillosis, 28 of 42 (67%) cases of disseminated candidiasis, 17 of 24 (71%) cases of zygomycosis, and 9 of 11 (82%) cases of fusariosis. Open-label ABLC was also effective in an emergency use study of children with invasive fungal infections.[174] In a prospective study comparing ABLC with conventional amphotericin B as treatment for hematogenous and invasive candidiasis, the two agents had similar efficacy, but ABLC was associated with reduced nephrotoxicity.[177]

AMPHOTERICIN B COLLOIDAL DISPERSION. ABCD is a complex of amphotericin B and cholesteryl sulfate forming a disc-like structure. In a dose-escalation study in BMT recipients with invasive fungal infections, infusion-related toxicities occurred in approximately 70% of patients; however, nephrotoxicity was not observed.[178] ABCD (4 mg/kg daily) was shown to be safe and to not exacerbate renal insufficiency in a retrospective series of 220 BMT recipients with invasive fungal infection.[179,180] In an open label compassionate use protocol in patients with invasive mycosis who either failed or were intolerant to conventional amphotericin B, the clinical response rate was approximately 50%, and nephrotoxicity was uncommon.[179] In a retrospective study, 82 patients with proven or probable aspergillosis treated with ABCD had increased survival (50% vs. 28%) and reduced nephrotoxicity compared with historical controls treated with amphotericin B.[181] ABCD as empiric therapy for prolonged neutropenic fever was associated with less nephrotoxicity but a greater frequency of infusion-related hypoxia and chills compared with conventional amphotericin B.[182]

WHEN TO CONSIDER A LIPID FORMULATION OF AMPHOTERICIN B. Clinical trials and a growing clinical experience suggest that lipid formulations of amphotericin B have comparable efficacy and reduced nephrotoxicity compared with conventional amphotericin B. However, the majority of treatment protocols for definite or probable invasive mycosis are limited by being open label and uncontrolled or using historical controls. The high cost of the lipid formulations of amphotericin B is an important consideration. However, in a retrospective study of 239 immunosuppressed patients receiving conventional amphotericin B for aspergillosis, serum creatinine greater than 2.5 mg/dL and BMT (autologous and allogeneic) were independently associated with subsequent requirement for dialysis and a higher mortality.[183] Seen in this light, lipid formulations of amphotericin B may reduce morbidity and cost in select patient groups.

A reasonable approach is to use a lipid preparation of amphotericin B as initial therapy when baseline renal insufficiency exists (e.g., creatinine clearance less than 50 mL/min) or a concomitant nephrotoxic agent is used (e.g., aminoglycoside, cyclosporin, foscarnet). Progressive deterioration of renal function despite adequate saline loading and severe infusion-related toxicities, such as high fever, rigors, and myalgias, inadequately controlled by premedication regimens clearly justify the use of a lipid preparation of amphotericin B. If maximal dosages of conventional amphotericin B do not adequately control infection, a lipid formulation may be considered as a salvage regimen. In the setting of invasive mycotic infections, the maximum recommended dosages of lipid formulations should be used.

Echinocandins

A large number of naturally produced antibacterial and antifungal peptides have been characterized.[24] These antimicrobial peptides have been isolated from mammals, amphibians, insects, and bacterial and fungal species. Antifungal peptides have two principal modes of action: (1) direct damage to the fungal membrane structure and (2) inhibition of synthesis of cell wall constituents. The latter group can in turn be divided into inhibitors of chitin and glucan synthesis.

The echinocandins are a family of cyclic lipopeptides that are noncompetitive inhibitors of (1,3)-β-D-glucan synthase, an enzyme complex that forms glucan polymers in fungal cell walls. Echinocandins have a broad spectrum of activity against *Candida* and *Aspergillus* species and *P carinii.* Three echinocandins are leading candidates for clinical trials: caspofungin (MK-0991), LY303366, and FK463. In a study of 400 blood stream isolates of *Candida* species, echinocandins were active against all isolates, including those that were resistant to fluconazole or itraconazole.[184] Echinocandins were effective in animal models of disseminated candidiasis and aspergillosis.[185,186]

Echinocandins have been used successfully in AIDS-associated mucosal and esophageal candidiasis.[187] Currently, caspofungin (Merck) and FK463 (Fujisawa Health Care) are being evaluated in phase III studies of hematogenous candidiasis and as prophylaxis in BMT recipients, respectively. Other echinocandin agents are in preclinical stages of development.

VIRAL INFECTIONS

HERPES VIRUSES

The herpes viruses are the most important viral pathogens in patients with cancer. Pathogens in this group include HSV 1 and 2, varicella zoster virus (VZV), CMV, EBV, and human herpesvirus 6 (HHV-6). These DNA viruses establish a latent phase after primary infection, in which the viral genome resides in target cells for the lifetime of the host, with the potential to reactivate. Host defense against these viruses is dependent on viral-specific helper and cytotoxic T lymphocytes, and thus both the likelihood of reactivation and the severity of disease are augmented during profound T-cell immunosuppression. Table 54-5 summarizes common antiviral agents used in persons with cancer (see reference 188 for an excellent review).

Herpes Simplex Virus

HSV differs from other members of the herpes virus group by predominantly affecting patients during profound neutropenia. Among seropositive patients, the incidence of HSV reactivation is approximately 70% to 80% after induction chemotherapy for leukemia[189] or conditioning for BMT[190] in seropositive patients. Among BMT recipients, HSV disease is most likely to occur within the first few weeks, but may occur in later stages during intense immunosuppression. Oropharyngeal HSV (usually caused by HSV-1) during neutropenia may be severe, causing gingival disease, stomatitis, and cheilitis, clinically indistinguishable from mucositis after cytotoxic chemotherapy. An oral swab culture for HSV detects viral shedding, suggesting that HSV is contributing to the mucosal disease. Local spread of HSV may cause esophagitis, and aspiration of mucosal HSV may occasionally lead to tracheitis and pneumonia. Documentation of pulmonary involvement requires a biopsy because respiratory secretions may be contaminated by oral mucosal HSV. Disseminated HSV disease may involve the skin abdominal organs (most notably, necrotizing hepatitis) and brain. HSV-2 disease is more likely to cause genital and anal disease.

Diagnosis of HSV disease is made by culture, by biopsy material, or both showing characteristic inclusions with positive immunohistochemistry. In patients with mucosal disease, it is safest to treat with intravenous acyclovir (5 mg/kg every 8 hours), switching to an oral regimen when the disease is abating. Milder HSV disease can be treated initially with an oral regimen (famciclovir, 500 mg three times a day, or valacyclovir, 1 g three times a day) under close observation. Disseminated HSV disease should be treated with intravenous acyclovir (10 mg/kg every 8 hours). Acyclovir prophylaxis during intensive myeloablative chemotherapy for acute leukemia[189] and during the early period of BMT[191] markedly reduces the incidence of HSV.

Cytomegalovirus and Prevention of Cytomegalovirus Disease

CMV is the most serious of the viral pathogens in BMT recipients, with seropositive recipients at the greatest risk of developing CMV disease. Before the widespread adoption of prophylaxis against CMV, approximately 50% of seropositive transplant recipients developed CMV disease. Seronegative recipients may acquire primary CMV infection from the bone marrow allograft from a seropositive donor or from infected blood products.

CMV disease most commonly occurs in the postengraftment period, between days 30 and 100 of transplantation. However, disease after day 100 is well documented. In patients with GVHD requiring intensive immunosuppressive therapy, T-cell immunity is

TABLE 54-5. Antiviral Agents Commonly Used in Immunocompromised Patients with Cancer

Disease	*Antiviral Therapy*[a]	*Comments*
Mucocutaneous herpes	Acyclovir, 5 mg/kg q8h IV	
Acyclovir-resistant	Foscarnet, 40 mg/kg 2–3 times daily	Antiviral testing available at reference laboratories
Prophylaxis	Acyclovir, 400 mg (oral) t.i.d.	
Herpes encephalitis	Acyclovir, 10–12 mg/kg q8h IV	Polymerase chain reaction of spinal fluid diagnostic method of choice
Chickenpox	Acyclovir, 10 mg/kg q8h IV	Varicella zoster immune globulin effective prophylaxis if given within 96 h of exposure
Varicella zoster virus	Acyclovir, 10 mg/kg q8h IV	
Cytomegalovirus disease	Ganciclovir, 5 mg/kg q12h IV Foscarnet, 60 mg/kg q8h IV	Use foscarnet for ganciclovir-resistant infection and consider in patients with borderline absolute neutrophil count (e.g., <1500/μL)
Prophylaxis (bone marrow transplant recipients)	Ganciclovir[b], 5–6 mg/kg IV 5–7 d/wk for 3 months, or acyclovir[c], 10 mg/kg IV q8h for first month, then 800 mg PO q.i.d. for at least 3 months	Initiate after myeloid recovery; many centers initiate cytomegalovirus prophylaxis on day 30
Influenza	Rimantadine, 200 mg PO q.d., or amantadine, 100 mg PO q.d.	Neuraminidase inhibitors recently licensed; have not been evaluated in highly immunocompromised persons
Respiratory syncytial virus	Ribavirin, 6 g/300 mL water, by aerosol 18 h/d	
Chronic hepatitis B	Interferon-α, 5 MIU q.d. or 10 MIU 3 times weekly, SC or IM; or lamivudine, 100 mg PO q.d.	
Chronic hepatitis C	Interferon-α, 3 MIU SC or IM 3 times weekly, along with ribavirin, 500–600 mg PO b.i.d.	

[a]Doses are for adults with normal renal function.
[b]Different strategies of ganciclovir prophylaxis in bone marrow transplant recipients have been employed (see text).
[c]Based on ref. 200.
(Adapted from ref. 188.)

suppressed, and the risk for CMV disease is consequently increased.[192] Antilymphocyte antibody preparations profoundly reduce the number of circulating T cells and likely further increase the risk of CMV reactivation. CMV disease is far less frequent in autologous BMT recipients, but can be lethal. CD34-selected autologous stem cell transplantation is associated with a greater risk of CMV disease than conventional nonselected peripheral stem cell transplantation.[193] The period of risk in autologous transplantation is generally confined to the first 3 months, corresponding to the period of reconstitution of T-cell immunity.[193]

CMV infection, either primary or reactivated, can have protean manifestations in the BMT recipient, ranging from asymptomatic viral shedding, to a self-limited mononucleosis-like syndrome, to life-threatening organ disease. Pulmonary disease typically manifests as an interstitial pneumonitis resembling PCP, associated with hypoxia and progression to respiratory failure. A definitive diagnosis of CMV pneumonitis requires a compatible clinical syndrome plus either the histologic documentation of characteristic CMV inclusions within parenchymal tissue or intracellular inclusions within epithelial cells obtained by bronchoalveolar lavage. Because CMV can be shed from pulmonary secretions without causing invasive disease, simple recovery of CMV from pulmonary secretions by culture, PCR, or antigen detection studies should not be considered evidence of CMV disease. However, in an allogeneic transplant recipient with a compatible chest radiograph, such documentation of CMV infection in the absence of cytologic or histologic evidence of disease should prompt anti-CMV therapy given the high likelihood of CMV disease in this setting. Both infectious and noninfectious processes may masquerade as, or occur in addition to, pulmonary CMV disease. In one study of late CMV pneumonia (occurring after day 100 of transplantation), approximately one-half of the cases were associated with concurrent pulmonary infections, including *P aeruginosa*, *Legionella*, *Aspergillus* species, *Mycobacteria* species, *Nocardia* species, toxoplasmosis, and respiratory viruses.[194] Therefore, diffuse interstitial disease in a BMT recipient should be evaluated early with bronchoalveolar lavage, and if feasible, transbronchial biopsy (see Pulmonary Infiltrates, later in this chapter). Treatment of CMV pneumonia consists of ganciclovir (5 mg/kg every 12 hours) plus immunoglobulin (normal or CMV hyperimmune). The expected mortality is between 30% and 50%, which is significantly improved compared with series in which ganciclovir alone was used.[195]

CMV disease can occur at any location within the gastrointestinal tract, although esophagitis and colitis are the most common sites. In the esophagus, ulcerations resembling HSV or candidal esophagitis occur. Differentiation of CMV from these causes relies on biopsy or cytology. CMV colitis is associated with abdominal pain and diarrhea. CMV involvement of enteric vessels may result in hemorrhage and infarction. However, in a randomized study, treatment of CMV gastroenteritis with ganciclovir produced similar results as placebo.[196]

CMV hepatitis should be considered in the setting of fever and elevations of liver transaminase enzymes. Other potential viral etiologies include HSV-1 and -2, hepatitis viruses, and EBV. A liver biopsy documenting CMV inclusions definitively establishes the diagnosis.

Less common sites of CMV disease in BMT recipients include pancreas, brain, spinal cord (transverse myelitis), and adrenals. CMV retinitis, the most common complication in patients with AIDS, is rare in transplant recipients. A CMV syndrome is associated with fever, pancytopenia, and CMV viremia and may precede the development of organ disease.

Because of the high mortality associated with CMV disease, much effort has been focused on prevention. CMV-seronegative blood transplant recipients should receive only CMV-seronegative blood products or leukocyte-depleted products to avoid primary CMV infection. The incidence of CMV infection in CMV-seronegative transplant recipients who had CMV-seronegative donors and were given only CMV-seronegative blood products was approximately 5% in three separate studies.[197–199] Use of CMV-seronegative blood products likely reduces the frequency of CMV infection in cases of CMV-seronegative recipients and seropositive donors, although the magnitude of protection varies widely with different series.[197–199]

Reactivation of latent CMV infection after transplantation occurs in approximately 70% of seropositive recipients who do not receive antiviral prophylaxis. Antiviral agents have been used successfully to reduce the rate of CMV disease. The following two preventive approaches have been evaluated in allogeneic BMT recipients.[195]

1. Prophylaxis: antiviral agents are administered to all CMV-seropositive BMT recipients (CMV-seronegative recipients receiving seropositive bone marrow were also candidates for antiviral prophylaxis in some studies).
2. Preemptive therapy: initiation of antiviral agents after detection of asymptomatic CMV infection by screening cultures or molecular detection methods.

Offering anti-CMV prophylaxis to all seropositive allogeneic transplant recipients has important advantages and shortcomings. In two studies, acyclovir prophylaxis was associated with increased survival, but the rates of CMV reactivation and disease were fairly high.[200,201] *In vitro,* ganciclovir, an acyclic nucleoside analog of guanosine, is approximately 50 times more active than acyclovir against CMV.[202] Two randomized placebo-controlled studies of ganciclovir prophylaxis for CMV-seropositive allogeneic transplant recipients produced similar results.[197,203] Ganciclovir prophylaxis was highly effective at suppressing CMV during the early transplant period, but was associated with higher rates of neutropenia, bacterial and opportunistic infections, and late CMV disease. Ganciclovir prophylaxis did not lead to an improvement in survival.

Nguyen et al.[194] retrospectively reviewed 541 adult allogeneic transplant recipients at the University of Texas M. D. Anderson Cancer Center who had received ganciclovir prophylaxis. Thirty-five episodes of CMV pneumonia were documented, 26 (74%) of which occurred after day 100. The mortality was approximately 75%. Almost all cases of late CMV pneumonia occurred in patients with GVHD or who had received T-cell–depleted transplants. Reconstitution of CMV-specific T-cell responses are delayed in allogeneic transplant recipients who received ganciclovir prophylaxis, thus, conceivably predisposing such patients to late CMV disease.[204] These observations provide a rationale for targeting patients at highest risk for CMV disease for antiviral therapy as opposed to administering prophylaxis to all seropositive patients.

Highly sensitive detection methods to identify subclinical CMV infection have been evaluated. These methods include detection of the CMV pp65 antigen from peripheral blood leukocytes and detection of CMV DNA by PCR from blood, serum, or plasma. Boeckh et al.[205,206] showed that preemptive ganciclovir based on detection of CMV antigenemia was associated with a similar rate of CMV disease and similar long-term survival rates as standard ganciclovir prophylaxis initiated at engraftment.

Einsele et al.[207] randomized allogeneic transplant recipients to receive preemptive ganciclovir therapy based on PCR detection of CMV from blood (PCR group) or a positive CMV culture from blood, urine, or throat washings (culture group). PCR screening led to earlier detection of subclinical CMV infection compared with culture. The PCR group had a reduced rate of CMV disease, duration of ganciclovir therapy, neutropenia, and nonviral infections compared with the culture group, and overall survival was superior. Discontinuing preemptive ganciclovir in patients whose blood became PCR negative appeared to be safe.

Foscarnet, an antiviral drug with activity against CMV, may have an advantage over ganciclovir in patients with delayed engraftment or with ganciclovir-associated neutropenia. Azotemia is the major toxicity associated with foscarnet. Moretti et al.[208] compared ganciclovir with foscarnet as preemptive therapy at the time of documentation of subclinical CMV antigenemia. There was a trend to more rapid clearance of CMV antigenemia in the foscarnet group. The major adverse effect was cytopenia in the ganciclovir group and azotemia in the foscarnet group. The study was not sufficiently powered to detect a difference in CMV disease or mortality.

Determination of optimal CMV preventive strategies will require additional prospective randomized studies. Newer, less toxic antiviral agents will need to be evaluated. Lowance et al.[209] showed that valacyclovir (a valine esterified analog of acyclovir with high oral bioavailability) was well tolerated and reduced CMV disease in renal transplant recipients. In addition, immune augmentation strategies (see Immune Augmentation Strategies, later in this chapter) may also be useful as preventive and treatment strategies.

Varicella Zoster Virus

Control of VZV infection is dependent on T-cell[210–212] and humoral immunity.[213] BMT recipients and patients receiving intensive corticosteroid therapy are at risk for life-threatening disseminated primary and reactivated VZV infection. Reactivated VZV disease is typically a late complication of BMT, usually occurring 3 months to more than a year after transplantation. Before the routine use of antiviral agents for prophylaxis against CMV infection, 17% of BMT recipients had an episode of reactivated VZV within the first year.[214] In one study of acyclovir prophylaxis for CMV, the rate of VZV at day 210 after transplantation was only 3% in patients receiving prolonged high-dose acyclovir.[200]

The major risk factor for developing VZV is acute and chronic GVHD requiring intensive immunosuppressive therapy.[214] In such immunocompromised patients, VZV infection may manifest with a multidermatomal or disseminated vesicular exanthem associated with hemorrhage and necrosis. Infection of visceral can cause hemorrhagic pneumonia, encephalitis, retinal necrosis, hepatitis, and small bowel disease. Secondary bacterial infections may occur in cutaneous VZV lesions. VZV infection can also be complicated by bleeding disorders, thrombocytopenia, vasculitis, disseminated intravascular coagulation, and fulminant purpura resembling bacterial sepsis.

The diagnosis of single dermatomal shingles can usually be made by visual inspection alone. In the immunosuppressed patient, multidermatomal or disseminated cutaneous disease may make the diagnosis on clinical grounds less certain. Immunofluorescent staining of material from an unroofed skin lesion or from a skin biopsy may establish the diagnosis within hours. A Tzanck's preparation confirms infection by a herpes virus, but is not specific for VZV. Viral culture should also be performed.

Intravenous acyclovir (10 mg/kg every 8 hours) is the established treatment for primary or reactivated VZV in immunosuppressed patients.[215] Early initiation of acyclovir reduces progression of disease and usually eliminates mortality in patients with reactivated disease. All BMT recipients with VZV infection should be treated initially as inpatients because of the potential for dissemination. Once clinical improvement has occurred (e.g., resolution of fever, healing of lesions), an oral regimen can be substituted and completed as an outpatient. The oral regimen may consist of acyclovir (800 mg five times per day), valacyclovir (1 g three times a day), or famciclovir (500 mg three times a day). Salicylates should not be used because of the risk of Reye's syndrome.

Lack of a clinical response to therapy should prompt reconsideration of the initial diagnosis, the possibility of a secondary infection, or VZV resistance to acyclovir. Streptococcal impetigo, dermatitis, and various noninfectious bullous diseases can mimic VZV. In such cases, a biopsy is required to establish the diagnosis. Severe streptococcal infections may occur after primary VZV infection. Resistance of VZV to acyclovir may be increased in BMT recipients who have received prolonged courses of acyclovir or ganciclovir as prophylaxis for CMV infection. However, in one study of acyclovir prophylaxis against CMV, the relatively small proportion (less than 10%) of patients who developed VZV disease were successfully treated with acyclovir, indicating that either antiviral resistance did not occur or could be overcome by intensification of the acyclovir regimen.[200] If VZV infection develops while receiving ganciclovir, foscarnet should be initiated because of the cross-resistance between acyclovir and ganciclovir.

Nosocomial transmission of VZV is well documented.[216] Patients with primary varicella (chicken pox), those with disseminated zoster, or immunocompromised patients with dermatomal zoster should be placed under contact and respiratory isolation (private negative-pressure room, air exhausted to outside, six or more air exchanges per hour). Varicella zoster immune globulin should be offered to immunosuppressed VZV-seronegative patients after exposures such as prolonged face-to-face contact, a household or playmate contact, or exposure to a roommate in a shared hospital room. Varicella zoster immune globulin is most effective when administered within 72 hours of exposure; its efficacy is unknown 96 hours after exposure.

The current varicella vaccine uses the live attenuated Oka strain (Merck). The vaccine is immunogenic and protective. The attenuated VZV can cause latent infection, and zoster caused by either the vaccine-type or wild-type VZV can occur months to years after vaccination.[217] This vaccine has been studied extensively in children with leukemia and has been shown to be safe and effective.[217,218]

The American Academy of Pediatrics states that the Oka vaccine is contraindicated in immunocompromised individuals, except for children with acute lymphoblastic leukemia to whom the vaccine may be administered in study conditions.[219] In families with immunocompromised persons, no precautions are required after vaccination of healthy children in whom a rash has not developed. If a rash does occur, direct contact with immunocompromised persons should be avoided. If inadvertent contact occurs, the use of varicella zoster immune globulin is not recommended because of the low transmission rate and the expectation that disease will be mild if it occurs.

Epstein-Barr Virus

In the United States, most adults have been infected by EBV. Primary infection is usually asymptomatic, but may cause a mononucleosis syndrome. Latent infection persists in B cells and produces no disease in the vast majority of people. EBV-specific cytotoxic T lymphocytes are the principal controllers of the replication of EBV-infected B cells.[220,221] EBV lymphoproliferative disorders are encountered in patients with severely impaired T-cell immunity,[222] such as AIDS or intensive and prolonged immunosuppressive therapy. EBV-induced posttransplant lymphoproliferative disorder (PTLD) is defined as an abnormal proliferation of B-lymphoid cells in transplant recipients. The lesions may be composed of a polyclonal or monoclonal population of transformed B cells. PTLD is most common during the first year of transplantation. Patients with GVHD treated with antilymphocyte immunoglobulins[223] and recipients of T-cell–depleted marrow from HLA-mismatched donors[224] are at highest risk for PTLD.

Clinical manifestations of PTLD are varied, and a high index of suspicion is required to make the diagnosis. Patients may have a mononucleosis-like syndrome with fever and localized adenopathy. Disseminated disease may manifest with generalized adenopathy and extranodal organ involvement, including the bowel, liver, bone marrow, and CNS. A CT scan of the head, chest, abdomen, and pelvis is useful in evaluating a high-risk patient with unexplained fever. Diagnosis of PTLD requires biopsy of an affected area showing a characteristic histologic appearance and evidence of EBV infection using immunohistochemical methods or by detecting EBV DNA.

In organ transplant recipients, most PTLD is of recipient origin. In BMT-associated PTLD, the abnormal clones are typically of donor origin.[223,224] Thus, in allogeneic BMT recipients, a balance is created between donor-derived B-cell clonal proliferation and the establishment of donor-derived cytotoxic T-cell immunity, which contain these proliferative responses. Whereas PTLD in organ transplant recipients typically responds to a reduction in the intensity of immunosuppression, PTLD in BMT recipients may not respond to such conservative measures. Adoptive immunotherapy is a promising strategy (see Immune Augmentation Strategies, later in this chapter).

Human Herpesvirus 6

HHV-6 was first isolated from peripheral blood from patients with lymphoproliferative disorders.[225] This virus was initially called *human B-lymphotrophic virus*, but it was later discovered that the virus is predominantly T-cell trophic.[226] HHV-6 has been recognized as an opportunistic pathogen in solid organ and BMT recipients. In BMT recipients, HHV-6 has been associated with a variety of syndromes: (1) fever and rash clinically resembling cutaneous GVHD; (2) an increased risk of GVHD; (3) bone marrow suppression; (4) encephalitis; and (5) pneumonitis. However, establishing a causal relationship between HHV-6 and these syndromes is made difficult by the fact that HHV-6 can be documented in approximately 50% of BMT recipients, usually between 2 and 4 weeks after transplantation.[227–229] The evidence supporting a link between HHV-6 infection and encephalitis[230] and interstitial pneumonitis[231] is the most persuasive, based on the *in situ* documentation of HHV-6 in the respective organs using immunohistochemistry, molecular detection methods, and culture.

Singh and Carrigan[232] proposed the following two criteria for the diagnosis of HHV-6 disease: (1) presence of bone marrow suppression, encephalitis, or pneumonitis and (2) documentation of active infection by culture, PCR from an acellular specimen (a positive PCR result from blood cannot distinguish active from latent infection), or immunohistochemistry. Comparative studies evaluating therapy for HHV-6 have not been performed, and it is therefore not possible to make definitive recommendations about therapy. HHV-6 is sensitive *in vitro* to ganciclovir and foscarnet, and it is reasonable to initiate therapy with either of these agents when HHV-6 disease is proven or strongly suspected. The role of screening for asymptomatic HHV-6 infection and prophylaxis with antiviral agents is uncertain.

COMMUNITY RESPIRATORY VIRUSES

Community respiratory viruses include members of the Orthomyxoviridae (influenza A, B, and C) and Paramyxoviridae [parainfluenza 1 through 4, respiratory syncytial virus (RSV), and measles] families, adenoviruses, and picornaviruses. These viruses are important causes of morbidity and mortality in immunocompromised patients.[233,234] With the progress in prophylaxis and treatment of CMV disease in BMT recipients, the relative proportion of pulmonary infections caused by community respiratory viruses is likely to grow. In contrast to CMV, these viruses are seasonal and are rapidly transmitted from one person to another by respiratory secretions, thus having the potential for nosocomial outbreaks.

Respiratory viruses may account for a significant proportion of undiagnosed or idiopathic pneumonias in BMT recipients in older series.[234] Their importance as pathogens in this population has been documented more recently by centers that routinely screen for community viral pathogens in patients with respiratory illnesses.

Respiratory Syncytial Virus

RSV infection is highly virulent in patients with leukemia and in BMT recipients. In patients with leukemia, progression to pneumonia and mortality are more common in the setting of neutropenia.[235] RSV infection can occur throughout the transplantation period, from the preengraftment stage to more than a year after transplantation. Upper respiratory symptoms (sinusitis, coryza, rhinorrhea) usually precede lower respiratory tract involvement (dyspnea, wheezing) and pneumonia, although upper airway symptoms may be absent. The historic mortality from RSV pneumonia in BMT recipients is approximately 80%.[236] At the University of Texas M. D. Anderson Cancer Center, patients who received aerosolized ribavirin and intravenous immunoglobulin containing high RSV-neutralizing titers at least 24 hours before respiratory failure had a 22% mortality compared with 100% mortality in patients who either did not receive therapy or in whom treatment was initiated after respiratory failure had occurred.[237]

Rapid diagnosis of RSV has been made possible by antigen detection methods. Englund et al.[238] showed that compared with culture, antigen detection had a sensitivity of 89% in bronchoalveolar lavage, 15% in nasal and throat washings, and 71% in endotracheal aspirates in symptomatic adult leukemia or BMT patients. The specificity was 97% to 100% from these sources. The lower sensitivity of antigen detection from the upper airway of adults is attributed to a lower viral burden. The low yield of upper airway cultures severely limits the value of these noninvasive tests in adults with respiratory disease.

A preliminary study of intravenous ribavirin for RSV pneumonia in BMT recipients who at enrollment did not require mechanical ventilation, was associated with an eventual 80% mortality.[239] In a second strategy, aerosolized ribavirin was administered to patients in whom RSV was isolated from nasopharyngeal washes without signs of lower respiratory tract involvement. Pneumonia developed in 8 of 25 (32%) patients, with a mortality of 29%.[236] These studies suggest that early diagnosis and treatment of RSV in this population may be life saving.

Parainfluenza

Parainfluenza viruses are important community respiratory viruses in leukemia and BMT patients. In a review of 45 cases of parainfluenza virus infection in BMT recipients, 26 (58%) patients had pneumonia, of whom 39% died.[240]

Therapy for parainfluenza infection has not been established. An uncontrolled retrospective series from the University of Minnesota showed that survival with and without aerosolized ribavirin was approximately 80% in BMT recipients with parainfluenza infection.[241] Ribavirin was generally begun late after onset of respiratory symptoms, which may have reduced its efficacy. The role of intravenous immunoglobulin against this organism merits further exploration.

Influenza Virus

Influenza virus is the most important respiratory virus globally and the most common cause of excess seasonal mortality in North America, accounting for approximately 20,000 deaths in the United States annually. During a winter outbreak period, influenza was diagnosed in approximately 30% of adult patients hospitalized for a respiratory illness at the M. D. Anderson Cancer Center.[240] Pneumonia occurred in 12 of 15 (80%) of patients with influenza, and four of these patients died. In other centers, the incidence of pneumonia and mortality associated with influenza virus infection was substantially lower.[236]

Amantadine and rimantadine are the most common agents used in treating influenza. These agents are only active against influenza A, not influenza B. In one center, resistance to these agents rapidly developed during therapy for influenza A among patients with leukemia and BMT recipients.[242] Ribavirin has activity against influenza A and B and has been used in patients with influenza virus infection.[243]

Two agents (zanamivir and oseltamivir) that inhibit the influenza virus neuraminidase have been licensed. These drugs are active against both influenza A and B and have been shown to be effective in reducing the duration of influenza illness[244] and to have a prophylactic benefit during community outbreaks.[245,246] The role of these agents as treatment or prophylaxis in immunocompromised patients with cancer has not been evaluated.

The Centers for Disease Control and Prevention recommend annual administration of the inactivated influenza vaccine to immunocompromised persons and their close contacts (e.g., health care workers and household members).[247] Immunocompromised persons are less likely to mount an adequate antibody response to immunization.[248] Immunization should be provided ideally 2 weeks before chemotherapy, or if given during chemotherapy, immunization is preferably administered between cycles. In one study, a two-step vaccination regimen enhanced the immune response in patients receiving chemotherapy for lymphoma.[249]

Adenovirus

The clinical manifestations of adenoviruses in BMT recipients include pneumonia, bronchiolitis, upper respiratory tract infection, renal parenchymal disease, hemorrhagic cystitis, hepatitis, small and large bowel disease, encephalitis, and disseminated infection.[250,251] Viral shedding from throat secretions, urine, and stool is common, occurring in approximately 5% to 20% of BMT recipients, and should not be equated with disease. In patients with definite invasive disease, long-term survival was poor. GVHD was the only significant risk factor in both studies.

Adenoviruses were cultured from 28 adult BMT recipients at the M. D. Anderson Cancer Center.[240] Seven of 12 patients with pneumonia and all six patients with disseminated disease died, whereas ten patients with upper respiratory tract infection survived. Risk factors for mortality included isolation of adenovirus from multiple sites and prolonged shedding. Ribavirin was not associated with benefit in this retrospective series. The role of intravenous immunoglobulin for management of adenovirus infection has not been established.

Measles

Kaplan et al.[252] conducted an extensive review of measles in immunocompromised patients. Of 40 patients (aged 3 months to 22 years) with malignancy, 16 (40%) had no rash whereas the remainder had either typical or atypical exanthemas. Twenty-three (58%) had pneumonitis, eight (20%) had encephalitis, six (20%) had both, and six (20%) had no complications. The overall fatality rate was 55%. The benefit of ribavirin could not be assessed.

Diagnosis of Respiratory Viruses

Rapid immunodiagnostic methods for common respiratory viruses have become widely used, and have resulted in reduced hospital stays, antibiotic use, and microbiologic investigations.[253] Such rapid methods also have additional potential benefits for early initiation of antiviral agents and implementation of appropriate infection control precautions. Cell culture is generally more sensitive than antigen detection methods, with the exception of RSV in children, in whom antigen detection is highly sensitive. Rapid antigen detection methods and cell culture are therefore complementary. PCR amplification methods are being evaluated and show promise.[254]

HEPATITIS VIRUSES

Liver test abnormalities are common in patients with cancer. Among BMT recipients, the differential diagnosis is broad and includes drug toxicity, GVHD, venoocclusive disease, recurrent malignancy, and infectious hepatitis. Patients who receive multiple transfusions of blood and pooled plasma products are at a higher risk for transfusion-associated viral hepatitis, despite the highly effective screening methods of blood products currently used. In addition, such patients are likely to be at higher risk for reactivation of latent viral infection during intensive immunosuppressive therapy and for developing life-threatening complications.

Hepatitis B

Reactivation of latent hepatitis B virus (HBV) infection in BMT recipients is an unpredictable but rare event. Although the hepatitis B surface antigen carrier state is not a contraindication to BMT, such patients appear to be at a higher risk for fulminant hepatitis as a result of reactivation.[255–257] In a prospective study of 100 Chinese patients who received induction chemotherapy for lymphoma, hepatitis developed in 67% of HBsAg-positive patients compared with 14% of HBsAg-negative patients.[258] Reactivation of HBV (as determined by serum levels of HBV DNA and HBeAg) was associated with icteric hepatitis, but infrequently with liver failure and mortality. Symptomatic hepatitis may manifest after withdrawal of immunosuppressive agents or between cycles of chemotherapy when recovery of immune responses occurs.[259,260]

Precore mutant HBV has been associated with cases of fulminant hepatic failure after cytotoxic chemotherapy and fibrosing cholestatic hepatitis.[261,262] This mutation results in failure to secrete HBeAg, and, therefore, this marker can not be used as an indicator of active viral replication.

Chronic HBV hepatitis has been reported in patients with negative serologic study results. Vergani et al.[263] reported 23 cases of histologically proven HBV infection in 23 children with leukemia and liver disease, none of whom had detectable HBV serum antigens or antibodies. In eight of the children, HBV markers subsequently appeared in the serum within 15 months of stopping chemotherapy. Bréchot et al.[264] documented HBV DNA in 59% of liver samples but in only 10% of serum samples among patients with chronic liver disease and negative test results for HBsAg.

Treatment of chronic HBV involves either the antiviral nucleoside analog lamivudine[265,266] or interferon-α (IFN-α).[267] The advantages of lamivudine include limited side effects and the fact that histologic improvement was documented in the majority of patients.[265] Favoring IFN-α is the limited duration of therapy and the absence of viral mutations that lead to resistance to therapy.[265]

Vaccination against HBV should be considered in seronegative patients with cancer. However, among BMT recipients, active immunization in the immediate pretransplant and posttransplant periods is often ineffective, most likely as a result of defective T-cell and B-cell function. Adoptive transfer of immunity to HBV can be achieved after allogeneic BMT from immune donors.[268]

Hepatitis C

Before routine blood screening began in 1991, BMT recipients were at significant risk for hepatitis C virus (HCV) infection. HCV infection can cause both early and late complications in BMT recipients. In a cohort study from Fred Hutchinson Cancer Research Center, pretransplant HCV infection plus an elevated serum aspartate transaminase level was predictive of severe venoocclusive disease (VOD) (relative risk, 9.6)[269]; HCV infection without elevated transaminases was not a significant risk factor for VOD. An acute flare of hepatitis occurred in about one-third of HCV-positive patients at a mean of 4 to 5 months after transplant and was usually self limited.[269] Frickhofen et al. also noted an association between pretransplant HCV infection and severe VOD in the early transplant period.[270]

Approximately one-half of HCV-positive transplant recipients at Fred Hutchinson continued to have mild to moderate elevations in liver enzymes 5 to 10 years following transplant.[269] However, HCV was not associated with increased mortality.[269] Cirrhosis was identified in 31 of 3721 patients surviving 1 or more years after BMT.[271] HCV infection was documented in 25 of the 31 (81%) patients, and cirrhosis was attributed to HCV infection in 15 of 16 (93%) patients presenting more than 10 years after transplantation.[271] To try to avoid cirrhosis, interferon-α and ribavirin therapy should be considered in transplant recipients with chronic HCV infection who have been off immunosuppressive agents for at least 6 months, have normal marrow recovery, and have no GVHD.[271a]

HCV is universally transmitted from HCV RNA-positive donors to their recipients.[271a] If an HCV-positive donor is the best available match, treatment of the donor with interferon-α and ribavirin before marrow or stem cell harvest may be considered to try to eliminate viremia (which can be monitored by PCR). Interferon should be stopped at least 1 week before harvest to avoid problems with engraftment in the recipient.[271a]

Significant hepatic dysfunction is uncommon in nontransplant HCV-positive patients receiving chemotherapy for hematologic malignancies.[271b] In a prospective study of 305 patients with lymphoma, the prevalence of HCV and HBV infection was 16% and 3.2%, respectively.[271c] No reactivation in HCV-positive patients occurred during chemotherapy. In contrast, HBV reactivation occurred in approximately 80% of HBV-infected patients, and was associated with a 37% mortality rate. Thus, HBV should be considered to be an opportunistic pathogen in heavily immunosuppressed persons with hematologic malignancies, whereas HCV is not.

Other Transfusion-Associated Hepatitis Viruses

Hepatitis G is a newly discovered transfusion-associated virus that can establish persistent infection in asymptomatic individuals. Surveillance studies have not established a role for this virus in non-A through E acute transfusion-related hepatitis or chronic liver disease.[273,274] TT virus is another virus capable of establishing persistent infection whose pathogenicity remains questionable.[275] In a Japanese study, TT virus DNA was detected with far greater frequency in BMT recipients than in blood donors, and, in one patient, was temporally associated with elevated serum hepatic enzymes.[276] Conceivably, these other transfusion-associated viruses yet to be discovered, may be agents of non-A through E hepatitis in heavily transfused persons with cancer.

PARASITIC INFECTIONS

PNEUMOCYSTIS CARINII

Pneumocystis carinii is more appropriately classified as a fungus than a protozoan based on gene sequence data and cell wall constituents. Defective T-cell immunity is the principal risk factor for PCP. Sepkowitz et al.[277–279] reported that corticosteroid use was associated with 204 of 227 (90%) cases of PCP in patients without AIDS at Memorial Sloan-Kettering Cancer Center between 1963 and 1992. The median time that patients received corticosteroids was 2 months, although a minority of patients had received corticosteroids for less than 1 month. Approximately 60% of patients had hematologic malignancies, 25% had solid tumors, 10% were BMT recipients, and 5% were receiving relatively mild immunosuppressive regimens.

The risk of PCP increases with the intensity of the immunosuppressive regimen. In a study of pediatric patients with acute lymphocytic leukemia, the risk of PCP was strikingly increased from less than 5% to 22% when cytosine arabinoside (Ara-C) was used.[280] Browne et al.[281] reported a 32% rate of PCP (probable plus definite) in patients with non-Hodgkin's lymphoma treated with an intensive regimen consisting of corticosteroids and multiple cytotoxic agents (methotrexate, doxorubicin, cyclophosphamide, etoposide, Ara-C, bleomycin, vincristine) as compared with no cases of PCP in patients who did not receive Ara-C and bleomycin.

Pneumocystis carinii can have a fulminant course, resembling a bacterial pneumonia with rapid progression to respiratory failure, or can be indolent.[282] Patients treated with corticosteroids may develop initial clinical manifestations of PCP only during corticosteroid taper. Bilateral interstitial infiltrates are most common in PCP, although unilateral or patchy infiltrates are also observed. Nodules, cavitary lesions, and pleural effusions are less common. In a minority of patients, the chest radiograph is normal. Extrapulmonary *P carinii* infection is rare in patients with cancer and has for the most part been reported only in patients with AIDS.

Diagnosis of PCP relies on visualization of the organism microscopically. Immunofluorescent staining using monoclonal antibodies is more sensitive than older staining methods, such as silver staining or Wright-Giemsa.[283] PCR-based detection of *P carinii* from induced sputum or blood is a promising experimental diagnostic method.[284]

Spontaneously expectorated sputum is generally unsatisfactory for diagnosis of PCP, but sputum induction using 3% sodium chloride solution in an ultrasonic nebulizer usually yields a satisfactory sample. In a small study of non-AIDS patients with PCP, the diagnostic sensitivity using this method was approximately 60%.[285] If sputum induction is nondiagnostic, bronchoscopy should be pursued.

Trimethoprim-sulfamethoxazole (trimethoprim 15 to 20 mg/kg daily divided into three to four doses) is the treatment of choice for *P carinii*. In patients intolerant of this agent, intravenous pentamidine, dapsone-trimethoprim, and clindamycin-primaquine are acceptable alternatives. In cases of a prior non–life-threatening reaction to a sulfonamide (e.g., a nonurticarial rash), experience with AIDS patients has shown that rechallenge with trimethoprim-sulfamethoxazole is safe under close medical observation,[286] although some investigators would opt for desensitization.[287] Patients without AIDS are less likely to have adverse reactions to trimethoprim-sulfamethoxazole.[282] In patients with moderate or severe PCP (PaO_2 less than 70 mm), corticosteroids should be added based on studies of patients with AIDS-associated PCP.[288] In patients who are not responding to therapy, repeat bronchoscopy should be performed to exclude additional pathogens that may have been missed or may not have been present initially.

Trimethoprim-sulfamethoxazole is highly effective as prophylaxis against PCP. In children with cancer at high risk for PCP, no case of PCP occurred in patients administered daily trimethoprim-sulfamethoxazole, compared with an approximately 20% incidence in the placebo arm.[289] Trimethoprim-sulfamethoxazole prophylaxis was also associated with a reduction in bacterial infections. In a subsequent study of children with acute lymphoblastic leukemia, trimethoprim-sulfamethoxazole administered either daily or on 3 consecutive days weekly was fully protective against PCP.[290]

Defining which patients with cancer will benefit from prophylaxis against PCP is often empiric given the absence of controlled studies in several high-risk groups. Children with acute lymphoblastic leukemia and allogeneic BMT recipients are known high-risk groups that should be offered prophylaxis. In BMT recipients, the peak risk of PCP is between 1 and 4 months after transplantation, corresponding to the period of most profound T-cell immunodeficiency. Prophylaxis is generally administered shortly after engraftment until 6 to 12 months after BMT, but should be reinitiated at later periods in the setting of GVHD requiring intensification of immunosuppressive agents. Adults with acute lymphoblastic leukemia,[291] patients with CNS tumors receiving high-dose corticosteroid therapy,[292,293] and patients receiving combination corticosteroid therapy with either myelotoxic agents or fludarabine are also at high risk for PCP, and prophylaxis should be considered.

TOXOPLASMOSIS

Reactivation of *Toxoplasma gondii* is associated with life-threatening disease primarily in patients with profound deficits in T-cell immunity. In a review of 128 reported cases of toxoplasmosis in patients with neoplastic disorders, 59 patients had Hodgkin's disease, 12 had non-Hodgkin's lymphoma, and 36 had acute or chronic leukemias.[294] Therapy with corticosteroids; cytotoxic agents, radiation therapy, or both; and poorly controlled malignancy are risk factors for toxoplasmas.[295]

Toxoplasmosis is an uncommon complication of BMT. In the largest series, toxoplasmosis was diagnosed in 12 of 3803 (0.3%) consecutive allogeneic BMT recipients and in none of 509 autologous transplant recipients at the Fred Hutchinson Cancer Center.[296] All 12 patients died; ten cases were diagnosed postmortem, and toxoplasmosis was believed to contribute to mortality in at least four patients. Toxoplasmosis manifested within the first 4 months of transplantation. Pretransplant seropositivity for *T gondii* and severe GVHD were the predominant risk factors.

CNS disease is most commonly observed. Altered mental status, coma, seizures, cranial nerve abnormalities, and motor weakness are the most common findings.[294] Cerebrospinal fluid is usually normal; however, a mononuclear pleocytosis and elevated protein level may be seen. Other organs involved may include the heart, lungs, liver, spleen, lymph nodes, bone marrow, pancreas, spleen, and skeletal muscle.

Definitive diagnosis of toxoplasmosis usually relies on demonstration of tachyzoites and cysts in histopathologic sections. Use of electron microscopy[297] and immunoperoxidase staining[298] may facilitate diagnosis. Visualization of the organism in cerebrospinal fluid using Giemsa staining is diagnostic of disease, but the sensitivity of this method is low.[299] Demonstration of local antibody production in cerebrospinal fluid[300] or aqueous humor[301] may facilitate the diagnosis of encephalitis and chorioretinitis, respectively. PCR is a promising diagnostic method available at specialized laboratories.

The treatment of choice for toxoplasmosis is oral sulfadiazine, 4 to 6 g/d, plus pyrimethamine (loading dose of 200 mg, followed by 50 to 75 mg daily). Folinic acid should be administered to reduce myeloid toxicity. Whether maintenance therapy is required after quiescence of disease is unknown. It is reasonable to continue a maintenance regimen (which may consist of sulfadiazine, 2 g/d, plus pyrimethamine, 50 mg/d) during periods of immunosuppressive therapy. In patients intolerant of sulfonamides, clindamycin and primaquine may be used instead.

ACANTHAMOEBA

Acanthamoeba species may cause an insidious granulomatous encephalitis in immunocompromised patients, such as those receiving high-dose corticosteroid therapy, solid organ transplant recipients, and patients with AIDS. Skin manifestations include persistent ulcers, nodules, or subcutaneous abscesses. BMT recipients may have a more fulminant course characterized by obtundation, coma, and seizures, associated with a necrotizing meningoencephalitis and hydrocephalus.[302] A necrotizing pneumonitis and adrenalitis may also be present. A diagnosis may be established by cerebrospinal fluid analysis or biopsy showing characteristic amebic trophozoites. The treatment of choice is parenteral pentamidine.

STRONGYLOIDES STERCORALIS

Strongyloides stercoralis is an intestinal nematode that can cause disseminated infection, or hyperinfection syndrome, in immunocompromised patients.[303] *S stercoralis* is particularly common in tropical and subtropical regions, but the parasite also is endemic in certain rural southern regions of the United States. Cross-infection between humans through contact with material soiled with feces appears to be likely in overcrowded and unsanitary conditions.[304] *S stercoralis* can establish an asymptomatic chronic gastrointestinal infection through internal autoinfection, with the hyperinfection syndrome occurring several years after the initial infection, frequently in the setting of immunosuppression. This underscores the need to obtain a thorough history about prior residence in endemic areas. Corticosteroid therapy with and without other agents appears to be associated with the highest risk of disseminated disease.[304] Among reported cases of hyperinfection syndrome associated with cancer, approximately 90% of patients had a hematologic malignancy.[304]

The hyperinfection syndrome results from penetration of filariform larvae through the intestinal mucosa, followed by dissemination. Sites of dissemination include the lungs, lymph nodes, brain, and abdominal organs. Secondary bacterial infection presumably results from passage of enteric bacteria through the bowel as a consequence of gastrointestinal strongyloidiasis, and may result in peritonitis, bacteremia, and meningitis.

Diagnosis of infection relies on visualization of larvae in feces, duodenal aspirates, sputum samples, or in other body fluids or tissue. Although uncommon, patients from endemic areas should be screened for *S stercoralis* carriage, ideally before receiving immunosuppressive agents. Obtaining multiple fresh stool samples increases the diagnostic yield. Patients with *S stercoralis* infection should be treated with thiabendazole or ivermectin.

EVALUATION AND MANAGEMENT OF FEBRILE NEUTROPENIA

Patients with cancer and neutropenic fever often have an established or an occult infection, and bacteremia is documented in approximately 20% of cases.[305] Because of the high likelihood of occult infection in a patient with febrile neutropenia without localizing symptoms or signs, and the potential for rapid progression to severe sepsis, prompt initiation of empiric antibiotics is essential. The likelihood of bacteremia is related to the intensity (with an ANC of less than 100/µL carrying the greatest risk) and the duration of neutropenia. A rapid decrease in the neutrophil count may also be a risk factor for infection, whereas evidence of marrow recovery even if the neutrophil count is still less than 500/µL, is a positive prognostic factor. For the purpose of this discussion, we use the following established criteria for neutropenic fever:

1. A single oral temperature of greater than 38.3°C (101°F) or greater than or equal to 38.0°C (100.4°F) over at least 1 hour.
2. ANC less than 500/µL or less than 1000/µL with predicted rapid decline to less than 500/µL.

Evaluation of the febrile neutropenic patient begins with a careful history and physical examination. A history of prior infectious complications associated with chemotherapy may be useful for risk stratification and selecting an empiric regimen. For example, a history of recent colitis caused by *Clostridium difficile* raises the likelihood of recurrent infection in a patient with fever and diarrhea. Prior invasive candidiasis or infection by one of the filamentous fungi may recur during subsequent neutropenic periods. The duration of neutropenia closely correlates with the risk of serious infectious complications, including the development of invasive fungal infections in patients with prolonged neutropenia (such as patients with leukemia and BMT recipients). Concomitant use of corticosteroid therapy raises the likelihood of opportunistic pathogens, such as *P carinii*, that characteristically afflict patients with defects in cell-mediated immunity. Epidemiologic exposures can provide useful clues for uncommon or rare pathogens. For example, swimming or fishing in fresh or brackish waters raises the possibility of infection by *Aeromonas hydrophilia*. Exposure to salt water increases the likelihood of infection by *Vibrio vulnificus*. Fever after a dog bite raisees the concern about infection by *Capnocytophaga canimorsus* (DF-2).

A meticulous physical examination is necessary, bearing in mind that typical signs of infection may be blunted or absent as a result of immunosuppression. Mucositis is commonly observed after chemotherapy and may be difficult to distinguish from gingivostomatitis caused by reactivation of HSV infection. The presence of thrush reflects compromise of cell-mediated immunity. In patients with prolonged neutropenia or who receive concomitant high-dose corticosteroid therapy, fungal infection of the palate, typically by Zygomycete or *Aspergillus* species, constitutes a surgical emergency. A black necrotic region is the most common sign of such infections. Palpation over the anterior sinuses and an ophthalmologic examination should be performed. A detailed inspection of the skin, including the nails, may disclose a lesion suggestive of systemic infection or a possible portal of entry. Examples include ecthyma gangrenosum caused by *P aeruginosa*, or erythematous papules caused by disseminated candidiasis. Catheter sites and sites of prior skin penetration (such as surgical wounds and biopsy sites) should be palpated. The perineum and perianal region are easily missed sources of infection that need careful inspection and palpation.

The initial evaluation should include the following: complete blood cell count and differential; serum chemistry, including liver associated enzymes; at least two sets of blood cultures from different sites (including from each lumen of the central venous catheter if one is present); a urine culture; and a chest radiograph. Potential sites of infection, such as skin lesions or sputum, should be obtained before instituting antibiotics. However, febrile neutropenia should be considered a medical emergency, and prompt initiation of empiric antibiotics should not be delayed if culture material is not immediately available. After the initial physical examination, it is critical to reevaluate the patient regularly to monitor the response to therapy and to identify evolving signs of infection that were not present during the initial encounter.

ANTIBIOTIC REGIMENS

In the early 1970s, Schimpff and colleagues conducted a nonrandomized study of 75 patients with cancer and febrile neutropenia who were treated empirically with carbenicillin and gentamicin.[306] Treated patients with *P aeruginosa* infection had dramatically improved survival rates compared with historic controls. This study established the rationale for empiric combination antibiotic therapy, based on the wide range of resistant profiles of *P aeruginosa* and enteric gram-negative rod isolates to carbenicillin. Empiric combination therapy increases the likelihood that at least one antibiotic will have activity against the isolate before the availability of susceptibility data. In addition, the β-lactam plus gentamicin combination has synergistic bactericidal activity *in vitro*. Since this early study, typical combination regimens for neutropenic fever have included an antipseudomonal penicillin plus an aminoglycoside with or without a drug with antistaphylococcal activity, such as a first-generation cephalosporin or vancomycin.

Since the mid-1980s, the development of broad-spectrum antipseudomonal antibiotics (ceftazidime and imipenem) with a high serum bactericidal level to minimal inhibitory concentration ratio has led to a reevaluation of the need for combination antibiotic therapy. Obviating the need for an aminoglycoside would be expected to reduce nephrotoxicity in a patient population frequently treated with nephrotoxic drugs, such as CSA, cisplatin, and amphotericin B. Pizzo et al.[307] conducted a randomized trial comparing ceftazidime monotherapy with a combination of cephalothin, gentamicin, and carbenicillin in 550 episodes of neutropenic fever in patients with cancer at the National Institutes of Health. Approximately 45% of patients had leukemias or lymphomas, and the remainder had solid tumors. The mean duration of neutropenia was 8 to 9 days. In patients with unexplained fever, 98% of patients in both groups survived by the time neutropenia resolved. Of the patients with documented infection, the survival rate was 89% in the monotherapy arm and 91% in the combination arm. Most patients with documented infections in both treatment arms required modifications in the initial antibiotic regimen, whereas the ini-

TABLE 54-6. Empirical Regimens for Neutropenic Fever

MONOTHERAPY
Ceftazidime
Cefepime
Imipenem
Meropenem
DUOTHERAPY
Ceftazidime plus an aminoglycoside
Cefepime plus an aminoglycoside
Antipseudomonal penicillin (e.g., piperacillin, ticarcillin, azlocillin) plus an aminoglycoside
Antipseudomonal penicillin plus ciprofloxacin
WHEN TO ADD VANCOMYCIN
Clinical instability
Isolation of a gram-positive pathogen from blood
β-Lactam allergy (can use vancomycin plus aztreonam; see text)
Severe mucositis (associated with cytosine arabinoside)[a]
Quinolone (ciprofloxacin, ofloxacin, norfloxacin) prophylaxis
Intravenous catheter-associated cellulitis or tunnel infection
Facilities with high prevalence of methicillin-resistant *Staphylococcus aureus*

[a]Vancomycin need not be added if a carbapenem is used, since these agents are highly active against oral gram-positive flora.

tial regimen was usually not modified in cases of no documented infection. This study was the first to establish that initial empiric monotherapy was safe and effective in this patient population. An important caveat is that patients must be closely monitored and the antibiotic regimen modified based on subsequent clinical and microbiologic data.

In a subsequent multicenter trial, De Pauw et al.[308] evaluated ceftazidime versus piperacillin plus tobramycin in approximately 800 episodes of neutropenic fever. The majority of patients had leukemia or were BMT recipients. The mean duration of neutropenia was 18 days. The two regimens were similar with regard to control of infections and infection-related mortality, but less adverse reactions occurred in the ceftazidime arm. This study confirmed that ceftazidime monotherapy is a viable empiric regimen in high-risk patients with febrile neutropenia. In a metaanalysis, ceftazidime monotherapy had similar efficacy as combination regimens for empiric treatment of neutropenic fever.[309]

Numerous studies of monotherapy and combination therapy have been conducted that further delineate the advantages and disadvantages of various empiric regimens for neutropenic fever. The Infectious Diseases Society of America (IDSA) has published evidence-based guidelines on antibiotic therapy for neutropenic fever without a documented source.[71] Initial antibiotic regimens are divided into three categories: (1) monotherapy, (2) duotherapy without vancomycin, and (3) vancomycin plus one or two drugs (Table 54-6).

MONOTHERAPY

The IDSA considered the following four antibiotics to be appropriate as empiric monotherapy for neutropenic fever: ceftazidime, cefepime, imipenem, and meropenem.[71] At the National Institutes of Health, ceftazidime monotherapy has been used since the 1980s in more than 1000 patients and has an excellent record in terms of efficacy and safety. Emergence of ceftazidime-resistant isolates has been infrequent. A disadvantage of ceftazidime monotherapy is the modest or absent activity against certain gram-positive pathogens (e.g., viridans streptococci, enterococci) and gram-negative pathogens with extended spectrum β-lactamases (most often encountered in *E coli* and *Klebsiella* species) and Bush group 1 β-lactamases (most commonly encountered in *Enterobacter, Serratia, Citrobacter*, and indole-positive *Proteus* species). The carbapenems (imipenem and meropenem) have a broader antibacterial spectrum that includes activity against these pathogens as well as potent activity against anaerobes.

In a randomized study of 399 episodes of neutropenic fever at the National Institutes of Health comparing ceftazidime with imipenem as initial therapy, the survival rate was approximately 98% for both regimens.[310] Forty-four percent of patients had leukemia or lymphoma, and the remainder had solid tumors. The mean duration of neutropenia was 9 days. Imipenem was associated with greater toxicity, including *Clostridium difficile*–associated diarrhea and nausea and vomiting.

In a study at M. D. Anderson Cancer Center, imipenem with and without amikacin was compared with ceftazidime with and without amikacin as initial therapy in 750 episodes of neutropenic fever.[311] The success rate (resolution of clinical and laboratory signs of infection without modification of the initial regimen) was poorest in the ceftazidime monotherapy arm (59%) but similar in the other three arms (71% to 76%). The majority of failures were due to coagulase-negative staphylococci and viridans streptococci. Nevertheless, overall mortality was less than 1%.

Cefepime is a fourth-generation cephalosporin with broad-spectrum activity appropriate for empiric therapy for neutropenic fever. In a study of activity of β-lactam antibiotics against gram-positive isolates from patients with cancer, cefepime had activity similar to imipenem and superior to ceftazidime.[312] Seventy-six percent of viridans streptococci were sensitive to cefepime versus 53% to ceftazidime. Ninety-eight percent of β-hemolytic streptococci were sensitive to cefepime versus 34% to ceftazidime. Cefepime has activity against greater than 95% of enteric aerobic gram-negative bacterial isolates harboring either Bush group 1 β-lactamases or extended spectrum β-lactamases.[313–315] In contrast, *Pseudomonas, Stenotrophomonas*, and *Acinetobacter* species resistant to ceftazidime are usually cross-resistant to cefepime.[315] Thus, in centers where ceftazidime-resistant Enterobacteriaceae are frequent, cefepime as empiric monotherapy for febrile neutropenia may be a viable option.

In a multicenter French study of 400 patients with neutropenic fever, empiric therapy with cefepime had similar survival compared with imipenem (95% vs. 98%, respectively), but caused less gastrointestinal toxicity.[316] In a study of 99 patients with febrile neutropenia, empiric cefepime therapy had similar efficacy compared with piperacillin plus gentamicin, but reduced nephrotoxicity.[317] Cefepime at a relatively high dose (2 g every 8 hours) is approved as monotherapy for empiric treatment of neutropenic fever.

Meropenem is a new carbapenem with a spectrum similar to that of imipenem, except for enhanced activity against gram-negative and less activity against gram-positive bacteria.[318] In a large multicenter study of 958 patients with febrile neutropenia, meropenem monotherapy was as effective as ceftazidime plus amikacin as initial empiric therapy.[319] The survival rate was 98% in the meropenem arm and 97% in the combination arm, and the proportion of adverse side effects was low in both groups. The mean duration of neutropenia, defined as an ANC less than 1000/μl, was 16 to 17 days. Bacteremia occurred in 10% of patients in the meropenem arm and in 7% of patients in the combination arm. Meropenem monotherapy was safe and effective for neutropenic fever in two other European studies compared with ceftazidime[320] and ceftazidime plus amikacin.[321] Meropenem appears to have less gastrointestinal toxicity than imipenem and a lower frequency of seizures. Thus, meropenem appears to be an appropriate alternative to imipenem in febrile neutropenic patients.

DUOTHERAPY WITHOUT VANCOMYCIN

The standard duotherapy regimen for empiric therapy of neutropenic fever is a broad-spectrum antipseudomonal β-lactam plus an aminoglycoside. The β-lactam/aminoglycoside synergy was thought to be important in effecting a rapid resolution of bacteremia. In addition, duotherapy increases the likelihood of the isolate being sensitive to at least one of the agents.

The hypothesis that a synergistic antibiotic regimen is superior to monotherapy as empiric treatment of neutropenic fever has not been validated in prospective clinical studies. In fact, ceftazidime singly has greater serum bactericidal activity against gram-negative bacteria compared with ticarcillin plus amikacin.[322]

Combination therapy using two β-lactam agents should generally not be used. The fact that some β-lactams may also be β-lactamase inducers raises concern about such combinations. This concern does not apply when an antistaphylococcal penicillin (e.g., oxacillin) is paired with an antipseudomonal β-lactam agent (e.g., ceftazidime).

Pairing an antipseudomonal β-lactam with a quinolone is yet another combination regimen used for neutropenic fever. The rationale of such a combination is to provide broad-spectrum activity against highly resistant gram-negative pathogens. In a small randomized study, piperacillin plus ciprofloxacin led to more rapid defervescence and reduced requirement for empiric amphotericin B compared with piperacillin plus gentamicin.[323] Other studies showed that azlocillin plus ciprofloxacin had similar efficacy compared with a β-lactam plus an aminoglycoside.[324,325]

An aminoglycoside as the sole agent active against gram-negative bacteria is not recommended because of the high failure rate. Ceftriaxone plus an aminoglycoside, which has the potential for single daily dosing, has been shown to be effective in some studies.[326–328] However, ceftriaxone does not have reliable activity against *P aeruginosa*. Therefore, in centers where this pathogen is encountered, the ceftriaxone plus aminoglycoside regimen may be suboptimal. In centers with a high frequency of Enterobacteriaceae resistant to third-generation cephalosporins, we advise against using empiric aztreonam as the sole agent active against gram-negative bacteria because of the likelihood of cross-resistance (see Table 54-3).

Today, with the availability of highly effective monotherapy regimens for neutropenic fever, initial empiric duotherapy regimens may be most appropriate in unstable patients and in institutions in which multidrug-resistant pathogens are frequently encountered.

WHEN TO ADD VANCOMYCIN

The rationale to add vancomycin to an empiric regimen for neutropenic fever stems from the increased proportion of infections by gram-positive bacteria. The change in the proportion of infections in neutropenic patients from predominantly gram-negative to gram-positive bacteria is associated with the widespread use of tunneled catheters in this patient population. Catheter-associated infection by coagulase-negative staphylococci has become the most common cause of bacteremia in patients with cancer.

Among the common gram-positive infections in neutropenic patients, the following are typically resistant to ceftazidime: MRSA, coagulase-negative *Staphylococcus* species, and *Enterococcus* species. In addition, although ceftazidime has *in vitro* activity against most viridans streptococci, serious infection by these pathogens has occurred in neutropenic patients receiving ceftazidime.[70,329]

Numerous studies have evaluated single and multiple drug regimens with and without vancomycin. In the largest study, ceftazidime plus amikacin with and without vancomycin were compared in 747 patients with febrile neutropenia in Europe and Canada.[330] The addition of vancomycin to the empiric regimen was not associated with any benefit with regard to duration of fever or morbidity or mortality related to gram-positive infections. Smaller studies of ceftazidime with or without an aminoglycoside also showed no benefit from adding vancomycin to the initial regimen.[331,332]

Because of the lack of efficacy of routine addition of vancomycin to empiric regimens for neutropenic fever, and because of the emergence of VRE in association with excessive vancomycin use, the IDSA guidelines have advised against the routine use of vancomycin as initial empiric therapy of neutropenic fever.[71] At institutions in which MRSA is common or if a patient is known to be colonized by MRSA, vancomycin should be included in the initial regimen for neutropenic fever. Erythema or tenderness at a catheter site requires the addition of vancomycin while awaiting culture results. Addition of vancomycin is reasonable in patients receiving prophylaxis with ciprofloxacin, which some studies have associated with breakthrough infections by viridans streptococci (see Viridans Streptococci, earlier in this chapter). The IDSA suggests the addition of vancomycin in patients with substantial mucosal damage from chemotherapy (such as regimens containing high-dose Ara-C) because of the added risk of infection by viridans streptococci. Empiric vancomycin should be discontinued after 2 days if the initial culture results are negative or show a pathogen, such as methicillin-sensitive *S aureus*, for which other antibiotics can be used.

In neutropenic febrile patients with allergies to β-lactams, empiric vancomycin should be combined with antibiotics active against aerobic gram-negative pathogens. In a clinically stable neutropenic patient, vancomycin plus aztreonam is a reasonable regimen[333,334] (see Table 54-6). Aztreonam monotherapy is not acceptable because it has no activity against gram-positive bacteria.

DURATION OF ANTIBACTERIAL THERAPY

Resolution of Fever within First 3 Days of Treatment and Persistent Neutropenia

If the fever rapidly abates after initiation of empiric therapy in a patient with an unremarkable physical examination and negative culture results, one should assume that an occult infection exists that has responded to antibiotics. Pizzo et al.[335] randomized patients with prolonged neutropenia and an undifferentiated fever to either discontinuing empiric antibiotics on day 7 of therapy or continuing therapy until resolution of neutropenia. Of patients who had become afebrile, 40% had recurrent fever after antibiotics were stopped, leading to the conclusion that day 7 of therapy was too early to stop antibiotics in the setting of persistent neutropenia. Discontinuation of antibiotics on day 14 of therapy is a reasonable practice among patients who remain afebrile during therapy, but who are still neutropenic.[336]

Since these early studies, attempts have been made to identify low-risk patients in whom early discharge on an oral regimen could be safely done while still neutropenic. In a retrospective series of 509 pediatric patients with neutropenic fever, lack of signs of sepsis on admission (chills, hypotension, requirement for intravenous hydration), ANC greater than 100 μL, and resolution of fever within 48 hours of therapy accurately distinguished patients who could be discharged on oral agents.[337] Buchanan's group reported that antibiotics could be safely discontinued and that early discharge was feasible in neutropenic pediatric patients who had become afebrile if there were no signs of infection, culture results were negative, and evidence of early marrow recovery existed.[338,339]

Based on these studies, the IDSA guidelines advise that low-risk patients with undifferentiated neutropenic fever who have become afebrile within 3 days of initiation of empiric parenteral antibiotics can be treated with an oral regimen (cefixime or quinolone) and discharged while still neutropenic.[71] In high-risk patients who become afebrile within 3 days, the IDSA recommends continuing parenteral antibiotics. If the high-risk patient remains afebrile and persistently neutropenic after 2 weeks of therapy, antibiotics can be stopped if no signs of infection exist.[71]

One difficulty in applying such guidelines is the lack of a uniform definition of low- and high-risk patients. The IDSA guidelines define low risk as appearing clinically well, absence of mucositis or unstable signs, and an ANC greater than 100/μL.[71] Several investigators consider whether the ANC is rising or falling and the anticipated rate of myeloid recovery to also be important predictors of risk. Talcott et al.[340,341] developed a risk prediction model to distinguish low- and high-risk groups with febrile neutropenia, which is further discussed in Outpatient Antibiotic Therapy for Neutropenic Fever, later in this chapter.

Persistent Fever in the Neutropenic Patient

After selection of an initial empiric regimen for neutropenic fever, close observation of the patient is necessary. Throughout the duration of neutropenic fever, daily physical examination should be performed. Modifications of the initial antibiotic regimen should be made on the basis of new physical examination findings pointing to a previously inapparent focus of infection, and radiographic and culture data.[342] If no source of infection is documented, the initial empiric antibacterial regimen need not be changed solely on the basis of persistent fever in a clinically stable patient (see Empiric Antifungal Therapy, later in this chapter). Antibiotic therapy should be continued for the duration of neutropenic fever.

New symptoms and signs of infection in neutropenic patients may be subtle and should be aggressively investigated (Table 54-7). A new erythematous papular lesion may provide initial evidence for isolated cutaneous or disseminated infection by bacterial or fungal pathogens, and biopsy and culture are necessary. Catheter exit sites, surgical wounds, and biopsy sites should be meticulously inspected and palpated for signs of infection. In the neutropenic patient, fever and local tenderness may be the only signs of infection. A diffuse maculopapular rash is suggestive of a drug etiology, but a culture should be performed to rule out an infectious etiology. Blurred vision may represent keratitis or endophthalmitis caused by bacterial, viral, or candidal species, or a CNS process. Careful optical evaluation, corneal scrapings, and aspiration of the vitreous may be needed to establish the diagnosis. Sinopulmonary symptoms in a persistently neutropenic patient (longer than 10 days) or in a patient receiving high-dose corticosteroid therapy are worrisome for a fungal infection. A CT scan is more sensitive and provides superior anatomic delineation of disease than plain radiographs. Aspiration or biopsy of lesions should be performed when feasible. Abdominal pain and tenderness, typically in the right lower quadrant, raises the possibility of typhlitis. Tenesmus suggests a rectal, perineal, or prostatic infection. In cases of suspected bowel or perianal infection, the antibiotic regimen should have broad-spectrum activity against anaerobes, such as imipenem or meropenem alone, or ceftazidime plus metronidazole. Because of the large differential diagnosis of causes of persistent fever in neutropenic patients, a systematic checklist of symptoms and signs should be evaluated daily. Table 54-6 summarizes the management of commonly encountered scenarios in neutropenic fever.

We suggest that two sets of blood cultures from different sites be obtained daily in patients with persistent neutropenic fever to avoid delay in making appropriate modifications to the antibiotic regimen in cases of superinfection during neutropenia. For pathogens that are not reliably isolated from the blood (such as fungal species), frequent collection of blood cultures may increase the likelihood of making an earlier diagnosis. In addition, the common use of deep, central catheters makes line infection an ever present and easily detected cause of fever.

TABLE 54-7. Diagnostic Evaluation and Modifications of Therapy during Neutropenia

Findings	*Evaluation and Modifications*
Persistent neutropenic fever (5–7 d)	Add empiric antifungal therapy (amphotericin B, 0.5–0.6 mg/kg/d, lipid formulation of amphotericin B or fluconazole 400mg/d). If fluconazole initially added, change to amphotericin B if neutropenic fever persists for 3 more days without a source.
Recurrent fever on day 14 or greater of neutropenia without a source and while receiving broad-spectrum antibacterial agents	Suspect fungal infection. Empirical amphotericin B (0.5–0.6 mg/kg/d) or lipid formulation. Consider chest computed tomographic scan to evaluate for fungal infection. If suggestive of mold infection, attempt to establish a culture diagnosis by sputum, BAL, or biopsy. If study results are not diagnostic, treat with amphotericin B (1.0–1.5 mg/kg/d) or lipid formulation.
Persistent or recurrent fever without a source at time of myeloid recovery	Consider hepatosplenic candidiasis (see text).
Blood culture obtained before starting empirical antibiotics for neutropenic fever	
Gram positive	Add vancomycin.
Gram negative	If patient stable, continue initial regimen; if unstable, replace ceftozidime (if used initially) with imipenem and add an aminoglycoside. Modify regimen once identification and sensitivities are known.

(continued)

TABLE 54-7. *(Continued)*

Findings	*Evaluation and Modifications*
Positive blood culture result while receiving antibacterial therapy	
Gram positive	Add vancomycin.
Gram negative	Suspect a resistant pathogen based on initial empiric regimen. If ceftazidime used initially, suspect extended spectrum β-lactamase or cephalosporinase; switch to imipenem and add an aminoglycoside. If imipenem used initially, consider *Stenotrophomonas maltophilia* or resistant *Pseudomonas* sp.; add a ciprofloxacin plus trimethoprim-sulfamethoxazole. Modify regimen once identification and sensitivities known.
Head and neck	
Necrotizing gingivitis	If ceftazidime or cefepime used in initial regimen, change to carbapenem for anaerobic coverage.
Oral ulcerative or vesicular lesions	Culture for herpes simplex virus. For documented or suspected mucocutaneous herpes simplex virus, acyclovir, 5 mg/kg q8h.
Sinus tenderness	Suspect aerobic gram-negative rod (Enterobacteriaceae and *Pseudomonas aeruginosa*). With prolonged neutropenia (greater than or equal to 10 days) or concomitant high-dose glucocorticosteroids, mold infections become more likely (*Aspergillus* sp., agents of zygomycosis, *Fusarium* sp.). Examine palate and nasal mucosa for signs of invasive infection. Computed tomographic scan if no improvement after 2–3 d of antibacterial agents to guide diagnostic and therapeutic drainage.
Respiratory tract	
Upper respiratory symptoms	Screen for community respiratory viruses.
New focal infiltrate after resolution of neutropenia	May be inflammatory response to old infection. If asymptomatic, observe; if symptomatic and not responding to antibacterial agents, consider BAL and biopsy.
New focal infiltrate while neutropenic	Suspect resistant bacteria or filamentous fungal infection. If sputum and BAL are nondiagnostic, start empiric amphotericin B (1.0–1.5 mg/kg/d) or lipid formulation.
Diffuse infiltrate	In patients receiving concomitant glucocorticosteroids, suspect *Pneumocystis carinii*. Community respiratory viruses, bacterial pneumonias, and noninfectious causes (e.g., hemorrhage, respiratory distress syndrome, drug toxicity) also possible. Urgent BAL recommended.
Gastrointestinal tract	
Retrosternal burning, odynophagia	Consider esophagitis. Suspect *Candida* and herpes simplex virus esophagitis. Bacterial esophagitis (and cytomegalovirus in bone marrow transplant recipients) also possible. Add fluconazole (400 mg oral or IV) and acyclovir (5 mg/kg q8h IV) empirically. If no response in 2–3 d, consider endoscopy.
Acute abdominal pain	Differential diagnosis includes same etiologies as in nonneutropenic patient (e.g., cholecystitis, appendicitis) plus typhlitis (neutropenic colitis). Ensure that antibiotic regimen has adequate anaerobic activity (e.g., ceftazidime or cefepime plus metronidazole; imipenem monotherapy). Bowel rest. Abdominal computed tomographic scan. Monitor need for surgical intervention (see text).
Perirectal tenderness	Broaden antibiotic regimen to include anaerobic activity. Local care. Monitor need for surgical drainage (see text).
Central venous catheter	
Exit site cellulitis	Add vancomycin.
Tunnel infection	Add vancomycin; remove catheter.
Collection around catheter	Incise and drain; if infected, add appropriate antibiotics and remove catheter.
Local infection by *Aspergillus* sp. or *Mycobacterium* sp.	Remove catheter. Local débridement. May require excision of tunnel tract. Add appropriate antimicrobial agents (see text).
Catheter-associated bacteremia	Add appropriate antibiotics. Remove catheter for infection by a highly resistant bacterial pathogen (e.g., *Bacillus* sp., *Corynebacterium* JK, *Mycobacterium* sp., possibly *Candida* sp.; see text). Catheter must be removed for infections refractory to antimicrobial agents or hemodynamic instability.

BAL, bronchoalveolar lavage.
(Modified from ref. 368.)

Empiric Antifungal Therapy

The rationale for empiric antifungal therapy for persistent febrile neutropenia is that meticulous clinical examination and collection of cultures are not sufficiently sensitive for early detection of fungal infections.[123] Before standard implementation of empiric antifungal therapy, there was a correlation between prolonged neutropenic fever and mortality in patients with cancer, and fungal infection was frequently found at autopsy. Two randomized prospective studies showed empiric amphotericin B was associated with fewer serious fungal infections in antibiotic-treated neutropenic patients with persistent fever.[343,344] Because fungal infections are uncommonly encountered in the first 7 days of neutropenic fever, empiric amphotericin B (0.5 to 0.6 mg/kg daily) is typically begun between days 4 and 7 of neutropenic fever (Table 54-7). Empiric antifungal therapy should be continued for the duration of neutropenia. The potential role of lipid formulations of amphotericin B and antifungal azoles are discussed in Antifungal Agents, earlier in this chapter.

Persistent Fever after Resolution of Neutropenia

In most cases, an undifferentiated fever that has persisted during neutropenia will resolve around the time of myeloid recovery. In a minority of patients, a fever of unknown origin persists for several days after myeloid recovery. Similar to the neutropenic period, evaluation of fever after myeloid recovery begins with a methodic evaluation of both noninfectious causes, such as drug fever (e.g., recombinant growth factors, β-lactam antibiotics), transfusion reactions, and deep venous thrombosis, as well as infectious causes.

A careful physical examination may show a site of infection that was inapparent during neutropenia, such as a perirectal process. A chest radiograph should be obtained because pulmonary infection may not be apparent radiographically during neutropenia. Blood and urine cultures, complete blood cell count, serum chemistry, and liver enzymes should be obtained. An elevated alkaline phosphatase should prompt consideration of hepatosplenic candidiasis, even if blood culture results were negative for *Candida* species. A CT scan, magnetic resonance imaging, and ultrasound are complementary imaging modalities and may show discrete bull's-eye lesions (see Candidiasis, earlier in this chapter).

In contrast to the neutropenic period, empiric antibiotics can be discontinued after resolution of neutropenia in patients who are stable with an undifferentiated fever and negative culture data. If a source of infection is known, then antibiotic therapy targeted to the specific pathogen(s), rather than broad-spectrum empiric regimens used for neutropenic fever, is advised.

OUTPATIENT ANTIBIOTIC THERAPY FOR NEUTROPENIC FEVER

Because of the high morbidity and mortality in febrile neutropenic patients and the need for emergent institution of systemic antibacterial therapy, hospital admission has been regarded as necessary, and inpatient observation was typically continued until resolution of neutropenia. More recent studies have shown that patients with febrile neutropenia can be stratified according to their risk of developing major or life-threatening infectious complications. Prospective randomized studies have suggested that patients in the lowest risk group are reasonable candidates for carefully monitored empiric outpatient antibiotic therapy.

Patients with a duration of neutropenia of 7 days or less are considered to be at low risk for serious infectious complications. In a study of 590 patients with neutropenia and an undifferentiated fever who had defervesced after initiation of empiric antibiotics, the risk for recurrent fever was directly related to the duration of neutropenia. Among patients with less than 7 days of neutropenia, only 0.6% developed a recurrent fever. The frequency of recurrent fever was 4% when the duration of neutropenia was 7 to 14 days and 38% when the duration of neutropenia exceeded 14 days.[345] Patients with neutropenia of 7 days or less were also far less likely to require modifications in the initial antibiotic regimen compared with patients with neutropenia lasting longer than 14 days.[346] Therefore, patients with long-duration neutropenia are less able to contain ongoing infections or are more likely to develop new infections (or both) after initiation of appropriate empiric antibiotics.[342]

Talcott et al.[340,341] developed a risk prediction model of serious complications and mortality in patients with febrile neutropenia based on a retrospective analysis of 261 patients and validated prospectively in 444 patients with cancer and febrile neutropenia. The following features predicted a high risk of substantial morbidity (25% to 40%) and mortality (12% to 18%): (1) inpatient status at time of fever and neutropenia (mostly made up of patients with hematologic malignancy or BMT recipients); (2) outpatients with concurrent comorbidity (hypotension, organ dysfunction, altered mentation, uncontrolled bleeding, and so forth); and (3) outpatients with uncontrolled progressive malignancy. In contrast, outpatients without significant comorbidity and with controlled malignancy had a low rate of morbidity (2% to 5%) and no infection-related mortality.

Talcott's group subsequently studied 30 low-risk patients with primarily hematologic malignancies and febrile neutropenia at the Dana Farber Cancer Center.[347] Standard intravenous antibiotics were administered for the initial 2 days as inpatients, followed by home antibiotic therapy with gentamicin plus either mezlocillin or ceftazidime. Patients with documented infections were excluded. Only 16 (53%) patients responded to the initial antibiotic regimen; nine (30%) patients were readmitted; and four (13%) patients had serious complications, including hypotension, renal failure, disseminated fungal infection, and coagulase-negative *Staphylococcus* bacteremia. No patient died, but the incidence of serious complications and the high admission rate in this pilot study suggested that criteria for selecting patients for outpatient therapy required further refinement.

Malik et al.[348] conducted a prospective, randomized study comparing oral ofloxacin with combination parenteral antibiotics (amikacin plus carbenicillin, cloxacillin, or piperacillin) in 122 hospitalized febrile neutropenic patients in Pakistan. This study was not confined to low-risk patients. Approximately two-thirds of patients had a hematologic malignancy or aplastic anemia, and the mean duration of neutropenia was 9 days. The overall response to antibiotics was 77% in the oral arm and 73% in the parenteral arm. Mortality in the oral group and parenteral groups were similar (7% and 10%, respectively).

This group subsequently compared oral ofloxacin administered in the outpatient versus the inpatient setting in 169 patients with febrile neutropenia.[349] Only low-risk patients as generally defined by the Talcott criteria were enrolled. Two-thirds of patients had solid tumors, and the remainder had hematologic malignancies. The mean duration of neutropenia was 5 days. Approximately 80% of outpatients and inpatients responded to ofloxacin monotherapy, and 20% of patients randomized to the outpatient group were subsequently admitted for parenteral antibiotics. Successful treatment with ofloxacin was more likely in cases in which no source of fever was documented by cultures or physical examination. Mortality in the group initially treated as outpatients was 4% versus 2% in the initial inpatient group.

Hidalgo et al.[350] compared outpatient-administered oral ofloxacin with inpatient-administered parenteral ceftazidime and amikacin in a prospective, randomized trial in 95 low-risk febrile neutropenic patients with solid tumors. The median duration of neutropenia was 3 to 4 days. Treatment failure, defined as fever persisting for 3 days or longer, a second febrile episode, or progression of infection, occurred in 10% and 8% of patients in the oral and parenteral arms, respectively. Eight patients in the oral arm were admitted for parenteral therapy, five because of treatment failure and three because of positive blood culture results. No death or serious complication occurred in those randomized to the oral arm, and one (2%) death occurred in the parenteral arm.

Rubenstein et al.[351] compared outpatient oral ciprofloxacin (750 mg three times a day) plus clindamycin with parenteral clindamycin and aztreonam in 83 low-risk febrile neutropenic patients with solid tumors or leukemia at M. D. Anderson Cancer Center. Patients were observed for 2 hours, then both oral and parenteral groups were sent home to complete therapy. The response rate (defined as resolution of clinical and laboratory evidence of infection) was 88% in the oral arm and 95% in the parenteral arm. Of the 20% in both groups who had bacteremia, five of seven in the oral arm and seven of eight in the parenteral arm responded to initial antimicrobial therapy. Six patients in the oral arm and none in the intravenous arm were admitted. No mortality or severe complications occurred in either group. The oral arm had additional renal toxicity, perhaps related to dehydration, the relatively high dose of ciprofloxacin, or both. The authors considered the parenteral regimen to have greater safety than the oral one.

Subsequently, the oral regimen was changed to ciprofloxacin (500 mg) plus amoxicillin/clavulanate (500 mg) every 8 hours, and the parenteral regimen was unchanged in a study of 179 patients with mostly solid tumors. Outcomes were similar, with 90% and 87% response rates in the oral and parenteral arms, respectively. Patients with solid tumors had higher response rates than those with hematologic malignancies. All patients survived without major infectious complications or antibiotic-related toxicity.

In general, these studies are encouraging about the safety of outpatient antibiotic therapy for low-risk patients with neutropenic fever (see references 352, 353, and 354 for more detailed reviews). However, important limitations exist in making broad conclusions. The prospective, randomized studies described previously individually each enrolled fewer than 200 patients, and therefore lacked sufficient power to detect small differences between treatment groups. Pooling data from different studies as a metaanalysis is made difficult by the differences in eligibility criteria, choice of antibiotics, criteria for hospital admission, and criteria for a successful outcome.

The National Cancer Institute and H. Lee Moffitt Cancer Center compared an oral regimen consisting of ciprofloxacin plus amoxicillin-clavulanate with intravenous ceftazidime alone in patients with febrile neutropenia in whom the expected duration of neutropenia was less than or equal to 10 days from the onset of fever.[355] All patients were hospitalized for the entire duration of neutropenic fever. A total of 116 episodes of neutropenic fever were evaluated. Approximately 75% of patients had solid tumors, and the remainder had leukemia or lymphoma. The mean duration of neutropenia in both groups was 3 to 4 days. Approximately two-thirds of febrile episodes were unexplained, and blood stream infections occurred in only 7% of episodes. Serious complications, such as hypotension or intraabdominal infection, were rarely encountered. Breakthrough infections associated with bacteremia, oral, or soft tissue infections were also rare in both groups and were controlled by modifications in the antibiotic regimen. There were no deaths.

In a European multicenter study of febrile neutropenia (defined as ANC less than 1000/μL), patients with an expected duration of neutropenia of less than or equal to 10 days were randomized to receive either oral ciprofloxacin plus amoxicillin-clavulanate or intravenous ceftriaxone plus amikacin.[356] A total of 312 patients were evaluated, approximately 70% with a solid tumor and the remainder with a hematologic malignancy. The median duration of neutropenia after antibiotics was 4 days. Two patients in the oral group and six patients in the intravenous group died of infection. At day 30 after randomization, survival was approximately 95% in both groups. Bacteremia occurred in less than 15% of patients in both groups. The duration of fever, duration of therapy, and need for modification of the initial regimen were similar in both groups.

These two well-designed studies clearly establish that for carefully selected patients with febrile neutropenia, an oral regimen consisting of ciprofloxacin plus amoxicillin-clavulanate is safe and effective. Both studies evaluated lower risk patients, but the inclusion of patients with hematologic malignancies and patients with an expected duration of neutropenia as high as 10 days after the onset of fever reflect more liberal criteria for risk stratification. Patients with comorbidities predictive of a higher risk of complications (e.g., hemodynamic instability; neurologic, hepatic, respiratory, or renal impairment; catheter infections; inability to take oral medications) were excluded. In addition, these studies were conducted in hospitalized patients and, therefore, extrapolations should not be made about the feasibility of this oral regimen in the outpatient setting.

The greatest concern about outpatient management of neutropenic fever relates to the possibility of life-threatening complications that may be reversible if detected early and appropriate interventions are made immediately (e.g., intravenous fluid, vasopressors, broadening of antibiotic coverage). Randomized clinical trials with sufficient statistical power are required to more precisely stratify patients for whom outpatient management of neutropenic fever is safe and to delineate optimal antibiotic regimens (oral versus parenteral) for different patient groups.

ANTIBACTERIAL PROPHYLAXIS IN AFEBRILE NEUTROPENIC PATIENTS

Despite improvements in antibacterial agents used in febrile neutropenia, persistent and profound neutropenia remains the most important predictor of life-threatening infections. Prophylactic agents administered at the onset of neutropenia therefore have potential appeal as a means of reducing the incidence of infections during this high-risk period. However, the concern for emergence of antibiotic-resistant bacteria plus the lack of a survival benefit associated with antibacterial prophylaxis led to the reasonable recommendation against routine prophylaxis in neutropenic patients by the IDSA.[71]

Today, antibacterial prophylaxis for neutropenia is largely restricted to quinolones and trimethoprim-sulfamethoxazole. These agents have activity against Enterobacteriaceae without significant activity against commensal intestinal anaerobes, thus providing selective decontamination of the gut. The rationale for selective, as opposed to global, suppression of gut flora is based on the concept of colonization resistance. In human studies, maintenance of the normal commensal intestinal flora provides a potent barrier to acquisition of pathogenic aerobic gram-negative rods.[357] Thus, it has been argued that an ideal prophylactic antibiotic regimen selectively targets aerobic gram-negative bacteria without inducing alterations in the normal intestinal microflora. Quinolones and trimethoprim-sulfamethoxazole have the added advantage of achieving high serum and tissue levels after oral administration, an important consideration given that multiple portals of bacterial invasion exist in neutropenic patients.

Two meta-analyses have been conducted on trials of fluoroquinolone prophylaxis in neutropenic patients.[358,359] The more recent study evaluated 18 trials with 1408 patients in which quinolones were compared with either placebo or trimethoprim-sulfamethoxazole.[358] Patients who received quinolones had 79% fewer gram-negative infections than those without prophylaxis, leading to an overall 46% reduction in total infections. The reduction in fever was small, and in blinded trials, was not significant. Quinolones were more effective than trimethoprim-sulfamethoxazole in preventing gram-negative infections. Prophylaxis with either agent did not affect mortality.

The frequencies of quinolone-resistant gram-negative isolates, gram-positive infections, and fungal infections were not significantly affected by quinolone prophylaxis in the metaanalysis.[358] However, a note of caution is required. Although quinolones have remained particularly effective at preventing gram-negative bacterial infections, quinolone-resistant gram-negative infections have developed during prophylaxis at several centers.[358] Among gram-positive pathogens, viridans streptococcal bacteremia is of particular concern in patients receiving quinolone prophylaxis (see Viridans Streptococci, earlier in this chapter).

To try to overcome the inadequate activity of quinolones against gram-positive bacteria, combination prophylactic regimens have been used. One large randomized study showed that addition of penicillin to a quinolone (pefloxacin) reduced the rate of bacteremia, especially that due to streptococcal species, compared with the quinolone alone.[360] Another randomized study showed that the combination of prophylactic ofloxacin and rifampin led to a reduction in gram-positive infections compared with ofloxacin alone.[361] However, addition of these agents to quinolone prophylaxis, of course, defeats the concept of selective decontamination. Newer generation quinolones with enhanced activity against streptococci are potential candidates for prophylaxis and warrant further study.

If prophylactic ciprofloxacin is used, vancomycin should be considered in the initial empiric regimen for neutropenic fever based on the high likelihood of breakthrough gram-positive infections. Vancomycin plus ceftazidime is a logical combination in this setting.

Trimethoprim-sulfamethoxazole as prophylaxis against *P carinii* in children with acute lymphocytic leukemia was also highly effective as prophylaxis against bacterial infections and sepsis.[289] More recent studies comparing trimethoprim-sulfamethoxazole with placebo have yielded inconsistent results. This discrepancy may reflect the emergence of resistant gram-negative bacteria during trimethoprim-sulfamethoxazole prophylaxis. In comparative studies, trimethoprim-sulfamethoxazole has, in general, been shown to be less effective than quinolones with regard to protection against gram-negative infections.[358] Other disadvantages of trimethoprim-sulfamethoxazole prophylaxis include lack of activity against *P aeruginosa*, potential suppression and delay of myeloid recovery, and hypersensitivity reactions. The main advantage of trimethoprim-sulfamethoxazole over quinolones relates to effective prophylaxis against *P carinii*. Although *P carinii* is rarely associated with isolated neutropenia, other comorbid conditions (such as AIDS) and regimens that contain intensive corticosteroid therapy predispose to infection by this organism (see *Pneumocystis carinii*, earlier in this chapter). Trimethoprim-sulfamethoxazole may also reduce the frequency of nocardiosis, listeriosis, and toxoplasmosis in persons with compromised T-cell immunity.

PROTECTED ENVIRONMENTS

The rationale for protective environments for neutropenic patients is derived from the same principle as selective decontamination by prophylactic antibiotics. By reducing the frequency of colonization by virulent bacteria, a germ-free environment was considered to be important in protecting neutropenic patients from infection.

However, it became clear that such stringent measures were not necessary for the majority of neutropenic patients. Nauseef and Maki[362] compared protective isolation (single room and use of gowns, gloves, and masks) with standard hospital care in hospitalized neutropenic patients with acute nonlymphocytic leukemia. Neither group received prophylactic antibiotics or sterilized food. The two groups were similar with respect to incidence of infection and days with fever. Paradoxically, the rate of bacteremia was higher in patients randomized to protective isolation. The availability of more effective antibacterial agents, the shift in predominance of infections from gram-negative to gram-positive pathogens in neutropenic patients, and the lack of evidence supporting the benefit of protective isolation have led to the adoption of less stringent methods of isolation at most centers. The cost and excess labor required to maintain stringent isolation and the additional emotional burden that patients and families must endure further militates against the routine use of such measures.

Isolation of aerobic gram-negative bacteria from food in hospitals is well known.[363] Uncooked vegetables often contain relatively large burdens of *E coli*, *Klebsiella* species, and *P aeruginosa*.[364] Thus, although not validated by controlled studies, it is reasonable to omit such foods from the diets of neutropenic patients. Similarly, tap water can harbor *P aeruginosa* and *Legionella* species. Careful hand washing before and after patient contacts remains the most effective method for preventing nosocomial infection.[365]

Laminar air flow units with high-efficiency particulate air filtration is the most effective means of removing aerosolized bacteria and fungal spores.[366] With more effective antimicrobial agents used today as empiric therapy for neutropenic fever, it is unclear that such protected environments are of benefit for most neutropenic patients. The high cost of maintaining such units makes them impractical for routine use for all neutropenic patients at most centers.[367] Today, the principal benefit of laminar air flow units is likely to be protection against *Aspergillus* species and other filamentous fungi. From a practical standpoint, they are usually restricted to patients at high risk for infection by molds (e.g., patients with leukemia and BMT recipients).

MANIFESTATIONS AND THERAPY OF INFECTIONS

BACTEREMIA

Bacteremia is a common complication of antineoplastic myeloablative chemotherapy. In a review of empiric antimicrobial regimens for neutropenic fever, the dominant risk factor for bacteremia was the duration of neutropenia.[305] Neutropenia lasting 1 to 5 days before trial entry was associated with a relative risk of bacteremia of 5.2 compared with no neutropenia; neutropenia of 6 to 15 days had a relative risk of 7.35. Patients with a hematologic disease and BMT recipients were also more likely to have bacteremia than patients with solid tumors. The presence of shock was highly predictive of bacteremia with a relative risk of 5.6.

In patients with suspected systemic infection, a meticulous physical examination and culture of all potential sources of infection should ideally be done before initiation of antibiotics. If it is not feasible to obtain all culture material at the time of initial evaluation, however, empiric antibiotic therapy should not be delayed. Cultures should be obtained from blood and urine, and depending on the clinical situation, from sputum, pleural fluid, and peritoneal fluid. Wounds and skin lesions should be aspirated or biopsied, and material submitted for culture. Particularly in neutropenic patients, the appearance of wounds may be deceptively benign without erythema or purulence.

Once a positive blood culture result is reported, the initial antibiotic therapy may need to be altered (see Table 54-7). Coagulase-negative *Staphylococcus* species and *Corynebacterium* (diphtheroid) species are common blood culture contaminants. However, patients with cancer often have indwelling intravenous catheters, which can be portals of entry for these bacteria, thereby increasing the risk of bacteremia. The likelihood of contamination is increased if these organisms are isolated from a single blood culture. It is therefore important to draw at least two sets of blood cultures from separate sites. *Corynebacterium jeikeium* is a virulent species associated with bacteremia and disseminated organ infection; isolation of this organism from a single blood culture requires prompt initiation of vancomycin therapy. Similarly, isolation of *S aureus* from a single blood culture (or from the urine in a febrile or septic appearing patient) should be considered to represent hematogenous infection.

If a gram-negative organism is isolated from a blood culture collected before the initiation of antibiotics, an appropriate parenteral regimen used empirically at the onset of neutropenic fever can be maintained while awaiting drug sensitivity data so long as the patient is clinically stable.[368] The rationale is that standard empiric antibiotic regimens for neutropenic fever and the specific regimen adopted at a given institution are selected to provide reliable coverage against all likely gram-negative pathogens. If the patient is not stable or if the gram-negative organism is isolated after initiation of antibiotics (i.e., breakthrough bacteremia), change to a new regimen is warranted (see Table 54-7 for specific suggestions). Once antibiotic susceptibilities are known, therapy should be tailored appropriately.

Shock and multiple organ dysfunction are dreaded complications of sepsis. In patients with neutropenia, prompt initiation of broad-spectrum antibiotics directed against commonly encountered blood-borne pathogens is essential (e.g., *S aureus*, viridans streptococci, Enterobacteriaceae, and *P aeruginosa*). Unlike the stable patient with neutropenic fever, there is likely not to be an opportunity to modify antibiotics based on culture data if the initial regimen does not provide adequate coverage. Combination vancomycin, imipenem, and an aminoglycoside is a reasonable empiric regimen. At centers in which carbapenem-resistant *P aeruginosa* is frequent, cefepime plus metronidazole may be used instead of imipenem. Modifications should be made once culture and sensitivity data are known.

In septic shock, several interventions should be made rapidly. When possible, removal of all indwelling catheters should be performed. If a nidus of infection is identified, surgical débridement should be performed emergently, and material sent for culture and staining for bacteria and fungi. Standard supportive measures include fluid resuscitation, oxygen, and invasive hemodynamic monitoring, and vasopressor agents should be instituted. In patients with documented or suspected adrenal insufficiency, stress dose corticosteroids (e.g., hydrocortisone, 50 to 100 mg every 8 hours) should be administered. Empiric corticosteroid administration for adrenal insufficiency is appropriate in patients who have received significant corticosteroid therapy within the last year, such as for the underlying malignancy or for GVHD. However, routine use of corticosteroids for severe sepsis and shock is not warranted.[369]

Numerous studies have evaluated therapy directed against specific mediators of septic shock, including antibodies against endotoxin and TNF-α and a recombinant IL-1 receptor antagonist. Other potential strategies include endotoxin vaccine, polyclonal hyperimmune serum (to neutralize bacterial toxins), bradykinin, cyclooxygenase, leukotriene, platelet-activating factor antagonists, pentoxifylline, endogenous antibacterial peptides (such as bactericidal permeability increasing protein), and inhibition of nitric oxide.[370] All such therapeutic modalities directed against mediators of the sepsis cascade should be considered to be experimental.

IMPLANTED VASCULAR CATHETERS

Tunneled, cuffed vascular catheters have been used extensively in patients with cancer, providing long-term central venous access for blood drawing and infusions. Catheter infections have been divided into several categories.[371] Greene[371] distinguished exit from tunnel infections based on whether inflammation extended greater than 2 cm from the exit site. Purulence from the exit site may be present, although in neutropenic patients, local erythema and tenderness may be the only signs of infection, making it difficult to distinguish from sterile inflammation associated with mild trauma. Tunnel infections manifest with inflammation extending along the subcutaneous tract through which the catheter was inserted. The third major category is catheter-related bacteremia or fungemia, which may occur in the presence or absence of signs of localized infection. A 5- to 10-fold greater organism recovery from blood drawn from the catheter compared with peripheral blood cultures is highly suggestive of a catheter source of septicemia. The fourth category is a septic thrombophlebitis in which a venous thrombus is documented in association with positive blood culture results.

Most exit site infections can be cured with antibiotics alone without catheter removal. At the University of Maryland Cancer Center, 160 exit site infections were identified out of 690 Hickman catheters placed, most caused by *S epidermidis* or *S aureus*.[372] Treatment was usually with vancomycin, and only 10 of 160 exit site infections resulted in catheter removal. In another study, 55 of 65 exit site infections were successfully treated with antibiotics and local care alone.[373]

In contrast to exit site infections, tunnel infections generally require catheter removal because of failure of antibiotic therapy alone. In cases of tunnel infection caused by the *Mycobacterium fortuitum* complex (*M fortuitum* and *M chelonae*), surgical excision of the tissue surrounding the tunnel may be required.[374]

Most cases of catheter-associated bacteremia can be cured without catheter removal, but certain situations should prompt catheter removal. Persistently positive blood culture results for longer than 3 days or recurrences of bacteremia by the same pathogen despite adequate antibiotic therapy are evidence of antibiotic failure and require catheter removal. In patients with severe sepsis (e.g., hypotension unresponsive to intravenous fluids), a new site of intravenous access should be established followed by immediate removal of all previous indwelling catheters. Certain pathogens (e.g., fungi, *M fortuitum* complex, *Bacillus* species, and antibiotic-resistant bacteria) are unlikely to clear or are prone to relapse without catheter removal.

In cases of septic thrombophlebitis, prompt catheter removal and initiation of antimicrobial therapy is essential. Anticoagulation is generally used, although its value has not been clearly established. Septic phlebitis of a central vein usually does not require surgical drainage if the catheter is removed. In cases in which a focus of infection exists in the soft tissue around the vein, surgical drainage may be necessary.[375]

Central catheters may be partially implanted, such as the Broviac or Hickman type in which the ports are exposed to the outside, or they may be entirely implanted. The totally implanted venous access devices have the advantage of being less likely to be traumatized or colonized by external skin flora and have fewer infections compared with catheters with external ports. In a study at Memorial Sloan-Kettering Cancer Center, 341 of 788 (43%) external tunneled catheters became infected compared with 57 of 680 (8%) completely implanted ports,[376] and external catheters were significantly more likely to be removed because of infection. It is possible that the more favorable infection rate associated with implanted ports is that such catheters are more likely used in patients with solid tumors who do not require multiple ports for intravenous access; the external catheters are in turn more likely to be used in patients who require more catheter manipulations, such as those with leukemia and BMT recipients.

The use of long-term tunneled catheters with a Dacron cuff to reduce entry of skin flora is generally associated with fewer infections than nontunneled catheters. However, at the M. D. Anderson Cancer Center, nontunneled silastic catheters were associated with long durability and a low infection rate comparable with tunneled catheters.[371] Such an approach requires meticulous catheter care, but has the advantage of reduced expense and morbidity associated with catheter insertion and easier catheter removal.

SKIN LESIONS AND SOFT TISSUE INFECTIONS

In the heavily immunocompromised patient with cancer, skin lesions can arise from several different etiologies (see reference 377 for an excellent review). Drug reactions are probably the most common noninfectious cause of cutaneous lesions. β-Lactam and sulfa antibiotics are relatively common offenders that are used extensively in this patient population. Cutaneous lesions may be manifestations of the underlying malignancy. For example, hematologic malignancies are associated with mixed cryoglobulinemia, which may produce cutaneous vasculitis. Sweet's syndrome is characterized by fever and skin lesions that may be papular, nodular, or ulcerative. These lesions may be misdiagnosed as cellulitis and be treated inappropriately with antibiotics. Histologically, a dense neutrophilic infiltrate located mostly in the mid and upper dermis is diagnostic. Sweet's syndrome is associated with hematologic malignancies and may occur during the neutropenic period. In the transplant recipient, GVHD typically presents as a diffuse maculopapular rash, and involvement of the gut and liver is common. Biopsy of skin lesions for histology and culture and staining for bacteria, fungi, mycobacteria, and viral infections is prudent to rule out infection.

Infections of the skin can either be localized or manifestations of systemic infection. Ecthyma gangrenosum is the most characteristic skin lesion associated with systemic *P aeruginosa* infection, but it is not pathognomonic (see Fig. 54-1). Ecthyma gangrenosum–like lesions can be caused by *S aureus*, enteric gram-negative rod infection, and by filamentous fungi, including *Aspergillus*, Zygomycete, and *Fusarium* species. Ecthyma gangrenosum begins as a raised erythematous papule or nodule that progresses to a bluish-black necrotic lesion within 12 to 24 hours. A central area of necrosis surrounded by erythema is typical. Hemorrhagic bullae may be observed. Pathologically, ecthyma gangrenosum is a necrotizing process in which masses of bacteria are often observed within the vessel wall. In neutropenic patients, infiltrating white cells may be absent.

Local soft tissue infection by *P aeruginosa* in the neutropenic patient can rapidly spread through fascial planes, causing extensive necrosis and fulminant sepsis.[378] The initial signs at the site of entry may be mild, pain and tenderness may be out of proportion to erythema, and purulence is likely to be absent. A needle aspiration of the lesion showing gram-negative bacilli establishes the diagnosis of invasive infection; however, a negative aspiration does not rule out the diagnosis. Prompt surgical débridement may be life saving in cases of localized disease.

Stenotrophomonas maltophilia can cause a variety of dermatologic infections, including mucocutaneous ulcerations, primary cellulitis, a metastatic nodular cellulitis, and ecthyma gangrenosum [see Stenotrophomonas (Xanthomonas) maltophilia, earlier in this chapter]. *Aeromonas hydrophilia* is a gram-negative rod that grows in fresh and brackish waters and can be acquired by nosocomial transmission. Immunocompromised persons are more susceptible to extensive soft tissue infections from direct penetration through the skin, leading to sepsis. In a patient exposed to fresh or brackish water preceding an episode of cellulitis, an antibiotic regimen with activity against *A hydrophilia* should be initiated. The organism is usually susceptible to fluoroquinolones, trimethoprim-sulfamethoxazole, third-generation cephalosporins, and imipenem.

Septicemia by viridans streptococci is associated with facial flushing and a rash in 60% of cases in a series from the M. D. Anderson Center in Texas.[65] The rash was usually maculopapular, started on the trunk, and extended to the face and extremities. Skin exfoliation occurred on the palms and soles in 25% of patients 2 weeks after the onset of the rash. These manifestations are likely the result of acquisition of a plasmid producing a toxin associated with a toxic shock syndrome.

Bacteremia caused by *C jeikeium* is associated with skin lesions in 30% to 50% of neutropenic patients. The skin lesions often occur at catheter sites and at sites of trauma, such as bone marrow aspiration, and may only become apparent after resolution of neutropenia.[72] The portal of entry is usually through the skin. The lesions may be cellulitic, ulcerative, or pustular. If diphtheroids are isolated from a skin lesion, the microbiology laboratory should be asked specifically to evaluate for *C jeikeium*. *Bacillus* species are rare causes of skin infection, but can be associated with impetiginous, ulcerative, and necrotic skin lesions. *C jeikeium* and *Bacillus* species are sensitive to vancomycin.

Clostridium species are gram-positive anaerobes that cause deep soft tissue infection involving the fascia and muscle (see Clostridium Species, earlier in this chapter). Typically, a small dusky or purplish lesion on the leg or abdominal wall rapidly expands, and as infection progresses, the lesions become necrotic, bullous, and hemorrhagic. Systemic toxicity, including fever, malaise, and mental status changes occur early. Because the infection occurs in the deep soft tissue, tenderness and evidence of vascular compromise typically precede the development of cellulitis. A rapidly progressive deep soft tissue infection with gas formation suggests clostridial myonecrosis (or polymicrobial necrotizing fascitis). Needle aspiration characteristically shows the organism in the setting of a mild or absent inflammatory response. Extensive surgical débridement may be life saving if initiated early, although at this stage of disease, most patients die.[86]

The characteristic skin lesions of disseminated candidiasis are raised erythematous discrete papules, measuring approximately 0.5 to 1.0 cm in diameter. The lesions are usually not tender. Concurrent myalgias raises the possibility of *Candida* myositis.[379] The yeast is cultured from skin lesions in approximately one-half the cases. Therefore, a negative culture result does not rule out the diagnosis. Biopsy and fungal staining of cutaneous lesions can provide an immediate clue to the diagnosis, prompting the early addition of antifungal therapy.

Trichosporon beigelii is a yeast that causes sepsis and disseminated infection in neutropenic patients.[144,145,380] Skin lesions occur in 30% of disseminated infections and are characterized by nontender erythematous nodules that may become necrotic. Histologically, budding yeast are present in the dermis, as distinguished from *Candida* species, which produce pseudohyphae. High-dose azole therapy is considered the treatment of choice.

Cutaneous infection by filamentous fungi may be primary or may represent systemic infection. Primary cutaneous infection with molds can occur in immunocompetent patients by traumatic inoculation. However, progression to angioinvasion, infarction, extension to the deep soft tissue fascia and muscle, and dissemination denote profound immunosuppression. Walmsley et al.[381] described 16 cases of primary cutaneous aspergillosis in children, most of whom had leukemia or lymphoma or had undergone BMT. Eleven cases were related to intravenous arm boards, and five cases were attributed to hematogenous dissemination. Clinically, these lesions resemble ecthyma gangrenosum associated with disseminated *P aeruginosa* infection. Histologically, hyphal elements are present and may cause angioinvasion and infarction.

Infection by *Fusarium* species is being observed with increasing frequency, predominantly in leukemia patients with prolonged neutropenia. Primary cutaneous fusariosis has a varied appearance, including cellulitis, paronychia, onychomycosis resembling dermatophyte infection, as well as papular and nodular lesions, and subcutaneous nodules[155] (see Fusarium Species, earlier in this chapter).

In the case of primary localized cutaneous infection with a mold, surgical resection is necessary and has an excellent prognosis.[382] In the neutropenic patient, the likelihood of subclinical systemic infection is high, and, therefore, high-dose amphotericin B (1.0 to 1.5 mg/kg daily) or a lipid formulation should be administered.

SINUSITIS

In immunocompetent patients, sinusitis results principally from inadequate drainage of mucous secretions from the sinus cavities. Respiratory bacterial pathogens, including *S pneumoniae, H influenzae,* and *M catarrhalis* predominate. In patients with neutropenia or otherwise highly immunocompromised patients, infections by *P aeruginosa,* Enterobacteriaceae, and molds are more commonly observed.

Treatment of sinusitis in immunocompetent patients with cancer involves a standard antibiotic regimen, such as trimethoprim-sulfamethoxazole, amoxicillin-clavulanate, or a cephalosporin with activity against respiratory pathogens. In cases of an obstructing tumor interfering with drainage from the maxillary sinuses, surgical creation of an antral window may be required to facilitate drainage.

In neutropenic patients with symptoms or signs suggestive of sinusitis, a regimen with activity against gram-negative bacteria (such as ceftazidime) should be administered. If no improvement occurs within 3 days, a CT scan of the sinuses with diagnostic aspiration of fluid collections is recommended. A sinus endoscopy may also be useful to visualize the upper airways and to obtain diagnostic material.

Infections by community respiratory viruses may initially manifest with sinus congestion or nonspecific upper airway symptoms. A high index of suspicion for such viruses is necessary for early therapy and prevention of nosocomial outbreaks. A nasopharyngeal or throat wash may rapidly establish the diagnosis (see Community Respiratory Viruses, earlier in this chapter).

Invasive fungal sinusitis in immunocompromised patients often has devastating results. Infection by *Aspergillus* species is most common in patients with persistent neutropenia (e.g., aplastic anemia) and in BMT recipients. The agents of mucormycosis are classically associated with rhinocerebral disease, leading to necrosis of the palate, and extension to surrounding structures. Sinusitis by emerging fungal pathogens, including *Fusarium* species, *Alternaria* species, dark-walled molds, and *Pseudallescheria boydii* are being recognized with increasing frequency.[154,383] A cluster of fungal sinusitis in a pediatric hospital was associated with soil reservoirs disturbed by hospital construction.[384]

Symptoms and signs suggestive of fungal sinusitis include fever, nasal congestion, headache, maxillary tenderness, and periorbital swelling. Sinus endoscopy may show necrotic material or ulceration. Hyphal invasion into blood vessels leads to tissue infarction and hemorrhage. Mental status changes are suggestive of involvement of the brain.

Therapy for invasive mold infections involves a combined medical and surgical approach. High-dose amphotericin B (1.5 mg/kg/d) or a lipid formulation of amphotericin B should be initiated. When feasible, surgical resection of involved tissue should be performed, as medical therapy alone is unlikely to contain infection in the setting of neutropenia or severe immunosuppression. Amphotericin B should be continued even if all of the visualized necrotic tissue is fully débrided, given the likelihood of inapparent local and disseminated disease. The most important predictor of a successful outcome is resolution of neutropenia.

PULMONARY INFILTRATES

In patients with cancer, pulmonary infiltrates pose a particularly difficult challenge. Numerous noninfectious causes of pulmonary infiltrates include congestive heart failure, pulmonary hemorrhage, infarction, drug-induced pneumonitis, radiation injury, tumor, and acute respiratory distress syndrome (Table 54-8). In addition, common processes can have atypical radiographic appearances, and two or more pulmonary processes can exist simultaneously in this patient population. Establishing an early diagnosis is crucial so that appropriate therapy can be instituted, and the toxicity of inappropriate therapy is avoided.

In heavily immunocompromised patients with cancer, such as those with leukemia and BMT recipients, pneumonia is com-

TABLE 54-8. Differential Diagnosis of Pulmonary Infiltrates in Patients with Cancer

Immune Status	*Radiographic Pattern*	*Pathogens*	*Noninfectious Causes*
No immunosuppressive therapy	Localized infiltrate	*Streptococcus pneumoniae*	Embolus
		Haemophilus influenzae	Hemorrhage
		Polymicrobial (aspiration)	Aspiration (sterile)
		Staphylococcus aureus (local infection or septic embolus)	Drugs
		Aerobic gram-negative rods[a]	Tumor
		Legionella sp.	
		Chlamydia sp.	
		Mycobacterium sp.	
		Dimorphic fungi (e.g., *Histoplasma capsulatum, Coccidioides immitis*)	
	Diffuse	Community respiratory viruses	Respiratory distress syndrome
		Bacterial pneumonia (hematogenous spread)	Congestive heart failure
		Mycoplasma sp.	Hypersensitivity reaction
		Chlamydia sp.	Drugs (e.g., methotrexate)
		Mycobacterium tuberculosis (miliary)	Tumor (lymphangitic spread)
			Hemorrhage
			Pulmonary leukostasis
Neutropenic (≤7 d)	Localized or diffuse	Aerobic gram-negative rods (Enterobacteriaceae, *Pseudomonas aeruginosa*)	As above
		Staphylococcus aureus	
		Community respiratory viruses	
Neutropenic (>7 d)	Localized or diffuse	Same as neutropenia ≤7 d plus filamentous fungi, principally *Aspergillus* sp.[b]	
Bone marrow transplantation (nonneutropenic)	Localized	*Aspergillus* sp.	As above
		Enterobacteriaceae	Graft-versus-host disease
		Pseudomonas aeruginosa	
		Staphylococcus aureus	
		Streptococcus pneumoniae	
		Legionella sp.	
		Mycobacterium sp.	
		Nocardia sp.	
		Cryptococcus neoformans	
		Dimorphic fungi	
	Diffuse	Cytomegalovirus	As above
		Pneumocystis carinii	Graft-versus-host disease
		Community respiratory viruses	
		Bacterial (hematogenous spread)	
		Herpes simplex virus	
		Varicella	
		Mycobacterium tuberculosis (miliary)	
		Dimorphic fungi (miliary)	
		Toxoplasma gondii	
		Strongyloides stercoralis	

[a]Aerobic gram-negative rods (Enterobacteriaceae and *Pseudomonas aeruginosa*) can cause severe community-acquired and nosocomial pneumonias in persons not treated with immunosuppressive or myelotoxic agents. Persons at risk include the elderly and those with comorbid illnesses, such as chronic pulmonary disease, alcohol abuse, and renal failure.

[b]The radiographic appearance of invasive mold infection (principally aspergillosis) is quite variable. In neutropenic patients, a computed tomographic scan may be required to detect nodular lesions. Nodular or patchy infiltrates indistinguishable from bacterial pneumonia are most common. Multifocal lesions are common. Cavitation with central necrosis (air crescent sign) is usually seen after myeloid recovery. Pulmonary hemorrhage complicating aspergillosis may produce a more diffuse alveolar pattern.

mon and is associated with a high mortality. Walsh and Pizzo[385] divided pulmonary infiltrates in neutropenic patients into four categories: (1) early, focal; (2) refractory, focal; (3) late, focal; and (4) interstitial or diffuse. Early infiltrates are defined as those that develop with the first onset of fever in a neutropenic patient. These infections are likely to be caused by Enterobacteriaceae, *P aeruginosa,* and *S aureus.* Because of neutropenia, physical findings of consolidation and sputum production may be absent. Two sets of blood cultures, a urine culture, a chest radiograph, and, if possible, a sputum for Gram's stain and culture should be obtained. Early in the course, the infiltrate is localized, but rapid progression to respiratory failure and sepsis is common. It is therefore essential to initiate appropriate empiric antibiotic therapy promptly and to closely monitor the response in an inpatient setting.

The optimal antibiotic regimen is controversial. The potential advantages of combination antibiotics include synergy and a reduced likelihood of the pathogen being resistant to all antibiotics in the initial regimen. An antipseudomonal penicillin (such as piperacillin or ticarcillin) or a third- (ceftazidime) or fourth- (cefepime) generation cephalosporin with activity against *P aeruginosa* may be combined with an aminoglycoside. If MRSA is common, empiric vancomycin should be added. Alternatively, standard monotherapy regimens for empiric treatment of febrile neutropenia, including ceftazidime, cefepime, imipenem, or meropenem, have sufficiently broad-spectrum activity to be used for treatment of acute bacterial pneumonia in neutropenic patients. The principle that a broad-spectrum antibiotic can be used as monotherapy for serious community-acquired and nosocomial pneumonias has gained widespread acceptance through well-designed prospective studies.[386,387] With regard to patients with cancer, ceftazidime monotherapy was shown to be equivalent to combination regimens as empiric therapy for neutropenic fever, including a subgroup of patients with pulmonary infiltrates. The rationale of monotherapy is to design a regimen with broad-spectrum activity against the most common pathogens and against the pathogens most likely to result in serious or life-threatening complications. Modifications of the initial regimen should be made on the basis of clinical response and microbiologic data. For this reason, use of a single antibiotic is probably not appropriate as empiric therapy for a fulminant pneumonia causing respiratory failure and sepsis, in which delay in the institution of appropriate antibiotics is likely to have disastrous consequences. The appropriateness of a particular empiric regimen for pneumonia, either monotherapy or combination therapy, depends on the frequency of isolates and their sensitivity profiles at a given institution.

If clinical improvement occurs within 48 to 72 hours, no further diagnostic measures are necessary, and antibiotic therapy should be continued until neutropenia resolves and for at least 10 to 14 days. Once neutropenia resolves, an appropriate oral antibiotic regimen could be administered for the remainder of the course.

In cases of refractory pneumonia, the possibility of a bacterial infection resistant to the empiric regimen as well as atypical causes of pneumonia become more likely. Examples of the latter group include *Legionella,*[388] *Chlamydia, Mycoplasma, P carinii, Nocardia,* and *Mycobacteria* species, as well as viral and fungal pathogens. Pneumonia and sepsis caused by enteric flora in a patient from an endemic area may result from a hyperinfection syndrome by *Strongyloides stercoralis.* A CT scan of the chest is useful in defining the location and morphology of the lesions, and an invasive diagnostic procedure (bronchoalveolar lavage, needle aspiration, open lung biopsy) may be warranted to establish the diagnosis.

Late onset of focal infiltrates applies to new pulmonary lesions developing on or after 7 days of empiric antibacterial therapy in persistently neutropenic patients. The likelihood of a fungal pneumonia in this setting is high. In contrast, development of a new pulmonary infiltrate after resolution of neutropenia is likely to represent a previous infection that was unrecognized during the neutropenic period; such infiltrates usually resolve without complications. *Aspergillus* species are the most common cause of pneumonia in persistently neutropenic patients. Less common fungal pathogens include *Trichosporon, Rhizopus, Fusarium* species, and dematiaceous molds. *Aspergillus* species and other filamentous fungi are angioinvasive and may cause pulmonary hemorrhage and infarction (see Aspergillosis, earlier in this chapter). Pleuritic chest pain may result from pulmonary infarction or direct invasion of chest wall structures. As is the case for refractory pneumonia, infection with resistant bacteria, viruses, and protozoa remain in the differential diagnosis.

Diffuse pulmonary infiltrates may be due to a variety of infectious causes, including progressive bacterial infection, *Legionella, P carinii, M tuberculosis* (miliary), atypical mycobacteria, *S stercoralis,* and fungal and viral pathogens. In the BMT recipient, CMV infection is the most common cause of pulmonary infiltrates in the postengraftment period, generally between 1 to 4 months after transplant. Respiratory viruses, including RSV, parainfluenza, influenza, and adenovirus can cause severe pulmonary infection in transplant recipients. In winter months, upper respiratory symptoms and bronchospasm favor the diagnosis of RSV. Diffuse necrotizing pneumonia by varicella and HSV are also encountered in transplant recipients. Patients receiving concomitant corticosteroid therapy in addition to myeloablative therapy are at particular risk for *P carinii* infection, and, to a lesser degree, histoplasmosis, coccidioidomycosis, cryptococcosis, and reactivation of tuberculosis.

Based on careful evaluation of the patient's level of immunosuppression, time course of the illness, epidemiologic exposures, physical examination, and radiographic and laboratory data, a preliminary differential diagnosis is established. For patients who are either not responding to antibacterial therapy or whose clinical course is not suggestive of an acute bacterial process, an aggressive and expeditious approach to establishing the diagnosis is indicated. Sputum induction with hypertonic saline is diagnostic of PCP in approximately 60% of cases in patients who not infected with human immunodeficiency syndrome.[285] Sputum induction is also of value in diagnosing tuberculosis. If sputum induction is not diagnostic, bronchoalveolar lavage has a high diagnostic yield in alveolar infiltrates such as pneumonia caused by *P carinii, M tuberculosis,* and respiratory viruses. The sensitivity of bronchoalveolar lavage for focal lesions such as nodules is variable. In lesions larger than 2 cm, the sensitivity of bronchoalveolar lavage ranges from 50% to 80%, but in smaller lesions, the diagnostic yield is usually approximately 15%.[385] Quantitative cultures from bronchoalveolar lavage or from a protected brush catheter may increase the specificity in the diagnosis of bacterial pneumonia as distinguished from oral flora. However, the diagnostic yield of such procedures is substantially reduced by prior antibiotic therapy.

Bronchoalveolar lavage is a relatively insensitive method for diagnosing aspergillosis, detecting only approximately 50% of cases.[389,390] In one study of patients with leukemia, bronchoalveolar lavage failed to document all nine cases of autopsy-proven pulmonary aspergillosis.[391] Percutaneous biopsy may increase the diagnostic yield, but in thrombocytopenic patients, the risk of bleeding may be unacceptably high. Open lung biopsy is the definitive diagnostic method in immunocompromised patients with pulmonary lesions. This procedure also allows for easier visualization and control of bleeding. False-negative results occur in approximately 5% of open lung biopsies as a result of sampling error in the case of patchy lesions.

CARDIAC INFECTIONS

Cardiac infections are relatively uncommon in patients with cancer. Infection can occur as a complication of thoracic surgery, such as a pneumonectomy, in which dehiscence of the bronchial stump can lead to a bronchopleural fistula and infection of the pleural space with extension to the pericardium. Meticulous and repeated débridements of infected tissue and repair of the fistula are necessary.

Endocarditis can occur as a complication of catheter-associated bacteremia[392] or a septic thrombophlebitis of the neck. In neutropenic patients, dental procedures should be avoided, but if they are necessary, antibiotic prophylaxis (amoxicillin) is reasonable to avoid secondary bacteremia. Evaluation by echocardiography is warranted in patients with bacteremia with signs suggestive of endocarditis, such as a new murmur or embolic phenomena.

Fungal endocarditis (principally *Candida* and *Aspergillus* species) may result from cardiac surgery and from illicit drug use.[393] Therapy for fungal endocarditis requires removal of the infected valve based on the poor penetration of antifungal agents into the valve, and the propensity for large vessel embolization. If valve surgery is not feasible, combination therapy generally consisting of high-dose amphotericin B (1.0 to 1.5 mg/kg/d) plus 5-flucytosine followed by prolonged fluconazole therapy has been successful in case reports of *Candida* endocarditis.[394,395] Rarely, filamentous fungi may also cause myocardial abscesses with direct extension to and destruction of the contiguous valve in profoundly immunosuppressed patients.[396]

Pericardial aspergillosis is a rare, but highly lethal complication in profoundly immunosuppressed patients with cancer.[397] In a review of 28 cases, pericardial involvement resulted from contiguous spread from the lungs or myocardium in all patients.[398] Patients with a hematologic malignancy are at highest risk for pericardial aspergillosis, reflecting the increased propensity for pulmonary *Aspergillus* infection. Clinical manifestations include chest pain, a pericardial friction rub, and pericardial constriction and tamponade.

Other pathogens associated with myopericarditis or endocarditis include *T gondii, C neoformans*, histoplasmosis, *Mycobacterium* species, nocardiosis, *Bartonella* species, and viral infections (e.g., HSV, CMV, influenza).

OROPHARYNGEAL INFECTIONS

Oropharyngeal infections in patients with cancer usually result from the combination of neutropenia and the breakdown of mucosal barriers related to cytotoxic chemotherapy and radiation therapy (see Mucosal Immunity, earlier in this chapter). A variety of oral manifestations may occur, including stomatitis, cheilitis, gingivitis, and periodontitis. Gingivitis is characterized by ulceration of the epithelium lining the gingival sulcus, resulting in a pocket between the gingiva and tooth. Necrotizing ulcerative gingivitis represents a severe end of the spectrum of this disease. In periodontitis, inflammation involves the supporting bone. The principal clinical sign of periodontal disease is bleeding through the ulcerated epithelium.[399]

Determining the incidence of oral bacterial infections in neutropenic patients is made difficult by the fact that the oral cavity is not a sterile site, making the distinction of chemotherapy-induced mucosal erosions from superimposed bacterial infection difficult. HSV is commonly shed in oral secretions and may produce mucosal ulcerations resembling chemotherapy-induced mucositis and necrotizing gingivitis. Oral mucosal candidiasis is most common in patients with profound T-cell deficiencies, such as those receiving high-dose corticosteroid therapy. Diagnosis is usually made by visual inspection alone, although in cases of uncertainty, a wet mount preparation showing pseudohyphal forms is confirmatory. A swab culture is not of diagnostic value because *Candida* species are commensals in the oral cavity. Filamentous fungi (e.g., *Aspergillus* and Zygomycete species) can cause invasive disease of the hard palate and other oral cavity structures, principally in patients with prolonged neutropenia.[400] The involved mucosa may initially have a dusky or violaceous appearance followed by necrosis, eschar formation, and ulceration. Surgical débridement of localized disease plus systemic antifungal therapy may be life saving.

Patients with oral mucosal disease may have difficulty eating because of pain. Malnourishment and dehydration may be severe if parenteral nutrition and fluid replacement are not initiated. Severe local infection with spread to adjacent tissue structures may occur, including paranasal sinusitis and septic thrombophlebitis. Disrupted oral mucosa may be a portal of entry for bacterial pathogens, leading to systemic infection.

If feasible, dental disease should be treated in advance of initiating chemotherapy and radiation therapy to allow for an adequate healing time. Plaque should be removed by scaling and curettage, and severely decayed or periapically infected teeth should be removed. A dentist experienced in the care of patients with malignancies should perform the initial clinical and radiographic evaluation and provide regular follow-up examinations through the course of antineoplastic therapy.

Chemical plaque control with agents such as chlorhexidine mouth rinses have been used routinely in patients with cancer, and different cancer centers use various rinsing protocols to enhance oral hygiene. Such rinses have lead to a reduction in microbial counts, but their value with regard to reducing oral disease and systemic infection remains unproved. (see reference 401 for review).

EPIGLOTTITIS

The diagnosis of epiglottitis should be considered in patients with fever and pain in the throat, odynophagia, difficulty handling upper airway secretions, and signs of upper airway compromise. In patients with cancer, the combination of neutropenia and mucotoxic chemotherapy and radiation therapy predisposes patients to epiglottitis.[402] Pathogens associated with epiglottitis in this population include common respiratory pathogens (such as *S pneumoniae* and *H influenzae*), as well as aerobic gram-negative rods and fungal pathogens. *Candida* epiglottitis is an unusual complication of neutropenia that may represent localized disease or disseminated infection.[403] Treatment with amphotericin B (1.0 mg/kg/d) is warranted for this potentially life-threatening infection.

If epiglottitis is considered, care should be taken to avoid unnecessary manipulations of the upper airway (e.g., probing the oral cavity with tongue depressors). Urgent consultation with an otolaryngologist should be obtained, and evaluation of the upper airway and obtaining culture material may be performed in the operating room. Tracheal intubation is required for impending upper airway obstruction.

ESOPHAGITIS

Esophagitis is encountered commonly in patients with cancer. A gradual onset of retrosternal chest pain or burning and odynophagia are the most common symptoms. The differential diagnosis includes candidiasis, HSV, CMV (principally in BMT recipients), bacterial infections, and aspergillosis. Radiation therapy to the chest may produce an erosive esophagitis clinically indistinguishable from the infectious etiologies.

The evaluation of presumed esophagitis requires consideration of the patient's immune status. Patients with prolonged neutropenia and BMT recipients are more likely to have an infectious etiology. In this population, *Candida* esophagitis is probably the most common etiology. More than one infectious cause may be present concomitantly. The presence of oral mucosal candidiasis increases the likelihood of *Candida* species as the etiology of esophagitis. However, the use of prophylactic topical antifungal agents (such as nystatin oral rinses) may protect against thrush while leaving the patient susceptible to esophageal candidiasis.

In highly immunocompromised patients with symptoms suggestive of esophagitis, two general strategies have been used. In the first, an endoscopy is performed initially. Whitish plaques are suggestive of candidiasis, whereas ulcerative lesions are more suggestive of viral infection. However, the gross endoscopic appearance is not specific enough to differentiate the various etiologies. Brushings and biopsy have the highest diagnostic yield. A brushing may suffice in lieu of a biopsy, which may carry the risk of bleeding, particularly in patients with thrombocytopenia.

In the second approach, empiric therapy is administered initially without an endoscopy. Fluconazole, with or without high-dose acyclovir (5 mg/kg every 8 hours), is administered as therapy for *Candida* and HSV, respectively. Alternatively, fluconazole may be administered initially, followed by acyclovir if no clinical response has occurred within 2 to 3 days. A history of oral HSV infections or presence of anti-HSV antibodies should prompt early initiation of acyclovir. In the setting of concurrent neutropenic fever, appropriate broad-spectrum antibacterial agents (e.g., vancomycin plus ceftazidime) with activity against oral flora should be added empirically. If symptoms do not rapidly abate, endoscopy should be performed.

Diagnosis of bacterial esophagitis relies on demonstration of bacterial invasion of the esophageal wall. Bacteria causing local disease include gram-positive cocci, gram-negative rods, and mixed infection.[404] Esophagitis may be complicated by bacteremia by predominantly gram-positive pathogens (viridans streptococci, *S aureus, Bacillus* species).[404] Erosive esophagitis may rarely lead to esophageal rupture or life-threatening bleeding.

INTRAABDOMINAL INFECTION

Intraabdominal infections present a unique set of challenges in patients with cancer. Incorporating clinical data related to the malignancy, therapy, and the immune status of the host is critical when evaluating a potential acute abdomen. Common causes of an acute abdomen in the general population (such as cholecystitis, pancreatitis, appendicitis, and diverticulitis) also occur in patients with malignancy. Intraabdominal tumors, depending on their location, may lead to an obstructive cholangitis (e.g., pancreatic and hepatobiliary tumors) or erosion through a viscus. In some instances, tumor may replace most of the bowel wall, with perforation after initiation of cytoreductive chemotherapy. An upright abdominal film showing air under the diaphragm in a patient who has not undergone recent abdominal surgery is likely to be indicative of a bowel perforation or an intraabdominal infection caused by gas-producing organisms.

Patients with prolonged neutropenia are at risk for a necrotizing enterocolitis, referred to as *neutropenic enterocolitis* or *typhlitis*. Typhlitis likely results from a combination of neutropenia and defects in the bowel mucosa related to cytotoxic chemotherapy. This disease is most common in patients with leukemia who have undergone intensive myeloablative chemotherapy. Pediatric patients appear to be at greater risk for typhlitis than adults. Rarely, typhlitis has been reported in patients with leukemia who have not received chemotherapy.[405] *P aeruginosa* is the principal pathogen associated with typhlitis, though clostridial species are implicated in a minority of cases. Pathologically, typhlitis is characterized by ulceration and necrosis of the bowel wall, hemorrhage, and masses of organisms. In the setting of neutropenia, inflammation may be sparse.

Presumptive diagnostic criteria for typhlitis include fever, abdominal pain and tenderness, and radiologic evidence of right-sided colonic inflammation in patients with neutropenia.[406] Nausea, vomiting, and diarrhea (often bloody) are the most common associated symptoms. Abdominal distension, tenderness, and a right lower quadrant fullness or mass reflecting thickened bowel or a pericecal collection may occur. Tenderness is usually localized to the right lower quadrant, but may become diffuse. Septicemia by aerobic gram-negative bacteria (*P aeruginosa* and Enterobacteriaceae) is common; prostration and hypotension may be presenting signs.[406] Septicemia may be due to polymicrobial pathogens, including anaerobes. Clostridial species are the most common anaerobic pathogens, and bacteremia may result in a devastating myonecrosis (see *Clostridium* Species, earlier in this chapter).

Diagnostic imaging by CT scans or ultrasonography should be performed in neutropenic patients with abdominal complaints. Positive findings are present in approximately 80% of cases[406] and include a right lower quadrant inflammatory mass, pericecal fluid, soft tissue inflammatory changes, localized bowel wall thickening and mucosal edema, and a paralytic ileus. Usually, disease is limited to the cecum, but more extensive involvement of the large bowel and disease of the terminal ileum may occur. Barium studies may show mucosal edema and effacement of the haustral markings, but are associated with a potential risk of bowel perforation.

Treatment of typhlitis involves administration of broad-spectrum antibiotics with activity against aerobic gram-negative rods and anaerobes. Imipenem or ceftazidime plus metronidazole are appropriate regimens. Supportive care, including intravenous fluids, bowel rest, and nasogastric decompression, should be instituted. Granulocyte transfusions and myeloid growth factors should be considered, as resolution of neutropenia is critical to a successful outcome.

The indications for surgery are derived from clinical experience rather than trials. Some older series suggest early surgical intervention[407] and others argue for a conservative approach except in situations of widespread necrosis of the colon.[408] Shamberger et al.[409] proposed the following criteria for surgical intervention: (1) persistent gastrointestinal bleeding after resolution of neutropenia, thrombocytopenia, and clotting abnormalities; (2) free intraperitoneal perforation; (3) uncontrolled sepsis despite fluid and vasopressor support; and (4) an intraabdominal process (such as an appendicitis) that would require surgery in the absence of neutropenia. Using these criteria, 20 of 25 pediatric patients with typhlitis were managed without surgery, and only one patient died of typhlitis. In cases of a localized peritonitis, a pericecal collection, or a suspected sealed off cecal perforation in a clinically stable neutropenic patient, surgical intervention may be delayed until resolution of neutropenia, given the increased surgical mortality during neutropenia. Surgical intervention involves resection of necrotic bowel, usually entailing a right hemicolectomy, ileostomy, and mucous fistula.[410]

Patients with cancer are at high risk for *C difficile*–associated colitis, probably in large measure due to prolonged hospitalization where environmental transmission is likely to occur, and to patients' receiving broad-spectrum antibiotics that alter the normal colonic flora and facilitate *C difficile* colonization. Hospitalized patients commonly become colonized with *C difficile*.[411] Clinical manifestations include asymptomatic carriage, colitis without pseudomembrane formation, pseudomembranous colitis, and fulminant colitis.[412] *C difficile* colitis may also increase the risk of bacteremia by enteric pathogens, including VRE.[413] In severe *C difficile* disease, patients may be septic. Paralytic ileus, toxic dilation of the colon, and bowel perforation may occur. An abdominal film typically shows a dilatated colon with mucosal edema (*thumbprinting*).

Oral metronidazole is the standard therapy for *C difficile* colitis. Because of the risk of selection for VRE, oral vancomycin should be reserved for refractory cases and for patients intolerant to metronidazole. Patients in whom oral agents cannot be administered should receive parenteral metronidazole, because biliary excretion of the drug and exudation from inflamed colon generally result in adequate luminal concentrations of the drug.[414] Intravenous vancomycin is of no value in this setting because of inadequate lumen levels. In cases involving toxic dilation of the colon or perforation, surgical management typically involving a subtotal colectomy and diverting ileostomy may be life saving.

Endoscopic diagnosis of pseudomembranous colitis relies on visualization of characteristic raised, adherent, yellow plaques on the colonic mucosa. A tissue culture cytotoxicity assay that detects *C difficile* toxin B in stool is the gold standard laboratory diagnostic method. Direct culture of *C difficile* does not distinguish toxin-producing from non–toxin-producing strains, and thus, by itself, is not a useful diagnostic method. Several commercial enzyme immunoassays are available that detect *C difficile* toxins A or B, with sensitivities of approximately 80% and specificities close to 100%.[415]

ANORECTAL INFECTIONS

Anorectal infections in patients with malignancy may be life-threatening. In some cases, infection may follow the development of an anal fissure. In other instances, tiny abrasions may be a portal of entry. Alternatively, infection may originate in the anal crypts. Once anorectal infection is established, fascial extension to the external genitalia, pelvic floor, retroperitoneum, and peritoneal cavity may occur. Anorectal infections, with or without extensive regional spread, may lead to septicemia and metastatic infections.

Patients with leukemia receiving intensive myeloablative chemotherapy are at greatest risk for anorectal infections. Recovery from neutropenia is the most important prognostic indicator for a positive outcome.[416] The most common pathogens isolated at surgery or from wound aspiration are the Enterobacteriaceae, anaerobes, group D streptococci, and *P aeruginosa*.[416,417] In most cases, the infection is polymicrobial.

The incidence of anorectal infections in patients receiving intensive myeloablative chemotherapy is approximately 5%.[416,418] Fever often precedes symptoms and signs suggestive of anorectal infection, and perirectal pain, often exacerbated by defecation, may initially occur in the absence of physical examination findings.[417] Therefore, serial examinations of the perianal region are necessary.

In one series, point tenderness and poorly demarcated induration were the most consistent signs of perianal infection.[417] Localized erythema and warmth were also observed. Advanced disease was heralded by soft tissue breakdown and necrosis and progressive extension to the adjacent perineal and pelvic structures.

Mild perianal infection characterized by slight tenderness or small fissures may respond to initial therapy for fever and neutropenia. The presence of significant local tenderness, swelling, or skin maceration should prompt early administration of antibiotics appropriate for neutropenic fever and with activity against anaerobes (such as ceftazidime plus metronidazole or imipenem monotherapy). Digital rectal examination should not be performed due to the risk of infection and bleeding. A pelvic CT scan may aid in assessing for perirectal infection. Stool softeners, sitz baths, warm compresses, and analgesics should be provided.

Most cases of anorectal infections can be managed with appropriate broad-spectrum antibiotics and supportive measures.[416,419] Indications for surgery include progression of disease locally or continued sepsis despite adequate antibiotics, obvious tissue necrosis, or fluctuance. With adequate surgical drainage, pain typically resolves within 2 days.[417] At surgery, perirectal lesions usually consist of necrotic cavities filled with tissue debris.[417]

CENTRAL NERVOUS SYSTEM INFECTIONS

CNS infections in patients with cancer can be divided into surgical and nonsurgical complications. Common surgical procedures include resection of tumor, insertion of a shunt for hydrocephalus, and insertion of a reservoir to facilitate delivery of chemotherapeutic agents and easy sampling of cerebrospinal fluid. Patients with cancer involving the brain typically receive high-dose corticosteroid and local radiation therapy, which may further increase the risk of neurosurgical infections.

Infections related to implanted hardware may manifest in a variety of ways. Infection of a shunt or an Ommaya reservoir may manifest with malfunction of the device. Overt signs of meningitis, such as meningismus and photophobia do not usually occur, but most patients have fever.[420] Change in mental status may be the only sign of infection. A CT scan may suggest meningitis, ventriculitis, or a brain abscess if the device is infected at the proximal end. Evaluation of the cerebrospinal fluid is required for a diagnosis. Infection may occur in the more distal region of the device manifesting as a soft tissue infection. In cases of ventriculoatrial shunts, a distal site of infection may cause persistently positive blood culture results, thrombophlebitis, right-sided endocarditis, or septic pulmonary emboli. Distal ventriculoperitoneal shunt infections are associated with peritonitis and intraabdominal collections.

Coagulase-negative staphylococci, *S aureus*, and *Propionibacterium acnes* are the most common organisms infecting intraventricular devices. Enterobacteriaceae and *P aeruginosa* account for approximately 10% of infections. Coagulase-negative staphylococci and *P acnes* usually cause indolent late postoperative infections.

When feasible, removal of the entire device should be performed and appropriate antibiotics administered.[420] Antibiotic therapy should be tailored to the specific pathogen isolated. In an acutely ill patient with suspected meningitis related to prior neurosurgery, empiric therapy with parenteral vancomycin should be administered to cover *Staphylococcus*, *Streptococcus*, and *Propionibacterium* species in combination with an agent with activity against Enterobacteriaceae and *P aeruginosa* (such as ceftazidime).

CNS infections unrelated to neurosurgery are relatively uncommon in patients with cancer. In two series, the incidence of CNS infections in BMT recipients was approximately 2%.[421,422] In a review of 58 cases of brain abscesses after BMT at the Fred Hutchinson Cancer Center, 92% were caused by fungi.[423] *Aspergillus* species accounted for approximately 60% of isolates and one-third were caused by *Candida* species. The remainder of fungal infections included agents of mucormycosis and *Scopulariopsis* and *Pseudallescheria* species. Approximately 90% of cases of CNS aspergillosis were associated with a pulmonary focus, whereas most cases of *Candida* brain abscess were associated with candidemia or neutropenia. Only 4 of 58 patients had a bacterial brain abscess, and one patient had cerebral toxoplasmosis. The mortality in this series was 97%.

The CNS is the most common target organ of hematogenous disseminated aspergillosis. Manifestations of CNS aspergillosis include focal seizures, hemiparesis, cranial nerve palsies, and hemorrhagic infarcts due to vascular invasion.[424] The presence of pulmonary infiltrates and focal neurologic deficits in an immunocompromised patient were significantly more predictive of CNS aspergillosis than for CNS candidiasis or cryptococcosis in a multivariate discriminant analysis of autopsy-proven fungal CNS infections.[425] *Aspergillus* brain abscesses are typically multiple, hypodense, and nonenhancing, with little mass effect. CT scans with contrast enhancement initially may reveal no focal lesions, but in a later stage may demonstrate focal ring-enhancing or hemorrhagic lesions. Magnetic resonance imaging may further facilitate early detection. Intermediate T2 signal surrounded by a rim of higher signal may be observed.[421] Biopsy of these lesions reveals the same pattern of vascular invasion and infarction similar to that seen in lung biopsy specimens. We suggest that CNS infections by *Candida* and *Aspergillus* species be treated with amphotericin B plus 5-flucytosine, which readily penetrates the blood–brain barrier.

Other less common causes of CNS infections in patients with cancer include members of the herpes virus family (HSV, VZV, CMV, EBV, and HHV-6), adenovirus, *L monocytogenes*, *Acanthamoeba*, *Nocardia* species, *Mycobacterium* species, and *T gondii*, which have been discussed earlier (see Bacterial Pathogens in Cancer Patients, Viral Infections, and Parasitic Infections, earlier in this chapter).

DEMENTIAS

Patients with cancer may develop a chronic dementia related to leukoencephalopathy, a debilitating complication of therapy for their malignancy. The combination of cranial radiation therapy and intrathecal or systemic methotrexate has been most closely linked with leukoencephalopathy, although other intrathecal regimens may produce similar findings.[426,427]

Progressive multifocal encephalopathy (PML) is a demyelinating disease associated with lytic infection of oligodendrocytes by the human polyomavirus JC virus. Patients may develop rapidly progressive dementia as well as focal motor or cerebellar findings. Today, this disease is most commonly seen in patients with advanced AIDS, reflecting the critical role of cell-mediated immunity in controlling this infection. Occasionally, PML is seen in heavily immunocompromised persons with hematologic malignancies and in BMT recipients.[428] Magnetic resonance imaging typically shows unilateral or bilateral white matter disease without mass effect or enhancement. Diagnosis is established by either brain biopsy or by detection of the JC virus in spinal fluid by PCR. There is no established therapy for PML. In patients with AIDS, highly active antiretroviral therapy has produced mixed results in patients with PML.[429–431] By extrapolation, it is logical to try to reduce immunosuppressive therapy in persons with cancer and PML as a means of augmenting cell-mediated immunity.

GENITOURINARY INFECTIONS

Patients with cancer may be at an increased risk of serious urinary tract infections as a result of breaches of the normal anatomy of the genitourinary system, colonization by pathogenic organisms, and defects in host defense. The most common mechanism of seeding the bladder is via the ascending route. Barriers to entry and proliferation of pathogens include the presence of normal perineal flora, urination, mucosal epithelial lining, phagocytes, and, possibly, immunoglobulin secretion (IgA and IgG).[432]

A bladder catheter greatly facilitates colonization of the normally sterile bladder. A strong correlation exists between precatheterization rectal and periurethral isolates and organisms subsequently isolated from the urinary tract after bladder catheterization.[432] Obstruction to urinary flow permits colonization and multiplication of bacteria. In patients with cancer, obstruction of urine flow may result from tumors originating within and outside of the genitourinary tract. Tumors associated with hypercalcemia or hyperuricemia predispose to urinary stones. Impaired bladder emptying resulting in urine stasis may result from tumors involving the spinal cord. Urinary intestinal diversions are associated with a high incidence of bacteriuria and may predispose to clinically significant infections after myeloablative chemotherapy.

The epithelial lining of the bladder and a layer of mucopolysaccharide form a protective barrier against bacterial colonization and invasion. Injury to the bladder mucosa by cytotoxic agents likely increases the risk of infection. In dogs, stripping of the bladder mucinous layer led to increased colonization of the bladder mucosa by bacteria.[433] During neutropenia, the genitourinary tract may be an important portal of entry for systemic infections. Alternatively, the kidney may be secondarily seeded as a consequence of hematogenous infection. Neutropenic patients with a urinary tract infection are less likely to have dysuria and pyuria and are far more likely to become bacteremic compared with nonneutropenic patients.[20]

Infection of the prostate, seminal vesicles, epididymis, and testes may represent localized disease or hematogenous seeding. Common bacterial infections include Enterobacteriaceae, *P aeruginosa, S aureus,* and enterococci. Less common pathogens include *Salmonella* species, tuberculosis (more likely to involve the kidneys and ureters), *Nocardia* species, *Candida* species, *Blastomyces dermatitidis,* and *C neoformans.*

Asymptomatic candiduria is common in patients with bladder catheters. Management of candiduria is limited by lack of knowledge about the natural history of this infection, specifically with regard to predicting in which patients systemic infection will occur. Fluconazole is effective in eradicating candiduria in the short term, but recurrent infection is likely.[434] Removal of indwelling bladder catheters and antibacterial agents frequently lead to clearing of candiduria. Therefore, routine treatment of candiduria in afebrile nonneutropenic patients with local or systemic antifungal agents does not appear to be warranted. Because of the risk of candidemia after genitourinary tract manipulations, candiduria should be treated before such procedures are performed.[435] Because of the increased risk of candidemia, neutropenic patients with candiduria should receive systemic antifungal therapy.

Hemorrhagic cystitis is a common consequence of cytotoxic regimens that cause direct bladder mucosal injury and thrombocytopenia. In BMT recipients with unexplained hematuria occurring beyond the early period (when it is an expected toxicity of the preparative regimen), a viral etiology should be considered. Adenovirus, the polyomavirus BK, and, rarely, CMV[436] have been associated with hemorrhagic cystitis. Childs et al.[437] reported adenovirus (four cases) or polyomavirus (four cases) in nine cases of hemorrhagic cystitis in patients receiving T-cell–depleted BMT.

Adenovirus can cause fatal disseminated infections in BMT recipients (see Viral Infections, earlier in this chapter). Detection of urinary shedding of this virus by PCR appears to be more sensitive than cell culture methods, and may, in some cases, be a harbinger of disseminated disease.[438]

BK virus is ubiquitous. Approximately one-half of BMT recipients shed BK virus in the urine.[439] Hemorrhagic cystitis occurred four times more frequently in patients with BK viruria, and BK shedding often preceded or occurred simultaneously with cystitis. In some patients, prolonged urinary BK shedding did not result in disease. Documentation of BK viruria can be made by electron microscopy of urinary sediments, PCR, and DNA hybridization. Treatment of BK virus–associated hemorrhagic cystitis is supportive and may include prolonged bladder irrigation to prevent clot retention as well as blood transfusions.[440]

IMMUNE AUGMENTATION STRATEGIES

GRANULOCYTE TRANSFUSIONS

The rationale for granulocyte transfusions is to buy time for the neutropenic patient with a life-threatening infection by augmenting the number of circulating neutrophils until native myeloid regeneration occurs.

In the 1970s, the technology for harvesting and infusing granulocytes became available. Controlled trials of granulocyte transfusions as adjuvant therapy in neutropenic patients produced mixed results.[441] In the 1980s, the enthusiasm for granulocyte transfusions waned as more effective antibiotics became available, survival from serious bacterial infections was improved, and recombinant growth factors reduced the duration of neutropenia. In addition, there were concerns about the toxicity of granulocyte transfusions, including pulmonary leukostasis, risk of HLA alloimmunization (complicating platelet transfusions and conceivably myeloid engraftment after BMT), and risk of transfusion-associated infections, which appeared to outweigh their perceived benefit.

Today, the impetus to take a second look at granulocyte transfusions in large part stems from improvements made in the mobilization methods.[442] Recombinant G-CSF with or without corticosteroids is now routinely administered to donors approximately 12 hours before apheresis. G-CSF is a potent stimulus for neutrophil production by mobilizing myeloid precursors from marrow reserves. Using a standard continuous flow centrifugation apparatus, the mean absolute neutrophil yield per collection typically exceeds 3×10^{10} cells.[443,444] The higher number of harvested neutrophils in turn correlates with a higher neutrophil count in the recipient after transfusion.[445] The increased neutropenia-free period may also be related to a prolonged circulating half-life of G-CSF–mobilized granulocytes.[444] The qualitative functions of G-CSF–mobilized and corticosteroid-mobilized neutrophils appear to be intact, as measured by *in vitro* bactericidal activity, respiratory burst, and *in vivo* migration to experimental skin chambers.[444] G-CSF–mobilized granulocytes have been shown to localize to sites of inflammation after transfusion in allogeneic BMT recipients.[446]

Successful outcomes using granulocyte transfusions have been described in patients with life-threatening fungal infections in small series and case reports. In one nonrandomized retrospective study, no benefit of granulocyte transfusions was documented in treating fungal infections in BMT recipients.[117] Obviously, such reports must be interpreted with caution and do not permit general recommendations. A more recent phase I/II clinical trial using G-CSF–mobilized transfusions for treatment of refractory fungal infections in neutropenic patients with hematologic malignancies reported favorable responses in 11 of 15 patients.[448] Adverse transfusion-related reactions were infrequent.

In the absence of modern, prospective, randomized studies, when might granulocyte transfusions be considered? Currently, there is no justification (outside of a clinical trial) to use granulocyte transfusions either as prophylaxis or in cases of documented infections that are likely to respond to conventional therapy. We reserve granulocyte transfusions for patients with prolonged neutropenia and life-threatening infections refractory to conventional therapy. Filamentous fungi are likely to constitute the majority of such refractory infections.

If granulocyte transfusions are used, several considerations are important. In neutropenic patients, it is likely that daily or every other day transfusions will be administered, depending on the length of the neutropenia-free period after transfusions. Granulocytes should be infused quickly after harvesting, given the short storage half-life. With modern apheresis methods, the number of harvested neutrophils should exceed 2×10^9 cells. Infusions of amphotericin B should be separated by several hours from granulocyte transfusions to avoid pulmonary toxicity.[449] Leukocyte compatibility should be established by HLA matching and, if available, by leukocyte cross-matching to avoid alloimmunization. In some highly alloimmunized patients, transfused granulocytes are rapidly consumed and are likely to have more toxicity than benefit. In CMV-seronegative BMT recipients, only seronegative donors should be used.

GROWTH FACTORS

Normal myelopoiesis requires the establishment of myeloid stem cells, which, under the influence of stem cell factor, IL-3, and GM-CSF, gives rise to a the colony-forming unit granulocyte-macrophage. G-CSF acts at a later stage in concert with other growth factors to specifically drive granulopoiesis.

Many potential applications exist for recombinant colony-stimulating factors in patients with cancer, the most obvious being a reduction in chemotherapy-induced neutropenia. We discuss the use of colony-stimulating factors in two specific settings: (1) prophylaxis (growth factor is administered around the time of initiation of the myeloablative regimen), and (2) adjunctive therapy for established infection.

Prophylaxis

Prophylactic G-CSF has been evaluated in several prospective, randomized studies. The most consistent benefit has been a reduction in the neutropenic period. In some studies of patients with acute myelogenous leukemia receiving potent myeloablative chemotherapy, the acceleration of myeloid recovery was associated with a reduction in the duration of fever, use of antibiotics, and hospitalization.[450,451] The frequency of infections and the number of fatal infections were unaffected by G-CSF.[450] In patients with small cell lung cancer, G-CSF led to a reduction of the neutropenic period, duration of hospitalization, and rate of confirmed infections.[452]

Use of G-CSF in patients with a short duration of neutropenia is associated with a reduction in the neutropenic period, but no effect on the rate and days of hospitalization, duration of parenteral antibiotics, and number of documented infections.[453] Prophylactic G-CSF had no benefit except for a modest reduction in the neutropenic period after preparative regimens for autologous stem cell transplantation.[454,455]

Prophylactic GM-CSF has been evaluated in two prospective, randomized studies of elderly patients with acute myelogenous leukemia.[456] In one study, GM-CSF was only administered to patients who had a hypocellular or remission marrow on day 10 of induction chemotherapy.[457] Patients who achieved complete remission received the same study drug (GM-CSF or placebo) for consolidation chemotherapy. The median time to neutrophil recovery was significantly reduced in the GM-CSF group as was the frequency of fatal fungal infections and early infection-related mortality. There was a trend toward increased complete remission in the GM-CSF group. Most important, the 6-month mortality was significantly reduced in the GM-CSF arm. To our knowledge, this is the only study that has shown a survival advantage attributed to a colony-stimulating factor. This study formed the basis for approval by the Food and Drug Administration of GM-CSF for patients with acute myelogenous leukemia. A larger study conducted by the International Oncology Study Group using a similar design is underway to evaluate prophylactic GM-CSF in older and younger patients with acute myelogenous leukemia.[456]

In another study of 388 elderly patients with acute myelogenous leukemia, prophylactic GM-CSF led to a modest reduction in the neutropenic period.[458] The incidence of serious infections, regrowth of leukemic cells, and treatment-related mortality was similar between the two groups. The authors concluded that GM-CSF should not be recommended for elderly patients with acute myelogenous leukemia.

The inconsistent results of studies of prophylactic colony-stimulating factors for chemotherapy-induced neutropenia are almost certainly due to important differences in the study population and in the study design. The populations differ with respect to the underlying malignancy and the chemotherapy regimen. Some studies are insufficiently powered to detect differences in morbidity between treatment arms. In addition, the timing and dosing of colony-stimulating factors vary among studies. In the case of GM-CSF, different formulations consisting of glycosylated and nonglycosylated products have been used in different trials.[459]

The American Society of Clinical Oncology has recommended that prophylactic colony-stimulating factors (G-CSF and GM-CSF) be used only in populations in which the frequency of febrile neutropenia is likely to exceed 40%.[460] The American Society of Clinical Oncology considered that certain patients receiving a relatively nonmyelosuppressive regimen may benefit from CSFs if they are at an unusually high risk for infectious complications. Such risk factors may include preexisting neutropenia, extensive prior chemotherapy or pelvic irradiation leading to a reduction in myeloid reserves, a history of recurrent febrile neutropenia associated with relatively nonmyelotoxic complications, or the presence of an open wound or an active infection. Patients with a history of a serious or life-threatening infection, such as typhlitis, or an invasive fungal infection should also be considered for CSF prophylaxis during subsequent chemotherapy cycles.

Colony Growth Factors in Established Infection

The rationale for colony-stimulating factors for established infections stems from both the quantitative and qualitative effects of these agents on phagocytic cells. In neutropenic patients with life-threatening infections, survival is strongly influenced by the rapidity of neutrophil recovery. Thus, colony-stimulating factors and granulocyte transfusions are used in these settings to augment the number of circulating neutrophils.

In addition to accelerating myelopoiesis, colony-stimulating factors augment phagocyte function. G-CSF, GM-CSF, and macrophage colony-stimulating factor (M-CSF) increase the fungicidal activity of phagocytes *in vitro* against *Candida* and *Aspergillus* species.[461–464] The action of G-CSF is specific to neutrophils. M-CSF increases phagocytosis, chemotaxis, and secondary cytokine production in monocytes and macrophages.[465] GM-CSF stimulates various neutrophil effector functions and prolongs neutrophil survival *in vitro*, increases antibody-dependent cytotoxicity of eosinophils, accelerates the proliferation of the monocyte-macrophage system, and is a potent activator of monocytes and macrophages (reviewed in reference 465). Thus, GM-CSF may have a theoretical advantage against pathogens such as *Candida* and *Aspergillus* species, in which host defense is dependent on both neutrophil and macrophage function.

At present, published data related to colony-stimulating factors as adjunctive therapy for established infection are limited to animal studies, case reports, and open-label pilot studies in humans. Nemunaitis et al.[465,466] suggested that among patients with candidiasis or aspergillosis, treatment with antifungal agents plus M-CSF was associated with enhanced survival compared with historical controls. In another pilot study of eight patients with established fungal infection, adjuvant GM-CSF appeared to be promising.[467] These initial studies are insufficient to permit conclusions about the efficacy of these agents.

INTERFERON-γ

IFN-γ is a macrophage-activating factor that is critical in host defense against intracellular infections such as *Leishmania* and *Mycobacteria* species. IFN-γ augments generation of microbicidal reactive oxidants in phagocytes and is also a potent activator of oxidant-independent mechanisms, including augmentation of TNF-α production, tryptophan metabolism, granule protein synthesis, and MHC II expression.[468] IFN-γ administered to normal volunteers was shown to increase expression of FcgR1 receptors on phagocytes, leading to enhanced phagocytosis, and to increased β_2-integrin expression on monocytes, which may improve phagocyte trafficking *in vivo*.[469] The combination of G-CSF and IFN-γ overcame the suppressive effects of corticosteroids on the *in vitro* fungicidal activity of neutrophils against *Aspergillus* hyphae.[25] These data suggest that IFN-γ may have a role in augmenting phagocyte function in immunosuppressed patients with cancer.

Currently, IFN-γ is licensed as a prophylactic agent in patients with chronic granulomatous disease, an inherited disorder of the phagocyte nicotinamide-adenine dinucleotide phosphate (reduced form) oxidase that renders phagocytes defective in generating superoxide anion and its downstream reactive oxidant metabolites.[470] Patients with chronic granulomatous disease experience recurrent life-threatening bacterial and fungal infections. The major cause of mortality in chronic granulomatous disease is from invasive aspergillosis.[471,472] Prophylactic IFN-γ reduced the number of serious infections by more than 70% in patients with chronic granulomatous disease.[470] In addition, IFN-γ in combination with antimycobacterial agents had a positive effect on patients with refractory atypical mycobacterial infection resulting from defective IFN-γ production.[473] It remains to be seen whether IFN-γ may have similar positive effects on patients with cancer with iatrogenic phagocytic disorders.

In certain experimental fungal infections, host defense was enhanced by augmentation of T cells committed to Th1 phenotype, reflecting cell-mediated immunity. IL-12 is generated by activated macrophages and drives uncommitted T-helper cells to the Th1 pole to produce IL-2 and IFN-γ.[474] This pathway appears to be critical in controlling various fungal infections. IL-12 reduced organism load in a murine cryptococcal model and acted synergistically when combined with fluconazole.[475] Improvement or worsening of experimental candidiasis correlated with administration of cytokines that stimulated a Th1 or Th2 T-cell response, respectively.[476] In a mouse model of invasive aspergillosis, administration of IFN-γ and TNF-α were protective.[477] These studies provide a scientific basis for evaluating combination immunotherapy and antimicrobial therapy in fungal infections in immunocompromised patients.

ADOPTIVE IMMUNOTHERAPY IN BONE MARROW TRANSPLANT RECIPIENTS

As discussed previously, the intensive preparative regimens used in allogeneic BMT result in a profound disruption of T-cell immunity. Reconstitution of T-cell immunity occurs over several months in uncomplicated cases and is further delayed in cases of GVHD requiring high-dose corticosteroid therapy and potentially antilymphocyte globulins. CMV and EBV are members of the herpes virus family that establish latent infection in normal hosts, and control of reactivation is largely mediated by CD8+ cytotoxic T lymphocytes. Cytotoxic T lymphocytes recognize intracellular proteins that are presented by surface MHC class I molecules on antigen-presenting cells.

Studies on immune reconstitution after allogeneic BMT have shown that recovery of CMV-specific cytotoxic T-lymphocyte responses confers protection from subsequent CMV disease,[204,478–480] and these protective responses are specific for the structural virion proteins.[204] Thus, one potential strategy for preventing CMV disease (aside from prophylaxis with antiviral agents) is by adoptive transfer of CMV-specific cytotoxic T-lymphocyte clones obtained from CMV-seropositive bone marrow donors and selectively expanded by *in vitro* culture. Such an approach has led to early reconstitution of CMV-specific immunity in allogeneic BMT recipients, which persisted for at least 12 weeks after infusion corresponding to the period of maximal risk for CMV disease.[481]

In allogeneic BMT recipients, the major risk of uncontrolled EBV infection is development of an aggressive EBV lymphoproliferative disease or lymphoma, which can be rapidly fatal. Infusions of unfractionated peripheral blood mononuclear cells from EBV-seropositive donors have been used to treat EBV lymphoproliferative disease in allogeneic BMT recipients.[482] However, alloreactive T cells in such unfractionated preparations may induce GVHD. A safer approach involves transfer of EBV-specific donor cytotoxic T-lymphocyte clones that have been selectively enriched *in vitro*.[483,484] This method has led to persistent cellular immune responses to EBV for as long as 18 months.[484]

Acknowledgments

The authors are grateful to Donna Ball, NP, for reviewing the chapter and making thoughtful suggestions and acknowledge the expert secretarial assistance provided by Jeanette Chase, Tracey Roth, Kimberly De Pasquale, and Kathleen Kingsbury.

REFERENCES

1. Zinner SH. Changing epidemiology of infections in patients with neutropenia and cancer: emphasis on gram-positive and resistant bacteria. *Clin Infect Dis* 1999;29:490.
2. Griffiths H, Lea J, Bunch C, Lee M, Chapel H. Predictors of infection in chronic lymphocytic leukaemia (CLL). *Clin Exp Immunol* 1992;89:374.
3. Weeks JC, Tierney MR, Weinstein MC. Cost effectiveness of prophylactic intravenous immune globulin in chronic lymphocytic leukemia. *N Engl J Med* 1991;325:81.
4. Savage DG, Lindenbaum J, Garrett TJ. Biphasic pattern of bacterial infection in multiple myeloma. *Ann Intern Med* 1982;96:47.
5. Cheson BD, Walker HS, Heath ME, Gobel RJ, Janatova J. Defective binding of the third component of complement (C3) to *Streptococcus pneumoniae* in multiple myeloma. *Blood* 1984;63:949.

6. Chapel HM, Lee M, Hargreaves R, Pamphilon DH, Prentice AG. Randomised trial of intravenous immunoglobulin as prophylaxis against infection in plateau-phase multiple myeloma. The UK Group for Immunoglobulin Replacement Therapy in Multiple Myeloma. *Lancet* 1994;343:1059.
7. Mackowiak PA, Demian SE, Sutker WL, et al. Infections of hairy cell leukemia. Clinical evidence of a pronounced defect in cell-mediated immunity. *Am J Med* 1980;68:718.
8. Fisher RI, DeVita VT Jr, Bostick F, et al. Persistent immunologic abnormalities in long-term survivors of advanced Hodgkin's disease. *Ann Intern Med* 1980;92:595.
9. Casazza AR, Duvall CP, Carbone PP. Summary of infectious complications occurring in patients with Hodgkin's disease. *Cancer Res* 1966;26:1290.
10. Graham BS, Tucker WS Jr. Opportunistic infections in endogenous Cushing's syndrome. *Ann Intern Med* 1984;101:334.
11. Walsh TJ, Mendelsohn G. Invasive aspergillosis complicating Cushing's syndrome. *Arch Intern Med* 1981;141:1227.
12. Tomonaga M. Adult T-cell leukemia and opportunistic infections. *Intern Med* 1999;38:83.
13. Walsh TJ, Meyers RAM, Herrington D, et al. Lemierre's postanginal septicemia: multidisciplinary management of severe fusobacterial infections. *Infect Med* 1985;2:83.
14. Heyman MR, Walsh TJ. Autoimmune neutropenia and Hodgkin's disease. *Cancer* 1987;59:1903.
15. Bodey GP, Buckley M, Sathe YS, Freireich EJ. Quantitative relationships between circulating leukocytes and infection in patients with acute leukemia. *Ann Intern Med* 1966;64:328.
16. Gerson SL, Talbot GH, Hurwitz S, et al. Prolonged granulocytopenia: the major risk factor for invasive pulmonary aspergillosis in patients with acute leukemia. *Ann Intern Med* 1984;100:345.
17. Weinberger M, Elattar I, Marshall D, et al. Patterns of infection in patients with aplastic anemia and the emergence of Aspergillus as a major cause of death. *Medicine (Baltimore)* 1992;71:24.
18. Walsh TJ, Hiemenz JW, Anaissie E. Recent progress and current problems in treatment of invasive fungal infections in neutropenic patients. *Infect Dis Clin North Am* 1996;10:365.
19. Rex JH, Walsh TJ, Anaissie EJ. Fungal infections in iatrogenically compromised hosts. *Adv Intern Med* 1998;43:321.
20. Sickles EA, Greene WH, Wiernik PH. Clinical presentation of infection in granulocytopenic patients. *Arch Intern Med* 1975;135:715.
21. Izutsu KT, Sullivan KM, Schubert MM, et al. Disordered salivary immunoglobulin secretion and sodium transport in human chronic graft-versus-host disease. *Transplantation* 1983;35:441.
22. Roy MJ, Walsh TJ. Histopathologic and immunohistochemical changes in gut-associated lymphoid tissues after treatment of rabbits with dexamethasone. *Lab Invest* 1992;66:437.
23. Ganz T, Weiss J. Antimicrobial peptides of phagocytes and epithelia. *Semin Hematol* 1997;34:343.
24. De Lucca AJ, Walsh TJ. Antifungal peptides: novel therapeutic compounds against emerging pathogens. *Antimicrob Agents Chemother* 1999;43:1.
25. Roilides E, Uhlig K, Venzon D, Pizzo PA, Walsh TJ. Prevention of corticosteroid-induced suppression of human polymorphonuclear leukocyte-induced damage of *Aspergillus fumigatus* hyphae by granulocyte colony-stimulating factor and gamma interferon. *Infect Immunol* 1993;61:4870.
26. Segal BH, Sneller MC. Infectious complications of immunosuppressive therapy in patients with rheumatic diseases. *Rheum Dis Clin North Am* 1997;23:219.
27. Fauci AS, Dale DC, Balow JE. Glucocorticosteroid therapy: mechanisms of action and clinical considerations. *Ann Intern Med* 1976;84:304.
28. Butler WT, Rossen RD. Effects of corticosteroids on immunity in man. I. Decreased serum IgG concentration caused by 3 or 5 days of high doses of methylprednisolone. *J Clin Invest* 1973;52:2629.
29. Staples PJ, Gerding DN, Decker JL, Gordon RS Jr. Incidence of infection in systemic lupus erythematosus. *Arthritis Rheum* 1974;17:1.
30. Ng TT, Robson GD, Denning DW. Hydrocortisone-enhanced growth of Aspergillus spp.: implications for pathogenesis. *Microbiology* 1994;140:2475.
31. Ferrazzini G, Klein J, Sulh H, et al. Interaction between trimethoprim-sulfamethoxazole and methotrexate in children with leukemia. *J Pediatr* 1990;117:823.
32. Kamel OW, van de Rijn M, Weiss LM, et al. Brief report: reversible lymphomas associated with Epstein-Barr virus occurring during methotrexate therapy for rheumatoid arthritis and dermatomyositis. *N Engl J Med* 1993;328:1317.
33. Kuhns DB, Young HA, Gallin EK, Gallin JI. Ca2+-dependent production and release of IL-8 in human neutrophils. *J Immunol* 1998;161:4332.
34. Ringden O, Backman L, Lonnqvist B, et al. A randomized trial comparing use of cyclosporin and methotrexate for graft-versus-host disease prophylaxis in bone marrow transplant recipients with haematological malignancies. *Bone Marrow Transplant* 1986;1:41.
35. Atkinson K, Biggs JC, Ting A, et al. Cyclosporin A is associated with faster engraftment and less mucositis than methotrexate after allogeneic bone marrow transplantation. *Br J Haematol* 1983;53:265.
36. Anaissie E, Kontoyiannis DP, Kantarjian H, et al. Listeriosis in patients with chronic lymphocytic leukemia who were treated with fludarabine and prednisone. *Ann Intern Med* 1992;117:466.
37. O'Brien S, Kantarjian H, Beran M, et al. Results of fludarabine and prednisone therapy in 264 patients with chronic lymphocytic leukemia with multivariate analysis-derived prognostic model for response to treatment. *Blood* 1993;82:1695.
38. Byrd JC, Hargis JB, Kester KE, et al. Opportunistic pulmonary infections with fludarabine in previously treated patients with low-grade lymphoid malignancies: a role for *Pneumocystis carinii* pneumonia prophylaxis. *Am J Hematol* 1995;49:135.
39. Klempner MS, Noring R, Mier JW, Atkins MB. An acquired chemotactic defect in neutrophils from patients receiving interleukin-2 immunotherapy. *N Engl J Med* 1990;322:959.
40. Molrine DC, Siber GR, Samra Y, et al. Normal IgG and impaired IgM responses to polysaccharide vaccines in asplenic patients. *J Infect Dis* 1999;179:513.
41. Doern GV, Pfaller MA, Erwin ME, Brueggemann AB, Jones RN. The prevalence of fluoroquinolone resistance among clinically significant respiratory tract isolates of *Streptococcus pneumoniae* in the United States and Canada—1997 results from the SENTRY Antimicrobial Surveillance Program. *Diagn Microbiol Infect Dis* 1998;32:313.
42. Chen DK, McGeer A, de Azavedo JC, Low DE. Decreased susceptibility of *Streptococcus pneumoniae* to fluoroquinolones in Canada. Canadian Bacterial Surveillance Network. *N Engl J Med* 1999;341:233.
43. Pers C, Gahrn-Hansen B, Frederiksen W. *Capnocytophaga canimorsus* septicemia in Denmark, 1982–1995: review of 39 cases. *Clin Infect Dis* 1996;23:71.
44. Lion C, Escande F, Burdin JC. *Capnocytophaga canimorsus* infections in human: review of the literature and cases report. *Eur J Epidemiol* 1996;12:521.
45. Rosner F, Zarrabi MH, Benach JL, Habicht GS. Babesiosis in splenectomized adults. Review of 22 reported cases. *Am J Med* 1984;76:696.
46. Clark RA, Johnson FL, Klebanoff SJ, Thomas ED. Defective neutrophil chemotaxis in bone marrow transplant patients. *J Clin Invest* 1976;58:22.
47. Sosa R, Weiden PL, Storb R, Syrotuck J, Thomas ED. Granulocyte function in human allogenic marrow graft recipients. *Exp Hematol* 1980;8:1183.
48. Winston DJ, Territo MC, Ho WG, et al. Alveolar macrophage dysfunction in human bone marrow transplant recipients. *Am J Med* 1982;73:859.
49. Lum LG. The kinetics of immune reconstitution after human marrow transplantation. *Blood* 1987;69:369.
50. Mackall CL, Gress RE. Pathways of T-cell regeneration in mice and humans: implications for bone marrow transplantation and immunotherapy. *Immunol Rev* 1997;157:61.
51. Matsue K, Lum LG, Witherspoon RP, Storb R. Proliferative and differentiative responses of B cells from human marrow graft recipients to T cell-derived factors. *Blood* 1987;69:308.
52. Winston DJ, Schiffman G, Wang DC, et al. Pneumococcal infections after human bone-marrow transplantation. *Ann Intern Med* 1979;91:835.
53. Kalhs P, Kier P, Lechner K. Functional asplenia after bone marrow transplantation [letter]. *Ann Intern Med* 1990;113:805.
54. Kalhs P, Panzer S, Kletter K, et al. Functional asplenia after bone marrow transplantation. A late complication related to extensive chronic graft-versus-host disease. *Ann Intern Med* 1988;109:461.
55. Seddik M, Seemayer TA, Lapp WS. T cell functional defect associated with thymic epithelial cell injury induced by a graft-versus-host reaction. *Transplantation* 1980;29:61.
56. Johanson WG, Pierce AK, Sanford JP. Changing pharyngeal bacterial flora of hospitalized patients. Emergence of gram-negative bacilli. *N Engl J Med* 1969;281:1137.
57. Woods DE. Role of fibronectin in the pathogenesis of gram-negative bacillary pneumonia. *Rev Infect Dis* 1987;9(Suppl 4):S386.
58. Schimpff SC, Young VM, Green WH, et al. Origin of infection in acute lymphocytic leukemia: significance of hospital acquisition of potential pathogens. *Ann Intern Med* 1972;77:707.
59. Edmond MB, Wallace SE, McClish DK, et al. Nosocomial bloodstream infections in United States hospitals: a three-year analysis. *Clin Infect Dis* 1999;29:239.
60. Smith TL, Pearson ML, Wilcox KR, et al. Emergence of vancomycin resistance in *Staphylococcus aureus.* Glycopeptide-intermediate *Staphylococcus aureus* Working Group. *N Engl J Med* 1999;340:493.
61. Sieradzki K, Roberts RB, Haber SW, Tomasz A. The development of vancomycin resistance in a patient with methicillin- resistant *Staphylococcus aureus* infection. *N Engl J Med* 1999;340:517.
62. Irish D, Eltringham I, Teall A, et al. Control of an outbreak of an epidemic methicillin-resistant *Staphylococcus aureus* also resistant to mupirocin. *J Hosp Infect* 1998;39:19.
63. Moellering RC, Linden PK, Reinhardt J, et al. The efficacy and safety of quinupristin/dalfopristin for the treatment of infections caused by vancomycin-resistant *Enterococcus faecium.* Synercid Emergency-Use Study Group. *J Antimicrob Chemother* 1999;44:251.
64. Noskin GA, Siddiqui F, Stosor V, Hacek D, Peterson LR. In vitro activities of linezolid against important gram-positive bacterial pathogens including vancomycin-resistant enterococci. *Antimicrob Agents Chemother* 1999;43:2059.
65. Elting LS, Bodey GP, Keefe BH. Septicemia and shock syndrome due to viridans streptococci: a case-control study of predisposing factors. *Clin Infect Dis* 1992;14:1201.
66. McWhinney PH, Patel S, Whiley RA, et al. Activities of potential therapeutic and prophylactic antibiotics against blood culture isolates of viridans group streptococci from neutropenic patients receiving ciprofloxacin. *Antimicrob Agents Chemother* 1993;37:2493.
67. Bochud PY, Calandra T, Francioli P. Bacteremia due to viridans streptococci in neutropenic patients: a review. *Am J Med* 1994;97:256.
68. Steiner M, Villablanca J, Kersey J, et al. Viridans streptococcal shock in bone marrow transplantation patients. *Am J Hematol* 1993;42:354.
69. Martino R, Manteiga R, Sanchez I, et al. Viridans streptococcal shock syndrome during bone marrow transplantation. *Acta Haematol* 1995;94:69.
70. Elting LS, Rubenstein EB, Rolston KV, Bodey GP. Outcomes of bacteremia in patients with cancer and neutropenia: observations from two decades of epidemiological and clinical trials. *Clin Infect Dis* 1997;25:247.
71. Hughes WT, Armstrong D, Bodey GP, et al. 1997 guidelines for the use of antimicrobial agents in neutropenic patients with unexplained fever. Infectious Diseases Society of America. *Clin Infect Dis* 1997;25:551.
72. van der Lelie H, Leverstein-Van Hall M, Mertens M, et al. *Corynebacterium* CDC group JK (*Corynebacterium jeikeium*) sepsis in haematological patients: a report of three cases and a systematic literature review. *Scand J Infect Dis* 1995;27:581.
73. Stamm WE, Tompkins LS, Wagner KF, et al. Infection due to *Corynebacterium* species in marrow transplant patients. *Ann Intern Med* 1979;91:167.
74. Henrickson KJ, Shenep JL, Flynn PM, Pui CH. Primary cutaneous bacillus cereus infection in neutropenic children. *Lancet* 1989;1:601.

75. McWhinney PH, Kibbler CC, Gillespie SH, et al. Stomatococcus mucilaginosus: an emerging pathogen in neutropenic patients. *Clin Infect Dis* 1992;14:641.
76. Swenson JM, Facklam RR, Thornsberry C. Antimicrobial susceptibility of vancomycin-resistant *Leuconostoc, Pediococcus,* and *Lactobacillus* species. *Antimicrob Agents Chemother* 1990;34:543.
77. Bush K, Jacoby GA, Medeiros AA. A functional classification scheme for beta-lactamases and its correlation with molecular structure. *Antimicrob Agents Chemother* 1995;39:1211.
78. Meyer KS, Urban C, Eagan JA, Berger BJ, Rahal JJ. Nosocomial outbreak of *Klebsiella* infection resistant to late-generation cephalosporins. *Ann Intern Med* 1993;119:353.
79. Bodey GP, Jadeja L, Elting L. *Pseudomonas* bacteremia. Retrospective analysis of 410 episodes. *Arch Intern Med* 1985;145:1621.
80. Livermore DM. Interplay of impermeability and chromosomal β-lactamase activity in imipenem-resistant *Pseudomonas aeruginosa. Antimicrob Agents Chemother* 1992;36:2046.
81. Khardori N, Elting L, Wong E, Schable B, Bodey GP. Nosocomial infections due to *Xanthomonas maltophilia* (*Pseudomonas maltophilia*) in patients with cancer. *Rev Infect Dis* 1990;12:997.
82. Vartivarian SE, Papadakis KA, Palacios JA, Manning JT Jr, Anaissie EJ. Mucocutaneous and soft tissue infections caused by *Xanthomonas maltophilia.* A new spectrum. *Ann Intern Med* 1994;121:969.
83. Villers D, Espaze E, Coste-Burel M, et al. Nosocomial *Acinetobacter baumannii* infections: microbiological and clinical epidemiology. *Ann Intern Med* 1998;129:182.
84. Rolston K, Guan Z, Bodey GP, Elting L. Acinetobacter calcoaceticus septicemia in patients with cancer. *South Med J* 1985;78:647.
85. Thaler M, Gill V, Pizzo PA. Emergence of *Clostridium tertium as* a pathogen in neutropenic patients. *Am J Med* 1986;81:596.
86. Bodey GP, Rodriguez S, Fainstein V, Elting LS. Clostridial bacteremia in cancer patients. A 12-year experience. *Cancer* 1991;67:1928.
87. Stevens DL, Maier KA, Laine BM, Mitten JE. Comparison of clindamycin, rifampin, tetracycline, metronidazole, and penicillin for efficacy in prevention of experimental gas gangrene due to *Clostridium perfringens. J Infect Dis* 1987;155:220.
88. Kurzrock R, Zander A, Vellekoop L, et al. Mycobacterial pulmonary infections after allogeneic bone marrow transplantation. *Am J Med* 1984;77:35
89. Roy V, Weisdorf D. Mycobacterial infections following bone marrow transplantation: a 20 year retrospective review. *Bone Marrow Transplant* 1997;19:467.
90. Aljurf M, Gyger M, Alrajhi A, et al. Mycobacterium tuberculosis infection in allogeneic bone marrow transplantation patients. *Bone Marrow Transplant* 1999;24:551.
91. Ip MS, Yuen KY, Woo PC, et al. Risk factors for pulmonary tuberculosis in bone marrow transplant recipients. *Am J Respir Crit Care Med* 1998;158:1173.
92. Skogberg K, Ruutu P, Tukiainen P, Valtonen V. Effect of immunosuppressive therapy on the clinical presentation and outcome of tuberculosis. *Clin Infect Dis* 1993;17:1012.
93. Aljada IS, Crane JK, Corriere N, Wagle DG, Amsterdam D. *Mycobacterium bovis* BCG causing vertebral osteomyelitis (Pott's disease) following intravesical BCG therapy. *J Clin Microbiol* 1999;37:2106.
94. Ward MS, Lam KV, Cannell PK, Herrmann RP. Mycobacterial central venous catheter tunnel infection: a difficult problem. *Bone Marrow Transplant* 1999;24:325.
95. Bennett C, Vardiman J, Golomb H. Disseminated atypical mycobacterial infection in patients with hairy cell leukemia. *Am J Med* 1986;80:891.
96. White MH, Papadopoulos EB, Small TN, Kiehn TE, Armstrong D. *Mycobacterium haemophilum* infections in bone marrow transplant recipients. *Transplantation* 1995;60:957.
97. Berkey P, Bodey GP. Nocardial infection in patients with neoplastic disease. *Rev Infect Dis* 1989;11:407.
98. Frazier AR, Rosenow ECD, Roberts GD. Nocardiosis. A review of 25 cases occurring during 24 months. *Mayo Clin Proc* 1975,50:657.
99. Young LS, Armstrong D, Blevins A, Lieberman P. *Nocardia asteroides* infection complicating neoplastic disease. *Am J Med* 1971;50:356.
100. van Burik JA, Hackman RC, Nadeem SQ, et al. Nocardiosis after bone marrow transplantation: a retrospective study. *Clin Infect Dis* 1997;24:1154.
101. Choucino C, Goodman SA, Greer JP, et al. Nocardial infections in bone marrow transplant recipients. *Clin Infect Dis* 1996;23:1012.
102. Pfaller MA, Jones RN, Messer SA, Edmond MB, Wenzel RP. National surveillance of nosocomial blood stream infection due to *Candida albicans*: frequency of occurrence and antifungal susceptibility in the SCOPE Program. *Diagn Microbiol Infect Dis* 1998;31:327.
103. Edwards JE Jr, Bodey GP, Bowden RA, et al. International Conference for the Development of a Consensus on the Management and Prevention of Severe Candidal Infections. *Clin Infect Dis* 1997;25:43.
104. Viscoli C, Girmenia C, Marinus A, et al. Candidemia in cancer patients: a prospective, multicenter surveillance study by the Invasive Fungal Infection Group (IFIG) of the European Organization for Research and Treatment of Cancer (EORTC). *Clin Infect Dis* 1999;28:1071.
105. Anaissie EJ, Kontoyiannis DP, O'Brien S, et al. Infections in patients with chronic lymphocytic leukemia treated with fludarabine. *Ann Intern Med* 1998;129:559.
106. Wingard JR. Importance of *Candida* species other than *C. albicans* as pathogens in oncology patients. *Clin Infect Dis* 1995;20:115.
107. Wingard JR, Dick JD, Merz WG, et al. Pathogenicity of *Candida tropicalis* and *Candida albicans* after gastrointestinal inoculation in mice. *Infect Immunol* 1980;29:808.
108. Wingard JR, Merz WG, Saral R. Candida tropicalis: a major pathogen in immunocompromised patients. *Ann Intern Med* 1979;91:539.
109. Berenguer J, Buck M, Witebsky F, et al. Lysis-centrifugation blood cultures in the detection of tissue-proven invasive candidiasis. Disseminated versus single-organ infection. *Diagn Microbiol Infect Dis* 1993;17:103.
110. Walsh TJ, Chanock SJ. Diagnosis of invasive fungal infections: advances in nonculture systems. *Curr Clin Top Infect Dis* 1998;18:101.
111. Lecciones JA, Lee JW, Navarro EE, et al. Vascular catheter-associated fungemia in patients with cancer: analysis of 155 episodes. *Clin Infect Dis* 1992;14:875.
112. Rex JH, Bennett JE, Sugar AM, et al. A randomized trial comparing fluconazole with amphotericin B for the treatment of candidemia in patients without neutropenia. Candidemia Study Group and the National Institute. *N Engl J Med* 1994;331:1325.
113. Anaissie EJ, Darouiche RO, Abi-Said D, et al. Management of invasive candidal infections: results of a prospective, randomized, multicenter study of fluconazole versus amphotericin B and review of the literature. *Clin Infect Dis* 1996;23:964.
114. Anaissie EJ, Vartivarian SE, Abi-Said D, et al. Fluconazole versus amphotericin B in the treatment of hematogenous candidiasis: a matched cohort study. *Am J Med* 1996;101:170.
115. Rex JH, Bennett JE, Sugar AM, et al. Intravascular catheter exchange and duration of candidemia. NIAID Mycoses Study Group and the Candidemia Study Group. *Clin Infect Dis* 1995;21:994.
116. Cole GT, Halawa AA, Anaissie EJ. The role of the gastrointestinal tract in hematogenous candidiasis: from the laboratory to the bedside. *Clin Infect Dis* 1996;22(Suppl 2):S73.
117. Thaler M, Pastakia B, Shawker TH, O'Leary T, Pizzo PA. Hepatic candidiasis in cancer patients: the evolving picture of the syndrome. *Ann Intern Med* 1988;108:88.
118. Walsh TJ, Whitcomb P, Piscitelli S, et al. Safety, tolerance, and pharmacokinetics of amphotericin B lipid complex in children with hepatosplenic candidiasis. *Antimicrob Agents Chemother* 1997;41:1944.
119. Walsh TJ, Whitcomb PO, Revankar SG, Pizzo PA. Successful treatment of hepatosplenic candidiasis through repeated cycles of chemotherapy and neutropenia. *Cancer* 1995;76:2357.
120. Wald A, Leisenring W, van Burik JA, Bowden RA. Epidemiology of *Aspergillus* infections in a large cohort of patients undergoing bone marrow transplantation. *J Infect Dis* 1997;175:1459.
121. McWhinney PH, Kibbler CC, Hamon MD, et al. Progress in the diagnosis and management of aspergillosis in bone marrow transplantation: 13 years' experience. *Clin Infect Dis* 1993;17:397.
122. Yuen KY, Woo PC, Ip MS, et al. Stage-specific manifestation of mold infections in bone marrow transplant recipients: risk factors and clinical significance of positive concentrated smears. *Clin Infect Dis* 1997;25:37.
123. Young RC, Bennett JE, Vogel CL, Carbone PP, DeVita VT. Aspergillosis. The spectrum of the disease in 98 patients. *Medicine (Baltimore)* 1970;49:147.
124. Yu VL, Muder RR, Poorsattar A. Significance of isolation of *Aspergillus* from the respiratory tract in diagnosis of invasive pulmonary aspergillosis. Results from a three-year prospective study. *Am J Med* 1986;81:249.
125. Kuhlman JE, Fishman EK, Burch PA, et al. Invasive pulmonary aspergillosis in acute leukemia. The contribution of CT to early diagnosis and aggressive management. *Chest* 1987;92:95.
126. Caillot D, Casasnovas O, Bernard A, et al. Improved management of invasive pulmonary aspergillosis in neutropenic patients using early thoracic computed tomographic scan and surgery. *J Clin Oncol* 1997;15:139.
127. Einsele H, Quabeck K, Muller KD, et al. Prediction of invasive pulmonary aspergillosis from colonisation of lower respiratory tract before marrow transplantation [letter]. *Lancet* 1998;352:1443.
128. Bretagne S, Costa JM, Bart-Delabesse E, et al. Comparison of serum galactomannan antigen detection and competitive polymerase chain reaction for diagnosing invasive aspergillosis. *Clin Infect Dis* 1998;26:1407.
129. Sutton DA, Sanche SE, Revankar SG, Fothergill AW, Rinaldi MG. In vitro amphotericin B resistance in clinical isolates of *Aspergillus terreus*, with a head-to-head comparison to voriconazole. *J Clin Microbiol* 1999;37:2343.
130. Pagano L, Ricci P, Nosari A, et al. Fatal haemoptysis in pulmonary filamentous mycosis: an underevaluated cause of death in patients with acute leukaemia in haematological complete remission. A retrospective study and review of the literature. Gimema Infection Program (Gruppo Italiano Malattie Ematologiche dell'Adulto). *Br J Haematol* 1995;89:500.
131. Offner F, Cordonnier C, Ljungman P, et al. Impact of previous aspergillosis on the outcome of bone marrow transplantation. *Clin Infect Dis* 1998;26:1098.
132. Karp JE, Burch PA, Merz WG. An approach to intensive antileukemia therapy in patients with previous invasive aspergillosis. *Am J Med* 1988;85:203.
133. Martino R, Lopez R, Sureda A, Brunet S, Domingo-Albos A. Risk of reactivation of a recent invasive fungal infection in patients with hematological malignancies undergoing further intensive chemo-radiotherapy. A single-center experience and review of the literature. *Haematologica* 1997;82:297.
134. Sugar AM. Mucormycosis. *Clin Infect Dis* 1992;14(Suppl 1):S126.
135. Diamond RD, Bennett JE. Prognostic factors in cryptococcal meningitis: a study of 11 cases. *Ann Intern Med* 1974;80:176.
136. Griffin FM Jr. Roles of macrophage Fc and C3b receptors in phagocytosis of immunologically coated *Cryptococcus neoformans. Proc Natl Acad Sci U S A* 1981;78:3853.
137. Kozel TR. Opsonization and phagocytosis of *Cryptococcus neoformans. Arch Med Res* 1993;24:211.
138. Dromer F, Mathoulin S, Dupont B, Brugiere O, Letenneur L. Comparison of the efficacy of amphotericin B and fluconazole in the treatment of cryptococcosis in human immunodeficiency virus-negative patients: retrospective analysis of 83 cases. French Cryptococcosis Study Group. *Clin Infect Dis* 1996;22(Suppl 2):S154.
139. Park MK, Hospenthal DR, Bennett JE. Treatment of hydrocephalus secondary to cryptococcal meningitis by use of shunting. *Clin Infect Dis* 1999;28:629.
140. Rex JH, Larsen RA, Dismukes WE, Cloud GA, Bennett JE. Catastrophic visual loss due to *Cryptococcus neoformans* meningitis. *Medicine (Baltimore)* 1993;72:207.
141. Bennett JE, Dismukes WE, Duma RJ, et al. A comparison of amphotericin B alone and combined with flucytosine in the treatment of cryptococcal meningitis. *N Engl J Med* 1979;301:126.
142. Saag MS, Cloud GA, Graybill JR, et al. A comparison of itraconazole versus fluconazole as maintenance therapy for AIDS-associated cryptococcal meningitis. National Institute of Allergy and Infectious Diseases Mycoses Study Group. *Clin Infect Dis* 1999;28:291.
143. van der Horst CM, Saag MS, Cloud GA, et al. Treatment of cryptococcal meningitis associated with the acquired immunodeficiency syndrome. National Institute of Allergy and Infectious Diseases Mycoses Study Group and AIDS Clinical Trials Group. *N Engl J Med* 1997;337:15.

144. Walsh TJ, Newman KR, Moody M, Wharton RC, Wade JC. Trichosporonosis in patients with neoplastic disease. *Medicine (Baltimore)* 1986;65:268.
145. Walsh TJ. Trichosporonosis. *Infect Dis Clin North Am* 1989;3:43.
146. Campbell CK, Payne AL, Teall AJ, Brownell A, Mackenzie DW. Cryptococcal latex antigen test positive in patient with *Trichosporon beigelii* infection [letter]. *Lancet* 1985;2:43.
147. Walsh TJ, Lee JW, Roilides E, Pizzo PA. Recent progress and current problems in management of invasive fungal infections in patients with neoplastic diseases. *Curr Opin Oncol* 1992;4:647.
148. Anaissie EJ, Hachem R, Karyotakis NC, et al. Comparative efficacies of amphotericin B, triazoles, and combination of both as experimental therapy for murine trichosporonosis. *Antimicrob Agents Chemother* 1994;38:2541.
149. Anaissie E, Gokaslan A, Hachem R, et al. Azole therapy for trichosporonosis: clinical evaluation of eight patients, experimental therapy for murine infection, and review. *Clin Infect Dis* 1992;15:781.
150. Martino P, Venditti M, Micozzi A, et al. *Blastoschizomyces capitatus*: an emerging cause of invasive fungal disease in leukemia patients. *Rev Infect Dis* 1990;12:570.
151. Redline RW, Dahms BB. *Malassezia* pulmonary vasculitis in an infant on long-term Intralipid therapy. *N Engl J Med* 1981;305:1395.
152. Vartivarian SE, Anaissie EJ, Bodey GP. Emerging fungal pathogens in immunocompromised patients: classification, diagnosis, and management. *Clin Infect Dis* 1993;17(Suppl 2):S487.
153. Dixon DM, Walsh TJ, Merz WG, McGinnis MR. Infections due to *Xylohypha bantiana* (*Cladosporium trichoides*). *Rev Infect Dis* 1989;11:515.
154. Segal BH, Walsh TJ, Liu JM, Wilson JD, Kwon-Chung KJ. Invasive infection with *Fusarium chlamydosporum* in a patient with aplastic anemia. *J Clin Microbiol* 1998;36:1772.
155. Boutati EI, Anaissie EJ. Fusarium, a significant emerging pathogen in patients with hematologic malignancy: ten years' experience at a cancer center and implications for management. *Blood* 1997;90:999.
156. Walsh TJ, Peter J, McGough DA, et al. Activities of amphotericin B and antifungal azoles alone and in combination against *Pseudallescheria boydii*. *Antimicrob Agents Chemother* 1995;39:1361.
157. Durkin MM, Connolly PA, Wheat LJ. Comparison of radioimmunoassay and enzyme-linked immunoassay methods for detection of *Histoplasma capsulatum* var. *capsulatum* antigen. *J Clin Microbiol* 1997;35:2252.
158. Deresinski SC, Stevens DA. Coccidioidomycosis in compromised hosts. Experience at Stanford University Hospital. *Medicine (Baltimore)* 1975;54:377.
159. Anaissie EJ, Vadhan-Raj S. Is it time to redefine the management of febrile neutropenia in cancer patients? *Am J Med* 1995;98:221.
160. Goodman JL, Winston DJ, Greenfield RA, et al. A controlled trial of fluconazole to prevent fungal infections in patients undergoing bone marrow transplantation. *N Engl J Med* 1992;326:845.
161. Slavin MA, Osborne B, Adams R, et al. Efficacy and safety of fluconazole prophylaxis for fungal infections after marrow transplantation—a prospective, randomized, double-blind study. *J Infect Dis* 1995;171:1545.
162. van Burik JH, Leisenring W, Myerson D, et al. The effect of prophylactic fluconazole on the clinical spectrum of fungal diseases in bone marrow transplant recipients with special attention to hepatic candidiasis. An autopsy study of 355 patients. *Medicine (Baltimore)* 1998;77:246.
163. Winston DJ, Chandrasekar PH, Lazarus HM, et al. Fluconazole prophylaxis of fungal infections in patients with acute leukemia. Results of a randomized placebo-controlled, double-blind, multicenter trial. *Ann Intern Med* 1993;118:495.
164. Rotstein C, Bow EJ, Laverdiere M, et al. Randomized placebo-controlled trial of fluconazole prophylaxis for neutropenic cancer patients: benefit based on purpose and intensity of cytotoxic therapy. The Canadian Fluconazole Prophylaxis Study Group. *Clin Infect Dis* 1999;28:331.
165. Wingard JR, Merz WG, Rinaldi MG, et al. Increase in *Candida krusei* infection among patients with bone marrow transplantation and neutropenia treated prophylactically with fluconazole. *N Engl J Med* 1991;325:1274.
166. Berenguer J, Ali NM, Allende MC, et al. Itraconazole for experimental pulmonary aspergillosis: comparison with amphotericin B, interaction with cyclosporin A, and correlation between therapeutic response and itraconazole concentrations in plasma. *Antimicrob Agents Chemother* 1994;38:1303.
167. Denning DW, Lee JY, Hostetler JS, et al. NIAID Mycoses Study Group Multicenter Trial of Oral Itraconazole Therapy for Invasive Aspergillosis [published erratum appears in *Am J Med* 1994 Nov;97:497]. *Am J Med* 1994;97:135.
168. Stevens DA, Lee JY. Analysis of compassionate use itraconazole therapy for invasive aspergillosis by the NIAID Mycoses Study Group criteria. *Arch Intern Med* 1997;157:1857.
169. Groll AH, Piscitelli SC, Walsh TJ. Clinical pharmacology of systemic antifungal agents: a comprehensive review of agents in clinical use, current investigational compounds, and putative targets for antifungal drug development. *Adv Pharmacol* 1998;44:343.
170. Louie A, Baltch AL, Franke MA, Smith RP, Gordon MA. Comparative capacity of four antifungal agents to stimulate murine macrophages to produce tumour necrosis factor alpha: an effect that is attenuated by pentoxifylline, liposomal vesicles, and dexamethasone. *J Antimicrob Chemother* 1994;34:975.
171. Rogers PD, Kramer RE, Chapman SW, Cleary JD. Amphotericin B-induced interleukin-1beta expression in human monocytic cells is calcium and calmodulin dependent. *J Infect Dis* 1999;180:1259.
172. MacGregor RR, Bennett JE, Erslev AJ. Erythropoietin concentration in amphotericin B-induced anemia. *Antimicrob Agents Chemother* 1978;14:270.
173. Hiemenz JW, Walsh TJ. Lipid formulations of amphotericin B: recent progress and future directions. *Clin Infect Dis* 1996;22(Suppl 2):S133.
174. Walsh TJ, Finberg RW, Arndt C, et al. Liposomal amphotericin B for empiric therapy in patients with persistent fever and neutropenia. National Institute of Allergy and Infectious Diseases Mycoses Study Group. *N Engl J Med* 1999;340:764.
174a. Prentice HG, Hann IM, Herbrecht R, et al. A randomized comparison of liposomal versus conventional amphotericin B for the treatment of pyrexia of unknown origin in neutropenic patients. *Br J Haematol* 1997;98:711.
175. Wingard JR, Hiemenz J, Anaissie EJ, et al. *A randomized study double blind safety study of AmBisome and Abelcet in febrile neutropenic patients* [abst]. Focus on Fungal Infections, 9, San Diego, CA, March 1999.
176. Walsh TJ, Hiemenz JW, Seibel NL, et al. Amphotericin B lipid complex for invasive fungal infections: analysis of safety and efficacy in 556 cases. *Clin Infect Dis* 1998;26:1383.
177. Anaissie EJ, White J, Uzun O, et al. Amphotericin B lipid complex (ABLC) versus amphotericin B (AMB) for treatment of hematogenous and invasive candidiasis: a prospective, randomized, multicenter trial. *Abstracts of the 35th Interscience Conference on Antimicrobial Agents and Chemotherapy, Washington, DC, 1995.* American Society for Microbiology.
178. Bowden RA, Cays M, Gooley T, Mamelok RD, van Burik JA. Phase I study of amphotericin B colloidal dispersion for the treatment of invasive fungal infections after marrow transplant. *J Infect Dis* 1996;173:1208.
179. Oppenheim BA, Herbrecht R, Kusne S. The safety and efficacy of amphotericin B colloidal dispersion in the treatment of invasive mycoses. *Clin Infect Dis* 1995;21:1145.
180. Noskin G, Pietrelli L, Gurwith M, Bowden R. Treatment of invasive fungal infections with amphotericin B colloidal dispersion in bone marrow transplant recipients. *Bone Marrow Transplant* 1999;23:697.
181. White MH, Anaissie EJ, Kusne S, et al. Amphotericin B colloidal dispersion vs. amphotericin B as therapy for invasive aspergillosis. *Clin Infect Dis* 1997;24:635.
182. White MH, Bowden RA, Sandler ES, et al. Randomized, double-blind clinical trial of amphotericin B colloidal dispersion vs. amphotericin B in the empiric treatment of fever and neutropenia. *Clin Infect Dis* 1998;27:296.
183. Wingard JR, Kubilis P, Lee L, et al. Clinical significance of nephrotoxicity in patients treated with Amphotericin B for suspected or proven aspergillosis. *Clin Infect Dis* 1999;29:1402.
184. Marco F, Pfaller MA, Messer SA, Jones RN. Activity of MK-0991 (L-743,872), a new echinocandin, compared with those of LY303366 and four other antifungal agents tested against blood stream isolates of *Candida* spp. *Diagn Microbiol Infect Dis* 1998;32:33.
185. Abruzzo GK, Flattery AM, Gill CJ, et al. Evaluation of the echinocandin antifungal MK-0991 (L-743,872): efficacies in mouse models of disseminated aspergillosis, candidiasis, and cryptococcosis. *Antimicrob Agents Chemother* 1997;41:2333.
186. Petraitiene R, Petraitis V, Groll AH, et al. Antifungal activity of LY303366, a novel echinocandin B, in experimental disseminated candidiasis in rabbits. *Antimicrob Agents Chemother* 1999;43:2148.
187. Arathoon E, Gotuzzo E, Noriega L, et al. *A randomized, double-blind, multicenter trial of MK-0991, an echinocandin antifungal agent, vs amphotericin B for the treatment of oropharyngeal candidiasis in adults.* Infectious Disease Society of America, Denver, CO, 1998.
188. Balfour HH Jr. Antiviral drugs. *N Engl J Med* 1999;340:1255.
189. Saral R, Ambinder RF, Burns WH, et al. Acyclovir prophylaxis against herpes simplex virus infection in patients with leukemia. A randomized, double-blind, placebo-controlled study. *Ann Intern Med* 1983;99:773.
190. Meyers JD, Flournoy N, Thomas ED. Infection with herpes simplex virus and cell-mediated immunity after marrow transplant. *J Infect Dis* 1980;142:338.
191. Wade JC, Newton B, Flournoy N, Meyers JD. Oral acyclovir for prevention of herpes simplex virus reactivation after marrow transplantation. *Ann Intern Med* 1984;100:823.
192. Miller W, Flynn P, McCullough J, et al. Cytomegalovirus infection after bone marrow transplantation: an association with acute graft-v-host disease. *Blood* 1986;67:1162.
193. Holmberg LA, Boeckh M, Hooper H, et al. Increased incidence of cytomegalovirus disease after autologous CD34-selected peripheral stem cell transplantation. *Blood* 1999;94:4029.
194. Nguyen Q, Champlin R, Giralt S, et al. Late cytomegalovirus pneumonia in adult allogeneic blood and marrow transplant recipients. *Clin Infect Dis* 1999;28:618.
195. Prentice HG, Kho P. Clinical strategies for the management of cytomegalovirus infection and disease in allogeneic bone marrow transplant. *Bone Marrow Transplant* 1997;19:135.
196. Reed EC, Wolford JL, Kopecky KJ, et al. Ganciclovir for the treatment of cytomegalovirus gastroenteritis in bone marrow transplant patients. A randomized, placebo-controlled trial. *Ann Intern Med* 1990;112:505.
197. Winston DJ, Ho WG, Bartoni K, et al. Ganciclovir prophylaxis of cytomegalovirus infection and disease in allogeneic bone marrow transplant recipients. Results of a placebo-controlled, double-blind trial. *Ann Intern Med* 1993;118:179.
198. Bowden RA, Sayers M, Flournoy N, et al. Cytomegalovirus immune globulin and seronegative blood products to prevent primary cytomegalovirus infection after marrow transplantation. *N Engl J Med* 1986;314:1006.
199. Miller WJ, McCullough J, Balfour HH Jr, et al. Prevention of cytomegalovirus infection following bone marrow transplantation: a randomized trial of blood product screening. *Bone Marrow Transplant* 1991;7:227.
200. Prentice HG, Gluckman E, Powles RL, et al. Impact of long-term acyclovir on cytomegalovirus infection and survival after allogeneic bone marrow transplantation. European Acyclovir for CMV Prophylaxis Study Group. *Lancet* 1994;343:749.
201. Meyers JD, Reed EC, Shepp DH, et al. Acyclovir for prevention of cytomegalovirus infection and disease after allogeneic marrow transplantation. *N Engl J Med* 1988;318:70.
202. Buhles WC Jr, Mastre BJ, Tinker AJ, Strand V, Koretz SH. Ganciclovir treatment of life- or sight-threatening cytomegalovirus infection: experience in 314 immunocompromised patients. *Rev Infect Dis* 1988;10(Suppl 3):S495.
203. Goodrich JM, Bowden RA, Fisher L, et al. Ganciclovir prophylaxis to prevent cytomegalovirus disease after allogeneic marrow transplant. *Ann Intern Med* 1993;118:173.
204. Li CR, Greenberg PD, Gilbert MJ, Goodrich JM, Riddell SR. Recovery of HLA-restricted cytomegalovirus (CMV)-specific T-cell responses after allogeneic bone marrow transplant: correlation with CMV disease and effect of ganciclovir prophylaxis. *Blood* 1994;83:1971.
205. Boeckh M, Gooley TA, Myerson D, et al. Cytomegalovirus pp65 antigenemia-guided early treatment with ganciclovir versus ganciclovir at engraftment after allogeneic marrow transplantation: a randomized double-blind study. *Blood* 1996;88:4063.
206. Boeckh M, Bowden RA, Gooley T, Myerson D, Corey L. Successful modification of a pp65 antigenemia-based early treatment strategy for prevention of cytomegalovirus disease in allogeneic marrow transplant recipients [letter]. *Blood* 1999;93:1781.

207. Einsele H, Ehninger G, Hebart H, et al. Polymerase chain reaction monitoring reduces the incidence of cytomegalovirus disease and the duration and side effects of antiviral therapy after bone marrow transplantation. *Blood* 1995;86:2815.
208. Moretti S, Zikos P, Van Lint MT, et al. Forscarnet vs ganciclovir for cytomegalovirus (CMV) antigenemia after allogeneic hemopoietic stem cell transplantation (HSCT): a randomised study. *Bone Marrow Transplant* 1998;22:175.
209. Lowance D, Neumayer HH, Legendre CM, et al. Valacyclovir for the prevention of cytomegalovirus disease after renal transplantation. International Valacyclovir Cytomegalovirus Prophylaxis Transplantation Study Group. *N Engl J Med* 1999;340:1462.
210. Huang Z, Vafai A, Lee J, Mahalingam R, Hayward AR. Specific lysis of targets expressing varicella-zoster virus gpI or gpIV by CD4+ human T-cell clones. *J Virol* 1992;66:2664.
211. Diaz PS, Smith S, Hunter E, Arvin AM. T lymphocyte cytotoxicity with natural varicella-zoster virus infection and after immunization with live attenuated varicella vaccine. *J Immunol* 1989;142:636.
212. Meyers JD, Flournoy N, Thomas ED. Cell-mediated immunity to varicella-zoster virus after allogeneic marrow transplant. *J Infect Dis* 1980;141:479.
213. Haumont M, Jurdan M, Kangro H, et al. Neutralizing antibody responses induced by varicella-zoster virus gE and gB glycoproteins following infection, reactivation or immunization. *J Med Virol* 1997;53:63.
214. Locksley RM, Flournoy N, Sullivan KM, Meyers JD. Infection with varicella-zoster virus after marrow transplantation. *J Infect Dis* 1985;152:1172.
215. Balfour HH Jr, Bean B, Laskin OL, et al. Acyclovir halts progression of herpes zoster in immunocompromised patients. *N Engl J Med* 1983;308:1448.
216. Williams WW. CDC guidelines for the prevention and control of nosocomial infections. Guideline for infection control in hospital personnel. *Am J Infect Control* 1984;12:34.
217. Hardy I, Gershon AA, Steinberg SP, LaRussa P. The incidence of zoster after immunization with live attenuated varicella vaccine. A study in children with leukemia. Varicella Vaccine Collaborative Study Group. *N Engl J Med* 1991;325:1545.
218. Gershon AA, Steinberg SP. Persistence of immunity to varicella in children with leukemia immunized with live attenuated varicella vaccine. *N Engl J Med* 1989;320:892.
219. Peter G. *1997 Red Book: Report of the Committee on Infectious Diseases.* Elk Grove Village, IL: American Academy of Pediatrics, 1997.
220. Rickinson AB, Moss DJ. Human cytotoxic T lymphocyte responses to Epstein-Barr virus infection. *Annu Rev Immunol* 1997;15:405.
221. Lucas KG, Small TN, Heller G, Dupont B, O'Reilly RJ. The development of cellular immunity to Epstein-Barr virus after allogeneic bone marrow transplantation. *Blood* 1996;87:2594.
222. Young L, Alfieri C, Hennessy K, et al. Expression of Epstein-Barr virus transformation-associated genes in tissues of patients with EBV lymphoproliferative disease. *N Engl J Med* 1989;321:1080.
223. Zutter MM, Martin PJ, Sale GE, et al. Epstein-Barr virus lymphoproliferation after bone marrow transplantation. *Blood* 1988;72:520.
224. Shapiro RS, McClain K, Frizzera G, et al. Epstein-Barr virus associated B cell lymphoproliferative disorders following bone marrow transplantation. *Blood* 1988;71:1234.
225. Salahuddin SZ, Ablashi DV, Markham PD, et al. Isolation of a new virus, HBLV, in patients with lymphoproliferative disorders. *Science* 1986;234:596.
226. Lusso P, Markham PD, Tschachler E, et al. In vitro cellular tropism of human B-lymphotropic virus (human herpesvirus-6). *J Exp Med* 1988;167:1659.
227. Wilborn F, Brinkmann V, Schmidt CA, et al. Herpesvirus type 6 in patients undergoing bone marrow transplantation: serologic features and detection by polymerase chain reaction. *Blood* 1994;83:3052.
228. Frenkel N, Katsafanas GC, Wyatt LS, Yoshikawa T, Asano Y. Bone marrow transplant recipients harbor the B variant of human herpesvirus 6. *Bone Marrow Transplant* 1994;14:839.
229. Drobyski WR, Dunne WM, Burd EM, et al. Human herpesvirus-6 (HHV-6) infection in allogeneic bone marrow transplant recipients: evidence of a marrow-suppressive role for HHV-6 in vivo. *J Infect Dis* 1993;167:735.
230. Drobyski WR, Knox KK, Majewski D, Carrigan DR. Brief report: fatal encephalitis due to variant B human herpesvirus-6 infection in a bone marrow-transplant recipient. *N Engl J Med* 1994;330:1356.
231. Carrigan DR, Drobyski WR, Russler SK, et al. Interstitial pneumonitis associated with human herpesvirus-6 infection after marrow transplantation. *Lancet* 1991;338:147.
232. Singh N, Carrigan DR. Human herpesvirus-6 in transplantation: an emerging pathogen. *Ann Intern Med* 1996;124:1065.
233. Whimbey E, Champlin RE, Couch RB, et al. Community respiratory virus infections among hospitalized adult bone marrow transplant recipients. *Clin Infect Dis* 1996;22:778.
234. Sable CA, Hayden FG. Orthomyxoviral and paramyxoviral infections in transplant patients. *Infect Dis Clin North Am* 1995;9:987.
235. Whimbey E, Couch RB, Englund JA, et al. Respiratory syncytial virus pneumonia in hospitalized adult patients with leukemia. *Clin Infect Dis* 1995;21:376.
236. Bowden R. Respiratory virus infections after marrow transplant: the Fred Hutchinson Cancer Research Center Experience. In Proceedings of a symposium: community respiratory infections in the immunocompromised host. *Am J Med* 1997;102:27.
237. Whimbey E, Champlin RE, Englund JA, et al. Combination therapy with aerosolized ribavirin and intravenous immunoglobulin for respiratory syncytial virus disease in adult bone marrow transplant recipients. *Bone Marrow Transplant* 1995;16:393.
238. Englund JA, Piedra PA, Jewell A, et al. Rapid diagnosis of respiratory syncytial virus infections in immunocompromised adults. *J Clin Microbiol* 1996;34:1649.
239. Lewinsohn DM, Bowden RA, Mattson D, Crawford SW. Phase I study of intravenous ribavirin treatment of respiratory syncytial virus pneumonia after marrow transplantation. *Antimicrob Agents Chemother* 1996;40:2555.
240. Whimbey E, Englund JA, Couch RB. Community respiratory virus infections in immunocompromised pateints with cancer. In Proceedings of a symposium: community respiratory infections in the immunocompromised host. *Am J Med* 1997;102:10.
241. Wendt CH, Weisdorf DJ, Jordan MC, Balfour HH Jr, Hertz MI. Parainfluenza virus respiratory infection after bone marrow transplantation. *N Engl J Med* 1992;326:921.
242. Englund JA, Champlin RE, Wyde PR, et al. Common emergence of amantadine- and rimantadine-resistant influenza A viruses in symptomatic immunocompromised adults. *Clin Infect Dis* 1998;26:1418.
243. Stein DS, Creticos CM, Jackson GG, et al. Oral ribavirin treatment of influenza A and B. *Antimicrob Agents Chemother* 1987;31:1285.
244. Hayden FG, Osterhaus AD, Treanor JJ, et al. Efficacy and safety of the neuraminidase inhibitor zanamivir in the treatment of influenzavirus infections. GG167 Influenza Study Group. *N Engl J Med* 1997;337:874.
245. Hayden FG, Atmar RL, Schilling M, et al. Use of the selective oral neuraminidase inhibitor oseltamivir to prevent influenza. *N Engl J Med* 1999;341:1336.
246. Monto AS, Robinson DP, Herlocher ML, et al. Zanamivir in the prevention of influenza among healthy adults: a randomized controlled trial. *JAMA* 1999;282:31.
247. Prevention and control of influenza: recommendations of the Advisory Committee on Immunization Practices (ACIP). *MMWR* 1999;48:1.
248. Gross PA, Gould AL, Brown AE. Effect of cancer chemotherapy on the immune response to influenza virus vaccine: review of published studies. *Rev Infect Dis* 1985;7:613.
249. Lo W, Whimbey E, Elting L, et al. Antibody response to a two-dose influenza vaccine regimen in adult lymphoma patients on chemotherapy. *Eur J Clin Microbiol Infect Dis* 1993;12:778.
250. Shields AF, Hackman RC, Fife KH, Corey L, Meyers JD. Adenovirus infections in patients undergoing bone-marrow transplantation. *N Engl J Med* 1985;312:529.
251. Flomenberg P, Babbitt J, Drobvski WR, et al. Increasing incidence of adenovirus disease in bone marrow transplant recipients. *J Infect Dis* 1994;169:775.
252. Kaplan LJ, Daum RS, Smaron M, McCarthy CA. Severe measles in immunocompromised patients. *JAMA* 1992;267:1237.
253. Woo PC, Chiu SS, Seto WH, Peiris M. Cost-effectiveness of rapid diagnosis of viral respiratory tract infections in pediatric patients. *J Clin Microbiol* 1997;35:1579.
254. Fan J, Henrickson KJ, Savatski LL. Rapid simultaneous diagnosis of infections with respiratory syncytial viruses A and B, influenza viruses A and B, and human parainfluenza virus types 1, 2, and 3 by multiplex quantitative reverse transcription- polymerase chain reaction-enzyme hybridization assay (Hexaplex). *Clin Infect Dis* 1998;26:1397.
255. Chen PM, Chiou TJ, Fan FS, et al. Fulminant hepatitis is significantly increased in hepatitis B carriers after allogeneic bone marrow transplantation. *Transplantation* 1999;67:1425.
256. Webster A, Brenner MK, Prentice HG, Griffiths PD. Fatal hepatitis B reactivation after autologous bone marrow transplantation. *Bone Marrow Transplant* 1989;4:207.
257. Pariente EA, Goudeau A, Dubois F, et al. Fulminant hepatitis due to reactivation of chronic hepatitis B virus infection after allogeneic bone marrow transplantation. *Dig Dis Sci* 1988;33:1185.
258. Lok AS, Liang RH, Chiu EK, et al. Reactivation of hepatitis B virus replication in patients receiving cytotoxic therapy. Report of a prospective study. *Gastroenterology* 1991;100:182.
259. Hoofnagle JH, Dusheiko GM, Schafer DF, et al. Reactivation of chronic hepatitis B virus infection by cancer chemotherapy. *Ann Intern Med* 1982;96:447.
260. Galbraith RM, Eddleston AL, Williams R, Zuckerman AJ. Fulminant hepatic failure in leukaemia and choriocarcinoma related to withdrawal of cytotoxic drug therapy. *Lancet* 1975;2:528.
261. McIvor C, Morton J, Bryant A, et al. Fatal reactivation of precore mutant hepatitis B virus associated with fibrosing cholestatic hepatitis after bone marrow transplantation. *Ann Intern Med* 1994;121:274.
262. Yoshiba M, Sekiyama K, Sugata F, et al. Reactivation of precore mutant hepatitis B virus leading to fulminant hepatic failure following cytotoxic treatment. *Dig Dis Sci* 1992;37:1253.
263. Vergani D, Locasciulli A, Masera G, et al. Histological evidence of hepatitis-B-virus infection with negative serology in children with acute leukaemia who develop chronic liver disease. *Lancet* 1982;1:361.
264. Bréchot C, Degos F, Lugassy C, et al. Hepatitis B virus DNA in patients with chronic liver disease and negative tests for hepatitis B surface antigen. *N Engl J Med* 1985;312:270.
265. Dienstag JL, Schiff ER, Wright TL, et al. Lamivudine as initial treatment for chronic hepatitis B in the United States. *N Engl J Med* 1999;341:1256.
266. Lai CL, Chien RN, Leung NW, et al. A one-year trial of lamivudine for chronic hepatitis B. Asia Hepatitis Lamivudine Study Group. *N Engl J Med* 1998;339:61.
267. Niederau C, Heintges T, Lange S, et al. Long-term follow-up of HBeAg-positive patients treated with interferon alfa for chronic hepatitis B. *N Engl J Med* 1996;334:1422.
268. Ilan Y, Nagler A, Adler R, et al. Adoptive transfer of immunity to hepatitis B virus after T cell-depleted allogeneic bone marrow transplantation. *Hepatology* 1993;18:246.
269. Strasser SI, Myerson D, Spurgeon CL, et al. Hepatitis C infection and bone marrow transplantation: a cohort study with a 10-year follow-up. *Hepatology* 1999;29:1893.
270. Frickhoken N, Wiesneth M, Jainto C, et al. Hepatitis C virus infection is a risk factor for liver failure from veno-occlusive disease after bone marrow transplantation. *Blood* 1994;83:1998.
271. Strasser SI, Sullivan KM, Myerson D, et al. Cirrhosis of the liver in long term marrow transplant survivors. *Blood* 1999;93:3259.
271a. Strasser SI, McDonald GB. Hepatitis viruses and hematopoietic cell transplantation: a guide to patient and donor management. *Blood* 1999; 93:1127.
271b. Zuckerman E, Zuckerman T, Douer D, et al. Liver dysfunction in patients infected with hepatitis C virus undergoing chemotherapy for hematologic malignancies. *Cancer* 1998;83:1224.
271c. Markovic S, Drozina G, Vovk M, Fidler-Jenko M. Reactivation of hepatitis B but not hepatitis C in patients with malignant lymphoma and immunosuppressive therapy. A prospective study in 305 patients. *Hepatogastroenterology* 1999;46:2925.
272. Davis GL, Esteban-Mur R, Rustgi V, et al. Interferon alfa-2b alone or in combination with ribavirin for the treatment of relapse of chronic hepatitis C. International Hepatitis Interventional Therapy Group. *N Engl J Med* 1998;339:1493.

273. Alter HJ, Nakatsuji Y, Melpolder J, et al. The incidence of transfusion-associated hepatitis G virus infection and its relation to liver disease. *N Engl J Med* 1997;336:747.
274. Alter MJ, Gallagher M, Morris TT, et al. Acute non-A-E hepatitis in the United States and the role of hepatitis G virus infection. Sentinel Counties Viral Hepatitis Study Team. *N Engl J Med* 1997;336:741.
275. Lefrere JJ, Roudot-Thoraval F, Lefrere F, et al. Natural history of the TT virus infection through follow-up of TTV DNA- positive multiple-transfused patients. *Blood* 2000;95:347.
276. Kanda Y, Tanaka Y, Kami M, et al. TT virus in bone marrow transplant recipients. *Blood* 1999;93:2485.
277. Sepkowitz KA, Brown AE, Telzak EE, Gottlieb S, Armstrong D. *Pneumocystis carinii* pneumonia among patients without AIDS at a cancer hospital. *JAMA* 1992;267:832.
278. Sepkowitz KA. *Pneumocystis carinii* pneumonia in patients without AIDS. *Clin Infect Dis* 1993;17(Suppl 2):S416.
279. Sepkowitz KA, Brown AE, Armstrong D. *Pneumocystis carinii* pneumonia without acquired immunodeficiency syndrome. More patients, same risk [editorial]. *Arch Intern Med* 1995;155:1125.
280. Hughes WT, Feldman S, Aur RJ, et al. Intensity of immunosuppressive therapy and the incidence of *Pneumocystis carinii* pneumonitis. *Cancer* 1975;36:2004.
281. Browne MJ, Hubbard SM, Longo DL, et al. Excess prevalence of *Pneumocystis carinii* pneumonia in patients treated for lymphoma with combination chemotherapy. *Ann Intern Med* 1986;104:338.
282. Kovacs JA, Hiemenz JW, Macher AM, et al. *Pneumocystis carinii* pneumonia: a comparison between patients with the acquired immunodeficiency syndrome and patients with other immunodeficiencies. *Ann Intern Med* 1984;100:663.
283. Kovacs JA, Ng VL, Masur H, et al. Diagnosis of *Pneumocystis carinii* pneumonia: improved detection in sputum with use of monoclonal antibodies. *N Engl J Med* 1988;318:589.
284. Lipschik GY, Gill VJ, Lundgren JD, et al. Improved diagnosis of *Pneumocystis carinii* infection by polymerase chain reaction on induced sputum and blood. *Lancet* 1992;340:203.
285. Masur H, Gill VJ, Ognibene FP, et al. Diagnosis of *Pneumocystis* pneumonia by induced sputum technique in patients without the acquired immunodeficiency syndrome. *Ann Intern Med* 1988;109:755.
286. Carr A, Penny R, Cooper DA. Efficacy and safety of rechallenge with low-dose trimethoprim- sulphamethoxazole in previously hypersensitive HIV-infected patients. *AIDS* 1993;7:65.
287. Koopmans PP, Burger DM. Managing drug reactions to sulfonamides and other drugs in HIV infection: desensitization rather than rechallenge? *Pharm World Sci* 1998;20:253.
288. Bozzette SA, Sattler FR, Chiu J, et al. A controlled trial of early adjunctive treatment with corticosteroids for *Pneumocystis carinii* pneumonia in the acquired immunodeficiency syndrome. California Collaborative Treatment Group. *N Engl J Med* 1990;323:1451.
289. Hughes WT, Kuhn S, Chaudhary S, et al. Successful chemoprophylaxis for *Pneumocystis carinii* pneumonitis. *N Engl J Med* 1977;297:1419.
290. Hughes WT, Rivera GK, Schell MJ, Thornton D, Lott L. Successful intermittent chemoprophylaxis for *Pneumocystis carinii* pneumonitis. *N Engl J Med* 1987;316:1627.
291. Lyytikainen O, Elonen E, Lautenschlager I, et al. *Pneumocystis carinii* pneumonia in adults with acute leukaemia: is there a need for primary chemoprophylaxis? [letter]. *Eur J Haematol* 1996;56:188.
292. Henson JW, Jalaj JK, Walker RW, Stover DE, Fels AO. *Pneumocystis carinii* pneumonia in patients with primary brain tumors. *Arch Neurol* 1991;48:406.
293. Slivka A, Wen PY, Shea WM, Loeffler JS. *Pneumocystis carinii* pneumonia during steroid taper in patients with primary brain tumors. *Am J Med* 1993;94:216.
294. Israelski DM, Remington JS. Toxoplasmosis in patients with cancer. *Clin Infect Dis* 1993;17(Suppl 2):S423.
295. Hakes TB, Armstrong D. Toxoplasmosis. Problems in diagnosis and treatment. *Cancer* 1983;52:1535.
296. Slavin MA, Meyers JD, Remington JS, Hackman RC. *Toxoplasma gondii* infection in marrow transplant recipients: a 20 year experience. *Bone Marrow Transplant* 1994;13:549.
297. Tang TT, Harb JM, Dunne WM Jr, et al. Cerebral toxoplasmosis in an immunocompromised host. A precise and rapid diagnosis by electron microscopy. *Am J Clin Pathol* 1986;85:104.
298. Conley FK, Jenkins KA, Remington JS. *Toxoplasma gondii* infection of the central nervous system. Use of the peroxidase-antiperoxidase method to demonstrate toxoplasma in formalin fixed, paraffin embedded tissue sections. *Hum Pathol* 1981;12:690.
299. Eggers C, Gross U, Klinker H, et al. Limited value of cerebrospinal fluid for direct detection of *Toxoplasma gondii* in toxoplasmic encephalitis associated with AIDS. *J Neurol* 1995;242:644.
300. Potasman I, Resnick L, Luft BJ, Remington JS. Intrathecal production of antibodies against *Toxoplasma gondii* in patients with toxoplasmic encephalitis and the acquired immunodeficiency syndrome (AIDS). *Ann Intern Med* 1988;108:49.
301. Kijlstra A, Luyendijk L, Baarsma GS, et al. Aqueous humor analysis as a diagnostic tool in toxoplasma uveitis. *Int Ophthalmol* 1989;13:383.
302. Anderlini P, Przepiorka D, Luna M, et al. Acanthamoeba meningoencephalitis after bone marrow transplantation. *Bone Marrow Transplant* 1994;14:459.
303. Cruz T, Reboucas G, Rocha H. Fatal strongyloidiasis in patients receiving corticosteroids. *N Engl J Med* 1966;275:1093.
304. Igra-Siegman Y, Kapila R, Sen P, Kaminski ZC, Louria DB. Syndrome of hyperinfection with *Strongyloides stercoralis*. *Rev Infect Dis* 1981;3:397.
305. Hann I, Viscoli C, Paesmans M, Gaya H, Glauser M. A comparison of outcome from febrile neutropenic episodes in children compared with adults: results from four EORTC studies. International Antimicrobial Therapy Cooperative Group (IATCG) of the European Organization for Research and Treatment of Cancer (EORTC). *Br J Haematol* 1997;99:580.
306. Schimpff S, Satterlee W, Young VM, Serpick A. Empiric therapy with carbenicillin and gentamicin for febrile patients with cancer and granulocytopenia. *N Engl J Med* 1971;284:1061.
307. Pizzo PA, Hathorn JW, Hiemenz J, et al. A randomized trial comparing ceftazidime alone with combination antibiotic therapy in cancer patients with fever and neutropenia. *N Engl J Med* 1986;315:552.
308. De Pauw BE, Deresinski SC, Feld R, Lane-Allman EF, Donnelly JP. Ceftazidime compared with piperacillin and tobramycin for the empiric treatment of fever in neutropenic patients with cancer. A multicenter randomized trial. The Intercontinental Antimicrobial Study Group. *Ann Intern Med* 1994;120:834.
309. Sanders JW, Powe NR, Moore RD. Ceftazidime monotherapy for empiric treatment of febrile neutropenic patients: a meta-analysis. *J Infect Dis* 1991;164:907.
310. Freifeld AG, Walsh T, Marshall D, et al. Monotherapy for fever and neutropenia in cancer patients: a randomized comparison of ceftazidime versus imipenem. *J Clin Oncol* 1995;13:165.
311. Rolston KV, Berkey P, Bodey GP, et al. A comparison of imipenem to ceftazidime with or without amikacin as empiric therapy in febrile neutropenic patients. *Arch Intern Med* 1992;152:283.
312. Diekema DJ, Coffman SL, Marshall SA, et al. Comparison of activities of broad-spectrum beta-lactam compounds against 1,128 gram-positive cocci recently isolated in cancer treatment centers. *Antimicrob Agents Chemother* 1999;43:940.
313. Jones RN, Pfaller MA, Doern GV, Erwin ME, Hollis RJ. Antimicrobial activity and spectrum investigation of eight broad-spectrum beta-lactam drugs: a 1997 surveillance trial in 102 medical centers in the United States. Cefepime Study Group. *Diagn Microbiol Infect Dis* 1998;30:215.
314. Pfaller MA, Jones RN, Marshall SA, et al. Inducible amp C beta-lactamase producing gram-negative bacilli from blood stream infections: frequency, antimicrobial susceptibility, and molecular epidemiology in a national surveillance program (SCOPE). *Diagn Microbiol Infect Dis* 1997;28:211.
315. Jones RN, Marshall SA. Antimicrobial activity of cefepime tested against Bush group I beta-lactamase-producing strains resistant to ceftazidime. A multilaboratory national and international clinical isolate study. *Diagn Microbiol Infect Dis* 1994;19:33.
316. Biron P, Fuhrmann C, Cure H, et al. Cefepime versus imipenem-cilastatin as empirical monotherapy in 400 febrile patients with short duration neutropenia. CEMIC (Study Group of Infectious Diseases in Cancer). *J Antimicrob Chemother* 1998;42:511.
317. Yamamura D, Gucalp R, Carlisle P, et al. Open randomized study of cefepime versus piperacillin-gentamicin for treatment of febrile neutropenic cancer patients. *Antimicrob Agents Chemother* 1997;41:1704.
318. Pfaller MA, Jones RN. A review of the in vitro activity of meropenem and comparative antimicrobial agents tested against 30,254 aerobic and anaerobic pathogens isolated world wide. *Diagn Microbiol Infect Dis* 1997;28:157.
319. Cometta A, Calandra T, Gaya H, et al. Monotherapy with meropenem versus combination therapy with ceftazidime plus amikacin as empiric therapy for fever in granulocytopenic patients with cancer. The International Antimicrobial Therapy Cooperative Group of the European Organization for Research and Treatment of Cancer and the Gruppo Italiano Malattie Ematologiche Maligne dell'Adulto Infection Program. *Antimicrob Agents Chemother* 1996;40:1108.
320. Equivalent efficacies of meropenem and ceftazidime as empirical monotherapy of febrile neutropenic patients. The Meropenem Study Group of Leuven, London and Nijmegen. *J Antimicrob Chemother* 1995;36:185.
321. Behre G, Link H, Maschmeyer G, et al. Meropenem monotherapy versus combination therapy with ceftazidime and amikacin for empirical treatment of febrile neutropenic patients. *Ann Hematol* 1998;76:73.
322. Standiford HC, Drusano GL, Fitzpatrick B, Tatem B, Schimpff SC. Bactericidal activity of ceftazidime in serum compared with that of ticarcillin combined with amikacin. *Antimicrob Agents Chemother* 1984;26:339.
323. Griggs JJ, Blair EA, Norton JR, et al. Ciprofloxacin plus piperacillin is an equally effective regimen for empiric therapy in febrile neutropenic patients compared with standard therapy. *Am J Hematol* 1998;58:293.
324. Philpott-Howard JN, Barker KF, Wade JJ, et al. Randomized multicentre study of ciprofloxacin and azlocillin versus gentamicin and azlocillin in the treatment of febrile neutropenic patients. *J Antimicrob Chemother* 1990;26(Suppl F):89.
325. Flaherty JP, Waitley D, Edlin B, et al. Multicenter, randomized trial of ciprofloxacin plus azlocillin versus ceftazidime plus amikacin for empiric treatment of febrile neutropenic patients. *Am J Med* 1989;87:278S.
326. Charnas R, Luthi AR, Ruch W. Once daily ceftriaxone plus amikacin vs. three times daily ceftazidime plus amikacin for treatment of febrile neutropenic children with cancer. Writing Committee for the International Collaboration on Antimicrobial Treatment of Febrile Neutropenia in Children. *Pediatr Infect Dis J* 1997;16:346.
327. Leoni F, Ciolli S, Pascarella A, et al. Ceftriaxone plus conventional or single-daily dose amikacin versus ceftazidime/amikacin as empiric therapy in febrile neutropenic patients. *Chemotherapy* 1993;39:147.
328. Gibson J, Johnson L, Snowdon L, et al. Single daily ceftriaxone and tobramycin in the empirical management of febrile neutropenic patients: a randomised trial. *Int J Hematol* 1993;58:63.
329. Kramer BS, Ramphal R, Rand KH. Randomized comparison between two ceftazidime-containing regimens and cephalothin-gentamicin-carbenicillin in febrile granulocytopenic cancer patients. *Antimicrob Agents Chemother* 1986;30:64.
330. Vancomycin added to empirical combination antibiotic therapy for fever in granulocytopenic cancer patients. European Organization for Research and Treatment of Cancer (EORTC) International Antimicrobial Therapy Cooperative Group and the National Cancer Institute of Canada-Clinical Trials Group [published erratum appears in *J Infect Dis* 1991 Oct;164:832]. *J Infect Dis* 1991;163:951.
331. Viscoli C, Moroni C, Boni L, et al. Ceftazidime plus amikacin versus ceftazidime plus vancomycin as empiric therapy in febrile neutropenic children with cancer. *Rev Infect Dis* 1991;13:397.
332. Ramphal R, Bolger M, Oblon DJ, et al. Vancomycin is not an essential component of the initial empiric treatment regimen for febrile neutropenic patients receiving ceftazidime: a randomized prospective study. *Antimicrob Agents Chemother* 1992;36:1062.
333. Raad II, Whimbey EE, Rolston KV, et al. A comparison of aztreonam plus vancomycin and imipenem plus vancomycin as initial therapy for febrile neutropenic cancer patients. *Cancer* 1996;77:1386.

334. Jones PG, Rolston KV, Fainstein V, et al. Aztreonam therapy in neutropenic patients with cancer. *Am J Med* 1986;81:243.
335. Pizzo PA, Robichaud KJ, Gill FA, et al. Duration of empiric antibiotic therapy in granulocytopenic patients with cancer. *Am J Med* 1979;67:194.
336. Pizzo PA, Commers J, Cotton D, et al. Approaching the controversies in antibacterial management of cancer patients. *Am J Med* 1984;76:436.
337. Lucas KG, Brown AE, Armstrong D, Chapman D, Heller G. The identification of febrile, neutropenic children with neoplastic disease at low risk for bacteremia and complications of sepsis. *Cancer* 1996;77:791.
338. Bash RO, Katz JA, Cash JV, Buchanan GR. Safety and cost effectiveness of early hospital discharge of lower risk children with cancer admitted for fever and neutropenia. *Cancer* 1994;74:189.
339. Aquino VM, Tkaczewski I, Buchanan GR. Early discharge of low-risk febrile neutropenic children and adolescents with cancer. *Clin Infect Dis* 1997;25:74.
340. Talcott JA, Finberg R, Mayer RJ, Goldman L. The medical course of cancer patients with fever and neutropenia. Clinical identification of a low-risk subgroup at presentation. *Arch Intern Med* 1988;148:2561.
341. Talcott JA, Siegel RD, Finberg R, Goldman L. Risk assessment in cancer patients with fever and neutropenia: a prospective, two-center validation of a prediction rule. *J Clin Oncol* 1992;10:316.
342. Freifeld AG, Walsh TJ, Pizzo PA. Infections in the cancer patient. In: DeVita VTJ, Hellman S, Rosenberg SA, eds. *Cancer: principles & practice of oncology.* Philadelphia: Lippincott–Raven, 1997:2659.
343. Pizzo PA, Robichaud KJ, Gill FA, Witebsky FG. Empiric antibiotic and antifungal therapy for cancer patients with prolonged fever and granulocytopenia. *Am J Med* 1982;72:101.
344. Empiric antifungal therapy in febrile granulocytopenic patients. EORTC International Antimicrobial Therapy Cooperative Group. *Am J Med* 1989;86:668.
345. Pizzo PA, Robichaud KJ, Wesley R, Commers JR. Fever in the pediatric and young adult patient with cancer. A prospective study of 1001 episodes. *Medicine (Baltimore)* 1982;61:153.
346. Pizzo PA. After empiric therapy: what to do until the granulocyte comes back. *Rev Infect Dis* 1987;9:214.
347. Talcott JA, Whalen A, Clark J, Rieker PP, Finberg R. Home antibiotic therapy for low-risk cancer patients with fever and neutropenia: a pilot study of 30 patients based on a validated prediction rule. *J Clin Oncol* 1994;12:107.
348. Malik IA, Abbas Z, Karim M. Randomised comparison of oral ofloxacin alone with combination of parenteral antibiotics in neutropenic febrile patients [published erratum appears in *Lancet* 1992 Jul 11;340:128]. *Lancet* 1992;339:1092.
349. Malik IA, Khan WA, Karim M, Aziz Z, Khan MA. Feasibility of outpatient management of fever in cancer patients with low-risk neutropenia: results of a prospective randomized trial. *Am J Med* 1995;98:224.
350. Hidalgo M, Hornedo J, Lumbreras C, et al. Outpatient therapy with oral ofloxacin for patients with low risk neutropenia and fever: a prospective, randomized clinical trial. *Cancer* 1999;85:213.
351. Rubenstein EB, Rolston K, Benjamin RS, et al. Outpatient treatment of febrile episodes in low-risk neutropenic patients with cancer. *Cancer* 1993;71:3640.
352. Freifeld AG, Pizzo PA. The outpatient management of febrile neutropenia in cancer patients. *Oncology* (*Huntingt*) 1996;10:599, 611; discussion 615.
353. Tice AD. Outpatient parenteral antibiotic therapy for fever and neutropenia. *Infect Dis Clin North Am* 1998;12:963.
354. Rolston KV. New trends in patient management: risk-based therapy for febrile patients with neutropenia. *Clin Infect Dis* 1999;29:515.
355. Freifeld A, Marchigiani D, Walsh T, et al. A double-blind comparison of empirical oral and intravenous antibiotic therapy for low-risk febrile patients with neutropenia during cancer chemotherapy. *N Engl J Med* 1999;341:305.
356. Kern WV, Cometta A, De Bock R, et al. Oral versus intravenous empirical antimicrobial therapy for fever in patients with granulocytopenia who are receiving cancer chemotherapy. International Antimicrobial Therapy Cooperative Group of the European Organization for Research and Treatment of Cancer. *N Engl J Med* 1999;341:312.
357. Buck AC, Cooke EM. The fate of ingested *Pseudomonas aeruginosa* in normal persons. *J Med Microbiol* 1969;2:521.
358. Engels EA, Lau J, Barza M. Efficacy of quinolone prophylaxis in neutropenic cancer patients: a meta-analysis. *J Clin Oncol* 1998;16:1179.
359. Cruciani M, Rampazzo R, Malena M, et al. Prophylaxis with fluoroquinolones for bacterial infections in neutropenic patients: a meta-analysis. *Clin Infect Dis* 1996;23:795.
360. Reduction of fever and streptococcal bacteremia in granulocytopenic patients with cancer. A trial of oral penicillin V or placebo combined with pefloxacin. International Antimicrobial Therapy Cooperative Group of the European Organization for Research and Treatment of Cancer. *JAMA* 1994;272:1183.
361. Bow EJ, Mandell LA, Louie TJ, et al. Quinolone-based antibacterial chemoprophylaxis in neutropenic patients: effect of augmented gram-positive activity on infectious morbidity. National Cancer Institute of Canada Clinical Trials Group. *Ann Intern Med* 1996;125:183.
362. Nauseef WM, Maki DG. A study of the value of simple protective isolation in patients with granulocytopenia. *N Engl J Med* 1981;304:448.
363. Shooter RA, Cooke EM, Faiers MC, Breaden AL, O'Farrell SM. Isolation of *Escherichia coli, Pseudomonas aeruginosa,* and *Klebsiella* from food in hospitals, canteens, and schools. *Lancet* 1971;2:390.
364. Remington JS, Schimpff SC. Occasional notes. Please don't eat the salads. *N Engl J Med* 1981;304:433.
365. Steere AC, Mallison GF. Handwashing practices for the prevention of nosocomial infections. *Ann Intern Med* 1975;83:683.
366. Bodey GP. Symposium on infectious complications of neoplastic disease (part II). Current status of prophylaxis of infection with protected environments. *Am J Med* 1984;76:678.
367. Fenelon LE. Protective isolation: who needs it? *J Hosp Infect* 1995;30(Suppl):218.
368. Pizzo PA. Management of fever in patients with cancer and treatment-induced neutropenia. *N Engl J Med* 1993;328:1323.
369. Bone RC, Fisher CJ Jr, Clemmer TP, et al. A controlled clinical trial of high-dose methylprednisolone in the treatment of severe sepsis and septic shock. *N Engl J Med* 1987;317:653.
370. Natanson C, Hoffman WD, Suffredini AF, Eichacker PQ, Danner RL. Selected treatment strategies for septic shock based on proposed mechanisms of pathogenesis. *Ann Intern Med* 1994;120:771.
371. Greene JN. Catheter-related complications of cancer therapy. *Infect Dis Clin North Am* 1996;10:255.
372. Newman KA, Reed WP, Schimpff SC, Bustamante CI, Wade JC. Hickman catheters in association with intensive cancer chemotherapy. *Support Care Cancer* 1993;1:92.
373. Press OW, Ramsey PG, Larson EB, Fefer A, Hickman RO. Hickman catheter infections in patients with malignancies. *Medicine (Baltimore)* 1984;63:189.
374. Raad II, Vartivarian S, Khan A, Bodey GP. Catheter-related infections caused by the *Mycobacterium fortuitum* complex: 15 cases and review. *Rev Infect Dis* 1991;13:1120.
375. Verghese A, Widrich WC, Arbeit RD. Central venous septic thrombophlebitis—the role of medical therapy. *Medicine (Baltimore)* 1985;64:394.
376. Groeger JS, Lucas AB, Thaler HT, et al. Infectious morbidity associated with long-term use of venous access devices in patients with cancer. *Ann Intern Med* 1993;119:1168.
377. Bodey GP. Dermatologic manifestations of infections in neutropenic patients. *Infect Dis Clin North Am* 1994;8:655.
378. Kusne S, Eibling DE, Yu VL, et al. Gangrenous cellulitis associated with gram-negative bacilli in pancytopenic patients: dilemma with respect to effective therapy. *Am J Med* 1988;85:490.
379. Kressel B, Szewczyk C, Tuazon CU. Early clinical recognition of disseminated candidiasis by muscle and skin biopsy. *Arch Intern Med* 1978;138:429.
380. Walsh TJ, Melcher GP, Rinaldi MG, et al. *Trichosporon beigelii,* an emerging pathogen resistant to amphotericin B. *J Clin Microbiol* 1990;28:1616.
381. Walmsley S, Devi S, King S, et al. Invasive *Aspergillus* infections in a pediatric hospital: a ten-year review. *Pediatr Infect Dis J* 1993;12:673.
382. Walsh TJ. Primary cutaneous aspergillosis—an emerging infection among immunocompromised patients. *Clin Infect Dis* 1998;27:453.
383. Iwen PC, Rupp ME, Hinrichs SH. Invasive mold sinusitis: 17 cases in immunocompromised patients and review of the literature. *Clin Infect Dis* 1997;24:1178.
384. Lueg EA, Ballagh RH, Forte V. Analysis of the recent cluster of invasive fungal sinusitis at the Toronto Hospital for Sick Children. *J Otolaryngol* 1996;25:366.
385. Shelhamer JH, Toews GB, Masur H, et al. NIH conference. Respiratory disease in the immunosuppressed patient. *Ann Intern Med* 1992;117:415.
386. Fink MP, Snydman DR, Niederman MS, et al. Treatment of severe pneumonia in hospitalized patients: results of a multicenter, randomized, double-blind trial comparing intravenous ciprofloxacin with imipenem-cilastatin. The Severe Pneumonia Study Group. *Antimicrob Agents Chemother* 1994;38:547.
387. Bartlett JG, Breiman RF, Mandell LA, File TM Jr. Community-acquired pneumonia in adults: guidelines for management. The Infectious Diseases Society of America. *Clin Infect Dis* 1998;26:811.
388. Schwebke JR, Hackman R, Bowden R. Pneumonia due to *Legionella micdadei* in bone marrow transplant recipients. *Rev Infect Dis* 1990;12:824.
389. Levine SJ. An approach to the diagnosis of pulmonary infections in immunosuppressed patients. *Semin Respir Infect* 1992;7:81.
390. Kahn FW, Jones JM, England DM. The role of bronchoalveolar lavage in the diagnosis of invasive pulmonary aspergillosis. *Am J Clin Pathol* 1986;86:518.
391. Saito H, Anaissie EJ, Morice RC, Dekmezian R, Bodey GP. Bronchoalveolar lavage in the diagnosis of pulmonary infiltrates in patients with acute leukemia. *Chest* 1988;94:745.
392. Martino P, Micozzi A, Venditti M, et al. Catheter-related right-sided endocarditis in bone marrow transplant recipients. *Rev Infect Dis* 1990;12:250.
393. Rubinstein E, Noriega ER, Simberkoff MS, Holzman R, Rahal JJ Jr. Fungal endocarditis: analysis of 24 cases and review of the literature. *Medicine (Baltimore)* 1975;54:331.
394. Nguyen MH, Nguyen ML, Yu VL, et al. *Candida* prosthetic valve endocarditis: prospective study of six cases and review of the literature. *Clin Infect Dis* 1996;22:262.
395. Zenker PN, Rosenberg EM, Van Dyke RB, Rabalais GP, Daum RS. Successful medical treatment of presumed *Candida* endocarditis in critically ill infants. *J Pediatr* 1991;119:472.
396. Walsh TJ, Hutchins GM. *Aspergillus* mural endocarditis. *Am J Clin Pathol* 1979;71:640.
397. Walsh TJ, Bulkley BH. *Aspergillus* pericarditis: clinical and pathologic features in the immunocompromised patient. *Cancer* 1982;49:48.
398. Le Moing V, Lortholary O, Timsit JF, et al. *Aspergillus* pericarditis with tamponade: report of a successfully treated case and review. *Clin Infect Dis* 1998;26:451.
399. Overholser CD, Peterson DE, Williams LT, Schimpff SC. Periodontal infection in patients with acute nonlymphocyte leukemia. Prevalence of acute exacerbations. *Arch Intern Med* 1982;142:551.
400. Myoken Y, Sugata T, Kyo TI, Fujihara M. Pathological features of invasive oral aspergillosis in patients with hematologic malignancies. *J Oral Maxillofac Surg* 1996;54:263.
401. Armstrong TS. Stomatitis in the bone marrow transplant patient. An overview and proposed oral care protocol. *Cancer Nurs* 1994;17:403.
402. Murray JC, Chiu JK, Dorfman SR, Ogden AK. Epiglottitis following preparation for allogeneic bone marrow transplantation. *Bone Marrow Transplant* 1995;15:997.
403. Walsh TJ, Gray WC. *Candida* epiglottitis in immunocompromised patients. *Chest* 1987;91:482.
404. Walsh TJ, Belitsos NJ, Hamilton SR. Bacterial esophagitis in immunocompromised patients. *Arch Intern Med* 1986;146:1345.
405. Paulino AF, Kenney R, Forman EN, Medeiros LJ. Typhlitis in a patient with acute lymphoblastic leukemia before the administration of chemotherapy. *Am J Pediatr Hematol Oncol* 1994;16:348.
406. Sloas MM, Flynn PM, Kaste SC, Patrick CC. Typhlitis in children with cancer: a 30-year experience. *Clin Infect Dis* 1993;17:484.

407. Varki AP, Armitage JO, Feagler JR. Typhlitis in acute leukemia: successful treatment by early surgical intervention. *Cancer* 1979;43:695.
408. Shaked A, Shinar E, Freund H. Neutropenic typhlitis. A plea for conservatism. *Dis Colon Rectum* 1983;26:351.
409. Shamberger RC, Weinstein HJ, Delorey MJ, Levey RH. The medical and surgical management of typhlitis in children with acute nonlymphocytic (myelogenous) leukemia. *Cancer* 1986;57:603.
410. Moir CR, Scudamore CH, Benny WB. Typhlitis: selective surgical management. *Am J Surg* 1986;151:563.
411. McFarland LV, Mulligan ME, Kwok RY, Stamm WE. Nosocomial acquisition of *Clostridium difficile* infection. *N Engl J Med* 1989;320:204.
412. Kelly CP, Pothoulakis C, LaMont JT. *Clostridium difficile* colitis. *N Engl J Med* 1994;330:257.
413. Roghmann MC, McCarter RJ Jr, Brewrink J, Cross AS, Morris JG Jr. *Clostridium difficile* infection is a risk factor for bacteremia due to vancomycin-resistant enterococci (VRE) in VRE-colonized patients with acute leukemia. *Clin Infect Dis* 1997;25:1056.
414. Bolton RP, Culshaw MA. Faecal metronidazole concentrations during oral and intravenous therapy for antibiotic associated colitis due to *Clostridium difficile*. *Gut* 1986;27:1169.
415. Doern GV, Coughlin RT, Wu L. Laboratory diagnosis of *Clostridium difficile*-associated gastrointestinal disease: comparison of a monoclonal antibody enzyme immunoassay for toxins A and B with a monoclonal antibody enzyme immunoassay for toxin A only and two cytotoxicity assays. *J Clin Microbiol* 1992;30:2042.
416. Glenn J, Cotton D, Wesley R, Pizzo P. Anorectal infections in patients with malignant diseases. *Rev Infect Dis* 1988;10:42.
417. Barnes SG, Sattler FR, Ballard JO. Perirectal infections in acute leukemia. Improved survival after incision and debridement. *Ann Intern Med* 1984;100:515.
418. Earle MF, Fossieck BE Jr, Cohen MH, et al. Perirectal infections in patients with small cell lung cancer. *JAMA* 1981;246:2464.
419. Cohen JS, Paz IB, O'Donnell MR, Ellenhorn JD. Treatment of perianal infection following bone marrow transplantation. *Dis Colon Rectum* 1996;39:981.
420. Schoenbaum SC, Gardner P, Shillito J. Infections of cerebrospinal fluid shunts: epidemiology, clinical manifestations, and therapy. *J Infect Dis* 1975;131:543.
421. Coley SC, Jager HR, Szydlo RM, Goldman JM. CT and MRI manifestations of central nervous system infection following allogeneic bone marrow transplantation. *Clin Radiol* 1999;54:390.
422. Graus F, Saiz A, Sierra J, et al. Neurologic complications of autologous and allogeneic bone marrow transplantation in patients with leukemia: a comparative study. *Neurology* 1996;46:1004.
423. Hagensee ME, Bauwens JE, Kjos B, Bowden RA. Brain abscess following marrow transplantation: experience at the Fred Hutchinson Cancer Research Center, 1984–1992. *Clin Infect Dis* 1994;19:402.
424. Walsh TJ, Hier DB, Caplan LR. Aspergillosis of the central nervous system: clinicopathological analysis of 17 patients. *Ann Neurol* 1985;18:574.
425. Walsh TJ, Hier DB, Caplan LR. Fungal infections of the central nervous system: comparative analysis of risk factors and clinical signs in 57 patients. *Neurology* 1985;35:1654.
426. Norrell H, Wilson CB, Slagel DE, Clark DB. Leukoencephalopathy following the administration of methotrexate into the cerebrospinal fluid in the treatment of primary brain tumors. *Cancer* 1974;33:923.
427. Ch'ien LT, Aur RJ, Verzosa MS, et al. Progression of methotrexate-induced leukoencephalopathy in children with leukemia. *Med Pediatr Oncol* 1981;9:133.
428. Seong D, Bruner JM, Lee KH, et al. Progressive multifocal leukoencephalopathy after autologous bone marrow transplantation in a patient with chronic myelogenous leukemia. *Clin Infect Dis* 1996;23:402.
429. De Luca A, Ammassari A, Cingolani A, Giancola ML, Antinori A. Disease progression and poor survival of AIDS-associated progressive multifocal leukoencephalopathy despite highly active antiretroviral therapy [letter]. *AIDS* 1998;12:1937.
430. Albrecht H, Hoffmann C, Degen O, et al. Highly active antiretroviral therapy significantly improves the prognosis of patients with HIV-associated progressive multifocal leukoencephalopathy. *AIDS* 1998;12:1149.
431. Tantisiriwat W, Tebas P, Clifford DB, Powderly WG, Fichtenbaum CJ. Progressive multifocal leukoencephalopathy in patients with AIDS receiving highly active antiretroviral therapy. *Clin Infect Dis* 1999;28:1152.
432. Korzeniowski OM. Urinary tract infection in the impaired host. *Med Clin North Am* 1991;75:391.
433. Parsons CL, Greenspan C, Moore SW, Mulholland SG. Role of surface mucin in primary antibacterial defense of bladder. *Urology* 1977;9:48.
434. Sobel JD. Management of asymptomatic candiduria. *Int J Antimicrob Agents* 1999;11:285.
435. Ang BS, Telenti A, King B, Steckelberg JM, Wilson WR. Candidemia from a urinary tract source: microbiological aspects and clinical significance. *Clin Infect Dis* 1993;17:662.
436. Spach DH, Bauwens JE, Myerson D, Mustafa MM, Bowden RA. Cytomegalovirus-induced hemorrhagic cystitis following bone marrow transplantation. *Clin Infect Dis* 1993;16:142.
437. Childs R, Sanchez C, Engler H, et al. High incidence of adeno- and polyomavirus-induced hemorrhagic cystitis in bone marrow allotransplantation for hematological malignancy following T cell depletion and cyclosporine. *Bone Marrow Transplant* 1998;22:889.
438. Echavarria MS, Ray SC, Ambinder R, Dumler JS, Charache P. PCR detection of adenovirus in a bone marrow transplant recipient: hemorrhagic cystitis as a presenting manifestation of disseminated disease. *J Clin Microbiol* 1999;37:686.
439. Arthur RR, Shah KV, Baust SJ, Santos GW, Saral R. Association of BK viruria with hemorrhagic cystitis in recipients of bone marrow transplants. *N Engl J Med* 1986;315:230.
440. Vogeli TA, Peinemann F, Burdach S, Ackermann R. Urological treatment and clinical course of BK polyomavirus-associated hemorrhagic cystitis in children after bone marrow transplantation. *Eur Urol* 1999;36:252.
441. Strauss RG. Granulocyte transfusion therapy. *Hematol Oncol Clin North Am* 1994;8:1159.
442. Chanock SJ, Gorlin JB. Granulocyte transfusions. Time for a second look. *Infect Dis Clin North Am* 1996;10:327.
443. Jendiroba DB, Lichtiger B, Anaissie E, et al. Evaluation and comparison of three mobilization methods for the collection of granulocytes. *Transfusion* 1998;38:722.
444. Dale DC, Liles WC, Llewellyn C, Rodger E, Price TH. Neutrophil transfusions: kinetics and functions of neutrophils mobilized with granulocyte-colony-stimulating factor and dexamethasone. *Transfusion* 1998;38:713.
445. Bensinger WI, Price TH, Dale DC, et al. The effects of daily recombinant human granulocyte colony-stimulating factor administration on normal granulocyte donors undergoing leukapheresis. *Blood* 1993;81:1883.
446. Adkins D, Goodgold H, Hendershott L, et al. Indium-labeled white blood cells apheresed from donors receiving G-CSF localize to sites of inflammation when infused into allogeneic bone marrow transplant recipients. *Bone Marrow Transplant* 1997;19:809.
447. Bhatia S, McCullough J, Perry EH, et al. Granulocyte transfusions: efficacy in treating fungal infections in neutropenic patients following bone marrow transplantation. *Transfusion* 1994;34:226.
448. Dignani MC, Anaissie EJ, Hester JP, et al. Treatment of neutropenia-related fungal infections with granulocyte colony-stimulating factor-elicited white blood cell transfusions: a pilot study. *Leukemia* 1997;11:1621.
449. Wright DG, Robichaud KJ, Pizzo PA, Deisseroth AB. Lethal pulmonary reactions associated with the combined use of amphotericin B and leukocyte transfusions. *N Engl J Med* 1981;304:1185.
450. Godwin JE, Kopecky KJ, Head DR, et al. A double-blind placebo-controlled trial of granulocyte colony-stimulating factor in elderly patients with previously untreated acute myeloid leukemia: a Southwest oncology group study (9031). *Blood* 1998;91:3607.
451. Heil G, Hoelzer D, Sanz MA, et al. A randomized, double-blind, placebo-controlled, phase III study of filgrastim in remission induction and consolidation therapy for adults with de novo acute myeloid leukemia. The International Acute Myeloid Leukemia Study Group. *Blood* 1997;90:4710.
452. Crawford J, Ozer H, Stoller R, et al. Reduction by granulocyte colony-stimulating factor of fever and neutropenia induced by chemotherapy in patients with small-cell lung cancer. *N Engl J Med* 1991;325:164.
453. Hartmann LC, Tschetter LK, Habermann TM, et al. Granulocyte colony-stimulating factor in severe chemotherapy-induced afebrile neutropenia. *N Engl J Med* 1997;336:1776.
454. Ojeda E, Garcia-Bustos J, Aguado M, et al. A prospective randomized trial of granulocyte colony-stimulating factor therapy after autologous blood stem cell transplantation in adults. *Bone Marrow Transplant* 1999;24:601.
455. Kawano Y, Takaue Y, Mimaya J, et al. Marginal benefit/disadvantage of granulocyte colony-stimulating factor therapy after autologous blood stem cell transplantation in children: results of a prospective randomized trial. The Japanese Cooperative Study Group of PBSCT. *Blood* 1998;92:4040.
456. Giles FJ. Monocyte-macrophages, granulocyte-macrophage colony-stimulating factor, and prolonged survival among patients with acute myeloid leukemia and stem cell transplants. *Clin Infect Dis* 1998;26:1282.
457. Rowe JM, Andersen JW, Mazza JJ, et al. A randomized placebo-controlled phase III study of granulocyte-macrophage colony-stimulating factor in adult patients (greater than 55 to 70 years of age) with acute myelogenous leukemia: a study of the Eastern Cooperative Oncology Group (E1490). *Blood* 1995;86:457.
458. Stone RM, Berg DT, George SL, et al. Granulocyte-macrophage colony-stimulating factor after initial chemotherapy for elderly patients with primary acute myelogenous leukemia. Cancer and Leukemia Group B. *N Engl J Med* 1995;332:1671.
459. Rowe JM. Treatment of acute myeloid leukemia with cytokines: effect on duration of neutropenia and response to infections. *Clin Infect Dis* 1998;26:1290.
460. American Society of Clinical Oncology. Recommendations for the use of hematopoietic colony-stimulating factors: evidence-based, clinical practice guidelines. *J Clin Oncol* 1994;12:2471.
461. Roilides E, Uhlig K, Venzon D, Pizzo PA, Walsh TJ. Enhancement of oxidative response and damage caused by human neutrophils to *Aspergillus fumigatus* hyphae by granulocyte colony-stimulating factor and gamma interferon. *Infect Immunol* 1993;61:1185.
462. Roilides E, Holmes A, Blake C, Venzon D, Pizzo PA. Antifungal activity of elutriated human monocytes against *Aspergillus fumigatus* hyphae: enhancement by granulocyte-macrophage colony-stimulating factor and interferon-gamma. *J Infect Dis* 1994;170:894.
463. Roilides E, Sein T, Holmes A, et al. Effects of macrophage colony-stimulating factor on antifungal activity of mononuclear phagocytes against *Aspergillus fumigatus*. *J Infect Dis* 1995;172:1028.
464. Roilides E, Holmes A, Blake C, Pizzo PA, Walsh TJ. Effects of granulocyte colony-stimulating factor and interferon-gamma on antifungal activity of human polymorphonuclear neutrophils against pseudohyphae of different medically important *Candida* species. *J Leukoc Biol* 1995;57:651.
465. Nemunaitis J. Use of macrophage colony-stimulating factor in the treatment of fungal infections. *Clin Infect Dis* 1998;26:1279.
466. Nemunaitis J, Meyers JD, Buckner CD, et al. Phase I trial of recombinant human macrophage colony-stimulating factor in patients with invasive fungal infections. *Blood* 1991;78:907.
467. Bodey GP, Anaissie E, Gutterman J, Vadhan-Raj S. Role of granulocyte-macrophage colony-stimulating factor as adjuvant therapy for fungal infection in patients with cancer. *Clin Infect Dis* 1993;17:705.
468. Gallin JI, Farber JM, Holland SM, Nutman TB. Interferon-gamma in the management of infectious diseases [clinical conference]. *Ann Intern Med* 1995;123:216.
469. Schiff DE, Rae J, Martin TR, Davis BH, Curnutte JT. Increased phagocyte Fc gammaRI expression and improved Fc gamma- receptor-mediated phagocytosis after in vivo recombinant human interferon-gamma treatment of normal human subjects. *Blood* 1997;90:3187.

470. A controlled trial of interferon gamma to prevent infection in chronic granulomatous disease. The International Chronic Granulomatous Disease Cooperative Study Group. *N Engl J Med* 1991;324:509.
471. Segal BH, DeCarlo ES, Kwon-Chung KJ, et al. *Aspergillus nidulans* infection in chronic granulomatous disease. *Medicine (Baltimore)* 1998;77:345.
472. Cohen MS, Isturiz RE, Malech HL, et al. Fungal infection in chronic granulomatous disease. The importance of the phagocyte in defense against fungi. *Am J Med* 1981;71:59.
473. Holland SM, Eisenstein EM, Kuhns DB, et al. Treatment of refractory disseminated nontuberculous mycobacterial infection with interferon gamma. A preliminary report. *N Engl J Med* 1994;330:1348.
474. Seder RA, Gazzinelli R, Sher A, Paul WE. Interleukin 12 acts directly on CD4+ T cells to enhance priming for interferon gamma production and diminishes interleukin 4 inhibition of such priming. *Proc Natl Acad Sci U S A* 1993;90:10188.
475. Clemons KV, Brummer E, Stevens DA. Cytokine treatment of central nervous system infection: efficacy of interleukin-12 alone and synergy with conventional antifungal therapy in experimental cryptococcosis. *Antimicrob Agents Chemother* 1994;38:460.
476. Stevens DA. Combination immunotherapy and antifungal chemotherapy. *Clin Infect Dis* 1998;26:1266.
477. Nagai H, Guo J, Choi H, Kurup V. Interferon-gamma and tumor necrosis factor-alpha protect mice from invasive aspergillosis. *J Infect Dis* 1995;172:1554.
478. Riddell SR, Watanabe KS, Goodrich JM, et al. Restoration of viral immunity in immunodeficient humans by the adoptive transfer of T cell clones. *Science* 1992;257:238.
479. Reusser P, Riddell SR, Meyers JD, Greenberg PD. Cytotoxic T-lymphocyte response to cytomegalovirus after human allogeneic bone marrow transplantation: pattern of recovery and correlation with cytomegalovirus infection and disease. *Blood* 1991;78:1373.
480. Quinnan GV Jr, Kirmani N, Rook AH, et al. Cytotoxic T cells in cytomegalovirus infection: HLA-restricted T-lymphocyte and non-T-lymphocyte cytotoxic responses correlate with recovery from cytomegalovirus infection in bone-marrow-transplant recipients. *N Engl J Med* 1982;307:7.
481. Walter EA, Greenberg PD, Gilbert MJ, et al. Reconstitution of cellular immunity against cytomegalovirus in recipients of allogeneic bone marrow by transfer of T-cell clones from the donor. *N Engl J Med* 1995;333:1038.
482. Papadopoulos EB, Ladanyi M, Emanuel D, et al. Infusions of donor leukocytes to treat Epstein-Barr virus-associated lymphoproliferative disorders after allogeneic bone marrow transplantation. *N Engl J Med* 1994;330:1185.
483. Rooney CM, Smith CA, Ng CY, et al. Use of gene-modified virus-specific T lymphocytes to control Epstein-Barr-virus-related lymphoproliferation. *Lancet* 1995;345:9.
484. Heslop HE, Ng CY, Li C, et al. Long-term restoration of immunity against Epstein-Barr virus infection by adoptive transfer of gene-modified virus-specific T lymphocytes. *Nat Med* 1996;2:551.

CHAPTER 55

Adverse Effects of Treatment

SECTION 1

ANN M. BERGER
REBECCA A. CLARK-SNOW

Nausea and Vomiting

NATURE OF THE PROBLEM

Chemotherapy-induced nausea and vomiting remain two of patients' most feared effects of cancer treatment. The incidence and severity of nausea or vomiting in patients receiving chemotherapy varies, depending on the type of chemotherapy given, dose, schedule, combinations of medications, and individual characteristics. Approximately 70% to 80% of all patients who receive chemotherapy experience nausea and vomiting.[1,2] Anticipatory nausea and vomiting are experienced by approximately 10% to 44% of patients who receive chemotherapy.[3–6]

The phenothiazines were the mainstay of antiemetic agents before the mid-1970s.[7,8] Currently, there are many efficacious antiemetic regimens for the nausea and vomiting produced by chemotherapeutic agents.[9] In a study conducted in 1983, cancer patients ranked nausea and vomiting as the first and second most severe side effects of chemotherapy, respectively.[10] After the emergence of new antiemetic agents and alterations in chemotherapeutic regimens, patients' perceptions of the most severe side effects were modified. In a 1993 study, 155 cancer patients receiving chemotherapy reported that they experienced an average of 20 physical and psychosocial symptoms: Nausea was ranked as the most severe symptom and vomiting as the fifth.[11] Therefore, nausea is also an important efficacy parameter when evaluating an antiemetic.

Use of these new antiemetic agents has decreased the incidence and severity of nausea and vomiting induced by chemotherapy; however, these agents have not totally prevented the problems. The consequences of not controlling the nausea and vomiting induced by cancer treatment may lead to medical complications, a failure of the patient to comply with the cancer therapy and follow-up, and a diminished quality of life.

PATHOPHYSIOLOGY OF NAUSEA AND VOMITING

The precise mechanisms by which chemotherapy induces nausea and vomiting are unknown; however, it appears probable that different chemotherapeutic agents act at different sites and that some chemotherapeutic agents act at multiple sites.[12] The fact that different chemotherapeutic agents cause nausea and vomiting by different mechanisms and that one chemotherapeutic agent may induce nausea and vomiting by more than one mechanism helps us to understand why there is no one antiemetic regimen that is effective all of the time.

Mechanisms by which chemotherapeutic agents cause nausea and vomiting are activation of the chemoreceptor trigger zone (CTZ) either directly or indirectly; peripheral stimulation of the gastrointestinal (GI) tract; vestibular mechanisms; cortical mechanisms; or alterations of taste and smell (Table 55.1-1). For the majority of the chemotherapeutic agents, the most common mechanism is thought to be activation of the CTZ.

The CTZ is located in the area postrema of the brain and can be reached by emetogenic chemicals via the cerebrospinal fluid or the blood. The thought is that the mechanisms of interaction between the CTZ and chemotherapy involve the release of various neurotransmitters that activate the vomiting center. Either one or a combination of these transmitters may induce vomiting.

TABLE 55.1-1. Mechanisms of Nausea and Vomiting after Chemotherapy

Stimulation of chemoreceptor trigger zone
Peripheral mechanisms
Damage of gastrointestinal mucosa
Stimulation of gastrointestinal neurotransmitter receptors
Cortical mechanisms
Direct cerebral activation
Indirect (psychogenic) mechanisms
Vestibular mechanisms
Alterations of taste and smell

Some of the neurotransmitters located in the area postrema of the brain that may be excited and lead to emesis include dopamine, serotonin, histamine, norepinephrine, apomorphine, neurotensin, angiotensin II, vasoactive intestinal polypeptide, gastrin, vasopressin, thyrotropin-releasing hormone, leucine-enkephalin, and substance P.[13] Other enzymes surround the CTZ, such as adenosine triphosphatase, monoamine oxidase, cholinesterase, and catecholamines; however, their role in chemotherapy-induced emesis is unknown.

Until recently, the neurotransmitter that appeared to be the most responsible for chemotherapy-induced nausea and vomiting was dopamine. Many effective antiemetics are dopamine antagonists that may bind specifically to the D_2 receptor. However, there is a high degree of variation in dopamine receptor binding affinity by these drugs.[14] The action of some drugs that cause nausea and vomiting is affected very little or not at all by dopamine antagonists. It is known that not all the important receptors in the CTZ are dopaminergic, as the effect of dopamine antagonists is not equal to surgical ablation of the CTZ.[15] It has also been noted that the degree of antiemetic activity of high-dose metoclopramide cannot be explained on the basis of dopamine blockade alone.[16]

Histamine receptors are found in abundance in the CTZ; however, H_2 antagonists do not work at all as antiemetics. H_1 antagonists alleviate nausea and vomiting induced by vestibular disorder and motion sickness but not nausea and vomiting induced by chemotherapy.[17,18]

Knowledge that opiate receptors are found in abundance in the CTZ, as well as the facts that narcotics have mixed emetic and antiemetic effects that are blocked by naloxone and that naloxone has emetic properties, have led to the proposal of opiates or enkephalins as an antiemetic. High doses of naloxone augments emesis induced by chemotherapy, and low doses of narcotic may reduce emesis.[19] Studies to date have shown that opiates can prevent chemotherapy-induced emesis in laboratory animals; however, both butorphanol and buprenorphine have not proven to be effective antiemetics in patients who received previous chemotherapy.[20,21] One study by Lissoni et al.[22] did demonstrate that Fk-33-824 was more effective as an antiemetic in patients who received cisplatin; however, it was ineffective for patients receiving cyclophosphamide or epirubicin.

Edwards et al.[23] found that arginine vasopressin levels rise to a greater extent in patients who vomit when they receive chemotherapy as compared to those who do not vomit.[23] It has been suggested that perhaps arginine vasopressin plays a role in nausea more than in the vomiting induced by chemotherapy. Dexamethasone, which is a known effective antiemetic, may work by reducing arginine vasopressin levels.[24] Another mechanism of action of corticosteroids as antiemetics may be related to modulation of prostaglandin release.[25]

Some evidence suggests that although no one neurotransmitter is responsible for all chemotherapy-induced nausea and vomiting, it appears that serotonin and 5-hydroxytryptamine (5-HT) receptors are particularly important in the pathophysiology of acute vomiting, whereas others may be more important in the pathophysiology of nausea and delayed emesis. The role of the 5-HT type 3 ($5\text{-}HT^3$) receptor in chemotherapy-induced emesis was recognized by examining the mechanism of action of high-dose metoclopramide in decreasing cisplatin-induced emesis. High-dose metoclopramide, unlike other D_2-receptor antagonists, has an exceptionally good capacity to decrease the emesis induced by cisplatin administration.[26] It has been recognized that metoclopramide has pharmacologic effects other than dopamine antagonism. Metoclopramide is a weak antagonist of peripheral $5\text{-}HT^3$ receptors[27] and can stimulate GI motility by increasing acetylcholine release from the cholinergic nerves of the GI tract.[28] To test whether $5\text{-}HT^3$-receptor blockade would decrease cisplatin-induced emesis, Miner and Sanger[29] took a substituted benzamide, BRL 24924, which has stimulatory effects on the GI tract and is a $5\text{-}HT^3$-receptor blocker, and demonstrated decreased emesis in ferrets that received cisplatin. This study was repeated with a nonbenzamide, selective $5\text{-}HT^3$-receptor blocker MDL 72222, which has no GI-stimulating activity. The study revealed that cisplatin-induced emesis was totally blocked by this compound.[30] The same conclusion was reached in another study using a different nonbenzamide, the selective $5\text{-}HT^3$ antagonist ICS 205-930.[31] These studies demonstrated the role of $5\text{-}HT^3$-receptor blockade in chemotherapy-induced emesis.

The precise mechanism of action of the 5-HT-receptor antagonists is unknown; however, they may have both a central and a peripheral effect. The GI tract contains 80% of the body's supply of serotonin, and it has been suggested that perhaps chemotherapy administration causes release of serotonin from the enterochromaffin cells of the GI tract, which then stimulates emesis via both the vagus and greater splanchnic nerve as well as stimulating the area postrema of the brain. After cisplatin administration, there is an increase in urinary excretion of 5-hydroxyindoleacetic acid, the main metabolite of serotonin, and this increase parallels the number of episodes of emesis.[32] Studies have shown that the $5\text{-}HT^3$-receptor antagonists decrease emesis from several chemotherapeutic agents, including cisplatin, cyclophosphamide, and doxorubicin.[33–36]

There has been new evidence regarding the potential role of substance P in emesis and new data about the use of neurokinin (NK1) antagonists in the management of emesis. Substance P, a neuropeptide found in the GI tract and the CTZ of the area postrema, exerts its emetic effects by binding to a specific neuroreceptor, NK1. A number of compounds that selectively block NK1 have been identified. These NK1 antagonists demonstrate a wide spectrum of antiemetic activity against numerous emetic stimuli in animal models, including several emetic stimuli that are not affected by serotonin and dopamine receptor antagonists. Studies in preclinical models have demonstrated that several NK1 antagonists have activity in the prevention of both acute and delayed cisplatin-induced nausea and vomiting. Two randomized double-blind studies have demonstrated that NK1 antagonists are beneficial in the prevention of delayed emesis.[37,38] These agents may also provide additional benefit in the prevention of acute nausea and vomiting when combined with a 5-HT^3 antagonist and dexamethasone.

The second most important mechanism whereby chemotherapy may induce emesis is peripheral effects that are thought to arise from the pharynx and the upper GI tract. Most likely, the chemotherapy does not directly stimulate the peripheral receptors. Rather, neurotransmitters probably are released as a result of local GI irritation or damage. GI tract serotonin, dopamine, opiate, histamine, and cholinergic receptors are most likely involved in the emesis induced by chemotherapy. The peripheral effects may be abolished by vagotomy, indicating that impulses from the GI tract may reach the vomiting center via the vagus and sympathetic nerves.[39]

Another mechanism that may be involved in chemotherapy-induced emesis could be the therapy's effect on the vestibular system. It is known that patients who have a history of motion sickness experience a greater severity, frequency, and duration of nausea and vomiting from chemotherapy than patients who do not experience motion sickness. The mechanism by which the vestibular system may lead to chemotherapy-induced emesis is unknown; however, it is postulated that sensory information that is received by the vestibular system is different from information that was expected.[40]

Some investigators believe that taste changes induced by chemotherapy may lead to nausea and vomiting. Some chemotherapeutic agents, such as cisplatin or gallium nitrate, can lead to loss of taste sensation or to a metallic taste in the mouth. A study conducted with patients receiving chemotherapy for malignant melanoma revealed that patients developed a more intense sense of taste for sweet, bitter, sour, and salt. After chemotherapy, the patients rated the highest concentration of sweet as lower, and the patients' discrimination between highest and lowest concentrations of sour, bitter, and sweet was decreased.[41] In another study of patients with breast carcinoma who received cyclophosphamide, methotrexate, and 5-fluorouracil, 36% reported a bitter taste in their mouth. One-third of the patients thought that the bitter taste caused vomiting.[42] The exact mechanism by which taste is changed by chemotherapy is unknown; however, it is thought that while the drugs are in the plasma or saliva, they have a direct effect on the oral mucosa or taste buds. Changes in taste may contribute both to nausea and vomiting as well as to anorexia.

Finally, chemotherapy-induced emesis may be induced by direct or indirect effects on the cerebral cortex. Animal studies have shown that nitrogen mustard partially causes emesis via direct stimulation of the cerebral cortex.[43] Studies demonstrate that the risk of nausea and vomiting is increased when a patient's roommate is experiencing nausea and vomiting. It is also known that the amount of sleep before receiving chemotherapy may influence whether a patient develops chemotherapy-induced emesis. In addition, large differences exist in the severity and incidence of nausea and vomiting from the same chemotherapeutic agents in different countries.[44] These studies indicate that indirect psychological effects can mediate chemotherapy-induced nausea and vomiting.

Aside from there being more than one mechanism by which each chemotherapeutic agent may induce emesis, chemotherapy induces emesis in a manner different from that of other classic emetic agents. Drugs such as apomorphine, levodopa, digitalis, pilocarpine, nicotine, and morphine cause vomiting almost immediately. Nitrogen mustard also may lead to emesis immediately; however, most chemotherapeutic agents and radiotherapy require a latency period before emesis begins. Also, most chemotherapeutic agents do not induce emesis in a monophasic way, as do the classic emetic agents. Chemotherapeutic agents induce emesis with a delayed onset, and the emesis has multiphasic time courses.[45] When managing chemotherapy-induced emesis, one should realize that there is most likely more than one mechanism involved, suggesting that there will not be one antiemetic regimen that will work for all patients all of the time.

EMETIC SYNDROMES

Patients undergoing therapy for the treatment and possible cure of cancer with chemotherapy often are faced with the distressing side effects of nausea and vomiting. Although advances in the 1990s have provided the clinician with an array of antiemetics and varied regimens, therapy-induced nausea and vomiting have yet to be totally eliminated. The goals of antiemetic therapy are as follows: (1) to achieve complete control in all settings, (2) to provide maximum convenience for patients and staff, (3) to eliminate potential side effects of the agents, and (4) to minimize the cost of treatment with antiemetic agents and drug administration.

As a result of antiemetic investigations, five distinct but related emetic syndromes have been identified: acute chemotherapy-induced emesis, delayed emesis, breakthrough nausea and vomiting, refractory emesis, and anticipatory emesis. Traditionally, acute nausea and vomiting are defined as occurring within the first 24 hours after administration of chemotherapy. Delayed nausea and vomiting have been arbitrarily defined as occurring 24 hours after chemotherapy administration. More recent observations of the pattern of emesis indicate that delayed emesis may begin as early as 16 hours after chemotherapy administration and that serotonin may not be the primary mediator of symptoms for delayed emesis. Breakthrough nausea and vomiting are nausea and vomiting that occur despite preventive therapy. Rescue therapy is the treatment administered to patients who have not responded to the prophylactic regimens prescribed for acute or delayed nausea and vomiting. Refractory emesis occurs during subsequent cycles when antiemetic prophylaxis or rescues (or both) have failed in earlier cycles.

Anticipatory vomiting is a learned or conditioned response that typically occurs before, during, or after the administration of chemotherapy. Patients receiving one or a combination of several of the agents must receive an antiemetic regimen that is tailored to the individual pattern and emetic potential of each agent. For example, patients receiving a combination of high doses of intravenous cyclophosphamide and doxorubicin (Adriamycin) would require antiemetic coverage for the early onset of emesis usually seen with Adriamycin, as well as continued protection from cyclophosphamide-induced emesis that does not begin until 9 to 18 hours after the drug's administration.[46] If patients are given the opportunity to receive the optimal antiemetic regimen during their initial course of chemotherapy, the likelihood of developing anticipatory emesis with subsequent cycles is greatly reduced. Other advantages for patients include increased tolerance of dose-intensified che-

TABLE 55.1-2. Emetic Potential of Chemotherapeutic Agents

Level 5 (>90% frequency)
Carmustine (>250 mg/m^2)
Cisplatin (>50 mg/m^2)
Cyclophosphamide (>1500 mg/m^2)
Dacarbazine (>500 mg/m^2)
Lomustine (60 mg/m^2)
Mechlorethamine
Pentostatin
Streptozocin
Level 4 (60% to 90% frequency)
Carboplatin
Carmustine (<250 mg/m^2)
Cisplatin (<50 mg/m^2)
Cyclophosphamide (>750 to <1500 mg/m^2)
Cytarabine (>1 g/m^2)
Dactinomycin (>1.5 mg/m^2)
Doxorubicin hydrochloride (>60 mg/m^2)
Irinotecan
Melphalan (intravenous)
Methotrexate (>1000 mg/m^2)
Mitoxantrone (15 mg/m^2)
Procarbazine (oral)
Level 3 (30% to 60% frequency)
Aldesleukin
Cyclophosphamide (intravenous <750 mg/m^2)
Dactinomycin (<1.5 mg/m^2)
Doxorubicin hydrochloride (20 to 60 mg/m^2)
Epirubicin hydrochloride (<90 mg/m^2)
Hycamtin
Idarubicin
Ifosfamide
Methenamine (oral)
Methotrexate (250 to 1000 mg/m^2)
Mitoxantrone (<15 mg/m^2)
Level 2 (10% to 30% frequency)
Asparaginase
Cytarabine (<1 g/m^2)
Docetaxel
Doxorubicin hydrochloride (<20 mg/m^2)
Etoposide
Fluorouracil (<1000 mg/m^2)
Gemcitabine
Methotrexate (>50 to <250 mg/m^2)
Mitomycin
Paclitaxel
Teniposide
Thiotepa
Topotecan
Level 1 (<10% frequency)
Androgens
Bleomycin
Busulfan (oral <4 mg/kg/d)
Chlorambucil
Cladribine
Corticosteroids
Fludarabine
Hydroxyurea
Interferon
Melphalan (oral)
Mercaptopurine
Methotrexate (<50 mg/m^2)
Thioguanine (oral)
Tretinoin
Vinblastine
Vincristine
Vinorelbine

(Adapted from refs. 47 and 48.)

motherapeutic regimens. In addition, through the prevention of emesis, patients are able to achieve an enhanced quality of life at a particularly difficult time.

Two reports, one by Hesketh et al.[47] and an expert consensus by the American Society of Health-System Pharmacists,[48] contain new guidelines for the classification of the acute emetogenicity of chemotherapy into five levels (Table 55.1-2). When the agents are combined, ratings are based on the combined emetogenicity of the individual agents. An algorithm for defining the emetogenicity of combination chemotherapy has been developed (Table 55.1-3).

CONTROL OF EMESIS AND PATIENT CHARACTERISTICS

The methodology used in antiemetic studies has identified several useful patient characteristics and prognostic factors that may affect antiemetic control. These indicators become important for tailoring antiemetic regimens as well as designing antiemetic trials. Careful studies have defined previous experience with chemotherapy, alcohol intake history, age, and gender as influencing patient outcomes. These references are listed below.

A patient's prior exposure to chemotherapy very often determines success or failure in controlling emesis with future treatment courses. Administration of the appropriate antiemetic during an initial course of chemotherapy can very often eliminate or significantly reduce the development of anticipatory emesis, in addition to decreasing the severity of delayed emesis.

Chronic and heavy alcohol usage—defined as more than 100 g of alcohol or five mixed drinks per day, whether in the past or currently—has been shown positively to affect the control of emesis. Ninety-three percent of patients in a prospective study who had a history of high alcohol intake were able to achieve a complete response, or no emesis, after receiving high doses of cisplatin with a combination antiemetic regimen.[49] The hypothesis is that chemotherapy-induced emesis may be decreased in patients with a high alcohol intake because of "burnout" of the CTZ. Although emesis may be easier to control in this setting, patients nonetheless must receive an appropriate and effective antiemetic regimen. As a result, this prognostic factor has been incorporated in many prospective trials for stratification purposes.

Age as a prognostic factor cannot predict patient response to antiemetic therapy. Some studies have indicated better control in older patients, while others have reported little difference among various age groups. Age is, however, an important factor in determining the potential for the occurrence of acute dystonic reactions. Patients aged 30 years and younger are

TABLE 55.1-3. Rules for Identifying the Emetogenicity of Combination Chemotherapy

The most highly emetogenic agent in the chemotherapeutic combination must first be identified.
Level 1 chemotherapeutic agents do not contribute to the emetogenicity of the regimen.
Adding one or more level 2 chemotherapeutic agents increases the emetogenicity of the combination by one level greater than the most emetogenic agent in the combination.
Adding level 3 and 4 agents increases the emetogenicity of the combination by one level per agent.

(Adapted from refs. 47 and 48.)

more prone to experience the acute dystonic reactions associated with the dopamine-receptor blocking agents, such as the phenothiazines, butyrophenones, and substituted benzamides. These side effects are usually characterized by trismus or torticollis. It is also important to remember that within this population of patients, chemotherapeutic agents that might necessitate antiemetics often are given over several consecutive days, increasing the possibility of the occurrence of acute dystonic reactions.[50] A distinct advantage for the use of the serotonin or 5-HT^3-blocking antiemetic agents is that they do not cause acute dystonic reactions, making them an especially beneficial treatment option for children and younger adults.

It has been difficult to explain the rationale for poorer control of emesis in some women receiving treatment for various malignancies. A possible explanation may be that women characteristically receive chemotherapeutic regimens that contain highly emetogenic agents, such as cisplatin and cyclophosphamide, usually given in combination, and are less likely than men to have a history of a high alcohol intake. Although these may be contributing factors, multivariate analyses in some larger studies have indicated that gender is an independent consideration that must be recognized in planning and analyzing clinical studies.

Other factors also have been reported possibly to affect the incidence of nausea and vomiting after chemotherapy. A patient may develop nausea and vomiting if he or she is anxious during the chemotherapy infusion, there is an expectation of severe side effects, or the patient's roommate is experiencing nausea and vomiting. Patients who are well motivated and have a good performance status may experience a decreased incidence of nausea and vomiting.[51,52] Food intake before chemotherapy and the amount of sleep a patient has had may influence the degree of nausea and vomiting.[53] Patients who are more likely to develop nausea and vomiting are those who have had severe emesis during pregnancy[54] and those who are prone to motion sickness (Table 55.1-4).[55,56]

TABLE 55.1-4. Factors Affecting the Control and Incidence of Nausea and Vomiting after Chemotherapy

Patient-specific factors
Previous emesis experience with chemotherapy
Alcohol intake
Age
Gender
Anxiety
Expectation of severe side effects
Roommate experiencing nausea and vomiting
Motivation level
Performance status
Food intake before chemotherapy
Amount of sleep before chemotherapy
Severe emesis during pregnancy
Motion sickness
Treatment-specific factors
Drug
Dose
Infusion rate

ANTIEMETIC AGENTS

MOST ACTIVE AGENTS

As outlined in the Pathophysiology of Nausea/Vomiting section, antagonism of the type 3 serotonin receptor (5-HT^3) is an important approach to controlling chemotherapy-induced emesis. Several agents are available that exert their efficacy in this manner. Metoclopramide, which was previously thought to block emesis by antagonism of a dopamine receptor (D_{23}), probably works primarily via the 5-HT^3 pathway at higher doses. This explains why higher doses of metoclopramide are more effective.[57] However, metoclopramide is not selective for the 5-HT^3 pathway, and development of highly selective antagonists of the 5-HT^3 receptor allowed for good antiemetic effect with a lower side effect profile.

Several selective 5-HT^3 antagonists are commercially available in many countries: dolasetron, granisetron, ondansetron, and tropisetron. Other similar agents are available in individual countries or under investigation. Many multiple, randomized, well-controlled studies have demonstrated that these agents have equivalent antiemetic activity and safety.[58–62]

Nonetheless, some differences do exist among these agents. The differences are primarily in their structure and pharmacokinetic profile; however, to date none of these differences has been shown to be of clinical importance. All agents work by the identical mechanism: antagonism of the 5-HT^3 receptor. All appear to accomplish this maximally, and differences among the relative potencies are unimportant at the recommended doses. There is no clear evidence that one of these agents will be effective when another is not. Half-lives in the serum vary from approximately 3 to 11 hours, but activity at the receptor appears to be similar in that single doses of all agents are equally effective. All agents have good bioavailability for oral administration. When tested, oral administration is as effective as is the intravenous route.[63–69]

Controversy remains concerning the optimal dose of the serotonin antagonists. From current trials, it appears that maximal benefit occurs once all relevant receptors are saturated. No matter what the emetic source, if the best results are to be achieved, an adequate dose should be given. Higher doses are not advantageous once all receptors have been saturated.[70,71] In that these are very safe and well-tolerated agents, it has been difficult to define the best dose regimens, and different doses have been mandated in different countries. Several international consensus guidelines have been published, including

TABLE 55.1-5. Doses, Schedules, and Classes of Commonly Administered Antiemetics

Antiemetic	*Dosage*
Serotonin receptor antagonists	
Ondansetron	8 mg IV × 1 24 mg PO × 1
Granisetron	10 μg/kg IV × 1 2 mg PO × 1
Dolasetron	1.8 mg/kg IV × 1 200 mg PO × 1
Tropisetron	5 mg IV × 1
Substituted benzamide	
Metoclopramide	1 to 3 mg/kg IV × every 3 hr
Phenothiazine	
Prochlorperazine	10 to 20 mg IV × 1 over 5 min 25-mg suppository PR q6h *or* 10 mg PO q4–6h *or* 15-mg spansule PO q8–12h
Butyrophenone	
Haloperidol	1 to 3 mg IV q4–6h 1 to 2 mg PO q4–6h
Corticosteroid	
Dexamethasone	10 to 20 mg IV × 1 over 5 min
Cannabinoid	
Dronabinol	2.5 to 5.0 mg PO q3–6h
Benzodiazepine	
Lorazepam	0.5 to 2.0 mg IV q4–6h 0.5 to 1.0 mg PO q4–6h

those from the subcommittee for antiemetics of the Multinational Association of Supportive Care in Cancer, those from the American Association of Clinical Oncology, and those from the American Society of Health-Systems Pharmacists. As a general rule, the lowest adequately tested dose should be assumed to be the best dose in all settings (Table 55.1-5).

Although some debate persists concerning the best dose of ondansetron, the majority of trials have indicated that the lower dose (8 mg) is as effective as the higher and far more expensive dose of 32 mg.[72,73] The latter dose was superior in only one trial and was troubled by a high inadequate treatment rate, indicating a poorly conducted trial.[74] The lower granisetron dose of 10 μg/kg is as effective in all circumstances as four times the dosage.[75,76] The same dose recommendations continue for single-agent or combination use.

The side effect profile of the 5-HT³ antagonists provides an advantage over such effective antiemetics as metoclopramide. Central nervous system effects, extrapyramidal reactions, and sedation are not observed with serotonin antagonists; this is particularly beneficial in younger patients. Common side effects include mild headaches usually not requiring treatment, transient transaminase elevations, and mild constipation with some agents.[77–80]

As indicated, the antiemetic activity of metoclopramide is likely as a serotonin antagonist, although it has substantial dopamine antagonist action as well. This latter mechanism explains the potential for extrapyramidal reactions. Studies have shown that higher doses are more effective.[81,82] A dose of 3 mg/kg given every 2 hours for two doses in a combination regimen has been found to be effective.[83,84] To date, metoclopramide appears to be at least as effective as serotonin antagonists in preventing delayed emesis and is far less expensive.[85–87]

Corticosteroids are valuable antiemetics. Dexamethasone is the best studied of all these agents, is available in oral and parenteral preparations and, in most countries, is very inexpensive. Although the best dose has not been established, it appears that a single 20-mg dose is adequate, with no clear indication that either higher or lower doses is preferred.[88] The other steroid that has been studied and that can be used is methylprednisolone. Caution must be used when treating diabetic patients or others with poor tolerance for corticosteroids. However, the short recommended course makes these agents very safe and easy to use. In preventing delayed emesis, adequate doses of corticosteroids currently are viewed as the starting point of treatment, with some studies showing advantage for metoclopramide combined with steroids.[89–91]

Efficacy for corticosteroids has been clearly outlined for cisplatin-containing regimens as well as other types of chemotherapy with lesser emetic potential.[92–98] The addition of a corticosteroid to 5-HT³ antagonists significantly improves antiemetic efficacy with each of the agents. This is seen with cisplatin chemotherapy[99,100] as well as with such drugs as anthracyclines, cyclophosphamide, and carboplatin.[101] Double-blind studies have shown that efficacy is raised in from 40% or 50% of patients having complete control with single agents to 75% or 85% of patients with a combination of 5-HT³ antagonist plus a corticosteroid.[102–104] This has led most investigators to advise that a corticosteroid should be added whenever the emetic source is thought to warrant a serotonin antagonist, unless a clearly documented reason for not using a corticosteroid in that patient has been demonstrated.

ANTIEMETICS OF LOWER ACTIVITY

Older agents, such as phenothiazines, butyrophenones, and cannabinoids, all have some degree of antiemetic efficacy. In general, this efficacy is substantially lower than that seen with the serotonin antagonists (including high-dose metoclopramide), and the side effects are greater.[105] When given intravenously, phenothiazines appear to be more active than when given by other routes but are associated with hypotension (especially orthostatic), which can be severe. Thus, these agents are not highly recommended. Oral forms of all three of these agents exhibit only modest activity and are of similarly low efficacy.

Several cannabinoids have been tested in chemotherapy-induced emesis and are of both historic and lay press interest. Semisynthetic agents, such as nabilone and levonantradol; tetrahydrocannabinol (or delta 9-THC), the active agent in marijuana; and inhaled marijuana, all appear to be of low and equal efficacy, with frequent autonomic side effects. These toxicities include dry mouth, hypotension, and dizziness.[106,107] Dronabinol may be useful as an adjuvant to other antiemetics.

Antianxiety agents, such as the benzodiazepine lorazepam, have little efficacy as single agents in carefully conducted trials.[108] However, they function well against anxiety in the emotionally charged atmosphere of receiving chemotherapy, although they add only a minor antiemetic effect to more active agents.[109] They should be regarded as adjuncts to antiemetics and, in that role, can be useful for many patients. Recommended doses range from 0.5 to 1.5 mg. It is not clear that there is any advantage in giving these agents parenterally

TABLE 55.1-6. Recommended Regimen for Delayed Emesis

Begin 16 to 24 hours after cisplatin:	
Days 1, 2	Metoclopramide 0.5 mg/kg PO q.i.d.
	plus
	Dexamethasone 8 mg PO b.i.d.
Days 3, 4	Dexamethasone 4 mg PO b.i.d.

1. Diphenhydramine should be given at the first sign of extrapyramidal symptoms and prophylactically to the young patient.
2. Regimen to be given for cisplatin >50 mg/m^2 or combination chemotherapy with an anthracycline and cyclophosphamide.
3. Oral 5-HT^3 antagonists can be substituted for metoclopramide.

5-HT^3, 5-hydroxytryptamine type 3.

rather than orally when given with the most effective antiemetics. Additionally, these drugs may be useful when given to patients with anticipatory emesis, starting one or more days before the next chemotherapy dosing. Side effects mainly concern sedation, which can be marked in some patients, especially if the drug is given intravenously (see Table 55.1-5).

DELAYED EMESIS

With the identification of useful antiemetics for the treatment of the acute emetic syndrome, it became apparent in patients receiving high total doses of cisplatin that, despite good control of emesis during the initial 24 hours after therapy, delayed emesis became an issue. To date, the pathophysiology of this especially difficult problem remains unclear. What is known, however, is that delayed emesis is a phenomenon observed in as many as 80% of patients, typically occurring 24 to 72 hours after high total doses of cisplatin (>100 mg/m^2) have been administered.[110] Delayed emesis may also be seen in a substantial number of patients who receive as little as 50 mg/m^2 cisplatin or a chemotherapy combination, including cyclophosphamide and an anthracycline. A study that outlined the natural history of delayed emesis concluded that although the emesis associated with this dilemma is less severe than that which is seen in the acute phase, it still poses significant problems with nutrition, hydration, and, possibly, a prolonged hospital course.

Initial studies revealed that delayed emesis could be controlled with a regimen of metoclopramide and dexamethasone (Table 55.1-6). Because of the possibility of extrapyramidal side effects, such as anxiety, akathisia, restlessness, torticollis, or oculogyric crisis, with metoclopramide, the patient should routinely be given a supply of diphenhydramine that should be taken at the first sign of an extrapyramidal symptom. In the younger patient, diphenhydramine should be given prophylactically.

Initial trials addressing the treatment of delayed emesis with the single-agent serotonin antagonist ondansetron were discouraging and labeled the serotonin antagonists as having low activity.[111,112] Two randomized studies, one with ondansetron and one with granisetron, indicated efficacy of the serotonin antagonists for delayed emesis in patients receiving chemotherapy of intermediate emetogenicity.[113,114]

As it is known from previous studies that a delayed antiemetic regimen with a substituted benzamide and dexamethasone controls the emesis, further research is needed to compare this standard regimen with a regimen of a serotonin antagonist and dexamethasone. One may need to differentiate between late-onset acute emesis (i.e., 18 to 48 hours after cyclophosphamide administration, for which oral granisetron and ondansetron have demonstrated benefit) versus true delayed emesis that is evident 2 to 7 days after cisplatin administration, for which the 5-HT^3 antagonists may not have a large advantage over standard metoclopramide-based regimens. It is likely that the mechanism of action for delayed emesis is very different from that for acute chemotherapy-induced emesis, and perhaps serotonin is not involved at all. This should be addressed further in carefully controlled clinical trials, as the cost of the serotonin antagonists is far more than the cost of a substituted benzamide.

Another group of agents that have a potential role in the prevention of delayed nausea and vomiting are the NK1 antagonists. Substance P, which is found in the GI tract and the central nervous system and can produce vomiting when injected into ferrets, exerts its effects by binding to the neuroreceptor NK1. Hesketh et al.[115] reported on a randomized phase II study of the NK1-receptor antagonist CJ-11,974 in the control of cisplatin-induced emesis in 61 patients. This exploratory trial revealed that CJ-11,974 was superior to placebo in controlling delayed emesis and may provide additive benefit in acute emesis and nausea control when combined with a 5-HT^3 antagonist and dexamethasone. In a multicenter, double-blind, placebo-controlled trial involving 159 patients who received a single dose of cisplatin, the NK1-receptor antagonist L-754,030 prevented delayed emesis and, in combination with granisetron plus dexamethasone, improved the prevention of acute emesis.[116]

Other agents that may be of benefit in the treatment of delayed emesis include benzodiazepines, especially lorazepam and alprazolam; the H_2 blockers cimetidine and ranitidine; and omeprazole. Studies are currently under way on the use of cisapride, a potent gastric prokinetic agent that does not affect the D_2 receptors and, therefore, does not lead to adverse extrapyramidal effects.

ANTICIPATORY NAUSEA AND VOMITING

Anticipatory nausea and vomiting usually occur approximately 24 hours before the patient begins chemotherapy. The symptoms may occur outside the hospital, in the clinic, when talking about chemotherapy, or when the patient perceives special tastes or odors.

Acute nausea and vomiting that occur with chemotherapy are thought to be secondary to the medication. The exact mechanism of posttreatment nausea and vomiting is unknown, though is most likely secondary to the chemotherapeutic agent itself; at times, it may also involve a psychological mechanism. Anticipatory nausea and vomiting always involve a psychological mechanism in that they are triggered by events that are not secondary to the direct administration of the chemotherapeutic agent itself.

The prevalence of anticipatory nausea and vomiting varies, depending on the study cited and whether nausea and vomiting are analyzed separately. A review by Morrow and Dobkin[117] summarized 28 surveys that were carried out in North America since 1979. The prevalence of anticipatory nausea ranged any-

TABLE 55.1-7. Factors Associated with an Increased Incidence of Anticipatory Nausea and Vomiting

Severe postchemotherapy side effects
Schedule of chemotherapy
Numerous chemotherapy cycles
Chemotherapeutic agents with high emetogenic potential
Age
History of motion sickness
Anxiety
Depression
Taste and odors

where from 14% to 63%, with a median of 33%. Many factors that appear to be associated with anticipatory nausea and vomiting have been studied (Table 55.1-7).

Numerous studies have revealed a relationship between severe postchemotherapy side effects and the development of anticipatory nausea and vomiting.[118–121] The schedule of chemotherapy also appears to be related to anticipatory symptoms. Anticipatory symptoms are related to the emetogenicity of the chemotherapeutic agents in most studies.[122–124] They also are related to the length of chemotherapy, in that patients who receive chemotherapy for longer periods have a higher incidence of anticipatory symptoms.[125–127]

Motion sickness is a risk factor for the development of postchemotherapy nausea and vomiting.[128] One study by Morrow[129] of 608 patients and another study by Morrow et al.[130] of 355 patients found a significant relationship between motion sickness and anticipatory nausea and vomiting. In some studies, age appears to be related to anticipatory symptoms. Anticipatory nausea and vomiting occur more often in patients younger than 45 to 50 years old.[131–134] Possibly, age is related to anticipatory symptoms in part because younger patients receive stronger emetogenic chemotherapeutic agents, which leads to increased postchemotherapy nausea and vomiting and, therefore, increased anticipatory nausea and vomiting. Another proposed explanation is that younger patients have a higher level of anxiety while receiving chemotherapy, which may lead to increases in anticipatory symptoms. Both of these explanations are plausible, though current data do not support either.[135]

Other factors that have been reported to be related to anticipatory nausea and vomiting include expectations. Those patients with anticipatory symptoms report the expectation of developing nausea and vomiting after chemotherapy.[136,137] Type and stage of cancer also are related.[138,139] Anticipatory symptoms have been found to be correlated with a patient's previous response of nausea and vomiting to different situations.[140] It has been noted that patients with anticipatory nausea and vomiting have higher levels of depression.[141] A relationship between anxiety and anticipatory nausea and vomiting has also been noted,[142,143] though, at this time, insufficient evidence is available to indicate the way that anxiety is related to anticipatory symptoms.[144]

Several retrospective reviews have indicated that taste and odors are related to anticipatory nausea and vomiting.[145–149] Though a prospective study did not reveal any relationship among taste, odors, and anticipatory nausea and vomiting, Bovbjerg et al.[150] reported a study in which they administered a beverage to patients before their receipt of chemotherapy. The investigators found a clear relationship between anticipatory nausea and a special taste. Blasco[151] suggested that taste and odors may be involved not only in anticipatory nausea and vomiting but perhaps with postchemotherapy nausea and vomiting. Indeed, the role of taste and smell is largely unknown; however, it may be involved in a spectrum of GI complaints experienced by the patient with cancer. Studies by Bernstein[152] suggest that a learned food aversion develops to specific tastes or food and occurs because of an association of the food with unpleasant symptoms, such as nausea and vomiting. This food aversion could partially explain the anorexia associated with cancer.

Antiemetics used in the treatment of acute nausea and vomiting induced by chemotherapy are ineffective in treating anticipatory nausea and vomiting. Many studies have indicated that behavioral techniques are effective in reducing anxiety as well as reducing or eliminating anticipatory nausea and vomiting. Behavioral techniques that have been studied and found to be effective include progressive relaxation with guided imagery, systematic desensitization, hypnosis, and cognitive and intentional distraction.[153–156]

In one report in the literature, a lemon solution given to a patient before the receipt of chemotherapy masked taste sensations so that the patient experienced decreased anticipatory nausea and vomiting.[157] It has also been suggested that the use of benzodiazepines, especially lorazepam, may be helpful in treating anticipatory nausea and vomiting. However, no formal studies have established lorazepam's effectiveness in this situation.

RADIATION-INDUCED NAUSEA AND VOMITING

The etiology of radiation-induced emesis, like chemotherapy-induced emesis, is not completely understood. However, it is clear that it is a complex, multifactorial event. The incidence, severity, and onset of radiation-induced emesis appear to be related to the size of the radiation field, the dose per fraction, and the site of irradiation. Radiation-induced emesis occurs acutely in more than 90% of patients who receive total body irradiation for bone marrow transplantation, within 30 to 60 minutes in more than 80% of patients who receive single high-dose or large-field hemibody irradiation (>500 cGy), and within 2 to 3 weeks in approximately 50% of patients who receive conventional fractionated radiotherapy (200 cGy per fraction) to the upper abdomen.[158] Radiation-induced emesis also occurs in those patients who receive radiosurgery to the area postrema in excess of 350 to 400 cGy in a single dose. The emesis usually occurs between 1 and 12 hours after the radiosurgery.

The exact mechanism of radiation-induced emesis remains unclear. However, as with chemotherapy-induced emesis, it is thought that it most likely is due to a peripheral mechanism in the GI tract or a central mechanism involving the CTZ. It has been proposed that several substances, including dopamine, catecholamines, and prostaglandins, are released and stimulate afferent visceral fibers, an action that then initiates sensory signals to the CTZ. As a result of both preclinical and clinical studies with serotonin antagonists, it has been suggested that serotonin may be released from enterochromaffin cells of the GI tract and may mediate emesis via mechanisms involving the 5-HT^3 receptors, visceral afferent fibers, and the CTZ. This mechanism is most likely involved when radiation is applied to the upper abdomen, hemibody, or total body. Radiosurgery to the area postrema most likely induces emesis from the release of serotonin in the CTZ.[159]

Clinical studies in the past using metoclopramide, nabilone (cannabinoid derivative), and chlorpromazine in the treatment of radiation-induced emesis revealed a response of 50% to 58%.[160,161] In a nonplacebo trial with domperidone, a dopamine antagonist, a response of 82% was reported.[162] A nonrandomized trial comparing ondansetron with other antiemetics reported response rates of 100% for ondansetron versus 43% for other antiemetics and 19% for no antiemetic treatment for patients who received middle to upper hemibody irradiation.[163] A randomized study by Priestman et al.[164] of patients who received radiotherapy to the abdomen, pelvis, and thoracolumbar spine reported response rates of 45% for metoclopramide versus 97% for ondansetron. A randomized, double-blind, placebo-controlled evaluation revealed oral ondansetron to be an effective therapy for the prevention of emesis induced by total body irradiation.[165] Ondansetron has been reported to be effective in radiotherapy-induced emesis in children[166] as well as for patients who receive radiosurgery to the area postrema.[167]

Data are available from two double-blind, randomized studies in the use of oral granisetron, 2 mg once daily, in radiation-induced nausea and vomiting. In a study involving patients undergoing fractionated upper abdominal radiation, patients who received oral granisetron had a significantly longer median time to first emesis than did those who received placebo (35 days vs. 9 days, respectively) and a longer median time to first nausea (11 days vs. 1 day, respectively).[168] In another study of patients undergoing total body irradiation, patients treated with oral granisetron had significantly greater complete control as compared to the historical control group over the entire 4-day treatment period (22% vs. 0%, respectively).[169]

Fauser et al.[170] reported on the use of oral dolasetron for the control of emesis during total body irradiation and high-dose cyclophosphamide in patients undergoing allogeneic bone marrow transplantation.

NAUSEA AND VOMITING SECONDARY TO COMORBID CONDITIONS

A number of comorbid conditions also may lead to nausea and vomiting, even though the majority of patients with cancer develop nausea and vomiting as a result of chemotherapy or radiotherapy (Table 55.1-8). Because the mechanism of the nausea and vomiting secondary to comorbid conditions is not usually well understood, it is difficult to know which antiemetics may be helpful. A study by Bruera et al.[171] revealed that controlled-release metoclopramide is safe and effective in managing chronic nausea in patients with advanced cancer. Future studies must be conducted to determine the optimal doses of metoclopramide as well as other antiemetics that may be used in drug combinations (e.g., metoclopramide plus corticosteroids) for the nausea and vomiting secondary to the malignancy itself.

TABLE 55.1-8. Comorbid Conditions That May Lead to Nausea and Vomiting

Central nervous system metastases
Peritonitis
Hepatic metastases
Uremia
Hypercalcemia
Volume depletion
Water intoxication
Adrenocortical insufficiency
Bowel obstruction
Deficiency of specific nutrients
Learned food aversion
Taste and smell alterations
Hunger satiety mechanisms
Narcotics
Psychological stress

COST AND BENEFIT OF ANTIEMETIC THERAPY

The important results of research that provide the medical community with additional chemotherapeutic choices and supportive care measures often translate into added health care costs for patients and families. With the increased use of expensive antiemetics and with managed care dictating the length of hospital stays, the emphasis is shifting to primary outpatient management of patient treatment courses. The challenge for physicians becomes one of providing a treatment plan in which patients are offered state-of-the-art and cost-effective therapy. This can be accomplished by applying certain guidelines.

Specifically addressing 5-HT^3 antagonist antiemetics and their associated cost, the choice among these agents should be made on the basis of acquisition costs and reimbursement differences. The 5-HT^3 antagonists all have demonstrated equivalent efficacy and side effects; therefore, once an effective dose has been established, there would be no advantage in exceeding this threshold dose. Ultimately, the 5-HT^3 antagonist of lowest cost should be selected for administration. Single-dose regimens given in combination with a corticosteroid provide an effective and convenient alternative in antiemetic therapy. Regimens that take advantage of a completely oral route of administration are easy and convenient for patients and are likely to reduce nursing and pharmacy costs; however, prolonged use of oral serotonin antagonists should be avoided, as there appears to be little or no value in this setting. In addition to these recommendations, adherence by physicians and nurses to established doses and schedules of antiemetics and their appropriate use can be cost-effective measures for patients and institutions.

Nolte et al.[172] discussed guidelines developed by the Memorial Sloan-Kettering Cancer Center for the cost-effective use of 5-HT^3 antagonists that resulted in substantial savings while treating more patients. The initial guidelines in 1993 were developed based on the premise that the dose of the intravenous 5-HT^3 antagonist ondansetron, 8 to 32 mg, could be adjusted on the basis of emetogenic potential of the chemotherapeutic regimen schema proposed by Hesketh et al.[95] Cost savings were documented without affecting the quality of life, as reported by the patients. The guidelines were modified in 1994 to include granisetron, 10 μg/kg, for moderately or highly emetogenic chemotherapy. When oral granisetron tablets were approved in 1995 for the prevention of highly emetogenic chemotherapeutic regimens, the guidelines were further modified to incorporate the use of oral granisetron instead of intravenous 5-HT3 antagonists for moderately to highly emetogenic chemotherapy. Additional cost savings were realized while the quality of life of the patients was unaffected.

The use of an oral form of a 5-HT3 antagonist for highly emetogenic chemotherapy, when data from well-controlled trials demonstrate comparable efficacy to the intravenous formulation, appears to be cost-effective.[173,174] One should take into consideration, when evaluating the results of these studies, whether a stringent efficacy end point was used. Some studies did not use "no nausea" as one of the criteria for a complete response. Because nausea was ranked as the most severe chemotherapy-related symptom according to a relatively recent survey, the effect of the agents on nausea should also be evaluated.

Economic considerations for the selection of antiemetic regimens should answer the following questions:

- Will the use of the regimens likely result in a reduced hospitalization?
- While receiving therapy, will patients be able to maintain their usual level of activity?
- Will nursing and pharmacy costs be reduced?
- Are there mandated restrictions on the use of an agent in hospital formularies and in clinical settings?
- Will the antiemetic regimen affect the patient's out-of-pocket expenses?

Extensive basic and clinical research has made it possible to control treatment-induced nausea and vomiting. With recognition and anticipation of nausea and vomiting, counseling of the patient and family, prophylactic intervention, flexibility in the therapeutic approach, and constant reassessment of the treatment plan, chemotherapy- and radiotherapy-induced nausea and vomiting can be managed effectively in 80% to 90% of patients. The progress made in the field of treatment-induced nausea and vomiting must be a paradigm for other symptoms faced by the cancer patient that lead to suffering and that affect the patient's quality of life.

REFERENCES

1. Jenns K. Importance of nausea. *Cancer Nurs* 1994;17:488.
2. Morran C, Smith DC, Anderson DA, et al. Incidence of nausea and vomiting with cytotoxic chemotherapy: a prospective randomized trial of antiemetics. *BMJ* 1979;1:1323.
3. Carey MP, Burish TG. Anxiety as a predictor of behavioral therapy outcome for cancer chemotherapy patients. *J Consult Clin Psychol* 1985;53:860.
4. Wilcox PM, Fetting JH, Nettesheim KM, et al. Anticipatory vomiting in women receiving cyclophosphamide, methotrexate, and 5-FU (CMF) adjuvant chemotherapy for breast carcinoma. *Cancer Treat Rep* 1982;66:1601.
5. Morrow GR, Lindke J, Black PM. Predicting development of anticipatory nausea in cancer patients: prospective examination of eight clinical characteristics. *J Pain Symptom Manage* 1991;6:2155.
6. Nesse RM, Carli T, Curtis GC, et al. Pretreatment nausea in cancer chemotherapy: a conditioned response? *Psychosom Med* 1980;42:33.
7. Moertel C, Reitemeir R, Gage R. A controlled clinical evaluation of antiemetic drugs. *JAMA* 1963;186:116.
8. Moertel C, Reitemeir R. Controlled clinical studies of orally administered antiemetic drugs. *Gastroenterology* 1989;57:262.
9. Ettinger DS. Preventing chemotherapy-induced nausea and vomiting: an update and review of emesis. *Semin Oncol* 1995;22:4[Suppl 10]:6.
10. Coates A, Abraham S, Kaye SB, et al. On the receiving end. Patient perceptions of the side-effects of cancer chemotherapy. *Eur J Clin Oncol* 1983;19:203.
11. Griffin AM, Butow PN, Coates AS, et al. On the receiving end: patient perceptions of the side effects of cancer chemotherapy. *Ann Oncol* 1996;7:189.
12. Stewart DJ. Nausea and vomiting in cancer patients. In: Kucharczyk J, Stewart DJ, Miller AD, eds. *Nausea and vomiting: recent research and clinical advances.* Boca Raton, FL: CRC Press, 1991:177.
13. Young RW. Mechanisms and treatment of radiation-induced nausea and vomiting. In: Davis CJ, Lake-Bakaar GV, Graham-Smith DG, eds. *Nausea and vomiting: mechanisms and treatment.* Berlin: Springer-Verlag, 1986:94.
14. Ison PJ, Peroutka SJ. Neurotransmitter receptor binding studies predict antiemetic efficacy and side effects. *Cancer Treat Rep* 1986;70:637.
15. McCarthy LE, Borison HL. Cisplatin-induced vomiting eliminated by ablation of the area postrema in cats. *Cancer Treat Rep* 1984;68:401.
16. Stewart DJ. Nausea and vomiting in cancer patients. In: Kucharczyk J, Stewart DJ, Miller AD, eds. *Nausea and vomiting: recent research and clinical advances.* Boca Raton, FL: CRC Press, 1991:190.
17. Fortner CL, Finley RS, Grove WR. Combination antiemetic therapy in the control of chemotherapy-induced drug emetogenic potential emesis. *Drug Intell Clin Pharm* 1985;19:21.
18. Price NM, Schmitt LG, McGuire J. Transdermal scopolamine in the prevention of motion sickness at sea. *Clin Pharmacol Ther* 1981;29:414.
19. Kobrinsky NL. Regulation of nausea and vomiting in cancer chemotherapy. *Am J Pediatr Hematol Oncol* 1988;10:209.
20. Hilliard D, Wilbur D, Camacho E. Butorphenol vs metoclopramide in the control of cisplatin-induced emesis. *Proc Am Soc Clin Oncol* 1985;4:274.
21. Dullemond-Westland AC, Neijt JP, Nortier JWR, et al. Buprenorphine versus domperidone in chemotherapy-induced emesis. A pilot study. *Radiother Oncol* 1986;6:127.
22. Lissoni P, Barni S, Crispino S, et al. Synthetic enkephalin analog in the treatment of cancer chemotherapy-induced vomiting. *Cancer Treat Rep* 1987;71:665.
23. Edwards C, Carmichael J, Baylis P, et al. Arginine vasopressin—a mediator of chemotherapy induced emesis? *Br J Cancer* 1989;59:467.
24. Kobrinsky NL. Regulation of nausea and vomiting in cancer chemotherapy. *Am J Pediatr Hematol Oncol* 1988;10:209.
25. Ettinger DS. Preventing chemotherapy-induced nausea and vomiting: an update and review of emesis. *Semin Oncol* 1995;22:4:[Suppl 10]:7.
26. Gralla RJ, Itri LM, Pisko SE, et al. Antiemetic efficacy of high-dose metoclopramide: randomized trials with placebo and prochlorperazine in patients with chemotherapy-induced nausea and vomiting. *N Engl J Med* 1981;305:905.
27. Fozard JR. Neuronal 5-HT receptors in the periphery. *Neuropharmacology* 1984;23:1473.
28. Sanger GJ. Mechanisms by which metoclopramide can increase gastrointestinal motility. In: Bennett A, Velo G, eds. *Mechanisms of gastrointestinal motility and secretion.* New York: Plenum Publishing, 1984:303.
29. Miner WD, Sanger GJ, Turner DH. Comparison of the effect of BRL 24924, metoclopramide and domperidone on cisplatin-induced emesis in the ferret. *Br J Pharmacol* 1986;88:374.
30. Miner WD, Sanger GJ. Inhibition of cisplatin-induced vomiting by selective 5-hydroxytryptamine M-receptor antagonism. *Br J Pharmacol* 1986;88:497.
31. Costall B, Domeney AM, Naylor RJ, et al. 5-Hydroxytryptamine M-receptor antagonism to prevent cisplatin-induced emesis. *Neuropharmacology* 1986;25:959.
32. Cubeddu L, Hoffman I, Fuenmayor N, et al. Efficacy of ondansetron (GR 38032F) and the role of serotonin in cisplatin-induced nausea and vomiting. *N Engl J Med* 1990;322:810.
33. Cubeddu LX, Hoffman IS, Fuenmayor N, et al. Antagonism of serotonin S3 receptors with ondansetron prevents nausea and emesis induced by cyclophosphamide-containing chemotherapy regimens. *J Clin Oncol* 1990;8:1721.
34. Khojasteh A, Sartiano G, Tapazoglou E, et al. Ondansetron for the prevention of emesis induced by high-dose cisplatin. A multi-center dose-response study. *Cancer* 1990;66:1101.
35. Carden PA, Mitchell SL, Waters KD, et al. Prevention of cyclophosphamide/cytarabine emesis with ondansetron in children with leukemia. *J Clin Oncol* 1990;8:1531.
36. Bonneterre J, Chevallier B, Metz R, et al. A randomized double-blind comparison of ondansetron and metoclopramide in the prophylaxis of emesis induced by cyclophosphamide, fluorouracil, and doxorubicin or epirubicin chemotherapy. *J Clin Oncol* 1990;8:1063.
37. Hesketh PJ, Gralla RJ, Webb W, et al. Randomized phase II study of the neurokinin 1 receptor antagonist CJ-11,974 in the control of cisplatin-induced emesis. *J Clin Oncol* 1999;17:338.
38. Navari RM, Reinhardt RR, Gralla RJ, et al. Reduction of cisplatin-induced emesis by a selective neurokinin-1-receptor antagonist. *N Engl J Med* 1999;340:190.
39. Harris JG. Nausea, vomiting and cancer treatment. *CA Cancer J Clin* 1978;28:194.
40. Morrow GR. The effect of a susceptibility to motion sickness on the side effects of cancer chemotherapy. *Cancer* 1985;55:2766.
41. Mulder NH, Smit JM, Kreumer WMI, et al. Effect of chemotherapy on taste sensation in patients with disseminated malignant melanoma. *Oncology* 1983;40:36.
42. Fetting JH, Wilcox PM, Sheidler VR, et al. Tastes associated with parenteral chemotherapy for breast cancer. *Cancer Treat Rep* 1985;69:1249.
43. Fortner CL, Finley RS, Grove WR. Combination antiemetic therapy in the control of chemotherapy-induced drug emetogenic potential emesis. *Drug Intell Clin Pharm* 1985;19:21.
44. Cassileth BR, Lusk EJ, Bodenheimer BJ, et al. Chemotherapeutic toxicity—the relationship between patient's pretreatment expectations and posttreatment results. *Am J Clin Oncol* 1985;8:419.
45. Borison HL, McCarthy LE. Neuropharmacology of chemotherapy-induced emesis. *Drugs* 1983;25[Suppl 1]:13.
46. Fetting JH, Grochow LB, Folstein MF, et al. The course of nausea and vomiting after high-dose cyclophosphamide. *Cancer Treat Rep* 1982;66:1487.
47. Hesketh P, Kris M, Grunberg SM, et al. Proposal for classifying the acute emetogenicity of cancer chemotherapy. *J Clin Oncol* 1997;15:103.
48. American Society of Health-Systems Pharmacists. Therapeutic guidelines on the pharmacologic management of nausea and vomiting in adult and pediatric patients receiving chemotherapy or radiation therapy or undergoing surgery. *Am J Health Syst Pharm* 1999;56:729.

49. D'Acquisto RW, Tyson LB, et al. Antiemetic trials to control delayed vomiting following high-dose cisplatin. *Proc Am Soc Clin Oncol* 1986;5:257.
50. Allen JC, Gralla RJ, Reilly C, et al. Metoclopramide dose-related toxicity and preliminary antiemetic studies in children receiving cancer chemotherapy. *J Clin Oncol* 1985;3:1136.
51. Holland JF, Frei E III, eds. *Cancer medicine,* 2nd ed. Philadelphia: Lea & Febiger, 1982:2332.
52. Jacobsen P, Andrykowski M, Redd W, et al. Nonpharmacologic factors in the development of posttreatment nausea with adjuvant chemotherapy for breast cancer. *Cancer* 1988;61:379.
53. Stewart DJ. Nausea and vomiting in cancer patients. In: Kucharczyk J, Stewart DJ, Miller AD, eds. *Nausea and vomiting: recent research and clinical advances.* Boca Raton, FL: CRC Press, 1991:177.
54. Martin M, Diaz-Rubio E. Emesis during pregnancy: a new prognostic factor in chemotherapy-induced emesis. *Ann Oncol* 1990;1:152.
55. Morrow GR. The effect of a susceptibility to motion sickness on the side effects of cancer chemotherapy. *Cancer* 1985;55:2766.
56. Guillem V, Aranda E, Carrato A, et al. Previous history of emesis during pregnancy and motion sickness as risk factors for chemotherapy-induced emesis. *J Clin Oncol* 1999;2280(18):590a(abst).
57. Gralla RJ, Itri LM, Pisko SE, et al. Antiemetic efficacy of high-dose metoclopramide: randomized trials with placebo and prochlorperazine in patients with chemotherapy-induced nausea and vomiting. *N Engl J Med* 1981;305:905.
58. American Society of Health-Systems Pharmacists. Therapeutic guidelines on the pharmacological management of nausea and vomiting in adult and pediatric patients receiving chemotherapy or radiation therapy or undergoing surgery. *Am J Health Syst Pharm* 1999;56:729.
59. Ettinger DS, Huber S, Kris MG, et al. NCCN antiemesis practice guidelines. *Oncology* 1997;11A:57.
60. Gralla RJ, Osoba D, Kris MG, et al. Recommendations for the use of antiemetics: evidence-based clinical practice guidelines. *J Clin Oncol* 1999;17:2971.
61. Multinational Association of Supportive Care in Cancer. Prevention of chemotherapy and radiotherapy-induced emesis: results of the Perugia consensus conference. *Ann Oncol* 1998;9:811.
62. Roila F, Ballatori, Tonato M, et. al. 5HT3 receptor antagonists: differences and similarities. *Eur J Cancer* 1997;33:1364.
63. Rubenstein E, Kalman L, Hainsworth J, et al. Dose-response trial across 4 oral doses of dolasetron for emesis prevention after moderately emetogenic chemotherapy. *Proc Am Soc Clin Oncol* 1995;14:527.
64. Palmer R, Moriconi W, Cohn J, et al. A double-blind comparison of the efficacy and safety of oral granisetron with oral prochlorperazine in preventing nausea and emesis in patients receiving moderately emetogenic chemotherapy. *Proc Am Soc Clin Oncol* 1995;14:528.
65. Gralla RJ, Rittenberg CN, Lettow L, et al. A unique all-oral, single-dose, combination antiemetic regimen with high efficacy and marked cost saving potential. *Proc Am Soc Clin Oncol* 1995;14:526.
66. Anthony LB, Krozely MG, Woodward NJ, et al. Antiemetic effect of oral versus intravenous metoclopramide in patients receiving cisplatin: a randomized double-blind trial. *J Clin Oncol* 1986;4(1):98.
67. Tyson LB, Gralla RJ, Kris MG, et al. Dose-ranging antiemetic trial of high-dose oral metoclopramide. *Am J Clin Oncol* 1989;12(3):239.
68. Krzakowski M, Graham, E, Goedhals L, et al. A multicenter, double-blind comparison of i.v. and oral administration of ondansetron plus dexamethasone for acute cisplatin-induced emesis. *Anticancer Drugs* 1998;9:593.
69. Lindley C, McCune J, Goodin S, et al. Efficacy of oral ondansetron and dexamethasone in prevention of nausea and vomiting associated with moderately high and highly emetogenic chemotherapy. *Proc Am Soc Clin Oncol* 1998;244:1763a(abst).
70. Kris MG, Gralla RJ, Clark RA, et al. Phase II trials of the serotonin antagonist GR38032F for the control of vomiting caused by cisplatin. *J Natl Cancer Inst* 1989;81:42.
71. Kris MG, Gralla RJ, Clark RA, et al. Dose ranging evaluation of the serotonin antagonist GR-C507/75 (GR38032F) when used as an antiemetic in patients receiving cancer chemotherapy. *J Clin Oncol* 1988;6:659.
72. Seynaeve C, Schuller J, Buser K, et al. Comparison of the anti-emetic efficacy of different doses of ondansetron given as either a continuous infusion or a single intravenous dose, in acute cisplatin-induced emesis. A multicentre, double-blind, randomized, parallel group study. *Br J Cancer* 1992;66:192.
73. Ruff P, Paska W, Goedhals L, et al. Ondansetron compared with granisetron in the prophylaxis of cisplatin-induced acute emesis: a multicenter double-blind, randomized, parallel group study. *Oncology* 1994;5:113.
74. Beck TM, Hesketh PJ, Madajewicz S, et al. Stratified, randomized, double-blind comparison of intravenous dose regimens in the prevention of cisplatin-induced nausea and vomiting. *J Clin Oncol* 1992;10(12):1969.
75. Navari R, Gandara D, Hesketh P, et al. Comparative clinical trial of granisetron and ondansetron in the prophylaxis of cisplatin-induced emesis. *J Clin Oncol* 1995;13:1242.
76. Perez EA, Gandara DR. The clinical role of granisetron (Kytril) in the prevention of chemotherapy-induced emesis. *Semin Oncol* 1994;21[Suppl 5]:15.
77. Gralla RJ, Itri LM, Pisko SE, et al. Antiemetic efficacy of high-dose metoclopramide: randomized trials with placebo and prochlorperazine in patients with chemotherapy-induced nausea and vomiting. *N Engl J Med* 1981;305:905.
78. Navari R, Gandara D, Hesketh P, et al. Comparative clinical trial of granisetron and ondansetron in the prophylaxis of cisplatin-induced emesis. *J Clin Oncol* 1995;13:1242.
79. DeMulder PHM, Seynaeve C, Vermorker JB, et al. Ondansetron compared with high-dose metoclopramide in prophylaxis of acute and delayed cisplatin-induced nausea and vomiting. A multicenter, randomized, double-blind, crossover study. *Ann Intern Med* 1990;113:834.
80. Navari R, Hesketh P, Grote T, et al. A double-blind, randomized, comparison intravenous study of single dose dolasetron versus ondansetron in preventing cisplatin-related emesis. *Proc Am Soc Clin Oncol* 1995;14:522.
81. Gralla RJ, Itri LM, Pisko SE, et al. Antiemetic efficacy of high-dose metoclopramide: randomized trials with placebo and prochlorperazine in patients with chemotherapy-induced nausea and vomiting. *N Engl J Med* 1981;305:905.
82. Basurto C, Roila F, Tonato M, et al. Antiemetic activity of high-dose metoclopramide combined with methylprednisolone versus metoclopramide alone in dacarbazine-treated cancer patients. A randomized double-blind study of the Italian Oncology Group for Clinical Research. *Am J Clin Oncol* 1989;12(3):235.
83. Kris MG, Gralla RJ, Clark RA, et al. Antiemetic control and prevention of side effects of anticancer therapy with lorazepam or diphenhydramine when used in conjunction with metoclopramide plus dexamethasone. A double-blind, randomized trial. *Cancer* 1987;69:1353.
84. Kris MG, Gralla RJ, Tyson LB, et al. Improved control of cisplatin-induced emesis with high dose metoclopramide and with combinations of metoclopramide, dexamethasone, and diphenhydramine. Results of consecutive trials in 255 patients. *Cancer* 1985;55:527.
85. Roila F, De Angelis V, Cognetti F, et al. Ondansetron vs. granisetron, both combined with dexamethasone in the prevention of cisplatin-induced emesis. *Proc Am Soc Clin Oncol* 1995;14:523.
86. DeMulder PHM, Seynaeve C, Vermorker JB, et al. Ondansetron compared with high-dose metoclopramide in prophylaxis of acute and delayed cisplatin-induced nausea and vomiting. A multicenter, randomized, double-blind, crossover study. *Ann Intern Med* 1990;113:834.
87. Kris MG, Gralla RJ, Tyson LB, et al. Controlling delayed vomiting: a double-blind, randomized trial comparing placebo, dexamethasone alone, and metoclopramide plus dexamethasone in patients receiving cisplatin. *J Clin Oncol* 1989;7:108.
88. Kris MG, Gralla RJ, Tyson LB, et al. Improved control of cisplatin-induced emesis with high dose metoclopramide and with combinations of metoclopramide, dexamethasone, and diphenhydramine. Results of consecutive trials in 255 patients. *Cancer* 1985;55:527.
89. Rittenberg CN, Gralla REJ, Lettow LA, Cronin MD, Kardinal CG. New approaches in preventing delayed emesis: altering the time of regimen initiation and use of combination therapy in a 109 patient trial. *Proc Am Soc Oncol* 1995;14:526.
90. Roila F, Tonato M, Cognetti F, et al. Prevention of cisplatin-induced emesis: a double-blind multicenter randomized crossover study comparing ondansetron and ondansetron plus dexamethasone. *J Clin Oncol* 1991;9:675.
91. Kris MG, Gralla RJ, Tyson LB, et al. Controlling delayed vomiting: a double-blind, randomized trial comparing placebo, dexamethasone alone, and metoclopramide plus dexamethasone in patients receiving cisplatin. *J Clin Oncol* 1989;7:108.
92. Navari R, Gandara D, Hesketh P, et al. Comparative clinical trial of granisetron and ondansetron in the prophylaxis of cisplatin-induced emesis. *J Clin Oncol* 1995;13:1242.
93. Kris MG, Grunberg SM, Gralla RJ, et al. Dose-ranging evaluation of the serotonin antagonist dolasetron mesylate in patients receiving high-dose cisplatin. *J Clin Oncol* 1994;12:1045.
94. Kris MG, Gralla RJ, Clark RA, et al. Phase II trials of the serotonin antagonist GR38032F for the control of vomiting caused by cisplatin. *J Natl Cancer Inst* 1989;81:42.
95. Hesketh PJ, Murphy WK, Lester RP, et al. GR38032F: a novel compound effective in the prevention of acute cisplatin-induced emesis. *J Clin Oncol* 1989;7:700.
96. Hainsworth J, Harvey W, Pendergrass K, et al. A single-blind comparison of intravenous ondansetron, a selective serotonin antagonist, with intravenous metoclopramide in the prevention of nausea and vomiting associated with high-dose cisplatin chemotherapy. *J Clin Oncol* 1991;9:721.
97. Kaplan HG, Jofthagen C. Use of granisetron to prevent platinol induced nausea and vomiting. *Proc Am Soc Oncol* 1991;10:339.
98. Schrnoll HJ. The role of ondansetron in the treatment of emesis induced by non-cisplatin-containing chemotherapy regimens. *Eur J Cancer* 1989;25[Suppl 1]:555.
99. Roila F, De Angelis V, Cognetti F, et al. Ondansetron vs. granisetron, both combined with dexamethasone in the prevention of cisplatin-induced emesis. *Proc Am Soc Clin Oncol* 1995;14:523.
100. Kris MG, Gralla RJ, Clark RA, et al. Dose ranging evaluation of the serotonin antagonist GR-C507/75 (GR38032F) when used as an antiemetic in patients receiving cancer chemotherapy. *J Clin Oncol* 1988;6:659.
101. The Italian Group for Antiemetic Trials. Dexamethasone, granisetron, or both for the prevention of nausea and vomiting during chemotherapy for cancer. *N Engl J Med* 1995;332:1.
102. Roila F, De Angelis V, Cognetti F, et al. Ondansetron vs. granisetron, both combined with dexamethasone in the prevention of cisplatin-induced emesis. *Proc Am Soc Clin Oncol* 1995;14:523.
103. Kris MG, Gralla RJ, Clark RA, et al. Antiemetic control and prevention of side effects of anticancer therapy with lorazepam or diphenhydramine when used in conjunction with metoclopramide plus dexamethasone. A double-blind, randomized trial. *Cancer* 1987;69:1353.
104. Dilly SG, Friedman C, Yocom K. Contribution of dexamethasone to antiemetic control with granisetron is greatest in patients at high risk of emesis. *Proc Am Soc Clin Oncol* 1994;13:436.
105. Gralla RJ, Itri LM, Pisko SE, et al. Antiemetic efficacy of high-dose metoclopramide: randomized trials with placebo and prochlorperazine in patients with chemotherapy-induced nausea and vomiting. *N Engl J Med* 1981;305:905.
106. Gralla RJ, Tyson LB, Borden LA, et al. Antiemetic therapy: a review of recent studies and a report of a random assignment trial comparing metoclopramide with delta-9-tetrahyrocannabinol. *Cancer Treat Rep* 1984;68:163.
107. Levitt M, Faiman C, Hawks R, et al. Randomized double-blind comparison of delta-9-tetrahydrocannabinol (THC) and marijuana as chemotherapy antiemetics. *Proc Am Soc Clin Oncol* 1984;3:91.
108. Lazlo J, Clark RA. Lorazepam in patients treated with cisplatin: a drug having antiemetic and anxiolytic effects. *J Clin Oncol* 1985;3:864.

109. Kris MG, Gralla RJ, Clark RA, et al. Antiemetic control and prevention of side effects of anticancer therapy with lorazepam or diphenhydramine when used in conjunction with metoclopramide plus dexamethasone. A double-blind, randomized trial. *Cancer* 1987;69:1353.
110. Kris MG, Gralla RJ, Clark RA, et al. Incidence, course, and severity of delayed nausea and vomiting following the administration of high-dose cisplatin. *J Clin Oncol* 1985;3:1379.
111. Kris MG, Tyson LB, Clark RA, et al. Oral ondansetron for the control of delayed emesis after cisplatin: report of a phase II study and a review of completed trials to manage delayed emesis. *Cancer* 1992;70:1012.
112. Grunberg SM, Groshen S, Stevenson LI, et al. Double-blind randomized study of two doses of oral ondansetron for the prevention of cisplatin-induced delayed nausea and vomiting. *Proc Am Soc Clin Oncol* 1990;9:327.
113. Kaizer L, Warr D, Hoskins P, et al. Effect of schedule and maintenance on the antiemetic efficacy of ondansetron combined with dexamethasone in acute and delayed nausea and emesis in patients receiving moderately emetogenic chemotherapy: a phase III trial by the National Cancer Institute of Canada Clinical Trials Group. *J Clin Oncol* 1994;12:1050.
114. Guillem V, Carrato A, Rifa J, et al. High efficacy of oral granisetron in the total control of cyclophosphamide-induced prolonged emesis. *Proc Am Soc Clin Oncol* 1998;17:46a(abst 177).
115. Hesketh PJ, Gralla RJ, Webb RT, et al. Randomized phase II study of the neurokinin 1 receptor antagonist CJ-11,974 in the control of cisplatin-induced emesis. *J Clin Oncol* 1999;17:338.
116. Navari RM, Reinhardt RR, Gralla RJ. Reduction of cisplatin induced emesis by a selective neurokinin-1-receptor antagonist. *N Engl J Med* 1999;340:190.
117. Morrow GR, Dobkin PL. Anticipatory nausea and vomiting in cancer patients undergoing chemotherapy treatment: prevalence, etiology, and behavioral interventions. *Clin Psychol Rev* 1988;8:517.
118. Fetting JH, Wilcox PM, Iwata BA, et al. Anticipatory nausea and vomiting in an ambulatory medical oncology population. *Cancer Treat Rep* 1983;67(12):1093.
119. Dolgin MJ, Katz ER, McGinty K, et al. Anticipatory nausea and vomiting in pediatric cancer pediatrics. *Pediatrics* 1985;75(3):547.
120. Morrow GR, Lindke J, Black PM. Anticipatory nausea development in cancer patients: replication and extension of a learning model. *Br J Psychol* 1991;82:61.
121. Wilcox PM, Fetting JH, Nettesheim KM, et al. Anticipatory vomiting in women receiving cyclophosphamide, methotrexate, and 5-FU (CMF) adjuvant chemotherapy for breast carcinoma. *Cancer Treat Rep* 1982;66(8):1601.
122. Dolgin MJ, Katz ER, McGinty K, et al. Anticipatory nausea and vomiting in pediatric cancer pediatrics. *Pediatrics* 1985;75(3):547.
123. Morrow GR. Prevalence and correlates of anticipatory nausea and vomiting in chemotherapy patients. *J Natl Cancer Inst* 1982;68(4):585.
124. Redd WH, Andrykowski MA. Behavioral intervention in cancer treatment: controlling aversion reactions to chemotherapy. *J Consult Clin Psychol* 1982;50(6):1018.
125. Andrykowski MA, Redd WH, Hatfield AK. Development of anticipatory nausea: a prospective analysis. *J Consult Clin Psychol* 1985;53(4):447.
126. Olafsdottir M, Sjoden PB, Wrestling B. Prevalence and prediction of chemotherapy-related anxiety, nausea and vomiting in cancer patients. *Behav Res Ther* 1986;24(1):59.
127. Alba E, Bastus R, De Andres L, et al. Anticipatory nausea and vomiting: prevalence and predictors in chemotherapy patients. *Oncology* 1989;46:26.
128. Morrow GR. The effect of a susceptibility to motion sickness on the side effects of cancer chemotherapy. *Cancer* 1985;55:2766.
129. Morrow GR. Susceptibility to motion-sickness and the development of anticipatory nausea and vomiting in cancer patients undergoing chemotherapy. *Cancer Treat Rep* 1984;68(9):1177.
130. Morrow GR, Lindke J, Black PM. Anticipatory nausea development in cancer patients: replication and extension of a learning model. *Br J Psychol* 1991;82:61.
131. Redd WH, Andrykowski MA. Behavioral intervention in cancer treatment: controlling aversion reactions to chemotherapy. *J Consult Clin Psychol* 1982;50(6):1018.
132. Morrow GR. Prevalence and correlates of anticipatory nausea and vomiting in chemotherapy patients. *J Natl Cancer Inst* 1982;68(4):585.
133. Fetting JH, Wilcox PM, Iwata BA, et al. Anticipatory nausea and vomiting in an ambulatory medical oncology population. *Cancer Treat Rep* 1983;67(12):1093.
134. Andrykowski MA, Redd WH, Hatfield AK. Development of anticipatory nausea: a prospective analysis. *J Consult Clin Psychol* 1985;53(4):447.
135. Watson M, Marvell C. Anticipatory nausea and vomiting among cancer patients: a review. *Psychol Health* 1992;6:97.
136. Andrykowski MA, Redd WH. Longitudinal analysis of the development of anticipatory nausea. *J Consult Clin Psychol* 1987;55(1):36.
137. Andrykowski MA, Jacobsen PB, Marks E, et al. Prevalence, predictors and course of anticipatory nausea in women receiving adjuvant chemotherapy for breast cancer. *Cancer* 1988;62:2607.
138. Fetting JH, Wilcox PM, Iwata BA, et al. Anticipatory nausea and vomiting in an ambulatory medical oncology population. *Cancer Treat Rep* 1983;67(12):1093.
139. Nesse RM, Carli T, Curtis GC, et al. Pretreatment nausea in cancer chemotherapy: a conditioned response? *Psychosom Med* 1980;42(1):33.
140. Andrykowski MA, Jacobsen PB, Marks E, et al. Prevalence, predictors and course of anticipatory nausea in women receiving adjuvant chemotherapy for breast cancer. *Cancer* 1988;62:2607.
141. Redd WH, Andrykowski MA. Behavioral intervention in cancer treatment: controlling aversion reactions to chemotherapy. *J Consult Clin Psychol* 1982;50(6):1018.
142. Andrykowski MA, Redd WH. Longitudinal analysis of the development of anticipatory nausea. *J Consult Clin Psychol* 1987;55(1):36.
143. Andrykowski MA, Redd WH, Hatfield AK. Development of anticipatory nausea: a prospective analysis. *J Consult Clin Psychol* 1985;53(4):447.
144. Andrykowski MA. The role of anxiety in the development of anticipatory nausea in cancer chemotherapy: a review and synthesis. *Psychosom Med* 1990;52:458.
145. Fetting JH, Wilcox PM, Iwata BA, et al. Anticipatory nausea and vomiting in an ambulatory medical oncology population. *Cancer Treat Rep* 1983;67(12):1093.
146. Olafsdottir M, Sjoden PB, Wrestling B. Prevalence and prediction of chemotherapy-related anxiety, nausea and vomiting in cancer patients. *Behav Res Ther* 1986;24(1):59.
147. Nerenz DR, Leventhal H, Easterling DV, et al. Anxiety and drug taste as predictors of anticipatory nausea in cancer chemotherapy. *J Clin Oncol* 1986;4(2):224.
148. Redd WH, Andrykowski MA. Behavioral intervention in cancer treatment: controlling aversion reactions to chemotherapy. *J Consult Clin Psychol* 1982;50(6):1018.
149. Andrykowski MA. Do infusion-related tastes and odors facilitate the development of anticipatory nausea? A failure to support hypothesis. *Health Psychol* 1987;6(4):329.
150. Bovbjerg DH, Redd WH, Jacobsen PB, et al. An experimental analysis of classically conditioned nausea during cancer chemotherapy. *Psychosom Med* 1992;54:623.
151. Blasco T. Anticipatory nausea and vomiting: are psychological factors adequately investigated? *Br J Clin Psychol* 1994;33:85.
152. Bernstein IL. Physiological and psychological mechanisms of cancer anorexia. *Cancer Res* 1982;42[Suppl]:715.
153. Burish TG, Shartner D, Lyles JN. Effectiveness of multiple site EMG biofeedback and relaxation in reducing the aversiveness of cancer chemotherapy. *Biofeedback Self-Reg* 1981;6:523.
154. Morrow GR, Morrell BS. Behavioral treatment for the anticipatory nausea and vomiting induced by cancer chemotherapy. *N Engl J Med* 1982;307:1476.
155. Redd WH, Andresen GV, Minagawa RY. Hypnotic control of anticipatory nausea in patients undergoing cancer chemotherapy. *J Consult Clin Psychol* 1982;50:14.
156. Redd WH, Jacobsen PB, Die-Trill M, et al. Cognitive/attentional distraction in the control of conditioned nausea in pediatric cancer patients receiving chemotherapy. *J Consult Clin Psychol* 1987;55:391.
157. Greene P, Seime R. Stimulus control of anticipatory nausea in cancer chemotherapy. *J Behav Ther Exp Psychiatry* 1987;18:61.
158. Scarantino CW, Ornitz RD, Hoffman LG, et al. Radiation-induced emesis: effects of ondansetron. *Semin Oncol* 1992;19(6)[Suppl 15]:38.
159. Bodis S, Alexander E, Kooy H, et al. The prevention of radiosurgery-induced nausea and vomiting by ondansetron: evidence of a direct effect on the central nervous system chemoreceptor trigger zone. *Surg Neurol* 1994;42:249.
160. Priestman TJ, Priestman SG. An initial evaluation of nabilone in the control of radiotherapy-induced nausea and vomiting. *Clin Radiol* 1984;35:265.
161. Lucraft HH, Palmer MK. Randomized clinical trial of levonantradol and chlorpromazine in the prevention of radiotherapy-induced vomiting. *Clin Radiol* 1982;33:621.
162. Reyntjens A. Domperidone as an anti-emetic: summary of research reports. *Postgrad Med J* 1979;55[Suppl]:50.
163. Scarantino CW, Ornitz RD, Hoffman LG, et al. Radiation-induced emesis: effects of ondansetron. *Semin Oncol* 1992;19(6)[Suppl 15]:38.
164. Priestman TJ, Roberts JT, Lucraft CH, et al. Results of a randomized, double-blind comparative study of ondansetron and metoclopramide in the prevention of nausea and vomiting following high dose upper abdominal irradiation. *Clin Oncol* 1990;2:71.
165. Spitzer TR, Bryson JC, Cirenza E, et al. Randomized double-blind, placebo-controlled evaluation of oral ondansetron in the prevention of nausea and vomiting associated with fractionated total-body irradiation. *J Clin Oncol* 1994;12(11):2432.
166. Jurgens H, McQuade B. Ondansetron as prophylaxis for chemotherapy and radiotherapy-induced emesis in children. *Oncology* 1992;49:279.
167. Bodis S, Alexander E, Kooy H, et al. The prevention of radiosurgery-induced nausea and vomiting by ondansetron: evidence of a direct effect on the central nervous system chemoreceptor trigger zone. *Surg Neurol* 1994;42:249.
168. Lanciano R, Sherman DM, Michalski J, et al. The efficacy and safety of Kytril Tablets (2 mg) once daily in patients receiving at least 10 fractions of upper abdominal radiation for malignancy. *Int J Radiat Oncol Biol Phys* 1998;42[Suppl]:159(abst).
169. Spitzer TR, Friedman C, Bushnell J, et al. Oral granisetron (Kytril) and ondansetron (Zofran) in the prevention of hyperfractionated total body irradiation induced emesis: the results of a double-blind, randomized parallel group study. *Blood* 1998;92[Suppl 1]:278a(abst).
170. Fauser AA, Russ W, Bischiff M. Oral dolasetron mesilate for the control of emesis during fractionated total-body irradiation and high-dose cyclophosphamide in patients undergoing allogenic bone marrow transplantation. *Support Care Cancer* 1997;5:219.
171. Bruera E, MacEachern TJ, Spachynski KA, et al. Comparison of the efficacy, safety and pharmacokinetics of controlled release and immediate release metoclopramide for the management of chronic nausea in patients with advanced cancer. *Cancer* 1994;74(31):7204.
172. Nolte MJ, Berkery R, Pizzo B, et al. Assuring the optimal use of serotonin antagonist antiemetics: the process for development and implementation of institutional antiemetic guidelines at Memorial Sloan-Kettering Cancer Center. *J Clin Oncol* 1998;16:771.
173. Gralla R, Navari RM, Hesketh P, et al. Single-dose oral granisetron has equivalent antiemetic efficacy to intravenous ondansetron for highly emetogenic cisplatin-based chemotherapy. *J Clin Oncol* 1998;16:1568.
174. Spector JI, Lester EP, Chevlon EM, et al. A comparison of oral ondansetron and intravenous granisetron for the prevention of nausea and emesis associated with cisplatin-based chemotherapy. *Oncologist* 1998;3:432.

SECTION 2 Oral Complications

ANN M. BERGER
THOMAS J. KILROY

In the discussion of orofacial complications and pain and its management for patients receiving chemotherapy or radiotherapy, we must consider and discuss many factors. In the brief space allocated to oral complications, we shall evaluate dentition, mucosa, and bone to understand the interrelationship of these organ systems and how they interface with orofacial pain.

Orofacial pain that develops during the course of oncologic therapy cannot simply be labeled *mucositis.* Although this is the term commonly applied to the presentation of oral symptoms that develop in an oncology patient during the course of therapy, mucositis is not simply the result of mucosal ulceration from chemotherapy or radiotherapy. We must examine the various etiologies of orofacial pain, as such pain arises from multiple origins (Table 55.2-1). The oral environment, when in a state of imbalance, poses a serious threat to the success of both chemotherapy and radiotherapy. A complex interrelationship exists among the oral microflora, occlusal pathology, dental restorations, and mucositis. In chemotherapy, bacteria play a major role in the morbidity associated with mucositis. For patients receiving radiotherapy, oral microorganisms and restorative dental procedures have a significant impact on both transient mucositis and long-term dental management.

TABLE 55.2-1. Etiologic Factors Contributing to Pain in the Oncology Patient

Dental
Root exposure secondary to periodontal (gum) attachment loss
Dental caries
Dentures
Denture sores
Occlusion
Overextension of borders
Fractured dentures or denture teeth
Denture hygiene
Orthodontic appliances
Soft tissue (mucosa)
Mucositis
Pericoronitis
Gingivitis
Periodontitis
Angular cheilosis
Epulis fissuratum
Bone
Osteomyelitis
Osteoradionecrosis
Denture-related dehiscence

Oral mucositis is a significant problem in patients receiving chemotherapy or radiotherapy. Estimates of oral mucositis incidence among cancer therapy patients range from 40% of those receiving standard chemotherapy to 76% of bone marrow transplant patients.[1] Virtually all patients who receive radiotherapy to the head and neck area develop oral complications. Mucositis not only is painful but also can limit adequate nutritional intake and decrease patients' willingness to continue treatment. Severe mucositis with extensive ulceration may necessitate costly hospitalizations, parenteral nutrition, and use of narcotics. Mucositis diminishes the quality of life and may result in serious clinical complications. A healthy oral mucosa serves to clear microorganisms and provides a chemical barrier that limits penetration of many compounds into the epithelium. A mucosal surface that is damaged increases the risk of a secondary infection and may even prove to be a nidus for systemic infection. Mucositis may result in the need to reduce the dosage of subsequent chemotherapy cycles or to delay radiotherapy, which ultimately may affect a patient's response to therapy.

Dentition, supporting tissue (both hard and soft), and fixed and removable prostheses must be thoroughly examined before commencement of therapy. Dental caries involving previous restorations or unrestored teeth will be a source of bacteria that can be implicated in the etiology of mucositis. The xerostomia associated with radiotherapy significantly increases plaque colonization on the surfaces of teeth and prostheses. Increases in bacterial volume are directly related to mucositis symptoms and elevated caries activity on the eroded and worn surfaces of the dentition.

DIRECT STOMATOTOXICITY

Normally, cells of the mouth undergo rapid renewal over a 7- to 14-day cycle. Both chemotherapy and radiotherapy interfere with cellular mitosis and reduce the regenerative ability of the oral mucosa. Cancer chemotherapeutic drugs that produce direct stomatotoxicity include the alkylating agents, antimetabolites, natural products, and other synthetic agents such as hydroxyurea and procarbazine hydrochloride.[2] Typical sequelae of these cytotoxic agents include epithelial hyperplasia, collagen and glandular degeneration, and epithelial dysplasia.[3] Mucositis is an inevitable side effect of irradiation. The severity of the mucositis depends on the type of ionizing radiation, the volume of irradiated tissue, the dose per day, and the cumulative dose. As the mucositis becomes more severe, pseudomembranes and ulcerations develop. Poor nutritional status further interferes with mucosal regeneration by decreasing cellular migration and renewal.[4]

Direct stomatotoxicity usually is seen 5 to 7 days after the administration of chemotherapy or radiotherapy. In the nonmyelosuppressed patient, oral lesions heal within 2 to 3 weeks.[5] The nonkeratinized mucosa is most affected. The most common sites include the labial, buccal, and soft palate mucosa, as well as the floor of the mouth and the ventral surface of the tongue. Clinically, mucositis presents with multiple complex symptoms: The condition begins with asymptomatic redness and erythema and progresses through solitary, white, elevated desquamative patches that are slightly painful to contact pressure, to large, contiguous, pseudomembranous,

TABLE 55.2-2. Four Phases in the Development of Mucositis

Phase 1. Inflammatory or vascular phase; day 0
Phase 2. Epithelial phase; days 4–5
Phase 3. Ulcerative or bacteriologic phase; days 6–12
Phase 4. Healing phase; days 12–16

(Adapted from ref. 6.)

acutely painful lesions with associated dysphagia and decreased oral intake. Histopathologically, edema of the rete pegs will be noted, along with vascular changes that demonstrate a thickening of the tunica intima and concomitant reduction in the size of the lumen and destruction of the elastic and muscle fibers of the vessel walls. The loss of basement membrane epithelial cells exposes the underlying connective tissue stroma with its associated innervation, which, as the mucosal lesions enlarge, contributes to increasing pain levels. Oral infections, which may be due to bacteria, viruses, or fungal organisms, can further exacerbate the mucositis and may lead to systemic infections. If the patient develops both severe mucositis and thrombocytopenia, oral bleeding may occur and may be very difficult to treat.

PATHOPHYSIOLOGY OF MUCOSITIS

Sonis et al.[6] proposed a hypothesis as to the mechanisms of the development and healing of mucositis. The hypothesis is based on both animal and clinical data, though it remains speculative to some degree. It describes mucositis as a complex biologic process that occurs in four phases: (1) the inflammatory or vascular phase, (2) the epithelial phase, (3) the ulcerative or bacteriologic phase, and (4) the healing phase (Table 55.2-2). Each phase is interdependent and is a consequence of the effect of the chemotherapy or radiotherapy on the epithelium, as well as actions mediated by cytokines, the status of the patient's bone marrow, and the oral bacterial flora.[6]

PHASE I: INFLAMMATORY OR VASCULAR PHASE

Cytokines such as tumor necrosis factor-α, interleukin-1 (IL-1), and perhaps interleukin-6, are released from the epithelial tissue and adjacent connective tissue shortly after the administration of chemotherapy or radiotherapy. Most likely, the initiating event in the development of mucositis is local tissue damage caused by the cytokines. Additional concentrations of cytotoxic drugs in the mucosa may result from the increased vascularity caused by IL-1. Also during this phase, increased submucosal vascularity occurs.

PHASE 2: EPITHELIAL PHASE

Reduced epithelial renewal, with atrophy and ulceration, occurs as a result of both radiotherapy and chemotherapy, particularly with drugs affecting the S phase of the cell cycle, whereby the impact is on dividing cells of the oral basal epithelium. The atrophy and ulceration that occurs is most likely exacerbated by locally produced cytokines as well as functional trauma. The first two phases usually occur from days 0 to 5 of therapy.

PHASE 3: ULCERATIVE OR BACTERIOLOGIC PHASE

The most complex and symptomatic phase is phase 3, during which localized areas of erosion often become covered with a fibrinous pseudomembrane. This phase usually coincides with the patient's period of maximum neutropenia. Secondary bacterial colonization, involving some gram-negative organisms, occurs, and the gram-negative organisms provide a source of endotoxin, which stimulates further cytokine release from the connective tissue around the cells. The patient's condition is exacerbated by the cytokines as well as the nitric oxide that is released. This phase usually occurs from days 6 to 12 of therapy.

PHASE 4: HEALING PHASE

The final phase usually consists of renewal in epithelial proliferation and differentiation, with normalization of the patient's peripheral white blood cell count and reestablishment of the local microbial flora. The healing phase usually takes place from days 12 to 16.

RISK FACTORS

Both direct and indirect factors appear to contribute to oropharyngeal mucositis. The direct factors include the chemotherapeutic agent, dosage, and schedule (Table 55.2-3), the total dose and days of radiotherapy, mucosal damage from such problems as ill-fitting dental prostheses, periodontal disease, microbial flora, salivary gland dysfunction, and patient susceptibility. Indirect factors include myelosuppression, immunosuppression, reduced secretory IgA, and bacterial, viral, or fungal infections.

A variety of patient-related factors have potential for affecting the development of mucositis after chemotherapy. It has been suggested that the repair of ill-fitting prostheses, extraction of offending teeth, elimination of periodontal disease, and effective oral hygiene reduce the incidence and severity of mucositis. A patient might develop more severe mucositis if his or her nutrition is poor, through impairment of mucosal regeneration. Xerostomia that develops as a result of irradiation or drug use contributes significantly to the development of oral mucositis. Drugs that can result in xerostomia include antidepressants, opiates, antihypertensives, antihistamines, diuretics, and sedatives. Although both alcohol and tobacco can impair salivary function, it has been suggested that tobacco has been associated with a decreased incidence of chemotherapy-induced stomatitis.[7] One recent study involving 332 outpatients receiving chemotherapy revealed no significant differences in the incidence of mucositis between patients who wore dental appliances, had a history of oral lesions and a history of smoking, and practiced different oral hygiene regimens, and those patients who did not.[8] These findings suggest that the risk factors for the development of chemotherapy-induced mucositis are many and complicated and that further research is needed.

Reports on the effects of age on chemotherapy-induced mucositis development are conflicting. In general, younger patients are at increased risk for developing mucositis.[7] Recent reports look at gender differences and the risk of mucositis. A metaanalysis of six North Central Cancer Treatment Group

TABLE 55.2-3. Chemotherapeutic Agents Commonly Producing Mucositis

Anthracyclines
Daunorubicin
Doxorubicin
Epirubicin
Alkylating agents
Cyclophosphamide
Busulfan
Procarbazine
Thiotepa
Mechlorethamine
Taxanes
Docetaxel
Paclitaxel
Vinca alkaloids
Vinblastine
Vincristine
Vinorelbine
Antimetabolites
Methotrexate
5-Fluorouracil
Hydroxyurea
Cytosine arabinoside
6-Mercaptopurine
6-Thioguanine
Antitumor antibiotics
Actinomycin D
Bleomycin
Mithramycin
Mitomycin
Amsacrine

(Adapted from ref. 7.)

(NCCTG) trials involving 731 patients (402 men and 329 women) revealed that women reported stomatitis both more often and of greater severity as compared with men.[9] In a pilot project using capsaicin for treating mucositis, data analysis revealed that women had a higher level of pain secondary to oral mucositis. It is also known that women are "supertasters" when tested with chemical relative phenylthiocarbamide/6-n-propylthiouracil (PROP); possibly, individuals who are supertasters and who therefore have more taste buds experience increased stomatitis (Table 55.2-4).[10,11]

ASSESSMENT OF THE ORAL MUCOSA

A mucositis grading system allows the physician to assess mucositis severity in terms of both pain and the patient's ability to maintain adequate nutrition, so that a treatment plan can be appropriately constructed. Many different grading systems exist, most of which are based on two or more clinical parameters, including erythema, pain, and problems with eating (Table 55.2-5). An example of a common grading system is that proposed by the National Cancer Institute, which uses a numbering scale from 0 to 4. Grade 0 indicates no mucositis; grade 1, the presence of painless ulcers, erythema, or mild soreness; grade 2, the presence of painful erythema, edema, or ulcers, but not interfering with the patient's ability to eat; and grade 4, symptoms so severe that the patient requires parenteral or enteral support.[12]

TABLE 55.2-4. Risk Factors Contributing to Mucositis

DIRECT FACTORS
Age
Gender
Preexisting dental hygiene
Nutritional status
Oral care during treatment
Radiation: dose, schedule
Chemotherapy: drug, dose, schedule
Xerostomia
INDIRECT FACTORS
Myelosuppression
Immunosuppression
Reduced secretory IgA
Infections: bacterial, viral, fungal

Recently, new scoring systems have been developed for the assessment of oral mucositis. Sonis et al.[13] reported on a scale that uses an objective measure of mucositis, evaluating ulceration and pseudomembrane formation and erythema. Subjective outcomes of mouth pain, ability to swallow, and function were measured. Analgesia use for mouth sensitivity was also recorded. In the study that was conducted in nine centers, there was high interobserver correlation, with objective mucositis scores demonstrating strong correlation with symptoms.

At the 1989 National Institutes of Health consensus conference on oral complications of cancer therapy, clinicians and researchers agreed that effective prevention of mucositis requires a comprehensive patient examination to identify potentially complicating oral disease before the cancer therapy begins.[14] Significant problems that must be corrected include poor oral hygiene, periapical pathology, third molar pathology, periodontal disease, dental caries, defective restorations, orthodontic appliances, ill-fitting prostheses, and other potential sources of infection. Bacterial and fungal surveillance cultures are not necessary, but prophylactic use of acyclovir should be considered in patients who are seropositive and at high risk for reactivating herpes simplex viral infection, such as those who undergo bone marrow transplant or who have prolonged and pronounced myelosuppression. If a diagnosis is made of a fungal, viral, or bacterial infection along with the mucosal lesions, prompt treatment is necessary to avoid the risk of systemic infection.

REMEDIES FOR THE PREVENTION AND TREATMENT OF MUCOSITIS

A standardized approach for the prevention and treatment of chemotherapy- and radiotherapy-induced mucositis is essential, although the efficacy and safety of most of the regimens have not been established. The prophylactic measures usually used for the prevention of mucositis include chlorhexidine gluconate (Peridex), saline rinses, sodium bicarbonate rinses, acyclovir, amphotericin, and ice. Regimens commonly used for the treatment of

TABLE 55.2-5. Mucositis Grading

Grade	*Criteria*
0	Mouth pink
	No bleeding
	Mucosa moist
	No edema or infection
	No limitation to eating or drinking
1	Slightly increased redness of mouth
	One to four oral lesions
	Thinning of mucosa
	No bleeding or infection
	Mucosa moist
	Mild discomfort, burning sensation
	Possible avoidance of hot, harsh, or spicy foods
2	Moderate increase in mouth redness
	More than four discrete oral lesions, not coalescing
	Mucosa bleeds with manipulation
	Mucosa slightly drier
	Saliva slightly thicker
	Moderate edema
	White or yellow patches, infection present
	Eating of only bland, soft foods
	Avoidance of hot, spicy, or acidic liquids
	Moderate continual pain, necessitating intermittent, usually topical analgesics
3	Severe redness throughout oral cavity
	Multiple confluent ulcers
	Possible total denudation of oral cavity
	Marked xerostomia
	Severe edema
	White, yellow, or purulent patches
	Inability to eat or drink
	Inability to swallow saliva
	Severe, constant pain, necessitating systemic analgesia

[Adapted from Western Consortium for Cancer Nursing Research, Development of a staging system for chemotherapy-induced stomatitis. *Cancer Nurs* 1991;14(1):6.]

mucositis and the associated pain include a local anesthetic such as lidocaine or dyclonine, magnesium-based antacids (Maalox, Mylanta), diphenhydramine (Benadryl), nystatin, or sucralfate. These agents are used either alone or in different combinations that compose a mouthwash. Other agents used less commonly include kaolin-pectin (Kaopectate), allopurinol, vitamin E, β-carotene, chamomile (Kamillosan) liquid, aspirin, antiprostaglandins, prostaglandins, MGI 209 (marketed as Oratect Gel), silver nitrate, and antibiotics. Oral and sometimes parenteral narcotics are used to relieve the pain caused by mucositis. A new method that uses capsaicin for such pain relief is currently being studied.

DIRECT CYTOPROTECTANTS

Sucralfate

Sucralfate, an aluminum salt of sucrose orasulfate, which has been used successfully to treat gastrointestinal ulceration, has been tested as a rinse for the prevention and treatment of mucositis. Sucralfate's mechanism of action appears to be by forming an ionic bond to proteins in an ulcer site, thereby creating a protective barrier.[15] Additionally, evidence points to an increase in the local production of prostaglandin E_2 (PGE_2), which results in an increase in mucosal blood flow, mucus production, mitotic activity, and surface migration of cells.[16,17]

Anecdotal experience suggests that sucralfate might be useful in the prevention and treatment of chemotherapy-induced mucositis; however, data from the studies are conflicting. Solomon[18] reported a 55% objective response rate in patients receiving chemotherapy (19 patients), which was defined as a decrease in one grade on the cancer and leukemia group B (CALGB) scale of oral toxicity. In 1984 and 1985, Ferraro and Mattern[19,20] reported encouraging results in the use of sucralfate for chemotherapy-induced mucositis. Two randomized, double-blind clinical trials also have evaluated sucralfate for the prevention of chemotherapy-induced mucositis. Pfeiffer et al.[21] found a significant reduction in edema, erythema, erosion, and ulceration in 23 of 40 evaluable patients receiving cisplatin and continuous infusion with 5-fluorouracil (5-FU) with or without bleomycin. Patient preference favored sucralfate, although this preference failed to reach statistical significance. Ten of the patients did not complete the study as the swishing of the sucralfate and the placebo aggravated chemotherapy-induced nausea. The authors suggested that, to help overcome this problem, the solution should have a neutral taste and should not be swallowed after swishing. In contrast, results from a similarly designed study, in which patients receiving remission-induction chemotherapy for acute nonlymphocytic leukemia were treated with sucralfate for mucositis, did not support the amelioration of mucositis.[22] The latter study also concluded that chronic administration of the sucralfate suspension had no effect on the incidence of gastrointestinal bleeding and ulceration. The authors did note that some patients reported pain relief from sucralfate.[22] A phase III study of sucralfate suspension versus placebo, recently completed by the NCCTG, revealed that of the 50 patients who developed stomatitis, the sucralfate suspensions provided no beneficial reduction in the duration or severity of 5-FU-induced mucositis.[23] In addition, the sucralfate induced considerable additional gastrointestinal toxicity.

Sucralfate has also been tested in patients receiving radiotherapy. One study compared 21 patients who received standard oral care to the head and neck with 24 patients who received sucralfate suspension four times daily.[24] Results revealed a significant difference in mucosal edema, pain, dysphagia, and weight loss in those patients receiving sucralfate. In a pilot study done by Pfeiffer et al.,[25] sequential patients who received radiotherapy to the head and neck received sucralfate at the onset of mucositis. The majority of patients had a decrease in pain after sucralfate use. A double-blind placebo-controlled study with sucralfate in 33 patients who received irradiation to the head and neck reported no statistically significant differences in mucositis; however, the sucralfate group reported less oral pain and, in these patients, other topical and systemic analgesics were started later in the course of radiation.[26]

A prospective double-blind study compared the effectiveness of sucralfate suspension to that of diphenhydramine syrup plus kaolin-pectin on radiotherapy-induced mucositis. Data on perceived pain, helpfulness of mouth rinses, weekly mucositis grade, weight change, and interruption of therapy were collected daily. Analysis of the two groups revealed no statistically significant differences between them. A retrospective comparison of a group of 15 patients who had not used daily oral rinses and the preceding two groups suggested that the use of a daily oral rinse with a mouth-coating agent may result in less pain, may reduce weight loss, and may help to prevent interruption of radiotherapy because of severe mucositis.[27]

Prostaglandins, Antiprostaglandins, and Nonsteroidal Agents

Prostaglandins are a family of naturally occurring eicosanoids, some of which have known cytoprotective activity. Dinoprostone, or PGE_2, has been reported to be beneficial in healing both gastric ulcers and chronic leg ulcers.[28,29] Pilot studies revealed the need for controlled clinical trials. In a pilot study undertaken by Kuhrer et al.,[30] five patients received topical dinoprostone for chemotherapy-induced mucositis. Four of the five patients reported pain relief, with healing of the ulcers within 3 to 7 days. Kuhrer's group then tested the prophylactic efficacy of dinoprostone by applying it topically to one patient who was receiving chemotherapy and who had developed previous episodes of mucositis, as well as to two patients receiving total body irradiation.[30] Only one of the patients who had received the dinoprostone and total body irradiation developed mucositis.

In a nonblinded study, ten patients who were receiving 5-FU and mitomycin with concomitant radiation for oral carcinomas were treated by Porteder et al.,[31] with dinoprostone four times daily during treatment. The control group consisted of 14 patients who were receiving identical treatment. Eight of the ten patients who received dinoprostone were evaluable, and none developed severe mucositis, as compared with six episodes in the control arm.

A third pilot study conducted with 15 patients who received radiotherapy of the head and neck found that an inflammatory reaction in the vicinity of the tumor could be detected in only 5 patients treated with topically applied PGE_2, and none of the patients developed any bullous or desquamating inflammatory lesions.[32] A double-blind, placebo-controlled study of PGE_2 in 60 patients undergoing bone marrow transplant revealed no significant differences in the incidence, severity, or duration of mucositis. It was noted that the incidence of herpes simplex virus was higher in those on the PGE_2 arm, and, in those patients who developed herpes simplex virus, there was an increase in the severity of the mucositis.[33]

Benzydamine is a nonsteroidal with analgesic, anesthetic, antiinflammatory, and antimicrobial properties. Epstein and Stevenson-Moore[34] found, in a double-blind, placebo-controlled trial, that benzydamine produced statistically significant relief of pain from radiation-induced mucositis. Positive responses to benzydamine were reported in at least two other studies.[35,36] The study conducted by Epstein and Stevenson-Moore[34] revealed not only a trend toward reduction in pain but also a statistically significant reduction in the total area of ulceration as well as the size of the ulcer. Another study demonstrated that when indomethacin, an antiprostaglandin, was given orally, it reduced the severity and delayed the onset of mucositis induced by radiotherapy.[37]

Corticosteroids

No placebo-controlled studies of the use of corticosteroids for chemotherapy-induced mucositis have been reported, though two reports have focused on pilot work conducted with patients who received radiotherapy. Abdelaal et al.[38] reported the use of a betamethasone and water mouthwash in five patients receiving radiotherapy whose mucosa remained virtually ulcer-free and who did not report any pain. The proposed mechanism of action of the steroid mouthwash was inhibition of leukotriene and prostaglandin production. Another pilot study compared 21 patients receiving radiotherapy who used an oral rinse consisting of hydrocortisone in combination with nystatin, tetracycline, and diphenhydramine with patients using a placebo rinse. Though only 12 of the 21 patients were evaluable, by the end of the radiotherapy cycles, there was a statistically significant difference in mucositis and a trend toward a reduction in pain. No patients in the treatment group needed to interrupt the radiotherapeutic regimen, whereas three patients in the control group did need to interrupt their radiotherapeutic care.[39]

Vitamins and Other Antioxidants

Vitamins in pharmacologic doses have been used to treat mucositis. Vitamin E has been tested in chemotherapy-induced mucositis because it can stabilize cellular membranes and may improve herpetic gingivitis, possibly through antioxidant activity.[40–42] The efficacy of vitamin E was demonstrated by Wadleigh et al.[43] in a randomized, double-blind, placebo-controlled study. Eighteen patients receiving chemotherapy were randomized to receive a topical application of vitamin E or a placebo. In the vitamin E–treated group, six of nine patients had complete resolution of their mucositis within 4 days of initiating therapy, whereas in the placebo group only one of nine had resolution of the lesions during the 5-day study period. This difference was statistically significant.[43] Because both sucralfate and vitamin E provide some effectiveness in mucositis, a phase III study of sucralfate versus vitamin E for treatment-induced mucositis is currently under way.

Other antioxidants that have been used clinically include vitamin C and glutathione. Another antioxidant tested in a pilot study, azelastine hydrochloride has been used in many allergic diseases and has been shown to be effective in the treatment of aphthous ulcers in Behçet's disease. Osaki et al.[44] reported on a study involving 63 patients who had head and neck tumors and received a combination of radiotherapy and concomitant chemotherapy. Twenty-six patients received regimen 1, which consisted of vitamins C and E and glutathione, whereas 37 patients received regimen 2, which consisted of everything in regimen 1 plus azelastine. At the completion of treatment, 21 of the patients in the azelastine arm remained at grade 1 or 2 mucositis, with 6 patients having grade 3 mucositis and 10 having grade 4 mucositis. In the control group, grade 3 or 4 mucositis was induced in 6 and 15 patients, respectively, with only 2 patients having grade 1 mucositis and 2 having grade 2 mucositis. The azelastine was shown to suppress neutrophil respiratory burst both *in vivo* and *in vitro,* as well as to suppress cytokine release from lymphocytes. The authors concluded that a regimen including azelastine, which suppresses reactive oxygen production and stabilizes cell membranes, may be useful for the prophylaxis of mucositis due to chemoradiotherapy.[44]

β-Carotene, a vitamin A precursor with known effects on cellular differentiation, has been used for mucositis induced by radiation. β-Carotene has been shown to produce regression of oral leukoplakia lesions.[45] Mills[46] reported on the use of β-carotene in treatment-induced mucositis. Ten patients receiving radiation interspersed with two cycles of chemotherapy were given β-carotene, 250 mg/d for the first 3 weeks of therapy and then 75 mg/d for the last 5 weeks of therapy. The control group consisted of ten patients with oral cancer who were receiving the identical treatment. At the end of treatment, there was a statistically significant difference in grade 3 to 4 mucositis in the β-carotene group; there was no difference in grades 1 and 2 mucositis.[46]

Silver Nitrate

Silver nitrate, a caustic agent, has been tested in radiation-induced mucositis. Because silver nitrate is known to stimulate cell division when it is applied to normal mucosa, it was thought that, if it were applied before cytotoxic therapy, it might enhance repair and replacement of mucosa that was damaged by cytotoxic therapy. Maciejewski et al.[47] reported on 16 patients who received radiotherapy to bilateral opposing fields. Silver nitrate 2% was applied to the left side of the oral mucosa three times daily for 5 days before radiotherapy and during the first 2 days of radiotherapy. The right side of the oral mucosa was unpainted and served as the control. The study revealed significantly less severe mucositis and a decrease in duration of mucositis on the mucosa that was treated with silver nitrate.[47] A second trial failed to confirm these results.[48] Silver nitrate has not been formally evaluated in the treatment of chemotherapy-induced mucositis.

Miscellaneous Cytoprotectants

An uncontrolled study involving 98 patients with different malignancies who were receiving different medical regimens with either chemotherapy or radiotherapy reported that Kamillosan liquid taken before and after the development of mucositis helped to prevent and decrease the duration of mucositis.[49] In a placebo-controlled trial conducted by NCCTG, patients were randomized to receive chamomile or placebo, along with an established oral cryotherapy regimen. This study revealed that chamomile mouthwash did not reduce stomatitis associated with 5-FU chemotherapy.[50]

Oshitani et al.[51] reported on the use of topical sodium alginate, an agent that has been shown to promote healing of esophageal and gastric mucosa, in radiation-induced mucositis. Thirty-nine patients with mucositis were randomized to receive either sodium alginate or placebo. Those who received sodium alginate had a reduction in both mucosal erosions and pain.[51] Other topical agents used clinically for treatment-induced mucositis include Kaopectate, Benadryl, saline, sodium bicarbonate, and gentian violet. Even though the previously mentioned agents are used clinically for treatment-induced mucositis, no controlled clinical trials have yet established their efficacy.

INDIRECT CYTOPROTECTANTS

Hematologic Growth Factors

Hematologic growth factors currently are standard in the treatment of patients receiving high-dose chemotherapy. The effect of the hematologic growth factors on decreasing the depth and duration of chemotherapy-induced neutropenia is well established. Lieschke et al.[52] examined the levels of neutrophil count and assessed whether oral neutrophil count correlated with oral mucositis. In the study, the researchers found that the oral neutrophil count, similar to circulating systemic neutrophils, diminished to undetectable levels but recovered earlier than did the systemic circulating neutrophils. In those patients receiving granulocyte colony-stimulating factor (G-CSF), the mean cumulative mucositis score was less than that in patients who did not receive G-CSF.[52]

Gabrilove et al.[53] reported on 27 patients receiving methotrexate, vinblastine, doxorubicin, and cisplatin for bladder carcinoma and escalating doses of G-CSF. The patients received the G-CSF on their first cycle of chemotherapy and did not receive it on their second chemotherapeutic cycle. Significantly less mucositis was seen during the cycle in which the patients received the G-CSF. In this study, a bias may have been inherent as there is perhaps cumulative chemotherapeutic toxicity such that with each cycle of chemotherapy, the severity of mucositis increases.

Bronchud et al.[54] treated 17 patients with breast or ovarian carcinoma who were receiving escalating doses of doxorubicin with G-CSF support. In this study, the G-CSF did not prevent severe mucositis. In a fourth study using G-CSF, 41 patients receiving chemotherapy for non-Hodgkin's lymphoma received G-CSF, whereas 39 received chemotherapy without G-CSF. In those patients who did not receive G-CSF, the main cause of treatment delay was neutropenia, whereas in those patients who did receive G-CSF, the main cause of treatment delay was mucositis.[55]

In a small prospective study, patients who received platinum, infused 5-FU, and leucovorin plus granulocyte-macrophage colony-stimulating factor (GM-CSF) had a decreased incidence of grade 3 mucositis.[56] In a study comparing patients undergoing bone marrow transplantation in whom GM-CSF was used to historical controls, recovery of neutrophils was more rapid in the GM-CSF group; however, there was no difference in the severity of mucositis nor in duration of hospitalization.[57] At this time, the use of colony-stimulating factors in the prevention or treatment of mucositis is investigational.

The effect of other biologically active factors on mucositis development is currently being studied. *In vitro* studies have shown that epidermal growth factor (EGF) not only is present in saliva but has the ability to affect growth, cell differentiation, and cell migration.[58,59] It is known that EGF induces chemotaxis of oral epithelial cells, indicating that it may be important in maintaining the integrity of the oral epithelium, especially in wound healing. Patients with peptic ulcers have been shown to have significantly lower levels of EGF in their saliva, suggesting that EGF may be involved in either protection or repair.[60] In an animal study in which the animals received either 5-FU with an infusion of EGF for 7 and 15 days or a placebo, the animals that received the EGF experienced increased mucosal breakdown. The results of the study indicate that chemotherapy-induced mucositis depends on the rate of epithelial cell growth. The timing of administration of the EGF in relation to the chemotherapy may determine whether the patient develops increased oral toxicity or repair of the mucosa.[61] In a study conducted by Sonis et al.,[62] hamsters received EGF versus placebo using four different treatment schedules. In this study, delayed exposure to EGF delayed the onset of mucositis, but it had no beneficial effects on the duration or severity of mucositis.

Tumor growth factor-β3 (TGF-β3) is an inhibitor of epithelial cell growth. In a study using Syrian hamsters done by Sonis et al.,[63] the topical application of TGF-β3 resulted in a decrease in the severity and duration of chemotherapy-induced mucositis. In another study performed by Spijkervet and Sonis[64] with Syrian hamsters, the topical application of TGF-β3 significantly reduced the severity and duration of ulcerative mucositis induced by 5-FU. In animal experiments, IL-1 and IL-11 demonstrated a cytoprotective effect.[65–67]

Antimicrobials

Many conflicting studies have been published on the use of chlorhexidine mouthwash for both alleviating mucositis and reducing oral colonization by gram-positive, gram-negative, and *Candida* species in patients receiving radiotherapy, chemotherapy, or bone marrow transplantation. In 1990, Ferretti et al.,[68] in a randomized, controlled trial, demonstrated that prophylactic chlorhexidine mouthwash reduces oral mucositis and microbial burden in cancer patients receiving chemotherapy. The majority of studies since that time have not demonstrated a reduction in mucositis in patients receiving intensive chemotherapy and using chlorhexidine mouthwash.[69–71] However, Weisdorf et al.[70] and Epstein et al.[71] did demonstrate a reduction in oral colonization by *Candida* species and oral candidiasis. Ferretti et al.[72] found that the use of chlorhexidine rinse for the prevention of mucositis was not effective, though there was a reduction in streptococcal counts. Spijkervet et al.,[73] in a placebo-controlled, double-blind study, revealed that the colonization index of viridans streptococci was reduced after 5 weeks of chlorhexidine treatment, though such therapy did not decrease the colonization of *Candida* species, *Streptococcus faecalis*, staphylococci, Enterobacteriaceae, Pseudomonadaceae, and Acinetobacter species, and there was no difference in the development and severity of mucositis. A recent randomized, double-blind study comparing chlorhexidine mouthwash to placebo in 25 patients receiving radiotherapy revealed that there was a trend toward more mucositis as well as mouthwash-induced discomfort, taste alteration, and teeth staining in the chlorhexidine arm.[74] The overall statistical data lead to the conclusion that chlorhexidine may result in improved oral hygiene, but the discomfort of using the rinse negates its minimal benefits.

The endotoxins of aerobic gram-negative bacilli are implicated in the etiology of mucositis. A study by Spijkervet et al.[75] postulated that lozenges containing 2 mg polymyxin E, 1.8 mg tobramycin, and 10 mg amphotericin (PTA) four times daily on the oropharyngeal flora would mediate and control mucositis. These researchers compared 15 irradiated patients using PTA and two other groups of 15 patients each, one of which was using 0.1% chlorhexidine and the other of which was using placebo. In the selectively decontaminated group, the severity and extent of mucositis was significantly reduced as compared with that in the chlorhexidine and placebo groups ($P < .05$). Clinically, all patients in the lozenge group showed erythema only, whereas 80% of both the placebo and chlorhexidine rinse patients experienced severe mucositis with extended pseudomembranes from the third week of irradiation. No nasogastric tube feedings were needed in the PTA group, as compared to 30% of patients in the other groups.[75] The potential role of PTA lozenges remains to be clarified.

IB-367, a broad-spectrum antimicrobial peptide found in porcine leukocytes, was tested in a hamster model.[76] The results indicated that mucositis scores were significantly lower in hamsters given topical IB-367 as compared to those receiving placebo. Though further study is needed, IB-367 might improve clinical outcomes in patients at risk for the development of mucositis.[76] Another antimicrobial, nystatin suspension, has been studied in the prophylaxis of candidiasis in leukemia and bone marrow transplantation patients. The majority of publications do not support the use of nystatin.[77–84]

Pharmacologic Modulation

Another agent that has been evaluated for the prevention and treatment of oral mucositis induced by 5-FU chemotherapy is allopurinol. The rationale for allopurinol mouthwash was based on data that systemic allopurinol was able to decrease 5-FU-induced toxicity by inhibiting the enzyme orotidylate decarboxylase and formation of the metabolites of fluorodeoxyuridine monophosphate (FdUMP) and fluorouridine (FUrd).[85] Two pilot studies support the use of allopurinol for oral mucositis. The study by Clark and Selvin[86] revealed that allopurinol mouthwash substantially decreased the incidence and severity of mucositis in six patients who received bolus 5-FU chemotherapy. Another pilot study, involving 16 patients receiving 5-day intravenous 5-FU infusions and using allopurinol mouthwashes four to six times daily, also found that the allopurinol alleviated the mucositis in all patients.[87] After the success of these pilot studies, the use of allopurinol became routine medical practice in many institutions. The efficacy of allopurinol was tested by the NCCTG and the Mayo Clinic in a randomized, double-blind clinical trial. Seventy-five patients were assigned to receive allopurinol mouthwash or placebo while they received their first 5-day course of 5-FU with or without leucovorin. This study demonstrated no protective effect against 5-FU-induced mucositis by the allopurinol regimen.[88]

Leucovorin has been used in combination with methotrexate to help decrease the oral mucositis that occurs with methotrexate. In a pilot study involving 19 patients who received edatrexate for non–small cell lung carcinoma, less mucositis was seen than was anticipated.[89] There is decreased mucositis when reduced folates are given systemically following methotrexate administration.[90] In a small crossover study, administration of leucovorin-hyaluronidase mouthwashes did not reduce the severity of mucositis induced by high-dose methotrexate.[91]

Glutamine administration in animal studies has been shown to lead to a reduction in both morbidity and mortality of animals who have received a variety of chemotherapeutic agents, including methotrexate. The glutamine both preserved the morphologic structure of the gastrointestinal tract and reduced the incidence of bacteremia.[92,93] In a randomized trial of 28 patients with gastrointestinal cancers who received 5-FU and folinic acid, no effect on oral mucositis was seen in the group who also received 16 g glutamine daily for 8 days as compared to the group who received a placebo. The authors concluded that perhaps both the dose and duration of exposure to the glutamine were not sufficient to show a decrease in mucositis.[94]

According to laboratory data, another agent that protects host tissues selectively from 5-FU's toxic effects without loss of antitumor effect is uridine.[95] A study was conducted involving 29 patients with advanced malignancies who received N-phosphoracetyl-disodium L-aspartic acid (PALA) and methotrexate, each at 250 mg/m^2, followed 24 hours later by increasing doses of 5-FU (600 to 750 mg/m^2), with a leucovorin rescue and uridine rescue for a 72-hour infusion. The uridine allowed dose escalation of 5-FU to 750 mg/m^2, with a decrease in all toxicities of the 5-FU except mucositis, which remained as the only significant chemotherapy-induced toxic effect.[96] Perhaps additional studies with oral uridine will reveal a reduction of the toxicity from mucositis.

A pilot study using propantheline, an anticholinergic agent that causes xerostomia, was performed to test whether the incidence of mucositis could be reduced when patients received etoposide.[97] It was hypothesized that the mucosal toxicity might be related to salivary excretion of etoposide after its systemic administration. Propantheline or placebo was given to 12 patients. The results revealed a decrease in the incidence and severity of mucositis in the patients who received the propantheline.[97]

CRYOTHERAPY

Cryotherapy, in the form of ice chips and flavored ice pops, has been used to prevent mucositis. The NCCTG and the Mayo Clinic undertook a controlled, randomized trial of oral cryotherapy for preventing 5-FU-induced mucositis and found that cryotherapy is helpful in reducing the severity of 5-FU-induced mucositis.[98,99] After this study had been completed, another was undertaken in which patients were randomized to receive 30 minutes versus 60 minutes of cryotherapy.[100] A total of 178 evaluable patients were studied. Both cryotherapy groups had similar degrees of mucositis. The conclusion was to continue to recommend the use of 30 minutes of oral cryotherapy for patients receiving bolus intensive courses of 5-FU-based chemotherapy.[100] An additional study, conducted after the original study reported by the NCCTG and the Mayo Clinic, once again confirmed that oral cryotherapy can reduce 5-FU-induced mucositis.[101]

LASER

Laser as a palliative methodology for mucositis has only recently begun to be investigated. The potential for lesion and pain control using laser was initially studied in an animal model. In a study of four groups of animals having a mucosal lesion, three groups received impulse laser exposure from 60 to 600 pulses, and one group remained untreated.[102] The only group that demonstrated more rapid resolution of the mucosal lesion (14 vs. 21 to 25 days) was the group that received the 600 pulsed exposures.

A preliminary report revealed that laser may be beneficial in reducing the severity and duration of mucositis. A study involving 20 patients, all having different cancers and chemotherapeutic protocols, who served as the controls and 16 patients who composed the treatment group and received laser revealed reduced duration of the mucosal lesions, from a mean of 19.3 days in the control arm to 8.1 days in the treatment arm.[103] At this time, double-blind, randomized trials are needed to verify these earlier reports.

ANESTHETIC COCKTAILS

Several anesthetic cocktails, made up of agents such as viscous lidocaine (Xylocaine) or dyclonine hydrochloride, have been used with some success.[104] The anesthetic agents relieve the patient's pain, but this relief is temporary and also prevents taste perception, which can further interfere with food intake. Other analgesics and mucosal coating agents that can control pain include kaolin-pectin, diphenhydramine, Orabase, and Oratect Gel. In a prospective, double-blinded study involving 18 patients, viscous lidocaine with cocaine 1%, dyclonine hydrochloride 1%, kaolin-pectin solution, diphenhydramine, and saline solution were compared with a placebo. The dyclonine hydrochloride 1% provided the most pain relief, whereas dyclonine hydrochloride with viscous lidocaine and cocaine 1% provided the longest pain relief.[105] Even though clinicians use many of the topical agents, little experimental evidence exists to establish the efficacy of many of them.[106]

CAPSAICIN

Capsaicin, the active ingredient in chili peppers, is a remedy that has been used for many different pain syndromes through the years and that may prove beneficial for mucositis pain induced by chemotherapy and radiotherapy. Several studies support the medical efficacy of locally applied capsaicin in a cream vehicle in neuropathic pain syndromes. A large, multicenter trial involving 277 patients demonstrated that topically applied capsaicin used for up to 8 weeks significantly reduced pain and improved quality of life in both postherpetic neuralgia and diabetic neuropathy.[107–109] Other neuropathic pain syndromes for which capsaicin has been shown to be effective include postmastectomy pain,[110] stump pain,[111] trigeminal neuralgia,[112] reflex sympathetic dystrophy,[113] and Guillain-Barré syndrome.[114] Topical capsaicin has also been shown to decrease the pain associated with rheumatoid and osteoarthritis,[115] and intranasal capsaicin spray has been shown to reduce the pain associated with cluster headaches.[116] Topical capsaicin has been shown to improve the rate of reepithelialization of wound healing in minipigs; thus, it may prove to be efficacious in wound healing in humans.[117]

In a pilot project, capsaicin in a candy vehicle (cayenne pepper candy) was given to patients with therapy-induced mucositis. Patients were instructed to allow the candy to dissolve in the mouth without chewing it. After the candy had dissolved, the burn produced by the candy was allowed to fade. The patients rated their pain before and after eating the candy. The reduction in pain was highly statistically significant.[10,11] A double-blinded, placebo-controlled study is under way to test the efficacy of oral capsaicin for pain control.

NARCOTICS

Many of the agents previously mentioned may have some value in preventing mucositis or palliating the pain; however, very few controlled clinical trials have established their efficacy. At present, no standard treatment has been defined for the prevention or treatment of mucositis. When mucositis is severe and interferes with nutritional intake and quality of life, it is appropriate to use any of the treatments that have already been cited, as well as oral, transmucosal or, if necessary, parenteral narcotics. Currently, a study is under way to investigate the usefulness of transmucosal fentanyl (Actiq) in the treatment of mucositis (Table 55.2-6). A recent article also reported on the successful use of topical opioids (morphine 0.08% gel, prepared with taste supplements) in treating oral mucositis in a patient who was terminally ill.[118] To discover an efficacious treatment, it is essential to continue studies of the treatments already available and to develop any promising new approaches.

TABLE 55.2-6. Formulary of Common Remedies for Oral Complications

PREVENTION OF MUCOSITIS	
Povidone iodine rinse 0.5%	Rinse two to four times daily. Do not swallow.
Chlorhexidine gluconate 0.12% oral rinse	Rinse twice daily for 30 seconds. Do not swallow.
$NAHCO_3$ powder: 3 tblsp or 11.6 g	Combine all ingredients. Rinse two to four times daily. Do not swallow.
NACI powder: 3 tblsp or 11.6 g	
Distilled water: 1 gal	
TREATMENT OF MUCOSITIS AND PAIN[a]	
Diphenhydramine (Benadryl), 12.5 mg/5 mL: 30 mL	Combine all ingredients. Rinse with 15 mL four to six times per day.
Viscous lidocaine 2%: 30 mL	
Maalox: 30 mL	
Diphenhydramine (Benadryl), 12.5 mg/5 mL: 30 mL	Combine all ingredients. Rinse with 15 mL four to six times per day.
Tetracycline or penicillin, 125 mg/5 mL suspension: 60 mL	
Nystatin oral suspension, 100,000 units/mL: 45 mL	
Viscous lidocaine (Xylocaine) 2%: 30 mL	
Hydrocortisone suspension, 10 mg/5 mL: 30 mL	
Sterile water for irrigation: 45 mL	
Carafate suspension	1 g four times daily.
Viscous lidocaine (Xylocaine) 2% solution *or* Dyclonine hydrochloride 0.5% or 1% solution	10–15 mL q2–3h.
Benadryl 12.5 mg/5 mL	Combine equal amounts of each. Swish 10–15 mL four to six times daily.
Kaopectate	
Benadryl 12.5 mg/5 mL: 30 mL	Combine all ingredients. Rinse with 15 mL four to six times per day.
Maalox: 30 mL	
Nystatin 100,000 units/mL: 30 mL	
Narcotics	May use oral or parenteral narcotics, such as patient-controlled analgesia. If oral analgesics are selected, use tablets. Do not use elixir, which has alcohol and will exacerbate mucositis. Transmucosal fentanyl (Actiq) currently being evaluated clinically.
Capsaicin candies	One candy q3–4h as needed. Currently being evaluated clinically.
XEROSTOMIA	
Saliva substitutes	
Xerolube	Rinse four to six times per day.
Salivart synthetic saliva spray	Spray four to six times per day.
Biotene chewing gum	Use as needed.
Pilocarpine	5 mg t.i.d.
Amifostine (Ethyol)	200 mg/m^2 daily, as a 3-minute IV infusion 15–30 minutes prior to radiotherapy. Hydrate adequately, monitor blood pressure, and administer antiemetics.

[a]Many of the medications listed have been used alone or in combination to treat mucositis.

ORAL COMPLICATIONS IN RADIOTHERAPY

Before one can discuss orofacial pain, one must understand the nature and necessity of a comprehensive dental examination and how its data interfaces with the treatment regimen. In accordance with the guidelines developed by the National Institutes of Health,[119] it is supremely important that the oncology patient be managed by a team. We recommend that a Preventive Dental Oncology Service be established for identification and management of patients receiving head and neck oncologic surgery, irradiation, and or chemotherapy. The objective of the Preventive Dental Oncology Service program is to evaluate the oncology patient for intraoral problems as related to the specific surgery, radiotherapy, or chemotherapy and to formulate a treatment plan for resolution of the intraoral symptoms associated with therapy.

Radiotherapy for the oncology patient carries a significant risk of mucositis. However, the long-term effects of the radiation are of greater concern to the clinical team than is the transient mucositis. The decrease in the numbers of osteocytes and the concomitant loss of vascularity in the maxillary or mandibular treatment fields precludes bone healing in the event of osseous surgery after therapy. The impaired, retarded, or nonhealing wound presents as an osteoradionecrosis (ORN), which requires specific management protocols (i.e., hyperbaric oxygen and intravenous antibiotics followed by osseous resection and additional hyperbaric oxygen and intravenous antibiotics). Second to the treatment of mucositis is xerostomia.

XEROSTOMIA

Xerostomia is a complex phenomenon that cannot be attributed to radiation damage to the salivary glands alone. To understand xerostomia and the radiotherapy patient more fully, one must review the mechanisms behind saliva production. Secretion of saliva is subject to reflex stimulation of not only a physical but of a psychic nature.[120] Physical stimulation of the salivary gland originates in the taste buds. The psychic stimulation of the salivary glands is via the sensory nerve receptors. Xerostomia presents with a twofold pathogenesis. First, the lack of a wetting medium reduces the ability of the chemoreceptors on the dorsum of the tongue and the palate to accept the stimuli presented with foods or liquids. This loss of physical stimulation (chemical) fails to trigger the neurogenic response to the salivary gland and the anticipated salivary response never occurs. The minimal, thickened, mucinous saliva produced by the affected glands coats the mucosa of the cheeks, tongue, and palate, forming an effective barrier that prevents physical contact of the taste buds by the dietary substances (chemophores) and diminishes the physical response to thermal and mechanical stimulation. The cumulative result of being unable to stimulate the taste buds physically has a direct corresponding effect on the psychic component of salivary gland secretions. Histopathologically, the mucosa on the dorsum of the tongue appears atrophied, the end result of which is decreased surface area on the taste buds.

In the xerostomic patient, the clinician notices a significant loss of appetite that occurs concomitantly with mucositis. The role of xerostomia, and not merely stomatitis, in weight loss must not be discounted. When the physical component of salivary stimulation is denigrated by mechanical (mucous) barriers, the anticipated taste sensation associated with specific food groups is altered. If the patient no longer can perceive what should be sour or sweet, he or she will be unable to elicit the correct sensory response through the neurogenic paths; consequently, the second component of salivary stimulation, the visual component, becomes ineffective and the xerostomia is exacerbated further. When patients no longer can achieve the sensory gratification normally associated with specific food groups, dietary intake decreases and weight loss becomes a significant factor in continuation of therapy. With the decrease of salivary enzymes necessary for the initial stages of digestion, a third factor presents itself in the weight loss arena—namely, inability to assimilate dietary nutrients efficiently. Xerostomia is compounded by other factors such as antidepressant therapy, diabetes, interstitial nephritis, aging, postmenopausal syndromes, antihypertensives, and diuretics. Vitamin A and nicotinic acid deficiencies also can affect salivary secretions.

The management of xerostomia is complex, requiring attention to the patient's medical history for drug interaction, provision of a diet that both physically and psychologically is able to stimulate the salivary responses, maintenance of excellent oral hygiene to provide physical access to the taste receptors, and monitoring of the vitamin A and nicotinic acid levels for deficiencies. Increased intake of nicotinic acid and vitamin A on a specific, monitored response-to-dose program can be effective in increasing saliva flow. Mechanical débridement of the dorsum of the tongue with a soft toothbrush and the use of a spray mister before and during meals assists in maintaining access to taste buds.

Early clinical pilot studies by Fox et al.[121] and Greenspan and Daniels[122] indicated that low doses of oral pilocarpine reduced radiation-induced xerostomia. Recently, a randomized, double-blind, placebo-controlled trial by Johnson et al.[123] found that pilocarpine improved saliva production and relieved symptoms of xerostomia after irradiation for cancer of the head and neck, with minor side effects that were predominantly limited to sweating.

A randomized, controlled trial of standard fractionated radiation with or without amifostine (Ethyol), administered at 200 mg/m^2 as a 3-minute IV infusion 15 to 30 minutes before each fraction of radiation, was conducted in 315 patients with head and neck cancer. Patients were required to have at least 75% of both parotid glands in the radiation field. The incidence of grade 2 or higher acute xerostomia (≤90 days from the start of radiotherapy) and late xerostomia (9 to 12 months after radiotherapy), as assessed by the Radiation Therapy Oncology Group Acute and Late Morbidity Scoring Criteria, was significantly reduced in patients receiving Ethyol. At 1 year after radiotherapy, whole saliva collection after irradiation showed that more patients given Ethyol produced 0.1 g of saliva (72% vs. 49%). In addition, the median saliva production at 1 year was higher in those patients who received Ethyol (0.26 g vs. 0.1 g). Stimulated saliva collections did not show a difference between treatment arms. These improvements in saliva production were supported by the patients' subjective responses to a questionnaire regarding oral dryness.[124]

With effective management of xerostomia, the thickened mucinous film that accumulates on the mucosa of the tongue, floor of mouth, palate, and buccal folds is eliminated. With this simple maintenance step that can be managed by the patient or support staff, a significant reduction in bacterial volume is achieved, which, in turn, will reduce the incidence of mucositis significantly. When xerostomia is not controlled, significant plaque and material will accumulate on the surfaces of prosthetic appliances. This bacterial film can contribute to denture irritation that will compound therapy-related mucositis and can lead to fenestration of the supporting mucosa and development of an osteonecrosis in the posttreatment patient. When xerostomia is not monitored or controlled, the clinical team can anticipate heavy plaque accumulation on the surfaces of the teeth. This plaque film is highly cariogenic and ultimately will cause dental complications involving the teeth (decay) and the supporting tissue (gingivitis and periodontitis). Patients with high plaque indices will not benefit from anticariogenic treatment using fluoride applicators, because the plaque is an effective barrier against fluoride absorption. It must be assumed that the elevated plaque matrix resulting from xerostomia poses the greatest risk in the postradiotherapy morbidity of ORN.

Because of this risk of ORN, it will be necessary for the clinical team not only to assess a patient's pretreatment periodontal health but also to query the patient regarding his or her intent to maintain adequate oral hygiene. If a patient is not psychologically prepared to play a role in his or her oral hygiene or if a patient is physically or mentally impaired and unable to manage an appropriate personal oral hygiene program, it will be prudent to consider oral surgery to remove all high-risk teeth, as a preventive measure. Amputation of a patient's dentition is a serious irreversible step and must be thoroughly planned by all members of the clinical team before proceeding.

From the dental examination, diagnostic models, and radiographs obtained before radiotherapy or chemotherapy, high-risk teeth can be identified and treated restoratively or surgically. The therapy team must recognize and identify teeth and other bone anatomy aberrations that would require posttreatment surgery. Because of the reduction in the vascular network and the permanent alteration of osteocytes in the bone in the treatment ports, it will be necessary to perform all prospective surgeries before the initiation of radiotherapy. This will minimize the potential for ORN in cases in which an operation must be performed after radiotherapy has been completed.

High-risk teeth and bone can be summarized as impacted third molars (both bony and soft tissue); teeth in which periodontal disease has been diagnosed and that will require mucosal flap surgery for treatment; unrestored endodontically treated teeth that are at high risk for traumatic fracture; teeth that have been surgically removed, endodontically treated, and reimplanted; teeth restored with dental implants; and teeth with root resorption secondary to orthodontic therapy. Supernumerary teeth and ossifications must also be evaluated.

After the dentition has been restored and appropriate surgeries have been completed, vacuum-formed vinyl fluoride applicators are made for home-care fluoride application. These applicators provide two functions: First, they help to prevent xerostomia-induced dental caries through fluoride induction into the tooth enamel and dentin. Second, the increased ambient fluoride levels on the tooth surface and the residual fluoride that remains in the oral cavity after each fluoride application reduces the level of oral bacteria and assists in microbial prophylaxis, which aids in the reduction of mucositis. In general, 0.04% stannous fluoride gel appears to be more effective than sodium fluoride 1.1%, as it reduces the levels of *Streptococcus mutans,* which causes caries.[125] In the use of fluoride applicators, Shenep et al.[125] recommend that a 0.04% stannous fluoride gel be placed into the applicators and that these be placed on the teeth and allowed to remain there for 3 minutes. After 3 minutes, the applicators should be removed and the excess fluoride expectorated, and the patient should not be allowed to rinse, eat, or drink for 30 minutes. For the week before initiation and for weeks 1 and 2 of radiotherapy, we recommend using the fluoride three times daily. This is in anticipation that we may discontinue fluoride therapy during the third, fourth, and fifth weeks of radiotherapy. For the first 3 months after radiotherapy, we recommend twice-daily fluoride. After 3 months and a thorough dental assessment, if the plaque indices are below 5%, we will maintain the patient on once-daily fluoride maintenance for life.

Before beginning radiotherapy, a protective radiation stent is fabricated. These stents are used during the radiotherapeutic sessions for all patients who have natural dentition. The purpose of the stents is to eliminate soft tissue contact with the surfaces of large dental restorations, thereby eliminating the secondary electron scatter from radiotherapy that will cause significant localized mucositis.

From the diagnostic examination and radiographs, the practitioner must ascertain whether the patient undergoing radiotherapy has had dental implants placed for prosthetic rehabilitation. Oral implantology is rapidly becoming commonplace in the prosthetic rehabilitation of missing teeth, support for cleft palate obturators, and support for facial muloges and prostheses. If it has been determined that implants are present, the dental oncologist must be prepared to fabricate the appropriate radiation shields and blocks to protect the areas of the bone supporting the implants, to minimize increased radiation dosimetry in those portions of the mandible or maxilla.

Keus et al.[126] reported on the effect of customized beam shaping on normal tissue complications in radiotherapy for parotid gland tumors. They evaluated a customized beam's-eye view as opposed to unblocked portals with field sizes defined by the largest target contour found in any computed tomographic slice and found that the volume of unnecessary exposed normal tissue that received more than 90% of the prescribed dose was reduced by a factor of 4% to 44%, on average, when the volume is expressed as a percentage of the target volume in each patient. For a tumor dose of 70 Gy, the average bone necrosis probability was reduced from 8.4% to 4.1%.

As regards patients with extensive implanted, supported, fixed or fixed removable prostheses, a very large volume of gold alloy is used in the fixed prostheses and in the framework of the fixed removable prostheses. For patients with dental implants, removal of the detachable portions of the prosthesis should be completed before radiotherapy, and beam-shaping blocks should be fabricated by the prosthodontist for protection of the mandible containing the titanium implant fixture. These precautions are necessary to reduce the risk of radiation-induced ORN.

OSTEORADIONECROSIS

ORN carries the greatest morbidity in any radiotherapy program involving osseous tissue. ORN is not an infection but nonhealing, acellular, avascular bone that may have been present for months or years before becoming clinically evident. Continuous monitoring of the radiotherapy patient by the dental oncologist on a 3-month recall basis is appropriate. This recall schedule will allow for evaluation of the plaque indices, monitoring of fluoride compliance, and maintenance of developing dental disease. Even with the best of diagnosis, planning, and staging, an osteonecrosis can develop spontaneously. Early osteonecrotic changes are subtle and difficult to detect. In many instances, ORN presents as asymptomatic dehiscence in the mucosa. As the necrosis progresses, the site can become more erythematous and painful. At this stage, it is not uncommon for the clinician to misdiagnose the signs as a minor infection and to place the patient on a regimen of antibiotics, which will minimize the symptoms but allow the necrosis to continue to progress. If teeth are present, the clinical symptoms are mobility, minimal to moderate pain, and ectopic eruption. In the early stages, routine dental radiographs are insufficient to provide an accurate diagnosis. As the necrosis advances, extraoral fistulas and intraoral antral fistulas will develop. Eventually, occlusion pathology becomes evident and, in many cases, pathologic fractures will occur.

Early definitive diagnosis using computed tomographic scans, dentiscans, bone density studies, and magnetic resonance imaging will aid in determining the extent of the necrosis so that a surgical template can be made. In very small, isolated, solitary lesions of less than 0.5 cm, surgical exposure and cautious débridement along with appropriate prophylactic antibiotics may suffice. This seldom is the case with ORN and, if remission and healing are not evident within the first 8 weeks, presurgical and postsurgical hyperbaric oxygen, intravenous antibiotics, and radical excision of the necrotic avascular bone will be necessary.

Myers and Marx[127] reported on the use of hyperbaric oxygen, which stimulates angiogenesis, leading to increased neovascularization and optimization of cellular levels of oxygen for osteoblast and fibroblast proliferation, collagen formation, and support of ingrowing blood vessels. The hypoxic, acellular matrix in the postirradiated field is changed to a hypercellular, hyperoxic or normally oxygenated situation. Oxygen is used as an adjunct to appropriate surgical intervention; by use of these two modalities in combination, the salvage rate for ORN and its complications of orocutaneous fistula, pathologic fractures, and severe bone loss can be increased dramatically.[127]

CONCLUSION

With accurate pretherapeutic diagnosis, appropriate treatment planning, and therapeutic staging by all members of the clinical team, the incidence of ORN and other oral complications can be minimized or eliminated. The medicolegal accountability, if such pretreatment protocols are not in place, is significant and economically devastating. For no reason should a patient be denied a thorough, comprehensive examination followed by a well-formulated and well-staged treatment plan. In summary, a total team effort is mandatory for the standard of care necessary to provide the oncology patient with a comprehensive treatment plan that encompasses all medical and dental health and rehabilitation issues.

REFERENCES

1. Sonis ST. Oral complications of cancer therapy. In DeVita VT, Hellman S, Rosenberg SA, eds. Cancer: *Principles and practice of oncology*, 4th ed. Philadelphia: JB Lippincott, 1993:2385.
2. Sonis ST. Oral complications of cancer therapy. In DeVita VT, Hellman S, Rosenberg SA, eds. Cancer: *Principles and practice of oncology*, 4th ed. Philadelphia: JB Lippincott, 1993:2389.
3. Peterson DE, Ambrosio JA. Diagnosis and management of acute and chronic oral complications of nonsurgical cancer therapies. *Dent Clin North Am* 1992;36:945.
4. Sonis ST. Oral complications of cancer therapy. In DeVita VT, Hellman S, Rosenberg SA, eds. Cancer: *Principles and practice of oncology*, 4th ed. Philadelphia: JB Lippincott, 1993:2385.
5. Sonis S, Clark J. Prevention and management of oral mucositis induced by antineoplastic therapy. *Oncology* 1991;5:11.
6. Sonis ST. Mucositis as a biological process: a new hypothesis for the development of chemotherapy-induced stomatotoxicity. *Oral Oncol* 1998;34(1):39.
7. Wilkes JD. Prevention and treatment of oral mucositis following cancer chemotherapy. *Semin Oncol* 1998;25:538.
8. Dodd MJ, Miaskowski C, Shiba GH, et al. Risk factors for chemotherapy-induced oral mucositis: dental appliances, oral hygiene, previous oral lesion, and a history of smoking. *Cancer Invest* 1999;17(4):278.
9. Sloan JA, Loprinzi CL, Novotny PJ, et al. Sex differences in fluorouracil-induced stomatitis. *J Clin Oncol* 2000;18(2):412.
10. Berger AM, Henderson M, Nadoolman W, et al. Oral capsaicin provides temporary relief for oral mucositis pain secondary to chemotherapy/radiation therapy. *J Pain Symptom Manage* 1995;10(3):243.
11. Berger AM, Bartoshuk LM, Duffy VB, et al. Capsaicin for the treatment of oral mucositis pain. *Principles Pract Oncol* 1995;9:1.
12. Oken MM, Creech RH, Tormey DC, et al. Toxicity and response criteria of the Eastern Cooperative Oncology Group. *Am J Clin Oncol* 1982;5:649.
13. Sonis ST, Eilers JP, Epstein JB. Validation of a new scoring system for the assessment of clinical trial research of oral mucositis induced by radiation or chemotherapy. *Cancer* 1999;85(10):2103.
14. Conference C. Oral complications of cancer therapies: diagnosis, prevention and treatment. *Conn Med* 1989;53:595.
15. Nagashima R, Hirano T. Selective binding of sucralfate to ulcer lesion: I. Experiments in rats with acetic acid–induced gastric ulcer receiving unlabeled sucralfate. *Arzneimittelforschung* 1980;30:80.
16. Nagashima R, Yoshida N, Terao N. Sucralfate, a basic aluminum salt of sucrose sulfate II. Inhibition of peptic hydrolysis as it results from sucrose sulfate interaction with protein substrate, serum albumins. *Arzneimittelforschung* 1979;29:73.
17. Ferraro JM, Mattern J. Sucralfate suspension for stomatitis. *Drug Intel Clin Pharm* 1984;18:153.
18. Solomon MA. Oral sucralfate suspension for mucositis. *N Engl J Med* 1986;315:459.
19. Ferraro JM, Mattern J. Sucralfate suspension for stomatitis [Letter]. *Drug Intel Clin Pharm* 1984;18:153.
20. Ferraro JM, Mattern J. Sucralfate suspension for mouth ulcers [Letter]. *Drug Intel Clin Pharm* 1985;19:480.
21. Pfeiffer P, Madsen EL, Hansen O, et al. Effect of prophylactic sucralfate suspension on stomatitis induced by cancer chemotherapy. A randomized, double-blind cross-over study. *Acta Oncol* 1990;29:171.
22. Shenep JL, Kalwihsky D, Hudson PR, et al. Oral sucralfate in chemotherapy-induced mucositis. *J Pediatr* 1988;113:753.
23. Loprinzi CL, Ghosh C, Camoriani J, et al. Phase III controlled evaluation of sucralfate to alleviate stomatitis in patients receiving fluorouracil-based chemotherapy. *J Clin Oncol* 1997;15:1235.
24. Scherlacher A, Beaufort-Spontin E. Radiotherapy of head-neck neoplasms: prevention of inflammation of the mucosa by sucralfate treatment. *HNO* 1990;38:24.
25. Pfeiffer P, Hansen O, Madsen EL, et al. A prospective pilot study on the effect of sucralfate mouth-swishing in reducing stomatitis during radiotherapy of the oral cavity. *Acta Oncol* 1990;29:471.
26. Epstein JB, Wong FLW. The efficacy of sucralfate suspension in the prevention of oral mucositis due to radiation therapy. *Int J Radiat Oncol Biol Phys* 1994;28:693.
27. Barker G, Loftus L, Cuddy P, et al. The effects of sucralfate suspension and diphenhydramine syrup plus kaolin-pectin on radiotherapy-induced mucositis. *Oral Surg Oral Med Oral Pathol* 1991;71:288.
28. Cohen MM, Clark L. Preventing acetylsalicylic acid damage to human gastric mucosa by the use of prostaglandin E_2. *Can J Surg* 1983;26:116.
29. Ericksson B, Johansson C, Aly A. Prostaglandin E_2 for chronic leg ulcers. *Lancet* 1986;1:905.
30. Kuhrer I, Kuzmits R, Linkesch W, et al. Topical PGE_2 enhances healing of chemotherapy-associated mucosal lesions. *Lancet* 1986;1:623.
31. Porteder H, Rausch E, Kment G, et al. Local prostaglandin E_2 in patients with oral malignancies undergoing chemo and radiotherapy. *J Craniomaxillofac Surg* 1988;16:371.
32. Matejka M, Nell A, Kment G, et al. Local benefit of prostaglandin E_2 in radiochemotherapy-induced oral mucositis. *Br J Oral Maxillofac Surg* 1990;28:89.
33. Labor B, Mrsic M, Pavleric A, et al. Prostaglandin E_2 for prophylaxis of oral mucositis following BMT. *Bone Marrow Transplant* 1993;11:379.
34. Epstein JB, Stevenson-Moore P. Benzydamine hydrochloride in prevention and management of pain in mucositis associated with radiation therapy. *Oral Surg Oral Med Oral Pathol* 1986;62:145.
35. Epstein JB, Stevenson-Moore P, Jackson S, et al. Prevention of oral mucositis in radiation therapy: a controlled study with benzydamine hydrochloride rinse. *Int J Radiat Oncol Biol Phys* 1989;16:1571.
36. Lever SA, Dupuis LL, Chan SL. Comparative evaluation of benzydamine oral rinse in children with antineoplastic-induced stomatitis. *Drug Intel Clin Pharm* 1987;21:359.
37. Pillsbury HC, Webster WP, Rosenman J. Prostaglandin inhibitor and radiotherapy in advanced head and neck cancer. *Arch Otolaryngol Head Neck Surg* 1986;112:552.
38. Abdelaal AS, Barker DS, Fergusson MM. Treatment for irradiation-induced mucositis. *Lancet* 1987;1:97.
39. Rothwell BR, Speltor WS. Palliation of radiation-related mucositis. *Spec Care Dentistry* 1990;10:21.
40. Starasoler S, Haber GS. Use of vitamin E oil in primary herpes gingivostomatitis in an adult. *NY State Dentistry* 1978;44:382.
41. Tampo Y, Yonaha M. Vitamin E and glutathione are required for preservation of microsomal glutathione S-transferase from oxidative stress in microsomes. *Pharmacology* 1990;66:259.
42. Regan V, Servinova E, Packer L. Antioxidant effects of ubiquinones in microsomes and mitochondria are mediated by tocopherol recycling. *Biochem Biophys Res Commun* 1990;169:851.
43. Wadleigh RG, Redman RS, Graham Ml, et al. Vitamin E in the treatment of chemo-induced mucositis. *Am J Med* 1992;92:481.
44. Osaki T, Ueta E, Yoneda K, et al. Prophylaxis of oral mucositis associated with chemoradiotherapy for oral carcinoma by Azelastine hydrochloride with other antioxidants. *Head Neck* 1994;16:331.
45. Garewal HS, Meyskens F. Retinoids and carcinoids in the prevention of oral cancer. A critical appraisal. *Cancer Epidemiol Biomarkers Prev* 1992;1:155.
46. Mills EE. The modifying effect of beta-carotene on radiation and chemotherapy induced oral mucositis. *Br J Cancer* 1988;57:416.
47. Maciejewski B, Zajusz A, Pilecki B, et al. Acute mucositis in the stimulated oral mucosa of patients during radiotherapy for head and neck cancer. *Radiother Oncol* 1991;22:7.
48. Dorr W, Jacubek A, Kummermehr J, et al. Effects of stimulated repopulation on oral mucositis during conventional radiotherapy. *Radiother Oncol* 1995;37:100.
49. Carl W, Emrich LS. Management of oral mucositis during local radiation and systemic chemotherapy. A study of 98 patients. *J Prosthet Dent* 1991;66:361.
50. Fidler P, Loprinzi CL, Lee JK, et al. A randomized clinical trial of chamomile mouthwash for prevention of 5-FU-induced oral mucositis. *Cancer* 1996;77:522.
51. Oshitani T, Okada K, Kushima T, et al. Clinical evaluation of sodium alginate on oral mucositis associated with radiotherapy. *J Jpn Soc Cancer Ther* 1990;25:1129.
52. Lieschke GT, Ramenghi U, O'Connor MP, et al. Studies of oral neutrophil levels in patients receiving G-CSF after autologous marrow transplantation. *Br J Haematol* 1992;82:589.
53. Gabrilove JL, Jakubowski A, Scher H, et al. Effect of granulocyte colony-stimulating factor on neutropenia and associated morbidity due to chemotherapy for transitional-cell carcinoma of the urothelium. *N Engl J Med* 1988;318:1414.
54. Bronchud MH, Howell A, Crowther D, et al. The use of granulocyte colony-stimulating factor to increase the intensity of treatment with doxorubicin in patients with advanced breast and ovarian cancer. *Br J Cancer* 1989;60:121.
55. Pettengell R, Gurney H, Radford JA, et al. Granulocyte colony-stimulating factor to prevent dose-limiting neutropenia in non-Hodgkin's lymphoma: a randomized controlled trial. *Blood* 1992;80:1430.

56. Chi KH, Chen CH, Chan WK, et al. Effect of granulocyte-macrophage colony-stimulating factor on oral mucositis in head and neck cancer patients after cisplatin, fluorouracil, and leucovorin. *J Clin Oncol* 1995;13:2620.
57. Atkinson K, Biggs JC, Downs K, et al. GM-CSF after allogeneic bone marrow transplantation—accelerated recovery of neutrophils, monocytes, and lymphocytes. *Aust NZ J Med* 1991;21:686.
58. Game SM, Stone A, Scully C, et al. Tumour progression in experimental oral carcinogenesis is associated with changes in EGF and TGF-beta receptor expression and altered responses to those growth factors. *Carcinogenesis* 1990;11:965.
59. Sundqvist K, Liu Y, Arvidson K, et al. Growth regulation of serum free cultures of epithelial cells from normal human buccal mucosa. *In Vitro Cell Dev Biol* 1991;27A:562.
60. Maccini DM, Veit BC. Salivary epidermal growth factor in patients with and without acid peptic disease. *Am J Gastroenterol* 1990;85:1102.
61. Sonis ST, Costa JW Jr, Evitts SM, et al. Effect of epidermal growth factor on ulcerative mucositis in hamsters that receive cancer chemotherapy. *Oral Surg Oral Med Oral Pathol* 1992;74:749.
62. Sonis ST, Tracey C, Shklar G, et al. An animal model for mucositis induced by cancer chemotherapy. *Oral Surg Oral Med Oral Pathol* 1990;69:437.
63. Sonis ST, Lindquist L, Vugt V, et al. Prevention of chemotherapy-induced ulcerative mucositis by TGF-β3. *Cancer Res* 1994;54:1135.
64. Spijkervet FK, Sonis ST. New frontiers in the management of chemotherapy-induced mucositis. *Curr Opin Oncol* 1998;10[Suppl 1]:S23.
65. Zaghloul MS, Dorie MJ, Kallman RF, et al. Interleukin 1 increases thymidine labeling index of normal tissue of mice, not the tumor. *Int J Radiat Oncol Biol Phys* 1994;29:805.
66. Sonis ST, Lindquist L, Vugt V, et al. Alteration in the frequency, severity, and duration of chemotherapy-induced mucositis in hamsters by interleukin-11. *Eur J Cancer* 1995;31B:261.
67. Sonis S, Edwards L, Lucey C. The biological basis for the attenuation of mucositis: the example of interleukin-11. *Leukemia* 1999;13:831.
68. Ferretti AG, Raybould TP, Brown AT, et al. Chlorhexidine prophylaxis for chemotherapy and radiotherapy-induced stomatitis: a randomized double-blind trial. *Oral Surg Oral Med Oral Pathol* 1990;69:1331.
69. Wahlin BY. Effects of chlorhexidine mouthrinse on oral health in patients with acute leukemia. *Oral Surg Oral Med Oral Pathol* 1989;68:279.
70. Weisdorf DJ, Bostrom B, Raether D, et al. Oropharyngeal mucositis complicating bone marrow transplantation: prognostic factors and the effect of chlorhexidine mouth rinse. *Bone Marrow Transplant* 1989;4:89.
71. Epstein JB, Vickais L, Spinelli J, et al. Efficacy of chlorhexidine and nystatin rinses in prevention of oral complications in leukemia and bone marrow transplantation. *Oral Surg Oral Med Oral Pathol* 1992;73:682.
72. Ferretti AG, Raybould TP, Brown AT, et al. Chlorhexidine prophylaxis for chemotherapy and radiotherapy-induced stomatitis: a randomized double-blind trial. *Oral Surg Oral Med Oral Pathol* 1990;69:1331.
73. Spijkervet FKL, Saene HKF, Panders AK, et al. Effect of chlorhexidine rinsing on the oropharyngeal ecology in patients with head and neck cancer who have irradiation mucositis. *Oral Surg Oral Med Oral Pathol* 1989;67:154.
74. Foote RL, Loprinzi CL, Frank AR, et al. Randomized trial of a chlorhexidine mouthwash for alleviation of radiation-induced mucositis. *J Clin Oncol* 1994;12:2630.
75. Spijkervet FK, Saene HK, van Saene JJ, et al. Effect of selective elimination of the oral flora on mucositis in irradiated head and neck cancer patients. *J Surg Oncol* 1991;46:167.
76. Loury DJ, Embree JR, Steinberg DA. Effect of local application of the antimicrobial peptide IB-367 on the incidence and severity of oral mucositis in hamsters. *Oral Surg Oral Med Oral Pathol Oral Radiol Endod* 1999;87:544.
77. Epstein JB, Vickais L, Spinelli J, et al. Efficacy of chlorhexidine and nystatin rinses in prevention of oral complications in leukemia and bone marrow transplantation. *Oral Surg Oral Med Oral Pathol* 1992;73:682.
78. Barrett AP. A long-term prospective clinical study of oral complications during conventional chemotherapy for acute leukemia. *Oral Surg Oral Med Oral Pathol* 1987;63:313.
79. DeGregorio MW, Lee WMF, Linker CA, et al. Fungal infections in patients with acute leukemia. *Am J Med* 1982;73:543.
80. Bender JF, Schimpff SC, Young VM, et al. A comparative trial of tobramycin vs gentamicin in combination with vancomycin and nystatin for alimentary tract suppression in leukemic patients. *Eur J Cancer* 1979;15:35.
81. Barrett AP. Evaluation of nystatin in prevention and elimination of oropharyngeal *Candida* in immunosuppressed patients. *Oral Surg Oral Med Oral Pathol* 1984;58:148.
82. William C, Whitehouse JMA, Lister TA, et al. Oral anticandidal prophylaxis in patients undergoing chemotherapy for acute leukemia. *Med Pediatr Oncol* 1977;3:275.
83. Carpentieri V, Haggard ME, Lockhart LH, et al. Clinical experience in prevention of candidiasis by nystatin in children with acute lymphocytic leukemia. *J Pediatr* 1978;92:593.
84. Hann IM, Prentice HG, Corringham R, et al. Ketoconazole versus nystatin plus amphotericin B for fungal prophylaxis in severely immunocompromised patients. *Lancet* 1982;1:826.
85. Schwartz PM, Dunigan JM, Marsh JC, et al. Allopurinol modification of the toxicity and antitumor activity of 5-fluorouracil. *Cancer Res* 1980;40:1885.
86. Clark PI, Selvin ML. Allopurinol mouthwash and 5-fluorouracil-induced oral toxicity. *Eur J Surg Oncol* 1985;11:267.
87. Tsavaris N, Caraglauris P, Kosmidus P. Reduction of oral toxicity of 5-fluorouracil by allopurinol mouthwashes. *Eur J Surg Oncol* 1988;14:405.
88. Loprinzi CI, Cianflone SG, Dose AM, et al. A controlled evaluation of an allopurinol mouthwash as prophylaxis against 5-fluorouracil induced stomatitis. *Cancer* 1990;65:1879.
89. Lee JS, Murphy WK, Shirinian MH, et al. Alleviation by leucovorin of the dose-limiting toxicity of edatrexate: potential for improved therapeutic efficacy. *Cancer Chemother Pharmacol* 1991;28:199.
90. Ackland SP, Schilsky RL. High-dose methotrexate: a critical reappraisal. *J Clin Oncol* 1987;5:2017.
91. Oliff A, Bleyer WA, Poplack DG. Methotrexate-induced oral mucositis and salivary methotrexate concentrations. *Cancer Chemother Pharmacol* 1979;2:225.
92. Fox AD, Kripke SA, Depaula JA, et al. Effect of a glutamine supplemented enteral diet on methotrexate-induced enterocolitis. *JPEN J Parenter Enteral Nutr* 1988;12:325.
93. O'Dwyer ST, Scott T, Smith RJ, et al. 5-Fluorouracil toxicity on small intestinal mucosa but not white blood cells is decreased by glutamine. *Clin Res* 1987;35:367A(abst).
94. Jebb SA, Osborne RJ, Maughan TS, et al. 5-Fluorouracil and folinic acid–induced mucositis: no effect of oral glutamine supplementation. *Br J Cancer* 1994;70:132.
95. Martin DS, Stolf RL, Sawyer RC, et al. High-dose 5-fluorouracil with delayed uridine rescue in mice. *Cancer Res* 1982;42:3964.
96. Seiter K, Kemeny N, Martin D, et al. Uridine allows dose escalation of 5-fluorouracil when given with N-phosphonacetyl-L-aspartate, methotrexate, and leucovorin. *Cancer* 1993;71(5):1875.
97. Ahmed T, Engelking C, Szalyga J, et al. Propantheline prevention of mucositis from etoposide. *Bone Marrow Transplant* 1993;12:131.
98. Dose AM, Mahoud DJ, Loprinzi CL. A controlled trial of oral cryotherapy for preventing stomatitis in patients receiving 5-fluorouracil plus leucovorin. A North Central Cancer Treatment Group and Mayo Clinic Study. *Proc Am Soc Clin Oncol* 1992;9:1242.
99. Mahoud DJ, Dose AM, Loprinzi CL, et al. Inhibition of fluorouracil-induced stomatitis by oral cryotherapy. *J Clin Oncol* 1991;9:449.
100. Rocke LK, Loprinzi CL, Lee JK, et al. A randomized clinical trial of two different durations of oral cryotherapy for prevention of 5-fluorouracil-related stomatitis. *Cancer* 1993;72(7):2234.
101. Cascinu S, Fedeli A, Fedeli SL, et al. Oral cooling (cryotherapy), an effective treatment for the prevention of 5-fluorouracil-induced stomatitis. *Oral Oncol Eur J Cancer* 1994; 30(4):234.
102. Bugai EP, Saprykina VA, Vakhtin VI, et al. The effect of light from a low intensity impulse laser on the processes of experimental inflammation and regeneration in the oral mucosa. *Stomatologiia* 1991;2:6.
103. Pourreau-Schneider N, Soudry M, Franquin JC, et al. Soft-laser therapy for iatrogenic mucositis in cancer patients receiving high-dose fluorouracil: a preliminary report. *J Natl Cancer Inst* 1992;84:358.
104. Poland J. Prevention and treatment of oral complications in the cancer patient. *Oncology* 1991;5:45.
105. Carnal SB, Blakeslee DB, Oswald SG, et al. Treatment of radiation- and chemotherapy-induced stomatitis. *Otolaryngol Head Neck Surg* 1990;102:326.
106. Miaskowski C. Management of mucositis during therapy. *Natl Cancer Inst Monogr* 1990;9:95.
107. Watson CPN, Evans RJ, Watt VR, et al. Post-herpetic neuralgia: 208 cases. *Pain* 1988;35:289.
108. Scheffler NM, Sheitel PL, Lipton MN. Treatment of painful diabetic neuropathy with capsaicin 0.075%. *J Am Podiatr Med Assoc* 1991;81:288.
109. Group CS. Treatment of painful diabetic neuropathy with topical capsaicin. A multicenter, double-blind, vehicle-controlled study. *Arch Intern Med* 1991;151:2225.
110. Watson CPN, Evans RJ, Watt VR. The post-mastectomy pain syndrome and the effect of topical capsaicin. *Pain* 1989;38:177.
111. Weintraub M, Golik A, Rubio A. Capsaicin for treatment of post-traumatic amputation stump pain. *Lancet* 1990;336:1003.
112. Fusco BM, Alessandri M. Analgesic effect of capsaicin in idiopathic trigeminal neuralgia. *Anesth Analg* 1992;74:375.
113. Cheshire WP, Snyder CR. Treatment of reflex sympathetic dystrophy with topical capsaicin: case report. *Pain* 1990;42:307.
114. Morgenlander JC, Hurwitz BJ, Massey EW. Capsaicin for the treatment of pain in Guillain-Barré syndrome. *Ann Neurol* 1990;28:199.
115. Deal CL, Schnitzer JJ, Lipstein E, et al. Treatment of arthritis with topical capsaicin. A double-blind trial. *Clin Ther* 1991;13:383.
116. Sicuteri F, Fusco BM, Marabini S. Beneficial effect of capsaicin application to the nasal mucosa in cluster headache. *Clin J Pain* 1989;5:49.
117. Watcher MA, Wheeland RG. The role of topical agents in the healing of full-thickness wounds. *J Dermatol Surg Oncol* 1989;15:1188.
118. Krajnik M, Zylicz Z, Finlay I, et al. Potential uses of topical opioids in palliative care—report of 6 cases. *Pain* 1999;80:121.
119. Conference C. Oral complications of cancer therapies: diagnosis, prevention and treatment. *Conn Med* 1989;53:595.
120. Thoma, Goldman. *Oral pathology.* St Louis: Mosby, 1960:892.
121. Fox PC, Atkinson JC, Macynski AA, et al. Pilocarpine treatment of salivary gland hypofunction and dry mouth (xerostomia). *Arch Intern Med* 1991;151:1149.
122. Greenspan D, Daniels TE. Effectiveness of pilocarpine in postradiation xerostomia. *Cancer* 1987;59:1123.
123. Johnson JT, Ferretti GA, Nethery J, et al. Oral pilocarpine for post-irradiation xerostomia in patients with head and neck cancer. *N Engl J Med* 1993;329:390.
124. Brizel DM, Wasserman TH, Strnad V, et al. Final report of a phase III randomized trial of amifostine as a radioprotectant in head and neck cancer. 41st annual meeting of the American Society for Therapeutic Radiology and Oncology. Texas, 1999 (abstract).
125. Shenep JL, Kalwihsky D, Hudson PR, et al. Oral sucralfate in chemotherapy-induced mucositis. *J Pediatr* 1988;113:758.
126. Keus R, Noach P, de Boer R, Lebesque J. The effect of customized beam shaping on normal tissue complications in radiation therapy of parotid gland tumors. *Radiother Oncol* 1991;21(3):211.
127. Myers RA, Marx RE. Uses of hyperbaric oxygen in postradiation head and neck surgery. *Natl Cancer Inst Monogr* 1990;9:151.

SECTION 3

DIANE E. STOVER
ROBERT J. KANER

Pulmonary Toxicity

Pulmonary disease can be caused by a wide spectrum of pathogenetic mechanisms in patients with cancer. These include a variety of infectious agents and neoplastic disorders as well as pulmonary thromboembolic disease, pulmonary hemorrhage, pulmonary edema (cardiogenic and noncardiogenic), and leukocyte agglutinin reactions. Pulmonary toxicity caused by antineoplastic agents is being recognized more frequently, and the number of drugs known or suspected to cause lung disease is steadily increasing. Because continued use of the offending agent may cause death and because withholding the agent may result in resolution of the pulmonary toxicity, it is important to recognize radiation- and drug-induced pulmonary disease. In this section, parenchymal lung disease caused by irradiation and chemotherapy is discussed. Mechanisms of lung injury, histopathologic findings, clinical and laboratory features, and diagnosis and treatment of the abnormalities produced by radiation therapeutic and chemotherapeutic agents are reviewed.

RADIATION-INDUCED PULMONARY TOXICITY

MECHANISM OF LUNG INJURY

Radiation can affect dividing and nondividing cells and can cause genetic and nongenetic damage.[1,2] In the lung, a hypothetical reconstruction of radiation injury might be as follows: Therapeutic radiation may result in nongenetic damage that is apparent in all cells, but capillary endothelial and type I cells (epithelial lining cells) appear to be most susceptible.[3] Many of these cells, whether dividing or not, undergo early necrobiosis and slough. The apoptotic pathway appears to be an important mechanism of cellular destruction after radiation. Specific signal transduction pathways are activated by radiation, including sphingomyelin hydrolysis, which generates ceramide as a second messenger and leads to apoptotic DNA degradation.[4] Nonlethal ionizing radiation also activates a stress response in cells, which leads to up-regulation of specific nuclear transcription factors such as NF-κB and transcription of such specific early-response genes as c-abl, c-jun, Egr-1, and c-fos.[5,6] This cellular activation initiates a repair process that involves cytokines and growth factors such as basic fibroblast growth factor,[7] as well as interleukin-1 and transforming growth factor-β (TGF-β).[8] Prostaglandin synthesis is also up-regulated.[9] Over time, capillaries regenerate, and the alveolar epithelium is repopulated by type II cells (surfactant-producing cells), because type I pneumocytes do not regenerate. Some of these type II cells redifferentiate into type I cells. If the initial injury is severe, extracellular matrix components of the lung, such as basement membrane glycoproteins and proteoglycans, are damaged. This can impede reconstruction of the delicate three-dimensional structure of the alveolar-capillary unit and result in functional derangement and scar formation, even if the cellular components are able to regenerate. Genetic damage to dividing cells, such as endothelial cells or type II pneumonocytes, can also occur. Depletion of these cells may result during successive mitoses, causing a loss of integrity of pulmonary capillaries and exudation of fluid into the alveoli. At the physiologic level, loss of compliance, abnormal gas exchange, and respiratory failure can occur owing to leakage of plasma proteins into the alveolar space. This type of genetic damage may also explain why pneumonitis may be seen so late after radiation. One might speculate that some endothelial cells initially remain normal but that, in the course of the next four cell divisions, chromosomal aberrations prevent further reduplication, which leads to loss of integrity of the capillary.[1]

Certain factors are critical to the development of classic radiation pneumonitis. In general, damage to the lung increases as the volume of lung tissue irradiated increases. There also appears to be a threshold effect, such that irradiation of at least 10% of the lung is required to produce significant pulmonary toxicity.[10] This threshold may be reached in the treatment of some patients with breast cancer, depending on the specifics of their individualized treatment program.[10] Also, the toxic effects of radiation, as measured by symptoms and signs, radiographic changes, and physiologic tests, are proportionate to the total amount delivered to the lung. Radiation pneumonitis after a single-dose whole lung irradiation shows a threshold level and a steep sigmoid dose-response curve.[11] Radiation pneumonitis seldom occurs with fractionated total doses of less than 20 Gy but is highly likely when doses exceed 60 Gy.[12] An unusual and dramatic demonstration of this principle is the use of therapeutic pneumothorax to protect the lung when high-dose external-beam radiation therapy is given for the treatment of chest wall tumors.[13]

Because local control of lung cancer is greater when higher doses are delivered to the tumor,[14] methods are being devised to give high doses to the target tissue while sparing normal surrounding lung. One such technique is called *three-dimensional treatment planning*.[15–18] To spare the lung further toxicity, *in situ* isolated lung perfusion for the treatment of unresectable pulmonary tumors, preceded or followed by high-dose irradiation, soon may be available.[19] Studies to evaluate the therapeutic activity of inhaled chemotherapeutic agents, such as doxorubicin, on metastasis to the lung are under way also.[20] Whether these treatment modalities will have a sparing effect on the lung or whether they will be associated with an increase in pulmonary toxicity is unknown.

Besides the total radiation dose, the number of fractions into which it is divided and, to a lesser extent, the time span over which it is delivered are important factors.[21] The greater the number of fractions in which the radiation is given, the lower is the damaging effect. However, the incidence of radiation pneumonitis still exhibits a threshold effect and a steep sigmoidal dose-response curve.[22] *Fractionation* is different from *dose rate*, which refers to output of the machine during radiation therapy. Dose rate certainly has an effect on lung tolerance: Radiation delivered as 5 cGy/minute is less damaging than radiation delivered at 30 cGy/minute, which in turn is less damaging than radiation delivered at 2 to 3 Gy/minute. The incidence and severity of radiation damage to the lungs thus are related principally to the volume of lung tissue irradiated, the total dose, the fractions into which the total dose is divided, and the quality of the radiation.

Genetic factors also influence the severity of response to lung irradiation in animals[23] and presumably may do so in humans as well, although there is no current method to evaluate this clinically.

HISTOPATHOLOGY

The histopathologic changes of radiation-induced pulmonary toxicity can be divided into early, intermediate, and late stages based on the time course and intensity of the radiation injury.[24] Early radiation damage (0 to 2 months after irradiation) is characterized by injury to small vessels and capillaries and subsequent development of vascular congestion and increased capillary permeability.[25] At this stage, a fibrin-rich exudate is present in the alveolar spaces. Hyaline membranes form on the alveoli, probably from condensation of the intraalveolar fibrin. After 1 month, an inflammatory infiltrate also is present, which may lead to a second course of increased permeability.[26] Abnormalities in the intermediate stage (2 to 9 months after irradiation) are characterized by obstruction of pulmonary capillaries by platelets, fibrin, and collagen. Alveolar-lining cells (primarily type II pneumonocytes) become hyperplastic, and the alveolar walls become infiltrated with fibroblasts and mast cells.[27] If the radiation injury is mild, these changes may subside entirely; however, when the injury is severe, a chronic phase (9 months or longer after irradiation) ensues that may persist or progress for months or years. In animal models, there is marked activation of genes that encode fibrillar collagens.[8] The histopathologic appearance then is dominated by dense fibrosis, thickening of the alveolar walls, vascular subintimal fibrosis, and luminal narrowing. In some instances, the lung may shrink to less than half its original size, with a thickened adherent pleura and scarred hilar structures.

In addition to this classic pattern of radiation pneumonitis, another syndrome of out-of-field pneumonitis, characterized by a hypersensitivity pneumonitis in areas of lung not directly irradiated, has been described. This syndrome, which occurs in a minority of patients, is characterized by a bilateral lymphocytic alveolitis of activated CD4+ T lymphocytes 4 to 6 weeks after strictly unilateral lung irradiation.[28]

CLINICAL FEATURES

Signs and Symptoms

The clinical syndrome of radiation pneumonitis develops in 5% to 15% of patients receiving high-dose external-beam radiation for treatment of lung cancer. Factors that can add to the development of radiation pneumonitis include concomitant chemotherapy, previous irradiation, and withdrawal of steroids. The incidence of radiation pneumonitis does not differ significantly between the young and the elderly, but the pneumonitis is inclined to be more severe in the latter group.[29] Underlying chronic obstructive pulmonary disease does not appear to potentiate radiation damage.

Symptoms of acute radiation pneumonitis usually become evident 2 to 3 months after the completion of therapy; rarely, they occur within the first month and, occasionally, as late as 6 months after irradiation. In general, the early onset of symptoms implies a more serious and more protracted clinical course. The cardinal symptom of radiation pneumonitis is dyspnea.[24] It may be self-limited or may progress to severe respiratory distress, depending on the extent and intensity of the injury. Patients may also have a nonproductive cough or a cough productive of small amounts of pinkish sputum. Frank hemoptysis early in the clinical course is distinctly uncommon; however, massive hemoptysis has been reported as a late complication of therapeutic pulmonary irradiation.[30] Fever is unusual but can be high and spiking; in severe cases, other constitutional symptoms may occur. Chest pain, which is rarely a prominent feature, may be due to fractured ribs, pleural changes, or coughing. Symptoms of airway obstruction can occur in the first few days of radiation therapy and usually are associated with swelling of a central bronchogenic carcinoma. Severe respiratory distress can result and may be prevented by the administration of steroids the day before and several days after the initiation of radiation therapy. Hemoptysis and other manifestations of radiation pneumonitis may also occur in patients given palliative endobronchial brachytherapy[31] or after surgical implantation of radioactive seeds.

On physical examination, signs of pulmonary involvement are minimal. Occasionally, moist rales, a pleural friction rub, or evidence of pleural fluid may be heard over the area of irradiation. In severe cases, tachypnea and cyanosis may be present and, occasionally, evidence of acute cor pulmonale appears, usually predicting a fatal outcome. Finger clubbing due to radiation is distinctly unusual and, if present, is most likely caused by the underlying malignancy. Skin changes corresponding to the ports of irradiation often are present but provide no clue as to the presence or severity of the pulmonary reaction beneath.

Although patients with acute pneumonitis may show complete resolution of signs and symptoms, most develop gradual, progressive fibrosis. In some cases, patients present with radiation fibrosis without a previous history of acute pneumonitis. The permanent changes of fibrosis evolve over 6 to 24 months but usually remain stable after 2 years. Patients with fibrosis may be asymptomatic or may have varying degrees of dyspnea. The major complications of radiation pneumonitis occur late in the disease and are secondary to persistent fibrosis of a large volume of lung. These include cor pulmonale and respiratory failure.

Diagnostic Imaging

Although radiographic abnormalities invariably are found concurrently with clinical radiation pneumonitis, these changes may be seen in asymptomatic patients as well. Early radiographic changes include a ground-glass opacification, diffuse haziness, or indistinct normal pulmonary markings over the irradiated area.[32] Later, the chest radiograph may show alveolar infiltrates or dense consolidation with or without air bronchograms. As the pneumonitis progresses to fibrosis, the radiographic appearance changes to that of linear streaks radiating from the area of pneumonitis and of contraction toward the hilar, the perimediastinal, or the apical areas. Pleural effusions, if present, are usually small and always coincident with the pneumonitis.[33] They can persist for long periods but often disappear spontaneously and never increase over a period of stability unless secondary complications occur, such as radiation-induced pericarditis. Mediastinal or hilar adenopathy and cavitation are almost always attributable to causes other than radiation pneumonitis.[2] Pneumothorax occasionally is associated with radiation fibrosis but not with acute pneumonitis.

One of the most characteristic features of radiation pneumonitis and fibrosis is that the radiologic changes are confined to the outlines of the field of radiation. In a few cases, extensive changes outside the field, even in the contralateral lung, have been observed. This syndrome of out-of-field pneumonitis is thought to represent a hypersensitivity response to the radiation.[34] Other possible explanations for this phenomenon include obstruction of lymphatic flow from radiation-induced mediastinal fibrosis[35] and absorption of x-rays by regions outside the irradiated ports.[36]

Some data suggest that computed tomographic scans of the chest and gallium 67 citrate imaging are more sensitive than chest radiography in the detection of radiation changes.[37,38] Correlation of abnormalities seen in these tests with the development of physiologic dysfunction and clinical toxicity requires clarification.

Pulmonary Function Tests

No gross physiologic changes occur in the lung until 4 to 8 weeks after completion of irradiation, usually coincident with the period of clinical pneumonitis. Then, one sees a decrease in lung volumes, which can progress.[39–42] These changes persist indefinitely, with little evidence of recovery.[41] Gas exchange abnormalities, which include a decrease in diffusing capacity and arterial hypoxemia, especially with exercise, occur about the same time but show some tendency toward recovery after 6 to 12 months.[40–42] A fall in compliance coincident with the clinical pneumonitis is seen in most subjects.[40] Accordingly, the elastic work of breathing is increased, and dyspnea, a result of the increased workload, ensues.[40] Air flow parameters remain nearly normal in most studies.[39–42]

DIAGNOSIS

The diagnosis of radiation pneumonitis can sometimes be made clinically on the basis of the timing of irradiation in relation to symptoms and the typical chest radiographic appearance (i.e., infiltrates corresponding to the margins of the irradiated portal). Differentiation from recurrent malignancy or infection often poses a problem, and then lung biopsy is necessary. Although histopathologic changes are nonspecific for radiation pneumonitis, when elements of the acute stages (fibrin exudate in the alveoli) are seen adjacent to the more chronic stages (alveolar fibrosis and subintimal sclerosis),[43] this entity can be diagnosed with reasonable certainty.

Biochemical markers that indicate radiation lung injury before the onset of clinical pathologic events would be valuable in the early diagnosis and management of patients with radiation toxicity. In irradiated animals, studies demonstrate that surfactant found in the serum may be a marker and predictor for later radiation pneumonitis.[44] Prospective studies are needed in humans to identify the sensitivity and specificity of monitoring serum surfactant levels as an early means of diagnosing clinical radiation toxicity. Though no standard tests currently are used to monitor patients for radiation pneumonitis (because most methods have little predictive value), some reports suggest that soluble intercellular adhesion molecule-1[45] or transforming growth factor-β[46] may be good candidates.

TREATMENT

Three treatment modalities have been used, prophylactically and therapeutically, for radiation-induced pneumonitis: corticosteroids, antibiotics, and anticoagulants. Of these, corticosteroid therapy is the most important.

Corticosteroid administration during irradiation in mice markedly improves the physiologic abnormalities and decreases mortality,[47,48] without exerting an effect on late pulmonary fibrosis.[49] No controlled clinical trials are available of the efficacy of steroid therapy in radiation pneumonitis in humans. Rubin and Casarett[2] collected data from eight studies on humans and categorized them according to whether corticosteroids were used prophylactically or therapeutically. Corticosteroids given prophylactically failed to prevent radiation pneumonitis but, when administered as clinical pneumonitis occurred, these agents prompted an objective response. In other reports, steroid therapy failed to ameliorate severe pneumonitis. Nonetheless, our practice is to begin prednisone, 1 mg/kg, as soon as the diagnosis is reasonably certain. The initial dose is maintained for several weeks and then reduced cautiously and slowly. It has been our experience that if steroids are tapered too rapidly, symptoms can be exacerbated, necessitating higher doses for longer periods. Similarly, if corticosteroids are part of a recent chemotherapeutic regimen, stopping them abruptly can precipitate clinically evident radiation pneumonitis. Which parameters, if any, to follow during the tapering schedule are not known, and no studies are available. Generally, decisions are based on the symptoms. Most authors agree that corticosteroids have no place in the treatment of radiation fibrosis.

In experimental and clinical reports, antibiotic administration has no effect on the course or outcome of radiation pneumonitis.[2,50] Although there is some rationale for the use of anticoagulants in view of the effects of irradiation on the vascular system, neither heparin injections nor oral anticoagulants have been found to be beneficial.[50] Captopril has been shown to be effective in animal studies,[51] but no human trials have been reported. The mechanism of action of captopril in this setting probably is not its inhibition of angiotensin-converting enzyme.[52] Pentoxifylline also has some effects on the late phase of pneumonitis in animal models.[53]

RADIATION-RELATED BRONCHIOLITIS OBLITERANS WITH ORGANIZING PNEUMONIA

Although bronchiolitis obliterans with organizing pneumonia (BOOP) is an unusual histopathologic pattern for drug-induced lung injury, radiation damage resulting in BOOP has been reported.[54] Patients with lung cancer usually receive the highest doses of radiation to the largest volume of lung tissue, which makes them more susceptible to radiation injury as compared with other patients receiving irradiation. Most of the cases of radiation-related BOOP, however, have occurred in patients receiving radiation to the breast. Whether the low dose or indirect radiation that these patients receive makes them more susceptible to this type of lung injury is not known. Besides the unusual pathologic pattern in these irradiated patients, clinical and radiologic differences are evident, as compared to conventional radiation pneumonitis. Whereas dyspnea is the hallmark of radiation-induced lung injury, fever and cough are the predominant features of radiation-related BOOP. Radiographically, the infiltrates can begin in the radiated areas but always progress outside the portal and, in approximately 40% of the cases, the radiographic abnormalities were observed on the side contralateral to the irradiated breast. Although patients respond dramatically to corticosteroid therapy with no obvious evidence of residual damage, there is a 67% relapse rate when the drug is tapered or discontinued. As with conventional radiation-induced pneumonitis, no studies are available on the minimal effective dose or duration of therapy but, in view of the high relapse rate, it seems prudent to taper corticosteroid therapy very slowly, with meticulous vigilance for clinical signs of relapse.

To spare the lung the toxic effects of chemotherapy, several unique treatment modalities are now being investigated. These include isolated lung perfusion (one or both lungs) with doxorubicin for either metastatic disease or bronchoalveolar carcinoma. In one study, six patients received the perfusate and, although no major responses were observed, the patients tolerated the procedure well and five of the six did not have any serious complications.[19] Antitumor efficacy in mice and dogs has been observed with inhaled chemotherapeutic agents[20]; clinical human testing now is under way in patients with metastatic lung disease using doxorubicin via nebulization.

CHEMOTHERAPY-INDUCED PULMONARY TOXICITY

The list of chemotherapeutic agents reported to cause cytotoxic drug-induced lung disease continues to grow (Table 55.3-1). Recently added agents are docetaxel and gemcitabine. An overview of the potential mechanisms of lung damage, a summary of the pathologic findings, and common clinical features of pulmonary toxicity are discussed in this section. Characteristics of pulmonary disease caused by some of these drugs are presented.

TABLE 55.3-1. Chemotherapeutic Agents Associated with Pulmonary Parenchymal Disease

ALKYLATING AGENTS
Busulfan
Cyclophosphamide
Chlorambucil
Melphalan
NITROSOUREAS
Carmustine (BCNU)
Lomustine (CCNU)
Semustine (methyl-CCNU)
Chlorozotocin (DCNU)
ANTIBIOTICS
Bleomycin
Mitomycin
Neocarzinostatin (zinostatin)
ANTIMETABOLITES
Methotrexate
Azathioprine
Mercaptopurine
Cytosine arabinoside
Gemcitabine
MISCELLANEOUS
Procarbazine
Vinblastine
Vindesine
VM-26
Retinoic acid
Etoposide
Paclitaxel

BCNU, bischloroethylnitrosourea; VM-26, teniposide.

MECHANISMS OF PULMONARY INJURY

The details of the pathophysiology of specific chemotherapeutic agents, except for bleomycin, generally are not known; however, several mechanisms of pulmonary toxicity mediated by these agents have been proposed. Certain cytotoxic drugs may induce pulmonary injury by triggering the formation of reactive oxygen metabolites, including the superoxide anion,[55] hydrogen peroxide, and hydroxyl radicals, primarily from activated neutrophils. Bleomycin induces reactive oxygen radicals by forming a complex with Fe^{3+}. Consistent with a direct pathologic role for this mechanism, iron chelators ameliorate the pulmonary toxicity of bleomycin in animal models.[56] Reactive oxygen species can produce direct toxicity through participation in redox reactions and subsequent fatty acid oxidation, which leads to membrane instability.[57] Oxidants can cause other inflammatory reactions within the lung. For example, the oxidation of arachidonic acid is an initial step in the metabolic cascade that produces immunologically active mediators, including prostaglandins and leukotrienes.[58] Cytokines such as interleukin-1, macrophage inflammatory protein-1 (MIP-1), monocyte chemoattractant protein-1 (MCP-1), and TGF-β are released from alveolar macrophages in animal models of bleomycin toxicity.[55,59–61] Cytotoxic drugs may also affect the local immune system. Because the lung is exposed to so many substances that can activate its immune system, there appears to be a pulmonary immune tolerance state to avoid unnecessary overreactions.[62] This tolerance state may, in part, be a result of effector and suppressor cell balance.

Cytotoxic drugs can alter the normal effector and suppressor balance, which may cause tissue damage.[63–65] Other homeostatic systems within the lung can be affected as well, such as the balance between collagen formation and collagenolysis.[62] Through modulation of fibroblast proliferation and phenotype,[66] excessive collagen deposition may result in severe, irreversible pulmonary fibrosis. Bleomycin is one cytotoxic agent that has this potential.[67–69] In addition, bleomycin may up-regulate collagen synthesis in fibroblasts by stimulating transcription directly through a TGF-β response element in the procollagen (I)α promoter as well as by an autocrine loop involving extracellular release of TGF-β.[69] Mast cells may also be involved in the inflammatory and fibrotic process.[70] Imbalance between the protease and antiprotease system has been implicated as well in a number of pulmonary disorders, including drug toxicities.[62] Bleomycin and cyclophosphamide produce substances that can inactivate the antiprotease system, enhancing the effects of proteolytic enzymes on the lung. Bleomycin also causes profound effects on the fibrinolytic system, altering the balance between fibrin deposition and fibrinolysis on the alveolar surface, leading to fibrin deposition.[71] Drugs may damage the lung through a variety of other mechanisms, and considerable investigation should be done to define and clarify the exact mechanism of lung injury for each chemotherapeutic drug.

One of the potential determinants of bleomycin toxicity is the cytoplasmic cysteine proteinase bleomycin hydrolase, which is the major enzyme responsible for metabolizing bleomycin to a nontoxic molecule.[72] In animal models, bleomycin hydrolase knockout mice are highly susceptible to bleomycin toxicity.[73] The two organs that are the most common targets for bleomycin toxicity—lung and skin—harbor the lowest levels of the enzyme.[74] With the cloning of the human gene encoding bleomycin hydrolase,[75] studies are needed to determine whether genetic variability of this enzyme can account for increased individual susceptibility to bleomycin pulmonary toxicity.

HISTOPATHOLOGY

The histopathologic changes of drug-induced pulmonary toxicity demonstrate common features. Similar to radiation-induced damage, abnormalities are seen in endothelial and epithelial cells. The vascular damage is characterized by endothelial swelling with exudation of fluid into the interstitium and the intraalveolar spaces. There is destruction and desquamation of type I pneumonocytes, with proliferation of type II pneumocytes. Mononuclear cell infiltration and fibroblast proliferation with fibrosis are common findings; the character of the inflammatory cellular infiltrate may be a feature that distinguishes the toxicity of one drug from another. Bronchoalveolar lavage studies in patients with methotrexate pulmonary toxicity have shown the presence of a T-lymphocytic alveolitis, whereas studies on some patients with bleomycin toxicity have revealed a polymorphonuclear alveolitis.[63,76] Eosinophil infiltration has been associated with drugs that cause apparent hypersensitivity reactions, such as methotrexate, procarbazine, and bleomycin.[62,63,77,78]

CLINICAL FEATURES

Table 55.3-2 lists predisposing factors associated with enhancement of drug-induced pneumonitis.[79–99] Because bleomycin toxicity is relatively common, it warrants special mention. Although it drastically increases with doses in excess of 450 to 500 mg, toxicity can occur with much lower doses, especially when other risk factors are present. One study described 9 of 45 patients (20%) who developed lung toxicity when they received bleomycin after cisplatin infusion.[95] Renal damage after cisplatin administration, with subsequent accumulation of bleomycin, was a likely cause of the high pulmonary toxicity and mortality rate of 67%. Extreme caution is recommended in the administration of combined bleomycin and cisplatin chemotherapy; if possible, bleomycin should precede cisplatin infusion to minimize the risk of lung toxicity. Some data suggest that continuous infusion of bleomycin may be associated with less pulmonary toxicity than bolus therapy[96]; however, these data are inconclusive, and further studies are warranted. Supplemental oxygen is a classic cofactor in bleomycin pulmonary toxicity.[97] An increased risk of pulmonary toxicity (4 of 12 patients, fatal in 75%) was described in a small, uncontrolled study of patients receiving granulocyte colony-stimulating factor in combination with bleomycin-containing combination chemotherapy [BACOP (bleomycin, Adriamycin, cyclophosphamide, Oncovin, prednisone)] for non-Hodgkin's lymphoma.[98] However, larger studies have not confirmed any increased risk of bleomycin toxicity with the use of granulocyte colony-stimulating factor.[99]

The interest in administration of several cycles of high-dose chemotherapy followed by peripheral stem cell rescue for treatment of breast cancer and lymphoma has led to reports of pulmonary toxicity of agents not previously thought to be highly toxic to the lung, such as etoposide.[100] Importantly, careful studies of pulmonary function after high-dose chemotherapy containing cyclophosphamide, cisplatin, and carmustine [1,3-Bis(2 chloroethyl)-1-nitrosourea (BCNU)], followed by autologous bone marrow transplant, for treatment of breast cancer show a delayed drop in diffusing capacity averaging 30% by week 18.[101] The majority of patients were symptomatic with dyspnea and responded well to systemic corticosteroids.[101] More of this type of toxicity can be anticipated in the future as this treatment modality becomes more common and new regimens for high-dose chemotherapy are studied.

Long intervals between drug administration and onset of clinical toxicity have been described. Late-onset pulmonary fibrosis has been reported many years after discontinuing cyclophosphamide[102] and carmustine.[103]

Signs and Symptoms

The cardinal symptom of drug-induced pulmonary toxicity is dyspnea. Nonproductive cough, fatigue, and malaise are other commonly associated complaints. Other characteristics of chemotherapy-induced pulmonary disease are outlined in Table 55.3-3. Although symptoms usually develop over a period of several weeks to months, hypersensitivity drug-induced lung disease can develop over hours. Fever may be a common finding with this type of toxicity. Chest pain has been reported during infusion of bleomycin[104] or immediately after therapy with methotrexate[105]; however, it is an unusual manifestation of toxicity. A syndrome of

TABLE 55.3-2. Factors Associated with Increased Risk of Drug-Induced Pneumonitis

Risk Factor	*Drugs*
Total dose	Bleomycin,[79,80] carmustine[89]
Age	Bleomycin,[80] carmustine[130]
Oxygen therapy	Bleomycin,[81–83,97–99] cyclophosphamide,[82] mitomycin[84]
Simultaneous or prior radiation therapy to lungs	Bleomycin,[85,86] busulfan,[87] mitomycin[88]
Increased toxicity when given with other drugs	Carmustine,[89] mitomycin,[90] cyclophosphamide,[92] bleomycin,[92,93] methotrexate,[91] etoposide[100]
Preexisting pulmonary disease	Carmustine[94]

TABLE 55.3-3. Characteristics of Pulmonary Disease Caused by Commonly Used Chemotherapeutic Agents

Drug	*Mechanics of Injury*	*Histopathology*	*Clinical Features*	*Chest Roentgenogram*	*Diagnosis*	*Treatment*
ALKYLATING AGENTS						
Busulfan (Myleran)[79,87,110,130–135]	No studies, but direct toxicity to epithelial lining cells is suggested	Pneumocyte dysplasia (degeneration of type I cells; atypical hyperplastic type II cells), atypical bronchial lining cells, mononuclear cell infiltration, fibrosis	Incidence, 4%; no direct dose-dependent toxicity; may be threshold dose (>500 mg); radiation and other alkylating agents may enhance toxicity insidious onset after 4 y (8 mo to 10 y). May contribute to toxicity after bone marrow transplant. Dyspnea, cough, weight loss, weakness, fever, crepitant basilar rales, pigmentation. Poor prognosis.	Most commonly bibasilar reticular pattern; rarely pleural effusion, pulmonary ossification, normal chest radiograph	Suggested by history and bizarre pneumocytes in sputum or lavage fluid. Definitive diagnosis by open lung biopsy.	Withdrawal of the drug; anecdotal reports of improvement with high-dose steroids. Mean survival after diagnosis, 5 mo.
Cyclophosphamide (Cytoxan)[79,82,127,136–139]	May be toxic through production of reactive oxygen species	Endothelial swelling, pneumocyte dysplasia, lymphocytic and histiocytic infiltration, fibrosis	Incidence, <1%; does not appear dose-dependent, but synergy with oxygen and other agents possible. Subacute onset 3 wk to 8 y after therapy discontinued. Cough, dyspnea, fever; basilar rales.	Commonly, basilar reticular pattern; diffuse pulmonary edema pattern also reported	Suggested by history and bizarre pneumocytes in sputum or lavage fluid. Definitive diagnosis by open lung biopsy.	Drug withdrawal; corticosteroids may hasten improvement but have no documented effect on mortality. Overall recovery, approximately 65%.
Chlorambucil[62,140]	Unknown	Similar to busulfan; fibrosis may predominate	Rare reports; subacute onset 6 mo to 3 y after therapy. Cough, dyspnea, anorexia; bibasilar rales.	Bibasilar reticular pattern; rarely, alveolar infiltrates not reported	Suggested by history and bizarre pneumocytes in sputum or lavage fluid. Definitive diagnosis by open lung biopsy.	Half of reported patients died despite cessation of drug and administration of steroids. Anecdotal reports of response to steroids.
Melphalan (Alkeran)[62,141,142]	Unknown	Similar to busulfan; pneumocyte dysplasia more common than fibrosis	Rare (five documented reports); appears 1 to 48 mo after therapy. Progressive dyspnea, productive cough, fever, malaise; bibasilar rales.	Reticular and alveolar infiltrates	Suggested by history and bizarre pneumocytes in sputum or lavage fluid. Definitive diagnosis by open lung biopsy.	Despite cessation of drug, three of five patients reported died of disease. In most cases, patients were receiving steroids for underlying disease.
ANTIBIOTICS						
Bleomycin[62,67–72,114,115,118,120,122,124,143–150]	Several possible mechanisms: (1) Direct toxicity through generation of reactive oxygen; (2) activation of metabolites, alveolar fibrin deposition; (3) leukocyte influx and lung injury from release of proteases; (4) increased synthesis directly and via TGF-β release	Endothelial blebbing; interstitial edema, necrosis of type I cells and metaplastic type II cells; inflammation with polymorphonuclear cells; fibroblast proliferation and fibrosis; occasionally, collagen eosinophilic infiltration	Incidence, 2% to 4%; age- and dose-related; synergy seen with oxygen therapy, radiation, and other agents. Occurs during and shortly after stopping therapy. Cough, dyspnea, fever; tachypnea, crepitant rales. Hypersensitivity pneumonitis variant.	Bibasilar reticular pattern; multiple nodules similar to metastatic disease; acinar pattern, especially with hypersensitivity reaction; rarely, localized infiltrate and cavitary nodules	Bronchoalveolar lavage might suggest diagnosis (polymorphonuclear alveolitis). Transbronchial or open lung biopsy required for diagnosis, especially to rule out other causes.	Drug withdrawal. In bleomycin hypersensitivity reactions, definite role for steroids; in other forms of bleomycin toxicity, efficacy less clear. Mortality estimated at 50% for latter forms.
Mitomycin[62,88,90,106,151–153]	Neutrophilia, alveolar macrophage activation and cytokine release	Similar to bleomycin in patients with microangiopathic hemolytic anemia, prominent vascular changes are present	Incidence, 3% to 12%; does not appear dose-related, but possible synergy with oxygen, radiation, and other agents. Dry cough, dyspnea; fever not seen; bibasilar rales. Acute dyspnea reaction in combination with vinca alkaloids.	Diffuse reticular pattern; pleural effusions seen; may be normal	Clinical picture suggestive; lung biopsy for definitive diagnosis.	Drug withdrawal; steroids may alter outcome. Mortality approaches 50%.
NITROSOUREAS[a]						
Carmustine (BCNU)[89,94,125,157–160]	Few studies; direct injury through generation of toxic oxidant molecules possible	Similar to bleomycin; fibrosis predominates	Incidence, 20% to 30%; dose-related; increased risk with preexisting lung disease and tobacco use; possible synergism with other agents; can be seen up to 17 y after drug is stopped. Dry cough, dyspnea, bibasilar rales.	Bibasilar reticular pattern; >10-y posttreatment peripheral fibrosis pattern in upper lung zones; may be normal	Lung biopsy for definitive diagnosis; no bronchoalveolar lavage studies reported.	Recognition and withdrawal of the drug; steroids not beneficial if patient already on steroids for intracranial processes when toxicity develops. Mortality reported between 24% and 90%. Steroids possibly beneficial acutely, after high-dose treatment.

TABLE 55.3-3 (Continued)

Drug	Mechanics of Injury	Histopathology	Clinical Features	Chest Roentgenogram	Diagnosis	Treatment
ANTIMETABOLITES						
Methotrexate[62,63,79,91,105,111]	Direct toxic effect may play a role, but mechanism not known; hypersensitivity suggested by occurrence of eosinophils and presence of increased T lymphocytes in lavage fluid	Interstitial and alveolar infiltration of lymphocytes, eosinophils, and plasma cells; occasionally, poorly formed, noncaseating granuloma; fibrosis unusual	Incidence, 8%; synergism with other agents possible; occurs 12 d to 18 y after beginning therapy. Fever, chills, malaise, headache a prodrome for days and weeks; cough, dyspnea, rales common. Skin rash in 17%, and blood eosinophilia in 40%.	Early interstitial infiltrates; later, alveolar infiltrates; hilar and mediastinal adenopathy, pleural effusions described; chest radiograph possibly normal	Clinical history suggestive; bronchoalveolar lavage might suggest diagnosis (increased T cells required for diagnosis).	Discontinue drug, but reports of reinstitution without recurrence of the abnormality. Dramatic responses to steroids reported. Mortality 1% looks favorable.
Cytosine arabinoside[161,162]	Unknown	Pulmonary edema; proteinaceous exudate with extravasation of red blood cells, no inflammatory cells	Abrupt onset of dyspnea; gastrointestinal toxicity coexists.	Diffuse interstitial and alveolar pattern	Clinical picture suggests diagnosis.	Supportive; no studies.
Gemcitabine[163]	Unknown	Rare reports—diffuse alveolar damage; findings resemble adult respiratory distress syndrome	Does not appear dose-dependent; dyspnea may be severe and progress to respiratory failure, chest tightness; dry cough.	Diffuse interstitial pulmonary infiltrates	Clinical suspicion; other causes should be excluded.	Drug withdrawal; corticosteroids.
MISCELLANEOUS						
Procarbazine (Matulane)[77,112,164]	Hypersensitivity	Mononuclear cell scattered foci of eosinophils; fibrosis in one case	Acute onset within hours to days of first dose. Nausea, fevers, chills, arthralgias, urticaria, dry cough, and dyspnea. Blood eosinophilia common.[6]	Interstitial infiltrates; pleural effusion	Clinical picture highly suggestive of diagnosis.	Rapid recovery after discontinuation of drug. Role of steroids not known.
Vinca alkaloids (vinblastine and vindesine)[90,106,126,165,166]	Unknown	Dysplasia of alveolar lining cells; interstitial and alveolar influx of inflammatory cells; fibrosis	Acute dyspnea during or shortly after the infusion, especially when given in combination with mitomycin. Wheezing may be prominent.	Diffuse interstitial and alveolar infiltrates with combination drugs; may be normal; normal chest radiograph with vinca alkaloid alone	Clinical history suggests diagnosis.	Drug withdrawal; steroids probably beneficial. Prognosis poor if pulmonary infiltrates develop.
Etoposide (VP-16)[100,167,168]	Unknown	Alveolar hemorrhage	Case report of fatal toxicity after oral use, after high-dose chemotherapy with bone marrow or stem cell transplant for breast cancer.	Interstitial and alveolar pattern; may be localized	Clinical picture suggestive.	Discontinue drug; some responses to steroids.
Paclitaxel (Taxol)[169]	Two types of reaction:					
	(1) Anaphylactoid hypersensitivity (AH): direct mast cell activation with histamine release	—	AH: Incidence, 3% to 10%; erythematous rash, urticaria, hypotension, dyspnea with or without bronchospasm in close proximity to infusion; rare reports and few data, no dose dependency known.	Normal chest radiograph	Clinical picture highly suggestive.	Slow infusion; pretreatment with corticosteroids; H_1 and H_2 histamine blockers.
	(2) Hypersensitivity pneumonitis (HP): mechanism not known; may be due to release of histamine or other vasoactive	—	HP: Dyspnea and/or cough several days to weeks after treatment; fever may occur; crepitant rales may be present.	Patchy reticular or nodular infiltrates	Clinical picture should raise suspicion; other causes (e.g., infection, progression of disease) should be excluded.	Can resolve on its own; if severe, corticosteroids; may not recur with rechallenge.

[a]Pulmonary toxicity has been reported with all other nitrosoureas, including lomustine (CCNU), semustine (methyl-CCNU), and chlorozotocin (DCNU).[154–156]

acute dyspnea, probably due to acute direct toxicity to the pulmonary vasculature, can occur during or shortly after vinca alkaloid infusion when given in combination with mitomycin for treatment of non–small cell lung cancer.[106] Because hemoptysis is an uncommon feature of drug-induced pulmonary toxicity, when it is present, other diagnoses should be considered. Physical examination of the lungs may be normal or may reveal end-inspiratory "Velcro" rales. Finger clubbing is distinctly unusual, but it may be related to the underlying malignancy.

All-*trans*-retinoic acid treatment of acute promyelocytic leukemia induces a distinct syndrome of respiratory distress, which are thought to be mediated by newly differentiated leukemia cells that are marginating into the pulmonary circulation, thereby increasing capillary permeability and releasing cytokines that induce neutrophil migration into the interstitium. High doses of corticosteroids are the most effective treatment.[107] Steroid prophylaxis of this syndrome has been reported to be useful.[108]

Paclitaxel (Taxol) and Docetaxel (Taxotere) cause bronchospasm and, in some cases, frank anaphylaxis or pulmonary edema, probably on the basis of a hypersensitivity reaction to the solvent needed to dissolve these agents. Prophylaxis with corticosteroids, administration of H_1 and H_2 histamine blockers, and slowing of the infusion rate are effective in reducing the incidence and severity of these reactions.

Diagnostic Imaging

The most common radiographic abnormality associated with drug-induced pulmonary toxicity is a reticulonodular pattern, which may be basilar or diffuse. Pleural effusions are uncommon but have occasionally been reported in association with mitomycin, busulfan, methotrexate, and procarbazine toxicity.[109–112] Hypersensitivity lung disease associated with methotrexate and procarbazine may present with bilateral acinar infiltrates that clear rapidly.[112] In some instances, the chest radiograph is normal, even in the presence of histologically proved pulmonary infiltration and fibrosis.[111,113] Most commonly, methotrexate and carmustine toxicity have been reported with normal chest radiographic findings. Hilar adenopathy is distinctly unusual and has been reported only with methotrexate toxicity.[111] Nodules with or without cavitation, simulating metastatic disease, have been seen with bleomycin toxicity.[114,115]

Both high-resolution, thin-section computed tomographic chest scans and gallium scintigraphy have been shown to be more sensitive techniques than chest radiography for detecting pulmonary parenchymal changes in association with drug toxicity.[116,117] Scintigraphy with technetium 99 aerosols appears to be highly sensitive for subtle capillary permeability defects in bleomycin toxicity.[118] The full relation of these changes to the development of functional or physiologic impairment is unclear, and further studies are needed. Magnetic resonance spectrometry may eventually be useful to differentiate among fibrosis, edema, and hemorrhage in the lung but, at present, it is not helpful in diagnosing interstitial lung disorders such as drug toxicity.[119]

Pulmonary Function Tests

The most common abnormalities associated with chemotherapy-induced pulmonary toxicity are a reduced diffusing capacity for carbon monoxide and a restrictive ventilatory defect.[62] Isolated gas transport abnormalities, manifested by a decrease in the diffusing capacity or arterial hypoxemia, especially with exercise, have been seen. Screening pulmonary function tests to predict which patients receiving chemotherapy are likely to develop toxicity would be helpful but have not been established for most pulmonary toxic agents. In bleomycin toxicity, changes in the diffusing capacity may be transient, whereas decreases in total lung capacity seem to correlate better with radiographic abnormalities.[120]

DIAGNOSIS

Although one might have a high clinical suspicion of drug-induced pulmonary toxicity, lung biopsy is usually necessary for a definitive diagnosis. Because pathognomonic pathologic changes associated with drug-induced pneumonitis often are not present, a biopsy is necessary to eliminate other specific diagnoses, such as opportunistic infection and malignancy. Through the use of bronchoalveolar lavage, several studies reported the presence of a characteristic or predominant cell associated with particular drugs.[63,76] Although these data might be of value in understanding the pathogenesis of drug-induced lung disorders, their usefulness in diagnosing drug toxicity is limited.

A serum marker for drug-induced pulmonary toxicity would be very useful. Though such a serum marker does not currently exist, initial studies of serum collagen type III N-propeptide in patients receiving neoadjuvant preoperative mitomycin, vinblastine, and cisplatin for stage III non–small cell lung cancer appear promising.[121] This peptide is elevated in serum after bleomycin treatment, but it does not correlate with toxicity.[122] Elevated levels of TGF-β in plasma after high-dose chemotherapy for breast cancer predicted an increased risk of pulmonary toxicity after autologous bone marrow transplantation.[123]

TREATMENT

The most effective way to manage pulmonary toxicity associated with chemotherapeutic agents is to prevent it. Animal studies of bleomycin toxicity showed a beneficial preventive effect of dietary supplementation with taurine and niacin; no comparable human studies have been reported. If toxicity occurs, withdrawal of the offending agent is the cornerstone of therapy. Although no controlled studies in humans have systematically examined the efficacy of corticosteroids, a trial of these agents probably is warranted in most cases.[124,125] The optimal dose and duration of therapy are not known; however, 1 mg/kg/d usually is initiated, with a slow and careful tapering schedule, because clinical deterioration after tapering has been reported.[126,127] One report described the case of a 23-year-old male patient who underwent a single lung transplantation because of presumed drug-induced pulmonary fibrosis 12 years after undergoing chemotherapy for acute lymphocytic leukemia.[128] The use of lung transplantation in the treatment of advanced drug-induced pulmonary fibrosis should be considered in appropriate patients, as more experience with successful lung transplantation in this setting is accumulating.[129]

REFERENCES

1. Gross NJ. The pathogenesis of radiation-induced lung damage. *Lung* 1981;159:115.
2. Rubin P, Casarett GW. *Clinical radiation pathology.* Philadelphia: WB Saunders, 1968.

3. Adamison ILR, Bowden DH, Wyatt JP. A pathway to pulmonary fibrosis: an ultrastructural study of mouse and rat following radiation to the whole body and hemithorax. *Am J Pathol* 1970;58:481.
4. Haimovitz-Friedman A, Kan CC, Ehleiter D, et al. Ionizing radiation acts on cellular membranes to generate ceramide and initiate apoptosis. *J Exp Med* 1994;180:525.
5. Weichselbaum RR, Hallahan D, Fuks Z, et al. Radiation induction of immediate early genes: effectors of the radiation-stress response [Review]. *Int J Radiat Oncol Biol Phys* 1994;30:229.
6. Kharbanda S, Ren R, Pandey P, et al. Activation of the c-Abl tyrosine kinase in the stress response to DNA-damaging agents. *Nature* 1995;376:785.
7. Haimovitz-Friedman A, Vlodavsky I, Chaudhuri A, et al. Autocrine effects of fibroblast growth factor in repair of radiation damage in endothelial cells. *Cancer Res* 1991;51:2552.
8. Rubin P, Johnston CJ, Williams JP, et al. A perpetual cascade of cytokines postirradiation leads to pulmonary fibrosis. *Int J Radiat Oncol Biol Phys* 1995;33:99.
9. Tsao C, Tsao FH, Taylor JM, et al. Annexin I concentration, phospholipase activity and thromboxane synthesis in irradiated rat lung. *Radiat Res* 1995;142:85.
10. Kimsey FC, Mendenhall NP, Ewald LM, et al. Is radiation treatment volume a predictor for acute or late effect on pulmonary function? A prospective study of patients treated with breast-conserving surgery and postoperative irradiation. *Cancer* 1994;73:2549.
11. VanDyk J, Keane T, Kan S, et al. Radiation pneumonitis following large single dose irradiation: a reevaluation based on absolute lung dose. *Int J Radiat Oncol Biol Phys* 1981;31:361.
12. Jennings FL, Arden A. Development of radiation pneumonitis: time and dose factors. *Arch Pathol* 1962;74:351.
13. Christie DR, Spry NA, Lamb DS, et al. Artificial pneumothorax can be used to prevent lung toxicity in chest wall radiotherapy. *Clin Oncol* 1993;5:257.
14. Perez C, Stanley K, Grundy C, et al. Impact of irradiation technique and tumor extent in tumor control and survival of patients with unresectable non-oat cell carcinoma of the lung. *Cancer* 1982;50:1091.
15. Goitein M, Abrams M, Rowell D, et al. Multidimensional treatment planning: beam's eye view back projection through CT sections. *Int J Radiol Oncol Biol Phys* 1983;9:789.
16. Emami B, Purdy JA, Manolis J, et al. Three dimensional treatment planning for lung cancer. *Int J Radiat Oncol Biol Phys* 1991;21:217.
17. Armstrong JG. Three-dimensional conformal radiotherapy: precision treatment of lung cancer [Review]. *Chest Surg Clin N Am* 1994;4:29.
18. Ling CC, Fuks Z. Conformal radiation treatment: a critical appraisal [Review]. *Eur J Cancer* 1995;5:799.
19. Johnston MR, Minchen RF, Dawson CA. Lung perfusion with chemotherapy in patients with unresectable sarcoma to the lung or diffuse bronchioloalveolar carcinoma. *J Thorac Cardiovasc Surg* 1995;110:368.
20. Tatsumura T, Koyama S, Stujimoto M, et al. Further study of nebulization chemotherapy, a new chemotherapeutic method in the treatment of lung carcinoma: fundamental and clinical. *Br J Cancer* 1993;68:1146.
21. Wara WM, Phillips TL, Margolis LW, et al. Radiation pneumonitis: a new approach to the deviation of time dose factors. *Cancer* 1973;32:547.
22. Mah K, Dyk JV, Keane T, et al. Acute radiation-induced pulmonary damage: a clinical study on the response to fractionated radiation therapy. *Int J Radiat Oncol Biol Phys* 1987;13:179.
23. Franko AJ, Sharplin J, Ward WF, et al. The genetic basis of strain-dependent differences in the early phase of radiation injury in mouse lung. *Radiat Res* 1991;126:349.
24. Gross NJ. Pulmonary effects of radiation therapy. *Ann Intern Med* 1977;86:81.
25. Maisin JR. The ultrastructure of the lung of mice exposed to a supralethal dose of ionizing radiation on the thorax. *Radiat Res* 1970;44:545.
26. Rosiello RA, Merrill WW, Rockwell S, et al. Radiation pneumonitis: bronchoalveolar lavage assessment and modulation by a recombinant cytokine. *Am Rev Respir Dis* 1993;148:1671.
27. Ward HE, Kemsley L, Davies L, et al. The pulmonary response to sublethal thoracic irradiation in the rat. *Radiat Res* 1993;136:15.
28. Roberts C, Foulcher E, Zaunders J, et al. Radiation pneumonitis: a possible lymphocyte-mediated hypersensitivity reaction. *Ann Intern Med* 1993;118:696.
29. Koga K, Kusumoto S, Watanabe K, et al. Age factor relevant to the development of radiation pneumonitis in radiotherapy of lung cancer. *Int J Radiat Oncol* 1988;14:367.
30. Isaacs RD, Wallie WJ, Wells UE, et al. Massive hemoptysis as a late complication of pulmonary irradiation. *Thorax* 1987;42:77.
31. Gustafson G, Vicini F, Freedman L, et al. High dose rate endobronchial brachytherapy in the management of primary and recurrent bronchogenic malignancies. *Cancer* 1995;75:2345.
32. Bate D, Guttman RJ. Changes in lung and pleura following two-million-volt therapy for carcinoma of the breast. *Radiology* 1957;73:679.
33. Bachman AL, Macken K. Pleural effusions following supervoltage radiation for breast carcinoma. *Radiology* 1959;72:699.
34. Smith JC. Radiation pneumonitis: case report of bilateral reaction after unilateral irradiation. *Am Rev Respir Dis* 1964;89:264.
35. Holt JAG. The acute radiation pneumonitis syndrome. *J Coll Radiol Aust* 1964;8:40.
36. Bennett DE, Million RR, Ackerman LV. Bilateral radiation pneumonitis: a complication of the radiotherapy of bronchogenic carcinoma. *Cancer* 1969;23:1001.
37. Ikezoe J, Takashima S, Morimoto S, et al. CT appearance of acute radiation-induced injury in the lung. *AJR Am J Roentgenol* 1988;150:765.
38. Kataoka M. Gallium-67 imaging for the assessment of radiation pneumonitis. *Ann Nucl Med* 1989;3:73.
39. Brady LW, German PA, Cander L. The effects of radiation therapy on pulmonary function in carcinoma of the lung. *Radiology* 1965;85:130.
40. Emirgil C, Heinemann HO. Effects of radiation of the chest on pulmonary function in men. *J Appl Physiol* 1961;16:331.
41. Prato FS, Kurdyak R, Saibil EA, et al. Regional and total lung function in patients following pulmonary irradiation. *Invest Radiol* 1977;12:224.
42. Wohl MEB, Griscom NT, Traggis DC, et al. Effects of therapeutic irradiation delivered in early childhood upon subsequent lung function. *Pediatrics* 1975;55:507.
43. Warren S, Spencer J. Radiation reaction in the lung. *AJR Am J Roentgenol* 1940;43:682.
44. Rubin P, McDonald S, Maasilta P, et al. Serum markers for prediction of pulmonary radiation syndromes. *Int J Radiat Oncol Biol Phys* 1989;17:553.
45. Ishii Y, Kitamura S. Soluble intercellular adhesion molecule-1 as an early detection marker for radiation pneumonitis. *Eur Respir J* 1999;13:733.
46. Anscher MS, Kong FM, Andrews K, et al. Plasma transforming growth factor beta-1 as a predictor of radiation pneumonitis. *Int J Radiat Oncol Biol Phys* 1998;41:1029.
47. Gross NJ, Narine KR. Experimental radiation pneumonitis: corticosteroids increase the replicative activity of aveolar type 2 cells. *Radiat Res* 1988;115:543.
48. Gross NJ, Narine KR, Wade R. Protective effect of corticosteroids on radiation pneumonitis. *Radiat Res* 1988;113:112.
49. Ward HE, Kemsley L, Davies L, et al. The effect of steroids on radiation-induced lung disease in the rat. *Radiat Res* 1993;136:22.
50. Moss WT, Haddy FJ, Sweany SK. Some factors altering the severity of acute radiation pneumonitis: variation with cortisone, heparin, and antibiotics. *Radiology* 1960;75:50.
51. Ward WF, Molteni A, Tsao CH, et al. Radiation pneumotoxicity in rats: modification by inhibitors of angiotensin converting enzyme. *Int J Radiat Oncol Biol Phys* 1992;22:623.
52. Nguyen L, Ward WF, Tsao CH, et al. Captopril inhibits proliferation of human lung fibroblasts in culture: a potential antifibrotic mechanism. *Proc Soc Exp Biol Med* 1994;205:80.
53. Koh WJ, Stelzer KJ, Peterson LM, et al. Effect of pentoxifylline on radiation-induced lung and skin toxicity in rats. *Int J Radiat Oncol Biol Phys* 1995;31:71.
54. Arbetter KR, Prakash VB, Tazelaar HD, et al. Radiation-induced pneumonitis in the "non-irradiated" lung. *Mayo Clin Proc* 1999;74:27.
55. Sakanashi Y, Takeya M, Yoshimura T, et al. Kinetics of macrophage subpopulations and expression of monocyte chemoattractant protein-1 (MCP-1) in bleomycin-induced lung injury of rats studied by a novel monoclonal antibody against rat MCP-1. *J Leukoc Biol* 1994;56:741.
56. Herman EH, Hasinoff BB, Zhang J, et al. Morphologic and morphometric evaluation of the effect of ICRF-187 on bleomycin-induced pulmonary toxicity. *Toxicology* 1995;98:163.
57. Freeman BA, Crapo JD. Biology of disease: free radicals and tissue injury. *Lab Invest* 1982;47:412
58. Lewis RA, Austen KF. The biologically active leukotrienes: biosynthesis, metabolism, receptors, functions and pharmacology. *J Clin Invest* 1984;73:889.
59. Khalil N, Whitman C, Zuo L, et al. Regulation of alveolar macrophage transforming growth factor-beta secretion by corticosteroids in bleomycin-induced pulmonary inflammation in the rat. *J Clin Invest* 1993;92:1812.
60. Smith RE, Strieter RM, Phan SH, et al. Production and function of murine macrophage inflammatory protein-1 alpha in bleomycin-induced lung injury. *J Immunol* 1994;153:4704.
61. Smith RE, Strieter RM, Zhang K, et al. A role for C-C chemokines in fibrotic lung disease [Review]. *J Leukoc Biol* 1995;57:782.
62. Cooper JAD, White DA, Matthay RA. Drug-induced pulmonary disease: I. Cytotoxic drugs. *Am Rev Respir Dis* 1986;133:321.
63. White DA, Rankin JR, Stover DE, et al. Methotrexate pneumonitis: lavage findings suggest an immune mediated disorder. *Am Rev Respir Dis* 1989;139:18.
64. Askenase PW, Hayden BJ, Gershon RK. Augmentation of delayed-type hypersensitivity by doses of cyclophosphamide which do not affect antibody responses. *J Exp Med* 1974;141:697.
65. L'Age-Stehr J, Diamanstein T. Induction of autoreactive T lymphocytes and their suppressor cells by cyclophosphamide. *Nature* 1978;27:1663.
66. Vyalov SL, Gabbiani G, Kapanci Y. Rat alveolar myofibroblasts acquire alpha-smooth muscle actin expression during bleomycin-induced pulmonary fibrosis. *Am J Pathol* 1933;143:1754.
67. Absher M, Hildebran J, Trombley L, et al. Characteristics of cultured lung fibroblasts from bleomycin-treated rats: comparison with in vitro exposed normal fibroblasts. *Am Rev Respir Dis* 1984;129:125.
68. Clark JG, Kostal KM, Marino BA. Bleomycin induced pulmonary fibrosis in hamsters: an alveolar macrophage product increases fibroblast prostaglandin E2 and cyclic adenosine monophosphate and suppresses fibroblast proliferation and collagen production. *J Clin Invest* 1983;72:2082.
69. King SL, Lichtler AC, Rowe DW, et al. Bleomycin stimulates pro-alpha 1 (I) collagen promoter through transforming growth factor beta response element by intracellular and extracellular signaling. *J Biol Chem* 1994;269:13156.
70. O'Brien-Ladner AR, Wesselius LJ, Stechschulte DJ. Bleomycin injury of the lung in a mast-cell-deficient model. *Agents Actions* 1993;39:20.
71. Olman MA, Mackman N, Gladson CL, et al. Changes in procoagulant and fibrinolytic gene expression during bleomycin-induced lung injury in the mouse. *J Clin Invest* 1995;96:1621.
72. Lazo JS, Humphreys CJ. Lack of metabolism as the biochemical basis of bleomycin induced pulmonary toxicity. *Proc Natl Acad Sci U S A* 1983;80:3064.
73. Schwartz DR, Homanics GE, Hoyt DG, et al. The neutral cysteine protease bleomycin hydrolase is essential for epidermal integrity and bleomycin resistance. *Proc Natl Acad Sci U S A* 1999;96:4680.
74. Sikic BI. Biochemical and cellular determinants of bleomycin cytotoxicity. *Cancer Surv* 1986;5:81.
75. Ferrando AA, Pendas AM, Llano E, et al. Gene characterization, promoter analysis, and chromosomal localization of human bleomycin hydrolase. *J Biol Chem* 1997;272:33298.
76. White DA, Kris MG, Stover DE. Bronchoalveolar lavage cell populations in bleomycin-induced pulmonary toxicity. *Thorax* 1987;42:551.
77. Jones SE, Moore M, Blank N, et al. Hypersensitivity to procarbazine (Matulane) manifested by fever and pleuropulmonary reaction. *Cancer* 1972;29:498.
78. Holoye PY, Luna MA, McKay B, et al. Bleomycin hypersensitivity pneumonitis. *Ann Intern Med* 1978;88:47.
79. Ginsberg SJ, Comis RL. The pulmonary toxicity of antineoplastic agents. *Semin Oncol* 1982;9:34.
80. Blum RH, Carter SK, Agre K. A clinical review of bleomycin: a new antineoplastic agent. *Cancer* 1973;31:903.

81. Goldiner PL, Carlon CC, Cvitkovic E, et al. Factors influencing postoperative morbidity and mortality in patients treated with bleomycin. *Br Med J* 1978;1:1664.
82. Hakkinen PJ, Whiteley JW, Witschi HR. Hyperoxia, but not thoracic x-irradiation, potentiates bleomycin and cyclophosphamide-induced lung damage in mice. *Am Rev Respir Dis* 1982;126:281.
83. Tryka AF, Codleski JJ, Brian JD. Differences in effects of immediate and delayed hyperoxia exposure on bleomycin-induced pulmonary injury. *Cancer Treat Rep* 1984;68:759.
84. Franklin R, Buroker TR, Vaishampayan W, et al. Combined therapies in esophageal squamous cell cancer. *Proc Am Assoc Cancer Res* 1979;20:223(abst).
85. Einhorn L, Krause M, Hornback N, et al. Enhanced pulmonary toxicity with bleomycin and radiotherapy in oat cell cancer. *Cancer* 1976;37:2414.
86. Samuels ML, Johnson DE, Holoye PY, et al. Large-dose bleomycin therapy and pulmonary toxicity: a possible role of prior radiotherapy. *JAMA* 1976;235:1117.
87. Soble AR, Perry H. Fatal radiation pneumonia following subclinical busulfan injury. *AJR Am J Roentgenol* 1977;128:15.
88. Buzdar AU, Legha SS, Luna MA, et al. Pulmonary toxicity of mitomycin. *Cancer* 1980;45:236.
89. Durant JR, Norgard MJ, Murad TM, et al. Pulmonary toxicity associated with *bis*-chloroethyl nitrosourea (BCNU). *Ann Intern Med* 1979;90:191.
90. Luedke D, Mclaughlin TT, Daughaday C, et al. Mitomycin C and vindesine associated pulmonary toxicity with variable clinical expression. *Cancer* 1985;55:542.
91. White DA, Orenstein M, Codwin TA, et al. Chemotherapy-associated pulmonary toxic reactions during treatment for breast cancer. *Arch Intern Med* 1984;144:953.
92. Skarin AT, Rosenthal DS, Maloney WC. The treatment of advanced non-Hodgkin's lymphoma (NHL) with bleomycin, adriamycin, cyclophosphamide, vincristine and prednisone. *Blood* 1977;49:759.
93. Bauer KA, Skarin AT, Balikian JP, et al. Pulmonary complications associated with combination chemotherapy programs containing bleomycin. *Am J Med* 1983;74:557.
94. Aronin PA, Mahaley MS, Rudnick SA, et al. Prediction of BCNU pulmonary toxicity in patients with malignant gliomas: an assessment of risk factors. *N Engl J Med* 1980;303:1983.
95. Rabinowits M, Souhami L, Gil RA, et al. Increased pulmonary toxicity with bleomycin and cisplatin chemotherapy combinations. *Am J Clin Oncol* 1990;13:132.
96. Cooper KR, Hong WK. Prospective study of the pulmonary toxicity of continuously infused bleomycin. *Cancer Treat Rep* 1981;65:419.
97. Ingrassia TB, Ryu JH, Trastek VF, et al. Oxygen-exacerbated bleomycin pulmonary toxicity [Review]. *Mayo Clin Proc* 1991;66:173.
98. Lei KI, Leung WT, Johnson PJ. Serious pulmonary complications in patients receiving recombinant granulocyte colony-stimulating factor during BACOP chemotherapy for aggressive non-Hodgkin's lymphoma. *Br J Cancer* 1994;70:1009.
99. Bastion Y, Reyes F, Bosly A, et al. Possible toxicity with the association of G-CSF and bleomycin [Letter; comment]. *Lancet* 1994;343:1221.
100. Crilley P, Topolsky D, Styler MJ, et al. Extramedullary toxicity of a conditioning regimen containing busulphan, cyclophosphamide and etoposide in 84 patients undergoing autologous and allogeneic bone marrow transplantation. *Bone Marrow Transplant* 1995;15:361.
101. Wilczynski SW, Erasmus JJ, Petros WP, Vredenburgh JJ, Folz RJ. Delayed pulmonary toxicity syndrome following high dose chemotherapy and bone marrow transplantation for breast cancer. *Am J Respir Crit Care Med* 1998;157:565.
102. Alvarado CS, Boat TF, Newman M. Late onset pulmonary fibrosis and chest deformity in two children treated with cyclophosphamide. *J Pediatr* 1978;92:443.
103. O'Driscoll BR, Hasleton PS, Taylor PM. Active lung fibrosis up to 17 years after chemotherapy with carmustine (BCNU) in childhood. *N Engl J Med* 1990;323:378.
104. White DA, Schwartzberg L, Kris MC, et al. Acute chest pain during bleomycin infusions. *Cancer* 1987;59:1582.
105. Walden PAM, Mitchell-Heggs PF, Coppin C, et al. Pleurisy and methotrexate treatment. *Br Med J* 1977;2:867.
106. Rivera MP, Kris MG, Gralla RJ, et al. Syndrome of acute dyspnea related to combined mitomycin plus vinca alkaloid chemotherapy. *Am J Clin Oncol* 1995;18:245.
107. Vahdat L, Maslak P, Miller W Jr, et al. Early mortality and the retinoic acid syndrome in acute promyelocytic leukemia: impact of leukocytosis, low-dose chemotherapy, PMN/RAR-alpha isoform, and CD13 expression in patients treated with all-*trans* retinoic acid [Review]. *Blood* 1994;84:3843.
108. Wiley JS, Firkin FC, Australian Leukaemia Study Group. Reduction of pulmonary toxicity by prednisolone prophylaxis during all-*trans* retinoic acid treatment of acute promyelocytic leukemia. *Leukemia* 1995;9:774.
109. Orwoll ES, Kiessling P, Patterson R. Interstitial pneumonia from mitomycin. *Ann Intern Med* 1978;89:352.
110. Smalley RV, Wall RL. Two cases of busulfan toxicity. *Ann Intern Med* 1966;64:154.
111. Sostman HD, Matthay RA, Putnam CE. Methotrexate-induced pneumonitis. *Medicine* 1976;55:371.
112. Ecker MD, May B, Keohane MF. Procarbazine lung. *AJR Am J Roentgenol* 1978;131:527.
113. Weiss RB, Poster DS, Penta JS. The nitrosoureas and pulmonary toxicity. *Cancer Treat Rev* 1981;8:111.
114. Glasier CM, Siegel MJ. Multiple pulmonary nodules: unusual manifestations of bleomycin toxicity. *AJR Am J Roentgenol* 1981;137:155.
115. Talcott JA, Garnick MB, Stomper PL, et al. Cavitary lung nodules associated with combination chemotherapy containing bleomycin. *J Urol* 1987;138:619.
116. Taylor CR. Diagnostic imaging techniques in the evaluation of drug-induced pulmonary disease. *Clin Chest Med* 1990;11:87.
117. Kuhlman JE. The role of chest computed tomography in the diagnosis of drug-related reactions [Review]. *J Thorac Imag* 1991;6:52.
118. Ugur O, Caner B, Balbay MD, et al. Bleomycin lung toxicity detected by technetium-99m diethylene triamine penta-acetic acid aerosol scintigraphy. *Eur J Nucl Med* 1993;20:114.
119. Vinitski S, Pearson MG, Karlik ST, et al. Differentiation of parenchymal lung disorders with in vivo proton nuclear magnetic resonance. *Magn Reson Med* 1986;3:120.
120. Wolkowicz J, Sturgeon J, Rawji M, et al. Bleomycin-induced pulmonary function abnormalities. *Chest* 1992;101:97.
121. Kaner R, McCaffrey T, Gerl M, et al. Serum connective tissue polypeptides are sensitive markers of matrix synthesis in iatrogenic pulmonary fibrosis. *Am J Respir Crit Care Med* 1994;149:A381.
122. Villani F, Bacchella L, Bulgheroni A, et al. Study of functional and biochemical indicators of subclinical lung damage in bleomycin-treated patients. *Respir Med* 1992;86:327.
123. Anscher MS, Peters WP, Reisenbichler H, et al. Transforming growth factor beta as a predictor of liver and lung fibrosis after autologous bone marrow transplantation for advanced breast cancer. *N Engl J Med* 1993;328:1592.
124. Kozielski J. Reversal of bleomycin lung toxicity with corticosteroids [Letter; comment]. *Thorax* 1994;49:290.
125. Kalaycioglu M, Kavuru M, Tuason L, et al. Empiric prednisone therapy for pulmonary toxic reaction after high-dose chemotherapy containing carmustine (BCNU). *Chest* 1995;107:482.
126. Gunstream SR, Seidenfeld JJ, Sobonya RE, et al. Mitomycin-associated lung disease. *Cancer Treat Rep* 1983;67:301.
127. Spector JI, Zimbler H, Ross JS. Cyclophosphamide and interstitial pneumonitis. *JAMA* 1980;243:1133.
128. Grossman RF, Frost A, Zamel N, et al. Results of single lung transplantation for bilateral pulmonary fibrosis. *N Engl J Med* 1990;322:727.
129. Levine SM, Anzueto A, Peters JI, et al. Single lung transplantation in patients with systemic disease. *Chest* 1994;105:837.
130. Locatelli F, Giorgiani G, Pession A, et al. Late effects in children after bone marrow transplantation: a review [Review]. *Haematologica* 1993;78:319.
131. Stover DE, Zaman MB, Hajdu SI, et al. Bronchoalveolar lavage in the diagnosis of diffuse pulmonary infiltrates in the immunosuppressed host. *Ann Intern Med* 1984;101:1.
132. Kuplic JB, Higley CS, Niewoehner DE. Pulmonary ossification associated with long-term busulfan therapy in chronic myeloid leukemia. *Am Rev Respir Dis* 1972;106:759.
133. Heard BE, Cooke RA. Busulfan lung. *Thorax* 1968;233:1987.
134. Burns WA, McFarland W, Matthews MJ. Busulfan-induced pulmonary disease: report of a case and review of the literature. *Am Rev Respir Dis* 1970;101:408.
135. Ghalie R, Reynolds J, Valentino LA, et al. Busulfan-containing pre-transplant regimens for the treatment of solid tumors. *Bone Marrow Transplant* 1994;14:437.
136. Collis CH. Lung damage from cytotoxic drugs. *Cancer Chemother Pharmacol* 1980;4:17.
137. Mark CJ, Lehimgar-Zadeh A, Ragsdale BD. Cyclophosphamide pneumonitis. *Thorax* 1978;33:89.
138. Alvarado CS, Boat TF, Newman M. Late onset pulmonary fibrosis and chest deformity in two children treated with cyclophosphamide. *J Pediatr* 1978;92:443.
139. Maxwell I. Reversible pulmonary edema following cyclophosphamide treatment. *JAMA* 1974;229:137.
140. Cole SR, Myers TJ, Kiatsky AU. Pulmonary disease with chlorambucil therapy. *Cancer* 1978;41:455.
141. Taetle R, Dickman PS, Feldman PS. Pulmonary histopathologic changes associated with melphalan therapy. *Cancer* 1978;42:1239.
142. Goucher C, Rowland V, Hawkins J. Melphalan-induced pulmonary interstitial fibrosis. *Chest* 1980;77:805.
143. Berend N. Protective effect of hypoxia on bleomycin lung toxicity in the rat. *Am Rev Respir Dis* 1984;130:307.
144. Frank L. Protection from O_2 toxicity by preexposure to hypoxia: lung antioxidant enzyme role. *J Appl Physiol* 1982;53:475.
145. Wesselius LJ, Catanzaro A, Wasserman SI. Neutrophil chemotactic activity generation by alveolar macrophages after bleomycin injury. *Am Rev Respir Dis* 1984;129:485.
146. Kelley J, Newman RA, Evans JN. Bleomycin-induced pulmonary fibrosis in the rat: prevention with an inhibitor of collagen synthesis. *J Lab Clin Med* 1980;96:954.
147. White DA, Stover DE. Severe bleomycin-induced pneumonitis: clinical features and response to corticosteroids. *Chest* 1984;86:723.
148. Luna MA, Bedrossian CWM, Uchtiger B, et al. Interstitial pneumonitis associated with bleomycin therapy. *J Clin Pathol* 1972;58:501.
149. DeLena M, Cuzzon A, Monfardim S, et al. Clinical, radiologic and histopathologic studies on pulmonary toxicity induced by treatment with bleomycin (NSC-125066). *Cancer Chemother Rep* 1972;56:343.
150. Jules KJ, White DA. Bleomycin-induced pulmonary toxicity. *Clin Chest Med* 1990;11:1.
151. Jolivet J, Giroux L, Laurin S, et al. Microangiopathic hemolytic anemia, renal failure, and noncardiogenic pulmonary edema: a chemotherapy-induced syndrome. *Cancer Treat Rep* 1983;67:429.
152. Kaner R, Garofano S, Rivera P, et al. Bronchoalveolar lavage findings after mitomycin combination chemotherapy for non–small cell lung cancer. *Am J Respir Crit Care Med* 1995;151:A201.
153. Castro M, Su J, Veeder M, et al. A prospective study of pulmonary function in patients receiving mitomycin-C. *Chest* 1996;109:939.
154. Cordonnier C, Vernant J-P, Mital P, et al. Pulmonary fibrosis subsequent to high doses of CCNU for chronic leukemia. *Cancer* 1983;51:1814.
155. Lee W, Moore RP, Wampler CL. Interstitial pulmonary fibrosis as a complication of prolonged methyl-CCNU therapy. *Cancer Treat Rep* 1978;62:1355.
156. Sordillo EM, Sordillo PP, Stover DE, et al. Chlorozotocin (DCNU)-induced pulmonary toxicity. *Cancer Clin Trials* 1981;4:397.
157. Nathan CF, Arrick BA, Murray HW, et al. Tumor cell antioxidant defenses: inhibition of the glutathione redox cycle enhances macrophage-mediated cytolysis. *J Exp Med* 1981;153:766.
158. Reznil-Schuller HM, Smith AC, Thenot JP, et al. Pulmonary toxicity of the anticancer drug, *bis*-chloroethyl nitrosourea (BCNU) in rats. *Toxicologist* 1984;4:29.
159. Selker RC, Jacobs SA, Moore PB. BCNU [1,3-bis (2-chloroethyl)-1-nitrosourea] induced pulmonary fibrosis. *Neurosurgery* 1980;7:560.

160. Taylor PM, O'Driscoll BR, Gattamaneni HR, et al. Chronic lung fibrosis following carmustine (BCNU) chemotherapy: radiological features. *Clin Radiol* 1991;44:299.
161. Haupt HM, Hutchins CM, Moore CW. Ara-C lung: noncardiogenic pulmonary edema complicating cytosine arabinoside therapy of leukemia. *Am J Med* 1981;70:256.
162. Hewlett RI, Wilson AF. Adult respiratory distress syndrome (ARDS) following aggressive management of extensive acute lymphoblastic leukemia. *Cancer* 1977;39:2422.
163. Vander Els N, Miller V. Successful treatment of gemcitabine toxicity with a brief course of oral corticosteroid therapy. *Chest* 1998;114:1779.
164. Lokich JJ, Moloney WC. Allergic reaction to procarbazine. *Clin Pharmacol Ther* 1972; 13:573.
165. Kris MC, Pablo D, Gralla RJ, et al. Dyspnea following vinblastine or vindesine administration in patients receiving mitomycin plus vinca alkaloid combination therapy. *Cancer Treat Rep* 1984;68:1029.
166. Konits PH, Aisner J, Sutherland J, et al. Possible pulmonary toxicity secondary to vinblastine. *Cancer* 1982;50:2771.
167. Sleijfer S, Van der Mark TW, Schraffordt Koops H, et al. Decrease in pulmonary function during bleomycin-containing combination chemotherapy for testicular cancer: not only a bleomycin effect. *Br J Cancer* 1995;71:120.
168. Dajczman E, Srolovitz H, Kreisman H, et al. Fatal pulmonary toxicity following oral etoposide therapy. *Lung Cancer* 1995;12:81.
169. Ramanathan RK, Reddy VV, Holbert JM. Pulmonary infiltrates following administration of paclitaxel. *Chest* 1996;110:289.

LAUREL J. STEINHERZ
JOACHIM YAHALOM

SECTION 4

Cardiac Toxicity

The treatment of cancer has been vastly improved by the expansion of chemotherapeutic agents and refinement of radiotherapy over the past three decades. However, many of the most effective antineoplastic agents and mediastinal irradiation produce toxic effects on the heart. This chapter describes some of these problems and discusses attempts at prevention and management.

CHEMOTHERAPY

ANTHRACYCLINES

The anthracyclines have been associated with cardiomyopathy since their introduction in the late 1960s. Early reports included isolated cases of unexplained cardiac failure in patients undergoing treatment with daunorubicin[1–3] and later, in the early 1970s with doxorubicin.[4–8] Lefrak et al.[9] reported a series in 1973 of 399 patients treated with doxorubicin. He found a 30% incidence of cardiac failure in the patients who received more than 550 mg/m^2 of doxorubicin, and a lower incidence in those who received less. This introduced the concept of increasing cardiotoxicity with cumulative doses above a *safe threshold* cumulative dose. In 1974, Halazun et al.[10] reported a series of children with acute lymphoblastic leukemia, in remission, treated with two different maintenance protocols, one including and one excluding daunorubicin. There was a 10% incidence of cardiac failure in the arm with daunorubicin and none in the arm without. This report clearly demonstrated the relationship of anthracycline treatment to the incidence of cardiac failure, while it excluded the influence of active malignancy or the stress of induction therapy as contributory factors. Von Hoff et al. demonstrated, in 5613 patients treated with daunorubicin[11] and in 4018 patients treated with doxorubicin,[12] a continuous, almost exponential increase of incidence of cardiac failure with increasing cumulative dose. Subsequently, Bristow et al.[13,14] used endomyocardial biopsy to show that pathologic lesions progressively worsened in a linear relationship to the increase in total cumulative dose, in contrast to the nonlinear increase in myocardial dysfunction. This contrast suggested a threshold of *tolerable myocardial damage* beyond which the administration of additional drug would result in clinical symptomatology. Both clinical and pathologic abnormalities increased at any dose level in patients who received mediastinal radiotherapy.[15]

Clinical Presentation

Anthracycline cardiomyopathy has been described as having three clinical presentations: acute, subacute, and late. The acute toxicity[16] presents as a myopericarditis and probably results from the combination of acute myocyte damage from drug exposure and the effects of the catecholamine and histamine[17] surge provoked by the administration of anthracyclines. This occurs within days of a dose and includes transient arrhythmias,[18,19] pericardial effusion, and myocardial dysfunction, sometimes leading to transient cardiac failure and occasionally death.[13,16] Histologically, acute myocyte disruption and sometimes infiltration of the myocardium by granulocytes, lymphocytes, and histiocytes[20] are seen.

The classic subacute presentation has a more insidious onset and appears from 0 to 231 days after the last dose (up to 30 months later),[21] with a peak onset of symptoms at 3 months from the last dose.[11] The clinical picture presents with increasing tachycardia and fatigue, progressing in some patients to tachypnea, dyspnea, and finally pulmonary edema, right-sided congestive signs, and low cardiac output. The mortality of patients actually manifesting congestive heart failure in these early series ranged up to 60%, although some patients could be stabilized with intensive cardiac treatment,[22,23] and many showed remarkable improvement of cardiac function over the first few years after chemotherapy.[23–26] However, evaluation of hemodynamics with exercise has revealed significant underlying abnormalities even in asymptomatic patients with normal resting parameters.[27] The pathology noted on endomyocardial biopsy and autopsy within the first 2 years after completion of anthracyclines includes disruption and loss of myofibrils, mitochondrial swelling, and disruption of the sarcoplasmic reticulum producing intramyocyte vacuolization.[15,28,29] With mild toxicity such damage is patchy, whereas with higher doses and toxicity it is found more extensively throughout the heart, with progression to myocyte necrosis and loss. Changes in children and adults are similar except for the more frequent appearance of lipid droplets within the myocytes of children younger than age 10.[30] While some authors have reported the finding of infiltrates of T lymphocytes in biopsy specimens otherwise indicative of subacute anthracycline cardiomyopathy,[31] classically a lymphocytic infiltrate is absent.[30] The biopsy findings after treatment with anthracycline analogues have been similar.[30] Later pathologic examination, 41 to 47 months from chemotherapy, reveals hypertrophy of the remaining myocytes without fibrosis, and diminution of vacuolization, suggesting healing and compensation.[32]

The late presentation of anthracycline cardiomyopathy has been described to occur 5 or more years after completion of anthracycline therapy.[33–51] It involves late clinical decompensation of patients who had recovered from subacute cardiac symptoms[33–35] (Fig. 55.4-1), or the occurrence of cardiac failure *de novo* in patients with no previous symptoms, 6 to 25 years after anthracycline therapy.[33–38,42] It has also been demonstrated subclinically, as abnormal systolic cardiac function in 23%,[33–35,42] abnormal myocardial mass in 52%,[38–41] and abnormal exercise response in up to 80% of patients.[43–45] While some authors have reported abnormalities of diastolic function[40,46] others have found no significant diastolic changes.[47,48] The conflicting results may reflect different sensitivity of different diastolic measurements used.[49] As with subacute toxicity, an increased incidence of late abnormalities correlates with increasing cumulative dose of anthracycline received, and mediastinal irradiation is an additive risk factor.[34,41,42,50] However, late abnormalities of resting echocardiography were found in patients treated with as little as 75 mg/m² of doxorubicin,[39] and late abnormalities of exercise response were seen in 55% of patients treated with low cumulative doses (median, 263 mg/m²).[45] A correlation of late cardiotoxicity with individual dose intensity has been reported.[41] Abnormalities of myo-

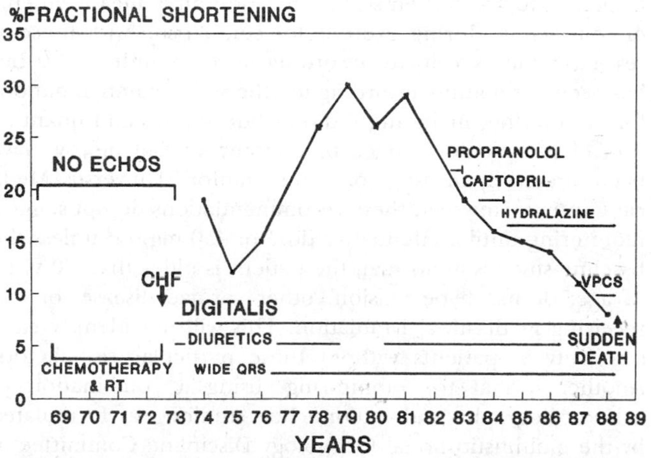

FIGURE 55.4-1. The clinical course of a patient after subclinical anthracycline cardiotoxicity. The initial increase and then progressive decrease of her fractional shortening on echocardiography and increasing requirements for therapeutic support of cardiac function can be seen. Despite an early fractional shortening of 11%, she gradually improved over the first 6 years. She discontinued diuretics, achieved modest exercise tolerance, and completed high school. Her fractional shortening on echocardiography reached 30% 6 years posttherapy. However, 8 years postdoxorubicin she required increasing amounts of diuretics for recurrent edema. Ten years postchemotherapy she had progressive deterioration of exercise tolerance and fractional shortening despite increasingly intensive medical management. During the last 2 years she was found to have moderately frequent premature ventricular contractions but no syncope or runs of ectopic ventricular beats. She was deemed unsuitable for cardiac transplant. Finally at 20 years post initial diagnosis and 17 years after her last anthracycline dose, she developed a tachy-bradyarrhythmia leading to sudden syncope and cardiac arrest. CHF, congestive failure; RT, radiotherapy; VPCS, ventricular premature contractions.

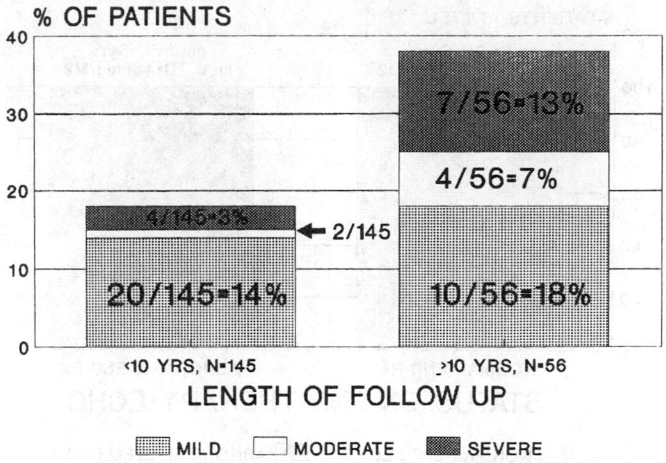

FIGURE 55.4-2. The percent of patients found to have abnormal echocardiogram results at the time of long-term follow-up is illustrated. Despite a similar cumulative anthracycline dose (495 vs. 420 mg/m²), 38% of those followed 10 years or longer had decreased fractional shortening (FS) as compared with 18% of those followed less than 10 years ($P < .004$). More than 50% of the abnormalities (11 of 21) seen in the 10 year or longer group were moderate (FS = 21% to 24%) or severe (FS ≤20%), while the degree of abnormality was mild (FS = 25% to 28%) in 77% (20 of 26) of the abnormal patients with shorter follow-up.

cardial mass are said, by some authors, to be more pronounced in patients treated in early childhood, implying a negative effect on myocardial growth.[39] Abnormalities of systolic function did not correlate with age during chemotherapy.[34] Measurements of systolic function[34,35] and myocardial wall thickness[39] deteriorate progressively with increasing time after anthracyclines as emphasized in reports including patients followed for more than 15 years after completion of anthracycline therapy[42] (Fig. 55.4-2). Serious arrhythmias have been identified in symptomatic and asymptomatic patients at late cardiac follow-up, including ventricular tachycardia and fibrillation and second-degree heart block.[34,35,37,45,51] Several young patients with late cardiomyopathy have experienced sudden death up to 15 years after chemotherapy.[34–37] The pathology found on biopsy and autopsy of patients with late cardiotoxicity is predominantly fibrosis and hypertrophy of remaining myocytes, with little remaining vacuolization.[34–37] Thus, even asymptomatic patients who have been treated with anthracyclines need long-term cardiac follow-up, and new symptoms suggestive of arrhythmia and especially syncope need vigorous investigation. Cardiac status on noninvasive testing during the year after completion of therapy is predictive for the likelihood of late abnormality (Fig. 55.4-3) and indicates the advisable frequency of follow-up.[34,35]

Mechanisms of Pathogenesis

An understanding of the mechanism of cardiotoxicity provides the basis for attempts at prevention. There are many mechanisms proposed and several may interact to cause the multiple sites of intracellular injury seen histologically. In the mitochondria, there is a deletion mutation of mitochondrial DNA that increases proportionate to dosage and duration of anthracycline exposure.[52] In addition, doxorubicin is found to bind to cardiolipin in the inner mitochondrial membrane[53,54] with two

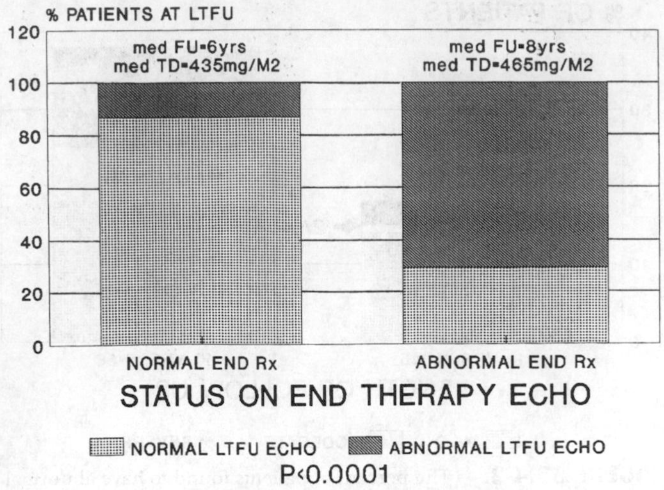

FIGURE 55.4-3. An echocardiogram (ECHO) taken after completion of anthracycline therapy has prognostic implications for cardiac function on late follow-up (LTFU). Eighty-seven percent of patients who had normal fractional shortening on echocardiography taken during the year posttherapy remained normal at LTFU, whereas only 29% of patients who were even mildly abnormal on end therapy echocardiography were normal at LTFU (P <.0001). FU, follow-up; TD, total dose.

deleterious results. The electron transfer in the respiratory chain, which is dependent on the binding of cardiolipin to cytochrome c for its interaction with cytochrome oxidase, and the activation by cardiolipin of the nicotinamide-adenine dinucleotide phosphate to cytochrome c oxidoreductase complex (complex I to III), for the synthesis of adenosine triphosphate (ATP), is disrupted. This leads to depletion of ATP and phosphocreatine concentrations and depression of contractility.[55] In addition, the doxorubicin-cardiolipin complex promotes transfer of electrons through doxorubicin, forming a doxorubicin free radicle that can reduce molecular oxygen, producing O_2^-. This induces the generation of free hydroxyl radicals and hydrogen peroxide, leading to mitochondrial membrane damage, further disruption of enzymatic respiration, and more extensive lipid peroxidation.[53,54] Oxidative damage is worsened by the concomitant decrease, during chemotherapy, in glutathione peroxidase, which normally serves as a free radical scavenger. Glutathione is especially important in myocytes, which lack catalase, which serves as a scavenger in other tissues. Free radical lipid peroxidation was identified[56,57] as an important mechanism of myocyte damage and has been found to depend, in the heart, on an iron-doxorubicin complex.[54,58,59] The resultant disruption of the sarcoplasmic reticulum and direct effects of the metabolite doxorubicinol[60,61] have been shown to cause disturbances of Ca^{2+} transport,[54,62] such as decrease in calcium release channels,[63] which is critical to regulation of cardiac action potentials, contraction, and relaxation.[64] Chronically, there is alteration of contractile proteins and their enzymes with a shift in the ratio of prevalent isomyosin types and decreased production of α myosin heavy chains, perhaps as an adaptation to chronic low-energy states.[65]

Prevention

MONITORING. Attempts at prevention of cardiomyopathy initially involved limitation of total cumulative dose below 450 to 550 mg/m². This limit was chosen to avoid the rapid increase in prevalence of clinical cardiac dysfunction, in excess of 30%, which occurs above that dose range. However, arbitrary dose limitation was inadequate because of variability of individual tolerance. Therefore, therapy has been modified according to serial monitoring of cardiac status, by various means, to identify increasing risk of unacceptable toxicity. Monitoring of systolic time intervals and of electrocardiography (ECG) for QRS voltage loss[66] or ST-T changes was too nonspecific or showed changes too late to direct prevention. Serial echocardiography has been helpful to identify changes in systolic and diastolic function, especially in children, in whom echo images are clear and more easily measurable.[67–73] The fractional shortening is the most frequent parameter followed, although some groups follow end-systolic wall stress and the relationship between wall stress and velocity of circumferential fiber shortening.[71] Early trends of rate of decrease in fractional shortening, at lower cumulative doses, have been reported to be predictive of eventual cardiac findings at end therapy, after higher cumulative doses.[73] Changes in posterior wall thickness appear to be more useful in late follow-up than for monitoring during chemotherapy.[73] Digitized echocardiography, with calculation of velocity of wall motion, thickening, and velocity of change of left ventricular chamber size in systole and diastole have been employed to enhance sensitivity. Radionuclide cardiac angiography has been used by many authors to follow systolic[74–77] and diastolic function,[78,79] and specific guidelines for modification of chemotherapy on the basis of radionuclide ejection fraction in adults, proposed by Schwartz et al., have gained wide acceptance.[74] Adherence to these guidelines reduced the incidence of cardiac failure from 21% to 3% in their study. The addition of measurements of contractility during exercise for comparison with those at rest has added sensitivity according to some authors,[75–77] but has been less helpful according to others.[80] Recommendations for monitoring, including radionuclide studies and quantitation of pathologic damage by endomyocardial biopsy, have been offered by investigators from Stanford University Medical Center.[77] However, these recommendations do not suggest monitoring until a cumulative dose of 450 mg/m² unless the baseline study is abnormal, the patient is older than 70 years of age, or has hypertension, other cardiac disease, or was receiving mediastinal irradiation. This will not identify early sensitivity in patients without those particular risk factors. Another format for monitoring, using a combination of echocardiography and radionuclide studies, was formulated by the multiinstitutional Cardiology Discipline Committee of the Children's Cancer Study Group.[67,68] These recommendations include cardiac evaluation before anthracyclines and further monitoring before every other course until a cumulative dose of 300 mg/m² and every course beyond this. Endomyocardial biopsy, which has proven to be safe and effective in experienced hands, with a complication rate of 1.5%,[81,82] is suggested to clarify abnormal or equivocal results.[67]

Although, not yet included in current routine monitoring, several newer modalities have been used for detection of toxicity. Tantalum 178 first-pass radionuclide imaging has allowed calculation of both right and left ventricular systolic function.[83] Indium-111-antimyosin scintigraphy[84,85] uses a monoclonal antibody labeled with ^{111}In that binds with cardiac myosin, which becomes exposed when cardiac myocytes are injured. Increasing uptake of ^{111}In during anthracycline therapy would imply increasing cardiac damage. Abnormalities of uptake of ^{111}In have been seen before a decrease in radionuclide ejection fraction[86] and could be used to compare damage from different methods of administration of conventional anthracyclines[86] or from different cardiotoxic agents.[87] This method was also reported to discriminate patients with sustained cardiotoxicity from those with transient decreases in ejection fraction or myocardial metastasis.[88] In studies in rats, the amount of cardiac ^{111}In uptake correlated with both histologic changes and end-diastolic pressure, and there was specific immunolocalization of the radiotracer in injured myocytes as opposed to normal neighboring ones microscopically.[89]

Another radionuclide, radioiodinated metaiodobenzylguanidine (^{123}I-MIBG), has been used to indicate early anthracycline cardiotoxicity. MIBG is an analogue of norepinephrine and reflects cardiac adrenergic neuron integrity that is disrupted with anthracycline damage. Animal studies[90] and clinic trials[91,92] demonstrated abnormalities of uptake and clearance of MIBG even before abnormalities of systolic and diastolic function are seen by echocardiography. These MIBG abnormalities were proportionate to severity of systolic dysfunction in patients with toxicity.

Positron emission tomography has been used to identify metabolic changes suggesting cardiac damage in patients receiving chemotherapy.[93] ^{31}P nuclear magnetic resonance spectroscopy has also demonstrated metabolic changes that correlate with the amount of doxorubicin-induced degeneration of myofibrils microscopically.[94]

Reports on the usefulness of monitoring serum levels of troponin T postmyocardial infarction, to detect limited myocardial necrosis, prompted investigation of this method's usefulness to detect early anthracycline damage. Although animal study results seem promising,[95] clinical trials are still in progress. Therefore, this method remains investigational and is not yet recommended for routine monitoring. Some investigators have reported that elevated serum natriuretic peptide, which is released in response to chronic or acute increase in atrial transmural pressure and stretch, may be a marker for anthracycline damage.[96]

Schwartz et al. correlated prolongation of the corrected QT interval (QTc) on 12-lead ECG with increasing anthracycline dose in both acute and chronic anthracycline cardiomyopathy.[97] Careful attention to concomitant electrolyte and calcium imbalance is clearly mandatory to avoid false results. Jakacki et al. suggested an algorithm combining measurement of QTc with fractional shortening on echocardiography and a history of exercise intolerance for screening.[98] Another new measurement from signal-averaged ECG, that of ventricular late potentials, may also have predictive value.[99]

SCHEDULE MODIFICATION. Other attempts to prevent cardiomyopathy involve decreasing the peak dose of anthracycline delivered to the heart by modification of schedules of delivery.[100–106] Legha et al. demonstrated that patients receiving continuous infusions of doxorubicin developed lower peak plasma levels the longer the time of the infusion.[100] Thus, levels with a 48-hour infusion were lower than with a 24-hour infusion and a 96-hour infusion of the same dose per course produced still lower levels. They proved by comparing endomyocardial biopsy scores in patients receiving doxorubicin that patients receiving their dose by 48- or 96-hour infusion had significantly lower biopsy scores, indicating less cardiomyopathy than patients receiving the dose by 20-minute bolus. In addition, the patients receiving 96-hour infusions had lower biopsy scores than those receiving 24-hour infusions. Infusions were administered through an indwelling intravenous line using a battery-powered portable pump. Currently, continuous infusion chemotherapy is usually given through a surgically implanted central venous access catheter. A study by Shapira et al., using radionuclide cardiac angiography to evaluate cardiotoxicity, demonstrated a decline in left ventricular ejection fraction (LVEF) of only 6% after a total cumulative dose of 400 mg/m^2 administered by only 6-hour continuous infusion, compared with a decrease of 21% in patients who received the same range of total doxorubicin dose by 20-minute bolus.[102] Casper et al. confirmed the cardioprotective effects of 72-hour infusion in a prospective randomized trial of 82 patients with soft tissue sarcoma.[101] The article suggested, however, that continuous infusion might have a negative effect on antitumor efficacy, although this was not conclusive since their infusion patients had tumors with worse prognostic features than their bolus patients. Other uncontrolled trials using continuous infusion for various solid tumors have shown no decrease in efficacy.[105] Reports of prospective randomized trials comparing infusion with bolus for treatment of leukemia, in which efficacy can be measured by percent cell kill on bone marrow sampling,[103] and in osteogenic sarcoma in which it is measured as histologic response of the surgically removed tumor after preoperative chemotherapy,[106] have shown no significant decrease in antitumor efficacy with continuous infusion. In fact, in the leukemia study, efficacy was better with infusion.[103] Schedules dividing the planned monthly doxorubicin dose into smaller weekly dosages have also decreased pathologic and physiologic abnormalities, allowing higher cumulative doses to be given.[107,108]

Cardioprotective Agents

Free radicle scavengers vitamin E,[109] ascorbic acid,[110] N-acetylcysteine,[111] and others[112,113] have shown promise in animals but no clear benefit in patients, although results of one study in rats using the lipid-lowering antioxidant agent probucol seem encouraging.[114] Similarly, trials of concomitant administration of verapamil,[115,116] prenylamine,[117] other calcium channel blockers, and β-adrenergic and histamine blockers[118,119] to prevent the effects of excessive vasoactive agents, antiinflammatory agents, carnitine, digoxin,[120] and amrinone[121] have not yet proven definitively useful in patients. Studies are ongoing examining the usefulness of coenzyme Q10[122] and amifostine.[123] Encapsulation of the anthracycline in liposomes and binding to agarose[124] were initially disappointing. However, the use of more stable liposomal complexes has provided some protection.[125,126]

Attempts to exploit the importance of the iron-doxorubicin complex appear to be more successful. The classic chelator deferoxamine did not prevent anthracycline cardiomyopathy in normal as opposed to iron overloaded cardiac cells.[127] However, 1-2-bis(3,5-dioxopiperazinyl-1-yl) propane, known as ICRF-187, ADR-529, or dexrazoxane and commercially as Zinecard or Cardioxane, an iron chelator that achieves better intracellular concentration, has been shown in various animals,[128–130] and several human studies to exhibit significant protection against anthracycline cardiomyopathy. Animal studies have demonstrated healing of lesions within 3 months after discontinuation of therapy in rabbits treated with ICRF.[131] Initial clinical trials included a pilot study of 12 patients with various solid tumors[132] and a randomized therapeutic trial in women with breast cancer.[133–135] Patients were evaluated both by radionuclide ejection fraction and myocardial biopsy. Incidence of clinical toxicity, degree of decrease of ejection fraction, and biopsy score were significantly less in the ICRF arm. These results have been confirmed in a large multicenter trial, in adults with breast cancer using fluorouracil, doxorubicin, and cyclophosphamide (FAC), and small cell lung cancer, using similar cardiac monitoring.[136–139] Smaller trials have been equally promising in pediatric patients.[140–143] The multicenter adult trial[136–139] and larger pediatric trials[143] have also attempted to examine the effect of ICRF on antimalignant efficacy, which seems, in most cases, to be preserved.[143] Investigators had hoped to combine the protective effects of infusion scheduling of doxorubicin and concomitant ICRF. To that end, studies of infusional ICRF are in progress.[144]

This agent appears to also provide cardiac protection for anthracycline analogues such as epirubicin[85,145,146] and mitoxantrone.[146–148]

NEW ANALOGUES. Analogues of daunorubicin and doxorubicin have been studied in clinical trials. Many agents that appear to have decreased cardiotoxicity in animal studies and even in early clinical trials eventually have been found to have similar toxicity to the parent compound. Patients treated with zorubicin experienced cardiotoxicity that was additive to prior anthracycline toxicity and some developed cardiac failure.[149,150] 4'Epi-doxorubicin is another analogue with cardiotoxicity similar to or possibly less[151–153] than doxorubicin. Incidences of atrioventricular block, ventricular fibrillation, decreased ejection fraction, and decreased velocity of circumferential fiber shortening[154,155] have been reported in phase I and II trials with another analogue, aclarubicin. Demethoxy daunorubicin (Idarubicin) has shown activity in patients whose malignancy has become resistant to daunorubicin. However, it is also cardiotoxic.[156,157] Its myelotoxicity is approximately four times that of daunorubicin milligram for milligram. When given in amounts of equivalent myelotoxicity, the cardiotoxicity is also similar.[157,158] Thus, careful monitoring of this agent would be warranted above a cumulative dose of 75 mg/m^2. Cardiac failure and subclinical decrease in ejection fraction occurred in patients treated with the analogue esorubicin. A 5% drop in mean LVEF was noted at 240 mg/m^2 and a 10% drop at 480 mg/m^2 of this agent.[159] Animal studies of 4'-deoxy-4'iodo-doxorubicinol indicate acute and chronic cardiotoxicity but possibly less than daunorubicin.[160] The ideal anthracycline has not yet been found.

Management

Clinical anthracycline cardiomyopathy needs to be managed with inotropic support and afterload reduction,[20] often initially by the intravenous route. Angiotensin-converting enzyme inhibitors have played an important role in stabilizing cardiac failure and delaying further myocardial deterioration.[37,51] Current reports suggest that selective β-receptor blockers, such as metoprolol[161] and more recently carvedilol,[162] may be useful in patients who do not improve with these modalities. Control of malignant arrhythmias may require intensive medical management with drugs such as amiodarone and mexiletine or placement of indwelling automatic cardioverters and pacemakers.[37,42,51] Most patients can be stabilized and show clinical improvement. Patients who have been refractory to treatment or have repeat bouts of pulmonary edema and are free of malignancy have benefited from cardiac transplantation.[163–167]

MITOXANTRONE

Mitoxantrone hydrochloride is an anthracenedione that is similar in structure to doxorubicin. It was found to be toxic to cardiac cells in culture despite a lack of production of free radical peroxidation.[147] The toxicity appeared to involve an interaction with iron similar to that of doxorubicin.[147] Animal studies revealed conflicting findings in different species. There were ECG abnormalities in treated monkeys and dose-related impairment of contractility in the rabbit heart,[168] but no ECG changes or progressive anthracycline-like lesions on endomyocardial biopsy specimens of Beagle hearts.[169] There were cases of cardiac failure and arrhythmia (mainly supraventricular) reported from the early phase I and II trials under the auspices of the National Cancer Institute.[170,171] The incidence of myocardial dysfunction and cardiac failure increased with increasing cumulative dose as with doxorubicin.[170,172] Significant decreases in ejection fraction occurred in these trials around 110 mg/m^2 [170] and a rapid increase in incidence of cardiac failure was noted at 160 mg/m^2.[172] Later studies have continued to detect cardiomyopathy and cardiac failure in patients with[173] and without[174] prior anthracycline therapy, and conduction delay, with prolongation of PR, QRS, and QT interval on ECG, was also reported.[175] A British patient trial reported a 46% incidence of abnormal LVEF, using radionuclide angiography during rest and cold pressor stress, in patients who received a wide range of doses.[176] A Greek cooperative study found decreases in ejection fraction of greater than or equal to 10% within normal range, in 10% of patients tested, and they reported minimal changes in echo systolic function and significant changes in systolic time intervals in the patient cohort as a whole, after receiving 60 mg/m^2 combined with cyclophosphamide and fluorouracil.[177] An Italian trial reported ECG abnormalities in 41%, echocardiographic abnormalities in 66%, and a greater than or equal to 15% decrease in radionuclide LVEF in almost 25% of patients receiving a cumulative dose of 28 to 84 mg/m^2.[178] The overall incidence, reported by Immunex Laboratories, of subclinical moderate to serious decrement in LVEF was 13%, and the incidence of cardiac failure, up to a cumulative dose of 140 mg/m^2, was 2.6%.[179]

AMSACRINE

Amsacrine (AMSA) is an acridine derivative used mainly in nonlymphoblastic leukemia. It has been associated with myocardial infarction[180] and ventricular and supraventricular arrhythmias including fatal ventricular fibrillation.[181–184] Many of these arrhythmias have been attributed to coexisting electrolyte abnormalities, particularly hypokalemia, and more recently AMSA has been safely administered even to patients with preexisting atrial[189] and ventricular[185] arrhythmias. Noninvasive monitoring of cardiac function during a prospective study of AMSA revealed reversible abnormalities on serial echocardiography in 18 of 27 patients and cardiac failure in 7 of 27 patients.[186,187] Echocardiographic abnormalities generally appeared within a week of AMSA therapy and resolved in most, once therapy was discontinued.

Four patients died with persistent cardiac failure. The incidence of echocardiographic abnormalities was related to total dose of AMSA, rate of AMSA administration, and the total dose of anthracyclines previously received. No patient who received less than 200 mg/m^2 AMSA in 48 hours, after having received less than 400 mg/m^2 of anthracyclines, had echocardiographic abnormalities. In contrast, all patients who received greater than or equal to 200 mg/m^2 of AMSA within 48 hours after having received greater than 400 mg/m^2 of anthracyclines exhibited echocardiographic abnormalities.[186] More recently, Arlin et al. treated 24 patients with preexisting myocardial dysfunction with AMSA greater than 200 mg/m^2/48 hours and reported no occurrences of cardiac failure in this group.[188] Nine of the patients had radionuclide ejection fractions determined after AMSA treatment and two of nine showed a further decrease of ejection fraction by more than 10%. It is not stated how soon after treatment the radionuclide angiograms were obtained. Therefore, it is possible that there were additional transient deficits that were not detected in this study. However, the absence of any clinical cardiac failure in these heavily treated patients is significant.

CYCLOPHOSPHAMIDE

There is still disagreement if doses of cyclophosphamide under 100 mg/kg/week contribute to cardiomyopathy,[13,24,107,189] and in our experience such doses do not. However, higher doses used for cytoreduction and immunosuppression before bone marrow transplantation can cause an acute hemorrhagic pancarditis. It was initially described in case reports,[190–192] animal studies,[193] and autopsy series[194,195] as involving a serosanguinous pericardial effusion, mural thickening with edema, and endocardial, myocardial, and epicardial hemorrhage. This results from endothelial capillary damage that allows extravasation of fluid and red cells into cardiac and pulmonary tissues. Reports of patient series[196–199] described the acute course, with an onset during the first week posttreatment, peak toxicity at 7 to 9 days, and improvement over the next 3 weeks. Abnormal findings of diastolic dysfunction, small to moderate pericardial effusion, restrictive cardiomyopathy, sometimes mimicking pericardial tamponade, and later systolic dysfunction, were found in more than one-half the patients.[197–199] The most frequent ECG change seen was decreased voltage, which did not necessarily correlate with impairment of function.[197–199] Abnormalities of T waves and ST segment and arrhythmias are seen,[200] including complete heart block[201] and ventricular tachyarrhythmias.[200] Some arrhythmias may be due to the infusion of the cryopreserved marrow graft.[202] The majority of patients remained asymptomatic.[197,199,203] Some had mild symptoms of fluid retention, edema, and tachypnea, and a few had an extremely fulminant course of cardiac failure shock and death that was resistant to even intensive treatment. Risk factors of previous anthracycline therapy and previous abnormal cardiac function were identified and the importance of dose and rate of delivery was stressed.[197,204] A weekly dose of 170 mg/kg over 4 days without anthracyclines and 120 mg/kg over 2 days after anthracyclines predicted risk for at least subclinical changes. More rapid delivery of 120 mg/kg over 24 hours produced fulminant cardiomyopathy in one patient.[192,194] Mildly symptomatic patients responded to diuretics and, if necessary, transient digitalization or intravenous inotropic agents. Those with the more fulminant course required prolonged intravenous inotropic support, respiratory assistance, and hemofiltration.[199] Pericardial drainage has not been helpful usually, although rare cases of true cardiac tamponade responding to pericardiocentesis have been reported.[205] In most cases the effusion can be managed with analgesics and corticosteroids.[206] To avoid this clinical cardiotoxicity, patients have been screened during the past decade with echocardiography or radionuclide studies to identify abnormal cardiac function and the pretransplant regimen adjusted for higher risk patients by administering the cyclophosphamide over additional days or using a preparative regimen without cyclophosphamide. A pretreatment radionuclide LVEF of less than 50%,[207,208] or even less than 55%,[209] has been correlated with increased risk of cardiotoxicity.[207–209] Studies have suggested that giving the cyclophosphamide by infusion or in smaller twice-a-day doses decreased the incidence of systolic dysfunction, although changes of myocardial mass were still seen.[208] Evaluation of patients' hemodynamics during exercise at least a year after transplant has shown significant abnormalities in children treated for malignancy before transplant with anthracyclines. However, the few children with aplastic anemia, who had not received anthracyclines, were normal.[210]

IFOSFAMIDE

Ifosfamide, an alkylating oxazaphosphorine related to cyclophosphamide, has been associated with atrial ectopy (including atrial fibrillation) and, less commonly, ST-T wave changes and bradycardia. These abnormalities were noted in patients who had received doses as high as 6.25 to 10.0 g/m^2 over 3 to 5 days.[211] One series reported an incidence of congestive heart failure in 9 of 52 patients enrolled in a phase I trial of high-dose ifosfamide with other agents with autologous marrow transplantation.[212] ECG abnormalities, negative inotropic effects, and pathologic myocardial damage were also found in animals who received high doses of ifosfamide.[213,214]

RETINOIC ACID

Trans-retinoic acid is an active agent for the treatment of acute promyelocytic leukemia. However, in more than 10% of patients, a syndrome is produced, known as *RA syndrome*, involving fever, dyspnea, pleural and pericardial effusion, pulmonary infiltrates, peripheral edema, and transient myocardial dysfunction and heart failure.[215] This is especially prevalent during the first 2 weeks of therapy and has responded to dexamethasone.

TAXANES

Paclitaxel (Taxol) has been described as causing abnormalities of cardiac rhythm, conduction, and function. In preclinical studies, paclitaxel produced arrhythmias and slowing of beat frequencies of rat cardiac cells growing *in vitro*.[216] Cases of clinically significant disturbances of cardiac rhythm and conduction were reported during phase I and II trials of this agent.[217] Significant sinus bradycardia (heart rate, 30 to 50 bpm) was common, occurring in up to 29% of patients in a phase II trial for ovarian cancer.[218] Several patients exhibited progressive although transient atrioventricular conduction delay from first-degree heart block, to complete heart block, to asystole[218] on continuous ECG monitoring during paclitaxel infusion as a single agent. Associated presyncope and syncope have been reported,[217] requiring temporary pacing. Episodes of sustained and nonsustained ventricular tachycardia have been reported with the combination of paclitaxel and cisplatin.[219] However, Markman et al. used this combination successfully in patients with significant preexisting cardiac risk factors.[220] Since few of their patients had significant preexisting conduction disorders, it is still recommended that patients with arrhythmia or abnormal conduction be monitored with continuous ECG during paclitaxel administration. The combination of paclitaxel with doxorubicin for the treatment of breast cancer has resulted in an increased incidence of clinically significant deterioration of left ventricular function at a lower cumulative dose of doxorubicin. It has been suggested that this is due to interaction between the two agents resulting in decreased elimination of the doxorubicin and that the cumulative doxorubicin dose should be limited to 340 to 380 mg/m^2 in this combination.[221] Preliminary experience with the synthetic analogue docetaxel (Taxatere) suggested similar potential for dysrhythmia; however, clinical trials have not shown cardiotoxicity of this agent or significant increase in doxorubicin toxicity when docetaxel and doxorubicin are combined.[222]

HOMOHARRINGTONINE

Homoharringtonine is an alkaloid from the Chinese *Cephalotaxus.* It is another drug that causes reversible atrioventricular block,[223] ventricular ectopy,[224] supraventricular tachycardia, and ST-T wave changes in animals[225] and patients.[223] It has also produced cardiac failure and hypotension, with vacuolar degeneration of the myocardium on pathologic examination.[223,225]

VINCRISTINE AND VINBLASTINE

Vincristine has been associated with cardiac autonomic dysfunction. One study demonstrated a loss of cyclic respiratory phase–related heart rate variation in nine children during vincristine treatment.[226]

Vincristine[227–229] and vinblastine[230] have also been associated with myocardial infarction. Angina pectoris was reported in up to 38% of patients during treatment with vinblastine combined with cisplatinum and bleomycin.[231] Another study of the same combination, reported angina with infarct-like ECG changes and apical akinesia occurring repeatedly, during multiple courses, in a 47-year-old patient with normal coronary angiography.[232] This seemed to clearly implicate the chemotherapy as the cause.

MITOMYCIN C

Mitomycin C has been reported to increase the incidence of anthracycline cardiotoxicity when these agents are combined[233] due to enhancement of formation of superoxide and hydrogen peroxide.[234] It has more recently been described as a cause of acute congestive heart failure in a woman who received a cumulative dose of 225 mg/m^2 of mitomycin as a single agent[235] and in another patient when 30 mg/m^2 of mitomycin was added to treatment with 150 mg/m^2 of doxorubicin.[236] The overall incidence of cardiotoxicity is said to be under 10% and limited to patients receiving a cumulative dose of at least 30 mg/m^2.[236,237]

5-FLUOROURACIL

The cardiotoxicity of 5-fluorouracil was first identified by Dent and McColl in 1975.[238] A survey of 1083 patients in 1982 reported cardiotoxicity in 1.1% of all patients, and 4.6% of patients with prior evidence of heart disease.[239] By 1990 there were more than 67 clinical cases described.[240] Since then, more frequent use of continuous infusion 5-fluorouracil increased awareness of the problem, and more sophisticated monitoring has increased the reported incidence. Thus, by 1991 another large cooperative series of 1145 patients included 31 patients with cardiac symptoms including four cardiotoxic deaths, an incidence of almost 3% of all patients.[241] An even higher incidence of cardiotoxicity of 7.6% was reported from a prospective study of high-dose continuous infusion in 1992.[242] An incidence of silent ischemic ECG changes, as high as 68%, was identified in patients monitored by continuous 24-hour ambulatory ECG during fluorouracil infusion.[243] The cardiotoxicity described has involved (1) precordial pain (both nonspecific and anginal)[240]; (2) ECG ST-T wave changes (nonspecific and ischemic)[240,243,244]; (3) acute myocardial infarction (rare)[244–246]; (4) atrial arrhythmias (including atrial fibrillation) and, less frequently, ventricular ectopy (including refractory ventricular tachycardia and fibrillation)[243–248]; (5) ventricular dysfunction (usually global, less frequently segmental); (6) cardiac failure, pulmonary edema, and cardiogenic shock (with and without ischemic symptoms)[246,248–252]; and (7) sudden death.[246,247] In most cases the arrhythmias were treatable and the *ischemia-like* symptoms and ECG changes disappeared if the infusion was discontinued, or responded to nitrates, allowing the infusion to continue. The abnormalities of segmental and global ventricular function reverted to normal within days to weeks of cessation of infusion. However, some patients needed intravenous inotropic and vasodilator support during the initial period.[248–250,252,253] In most cases with chest pain with or without ECG changes, the creatine phosphokinase (CPK) MB fraction remained normal.[240,246,249,251] Most frequently, patients developed cardiac toxicity during the second or later course of treatment, but some experienced problems during the first course.[240] Those who developed cardiac toxicity and recovered, usually had symptoms again when rechallanged with another infusion.[240,246,248] Some investigators reported success in preventing cardiotoxicity with calcium blockers such as nifedipine and diltiazem,[254] whereas others had less success.[251,255] There was no influence of age or sex on incidence.[240] Symptoms were reported in a 38-year-old man[252] and several women in their 40s[240,249,250] with no prior cardiac history. Cardiac findings have occurred when 5-fluorouracil was given by infusion or bolus, as a single agent, or with cisplatin and other drugs.[240,244] While some believed that cardiac irradiation[256] and preexisting heart disease[239,243] were risk factors, others did not.[240,257] Several investigators have documented normal coronary arteries in patients with severe symptoms.[246,250] One investigator excluded increased proclivity for coronary vasospasm by challenging a patient, who had previous angina during fluorouracil infusion, with ergonovine during a posttreatment coronary study.[246] Findings on autopsy and endomyocardial biopsy have shown diffuse, interstitial edema, intracytoplasmic vacuolization of myocytes, and no inflammatory infiltrate.[258] Acute infarcts have been demonstrated pathologically in some, but not all, patients with clinical infarction.[240]

The ischemic-like pain and ECG findings, with lack of CPK MB changes, with frequent response to nitrates and at times to calcium channel blockers, in the setting of anatomically normal coronary angiograms plus reversible contractility deficits, would suggest coronary vasospasm as a mechanism for fluorouracil cardiotoxicity. However, the global dysfunction, possibly due to *stunned myocardium*, and lack of universal response to coronary vasodilators leaves some questions about this hypothesis and some postulate a myocarditis or myocardiopathy etiology.[259–261]

Although the mechanism is still uncertain, it seems clear that careful observation for cardiac symptoms and arrhythmias is warranted during drug infusion, especially in patients who have been symptomatic in prior courses.

CISPLATIN

Cisplatin has been associated with arrhythmias such as atrial fibrillation[262] and with angina and ST-T wave changes on ECG.[263–266] These may be caused or exacerbated by electrolyte imbalances from the excessive hydration and forced diuresis required for the drug's administration.

INTERFERON

Cardiotoxicity has been identified in 44 of 432 patients from 15 phase I clinical trials of interferon-α, α_2, β, and γ.[267] Significant abnormalities of cardiac rhythm and conduction,[267–270] ischemia and infarction,[267,271–274] and cardiomyopathy[267,274–276] were observed. These problems were identified with all types of interferon used except interferon-β, which was used in only a small subset of the patients.[267] No correlation with patient age, individual dose, or cumulative dose was identified although some patients had less toxicity when retreated at doses lower than the dose producing toxicity.[267,275] Cardiomyopathy was seen in patients after more prolonged treatment,[275] but the other forms of toxicity were seen frequently during the first 5 weeks of treatment, even within 1 to 7 days of initiation of therapy.[267] The occurrence of ischemia and infarction was definitely related to a prior history of ischemic heart disease and may have related to increased myocardial oxygen demand from the fever and stress of the flu-like syndrome accompanying treatment or to peripheral and coronary arterial constriction.[267] The arrhythmias were less clearly related to prior heart disease but may have been exacerbated by the features of this flu-like syndrome as well. Arrhythmias and ischemic ECG changes were identified in mice treated with interferon-α with no myocardial lesions on necropsy, suggesting mediation by peripheral effects.[270] Arrhythmias have been seen in up to 20% of patients in clinical trials.[269] The arrhythmias observed include fatal[277] and reversible[278] ventricular fibrillation, ventricular tachycardia,[268,269] atrial flutter and fibrillation, atrioventricular block, and less severe atrial and ventricular ectopy.[267] Sudden death was seen in two patients.[267] Cardiomyopathy, presenting as cardiac failure, with severe decrease in radionuclide ejection fraction to 10% to 33%, was seen in seven patients during prolonged administration of interferon-α or interferon-α_2.[275,276,279,280] The cardiomyopathy was reversible in four of the patients after cessation of interferon, with and without inotropic, diuretic, and afterload reduction therapy. Congestive symptoms disappeared and ejection fractions improved to 29% to 46%. Two patients were able to be retreated with lower doses of interferon without return of failure. Three of the patients with reversible cardiomyopathy had acquired immunodeficiency syndrome (AIDS) with Kaposi's sarcoma.[275] However, AIDS-associated cardiomyopathy is not reversible. Two others had chronic myelogenous leukemia[279] and hairy cell leukemia,[276] and two more patients had other cancer.[280] Myocardial biopsy in one patient revealed only mild focal intramyocyte vacuolization.[275] The etiologic mechanism is unknown. *In vitro* studies have been conflicting. One study in isolated rat cardiac myocytes, incubated with interferon, showed inhibition of contractility and depletion of ATP,[281] while another similar study did not.[282] Some postulate an interaction between interferon and noradrenaline.[267,283] Cautious observation for cardiac symptoms and monitoring of rhythm appear to be warranted for these agents with reduction in dose for significant abnormalities.

OTHER BIOLOGIC AGENTS

Interleukin-2 and tumor necrosis factor produced no reduction of ATP or decrease in contractility when incubated with isolated rat cardiac myocytes for 24 to 48 hours.[282] However, a major reduction of ventricular stroke work index was found in patients with a variety of solid tumors monitored with indwelling arterial and pulmonary catheters during interleukin-2 treatment.[284] This resulted from a poor increase in cardiac index in comparison with the decrease in peripheral resistance. All patients developed a capillary leak syndrome[285] requiring dopamine and crystalloid support. Deleterious effects on blood pressure, systemic resistance, and stroke work appeared to peak at approximately 4 hours after individual doses and to worsen with subsequent doses.[284] In addition, there has been a significant (4% to 30% in various trials) incidence of apparent myocardial infarction with this agent.[274,284–290] One patient with elevated CPK MB fraction, focal injury pattern on ECG, and segmental wall motion abnormality on radionuclide angiography underwent coronary angiography, revealing normal coronary arteries.[291] This suggested a pathogenesis involving coronary vasospasm or focal myocarditis. A series of 199 patients had an incidence of 6% arrhythmias including ventricular tachycardia, 53% hypotension, and 25% elevated CPK MB.[292] Another biologic agent, interleukin-4, has been associated with myocarditis.[293]

A new biologic agent OK432 derived from *Streptococcus* was suspected of inducing an autoimmune cardiomyopathy. However, it was shown not to provoke the formation of antiheart antibody or ECG changes in rabbits or human patients.[294] Continued evidence of lack of cardiotoxicity should remove an obstacle toward its development as an active anticancer agent.

Transtuzumab (Herceptin), a humanized monoclonal antibody developed to target the HER2 receptor (an epidermal growth factor receptor that is overexpressed in many types of tumor cells), has been associated with cardiotoxicity in several clinical trials.[295–297] The toxicity was manifested as deteriorating systolic function with either asymptomatic decrease in ejection fraction or congestive heart failure similar to anthracycline toxicity. This was observed, however, mainly in patients who had previously received anthracyclines or were concomitantly receiving anthracyclines.[296] Therefore, it is not clear that transtuzumab is itself cardiotoxic or rather potentiates the cardiotoxicity from the previous or ongoing anthracycline therapy. The mechanism of the cardiotoxicity is unknown and histologic information from endomyocardial biopsy is not available. However, clinical and noninvasive evidence of abnormal systolic function was seen more than four times as frequently in patients treated with doxorubicin plus transtuzumab (27%) as in patients treated with doxorubicin alone (6%) in a phase III clinical trial.[295,296] In another randomized clinical trial there was more congestive heart failure in patients treated with paclitaxel and transtuzumab (11%) than in patients treated with paclitaxel alone (1%).[297] In a third trial, a single-arm study, there was a 7% incidence of congestive failure in 213 patients receiving transtuzumab alone.[297] Clearly the cardiotoxic potential of this promising agent will require further investigation, and patients treated with both transtuzumab and an anthracycline need careful monitoring.

OTHER AGENTS

Case reports have attributed cardiotoxicity to several other agents. Melphalan,[298] Bis(helenal)malonate,[299] mithramycin,[300] and bis[1,2-bis(diphenylphosphino)ethane] gold (I) chloride (a cytotoxic antineoplastic drug containing gold),[301] teniposide,[302] etoposide,[303] busulfan,[304] and deoxycoformycin[305] have been implicated in this respect.

AGENTS USED FOR SUPPORTIVE CARE

Patients undergoing therapy for cancer usually receive various medications, in addition to their chemotherapeutic agents, especially for supportive care and treatment of toxicity. Some of these may also have cardiotoxic effects. For example, granisetron, an antiemetic, has been associated with sinus bradycardia, atrioventricular block varying from increased PR interval to Wenckebach's and junctional rhythm.[306] The cytokines, granulocyte colony-stimulating factor and granulocyte-macrophage colony-stimulating factor, have been associated with pericardial effusion.

RADIATION-INDUCED HEART DISEASE

Cardiac complications resulting from mediastinal irradiation were considered rare and insignificant for a long period in the history of radiotherapy.[307,308] Since the mid-1960s, when follow-up information on a large number of patients who had been cured of Hodgkin's disease (HD) with higher doses of radiation became available, the heart has no longer been considered radioresistant.[309] Radiation-induced heart disease has now been characterized[310–312] and investigated in experimental animals,[313–317] and the pathologic features of the damage have been described with regard to the coronary arteries and all three layers of the heart.[318–323]

Pericarditis and pericardial effusion have been regarded as the most common side effects of cardiac irradiation.[310] However, modern techniques of irradiation, dose fractionation, and reduction of the heart volume irradiated in most malignancies have substantially reduced the frequency of this complication during the last decade.[324] At the same time, evidence has accumulated to suggest that ischemic heart disease resulting from radiation-induced CAD is the most concerning long-term risk of cardiac irradiation, particularly in high-risk patients.[325–329]

The clinical spectrum of radiation-induced heart disease involves most structures of the heart and is summarized as follows:

- Pericardial disease
- Acute pericarditis during irradiation
- Delayed acute pericarditis
- Pericardial effusion
- Constrictive pericarditis
- Myocardial dysfunction
- Valvular heart disease
- Electrical conduction abnormalities
- Coronary artery disease

Although the pathologic and clinical manifestations of radiation-induced heart disease may overlap in many patients, they are discussed separately in the following paragraphs.

PERICARDIAL DISEASE

Incidence

The risk of radiation-induced pericardial disease depends on both the dose given and on the volume of the heart irradiated.[310,312,322,330,331] Even when a large volume of the heart (60% or more) is irradiated at or below 40 Gy, the risk for mild pericarditis is below 5%, and severe pericarditis is rare.[324] Smaller heart volumes (20% to 30%) may tolerate up to 60 Gy, with an expected 2% risk of mild pericarditis. The importance of both volume and dose in the production of radiation pericarditis in HD was demonstrated in an analysis of mantle field radiotherapy practices at Stanford.[332] In instances in which the whole pericardium was irradiated, the pericarditis incidence was 20%, but when most of the left ventricle was excluded, it was reduced to 7%. When an additional block was implemented to shield most of the heart after 30 Gy, the incidence was reduced to only 2.5%. An update of the Stanford data corroborated this finding, demonstrating a sharp decrease in the risk of death from cardiac complications other than acute myocardial infarction for patients who received mediastinal irradiation after 1972.[326] Indeed, all series that showed a high risk of pericarditis[333–335] are of patients treated with a radiation technique, energy, and fractionation schedules that are no longer considered to be an acceptable standard of care in most centers.[329] With current radiotherapy techniques for HD and breast cancer, pericarditis is an infrequent event.[329,331,336,337]

Pathology

Clinical and pathologic changes involving the pericardium are the most common abnormalities described after cardiac irradiation.[317,323] The macroscopic abnormalities consist of pericardial thickening and effusion.[310] Collagen replaces the normal adipose tissue, fibrinous exudate is present on the surface and interstitially, and proliferation of small blood vessels can be observed microscopically.[310] The pericardial fluid is protein rich and may contain strands of fibrin. The fluid ranges in appearance from serous to grossly sanguineous.[311] Over time, the fibrinous exudate may organize with the fibrotic pericardium and epicardium to develop into constrictive pericarditis. The mechanism for pericardial fibrosis and effusion is not clear. It may result from increased capillary permeability and inhibition of the local fibrinolytic mechanism.[310,338] Radiation-induced hypothyroidism should also be considered in the etiology of pericardial effusion after mediastinal irradiation.[339]

Acute Pericarditis during Radiation

Acute pericarditis during the course of radiotherapy is rare. It is almost always associated with massive mediastinal tumors adjacent to the heart. The signs and symptoms are of acute nonspecific pericarditis with chest pain, fever, and often ECG abnormalities. It does not lead to a significant risk of late pericardial damage and is not an indication for interrupting the radiation course.[310,312,327]

Delayed Pericarditis

Radiation-induced pericarditis typically occurs within the first year after mediastinal irradiation. The common range is between 4 months to several years after treatment.[310,312,335,340-342] Pericardial disease presents either as an acute pericarditis, as a pericardial effusion that may be asymptomatic, or as a combination of both. The symptoms of delayed acute pericarditis are indistinguishable from those of other types of pericarditis and usually consist of fever, pleuritic chest pain, pericardial friction rub, ST-T segment changes, and a decrease of the QRS voltage in the ECG.[310,311,335]

Pericardial effusion may be large and manifest as an enlarged cardiac silhouette.[343] The differential diagnosis of pericardial effusion after radiation includes recurrent malignancy, idiopathic pericarditis, myxedema, and pericardial abscess.[311,344,345] It is estimated that 10% to 30% of patients with radiation-related pericardial effusion develop tamponade and require pericardiocentesis.[334,346,347] Most cases of radiation-induced pericarditis and pericardial effusion resolve spontaneously, usually within 16 months.[347] Approximately 20% of patients with delayed pericarditis progress within 5 to 10 years to develop symptomatic constriction requiring pericardiectomy.[348]

Treatment

Careful cardiac evaluation and monitoring with echocardiography and radionuclide ventriculography should be performed whenever radiation-induced heart disease is suspected.[340,343] Patients with mild symptoms and no hemodynamic compromise may be followed without treatment or may receive symptomatic therapy with salicylates or other nonsteroidal antiinflammatory agents.[310,311] There are reports of a few patients who have received corticosteroids with apparent improvement.[349] However, relapse of symptoms or unmasking of latent radiation injury following rapid withdrawal of corticosteroid therapy has been reported.[350,351] Symptomatic pericardial effusion or clinical evidence for hemodynamic compromise warrants a drainage procedure. Pericardiocentesis with or without percutaneous placement of an indwelling catheter is successful in the majority of patients.[337,352] Failure to relieve tamponade with pericardiocentesis, recurrence of effusion, or the presence of symptomatic constrictive pericarditis requires pericardiectomy.[314,335,353] The mortality of this procedure in patients with postradiation pericarditis is high. Cameron and colleagues[354] reported a postoperative mortality of 21%, and a review by Ni and associates[355] showed an early mortality of 22% in patients operated on for radiation-induced pericarditis and a late mortality (after 30 days or more) of 35%. The high rate of complication in previously irradiated patients is attributed to the existence of additional radiation injury to other cardiac and thoracic structures. Occult constrictive pericarditis requires no surgical intervention and usually has a good prognosis.[311]

MYOCARDIAL DYSFUNCTION

When myocardial dysfunction is detected after standard-dose mediastinal irradiation, it is typically mild or subclinical.[311,329,356,357] Impaired exercise capacity in asymptomatic postradiation patients has been reported.[358,359] In patients who were studied 15 days after mediastinal irradiation, a transient decrease in LVEF was observed. Complete recovery of ejection fraction 2 months after irradiation and no additional change in patients who were also receiving doxorubicin was documented in this study.[360] Noninvasive studies using echocardiography and radionuclide angiogram detected subtle left ventricular dysfunction in HD patients evaluated a few years after mediastinal irradiation.[334,353,355] The majority of patients with abnormal ventricular function findings, however, do not have clinical heart failure.[351]

The magnitude of the potential contribution of cardiac irradiation to the risk of doxorubicin-induced cardiomyopathy is not well established. But some data suggest potentiation of anthracycline-induced cardiotoxicity when combined with radiotherapy.[11,15,22,356–358] The histopathologies of radiation heart disease and anthracycline heart disease are different,[359] and the combined effects are probably additive rather than synergistic.[307,359,360] Reducing the doxorubicin dose to 300 to 350 mg/m^2 in the setting of cardiac irradiation has been recommended.[11] In programs of combined modality therapy for HD that included relatively low doses of doxorubicin (up to 250 mg/m^2) and mediastinal irradiation of 20 to 40 Gy, no significant clinical myocardial dysfunction was detected.[361–369] However, longer follow-up is required to fully appreciate the potential risk of combined modality cardiac toxicity.[34]

Symptomatic myocardial dysfunction after a radiation dose that does not exceed 60 Gy is rare.[310] The few cases described with intractable heart failure had myocardial fibrosis as part of pancarditis, a generalized process with damage to all three layers of the heart. The hemodynamic pattern is usually of restrictive cardiomyopathy and is difficult to distinguish from constrictive pericarditis.[310,311,338] Its coexistence with pericarditis explains the poor outcome of pericardiectomy when attempted under these circumstances.[310,355] In a pathologic analysis of cardiac tissue from patients with radiation-induced heart disease, interstitial fibrosis (of various degrees) of the myocardium was mostly pericellular and perivascular. The degree of fibrosis was proportional to the radiation dose and was not enhanced in cases in which doxorubicin therapy was also administered.[323]

VALVULAR DISEASE

Clinically significant valvular heart disease resulting from mediastinal irradiation is rare.[310,311,370,371] In a review of radiation-associated valvular disease, only ten patients with symptomatic postradiation valvular disease could be found.[370] Analysis of 635 patients treated for HD before the age of 21 years revealed 29 patients who developed new murmurs of indeterminate significance. Of those, 14 received mediastinal doses of 44 Gy or more, and two patients who received high-dose irradiation died of valvular heart disease.[326,327] When echocardiographic studies were performed in asymptomatic HD patients more than 7 years after mediastinal irradiation, valvular abnormalities were detected in 25% to 33% of the patients, although there was rarely any clinical significance. Of interest is a report from Norway that showed a significantly higher risk of cardiopulmonary complications for female subjects after radiation for HD.[357,372–374] Most of the changes were found in the mitral or aortic valve and consisted of thickening or regurgitation.[323,357,370,372,375] In one series,[358] mild pulmonary stenosis was detected in three patients 6 to 12 years after radiotherapy. Fibrous thickening of the valvular endocardium was found at autopsy in 13 of 16 young patients who received over 35 Gy to the heart, but none of them had apparent valvular dysfunction.[318] The mean interval from irradiation to detection of valvular disease in asymptomatic and symptomatic patients was 11.5 and 16.5 years, respectively.[370] The contribution of irradiation to clinically significant valvular disease appears to be small.[323,329]

ELECTRICAL ABNORMALITIES

Many ECG abnormalities were recorded years after mediastinal irradiation, the most common clinically significant abnormality being complete atrioventricular block.[340,358,376–383] Slama and colleagues[380] reported that radiation-related atrioventricular block was typically infranodal and occurred at long intervals (mean of 12 years), after radiation doses above 40 Gy, most frequently in patients with abnormal conduction on ECG before the advent of complete block, and who had other radiation-related cardiac abnormalities. At postmortem examination, fibrosis of the conduction system has been reported.[377,380]

Another aspect of radiation therapy and heart disease relates to the management of patients with implanted cardiac pacemakers.[386] Although transient interference from electromagnetic noise (with the exception of betatrons) is not a problem in properly functioning radiotherapy equipment, pacemaker-dependent patients should be closely observed during the first treatment with a linear accelerator.[385] Placing the pacemaker in an unshielded radiotherapy field may cause cumulative damage to the pacemaker components.[384] The absorbed dose to the pacemaker should be estimated before treatment. If the total dose to the pacemaker might exceed 2 Gy, the pacemaker function should be checked weekly to detect any indicator of damage that may require replacement of the device.[384]

CORONARY ARTERY DISEASE

Experiments in laboratory animals,[313–316,386–388] analysis of pathologic specimens,[318] clinical observations,[333,389–391] and, in the 1990s, long-term risk analysis in large series of patients treated for HD[325–327,392–394] all indicate that mediastinal irradiation may facilitate the development of CAD.

Studies in rabbits on an atherogenic diet and exposed to radiation showed extensive atherosclerotic coronary damage to a degree disproportionately higher than what might have been expected from the summation of the changes induced by radiation alone and by high-cholesterol diet alone.[387] Similar observations have been made in other experimental animals.[388,389]

An autopsy study in 16 young patients (aged 15 to 33 years) who received over 35 Gy to the heart showed that 16 of 64 (25%) major coronary arteries had significant stenosis (greater than 76% obstruction) compared with only 1 of 40 (2.5%) obstructed coronary arteries in a group of age- and sex-matched controls.[318] In this study, the proximal portion of the arteries had significantly more narrowing than the distal parts. McEniery and coworkers[391] described coronary angiograms of 15 patients with CAD after chest irradiation. Eight of these 15 had significant narrowing (more than 50% diameter) of the left main coronary artery, and four had severe ostial stenosis of the right coronary artery. Stenosis at the origin of the coronary arteries appears to be a common finding for radiation-associated CAD.[328,395–398] After mediastinal irradiation, there is a greater likelihood for right coronary or left main or left anterior descending coronary artery lesions as opposed to circumflex lesions, which might be due to the fact that the former vessels, particularly at their origin, receive more radiation.[399] Coronary spasm following radiotherapy has also been documented in patients who developed acute myocardial infarction with patent coronary arteries.[391,400]

Reports of CAD in young patients who had received mediastinal irradiation for HD have long indicated that radiation is a facilitating factor in this multifactorial disease process.[311,318,389–391,399] However, only more recently could analyses of large databases of patients with HD demonstrate a significantly increased risk of mortality from myocardial infarction after mediastinal irradiation. These studies are summarized in Table 55.4-1. Although only approximately 1% to 2% of HD patients in these series died of myocardial infarction, the observed risk in all six series was still higher than expected.[325–329,336,392,393] Boivin and associates[392] analyzed the risk of mortality from CAD in 4665 patients treated for HD and followed for an average of 7 years. The age-adjusted relative risk of death with myocardial infarction after mediastinal irradiation was 2.6 and was even higher (relative risk, 4.0) when myocardial infarction was considered as

TABLE 55.4-1. Relative Risk of Mortality from Myocardial Infarction after Mediastinal Irradiation for Hodgkin's Disease

Source	*Center*	*Patients*	*Lethal Myocardial Infarctions*	*Relative Risk*	*95% Confidence Interval*
Boivin[392]	Multiple	4665	68	2.6	1.1–5.9
Hancock[326]	Stanford	2232	55	3.2	1.5–5.8
Henry-Amar[393]	European Organization for Treatment and Research on Cancer	1449	17	8.8	5.1–14.1
Mauch[325]	Joint Center for Radiation Therapy (Boston)	636	15[a]	2.2[a]	1.2–3.6
Glanzmann[329]	Zurich	352	8	4.2	1.8–8.3
Reinders[328]	Rotterdam	258	12[b]	5.3	2.7–9.3

[a]Includes one patient who died of cardiomyopathy.
[b]Myocardial infarction or sudden death.

a direct cause of death. In this study, the onset of increased risk was rapid, within the first 5 years of observation. None of the risk factors for CAD significantly altered the relative risk estimates.

Current mantle radiotherapy techniques, better fractionation schemes, and modern equipment deliver smaller doses of radiation to the coronary arteries and may have a lower risk of promoting CAD.[331] In the study by Boivin and colleagues,[392] the relative risk of acute myocardial infarction was reduced from 6.33 for patients treated during the years 1940 to 1966 to 1.97 (with no significant difference from unity) for patients irradiated from 1967 to 1985.

Hancock and coworkers[326,327] analyzed the risk of cardiac disease in patients with HD who were treated at Stanford from 1961 to 1991. The analysis that was limited to children and adolescents younger than age 21 years at the time of treatment showed that the relative risk for death from acute myocardial infarction in this age group was 41.5 (95% CI, 18.1 to 82.1) and that the actuarial risk of fatal or nonfatal myocardial infarction at 22 years was 8.1%.[327] Of note, all deaths in this study occurred in patients who received relatively high doses of radiation (42 to 45 Gy) to the mediastinum. When the Stanford analysis was extended to include 2232 HD patients of all age groups, the relative risk for death from acute myocardial infarction was 3.2 (95% CI, 1.5 to 5.8).[326] This study showed that patients younger than 20 years who received high-dose irradiation had the highest relative risk, the risk decreases with increasing age, and patients older than 50 years of age had no increased risk. However, these results contrast with data published by other investigators,[325,328,392] suggesting an increased risk of acute myocardial infarction for the older age groups. The small number of patients in the Stanford study who received radiation doses of less than 30 Gy did not allow an adequate analysis of the dose effect. The average interval between HD treatment and death from acute myocardial infarction was 10.3 years, but risk was already significant during the first 5 years following treatment and remained elevated throughout the follow-up period (more than 20 years).[326]

Two European studies analyzed the ischemic heart disease in HD patients who received standard fractions and dose (30 to 42 Gy) of mediastinal irradiation.[328,329] Both studies demonstrated an increase of ischemic heart disease after mediastinal irradiation. The study from Rotterdam, with a median follow-up of 14 years, reported that 12% of the patients experienced ischemic heart disease, with death rate of 4.7% (from myocardial infarction or sudden death).[328] When compared with expected incidence, the standardized mortality ratio was 5.3 (CI 2.7 to 9.3). Of importance, a multivariate analysis of risk factors in the Rotterdam study showed that increasing age, gender (male), and a pretreatment cardiac medical history were significant for developing ischemic heart disease. Treatment-related parameters did not affect the risk.[328] In a study from Zurich, a detailed analysis of the effect of other CAD risk factors on the radiation-induced risk was performed. The study showed that while the risk of CAD after irradiation increased by 4.2 for all patients, in irradiated female patients and in all irradiated patients without other cardiovascular risk factors (smoking, hypertension, obesity, hypercholesterolemia, diabetes), the risk remained as expected in the normal population.[329]

Long-term mortality data from three trials, which randomized breast cancer patients to receive postmastectomy radiotherapy as opposed to no additional treatment, demonstrated a higher incidence of cardiac death in the irradiated group.[401–403] The excess in mortality did not appear until after 10 years post-treatment.[402,403] In one study, the increase in mortality risk was significant only in women who were irradiated for tumors in the left breast.[403] It was also increased in patients treated with orthovoltage irradiation as opposed to those treated with more modern supervoltage equipment.[403]

These data demonstrate the risk associated with coronary artery irradiation. It should be emphasized that the old breast irradiation techniques used in these particular studies delivered high doses of radiation to the heart.[331,404] These techniques are no longer in use in most centers. Long-term follow-up of patients in similar randomized trials who were treated with heart-sparing techniques did not show increased cardiovascular morbidity.[405–407] Prophylactic irradiation of the internal mammary nodes using a single anterior photon beam (*hockey stick technique*), which may deliver a high dosage to the heart, is not indicated in most patients irradiated for breast conservation or postmastectomy.[408,409] Breast cancer patients irradiated with modern techniques, energies, and fractionation schedules are unlikely to receive a significant dose of radiation to the coronary arteries.[404,410–412]

Conventional-dose doxorubicin-containing chemotherapy used as adjuvant in combination with locoregional irradiation was not associated with a significant increase in the risk of cardiac events. However, higher doses of adjuvant doxorubicin were associated with a threefold to fourfold increased risk of cardiac events. This appears to be especially true in patients treated with higher dose volumes of cardiac irradiation.[413]

The radiation threshold for an increased risk of CAD has not been determined. Lederman and associates[414] reported that patients with seminoma who received a relatively low dose of mediastinal irradiation (median, 24 Gy) had more ischemic heart disease compared with a similar group of patients whose mediastinums were not irradiated. It should be noted, however, that the observed cardiac risk in the irradiated group did not differ significantly from the expected risk of a comparable normal population.

Monitoring and reduction of other contributing CAD factors in patients who received mediastinal irradiation should be part of the follow-up of patients who underwent mediastinal irradiation. However, the value of routine noninvasive or invasive cardiac studies in asymptomatic patients has not been determined.[329,373,415–418] Still, early detection of CAD should be encouraged, particularly in irradiated patients with other CAD risk factors,[329] because angioplastic or surgical intervention may be indicated in special anatomic or clinical situations. Successful treatment of radiation-induced coronary disease with bypass surgery and with angioplasty has been reported.[391,419,420] In some cases, surgery may be technically difficult because of mediastinal and pericardial fibrosis.[391]

Although the mechanism of radiation-induced coronary heart disease remains unclear, insult to the endothelial cell is considered to be a central event in the pathogenesis of damage to the coronary arteries.[397] Research indicates that programmed cell death (apoptosis) is the underlying mechanism for postradiation endothelial cell death.[421] Growth factors that interfere with the apoptotic pathway, such as bFGF, may prevent radiation-induced death of endothelial cells, as in the study by Fuks and colleagues,[421] who demonstrated that treatment with bFGF during chest irradiation of experimental animals decreased postradiation blood vessel stenosis and significantly increased the survival of the bFGF-treated animals following radiation. These findings provide a basis for future interventions that may decrease the risk of radiation-induced heart disease.

CONCLUSION

It is hoped that increased awareness and knowledge about potential cardiotoxicity from chemotherapy and radiotherapy will enable physicians to adequately monitor patients and modify therapy so as to minimize serious acute and chronic cardiac sequelae. The growing information about late cardiac effects should facilitate early diagnosis and therapeutic intervention for the benefit of previously treated patients.

REFERENCES

1. Tan CT, Tasaka H, Yu KP, et al. Daunomycin an antitumor antibiotic in the treatment of neoplastic disease. *Cancer* 1967;20:333.
2. Malpas JS, Scott RB. Rubidomycin in acute leukaemia in adults. *BMJ* 1968;3:227.
3. Marmont AM, Damasio E, Rossi F. Cardiac toxicity of daunorubicin. *Lancet* 1969;1:837.
4. Bonadonna G, Monfardini S, De Lena M, et al. Phase I and preliminary phase II evaluation of adriamycin. *Cancer Res* 1970;30:2572.
5. Tan C, Etcubans E, Wollner N, et al. Adriamycin an antitumor antibiotic in the treatment of neoplastic disease. *Cancer* 1973;32:9.
6. O'Bryan RM, Luce JK, Tally RW, et al. Phase II evaluation of adriamycin in human neoplasia. *Cancer* 1973;32:1.
7. Blum RH, Carter SK. Adriamycin, a new anticancer drug with significant clinical activity. *Ann Intern Med* 1974;80:249.
8. Gilladoga AC, Manuel C, Tan CT, et al. Cardiotoxicity of adriamycin in children. *Cancer Chemother Rep* 1975;6:75.
9. Lefrak EA, Pitha J, Rosenheim S, et al. A clinicopathologic analysis of adriamycin cardiotoxicity. *Cancer* 1973;32:302.
10. Halazun JF, Wagner HR, Gaeta JF, et al. Daunorubicin cardiac toxicity in children with acute lymphocytic leukemia. *Cancer* 1974;33:545.
11. Von Hoff DD, Layard M, Basa P. Risk factors for doxorubicin induced congestive heart failure. *Ann Intern Med* 1979;91:701.
12. Von Hoff DD, Rozencweig M, Layard M, et al. Daunomycin-induced cardiotoxicity in children and adults. *Am J Med* 1977; 62:200.
13. Bristow MR, Billingham ME, Mason JW, et al. Clinical spectrum of anthracycline cardiotoxicity. *Cancer Treat Rep* 1978;62:873.
14. Bristow MR. Pathophysiologic basis for cardiac monitoring in patients receiving anthracyclines. In: Crooke ST, Reich SD, eds. *Anthracyclines: current status and new developments.* New York: Academic Press, 1980:255.
15. Billingham ME, Bristow MR, Glastein E, et al. Adriamycin cardiotoxicity: endomyocardial biopsy evidence of enhancement by irradiation. *Am J Surg Pathol* 1977;1:17.
16. Bristow MR, Thompson PD, Martin RP, et al. Early anthracycline cardiotoxicity. *Am J Med* 1978;65:823.
17. Bristow MR, Minobe WA, Billingham ME, et al. Anthracycline-associated cardiac and renal damage in rabbits. Evidence for mediation by vasoactive substances. *Lab Invest* 1981;45:157.
18. Wortman JE, Lucas VS, Schuster E, et al. Sudden death during doxorubicin administration. *Cancer* 1979;44:1588.
19. Dindogru A, Barcos M, Henderson ES, et al. Electrocardiographic changes following Adriamycin treatment. *Med Pediatr Oncol* 1978;5:65.
20. Porembka DT, Lowder JN, Orlowski JP, Bastulli J, Lockrem J. Doxorubicin cardiotoxicity. *Crit Care Med* 1989;17:569.
21. Gottlieb SL, Edmiston WA, Haywood LJ. Late, late doxorubicin cardiotoxicity. *Chest* 1980;78:880.
22. Gilladoga AC, Manuel C, Tan CTC, et al. The cardiotoxicity of adriamycin and daunomycin in children. *Cancer* 1976;37:1070.
23. Goorin AM, Borow KM, Goldman A, et al. Congestive heart failure due to adriamycin cardiotoxicity: it's natural history in children. *Cancer* 1981;47:2810.
24. Alexander J, Dainiak N, Berger HJ, et al. Serial assessment of doxorubicin cardiotoxicity with quantitative radionuclide angiocardiography. *N Engl J Med* 1979;300:278.
25. Cohen M, Kronzon I, Lebowitz A. Reversible doxorubicin-induced congestive heart failure. *Arch Intern Med* 1982;142:1570.
26. Saini J, Rich MW, Lyss AP. Reversibility of severe left ventricular dysfunction due to doxorubicin cardiotoxicity. *Ann Intern Med* 1987;106:814.
27. Yeung ST, Yoong C, Spink J, Galbraith A, Smith PJ. Functional myocardial impairment in children treated with anthracyclines for cancer. *Lancet* 1991;337:816.
28. Bristow MR, Mason JW, Billingham ME, Daniels JR. Doxorubicin cardiomyopathy: evaluation by phonocardiography, endomyocardial biopsy, and cardiac catheterization. *Ann Intern Med* 1978;88:168.
29. Billingham ME, Mason JW, Bristow MR, et al. Anthracycline cardiomyopathy monitored by morphologic changes. *Cancer Treat Rep* 1978;62:865.
30. Billingham ME, Masek MA. The pathology of anthracycline cardiotoxicity in children, adolescents, and adults. In: Bricker JT, Green DM, D'Angio GJ, eds. *Cardiac toxicity after treatment for childhood cancer.* New York: Wiley-Liss, 1993:17.
31. Gaudin PB, Hruban RH, Beschorner WE, et al. Myocarditis associated with doxorubicin cardiotoxicity. *Am J Clin Pathol* 1993;100:158.
32. Koh E, Imashuku S, Kiyosawa N, Sawada T. Anthracycline-induced congestive heart failure in two pediatric leukemia cases and long-term follow-up. *Pediatr Hematol Oncol* 1988;5:245.
33. Steinherz L, Murphy ML, Steinherz P, et al. Long-term cardiac follow up 4-13 years post anthracycline therapy. In: Doyle E, Engle MA, Gersony W, Rashkin W, Talner N, eds. *Pediatric cardiology.* New York: Springer Verlag, 1986:1058.
34. Steinherz LJ, Steinherz PG, Tan CTC, Heller G, Murphy ML. Cardiotoxicity 4-20 years after completing anthracycline therapy. *JAMA* 1991;266:1672.
35. Steinherz LJ, Steinherz PG. Delayed anthracyclines cardiac toxicity. In: DeVita VT, Hellman S, Rosenberg SA, eds. *Cancer: principles and practice of oncology, PPO updates.* 1991;5:1.
36. Steinherz L, Steinherz P. Cardiac failure more than six years post anthracyclines. *Am J Cardiol* 1988;62:505.
37. Steinherz LJ, Steinherz PG, Tan C. Cardiac failure and dysrhythmias 6-19 years after anthracycline therapy: a series of 15 patients. *Med Pediatr Oncol* 1995;24:352.
38. Krischer JP, Epstein S, Cuthbertson DD, et al. Clinical cardiotoxicity following anthracycline treatment for childhood Cancer: the Pediatric Oncology Group Experience. *J Clin Oncol* 1997;15:1544.
39. Lipshultz SE, Colan SD, Gelber RD, et al. Late cardiac effects of doxorubicin in childhood lymphoblastic leukemia. *N Engl J Med* 1991;324:808.
40. Hausdorf G, Morf G, Beron G, et al. Long-term doxorubicin cardiotoxicity in childhood: non-invasive evaluation of the contractile state and diastolic filling. *Br Heart J* 1988; 60:309.
41. Sorenson K, Levitt G, Sebag-Montefiore D, Bull C, Sullivan I. Cardiac function in Wilms' tumor survivors. *J Clin Oncol* 1995;13:1546.
42. Steinherz LJ. Anthracycline-induced cardiomyopathy. *Ann Intern Med* 1996;126:827.
43. Pihkala J, Happonen JM, Virtanen K, et al. Cardiopulmonary evaluation of exercise tolerance after chest irradiation and anticancer chemotherapy in children and adolescents. *Pediatrics* 1995;95:722.
44. Weesner KM, Bledsoe M, Chauvenet A, Wofford M. Exercise echocardiography in the detection of anthracycline cardiotoxicity. *Cancer* 1991;68:435.
45. Jakacki RI, Larsen RL, Barber G, Goldwein JW, Silber JH. Cardiac function following cardiotoxic therapy during childhood: assessing the damage. In: Bricker JT, Green DM, D'Angio GJ, eds. *Cardiac toxicity after treatment for childhood cancer.* New York: Wiley-Liss, 1993:87.
46. Stoddard MF, Seeger J, Liddell NE, Hadley TJ, Sullivan DM, Kupersmith J. Prolongation of isovolumetric relaxation time as assessed by Doppler echocardiography predicts doxorubicin-induced systolic dysfunction in humans. *J Am Coll Cardiol* 1992;20:62.
47. Kreuser ED, VollerH, Behlers C, et al. Evaluation of late cardiotoxicity with pulsed Doppler echocardiography in patients treated for Hodgkin's disease. *Br J Haematol* 1993;84:615.
48. Ewer MS, Ali MK, Gibbs HR, et al. Cardiac diastolic function in pediatric patients receiving doxorubicin. *Acta Oncol* 1994;33:645.
49. Fukazawa R, Ogawa S, Hirayama T. Early detection of anthracycline cardiotocixity in children with acute leukemia using exercise-based echocardiography and Doppler echocardiography. *Jpn Circ J* 1994;58:625.
50. Steinherz LJ, Steinherz PG, Heller G. Anthracycline-related cardiac damage. In: Bricker JT, Green DM, D'Angio GJ, eds. *Cardiac toxicity after treatment for childhood cancer.* New York: Wiley-Liss, 1993:63.
51. Hausdorf G. Late effects of anthracycline therapy in childhood: evaluation and current therapy. In: Bricker JT, Green DM, D'Angio GJ, eds. *Cardiac toxicity after treatment for childhood cancer.* New York: Wiley-Liss, 1993:73.
52. Adachi K, Fujiura Y, Mayumi F, et al. A deletion of mitochondrial DNA in murine doxorubicin-induced cardiotoxicity. *Biochem Biophys Res Comm* 1993;195:945.
53. Goormaghtigh E, Huart P, Praet M, Brasseur R, Ruysschaert JM. Structure of the adriamycin-cardiolipin complex role in mitochondrial toxicity. *Biophys Chem* 1990;35:247.
54. Fu LX, Waagstein F, Hjalmarson A. A new insight into adriamycin-induced cardiotoxicity. *Int J Cardiol* 1990;29:15.
55. Kapelko VI, Saks VA, Novikova NA, et al. Adaptation of cardiac contractile functions to conditions of chronic energy deficiency. *J Mol Cell Cardiol* 1989;21:79.
56. Myers CE, McGuire WP, Liss RH, et al. Adriamycin: the role of lipid peroxidation in cardiac toxicity and tumor response. *Science* 1977;197:165.
57. Rajagopalan S, Politi PM, Sinha BK, Myers CE. Adriamycin-induced free radical formation in the perfused rat heart: implications for cardiotoxicity. *Cancer Res* 1988;48:4766.
58. Myers CE, Gianna L, Simone CB, Klecker R, Greene R. Oxidative destruction of erythrocyte ghost membranes catalyzed by the doxorubicin-iron complex. *Biochemistry* 1982;21:1707.
59. Gutteridge JM. Lipid peroxidation and possible hydroxyl radical formation stimulated by the self-reduction of a doxorubicin-iron (III) complex. *Biochem Pharmacol* 1984;33:1725.
60. Olson RD, Mushlin PS, Brenner DE, et al. Doxorubicin cardiotoxicity may be caused by its metabolite doxorubicinol. *Proc Natl Acad Sci U S A* 1988;85:3585.
61. Cusack BJ, Mushlin PS, Voulelis LD, et al. Daunorubicin-induced cardiac injury in the rabbit: a role for daunorubicinol? *Toxicol Appl Pharmacol* 1993;118:177.
62. Pessah IN, Durie EL, Schiedt MJ, Zimanyi I. Anthraquinone-sensitized Ca^{2+} release channel from rat cardiac sarcoplasmic reticulum: possible receptor-mediated mechanism of doxorubicin cardiomyopathy. *Mol Pharmacol* 1990;37:503.
63. Dodd DA, Atkinson JB, Olson RD, et al. Doxorubicin cardiomyopathy is associated with a decrease in calcium release channel of the sarcoplasmic retuculum in a chronic rabbit model. *J Clin Invest* 1993;91:1697.
64. Shenasa H, Calderone A, Vermeulen M, et al. Chronic doxorubicin induced cardiomyopathy in rabbits: mechanical, intracellular action potential, and beta adrenergic characteristics of the failing myocardium. *Cardiovasc Res* 1990;24:591.

65. Cappelli V, Moggio R, Monti E, et al. Reduction of myofibrillar ATPase activity and isomyosin shift in delayed doxorubicin cardiotoxicity. *J Mol Cell Cardiol* 1989;21:93.
66. Minow RA, Benjamin RS, Lee ET, et al. QRS voltage change with adriamycin administration. *Cancer Treat Rep* 1978;62:931.
67. Steinherz LJ, Graham T, Hurwitz R, et al. Guidelines for cardiac monitoring of children during and after anthracycline therapy: report of the Cardiology Committee of the Childrens Cancer Study Group. *Pediatrics* 1992;89:942
68. Iacuone J, Steinherz LJ, Oblender M, Barnard D, Ablin AR. Modifications for toxicity. In: Ablin AR, ed. *Supportive care of children with cancer: current therapy and guidelines from the Childrens Cancer Group*, 2nd ed. Baltimore: Johns Hopkins University Press, 1997:79.
69. Bloom K, Bini R, Williams C, et al. Echocardiography in adriamycin cardiotoxicity. *Cancer* 1978;41:1265.
70. Biancaniello T, Meyer RA, Wong KY, et al. Doxorubicin cardiotoxicity in children. *J Pediatr* 1980;97:45.
71. Borow K, Henderson I, Neuman A, et al. Assessment of left ventricular contractility in patients receiving doxorubicin. *Ann Intern Med* 1983;99:750.
72. Steinherz LJ, Wexler LH. The prevention of anthracycline cardiomyopathy. *Prog Pediatr Cardiol* 1998;8:97.
73. Bu'Lock FA, Martin RP, Oakhill A, Mott MG. Early identification of anthracycline cardiomyopathy: possibilities and implications. *Arch Dis Child* 1996;75:1416.
74. Schwartz RG, McKenzie WB, Alexander S, et al. Congestive heart failure and left ventricular dysfunction complicating doxorubicin therapy: a seven year experience using serial radionuclide angiocardiography. *Am J Med* 1987;82:1109.
75. Gottdiener JS, Mathisen DJ, Borer JS, et al. Doxorubicin cardiotoxicity: assessment of late left ventricular dysfunction by radionuclide cineangiography. *Ann Intern Med* 1981;94:430.
76. Palmeri ST, Bonow RO, Myers CE, et al. Prospective evaluation of doxorubicin cardiotoxicity by rest and exercise radionuclide angiography. *Am J Cardiol* 1986;58:607.
77. McKillop JH, Bristow MR, Goris ML, et al. Sensitivity and specificity of radionuclide ejection fractions in doxorubicin cardiotoxicity. *Am Heart J* 1983;106:1048.
78. Lee BH, Goodenday LS, Muswick GJ, et al. Alterations in left ventricular diastolic function with doxorubicin therapy. *J Am Coll of Cardiol* 1987;9:184.
79. Ganz WI, Sridhar KS, Forness TJ. Detection of early anthracycline cardiotoxicity by monitoring the peak filling rate. *Am J Clin Oncol* 1993;16:109.
80. Iarussi D, Auricchio U, Agretto A, et al. Protective effect of coenzyme Q10 on anthracycline cardiotoxicity: control study in children with acute lymphoblastic leukemia and non-Hodgkin's lymphoma. *Mol Asp Med* 1994;15:207.
81. Ewer MS, Carrasco CH, Mackay B, Ali MK, Benjamin RS. Cardiac biopsy procedures at a cancer center. *Proc Ann Meet Am Soc Clin Oncol* 1991;10:A1189.
82. Siveski-Iliskovic N, Hill M, Chow DA, Singal PK. Probucol protects against Adriamycin cardiomyopathy without interfering with its antitumor effect. *Circulation* 1995;91:10.
83. Dreyer Z, Guidry G, Mahoney D, et al. Tantalum-178 first pass radionuclide imaging (TaRNA) sensitive early detection of cardiac dysfunction (CD) in anthracycline (ANTH) treated pediatric patients. *Proc Ann Meet Am Soc Clin Oncol* 1994;13:A1499.
84. Estorch M, Carrio I, Berna L, et al. Indium-111-antimyosin scintigraphy after doxorubicin therapy in patients with advanced breast cancer. *J Nucl Med* 1990;31:1965.
85. Lopez M, Vici P, Di Lauro K, et al. Randomized prospective clinical trial of high-dose epirubicin and dexrazoxane in patients with advanced breast cancer and soft tissue sarcomas. *J Clin Oncol* 1998;16:86.
86. Carrio I, Lopez-Pousa A, Estorch M, et al. Detection of doxorubicin cardiotoxicity in patients with sarcomas by indium-111-antimyosin monoclonal antibody studies. *J Nucl Med* 1993;34:1503.
87. Estorch M, Carrio I, Martinez-Duncker D, et al. Myocyte cell damage after administration of doxorubicin or mitoxantrone in antibody studies. *J Clin Oncol* 1993;11:1264.
88. Fountzilas G, Afthonidis D, Geleris P, et al. Cardiotoxicity evaluation in patients treated with a mitoxantrone combination as adjuvant chemotherapy for breast cancer. *Anticancer Res* 1992;12:231.
89. Hiroe M, Ohta Y, Fujita N, et al. Myocardial uptake of Indium 111 in monoclonal antimyosin Fab in detecting doxorubicin cardiotoxicity in rats. Morphological and hemodynamic findings. *Circulation* 1992;86:1965.
90. Wagasugi S, Fischman AJ, Babich JW, et al. Metaiodobenzylgaunidine: evaluation of its potential as a tracer for monitoring doxorubicin cardiomyopathy. *J Nucl Med* 1993;34:1282.
91. Valdes Olmos RA, ten Bokkel Huinink WW, Greve JC, Hoefnagel CA. I-123 MIBG and serial radionuclide angiocardiography in doxorubicin-related cardiotoxcity. *Clin Nucl Med* 1992;17:163.
92. Takeishi Y, Sukekawa H, Sakurai T, et al. Noninvasive identification of anthracycline cardiotoxicity: comparison of 123I-MIBG and 123I-BMIPP imaging. *Ann Nucl Med* 1994;8:177.
93. Gardner SF, Lazarus HM, Bednarczyk EM, et al. High-dose cyclophosphamide-induced myocardial damage during BMT: assessment by position emission tomography. *Bone Marrow Transplant* 1993;12:139.
94. Thompson RT, Marsh GD, Butland T, et al. An in vivo animal model to study chronic adriamycin cardiotoxocity: a F-31-nuclear magnetic resonance spectroscopy investigation. *In Vivo* 1991;5:13.
95. Herman EH, Lipshultz SE, Rifai N, et al. Use of cardiac troponin T levels as an indicator of doxorubicin-induced cardiotoxicity. *Cancer Res* 1998;58:195.
96. Bauch M, Ester A, Kimura B, et al. Atrial natriuretic peptide as a marker for doxorubicin-induced cardiotoxic effects. *Cancer* 1992;69:1492.
97. Schwartz CL, Hobbie WL, Truesdell A. Corrected QT interval prolongation in anthracycline treated survivors of childhood cancer. *J Clin Oncol* 1993;11:1906.
98. Jakacki R, Larsen RL, Barber G, et al. Comparison of cardiac function tests after anthracycline therapy in childhood. *Cancer* 1993;72:2739.
99. Foltinova A, Sejnova D, Mladosievicova B, Hulin I. Anthracycline-related abnormalities on signal-averaged ECG in survivors of childhood cancer. *Med Pediatr Oncol* 1999;33:247(abst).
100. Legha SS, Benjamin RS, Mackay B, et al. Reduction of doxorubicin cardiotoxicity by prolonged continuous intravenous infusion. *Ann Intern Med* 1982;96:133.
101. Casper ES, Gaynor JJ, Hajdu SI, et al. A prospective randomized trial of adjuvant chemotherapy with bolus versus continuous infusion of doxorubicin in patients with high-grade extremity soft tissue sarcoma and an analysis of prognostic factors. *Cancer* 1991;68:1221.
102. Shapira J, Gotfried M, Lishner M, Ravid M. Reduced cardiotoxicity of doxorubicin by a 6-hour infusion regimen. *Cancer* 1990;65:870.
103. Steinherz P, Redner A, Steinherz L, et al. Intensive therapy for acute lymphoblastic leukemia (ALL) in children at increased risk of early relapse—the MSK-NY-II protocol. *Cancer* 1993;72:3120.
104. Ewer M, Benjamin R. Prevention of cardiac damage due to adriamycin: modification of method of administration. In: Bricker JT, Green DM, D'Angio GJ, eds. *Cardiac toxicity after treatment for childhood cancer.* New York: Wiley-Liss, 1993:109.
105. Bielack SS, Erttmann R, Winkler K, Landbeck G. Doxorubicin: effect of different schedules on toxicity and antitumour efficacy. *Eur J Cancer Clin Oncol* 1989;25:873.
106. Bielack SS, Erttmann R, Kempf-Bielack B, Winkler K. Impact of scheduling on toxicity and clinical efficacy of doxorubicin: what do we know in the mid-nineties? *Eur J Cancer* 1996;32A:1652.
107. Torti FM, Bristow MR, Howes AE, et al. Reduced cardiotoxicity of doxorubicin delivered on a weekly schedule: assessment by endomyocardial biopsy. *Ann Intern Med* 1983;99:745.
108. Weiss A, Manthel RW. Experience with the use of adriamycin in combination with other anti cancer agents using a weekly schedule with particular reference to lack of cardiac toxicity. *Cancer* 1977;40:2046.
109. Sonneveid P. Effect of α-tocopherol on the cardiotoxicity of Adriamycin in the rat. *Cancer Treat Rep* 1978;62:1033.
110. Shimpo K, Nagatsu T, Yamada K, et al. Ascorbic acid and adriamycin toxicity. *Am J Clin Nutr* 1991;54(6 Suppl):1298S.
111. Villani F, Galimberti M, Monti E, et al. Effect of glutathione and N-acetylcysteine on in vitro and in vivo cardiac toxicity of doxorubicin. *Free Radic Res Commun* 1990;11:145.
112. Perletti G, Monti E, Paracchini L, Piccinini F. Effect of trimetazidine on early and delayed doxorubicin myocardial toxicity. *Arch Int Pharmacodyn Ther* 1989;302:280.
113. Buc-Calderon P, Praet M, Ruysschaert JM, Roberfroid M. Increasing therapeutic effect and reducing toxicity of doxorubicin by N-acyl dehydroalanines. *Eur J Cancer Clin Oncol* 1989;25:679.
114. Siveski-Iliskovic N, Hill M, Chow DA, Singal PK. Probucol protects against adriamycin cardiomyopathy without interfering with its antitumor effect. *Circulation* 1995;91;10.
115. Kraft J, Grille W, Appelt M, et al. Effects of verapamil on anthracycline-induced cardiomyopathy: preliminary results of a prospective multicenter trial. *Hamatol Bluttransfus* 1990;33:566.
116. Akimoto H, Bruno NA, Slate DL, et al. Effect of verapamil on doxorubicin cardiotoxicity: altered muscle gene expression in cultured neonatal rat cardiomyocytes. *Cancer Res* 1993;53:4658.
117. Milei J, Vazquez A, Boveris A, et al. The role of prenylamine in the prevention of adriamycin-induced cardiotoxicity. A review of experimental and clinical findings. *J Int Med Res* 1988;16:19.
118. Bartoli KF, Decorti G, Candussio L, et al. Effect of ketotifen on adriamycin toxicity: role of histamine. *Cancer Lett* 1988;39:145.
119. Harman GS, Craig JB, Kuhn JG, et al. Phase I and clinical pharmacology trial of crisnatol (BWA770u mesylate) using a monthly single-dose schedule. *Cancer Res* 1988;48:4706.
120. Reeves WC, Griffith JW, Wood MA, Whitesell L. Exacerbation of doxorubicin cardiotoxicity by digoxin administration in an experimental rabbit model. *Int J Cancer* 1990;45:731.
121. Villani F, Manzotti C, Mella M, et al. Effect of amrinone on anthracycline-induced lethal and cardiac toxicity in mice and rats. *Med Oncol Tumor Pharmacother* 1990;7:227.
122. Iarussi D, Auricchio U, Agretto A, et al. Protective effect of coenzyme Q10 on anthracycline cardiotoxicity: control study in children with acute lymphoblastic leukemia and non-Hodgkins lymphoma. *Mol Asp Med* 1994;15:207.
123. Nazeyrollas P, Prevost A, Baccard N, et al. Effects of amifostine on perfused isolated rat heart and on acute doxorubicin-induced cardiotoxicity. *Cancer Chemother Pharmacol* 1999;43:227.
124. Hacker MP, Lazo JS, Pritsos CA, Tritton TR. Immobilized adriamycin: toxic potential in vivo and in vitro. *Sel Cancer Ther* 1989;5:67.
125. Berry G, Billingham M, Alderman E, et al. The use of cardiac biopsy to demonstrate reduced cardiotoxicity in AIDS Kaposi's sarcoma patients treated with pegylated liposomal doxorubicin. *Ann Oncol* 1998;9:711.
126. Speyer J, Wasserheit C. Strategies for reduction of anthracycline cardiac toxicity. *Semin Oncol* 1998;25:525.
127. Hershko C, Link G, Tzahor M, et al. Anthracycline toxicity is potentiated by iron and inhibited by deferoxamine: studies in rat heart cells in culture. *J Lab Clin Med* 1993;122:245.
128. Herman EH, Ferrans VJ. Reduction of chronic doxorubicin cardiotoxicity in dogs by pretreatment with (+) -1,2-bis(3,5-dioxopiperazinyl-l-yl) propane (ICRF-187). *Cancer Res* 1981;41:3436.
129. Herman EG, Ferrans VJ, Jordan W, Ardalan B. Reduction of chronic daunorubicin cardiotoxicity by ICRF-187 in rabbits. *Res Comm Chem Pathol Pharmacol* 1981;31:85.
130. Alderton P, Gross J, Green MD. Role of (+)-1,2-Bis(3,5-dioxo-piperazinyl-1-yl-propane (ICRF-187) in modulating free radical scavenging enzymes in doxorubicin-induced cardiomyopathy. *Cancer Res* 1990;50:5136.
131. Herman EH, Ferrans VJ. Animal models of anthracycline cardiotoxicity: basic mechanisms and cardioprotective activity. *Prog Pediatr Cardiol* 1997;8:49.
132. Belt RJ. Prevention of Adriamycin-induced cardiotoxicity by ICRF-187 (NSC-169780). *Proc Am Soc Clin Oncol* 1984;3:27.
133. Speyer JL, Green MD, Kramer E, et al. Protective effect of the bispiperazinedione ICRF-187 against doxorubicin-induced cardiac toxicity in women with advanced breast cancer. *N Engl J Med* 1988;319:745.

134. Speyer JL, Green MD, Sanger J, et al. A prospective randomized trial of ICRF-187 for prevention of cumulative doxorubicin-induced cardiac toxicity in women with breast cancer. *Cancer Treat Rev* 1990;17:161.
135. Green MD, Alderton P, Sobol MM, et al. ICRF-187 (ADR-529) cardioprotection against anthracycline-induced cardiotoxicity: clinical and preclinical studies. *Cancer Treat Res* 1991;58:101.
136. Swain SM, Whaley FS, Gerber MC, et al. Cardioprotection with dexrazoxane for doxorubicin-containing therapy in advanced breast cancer. *J Clin Oncol* 1997;15:1318.
137. Rosenfeld CS, Weisberg SR, York RM, et al. Prevention of adriamycin cardiomyopathy with dexrazoxane (ADR-529, ICRF-87). *Proc Ann Meet Am Soc Clin Oncol* 1992;11:A74.
138. Swain SM, Whaley FS, Gerber MC, et al. Delayed administration of dexrazoxane provides cardioprotection for patients with advanced breast cancer treated with doxorubicin-containing therapy. *J Clin Oncol* 1997;15:1333.
139. Swain SM. Adult multicenter trials using dexrazoxane to protect against cardiac toxicity. *Semin Oncol* 1998;25:43.
140. Bu'Lock FA, Gavriel H, Oakhill A, Mott GM, Martin RP. Cardioprotection by ICRF187 against high dose anthracycline toxicity in children with malignant disease. *Br Heart J* 1993;70:185.
141. Rubio ME, Wiegman A, Naeff MSJ, et al. ICRF-187 protection against doxorubicin induced cardiomyopathy in paediatric osteosarcoma patients (SIOP XXVII Meeting Abstract). *Med Pediatr Oncol* 1995;25:292.
142. Schiavetti A, Castello MA, Clerico A, et al. Use of ICRF-187 for prevention of anthracycline cardiotoxicity in children: preliminary results. (SIOP XXVII Meeting Abstract). *Med Pediatr Oncol* 1995;25:293.
143. Wexler LH, Andrich MP, Venzon D, et al. A randomized trial of the cardioprotective agent, ICRF-187, in pediatric sarcoma patients treated with doxorubicin. *J Clin Oncol* 1996;14:362.
144. Synold TW, Tetef ML, Doroshow JH. Antineoplastic activity of continuous exposure to dexrazoxane: potential new role as a novel topoisomerase II inhibitor. *Semin Oncol* 1998;25:93.
145. Venturini M, Michelotti A, Del Mastro L, et al. Multicenter randomized controlled clinical trial to evaluate cardioprotection of dexrazoxane versus no cardioprotection in women receiving epirubicin chemotherapy for advanced breast cancer. *J Clin Oncol* 1996;14:3112.
146. Alderton PM, Gross J, Green MD. Comparative study of doxorubicin, mitoxantrone, and epirubicin in combination with ICRF-187 (ADR-529) in a chronic cardiotoxicity animal model. *Cancer Res* 1992;52:194.
147. Lemez P, Maresova J. Efficacy of dexrazoxane as a cardioprotective agent in patients receiving mitoxantrone- and daunorubicin-based chemotherapy. *Semin Oncol* 1998;25(Suppl 10):61.
148. Shipp NG, Dorr RT, Alberts DS, Dawson BV, Hendrix M. Characterization of experimental mitoxantrone cardiotoxicity and its partial inhibition by ICRF-187 in cultured neonatal rat heart cells. *Cancer Res* 1993;53:550.
149. Tan C, Mitta SK, Steinherz L, Miller DR. Phase I trial of Rubidazone (NSC-164011) in children with cancer. *Med Pediatr Oncol* 1981;9:347.
150. Benjamin RS, Mason JW, Billingham ME. Cardiac toxicity of adriamycin-DNA complex and rubidazone: evaluation by electrocardiogram and endomyocardial biopsy. *Cancer Treat Rep* 1978;62:935.
151. Tan CTC, Hancock C, Steinherz LJ. Preliminary results of epirubicin in children with acute leukemia. In: Bonadonna G, ed. *Advances in anthracycline chemotherapy: epirubicin.* Milan: Masson Italia Editori, 1984:129.
152. Nielsen D, Jensen JB, Dombernowsky P, et al. Epirubicin cardiotoxicity: a study of 135 patients with advanced breast cancer. *J Clin Oncol* 1990;8:1806.
153. Ryberg M, Nielson D, Skovsgaard T, et al. Epirubicin cardiotoxicity: an analysis of 469 patients with metastatic breast cancer. *J Clin Oncol* 1998;16:3502.
154. Mortensen SA. Aclarubicin: preclinical and clinical data suggesting less chronic cardiotoxicity compared with conventional anthracyclines. *Eur J Heametol* 1987;47(Suppl):21.
155. Wojnar J, Mandecki M, Wnuk-Wojnar AM, Holowiecki J. Clinical studies on aclacinomycin A cardiotoxicity in adult patients with acute non lymphoblastic leukemia. *Folia Haematol, Leipsiz* 1989;116:S.297.
156. Carella AM, Berman E, Maraone MP, Ganzina F. Idarubicin in the treatment of acute leukemias. An overview of preclinical and clinical studies. *Haematology* 1990;75:159.
157. Tan CT, Hancock C, Steinherz P, et al. Phase I and clinical pharmacological study of 4-demethoxydaunorubicin (Idarubicin) in children with advanced cancer. *Cancer Res* 1987;47:2990.
158. Feig SA, Krailo MD, Harris RE, et al. Determination of the maximum tolerated dose of idarubicin when used in a combination chemotherapy program of reinduction of childhood ALL at first marrow relapse and a preliminary assessment of toxicity compared with that of daunorubicin: a report from the Children's Cancer Study Group. *Med Pediatr Oncol* 1992;20:124.
159. Ringenberg QS, Propert KJ, Muss HB, et al. Clinical cardiotoxicity of esorubicin (4'-deoxydoxorubicin DxDy): prospective studies with serial gated heart scans and reports of selected cases. *Invest New Drugs* 1990;8:221.
160. Danesi R, Marchetti A, Bernardini N, et al. Cardiac toxicity and antitumor activity of 4'-deoxy-4'-iodo-doxorubicinol. *Cancer Chemother Phamacol* 1990;26:403.
161. Shaddy RE, Olsen SI, Bristow MR, et al. Efficacy and safety of metoprolol in the treatment of doxorubicin-induced cardiomyopathy in pediatric patients. *Am Heart J* 1995;129:197.
162. Fazio S, Palmieri EA, Ferravante B, et al. Doxorubicin-induced cardiomyopathy treated with carvedilol. *Clin Cardiol* 1998;21:777.
163. Musci M, Loebe M, Grauhan O, et al. Heart transplantation for doxorubicin-induced congestive heart failure in children and adolescents. *Transplant Proc* 1997;29:578.
164. Arico M, Pedroni E, Nespoli L, et al. Long-term survival after heart transplantation for doxorubicin induced cardiomyopathy. *Arch Dis Child* 1991;66:985.
165. Levitt G, Bunch K, Rogers CA, Whitehead B. Cardiac transplantation in childhood cancer survivors in Great Britian. *Eur J Cancer* 1996;32A:826.
166. Schaison G, Sommelet D, Le Bidois J, et al. Good results of heart transplantation for anthracycline (A) (+/- mediastinal radiotherapy (RY)) related cardiomyopathy in cancer in childhood. *Proc Ann Meet Am Soc Clin Oncol* 1996;15:A1432(abst).
167. Edwards BS, Hunt SA, Fowler MB, et al. Cardiac transplantation in patients with preexisting neoplastic diseases. *Am J Cardiol* 1990;65:501.
168. Tumminello FM, Leto G, Gebbia N, et al. Acute myocardial effects of mitoxantrone in the rabbit. *Cancer Treat Rep* 1987;71:529.
169. Sparano BM, Gordon G, Hall C, Iatropoulos MJ, Noble FJ. Safety assessment of a new anticancer compound, mitoxantrone, in beagle dogs. Comparison with doxorubicin. II Histologic and ultrastructural pathology. *Cancer Treat Rep* 1982;66:1145.
170. Saletan S. Mitoxantrone: an active, new antitumor agent with an improved therapeutic index. *Cancer Treat Rev* 1987;14:297.
171. Shenkenberg TD, Von Hoff DD. Mitoxantrone: a new anticancer drug with significant clinical activity. *Ann Intern Med* 1986;105:67.
172. Posner LE, Dukart G, Goldberg J, Bernstein T, Cartwright K. Mitoxantrone: an overview of safety and toxicity. *Invest New Drugs* 1985;3:123.
173. Janmohammed R, Milligan DW. Mitoxantrone induced congestive heart failure in patients previously treated with anthracyclines. *Br J Haematol* 1989;71:292.
174. Pai GR, Reed NS, Ruddell WS. A case of mitozantrone-associated cardiomyopathy without prior anthracycline therapy. *Br J Radiol* 1987;60:1125.
175. Ewer MS, Ali MK, Abraham K, et al. Electrocardiographic (ECG) changes in patients receiving mitoxantrone previously treated with adriamycin. *Proc Am Soc Clin Oncol* 1990;9:315.
176. Cassidy J, Merrick MV, Smyth JF, Leonard RC. Cardiotoxicity of mitozantrone assessed by stress and resting nuclear ventriculography. *Eur J Cancer Clin Oncol* 1988;24:935.
177. Fountzilas G, Afthonidis D, Geleris P, et al. Cardiotoxicity evaluation in patients treated with a mitoxantrone combination as adjuvant chemotherapy for breast cancer. *Anticancer Res* 1992;12:231.
178. Villani F, Galimberti M, Crippa F. Evaluation of ventricular function by echocardiography and radionuclide angiography in patients treated with mitoxantrone. *Drugs Exp Clin Res* 1989;15:501.
179. *Physicians Desk Reference.* 50th ed. 1996:1280.
180. Lindpaintner K, Lindpaintner LS, Wentworth M, et al. Acute myocardial necrosis during administration of amsacrine. *Cancer* 1986;57:1284.
181. Legha SS, Latreille J, McCredie KB, et al. Neurologic and cardiac rhythm abnormalities associated with 4'-(9-acridinylamino) methanesulfon-m-anisidide (AMSA) therapy. *Cancer Treat Rep* 1979;63:2001.
182. Von Hoff DD, Elson D, Polk G, et al. Acute ventricular fibrillation and death during infusion of 4'-(9-acridinylamino) methanesulfon-m-anisidide (AMSA) [letter]. *Cancer Treat Rep* 1980;64:356.
183. Falkson G. Multiple ventricular extrasystoles following administration of 4'-(9-acridinylamino) methanesulfon-m-anisidide (AMSA). *Cancer Treat Rep* 1980;64:358.
184. Arlin Z, Mehta R, Feldman E, Sullivan P, Pucillo A. Amsacrine treatment of patients with supraventricular arrhythmias and acute leukemia. *Cancer Chemother Pharmacol* 1987;19:163.
185. Puccio CA, Feldman EJ, Arlin ZA. Amsacrine is safe in patients with ventricular ectopy. *Am J Hematol* 1988;28:197.
186. Steinherz LJ, Steinherz PG, Mangiacasale D, Tan C, Miller DR. Cardiac abnormalities after AMSA administration. *Cancer Treat Rep* 1982;66:483.
187. Tan CTC, Hancock C, Steinherz PG, et al. Phase II study of 4'-(9-acridinylamino) methanesulfon-m-anisidide (NSC 249992) in children with acute leukemia and lymphoma. *Cancer Res* 1982;42:1579.
188. Arlin ZA, Feldman EJ, Mittelman A, et al. Amsacrine is safe and effective therapy for patients with myocardial dysfunction and acute leukemia. *Cancer* 1991;68:1198.
189. Praga C, Beretta G, Vigo PL, et al. Adriamycin cardiotoxicity: a survey of 1273 patients. *Cancer Treat Rep* 1979;63:827.
190. Santos GW, Sensenbrenner LL, Burke PJ, et al. Marrow transplants in man using cyclophosphamide summary of Baltimore experience. *Exp Hematol* 1970;20:78.
191. Buckner CD, Rudolph RH, Fefer A, et al. High-dose cyclophosphamide therapy for malignant disease (toxicity, tumor, response, and the effects of stored autologous marrow). *Cancer* 1972;29:357.
192. Mullins GM, Anderson PN, Santos GW. High dose cyclophosphamide therapy in solid tumors. Therapeutic, toxic and immunosuppressive effects. *Cancer* 1975;36:1950.
193. Storb R, Buckner CS, Dillingham LA, et al. Cyclophosphamide regimens in rhesus monkeys with and without marrow infusion. *Cancer Res* 1970;30:2195.
194. Slavin RE, Millan JC, Mullins GM. Pathology of high dose intermittent cyclophosphamide therapy. *Hum Pathol* 1975;6:693.
195. Buja LM, Ferrans VJ, Graw RG. Cardiac pathologic findings in patients treated with bone marrow transplantation. *Hum Pathol* 1976;7:17.
196. Applebaum FR, Strauchen JA, Graw RG, et al. Acute lethal carditis caused by high dose combination chemotherapy. A unique clinical and pathological entity. *Lancet* 1976;1:58.
197. Steinherz L, Steinherz P, Mangiacasale D, et al. Cardiac changes with cyclophosphamide. *Med Pediatr Oncol* 1981;9:417.
198. Lee CK, Harman GS, Hohl RJ, Gingrich RD. Fatal cyclophosphamide cardiomyopathy: its clinical course and treatment. *Bone Marrow Transplant* 1996;18:573.
199. Steinherz LJ, Steinherz PG. Cyclophosphamide cardiotoxicity. *Cancer Bull* 1985;37:231.
200. Kupari M, Volin L, Suokas A, et al. Cardiac involvement in bone marrow transplantation: electrocardiographic changes, arrhythmias, heart failure and autopsy findings. *Bone Marrow Transplant* 1990;5:91.
201. Ramireddy K, Kane KM, Adhar GC. Acquired episodic complete heart block after high-dose chemotherapy with cyclophosphamide and thiotepa. *Am Heart J* 1994;127:701.
202. Lopez-Jimenez J, Cervero C, Munoz A, et al. Cardiovascular toxicities related to the infusion of cryopreserved grafts: results of a controlled study. *Bone Marrow Transplant* 1994;13:789.
203. Kupari M, Volin L, Suokas A, Hekali P, Ruutu T. Cardiac involvement in bone marrow transplantation: serial changes in left ventricular size, mass and performance. *J Int Med* 1990;227:259.
204. Isberg B, Paul C, Johsson L, Svahn U. Myocardial toxicity of high-dose cyclophosphamide in rabbits treated with daunorubicin. *Cancer Chemother Pharmacol* 1991;28:717.

205. Angelucci E, Mariotti E, Lucarelli G, et al. Sudden cardiac tamponade after chemotherapy for marrow transplantation in thalassaemia. *Lancet* 1992;339:287.
206. Veys PA, McAvinchey R, Rothman MT, Mair GHM, Newland AC. Pericardial effusion following conditioning for bone marrow transplantation in acute leukemia. *Bone Marrow Transplant* 1987;2:213.
207. Bearman SI, Petersen FB, Schor RA, et al. Radionuclide ejection fractions in the evaluation of patients being considered for bone marrow transplantation: risk for cardiac toxicity. *Bone Marrow Transplant* 1990;5:173.
208. Braverman AC, Antin JH, Plappert MT, Cook EF, Lee RT. Cyclophosphamide cardiotoxicity in bone marrow transplantation: a prospective evaluation of new dosing regimens. *J Clin Oncol* 1991;9:1215.
209. Hertenstein B, Stefanic M, Schmeiser T, et al. Cardiac toxicity of bone marrow transplantation: preventive value of cardiologic evaluation before transplant. *J Clin Oncol* 1994;12:998.
210. Larsen RL, Barber G, Heise CT, August CS. Exercise assessment of cardiac function in children and young adults before and after bone marrow transplantation. *Pediatrics* 1992;89:722.
211. Kandylis K, Vassilomanolakis M, Tsoussis S, Efremidis AP. Ifosfamide cardiotoxicity in humans. *Cancer Chemother Pharmacol* 1989;24:395.
212 Quezado ZM, Wilson WH, Cunnion RE, et al. High-dose ifosfamide is associated with severe, reversible cardiac dysfunction. *Ann Intern Med* 1993;118:31.
213. Herman EM, Mhatre RM, Warardekar VS, Lee IP. Comparison of the cardiovascular actions of NSC-109, 824 (ifosfamide) and cyclophosphamide. *Toxicol Appl Pharmacol* 1972;23:178.
214. O'Connel TX, Berenbaum MC. Cardiac and pulmonary effects of high doses of cyclophosphamide and isophosphamide. *Cancer Res* 1974;34:1586.
215. De Botton S, Dombret H, Sanz M, et al. Incidence, clinical features, and outcome of all trans-retinoic acid syndrome in 413 cases of newly diagnosed acute promyelocytic leukemia. The European APL Group. *Blood* 1998;92:2712.
216. Brouty-Boye D, Kolonias D, Lampidis TJ. Antiproliferataive activity of taxol on human tumor and normal breast cells vs. effects on cardiac cells. *Int J Cancer* 1995;60:571.
217. Rowinsky EK, McGuire WP, Guarnieri T, et al. Cardiac disturbances during the administration of Taxol. *J Clin Oncol* 1991;9:1704.
218. McGuire WP, Rowinsky EK, Rosenshein NB, et al. Taxol: a unique antineoplastic agent with significant activity in advanced ovarian epithelial neoplasms. *Ann Intern Med* 1989;111:273.
219. Rowinsky EK, Bilbert MR, McGuire WP, et al. Sequences of taxol and cisplatin: a phase I and pharmacologic study. *J Clin Oncol* 1991;9:1692.
220. Markman M, Kennedy A, Webster K, et al. Paclitaxel administration to gynecologic cancer patients with major cardiac risk factors. *J Clin Oncol* 1998;16:3483.
221. Perez EA. Paclitaxel and cardiotoxicity. *J Clin Oncol* 1998;16:3481.
222. Aapro MS. Combining new agents with anthracyclines in metastatic breast cancer: an overview of recent findings. *Semin Oncol* 1999;26(Suppl 3):17.
223. Tan CTC, Luks E, Bacha DM, et al. Phase I trial of homoharringtonine (NSC 141633) in children with refractory leukemia. *Cancer Treat Rep* 1987;71:1245.
224. Ajani JA, Dimery I, Chawla SP, et al. Phase II studies of homoharringtonine in patients with advanced malignant melanoma: sarcoma and head and neck, breast and colorectal carcinomas. *Cancer Treat Rep* 1989;70:375.
225. Jongii L, Hui Y, Xueying L, et al. Experimental studies on the toxicity of harringtonine and homoharringtonine. *Chin Med J* 1979;92:175.
226. Hirvonen HE, Salmi TT, Heinonen E, Antila KJ, Valimaki IA. Vincristine treatment of acute lymphoblastic leukemia induces transient autonomic cardioneuropathy. *Cancer* 1989;64:801.
227. Mandel EM, Lewinski U, Djadetti M. Vincristine-induced myocardial infarction. *Cancer* 1975;36:1979.
228. Cargill RI, Boyter AC, Lipworth BJ. Reversible myocardial ischaemia following vincristine containing chemotherapy. *Respir Med* 1994;88:709.
229. House KW, Simon SR, Pugh RP. Chemotherapy-induced myocardial infarction in a young man with Hodgkin's disease. *Clin Cardiol* 1992;15:122.
230. Lejonc JL, Vernant JP, Macquin I, et al. Myocardial infarction following vinblastine treatment. *Lancet* 1980;2:692.
231. Stefenelli T, Kuzmits R, Ulrich W, Glogar D. Acute vascular toxicity after combination chemotherapy with cisplatin, vinblastine, and bleomycin for testicular cancer. *Eur Heart J* 1988;9:552.
232. Zeymer U, Neuhaus KL. Infarct-typical changes in the electrocardiogram following chemotherapy with vinblastine. *Dtsch Med Wochenschr* 1989;114:589.
233. Buzdar AR, Leghe SS, Tashimal CK, et al. Adriamycin and mitomycin C: possible synergistic toxicity. *Cancer Treat Rep* 1978;62:1005.
234. Doroshow JH. Mitomycin-C enhanced superoxide and hydrogen peroxide in the rat heart. *J Pharmacol Exp Ther* 1981;218:206.
235. Sivanesaratnam V. FRCOG Mitomycin-C cardiotoxicity. *Med J Aust* 1989;151:300.
236. Verweij J, Funke-Kupper AJ, Teule GJJ, Pinedo HM. A prospective study on the dose dependency of cardiotoxicity induced by mitomycin C. *Med Oncol Tumor Pharmacother* 1988;5:159.
237. Verweij J, Van Der Burg ME, Pinedo HM. Mitomycin C-induced hemolytic uremic syndrome. Six case reports and review of the literature on renal, pulmonary and cardiac side effects of the drug. *Radiother Oncol* 1987;8:33.
238. Dent R, McColl I. 5-fluorouracil and angina. *Lancet* 1975;1:347.
239. Labianca R, Beretta G, Clerici M, Fraschini P, Luporini G. Cardiac toxicity of 5-fluorouracil: a study of 1083 patients. *Tumori* 1982;68:505.
240. Lomeo AM, Avolio C, Iacobellis G, Manzione L. 5-Fluorouracil cardiotoxicity. *Eur J Gynaecol Oncol* 1990;3:237.
241. Clavel M, Sorbette F, David M, Vignoud J, Hauchecorne J. 5-Fluorouracil (5FU) cardiotoxicity. 33 events out of 1145 consecutive patients. *Proc Ann Meet Am Soc Clin Oncol* 1991;10:A346.
242. de Forni M, Malet-Martino MC, Jaillais P, et al. Cardiotoxicity of high-dose continuous infusion fluorouracil: a prospective clinical study. *J Clin Oncol* 1992;10:1795.
243. Rezkalla S, Kloner RA, Ensley J, et al. Continuous ambulatory ECG monitoring during fluorouracil therapy: a prospective study. *J Clin Oncol* 1989;7:509.
244. Keefe DL, Roistacher N, Pierri MK. Clinical cardiotoxicity of 5-fluorouracil. *J Clin Pharmacol* 1993;33:1060.
245. Collins C, Weiden PL. Cardiotoxicity of 5-fluorouracil. *Cancer Treat Rep* 1987;71:733.
246. Freeman NJ, Costanza ME. 5-Fluorouracil-associated cardiotoxicity. *Cancer* 1988;61:36.
247. Eskilsson J, Albertsson M, Mercke C. Adverse cardiac effects during induction chemotherapy treatment with cis-platin and 5-fluorouracil. *Radiother Oncol* 1988;13:41.
248. Weidmann B, Jansen W, Heider A, Niederle N. 5-Fluorouracil cardiotoxicity with left ventricular dysfunction under different dosing regimens. *Am J Cardiol* 1995;75:194.
249. Jakubowski AA, Kemeny N. Hypotension as a manifestation of cardiotoxicity in three patients receiving cisplatin and 5-fluorouracil. *Cancer* 1988;62:266.
250. McKendall GR, Shurman A, Anamur M, Most AS. Toxic cardiogenic shock associated with infusion of 5-fluorouracil. *Am Heart J* 1989;118:184.
251. Patel B, Kloner RA, Ensley J, Al-Sarraf M, Kish J, Wynne J. 5-Fluorouracil cardiotoxicity: Left ventricular dysfunction and effect of coronary vasodilators. *Am J Med Sci* 1987;294:238.
252. Misset B, Escudier B, Leclercq B, et al. Acute myocardiotoxicity during 5-fluorouracil therapy. *Intensive Care Med* 1990;16:210.
253. Coronel B, Madonna O, Mercatello A, Caillette A, Moskovtchenko JF. Myocardiotoxicity of 5 fluorouracil. *Intensive Care Med* 1988;14:429.
254. Kleiman NS, Lehane DE, Geyer CE Jr, Pratt CM, Young JB. Prinzmetal's angina during 5-fluorouracil chemotherapy. *Am J Med* 1987;82:566.
255. Burger AJ, Mannino S. 5-Fluorouracil-induced coronary vasospasm. *Am Heart J* 1987;114:433.
256. Pottage A, Holt S, Ludgate S, Langlands A. Fluorouracil cardiotoxicity. *BMJ* 1978;1:1547.
257. Jeremic B, Jevremovic S, Djuric L, Mijatovic L. Cardiotoxicity during chemotherapy treatment with 5-fluorouracil and cisplatin. *J Chemother* 1990;2:264.
258. Martin M, Diaz-Rubio E, Furio V, et al. Lethal cardiac toxicity after cisplatin and 5-fluorouracil chemotherapy. Report of a case with necropsy study. *Am J Clin Oncol* 1989;12:229.
259. Liss RH, Chadwick M. Correlation of 5-fluorouracil distribution in rodents with toxicity and chemotherapy in man. *Cancer Chemother Rep* 1974;58:777.
260. Suzuki T, Nakanishi H, Hayashi A, et al. Cardiac toxicity of 5-fluorouracil in rabbits. *Jpn J Pharmacol* 1972;27:(Suppl)137.
261. Matsubara I, Kamiya J, Imai S. Cardiotoxicity effects of 5-fluorouracil in the guinea pig. *Jpn J Pharmacol* 1980;30:871.
262. Menard O, Martinet Y, Lamay P. Cis-platin-induced atrial fibrillation. *J Clin Oncol* 1991;9:192.
263. Fassio T, Canobbio L, Gasparini G, Villani F. Paroxymal supraventricular tachycardia during treatment with cisplatin and etoposide combination. *Oncology* 1986;43:219.
264. Talley RW, O'Bryan RM, Gutterman JV, Brownlee RW, McGredie KB. Clinical evaluation of toxic effects of cis-diammine dichloroplatinum (NSC-119875). Phase I clinical study *Cancer Chemother Rep* 1973;57:465.
265. Tomirotti M, Riundi R, Pulici S, et al. Ischemic cardiopathy from cis-diamminedichloroplatinum (CDDP). *Tumori* 1984;70:235.
266. Doll DC, List AF, Greco A, et al. Acute vascular ischemic events after cisplatin-based combination chemotherapy for germ-cell tumors of the testis. *Ann Intern Med* 1986;105:48.
267. Sonnenblick M, Rosin A. Cardiotoxicity of interferon. A review of 44 cases. *Chest* 1991;99:557.
268. Friess GG, Brown TD, Wrenn RC. Cardiovascular rhythm effects of gamma recombinant DNA interferon. *Invest New Drugs* 1989;7:275.
269. Martino S, Ratanatharathorn V, Karanes C, et al. Reversible arrhythmias observed in patients treated with recombinant alpha 2 interferon. *J Cancer Res Clin Oncol* 1987;113:376.
270. Zbinden G. Effects of recombinant human alpha-interferon in a rodent cardiotoxicity model. *Toxicol Lett* 1990;50:25.
271. Dickson D. Death halts interferon trials in France. *Science* 1982;218:772.
272. Foon KA, Sherwin SA, Abrams PG, et al. Treatment of advanced non-Hodgkin's lymphoma with recombinant leukocyte A interferon. *N Engl J Med* 1984;311:1148.
273. Brown TD, Koeller J, Beougher K, et al. A phase I clinical trial of recombinant DNA gamma interferon. *J Clin Oncol* 1987;5:790.
274. Kruit WH, Punt KJ, Goey SH, et al. Cardiotoxicity as a dose-limiting factor in a schedule of high dose bolus therapy with interleukin-2 and alpha-interferon. *Cancer* 1994;74:2850.
275. Deyton LR, Walker RE, Kovacs JA, et al. Reversible cardiac dysfunction associated with interferon Alfa therapy in AIDS patients with Kaposi's sarcoma. *N Engl J Med* 1989;321:1246.
276. Sonnenblick M, Rosenmann D, Rosin A. Reversible cardiomyopathy induced by interferon. *BMJ* 1990;300:1174.
277. Budd GT, Bukowski RM, Miketo L, Yen-Lieberman B, Proffitt MR. Phase I trial of ultrapure human leukocyte interferon in human malignancy. *Cancer Chemother Pharmacol* 1984;12:39.
278. Grunberg SM, Kempf RA, Itri LM, et al. Phase II study of recombinant alpha interferon in the treatment of advanced non-small cell lung carcinoma. *Cancer Treat Rep* 1985;69:1031.
279. Cohen MC, Huberman MS, Nesto RW. Recombinant alpha-2 interferon related cardiomyopathy. *Am J Med* 1988;85:549.
280. Sherwin SA. The interferons. *Ann Intern Med* 1987;106:425.
281. Lampidis TJ, Brouty-Boye D. Interferon inhibits cardiac cell function in vitro (41043). *Proc Soc Exp Biol Med* 1981;166:181.
282. Dorr RT, Shipp NG. Effect of interferon, interleukin-2 and tumor necrosis factor on myocardial cell viability and doxorubicin cardiotoxicity in vitro. *Immunopharmacology* 1989;18:31.
283. Bialock JE, Stanton JD. Common pathways of interferon and hormonal action. *Nature* 1980;283:406.
284. Nora R, Abrams JS, Tait NS, Hiponia DJ, Silverman HJ. Myocardial toxic effects during recombinant interleukin-2 therapy. *J Natl Cancer Inst* 1989;81:59.
285. Schechter D, Nagler A. Recombinant interleukin-2 and recombinant interferon α immunotherapy cardiovascular toxicity. *Am Heart J* 1992;123:1736.
286. Rosenberg SA, Lotze MT, Muul LM, et al. A progress report on the treatment of 157 patients with advanced cancer using lymphokine-activated killer cell and interleukin-2 or high dose interleukin alone. *N Engl J Med* 1987;316:889.
287. Nora R, Belani C, Silverman H, et al. Immunotherapy of advanced cancer [letter]. *N Engl J Med* 1987;316:275.

288. Nora R, Abrams J, Silverman HJ. Myocardial infarction (MI) in patients receiving high dose recombinant interleukin-2 (rIL-2). *Proc Am Soc Clin Oncol* 1987;6:245.
289. Fisher RI, Coltman CA, Doroshow JH, et al. Metastatic renal cancer treated with interleukin-2 and lymphokine-activated killer cells. A phase II clinical trial. *Ann Int Med* 1988; 108:518.
290. Dutcher JP, Creekmore S, Weiss GR, et al. Phase II study of interleukin-2 and lymphokine-activated killer cells in patients with metastatic malignant melanoma. *J Clin Oncol* 1989;7:477.
291. Osanto S, Cluitmans FGM, Franks CR, et al. Myocardial injury after interleukin-2 therapy. *Lancet* 1988;2:48.
292. White RL, Schwartzentruber DJ, Guleria A, et al. Cardiopulmonary toxicity of treatment with high dose interleukin-2 in 199 consecutive patients with metastatic melanoma or renal cell carcinoma. *Cancer* 1994;74:3212.
293. Trehu EG, Isner JM, Mier JW, Karp DD, Atkins MB. Possible myocardial toxicity associated with interleukin-4 therapy. *J Immunother* 1993;14:348.
294. Torisu M, Goya T, Hayashi Y, et al. Electrocardiogram studies on cancer patients treated with OK-432, a streptococcal preparation with potent biological response modifier activities. *J Biol Res Mod* 1989;8:665.
295. Slamon D, Leyland-Jones B, Shak S, et al. Addition of Herceptin (humanized anti-HER2 antibody) to first line chemotherapy for HER2 overexpressing metastatic breast cancer (HER2+/MBC) markedly increases anticancer activity: A randomized, multinational controlled phase III trial. *Proc Am Soc Clin Oncol* 1998;17:98a.
296. Ewer MS, Gibbs HR, Swafford J, Benjamin RS. Cardiotoxicity in patients receiving trastuzumab (Herceptin): primary toxicity, synergistic or sequential stress, or surveillance artifact? *Semin Oncol* 1999;26:96.
297. Jerian S, Keegan P. Cardiotoxicity associated with paclitaxel/trastuzumab combination therapy. *J Clin Oncol* 1999;17:1647.
298. Sanz Manrique N, Valcarce Perez J, Broto Escapa P, et al. Enhancing factors in the cardiotoxicity of anthracyclines. *Anales Espanoles de Pediatria* 1990;32:11.
299. Hall IH, Grippo AA, Holbrook DJ, et al. Renal, hepatic, cardiac and thymic acute toxicity afforded by bis(helenalinyl)malonate in BDF1 mice. *Toxicity* 1990;64:205.
300. Bashir Y, Tomson CR. Cardiac arrest associated with hypokalaemia in a patient receiving mithramycin. *Postgrad Med J* 1988;64:228.
301. Hoke GD, Macia RA, Meunier PC, et al. In vivo and in vitro cardiotoxicity of a gold-containing antineoplastic drug candidate in the rabbit. *Toxicol Appl Pharmacol* 1989;100:293.
302. Gebbia N, Flandina C, Leto G, Tumminello FM, et al. The roleof histamine in doxorubicin and teniposide-induced cardiotoxicity in dog and mouse. *Tumori* 1987;73:279.
303. Schecter JP, Jones SE. Myocardial infarction in a 27 year old woman: possible complication of treatment with VP-16-213 (NSC-141540), mediastinal irradiation or both. *Cancer Chemother Rep* 1975;59:887.
304. Winberger A, Pinkhas J, Sandbank U, et al. Endocardial fibrosis following busulfan treatment. *JAMA* 1975;231:495.
305. Grem JL, King SA, Chun HG, Grever MR. Cardiac complications observed in elderly patients following 2'-deoxycoformycin therapy. *Am J Hematol* 1991;38:245.
306. Watanabe H, Hasegawa A, Shinozaki T, Arita S, Chigira M. Possible cardiac side effects of granisetron, an antiemetic agent, in patients with bone and soft-tissue sarcomas receiving cytotoxic chemotherapy. *Cancer Chemother Pharmacol* 1995;35:278.
307. Desjardins AU. Action of roentgen rays and radium on the heart and lungs. *Am J Roentgenol* 1932;27:153, 303, 447.
308. Leach JEL. Effect of roentgen therapy on the heart: clinical study. *Arch Intern Med* 1943;72:715.
309. Cohn KE, Stewart JR, Fajardo LF, et al. Heart disease following radiation. *Medicine* 1967;46:281.
310. Stewart JR, Fajardo LF. Radiation-induced heart disease: an update. *Prog Cardiovasc Dis* 1984;27:173.
311. Arsenian MA. Cardiovascular sequelae of therapeutic thoracic radiation. *Prog Cardiovasc Dis* 1991;33:299.
312. Benoff LJ, Schweitzer P. Radiation therapy-induced cardiac injury [Review]. *Am Heart J* 1995;129:1193.
313. Stewart JR, Fajardo LF, Cohn KE. Experimental radiation-induced heart disease in rabbits. *Radiology* 1968;91:814.
314. Fajardo LF, Stewart JR. Experimental radiation-induced heart disease. I. Light microscopic studies. *Am J Pathol* 1970;59:299.
315. Lauk S, Kiszel Z, Buschmann J, et al. Radiation-induced heart disease in rats. *Int J Radiat Oncol Biol Phys* 1985;11:801.
316. Gillette EL, McChesney SL, Hoopes PJ. Isoeffect curves for radiation-induced cardiomyopathy in the dog. *Int J Radiat Oncol Biol Phys* 1985;11:2091.
317. Schultz-Hector S. Radiation-induced heart disease: review of experimental data on dose response and pathogenesis [Review]. *Int J Radiat Biol* 1992;61:149.
318. Brosius FC, Waller BF, Robert WG. Radiation heart disease: analysis of 16 young (aged 15 to 33 years) necropsy patients who received over 3,500 rads to the heart. *Am J Med* 1981; 70:519.
319. Fajardo LF, Stewart JR, Cohn KE. Morphology of radiation-induced heart disease. *Arch Pathol* 1968;86:512.
320. Fajardo LF, Stewart JR. Pathogenesis of radiation-induced myocardial fibrosis. *Lab Invest* 1973;29:244.
321. Fajardo LF. In: Stemberg S, ed. *Pathology of radiation injury.* New York: Masson, 1982.
322. Stewart JR, Fajardo L, Gillette S, et al. Radiation injury to the heart. *Int J Radiat Oncol Biol Phys* 1995;31:1205.
323. Veinot JP, Edwards WD. Pathology of radiation-induced heart disease: a surgical and autopsy study of 27 cases. *Hum Pathol* 1996;27:766.
324. Stewart JR. Normal tissue tolerance irradiation of the cardiovascular system. *Front Radiat Ther Oncol* 1989;23:302.
325. Mauch P, Kalish L, Marcus KC, et al. Long-term survival in Hodgkin's disease. *Cancer J Sci Am* 1995;1:33.
326. Hancock SL, Tucker MA, Hoppe RT. Factors affecting late mortality from heart disease after treatment of Hodgkin's disease. *JAMA* 1993;270:1949.
327. Hancock SL, Donaldson SS, Hoppe RT. Cardiac disease following treatment of Hodgkin's disease in children and adolescents. *J Clin Oncol* 1993;1:1208.
328. Reinders JG, Heijmen BJ, Olofsen-van Acht MJ, et al. Ischemic heart disease after mantle-field irradiation for Hodgkin's disease in long-term follow-up. *Radiother Oncol* 1999;51:35.
329. Glanzmann C, Kaufmann P, Jenni R, et al. Cardiac risk after mediastinal irradiation for Hodgkin's disease. *Radiother Oncol* 1998;46:51.
330. Stewart JR, Fajardo LF. Dose response in human and experimental radiation-induced heart disease: application of the nominal standard dose (NSD) concept. *Radiology* 1971;99:403.
331. Corn BW, Trock BJ, Goodman RL. Irradiation-related ischemic heart disease. *J Clin Oncol* 1990;8:741.
332. Carmel RJ, Kaplan HS. Mantle irradiation in Hodgkin's disease. *Cancer* 1976;37:2813.
333. Appelfeld MM, Slawson RG, Spicer KM, et al. Long-term cardiovascular evaluation of patients treated by thoracic mantle radiation therapy. *Cancer Treat Rep* 1982;66:1003.
334. Appelfeld MM, Wiernik PH. Cardiac disease after radiation therapy for Hodgkin's disease: analysis of 48 patients. *Am Heart J* 1983;51:1679.
335. Ruckdeschel JC, Chang P, Martin RG, et al. Radiation-related pericardial effusions in patients with Hodgkin's disease. *Medicine* 1975;54:245.
336. Tarbell NJ, Thompson L, Mauch P. Thoracic irradiation in Hodgkin's disease: disease control and long-term complications. *Int J Radiat Oncol Biol Phys* 1990;18:275.
337. Harris JR, Recht A. In: Harris JR, Hellman S, Henderson IC, Kinne DW, eds. *Breast diseases,* 2nd ed. Philadelphia: Lippincott, 1991:406.
338. Fleming WH, Szakacs TE, King ER. The effects of gamma radiation on the fibrinolytic system of the dog lung and its modification by certain drugs: relationship to radiation pneumonitis and hyaline membrane formation in the lung. *J Nucl Med* 1962;3:34.
339. Blayney DW, Longo D. Radiation-induced pericarditis. *N Engl J Med* 1982;306:550.
340. Gottdeiner JS, Katin MJ, Borer JS, et al. Late cardiac effects of therapeutic mediastinal irradiation: assessment by echocardiography and radionuclide angiography. *N Engl J Med* 1983;308:569.
341. Totterman KJ, Personen E, Siltanen P. Radiation-related chronic heart disease. *Chest* 1983;83:875.
342. Gomm SA, Stretton TB. Chronic pericardial effusion after mediastinal radiotherapy. *Thorax* 1981;36:149.
343. Loyer EM, Delpassand ES. Radiation-induced heart disease: imaging features [Review]. *Semin Roentgenol* 1993;28:321.
344. Posner MR, Cohen GI, Skarin AT. Pericardial disease in patients with cancer. *Am J Med* 1981;71:407.
345. Carey RW, Sawicka JM, Choi NC. Cytologically negative pericardial effusion complicating combined modality therapy for localized small-cell carcinoma of the lung. *J Clin Oncol* 1987;5:818.
346. Stewart JR, Fajardo LF. Radiation-induced heart disease. *Radiol Clin North Am* 1971;3:511.
347. Martin RG, Ruckdeschel JC, Chang P, et al. Radiation-related pericarditis. *Am J Cardiol* 1975;35:216.
348. Fajardo LF, Stewart JR. Radiation-induced heart disease: human and experimental observations. In: Bristow MR, ed. *Drug-induced heart disease.* Amsterdam: Elsevier North-Holland, 1980:291.
349. Keelan MH, Rudders RA. Successful treatment of radiation pericarditis with corticosteroids. *Arch Intern Med* 1974;134:145.
350. Castellino RA, Glatstein E, Turbow MM, et al. Latent radiation injury of lungs or heart activated by steroid withdrawal. *Ann Intern Med* 1974;80:593.
351. Biran S. Corticosteroids in radiation-induced pericarditis. *Chest* 1978;74:96.
352. Krikorian JG, Hancock EW. Pericardiocentesis. *Am J Med* 1978;65:808.
353. Morton DL, Glancy L, Joseph WL, et al. Management of patients with radiation-induced pericarditis with effusion: a note on the development of aortic regurgitation in two of them. *Chest* 1973;64:291.
354. Cameron J, Osterle SN, Baldwin JC, et al. The etiologic spectrum of constrictive pericarditis. *Am Heart J* 1987;113:354.
355. Ni Y, von Segesser LK, Turina M. Futility of pericardiectomy for postirradiation constrictive pericarditis? *Ann Thorac Surg* 1990;49:445.
356. Savage DE, Constine LS, Schwartz RG, Rubin P. Radiation effects of left ventricular function and myocardial perfusion in long-term survivors of Hodgkin's disease. *Int J Radiat Oncol Biol Phys* 1990;19:721.
357. Perrault DJ, Levy M, Herman JD, et al. Echocardiographic abnormalities following cardiac radiation. *J Clin Oncol* 1985;3:546.
358. Pohjola-Sintonen S, Totterman KJ, Salmo M, et al. Late cardiac effects of mediastinal radiotherapy in patients with Hodgkin's disease. *Cancer* 1987;60:31.
359. Burns RJ, Bar-Shlomo B, Druck MN, et al. Detection of radiation cardiomyopathy by gated radionuclide angiography. *Am J Med* 1983;74:297.
360. Lagrange JL, Darcourt J, Benoliel J, et al. Acute cardiac effects of mediastinal irradiation: assessment by radionuclide angiography. *Int J Radiat Oncol Biol Phys* 1992;22:897.
361. Gomez GA, Park JJ, Panahon AM, et al. Heart size and function after radiation therapy to the mediastinum in patients with Hodgkin's disease. *Cancer Treat Rep* 1983;67:1099.
362. Merrill J, Greco FA, Zimbler H, et al. Adriamycin and radiation: synergistic cardiotoxicity. *Ann Intern Med* 1975;82:122.
363. Kinsella TJ, Ahmann DL, Giuliani ER, et al. Adriamycin cardiotoxicity in stage IV breast cancer: possible enhancement with prior left chest radiation therapy. *Int J Radiat Oncol Biol Phys* 1979;5:1997.
364. Mayer EG, Poulter CA, Aristizabal SA. Complications of irradiation related to apparent drug potentiation by Adriamycin. *Int J Radiat Oncol Biol Phys* 1976;1:1179.

365. Eltringham JR, Fajardo LF, Stewart JR, et al. Investigation of cardiotoxicity in rabbits from Adriamycin and fractionated cardiac irradiation: preliminary results. *Front Radiat Ther Oncol* 1979;13:21.
366. Petrovic D, Brown SM, Yatvin MB. Effects of Adriamycin and irradiation on beating of rat heart muscle cells in culture. *Int J Radiat Oncol Biol Phys* 1977;2:505.
367. LaMonte CS, Yeh SDJ, Straus DJ. Long-term follow-up of cardiac function in patients with Hodgkin's disease treated with mediastinal irradiation and combination chemotherapy including doxorubicin. *Cancer Treat Rep* 1986;70:439.
368. Santoro A, Bonadonna G, Valagusso P, et al. Long-term results of combined chemotherapy-radiotherapy approach in Hodgkin's disease: superiority of ABVD plus radiotherapy versus MOPP plus radiotherapy. *J Clin Oncol* 1987;5:27.
369. Brice P, Tredaniel J, Monsuez JJ, et al. Cardiopulmonary toxicity after three courses of ABVD and mediastinal irradiation in favorable Hodgkin's disease. *Ann Oncol* 1991; 2(Suppl 2):73.
370. Carlson RG, Mayfield WR, Normann S, Alexander JA. Radiation-associated valvular disease. *Chest* 1991;99:538.
371. Glanzmann C, Huguenin P, Lutolf UM, et al. Cardiac lesions after mediastinal irradiation for Hodgkin's disease. *Radiother Oncol* 1994;30:43.
372. Kadota RP, Burgert EO Jr, Driscoll DJ, et al. Cardiopulmonary function in long-term survivors of childhood Hodgkin's lymphoma: a pilot study. *Mayo Clin Proc* 1988;63:362.
373. Gustavsson A, Eskilsson J, Landberg T, et al. Late cardiac effects after mantle radiotherapy in patients with Hodgkin's disease. *Ann Oncol* 1990;1:355.
374. Lund MB, Kongerud J, Boe J, et al. Cardiopulmonary sequelae after treatment for Hodgkin's disease: increased risk in females? *Ann Oncol* 1996;7:257.
375. Warda M, Khan A, Massumi A, et al. Radiation-induced valvular dysfunction. *J Am Coll Cardiol* 1983;2:180.
376. Cohen SL, Bharati S, Glass J, et al. Radiotherapy as a cause of complete atrioventricular block in Hodgkin's disease. *Arch Intern Med* 1981;141:676.
377. Mary-Rabine L, Waleffe A, Kulbertius HE. Severe conduction disturbances and ventricular arrhythmias complicating mediastinal irradiation for Hodgkin's disease: a case report. *PACE* 1980;3:612.
378. Tzivoni D, Ratzkowski E, Biran S, et al. Complete heart block following therapeutic irradiation of the left side of the chest. *Chest* 1977;71:231.
379. Kereiakes DJ, Morady F, Ports TA. High degree atrioventricular block after radiation therapy. *Am J Cardiol* 1983;51:1233.
380. Slama M-S, LeGuludec D, Sebag C, et al. Complete atrioventricular block following mediastinal irradiation: a report of six cases. *PACE* 1991;14:1112.
381. Strender LE, Lindahl J, Larsson LE. Incidence of heart disease and functional significance of change in the electrocardiogram 10 years after radiotherapy for breast cancer. *Cancer* 1986;57:929.
382. Watchie J, Coleman CN, Raffin TA, et al. Minimal long-term cardiopulmonary dysfunction following treatment for Hodgkin's disease. *Int J Radiat Oncol Biol Phys* 1987;13:513.
383. Orzan F, Brusca A, Gaita F, et al. Associated cardiac lesions in patients with radiation-induced complete heart block [Review]. *Int J Cardiol* 1993;39:151.
384. Marbach JR, Sontag MR, Van DJ, et al. Management of radiation oncology patients with implanted cardiac pacemakers: report of AAPM Task Group No. 34. American Association of Physicists in Medicine. *Med Phys* 1994;21:85.
385. Souliman SK, Christie J. Pacemaker failure induced by radiotherapy. *Pacing Clin Electrophysiol* 1994;17:270.
386. Amronim GD, Solomon RD. Production of arteriosclerosis in the rabbit: a quantitative assessment. *Arch Pathol* 1965;75:219.
387. Gold H. Production of arteriosclerosis in the rat: effect of X-ray and high-fat diet. *Arch Pathol* 1961;71:268.
388. Artom C, Lofton HB, Clarkson TB. Ionizing radiation atherosclerosis and lipid metabolism in pigeons. *Radiat Res* 1965;26:165.
389. Kopelson G, Herwig KJ. The etiologies of coronary artery disease in cancer patients. *Int J Radiat Oncol Biol Phys* 1978;4:895.
390. Yahalom J, Hasin Y, Fuks Z. Acute myocardial infarction with normal coronary arteriogram after mantle field radiation therapy for Hodgkin's disease. *Cancer* 1983;52:637.
391. McEniery PT, Dorosti K, Schiavone WA, et al. Clinical and angiographic features of coronary artery disease after chest irradiation. *Am J Cardiol* 1987;60:1020.
392. Boivin JF, Hutchison GB, Lubin JH, Mauch P. Coronary artery disease mortality in patients treated for Hodgkin's disease. *Cancer* 1992;69:1241.
393. Henry-Amar M, Hayat M, Meerwaldt JH. Causes of death after therapy for early stage Hodgkin's disease entered on EORTC protocols. *Int J Radiat Oncol Biol Phys* 1990;19:1155.
394. Cosset JM, Henry-Amar M, Meerwaldt JH. Long-term toxicity of early stages of Hodgkin's disease therapy: the EORTC experience. *Am Oncol* 1991;2(Suppl 2):77.
395. Handler CE, Livesey S, Lawton PA. Coronary ostial stenosis after radiotherapy: angioplasty or coronary artery surgery? *Br Heart J* 1989;61:208.
396. Grollier G, Commeau P, Mercier V, et al. Post-radiotherapeutic left main coronary ostial stenosis: clinical and histiological study. *Eur Heart J* 1988;9:567.
397. Om A, Ellahham S, Vetrovec GW. Radiation-induced coronary artery disease [Review]. *Am Heart J* 1992;124:1598.
398. Orzan F, Brusca A, Conte MR, et al. Severe coronary artery disease after radiation therapy of the chest and mediastinum: clinical presentation and treatment. *Br Heart J* 1993;69:496.
399. Annest LS, Anderson RP, Li W, et al. Coronary artery disease following mediastinal radiation therapy. *J Thorac Cardiovasc Surg* 1983;85:257.
400. Miller DD, Waters DD, Dangoisse V, et al. Symptomatic coronary artery spasm following radiotherapy for Hodgkin's disease. *Chest* 1983;83:284.
401. Host H, Brennhoud IO, Loeb M. Post-operative radiotherapy in breast cancer: long-term results from the Oslo study. *Int J Radiat Oncol Biol Phys* 1986;12:727.
402. Jones JM, Ribeiro GG. Mortality patterns over 34 years of breast cancer patients in a clinical trial of post-operative radiotherapy. *Clin Radiol* 1989;40:204.
403. Haybittle JL, Brinkley D, Houghton J, et al. Postoperative radiotherapy and late mortality: evidence from the Cancer Research Campaign trial for early breast cancer. *BMJ* 1989;298:1611.
404. Levitt SH, Fletcher GH. Trials and tribulations: do clinical trials prove that irradiation increases cardiac and secondary cancer mortality in the breast cancer patient? *Int J Radiat Oncol Biol Phys* 1991;20:523.
405. Wallgren A, Arner O, Bergstrom J, et al. Radiation therapy in operable breast cancer: results from the Stockholm trial in adjuvant radiotherapy. *Int J Radiat Oncol Biol Phys* 1986;12:533.
406. Stender LE, Lindahl J, Larsson LE. Incidence of heart disease and functional significance of changes in the electrocardiogram 10 years after radiotherapy for breast cancer. *Cancer* 1986;57:929.
407. Cuzick J, Stewart H, Rutqvist L, et al. Cause-specific mortality in long-term survivors of breast cancer who participated in trials of radiotherapy. *J Clin Oncol* 1994;12:447.
408. Harris JR, Hellman S. Put the "hockey stick" on ice. *Int J Radiat Oncol Biol Phys* 1988;15:497.
409. Marks LB, Hebert ME, Bentel G, et al. To treat or not to treat the internal mammary nodes: an opposible compromise. *Int J Radiat Oncol Biol Phys* 1994;29:903.
410. Gustavsson A, Bendahl PO, Cwikeil M, et al. No serious late cardiac effects after adjuvant radiotherapy following mastectomy in premenopausal women with early breast cancer. *Int J Radiat Oncol Biol Phys* 1999;43:745.
411. Nixon AJ, Manola J, Gelman R, et al. No long-term increase in cardiac-related mortality after breast-conserving surgery and radiation therapy using modern techniques. *J Clin Oncol* 1998;16:1374.
412. Rutqvist LE, Leidberg A, Hammar N, Dalhberg K. Myocardial infarction among women with early-stage breast cancer treated with conservative surgery and breast irradiation. *Int J Radiat Oncol Biol Phys* 1998;40:359.
413. Shapiro CL, et al. Cardiac effects of adjuvant doxorubicin and radiation therapy in breast cancer patients. *J Clin Oncol* 1998;16:3493.
414. Lederman GS, Sheldon TA, Chaffey JT, et al. Cardiac disease after mediastinal irradiation for seminoma. *Cancer* 1987;60:772.
415. Savage DE, Constine LS, Schwartz RG, et al. Radiation effects on left ventricular function and myocardial perfusion in long-term survivors of Hodgkin's disease. *Int J Radiat Oncol Biol Phys* 1990;19:721.
416. Pierga JY, Maunoury C, Valette H, et al. Follow-up thallium-201 scintigraphy after mantle field radiotherapy for Hodgkin's disease. *Int J Radiat Oncol Biol Phys* 1993;25:871.
417. Pihkala J, Happonen JM, Virtanen K, et al. Cardiopulmonary evaluation of exercise tolerance after chest irradiation and anticancer chemotherapy in children and adolescents. *Pediatrics* 1995;95:755.
418. Piovaccari G, Ferretti RM, Prati F, et al. Cardiac disease after chest irradiation for Hodgkin's disease: incidence in 108 patients with long follow-up. *Int J Cardiol* 1995;49:39.
419. Reber D, Birnbaum DE, Tollenaere P. Heart disease following mediastinal irradiation: surgical management. *Eur J Cardiothorac Surg* 1995;9:202.
420. Van Son JA, Noyez L, van Asten WN. Use of internal mammary artery in myocardial revascularization after mediastinal irradiation. *J Thoracic Cardiovasc Surg* 1992;104:1539.
421. Fuks Z, Persaud RS, Alfieri A, et al. Basic fibroblast growth factor protects endothelial cells against radiation-induced programmed cell death in vitro and in vivo. *Cancer Res* 1994;54:2582.

SECTION 5

CLAUDIA A. SEIPP

Hair Loss

Alopecia is a psychologically distressing but common side effect of many chemotherapeutic agents and radiation therapy. As patients embark on new therapies, hair loss can induce a negative body image, cause depression and alter interpersonal relationships, and arouse enough anxiety to cause some patients to reject potentially curative treatment. In one study, 88% of women who received perioperative chemotherapy for early breast cancer considered alopecia to be the most traumatic aspect of therapy.[1] Adolescents have particular difficulty in coping with hair loss during a time of adjustment to the diagnosis of cancer.[2]

Frank discussion of the problem by clinicians and oncology nurses, with recognition of patients' stress and personal loss of self-esteem, is helpful in preparing affected patients to confront this event.[3] Although not all patients are entirely satisfied by current methods for the prevention of total scalp hair loss or the use of wigs after hair loss, care-givers can offer supportive listening, some practical suggestions, and identification of resources. Often, the presence of a spouse, family member, or friend during such a discussion with patients is helpful to place the problem in perspective and to aid affected families and patients in adapting.[4]

The hair loss caused by scalp irradiation is unpredictable. Epilation can begin at doses of 500 cGy and generally progresses, causing spotty areas of baldness as the course of treatment continues. The prospects for hair regrowth diminish with increasing doses.[5] Irradiation ports on extremities have been noted to be hair-free 10 years after radiation therapy and may never have hair regrowth. In lower-dose ranges, regrowth begins 8 to 9 weeks after cessation of therapy. Patients should be cautioned that new hair may be different in character from pretreatment hair.[6]

The extent of body hair loss by patients in any chemotherapeutic program is both drug- and dose-dependent and is related to the frequency of cycle repetition. Often, it is caused by more than one drug used concurrently (Table 55.5-1). Long-term therapy may result in loss of pubic, axillary, and facial hair in addition to scalp hair. Often, the loss of scalp hair occurs in an acute episode while washing. It should be emphasized to patients that alopecia from chemotherapy is reversible, with hair regeneration beginning 1 to 2 months after therapy is discontinued. Alterations in color and texture of hair may occur: Shade of hair may be lighter or darker and often is curlier as it regrows.[7] Hair loss may begin 1 to 2 weeks after a single chemotherapeutic dose and reaches maximum loss within 2 months in most drug sequences. Doxorubicin and cyclophosphamide are common cytologic agents known to cause epilation after two cycles at doses of doxorubicin greater than 50 mg/m^2 and cyclophosphamide greater than 500 mg/m^2. Although agents differ in degree to which they cause hair loss, alopecia may be expected with other single-agent antibiotics, alkylators, nitrosoureas, and especially their combinations.[8]

TABLE 55.5-1. Single Agents with Potential to Induce Reversible Alopecia

Actinomycin
Amsacrine
Bleomycin
Cyclophosphamide
Dactinomycin
Daunorubicin
Doxorubicin
Epirubicin
Etoposide
5-Fluorodeoxyuridine
5-Fluorouracil
Hydroxyurea
Ifosfamide
Methotrexate
Mitoxantrone
Mitomycin
Melphalan
Paclitaxel
Taxol
Vinblastine
Vincristine

Note: The degree or onset of alopecia is inversely proportional to dose, schedule of sequences, rate and route of delivery, and various combinations of agents used concurrently.[8]

HEAD COVERING

Most patients will choose to cover their heads during periods of hair loss. Nurses and clinicians can suggest wigs or head covering with stylish scarves, turbans, or hats. Wigs should be selected before hair loss begins so that the patient is prepared when alopecia occurs and so that hair color and style can be matched. Hairpieces are tax-deductible medical expenses and are covered by some medical insurance policies. The American Cancer Society (ACS) can provide wigs free of charge through their "wig bank" program. Several small private businesses have been developed by former patients who distribute or sell head coverings of various designs. An ACS patient service called *Look Good, Feel Better* has been developed in partnership with the National Cosmetology Association and the Cosmetic, Toiletry, and Fragrance Association Foundation. This service specifically assists women in compensating for hair loss and skin changes to enhance self-image during cancer treatment.[9] Volunteer beauticians and cosmetologists help women to improve their appearance and to feel more comfortable with changes in appearance, such as dry, discolored, or blotching skin; loss of eyebrows and eyelashes; discolored nails; and alopecia. Such volunteers provide instruction with makeup and give advice about wigs and other types of head coverings. Information about group programs and their location is available through an ACS toll-free telephone number, 1-800-395-LOOK, 24 hours daily, 7 days per week. The support program is active in all 50 states and Puerto Rico, with groups designed especially for teenagers in limited areas around the country. The program celebrated its tenth anniversary in 1999, having provided this service to more than 250,000 women.

PREVENTION OF ALOPECIA

Since 1966, interventions have been proposed to prevent scalp hair loss from chemotherapy.[9] The rationale for these procedures is to prevent drug circulation to the hair follicles by causing temporary vasoconstriction and decreasing tissue metabolism at the time of peak plasma drug level, with either an occlusive scalp tourniquet or localized hypothermia. The pharmacokinetic profiles of the drugs to be used should be understood before either of these methods is considered. Scalp-cooling systems must maintain temperatures below 22°C to have any effect. Occlusion of the superficial scalp veins must begin before the drugs are given and, to be effective, must be extended beyond the time of the peak plasma drug levels.[9–11]

Various types of scalp-icing devices have been manufactured by several different American companies. Although the U.S. Food and Drug Administration (FDA) initially had approved the marketing of cooling caps intended to cause localized scalp hypothermia, early in 1990 the FDA reviewed these applications and became concerned that the safety and efficacy of these devices had not been substantiated by adequate clinical data.[12–16] Regulatory action was initiated to address the following concerns:

- The potential for scalp metastasis posed by the use of these devices.
- The potential for reducing drug circulation to other anatomic sites beyond the scalp, such as the skull and possibly the brain.
- The effectiveness of preventing hair loss and effects of specific cytologic doses and other variables on the results achieved.

On the basis of these factors, the FDA halted the commercial distribution of these devices. Five years after their withdrawal, no company has come forward with supporting clinical evidence of reasonable safety and effectiveness, according to Frances Moreland Curtis of the FDA's Division of General and Restorative Devices (written communication, August 1995).

Though indications demonstrate that continuous-flow systems with thermostatically controlled cooling caps still are used in Europe, they seem to be limited to regimens containing a single anthracycline alopecia-inducing agent.[16] Limitations of safety and inconclusive and conflicting reports of the results of the usefulness of scalp hypothermia should be factors discussed with patients seeking information about these devices and hair preservation techniques.

REFERENCES

1. Kiebert GM, Hanneke CJM de Haes, Kievit J, van de Verde CJH. Effect of perioperative chemotherapy on quality of life of patients with early breast cancer. *Eur J Cancer* 1990;26:1038.
2. Pickard-Holley S. The symptom experience of alopecia. *Semin Oncol Nurs* 1995;11:235.
3. Williams J, Wood C, Cunningham-Warburton P. A narrative study of chemotherapy-induced alopecia. *Oncol Nurs Forum* 1999;26(9):1463.
4. Freedman T. Social and cultural dimensions of hair loss in women treated for breast cancer. *Cancer Nurs* 1994;17(4):334.
5. Moss WT, Brand WN, Battiford H. *Radiation oncology: rationale, techniques, results*, 5th ed. St. Louis: Mosby, 1979:57.
6. Nordstrom RE, Holsti LR. Hair transplantation in alopecia due to radiation. *Plast Reconstr Surg* 1983;72:454.
7. Cancer, cancer therapy, and hair [Editorial]. *Lancet* 1983;2:1177.
8. Cline BW. Prevention of chemotherapy-induced alopecia: a review of the literature. *Cancer Nurs* 1984;7:221.
9. Satterwaite B, Zimm S. The use of scalp hypothermia in the prevention of doxorubicin-induced hair loss. *Cancer* 1984;54:34.
10. Robinson MH, Jones AC, Durant KD. Effectiveness of scalp cooling in reducing scalp alopecia caused by epirubicin treatment in breast cancer. *Cancer Treat Rep* 1987;71:913.
11. Middleton J, Franks D, Buchanan RB, et al. Failure of scalp hypothermia to prevent hair loss when cyclosphosphamide is added to doxorubicin and vincristine. *Cancer Treat Rep* 1985;69:337.
12. Wheelock JB, Myers MB, Krebs HB, et al. Ineffectiveness of scalp hypothermia in the prevention of alopecia in patients treated with doxorubicin and cis-platin combinations. *Cancer Treat Rep* 1984;68:1387.
13. Seipp CA. Scalp hypothermia: indicators for precaution [Letter]. *Oncol Nurs Forum* 1983;10:12.
14. Whitman G, Cadman E, Chen M. Misuse of scalp hypothermia. *Cancer Treat Rep* 1981;65:507.
15. Camp-Sorrell D. Scalp hypothermia devices: current status. *ONS News* 1991;7:1.
16. Tollenaar RAEM, Liefors GJ, Repelaer van Driel OJ, van de Velde CJH. Scalp cooling has no place in the prevention of alopecia in adjuvant chemotherapy for breast cancer. *Eur J Cancer* 1994;10:1448.

MARVIN L. MEISTRICH
RENA VASSILOPOULOU-SELLIN
LARRY I. LIPSHULTZ

SECTION **6**

Gonadal Dysfunction

For young adults who have cancer, the success of treatment with regimens that are toxic to gonadal function has made infertility an important problem. When the cancer is controlled, quality of life then becomes a major issue. To many of these young men and women, a major quality-of-life issue is the ability to have a normal child.

Both neoplastic disease and its treatment can interfere with normal sexual and reproductive function (Table 55.6-1). Testicular and ovarian cancer directly involves the gonad, and prostate, endometrial, and cervical cancer directly involves the reproductive tract. Surgical treatment for any of these diseases results by necessity in the loss of these important reproductive organs. Retroperitoneal lymph node dissection (RPLND) for testicular and colon cancer, as well as prostatectomy and surgery involving the bladder neck, may result in loss of the ability to ejaculate. Primary and metastatic tumors in the hypothalamus and pituitary can directly affect gonadotropin secretion, resulting in secondary hypogonadism. Both chemotherapy and radiation can cause a variety of toxic effects on the male and female gonads. Cytotoxic therapies delivered to women during pregnancy might have teratogenic effects on the fetus.[1,2] If fertility is maintained or returns, there remains the concern about the heritability of cancer and at least a theoretical risk of mutagenic alterations to germ cells caused by cytotoxic therapies.

The reproductive consequences of cancer therapy affect many people. In the United States, 17,000 men 15 to 45 years old are diagnosed each year with Hodgkin's disease, lymphoma, bone and soft tissue sarcomas, testicular cancer, or leukemia.[3,4] Of these, more than 3000 are treated with doses of alkylating agents, platinum drugs, or radiation sufficient to induce prolonged azoospermia. Similarly, 35,000 women aged

TABLE 55.6-1. Impact of Cancer and Cancer Therapy on the Reproductive System

Tumor	Direct gonadal involvement
	Reproductive tract involvement
	Hypothalamic and pituitary involvement
	Concern about heritability of cancer susceptibility
Surgery	Removal of gonad
	Genital mutilation
	Failure of emission and retrograde ejaculation
	Impotence and loss of orgasm
Radiotherapy or chemotherapy	Germ cell depletion
	Loss of gonadal hormones
	Mutagenic changes in germ cells
	Teratogenic effects on fetus
Chemotherapy	Seminal transmission of drug
Radiotherapy (cranial)	Loss of gonadotropic hormones

15 to 45 years old are treated for breast cancer (mostly), Hodgkin's disease, lymphoma, and leukemia; at least 80% of these patients receive radiation or alkylating agent–based cytotoxic therapies. These treatments cause not only sterility but also premature menopause and the associated estrogen deficiency in nearly 20,000 women. In addition, 12,000 children younger than 15 years are diagnosed each year with cancer, including leukemia, nervous system tumors, lymphomas, and other solid tumors.[5] Survival is approaching 80%, and because 85% of patients receive chemotherapy or gonadal or pituitary irradiation, reproductive dysfunction is a significant concern.

EFFECTS OF CYTOTOXIC AGENTS ON ADULT MEN

BIOLOGIC CONSIDERATIONS

The sensitivities of the seminiferous (or germinal) epithelium and the endocrine components of the testis to killing by cytotoxic therapies are related to the relative proliferation rates of the different cells.[6] The germ cells consist of stem spermatogonia, differentiating spermatogonia, spermatocytes, spermatids, and sperm. Among the germ cells, which are within the seminiferous epithelium, the differentiating spermatogonia proliferate most actively and are extremely susceptible to cytotoxic agents. In contrast, the Leydig cells, which are in the interstitium and produce the androgens, and the Sertoli cells, which provide support and regulatory factors to the germ cells, do not proliferate in adults and so survive most cytotoxic therapies. These cells may, however, suffer functional damage. Frequently after cytotoxic therapies, germinal tissue appears completely absent, a state described as *germinal aplasia,* and only the Sertoli cells remain lining the tubules. This could be a result of killing of the spermatogenic stem cells, the loss of the ability of the somatic cells to support the differentiation of a few surviving stem cells, or a combination of both.

After cytotoxic treatment, sperm count diminishes with a time course that depends on the sensitivities of the different spermatogenic cells and their kinetics of maturation to sperm. Because the later-stage germ cells (spermatocytes onward) are relatively insensitive to killing and progress with invariant kinetics, sperm count is not immediately affected. However, these cells are susceptible to the induction of mutagenic damage, and studies in rodents have shown they can become spermatozoa and transmit mutations induced in their DNA to the next generation.[7] The eventual recovery of sperm production depends on the survival of the spermatogonial stem cells and their ability to differentiate. In both rats and humans, surviving stem cells may fail to produce differentiating germ cells for a year or more after cytotoxic insult.[8,9]

The loss of germinal cells has secondary effects on the endocrine function of the testis and the hypothalamic-pituitary-gonadal axis. Inhibin secretion by the Sertoli cells declines and, as inhibin limits follicle-stimulating hormone (FSH) secretion by the pituitary, serum FSH rises. Because germinal aplasia reduces testis size and there is a concomitant reduction in testicular blood flow,[10] less testosterone is distributed into the circulation, and as testosterone inhibits pituitary luteinizing hormone (LH) secretion, serum LH increases. Conversely, LH is the primary stimulator of Leydig cell testosterone synthesis, and the reduced blood flow also lessens Leydig cell exposure to circulating LH. These alterations of pituitary-gonadal feedback could elevate serum LH and reduce serum testosterone levels even in the absence of any Leydig cell injury.

CHARACTERISTICS OF GONADAL TOXICITY

Although subnormal semen profiles, ejaculatory dysfunction, and low libido in treated patients are most likely a result of treatment, other causes must be considered, too. A sexual and reproductive history should include developmental factors such as age of testicular descent and puberty; surgery or injury to the genitals; diseases that might affect reproduction; drug, chemical, or heat exposure; and pretreatment fertility and libido status. A physical examination should consist of examination of the testicles and secondary sexual characteristics such as beard and hair distribution pattern. Laboratory tests entail semen analysis and a hormone profile. Normal values and those associated with germinal aplasia are outlined in Table 55.6-2.

During the first 2 months of cytotoxic therapy, sperm counts may remain normal or be only moderately reduced. Some regimens cause azoospermia 2 to 3 months after the initiation of therapy,[11,12] corresponding to the interval during which the sensitive differentiating spermatogonia become sperm. With other regimens, oligospermia or even normospermia may be maintained.[13]

Increases in FSH are associated with germinal aplasia. Although FSH measurements have sometimes been used as a surrogate for sperm count, they only show an imperfect correlation,[14] in part because of interpatient variability in baseline FSH levels.[15] After cytotoxic therapy, LH tends to be elevated and serum testosterone levels in the low normal range.[16] This has been interpreted as indicating subclinical, compensated Leydig cell failure; however, changes in testicular blood flow can also explain these observations.[10] The only treatment that produces testosterone insufficiency in a high proportion of adult patients is high-dose (30 Gy) radiation direct to the testes, which directly damages Leydig cell function.[17]

The induced azoospermia can be either temporary or prolonged, depending on the ability of surviving stem sper-

TABLE 55.6-2. Typical Clinical and Laboratory Features for Diagnosis of Male Reproductive Dysfunction

	Testis Size			*Serum Hormone Levels*		
	Length × Width (cm)	Volume (mL)	*Sperm Count (millions/mL)*	Follicle-Stimulating Hormone (mIU/mL)	Luteinizing Hormone (mIU/mL)	Testosterone (ng/dL)
Normal men	5.0 × 3.0	15–25	20– >100	1–12	2–12	300–1200
Germinal aplasia	3.7 × 2.3	8–15	0	>20	>12	200–700

matogonia to proliferate, differentiate, and produce spermatozoa, which in turn depends on the nature of the cytotoxic agent and dose (Table 55.6-3). If treatment is limited to the cytotoxic agents that do not kill stem spermatogonia or block their differentiation into spermatozoa, normospermic levels are usually restored within 3 months after the cytotoxic therapy. However, if agents that inactivate stem spermatogonia or affect differentiation are used, longer periods of azoospermia ensure. At lower doses of these agents, recovery to normospermic levels can occur within 1 to 3 years, but at higher doses, azoospermia can be more prolonged or even permanent. The probability that spermatogenesis will recover decreases with the duration of azoospermia.[12,18] However, in a few men spermatogenesis recovered after as long as 20 years of azoospermia.[19] FSH levels drop to normal when sperm production recovers. When sperm count recovers after cytotoxic therapy, sperm motility appears to be normal,[12,18,20] and fertility is generally restored. However, when the duration of azoospermia is long, recovery may sometimes plateau at less than 1 million/mL,[12] which may not be compatible with fertility.

To evaluate the effects of cytotoxic therapy, the initial gonadal status must be considered. Men with both seminomas and nonseminomatous germ cell tumors have impaired semen quality even before cytotoxic therapy is instituted. Approximately 65% are oligospermic (counts less than 20 million/mL), 50% have less than 10 million/mL, and 13% are azoospermic,[21,22] compared with values of 9%, 5%, and 1%, respectively, in control populations.[23] In approximately 40% of the patients with reduced semen quality, this impaired testicular function is a result of irreversible abnormalities associated with the uninvolved gonad (e.g., carcinoma *in situ* or a history of cryptorchidism) that predate the onset of cancer.[24] In the other 60%, it may be a result of reversible factors such as elevated chorionic gonadotropin produced by the tumor with resulting increases in estradiol.[25] In addition, emission and ejaculation may have been compromised by earlier RPLND so that the sperm density may not accurately reflect gonadal function.[26] In contrast to the severe dysfunction in testicular cancer, in Hodgkin's disease only 21% of Hodgkin's disease patients are oligospermic and 2% are azoospermic, and the distribution of counts in the remainder is not significantly different from normal.[27] The presence of low-grade fever and B symptoms was not predictive for poor semen quality.[27,28] Similarly, in other lymphomas and sarcomas, pretreatment sperm counts tend to be normal except for a trend toward an increase in the incidence of oligospermia.[12,18,20]

Age at treatment is not a major factor in recovery from gonadal damage in men. Two studies indicate increased inci-

TABLE 55.6-3. Effects of Different Antitumor Agents on Sperm Production in Men

Agents (Cumulative Dose for Effect)	*Effect*
Radiation (2.5 Gy to testis) Chlorambucil (1.4 g/m^2) Cyclophosphamide (19 g/m^2) Procarbazine (4 g/m^2) Cisplatin (500 mg/m^2)	Prolonged azoospermia
Busulfan (≥600 mg/kg) Carboplatin (>2 g/m^2) Ifosfamide (>30 g/m^2) Carmustine (1 g/m^2), lomustine (500 mg/m^2)	Prolonged azoospermia likely, but conclusive data not available
Nitrogen mustard Melphalan, actinomycin D	Unknown because always given with other highly sterilizing agents
Adriamycin (770 mg/m^2) Cytosine arabinoside (1 g/m^2) Vinblastine (50 g/m^2) Vincristine (8 g/m^2)	Can be additive with above agents in causing prolonged azoospermia, but cause only temporary reductions in sperm count when not combined with above agents
Amsacrine, bleomycin, dacarbazine, daunorubicin, epirubicin, etoposide, 5-fluorouracil, 6-mercaptopurine, methotrexate, mitoxantrone, thioguanine, thiotepa	Only temporary reductions in sperm count at doses used in conventional regimens, but additive effects are possible
Prednisone	Unlikely to affect sperm production
Interferon-α	No effects on sperm production

dence of testicular damage after cytotoxic therapy in older men,[29,30] but others fail to indicate any effect.[12,18,31]

INDIVIDUAL DRUGS

The most sterilizing drugs are the alkylating agents and cisplatin, all of which form adducts and/or cross-links on DNA. Only two of these, chlorambucil[32] and cyclophosphamide,[33] have been demonstrated to induce prolonged azoospermia when given alone. Evidence from combination chemotherapy regimens demonstrates that procarbazine[34,35] and cisplatin in high doses[20,36] are also highly sterilizing. Table 55.6-3 lists the cumulative doses of these drugs at which recovery of sperm production is unlikely. The cumulative dose appears to be more important than the dose rate.[12] Some doses are based on data from combination chemotherapy regimens and do not account for possible additive contributions from other drugs in the regimen.

The evaluations of other individual alkylating agents have been obtained from combination chemotherapy regimens. Busulfan has an additive effect on the sterility in men resulting from cyclophosphamide treatment,[37] but there are no studies on busulfan in the absence of highly sterilizing agents. Carboplatin, an analogue of cisplatin, is expected to produce sterility, but in clinical studies it appeared to be less sterilizing than cisplatin.[21] The addition of the cyclophosphamide analogue ifosfamide to cisplatin-containing chemotherapy regimens failed to produce significant levels of additional prolonged azoospermia.[38] Treatment of boys with carmustine and lomustine did produce prolonged azoospermia,[39] and it is likely, but not proven, that the same would occur in adults.

The list of agents that only have temporary effects (see Table 55.6-3) includes some that have been used as single agents. However, most were used in regimens that do not cause prolonged azoospermia or were not independent prognostic factors in the prediction of recovery in variably sterilizing regimens.[18]

In addition to cytotoxic agents, hormonal and biologic agent therapies are also used in treatment of cancer.[40] Any reproductive effects of hormones should generally be reversible. However, only the corticosteroid prednisone and the cytokine interferon-α have been studied, and there are no indications of negative effects on male gonadal function of these agents.[18,41]

RADIATION THERAPY

The effects of radiation on the testes are dependent on the fractionation regimen: Doses given in 3- to 7-week fractionated courses cause more gonadal damage than do single doses.[42] In contrast, in all other organ systems fractionation of radiation reduces the damage. Doses of radiation to the testes above 0.15 Gy diminish sperm count after a lag period of approximately 6 weeks.[43] Fractionated doses between 0.15 and 0.5 Gy only cause oligospermia. The nadir of sperm count is at 4 to 6 months after the end of treatment, but 10 to 18 months are required for complete recovery.[44] At doses above 0.6 Gy, azoospermia occurs. The duration of azoospermia is dose dependent, and recovery can begin within 1 year after doses of less than 1 Gy,[45] but requires 2.0 to 3.5 years at approximately 2 Gy.[30] Cumulative doses of fractionated radiotherapy of 2.5 Gy and higher generally result in prolonged and likely permanent azoospermia.[46] Likewise, single testicular doses of 8 Gy or fractionated doses of 12 Gy, given as total body irradiation in preparation for bone marrow transplantation, generally produce permanent azoospermia. However, spermatogenesis does recover in 17% of these men after a median follow-up time of 5 years,[37] but the recovery is only 10% when cyclophosphamide (4.5 g/m^2) is added to the conditioning regimen.[47]

Direct testicular radiation is the only treatment that consistently produces clinically significant reductions in testicular androgen production in the adult. Doses of 30 Gy for treatment of testicular carcinoma *in situ* significantly reduce testosterone levels,[17] but doses of less than 20 Gy do not appear to have clinically significant effects on testosterone levels.[48] Furthermore, the gonadal scatter doses of 2 to 6 Gy during treatment for prostate cancer also do not produce clinically significant reductions in testosterone levels[49]; the radiation-associated impotence after such treatments is likely a result of vascular damage.[50]

COMBINATION REGIMENS

The sterilizing potential of different combinations depends on the individual agents and the dose given. Although interindividual variation makes it impossible to predict whether sperm production in any given man will recover, the probability of inducing prolonged azoospermia has been determined for many combinations (Table 55.6-4).

The sterilizing potentials of combination chemotherapy and chemotherapy plus radiotherapy regimens are additive; there is no evidence for synergistic interactions between the agents. The listing in Table 55.6-3 and the results with similar regimens can be used to predict the sterilizing potential of regimens not presented here. The additive effects of multiple agents can be seen in the case of cyclophosphamide, which when given alone requires 19 g/m^2 to produce prolonged sterility in one-half the men. However, the prolonged azoospermia observed in one-half the men after a median cyclophosphamide dose of only 10.6 g/m^2 in the CY(V)ADIC regimen, which had a median doxorubicin dose of 880 g/m^2, can be explained by additive effects from other drugs, particularly doxorubicin.[12,18] The absence of azoospermia after 5.1 g/m^2 of cyclophosphamide given for treatment of leukemia[57] may be a result of the extreme fractionation, as the drug was given once every 20 weeks over 3.5 years. Two cycles of Mustargen, Oncovin, procarbazine, and prednisone (MOPP) and pelvic radiotherapy had additive effects on the induction of prolonged azoospermia,[34] but the gonadal toxicity of mitoxantrone, vincristine, vinblastine, and prednisone (NOVP) was insufficient to produce noticeable enhancement of the sterilizing effects of pelvic radiotherapy.[60]

EFFECTS OF CYTOTOXIC AGENTS ON ADULT WOMEN

BIOLOGIC CONSIDERATIONS

Gonadal cell kinetics in women are opposite of those in men, as the germ cells are nonproliferative whereas the somatic cells proliferate. Prenatally, female germ cells proliferate as oogonia and become arrested at the oocyte stage. At birth, a woman has 1 million oocytes, which are reduced to 300,000 at puberty. These are progressively lost by atresia, development, and ovulation, until almost all are lost and menopause is reached at approximately age 50 years.

TABLE 55.6-4. Probability of Germinal Aplasia in Men Treated with Different Combination Chemotherapy Regimens

Regimen	*Disease*	*Courses or Dose*	*Patients with Prolonged Azoospermia (%)*	*References*
HIGH-DOSE ALKYLATING AGENT				
MOPPd or MVPPd	Hodgkin's disease	≥6 courses	85	51,34
COPPd	Hodgkin's disease	4–9 courses	100	35
BuCy + HSCT	Leukemia, lymphoma	Bu = 600 mg/m^2	83	37
		Cy = 7.4 g/m^2		
BcECaMl + HSCT	Lymphoma	Bc = 300 mg/m^2	100	47
		Ml = 140 mg/m^2 + prior treatment		
MODERATELY HIGH-DOSE ALKYLATING AGENT				
MOPPd/ABVD	Hodgkin's disease	6–9 courses	50	28
COPPd/ABVD, X	Hodgkin's disease	6–9 courses	85	52
ChlVPPd/EVA	Hodgkin's disease	6–8 courses	95	53
CHOPd-bleomycin	Lymphoma	Cy <9.5 g/m^2	17	18
		Cy >9.5 g/m^2	53	
CyVAD or CyAD	Sarcoma	Cy <7.5 g/m^2	30	12
		Cy >7.5 g/m^2	90	
Cy, A, Mx	Sarcoma	Cy = 5.6 g/m^2	18	54
VACAd, X	Testicular cancer	Cy = 5.8 g/m^2	62	55
NONALKYLATING OR LOW-DOSE ALKYLATING AGENT				
MOPPd	Hodgkin's disease	2 courses	0	34
ABVD, X	Hodgkin's disease	6 courses	0	13
NOVPd, X	Hodgkin's disease	3 courses	0	56
Bc, Cy, Ca, L, Mp, TG	Leukemia	Cy = 5.1 g/m^2	0	57
A, Cy, Ca, Dn, Mx, Mp, Pd, TG, V	Leukemia	Cy = 2.6 g/m^2	0	58
PLATINUM				
PlVB	Testicular cancer	Pl ≤400 mg/m^2	10	21
		Pl >400 mg/m^2	50	
PlEB	Testicular cancer	Pl ≤300 mg/m^2	0	59
		Pl = 400 mg/m^2	25	
CbEB	Testicular cancer	≤4 courses	0	21
		>4 courses	10	
Pl A, D	Osteosarcoma	Pl <600 mg/m^2	5	20
		Pl ≥600 mg/m^2	57	

A, doxorubicin (Adriamycin); Ad, actinomycin D; B, bleomycin; Bc, BCNU (carmustine); Bu, busulfan; Ca, cytosine arabinoside; Cb, carboplatin; Chl, chlorambucil; Cy, cyclophosphamide; D, dacarbazine; Dn, daunorubicin; E, etoposide; F, 5-fluorouracil; HSCT, hematopoietic stem cell transplant; I, ifosfamide; L, L-asparaginase; M, mechlorethamine (nitrogen mustard); Ml, melphalan; Mp, 6-mercaptopurine; Mx, methotrexate; N, mitoxantrone (Novantrone); O, vincristine (Oncovin); P, procarbazine; Pd, prednisone; Pl, cisplatin; TG, thioguanine; V, vinblastine; X, radiotherapy.

Before recruitment to the process leading to ovulation, oocytes are found in primordial follicles with few pregranulosa cells, surrounded by thecal cells of the ovarian stroma. The stimulus for the initiation of follicular maturation, which occurs in the absence of gonadotropic hormones, is unknown, but a role for gonadotropins cannot be excluded.[61] Once a follicle is recruited into growth, it develops until it either degenerates or ovulates. Follicular maturation is characterized by proliferation of granulosa cells and the development of steroidogenic potential of both the thecal and granulosa cells. Estrogens, produced by biosynthetic steps in both the thecal and the granulosa cells under LH and FSH stimulation, cause the LH surge that triggers ovulation. The day-to-day sequential variations in FSH, LH, and estradiol are essential for menstrual cyclicity and the female reproductive processes. The close interaction between granulosa cells and oocytes makes it difficult to identify which type of cell is the target of cytotoxic agents; death of either results in atrophy of the other. Because destruction of oocytes results in loss of follicles and steroidogenesis, germ cell loss leads directly to estrogen insufficiency.

The time between recruitment of follicles and their ovulation is approximately 85 days. When maturing follicles are destroyed by cytotoxic therapy, temporary amenorrhea results. If primordial follicles are reduced below the minimum number necessary for menstrual cyclicity, irreversible ovarian failure occurs and the amenorrhea is permanent. Different species of experimental animals have yielded conflicting information regarding the sensitivity of primordial follicles to radiation[62] and cyclophosphamide[63,64] and do not yet allow prediction of response in women.

CHARACTERISTICS OF GONADAL TOXICITY

Because the size of the germ cell population in women cannot be estimated, menstrual and reproductive histories are important in

TABLE 55.6-5. Typical Laboratory Features for Diagnosis of Ovarian Failure

Menstrual Phase	*Follicle-Stimulating Hormone (mIU/mL)*	*Luteinizing Hormone (mIU/mL)*	*Estradiol (pg/mL)*
Prepubertal	0–3	0–2	0–40
Follicular	3–20	2–15	10–200
Midcycle	5–16	50–150	200–700
Luteal	1–12	0.6–19.0	15–260
Ovarian failure	18–153	16–64	<50

assessing the effects of cytotoxic therapy on ovarian function. Information on the patient's menstrual cycle during and after therapy, as well as oral contraceptive use, should be noted. To determine if effects are related to cytotoxic therapy, pretherapy ovarian function should be evaluated from the history of menarche, menses, pregnancies, and oral contraceptive use. The occurrence of symptoms of recent primary ovarian failure, including hot flashes, night sweats, insomnia, mood swings, irritability, vaginal dryness, dyspareunia, decreased libido, and bladder infection, should be recorded. Laboratory measurements of hormone levels are most definitive in the diagnosis of primary ovarian failure; FSH is the most sensitive, but LH and estradiol levels are also useful (Table 55.6-5). The symptoms of ovarian failure may be masked and the hormone levels altered if the woman is taking oral contraceptives.

Some of the variability reported in the literature regarding the incidence of ovarian failure after cytotoxic therapy is a result of the lack of consistent definitions.[65] Menopause should be defined as more than 12 months without a menstrual period, treatment-related amenorrhea as at least 6 months without menstrual periods in a premenopausal patient, and oligomenorrhea as a reduction in the frequency of menses to between 40 days and 6 months. Because the mechanisms of temporary and irreversible treatment-related amenorrhea may be different, posttreatment follow-up time should be given, and they should be distinct outcomes.

Cytotoxic therapy often induces temporary amenorrhea, which may last a few months or up to 7 years.[66] Some of this temporary amenorrhea is a result of direct ovarian damage, causing failure of follicular recruitment or loss of maturing follicles. Alternatively, stress and malnutrition or weight loss can also cause temporary gonadal dysfunction by altering hypothalamic activity and estrogen metabolism.[67] The destruction of growing follicles and the resulting temporary amenorrhea during treatment appear to be independent of age.[68] Although some patients with treatment-induced temporary amenorrhea do display menopausal symptoms, these symptoms are usually indicative of permanent ovarian failure. In contrast, permanent treatment-induced amenorrhea, which is equivalent to ovarian failure, dramatically increases in an apparently continuous manner with age at treatment[69,70]; examples are given in Tables 55.6-6 and 55.6-7. This trend is expected as the number of follicles decreases with increasing age. The permanent amenorrhea may begin during chemotherapy or subsequently after several years of oligomenorrhea.[71,72]

If cytotoxic therapy depletes the pool of primordial follicles, premature ovarian failure should occur even in young women who continue menstruating after cytotoxic therapy.[71,73] In women aged 13 to 19 years at diagnosis treated with alkylating agent chemotherapy and radiotherapy below the diaphragm, the median age at menopause is 32 years, compared with 44 years for women treated with radiotherapy or chemotherapy alone, and 49 years for controls.[74] The degree of acceleration of menopause in these women correlated with the probability of induction of primary ovarian failure by the different therapies.[75]

Cytotoxic therapy-induced ovarian failure and premature menopause can accelerate bone density loss.[76] However, when only chemotherapy is used, some residual ovarian function may be present and can ameliorate the loss.[77]

INDIVIDUAL DRUGS

As in men, only alkylating agents appear to produce permanent gonadal failure in women (see Table 55.6-6), and the cumulative dose appears to be more important than the dose rate. Administration of low daily doses of cyclophosphamide over several months[78] is only slightly less effective at inducing permanent ovarian failure than is a high dose in 4 days.[73] Melphalan, chlorambucil, busulfan, mitomycin C, and doses of cisplatin of 600 mg/m^2 or higher[87] also produce permanent ovarian failure. Procarbazine is likely to be highly sterilizing inasmuch as permanent ovarian failure is observed in all procarbazine-containing combinations and, in the case of cyclophosphamide, Oncovin, procarbazine, and prednisone (COPP), the dose of cyclophosphamide is insufficient to cause this effect (see Table 55.6-7).

Other agents studied do not induce permanent ovarian failure. 5-Fluorouracil up to 30 g did not induce amenorrhea in women with a median age of 35.[78] Methotrexate (200 g) plus vincristine (40 g),[92] etoposide (5 g),[93] and cisplatin (less than 450 mg/m^2) plus doxorubicin (less than 400 mg/m^2)[87] failed to produce permanent ovarian failure in women 15 to 30 years of age. Doxorubicin, bleomycin, vincristine, and dacarbazine (ABVD), must not induce ovarian failure because none is observed after treatment of women up to age 41.[94] Reproductive effects of hormonal agents, such as tamoxifen, which interferes with pregnancy in animals,[95] should be reversible.

RADIATION THERAPY

Radiation is highly effective at inducing permanent ovarian failure with a marked age-dependence in sensitivity[96] (see Table 55.6-6). In adult women, irradiation of the ovaries occurs in the treatment of Hodgkin's disease and during total body irradiation in preparation for hematopoietic stem cell transplantation. Irradiation of the paraaortic nodes results in cumulative doses of only 1.5 Gy to the ovaries and does not appear to interfere with menstruation in most patients.[88,97] When total nodal irradiation for Hodgkin's disease or pelvic radiation for cervical cancer is given, and the ovarian dose can be reduced to 4 to 5 Gy by translocation (oophoropexy) and shielding of the ovaries, a partial preservation of fertility

TABLE 55.6-6. Effects of Different Cytotoxic Agents on Ovarian Function

Agent	*Prepubertal*	*Age 20 Y*	*Age 35 Y*	*Age 45 Y*	*References*
CUMULATIVE DOSES TO CAUSE PERMANENT OVARIAN FAILURE					
Cyclophosphamide (g)	>48	20–50	6–8	5	54,73,78–80
Melphalan (mg/m²)	—	>240	>510	340	81–83
Busulfan (mg/m²)	600	<600	<600	—	37,66
Chlorambucil (g)	>3	>1.5	>1	1	32,84
Mitomycin C (g)	—	—	≥30	≥30	78
Radiation (Gy)	12	7	3	<2	85
INCIDENCE OF PERMANENT OVARIAN FAILURE (%)					
Cyclophosphamide (7.4 g/m²)	0	0	60	—	73
Radiation (pelvic; 4–5 Gy)	<10	40	90	95	70,86
Radiation (total body irradiation; 10 Gy)	40	75	100	100	73,85

in younger women results.[70,98] Total body irradiation in preparation for bone marrow transplantation delivers 8 to 12 Gy to the gonads, which destroys ovarian function in all adult women, even the young ones.[73,85] Fractionation appeared not to spare the ovary, as 27% of women receiving 10 Gy in a single fraction recovered ovarian function as opposed to only 10% of those receiving 12 Gy in 6 days.[37]

COMBINATION REGIMENS

All combinations that include procarbazine or high doses of other alkylating agents [e.g., mechlorethamine, vinblastine, procarbazine, and prednisone (MOPP); COPP; and chlorambucil, vinblastine, procarbazine, and prednisone (ChlVPP)] induce ovarian failure in almost all older women and even in some younger ones (see Table 55.6-7). Recovery is better when the dose of procarbazine is reduced by using the MOPP/ABVD regimen.[90] Radiation and MOPP chemotherapy clearly have an additive (but not synergistic) effect, and the combination results in a higher incidence of ovarian failure than either modality alone.[70]

Similarly, regimens using high doses of cyclophosphamide, as used in treatment of breast cancer, also produce ovarian failure; however, the age dependence obscures any possible dose dependence.[69,79,91] Lower doses of cyclophosphamide usually given along with antimetabolites and other agents for treatment of leukemia do not destroy primordial follicles nor produce permanent

TABLE 55.6-7. Probability of Ovarian Failure in Postmenarchal Women with Combination Chemotherapy Regimens Containing Alkylating Agents

Regimen	*Disease*	*Courses or Doses*	*Age (y)*	*Incidence of Permanent Ovarian Failure (%)*	*References*
MOPPd or MVPPd	Hodgkin's disease	Approximately 6 courses	25	15	71,88,89
		P approximately 6 g/m²	35	85	
MOPPd/ABVD	Hodgkin's disease	6 courses	25	0	90
		P = 4.2 g/m²			
COPPd	Hodgkin's disease	Cy = 8 g/m²	<24	28	35
		P = 8 g/m²	>24	86	
ChlVPPd/EVA	Hodgkin's disease	6–8 courses	25	0	53
		P = 4 g/m²	36	100	
		Chl = 300 mg/m²			
Cy (alone) + HSCT	Aplastic anemia	Cy = 7.4 g/m²	13–58	50	37,66
BuCy + HSCT	Leukemia	Bu = 600 mg/m²	14–57	99	37
		Cy = 7.4 g/m²			
FAC	Breast cancer	Cy = 13 g/m²	<34	0	91
			>39	100	
CMxF	Breast cancer	Cy = 34 g/m²	<30	0	79
			>35	100	
CAMx	Sarcoma	Cy = 5.3 g/m²	<35	0	54
			>40	100	
A, Cy, Ca, Dn, Mx, Mp, Pd, TG, V	Leukemia	Cy = 2.6 g/m²	14–36	0	58

A, doxorubicin (Adriamycin); B, bleomycin; Bu, busulfan; Ca, cytosine arabinoside; Cb, carboplatin; Chl, chlorambucil; C and Cy, cyclophosphamide; D, dacarbazine; Dn, daunorubicin; E, etoposide; F, 5-fluorouracil; HSCT, hematopoietic stem cell transplant; M, mechlorethamine (nitrogen mustard); Mp, 6-mercaptopurine; Mx, methotrexate; O, vincristine (Oncovin); P, procarbazine; Pd, prednisone; TG, thioguanine; V, vinblastine.

ovarian failure.[35,68] Combination chemotherapy regimens without alkylating agents tend not to produce ovarian failure.

EFFECTS OF CYTOTOXIC AGENTS ON CHILDREN

BIOLOGIC CONSIDERATIONS IN BOYS

In the prepubertal testis, the immature Sertoli cells are the most numerous cells in the seminiferous tubules.[99] They proliferate at an extremely low level in the prepubertal period, only increasing twofold in numbers, but there is a marked increase during puberty. Spermatogonia are the only germ cells present and transform from an appearance of fetal germ cells to that of adult spermatogonia. They proliferate at a low level, increasing sixfold from birth to 10 years. Leydig cells cannot be identified in the interstitial spaces from shortly after birth until puberty. At puberty, new Leydig cells are formed from mesenchymal cells already in the interstitium, involving extensive proliferation of the precursors.[100] The appearance of the Leydig cells elevates secretion of testosterone, which, along with enhanced FSH levels, initiates spermatogenesis at a median age of 13.

EXTENT OF GONADAL TOXICITY IN BOYS

The germinal epithelium in the prepubertal testis does not appear to be any more resistant to cytotoxic therapy than that in the adult. The concept that prepubertal are less sensitive than adult testes[101] derived from comparison of cyclophosphamide doses given on a milligram per kilogram basis and the failure of prepubertal boys to show elevation of FSH after chemotherapy.[102] But when treated patients are followed after puberty by sperm count and hormone evaluation, the sensitivity of the prepubertal testis to a variety of cytotoxic regimens is apparent. Appropriately expressing chemotherapy doses to boys on a milligram per square meter basis and using calculated radiation doses, the sterilizing effects of a variety of chemotherapy regimens[103–107] and radiotherapy[86,108] can be predicted on the basis of the sensitivity of the adult testis (see Tables 55.6-3 and 55.6-4).

As in adults, radiation and alkylating agents, such as procarbazine, cyclophosphamide, and chlorambucil, are the most sterilizing and produce prolonged and sometimes permanent azoospermia. The nitrosoureas (carmustine, lomustine), which are also alkylating agents, and cisplatin likewise produce prolonged germinal aplasia.[39,87] In addition, high doses of doxorubicin and cytosine arabinoside appear to be additive with the preceding agents in producing gonadal damage.[109] In general, regimens lacking alkylating agents, such as some used for acute lymphocytic leukemia, allow pubertal progression of spermatogenesis even during treatment[110] and do not appear to affect postpubertal sperm counts[111] or fertility.[75]

Chemotherapy does not have major effects on Leydig cell function, and hence the timing of pubertal development and postpubertal testosterone levels are generally normal.[112] There is one report that treatment with MOPP chemotherapy during puberty results in gynecomastia[102]; however, other studies indicate that this incidence is not above background levels.[107,113] Preliminary data do indicate, however, that approximately 30% of boys treated with busulfan plus cyclophosphamide show delayed puberty.[66] In contrast, direct testicular irradiation, used in treatment of leukemia or sarcomas, produces dramatic Leydig cell damage. There is significant age dependence, as children are more sensitive than adults[114] and within the prepubertal period, the youngest are most sensitive.[115] The incidence of extremely low testosterone levels and failure to complete puberty rises from 0% at 7.5 Gy,[116] to 0% to 50% at 12 Gy,[66,117] 75% at 24 Gy,[118,119] and 100% at 27 to 30 Gy.[114]

BIOLOGIC CONSIDERATIONS IN GIRLS

Despite the low levels of circulating gonadotropins, the immature ovary is far from quiescent. In addition to primordial follicles, maturing follicles up to and including the large antral stage appear within a few months after birth.[120] After 6 years of age, FSH levels, the numbers and diameters of large antral follicles, and estrogen levels all increase. The lack of gonadotropin support prevents full follicular development or ovulation before menarche.

EXTENT OF GONADAL TOXICITY IN GIRLS

Prepubertal girls appear to be even less susceptible than young postpubertal women to ovarian failure induced by cytotoxic therapy (see Table 55.6-6). Furthermore, girls treated between the ages of 0 and 12 do not appear to experience premature menopause during their 20s and 30s as is the case with those treated at ages 13 to 19.[74] However, additional numbers and longer follow-up are needed.

Radiation is the most damaging agent to the prepubertal ovary. Doses of approximately 20 to 30 Gy induce permanent ovarian failure in nearly all girls.[121,122] Doses of 8 to 15 Gy, given as single doses or in a few fractions, usually with some cyclophosphamide in preparation for bone marrow transplantation, cause permanent ovarian failure and failure of pubertal development in only 50% of girls, with those at younger ages being less sensitive than older ones.[66,115] Fractionated doses of up to 7 Gy cause little failure of ovarian function or pubertal development,[86,123] although there can be additive detrimental effects of chemotherapy.

Most chemotherapy regimens, including high doses of cyclophosphamide up to 48 g,[80] do not cause failure of pubertal development and menarche. Although various combination chemotherapy regimens used for treatment of leukemia and Hodgkin's disease reduce the number of growing follicles, no significant change in numbers of primordial follicles could be measured,[124] and puberty and associated ovarian function develop normally.[112,125] Even with the standard MOPP chemotherapy for Hodgkin's disease, 90% of prepubertal girls develop normally.[86,126] However, regimens with high doses of certain alkylating agents can produce detectable ovarian damage in a significant percentage of prepubertal girls. ChlVPP (30% failure)[127] and carmustine or lomustine (greater than 90% failure)[128] produce transient biochemical evidence of ovarian failure, but there is no evidence that they interfere with pubertal development. In contrast, busulfan plus cyclophosphamide actually inhibits puberty in 50% of girls.[66]

GONADAL DYSFUNCTION AFTER CRANIAL IRRADIATION

Whereas gonadal irradiation causes primary hypogonadism, cranial irradiation is associated with secondary hypogonadism due to damage to the hypothalamus, gonadotrophs in the pituitary, or both. In patients with pituitary or suprasellar lesions, gonadotropin deficiency is often present before antineoplastic therapy; however, patients with nasopharyngeal cancer or brain tumors have normal hypothalamic-pituitary-gonadal axes until they receive therapeutic irradiation with fields encompassing the hypothalamic-pituitary areas. There is no convincing evidence that any of the cytotoxic drugs directly impair hypothalamic and anterior pituitary function.

In children, prophylactic cranial irradiation with 24 Gy for leukemia does not affect LH or FSH pulsatile secretion in the first 6 years.[129] Irradiation of children for cranial tumors with doses of 25 to 55 Gy to the hypothalamic-pituitary region decreased LH and FSH secretion in 11% of cases within 6 years in one study.[130] However, in some cases radiation doses between 18 and 47 Gy, sometimes combined with chemotherapy, may not inactivate the mechanisms necessary for gonadotropin production and secretion, but indirectly stimulate this process before puberty, and hence increase LH and FSH levels and cause precocious puberty.[131,132] Because growth hormone deficiency is common in these patients, precocious puberty further exacerbates the risk of adult shortness.

In adults, decreased LH and FSH secretion, measured after gonadotropin-releasing hormone (GnRH) stimulation, is observed after cranial irradiation. The damage increases with treatment dose[133] and time interval since treatment.[134] LH and FSH deficiency is observed in 33% of patients 5 years after treatment with 20 Gy, but 66% are affected 5 years after 35 to 49 Gy, progressing to 100% by 10 years.[135] This results in oligomenorrhea in women and low testosterone in men; hyperprolactinemia might mediate the observed gonadal dysfunction is some cases.[136,137]

In many patients who receive multimodality treatment, complex hormonal dysregulation may develop; although cranial irradiation, for example, may affect the hypothalamus and pituitary, total body or abdominal irradiation and concomitant chemotherapy may induce primary gonadal failure.

PRESERVATION OF FERTILITY, HORMONE LEVELS, AND SEXUAL FUNCTION

CHOICE OF REGIMENS

It is sometimes possible to choose between nearly equally curative regimens on the basis of their sterilizing potentials. The principle is to minimize the doses of the agents in Tables 55.6-3 and 55.6-6 that are most sterilizing. A classic example is to use ABVD instead of MOPP to treat Hodgkin's disease.[13] In the treatment of non-Hodgkin's lymphoma, regimens that minimize the dose of cyclophosphamide, such as VAPEC-B, produce less gonadal failure in men than does cyclophosphamide, hydroxydaunorubicin (Adriamycin), Oncovin, prednisone, and bleomycin (CHOP-Bleo).[138]

GONADAL SHIELDING

Except when they must be irradiated because of neoplastic involvement or anatomic inclusion within the irradiated target, the gonads are outside or are shielded from the direct radiation beam. Nevertheless, an appreciable radiation dose from the accelerator head, collimator scatter, or internal lateral scatter may reach the gonads. Even at moderately low radiation doses, the possibilities of additive effects from chemotherapy and genetic damage to the sperm make it desirable to further minimize the radiation dose.

Gonadal dose depends on distance from the field edge, field size, and photon energy; it can vary from 0.1% to 10.0% of the prescribed dose within the field.[139] Pelvic radiation fields result in significant doses to the testis. Clamshell type shields[139,140] and beam blocking can reduce testicular doses approximately fivefold to approximately 2 Gy for the inverted Y field used for Hodgkin's disease and approximately 0.5 Gy for the hemipelvic field used for seminoma. When treatment of the hemiscrotum after unilateral orchiectomy for testicular cancer is indicated, a special positioning device to retract the remaining testicle out of the treatment field and provide shielding above the area[141] can reduce the dose to the gonad to 0.6 Gy.[142]

To shield the ovaries, an oophoropexy, in which the ovaries are surgically translocated, usually to the midline behind the uterus, must be performed. That region is then shielded from the direct radiation beam using lead blocks. Some investigators report reductions in cumulative ovarian doses to approximately 4 to 5 Gy during total nodal irradiation[143] and good preservation of fertility in younger women[86] (see Table 55.6-6); however, others report higher doses and poorer recoveries.[97]

MALE GERM CELL CRYOPRESERVATION

Semen cryopreservation is an extremely important procedure for men who want to preserve their fertility potential after cytotoxic treatment for cancer. The significance of notifying the patient of the potential risk of iatrogenic sterility as early as possible cannot be overemphasized. Physicians often are aware early during the diagnostic process that the patient will most likely need to receive potentially sterilizing cytotoxic therapy, although the exact diagnosis, stage, and treatment regimen have not yet been decided. This time should be used to initiate and complete the cryopreservation procedure. The banking of at least three semen samples with at least a 48-hour period of abstinence between samples is recommended. This usually requires 5 to 8 days to complete. Additional samples (four) and longer abstinence periods (72 hours) to achieve higher total sperm counts may be considered. But fewer samples with shorter times are often obtained because of the need to initiate anticancer therapy quickly, and it is important to avoid possible increased genetic damage in sperm collected after the start of therapy.[7] It is even possible to obtain semen with normal characteristics from 14- to 17-year-old boys.[144] In boys unable to obtain samples by masturbation, penile vibratory stimulation or electroejaculation have been used.[145]

Because of the low overall success rate with artificial insemination using banked semen in the past, it had been recommended that only samples with high sperm counts and motilities be stored. Currently, the success of *in vitro* fertilization (IVF) and intracytoplasmic sperm injection (ICSI) make cryopreservation of all samples containing any live sperm appropriate. The cost of sperm banking three samples, including analysis and storage for 5 years, is approximately $1200 at a university medical school clinic, although it may be higher at private sperm banks. The patient should be made aware that conception rates are only 30% with interuterine insemination (cost per cycle, approximately $250). If the sperm count or motility are significantly impaired, more complicated assisted reproductive technologies may be necessary. The average cost of IVF without ICSI, including the drugs used, is $10,000 per cycle and with ICSI it is approximately an additional $1200 per cycle.

The transplantation of a population of testicular cells, including stem spermatogonia from a donor mouse to a recipient mouse, in which endogenous stem spermatogonia were killed with busulfan, restored spermatogenesis and fertility.[146] Restoration of spermatogenesis is also possible with cryopreserved cells.[147] This suggests the possibility that testicular tissue may be harvested from men before sterilizing cytotoxic therapy and cryopreserved as a cell suspension, for later injection back into the testis after the completion of chemotherapy. Currently, a trial is underway at the Christie Hospital, Manchester, England.[148] This technique would be most valuable for boys, who may be too young to produce sperm, especially because the prepubertal testis is enriched in spermatogonia.[146]

FEMALE GERM CELL CRYOPRESERVATION

Freezing oocytes, unlike sperm, is currently still experimental. There have been offspring born using frozen human oocytes in IVF procedures[149]; however, the success rate is low. In addition, currently used procedures for freezing human and animal oocytes may increase chromosomal aberrations.[150] Furthermore, obtaining mature oocytes is limited to patients in whom there are no contraindications to hormone-induced superovulation. It is also possible to freeze embryos obtained by IVF or by uterine lavage after natural coitus,[151] but these methods are rarely practical with cancer patients, especially when cytotoxic therapy must be initiated without much delay.

Another alternative under active investigation is the surgical removal of ovarian tissue, cryopreservation of tissue slices, and grafting back to the remaining vessels after chemotherapy. This procedure restored ovarian endocrine function and fertility in sheep.[152] Follicular development has been observed in human ovarian tissue implanted into immunodeficient mice.[153] Restoration of hormone production and follicular growth after transplantation of cryopreserved ovarian tissue has been reported,[154] but the true long-term success of this technique remains to be determined.[148] One limitation is the concern that the technique may reintroduce malignant cells to patients in remission.[155] Isolating a follicle from the thawed tissue and maturing an oocyte *in vitro* would be a preferable option, but at present the technique has only been developed in the mouse.

ASSISTED REPRODUCTIVE TECHNOLOGIES

Assisted reproductive technologies have and still are undergoing rapid advances, providing new options for survivors of cancer with gonadal damage to achieve fertility.[156] Previously, intrauterine artificial insemination, often using controlled ovarian hyperstimulation, had been the only method available. Only approximately 30% of women whose partners were cancer patients were able to achieve pregnancy,[157] because of the limited number of samples, poor semen quality in some patients, and loss of motility during freezing and thawing.

Currently, IVF, and especially IVF with ICSI, either as the primary modality or after unsuccessful attempts with artificial insemination, are important in achieving pregnancies from stored semen after the completion of cytotoxic therapy. In IVF, only approximately 100,000 motile sperm are placed in a small droplet of medium with an oocyte, and fertilization is allowed to occur. In ICSI, one spermatozoon is selected with a micropipette and microinjected into the cytoplasm of an oocyte.[158] In both procedures, the oocytes are examined for fertilization and embryo cleavage, and multiple embryos are reimplanted into the uterine cavity. Multiple oocytes can be fertilized in a single IVF cycle, and the embryos that are not transferred can be frozen for implantation at a later time. IVF, however, requires hormonal induction of multiple ovulations, and the implantation of several embryos increases the risks of fetal loss and multiple births.

Because freezing and thawing may result in complete loss of sperm motility, IVF may not be possible in some cases, but IVF with ICSI can still be used.[158] ICSI can be performed with semen samples with 0% motility as long as the sperm are viable.[158] It is possible to select sperm for injection from individuals with exceptionally low counts (e.g., 100 per ejaculate) and even from the testis (testicular sperm extraction).[159,160]

If the number and quality of the sperm meet standards set by a given clinic, IVF alone is used. However if the standards are not met or if IVF has failed, IVF with ICSI is then used. With ICSI, the fertilization rate is 50% to 60%. The success rate of IVF or IVF is ICSI is 22% per initiated cycle and 26% per completed cycle.[161] When multiple cycles are used, these procedures offer couples a success rate of 80% to 100% for achieving a pregnancy.[157,162]

There appear to be no increases in congenital malformations in the offspring from IVF or ICSI; however, there is a small increase in the incidence of chromosomal abnormalities, mostly in the numbers of sex chromosomes.[163] Some of the chromosome abnormalities observed after the use of ICSI for primary male infertility are not caused by ICSI but are already in the spermatozoa of the infertile patient[164]; the latter should not be a factor in cryopreserved sperm from cancer patients.

HORMONAL METHODS OF PRESERVING FERTILITY

Although hormone treatments have been used to enhance the survival of germ cells and their ability to recover after cytotoxic treatments, there currently are no reliable methods for hormonal protection of gonadal function in humans.

Pretreatment of male rats with gonadal steroids,[165] GnRH analogues,[166] or GnRH analogues combined with antiandrogens,[167] all of which suppress gonadotropin and testosterone levels and action, enhance recovery of spermatogenesis and fertility after procarbazine, irradiation, or cyclophosphamide. The original proposal that these treatments protect the spermatogonia from killing by suppressing their proliferation[168] is incorrect, as the protective hormone treatments neither suppress spermatogonial proliferation[169] nor enhance stem spermatogonial survival.[170] Rather, the hormones appear to act via suppression of testosterone levels to protect the subsequent ability of the somatic cells of the testis to support the recovery of spermatogenesis from surviving stem spermatogonia. In rats, stem spermatogonia survive some cytotoxic therapies but are unable to differentiate,[171,172] and hormone treatment, even given after the cytotoxic treatment, can stimulate recovery of spermatogenesis.[171] The presence of stem spermatogonia in testes of cancer patients during prolonged periods of iatrogenic azoospermia suggests that this procedure may be applicable to humans as well. Only one out of eight clinical trials has been able to demonstrate protection of spermatogenesis in humans by hormone treatment before and during cytotoxic therapy.[173–175] The failures may, in part, be attributed to the administration, along with the GnRH agonist (GnRH-Ag), of testosterone, which has been shown in the rat to reduce the recovery of spermatogenesis. The continuation of testosterone-suppressive treatment after completion of cytotoxic therapy, which was successful in the rat,[176] has not been tested in humans.

In the female rat, there is one convincing study showing protection of ovarian function. The number of developing follicles several months after cyclophosphamide treatment was enhanced when GnRH-Ag had been given along with cyclophosphamide.[177] It is not apparent how GnRH-Ag worked as recruitment of primordial follicles is gonadotropin independent. However, GnRH-Ag also inhibits the normal physiologic loss of primordial follicles by recruitment and atresia.[178] Thus, GnRH-Ag treatment for several months might prolong fertility in rodents because it could be given for an appreciable fraction of their reproductive lifetime, but if this were the mechanism, it would not have a significant effect in women, who have a 40-year interval from menarche to menopause. Clinical studies attempting to protect ovarian function in women with GnRH-Ag[179,180] or oral contraceptives[181,182] during treatment for Hodgkin's disease have yielded contradictory results.

Despite clinical symptoms of ovarian failure, there may be some residual ovarian function remaining after chemotherapy; the possibility is less likely after gonadal radiation.[77] It is possible to stimulate ovulation and fertility after apparent chemotherapy-induced ovarian failure, at least for a short time, with a brief course of gonadotropin treatment[183] or with steroid hormone replacement therapy.[85]

OPTIMIZATION OF FERTILITY AFTER TREATMENT

Men whose sperm count recovers after cancer therapy usually achieve normospermic levels, but some remain oligospermic for extended periods. Although controlled studies have not been done, these men appear to have normal fertility based on their sperm count, and the incidence of infertility in these patients does not appear to be any higher than the 15% rate among couples in the general population. In contrast, cancer patients with recovered sperm counts ranging from below 1 to 10 million/mL, levels associated with subfertility when they occur in the general population, are able to successfully father children.[14,43,51] In cases of infertility with oligospermic counts, management of the patient should be the same as in those from a normal population with male factor infertility. Of the various procedures, IVF and IVF with ICSI appear to offer the most promise.[184]

In most women who continue to have menstrual function after cytotoxic therapy for cancer, infertility should generally be treated as in a normal population. The one major exception is those who received high doses of abdominal radiation (10 to 16 Gy for hematopoietic stem cell transplantation and more than 20 Gy for Wilms' tumor), particularly in childhood. These patients have increased rates of adverse pregnancy outcomes, including fetal or neonatal deaths, premature deliveries, low-birth-weight babies, and neonatal deaths, and hence these pregnancies must be closely monitored.[37,185]

HORMONE REPLACEMENT THERAPY

It is important to test for ovarian failure and to start hormone replacement therapy rapidly because, in some cases, a 2- to 3-year delay in administering estrogen replacement therapy may result in an irreversible loss of bone mass and increased risk of osteoporosis.[76] In addition, estrogen deficiency places women at increased risk for morbidity and mortality from cardiovascular disease and causes sexual dysfunction.[186] Estrogen replacement can be provided orally, transdermally, or by injection.[187] If a patient has an intact uterus, estrogen should generally be combined with progesterone to prevent endometrial hyperplasia and cancer.[188]

In male subjects, germinal aplasia is often associated with testosterone levels in the low to normal range, and they may experience reduced bone mineral density.[16] Some of these men with reduced libido after chemotherapy report improvement after testosterone treatment.[53] Testosterone replacement is important in cases of overt Leydig cell failure in prepubertal boys to promote secondary sexual characteristics, growth, and bone density. It can be provided transdermally or by injection[188]; the use of oral anabolic preparations should be discouraged.

MODIFIED NERVE-SPARING SURGERY

Ejaculation of semen involves emission, by which semen is deposited in the posterior urethra by contractions of the vas deferens, seminal vesicles, and prostate, and antegrade ejaculation, which requires coordinated tightening of the bladder neck, relaxation of the external sphincter, and expulsion of semen. Most of these processes are controlled by nerve fibers that arise from the lumbar ganglia at L1 to L4 and then course anteriorly over the aorta and coalesce into multiple trunks, forming the hypogastric plexus overlying the aorta and sacrum below the origin of the inferior mesenteric artery.[24]

Surgery in the treatment of testicular, prostate, and bladder cancer can produce neurologic dysfunction resulting in failure of emission, retrograde ejaculation, impotence, and loss of orgasm. However, improvements in surgical techniques have reduced these adverse outcomes without diminishing the efficacy of treating the cancer.

RPLND has an important role in the treatment of nonseminomatous testicular germ cell tumors. Procedures for radical RPLND that were standard before 1972 almost always produced failures of emission and ejaculation. Based on the location of positive nodes, a modified template of dissection (unilateral dissection below the inferior mesenteric artery), which avoids disturbance of the lumbar sympathetic fibers, particularly at the hypogastric plexus, was developed,[24] preserving ejaculation of semen in 50% to 85% of men. The RPLND technique has been further refined by identifying the postganglionic fibers and retracting them from the lymph nodes over and around the aorta, which are then dissected out and removed in multiple small packages, sparing the nerve fibers,[189] preserving ejaculation of semen in 89% of men.[190]

Improved surgical techniques also preserve sexual function in many men undergoing surgery for prostate and bladder cancer.[191] By avoiding damage to the nerve fibers that are located in neurovascular bundles that innervate the penile corpora cavernosa, sexual function, including the ability to have an erection sufficient for vaginal penetration and orgasm, is maintained in 70% to 80% of men undergoing radical prostatectomy for localized prostate cancer or radical cystoprostatectomy for invasive bladder cancer. In addition, a promising technique for those patients who do require nerve excision with the prostate is that of bilateral sural nerve grafts.[192] It is too early to quantify the true effectiveness of this technique, but the results are encouraging.

MANAGEMENT OF RETROGRADE EJACULATION

In patients with ejaculatory dysfunction after RPLND, sympathomimetic agents may enhance seminal emission and partially or completely convert the patient to antegrade ejaculation.[26] Drugs, such as pseudoephedrine HCl, ephedrine sulfate, phenylpropanolamine HCl, or imipramine HCl, should be given sequentially as 2-week trials until improvements in semen volume and sperm count are observed. Pregnancies have been reported but, in general, medical therapy must be combined with some additional techniques to use sperm from retrograde ejaculation.

When retrograde ejaculation is present, sperm may be recovered from the bladder by direct voiding or by catheterization with irrigation.[193] For greater sperm survival, it is important to ensure a dilute, slightly alkaline urine and then to dilute the voided semen-urine mixture with buffering media to reduce harmful urine components.

When medical treatment is not successful at producing emission and ejaculation, electroejaculation has been successful in more than 70% of patients.[194] After administration of general anesthesia, a rectal probe is used to electrically stimulate sympathetic efferent fibers and smooth muscle. Although most patients have some antegrade ejaculate, catheterization should always be done to collect the retrograde semen. Sperm motility tends to be low after electroejaculation, and the fecundity per cycle is at most 9% using artificial insemination. IVF with ICSI is now being used to enhance pregnancy rates.[184]

GENETIC CONCERNS

BIOLOGIC CONSIDERATIONS

Many anticancer agents damage DNA and interfere with DNA replication, DNA repair, and chromosome segregation in both animal and human cells. They induce mutations in germ cells of animals that cause genetic disease.[195] Because the studies that have been or can be done in humans are limited, risk estimates are derived from the induction of single-gene mutations and chromosomal aberrations, both of which contribute significantly to human genetic disease in the mouse.[196]

Radiation, procarbazine, melphalan, and mitomycin C produce single-gene mutations in murine spermatogonia, whereas seven other tested chemotherapeutic drugs do not.[195,197] Risk can be estimated by using the doubling dose (i.e., dose to produce twice the background rate of mutation) from the mouse and the incidence of clinically significant dominant genetic traits in human liveborn due to new mutations.[196] Doubling doses for single-gene mutations in mouse spermatogonial mutations are 1 Gy for subchronic radiation and 0.4 g/m^2 for procarbazine.[198] At the mouse doubling dose, the incidence of dominant mutations in humans should be increased by 0.2%; however, data from offspring of atomic bomb survivors indicate that estimates based on the mouse may overestimate the human genetic risk.[199]

Radiation is the only agent that effectively induces stable reciprocal chromosomal translocations in stem spermatogonia that can be visualized in spermatocytes or in offspring.[196] Although the mouse data indicate that a fractionated dose of 1 Gy would induce translocations in 0.06% of the offspring, the induction of translocations in human germ cells appears to be higher than in the mouse.[200]

In male rodents, meiotic and postmeiotic germ cells are more sensitive to induction and transmission of mutations than are stem spermatogonia.[7] Therefore, mutational risks are highest when a pregnancy occurs within one spermatogenic cycle (time for stem cell to become sperm) after the man is exposed to the damaging agent. In men, this higher risk period extends from the start of cytotoxic therapy until 3 months after the last course. (In practice, waiting 6 months after therapy to effect a pregnancy is recommended for safety.) After this time, the incidence of mutations is at the lower level found in sperm that were exposed to the mutagen as stem cells, which determines the genetic risk for the remainder of the reproductive lifetime.

Fewer studies of the mutagenicity of cytotoxic agents have been done in the female subject. Single-gene and chromosomal mutations are induced by radiation in the developing oocytes of female mice at a similar rate as in stem spermatogonia.[196] Procarbazine induces a similar level of specific-locus mutations in primordial oocytes as in stem spermatogonia.[201] Most alkylating agents and a variety of other drugs induce chromosome aberrations or mutations in oocytes in growing follicles, resulting in embryonic death.[195,197] Although there are insufficient data to determine whether growing oocytes are more sensitive to induction of mutations than primordial oocytes, it is still prudent for a woman to wait at least 3 months after cytotoxic treatment before conceiving.

These animal studies show that there are theoretical genetic risks to the offspring of treated patients of both sexes. Calculations predict that the incidence of congenital abnormalities would be increased by less than 2%, even at the highest doses of cytotoxic therapies and, hence, large-scale controlled studies will be required to measure effects in human populations.

GAMETE GENOMIC ANALYSIS

Because epidemiologic studies of genetic damage in humans require large numbers of offspring, direct analysis of the genetic material of gametes has potential advantages for identifying mutations in human germ cells. Such analyses are practical only in the male subject because harvest of female gametes is impractical. Several assays have been developed and new methods are under investigation (Table 55.6-8).

Sperm karyotyping has demonstrated the persistence of structural and numeric chromosomal abnormalities several years after radiation or chemotherapy.[204,207] Currently, the more efficient technique of fluorescence *in situ* hybridization of sperm is being used to measure the rates of aneuploidy and chromosome breakage. There was a significant sixfold increase in aneuploidy[208] and chromosome structural aberrations[209] during mitoxantrone, vincristine, vinblastine, and prednisone (NOVP) chemotherapy, demonstrating that there are genetic risks if conception or storage of sperm occurs during cytotoxic therapy. Fluorescence *in situ* hybridization failed to show any significant persistence of the increase in aneuploidy 6 months after the completion of NOVP or cisplatin, etoposide, and bleomycin (PEB) chemotherapy,[205,210] but increases after MOPP chemotherapy did persist.[209]

Minisatellite repeat number mutations in human spermatozoa[202] could also be a useful marker for detecting mutations. Minisatellite mutations were increased in offspring of men

TABLE 55.6-8. Mutational End Points Used in Human Germ Cells

Mutation/Method	*Description*
Single locus	
Analysis of DNA sequences in offspring and gametes	Southern blot analysis of polymerase chain reaction–amplified, highly mutable minisatellite sequences from small pools of individual sperm[202]
Chromosomal abnormality	
Chromosome aberrations at meiosis	Reciprocal translocations in spermatocytes obtained by testicular biopsy[203]
Sperm karyotype	Interspecific fusion of sperm with hamster oocytes followed by cytogenetic analysis at first cleavage metaphase[204]
Fluorescence *in situ* hybridization of sperm	Centromeric probes for chromosome number and multiple probes per chromosome for structural aberrations[205,206]

exposed to radioactive fallout from Chernobyl.[211] However, studies so far have not detected any significant induction of these mutations by radiotherapy or chemotherapy for cancer.[212]

PREGNANCY OUTCOME

Nearly all of the case reports, small series, and a few large retrospective case studies of the outcomes of pregnancies in, or produced by, survivors of cancer indicated no significant increase in birth defects or genetic disease, above the background in the general population of approximately 4%, in offspring conceived after cytotoxic treatment.[213] The results from the atomic bomb studies in Japan also show no significant increase in genetic damage in 30,000 offspring born to radiation-exposed parents.[199] These observations should reassure those who wish to have children after treatment for cancer. However, they do not rule out the possibility of a small genetic risk.

The largest published studies involved patients who were children or adolescents at the time of treatment.[214,215] A total of 630 offspring from patients receiving potentially mutagenic therapy (radiation proximal to the gonads or alkylating agents) showed no significant increases in birth defects or other genetic diseases. A study of incidence of cancer in offspring of patients treated with potentially mutagenic therapies also found no increase above control populations in the induction of cancer (excluding highly heritable cancers).[216] There was, however, a fourfold increase in adverse reproductive outcomes observed in women who received more than 20 Gy abdominal radiation in childhood, primarily for Wilms' tumor.[185] The cause of this increase appears not to be genetic but rather irreversible radiation damage to the uterine musculature and blood flow.[217]

The largest study of offspring from adults treated with cytotoxic therapies involved 368 conceptions in women treated with methotrexate alone or in combination for choriocarcinoma or invasive mole; there were no significant increases in miscarriages, stillbirths, neonatal deaths, or congenital abnormalities.[218] In male subjects, a study of 70 offspring from testicular cancer patients treated with radiotherapy, chemotherapy, or both revealed no apparent increase in congenital malformations; the power of the study was sufficient to rule out an increase greater than threefold.[219] In a large case-control study (parents of children with a congenital anomaly versus parents of normal children), the relative risk that treatment with mutagenic therapy would cause congenital abnormalities was close to 1, and the upper confidence limits were approximately 2.[220]

The lack of observable increases in birth defects or genetic diseases in nearly all studies makes it highly probable that there is less than a twofold increase in genetic risk after radiotherapy or chemotherapy of both adults and children. However, larger studies will be required to determine whether that limit can be further reduced, and further research is needed to evaluate new chemotherapeutic agents.

There are limited reports of outcomes of pregnancies in which conception occurred while the father was undergoing cytotoxic therapy. No significant increases in untoward pregnancy outcomes or birth defects were reported in a review of nine conceptions.[221] However, one child with trisomy was conceived shortly after the completion of therapy,[222] and this aneuploidy might be attributable to mutagenesis in maturing germ cells. If conception does occur during these times, the couple should be informed of the risks, which may only be moderate, to evaluate the continuation of the pregnancy.

The teratogenic risk from cytotoxic therapy delivered to a woman during pregnancy can be much higher than mutagenic risk from prior exposure. The decisions of whether to initiate, continue, modify, or withhold therapy and whether to continue or terminate the pregnancy are extremely complex.[1] There are documented risks from fetal radiation doses as low as 0.2 Gy in the first trimester and from somewhat higher doses in the second trimester.[223] All of the cytotoxic chemotherapeutic agents are classified as teratogens[224]; however, some may be given in the second and third trimester of pregnancy. Treatment with fluorouracil, doxorubicin, and cyclophosphamide during this period did not result in any pregnancy complications, congenital abnormalities, or immediate postpartum deficits; methotrexate was deliberately excluded from the combination.[2]

COUNSELING

Cancer patients should be informed by their physician about the possibilities of sterility and genetic risk from the disease and treatment (Table 55.6-9). They should also be told about psychological and physical effects on sexual desire, erectile function, and the ability to achieve orgasm.

During treatment, sexual relations between partners may continue, but reliable contraception should be used. The genetic and teratogenic risk of conception when either partner is undergoing treatment should be outlined. In addition, the seminal transmission of chemotherapeutic drugs should be mentioned, and the use of condoms when sexual intercourse occurs within 24 hours of administration of a chemotherapeutic agent to the man should be recommended.

TABLE 55.6-9. Guidelines for Reproductive and Genetic Counseling of Couples Seeking Pregnancy after Cancer Diagnosis and Treatment

Discuss risk of infertility after cancer treatment, the option of sperm banking, and the possibility of healthy children if fertility is preserved.
Explain options for gamete or embryo cryopreservation.
Inquire about family history of cancer.
Strongly encourage birth control during cancer treatment up to 6 months after the end of treatment; becoming pregnant or producing a pregnancy is contraindicated.
Discuss theoretical concerns about mutational damage.
Discuss the limited data for humans regarding congenital malformations and genetic disease, which indicate no measurable excess above the background level 4% risk for any pregnancy.
Recommend that any pregnancy after therapy should be monitored with ultrasound and amniocentesis offered because of the theoretically increased genetic risk.

The probability that sterility will result from the planned cytotoxic therapy should be calculated from the cumulative doses of agents and combinations that cause prolonged azoospermia (see Tables 55.6-3 and 55.6-4) and ovarian failure (see Tables 55.6-6 and 55.6-7). This risk should be communicated to the patient.

Pretreatment sperm banking should be offered to all male patients interested in having children after the completion of cytotoxic therapy. The risks of sterility from a given treatment and the probability that more aggressive, highly sterilizing treatment may be needed before there is another opportunity for semen storage should be considered in making the decision on sperm banking. The costs of semen cryopreservation and other assisted reproductive technologies should be presented, and the patient should be reminded that these are not standard benefits in the majority of health insurance programs in the United States.

Female patients should be told that the use of cryopreserved ovarian tissue is experimental at this time. If therapy can be delayed for several months and the woman has a partner, embryo cryopreservation may be possible. Women should also be told about the risks of chemotherapy-induced premature menopause. If this does occur, it is important to present a balanced discussion of potential benefits of prompt initiation of hormone replacement therapy versus the risk (e.g., possibly endometrial and breast cancers) so that an individually appropriate decision may be reached.

REFERENCES

1. Allen HH, Nisker JA, eds. *Cancer in pregnancy.* Mt. Kisco, NY: Futura, 1986.
2. Berry DL, Theriault RL, Holmes FA, et al. Management of breast cancer during pregnancy using a standardized protocol. *J Clin Oncol* 1999;17:855.
3. Ries LA, Hankey BF, Edwards BK. *Cancer statistics review, 1973–1987.* Bethesda, MD: U.S. Department of Health and Human Services, 1991.
4. Landis SH, Murray T, Bolden S, Wingo PA. Cancer statistics, 1999. *CA Cancer J Clin* 1999;49:8.
5. Bleyer WA. Impact of childhood cancer on the United States and the world. *CA Cancer J Clin* 1990;40:355.
6. Meistrich ML. Relationship between spermatogonial stem cell survival and testis function after cytotoxic therapy. *Br J Cancer* 1986;53(Suppl VII):89.
7. Meistrich ML. Potential genetic risks of using semen collected during chemotherapy. *Hum Reprod* 1993;8:8.
8. Kangasniemi M, Huhtaniemi I, Meistrich ML. Failure of spermatogenesis to recover despite the presence of A spermatogonia in the irradiated $LBNF_1$ rat. *Biol Reprod* 1996;54:1200.
9. Clifton DK, Bremner WJ. The effect of testicular X-irradiation on spermatogenesis in man. A comparison with the mouse. *J Androl* 1983;4:387.
10. Wang J, Galil KAA, Setchell BP. Changes in testicular blood flow and testosterone production during aspermatogenesis after irradiation. *J Endocrinol* 1983;98:35.
11. Chapman RM, Sutcliffe SB, Malpas JS. Male gonadal dysfunction in Hodgkin's disease. A prospective study. *JAMA* 1981;245:1323.
12. Meistrich ML, Wilson G, Brown BW, da Cunha MF, Lipshultz LI. Impact of cyclophosphamide on long-term reduction in sperm count in men treated with combination chemotherapy for Ewing's and soft tissue sarcomas. *Cancer* 1992;70:2703.
13. Viviani S, Santoro A, Ragni G, et al. Gonadal toxicity after combination chemotherapy for Hodgkin's disease. Comparative results of MOPP vs ABVD. *Eur J Cancer Clin Onc* 1985;21:601.
14. Marmor D, Duyck F. Male reproductive potential after MOPP therapy for Hodgkin's disease: a long-term survey. *Andrologia* 1995;27:99.
15. Kinsella TJ, Trivette G, Rowland J, et al. Long-term follow-up of testicular function following radiation therapy for early-stage Hodgkin's disease. *J Clin Oncol* 1989;7:718.
16. Holmes SJ, Whitehouse RW, Clark ST, et al. Reduced bone mineral density in men following chemotherapy for Hodgkin's disease. *Br J Cancer* 1994;70:371.
17. Shalet SM. Effect of irradiation treatment on gonadal function in men treated for germ cell cancer. *Eur Urol* 1993;23:148.
18. Pryzant RM, Meistrich ML, Wilson E, Brown B, McLaughlin P. Long-term reduction in sperm count after chemotherapy with and without radiation therapy for non-Hodgkin's lymphomas. *J Clin Oncol* 1993;11:239.
19. Marmor D, Grob-Menendez F, Duyck F, Delafontaine D. Very late return of spermatogenesis after chlorambucil therapy: case reports. *Fertil Steril* 1992;58:845.
20. Meistrich ML, Chawla SP, da Cunha MF, et al. Recovery of sperm production after chemotherapy for osteosarcoma. *Cancer* 1989;63:2115.
21. Lampe H, Horwich A, Norman A, Nicholls J, Dearnaley DP. Fertility after chemotherapy for testicular germ cell cancers. *J Clin Oncol* 1997;15:239.
22. Pont J, Albrecht W. Fertility after chemotherapy for testicular germ cell cancer. *Fertil Steril* 1997;68:1.
23. Lipshultz LI, Ross CE, Whorton D, et al. Dibromochloropropane and its effect on testicular function in man. *J Urol* 1980;124:464.
24. Lange PH, Narayan P, Fraley EE. Fertility issues following therapy for testicular cancer. *Semin Urol* 1984;11:264.
25. Morrish DW, Venner PM, Siy O, et al. Mechanisms of endocrine dysfunction in patients with testicular cancer. *J Natl Cancer Inst* 1990;82:412.
26. Narayan P, Lange PH, Fraley EE. Ejaculation and fertility after extended retriperitoneal lymph node dissection for testicular cancer. *J Urol* 1982;127:685.
27. Redman JR, Bajorunas DR, Goldstein MC, Evenson DP. Semen cryopreservation and artificial insemination for Hodgkin's disease. *J Clin Oncol* 1987;5:233.
28. Viviani S, Ragni G, Santoro A, et al. Testicular dysfunction in Hodgkin's disease before and after treatment. *Eur J Cancer* 1991;27:1389.
29. Shamberger RC, Sherins RJ, Rosenberg SA. The effects of postoperative adjuvant chemotherapy and radiotherapy on testicular function in men undergoing treatment for soft tissue sarcoma. *Cancer* 1981;47:2368.
30. Hansen PV, Trykker H, Svennakjaer IL, Hvolby J. Long-term recovery of spermatogenesis after radiotherapy in patients with testicular cancer. *Radiother Oncol* 1990;18:117.
31. Drasga RE, Einhorn LH, Williams SD, Patel DN, Stevens EE. Fertility after chemotherapy for testicular cancer. *J Clin Oncol* 1983;1:179.
32. Marina S, Barcelo P. Permanent sterility after immunosuppressive therapy. *Int J Androl* 1979;2:6.
33. Buchanan JD, Fairley KF, Barrie JV. Return of spermatogenesis after stopping cyclophosphamide therapy. *Lancet* 1975;2:156.
34. da Cunha MF, Meistrich ML, Fuller LM, et al. Recovery of spermatogenesis after treatment for Hodgkin's disease: limiting dose of MOPP chemotherapy. *J Clin Oncol* 1984;2:571.
35. Kreuser ED, Xiros N, Hetzel WD, Heimpel H. Reproductive and endocrine gonadal capacity in patients treated with COPP chemotherapy for Hodgkin's disease. *J Cancer Res Clin Oncol* 1987;113:260.
36. Hansen PV, Trykker H, Helkjaer PE, Andersen J. Testicular function in patients with testicular cancer treated with orchiectomy alone or orchiectomy plus cisplatin-based chemotherapy. *J Natl Cancer Inst* 1989;81:1246.
37. Sanders JE, Hawley J, Levy W, et al. Pregnancies following high-dose cyclophosphamide with or without high-dose busulfan or total-body irradiation and bone marrow transplantation. *Blood* 1996;87:3045.
38. Brennemann W, Stoffel-Wagner B, Helmers A, et al. Gonadal function of patients treated with cisplatin based chemotherapy for germ cell cancer. *J Urol* 1997;158:844.
39. Ahmed SR, Shalet SM, Campbell RHA, Deakin DP. Primary gonadal damage following treatment of brain tumors in childhood. *J Pediatr* 1983;103:562.
40. Vassilopoulou-Sellin R. Endocrine effects of cytokines. *Oncology* 1994;8:43.
41. Schilsky RL, Davidson HS, Magid D, Daiter S, Golomb HM. Gonadal and sexual function in male patients with hairy cell leukemia: lack of adverse effects of recombinant α2-interferon treatment. *Cancer Treat Rep* 1987;71:179.
42. Meistrich ML, van Beek MEAB. Radiation sensitivity of the human testis. In: Lett JR, Altman KI, eds. *Advances in radiation biology.* New York: Academic Press, 1990:227.
43. Sandeman TF. The effects of X irradiation on male human fertility. *Br J Radiol* 1966;39:901.
44. Gordon W, Siegmund K, Stanisic TH, et al. A study of reproductive function in patients with seminoma treated with radiotherapy and orchidectomy: (SWOG-8711). *Int J Radiat Oncol Biol Phys* 1997;38:83.
45. Schlappack OK, Kratzik C, Schmidt W, Spona J, Schuster E. Response of the seminiferous epithelium to scattered radiation in seminoma patients. *Cancer* 1988;62:1487.
46. Centola GM, Keller JW, Henzler M, Rubin P. Effect of low-dose testicular irradiation on sperm count and fertility in patients with testicular seminoma. *J Androl* 1994;15:608.

47. Jacob A, Barker H, Goodman A, Holmes J. Recovery of spermatogenesis following bone marrow transplantation. *Bone Marrow Transplant* 1998;22:277.
48. Giwercman A, von der Maase H, Berthelsen JG, et al. Localized irradiation of testes with carcinoma *in situ:* effects on Leydig cell function and eradication of malignant germ cells in 20 patients. *J Clin Endocrinol Metab* 1991;73:596.
49. Zagars GK, Pollack A. Serum testosterone levels after external beam radiation for clinically localized prostate cancer. *Int J Radiat Oncol Biol Phys* 1997;39:85.
50. Goldstein I, Feldman MI, Deckers PJ, Babayan RK, Krane RJ. Radiation-associated impotence. A clinical study of its mechanism. *JAMA* 1984;251:903.
51. Chapman RM, Sutcliffe SB, Rees LH, Edwards CRW, Malpas JS. Cyclical combination chemotherapy and gonadal function. A retrospective study in males. *Lancet* 1979;1:285.
52. Kulkarni SS, Sastry PS, Saikia TK, et al. Gonadal function following ABVD therapy for Hodgkin's disease. *Am J Clin Oncol* 1997;20:354.
53. Clark ST, Radford JA, Crowther D, Swindell R, Shalet SM. A comparative study of MVPP and a seven-drug hybrid regimen. *J Clin Oncol* 1995;13:134.
54. Shamberger RC, Sherins RJ, Ziegler JL, Glatstein E, Rosenberg SA. Effects of postoperative adjuvant chemotherapy and radiotherapy on ovarian function in women undergoing treatment for soft tissue sarcoma. *J Natl Cancer Inst* 1981;67:1213.
55. Fossa SD, Klepp O, Norman N. Lack of gonadal protection by medroxyprogesterone acetate-induced transient medical castration during chemotherapy for testicular cancer. *Br J Urol* 1988;62:449.
56. Meistrich ML, Wilson G, Mathur K, et al. Rapid recovery of spermatogenesis after mitoxantrone, vincristine, vinblastine, and prednisone chemotherapy for Hodgkin's disease. *J Clin Oncol* 1997;15:3488.
57. Evenson DP, Arlin Z, Welt S, Claps ML, Melamed MR. Male reproductive capacity may recover following drug treatment with the L-10 protocol for acute lymphocytic leukemia. *Cancer* 1984;53:30.
58. Kreuser ED, Hetzel WD, Heit W, et al. Reproductive and endocrine gonadal functions in adults following multidrug chemotherapy for acute lymphoblastic or undifferentiated leukemia. *J Clin Oncol* 1988;6:588.
59. Stephenson WT, Poirier SM, Rubin L, Einhorn LH. Evaluation of reproductive capacity in germ cell tumor patients following treatment with cisplatin, etoposide, and bleomycin. *J Clin Oncol* 1995;13:2278.
60. Dubey P, Wilson G, Mathur KK, et al. Recovery of sperm production following radiation therapy for Hodgkin's disease after induction chemotherapy with mitoxantrone, vincristine, vinblastine and prednisone (NOVP). *Int J Radiat Oncol Biol Phys* 2000;46:609.
61. Greenwald GS, Roy SK. Follicular development and its control. In: Knobil E, Neill JD, eds. *The physiology of reproduction.* 2nd ed. New York: Raven Press, 1994:629.
62. Dobson RL, Felton JS. Female germ cell loss from radiation and chemical exposures. *Am J Ind Med* 1983;4:175.
63. Plowchalk DR, Mattison DR. Reproductive toxicity of cyclophosphamide in the C57BL/6N mouse: 1. Effects on ovarian structure and function. *Reprod Toxicol* 1991;6:411.
64. Jarrell J, YoungLai EV, Barr R, et al. Ovarian toxicity of cyclosphosphamide alone and in combination with ovarian irradiation in the rat. *Cancer Res* 1987;47:2340.
65. Bines J, Oleske DM, Cobleigh MA. Ovarian function in premenopausal women treated with adjuvant chemotherapy for breast cancer. *J Clin Oncol* 1996;14:1718.
66. Sanders JE. Growth and development after hematopoietic cell transplantation. In: Thomas ED, Blume KG, Forman SJ, eds. *Hematopoietic cell transplantation.* 2nd ed. Malden, MA: Blackwell, 1999:764.
67. Speroff L, Glass RH, Kase NG. Amenorrhea. In: Speroff L, Glass RH, Kase NG, eds. *Clinical gynecologic, endocrinology, and infertility.* Baltimore: Williams & Wilkins, 1994:401.
68. Kuhajda FP, Haupt HM, Moore GW, Hutchins GM. Gonadal morphology in patients receiving chemotherapy for leukemia. Evidence for reproductive potential and against a testicular tumor sanctuary. *Am J Med* 1982;72:759.
69. Hortobagyi GN, Buzdar AU, Marcus CE, Smith TL. Immediate and long-term toxicity of adjuvant chemotherapy regimens containing doxorubicin in trials at M.D. Anderson Hospital and Tumor Institute. *NCI Monogr* 1986;1:105.
70. Horning SJ, Hoppe RT, Kaplan HS, Rosenberg SA. Female reproductive potential after treatment for Hodgkin's disease. *N Engl J Med* 1981;304:1377.
71. Schilsky RL, Sherins RJ, Hubbard SM, et al. Long-term follow-up of ovarian function in women treated with MOPP chemotherapy for Hodgkin's disease. *Am J Med* 1981;71:552.
72. Chapman RM, Sutcliffe SB, Malpas JS. Cytotoxic-induced ovarian failure in women with Hodgkin's disease. I. Hormone function. *JAMA* 1979;242:1877.
73. Sanders JE, Buckner CD, Amos D, et al. Ovarian function following marrow transplantation for aplastic anemia or leukemia. *J Clin Oncol* 1988;6:813.
74. Byrne J, Fears TR, Gail MH, et al. Early menopause in long-term survivors of cancer during adolescence. *Am J Obstet Gynecol* 1992;166:788.
75. Byrne J, Mulvihill JJ, Myers MH, et al. Effects of treatment on fertility in long-term survivors of childhood or adolescent cancer. *N Engl J Med* 1987;317:1315.
76. Kreuser ED, Felsenberg D, Behles C, et al. Long-term gonadal dysfunction and its impact on bone mineralization in patients following COPP/ABVD chemotherapy for Hodgkin's disease. *Ann Oncol* 1992;3:S105.
77. Howell SJ, Berger G, Adams JE, Shalet SM. Bone mineral density in women with cytotoxic-induced ovarian failure. *Clin Endocrinol* 1998;49:397.
78. Koyama H, Wada T, Nishizawa Y, Iwanaga T, Aoki Y. Cyclophosphamide-induced ovarian failure and its therapeutic significance in patients with breast cancer. *Cancer* 1977;39:1403.
79. Dnistrian AM, Schwartz MK, Fraccia AA, et al. Endocrine consequences of CMF adjuvant therapy in premenopausal and postmenopausal breast cancer patients. *Cancer* 1983;51:803.
80. Watson AR, Taylor J, Rance CP, Bain J. Gonadal function in women treated with cyclophosphamide for childhood nephrotic syndrome: a long-term follow-up study. *Fertil Steril* 1986;46:331.
81. Rose DP, Davis TE. Ovarian function in patients receiving adjuvant chemotherapy for breast cancer. *Lancet* 1977;1:1174.
82. Fisher B, Sherman B, Rockette H, et al. L-phenylalanine mustard (L-PAM) in the management of premenopausal patients with primary breast cancer. Lack of association of disease-free survival with depression of ovarian function. *Cancer* 1979;44:847.
83. Singhal S, Powles R, Treleaven J, et al. Melphalan alone before allogeneic bone marrow transplantation from HLA-identical sibling donors for hematologic malignancies: alloengraftment with potential preservation of fertility in women. *Bone Marrow Transplant* 1996;18:1049.
84. Freckman HA, Fry HL, Mendez FL, Maurer ER. Chlorambucil-prednisolone therapy for disseminated breast carcinoma. *JAMA* 1964;189:111.
85. Spinelli S, Chiodi S, Bacigalupo A, et al. Ovarian recovery after total body irradiation and allogeneic bone marrow transplantation: long-term follow up of 79 females. *Bone Marrow Transplant* 1994;14:373.
86. Sy Ortin TT, Shostak CA, Donaldson SS. Gonadal status and reproductive function following treatment for Hodgkin's disease in childhood: the Stanford experience. *Int J Radiat Oncol Biol Phys* 1990;19:873.
87. Wallace WHB, Shalet SM, Crowne EC, et al. Gonadal dysfunction due to cisplatinum. *Med Pediatr Oncol* 1989;17:409.
88. Specht L, Hansen MM, Geisler C. Ovarian function in young women in long-term remission after treatment for Hodgkin's disease stage I and II. *Scand J Hematol* 1984;32:265.
89. Andrieu JM, Ochoa-Molina ME. Menstrual cycle, pregnancies and offspring before and after MOPP therapy for Hodgkin's disease. *Cancer* 1983;52:435.
90. Longo DL, Glatstein E, Duffey PL, et al. Alternating MOPP and ABVD chemotherapy plus mantle-field radiation therapy in patients with massive mediastinal Hodgkin's disease. *J Clin Oncol* 1997;15:3338.
91. Samaan NA, deAsis DN, Buzdar AU, Blumenschein GR. Pituitary-ovarian function in breast cancer patients on adjuvant chemoimmunotherapy. *Cancer* 1978;41:2084.
92. Shamberger RC, Rosenberg SA, Seipp CA, Sherins RJ. Effects of high-dose methotrexate and vincristine on ovarian and testicular functions in patients undergoing postoperative adjuvant treatment for osteosarcoma. *Cancer Treat Rep* 1981;65:739.
93. Choo YC, Chan SYW, Wong LC, Ho K. Ovarian dysfunction in patients with gestational trophoblastic neoplasia treated with short intensive courses of etoposide (VP-16-213). *Cancer* 1985;55:2348.
94. Bonadonna G, Santoro A, Viviani S, Lombardi C, Ragni G. Gonadal damage in Hodgkin's disease from cancer chemotherapy regimens. *Arch Toxicol* 1984;7(Suppl):140.
95. Wisel MS, Datta JK, Saxena RN. Effects of anti-estrogens on early pregnancy in guinea pigs. *Int J Fertil Menopausal Stud* 1994;39:156.
96. Ash P. The influence of radiation on fertility in man. *Br J Radiol* 1980;53:271.
97. Thomas PRM, Winstantly D, Peckham M, et al. Reproductive and endocrine function in patients with Hodgkin's disease: effects of oophoropexy and irradiation. *Br J Cancer* 1976;33:226.
98. Chambers SK, Chambers JT, Kier R, Peschel RE. Sequelae of lateral ovarian transposition in irradiated cervical cancer patients. *Int J Radiat Oncol Biol Phys* 1991;20:1305.
99. Muller J, Skakkebaek NE. The prenatal and postnatal development of the testis. *Ballieres Clin Endocrinol Metab* 1992;6:251.
100. Teerds KJ, de Rooij DG, Rommerts FFG, Wensing CJG. Development of a new Leydig cell population after the destruction of existing Leydig cells by ethane dimenthane sulphonate in rats: an autoradiographic study. *J Endocrinol* 1990;126:229.
101. Rivkees SA, Crawford JD. The relationship of gonadal activity and chemotherapy-induced gonadal damage. *JAMA* 1988;259:2123.
102. Sherins RJ, Olweny CLM, Ziegler JL. Gynecomastia and gonadal dysfunction in Hodgkin's disease: a prospective study. *N Engl J Med* 1978;229:12.
103. Jaffe N, Sullivan MP, Ried H, et al. Male reproductive function in long-term survivors of childhood cancer. *Med Pediatr Oncol* 1988;16:241.
104. Aubier R, Flamant F, Brauner R, et al. Male gonadal function after chemotherapy for solid tumors in childhood. *J Clin Oncol* 1989;7:304.
105. Bramswig JH, Heimes U, Heiermann E, et al. The effects of different cumulative doses of chemotherapy on testicular function. Results in 75 patients treated for Hodgkin's disease during childhood and adolescence. *Cancer* 1990;65:1298.
106. Dhabhar BN, Malhotra H, Joseph R, et al. Gonadal function in prepubertal boys following treatment for Hodgkin's disease. *Am J Pediatr Hematol Oncol* 1993;15:306.
107. Whitehead E, Shalet SM, Morris-Jones PH, Beardwell CG, Deakin DP. Gonadal function after combination chemotherapy for Hodgkin's disease in childhood. *Arch Dis Child* 1982;47:287.
108. Shalet SM, Beardwell CG, Jacobs HS, Pearson D. Testicular function following irradiation of the human prepubertal testis. *Clin Endocrinol* 1978;9:483.
109. Siimes MA, Dunkel L, Rautonen J. Risk factors for endocrine testicular dysfunction in adolescent and adult males who have survived malignancies in childhood. *Cancer Journal* 1992;5:28.
110. Muller J, Skakkebaek NE, Hertz H. Initiation of spermatogenesis during chemotherapy for leukemia. *Acta Paediatr Scand* 1985;74:956.
111. Blatt J, Poplack DG, Sherins RJ. Testicular function in boys after chemotherapy for acute lymphoblastic leukemia. *N Engl J Med* 1981;304:1121.
112. Quigley C, Cowell C, Jiminez M, et al. Normal or early development of puberty despite gonadal damage in children treated for acute lymphoblastic leukemia. *N Engl J Med* 1989;321:143.
113. Green DM, Brecher ML, Lindsay AN, et al. Gonadal function in pediatric patients following treatment for Hodgkin disease. *Med Pediatr Oncol* 1981;9:235.
114. Shalet SM, Tsatsoulis A, Whitehead E, Read G. Vulnerability of the human Leydig cell to radiation damage is dependent upon age. *J Endocrinol* 1989;120:161.
115. Sarafoglou K, Boulad F, Gillio A, Sklar C. Gonadal function after bone marrow transplantation for acute leukemia during childhood. *J Pediatr* 1997;130:210.
116. Sklar CA, Kim TH, Ramsay NKC. Testicular function following bone marrow transplantation performed during or after puberty. *Cancer* 1984;53:1498.
117. Castillo LA, Craft AW, Kernahan J, Evans RG, Aynsley-Green A. Gonadal function after 12-Gy testicular irradiation in childhood acute lymphoblastic leukaemia. *Med Pediatr Oncol* 1990;18:185.

118. Brauner R, Czernichow P, Cramer P, Schaison G, Rappaport R. Leydig-cell function in children after direct testicular irradiation for acute lymphoblastic leukemia. *N Engl J Med* 1983;309:25.
119. Blatt J, Sherins RJ, Niebrugge D, Bleyer WA, Poplack DG. Leydig cell function in boys following treatment for testicular relapse of acute lymphocytic leukemia. *J Clin Oncol* 1985;3:1227.
120. Peters H, Himelstein-Braw R, Faber M. The normal development of the ovary in childhood. *Acta Endocrinol* 1976;82:617.
121. Himelstein-Braw R, Peters H, Faber M. Influence of irradiation and chemotherapy on the ovaries of children with abdominal tumours. *Br J Cancer* 1977;36:269.
122. Stillman RJ, Schinfeld JS, Schiff I, et al. Ovarian failure in long-term survivors of childhood malignancy. *Am J Obstet Gynecol* 1981;139:62.
123. Thibaud E, Ramirez M, Brauner R, et al. Preservation of ovarian function by ovarian transposition performed before pelvic irradiation during childhood. *J Pediatr* 1992;121:880.
124. Nicosia SV, Matus-Ridley M, Meadows AT. Gonadal effects of cancer therapy in girls. *Cancer* 1985;55:2364.
125. Fryer CJ, Hutchinson RJ, Krailo M, et al. Efficacy and toxicity of 12 courses of ABVD chemotherapy followed by low-dose regional radiation in advanced Hodgkin's disease in children: a report from the Children's Cancer Study Group. *J Clin Oncol* 1990;8:1971.
126. Donaldson SS, Kaplan HS. Complications of treatment of Hodgkin's disease in children. *Cancer Treat Rep* 1982;66:977.
127. Mackie EJ, Radford M, Shalet SM. Gonadal function following chemotherapy for childhood Hodgkin's disease. *Med Pediatr Oncol* 1996;27:74.
128. Clayton PE, Shalet SM, Price DA, Jones PH. Ovarian function following chemotherapy for childhood brain tumors. *Med Pediatr Oncol* 1989;17:92.
129. Mauras N, Sabio H, Rogol QD. Neuroendocrine function in survivors of childhood acute lymphocytic leukemia and non-Hodgkins lymphoma: a study of pulsatile growth hormone and gonadotropin secretion. *Am J Pediatr Hematol Oncol* 1988;10:9.
130. Rappaport R, Brauner R, Czernichow P, et al. Effect of hypothalamic and pituitary irradiation on pubertal development in children with cranial tumors. *J Clin Endocrinol Metab* 1982;54:1164.
131. Rappaport R, Brauner R. Growth and endocrine disorders secondary to cranial irradiation. *Pediatr Res* 1989;25:561.
132. Lannering B, Jansson C, Rosberg S, Albertsson-Wikland K. Increased LH and FSH secretion after cranial irradiation in boys. *Med Pediatr Oncol* 1997;29:280
133. Chen MS, Lin FJ, Huang MJ, et al. Prospective hormone study of hypothalamic-pituatary function in patients with nasopharyngeal carcinoma after high-dose irradiation. *Jpn J Clin Oncol* 1989;19:265.
134. Samaan NA, Schultz PN, Yang KPP, et al. Endocrine complications after radiotherapy for tumors of the head and neck. *J Lab Clin Med* 1987;109:364.
135. Littley MD, Shalet SM, Beardwell CG, Robinson EL, Sutton ML. Radiation-induced hypopituitarism is dose-dependent. *Clin Endocrinol* 1989;31:363.
136. Lam KS, Tse VK, Wang C, Yeung RT, Ho JH. Effects of cranial irradiation on hypothalamic-pituitary function: a 5-year longitudinal study in patients with nasopharyngeal carcinoma. *Q J Med* 1991;78:165.
137. Constine LS, Woolf PD, Cann D, et al. Hypothalamic-pituitary dysfunction after radiation for brain tumors. *N Engl J Med* 1993;328:87.
138. Radford JA, Clark S, Crowther D, Shalet SM. Male fertility after VAPEC-B chemotherapy for Hodgkin's disease and non-Hodgkin's lymphoma. *Br J Cancer* 1994;69:379.
139. Fraass BA, Kinsella TJ, Harrington FS, Glatstein E. Peripheral dose to the testes: the design and clinical use of a practical and effective gonadal shield. *Int J Radiat Oncol Biol Phys* 1985;11:609.
140. Kubo H, Shipley WU. Reduction of the scatter dose to the testicle outside the radiation treatment fields. *Int J Radiat Oncol Biol Phys* 1982;8:1741.
141. Harter DJ, Hussey DH, Delclos L, Eagle DF, Moore EB. Device to position the testicle during irradiation. *Int J Radiat Oncol Biol Phys* 1976;1:361.
142. Zagars GK. Management of stage I seminoma: radiotherapy. In: Horwich A, ed. *Testicular cancer.* London: Chapman & Hall, 1994:83.
143. Le Floch O, Donaldson SS, Kaplan HS. Pregnancy following oophoropexy and total nodal irradiation in women with Hodgkin's disease. *Cancer* 1976;38:2263.
144. Kliesch S, Behre HM, Jurgens H, Nieschlag E. Cryopreservation of semen from adolescent patients with malignancies. *Med Pediatr Oncol* 1996;26:20.
145. Schmiegelow ML, Sommer P, Carlsen E, et al. Penile vibratory stimulation and electroejaculation before anticancer therapy in two pubertal boys. *J Pediatr Hematol Oncol* 1998;20:429.
146. Brinster RL, Avarbock MR. Germline transmission of donor haplotype following spermatogonial transplantation. *Proc Natl Acad Sci U S A* 1994;91:11303.
147. Avarbock MR, Brinster CJ, Brinster RL. Reconstitution of spermatogenesis from frozen spermatogonial stem cells. *Nat Med* 1996;2:693.
148. Radford J, Shalet S, Lieberman B. Fertility after treatment for cancer. Questions remain over ways of preserving ovarian and testicular tissue. *BMJ* 1999;319:935.
149. Chen C. Pregnancy after human oocyte cryopreservation. *Lancet* 1986;1:884.
150. Bouquet M, Selva J, Auroux M. Cryopreservation of mouse oocytes: mutagenic effects in the embryo. *Biol Reprod* 1993;49:764.
151. Buster JE, Bustillo M, Rodi IA, et al. Biologic and morphologic development of donated human ova recovered by nonsurgical uterine lavage. *Am J Obstet Gynecol* 1985;153:211.
152. Baird DT, Webb R, Campbell BK, Harkness LM, Gosden RG. Long-term ovarian function in sheep after ovariectomy and transplantation of autografts stored at -196 C. *Endocrinology* 1999;140:462.
153. Oktay K, Newton H, Mullan J, Gosden RG. Development of human primordial follicles to antral stages in SCID/hpg mice stimulated with follicle stimulating hormone. *Hum Reprod* 1998;13:1133.
154. Oktay K, Karlikaya G, Gosden R, Schwartz R. Ovarian function after autologous transplantation of frozen-banked human ovarian tissue. *Fertil Steril* 1999;72:s21(abst).
155. Shaw JM, Bowles J, Koopman P, Wood EC, Trounson AO. Fresh and cryopreserved ovarian tissue samples from donors with lymphoma transmit the cancer to graft recipients. *Hum Reprod* 1996;11:1668.
156. Pfeifer SM, Coutifaris C. Reproductive technologies 1998: options available for the cancer patient. *Med Pediatr Oncol* 1999;33:34.
157. Sanger WG, Olson JH, Sherman JK. Semen cryobanking for men with cancer-criteria change. *Fertil Steril* 1992;58:1024.
158. Palermo GD, Cohen J, Alikani M, Adler A, Rosenwaks Z. Intracytoplasmic sperm injection: a novel treatment for all forms of male factor infertility. *Fertil Steril* 1995;63:1231.
159. Sherins RJ, Thorsell LP, Dorfmann A, et al. Intracytoplasmic sperm injection facilitates fertilization even in the most severe forms of male infertility: pregnancy outcome correlates with maternal age and number of eggs available. *Fertil Steril* 1995;64:369.
160. Rosenlund B, Sjoblom P, Tornblom M, Hultling C, Hillensjo T. In-vitro fertilization and intracytoplasmic sperm injection in the treatment of infertility after testicular cancer. *Hum Reprod* 1998;13:414.
161. Anonymous. Assisted reproductive technology in the United States and Canada: 1994 results generated from the American Society for Reproductive Medicine/Society for Assisted Reproductive Technology Registry. *Fertil Steril* 1996;66:697.
162. Tournaye H, Camus M, Bollen N, et al. In vitro fertilization techniques with frozen-thawed sperm: a method for preserving the progenitive potential of Hodgkin patients. *Fertil Steril* 1991;55:443.
163. Bonduelle M, Wilikens A, Buysse A, et al. Prospective follow-up study of 877 children born after intracytoplasmic sperm injection (ICSI), with ejaculated epididymal and testicular spermatozoa and after replacement of cryopreserved embryos obtained after ICSI. *Hum Reprod* 1996;11(Suppl 4):131.
164. Pfeffer J, Pang MG, Hoegerman SF, et al. Aneuploidy frequencies in semen fractions from ten oligoasthenoteratozoospermic patients donating sperm for intracytoplasmic sperm injection. *Fertil Steril* 1999;72:472.
165. Delic JI, Bush C, Peckham MJ. Protection from procarbazine-induced damage of spermatogenesis in the rat by androgen. *Cancer Res* 1986;46:1909.
166. Ward JA, Robinson J, Furr BJA, Shalet SM, Morris ID. Protection of spermatogenesis in rats from the cytotoxic procarbazine by the depot formulation of Zoladex, a gonadotropin-releasing hormone agonist. *Cancer Res* 1990;50:568.
167. Meistrich ML, Parchuri N, Wilson G, Kurdoglu B, Kangasniemi M. Hormonal protection from cyclophosphamide-induced inactivation of rat stem spermatogonia. *J Androl* 1995;16:334.
168. Glode LM, Robinson J, Gould SF. Protection from cyclophosphamide-induced testicular damage with an analogue of gonadotropin-releasing hormone. *Lancet* 1981;1:1132.
169. Meistrich ML, Wilson G, Zhang Y, Kurdoglu B, Terry NHA. Protection from procarbazine-induced testicular damage by hormonal pretreatment does not involve arrest of spermatogonial proliferation. *Cancer Res* 1997;57:1091.
170. Meistrich ML, Wilson G, Kangasniemi M, Huhtaniemi I. Mechanism of "protection" of rat spermatogenesis by hormonal pretreatment: stimulation of spermatogonial differentiation after irradiation. *J Androl* 2000;21:464.
171. Meistrich ML, Wilson G, Huhtaniemi I. Hormonal treatment after cytotoxic therapy stimulates recovery of spermatogenesis. *Cancer Res* 1999;59:3557.
172. Meistrich ML. Hormonal stimulation of the recovery of spermatogenesis following chemo- or radiotherapy. *APMIS* 1998;106:37.
173. Morris ID, Shalet SM. Protection of gonadal function from cytotoxic chemotherapy and irradiation. *Ballieres Clin Endocrinol Metab* 1990;4:97.
174. Kreuser ED, Klingmuller D, Thiel E. The role of LHRH-analogues in protecting gonadal functions during chemotherapy and irradiation. *Eur Urol* 1993;23:157.
175. Masala A, Faedda R, Alagna S, et al. Use of testosterone to prevent cyclophosphamide-induced azoospermia. *Ann Intern Med* 1997;126:292.
176. Pogach LM, Lee Y, Gould S, Giglio W, Huang HFS. Partial prevention of procarbazine induced germinal cell aplasia in rats by sequential GnRH antagonist and testosterone administration. *Cancer Res* 1988;48:4354.
177. Bokser L, Szende B, Schally AV. Protective effects of D-Trp^6-luteinising hormone-releasing hormone microcapsules against cyclophosphamide-induced gonadotoxicity in female rats. *Br J Cancer* 1990;61:861.
178. Ataya KM, Tadros M, Ramahi A. Gonadotropin-releasing hormone agonist inhibits physiologic ovarian follicular loss in rats. *Acta Endocrinol* 1989;121:55.
179. Waxman JH, Ahmed R, Smith D, et al. Failure to preserve fertility in patients with Hodgkin's disease. *Cancer Chemother Pharmacol* 1987;19:159.
180. Blumenfeld Z, Avivi I, Linn S, et al. Prevention of irreversible chemotherapy-induced ovarian damage in young women with lymphoma by a gonadotrophin-releasing hormone agonist in parallel to chemotherapy. *Hum Reprod* 1996;11:1620.
181. Whitehead E, Shalet SM, Blackledge G, et al. The effect of combination chemotherapy on ovarian function in women treated for Hodgkin's disease. *Cancer* 1983;52:988.
182. Chapman RM, Sutcliffe SB. Protection of ovarian function by oral contraceptives in women receiving chemotherapy for Hodgkin's disease. *Blood* 1981;58:849.
183. Chatterjee R, Goldstone AH. Gonadal damage and effects on fertility in adult patients with haematological malignancy undergoing stem cell transplantation. *Bone Marrow Transplant* 1996;17:5.
184. Chung PH, Palermo G, Schlegel PN, et al. The use of intracytoplasmic sperm injection with electroejaculates from anejaculatory men. *Hum Reprod* 1998;13:1854.
185. Li FP, Gimbrere K, Gelber RD, et al. Outcome of pregnancy in survivors of Wilms' tumor. *JAMA* 1987;257:216.
186. Syrjala KL, Roth-Roemer SL, Abrams JR, et al. Prevalence and predictors of sexual dysfunction in long-term survivors of marrow transplantation. *J Clin Oncol* 1998;16:3148.
187. Apperley JF, Reddy N. Mechanism and management of treatment-related gonadal failure in recipients of high dose chemoradiotherapy. *Blood Rev* 1995;9:93.
188. Mulder JE. Benefits and risks of hormone replacement therapy in young adult cancer survivors with gonadal failure. *Med Pediatr Oncol* 1999;33:46.

189. Donohoe JP. Nerve-sparing retroperitoneal lymphadenectomy with preservation of ejaculation. *J Urol* 1990;144:287.
190. Jacobsen KD, Ous S, Waehre H, et al. Ejaculation in testicular cancer patients after post-chemotherapy retroperitoneal lymph node dissection. *Br J Cancer* 1999;80:249.
191. Walsh PC, Mostwin JL. Radical prostatectomy and cystoprostatectomy with preservation of potency. Results using a new nerve-sparing technique. *Br J Urol* 1984;56:694.
192. Kim ED, Scardino PT, Hampel O, et al. Interposition of sural nerve restores function of cavernous nerves resected during radical prostatectomy. *J Urol* 1999;161:199.
193. Gilja I, Parazajder J, Radej M, Cvitkovic P, Kovacic M. Retrograde ejaculation and loss of emission: possibilities of conservative treatment. *Eur Urol* 1994;25:226.
194. Ohl DA, Denil J, Bennett CJ, et al. Electroejaculation following retroperitoneal lymphadenectomy. *J Urol* 1991;145:980.
195. Witt KL, Bishop JB. Mutagenicity of anticancer drugs in mammalian germ cells. *Mutat Res* 1996;355:209.
196. BEIR (Committee on Biological Effects of Ionizing Radiation). *Health effects of exposure to low levels of ionizing radiation (BEIR V)*. Washington, DC: National Academy Press, 1990.
197. Shelby MD, Bishop JB, Mason JM, Tindall KR. Fertility, reproduction, and genetic disease: studies on the mutagenic effects of environmental agents on mammalian germ cells. *Environ Health Perspect* 1993;100:283.
198. Ehling UH, Neuhauser A. Procarbazine-induced specific locus mutations in male mice. *Mutat Res* 1979;59:245.
199. Neel JV, Schull WJ, Awa AA, et al. The children of parents exposed to atomic bombs: estimates of the genetic doubling dose of radiation for humans. *Am J Hum Genet* 1990;46:1053.
200. Searle AG. Radiation—the genetic risk. *Trends Genet* 1987;3:152.
201. Ehling UH, Neuhauser-Klaus A. Induction of specific-locus mutation in female mice by 1-ethyl-1-nitrosourea and procarbazine. *Mutat Res* 1988;202:139.
202. Jeffreys AJ, Tamaki K, MacLeod A, et al. Complex gene conversion events in germline mutation at human minisatellites. *Nat Genet* 1994;6:136.
203. Brewen JG, Preston RJ, Gengozian N. Analysis of x-ray-induced chromosomal translocations in human and marmoset spermatogonial stem cells. *Nature* 1975;253:468.
204. Brandriff BF, Meistrich ML, Gordon LA, Carrano AV, Liang JC. Chromosomal damage in sperm of patients surviving Hodgkin's disease following MOPP therapy with and without radiotherapy. *Hum Genet* 1994;93:295.
205. Robbins WA, Meistrich ML, Moore D, et al. Chemotherapy induces transient sex chromosomal and autosomal aneuploidy in human sperm. *Nat Genet* 1997;16:74.
206. Baumgartner A, Van Hummelen P, Lowe XR, Adler ID, Wyrobek AJ. Numerical and structural chromosomal abnormalities detected in human sperm with a combination of multicolor FISH assays. *Environ Mol Mutagen* 1999;33:49.
207. Martin RH, Rademaker A, Hildebrand K, et al. A comparison of chromosomal aberrations induced in vivo by radiotherapy in human sperm and lymphocytes. *Mutat Res* 1989;226:21.
208. Robbins WA, Meistrich ML, Cassel MJ, Wyrobek AJ. Aneuploidy in sperm of Hodgkin's disease patients receiving NOVP chemotherapy. *Am J Hum Genet* 1994;55(Suppl):A68(abst).
209. Van Hummelen P, Lowe X, Meistrich ML, Wyrobek AJ. A novel multi-probe FISH procedure for the simultaneous detection of chromosomal aberrations, disomy, and diploidy in sperm of Hodgkin patients receiving chemotherapy. *Am J Hum Genet* 1995;57(Suppl):A79(abst).
210. Martin RH, Ernst S, Rademaker A, et al. Chromosomal abnormalities in sperm from testicular cancer patients before and after chemotherapy. *Hum Genet* 1997;99:214.
211. Dubrova YE, Nesterov VN, Krouchinsky NG, et al. Further evidence for elevated human minisatellite mutation rate in Belarus eight years after the Chernobyl accident. *Mutat Res* 1997;381:267.
212. Armour JA, Brinkworth MH, Kamischke A. Direct analysis by small-pool PCR of MS205 minisatellite mutation rates in sperm after mutagenic therapies. *Mutat Res* 1999;445:73.
213. Blatt J. Pregnancy outcome in long-term survivors of childhood cancer. *Med Pediatr Oncol* 1999;33:29.
214. Hawkins MM. Is there evidence of a therapy-related increase in germ cell mutation among childhood cancer survivors? *J Natl Cancer Inst* 1991;83:1643.
215. Byrne J, Rasmussen SA, Steinhorn SC, et al. Genetic disease in offspring of long-term survivors of childhood and adolescent cancer. *Am J Hum Genet* 1998;62:45.
216. Hawkins MM, Draper GJ, Smith RA. Cancer among 1,348 offspring of survivors of childhood cancer. *Int J Cancer* 1989;43:975.
217. Critchley HO. Factors of importance for implantation and problems after treatment for childhood cancer. *Med Pediatr Oncol* 1999;33:9.
218. Rustin GJ, Booth M, Dent J, et al. Pregnancy after cytotoxic chemotherapy for gestational trophoblastic tumours. *BMJ* 1984;288:103.
219. Senturia YD, Peckham CS, Peckham MJ. Children fathered by men treated for testicular cancer. *Lancet* 1985;2:766.
220. Dodds L, Marrett LD, Tomkins DJ, Green B, Sherman G. Case-control study of congenital anomalies in children of cancer patients. *BMJ* 1993;307:164.
221. Carson SA, Gentry WL, Smith AL, Buster JE. Feasibility of semen collection and cryopreservation during chemotherapy. *Hum Reprod* 1991;6:992.
222. Gulati SC, Vega R, Gee T, Koziner B, Clarkson B. Growth and development of children born to patients after cancer therapy. *Cancer Invest* 1986;4:197.
223. Yamazaki JN, Schull WJ. Perinatal loss and neurological abnormalities among children of the atomic bomb. Nagasaki and Hiroshima revisited, 1949 to 1989. *JAMA* 1990;264:605.
224. Wiebe VJ, Sipila PE. Pharmacology of antineoplastic agents in pregnancy. *Crit Rev Oncol Hematol* 1994;16:75.

SECTION 7

FLORA E. VAN LEEUWEN
LOIS B. TRAVIS

Second Cancers

Modern chemotherapy and radiotherapy have increased substantially the survival of patients with cancer. In particular, cure rates have shown dramatic improvement for patients with Hodgkin's disease, testicular cancer, and pediatric malignancies. Less impressive, but nonetheless convincing, improvements in survival also have been achieved for patients with breast cancer, non-Hodgkin's lymphoma (NHL), and several other tumors. Now that substantial numbers of cancer patients experience such a favorable prognosis, it becomes increasingly important to evaluate the long-term complications of treatment. Because the survival benefits associated with modern treatments have been greatest for those cancers that occur at relatively young ages, cured patients are subject to long-term side effects, which may not emerge until several decades after treatment. Paradoxically, research conducted since the late 1970s has clearly demonstrated that some of the modalities used to treat cancer have the potential to induce new (second) primary malignancies. Of the many late complications of treatment, second cancers are generally considered to be the most serious, because they not only cause substantial morbidity but also considerable mortality. For example, among 15-year survivors of Hodgkin's disease, second cancer deaths have been reported to be the largest contributor to the substantial excess mortality that these patients experience.[1] Increased risks of second cancers have been observed after radiotherapy, chemotherapy, or combined modality treatment.

In any discussion of treatment-related second malignancies, it is of primary importance to remember that not all second cancers are due to therapy. The occurrence of two primary malignancies in the same individual may reflect the operation of numerous influences. Multiple primary cancers may result from host susceptibility (genetic predisposition or immunodeficiency), common carcinogenic influences, a clustering of risk factors, treatment for the first tumor, diagnostic surveillance, a chance event, or the interaction of these factors. In view of the high prevalence of cancer in the general population and the increasing incidence of most cancers with age, it is important to exclude the role of chance in the development of second cancers. To this end, comparison with cancer incidence statistics derived from the general population is crucial. If a second malignancy is demonstrated to occur in excess, the contributions of other risk factors need to be ruled out convincingly before the increased risk can be attributed to treatment. The temporal trend of excess second cancer risk may provide an important initial clue to etiology; for example, the risk of solid tumors after radiotherapy generally increases with time since exposure. The evaluation of the carcinogenic effects of therapy, however, is complicated by the fact that therapeutic agents are frequently given in combination. Appropriate epidemiologic and statistical methods are required to quantify the excess risk and to unravel the role of treatment and other factors.

Whenever interpreting results of second cancer studies, it must be kept in mind that the problem of treatment-induced malignancies has arisen by virtue of the success of cancer therapy. As more becomes known about the influence of various treatment factors on second cancer risk, therapies may be modified to decrease the risk while maintaining equal levels of therapeutic effectiveness.

The major aspects of second malignancy risk in relation to cancer treatment are addressed in this chapter. After a discussion of methods used for the assessment of second cancer risk, an overview of the carcinogenic effects of radiotherapy and chemotherapy is presented. Subsequently, the risk of second malignancies after treatment for Hodgkin's disease, NHL, testicular cancer, breast cancer, ovarian cancer, and pediatric malignancies is reviewed. Emphasis is on large studies that have been published most recently.

METHODS TO ASSESS SECOND CANCER RISK

Estimates of second cancer risk after treatment of various primary malignancies derive from several sources, including population-based cancer registries, hospital-based cancer registries, or clinical trial series.[2] The epidemiologic study designs generally used are the cohort study and the case-control study.

In a cohort study, a large group of patients with a specified first malignancy (the cohort) is followed for a number of years to determine the incidence of second cancers. To evaluate whether second cancer risk in the cohort is increased compared with cancer risk in the general population, the observed number of second cancers in the cohort is compared with the number expected on the basis of age-, gender-, and calendar year–specific cancer incidence rates in the general population. The analysis takes into account the observation period of individual patients (person-years).[3] The relative risk of developing a second cancer is estimated by comparing the ratio of the observed number of second cancer cases in the cohort to the number expected. When the relative risk is increased, the question arises as to whether the excesses are due to therapy. This issue can be evaluated by comparing risks between treatment groups, preferably within specified follow-up intervals and, when possible, with a reference group of patients not treated with radiotherapy and chemotherapy. Second cancer risk in the cohort (and in different treatment groups) can also be expressed by the cumulative (actuarial estimated) risk,[4] which yields the proportion of patients alive at time t (e.g., 5 years from diagnosis) who can be expected to develop a second malignancy. When the cohort's death rate due to causes other than second malignancy is high, the assumptions underlying the actuarial method may not be valid, and competing risk techniques should be considered to estimate cumulative risk.[5,6] Because many treatment-related cancers are rare in the general population (e.g., leukemia, sarcoma), a high relative risk (compared to the population) may still translate into a rather low cumulative risk. Absolute excess risk, which estimates the excess number of second malignancies per 10,000 patients per year, perhaps best reflects the second cancer burden in a cohort. This risk measure is also the most appropriate one by which to identify those second malignancies that contribute the most to elevated risks.

Each of the data sources used to construct a cohort has its own set of advantages and disadvantages. Population-based cancer registries frequently have large numbers of patients available, which allows the detection of even small increases in the site-specific risk of second cancers.[7] An additional advantage is that the observed and expected numbers of cancers derive from the same reference population. Disadvantages of this approach include the limited availability of treatment data, underreporting of second cancers[8,9] (in particular hematologic malignancies and bilateral cancers in paired organs), and different diagnostic criteria for second cancers. Population-based registries differ greatly in these aspects and, hence, in their usefulness for second cancer studies. If treatment data are not available, it is impossible to determine whether excess risk for a second malignancy is related to treatment or to shared etiology with the first cancer. Despite their disadvantages, population-based registries are especially well suited to broadly evaluate which second cancers occur in excess after a wide spectrum of different first primary malignancies. They also provide a valuable starting point for case-control studies that evaluate treatment effects in detail (see later in this section).

A major strength of clinical trial databases is that detailed treatment data on all patients are available. Comparison of second cancer risk between the treatment arms of the trial controls for any intrinsic risk for a second malignancy associated with the first cancer. Limitations of most trials include the small number of patients involved and the frequent lack of data on subsequent therapy. The dearth of large numbers becomes more serious when the second cancer of interest has a low background incidence (e.g., leukemia). Furthermore, the end points of interest in the majority of clinical trials include only treatment response and survival, not the development of second cancers. Therefore, many clinical trials do not routinely collect information on second malignancies, and some do not collect any data beyond 5 years. Routine reporting and assessment of second malignancy risk should become an integral part of clinical trial research.[10]

Many large cancer treatment centers maintain registries of all admitted patients. Most of these registries have been in existence for decades and collect extensive data on treatment and follow-up. As compared with trial data, hospital registries provide larger patient numbers and a wider variety of treatments and dose levels, which may yield important information on drug and radiation carcinogenesis. Most studies of second cancer risk after Hodgkin's disease have been based on data accrued from hospital registries.[11–13]

The cohort study is not an efficient design when examining detailed treatment factors (e.g., cumulative dose of alkylating agents) in relation to second cancer risk. Most cohorts are fairly large (to yield reliable estimates of second cancer risk), rendering the collection of detailed treatment data for all patients prohibitively expensive and time-consuming. In such instances, the so-called nested case-control study within an existing cohort is the preferred approach. The case group consists of all patients identified with the second cancer of interest, whereas the controls are a matched sample of all patients in the cohort who did not develop the cancer concerned, although they experienced the same amount of follow-up time. Matching factors typically include age, gender, and calendar year of diagnosis of the first cancer. Even when the control group is three times as large as the case group, detailed treatment data need only be collected for a small proportion of the total cohort. In each case-control investigation, it is critical to the validity of the study that the controls are truly representative of all patients who did not contract the second cancer of interest. In data analysis, treatment factors are compared between cases and controls, and the risk associated with specific therapies is estimated relative to the risk in patients who received other treatments. The cumulative risk of developing a second malignancy cannot be derived from a case-control study. Treatment-specific absolute excess risks can be estimated, however, when the case-control study follows a cohort analysis. Although case-control methodology has not been applied to the investigation of second cancer risk for a long period,[14,15] several landmark studies have already demonstrated its strengths.[8,16–22]

CARCINOGENICITY OF INDIVIDUAL TREATMENT MODALITIES

RADIOTHERAPY

The carcinogenic potential of ionizing radiation was first recognized in the mid-twentieth century,[23–25] and comprehensive reviews have now been published.[26–28] Much of the data with regard to radiation effects in humans has derived from epidemiologic studies of the atomic bomb survivors in Japan,[29–32] occupationally exposed workers,[33,34] patients given large amounts of diagnostic radiation,[35,36] and patients treated with radiotherapy for malignant[16,19,37–39] and nonmalignant diseases.[40–44] Most types of cancer, with the exception of chronic lymphocytic leukemia, can be caused by exposure to ionizing radiation.[26,30,45] Boice et al.[28] have ranked various body tissues with regard to cancer induction by radiation; certain sites, such as the thyroid, female breast, and bone marrow, clearly are more radiosensitive than others.

The excess risk of leukemia attributable to irradiation is observed within a few years after exposure, with a peak at 5 to 9 years, and a slow decline thereafter.[16,27,30,40,41] Some controversy exists as to whether, and when, leukemia risk decreases to background levels in the population.[16,30,41,46,47] In the atomic bomb survivors, risk declined more rapidly for those exposed earlier in life.[30] Increased risks of solid tumors have been shown to emerge much later. After a minimum induction period of 5 to 10 years,[12,13,37,40,41,48] solid tumor risk appears to follow a time-response model consistent with a multiplicative relationship with the underlying incidence in the population—that is, risk after exposure is proportional to the background incidence of cancer over time.[27,41] Data are inconsistent as to whether the risk remains elevated throughout life. Studies in the atomic bomb survivors[31] and in women treated for benign gynecologic disorders[41,49] have shown that the excess relative risk per Gray (Gy) tends to be fairly stable over time for at least 30 years after radiation. However, the last update of the mortality experience of ankylosing spondylitis patients showed that, 25 years after irradiation, risk had decreased for a number of malignancies.[40] In the few studies of second cancer risk in which the time course beyond 20 years from first treatment was evaluated, the relative risks of solid tumor development tended to decrease in very long-term survivors.[50,51] The most recent cancer incidence report on the Japanese atomic bomb survivors, with 42 years of follow-up, indicated that the excess relative risk decreased with time for the younger age-at-exposure groups and remained virtually constant for the older cohorts.[31] Cancer incidence data from the atomic bomb survivors and five other groups exposed to radiation have been analyzed to specifically address the evolution of risk with increasing time since exposure in childhood.[52] Ten to 15 years after radiation exposure, the relative risk of solid tumors decreased with increasing follow-up time (5.7% to 6.1% per year). The excess absolute risk, however, significantly increased with time since exposure.[52]

An important part of our knowledge of radiation carcinogenesis derives from populations exposed to relatively low levels of radiation, such as the atomic bomb survivors. For solid tumors, convincing evidence for a strongly linear radiation dose-response in the lower dose ranges (up to approximately 5 Gy) has emerged.[31,35,40] The results for leukemia are less consistent, but data from most studies are compatible with a linear trend for doses of less than 1.5 to 2.0 Gy.[16,30,45] Extrapolation of radiation effects from low doses to the high-dose ranges used therapeutically cannot be done with certainty, because of the possibility of cell killing at high doses. Therefore, more recent studies of second cancer risk have focused on the shape of the radiation dose-response curve in the high-dose range.

Radiation-related leukemia risk depends on a number of parameters, such as radiation dose to the active bone marrow, dose rate, and percentage of marrow exposed. Consistent evidence indicates that the excess risk of leukemia per unit radiation dose is much higher at low doses than at the high doses administered for the treatment of malignant disease.[16,30,45,47] This phenomenon has been attributed to cell killing or inactivation of potentially leukemic cells at the higher radiation doses.[16,27] Many studies in cancer patients have shown that high radiation doses to a limited field confer very little or no increased risk of leukemia.[8,17,18,20] Both in the atomic bomb survivors and in patients who received radiotherapy for cervical cancer, leukemia risk appeared to increase with increasing average dose to the bone marrow until approximately 4 Gy, above which leukemia risk was progressively reduced with increasing dose.[16,30] However, leukemia risk in survivors of uterine cancer showed little evidence for a downturn in risk at bone marrow doses as high as 6 to 14 Gy[45]; at more than 1.5 Gy, the dose-response pattern was more or less flat, and the risk after continuous exposures from brachytherapy at comparatively low doses was similar to that after fractionated exposures at much higher doses from external beam radiotherapy. Clearly, more research is needed into the effects of dose fractionation and portion of bone marrow irradiated. Age at exposure to irradiation does not appear to greatly influence the risk of radiation-induced leukemia,[30,41,45,53] although decreasing relative risk with increasing age at exposure has been reported for one radiogenic leukemia subtype [acute lymphocytic leukemia (ALL)].[47]

In contrast, studies of radiogenic breast cancer have demonstrated that age at exposure is a major determinant of risk, with the greatest risk for those irradiated as children and adolescents.[32,50,54] Irradiation may thus affect cells of the mammary ducts before full organ development begins. Atomic bomb survivors who were younger than 10 years old at the time of the bombing had an excess relative risk per Gy five times that of women who were older than 40 years when exposed. A strong trend of increasing breast cancer risk with decreasing age at exposure was also observed in patients irradiated for Hodgkin's disease,[13,39,50,55] with no excess breast cancer risk apparent among women irradiated at 40 years or older.[13,22,35,39,55] In two studies, increased breast cancer risk after radiation exposure in childhood emerged at an early age (younger than 40), before the peak incidence in the population.[50,56] In the low-dose range, breast cancer risk increases linearly with radiation dose.[35,36,44] For a specified dose, the age-specific excess rates of breast cancer were found to be remarkably similar across studies in the Japanese atomic bomb survivors and in medically irradiated populations in the United States.[32,35] Very few studies have examined whether linear dose-response extends to the higher dose ranges used therapeutically. However, long-term survivors of Hodgkin's disease who were younger than 20 years when they received breast doses between 4 and 45 Gy from mantle field irradiation were reported to have a 40- to 75-fold increased risk of breast cancer.[13,39,57] One study found that a higher radiation dose to the mantle region (20 Gy or more vs. less than 20 Gy) was associated with a significantly greater increase of breast cancer risk.[57]

Risk of lung cancer also rises with increasing radiation dose in the lower dose range,[31,40] but studies in survivors of Hodgkin's disease[38] and breast cancer[58] suggest that the risk may level off at doses higher than 9 to 10 Gy. A similar leveling of risk at doses of 10 Gy or more has been observed for radiation-induced thyroid cancer.[59,60] However, even at thyroid doses up to 60 Gy, the risk of thyroid cancer did not decrease.[60] For bone sarcoma, two studies in survivors of childhood cancer[19,61] show no evidence of increased risk for doses less than 10 Gy to the site of the bone tumor. Beyond 10 Gy, risk for bone sarcoma rose sharply with increasing dose, reaching more than 90-fold at doses of 30 to 50 Gy.[61] Importantly, studies have shown that, also for solid tumors other than breast cancer, the excess relative risk due to radiation is much greater for children and adolescents than for adults.[12,31,50,59,62,63] Significantly greater relative risks with younger age at radiation exposure have been reported for lung cancer,[63] thyroid cancer,[31] bone sarcoma,[12,62] and gastrointestinal cancer.[50,63] After radiation in childhood, the excess relative risk per Gy for thyroid cancer [RR, 7.7; 95% confidence interval (CI), 2.1 to 28.7] is higher than for any other solid malignancy.[31]

For radiogenic lung cancer, the interaction of radiation with other risk factors, such as smoking, has been examined. Studies in uranium and tin miners exposed to radon have indicated that smoking and radiation may act multiplicatively (or at least supraadditively) in the causation of lung cancer,[64–66] implying that the absolute risk of developing radon-induced cancer is much higher in smokers than in nonsmokers. In Hodgkin's disease patients, the combined effects of smoking and high-dose radiotherapy for Hodgkin's disease were significantly stronger than multiplicative.[38,67] In the latter study, the increase in lung cancer risk with increasing radiation dose was significantly greater among patients who continued to smoke after diagnosis of Hodgkin's disease than among those who refrained from smoking. As discussed more extensively in the previous edition of this text,[68] interaction models accounting for the sequencing of radiation and smoking suggest that radiation may act as a powerful promoter of cells initiated by smoking.

The carcinogenic effects of therapeutic irradiation deserve much more study. Issues to be clarified include the shape of the radiation dose-response curve in the higher dose range, the duration of radiation-induced cancer risk and, importantly, the interaction of radiotherapy with environmental carcinogens (e.g., smoking) and genetic susceptibility. Increasing evidence suggests that genetic factors contribute to the development of radiation-induced cancers. This is perhaps best demonstrated in survivors of hereditary retinoblastoma who harbor a heterozygous germline mutation in the RB1 tumor suppressor gene, and who have a much greater risk of developing osteosarcomas within the radiation field than children irradiated for nonhereditary retinoblastoma.[69] In addition, two studies showed that patients with a positive family history of cancer are more likely to develop radiation-associated second malignancies.[70,71] In view of the postulated radiation sensitivity of heterozygous carriers of the mutated ataxia-telangiectasia (ATM) gene, it has been speculated that AT heterozygotes (approximately 1.0% of the population) may have an increased risk of radiation-induced cancer, specifically breast cancer.[72,73] In two studies, however, no ATM mutations were found in a total of 56 women who had developed breast cancer after radiotherapy for Hodgkin's disease.[71,74] Further studies should focus on the identification of other genes that may influence susceptibility to the DNA damaging effects of radiation. Such research will provide more insight into the mechanisms underlying radiation carcinogenesis and will also be of clinical benefit in minimizing radiation exposure to the most susceptible subgroups of the population.

CHEMOTHERAPY

The development of acute myeloid leukemia (AML) after chemotherapy for malignant disease was reported as early as 1970 by Kyle et al.[75] In the following three decades, the occurrence of this late effect has increased to the extent that, in some institutions, treatment-related AML now comprises up to 10% to 20% of all such entities.[76] Moreover, it is now established that the spectrum of treatment-related leukemia extends beyond AML. ALL, for example, is increasingly recognized as therapy-related[77,78] and may comprise 5% to 10% of all secondary acute leukemias.[78] Chronic granulocytic leukemia accounts for a small percentage of secondary leukemia,[77,79] and has been included in numerous analytic studies in which associations with prior chemotherapy have been evaluated,[8,17,18,20,80,81] although separate risk estimates have not been presented. To date, only chronic lymphocytic leukemia has not been convincingly associated with prior exposure to chemotherapy.

Chemotherapy is far more potent than radiotherapy in inducing leukemia. It has become evident that at least two major syndromes of treatment-related leukemia may exist[82,83]: "classic" alkylating agent–induced AML and acute leukemia related to the topoisomerase II inhibitors. Risk of alkylating agent–related leukemia typically begins to increase 1 to 2 years after the start of chemotherapy, peaks in the 5- to 10-year follow-up period, and decreases afterward.[8,13,17,20,84] Even in large patient series, the number of long-term survivors has typically been too small to determine whether 15 to 20 years after chemotherapy the risk of leukemia returns to the background level of the population.[13] Although one registry-based study indicates that leukemia risk might persist among 15-year survivors of testicular cancer,[85] it is not clear whether these late excesses might reflect the influence of salvage therapy. More than 50% of leukemias after alkylating agent therapy present initially as myelodysplastic syndromes (MDS), whereas *de novo* AML is preceded by MDS much less frequently.[77] Most cases of MDS progress to AML within 1 year.[77] Cytogenetic studies of alkylating agent–related AML/MDS have shown unbalanced chromosome aberrations, typically with loss of whole chromosomes 5 or 7 (or both), or various parts of the long arms of these chromosomes.[86] Morphologically, alkylating agent–related AML most commonly consists of French-American-British (FAB) subtypes M1/M2, but most subtypes,[77] including erythroleukemia,[20] have been observed. Survival after secondary AML is generally quite poor, typically only several months.[87]

Alkylating agents with known leukemogenic effects in humans include mechlorethamine, chlorambucil, cyclophosphamide, melphalan, semustine, lomustine, carmustine, prednimustine, busulfan, and dihydroxybusulfan.[20,77,82,88–90] Controversial findings have been reported with regard to procarbazine,[89,91] which demonstrates an underlying mechanism of action similar to alkylating agents. Few studies have addressed the relative leukemogenicity of the various alkylating drugs, but a strong body of evidence to date suggests that, at doses of equal therapeutic effect, cyclophosphamide is substantially less leukemogenic than melphalan, mechlorethamine, chlorambucil, lomustine, and thiotepa.[8,17,20,89,90,92] The risk of alkylating agent–related AML has been shown to increase with increasing cumulative dose or duration of therapy.[20,89,90] Few studies have attempted to separate the effects of cumulative dose, duration of treatment, and dose intensity, which tend to be highly correlated, but limited evidence to date suggests that cumulative dose may be a pivotal determinant of risk[20,89] (discussed later in Hodgkin's Disease).

The platinating agents cisplatin and carboplatin are among the most important cytotoxic drugs introduced since the 1960s and are widely used to treat many cancers. The platinum compounds, however, demonstrate carcinogenicity *in vitro* and in laboratory animals,[10] forming intrastrand and interstrand DNA cross-links similar to bifunctional alkylating agents. In a population-based study of women with ovarian cancer,[81] cisplatin-based combination chemotherapy was linked to significantly increased risks of leukemia (P trend for cumulative dose $<.001$) in a multivariate model adjusted for other treatment parameters (discussed later in Ovarian Cancer). Future studies should evaluate whether other drug combinations that include platinum might also be linked to elevated risks of leukemia, because it is not clear whether cisplatin acts as a human leukemogen only in combination with selected cytotoxic agents.

The topoisomerase II inhibitors, especially the epipodophyllotoxins, have been implicated in the development of a clinically and cytogenetically distinct type of AML. The International Agency for Research on Cancer (IARC) has concluded that the epipodophyllotoxins etoposide and teniposide are probably carcinogenic to humans.[93] Ratain and coworkers[94] were the first to recognize the potentially leukemogenic properties of etoposide-containing regimens in patients with non–small cell lung cancer, which also has been documented for patients with other types of malignancies.[95–97] As compared with "classic" alkylating agent–induced AML, epipodophyllotoxin-related AML has a shorter induction period (median, 2 to 3 years) and generally lacks a preceding phase of MDS. Furthermore, this type of AML appears to be characterized by balanced translocations involving chromosome bands 11q23, 21q22, and 3q23,[93,98] as well as morphologic features consistent with acute monoblastic or myelomonocytic leukemia (M4 or M5 according to the FAB criteria).[82,99,100] It is unclear whether epipodophyllotoxin-related AML has a better prognosis than "classic" alkylating agent–related AML, which is notoriously resistant to antileukemic treatment.[86,97]

Evidence has accumulated that the anthracyclines doxorubicin and 4-epi-doxorubicin, which are intercalating topoisomerase II inhibitors, may induce a similar type of AML as the one related to epipodophyllotoxin treatment.[17,101,102] In 1987, the IARC concluded that doxorubicin was probably carcinogenic to humans, based on a review of limited data.[88] As with many cytotoxic drugs, an evaluation of the carcinogenic potential of doxorubicin is complicated, because it is typically given in combination with other chemotherapeutic agents, including alkylators.[17,101–103] Curtis et al.[20] found no increase in the risk of leukemia associated with doxorubicin therapy for breast cancer, after adjusting for the effects of alkylating agents and radiotherapy. Although increasing dose of doxorubicin to treat childhood cancer seemed weakly associated with an increased risk of leukemia after adjustment for alkylating agents,[18] the investigators concluded that the excess risk was almost completely attributable to alkylators. In a study of children with Wilms' tumor,[104] the relative risk of leukemia (six cases) after doxorubicin-containing regimens was approximately 14-fold; however, because a relatively constant dose (300 mg/m^2) of doxorubicin was used and data for treatment of relapse were incomplete, evaluation of a dose-response relation was not possible.

The relative leukemogenicity of the anthracyclines and different epipodophyllotoxins is not known. Furthermore, it is unclear whether the schedule of administration or the cumulative dose is the major determinant of leukemia risk (discussed in more detail later in the sections Testicular Cancer and Pediatric Malignancies).[95–97,105,106] In view of the widespread use of epipodophyllotoxins and anthracyclines in curative treatments, continued evaluation of the leukemogenic potential of these agents is urgently needed.[83,106] Detailed descriptions of molecular mechanisms involved in the development of AML after administration of these cytotoxic drugs have been provided elsewhere.[82,83,107–109] As postulated by Pedersen-Bjergaard and Rowley,[82] cytostatic drugs with different mechanisms of action [i.e., direct binding to DNA (alkylating agents) and inhibition of DNA-topoisomerase II (epipodophyllotoxins and anthracyclines)] may have a synergistic effect in leukemogenesis.

The antimetabolites have generally not been regarded as carcinogenic,[88] and Cheson et al.[110] observed that nucleoside analogue therapy for chronic lymphocytic leukemia did not appear to confer a significantly increased risk of second cancer. However, in a report[111] from St. Jude's Children's Research Hospital, it was shown that children with ALL who received cranial irradiation and who had wild-type thiopurine methyltransferase phenotype had an 8.3% cumulative risk of brain cancer, while children with ALL who received irradiation and had a defective phenotype had a 42% risk ($P = .0077$). Patients also had received concurrent systemic chemotherapy with high-dose (75 mg/m^2) 6-mercaptopurine plus high-dose methotrexate. It was hypothesized that the defective thiopurine methyltransferase activity resulted in higher exposures to thioguanine nucleotide metabolites of 6-mercaptopurine during the period of radiation.

Just as the pharmacology of effective cancer chemotherapy is impacted by underlying principles of pharmacokinetics and pharmacodynamics (see Chapter 19.1), these influences likely contribute to the development of secondary leukemia. The possible role of polymorphisms in drug-metabolizing genes, including the cytochrome P-450 enzymes, glutathione S-transferases, and arylamine

N-acetyltransferases in chemotherapy-related leukemias has been reviewed.[112] Felix et al.[113] described an association between CYP3A4 genotype and treatment-related leukemia. Other factors in the development of chemotherapy-related leukemias may include interindividual differences in repair of DNA damage,[114,115] germline mutations in tumor suppressor genes,[76,112] administration of concomitant medications, and interpatient variation in renal and hepatic function. Clarification of the important interrelationships between these factors are critical to a better understanding of individual susceptibility to secondary leukemia. Because cancer patients frequently receive large doses of cytotoxic drugs, interindividual differences in drug absorption, distribution, metabolism, and excretion are accentuated. Until these influences and their interrelationships are better understood, empiric end points, such as the development of acute hematopoietic toxicity after chemotherapy, might be explored for their value as possible surrogate markers of secondary leukemia risk.[89] For cytotoxic agents for which both oral and intravenous formulations are available, the route of administration in describing dose-response associations with secondary leukemia risk should also be taken into account.[81] Whether chemoprotectants such as amifostine (WR-2721), which ameliorates the myelosuppressive effects of alkylating agents[116] and platinum compounds,[117] might possibly contribute to decreased risks of second leukemias should be examined.

Many chemotherapeutic agents are known mutagens and animal carcinogens,[88] and the induction period of solid tumors may be longer than the observation period available in published research. Thus, the question of whether the increased risks of leukemia after chemotherapy might be later followed by excess solid tumors is important. To date, the causal link between cyclophosphamide and bladder cancer represents one of the few established relationships between a specific cytostatic drug and a solid tumor (reviewed later in Non-Hodgkin's Lymphoma).[21,118,119] Elevated risks of bone sarcomas[19,61] and possibly lung cancers[120,121] also have been observed after alkylating agent chemotherapy. The contribution of chemotherapy to radiation-induced solid tumors[50,55,104,111,122] should also be investigated. For example, as discussed in the section Pediatric Malignancies, doxorubicin has been found to potentiate the development of second solid tumors after radiation for Wilms' tumor.[104] The investigators of this study[104] hypothesized that doxorubicin may inhibit the repair of radiation-induced damage, likely through its interaction with DNA topoisomerase II. Newton et al.[123] reported a significantly shorter time to bone sarcoma in children given both anthracyclines and radiation to treat cancer. The radiation enhancement properties of other cytotoxic drugs (e.g., platinum, hydroxyurea, and 5-fluorouracil) have been well described[124]; whether these features might be correlated with increased risk of solid tumors in cancer patients who survive long term after radiotherapy might also be explored.

RISK OF SECOND MALIGNANCY IN PATIENTS WITH SELECTED PRIMARY CANCERS

HODGKIN'S DISEASE

In view of the excellent cure rates that are currently achieved in the relatively young population of Hodgkin's disease patients, it has become increasingly important to evaluate how the occurrence of second cancers affects their long-term survival. Since the first reports of increased second cancer risk in Hodgkin's disease patients in the early 1970s,[125,126] nearly all major treatment centers have evaluated second cancer risk in their patients. An excess of AML in chemotherapy-treated patients and an increased risk of solid tumors in radiotherapy-treated patients have been reported consistently in the literature.[127] The overall risk of selected second malignancies compared with the general population is given in Table 55.7-1, based on a combined analysis of three studies that included a total of 9618 patients.[50,63,128]

The largest relative risk (95-fold) is observed for AML, followed by a 19-fold increased risk for NHL, tenfold excesses for connective tissue and bone cancers, and a ninefold elevated risk for thyroid cancer. Moderately increased risks (two- to five-fold) are observed for a number of solid tumors, such as cancers of the lung, stomach, colon, breast, mouth, and pharynx, as well as melanoma. Because AML and NHL are diseases with a low incidence in the general population, even a high relative risk compared to the population may translate into a low cumulative (actuarial) risk. As shown in Figure 55.7-1, for the entire follow-up period, the cumulative risk of solid tumors far exceeds that of leukemia or NHL.[50] Absolute excess risk is the best measure to judge which subsequent tumors contribute most to the second cancer burden. Table 55.7-1 shows that, compared with the general population, Hodgkin's disease patients experience an excess of 62 malignancies per 10,000 person-years of observation. Solid tumors account for the majority of excess cancers (38 per 10,000 patients per year), with lung cancer contributing 13 excess cases per 10,000 person-years. Leukemia and NHL each account for approximately 12 cases per 10,000 person-years.

The evolution of second malignancy risk over follow-up time varies by tumor site. In the majority of studies, increased leukemia risk is observed as early as 2 to 4 years after initiation of chemotherapy, with peak occurrence between 5 and 9 years and decreasing risks thereafter.[8,13,48,50,57,63] In studies with large numbers of long-term survivors, significantly increased relative risks are still observed for 15 years after first treatment.[13,50,63] The relative risk of NHL is already greatly increased in the first 5 years after treatment. In some studies, the risk remains rather constant over time,[48,55] whereas others report that risk increases with time since treatment.[12,13] The relative risk of solid tumors is minimally elevated in the 1- to 4-year follow-up period and increases steadily with increasing follow-up time from 5 years since first treatment.[12,13,48,50,55,63,84] For several tumor sites (breast, thyroid), the excess risk does not become apparent until after 10 or even 15 years of observation. In the few studies that include data on 20-year survivors, the relative risk of solid tumors continued to increase through the 15- to 20-year follow-up period.[13,39,50,55,57,63,84,122] Almost no data are available on the time course of risk 20 or more years after treatment. In a study of patients diagnosed with Hodgkin's disease before age 40 in the Netherlands, the relative risk of solid tumor development in 25-year survivors was somewhat lower than in the 15- to 24-year follow-up period (RRs of 5.3 and 8.8, respectively; $P = .29$), suggesting that relative risk may decrease in very long-term survivors.[50] In this study, the 25-year risk of developing any second malignancy was 27.7% (95% CI, 23.1% to 32.8%), compared with 4% in the general population (see Fig. 55.7-1).[50] Because the relative risks of leukemia, NHL, and solid tumors each show a distinctive pattern with

TABLE 55.7-1. Relative Risk of Second Cancers after Hodgkin's Disease: Combined Results from Three Large Studies in 9618 Patients

Site or Type	*Observed Cases*	*Expected Cases*	*Relative Risk (O/E Cases)*	*95% Confidence Interval*	*Absolute Excess Risk per 10,000 Patients per Year*
All cancers	747	195.0	3.8	3.6–4.1	62.2
Leukemia	116	5.2	22.3	18.4–26.7	12.5
Acute nonlymphocytic leukemia[a]	63	0.7	94.8	72.9–121	14.9
Non-Hodgkin's lymphoma	112	6.0	18.5	15.2–22.3	12.0
Solid tumors	519	183.8	2.8	2.6–3.1	37.9
Lung	155	36.1	4.3	3.6–5.0	13.4
Mouth and pharynx	18	4.8	3.7	2.2–5.9	1.5
Stomach	29	10.4	2.8	1.9–4.0	2.1
Colon	46	24.3	1.9	1.4–2.5	2.4
Bone	7	0.7	10.1	4.0–20.8	0.7
Connective tissue	15	1.5	9.8	5.5–16.2	1.6
Melanoma	21	5.1	4.1	2.5–6.3	1.8
Female breast	76	28.5	2.7	2.1–3.3	13.2
Bladder	10	9.3	1.1	0.5–2.0	0.1
Thyroid	14	1.5	9.2	5.0–15.4	1.4
Pancreas	8	4.8	1.7	0.7–3.3	0.4
Liver	6	0.9	6.5	2.4–14.2	0.7
Cervix	11	4.3	2.6	1.3–4.6	2.5
Prostate	8	7.3	1.1	0.5–2.1	0.2
All solid tumors except lung cancer	364	147.7	2.5	2.2–2.7	24.4
Gastrointestinal tract	115	48.6	2.4	2.0–2.8	7.0

O/E, observed/expected.
[a]Reported only in refs. 50 and 128.
(Based on results from refs. 50, 63, and 128.)

time since first treatment, the absolute excess risks in 10-year survivors differ greatly from those observed in the entire patient population. Based on combined estimates from two of the studies included in Table 55.7-1,[50,63] lung cancer contributes most to the absolute excess risk in 10-year survivors, with 22 excess cases per 10,000 patients per year, followed by NHL (16 per 10,000 per year), gastrointestinal tract tumors (15 per 10,000 per year), and leukemia (7 per 10,000 per year). In females, breast cancer accounts for most of the absolute excess risk in 10-year survivors (58 per 10,000 per year).[39,50]

For several second malignancies, the association with treatment factors has been investigated in detail. Leukemia after Hodgkin's disease is certainly the most studied malignancy

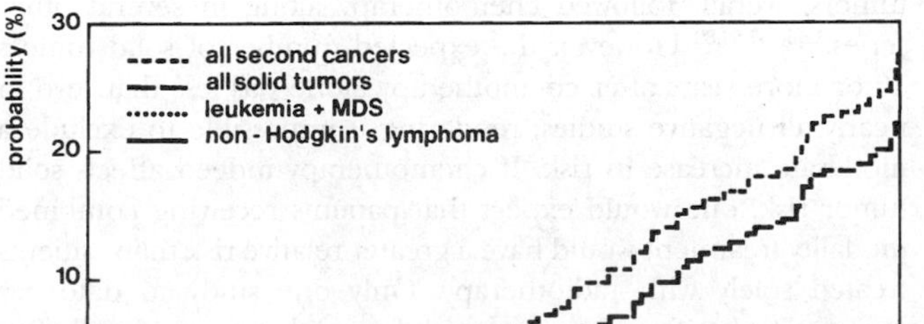

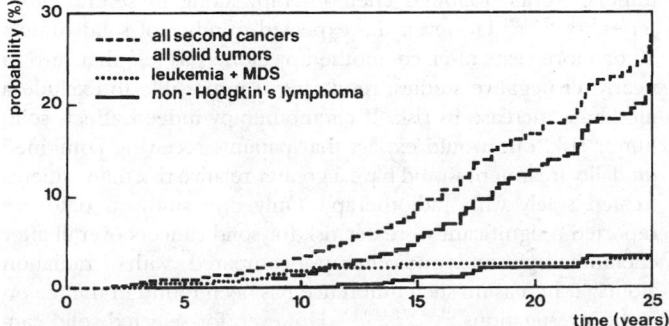

FIGURE 55.7-1. Cumulative risk of second cancers in 1253 patients with Hodgkin's disease diagnosed younger than 40 years of age. MDS, myelodysplastic syndromes. (From ref. 50, with permission.)

induced by treatment, and extensive knowledge of its risk factors has emerged.[127] Radiotherapy alone is associated with very little or no increased risk of leukemia,[12,48,63,84,89] whereas alkylating agent chemotherapy is linked with greatly elevated risk. Several studies have compared the leukemogenicity of different chemotherapy regimens. Risk of AML rises sharply with an increasing number of mechlorethamine, vincristine, procarbazine, and prednisone (MOPP or MOPP-like) cycles.[8,89] The risk associated with 10 to 12 MOPP cycles appears to be approximately three to five times higher than the risk after six MOPP cycles.[8,89] Since the 1980s, MOPP-only chemotherapy has been gradually replaced by doxorubicin, bleomycin, vinblastine, and dacarbazine [ABV(D)]-containing regimens in many centers. Only a few reports have described AML occurrence after ABV(D) alone. Patients treated with ABVD in the Milan Cancer Institute, where this regimen was designed, were shown to have a significantly lower risk of AML than MOPP-treated patients (15-year cumulative risks of 0.7% and 9.5%, respectively).[129] Another study showed that Hodgkin's disease patients treated with MOPP/ABV(D)-containing regimens in the 1980s had a substantially lower risk of AML/MDS than patients treated in the 1970s with MOPP alone (10-year cumulative risks of 2.1% and 6.4%, respectively, $P = .07$).[13] The German-Austrian Pediatric Hodgkin's Disease Group observed a low risk of AML (1.1% at 15 years) after regimens that contained relatively low doses of procarbazine, doxorubicin, and cyclophosphamide, without mechlorethamine.[130]

An important question is whether radiotherapy adds to the leukemia risk associated with chemotherapy. Evidence that combined modality treatment results in greater risk than chemotherapy alone is provided by several reports,[84,129,131] whereas other large series indicate that the risk of AML after combined treatment is comparable to that after chemotherapy alone.[8,12,13,48,57,63,89,91] These inconsistent results may be due partly to differences in treatment regimens between studies but also to lack of adjustment for type and amount of chemotherapy in some reports. The interaction between radiotherapy and chemotherapy could be evaluated most rigorously in the large case-control study by Kaldor and associates,[8] which included 163 cases of leukemia after Hodgkin's disease. When examining the combined effects of radiation dose to the active bone marrow and number of mechlorethamine-procarbazine containing cycles, it was found that, for each category of radiation dose (less than 10, 10 to 20, and more than 20 Gy to the marrow), leukemia risk clearly increased with the number of chemotherapy cycles. In contrast, among patients with a given number of chemotherapy cycles, risk of leukemia did not consistently increase with higher radiation dose. Taken together, the preponderance of available data does not support the hypothesis that the combination of chemotherapy and radiotherapy confers a higher risk of leukemia than chemotherapy alone.

Several studies have identified splenectomy as an independent risk factor for the development of AML,[8,84,91,129,132] with an approximate twofold difference in risk between patients who did and did not undergo a splenectomy. In other reports, however, splenectomy was either not linked or was only weakly related to leukemia risk.[57,131] The mechanism underlying the association with splenectomy remains unclear, but a relationship with immunologic function of the spleen seems likely.[89]

The modifying effect of host-related factors, such as age, on leukemia risk in Hodgkin's disease survivors has been examined in a number of studies and has been reviewed elsewhere.[127] The reported higher *cumulative* risk of AML in older Hodgkin's disease patients as compared to younger ones simply reflects the higher baseline incidence of the disease in older persons. In the few studies that have analyzed *relative* risk of leukemia by age, based on comparisons to general population expectations, no differences between age groups were observed,[12,50,55] or the relative risk of AML was even significantly greater at younger ages than at older ages.[8,63] The risk of AML in relation to treatment-associated acute and chronic bone marrow toxicity has been examined in only one study to date.[89] Significantly increased risks of leukemia were found among patients who developed thrombocytopenia, either in response to initial therapy or during follow-up. After adjustment for type and amount of chemotherapy, patients who showed a decrease of 70% or more in platelet counts after initial treatment had an approximately fivefold higher risk of developing leukemia than patients who showed a decrease of 50% or less. Severe acute thrombocytopenia may indicate greater bioavailability of cytotoxic drugs, which would likely contribute to the development of leukemia.

Although increased risks of NHL after Hodgkin's disease are consistently reported, the causes of the excess risk are not well understood.[127] Because increased risks of NHL occur in immunosuppressed patients, such as transplantation recipients,[133] and because Hodgkin's disease may be accompanied by immunosuppression,[134] several investigators have argued that the elevated risk of NHL may be attributed to Hodgkin's disease itself rather than to its treatment. This view is supported by several studies in which risk did not vary appreciably between treatments.[12,48,55,63] In other studies, however, the risk of NHL was found to be lowest among patients treated with radiotherapy alone and highest among patients who received intensive combined modality treatment, both initially and for relapse.[13,84,135,136] The inconsistent results regarding the relationship with treatment may be partly attributed to diagnostic misclassification—that is, misdiagnosis of the primary tumor as Hodgkin's disease, whereas NHL was represented according to modern lymphoma classification schemes.[127] In only very few studies were diagnostic pathology slides of the second NHL and original Hodgkin's disease reviewed to avoid such misclassification.[13,48] Although transformation to NHL may be part of the natural history of some types of Hodgkin's disease, the role of intensive combined modality treatment and its associated immunosuppression should be explored further.

Increased risks of solid cancers after Hodgkin's disease generally have been attributed to radiotherapy.[12,13,39,48,50,55,57,84,122,127,137] Excesses of melanoma, however, are more likely to be related to immunosuppression accompanying Hodgkin's disease or its treatment, because elevated risks appear as early as in the 1- to 4-year follow-up interval.[63,138] The other sites for which excess solid cancers have been reported (lung, breast, gastrointestinal tract, thyroid, bone, connective tissue) are those for which elevated risks also have been described in other radiation-exposed cohorts.[26,28] One case-control study examined lung cancer risk in relation to the radiation dose to the affected lung area, as well as the modifying effect of the patient's smoking habits.[38] Based on 30 cases of lung cancer in a cohort of 1939 patients with Hodgkin's disease, it was observed that lung cancer risk rose with increasing radiation dose (P trend = .01), with a relative risk of 9.6 (95% CI, 0.93 to 98.0) for patients who received 9 Gy or more as compared to those who received less than 1 Gy. The increase in risk of lung cancer with increasing radiation dose was significantly greater among patients who smoked after diagnosis of Hodgkin's disease than among those who refrained from smoking.

A very important question is whether chemotherapy for Hodgkin's disease can also induce solid cancers, and if so, at which sites. A few studies have raised concern about a possible long-term effect of chemotherapy on lung cancer risk.[48,63,120] The British National Lymphoma Investigation cohort study of 2846 patients[48] showed a significantly increased risk of lung cancer after chemotherapy alone, with the relative risk (4.2; 95% CI, 2.2 to 7.3) of similar magnitude as that observed in patients treated with either extensive radiotherapy or combined modality treatment. A similar excess risk of lung cancer in patients given chemotherapy, but no radiotherapy, was found in a more recent expansion and update of this study.[63] No increased risk of lung cancer, or solid tumors overall, followed chemotherapy alone in several other series.[12,50,57,84,89] However, the expected number of solid tumors 10 or more years after chemotherapy alone was less than two in nearly all negative studies, rendering it impossible to exclude a moderate increase in risk. If chemotherapy indeed affects solid tumor risk, one would expect that patients receiving combined modality treatment would have a greater relative risk than patients treated solely with radiotherapy. Only one study to date has reported a significantly greater risk for solid cancers overall after chemotherapy and radiotherapy compared with irradiation alone,[55] whereas no such difference has been found in the majority of investigations.[12,48,57,84,89,128] However, for selected solid cancer sites (e.g., gastrointestinal tract), larger risks were observed after combined modality treatment than after irradiation alone.[50,63,122] For lung cancer risk in irradiated patients, two case-control studies showed no association with chemotherapy overall, the number of cycles, or the cumulative doses of mechlorethamine and procarbazine,[38,120] which argues against an important contribution of chemotherapy to lung cancer risk.

The inconsistent results reported with regard to the influence of chemotherapy on solid tumor risk may be partly related to the fact that most studies considered all solid tumors combined, whereas chemotherapy may differentially affect the risk of tumors at disparate sites. A study from the Netherlands Cancer Institute demonstrated that the addition of salvage chemotherapy to initial radiotherapy, as compared to initial irradiation alone, did not influence the risk of solid cancers overall but significantly increased the risk of solid tumors other than breast cancer (RR, 9.4, compared to 4.7 for initial irradiation alone).[50] Conversely, patients who received salvage chemotherapy were found to experience significantly lower risks of breast cancer than patients treated with radiotherapy alone (RRs of 2.8 and 7.6, respectively), possibly related to premature ovarian failure due to intensive chemotherapy.[50] Additional studies are warranted to examine which cytotoxic drugs might be responsible for site-specific increased risks of solid tumors.

The strongly elevated risk of breast cancer after radiotherapy for Hodgkin's disease has become a major concern for female survivors.[139–141] In a Dutch study, 27 cases of breast cancer were observed in 544 female patients diagnosed with Hodgkin's disease during adolescence or young adulthood and were followed for an average of 14 years.[50] Women with follow-up equal to or exceeding 15 years had 9.4-fold increased risk of breast cancer as compared with the general population. The risk of developing breast cancer increased dramatically with younger age at first irradiation. Fifteen-year survivors who had radiation treatment before 20 years of age had an 18-fold increased risk of breast cancer; women irradiated at ages 20 to 29 had a sixfold increased risk; and a small, nonsignificant increase was observed for women irradiated at age 30 or older (RR, 1.7). A similar trend, with even larger relative risks, has been reported from Stanford University.[39] An approximately 100-fold increase of breast cancer risk has been observed after treatment at younger than 16 years of age, with relative risks ranging from 17 to 458.[39,55,57,142] This huge variation in estimated risk is not surprising in view of the large differences between series in important variables such as proportion of patients irradiated, duration of follow-up, and completeness of follow-up. Generally, surveys with more complete follow-up have found lower relative risks of breast cancer[50,63,142,143] than those in which completeness of follow-up was less satisfactory or not addressed.[55,57,144] Incomplete follow-up may lead to overestimation of second malignancy risk if patients who remain well lose contact with clinical follow-up, whereas those with second cancer come to attention because of this. The very high *actuarial* risks reported in two U.S. studies (34% at 25 years after first treatment for women treated at younger than 20 years of age,[144] and 35% at 40 years of age for those treated when younger than 16 years[57]) are likely to be exaggerated estimates, not only because of losses to follow-up, but also because the actuarial method is less appropriate when including events that occur at follow-up intervals later than those at which data for most of the patients were censored.[139] In the more recently published Dutch study, with (nearly) complete follow-up, the 25-year actuarial risk of breast cancer amounted to 16%, both for women first treated before the age of 20 and at ages 20 to 30.[50] In two studies, the majority of breast cancers arose within or at the margin of the anterior radiation field, in breast tissue that had received a treatment dose of 40 to 46 Gy.[39,57] Because it is not known whether breast cancer risk is linearly related to radiation dose in the therapeutic dose range, it will be of interest to see whether the reduced mantle field doses in current treatment protocols will result in lower breast cancer risk.

Several studies have demonstrated that age at treatment for Hodgkin's disease is also a crucial determinant of increased relative risks for solid malignancies other than breast cancer.[50,63,122] Van Leeuwen and colleagues[50] reported that the relative risks of nonbreast solid tumors were 4.9, 6.9, and 12.7 for patients first treated at ages 31 to 39, 21 to 30, and 20 or younger, respectively (Table 55.7-2). Data from Stanford University and the United Kingdom show that the highest relative risks for gastrointestinal cancers (approximately eightfold)[63,122] and thyroid cancer[63] occur among patients treated before age 25, with no excesses observed for those treated after 45 years of age. Importantly, Table 55.7-2 demonstrates that the *absolute excess risk* of developing a solid cancer does not show much variation by age at first treatment, probably because the increasing background incidence of solid tumors with age in the population at large outweighs the stronger increase of *relative* risk at younger ages.

The strongly increased relative risks of solid tumors in patients treated for Hodgkin's disease at a young age only become manifest after an extended follow-up period. This might point to a prolonged induction period, but it may also be due to this young patient group reaching an age at which solid tumor incidence begins to rise in the general population. Although a few studies addressed the relative risk of solid malignancies according to attained age,[39,50,122] only one study distinguished the separate contributions of age at first treatment and attained age.[50] Solid tumor risk was greatest among patients treated at a young age (20 years or younger), but the largest relative risk emerged *before* the patients attained the age range at which solid tumors normally occur. Among patients first treated at age 20 or before, the relative risk of developing a solid tumor at ages 40 to 49 was significantly lower than the relative risk of solid tumor development before age 40 (RR, 4.2 vs. 27.9; $P = .0001$). It is notable that a similar finding has been reported with regard to breast cancer risk among atomic bomb survivors in Japan.[145]

In conclusion, the occurrence of treatment-related second cancers is a major problem in survivors of Hodgkin's disease. The substantial increase in solid tumor risk with time since Hodgkin's disease diagnosis necessitates careful, lifelong medical surveillance of all patients. The greatly increased risk of NHL throughout follow-up demonstrates the importance of performing biopsies in recurrent Hodgkin's disease. Because smokers experience a significantly greater risk of lung cancer attributable to radiotherapy than nonsmokers, physicians should make a special effort to dissuade Hodgkin's disease patients from smoking, even before treatment starts. Women treated with mantle field irradiation before age 30 are at greatly increased risk of breast cancer. The importance of regular breast examinations should be explained to them, and they should be taught to perform monthly breast self-examination. From 8 years after irradiation, the follow-up program of these women should include yearly breast palpation and mammography. Physicians should also be alert to the higher risk of gas-

TABLE 55.7-2. Relative and Absolute Excess Risks of Second Cancer in 1253 Patients with Hodgkin's Disease, According to Age at Start of Treatment

Type of Second Cancer and Age at Diagnosis of Hodgkin's Disease	*Observed Cases*	*Relative Risk*	*95% Confidence Interval*	*Absolute Excess Risk per 10,000 Patients per Year*
All malignancies				
≤20	28	13.3	8.8–19.2	58.3
21–30	61	8.2	6.3–10.5	72.2
31–39	48	4.9	3.6–6.4	86.6
Solid tumors				
≤20	25	13.9	9.0–20.6	52.3
21–30	43	6.5	4.7–8.8	49.1
31–39	38	4.2	3.0–5.8	65.9
Breast cancer				
≤20	9	16.9	7.8–32.2	37.8
21–30	12	5.6	2.9–9.8	29.6
31–39	6	2.4	0.9–5.2	18.9
Non-breast solid tumors				
≤20	16	12.7	7.2–20.6	33.2
21–30	31	6.9	4.7–9.8	35.8
31–39	32	4.9	3.4–7.0	57.9
Gastrointestinal cancer				
≤20	7	35.7	14.4–73.6	15.3
21–30	11	10.5	5.3–18.9	13.4
31–39	8	4.3	1.9–8.5	14.0
Non-Hodgkin's lymphoma				
≤20	1	10.3	0.3–57.6	2.0
21–30	6	19.5	7.1–42.4	7.7
31–39	9	26.4	12.1–50.2	19.7
Leukemia				
≤20	2	27.6	3.3–99.5	4.3
21–30	14	73.0	39.9–123	18.6
31–39	2	9.3	1.1–33.4	4.1

(From ref. 50, with permission.)

trointestinal cancers in patients who received paraaortic and pelvic radiation fields. Thorough examination of gastrointestinal complaints is indicated. An important question to be answered in future research is whether, in long-term survivors, chemotherapy contributes to the risk of solid tumors, and if so, which cytotoxic drugs are responsible for the excess risk. The most devastating second malignancy to occur among patients cured of Hodgkin's disease remains chemotherapy-related leukemia. Because the poor prognosis of this complication cannot be changed by early diagnosis, it is promising that leukemia risk has decreased dramatically with the introduction of ABV-based regimens in the 1980s. It is hoped that current treatment protocols that limit the dose and fields of radiotherapy will similarly reduce the late risk of solid cancers.

NON-HODGKIN'S LYMPHOMA

Although surveys in the past[146,147] concluded that NHL patients are not at increased risk for second solid tumors, most either predated the advent of modern therapeutic approaches or lacked sufficient statistical power to detect all but very high risks. Due largely to the introduction of effective treatment, NHL patients now demonstrate a 5-year relative survival rate of approximately 51%.[148] Commensurate with improvements in life expectancy, several large follow-up studies of NHL patients reported significantly increased risks of second cancers.[149,150] In the largest published study to date, the incidence of second malignancies was estimated in 29,153 patients diagnosed with NHL between 1973 and 1987 in one of nine population-based areas participating in the National Cancer Institute's Surveillance, Epidemiology and End Results (SEER) program.[149] Significantly increased risks were observed for all second cancers taken together (observed/expected [O/E] = 1.2; O = 1231), with excesses increasing with follow-up time to reach 1.8 in 10-year survivors. A subsequent international survey of 6171 2-year survivors of NHL confirmed the increased risk of second cancer and showed that significant excesses persisted for two decades.[150] In an update of the SEER program data, which included more than 48,000 patients diagnosed with NHL between 1973 and 1993, significantly increased site-specific risks were observed for cancers of lip (O/E = 2.0), lung (O/E = 1.4), kidney (O/E = 1.3), bladder (O/E = 1.4), thyroid (O/E = 2.0), and bone (O/E = 4.1), as well as AML (O/E = 3.6) (L. Travis, unpublished observations). Although registry-based treatment data are incomplete, it appeared that chemotherapy was related to subsequent AML and to bladder cancer and that

TABLE 55.7-3. Risk of Bladder Cancer According to Cumulative Dose and Duration of Cyclophosphamide Therapy

Cyclophosphamide	*Median Dose or Duration*[a]	*Cases*	*Controls*	*Matched Relative Risk*[b]	*95% Confidence Interval*
CUMULATIVE DOSE					
<20 g[c]	10.0 g	8	22	2.4	0.7–8.4
20–49 g	34.0 g	5	6	6.3[d]	1.3–29.0
≥50 g	87.7 g	5	2	14.5[d,e]	2.3–94.0
DURATION OF THERAPY					
<1 y	6 mo	8	20	2.5	0.7–9.0
1–2 y	18 mo	3	6	3.7	0.6–22.0
>2 y	51 mo	7	4	11.8[d,e]	2.3–61.0

[a]Median cumulative dose of cyclophosphamide or median duration of therapy among all patients within the specified category.
[b]The referent group consists of six case subjects and 42 control subjects who were not treated with cyclophosphamide and who received a radiation dose to the bladder of 0.5 Gy or less. The multivariate model also included terms for patients who received radiotherapy without cyclophosphamide (six case subjects and 16 control subjects).
[c]The minimum cumulative dose of cyclophosphamide in this group was 2.1 g.
[d]$P<.05$.
[e]P for trend <.005.
(From ref. 21, with permission.)

radiotherapy was associated with AML and, possibly, cancers of lung, bladder, and bone.

The excesses of second genitourinary cancers[21,118] and AML[14,90,151–155] have been examined in relationship to treatment for NHL. The largest investigation[21] of secondary bladder tumors was set within a cohort of 6171 2-year survivors of NHL and included 31 patients with transitional cell carcinoma, along with 17 cases of kidney cancer. Detailed information on chemotherapeutic drugs and cumulative dose was collected for all subjects, and radiation dose to the target organ was estimated from individual radiotherapy records. A significant 4.5-fold risk of bladder cancer followed therapy with cyclophosphamide, with risk strongly dependent on cumulative dose (Table 55.7-3).

Significantly elevated sixfold and 14.5-fold risks followed cumulative doses of 20 to 50 g and 50 g or more, respectively (P trend = .004). Neither radiotherapy nor cyclophosphamide was associated with excess kidney cancers. The absolute risk of bladder cancer predicted during 15 years of follow-up was on the order of three excess cancers per 100 NHL patients who had been given cumulative doses of between 20 and 50 g. At cumulative doses of 50 g or more, the excess risk increased to approximately seven bladder cancers per 100 NHL patients.

NHL treatment has been linked to excess risks of AML in several studies,[14,90,151–155] which have been reviewed.[155] Because leukemic progressions of NHL (lymphocytic leukemias) are relatively frequent, histopathologic confirmation of AML diagnosis has been an essential part of all series in which leukemia risk was examined. The largest investigation to date[90] included 11,386 2-year survivors of NHL, among whom 35 cases of AML or MDS were identified. The risk of AML was only weakly associated with the use of cyclophosphamide-containing regimens (RR, 1.8; 95% CI, 0.7 to 4.9) and did not increase with increasing cumulative dose or duration of treatment. However, the median cumulative dose of cyclophosphamide was only 12.5 g, which is considerably lower than in previous studies[14,152] in which nine leukemia cases each were included and substantially higher risks (RR, 105 and 76, respectively) were reported. The weak association between cyclophosphamide at lower dose levels and AML,[90] however, supports other evidence that the drug has a low leukemogenic potential.[8,20,92] Among 10,000 NHL patients treated for 6 months with chemotherapy regimens containing low cumulative doses of cyclophosphamide, an excess of four AMLs might develop in 10 years of follow-up.[90] This is an important conclusion in view of the frequent use of cyclophosphamide-containing regimens in current treatment regimens for NHL. Risk of AML after alkylating agent therapy did not vary significantly by age at NHL diagnosis or gender when evaluated by multivariate methods.

Low-dose total body irradiation (TBI), as used in past treatment approaches for NHL, seems linked with an unusually high occurrence of secondary leukemias.[155,156] This treatment modality used very low individual TBI fraction sizes (most commonly 10 to 15 cGy) given several times a week until a cumulative dose of approximately 150 cGy was administered. The risk of leukemia after low-dose TBI was quantified in a study of 61 2-year NHL survivors who received low-dose TBI as primary therapy.[155] Four patients developed AML (RR, 117 compared with population rates; 95% CI, 31.5 to 300.0). A fifth patient was diagnosed with MDS. All five patients with secondary hematologic malignancies had received salvage treatment with either alkylating agents alone or combined modality therapy. It is noteworthy that the excess risk of AML after low-dose TBI[155] was much greater than the risk observed in the larger international investigation of AML after NHL,[90] although similar chemotherapy regimens were used. Other types of NHL treatment that combine high-dose, large-field radiotherapy with alkylating agents also have been associated with very large risks (100- to 1000-fold) of AML.[14,151] It is likely that the chemotherapy contributed to the excess risk of leukemia, either directly or by enhancing the effect of low-dose TBI.[155] Studies of laboratory animals suggest that low-dose TBI may expand the number of bone marrow stem cells subject to potential transformation by alkylating agents.[157]

Estimates of the cumulative risk of secondary MDS/AML 5 to 6 years after autologous bone marrow transplantation (ABMT) for NHL range from 4% to 18%.[6,158,159] Based on long-term follow-up of a large cohort, Friedberg et al.[160] reported that the actuarial risk at 10 years was approximately 20%, with no evidence of a plateau. Because most lymphoma patients tend to be intensively treated, even before ABMT,[158,159] the roles of prior therapy and the preparative regimen for transplantation in the development of leukemia are difficult to distinguish.[6,158,159] In a review, Traweek et al.[161] concluded that although the available evidence suggests that prior therapy makes a pivotal contribution to risk of secondary leukemia, an ancillary role for the transplantation procedure itself can not be excluded. The investigators[161] suggested that the incidence of leukemia after ABMT for lymphoma might be reduced by earlier transplantation or stem cell harvest (or both) and the screening of bone marrow for karyotypic abnormalities before autologous grafting. Based on analyses of pretransplant specimens, Abruzzese and colleagues[162] suggested that, in many cases of MDS after ABMT, stem cell damage results from prior chemotherapy.

In conclusion, survivors of NHL are at increased risk for a number of second malignancies, albeit much less so than patients with Hodgkin's disease. To date, the excess risks of AML and bladder cancer have been demonstrated to be treatment-related. To assess risk factors for leukemia after ABMT, there is a strong need for a large study with data on prior therapy, the transplant preparative regimen, and the transplantation procedure itself.

TESTICULAR CANCER

The introduction of cisplatin into chemotherapy protocols for testicular cancer represents one of the landmark accomplishments of modern cancer treatment.[163] Testicular cancer is now largely curable, with a 5-year relative survival rate of approximately 95%.[148] Although effective therapy for early-stage seminoma with infradiaphragmatic radiotherapy has been used for many decades, treatment with platinum-based chemotherapy for nonseminoma and advanced seminoma was not widely available until the late 1970s. In the interim period, radiotherapy fields to treat testicular cancer have decreased in size and smaller doses are used,[164] but patients treated with earlier, more aggressive approaches remain at risk for possible late sequelae. Few studies have addressed the long-term risks of second cancers among a sizable number of survivors[85,165–167] that also take into account the histologic type of testicular tumor.[85] The largest study of second malignant neoplasms after testicular cancer included 28,843 1-year survivors diagnosed with a first primary cancer of the testis between 1935 and 1993 and reported to 16 population-based cancer registries in North America and Europe.[85] More than 3300 testicular cancer patients survived more than 20 years after diagnosis. Second cancers, excluding contralateral testis, developed in 1406 patients (O/E = 1.43; 95% CI, 1.36 to 1.51) (Table 55.7-4).

The absolute risk was 16 excess cancers per 10,000 men per year. Significantly elevated risks were observed for all second solid tumors (O/E = 1.4; O = 1251), with significant site-specific excesses for ALL, acute nonlymphocytic leukemia, melanoma, NHL, and cancers of the stomach, colon, rectum, pancreas, prostate, kidney, bladder, thyroid, and connective tissue. Second cancer risk was similar after seminomas (O/E = 1.4) and nonseminomatous tumors (O/E = 1.5), with little variation in site-specific patterns. Increased risks for cancers of small intestine (O/E = 4.4) and rectum (O/E = 1.6) were observed only for seminomas, whereas patients with nonseminomatous germ cell tumors (GCT) showed elevated twofold risks for hepatobiliary cancer. Risk of solid tumors increased with time since diagnosis of testicular cancer to reach 1.5 after 20 years (*P* trend = .00002). Among 20-year survivors, 369 (O/E = 1.5) solid tumors were reported, with significant excesses for cancers of stomach (O/E = 2.3), colon (O/E = 1.7), pancreas (O/E = 3.2), prostate (O/E = 1.4), kidney (O/E = 2.3), bladder (O/E = 2.8), and connective tissue (O/E = 4.7).[85] The actuarial risks of developing any second cancer, excluding contralateral testicular tumors, were 15.7% and 22.6%, respectively, 25 and 30 years after testicular cancer diagnosis. The corresponding population expected risks were 9.3% and 13.1%, respectively. The somewhat higher cumulative risk of second cancer at 25 years for men with seminomas (Fig. 55.7-2) reflects the younger mean age of the patients with nonseminomatous tumors, because the excess cumulative risks were comparable.

Increased risks for cancers of the stomach, bladder and, possibly, pancreas seemed associated with antecedent radiotherapy, whereas leukemia was linked with both prior radiation and chemotherapy. In the past, large doses (mean, 13 to 26 Gy) of radiation could be delivered to the stomach during irradiation of paraaortic lymph nodes for testicular cancer.[85] In prior smaller surveys, a significant eightfold risk of stomach cancer (n = 2) was associated with infra- and supradiaphragmatic irradiation for testicular tumors,[165] and a four- to fivefold risk with was associated with abdominal radiotherapy (n = 10).[166] The study by Travis et al.[85] demonstrated that the increased risks for stomach cancer persisted for at least two decades after diagnosis of testicular cancer. After irradiation for peptic ulcer disease, significant excesses of stomach cancer extend beyond 30 years.[168] A pattern of increasing risk of pancreas cancer with time in the international study,[85] with excesses mainly in testicular cancer patients who received initial radiotherapy, was suggestive of a radiogenic effect, consistent with the location of the pancreas in the radiation field (mean organ dose, 17 to 34 Gy) during therapy for testicular cancer. The pancreas is not considered particularly susceptible to the carcinogenic effects of ionizing radiation,[26] except when very high doses (e.g., on the order of 13 Gy) are given.[168]

Few large, comprehensive studies that quantify the high risk of contralateral testicular cancer (CLTC) have been published,[166,169] which has historically been attributed to common predisposing factors, such as cryptorchism or atrophic testis. Van Leeuwen and colleagues[166] assessed the risk of all second malignancies, including CLTC, in a population-based cohort of 1909 testicular cancer patients for whom complete treatment data and nearly complete follow-up information were available. With a median follow-up of 7.7 years, 20 CLTCs were observed (RR, 35.7; 95% CI, 21.8 to 55.2). Importantly, it appeared that chemotherapy may have reduced the risk of CLTC compared with patients who received radiation or surgery alone.

The increased risk of leukemia after testicular cancer is an order of magnitude lower than that observed in patients with

TABLE 55.7-4. Observed and Expected Numbers of Selected Second Malignant Neoplasms among 1-Year Survivors of Testicular Cancer[a]

	Observed	*Observed to Expected Ratio*	*95% Confidence Interval*
All second cancers[b]	1406	1.4[c]	1.4–1.5
All solid tumors[b]	1251	1.4[c]	1.3–1.4
Esophagus	20	1.3	0.8–2.1
Stomach	93	2.0[c]	1.6–2.4
Small intestine	12	3.2[c]	1.6–5.6
Colon	105	1.3[c]	1.0–1.5
Rectum	77	1.4[c]	1.1–1.8
Liver, gallbladder	26	1.5	1.0–2.1
Pancreas	66	2.2[c]	1.7–2.8
Lung	201	1.0	0.9–1.2
Prostate	164	1.3[c]	1.1–1.5
Kidney	55	1.5[c]	1.1–2.0
Bladder	154	2.0[c]	1.7–2.4
Melanoma	58	1.7[c]	1.3–2.2
Thyroid	19	2.9[c]	1.8–4.6
Bone	6	2.4	0.9–5.3
Connective tissue	22	3.2[c]	2.0–4.8
Non-Hodgkin's lymphoma	68	1.9[c]	1.5–2.4
All leukemia	64	2.1[c]	1.6–2.7
Acute lymphoblastic leukemia	9	5.2[c]	2.4–9.9
Acute nonlymphocytic leukemia	27	3.1[c]	2.0–4.5
Chronic lymphocytic leukemia	7	0.6	0.2–1.2
Chronic granulocytic leukemia	9	0.9	0.4–1.8

[a]Includes 28,843 patients diagnosed with a first primary cancer of the testis who survived 1 or more years.
[b]Numbers exclude contralateral testicular cancers. Category of all solid tumors also excludes lymphohematopoietic disorders.
[c]*P*<.05.
(From ref. 85, with permission.)

Hodgkin's disease. Moderately elevated risks have been observed after chemotherapy,[95,96] but also after irradiation alone.[165,166] Mediastinal nonseminomatous GCTs are known to be associated with an inherent predisposition to develop secondary leukemias,[170] however, such a relationship has not been reported for testicular tumors. In men with mediastinal GCT

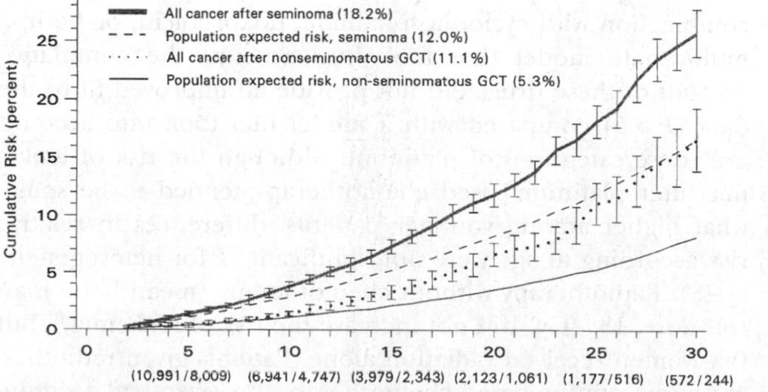

FIGURE 55.7-2. Cumulative risk of second malignant neoplasms among 28,010 1-year survivors of testicular germ cell tumors (GCT). Percentages in parentheses indicate the actuarial risk at 25 years. Within the figure, 95% confidence intervals for point estimates are shown by vertical bars. (From ref. 85, with permission.)

and leukemia, both cancers contain the cytogenetic abnormality *i(12p)* pathognomonic of GCT,[171] consistent with a common derivation.[170] In contrast, cytogenetic studies of leukemias that follow testicular cancer have displayed alterations characteristic of treatment-related AML.[172–174] Analytic studies that have examined the risk of leukemia after testicular cancer have typically excluded mediastinal GCT.

In the early years of platinum-based chemotherapy, the majority of patients received the PVB regimen (cisplatin, vinblastine, bleomycin). The absence of excess leukemia risk after this regimen has been documented in several large studies.[95,166,175–177] In contrast, a number of studies have reported a 20- to 330-fold increased risk of AML after etoposide-containing regimens, which were introduced for the treatment of testicular cancer in the early 1980s.[95,96,172,174] In most of these schedules, etoposide is combined with a platinum compound and other active drugs (bleomycin), but classical alkylating drugs are generally not used. More recently, the IARC concluded that sufficient evidence indicates that etoposide in combination with cisplatin and bleomycin is carcinogenic to humans.[93]

The report by Pedersen-Bjergaard and colleagues[95] was one of the first to note that leukemias induced by epipodophyllotoxins were cytogenetically distinct from classical alkylating agent–related AML. All five cases of AML/MDS were observed in the subgroup of 82 patients who had received cumulative doses of more than 3000 mg/m^2 of etoposide (most patients had three 3-weekly cycles with etoposide, 200 mg/m^2 daily, for 5 days, resulting in a cumulative dose of 3000 mg/m^2). Most etoposide-containing treatment regimens for testicular cancer have used lower cumulative doses of etoposide (up to 2000 mg/m^2) and also a lower dose intensity (100 to 120 mg/m^2). On the basis of the combined data from five studies, Bokemeyer and Schmoll[167] estimated that the relative risk for AML was approximately 20-fold increased in patients treated with conventional etoposide-containing regimens (cumulative dose less than 2000 mg/m^2). Because of the low background incidence of AML in the population, this rather high relative risk translates to a low cumulative risk of 0.6% (95% CI, 0.3 to 0.9%) at 5 years.

In conclusion, patients treated for testicular cancer have less than one-third of the excess risk of second malignancy experienced by patients with Hodgkin's disease. The increased risk of stomach cancer should alert clinicians to the importance of thorough examination of gastrointestinal complaints in patients who received radiotherapy to the paraaortic lymph nodes. Because all reports of increased risks of gastrointestinal cancer have derived from studies in which patients were treated with high doses of radiation, it is important to determine whether smaller risks will follow the lower doses (20 to 25 Gy) that are currently used. Reassuringly, PVB chemotherapy seems to carry a negligible risk of leukemia. Although high-dose etoposide therapy (more than 2000 mg/m^2 in combination regimens) is associated with substantial excess leukemia, cumulative risk after conventional-dose etoposide-containing regimens is low. Radiotherapy regimens for testicular cancer have been modified with the introduction of smaller fields, lower doses, and elimination of prophylactic mediastinal radiation, but the late sequelae of therapy given decades ago continue to emerge. In the future, radiation dose to second cancer sites for which risks are elevated should be estimated in individual patients, along with specific chemotherapeutic agents to further delineate the contribution of treatment factors. Long-term follow-up studies are also needed to evaluate the risk of second solid tumors among testicular cancer patients treated with modern cisplatin-based chemotherapy.[10,81]

OVARIAN CANCER

Because survival for ovarian cancer patients has improved significantly within the last two decades,[148] the study of second primary cancers has assumed increasing clinical importance.[178] The site-specific risk of solid tumors after ovarian cancer has been quantified in a large population-based study of more than 32,000 women with ovarian cancer, including 4402 10-year survivors.[178] Almost 1300 second cancers (n = 1296) were reported, representing a significantly increased risk (O/E = 1.3; 95% CI, 1.2 to 1.4). Significant excesses were observed for cancers of colon (O/E = 1.3), rectum (O/E = 1.4), breast (O/E = 1.2), and bladder (O/E = 2.1), as well as leukemia (O/E = 4.2). Ocular melanoma (O/E = 4.5) was also significantly increased. Secondary leukemia appeared to be linked with antecedent chemotherapy, whereas radiotherapy was associated with cancers of connective tissue, bladder and, possibly, pancreas. The risk of solid tumors was elevated during all follow-up intervals, including 10 to 14 years (O/E = 1.3) and 15 years or more (O/E = 1.3) after ovarian cancer. Fifteen-year survivors experienced significant excesses of cancers of pancreas, bladder, and connective tissue. The cumulative risk of second cancers at 20 years was 18.2% compared with a population-expected risk of 11.5% (Fig. 55.7-3).

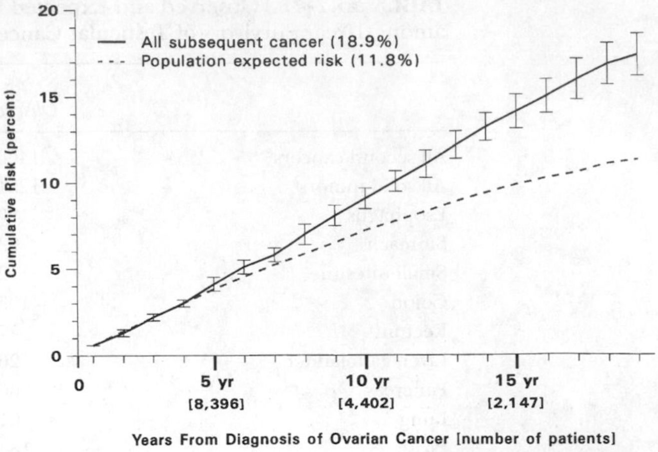

FIGURE 55.7-3. Cumulative risk of second malignant neoplasms among 32,251 2-month survivors of ovarian cancer. Percentages in parentheses are actuarial risk at 20 years. Within the figure, 95% confidence intervals for point estimates are shown by vertical bars. (From Travis LB, Curtis RE, Boice JD Jr, et al. Second malignant neoplasms among long-term survivors of ovarian cancer. *Cancer Res* 1996;56:1564, with permission.)

In an analytic study of bladder cancer after ovarian cancer, Kaldor et al.[119] found increased risks after radiotherapy only (RR, 1.9; 95% CI, 0.8 to 4.9) compared with patients treated with surgery alone. Cyclophosphamide-based chemotherapy, with or without radiotherapy, was associated with a fourfold risk.

Large risks of AML and preleukemia have been documented after ovarian cancer, and they have been linked to therapy with melphalan,[17,92] cyclophosphamide,[17,80,92] and chlorambucil.[17,179] In one large population-based study of more than 28,000 ovarian cancer patients in whom 96 leukemias were diagnosed, platinum-based combination chemotherapy was associated with a significantly increased fourfold risk compared with women who received neither alkylating drugs nor radiotherapy.[81] Excesses of leukemia increased with increasing cumulative platinum dose (P trend for dose <.001) (Table 55.7-5).

Although the platinating agents were frequently given in combination with cyclophosphamide, doxorubicin, or both, a multivariate model that took into account the cumulative amount of these drugs did not provide an improved fit to the data (P >.5) compared with a model that took into account only dose categories of platinum. Although the risk of leukemia after platinum-based chemotherapy tended to be somewhat higher among younger patients, differences in relative risk according to age were not significant (P for heterogeneity = .48). Radiotherapy without chemotherapy (mean bone marrow dose, 13.4 Gy) did not increase the risk of leukemia,[81] but few women received radiation alone. Patients given radiotherapy and platinum-based chemotherapy, however, had a significantly (P = .006) higher risk of leukemia than those who received platinum-based chemotherapy alone in a multivariate model adjusted for cumulative amount of the drug. A dose response was observed for platinum among women treated and not treated with radiotherapy, with risks higher within the radi-

TABLE 55.7-5. Risk of Leukemia According to the Cumulative Dose of Platinum, Duration of Therapy, and Specific Drug[a]

Dose and Duration	*Number of Patients with Leukemia*	*Number of Matched Control Patients*	*Median Value in Controls*[b]	*Relative Risk (95% Confidence Interval)*[c]
All platinum drugs				
Dose[d]				
<500 mg	4	30	418 mg	1.9 (0.5–7.9)
500–749 mg	5	28	600 mg	2.1 (0.6–8.0)
750–999 mg	7	25	896 mg	4.1 (1.1–14.8)
>1000 mg	11	20	1230 mg	7.6 (2.3–25.3)[e]
Duration				
<6 mo	3	36	5.4 mo	1.2 (0.3–5.5)
6–12 mo	16	49	8.5 mo	4.3 (1.4–12.9)
>12 mo	8	18	14.2 mo	7.0 (1.8–26.6)[f]
Specific drug				
Cisplatin	19	85	600 mg	3.3 (1.1–9.4)
Carboplatin	3	9	3300 mg	6.5 (1.2–36.6)
Both	5	9		9.0 (2.2–37.6)
Cisplatin			720 mg	
Carboplatin			2200 mg	

[a]The data are limited to 27 patients with leukemia and 103 controls who receive platinum-based chemotherapy without melphalan.
[b]The values shown are median cumulative doses of platinum and the median duration of therapy among controls.
[c]The reference group consisted of six patients with leukemia and 94 controls who were not exposed to platinum derivatives of other alkylating drugs.
[d]Cumulative amounts of carboplatin were divided by 4 to convert them to cisplatin-equivalent doses.
[e]*P* for trend <.001.
[f]*P* for trend = .001.
(From ref. 81, with permission.)

ation group; in all of the latter patients, radiotherapy had been given as part of initial treatment. It is unlikely that women newly diagnosed with ovarian cancer would receive both platinum and radiotherapy in view of modern treatment recommendations.[180] However, the possibility that the risk of leukemia after treatment with platinum might be increased by radiotherapy should be investigated among patients with other cancers, especially cancers of bladder and head and neck, given therapeutic strategies to increase dose intensities of both modalities in the treatment of these tumors.[181]

The risk of leukemia associated with the cumulative dose of melphalan[17,92] and, importantly, route of administration[81] also has been evaluated among women with ovarian cancer. In the largest study to date,[81] significant excesses of leukemia followed intravenous (RR, 22.9) and oral (RR, 9.0) melphalan, and risks increased with increasing cumulative dose and duration of therapy. Intravenous melphalan was six times more leukemogenic than platinum.

In conclusion, survivors of ovarian cancer experience significantly increased risks of secondary leukemias and solid tumors. Despite the elevated relative risk of leukemia after modern platinum-based chemotherapy for ovarian cancer, the absolute risk is small.[81] Of 10,000 ovarian cancer patients treated for 6 months with cumulative doses of cisplatin between 500 and 1000 mg or 1000 mg or more and followed for one decade, an excess of 21 and 71 leukemias, respectively, was predicted based on observed risks.[81] Thus, Travis and colleagues[81] concluded that the significant improvement in clinical response provided by platinum-based treatment for advanced ovarian cancer, with 5-year survival rates of up to 20% to 30%,[180,182] far exceeded the relatively small excesses of leukemia. Further interdisciplinary investigations are needed to elucidate the carcinogenic risks associated with modern therapies for ovarian cancer and with shared susceptibility mechanisms, including genetic and reproductive factors. Meanwhile, in proposing recommendations for the follow-up and management of women with ovarian cancer,[180] it is important to recognize their long-term predisposition to an array of second cancers.

BREAST CANCER

Numerous studies have demonstrated that women with breast cancer are at a three- to fourfold increased risk of developing a new primary cancer in the contralateral breast.[183,184] Significant excesses relative to the general population also have been observed for cancers of the ovary,[183,185] uterus,[183,186,187] lung,[58,183,185,188,189] esophagus,[190] colon-rectum,[183,185,187] connective tissue,[183,189,191–193] and thyroid,[183,185] as well as melanoma[183,189] and leukemia.[101,185,189,194] For some of these cancers, such as those of the contralateral breast, ovary, and uterus, and possibly melanoma, the excesses may be fully or partly explained by a common etiology (e.g., genetic predisposition or hormonal risk factors). Other excess risks may be treatment-related or reflect the interaction of several factors. Adjuvant chemotherapy, hormonal treatment, and radiotherapy, and combinations of these modalities, are being administered to a growing proportion of breast cancer patients. In view of the proven therapeutic benefit of these treatments[195,196] and the prolonged life expectancy of those treated, it has become exceedingly important to evaluate the carcinogenic potential of adjuvant treatment.

Contralateral breast cancer accounts for 40% to 50% of all second tumors in women with breast cancer,[183] and the 15-year cumulative risk of developing contralateral disease amounts to 10% to 13%.[197,198] With this high risk, even small effects of treatment may have a large impact in terms of absolute numbers of contralateral breast cancers. The effect of radiation treatment for the initial breast cancer was evaluated in two large case-control studies in Connecticut and Denmark that involved 655 and 529 women with contralateral breast cancer, respectively. The mean radiation doses to the contralateral breast were estimated at 2.8 and 2.5 Gy, respectively.[22,199] Both studies found that radiotherapy did not contribute to the high risk of contralateral disease among women treated after the age of 45. In the Connecticut study, however, significantly elevated risks were observed for women who underwent irradiation before the age of 45, with a radiation-associated relative risk of 1.9 among those who survived for at least 10 years.[22] Significant excess risk in women irradiated at a young age was not found in the Danish study, possibly because it included fewer women younger than 45 years of age.[199] Based on the Connecticut study, Boice and associates[22] estimated that approximately 11% of all second breast cancers in women irradiated before age 45 could be attributed to radiotherapy.

Several large studies have shown that hormonal treatment with tamoxifen reduces the risk of contralateral breast cancer by approximately 40%.[186,187,195,200,201] Data collected by the Early Breast Cancer Trialists' Collaborative Group (EBCTCG), based on 37,000 women from 55 trials, demonstrated that longer durations of tamoxifen use were associated with greater reductions in risk, such that 1 year, 2 years, and 5 years of treatment produced risk reductions of 13%, 26%, and 47%, respectively.[195] It is not yet known whether the protective effect of tamoxifen against contralateral disease persists over prolonged follow-up periods (more than 10 years). Some studies have provided evidence that adjuvant chemotherapy may also reduce the risk of contralateral breast cancer, a phenomenon that is likely to be mediated through drug-induced premature ovarian failure.[153,196,202]

Several studies have assessed the risk of leukemia after adjuvant chemotherapy and radiotherapy for breast cancer. The relationship between AML risk and drug dose was examined in detail in the large case-control study by Curtis and associates.[20] These investigators identified 90 cases of leukemia or MDS among 82,700 women diagnosed with breast cancer between 1973 and 1985 in five areas of the United States. Compared with patients treated without alkylating agents and irradiation, the risk of AML was significantly elevated after locoregional radiotherapy alone (RR, 2.4), after treatment with alkylating agents alone (RR, 10.0) and after treatment with alkylating agents in combination with radiotherapy (RR, 17.4). The risk of AML associated with combined modality treatment was significantly greater than that for alkylating agents alone ($P = .02$). The study included large numbers of women who had been treated with only one alkylating agent, including cyclophosphamide. Cumulative cyclophosphamide doses of less than 20 g were associated with an approximately twofold, nonsignificant increase in risk (compared with women not exposed to alkylating agents), whereas women treated with 20 g or more had a 5.7-fold risk of AML (95% CI, 1.6 to 20.6). Women who received melphalan experienced tenfold risks of AML compared with women treated with cyclophosphamide ($P < .001$). After adjustment for the effects of chemotherapy, the risk of AML increased significantly with higher doses of radiation to the active bone marrow, with a sevenfold risk increase for patients who received 9 Gy or more (compared to patients not treated with radiotherapy).

Present-day adjuvant treatment of early breast cancer is in several ways different from the treatments evaluated in this large study by Curtis et al.[20] In the 1980s, the cumulative doses of cyclophosphamide were reduced [approximately 12 to 15 g with six standard cycles of CMF (cyclophosphamide, methotrexate, and fluorouracil) or FAC (fluorouracil, doxorubicin, and cyclophosphamide)]. Regional radiotherapy is less frequently used. On the basis of their data, Curtis and associates[20] estimated that, among 10,000 patients with breast cancer treated for 6 months with a cyclophosphamide-based regimen and followed for 10 years, an excess of only five cases of treatment-related AML would be expected to develop.

The low risk of AML after CMF-based chemotherapy was confirmed by the Milan Cancer Institute[203] and the Eastern Cooperative Oncology Group,[204] with cumulative risks of AML of 0.23% at 15 years and 0.18% at 7 years, respectively. Thirty-nine percent of women treated with CMF-based chemotherapy in the Milan series[203] also received doxorubicin, and no clear evidence indicated a synergistic effect of cyclophosphamide and doxorubicin on leukemia risk. Radiation therapy (applied only after breast-conserving surgery) did not add to the risk of AML. The University of Texas M. D. Anderson Cancer Center has reported a higher risk of leukemia after standard dose–intensity FAC treatment. Fourteen cases of leukemia were observed among 1474 patients, for an estimated cumulative risk of 1.5% (95% CI, 0.7 to 2.9) at 10 years. The risk of AML was significantly higher when chemotherapy was given in combination with radiotherapy (2.5% vs. 0.5%).[103]

There has been an increasing trend toward the use of dose intensification strategies in chemotherapy protocols for breast cancer. Typically, these regimens contain high-dose cyclophosphamide in combination with one of the anthracyclines (doxorubicin or 4-epidoxorubicin) and other active drugs. The risk of AML associated with such dose-intensive chemotherapy has not yet been quantified, but evidence suggests that the combination of anthracyclines and alkylating agents (including cisplatin) may be leukemogenic.[101] With the increasing tendency to administer high doses of cytotoxic drugs accompanied by bone marrow support, there is certainly a strong need to closely monitor the subsequent risk of AML.

Patients treated with CMF-based chemotherapy have not been reported to be at increased risk of solid tumors.[203,205] More prolonged follow-up, however, is needed to evaluate possible carcinogenic effects 15 years or more after treatment.

Conclusive evidence has emerged that tamoxifen is associated with a moderately increased risk of endometrial cancer.[186,187,195,200,206–210] The consistent results across studies with different designs, the duration-response relationship observed in several investigations,[206,207,209,211,212] and the established estrogen-agonist effects of tamoxifen on the endometrium[213–215] strongly support a causal relationship.[208] The individual studies, which are summarized in Table 55.7-6, show that the use of tamoxifen for 2 years is associated with an approximately twofold increased risk of endometrial cancer, whereas use for 5 or more years produces four- to eightfold excess risks. Although the risk estimates in some studies may be affected by a certain degree of detection bias as a result of gynecologic examinations in women with side effects from tamoxifen, the magnitude of the observed risk is unlikely to be explained by such bias.[208] Furthermore, the analysis of the EBCTCG not only shows increased incidence of endometrial cancer in women randomized to tamoxifen treatment (as compared to women not randomized to tamoxifen) but also significantly increased

TABLE 55.7-6. Risk of Endometrial Cancer after Tamoxifen Therapy in Women with Breast Cancer

Author[a]; Design	*Number of Breast Cancers*	*Number of Endometrial Cancers (Number in Tamoxifen Users)*	*Dosage Evaluated*	*Duration of Tamoxifen Use*	*Relative Risk (95% Confidence Interval)*
Fisher et al. 1994[186]; clinical trial	4063	24 (23)	20 mg	Planned: ≥5 y	Tamoxifen vs. control: 7.5 (1.7–32.7) Tamoxifen vs. general population: 2.2[b] Tamoxifen vs. control other trial: 2.3[b]
Rutqvist et al. 1995[187]; clinical trial	4914	42 (34)	30–40 mg	48 wk–5 y	Any: 4.1 (1.9–8.9)
EBCTCG 1998[195]; clinical trials	36,689	124 (92)	Mostly 20 mg	1, 2, or 5 y	Ever use: 2.6 (2.2–2.9) 5 y: 4.2 (*P*<.001)
Fisher et al. 1998[210]; prevention trial	13,388	51 (36)	20 mg	1–5 y	Any: 2.5 (1.4–5.0)
Curtis et al. 1996[200]; cohort (SEER-based)	87,323	457 (73)	Unknown	Unknown	Any tamoxifen vs. general population: 2.0 (1.6–2.6) No tamoxifen vs. general population: 1.2 (1.1–1.4)
Sasco et al. 1996[207]; case-control	NA	43 (29)	Mostly 20 mg	Varied	Any: 1.4 (0.6–3.5) ≥5 y: 3.5 (0.9–12.7) Trend with duration: *P*=.0001
Mignotte et al. 1998[212]; case-control	NA	135 (91)	20–40 mg	Varied	Ever use: 3.1 (1.1–8.7) ≥5 y: 10.7 (3.4–34) Trend with duration: *P*=.0001
Bernstein et al. 1999[209]; case-control	NA	324 (146)	Mostly 20 mg	Varied	Ever use: 1.5 (1.1–2.2) ≥5 y: 4.1 (1.7–9.5) Trend with duration: *P*=.0002
Bergman et al. 1998[211]; case-control	NA	299 (108)	20–40 mg	Varied	Ever use: 1.5 (1.1–2.0) ≥5 y: 6.6 (2.2–19.7) Trend with duration: *P*<.001

EBCTCG, Early Breast Cancer Trialists' Collaborative Group; NA, not available; SEER, Surveillance, Epidemiology and End Results.
[a]Several early reports are not presented because the data are included in larger or updated studies presented here.[187,209,211]
[b]Because the incidence of endometrial cancer appeared to be unexpectedly low among placebo-treated women, the investigators reestimated the risk associated with tamoxifen, using population-based rates and information from another trial. However, the resulting risk estimates of 2.2 and 2.3, respectively, are less valid than the estimate based on the endometrial cancer rate in placebo-allocated controls (relative risk, 7.5) because (a) regardless of treatment, a population of breast cancer patients entered into a clinical trial may have different endometrial cancer rates than the general population; and (b) the rates used were from a different geographic area, a different period, or both.[208]

mortality due to endometrial cancer.[195] From Table 55.7-6, it is clear that elevated risks of endometrial cancer have been observed after daily tamoxifen dosages of 20 mg, 30 mg, or 40 mg. In the Netherlands case-control study, which included different dose intensities, daily dosage did not affect endometrial cancer risk in a model accounting for duration of use, and the duration-response trends were similar, with daily doses of 40 mg, or 30 mg or less.[211] Very few studies have addressed the risk for ex-users. In three investigations,[209,211,212] recent and former users of tamoxifen were found to experience very similar increases in risk; however, only a few patients had discontinued tamoxifen more than 2 years before the diagnosis of endometrial cancer.

Only two studies have addressed the combined effects of tamoxifen and other risk factors for endometrial cancer.[209,211] In the largest study conducted to date, Bernstein and colleagues[209] reported that women who previously used estrogen replacement therapy experienced greater increases in endometrial cancer risk associated with tamoxifen use than women not exposed to estrogen replacement therapy. Furthermore, the effects of tamoxifen on endometrial cancer risk were stronger among heavy women than among thin women. In the Dutch study, however, body weight did not modify the increased risk associated with tamoxifen use.[211]

An important question is whether the clinicopathologic characteristics and ultimate prognosis of endometrial cancers after tamoxifen treatment are different from those in patients not treated with tamoxifen. In four small studies, the stage distribution and histologic features of endometrial cancers in tamoxifen-treated women were not remarkably different from those diagnosed in nontreated women.[186,200,206,216] Magriples and colleagues,[217] however, reported a higher frequency of poorly differentiated and high-grade tumors with a poor prognosis in tamoxifen-treated patients. In the Dutch study, which included 309 patients with endometrial cancer after breast cancer, endometrial tumors of FIGO stage III and IV occurred

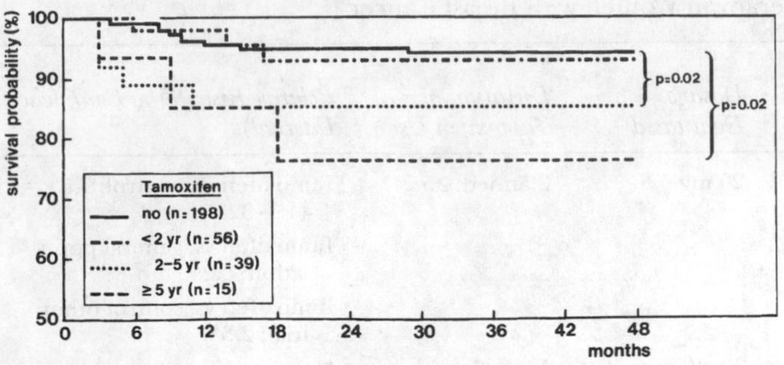

FIGURE 55.7-4. Actuarial endometrial cancer–specific survival according to duration of tamoxifen use. (From ref. 211, with permission.)

more frequently among long-term tamoxifen users (2 or more years) than in nonusers (17% vs. 5%, $P = .006$). Based on a centralized review of diagnostic pathology slides, long-term tamoxifen users more often developed malignant mixed mesodermal tumors or sarcomas of the endometrium than did nonusers (15% vs. 3%, $P = .02$). Furthermore, the tumors diagnosed among long-term tamoxifen users were more often p53-positive and estrogen receptor–negative. Figure 55.7-4 shows that the 3-year actuarial endometrial cancer–specific survival in this study was significantly worse for long-term tamoxifen users than for nonusers, largely due to the less favorable tumor characteristics associated with tamoxifen use.[211] The association between tamoxifen use and specific clinicopathologic and molecular characteristics of subsequent endometrial cancer deserves further investigation in large studies.

Animal experiments have shown that tamoxifen can act as a hepatic carcinogen in rats.[218,219] However, no increased risk of hepatocellular cancer in tamoxifen-treated patents has been observed to date.[186,187,195,200] In the large metaanalysis of the EBCTCG, women randomized to tamoxifen had a slightly lower mortality from primary liver cancer than the control group.[195] The joint analysis of Scandinavian tamoxifen trials showed an elevated risk of gastrointestinal cancer after tamoxifen use (RR, 1.9; 95% CI, 1.2 to 2.9)[187]; however, the excess risk was due to colorectal and stomach cancer, not liver cancer. Furthermore, a study from the SEER program found that tamoxifen was associated with a 50% increased risk of colorectal cancer in the period 5 or more years after diagnosis.[220] No such risk increase was observed in the EBCTCG data.[195]

Increased risks of lung cancer after breast cancer have been largely attributed to radiotherapy.[58,188,221] No appreciable risk increase has been observed within 10 years of treatment, but two- to threefold elevated risks have been reported in 10-year survivors.[58,188,189] The association between breast radiotherapy and subsequent lung cancer risk was found to be stronger for the ipsilateral lung, which supports a radiogenic effect.[188,221] Using individual patient dosimetry, Inskip and associates[58] assessed the effect of radiation dose to the lung in a case-control study of lung cancer after breast cancer. Sixty-one lung cancers were identified among 8976 10-year survivors of breast cancer treated in Connecticut between 1935 and 1971. Mean radiation dose was 15 Gy to the ipsilateral lung and 4.6 Gy to the contralateral lung. A nonsignificant increase in lung cancer risk was noted with increasing radiation dose to the affected lung, with an approximate threefold excess risk for patients who received 5 to 10 Gy. Risk seemed to level off at doses higher than 10 Gy, as has been observed in a similar study of lung cancer after Hodgkin's disease.[38] The results were used to predict that, among 10,000 10-year survivors of breast cancer who received an average lung dose of 10 Gy, approximately nine radiogenic lung cancers would be expected to develop per year. Current radiotherapy practices for breast cancer involve high-energy megavoltage treatment to localized radiation fields, which results in considerably lower lung doses than the orthovoltage and cobalt-60 radiation treatments used in the studies described above. The risk of radiogenic lung cancer should be correspondingly lower (i.e., approximately one excess lung cancer per 10,000 women-years per Gy) beginning 10 years after radiotherapy.[58] In one study, smokers were found to be at greater risk of radiation-associated lung cancer than nonsmokers.[221,222]

Heightened concern with regard to the subsequently increased risk of angiosarcomas in the irradiated conserved breast has been expressed.[192,193] In a nationwide study, 21 Dutch patients with angiosarcoma of the breast after breast-conserving treatment and localized radiation were reported, with a median latency of 6 years.[193] The incidence of angiosarcoma in the breast was estimated at 1.6 per 1000 patients treated with breast conservation per year. Although the absolute excess risk is small, the relative risk is more than 1000-fold increased in comparison with the incidence of this very rare disease in the general population. In a nationwide case-control study in Sweden[191] of 116 women with soft tissue sarcoma after a diagnosis of breast cancer between 1958 and 1992, it was found that the risk of sarcomas other than angiosarcoma increased with the amount of radiation, but stabilized at high doses. The study included 40 angiosarcomas (located mostly in the ipsilateral arm, with only two cases in conserved breasts). The risk of angiosarcoma was 9.5-fold increased in women with lymphoedema of the arm, but radiotherapy was not a risk factor.

In conclusion, only part of the elevated risk of second malignancies after breast cancer is due to treatment. The intrinsically increased risk of developing a contralateral tumor is unlikely to be meaningfully affected by current radiotherapy for the initial breast cancer, whereas tamoxifen reduces the risk of contralateral disease. Standard dose–intensity CMF treatment is associated with a low excess risk of leukemia, whereas conventional FAC treatment may be associated with a somewhat higher risk. Whether the risk of leukemia will increase further with the introduction of dose-intensification strategies should be explored. Although tamoxifen causes a moderate increase in endometrial cancer risk, the proven clinical benefit of this drug in controlling breast cancer[195] far outweighs the excess morbidity and mortality due to endometrial cancer. Clinicians should be alert to signs and symptoms in women taking tamoxifen, and long-term users should be advised to seek prompt gynecologic evaluation on the development of symptoms. The effectiveness of screening for endometrial cancer has not been demonstrated. Consequently, outside of research settings, there is no basis for regular gynecologic examinations in asymptomatic patients taking tamoxifen. The absolute excess risk of lung cancer is likely to be small with current radiotherapy techniques for breast cancer. Nevertheless, there is ample reason to advise breast cancer patients to stop smoking when they receive radiation treatment.

PEDIATRIC MALIGNANCIES

Survival rates for children with cancer have improved substantially since the late 1970s. Consequently, a rapidly growing young population is subject to the late effects of cancer treatment for life. The overall pattern of second cancer risk in the population of childhood cancer survivors has been described in several large studies.[51,62,223–225] Most recently, de Vathaire and colleagues[51] reported on the long-term risk of second cancer in a cohort of 4400 3-year survivors of childhood cancer (excluding patients with leukemia) treated in eight centers in France and the United Kingdom. The risk of second solid malignancies was increased 9.2-fold compared to the general population (95% CI, 7.6 to 11.0), and the absolute excess risk was 188 cases per 10,000 patients per year. The 30-year cumulative risk was 7.7% (95% CI, 5.0 to 8.2%). Olsen and collaborators[223] observed a 3.6-fold increased risk of second malignancy (95% CI, 3.1 to 4.1) in 30,880 children diagnosed with cancer and reported to the population-based cancer registries of five Nordic countries between 1943 and 1987. The cumulative risks of developing a second tumor within 25 years were 3.7% and 3.5%, respectively. Among 9170 2-year survivors of childhood cancer who were treated by members of the U.S. Late Effects Study Group (LESG), the risk of developing a second malignancy was increased 15-fold compared to the general population (95% CI, 13 to 17), with a cumulative incidence of 12.1% at 25 years.[62] The lower risks in the European studies may be related to their population-based nature (less selection),[223,224] to treatment differences between Europe and the United States, and to differences between the study populations with respect to calendar years of diagnosis and length of follow-up. In all studies, the largest relative risks were found for second primary bone tumors (133-fold and 43-fold increased risks in the LESG[225] and British cohort,[224] respectively) and second soft tissue sarcoma. Large risks were also observed for second thyroid cancer, gastrointestinal cancers, brain tumors, and leukemia. Retinoblastoma is the initial malignancy that has been consistently associated with the highest risk of subsequent tumors.[51,62,223,224]

Only a portion of the excess second cancer risk in survivors of childhood cancer is related to treatment. Retinoblastoma is the prototype of an initial malignancy in which genetic factors are responsible for a large part of subsequent cancers. Familial retinoblastoma is caused by inherited mutations of the RB1 tumor suppressor gene, which has been localized to the long arm of chromosome 13q14.[226,227] Approximately 80% of hereditary retinoblastoma patients have bilateral disease. In a long-term follow-up study of 1604 1-year survivors of retinoblastoma diagnosed between 1914 and 1984 (median follow-up, 20 years), the incidence of second cancers as well as risk factors for second malignancy were evaluated.[69] Overall, the risk of second malignancy was increased 17-fold compared to the general population expectation. The excess risk was restricted to the 961 patients with hereditary retinoblastoma (RR, 30; 95% CI, 26 to 47), with strongly increased relative risks for cancers of the bone, soft tissues, nasal cavities, and brain, and for melanoma (relative risks of 446, 103, more than 100, 14, and 51, respectively). No significantly increased risk of second malignancy was observed among 643 nonhereditary retinoblastoma patients (RR, 1.6; 95% CI, 0.7 to 3.1). Fifty years after retinoblastoma diagnosis, the cumulative risk of second primary cancer was 51.0% (± 6.2%) in hereditary cases, and only 5.0% (± 3.0%) in nonhereditary cases. As shown in Figure 55.7-5, radiotherapy significantly increased the risk of second cancers in patients with hereditary retinoblastoma (50-year cumulative risk of 58% vs. 27% in nonirradiated hereditary patients). Radiotherapy did not significantly affect risk in nonhereditary retinoblastoma patients.[69] In a case-control investigation that included 52 patients with bone sarcoma, 31 with soft tissue sarcoma, and 89 controls without sarcoma, Wong and associates[69] also collected individual radiation dosimetry data. For all sarcomas combined, risk was significantly elevated at all dose levels, even at 5.0 to 9.9 Gy, and a significant increase in risk was observed with increasing radiation dose to the site of tumor (relative risk of 11 for doses of 60 Gy or more as compared with doses of 0 to 4.9 Gy) For the first time in humans, a radiation dose-response relationship was also demonstrated for soft tissue sarcoma, with a 12-fold risk increase at doses of 60 Gy or greater. Osteosarcomas and soft tissue sarcomas developing after hereditary retinoblastoma harbor similar RB1 mutations as those found in retinoblastoma.[228,229] Radiation is thus likely to cause somatic mutations needed to produce sarcomas in carriers of germline RB1 mutations.

Wilms' tumor is another example of an initial malignancy in which genetic predisposition contributes to the excess risk of second cancers.[225] The National Wilms' Tumor Study Group reported on the second malignancy experience of 5278 patients followed for an average of 7.5 years.[104] Forty-three second malignancies were observed, with an overall relative risk of 8.4 (95% CI, 6.1 to 11.4). The 15- and 20-year cumulative risks of developing a second tumor were 1.6% and 3.8%, respectively. Significant excesses were seen for leukemia (RR, 7.0), lymphoma (RR, 9.0), osteosarcoma (RR, 19), soft tissue sarcoma (RR, 22), and hepatocellular carcinoma (RR, 56)[104] (N. E. Breslow, written communication, April 1996). Among patients not treated with radiation or doxorubicin, risk of second malignancy was increased threefold, reflecting genetic predisposition.[104] Each 10 Gy of abdominal irradiation was found to increase second malignancy risk by 43% in the absence of doxorubicin and by 78% in its presence. Treatment with both doxorubicin and more than 35 Gy of abdominal irradiation was associated with a relative risk of 36 (95% CI, 16 to 72).[104] Because the small numbers of individual second malignancies precluded an analysis by site, it is unclear whether these results apply equally for leukemia, sarcoma, and other tumors.

ALL, the most common malignancy in childhood, is also associated with an increased risk of subsequent cancer. In a series of 9720 childhood ALL patients treated in trials of the Children's Cancer Study Group between 1972 and 1988, the risk of developing a second malignancy was increased 6.9-fold as compared with the general population.[230] The associated 10- and 15-year cumulative risks were 1.5% and 2.5%, respectively. In a multicenter Italian study including 1664 ALL patients, the relative risk of all second cancers was 13.6, with cumulative risks of 2.6% and 4.5%, respectively, at 10 and 15 years since the completion of initial treatment.[231] In both studies, the largest excess was observed for central nervous system tumors, with

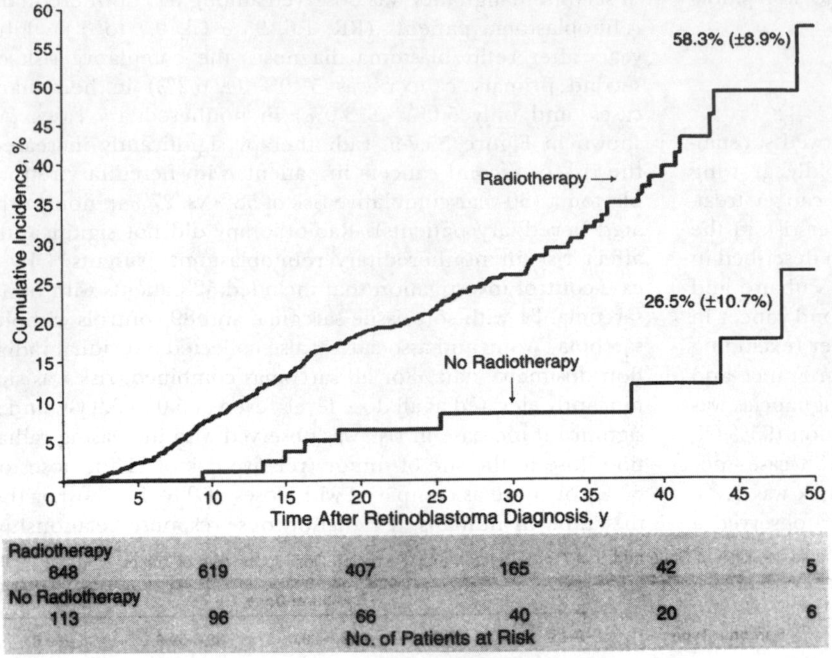

FIGURE 55.7-5. Cumulative incidence (± s.e.) of second cancers after diagnosis of retinoblastoma in 961 patients with hereditary disease, by radiation treatment. (From ref. 69, with permission.)

relative risks of 22[230] and 52.[231] Most brain tumors were high-grade astrocytomas or glioblastomas, and all occurred in children who had previously received radiotherapy, mostly cranial irradiation with doses ranging from 18 to 24 Gy. A study of 1612 patients with ALL from St. Jude Children's Research Hospital, with long-term follow-up data (median follow-up, 16 years), demonstrated an excess of high-grade gliomas during early follow-up (up to 10 years after diagnosis), whereas an increased risk of low-grade brain tumors was observed at later follow-up intervals.[232] The risk of developing a brain tumor was significantly increased with increasing cranial radiation dose, with 20-year cumulative risks of 1.0%, 1.7%, and 3.2% for patients who received radiation doses of 10 to 21 Gy, 21 to 30 Gy, and 30 Gy or more, respectively.

During the 1990s, prophylactic cranial radiotherapy has been largely replaced by intrathecal methotrexate. The number of intrathecal methotrexate administrations was not related to the risk of brain tumors,[232] but few children treated without cranial radiation were followed for more than 15 years. In two studies,[230,232] risk of central nervous system tumors was significantly higher in children 5 years of age or younger at first treatment.

Several very large studies of ALL survivors have reported negligible risks of AML after chemotherapy regimens that contain cyclophosphamide, anthracyclines, or both.[230,231,233] In contrast, very high risks of AML have been reported for children treated with epipodophyllotoxin-containing regimens. Pui and associates[97] were the first to report on the risk of AML in 734 children with ALL who received maintenance treatment according to different schedules of epipodophyllotoxin administration at St. Jude Children's Research Hospital. AML developed in 21 children, with an overall cumulative risk of 3.8% at 6 years follow-up. The schedule of epipodophyllotoxin treatment appeared to be a crucial factor in determining AML risk. Patients who received weekly or twice-weekly doses of teniposide (with or without etoposide), were at an approximately 12 times greater risk of AML than patients treated only during remission induction, or every 2 weeks during maintenance treatment. Several subgroups of patients in this study were exposed to other potentially leukemogenic factors, such as cyclophosphamide and cranial irradiation. The strongest evidence that the excess risk of AML was due to epipodophyllotoxin treatment came from comparing two subgroups that differed only in schedule of epipodophyllotoxin administration. Among 84 patients who received epipodophyllotoxins weekly, the risk of AML was clearly and significantly increased (12.4% at 6 years; 95% CI, 6.1% to 24.4%) compared with 148 patients who received the agents every other week (1.6% at 6 years; 95% CI, 0.4% to 6.1%; $P = .01$). Cumulative dose did not show enough variation within the study groups to reliably assess its effect. Compelling evidence for a causal link between epipodophyllotoxin therapy for ALL and the development of AML was also provided by Winick and associates.[234]

Elevated risk of AML also has been reported after a number of other childhood malignancies, especially lymphomas.[57,62,105,223,235,236] Two case-control studies addressed the effects of radiation dose and amount of chemotherapy on the risk of AML in children treated for various malignancies.[18,105] A significant dose-response relationship between total dose of alkylating agents and AML risk was observed in both studies. The Late Effects Study Group[18] found no association between leukemia risk and radiation dose to active bone marrow. In contrast, using similar methods of estimating bone marrow dose, Hawkins and colleagues[105] observed a highly significant trend, with an approximately 20-fold increased risk for patients receiving 15 Gy or more (compared to patients not treated with radiotherapy). These discrepant results may be explained by differences between the studies in the pattern of first cancers and in therapeutic practices. It is possible that the patients in the British study received lower radiation doses to larger vol-

TABLE 55.7-7. A Case-Control Study of Second Primary Bone Cancer in Relation to Radiation Dose and Cumulative Exposure to Alkylating Agents

Radiation Dose, cGy	*Number of Patients* Cases (n = 59)	Controls (n = 220)	*Relative Risk (95% CI) Adjusted for Alkylating Agent Exposure*	*P Value*
0	10	61	1.0	—
1–999	13	79	0.7 (0.2–2.2)	*P* = .537
1000–2999	7	15	12.4 (0.9–163.3)	*P* = .055
3000–4999	15	7	93.4 (6.8–1285.4)	*P*<.001
≥5000	5	6	64.7 (3.8–1103.4)	*P* = .004
Incomplete information	9	52	—	—
Test for linear trend	—	—	—	*P*<.001
Total Cumulative Exposure to Alkylating Agents, mg/m²	*Number of Patients* Cases (n = 59)	Controls (n = 220)	*Relative Risk (95% CI) Adjusted for Radiation Exposure*	*P Value*
0	37	164	1.0	—
1–9999	6	21	1.3 (0.3–6.0)	*P* = .698
10,000–19,999	7	20	3.0 (0.4–21.7)	*P* = .278
≥20,000	7	8	3.3 (0.8–13.8)	*P* = .107
Incomplete information	2	7	—	—
Test for linear trend	—	—	—	*P* = .080

CI, confidence interval.
(Adapted from ref. 61, with permission.)

umes of bone marrow, which, for a specified dose, might result in less cell kill and a greater susceptibility to leukemogenic transformation.[105] The case-control study in the United Kingdom[105] included ten cases of secondary AML after epipodophyllotoxin treatment, mostly for pediatric NHL. It is of interest that, at much lower cumulative doses than used in the St. Jude Children's Research Hospital study,[97] a steep increase in AML risk was noted with increasing dose of epipodophyllotoxins. Another striking difference between the two studies was that the strong dose-response relationship in the British study was observed for regimens in which the epipodophyllotoxins were given less frequently than weekly.

The Cancer Therapy Evaluation Program of the National Cancer Institute has developed a monitoring plan to better quantify the risk of AML after epipodophyllotoxin treatment. Smith and colleagues[106] reported results for patients included in trials that used epipodophyllotoxins at low (less than 1.5 g/m²), moderate (1.5 to 2.9 g/m²), or higher (3 g/m² or more) cumulative etoposide doses. The 6-year cumulative risks for AML (including MDS) with the low, moderate, and higher cumulative dose groups were 3.3% (based on eight AML cases in 451 patients), 0.7% (based on four AML cases in 1270 patients), and 2.2% (based on five AML cases in 570 patients), respectively. This result does not appear to provide support for a cumulative-dose effect for the leukemogenic activity of the epipodophyllotoxins, at least not within the cumulative-dose range and with the treatment schedules encompassed by the monitoring plan (cumulative etoposide dose of 5.0 g/m² or less, on daily times 2- to 5 schedules). A limitation of this study, however, is that the three treatment strata according to cumulative etoposide dose also differed with respect to other cytotoxic drugs received, primary tumor, and age. These differences and the administration of radiotherapy were not accounted for in the analysis.[93] Smith and associates[106] suggested that the much larger AML risk observed in earlier investigations might be due to the higher cumulative epipodophyllotoxin doses used in those studies (as high as 9 to 19 g/m²)[97,234,235] or, alternatively, to their schedule of weekly or twice-weekly administration. This intermittent exposure schedule, which is not commonly used in current treatment regimens, has been associated with increased leukemogenicity *in vitro*.[237] In view of several inconsistencies between the studies conducted to date, final conclusions regarding the leukemogenicity of different epipodophyllotoxin-based regimens cannot yet be drawn.

Hawkins and associates[61] addressed the quantitative relationship between radiation dose, alkylating agent therapy, and risk of bone sarcoma in a case-control study within a British cohort of 13,175 3-year survivors of childhood cancer. Risk of bone cancer was strongly increased in all follow-up intervals beyond 3 years, with no apparent trend of increasing or decreasing relative risks up to 25 years after diagnosis of primary cancer. As in an earlier study,[19] no increased risk was observed for radiation doses to the site of the bone tumor of less than 10 Gy. At more than 10 Gy, risk for bone sarcoma rose sharply with increasing radiation dose, with a relative risk of 93 for patients who received 30 to 50 Gy as compared to those not treated with radiation. At higher radiation doses, however, the risk appeared to decline somewhat (Table 55.7-7). Such a downturn in relative risk at very high doses was also observed in a smaller case-control study of osteosarcoma after childhood cancer[238] but was not found in the large case-control investigation nested in the LESG cohort.[19] In the latter study, Tucker and colleagues[19] showed that the pattern of risk increase in relation to radiation dose was similar in patients treated for retinoblastoma and those treated for other initial malignancies. Thus, although patients with retinoblastoma have a higher intrinsic risk for sarcoma development, their relative responses to radiation treatment do not appear to be different from patients with other childhood cancers. Importantly, the study by Hawkins and colleagues[61] also showed that the relative risk of bone sarcoma increases with increasing cumulative exposure to alkylating agents, even after adjustment for radiation therapy (see Table 55.7-7). It is clear, however, that the effect of radiotherapy on sarcoma risk is stronger than that of chemotherapy. An association between chemotherapy and risk of bone sarcoma also has been observed in other studies[19,91,238,239]; an effect of alkylating chemotherapy on sarcoma risk in the absence of radiotherapy was found only in the LESG study.[19] Comparative studies of children and adults irradiated for Hodgkin's disease have shown that children experience a much higher relative risk of developing bone sarcomas than adults, probably because of greater radiosensitivity of growing bone.[12,62]

The risk of thyroid cancer after radiotherapy for childhood malignancies was assessed in the LESG cohort.[60] High relative risks compared with general population rates were observed for thyroid malignancies after treatment of neuroblastoma (RR, 350), Wilms' tumor (RR, 132), and Hodgkin's disease (RR, 67). The relative risk increased significantly with time since treatment throughout the observation period (more than 20 years). In a case-control study, radiation dose to the thyroid was estimated for 23 thyroid cancer cases and 89 matched controls. Radiation doses of 2 Gy or more carried 13 times greater risk than doses of less than 2 Gy ($P < .05$). Because all patients with thyroid cancer had been exposed to at least 1 Gy of radiation to the thyroid, the risk associated with doses less than 2 Gy could not be reliably determined in this study. However, the investigators estimated that the risk associated with doses of 2 Gy or more was increased approximately 130-fold compared to nonirradiated patients.[60] Unexpectedly, the dose-response relationship was more or less flat at radiation doses beyond 2 Gy; even at doses as high as 60 Gy, no decrease in thyroid cancer risk was observed. A pooled analysis of seven large studies of thyroid cancer after various radiation exposures demonstrated that the risk decreases significantly with increasing age at exposure and is highest for persons with radiation exposure before age 5 years.[59]

In conclusion, survivors of childhood cancer are at substantially elevated risk to develop new malignancies. The magnitude of this risk depends on the type of the initial malignancy, because some childhood cancers, such as bilateral retinoblastoma, carry a high intrinsic risk for second cancer occurrence. Long-term survival after various types of childhood cancer has become possible through therapies introduced from the early 1970s onwards. Consequently, the growing population of cured patients is just beginning to enter the ages at which adult cancers typically occur, so the full spectrum of second malignancies has not yet been encountered. It is therefore imperative that survivors of childhood cancer be carefully monitored to assess the long-term risks of various types of second cancers. Bone sarcoma has consistently been identified as the second malignancy for which the excess risk is highest. Of much interest is the potential interaction between genetic susceptibility and treatment in second cancer development. The leukemogenic potential of epipodophyllotoxin-containing regimens that vary in cumulative dose and schedule of administration should continue to be rigorously assessed. As quantitative risk information from more studies becomes available, it will be possible to carefully weigh the benefits derived from epipodophyllotoxin treatment against the risks. Second cancers among survivors of childhood cancer are associated with a poor prognosis.[97,230,232,240,241] Hence, the need is pressing to develop therapeutic strategies with less oncogenic potential, without compromising the excellent cure rates that have been achieved.

CONCLUSION

The results described in this chapter have multiple clinical implications. Knowledge of risk factors for second malignancy has made it possible to identify patient groups at high risk of developing second cancers due to treatments that they received in the past. Whenever effective screening methods are available, these should be implemented in the patients' follow-up program to improve their survival after diagnosis of second malignancy. In some cases, preventive strategies (e.g., smoking cessation) may reduce substantially the risk of developing a treatment-related cancer. The issue of treatment-induced second cancers must always be viewed in relation to the sometimes dramatic improvement in survival rates for patients with various malignancies. The risks associated with various treatments should be weighed carefully against the consequences of not using such treatments. Clinical research should focus on the development of therapeutic regimens with less carcinogenic potential. However, the arbitrary alteration of a successful therapy to mitigate second cancer risk is unwarranted. It is of the utmost importance that changes in therapy to reduce the risk of late complications be made only in the context of carefully designed clinical trials that evaluate whether the overall efficacy of treatment is maintained.

For many cancer treatments, the long-term effects on second malignancy risk are not yet known. In addition, new therapies are being introduced continuously, and the associated risks of late sequelae must be evaluated. Whenever possible, future studies of second cancer risk should incorporate investigations at the molecular level. Results of these laboratory analyses may clarify the influence of genetic susceptibility on treatment-related risk and contribute important data for the elucidation of mechanisms underlying drug- and radiation-induced carcinogenesis.

REFERENCES

1. Hoppe RT. Hodgkin's disease: complications of therapy and excess mortality. *Ann Oncol* 1997;8[Suppl 1]:115.
2. Kaldor JM, Day NE, Shiboski S. Epidemiological studies of anticancer drug carcinogenicity. *IARC Sci Publ* 1986;78:189.
3. Makuch R, Simon R. Recommendations for the analysis of the effect of treatment on the development of second malignancies. *Cancer* 1979;44:250.
4. Kaplan EL, Meier P. Non-parametric estimation from incomplete observations. *J Am Stat Assoc* 1958;53:457.
5. Pepe MS, Mori M. Kaplan-Meier, marginal or conditional probability curves in summarizing competing risks failure time data? *Stat Med* 1993;12:737.
6. Darrington DL, Vose JM, Anderson JR, et al. Incidence and characterization of secondary myelodysplastic syndrome and acute myelogenous leukemia following high-dose chemoradiotherapy and autologous stem-cell transplantation for lymphoid malignancies. *J Clin Oncol* 1994;12:2527.
7. Boice JD Jr, Day NE, Andersen A, et al. Second cancers following radiation treatment for cervical cancer. An international collaboration among cancer registries. *J Natl Cancer Inst* 1985;74:955.
8. Kaldor JM, Day NE, Clarke EA, et al. Leukemia following Hodgkin's disease. *N Engl J Med* 1990;322:7.
9. Storm HH, Prener A. Second cancer following lymphatic and hematopoietic cancers in Denmark, 1943–80. *Natl Cancer Inst Monogr* 1985;68:389.
10. Greene MH. Is cisplatin a human carcinogen? [Review]. *J Natl Cancer Inst* 1992;84:306.
11. Coleman CN, Williams CJ, Flint A, et al. Hematologic neoplasia in patients treated for Hodgkin's disease. *N Engl J Med* 1977;297:1249.

12. Tucker MA, Coleman CN, Cox RS, Varghese A, Rosenberg SA. Risk of second cancers after treatment for Hodgkin's disease. *N Engl J Med* 1988;318:76.
13. van Leeuwen FE, Klokman WJ, Hagenbeek A, et al. Second cancer risk following Hodgkin's disease: a 20-year follow-up study. *J Clin Oncol* 1994;12:312.
14. Greene MH, Young RC, Merrill JM, DeVita VT. Evidence of a treatment dose response in acute nonlymphocytic leukemias which occur after therapy of non-Hodgkin's lymphoma. *Cancer Res* 1983;43:1891.
15. Ewertz M, Machado SG, Boice JD Jr, Jensen OM. Endometrial cancer following treatment for breast cancer: a case-control study in Denmark. *Br J Cancer* 1984;50:687.
16. Boice JD Jr, Blettner M, Kleinerman RA, et al. Radiation dose and leukemia risk in patients treated for cancer of the cervix. *J Natl Cancer Inst* 1987;79:1295.
17. Kaldor JM, Day NE, Pettersson F, et al. Leukemia following chemotherapy for ovarian cancer. *N Engl J Med* 1990;322:1.
18. Tucker MA, Meadows AT, Boice JD Jr, et al. Leukemia after therapy with alkylating agents for childhood cancer. *J Natl Cancer Inst* 1987;78:459.
19. Tucker MA, D'Angio GJ, Boice JD Jr, et al. Bone sarcomas linked to radiotherapy and chemotherapy in children. *N Engl J Med* 1987;317:588.
20. Curtis RE, Boice JD Jr, Stovall M, et al. Risk of leukemia after chemotherapy and radiation treatment for breast cancer. *N Engl J Med* 1992;326:1745.
21. Travis LB, Curtis RE, Glimelius B, et al. Bladder and kidney cancer following cyclophosphamide therapy for non-Hodgkin's lymphoma. *J Natl Cancer Inst* 1995;87:524.
22. Boice JD Jr, Harvey EB, Blettner M, Stovall M, Flannery JT. Cancer in the contralateral breast after radiotherapy for breast cancer. *N Engl J Med* 1992;326:781.
23. Court-Brown WM, Doll R. *Leukaemia and aplastic anaemia in patients irradiated for ankylosing spondylitis.* London: Her Majesty's Stationary Office, 1957.
24. Upton AC. Physical carcinogenesis: radiation, history and sources. In: Becker FF, ed. *Cancer: a comprehensive treatise.* New York: Plenum Press, 1975:387.
25. Martland HS. The occurrence of malignancy in radioactive persons: a general review of data gathered in the study of the radium dial painters, with special reference to the occurrence of osteogenic sarcoma and the interrelationship of certain blood diseases. *Am J Cancer* 1931;15:2435.
26. United Nations Scientific Committee on the Effects of Atomic Radiation. *Sources and effects of ionizing radiation: UNSCEAR 1994 report to the general assembly with scientific annexes.* New York: United Nations, 1994.
27. Boice JD Jr. Carcinogenesis—a synopsis of human experience with external exposure in medicine [Review]. *Health Phys* 1988;55:621.
28. Boice JD Jr, Land CE, Preston DL. Ionizing radiation. In: Schottenfeld D, Fraumeni JF Jr, eds. *Cancer epidemiology and prevention.* New York: Oxford University Press, 1996:319.
29. Heyssel R, Brill AB, Woodbury L, et al. Leukemia in Hiroshima atomic bomb survivors. *Blood* 1960;15:313.
30. Preston DL, Kusumi S, Tomonaga M, et al. Cancer incidence in atomic bomb survivors. Part III. Leukemia, lymphoma and multiple myeloma, 1950–1987 [published erratum appears in *Radiat Res* 1994;139:129]. *Radiat Res* 1994;137:S68.
31. Thompson DE, Mabuchi K, Ron E, et al. Cancer incidence in atomic bomb survivors. Part II: Solid tumors, 1958–1987 [published erratum appears in *Radiat Res* 1994;139:129]. *Radiat Res* 1994;137:S17.
32. Tokunaga M, Land CE, Tokuoka S, et al. Incidence of female breast cancer among atomic bomb survivors, 1950–1985. *Radiat Res* 1994;138:209.
33. Smith PG, Doll R. Mortality from cancer and all causes among British radiologists. *Br J Radiol* 1981;54:187.
34. Wang JX, Inskip PD, Boice JD Jr, et al. Cancer incidence among medical diagnostic x-ray workers in China, 1950 to 1985. *Int J Cancer* 1990;45:889.
35. Boice JD Jr, Preston D, Davis FG, Monson RR. Frequent chest x-ray fluoroscopy and breast cancer incidence among tuberculosis patients in Massachusetts. *Radiat Res* 1991;125:214.
36. Miller AB, Howe GR, Sherman GJ, et al. Mortality from breast cancer after irradiation during fluoroscopic examinations in patients being treated for tuberculosis. *N Engl J Med* 1989;321:1285.
37. Boice JD Jr, Engholm G, Kleinerman RA, et al. Radiation dose and second cancer risk in patients treated for cancer of the cervix. *Radiat Res* 1988;116:3.
38. van Leeuwen FE, Klokman WJ, Stovall M, et al. Roles of radiotherapy and smoking in lung cancer following Hodgkin's disease. *J Natl Cancer Inst* 1995;87:1530.
39. Hancock SL, Tucker MA, Hoppe RT. Breast cancer after treatment of Hodgkin's disease. *J Natl Cancer Inst* 1993;85:25.
40. Weiss HA, Darby SC, Doll R. Cancer mortality following x-ray treatment for ankylosing spondylitis. *Int J Cancer* 1994;59:327.
41. Darby SC, Reeves G, Key T, Doll R, Stovall M. Mortality in a cohort of women given x-ray therapy for metropathia haemorrhagica. *Int J Cancer* 1994;56:793.
42. Hildreth NG, Shore RE, Hempelmann LH, Rosenstein M. Risk of extrathyroid tumors following radiation treatment in infancy for thymic enlargement. *Radiat Res* 1985;102:378.
43. Karlsson P, Holmberg E, Lundberg LM, Nordborg C, Wallgren A. Intracranial tumors after radium treatment for skin hemangioma during infancy—a cohort and case-control study. *Radiat Res* 1997;148:161.
44. Lundell M, Mattsson A, Karlsson P, et al. Breast cancer risk after radiotherapy in infancy: a pooled analysis of two Swedish cohorts of 17,202 infants. *Radiat Res* 1999;151:626.
45. Curtis RE, Boice JD Jr, Stovall M, et al. Relationship of leukemia risk to radiation dose following cancer of the uterine corpus. *J Natl Cancer Inst* 1994;86:1315.
46. Inskip PD, Monson RR, Wagoner JK, et al. Leukemia following radiotherapy for uterine bleeding. *Radiat Res* 1990;122:107.
47. Little MP, Weiss HA, Boice JD Jr, et al. Risks of leukemia in Japanese atomic bomb survivors, in women treated for cervical cancer, and in patients treated for ankylosing spondylitis. *Radiat Res* 1999;152:280.
48. Swerdlow AJ, Douglas AJ, Hudson GV, et al. Risk of second primary cancers after Hodgkin's disease by type of treatment: analysis of 2846 patients in the British National Lymphoma Investigation. *BMJ* 1992;304:1137.
49. Inskip PD, Monson RR, Wagoner JK, et al. Cancer mortality following radium treatment for uterine bleeding [published erratum appears in *Radiat Res* 1991;128:326]. *Radiat Res* 1990;123:331.
50. van Leeuwen FE, Klokman WJ, Veer MB, et al. Long-term risk of second malignancy in survivors of Hodgkin's disease treated during adolescence or young adulthood. *J Clin Oncol* 2000;18:487.
51. de Vathaire F, Hawkins M, Campbell S, et al. Second malignant neoplasms after a first cancer in childhood: temporal pattern of risk according to type of treatment. *Br J Cancer* 1999;79:1884.
52. Little MP, de Vathaire F, Charles MW, Hawkins MM, Muirhead CR. Variations with time and age in the risks of solid cancer incidence after radiation exposure in childhood. *Stat Med* 1998;17:1341.
53. Darby SC, Doll R, Gill SK, Smith PG. Long term mortality after a single treatment course with x-rays in patients treated for ankylosing spondylitis. *Br J Cancer* 1987;55:179.
54. Hildreth NG, Shore RE, Dvoretsky PM. The risk of breast cancer after irradiation of the thymus in infancy. *N Engl J Med* 1989;321:1281.
55. Mauch PM, Kalish LA, Marcus KC, et al. Second malignancies after treatment for laparotomy staged IA-IIIB Hodgkin's disease: long-term analysis of risk factors and outcome. *Blood* 1996;87:3625.
56. Land CE, Hayakawa N, Machado SG, et al. A case-control interview study of breast cancer among Japanese A-bomb survivors. II. Interactions with radiation dose. *Cancer Causes Control* 1994;5:167.
57. Bhatia S, Robison LL, Oberlin O, et al. Breast cancer and other second neoplasms after childhood Hodgkin's disease. *N Engl J Med* 1996;334:745.
58. Inskip PD, Stovall M, Flannery JT. Lung cancer risk and radiation dose among women treated for breast cancer. *J Natl Cancer Inst* 1994;86:983.
59. Ron E, Lubin JH, Shore RE, et al. Thyroid cancer after exposure to external radiation: a pooled analysis of seven studies. *Radiat Res* 1995;141:259.
60. Tucker MA, Jones PH, Boice JD Jr, et al. Therapeutic radiation at a young age is linked to secondary thyroid cancer. The Late Effects Study Group. *Cancer Res* 1991;51:2885.
61. Hawkins MM, Wilson LM, Burton HS, et al. Radiotherapy, alkylating agents, and risk of bone cancer after childhood cancer. *J Natl Cancer Inst* 1996;88:270.
62. Tucker MA, Meadows AT, Boice JD Jr, Hoover RN, Fraumeni JF Jr. Cancer risk following treatment of childhood cancer. In: Boice JD, Fraumeni JF, eds. *Radiation carcinogenesis: epidemiology and biological significance.* New York: Raven Press, 1984:211.
63. Swerdlow AJ, Barber JA, Hudson GV, et al. Risk of second malignancy after Hodgkin's disease in a collaborative British cohort: the relation to age at treatment. *J Clin Oncol* 2000;18:498.
64. National Research Council. *Health risks of radon and other internally deposited alpha-emitters.* Washington, DC: National Academy Press, 1988.
65. Moolgavkar SH, Luebeck EG, Krewski D, Zielinski JM. Radon, cigarette smoke, and lung cancer: a re-analysis of the Colorado Plateau uranium miners' data. *Epidemiology* 1993;4:204.
66. Yao SX, Lubin JH, Qiao YL, et al. Exposure to radon progeny, tobacco use and lung cancer in a case-control study in southern China. *Radiat Res* 1994;138:326.
67. van Leeuwen FE, Klokman WJ. Re: Smoking, treatment for Hodgkin's disease, and subsequent lung cancer risk. *J Natl Cancer Inst* 1996;88:209.
68. van Leeuwen FE. Second cancers. In: DeVita VT, Hellman S, Rosenberg SA, eds. *Cancer: principles and practice of oncology.* Philadelphia: Lippincott, 1997:2773.
69. Wong FL, Boice JD Jr, Abramson DH, et al. Cancer incidence after retinoblastoma. Radiation dose and sarcoma risk. *JAMA* 1997;278:1262.
70. Kony SJ, de Vathaire F, Chompret A, et al. Radiation and genetic factors in the risk of second malignant neoplasms after a first cancer in childhood. *Lancet* 1997;350:91.
71. Nichols KE, Levitz S, Shannon KE, et al. Heterozygous germline ATM mutations do not contribute to radiation-associated malignancies after Hodgkin's disease. *J Clin Oncol* 1999;17:1259.
72. Easton DF. Cancer risks in A-T heterozygotes [Review]. *Int J Radiat Biol* 1994;66:S177.
73. Swift M, Morrell D, Massey RB, Chase CL. Incidence of cancer in 161 families affected by ataxia-telangiectasia. *N Engl J Med* 1991;325:1831.
74. Broeks A, Russell NS, Floore AN, et al. Increased risk of breast cancer following irradiation for Hodgkin's disease is not a result of ATM germline mutations. *Int J Radiat Biol* 2000;76:693.
75. Kyle RA, Pierre RV, Bayrd ED. Multiple myeloma and acute myelomonocytic leukemia. *N Engl J Med* 1970;283:1121.
76. Smith MA, McCaffrey RP, Karp JE. The secondary leukemias: challenges and research directions [Review]. *J Natl Cancer Inst* 1996;88:407.
77. Levine EG, Bloomfield CD. Leukemias and myelodysplastic syndromes secondary to drug, radiation, and environmental exposure [Review]. *Semin Oncol* 1992;19:47.
78. Hunger SP, Sklar J, Link MP. Acute lymphoblastic leukemia occurring as a second malignant neoplasm in childhood: report of three cases and review of the literature [Review]. *J Clin Oncol* 1992;10:156.
79. Whang-Peng J, Young RC, Lee EC, et al. Cytogenetic studies in patients with secondary leukemia/dysmyelopoietic syndrome after different treatment modalities. *Blood* 1988;71:403.
80. Haas JF, Kittelmann B, Mehnert WH, et al. Risk of leukaemia in ovarian tumour and breast cancer patients following treatment by cyclophosphamide. *Br J Cancer* 1987;55:213.
81. Travis LB, Holowaty EJ, Bergfeldt K, et al. Risk of leukemia after platinum-based chemotherapy for ovarian cancer. *N Engl J Med* 1999;340:351.
82. Pedersen-Bjergaard J, Rowley JD. The balanced and the unbalanced chromosome aberrations of acute myeloid leukemia may develop in different ways and may contribute differently to malignant transformation [Review]. *Blood* 1994;83:2780.
83. Smith MA, Rubinstein L, Ungerleider RS. Therapy-related acute myeloid leukemia following treatment with epipodophyllotoxins: estimating the risks [Review]. *Med Pediatr Oncol* 1994;23:86.
84. Henry-Amar M. Second cancer after the treatment for Hodgkin's disease: a report from the International Database on Hodgkin's Disease. *Ann Oncol* 1992;3[Suppl 4]:117.

85. Travis LB, Curtis RE, Storm H, et al. Risk of second malignant neoplasms among long-term survivors of testicular cancer. *J Natl Cancer Inst* 1997;89:1429.
86. Pedersen-Bjergaard J, Philip P, Larsen SO, Jensen G, Byrsting K. Chromosome aberrations and prognostic factors in therapy-related myelodysplasia and acute nonlymphocytic leukemia. *Blood* 1990;76:1083.
87. Neugut AI, Robinson E, Nieves J, Murray T, Tsai WY. Poor survival of treatment-related acute nonlymphocytic leukemia. *JAMA* 1990;264:1006.
88. Overall evaluations of carcinogenicity: an updating of IARC Monographs volumes 1 to 42. *IARC Monogr Eval Carcinog Risks Hum Suppl* 1987;7:1.
89. van Leeuwen FE, Chorus AM, van den Belt-Dusebout AW, et al. Leukemia risk following Hodgkin's disease: relation to cumulative dose of alkylating agents, treatment with teniposide combinations, number of episodes of chemotherapy, and bone marrow damage. *J Clin Oncol* 1994;12:1063.
90. Travis LB, Curtis RE, Stovall M, et al. Risk of leukemia following treatment for non-Hodgkin's lymphoma. *J Natl Cancer Inst* 1994;86:1450.
91. Boivin JF, Hutchison GB, Zauber AG, et al. Incidence of second cancers in patients treated for Hodgkin's disease. *J Natl Cancer Inst* 1995;87:732.
92. Greene MH, Harris EL, Gershenson DM, et al. Melphalan may be a more potent leukemogen than cyclophosphamide. *Ann Intern Med* 1986;105:360.
93. Some antiviral and antineoplastic drugs, and other pharmaceutical agents. *IARC Monogr Eval Carcinog Risks Hum* 2000;76:177.
94. Ratain MJ, Kaminer LS, Bitran JD, et al. Acute nonlymphocytic leukemia following etoposide and cisplatin combination chemotherapy for advanced non-small-cell carcinoma of the lung. *Blood* 1987;70:1412.
95. Pedersen-Bjergaard J, Daugaard G, Hansen SW, et al. Increased risk of myelodysplasia and leukaemia after etoposide, cisplatin, and bleomycin for germ-cell tumours. *Lancet* 1991;338:359.
96. Boshoff C, Begent RH, Oliver RT, et al. Secondary tumours following etoposide containing therapy for germ cell cancer. *Ann Oncol* 1995;6:35.
97. Pui CH, Ribeiro RC, Hancock ML, et al. Acute myeloid leukemia in children treated with epipodophyllotoxins for acute lymphoblastic leukemia. *N Engl J Med* 1991;325:1682.
98. Pedersen-Bjergaard J, Pedersen M, Roulston D, Philip P. Different genetic pathways in leukemogenesis for patients presenting with therapy-related myelodysplasia and therapy-related acute myeloid leukemia. *Blood* 1995;86:3542.
99. Pedersen-Bjergaard J, Philip P. Balanced translocations involving chromosome bands 11q23 and 21q22 are highly characteristic of myelodysplasia and leukemia following therapy with cytostatic agents targeting at DNA-topoisomerase II [Letter]. *Blood* 1991;78:1147.
100. Rubin CM, Arthur DC, Woods WG, et al. Therapy-related myelodysplastic syndrome and acute myeloid leukemia in children: correlation between chromosomal abnormalities and prior therapy. *Blood* 1991;78:2982.
101. Pedersen-Bjergaard J, Sigsgaard TC, Nielsen D, et al. Acute monocytic or myelomonocytic leukemia with balanced chromosome translocations to band 11q23 after therapy with 4-epi-doxorubicin and cisplatin or cyclophosphamide for breast cancer. *J Clin Oncol* 1992;10:1444.
102. Sandoval C, Pui CH, Bowman LC, et al. Secondary acute myeloid leukemia in children previously treated with alkylating agents, intercalating topoisomerase II inhibitors, and irradiation. *J Clin Oncol* 1993;11:1039.
103. Diamandidou E, Buzdar AU, Smith TL, et al. Treatment-related leukemia in breast cancer patients treated with fluorouracil-doxorubicin-cyclophosphamide combination adjuvant chemotherapy: the University of Texas M. D. Anderson Cancer Center experience. *J Clin Oncol* 1996;14:2722.
104. Breslow NE, Takashima JR, Whitton JA, et al. Second malignant neoplasms following treatment for Wilms' tumor: a report from the National Wilms' Tumor Study Group. *J Clin Oncol* 1995;13:1851.
105. Hawkins MM, Wilson LM, Stovall MA, et al. Epipodophyllotoxins, alkylating agents, and radiation and risk of secondary leukaemia after childhood cancer. *BMJ* 1992;304:951.
106. Smith MA, Rubinstein L, Anderson JR, et al. Secondary leukemia or myelodysplastic syndrome after treatment with epipodophyllotoxins. *J Clin Oncol* 1999;17:569.
107. Anderson RD, Berger NA. International Commission for Protection Against Environmental Mutagens and Carcinogens. Mutagenicity and carcinogenicity of topoisomerase-interactive agents [Review]. *Mutat Res* 1994;309:109.
108. Rivera GK, Pui CH, Santana VM, Pratt CB, Crist WM. Epipodophyllotoxins in the treatment of childhood cancer [Review]. *Cancer Chemother Pharmacol* 1994;34[Suppl]:S89.
109. Davies SM. Mechanisms of cytotoxicity and leukemogenesis: topoisomerase II inhibitors and alkylating agents. Proceedings of the American Society of Clinical Oncology Educational Symposia 31st annual meeting, Los Angeles, May 20–23, 1995. Los Angeles: American Society of Clinical Oncology, 1995:204.
110. Cheson BD, Vena DA, Barrett J, Freidlin B. Second malignancies as a consequence of nucleoside analog therapy for chronic lymphoid leukemias. *J Clin Oncol* 1999;17:2454.
111. Relling MV, Rubnitz JE, Rivera GK, et al. High incidence of secondary brain tumours after radiotherapy and antimetabolites. *Lancet* 1999;354:34.
112. Felix CA. Chemotherapy-related second cancers. In: Neugut AI, Meadows AT, Robinson E, eds. *Multiple primary cancers*. Philadelphia: Lippincott Williams & Wilkins, 1999:137.
113. Felix CA, Walker AH, Lange BJ, et al. Association of CYP3A4 genotype with treatment-related leukemia. *Proc Natl Acad Sci U S A* 1998;95:13176.
114. Ben-Yehuda D, Krichevsky S, Caspi O, et al. Microsatellite instability and p53 mutations in therapy-related leukemia suggest mutator phenotype. *Blood* 1996;88:4296.
115. Zhu YM, Das-Gupta EP, Russell NH. Microsatellite instability and p53 mutations are associated with abnormal expression of the MSH2 gene in adult acute leukemia. *Blood* 1999;94:733.
116. Alberts DS. Protection by amifostine of cyclophosphamide-induced myelosuppression [Review]. *Semin Oncol* 1999;26[Suppl 7]:37.
117. Castiglione F, Dalla Mola A, Porcile G. Protection of normal tissues from radiation and cytotoxic therapy: the development of amifostine [Review]. *Tumori* 1999;85:85.
118. Pedersen-Bjergaard J, Ersboll J, Hansen VL, et al. Carcinoma of the urinary bladder after treatment with cyclophosphamide for non-Hodgkin's lymphoma. *N Engl J Med* 1988;318:1028.
119. Kaldor JM, Day NE, Kittelmann B, et al. Bladder tumours following chemotherapy and radiotherapy for ovarian cancer: a case-control study. *Int J Cancer* 1995;63:1.
120. Kaldor JM, Day NE, Bell J, et al. Lung cancer following Hodgkin's disease: a case-control study. *Int J Cancer* 1992;52:677.
121. Tucker MA, Murray N, Shaw EG, et al. Second primary cancers related to smoking and treatment of small-cell lung cancer. Lung Cancer Working Cadre. *J Natl Cancer Inst* 1997;89:1782.
122. Birdwell SH, Hancock SL, Varghese A, Cox RS, Hoppe RT. Gastrointestinal cancer after treatment of Hodgkin's disease. *Int J Radiat Oncol Biol Phys* 1997;37:67.
123. Newton WA Jr, Meadows AT, Shimada H, Bunin GR, Vawter GF. Bone sarcomas as second malignant neoplasms following childhood cancer. *Cancer* 1991;67:193.
124. Schilsky RL. Biochemical pharmacology of chemotherapeutic drugs used as radiation enhancers [Review]. *Semin Oncol* 1992;19[Suppl 11]:2.
125. Arseneau JC, Sponzo RW, Levin DL, et al. Nonlymphomatous malignant tumors complicating Hodgkin's disease. Possible association with intensive therapy. *N Engl J Med* 1972;287:1119.
126. Bonadonna G, De Lena M, Banfi A, Lattuada A. Secondary neoplasms in malignant lymphomas after intensive therapy. *N Engl J Med* 1973;288:1242.
127. van Leeuwen FE, Swerdlow AJ, Valagussa P, Tucker MA. Second cancers after treatment of Hodgkin's disease. In: Mauch PM, Armitage JO, Diehl V, Hoppe RT, Weiss LM, eds. *Hodgkin's disease*. Philadelphia: Lippincott Williams & Wilkins, 1999:607.
128. Hancock SL, Hoppe RT. Long-term complications of treatment and causes of mortality after Hodgkin's disease. *Semin Radiat Oncol* 1996;6:225.
129. Valagussa PA, Bonadonna G. Carcinogenic effects of cancer treatment. In: Peckham M, Pinedo H, Veronesi U, eds. *Oxford textbook of oncology*. Oxford: Oxford University Press, 1995:2348.
130. Schellong G, Riepenhausen M, Creutzig U, et al. Low risk of secondary leukemias after chemotherapy without mechlorethamine in childhood Hodgkin's disease. German-Austrian Pediatric Hodgkin's Disease Group. *J Clin Oncol* 1997;15:2247.
131. Andrieu JM, Ifrah N, Payen C, et al. Increased risk of secondary acute nonlymphocytic leukemia after extended-field radiation therapy combined with MOPP chemotherapy for Hodgkin's disease [Review]. *J Clin Oncol* 1990;8:1148.
132. van Leeuwen FE, Somers R, Hart AA. Splenectomy in Hodgkin's disease and second leukaemias [Letter]. *Lancet* 1987;2:210.
133. Penn I. Cancers complicating organ transplantation [Editorial; comment]. *N Engl J Med* 1990;323:1767.
134. van Rijswijk RE, Sybesma JP, Kater L. A prospective study of the changes in immune status following radiotherapy for Hodgkin's disease. *Cancer* 1984;53:62.
135. Krikorian JG, Burke JS, Rosenberg SA, Kaplan HS. Occurrence of non-Hodgkin's lymphoma after therapy for Hodgkin's disease. *N Engl J Med* 1979;300:452.
136. Prosper F, Robledo C, Cuesta B, et al. Incidence of non-Hodgkin's lymphoma in patients treated for Hodgkin's disease. *Leuk Lymphoma* 1994;12:457.
137. Hancock SL, Cox RS, McDougall IR. Thyroid diseases after treatment of Hodgkin's disease. *N Engl J Med* 1991;325:599.
138. Tucker MA, Misfeldt D, Coleman CN, Clark WH Jr, Rosenberg SA. Cutaneous malignant melanoma after Hodgkin's disease. *Ann Intern Med* 1985;102:37.
139. Donaldson SS, Hancock SL. Second cancers after Hodgkin's disease in childhood [Editorial; comment]. *N Engl J Med* 1996;334:792.
140. Goss PE, Sierra S. Current perspectives on radiation-induced breast cancer [Review]. *J Clin Oncol* 1998;16:338.
141. Wolf J, Schellong G, Diehl V. Breast cancer following treatment of Hodgkin's disease—more reasons for less radiotherapy? [Editorial; comment]. *Eur J Cancer* 1997;33:2293.
142. Sankila R, Garwicz S, Olsen JH, et al. Risk of subsequent malignant neoplasms among 1,641 Hodgkin's disease patients diagnosed in childhood and adolescence: a population-based cohort study in the five Nordic countries. Association of the Nordic Cancer Registries and the Nordic Society of Pediatric Hematology and Oncology. *J Clin Oncol* 1996;14:1442.
143. Wolden SL, Lamborn KR, Cleary SF, Tate DJ, Donaldson SS. Second cancers following pediatric Hodgkin's disease. *J Clin Oncol* 1998;16:536.
144. Aisenberg AC, Finkelstein DM, Doppke KP, et al. High risk of breast carcinoma after irradiation of young women with Hodgkin's disease. *Cancer* 1997;79:1203.
145. Land CE. Studies of cancer and radiation dose among atomic bomb survivors. The example of breast cancer. *JAMA* 1995;274:402.
146. Zarrabi MH. Association of non-Hodgkin's lymphoma (NHL) and second neoplasms. *Semin Oncol* 1980;7:340.
147. MacDougall BK, Weinerman BH, Kemel S. Second malignancies in non-Hodgkin's lymphoma. *Cancer* 1981;48:1299.
148. *SEER cancer statistics review, 1973–1994*. Bethesda, MD: National Cancer Institute, 1997.
149. Travis LB, Curtis RE, Boice JD Jr, Hankey BF, Fraumeni JF Jr. Second cancers following non-Hodgkin's lymphoma. *Cancer* 1991;67:2002.
150. Travis LB, Curtis RE, Glimelius B, et al. Second cancers among long-term survivors of non-Hodgkin's lymphoma. *J Natl Cancer Inst* 1993;85:1932.
151. Gomez GA, Aggarwal KK, Han T. Post-therapeutic acute malignant myeloproliferative syndrome and acute nonlymphocytic leukemia in non-Hodgkin's lymphoma. *Cancer* 1982;50:2285.
152. Pedersen-Bjergaard J, Ersboll J, Sorensen HM, et al. Risk of acute nonlymphocytic leukemia and preleukemia in patients treated with cyclophosphamide for non-Hodgkin's lymphomas. Comparison with results obtained in patients treated for Hodgkin's disease and ovarian carcinoma with other alkylating agents. *Ann Intern Med* 1985;103:195.
153. Lavey RS, Eby NL, Prosnitz LR. Impact on second malignancy risk of the combined use of radiation and chemotherapy for lymphomas. *Cancer* 1990;66:80.
154. Lishner M, Slingerland J, Barr J, et al. Second malignant neoplasms in patients with non Hodgkin's lymphoma. *Hematol Oncol* 1991;9:169.

155. Travis LB, Weeks J, Curtis RE, et al. Leukemia following low-dose total body irradiation and chemotherapy for non-Hodgkin's lymphoma. *J Clin Oncol* 1996;14:565.
156. Mendenhall NP, Noyes WD, Million RR. Total body irradiation for stage II–IV non-Hodgkin's lymphoma: ten-year follow-up. *J Clin Oncol* 1989;7:67.
157. Rubin P, Constine LS III, Scarantino CW. The paradoxes in patterns and mechanism of bone marrow regeneration after irradiation. II. Total body irradiation. *Radiother Oncol* 1984;2:227.
158. Miller JS, Arthur DC, Litz CE, et al. Myelodysplastic syndrome after autologous bone marrow transplantation: an additional late complication of curative cancer therapy. *Blood* 1994;83:3780.
159. Stone RM, Neuberg D, Soiffer R, et al. Myelodysplastic syndrome as a late complication following autologous bone marrow transplantation for non-Hodgkin's lymphoma. *J Clin Oncol* 1994;12:2535.
160. Friedberg JW, Neuberg D, Stone RM, et al. Outcome in patients with myelodysplastic syndrome after autologous bone marrow transplantation for non-Hodgkin's lymphoma. *J Clin Oncol* 1999;17:3128.
161. Traweek ST, Slovak ML, Nademanee AP, et al. Myelodysplasia and acute myeloid leukemia occurring after autologous bone marrow transplantation for lymphoma [Review]. *Leuk Lymphoma* 1996;20:365.
162. Abruzzese E, Radford JE, Miller JS, et al. Detection of abnormal pretransplant clones in progenitor cells of patients who developed myelodysplasia after autologous transplantation. *Blood* 1999;94:1814.
163. Einhorn LH. Testicular cancer as a model for a curable neoplasm: The Richard and Hinda Rosenthal Foundation Award Lecture. *Cancer Res* 1981;41:3275.
164. Fossa SD, Horwich A, Russell JM, et al. Optimal planning target volume for stage I testicular seminoma: a Medical Research Council randomized trial. *J Clin Oncol* 1999;17:1146.
165. Fossa SD, Langmark F, Aass N, et al. Second non–germ cell malignancies after radiotherapy of testicular cancer with or without chemotherapy. *Br J Cancer* 1990;61:639.
166. van Leeuwen FE, Stiggelbout AM, van den Belt-Dusebout AW, et al. Second cancer risk following testicular cancer: a follow-up study of 1,909 patients. *J Clin Oncol* 1993;11:415.
167. Bokemeyer C, Schmoll HJ. Treatment of testicular cancer and the development of secondary malignancies [Review]. *J Clin Oncol* 1995;13:283.
168. Griem ML, Kleinerman RA, Boice JD Jr, et al. Cancer following radiotherapy for peptic ulcer. *J Natl Cancer Inst* 1994;86:842.
169. Osterlind A, Berthelsen JG, Abildgaard N, et al. Risk of bilateral testicular germ cell cancer in Denmark: 1960–1984. *J Natl Cancer Inst* 1991;83:1391.
170. Nichols CR, Roth BJ, Heerema N, Griep J, Tricot G. Hematologic neoplasia associated with primary mediastinal germ-cell tumors. *N Engl J Med* 1990;322:1425.
171. Oliver RT. Testicular cancer [Review]. *Curr Opin Oncol* 1994;6:285.
172. Nichols CR, Breeden ES, Loehrer PJ, Williams SD, Einhorn LH. Secondary leukemia associated with a conventional dose of etoposide: review of serial germ cell tumor protocols. *J Natl Cancer Inst* 1993;85:36.
173. Bajorin DF, Motzer RJ, Rodriguez E, Murphy B, Bosl GJ. Acute nonlymphocytic leukemia in germ cell tumor patients treated with etoposide-containing chemotherapy. *J Natl Cancer Inst* 1993;85:60.
174. Bokemeyer C, Schmoll HJ, Kuczyk MA, Beyer J, Siegert W. Risk of secondary leukemia following high cumulative doses of etoposide during chemotherapy for testicular cancer [Letter]. *J Natl Cancer Inst* 1995;87:58.
175. Bokemeyer C, Schmoll HJ. Secondary neoplasms following treatment of malignant germ cell tumors. *J Clin Oncol* 1993;11:1703.
176. Roth BJ, Greist A, Kubilis PS, Williams SD, Einhorn LH. Cisplatin-based combination chemotherapy for disseminated germ cell tumors: long-term follow-up. *J Clin Oncol* 1988;6:1239.
177. Ozols RF, Ihde DC, Linehan WM, et al. A randomized trial of standard chemotherapy vs a high-dose chemotherapy regimen in the treatment of poor prognosis nonseminomatous germ-cell tumors. *J Clin Oncol* 1988;6:1031.
178. Travis LB, Curtis RE, Boice JD Jr, et al. Second malignant neoplasms among long-term survivors of ovarian cancer. *Cancer Res* 1996;56:1564.
179. Greene MH, Boice JD Jr, Greer BE, Blessing JA, Dembo AJ. Acute nonlymphocytic leukemia after therapy with alkylating agents for ovarian cancer: a study of five randomized clinical trials. *N Engl J Med* 1982;307:1416.
180. NIH consensus conference. Ovarian cancer. Screening, treatment, and follow-up. NIH Consensus Development Panel on Ovarian Cancer [Review]. *JAMA* 1995;273:491.
181. Vokes EE, Weichselbaum RR. Concomitant chemoradiotherapy: rationale and clinical experience in patients with solid tumors [published erratum appears in *J Clin Oncol* 1990;8:1447]. *J Clin Oncol* 1990;8:911.
182. Neijt JP. New therapy for ovarian cancer [Editorial; comment]. *N Engl J Med* 1996;334:50.
183. Harvey EB, Brinton LA. Second cancer following cancer of the breast in Connecticut, 1935–82. *Natl Cancer Inst Monogr* 1985;68:99.
184. Adami HO, Bergstrom R, Hansen J. Age at first primary as a determinant of the incidence of bilateral breast cancer. Cumulative and relative risks in a population-based case-control study. *Cancer* 1985;55:643.
185. Teppo L, Pukkala E, Saxen E. Multiple cancer—an epidemiologic exercise in Finland. *J Natl Cancer Inst* 1985;75:207.
186. Fisher B, Costantino JP, Redmond CK, et al. Endometrial cancer in tamoxifen-treated breast cancer patients: findings from the National Surgical Adjuvant Breast and Bowel Project (NSABP) B-14 [Prior annotation incorrect]. *J Natl Cancer Inst* 1994;86:527.
187. Rutqvist LE, Johansson H, Signomklao T, et al. Adjuvant tamoxifen therapy for early stage breast cancer and second primary alignancies. Stockholm Breast Cancer Study Group. *J Natl Cancer Inst* 1995;87:645.
188. Neugut AI, Robinson E, Lee WC, et al. Lung cancer after radiation therapy for breast cancer. *Cancer* 1993;71:3054.
189. Ewertz M, Mouridsen HT. Second cancer following cancer of the female breast in Denmark, 1943–80. *Natl Cancer Inst Monogr* 1985;68:325.
190. Ahsan H, Neugut AI. Radiation therapy for breast cancer and increased risk for esophageal carcinoma. *Ann Intern Med* 1998;128:114.
191. Karlsson P, Holmberg E, Samuelsson A, Johansson KA, Wallgren A. Soft tissue sarcoma after treatment for breast cancer—a Swedish population-based study. *Eur J Cancer* 1998;34:2068.
192. Wijnmaalen A, van Ooijen B, van Geel BN, Henzen-Logmans SC, Treurniet-Donker AD. Angiosarcoma of the breast following lumpectomy, axillary lymph node dissection, and radiotherapy for primary breast cancer: three case reports and a review of the literature [Review]. *Int J Radiat Oncol Biol Phys* 1993;26:135.
193. Strobbe LJ, Peterse HL, van Tinteren H, Wijnmaalen A, Rutgers EJ. Angiosarcoma of the breast after conservation therapy for invasive cancer, the incidence and outcome. An unforseen sequela. *Breast Cancer Res Treat* 1998;47:101.
194. Fisher B, Rockette H, Fisher ER, et al. Leukemia in breast cancer patients following adjuvant chemotherapy or postoperative radiation: the NSABP experience. *J Clin Oncol* 1985;3:1640.
195. Tamoxifen for early breast cancer: an overview of the randomised trials. Early Breast Cancer Trialists' Collaborative Group. *Lancet* 1998;351:1451.
196. Polychemotherapy for early breast cancer: an overview of the randomised trials. Early Breast Cancer Trialists' Collaborative Group. *Lancet* 1998;352:930.
197. Chaudary MA, Millis RR, Hoskins EO, et al. Bilateral primary breast cancer: a prospective study of disease incidence. *Br J Surg* 1984;71:711.
198. Kurtz JM, Amalric R, Brandone H, Ayme Y, Spitalier JM. Contralateral breast cancer and other second malignancies in patients treated by breast-conserving therapy with radiation. *Int J Radiat Oncol Biol Phys* 1988;15:277.
199. Storm HH, Andersson M, Boice JD Jr, et al. Adjuvant radiotherapy and risk of contralateral breast cancer. *J Natl Cancer Inst* 1992;84:1245.
200. Curtis RE, Boice JD Jr, Shriner DA, Hankey BF, Fraumeni JF Jr. Second cancers after adjuvant tamoxifen therapy for breast cancer: brief communication. *J Natl Cancer Inst* 1996;88:832.
201. O'Regan R, Jordan VC, Gradishar WJ. Tamoxifen and contralateral breast cancer. *J Am Coll Surg* 1999;188:678.
202. Bernstein JL, Thompson WD, Risch N, Holford TR. Risk factors predicting the incidence of second primary breast cancer among women diagnosed with a first primary breast cancer. *Am J Epidemiol* 1992;136:925.
203. Valagussa P, Moliterni A, Terenziani M, Zambetti M, Bonadonna G. Second malignancies following CMF-based adjuvant chemotherapy in resectable breast cancer. *Ann Oncol* 1994;5:803.
204. Tallman MS, Gray R, Bennett JM, et al. Leukemogenic potential of adjuvant chemotherapy for early-stage breast cancer: the Eastern Cooperative Oncology Group experience. *J Clin Oncol* 1995;13:1557.
205. Castiglione M, Goldhirsch A. Second tumours after breast cancer: is it still too soon to tell? [Editorial]. *Ann Oncol* 1994;5:785.
206. van Leeuwen FE, Benraadt J, Coebergh JW, et al. Risk of endometrial cancer after tamoxifen treatment of breast cancer. *Lancet* 1994;343:448.
207. Sasco AJ, Chaplain G, Saez S, Amoros E. Case-control study of endometrial cancer following breast cancer: effect of tamoxifen and radiotherapeutic castration. *Epidemiology* 1996;7:9(abst).
208. Some pharmaceutical drugs. *IARC Monogr Eval Carcinog Risks Hum* 1996;66:35.
209. Bernstein L, Deapen D, Cerhan JR, et al. Tamoxifen therapy for breast cancer and endometrial cancer risk. *J Natl Cancer Inst* 1999;91:1654.
210. Fisher B, Costantino JP, Wickerham DL, et al. Tamoxifen for prevention of breast cancer: report of the National Surgical Adjuvant Breast and Bowel Project P-1 Study. *J Natl Cancer Inst* 1998;90:1371.
211. Bergman L, Beelen MLR, Gallee MPW, Benraadt J, van Leeuwen FE. The effect of tamoxifen on the risk and prognosis of endometrial cancer following breast cancer: a study with 309 cases. *Lancet* 2000 (in press).
212. Mignotte H, Lasset C, Bonadona V, et al. Iatrogenic risks of endometrial carcinoma after treatment for breast cancer in a large French case-control study. Federation Nationale des Centres de Lutte Contre le Cancer (FNCLCC). *Int J Cancer* 1998;76:325.
213. Gottardis MM, Robinson SP, Satyaswaroop PG, Jordan VC. Contrasting actions of tamoxifen on endometrial and breast tumor growth in the athymic mouse. *Cancer Res* 1988;48:812.
214. Nayfield SG, Karp JE, Ford LG, Dorr FA, Kramer BS. Potential role of tamoxifen in prevention of breast cancer [Review]. *J Natl Cancer Inst* 1991;83:1450.
215. De Muylder X, Neven P, De Somer M, et al. Endometrial lesions in patients undergoing tamoxifen therapy. *Int J Gynaecol Obstet* 1991;36:127.
216. Fornander T, Hellstrom AC, Moberger B. Descriptive clinicopathologic study of 17 patients with endometrial cancer during or after adjuvant tamoxifen in early breast cancer. *J Natl Cancer Inst* 1993;85:1850.
217. Magriples U, Naftolin F, Schwartz PE, Carcangiu ML. High-grade endometrial carcinoma in tamoxifen-treated breast cancer patients. *J Clin Oncol* 1993;11:485.
218. Greaves P, Goonetilleke R, Nunn G, Topham J, Orton T. Two-year carcinogenicity study of tamoxifen in Alderley Park Wistar-derived rats. *Cancer Res* 1993;53:3919.
219. Williams GM, Iatropoulos MJ, Djordjevic MV, Kaltenberg OP. The triphenylethylene drug tamoxifen is a strong liver carcinogen in the rat. *Carcinogenesis* 1993;14:315.
220. Newcomb PA, Solomon C, White E. Tamoxifen and risk of large bowel cancer in women with breast cancer. *Breast Cancer Res Treat* 1999;53:271.
221. Neugut AI, Murray T, Santos J, et al. Increased risk of lung cancer after breast cancer radiation therapy in cigarette smokers. *Cancer* 1994;73:1615.
222. Inskip PD, Boice JD Jr. Radiotherapy-induced lung cancer among women who smoke [Editorial; comment] [published erratum appears in *Cancer* 1994;73:2456]. *Cancer* 1994;73:1541.
223. Olsen JH, Garwicz S, Hertz H, et al. Second malignant neoplasms after cancer in childhood or adolescence. Nordic Society of Paediatric Haematology and Oncology Association of the Nordic Cancer Registries. *BMJ* 1993;307:1030.
224. Hawkins MM, Draper GJ, Kingston JE. Incidence of second primary tumours among childhood cancer survivors. *Br J Cancer* 1987;56:339.

225. Meadows AT, Baum E, Fossati-Bellani F, et al. Second malignant neoplasms in children: an update from the Late Effects Study Group. *J Clin Oncol* 1985;3:532.
226. Friend SH, Bernards R, Rogelj S, et al. A human DNA segment with properties of the gene that predisposes to retinoblastoma and osteosarcoma. *Nature* 1986;323:643.
227. Knudson AG Jr, Meadows AT, Nichols WW, Hill R. Chromosomal deletion and retinoblastoma. *N Engl J Med* 1976;295:1120.
228. Brachman DG, Hallahan DE, Beckett MA, Yandell DW, Weichselbaum RR. p53 gene mutations and abnormal retinoblastoma protein in radiation-induced human sarcomas. *Cancer Res* 1991;51:6393.
229. Weichselbaum RR, Beckett M, Diamond A. Some retinoblastomas, osteosarcomas, and soft tissue sarcomas may share a common etiology. *Proc Natl Acad Sci U S A* 1988;85:2106.
230. Neglia JP, Meadows AT, Robison LL, et al. Second neoplasms after acute lymphoblastic leukemia in childhood. *N Engl J Med* 1991;325:1330.
231. Rosso P, Terracini B, Fears TR, et al. Second malignant tumors after elective end of therapy for a first cancer in childhood: a multicenter study in Italy. *Int J Cancer* 1994;59:451.
232. Walter AW, Hancock ML, Pui CH, et al. Secondary brain tumors in children treated for acute lymphoblastic leukemia at St Jude Children's Research Hospital. *J Clin Oncol* 1998;16:3761.
233. Kreissman SG, Gelber RD, Cohen HJ, et al. Incidence of secondary acute myelogenous leukemia after treatment of childhood acute lymphoblastic leukemia. *Cancer* 1992; 70:2208.
234. Winick NJ, McKenna RW, Shuster JJ, et al. Secondary acute myeloid leukemia in children with acute lymphoblastic leukemia treated with etoposide. *J Clin Oncol* 1993;11:209.
235. Sugita K, Furukawa T, Tsuchida M, et al. High frequency of etoposide (VP-16)-related secondary leukemia in children with non-Hodgkin's lymphoma. *Am J Pediatr Hematol Oncol* 1993;15:99.
236. Heyn R, Khan F, Ensign LG, et al. Acute myeloid leukemia in patients treated for rhabdomyosarcoma with cyclophosphamide and low-dose etoposide on Intergroup Rhabdomyosarcoma Study III: an interim report. *Med Pediatr Oncol* 1994;23:99.
237. Chen CL, Fuscoe JC, Liu Q, et al. Relationship between cytotoxicity and site-specific DNA recombination after *in vitro* exposure of leukemia cells to etoposide. *J Natl Cancer Inst* 1996;88:1840.
238. Le Vu B, de Vathaire F, Shamsaldin A, et al. Radiation dose, chemotherapy and risk of osteosarcoma after solid tumours during childhood. *Int J Cancer* 1998;77:370.
239. Strong LC, Herson J, Osborne BM, Sutow WW. Risk of radiation-related subsequent malignant tumors in survivors of Ewing's sarcoma. *J Natl Cancer Inst* 1979;62:1401.
240. Smith MB, Xue H, Strong L, et al. Forty-year experience with second malignancies after treatment of childhood cancer: analysis of outcome following the development of the second malignancy. *J Pediatr Surg* 1993;28:1342.
241. Sandler ES, Friedman DJ, Mustafa MM, et al. Treatment of children with epipodophyllotoxin-induced secondary acute myeloid leukemia. *Cancer* 1997;79:1049.

SECTION **8**

RAYMOND B. WEISS

Miscellaneous Toxicities

NEUROTOXICITY

VINCRISTINE, VINBLASTINE, AND VINORELBINE

The first drug class to be recognized as having neurotoxicity was the vinca alkaloids, especially vincristine. Vincristine is unique among the antitumor agents in that neurotoxicity is the sole dose-limiting problem. The neurologic injury can occur in the peripheral, central, or autonomic nervous systems.[1,2]

The most common and initial manifestations of neurotoxicity are depression of the deep tendon reflexes and paresthesias of the distal extremities. The Achilles' tendon reflexes and the fingertips are the usual respective initial sites of abnormalities. Loss of the tendon reflexes is usually asymptomatic. The paresthesias commonly progress proximally as vincristine therapy is continued and may involve the entire hands or feet. Despite the presence of peripheral paresthesias, vibration sense, position sense, pinprick sensation, and two-point discrimination are generally unaffected.

Motor dysfunction and gait disorders are initially manifested as lower extremity weakness. Footdrop may ensue, and if vincristine is continued, weakness to the point of paraparesis may develop. However, when vincristine and corticosteroids are administered together, steroid myopathy often occurs and causes similar symptoms of weakness, which should not be ascribed to vincristine neurotoxicity and result in a dose modification of the wrong drug.[3] Patients with hereditary neuropathies are especially prone to the additive effects of vincristine neuropathy.[4] Severe bone pain (especially in the mandible) may occur acutely a few hours after drug administration but usually subsides after a few days.[5]

Cranial nerves may be affected and cause ophthalmoplegia and facial palsy. Toxicity to the parasympathetic nervous system is manifested by constipation and difficult micturition, which can progress to paralytic ileus and bladder atony. Autonomic neuropathy can produce orthostatic hypotension (which can be symptomatic or clinically silent[6]) and erection/ejaculatory dysfunction.[7] Other rare, but severe, neurotoxic manifestations observed from vincristine include cortical blindness[8] and laryngeal nerve (with vocal cord) paralysis,[9] resulting in dysphonia and even aphonia.

Neurotoxicity from the vinca alkaloids, especially vincristine, is both an individual dose and a cumulative dose phenomena. The usual practice in adults is to limit an individual dose of vincristine to 2 mg. Studies of higher vincristine dosing[7] have shown a very high rate of neurotoxicity. No effective prevention or treatment has been developed except to stop therapy and wait for neurologic recovery. The neuropathy symptoms may persist as long as 3 or 4 years after cessation of therapy, but they usually wane to a point where they are no longer troublesome to the patient.[10] Empiric vitamin therapy is ineffective. Intestinal dysfunction from autonomic neuropathy may be improved by metoclopramide therapy.[11]

Vincristine binds to the B subunit of tubulin, causing disruption of microtubule function in neuronal axons. Electrophysiologic studies indicate distal axonal dysfunction, and nerve conduction testing shows sensory nerves are most affected with a reduced amplitude of nerve action potentials. Histologic changes are generally those of axonal degeneration.

The vincristine analogues vinblastine and vinorelbine also have neurotoxicity potential. The primary dose-limiting toxicity of both vinblastine and vinorelbine is myelosuppression, and neurotoxicity is less common than that occurring from vincristine. The form and range of neurotoxicity manifestations from these analogues are similar to those of vincristine, and again, the degree of dysfunction is related to both individual and cumulative drug doses. However, vinblastine and vinorelbine seem to produce more autonomic effects, resulting in severe constipation and paralytic ileus.[12]

Concurrent use of two neurotoxic agents has been reported to cause enhanced neurotoxicity or no such toxicity, depending on the drug involved. The combination of vinorelbine and cisplatin seems not to increase the incidence or severity of neuropathy.[13] However, when vinorelbine is used either in combination with, or sequentially after, paclitaxel, there is more potential for severe neuropathy.[14,15] In addition, the combination of vincristine and a granulocyte growth factor may precipitate a severe neuropathy involving primarily the legs.[16]

CISPLATIN AND OXALIPLATIN

Although nephrotoxicity is a major and cumulative dose-limiting toxicity of cisplatin, neurotoxicity is also a common problem and can be dose-limiting for both single and cumulative doses, but primarily the latter.[17–20] Cisplatin-induced neuropathy can be manifested as sensory peripheral neuropathy, Lhermitte's sign, autonomic neuropathy, grand mal or focal seizures, encephalopathy, transient cortical blindness, retrobulbar neuritis, and retinal injury.[17,21,22]

The incidence of neurotoxicity ranges up to 100%, depending on individual and cumulative drug dose, treatment duration, concurrent or prior neurotoxic drugs used, the presence of other medical conditions, and possibly gender (women being more sensitive).[17,18] A cumulative cisplatin dose of 300 to 500 mg/m^2 is the range in which toxicity most often occurs.[17,20]

Peripheral neuropathy similar to that induced by vincristine is the most common form of cisplatin neurotoxicity. Vincristine produces initial paresthesias in the fingers, whereas cisplatin most often affects the toes and feet.[23] Loss of the Achilles' tendon reflexes is an early sign, and continued treatment leads to sensory ataxia and loss of proximal deep tendon reflexes and vibration sense. Although muscle cramps are a common symptom, motor function is usually not affected.

The pathophysiology of cisplatin neurotoxicity is not known, but it is probably related to the accumulation of inorganic platinum within neurons, which may be irreversible. An autopsy study[24] of platinum concentrations and histopathologic changes in the dorsal root ganglia of cisplatin-treated patients demonstrated a correlation of the tissue level of platinum with neuronal histologic changes and clinical neurotoxicity.

Treatment is discontinuation of therapy, but neurotoxic symptoms may last for months after cisplatin therapy is discontinued. The electrophysiologic test abnormalities may last for several years and perhaps indefinitely. The symptoms and signs may even progress despite discontinuing treatment.[25] Amitriptyline has been used as treatment for the neuropathies related to use of antitumor agents, but no clinical trials in this clinical setting evaluating efficacy in double-blind fashion have been performed. Because treatment of neurotoxicity is of limited benefit, prevention using protective agents has been extensively explored.[26] Amifostine, a nephrotoxicity protectant, also provides significant protection against peripheral neuropathy when used in conjunction with cisplatin.[27] Dimesna is a new drug with exceptional promise as a neuroprotective agent and is in advanced clinical development for this indication.[28]

Concurrent use of cisplatin with paclitaxel has demonstrated an enhanced potential for neurotoxicity, although variability exists, probably related to the drug doses and schedules employed. At the doses of these two drugs that are commonly used, more than 50% of patients may develop neuropathy, and this problem is often dose-limiting.[29,30] When patients receiving this drug combination are closely monitored, neurotoxicity may be evident after just two cycles in nearly all cases.[30]

Neuropathy is the most common toxicity of the cisplatin analogue oxaliplatin, and cumulative neurotoxicity is usually dose-limiting. The manifestations are peripheral sensory neuropathy and muscle cramps similar to that of cisplatin, but pharyngolaryngeal dysesthesias (presenting as dyspnea and dysphagia) are a unique symptom seen with this drug.[31] These neuropathic problems may be triggered by touching cold surfaces (finger paresthesias) or drinking cold liquids (pharyngolaryngeal symptoms). Most patients have a nearly full recovery within 6 months after discontinuing therapy.[32]

CYTARABINE

Cytarabine is administered both intravenously and intrathecally, and both routes can produce neurotoxicity. Manifestations include cerebellar dysfunction, seizures, generalized encephalopathy, peripheral neuropathy, necrotizing leukoencephalopathy, spinal myelopathy, basal ganglia necrosis, and pseudobulbar palsy.[33]

The highest incidence (15% to 37%) occurs in patients receiving high-dose cytarabine therapy (i.e., more than 1 g/m^2 in multiple doses).[33,34] The toxicity is generally acute and not related to cumulative drug doses, in contrast to neuropathy associated with cisplatin and vincristine. Risk factors for neurotoxicity are age older than 50 years, drug dose, prior cytarabine treatment, and renal dysfunction.[33,35]

Cerebellar effects (dysarthria, ataxia, and dysmetria) are the most common form of neurotoxicity. These symptoms often occur within days of first treatment and are accompanied by headache, altered mentation, memory loss, and somnolence. Seizures have rarely occurred. Peripheral neuropathy can also occur but is rare. Symptoms range from a purely sensory neuropathy to sensorimotor polyneuropathies in a glove-stocking distribution.[33] The neuropathy can even progress to a quadriparesis, with ventilatory support being necessary.[36] Intrathecal cytarabine can produce an ascending myelopathy.[37] All of these neurologic abnormalities (even the peripheral neuropathy) can progress to coma and death.[33,35,38]

Recovery from the neurologic effects usually occurs within a few days after discontinuing cytarabine therapy. There is no known treatment. Serial radiographic studies of the brain have shown improvement in cerebellar abnormalities after discontinuing treatment,[39] but progressive atrophy may also occur after a few months and is associated with persistent symptoms.[40] Instances[41] have been reported of ascending myelopathy with paraplegia from intrathecal cytarabine in which complete recovery took place within 1 hour after onset.

The mechanism of such neurotoxicity is not known. When high drug doses are used, cytotoxic concentrations of cytarabine reach the cerebrospinal fluid, but parent drug and metabolites are cleared more slowly from spinal fluid than blood, a likely explanation for the dose relationship of this toxicity.[42] Neuron function and survival appears to be inhibited by cytarabine through blocking of an essential deoxynucleoside.[43] Why the Purkinje cells of the cerebellum are particularly prone to injury from intravenous cytarabine, even in experimental animals,[44] is unknown.

IFOSFAMIDE

Ifosfamide and cyclophosphamide have similar chemical structures, but ifosfamide induces neurotoxicity (as it does nephrotoxicity), whereas cyclophosphamide does not. Acute symptoms are visual and auditory hallucinations, vivid dreams, logorrhea, incontinence, dizziness, palilalia, confusion, perseveration, agitation, personality changes, somnolence, cerebellar and cranial nerve dysfunction, hemiparesis, seizures, coma, and occasionally death.[45–48] Peripheral neuropathy and extrapyramidal abnormalities, such as myoclonus and muscular spasticity, also have been reported. The onset is acute up to 5 days after beginning ifosfamide, and recovery usually occurs within a few days after discontinuing therapy. Memory and affect disorders may occasionally persist. No cumulative-dose neurotoxic effects have been reported, but re-treatment with ifosfamide may again precipitate the same acute toxicity manifestations.

Significant neurotoxic abnormalities occur in approximately 10% of patients treated with ifosfamide. The incidence varies depending on how carefully patients are monitored for this problem, the ifosfamide dose and method of administration used, and the presence of various risk factors. Such risk factors are low serum albumin, any degree of renal dysfunction, prior administration of cisplatin (probably resulting in subclinical renal dysfunction), poor performance status, the presence of central nervous system tumor, and age (children being more susceptible than adults).[45,48,49] High doses may accentuate symptoms of an underlying mild neuropathy and cause severe and painful paresthesias.[50] For unknown reasons, oral administration of ifosfamide has more neurotoxic potential than the intravenous route.[51]

The etiology of this neurotoxicity is probably multifactorial and is due to one or more metabolites of ifosfamide that are produced in high quantities.[52] Cyclophosphamide may not produce neurotoxicity because metabolites with encephalopathic potential are a minor component of its degradation. Effective treatment (besides discontinuing the ifosfamide) has been intravenous diazepam[53] and methylene blue.[52,54] Such treatment can produce dramatic reversal of the neurotoxic manifestations. Means of prevention include a continuous infusion schedule of drug administration and concurrent use of methylene blue.[54]

5-FLUOROURACIL

5-Fluorouracil (5-FU) has been known to cause neurotoxicity since the earliest clinical trials were conducted with this drug. Cerebellar dysfunction with findings of gait ataxia, nystagmus, dysmetria, and dysarthria is the most common form of neurotoxicity, but confusion, somnolence, seizures, coma, and peripheral neuropathy also have been observed.[55–57] The incidence is approximately 5%, and it may occur with any of the administration schedules in common use. Neurotoxicity from this drug is acute in onset, and a cumulative-dose effect has not been observed. It is now common practice to administer leucovorin in combination with 5-FU to enhance antitumor activity. Leucovorin may itself be the etiology[58] of some of the instances of seizures occurring in conjunction with administration of these two drugs.

The combination of 5-FU and levamisole may produce a multifocal leukoencephalopathy manifested by agitation, confusion, short-term memory loss, diplopia, cerebellar dysfunction, and expressive aphasia.[59] Magnetic resonance imaging of the brain shows multiple, enhanced, white matter lesions (sometimes ring-enhanced) in the cerebrum, and histologic examination shows focal demyelination. Such toxicity has not been reported when 5-FU has been used alone, but it has occurred with use of levamisole alone.[60] Therefore, the levamisole in this adjuvant therapy combination is probably the most culpable in producing these cerebral effects.

The etiology of 5-FU neurotoxicity is not well understood. 5-FU metabolites have been shown to have neuropathic action in experimental animals.[61] However, it may also be due to parent drug, and not metabolites, because patients have been reported who developed severe toxic symptoms due to a genetic deficiency of the initial enzyme necessary for catabolizing 5-FU.[62] Patients with complete or partial deficiency of this enzyme, dihydropyrimidine dehydrogenase, appear particularly subject to 5-FU toxicity of all kinds including neuropathy.

METHOTREXATE

Neurotoxicity from methotrexate can manifest as meningeal irritation, transient paraparesis, or encephalopathy. When the drug is administered intrathecally (IT), it can cause headache, nausea and vomiting, lethargy, nuchal rigidity, and other features of meningeal irritation.[63] A subacute set of abnormalities include paraparesis, hemiparesis, somnolence, cranial nerve dysfunction, cerebellar symptoms, and seizures, which can develop days to several weeks after therapy. Such encephalopathy symptoms may occur more commonly when both IT and intravenous high-dose methotrexate are administered.[64] When IT methotrexate is given repetitively (especially if it is administered via an intraventricular device), progressive necrotizing leukoencephalopathy may develop. Although acute onset with resultant death has occurred,[65] the usual symptoms include initial memory loss with occasional later progression to severe dementia, gait disturbance, dysphasia, and seizures.[66] Even if serious neuropathy does not occur, subtle cognitive deficits may develop months to years later, especially in children.[67] Risk factors for such problems are cranial irradiation, presence of neoplastic cells in the spinal fluid, and cumulative drug dose. The neurotoxic effect is probably a direct consequence of high drug dose concentrations in the cerebrospinal fluid.

Intravenous methotrexate also can produce encephalopathy, especially if high doses and leucovorin rescue are used.[68] The manifestations and risk factors are similar to those of IT methotrexate. The neurologic dysfunction may be acute and transient or delayed in onset with personality changes. Magnetic resonance imaging can show white matter abnormalities in asymptomatic patients that are probably subclinical manifestations of neurotoxicity.[69] However, it has been argued that such findings do not necessarily correlate with subsequent intellectual dysfunction and therefore may be inconsequential.[70] Treatment consists of active hydration to facilitate methotrexate clearance and leucovorin to circumvent the enzyme inhibition of methotrexate.

It has been postulated that this toxicity arises from methotrexate-related impairment of synthesis of neurotransmitters and accumulation of adenosine and homocysteine.[71] Based on this hypothesis that the neurotoxicity is related to brain accumulation of adenosine, aminophylline (an adenosine receptor antagonist) has been used successfully to reverse the neurologic effects of methotrexate.[72]

PACLITAXEL AND DOCETAXEL

The two analogues paclitaxel and docetaxel cause neurotoxicity similar to that of cisplatin and vincristine in the form of a peripheral neuropathy that can be a treatment-limiting effect.[73–77] The clinical manifestations are glove-stocking or perioral paresthesias and/or burning pain, loss of vibration sense, loss of deep tendon reflexes, Lhermitte's sign, and orthostatic hypotension. Motor dysfunction in the form of both proximal and distal extremity weakness also has been observed.[78] However, it is impossible to determine how much taxane-associated myopathy might be due to the antitumor drug and how much to the intermittent, but large, doses of corticosteroids that are used concurrently with the taxanes to minimize the risk of hypersensitivity reactions. Transient scintillating scotomata and visual deficits due to optic neuropathy[79] and encephalopathy[80] in the form of confusion and behavioral changes also have been reported. A possible risk factor for initiating or enhancing the neural dysfunction from these drugs is an underlying neuropathy from other conditions such as diabetes mellitus and ethanol abuse.[73] However, one study[81] has shown that patients with diabetes may be treated with standard doses of paclitaxel, and they do not develop neurotoxicity to a greater degree than expected.

Both a single-dose and cumulative-dose relationship is noted for paclitaxel. Single doses of more than 175 mg/m^2 given at 3-week intervals produce a higher rate of neurotoxicity than lesser doses, and at 250 mg/m^2, neurotoxicity is dose-limiting in as many as 70% of patients.[74] When paclitaxel is given weekly in 1-hour infusions, severe neurotoxicity occurs at doses of more than 100 mg/m^2.[82] Cumulative dosing also increases the frequency of neurotoxicity, but there is no neurotoxic dose threshold. Depending on the drug dose used, the onset of these problems can be within a few days of receiving the first dose or after several cycles of therapy. A docetaxel dose of 100 mg/m^2 also induces mild to moderate neurotoxic symptoms in as many as 50% of patients after five cycles of therapy.[76,77] A cumulative docetaxel dose of 400 mg/m^2 can produce severe symptoms and electrophysiologic changes in nerves,[77] but as with paclitaxel, there is no threshold dose. Concurrent or prior use of other neurotoxic agents (cisplatin,[30,83,84] oxaliplatin,[85] or vinorelbine[14]) enhances the risk and degree of neurotoxicity manifestations from both of the taxanes.

The mechanism of taxane neurotoxicity is likely a drug effect on neuronal microtubules, causing axonal degeneration and demyelination. Neurometric testing demonstrates decreased nerve conduction velocities and absent sural nerve action potentials from both taxanes.[73,76,77]

The only effective treatment, as with the other neurotoxic antitumor agents, is discontinuing therapy and allowing the symptoms to wane over time (which they usually, but not always, do). Amitriptyline may or may not help with symptom relief. With this toxicity being so prevalent and often dose-limiting with these two potent antitumor agents, development of an efficacious neuroprotectant is a high priority. Amifostine has not demonstrated efficacy as a neurotoxicity protectant for paclitaxel.[86] Dimesna is a new agent in clinical development as a protectant for both paclitaxel-induced[87] and cisplatin-induced[28] neurotoxicity.

ALTRETAMINE (HEXAMETHYLMELAMINE)

Altretamine (hexamethylmelamine) causes a variety of peripheral and central nervous system toxicities. Peripheral neuropathy is the most common form and manifests as paresthesias, hyperesthesia, hyporeflexia, and diminished proprioception.[88] Central nervous effects are confusion, dysphagia, personality changes, ataxia, somnolence, seizures, respiratory dyskinesia, and parkinsonian tremors.[88]

Neurotoxicity is related to both individual and cumulative doses. Intermittent dosing schedules help reduce this side effect. The incidence varies depending on the dose but can be as high as 40%. Altretamine can be safely administered to patients who have been treated previously with cisplatin, but if significant cisplatin neuropathy is present, the neurotoxic manifestations may worsen.[89]

PROCARBAZINE

Neurotoxicity from procarbazine has been known since it was first used clinically.[90] Both central and peripheral neurotoxicity symptoms can occur. Cerebral symptoms predominate and consist of lethargy, depression, confusion, hallucinations, agitation and, rarely, psychosis. Extremity paresthesias and depressed deep tendon reflexes are the manifestations of peripheral neuropathy.

Procarbazine is most commonly used in combination with the vinca alkaloids, so it is difficult to determine which agent is causing peripheral neuropathy symptoms. The incidence of neuropathy induced by procarbazine alone is 20% or less. It is much higher when procarbazine and vincristine are used concurrently. Treatment is discontinuation of therapy. Cerebral symptoms usually resolve promptly, but peripheral neuropathy may last for weeks to months.

ALDESLEUKIN (INTERLEUKIN-2)

The biologic antitumor agent aldesleukin (interleukin-2) has many toxicities precipitated by increased vascular permeability. Neurotoxicity in the form of hallucinations, disorientation, agitation, combativeness, seizures, and coma may also occur.[91,92] A neurotoxic manifestation unique to this drug is carpal tunnel syndrome, which appears to be a consequence of interstitial edema (due to the vascular leak), causing pressure on the median nerve.[93]

FLUDARABINE, CLADRIBINE, AND PENTOSTATIN

When fludarabine was tested in phase I and II trials, central nervous toxicity was so severe that the studies had to be closed prematurely. Altered mental status, photophobia, amaurosis, generalized seizures, dementia, spastic or flaccid paralysis, quadriparesis, and coma occurred at doses of more than 90 mg/m^2 given for 5 to 7 days.[94] Despite discontinuing therapy, some patients had progressive neurologic abnormalities and died. At autopsy, leukoencephalopathy was present in the occipital lobes. Because such severe toxicity is clearly dose-related, the recommended fludarabine dose is 25 mg/m^2 daily for 5 days at monthly intervals. This dose usually causes no more than mild and uncommon (incidence of approximately 15%) neurotoxicity symptoms, but sporadic cases of severe (and even fatal) neurotoxicity have occurred, some of which even developed a few months after fludarabine therapy was stopped.[95–97]

Both cladribine and pentostatin can cause severe, and fatal, neurotoxicity when administered at doses producing marked myelosuppression. The manifestations are similar to those of fludarabine.[95] However, like fludarabine, drug doses in the range recommended for usual therapy produce only rare instances of severe neurotoxicity.[95]

TABLE 55.8-1. Antitumor Agents That Cause Neurotoxicity

HIGH POTENTIAL FOR NEUROTOXICITY
Altretamine
L-Asparaginase
Carboplatin
Cisplatin
Cytarabine
Docetaxel
Fludarabine
5-Fluorouracil
Ifosfamide
Interferons (in high doses)
Methotrexate
Oxaliplatin
Paclitaxel
Pentostatin
Procarbazine
Suramin
Tretinoin
Vinblastine
Vincristine
Vinorelbine
OCCASIONAL IRREVERSIBLE NEUROTOXICITY
Cisplatin
Cytarabine
Docetaxel
5-Fluorouracil (with levamisole)
Ifosfamide
Paclitaxel
Suramin
ISOLATED INSTANCES OF NEUROTOXICITY
Aldesleukin
Busulfan (in stem cell transplant doses)
Chlorambucil
Dacarbazine
Etoposide (in stem cell transplant doses)
Gemcitabine
Interferons (in low doses)
Teniposide

OTHER AGENTS

Table 55.8-1 lists other antitumor drugs that can produce neurotoxicity and categorizes them based on the risk for this effect. The manifestations are similar to those described for the individual drugs. Certain ones (e.g., busulfan[98]) produce problems such as seizures only when very high doses are administered in the stem cell transplantation setting, even despite the use of prophylactic anticonvulsant medication.

NEPHROTOXICITY

The kidneys are the elimination pathway of many antitumor drugs and their metabolites and, therefore, are vulnerable to injury. The entire anatomic pathway from glomerulus to distal tubule is at risk, depending on the drug involved. The symptoms vary from an asymptomatic rise in serum creatinine or mild proteinuria to acute renal failure with anuria requiring dialysis.

CISPLATIN AND CARBOPLATIN

The nephrotoxicity of cisplatin has been well known since it was first used clinically in the early 1970s. This obstacle to its clinical use has been so profound that several thousand cisplatin analogues have subsequently been synthesized in hopes of finding a less nephrotoxic compound with equivalent antitumor efficacy. A means of avoiding nephrotoxicity by forcing diuresis and enhancing cisplatin excretion was first reported in 1977.[99] This seminal work allowed safer use of this drug with its wide spectrum of antitumor efficacy.

Cisplatin renal toxicity is dose-related, cumulative, and manifested primarily by a decrease in the glomerular filtration rate, which is clinically approximated by increases in the serum creatinine and decreases in the creatinine clearance. Single drug doses of less than 50 mg/m^2 usually cause little renal injury, but higher doses require aggressive hydration, otherwise abrupt, irreversible renal failure may ensue.[100] Hydration reduces cisplatin concentration and the time it is in contact with the tubular epithelium, which helps to limit the tubular injurious effect of the drug. The hydration used most successfully is normal saline because the high chloride inhibits cisplatin hydrolysis in the tubules, which seems to add to the nephrotoxicity-protection effect of diuresis. Mannitol also is used to enhance diuresis, but no evidence indicates that mannitol is necessary. Concurrent use of furosemide to enhance diuresis further is unnecessary and may even be harmful, as it was in animal experiments.[101] A urine output of at least 100 mL/hour for 2 to 4 hours before and 4 to 6 hours after cisplatin doses of 50 to 75 mg/m^2 reduces, but does not eliminate, nephrotoxicity. More intensive hydration schedules are necessary when higher cisplatin doses are used.

The pathologic lesion of cisplatin nephrotoxicity is seen primarily in the proximal and distal tubules but also may involve the collecting ducts, whereas the glomeruli are unaffected.[102] The extent of tubular injury helps to explain why electrolyte abnormalities, such as hyponatremia and hypomagnesemia, are so common after cisplatin administration.[103,104] The hypomagnesemia is symptomatic only in approximately 10% of patients, but it can last months to years after completing therapy.[105] Magnesium supplementation in conjunction with cisplatin administration can minimize, but does not eliminate, hypomagnesemia.[106] The hyponatremia has been reported to cause persistent orthostatic hypotension.[104]

The mechanism of the tubular injury is not fully understood. It is not simply the tubular handling of a heavy metal, because the *trans* isomer of cisplatin is not nephrotoxic. Cisplatin produces DNA intrastrand cross-links as one of its mechanisms of antitumor effect, and the same effect perhaps occurs on DNA in tubule cells, causing defects in tubular (especially proximal) resorption.

A variety of substances have been evaluated for minimizing cisplatin nephrotoxicity in the hope that the cumbersome process of hydration can be circumvented. These include sodium thiosulfate, amifostine, probenecid, diethyldithiocarbamate, superoxide dismutase, hypertonic saline, glutathione, bismuth compound, and mesna.[107] Only one of these many compounds (amifostine) has provided sufficient protective benefits to become accepted for routine use. Amifostine demonstrated statistically significant protection against cisplatin-induced nephrotoxicity[27,108] and is now marketed for this indication. However, amifostine has its own toxicities that can be an obstacle to convenient use, such as hypotension and nausea and vomiting. One simple technique for nephrotoxicity protection besides hydration is to administer cisplatin in the evening to take advantage of circadian rhythm effects that have been shown to reduce renal injury,[109] although this timing may be impractical in the outpatient setting. A final measure of protection is to be certain that renal function is normal by performing a pretreatment 24-hour, measured creatinine clearance. A result of less than 70 mL/min, especially in patients older than 60 years of age, may preclude cisplatin use without a significant risk of nephrotoxicity.[110] In addition, other renal tubular toxins, such as aminoglycoside antibiotics, should be avoided whenever possible to prevent additive tubular damage.

Carboplatin was synthesized as a cisplatin alternative with less nephrotoxicity and without a requirement of hydration for safe administration. It is definitely less nephrotoxic, but it is not free of potential for renal injury, especially in patients who have previously received nephrotoxins, or when given in high doses in the stem cell transplantation setting.[111,112] Carboplatin-related renal dysfunction is usually detectable only by means of sensitive kidney function tests, such as urine tubular enzyme excretion or glomerular filtration rate, and is transient.[113,114] The serum creatinine and creatinine clearance are rarely affected.

Life-threatening hemolytic-uremic syndrome has been reported as a rare form of acute renal dysfunction related to cisplatin and carboplatin.[115,116] Many of the reported instances related to cisplatin have involved combined use of cisplatin and bleomycin,[117] so it is unclear which drug is most culpable in initiating this fulminant toxicity.

MITOMYCIN

The capacity of mitomycin to produce renal toxicity has been known for many years, and it can be life-threatening. The clinical manifestations vary from a chronic, progressive rise in serum creatinine to fulminant onset of microangiopathic hemolytic anemia (MAHA). The latter problem has been reported in a large number of anecdotal cases,[118,119] but in one study of adjuvant therapy with mitomycin, a 10.7% incidence occurred.[120] It was also observed[121] in 10% of patients treated with a combination of mitomycin and tamoxifen, and the authors of this study suggested some interaction between the two drugs might have contributed to the development of this toxicity.

The MAHA toxicity is cumulative dose–related, but even only several mitomycin doses can initiate it. It also can develop a few months after mitomycin has been discontinued.[118,122] The risk of developing MAHA increases when the cumulative mitomycin dose exceeds 60 mg.[122]

The clinical presentation of MAHA is an abrupt and often severe hemolytic anemia that usually precedes the renal dysfunction by 1 or 2 weeks. The peripheral blood smear shows schistocytes, and thrombocytopenia becomes apparent as renal failure develops. Other manifestations are rash, fever, arterial hypertension, central neurologic dysfunction, pericarditis, interstitial pneumonitis, pulmonary hemorrhage, hematuria, and proteinuria.[118,122] A high rate (65%) of patients have noncardiogenic pulmonary edema.[122] A prominent feature is the fact the MAHA is often precipitated or worsened by blood transfusions, suggesting that blood product administration should be avoided as much as possible when treating patients with mitomycin. The outcome is often (more than 50% of the time) death, despite vigorous treatment, although a few long-term survivors (who have persistent mild renal dysfunction) have been reported.[122,123]

Treatment includes hemodialysis and plasmapheresis. The most successful treatment has been plasma perfusion over filters containing staphylococcal protein A, a method of extracting circulating immune complexes.[124]

The pathogenesis of this acute nephropathy is not certain. When injected directly into the renal arteries of rats, mitomycin caused glomerular endothelial damage,[125] and increases in vascular endothelial cell markers in plasma have been observed in patients who developed MAHA related to mitomycin.[126] This vascular injury probably activates platelets and leads to fibrin thrombi deposition in the microvasculature of the kidney, thus initiating renal dysfunction and a mechanical shearing of red blood cells with resultant hemolysis.

METHOTREXATE

When methotrexate is administered in conventional oral or intravenous doses, nephrotoxicity is only an occasional problem. If high doses with folinic acid rescue are used, acute nephrotoxicity can pose a greater danger.

Methotrexate is excreted rapidly in the urine whether it is administered orally or parenterally. Both the parent compound and the major metabolite, 7-hydroxymethotrexate, are filtered by the glomeruli and actively secreted by the tubules. At physiologic pH, the drug is fully ionized, but in acidified form (pH less than 5.7), the parent drug and main metabolite are less ionized and may precipitate. During urinary excretion, drug precipitation occurs as the urine is concentrated and acidified in the tubules. The solubility of 7-hydroxymethotrexate is only one-fourth that of the parent drug, thus providing further potential for drug precipitation within tubules and resultant acute renal dysfunction.

Acute methotrexate nephrotoxicity produces abrupt renal insufficiency. The serum creatinine rises rapidly, and costovertebral angle pain (from renal swelling) may occur. Dehydration, oliguria, and even anuria may develop.

Methotrexate-induced renal insufficiency is primarily a physical process of tubular drug precipitation. It can be largely prevented by methods designed to hinder this precipitation of drug in the tubules: hydration and urine alkalinization.[127] Whenever a drug dose high enough to require leucovorin rescue is being given, the urine should be kept alkaline (pH higher than 8) with sodium bicarbonate administration, and a urine output of 100 mL/hour should be maintained. Serial serum methotrexate levels should be monitored until the drug concentration declines to 10^{-8} molar or less, 24 to 48 hours after administration.[127]

If methotrexate clearance is impaired by renal dysfunction already present or initiated by concurrently administered drugs, nephrotoxicity can develop or be enhanced. For example, prior therapy with cisplatin may contribute to methotrexate nephrotoxicity,[128] and concurrent administration of nonsteroidal antiinflammatory drugs may engender serious, and even fatal, renal dysfunction from methotrexate. Indomethacin, ketoprofen, diclofenac, and naproxen all have been reported to intensify renal dysfunction from methotrexate, whether it is being given in high doses[129] or low doses.[130] This enhanced toxicity is probably mediated by a reduction in methotrexate clearance caused by the concurrent drug administration.

Sequential hemodialysis and charcoal hemofiltration[131] have been used as treatment of acute nephrotoxicity from high methotrexate doses. A highly successful therapy has been administration of a combination of thymidine, leucovorin, and the recombinant form of the bacterial enzyme carboxypeptidase G_2,[132] which quickly converts methotrexate to a harmless metabolite. Both thymidine and carboxypeptidase are available on a compassionate-use basis from the National Cancer Institute for treating this life-threatening toxicity.[132]

STREPTOZOCIN, CARMUSTINE, AND LOMUSTINE

Streptozocin has the most potential for nephrotoxicity in the nitrosourea drug class, and renal damage is its dose-limiting toxicity.[133] Prolonged drug administration increases the risk of such toxicity, and most patients eventually display it if therapy continues.

The kidneys are the major excretion pathway for both parent drug and its metabolites, the probable main factor in the pathogenesis of the nephrotoxicity. Streptozocin injury occurs in both the glomeruli and tubules (primarily the proximal), where histologic changes have been observed, but the mechanism is unknown. Hyperphosphatemia and proteinuria are early indicators of renal effect. Renal tubular acidosis is a frequent occurrence, manifested by glycosuria, acetonuria, hyperchloremia, and aminoaciduria.[133] If streptozocin is discontinued, these findings usually resolve. A rising serum creatinine is a later, and sometimes irreversible, finding. Hydration and diuresis during therapy have occasionally minimized the renal dysfunction.[134]

The other two nitrosoureas in wide clinical use (carmustine and lomustine) are much less nephrotoxic. Carmustine usually causes interstitial pneumonitis toxicity before it affects the kidneys. Lomustine has produced only rare instances of nephrotoxicity when unusually large cumulative doses have been administered.[135]

IFOSFAMIDE

Cyclophosphamide and ifosfamide are analogues with similar chemical structures. Both produce the metabolite acrolein, which can cause hemorrhagic cystitis during urinary excretion. Despite their similarities in chemical structure, toxicity, and antitumor efficacy, they differ significantly in their ability to cause nephrotoxicity. Cyclophosphamide produces no renal toxicity of any clinical consequence, whereas ifosfamide initiates a variety of renal abnormalities that may in some instances result in death or irreversible renal failure requiring chronic hemodialysis or renal transplantation, especially in children who are at higher risk for this problem.[136,137] Hypotheses regarding the mechanism of ifosfamide nephrotoxicity and why cyclophosphamide does not have such effect have been formulated based on the differences in metabolism of these two drugs (ifosfamide produces much more chloracetaldehyde) and the unique effect of ifosfamide on proximal renal tubule cells.[138,139]

Initial clinical studies of ifosfamide showed that single high doses could precipitate acute tubular necrosis and renal failure within a few days of administration. This severe toxicity was one reason a fractionated dose schedule was developed for this drug. Administration over 5 consecutive days reduced both renal and bladder toxicity, but the most effective measure for reducing urinary tract problems was the development of mesna as a means of protection against the drug-induced cystitis. Mesna is now a standard accompaniment to ifosfamide use, but it limits the cystitis, *not* the nephrotoxicity.[140] There is no known means of preventing ifosfamide renal toxicity.

The incidence of renal toxicity varies from 5% up to 30%. Besides young age (especially younger than 5 years),[137] risk factors are drug dose (cumulative doses of more than 60 g/m^2), unilateral nephrectomy, prior renal irradiation, presence of retroperitoneal masses, and prior cisplatin treatment.[141–143] Clinical manifestations include tubular dysfunction, Fanconi's syndrome, and a rising serum creatinine. The tubular injury is indicated by aminoaciduria, glycosuria, renal tubular acidosis, hypokalemia, proteinuria, and phosphaturia with hypophosphatemia.[138] These abnormalities can even result in renal rickets and growth retardation, which require long-term therapy.[137,141,144] Once acute renal dysfunction from this drug becomes evident, it may or may not be reversible, so frequent monitoring of renal and tubular function during ifosfamide therapy is important, with prompt treatment when dysfunction occurs.[138] Progression to renal failure is generally not a problem in children,[144] but such failure may occur in adults, even with only moderate cumulative doses of ifosfamide.[145] Renal abnormalities may not become evident until long after ifosfamide therapy has been completed.[146]

OTHER AGENTS

Table 55.8-2 lists the antitumor agents that have been reported to cause renal injury. They are categorized by the risk of such toxicity from those drugs with an occasional anecdotal report to those with high risk for severe damage.

Not only can individual drugs cause nephrotoxicity, but combinations of agents can occasionally precipitate serious reactions, such as hemolytic uremic syndrome from cisplatin and bleomycin.[117] In addition, the intensive doses of chemotherapy used in conditioning for stem cell transplantation can induce hemolytic uremic syndrome with an acute or delayed onset and sometimes fatal outcome.[147]

HEPATOTOXICITY

A number of antitumor agents cause hepatic toxicity (Table 55.8-3). This toxicity takes three main forms: hepatocellular dysfunction and chemical hepatitis, venoocclusive disease (VOD), and chronic fibrosis.

HEPATOCELLULAR DYSFUNCTION

Hepatocellular dysfunction usually is caused by a direct effect of either the parent drug or a metabolite and is an acute event. Serum hepatic enzymes rise as cellular damage occurs. Fatty infiltration and cholestasis may occur as the toxic effect progresses. Hepatic metastases, viral hepatitis, and drugs administered for other therapeutic purposes (e.g., antiemetics) can cause similar enzymatic abnormalities. Thus, the clini-

TABLE 55.8-2. Antitumor Agents That Cause Nephrotoxicity

HIGH POTENTIAL FOR NEPHROTOXICITY
Aldesleukin (interleukin-2)
Azacitidine
Cisplatin
Gallium nitrate
Ifosfamide
Methotrexate (in high doses)
Mitomycin
Plicamycin
Streptozocin
AZOTEMIA WITHOUT NEPHROTOXICITY
L-Asparaginase
Dacarbazine
OCCASIONAL IRREVERSIBLE NEPHROTOXICITY
Cisplatin
Fludarabine
Gallium nitrate
Ifosfamide
Interferons
Lomustine
Mitomycin
Pentostatin
Streptozocin
ISOLATED INSTANCES OF NEPHROTOXICITY
Carboplatin
6-Mercaptopurine
Methotrexate (in low doses)

TABLE 55.8-3. Antitumor Agents That Cause Hepatotoxicity

HIGH POTENTIAL FOR HEPATOTOXICITY
L-Asparaginase
Cytarabine
Interferons (in high doses)
Methotrexate (long-term therapy)
Streptozocin
HIGH POTENTIAL FOR HEPATOTOXICITY WITH HIGH DOSES
Busulfan
Carmustine
Cyclophosphamide
Cytarabine
Dactinomycin
Methotrexate
Mitomycin
OCCASIONAL IRREVERSIBLE HEPATOTOXICITY
Busulfan (in high doses)
Carmustine (in high doses)
Cytarabine
Dacarbazine
Methotrexate
Mitomycin
ISOLATED INSTANCES OF HEPATOTOXICITY
Dacarbazine
Hydroxyurea
Interferons (in low doses)
6-Mercaptopurine
Pentostatin
6-Thioguanine
Vincristine

cal picture, appropriate laboratory or radiologic studies, and the pattern of abnormal liver function tests must be analyzed to identify the cause of the hepatic changes.

The drugs most likely to cause enzymatic abnormalities are L-asparaginase, carmustine in high doses, cytarabine, dactinomycin, etoposide, levamisole in combination with 5-FU, 6-mercaptopurine, methotrexate in high doses, streptozocin, and vincristine. These drugs can cause rises in the serum glutamic-oxaloacetic transaminase, serum glutamic-pyruvic transaminase, and serum bilirubin.

L-Asparaginase causes the widest spectrum of liver abnormalities and has the highest incidence of hepatotoxicity. It produces changes in liver enzymes and in hepatic protein synthesis, resulting in low plasma levels of albumin, lipoproteins, and clotting factors. Prolongation of the prothrombin and thrombin times occurs as a result. Fatty metamorphosis is commonly seen, and these changes may persist for several months after discontinuing treatment.[148]

The combination of levamisole and 5-FU, used as adjuvant therapy for colon cancer, also frequently produces reversible hepatic enzyme and serum bilirubin changes.[149] These abnormalities are due to fatty infiltration of the liver, and in some cases the degree of liver abnormality may be sufficient to mimic liver metastases on radiographic studies.[150]

Cytarabine hepatotoxicity is a common event in the treatment of acute leukemia, especially when high doses are used.[151] Because patients with acute leukemia are subject to transfusion-related hepatitis and receive a variety of potentially hepatotoxic drugs, it is always difficult to establish cytarabine as the sole hepatotoxin. However, hyperbilirubinemia developing in temporal relation to cytarabine administration, accompanied by histologic abnormalities on liver biopsy, has confirmed the hepatotoxicity potential of this drug.[152]

6-Mercaptopurine has been known since the 1950s to cause hepatotoxicity, which may even be rarely fatal.[153] Intrahepatic cholestasis is the most common abnormality, and liver function usually returns to normal with discontinuation of therapy.

Hepatic dysfunction from dactinomycin may occur in up to 10% of patients with Wilms' tumor treated with this drug, but it is very uncommon when used for treatment of other malignancies. Hepatomegaly, enzyme abnormalities, and jaundice may occur.[154] Fever is also common, and thrombocytopenia may occur. Most cases appear to be associated with Wilms' tumors occurring in the right kidney, so the tumor mass effect present in the liver region may play a precipitating role in this toxic manifestation.[155]

VENOOCCLUSIVE DISEASE

VOD results from blockage of venous outflow in the small centrilobular and sublobular hepatic vessels. Antitumor drugs known to produce this form of hepatotoxicity are cytarabine, cyclophosphamide, dacarbazine, 6-mercaptopurine, mitomycin, and 6-thioguanine. In addition, high doses of busulfan, carmustine, cyclophosphamide, and mitomycin given in the stem cell transplantation setting can cause VOD.

The clinical features of VOD are painful hepatomegaly, ascites, peripheral edema, marked elevations in serum enzymes and bilirubin, and hepatic encephalopathy. The onset is often abrupt, occurring during the first posttransplant week, and the clinical course is fulminant. It is caused by damage to endothelial cells, sinusoids, and hepatocytes in the area of the liver surrounding the central vein.[156] Thrombosis is precipitated, causing ischemia and hepatocellular necrosis. A component of hepatocellular injury may also be directly related to the high doses of drugs and not mediated by thrombosis. VOD occurring in the transplantation setting may be irreversible and lead to death with multiorgan failure in 25% to 50% of the patients developing it.[156] All of the drugs reported to induce VOD at high doses have been alkylating agents. This situation may not be because of any unusual tendency of alkylating agents to cause VOD, but rather to the fact that these are the drugs used in very large doses in the stem cell transplantation setting.

Conventional doses of certain antitumor agents (e.g., dacarbazine, 6-mercaptopurine, 6-thioguanine) can also cause hepatic VOD. Dacarbazine has been most frequently implicated in this form of hepatotoxicity, but only sporadic cases have been reported, both from dacarbazine alone and in combination with other drugs.[157] Why only some patients develop this life-threatening complication of dacarbazine is unknown. It may be some sort of idiosyncratic or hypersensitivity reaction.

CHRONIC FIBROSIS

Methotrexate used for cancer treatment can produce acute and reversible hepatocellular injury and elevation of serum enzymes. The intermittent dosing schedules seem to obviate any chronic hepatotoxicity from this drug. However, long-term use of methotrexate for the treatment of nonmalignant disease (e.g., rheumatoid arthritis) poses a hazard for the development of irreversible hepatic fibrosis.[158] Because patients with autoimmune diseases may already have underlying liver abnormalities, methotrexate may not be the sole etiologic factor in the development of this chronic toxicity.

HYPERSENSITIVITY REACTIONS

Most of the available antitumor agents can produce hypersensitivity reactions, and a substantial minority cause such reactions in 5% or more of patients treated. Several drugs (e.g., L-asparaginase and the taxanes) cause hypersensitivity reactions that are frequent enough to be a major treatment-limiting toxicity. Most of the other antitumor drugs produce such reactions only sporadically. The mechanism of these reactions is often unknown or evaluated only in a single patient. Premedication regimens designed to prevent or minimize reactions from the taxanes and a new formulation of L-asparaginase (pegaspargase) created to minimize reactions from this drug have been successful in reducing the frequency and severity of this toxicity.

L-Asparaginase produces hypersensitivity reactions in 10% to 20% of patients treated, which can be immediate and life-threatening, with all the components of anaphylaxis. This high rate is related to the fact L-asparaginase is a polypeptide of bacterial origin, displaying multiple antigenic sites that can stimulate production of immunoglobulin E (IgE) or other immunoglobulins. These immunoglobulins can then mediate an acute anaphylactic reaction.

The clinical manifestations are typical of type I reactions, with acute onset of wheezing, pruritus, rash, angioedema, extremity pain, agitation, and hypotension.[159,160] The mechanism of L-asparaginase reactions appears to be mediated by an IgE antibody in at least some cases. Complement activation also occurs, perhaps induced by specific IgG or IgM antibodies. A number of factors increase the risk for hypersensitivity reactions, including a history of atopy or other drug allergy, prior L-asparaginase therapy (including even several years previously), high drug doses, and the intravenous route of administration. Intramuscular administration often reduces the severity of reactions,[161] but they can still occur and may do so several hours after the drug is given. Concurrent treatment with prednisone and vincristine (for the acute leukemia being treated) also appears to reduce the risk of reactions.[159]

No reliable method has been found that can indicate who will have a reaction to any dose of L-asparaginase. Intradermal skin testing may give either false-negative or false-positive results, and test doses of the drug are valueless.[159] Therefore, one must approach each dose of L-asparaginase as the one that could initiate a hypersensitivity reaction and be prepared to treat it. Antianaphylaxis medication must be at hand, and the patient should be observed for approximately 1 hour after the drug is administered.

When a hypersensitivity reaction occurs with the *Escherichia coli* source of L-asparaginase, one can substitute the *Erwinia chrysanthemia* form and continue therapy without a loss of efficacy of this important drug for the treatment of acute lymphoblastic leukemia.[160] This drug form is immunologically distinct and appears to have a lower degree of immunogenicity. Patients may still sustain a hypersensitivity reaction from the substitute, but most (more than 75%) do not and can complete the planned therapy.[160] Precautions for treating anaphylaxis are necessary no matter the origin of the L-asparaginase. A third form of L-asparaginase (pegaspargase[162]) provides another alternative for the patient who is reactive to either of the other asparaginases. This form is a conjugate of polyethylene glycol with the enzyme. It may be the least immunogenic of all three forms of this drug, but hypersensitivity reactions are still possible. Because this drug has a prolonged serum half-life compared to the other two, it is administered only once or twice per week.

Paclitaxel has high potential for initiating a hypersensitivity reaction, and because of this fact, it is necessary to administer prophylaxis therapy before each dose.[163] The Cremophor EL excipient used to maintain solubility of paclitaxel has long been suspected of being the initiator of these reactions. When docetaxel was first evaluated in clinical trials, it was assumed that premedication to prevent hypersensitivity reactions was unnecessary, because docetaxel is formulated with Tween 80 (instead of Cremophor EL), and thus reactions would be unlikely to occur. This assumption proved incorrect, because docetaxel can initiate reactions with the same manifestations and with approximately the same frequency (5%) as paclitaxel.[164] The signs and symptoms can occur even despite premedication, although the intensity may be diminished.[164] The etiology appears to be either the two taxanes themselves or that Cremophor EL and Tween 80 are equally capable of causing reactions, with the former explanation being more likely. The

TABLE 55.8-4. Antitumor Agents That Cause Hypersensitivity Reactions

HIGH POTENTIAL FOR HYPERSENSITIVITY REACTIONS
L-Asparaginase
Docetaxel
Elliptinium
Paclitaxel
Procarbazine
Teniposide
OCCASIONAL INSTANCES OF HYPERSENSITIVITY REACTIONS
Aldesleukin
Anthracyclines
Bleomycin
Carboplatin
Chlorambucil
Cisplatin
Cyclophosphamide
Cytarabine
Dacarbazine
Etoposide
5-Fluorouracil
Hydroxyurea
Ifosfamide
Interferons
Mechlorethamine
Melphalan
6-Mercaptopurine
Methotrexate
Mitomycin
Mitoxantrone
Pegaspargase
Pentostatin
Vinca alkaloids

mechanism of these reactions has not been well studied. Although a few reported cases have occurred from later drug cycles,[165] the fact that they most often (more than 70% of the time) occur with the first drug dose[163,164] suggests a nonimmunologic mechanism.

The clinical manifestations are those of any type I hypersensitivity reaction and include bronchospasm and wheezing, agitation, chest and back pain, rash, angioedema, and hypotension. The onset is usually within minutes of starting a drug infusion, and even very small drug doses are capable of initiating a reaction. A form of apparent hypersensitivity that may be delayed in onset is pulmonary infiltrates typical of a hypersensitivity pneumonitis that may either resolve spontaneously or after corticosteroid therapy.[166]

To prevent or assuage these reactions, paclitaxel is usually infused over 1 to 3 hours. Infusion in any interval shorter than 1 hour may precipitate an unacceptable frequency of reactions.[167] Premedication with corticosteroids and antihistamines is standard procedure. Docetaxel is given over 1 hour, and premedications must also be used. Such measures reduce the frequency and perhaps the intensity of reactions but do not fully prevent them.

A number of other chemotherapeutic agents (Table 55.8-4) are known to produce hypersensitivity reactions in at least sporadic instances. Most of these reactions have the features of a type I hypersensitivity, whether mediated by IgE or nonimmunologically. Hemolytic anemia (a type II reaction) is an uncommon form of such toxicity. Some drugs, such as procarbazine and methotrexate, may produce acute episodes that are typical of a type III reaction and cause interstitial pneumonitis and vasculitis.

In most instances of hypersensitivity reactions from antitumor drugs, only isolated cases are studied adequately to define the cause of the reaction, and it is not possible to exclude the excipients used in drug formulation (e.g., benzyl alcohol, dimethyl acetamide) or other drugs given concurrently (e.g., mesna, mannitol, white blood cell growth factors) as the source of the reactivity. When such reactions occur from one drug, it is often possible to continue therapy by either substituting another drug in the same class or administering premedication as prophylaxis.

VASCULAR TOXICITY

Four main forms of vascular toxicity are produced by cancer chemotherapeutic agents: VOD, thrombotic microangiopathy with hemolytic uremic syndrome, venous or arterial thrombosis, and vascular ischemia (involving cerebral, myocardial, or extremity arterial vessels).[168] VOD of hepatic vessels (see the section Venoocclusive Disease) and microangiopathy (see the section Mitomycin) were discussed earlier in this chapter.

Venous thrombosis in association with metastatic cancer has long been recognized (Trousseau's syndrome). Chemotherapeutic agents can also induce venous thrombosis in the form of extremity thromboses and pulmonary emboli, even in the absence of demonstrable metastatic cancer.[169,170] Although they are less common, thromboses of cerebral, coronary, and extremity arteries can also be initiated by chemotherapy, again in the absence of demonstrable cancer.[171,172] These events are not limited to one form of cancer. They have occurred in a variety of cancers as disparate as stage II breast cancer, testicular cancer, and lymphomas. One drug associated with such thrombotic episodes more than others is cisplatin,[173] and a combination of chemotherapy with tamoxifen seems to produce a higher rate of such thrombotic episodes than either one alone.[170]

Arterial ischemia without thrombosis can be induced by chemotherapy in major coronary or cerebral vessels and in the small vessels of the extremities. Myocardial ischemia and infarction occur in patients who receive continuous infusions of 5-FU, and precipitous heart failure and sudden death have occurred.[174] Such events may occur in patients who have no known underlying coronary vessel disease, and they develop a few days after the start of the first infusion of 5-FU. The pathogenesis seems to be induction of coronary spasm by 5-FU, but the physiologic mechanism is not known. Anginal symptoms are often a precursor, which can be relieved by discontinuing the 5-FU therapy. Raynaud's phenomenon occurs as a chronic toxicity in approximately 40% of young men treated with cisplatin-bleomycin regimens for testicular cancer.[175] Cigarette smoking increases the risk for this toxicity. Clinical manifestations are painful digits and paresthesias, which may last indefinitely for years after the chemotherapy is completed. The mechanism appears to be vasospasm, without thrombosis, in the terminal arterioles of the fingers due to impaired smooth muscle function.[176] Bleomycin is the most likely etiology of this toxicity, because it can cause Raynaud's phenomenon when administered alone.[177] In similar fashion to causing vasoconstriction in coronary arteries, a continuous infusion of 5-FU may also engender digital arterial spasm and Raynaud's phenomenon.[178]

REFERENCES

1. Weiden PL, Wright SE. Vincristine neurotoxicity. *N Engl J Med* 1972;286:1369.
2. Casey EB, Jellife AM, Le Quesne PM, Millett YL. Vincristine neuropathy. Clinical and electrophysiologic observations. *Brain* 1973;96:69.
3. DeAngelis LM, Gnecco C, Taylor L, Warrell RP. Evolution of neuropathy and myopathy during intensive vincristine/corticosteroid chemotherapy for non-Hodgkin's lymphoma. *Cancer* 1991;67:2241.
4. Graf WD, Chance PF, Lensch MW, et al. Severe vincristine neuropathy in Charcot-Marie-Tooth disease type 1A. *Cancer* 1996;77:1356.
5. McCarthy GM, Skillings JR. Jaw and other orofacial pain in patients receiving vincristine for the treatment of cancer. *Oral Surg Oral Med Oral Pathol* 1992;74:299.
6. Roca E, Bruera E, Politi PM, et al. Vinca alkaloid–induced cardiovascular autonomic neuropathy. *Cancer Treat Rep* 1985;69:149.
7. Haim N, Epelbaum R, Ben-Shahar M, et al. Full dose vincristine (without 2-mg dose limit) in the treatment of lymphomas. *Cancer* 1994;73:2515.
8. Merimsky O, Loewenstein A, Chaitchik S. Cortical blindness—a catastrophic side effect of vincristine. *Anti-Cancer Drugs* 1992;3:371.
9. Burns BV, Shotton JC. Vocal fold palsy following vinca alkaloid treatment. *J Laryngol Otol* 1998;112:485.
10. Postma TJ, Benard BA, Huijgens PC, Ossenkoppele GJ, Heimans JJ. Long term effects of vincristine on the peripheral nervous system. *J Neurooncol* 1993;15:23.
11. Garewal HS, Dalton WS. Metoclopramide in vincristine-induced ileus. *Cancer Treat Rep* 1985;69:1309.
12. Lonardi F, Pavanato G, Ferrari V, et al. Neurotoxicity after chemotherapy with vinorelbine. *Eur J Cancer* 1993;29A:1794.
13. Le Chevalier T, Brisgand D, Douillard JY, et al. Randomized study of vinorelbine and cisplatin versus vindesine and cisplatin versus vinorelbine alone in advanced non-small-cell lung cancer: results of a European multicenter trial including 612 patients. *J Clin Oncol* 1994;12:360.
14. Parimoo D, Jeffers S, Muggia FM. Severe neurotoxicity from vinorelbine-paclitaxel combinations. *J Natl Cancer Inst* 1996;88:1079.
15. Fazeny B, Zifki U, Meryn S, et al. Vinorelbine-induced neurotoxicity in patients with advanced breast cancer pretreated with paclitaxel—A phase II study. *Cancer Chemother Pharmacol* 1996;39:150.
16. Weintraub M, Adde MA, Venzon DJ, et al. Severe atypical neuropathy associated with administration of hematopoietic colony-stimulating factors and vincristine. *J Clin Oncol* 1996;14:935.
17. Cersosimo RJ. Cisplatin neurotoxicity. *Cancer Treat Rev* 1989;16:195.
18. Gerritsen van der Hoop R, van der Burg MEL, ten Bokkel Huinink WW, van Houweligen JC, Neijt JP. Incidence of neuropathy in 395 patients with ovarian cancer treated with or without cisplatin. *Cancer* 1990;66:1697.
19. Cavaletti G, Marzorati L, Bogliun G, et al. Cisplatin-induced peripheral neurotoxicity is dependent on total dose intensity and single-dose intensity. *Cancer* 1992;69:203.
20. Hilkens PHE, van der Burg MEL, Moll JWB, et al. Neurotoxicity is not enhanced by increased dose intensities of cisplatin administration. *Eur J Cancer* 1995;31A:678.
21. van Gelder T, Geurs P, Kho GS, et al. Cortical blindness and seizures following cisplatin treatment: Both of epileptic origin. *Eur J Cancer* 1993;29A:1497.
22. Wilding G, Caruso R, Lawrence TS, et al. Retinal toxicity after high-dose cisplatin therapy. *J Clin Oncol* 1985;3:1683.
23. Thompson SW, Davis LE, Kornfeld M, Hilgers RD, Standefer JC. Cisplatin neuropathy: Clinical, electrophysiologic, morphologic, and toxicologic studies. *Cancer* 1984;54:1269.
24. Gregg RW, Molepo JM, Monpetit VJA, et al. Cisplatin neurotoxicity: The relationship between dosage, time, and platinum concentration in neurologic tissues, and morphologic evidence of toxicity. *J Clin Oncol* 1992;10:795.
25. Siegal T, Haim N. Cisplatin-induced peripheral neuropathy: Frequent off-therapy deterioration, demyelinating syndromes, and muscle cramps. *Cancer* 1990;66:1117.
26. Alberts DS, Noel JK. Cisplatin-associated neurotoxicity: Can it be prevented? *Anti-Cancer Drugs* 1995;6:369.
27. Kemp G, Rose P, Lurain J, et al. Amifostine pretreatment for protection against cyclophosphamide-induced and cisplatin-induced toxicities: Results of a randomized control trial in patients with advanced ovarian cancer. *J Clin Oncol* 1996;14:2101.
28. Hausheer F, Cavalletti E, Cavaletti G, et al. Oral and intravenous BNP7787 protects against platinum neurotoxicity without in vitro or in vivo tumor protection. *Proc Am Assoc Cancer Res* 1999;40:398.
29. Wasserheit C, Frazein A, Oratz R, et al. Phase II trial of paclitaxel and cisplatin in women with advanced breast cancer: an active regimen with limiting neurotoxicity. *J Clin Oncol* 1996;14:1993.
30. Berger T, Malayeri R, Doppelbauer A, et al. Neurological monitoring for neurotoxicity induced by paclitaxel/cisplatin chemotherapy. *Eur J Cancer* 1997;33:1393.
31. Becouarn Y, Ychou M, Ducreux M, et al. Phase II trial of oxaliplatin as first-line chemotherapy in metastatic colorectal cancer patients. *J Clin Oncol* 1998;16:2739.
32. Gilles-Amar V, Garcia ML, Seille A, et al. Evolution of severe sensory neuropathy with oxaliplatin combined to the bimonthly 48h leucovorin (LV) and 5-fluorouracil (5FU) regimens (FOLFOX) in metastatic colorectal cancer. *Proc Am Soc Clin Oncol* 1999;18:246a.
33. Baker WJ, Royer GL, Weiss RB. Cytarabine and neurologic toxicity. *J Clin Oncol* 1991;9:679.
34. Graves T, Hooks MA. Drug-induced toxicities associated with high-dose cytosine arabinoside infusions. *Pharmacotherapy* 1989;9:23.
35. Rubin EH, Anderson JW, Berg DT, et al. Risk factors for high-dose cytarabine neurotoxicity: an analysis of a Cancer and Leukemia Group B trial in patients with acute myeloid leukemia. *J Clin Oncol* 1992;10:948.
36. Openshaw H, Slatkin NE, Stein AS, Hinton DR, Forman SJ. Acute polyneuropathy after high dose cytosine arabinoside in patients with leukemia. *Cancer* 1996;78:1899.
37. Resar LMS, Phillips PC, Kastan MB, et al. Acute neurotoxicity after intrathecal cytosine arabinoside in two adolescents with acute lymphoblastic leukemia of B-cell type. *Cancer* 1993;71:117.
38. Paul M, Joshua D, Rahme N, et al. Fatal peripheral neuropathy associated with axonal degeneration after high-dose cytosine arabinoside in acute leukemia. *Br J Haematol* 1991;79:521.
39. Patel AG, Rao R. Transient ara-C leukoencephalopathy: MR findings. *J Comput Tomogr* 1996;20:161.
40. Miller L, Link MP, Bologna S, Parker BR. Cerebellar atrophy caused by high-dose cytosine arabinoside: CT and MR findings. *AJR Am J Roentgenol* 1989;152:343.
41. Dunkelman H, Earl HM, Twelves C. Acute reversible neurological deficit following intrathecal chemotherapy. *Cancer Chemother Pharmacol* 1991;27:329.
42. DeAngelis LM, Kreis W, Chan K, Dantis E, Akerman S. Pharmacokinetics of ara-C and ara-U in plasma and CSF after high-dose administration of cytosine arabinoside. *Cancer Chemother Pharmacol* 1992;29:173.
43. Wallace TL, Johnson EM. Cytosine arabinoside kills postmitotic neurons: evidence that deoxycytidine may have a role in neuronal survival that is independent of DNA synthesis. *J Neurosci* 1989;9:115.
44. Ono K, Mizukawa K, Yangihara M, Tokunaga A. Morphological changes of astroglia in the cerebellar cortex of developing mice after neonatal administration of cytosine arabinoside. *GLIA* 1990;3:311.
45. Weiss RB. Ifosfamide vs cyclophosphamide in cancer therapy. *Oncology (Huntingt)* 1991;5:67.
46. Merimsky O, Inbar M, Reider-Grosswasser I, Scharf M, Chaitchik S. Ifosfamide-related acute encephalopathy: clinical and radiological aspects. *Eur J Cancer* 1991;27:1188.
47. Miller LJ, Eaton VE. Ifosfamide-induced neurotoxicity: a case report and review of the literature. *Ann Pharmacother* 1992;26:183.
48. Chastagner P, Sommelet-Olive D, Kalifa C, et al. Phase II study of ifosfamide in childhood brain tumors: a report by the French Society of Pediatric Oncology (SFOP). *Med Pediatr Oncol* 1993;21:49.
49. Cerny T, Kupfer A. The enigma of ifosfamide encephalopathy. Ann Oncol 1992;3:679.
50. Patel SR, Forman AD, Benjamin RS. High-dose ifosfamide-induced exacerbation of peripheral neuropathy. *J Natl Cancer Inst* 1994;86:305.
51. Manegold C, Drings P, Pawinski A, et al. Oral ifosfamide/mesna versus intravenous ifosfamide/mesna in non–small cell lung cancer: a randomized phase II trial of the EORTC Lung Cancer Cooperative Group. *Ann Oncol* 1996;7:637.
52. Kupfer A, Aeschlimann C, Cerny T. Methylene blue and the neurotoxic mechanisms of ifosfamide encephalopathy. *Eur J Clin Pharmacol* 1996;50:249.
53. Simonian NA, Gilliam FG, Chiappa KH. Ifosfamide causes a diazepam-sensitive encephalopathy. *Neurology* 1993;43:2700.
54. Kupfer A, Aeschlimann C, Wermuth B, Cerny T. Prophylaxis and reversal of ifosfamide encephalopathy with methylene-blue. *Lancet* 1994;343:763.
55. Bygrave HA, Geh JI, Jani Y, Glynne-Jones R. Neurological complications of 5-fluorouracil chemotherapy: case report and review of the literature. *Clin Oncol (R Coll Radiol)* 1998;10:334.
56. Langer CJ, Hageboutros A, Kloth DD, Roby D, Shaer AH. Acute encephalopathy attributed to 5-FU. *Pharmacotherapy* 1996;16:311.
57. Stein ME, Drumea K, Yarnitsky D, Benny A, Tzuk-Shina T. A rare event of 5-fluorouracil-associated peripheral neuropathy: a report of two patients. *Am J Clin Oncol* 1998;21:248.
58. Meropol NJ, Creaven PJ, Petrelli NJ, White RM, Arbuck SG. Seizures associated with leucovorin administration in cancer patients. *J Natl Cancer Inst* 1995;87:56.
59. Fassas ABT, Gattani AM, Morgello S. Cerebral demyelination with 5-fluorouracil and levamisole. *Cancer Invest* 1994;12:379.
60. Lucia P, Pocek M, Passacantando A, Sebastiani ML, De Martinis C. Multifocal leucoencephalopathy induced by levamisole. *Lancet* 1996;348:1450.
61. Okeda R, Shibutani M, Matsuo T, et al. Experimental neurotoxicity of 5-fluorouracil and its derivatives is due to poisoning by the monofluorinated organic metabolites, monofluoroacetic acid and α-fluoro-β-alanine. *Acta Neuropathol (Berl)* 1990;81:66.
62. Milano G, Etienne MC, Vierrefite V, et al. Dihydropyrimidine dehydrogenase deficiency and fluorouracil-related toxicity. *Br J Cancer* 1999;79:627.
63. Nelson RW, Frank JT. Intrathecal methotrexate-induced neurotoxicities. *Am J Hosp Pharm* 1981;38:65.
64. Rubnitz JE, Relling MV, Harrison PL, et al. Transient encephalopathy following high-dose methotrexate treatment in childhood acute lymphoblastic leukemia. *Leukemia* 1998;12:1176.
65. Shore T, Barnett MJ, Phillips GL. Sudden neurologic death after intrathecal methotrexate. *Med Pediatr Oncol* 1990;18:159.
66. Lovblad KO, Kelkar P, Ozdoba C, et al. Pure methotrexate encephalopathy presenting with seizures: CT and MRI features. *Pediatr Radiol* 1998;28:86.
67. Brown RT, Madan-Swain A, Walco GA, et al. Cognitive and academic late effects among children previously treated for acute lymphocytic leukemia receiving chemotherapy as CNS prophylaxis. *J Pediatr Psych* 1998;23:333.

68. Kiu MC, Liaw CC, Yang TS, et al. Transient neurological disturbances induced by the chemotherapy of high-dose methotrexate for osteogenic sarcoma. *Anti-Cancer Drugs* 1994;5:480.
69. Lien HH, Blomlie V, Saeter G, Solheim O, Fossa SD. Osteogenic sarcoma: MR signal abnormalities of the brain in asymptomatic patients treated with high-dose methotrexate. *Radiology* 1991;179:547.
70. Bleyer WA. Leukoencephalopathy detectable by magnetic resonance imaging: much ado about nothing? *Int J Radiat Oncol Biol Phys* 1995;32:1251.
71. Quinn CT, Griener JC, Bottiglieri T, et al. Elevation of homocysteine and excitatory amino acid neurotransmitters in the CSF of children who receive methotrexate for the treatment of cancer. *J Clin Oncol* 1997;15:2800.
72. Bernini JC, Fort DW, Griener KC, et al. Aminophylline for methotrexate-induced neurotoxicity. *Lancet* 1995;345:544.
73. Rowinsky EK, Chaudhry V, Cornblath DR, Donehower RC. Neurotoxicity of Taxol. *Monog Natl Cancer Inst* 1993;15:107.
74. Postma TJ, Vermoken JB, Liefting AJM, Pinedo HM, Heimans JJ. Paclitaxel-induced neuropathy. *Ann Oncol* 1995;6:489.
75. Forsyth PA, Balmaceda C, Peterson K, et al. Prospective study of paclitaxel-induced peripheral neuropathy with quantitative sensory testing. *J Neurooncol* 1997;35:47.
76. Hilkens PHE, Verweij J, Vecht CJ, Stoter G, van den Bent MJ. Clinical characteristics of severe peripheral neuropathy induced by docetaxel (Taxotere). *Ann Oncol* 1997;8:187.
77. New PZ, Jackson CE, Rinaldi D, Burris H, Barohn RJ. Peripheral neuropathy secondary to docetaxel (Taxotere). *Neurology* 1996;46:108.
78. Freilich RJ, Balmaceda C, Seidman AD, Rubin M, DeAngelis LM. Motor neuropathy due to docetaxel and paclitaxel. *Neurology* 1996;47:115.
79. Capri G, Munzone E, Trarenzi E, et al. Optic nerve disturbances: a new form of paclitaxel neurotoxicity. *J Natl Cancer Inst* 1994;86:1099.
80. Perry JR, Warner E. Transient encephalopathy after paclitaxel (Taxol) infusion. *Neurology* 1996;46:1596.
81. Gogas H, Shapiro F, Aghajanian C, et al. The impact of diabetes mellitus on the toxicity of therapy for advanced ovarian cancer. *Gynecol Oncol* 1996;61:22.
82. Seidman AD, Hudis CA, McCaffrey J, et al. Dose-dense therapy with paclitaxel via weekly 1-hour infusion: preliminary experience in the treatment of metastatic breast cancer. *Semin Oncol* 1997;24[Suppl 17]:S17.
83. Connelly E, Markman M, Kennedy A, et al. Paclitaxel delivered as a 3-hr infusion with cisplatin in patients with gynecologic cancers: unexpected incidence of neurotoxicity. *Gynecol Oncol* 1966;62:166.
84. Cavaletti G, Boglium G, Marzorati L, et al. Peripheral neurotoxicity of Taxol in patients previously treated with cisplatin. *Cancer* 1995;75:1141.
85. Faivre S, Kalla S, Cvitkovic E, et al. Oxaliplatin and paclitaxel combination in patients with platinum-pretreated ovarian carcinoma: an investigator-originated compassionate-use experience. *Ann Oncol* 1999;10:1125.
86. Gelman K, Eisenhauer E, Bryce C, et al. Randomized phase II study of high-dose paclitaxel with or without amifostine in patients with metastatic breast cancer. *J Clin Oncol* 1999;17:3038.
87. Cavalletti E, Cavaletti G, Tredici G, et al. Oral and intravenous BNP7787 protects against paclitaxel-mediated neurotoxicity in Wistar rats. *Proc Am Assoc Cancer Res* 1999;22:398.
88. Weiss RB. The role of hexamethylmelamine in advanced ovarian carcinoma treatment. *Gynecol Oncol* 1981;12:141.
89. Manetta A, MacNeill C, Lyter JA, et al. Hexamethylmelamine as a single second-line agent in ovarian cancer. *Gynecol Oncol* 1990;36:93.
90. Brunner KW, Young CW. A methylhydrazine derivative in Hodgkin's disease and other malignant neoplasms: therapeutic and toxic effects studied in 51 patients. *Ann Intern Med* 1965;63:69.
91. Siegel JP, Puri RK. Interleukin-2 toxicity. *J Clin Oncol* 1991;9:694.
92. Fenner MH, Hanninen EL, Kirchner HH, Poliwoda H, Atzpodien J. Neuropsychiatric symptoms during treatment with interleukin-2 and interferon-α. *Lancet* 1993;341:372.
93. Puduvalli VK, Sella S, Austin SF, Forman AD. Carpal tunnel syndrome associated with interleukin-2 therapy. *Cancer* 1996;77:1189.
94. Chun HG, Leyland-Jones BR, Caryk SM, Hoth DF. Central nervous system toxicity of fludarabine phosphate. *Cancer Treat Rep* 1986;70:1225.
95. Cheson BD, Vena DA, Foss FM, Sorenson JM. Neurotoxicity of purine analogs: a review. *J Clin Oncol* 1994;12:2216.
96. Johnson PWM, Fearnley J, Domizio P, et al. Neurological illness following treatment with fludarabine. *Br J Cancer* 1994;70:966.
97. Zabernigg A, Maier H, Thaler J, Gattringer C. Late-onset fatal neurological toxicity of fludarabine. *Lancet* 1994;344:1780.
98. Kobayashi R, Watanabe N, Iguchi A, et al. Electroencephalogram abnormality and high-dose busulfan in conditioning regimens for stem cell transplantation. *Bone Marrow Transplant* 1998;21:217.
99. Hayes DM, Cvitkovic E, Golbey RB, et al. High dose *cis*-platinum diammine dichloride. Amelioration of renal toxicity by mannitol diuresis. *Cancer* 1977;39:1372.
100. Higby DJ, Wallace HJ, Albert DJ, Holland JF. Diaminedichloroplatinum: a phase I study showing responses in testicular and other tumors. *Cancer* 1974;33:1219.
101. Pera MF, Zook BC, Harder HC. Effects of mannitol or furosemide diuresis on the nephrotoxicity and physiologic distribution of *cis*-dichlorodiammineplatinum-(II) in rats. *Cancer Res* 1979;39:1269.
102. Tanaka H, Ishikawa E, Teshima S, et al. Histopathological study of human cisplatin nephropathy. *Toxicol Pathol* 1986;14:247.
103. Lajer H, Daugaard G. Cisplatin and hypomagnesemia. *Cancer Treat Rev* 1999;25:47.
104. Hutchison FN, Perez EA, Gandara DR, Lawrence HJ, Kaysen GA. Renal salt wasting in patients treated with cisplatin. *Ann Intern Med* 1988;108:21.
105. Markman M, Rothman R, Reichman B, et al. Persistent hypomagnesemia following cisplatin chemotherapy in patients with ovarian cancer. *J Cancer Res Clin Oncol* 1991;117:89.
106. Evans TRJ, Harper CL, Beveridge IG, Wastnage R, Mansi JL. A randomized study to determine whether routine intravenous magnesium supplements are necessary in patients receiving cisplatin chemotherapy with continuous infusion 5-fluorouracil. *Eur J Cancer* 1995;31A:174.
107. Pinzani V, Bressolle F, Haug IJ, et al. Cisplatin-induced renal toxicity and toxicity-modulating strategies: a review. *Cancer Chemother Pharmacol* 1994;35:1.
108. Tannehill SP, Mehta MP, Larson M, et al. Effect of amifostine on toxicities associated with sequential chemotherapy and radiation therapy for unresectable non-small-cell cancer: results of a phase III trial. *J Clin Oncol* 1997;15:2850.
109. Hrushesky WJM. Circadian timing of cancer chemotherapy. *Science* 1985;228:73.
110. Hargis JB, Anderson JR, Propert KJ, et al. Predicting genitourinary toxicity in patients receiving cisplatin-based combination chemotherapy: a Cancer and Leukemia Group B study. *Cancer Chemother Pharmacol* 1992;30:291.
111. McDonald BR, Kirmani S, Vasquez M, Mehta RL. Acute renal failure associated with the use of intraperitoneal carboplatin: a report of two cases and review of the literature. *Am J Med* 1991;90:386.
112. Frenkel J, Kool G, de Kraker J. Acute renal failure in high-dose carboplatin chemotherapy. *Med Pediatr Oncol* 1995;25:473.
113. Sleijfer DT, Smit EF, Meijer S, Mulder NH, Postmus PE. Acute and cumulative effects of carboplatin on renal function. *Br J Cancer* 1989;60:116.
114. Hardy JR, Tan S, Fryatt I, Wiltshaw E. How nephrotoxic is carboplatin? *Br J Cancer* 1990;61:644.
115. Palmisano J, Agraharkar M, Kaplan AA. Successful treatment of cisplatin-induced hemolytic uremic syndrome with therapeutic plasma exchange. *Am J Kidney Dis* 1998;32:314.
116. Walker RW, Rosenblum MK, Kempin SJ, Christian MC. Carboplatin-associated thrombotic microangiopathic hemolytic anemia. *Cancer* 1989;64:1017.
117. Gardner G, Mesler D, Gitelman HJ. Hemolytic uremic syndrome following cisplatin, bleomycin, and vincristine chemotherapy: a report of a case and a review of the literature. *Renal Failure* 1989;11:133.
118. Doll DC, Weiss RB. Hemolytic anemia associated with antineoplastic agents. *Cancer Treat Rep* 1985;69:777.
119. Wu DC, Liu JM, Chen YM, et al. Mitomycin-C induced hemolytic uremic syndrome: a case report and literature review. *Jpn J Clin Oncol* 1997;27:115.
120. Allum WH, Hallissey MT, Kelly KA, for the British Stomach Cancer Group. Adjuvant chemotherapy in operable gastric cancer. *Lancet* 1989;1:571.
121. Montes A, Powles TJ, O'Brien MER, et al. A toxic interaction between mitomycin C and tamoxifen causing the haemolytic uraemic syndrome. *Eur J Cancer* 1993;29A:1854.
122. Lesesne JB, Rothschild N, Erickson B, et al. Cancer-associated hemolytic-uremic syndrome: analysis of 85 cases from a national registry. *J Clin Oncol* 1989;7:781.
123. Motoo Y, Sawabu N, Ikeda K, et al. Long-term follow-up of mitomycin C nephropathy. *Intern Med* 1994;33:180.
124. Snyder HW, Mittelman A, Oral A, et al. Treatment of cancer chemotherapy–associated thrombotic thrombocytopenic purpura/hemolytic uremic syndrome by protein A immunoadsorption of plasma. *Cancer* 1993;71:1882.
125. Cattell V. Mitomycin-induced hemolytic uremic kidney: an experimental model in the rat. *Am J Pathol* 1985;121:88.
126. Nagaya S, Wada H, Oka K, et al. Hemostatic abnormalities and increased vascular endothelial cell markers in patients with red cell fragmentation syndrome induced by mitomycin C. *Am J Hematol* 1995;50:237.
127. Ackland SP, Schilsky RL. High-dose methotrexate: a critical reappraisal. *J Clin Oncol* 1987;5:2017.
128. Goren MP, Wright RK, Horowitz ME, Meyer WH. Enhancement of methotrexate nephrotoxicity after cisplatin therapy. *Cancer* 1986;58:2617.
129. Thyss A, Kubar J, Milano G, Namer M, Schneider M. Clinical and pharmacokinetic evidence of life-threatening interaction between methotrexate and ketoprofen. *Lancet* 1986;1:256.
130. Singh RR, Malaviya AN, Pandey JN, Guleria JS. Fatal interaction between methotrexate and naproxen. *Lancet* 1986;1:1390.
131. Molina R, Fabian C, Cowley B. Use of charcoal hemoperfusion with sequential hemodialysis to reduce serum methotrexate levels in a patient with acute renal insufficiency. *Am J Med* 1987;82:350.
132. Widemann BC, Balis FM, Murphy RF, et al. Carboxypeptidase-G_2, thymidine, and leucovorin rescue in cancer patients with methotrexate-induced renal dysfunction. *J Clin Oncol* 1997;15:2125.
133. Weiss RB. Streptozocin: a review of its pharmacology, efficacy, and toxicity. *Cancer Treat Rep* 1982;66:427.
134. Tobin MV, Warenius HM, Morris AI. Forced diuresis to reduce nephrotoxicity of streptozotocin in the treatment of advanced metastatic insulinoma. *BMJ* 1987;294:1128.
135. Ellis ME, Weiss RB, Kuperminc M. Nephrotoxicity of lomustine: a case report and literature review. *Cancer Chemother Pharmacol* 1985;15:174.
136. Berns JS, Haghighat A, Staddon A, et al. Severe, irreversible renal failure after ifosfamide treatment. A clinicopathologic report of two patients. *Cancer* 1995;76:497.
137. Loebstein R, Atanackovic G, Bishai R, et al. Risk factors for long-term outcome of ifosfamide-induced nephrotoxicity in children. *J Clin Pharmacol* 1999;39:454.
138. Skinner R, Sharkey IM, Pearson ADJ, Craft AW. Ifosfamide, mesna, and nephrotoxicity in children. *J Clin Oncol* 1993;11:173.
139. Rossi R. Nephrotoxicity of ifosfamide—moving towards understanding the molecular mechanisms. *Nephrol Dial Transplant* 1997;12:1091.
140. Sangster G, Kaye SB, Calman KC, Dalton JF. Failure of 2-mercaptoethane sulphonate sodium (mesna) to protect against ifosfamide nephrotoxicity. *Eur J Cancer Clin Oncol* 1984;20:435.
141. Rossi R, Godde A, Kleinebrand A, et al. Unilateral nephrectomy and cisplatin as risk factors of ifosfamide-induced nephrotoxicity: analysis of 120 patients. *J Clin Oncol* 1994;12:159.
142. Skinner R, Pearson ADJ, English MW, et al. Risk factors for ifosfamide nephrotoxicity in children. *Lancet* 1996;348:578.
143. Le Cesne A, Antoine E, Spielmann M, et al. High-dose ifosfamide: circumvention of resistance to standard-dose ifosfamide in advanced soft tissue sarcomas. *J Clin Oncol* 1995;13:1600.

144. Rossi R, Pleyer J, Schafers P, et al. Development of ifosfamide-induced nephrotoxicity: prospective follow-up in 75 patients. *Med Pediatr Oncol* 1999;32:177.
145. Kramer A, Goldschmidt H, Hahn U, Andrassy K. Progressive renal failure in two breast cancer patients after high-dose ifosfamide. *Lancet* 1994;344:1569.
146. Friedlaender MM, Haviv YS, Rosenmann E, Peylan-Ramu N. End-stage renal interstitial fibrosis in an adult ten years after ifosfamide therapy. *Am J Nephrol* 1998;18:131.
147. van der Lelie H, Baars JW, Rodenhuis S, et al. Hemolytic uremic syndrome after high dose chemotherapy with autologous stem cell support. *Cancer* 1995;76:2338.
148. Pratt CB, Johnson WW. Duration and severity of fatty metamorphosis of the liver following L-asparaginase therapy. *Cancer* 1971;28:361.
149. Moertel CG, Fleming TR, Macdonald JS, Haller DG, Laurie JA. Hepatic toxicity associated with fluorouracil plus levamisole adjuvant therapy. *J Clin Oncol* 1993;11:2386.
150. Norum J. 5-Fluorouracil/levamisole induced intrahepatic fat infiltration imitating liver metastasis. *Acta Oncol* 1995;34:971.
151. Herzig RH, Wolff SN, Lazarus HM, et al. High-dose cytosine arabinoside therapy for refractory leukemia. *Blood* 1983;62:361.
152. Pizzuto J, Aviles A, Ramos E, Cervera J, Aguirre J. Cytosine arabinoside induced liver damage: histopathologic demonstration. *Med Pediatr Oncol* 1983;11:287.
153. Laidlaw ST, Reilly JT, Suvarna SK. Fatal hepatotoxicity associated with 6-mercaptopurine therapy. *Br J Haematol* 1999;105:316.
154. Raine J, Bowman A, Wallendszus K, Pritchard J. Hepatopathy-thrombocytopenia syndrome—a complication of dactinomycin therapy for Wilms' tumor: a report from the United Kingdom Childrens Cancer Study Group. *J Clin Oncol* 1991;9:268.
155. Davidson A, Pritchard J. Actinomycin D, hepatic toxicity, and Wilms' tumor—a mystery explained? *Eur J Cancer* 1998;34:1145.
156. Richardson P, Bearman SI. Prevention and treatment of hepatic venoocclusive disease after high-dose cytoreductive therapy. *Leuk Lymphoma* 1998;31:267.
157. Marsh JC. Hepatic vascular toxicity of dacarbazine (DTIC): not a rare complication. *Hepatology* 1989;9:790.
158. West SG. Methotrexate hepatotoxicity. *Rheum Dis Clin North Am* 1997;23:883.
159. Evans WE, Tsiatis A, Rivera G, et al. Anaphylactoid reactions of *Escherichia coli* and *Erwinia* asparaginase in children with leukemia and lymphoma. *Cancer* 1982;49:1378.
160. Larson RA, Fretzin MH, Dodge RK, Schiffer CA. Hypersensitivity reactions to L-asparaginase do not impact on the remission duration of adults with acute lymphoblastic leukemia. *Leukemia* 1998;12:660.
161. Eden OB, Shaw MP, Lilleyman JS, Richards S. Non-randomized study comparing toxicity of *Escherichia coli* and *Erwinia* asparaginase in children with leukaemia. *Med Pediatr Oncol* 1990;18:497.
162. Pegaspargase for acute lymphoblastic leukemia. *Med Lett Drugs Ther* 1995;37:23.
163. Weiss RB, Donehower RH, Wiernik PH, et al. Hypersensitivity reactions from Taxol. *J Clin Oncol* 1990;8:1263.
164. Tyson LB, Kris MG, Corso DM, Choy E, Timoney JP. Incidence, course, and severity of taxoid-induced hypersensitivity reaction in 646 oncology patients. *Proc Am Soc Clin Oncol* 1999;18:585a.
165. van Herpen CML, van Hoesel QGCM, Punt CJA. Paclitaxel-induced severe hypersensitivity reaction occurring as a late toxicity. *Ann Oncol* 1995;6:852.
166. Ramanathan RK, Reddy VV, Holbert JM, Belani CP. Pulmonary infiltrates following administration of paclitaxel. *Chest* 1996;110:289.
167. Tsavaris NB, Kosmas C. Risk of severe acute hypersensitivity reactions after rapid paclitaxel infusion of less than 1-h duration. *Cancer Chemother Pharmacol* 1998;42:509.
168. Doll DC, Yarbro JW. Vascular toxicity associated with antineoplastic agents. *Semin Oncol* 1992;19:580.
169. Weiss RB, Tormey DC, Holland JF, Weinberg VE. Venous thrombosis during multimodal therapy of primary breast carcinoma. *Cancer Treat Rep* 1981;65:677.
170. Pritchard KI, Paterson AHG, Paul NA, et al. Increased thromboembolic complications with concurrent tamoxifen and chemotherapy in a randomized trial of adjuvant therapy for women with breast cancer. *J Clin Oncol* 1996;14:2731.
171. Wall JG, Weiss RB, Norton L, et al. Arterial thrombosis associated with adjuvant chemotherapy for breast carcinoma: a Cancer and Leukemia Group B study. *Am J Med* 1989;87:501.
172. Gerl A. Vascular toxicity associated with chemotherapy for testicular cancer. *Anti-Cancer Drugs* 1994;5:607.
173. Czaykowski PM, Moore MJ, Tannock IF. High risk of vascular events in patients with urothelial transitional cell carcinoma treated with cisplatin based chemotherapy. *J Urol* 1998;160:2021.
174. Meyer CC, Calis KA, Burke LB, Walawander CA, Grasela TH. Symptomatic cardiotoxicity associated with 5-fluorouracil. *Pharmacotherapy* 1997;17:729.
175. Berger CC, Bokemeyer C, Schneider M, Kuczyk MA, Schmoll HJ. Secondary Raynaud's phenomenon and other late vascular complications following chemotherapy for testicular cancer. *Eur J Cancer* 1995;31A:2229.
176. Hansen SW, Olsen N, Rossing N, Rorth M. Vascular toxicity and the mechanism underlying Raynaud's phenomenon in patients treated with cisplatin, vinblastine and bleomycin. *Ann Oncol* 1990;1:289.
177. Epstein E. Intralesional bleomycin and Raynaud's phenomenon. *J Am Acad Dermatol* 1991;24:785.
178. Papmichael D, Amft N, Slevin ML, D'Cruz D. 5-fluorouracil-induced Raynaud's phenomenon. *Eur J Cancer* 1998;34:1983.

CHAPTER 56

Supportive Care and Quality of Life

SECTION 1

KATHLEEN M. FOLEY

Management of Cancer Pain

Advances in the diagnosis and treatment of cancer, coupled with advances in our understanding of the anatomy, physiology, pharmacology, and psychology of pain perception, have led to improved care of the patient with pain of malignant origin.[1] Specialized methods of cancer diagnosis and treatment provide the most direct approach to treating cancer pain by treating the cause of the pain. However, before the introduction of successful antitumor therapy, when treatment of the cause of the pain has failed, or when injury to bone, soft tissue, or nerve has occurred as a result of therapy, appropriate pain management is essential. Patients with cancer are managed most effectively by a multidisciplinary approach, using the expertise of a wide range of health care professionals. The goal of pain therapy for patients receiving active treatment is to provide them with sufficient relief to tolerate the diagnostic and therapeutic approaches required to treat their cancer. For patients with advanced disease, pain control should be sufficient to allow them to function at a level they choose and to die relatively free of pain.[2] The management of the symptom of pain is only one component of a broad palliative care approach for cancer patients.[3] Control of other symptoms, treatment of psychological distress, and attention to the religious, spiritual, and existential dimensions of the patient's illness experience should be concurrently addressed to maintain the patient's quality of life throughout the cancer illness course from diagnosis to death.[4]

EPIDEMIOLOGY

Existing studies based on numerous national and international surveys and World Health Organization (WHO) estimates suggest that moderate to severe pain is experienced by one-third of cancer patients receiving active therapy and by 60% to 90% of patients with advanced disease.[5–9] There are 17 million new cases of cancer diagnosed worldwide each year and 5 million cancer deaths, accounting for large numbers of patients who suffer from cancer pain.[9] Pain associated with direct tumor involvement is the most common cause of cancer pain, occurring in as many as 85% of patients reported from a pain service study, to 65% from an outpatient cancer center pain clinic survey.[5] Bone pain is the most common type, with tumor infiltration of nerve and hollow viscus as the second and third most common pain locations. Cancer therapy causes pain in approximately 15% to 25% of patients receiving chemotherapy, surgery, or radiation therapy. Three percent to 10% of patients with cancer have pain caused by non–cancer-related problems, with pain syndromes reflecting the common causes of pain in the general population.

Patients with cancer often have multiple causes of pain and multiple sites of pain.[6] Based on a variety of survey data, up to one-third of patients had more than one pain and 81% of patients reported two or more distinct pain complaints; 34% reported three pains. Cross-cultural studies from India, Thailand, Vietnam, Germany, France, Taiwan, the Philippines, and

China report a similar prevalence of cancer pain in patients in active therapy and advanced disease.[10–12]

Studies have focused not only on the prevalence of pain but on its intensity, degree of pain relief, and the effect of pain on quality of life in patients with various cancers including lung, colon, ovarian, and pancreatic cancers.[13–15] In one study of lung and colon cancer ambulatory patients, the median pain duration was 4 weeks and the average pain intensity was moderate. Ninety percent experienced pain more than 25% of the time, and 50% reported that pain interfered moderately or more with their general activity or work.[13] In the Netherlands, 60% of all outpatients seen at an oncology clinic were in pain and 20% of this group reported moderate to severe pain.[16] In a 1999 survey of cancer outpatients, Weber and Huber reported inadequate documentation of pain severity, opioid dose, and rescue doses, observing that lack of documentation is a significant barrier to providing effective pain control.[17] Cleeland et al., in a study of patients who were followed by the Eastern Cooperative Oncology Group, reported that 56% of patients reported moderate to severe pain 50% of the time.[18] Numerous studies point out the fact that pain is prevalent in ambulatory patients, as well as hospitalized patients, and compromises function in approximately one-half of the patients who experience it.

A series of studies have focused on the seriously ill and nursing home cancer population and have identified a high prevalence of pain in these populations. The Study to Understand Prognoses and Preferences for Outcomes and Risks of Treatments showed that 50% of adults who die in the hospital experience moderate to severe pain in the last 3 days of life.[19] A study of 4000 elderly nursing home residents with cancer revealed that 24%, 29%, and 38% of those over age 85, 74 to 84, and 65 to 74, respectively, reported daily pain.[20] Twenty-six percent in daily pain did not receive any medication. Those over 85 who reported pain were most likely to receive no analgesic.[20]

Such studies have led to an assessment of the factors that influence the prevalence of cancer pain. Primary tumor type is one factor. Tumors that commonly metastasize to bone such as breast or prostate have a higher incidence of pain (60% to 80%) as compared with patients with lymphoma and leukemia. Stage of disease is a contributing factor, with increasing pain prevalence with disease progression. For example, less than 15% of patients with nonmetastatic disease report pain. Tumors that occur in close proximity to neural structures also have a greater incidence of pain. Patient variables such as anxiety, depression, and history of previous substance abuse influence the patient's report and experience of pain.[21]

Several studies have detailed the characteristics of patient populations followed by pain services and palliative and hospice care programs, providing further data on the magnitude of the cancer pain problem.[18,22–27] A 10-year experience of a German anesthesiology-based pain service associated with a palliative care program reported on the course of treatment of 2118 patients over a period of 140,478 treatment days.[27] Table 56.1-1 lists the primary tumors and pain localization etiology and type of pain syndrome. In their survey, gastrointestinal and head and neck cancers were the most common types, with the majority (85%) caused by tumor involvement. Pain intensity data were collected through the course of treatment. Eighty-two percent of patients had moderate to very severe pain at the beginning of treatment, with only 7% reporting such high intensity at the completion of treatment.

TABLE 56.1-1. Sites of Cancer Pain and Localization, Etiology, and Type of Pain Syndromes

	No. (%) of Patients (n = 2118)
SITES OF CANCER PAIN	
Head and neck region	347 (16)
Gastrointestinal tract	619 (29)
Respiratory system	206 (10)
Breast	210 (10)
Genitourinary system	363 (17)
Lymphatic-hematopoietic system	109 (5)
Skin, bones, connective tissue	112 (5)
Others or more than one	152 (7)
LOCALIZATION, ETIOLOGY, AND TYPE OF PAIN SYNDROMES	
Localization[a]	
Head, face, mouth	364 (17)
Cervical region	244 (12)
Upper shoulder, upper limbs	238 (11)
Thoracic region	499 (24)
Abdominal region	571 (27)
Lower back, lumbar spine, sacrum, coccyx	764 (36)
Lower limbs	457 (22)
Pelvic region	335 (16)
Anal, perianal, genital region	141 (7)
Missing value	4 (0)
Etiology	
Caused by cancer	1800 (85)
Caused by treatment	360 (17)
Associated with cancer disease	184 (9)
Unrelated to cancer or treatment	181 (9)
Missing value	71 (3)
Pathophysiologic type	
Somatic (bone or soft tissue)	744 (35)
Visceral	354 (17)
Neuropathic	185 (9)
Somatic and visceral	273 (13)
Somatic and neuropathic	444 (21)
Visceral and neuropathic	39 (2)
Somatic, visceral, and neuropathic	36 (2)
Missing value	43 (2)

[a]Multiple selections possible.
(From ref. 27, with permission.)

Several studies have also addressed the epidemiology and ethnography of pain treatment. In a study to assess the effect of a comprehensive medical and neurologic evaluation of pain in the cancer patient, 64% of patients had a lesion newly identified by the pain consultant.[28] Of note, more than 50% were neurologic in origin and, in 19% of patients further anticancer therapy combined with analgesic approaches were recommended. Further studies have observed that neurologic lesions make up a substantial portion of painful lesions in the cancer population. In a prospective study of neurologic symptoms, neurologic diagnoses, and primary tumors in all patients with a history with systemic cancer referred to Memorial Sloan-Kettering Cancer Center Neurology Consultation Service, the three most common symptoms in 851 patients were back pain

(18.2%), altered mental status (17.1%), and headache (15.4%).[29] The most common neurologic diagnosis was brain metastases (15.9%), followed by metabolic encephalopathy (10.2%), pain associated with bone metastases only (9.9%), and epidural extension or metastases of tumor (8.4%).[29]

In studies of patients with far-advanced disease cared for in palliative care programs, pain is the most common physical symptom. Of note, pain treatment significantly reduced this symptom but several other prominent symptoms including anxiety, fatigue, weakness, anorexia, nausea and vomiting, and dyspnea were less effectively managed.[30] This observation supports the critical need to evaluate, prioritize, and treat all symptoms to improve cancer pain patients' quality of life.

DEFINITION AND TYPES OF CANCER PAIN

DEFINITION OF PAIN

The definition of pain proposed by the International Association for the Study of Pain is "an unpleasant sensory and emotional experience associated with actual or potential tissue damage or described in terms of such damage."[31] Because pain is a subjective complaint, there is no definitive way to distinguish pain occurring in the absence of tissue damage from pain resulting from such damage. Pain as a somatic delusion or masked depression is rare in cancer patients and the presence of pain usually implies a pathologic process.

ANATOMY AND PHYSIOLOGY OF PAIN

Extensive investigations over the last 30 years have expanded our knowledge of ascending and descending central nervous system pathways that process and modulate nociceptive information. These advances provide a scientific rationale for the use of new and improved methods of cancer pain treatment.[1,32–34] A brief review of the neuroanatomy, physiology, and pharmacology of pain provides a background for the later discussions of specific drug, anesthetic, and neurosurgical approaches. Detailed information now supports the theory that activation of peripheral receptors in both superficial and deep structures as well as viscera by mechanical and chemical stimuli excites afferent discharges. Nonnociceptive messages are transmitted through rapidly conducting A-beta fibers and nociceptive information is signaled through slowly conducting A-delta and C-fiber afferents. The receptor endings of A-delta fibers most often respond to one sensory stimulus, whereas most C-fiber receptors are multimodal and respond to multiple high-threshold stimuli. These primary sensory afferents have their cell bodies in the dorsal root ganglion, and their axons enter the spinal cord via the dorsal root. The synaptic connections of these primary afferents with the corresponding second-order nociceptive neurons in the spinal dorsal horn are the initial site of processing for sensory information and act as a relay in transmitting noxious signals to the central nervous system.[34,35]

They ascend or descend from one or two segments in Lissauer's tract and synapse in specific lamina in the dorsal horn, lamina I and lamina II. Evidence suggests that myelinated nociceptors project to lamina I and V and unmyelinated nociceptors to lamina II and possibly lamina I, and nonnociceptive myelinated afferents project to only deep lamina. The dorsal horn is a critical site for modulating sensory input. Sensory transmission is mediated through excitatory amino acids (EAAs), predominantly glutamate.[36] The EAA aspartate and the neuropeptides substance P and calcitonin gene-related peptide are also involved. Excitatory synaptic transmission from the primary afferent is also modulated by the N-methyl-D-aspartate (NMDA) receptor as well as non-NMDA receptors.[34] Following EAA-NMDA receptor interaction, intracellular calcium influx and mobilization of intracellular calcium lead to subsequent changes in second messenger systems. One second messenger system activated following EAA-NMDA receptor interaction is the generation of nitric oxide via the enzyme nitric oxide synthase. There is also an increase in transcription of immediate early gene c-fos, which may regulate the subsequent expression of endogenous opioid genes, preproenkephalin and preprodynorphin. NMDA receptor activation initiates and maintains central sensitization and the component known as *windup*. These phenomena are manifestations of persistent signaling from primary sensory afferents. Central sensitization is thought to be the major mechanism underlying neuropathic pain and accounts for the hyperpathia and enlarged cutaneous receptor fields that occur following nerve injury.

At the level of the second-order neurons in the dorsal horn, sensory processing occurs through interactions among neurochemical transmitters released by primary afferents including gamma-aminobutyric acid, glycine, adenosine, bombesin, cholecystokinin, dynorphin, enkephalin, neuropeptide Y, neurotensin, substance P, somatostatin, and vasoactive intestinal polypeptide.

Several ascending pathways arise from these second-order neurons and decussate in the central gray of the spinal cord to become the neospinothalamic and paleospinothalamic tracts. These tracts project to discrete regions of the thalamus and cortex. The neospinothalamic pathway subserves pain intensity and localization, whereas the phylogenetically older paleospinothalamic pathway subserves the arousal and emotional component of pain. Descending pathways, the most important of which originate from the periaqueductal gray nuclei of the midbrain, synapse in the raphae magnus nucleus of the medulla. From this nucleus a medial pathway, the dorsal longitudinal fasciculus, projects to the dorsal horn to modulate pain transmission. This pathway represents an important descending inhibitory pathway. A more laterally placed descending pathway from the locus ceruleus to the dorsal horn also plays a role on pain modulation at the spinal cord level.

Opiate receptors, stereospecific binding sites on the end of free nerve endings that bind exogenous opioids, are localized in the ascending and descending pain pathways. These receptors mediate the multiple pharmacologic effects of the opioid analgesics. Subpopulations of opioid receptors including high-affinity and low-affinity μ receptors and γ, κ, and δ receptors are localized to specific areas of the brain and spinal cord. More recently, several opioid receptor subtypes have been cloned and quantitative changes in the messenger RNA for these receptors determined in experimental models. The cloning of these subtypes of receptors that mediate different pharmacologic effects and then are located in specific cerebral and spinal sites offers the possibility of developing new analgesics targeted for specific receptors.[37] For example, μ receptors modulate predominantly supraspinal analgesia, whereas δ and κ receptors are important in modulating analgesia at the spinal cord level. The periaqueductal gray region in the midbrain and dorsal horn in the spinal cord are rich in these receptors and are the supraspinal and spinal sites that mediate opioid analgesia. The use of brainstem stimulation and the administration of opioid analgesics directly into the cerebrospinal fluid bathing the selective opioid sites in animals and cancer patients with pain are procedures based on this knowledge.[38] Pain transmission at the spinal cord level can be inhibited by the direct application of morphine, and these studies have led to the use of spinal opioid analgesia in clinical pain states.[39,40] There is now increasing information about the molecular basis of opioid tolerance development. A variety of NMDA receptor antagonists have been demonstrated both to attenuate and to reverse experimental opioid analgesic tolerance.[41] Therefore, the confluence of NMDA receptors in pain transmission and their role in the development of tolerance have provided new insights into the role of opioid receptors in analgesia.

These advances in our understanding of pain modulatory systems and their neuroanatomic and neuropharmacologic correlates have had a major effect on the management of patients with pain. A better understanding of the molecular biology of both nociceptive and neuropathic pain is facilitating the wide application of a variety of agents including the NMDA antagonists, calcium channel agonists and antagonists, and topical and local systemic anesthetics and opioids.[34,35]

TYPES OF PAIN

Three types of pain have been described based on the neuroanatomy and the neurophysiology of pain pathways: somatic, visceral, and neuropathic pain. Each type results from activation and sensitization of nociceptors and mechanoreceptors in the periphery by either mechanical (tumor compression or infiltration) or chemical (epinephrine, serotonin, bradykinin, prostaglandin, histamine, and so forth) stimuli.

SOMATIC PAIN

When nociceptors are activated in cutaneous or deep tissues, somatic pain results, typically characterized by a dull or aching but well-localized pain. Metastatic bone pain, postsurgical incisional pain, and myofascial and musculoskeletal pain are common examples of somatic pain.

VISCERAL PAIN

Visceral pain results from activation of nociceptors from infiltration, compression, extension, or stretching of the thoracic, abdominal, or pelvic viscera. This typically occurs in patients with intraperitoneal metastases and is common with pancreatic cancer. This type of pain is poorly localized; is often described as deep, squeezing, and pressure-like; and when acute is often associated with significant autonomic dysfunction, including nausea, vomiting, and diaphoresis. Visceral pain is often referred to cutaneous sites that may be remote from the site of the lesion (e.g., shoulder pain with diaphragmatic irritation). It may be associated with tenderness in the referred cutaneous site. Increasing data have demonstrated the role of κ opioid receptors in modulating visceral pain.[42]

NEUROPATHIC PAIN

Neuropathic pain results from injury to the peripheral or central nervous system as a consequence of tumor compression or infiltration of peripheral nerves or the spinal cord, or from chemical injury to the peripheral nerve or spinal cord caused by surgery, radiation therapy, or chemotherapy. Examples of neuropathic pain include both metastatic and radiation-induced brachial and lumbosacral plexopathies, chemotherapy-induced peripheral neuropathies, paraneoplastic peripheral neuropathies, and postmastectomy, postthoracotomy, and phantom limb pain.[34,43] Pain from nerve injury is often severe and is described as burning or dysesthetic, with a vice-like quality. The pain is typically most common in the site of sensory loss and may be associated with hypersensitivity to nonnoxious (allodynia) and noxious stimuli. Intermittently, patients complain of paroxysms or burning or electric shock–like sensations. The latter symptoms result from the phenomenon of central sensitization.

These three types of pain may occur alone or combined in the same patient. These different types of pain account for different responses to drug and nondrug approaches. For instance, the nonsteroidal antiinflammatory drugs (NSAIDs) reduce chemical activation of nociceptors peripherally (e.g., bone pain), whereas anesthetic approaches suppress the pain transmission in peripheral nerves. Management of both somatic and visceral pain suggests that these types of pain respond to a wide variety of approaches. The management of neuropathic pain is more complicated: Changes in the peripheral nervous system and the central nervous system make this type of pain less responsive to a wide variety of pharmacologic, anesthetic, and neurosurgical approaches.

Evidence suggests that most cancer patients have both somatic and visceral pain, with neuropathic pain representing 15% to 20% of the significant pain problems in this population.[1,32] Certain adjuvant drugs appear to be more appropriate in the management of neuropathic pain; these issues are discussed in a later section (see Adjuvant Analgesics for Neuropathic Pain).

TEMPORAL ASPECTS OF PAIN

ACUTE PAIN

Acute pain is characterized by a well-defined temporal pattern of pain onset, generally associated with subjective and objective physical signs and with hyperactivity of the autonomic nervous system. These signs provide the physician with objective evidence that substantiates the patient's complaint of pain. Acute pain is usually self-limited and responds to treatment with analgesic drug therapy and to treatment of its precipitating cause. It can be further subdivided into subacute and episodic. Subacute pain comes on over several days, often with increasing intensity, and represents a pattern of progressive pain symptomatology. Episodic or intermittent pain occurs during confined periods of time on a regular or irregular basis. All of the pains in this category of acute pain have associated autonomic hyperactivity.

CHRONIC PAIN

Chronic pain is the persistence of pain for more than 3 months, with a less well-defined temporal onset. The autonomic nervous system adapts, and chronic pain patients lack the objective signs common to those with acute pain. Chronic pain leads to significant changes in personality, lifestyle, and functional ability. Treatment of chronic pain in the cancer patient is especially challenging because it requires a careful assessment of not only the intensity of the pain but its broad multidimensional aspects.[21] Evidence suggests that the persistence of pain plays a major negative role in the quality of life of patients with pain and cancer.

Investigators have developed a nomenclature to describe a series of specific pains in cancer patients with both acute and chronic pain states. *Baseline pain* is the average pain intensity experienced for 12 or more hours during a 24-hour period. *Breakthrough pain* is a transient increase in pain to greater than moderate intensity occurring on a baseline pain of moderate intensity or less. In a study of 70 adult inpatient cancer patients, 65% reported breakthrough pain.[44] The median number of reported pains was four, with a wide range. Most pains had a rapid onset and a brief duration. Breakthrough pain has a diversity of characteristics. Some authors have detailed the prevalence of such transitory flares of pain.[45] In a study of 613 consecutive cancer patients, 39% reported transitory flares that were severe or worse in 92% of patients. There were no correlations with gender, age, tumor site, stage, and therapy. The pain was somatic in 39%, visceral in 22%, and neuropathic in 36%. In this and other series, the transitory increase in pain marks the onset or worsening of pain at the end of the dosing interval or the regularly scheduled analgesic. In other patients, it is caused by an action of the patient, referred to as *incident pain*; sometimes the incident pain has a nonvolitional precipitant, such as flatulence. Most breakthrough or transitory pains are thought to be associated with a known malignant cause from direct tumor infiltration. Clinical trials with an oral transmucosal fentanyl preparation have focused attention on the clinical management of such episodes of worsening pain.[46]

INTENSITY OF PAIN

Pain may also be defined on the basis of intensity, but there are limitations to a concept of pain based solely on intensity. Specific categoric scales of pain intensity have been used in which patients are asked to describe their pain as mild, moderate, severe, or excruciating.[47] Visual analog scales (VAS) have also been used. These are often a 10-cm line anchored on either end by two points, signifying *no pain* and *worst possible pain*. The patient is asked to mark the intensity of the pain on the line. Numeric scales are also commonly used, asking patients to rate their pain between 1 (no pain) and 10 (worst possible pain). These scales have their limitations, but they are part of a series of validated instruments that include a measure of pain intensity as one of the components of the pain experience to be defined.[47] In a study of physicians' and nurses' understanding of the language to describe pain, there was a close correlation among them of the level of intensity meant by the terms *ache*, *hurt*, or *pain*.[48] Although health care professionals may understand the common language of pain, there is an enormous discrepancy between their assessment and the patient's report of pain, particularly when the patient reports pain as moderate or severe. They compared the ratings of pain severity by patients with those by physicians and found that patients tended to rate their pain as more intense than did physicians. In a study by Grossman and associates, the cancer patients' report of pain and the physicians' concurrent observation had a close correlation when patients reported mild pain.[49] However, when patients reported moderate to severe pain, the correlation of the nurse, house officer, and oncology fellow differed significantly from that of the patient: The concordance dropped from 78% for patients with mild pain to 20% for those with moderate to severe pain.

MEASUREMENT OF PAIN

These problems in communication about pain intensity strongly support the argument that multiple dimensions of the pain experience should be used to assess it adequately. Several validated instruments for pain measurement attempt to look at it in a multidimensional nature. The use of such methods can provide rapid evaluation in clinical settings of the major aspects of the pain experienced by cancer patients. Growing evidence suggests that they should be integrated into clinical trials and should be available for use on a routine basis to better define the pain symptomatology and to study the effect on pain by various treatment approaches.

BRIEF PAIN INVENTORY (BPI)

The Wisconsin Brief Pain Questionnaire (BPI) is a self-administered, easily understood, brief method to assess pain.[50] It addresses the relevant aspects of pain (history, intensity, location, and quality) and the pain's ability to interfere with the patient's activities and helps to provide an understanding of its cause. The history of pain and its relation to the patient's disease are assessed initially. If the patient admits to pain in the last month, he or she answers questions about current manifestations of pain. If the patient has no pain, he or she skips to the end of the questionnaire to complete demographic information. For patients with pain, a human figure drawing is provided for the patient to shade the area corresponding to the pain. Patients are asked to rate their pain at its worst, usual pain, and pain now. The pain scales consist of numbers from 0 to 10; 0 is labeled *no pain* and 10 is labeled *pain as bad as you can imagine*. Patients are asked to report the medications or treatments they receive for pain, the percent relief that these medications or treatment provide, and their belief about the cause of their pain. Finally, they are asked to rate how much the pain interferes with their mood, relations with other people, and functional ability (walking, sleeping, working, enjoying life). All patients, including those without pain, are asked for basic demographic information about marital status, education, occupation, spouse's occupation, and months since diagnosis.

This inventory has been translated into numerous languages and has been used to assess pain in cancer patients in such diverse settings as Vietnam, Mexico, the Philippines, China, and the University of Wisconsin Cancer Center. Data from these studies suggest that cancer pain patients from widely different cultural and linguistic backgrounds respond in a similar fashion to rating the severity of their cancer-related pain and the interference caused by the pain.

MCGILL PAIN QUESTIONNAIRE

The McGill Pain Questionnaire (MPQ) is an extensively used pain assessment instrument that produces scores on four empirically derived dimensions, as well as several summary

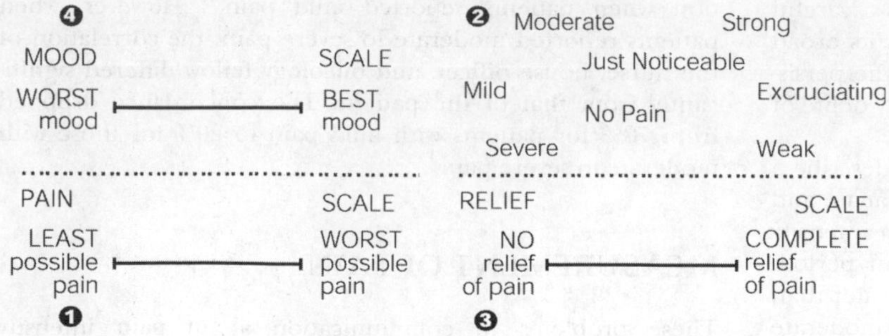

FIGURE 56.1-1. Memorial Pain Assessment Card, front (1 and 4) and back (2 and 3) sides. The card is folded along the broken line, and each measure is presented to the patient separately, in the numbered order. (1) Visual analog scale (VAS) of pain intensity; (2) modified Tursky pain descriptors scale; (3) VAS pain relief; (4) VAS mood. (From ref. 52, with permission.)

scores.[51] The instrument consists of 78 adjectives that cluster in 20 categories. Within each category, the adjectives are arranged in order of intensity from low to high. The categories are divided into four dimensions: sensory, affective, evaluative, and miscellaneous. The patient is asked to choose one adjective from each applicable category that describes an aspect of his or her current pain, and the score for each dimension is obtained by adding the rank values of the selected adjectives. A total summary score is derived by adding the scores across the four dimensions, and a total word count is also obtained. Finally, a rating of present pain intensity is made on a five-point scale. Studies with this instrument have demonstrated that the factors derived reflect specific sensory qualities and combined emotional and sensory dimensions. This tool has also been used to assess distinct score profiles according to the nature of pain. For instance, patients with acute pain tend to use more sensory words, but patients with chronic pain tend to use more affective and reaction word subgroups. The MPQ offers a methodologic approach to assess the sensory, affective, and evaluative components of pain, but it may be more difficult and cumbersome for patients to understand and complete and may be limited by its language constraints.

MEMORIAL PAIN ASSESSMENT CARD

The Memorial Pain Assessment Card (MPAC) (Fig. 56.1-1) was initially developed by the Analgesic Studies Section of the Memorial Sloan-Kettering Cancer Center to assess the relative potency of new and standard analgesic drugs. In that context, this method was found repeatedly to be a valid, reliable, efficient, and sensitive measure.[52] The MPAC consists of three VAS that measure pain intensity, pain relief, and mood, and a set of pain severity descriptors adapted from the Tursky rating scale. The card is 8.5 by 11 inches and is folded in the middle so that the four sides can be quickly presented to the patient. Three sides are imprinted with the 100-mm long VAS scale; the fourth side is the set of Tursky adjectives. The pain intensity VAS is anchored by the terms *least possible pain* and *worst possible pain.* The patient is asked to place a mark along the line to indicate his or her subjective judgment of pain intensity. The score on this and the other VAS is obtained by measuring in millimeters the distance between the left end of the line and the patient's mark. The Tursky pain adjective scale is a categorical measure of pain intensity. Eight intensity descriptors, ranging from *no pain* to *excruciating,* are printed in a random arrangement and the patient is asked to circle the adjective that describes his or her subjective experience of pain severity. Side 3 of the MPAC is a pain-relief VAS. Patients are asked to indicate with a mark the degree of pain reduction they experience after the most recent intervention, which is usually the administration of an analgesic drug. On side 4 the VAS measures the subjective experience of mood; on this side patients are asked to rate their current feeling, from *worst* to *best.* The instructions for administration of these scales are simple and readily understood, and an experienced patient can complete the four ratings in less than 20 seconds.

The MPAC has been compared with the MPQ, the Profile of Mood States Questionnaire (a standardized self-report instrument that measures six dimensions of mood, reflecting degree and type of psychological distress), the Hamilton Rating Scale for Depression (an interviewer-rated scale evaluating the presence and severity of 17 symptoms typical of clinical depression), and the Zung Anxiety Scale (a standardized self-report scale that reports the presence and severity of various symptoms of anxiety). The MPAC and the MPQ both provide reasonably equivalent assessments of the intensity dimension of pain. However, the evaluative scales of the MPQ did not correlate significantly with any of the measures of the MPAC, suggesting that the cognitive judgmental dimension of pain may be independent of the experiences of intensity, relief, and mood. None of the MPQ subscales correlated significantly with the VAS ratings of mood and pain relief.

These observations have led to the conclusion that the VAS mood scale on the MPAC represents a much more global assessment of general psychological distress rather than a specific pain-related affect. This would suggest that the MPAC provides a broader assessment of the patient by its use of the mood scale, whereas the MPQ has a more narrow focus of simply representing pain-related emotional distress. What was particularly impressive was that in the use of any of the available scales, patients could differentiate pain and mood when they were explicitly asked. The perceptions of pain intensity and pain relief have different weights as components of psychological distress. The existence of such distinctions has important clinical and theoretical significance. Although the perception of pain intensity was found to contribute significantly to subjective distress, the perception of inadequate pain relief was a more important factor. The MPAC provides valid, multidimensional information for the evaluation of pain and distress in cancer patients. It can distinguish pain intensity from pain relief and from global suffering, and it can be used to study the subtle interactions of these factors. With repeated administration it has now been demonstrated to be valid, reliable, easy to use, and nondisruptive. The MPAC and the BPI are the tools recommended for use in the clinical evaluation of individual patients and as an outcome measure in clinical trials.[53]

MEMORIAL SYMPTOM ASSESSMENT SCALE

The Memorial Symptom Assessment Scale (MSAS) is a validated, patient-rated measure that provides multidimensional information about a diverse group of common symptoms.[30] Thirty-two physical and psychological symptoms are characterized in terms of intensity, frequency, and distress. The MSAS provides a Global Distress Index (MSAS-GDI), a ten-item subscale that reflects global symptom distress and separate subscales that measure physical (MSAS-Phys) and psychological (MSAS-Psych) symptom distress, respectively. Ongoing studies have confirmed its value in patients with various types of cancer, and studies of its reliability and validity with repeated administration are currently under way. The use of the MSAS allows the concurrent measurement of pain with various other symptoms, psychological distress, and psychological factors and represents overall a useful, patient-accepted method to measure the multidimensional issues facing cancer patients with pain.[53] Newer studies have identified the usefulness of a short form for rapid assessment.[54]

QUALITY IMPROVEMENT GUIDELINES FOR THE TREATMENT OF CANCER PAIN

The American Pain Society Quality of Care Committee has strongly advocated pain measurement as an integral part of any continuous quality-improvement program.[55] They have argued that such quality-improvement programs should include five key elements: (1) ensuring that a report of unrelieved pain raises a red flag that attracts clinicians' attention; (2) making information about analgesics convenient where orders are written; (3) promising patients responsive analgesic care and urging them to communicate pain; (4) implementing policies and safeguards for the use of modern analgesic technologies; and (5) coordinating and implementing these measures. They have argued formally for there to be methods in place to chart and display patients' self-reported pain in a way that makes it highly visible and facilitates regular review by members of the health care team. Such information should be incorporated in the patient's permanent record. Figure 56.1-2 is an example of recording pain data as a fifth vital sign to be available on a page at the front of the patient's record. Unrelieved pain then should be a red flag that promptly turns attention to the problem. National programs have supported the development of broad institutional programs to improve pain management. The Veterans Administration has instituted a quality-improvement program in a wide effort to include pain as the fifth vital sign. The Joint Commission on Accreditation of Hospitals has similarly adopted clear guidelines for hospitals to improve pain management. Both of these programs, although not specifically focused on the cancer patient, are evidence of a broad commitment to reduce the barriers to effective pain management at institutional levels by instituting routine quality indicators of pain management. DuPen and colleagues have focused attention on the need to improve outpatient pain management, and through the use of a specific algorithm and nurse and chart reminders have demonstrated improved pain management for outpatient cancer patients using a specific algorithm.[56]

MEMORIAL SYMPTOM ASSESSMENT SCALE

NAME: DATE:

SECTION 1:

INSTRUCTIONS: We have listed 24 symptoms below. Read each one carefully. If you have had the symptom during this past week, let us know how OFTEN you had it, how SEVERE it was usually and how much it DISTRESSED OR BOTHERED you by circling the appropriate number. If you DID NOT HAVE the symptom, make an "X" in the box marked "DID NOT HAVE".

DURING THE PAST WEEK, Did you have any of the following symptoms?	DID NOT HAVE	IF YES, How OFTEN did you have it?				IF YES, How SEVERE was it usually?				IF YES, How much did it DISTRESS or BOTHER you?				
		Rarely	Occasionally	Frequently	Almost Constantly	Slight	Moderate	Severe	Very Severe	Not At All	ALittle Bit	Somewhat	Quite A Bit	Very Much
Difficulty concentrating		1	2	3	4	1	2	3	4	0	1	2	3	4
Pain		1	2	3	4	1	2	3	4	0	1	2	3	4
Lack of energy		1	2	3	4	1	2	3	4	0	1	2	3	4
Cough		1	2	3	4	1	2	3	4	0	1	2	3	4
Feeling nervous		1	2	3	4	1	2	3	4	0	1	2	3	4
Dry mouth		1	2	3	4	1	2	3	4	0	1	2	3	4
Nausea		1	2	3	4	1	2	3	4	0	1	2	3	4
Feeling drowsy		1	2	3	4	1	2	3	4	0	1	2	3	4
Numbness/tingling in hands/feet		1	2	3	4	1	2	3	4	0	1	2	3	4
Difficulty sleeping		1	2	3	4	1	2	3	4	0	1	2	3	4
Feeling bloated		1	2	3	4	1	2	3	4	0	1	2	3	4
Problems with urination		1	2	3	4	1	2	3	4	0	1	2	3	4

FIGURE 56.1-2. Memorial Sloan-Kettering Observation Chart with patient-rated pain intensity and relief measures. (From ref. 53, with permission.)

TABLE 56.1-2. Types of Patients with Pain from Cancer

I. Patients with acute cancer-related pain
  a. Associated with the diagnosis of cancer
  b. Associated with cancer therapy (surgery, chemotherapy, or radiation)
II. Patients with chronic cancer-related pain
  a. Associated with cancer progression
  b. Associated with cancer therapy (surgery, chemotherapy, or radiation)
III. Patients with preexisting chronic pain and cancer-related pain
IV. Patients with a history of drug addiction and cancer-related pain
  a. Actively involved in illicit drug use
  b. In methadone maintenance program
  c. With a history of drug abuse
V. Dying patients with cancer-related pain

CLASSIFICATION OF PATIENTS WITH CANCER PAIN

Five types of cancer pain patients can be identified, exemplifying the distinctions between acute and chronic pain (Table 56.1-2). Although these categories are fluid, they serve as a useful preamble for discussion of the specific therapeutic approaches to the management of cancer patients.

GROUP I: ACUTE CANCER-RELATED PAIN

Group I, patients with acute cancer-related pain, can be subdivided further according to etiology.

GROUP IA: TUMOR-ASSOCIATED PAIN

For group IA patients, with tumor-associated pain, pain is the major symptom prompting medical consultation and the diagnosis of cancer. In addition, pain has a special significance as the harbinger of the patient's illness. Recurrent pain during the course of the illness or after successful therapy has the immediate implication of recurrent disease. Defining the cause of the pain may present a diagnostic problem, but effective treatment of its cause (e.g., radiation therapy for bone metastases) is usually associated with dramatic pain relief in most patients.

GROUP IB: PAIN ASSOCIATED WITH CANCER THERAPY

Group IB patients have postoperative pain, pain secondary to oral ulceration from chemotherapy, or myalgias secondary to corticosteroid withdrawal. The cause of the pain is readily identifiable, and its course is predictable and self-limiting (Table 56.1-3). These patients do not represent difficult diagnostic problems. Pain treatment directed at the cause of the pain is used to manage the transient symptoms. These patients endure significant pain for the promise of a successful outcome.

GROUP II: CHRONIC CANCER-RELATED PAIN

Group II patients, those with chronic cancer-related pain, represent difficult diagnostic and therapeutic problems, in contrast to patients with acute cancer-related pain. They can be

TABLE 56.1-3. Cancer-Related Acute Pain Syndromes

ACUTE PAIN ASSOCIATED WITH DIAGNOSTIC AND THERAPEUTIC INTERVENTIONS
Acute pain associated with diagnostic interventions
Lumbar puncture headache
Arterial or venous blood sampling
Bone marrow biopsy
Lumbar puncture
Colonoscopy
Myelography
Percutaneous biopsy
Thoracocentesis
Acute postoperative pain
Acute pain caused by other therapeutic interventions
Pleurodesis
Tumor embolization
Suprapubic catheterization
Intercostal catheter
Nephrostomy insertion
Acute pain associated with analgesic techniques
Injection pain
Opioid headache
Spinal opioid hyperalgesia syndrome
Epidural injection pain
ACUTE PAIN ASSOCIATED WITH ANTICANCER THERAPIES
Acute pain associated with chemotherapy infusion techniques
Intravenous infusion pain
Venous spasm
Chemical phlebitis
Vesicant extravasation
Anthracycline-associated flare reaction
Hepatic artery infusion pain
Intraperitoneal chemotherapy abdominal pain
Acute pain associated with chemotherapy toxicity
Mucositis
Corticosteroid-induced perineal discomfort
Corticosteroid pseudorheumatism
Painful peripheral neuropathy
Headache
  Intrathecal methotrexate meningitic syndrome
  L-Asparaginase associated dural sinus thrombosis
  Trans-retinoic acid headache
Diffuse bone pain
  Trans-retinoic acid
  Colony-stimulating factors
5-Fluorouracil-induced anginal chest pain
Postchemotherapy gynecomastia
Acute pain associated with hormonal therapy
Luteinizing hormone–releasing factor tumor flare in prostate cancer
Hormone-induced pain flare in breast cancer
Acute pain associated with immunotherapy
Interferon-induced acute pain
Acute pain associated with radiotherapy
Incident pain associated with positioning
Oropharyngeal mucositis
Acute radiation enteritis and proctocolitis
Early-onset brachial plexopathy
Subacute radiation myelopathy
ACUTE PAIN ASSOCIATED WITH INFECTION
Acute herpetic neuralgia

(From ref. 64, with permission.)

divided for discussion purposes into two groups: those with chronic pain from tumor progression, and those with chronic pain related to cancer treatment. Both groups share the characteristic of a pain symptom that has persisted for more than 3 months.

GROUP IIA: CHRONIC PAIN FROM TUMOR PROGRESSION

In patients with chronic pain associated with progression of disease (e.g., patients with carcinoma of the pancreas, metastatic melanoma to bone, or Pancoast's syndrome), the pain escalates in intensity secondary to tumor infiltration of adjacent bone, nerve, or soft tissue. Combinations of antitumor therapy, analgesic drug therapy, anesthetic blocks, and behavioral approaches are all applied with varying degrees of success. Psychological factors play a significant role in this group of patients, in whom palliative cancer therapy may be of little value and is physically debilitating. The sense of hopelessness and fear of impending death may further add to and exaggerate the pain complaint; pain then becomes an aspect of the global *suffering* component.[57] Identifying both the pain and the suffering component is essential to the development of adequate therapy for these patients. Management approaches must be directed to controlling the pain and identifying and developing treatment strategies for each of the components of the patient's symptoms and psychological distress. Analgesic therapy combined with a wide range of alternative approaches is necessary to provide adequate analgesia. Such patients are appropriate candidates for palliative care programs to address the broader aspects of symptom management and psychological support.[2,4,58]

GROUP IIB: CHRONIC PAIN ASSOCIATED WITH CANCER THERAPY

Group IIB includes patients with chronic pain associated with cancer therapy, such as patients who develop pain after mastectomy, thoracotomy, or limb amputation (phantom limb). The nature of pain in these patients is secondary to nerve injury (neuropathic pain) with the development of a traumatic neuroma. Treatment of the pain for these patients is limited by the lack of available methods to remove the cause of the pain. Again, treatment is directed at the symptoms, not the cause. These patients closely parallel those in the general population with chronic intractable pain syndromes. Psychological factors play a significant role in how these patients adapt to and function with chronic pain. Defining this group is imperative: Identifying the cause of the pain as not directly related to tumor markedly alters the patient's therapy, prognosis, and psychological state. Each of the primary modalities of cancer therapy is associated with a series of specific chronic pain syndromes with characteristic pain patterns and clinical presentations (Tables 56.1-4, 56.1-5, and 56.1-6). Although it is consoling to both the patient and the physician to realize that the pain does not represent recurrent or progressive disease, the persistence of the pain is a constant reminder of the previous diagnosis of cancer.

In these patients, all approaches aimed at maintaining the patient's functional status should be used. Alternative methods of therapy, in contrast to drug therapy, represent the major management approach. This group of patients with neuropathic pain is increasing in number and accounts for 15% to 25% of patients referred to a medical pain clinic.

TABLE 56.1-4. Treatment-Related Chronic Pain Syndromes

POSTCHEMOTHERAPY PAIN SYNDROMES
Chronic painful peripheral neuropathy
Avascular necrosis of femoral or humeral head
Plexopathy associated with intraarterial infusion
CHRONIC PAIN ASSOCIATED WITH HORMONAL THERAPY
Gynecomastia with hormonal therapy for prostate cancer
CHRONIC POSTSURGICAL PAIN SYNDROMES
Postmastectomy pain syndrome
Postradical neck dissection pain
Postthoracotomy pain
Postoperative frozen shoulder
Phantom pain syndromes
Phantom limb pain
Phantom breast pain
Phantom anus pain
Phantom bladder pain
Stump pain
Postsurgical pelvic floor myalgia
CHRONIC POSTRADIATION PAIN SYNDROMES
Plexopathies
Radiation-induced brachial and lumbosacral plexopathies
Radiation-induced peripheral nerve tumors
Chronic radiation myelopathy
Chronic radiation enteritis and proctitis
Burning perineum syndrome
Osteoradionecrosis

(From ref. 64, with permission.)

GROUP III: PREEXISTING CHRONIC PAIN AND CANCER-RELATED PAIN

Group III includes patients with a history of chronic nonmalignant pain who develop cancer and pain. Psychological factors play a significant role in this group of patients, whose psychological and functional status is already compromised by their chronic nonmalignant pain state. These patients are at high risk of developing further functional incapacity and escalating chronic pain symptoms. However, their history should not be used in a punitive way to minimize or deny their complaints. Identifying this group of patients as a high-risk group helps to improve their psychological assessment and intervention.

GROUP IV: PATIENTS WITH A HISTORY OF DRUG ADDICTION AND PAIN

Group IV includes patients with a history of drug addiction who have cancer-related pain. Three subgroups can be identified: patients actively involved in illicit drug use and drug-seeking behavior, those receiving methadone in a maintenance program, and those who have not used drugs for several years. Undertreatment with analgesic drugs occurs most commonly in this group of patients. Assessment of reported pain by physicians and nurses is colored by the fact that the pain symptoms are confused with drug-seeking behavior. Attention to the

TABLE 56.1-5. Tumor-Related Chronic Pain Syndromes

BONE PAIN
Multifocal or generalized bone pain
 Multiple bony metastases
 Marrow expansion
Vertebral syndromes
 Atlantoaxial destruction and odontoid fractures
 C-7 to T-1 syndrome
 T-12 to L-1 syndrome
 Sacral syndrome
Back pain and epidural compression
Pain syndromes of the bony pelvis and hip
 Hip joint syndrome

HEADACHE AND FACIAL PAIN
Intracerebral tumor
Leptomeningeal metastases
Base of skull metastases
 Orbital syndrome
 Parasellar syndrome
 Middle cranial fossa syndrome
 Jugular foramen syndrome
 Clivus syndrome
 Sphenoid sinus syndrome
Painful cranial neuralgias
 Glossopharyngeal neuralgia
 Trigeminal neuralgia

TUMOR INVOLVEMENT OF THE PERIPHERAL NERVOUS SYSTEM
Tumor-related radiculopathy
 Postherpetic neuralgia
Cervical plexopathy
Brachial plexopathy
 Malignant brachial plexopathy
 Idiopathic brachial plexopathy associated with Hodgkin's disease
Malignant lumbosacral plexopathy
Tumor-related mononeuropathy
Paraneoplastic painful peripheral neuropathy
 Subacute sensory neuropathy
 Sensorimotor peripheral neuropathy

PAIN SYNDROMES OF THE VISCERA AND MISCELLANEOUS TUMOR-RELATED SYNDROMES
Hepatic distension syndrome
Midline retroperitoneal syndrome
Chronic intestinal obstruction
Peritoneal carcinomatosis
Malignant perineal pain
 Malignant pelvic floor myalgia
Ureteric obstruction

PARANEOPLASTIC NOCICEPTIVE PAIN SYNDROMES
Tumor-related gynecomastia

(From ref. 64, with permission.)

medical and psychological needs of these patients requires individualized assessment and consultation with experts in drug-related problems. The first subgroup represents a major management problem, straining the most tolerant of medical care systems. Pain in the other two subgroups is readily managed, with the recognition that the psychological stresses consequent to the pain and cancer may place the patient at a high risk for recidivism. There is increasing expertise to address the need of this patient population with experts in addiction medicine and cancer pain working together to provide a coordinated system of care.[59]

GROUP V: DYING PATIENTS WITH PAIN

In dying patients in pain, diagnostic and therapeutic considerations are directed at maintaining the patient's comfort. This group is identified separately from group II patients, because the psychological factors further compound adequate pain management. The issues of hopelessness and coping with death and dying become more prominent, and the suffering component must be addressed.[57,60,61] Inadequate control of pain in the dying patient exacerbates the suffering component and demoralizes the family and the caregivers, who feel that they have failed in treating the patient's pain at a time when adequate treatment may matter the most. Rapid escalation of analgesic drug therapy, usually by the parenteral route (intravenous, subcutaneous, or transdermal), and amelioration of psychological symptoms should be attempted. The risk-to-benefit ratios in analgesic approaches become less of an issue when the goal of pain therapy is the patient's comfort. It is now widely recognized that it is the role and the responsibility of the physician to treat pain and suffering in this population of patients. Defined guidelines for the care of the dying have been published.[2,61,62] Good physician–patient communication, which include issues of truth telling and the assault of truth; respect for patients' religious, cultural, and spiritual needs; and clearly defining goals of care can improve the care of this population of patients.[58]

COMMON PAIN SYNDROMES

Pain in the cancer patient results from direct tumor infiltration and from the various cancer treatments and can occur unrelated to the cancer and cancer therapy. Tables 56.1-3, 56.1-4, and 56.1-5 list the common acute and chronic pain syndromes that occur in patients with cancer. These lists are a compendium of various sources, but serve to summarize the broad and now well-recognized pain syndromes that occur often uniquely in this population of patients.[32,33,64,65]

CLINICAL ASSESSMENT OF PAIN

Certain general principles should be followed in evaluating cancer patients who complain of pain. Lack of attention to these general principles is the major cause for misdiagnosis of a specific pain syndrome. Adequate assessment is a critical component for defining the appropriate therapeutic strategy for each patient. The general principles are presented here:

Believe the patient's complaint of pain.
Take a careful history of the patient's pain complaint.
Evaluate the patient's psychological state.

TABLE 56.1-6. Causes of Brachial Plexopathy in Patients with Breast Cancer: Distinguishing Clinical Features

Feature	*Tumor Infiltration*	*Radiation Fibrosis*	*Transient Radiation Injury*	*Acute Ischemic Injury*
Incidence of pain	80%	18%	40%	Painless
Location of pain	Shoulder, upper arm, elbow, fourth and fifth fingers	Shoulder, wrist, hand	Hand, forearm	Hand, forearm
Nature of pain	Dull ache in shoulder, lancinating pains in elbow and ulnar aspect of hand; occasional paresthesias and dysesthesias	Ache in shoulder; prominent paresthesias in C-5 to C-6 distribution of hand and arm	Ache in shoulder; prominent paresthesias in C-5 to C-6 distribution of hand and arm	Paresthesias in C-5 to C-6 distribution of hand and arm
Severity	Moderate to severe (severe in 98%)	Usually mild to moderate (severe in 20–30%)	Mild	Mild
Course	Progressive neurologic dysfunction: atrophy and weakness in C-7 to T-1 distribution, persistent pain; occasional Horner's syndrome	Progressive weakness; panplexus or upper plexus distribution; Horner's syndrome uncommon	Transient weakness with complete resolution	Acute nonprogressive weakness and sensory loss
Study findings				
Magnetic resonance imaging	High-signal intensity mass on T2-weighted images; may enhance with gadolinium	Low-signal intensity lesion on T2-weighted images; generally nonenhancing with gadolinium	No data	Normal
Computed tomography	Mass: circumscribed or diffuse tissue infiltration	Diffuse tissue infiltration	Normal	Angiography demonstrates subclavian artery
Electromyography	Segmental slowing	Diffuse myokymia	Segmental slowing	Segmental slowing

From Cherny NI, Foley KM. Brachial plexopathy in patients with breast cancer. In: Harris JR, Hellman S, Henderson IC, Kinne D, eds. *Diseases of the breast,* 2nd ed. Philadelphia: Lippincott, 1996:796, with permission.

Perform a careful medical and neurologic examination.
Order and personally review the appropriate diagnostic studies.
Treat the pain to facilitate the appropriate workup.
Reassess the patient's response to therapy.
Individualize the diagnostic and therapeutic approaches.
Clearly define the goals of care.
Discuss advance directives with the patient and the family.

BELIEVE THE PATIENT'S COMPLAINT OF PAIN

Critical to the management of the patient with cancer pain is the establishment of a trusting relationship with the physician. The complaint of pain is a symptom, not a diagnosis. Pain perception is not simply a function of the amount of physical injury sustained by the patient, but is a complex state determined by multiple factors. The diagnosis of a specific pain syndrome and a complete understanding of the patient's psychological state is not always made during the initial evaluation. In fact, it may take several weeks to define its nature because of the lack of radiologic or pathologic verification. It may take a similar period to fully comprehend each patient's psychological makeup. Numerous examples in the assessment of patients with pain and cancer highlight the limitation of the diagnostic process. It is not uncommon for patients with tumor infiltration of the brachial plexus from either lung or breast cancer to have pain for several weeks or months before the onset of objective radiologic and neurologic findings. A comprehensive evaluation involves taking a careful history; performing a detailed medical, neurologic, and psychological evaluation; developing a series of diagnosis-related hypotheses; and ordering the appropriate diagnostic studies.

TAKE A CAREFUL HISTORY OF THE PATIENT'S PAIN COMPLAINT

A careful history of the patient's pain complaint should include the patient's description of site of pain, quality of pain, exacerbating and relieving factors, temporal pattern, exact onset, associated symptoms and signs, interference with activities of daily living, effect on the patient's psychological state, and response to previous and current analgesic therapies. Multiple pain complaints are common in patients with advanced disease and must be ranked and classified.

EVALUATE THE PATIENT'S PSYCHOLOGICAL STATE

The patient's current level of anxiety and depression must be clarified and his or her past history of such symptoms must be defined. Knowledge of the patient's previous psychiatric history and need for past hospitalization for psychiatric care helps to clarify the patient's potential psychological risk. Information on how the patient has handled previous painful events may provide insight into whether the patient has demonstrated chronic illness behavior or has a past history of a chronic pain syndrome. It is important to know about a personal or family history of alcohol or drug dependence, to understand why the patient may be fearful or refuse to take opioid drugs.

Because each patient has his or her own understanding of the meaning of pain, it is useful to have the patient elaborate this meaning.[21,57,63,66] Does he or she think it represents recurrent tumor, or is he or she convinced it is simply arthritis? Evidence suggests that when patients have a clear understanding of the meaning of their pain as representing recurrent tumor, they have increased psychological distress.

The importance of defining the psychological makeup of the patient with pain is supported by a variety of studies that have focused on the effect of suffering in patients with pain.[2,57] Psychological factors play a significant role in accounting for the differences in pain experiences in cancer patients. A series of psychiatric syndromes have been described for cancer patients, with depression occurring in as many as 25% of patients.[21] The depression presents either as an acute stress response or as a major depression. Awareness of the common psychiatric syndromes when evaluating the pain complaint expands the physician's understanding of such a complaint.

Although it is critical to know as much as possible about each patient with pain, some information may not be readily available in the first interview; in some instances it may never be available because of the lack of intellectual competence on the patient's part to define clearly the various components of the pain complaint. It is often necessary to verify the history from a family member who may provide information that the patient is unable or unwilling to provide. The family may be more objective in assessing a disability of a patient who underreports his or her symptoms. Similarly, in a patient who is a poor historian, the family member may be able to provide essential information that may alter the diagnostic approach. All attempts should be made to compile a careful history and define the medical, neurologic, and psychological profile of the pain complaint.

It is also useful to define for the patient the goal of treatment. Some patients may have unreasonable expectations for adequate pain control, whereas others fail to critically consider the various options available to them. Before starting any new procedure, review carefully with the patient the risks and benefits to provide them with their expectation of the potential outcome of the therapeutic approach. As patients become more active in defining advance directives and as they focus on the quality of life, it is critical to ask patients to define what they would do if the pain were intractable or intolerable.[67] Did the patient have a family member who died a painful death? From our experience, patients who have had such an experience are particularly fearful of their own deaths. Does the patient have suicidal thoughts or a pact with a family member? Does the patient have a family history of suicide? Does the patient have drugs in reserve or a gun in the house that he or she might use in desperation?[67] In a study by Chochinov et al., pain alone did not correlate with patients' suicidal ideation.[68] Significant depression appeared to be the major correlating factor, although pain clearly played a role in the development of depression in some patients. This series of questions allows patients to discuss openly their fears of death and their intention to take matters into their own hands rather than trust the health care professional. Such open discussions can allow the physician to better define for the patient the options for care and to reassure the patient of the physician's commitment to care. Because patients rarely offer this information unless requested, it is critical to develop specific questions that can be readily integrated into the initial history taken by the physician. Discussing with the patient how they would die and engaging the patient in a discussion of his or her concerns and wants can address the commonly heard quote of patients, "I have never died before, how do I do it?"

PERFORM A CAREFUL MEDICAL AND NEUROLOGIC EXAMINATION

A medical and neurologic examination helps provide the necessary data to substantiate the history. It also provides a direct assessment of the cognitive status of the patient. Knowledge of the referral patterns of pain and the common cancer pain syndromes can direct the examination. The commonly described pain syndromes in cancer patients associated with a postmastectomy pain syndrome can readily be defined as separate from tumor infiltration of the brachial plexus[5,69] (see Table 56.1-6).

The physical and neurologic examination allows the physician to visually inspect and palpate the site of pain and to look for the associated physical and neurologic signs that might help to better define the nature of the pain symptom. Defining the degree of motor or sensory changes can help define the specific site in the nervous system that may be involved. Similarly, in patients with sensory loss, the presence of allodynia and hyperesthesia can further define the nature of the sensory problem and define a neuropathic pain syndrome. Moreover, the degree of muscle spasm, gait instability, and impaired coordination can only be fully assessed by such an evaluation.

ORDER AND PERSONALLY REVIEW THE APPROPRIATE DIAGNOSTIC STUDIES

Diagnostic studies confirm the diagnosis and define in patients with metastatic disease the site and extent of tumor infiltration. Computed tomography and magnetic resonance imaging (MRI) are the most useful diagnostic procedures in evaluating cancer patients with pain.[70] The positron emission tomography scan is increasingly being used to further define tumor and to differentiate tumor from radiation injury. The bone scan is a useful screening device and is more sensitive for demonstrating abnormalities in the bone before changes appear on plain radiography. However, a negative bone scan does not rule out bony metastatic disease, nor does a positive bone scan confirm the diagnosis of metastatic tumor. In patients with collapsed vertebral bodies, an MRI can distinguish osteoporotic from tumor-induced bony changes. The physician should review the results personally with the radiologist to correlate any pathologic change with the site of pain.

Evaluation of the extent of metastatic disease may help to discover the relation of the pain complaint to possible recurrent disease. The use of tumor markers such as carcinoembryonic antigen, CA 125, CA 15-3, and prostate-specific antigen can be useful in a patient in whom recurrent tumor is suspected. In certain pain syndromes the presence of recurrent disease is closely associated with the onset of pain (e.g., in the appearance of late postthoracotomy pain syndrome in a patient after initial resolution of the postoperative pain).

TREAT THE PAIN TO FACILITATE THE APPROPRIATE WORKUP

No patient should be evaluated inadequately because of a significant pain problem. Early management of the pain while investigating the source markedly improves the patient's ability to

TABLE 56.1-7. Reasons for Referral to the Pain Service (n=100)

Reason for Referral[a]	*No. of Referrals*
Uncontrolled chronic pain despite analgesic therapy	73
Excessive side effects without adequate analgesia	24
Difficulties in assessment	22
Uncontrolled acute pain despite analgesic therapy	12
Change route of opioid administration	8
Concern regarding drug-seeking behavior or possibility of addiction	8
Excessive side effects with adequate analgesia	5
Manage preexistent route of drug administration	2
Concern that the patient's analgesic regimen involves too many pills	2
Concern that pain is disproportionate for extent of disease	1
Concern that patient is using excessive opioid therapy	1

[a]Physicians were asked to record one or more reasons for referral. The three reasons that were never cited included uncontrolled pain in a patient not on analgesic therapy, concern that the patient is receiving too many drugs, or concern that the treatment is too expensive.
(From ref. 26, with permission.)

participate in the necessary diagnostic procedures. Table 56.1-7 lists the reasons for a pain consultation at Memorial Sloan-Kettering Cancer Center. During the initial evaluation of the pain complaint, early consideration of the use of alternative methods of pain control, including anesthetic and neurosurgical approaches, should be considered (e.g., the temporary use of a local anesthetic via an epidural catheter to manage sacral pain).

REASSESS THE PATIENT'S RESPONSE TO THERAPY

Continual reassessment of the response of the patient's pain complaint to the prescribed therapy provides the best method to validate the initial diagnosis as correct. If relief is less than predicted or if the pain worsens, reassessment of the treatment approach or a search for a new cause of the pain should be considered. A common example is the patient with epidural cord compression who develops a second block proximal to the one being radiated, with neurologic signs mimicking the original one.[71]

INDIVIDUALIZE THE DIAGNOSTIC AND THERAPEUTIC APPROACH

Evaluation of the patient must be closely linked to the patient's level of function, ability to participate in the diagnostic workup, willingness to undergo the necessary diagnostic approaches, objective evidence that treatment approaches may be beneficial, and life expectancy. Careful judgment is required to select diagnostic approaches that will have a direct effect on the choice of the therapeutic strategy or will answer a specific question. The random use of diagnostic procedures in these patients, particularly those with advanced cancer and significant pain, is inappropriate because it may have an adverse effect on their quality of life. Open discussion with the patient about the need for assessment as well as the therapeutic options is critical to allow the patient to be part of the decision-making process. In some patients, diagnostic procedures such as MRI are inappropriate because they simply confirm the existence of a disease for which no treatment is available or for which the treatment would be a major surgical procedure (e.g., vertebral body resection) that would be inappropriate for a dying patient. Patient refusal of evaluation or treatment must be respected when the physician has fully explained the options and is convinced that the patient has an accurate understanding of the implications of no further workup or treatment.[72]

DISCUSS ADVANCE DIRECTIVES WITH THE PATIENT AND FAMILY

When developing approaches for treatment, there must be an open discussion about advance directives so that the physician has a clear understanding of the patient's goal for therapy or his or her ambivalence in developing a therapeutic strategy. The physician must have unconditional positive regard for the patient, placing the control of symptoms of pain and treatment of psychological distress in the highest regard. Knowledge of the patient's decisions about resuscitation, living wills, and symptom management should he or she become incompetent improves the physician's ability to appropriately and humanely care for the dying patient with advanced disease.[61] In a study of Memorial Sloan-Kettering Cancer Center patients evaluated by the Pain and Palliative Care Service, patients reported reluctance to discuss end-of-life care issues with their physicians, preferring to discuss their concerns with family and friends.[73] Such data emphasize the need for education of families in the continuum of cancer care including issues of pain management and the role of sedation in patients whose lives are ending.

MANAGEMENT OF CANCER PAIN

The management of cancer pain incorporates treatment of the primary disease with analgesic drug therapy and aesthetic, neurosurgical, rehabilitative, psychological (cognitive behavioral), and psychiatric methods. Individualizations of the treatment strategy and titration to effective pain relief are the hallmarks of this therapeutic approach. Increasing sophistication in the use of analgesic drugs, coupled with advances in research on the underlying mechanisms of pain, have provided the scientific rationale for the more effective use of standard analgesic drug therapy (nonopioid, opioid, and adjuvant drugs), including the use of novel routes of drug administration (transdermal and transmucosal), the use of novel methods (bisphosphonates and calcitonin for bone pain, antidepressants and anticonvulsants for neuropathic pain), and the indication for the use of anesthetic, neurosurgical, psychological, and psychiatric approaches concurrently applied in the overall continuum of care.

Pain management is only one aspect of a broad palliative care approach, but it serves as a model for the scientific rigor and clinical trials that have defined cancer pain treatment as a specific strategic focus. The full impact of such a comprehensive approach has not been fully determined. From data evaluating the use of analgesic drug therapy to cancer pain alone, 70% to 90% of patients report adequate analgesia. Studies from various pain services, hospices, and palliative care programs report results as high as 95% of patients receiving effective analgesia.

To develop appropriate outcome assessment methods and to provide a basis for comparison of treatment strategies, Bruera and Wantanabe have developed the Edmonton Staging System for cancer pain, patterning it to the various staging systems for different primary tumors. Stage I (good prognosis), stage II (intermediate prognosis), and stage III (poor prognosis) are based on five prognostic features, including the presence or absence of neuropathic pain, incident pain, psychological distress, rapid tolerance development, and a history of drug addiction or alcohol abuse.[74] This methodology, in preliminary studies, has been validated as a way to compare different patient populations with different primary tumors in clinical trials and outcome assessments of cancer pain therapy.[75]

ANALGESIC DRUG THERAPY

Numerous guidelines for the management of cancer pain have been issued by various organizations and researchers.[3,76,77] All of these guidelines have emphasized that analgesic drug therapy is the mainstay of treatment and have focused on the aims of drug therapy to achieve adequate pain relief safely within an acceptable time frame, minimize side effects of treatment, and provide ongoing analgesic therapy by the most convenient and least noxious means available. More recently, detailed descriptions of the decision-making process implemented during the treatment of patients with pain have provided further data on the rationale and outcomes of specific decisions and have detailed a series of principles in the selection of opioid drug and route of administration.[26,78] In the following section, guidelines for the rational use of analgesics in the management of cancer pain are detailed. These guidelines are based on clinical pharmacologic principles, clinical trials, available metaanalyses of analgesic studies, and the clinical experience developed by the Pain Service at Memorial Sloan-Kettering Cancer Center. Table 56.1-7 lists the reasons why patients with pain were referred to an inpatient consultation service at Memorial Sloan-Kettering Cancer Center. These reasons for referral point out the complexity that has now developed in providing individualized pharmacotherapy for patients with pain. These data also point out the need for physicians and nurses to be knowledgeable in the use of these guidelines to provide patients with effective analgesia. These data, from 100 consecutive inpatients who were referred over a 14-week period to Memorial Sloan-Kettering Cancer Center Pain Service had 158 reasons for referral.[26] The two most common reasons were uncontrolled chronic pain, which occurred in 73 patients, and excessive side effects without adequate analgesia, despite analgesic therapy, which occurred in 24 patients. The most common reasons included difficulties in pain assessment and poorly controlled acute pain. At the time of initial evaluation, 77 patients had a pain intensity of 7 out of 10, and 18 patients had a pain intensity of 4 to 6 out of 10. After initial evaluation by the Pain Service physicians, the therapeutic intent of analgesic therapy was to provide comfort and function for 87 patients and comfort only for 13 patients. Comfort and function were the therapeutic intent of analgesic therapy for 75 of the patients discharged (92%) and comfort only for 17 patients who died (94%). After initial evaluation, the Pain Service physicians changed the opioid drug, the route of administration, or both for 58 patients. Of 42 patients whose regimens were not changed, 17 were discharged, 3 died, and 22 required subsequent changes in either drug or route of administration. In short, a total of 80 patients required changes in opioid therapy before death or discharge. Sixty-four patients required more than one change in therapy. Forty-four patients required one or more changes, and 20 patients required two or more changes. These data are particularly important to point out the complexity of analgesic drug therapy in this population of patients. Side effects were problematic in providing patients with a balance between adequate analgesia and excessive side effects. It is critical, then, that the goals of care for an individual patient be recognized and help provide the essential context for therapeutic decision making. When patients prioritize optimal comfort and function equally, the therapeutic attempt is to achieve an adequate degree of relief without compromising cognitive and physical function. When comfort is the overriding goal of care, there is a willingness to use whatever analgesic therapy is necessary to achieve relief, even if function is diminished in the process. To achieve the goal of care as comfort and function, substantial effort is necessary to optimize a balance between relief and side effects through dose adjustment, sequential trials of opioid drugs, coadministration of adjuvant medications, and the use of spinal analgesic techniques. Increasing attention has focused on the need to switch patients from one opioid to another. Several studies have outlined the need for opioid rotation and substitution.[78–82]

In the following section, detailed guidelines for the rational use of analgesics in the management of cancer pain are provided (Table 56.1-8). The use of drug therapy should be within the armamentarium of any physician or nurse who cares for patients with pain in cancer. Similarly, the integration of some of the psychological and psychiatric approaches should be widely available. The use of specific anesthetic and neurosurgical techniques will often require the services of trained medical personnel who have clinical experience in managing cancer pain, but such approaches may require referral to a specialty center.

WORLD HEALTH ORGANIZATION THREE-STEP ANALGESIC LADDER

As part of a global program of WHO, the Cancer and Palliative Care Unit has created a Cancer Pain Relief Program, and through a series of expert panels, has developed guidelines for the treatment of cancer pain.[7,83,84] This program has achieved a broad international consensus, based on the concept that analgesic drug therapy is the mainstay for the majority of patients with cancer pain. As previously stated, field testing of the WHO guidelines, in conjunction with clinical experience, has shown that 70% to 90% of cancer patient's pain can be controlled using a simple and inexpensive method described as the *three-step analgesic ladder*.[83] This approach is based on the use of a combination of nonopioid, opioid, and adjuvant drugs, titrated to the individual needs of the patient according to the severity of pain and its pathophysiology (Tables 56.1-9, 56.1-10, and 56.1-11). Implementation of the analgesic guidelines, assurance of drug availability (specifically opioids), the education of health care professionals, and designating cancer pain as a priority for all national cancer control programs are the major goals of the WHO effort.[84]

Step 1

Step 1 of the analgesic ladder focuses on analgesic drug therapy for patients with mild to moderate cancer pain. Such patients

TABLE 56.1-8. Guidelines for the Rational Use of Analgesics in the Management of Cancer Pain

Start with a specific drug for a specific type of pain
Know the pharmacology of the drug prescribed
Know the relative potency of the drug
Know the duration of the analgesic effect
Know the pharmacokinetics of the drug
Know the equianalgesic doses for the drug and its route of administration
Administer analgesic on a regular basis
Gear the route of administration to the patient's needs
Oral
Buccal
Rectal
Subcutaneous
Intrathecal
Sublingual
Transmucosal
Transdermal
Intravenous
Intraventricular
Use a combination of drugs to provide additive analgesia
Narcotic plus nonnarcotic (aspirin, acetaminophen, nonsteroidal antiinflammatory drugs)
Narcotic plus adjuvants
Anticipate and treat side effects
Sedation
Respiratory depression
Nausea and vomiting
Constipation
Multifocal myoclonus and seizures
Management of the tolerant patient
Use combinations of nonopioid and opioid drugs
Use combinations of drug therapy, anesthetic, and neurosurgical procedures
Switch to an alternative opioid analgesic starting with one-half the equianalgesic dose
Use epidural local anesthetics
Reassess the nature of the pain
Prevent and treat acute withdrawal
Taper drugs slowly
Anticipate complications
Overdose
Psychological dependence

should be treated with a nonopioid analgesic that may or may not be combined with an adjuvant drug, depending on the specific pain pathophysiology. For example, in a patient with mild pain from bone metastases, the use of acetaminophen, aspirin, or one of the NSAIDs would be appropriate. In a patient with mild pain from a peripheral neuropathy, the combination of a nonopioid with a tricyclic antidepressant drug, such as amitriptyline, would be an appropriate combination.

Step 2

Step 2 focuses on patients with moderate pain who failed to achieve adequate relief after a trial of a nonopioid analgesic. They are candidates for a combination of a nonopioid (e.g., aspirin or acetaminophen) and an opioid such as codeine, oxycodone, propoxyphene, buprenorphine, or tramadol. Dependent on the pain pathophysiology, adjuvant drugs should be used as well.

Step 3

Step 3 is for those patients who fail to achieve adequate relief following appropriate administration of drugs on the second rung of the analgesic ladder. Nonopioids are often used in combination to spare the opioid effect and adjuvants are used dependent on the pain pathophysiology or the need to control other concurrent symptoms in the individual patient.

In short, the analgesic drug ladder of the WHO simply defines a method for using drug combinations and is based on previously well-tested pharmacologic principles. It is well recognized that nonopioid drugs such as aspirin and acetaminophen when combined with opioids provide additive analgesia. It is also well recognized that drugs such as morphine, methadone, fentanyl, levorphanol, and so forth are most effective for severe pain, whereas drugs such as codeine, oxycodone, and tramadol are more effective in a range of pain intensity of mild to moderate. What continues to be controversial in the application of the WHO ladder is the choice of the analgesic drug for the individual patient. Such controversies are discussed within the framework of the current application of the guidelines for rational use.[78,85–88] Critical assessment of the WHO ladder has raised challenging questions to the selection of specific drugs. A metaanalysis of the role of NSAIDs in bone pain did not define them as any more or less effective than opioids.[89]

CLASSES OF DRUGS

NONOPIOID ANALGESICS

The nonopioid analgesics include acetaminophen and the NSAIDs, of which aspirin is the prototypic agent. These compounds are most commonly used orally and their analgesia is limited by a ceiling effect, so that increasing the dose beyond a certain level (900 to 1300 mg/dose of aspirin) produces no increase in peak effect. Tolerance and physical dependence do not occur with repeated administration. Aspirin and the other NSAIDs have analgesic, antipyretic, antiinflammatory, and antiplatelet actions. Some NSAIDs lack the antiplatelet effects of aspirin, such as choline, magnesium trisalicylate. Others appear to produce fewer gastrointestinal side effects than aspirin (ibuprofen). Two new drugs within the NSAID class are the cyclooxygenase enzyme inhibitors and include rofecoxib (Vioxx) and celecoxib (Celebrex). Neither drug has been studied in cancer patients, and the current indications for use are based on their current approval by the Food and Drug Administration; rofecoxib for acute pain management and osteoarthritis and celecoxib for osteoarthritis and rheumatoid arthritis.[90] Although these drugs offer the unique advantage of less gastrointestinal and renal toxicity, their specific role remains undefined. Acetaminophen, which is equipotent to aspirin, is an analgesic and antipyretic. It is much less effective as an antiinflammatory agent and does not interfere with platelet function. In general, this class of drugs is thought to produce analgesia by inhibiting activation of peripheral nociceptors through their prevention of the formation of prostaglandin E_2, a known sensitizer of peripheral receptors to nociceptive stimulation from tissue injury. Evidence suggests

TABLE 56.1-9. Nonopioid Analgesic Drugs in the Management of Cancer Pain

Class/Drug	*Indications*	*Starting Oral Dose (mg) and Range/24 H*	*Comments*
Nonsteroidal antiinflammatory drugs			
Aspirin	Soft-tissue and metastatic bone pain	650, 650–1000	Used together with opioids, gastrointestinal and hematologic effects; avoid combination with corticosteroids
Acetaminophen	Like aspirin	650, 650–1000	Fewer gastrointestinal effects, no effects on platelet function, no significant antiinflammatory effects
Ibuprofen		400, 200–800	Higher analgesic potential than aspirin, fewer gastrointestinal and hematologic effects than aspirin
Choline magnesium trisalicylate	Like aspirin	1500, 1000–4000	Antiinflammatory and analgesic effects, similar to aspirin without hematologic effects
Fenoprofen	Like aspirin	200, 200–400	Like ibuprofen
Diflunisal	Like aspirin	500, 500–1000	Longer duration of action than ibuprofen, higher analgesic potential than aspirin
Naproxen	Like aspirin	240, 240–500	Like diflunisal

that central mechanisms augment the peripheral effects of these drugs via inhibition of neural activity induced by EAAs such as glutamate or tachykinins (such as substance P). The NSAIDs differ from each other both in duration of analgesic action and in their pharmacokinetic profile. Ibuprofen and fenoprofen have short half-lives and the same duration of action as aspirin, whereas diflunisal and naproxen have longer half-lives and are longer acting. These drugs are thought to have a special role to play in the management of bone pain because numerous studies have shown that aspirin inhibits tumor growth in an animal model of metastatic bone tumor. A metaanalysis of NSAIDs in bone pain did not demonstrate them to be more effective than weak opioids such as codeine, oxycodone, and propoxyphene.[89] From clinical experience, some patients respond better to one NSAID than to another, and each patient should be given an adequate trial of one drug on a regular basis before switching to another. Survey data from the WHO demonstration projects suggest that 20% to 40% of patients obtain pain relief with the use of nonopioid analgesics alone.[91]

Numerous studies have elucidated the major risk factors for gastrointestinal toxicity associated with NSAID use. Various factors contribute to the high risk of ulcer complications including advanced age, use of higher doses, concomitant administration of corticosteroids, and a history of either ulcer disease or previous gastrointestinal complications from NSAIDs. The empiric use of various prophylactic therapies to prevent gastrointestinal complications is controversial. Except for misoprostol, there is no evidence that any of these approaches reduces the risk of serious gastrointestinal toxicity. The empiric approach at this time is to administer misoprostol to all patients who have significant risk factors for gastrointesti-

TABLE 56.1-10. Opioid Drugs Commonly Used in Cancer Pain Management

Drug[a]	*Intramuscular (mg)*	*Oral (mg)*	*Half-Life (h)*	*Duration of Action (h)*
Codeine	130	200	2–3	2–4
Dihydrocodeine		200	2–3	2–4
Oxycodone	15	30	2–3	2–4
Propoxyphene	50	100	2–3	2–4
Morphine	10	30 (repeated dose) 60 (single dose)	2–3	3–4
Hydromorphone	1.5	7.5	2–3	2–4
Methadone	10	20	15–190	4–8
Meperidine	75	300	2–3	2–4
Oxymorphone	1	10 (per rectum)	2–3	3–4
Levorphanol	2	4	12–15	4–8
Fentanyl (parenteral)	0.1	—	1–2	1–3
Fentanyl (transdermal system)[b]				48–72
Fentanyl (transmucosal)			1–2	1–2

[a]Oxycodone, hydromorphone, and morphine available in slow-release preparations.
[b]Transdermal fentanyl, 100 μg/h; morphine, 4 mg/h.

TABLE 56.1-11. Adjuvant Analgesics in the Management of Cancer Pain

ADJUVANT DRUGS FOR NEUROPATHIC PAIN
Antidepressants
Anticonvulsants
Oral and cutaneous local anesthetics
Corticosteroids
Clonidine
Benzodiazepines
Neuroleptics
α_2-Adrenergic agonist drugs
N-methyl-D-aspartate antagonists
Calcitonin
ADJUVANT DRUGS FOR BONE PAIN
Bisphosphonates
Gallium nitrate
Calcitonin
Strontium 89
ADJUVANTS TO TREAT SIDE EFFECTS
Antiemetics
Compazine
Metoclopramide
Ondansetron
Psychostimulants
Caffeine
Methylphenidate
Dextroamphetamine
Laxatives
Senna
ADJUVANTS TO ENHANCE ANALGESIA
Acetaminophen
Nonsteroidal antiinflammatory drugs
Hydroxyzine

TABLE 56.1-12. Types of Anesthetics Procedures Commonly Used in Cancer Pain

Type of Procedure	*Most Common Indications*
Inhalation therapy with nitrous oxide	Breakthrough pain, incidental pain in patients with diffuse poorly controlled pain
Intravenous barbiturates (sodium pentobarbital)	Diffuse body pain and suffering inadequately controlled by systemic opioids
Local anesthetic by intravenous, subcutaneous, or transdermal application	Neuropathic pain in any site with local application to the area of hyperesthesia or allodynia
Trigger point injections	Focal muscle pain
Nerve block	
Peripheral	Pain in discrete dermatomes in chest and abdomen or in distal extremities
Epidural	Unilateral lumbar or sacral pain; midline perineal pain; bilateral lumbosacral pain
Intrathecal	Midline perineal pain; bilateral lumbosacral pain
Autonomic	
Stellate ganglion	Reflex sympathetic dystrophy
Lumbar sympathetic	Reflex sympathetic dystrophy of the lower extremities; lumbosacral plexopathy; vascular insufficiency of the lower extremity
Celiac plexus	Midabdominal pain from tumor infiltration
Intermittent or continuous epidural infusion with local anesthetics	Unilateral and bilateral lumbosacral pain; midline perineal pain; neuropathic pain from the midthoracic region down
Intermittent or continuous epidural or intrathecal with local opioid analgesics	Unilateral and bilateral pain below the midthoracic region: often combined with local anesthetics
Intermittent or continuous intraventricular infusions with opioid analgesics	Head and neck pain and upper chest
Chemical hypophysectomy	Diffuse bone pain

nal complications.[92] Many of these data have been accumulated in the general literature and have not been specifically analyzed for the patient with cancer. Several NSAIDs have been approved by the Food and Drug Administration for use as analgesics for mild to moderate pain and are listed in Table 56.1-12. Guidelines for the use of NSAIDs in patients with cancer are largely empiric. This class of drugs represents the first-line approach, but the choice and use of the nonopioid need to be individualized. Each patient should be given an adequate trial of one nonopioid analgesic before switching to an alternative one. Such a trial should include administration of the drug to maximum levels at regular intervals. Because there is a great variability among patient responses to different drugs, patients may require trials with several NSAIDs before finding an effective drug and dose regimen. If pain relief is not obtained, adding an opioid to a nonopioid provides additive analgesia. Combinations of codeine, oxycodone, and propoxyphene are available, but these combinations often contain less than the full dose of 650 mg of aspirin or acetaminophen. Prescribing each drug separately provides a better method for individualizing pain control. This is particularly important when the patient requires escalation of the combination to provide analgesia, in which case the additional dosage of the NSAID or acetaminophen may become excessive.

OPIOID DRUGS

The opioid analgesics, of which morphine is the prototype, vary in potency, efficacy, and adverse effects. These drugs produce their analgesic effects by binding to discrete opiate receptors in the peripheral and central nervous systems. This group also includes a series of heterogeneous substances with varying chemical structures. In contrast to the nonopioid analgesics, opioid analgesics, at least the opioid pure agonist, do not appear to have a ceiling effect (i.e., as the dose is escalated on a log scale, the increment in analgesia is linear to the point of loss of consciousness). There are also series of drugs that are pure antagonists (i.e., they block the effect of morphine at the receptor). The drug most commonly used in clinical practice is naloxone, which is used to reverse respiratory depression and other complications associated with opioid overdose.

Effective use of the opioid drugs requires the balancing of the most desirable effects of pain relief with the undesirable effects of nausea, vomiting, mental clouding, sedation, constipation, tolerance, and physical dependence. These undesirable effects impose a practical limit on the dose useful for a particular patient and have led to the concept of opioid responsiveness (see Principles of Opioid Drug Therapy, later in this chapter).

The use of opioids in the management of cancer pain remains a controversial issue.[85–87] Some of the controversies include their role in the management of neuropathic pain, which has been suggested for the *opioid resistant,* the specific choice of opioid drug, the use of sequential trials of opioids, routes of administration, development of tolerance, economic factors influencing these controversies, and the concern that opioids are agents of physician-assisted suicide and euthanasia.[93–96] When appropriate, these controversies are addressed in the following discussion of the principles of opioid drug therapy.

PRINCIPLES OF OPIOID DRUG THERAPY

START WITH A SPECIFIC DRUG FOR A SPECIFIC TYPE OF PAIN

As defined by the three-step analgesic ladder, the specific drug chosen is dependent in part on the degree of pain intensity. As previously noted, cancer patients commonly have multiple sites and types of pain. It has been suggested that neuropathic pain, which accounts for 10% to 20% of pain problems that are difficult to manage, is opioid resistant, and that opioid drugs should not be used in this population.[88] Studies in cancer patients with both nociceptive and neuropathic pain, as well as controlled studies in nonmalignant neuropathic pain, demonstrate the variable responsiveness of neuropathic pain to opioid analgesics.[88] The concept of a continuum of opioid responsiveness, rather than an all or none quantal phenomenon, has been clearly observed. *Opioid responsiveness* is defined as the degree of analgesia achieved during dose escalation to either intolerable side effects or adequate analgesia. Patient characteristics, pain-related factors, as well as drug-selective effects influence this variable response.

A wide range of adjuvant analgesics has been suggested to provide analgesia alone or in combination with opioid drug therapy, and there are specific adjuvants for bone pain and neuropathic pain. Not only pain intensity and type of pain dictate the choice of a specific drug, but also the patient's prior opioid exposure, history of allergy, and history of side effects.

The WHO Cancer Pain Guidelines designated morphine as the drug of choice in its Cancer Pain Relief Program. The choice was based on practical, not scientific, considerations. The introduction of the WHO program rapidly demonstrated the limited availability of morphine worldwide for oral treatment of chronic cancer pain.[97] Morphine consumption worldwide is now used as an indicator of the success of the WHO Cancer Pain Relief Program. For example, in Japan following a nationwide program to improve cancer pain management, a 17-fold increase in morphine consumption has been reported. The expanded use of morphine, combined with new formulations and new information about the analgesic activities of its metabolites, focuses renewed attention on its clinical pharmacology with recognition of morphine-6-glucuronide (M6G) as an active metabolite.[98] Human studies have shown that M6G is analgesic in humans and appears in the plasma and cerebrospinal fluid of patients receiving morphine systemically.[99] In renal dysfunction, M6G has an increased elimination half-life and decreased clearance, confirming a true delay in elimination of the compound, leading to an increase in the M6G to morphine ratio during chronic therapy.[100] Adverse effects (nausea and respiratory depression) have been attributed to plasma concentration of the metabolite, particularly in patients with renal failure.[101] However, attempts to correlate M6G to morphine ratio or M6G to M3G ratio with side effects such as cognitive impairment or myoclonus have not been possible.[102,103] Various factors may influence the levels of both M6G and M3G, including route (increased M6G following oral administration), age (increased M3G and M6G if greater than 70 years), male sex (decreased morphine and M6G plasma concentrations), concurrent use of tricyclic antidepressants (increased M3G), and use of ranitidine (increased morphine). Controlled-release oral morphine is currently available in a wide range of doses from 50 to 200 mg for every 8-, 12-, and 24-hour administration. These preparations provide comparable analgesia with immediate release forms and offer increased convenience, improved compliance, and a reduction in duration of pain.

The increasing need for a wide range of opioids to manage cancer pain has led to the wide use of a series of alternative opioids to morphine, including hydromorphone, oxycodone, oxymorphone, and levorphanol, all congeners of morphine. Hydromorphone has poor oral availability and a short half-life. It is highly soluble and available in a high-potency parenteral form (10 mg/mL), making it a useful choice for chronic subcutaneous administration. Because of its short half-life, it is commonly used in the elderly patient. Myoclonus has been reported following high doses possibly due to accumulation of its metabolites (3-0 methyl or a 6-glucuronide).[104] When compared in a double-blind trial of patient-controlled analgesia, no differences in analgesia or side effects were noted between morphine and hydromorphone. Although cognitive performance was poorer in the hydromorphone group, patients reported better mood as compared with morphine.[105] Hydromorphone is available in slow-release preparations.

Oxycodone, which is commonly used at a 5-mg dose in the second step of the WHO analgesic ladder, can also be used in the third step at higher doses. It is now available in a slow-release preparation.[106] Its half-life is approximately 3 to 4 hours. Oxymorphone is its active metabolite. Oxymorphone is currently only available by the intravenous and rectal routes and serves as an alternative to morphine and its other congeners. Oxymorphone has less of a histamine effect and may be of use in those patients who complain of headache or itch following other opioid administration.

Levorphanol has good bioavailability but a long plasma half-life (12 to 16 hours). It should be used cautiously because with repeated administration, accumulation may occur.

The role of methadone in cancer pain also remains controversial.[79–82] Methadone represents a second-line drug for cancer pain patients who have had prior exposure to opioids. It is a relatively inexpensive oral analgesic, but its name has negative connotations for cancer patients who view methadone as a drug used to treat addicts. The bioavailability of methadone is higher than that of morphine (85% vs. 35%, respectively). Its analgesic potency also differs with a parenteral to oral ratio of 1:2 in contrast to 1:6 with morphine. Moreover, the plasma half-life of methadone is 17 to 24 hours, with reports of up to 50 hours in some cancer patients, but with a duration of analgesia of only 4 to 8 hours. Significant adverse effects have been reported in cancer patients receiving methadone by various routes. The discrepancy between analgesic duration and plasma half-life of methadone have made it a difficult drug to use in the naïve patient because of the need for careful titration.

A number of case reports have highlighted the possible greater analgesic potency of methadone than the often quoted 1:1 equivalency with morphine.[79–82] Studies of interindividual differences in response to opioid analgesics demonstrate dramatically reduced doses of methadone required to produce analgesia in patients chronically taking morphine or hydromorphone. Several authors have shown marked reductions in the equianalgesic dose of methadone when patients with either uncontrolled pain or extreme side effects were switched. These clinical survey studies suggested up to a 75% reduction in the methadone equianalgesic dose. In the only perspective study, Ripamonti et al. developed a specific dose ratio based on the patient's morphine doses.[80] For patients on 30 to 90 mg of morphine, the dose ratio is 4:1; for those on 90 to 300 mg daily, the dose ratio is 6:1; and for those on 300 mg or more, the dose ratio is 8:1. Bruera et al. developed a similar ratio for hydromorphone based on survey data.[79] In patients receiving more than 330 mg of hydromorphone, the dose ratio is 1.6:1; and less than 300 mg, the dose ratio is 0.95:1.

In general, a good rule is to reduce the calculated equianalgesic dose by 75% and titrate the patients to effective pain relief. These reports have pointed out the need to use one-fourth to one-third the equianalgesic dose of methadone when switching from other opioids to this regimen. This observation relates in part to significant incomplete cross-tolerance with methadone and other factors that have not been fully assessed. Methadone can be administered by a variety of routes, but the subcutaneous route is associated with adverse effects including cutaneous hypersensitivity.[107] Due to its long half-life, some offer the suggestion that methadone be used on a every 8 to 12 hour basis, whereas others have demonstrated analgesic efficacy and safety in acute 3- to 4-hour dosing intervals. Ongoing studies are attempting to elucidate better the clinical pharmacology of methadone to facilitate its broader use.

Meperidine is a drug that should not be used chronically in the management of patients with cancer pain. Meperidine has a poor parenteral to oral ratio (1:4). It is available in oral and intramuscular routes but repetitive intramuscular administration is associated with local tissue fibrosis and sterile abscess. Repetitive dosing of meperidine (greater than 250 mg/d) can lead to normeperidine accumulation, an active metabolite that can produce central nervous system hyperexcitability.[108] This hyperirritability is characterized by subtle mood effects followed by tremors, multifocal myoclonus, and occasional seizures. It occurs most commonly in patients with renal disease, but can also occur following repeated administration in patients with normal renal function. Naloxone does not reverse meperidine-induced seizures and its use in meperidine toxicity is controversial; there have been some case reports that the use of naloxone has precipitated generalized seizures in individual patients. In rare instances, central nervous system toxicity characterized by hyperpyrexia, muscle rigidity, and seizure have been reported following the administration of a single dose of meperidine to patients receiving treatment with monoaminoxidase inhibitors.

With the development of a novel transdermal patch, fentanyl is an opioid analgesic used effectively in cancer pain patients for management of both acute and chronic pain.[109] The half-life of fentanyl is 1 to 2 hours. Its relative potency compared with parenteral morphine is 1 to 20 in intolerant acute pain patients. In chronic cancer pain, relative potency comparisons have not been fully established but the common dosing guideline is that 4 mg of intravenous morphine is equivalent to 100 μg of intravenous fentanyl. The uniqueness of this preparation facilitates the management of patients who are unable to take drugs by mouth by providing them with continuous opioid analgesia. Patches are currently available in 25 to 100 μg/h doses. Fentanyl can also be used as an anesthetic premedication, as well as intravenously and epidurally for pain control. Oral transmucosal formulations have demonstrated effectiveness in breakthrough pain in cancer patients.[45] Fentanyl (Actiq) is available in a range of dosages from 200 to 1600 μg. Twenty-five percent of the preparations in a lozenge formulation in a stylet is absorbed transmucosally over a 15-minute period and an additional 25% is absorbed via the gastrointestinal tract over the following 90 minutes. Onset of relief occurs in 5 minutes. Oral transmucosal fentanyl citrate in dose titration trials is shown to be safe and effective with the effective dose being a variable requiring titration in the majority of patients.

KNOW THE EQUIANALGESIC DOSE OF THE DRUG AND ITS ROUTE OF ADMINISTRATION

Knowing the equianalgesic dose can ensure more appropriate drug use. Lack of attention to these differences in drug dose is the most common cause of undermedication of pain patients. These doses have been derived from assessment of the relative analgesic potency of a drug. *Relative potency* is the ratio of the doses of two analgesics required to produce the same effect. Estimates of relative potency allow calculation of the equianalgesic dose, which provides the basis for selecting the appropriate dose when switching drugs or route of administration of the same drug. The values in Table 56.1-10 are based on studies in which 10 mg of morphine was the standard dose.[110] The equianalgesic dose is the recommended starting dose, with the optimal dose for each patient determined by dose adjustment. There is now evidence to suggest that relative potency may differ in single-dose and repeated dose studies. For example, for morphine, a 1:6 relative analgesic potency ratio should be used for patients with acute pain, whereas a 1:2 or 1:3 ratio in patients treated with repeated doses on a chronic basis is more appropriate. For methadone, the equianalgesic dose ratios vary with the degree of prior exposure as previously discussed.[80]

ADMINISTER ANALGESICS REGULARLY AFTER INITIAL TITRATION

Medication should be given regularly in order to maintain the plasma level of the drug above the minimum effective concentration for pain relief. In the initial titration, patients should be advised to take their medication as needed to determine their total 24-hour requirements. This is also the time frame for reaching the steady-state level of drug, which depends on the drug's half-life. For morphine, steady state can be reached in 24 hours; with methadone it may take up to 5 to 7 days to reach steady state. In patients on a fixed schedule, rescue medications equivalent to one-half of the standing dose should be available to patients for breakthrough pain.

Continuous intravenous and subcutaneous opioid infusions to manage both acute and chronic cancer pain are commonly used with a patient-controlled analgesic pump programmed to the patient's need with a set *lock-out time* to prevent overdosing. This method of drug administration is especially useful to manage patients with breakthrough pain. It is a significant advance in facilitating adequate titration of analgesics in chronic cancer patients, allowing discharge to home and hospice settings.

GEAR THE ROUTE OF ADMINISTRATION TO THE PATIENT'S NEEDS

Various methods of drug delivery of opioids have been developed in an attempt to maximize pharmacologic effects and minimize side effects. Most patients require at least two routes of drug administration, and 20% need up to four approaches during the course of their cancer pain treatment, from diagnosis to death.

The oral route is preferable and easy. Orally administered drugs have a slower onset of action, delayed peak time, and longer duration of effect; drugs given parenterally have a rapid onset of action but a shorter duration of effect. Slow-release preparations of morphine, hydromorphone, and oxycodone allow more convenient dosing of cancer pain patients every 8 to 12 hours or 24 hours.

For cancer pain management by the sublingual route, these are drugs that are well absorbed sublingually including both fentanyl and methadone.[111] As discussed there is now an oral transmucosal fentanyl citrate preparation that has been widely studied for the management of breakthrough pain and is absorbed transmucosally.

For the rectal route, oxymorphone, hydromorphone, and morphine are available in suppository form. Oxymorphone suppositories produce analgesia equivalent to 10 mg of parenteral morphine. Slow-release oxycodone and morphine preparations have also been demonstrated to be effective rectally and ongoing studies with rectal methadone suggest that this drug is well absorbed by the rectal route.

The transdermal route is a convenient way to deliver a potent short-acting opioid on a continuous basis. Drug is released through the skin patch at a nearly constant amount per unit time with a concentration gradient from patch to skin. Serum fentanyl concentrations increase and steady-state levels are approached at 12 to 24 hours.[109] After patch removal, the drug persists in the skin, with falling blood levels over 24 hours. In calculating the equianalgesic dose, 4 mg of intravenous morphine is equivalent to 100 μg of fentanyl transdermally. Innovative transdermal delivery systems are in development, which include systems for immediate-dose delivery using iontophoresis and drug reservoirs. Iontophoresis is the transfer of ionic solutes through biologic membranes under the influence of an electric field. It offers an alternative system for parenteral administration and has been shown to allow for comparatively rapid achievement of fentanyl dose levels using a transdermal system.[112]

Various parenteral routes include intermittent and continuous subcutaneous, intravenous, epidural, intraventricular, and intrathecal infusions. The use of intermittent and continuous subcutaneous infusions is most useful in patients who cannot tolerate oral analgesics because of gastrointestinal obstruction or intractable nausea and vomiting and do not have intravenous access. The usefulness of this technique has been demonstrated using morphine, heroin, hydromorphone, levorphanol, and fentanyl. Methadone by this route is associated with the development of a cutaneous hypersensitivity syndrome.[107]

Patient-controlled analgesic pumps designed to infuse continuously but with options for bolus administration are connected to a 27-gauge butterfly needle that the patient can insert into a new subcutaneous site every third to sixth day. Limited pharmacokinetic studies have demonstrated that systemic absorption of the drug from subcutaneous sites at steady state has an 87% bioavailability with hydromorphone, for example.[112]

Intermittent and continuous intravenous infusions are used if intravenous access is available and more commonly in the patient who is hospitalized. Specific guidelines for the use of continuous infusions have been developed.[113]

Intermittent and continuous epidural and intrathecal opioid infusions are based on the demonstration of opioid receptors in the dorsal horn of the spinal cord and the availability of opioid drugs to suppress noxious stimuli at the spinal cord level.[34,35] Localized selective analgesia is produced without motor or sensory blockade. The pharmacokinetics of epidural opioid administration demonstrate that there is significant systemic uptake after epidural injection, comparable with an intramuscular injection of the same drug and dose. However, distribution of the drug directly into the cerebrospinal fluid is 10 to 100 times greater. Existing studies demonstrate that approximately 10% of cancer patients use this approach to maximize analgesia and minimize side effects. This technique is commonly used in patients who have mixed nociceptive neuropathic pain syndromes and in whom combinations of local anesthetics and opioids are administered epidurally.

Rarely, intraventricular opioid infusion has been used to manage patients with pain in the cervical and craniofacial region from tumor infiltration.[114] Doses between 1.0 and 7.5 mg/24 hours have been used and patients have reported 70% excellent results. At present, there is not a clear indication that this intraventricular route offers special advantages over systemic opioids.[114]

USE A COMBINATION OF DRUGS

The use of a combination of drugs enables a physician to increase analgesic effects without escalating the opioid dose. Combinations that produce additive analgesic effects include an opioid plus a nonopioid, an opioid plus an antihistamine (100 mg of intramuscular hydroxyzine), and an opioid plus an amphetamine (10 mg of intramuscular dextroamphetamine).[115–117] Trials with opioids combined with dextromethorphan demonstrate additive analgesia and such combinations are now under study for their role in cancer pain patients.[118]

ANTICIPATE AND TREAT SIDE EFFECTS

The side effects of the opioid analgesics often limit their effective use. The most common side effects are sedation, respiratory depression, nausea, vomiting, constipation, and multifocal myoclonus and seizures.

Sedation and drowsiness vary with the drug and dose and may occur after both single and repeated administration. They are mediated through activation of opiate receptors in the reticular formation and diffusely throughout the cortex. Management of these effects includes reducing the individual drug dose but prescribing the drug more frequently, or switching to an analgesic with a shorter plasma half-life. Amphetamine, methylphenidate, and caffeine can be used to counteract these sedative effects.[116,117,119] It is important to discontinue all other drugs that might exacerbate the sedative effects of the opioid analgesic, including a wide variety of medications such as cimetidine, barbiturates, and other anxiolytic medications.

Respiratory depression is the most serious adverse effect of the opioid drugs. It occurs most commonly after short-term administration of an opioid and is usually associated with other signs of central nervous system depression, including sedation and drowsiness. The opioid-agonist drugs act on brainstem respiratory centers to produce, as a function of dose, increasing respiratory depression to the point of apnea. Tolerance to this effect develops rapidly with repeated drug administration, thereby allowing prolonged use without significant risk of respiratory depression.

Respiratory depression can be reversed by giving the short-acting opioid antagonist naloxone (suggested dose, 0.4 mg/mL). Repeated administration, including an intravenous drip, may be necessary to prevent respiratory arrest in such patients. In patients receiving opioids for prolonged periods who develop respiratory depression, diluted doses of naloxone (0.4 mg in 10 mL of saline) should be titrated carefully to prevent the precipitation of severe withdrawal symptoms while reversing the respiratory depression. A useful dosing normogram for continuous intravenous infusion of naloxone has been developed in which two-thirds of the initial bolus is started on an hourly basis and titrated against the patient's symptoms.[120]

In some patients the use of naloxone to reverse drug-induced respiratory depression can be dangerous. An endotracheal tube should be placed in the comatose patient before giving naloxone to prevent aspiration from excessive salivation and bronchial spasm induced by naloxone administration. In patients receiving meperidine over a longer period, naloxone may precipitate seizures by lowering the seizure threshold and by allowing the convulsant activity of the active metabolite, normeperidine, to become evident. In this instance, special attention must be given to the potential seizure effect of naloxone. If naloxone is used, diluted doses, slow titration, and appropriate seizure precautions are advised. There is insufficient clinical evidence to make more specific recommendations. If respiratory support can be effected by other means (i.e., continuous stimulation to maintain the patient's wakefulness), such an approach may place the patient at less risk and clearly in less discomfort.

The opioid analgesics produce nausea and vomiting by an action limited to the medullary chemoreceptor trigger zone. The incidence of nausea and vomiting is markedly increased in ambulatory patients. Tolerance develops to these side effects with repeated administration. Nausea with one drug does not mean that all drugs will produce it.[121] Switching to alternative opioid analgesics or using an antiemetic together with the opioid analgesic are ways to obviate this effect. Lack of controlled trials to identify a specific first-line agent has supported the practice of using sequential trials of agents beginning with prochlorperazine (Compazine) concurrently with the opioid to clarify a useful regimen. Droperidol has also been noted to be effective in opioid-induced nausea and vomiting.

Constipation results from the action of these drugs at multiple sites in the gastrointestinal tract and in the spinal cord to produce a decrease in the intestinal secretions and peristalsis, resulting in a dry stool and constipation. When opioid analgesics are started, a regular bowel regimen, including cathartics and stool softeners, should also be instituted. Several bowel regimens have been suggested because of their specific ability to counteract the effects of the opioid drugs, but none has been studied in a controlled way.[122] Anecdotal surveys suggest that doses far above those used for routine bowel management are needed, that senna derivatives are effective, and that careful attention to dietary factors along with the use of a bowel regimen can reduce patient complaints dramatically. Tolerance to this effect develops over time, but relatively slowly. Oral naloxone has been shown to be effective in treating constipation, but its use is variable depending on the degree of opioid exposure of the patient.[123]

Multifocal myoclonus may occur with high doses of all of the opioid drugs. Multifocal myoclonus and seizures have been reported in patients receiving multiple doses of meperidine (250 mg or more per day), although signs and symptoms of central nervous system hyperirritability may occur with toxic doses of all the opioid analgesics. In a series of cancer patients receiving meperidine, accumulation of the active metabolite normeperidine was associated with these neurologic signs and symptoms. However, in a similar group of cancer patients with pain, subtle mood effects were noted after meperidine administration, which suggests a spectrum of central nervous system effects. Management of this hyperirritability includes discontinuing the meperidine, using intravenous diazepam if seizures occur, and substituting morphine to control the persistent pain. Because the half-life of normeperidine is 16 hours, it may take 2 or 3 days for the signs of central nervous system hyperirritability to clear completely. Meperidine is contraindicated in patients with chronic renal disease, but these complications noted in cancer pain occurred in patients with normal renal function.[108] Morphine and hydromorphone at high doses produce myoclonus, which has not been directly associated with their known active metabolite such as M6G and hydromorphone-6-glucuronide. In dying patients with myoclonus, the use of benzodiazepines or barbiturates has been reported anecdotally to suppress this sign, improving the patient's comfort.

Opioid hyperexcitability and hyperalgesia have been reported with the use of increasing opioid doses by the parenteral acute and epidural routes. It has most often been observed in patients on high doses of morphine and hydromorphone and is characterized by uncontrolled pain, hypervigilance, total body hyperalgesia, and allodynia. It is best managed by rapid dose reduction and substitution with an alternative opioid such as methadone. The mechanism of action is unclear.[103]

In animal studies with morphine it is thought to be related to M3G, which in animals is associated with allodynia and hyperalgesia following intracerebroventricular administration. This action of M3G is mimicked by strychnine, a glycine agonist. Glycine medicates postsynaptic inhibition on dorsal horn neurons. It is suggested that high doses of morphine or its metabolites may act via a spinal antiglycinergic effect, reducing postsynaptic inhibition causing allodynia and myoclonus.

MANAGE TOLERANCE

The earliest sign of the development of tolerance is the patient's complaint that the duration of effective analgesia has decreased. For reasons not yet understood, the rate of development of tolerance varies greatly among cancer patients. Some demonstrate tolerance within days of initiating opioid therapy; others remain controlled for many months on the same dose. Studies in an outpatient clinic population, a hospitalized population, and a home care population revealed three patterns of drug use: those who rapidly increase their opioid requirements, those who stabilize at one dose for several weeks or months, and those who decrease or eliminate opioids.[124] Increased opioid requirements are most commonly associated with disease progression rather than tolerance alone. With the development of tolerance, increases in the frequency of the dose of the opioid are required to provide continued pain relief. Because the analgesic effect is a logarithmic function of the dose of opioid, a doubling of the dose may be needed to restore full analgesia. There appears to be no limit to the development of tolerance, and with appropriate dose adjustments patients can continue to obtain pain relief. Cross-tolerance among the opioid analgesics is not complete; therefore, it is advantageous to change to an alternative opioid, selecting half the predicted equianalgesic dose as the starting dose.

The use of analgesic combinations can reduce the amount of opioid required. Similarly, the use of bolus or continuous epidural local anesthesia in patients with perineal pain can dramatically reduce the need for systemic opioids and reverse tolerance.

TAPER DRUGS SLOWLY

The long-term administration of opioid analgesics is associated with the development of physical dependence, a state in which the sudden cessation of the opioid analgesic produces signs and symptoms of withdrawal: agitation, tremors, insomnia, fear, marked autonomic nervous system hyperexcitability, and exacerbation of pain. Slowly tapering the dose of the opioid analgesic prevents such symptoms. The appearance of abstinence symptoms from the time of drug withdrawal is related to the elimination half-life for the particular drug. The type of abstinence syndrome similarly varies with the drug. For example, with morphine, withdrawal symptoms occur within 6 to 12 hours after drug cessation. Reinstituting the drug in doses of approximately 25% of the previous daily dose suppresses these symptoms.

ANTICIPATE COMPLICATIONS

Overdose with opioid analgesics occurs either intentionally, when a patient takes an excessive amount of drug in a suicide attempt, or unintentionally, when the recommended dosage accidentally produces excessive sedation and respiratory depression. In both instances, the complication can be treated effectively with naloxone. Intentional overdose in cancer patients occurs rarely, and concern for this is overemphasized. Overdose in patients previously stabilized on a opioid regimen for cancer pain rarely is caused by drug intake alone. More commonly, it is the medical deterioration of the patient with a superimposed metabolic encephalopathy. Eagel studied the use and misuse of naloxone and identified that sedation was the most common reason for naloxone use.[125] Of note, in this study of naloxone use in 34 patients over 1 year in a cancer center, 71% of patients had a medical reason other than opioid dose escalation as an explanation for the change in medical condition prompting naloxone use. Following naloxone administration, 64% of patients experienced significant side effects; 42% had increased pain and 14% had increased agitation. Patients were given intravenous boluses of 0.4 mg of naloxone rather than titrated with diluted naloxone as has been recommended.[126] Reducing the opioid drug dosage and carefully assessing the patient's metabolic status usually provide the differential diagnosis. Patients who have taken an unintentional drug overdose should be scrutinized carefully to rule out other causes of excessive sedation, confusion, or respiratory depression. In such cases a reversal of these effects with naloxone is more therapeutic than diagnostic.

Psychological dependence or addiction is characterized by a concomitant behavioral pattern of drug abuse evidenced by craving a drug for other than pain relief and overwhelming involvement in the use and procurement of the drug. This is a state distinct from tolerance and physical dependence, which are responses to the pharmacologic effects of long-term opioid administration. The profound fear of causing psychological dependence plays a major role in a physician's reluctance to prescribe opioid analgesics, particularly in cancer patients in the early phase of their disease. Patients may share this fear, consistently taking less analgesic drug than is effective to control their pain. Increasing evidence suggests that cancer patients with pain can take opioid analgesics for prolonged periods but can discontinue such drugs when adequate pain relief is achieved from other approaches. In almost all instances, dramatic escalation of drug intake is associated with progression of disease and subsequent death. Few patients with cancer and pain become psychologically dependent on the drugs and participate in drug-seeking and illicit drug use. Careful evaluation of patients who might be at risk for this complication is necessary, but such concern should not be punitive to the patient with severe cancer pain.

Out-of-control aberrant drug taking among oncology patients with or without a prior history of substance abuse represents a serious and complex clinical occurrence. Passik and Portenoy have developed guidelines to manage such patients.[59] The most difficult situations present themselves in the patient who is actively abusing illicit or prescription drugs or alcohol while concurrently receiving medical therapies. Such patients need a multidisciplinary approach usually focused on a harm-reduction concept that attempts to enhance social support for the patient to maximize treatment compliance. Passik and Portenoy have outlined a series of approaches to maximize a number of strategies for promoting compliance, including the consideration of a written contract between the team and patient, the inclusion of spot urine toxicology screens to assess compliance, set expectations regarding attendance in clinic, and the patient's management of medication supplies. It is often most useful to see the patient on a regular basis, often every several days, and to limit prescribing of opioids to that basis until the patient has demonstrated his or her willingness to be compliant and to follow an appropriate drug regimen. Other approaches include the use and encouragement for the patient to attend a 12-step program and to engage the patient's family members and friends to further bolster social support and functioning. Such approaches can be helpful on an outpatient basis, but on an inpatient basis when patients demonstrate manipulative behaviors in the inappropriate use of medication, direct discussion with the patient about the drug use in an open manner is a first step. Providing the patient with a private room near the nurses' station to monitor the patient and discourage attempts to leave the hospital for purchase of illicit drugs and requiring visitors to check in with the nursing staff before visitation are additional steps. As well, the use of daily urine specimens is another method to evaluate compliance. Underlying all of this is the attempt to provide the patient with a supportive environment that respects the patient's pain symptomatology and serious medical illness and attempts to limit harm to the patient or others by the aberrant drug use and behaviors.

ADJUVANT DRUGS

Adjuvant drugs are used to enhance opioid analgesia, provide analgesia for certain types of pain (e.g., neuropathic pain, bone pain, and visceral pain), and treat opioid side effects or other symptoms associated with pain.[127] They are an integral part of the WHO three-step analgesic ladder. Because of the lack of well-defined guidelines for their use, sequential drug trials are necessary to identify the most useful drug and dose titration to find a safe effective dose. Table 56.1-11 lists the commonly used adjuvants and their therapeutic categories.

Adjuvants to Enhance Analgesia

Adjuvants to enhance analgesia have been previously discussed in the section on combinations of drugs (see Use a Combination of Drugs, earlier in this chapter). Acetaminophen, NSAIDs, hydroxyzine, and dextromethorphan have been demonstrated to provide additive analgesia to patients chronically receiving opioids.

Adjuvant Analgesics for Neuropathic Pain

The common neuropathic pain syndromes in patients with cancer include injury to peripheral nerves and plexus by tumor invasion, chemotherapy, surgery, or viral agents. Depending on the intensity of pain, nonopioid and opioid analgesics are the first-line agents. However, as previously discussed, there is evidence to suggest that such neuropathic pains are less responsive to nonopioid and opioid approaches. Some of the commonly used adjuvant drugs for managing this population of patients are described in the following sections.

Antidepressants

The tricyclic antidepressants may be the most useful group of psychotropic drugs used in pain management.[128,129] Their analgesic effects are mediated by enhancement of serotonin activity. Data from controlled trials indicate that both the tertiary amine tricyclic antidepressants (amitriptyline, doxepin, imipramine and clomipramine), and the secondary amine compounds (desipramine and nortriptyline) have analgesic effects. More recently, one of the serotonin selective reuptake inhibitors, paroxetine, has also been shown to have analgesic properties in patients with neuropathic pain.[130] These drugs have been reported to be effective in treating continuous dysesthesias, as well as intermittent lancinating dysesthetic pain. The doses used for analgesia are far below those needed to produce an antidepressant effect. The analgesic properties of these drugs appear to occur independent of their mood-altering effects. Patients should be started on low doses of 10 to 25 mg and titrated up to achieve adequate analgesia in a 2- to 4-week trial. Blood levels should be measured to determine both patient compliance and drug absorption, because of wide individual variation. Patients who are unable to tolerate amitriptyline, or who are predisposed to its sedative, anticholinergic or hypotensive effects, should be considered for a trial with a secondary amine tricyclic antidepressant, or a serotonin selective reuptake inhibitor such as paroxetine. In the management of cancer patients with pain, the antidepressant drugs are the first-line therapeutic approach for neuropathic pain, and every attempt should be made to provide the patient with a several-week trial before discontinuing these drugs.

Anticonvulsants

The role of anticonvulsants in the management of patients with neuropathic pain is based, in part, on the fact that the mode of action is to stabilize membranes and alter sodium and calcium influx.[130,131] Many patients with neuropathic pain complain of paroxysmal, brief lancinating pains. To date, clinical experience with the anticonvulsants has been positive. The drugs most commonly used include gabapentin, carbamazepine, phenytoin, valproate, and clonazepam. Gabapentin is considered the first-line anticonvulsant to manage neuropathic pain. Controlled trials in diabetic neuropathy, postherpetic neuralgia, and acquired immunodeficiency syndrome neuropathy demonstrate the effectiveness of this agent in reducing pain. Doses range from 900 to 1800 mg/d.[131] The major drug side effect is sedation. Patients should be started at 300 mg/d and rapidly titrated to 900 mg. Pain relief up to 30% to 50% of patients has been suggested. Clinical studies with carbamazepine demonstrate efficacy, but the utility of this drug in the cancer population is limited by its potential to produce bone marrow suppression, particularly leukopenia. The dosing guidelines used for the treatment of seizures are suggested in managing neuropathic pain. Each of the drugs should be initiated at low doses and gradually titrated upward. There is anecdotal experience to suggest that using intravenous loading doses of phenytoin for patients in an acute crisis with severe lancinating pain may be of clinical value. Gabapentin was not effective in drug trials in neuropathic pain. Both valproate and clonazepam have been reported anecdotally to be useful in neuropathic pain, but these are considered third-line agents in this patient population. Currently, there are no data to relate the plasma level and pain relief with any of these drugs. As previously stated, sequential trials are necessary to identify the most useful agent. With the use of baclofen, which is generally well tolerated, doses should begin at 5 mg two or three times a day, with titrations upward, with the highest reported doses between 100 to 150 mg/d titrated to the individual responses of the patient.[132]

Local Anesthetics

The use of both brief intravenous local anesthetic infusions (lidocaine), as well as maintenance oral anesthetic drugs, have demonstrated some efficacy in the management of chronic neuropathic pain, particularly in those patients with both lancinating and continuous dysesthesias. Mexiletine is the oral local anesthetic for which there are pilot data to support its analgesic efficacy.[133] The initial dose of mexiletine is low, at 150 mg/d, with gradual upward dose titration. Electrocardiograms should be monitored at higher doses, and blood levels of mexiletine may be useful to prevent toxicity. Currently, there are no good data available to predict what patient might respond to the use of oral local or intravenous anesthetics, as have been done in the use of brief local anesthetic infusions to determine control of cardiac arrhythmias.

Epidural local anesthetics (bupivacaine, lidocaine) have been most widely used to manage neuropathic pain either alone or in combination with opioid. Alternatively, the use of brief intravenous infusions of lidocaine may be helpful in patients who have an opioid-refractory continuous dysesthesia that has not responded to an antidepressant or anticonvulsant.[134] These drugs clearly serve as a second-line approach, with individualized therapy the rule.

CUTANEOUS LOCAL ANESTHETICS. The use of cutaneous anesthesia has been suggested to be most helpful in patients who have significant allodynia and marked hyperesthesia. The use of the topical application of a local anesthetic, such as a eutectic mixture of local anesthetics, has been demonstrated to be efficacious in patients with postherpetic neuralgia.[135] The cream should be applied under an occlusive dressing, to increase skin penetration and augment analgesic efficacy. The use of high-concentration lidocaine (5% and 10%) has also been reported to be effective in this population of patients.[136]

Corticosteroids

A series of controlled and uncontrolled surveys have demonstrated that the use of chronic corticosteroid therapy to reduce pain in patients with breast and prostate cancer improves quality of life.[70,137,138] In a controlled study of corticosteroid use in patients with far-advanced disease, transient improvement in appetite, analgesia, and mood were noted, but they were not sustained after the initial effect.[139] The major indications for corticosteroid use include refractory neuropathic pain, bone pain, pain associated with capular expansion or duct obstruction, and headache due to increased intercranial pressure. In certain cancer pain syndromes, such as epidural cord compression, 85% of patients receiving 100 mg of dexamethasone as part of their radiation therapy protocol reported significant pain relief associated with marked reduction in analgesic requirements.[70] Similarly, in patients with tumor infiltration of the brachial and lumbosacral plexus, corticosteroids provided additive analgesic effects. The risk of adverse effects associated with corticosteroid therapy varies with the duration. Long-term use may be associated with gastrointestinal toxicity and acute psychosis. A wide range of doses have been suggested, including doses of 30 mg/d in patients with prostate cancer, which was effective in providing improved quality of life and reduced pain. As stated, with epidural cord compression, initial doses of 100 mg with maintenance doses of 16 mg have been associated with effective analgesia. In our experience, the use of 16 mg as a loading bolus and rapid titration to lower doses of approximately 4 mg/d is one approach commonly used in the refractory chronic pain patient with advanced disease.

Other Adjuvant Drugs

There are a wide variety of other drugs that have been used to manage neuropathic pain, including benzodiazepines, neuroleptics, α_2-adrenergic agonist drugs, NMDA antagonists, and peptides. Of the benzodiazepines, clonazepam is commonly used in patients with lancinating or paroxysmal pain.[140] The use of these drugs must be balanced with their potential for somnolence and cognitive impairment. They serve as second- to third-line therapy in patients who have not responded to antidepressant or anticonvulsant drug therapy. Of the neuroleptics, pimozide has been reported to be analgesic in patients with trigeminal neuralgia.[141] Methotrimeprazine has been demonstrated to have analgesic properties comparable with morphine.[142] This drug has sedative, anxiolytic, and antiemetic properties and is commonly used in patients who have excessive opioid side effects. It provides analgesia by a nonopioid mechanism.

Coadministration of these drugs with opioids can often be effective in patients with neuropathic pain. Of the α_2-adrenergic agonist drugs, clonidine has been demonstrated to be analgesic in controlled trials.[143] It can be used by either the oral or transdermal route and has been reported to be specifically effective in patients with dysesthetic pain, who demonstrate sympathetic hyperactivity. Following intrathecal administration, clonidine was reported to improve pain in patients with intolerable neuropathic pain. Dextromethorphan and ketamine are two commercially available NMDA antagonists. Both have been shown to have analgesic effects in controlled studies.[144,145] The mechanism of action relates to the fact that the NMDA receptor reduces the development of the windup phenomenon, which occurs as a result of changes in the response of central dorsal horn neurons with neuropathic pain. Case reports have suggested that dextromethorphan has been beneficial in selected patients, although a controlled trial of low-dose dextromethorphan had negative results.[145] The drug may be initiated at doses of 40 to 60 mg daily and gradually escalated. Doses of 1 g have been administered safely, at least in the short-term. Studies of dextromethorphan combined with opioids demonstrated added analgesia, suggesting an opioid-sparing effect of the drug. The use of ketamine infusions have been previously well established to produce analgesia, and they have been reintroduced into clinical use as brief infusions for the management of patients with refractory neuropathic pain. Further studies are necessary to demonstrate the safety and efficacy of these treatment approaches in long-term management for chronic neuropathic pain. Oral ketamine in case reports has demonstrated efficacy in cancer patients with pain uncontrolled by other approaches.

Calcitonin has been reported to provide analgesia in patients with sympathetically maintained pain and in the management of acute phantom pain.[146] The mechanism underlying these analgesic effects is unknown, but it has suggested the empiric use of calcitonin in patients with refractory neuropathic pain. The clinical, anecdotal literature suggests that patients be treated initially with a low dose, after initial skin testing to rule out hypersensitivity to this agent, with gradual escalation to a range of 100 to 200 IU/d. Its use chronically has not been assessed, and further studies are necessary to define its place in the treatment of patients with neuropathic pain.

Adjuvants for Bone Pain

Metastatic disease to bone is the most common cause of pain in patients with cancer. Analgesic drug therapy is commonly used to manage the pain during the initial treatment with either chemotherapy or radiation therapy. Numerous investigators have identified a management approach for bone pain, which includes the use of specific surgical palliative approaches, radiotherapeutic approaches, hormonal therapies, and bone resorption inhibitors. Multifocal metastatic bone disease that is refractory to routine treatments may benefit from the use of a series of agents, including the bisphosphonate compounds, gallium nitrate, calcitonin, and strontium 89. The current bisphosphonates most widely studied for the treatment of bone pain include pamidronate and clonidronate.[147–149] Pamidronate is usually administered as a brief infusion in a starting dose of 60 to 120 mg. Analgesia, if it occurs, usually appears within days, but may accrue for many weeks with repeated infusions. In two studies patients receiving pamidronate in doses of 30 to 60 mg every 2 weeks showed relief of pain in 30% to 60% of patients. Bisphosphonates' analgesic effect appears to be dose dependent. Current recommendations include a regimen of intravenous pamidronate, 60 mg every 2 weeks for at least two or three treatments. If no response, therapy can be discontinued. If effective, a biweekly regimen can be continued. A study of pamidronate, 120 mg intravenously, versus placebo in patients with painful bone metastases revealed a correlation between analgesic response and collagen cross-links suggesting such peptide cross-links may be used to select those patients more likely to achieve improvement in pain with bisphosphonate therapy. The major indication of these drugs is to prevent skeletal morbidity, with data in breast cancer patients and patients with multiple myeloma showing efficacy in reduction of fractures and reduction in bone pain. Clonidronate may be administered orally and has been demonstrated to be efficacious in patients with breast cancer and multiple myeloma.

Calcitonin has also been reported anecdotally to be useful in patients with malignant bone pain, but the appropriate dose and dosing frequency have not been well defined.[150] Gallium nitrate has also been used with some efficacy in patients with metastatic bone pain, but the limited experience has not well defined the appropriate dosing guidelines, and nephrotoxicity has been reported.[151] Strontium 89 is a bone-seeking radiopharmaceutical, recognized as useful in the treatment of bone pain secondary to metastatic disease.[152,153] It is indicated in patients with refractory multifocal pain due to osteoblastic lesions who have a life expectancy greater than 3 months, who have sufficient bone marrow reserve (i.e., a platelet count above 60,000 and a white blood cell count above 2400), and for whom there is no further planned myelosuppressive chemotherapy. The onset of effect is slow and may require several weeks, with peak effects at 2 to 3 months. Bone marrow suppression is the major adverse effect, with irreversible thrombocytopenia.

The selection of any one of these treatments in metastatic bone pain needs to be individualized, with evidence that both the bisphosphonates and strontium 89 have clearly demonstrated efficacy in certain patients.

Adjuvants to Treat Side Effects

Nausea and vomiting, confusion, sedation, and constipation are common opioid-induced side effects. The use of drugs to manage these have been previously discussed (discussed earlier, in Anticipate and Treat Side Effects). The use of caffeine, methylphenidate, and dextroamphetamine have all been demonstrated in clinical trials to reduce opioid-induced sedation. Haloperidol is the treatment of choice to manage hallucinations and agitated delirium in patients receiving opioid analgesics. The use of bowel regimens to manage depressed gastrointestinal motility have also been discussed.

PSYCHOLOGICAL APPROACHES

Psychological approaches should be an integral part of the care of the cancer patient with pain. A series of psychological variables contribute to the cancer pain experience and suffering, such as perception of control, the meaning of pain, fear of death, depressed mood, and hopelessness. The level of psychological distress experienced by each patient varies depending on personality, coping ability, social support, and medical factors. Pain has a profound effect on levels of emotional distress, and psychological factors such as depression and anxiety intensify the pain experience. Measures of emotional disturbance have been reported to be predictors of pain in advancing later stages of cancer. The incidence of pain, depression, and delirium increases with high levels of physical debilitation in advanced disease. Approximately 25% of all cancer patients experience severe depressive symptoms, with the prevalence increasing to 77% in those with advanced illness. Uncontrolled pain is a major factor in cancer suicide.[21]

Various psychological interventions have been advocated for patients with cancer pain. Optimal treatment is multimodal and requires pharmacologic, psychotherapeutic, and cognitive-behavioral approaches. The roles of the psychiatrist, psychologist, and social worker in cancer pain management are well described in the literature.

The goals of short-term psychotherapy are to provide emotional support, continuity, and information and to assist patients in adapting to the crisis. Communication skills are of paramount importance for patient and family, particularly about pain and analgesic issues. The needs of the patient and family must be addressed. Psychotherapy in the cancer pain setting is primarily nonanalytic and focuses on current issues and exploration of reactions to cancer, which often provides insight into other life issues. Group interventions may also be helpful.

A specialized approach called cognitive-behavioral therapy has been used to treat pain disorders, including cancer pain.[154] This approach uses short-term therapeutic interventions based on theoretically and empirically derived principles that can be adapted to each patient's problems and needs. It includes a set of systematic mental and behavioral techniques designed to modify specific emotional, behavioral, and social problems as well as the global experience of pain and distress. Its major goal is to enhance the sense of personal control or self-efficacy. In a multidisciplinary approach to cancer pain, not every patient needs referral for this therapy, but it is useful if all members of the pain team follow a cognitive-behavioral model. Because cognitive-behavioral therapy is a commonsense psychological approach consisting of specific techniques, it can be learned and practiced by any interested clinician, nurse, or social worker who can gain practical training in the use of these techniques and apply them effectively.

Various intervention methods have been developed and are arbitrarily divided into behavioral and cognitive methods for discussion purposes. These approaches must be targeted to each patient's needs.

Behavioral techniques include ways to modify physiologic pain reactions and pain behaviors. Relaxation training can be used by all caregivers who manage patients with pain and cancer. Its mechanism of action includes the reduction of muscle tension, and it can provide the patient with a sense of improved self-control and a calming diversion of attention, breaking the associated pain-anxiety-tension cycle. Techniques range from simple deep-breathing exercises to more specialized methods of biofeedback and hypnosis. Contingency management is another behavioral approach designed to modify dysfunctional pain behaviors and replace them with *well* behaviors.

Cognitive techniques are designed to modify dysfunctional mental processes or to teach adaptive coping strategies. Cognitive coping and cognitive modification are approaches in which distraction, focusing, and perception and interpretation of the meaning of pain are assessed.

ANESTHETIC AND NEUROSURGICAL APPROACHES

Anesthetic and neurosurgical approaches are most effective in treating patients with well-defined localized pain. Tables 56.1-12 and 56.1-13 outline the indications for their use. Approximately 10% to 20% of cancer pain patients require these approaches, together with pharmacologic approaches, to provide adequate analgesia.

In a prospective study, Ventafridda and colleagues evaluated two groups of patients for 3 months who presented with intractable cancer pain not responsive to specific anticancer therapies.[22] One group was treated with sequential pharmacologic approaches using the analgesic ladder. The second group was treated with a multimodal approach of analgesic therapy followed by the use of neurolytic blocks or chronic spinal opioid administration. Patients treated with neurolytic procedures combined with pharmacologic therapy showed a statistically significant degree of greater pain relief than those treated with drugs alone by the third week of therapy. However, by 6 weeks, there was no statistical difference between the two groups. Complete pain relief without the need for analgesic drug therapy persisted to 3 months in 29% of the patients who received spinal opiates, 25% treated with celiac ganglion neurolytic block, 24% with percutaneous cordotomy, 12% with chemical rhizotomy, and 7% with gasserian thermorhizotomy. This study demonstrated that although analgesic therapy is the mainstay of treatment, anesthetic and neurosurgical procedures provide an important, but limited, contribution to adequate analgesia. Cherny et al. reported that 17% of patients in a prospective study of 100 cancer patients involved at Memorial Sloan-Kettering Cancer Center were evaluated for anesthetic and neurosurgical approaches with 10% requiring such approaches. One study assessed attitudes of oncologists toward interventional cancer pain treatments. Eighty-one percent of oncologists reported patient referral to pain specialists, yet their familiarity with intrathecal therapy was low, with only 46% referring patients for intrathecal therapy in the previous 6 months, citing the invasive nature of device placement as a drawback by 42% of physicians.[26]

Several factors are important in selecting the appropriate procedure for each patient. Because diffuse pain problems are common in cancer patients and most of the procedures are useful for well-defined localized pain, the role of these approaches is limited at best. Further complicating their use is the limited number of professionals who have expertise in these procedures. As patients become more cognizant of their disease and treatment options, they are often hesitant to

TABLE 56.1-13. Neuroablative and Neurostimulatory Procedures for Relief of Pain from Cancer

Site	*Procedure*	*Indications*
NEUROABLATIVE PROCEDURES		
Nerve root	Rhizotomy	Useful in somatic and neuropathic pain from tumor infiltration of the cranial and rarely intercostal nerves.
Spinal cord	Dorsal root entry zone lesion	Useful in unilateral neuropathic pain from brachial, intercostal, and lumbosacral plexopathy and postherpetic neuralgia.
	Cordotomy	Useful in unilateral pain below the waist. Often combined with local neurolytic blocks in perineal and bilateral lumbosacral plexopathy; may be performed bilaterally.
	Myelotomy	Useful in midline pain below the waist but rarely used because it involves extensive surgery.
Brainstem	Mesencephalic tractomy	Useful in pain in the nasopharynx and trigeminal region.
Thalamus	Thalamotomy	Useful in unilateral neuropathic pain in the chest and lower extremity.
Cortex	Cingulotomy	Useful through a stereotactic approach for diffuse pain.
Pituitary	Transsphenoidal hypophysectomy	Useful in pain control of bone metastases in endocrine-dependent tumors, breast, and prostate.
NEUROSTIMULATORY PROCEDURES		
Peripheral nerve	Transcutaneous and percutaneous electrical nerve stimulation	Useful in reducing painful dysesthesias from tumor infiltration of nerve or trauma (e.g., neuroma).
Spinal cord	Dorsal column stimulation	Of limited use in neuropathic pain in the chest, midline, and lower extremities.
Thalamus	Thalamic stimulation	Of rare use in neuropathic pain in the chest, midline, or lower extremity.

undergo neurodestructive procedures. Patients often consider their pain to be an important marker for their disease and are frightened of the potential, although unlikely, complications of these procedures. As a result, these procedures are often performed late in the illness, and full evaluation of their effectiveness and duration of action is limited by the patient's overriding medical problems.

These procedures are often not very effective in managing neuropathic pain, except for the use of local anesthetics, and are most helpful in managing most types of somatic and visceral pain. However, cancer patients often have a mixed somatic, visceral, and neuropathic pain syndrome. We advocate early consideration for the use of some of these anesthetic and neurosurgical procedures in patients to improve their quality of life through adequate pain management.

LOCAL ANESTHETICS

Anecdotal reports and several controlled studies support the use of cutaneous, subcutaneous, intravenous, intrapleural, and epidural local anesthetics in the management of patients with somatic, visceral, and neuropathic pain.[37]

Intravenous lidocaine should be considered as both a diagnostic and therapeutic approach in patients with neuropathic pain.[155] If such patients obtain an analgesic response, a trial of oral mexiletine or the use of continuous subcutaneous lidocaine should be considered to determine whether prolonged relief may be possible. Although no studies have confirmed that the response to lidocaine predicts a response to mexiletine for pain, a comparable predictive value exists in the cardiac literature, in which intravenous lidocaine's effectiveness in controlling ventricular arrhythmias predicts the usefulness of mexiletine for this same disorder.

Brose and Cousins reported the use of continuous subcutaneous infusions in two patients with cancer-related neuropathic pain, advocating this approach as an alternative in patients who do not respond to standard opioid and adjuvant treatments as well as anesthetic approaches for neuropathic pain.[134]

Intrapleural local anesthetics have been used for acute pain in the chest wall and have been adapted for the management of chronic cancer pain.[156] A subcutaneously tunneled intrapleural catheter offered long-term relief of right upper quadrant pain from hepatic metastases in a patient with significant pain from tumor infiltration of the liver. This novel method offers an alternative approach for patients with local regional pain in the pleural and abdominal regions.

Epidural local anesthetics are used to manage patients with localized pain syndromes, usually below the waist. Intermittent and continuous epidural infusions of local anesthetics have been used to manage the difficult chronic pain associated with metastatic disease below the waist, often involving the sacrum and lumbosacral plexus.[157] This method consists of infusing a local anesthetic via a subcutaneous infusion pump or Ommaya reservoir to a catheter, temporarily or permanently placed in the epidural space. If the amount and concentration of the anesthetic are varied, effective pain relief can be achieved without interrupting significant motor or autonomic function. The risk of infection is minimized because local anesthetics have antimicrobial effects. The use of continuous low-dose infusions of local anesthetics is associated with minimal systemic side effects. Further studies on the use of this technique in comparison with standard therapies are needed to define its place in the management of the cancer patient. Its major advantages are that the resultant analgesia is not cross-tolerant with the analgesic produced by the opioid analgesic, and that temporary use of this technique allows for reduction in the amount of systemic opiate drugs, therefore partially reversing tolerance. This has been a useful preliminary approach in patients for whom the use of spinal opiate analgesia is considered, but who have developed tolerance from large doses of systemic opiates. Because tolerance develops to these analgesic effects, this approach is temporary (days to weeks) rather than long-term. This approach is most useful in patients who experience an acute pain crisis, such as the patient with a pathologic hip fracture who is not a surgical candidate; this approach would allow the patient to move about in bed. In patients with chronic cancer neuropathic pain, local anesthetics combined with opioids are used.

PERIPHERAL NERVE BLOCKS

Peripheral nerve blocks are used both diagnostically to localize the nerve distribution and therapeutically to interrupt pain transmission within a determined nerve distribution. This technique is limited to areas of the body in which the interruption of both motor and sensory function will not interfere with the patient's functional status. This approach is most commonly used with patients who have pain in the head, chest, or abdomen.[158,159] This technique is also limited by the fact that each peripheral nerve subserves sensory function over many levels, and usually several nerves must be blocked to provide adequate analgesia. These techniques are most useful in patients with somatic pain; neuropathic pain is rarely controlled by peripheral nerve blocks alone. Examples of successful blocks include gasserian ganglion block for craniofacial pain, intercostal blocks for chest wall infiltration from tumor, and paravertebral blocks for radicular pain.

In patients with somatic pain who respond to a local anesthetic block, neurolytic blockade with either alcohol or phenol may provide more prolonged relief. A block produced by phenol tends to be less profound and of shorter duration than that produced by alcohol. Phenol has local anesthetic as well as neurolytic effects.

The most common peripheral neurolytic block is a paravertebral block for localized intercostal pain. From our experience in treating patients with chest wall pain, we advise that this procedure be done under fluoroscopic control or computed tomographic localization to accurately interrupt the individual intercostal nerve.

Epidural and intrathecal neurolytic blocks have been used primarily to manage patients with far-advanced disease whose pain is either unilateral in the chest or abdomen or midline in the perineum. These approaches are less useful in managing upper and lower limb pain associated with brachial and lumbosacral plexopathy because of the high risk of motor weakness associated with effective neurolytic blockade by this route. Epidural phenol blocks are useful in chest wall pain over several dermatomes. Such an approach obviates the need for multiple paravertebral injections. Phenol is injected in small increments (1 to 2 mL per segment) over 2 or 3 days by an epidural catheter, and preliminary data demonstrate 80% pain relief in patients with documented somatic pain. Epidural and intrathecal phenol blocks have been used to manage perineal pain, but no studies have delineated the superiority of one approach over the other.[159]

A review of a large number of alcohol subarachnoid blocks reports an average of 60% good relief, 21% fair relief, and 18% poor relief.[70] Because the duration of pain relief has seldom been documented with careful follow-up studies, the overall estimate for relief of pain with both subarachnoid alcohol and phenol blocks suggests a mean duration of pain relief of between 2 weeks and 3 months.

Complications are of two kinds. With intrathecal injection, a self-limiting spinal headache may occur. Complications that result from the action of neurolytic substances on nerve fibers include motor paresis, loss of sphincter function, impairment of touch and proprioception, and troublesome dysesthesias. Injection in the thoracic region has a low complication rate. In our experience, many cancer patients already have both motor and autonomic dysfunction before the use of neurolytic blockade; these often remain the same or may worsen. Patients should be informed of the risk of these procedures, with particular attention to the fact that they may develop motor paresis and bladder dysfunction, specifically incontinence, after the blockade.

The selection of patients for management with epidural or intrathecal neurolytic agents should be based on the following criteria: exhaustion of appropriate antitumor approaches; clear clinical and radiologic definition of the pain; poor candidacy for percutaneous cordotomy; failure of nonopioid, opioid, and adjuvant analgesics to produce adequate analgesia without significant side effects; a favorable response to diagnostic or epidural or intrathecal blocks, producing at least 75% pain relief; and MRI of the spine or myelography done before the procedure to rule out tumor infiltration of the subarachnoid space.

AUTONOMIC NERVE BLOCK

Sympathetic block is effective in conditions with vasomotor or visceromotor hyperactivity. This hyperactivity accompanies many of the cancer-related pain syndromes such as visceral pain or plexopathies. The most commonly used sympathetic block is that of the celiac ganglion for pain due to abdominal malignancy, including cancer of the pancreas, stomach, duodenum, liver, gallbladder, adrenal gland, and colon. Nociceptive fibers of the splanchnic, sympathetic, vagal, phrenic, and somatic nerves converge on the celiac ganglion, which is amenable to a regional block that is successful in from 70% to 85% of patients treated.[158]

Standardized approaches for the use of this technique have been described using computed tomography monitoring or fluoroscopic control. After placement of the needle, 25 mg of absolute alcohol mixed with local anesthetic and contrast is injected. Bilateral needle placement has been reported to provide the best results, but anecdotal reports suggest that unilateral needle placement on the right provides comparable analgesia. The major side effect of the procedure is transient hypotension, and patients must be well hydrated and monitored carefully during the procedure and for 4 to 6 hours afterward. Significant neurologic complications occur in less than 1% of patients if proper technique is used. Complications include paraparesis, postural hypotension, and urinary difficulties.

Although there has been debate about the usefulness of this procedure in patients with pancreatic cancer, it should be considered as one of the approaches, together with pharmacologic approaches, in managing these patients.

Lumbar sympathetic block may provide significant relief of intractable urogenital pain or pain due to carcinomatous invasion of local nerves and plexus in the perineum and lower extremity.[159] This ganglion conveys visceral nociceptive afferents from the pelvic viscera. Pain caused by cancer of the sigmoid colon or rectum may be relieved by bilateral lumbar sympathetic block if the disease is confined to those viscera. Pain caused by cancer of the seminal vesicles or prostate may sometimes be relieved by bilateral lumbar sympathetic block. Similarly, pain caused by uterine cancer may be relieved if the disease is confined to the body of the uterus. In many instances, however, the block must be extended to the T-12 ganglion. Good evidence suggests that lumbar sympathetic block alone is not useful in patients with lumbosacral plexopathy; therefore, the role of this procedure is limited to specific anatomic sites of pain.

Stellate ganglion block may sometimes be useful for pain in the face, upper neck, ear, and hemicranium. However, the potential complications of stellate ganglion block limit the use of this technique with neurolytic solution, as there is a high risk of spillage of the neurolytic material into the brachial plexus, with secondary nerve injury and focal pain.

NEUROADENOLYSIS OF THE PITUITARY

Chemical hypophysectomy is a special use of a neurolytic method. Several early studies suggest that 35% to 95% of patients undergoing this approach report pain relief, with a median duration of 6 to 7 weeks and a maximum duration of 20 weeks.[160] The mechanism by which analgesia is produced may result from alcohol tracking up the pituitary stalk into the hypothalamus, with consequent disruption of the hypothalamic-thalamic endorphinergic pain pathways. Side effects include diabetes insipidus, cranial nerve palsies, cerebrospinal fluid leakage, and rarely meningitis. The lack of detailed clinical data limits critical assessment of these studies. This technique is rarely if ever used in patients with diffuse pain.

NEUROSURGICAL APPROACHES

Neurosurgical approaches for cancer pain can be divided into two major categories, antitumor and antinociceptive. These approaches are often used alone or in combination by neurosurgeons to provide improved pain relief.[161,162]

ANTITUMOR APPROACHES

Antitumor approaches are often more acceptable to patients because they focus on cancer treatment, offering the hope of prolonged survival. The major procedures are listed in Table 56.1-8 and include tumor removal from the spine, epidural space, or adjacent plexus; stabilization procedures for spinal fracture, instability, and subluxation; and implantation of regional delivery devices for epidural, intrathecal, and intraventricular opioid drugs.

Tumor removal through resection of spinal metastases is associated with dramatic improvements in pain in 70% to 90% of patients.[163,164] With the use of improved methods of internal fixation with methyl methacrylate and improved stabilizing procedures, the use of this approach has increased in patients with intractable continuous or incidental back and neck pain. Patients may also have an associated segmental instability associated with a pathologic fracture of the vertebral body or subluxation, syndromes that place patients at significant risk for neurologic dysfunction. Careful radiologic workup is necessary to define the specific anatomic basis for the spinal pain, but aggressive surgical approaches have improved the quality of life for many patients bedridden by uncontrolled pain. In patients with epidural cord compression, the indications for surgery include uncontrolled pain in a patient with a pathologic fracture or a solitary relapse in the epidural space or vertebral body from a radioresistant tumor. In patients with radiosensitive tumors who relapse after radiation therapy, spinal surgery should be considered as a reasonable approach and is specifically indicated in the patient with an acute neurologic deterioration during radiation therapy. When percutaneous or open vertebral body biopsy is impossible, surgical resection should be strongly considered to define the primary tumor type in patients with undiagnosed lesions; this serves as both a diagnostic and therapeutic procedure.

In patients with paraspinal tumor or tumor infiltration of the plexus, *en bloc* resection of tumor has successfully provided pain relief and has served as a debulking antitumor procedure. In patients with Pancoast's syndrome, invasion of the spine or epidural extension is present in 20% at initial presentation and is associated with a significant morbidity in up to 50% of patients when local treatment is ineffective. In the good-risk patient with plexopathy and spinal invasion, Sundaresan et al. recommend surgery in which tumor is removed from the lower plexus, C-8 to T-1, and the vertebral body is resected, with brachytherapy to provide further tumor control.[164]

In patients with tumor invasion of the paraspinal area (specifically the psoas and iliacus), radical resection of these tumor masses concurrent with spinal surgery, followed by brachytherapy, combines antitumor and antinociceptive therapies.

When considering the use of these neurosurgical procedures to provide palliative surgery with an antinociceptive component, the patient's extent of disease, performance score, prognosis, and ability to tolerate the surgery must be weighed.

ANTINOCICEPTIVE PROCEDURES

Antinociceptive procedures include neuroablative, neurostimulatory, and neuropharmacologic approaches.

Neuroablative Procedures

Neuroablative procedures involve the production of a surgical or radiofrequency lesion along the nociceptive neural pathway. Sectioning on the posterior roots (rhizotomy), lesioning the lateral dorsal horn (dorsal root entry zone lesion), and interrupting the ascending neospinothalamic pathway (cordotomy) or the crossing interneuronal fibers (myelotomy) in the spinal cord are examples of neuroablative procedures performed for pain relief.

Cordotomy, either percutaneous or open, is the most common neuroablative procedure used to manage cancer pain.[162–167] It is the neurosurgical procedure of choice for patients with unilateral pain below the waist and with a relatively short life expectancy. Cordotomy is usually effective for 1 to 3 years, with dysesthesias substituting for analgesia in patients living longer than 3 years. Pain in the chest wall or upper extremity may be successfully treated initially with cordotomy, but extensive data demonstrate that, with time, the level of analgesia drops, limiting the effectiveness of this approach. Somatic pain appears to be the most responsive to cordotomy; visceral and neuropathic pain are less responsive for reasons that are not fully understood.

Percutaneous cordotomy is performed in a supine, awake patient through a lateral C-1 to C-2 approach.[162,165] A needle is advanced under fluoroscopic control until cerebrospinal fluid is obtained. A minimyelogram is done to identify the dentate ligament. A cordotomy electrode is passed through the spinal needle and the spinal cord is punctured with the aid of impedance monitoring. Electrophysiologic stimulation is done to identify the spinothalamic tract and then a radiofrequency lesion is made in the appropriate painful site. Such a lesion interrupts pain and temperature on the contralateral side of the lesioned site. Patients typically report spontaneous relief of pain in this lesioned area.

The anatomic area at the lesion site includes fibers mediating respiration and autonomic function. These fibers are adjacent to the anterior horn and the cervical spinothalamic fibers. Near the lumbar spinothalamic tract are the fibers governing the intercostal muscles. This quadrant of the spinal cord also contains the sacral fibers to and from the bladder, which are closer to the spinothalamic fibers. These anatomic relations explain some of the complications associated with cordotomy: bladder dysfunction, respiratory compromise, and ipsilateral motor weakness.

From the literature that does not provide comparative studies in cancer patients with pain, pain relief can be obtained in 60% to 80% of patients immediately after cordotomy; results at 6 to 12 months are 40% to 50%.[162–165] In a retrospective survey of 40 percutaneous cordotomies in patients with predominant unilateral pain below the waist, 70% of patients obtained complete relief with continued use of some supplemental analgesics, 16% had moderate relief, and 13% did not benefit from this procedure.[167] In another study, Arbit reported that 16% of patients referred for percutaneous cordotomy could not undergo the procedure because of difficulty in positioning or with participating in the procedure, even with the use of increased analgesic drug doses and anesthetic assistance.[162] Careful patient selection is necessary for this procedure.

Open cordotomy is usually done below the cervicothoracic junction through a hemilaminectomy or full laminectomy. Open cordotomy should be reserved for the patient who cannot tolerate a percutaneous approach or for the patient with limited motor or sensory dysfunction from tumor infiltration below the waist in whom bilateral cordotomy is to be done for bilateral or midline pain.

The complications of cordotomy vary with the type of procedure (percutaneous or open) and are also strongly influenced by the patient's premorbid neurologic condition. Many patients have borderline bladder function and mild paresis from tumor infiltration that is transiently or permanently exacerbated by these procedures. In our series at Memorial Sloan-Kettering Cancer Center, 45% of patients had transient or permanent urinary retention.[167] After cordotomy there is often an unmasking of pain ipsilateral to the cordotomy site. This pain was reported in 22% of patients in our series.[162] In some patients it was difficult to clarify if this nerve pain was caused by unidentified tumor and really represented mirror pain or was caused by the unmasking of tumor-related pain. In 60% of patients in the Arbit series, unmasking of pain on the contralateral side occurred because of bilateral lumbosacral plexopathy. Dysesthesias characterized by burning pain in the area of sensory loss are reported in 1% to 2% of patients after a delay of several months to 2 years after the procedure. Ipsilateral motor weakness results from an inadvertent anterior extension of the lesion to involve the corticospinal tract. In our series, 7% of patients had transient paresis and 22% had permanent paresis. Most series report motor paresis in 10% to 20% of patients.

Respiratory complications occur in patients with a dysfunctional lung contralateral to the site of the cordotomy. This is a predictable risk when patients undergo cordotomy on the same side as their only functioning lung: Interruption of the reticulospinal fibers controlling the intercostal muscles and of the phrenic nerve may occur because of their proximity to the lateral spinothalamic tract in this spinal cord quadrant.

Several other complications, including headache, fever, and meningismus, are associated with the percutaneous procedure, as well as a Horner's syndrome because of interruption of the sympathetic tract.

In our series, 30% of patients demonstrated a profound depressive syndrome associated with significant pain relief.[167] Patients should be warned about this complication, but the factors contributing to its development have not been fully clarified. Rapid reduction in opioids, realization that with pain relief they must face their terminal illness, and other factors, including exhaustion, depression, and preexisting psychopathology, may all play a role in the appearance of this problematic complication. Psychological intervention and the use of tricyclic antidepressants have been effective in managing these patients.

Dorsal rhizotomy is the next most common neuroablative procedure used for cancer pain. It is performed by sectioning the posterior sensory rootlets, and a specific localized dermatomal pain level can be identified. It can be performed by an operative section of the nerve, or as previously discussed, by a neurolytic block. In patients with chest wall pain from tumor invasion, improved analgesia in 50% to 80% has been reported with dorsal rhizotomy.[168] Arbit et al. have adapted this procedure to manage patients with significant chest wall pain.[169]

Rhizotomies of the trigeminal nerve, nervus intermedius, glossopharyngeal nerve, and portions of the vagus nerve are effective in controlling pain from head and neck tumors that invade the base of the skull.[170] Bilateral sacral rhizotomy has been reported to treat sacral or perineal pain involving the sacral plexus at the S-2 and S-3 levels. However, these patients have often had extensive radiation therapy, and wound closure in the irradiated skin over the sacrum may complicate recovery and increase the risk-to-benefit ratio. A neurolytic, epidural, or subarachnoid block is usually considered before surgical sacral rhizotomy.

The use of a dorsal root entry zone lesion is based on the recognition that nociceptive fibers enter laminae I and II at the dorsal horn; interruption of this anterior lateral site has been associated with reduction in neuropathic pain in experimental animals. This approach has been used most commonly in avulsion of the brachial plexus, postherpetic neuralgia, and postradiation plexopathy. Because this approach has not been widely used in cancer pain, its usefulness for brachial and lumbosacral plexopathy is not established, but it is an interesting approach for such patients.[171] The procedure requires a laminectomy of several levels to provide an adequate approach to this anatomic site, and this may be too extensive a procedure for the cancer patient with advanced disease. Further studies are necessary to determine its usefulness.

The midline commissural myelotomy approach has been used in patients with midline perineal or coccygeal pain or bilateral pain in the lower extremities. Using a limited midline myelotomy, Gildenberg and Hirschberg reported satisfactory pain relief in 10 to 14 patients with midline pain below the waist from cancer.[172] This procedure is based on the fact that nociceptive fibers cross in the anterior commissure from the dorsal horn to the contralateral spinothalamic pathway. This approach is used rarely, if ever, in patients with bilateral pain.

Cingulotomy has received attention in the treatment of some patients with cancer pain, using a stereotactic procedure with MRI to permit a radiofrequency lesion. Four patients with pain from widely metastatic, diffuse bone disease who were receiving opioid analgesics reported immediate pain relief with bilateral cingulate lesions.[173] The pain relief persisted until death in 2 to 6 weeks. This procedure was previously used to treat psychiatric illness and has a long history of use in severe chronic pain from a variety of neuropathic syndromes. The literature suggests that up to 50% of cancer patients have had moderate, marked, or complete relief for 3 months after the procedure. The extent to which the development of this improved method will alter the use of this technique needs to be clarified.

Neurostimulatory Procedures

Neurostimulatory procedures involving the peripheral nerve and spinal cord are generally based on the gate theory of pain. The original theory suggests that there is a neurophysiologic gating mechanism in the spinal cord, probably within the substantia gelatinosa. Noxious sensation is conducted via small-diameter peripheral nerve fibers and nonnoxious sensation via large-diameter fibers, and both send collaterals to the substantia gelatinosa and up the spinal dorsal columns. Stimulation of the small fibers tends to promote pain, or *open the gate*, whereas stimulation of the large fibers tends to inhibit pain or *close the gate.* Because the large nerve fibers ascend in a compact bundle through the dorsal columns, they are accessible to selected electric stimulation. Retrograde firing of the large fibers ensues, and pain sensation is inhibited at multiple levels of the spinal cord below that being stimulated.

Based on reports that high-frequency (50 to 100 Hz) percutaneous electrical nerve stimulation relieved chronic neurogenic pain, the use of transcutaneous electrical nerve stimulation (TENS) was reported effective in treating neuropathic pain. Although control studies are lacking, numerous clinical surveys suggest that this approach is useful for nociceptive and neuropathic pain. With the advent of sophisticated electronic devices, various patterns of electric stimulation are currently in use transcutaneously, including pulsed (burst), modulation (ramped), random, and complex wave forms, all designed to improve efficacy. Patients are instructed on proper electrode placement in a dermatomal pattern and are instructed to try both intermittent and continuous stimulation. By trial and error, analgesic effects should be observed either immediately or, in some cases, after the stimulation is discontinued.

TENS is used for a wide variety of pains and serves as a safe, noninvasive approach. Clinical experience suggests its usefulness in some patients with peripheral nerve pain. Several investigators have reported that it is useful in cancer pain for a wide variety of tumor-related and neuropathic pain syndromes.[174] Further studies are necessary to define the usefulness of TENS in the cancer patient with pain.

The dorsal column stimulation technique involves the introduction of an electrode into the epidural or intrathecal space and advancing it to the appropriate level overlying the dorsal columns. The main indications for placement of a dorsal column stimulator are intractable dysesthetic or deafferentation pain of the limbs or trunk, such as radiation-induced brachial or lumbosacral plexopathy. This procedure is effective in 43% to 75% of patients and carries a low morbidity. The most common complication is failure of the device itself, which occurs in approximately 10% of patients annually. Other complications include infection, cerebrospinal fluid fistula, allergic or rejection response to the device material, and changes in stimulation over time, which may be related to cellular changes around the electrode or shifts in its position.

Thalamic stimulation involves the placement of electrodes in the medial thalamus and has been reported to be most useful for managing neuropathic pain from lesions in the central and peripheral nervous system. There are a series of reports on the usefulness of this technique in patients with head and neck cancer and prominent cranial neuropathic pain, but the limited use of this technique in these patients makes it difficult to define its specific role.[175,176]

Neuropharmacologic Approaches

Epidural and intraspinal analgesia using opioids alone or in combination with local anesthetics, clonidine, or both or experimental agents are used to manage chronic cancer pain in patients with a reasonable (1 year) prognosis. In all instances, patients should have a trial of an epidural or intraspinal drug combination before permanent implementation is considered. It is advised that patients have as continuous intrathecal trial lasting as long as possible before permanent implementation, and Figure 56.1-3 provides an algorithm for the use of opioid intrathecal alone or with clonidine in a patient with a mixed somatic-neuropathic pain syndrome inadequately managed by systemic opioids.[177] A wide array of external and implantable catheters and pumps are available with specific indicators and uses. Both computer-controlled battery-operated pumps and continuous fixed infusion pumps are used. Cost of the pumps and the patient's psychosocial status and social support systems and ability to care for the pump and port are important considerations in selecting the use of such devices. No studies have clearly defined the efficacy of this approach as compared with systemic treatment, and longitudinal surveys have identified complication rates that vary from 10% to 50%, with meningitis as a serious complication. With long-term epidural catheter use, 5% to 15% infection rates have been reported.

TRIGGER POINT INJECTION

The use of trigger point injections is within the scope of the practicing physician.[178] Patients with significant musculoskeletal pain often describe specific, tender trigger point areas that, when injected with either saline or local anesthetic, are associated with significant pain relief. Effective relief of pain from trigger point injections, however, is not diagnostic of musculoskeletal pain alone, and an evaluation of the cause of the pain is still necessary to rule out the specific etiology.

Acupuncture has been used to treat both acute and chronic pain. The selected acupuncture points are manually or electrically stimulated with a needle until the patient feels the sensation. A wide variety of acupuncture techniques are available, ranging from a traditional Chinese approach to a Western adaptation. Laser acupuncture with external laser probes has also been used. The studies in cancer patients with pain represent large, uncontrolled, retrospective surveys. Minimal stimulation in manual acupuncture was used in all cases, and three acupuncture treatments represented an adequate trial. Fifty-two percent and 56% of patients reported some pain improvement for at least 7 days; an additional 30% and 22% had pain relief for 2 days or less or reported increased mobility alone.[179] A lack of detailed pain assessment in specific acupuncture techniques or a critical review of the patient population make it difficult to interpret these observations. Based on its current empiric use, this approach is relatively safe, but its benefit in cancer patients with pain remains undefined.

PHYSIATRIC APPROACHES

Rehabilitation medicine plays an important role in the multidisciplinary approach to the patient with cancer pain. Physiatrists are concerned with a patient's physical functioning and provide expertise in assessing how impairment in a patient's physical capacity affects his or her ability to function. A wide variety of interventions are available, including TENS, diathermy (heating pads, ultrasound, hydrotherapy), and cryotherapy (ice and vapo-coolants). Assistive device and braces, as well as therapeutic exercise and massage, are important. Trigger point injections and acupuncture have also been used. These interventions are commonly used in combination with other pain-therapy approaches, particularly behavioral and pharmacologic approaches. Rehabilitation approaches are discussed throughout the text specific to cancer patients' needs.

A large body of data supports the use of rehabilitative interventions in acute and chronic nonmalignant pain, but similar studies have not addressed the rehabilitation needs of the cancer pain patient. From our experiences, neurologic dysfunction is one of the common components in patients with cancer pain, and aggressive neurorehabilitation is necessary to ambulate these patients and provide them with functional independence.

SEDATION IN THE IMMINENTLY DYING

NITROUS OXIDE

Nitrous oxide has analgesic properties and has been used in the management of patients with far-advanced disease to provide added analgesia. It is administered with oxygen through a nonrebreathing face mask in concentrations from 25% to 75%. Its use in combination with systemic opioid analgesics is associ-

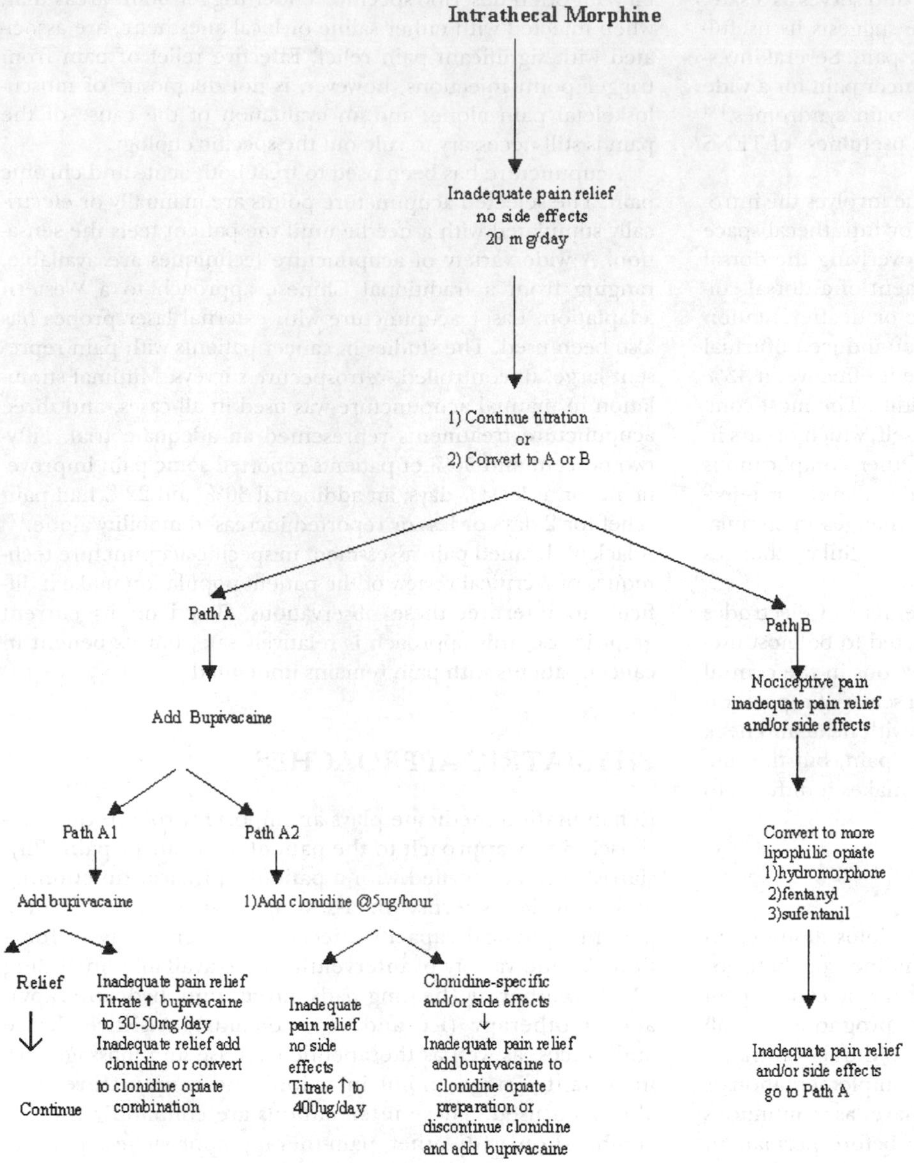

FIGURE 56.1-3. In intrathecal analgesic titration, doses are usually increased to about 20 mg/day of morphine and sometimes higher. Alternative therapies for when intraspinal morphine is failing are shown.

ated with improvement of symptoms of pain and anxiety and a demonstrable improvement in alertness.[180] This anesthetic approach should be considered in patients with breakthrough pain or incident pain to provide adequate analgesia to facilitate their care.

INTRAVENOUS BARBITURATES

This approach has been advocated to manage dying patients who have inadequate analgesia or uncontrolled symptoms, who ask to be maintained in a sedated state. Intravenous thiopental titrated to a level of sedation was the approach advocated in a series of 17 terminally ill patients.[181] The authors suggested that the value of this approach is based on the use of one agent to treat both physical and psychological symptoms. This approach may be seen as a more generalized one to palliative care and should be considered only if the standard approaches with opioid analgesics and adjuvant drugs fail to provide adequate analgesia with minimum side effects. However, because it is the physician's responsibility to manage not only pain but also suffering, this may be a reasonable approach, particularly in the dying patient with profound dyspnea, myoclonus, or agitation. Further studies are needed to clarify the usefulness of this approach. In the published study, 13 of 17 patients developed somnolence and died; the somnolence lasted from 2 hours to 4 days, with an average of 23 hours. Four patients died without being somnolent.

Several problematic symptoms often arise in the management of the dying patient, including intractable vomiting, profound dyspnea, extreme agitation and anxiety, and uncontrolled pain. Several authors have reported that most cancer patients have crescendo symptoms before death, requiring somnolence.[182–184] This approach offers one method to manage these difficult patients.

Whatever pain management techniques are used, the physician is responsible for providing continuing care, constantly reassessing both the diagnosis and the treatment to achieve optimal relief of pain and suffering for both patient and family.

The care of patients with cancer and chronic pain strains the resources of a single physician, especially after the patient's discharge from the hospital. Various supportive care and continuing care programs have been developed to manage dying patients, both in the hospital and at home. In these patients the focus of treatment shifts to symptom control and palliative comfort care. Palliative care services, home- and hospital-based hospices, and high-technology home care programs are some of the approaches to care for patients with terminal illness.

The program at Memorial Sloan-Kettering Cancer Center centers on the patient and family and is coordinated by a nurse, physician, and social worker.[185] The nurse is responsible for day-to-day management of the patient's pain and works with the patient, family, and community physicians and nurses on symptom control and supportive care. Community health professionals work with the patient at home, and the team is available to the patient, family, and community health workers on a 24-hour-a-day basis.

ALGORITHM FOR CANCER PAIN MANAGEMENT

An algorithm has been developed that integrates all of these management approaches for cancer pain. It attempts to integrate assessment techniques, drug therapy, behavioral approaches, and anesthetic and neurosurgical approaches and stresses continuity of care. Treatment begins with a diagnostic evaluation that addresses the medical, psychological, and social components of pain. A plan is developed to treat the cancer and pain. If the anticancer treatment is effective, pain relief usually occurs and the drugs used for analgesia can be discontinued without difficulty. Pain treatment begins with the use of analgesic drugs, starting with nonopioid drugs alone or in combination. If they are successful, no further therapy is necessary. If severe persistent pain does not respond to analgesic drugs or if the side effects of the drugs are not tolerated, the physician should consider switching analgesics (e.g., from oral morphine to methadone), changing the route of administration (e.g., from oral to subcutaneous), or performing a cordotomy for localized pain. A trial of an adjuvant drug together with the opioid and nonopioid drug would also be appropriate. In patients with excessive sedation or confusion, the use of a neurostimulant or haloperidol provides adequate treatment of the side effects of the opioid drugs and maintains the patient's analgesia while markedly reducing concurrent side effects. Alternatively, epidural or intrathecal opioids may be considered if systemic analgesics produce excessive side effects such as confusion or sedation. If the pain is localized (e.g., intercostal pain from tumor infiltration of the chest wall), neurolytic blocks are indicated. If the pain is unilateral and below the waist, cordotomy should be considered. For diffuse pain, nitrous oxide inhalation may be tried. Cognitive-behavioral approaches must be integrated from the onset of treatment and should be used along with the medical and surgical approaches.

FUTURE DIRECTIONS

The study of pain in cancer patients offers a unique opportunity to use clinical observations to advance our biologic knowledge. There is a critical need to expand both the research and educational efforts in cancer pain to improve the control of pain in these patients. Information on the basic mechanisms of pain modulation can be culled only from a careful study of these clinical pain problems. These patients can teach us the physiologic and psychological differences between acute and chronic pain problems, the importance of the evolution of psychological factors, the difference between pain and suffering, the clinical pharmacology of analgesic drugs, and the behavioral mechanisms humans use to suppress pain. The use of innovative approaches based on sound scientific principles and advanced on research technology offers the opportunity to understand the complex phenomenon of pain.

REFERENCES

1. Foley KM. Advances in cancer pain. *Arch Neurol* 1999;56:413.
2. Foley KM. Clinical crossroads: a 44-year old woman with severe pain at the end of life. *JAMA* 1999;281:1937.
3. Doyle D, Hanks GWC, MacDonald N, eds. *Oxford textbook of palliative medicine,* 2nd ed. New York: Oxford University Press, 1998.
4. MacDonald N. The interface between oncology and palliative medicine. In: Doyle D, Hanks GWC, MacDonald N, eds. *Oxford textbook of palliative medicine,* 2nd ed. New York: Oxford University Press, 1998:11.
5. Foley KM. Pain syndromes in patients with cancer. In: Bonica JJ, Ventafridda V, eds. *Advances in pain research and therapy.* New York: Raven Press, 1979:59.
6. Twycross RG, Fairfield S. Pain in far-advanced cancer. *Pain* 1982;14:303.
7. World Health Organization. *Cancer pain relief,* 2nd ed. Geneva: World Health Organization, 1996.
8. Daut RL, Cleeland CS. The prevalence and severity of pain in cancer. *Cancer* 1982;50:1913.
9. Stjernsward J. Pampallona palliative medicine: a global perspective. In: Doyle D, Hanks GWC, MacDonald N, eds. *Oxford textbook of palliative medicine.* New York: Oxford University Press, 1998:1127.
10. Cleeland CS, Ladinsky JL, Serlin RC, Thuy NC. Multidimensional measurement of cancer pain: comparisons of US and Vietnamese patients. *J Pain Symptom Manage* 1988;3:23.
11. Cleeland CS. Assessment of pain in cancer: measurement issues. In: Foley KM, Bonica JJ, Ventafiridda V, eds. *Advances in pain research and therapy.* New York: Raven Press, 1990:47.
12. Foley KM, Portenoy RK. WHO and IASP: joint programs in pain and palliative care. *J Pain Symptom Manage* 1993;8:335.
13. Portenoy RK, Miransky J, Thaler HT, et al. Pain in ambulatory patients with lung or cancer: prevalence, characteristics and impact. *Cancer* 1992;70:1616.
14. Portenoy RK, Thaler HT, Kornblith AB, et al. Pain in ovarian cancer: prevalence, characteristics, and associated symptoms. *Cancer* 1994;74:907.
15. Kelsen D, Portenoy RK, Thaler HT, et al. Pain and depression in patients with newly diagnosed pancreas cancer. *J Clin Oncol* 1995;13:748.
16. Schuit KW, Sleijfer DT, Meijler WJ, et al. Symptoms and functional status of patients with disseminated cancer visiting outpatient departments. *J Pain Symptom Manage* 1998;16:290.
17. Weber M, Huber C. Documentation of severe pain, opioid doses, opioid related side effect with patients with cancer: a retrospective study. *J Pain Symptom Manage* 1999;17:49.
18. Cleeland CS, Gonin R, Hatfield AK, et al. Pain and its treatment in outpatient with metastatic cancer. *N Engl J Med* 1994;330:592.
19. The SUPPORT principal investigators. A controlled trial to improve care for seriously ill hospitalized patients: the study to understand prognosis and preferences for outcomes and risks of treatments. *JAMA* 1995;274:1591.
20. Bernabei R, Gambassi G, Lapane K, et al. Management of pain in elderly patients with cancer. *JAMA* 1998;279:1877.
21. Chochinov HM, Breithart WS, eds. *Handbook of psychiatry in palliative medicine.* New York: Oxford University Press, 1999.
22. Ventafridda V, DeConno F, Riparnonti C, Gamba A, Tamburini M. Quality-of-life assessment during a palliative care programme. *Ann Oncol* 1990;1:415.
23. Coyle N, Adelhardt J, Foley KM, Portenoy RK. Character of terminal illness in the advanced cancer patient: pain and other symptoms during the last 4 weeks of life. *J Pain Symptom Manage* 1990;5:83.
24. Ventafridda V, Ripamonti C, DeConno F, Tamburini M. Symptom prevalence and control during cancer patients' last days of life. *J Palliative Care* 1990;6:7.
25. Moulin DE, Foley KM. A review of a hospital-based pain service. In: Foley KM, Bonica JJ, Ventafridda V, eds. *Advances in pain research and therapy.* New York: Raven Press, 1990:413.
26. Cherny NI, Chang V, Frager G, et al. Opioid pharmacotherapy in the management of cancer pain. *Cancer* 1995;76:1283.
27. Zech DL, Grond S, Lynch J, Hertel D, Lehman KA. Validation of World Health Organization guidelines for cancer pain relief: a 10 year prospective study. *Pain* 1995;63:65.
28. Gonzales GR, Elliott KJ, Portenoy RK, Foley KM. Impact of a comprehensive evaluation in the management of cancer pain. *Pain* 1991;47:141.
29. Clouston P, DeAngelis L, Posner JB. The spectrum of neurologic disease in patients with systemic cancer. *Ann Neurol* 1992;31:268.

30. Portenoy RK, Thaler HT, Kornblith AB, et al. Symptom prevalence, characteristics and distress in a cancer population. *Quality of Life Research* 1994;3:183.
31. IASP Subcommittee on Taxonomy. Pain terms: a list with definitions and notes on usage. *Pain* 1980;8:249.
32. Portenoy RK, Lesage P. Management of cancer pain. *Lancet* 1999;353:1695.
33. Levy MH. Pharmacologic treatment of cancer pain. *N Engl J Med* 1996;335:1124.
34. Woolf CJ, Mannion RJ. Neuropathic pain: etiology, mechanisms and management. *Lancet* 1999;353:1959.
35. Besson JM. The neurobiology of pain. *Lancet* 1999;353:1610.
36. Pasternak GW. Multiple morphine and encephalin receptors and the relief of pain. *JAMA* 1988;259(9):1362.
37. Swarm RA, Cousins MJ. Anesthetic techniques for pain control. In: Doyle D, Hanks GWC, MacDonald N, eds. *Oxford textbook of palliative medicine,* 2nd ed. New York: Oxford University Press, 1998:390.
38. Max MB, Inturrisi CE, Kaiko RF, Grabinski PY, Li CH, Foley KM. Epidural and intrathecal opiates: distribution in CSF and plasma and analgesic effects in patients with cancer. *Clin Pharm Ther* 1985;38:631.
39. Onofrio BM, Yaksh TL. Long-term pain relief: intrathecal morphine infusion in 53 patients. *J Neurosurg* 1990;72:200.
40. Elliott KJ, Brodsky M, Hynansky A, Foley KM. Dextromethorphan suppresses the formalin-induced increase in spinal cord C-fos mRNA. *Soc Neurosci* 1994;568:1391.
41. Cervero F, Laird JMA. Pain: visceral pain. *Lancet* 1999;353:2145.
42. Elliott K, Foley KM. Neurologic pain syndromes in patients with cancer. *Crit Care Clin* 1990;6:393.
43. Portenoy RK, Hagen NA. Breakthrough pain: definition, prevalence, and characteristics. *Pain* 1990;41:273.
44. Petzke F, Radbruch L, Zech D, Loick G, Grong S. Temporal presentation of chronic cancer pain: transitory pains on admission to a multidisciplinary pain clinic. *J Pain Symptom Manage* 1999;17:391.
45. Portenoy RK, Payne R, Coluzzi P, et al. Oral transmucosal fentanyl citrate (OTFC) for the treatment of breakthrough pain in cancer patients, a controlled dose titration study. *Pain* 1999;79:303.
46. Wallenstein SL. Measurement of pain and analgesia in cancer patients. *Cancer* 1984;53:2217.
47. Foley KM. Pain assessment and cancer pain syndromes. In: Doyle D, Hanks GW, MacDonald RN, eds. *Oxford textbook of palliative medicine,* 2nd ed. New York: Oxford University Press, 1998:310.
48. McGrath PJ, Beyer J, Cleeland CS, et al. Report of a subcommittee on assessment and methodologic issues in the management of childhood cancer. *Pediatrics* 1990;86:813.
49. Grossman SA, Sheidler VR, Swedeen K, Mucenski J, Pianladosi S. Correlation of patient and caregiver ratings of cancer pain. *J Pain Symptom Manage* 1991;6:53.
50. Daut RL, Cleeland CS, Flanery RC. The development of the Wisconsin Brief Pain Questionnaire to assess pain in cancer and other diseases. *Pain* 1983;1:197.
51. Graham C, Bond SS, Gertrovitch MM, Cook MR. Use of the McGill Pain Questionnaire in the management of cancer pain-replicability and consistency. *Pain* 1980;8:377.
52. Fishman B, Pasternak S, Wallenstein SL, et al. The Memorial Pain Assessment Card: a valid instrument for the assessment of cancer pain. *Cancer* 1986;60:1151.
53. Ingham JM, Portenoy RK. Symptom assessment. *Hematol Oncol Clin North Am* 1996;10:21.
54. Chang VT, Hwang SS, Feuerman M, et al. Symptom and quality of life survey of medical oncology patients at a Veterans Affairs Medical Center. A role for symptom assessment. *Cancer* 2000;88:1175.
55. American Pain Society Quality of Care Committee. Quality improvement guidelines for the treatment of acute pain and cancer pain. *JAMA* 1995;274:1874.
56. DuPen SL, DuPen AR, Palissar N, et al. Implementation of guidelines for cancer pain management: results of a randomized controlled clinical trial. *J Clin Oncol* 1999;17:361.
57. Cherny NI, Coyle N, Foley KM. Suffering in the advanced cancer patient. Part I: a definition and taxonomy. *J Palliat Care* 1994;10:57.
58. Cherny NI, Catane R. Palliative medicine and the medical oncologist: defining the purview of care. *Hematol Oncol Clin North Am* 1996;10:1.
59. Passik SD, Portenoy Rk. Substance abuse issues in palliative care. In: Berger A, et al., eds. *Principles and practices of supportive oncology.* Philadelphia: Lippincott–Raven, 1998.
60. Foley KM. The relationship of pain and symptom management to patient requests for physician-assisted suicide. *J Pain Symptom Manage* 1991;6:289.
61. Cherny NI, Coyle N, Foley KM. Guidelines in the care of the dying cancer patient. *Hematol Oncol Clin North Am* 1996;10:261.
62. Cassem NH. The dying patient. In: Cassem NH, ed. *Massachusetts General Hospital handbook of general hospital psychiatry.* St Louis: Mosby–Year Book, 1991:343.
63. Buckman R. Communication in palliative care: a practical guide. In: Doyle D, Hanks GW, MacDonald N, eds. *Oxford textbook of palliative medicine.* Oxford, England: Oxford University Press, 1993:47.
64. Cherny NI, Portenoy RK. Cancer pain: principles of assessment and syndromes. In: Wall PK, Melzack R, eds. *Textbook of pain.* London: Churchill Livingstone, 1994:787.
65. Foley KM. The treatment of cancer pain. *N Engl J Med* 1985;313:84.
66. Cassell EJ. The nature of suffering and the goals of medicine. *N Engl J Med* 1982;306:639.
67. Roth AJ, Breitbart W. Psychiatric emergencies in terminally ill cancer patients. *Hematol Oncol Clin North Am* 1996;10:235.
68. Chochinov HM, Wilson KG, Enns M, et al. Desire for death in the terminally ill. *Am J Psychiatry* 1995;152:1185.
69. Cherny NI, Foley KM. Brachial plexopathy in patients with breast cancer. In: Harris JR, Hellman S, Henderson IC, Kinne D, eds. *Breast diseases,* 2nd ed. Philadelphia: Lippincott, 1996:796.
70. Hewitt JD, Foley KM. Neuro-imaging. In: Greenberg J, ed. *A companion to Adams and Victors principles of neurology.* New York: McGraw-Hill, 1995:4182.
71. Posner JB. *Neurologic complications of cancer.* Philadelphia: F.A. Davis, 1995.
72. Emmanuel EJ. Pain and symptom control: patient rights and physician responsibilities. *Hematol Oncol Clin North Am* 1996;10:41.
73. Constantini-Ferrando M, Foley KM, Rapkin BD. Communicating with patients about advanced cancer. *JAMA* 1998;280:1403.
74. Bruera E, Wantanabe S. New developments in the assessment of pain in cancer patients. *Supportive Cancer Care* 1994;2:312.
75. Chang VT, Hwang S, Feuerman M. Validation of the Edmonton symptom assessment scale. *Cancer* 2000;88:2164.
76. American Pain Society. *Principles of analgesic use in the treatment of acute pain and cancer pain,* 3rd ed. Skokie, IL: American Pain Society, 1992.
77. Management of cancer pain guideline panel. *Management of cancer pain: clinical practice guideline.* AHCPR Pub. No. 94-0592. Rockville, MD: US Public Health Service, Agency for Health Care Policy and Research, 1994.
78. McQuay H. Opioids in pain management. *Lancet* 1999;353:2229.
79. Bruera E, Pereira J, Watanabe S, et al. Opioid rotation in patients with cancer pain. A retrospective comparison of dose ratios between methadone, hydromorphone, and morphine. *Cancer* 1996;78:852.
80. Ripamonti C, Groff L, Bernelli C, et al. Switching from morphine to oral methadone in treating cancer pain: what is the equianalgesic dose ratio? *J Clin Oncol* 1998;16:3216.
81. Mercadante S, Casuccio A, Aguello A, et al. Morphine versus methadone in the pain treatment of advanced cancer patients followed up at home. *J Clin Oncol* 1998;16:3656.
82. Mercadante S, Casuccio A, Calderone L. Rapid switching from morphine to methadone in cancer patients with poor response to morphine. *J Clin Oncol* 1999;17:3307.
83. Ventafridda V, Caraceni A, Gamba A. Field-testing of the WHO Guidelines for Cancer Pain Relief: summary report of demonstration projects. In: Foley KM, Bonica JJ, Ventafridda V, Callaway MV, eds. *Second International Congress on Cancer Pain. Advances in Pain Research and Therapy,* Vol. 16. New York: Raven Press, 1990;451.
84. World Health Organization. *Cancer pain relief and palliative care.* Geneva: World Health Organization, 1990.
85. Foley KM. Controversies in cancer pain—medical perspective. *Cancer* 1989;63:2266.
86. Foley KM. Current controversies in the management of cancer pain. *NIDA Research Monograph Series* 1981;36:169.
87. Jadad AR, Bowman GP. The WHO analgesic ladder for cancer pain management. Stepping up the quality of its evaluation. *JAMA* 1996;274:1870.
88. Portenoy RK, Foley KM, Inturrisi CE. The nature of opioid responsiveness and its implications for neuropathic pain: new hypotheses derived from studies of opioid infusions. *Pain* 1990;43:273.
89. Eisenberg E, Berkey CS, Carr DB, Mosteller F, Chalmers TC. Efficacy and safety of nonsteroidal antiinflammatory drugs for cancer pain: a meta-analysis. *J Clin Oncol* 1994;12:2756.
90. Lane NE. Pain management in osteoarthritis: the role of Cox-2 inhibitors. *J Rheumatol* 1997;24:20.
91. Ventafridda V, DeConno F, Panerai AE, et al. Non steroidal anti-inflammatory drugs as the first step in cancer pain therapy; double-blind, within-patient study comparing nine drugs. *J Intl Med Res* 1990;18:21.
92. Langman MJS. Treating ulcers in patients receiving anti-arthritic drugs. *Q J Med* 1989;73:1089.
93. Foley KM. Changing concepts of tolerance to opioids. What the cancer patient has taught us. In: Chapman CR, Foley KM, eds. *Current & emerging issues in cancer pain: research & practice.* New York: Raven Press, 1993:331.
94. Ferrell BR, Griffith H. Cost issues related to pain management: report from the cancer pain panel of the Agency for Health Care Policy and Research. *J Pain Symptom Manage* 1994;9:221.
95. Foley KM. Competent care for the dying instead of physician-assisted suicide. *N Engl J Med* 1997;336:54.
96. Foley KM. For more rhetoric and less regulation. *Pain Forum* 1995;4:197.
97. Joranson DE. Availability of opioids for cancer pain relief: recent trends, assessment of symptom barriers, New York health organization guidelines, and the risk of diversion. *J Pain Symptom Manage* 1993;8:353.
98. Paul D, Standifier KM, Inturrisi CE, Pasternak GW. Pharmacological characterization of morphine-6-glucuronide, a very potent morphine metabolite. *J Pharmacol Exp Ther* 1989;251:477.
99. Portenoy RK, Thaler HT, Inturrisi CE, Friedlander-Klar H, Foley KM. Metabolite, morphine-6-glucuronide, contributes to the analgesia produced by morphine infusion in pain patients with normal renal function. *Clin Pharmacol Ther* 1992;51:422.
100. Portenoy RK, Foley KM, Stuhnan J, et al. Plasma morphine and morphine-6-glucuronide during chronic morphine therapy for cancer pain: plasma profiles, steady-state concentrations and the consequences of renal failure. *Pain* 1991;47:13.
101. Hagen N, Foley KM, Cebrone DJ, Portenoy RK, Inturrisi CE. Chronic nausea and morphine-6-glucuronide. *J Pain Symptom Manage* 1991;6:125.
102. Tiseo PJ, Thaler HT, Lapin J, et al. Morphine-6-glucuronide concentrations and opioid-related side effects: a survey in cancer patients. *Pain* 1995;61:47.
103. Sjogren P. Clinical implications of morphine metabolites. In: Portenoy RK, Bruera E, eds. *Topics in palliative care,* Vol. 1. New York: Oxford University Press, 1997:163.
104. Babul N, Darke AC, Hagen N. Hydromorphone metabolite accumulation in renal failure. *J Pain Symptom Manage* 1995;10:184.
105. Moulin DE, Kreeft JH, Murray-Parsons N, et al. Comparison of continuous subcutaneous and intravenous hydromorphine infusions for management of cancer pain. *Lancet* 1991;337:465.
106. Kaiko BF, Benziger DP, Fitzmartin RD, et al. Pharmacokinetic-pharmacodynamic relationships of controlled-release oxycodone. *Clin Pharmacol Ther* 1995;59:50.
107. Bruera E, Fainsinger R, Moore M, et al. Local toxicity with subcutaneous methadone. *Pain* 1991;45:141.
108. Kaiko RR, Foley KM, Grabinski PY, et al. Central nervous system excitatory effects of meperidine in cancer patients. *Ann Neurol* 1983;13:180.

109. Portenoy RK, Southam MA, Gupta SK, et al. Transdermal fentanyl for cancer pain: repeated dose pharmacokinetics. *Anesthesiology* 1993;78:36.
110. Houde RW. Methods for measuring clinical pain in humans. *Acta Anaesthesiol Scand* 1982;74(Suppl):25.
111. Weinberg DS, Inturrisi CE, Reidenberg B, et al. Sublingual absorption of selected opioid analgesics. *Clin Pharmacol Ther* 1988;44:335.
112. Moulin DE, Kreeft JH, Murray-Parsons N, Bouquillon AL. Comparison of continuous subcutaneous and intravenous hydromorphone infusions for management of cancer pain. *Lancet* 1991;337:465.
113. Portenoy RK, Moulin DE, Rogers A, Inturrisi CE, Foley KM. Infusion of opioids in cancer pain: clinical review and guidelines for use. *Cancer Treat Rep* 1985;70:575.
114. Dennis CG, DeWitty RL. Long-term intraventricular infusion of morphine for intractable pain in cancer of the head and neck. *Neurosurgery* 1990;26:404.
115. Beaver WT. Comparison of analgesic effects of morphine sulfate, hydroxyzine and other combinations in patients with postoperative pain. In: Bonica JJ, Ventafridda V, eds. *Advances in pain research and therapy.* New York: Raven Press, 1976:553.
116. Forrest WH, Brown B, Brown C, et al. Dextroamphetamine with morphine for the treatment of postoperative pain. *N Engl J Med* 1977;296:712.
117. Bruera E, Chadwich S, Brenneis C, et al. Methylphenidate associated with narcotics for the treatment of cancer pain. *Cancer Treat Rep* 1987;71:67.
118. Mercandante S, Casuccio A, Genovese G. Ineffectiveness of dextromethorphan in cancer pain. *J Pain Symptom Manage* 1998;16:317.
119. Laska EM, Sunshine A, Mueller F, et al. Caffeine as an analgesic adjuvant. *JAMA* 1984;251:1711.
120. Goldfrank L, Weisman RS, Enick JK, Lo MW. A normogram for continuous intravenous naloxone. *Ann Emerg Med* 1986;1:566.
121. Lichter J. Nausea and vomiting in patients with cancer. *Hematol Oncol Clin North Am* 1996;10:207.
122. Derby S, Portenoy RK. Assessment and management of opioid-induced constipation. In: Portenoy RK, Bruera E, eds. *Topics in palliative care,* Vol. 1. New York: Oxford University Press, 1997;1:95.
123. Yuan CS, Foss JF, O'Connor M, et al. Methylnaltrexone for reversal of constipation due to chronic methadone use: a randomized controlled trial. *JAMA* 2000;283:367.
124. Kanner RM, Foley KM. Patterns of narcotic drug use in a cancer pain clinic. *Ann NY Acad Sci* 1981;362:161.
125. Eagel B, Portnoy R, Foley KM. Use and misuse of naloxone. *J Pain Symptom Manage* 2000 (*in press*).
126. Manfredi PL, Ribeiro S, Chandler SW, Payne R. Inappropriate use of naloxone in cancer patients with pain. *J Pain Symptom Manage* 1996;11:131.
127. Portenoy RK. Adjuvant analgesic agents. *Hematol Oncol Clin North Am* 1996;10:103.
128. Max MB, Culnane M, Schafer SC, et al. Amitriptyline relieves diabetic neuropathy pain in patients with normal or depressed mood. *Neurology* 1987;37:589.
129. Max MB, Schafer SC, Culnane M, et al. Association of pain relief with drug side effects in postherpetic neuralgia: a single dose study of clonidine, codeine, ibuprofen, and placebo. *Clin Pharmacol Ther* 1988;43:363.
130. Sindrup SH, Gram LF, Brosen K, et al. The selective serotonin reuptake inhibitor paroxetine is effective in the treatment of diabetic neuropathy symptoms. *Pain* 1990;42:135.
131. Backonja M, Beydoun A, Edwards KR, et al. Gabapentin for the symptomatic treatment of painful neuropathy in diabetes mellitus, a randomized controlled trial. *JAMA* 1998;280:1831.
132. Fromm GH, Terence CR, Chatta AS. Baclofen in the treatment of trigeminal neuralgia. *Ann Neurol* 1984;15:240.
133. Dejgard A, Petersen P, Kastrup J. Mexiletine for treatment of chronic painful diabetic neuropathy. *Lancet* 1988;1:9.
134. Brose WG, Cousins MJ. Subcutaneous lidocaine for treatment of neuropathic cancer pain. *Pain* 1991;45:141.
135. Ehrenstrom GME, Reiz SLA. EMLA—a eutectic mixture of local anesthetics for topical anesthesia. *Acta Anaesthesiol Scand* 1982;26:596.
136. Rowbotham MC, Davies PS, Fields HL. Topical lidocaine relieves postherpetic neuralgia. *Ann Neurol* 1995:37:246.
137. Tannock I, Gospodarowicz M, Meakin W, et al. Treatment of metastatic prostate cancer with low-dose prednisone—evaluation of pain and quality of life as prognostic indices of response. *J Clin Oncol* 1989;7:590.
138. Bruera E, Roca E, Cedaro L, Carraro S, Chacon R. Action of oral methylprednisolone in terminal cancer patients: a prospective randomized double-blind study. *Cancer Treat Rep* 1985;69:751.
139. Weissman DE. Glucocorticoid treatment for brain metastases and epidural spinal cord compressions review. *J Clin Oncol* 1988;6:543.
140. Fernandez F, Adams F, Holmes VF. Analgesic effect of alprazolam in patients with chronic, organic pain of malignant origin. *J Clin Psychopharmacol* 1987;7:167.
141. Lechin F, vander Dijs B, Lechin ME, et al. Pimozide therapy for trigeminal neuralgia. *Arch Neurol* 1989;9:960.
142. Beaver WT, Wallenstein SM, Houde RW, et al. A comparison of the analgesic effects of methotrimeprazine and morphine in patients with cancer. *Clin Pharmacol Ther* 1966;7:436.
143. Eisenach JC, Dewan DM, Rose JC, et al. Epidural clonidine produces antinociception, but not hypotension, in sheep. *Anesthesiology* 1987;66:496.
144. Persson J, Axelsson G, Hallin RG, et al. Beneficial effects of ketamine in a chronic pain state with allodynia, possibly due to central sensitization. *Pain* 1995;60:217.
145. McQuay HJ, Carrol D, Jadad AR, et al. Dextromethorphan for the treatment of neuropathic pain: a double-blind, randomised controlled crossover trial with integral n-of-1 design. *Pain* 1994;59:127.
146. Jaeger H, Maier C. Calcitonin in phantom limb pain: a double blind study. *Pain* 1992;48:21.
147. Ernst DS, MacDonald RN, Paterson AH, et al. A double-blind, crossover trial of intravenous clodronate in metastatic bone pain. *J Pain Symptom Manage* 1992;7:4.
148. Thiebaud D, Leyvraz S, von Fliedner V, et al. Treatment of bone metastases from breast cancer and myeloma with pamidronate. *Eur J Cancer* 1991;27:37.
149. Glover D, Lipton A, Keller A, et al. Intravenous pamidronate disodium treatment: bone metastases in patients with breast cancer. *Cancer* 1994;74:2949.
150. Roth A, Kolaric K. Analgesic activity of calcitonin in patient with painful osteolytic metastases of breast cancer: results of a controlled randomized study. *Oncology* 1986;43:283.
151. Warrel RP, Lovett D, Dilmanian FA, et al. Low-dose gallium nitrate for prevention of osteolysis in myeloma: results of a pilot randomized study. *J Clin Oncol* 1993;11:2443.
152. Porter AT, McEwan AJ, Powe JE, et al. Results of a randomized phase-III trial to evaluate the efficacy of strontium-89 adjuvant to local field external beam irradiation in the management of endocrine resistant metastatic prostate cancer. *Int J Radiat Oncol Biol Phys* 1993;25:805.
153. Berna L, Carrio J, Alinso C, et al. Bone pain palliation with strontium 89 in breast cancer patients with bone metastases with refractory bone pain. *Eur J Nucl Med* 1995;22:1101.
154. Loscalzo M, Amendola J. Psychosocial and behavioral management of cancer pain: the social work contribution. In: Foley KM, Bonica JJ, Ventafridda V, eds. *Advances in pain research and therapy.* New York: Raven Press, 1990:429.
155. Edwards WT, Habib F, Burney RG, Begin G. Intravenous lidocaine in the management of various chronic pain states. *Reg Anesth* 1985;10:1.
156. Waldman SD, Cronen MC. Thoracic epidural morphine in the palliation of chest wall pain secondary to relapsing polychondritis. *J Pain Symptom Manage* 1989;4:38.
157. Cherny NI, Arbit E, Jain S. Invasive techniques in the management of cancer pain. *Hematol Oncol Clin North Am* 1996;10:121.
158. Patt R. Peripheral neurolysis and the management of cancer pain. In: Patt R, ed. *Cancer pain.* Philadelphia: Lippincott, 1993:359.
159. Robertson DH. Transsacral neurolytic nerve block. An alternative approach to intractable perineal pain. *Br J Anaesth* 1983;55:873.
160. Gianasi C. Neuroadenolysis of the pituitary: an overview of development, mechanisms, technique and results. In: Benedetti C, Chapman CR, Moricca G, et al., eds. *Advances in pain research and therapy.* New York: Raven Press, 1984:647.
161. Sundaresan N, DiGiacinto GV, Hughes EO. Neurosurgery in the treatment of cancer pain. *Cancer* 1989;63:2365.
162. Arbit E. Neurosurgical management of cancer pain. In: Foley KM, Bonica JJ, Ventafridda V, eds. *Advances in pain research and therapy.* New York: Raven Press, 1990:289.
163. Sundaresan N, Galicich JH, Lane JM, Scher H. Stabilization of the spine involved by cancer. In: Dunsker DB, Schmidek HH, eds. *The unstable spine.* Orlando: Grune & Stratton, 1986:249.
164. Sundaresan N, Hilaris BS, Martini N. The combined neurosurgical-thoracic management of superior sulcus tumors. *J Clin Oncol* 1987;5:1739.
165. Lahuerta T, Lipton SA, Wells JD. Percutaneous cervical cordotomy: results and complications in a recent series of 100 patients. *Ann R Coll Surg Exp* 1985;67:41.
166. Ischia S, Luzzani A, Ischia A, et al. Subarachnoid neurolytic block (L5, S1) and unilateral percutaneous cervical cordotomy for the treatment of neoplastic vertebral pain. *Pain* 1984;19:123.
167. Macaluso C, Arbit E, Foley KM. Cordotomy for lumbosacral, pelvic, and lower extremity pain of malignant origin: safety and efficacy. *Neurology* 1988;38:110.
168. Barrash JM, Milan EL. Dorsal rhizotomy for the relief of pain of malignant tumor origin. *J Neurosurg* 1973;38:755.
169. Arbit E, Galicich JH, Burt M, et al. Modified open thoracic rhizotomy for treatment of intractable chest wall pain of malignant etiology. *Ann Thorac Surg* 1989;48:820.
170. Giorgi C, Broggi G. Surgical treatment of glossopharyngeal neuralgia and pain from cancer of the nasopharynx. *J Neurosurg* 1984;61:952.
171. Nashold BS, Ostdahl RH. Dorsal root entry zone lesions for pain relief. *J Neurosurg* 1979;51:59.
172. Gildenberg PL, Hirschberg RM. Limited myelotomy for the treatment of intractable cancer pain. *J Neurol Neurosurg Psychiatry* 1984;47:94.
173. Hassenbusch SJ, Pillay PK, Barnett GH. Radiofrequency cingulotomy for intractable cancer pain using stereotaxis guided by magnetic resonance imaging. *Neurosurgery* 1990;27:220.
174. Thompson JW, Filshie J. In: Doyle D, Hanks G, MacDonald N, eds. *Transcutaneous electrical nerve stimulation and acupuncture in palliative care medicine.* New York: Oxford University Press, 1992.
175. Levy RM, Lamb S, Adams JE. Treatment of chronic pain by deep brain stimulation: long-term followup and review of the literature. *Neurosurgery* 1987;21:885.
176. Young RF, Brechner T. Electrical stimulation of the brain for relief of intractable pain due to cancer. *Cancer* 1986;57:1266.
177. Staats P. Neuraxial infusion for pain control: when, why and what to do after the implant. *Oncology* 1999;13:58.
178. Travell JG, Simons DG. *Myofascial pain and dysfunction: the trigger-point manual.* Baltimore: Williams & Wilkins, 1983.
179. Filshle J. Acupuncture and malignant pain problems. *Acupuncture in Medicine* 1990;8:38.
180. Fosburg MT, Crone RK. Nitrous oxide analgesia for refractory pain in the terminally ill. *JAMA* 1983;250:511.
181. Green VFR, David WH. Titrated intravenous barbiturates in the control of symptoms in patients with terminal cancer. *South Med J* 1991;84:332.
182. Cherny NI, Portenoy RK. Sedation in the management of refractory symptoms: guidelines for evaluation and treatment. *J Palliat Care* 1994;10:31.
183. Roy D. Need they sleep before they die? *J Palliat Care* 1990;6:3.
184. Ventafridda V, Ripamonti C, De Conno F, et al. Symptom prevalence and control during cancer patients' last days of life. *J Palliat Care* 1990;6:7.
185. Coyle N. A model of continuity of care for cancer patients with chronic pain. *Med Clin North Am* 1987;71:24.

SECTION 2

J. STANLEY SMITH
WILEY W. SOUBA

Nutritional Support

Malnutrition is common in cancer patients and is frequently referred to as *cancer cachexia.* Although this is a true malnutrition syndrome, it differs from the protein-calorie malnutrition seen in starvation. Further, the etiology of this clinically obvious problem is not entirely clear, but investigations delineating the role of cytokines and other substances responsible for mediating the cachexia of cancer have increased our knowledge of the causes of malnutrition in these patients with advanced malignant disease. Studies have also provided insight into why it is difficult or impossible to gain lean body mass in cachectic cancer patients even when aggressive feeding regimens are implemented. Now and in the future, nutritional therapy may be most effective in cancer patients when used in combination with other forms of metabolic intervention.

While cancer patients can develop deficiencies in vitamins and trace minerals, the most common form of nutritional depletion is that of protein-calorie malnutrition, manifested as a loss of body cell mass. Severe protein-calorie malnutrition is associated with increases in postoperative complications in cancer patients, and it has been shown to have adverse effects on immune function and treatment tolerance to anticancer treatments. Since intuition would indicate the well-nourished patient should tolerate aggressive antineoplastic therapy better than the malnourished individual, numerous studies have tried to define the role of nutritional support in patients with malignant disease. Moreover, the observation that this commonly occurring weight loss is a predictor of therapeutic response and survival has led to aggressive attempts to restore nutritional integrity. The rationale for providing nutritional support to selected patients is to prevent or reverse host tissue wasting, broaden the spectrum of therapeutic options, improve the clinical course, and ultimately prolong patient survival.

More recent developments have increased our understanding of the relationship between nutrition and metabolism in cancer patients, and it is clear that limited weight loss in cancer patients is acceptable because short-term undernutrition does not appear to adversely affect treatment tolerance. However, many cancer patients do develop significant malnutrition such that some form of nutritional support or metabolic intervention appears to be indicated. Cancer patients often require chemotherapy, radiation therapy, or both in combination with surgery, and these treatments can further compromise an already fragile nutritional status and further reduce treatment tolerance. Not only may the anticancer treatments directly affect nutrition and reduce the urge to eat, but they may affect the ability to chew, swallow, or absorb food. Accordingly, oncologists need to become familiar with the changes in body metabolism developing during malignancy and with the indications and delivery of nutritional or metabolic support to the cancer patient. Although the need for well-designed prospective randomized trials examining the role of nutritional support as adjunctive therapy in cancer patients continues to exist, it is clear that patients with a functioning gut deserve enteral nutrition as the route of preference for feeding. Parenteral nutrition should be reserved for patients who have unusable gastrointestinal tracts.

The purpose of this chapter is to examine the etiologies and metabolic alterations in cancer cachexia, to establish a rationale for metabolic treatment and support in the malnourished cancer patient, and to define the indications for and the effect of nutritional support in patients with malignant disease. Portions of this review have been previously published.[1–4]

CLINICAL MANIFESTATIONS OF CANCER CACHEXIA

WEIGHT LOSS

The most obvious clinical manifestation of cancer cachexia is the depletion of host tissues that becomes quite apparent to the casual observer as weight loss. Most patients lose weight at some point during the course of their disease and nearly one-half of all cancer patients have weight loss at the time of initial diagnosis. Warren and colleagues in 1932 reported that 22% of deaths were due to inanition, and two-thirds of all tumor-bearing patients in their series developed some degree of cachexia.[5] A large study from the Eastern Cooperative Oncology Group showed significantly shorter survival if weight loss was present. Further, the amount of weight loss was dependent on the type and site of the tumor. Non-Hodgkin's lymphomas, breast cancers, acute nonlymphocytic leukemias, and sarcomas had the least weight loss. Colon, prostate, and lung cancers had a moderate weight loss, whereas pancreatic and gastric cancers had the most.[6]

DeWys and colleagues[6] reported that patients who presented without weight loss had a significantly prolonged survival following therapy than similarly treated patients who had weight loss at presentation. These findings suggest that weight loss adversely affects survival following antineoplastic therapy and imply that appropriate nutritional therapy may be beneficial to certain patient groups (Table 56.2-1). In both animals and patients with cancer, it is apparent that weight loss is dependent on the presence of the tumor since curative surgical resection (or nonsurgical ablation) of the malignancy is almost invariably associated with a return of normal food intake and normal body weight, whereas palliative resection is not. In fact, in patients not regaining their weight following supposedly curative surgical resection, the presence of metastatic or recurrent disease should be suspected. As a general rule, cancer patients with significant weight loss do not tolerate treatment regimens as well as well-nourished patients.

Nutritional support therapy has attempted to reverse this cachexia and, although some weight loss has been halted, restoration of the protein and caloric intake has not reversed the abnormalities of energy, protein, carbohydrate, and fat metabolism, showing that something else must be added.[7,8]

LOSS OF APPETITE

Loss of appetite resulting in a reduction in voluntary food intake is a central component of the syndrome of cancer

TABLE 56.2-1. Extent of Weight Loss in Cancer Patients at the Time of Initial Diagnosis and Its Effect on Survival After Antineoplastic Therapy

Type of Cancer (Diagnosis)	*No. of Patients*	*Percentage of Patients with Weight Loss at Diagnosis*	*Survival of Patients with Weight Loss (wk)*	*Survival of Patients without Weight Loss (wk)*
Breast	289	36	45	70[a]
Colon	307	54	21	43[a]
Prostate	78	56	24	46[a]
Sarcoma	189	39	25	46[a]
Lung	590	61	14	20[a]
Small cell (lung)	436	60	27	34
Stomach	179	83	27	41[a]

[a]$P < .05$ versus patients with weight loss.
(From ref. 6, with permission.)

cachexia. Careful studies in numerous animal models of cancer cachexia have documented a decline in food intake.

Appetite is strongly controlled by various neurotransmitters such as serotonin, catecholamines, and opiates.[9] Any serotonergic agonist decreases appetite. In animal studies, there is evidence of increased brain tryptophan and serotonin turnover in the tumor-bearing host.[10,11] Inhibition of serotonin synthesis increases food intake. However, serotonin antagonists demonstrate no effect on tumor anorexia. Further, there may be a serum factor responsible since rats receiving serum from tumor-bearing rats become anorectic.[12]

At some point during the course of their disease, most patients report a loss of appetite including alterations in taste and smell plus the loss of the appeal of most foods. Moreover, some patients exhibit an increase in resting energy expenditure (REE) that is seldom accompanied by a compensatory increase in calorie intake. The combination of a decrease in voluntary food intake with an increase in energy expenditure further contributes to weight loss and negative calorie and nitrogen balance.

There may also be anatomic factors including the location of the tumor affecting the ability to eat. Sometimes the malignant process may even involve the digestive tract, leading to pain, early satiety, mechanical obstruction, or nausea. Head and neck cancers and the treatments used for them may cause dysphagia, mucositis, and stomatitis, with the resultant inability to take oral feeds. Gastric and pancreatic cancers cause obstruction, early satiety, or pain with eating and notoriously present late with marked metabolic changes and weight loss. Early provision of enteral routes for feeding need to be considered along with any other types of treatment and should be performed with the primary surgery or early in the course of radiation therapy. With today's minimally invasive procedures for tube placements, there is no excuse for delay in provision of enteral feeds.

WEAKNESS

Secondary to loss of body cell mass and treatment regimens, cancer patients almost invariably develop a reduction in strength and a diminished physical capacity for work. Evidence for a central role of the tumor in the etiology of this weakness is derived from the clinical observation that cure of the cancer almost always results in a return to preillness strength and work capacity.

CAUSES AND CONSEQUENCES OF CANCER CACHEXIA

Many of the physiologic changes seen in cancer cachexia resemble those of simple starvation, but it is clear that more derangement is involved since few studies have documented that aggressive feeding of cachectic cancer patients completely restores lean body mass[7] (Table 56.2-2). Rather, such patients tend to primarily gain water and fat. Although the substrate demand of the tumor may account for the tumor behaving as a nitrogen trap, the actual energy and nitrogen demands of human tumors cannot account for the profound weight loss generally observed. It is unusual for the total mass of the tumor to exceed 1% or 2% of total body weight, yet patients with much smaller tumors are often markedly cachectic. Studies in the last decade suggest that circulating factors are the major cause of cancer cachexia and that appropriate therapy for this detrimental syndrome of weight loss and wasting will require a better understanding of these mediators.

The term *cancer cachexia* is used to describe a complex metabolic syndrome composed of weight loss, anorexia, and wasting of host lean body mass secondary to the growing malignancy. No consistent or clear-cut association with duration of illness, stage of disease, or tumor histology has been demonstrated. Although the exact prevalence of cancer cachexia is unknown, many studies have shown a high frequency of nutritional

TABLE 56.2-2. Metabolic Differences between the Response to Simple Starvation and Advanced Malignant Disease

	Simple Starvation	*Advanced Malignant Disease*
Basal metabolic rate	– or decreased	–, increased, or decreased
Presence of mediators	–	+++
Hepatic ureagenesis	+	+++
Negative nitrogen balance	+	+++
Gluconeogenesis	+	+++
Muscle proteolysis	+	+++
Hepatic protein synthesis	+	+++
Lipolysis	+	+++

–, indicates normal; +, indicates slightly increased; +++, indicates a substantial increase.

derangements in cancer patients. These studies have focused on findings such as weight loss or hypoproteinemia as indicators of cancer cachexia. Consequently, the prevalence of cancer cachexia may be underestimated, since it is likely that subtle metabolic alterations precede these clinically apparent changes manifested by the weight and lean tissue loss.

Since many cancer-related deaths are a consequence of malnutrition and host depletion, understanding the mechanism of cancer cachexia is imperative, as the syndrome always results in death if oncologic therapy is not administered. Many etiologies for the cancer cachexia syndrome have been proposed, but no clear explanation exists. Therefore, the etiology seems to be multifactorial. Causes can be broadly categorized into anorexia of malignancy, anorexia of therapy, and abnormalities in host intermediary metabolism.

ANOREXIA OF MALIGNANCY

As mentioned previously, the *anorexia of malignancy* refers to the decrease in voluntary food intake that occurs in cancer patients. Although this anorexia comes eventually in all patients with advanced cancer, it may sometimes develop early in the course of the disease when the tumor is quite small. Weight loss is common in patients with gastrointestinal tumors, but dysfunction of the digestive tract cannot solely explain this phenomenon, since significant cachexia is also noted in patients with cancers that originate outside the abdominal cavity. Proposed mechanisms include local effects of the tumor, alterations in taste or palatability, hypothalamic dysfunction, modification of satiety mechanisms, and learned food aversion. Many of these effects seem to be mediated by circulating factors.

ANOREXIA OF THERAPY

Oncologic therapies may often initiate or worsen anorexia. Many chemotherapeutic agents can cause nausea, vomiting, mucositis, gastrointestinal dysfunction, or all of these symptoms for varying periods of time that may result in anorexia and weight loss. Radiation therapy is often associated with similar acute side effects and may lead to stricture formation in the bowel. After surgery, causes of weight loss range from routine postoperative ileus to the hypermetabolism associated with sepsis. An important consideration for the clinician to remember is that, in the midst of a diagnostic workup, hospitalized cancer patients are often restricted from taking adequate nutrition. As a result, the patient may become iatrogenically malnourished before even the initiation of oncologic treatment.

CACHEXIA SECONDARY TO ALTERATIONS OF HOST INTERMEDIARY METABOLISM

A number of metabolic abnormalities are characteristic of the tumor-bearing host (Table 56.2-3). REE is variably affected by the presence of a tumor. Knox and coworkers studied 200 malnourished cancer patients using indirect calorimetry and found that 41% had normal basal metabolic rates, 33% had decreased expenditures, and 25% had increased expenditures.[13] Even patients with no increase in metabolic rate can develop weight loss and negative nitrogen balance despite a normal food intake and a small tumor burden. Fearon and coworkers demonstrated that whole body protein turnover was increased 50% in solid tumor-bearing patients, despite having no change in REE.[14] Other studies have shown that, unlike simple starvation, REE remains elevated even in the face of reduced intake.[15] But, even for tumors with elevated REE, the increased energy expenditure is not enough to explain the weight loss. Curative resections return the REE to normal, but palliation does not.[16–18] Further, rebound in the REE indicates a recurrence of the tumor.

TABLE 56.2-3. Metabolic Abnormalities in Animal and Human Cancer Cachexia

Substrate	*Clinical Parameter*	*Observation*
Water	Total body water	Increased
Energy	Energy balance	Negative
	Energy stores	Diminished
Lipid	Body fat mass	Decreased
	Lipoprotein lipase activity	Decreased
	Fat breakdown	Increased
	Serum lipid levels	Increased
Carbohydrate	Gluconeogenesis	Increased
	Insulin resistance	Present
	Body glucose consumption	Increased
	Hepatic glucose production	Increased
Protein	Muscle mass	Diminished
	Muscle proteolysis	Increased
	Muscle amino acid release	Increased
	Hepatic protein synthesis	Increased
	Hepatic amino acid transport	Increased
	Nitrogen balance	Negative

Glucose metabolism is also abnormal in cancer patients secondary to increased whole body glucose turnover. There is decreased glucose use by skeletal muscle, increased hepatic glucose production, and increased production of glucose from lactate through Cori's cycle.[19,20] There is also increased glucose use by the tumor as the tumor switches to glucose as its primary fuel source. Shaw and Wolfe demonstrated that hepatic gluconeogenesis in patients with gastrointestinal malignancies was elevated proportional to tumor burden.[20] Patients with the largest tumors even failed to suppress endogenous glucose production during glucose infusion, a response attributed to insulin resistance.[20–22] This glucose intolerance and hyperglycemia in cancer patients has been recognized for a long time.[23] Lundholm et al. showed that the beta cell receptor in the pancreas may have diminished sensitivity to glucose loading,[24] indicating that the tumor-bearing host may be in a type II diabetic-like state. However, this insulin resistance also shares elements similar to the stress state. Overall, there is a combination of a significant decrease in metabolized and cleared glucose in both the weight-stable and weight-losing cancer patients. Since the insulin resistance may decrease after complete tumor resection, it appears to be related to the tumor itself, rather than the associated malnutrition.[25] This could contribute significantly to tissue wasting, since insulin is important for tissue anabolism.

Protein and amino acid metabolism are also altered in the tumor-bearing host. Jeevanandam et al. compared tumor-bearing patients with both malnourished non–tumor-bearing patients and healthy controls to find elevated levels of protein turnover in the cancer group.[26–28] Patients with non–small cell lung cancer have increased whole body protein turnover, elevated 3-methylhistidine excretion, and increased muscle proteolysis.[29] In tumor-bearing rats, whole body nitrogen turnover and liver protein fractional synthetic rates increase, and the animal cannot adapt to starvation by diminishing the rate of muscle amino acid release. Further, skeletal muscle synthesis of new protein decreases. Norton et al. measured arteriovenous differences of amino acids across a sarcoma-bearing limb in patients using the non–tumor-bearing limb as a control.[30] Compared with the non–tumor-bearing extremity, the tumor-bearing limb released lesser amounts of every amino acid, consistent with the tumor's requirement for amino acids to support neoplastic growth. Further work by Fischer et al. has shown the primary amino acid for tumor protein synthesis is glutamine.[34]

Lipid metabolism is also altered in the host with cancer. Shaw and Wolfe studied glycerol and fatty acid kinetics using radioisotopes and found cancer patients with weight loss have increased glycerol and fatty acid turnover compared with weight-stable patients.[20] These weight-losing patients may be incapable of oxidizing endogenous fatty acids or intravenous lipids at normal rates and fail to suppress lipolysis during glucose infusion. In fact, there is increased lipid mobilization from peripheral fat stores and decreased serum lipid clearance, leading to depletion of body fatty tissue. There have now been a number of studies suggesting a transmissible fat-mobilizing substance [lipid-mobilizing proteoglycan (LMF), *azaftig*] in the serum of cancer patients that increases lipid breakdown and decreases fat synthesis.[31–33] This lipid-mobilizing factor is a 24-kD zinc α_2-glycoprotein that has been isolated from the urine of tumor-bearing animals and patients. It has been found in the urine of pancreas, lung, breast, and ovarian cancer patients. The N-terminal amino acid sequence is different from that of any of the known cytokines. Administration of this material shows significant reduction in body weight and decrease in both fat and lean body mass and can be neutralized by administration of monoclonal or polyclonal antibodies.

GLUTAMINE AND CANCER CACHEXIA

Glutamine metabolism in the tumor-bearing host has been extensively studied for four principal reasons: (1) glutamine is the principal amino acid used by many cancers,[36] (2) it is the most abundant amino acid in the body, (3) its stores are quite labile, and (4) studies indicate that glutamine is a conditionally essential amino acid. Glutamine appears to be an unusually good substrate for use by the tumor. In fibrosarcoma cells, glutamine oxidation is decreased and the glutamine is shunted into protein synthesis while the tumor switches to glucose for energy.[34] Circulating glutamine extraction by the tumor is 50% greater than the rate of glutamine extraction for any normal healthy organ. Because tumors must compete with host tissues for plasma amino acids and are often poorly vascularized, they must possess efficient mechanisms for their extraction, especially in an environment (e.g., intratumoral space) in which levels of these nutrients may be diminished compared with plasma levels. Studies[35] in a variety of different solid tumor cell lines, regardless of tissue origin, indicate a single efficient high-affinity carrier-mediated Na^+-dependent glutamine transport. There was a range of kinetic parameters for the glutamine transporter in each cell type, but the amino acid inhibition profiles were nearly identical, consistent with uptake by the system ASC family of transporters. Rates of cell growth, DNA and protein synthesis, and thymidine transport correlated with the glutamine concentration in the culture media, indicating the central role of this amino acid in regulating cellular proliferation.

The methylcholanthrene-induced sarcoma (MCA tumor) rat model has been used by several investigators to study glutamine metabolism.[35] One of the most reproducible observations in rats bearing the MCA tumor is a progressive decrease in plasma glutamine concentrations that correlates with tumor size. With time, blood glutamine levels decrease to less than 50% of normal, indicating an imbalance between rates of glutamine production and consumption expressed by the various organs of the body. This reduction in circulating levels occurs despite an increase in the rate of muscle glutamine release because the accelerated glutamine consumption by tumor and other tissues exceeds the net rate of glutamine uptake into the blood stream. Concomitant temporally with the tumor-induced alterations in muscle glutamine metabolism are marked increases in tumor and hepatic glutamine uptake. Thus, with progressive tumor growth, glutamine depletion gradually becomes more severe. This low glutamine level may serve as a signal to induce net proteolysis.

Since glutamine uptake by the tumor is increased, the assumption might be made that providing exogenous glutamine would promote tumor growth. However, glutamine-enriched total parenteral nutrition (TPN) seems to be more beneficial to the host than the tumor.[36] In fact, dietary glutamine improves the immune status of rats recovering from chemotherapy in a dose-dependent manner and becomes more pronounced after a longer duration of intake.[37]

CYTOKINES: MEDIATORS OF CANCER CACHEXIA

Cytokines, polypeptide signalers produced by the host's cells in response to a growing tumor, regulate many of the nutritional and metabolic derangements that occur in the host with cancer (Table 56.2-4). The recognition that cytokines are important mediators of the body's response to the growing tumor has allowed investigators to focus research efforts on finding common mechanisms responsible for the development of the cancer cachexia. These studies will likely lead to the incorporation of nutritional strategies designed to optimize the metabolic and immunologic integrity of the host while simultaneously allowing tumor-directed therapies to be maximally effective.

Elevated concentrations of tissue and circulating cytokines have been demonstrated in the host with cancer,[38] and enhanced hepatic cytokine gene expression has been demonstrated in

TABLE 56.2-4. Some Effects of Cytokines on Nutrition and Metabolism in the Tumor-Bearing Host

Reduce appetite
Stimulate basal metabolic rate
Stimulate glucose uptake
Stimulate mobilization of fat and protein stores
Reduce adipocyte lipoprotein lipase activity
Enhance muscle amino acid release
Stimulate hepatic amino acid transport activity

tumor-bearing animals. Cytokines can regulate both energy intake (appetite) and energy expenditure (metabolic rate). Administration of tumor necrosis factor (TNF) to rodents and humans decreases food intake, but the effect appears to be short lived. In rats treated with chronic injections of TNF, voluntary food intake was markedly reduced for 2 days but had normalized by the sixth day of TNF administration.[39] In patients receiving TNF, food intake was also diminished, but nitrogen losses were not accelerated, indicating that the resultant negative nitrogen balance was due to something other than TNF alone. Interleukin-1 (IL-1) also suppresses food intake, and its effect, like that of TNF, appears to be directly on the central nervous system. Darling and associates[40] suggest that when TNF is given via a constant infusion, the anorexic effects are sustained as opposed to the tolerance that develops when the cytokine is given by bolus injection. Further evidence for a role for TNF and IL-1 in mediating appetite suppression during critical illness comes from additional studies that demonstrate that treatment of tumor-bearing mice with anticytokine antibodies improves food intake and attenuates weight loss.[41] Even mice whose tumors were injected with inhibitors to TNF and IL-1 resulted in the attenuation of weight loss, an increase in food intake, a decrease in serum triglyceride and glucose, and an increase in total protein.[42] Mice implanted with tumors that secreted TNF showed marked reductions in weight compared with animals with non–TNF-secreting tumors.[43] Therefore, the effects of TNF on food intake and body composition are unlikely to be due to partial starvation alone, but rather may be due to the ability of TNF to stimulate basal metabolic rate (oxygen consumption). In patients receiving injections of TNF, metabolic rates were noted to increase by 30%.[44]

In addition to stimulating anorexia and thermogenesis, cytokines can also stimulate mobilization of fat and protein stores *in vivo*. Accordingly, TNF was first identified as a mediator of cachexia and was termed *cachectin*. Although few clinical studies demonstrate weight loss in subjects receiving TNF, it is likely that these cytokines cause fluid retention. It is clear that TNF can alter the vascular endothelium and lead to an increase in capillary permeability.

Other cytokines have been shown to have effects as well, particularly IL-6. IL-6 is increased in lung cancer patients and is correlated with poor nutritional status and shorter survival.[45] Further, IL-6 levels decrease in treatment responders and do not change or may even increase in nonresponders. IL-12 may also increase secretion of interferon-γ, which may enhance TNF production and subsequent cytokine-induced cachexia.[46] Serum levels of soluble TNF receptors have also been measured and found to correlate with the extent of disease, degree of cachexia, and inversely with nutritional parameters.[47] But the cachexia of cancer does not depend on cytokines alone. Other mediators that have been investigated include corticosteroids, β-agonists, and insulin-like growth factors. Glucocorticoids appear to have additive effects to cytokines in the development of cachexia and may be the missing factor for the cachectic effects of cytokines.[48] In the presence of dexamethasone, there is an up-regulation of IL-6 receptors that seems to prime liver cells for subsequent stimulation by cytokines.[49] There may also be an effect from the autonomic nervous system. One study has shown increased renal sympathetic nerve activity in cachexia, and another has shown improvement in dietary intake with the use of propranolol to block the elevation of REE from this autonomic dysfunction.[50,51] Insulin-like growth factor and insulin have also been studied in an attempt to attenuate cancer cachexia and although they induced weight gain in other mice, they could not do so in those with colon tumors.[52] Some of the most promising effects on cachexia may come from eicosanoids and progestogens (see Nutritional Support of the Cancer Patient, later in this chapter).

Effects on Glucose Metabolism

Studies evaluating the effects of cytokine administration on the circulating glucose concentration indicate that the plasma glucose level rises or falls depending on the dose of cytokine administered, the temporal nature of the measurement, and the specific cytokine given. In rats, sublethal doses of TNF that do not produce hemodynamic changes result in the development of hyperglycemia within 1 hour of administration.[53] The increase in plasma glucose was only mild, however (20%), and was associated with an increase in the circulating concentration of glucagon, adrenocorticotropic hormone, corticosterone, and epinephrine, all of which can cause hyperglycemia. Further, incubation of adrenocortical cells with TNF stimulated cortisol secretion to the same extent, as did adrenocorticotropic hormone. Blood glucose was unchanged when a lower dose of TNF was used.[54] Similar changes in blood glucose levels are observed after IL-1 administration. At higher IL-1 doses, Fischer and colleagues[55] reported a rapid increase in blood glucose from 100 to 140 mg/dL within 1 hour. However, this increase was transient, with a return to baseline levels by 2 hours. Simultaneously, there was a several-fold increase in hindquarter (most likely skeletal muscle) glucose consumption that was also transient. In cultured muscle cells (L6 cell line), TNF-α stimulates glucose transport via a mechanism that involves *de novo* synthesis of glucose transporters that are inserted into the plasma membrane.[56] Simultaneously, there is depletion of cellular glycogen stores and an increase in lactate efflux, all of which are consistent with stimulation of anaerobic glycolysis.

Meszaros and colleagues[57] have studied tissue glucose utilization *in vivo* using the 2-deoxyglucose tracer technique in rats following infusion of a nonlethal dose of TNF. Glucose uptake was increased by 80% to 100% in liver, kidney, and spleen, skin (60%), lung (30% to 40%), and ileum (30% to 40%). The largest increase was observed in diaphragm (150%). No significant increase was observed in skeletal muscle, testis, or brain. These data indicate a marked increase in whole body glucose use following TNF administration. Acute exposure of pancreatic islets to IL-1β results in no change in glucose uptake but diminishes the rate of mitochondrial glucose oxidation, a response that is potentiated by TNF.[58] In response to IL-1β, islets exhibit an increase in insulin release in the presence of high glucose concentrations.

Effect on Fat Metabolism

Altered fat metabolism is apparent clinically in catabolic patients from the observation that fat stores are diminished in association with weight loss. It is likely that the loss of fat stores in cancer patients is due to the ability of TNF, IL-1, and LMF to mobilize fat stores. Bolus administration of TNF to rats causes an increase in serum triglyceride levels within 2 hours.[50] Greenberg and colleagues investigated the possible role of IL-6 and TNF in mediating the depleted fat stores that occur with malignancy-associated cachexia.[59] Injection of IL-6 and TNF each reduced adipose tissue lipoprotein lipase activity by more than 50%. Similarly, both IL-6 and TNF reduced heparin-releasable lipoprotein lipase activity in 3T3-L1 adipocytes in a dose-dependent manner by 50% to 70%. In addition to a reduction in adipocyte lipoprotein lipase activity, the increase in serum triglyceride levels that is observed after TNF administration is also due to stimulation of hepatic lipid secretion.[60–61]

The discovery of the LMF may either add to the lipid-mobilizing effects or be stimulated by the cytokines. Further study of this factor is needed to elucidate its full effects in cancer cachexia.

Regulation of Protein and Amino Acid Metabolism

Marked changes in protein and amino acid metabolism are characteristic of cancer patients, and a number of published studies have evaluated the effects of cytokines on muscle protein metabolism with conflicting results. When recombinant TNF was infused into cancer patients, forearm amino acid efflux was accelerated, consistent with net skeletal muscle proteolysis, although this accelerated nitrogen release could have been due to starvation effects.[58] Similarly, when Flores and colleagues infused radiolabeled leucine into rats receiving TNF, IL-1, or both using tracer methodology techniques, they found an increase in muscle protein degradation in cytokine-treated animals.[62] However, when the IL-1 activity in activated monocyte supernatants was blocked with specific anti–IL-1 antibodies, the accelerated protein breakdown was not attenuated, indicating a major role for other mediators.[63,64] Thus, although it is generally agreed that cytokine administration *in vivo* (at sufficient doses) stimulates net muscle proteolysis, it is unclear which distal mediators in the cytokine cascade are the key players (IL-6, LMF).

In contrast to whole animal studies, the majority of which indicate that *in vivo* administration of TNF or IL-1 results in net muscle proteolysis, *in vitro* studies have yielded negative results. In studies evaluating the effects of corticosterone on muscle protein breakdown, this glucocorticoid was noted to accelerate protein degradation and diminish protein synthesis. In combination with TNF, these steroid-mediated effects were augmented, but TNF alone did not alter protein turnover, indicating a helping role for the corticosteroid.[65]

In vitro and *in vivo* studies demonstrate that cytokines occupy an important role in mediating the hepatic metabolic response to malignant disease. Tumor-bearing rats display a global increase in Na^+-dependent amino acid transport, a response that can be attenuated by treatment with anti-TNF antibody.[66] Similar observations were made in animals treated with a single dose of TNF: Stimulation of hepatic amino acid transport systems A, ASC, and N were noted within 4 hours of TNF administration.[67,68] The increase in transport activity was due to an increase in carrier maximal transport velocity, consistent with the appearance of increased numbers of transport protein molecules in the plasma membrane. IL-6 and glucocorticoids have also been shown to work in a coordinated fashion to stimulate hepatic amino acid transport *in vivo*.[69] Moreover, these cytokines stimulate amino acid transport activity in cultured hepatocytes.[70]

NUTRITIONAL SUPPORT OF THE CANCER PATIENT

RATIONALE

Malnutrition is defined as any nutritional deficit that is associated with an increased risk of morbidity and mortality. There is a diminished risk of such events when the nutritional deficiency is corrected. Although it seems apparent that the provision of nutritional support to the malnourished patient with cancer is essential and would be beneficial, evidence indicating that currently available nutritional formulae *alone* can maintain or reverse malnutrition in the patient with advanced malignant disease is lacking. This observation suggests that many patients with cancer exhibit ongoing catabolism of body cell mass that persists and is refractory to nutritional repletion. Despite diminished food intake, the tumor-bearing host does not adapt to partial starvation by conserving lean body mass. Instead, the host continues to deplete its own muscle mass to provide amino acids taken up by the tumor to support growth and by the liver to support gluconeogenesis and biosynthesis of important defense proteins. The rationale behind the provision of specialized nutritional support, whether it be enteral or parenteral, is the belief that such support will preferentially benefit the patient rather than stimulate tumor growth. From a more practical standpoint, nutritional support would not be indicated if it clearly demonstrated no favorable effect on the response to antineoplastic therapies, no lengthening of the disease-free survival, or no improvement in the quality of life. Interestingly, a consensus of opinion regarding the role and efficacy of nutritional support in patients with cancer is lacking. Nonetheless, several well-designed clinical studies have allowed us to generate guidelines for the use of enteral and parenteral nutrition in patients with cancer, and most physicians and surgeons who care for patients with cancer continue to use nutritional support aggressively under specific circumstances.

Several studies have suggested additional therapies can be used along with nutritional support to alleviate the tumor cachexia. The synthetic progestogens, megestrol acetate (MA) and medroxyprogesterone acetate, may be helpful in high doses in the non–hormone-sensitive cancer with associated cachexia syndrome to decrease production of cytokines, particularly TNF and IL-6, as well as serotonin. These agents have been able to improve appetite, well-being, and quality of life as well as decreasing nausea and vomiting. MA has also been shown to increase body nonfluid weight gain although primarily with fat. Patients have been reported to respond with only 15 days of therapy with MA, and it may be discontinued after just 2 weeks of therapy. However, MA may be associated with more thromboembolic complications and there may have been less response to chemotherapeutic regimens.[71–80]

Other agents associated with a beneficial effect on the cachexia syndrome include eicosanoids and melatonin. Tisdale reported eicosapentaenoic acid, a component of fish oil, attenuated the action of cachectic factors and stabilized the weight loss and energy expenditure in patients with pancreatic cancer.[81] Reports from Japan show that maintained body weight was significantly greater in groups of mice treated with two different eicosanoids, docosahexanoic acid and eicosapentaenoic acid.[82] McMillan et al. reported that patients with advanced gastrointestinal cancers given ibuprofen, 1200 mg/d, in addition to MA, 480 mg/d, had an increase in body weight and no change in body water.[83] Lissoni et al. reported that melatonin has also been shown to decrease levels of TNF and lead to decreased weight loss in untreatable metastatic tumor patients and may therefore be helpful in treating cancer cachexia.[84] Gagnon and Bruera reviewed other treatment modalities for cancer cachexia and suggested drugs such as thalidomide and melatonin may be useful because of their effects on TNF. They also suggested β-adrenergic agonists might help as well because of their effect on muscle metabolism.[85]

NUTRITIONAL ASSESSMENT OF THE CANCER PATIENT

In order to determine the best strategies for treatment of the cancer patient, the nutritional status must first be determined. This is done by a careful history and physical examination followed by additional tests to confirm the clinical impression. The history should include inquiries about appetite, preferred foods, and weight loss. The physical examination can establish the diagnosis of muscle wasting and specific nutrient deficiencies. Anthropometric measurements should be done including measurement of body weight and height, skinfold thickness, and a 24-hour urine collection for the measurement of nitrogen. Peripheral blood lymphocyte count and skin testing to common antigens for assessment of delayed hypersensitivity have been used as indicators of immunocompetence in the cancer patient. Altered immunologic responses are not specific for nutritional deficiencies and are often observed even in patients with advanced malignant disease who are well nourished. Serum albumin and transferrin are the most common serum proteins measured. Other laboratory studies useful in nutritional assessment include red blood cell indices to determine iron and micronutrient deficiencies, plasma glucose to assess insulin resistance, blood urea nitrogen to determine renal status, and liver function tests to evaluate hepatic function.

NUTRITION AND TUMOR GROWTH

With the introduction of specialized enteral and parenteral feeding regimens into clinical medicine, aggressive nutritional support can be provided to cancer patients who previously could not or would not eat. However, concerns over the stimulation of tumor growth have existed for many years. While animal studies indicate that tumor growth can be enhanced with a high-protein diet and diminished by protein-depleted diets, studies in cancer patients are less clear. Baron and coworkers studied 14 malnourished patients with untreated head and neck squamous cell carcinoma who underwent biopsies of both normal and malignant tissues.[86] The patients were then randomized to either a control or TPN group. Cell-cycle kinetics were analyzed using flow cytometry after 3 to 17 days of TPN. After TPN, the percentage of hyperdiploid cells in malignant tissue was significantly increased over controls. It is likely that species differences exist and that different tumors respond dissimilarly to nutrient manipulation. If tumor growth is stimulated by nutritional or metabolic support, this could potentially be exploited with cycle-specific chemotherapeutic agents.

ENTERAL NUTRITION IN CANCER PATIENTS

Numerous clinical trials have evaluated the use of aggressive enteral nutritional support as adjunctive therapy during the administration of antineoplastic regimens to cancer patients, but well-designed studies make up a small fraction of these. Although these trials do not demonstrate any consistent benefits of enteral nutrition, most authorities would agree that enteral nutrition is always the preferred route of feeding cancer patients when the gastrointestinal tract is functional (Table 56.2-5). This can be accomplished by using in-between meal supplements, inserting soft comfortable nasogastric feeding tubes, or inserting gastrostomy or jejunostomy feeding catheters. Some of the better enteral clinical trials in cancer patients[87–98] are listed in Tables 56.2-6, 56.2-7, and 56.2-8. Commonly used enteral formulas are listed in Table 56.2-9. A physician order form for enteral nutrition is presented in Figure 56.2-1.

TABLE 56.2-5. Proposed Benefits of Oral and Enteral Nutrition versus Parenteral Nutrition

Maintain gut mucosal mass
Maintain brush border enzyme activity
Support gut immune function
Preserve gut mucosal barrier function
Maintain a balanced luminal microflora environment
Improve outcome after chemotherapy and radiation therapy

TOTAL PARENTERAL NUTRITION IN THE CANCER PATIENT: GENERAL RECOMMENDATIONS

Although the initial enthusiasm for the use of TPN in cancer patients was considerable, it is now clear that TPN should only be provided to selected patients. Because of the failure of numerous clinical trials to yield a consensus with regard to the efficacy of TPN in cancer patients[89,99–123] (see Tables 56.2-6, 56.2-7, and 56.2-8), more recently published articles have used metaanalysis to review these studies collectively and generate feeding guidelines. The general conclusion has been that parenteral nutrition appears to be of little benefit in most cancer populations. In some patients, the use of TPN was associated with an increase in complications. However, the most important factor to consider when making decisions about the use of TPN in patients with cancer is the response of the tumor to antineoplastic therapy. It is anticipated that the guidelines listed in Table 56.2-10 will undergo future revision, as more effective antitumor regimens become clinically available.

SPECIFIC INDICATIONS FOR THE USE OF TOTAL PARENTERAL NUTRITION IN THE CANCER PATIENT

Patients with Enterocutaneous Fistulas

Patients with cancer who undergo major gastrointestinal surgery occasionally develop enterocutaneous fistulas that preclude the use of the gastrointestinal tract for nutritional support. In such patients, enteral nutrition often stimulates fistula output and can result in metabolic disturbances and dehydration. TPN can affect the course of disease in cancer patients with gastrointestinal fistulas. Studies indicate that TPN increases the spontaneous closure rate of enterocutaneous fistulas, although fistulas that originate from radiated or neoplastic bowel have a much lower rate of spontaneous closure. In such patients, aggressive early surgical treatment is generally indicated. Provision of TPN maintains the nutritional status of the cancer patient who develops an enterocutaneous fistula such that he or she better tolerates operative intervention if closure does not occur. Perhaps insulin-like growth factor or a progestogen may help in this situation.

Patients with Hepatic or Renal Failure

Patients with cancer occasionally develop liver failure after major surgery or from cytotoxic chemotherapy. Because of liver damage and portasystemic shunting, these patients

TABLE 56.2-6. Results of Major Prospective Randomized Controlled Trials Evaluating Perioperative Nutrition

			No. of Patients		*Major Complications (%)*		*Perioperative Mortality (%)*	
Author	*Tumor Type*	*Total Parenteral Nutrition Course*	Total Parenteral Nutrition	Control	Total Parenteral Nutrition	Control	Total Parenteral Nutrition	Control
PARENTERAL NUTRITION								
Holter and Fischer[99]	Gastrointestinal	3 d preoperative 10 d postoperative	30	26	4 (13)	5 (19)	2 (7)	2 (8)
Heatley et al.[100]	Esophageal, gastric	7–10 d preoperative	38	36	2 (5) 3 (8) 9 (24)	3 (8) 11 (31) 16 (44)	6 (16)	8 (22)
Yamada et al.[101]	Gastric	18 d postoperative	18	16	1 (6)	5 (31)	0 (0)	1 (6)
Askanazi et al.[102]	Bladder	7 d postoperative	22	13	1 (5)	0 (0)	0 (0)	2 (15)
Müller et al.[103]	Esophageal	10 d preoperative	58	55	8 (14)	17 (31)	4 (7)	11 (20)
Bellantone et al.[104,105]	Gastrointestinal	7 d preoperative	49	51	13 (27)	18 (35)	1 (2)	2 (4)
Woolfson and Smith[106]	Oropharyngeal, esophageal, gastric, bladder	6 d postoperative	62	60	12	7	8 (13)	8 (13)
Buzby et al.[107,130]	Gastrointestinal Lung	7–15 d preoperative 3 d postoperative	192	203	49 (26)	50 (25)	16 (8)	12 (6)
Sandstrom et al.[108]	Gastrointestinal, bladder	Postoperative	150	150	227	163	12 (8)	10 (7)
von Meyenfeldt et al.[89]	Gastric, colorectal	10 d preoperative	51	50	5 (10)	8 (16)	NR	NR
Sclafani et al.[109]	Pancreas	5–20 d postoperative	24	27	9 (38)	12 (44)	2 (8)	
ENTERAL NUTRITION								
Shukla et al.[87]	Gastrointestinal, breast, oropharyngeal	10 d nasogastric feeding preoperative	67	43	7 (10)	16 (37)	4 (6)	5 (12)
Smith et al.[88]	Gastrointestinal	10 d needle catheter jejunostomy feeding postoperative	25	25	11 (44)	9 (36)	4 (17)	1 (4)
Foschi et al.[131]	Upper gastrointestinal	12 d ND feeding postoperative	28	32	5 (18)	15 (47)	1 (4)	4 (13)
von Meyenfeldt et al.[89]	Gastric, colorectal	10 d preoperative	50	50	6 (12)	8 (16)	NR	NR

ND, nasoduodenal; NR, not reported.

develop derangements in their circulating levels of amino acids. The plasma aromatic to branched chain amino acid ratio is increased. Transport of amino acids across the blood–brain barrier favors the aromatic amino acids such as tryptophan, precursors for *false neurotransmitters* such as serotonin, which contribute to lethargy and encephalopathy. Treatment of individuals with liver failure with solutions enriched in branched chain amino acids and deficient in aromatic amino acids may result in improved tolerance to the administered protein and clinical improvement in the encephalopathic state.

TPN with amino acids of high biologic value may also be of value in patients with acute renal failure. Presumably, provision of only essential amino acids allows the body to maximally reuse nitrogen for the synthesis of nonessential amino acids and thereby helps prevent rapid increases in blood urea nitrogen. If the hypermetabolic cancer patient is receiving dialysis, there appears to be no advantage to using an essential amino acid solution and therefore a balanced standard amino acid formulation is recommended. Solutions containing branched chain amino acids or just essential amino acids are expensive and probably not worth the cost except in specific patients in whom adjusted standard formulas are not tolerated.

Acute Radiation and Chemotherapy Enteritis

Cancer patients who receive abdominal or pelvic irradiation or chemotherapy may develop severe and prolonged mucositis and enterocolitis, precluding use of the gastrointestinal tract for nutritional support. Under these circumstances, TPN should be provided to malnourished patients until the enteritis resolves and oral feeding can be resumed. Moreover, under circumstances in which chemotherapy has been contraindicated secondary to severe malnutrition, TPN may be beneficial in optimizing nutritional status and allowing the initiation of the chemotherapeutic regimen. When enteral nutrition is feasible in such patients, TPN has not demonstrated a treatment advantage. When studies have been performed using well-nourished patients, the effects of TPN predictably have not been beneficial.

Patients undergoing radiation treatment may also develop malnutrition secondary to inadequate nutritional intake from

TABLE 56.2-7. Results of Prospective Randomized Controlled Trials in Patients Treated with Radiation Therapy

Author	Tumor Type	No. of Patients		Survival		Treatment Toxicity	
		NS	Control	NS	Control	Heme	Gastrointestinal
PARENTERAL NUTRITION TRIALS							
Solassol et al.[110]	Ovarian	42	39	9 mo	8 mo (median)	Not reported	Better
Kinsella et al.[111]	Pelvic	17	15	47%	47%	Not reported	Not reported
Ghavimi et al.[112]	Childhood	14	14	27%	29%	Worse	Worse
Donaldson et al.[113]	Childhood	12	13	8%	8% (posttherapy)	Not reported	Worse
ENTERAL NUTRITION TRIALS							
Douglass et al.[90]	Gastrointestinal	13	17	62%	76%	No difference	Not reported
Brown et al.[91]	Pelvic	30	17	Not reported	Not reported	Better	No difference
Bounous et al.[92]	Abdomen/pelvic	9	9	Not reported	Not reported	Better	Better
Daly et al.[93]	Head and neck	22	18	Not reported	Not reported	Not reported	Worse
Moloney et al.[94]	Various	42	42	36%	38%	Not reported	Not reported

NS, nutritional support.

an inability to eat. The potential side effects from radiotherapy are broad and include nausea, vomiting, malnutrition, mucositis, xerostomia, dysphagia, diarrhea, and anorexia. Whenever possible, the enteral route is preferable for nutritional support. However, in cases involving severe dysfunction of the gastrointestinal tract, TPN is indicated. TPN can be useful in allowing the malnourished, poor-risk patient to complete radiotherapy with less morbidity. Patients undergoing irradiation of the head, neck, or chest need to be considered for early tube placement so enteral nutrition can be used.

Use of Perioperative Total Parenteral Nutrition in Cancer Patients

One of the best studies to date evaluating the effects of preoperative TPN was published by the Veterans Affairs Total Parenteral Nutrition Cooperative Study Group.[107] More than 3500 patients, many of whom had cancer, were entered into this prospective randomized trial. The patients were divided into one of four groups: well-nourished, borderline malnourished, moderately malnourished, or severely malnourished. Patients in each malnourished category were randomized to at least 7 days of preoperative TPN or immediate operation. Patients randomized to receive TPN received 1000 kcal/d in excess of calculated caloric requirements. Lipid was provided on a daily basis. One criticism of this study was that patients were allowed to eat in addition to receiving parenteral feedings. Analysis of the data from this study indicated that there was no difference in short-term or long-term survival among groups. Infectious complications including pneumonia, abscess, and line sepsis were statistically significantly higher in patients receiving TPN. Noninfectious complications (impaired wound healing) were significantly lower only in those patients receiving TPN who were in the severely malnourished group (greater than 15% weight loss and serum albumin less than 2.8 mg%). This study strongly suggests that preoperative TPN should be limited to the severely malnourished patient. Therefore, contraindications to the use of preoperative TPN should include patients requiring emergency operation and those who are only mildly or moderately malnourished.

In the few patients who are candidates for preoperative nutritional support, we recommend instituting TPN only if the gastrointestinal tract cannot be used for tube feedings. In most patients undergoing major abdominal surgery, feeding tubes may be placed intraoperatively if resumption of oral feedings is not anticipated for relatively lengthy periods of time (7 to 10 days) after surgery. TPN may also be required in the well-nourished cancer patient who develops a postoperative complication that precludes enteral support. For example, some cancer patients develop a prolonged ileus after an abdominal procedure that precludes the use of the intestinal tract as a route of feeding. Such an occurrence is generally unpredictable and the cause of the ileus is often not demonstrated. If the patient is unable to eat by postoperative day 7, TPN should be considered. The ileus may persist for several weeks, especially in gastric or pancreatic cancer patients. Although provision of TPN does not influence the disease process per se, it is beneficial because it prevents further erosion of lean body mass.

Two prospective studies have helped to further clarify both the indications and contraindications for the use of TPN in the surgical patient with cancer. Brennan and colleagues[124] examined the use of routine postoperative TPN following major pancreatic resection. In patients randomized to receive TPN starting on postoperative day 1, the investigators found a statistically significant increase in the incidence of intraabdominal abscesses as well as a tendency toward an increased incidence of peritonitis and bowel obstruction. The control group received a peripheral infusion of dextrose rather than luminal nutrition, suggesting that the increase in complications was not due to the absence of luminal nutrients but rather to some toxic effect of the TPN. The authors concluded that routine use of postoperative TPN was not indicated and may in fact have harmful side effects. It should be noted that many surgeons would elect to place a feeding jejunostomy in such patients.

In contrast to the Brennan study, Fan and colleagues[125] studied the use of perioperative (starting 7 days before the planned procedure) TPN for patients undergoing hepatectomy for hepatocellular carcinoma. They found that patients

TABLE 56.2-8. Results of Prospective Randomized Controlled Trials Evaluating Nutritional Therapy in Patients Receiving Chemotherapy

Author	*Tumor Type*	*No. of Patients*		*Survival*		*Tumor Response (%)*		*Treatment Toxicity*		*Infection Rate (%)*	
		TPN/EN	Control	TPN/EN	Control	TPN/EN	Control	Heme	Gastrointestinal	TPN/EN	Control
PARENTERAL NUTRITION											
Nixon et al.[114,115]	Colorectal	20	25	79	308 (mean)	15	12	Worse	No difference	5	4
Samuels et al.[116]	Testicular	16	14	72%	77% (2.5 y)	63	79	Better	No difference	17	4
Shamberger et al.[117,118]	Sarcoma	14	18	13%	44% (4 y)	14	50	No difference	No difference	42	33
Valdivieso et al.[119,120]	Small cell lung	30	35	11 mo	12 mo (median)	43	66	No difference	Worse	27	18
Clamon et al.[121]	Small cell lung	57	62	51%	57% (1 y)	48	43	Better	N/A	35	5
Issell et al.[122]	Squamous cell lung	13	13	NR	NR	31	8	Better	Better	N/A	N/A
Jordan et al.[123]	Adenocarcinoma lung	19	24	22 wk	40 wk (median)	12	30	Worse	No difference	32	8
ENTERAL NUTRITION											
Elkort et al.[95]	Breast	24	23	84%	87% (1 y)	No difference		No difference	No difference		
Evans et al.[96]	Non–small cell	30	36	8 mo	6 mo (median)	28	15	NR	NR		
	Lung	30		7 mo		20		NR			
Evans et al.[96]	Colorectal	21	33	9 mo	24 mo (median)	10	16	NR	No difference		
Tandon et al.[97]	Gastrointestinal	31	39	94%	85%	35	21	NR	Better		
Bounous et al.[98]	Metastatic	9	12	NR	NR	56	64	No difference	No difference		

EN, enteral nutrition; NR, not reported; TPN, total parenteral nutrition.

TABLE 56.2-9. Adult Nutrition: Physician Order Form for Tube Feedings[a]

	Adult Nutrition Enteral Products Formulary								
	Tube Feedings, Lactose Free					*Modular Supplements (Tube Feeding or Oral)*			
	Standard Isotonic with Fiber	High Protein	Very High Protein with Fiber	High Calorie, Low Volume	Semielemental	Carbohydrate Module	Fat, Medium-Chain Triglyceride Module	Fat, Long-Chain Triglyceride Module	Protein Module
Description per L	(Nutren 1.0 with fiber)	(Probalance)	(Replete with fiber)	(Deliver 2.0)	(Peptamen VHP)	(Polycose, per oz)	(MCT oil, per oz)	(Microlipid, per oz)	(Pro Mod, per Scoop[b])
Protein (g)/kcal (nonprotein)	40/840	54/984	63/750	75/1700	63/750	0/60	0/230	0/135	5/8
Nonprotein kcal:N ratio	131:1	114:1	75:1	145:1	75:1	N/A	N/A	N/A	N/A
Volume (mL) to meet recommended daily allowance	1500	1000	1000	1000	1500	N/A	N/A	N/A	N/A
Caloric density (kcal/mL)	1.0	1.2	1.0	2.0	1.0	2.0	7.7	4.5	N/A
Carbohydrate (g)/% kcal (nonprotein)	127/60% (14 g dietary fiber)	156/63%	113/60% (14 g dietary fiber)	200/47%	104/55%	15/100%	0/0%	0/0%	(0.7 g)
Fat (g)/% kcal (nonprotein)	38/40%	41/37%	34/40%	102/53%	39/45%	0/0%	28/100%	15/100%	(0.6 g)
Protein composition	Calcium and potassium caseinate	Calcium and potassium caseinate	Calcium and potassium caseinate	Calcium and sodium caseinate	Enzymatically hydrolyzed whey	N/A	N/A	N/A	Whey
Fat composition	Canola oil, MCT oil (24%), corn oil	Canola oil, MCT (20%), corn oil	Canola oil, MCT oil (25%)	Soybean oil, MCT oil (30%)	MCT oil (70%), soy oil	N/A	MCT oil (>96%)	Safflower oil	N/A
Carbohydrate composition	Maltodextrins, corn syrup solids, soy polysaccharides	Maltodextrin, corn syrup solids, sucrose	Maltodextrin sucrose, soy, polysaccharides	Corn syrup	Maltodextrin, sucrose, starch	Hydrolyzed cornstarch	N/A	N/A	0.3 g lactose
Sodium (mg/mEq)	876/38	759/33	876/38	800/35	560/24	21/<1	0	N/A	15/1
Potassium mg/mEq	1248/32	1521/39	1500/38	1700/43	1500/38	2/<1	0	N/A	66/2
Phosphorus (mg/mm)	668/21	1000/32	1000/32	1000/32	700/22	1/<1	0	N/A	30/1
Magnesium (mg)	268	400	400	400	296	0	0	N/A	0
Vitamin K (μg)	50	80	50	250	80	0	0	N/A	0
Percent free water	84	82	84	71	84	70	0	44	N/A
Osmolality (mOsm/kg)	303	590	390	640	430	630	0	80	30

	Oral Supplements, Lactose Free				*Oral Supplements, Lactose Containing*			
	High Calorie	Elemental	Hi-Pro Liquid	Hi-Pro Gelatin	Hi-Cal Milkshake	Hi-Pro Sugar Free	Low-Pro, Lo-Electrolyte	Hi-Pro Pudding
Description per L	(Nutren 1.5)[c]	(Vivonex TEN)[e]	(Sustacal, per 240-mL serving)	(Delmark, per 4-oz serving)	(Shake-up Plus, per 6-oz serving)[c]	Instant Breakfast, per 9-oz serving[c]	(Renal Shake, per 400-mL serving)	(Delmark, per 5-oz serving)
Protein (g)/ kcal (nonprotein)	60/1260	38/847	15/185	12/104	9/214	12/171	2/569	9/212

Nonprotein kcal: N ratio	131:1	149:1	78:1	56:1	149:1	89:1	1778:1	149:1
Volume (mL) to meet recommended daily allowance	1000	2000	1080	Incomplete feeding	Incomplete feeding	Incomplete feeding	Incomplete feeding	750
Caloric density (kcal/mL)	1.5	1.0	1.0	1.3	1.4	0.8	1.2	1.7
Carbohydrate (g)	169	206	33	26	40	24	95	35
Fat (g)	68	3	6	<1	6	8[d]	21	8
Protein composition	Calcium and potassium caseinate	Free amino acids	Sodium and calcium caseinate, soy protein isolate	Egg albumin, gelatin	Nonfat and whole milk, calcium caseinate	Nonfat and whole milk	Milk solids, whey	Nonfat dry milk, sodium caseinate
Fat composition	MCT oil (48%), canola oil, corn oil	Safflower oil	Soy oil	Vegetable oil	Whole milk, cream	Whole milk[d]	Soy oil, milk fat	Partially hydrogenated soy oil
Carbohydrate composition	Maltodextrin, corn syrup solids	Maltodextrin, modified starch	Sucrose, corn syrup	Maltodextrin, sucrose	High fructose corn syrup, lactose	Maltodextrin, lactose, aspartame	Sucrose, lactose hydrolyzed corn starch, fructose, corn sweeteners	Sucrose dextrose modified food starch, lactose
Sodium (mg/mEq)	1170/51	460/20	220/10	120/5	135/6	210/9	108/5	140/6
Potassium (mg/mEq)	1872/48	782/20	490/13	140/4	350/9	590/15	130/3	725/19
Phosphorus (mg/mm)	1002/31	500/16	220/7	140/5	300/10	338/11	73/2	250/8
Magnesium (mg)	400	200	90	N/A	100	113	N/A	N/A
Vitamin K (μg)	75	22	56	Trace	N/A	N/A	N/A	N/A
Free water	78	85	84	N/A	N/A	N/A	N/A	N/A
Osmolality (mOsm/kg)	510	630	650	711	N/A	N/A	N/A	N/A

[a]Note to physicians: Most patients can tolerate initial tube feedings with full-strength standard isotonic with fiber formula at 30 to 50 mL/hr × 24 hours.
[b]Scoop = 6.6 g.
[c]Nutrient analysis for vanilla flavor, other flavors available.
[d]Fat source is whole milk; if mixed with skim milk, vanilla contains 0 g fat; other flavors vary.
[e]Mixed according to package instructions.
MCT, medium-chain triglyceride.

PennState Health System

The Milton S. Hershey Medical Center

ADULT NUTRITION: PHYSICIAN ORDER FORM
TUBE FEEDINGS

Instructions to physician:

Complete this form to initiate tube feedings or change formula type. Changes in rate and strength may be made directly on the physician order sheet.

Formula type: (Check below)
See reverse of the order form or current Adult Nutrition Enteral Products Formulary for brand name and nutrient content of specific products.

- ☐ Standard Isotonic with Fiber
- ☐ High Protein with Fiber
- ☐ Very High Protein with Fiber
- ☐ High Calorie, Low Volume
- ☐ High Calorie
- ☐ 1:1 mixture of specified products (Select 2)
- ☐ Elemental
- ☐ Semi-Elemental
- ☐ Other:____________

MANDATORY NUTRITION SUPPORT TEAM CONSULT WITH HIGHLIGHTED FORMULAS

Additives:
- ☐ Carbohydrate module:_______ml/liter or _______ml/day
- ☐ Fat - LCT module:_______ml/liter or _________ml/day
- ☐ Protein module:_______scoops/liter or _______scoops/day

Prescription: (Check one)
- ☐ *Continuous or cyclic infusion_______strength at_______ml/hr x _______hrs/day*
- ☐ *Intermittent or bolus infusion_______ml over_______hrs_______times daily*

Route of Administration: (Check one)
- ☐ Oro/Nasogastric
- ☐ Transpyloric
- ☐ Gastrostomy
- ☐ Jejunostomy
- ☐ Other

Infusion Method: (Check one)
- ☐ Enteral feeding pump
- ☐ Gravity drip
- ☐ Bolus

Verify tube placement via KUB before use: (Complete x-ray form for KUB)
Consult Clinical Nutrition for nutrition assessment.
Oral diet in addition to Tube Feeding:______________________________
Other Orders: (Check as needed)
- ☐ Aspiration precautions: (for gastric feedings) Check residuals q 4 hrs. Tolerate residual to 150 ml. Hold feeding for 1 hr. if residual > than 150 ml, resume feedings when residual <150 ml. Elevate head of bed 30-40° or reverse Trendelenburg position unless contraindicated. Add blue food coloring to tube feeding solution.
- ☐ Flush feeding tube with 15 ml tap water before and after medication administration per feeding tube and before and after residual checks.
  - ☐ For continuous feedings: Flush feeding tube with _______ml tap water q 8 hours
  - ☐ For intermittent feedings: Flush feeding tube with _______ml tap water before and after feeding administration.
- ☐ Check labs with next lab draw: Albumin, transferrin, prealbumin, phosphorus, and magnesium.
- ☐ Concurrent phenytoin (Dilantin) administration p.o. or per feeding tube: Hold continuous tube feeding 1 hour before and after phenytoin administration.
- ☐ Initiate discharge teaching for home tube feeding.

FIGURE 56.2-1. Enteral order sheet. KUB, kidney, ureter, bladder; LCT, long-chain triglyceride.

randomized to receive perioperative TPN had a statistically significant reduction in infectious complications and a decreased diuretic requirement compared with similar patients who did not receive TPN. The significance of this study is that it is only one of two studies that show a benefit to the use of routine perioperative TPN in patients not suffering from severe malnutrition. In addition, it establishes a distinct group of patients in whom routine perioperative TPN may be of benefit. The mechanism by which TPN is of value in these patients is not known.

Patients with Short Bowel Syndrome

Cancer patients may develop short bowel syndrome secondary to multiple bowel resections or massive resection of infarcted

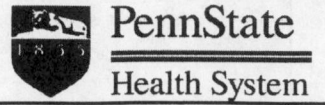

TABLE 56.2-10. Indications for the Use of Total Parenteral Nutrition in the Cancer Patient

A. TPN for brief, inhospital periods (7–10 days)
   1. TPN is not indicated:
      a. In well-nourished or mildly malnourished patients undergoing chemotherapy, radiation therapy, or surgery.
      b. In patients with rapidly progressive malignant disease who fail to respond to treatment and in those patients who have evidence of terminal disease and are not candidates for further antitumor therapy.
   2. TPN is indicated:
      a. In severely malnourished patients who are responding to chemotherapy or in those in whom gastrointestinal or other toxicities preclude adequate enteral intake for 7–10 days or a longer period. Available evidence would suggest that patients who are candidates for TPN under these circumstances should, when feasible, receive TPN before or in conjunction with the institution of therapy.

B. Prolonged periods of inhospital TPN or home TPN
   1. TPN is not indicated:
      a. In patients with rapidly progressive tumor growth that is unresponsive to therapy.
   2. TPN is indicated:
      a. In those patients for whom treatment-associated toxicities preclude the use of enteral nutrition and represent the primary impediment to the restoration of performance status. Such patients usually respond to antitumor therapy.
      b. In selected malnourished cancer patients in whom the natural history of the disease can be expected to permit a period of normal or near normal performance status. Such patients should be receiving antitumor therapy with a reasonable anticipation of response, or the natural history of the untreated tumor is such that a reasonable quality of life can be expected (survival greater than 6–12 months).

TPN, total parenteral nutrition.

bowel. Most of these patients, if cured of their cancer, can now survive for long periods on home TPN. Due to the duration of therapy involved, these patients are at risk for developing long-term problems such as micronutrient deficiency, bone demineralization, or line sepsis. Studies by Wilmore and colleagues[126] have demonstrated that the requirement for TPN could be decreased or even eliminated in patients with short gut syndrome by providing a nutritional regimen consisting of supplemental glutamine, growth hormone, and a modified oral high-carbohydrate, low-fat diet. There was a marked improvement in the absorption of nutrients with this combination therapy and a decrease in stool output. In addition, TPN requirements were reduced by 50%, as were the costs associated with care of these individuals. Discontinuation of the growth hormone did not increase TPN needs in these patients once they had undergone successful gut rehabilitation.

COMPOSITION OF TOTAL PARENTERAL NUTRITION FORMULATIONS

TPN solutions are administered through a central venous catheter that is generally inserted into the subclavian vein. TPN solutions are hyperosmolar and calorie dense (1 kcal/mL), and the infusion of 2.0 to 2.5 L/d provides 2000 to 2500 kcal/d. The addition of minerals, vitamins, and electrolytes completes the basic composition of the solution (Table 56.2-11). Solutions must be prepared under sterile conditions. Because of the hyperosmolarity of such solutions, they must be delivered into a high flow system to prevent venous sclerosis. As a general rule, 65% of total nonprotein calories should be provided as dextrose and 35% in the form of an intravenous fat emulsion. Patients receiving TPN should be monitored regularly by measuring blood sugar, serum electrolytes, triglycerides, and liver function test results. The amounts of the various electrolytes provided to cancer patients receiving TPN may vary depending on factors such as previous nutritional and hydration status. Careful monitoring is critical because severe hypokalemia or hypophosphatemia can develop with aggressive feedings. Hypophosphatemia may develop in the chronically malnourished cachectic cancer patient given dextrose infusion who uses the phosphate to make adenosine triphosphate. This is referred to as the *refeeding syndrome.* These electrolyte disturbances can develop rapidly and are much more life-threatening than hyponatremia. Critical drops in serum phosphate levels below 1.5 mmol/dL can lead to an irreversible cardiac arrest.

TABLE 56.2-11. Composition of a Standard Central Venous Solution

Volume	
Amino acids	500 mL
Dextrose	300 mL (50%)
Fat emulsion 20%	125 mL
Electrolytes + vitamins + minerals	Approximately 50 mL
Total volume	Approximately 1000 mL
Composition	
Amino acids	50 g
Dextrose	600 kcal (150 g)
Fat	250 kcal
Total nitrogen	50/6.25 = 8 g
mOsm/L	Approximately 2000
Standard electrolytes	
Na	37 mEq
K	30 mEq
Ca	5 mEq
Mg	5 mEq
Cl	30 mEq
Acetate	35 mEq
Phosphate	9 mmol
General rules	
Protein	1.0–1.5 g/kg/d
Volume	10 mL/g
Nonprotein calories	25 kcal/kg/d
Minimum volume	0.5 mL/kcal
Dextrose	65% of calories (must be at least 40%)
Fat	35% of calories

TABLE 56.2-12. Complications Associated with the Use of Total Parenteral Nutrition

Complication	*Cause*	*Treatment*
MECHANICAL		
Pneumothorax	Puncture/laceration of lung pleura	Serial radiographs; chest tube if indicated
Subclavian artery injury	Penetration of subclavian artery during needle stick	Radiography; serial monitoring of vital signs
Air embolism	Aspiration of air into the vein and right-sided heart	Place patient in Trendelenburg subclavian left lateral decubitus; aspirate air
Catheter embolization	Shearing off the tip when withdrawing catheter	Retrieve catheter transvenously under fluoroscopic guidance
Venous thrombosis	Clot formation in great vein secondary to catheter	Heparinization if clinically significant
Catheter malposition	Tip of catheter directed into internal jugular or opposite subclavian	Reposition under fluoroscopy
METABOLIC		
Hyperglycemia	Excessive glucose calories or glucose intolerance	Decrease glucose calories; administer insulin
Hypoglycemia	Sudden cessation of total parenteral nutrition	Bolus 50% glucose solution, monitor blood glucose
Carbon dioxide retention	Infusion of glucose calories in excess of energy needs	Decrease glucose calories and replace with fat
Hyperglycemic, hyperosmolar, nonketotic coma	Dehydration from excessive diuresis, excess Na administration	Discontinue total parenteral nutrition immediately; give insulin; monitor glucose/lytes
Hyperchloremic metabolic acidosis	Excessive chloride administration	Give Na and K as acetate salts
Azotemia	Excessive amino acid administration with inadequate calories	Decrease amino acids; increase glucose calories
Essential fatty acid deficiency	Inadequate essential fatty acid administration	Administer fat solution
Hypertriglyceridemia	Rapid fat infusion or decreased fat clearance	Slow rate of fat infusion
Hypophosphatemia, hypocalcemia, hypomagnesemia, hypokalemia	Inadequate administration of electrolyte in question	Increase administration
Bleeding	Vitamin K deficiency	Administer vitamin K
SEPTIC		
Line sepsis	Catheter tip infected	Remove catheter; antibiotics
Infection at skin site	Bacteria at site of catheter entry into skin	Remove catheter; local wound care

POTENTIAL COMPLICATIONS OF TOTAL PARENTERAL NUTRITION

Advances in technology, monitoring, and catheter care have greatly reduced the incidence of complications associated with the use of TPN. The establishment of a nutritional support team (physician, dietitian, nurse, and pharmacist) and the recognition of such a team as an important part of overall patient care have also been key factors in reducing complications. Complications of TPN that occur in cancer patients can be divided into three types: (1) mechanical (i.e., pneumothorax, laceration of the subclavian artery, air embolism, catheter embolism); (2) metabolic (hyperglycemia, electrolyte abnormalities, abnormalities in liver enzymes); and (3) infectious (catheter sepsis). These complications are listed in Table 56.2-12. The management of the patient who develops signs and symptoms of catheter sepsis is shown in Figure 56.2-2.

EFFECTS OF TOTAL PARENTERAL NUTRITION ON THE GASTROINTESTINAL TRACT

Although the intestinal tract had long been considered an organ of inactivity in critically ill patients, this concept has clearly been shown to be invalid. Disuse of the gastrointestinal tract, either via starvation or nutritional support by TPN, may lead to numerous physiologic derangements as well as changes in gut microflora, impaired gut immune function, and disruption of the integrity of the mucosal barrier. Thus, maintaining gut function in the cancer patient who is receiving vigorous therapy may be essential in order to minimize septic complications and organ failure.

The majority of studies that have examined the effects of TPN on intestinal function and immunity have been done in animals. These studies clearly demonstrate that TPN is detrimental and related to intestinal disuse. In rats receiving TPN, villous atrophy develops and there appears to be a breakdown in the gut mucosal barrier. TPN results in significant disruption of the intestinal microflora and bacterial translocation from the gut lumen to the mesenteric lymph nodes. In addition, when insults such as chemotherapy or radiation are introduced into these models, animals on TPN have a much higher mortality. This body of literature suggests that under certain circumstances, TPN may predispose patients to an increase in gut-derived infectious complications. Whether these are related to bacterial translocation or just absorption of endotoxin or cytokines is still debated.

IMPROVING THE EFFICACY OF CURRENT FEEDING REGIMENS

Role of Ambulation

Patients with cancer may be bedridden, but should be encouraged to ambulate as much as is feasible. Exercise can increase functional aerobic capacity, stimulate skeletal muscle amino acid

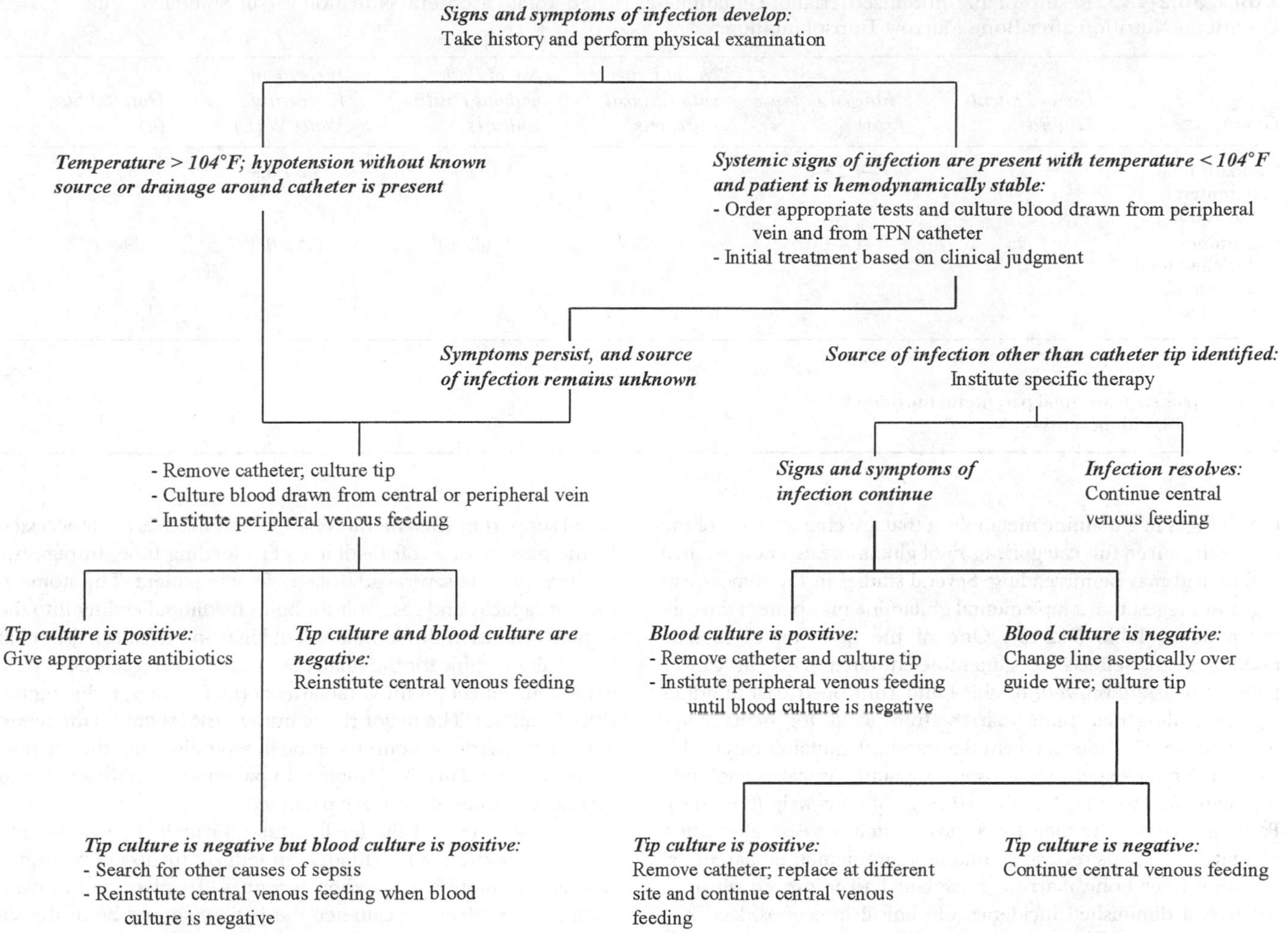

FIGURE 56.2-2. Algorithm for the evaluation of a cancer patient on total parenteral nutrition (TPN) who develops signs and symptoms of sepsis.

uptake, and reduce proteolysis in normal individuals receiving TPN. It is unclear whether higher exercise thresholds are necessary to induce anabolism in nutritionally depleted cancer patients, although a higher threshold does seem to reduce fatigue.

Pharmacologic and Hormonal Therapy

The potential beneficial effects of the administration of insulin, the primary anabolic hormone in the body, to the tumor-bearing host has been studied because of its role in stimulating muscle amino acid uptake and protein synthesis. Studies indicate that treatment with insulin stimulates food intake and nitrogen retention without stimulating tumor growth. Likewise, administration of insulin in combination with the glutamine antimetabolite acivicin to tumor-bearing rats on TPN preserved lean body mass and retarded tumor growth. Whether these observations can be extrapolated to the clinical arena is unknown.

The availability of recombinant human growth hormone has led investigators to examine the role of this anabolic agent in patients. The present data indicate that growth hormone is capable of promoting accrual of lean body mass in healthy individuals. It is unclear whether this anabolism will be observed in cachectic cancer patients. A potential downside to the use of growth hormone in patients is its association with the development of lymphoid malignancies. In tumor-bearing rats, treatment with exogenous growth hormone has been shown to increase carcass weight and improve the host immune response. Additional studies that examine the effects of growth hormone on tumor growth parameters are necessary before clinical use of this drug is justifiable.

Additional research using the progestogens MA and medroxyprogesterone acetate, as well as melatonin, is needed to assess the value of their use in treating or preventing cancer cachexia. Current recommendations for MA are 480 mg/d in addition to nutritional support.

Use of Glutamine and Arginine

The classification of glutamine as a nonessential or nutritionally dispensable amino acid implies that, in its absence from the diet, it can be synthesized in adequate quantities from other amino acids and precursors. For this reason, and because of the relative instability and short shelf life of glutamine compared with other amino acids, it has not been considered necessary to include glutamine in nutritional formulas. Glutamine has been eliminated from TPN solutions and with few exceptions, glutamine is present in oral and enteral diets only at the relatively low levels characteristic of its concentration in most dietary proteins. Based on our knowledge of

TABLE 56.2-13. Results of a Randomized Trial of Glutamine-Enriched Total Parenteral Nutrition versus Standard Total Parenteral Nutrition after Bone Marrow Transplantation[a]

Group	*No. of Patients Studied*	*Nitrogen Balance (g/d)*	*No. of Patients with Clinical Infections*	*No. of Patients without Positive Cultures*	*Increase in Extracellular Water W (L)*	*Hospital Stay (d)*
Standard total parenteral nutrition	21	−4.2 ± 1.2	9 (43%)	1 (5%)	3.2 ± 0.9	36 ± 2
Glutamine-enriched total parenteral nutrition	25	−1.4 ± 0.5[c]	3(12%)[b]	0 (42%)[b]	0.4 ± 0.9[b]	29 ± 1[b]

[a]Data analysis by unpaired t-test or Fisher's exact test.
[b]$P<.05$.
[c]$P<.01$ versus standard total parenteral nutrition.
(From ref. 79, with permission.)

the changes in glutamine metabolism that are characteristic of the host with cancer, this categorization of glutamine as a nonessential amino acid may be misleading. Several studies in the tumor-bearing host suggest that supplemental glutamine may benefit the cancer patient (Table 56.2-13). One of the best studies to date evaluating the effects of glutamine-enriched TPN in cancer patients is a randomized, double-blind controlled trial in adults receiving allogeneic bone marrow transplants for hematologic malignancies.[127] Patients received a standard, glutamine-free TPN solution or an experimental isonitrogenous, isocaloric solution supplemented with L-glutamine (0.57 g/kg body weight per day). Patients received the diets for approximately 4 weeks after transplantation. Patients receiving glutamine-supplemented parenteral nutrition after bone marrow transplant had improved nitrogen balance, a diminished incidence of clinical infections, less fluid accumulation, and a shortened hospital stay (see Table 56.2-13). In a more recent study, glutamine-enriched TPN was shown to prevent the increase in gut mucosal permeability that develops with the administration of commercially available glutamine-free TPN. Van der Hulst and associates[128] randomized surgical patients requiring parenteral feedings to either receive standard TPN or glutamine-enriched TPN for 10 to 14 days. Duodenal mucosal biopsies and gut permeability studies were performed at the start and completion of TPN. The investigators found no change in either villous height or gut permeability in the group receiving glutamine-enriched TPN, whereas the control group showed both loss of villous height and increased gut permeability. This study provides strong evidence in favor of a gut-protective effect of glutamine. Similarly, arginine, because of its immunomodulatory properties may be useful as a dietary supplement in cancer patients, but further work is necessary to more clearly define the potential role of these two amino acids in the nutritional care of the cancer patient.

TECHNIQUES OF PROVIDING NUTRITIONAL SUPPORT

TRANSNASAL (NASOGASTRIC AND NASODUODENAL) FEEDING CATHETERS

The use of transnasal feeding catheters for intragastric feeding or for duodenal intubation is a popular adjunct for providing nutritional support by the enteral route. The stomach is easily accessed by the passage of a soft flexible (8 Fr.) feeding tube. Intragastric feedings provide several advantages for the patient. The stomach has the capacity and reservoir for bolus feedings. Feeding into the stomach results in the stimulation of biliary-pancreatic axis, which is probably trophic for the small bowel, and gastric secretions have a dilutional effect on the osmolarity of the feedings, reducing the risk of diarrhea. The major risk of intragastric feeding is the regurgitation of gastric contents resulting in aspiration into the tracheobronchial tree. This risk is highest in patients who have an altered mental sensorium or who are paralyzed.

The placement of the feeding tube through the pylorus into the fourth portion of the duodenum reduces the risk of regurgitation and aspiration of feeding formulas. To place a transnasal intraduodenal feeding catheter, the patient should be in the sitting position with the neck slightly flexed. This allows for the passage of a lubricated 8-Fr. polyurethane feeding catheter (with a stylette in place) through the patient's nose in a posterior and inferior direction, bringing the catheter to the level of the pharynx. The head is brought back to a neutral position and the patient is instructed to swallow while the feeding catheter is simultaneously passed down into the esophageal lumen. The advancement of the catheter is continued for a distance of about 45 to 50 cm. Once the catheter is confirmed to be in the stomach by injecting air while listening over the epigastrium, the patient is laid on the right side and the tube is advanced another 15 to 20 cm. This should position the tube into the duodenum and can be confirmed by listening over the right upper quadrant while advancing the tube. The stylette is removed and the position of the catheter is confirmed radiographically before the initiation of feedings. Tubes can be positioned fluoroscopically if necessary.

Gastric feedings are initiated by a bolus test volume of saline, representing the hourly feeding volume infused over 1 hour, into the stomach. The tube is clamped for 30 minutes and then checked for residual volume. If less than 50% of the volume load returns, then the selected volume is appropriate. In general, duodenal feedings can be started at 25 mL/hr at full-strength concentration unless the patient has been at bowel rest for several days, in which case the formula should be diluted to one-fourth strength. In such patients, we generally increase the rate of infusion before increasing the concentration. Despite these precautions, approximately 10% to 20% of patients receiving enteral feedings develop some degree of diarrhea secondary to malabsorption and the osmotic load of the feedings. When this occurs, decrease the rate of feeding by 50% rather than stopping the feedings altogether. The rate of feedings is then increased as tolerated over the next 3 to 4 days.

GASTROSTOMY TUBE FEEDINGS

A feeding gastrostomy should be considered in patients requiring long-term enteral nutrition and in patients with unresectable carcinomas of the head and neck or esophagus. In patients with an unresectable esophageal carcinoma who are not surgical candidates or in individuals who are unable to maintain caloric needs, a permanent gastrostomy should be considered. A temporary Stamm gastrostomy is a popular method for access to the gastric lumen that can be performed at the time of any major abdominal procedure. The surgical technique is relatively simple and straightforward.[4] After placement, the gastrostomy tube is placed to gravity drainage for 3 days and then is elevated. If the patient tolerates catheter elevation, we advance enteral feedings as described previously.

Percutaneous endoscopic gastrostomy to provide access for gastric feedings can be performed without a laparotomy or general anesthesia. This technique involves the safe passage of an endoscope into the stomach. The stomach is then dilated by the insufflation of air via the endoscope. Transabdominal illumination with the endoscopic light source selects an area on the anterior abdominal wall, usually halfway between the costal margin and the umbilicus. Local anesthesia is injected over the site followed by the insertion of an Angiocath percutaneously into the stomach. A wire is passed through the Angiocath, grabbed by a snare that has been passed through the endoscope, and pulled back with the endoscope out of the mouth. A standard percutaneous gastrostomy tube with a wire loop is attached to the guidewire and pulled back down the esophagus and out through the abdominal wall. The endoscope is passed back with the tube and the catheter is pulled under direct visualization until taut and then sutured to the abdominal wall. Inability to pass the endoscope safely or to identify the transabdominal illumination of the endoscope tip within the dilated stomach are contraindications to the procedure. Ascites, coagulopathies, and intraabdominal infections are relative contraindications as well.

FEEDING CATHETER JEJUNOSTOMY PLACEMENT AND WITZEL JEJUNOSTOMY

A feeding catheter jejunostomy should be placed following any major upper abdominal oncologic procedure if prolonged enteral nutrition support is anticipated, especially after gastric or pancreatic cancer surgery. The simplest method is a needle catheter jejunostomy, which can be performed fairly quickly at the end of the definitive operation. The entire length of a 14-gauge needle is used to create a subserosal tunnel approximately 30 to 40 cm distal to the ligament of Treitz and then the needle tip is introduced into the jejunal lumen. A 16-gauge feeding catheter is inserted through the needle and advanced 30 to 40 cm distally into the bowel lumen and the needle is withdrawn. The catheter is secured to the jejunal wall with sutures and then the loop of jejunum is anchored to the parietal peritoneum. The catheter is then secured to the skin with nylon sutures. The needle catheter jejunostomy is generally removed 2 to 4 weeks postoperatively when no longer needed.

A more permanent form of feeding jejunostomy employs the use of a 14-Fr. red rubber catheter for feeding. The placement technique is simple Witzel tunnel[128] and takes only 10 to 15 minutes. Jejunal feeding catheters can be used immediately for feeding purposes following the operation. Catheter care is essential to maintain patency, and the nursing staff need to flush the catheter with saline every 8 hours to ensure adequate patency. The catheter can be removed at the patient's bedside at the desired time by simple traction and the resulting fistula should close quickly.

PERIPHERAL INTRAVENOUS FEEDINGS

Peripheral veins may be used for infusion of glucose, amino acid solutions, and fat emulsions. However, these solutions must be nearly isotonic to avoid peripheral vein sclerosis. Ten percent glucose solutions may be used to increase the efficacy of amino acid use. Fat emulsions can be administered simultaneously with glucose and amino acid solutions, because they provide an efficient fuel source and isotonic. The major disadvantage of these peripherally administered mixtures is limited caloric delivery to meet catabolic demands within tolerated fluid volumes. Patients with renal and cardiac diseases may not tolerate the additional fluid load. Indications for peripheral vein feeding include the following: (1) as a supplement when enteral feedings can only be partially tolerated because of gastrointestinal dysfunction; (2) as a method of nutritional support when the gastrointestinal tract must be kept relatively empty for short periods during diagnostic workup; and (3) as preliminary feedings before subclavian catheter insertion in patients requiring TPN.

CENTRAL VENOUS TOTAL PARENTERAL NUTRITION

The preferred method of access to the superior vena cava is by percutaneous cannulation of the subclavian vein. Alternate sites include the internal and external jugular vein, but with the catheter exiting in the neck region this makes it more difficult to secure and maintain a sterile dressing site. Thus, long-term indwelling catheters should not be placed in this location because of an increased risk of catheter infections.

An individual who is experienced in the technique should perform the placement of a central venous catheter. To reduce the risk of hemostatic complications, patients with a platelet count below 50,000 should receive fresh platelets before catheter insertion. The procedure is performed using aseptic technique; the surgeon should wear a hat, mask, gown, and gloves. The patient is placed in Trendelenburg's position with both arms at the sides and the head turned away from the site of insertion. The chest is shaved, prepped, and draped in a sterile fashion. Local anesthesia is infiltrated near the insertion site and the underlying tissues along the inferior border of the clavicle. A standard subclavian insertion tray is used for catheter insertion via the Seldinger technique. The tip of the needle is inserted into the skin and subcutaneous tissues at the midpoint of the clavicle aiming for the suprasternal notch. The needle is directed parallel to the patient's bed, inserting beneath the clavicle with negative pressure applied at all times to the syringe. The prompt inflow of blood into the syringe indicates entrance into the subclavian vein, and the needle is advanced a few millimeters to ensure the bevel is within the lumen of the vessel. The patient is instructed to perform a gentle

Valsalva maneuver to prevent an air embolism, the syringe is disconnected from the needle and the guidewire is passed through the needle lumen, and the needle is then withdrawn over the guidewire. The passage of the wire through the needle should be met with minimal resistance and the needle should be removed only after 15 cm of the wire has been passed into the vessel. A small incision is made at the guidewire exit site and a dilator is passed over the wire. The dilator is then removed over the wire and is replaced by the catheter that is fully advanced. The wire is withdrawn and the catheter is flushed with sterile saline. The catheter is then sutured into position, the insertion site cleaned, and a sterile dressing placed. A portable chest radiograph is taken to confirm placement of the catheter. Chest films are inspected for location of the catheter tip and to search for evidence of pneumothorax and hemothorax.

Complications from long-term central venous catheterization in the cancer patient population include venous thrombosis and catheter-related infections. Thrombosis of the central vessels is a complication that may be often overlooked. The clinical suspicion of subclavian vein thrombosis is only approximately 3%, whereas studies that use phlebography or radionuclide venography indicate that the incidence is as high as 35%. Febrile episodes are not uncommon in the cancer patient population, particularly in the neutropenic individual. If primary catheter sepsis is confirmed, the catheter must be removed immediately. The tip of the catheter is sent to the laboratory for culture and compared with the blood cultures drawn from the patient. Appropriate antibiotics are administered and a new catheter is inserted when the patient's repeat blood culture results are negative.

NUTRITION SUPPORT FOR CANCER PATIENTS AND HEALTH CARE REFORM

The effect of corporate medicine on nutrition support has been addressed.[129] With the introduction of health care reform, nutrition support teams and the services they provide are now considered a cost center rather than a revenue center and both the role and existence of the traditional team is being threatened. Formal nutrition support teams began to form in the 1970s when TPN gained widespread clinical acceptance in the cancer. Although the indications for TPN in the cancer patient are few, the risk to these patients is that issues of cost may override those of access to and quality of nutritional support.

The challenge to nutrition support professionals is to coordinate efficient and early intervention and to document its efficacy and outcome. In the absence of any documented efficacy, many people argue, there is no need for formal nutrition support or the team in charge of that service. Therefore, it becomes imperative that the team justifies its importance to the hospital and convinces the administration that a formal nutrition support team provides quality control and polices the administration of nutritional support. To do this, nutrition support units must (1) identify specific patient populations who will benefit from nutrition support, (2) establish clinical pathways (guidelines), and (3) develop and implement measurements of efficacy (outcomes). In capitated models of health care, it is in the best interest of all caregivers to provide cost-effective care.

In the past, the costs required to pay the members of the nutrition support team have been more than offset by the reimbursements for the services provided, particularly for the delivery of TPN. The danger of this approach in the nutritional support of hospitalized patients, particularly patients with complicated problems and complex diseases, is that the withholding of nutritional and metabolic support from certain patients may result in serious consequences. Aggressive early feeding may be the best approach if it reduces complications in the long run. Methods of ensuring that nutrition support is cost effective have been suggested.[129]

REFERENCES

1. Souba WW, Wilmore DW. Diet and nutrition in the care of the patient with surgery, trauma, and sepsis. In: Shils M, Young V, eds. *Modern nutrition in health and disease,* 8th ed. Philadelphia: Lea & Febiger, 1994:1202.
2. Souba WW. Total parenteral nutrition. In: Copeland EM III, Levine BA, Howard RJ, et al., eds. *Current practice of surgery.* New York: Churchill Livingstone, 1993.
3. Souba WW. Cytokines: key regulators of the nutritional/metabolic response to critical illness. *Curr Probl Surg* 1994;31:577.
4. Hautamaki RD, Souba WW. Principles and techniques of nutritional support in the cancer patient. In: Karakousis CP, Copeland EM, Bland KI, eds. *Atlas of surgical oncology.* Philadelphia: WB Saunders,1995:740.
5. Warren S. The immediate causes of death in cancer. *Am J Med Sci* 1932;184:610.
6. DeWys WD, Begg D, Lavin PT, et al. Prognostic effect of weight loss before chemotherapy in cancer patients. *Am J Med* 1980; 69:491.
7. Espat NJ, Moldawer LL, Copeland EM III. Cytokine-mediated alterations in host metabolism prevent nutritional repletion in cachectic cancer patients. *J Surg Oncol* 1995;58:77.
8. Mercadente S. Parenteral versus enteral nutrition in cancer patients: indications and practice. *Supportive Care in Cancer* 1998;6:85.
9. Bernstein IL, Bernstein ID. Learned food aversion and cancer anorexia. *Cancer Treat Rep* 1981;65(Suppl 5):37.
10. Nelson KA, Walsh D, Sheehan FA. The cancer anorexia-cachexia syndrome. *J Clin Oncol* 1994;12:213.
11. Wesdorf RIC, Krause R, von Meyenfeldt MF. Cancer cachexia and its nutritional implications. *Br J Surg* 1983;70:352.
12. Norton JA, Moley JF, Green MV, Carson RE, Morrison SD. Parabiotic transfer of cancer anorexia/cachexia in male rats. *Cancer Res* 1985;45:5547.
13. Knox LS, Crosby LO, Feurer ID, et al. Energy expenditure in malnourished cancer patients. *Ann Surg* 1983;197:152.
14. Fearon KCH, Hansell DT, Preston T, et al. Influence of whole body protein turnover rate on resting energy expenditure on patients with cancer. *Cancer Res* 1988;48:2590.
15. Brennan MF. Uncomplicated starvation versus cancer cachexia. *Cancer Res* 1977;37:2359.
16. Arbeit JM, Lees DE, Corsey R, Brennan MF. Resting energy expenditure in controls and cancer patients with localized and diffuse disease. *Ann Surg* 1984;199:292.
17. Frederix EWHM, Soeters PB, Wouters EFM, et al. Effect of different tumor types on resting energy expenditure. *Cancer Res* 1991;61:38.
18. Luketich JD, Mullen JL, Feurer ID, Sternleib J, Fried RC. Ablation of abnormal energy expenditure by curative tumor resection. *Arch Surg* 1990;125:337.
19. Kolal WA, McCulloch A, Wright PD, Johnston IDA. Glucose turnover and recycling on colorectal cancer. *Ann Surg* 1983;198:601.
20. Shaw JHF, Wolfe RR. Glucose and urea kinetics in patients with early and advanced gastrointestinal cancer: the response to glucose infusion, parenteral feeding, and surgical resection. *Surgery* 1986;101:181.
21. Shaw JHF, Humberstone DM, Wolfe RR. Energy and protein metabolism in sarcoma patients. *Ann Surg* 1988; 203:283.
22. Humberstone DM, Shaw JHF. Metabolism in hematologic malignancy. *Cancer* 1988;62:1619.
23. Glickman AS, Rawson RW. Diabetes and altered carbohydrate metabolism in patients with cancer. *Cancer* 1956;9:1127.
24. Lundholm K, Edstrom S, Karlberg I, et al. Glucose turnover, gluconeogenesis from glycerol, and estimation of net glucose cycling in cancer patients. *Cancer* 1982;50:1142.
25. Yoshikawa T, Noguchi Y, Matsumoto A. Effects of tumor removal and body weight loss on insulin resistance in patients with cancer. *Surgery* 1994;116:62.
26. Jeevanandam M, Lowry SF, Horowitz GD, et al. Cancer cachexia and protein metabolism. *Lancet* 1984;1:1423.
27. Goodlad GAJ, Clark CM. The action of the Walker 256 carcinoma and toxohormone on amino acid incorporation into diaphragm protein. *Eur J Cancer* 1973;9:139.
28. Lundholm K, Edstrom S, Ekman L, et al. A comparative study of the influence of malignant tumor on host metabolism in mice and man. *Cancer* 1978;42:453.
29. Heber D, Chlebowski RT, Ishibashi DE, et al. Abnormalities in glucose and protein metabolism in noncachectic lung cancer patients. *Cancer Res* 1982;42:4815.
30. Norton JA, Burt ME, Brennan MF. In vivo utilization of substrate by human sarcoma bearing limbs. *Cancer* 1980;45:29.
31. Cariuk P, Lorite MJ, Todorov PT, et al. Induction of cachexia in mice by a product isolated from the urine of cachectic cancer patients. *Br J Cancer* 1997;76:606.
32. Todoruv PT, McDevitt TM, Meyer DJ, et al. Purification and characterization of a tumor lipid-mobilizing factor. *Cancer Res* 1998;58:2353.
33. Choudhary G, Chakel J, Hancock W, et al. Investigation of the potential of capillary electrophoresis with off-line matrix-assisted laser desorption/ionization time-of-flight mass

spectrometry for clinical analysis: examination of a glycoprotein factor associated with cancer cachexia. *Analytical Chem* 1999;71:855.
34. Fischer CP, Bode BP, Souba WW. Adaptive alterations in cellular metabolism with malignant transformation. *Ann Surg* 1998;227:627.
35. Wasa M, Bode B, Abcouwer S, Tanabe K, Souba WW. Glutamine as a regulator of DNA and protein biosynthesis in human solid tumor cell lines. *Ann Surg* 1996;224:189.
36. Souba WW. Glutamine and cancer. *Ann Surg* 1993;218:715.
37. Lin CM, Abcouwer SF, Souba WW. Effect of dietary glutamate on chemotherapy-induced immunosuppression. *Nutrition* 1999;15:687.
38. Balkwill F, Osborne R, Burke F, et al. Evidence for tumor necrosis factor/cachectin production in cancer. *Lancet* 1987;2:1229.
39. Michie HR, Sherman ML, Spriggs DR, et al. Chronic TNF infusion causes anorexia but not accelerated nitrogen loss. *Ann Surg* 1989;209:19.
40. Darling G, Fraker DL, Jensen C, et al. Cachectic effects of recombinant human tumor necrosis factor in rats. *Cancer Res* 1990;50:4008.
41. Sherry BA, Gelin J, Fong Y, et al. Anticachectin/tumor necrosis factor-a antibodies attenuate development of cachexia in tumor models. *FASEB J* 1989;3:1956.
42. Yamamoto N, Kawamura I, Nishigaki F, et al. Effect of FR143430, a novel cytokine suppressive agent, on adenocarcinoma colon 26-induced cachexia in mice. *Anticancer Res* 1998;18:139.
43. Oliff A, Defeo-Jones D, Boyer M, et al. Tumors secreting human TNF/cachectin induce cachexia in mice. *Cell* 1987;50:555.
44. Starnes HF, Warren RS, Jeevanandem M, et al. Tumor necrosis factor and the acute metabolic response to injury in man. *J Clin Invest* 1988;82:1321.
45. Martin F, Santolaria F, Batista N, et al. Cytokine levels (IL-6 and IFN-gamma), acute phase response and nutritional status as prognostic factors in lung cancer. *Cytokine* 1999;11:80.
46. Uno K, Setoguchi J, Tanigawa M, et al. Differential IL-12 responsiveness for interferon-gamma production in advanced stages of cancer patients correlates with performance status. *Clin Cancer Res* 1998;4:2425.
47. Shibata M, Takekawa M, Amano S. Increased serum concentrations of soluble tumor necrosis factor receptor I in non-cachectic and cachectic patients with advanced gastric and colorectal cancer. *Surg Today* 1998;28:884.
48. Argiles JM, Lopez-Soriano FJ. The role of cytokines in cancer cachexia. *Med Res Rev* 1999;19:223.
49. Fischer CP, Bode BP, Takahashi K, Tanabe KK, Souba WW. Glucocorticoid-dependent induction of IL-6 receptor expression in human hepatocytes facilitates IL-6 stimulation of amino acid transport. *Ann Surg* 1996;223:610.
50. Gambardella A, Tortoriello R, Pesce L, et al. Intralipid infusion combined with propranolol administration has favorable metabolic effects in elderly malnourished cancer patients. *Metabol Clin Exp* 1999;48:291.
51. Mimura Y, Kanauchi H, Ogawa T, Oohara T. Resistance to natriuresis in patients with peritoneal carcinomatosis. *Horm Metab Res* 1996;28:183.
52. Lazarus DD, Kambayashi T, Lowry SF, Strassman G. The lack of an effect by insulin or insulin-like growth factor-1 in attenuating colon-26 mediated cancer cachexia. *Cancer Lett* 1996;103:71.
53. Darling G, Goldstein DS, Stull R, et al. Tumor necrosis factor: immune endocrine interaction. *Surgery* 1989;106:1155.
54. Arbos J, Lpoz-Soriano FJ, Carbo N, et al. Effects of tumor necrosis factor-a (cachectin) on glucose metabolism in the rat. *Mol Cell Biochem* 1992;112:53.
55. Fischer E, Marano M, Barber AE, et al. Comparison between effects of interleukin-1a administration and sublethal endotoxemia in primates. *Am J Physiol* 1991;261:R442.
56. Lee MD, Zentella A, Pekala PH, et al. Effect of endotoxin-induced monokines on glucose metabolism in the muscle cell line L6. *Proc Natl Acad Sci U S A* 1987;84:2590.
57. Meszaros K, Lang CH, Bagby GJ. Tumor necrosis factor increases in vivo glucose utilization of macrophage-rich tissues. *Biochem Biophys Res Commun* 1987;149:1.
58. Eisirik DL. Interleukin-1 induced impairment in pancreatic islet oxidative metabolism of glucose is potentiated by tumor necrosis factor. *Acta Endocrinol* 1988;119:321.
59. Greenberg AS, Nordan RP, McIntosh J, et al. Interleukin 6 reduces lipoprotein lipase activity in adipose tissue of mice in vivo and in 3T3-L1 adipocytes: a possible role for interleukin 6 in cancer cachexia. *Cancer Res* 1992;52:4113.
60. Memon RA, Feingold KR, Moser AH, et al. Differential effects of interleukin-1 and tumor necrosis factor on ketogenesis. *Am J Physiol* 1992;263:E301.
61. Warren RS, Starnes HF, Gabrilove JL, et al. The acute metabolic effects of tumor necrosis factor administration in humans. *Arch Surg* 1987;122:1396.
62. Flores EA, Bistrian BR, Pomposelli JJ, et al. Infusion of tumor necrosis factor/cachectin promotes muscle catabolism in the rat. *J Clin Invest* 1989;83:1614.
63. Fong Y, Moldawer LL, Marano M, et al. Cachectin/TNF or IL-1a induces cachexia with redistribution of body proteins. *Am J Physiol* 1989;256:R659.
64. Moldawer LL, Svanninger G, Gelin J, et al. Interleukin-1 and tumor necrosis factor do not regulate protein balance in skeletal muscle. *Am J Physiol* 1987;253:C766.
65. Hall-Angeras M, Angeras U, Zamir O, et al. Interaction between corticosterone and tumor necrosis factor stimulated protein breakdown in rat skeletal muscle, similar to sepsis. *Surgery* 1990;108:460.
66. Inoue Y, Bode B, Copeland EM, Souba WW. Tumor necrosis factor mediates tumor-induced increases in hepatic amino acid transport. *Cancer Res* 1995;55:3525.
67. Hummel RP, Warner B, Pedersen P, et al. In vitro effects of TNF, IL-1a, and other monokines on skeletal muscle amino acid uptake and protein degradation. *Surg Forum* 1987;38:13.
68. Pacitti AJ, Inoue Y, Souba WW. Tumor necrosis factor stimulates Na^+-dependent amino acid uptake in plasma membrane vesicles. *J Clin Invest* 1993;91:474.
69. Watkins K, Souba WW. Coordinated regulation of hepatic amino acid transport by interleukin-6 and glucocorticoids. *J Trauma* 1994;36:523.
70. Fischer CP, Bode BP, Souba WW. Glucocorticoids exert a permissive effect on cytokine-stimulated glutamine transport in cultured hepatocytes. *Surg Forum* 1995;46:546.
71. McMillan DC, O'Gorman P, Fearon KC, McArdle CS. A pilot study of megestrol acetate and ibuprofen in the treatment of cachexia in gastrointestinal cancer patients. *Br J Cancer* 1997;76:788.
72. Von Roenn JH, Knopf K. Anorexia/cachexia in patients with HIV: lessons for the oncologist. *Oncology* 1996;10:1049.
73. Vansteenkiste JF, Simons JP, Wouters EF, Demedts MG. Hormonal treatment in advanced non-small cell lung cancer: fact or fiction? *Eur Respir J* 1996;9:1707.
74. Strang P. The effect of megestrol acetate on anorexia, weight loss and cachexia in cancer and AIDS patients. *Anticancer Res* 1997;17:657.
75. Vadell C, Segui MA, Gimenez-Arnau JM, et al. Anticachectic efficacy of megestrol acetate at different doses and versus placebo in patients with neoplastic cachexia. *Am J Clin Oncol* 1998;21:347.
76. Bruera E, Ernst S, Hagen N, et al. Effectiveness of megestrol acetate in patients with advanced cancer: a randomized, double-blind, crossover study. *Cancer Prev Control* 1998;2:74.
77. De Conno F, Martini C, Zecca E, et al. Megestrol acetate for anorexia in patients with far-advanced cancer: a double-blind controlled clinical trial. *Eur J Cancer* 1998;34:1705.
78. Kurebayashi J, Yamamoto S, Otsuki T, Sonoo H. Medroxyprogesterone acetate inhibits IL-6 secretion from KPL-4 human breast cancer cells both in vitro and in vivo: a possible mechanism of the anticachectic effect. *Br J Cancer* 1999;79:631.
79. Mantovani G, Maccio A, Esu S, et al. Medroxyprogesterone acetate reduces the invitro production of cytokines and serotonin involved in anorexia/cachexia and emesis by peripheral blood mononuclear cells of cancer patients. *Eur J Cancer* 1997;33:602.
80. Simons JP, Schols AM, Hoefnagels JM, et al. Effects of medroxyprogesterone acetate on food intake, body composition, and resting energy expenditure in patients with advanced, non-hormone sensitive cancer: a randomized, placebo-controlled trial. *Cancer* 1998;82:553.
81. Tisdale MJ. Biology of cachexia. *J Natl Cancer Inst* 1997;89:1763.
82. Ohlra T, Nishio K, Ohe Y, et al. Improvement by eicosanoids in cancer cachexia induced by LLC-IL6 transplantation. *J Cancer Res Clin Oncol* 1996;122:711.
83. McMillan DC, O'Gorman P, Fearon KC, McArdle CS. A pilot study of megestrol acetate and ibuprofen in the treatment of cachexia in gastrointestinal cancer patients. *Br J Cancer* 1997;76:788.
84. Lissoni P, Paolorossi F, Tancini G, et al. Is there a role for melatonin in the treatment of neoplastic cachexia? *Eur J Cancer* 1996;32A:1340.
85. Gagnon B, Bruera E. A review of drug treatment of cachexia associated with cancer. *Drugs* 1998;55:675.
86. Baron PL, Lawrence W, Chan WM, et al. Effects of parenteral nutrition on cell cycle kinetics of head and neck cancer. *Arch Surg* 1986;121:1282.
87. Shukla HS, Rao RR, Banu N, et al. Enteral hyperalimentation in malnourished surgical patients. *Indian J Med Res* 1984;80:339.
88. Smith RC, Hartemink RJ, Holinshead JW, et al. Fine bore jejunostomy feeding following major abdominal surgery: a controlled randomized clinical trial. *Br J Surg* 1985;72:458.
89. von Meyenfeldt MF, Meyerink WJ, Soeters PB, et al. Perioperative nutritional support results in a reduction of major postoperative complications especially in high risk patients. *Gastroenterology* 1991;100:A553(abst).
90. Douglass HO, Milliron S, Nava H, et al. Elemental diet as an adjuvant for patients with locally advanced gastrointestinal cancer receiving radiation therapy: a prospectively randomized study. *JPEN* 1978;2:682.
91. Brown MS, Buchanan RB, Karran SJ. Clinical observations on the effects of elemental diet supplementation during irradiation. *Clin Radiol* 1980;31:19.
92. Bounous G, LeBel E, Shuster J, et al. Dietary protection during radiation therapy. *Strahlentherapie* 1975;149:476.
93. Daly JM, Hearne B, Dunaj J, et al. Nutritional rehabilitation in patients with advanced head and neck cancer receiving radiation therapy. *Am J Surg* 1984;148:514.
94. Moloney M, Moriarty M, Daly L. Controlled studies of nutritional intake in patients with malignant disease undergoing treatment. *Hum Nutr Appl Nutr* 1983;37A:30.
95. Elkort RJ, Baker FL, Vitale JJ, et al. Long-term nutritional support as an adjunct to chemotherapy for breast cancer. *JPEN* 1981;5:385.
96. Evans WK, Nixon DW, Dlay JM, et al. A randomized study of oral nutritional support versus ad lib nutritional intake during chemotherapy for advanced colorectal and non-small cell lung cancer. *J Clin Oncol* 1987;5:113.
97. Tandon SP, Gupta SC, Sinha SN, et al. Nutritional support as an adjunct therapy of advanced cancer patients. *Indian J Med Res* 1984;80:180.
98. Bounous G, Gentile JM, Hugon J. Elemental diet in the management of the intestinal lesion produced by 5-fluorouracil in man. *Can J Surg* 1971;14:312.
99. Holter AR, Fischer JE. The effects of perioperative hyper-alimentation complications in patients with carcinoma and weight loss. *J Surg Res* 1977;23:31.
100. Heatley RV, Williams RH, Lewis MH. Pre-operative intravenous feeding: a controlled trial. *Postgrad Med J* 1979;55:541.
101. Yamada N, Koyama H, Hioki K, et al. Effect of postoperative total parenteral nutrition (TPN) as an adjunct to gastrectomy for advanced gastric carcinoma. *Br J Surg* 1983;70:267.
102. Askanazi J, Hensle TW, Starker PM, et al. Effect of immediate postoperative nutritional support on length of hospitalization. *Ann Surg* 1986;203:236.
103. Müller JM, Keller HW, Brenner U, et al. Indications and effects of preoperative parenteral nutrition. *World J Surg* 1986;10:53.
104. Bellantone R, Doglietto GB, Bossola M, et al. Preoperative parenteral nutrition in the high risk surgical patient. *JPEN* 1988;12:195.
105. Bellantone R, Doglietto G, Bossola M, et al. Preoperative parenteral nutrition of malnourished surgical patients. *Acta Chir Scand* 1988;154:249.
106. Woolfson AM, Smith JA. Elective nutritional support after major surgery: a prospective randomized trial. *Clin Nutr* 1989;8:15.
107. Buzby GP. The Veterans Affairs Total Parenteral Nutrition Cooperative Study Group. Perioperative total parenteral nutrition in surgical patients. *N Engl J Med* 1991;325:525.

108. Sandstrom R, Drott C, Hyltander A, et al. The effect of postoperative intravenous feeding (TPN) on outcome following major surgery evaluated in a randomized study. *Ann Surg* 1993;217:185.
109. Sciafani LM, Shike M, Quesada E, et al. A randomized prospective trial of TPN following major pancreatic resection or radioactive implant for pancreatic cancer. Presented at the Society of Surgical Oncology, March 1991, Orlando, FL.
110. Solassol C, Joyeux J, Dubois JB. Total parenteral nutrition (TPN) with complete nutritive mixtures: an artificial gut in cancer patients. *Nutr Cancer* 1979;1:13.
111. Kinsella TJ, Malcolm AW, Bothe A, et al. Prospective study of nutritional support during pelvic irradiation. *Int J Radiat Oncol Biol Phys* 1981;7:543.
112. Ghavimi F, Shils ME, Scott BF, et al. Comparison of morbidity in children requiring abdominal radiation and chemotherapy, with and without total parenteral nutrition. *J Pediatr* 1982;101:530.
113. Donaldson SS, Wesley MN, Ghavimi F, et al. A prospective randomized clinical trial of total parenteral nutrition in children with cancer. *Med Pediatr Oncol* 1982;10:129.
114. Nixon DW, Moffitt S, Lawson DH, et al. Total parenteral nutrition as an adjunct to chemotherapy of metastatic colorectal cancer. *Cancer Treat Rep* 1981;65(Suppl 5):121.
115. Nixon DW, Heymsfield SB, Lawson DH, et al. Effect of total parenteral nutrition on survival in advanced colon cancer. *Cancer Detect Prev* 1981;4:421.
116. Samuels ML, Selig DE, Ogden S, et al. IV hyperalimentation and chemotherapy for stage II testicular cancer: a randomized study. *Cancer Treat Rep* 1981;65:615.
117. Shamberger RC, Brennan MF, Goodgame JT, et al. A prospective, randomized study of adjuvant parenteral nutrition in the treatment of sarcoma: results of metabolic and survival studies. *Surgery* 1984;96:1.
118. Shamberger RC, Pizzo PA, Goodgame JT, et al. The effect of total parenteral nutrition on chemotherapy-induced myelosuppression. *Am J Med* 1983;74:40.
119. Valdivieso M, Frankmann C, Murphy WK, et al. Long-term effects of intravenous hyperalimentation administered during intensive chemotherapy for small cell bronchogenic carcinoma. *Cancer* 1987;59:362.
120. Valdivieso M, Bodey GP, Benjamin RS, et al. Role of intravenous hyperalimentation as an adjunct to intensive chemotherapy for small cell bronchogenic carcinoma. *Cancer Treat Rep* 1981;65(Suppl 5):145.
121. Clamon GH, Feld R, Evans WK, et al. Effect of adjuvant central IV hyperalimentation on the survival and response to treatment of patients with small cell lung cancer: a randomized trial. *Cancer Treat Rep* 1985;69:167.
122. Issell BF, Valdivieso MD, Zaren HA, et al. Protection against chemotherapy toxicity by IV hyperalimentation. *Cancer Treat Rep* 1978;62:1139.
123. Jordan WM, Valdivieso M, Frankman C, et al. Treatment of advanced adenocarcinoma of the lung with ftorafur, doxorubicin, cyclophosphamide, and cisplatin (FACP) and intensive IV hyperalimentation. *Cancer Treat Rep* 1981;65:197.
124. Brennan MF, Pisters PWT, Posner M, et al. A prospective randomized trial of total parenteral nutrition after major pancreatic resection for malignancy. *Ann Surg* 1994;220:436.
125. Fan ST, Lo CM, Lai ECS, et al. Perioperative nutritional support in patients undergoing hepatectomy for hepatocellular carcinoma. *N Engl J Med* 1994;331:1547.
126. Wilmore DW, Byrne TA, Young LS, et al. A new treatment for patients with the short bowel syndrome: growth hormone, glutamine, and a modified diet. *Ann Surg* 1995;222:243.
127. Ziegler TR, Young LS, Benfell K, et al. Glutamine-supplemented parenteral nutrition improves nitrogen retention and reduces hospital mortality versus standard parenteral nutrition following bone marrow transplantation: a randomized, double-blind trial. *Ann Intern Med* 1992;116:821.
128. van der Hulst RRWJ, van Kreel BK, von Meyenfeldt MF, et al. Glutamine and the preservation of gut integrity. *Lancet* 1993;341:1363.
129. Nelson J. The impact of health care reform on nutrition support—the practitioner's perspective. *Nutr Clin Pract* 1995;4:1.
130. Buzby GP. Overview of randomized clinical trials of total parenteral nutrition for malnourished surgical patients. *World J Surg* 1993;17:173.
131. Foschi D, Cavagna G, Callioni F, et al. Hyperalimentation of jaundiced patients on percutaneous biliary drainage. *Br J Surg* 1986;73:716.

PATRICIA A. GANZ
MARK S. LITWIN
BETH E. MEYEROWITZ

SECTION **3**

Sexual Problems

To understand the impact of a cancer diagnosis and its treatment on sexual health and functioning, it is useful to have some knowledge about what is "normal," as well as the range of sexual problems that occur in the general population not affected by cancer. This background is essential for understanding the unique contribution that cancer and its treatments play in exacerbating what are often premorbid sexual difficulties. Table 56.3-1 describes a broad range of factors that influence sexual functioning before a cancer diagnosis (e.g., age, gender, anxiety, chronic disease), and these preexisting factors strongly influence sexual functioning after a cancer diagnosis. Other naturally occurring events that may coincide with cancer are age-related changes in sexual functioning, such as erectile dysfunction in men and menopause-related changes in women. Cancer treatments, however, cause unique side effects not usually experienced in other patient populations (e.g., body image changes, infertility, fatigue, and pain). Sexual problems can also be exacerbated by the uncertain prognosis associated with a cancer diagnosis. In this chapter, we provide some background about normal sexual health and functioning to provide a context for the changes associated with a cancer diagnosis. We then discuss general changes in sexuality associated with cancer, as well as treatment and site-specific changes.

SEXUAL HEALTH AND PHYSIOLOGY

HUMAN SEXUAL RESPONSE CYCLE

The human sexual response cycle (HSRC), as detailed by Masters and Johnson,[1] involves the physiologic changes that occur when individuals receive adequate sexual stimulation. The HSRC consists of four, somewhat arbitrary, phases—*excitement, plateau, orgasm,* and *resolution.* In Table 56.3-2 we have listed some of the key responses in each phase, with a focus on those that might be affected by cancer and its treatments. The disease and treatment can disrupt the response cycle entirely or can lead to changes in sensation and experience during the response cycle. The response cycle is similar for women and men, with parallel processes for homologous tissues.

Although Masters and Johnson's research advanced our knowledge of the psychophysiology of human sexual response, the four-phase model of the HSRC has been criticized on both conceptual and methodologic grounds.[2,3] In a triphasic model of human sexuality, Kaplan[4] addressed two of the primary concerns—the characterization of the phases of sexual responding as sequential and interdependent and the inattention to motivational aspects of sexuality. The triphasic model is characterized by separate *desire, excitement,* and *orgasm* phases. Kaplan proposed that these are discrete phases controlled by distinct neurophysiologic mechanisms. Thus, she suggests that different etiologic factors and treatment approaches should be considered, depending on the phase in which difficulties occur.[5] However, the extent to which responses in each of these phases is mediated through different pathways has not been documented empirically.[2] The fact that individuals often report dysfunction in more than one phase argues against assuming unrelated etiologies.[6]

TABLE 56.3-1. Factors Affecting Sexual Functioning before and after a Cancer Diagnosis

Before Cancer	*After Cancer*
Demographic factors	Unchanged
Age	
Gender	
Ethnicity	
Psychological status	Unchanged, better, or worse; *new* fear of recurrence, increased sense of vulnerability
Anxiety disorders	
Depressive disorders	
Chronic health problems	Unchanged or worse
Diabetes	
Hypertension	
Cardiovascular disease	
Arthritis	
Partnership factors	Better, worse, or unchanged
Availability of a partner	
Quality of the relationship	
Partner's health and physical problems	
Body image	Likely to change, probably worse
Sexual attractiveness	
Self-esteem	
Gender-specific factors	
Menopause-related changes (women)	Likely to change, probably worse, especially if estrogen is prohibited; premature menopause
Vaginal dryness	
Decreased sexual interest	
Erectile dysfunction (men)	Unchanged or worse, especially if pelvic surgery or androgen ablative therapy performed
Age-related	
Psychogenic	
Neurovascular changes	
Cancer-specific factors	Cancer-related symptoms: pain, fatigue, nausea; treatment toxicities; infertility; severity and degree of influence related to stage of disease and treatment goals
Occasionally may precede diagnosis	

TABLE 56.3-2. Human Sexual Response Cycle

- Excitement phase
  - Women
    - Vaginal lubrication begins
    - Heart rate and muscle tension increase
    - Uterus enlarges and elevates
    - Labia majora separate and elevate
    - Clitoris and breasts swell and nipples become erect
    - Vaginal canal lengthens
  - Men
    - Penile erection begins
    - Heart rate and muscle tension increase
    - Testes enlarge
    - Scrotum thickens
- Plateau phase
  - Women
    - Pelvic vasocongestion and generalized myotonia reach peak
    - Labia minora swell and darken
    - Uterus elevates and pulls away from vaginal canal
    - Outer vaginal canal swells such that sides are touching
    - Inner vaginal canal widens such that sides balloon open
    - Clitoris retracts under clitoral hood
    - Breasts swell such that areola masks nipple erection
  - Men
    - Pelvic vasocongestion and generalized myotonia reach peak
    - Testes enlarge further and elevate close to perineum
    - Urethra increases in diameter
    - Cowper's gland secretes fluid into urethra
    - Point of "ejaculatory inevitability" is reached with full testicular elevation
- Orgasm phase
  - Women
    - Contractions of circumvaginal and perineal muscles
    - Multiple orgasms for some women
  - Men
    - Contractions of penile urethra and perineal and bulbocavernous muscles (emission)
    - Expulsion of seminal fluid and sperm through urethra (ejaculation)
- Resolution phase
  - Women
    - Thin film of perspiration covers body
    - Pelvic region and breasts return to prearousal state
    - Sensation of relaxation and calm
  - Men
    - Thin film of perspiration covers body
    - Body gradually returns to prearousal state
    - Sensation of relaxation and calm
    - Gradual detumescence of partial erection
    - Refractory period during which sexual arousal is not possible

SEXUAL DYSFUNCTIONS AND PROBLEMS

The nomenclature for diagnosing sexual dysfunctions[7] uses the triphasic model of sexuality—involving disturbances in desire, excitement, or orgasm—or by pain associated with sexual intercourse. For patients to be diagnosed with a sexual dysfunction, their disturbance or pain must cause marked distress or interpersonal difficulties, must be persistent or recurrent, and cannot be due to another psychiatric disorder (such as mood or personality disorders). The diagnosis also includes reference to etiologic factors. If the dysfunction is due exclusively to one set of factors (psychological causes, general medical conditions, or substance use), the diagnosis so indicates. In the case of many cancer patients, sexual dysfunctions may be diagnosed as "due to combined factors," indicating a more complex etiology in which multiple causes contribute to the dysfunction. Table 56.3-3 provides a list of the diagnostic categories given in the *Diagnostic and Statistical Manual of Mental Disorders, Fourth Edition.*[7]

In addition to these diagnosable disorders, many patients experience disruptions that are less intense in nature but that, nonetheless, cause decreases in previously enjoyable sexual activities and reduce global satisfaction with sexuality. The subjective experience that one has a satisfying sex life may or may not be associated with the ability to progress through the phases of the HSRC. Some individuals with no diagnosable dysfunction can be dissatisfied with factors such as the frequency or variety of sexual behavior, whereas some individuals with organically based dysfunctions can enjoy other forms of sexual and intimate contact. Also, as indicated in Table 56.3-1, cancer can have an indirect

TABLE 56.3-3. Diagnostic Categories for Sexual Dysfunctions

Desire disorders	
Hypoactive sexual desire disorder	Deficiency or absence of sexual fantasies and desire
Sexual aversion disorder	Aversion to and avoidance of genital sexual contact with a partner
Arousal disorders	
Female sexual arousal disorder	Inability to attain or maintain adequate lubrication-swelling response of sexual excitement until completion of sexual activity
Male erectile disorder	Inability to attain or maintain adequate erection until completion of sexual activity
Orgasmic disorders	
Female orgasmic disorder	Delay in or absence of orgasm after a normal sexual excitement phase
Male orgasmic disorder	Delay in or absence of orgasm after a normal sexual excitement phase
Premature ejaculation	Orgasm and ejaculation with minimal sexual stimulation before, on, or shortly after penetration and before the person wishes it
Pain disorders	
Dyspareunia	Genital pain associated with sexual intercourse
Sexual pain disorder in females (vaginismus)	Involuntary contraction of the perineal muscles with vaginal penetration

(Adapted from ref. 7, with permission.)

influence on sexuality through disruptions in partnership factors, body image, and overall psychological well-being.

SEXUAL PROBLEMS AND THEIR PREVALENCE AMONG THE GENERAL POPULATION

PREVALENCE OF SEXUAL DYSFUNCTIONS AND PROBLEMS

Sexual problems are common, even among community samples of happily married couples.[8,9] In a large and extensive national survey of sexuality of 18 to 59 year olds in the United States, 43% of women and 31% of men reported dysfunction in one of the diagnostic categories during the previous year.[10] Among men, premature ejaculation was the most common complaint (28.5%), followed by anxiety about performance (17.0%), lack of interest in sex (15.8%), and inability to keep an erection (10.4%).[8] Women most frequently reported lack of interest in sex (33.4%), inability to reach orgasm (24.1%), not finding sex pleasurable (21.2%), difficulty becoming lubricated (18.8%), and pain during intercourse (14.4%). Individuals who experienced emotional or stress-related problems or who were victims of adult-child sexual contact were significantly more likely to report sexual dysfunction. Other predictors varied somewhat between men and women, with poor health being particularly salient for men and falling household income and low sexual activity being important for women. Despite these difficulties, most respondents indicated that sex was emotionally satisfying and was associated with very positive feelings.

Although specific prevalence rates vary somewhat in other studies,[11–17] depending on study sample and methodology, the general conclusions are similar. Sexual dysfunction is a common experience, with most individuals experiencing difficulty at some points in their lives. However, sexual dysfunction need not result in dissatisfaction with sexuality or loss of intimacy. Sexuality after cancer should be viewed within this larger context.

SEXUALITY AND AGING

Normal aging is associated with decreases in both physiologic functioning and behavioral aspects of sexuality. With regard to the phases of the HSRC, response slows and decreases in intensity with age for both men and women.[1] For example, vasocongestion during arousal occurs more slowly, extending the time required for penile erection and vaginal lubrication. More intense and direct tactile stimulation typically is required for arousal and orgasm than is needed in younger men and women. As most men age, erections are less rigid, ejaculation is less forceful, and the refractory period lasts longer (often for many hours). In addition to the anatomic changes associated with menopause, women experience decreased lubrication and, in some cases, reduced intensity of orgasm. Chronic medical conditions and general ill-health can exacerbate the natural slowing of sexual response.[18]

The prevalence of some diagnosable sexual disorders varies with age, although little research has been done on very old populations to provide specific information. Sexual desire and the frequency of sexual thoughts appear to decline with age, particularly for men, although sexual interest does remain present.[2,10,19,20] Researchers consistently have found that erectile functioning also worsens with age, with increases in dysfunction beginning in middle age and increasing gradually over the rest of the lifespan.[10,21,22] For example, the Massachusetts Male Aging Study[22] demonstrated that rates of complete erectile dysfunction triple from 5% to 15% between the ages of 40 and 70. For women, the prevalence of arousal disorders, as indicated by difficulty lubricating, increases with age.[2,10] Findings regarding the rates of other disorders in women are inconsistent, with different studies reporting that problems can increase, decrease, or remain stable.[10,14,15,18,21]

Sexual activity decreases with age for both women and men.[8,14,15,21,23] In some cases, this decrease results from the absence of a partner, coupled with an unwillingness to engage in self-pleasuring activities, especially among very old women.[10,13,23] Even among older married couples, rates of intercourse decrease.[8,21] Nonetheless, many older individuals do consider sex an important part of their lives and have satisfying sex lives.[8,24] Age alone should not be viewed as an adequate explanation for serious sexual dysfunction or inactivity among interested older adults.

MENOPAUSE AND SEXUAL FUNCTIONING

Menopause is clinically diagnosed when a previously menstruating woman with an intact uterus has amenorrhea for at least 12 months. The average age of menopause in North American women is 51 years.[25] Secondary forms of amenorrhea may be related to endocrine disorders or conditions such as anorexia nervosa; however, cancer treatment–induced secondary amenorrhea is the most relevant for our purposes. Hysterectomy can complicate the evaluation of woman's menopausal status, because menstrual bleeding can no longer be used to classify her status. If a woman's ovaries are removed as a result of surgery, she experiences a surgically induced menopause.

The menopausal transition is characterized by a decreased responsiveness of the ovaries to luteinizing hormone and follicle-stimulating hormone. Gradually, over time, the estradiol levels fall as the ovarian follicles are depleted and there is no further response to the pituitary gonadotropins luteinizing hormone and follicle-stimulating hormone. It is with these changes that the clinical symptoms of estrogen deficiency begin to occur. Lowered levels of estradiol affect various target tissues, including the vagina, skin, bone, vascular endothelium, and smooth muscle, as well as the hypothalamic temperature-regulating centers.[26] The ovaries are the primary source of androgens in women, even into postmenopause, and decreased production of ovarian androgens may account for changes in libido during this time. Many women who become menopausal experience symptoms associated with estrogen deficiency, including vasomotor symptoms (hot flashes, sweats, palpitations), urinary incontinence, and vaginal dryness. Vasomotor symptoms are most frequent (up to 75% of menopausal women experience these at some point) and are among the earliest symptoms of menopause, with urinary incontinence and vaginal dryness increasing slowly during the later postmenopausal years.[26]

The impact of menopause on sexual health is controversial, because many women remain sexually active into old age. Several population-based studies of perimenopausal and menopausal women have documented that most women who have partners are sexually active[13]; however, changes can occur in sexual functioning (desire, arousal, orgasm) that are age related[23,27] and to which menopause may contribute. The relation between menopause, sex steroids, and sexual motivation ("libido") remain controversial.[26] Research suggests that, in postmenopausal women, a variety of factors are potential moderators of the components of sexual functioning (e.g., psychological distress, quality of the partner relationship, physical activity, body mass index).[13] Without sufficient levels of endogenous estrogen, the vaginal epithelium may become atrophic, leading to clinical symptoms of vaginal dryness and dyspareunia. With chronic or untreated symptoms of vaginal dryness, postmenopausal women may choose to avoid sexual intercourse completely. However, this may not preclude other forms of sexual activity. In a volunteer sample of healthy postmenopausal women who were not on hormone replacement therapy, vaginal dryness was reported by 37% of women 45 to 64 years of age.[13] Hormone replacement therapy is effective in managing menopausal symptoms, such as hot flashes and vaginal dryness, but does not appear to improve sexual functioning.[28,29]

Premature menopause and vaginal dryness that cannot be treated with estrogen after cancer can contribute to dyspareunia, thus affecting both desire and arousal in women with cancer (see Chemotherapy, later in this chapter). If one adds to this the variety of physical, psychosocial, and treatment-related factors associated with cancer treatment, a menopausal woman may certainly experience sexual dysfunction. Nevertheless, the menopause per se may not be the culprit.

ERECTILE DYSFUNCTION IN HEALTHY AGING MEN

Erectile function may be impaired by a number of conditions, both physical and psychological, and it declines with advancing age. As healthy men age, androgen levels begin to decline. Although these changes do not occur as precipitously as in menopause, a steady, age-related diminution is noted in most men. This can result in declining libido, which in turn tends to decrease erectile function. A notable variation in this pattern exists, and it is not uncommon for men to remain libidinous and potent well into advanced years. Peripheral circulatory problems and degenerative neuromuscular conditions also become more common, both increasing the incidence of vasculogenic and neurogenic erectile dysfunction (see Table 56.3-1).[30]

IMPACT OF CANCER AND ITS TREATMENT ON SEXUAL HEALTH

PSYCHOLOGICAL DISTRESS

Symptoms of anxiety or depression are frequent, and often appropriate, among cancer patients.[31–33] Psychological distress affects sexual functioning in healthy individuals, and this can be an important problem for patients with cancer. The literature suggests that patients with higher levels of psychological distress experience more sexual dysfunction.[31–35] For example, in a study of 227 newly diagnosed breast cancer patients, Schag et al.[31] found that patients who were classified by a social worker at 1 month after surgery as being "at-risk" for psychosocial distress were found to have more sexual difficulties than a comparison "low-risk" group, both at 1 month after surgery and 1 year later. Sexual problems that were increased included not being interested in having sex, difficulty in being sexually aroused, and difficulty reaching orgasm.[31] In a comprehensive follow-up study of advanced Hodgkin's disease and acute leukemia survivors, Kornblith et al.[33] found higher levels of distress in the Hodgkin's disease survivors, which was associated with significantly poorer sexual functioning than in the acute leukemia survivors. In a study of patients with early-stage cervical cancer, psychological as well as physical problems were highly correlated with sexual outcome.[34] In a study of long-term survivors of acute leukemia, no difference was found in psychosexual outcomes for patients treated with bone marrow transplantation compared to conventional therapy; however, those survivors who reported decreased sexual frequency and satisfaction and poorer body image were more likely to demonstrate greater psychological distress and decreased energy.[44] Thus, psychological distress, often manifested as increased symptoms of anxiety or depression, is an important variable that influences sexual outcomes, both acutely and chronically, in cancer patients.

BODY IMAGE CHANGES

One prominent cause of distress among cancer patients is change in body image. The changes associated with cancer and its treatment are often dramatic, ranging from surgical defects and deformities (e.g., limb amputation, loss of a breast, radical neck dissection) to total body alopecia from chemotherapy (e.g., loss of scalp hair, eyebrows, eyelashes, pubic and axillary hair) to more subtle changes (e.g., weight loss secondary to disease or treatment, weight gain from corticosteroids). All of these alterations can influence the patient's sense of sexual attractiveness and self-esteem.[36]

For women with breast cancer, the major advantage of breast-conserving surgery is the preservation of body image.[37–40] Patients with head and neck cancer often experience a range of physical and psychosocial problems related to disfiguring surgery, with consequent effects on sexual functioning.[41] Patients with colorectal cancer and stomas experience more body image problems than nonstoma patients and have poorer sexual functioning.[42] Thus, contemporary treatments that set organ preservation as a goal or provide immediate reconstructive surgery may well spare cancer patients the added burden of poorer body image. In one study, more favorable body image was a significant predictor of sexual interest in breast cancer survivors.[43] Nevertheless, the complexity of contemporary combined modality treatment (surgery, radiation therapy, and chemotherapy) aimed at organ preservation may also contribute to poorer body image through weight loss and hair loss, which may have a temporary or long-term adverse effect on body image.[35,44,45] In a study of long-term survivors of Hodgkin's disease (median time since treatment, 9 years), Fobair et al.[45] found that 26% of these survivors felt that their physical attractiveness had decreased, which was attributed to the diagnosis or treatment of the disease. More research is needed to determine the mechanisms through which body image disruption affects sexual functioning.

For some patients, weight gain is an important consequence of treatment that can interfere with body image. This effect has been particularly noted for women receiving adjuvant chemotherapy for breast cancer.[46–49] Goodwin et al.[49] followed an inception cohort of 535 women with newly diagnosed locoregional breast cancer and performed anthropometric measurements at baseline and 1 year later. Mean weight gain overall was 1.6 kg, with an average 2.5 kg gain in women receiving chemotherapy, 1.3 kg in those receiving tamoxifen, and 0.6 kg in those receiving no adjuvant treatment. In a multivariate analysis, onset of menopause and chemotherapy administration were each independent predictors of weight gain. Weight gain was not explained by increased caloric intake or decreased physical activity.[49] Thus, in addition to the effects of chemotherapy on energy, nausea, vomiting, and alopecia, weight gain must be added to the list, potentially decreasing self-esteem and sexual attractiveness.

DETERIORATING PHYSICAL FUNCTION, FATIGUE, AND PAIN

Declining physical functioning and the symptoms of fatigue and pain negatively influence sexual functioning. In a cross-sectional evaluation of 779 patients with colorectal, lung, and prostate cancers at all phases of disease (i.e., no evidence of disease, localized, and metastatic), sexual functioning was poorest for patients with advanced metastatic disease, who concomitantly experienced more frequent and severe physical problems associated with the cancer.[50] This finding was most significant for the patients with colorectal and lung cancer, whereas sexual problems were important for prostate cancer patients independent of stage and physical symptoms, likely due to the local effects of treatment on sexual functioning for all stages of the disease.[50]

Fatigue has begun to emerge as an important symptomatic problem for cancer patients and survivors.[51–53] Although this may be the result of clinical problems, such as anemia, which can be managed medically with transfusions or growth factors, chronic fatigue after cancer treatment may be multifactorial and represent late effects of chemotherapy and radiation, as well as be manifestations of both pain and depression. Fatigue has been most dramatically noted in patients treated for Hodgkin's disease,[45,53] in which the impact of fatigue on quality of life is multifaceted but includes sexual dysfunction as well. Treatment of the underlying causes of the fatigue, whether medically or psychologically, may have important benefits in terms of psychological functioning.

Other studies have begun to examine fatigue in breast cancer survivors.[51,52,54] In an analysis reported by Bower et al.[54] in almost 2000 breast cancer survivors, the strongest predictors of fatigue were pain and depression—both treatable problems. In that study sample, fatigue was significantly correlated with poorer sexual functioning ($r = -0.265$, $P = .0001$); when fatigue scores were used to classify the patients as either high or low energy, a significant difference was found in sexual functioning scores ($P = .0001$).[55] Interestingly, specific treatments (chemotherapy, radiation, tamoxifen) were not significantly associated with fatigue in the predictive model.[54]

Similarly, uncontrolled pain can be an important contributor to sexual dysfunction in cancer patients and survivors. Uncontrolled pain is associated with psychological distress, poor appetite, and lack of sleep, all of which can decrease sexual interest. Surprisingly, little empiric research has been conducted in this area. However, one study demonstrated the association of pain with decreased sexual functioning after high dose chemotherapy and autologous bone marrow support.[56] Another study that examined breast cancer patients with upper extremity lymphedema found that the presence of associated pain predicted psychological distress, but it did not independently predict sexual dysfunction.[57]

PARTNER RELATIONSHIPS

The literature suggests that the presence of a partner plays an important role in the maintenance of an active sex life for both men and women.[8,10,13,23] Problems in the marital relationship after cancer most often reflect preexisting stresses and strains, such that marital dissolution as a result of cancer is probably less common than once thought.[58] Often, cancer patients cite improvement in their love relationships rather than deterioration.[59] In a study of prostate cancer survivors compared with aged matched health controls, marital function did not differ between treatment groups and controls.[60]

The presence of a spouse or partner is invaluable for patients facing the possibility of sexual dysfunction from cancer or its treatments. Not only can spouses provide much needed emotional support, but they may also contribute to the clinical decision-making process. Physicians must be aware that the spouse often does not agree with the patient when assessing the relative value of sexual function versus survival. In fact, studies comparing husbands and wives suggest that the latter are much more willing to give up sexual function for a chance at longer survival.[61,62] Ultimately, the right choice of treatment must emanate from the patients themselves, but involvement of spouses can facilitate this process.

In addressing the partner relationship, it is also important never to assume that the patient is heterosexual, especially when the patient is alone for tests, consultations, and follow-up visits. The astute clinician should probe in a nonjudgmental way about the patient's partnership status and ensure that a same-gender partner is included, as appropriate, in medical decision making. Gay and lesbian couples enjoy long-term relationships that are emotionally equivalent to heterosexual marriage, yet given the degree of societal homophobia, they may fear being honest, even with their physicians. A few words of candid support may go a long way in allowing patients to feel better about involving their same-gender partner.

The literature does suggest that survivors of childhood and adolescent cancers are at increased risk for marital difficulties. In a large study of long-term survivors of childhood cancers compared with sibling controls, Byrne and colleagues[63] noted that both male and female survivors were less likely to marry than sibling controls and that the marriage deficit was particularly pronounced for survivors of brain and central nervous system tumors. In addition, the average length of first marriages was shorter for survivors than controls.[63] Men who had survived central nervous system tumors before the age of 10 years and male survivors of retinoblastoma had substantially higher divorce rates than controls (relative risk, 2.9 and 1.9, respectively). As noted by this study's authors, the treatment intensity for the patients studied in this cohort was much less intense than contemporary therapies, thus making altered marriage practices an important concern among adult survivors of pediatric brain tumors.[63] These findings have largely been confirmed in a preliminary report from a successor cohort study, the Childhood Cancer Survivor Study, in which rates of marriage have been compared to U.S. population census data and are found to be reduced.[64] Survivors were less likely to have married, particularly women and whites, but once married, they were less likely to divorce or separate. As in the study of Byrne et al.,[63] pediatric brain tumor survivors, particularly men, were less likely to have married and more likely to divorce or separate compared to those with other cancer diagnoses and the general population.[64] Other single-institution, detailed investigations of childhood survivors support these findings,[65] with the observation that many former patients indicate their diagnosis and treatment for childhood cancer influenced their own personal decision to have children and that this decision may play a role in the marital relationship. These findings may have important long-term implications for the sexual functioning of these long-term survivors, warranting more detailed inquiry.

SPECIFIC TREATMENTS

Surgery in General and Pelvic Surgery

Surgical treatment usually involves hospitalization, general or local anesthetic, and exploration of body cavities (thoracic, abdominal, pelvic), with adjacent organ dysfunction and the need to recover from the treatment insult. Postoperative pain and fatigue are important factors that limit recovery of sexual functioning for several weeks after surgery. Surgical treatments with the most significant impact on sexual functioning are those involving the pelvis, such as radical prostatectomy, radical cystectomy, abdominal-perineal resection for rectal cancer, and radical hysterectomy for gynecologic cancers. When radiation is added to surgical treatments, additional nerve and tissue injury may occur, with fibrosis and occasional pelvic pain syndromes. Changes in body image may occur as a result of surgery, especially when it is disfiguring and visible to others, but even hidden body scars may present a difficulty for some patients.

In men, pelvic surgery for prostate, bladder, or rectal cancer can easily damage the parasympathetic sacral fibers that are responsible for penile erection. These nerves course posterolateral to the prostate and anterolateral to the rectum and are intimately associated with both structures, especially at the apex of the prostate just anterior to the rectal wall. Although techniques have been developed for identification and preservation of these neurovascular bundles during radical prostatectomy,[66] such preservation is much more difficult during abdominal-perineal resection of the rectum.[67,68] These nerves do not need to be cut to disrupt their function. The mere trauma of dissection to separate them from the prostate or rectum may also lead to their permanent failure. The effect is immediate, and neuronal recovery is slow, often lasting months or years. Pelvic surgery for bladder or rectal cancer may also result in female sexual dysfunction, largely due to scarring, shortening, and stenosis of the vagina.[69,70] Despite initial dyspareunia, many women who are treated for bladder cancer with surgery and radiation ultimately do enjoy a return of sexual function.[71]

Retroperitoneal lymphadenectomy in men with testis cancer does not interfere with erections, but it may cause retrograde ejaculation. The primary landing site for lymphatic spread from the testes is located in the interaortocaval region for right-sided tumors and in the paraaortic region for left-sided tumors. From here, metastatic deposits can extend cephalad or caudad alongside the great vessels. Intertwined with these lymphatic channels are the lumbar sympathetic fibers that are responsible for normal antegrade ejaculation. If these are damaged during surgery, patients may experience a failure of both seminal emission and bladder neck closure. This in turn results in retrograde ejaculation. Although the patient is able to enjoy the pleasure of orgasm, it is dry and fluidless. Techniques to preserve these nerve fibers by using template dissections have been popularized and are largely successful at maintaining antegrade ejaculation in most men undergoing retroperitoneal lymphadenectomy.[72–75]

The effects of pelvic and genital surgery on sexual response in men and women vary depending on the organs involved and are summarized in Tables 56.3-4 and 56.3-5. Schover and Fife[76] provide an excellent overview of the components of the sexual response that are affected by these various surgical procedures. The amount of dysfunction depends on the extent of injury to the sacral plexus (especially for erectile functioning in men), and for women, vaginal lubrication may be strongly influenced by oophorectomy and the loss of estrogen, as well as the prohibition against estrogen replacement therapy. Dry orgasms occur in men after radical prostatectomy and radical cystectomy through surgical removal of the prostate and seminal vesicles. For women, vaginal shortening and anatomic changes that result from several of the surgical procedures leads to dyspareunia and the need to use lubricants and vaginal dilators.

The goals of contemporary multimodal therapies for cancer have focused on limiting the extent of surgery, with the addition of chemotherapy and radiation to control local and distant disease. Excellent examples of this trend are primary radiation therapy for prostate cancer, bladder-conserving surgery with radiation and chemotherapy, and sphincter preservation treatment of anal and rectal cancer. These approaches still have associated sexual dysfunctions, but the time course and specific problems may differ from surgery alone. In addition, patients may have to deal with the morbidity of the additional

TABLE 56.3-4. Effects of Surgery for Pelvic or Genital Cancer on Male Sexual Physiology

Procedure	*Desire*	*Pleasure from Touch*	*Ability to Have Erection*	*Orgasm*	*Ejaculation*	*Pain with Intercourse*
Radical prostatectomy	No change	No change	Decreased functioning that is age-dependent	No change or some decreased intensity	Dry orgasm	Rare
Radical cystectomy	No change	No change	Decreased functioning that is age-dependent	No change or some decreased intensity	Dry orgasm	Rare, but more likely after complete urethrectomy
Abdomino-perineal resection	No change	No change	Some impairment but less than radical prostatectomy	No change or some decreased intensity	Dry orgasm	Rare, but some perineal pain or phantom rectal sensations
Total pelvic exenteration	No change	No change	Almost always impaired	No change or some decreased intensity	Dry orgasm	Rare; possible genital edema from groin dissection
Partial penectomy	No change	Erotic sensation in remaining genital area	No change	No change	No change	Rare; possible genital edema from groin dissection
Total penectomy	No change	Erotic sensation in remaining genital area	Not possible	No change; need to identify erotic zones	No change; semen comes out perineal urethrostomy	Occasional; genital edema from groin dissection

(Adapted from ref. 84, with permission.)

therapies. Other procedures, such as bladder replacement with a continent reservoir, may avoid the embarrassment of external stomas and appliances, but this may not necessarily have a positive impact on sexual functioning.[77]

Chemotherapy

The effects of systemic chemotherapy on sexual functioning can be conceptualized as acute and chronic, with somewhat different risks for men and women. Acutely, and dependent on the type of chemotherapeutic agent, many patients experience nausea, vomiting, fatigue, hair loss, and mucositis. All of these factors contribute to a decrease in well-being and less interest in sexual activity. Women may experience vaginal and perineal mucositis from some agents, with some data suggesting decreased vaginal lubrication as a late effect of chemotherapy.[78,79] Loss of body hair decreases sexual attractiveness for most individuals, and extra effort may be required to maintain this aspect of sexuality. All of these effects are intensified in those receiving high-dose chemotherapy regimens.[80] Protracted fatigue may be a significant contributor to sexual dysfunction in bone marrow transplantation survivors.[56]

For women, one of the most dramatic consequences of chemotherapy treatment is the cessation of menses and the onset of menopause, with the consequent loss of fertility. This effect also has been reviewed for breast cancer treatments.[81,82] In a prospective study of a cohort of 183 early-stage breast cancer patients receiving no adjuvant therapy, either chemotherapy or tamoxifen adjuvant therapy, or both chemotherapy and tamoxifen,[83] age and systemic chemotherapy (in this case cyclophosphamide, methotrexate, or epirubicin, plus 5-fluorouracil) were the strongest predictors of menopause in women with locoregional disease, with tamoxifen making a small contribution (Fig. 56.3-1). As Figure 56.3-1 demonstrates, the probabil-

TABLE 56.3-5. Effects of Surgery for Pelvic or Genital Cancer on Female Sexual Physiology

Procedure	*Desire*	*Pleasure from Touch*	*Vaginal Lubrication*	*Ease of Orgasm*	*Orgasm*	*Pain with Intercourse*
Radical hysterectomy	No change	No change	May need ERT	No change	No change	Rare; shorter vagina
Radical cystectomy	No change	No change	Reduced, may need ERT	No change	No change	Frequent, but can be treated
Abdominoperineal resection	No change	No change	May need ERT	Probably no change	No change	Frequent, but can be treated
Total pelvic exenteration and vaginal reconstruction	No change	Some loss of erotic zones	Lost	Need to relearn how to reach orgasm	No change or mild decreased intensity	Occasional
Radical vulvectomy	No change	Some loss of erotic zones	No change	Need to relearn how to reach orgasm	?	Frequent, but can be treated

ERT, estrogen replacement therapy.
(Adapted from ref. 84, with permission.)

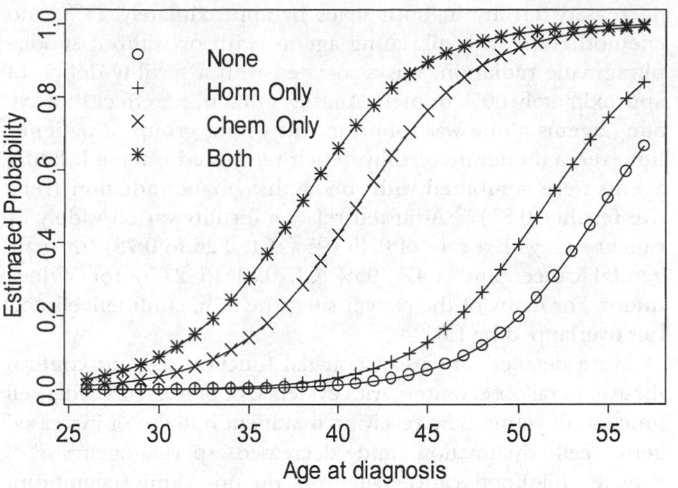

FIGURE 56.3-1. Probability of menopause during the first year after the diagnosis and adjuvant treatment of breast cancer. Horm, hormone; Chem, chemotherapy. (From ref. 90, with permission.)

ity of menopause with chemotherapy begins to rise at approximately 35 years of age, with more than 40% of women at age 40 predicted to become amenorrheic. The closer a woman was to the age of natural menopause (age 51), the greater her risk of amenorrhea.[83] Because this study only followed women for 1 year after treatment, however, some small proportion of women may have resumed menses after that time. Because some evidence suggests that amenorrhea may be beneficial in preventing breast cancer recurrence, it may be an acceptable consequence of treatment for some women. Nevertheless, the effects of menopause on sexual functioning, especially vaginal dryness, may contribute to sexual dysfunction in breast cancer survivors.[43]

Preservation of fertility is very important for younger patients treated for leukemia, testicular cancer, lymphoma, and Hodgkin's disease. Although current regimens for Hodgkin's disease that avoid alkylating agent therapy [e.g., Adriamycin, bleomycin, vinblastine, and dacarbazine (ABVD)] may spare ovarian and testicular function in terms of fertility and premature menopause, their value in preservation of sexual functioning may be more limited.[84] In Kornblith et al.'s study[84] examining the late effects of ABVD in comparison to Mustargen, Oncovin, procarbazine, and prednisone (MOPP) or MOPP/ABVD, no difference was found in sexual functioning by treatment arm. However, the small sample size of this study (93 disease-free survivors) across three treatment arm comparisons may have made it difficult to detect significant differences in outcomes. In another study comparing survivors of advanced-stage Hodgkin's disease and acute leukemia survivors treated on a variety of chemotherapy protocols, Kornblith et al.[33] found that Hodgkin's disease survivors experienced significantly poorer sexual relationships than the leukemia survivors. Thus, the specific type of chemotherapy regimen and its duration can have differing effects on sexual functioning.

Radiation Therapy

The acute effects of radiation include fatigue, nausea, skin changes, and hair loss, with local changes limited to the area of the radiation port. As already discussed, fatigue can interfere with sexual functioning, and hair loss and skin changes can affect sexual functioning through changes in body image. Long-lasting effects on skin and hair may occasionally occur, especially when combined modality therapies are used. Radiation injury to the pelvis can lead to fibrosis of soft tissue, as well as nerve damage, with loss of sexual functioning attributable to treatment. This is especially an issue when high-dose primary therapy is given, as for prostate cancer, bladder-conservation treatment, cervical cancer, and rectal cancers. In addition, injury to adjacent normal tissues (rectum, bladder, vagina) can lead to symptomatic problems (proctitis, cystitis, vaginal stenosis) that can detract from sexual activities.

Primary pelvic irradiation for prostate or bladder cancer may be as damaging to the erectile nerves as surgery. Radiation also damages the small blood vessels that supply and drain the corpora cavernosa.[85] The primary difference is the time course over which the effect is seen. Whereas surgical nerve injury reveals itself immediately, radiation injury to the nerves and vessels often does not manifest itself for many months. Because the mechanism of radiation tissue damage is to induce scarring over time, the pelvic vessels and erectile nerves may retain normal function initially and then decline fairly rapidly as long as 18 to 36 months after the completion of treatment.[86] The advent of three-dimensional conformal therapy has improved the radiation oncologist's ability to focus the beam at the center of the prostate and decrease the dose delivered to its periphery, where the nerves are located.[87] To treat prostate cancer effectively, however, an adequate dose must be administered to the entire gland, and this can certainly cause subsequent nerve damage. Proton-beam therapy, a variation of external-beam radiotherapy, is heavily marketed as causing fewer erectile complications in prostate cancer patients; however, no published evidence supports this claim.

Brachytherapy, the implantation of radioactive seeds into the prostate, has gained national prominence because it, too, is reputed to cause fewer complications than external-beam therapy. However, no reliable and valid longitudinal measurements of erectile function have yet been reported in patients who undergo this form of treatment. More information is needed before it can be established whether brachytherapy preserves erectile function in men treated for prostate cancer.

Hormonal Treatments

Hormonal treatments used in the management of endocrine-sensitive cancers may have important effects on sexual functioning. Tamoxifen, an antiestrogen, increases the rate of vaginal discharge and vasomotor symptoms in a proportion of breast cancer patients[79] and in those women taking this therapy for breast cancer prevention.[88] Although rates of sexual activity did not appear to differ between the women taking tamoxifen and those taking a placebo in the now completed Breast Cancer Prevention Trial, subtle differences in sexual functioning for women taking tamoxifen were noted (see Breast Cancer, later in this chapter).[88] In a small study that examined the effect of tamoxifen and sexual functioning in patients with breast cancer, Mortimer et al.[89] found that the desire, arousal, and orgasmic problems were not increased in their patient sample, but that more than one-half of patients complained of pain, burning, or discomfort with intercourse and that the majority of those with these symptoms routinely used a vaginal lubricant with intercourse. Vaginal cytology was examined in these women, and the presence of an estrogen effect was associated with negative reactions during sex ($P = .02$) and vaginal dryness or tightness ($P = .046$), but it was not associated with other aspects of sexual functioning.[89]

Weight gain is an important side effect with megestrol acetate, which is often used in the treatment of metastatic breast and endometrial cancers. This weight gain may contribute to a poorer body image in these patients and potentially affect sexual functioning.[90] Since the 1990s, interest has been renewed in ovarian ablation for women with breast cancer, either with surgical oophorectomy or with use of gonadotropin-releasing hormone analogues. As already mentioned, the precipitation of premature menopause in these women may cause substantial disruption in sexual functioning.

For men with advanced prostate cancer, the mainstay of therapy is androgen ablation,[91] which can be accomplished by either surgical or medical castration. Historically, the medical approach involved an oral estrogen, such as diethylstilbestrol, which inhibits the release of luteinizing hormone from the anterior pituitary and, in turn, decreases testicular androgen production. More recently, chemical castration is achieved with gonadotropin-releasing hormone blockers with or without the addition of antiandrogens to eliminate the effect of adrenal androgens. Other agents, such as aminoglutethimide or ketoconazole, may also be used for the same effect. Men who participate actively in the selection of their androgen ablation option tend to be happier with their decisions.[92]

The primary sexual side effect of androgen ablation is loss of libido. Many men report the ability to have erections and ejaculations despite the absence of testosterone, although decline in libido is universal. As a result, men who are sexually active and asymptomatic from the cancer (e.g., those who have a rising prostate-specific antigen level without documented metastatic disease) often choose to delay hormone therapy. For men who are experiencing clinical progression of metastatic prostate cancer, sexual function may already have declined or disappeared as their constitutional symptoms have advanced. For these individuals, androgen ablation may not have a great impact on erectile function, which is already greatly reduced.[93]

CONCERNS ABOUT FERTILITY

Preservation of fertility is an important aspect of treatment, especially for those individuals who have not had children. This issue pertains in particular to children and young adults with cancers who are treated with curative intent. As noted by Laufer,[94] it is increasingly useful to know the reproductive health outcomes for specific types of cancer treatments and "to differentiate between sex steroid production and fertility or reproductive function." In one of the largest studies of the effects of treatment on fertility in long-term survivors of childhood or adolescent cancer, Byrne and colleagues[95] estimated the risk of infertility after treatment in a retrospective cohort study of survivors of cancer and controls. The cancer patients, who were diagnosed before the age of 20 years, were treated between 1945 and 1975 at five cancer centers in the United States. Cancer survivors who married were less likely than their sibling controls to have ever begun a pregnancy [relative fertility, 0.85; 95% confidence interval (CI), 0.78 to 0.92]. With regard to therapy, radiation directed below the diaphragm decreased fertility in both sexes by approximately 25%, and chemotherapy with alkylating agents, with or without subdiaphragmatic radiation, was associated with a fertility deficit of approximately 60% in men. Among women, no effect of alkylating agents alone was found in this young group of patients; however, a moderate fertility deficit was noted when alkylating agents were combined with subdiaphragmatic radiation (relative fertility, 0.81).[95] Adjusted relative fertility varied widely by cancer site, with a rate of 0.45 (95% CI, 0.26 to 0.78) for male genital cancer and 1.47 (95% CI, 0.81 to 2.65) for Wilms' tumor. For many of the cancer sites, the 95% confidence intervals overlapped by 1.0.[95]

More detailed studies of gonadal function tend to confirm these general observations, with evidence of preserved Leydig cell function in young boys receiving treatment but also of increased germ cell dysfunction and decreased spermatogenesis.[96,97] Female childhood cancer survivors do not exhibit significant changes in gonadal function with contemporary treatments[97]; however, in the earlier era of extensive craniospinal and abdominal radiation used in the treatment of childhood acute lymphoblastic leukemia, lack of pubertal development and delayed onset of menses was common.[98] Even in young women treated for ovarian dysgerminoma, reproductive function can be preserved with conservative surgery and contemporary chemotherapy treatment regimens.[99]

For young adults with cancer, strategies to conserve fertility are often used and are highly dependent on the type of cancer and available treatments.[100] ABVD has largely replaced MOPP chemotherapy for Hodgkin's disease because of a more limited risk of infertility.[101] In general, however, diseases that require treatment with alkylating agents are likely to put both men and women at risk for infertility.[100] The risk for women begins to rise after 30 years of age, and for men the risk increases at any age. Cryopreservation of sperm is a strategy used to preserve fertility in men. Newer approaches to ovarian tissue preservation and subsequent reimplantation are on the horizon for women.[102,103]

A past history of cancer, uncertainty related to reproductive potential, and changes in sense of self-esteem and attractiveness may impair dating and sexual function in young adults with a history of cancer. Often, young adults who were treated for cancer as a child may have limited awareness of their past treatment, and they may be confronting this aspect of their health for the first time as they marry and attempt to start a family. Importantly, these individuals can be reassured that their offspring are unlikely to experience adverse consequences as a result of past parental treatments for cancer.[104,105]

SEXUAL PROBLEMS ASSOCIATED WITH SPECIFIC CANCERS

BREAST CANCER

Among specific cancer sites, breast cancer has been one of the most frequently studied regarding sexual functioning because of the surgical trauma to the breast and the severe disruption in body image associated with mastectomy. The important role of the breast in terms of femininity and sexual identity, and as an organ involved in sexual activity, has made sexual health after breast cancer an important issue. All of these concerns point to the potential impact of the type of surgical treatment on sexual functioning. However, as adjuvant treatment for breast cancer has expanded to earlier stages of disease, including noninvasive cancer, the impact of chemotherapy and hormonal therapy (e.g., tamoxifen, oophorectomy, gonadotropin-releasing hormone analogues) must also be considered. As already noted, each of these adjuvant therapies may induce premature menopause, lead to vaginal dryness, and may have other specific effects that can influence sexual health. These issues take on increasing importance in treatment decision making, because women with very early-stage breast cancer can expect survival that is equivalent to women without a cancer diagnosis.

One of the most investigated questions in breast cancer patients has been the impact of type of surgery on sexual health and quality of life.[40,106–108] Several large reviews of this topic[37–39,109] address the potential differences in outcomes for women treated with modified radical mastectomy compared to breast-conserving surgery with radiation. In only a few studies were women randomly assigned to the type of surgical treatment; most have been observational cohort studies in which patient choice or preference for treatment likely occurred. Thus, some bias could be influencing the results. Nevertheless, the consistency of findings across so many studies and countries suggests that the findings are real. There is consensus that breast-conserving surgery offers a better sense of body image to women after breast cancer but only limited differences in other dimensions of quality of life (physical, emotional, or social functioning). In studies that have specifically addressed sexual functioning,[40,107,109,110] little difference was found between the two types of surgery, although in the one randomized treatment trial,[110] some evidence suggested better sexual functioning in women with conservation surgery.

In a study comparing women with breast conservation treatment to those receiving mastectomy with reconstruction, Schover et al.[111] found that the two groups did not differ in body image, satisfaction with relationships, or sexual life. However, the authors did find that women with breast reconstruction experienced less caressing of the breast in lovemaking than women with partial mastectomy.[111] In a study of sexual health and functioning in breast cancer survivors,[43] body image influenced sexual interest, but the type of surgery did not predict any aspect of sexual health after breast cancer. Thus, although total loss of the breast may negatively influence a woman's body image, it does not necessarily impact her sexual health and functioning. As has been shown in healthy women without breast cancer[13] and in breast cancer survivors,[43] other factors may play a more important role in influencing sexual health in middle-age women (e.g., presence of a partner, vaginal dryness, emotional well-being, quality of the partnered relationship).

The etiology of sexual dysfunction in breast cancer survivors has not been well studied. As with other patients, multiple predisposing factors are involved, including preexisting sexual problems, negative sexual self-schemas, and normal age-related changes in sexual functioning.[14,15,112,113] In addition, induction of premature menopause by chemotherapy can result in an estrogen deficiency state that increases the likelihood of hot flashes and poor vaginal lubrication that may contribute to sexual dysfunction.[81,114–116] These symptoms are also a potential problem for older patients for whom hormone replacement therapy is discontinued at the time of a breast cancer diagnosis. Furthermore, these symptoms may be exacerbated by tamoxifen adjuvant therapy.[117] The results from the newly completed Breast Cancer Prevention Trial[88] suggest that, overall, tamoxifen has minimal effects on sexual functioning in healthy high-risk women. Comparing women taking tamoxifen to those taking placebo,[88] over the course of 3 years of follow-up, no difference was found in the number of women who were sexually active, although both groups showed a subtle decline in sexual activity over time. There was an increase in vaginal discharge, genital itching, and pain with intercourse in women taking tamoxifen, as well as very subtle changes in some aspects of sexual functioning (sexual interest, sexual arousal, orgasm).[88]

Multiple studies suggest an important role for chemotherapy in increasing sexual dysfunction in women with breast cancer.[78,79,115,118,119] This effect may be working through the precipitation of premature menopause and loss of both estrogens and androgens from the ovary.[119] However, chemotherapy may also have a direct effect on the vaginal epithelium, causing vaginal dryness, because postmenopausal women also experience poorer sexual functioning after chemotherapy.[78]

An increasing body of literature has examined sexual functioning in long-term survivors of breast cancer, with comparative information on women without a cancer diagnosis.[78,120–122] In a cross-sectional study of more than 800 breast cancer survivors between 1 and 5 years after diagnosis, Ganz et al.[78] found that approximately 60% of the study sample had been sexually active with a partner in the past 6 months, with the most common reason for inactivity being lack of a partner, lack of interest, her partner's lack of interest, or the partner's physical health problems.[78] Sexual functioning data from two standardized instruments showed a decline in sexual functioning with age, especially in the areas of arousal and orgasm. Overall, the responses of the breast cancer survivors were comparable to an age- and menopause-matched sample of healthy women who participated in the Postmenopausal Estrogen Progestins Intervention Trial and were not on hormone replacement therapy.[13] Overall, the breast cancer survivors reported fairly high levels of satisfaction with their sexual relationships.[78,121] Nevertheless, in a more detailed analysis, this study's authors found that one-third of women reported that breast cancer had had a negative impact on their sex life, and most reported negative changes in at least some areas (e.g., frequency of sexual activity, awareness of decreased lubrication in vagina with sexual activity, pain in genital area during sexual activity, discomfort when touching breast cancer surgery area).[121] Women who were most likely to report a negative impact were significantly more likely to report relationship difficulties, to have experienced changes in hormonal levels because of breast cancer (premature menopause or discontinuation of hormone replacement), and to be bothered by vaginal dryness.[121] These findings are similar to those obtained in smaller samples of breast cancer survivors.[120,122]

PROSTATE CANCER

The effect of erectile dysfunction on sexual functioning after treatment for prostate cancer has been studied extensively with a variety of experimental designs. All studies have shown that men undergoing radical prostatectomy or pelvic irradiation have more sexual impairment than age-matched controls.[123,124] Despite consistent reports of better outcomes with nerve-sparing techniques in centers of excellence, rates of sexual dysfunction in random, national, population-based samples reveal that erectile dysfunction remains common after surgery[125,126] or radiation[127] for early-stage prostate cancer.

Talcott[128] examined a group of men who underwent nerve-sparing radical prostatectomy and compared them with men who underwent non–nerve-sparing radical prostatectomy. Talcott found that patients who underwent nerve-sparing surgery had low levels of sexual function that were not significantly different from men who underwent non–nerve-sparing procedures. However, when the nerve-sparing population was broken down into one or both nerves spared, the bilateral nerve-sparing group reported significantly better potency at 1 year when compared to those who underwent non–nerve-sparing surgery. In a longitudinal follow-up study, Talcott et al.[129] confirmed that nerve-sparing appears to improve postoperative sexual function to a lesser extent than previously reported. Talcott et al.[86] also published the first prospective cohort study of patients treated with either surgery or radiotherapy, in which 279 patients were assessed with validated quality-of-life instruments before treatment and at 3 and 12 months afterward. Initially, surgery patients had more impotence; however, over time, sexual function declined in the radiotherapy group and improved in the surgery group. Hence, with longer follow-up, treatment group differences in sexual function continued to narrow. Other studies also have shown that the incidence of impotence increases to at least 35% to 40% during the 2 to 3 years after radiation therapy for localized prostate cancer.[130,131]

In a more recent longitudinal study of 438 men treated with surgery or radiation for early-stage prostate cancer,[132] sexual function after treatment for prostate cancer appeared to improve over time. Although sexual function was significantly better in radiation than surgery patients immediately after treatment, both groups improved at comparable rates during the first year. In the second year, radiation patients began to show a modest but statistically significant decline in sexual function, whereas surgery patients continued to improve. Both nerve-sparing and postsurgical erectile aids improved sexual function after prostatectomy. Given the decline in sexual function during the second year after radiation, these factors ultimately serve to equalize sexual function in the postsurgical and postradiation settings. The most elderly men experienced a posttreatment sexual function course that differed greatly from the youngest men. This finding validates the clinical observation that older men are much less likely than younger men to regain sexual function after treatment. In particular, octogenarians who choose radiotherapy can expect significant declines in sexual function without apparent recovery.

TESTIS CANCER

Therapy for testicular cancer, including orchiectomy, retroperitoneal lymphadenectomy, and radiation therapy, can cause a variety of physical and psychological sequelae.[133] Rieker et al.[134,135] showed that these patients express distress over poor sexual performance and infertility, although not with decreased libido. Those with ejaculatory dysfunction note more strained intimate relationships and more psychological problems. Compared with healthy controls, testis cancer patients as a group do not reveal any more difficulty with relationships, employment, divorce, or overall mental outlook. Bloom et al.[136] compared a sample of men treated for testis cancer with an age-matched sample treated for Hodgkin's disease. Those with testicular cancer were significantly more likely to report decreased sexual enjoyment; however, they were also more likely to report their health as excellent when compared to the lymphoma group, leading the authors to conclude that the response to testicular cancer is more site-specific.

After radiation therapy for seminoma, most men marry within a few years; however, a significant proportion of patients continue to report ejaculatory dysfunction and anxiety about fertility.[137] Gritz et al.[44,138] compared the outlooks of patients and their wives several years after testicular cancer treatment. Compared to their wives, patients reported higher levels of anxiety over sexual performance. Long-term psychosocial adjustment was good in both groups, however.

BLADDER CANCER

The overwhelming majority of men who undergo cystectomy for bladder cancer either report difficulties before treatment or develop erectile dysfunction after treatment. Despite this observation, at least 50% of these patients continue to enjoy some form of sexual stimulation other than coitus after recuperation from surgery,[139] and at least 75% maintain their libido.[140] For women, changes may occur that are associated with decreased vaginal lubrication if women are estrogen deficient,[76] and similar issues face both men and women if a stoma is created. Mansson and colleagues[77] administered a quality-of-life instrument to patients undergoing cystectomy and compared those reconstructed by continent cutaneous ileocecal diversion with those undergoing simple conduit diversion. Patients in both groups experienced equivalent declines in quality of life related to sexual problems, disturbed partner relationships, and emotional dysfunction.[77] In a similar study, Boyd and colleagues[141] demonstrated that, postoperatively, ileal conduit patients had the poorest self-image, as defined by a decrease in sexual desire and in all forms of physical contact (sexual and nonsexual). Those who later underwent conversion from ileal conduit diversions to continent cutaneous Kock pouches were the most physically and sexually active. Gerharz et al.[142] found that, after cystectomy, patients receiving an ileal conduit had worse scores than continent reservoir patients in sexual activity and general quality-of-life domains. Hart et al.[143] reported more optimistic findings, showing that general quality of life was not differentially affected by the choice of urinary diversion method after cystectomy in either women or men.

GYNECOLOGIC CANCERS

Cancer involving the female genital organs immediately evokes concerns about sexual dysfunction related to cancer-related symptoms that predate the diagnosis,[144] as well as treatments that may be required to extirpate the cancer. Cancers of the uterine corpus and cervix make up the majority of gynecologic cancers (roughly 70%), and these primarily localized cancers are treated with surgery or radiotherapeutic approaches, or both. Rarer cancers, such as vulvar cancer, may be treated with a variety of local or extensive surgical modalities, with some use of topical therapies. Nevertheless, the visible and disfiguring aspects of perineal surgery has its own serious sexual consequences. Other gynecologic cancers (ovarian cancer, trophoblastic disease, uterine sarcomas) are treated with combinations of chemotherapy, surgery and, sometimes, radiotherapy. The more disseminated nature of these cancers and the severity of the disease lead to different patterns of sexual dysfunction. For all gynecologic cancers, the age, partnership status, menopausal status, and preexisting sexual functioning of a woman play an important role in her sexual rehabilitation after cancer treatment (see Table 56.3-1 and review by Andersen[145]).

Because of the involvement of the genital organs with gynecologic cancers, changes in sexual functioning may often take place before the diagnosis of cancer. In a comparison of healthy control subjects and women with early-stage cervical and uterine cancer, Andersen et al.[144] found few differences in aspects of the sexual response cycle reported before the onset of signs or symptoms of the cancer. However, a substantial number of the gynecologic cancer patients reported a disruption in sexual responsiveness with the onset of symptoms, including changes in desire, excitement, orgasm, and resolution and a global deterioration in sexual functioning.[144] These changes were most often associated with symptoms of fatigue, postcoital bleeding, and multiple other signs and symptoms.

Sexual functioning outcomes in patients with gynecologic cancers often have been reported in small case series. Andersen and colleagues[146] prospectively studied 47 women with early-stage gynecologic cancers (cervix, n = 33; endometrium, n = 9; ovary, n = 5) and benign gynecologic disease before treatment, and then interviewed them again at 4, 8, and 12 months posttreatment. Women treated for disease, whether benign or malignant, reported similar declines in frequency of intercourse, decreased sexual excitement, and a less positive global evaluation of their sexual life. In addition, a three- to sixfold increase in the incidence of sexual dysfunction diagnoses was found in comparison to the rates in healthy women.[146] Pain with intercourse, prominent early in the recovery period in treated women, improved with time but remained more frequent in the cancer patients. Although both treated groups experienced increased sexual dysfunctions posttreatment, the cancer patients experienced a higher incidence of inhibited excitement. As discussed by Andersen et al.,[146] these particular changes can be a manifestation of increased anxiety associated with the cancer diagnosis.

Looking more specifically at the impact of cervical cancer and its treatment on sexual functioning, several other small, descriptive studies are relevant. Schover et al.[147] examined sexual frequency, function, and behavior in 61 women with early-stage invasive carcinoma of the cervix. The impact of treatment (radical hysterectomy alone, radiotherapy with or without surgery) was examined in this study. Sexual satisfaction, capacity for orgasm, and frequency of masturbation remained stable over 12 months of observation posttreatment; however, frequency of sexual activity with a partner and the range of sexual practices decreased significantly over the course of the year of follow-up. Although at 6 months few differences were noted between those who had received irradiation and those who had not, at the 12-month assessment, the women receiving radiotherapy had more dyspareunia (as well as an abnormal vaginal examination) and had more problems with sexual desire and arousal.[147] Treatment modality had no effect on marital happiness or stability.

These findings suggest an additional complication from irradiation of the pelvis, which is vaginal stenosis or foreshortening. Several other studies have documented this problem,[148,149] with level of sexual activity being lowest at the completion of radiotherapy. The finding of progressive dyspareunia and vaginal shortening[147] suggests the need for active intervention in these women, with the need for early use of vaginal lubricants, resumption of sexual activity, or use of dilators to maintain vaginal length and elasticity. In one small study,[150] women who did not follow advice regarding use of vaginal dilators and did not resume the same level of sexual intercourse as before their illness were more likely to develop physical and sexual changes.

These small descriptive studies shed some light on the mechanisms of sexual dysfunction and the range of sexual problems in the first year after treatment for cervical cancer. However, the late sexual effects of treatment for cervical cancer are important, because this is a group of women who are likely to be cured of their disease and be long-term cancer survivors. A report by Bergmark et al.[151] provides important new information on vaginal changes and sexuality in a large sample of Swedish cervical cancer survivors (n = 256) and a concurrent control sample (n = 350). The cancer survivors had been treated, on average, approximately 5 years earlier and were a mean age of 51 years at the time they responded to the study questionnaire. Significant differences were found between the two groups in problems with vaginal lubrication (26% of the women with cancer vs. 11% of the controls), reporting of a short vagina (26% of the women with cancer vs. 3% of the controls), and decreased vaginal elasticity (23% of the women with cancer vs. 4% of the controls). In spite of these significant changes associated with the treatment of cervical cancer, no differences were noted in sexual interest, desire, frequency of vaginal intercourse, or orgasm; however, there was much distress related to the frequency of vaginal intercourse and problems during vaginal intercourse (dyspareunia, vaginal bleeding) among the women with a history of cervical cancer.[151]

Treatment with surgery alone was associated with decreased vaginal lubrication, vaginal shortness, and decreased vaginal elasticity.[151] When surgery was combined with radiotherapy or when radiotherapy was given alone, no apparent differences in these vaginal outcomes were found when compared to surgery alone, except for some decreased sexual interest among those treated with radiotherapy alone. Interestingly, treatment for cervical cancer negatively influenced feelings of femininity and attractiveness among the cervical cancer survivors but did not seem to influence sexual satisfaction. Importantly, the authors observed no age above which sexual function was not important to women, and they suggest that efforts to prevent vaginal changes or relieve them after therapy should be considered in all women who are treated for cervical cancer.[151] Finally, it should be noted that the use of a healthy control group in this study was important, in that 41% of both patients and controls reported little or no interest in sex in the previous 6 months, with more than 50% reporting reduced sexual desire in the previous 5 years. Without such a control group, these findings might have been attributed to the history of cancer.

Although rare, other gynecologic cancers can have profound effects on sexual functioning. In spite of being the third most common gynecologic cancer, ovarian cancer patients have been less frequently studied.[152] Most experience all of the physical changes associated with the treatment of uterine and cervical cancer due to surgical removal of the uterus and ovaries. However, treatment of these patients is often dominated by the use of systemic or intraperitoneal chemotherapy and the side effects of this treatment, especially decreased physical functioning, fatigue, pain, and abdominal discomfort. Symptoms of advanced cancer significantly impact sexual functioning in these women.

Sexual functioning after vulvar cancer has been examined in two series.[153,154] In Andersen et al.'s study,[153] women with *in situ* vulvar cancer were compared with a matched sample of gynecologically healthy women. They found a higher rate of inhibited sexual excitement and inhibited orgasm among the women with cancer, as well as an increasing rate of sexual inactivity over time, compared with the healthy women. As might be predicted, the wider the surgical excision, the greater the magnitude of sexual disruption.[153] In a prospective study of ten couples, with the women being treated for vulvar cancer with radical vulvectomy, Weijmar Schultz et al.[154] found a postoperative decline in functioning with gradual recovery over 2 years. However, genital symptoms of sexual arousal and satisfaction were diminished in the cancer group and did not return to levels of those found in the control group.[154] Importantly, general satisfaction with sexual interaction with the partner hardly changed over a 2-year period of observation.[154]

HODGKIN'S DISEASE

As a group, patients with Hodgkin's disease can anticipate long-term survival and cure. Therefore, the impact of disease and treatment on sexual functioning is an important consideration. Several groups have studied the long-term psychosocial outcomes for this group of patients.[32,45] Hodgkin's disease survivors in one study[32] (n = 273) were found to have elevated levels of psychological distress, on average, compared to healthy controls, and those survivors in greater distress reported more problems in other areas of functioning, including sexual problems. When survivors rated their overall current sexual satisfaction, the median scores were similar to healthy subjects. However, when asked to consider the effect of cancer on their sexual life, 37% reported one or more sexual problems, primarily because of decreased sexual satisfaction (31%), interest (21%), and activity (18%). Of these survivors, 26% had been tested and were told they were infertile, and an additional 27% believed that they were infertile.[32] In addition, all survivors who were not currently married experienced higher distress than those who were married, and 56% of those who were separated or divorced attributed their marital status to having had cancer.[32] Although these data are not controlled, from the patient perspective, the disease and its treatment has had a substantial effect on sexual functioning. However, in a comparative study of survivors of acute leukemia,[33] the same investigators found substantially more psychological distress and poorer sexual functioning among the Hodgkin's disease survivors than those with leukemia. These authors suggest that the risk of second malignancies, relapse, and infertility are likely contributors to the greater problems in adjustment among the Hodgkin's disease survivors.[33]

In another comparative study, Bloom et al.[136] examined the psychosocial outcomes of testicular cancer and Hodgkin's disease to test the hypothesis that more specific dysfunction and less hiding of symptoms would be found among the testicular cancer patients. The main differences were in physical activity, fatigue, and vigor (worse for Hodgkin's disease) and decrease in quality of orgasm (worse for testicular cancer), with no difference in psychological distress between the two groups of patients. In addition, no differences between the two sites were found in terms of body image.[136] As noted by these authors,[136] without concurrent data on healthy controls, it is uncertain how much sexual dysfunction may be specifically related to the disease, its treatment, age, or other unmeasured variables.

COLORECTAL CANCER

Colorectal cancer is a disease of older individuals, with most cancers occurring in persons older than 60 years of age. There is a paucity of specific literature on sexual dysfunction in this population, but the information that is available focuses on the consequences of abdominoperineal resection and ostomies. In a review of sexual functioning in women after radical surgery for rectal cancer,[155] prospective studies of small samples suggest a decline in sexual activity postoperatively, with declines in interest, lubrication, and orgasmic activity. In a study comparing abdominoperineal resection with colostomy and low anterior resection, sexual functioning was preserved at a higher rate with low anterior resection. Overall, the prognostic variables most influencing posttreatment sexual functioning include the woman's age at surgery, the magnitude of the surgical intervention, handmade versus stapled anastomoses, and the number of autonomic nerves present in the surgical specimen.[155]

For men, similar issues pertain; however, erectile dysfunction is a more salient issue.[156] In a study of 60 sexually active men surgically treated for colorectal cancer, Koukouras et al.[156] found that sexual activity was decreased in 32% of patients. The distribution of difficulties among those affected were dry ejaculate (25%), erection not firm enough for penetration (45%), and complete absence of erection (25%). The decreases in sexual functioning occurred in all groups of patients, from high anterior resection to low anterior resection to abdominoperineal resection, but were most frequent in those with abdominoperineal resection.[156]

In another report, Sprangers et al.[42] reviewed the quality of life in colorectal cancer according to whether a sphincter-preserving procedure was performed. They found that stoma patients reported higher levels of psychological distress than nonstoma patients and that sexual functioning of male and female stoma patients is consistently more impaired than that of patients with intact sphincters. Both groups, however, are troubled by frequent and irregular bowel function that can increase psychological distress and affect sexual functioning.[42]

STRATEGIES FOR ASSESSMENT AND INTERVENTION

ASSESSMENT

A comprehensive assessment of sexual difficulties requires an interdisciplinary and multifaceted approach that is often beyond the scope of the oncology team. Depending on the particular problem(s), it can be important to consider hormonal, physiologic, anatomic, psychological, cognitive, behavioral, relational, and cultural factors in a biopsychosocial model[6] (see Table 56.3-1). To provide a differential diagnosis, it also is necessary to assess for psychopathology, medical conditions, substance abuse, and relationship difficulties as primary etiologic factors. Modes of assessment include open-ended conversations, structured diagnostic interviews, standardized self-report questionnaires, medical examination, and laboratory studies. Several volumes are available for readers who wish to learn about specific assessment procedures.[2,4,17,157]

Although a comprehensive assessment is unrealistic within the constraints of an oncology practice, a preliminary review of sexual difficulties *is essential* to providing optimal care to the cancer patient. Patients regularly report that they would like to discuss sexual issues with their physicians but feel reluctant to do so.[24,114] Therefore, it is up to the medical team to broach the issue and open lines of communication. Straightforward questions about each of the four categories of sexual dysfunction—desire, arousal, orgasm, and pain—and questions about sexual activity and satisfaction generally provide sufficient information to determine the need for further testing or referral.[11,158] One member of the team could be identified as a primary resource for assessment and referral.

COUNSELING, INTERVENTION, AND REFERRAL

After a member of the oncology team has raised the issue of sexuality and made a preliminary assessment of reported problems, a decision must be made regarding the level and type of intervention that is needed.[159] In some cases, the specific concerns that arise can be addressed directly by a member of the team who has developed expertise in sexuality and cancer. Providing patients and (when appropriate) their partners with information about sexual functioning, aging, and sexual problems related to the cancer experience can help to normalize the concerns that arise for some patients. Patients also can benefit from receiving written materials, such as those available from the National Cancer Institute and the American Cancer Society or produced by other experts.[160] They may also benefit from learning about local resources for cancer patients and survivors. For limited problems, specific suggestions or a brief course of sexual counseling may be sufficient. For example, for a woman with vaginal dryness who cannot use estrogen, a vaginal lubricant or moisturizer might be extremely effective. Schover and colleagues[16] found that 63.5% of cancer patients who received brief sexual counseling within a cancer center reported improvement. Patients who were depressed or in conflicted marriages were least likely to benefit.

When the patient has more complex problems, it may be necessary to provide a referral to a mental health professional with special training in sex therapy, marital therapy, or individual psychotherapy with cancer patients. The oncologist can play a pivotal role in ensuring successful treatment by making appropriate referrals that normalize the need for therapy. In addition, specific medical interventions such as those detailed in the next two sections may be helpful.

MEDICAL INTERVENTIONS FOR WOMEN

One of the most important targets for intervention in women is vaginal dryness. This problem is common for women as they age, independent of cancer treatment, and is usually managed with some form of estrogen therapy. In women who can receive estrogen therapy after cancer, this treatment is the most effective therapeutic remedy, and it can be used topically or systemically. The role of hormone replacement in addressing sexual functioning after intensive chemotherapy should not be underestimated. In a study of the prevalence and predictors of sexual dysfunction in long-term survivors of bone marrow transplantation, Syrjala et al.[161] found that women reported significantly more sexual dysfunction than men. The number of women with lubrication problems increased from 30% before transplantation to 49% at 1 year posttransplantation and 52% at 3 years posttransplantation.[161] This finding was associated with a doubling in the rate of women reporting pain with intercourse, from 14% at pretransplantation to approximately 34% posttransplantation. In addition, this study's authors found a significant difference in sexual satisfaction at 3 years for those who had received hormone replacement therapy by 1 year compared to the 15% of women who had not. Changing hormone replacement therapy after 1 year, either by starting therapy or electing to stop hormone therapy, did not show a measurable influence on reported sexual satisfaction at 3 years.[161] This finding suggests that once sexual problems are established early after cancer treatment (vaginal dryness, dyspareunia), it may be more difficult to restore satisfactory sexual activity. Thus, early intervention with hormonal therapy should be considered for patients receiving chemotherapy if it is not otherwise contraindicated.

In breast cancer patients and survivors, the use of hormone replacement therapy is much more controversial (see discussion of menopause earlier in Menopause and Sexual Functioning). As a result, nonestrogen alternatives are often considered first in the management of vaginal dryness. One randomized controlled trial comparing estrogen to the vaginal moisturizer Replens has demonstrated improvement in vaginal cytology with this preparation in healthy women.[162] The North Central Cancer Treatment Group has tested the efficacy of Replens for the management of vaginal dryness and dyspareunia in a placebo-controlled trial.[163] They found this product to be effective in relieving symptoms; however, similar results were seen with the placebo (K-Y Jelly), which was apparently not an inert substance. A discussion of these nonestrogen alternatives is reviewed elsewhere.[164–166] If these therapies do not work, the use of the estrogen-impregnated product Estring can be considered for topical relief of symptoms without significant systemic absorption.[167]

In a study addressing menopausal symptoms in breast cancer survivors, Ganz et al.[168] found that most of the women who wanted some form of treatment were highly symptomatic, with more than 80% having two of three symptoms (hot flashes, vaginal dryness, urinary incontinence). Using education, counseling, lifestyle modifications, and several pharmacologic agents (Bellergal-S, clonidine patch, megestrol acetate, Replens), after a 4-month period of intervention, a significant improvement in the target menopausal symptoms and sexual functioning in the women assigned to treatment was demonstrated, compared to a no-treatment control group. Unlike the single-agent pharmacologic trials, this study tried to address all three symptoms simultaneously, as well as tailor the treatment strategies to the individual's needs and her willingness or unwillingness to take a medication.

Other important strategies to consider are the treatment of psychological distress and marital or partner difficulties. In both healthy women and women with breast cancer,[13,43] distress in these domains has been shown to influence sexual functioning and satisfaction. Control of pain and other symptoms may also be critical for assuring sufficient relaxation to allow women to engage in meaningful sexual activities.

MEDICAL AND SURGICAL INTERVENTIONS FOR MEN

The clinical management of cancer patients with erectile dysfunction should follow the same algorithms used in men presenting primarily for evaluation of impotence. Even when other interventions are prescribed, brief sexual counseling in the primary oncology setting can play a critical role in the care of the patient.[169] The model currently used in the management of patients with erectile dysfunction involves a stepwise approach.[169] First-line therapies are selected based on their ease of administration, reversibility, and noninvasiveness. Oral erectogenic agents, such as sildenafil, yohimbine, trazodone, and phentolamine, have gained widespread popularity, largely because of the convenience and effectiveness of sildenafil.[170] Sildenafil works in most forms of erectile dysfunction and has few side effects. It is a selective type 5 phosphodiesterase inhibitor, which increases penile cyclic guanosine monophosphate, thus enhancing the effect of nitric oxide in response to sexual stimulation. In the penis, the effect of sildenafil is to increase cavernosal smooth muscle dilation, a requisite component of erection. At doses of 25, 50, or 100 mg taken 30 to 60 minutes before sex, it is successful in approximately 70% of impotent men. Side effects are minor and may include mild headache, facial flushing, rhinitis, dyspepsia, or blue-hued vision.[171] Sildenafil is thought to have been partially responsible for mortality in a very small percentage of cases by interacting with medicinal or recreational nitrates or by allowing sexual overexertion in men with severe cardiac disease. It should never be used concomitantly with nitrates. Apomorphine, another oral erectogenic whose U.S. Food and Drug Administration approval is reportedly imminent, is thought to work by interacting with central and peripheral dopaminergic pathways in impotent men.[172]

Another noninvasive technique is the penile vacuum erection device (VED).[173–175] Although it is somewhat more cumbersome and requires training, a substantial minority of patients prefer the VED for its simplicity, safety, and effectiveness. A clear, plastic, hollow cylinder is placed around the penis and sealed at the skin with lubricant. A small handheld pump, attached by a rubber tube to the tip of the cylinder, is activated, creating a vacuum around the penis within the cylinder. This draws blood into the erectile bodies and creates an erection. Once the penis becomes tumescent, a rubber constriction band is placed around the base of the penis to retain the erection, and the cylinder is removed. After sex, the band is removed, allowing the penile blood to drain. Few risks are associated with use of the VED.

Second-line therapies involve the administration of pharmacologic vasodilators, either by direct intracavernosal needle injection[176] or by intraurethral suppository.[177] Injections typically include prostaglandin E_1 alone (marketed as Caverject or Edex) or in combination with papaverine or phentolamine. The intraurethral suppository (marketed as Muse) contains prostaglandin E_1 alone in doses of 5, 10, or 20 μg. Both methods function by producing dilation of the cavernosal smooth muscle, enhancing the vascular component of penile erection. Intracavernosal injection is much more effective than intraurethral administration, but it also carries a greater short-term risk of priapism or pain and the long-term risk of corporal scarring at the injection sites. With intracavernosal medication, the patient is trained to draw up the drug in a tuberculin syringe and inject it into the penis. The patient must take care to place the needle perpendicular to the long axis of the penis and advance it all the way through the subcutaneous fat into the corpus cavernosum. Because of intercavernosal connections, only one corpus needs to be injected to induce erection. The patient must be careful to avoid the nerve bundle dorsally and the urethra ventrally. He must also rotate injection sites and apply 2 to 3 minutes of pressure after injection to avoid bruising. The intraurethral medication is sold as a suppository of 250, 500, or 1000 μg loaded into a small applicator that the patients inserts into his urethral meatus. Once in position, he pushes the medicated pellet out by advancing a small probe. The medication is packaged with pictorial instructions that facilitate patient teaching. With either penile vasodilator, the dose must be individually titrated.

Third-line therapies include the surgical implantation of semirigid or inflatable penile prostheses.[178] The operation is usually performed on an outpatient basis and involves a single, small dorsal or ventral incision at the base of the penis. After dissecting and entering the corpora cavernosa, their internal spongy tissue is compressed with dilators and their size calibrated. The appropriate length prostheses are inserted into both corpora. Semirigid prostheses may contain malleable metal rods encased in silicone, or they may be made of solid silicone. After recovery from surgery, the semirigid penile prosthesis requires no training and is ready for use approximately 8 to 12 weeks postoperatively. Inflatable prostheses contain pliable hollow tubes that are filled with saline from a nearby reservoir by activating a pump. In the three-piece versions, the reservoir is implanted through the groin in the perivesical space, and the pump is implanted subcutaneously in the scrotum. These components are connected to each other and to the cylinders with silicone tubing. A two-piece version is also available, in which the pump and reservoir are combined into one scrotal component. Self-contained inflatable prostheses have the cylinders, reservoir, and pump all located in one structure. These have become the preferred choice because of easier surgical implantation. After recovery, the inflatable prosthesis requires detailed training before the patient becomes comfortable with its use. The primary advantage of the inflatable version is that it appears flaccid when not in use; however, it is also associated with a greater chance of mechanical problems, which may require further surgery. Both semirigid and inflatable prostheses carry some risk of infection, but this complication is uncommon. Placement of a penile prosthesis is an invasive maneuver, in which any residual existing erectile capacity is lost. This option is reserved for the most severe and refractory cases of erectile dysfunction. If the devices ever require removal, natural erections are unlikely to return.

CONCLUSIONS

It is important to recognize that sexual problems are prevalent in the general population and that age-related changes in sexual interest and responsiveness occur naturally. When one adds a cancer diagnosis and its treatments to this background environment, existing sexual problems can be exacerbated, and an active sex life may cease for some cancer patients. Understanding the natural history of sexual problems associated with specific treatments and cancers can enhance the ability of clinicians to detect sexual problems in the patients under their care. Because patients seldom directly express sexual concerns to their health care provider either before or after cancer treatment, it is essential that these issues be brought up with patients in a routine and matter-of-fact way. The treating oncologist should find a comfortable way to ask, "How is your sex life going?" Often, a good time to ask this question is somewhere in the middle or toward the end of a treatment course. This can serve as a "check-in" to let the patient know the oncologist is willing to talk about these issues. If the patient has no problems or is not interested in talking, the conversation ends there.

However, patients know that they can bring up the topic in the future if they wish. Similarly, patients who are anxious to share concerns about sexual functioning appreciate the opportunity to discuss the specific problems. The health care professional can often provide information, reassurance, referrals, and specific remedies (e.g., treatment for vaginal dryness, medication of erectile dysfunction, treatment of pain).

Another perspective that is often overlooked is that of the young adult with cancer. Even more challenging than when a spouse is present is the young man with testis cancer, the young woman with breast cancer, or the teenager with lymphoma. With less experience and self-confidence, these individuals may be even shyer about bringing up the topic of sexuality with their oncologists. For the young adult with cancer, it is especially incumbent upon the clinician to talk about sex during and after treatment. In these situations, the difficult questions may be, for example, "Should I tell a new romantic interest about the cancer on the first date, or should I wait?" Of course, these problems are relevant for the single patient at any age.

With the increasing media attention given to sexual health in the general population, patients now expect their physicians to be well informed and receptive to discussing these issues. The very privileged relationship that oncologists have with their patients with cancer, guiding them through treatment decisions for a life-threatening condition, should permit the physician to assist the patient with this aspect of health and recovery. We are fortunate that a growing body of research on sexual health after cancer now exists, which can inform and guide those discussions.

REFERENCES

1. Masters WH, Johnson VE. *Human sexual response.* Boston: Little, Brown and Company, 1966.
2. Bancroft J. *Human sexuality and its problems.* Edinburgh, Scotland: Churchill Livingstone, 1989.
3. Tiefer L. The medicalization of sexuality: conceptual, normative, and professional issues. *Ann Rev Sex Res* 1996;7:252.
4. Kaplan HS. *Disorders of sexual desire: the new sex therapy.* New York: Brunner/Mazel, 1979.
5. Kaplan HS. *The evaluation of sexual disorders: psychological and medical aspects.* New York: Brunner/Mazel, 1983.
6. Rosen RC, Leiblum SR. Treatment of sexual disorders in the 1990s: an integrated approach. *J Consult Clin Psychol* 1995;63:877.
7. American Psychiatric Association. *Diagnostic and statistical manual of mental disorders,* 4th ed. Washington, DC: American Psychiatric Association, 1994.
8. Laumann EO, Gagnon JH, Michael RT, Michaels S. *The social organization of sexuality: sexual practices in the United States.* Chicago: University of Chicago Press, 1994.
9. Frank E, Anderson C, Rubinstein D. Frequency of sexual dysfunction in "normal" couples. *N Engl J Med* 1978;299:111.
10. Laumann EO, Paik A, Rosen RC. Sexual dysfunction in the United States: prevalence and predictors. *JAMA* 1999;281:537.
11. Ackerman MD, Carey MP. Psychology's role in the assessment of erectile dysfunction: historical precedents, current knowledge, and methods. *J Consult Clin Psychol* 1995;63:862.
12. Beck JG. Hypoactive sexual desire disorder: an overview. *J Consult Clin Psychol* 1995;63:919.
13. Greendale GA, Hogan P, Shumaker S, for the Postmenopausal Estrogen/Progestin Interventions (PEPI) Trial investigators. Sexual functioning in postmenopausal women: the postmenopausal estrogen/progestin interventions (PEPI) trial. *J Womens Health* 1996;5:445.
14. Hawton K, Gath D, Day A. Sexual function in a community sample of middle-aged women with partners: effects of age, marital, socioeconomic, psychiatric, gynecological, and menopausal factors. *Arch Sex Behav* 1994;23:375.
15. Rosen RC, Taylor JF, Leiblum SR, Bachmann GA. Prevalence of sexual dysfunction in women: results of a survey study of 329 women in an outpatient gynecology clinic. *J Sex Marital Ther* 1993;19:171.
16. Schover LR, Evans RB, von Eschenbach AC. Sexual rehabilitation in a cancer center: diagnosis and outcome in 384 consultations. *Arch Sex Behav* 1987;16:445.
17. Wincze JP, Carey MP. *Sexual dysfunction: a guide for assessment and treatment.* New York: Guilford Press, 1991.
18. Bachmann GA. Sexual function in the perimenopause. *Obstet Gynecol Clin North Am* 1993; 20:379.
19. Schiavi RC, Schreiner-Engel P, Mandeli J, Schanzer H, Cohen E. Healthy aging and male sexual function. *Am J Psychiatry* 1990;147:766.
20. Mulligan T, Moss CR. Sexuality and aging in male veterans: a cross-sectional study of interest, ability, and activity. *Arch Sex Behav* 1991;20:17.
21. Dionko AC, Brown MB, Herzog AR. Sexual function in the elderly. *Arch Intern Med* 1990;150:197.
22. Feldman HA, Goldstein I, Hatzichristou DG, Krane RJ, McKinlay JB. Impotence and its medical and psychosocial correlates: results of the Massachusetts Male Aging Study. *J Urol* 1994;151:54.
23. Thirlaway K, Fallowfield L, Cuzick J. The Sexual Activity Questionnaire: a measure of women's sexual functioning. *Qual Life Res* 1996;5:81.
24. Loehr J, Verma S, Seguin R. Issues of sexuality in older women. *J Womens Health* 1997;6:451.
25. McKinlay SM. The normal menopause transition: an overview. *Maturitas* 1996;23:137.
26. Greendale GA, Lee NP, Arriola ER. The menopause. *Lancet* 1999;353:571.
27. Ganz PA, Day R, Ware JE, et al. Base-line quality-of-life assessment in the National Surgical Adjuvant Breast and Bowel Project Breast Cancer Prevention Trial. *J Natl Cancer Inst* 1995;87:1372.
28. Myers LS, Dixen J, Morrissette D, Carmichael M, Davidson JM. Effects of estrogen, androgen, and progestin on sexual psychophysiology and behavior in postmenopausal women. *J Clin Endocrinol Metab* 1990;70:1124.
29. Sherwin BB. The impact of different doses of estrogen and progestin on mood and sexual behavior in postmenopausal women. *J Clin Endocrinol Metab* 1991;72:336.
30. Helgason AR, Adolfsson J, Dickman P, et al. Factors associated with waning sexual function among elderly men and prostate cancer patients. *J Urol* 1997;158:155.
31. Schag CAC, Ganz PA, Polinsky ML, et al. Characteristics of women at risk for psychosocial distress in the year after breast cancer. *J Clin Oncol* 1993;11:783.
32. Kornblith AB, Anderson J, Cella DF, et al. Hodgkin disease survivors at increased risk for problems in psychosocial adaptation. *Cancer* 1992;70:2214.
33. Kornblith AB, Herndon JE II, Zuckerman E, et al. Comparison of psychosocial adaptation of advanced stage Hodgkin's disease and acute leukemia survivors. Cancer and Leukemia Group B. *Ann Oncol* 1998;9:297.
34. Cull A, Cowie VJ, Farquharson DI, et al. Early stage cervical cancer: psychosocial and sexual outcomes of treatment. *Cancer* 1993;68:1216.
35. Mumma GH, Mashberg D, Lesko LM. Long-term psychosexual adjustment of acute leukemia survivors: impact of marrow transplantation versus conventional chemotherapy. *Gen Hosp Psychiatry* 1992;14:43.
36. Wood JD, Tombrink J. Impact of cancer on sexuality and self-image: a group program for patients and partners. *Soc Work Health Care* 1983;8(4):45.
37. Kiebert GM, de Haes JCJM, van de Velde CJH. The impact of breast-conserving treatment and mastectomy on the quality of life of early-stage breast cancer patients: a review. *J Clin Oncol* 1991;9:1059.
38. Hall A, Fallowfield L. Psychological outcome of treatment for early breast cancer: a review. *Stress Med* 1989;5:167.
39. Moyer A. Psychosocial outcomes of breast-conserving surgery versus mastectomy: a meta-analytic review. *Health Psychol* 1997;16:284.
40. Ganz PA, Schag CAC, Lee JJ, Polinsky ML, Tan SJ. Breast conservation versus mastectomy: is there a difference in psychological adjustment or quality of life in the year after surgery? *Cancer* 1992;69:1729.
41. DeBoer MF, McCormick LK, Pruyn JF, Ryckman RM, van den Borne BW. Physical and psychosocial correlates of head and neck cancer: a review of the literature. *Otolaryngol Head Neck Surg* 1999;120:427.
42. Sprangers MA, Taal BG, Aaronson NK, te Velde A. Quality of life in colorectal cancer. Stoma vs. nonstoma patients. *Dis Colon Rectum* 1995;38:361.
43. Ganz PA, Desmond KA, Belin TR, Meyerowitz BE, Rowland JH. Predictors of sexual health in women after a breast cancer diagnosis. *J Clin Oncol* 1999;17:2371.
44. Gritz ER, Wellisch DK, Wang HJ, et al. Long-term effects of testicular cancer on sexual functioning in married couples. *Cancer* 1989;64:1560.
45. Fobair P, Hoppe RT, Bloom J, et al. Psychosocial problems among survivors of Hodgkin's disease. *J Clin Oncol* 1986;4:805.
46. Knobf MK, Mullen JC, Xistris D, et al. Weight gain among women with breast cancer receiving adjuvant chemotherapy. *Oncol Nurs Forum* 1983;10:28.
47. Goodwin PJ, Panzarella T, Boyd NF. Weight gain in women with localized breast cancer: a descriptive study. *Breast Cancer Res Treat* 1988;11:59.
48. Demark-Wahnefried W, Rimer BK, Winer EP. Weight gain in women diagnosed with breast cancer. *J Am Diet Assoc* 1997;97:519.
49. Goodwin PJ, Ennis M, Pritchard KI, et al. Adjuvant treatment and onset of menopause predict weight gain after breast cancer diagnosis. *J Clin Oncol* 1999;17:120.
50. Ganz PA, Lee JJ, Schag CAC, Sim MS. The CARES: a generic measure of health-related quality of life for patients with cancer. *Qual Life Res* 1992;1:19.
51. Hann DM, Jacobsen P, Azzarello LM, et al. Measurement of fatigue in cancer patients: development and validation of the Fatigue Symptom Inventory. *Qual Life Res* 1998;7:301.
52. Andrykowski MA, Curran SL, Lighner R. Off-treatment fatigue in breast cancer survivors: a controlled comparison. *J Behav Med* 1998;21:1.
53. Loge JH, Abrahamsen AF, Ekeberg O, Kaasa S. Hodgkin's disease survivors more fatigued than the general population. *J Clin Oncol* 1999;17:253.
54. Bower JE, Ganz PA, Desmond KA, et al. Fatigue in breast cancer survivors: occurrence, correlates, and impact on quality of life. *J Clin Oncol* 2000;18:743.
55. Ganz PA, unpublished data, 1999.
56. Winer EP, Lindley C, Hardee M, et al. Quality of life in patients surviving at least 12 months following high dose chemotherapy with autologous bone marrow support. *Psychooncology* 1999;8:167.
57. Passik SD, Newman ML, Brennan M, Tunkel R. Predictors of psychological distress, sexual dysfunction and physical functioning among women with upper extremity lymphedema related to breast cancer. *Psychooncology* 1995;4:255.

58. Dorval M, Maunsell E, Taylor-Brown J, Kilpatrick M. Marital stability after breast cancer. *J Natl Cancer Inst* 1999;91:54.
59. Andrykowski MA, Curran SL, Studts JL, et al. Psychosocial adjustment and quality of life in women with breast cancer and benign breast problems: a controlled comparison. *J Clin Epidemiol* 1996;49:827.
60. Litwin MS, Hays RD, Fink A, et al. Quality-of-life outcomes in men treated for localized prostate cancer. *JAMA* 1995;273:129.
61. Barry HC. Do husbands and wives agree on prostate cancer screening? *J Fam Pract* 1997;44:443.
62. Volk RJ, Cantor SB, Spann SJ, et al. Preferences of husbands and wives for prostate cancer screening. *Arch Fam Med* 1997;6:72.
63. Byrne J, Fears TR, Steinhorn SC, et al. Marriage and divorce after childhood and adolescent cancer. *JAMA* 1989;262:2693.
64. Rauck AM, Green DM, Yasui Y, Mertens A, Robison LL. Marriage in the survivors of childhood cancer: a preliminary description from the Childhood Cancer Survivor Study. *Med Pediatr Oncol* 1999;33:60.
65. Green DM, Zevon MA, Hall B. Achievement of life goals by adult survivors of modern treatment for childhood cancer. *Cancer* 1991;67:206.
66. Walsh PC, Donker PJ. Impotence following radical prostatectomy: insight into etiology and prevention. *J Urol* 1982;128:492.
67. Fegiz GA, Trenti A, Bezzi M, et al. Sexual and bladder dysfunctions following surgery for rectal carcinoma. *Ital J Surg Sci* 1986;16:103.
68. Kinn AC, Ohman U. Bladder and sexual function after surgery for rectal cancer. *Dis Colon Rectum* 1986;29:43.
69. Jhaveri FM, Whitesides EW, Sackett CK, Bissada NK, Mohler JL. Preservation of sexual function in women after anterior exenteration for bladder cancer. *Br J Urol* 1998;81:312.
70. van Driel MF, Weymar Schultz WC, van de Wiel HB, Hahn DE, Mensink HJ. Female sexual functioning after radical surgical treatment of rectal and bladder cancer. *Eur J Surg Oncol* 1993;19:183.
71. Schover LR, von Eschenbach AC. Sexual function and female radical cystectomy: a case series. *J Urol* 1985;134:465.
72. Coogan CL, Hejase MJ, Wahle GR, et al. Nerve sparing post-chemotherapy retroperitoneal lymph node dissection for advanced testicular cancer. *J Urol* 1996;156:1656.
73. Donohue JP, Foster RS, Rowland RG, et al. Nerve-sparing retroperitoneal lymphadenectomy with preservation of ejaculation. *J Urol* 1990;144:287; discussion, 291.
74. Donohue JP, Foster RS. Retroperitoneal lymphadenectomy in staging and treatment. The development of nerve-sparing techniques. *Urol Clin North Am* 1998;25:461.
75. Donohue JP. Nerve-sparing retroperitoneal lymphadenectomy for testis cancer. Evolution of surgical templates for low-stage disease. *Eur Urol* 1993;23:44.
76. Schover LR, Fife M. Sexual counseling of patients undergoing radical surgery for pelvic or genital cancer. *J Psychosoc Oncol* 1985;3:21.
77. Mansson A, Johnson G, Mansson W. Quality of life after cystectomy. Comparison between patients with conduit and those with continent caecal reservoir urinary diversion. *Br J Urol* 1988;62:240.
78. Ganz PA, Rowland JH, Desmond K, Meyerowitz BE, Wyatt GE. Life after breast cancer: understanding women's health-related quality of life and sexual functioning. *J Clin Oncol* 1998;16:501.
79. Ganz PA, Rowland JH, Meyerowitz BE, Desmond KA. Impact of different adjuvant therapy strategies on quality of life in breast cancer survivors. *Recent Results Cancer Res* 1998;152:396.
80. Neitzert CS, Ritvo P, Dancey J, et al. The psychosocial impact of bone marrow transplantation: a review of the literature. *Bone Marrow Transplantation* 1998;22:409.
81. Bines J, Oleske DM, Cobleigh MA. Ovarian function in premenopausal women treated with adjuvant chemotherapy for breast cancer. *J Clin Oncol* 1996;14:1718.
82. Knobf MT. Natural menopause and ovarian toxicity associated with breast cancer therapy. *Oncol Nurs Forum* 1998;25:1519.
83. Goodwin PJ, Ennis M, Pritchard KI, Trudeau M, Hoo N. Risk of menopause during the first year after breast cancer diagnosis. *J Clin Oncol* 1999;17:2365.
84. Kornblith AB, Anderson J, Cella DF, et al. Comparison of psychosocial adaptation and sexual function of survivors of advanced Hodgkin disease treated by MOPP, ABVD, or MOPP alternating with ABVD. *Cancer* 1992;70:2508.
85. Goldstein I, Feldman MI, Deckers PJ, Babayan RK, Krane RJ. Radiation-associated impotence. A clinical study of its mechanism. *JAMA* 1984;251:903.
86. Talcott JA, Rieker P, Clark JA, et al. Patient-reported symptoms after primary therapy for early prostate cancer: results of a prospective cohort study. *J Clin Oncol* 1998;16:275.
87. Beard CJ, Propert KJ, Rieker PP, et al. Complications after treatment with external-beam irradiation in early-stage prostate cancer patients: a prospective multiinstitutional outcomes study. *J Clin Oncol* 1997;15:223.
88. Day R, Ganz PA, Costantino JP, et al. Health-related quality of life and tamoxifen in breast cancer prevention: a report from the National Surgical Adjuvant Breast and Bowel Project P-1 study. *J Clin Oncol* 1999;17:2659.
89. Mortimer JE, Boucher L, Baty J, et al. Effect of tamoxifen on sexual functioning in patients with breast cancer. *J Clin Oncol* 1999;17:1488.
90. Kornblith AB, Hollis DR, Zuckerman E, et al. Effect of megestrol acetate on quality of life in a dose-response trial in women with advanced breast cancer. The Cancer and Leukemia Group B. *J Clin Oncol* 1993;11:2081.
91. Huggins C, Hodges CV. Studies in prostate cancer. 1. The effects of castration, of estrogen and androgen injection on serum phosphatases in metastatic carcinoma of the prostate. *Cancer Res* 1941;1:293.
92. Cassileth BR, Hait HI, Kennealey GT, et al. Patients' choice of treatment in stage D prostate cancer. *Urology* 1989;33:57.
93. Cassileth BR, Soloway MS, Vogelzang NJ, et al. Quality of life and psychosocial status in stage D prostate cancer. Zoladex Prostate Cancer Study Group. *Qual Life Res* 1992;1:323.
94. Laufer MR. Reproductive issues for cancer patients/survivors. *J Clin Oncol* 1999;17:2631.
95. Byrne J, Mulvihill JJ, Myers MH, et al. Effects of treatment on fertility in long-term survivors of childhood or adolescent cancer. *N Engl J Med* 1987;317:1315.
96. Sklar CA, Robison LL, Nesbit ME, et al. Effects of radiation on testicular function in long-term survivors of childhood acute lymphoblastic leukemia: a report from the Children Cancer Study Group. *J Clin Oncol* 1990;8:1981.
97. Müller HL, Klinkhammer-Schalke M, Seelbach-Göbel B, Hartman AA, Kühl J. Gonadal function of young adults after therapy of malignancies during childhood or adolescence. *Eur J Pediatr* 1996;155:763.
98. Hamre MR, Robison LL, Nesbit ME, et al. Effects of radiation on ovarian function in long-term survivors of childhood acute lymphoblastic leukemia: a report from the Children's Cancer Study Group. *J Clin Oncol* 1987;5:1759.
99. Brewer M, Gershenson DM, Herzog CE, et al. Outcome and reproductive function after chemotherapy for ovarian dysgerminoma. *J Clin Oncol* 1999;17:2670.
100. Kreuser ED, Hetzel WD, Billia DO, Thiel E. Gonadal toxicity following cancer therapy in adults: significance, diagnosis, prevention and treatment. *Cancer Treat Rev* 1990;17:169.
101. Viviani S, Santoro A, Ragni G, et al. Gonadal toxicity after combination chemotherapy for Hodgkin's disease. Comparative results of MOPP vs ABVD. *Eur J Cancer Clin Oncol* 1985;21:601.
102. Opsahl MS, Fugger EF, Sherins RJ, Schulman JD. Preservation of reproductive function before therapy for cancer: new options involving sperm and ovary cryopreservation. *Cancer J* 1997;3:189.
103. Oktay K, Newton H, Aubard Y, Salha O, Gosden RG, Cryopreservation of immature human oocytes and ovarian tissue: an emerging technology? *Fertil Steril* 1998;69:1.
104. Janov AJ, Anderson J, Cella DF, et al. Pregnancy outcome in survivors of advanced Hodgkin disease. *Cancer* 1992;70:688.
105. Mulvihill JJ, McKeen EA, Rosner F, Zarrabi MH. Pregnancy outcome in cancer patients. Experience in a large cooperative group. *Cancer* 1987;60:1143.
106. Maunsell E, Brisson J, Deschennes L. Psychological distress after initial treatment for breast cancer: a comparison of partial and total mastectomy. *J Clin Epidemiol* 1989;42:765.
107. Wolberg WH, Romsaas EP, Tanner MA, Malec JF. Psychosexual adaptation to breast cancer surgery. *Cancer* 1989;63:1645.
108. Shimozuma K, Ganz PA, Petersen L, Hirji K. Quality of life in the first year after breast cancer surgery: rehabilitation needs and patterns of recovery. *Breast Cancer Res Treat* 1999;56:45.
109. Fallowfield LJ, Hall A. Psychosocial and sexual impact of diagnosis and treatment of breast cancer. *Br Med Bull* 1991;47:388.
110. Schain WS, d'Angelo TM, Dunn ME, Lichter AS, Pierce LJ. Mastectomy versus conservative surgery and radiation therapy. Psychosocial consequences. *Cancer* 1994;73:1221.
111. Schover LR, Yetman RJ, Tuason LJ, et al. Partial mastectomy and breast reconstruction. A comparison of their effects on psychosocial adjustment, body image, and sexuality. *Cancer* 1995;75:54.
112. Sarrel PM. Sexuality and menopause. *Obstet Gynecol* 1990;75:26S.
113. Cyranowski JM, Andersen BL. Schemas, sexuality and romantic attachment. *J Pers Soc Psychol* 1998;74:1364.
114. Kaplan HS. A neglected issue: the sexual side effects of current treatments for breast cancer. *J Sex Marital Ther* 1992;18:3.
115. Schover LR. The impact of breast cancer on sexuality, body image, and intimate relationships. *CA Cancer J Clin* 1991;41:112.
116. Cobleigh MA, Berris RF, Bush T, et al. Estrogen replacement therapy in breast cancer survivors. A time for change. *JAMA* 1994;272:540.
117. Love RR, Cameron L, Connell BL, Leventhal H. Symptoms associated with tamoxifen treatment in postmenopausal women. *Arch Intern Med* 1991;151:1842.
118. Young-McCaughan S. Sexual functioning in women with breast cancer after treatment with adjuvant therapy. *Cancer Nurs* 1996;19:308.
119. Schover LR. Sexuality and body image in younger women with breast cancer. *Monogr Natl Cancer Inst* 1994;16:177.
120. Dorval M, Maunsell E, Deschênes L, Brisson J, Mâsse B. Long-term quality of life after breast cancer: comparison of 8-year survivors with population controls. *J Clin Oncol* 1998;16:487.
121. Meyerowitz BE, Desmond KE, Rowland JH, Wyatt GE, Ganz PA. Sexuality following breast cancer. *J Sex Marital Ther* 1999;25:237.
122. Lindley C, Vasa S, Sawyer WT, Winer EP. Quality of life and preferences for treatment following systemic adjuvant therapy for early-stage breast cancer. *J Clin Oncol* 1998;16:1380.
123. Fransson P, Widmark A. Self-assessed sexual function after pelvic irradiation for prostate carcinoma. Comparison with an age-matched control group. *Cancer* 1996;78:1066.
124. Widmark A, Fransson P, Tavelin B. Self-assessment questionnaire for evaluating urinary and intestinal late side effects after pelvic radiotherapy in patients with prostate cancer compared with an age-matched control population. *Cancer* 1994;74:2520.
125. Fowler FJ Jr, Barry MJ, Lu-Yao GL, et al. Patient-reported complications and follow-up treatment after radical prostatectomy. *Urology* 1993;42:622.
126. Fowler FJ Jr, Barry MJ, Lu-Yao G, et al. Effect of radical prostatectomy for prostate cancer on patient quality of life: results from a Medicare survey. *Urology* 1995;45:1007.
127. Fowler FJ Jr, Barry MJ, Lu-Yao G, Wasson JH, Bin L. Outcomes of external-beam radiation therapy for prostate cancer: a study of Medicare beneficiaries in three Surveillance, Epidemiology, and End Results areas. *J Clin Oncol* 1996;14:2258.
128. Talcott JA. Quality of life in early prostate cancer. Do we know enough to treat? *Hematol Oncol Clin North Am* 1996;10:691.
129. Talcott JA, Rieker P, Propert KJ, et al. Patient-reported impotence and incontinence after nerve-sparing radical prostatectomy. *J Natl Cancer Inst* 1997;89:1117.
130. Crook J, Esche B, Futter N. Effect of pelvic radiotherapy for prostate cancer on bowel, bladder, and sexual function: the patient's perspective. *Urology* 1996;47:387.
131. Turner SL, Adams K, Bull CA, Berry MP. Sexual dysfunction after radical radiation therapy for prostate cancer: a prospective evaluation. *Urology* 1999;54:124.

132. Litwin MS, Flanders SC, Pasta DJ, et al. Sexual function and bother after radical prostatectomy or radiation for prostate cancer: multivariate quality-of-life analysis from CaPSURE. Cancer of the Prostate Strategic Urologic Research Endeavor. *Urology* 1999;54:503.
133. Schover LR. Sexuality and fertility in urologic cancer patients. *Cancer* 1987;60:553.
134. Rieker PP, Edbril SD, Garnick MB. Curative testis cancer therapy: psychosocial sequelae. *J Clin Oncol* 1985;3:1117.
135. Rieker PP, Fitzgerald EM, Kalish LA, et al. Psychosocial factors, curative therapies, and behavioral outcomes. A comparison of testis cancer survivors and a control group of healthy men. *Cancer* 1989;64:2399.
136. Bloom JR, Fobair P, Gritz E, et al. Psychosocial outcomes of cancer: a comparative analysis of Hodgkin's disease and testicular cancer. *J Clin Oncol* 1993;11:979.
137. Schover LR, Gonzales M, von Eschenbach AC. Sexual and marital relationships after radiotherapy for seminoma. *Urology* 1986;27:117.
138. Gritz ER, Wellisch DK, Siau J, Wang HJ. Long-term effects of testicular cancer on marital relationships. *Psychosomatics* 1990;31:301.
139. Schover LR, Evans R, von Eschenbach AC. Sexual rehabilitation and male radical cystectomy. *J Urol* 1986;136:1015.
140. Oishi K, Arai Y, Hashimura T, et al. [Quality of life of the patients with continent urinary reservoir]. *Hinyokika Kiyo* 1993;39:7.
141. Boyd SD, Feinberg SM, Skinner DG, et al. Quality of life survey of urinary diversion patients: comparison of ileal conduits versus continent Kock ileal reservoirs. *J Urol* 1987;138:1386.
142. Gerharz EW, Weingartner K, Dopatka T, et al. Quality of life after cystectomy and urinary diversion: results of a retrospective interdisciplinary study [published erratum appears in *J Urol* 1997;158:2253]. *J Urol* 1997;158[3 Pt 1]:778.
143. Hart S, Skinner EC, Meyerowitz BE, et al. Quality of life after radical cystectomy for bladder cancer in patients with an ileal conduit, cutaneous or urethral Kock pouch. *J Urol* 1999;162:77.
144. Andersen BL, Lachenbruch PA, Anderson B, DeProsse C. Sexual dysfunction and signs of gynecological cancer. *Cancer* 1986;57:1880.
145. Andersen BL. Sexual functioning complications in women with gynecologic cancer. Outcomes and directions for prevention. *Cancer* 1987;60:2123.
146. Andersen BL, Anderson BA, DeProsse C. Controlled prospective longitudinal study of women with cancer. I. Sexual functioning outcomes. *J Consult Clin Psychol* 1989;57:683.
147. Schover LR, Fife M, Gershenson DM. Sexual dysfunction and treatment for early stage cervical cancer. *Cancer* 1989;63:204.
148. Bruner DW, Lanciano R, Keegan M, et al. Vaginal stenosis and sexual function following intracavitary radiation for the treatment of cervical and endometrial carcinoma. *Int J Radiat Oncol Biol Phys* 1993;27:825.
149. Flay LD, Matthews JH. The effects of radiotherapy and surgery on the sexual function of women treated for cervical cancer. *Int J Radiat Oncol Biol Phys* 1995;31:399.
150. Krumm S, Lamberti J. Changes in sexual behavior following radiation therapy for cervical cancer. *J Psychosom Obstet Gynaecol* 1993;14:51.
151. Bergmark K, Åvall-Lundqvist E, Dickman PW, Henningsohn L, Steineck G. Vaginal changes and sexuality in women with a history of cervical cancer. *N Engl J Med* 1999;340:1383.
152. Ganz PA. Overview—quality of life and psychosocial issues. In: Sharp F, Blackett T, Berek J, Bast R, eds. *Ovarian cancer 5.* Oxford: Isis Medical Media, 1998:409.
153. Andersen BL, Turnquist D, LaPolla J, Turner D. Sexual functioning after treatment of *in situ* vulvar cancer: preliminary report. *Obstet Gynecol* 1988;71:15.
154. Weijmar Schultz WC, van de Wiel HB, Bouma J, Janssens J, Littlewood J. Psychosexual functioning after the treatment of cancer of the vulva. A longitudinal study. *Cancer* 1990;66:402.
155. van Driel MF, Weymar Schultz WC, van de Wiel HB, Hahn DE, Mensink HJ. Female sexual functioning after radical surgical treatment of rectal and bladder cancer. *Eur J Surg Oncol* 1993;19:183.
156. Koukouras D, Spilotis J, Scopa CD, et al. Radical consequence in the sexuality of male patients operated for colorectal carcinoma. *Eur J Surg Oncol* 1991;17:285.
157. Schover LR, Jensen SB. *Sexuality and chronic illness: a comprehensive approach.* New York: Guilford Press, 1988.
158. Taylor JF, Rosen RC, Leiblum SR. Self-report assessment of female sexual function: psychometric evaluation of the brief index of sexual functioning for women. *Arch Sex Behav* 1994;23:627.
159. Annon J. *Behavioral treatment of sexual problems.* Honolulu: Enabling Systems, 1974.
160. Schover LR. *Sexuality and fertility after cancer.* New York: John Wiley & Sons, 1997.
161. Syrjala KL, Roth-Roemer SL, Abrams JR, et al. Prevalence and predictors of sexual dysfunction in long-term survivors of marrow transplantation. *J Clin Oncol* 1998;16:3148.
162. Nachtigall LE. Comparative study: Replens versus local estrogen in menopausal women. *Fertil Steril* 1994;61:178.
163. Loprinzi CL, Abu-Ghazaleh S, Sloan JA, et al. Phase III randomized double-blind study to evaluate the efficacy of a polycarbophil-based vaginal moisturizer in women with breast cancer. *J Clin Oncol* 1997;15:969.
164. Cass I, Runowicz CD. Nonhormonal alternative to treating menopausal symptoms. *Am J Managed Care* 1998;4:732.
165. Boar's Head Workshop Conference Consensus Statement. Treatment of estrogen deficiency symptoms in women surviving breast cancer. *J Clin Endocrinol Metab* 1998;83:1993.
166. The consensus conference on treatment of estrogen deficiency symptoms in women surviving breast cancer. *Obstet Gynecol Surv* 1998;53(10)[Suppl]:S1.
167. Holmgren PA, Lindskog M, von Schoultz B. Vaginal rings for continuous low-dose release of oestradiol in the treatment of urogenital atrophy. *Maturitas* 1989;11:55.
168. Ganz PA, Greendale GA, Petersen L, et al. Managing menopausal symptoms in breast cancer survivors: results of a randomized controlled trial. *J Natl Cancer Inst* 2000; 92:1054
169. Schover LR. Sexual rehabilitation after treatment for prostate cancer. *Cancer* 1993; 71[Suppl]:1024.
170. Meinhardt W, Kropman RF, Vermeij P. Comparative tolerability and efficacy of treatments for impotence. *Drug Safety* 1999;20:133.
171. Goldstein I, Lue TF, Padma-Nathan H, et al. Oral sildenafil in the treatment of erectile dysfunction. Sildenafil Study Group [see comments] [published erratum appears in *N Engl J Med* 1998;339:59]. *N Engl J Med* 1998;338:1397.
172. O'Sullivan JD, Hughes AJ. Apomorphine-induced penile erections in Parkinson's disease. *Mov Disord* 1998;13:536.
173. Earle CM, Seah M, Coulden SE, Stuckey BG, Keogh EJ. The use of the vacuum erection device in the management of erectile impotence. *Int J Impot Res* 1996;8:237.
174. Opsomer RJ, Wese FX, De Groote P, Van Cangh PJ. The external vacuum device in the management of erectile dysfunction. *Acta Urol Belg* 1997;65:13.
175. Turner LA, Althof SE, Levine SB, et al. Treating erectile dysfunction with external vacuum devices: impact upon sexual, psychological and marital functioning. *J Urol* 1990;144:79.
176. Godschalk MF, Chen J, Katz PG, Mulligan T. Treatment of erectile failure with prostaglandin E1: a double-blind, placebo-controlled, dose-response study. *J Urol* 1994;151:1530.
177. Padma-Nathan H, Hellstrom WJ, Kaiser FE, et al. Treatment of men with erectile dysfunction with transurethral alprostadil. Medicated Urethral System for Erection (MUSE) Study Group. *N Engl J Med* 1997;336:1.
178. Montague DK. Penile prostheses. An overview. *Urol Clin North Am* 1989;16:7.

SECTION 4

ELLEN T. MATLOFF
ALLEN E. BALE

Genetic Counseling

The availability of clinically based genetic testing has brought with it a growing demand for accurate risk assessment and cancer genetic counseling. Extensive coverage of this topic by the media and widespread advertising by commercial testing laboratories has further fueled the demand for counseling and testing.

The field of cancer genetic counseling is evolving rapidly to meet the newfound needs of patients and the medical community. Cancer genetic counseling is a communication process between health care professionals and individuals concerning cancer occurrence and risk in their family.[1] The process, which may include the entire family through a blend of genetic, medical, and psychosocial assessment and intervention, has been described as a bridge between the fields of traditional oncology and genetic counseling.[1]

The goals of this process include providing clients with an assessment of individual cancer risk while offering the emotional support needed to understand and cope with this information.[2] The process also involves deciphering whether the cancers in a family are likely to be caused by a mutation in a cancer gene and, if so, which one. To achieve the informed consent crucial to the testing process, each patient is thoroughly counseled about the associated risks, benefits, and limitations of testing. If the patient is interested in pursuing testing, the counselor will identify a laboratory that offers appropriate genetic testing and will facilitate sample collection and shipping and result interpretation. The result session will include detailed counseling about medical management options for early detection and risk reduction counseling and may include referrals to prevention trials, surveillance programs, and medical specialists.

Counselors find that this process differs from traditional genetic counseling in several ways. Clients seeking cancer genetic counseling are rarely concerned with reproductive decisions and risks that are often the primary focus in traditional genetic counseling but are instead seeking information about their own and other relatives' chances of developing cancer.[3,4] Additionally, the risks given are not absolute but change over time as the family and personal history changes and the patient ages. Perhaps the greatest divergence from traditional genetic counseling is the departure from nondirectiveness. *Nondirectiveness,* one of the cornerstones of traditional genetic counseling, can be loosely defined as the tenet of presenting clients with accurate genetic and medical information, providing them with their options, helping them to choose the option that best fits their needs (free of coercion from the counselor regarding which choices are "right" or "wrong"), and then supporting their decision. Nondirectiveness is not always appropriate in cancer genetic counseling. Standard screening guidelines and prevention strategies are presented as recommendations,[5] and the counselor is often proactive in promoting behavioral changes that could reduce the risk of developing cancer.[3] Counseling for susceptibility testing is based on the nondirective framework, although some data indicate that patients desire more assistance in decision making than their health care providers offer.[6] Helping patients reach the decision that is most consistent with their personal values and goals and that is best suited to their personal situation is the ultimate goal of genetic counseling.

Why is cancer genetic counseling necessary? The advances in cancer genetics bring with them new issues involving the medical, psychological, discriminatory, and ethical side effects of genetic testing for cancer predisposition.[7] Potential clients must be made aware of these risks before testing and, when possible, assisted in avoiding pitfalls. Additionally, the public demands this resource.[8] Several studies have documented a high level of interest in genetic testing among people who have one first-degree relative with diagnosed cancer.[9–13] Although anticipated interest in testing generally overestimates actual uptake,[14–17] the need for cancer genetic counseling is great and is bound to grow as more genes are cloned.

At present, a limited number of referral centers across the country specialize in cancer genetic counseling. Graduate programs in genetic counseling are actively integrating this new body of knowledge into their curricula and are producing more counselors who can provide cancer services. However, some experts insist that the only way to keep up with the overwhelming demand for counseling will be to educate more physicians and nurses in cancer genetics.[18,19] The feasibility of adding another time- and energy-consuming task to the clinical burden of these professionals is questionable. A more practical goal may be to educate primary care providers better in the area of generalized risk assessment so that they can screen their patient populations for individuals at high risk for hereditary cancer and refer them to comprehensive counseling and testing programs.

WHO IS A CANDIDATE FOR CANCER GENETIC COUNSELING?

Only 5% to 10% of most cancers are due to mutations within inherited cancer susceptibility genes.[20] The key for the clinician is to determine which patients are at greatest risk to carry one of these mutations. Six risk factors that are common among hereditary cancer families have been identified (Table 56.4-1). The first is early age of cancer onset. This risk factor, even in the absence of a family history, has been shown to be associated with an increased frequency of germline mutations in many types of cancers.[21–26] The second risk factor is the presence of the same cancer in multiple affected relatives on the same side of the pedigree that are consistent with autosomal dominant inheritance. These cancers do not necessarily have to be of similar histologic type to be caused by a single mutation. The third risk factor is the clustering of cancers known to be caused by a single gene mutation in one family. Examples include breast-ovarian cancer, pancreatic cancer–melanoma, and colon-ovarian-uterine cancers. The fourth risk factor is the occurrence of multiple primary cancers in one individual. This includes multiple primary breast cancers, colon cancers, and melanomas and a single individual with separate cancers known to be caused by a single gene mutation (e.g., breast and ovarian cancer in a single individual). Ethnicity also plays a role in determining who is at greatest risk to carry a hereditary cancer mutation. Individuals of Jewish ancestry are at increased risk to carry three specific BRCA1/2 mutations[27] and the I1307K APC allele.[28] Founder BRCA1/2 mutations have also been discovered in families of French Canadian descent, and mutations in cancer susceptibility genes are likely to be identified in other ethnicities as more subpopulations are studied.[29–32] The final risk factor for a hereditary cancer syndrome is the presence of a cancer that presents unusually, the prime example of which is breast cancer in a man. These risk factors should be viewed in the context of the entire family history and must be weighed in proportion to the number of individuals who have not developed cancer.

TABLE 56.4-1. Risks Factors for Hereditary Cancer Syndromes

Early age of onset
Presence of the same cancer in multiple family members on the same side of the pedigree
Clustering of cancers known to be caused by a single gene mutation (e.g., breast-ovarian cancers, colon-uterine-ovarian cancers)
Multiple primary cancers in one individual
Ethnicity (e.g., Jewish ancestry for breast-ovarian cancer syndrome)
Unusual presentation of cancer (e.g., breast cancer in a man)

A less common but extremely important finding is the presence of birth defects or unusual medical findings that are known to be associated with rare hereditary cancer syndromes. Examples include benign skin findings and thyroid disorders in Cowden syndrome, sebaceous skin tumors in Muir-Torre syndrome, and supernumerary teeth in familial adenomatous polyposis (FAP).[33]

Another class of candidates for genetic counseling are those patients who are very concerned about their risks for cancer, even in the absence of a strong family history. Many patients overestimate their risks to develop cancer. This inaccurate perception of risk may have a profound effect on a patient's anxiety level and quality of life and may have a negative impact on his or her surveillance patterns.[34] Such patients may gain reassurance and empowerment from learning their actual—as compared to their anticipated—risks for developing cancer and their options to reduce those risks.

At present, breast-ovarian cancer syndrome referrals account for the majority of patients seen in the average cancer genetic counseling clinic. In this chapter, the breast-ovarian cancer counseling session will serve as a paradigm that all other sessions may follow broadly.

COMPONENTS OF THE CANCER GENETIC COUNSELING SESSION

PRECOUNSELING INFORMATION

Before coming in for genetic counseling, the counselee should be given some basic information about the process. This information, which can be imparted by telephone or in the form of written material, should outline what the counselee can expect at each session and what information he or she should collect before the first visit. The counselee can then begin to collect medical and family history information that will be essential for the genetic counseling session.

FAMILY HISTORY

An accurate family history is undoubtedly one of the most essential components of the cancer genetic counseling session. Despite its importance, the thorough family cancer history has been called "the most severely neglected portion of the patient's medical evaluation,"[35] possibly reflecting a lack of emphasis placed on the family history during the primary and postgraduate education of physicians.[36] It may also be due, in part, to the lack of knowledge about what to do with the information once it has been collected.

A thorough family history should include at least two, optimally three, generations.[37] For each individual affected with cancer, it is important to document the exact diagnosis, age at diagnosis, treatment strategies, and environmental exposures (i.e., occupational exposures, cigarettes, other agents).[5] The current age of the individual and laterality and occurrence of any other cancers must also be documented.[3] Individuals should be asked whether there are any consanguineous (inbred) relationships in the family, whether any relatives were born with birth defects or mental retardation, and whether other genetic diseases run in the family, as these pieces of information could prove important in reaching a diagnosis and in counseling.

It is advised that cancer diagnoses be documented with pathology reports, hospital summaries, or other medical records to maintain accuracy.[3] A study by Love et al.[38] revealed that individuals accurately reported the primary site of cancer only 83% of the time in their first-degree relatives with cancer and 67% and 60% of the time in second- and third-degree relatives, respectively. It is common for patients to report a uterine cancer as an ovarian cancer or a colon polyp as an invasive colorectal cancer. These differences, although seemingly subtle to the patient, can make a tremendous difference in risk assessment.

The most common misconception in family history taking is that somehow a maternal family history of breast, ovarian, or uterine cancer is more significant than a paternal history. Conversely, many still believe that a paternal history of prostate cancer is more significant than a maternal history. Few of the cancer genes discovered thus far are located on the sex chromosomes; therefore, both maternal and paternal history are significant and must be explored thoroughly.

DYSMORPHOLOGY SCREENING

Congenital anomalies, benign tumors, and unusual dermatologic features occur in a large number of hereditary cancer predisposition syndromes. Examples include osteomas of the jaw in FAP, palmar pits in Gorlin syndrome, and papillomas of the lips and mucous membranes in Cowden syndrome. Obtaining an accurate medical history of benign lesions and birth defects and screening for such dysmorphology can have a great impact on diagnosis and counseling. For example, BRCA1/2 testing is unnecessary in a patient with breast cancer who has a family history of thyroid cancer and the orocutaneous manifestations of Cowden syndrome.

RISK ASSESSMENT

Risk assessment is one of the most complicated components of the genetic counseling session. It is crucial to remember that risk assessment changes over time as the person ages and as the health status of family members changes.[3] Risk assessment can be broken down into three separate components: What is the chance that the counselee will develop the cancer observed in his or her family (or a genetically related cancer)? What is the chance that the cancers in this family are caused by a single gene mutation? What is the chance that we can identify the gene mutation in this family with our current knowledge and laboratory techniques?

Cancer clustering in a family may be due to genetic or environmental factors (or both) or may be coincidental because some cancers are common in the general population. Although inherited factors may be the primary cause of cancers in some families, in others cancer may develop because an inherited factor increases the individual's susceptibility to environmental carcinogens.[39] It is also possible that members of the same family may be exposed to similar environmental exposures, owing to shared geography or patterns in behavior and diet that may increase the risk of cancer.[40] Therefore, it is important to distinguish the difference between a familial pattern of cancer (due to environmental factors or chance) and a hereditary pattern of cancer (due to a shared genetic mutation).

Several models are available to calculate the chance that a woman will develop breast cancer. Each model has its strengths and weaknesses, and the counselor must decide which model is most appropriate for each individual family. The Gail model for calculating risk takes into account current age, age of first menses, age at first live birth, and number of previous biopsies.[41] This model may be problematic for women who cannot recall their exact age at menses and who are followed more aggressively than women without a positive family history and, therefore, may be subjected to biopsy more frequently. Biopsy results are not considered in this model, so a normal biopsy is weighed equally with a result of atypical hyperplasia. It has also been suggested that the importance of general risk factors for breast cancer, such as age at first menses and first live birth, may vary in hereditary cancer families.[42] A modified form of the Gail model was used to determine entry into the National Surgical Adjuvant Breast and Bowel Project (NSABP) Breast Cancer Prevention Trial and will also be used for entry into the

NSABP P-2 STAR trial.[43] Although this model has utility in determining entry for trials and may be of use for women in the general population who receive frequent breast screening, it is not appropriate in families in which there is a question of a hereditary cancer syndrome. The Gail model considers only first-degree relatives in its calculations and, therefore, does not take into account paternal family history and extended family members. It does not weigh ovarian cancer, Jewish ancestry, male breast cancer, and other factors essential in hereditary risk assessment and is, therefore, not the appropriate tool when hereditary cancer is in question.

Claus et al.[44] created a model that considers limited paternal and maternal family history as well as age of onset of affected relatives in determining empiric cancer risk. This model allows calculation of individual risk by decade and by lifetime, which is useful in helping women understand that their risk accumulates over time and is not clumped at their current age. This model does not take ancestry, ovarian cancer, or extended family history into account and is, therefore, not useful in families in which there appears to be a genetic mutation. Of course, all empiric risks are superseded in families in which DNA testing has revealed a mutation for cancer predisposition.

When the BRCA1 gene was mapped, risk tables were created based on linkage data from high-risk breast and ovarian cancer families. These tables estimated the chance that the cancers found in hereditary breast-ovarian cancer families were due to mutations in BRCA1, and these estimates were fairly high.[45] When direct mutation analysis for BRCA1 became available, the number of families found to carry a mutation was significantly smaller than predicted by linkage studies. This finding suggests that current techniques do not detect all mutations within the gene. More recent tables reflect the chance of actually finding a mutation within BRCA1.[46] Parmigiani et al.[47] have developed a more sophisticated computer model that calculates the probability of finding a BRCA1 or 2 mutation in a family using a variety of risk factors. This model is being validated.

DNA TESTING

DNA testing is available for a variety of hereditary cancer syndromes [e.g., breast-ovarian cancer syndrome, hereditary nonpolyposis colon cancer (HNPCC), and hereditary melanoma]. However, despite misrepresentation by the media,[48] testing is feasible for only a small percentage of individuals with cancer. DNA testing offers the obvious and important advantage of presenting clients with actual risks instead of the empiric risks derived from risk calculation models.

The results of DNA testing are generally provided in person in a result disclosure session. It is recommended that patients bring a close friend or relative with them to this session who can provide them with emotional support and who can help them to listen to and process the information provided.

One of most crucial aspects of DNA testing is accurate result interpretation. One study found that test results for the hereditary colon cancer syndrome FAP were misinterpreted more than 30% of the time by those ordering the testing.[49] The potential impact of test results on the patient and his or her family is great; therefore, accurate interpretation of the results is paramount.

Results of genetic testing fall into three categories: true positive, whereby an individual is found to carry a mutation that is known to be deleterious; true negative, whereby an individual does not carry the deleterious mutation found in their family and, therefore, the cancer risks are reduced to the population risks; and indeterminate, whereby a mutation cannot be identified in the affected family members or a genetic change is identified with unknown significance. This result category is currently the most common outcome.

To pinpoint the mutation in a family, an affected individual likely to carry a mutation should be tested first. This is most often a person affected with the cancer in question (i.e., the proband). Test subjects should be selected with care, as it is possible for a person to develop sporadic cancer in a hereditary cancer family. If a mutation is detected in an affected relative, other unaffected family members can be tested for the same mutation with a great degree of accuracy. Family members who do not carry the mutation found in their family are deemed to be true negative. Those who are found to carry the mutation in their family will have more definitive information about their risks to develop cancer. This information can be crucial in assisting patients in decision making regarding surveillance and risk reduction.

If a mutation is not identified in the affected relative, it usually means either that the cancers in the family are not caused by a single genetic mutation or that the mutation in the family is undetectable by current methods. Such results are indeterminate, and other family members cannot be offered accurate predisposition testing. In some such cases, DNA banking should be offered to the proband for a time in the future when improved testing may become available. A notarized letter indicating exactly who in the family has access to the DNA should accompany the banked sample.

The result stated as "genetic variant of uncertain significance" must be interpreted with caution. Sometimes, other affected family members can be tested to see whether the variant segregates with disease in the family. Most of the time, the significance of the variant remains unknown until functional studies are conclusive or further data are available.

The penetrance of mutations in cancer susceptibility genes is also difficult to interpret. Initial estimates derived from high-risk families provided very high cancer risks for BRCA1 and BRCA2 mutation carriers.[45] More recent studies of populations that were not selected for family history have revealed lower penetrances.[27] Some have interpreted these population-based data as being "more accurate" and have suggested that they apply to all families. In fact, the higher range of risk may be more accurate for families who present with strong histories of breast and ovarian cancer. Because exact penetrance rates cannot be determined for individual families at this time, it is prudent to provide patients with a range of cancer risk and to explain that their risk probably falls somewhere within this spectrum.[50,51]

Female carriers of BRCA1 and BRCA2 mutations have a 50% to 85% lifetime risk of developing breast cancer and between a 15% to 60% lifetime risk of developing ovarian cancer.[27,45,52–57] Carriers of HNPCC mutations have a 65% to 85% lifetime risk of developing colon cancer, and female carriers have a 30% to 40% lifetime risk of uterine cancer and as great as a 10% risk of ovarian cancer.[58,59]

OPTIONS FOR SURVEILLANCE AND RISK REDUCTION

The cancer risk counseling session is a forum to provide counselees with choices, options, and hope (Table 56.4-2). Mutation

TABLE 56.4-2. Methods for Surveillance and Risk Reduction for Selected Hereditary Cancers

Cancer Type	*Clinical Genetic Testing*	*Surveillance*	*Risk Reduction*
Breast	BRCA1, BRCA2	Breast self-examinations, clinical breast examinations, mammography	Prophylactic bilateral mastectomies; tamoxifen,[a] raloxifene[a]
Ovary	BRCA1, BRCA2, MLH1, MSH2	CA-125, transvaginal ultrasonography	Prophylactic oophorectomy, oral contraceptives
Colon	MLH1, MSH2, APC	Colonoscopy	Prophylactic colectomy, nonsteroidal antiinflammatory drugs[a]
Melanoma	CDKN2, CDK4	Skin self-examinations, clinical skin examinations	Avoidance of ultraviolet light exposure, use of sunscreen and protective clothing

[a]Investigative.
Note: Diet and lifestyle recommendations for cancer prevention are available through national cancer organizations.

carriers can be offered earlier and aggressive surveillance, chemoprevention plus surveillance, or prophylactic surgery.

It is recommended that individuals at increased risk for breast cancer have annual mammograms beginning between ages 25 and 35 years and annual or semiannual clinical breast examinations, and that they perform monthly breast self-examinations.[60] BRCA1/2 carriers may take tamoxifen in hopes of reducing their risks of developing breast cancer. However, although tamoxifen has proven effective in women at risk due to a positive family history of breast cancer, the efficacy of this intervention in BRCA1/2 carriers is still unknown.[61] The results of preliminary studies indicate that a second chemopreventive agent, raloxifene (EVISTA), may also be effective in reducing the risk of breast cancer in healthy postmenopausal women.[62] However, this medication is approved by the U.S. Food and Drug Administration only for the prevention of osteoporosis and has not been studied in BRCA1/2-positive women. A current study, the NSABP P-2 STAR trial, is examining the role of this drug in women at high risk for breast cancer. Data should be available by 2006. Prophylactic bilateral mastectomy is believed to reduce the risk of breast cancer by more than 90% in women at high risk for the disease[63]; however, the efficacy of this procedure specifically in BRCA mutation carriers is unknown. Before genetic testing was available, it was not uncommon for entire generations of cancer families to have their at-risk organs removed without knowing whether they were personally at increased risk for their familial cancer. Fifty percent of individuals in hereditary cancer families do not carry the inherited predisposition gene and can be spared prophylactic surgery or invasive high-risk surveillance regimens. Therefore, it is no longer appropriate to offer prophylactic surgery until a patient is referred for genetic counseling and, if possible, testing (Table 56.4-3).[64]

Women who carry BRCA1/2 mutations are also at increased risk for developing second contralateral and ipsilateral primary tumors of the breast.[65] These data bring into question the option of breast-conserving surgery in women at high risk to develop a second primary tumor within the same breast. For this reason, BRCA1/2 carrier status may have a profound impact on surgical decision making in the future.[64]

Women who carry BRCA1/2 mutations are also at increased risk for developing ovarian cancer, even if no one in their family has developed this cancer. Surveillance for ovarian cancer is complex, with the recommended interventions being annual transvaginal ultrasonography and tests of CA-125 levels beginning between the ages of 25 and 35 years.[60] The effectiveness of such surveillance in detecting ovarian cancers at early and more treatable stages has not been proven in any population. Oral contraceptives have been shown to reduce the risk of ovarian cancer in women carrying BRCA mutations.[66] The impact of this intervention on breast cancer risk is not known. However, it is possible that, given the likelihood of mortality from breast versus ovarian cancer, a risk-benefit analysis would favor the use of oral contraceptives in carriers of BRCA1/2 mutations.[40] Prophylactic oophorectomy is the most effective means to reduce the risk of ovarian cancer,[67] but even women who have had this procedure may develop primary peritoneal carcinoma.[68,69] This condition is clinically and histologically similar to ovarian cancer but appears to arise from the cells lining the peritoneal cavity. Some data indicate that BRCA1 carriers who opt for prophylactic oophorectomy also have a reduced chance of developing a subsequent breast cancer, particularly if they have this surgery before menopause.[70] Premenopausal women who opt for oophorectomy and, therefore, experience premature surgical menopause may be candidates for hormone replacement therapy (HRT) with the lowest dose of estrogen possible.[40] This may provide some of the benefits of HRT while minimizing the potential breast cancer–related risks. Preliminary data suggest that premenopausal BRCA1 carriers who have oophorectomies followed by HRT still have a reduced risk of future breast cancers.[70]

The standard surveillance method in carriers of HNPCC mutations is full colonoscopy to the cecum every 1 to 3 years beginning between the ages of 20 and 25 years.[71] Although sev-

TABLE 56.4-3. Cancer Genetic Counseling and Testing Resources

CancerNet
(800) 4-CANCER
http://cancernet.nci.nih.gov/index.html
Provides a free service designed to locate providers of cancer risk counseling and testing services in the context of both research and clinical fee-for-service programs

GeneTests: Genetic testing resource
(206) 527-5742
http://www.genetests.org
Offers current information on testing availability for specific conditions and sites that offer such testing

National Society of Genetic Counselors
(610) 872-7608
http://www.nsgc.org
Offers a listing of genetic counselors in user's geographic area who specialize in cancer

eral studies are investigating chemopreventive options for colorectal cancer, no agents are currently approved for clinical use. Prophylactic subtotal colectomy with ileorectal anastomosis is an option for HNPCC carriers, and a decision analysis revealed that this procedure may offer slightly greater gains in life expectancy for young HNPCC carriers than surveillance alone.[72,73]

Options for endometrial cancer surveillance include endometrial aspirate and transvaginal ultrasonography beginning between the ages of 25 and 35 years. The efficacy of such surveillance in HNPCC carriers is unknown. Oral contraceptives are known to reduce the risk of endometrial cancer in the general population,[74] but the impact of this intervention in HNPCC carriers is currently unknown. Prophylactic transabdominal hysterectomy is also an option. Although this option is likely to reduce risk of uterine cancer significantly, long-term prospective studies of the impact of this intervention on HNPCC carriers have not been performed. Women who carry HNPCC mutations are also at risk for ovarian cancer and should, therefore, be offered the aforementioned surveillance and risk reduction options for ovarian cancer.

Management of hereditary melanoma patients involves frequent full-body examination by a dermatologist familiar with pigmented lesions. Semiannual appointments typically include photography of the entire body, to allow for objective determination of differences in size or appearance of moles, and subsequent excision of any suspicious lesions. Avoidance of sunlight exposure is recommended. Melanoma is often curable when diagnosed and treated in an early stage.

Genetic counseling and testing are also available for many rare cancer syndromes, including von Hippel-Lindau syndrome, multiple endocrine neoplasia, and FAP. Surveillance and risk reduction for patients who are known mutation carriers for such conditions may decrease the associated morbidity and mortality of these syndromes.

FOLLOW-UP

A follow-up letter to the patient is a concrete means of documenting the information conveyed in the sessions so that the patient and his or her family members can review it over time. (It is crucial that this letter be sent only to the patient and health care professionals to whom the patient has granted access to this information; in most cases, it should not be placed in the patient's general medical records.) A follow-up phone call is also helpful, particularly in the case of a positive test result. Some programs provide patients with an annual or biannual newsletter updating them on new information in the field of cancer genetics. A small proportion of patients may return for a follow-up counseling session months, or even years, after their initial consult to discuss the emergence of new family history data and new clinical issues or because they are now ready to move forward with genetic testing.

ISSUES IN CANCER GENETIC COUNSELING

PSYCHOSOCIAL ISSUES

The psychosocial impact of cancer genetic counseling cannot be underestimated. Just the process of scheduling a cancer risk counseling session may be fairly difficult for some individuals with a family history who are not only frightened about their own cancer risk but are reliving painful experiences associated with the cancer of their loved ones.[2] Counselees may be faced with an onslaught of emotions, including anger, fear of developing cancer, fear of disfigurement and dying, grief, lack of control, negative body image, and a sense of isolation.[5] Their feelings about cancer will also vary depending on how close they have been to affected individuals, both emotionally and in geographic proximity, and how often they saw these relatives. Some counselees are wrestling with the fear that insurance companies, employers, family members, and even future partners will react negatively to their cancer risks. For many, it is a double-edged sword as they balance their fears and apprehensions about dredging up these issues with the possibility of obtaining reassuring news and much-needed information.

A person's perceived cancer risk is often dependent on many "nonmedical" variables. They may estimate that their risk is higher if they resemble an affected individual or share some of that individual's personality traits.[5] Their perceived risks will vary depending on whether their relatives were cancer survivors or died painful deaths from the disease. Many people wonder not *whether* they are going to get cancer but *when.* Some first-degree relatives of women with breast cancer said they felt as though they were living with a sword over their heads or that they were walking time bombs.[75]

In their study of women with a first-degree relative who had breast cancer, Lerman et al.[76] found that more than one-half of their respondents reported having intrusive thoughts and waves of feelings about breast cancer. More than one-third of these nonaffected women reported breast cancer images and associations that intruded on their awareness, and 20% had difficulty in sleeping because of their breast cancer concerns. Importantly, these authors found that genetic counseling was significantly less effective among women with higher baseline levels of breast cancer preoccupation. Therefore, they concluded that efforts to provide individuals with cancer genetic counseling are not likely to be effective unless their cancer anxieties and feelings are also addressed.[76]

It might be assumed that fear of cancer motivates individuals to increase their cancer awareness and prevention strategies. On the contrary, Kash et al.[34] found that women who perceived their breast cancer risks as high were engaged in *fewer* general preventive health care behaviors (including breast self-examinations and regular clinical breast examinations) than those women who perceived their risks as only moderate. It is theorized that perhaps these individuals believe that they will definitely develop breast cancer and are helpless in decreasing their risks, or perhaps they are completely immobilized by their fear or denial. Whatever the reason for these behaviors, it is obvious that psychological and educational interventions should be a component of cancer genetic counseling.

The counseling session is an opportunity for individuals to express why they believe that they have developed cancer or why their family members have cancer. Some explanations may revolve around family folklore, and it is important to listen to and address these explanations rather than to dismiss them.[5] In doing this, the counselor will allow the clients to alleviate their greatest fears and to give more credibility to the "medical" theory. For patients who are moving forward with DNA testing, a referral to a mental health care professional who can help to facilitate the process is often very helpful.

To date, studies conducted in the setting of pre- and post-genetic counseling have revealed that, at least in the short term, most patients do not experience adverse psychological outcomes after receiving their test results.[77,78] In fact, preliminary data have revealed that individuals in families with known mutations who seek testing seem to fare better psychologically at 6 months than those who avoid testing.[79] Although these data are reassuring, it is important to recognize that genetic testing is an individual decision and will not be right for every patient or every family.

PRESYMPTOMATIC TESTING OF CHILDREN

Presymptomatic testing of children has been widely discussed, and most concur that it is appropriate only when the onset of the condition regularly occurs in childhood or there are useful interventions that can be applied.[80] For example, DNA-based diagnosis of children and young adults at risk for hereditary medullary thyroid carcinoma has improved the management of these patients.[81–83] DNA-based testing for RET mutations is virtually 100% accurate and allows at-risk family members to make informed decisions about prophylactic thyroidectomy. FAP is a disorder that occurs in childhood and in which mortality can be reduced if detection is presymptomatic.[84,85] Testing is clearly indicated in these instances.

Predisposition testing may also be appropriate if it will be useful to the minor child in making reproductive decisions now or in the near future.[86] Early observations by Malkin et al.[87] indicated an interest among parents in cancer-predictive testing for their children. Their willingness to have their children undergo testing appeared to be dependent on the accuracy of the test and the availability of preventive or curative options. Questions have been raised about parents' right to demand testing for adult-onset diseases. Parents may have a constitutionally protected right to demand that unwilling physicians order this test, but there is little risk for liability for damages unless the child experiences physical harm as a direct result of this refusal.[80] The child's right not to be tested must be considered. Whenever childhood testing is not medically indicated, it is preferable that testing decisions be postponed until the children are adults and can decide for themselves whether to be tested. However, the argument has been made that if a child younger than 18 years is able to appreciate not only the genetic facts but also the emotional and social consequences, he or she should be allowed to have genetic testing.[88] This subject is highly controversial and will likely continue to be debated.

CONFIDENTIALITY

The level of confidentiality surrounding cancer genetic testing is paramount, owing to concerns of genetic discrimination. Many programs are opting to keep shadow files separate from the general hospital charts. Patient-identifying data are generally not entered into computer databases that are accessible by modem or a network of users. Some counseling programs are submitting DNA samples to laboratories by coded number only in an attempt to increase the level of confidentiality. Special precautions to protect confidentiality should be taken when leaving voice mail messages, at home and at work, regarding patient appointments. Conversations with patients or other colleagues via E-mail that include patient names are discouraged, as the Internet is not secure. Additionally, genetic counseling summary letters are sent directly to patients and are copied to the referring physicians only with the explicit permission of the patient. These measures are taken because confidentiality and genetic discrimination are a grave concern for many of the patients seen in the cancer genetic counseling clinic.[15,74,89]

Confidentiality of test results within a family can also be an issue, as genetic counseling and testing often reveal the risk status of family members other than the patient. Under confidentiality codes, the patient should grant permission before at-risk family members can be contacted. It has been questioned whether family members could sue a health care professional for negligence if they were identified as at high risk yet not informed.[90] Most recommendations have stated that the burden of confidentiality lies between the provider and the patient. However, more recent recommendations state that confidentiality should be violated if the potential harm of not notifying other family members outweighs the harm of breaking a confidence to the patient.[91] There is no patent solution for this difficult dilemma, and situations must be considered on a case-by-case basis with the assistance of the in-house legal department and ethics committee.

Patients should be counseled about the benefits to other family members of knowing testing results but, at present, the decision is ultimately the patient's. Extended family members who are notified with the patient's consent may not always be grateful to receive this information and may think that their privacy has been invaded by being contacted.

INSURANCE ISSUES

Insurance companies are, understandably, in the business of making money. Before issuing health insurance policies, some companies determine the risk that an individual carries and adjust the premium to match that risk.[92] Information regarding family history, genetic information, and prior diagnostic testing may very well be used in calculating this risk. This should be clearly conveyed to the patient in the precounseling interview, as it may change the method by which he or she chooses to pay for the session or for testing. These issues should be discussed in detail again in the counseling session. Although individuals and counselors can attempt to keep records and results confidential, there is always a risk that this information will reach insurers.

More and more patients are choosing to submit their genetic counseling or testing charges to their health insurance companies. In the last few years, more insurance companies have agreed to pay for counseling or testing (or both),[93] perhaps in light of decision analyses that show these services and subsequent prophylactic surgeries to be cost-effective.[94] Letters of justification are often required for insurance companies to cover the charges for testing. These letters must clearly delineate the impact of testing on the short- and long-term management of the patient being tested. Justification of testing based on assisting other, unaffected family members is rarely helpful.

DISCRIMINATION

Many health care providers and patients fear that genetic discrimination by health, life, and disability insurance companies resulting from a positive test is a potential hazard of genetic testing.[95,96] Fear of genetic discrimination by patients has been cited as a major deterrent to genetic testing.[15,74,89] Some data indicate that consumer fear of genetic discrimination is out of proportion with the actual amount of discrimination experienced[97]; however, it is well known that current legislation aimed at protecting individuals from genetic discrimination is not without loopholes.[98] Patients should be informed of local and national legislation on genetic discrimination as well as the limitations of these laws.

FUTURE DIRECTIONS

The field of cancer genetic counseling and testing grew tremendously in the late 1990s. Although cancer genetic counseling is targeted at individuals with strong personal or family histories of cancer, it is clear that this focus will broaden over the next decade. Genetic testing may be used to guide surgical decision making, as the risk of new primary tumors is greater in individuals who carry germline mutations.[64,65] Data showing that germline mutations are more frequent in individuals with early-onset breast and colon cancers, even in the absence of a family history of these diseases, will expand the criteria for genetic testing.[21–26] Specific histologic tumor types may indicate that a patient is at increased risk to carry a germline mutation[99] and may prompt a referral to genetic counseling. The U.S. Food and Drug Administration approval of tamoxifen as a method of breast cancer risk reduction for women at moderately increased risk of the disease will likely bring an onslaught of genetic counseling referrals. These patients will need to know their personal risks of developing breast cancer, and the counseling session will include a detailed discussion of their personal risks for osteoporosis, coronary heart disease, menopausal symptoms, and cognitive deficiencies and the pros and cons of HRT versus selective estrogen receptor modulators, such as tamoxifen. The discovery of modifying genes[100] and specific environmental factors that affect the lifetime risks of cancer associated with current susceptibility genes will render it possible to refine lifetime cancer risks in individual families.

Perhaps the most profound new direction in cancer genetics will be the integration of genetic testing for high-prevalence, low-penetrance mutations, such as the APC mutation I1307K. I1307K is a common mutation among Ashkenazi Jews that is associated with an increased, but relatively modest, risk of colorectal cancer.[28] The utility of such testing among Jews with a family history of colon cancer has been questioned, as increased surveillance is recommended, owing to the family history, regardless of the test result. Gruber et al.[101] described that Ashkenazi Jewish individuals with no family history of colon cancer may actually derive the most benefit from such testing, as a positive test result would elucidate which patients in that population would benefit from increased colorectal surveillance. This shift in emphasis from rare, high-risk mutation screening to broad screening for lower-penetrance mutations could change the face of the field of cancer genetic counseling.

The combination of technologic advances in genetic testing, new pharmacologic developments for cancer risk reduction, and increased utility for testing in high- and moderate-risk populations will result in a significant expansion in the field of cancer genetic counseling. Maintenance of high standards for thorough genetic counseling, informed consent, and accurate result interpretation will be paramount in reducing potential risks and maximizing the benefits of this technology in the next century.

Acknowledgments

Special thanks to Beth N. Peshkin, MS, for her insightful review of this chapter.

REFERENCES

1. Peters J. Breast cancer genetics: relevance to oncology practice. *Cancer Control* 1995;May/June:195.
2. Kelly PT. Informational needs of individuals and families with hereditary cancers. *Semin Oncol Nurs* 1992;8:288.
3. Peters JA. Familial cancer risk: 1. Impact on today's oncology practice. *J Oncol Manage* 1994;Sept/Oct:18.
4. Kelly PT. Genetic counseling with the cancer patient's family. *Curr Probl Cancer* 1983;7:15.
5. Schneider KA. *Counseling about cancer: strategies for genetic counselors*. Boston: Dana-Farber Cancer Institute, 1994.
6. Geller G, Bernhardt BA, Doksum T, et al. Decision making about breast cancer susceptibility testing: How similar are the attitudes of physicians, nurse practitioners, and at-risk women? *J Clin Oncol* 1998;16:2868.
7. Lerman C, Rimer BK, Engstrom PF. Cancer risk notification: psychosocial and ethical implications. *J Clin Oncol* 1991;9:1275.
8. Peters JA. Familial cancer risk: II. Breast cancer risk counseling and genetic susceptibility testing. *J Oncol Manage* 1994;Nov/Dec:14.
9. Lerman C, Seay J, Balshem A, Audrain J. Interest in genetic testing among first-degree relatives of breast cancer patients. *Am J Med Genet* 1995;57:385.
10. Benkendorf JL, Reutenauer JE, Hughes CA, et al. Patients' attitudes about autonomy and confidentiality in genetic testing for breast-ovarian cancer susceptibility. *Am J Med Genet* 1997;73:296.
11. Durfy SJ, Bowen DJ, McTiernan A, et al. Attitudes and interest in genetic testing for breast and ovarian cancer susceptibility in diverse groups of women in western Washington. *Cancer Epidemiol Biomarkers Prev* 1999;8:369.
12. Glanz K, Grove J, Lerman C, et al. Correlates of intentions to obtain genetic counseling and colorectal cancer gene testing among at-risk relatives from three ethnic groups. *Cancer Epidemiol Biomarkers Prev* 1999;8:329.
13. Smith KR, Croyle RT. Attitudes toward genetic testing for colon cancer risk. *Am J Public Health* 1995;85:1435.
14. Lerman C, Narod S, Schulman K, et al. *BRCA1* testing in families with hereditary breast-ovarian cancer. A prospective study of patient decision making and outcomes. *JAMA* 1996;275:1885.
15. Lynch HT, Lemon SJ, Durham C, et al. A descriptive study of *BRCA1* testing and reactions to disclosure of test results. *Cancer* 1997;79:2219.
16. Croyle RT, Lerman C. Interest in genetic testing for colon cancer susceptibility: cognitive and emotional correlates. *Prev Med* 1993;22:284.
17. Lerman C, Hughes C, Trock BJ. Genetic testing in families with hereditary nonpolyposis colon cancer. *JAMA* 1999;281:1618.
18. Cotton P. Prognosis, diagnosis, or who knows? Time to learn what gene tests mean. *JAMA* 1995;273:93.
19. Collins FS. Preparing health professionals for the genetic revolution. *JAMA* 1997; 278(15):1285.
20. Claus EB, Schildkraut JM, Thompson WD, et al. The genetic attributable risks of breast and ovarian cancer. *Cancer* 1996;77:2318.
21. FitzGerald MG, MacDonald DJ, Krainer M, et al. Germ-line BRCA1 mutations in Jewish and non-Jewish women with early-onset breast cancer. *N Engl J Med* 1996;334:143.
22. Langston AA, Malone KE, Thompson JD, et al. BRCA1 mutations in a population-based sample of young women with breast cancer. *N Engl J Med* 1996;334:137.
23. Krainer M, Silva-Arrieta S, FitzGerald MG, et al. Differential contributions of BRCA1 and BRCA2 to early-onset breast cancer. *N Engl J Med* 1997;336:1416.
24. Farrington SM, Lin-Goerke J, Ling J, et al. Systematic analysis of hMSH2 and hMLH1 in young colon cancer patients and controls. *Am J Hum Genet* 1998;63:749.
25. Syngal S, Fox EA, Li C, et al. Interpretation of genetic test results for hereditary nonpolyposis colorectal cancer: implications for clinical predisposition testing. *JAMA* 1999;282:247.
26. Peto J, Collins N, Barfoot R, et al. Prevalence of BRCA1 and BRCA2 gene mutations in patients with early-onset breast cancer. *J Natl Cancer Inst* 1999;91:943.
27. Struewing JP, Hartge P, Wacholder S, et al. The risk of cancer associated with specific mutations of BRCA1 and BRCA2 among Ashkenazi Jews. *N Eng J Med* 1997;336:1401.
28. Gryfe R, Nicola ND, Lal G, Gallinger S, Redston M. Inherited colorectal polyposis and cancer risk of the APC I1307K polymorphism. *Am J Hum Genet* 1999;64:378.
29. Tonin PT, Mes-Masson A-M, Futreal PA, et al. Founder BRCA1 and BRCA2 mutations in French Canadian breast and ovarian cancer families. *Am J Hum Genet* 1998;63:1341.
30. Santarosa M, Viel A, Dolcetti R, et al. Low incidence of BRCA1 mutations among Italian families with breast and ovarian cancer. *Int J Cancer* 1998;78:581.
31. Tang NLS, Pang C-P, Yeo W, et al. Prevalence of mutations in the BRCA1 gene among Chinese patients with breast cancer. *J Natl Cancer Inst* 1999;91(10):882.
32. Weber TK, Chin H-M, Rodriguez-Bigas M, et al. Novel hMLH1 and hMSH2 germline mutations in African Americans with colorectal cancer. *JAMA* 1999;281:2316.
33. Lindor NM, Greene MH. The Mayo Familial Cancer Program. *J Natl Cancer Inst* 1998;90(14):1039.
34. Kash KM, Holland JC, Halper MS, Miller DG. Psychological distress and surveillance behaviors of women with a family history of breast cancer. *J Natl Cancer Inst* 1992;84:24.

35. Lynch HT. Cancer and the family history trail. *NY State J Med* 1991;91:145.
36. Lynch HT, Kullander S. Introduction to cancer genetics in women. In: Lynch HT, Kullander S, eds. *Cancer genetics in women*, vol 1. Boca Raton, FL: CRC Press, 1987.
37. Eng C, Stratton M, Ponder B, et al. Familial cancer syndromes. *Lancet* 1994;343:709.
38. Love RR, Evan AM, Josten DM. The accuracy of patient reports of a family history of cancer. *J Chronic Dis* 1985;38:289.
39. Hodgson SV, Maher ER. *A practical guide to human genetics*. Cambridge: Cambridge University Press, 1993.
40. Olopade OI, Weber BL. Breast cancer genetics: toward molecular characterization of individuals at increased risk for breast cancer: II. *PPO Updates* 1998;12(11):1.
41. Gail MH, Brinton LA, Byar DP, et al. Projecting individualized probabilities of developing breast cancer for white females who are being examined annually. *J Natl Cancer Inst* 1989;81:1879.
42. Colditz GA, Rosner BA, Speizer FE. Risk factors for breast cancer according to family history of breast cancer. *J Natl Cancer Inst* 1996;88:365.
43. Anderson SJ, Ahnn S, Duff K. NSABP breast cancer prevention trial risk assessment program, version 2 [Technical Report]. Pittsburgh, PA: National Surgical Adjuvant Breast and Bowel Project Biostatistical Center, 1992.
44. Claus EB, Risch N, Thompson WD. Autosomal dominant inheritance of early-onset breast cancer. *Cancer* 1994;73:643.
45. Ford D, Easton DF, Bishop DT, et al. Risks of cancer in BRCA1-mutation carriers. *Lancet* 1994;343:692.
46. Couch FJ, DeShano ML, Blackwood A, et al. BRCA1 mutations in women attending clinics that evaluate the risk of breast cancer. *N Engl J Med* 1997;336(20):1409.
47. Parmigiani G, Berry DA, Agilar O. Determining carrier probabilities for breast cancer susceptibility genes BRCA1 and BRCA2. *Am J Hum Genet* 1998;62:145.
48. Richards MPM, Hallowell N, Green JM, Murton F, Statham H. Counseling families with hereditary breast and ovarian cancer: a psychosocial perspective. *J Genet Couns* 1995;4:219.
49. Giardiello FM, Brensinger JD, Petersen GM, et al. The use and interpretation of commercial APC gene testing for familial adenomatous polyposis. *N Engl J Med* 1997;336:823.
50. Lynch HT, Watson P, Tinley S, et al. An update on DNA-Based *BRCA1/BRCA2* genetic counseling in hereditary breast cancer. *Cancer Genet Cytogenet* 1999;109:91.
51. Easton DF, Ford D, Bishop T, et al. Breast and ovarian cancer incidence in *BRCA1*-mutation carriers. *Am J Hum Genet* 1995;56:265.
52. Easton DF, Steele L, Fields P, et al. Cancer risks in two large breast cancer families linked to *BRCA2* on chromosome 13q12-13. *Am J Hum Genet* 1997;61:120.
53. Struewing JP, Brody LC, Erdos MR, et al. Detection of eight *BRCA1* mutations in 10 breast/ovarian cancer families, including 1 family with male breast cancer. *Am J Hum Genet* 1995;57:1.
54. Friedman LS, Gayther SA, Kurosaki T, et al. Mutation analysis of *BRCA1* and *BRCA2* in a male breast cancer population. *Am J Hum Genet* 1997;60:313.
55. Serova OM, Mazoyer S, Puget N, et al. Mutations in *BRCA1* and *BRCA2* in breast cancer families: Are there more breast cancer-susceptibility genes? *Am J Hum Genet* 1997;60:486.
56. Phelan CM, Lancaster JM, Tonin P, et al. Mutation analysis of the *BRCA2* gene in 49 site-specific breast cancer families. *Nat Genet* 1996;13:120.
57. Wooster R, Bignell G, Lancaster J, et al. Identification of the breast cancer susceptibility gene BRCA2. *Nature* 1995;378:789.
58. Marra G, Boland CR. Hereditary nonpolyposis colorectal cancer. *J Natl Cancer Inst* 1995;87:1114.
59. Aarnio M, Mecklin J-P, Aaltonen LA, et al. Lifetime risk of different cancers in hereditary non-polyposis colorectal cancer (HNPCC) syndrome. *Int J Cancer* 1995;64:430.
60. Burke W, Daly M, Garber J, et al. Recommendations for follow-up care of individuals with an inherited predisposition to cancer: II. BRCA1 and BRCA2. *JAMA* 1997;277:997.
61. Fisher B, Costantino JP, Wickerman DL, et al. Tamoxifen for the prevention of breast cancer: report of the National Surgical Adjuvant Breast and Bowel Project P-1 study. *J Natl Cancer Inst* 1998;90:1371.
62. Cummings SR, Eckert S, Krueger KA, et al. The effect of raloxifene on risk of breast cancer in postmenopausal women: results from the MORE randomized trial. *JAMA* 1999;281:2189.
63. Hartmann LC, Schaid DJ, Woods JE, et al. Efficacy of bilateral prophylactic mastectomy in women with a family history of breast cancer. *N Engl J Med* 1999;340:77.
64. Matloff ET, Peshkin BN, Ward BA. The impact of genetic screening on surgical decision making in breast cancer. In: Szabo Z, Lewis JE, Fantini GA, Savalgi RS, eds. *Surgical technology international VII: international developments in surgery and surgical research*. San Francisco: Universal Medical Press, 1998.
65. Turner BC, Harold E, Matloff E, et al. BRCA1/BRCA2 germline mutations in locally recurrent breast cancer patients after lumpectomy and radiation therapy: implications for breast-conserving management in patients with BRCA1/BRCA2 mutations. *J Clin Oncol* 1999;10:3017.
66. Narod SA, Risch H, Moslehi R, et al. Oral contraceptives and the risk of hereditary ovarian cancer. *N Engl J Med* 1998;339:424.
67. American College of Obstetrics and Gynecology. Committee opinion: breast-ovarian cancer screening. *Am J Obstet Gynecol* 1996;176:1.
68. Piver MS, Jishi MF, Tsukada Y, et al. Primary peritoneal carcinoma after prophylactic oophorectomy in women with a family history of ovarian cancer. *Cancer* 1993;71:2751.
69. Struewing JP, Watson P, Easton DF, et al. Prophylactic oophorectomy in inherited breast/ovarian cancer families. *J Natl Cancer Inst Monogr* 1995;17:33.
70. Rebbeck TR, Levin AM, Eisen A, et al. Breast cancer risk after bilateral prophylactic oophorectomy in BRCA1 mutation carriers. *J Natl Cancer Inst* 1999;91(17):1475.
71. Burke W, Petersen G, Lynch P, et al. Recommendations for follow-up care of individuals with an inherited predisposition to cancer. Hereditary nonpolyposis colon cancer. *JAMA* 1997;277:915.
72. DeCosse JJ. Surgical prophylaxis of familial colon cancer: prevention of death from familial colorectal cancer. *J Natl Cancer Inst Monogr* 1995;17:31.
73. Syngal S, Weeks JC, Schrag D, et al. Benefits of colonoscopic surveillance and prophylactic colectomy in patients with hereditary nonpolyposis colorectal cancer mutations. *Ann Intern Med* 1998;129:787.
74. Silverberg SG, Makowski EL. Endometrial carcinoma in young women taking oral contraceptive agents. *Obstet Gynecol* 1975;46:503.
75. Kelly PT. Breast cancer risk analysis: a genetic epidemiology service for families. *J Genet Couns* 1992;1:155.
76. Lerman C, Lustbader E, Rimer B, et al. Effects of individualized breast cancer risk counseling: a randomized trial. *J Natl Cancer Inst* 1995;87:286.
77. Lerman C, Narod S, Schulman K, et al. BRCA1 testing in families with hereditary breast-ovarian cancer: a prospective study of patient decision making and outcomes. *JAMA* 1996;275(24):1885.
78. Croyle RT, Smith KR, Botkin JR, et al. Psychological responses to BRCA1 mutation testing: preliminary findings. *Health Psychol* 1997;16:63.
79. Lerman C, Hughes C, Lemon SJ, et al. What you don't know can hurt you: adverse psychologic effects in members of BRCA1-linked and BRCA2-linked families who decline genetic testing. *J Clin Oncol* 1998:16:1650.
80. Clayton EW. Removing the shadow of the law from the debate about genetic testing of children. *Am J Med Genet* 1995;57:630.
81. Ledger GA, Khosia S, Lindor NM, Thibodeau SN, Gharib H. Genetic testing in the diagnosis and management of multiple endocrine neoplasia type II. *Ann Intern Med* 1995;122:118.
82. Lips CJ, Landsvater RM, Hoppener JW, et al. Clinical screening as compared with DNA analysis in families with multiple endocrine neoplasia type 2A. *N Engl J Med* 1994;331:828.
83. Wells SA Jr, Chi DD, Toshima K, et al. Predictive DNA testing and prophylactic thyroidectomy in patients at risk for multiple endocrine neoplasia type 2A. *Ann Surg* 1994;220:237.
84. Rhodes M, Bradburn DM. Overview of screening and management of familial adenomatous polyposis. *Gut* 1992;33:125.
85. Lerman C, Marshall J, Audrain J, et al. Genetic testing for colon cancer susceptibility: anticipated reactions of patients and challenges to providers. *Int J Cancer* 1996;69:58.
86. Wertz DC, Fanos JH, Reilly PR. Genetic testing for children and adolescents: Who decides? *JAMA* 1994;272:875.
87. Malkin D, Australie K, Shuman C, Barrera M, Weksberg R. Childhood cancer: parental attitudes to genetic counseling and predictive testing. *Am J Hum Gen* 1995;57:A156(abst).
88. Dickenson DL. Can children and young people consent to be tested for adult onset genetic disorders? *BMJ* 1999;318:1063.
89. Bluman LG, Rimer BK, Berry DA, et al. Attitudes, knowledge, and risk perceptions of women with breast and/or ovarian cancer considering testing for BRCA1 and BRCA2. *J Natl Cancer Inst* 1999;17:1040.
90. Tsoucalas CL. Legal aspects of cancer genetics—screening, counseling, and registers. In: Lynch HT, Kullander S, eds. *Cancer genetics in women*, vol 1. Boca Raton, FL: CRC Press, 1987:9.
91. The American Society of Human Genetics Social Issues Subcommittee on Familial Disclosure. ASHG statement: professional disclosure of familial genetic information. *Am J Hum Genet* 1998;62:474.
92. ASHG Ad Hoc Committee on Insurance Issues in Genetic Testing. Background statement: genetic testing and insurance. *Am J Hum Genet* 1995;56:327.
93. Manley SA, Pennell RL, Frank TS. Insurance coverage of BRCA1 and BRCA2 sequence analysis. *J Genet Couns* 1998;7(6):A462.
94. Grann VR, Whang W, Jacobson JS, et al. Benefits and costs of screening Ashkenazi Jewish women for BRCA1 and BRCA2. *J Clin Oncol* 1999;17:494.
95. Lapham EV, Kozma C, Weiss JO. Genetic discrimination: perspectives of consumers. *Science* 1996;274:621.
96. Billings PR, Kohn MA, de Cuevas M, et al. Discrimination as a consequence of genetic testing. *Am J Hum Genet* 1992;50:476.
97. Wingrove KJ, Norris J, Barton PL, et al. Experiences and attitudes concerning genetic testing and insurance in a Colorado population: a survey of families diagnosed with fragile X syndrome. *Am J Med Genet* 1996;64:378.
98. Smetanka SL. The asymptomatic ill and genetic discrimination: 2. *Health Care Law Monogr* 1998;9:3.
99. Eisinger F, Jacquemier J, Charafe-Jauffret E, et al. More about multifactorial analysis of difference between sporadic breast cancers and cancers involving BRCA1 and BRCA2 mutations. *J Natl Cancer Inst* 1999;91(16):1421.
100. Rebbeck TR, Kantoff PW, Krithivas K, et al. Modification of BRCA1-associated breast cancer risk by the polymorphic androgen-receptor CAG repeat. *Am J Hum Genet* 1999;64:1371.
101. Gruber SB, Petersen GM, Kinzler KW, Vogelstein B. Cancer, crash sites, and the new genetics of neoplasia. *Gastroenterology* 1999;116(1):210.

MARY JANE MASSIE
LISA CHERTKOV
ANDREW J. ROTH

SECTION 5

Psychological Issues

PSYCHIATRIC DISORDERS IN CANCER PATIENTS

One-third of patients with cancer report a degree of anxiety or depression that requires psychiatric treatment.[1,2] In the past, symptoms of emotional distress were often unrecognized, undetected and, as a result, untreated. In this chapter, we review the normal responses to cancer; the most frequently encountered psychiatric disorders; and psychotherapeutic, pharmacologic, and behavioral management of these disorders.

There are characteristic normal responses to receiving a diagnosis of cancer. A period of initial disbelief, denial, or despair is common and generally lasts only a few days. Subsequently, many have a dysphoric mood, with anxiety symptoms, depressed mood, anorexia, insomnia, or irritability lasting a few weeks. The ability to concentrate and to carry out usual daily activities is impaired, and intrusive thoughts of the illness and uncertainty about the future are present. Adaptation usually begins after several weeks and continues for months to years as most patients integrate new information, confront reality issues, find reasons for optimism, and resume activities.[3]

The patient's ability to successfully manage a cancer diagnosis depends on medical, psychological, and social factors and commonly changes over the course of the illness. These factors include the disease itself (i.e., site, symptoms, clinical course, prognosis, type of treatments required); prior level of adjustment, especially to medical illness; the threat that cancer poses to attaining age-appropriate developmental tasks and goals (i.e., adolescence, career, family, retirement); cultural, spiritual, and religious attitudes; the presence of emotionally supportive persons in the patient's environment; the patient's potential for physical and psychological rehabilitation; the patient's own personality and coping style; prior experience with cancer; and history of losses.

PREVALENCE

There have been many assumptions about the psychological state of cancer patients, varying between the assumption that all patients must be depressed and need help and the opposite assumption that most manage well and few need psychiatric intervention. Prevalence studies counter these extreme attitudes. In the first comprehensive study, the Psychosocial Collaborative Oncology Group reported that of 215 randomly selected hospitalized and ambulatory patients at three major cancer centers, 47% met criteria for a psychiatric disorder.[4] Of the cancer patients who had an identified psychiatric disorder, 68% had an adjustment disorder with depressed, anxious, or mixed mood; 13% had major depression; 8% had an organic mental disorder (i.e., delirium); 7% had a personality disorder; and 4% had an anxiety disorder. Depressive disorders accounted for the majority of diagnoses. Nearly 90% of the psychiatric disorders observed were either reactions to, or manifestations of, disease or treatment. Only 11% of patients had prior psychiatric illness. Patients with cancer are thus largely psychologically healthy individuals who have emotional distress related to illness. However, there is a significant incidence of psychiatric illness, as approximately 25% of all cancer patients experience significant depression, irrespective of their hospital and physical status.[5]

DEPRESSION

Depression is clearly the most prevalent psychiatric symptom in cancer patients. Depression can be distinguished from normal sadness and anticipatory grieving based on the nature and severity of the symptoms, their duration and intensity, and their impact on functioning. Depression in cancer patients results from (1) stress related to the cancer diagnosis and treatment; (2) medications (Table 56.5-1); (3) underlying neurologic or medical problems, such as nutritional deficiencies (folate, vitamin B_{12}), endocrine disturbances (thyroid abnormalities, adrenal insufficiency), brain metastases, and leptomeningeal disease; or (4) recurrence of a preexisting depressive syndrome or bipolar mood disorder. The emotional stress of the cancer experience and medications are the most common causes of depression. Whereas the diagnosis of depression in physically healthy patients depends heavily on the somatic symptoms of anorexia, fatigue, and weight loss, these indicators are of lesser value in the assessment of a cancer patient, since they are common to both cancer and depression. Diagnosis must rest on psychological or cognitive symptoms: anhedonia, dysphoric mood, feelings of hopelessness-helplessness-worthlessness-guilt, poor self-esteem, or suicidality. Cancer patients are at higher risk for depression if they are in poor physical condition, have inadequately controlled pain, are in the advanced stages of illness, have a history of depression, or have other significant life stresses or losses.[5] An increased risk has also been associated with pancreatic, head and neck, and lung cancer.

Early detection and aggressive treatment of depression is essential in cancer patients. Psychoeducation about normal responses to coping with the stresses of cancer and identification of symptoms requiring treatment is the first step. Despite tremendous advances in efforts to destigmatize psychiatric illness and treatment, many patients continue to be reluctant to seek counseling or to consider psychotropic medications. The oncologist and nursing staff play essential roles in communicating the importance of treating the whole person, and attending to the psychological distress that many patients experience. Referral for psychiatric evaluation when indicated is a significant opportunity to validate the patient's feelings of distress and provide supportive counseling. A recent report by Watson et al.[6] that a high helplessness-hopelessness score has a detrimental effect on 5-year survival in women with early breast cancer and that a high score for depression is linked to a significantly reduced chance of survival is provocative and calls for more research in the identification and treatment of the depressed cancer patient. Currently, a range of psychopharmacologic and psychotherapeutic treatments is available for depression (Table 56.5-2).

Selective Serotonin Reuptake Inhibitors and Other New Antidepressants

The selective serotonin reuptake inhibitors (SSRIs) are the first-line antidepressants prescribed in cancer settings because

TABLE 56.5-1. Medications That Can Cause Depression in Cancer Patients

Glucocorticoids
Interferon and interleukin-2
Acyclovir
Narcotics
Barbiturates and other anticonvulsants
Propranolol
Some antibiotics (amphotericin B)
Some chemotherapeutic agents
Vincristine
Vinblastine
Procarbazine
L-Asparaginase

they are effective, with few side effects and few drug interactions. The SSRIs (e.g., fluoxetine, sertraline, paroxetine, and citralopram) have proven as effective as tricyclic antidepressants (TCAs) but with less sedative and autonomic effects. The most common side effects are mild nausea, gastrointestinal disturbance, headache, somnolence or insomnia, and a brief period of increased anxiety. SSRIs can cause sexual dysfunction in both men and women, a side effect that often leads to cessation of the drug, although there are a number of interventions that may address this symptom. There has been contradictory information about the potential for appetite suppression with SSRIs as they have been demonstrated to cause transient anorexia but have also been successfully used in patients with eating disorders to improve food intake. Some cancer patients experience transient weight loss; however, weight usually returns to baseline level, and the anorectic properties of these drugs have not been a limiting factor in this population. The SSRIs do vary in their metabolism, with paroxetine having no active metabolites and sertraline having relatively few and both paroxetine and sertraline having short half-lives. The newest SSRI, citalopram, may be less likely to cause gastrointestinal symptoms and anxiety. Fluoxetine, sertraline, and paroxetine have been used to reduce both the number and intensity of hot flashes in non-depressed women who become menopausal after chemotherapy for breast cancer.

Bupropion and trazodone are prescribed less frequently than the SSRIs for individuals with cancer. Bupropion's activating profile makes it useful in lethargic patients, but it is associated with anorexia and increased seizure risk and should be avoided in patients with a history of seizures or brain tumor and in those who are malnourished. Bupropion has been demonstrated to improve the chances of success for patients attempting to quit smoking tobacco and thus may be especially important in patients with lung or head and neck cancers. Trazodone is strongly sedating and in low doses (25 to 100 mg q.h.s.) is helpful in the treatment of the depressed cancer patient with insomnia. Trazodone has been associated with priapism and should, therefore, be used with caution in male patients. The use of venlafaxine, nefazodone, and mirtazapine has not been studied in cancer patients. Venlafaxine affects both norepinephrine and serotonin neurotransmitter systems, but it does not produce the same uncomfortable antimuscarinic and antiadrenergic side effects as the tricyclic antidepressants. Hypertensive side effects

TABLE 56.5-2. Antidepressants Commonly Prescribed for Cancer Patients

Drug Name	*Starting Dose (mg)*	*Therapeutic Dose (mg/d)*
Newer antidepressants		
SSRIs		
Citalopram (Celexa)	10–20 q.d.	20–60
Fluoxetine (Prozac)	20 q.d.	10–80
Paroxetine (Paxil)	10 q.d.	10–50
Sertraline (Zoloft)	25–50 q.d.	50–200
Others		
Bupropion (Wellbutrin)	50–75 b.i.d.	300–450
Nefazodone (Serzone)	100 t.i.d.	100–600
Trazodone (Desyrel)	50 q.h.s.	50–300
Venlafaxine (Effexor)	37.5 b.i.d.	75–375
Mirtazapine (Remeron)	15 q.h.s.	15–45
TCAs		
Amitriptyline (Elavil)	10–25 q.h.s.	50–300
Desipramine (Norpramin)	10–25 q.h.s.	50–300
Doxepine (Sinequan)	10–25 q.h.s.	75–300
Imipramine (Tofranil)	10–25 q.h.s.	50–300
Nortriptyline (Pamelor)	10–25 q.h.s.	50–200
Psychostimulants		
Dextroamphetamine (Dexedrine)	2.5 b.i.d. (a.m. & 2 p.m.)	5–20
Methylphenidate (Ritalin)	2.5 b.i.d. (a.m. & 2 p.m.)	5–20
Pemoline (Cylert)	18.75 every a.m.	37.5–112.5

SSRI, selective serotonin reuptake inhibitor; TCA, tricyclic antidepressant.

at higher doses can be problematic in medically ill patients. Nefazodone also affects serotonin and norepinephrine systems and is useful in those with agitated depression or insomnia. Mirtazapine, another sedating antidepressant, is similarly efficacious for patients with agitated depression and insomnia and is currently under study for its potential analgesic and antiemetic effects. Bupropion, nefazodone, and mirtazapine are less likely to cause sexual dysfunction than the SSRIs and venlafaxine.

Tricyclic Antidepressants

The tricyclic antidepressants are still used to treat depression in adults and children with cancer. Nortriptyline and desipramine have the most favorable side effect profiles for cancer patients, with less anticholinergic and sedating symptoms. For reasons that are unclear, depressed cancer patients often show a therapeutic response to a tricyclic at much lower doses (75 to 125 mg/d) than are usually required in physically healthy depressed patients (150 to 300 mg/d). Obtaining serum levels of the medications is helpful in titrating dosages and monitoring toxicity. The beneficial effects on appetite and sleep are frequently immediate, while the effects on mood may be delayed. Tricyclic antidepressants have been favored in medical settings because of their demonstrated analgesic effects in some patients. However, they are notorious for their side effects, such as hypotension and cardiac conduction disturbances.

Psychostimulants

In cancer patients, low doses of psychostimulants (i.e., dextroamphetamine, methylphenidate, and pemoline) promote a sense of well-being, decrease fatigue, and stimulate appetite. Psychostimulants offer clear benefits, especially in terminally medically ill patients, as there may be an improvement in symptoms within hours to days.

Psychostimulants can also potentiate the analgesic effects of opioid analgesics and are commonly used to counteract opioid-induced sedation. As tolerance develops, an adjustment of the dose is necessary. Side effects at low doses include insomnia, tachycardia, euphoria, and mood lability. High doses and long-term use may produce nightmares, insomnia, and paranoia. Patients should be cardiologically and neurologically stable before starting a stimulant.

Psychostimulant dosing is usually at 8 a.m. and noon to avoid any potential for sleep disturbance. Pemoline, a gentler psychostimulant available in chewable form with buccal absorption, may be chosen for more frail, debilitated patients or for those who cannot swallow. However, pemoline should be used with caution in patients with renal impairment; liver and renal function tests should be monitored periodically. Typically, patients are maintained on a psychostimulant for 1 to 2 months, after which time many can discontinue these medications without a recurrence of depressive symptoms. Those who experience further depressive symptoms can be maintained on a psychostimulant for longer periods, and tapering may be aided by concurrent use of another antidepressant.

Mood Stabilizers

Patients with a history of bipolar disorder (manic-depressive illness) maintained on mood stabilizers must be continued on their medications throughout treatment. They may require close psychiatric monitoring, as the stresses of their illness and treatment place them at high risk for episodes of severe affective illness. There are few studies of the use of mood stabilizers during cancer treatment. Patients who have been treated with lithium carbonate should be maintained on it throughout their cancer treatment, but close monitoring is necessary, as patients are vulnerable to toxicity in the setting of fluid and electrolyte imbalances, such as during perioperative periods, in critically ill patients with renal dysfunction, or in those receiving potentially nephrotoxic drugs. Use of carbamazepine as a mood stabilizer can be problematic in cancer patients because of its marrow-suppressing properties. Valproic acid, on the other hand, is better tolerated and considered to be quite efficacious. Gabapentin is currently under study as a mood stabilizer. It is well tolerated with few side effects and has a growing role in the treatment of neuropathic pain.

Monoamine Oxidase Inhibitors

If a patient has responded well to a monoamine oxidase inhibitor (MAOI) for depression before treatment for cancer, its continued use is warranted. Most psychiatrists, however, are reluctant to start depressed cancer patients on MAOIs because of the difficulty of maintaining dietary restrictions in patients who may already be confronting nutritional problems due to their illness and treatment. These drugs may also be contraindicated in patients receiving the antineoplastic procarbazine, because it has some monoamine oxidase inhibitory activity. Although MAOIs have demonstrated efficacy in the treatment of depression, the risk of hypertensive crisis and serotonin syndrome due to drug interactions (i.e., meperidine) has led to substantial concern about their safety.

Electroconvulsive Therapy

Electroconvulsive therapy is one of the most effective treatments for depression in patients who are medically ill and unable to tolerate psychotropic medications. Electroconvulsive therapy continues to be a viable option for patients who are refractory to antidepressants, for whom medications are medically contraindicated, or for those with psychotic features, dangerous suicidality, or self-injurious behavior. The most common side effects include anterograde amnesia that usually improves within days to weeks of the treatment.

CANCER-RELATED SUICIDE

Although few cancer patients commit suicide, they may be at a somewhat greater risk than the general population. Passive suicidal thoughts are relatively common; confronting mortality while battling a life-threatening illness leads many to contemplate suicide. Consideration of death and dying is complex for patients who are faced with substantial suffering and are struggling to assess quality-of-life concerns. Suicide may transiently appear to be a means of maintaining a sense of control and a reassuring theoretic alternative for patients overwhelmed by uncertainty, feelings of helplessness, and fears of suffering. The actual suicide rate in cancer patients is difficult to confirm as death certificates may reflect an underreporting of suicide in patients with advanced illness. The degree to which noncompliance or treatment refusal represents a deliberate decision to end life is unknown.

Factors associated with an increased risk of suicide in cancer patients include being male, having tumors associated with alcohol and tobacco abuse, advanced stage of disease, poor prognosis, delirium with poor impulse control, inadequately controlled pain, depression, history of psychiatric illness, current or previous alcohol or substance abuse, previous suicide attempts, physical and emotional exhaustion, and social isolation.[5,7] Suicidal depression has been associated with chemotherapy treatment.[8]

Frank discussion of suicidal ideation is important. Although such discussion is often feared by clinicians, there is no evidence that talking about suicide encourages attempts. Assessment of severity of suicide risk depends on the clinical circumstances, identification of factors that may increase impulsivity or impair judgment (e.g., active substance abuse or delirium), and review of the patient's intent and plan. Emergent psychiatric evaluation is indicated when there is a risk of injury to self or others. Identifying and treating depression among patients with cancer has been shown to decrease morbidity and mortality.[9,10]

ANXIETY

Anxiety is a normal reaction to the emotionally stressful, even traumatic, experience of cancer. Cancer may force changes in social roles, disrupt personal relationships, cause bodily dysfunction, and alter appearance, in addition to posing a threat of death or significantly shortened life.[11] Anxiety is common at crisis points, such as the time of diagnosis, before the start of any new treatment, when recurrent disease is diagnosed, and when the patient progresses to advanced and terminal illness stages. After initial shock and disbelief, patients may develop symptoms of anxiety, accompanied by irritability, loss of appetite, insomnia, intrusive thoughts about their prognosis, and decreased ability to concentrate and carry on usual activities. Anxiety that persists and causes impairment is considered pathologic. Anxiety disorders may present with a variety of symptoms, including phobias, obsessive-compulsive symptoms, panic attacks, generalized anxiety, or somatic complaints. Severe anxiety can contribute to denial and noncompliance with treatment, disabling anticipatory nausea and vomiting before chemotherapy, avoidance of tests and procedures, panic attacks, and overwhelming distress. Untreated anxiety increases the risk of alcohol and substance abuse. Multiple organic factors may give rise to anxiety disorders in cancer patients, including poorly controlled pain, altered metabolic states (e.g., hypoxia, hypotension), sepsis, neurologic disorders, endocrine disturbances (e.g., thyroid dysfunction), hormone-secreting tumors, and medications (e.g., steroids).

The management of anxiety symptoms begins with the provision of emotional support and information to the patient and family. Patient education may offer substantial relief through identification of anxiety symptoms, explanation of the interplay of psychological and somatic symptoms, and reassurance that severe distress is treatable. Often the physical symptoms, such as sweating, tremor, dyspnea, or chest tightness, cause even greater anxiety in cancer patients who may already be somatically preoccupied. There are many possible psychotherapeutic and psychopharmacologic interventions available for the treatment of anxiety symptoms.

Many patients are helped through behavioral techniques, such as relaxation, distraction, and cognitive reframing.[12] In addition to behavioral treatments, individual psychotherapy and group interventions have been demonstrated as effectively reducing anxiety in cancer patients. Studies of group interventions that included education, emotional support, and behavioral training demonstrated benefits of less tension and fewer phobias (trend) than was found in the control groups.[13] Many patients with intermittent anxiety or simple phobias find relaxation therapy and distraction techniques helpful. When the need for a diagnostic procedure or treatment is urgent, benzodiazepines should be used.

Phobias related to medical procedures are common in children with cancer and also are problematic in some adults. While careful attention to preparation of children in advance of painful procedures (e.g., role playing) may limit the incidence of anxiety, specific behavioral interventions, including relaxation training and distraction, may be indicated for some symptoms.[14] Self-hypnosis is a highly effective treatment for both generalized anxiety and specific phobias in children and adolescents.

Before being treated with an anxiolytic, all patients should be screened for depressive symptoms as well as for other symptoms in the anxiety disorder spectrum, such as posttraumatic stress disorder and obsessive-compulsive disorder. Anxiety and its associated somatic complaints often accompany depression, and effective treatment, therefore, may require use of an antidepressant in conjunction with, or instead of, a short trial of a benzodiazepine. The experience of cancer treatment may reawaken longer-standing problems in patients who have been the victims of previous trauma, increasing their risk of anxiety and depressive symptoms.

Benzodiazepines (lorazepam, alprazolam, and clonazepam) are the drugs of choice for acute anxiety states. Table 56.5-3 lists the usual initial dose of benzodiazepines, approximate dose equivalent, half-life, and presence or absence of active metabolites. The dosing schedule depends on the patient's tolerance and the anxiolytic's duration of action. The shorter-acting benzodiazepines may be given four or more times a day. Lorazepam and alprazolam are favored in the acute setting due to their rapid onset of action and thus are efficacious when prescribed on an as-needed basis. Lorazepam is available in both oral and parenteral forms and has both antiemetic and anxiolytic properties.[15] Clonazepam is substantially longer-acting, offering the benefit of ease of administration as well as avoiding the potential for recurrent anxiety between doses and rebound symptoms of worsened anxiety. It is best to increase the dose before switching to another agent in patients with persistent symptoms, as there is substantial variability in patient tolerance of the benzodiazepines and in effective dosages. The most common side effects of the benzodiazepines are dose-dependent and include drowsiness, confusion, and poor motor coordination. These occur more frequently in older patients and in those with impaired liver function. The synergistic effects of the benzodiazepines with other medications with central nervous system depressant properties, such as narcotics and some antidepressants, can contribute to excess sedation. When the dose is lowered, uncomfortable sedation often disappears, while the antianxiety effects continue. Lorazepam is renally excreted and, hence, is better tolerated by patients with impaired hepatic function and by those taking other medications with sedative effects (e.g., analgesics). There are effective alternatives to benzodiazepines, includ-

TABLE 56.5-3. Benzodiazepines Commonly Prescribed for Cancer Patients

Drug Name	*Approximate Dose Equivalent*	*Initial Dosage (mg PO)*	*Elimination Half-Life Drug Metabolites (h)*	*Active Metabolite*
Short-acting				
Alprazolam	0.5	0.25–0.5 t.i.d.	10–15	Yes
Lorazepam[a]	1.0	0.5–2.0 t.i.d.	10–20	No
Temazepam[b]	15.0	15–30 q.h.s.	10–15	No
Triazolam[b]	0.25	0.125–0.25 q.h.s.	1–5	No
Long-acting				
Clonazepam	0.5	0.25–1 b.i.d.	18–50	No
Diazepam	5.0	5–10 b.i.d.	20–100	Yes
Clorazepate	7.5	7.5–15 b.i.d.	30–200	Yes

[a]Lorazepam can also be administered parenterally.
[b]Hypnotic agent.

ing other anxiolytics, such as buspirone. In addition, antidepressants with more calming-sedating side effects, such as nefazadone, mirtazapine, and paroxetine, have also been found to be beneficial in the treatment of anxiety. Low doses of neuroleptics (i.e., olanzapine, haloperidol, or thioridazine) are effective in patients with severe anxiety that is not controlled with maximal therapeutic doses of benzodiazepines, in patients whose anxiety leads to frank agitation, and for those who cannot tolerate benzodiazepines due to respiratory problems.

DELIRIUM

Delirium is common in cancer as a result of direct central nervous system involvement by tumor, paraneoplastic syndromes, and the indirect effects of toxic-metabolic sequelae of the disease and treatment (Table 56.5-4).[16] The hallmark of delirium is impairment of consciousness, usually accompanied by global cognitive dysfunction, and abnormalities of mood, behavior, and perception. The onset is often rapid, and the course is usually fluctuating. The prevalence of delirium in cancer patients ranges from 5% to 25% in various studies and is substantially higher in terminal stages of illness.[17]

TABLE 56.5-4. Chemotherapeutic Drugs That Can Cause Delirium

Methotrexate (intrathecal)
Vincristine, vinblastine
Asparaginase
Carmustine
Bleomycin
Fluorouracil
Cisplatinum
Hydroxyurea
Procarbazine
Cytosine arabinoside
Hexylmethylamine
Ifosfamide
Prednisone
Interferon
Interleukin

Delirium is a syndrome of symptoms with multiple possible etiologies. Changes in mental status may be subtle or extreme, ranging from an appearance of mild depression or social withdrawal to severe agitation or hallucinations. Early symptoms of delirium are often unrecognized or misdiagnosed by medical or nursing staff as depression. Yet, early recognition of delirium is essential, since the underlying etiology may be a treatable complication of cancer. When faced with an abrupt behavior change in a cancer patient, the physician must investigate a number of potential causes of delirium. Particularly frequent metabolic causes include hyponatremia, hypercalcemia, malnutrition, and liver failure. Altered thyroid or adrenal status may cause delirium. Infections and brain metastases commonly cause delirium. Patients with hematologic malignancies are at especially high risk for opportunistic infection. Other cancers, such as those of the lung and the breast, frequently metastasize to the brain. Head and neck cancer patients undergoing surgery are at high risk for delirium because of their generally older age and the high prevalence of alcohol abuse and withdrawal syndromes. Many antineoplastic and immunotherapeutic agents (i.e., interleukin)[18] can cause delirium and other changes in mental status.[19] Corticosteroids can cause confusion, depression, mania, and anxiety. Antibiotics and antifungals, such as amphotericin B, can cause delirium, particularly with intrathecal administration. In seriously ill cancer patients, the etiology of delirium is often multifactorial. The delirium workup is tailored to the patient's specific cancer and medical condition at the time that the symptoms develop.

The management of delirium includes identification and correction of its underlying causes while symptomatic and supportive therapies are initiated. Symptomatic treatment measures include reassurance and support for the patient and family, manipulation of the environment to provide a reorienting safe milieu, and appropriate use of pharmacotherapy. Measures to help reduce anxiety and mild disorientation include a quiet, well-lit room with familiar objects, a visible clock or calendar, and the presence of family, as these increase structure and familiarity. Judicious use of physical restraints to prevent self-harm, along with one-to-one nursing observation, may also be necessary. Often, these supportive techniques alone are not sufficient, and symptomatic treatment with neuroleptic or sedative medications is necessary.

As with other medically ill patients, neuroleptics are the mainstay in the management of delirium in cancer patients.

Haloperidol is particularly useful because of its low incidence of cardiovascular and anticholinergic effects and its availability in parenteral and oral forms. Relatively low doses of haloperidol (1 to 3 mg/d) are usually effective in treating agitation, hallucinations, paranoia, and fear, and most cancer patients respond to less than 20 mg in divided doses over 24 hours. The more common side effects of haloperidol include akathisia and extrapyramidal side effects (cog-wheeling, masked facies, and gait disturbances). Dystonic reactions are treated with anticholinergic medications. Newer neuroleptics, such as risperidone and olanzapine, have not been studied in cancer patients; however, they appear to be well tolerated, with lower incidences of extrapyramidal side effects than haloperidol. They are not yet available in parenteral form. Methotrimeprazine (available in intravenous or subcutaneous form) and midazolam have been used to control confusion and agitation in terminal delirium.[20]

PSYCHIATRIC SYMPTOMS IN CANCER PATIENTS WITH PAIN

There is clearly an increased incidence of depression and anxiety in patients experiencing severe pain. In the Psychosocial Collaborative Oncology Group study, 39% of patients with a psychiatric diagnosis experienced significant pain. In more than 80% of these patients, a depressive syndrome was diagnosed. In contrast, only 19% of patients who did not receive a psychiatric diagnosis had significant pain.[4]

The psychiatric symptoms of patients who are in significant pain must initially be considered a consequence of their uncontrolled pain. Acute anxiety, depression with despair (especially when the patient believes the pain means disease progression), agitation, irritability, lack of cooperation, anger, and insomnia may be the emotional or behavioral concomitants of pain. These symptoms are not labeled as a psychiatric disorder unless they persist after pain is adequately controlled. Undertreatment of pain is a major problem in both adult and pediatric settings. Aggressive pain management strategies, including narcotics, are essential to the emotional care of both physically ill children and adults. Long-term psychiatric sequelae of cancer are less likely in children whose pain is well treated. There is no evidence of increased risk of subsequent drug abuse in cancer patients receiving narcotic analgesia. In fact, most patients associate the narcotic effects with the unpleasant aspects of the illness and seek to avoid narcotics during their recovery.[21] Effective pain management often requires substantial patient education and has been facilitated by recent advances, such as the growing emphasis on the use of adequate regimens of standing doses of analgesics with as-needed rescue dosing for breakthrough pain, and the advent of patient-controlled analgesia. Collaborative efforts between doctor and patient to identify problematic symptoms and negotiate treatment strategies depend on open communication about pain and its psychological sequelae. A full discussion of issues in pain management is available in Chapter 56.1.

UNCONVENTIONAL CANCER TREATMENTS

The alternative therapies ranging from herbal treatments and spiritual teachers to acupuncture, physical manipulation, and mental imaging proliferated in the 1990s, and many "traditional" Western doctors are seeking to understand these modalities. Recent surveys suggest that 30% to 40% of the U.S. public use what are described as alternative or complementary therapies.[22] The field is broad and encompasses many modalities and ideas. However, due to the lack of clinical trials of many of these therapies, conventional practitioners and alternative healers exist on opposite ends of the spectrum, often leaving patients confused about how to integrate these differing perspectives. Despite this, the demand for these therapies has led insurers to offer some expanded benefits for alternative medicine.

The overlap of traditional and alternative therapies is particularly complex in the provision of psychosocial and behavioral treatments to cancer patients. Some of the psychological and behavioral methods that are used in medicine (i.e., psychological support, visual imagery, hypnosis, and relaxation exercises) for enhancing quality of life and symptom control are also included in unconventional therapies that promise cancer cure or extended survival. A recent study of 480 women with newly diagnosed early-stage breast cancer found 28% used alternative medicine as a complimentary therapy.[23] Interestingly, the use of alternative medicine was independently associated with depression, fear of recurrence of cancer, lower scores for mental health and sexual satisfaction, and more physical symptoms as well as symptoms of greater intensity. The study suggests that patients seeking alternative medicine therapies may be experiencing anxiety, depression, or physical symptoms that should be addressed by the "traditional" medical system. Further, the study demonstrated that the use of these therapies does not always provide the sought-after panacea.

The urgency with which many cancer patients and families feel the need to seek any potentially beneficial or hopeful treatment option leads many to try any promising therapy that is offered. In the setting of tremendous fear and uncertainty, it is difficult for patients even to choose between conflicting traditional biomedical opinions, much less to navigate the uncharted waters of alternative treatments. Many patients elect untried or unproven therapies in their desperate search for a cure or for a more acceptable quality of life, attempting any therapy "as long as it doesn't hurt."

There are real challenges for the clinician attempting to advise patients about the use of unconventional therapies. Many conflicts are born of the desire not to take away hope but also not to condone unproven treatments. There has been concern that some therapies that suggest that personality and behavior are the vehicle for recovery or tumor progression place undue burden on patients who may hold themselves responsible for a negative outcome. Some patients feel empowered in the hopeful "heroic warrior" stance described by Gray and Doan[24] and should be encouraged to maintain it. These patients benefit from the oncologist's admission that there are still many unknowns and encouragement of their use of self-help books, visualization, efforts to improve mental attitude, and diet regimens, insofar as they find them to be helpful. However, there are other patients for whom the warrior myth is a distressing burden, leading to self-criticism and a sense of guilt because they cannot fight hard enough and will be responsible for their own death. Families may contribute to the patient's guilt about illness, offering unrealistic advice and remedies in an effort to overcome their own feelings of helplessness and expressing frustration and anger with the patient's failure to live up to their expectations and to fight hard enough. Further study of alternatives is important, as current research does not support the assertion that unconventional therapies prolong survival.[25,26] However, there is no question that alternative therapies may play a substantial role in the patient's experience of illness and quality of life.

PSYCHOTHERAPEUTIC INTERVENTIONS WITH CANCER PATIENTS

INDIVIDUAL PSYCHOTHERAPY

Although psychological interventions for patients with cancer were slow to develop, since the 1950s efforts to implement interventions have grown steadily because of a greater emphasis on quality-of-life concerns. The types of interventions most commonly used by health professionals working with cancer patients are education, behavioral training, groups, and individual psychotherapy. Fawzy et al.[27] have provided a critical review of psychosocial interventions in cancer care that should be read by all individuals who are preparing to establish psychosocial support services for cancer patients.

Although some enthusiasts have advocated offering counseling to all patients on the assumption that they can benefit from help and will take advantage of it, many patients reject the offer of psychological help. In one study, only two-thirds of the patients identified as high-risk accepted counseling.[28] Those who refused had a positive outlook, minimized the implications of their diagnosis, and viewed the offer of therapy as a threat to their emotional equilibrium. Patients who accepted counseling were less able to deny the diagnosis and its implications; they were less hopeful and were more apt to experience their situation in religious or existential terms. Stam et al.[29] found that 20% of 449 ambulatory cancer patients seen in a single cancer center in Canada were referred and seen for psychological counseling over a 1-year period. Family and personal problems were the most common reasons for seeking help. Interventions most commonly applied are either educational or psychotherapeutic, including supportive, insight-oriented, interpersonal, and cognitive behavioral therapies.[30–32]

Sourkes et al.[33] have described the focus of psychotherapy with the cancer patient as the emotional stress engendered by the illness, rather than the more general intrapsychic and interpersonal concerns of the physically healthy person.[33] The therapist who is outside of the friend and kinship circle plays a useful role by encouraging exploring emotions, which are otherwise unexpressed. Because of the strong bond felt by families for the therapist who took care of their relative over the course of a long illness, families often enter into a one- to ten-session bereavement counseling with the patient's therapist after the patient's death to provide a healing conclusion to a long illness.

GROUP PSYCHOTHERAPY

Group therapy may be advantageous for cancer patients, allowing them to receive support from others who have experienced and conquered similar problems of medical illness.[34,35] The cancer patient, in a group setting, learns that there is a range of normal reactions to illness and a range of healthy adaptive coping styles and strategies that others have used to make adjustment to illness easier. Group participation helps decrease the sense of isolation and alienation because the patient and the family can see that they are not alone in adjusting to illness. Groups for cancer patients or families (or both) are often disease-specific or targeted for patients at the same stage of different diseases. In the past, doctors had some concern about having the dying patient in a group with patients who recently were given diagnoses or whose prognosis was good, but when directed by skilled leaders, these groups can be highly rewarding.[13] The Spiegel et al.[36] report of greater longevity in a small number of women with advanced breast cancer undergoing group psychotherapy remains controversial, and replication with larger samples is needed.[37,38]

SELF-HELP AND MUTUAL SUPPORT PROGRAMS

Self-help and mutual support programs are additional potential supports for patients and families. Life crises, such as life-threatening illness and bereavement, often are the impetus for individuals to seek emotional support from others experiencing the same trauma. Uniquely American in their inception, most self-help support networks work closely with professional medical services, thereby offering social support as an adjunct to medical care. Self-help groups or visitation programs help decrease the sense of alienation and isolation of patients because of the unique knowledge and sensitivity that volunteers bring from personal experience. Veteran patients facilitate coping by being a source of credible information about the needs of cancer patients, demonstrating constructive ways of managing and living despite illness, providing the motivation for rehabilitation and enhancement of self-worth, and encouraging patients to participate in their own treatment.[39]

SURVIVOR ISSUES

Advances in the treatment of cancer in the last 30 years have led to improvement in both prognosis and quality of life, resulting in a rapidly growing population of more than 5 million long-term survivors, many of them children and young adults. Psychiatric sequelae of cancer include those related to the direct effects of the disease as well as those that are consequences of the treatments, of family factors, and of the individual psychology of the person. The long-term adjustment of survivors of childhood cancer appears to be largely unimpaired. Cured cancer patients have special medical and psychiatric concerns, including fears of termination of treatment, preoccupation with disease recurrence, and minor physical problems; a sense of greater vulnerability to illness (the Damocles syndrome); pervasive awareness of mortality and difficulty with reentry into normal life (the Lazarus syndrome); persistent guilt (the survivor syndrome); difficult adjustment to physical losses and handicaps; a sense of physical inferiority; diminished self-esteem or confidence; perceived loss of job mobility, and fear of insurance discrimination. A recent book by Landay[40] teaches patients how to handle many "nuts and bolts" issues of coping, such as insurance, career issues, estate planning, advanced directives, and home and hospice care. Concerns about infertility, often understandably submerged at the time of diagnosis and treatment, reappear when rigorous treatment concludes. The survivor's intellectual functioning is also a major concern. Children and adults with brain tumors or central nervous system involvement and those undergoing bone marrow transplant are at risk from both their disease and their treatment. Most have residual deficits with neuropsychological impairment, including compromised motor and cognitive test performance.[41]

In coping with a variety of physical, social, sexual, employment, and insurance problems, survivors often report psychological distress at subsyndromal levels. The severity of these symptoms may vary by premorbid adjustment personality traits and site of cancer and treatment (i.e., bone marrow transplantation), but they usually do not interfere with reentry to family, social, or employment networks.[41] Survival may be associated with an increased risk for delayed medical complications, including organ failure, central nervous system dysfunction, sterility, secondary malignancies, and decreased physical stamina.[42,43] Sociodemographic, disease-treatment, and psychological distress variables only partially explain the wide variability in survivors' psychosocial dysfunction.[44]

Special attention to identifying adolescent and young adult survivors most at risk for psychosocial dysfunction is needed. Adolescents who have been treated for cancer not only have the substantial physical, cognitive, emotional, and interpersonal tasks faced by all adolescents but have the added burden of integrating a life-threatening disease into their experiences. Persistent body image concerns, somatic preoccupation, disruptions in sexual relationships, and deficits in social competence are not uncommon.[45] Fritz and Williams[46] assessed 52 survivors of childhood cancer and their families who were more than 2 years past treatment. Two-thirds of the patients studied had excellent psychosocial functioning without serious social issues. Many expressed a positive effect of their illness and reported little depression. Illness variables were not predictive of psychosocial outcome, unlike some psychosocial variables, such as communication patterns and peer support. The National Coalition of Cancer Survivorship is an outgrowth of survivors' need for support. The political issues surrounding health and life insurance are a prime example of an area where research is needed to delineate problems, and advocacy is needed to encourage societal solutions.

Acknowledgment

The authors thank Robert F. Quigley and Theresa A. Carpenter for their assistance in the preparation of this manuscript.

REFERENCES

1. Roth AJ, Kornblith AB, Barel-Copel L, et al. Rapid screening for psychological distress in men with prostate carcinoma: a pilot study. *Cancer* 1998;82:1904.
2. Payne DK, Hoffman RG, Theodoulou M, Dosik M, Massie MJ. Screening for anxiety and depression in women with breast cancer. *Psychosomatics* 1999;40:64.
3. Roth AJ, McClear KZ, Massie MJ. Oncology. In: Stoudemire A, Fogel BS, Greenberg D, eds. *Psychiatric care of the medical patient.* New York: Oxford University Press, 2000:733.
4. Derogatis LR, Morrow GR, Fetting JH, et al. The prevalence of psychiatric disorders among cancer patients. *JAMA* 1983;249:751.
5. Massie MJ, Popkin M. Depressive disorders. In: Holland JC, ed. *Psycho-oncology.* New York: Oxford University Press, 1998;518.
6. Watson M, Haviland JS, Greer S, Davidson J, Bliss JM. Influence of psychological response on survival in breast cancer: a population-based cohort study. *Lancet* 1999;40:64.
7. Henderson JM, Ord RA. Suicide in head and neck cancer patients. *J Oral Maxillofac Surg* 1997;55:1217.
8. Cousins JP, Harper G. Neurobiochemical changes from Taxol/Neupogen chemotherapy for metastatic breast carcinoma corresponds with suicidal depression. *Cancer Lett* 1996;110:163.
9. Chochinov HM, Wilson KG, Enns M, et al. Desire for death in the terminally ill. *Am J Psychiatry* 1995;152:1185.
10. Valente SM, Saunders JM. Diagnosis and treatment of major depression among people with cancer. *Cancer Nurs* 1997;20:168.
11. Noyes R, Holt CS, Massie MJ. Anxiety disorders. In: Holland JC, ed. *Psycho-oncology.* New York: Oxford University Press, 1998;548.
12. Payne DK, Massie MJ. Anxiety and depression. In: Berger A, Levy MH, Portenoy RK, Weissman DE, eds. *Principles and practice of supportive oncology.* Philadelphia: JB Lippincott Co, 1997:497.
13. Spiegel D, Bloom J, Yalom I. Group support for patients with metastatic cancer. *Arch Gen Psychiatry* 1981;455:333.
14. Redd WH, Adresen GV, Minagawa Y. Hypnotic control of anticipatory emesis in patients receiving cancer chemotherapy. *J Consult Clin Psycho* 1989;50:14.
15. Greenberg DB. Strategic use of benzodiazepines in cancer patients. *Oncology* 1991;5:83.
16. Patchel RA, Posner JB. Cancer and the nervous system. In: Holland JC, Rowland J, eds. *Handbook of psycho-oncology.* New York: Oxford University Press, 1989:314.
17. Fleishman S, Lesko L, Breitbart WS. Treatment of organic mental disorders in cancer patients. In: Breitbart WS, Holland JC, eds. *Psychiatric aspects of symptom management in cancer patients.* Washington, DC: American Psychiatric Press, 1993:23.
18. Smith MJ, Mougwad R, Vuillemin E, et al. Psychological side effects induced by interleukin-2/alpha interferon treatment. *Psychooncology* 1994;3:289.
19. Brown TM, Stoudemire A. Antineoplastic agents. In: Brown TM, Stoudemire A, eds. *Psychiatric side effects of prescription and over-the-counter medications.* Washington, DC: American Psychiatric Press, 1998:239.
20. Ramani S, Karnard AB. Long term subcutaneous infusion of midazolam for refractory delirium in terminal breast cancer. *South Med J* 1996;89:1101.
21. Caraceni A, Cheville A, Portenoy RK. Pain management: pharmacological and nonpharmacological treatments. In: Massie MJ, ed. Pain: what psychiatrists need to know (Review of Psychiatry Series, Vol. 19, No. 2; Oldham JO, Riba MB, series eds.) Washington, DC, American Psychiatric Press, 2000.
22. Eisenberg DM. Advising patients who seek alternative medical therapies. *Ann Intern Med* 1997;127:61.
23. Burnstein HJ, Gelber S, Guadagnoli E, Weeks JC. Use of alternative medicine by women with early stage breast cancer. *N Engl J Med* 1999;340:1733.
24. Gray RE, Doan BD. Heroic self-healing and cancer: clinical issues for the health professions. *J Palliat Care* 1990;6:32.
25. Bagenal FS, Easton DF, Harris E, Chilvers CE, McElwain TJ. Survival of patients with breast cancer attending Bristol Cancer Help Centre. *Lancet* 1990;336:606.
26. Morgenstern H, Gellert GA, Walter SD, Ostfeld AM, Siegel BS. The impact of a psychosocial support program on survival with breast cancer: the importance of selection bias in program evaluation. *J Chronic Dis* 1984;37:273.
27. Fawzy FI, Fawzy NW, Arndt LA, Pasnau RO. Critical review of psycho-social interventions in cancer care. *Arch Gen Psychiatry* 1995;52:100.
28. Worden JW, Weisman AD. Preventive psychosocial intervention with newly diagnosed cancer patients. *Gen Hosp Psychiatry* 1984;6:243.
29. Stam HJ, Bultz BP, Pittman CA. Psychosocial problems and interventions in a referred sample of cancer patients. *Psychosom Med* 1986;48:563.
30. Moynihan C, Bliss JM, Davidson J, Burchell L, Horwich A. Evaluation of adjuvant psychological therapy in patients with testicular cancer: randomized controlled trial. *Br Med J* 1998;316:429.
31. Lovejoy NC, Matteis M. Cognitive-behavioral interventions to manage depression in patients with cancer: research and theoretical initiatives. *Cancer Nurs* 1997;20:155.
32. Kissane DW, Bloch S, Miach P, et al. Cognitive-existential group therapy for patients with primary breast cancer-techniques and themes. *Psychooncology* 1997;6:25.
33. Sourkes B, Massie MJ, Holland JC. Psycho-therapeutic issues. In: Holland JC, ed. *Psycho-oncology.* New York: Oxford University Press, 1998:694.
34. Bottomley A. Where are we not? Evaluating two decades of group interventions with adult cancer patients. *J Psychiatr Ment Health Nurs* 1997;4:251.
35. Cunningham AJ. Group psychological therapy for cancer patients. A brief discussion of indications for its use, and the range of interventions available. *Support Care Cancer* 1995;3:244.
36. Speigel D, Bloom JR, Kraemer HJC, Gottheil E. Effect of psychosocial treatment on survival of patients with metastatic breast cancer. *Lancet* 1989;14:888.
37. Fox BH. A hypothesis about Spiegel et al.'s 1989 paper on psychological intervention and breast cancer survival. *Psychooncology* 1998;7:361.
38. Cunningham AJ, Edmonds CV, Jenkens GP, et al. A randomized controlled trial of the effects of group psychological therapy on survival in women with metastatic breast cancer. *Psychooncology* 1998;7:508.
39. Mastrovito R, Moynahan R. Self-help and mutual support programs in cancer. In: Holland JC, Rowland JH, eds. *Handbook of psycho-oncology.* New York: Oxford University Press 1989:502.
40. Landay DS. *Be prepared.* New York: St. Martin Press, 1998.
41. Kornblith AB. Psychological adaptation to cancer: cancer survivor's adaptation. In: Holland JC, ed. *Psycho-oncology.* New York: Oxford University Press, 1998:223.
42. Meadows A, Silber J. Delayed consequences of therapy for childhood cancer. *Cancer* 1985;58:524.
43. Meadows A, Hobbie N. The medical consequences of cure. *Cancer* 1986;58:524.
44. Lesko LM, Ostroff JS, Mumma GH, Mashberg DE, Holland JC. Long-term psychological adjustment of acute leukemia survivors: impact of bone marrow transplantation vs. chemotherapy. *Psychosom Med* 1992;54:30.
45. Mulhern R, Wasserman A, Friedman A, Fairclough D. Social competence and behavioral adjustment of children who are long-term survivors of cancer. *Pediatrics* 1989;83:18.
46. Fritz B, Williams J. Issues of adolescent development for survivors of childhood cancer. *J Am Acad Child Adolesc Psychiatry* 1988;27:712.

SECTION **6**

BONNIE A. INDECK
PHYLLIS M. SMITH

Community Resources

The impact of changes in the health care system has caused greater numbers of patients to be treated in an ambulatory setting. Services in this setting range from maintenance of central lines to chemotherapy, nutritional support, pain control, intravenous antibiotics, and blood support. Patients are not usually admitted to the hospital unless their condition is so serious that it meets an acute level of care. Ever-changing reimbursement issues along with an ever-increasing number of cancer survivors[1] have placed yet a greater burden on the community to provide services for this often chronically ill population.[2]

Resource directories are regularly updated to include the latest evolving information. The American Cancer Society (ACS) and Cancer Care are just two sources that publish a comprehensive listing of services.[3,4] These guides may be cross-referenced from the general to specific site of cancer and often provide information on a variety of services, including emotional support, financial assistance, and transportation resources. Additionally, increasing access to personal computers and the World Wide Web have allowed individuals to gather information in an unprecedented manner. Rimer points out that "communication is central to effective cancer control, from primary prevention to survivorship."[5] Although this information, along with the increasing fingertip access to the most current information, should theoretically allow patients to gather the assistance they require to live with their illness, a gap still remains between availability of these resources and specific individual needs. These gaps in provision of service occur across many communities and insurance carriers.

The individual diagnosed with cancer undergoes an experience that is intensely personal, that calls into question basic assumptions and expectations about life, and that somehow must be integrated into a sense of self, and thus involves the complexities of individual personalities. To deliver effective service, those who are working with this population must understand the adaptation that occurs. This adaptation involves incorporating a new sense of self after living through the crisis of diagnosis, initial treatment, potential side effects, and emotional impact on one's self and one's family. In addition to discussing individual adjustment, this chapter discusses different types of support and resources that may be beneficial to the patient and family, computer trends, the impact of an evolving health care delivery and reimbursement system, and survivorship issues, and concludes with a list of available resources.

INITIAL DIAGNOSIS OF CANCER

Cancer is the third major cause of mortality.[6] More than 1 million people are estimated to have been diagnosed with cancer in 1999, and 564,000 people will survive their disease.[1] Although these statistics present an increase in survivorship, the reality of living with cancer represents something quite different. Concerns must be broadened to view cancer as a chronic or curable illness.[7] The majority of those 1 million people diagnosed with cancer must face their own mortality, but they then move from focusing on their mortality to dealing with their illness. It is incumbent on medical providers to help the patient participate in a plan to develop adequate internal and external resources for living with cancer.

The spectrum of reactions includes fear, shock, despair, anger, anxiety and, sometimes, total insensibility.[8] In the 1970s, Weisman and Worden identified the immediate coping response of denial as appropriate, albeit temporarily.[9] This is still valid today, but given the changing nature of today's medical delivery system, we may need to help patients progress from denial to mastery in a more expeditious fashion. Although today's cancer patients experience distress that is often not considered or reflected in the economics of treatment, they still desire and need psychosocial intervention to cope with their cancer. The medical system has resources that can address these emotions and enable a person to function more effectively. The physician may call on members of the team, such as the oncology social worker or oncology nurse, to assist in presenting the diagnosis. These team members can facilitate the understanding of the diagnosis in many distinct ways. The professional oncology team helps the patient move toward a sense of mastery over the situation. Assistance is provided so that a patient moves along a continuum through which control is gained and progress is made from a passive to an active state. This movement promotes an active course of treatment.

SOCIAL SUPPORT NETWORK

During the 1980s, the literature identified and recognized the importance of a social support network. Research has consistently found that people coping with cancer have difficulty with interpersonal relationships and that one's social support system can alleviate these stressors.[7] Although this network may not prolong the life of a cancer patient, it has been shown to enhance the quality of life one experiences. The providers in a social support network may be professionals from the community, family, friends, significant others, organizations, and agencies. These providers enable the cancer patient to enhance their coping skills so that they may function in an effective, competent, and proficient manner. The literature continues to report that this social support network impacts positively on the psychological well-being of the cancer patient.[10,11] The constructs of the social support system identified as emotional, informational, or instrumental as defined by Wortman[12] is the structure in which we define support and resources for the cancer patient.

EMOTIONAL SUPPORT

Psychosocial interventions have consistently contributed to a positive outcome on the emotional adjustment of a person coping with cancer,[13] and emotional support is frequently considered to be one of the most essential interventions. Family, friends, and those closest to the patient frequently provide emotional support. Dunkel-Schetter[14] surveyed 79 cancer patients and found that 81% defined emotional support as most helpful, followed by informational support (41%) and instrumental aid (6%).

ASSESSMENT AND EVALUATION OF COPING SKILLS

Individuals deal with problems in diverse ways. It is important that the medical team identify an individual's ability to cope with stress so that they have some indication of how the patient will deal with their cancer. An assessment of other crises endured and how those were handled is particularly helpful in an assessment and evaluation. Studies have led to development of a profile of predictors of poor coping.[15] Some indicators of the inability to cope with crises are character traits such as rigidity of behavior or morose, gloomy outlook on life. This type of patient may not be amenable to the support received or may need more intense intervention. Substance abuse, recent losses, social isolation, unemployment, or other debilitating illnesses may be warning signs that an individual may be more emotionally overwhelmed. Cancer causes much emotional distress in a person's life, and disruptions in routine functioning are normal. Some of these disruptions may have lingering effects and cause enduring problems.[16] Traditional emotional support may not be enough for such individuals. Specialized or very individualized emotional support may be necessary for these patients to cope with cancer.

FAMILY AS EMOTIONAL SUPPORT

As the person diagnosed with cancer enters the health care system it is important for the professionals to recognize that this person rarely functions alone. The person who receives a diagnosis of cancer usually summons his or her closest family to become the immediate support system. As healthcare professionals, we must recognize the significance of including the family at times of diagnosis, recurrence, change in treatment plans, and terminal illness.[17] The family system changes when the diagnosis is made. All members who interact with the patient should be aware of the potential changes and the subsequent impact on the family.

The family value and belief system must be identified so that help can be provided within the context of the sociocultural system. Fears are minimized and coping skills enhanced if understanding is provided within a familiar context. It must be recognized that cancer is not openly discussed in all cultural groups. Certain cultural groups may need special assistance to contend with a health care system in which the patient is expected to be an active participant. Roles within the family frequently change when a diagnosis of cancer is made. Family members may need help in evaluating whether these role changes are comfortable for them. In addition, a family member who is also a health care professional, and particularly an oncology health care professional, may need help in maintaining the role of a family member rather than becoming the resource person. The alacrity to help is frequently seen during the initial crisis of diagnosis. This is the time a family pulls itself together and offers whatever resources they can provide for the newly diagnosed patient. As the illness extends over time and sometimes becomes chronic, family support may wane and become difficult to sustain. It is at this time that patients and families may need to find resources outside the immediate family system.

EMOTIONAL SUPPORT OUTSIDE THE FAMILY SYSTEM

The social support network, as identified earlier, includes friends, neighbors, both self-help and professionally facilitated support groups, religious groups, community agencies, and health care professionals.[15] A review of the literature has indicated that making use of emotional support, whether informal or formal, can relieve distress.[13] It is important that there be some commonality perceived in the support system. People undergoing similar experiences may find it easier to relate to each other because the cancer is accepted more easily. If the perception is that a situation is understood, empathy can be accepted and emotional support to the patient becomes positive. The validity of the cancer patient's experiences must be recognized by the support system for support to be effective. A member of a support system who truly does not understand the trauma cannot minimize the anxieties and fears of the cancer patient. Support is not effective in a situation in which real feelings are not recognized.

VISITATION GROUPS

The changing scene of health care delivery has affected visits by volunteers. The ACS has many groups maintained by volunteers who have had cancer experiences. Reach to Recovery, Cansurmount, and the ostomy programs all have volunteers who have undergone some type of cancer experience. In the past, these volunteers were able to visit with newly diagnosed patients in the hospital. In today's health care system, patients are admitted and discharged quickly, and frequently their procedures are performed in 1-day surgery centers, so there may not be time for these volunteers to visit. Health care professionals must take special care in providing patients with information about these groups, and patients must be encouraged to become proactive and make the first contact themselves. The health care professional that one meets in the hospital or surgical center is an invaluable source of information. Cancer Information Service, reachable at 1-800-4-CANCER, can also help patients with local resources.

SELF-HELP GROUPS

An extensive network of self-help groups exists for the cancer patient. Self-help groups are frequently formed by people with similar interests or concerns, and many of these groups are disease specific. They may meet weekly, biweekly, or monthly. These groups are not professionally led; rather, they are a gathering led by the peer participants, although medical professionals may be invited to present their particular expertise. Information about self-help groups can be accessed through the National Self-Help Network. This organization is listed individually in each state.

SUPPORT GROUPS

Support groups are available in most communities and are facilitated by health care professionals. The professional has the responsibility of establishing a group that is cohesive and has the goals of providing educational and emotional support. Groups may be established for patients, for family members and significant others, or for patients and family together. Although no positive correlation has been made that support groups have cured disease, improved survival of patients in support groups has been found.[18]

Although emotional support and social support are separated for descriptive purposes here, they are frequently intertwined and inseparable. The family member who transports a cancer patient for daily radiation treatments is both part of the social support system and is also providing the necessary emotional support.

ROLE OF THE MEDICAL TEAM IN EMOTIONAL SUPPORT

The medical team is comprised of a number of people who can assist the cancer patient. Social workers, clinical nurse specialists, psychologists, psychiatrists, and nutritionists are often available to provide services. Although these professionals may not be immediately available in every setting, referrals can be made for consultation. Ancillary personnel have become more important in today's system of health care delivery. Many concerns cannot be addressed in the leisurely manner of years ago. Specialized health care professionals can also help a patient navigate the health care system with greater ease and less stress.

INFORMATIONAL SUPPORT

It is axiomatic that knowledge is power and that cancer patients and families who know more about the illness and are actively involved in treatment decisions cope better than do those who are more passive. It is this demand for knowledge and information that helps such individuals feel less powerless and helpless and more in control of the situation. The need for information depends not only on individual preference for control, but on a person's educational, cultural, and financial background.[19] In the past, initial cancer information was obtained in the physician's office or hospital. Today, 22 million adults use the Internet to find health information, and 70% search for information before even meeting with a physician.[20] Dr. Gaisser, of the Cancer Information Service in Heidelberg, Germany, analyzed when inquiries were made to the service. Forty-three percent of the requests in 1996 occurred before the patient's second treatment, illustrating the patient's need for earlier information.[21]

According to Fernsler and Cannon[22] "patients with cancer benefit from education in terms of their ability to care for themselves, enhanced self-image and self-esteem, improved symptom management, reduced anxiety and reduced disruption in daily life." Other benefits of education include increased participation in treatment decisions and improved understanding of the disease process and treatment options. There may be some inherent differences for some individuals in obtaining information because of personality style. Too much information can increase anxiety for some people and cause greater difficulty in coping. It is therefore important to first assess a person's readiness to receive information by reviewing their cultural and socioeconomic background, literacy, educational level, psychological adjustment, and personal preferences for control.

Because culture influences the very meaning of the disease to the individual, it is imperative to understand that person's background, values, and beliefs. Communities also vary by culture, implying that culturally sensitive material must be developed. Providers must explore the patient's educational level and determine how to maximize both comprehension and retention of material while encouraging greater patient participation in decision making and encouraging greater dialogue with the health care team. Harris[19] talks about individuals with poor reading skills having greater difficulty understanding instructions and integrating them into their activities of daily living. As already mentioned, a diagnosis of cancer is a psychologically traumatic event. One's disposition affects how well the information is integrated and remembered. It has been suggested that individuals who try to maintain self-control are more likely to be compliant with health care regimens. They also tend to seek more detailed information and are therefore more involved in treatment decisions. Those individuals who give more control to the team are more of a challenge to educate and are not as receptive to the information. Lastly, a patient's financial situation directly impacts his or her ability to obtain information.

In summary, the best education occurs when there is open communication, awareness of the patient's needs, minimization of the patient's stress level, and a caring attitude on the part of the professionals. Patients are sensitive to the health professional's voice, body language, eye contact and proximity. It is crucial to meet and talk at an appropriate time and place while being supportive, encouraging, and personal in style. Print materials are often helpful, particularly those endorsed by the physician; however, screening for low-literacy populations is mandatory. Social workers can often remove barriers that may hinder education by facilitating communication or by connecting to community resources whose main goal it is to educate the public.

INTERNET

The Internet can increase knowledge and hasten the pace of obtaining this knowledge via the following online services[23]:

E-mail: Messages are posted electronically, facilitating instant communication. By 1998, 1,300,000 pieces of e-mail per week were being processed by the cancer-related listservs hosted by the Association of Cancer Online Resources. That same year, 22.3 million Americans performed online searches for medical and health information.[5]

Mailing lists and listservs: Through e-mail, one can subscribe to specific mailing lists, through which information is shared regarding similar interests.

World Wide Web: The Web allows easy access to an unlimited amount of information. One can research particular interests via search engines such as Yahoo, Excite, AltaVista, or a host of others.

Bulletin boards: Electronic message boards allow one to post a message concerning a specific topic while not needing to be on the computer simultaneously with others.

Chat rooms: In these forums, one can participate in "live" conversation, usually in regard to specific topics. These gatherings may be formalized with a facilitator or be used for informal discussion purposes.

Professionals, patients, and caregivers are using these Internet resources regularly. In the past, information was unidirectional, from health professionals to patients; now many patients are seeking out this information for themselves. Although access to this information is valuable, it is not without issue. People on the Internet are not always as they present themselves, and information obtained may be inaccurate or misleading. Because material can be posted on the Internet without proper oversight or professional review and because people have a tendency to believe what they read, reliance on the Internet for information can cause potential harm. Web sites should be evaluated by the same five criteria generally used for printed material, including evaluation of the authority, accuracy, objectivity, currency and coverage, and intended audience of the information.[20] Is an author listed? What are the author's qualifications? How reliable is the information? Has the material been reviewed by editors? Is the information provided without bias? Is the content up-to-date with date listed (of both creation and revision)? To what depth are the topics explored? It is extremely important for health care professionals to encourage access to this new technology but also give caution about the potential pitfalls. In general, it is advisable to encourage patients and family members to start their searches with reputable sites. C. Everett Koop, former Surgeon General, has a Web site (World Wide Web URL: http://www.drkoop.com) that rates approximately 10% of the 15,000 health-related sites on the Internet for credibility, content, and opportunity for feedback. A list of cancer-related Web sites appears in the appendix at the end of this chapter.

COMPUTER GROUPS

Groups have been long cited in the literature as an effective means of treating individuals with cancer.[24,25] These groups often provide information, education, and support that illustrates positive survival outcomes,[26] but today the strain of diagnosis and the rigors of treatment combined with concerns about confidentiality often discourage patients from attending these groups. In the past, people had to physically leave their homes and go to hospitals, physicians' offices, religious houses of worship, or community centers to attend a support group. With the advent of personal computers, Internet support groups have become popular.[27,28] In 1998, more than 40% of households owned a computer. The ability to use computer technology has assisted individuals in overcoming barriers to group participation, such as groups that meet at an inconvenient time, transportation difficulties, physical ill health, inclement weather, or the stigma that may be associated with attending the group. Computer networks have been described as a "support group without walls."[30] Advantages to computer group membership include increased patient control of both time of participation and of information disclosed or obtained, safety to discuss difficult issues, availability of information, and subsequent support. The system also has been described as empowering.[31] These groups also benefit individuals with hearing or speech disabilities.[32] Logistical obstacles, such as time spent in the assembly of the group or in travel, cost of transportation, facility costs, and scheduling problems, are overcome. An additional important benefit is anonymity. Anonymity may lead to greater self-disclosure, honesty, and intimacy while allowing specific issues to be more quickly discussed as well as discussion of taboo topics that might otherwise not arise. One of the major disadvantages is decreased interpersonal relationships. Although anonymity may be an advantage, the inability to see individuals, hear their voices, or read their body language may encourage isolation or interfere with empathy. Technological problems have been noted, including computer malfunction, cost of telephone lines and computers, access to such equipment, illiteracy, and patient discomfort with technology. Another challenge has been to facilitate group process. Individuals who are less verbal may not be encouraged to participate as much as in a face-to-face group. Trust may take longer to develop, and bonding may be more gradual. Because one must wait for feedback (and some individuals do not have good typing skills), response rate may be altered. The group leader may have more difficulty interpreting, limit setting, and tracking patterns. More recent technological advances now allow individuals to actually "speak" to each other online. The Internet site Yahoo! (http://www.yahoo.com) allows individuals with the use of a microphone to download their software for free, thus enabling them to talk and hear others. A "conference" across the Internet can occur, which may counteract decreased proficiency with typing and other discomforts that the patient may have.

Fernsler and Manchester[28] evaluated the use of a computer network (CompuServe Information Service's Cancer Forum) both by individuals and those supporting them. They found that respondents began using the network within 4 months of diagnosis and continued through all stages of the diagnosis. They concluded that "information seeking is a common coping strategy, both initially and throughout the cancer experience." Both patients and caregivers were positive about the information and support received via the computer, and this may be a "convenient alternative to traditional information and support services."[28]

INSTRUMENTAL SUPPORT

As health care delivery evolved during the 1990s, emphasis shifted to ambulatory care. Most medical care is now provided on an outpatient basis, which can create additional stressors for the patient and support system. In a study done by Emanuel et al.,[33] more than 86% of the population surveyed indicated a need for assistance. Sixty-two percent indicated a need for transportation assistance, and 55% indicated a need for homemaking assistance.

Transportation can sometimes emerge as a barrier to quality treatment. Medications that were previously administered in the hospital are now given on an outpatient basis and may not be covered by insurance. Home care and medical equipment needs may be intensified as hospital stays have become abbreviated.

FINANCES

The cost of the illness and the financial impact on the patient and family has been well documented. The direct cost of the illness as well as incidental expenses such as transportation, parking, and child care can be overwhelming to patients. Mor and associates[34] interviewed 217 people with cancer and found that 87% had experienced a significant increase in monthly expenses directly related to the disease. Wang et al.[35] indicated that minorities had more concerns about finances than whites. For the elderly and others on fixed incomes, the uninsured, and the unemployed, these expenses become significant barriers to continuing treatment.

Patients are often reluctant to discuss their finances with physicians and may feel more comfortable with another member of the medical team. A social worker can do an in-depth financial assessment, including a full discussion of insurance coverage and subsequent referral to available resources. Constant reevaluation of insurance coverage is necessary as insurance changes with employment changes, managed care providers differ in services offered, and family income changes. Patients may feel pressure, either self-imposed or by hospital and physicians' offices, for prepayment or payment of outstanding bills,[36] all adding to the stress of contending with cancer.

Coverage for medical care costs in the United States comes from four main sources: the federal government, employers and private health insurance, state and local government, and private households.[37] Exploration of privately funded sources should be made with the assistance of the social worker. Cancer Care is an agency that frequently assists with finances. Hospital and communities may have funds established from donations that help with finances for the cancer patient.

The federal government funds the Medicare program and the Social Security Disability program. Eligibility is governed by age or permanent disability for Medicare application and by work history for Social Security Disability. Eligibility for Medicaid and local welfare programs always involves a means test, although this test differs regionally. Application for Medicaid programs is made through the state department of social services. Local aid is available through individual towns to those who have state applications pending or do not meet a particular state's eligibility requirements. A newly diagnosed, unemployed, uninsured person might be eligible for these entitlements.

TRANSPORTATION

Patients often live at great distances from treatment centers or are too debilitated to drive themselves. Transportation becomes a major issue in accessing proper care. Family members, although well meaning and caring, may not be able to devote as much time as they wish to provide transportation. Transportation to doctor appointments or home from the hospital is infrequently covered by insurance. In a study of the terminally ill,[33] it was found that 62% of patients indicated a need for help with transportation. Transportation needs for economically disadvantaged patients were particularly troublesome.[38]

The ACS, the American Red Cross, and the Leukemia Society are agencies that exist nationwide and assist in transporting patients to medical care. In many areas, local towns or regional districts provide transportation to medical appointments. Resources change frequently, and it is necessary to investigate local services to assess availability.

HOME HEALTH CARE

Home health care provides for those patients who do not require hospitalization, and it is the most rapidly expanding segment of the health care industry today. Agencies, visits, and services have multiplied exponentially due to two major influences—demographic changes and managed care. Each year, almost 500,000 new senior citizens are added to the census,[39] and there is steadily increasing pressure from insurance companies and managed care programs to search for the least expensive treatment method and to emphasize the lowest appropriate level of care, low-cost alternatives, and early discharge from hospitals and other health care facilities. As the trend toward home care has grown, patients are becoming more familiar with the concept of this type of care in today's health care delivery system.

To be eligible for home care services, a patient must be homebound and require skilled nursing services. Short-term custodial services are provided after the these criteria are met. The value of home health care to both patient and family has been confirmed in a study by Groebe and colleagues.[40] Home health care also provides for continuity of care between physician visits.

HOSPICE

Hospice home care is available for patients living at home and requiring nursing care who have a prognosis of 6 months or less. The first hospice was organized in Connecticut in 1974; in 1996, more than 3000 hospice programs were caring for close to 500,000 dying patients in the United States.[41] A patient can be eligible for hospice home care even while receiving chemotherapy or radiation outpatient services. In addition to providing nursing care, emphasis also is placed on patient and family support. Physicians, nurses, social workers, clergy, volunteers, aides, and other ancillary personnel work together to provide services to patients and families from diagnosis through bereavement. This service can be invaluable for those dealing with a terminal illness.

BARRIERS TO EFFECTIVE HOME CARE

Home care should provide the support, reassurance, and medical assistance necessary to help patients function while remaining in the comfort of their own home environment. The success of a good home care plan depends on the skills of the professional responsible for planning this service before patient discharge from the hospital. A serviceable home care plan also relies heavily on family support and family caregivers. Most insurance companies follow Medicare guidelines and usually provide for a maximum of 2 to 3 hours of home care daily.

The burden of home care usually becomes the responsibility of the primary caregiver, who, although frequently willing to provide care on a time-limited basis, cannot continue to do so for an extended period. Patients may lack knowledge regarding the available services or may be unable to afford services to supplement insurance-covered home care. In some areas, geographic limitations exist, and not all services are available in all areas. Rural regions, in particular, usually have a dearth of available services.[42]

The growing number of home health care agencies, although ensuring a degree of competition, can make it more difficult for patients to select the agency that is most appropriate for them. Selection may be based on availability, patient and family needs, reimbursement, cost, or insurance dictates. Agencies that provide home care services may be Medicare certified, public health departments, and proprietary agencies, both profit and nonprofit. Services offered can include nursing, home health aides, social work, physical therapy, occupational therapy, speech therapy, nutritional assessment and monitoring, laboratory work, and intravenous therapy.

In caring for a patient at home, the caregivers must provide various levels of support. Needs may range from the highly technical to simple companionship and monitoring for safety. Technical support can be received from a home health care agency, whereas less technical support, such as housecleaning, shopping, or cooking, may be available from church or synagogue groups or senior center groups.

MEDICAL EQUIPMENT

At various times during the course of treatment for cancer, a patient may need special medical equipment or require modification to their home. The medical team should make this assessment before discharge from the hospital or during the course of treatment. Home health care personnel can also complete a safety evaluation. Insurance may cover these items, but only when prescribed by a physician. The ACS and Visiting Nurses Association often have loan closets in which equipment owned by such agencies is stored and available, usually free of charge. It is critical that the patient and those providing care be given ample instruction in the care and use of any equipment, including emergency access numbers for urgent problems.

Case managers now have access to a remote patient monitoring system called a *telemedicine system.* Images are transmitted via telephone lines and a video camera to allow various segments of the health care community, including physicians, clinic staff, and home care companies, to view patient images. More than 250,000 diagnostic teleradiology readings were done in the United States in 1997, and most commonly, telemedicine is used to monitor vital signs. Dr. Ace Allen, editor of *Telemedicine Today,* stated that patients with chronic diseases could be better managed if they received ongoing monitoring at home.[43] Despite the expansion of telemedicine, the volume of patients receiving services that use this technology remains relatively low (approximately 21,000 in 1996).[44] Currently, the evaluative data on telemedicine consultations are not definitive and need further exploration, particularly in the areas of insurance coverage, cost-effectiveness, and state-of-the-art evaluation.[45]

TRENDS AFFECTING DEMAND FOR COMMUNITY SERVICES

Because significant changes in the health care environment affect the need for specific resources, it is necessary to discuss them even though they remain in a continual state of flux. The maelstrom of public debate early in the 1990s swirled around the concerns of escalating medical spending[46,47] and suboptimal care,[48,49] along with increasing awareness that a significant contingent of Americans has no health insurance or inadequate insurance.[50] Since Congress rejected President Clinton's proposal for health care reform, the most significant issue has been how to protect consumers from restrictions or access to care by managed care organizations. All states have a contact for health insurance complaints at the National Association of Insurance Commissioners (http://www.naic.org/consumer/state/usamap.htm).

The percentage of health maintenance organization (HMO) members in for-profit organizations increased from 12% in 1981 to 62% in 1998.[51] Typical issues that have arisen include the fact that the number of Americans without insurance increased to 16.1% in 1997[52] and that 100,000 Americans lose their health insurance each month.[53] According to the latest U.S. census report, a total of 44.3 million Americans were uninsured in 1998,[54] which was 1 million more than just a year earlier. Children, Hispanics, and part-time workers were affected the most by these insurance losses. Kuttner[50] also states that the number of inadequately insured people is growing even faster. This development is related to several trends in coverage,[55] namely the deterioration of employer-provided coverage that insures two out of three Americans. Employers have streamlined employee choice of plans while shifting the costs to the employee and sometimes terminating coverage because of the high cost of premiums. Some plans limit benefits, such as prescription coverage, or charge higher copayments and deductibles. In addition, "casual" employees and part-time workers rarely receive insurance coverage, yet these groups accounted for approximately 29% of working Americans in 1997.[51] Americans with the broadest choice of plans are either government workers or those insured by Medicare or Medicaid.[56]

The 1985 Consolidated Omnibus Budget Reconciliation Act (COBRA) allows people to leave their jobs and pay privately for their insurance, but it does not consider the expense involved. Although the Health Insurance Portability and Accountability Act (HIPAA) prohibits denial of those with preexisting conditions, this cost is so exorbitant that it becomes self-limiting, protecting only a few hundred thousand people instead of the potential 25 million who have lost insurance. A 1998 study by the Lewin Group for Consumers Union[29] found that one in eight families spend 10% of their income on premiums and out-of-pocket expenses, but the number increased to two in ten in families with a family member between the ages of 55 and 64, and to five in ten with a family member older than 65. Thirty-four percent of insured adults have been enrolled in their plan for less than 2 years,[51] which results in lack of continuity of care and inability to track patterns, pointing to additional problems with managed care and needed resources.

Congress has considered patient protection legislation, including allowing subscribers to bring suit against their HMO. Managed care forces practitioners to search for the least expensive treatment method and emphasizes the lowest appropriate level of care. In addition to these issues, it has been determined that trust and confidence in managed care plans decreased 12% from 1998 to 1999 (42% to 30%) in a survey of 160,000 households in 1999 by the National Research Corporation.[57] A Kaiser Family Foundation survey found that physicians overwhelmingly report that HMOs have denied coverage, resulting in a decline in patient health. A Maryland state audit of denial for hospital services concluded that questionable judgment is used in denying care, and a Washington state study found a pattern of improper denials for emergency room treatment.[57] However, according to Karen Ignagni, chief executive officer of the American Association of Health Plans, health plans have heard the public's concerns and have subsequently developed "point of service" plans and grievance procedures and are incorporating independent external review. She believes that if Congress continues down its current path of allowing managed care organization decisions to be questioned in the courtroom,

HMOs will not be able to challenge the dangerous levels of misuse of health care resources and that continued variations in medical practice may threaten patient safety.[57] Nonetheless, these coverage denials have placed an all-encompassing burden on the general public, adding the emotional burden of having to advocate for themselves while they are physically compromised and financially vulnerable.

As prescription costs continue to increase, many of the elderly are flocking to "managed Medicare" policies, because traditional Medicare does not cover this service. Although the managed care plans may be enticing, patients may not realize the involved restrictions that are imposed. Many professionals are advocates for the effort to "shift power not from physicians and hospitals to patients but from managed care companies, insurance companies and health care facilities to patients and their physicians."[58] In 1999, a for-profit managed care company hired a liaison to "quell a mounting rebellion by doctors upset with new rules the insurer is trying to impose on them,"[59] including finding the cheapest way to treat patients, even if another treatment would be more beneficial, and penalizing physicians who refer to out-of-network providers, even if the patient requires the specialist services. It is precisely these types of restrictions from which the public must be protected.

Between 1998 and 2002, hospitals nationwide are expecting a $71 billion reduction in Medicare payments resulting from the Balanced Budget Act of 1997.[60] These reductions, combined with Medicaid shortfalls, will potentially compromise the current level of care provided by hospitals. Because individuals are now hospitalized for shorter periods, the multidisciplinary team often is no longer able to help patients adjust to a new diagnosis while anticipating the next phase of the illness and adaptation to its demands. Often, a social worker or discharge planner assisted the patient and family with transition to the community and assessed the barriers to care and, subsequently, planned for appropriate intervention. Although reimbursable services are obtainable, a wide gap in financial assistance faces patients without adequate coverage. Because of the these concerns, many suggestions have been put forward for a universal health policy,[53,61] thereby allowing greater access for a majority of Americans.

SURVIVORSHIP

The National Coalition of Cancer Survivorship defines survivors as living through and beyond a cancer diagnosis.[62] Today, approximately 8 million cancer survivors are alive,[63] and for the first time since the 1930s, the death rate of this disease has decreased and is leveling off or declining in all major body sites.[1] These statistics are mainly true for the nonminority community. According to McDonald,[64] African Americans continue to have higher incidence rates and are at greater risk of dying from cancer than any other racial or ethnic group.

Dow et al.[65] sent surveys to 1200 National Coalition of Cancer Survivorship members to explore quality-of-life issues for survivors. In a sample of nearly 700 people, the top emerging quality-of-life themes related to fatigue and pain, menopausal symptoms, and reproductive and fertility concerns, as well as to fears related to recurrence and immobility after treatment. Issues such as these encouraged the National Cancer Institute (NCI) to create the Office of Cancer Survivorship in July 1996. Additional issues reported by the NCI include fear of recurrence, late effects of treatment, the economic burden of the disease, physiological difficulties, depression, and sexual problems. Psychosocial difficulties occur more often with those who have had more aggressive initial treatment and those who have experienced a relapse. Additional concerns include cognitive deficits, such as in memory and concentration. Cases of discrimination in the workplace also have been reported, with their subsequent economic burdens. Klausner, director of the NCI, has stated that "the NCI has a responsibility to direct its efforts to issues that concern the many individuals who have survived cancer and their quality of life beyond treatment." The ACS also directs part of its mission toward the needs of cancer survivors, and organizations such as the Leukemia Society are following suit.[66] Continuing assessment of quality-of-life issues, along with appropriate interventions in the community, can enhance the lives of the ever-increasing number of cancer survivors. New and creative resources must be developed to meet the needs of this growing population, such as the technology that now allows for removal, freezing, and reimplantation of a woman's ovary to restore fertility.[57]

APPENDIX: COMMON RESOURCES

This appendix lists the most commonly used and helpful resources, to which most of the populace can gain easy access.

BONE MARROW TRANSPLANTATION

- Barbara Ann DeBoer Foundation: Identifies and makes use of resources in the patient's community to raise the funds necessary for the procedure. 1-800-895-8478.
- Blood and Marrow Transplant Newsletter: Provides a newsletter, resource directory, and patient support through telephone or e-mail. Keeps a list of attorneys who advocate for patients where insurance coverage has been difficult. 1-888-597-7674.
- Bone Marrow Transplant Link: Provides educational booklets, resource guides, and peer support via the telephone. 1-800-LINK-BMT.
- Bone Marrow Transplant Family Support Network: Provides support for newly diagnosed patients with recovered bone marrow transplantation patients. Offers counseling, groups, and insurance assistance. 1-800-826-9376.
- Caitlin Raymond International Registry: An international search coordinating center that assists individuals in finding compatible bone marrow donors. 1-800-726-2824.
- National Children's Cancer Society: Provides financial assistance for children diagnosed before 18 years of age in need of a bone marrow transplantation. Assists with fund-raising efforts and provides education, information, and patient advocacy. 1-800-882-6227.
- National Marrow Donor Program: Central registry facilitating searches and matches of donors and recipients. 1-800-654-1247.
- National Transplant Assistance Fund: Helps individuals raise funds for medically related transplantation expenses. Offers direct financial assistance in the form of grants to eligible candidates. 1-800-642-8399.
- Childrens' Organ Transplant Association: Helps families to raise funds for transplantation-related expenses. 1-800-366-2682.

- The Bone Marrow Foundation: Provides limited financial assistance for adjunct costs associated with bone marrow transplantation. 1-800-365-1336.

CAMPS

Contact the local ACS (1-800-ACS-2345), Cancer Information Service (1-800-4-CANCER), or Children's Oncology Camps of America (803-434-3503) for a listing of local camps.

CARE FACILITIES

Care facilities provide for the continuous health-related care of patients who are temporarily or permanently no longer able to manage living in their home. Various levels of care are available, and patients should explore these services with their physician or social worker to ascertain the most appropriate level of care. Patients should also confer with their insurance company to determine coverage.

Licensed boarding home: Provides a room and meals to fairly independent individuals. Health aides are often on staff.

Intermediate care facility: Provides limited nursing supervision and care.

Skilled nursing facility: Provides medical and continuous nursing and health-related services to patients who are not in the acute phase of an illness but who require an inpatient setting.

Subacute facility: Provides continuous medical, nursing, and health-related services to patients in a semiacute phase of their illness. These patients usually require high-tech care, such as total parenteral nutrition and intravenous antibiotics.

Hospice: Provides supportive care, terminal care, or symptom control to patients in various stages of cancer.

Rehabilitation: Provides services to patients with the goal of restoring them to an adequate level of functioning.

CHILDHOOD RESOURCES

Candlelighters Childhood Cancer Foundation: Provides information, support, and advocacy to families of children with cancer, survivors of childhood cancer, and professionals who work with these populations. 1-800-366-2223.

Childhood Leukemia Foundation: 1-732-840-4533.

Children's Hospice International: Provides support, education, resources, information, and referrals for the care of ill children and the professionals who work with them. 1-800-242-4453.

Compassionate Friends: Provides assistance with bereavement issues after the death of a child. 630-990-0010.

Many people coping with a diagnosis of cancer now turn to their computers for cutting-edge information. When researching these databases, patients should always be aware of the source of information. Is it an informed oncology professional organization or credible institution? The following is a representative listing of the numerous commercial databases that can assist in accessing oncology information. Many databases and associated links exist for specific cancers. To obtain a more comprehensive list, search engines can be used, such as About.com, Achoo, AtCancer, CiteLine, Physicians' Choice, MedNets, Medscape, Medical Matrix, Medsite, and Yahoo!.

Organizations with Online Services	
American Association for Cancer Research	http://www.aacr.org
American Brain Tumor Association	http://www.abta.org
American Cancer Society	http://www.cancer.org
American Institute for Cancer Research	http://www.aicr.org
American Lung Association	http://www.lungusa.org
BMT Newsletter	http://www.bmtnews.org
Cancer Care	http://www.cancercare.org
Cancer Guide	http://www.cancerguide.org
Cancer Information Service	http://cis.nci.nih.gov
Candlelighters Childhood Cancer Foundation	http://www.candlelighters.org
Coping Magazine	E-mail: copingmag@aol.com
Compassionate Friends	http://www.compassionatefriends.org
Cure for Lymphoma Foundation	http://www.cfl.org
Friends Network/Fun Letters	http://www.friendsnetwork.org
Gillette Women's Cancer Connection	http://www.gillettecancerconnect.org
International Myeloma Foundation	http://www.myeloma.org
Kidney Cancer Association	http://www.nkca.org
Kids Konnected	http://www.kidskonnected.org
Susan B. Komen Breast Cancer Foundation	http://www.breastcancer-info.com
Leukemia Society of America	http://www.leukemia.org
Lymphoma Research Foundation	http://www.lymphoma.org
National Alliance of Breast Cancer Organizations	http://www.nabco.org
National Bone Marrow Transplant Link	http://comnet.org/nbmtlink
National Brain Tumor Foundation	http://www.braintumor.org
National Cancer Institute	http://cancernet.nci.nih.gov
National Childhood Cancer Foundation	http://www.nccf.org
National Coalition for Cancer Survivorship	http://www.cansearch.org
National Hospice Organization	http://www.nho.org
National Lymphedema Network	http://www.lymphnet.org
National Marrow Donor Program	http://www.marrow.org
National Ovarian Cancer Coalition	http://www.ovarian.com
National Patient Air Transport Helpline	http://www.npath.org
National Prostate Cancer Coalition	http://www.4npcc.org
Patient Advocate Foundation	http://www.patientadvocate.org
R. A. Bloch Cancer Foundation, Inc.	http://www.blochcancer.org
Ronald McDonald House Charities	http://www.rmhc.com
Support for People with Oral and Head and Neck Cancer	http://www.spohnc.org
The Brain Tumor Society	http://www.tbts.org
The Wellness Community	http://www.thewc.com
United Ostomy Association, Inc.	http://www.uoa.org
US TOO! International, Inc.	http://www.ustoo.com
Vital Options Telesupport Cancer Network	http://www.vitaloptions.org
Y-ME National Breast Cancer Organization	http://www.y-me.org

Oncology Web Sites	
CancerDirectory.com	Assists in providing products and services to accommodate needs resulting from cancer and related treatment
CancerEducation.com	Improves cancer care through the dissemination of information
CancerFacts.com	Provides information to help patients make treatment choices
CancerGroup.com	Cancer Group Institute
CancerHelp.com	Provides comprehensive cancer resources
Cancer-info.com	Cancer Information and Support International
CancerLinksUSA.com	Provides support and information
CancerNews.com	Offers information on diagnosis, treatment, and prevention
CancerPage.com	Provides assistance to becoming informed, connected, and empowered
CancerResources.com	Guide to information, resources, and organizations
CancerSource.com	Provides comprehensive, reliable, and personalized information by internationally known health professionals
Nocr.com	Network for Oncology Communication and Research
Oncology.com	Provides oncology news and information
OncoLink.com	Provides assistance in obtaining accurate oncology information
Meds.com	Provides medical information and education
Patientsupport.com	Provides general cancer information

EMOTIONAL SUPPORT

In the cancer experience, stress commonly occurs at the time of diagnosis, during the treatment phase, at the end of treatment, at time of relapse, or during the terminal phase. To adequately cope with the impact of cancer, emotional support is essential for both the patient and the caregiver. Although some individuals may choose to procure support from intimate sources, others look to the community for support. Community services include self-help, professional, individual, or group modalities. Ambulatory and hospital-based settings may provide social work, psychiatric therapy, and pastoral care services.

- American Cancer Society: The ACS sponsors the following programs. Contact your local ACS at 1-800-ACS-2345, as programs may vary.
  - Cancer Survivors Network: Provides one-to-one telephone or computer support to cancer survivors.
  - I Can Cope: Support group for individuals with cancer and their families.
  - Look Good Feel Better: Provides assistance to individuals with cancer regarding skin and hair changes.
  - Man to Man: Support for men with prostate cancer.
  - Reach to Recovery: Provides support, information, and education to women who have been diagnosed with breast cancer.
  - Road to Recovery: Provides volunteer drivers to assist with transportation to and from physicians' offices or hospitals.
  - Taking Charge of Money Matters Workshop: Provides education about financial concerns during the treatment of cancer, regardless of insurance status.
- American Chronic Pain Association: A self-help organization that offers education and peer support to help people live with chronic pain.
- Cancer Care: Offers free support services, education, information, and referrals. 1-800-813-HOPE.
- Family service agencies: Provides information, emotional support, and psychological assistance.
- International Association of Laryngectomies: Works toward the rehabilitation of the laryngectomy patient by providing support to those individuals who have lost their voice box as a result of cancer. 301-983-9323.
- Leukemia Society of America: Provides support, education, and limited financial assistance. 1-800-955-4572.
- National Self-Help Clearinghouse: Refers individuals to self-help groups in their community. 212-817-1822.
- Private practitioners: Provide emotional support and psychological interventions. Many insurance companies have a preferred provider list, which should be consulted for reimbursement purposes.
- Bloch Cancer Foundation: Provides information, peer counseling, and support groups. 1-800-433-0464.
- Religious organizations: Provide emotional support, pastoral care, and spiritual guidance.
- Us Too International: Provides support to men with prostate cancer and their families.
- Well Spouse Foundation: Provides support groups and newsletters to partners and caregivers of the chronically ill. 1-800-838-0879.
- Y-Me: Provides peer support to women with breast cancer. 1-800-221-2141.

FINANCIAL ASSISTANCE

INCOME-RELATED ASSISTANCE

- Short-term disability: Some employers offer short-term disability income with proof of medical necessity.
- Social Security Administration: 1-800-772-1213.
  - Supplemental Security Income (SSI): A federally funded income maintenance program for the elderly, blind, or disabled. SSI has restrictions on income and asset allotments.
  - Social Security Disability: A federally funded program for the disabled and for survivors of a deceased wage earner.
- City, state, or federal assistance
  - Aid to Dependent Children: Provides financial assistance, medical insurance, and food stamps for eligible families with dependent children.
  - General assistance/city or town welfare: Financial assistance program for eligible individuals who do not have enough resources to meet basic needs.
  - Food stamps: A program designed to assist eligible individuals or families to purchase food.

TREATMENT-RELATED ASSISTANCE

State departments on insurance can provide information about local insurance carriers. Once cancer is diagnosed, it is often difficult for patients to obtain commercial insurance, except with an exclusionary clause.

Medicare: A federally funded insurance program for the elderly or disabled. To be eligible as the latter, one must be on Social Security Disability for 2 years. Hospital coverage is called *Part A* and covers the costs of hospitalization, except for the deductible, skilled nursing facility, and home health care. Medical coverage is called *Part B* and pays for a share of the cost for physician, outpatient, and hospital services; ambulance transportation; and physical and occupational therapy. One must be enrolled in Part B and pay monthly for this coverage. Social Security can be contacted at 1-800-772-1213 for more details.

Medicare health maintenance organizations: Similar benefits to Medicare but "managed" differently and may include additional benefits, such as prescription coverage. A preferred provider list is used.

Medicaid: A state program that provides coverage for medical expenses and financial entitlements to eligible individuals. The Department of Social Services can be contacted for more information. Check local phone listings.

Hill Burton: Federal funds are provided to some institutions to cover the cost of care for individuals who are ineligible for other entitlements. Financial restrictions apply. 1-800-638-0742.

American Association of Retired Persons: Organization that assists persons 50 years of age and older. Provides information and supplemental insurance options. Fees vary based on policy choice. 202-434-2277.

Pharmaceutical assistance: Some states offer programs that assist with the cost of prescription drugs for the elderly or disabled who meet financial criteria. Most pharmaceutical companies offer drugs at no cost to people who cannot afford them; however, stringent criteria apply and application is required. A listing can be obtained through PhRMA (America's Pharmaceutical Research Companies; http://www.phrma.org).

Transportation reimbursement: Can be obtained through various agencies, such as the Leukemia Society.

HOME HEALTH CARE

Resources can be provided through hospital departments of social work or discharge planning, as well as physicians' offices or ambulatory settings.

Visiting nurse/public health nurse: Provides skilled care, nurses aides, and ancillary staff to eligible individuals. Requires physician's orders and, often, preauthorization. Can also provide information about local resources to supplement these programs.

Hospice: Provides comprehensive home care services, including the use of volunteers, to individuals with a limited prognosis. Requires physician's orders and, often, preauthorization.

Home medical equipment: Usually reimbursed by insurance and is available through local suppliers. Some local agencies, such as the ACS or the Visiting Nurse Association, may have a loan closet.

Proprietary home care agencies: Can provide high-tech services in the home, such as home chemotherapy, total parenteral nutrition, and intravenous administration of antibiotics or other drugs. Preauthorization is needed.

Meals on Wheels: Meals are prepared and delivered to eligible homebound elderly or disabled people. A fee is often charged.

Friendly Visiting: A community outreach program offered through towns, agencies, and religious organizations in many areas.

HOUSING

Ronald McDonald House: Provides housing for families of out-of-town pediatric patients. Some facilities can occasionally accept adult patients on a priority basis. Contact local hospital social work departments or physicians' offices for referral.

Westin Hotels: Some of these hotels offer free accommodations to ambulatory patients and their family members. Contact the hotel directly or the ACS.

National Association of Hospital Hospitality Houses: Provides a resource directory of no-cost accommodation. 1-800-542-9730.

SURVIVORSHIP

Cancervive: Assists cancer survivors to face and overcome the challenges of having cancer. 310-203-9232.

Coping magazine: Publication for individuals involved with cancer. 615-790-2400.

National Cancer Survivors Day: National annual celebration of life for cancer survivors.

National Coalition for Cancer Survivorship: Provides information regarding the issues of survivorship and provides peer support. 877-622-7937.

The Wellness Community: Provides psychosocial support to individuals recovering from cancer. 310-314-2555.

TRANSPORTATION

Airlifeline: A nonprofit association of pilots who donate their time, fuel, and aircraft to provide medical transportation to ambulatory patients. 1-800-446-1231.

Ambulance/chair cars (Handivans): Can be arranged for medical appointments and sometimes are covered by insurance. Preauthorization is necessary, except in emergency.

American Airlines Miles for Kids in Need: Provides free transportation to children who demonstrate need. 817-963-8118.

Corporate Angel Network: A nonprofit organization that provides free plane transportation. 914-328-1313.

National Patient Transport Helpline: Assists patients in finding the most economical way of being transported to a medical facility. 1-800-296-1217.

Southwest Airlines: Provides no-cost transportation to medical destinations to patients in medical need. 214-792-4103.

VETERANS BENEFITS

U.S. Department of Veteran Affairs: Provides benefit information to veterans regarding educational assistance, disability compensation, medical care, life insurance, burial benefits, and dependent benefits. Some states may offer local benefits.

WISH FOUNDATIONS

A Wish with Wings: Grants wishes to children with life-threatening illness. 817-469-WISH.

Brass Ring Society: Grants wishes to children with life-threatening illness. 1-800-666-9474.

Dream Factory: Grants wishes to children ages 3 to 13 with life-threatening illness in cities where there are chapters. 502-637-8700.

Make-a-Wish Foundation: Grants wishes to children with life-threatening illness. 1-800-722-9474.

REFERENCES

1. Landis SH, Murray T, Bolden S, Wingo PA. Cancer statistics, 1999. *CA Cancer J Clin* 1999;49:8.
2. Dehgan A, Mellody P, Owen M. Keys to managing oncology care. *Case Manag* 1999;May/June:68.
3. *ACS resource directory. Community connection: resources, information and guidance.* Atlanta, American Cancer Society, 1995.
4. *"A helping hand"—the resource guide for people with cancer,* 2nd ed. New York: Cancer Care Inc., 1998.
5. Rimer B. Future directions in cancer patient education: using new media to enhance cancer communications. National Cancer Institute, Cancer Patient Education Network meeting, Tampa, Florida, September 23, 1999.
6. Iacovino V, Recsor K. Literature on interventions to address cancer patients' psychosocial needs: what does it tell us? *J Psychosoc Oncol* 1997;15:47.
7. Holland J. Historical overview. In: Holland JC, Rowland JH, eds. *Handbook of psychooncology.* New York: Oxford University Press, 1989:3.
8. Zabora JR, Blanchard CG, Smith ED, et al. Prevalence of psychological distress among cancer patients across the disease continuum. *J Psychosoc Oncol* 1997;15:73.
9. Weisman AD, Worden JW. The existential plight in cancer: significance of the first 100 days. *Int J Psychiatry Med* 1976;7:1.
10. Gotay CC, Wilson MG. Social support and screening in African American Hispanic and Native American women. *Cancer Pract* 1998;6:31.
11. Guidry JJ, Aday LA, Zhang D, Winn RJ. The role of informal and formal social support networks for patients with cancer. *Cancer Pract* 1997;5:241.
12. Wortman CB. Social support and the cancer patient. *Cancer* 1984;5[Suppl]:2339.
13. Cwikel JG, Behar LC, Zabora JR. Psychosocial factors that affect the survival of adult cancer patients: a review of research. *J Psychosoc Oncol* 1997;15:1.
14. Dunkel-Schetter C. Social support and cancer: findings based on patient interviews and their implications. *J Soc Issues* 1984;40:77.
15. Rowland JH. Intrapersonal resources: coping. In: Holland JC, Rowland JH, eds. *Handbook of psychooncology.* New York: Oxford University Press, 1989:58.
16. Nezu CM, Nezu AM, Friedman SH, et al. Cancer and psychological distress: two investigations regarding the role of social problem solving. *J Psychosoc Oncol* 1999;16:27.
17. Ey S, Compas BE, Epping-Jordan JE, Worsham N. Stress responses and psychological adjustment in patients with cancer and their spouses. *J Psychosoc Oncol* 1998;16:59.
18. Spiegel D. Facilitating emotional coping during treatment. *Cancer* 1990;16[Suppl]:1422.
19. Harris KA. The informational needs of patients with cancer and their families. *Cancer Pract* 1998;6:39.
20. Brown-McCormack K. Evaluation of cancer-related websites on the WWW. National Cancer Institute, Cancer Patient Education Network meeting, Tampa, Florida, September 23, 1999.
21. Improving doctor-patient communication. Presented at the European Cancer Conference, September 14–18, 1997.
22. Fernsler JI, Cannon CA. The whys of patient education. *Semin Oncol Nurs* 1991;7:79.
23. Giffords ED. Social work on the Internet: an introduction. *Social Work* 1998;43:243.
24. Baumans IJ, Gervey R, Siegel K. Factors associated with cancer patients' participation in support groups. *J Psychosoc Oncol* 1992;10:1.
25. Cella DF, Yellen SB. Cancer support groups: the state of the art. *Cancer Prac* 1993;1:56.
26. Spiegel D, Bloom JR, Kraemer HC, Gotthell E. Effect of psychosocial treatment on survival of patients with metastatic breast cancer. *Lancet* 1989;2:888.
27. "Internet patients" turn to support groups to guide medical decisions. *J Natl Cancer Inst* 1998;90:1695.
28. Fernsler JI, Manchester LJ. Evaluation of a computer-based cancer support network. *Cancer Pract* 1997;5:46.
29. Shearer G. *Hidden from view: the growing burden of health care costs.* Washington DC: Consumers Union, 1998:3.
30. Brennan PF, Ripich S, Moore SM. The use of home-based computers to support persons living with AIDS/ARC. *J Community Health Nurs* 1991;8:3.
31. Gustafson D, Wise M, McTavish P, et al. Development and pilot evaluation of a computer-based support system with women with breast cancer. *J Psychosoc Oncol* 1993;11:69.
32. Galinsky MJ, Schopler JH, Abell MD. Connecting group members through telephone and computer groups. *Health Soc Work* 1997;22:181.
33. Emanuel EF, Fairclough DL, Slutsman J, et al. Assistance from family members, friends, paid caregivers, and volunteers in the care of terminally ill patients. *N Engl J Med* 1999;13:956.
34. Mor V, Guadagnoli E, Wood M. The role of concrete services in cancer care. *Adv Psychosom Med* 1988;18:102.
35. Wang X, Cosby LG, Harris MG, Liv T. Major concerns and needs of breast cancer patients. *Cancer Nurs* 1999;22:157.
36. Glajchen M. Psychosocial consequences of inadequate health insurance for patients with cancer. *Cancer Pract* 1994;2:115.
37. Ginzberg E, Ostow M. *The road to reform: the future of health care in America.* New York: Macmillan, 1994.
38. Guidry JJ, Aday LA, Zhang D, Winn RJ. Transportation as a barrier to cancer treatment. *Cancer Pract* 1997;5:361.
39. Thomas RK. Healthcare's changing face. *Home Health Care Dealer* 1995;7:135.
40. Groebe ME, Ahmann DL, Ilstrup DM. Needs assessment for advanced cancer patients and their families. *Oncol Nurs Forum* 1982;9:26.
41. Horne BK. Partners at the end of life. *Case Manag* 1998;Sept–Oct:59.
42. Buehler JA, Lee HL. Exploration of homecare resources for rural families with cancer. *Cancer Nurs* 1992;15:299.
43. Talking technology: telemedicine update for case managers. *Case Manag* 1998;Sept-Oct:55.
44. Grigsby J, Sanders JH. Telemedicine: where it is and where it's going. *Ann Intern Med* 1998;129:138.
45. Sanders JH. Moving forward, looking back: telemedicine in the year ahead. *Telemed Telehealth Netw* 1998;4:28.
46. Igelhart JK. The American health care system—expenditures. *N Engl J Med* 1999;340:70.
47. Smith S, Freeland M, Heffler S, McKusick D. The next ten years of health spending: what does the future hold? *Health Aff (Millwood)* 1998;17:128.
48. The President's Advisory Commission on Consumer Protection and Quality in the Health Care Industry. Quality first: better health care for all Americans: final report to the President of the United States. Washington, D.C.: Government Printing Office, 1998.
49. Brook RH, McGlynn EA, Cleary PD. Measuring quality of care. *N Engl J Med* 1996; 335:966.
50. Kuttner R. The American health care system—health insurance coverage. *N Engl J Med* 1999;340:163.
51. Kuttner R. Must good HMOs go bad? Part I. The commercialization of prepaid group health care. *N Engl J Med* 1998;338:1558.
52. Igelhart JK. The American health care system—Medicare. *N Engl J Med* 1999;340:403.
53. Light DW. Good managed care needs universal health insurance. *Ann Intern Med* 1999;130:686.
54. *Los Angeles Times,* October 4, 1999.
55. Fronstin P. Features of employment based health plans. Washington, D.C.: Employee Benefit Research Institute, 1998.
56. Kuttner R. Must good HMOs go bad? Part II. The search for checks and balances. *N Engl J Med* 1998;338:1635.
57. "Confidence in HMOs sinks, but Congress is still offering placebos." *USA Today,* September 24, 1999.
58. Annas GJ. A national bill of patients' rights. *N Engl J Med* 1998;338:695.
59. *New Haven Register,* October 2, 1999.
60. *Bulletin—The Newsletter of Yale-New Haven Hospital,* vol 22, August 12, 1999.
61. Blumenthal D. Sounding board—health care reform at the close of the 20th century. *N Engl J Med* 1999;340:1916.
62. Clark EJ, Stovall E, Leigh S, et al. *Imperatives for quality cancer care: access, advocacy, action and accountability.* Silver Spring, MD: National Coalition of Cancer Survivorship, 1996.
63. *Facts and figures 1999.* Atlanta: American Cancer Society, 1999.
64. McDonald CJ. Cancer statistics, 1999: challenges in minority populations. *CA Cancer J Clin* 1999;49:6.
65. Dow KH, Ferrell BR, Haberman MR, Eaton L. The meaning of quality of life in cancer survivorship. *Oncol Nurs Forum* 1999;26:519.
66. "Survivorship program set for nationwide roll out." *Leukemia Society of America Newsline,* Fall 1999.

SECTION 7

FREDERICK A. FLATOW
SCOTT LONG

Specialized Care of the Terminally Ill

The functions of medicine are threefold: to relieve pain, to reduce the violence of disease and to refrain from trying to cure those whom disease has conquered, acknowledging that in such cases medicine is powerless.[1]

Hippocrates

Although Hippocrates called for restraint in the presence of terminal illness, research has documented substantial shortcomings in the contemporary care of terminally ill patients. The Study to Understand Prognoses and Preferences for Outcomes and Risks of Treatments (SUPPORT), involving more than 9000 patients hospitalized in five U.S. medical centers, found that end-of-life treatments were overly aggressive and too often not in accordance with patients' wishes. Furthermore, 50% of conscious patients dying in the hospital were reported by their surviving family members to have been in moderate to severe pain in the last week of life.[2] Among 913 Canadian outpatients "respondents were more likely to be dissatisfied with their treatments for their symptoms than for their cancer,"[3] which were similar to findings in Italy.[4] Reasons for inadequate care of the seriously ill range from a basic lack of medical education and experience in palliative care to a professional ideology that precludes the acceptance of death as an outcome of care.

Organized efforts to promote palliative care in the United States are relatively recent. Several U.S. organizations have funded studies and developed programs to promote palliative care (Table 56.7-1). The Robert Wood Johnson Foundation, through Last Acts, has sponsored several initiatives in end-of-life care, and the Open Society Institute's Project on Death in America supports clinicians active in this area of medicine. The American Medical Association has now launched the Education for Physicians on End-of-Life Care (EPEC) Project.

These programs promote integration of palliative care standards into our major health care delivery systems, as well as education for consumers about options at the end of life. Changes in medical education are also occurring.[5] Publishers of medical and nursing textbooks are incorporating new content on end-of-life care. The fifth edition of this textbook received the award for "Best Chapter with End-of-Life Care Content in a Specialty Textbook," sponsored by the Robert Wood Johnson Foundation.

OVERVIEW OF HOSPICE CARE

A BRIEF HISTORY

In the second half of the nineteenth century, the Irish Sisters of Charity in Dublin, Ireland, and a group of "pious widows" in Lyon, France, began to provide care specifically dedicated to the dying. In 1905, the Irish nuns opened St. Joseph's Hospice in Hackney, where Cicely Saunders (now Dame Cicely in honor of this achievement) began her work in developing the principles of modern hospice and palliative care. With formal training in social work, nursing, and medicine, Dr. Saunders has continued these efforts at St. Christopher's in Sydenham outside London since 1967. The concept of around-the-clock analgesia, consideration of "total pain," and comprehensive care through the integrated work of an interdisciplinary team (IDT) are hers.

Inspired by visits from Dr. Saunders to the Yale School of Medicine in the early 1960s, a group of forward-looking health care practitioners from several clinical disciplines developed a hospice program that received state regulatory approval. The home hospice served its first patient and family in early 1974, followed by the opening of the first American inpatient facility in Branford, Connecticut, in 1980.

In 1978, the U.S. government established a Hospice Task Force to examine the potential role of the federal government in the development of hospice care. The Health Care Financing Administration funded a project to assess cost and quality of service provided by hospices.[6]

ORGANIZATION AND FINANCING

The National Hospice Education Project, the political arm of the hospice movement, crafted legislation that eventually became part of the Tax Equity and Fiscal Responsibility Act of August 1982.[7] In 1983, terminally ill patients older than 65 years of age became eligible for hospice services under the Hospice Benefit of the Medicare program. To qualify for the benefit, a patient must be certified by both the referring physician and the hospice physician as having a terminal illness with life expectancy of 6 months or less. Services were limited by time and a financial cap. Eighty percent of patient care costs for each hospice were allocated to home care services to reduce expenditures for institutional care. Patients receiving services reimbursed by Medicare under the Hospice Benefit relinquished their Part A coverage for any active treatment of their terminal illness. If patients wish to return to active treatment, they may revoke the Hospice Benefit at any time. In later years, Medicaid coverage was approved by the Health Care Financing Administration as a state option. At present, Medicaid covers hospice care in 43 states and the District of Columbia.[8]

THE ORGANIZATION AND PHILOSOPHY OF HOSPICE TODAY

In 1999, the National Hospice Organization estimated that more than 3000 hospices are operating in the fifty states, Washington D.C., and Puerto Rico. Approximately 540,000 patients and families received hospice care in 1998. Although hospices may exist within institutions, such as a hospice wing in a hospital, or as free-standing hospices, the majority of care is provided as home care.[8]

No standard definition of hospice care exists, but several core principles govern its practice: (1) Hospice work is meant to enhance the quality of remaining life, not to hasten death or prolong life. The goal is to maintain for patients and families the level of comfort and calm that they wish and to offer education and guidance concerning their options at various stages of disease. (2) Delivery of care to patients and family is provided by an IDT that includes nurses, physicians, social workers, pastoral care givers, and volunteers. Often, additional members

TABLE 56.7-1. Selected Web Sites in Palliative Care

Organization	*World Wide Web URL*
American Alliance of Cancer Pain Initiatives	http://www.aacp.org
American Medical Association Education of Physicians on End-of-Life Care	http://www.ama-assn.org/ethic/epec
American Academy of Hospice and Palliative Medicine	http://www.aahpm.org
Americans for Better Care of the Dying	http://www.ABCD-CARING.com
Choice in Dying	http://www.choices.org
Edmonton Palliative Care Program	http://www.palliative.org
Last Acts Campaign to Improve End-of-Life Care	http://www.lastacts.org
National Hospice Organization	http://www.nho.org
Project on Death in America	http://www.soros.org/death.html

contribute through the arts, physical therapy, dietary consultations, and alternative therapies. (3) The patient and family group is considered the primary focus of care, not just the patient and not just the disease. After a patient's death, hospice provides bereavement services.

DIAGNOSES, ADMISSION GUIDELINES, AND ESTIMATING PROGNOSIS

The life-threatening illness most identified with hospice is cancer. In 1995, however, the National Hospice Organization census reported that malignant disease accounted for only 60% of hospice patients.[8] From its beginnings, hospice services have been available to patients with other terminal illnesses, and criteria for admission to hospice with these diagnoses were formulated and, in 1998, accepted by Medicare.[9] Most hospice patients are covered by Medicare under the Hospice Benefit.

Prognosis is generally taken in medicine to indicate whether a given disease is life-threatening and, if so, how long the patient can expect to live. Establishing a prognosis for an individual cancer patient is much more difficult than doing so for a population of such patients.

Three studies that included large numbers of patients with cancer at all stages[10–12] found that functional or performance status was the most accurate predictor of survival. Decline in activities of daily living, including bathing, continence, dressing, and transfer, were very strongly associated with decreased survival. The Karnofsky performance status is another useful measure of prognosis, and it clearly differentiates the survival time of patients with terminal cancer. The median length of survival for three groups with Karnofsky scores of 10 to 20, 30 to 40, and 50 or higher were 17, 50, and 86 days, respectively. This predictive score was strengthened by five common findings: anorexia, weight loss within 2 weeks, dry mouth, shortness of breath, and dysphagia.[11] Deteriorating mental status and cognitive ability are also predictors of shortened survival in cancer patients.[13]

A model of survival at 2 and 6 months for seriously ill hospitalized patients has been developed as part of the SUPPORT study. This model uses primarily demographic, diagnostic, and physiologic variables as opposed to the symptom-based models. However, addition of a physician's prognosis improved the model's performance.[14]

All authors agree that accurate prognosis for cancer patients is both important and difficult for physicians, patients, and families. Physician prognoses are often too optimistic[15,16] (but not always).[17] Overoptimistic prognoses can inappropriately commit the patient to futile interventions, thereby increasing the anguish of patient and family, and also increase the expenditure of valuable time and resources. In addition, unexpectedly short survival times and resulting late referrals to hospice programs deprive patients and families of available support and of time to settle affairs and achieve closure.[18] More research is needed to improve the accuracy of predicting life expectancy. The ultimate decision to seek admission to hospice must rest on the patient's, family's, and physician's acceptance of the futility of further curative treatments.

FUTILITY AND THE DECISION TO SEEK PALLIATIVE CARE

In the progression of most serious illnesses, therapeutic response eventually diminishes or disappears; risks begin to outweigh benefits as further therapy becomes futile.

Jecker and Schneiderman[19] identify four common sources for the current debate over futility and health care: (1) Increasing costs raise societal concerns about equitable delivery and possible rationing of health care. (2) Expensive technical innovations make it possible to extend life in ways that only recently seemed impossible. (3) The aging of the population raises concerns about future costs during years of longer life in this increasingly numerous group. (4) The concept of patient autonomy is being challenged as society confronts the new concerns just mentioned. Physicians must be better prepared to educate patients and families about the options of palliative care as a desirable option in progressive terminal illness.

Acknowledgment of futility is a moment when optimal care of the patient shifts from a focus of cure and care to a palliative one of care only. Jonsen[20] has formulated the following situations in which futility should be considered: (1) *futility in process,* in which a long and difficult course continues without any improvement; (2) *futility in prognosis,* when patients start treatment that has rarely or never proved useful in similar cases; (3) *futility in result,* when treatment is technically successful but the resulting quality of life is undesirable. Each of these decision points is frequently encountered by oncologists.

Recognizing these junctures and communicating them to patients and families requires physician sensitivity to the philosophy and practice of palliative care. The patient's concerns, fears, and goals can be elicited by using open-ended questions and probing the patient's response.[21] Some patients sincerely question the advisability of pursuing or initiating new active therapy, thereby providing an opportunity for discussing other options.

During such discussions, the physician can state that cure or control of disease is no longer possible. The choice of "no therapy" can hold the same stature as the alternative. Each physician must use his or her experience to influence the proper choice, always supporting the patient in the final decision and never implying disappointment, anger, or abandonment. Where patient and family insist on or demand futile treatments, it is incumbent upon the physician to begin discussion of palliative care as an acceptable option. Furthermore, the possibility for hope and the new goal of maintaining quality of life through palliative care are emphasized. Patients and families should understand that their role in developing symptom management may be greater than their role in directing curative therapies. This shift in goals and participation is a significant part of the process for patients and families in dealing with the end of life.

Many patients have fears and beliefs that make it difficult for them to accept palliative rather than curative care. Patients may fear that accepting death means that they will experience abandonment and isolation as both their families and medical care givers "give up" on them. They may foresee uncontrolled pain and suffering and devaluation of their personhood. Physicians should be mindful that these concerns may hinder patients from finding hope in the decision to seek palliative care, and they should openly discuss the support provided by palliative care programs.[22] The decision for palliative care usually involves the opening of many other emotional, interpersonal, and spiritual opportunities for patients and families. Patients may use this decision point to resolve these interpersonal issues and to seek closure. Hospice caregivers are trained to assist patients in reviewing their lives, thereby affirming self-worth. The IDT includes the pastoral care staff whose members can help patients and families find spiritual meaning as they face the end of the patient's life.

From the physician's perspective, providing palliative care rather than therapy with curative intent implies a change in his or her role with respect to patient and family. Within hospice, the physician is only one member of the IDT. The physician receives support from that team and, in turn, can help empower patients to see their medical care and symptom management as part of a more comprehensive approach to terminal illness.

The following section describes in greater detail the most common symptoms encountered at the end of life and the options available to physicians, patients, and families.

SYMPTOM MANAGEMENT

SYMPTOM PREVALENCE IN HOSPICE PATIENTS

Table 56.7-2 lists symptom prevalence as percent of patients affected in the surveyed populations; other comparable studies exist.[11,23] The results allow a few clear-cut conclusions: (1) Weakness, fatigue, pain, dyspnea, nausea, and vomiting remain important symptoms throughout much of the course of the disease. As cancer progresses, some decrease in pain may be due to adequate palliation. Others have noted increasing prevalence of dyspnea at the very end of life.[24,25] (2) Weight loss, anorexia, and insomnia become irrelevant in the last stages of disease, despite earlier importance. (3) Troublesome oral and respiratory secretions ("chesty" symptoms), drowsiness, and myoclonus become prominent in the last days of life.

TABLE 56.7-2. Symptom Prevalence in Cancer Patients at Various Stages of Disease

	Prevalence (%)		
Symptoms	2-Mo Median Survival[a]	During Week before Death[b]	24–48 H before Death[c]
Weakness	47	71	—
Pain	67	50[d]	38
Fatigue	48	52	—
Anorexia	46	55	—
Confusion and hazy thinking	20	50[d]	10
Dyspnea	28	42[d]	24
Nausea and vomiting	26	34[d]	10
Weight loss	44	—	—
Anxiety	11	36	—
Insomnia	29	21	—
Depression	21	27	—
"Chesty"	—	6	55
Drowsy	—	57	47
Myoclonus	—	—	10

[a]Data from ref. 27: prospective study of 1000 hospitalized cancer patients seen by palliative care consultation team; median survival, approximately 2 months (range 0.5–33.0).

[b]Data from ref. 24: retrospective study of 90 consecutive cancer patients referred to supportive care team for home care; ref.117: retrospective study of 100 consecutive cancer patients admitted to palliative care unit; and ref. 29: prospective study of 176 cancer patients cared for at home, in hospice unit, or in hospital by palliative care team.

[c]Data from ref. 32: retrospective study of 200 patients in hospice unit; and ref. 33: prospective study of 200 patients in hospice care at home or in inpatient ward. These two reports do not classify patients specifically as cancer patients.

[d]Prevalences based on all three reports in refs. 24, 117, and 29. All other prevalences in this column are based on refs. 24 and 29 only.

Several important points about symptom prevalence are not evident from Table 56.7-2: (1) Most cancer patients have multiple symptoms.[24,26–30] (2) The most common symptoms are often the most severe.[3,27,28] (3) The constellation of symptoms shows some variation with the site of primary disease.[25–27,31,32] For example, dyspnea is especially common in lung cancer[25,27]; nausea and vomiting in carcinoma of pulmonary, gastrointestinal, and gynecologic origins[26,27]; dysphagia in carcinoma of head and neck and of esophagus[27]; and pain in bony metastases of any origin and in primary lung, gynecologic, and prostate cancers.[26,27,31] (4) Some symptoms either worsen or recur, and new ones appear as cancer progresses. In one study of the last 48 hours of life, 22% of patients had worsening of previously controlled pain, and 30% had new pain.[33] (5) Older patients tend, as a group, to have less pain than younger patients.[27,31]

In the following sections, palliation of many of these symptoms is discussed; others are treated more fully in Chapters 55.1, 56.1, 56.2, and 56.5. Readers should consult the review by Ingham and Portenoy[34] for extended discussion of symptom assessment tools.

FAILURE TO THRIVE

The effects of cancer disrupt normal anatomy and physiology, locally in the vicinity of the tumor or its metastases and globally in sites far removed from the tumor. The latter global effects may also be called *constitutional* or *paraneoplastic.* The signs and symptoms of failure to thrive are a prime example of constitutional change and occur in many (and probably most) cancers.[3,35,36] The phrase *failure to thrive* incorporates many terms, including anorexia, asthenia, cachexia, fatigue, lethargy, and weakness, which overlap in etiology and manifestations. *Weakness* implies generalized physical debility and *lethargy* refers to the inability to maintain normal physical and mental effort. In this discussion, fatigue is comprised of weakness and lethargy. Failure to thrive is defined as a symptom complex of anorexia and fatigue.

The intensity of the components of failure to thrive is not necessarily related to tumor size, tissue origin, cell type, or degree of differentiation.[37] Evidence now implicates tumor-associated cytokines and their interaction with normal components of the immune system creating these signs and symptoms.[38]

Anorexia occurs in most patients with cancer at some time.[30,36,39] The goal of its treatment in hospice care is patient satisfaction and, in some cases, nonfluid weight gain.

Pharmacologic therapy can promote nutrition by increasing appetite, controlling nausea and vomiting, improving gastric reflux, and sometimes by relieving obstruction. Clear-cut improvement in anorexia has been documented with progestational drugs, especially megestrol acetate. At 800 mg/d, patients showed improved appetite, nonfluid weight gain, and reduction in nausea and vomiting.[40–42] Doses of more than 800 mg/d are not more effective. In a trial of chemotherapy with and without megestrol in patients with extensive small cell lung cancer,[42] however, neither quality of life nor survival time was improved with megestrol. Corticosteroids may also be helpful in stimulating appetite and improving mood. Corticosteroids are less expensive than progestational agents but also have more significant side effects.[43] Other agents are being studied as therapy for anorexia and wasting. For surveys of these medications, the reader should consult available reviews.[38,39,44]

Nonpharmacologic maneuvers may be helpful in treating anorexia and promoting nutrition. These maneuvers include mouth care, maintenance of regular bowel movements, and stressing patient choice in food preparation. Meals should consist of small portions served at the proper temperature, usually course by course, and seasoned to the patient's taste. Family and friends eating with the patient creates a shared experience that may be beneficial to all.[45] Mouth care involves simple measures such as gentle cleansing of the tongue, teeth, and gums; moistening with artificial saliva or ice chips; and promoting salivation with tart foods such as lemon ice. On occasion, oral comfort entails more intensive therapy to treat mucositis due to antitumor therapy or oral thrush.[46]

In late stages of cancer, most patients neither wish nor profit from interventions to treat anorexia pharmacologically. Similarly, forced feedings or nutritional supplements urged on the patient by well-meaning clinicians and family often offer more risk (e.g., aspiration, anxiety) than benefit. Enteral and parenteral nutrition have not been shown to be helpful in improving the quality of life or prolonging survival of cancer patients at the end of life.[47,48]

Fatigue is a major symptom in the failure to thrive of progressive illness.[3,24,35,36] The components of weakness and lethargy are multifactorial and appear to be driven by direct effects of tumor products creating deleterious changes in skeletal muscle and the central nervous system.[38] Many common elements of cancer and its treatment may contribute to fatigue: fluid and electrolyte imbalance, infection, anemia, paraneoplastic disorders, side effects of chemotherapy, radiation, other medications, and psychological reactions to disease and therapy.

In evaluation of fatigue, one monitors the patient for potentially correctable causes, such as anemia, dehydration, hyponatremia, hypokalemia, hypercalcemia, hypoglycemia, and renal and hepatic function. Medications that contribute to fatigue, including the opioids, sedatives, antidepressants, and muscle relaxants, can be adjusted by choosing agents for better side effect profiles. Rotation of opioids can maintain analgesia while decreasing side effects. Other medications can be discontinued if not important to comfort.

Nonpharmacologic approaches to improving fatigue include budgeting energy, delegating some daily tasks to others, and rescheduling activities to allow time for rest. Reassessment of goals in everyday life is necessary to form realistic expectations of physical abilities and energy capacity. Controlled programs of exercise and the use of physical and occupational therapy can improve a patient's tolerance of everyday activities.[49]

Medications used to alleviate fatigue include psychostimulants and steroids. Psychostimulants such as methylphenidate[50,51] and pemoline[52] are used in palliative care to counter the sedative effects of opioid analgesia and as antidepressants.[52,53] Steroid therapy has shown some improvement in asthenia,[43] although the beneficial effect seems to diminish 2 to 3 weeks after initial use. As was noted with anorexia, total parenteral nutrition does not reverse fatigue.[47]

Finally, although the emphasis in palliative medicine is symptom control rather than curative therapy, palliative antineoplastic therapy is the most global means of controlling the cancer and its underlying pathophysiology and improving failure to thrive.

PAIN

Pain pervades the physical being, social relationships, and spiritual dimensions of those who live with it. The presence or recurrence of pain is perceived as a sign of persistent disease and creates fear and anxiety. However, its treatment by physicians is often inadequate[2,54,55] (see Chapter 56.1 for an extensive discussion of pain and its treatment). Twelve important considerations in pain management relative to the terminally ill patient are emphasized in this chapter:

1. Assess pain carefully and reassess frequently. Believe the patient and treat pain promptly. Successful analgesia is possible in 85% to 95% of cancer patients using basic pain management techniques.[56]
2. The World Health Organization ladder is used to start treatment at the level most appropriate to the degree of pain, with escalation as necessary.[57]
3. Morphine is the standard of opioid therapy for severe pain.
4. The oral route for opioids is preferred whenever possible.
5. Alternative preparations and routes of administration are available, including rectal suppositories, transdermal patches, and both subcutaneous and intravenous parenteral preparations. A percutaneous button for multiple injections provides a single subcutaneous route lasting 3 to 4 days before change of site is needed. Compact portable pumps can deliver medication by both intravenous and subcutaneous infusion.
6. Around-the-clock analgesia controls pain best, with breakthrough doses available as needed.
7. A good command of equianalgesic doses and oral-parenteral ratios of the available opioids is essential. Methadone is gaining more acceptance for chronic pain therapy.[58] Note that the equianalgesic ratio, published as 1:1, may be much smaller, implying that methadone is more potent than anticipated.[59] When switching to methadone, approximately 10% to 30% of the equivalent daily morphine dose should be used.[60]
8. Rotation of opioids can be helpful in controlling side effects.[61] The cross-tolerance of opioids is incomplete, and using one-half to two-thirds of the equianalgesic dose of an alternate opioid can result in the same level of pain control with fewer side effects.
9. Avoid chronic use of inappropriate opioids. Accumulation of the active metabolite of meperidine, normeperidine, can produce central nervous system hyperexcitability with myoclonus and generalized seizures.[62] The mixed agonist-antagonist analgesics have a ceiling dose for pain control and can block the pure agonists at the mu opioid receptor sites.
10. Use adjuvant medications in combination with opioids, particularly for neuropathic pain and pain due to bone metastases.
11. Always begin medications for bowel care when opioid therapy starts.
12. Understand tolerance, dependence, and addiction. Psychological dependence or addiction is extremely rare in the patient with cancer and chronic pain.[63,64] This consideration should never be a barrier to good pain control in cancer patients, including those with a history of illicit drug use.

DYSPNEA

Dyspnea is the uncomfortable sensation of labored breathing. Shortness of breath can be a terrifying experience, and it frequently increases at the end of life.[24,25] Pain, anxiety, and fear complicate its clinical presentation. For patients with terminal illness but months to live, proper evaluation of dyspnea may lead to at least temporary control of its underlying cause or causes. For those with days or weeks of life remaining and who are unable or unwilling to undergo further testing, one should proceed directly to symptom control.

Dyspnea can be multifactorial in many cancer patients. Investigation of dyspnea is often limited by patient tolerance. Full pulmonary function tests are not usually necessary. However, measuring the forced expiratory volume with and without bronchodilators, standard chest x-rays, ultrasound, and ventilation/perfusion scans are not invasive and can detect abnormalities that respond to tolerable remedies.

Therapy for dyspnea requires addressing both malignant and nonmalignant causes in cancer patients. Treatment of chronic lung disease, pulmonary infection, cardiac failure, and arrhythmias can improve the patient's comfort. Venous thrombosis and pulmonary embolism are common in malignant disease and, barring major contraindication, can be managed with oral or subcutaneous anticoagulants. Thoracentesis and paracentesis can be bedside procedures in a hospice inpatient setting. However, thoracentesis can result in pneumothorax, and the risks must be discussed, particularly when tube thoracostomy is not immediately at hand. For the dyspnea of obstructing pulmonary lesions with atelectasis, a short course of palliative chest radiation may be appropriate.[65] Aspiration of a pericardial effusion can bring dramatic relief of dyspnea, but proceeding to a pericardial window requires careful consideration of benefits to the patient. Maximal supportive care may be more appropriate. Similarly, laser therapy of obstructing pulmonary lesions and endobronchial stents[66] are available for patients who can tolerate the procedures. High-dose corticosteroids can temporarily improve the dyspnea of metastatic pulmonary lesions, especially that of the lymphangitic type. Steroids also are effective in treating superior vena cava syndrome and, to a lesser extent, radiation pneumonitis.

Respiratory sedatives must be considered for those patients very near the end of life who are in respiratory distress and cannot tolerate the treatments just mentioned. The benefit of these medications, including alcohol, barbiturates, benzodiazepines, phenothiazines, and opioids, comes from suppression of respiratory awareness. Parenteral opioids have become an established treatment of dyspnea in cancer patients, without causing significant deterioration in respiratory function.[67,68] Morphine sulfate, 2.5 to 5.0 mg, subcutaneously as a single dose can be effective in the opioid naïve patient or in patients receiving only intermittent analgesia. It may be necessary to repeat two or three doses at 20- to 30-minute intervals for satisfactory relief. For those patients already receiving opioids for pain on a regular basis, a larger dose is needed, one that is 1.5 to 2.5 times the patient's q4h dose. Morphine for dyspnea is usually prescribed on an as-needed basis, but for chronic dyspnea, administration is needed every 4 hours.

Nebulized morphine has been proposed as an alternative route of administration for therapy of dyspnea. Its use has been reported in both cancer patients[69–71] and those with nonmalignant chronic lung disease.[72–74] Although several authors report relief with nebulized opioids, the studies are uncontrolled case reports and retrospective chart reviews. Morphine and hydromorphone were the most commonly used medications. A subset of patients responded to this treatment, but additional randomized and controlled studies are needed.

Morphine is prepared for inhalation by addition of 5 mg of the standard parenteral product to 3 mL of normal saline as a starting dose. Doses as high as 50 mg have been used without undue side effects.[70,71] In both normal volunteers and patients at surgery, systemic bioavailability of morphine after inhalation is only 5% to 35% of the comparable parenteral dose.[75] Patients familiar with nebulizer therapy may prefer this route. Nebulizer therapy is easily used at home and is inexpensive. However, a word of caution is necessary. Rarely, inhaled morphine can induce bronchospasm, possibly related to the preservatives present.[69] The first dose by inhalation should be administered in a controlled situation. In some patients, severe unremitting cough can contribute to breathlessness, and relief can be obtained with nebulized anesthetics. Nebulized lidocaine can be an effective cough suppressant.

Audible congestion in the last hours of life, the death rattle, is very disturbing to caregivers and family, if not the patient. Scopolamine can reduce secretions and control noisy respiration. A scopolamine patch may be sufficient, but a subcutaneous dose of 0.4 to 0.8 mg of scopolamine every 2 hours as needed is more potent and more rapid in onset. Scopolamine is sedating and may not be appropriate in some situations.

NAUSEA AND VOMITING

Increasingly, interest in nausea and vomiting has been directed toward terminally ill cancer patients not receiving chemotherapy.[76] Prevalence can be as high as 40% to 46% in the last 6 weeks of life[77] and, in the final days, may be so refractory that patients require sedation. The physiology of nausea and vomiting and appropriate therapies are reviewed in Chapter 55.1, especially as related to chemotherapy.

Workup of this problem in a terminally ill patient begins with a history and physical examination. Diagnostic studies must be consistent with the patient's condition and goals of palliative care. Invasive diagnostic studies may not be appropriate when no primary therapy exists.

Four anatomic centers initiate stimuli that produce nausea and vomiting: the central nervous system, the vestibular apparatus, the chemoreceptor trigger zone, and the viscera.[78]

Recurrent primary or metastatic brain tumors often cause emesis. Dexamethasone up to 30 mg/d may relieve symptoms associated with increased intracranial pressure due to either primary or metastatic tumors. Fear, anxiety, and pain can cause nausea and vomiting, and can be controlled by benzodiazepines and analgesics, respectively.

Vestibular causes may respond to anticholinergics (scopolamine), antihistamines (meclizine), and phenothiazines with H_1 antagonism (promethazine).

Relief of nausea and vomiting due to stimulation of the chemoreceptor trigger zone requires adjustment or replacement of medications. Chronic medications previously tolerated may become toxic because of altered drug metabolism or excretion as cancer progresses. Evaluation of metabolic abnormalities, such as hypercalcemia and uremia, may reveal correctable causes of nausea and vomiting.

The most problematic and refractory causes of emesis in advanced cancer patients result from gastrointestinal or visceral disease. If gastric irritation is suspected, as from nonsteroidal antiinflammatory drugs, cytoprotectants and acid-blocking agents can be effective without the need for antiemetics. New medications time-related to onset of nausea and vomiting can be stopped or replaced.

Overfeeding can lead to vomiting; and small feedings satisfy anorexic patients. At the end of life, tube feedings are associated with large gastric residuals, gastric distension, vomiting, and increased risk of aspiration.[48] Prokinetics, such as metoclopramide, may be helpful, but it is often appropriate to reduce or discontinue feeding. Effective bowel care controls nausea and vomiting associated with constipation. Laxatives must accompany routine opioid use. Urinary catheterization with relief of retention can end nausea, agitation, and restlessness.

The pain and nausea of hepatic metastases presumably caused by stretching of the liver capsule are relieved by nonsteroidal antiinflammatory drugs and corticosteroids with gastroprotection. Paracentesis for tense ascites controls one cause of the "squashed stomach syndrome," with restricted gastric volume, early satiety, and nausea.

Gastrointestinal obstruction, commonly due to ovarian, colonic, pancreatic, and gastric carcinomas, results in nausea and vomiting[79]; metastases from extraabdominal cancers, such as lung and breast carcinoma and melanoma, can also obstruct.[80] Gastric outlet obstruction from benign or malignant causes produces large-volume vomiting. A percutaneous endoscopic gastrostomy (PEG) tube allows gastric drainage and relieves vomiting, while a jejunostomy tube provides feeding and medication.[81,82]

Obstruction of both small and large bowel is a frequent terminal event in cancer patients. Obstruction may be partial or complete at single or multiple sites and may be due to benign causes (adhesions, radiation bowel damage, hernia) or malignant causes (new or recurrent tumor, abdominal carcinomatosis).[80] Tumor infiltration of mesentery or bowel wall and, occasionally, of celiac plexus, may cause mechanical obstruction of the lumen or paralytic ileus. Common symptoms include intestinal colic, abdominal pain, and vomiting.

Surgical treatment of bowel obstruction remains controversial. Review of therapies for gastrointestinal obstruction compared exploratory laparotomy with bowel bypass and more conservative therapy with gastrostomy drainage. The authors[83] concluded that intestinal obstruction due to chemotherapy-resistant tumors and peritoneal carcinomatosis associated with ascites or palpable masses should not be treated surgically, and neither should patients with intestinal paralysis secondary to tumor involvement of the mesentery. PEG tube placement was a simple procedure for drainage, and it improved quality of life without other surgical intervention.[83] Consideration for surgical palliation of malignant obstruction requires careful individual patient evaluation.

The goal of medical management of bowel obstruction is relief of abdominal pain and vomiting in patients in whom surgical intervention is contraindicated.[79,80] In partial obstruction, clear liquid diet, corticosteroids (dexamethasone, 12 to 24 mg/d) to reduce peritumoral edema, and bisacodyl suppositories to decompress the colon can improve intestinal passage. The steroid dose can be tapered and the diet advanced if bowel function resumes. In complete obstruction, drainage by PEG tube is the most important intervention to relieve nausea and vomiting, but antiemetics (haloperidol or prochlorperazine) may be needed. Intestinal colic is controlled with scopolamine (0.15 to 0.30 mg subcutaneously every 6 to 8 hours as needed), and abdominal pain is controlled with opioids. Octreotide (0.1

TABLE 56.7-3. Medications for Nausea and Vomiting with Associated Neurotransmitter Receptors

Medication (Receptor)	*Dose*
Scopolamine (M)	0.15 mg SQ q6–8h; transdermal patch 0.5 mg q72h
Meclizine (H1)	12.5–25.0 mg PO b.i.d.
Promethazine (H1, M, D2)	12.5–25.0 mg PO, IM, PR q4–6h
Haloperidol (H1, D2)	0.5–3.0 mg PO, SQ q6–8h
Prochlorperazine (D2, H1, M)	5–10 mg PO, IM q6–8h; 25 mg PR q8–12h
Chlorpromazine (D2, H1, M)	10–25 mg PO, IM q4–6h; 25–50 mg PR q6–8h
Hydroxyzine (H1)	25–50 mg PO, IM q4–6h
Metoclopramide (H1, D2)	10–15 mg PO, IM q.i.d. (before meals, at bedtime)
Ondansetron (5-HT3)	32 mg IV × 4 days, then 8 mg PO, SQ q8–12h
Dexamethasone	4–8 mg PO, SQ q8–12h

to 0.2 mg every 8 to 12 hours subcutaneously) reduces intestinal epithelial electrolyte and water secretion.[84,85] This reduces bowel distention, vomiting, and pain and may preclude the need for gastric drainage.

Research has revealed four major neurotransmitter receptor systems involved in emesis: muscarinic (M, one of the cholinergic subclasses), dopaminergic (D_2), histaminic (H_1), and serotonergic (5-HT_3). No one broad spectrum antiemetic is effective in all pathways[78] despite the fact that many antiemetics affect more than one neurotransmitter pathway as shown in Table 56.7-3.[86] Furthermore, nausea and vomiting in a patient may have more than one cause. When the probable causes of nausea and vomiting are established, the most effective medication should be selected from the appropriate class of medications.

Among commonly used antiemetics, phenothiazines such as perchlorperazine and chlorpromazine have a broad range (i.e., affect several pathways) and offer several routes of administration; chlorpromazine, however, is sedating and may cause hypotension. Haloperidol is available in concentrated solution (5 mg/mL) so that effective doses can be given subcutaneously in small injected volumes. Metoclopramide promotes gastric emptying. In severe nausea and vomiting, 5-HT_3 antagonists such as ondansetron, granisetron, and dolasetron can bring relief. One protocol for ondansetron is given in Table 56.7-3. In addition to control of intracranial pressure, adjuvant corticosteroids (dexamethasone) empirically enhance many antiemetics.

FLUIDS AND NUTRITION

Provision of fluids and nutrition to terminally ill patients may be a contentious issue between families and hospice caregivers.[87] Families often feel that fluids and nutrition prevent suffering by reducing dehydration and starvation. The issue often intensifies as patients begin to lose the ability to take sustenance and medications orally. Even a balanced discussion of not starting artificial fluid and nutritional support may cast the caregivers in the eyes of the family as threats to the patient's comfort. At the same time, hospice caregivers differ personally and professionally concerning provision of nonoral fluids and about the degree of suffering resulting from thirst.[88,89]

Estimation of the prevalence of thirst and dry mouth among cancer patients in palliative care ranges from 28%[90] to 83%.[91] Clinical concerns favoring provision of fluids include protection of patients from bed sores, constipation, nausea, delirium, myoclonus, and accumulation of drug metabolites with significant risk to patient comfort. Commonly used palliative medications (e.g., opioids, tricyclic antidepressants, phenothiazines, some antiemetics) all promote dry mouth. In some cases, intravenous fluids are delivered because the benefits to the family outweigh any risks.[87]

On the other hand, intravenous hydration and nutrition may prolong life so that patients die from other less comfortable causes. They may cause prolonged suffering from other symptoms, including increased respiratory and gastrointestinal secretions, phlebitis at the intravenous site, ascites and edema, and need for a urinary catheter with its accompanying risks and discomfort. Some of these objections may be avoided by using subcutaneous delivery of fluids by hypodermoclysis.[89,92,93]

The symptom of thirst is not identical to dry mouth or other signs of dehydration, often defined clinically as serum sodium, osmolality, and azotemia above normal values. Thirst is best assessed by patient report. Substituting a workup of dehydration by physical and laboratory examinations may be misleading.

It is difficult to draw firm conclusions about the relations among thirst, dry mouth, dehydration, and suffering from the few clinical studies published.[94] As a group, these studies[90,91,95–97] support but do not prove the following statements:

1. Thirst, dry mouth, and fluid retention are not closely associated with demonstrable dehydration.[95,96]
2. Intravenous fluids do not uniformly alleviate dehydration or thirst nor improve awareness.[96,97]
3. Assiduous mouth care and small amounts of ice chips or fluid may or may not relieve dry mouth or thirst.[90,91]
4. Dehydration is associated with decreased awareness and may not be improved by intravenous fluids.[97] In contrast, in a large study of a palliative care center,[61] decreased prevalence of delirium was associated with increasing use of hydration and opioid rotation.
5. Thirst was not significantly related to length of survival in one study,[95] although taken together, the studies cited show increasing prevalences of thirst and dehydration as patients approach death. Of note, these studies do not define subgroups of patients whose symptoms improve with hydration.

In hospice care, no single approach to provision of fluid by nonoral routes is used. Most caregivers would agree that the patient's choice is paramount. At the same time, institutional preferences for providing or withholding nonoral fluids exist and have been discussed.[89] The scientific basis for such patterns is still not clear and needs more study.

The issues surrounding nutrition in terminally ill patients are simpler than those concerning fluids. As cancer progresses, patients become increasingly anorexic rather than hungrier. Fewer than one-third of patients admitted to the hospice unit complained of hunger, and that occurred only during the first quarter of their stay.[90] The issue of hunger is rarely mentioned among symptoms in patients in the last 24 to 48 hours of life. Furthermore, little or no evidence shows that enteral feeding by either nasogastric or by gastrostomy and jejunostomy tubes prevents malnutrition, infections, or pressure ulcers or that it improves functional status or survival compared to patients without feeding tubes.[48] Conservative measures may be helpful to the patient and family without subjecting the patient to what appears to be a futile intervention in most cases, especially in the terminal phases of illness. Such measures involve frequent, careful feeding of small bites or boluses (generally less than a teaspoon) placed carefully into the mouth, encouragement to chew and to swallow, use of a patient's favorite foods, use of flavorful food and fluids, diets ad lib enriched with cream and fats, and the company of family and friends when desired.[48]

PSYCHIATRIC SYMPTOMS

The major psychiatric complications in terminally ill cancer patients are anxiety, depression, and delirium. Uncontrolled physical symptoms, especially pain, increase their prevalence and intensity.[98]

Anxiety

In many cancer patients, anxiety is a pervasive feeling of dread for themselves and others in their lives. Beginning in some patients before diagnosis, anxiety produces easy distraction, poor attention and concentration, and physical signs of autonomic activation. At times, anxiety may escalate into panic. Control is important for patient comfort and for adequate calm so that the patient can understand and cooperate with caregivers during workup and treatment of physical illness and psychosocial issues.

Diagnosis is based primarily in observing and talking to the patient and family; the goal is to elicit any previous history of anxiety disorders and treatment, as well as current history and symptoms. We ask the patient to describe the major sources of anxiety so that we can respond to them. Anxiety commonly concerns both self and others. The physical examination may reveal anxious facies; tics; and signs of autonomic hyperactivity, such palpitations, tachycardia, dyspnea, sweating, nausea and vomiting, diarrhea, and paresthesias.

Some patients calm adequately in response to information and to empathic support from members of the IDT and from family and friends. Others require therapies and medications designed to control anxiety. Nonpharmacologic therapies include relaxation techniques such as meditation, biofeedback, and guided imagery, as well as "talk therapy."[99,100] Such therapy should be tried, but success may depend on addition of medication, usually a benzodiazepine. A wide variety of benzodiazepines is available with differences in duration of action, metabolites, timing of onset, and routes.

In urgent situations, short-acting benzodiazepines, such as alprazolam and lorazepam, are used; the latter can be given intramuscularly or by slow intravenous push as well as by mouth. Shorter acting benzodiazepines provide easier titration of the medication. Longer acting benzodiazepines, such as diazepam and clonazepam, are used for routine control of anxiety and may be given two or three times a day.

Selective use of benzodiazepines depends on the clinical situation. Anxiety due to ongoing pain should be addressed first with analgesics. Anticipated pain can be treated with both analgesia and a benzodiazepine; lorazepam in this situation not only acts as an anxiolytic and adjuvant analgesic but also provides anterograde amnesia. Similarly, lorazepam given before chemotherapy works to relieve anxiety as well as nausea and vomiting.[100]

Anxiety is a concomitant of dyspnea. Relief of dyspnea with oxygen and, in some cases, morphine may relieve anxiety. If not, trial of an antihistamine such as hydroxyzine may be effective and prevent the use of benzodiazepines, which can interact with opioids to depress respiration. Opioids and benzodiazepines used together for rapid relief of dyspnea are appropriate at the very end of life when more concern is focused on providing dying patients with calm and comfort during this irreversible process and less on drug interactions.

Benzodiazepines protect patients during withdrawal from habit-forming substances (e.g., barbiturates, alcohol, opioids, and other benzodiazepines). After 2 to 4 weeks of routine use, benzodiazepines should be tapered to prevent physiologic withdrawal.

On occasion, the clinical situation suggests that other medications be used to treat anxiety or supplement the benzodiazepines already used. Butyrophenones such as haloperidol or a lower potency phenothiazine such as thioridiazine may be appropriate, especially in anxious patients with psychotic features of hallucinations and delusions. More sedating drugs, such as thioridazine and chlorpromazine, are helpful in agitated or insomniac patients. Methotrimeprazine is a phenothiazine that combines relief of both pain and anxiety. Like chlorpromazine, however, it is associated with sedation, hypotension and orthostasis, and the anticholinergic side effects. Anxiety escalating into panic attacks can be treated with tricyclics such as imipramine, the benzodiazepine clonazepam or a selective serotonin reuptake inhibitor such as paroxetine.[100,101]

Depression

Diagnosis of depression in cancer patients relies heavily on psychological and cognitive signs and symptoms (e.g., feelings of guilt, worthlessness, futility, suicidal ideation) because many of its physical signs and symptoms (e.g., fatigue, anorexia, weight loss) can result from underlying cancer and its treatments.[102] Prevalence of self-reported depression in cancer patients is near 25%[103] and increases with poor symptom control.[98] Among hospitalized cancer patients referred for psychiatric consultations, almost 60% were seen for depression, suicidal ideation, or both.[104]

Diagnosis and treatment for depression in early stages of cancer have been reviewed[105] and are discussed in Chapter 56.5. In this chapter, we concentrate on depression in the last stages of disease, when patients and families cannot wait weeks for therapeutic response.

Psychostimulants such as dextroamphetamine, methylphenidate, and pemoline may improve depression in a few days, as well as counteract sedative side effects of opioids and promote appetite and concentration[51,53]; in the presence of opioids, they also provide adjuvant analgesia.[51,106] Initial dosing of methylphenidate is 2.5 mg at breakfast and lunch. The dose is increased every 3 to 4 days until relief of depression or unacceptable side effects (e.g. anxiety, autonomic hyperactivity, confusion) intervene; it is rarely necessary to go beyond 30 mg/d. Relief of depression is usually evident in a few days, as opposed to the few weeks with tricyclics and selective serotonin reuptake inhibitors. Pemoline is reported to be as effective as dextroamphetamine and methylphenidate and has fewer sympathomimetic side effects, although it should be used with caution in patients with liver dysfunction.[52]

Patients with poor symptom control, especially pain and depression, are at high risk for suicidal ideation. Members of the IDT must be alert to protect them through symptom control, counseling, and pharmacotherapy.[101]

Delirium

Clinically, confusion is most often divided into delirium and dementia, although other categories of cognitive disorders exist. *Delirium* refers to a fluctuating complex of mental states of "altered alertness and impaired cognition,"[107] including some or all of the following presentations: variable attention, shifting awareness, disturbed sleeping patterns, disorientation, hallucinations, and difficulties of memory and speech.[101] In delirium, changes in mental status occur over hours to 1 or 2 weeks, which is much more rapidly than in dementia. Fluctuations of mental status and, in some cases, reversibility of delirium also distinguish it from dementia. Differentiation of dementia and delirium is especially difficult when they coexist, as they commonly do in older patients.

Prevalence of delirium increases as cancer progresses, estimated variously at 10% to 27% early in the course to 85% near death.[103,108,109] At the very end of life, it may be a major component of terminal restlessness or terminal agitation. The inability of patients to communicate with families and caregivers is frustrating. Stress created by a delirious patient can produce the "destructive triangle"[110]: a distressed family creates pressure for relief on the nurse who then adds his or her own distress to the pressure transmitted to the prescribing physician who may treat by sedating the patient without an appropriate workup. At the very end of life, however, proceeding directly to sedation may be the most effective and appropriate help.

A wide range of etiologies exists for what is called by the single name *delirium,* and Table 56.7-4 lists some of these. In earlier stages of disease, when a desirable quality of life can potentially be restored, search for and treatment of causes related to both cancer and to comorbid conditions is appropriate. Causes may not be found, even in this multifactorial condition. In one study of confused terminally ill patients, only 44% had identifiable causes of confusion.[13]

Several tools exist to aid in predicting, diagnosing, and following the evolution of delirium.[111,112] The Mini-Mental State Examination measures cognitive function and has the advantage that it can be administered in a few minutes by caregivers without special training. Other instruments may be used to measure aspects of delirium other than cognitive failure and to check the validity of the Mini-Mental State Examination if in doubt.[111]

Treatment of delirium, usually begun during workup, involves several steps: stabilization of the environment, modification of medications, and correction of contributory conditions when appropriate.[113]

At all stages of disease, a stable environment minimizes delirium (e.g., the presence of trusted family and friends at the bedside, use of consistent and trusted caregivers, a well-lighted environment with date and time readily available). Efforts to engage patients in conversation help to reorient and to distract them from distressing thoughts and hallucinations. Personal observation is usually better than physical restraints in maintaining patients' safety.

TABLE 56.7-4. Delirium in Cancer Patients: Etiologies and Facilitators

Primary cancer and metastases
Neoplasms of central nervous system
Cerebral and meningeal metastases, especially lung and breast primaries
Antineoplastic therapies
Chemotherapeutic agents: asparaginase, vinca alkaloids, intrathecal methotrexate, bleomycin, 5-fluorouracil, cisplatinum, cytosine arabinoside, ifosfamide, procarbazine, whole brain radiation therapy for primary tumors or metastatic disease
Corticosteroids
Postsurgical recovery
Constitutional and comorbid states
Age
Nonmalignant cerebral disease (e.g., dementias)
Organ insufficiency (e.g., lung disease promoting hypoxia, renal and hepatic disease distorting metabolism of medications)
Sepsis
Some antibiotics (e.g., amphotericin B, acyclovir)
Electrolyte imbalance, especially hyponatremia, hypercalcemia
Hypo- or hyperglycemia
Anemia
Palliative medications
Opiate analgesics
Phenothiazines
Antiemetics
Anticholinergics
Antihistamines
Corticosteroids

All patients should have medications reviewed to eliminate unneeded medications and substitute others less harmful whenever possible, including rotation of opioids to take advantage of partial cross-tolerance. Hydration and rotation of opioids may produce or contribute to clearing of mental status.[61]

Pharmacotherapy for delirium varies depending on the stage of illness. Haloperidol has the advantage for some patients of being less sedating than other phenothiazines. Because haloperidol administered parenterally has a faster onset and is approximately twice as potent as the same dose orally, it is used intravenously or subcutaneously in urgent cases. For agitated delirium, the initial dose is 2 to 5 mg, preferably by the intravenous route, repeated every 15 to 30 minutes with a maximal dose of 5 mg every 15 minutes. For calmer patients, starting doses are 0.5 to 1.0 mg orally or parenterally, then titrated up every 45 to 60 minutes as necessary.[101] Ultimately, most patients receive 0.5 to 3.0 mg three times a day by mouth or parenterally. Side effects of haloperidol and other phenothiazines include extrapyramidal effects, including akathisia and, rarely, neuroleptic malignant syndrome.

At times, confused patients may be aided by a sedating benzodiazepine used with haloperidol (e.g., lorazepam, which has no active metabolites), initially started at 0.5 to 1.0 mg every 1 to 2 hours by mouth, intravenously, or intramuscularly. Effective doses of these two drugs are then adjusted so that haloperidol is given every 8 hours and lorazepam every 6 hours.

Alternatively, the sedating phenothiazine chlorpromazine is usually successful in calming an agitated patient at doses of 12.5 to 50.0 mg given by mouth, intravenously, or intramuscularly every 4 to 12 hours.[102] As death nears, the benefit of imposing calm outweighs the risk of hypotension associated with chlorpromazine. In dying patients with poorly controlled agitation, a very short-acting benzodiazepine with rapid onset, midazolam, is used intravenously or subcutaneously for sedation; it does not correct disordered thought. Initially, midazolam is started at 0.4 mg/hr and is titrated up to control agitation, usually in the range of 20 to 60 mg/d, although higher doses up to 200 mg/d have been used.[114,115]

ACTIVELY DYING PATIENTS: CALM, COMFORT, AND REFRACTORY SYMPTOMS AT THE END OF LIFE

Several groups have confirmed significant improvement in symptom control, especially pain, during hospice care.[24,25,29,116] Good control of overall symptom distress increased from 64% of patients on admission to a palliative care unit to 84% on the day of death,[117] and Saunders notes that only 2% did not die peacefully in her survey.[32] In contrast, the National Hospice Study showed that only 19% of patients were pain free at the time of last pain measurement before death, whereas 18% had persistent pain.[31]

Management of refractory symptoms was sharply focused in 1990 by a prospective study of 120 Italian home care hospice patients with cancer, 52% of whom had such severe symptoms that only sedation provided comfort.[28] Subsequent reviews reported a range of 18% to 48% of hospice patients with refractory symptoms.[117–119] The most common symptoms requiring sedation were dyspnea, pain, delirium, and nausea. Time from starting sedation to death was, on average, 2 to 4 days.[28,118,119]

Refractory symptoms, as thoughtfully discussed by Cheney and Portenoy,[120] are those for which no adequate relief can be found despite rational and thorough trials of conventional approaches. In addition, other options cannot be effected in an acceptable length of time or may cause further suffering in trying them. These authors discuss efforts to control terrible pain as a guide to the workup of other symptoms before their classification as "refractory." The emphasis on interdisciplinary teamwork is further stressed in a brief discussion of intolerable psychological or existential suffering.

In the studies cited, the most common medications used to produce sedation were midazolam (more than any other benzodiazepines); neuroleptics, such as haloperidol and chlorpromazine; opioids; and barbiturates. Choice of sedating medications depends in part on the symptom to be controlled—for example, opioids for pain, opioids and benzodiazepines for dyspnea, and neuroleptics for agitated delirium. In some cases, higher doses entrain unacceptable side effects (e.g., myoclonus with opioids); in this particular case, rotation of opioids may be helpful. Additional medication may be needed. At the beginning of sedation, medications with shorter half-lives provide physicians with better control, which is especially important when varying degrees of sedation may be sought. Among benzodiazepines, midazolam offers not only a short half-life but also a variety of routes. Special attention has been given to primary use of chlorpromazine[121] and of barbiturates[122,123] as agents of sedation for refractory symptoms.

Among the most difficult of all tasks for caregivers are withdrawal of life support[124,125] and sedation for refractory symptoms to provide patients with calm and comfort as they die. Both professionally and personally, caregivers often feel frustrated and threatened by not being able to provide adequate comfort; this frustration can lead to a sense of division among members of the caregiving team. Some clinicians may have qualms that symptom control may hasten the patient's death rather than preserving or improving the quality of life. The principle of the "double effect" provides comfort to some caregivers. The double effect refers to the fact that medication given for the purpose of symptom relief carries foreseeable risk and may unintentionally hasten a patient's death. This principle recognizes the ethical desirability of promoting symptom relief and is meant to protect caregivers so long as they have sought comfort for their patients and not their deaths. These situations are often complex, however, and a simple statement of benign intent may not encompass all components of decision.[126] Clinicians unable to accept the distinction between intended benefit and an unavoidable risk of death for the treated patient may need to transfer the patient's care to another colleague.

CONCLUSION

Although still relatively recent in American medical history, hospice is becoming accepted practice in caring for the terminally ill. Insurers, providers, and patients and their families are increasingly aware that hospice is available to them and that it is often the best choice for care at the end of life. Nevertheless, hospice and palliative care practice standards remain outside the mainstream of medicine and are only now being included in medical education curricula at all levels of training from medical school to oncology fellowships.

Practitioners, researchers, and funders are beginning to establish a clinical knowledge base, which can be used to guide the practice of palliative medicine that will grow with experience and systematic research. However, the practice of hospice care will face many challenges as well. Hospice stays have been shortening in many programs, suggesting that patients may be referred to hospice later than is desirable.[18] Research is needed to understand better the sources of this shift, including problems with prognosis, institutional barriers, physician knowledge and attitudes, and the views of families and patients. Better understanding of the underuse of hospice can inform a variety of approaches, including policy changes, health education interventions, and professional training resources. The desired outcome is continuing growth of knowledge and training in palliative care and its expanded use for patients with terminal illness.

REFERENCES

1. Hippocratic Corpus. In: Jones WHS, trans. *The art.* Cambridge, MA: 1959;11,193.
2. SUPPORT Principal Investigators. A controlled trial to improve care for the seriously ill hospitalized patients: the study to Understand Prognoses and Preferences for Outcomes and Risks of Treatments (SUPPORT). *JAMA* 1995;274:1591.
3. Ashbury FD, Findlay H, Reynolds B, McKerracher K. A Canadian survey of cancer patients' experiences: are their needs being met? *J Pain Symptom Manage* 1998; 16:298.
4. Morasso G, Capelli M, Viterbori P, et al. Psychological and symptom distress in terminal cancer patients with met and unmet needs. *J Pain Symptom Manage* 1999;17:402.
5. Billings JA, Block S. Palliative care in undergraduate medical education. Status report and future directions. *JAMA* 1997:278:733.
6. Hoyer T. A history of the Medicare hospice benefit. *Hospice J* 1998;13(2):61.
7. Bayer R, Feldman E. Hospice under the Medicare wing. *Hastings Center Rep* 1982;12(6):5.
8. National Hospice Organization. *NHO fact sheet.* World Wide Web URL: www.nho.org, Spring 1999.
9. National Hospice Organization. Medical guidelines for determining prognosis in selected non-cancer diseases. *Hospice J* 1996;11:47.

10. Loprinzi CL, Laurie JA, Wieand HS, et al. Prospective evaluation of prognostic variables from patient-completed questionnaires. *J Clin Oncol* 1994;12:601.
11. Reuben DB, Mor V, Hiris J. Clinical symptoms and length of survival in patients with terminal cancer. *Arch Intern Med* 1988;148:1586.
12. Allard P, Dionne A, Potvin D. Factors associated with length of survival among 1081 terminally ill cancer patients. *J Palliat Care* 1995;11:20.
13. Bruera E, Miller L, McCallion J, et al. Cognitive failure (CF) in patients with terminal cancer: a prospective study. *J Pain Symptom Manage* 1992;7:192.
14. Knaus WA, Harrell FE, Lynn J, et al. The SUPPORT prognostic model. Objective estimates of survival for seriously ill hospitalized adults. *Ann Intern Med* 1995;122:191.
15. Forster LE, Lynn J. Predicting life span for applicants to inpatient hospice. *Arch Intern Med* 1988;148:2540.
16. Lamont EB, Christakis NA. Some elements of prognosis in terminal cancer. *Oncology* 1999;13:1165.
17. Zhong Z, Lynn J. The Lamont/Christakis article reviewed. *Oncology* 1999;12:1172.
18. Christakis N, Escarce JJ. Survival of Medicare patients after enrollment in hospice programs. *New Engl J Med* 1996;335:172.
19. Jecker NS, Schneiderman LJ. Futility and rationing. *Am J Med* 1992;92:189.
20. Jonsen AR. Intimations of futility. *Am J Med* 1994;96:107.
21. Lo B, Quill T, Tulsky J. Discussing palliative care with patients. *Ann Intern Med* 1999;130:744.
22. Herth K. Fostering hope in terminally ill people. *J Adv Nurs* 1990;15:1250.
23. Brescia FJ, Adler D, Gray G, et al. Hospitalized advanced cancer patients: a profile. *J Pain Symptom Manage* 1990;5:221.
24. Coyle N, Adelhardt J, Foley KM, Portenoy RKP. Character of terminal illness in the advanced cancer patient: pain and other symptoms during the last four weeks of life. *J Pain Symptom Manage* 1990;5:83.
25. Higginson J, McCarthy M. Measuring symptoms in terminal cancer: are pain and dyspnea controlled? *J Royal Soc Med* 1989;82:264.
26. Bedard K, Dionne A, Dionne L. The experience of La Maison Michel Sarrazin (1985–1990): profile analysis of 952 terminal-phase cancer patients. *J Palliat Care* 1991;7:42.
27. Donnelly S, Walsh D, Rybicky L. The symptoms of advanced cancer: identification of clinical and research priorities by assessment of prevalence and severity. *J Palliat Care* 1995;11:27.
28. Ventafridda V, Ripamonti C, de Conno F, Tamburini M. Symptom prevalence and control during cancer patients' last days of life. *J Palliat Care* 1990;6:7.
29. Connill C, Verger E, Henriquez I, et al. Symptom prevalence in the last week of life. *J Pain Symptom Manage* 1997;14;328.
30. Schuit KW, Sleijfer DT, Meijler WJ, et al. Symptoms and functional status of patients with disseminated cancer visiting outpatient departments. *J Pain Symptom Manage* 1998;16:290.
31. Morris JN, Mor V, Goldberg RJ, et al. The effect of treatment setting and patient characteristics on pain in terminal cancer patients: a report from the National Hospice Study. *J Chronic Dis* 1986;39:27.
32. Saunders C. Pain and impending death. In: Wall PD, Melzack R, eds. *Textbook of pain.* London: Churchill Livingstone, 1989:624.
33. Lichter I, Hunt E. The last 48 hours of life. *J Palliat Care* 1990;6:7.
34. Ingham J, Portenoy RK. The measurement of pain and other symptoms. In: Doyle D, Hanks GWC, MacDonald N, eds. *The Oxford textbook of palliative medicine,* 2nd ed. Oxford: Oxford University Press, 1998:203.
35. Neuenschwander H, Bruera E. Asthenia. In: Doyle D, Hanks GWC, MacDonald N, eds. *The Oxford textbook of palliative medicine,* 2nd ed. Oxford: Oxford University Press, 1998:573.
36. Vachon MS, Kristjanson L, Higginson I. Psychosocial issues in palliative care: the patient, the family and the process and outcome of care. *J Pain Symptom Manage* 1995;10:142.
37. DeWys WD, Begg C, Lavin PT, et al. Prognostic effect of weight loss prior to chemotherapy in cancer patients. *Am J Med* 1980;69;491.
38. Loprinzi L, Goldberg RM, Peethambaram PP. Cancer anorexia/cachexia. In: Berger A, Portenoy RK, Weissman DE, eds. *Principles and practice of supportive oncology.* Philadelphia: Lippincott–Raven, 1998:133.
39. Bruera E, Fainsinger RL. Clinical management of cachexia and anorexia. In: Doyle D, Hanks GWC, MacDonald N, eds. *The Oxford textbook of palliative medicine,* 2nd ed. Oxford: Oxford University Press, 1998:548.
40. Bruera E, Macmillan K, Kuehn N, Hansen J, MacDonald RN. A controlled trial of megestrol acetate on appetite, caloric intake, nutritional status, and other symptoms in patients with advanced cancer. *Cancer* 1990;66:1279.
41. Loprinzi CL, Schaid DJ, Dose AM, Burnham NL, Jensen MD. Body composition changes in patients who gain weight while receiving megestrol acetate. *J Clin Oncol* 1993;11:152.
42. Rowland KM Jr, Loprinzi CL, Shaw EG, et al. Randomized, double-blind, placebo-controlled trial of cisplatin and etoposide plus megestrol acetate/placebo in extensive stage small cell lung cancer: a North Central Cancer Treatment Group Study. *J Clin Oncol* 1996;14:135.
43. Bruera E, Roca E, Cedaro L, Carraro S, Chacon R. Action of oral methylprednisolone in terminal cancer patients: a prospective randomized double-blind study. *Cancer Treat Rep* 1985;69:751.
44. Bruera E. Recent research in pain and cachexia in advanced cancer and AIDS. In: Eguchi K, Klastersky J, Feld R, eds. *Current perspectives and future directions in palliative medicine.* Tokyo: Springer-Verlag, 1998:3.
45. World Health Organization. *Symptom relief in terminal illness.* Geneva: World Health Organization, 1998.
46. Berger A, Kilroy TJ. Oral complications of cancer therapy. In: Berger A, Portenoy RK, Weissman DE, eds. *Principles and practice of supportive oncology.* Philadelphia: Lippincott–Raven, 1998:223.
47. American College of Physicians. Parenteral nutrition and the cancer patient. *Ann Intern Med* 1989;110:734.
48. Finucane TE, Christmas C, Travis K. Tube feeding in patients with advanced dementia. A review of the evidence. *JAMA* 1999;282:1365.
49. O'Gorman B. Physiotherapy in palliative medicine. In: Saunders C, Sykes N, eds. *The management of terminal malignant disease,* 3rd ed. London: Edward Arnold, 1993:168.
50. Bruera E, Watanabe S. Psychostimulants as adjuvant analgesics. *J Pain Symptom Manage* 1994;9:412.
51. Bruera E, Miller MJ, Macmillan K, Kuehn N. Neuropsychological effects of methylphenidate in patients receiving a continuous infusion of narcotics for cancer pain. *Pain* 1992;48:163.
52. Breitbart W, Mermelstein H. Pemoline. An alternative psychostimulant for the management of depressive disorders in cancer patients. *Psychosomatics* 1992;33:352.
53. Rosenberg PB, Ahmed I, Hurwitz S. Methylphenidate in depressed medically ill patients. *J Clin Psychiatry* 1991;52:263.
54. Weisman SJ, ed. Pain management in children. *Child Adolesc Psychiatr Clin North Am* 1997;6(4):687.
55. Wolfe J, Grier HE, Klar N, et al. Symptoms and suffering at the end of life in children with cancer. *N Engl J Med* 2000;342:326.
56. Levy MH. Pharmacologic treatment of pain. *New Engl J Med* 1996;335:1124.
57. Jacox A, Carr DB, Payne R, et al. *Management of cancer pain: clinical practice guideline no. 9.* Rockville, MD: Agency for Health Care Policy and Research, U.S. Department of Health and Human Services, Public Health Service, March 1994. AHCPR publication 94-0592.
58. Bruera E, Neumann CM. Role of methadone in the management of pain in cancer patients. *Oncology* 1999;13:1275.
59. Ripamonti C, Groff L, Brunelle C, et al. Switching from morphine to oral methadone in treating cancer pain: what is the equianalgesic dose ratio? *J Clin Oncol* 1998;16:3216.
60. Lawlor PG, Turner KS, Hanson J, Bruera E. Dose ratio between morphine and methadone in patients with cancer pain: a retrospective study. *Cancer* 1998;82:1167.
61. Bruera E, Franco JJ, Maltoni M, Watanabe S, Suarez-Almazor M. Changing pattern of agitated impaired mental status in patients with advanced cancer: association with cognitive monitoring, hydration and opioid rotation. *J Pain Symptom Manage* 1995;10:287.
62. Kaiko RF, Foley KM, Grabinski PY, et al. Central nervous system excitatory effects of meperidine in cancer patients. *Ann Neurol* 1983;13:180.
63. Porter J, Jick H. Addiction rare in patients treated with narcotics [Letter]. *New Engl J Med* 1980;302:123.
64. Perry S, Heidrich G. Management of pain during debridement: a survey of U.S. burn units. *Pain* 1982;13:267.
65. Medical Research Council. Lung cancer: a Medical Research Council randomized trial of palliative radiotherapy with two fractions or ten fractions. *Br J Cancer* 1991;63:265.
66. Pierce RJ. Lasers, brachytherapy and stents—keeping airways open. *Respir Med* 1991;85:263.
67. Bruera E, MacEachern T, Ripamonti C, Hanson J. Subcutaneous morphine for dyspnea in patients. *Ann Intern Med* 1993;119:906.
68. Allard P, Lamontagne C, Bernard P, Tremblay C. How effective are supplementary doses of opioids for dyspnea in terminally ill cancer patients? A randomized continuous sequential clinical trial. *J Pain Symptom Manage* 1999;17:256.
69. Farncombe M, Chater S, Gillin A. The use of nebulized opioids for breathlessness: a chart review. *Palliat Med* 1994;8:306.
70. Quelch PC, Faulkner DE, Yun JWS. Nebulized opioids in the treatment of dyspnea. *J Palliat Care* 1997;13(3):48.
71. Davis C. The role of nebulized drugs in palliating respiratory symptoms of malignant disease. *Eur J Palliat Care* 1995;2:9.
72. Davis CL, Hodder C, Love S, et al. Effect of nebulized morphine and morphine 6-glucuronide on exercise endurance in patients with chronic obstructive airways disease. *Thorax* 1989;44:387.
73. Beauford W, Saylor TT, Stansbury D, Avalos K, Light R. Effects of nebulized morphine sulfate on the exercise tolerance of the ventilatory limited COPD patient. *Chest* 1993;104:175.
74. Young IH, Daviskas E, Keena VA. Effect of low dose nebulized morphine on exercise endurance in patients with chronic lung disease. *Thorax* 1989;44:387.
75. Davis CL, Lam W, Butcher M, Joel SP, Slevin ML. Low systemic bio-availability of nebulized morphine: potential therapeutic role for the relief of dyspnea. *Br J Cancer* 1992;[Suppl 16]:S12.
76. Fallon BG. Nausea and vomiting unrelated to cancer treatment. In: Berger A, Portenoy RK, Weissman DE, eds. *Principles and practice of supportive oncology.* Philadelphia: Lippincott–Raven, 1998:179.
77. Wachtel T, Allen-Masterson S, Reuben D, Goldberg R, Mor V. The end stage cancer patient: terminal common pathway. *Hospice J* 1988;4:43.
78. Lichter I. Which antiemetic? *J Palliat Care* 1993;9:42.
79. Baines M, Oliver DJ, Carter RL. Medical management of intestinal obstruction in patients with advanced malignant disease. *Lancet* 1985;2:990.
80. Ripamonti C, DeConno F, Ventrafridda V, Rossi B, Baines MJ. Management of bowel obstruction in advanced and terminal cancer patients. *Ann Oncol* 1993;4:15.
81. Stellato TA, Gauderer MW. Percutaneous endoscopic gastrostomy for gastrointestinal decompression. *Ann Surg* 1987;205:119.
82. Gilbar PJ. A guide to enteral drug administration in palliative care. *J Pain Symptom Manage* 1999;17:197.
83. van Ooijen B, van der Burg MEL, Planting AS, Siersema PD, Wiggers T. Surgical treatment or gastric drainage only for intestinal obstruction in patients with carcinoma of the ovary or peritoneal carcinomatosis of other origin. *Surg Gynecol Obstet* 1993;176:469.
84. Marks WH, Perkal MF, Schwartz PE. Percutaneous endoscopic gastrostomy for gastric decompression in metastatic gynecologic malignancies. *Surg Gynecol Obstet* 1993;177:573.
85. Mercadante S, Maddaloni S. Octreotide in the management of inoperable gastrointestinal obstruction in terminal cancer patients. *J Pain Symptom Manage* 1992;7:496.
86. Lichter I. Results of antiemetic management in terminal illness. *J Palliat Care* 1993;9(2):19.

87. Parkash R, Burge F. The family's perspective on issues of hydration in terminal care. *J Palliat Care* 1997;13:23.
88. Collaud T, Rapin CH. Dehydration in dying patients: study with physicians in French-speaking Switzerland. *J Pain Symptom Manage* 1991;6:230.
89. Fainsinger R, Bruera E. The management of dehydration in terminally ill patients. *J Palliat Care* 1994;10:55.
90. McCann RM, Hall WJ, Groth-Juncker A. Comfort care for terminally ill patients. The appropriate use of nutrition and hydration. *JAMA* 1994;272:1263.
91. Ellershaw JE, Sutcliffe JM, Saunders CM. Dehydration and the dying patient. *J Pain Symptom Manage* 1995;10:192.
92. Fainsinger RL, MacEachern T, Miller MJ, et al. The use of hypodermoclysis (HDC) for rehydration in terminally ill cancer patients. *J Pain Symptom Manage* 1994;9:298.
93. Centeno C, Bruera E. Subcutaneous hydration with no hyaluronidase in patients with advanced cancer. *J Pain Symptom Manage* 1999;17:305.
94. Viola RA, Wells GA, Peterson J. The effects of fluid status and fluid therapy on the dying: a systematic review. *J Palliat Care* 1997;13:41.
95. Burge FI. Dehydration symptoms of palliative care cancer patients. *J Pain Symptom Manage* 1993;8:454.
96. Musgrave CF, Bartal N, Opstad J. The sensation of thirst in dying patients receiving IV hydration. *J Palliat Care* 1995;11:17.
97. Waller A, Hershkowitz M, Adunsky A. The effect of intravenous fluid infusion on blood and urine parameters of hydration and on state of consciousness in terminal cancer patients. *Am J Hosp Palliat Care* 1994;11:22.
98. Derogatis LR, Morrow GR, Fetting J, et al. The prevalence of psychiatric disorders among cancer patients. *JAMA* 1983;249:751.
99. Fawzy FI, Fawzy WW, Arndt LA, Pasnau RO. Critical review of psychosocial interventions in cancer care. *Arch Gen Psychiatry* 1995;52:100.
100. Noyes R Jr, Holt CS, Massie MJ. Anxiety disorders. In: Holland JC, ed. *Psycho-oncology.* New York: Oxford University Press, 1998:548.
101. Roth AJ, Breitbart W. Psychiatric emergencies in terminally ill cancer patients. *Hematol Oncol Clin North Am* 1996;10:235.
102. Breitbart W, Jacobsen PB. Psychiatric symptom management in terminal care. *Clin Geriatr Med* 1996;12:329.
103. Massie MJ, Holland JC. The cancer patient with pain: psychiatric complications and their management. *J Pain Symptom Manage* 1992;7:99.
104. Massie MJ, Holland JC. The cancer patient with pain: psychiatric complications and their management. *Med Clin North Am* 1987;71:243.
105. Block SD. Assessing and managing depression in the terminally ill patient. *Ann Intern Med* 2000;132:209.
106. Bruera E, Chadwick S, Brenneis C, Hanson J, MacDonald RN. Methylphenidate associated with narcotics for the treatment of cancer pain. *Cancer Treat Rep* 1987;71:67.
107. Ingham J, Caraceni AT. Delirium. In: Berger A, Portenoy RK, Weissman DE, eds. *Principles and practice of supportive oncology.* Philadelphia: Lippincott–Raven, 1998:477.
108. Pereira J, Hanson J, Bruera E. The frequency and clinical course of cognitive impairment in patients with terminal cancer. *Cancer* 1997;69:835.
109. Massie MJ, Holland J, Glass E. Delirium in terminally ill cancer patients. *Am J Psychiatry* 1983;140:1048.
110. Fainsinger RL, Tapper M, Bruera E. A perspective on the management of delirium in terminally ill patients on a palliative care unit. *J Palliat Care* 1993;9:4.
111. Smith MJ, Breitbart WS, Platt MM. A critique of instruments and methods to detect, diagnose, and rate delirium. *J Pain Symptom Manage* 1995;10:35.
112. Inouye SK, Van Dyck CH, Alessi CA, et al. Clarifying confusion: the confusion assessment method. *Ann Intern Med* 1990;113:941.
113. de Stoutz ND, Tapper M, Fainsinger RL. Reversible delirium in terminally ill patients. *J Pain Symptom Manage* 1995;10:249.
114. DeSousa E, Jepson A. Midazolam in terminal care. *Lancet* 1988;1:67.
115. Bottomley DM, Hanks GW. Subcutaneous midazolam infusion in palliative care. *J Pain Symptom Manage* 1990;5:259.
116. Twycross R, Lichter I. The terminal phase. In: Doyle D, Hanks GWC, MacDonald N, eds. *The Oxford textbook of palliative medicine,* 2nd ed. Oxford: Oxford University Press, 1998:977.
117. Fainsinger R, Miller MJ, Bruera E, Hanson J, MacEachern T. Symptom control during the last week of life on a palliative care unit. *J Palliat Care* 1991;7:5.
118. Fainsinger RL, Landman W, Hoskings M, Bruera E. Sedation for uncontrolled symptoms in a South African hospice. *J Pain Symptom Manage* 1998;16:145.
119. Morita T, Inoue S, Chihara S. Sedation for symptom control in Japan: the importance of intermittent use and communication with family members. *J Pain Symptom Manage* 1996;12:32.
120. Cheney NI, Portenoy RK. Sedation in the management of refractory symptoms: guidelines for evaluation and treatment. *J Palliat Care* 1991;10:31.
121. MacIver B, Walsh D, Nelson K. The use of chlorpromazine for symptom control in dying cancer patients. *J Pain Symptom Manage* 1994;9:341.
122. Truog RD, Berde CB, Mitchell C, Grier HE. Barbiturates in the care of the terminally ill. *N Engl J Med* 1992;327:1678.
123. Stirling LC, Kurowska A, Tookman A. The use of phenobarbitone in the management of agitation and seizures at the end of life. *J Pain Symptom Manage* 1999;17:363.
124. Dickey N. Withholding or withdrawing life-prolonging medical treatment. *JAMA* 1986;256:471.
125. Brody H, Campbell ML, Faber-Langendoen K, Ogle KS. Withdrawing intensive life-sustaining treatment—recommendations for compassionate clinical management. *New Engl J Med* 1997;336:652.
126. Quill TE. The ambiguity of clinical intentions. *New Engl J Med* 1993;329:1039.

Lynn Gerber
Jeanne Hicks
Jay Shah

CHAPTER 57

Rehabilitation of the Cancer Patient

The American Cancer Society predicts 1.2 million new cases of cancer diagnosed in 1999 and 8 million cancer survivors requiring care for cancer-related problems.[1] These patients are likely to be older, will survive for years with their cancers, and will present considerable challenge to health professionals.

The incidence of cancer climbs appreciably with each decade of life, and the population is aging.[2] The 5-year survival has improved over the last 20 years, such that more than 50% of those with cancer of the prostate, colon, bladder, breast, uterus, thyroid, and some lymphomas will survive 5 years.[2]

Patients with cancer, in part because of the likelihood that they are older and have preexisting medical conditions, are likely to present significant challenges and complex management decisions. They are complex because, often, cancer has many phases and may recur and remit throughout multiple life stages. The illness may not be stable, and the functional impact may vary with disease stage and may change with remote effects of treatments. Table 57-1 outlines one scheme for conceptualizing this view of cancer management needs.

The pretreatment and treatment phases should include a functional assessment to help to identify what the patient is able and wishes to do and to predict what is likely to influence function subsequently. A systematic evaluation of the neuromusculoskeletal system is essential for targeting areas likely to need intervention for maintaining or restoring function. Often, instruction in the use of gait aides can best be given before treatment, when pain and mobility loss have not occurred. Prosthetic and orthotic devices can be planned and provided intraoperatively when needed.

The post–definitive treatment phase is an opportunity for initiating preventive measures. Early mobilization, the use of wraps, and limb massage may help to mitigate disuse and deconditioning or control lymphedema and limb swelling. This phase usually includes preparing the patient and family for discharge and educating them about what the course is likely to be and what they (collectively) should be doing to keep the functional level high.

The intercurrent period, when the definitive treatment has been complete, may be psychologically difficult and require guidance to assist patients and family to enter or reenter an active and healthy life program and resume usual activities, when possible. Patients may need to plan for adjusting to late neurologic sequelae (plexopathies, neuropathies) or musculoskeletal sequelae (fibrosis, atrophy) of disease or treatment. Chronic pain, weakness, fatigue, and lymphedema may require ongoing and intensive therapy.

Recurrence may require that the cycle of assessment and treatment begin anew. This process may be fairly psychologically demanding and anxiety-provoking. The goals of rehabilitation management are to provide education about problem solving for issues relating to functional loss.

Rehabilitation professionals also have significant contributions to make at the end of life. During this phase, rehabilitation professionals can assist in answering questions pertaining to nonpharmacologic treatments for pain control and strategies for enhancing quality activities and independence and can help families, friends, and patients address issues at the end of life.

TABLE 57-1. Rehabilitation Support throughout Phases of Cancer

Phase of Disease	*Issues to Address*
Diagnosis to treatment planning	Anticipating the impact of cancer treatment on function; understanding and preserving function; using comprehensive pretreatment rehabilitation (e.g., ROM, ADL, strength)
Treatment	Evaluating effects of treatments on function (surgical therapy, chemotherapy, radiotherapy, biologic agents); preserving and restoring function through exercise, edema management, and increased activity; controlling pain using heat, cold, and TENS
Posttreatment	Developing and supporting a program to help to restore daily routines and to promote a healthy lifestyle; educating patients about what to self-monitor (strength, ROM, edema, pain, etc.); supervising a maintenance program of exercise, edema management, and mobility
Recurrence	Educating patients about impact of recurrence and its effect on function; educating patients about what to monitor in the context of new clinical status; supervising patients in an appropriate program to restore function or prevent its decline; assisting patients in maintaining activity and quality of life
End of life	Educating patients and families about mobility training, good body mechanics, and assistive devices; managing pain (nonpharmacologic treatment) and controlling symptoms; and maintaining independence and quality of life

ADL, activities of daily living; ROM, range of motion; TENS, transcutaneous electrical nerve stimulation.

Cancer is common, chronic, and complex. Decision making about primary cancer treatment often factors elements reflective of these features. In fact, patients (our consumers) are not only requesting participation in decision making, they are asking for information about the impact of the tumor and its treatments on function and their quality of life. Patients, especially cancer patients, fear disability and have identified a host of concerns that include fatigue, independence, and pursuit of valued activity, in addition to mortality, that influence their ultimate treatment choices.[3] Many concerns and needs of patients throughout the phases of cancer treatment can be ameliorated by rehabilitation professionals. Table 57-2 describes the functional areas affected by various symptoms and in need of rehabilitation.

CANCER REHABILITATION TEAM

Rehabilitation specialists most frequently involved in treatment of the cancer patient include physiatrists; occupational, physical, and recreation therapists; speech-language pathologists; audiologists; and vocational counselors. Other health care professionals join the team as needed for particular problems (e.g., orthotists-prosthetists, psychologists, dietitians).

Physiatrists are trained in the specialty practice of physical medicine and rehabilitation. This training enables them to assess functional ability, relative strength and stamina, the basics of human mobility (biomechanics), the design and appropriate use of adaptive equipment, and orthotics and prostheses. Physiatrists often combine information about disease and its treatment with the impact it is likely to have on function. It is usually physiatrists that coordinate rehabilitation services and prepare a comprehensive plan for treatment and follow-up.

Occupational therapy is an integral part of the rehabilitation of the cancer patient. Therapists evaluate the impact of disease or treatment on function, roles and daily routines, and the coping strategies needed to compensate for changes in a person's ability to participate as fully as possible in activity. Occupational therapists (OTs) determine which strengths and support networks are available to a person and identify interventions that are critical to potentiate quality of life for those who are terminally ill. Adaptive device training and safety training for activities of daily living (ADL); fabrication of splints or prosthetic training to maximize upper extremity function; counseling for the development of coping strategies; fracture risk education and assistance with mobility; and seating and environmental adaptations are examples of interventions that an OT can provide. Preparation for discharge requires input from an OT, with concentration on environmental safety (e.g., home, bathroom) and functional independence (Table 57-3).

Physical therapists (PTs) provide evaluation and treatment of human motion. Treatments include strategies and exercises to improve mobility, strength, and stamina. Therapists often help to relieve painful musculoskeletal symptoms using nonpharmacologic modalities and postural treatment. If therapy is instituted early, it can prevent muscle atrophy and joint contractures and maintain or promote fitness. Typically, PTs assess range of motion (ROM), muscle strength, exercise tolerance, gait, shoulder and trunk strength, and balance. PTs usually apply orthotics and prostheses for the lower extremities, apply modalities of heat and cold, and help to manage peripheral edema using compression pumps and stockings. Standardized evaluations are listed in Table 57-4.

TABLE 57-2. Patient Functional Areas Affected by Cancer Symptoms in Various Phases of Disease

Phase of Cancer	*Symptom*	*Functional Areas Affected*
Pretreatment and evaluation	Pain, anxiety, depression	Daily routines, sleep, fatigue
Treatment	Pain, anxiety, loss of mobility, wound and skin care, speech and swallowing	Daily routines, sleep, stamina, self-care, cosmesis, communication
Posttreatment	Pain, weakness, anxiety, depression, loss of mobility, edema, fatigue, stamina	Sleep, fatigue, ADL, vocational and avocational concerns, cosmesis
Recurrence	Pain, weakness, anxiety, depression, fatigue, stamina, edema, bony instability, anorexia	Sleep, fatigue, disability, disruption of routines, cosmesis, vocational and avocational concerns
End of life	Pain, fatigue, anorexia	Dependence, immobility

ADL, activities of daily living.

TABLE 57-3. Occupational Therapy: Evaluation and Treatment

Self-care, activities of daily living
Exploration of important roles, daily routines, personal values
Adaptive device training and environmental adaptations
Mobility and transfer safety
Wheelchairs, scooters, customized seating
Orthoses and prostheses
Fracture risk education
Help for pain, edema, sensory changes, and weakness
Joint contracture prevention
Psychosocial issues, coping
Family education and support system development

Rehabilitation counseling addresses the educational-vocational issues of the cancer patient. Table 57-5 summarizes this information.

Recreation therapists (RTs) are part of a comprehensive cancer rehabilitation program. RTs evaluate whether areas of function that have been adversely affected by disease or its treatment are amenable to interventions aimed at enhancing leisure activity. Interventions designed to address the primary and secondary symptoms and side effects related to cancer and cancer treatment include behavioral and cognitive strategies for pain, anxiety, and stress management; recreational activities for fine and gross motor function and stamina building; games for cognitive stimulation; age- and developmentally appropriate activities to ensure normalized experiences for hospitalized children and adolescents; and creative and expressive outlets for thoughts and feelings. Further, RTs assist patients in identifying opportunities for developing interpersonal and social supports through avocational activities; in enhancing patient management by providing clinical information; in motivating patient compliance; and in educating the patient and significant others about strategies for coping and maintaining quality of life. A summary of what RTs provide is found in Table 57-6.

Speech-language pathology provides oral motor evaluation of speech and swallowing and assessment of cognition for patients with cancer diagnoses, as needed. Specifically, patients with central nervous system (CNS) tumors or head and neck tumors are evaluated for communication skills, comprehension, and memory. Speech pathologists assess functional integrity and compensatory ability of structures and mechanisms needed to achieve adequate communication, deglutition, and cognition. They evaluate dysphagia and work with gastroenterologists to identify its causes. They frequently collaborate with maxillofacial prosthetists in the restoration of facial appearance and oral function.

TABLE 57-4. Physical Therapy: Evaluation and Treatment

Range of motion and strength assessment
Bed mobility and transfers
Gait evaluation
Prostheses, orthoses, and assistive devices
Pain and edema management (compression garments, compression units)
Modalities (heat, cold, electrical stimulation)
Exercise and endurance
Contracture prevention

TABLE 57-5. Rehabilitation Counseling: Evaluation and Treatment

Educational, vocational, avocational functioning
Psychosocial issues, adjustment, coping
Vocational and career counseling
Vocational testing and assessment
Work adjustment
Résumé, job seeking, interviewing
Essential functions of a job
Job analysis
Job accommodation
Job modifications
Community resource development and referral
Volunteer work
Disability laws and legislation

FUNCTIONAL ASSESSMENT

There has been substantial improvement in the ability to assess function, its limitations, and quality of life during the last decade. Measures are available to quantitate performance and activity of daily routines and assess changes in social and psychocognitive function.[4–7] When these assessments, which incorporate multiple domains, add measures of value, they are termed *quality-of-life measures.* Many of these have been developed specifically for those with cancer diagnoses.[8,9]

COMMON FUNCTIONAL IMPAIRMENTS IN ONCOLOGY

IMMOBILITY AND ITS IMPACT

One of the most significant problems facing cancer patients is the impact of relative or absolute immobility. Bed rest in cancer patients is associated with numerous metabolic and physiologic changes that may impair the patient's medical and

TABLE 57-6. Recreation Therapy: Evaluation and Treatment

Leisure function and satisfaction assessment
Treatment tolerance and protocol compliance
Coping and behavioral strategies for psychosocial sequelae
Management strategies for pain, edema, sensory changes, and other secondary symptoms
Relationship issues and identification and development of social support
Exploration and clarification of roles, habits, and values
Developmental and age-appropriate activities
Leisure education and counseling (individual, family)
Avocational interest and leisure skill development
Medical play
Activity adaptation
Community reintegration

functional recovery.[10] Bone loss is well documented and, in extreme cases, may lead to hypercalcemia.[11–13] In patients who are already osteoporotic or who have metastatic involvement of the skeletal system, this may predispose to pathologic fractures and further disability. Muscle atrophy can be fairly rapid, often leading to an inability to walk in as short a time as a week. Decreased activity may result in contractures and changes in muscle and joint physiology.[14,15] Lack of mobility can also lead to the development of deep venous thrombosis and pulmonary embolus.[16] Changes in muscle physiology and fiber type have been documented as well.[17,18] This is particularly true of patients with gastroenterologic tumors in which weight loss, anorexia, and inflammatory cytokine production negatively impact on function and quality of life.[19,20] As muscle mass becomes reduced, the amount of soft tissue covering bony prominences can become marginal, predisposing to the development of pressure (decubitus) ulcers. In this state, pressure over peripheral nerves, especially as it crosses bony prominences, may lead to a neuropraxia. All these factors can significantly reduce mobility and independence.

MUSCLE WASTING AND CACHEXIA

Patients with a variety of tumors, including gastrointestinal tract, breast, colon, prostate, lung, small cell, and the like, may develop muscle wasting and cachexia. Cachexia is a condition characterized by weight loss, anorexia, weakness, loss of functional capacity, and fundamental changes in metabolic processes.[21]

Some of these changes include presence of inflammatory cytokines (tumor necrosis factor-α, interleukin-6), severe negative nitrogen balance, increased proteolysis, and gluconeogenesis. Muscle mass, body fat mass, and energy stores all are decreased. Interestingly, parenteral nutrition seems to maintain body hydration and fat stores but has little effect on loss or restoration of lean mass and, as such, cannot reverse muscle wasting.

Exercise, long used to build lean mass, is often ineffective in this population. In the setting of cachexia, the effects of exercise on nitrogen balance and other metabolic abnormalities are fairly modest. Rigor of exercise is significantly curtailed, in part limited by symptoms of pain, fatigue, depression, and aesthenia.[22]

GENERALIZED DECONDITIONING

As a rule, each week of immobility requires as much as a month of rehabilitation to regain functional mobility. Complications such as pathologic fractures and pressure ulcers can further delay recovery. Although it is sometimes impossible to fully mobilize a patient receiving chemotherapy or major surgery, some degree of mobilization under a PT's supervision may significantly reduce morbidity. For the patient who is mildly restricted by disease or treatment, active ambulation at least once or twice daily is strongly encouraged. If this is not possible, an exercise program in bed may be started, using resistance against gravity or against an elastic band. A tilt table may be used to maintain sympathetic tone, reduce orthostatic hypotension, or restore cardiovascular conditioning in the patient who is unable to stand. This also helps to minimize heel cord contractures, increase muscular tone, and facilitate venous compression and helps to maintain cardiovascular volume. In patients with severe dependent edema, compressive garments or manual therapy, such as massage and lymph drainage, may help to maintain the vascular volume and to reduce the degree of the edema while facilitating ambulation. Passive or active assistive stretching may be needed to maintain joints in functional alignment.

SKIN BREAKDOWN

Prevention of skin breakdown is critical for the bed-bound patient. Above all else, the patient must not be allowed to remain in a single position for more than 2 hours. If patients are unable to position themselves in bed, repositioning should be done with pillows or cushions, taking care not to encourage the development of contractures by, for example, persistently flexing the neck, hips, or knees. Air-cushioned beds can help to reduce the incidence of pressure injuries.

Shear forces and direct pressure are important in the development of decubitus ulcers. Care should be taken, therefore, to avoid dragging patients across sheets or examination tables.

If skin becomes dry, aqueous remoisturizing creams should be applied. Healing is promoted in a moist wound environment. Greasy agents can predispose to maceration and breakdown. Irradiated skin is of particular concern, due to the loss of normal resilience and healing capacity. Hygiene is important with irradiated skin, and all open cuts and abrasions should receive scrutiny, because they can easily become infected.

When complications arise, they should be treated promptly. Areas of skin redness that do not blanch should be considered early pressure ulcers (stage 1) and treated by removing pressure over the affected area. Most tissue damage in pressure ulcers occurs in the deep layers of the dermis and underlying tissues, such that the visible portion of the ulcer may represent only a fraction of the total extent. In many instances, hydrotherapy (whirlpool) can aid in the process of debridement and cleansing.

Packing the wound with an antiseptic solution should be done only when proven infection is present. In the case of noninfected small lesions, absorptive hydrocolloid occlusive dressings can be effective in promoting healing, provided that they are used in accordance with the manufacturer's recommendations. The use of occlusive dressings with larger wounds is controversial. Management should include mechanical and enzymatic débridement when necrotic tissue is present. Although we have seen many cases of complete resolution with the use of absorptive granules and occlusive dressings in deeper wounds, the potential exists for developing a superinfection. Occlusive dressings cannot be used as a substitute for adequate nursing care.

CONTRACTURES

In cases of prolonged disuse or fixed joint positions, collagen fibers within muscles, tendons, and ligaments shorten, leading to contractures. Shoulder, heel cord, hamstring, and hip flexor contractures are most common.

ROM exercises should be practiced actively by the debilitated patient or passively by nursing or by the family at least two to three times each day, moving all major joints through their full ROM in all directions. In the case of the shoulder, this includes external and internal rotation, full abduction, and flexion. If flexion and abduction need to be limited, (e.g., in

TABLE 57-7. Upper Extremity Orthoses

Static splints	
	Fracture stabilization
	Joint immobilization
	Contracture prevention
	Functional positioning (wrist, thumb, fingers)
	Compensation (weakness, sensory loss)
Dynamic splints	
	Joint and soft tissue mobilization
	Contracture reduction and prevention
	Functional positioning (wrist, thumb, fingers)
	Compensation (weakness, sensory loss)

the patient after mastectomy or axillary lymph node dissection), internal and external rotation should be performed to stretch the joint capsule.[23] Splinting may be used to maintain functional hand and foot position.

The role of upper extremity bracing during the acute or chronic stages of disease or treatment should not be overlooked. Because of the complexities of movement patterns and compensatory adjustments, patients can continue to manipulate objects despite progressive changes that, if left unattended, may render them nonfunctional. Splints are designed to maintain soft tissue length, place joints in functional positions, and align hands and wrists to prepare for grasp and release activities. Thumbs can be positioned to oppose fingers for pinch, fingers can be pulled into extension with dynamic forces to compensate for weakness, wrists can be supported to allow for better mechanical advantage of forearm finger tendon function, and elbows or shoulders can be positioned by slings or splints to aid in the prevention of joint subluxation and ligamentous laxity. Rehabilitation goals are to prevent contractures, when possible. Uses for splinting devices are summarized in Table 57-7.

When neuropathy from disease or treatment results in dysfunction, splints can be applied to hand and wrist to compensate for loss of proprioception. If sensory loss is severe, splint design can foster safety as well as positioning during manipulation. When weakness is severe or prolonged, splints aid by preventing or improving contractures. Long finger flexors contract quickly; thus, night resting splints are indicated to position the wrist and fingers in a functional position (i.e., 30 degrees wrist extension, 50 degrees metacarpophalangeal joint flexion and 20 degrees proximal interphalangeal joint flexion, and 10 degrees distal interphalangeal joint flexion, with the thumb opposed).

When neuropathy, immobility, weakness, pain, or the disease process itself has an impact on hand and wrist manipulation, appropriately designed splints need to be applied immediately, adjusted over time in accordance with the condition of the individual, and monitored for effectiveness. They also need to be used in conjunction with exercises and education regarding wearing schedules and precautions. When used appropriately and in a timely fashion, splints can make a difference in the functional outcome of patients and help to preserve alignment.

Radiation may potentiate fibrosis and the development of joint contractures. The effect of radiation on soft tissues is often long term, rendering recovery of ROM especially difficult. The rehabilitation team should instruct the patient in a home stretching program when radiation is initiated, and it should be continued for the life of the patient because of the tendency for irradiated tissues to develop persistent fibrosis.

If contractures do occur, affected areas may require months of therapy to regain full or functional motion or they may never achieve this. Stretching exercises should be performed at least once or twice daily under the guidance of a PT. This may be supplemented by the use of superficial or deep heating modalities, particularly ultrasonography, which can help to increase the distensibility of collagen, facilitating stretching. However, ultrasonography is contraindicated in an area of tumor. It has been shown to increase blood flow and tumor size and may increase the tendency for metastasis.[24] In extreme conditions of fixed, painful, and unresponsive contractures, surgical release or manipulation under anesthesia may be considered.

TUMOR-ASSOCIATED MYOPATHY

Tumor-associated myopathy may result in immobility and ADL deficits. The myopathy may be a result of direct tumor invasion of muscle and other soft tissues, paraneoplastic syndrome, carcinomatous myopathy, steroid myopathy, or carcinomatous neuromyopathy.

PARANEOPLASTIC SYNDROME

Nonmetastatic paraneoplastic syndromes of malignancy have been recognized with polymyositis and dermatomyositis. Malignancy occurs primarily in association with dermatomyositis rather than with polymyositis.[25] The incidence is thought to be higher in men older than 50 years.[26] A study by Lakhanpal et al.[27] mentions a 25% incidence of malignancy in a polymyositis and dermatomyositis group and a 17% incidence in the control group. Breast cancers (18%) and lung cancers (16%) are most frequently associated with polymyositis and dermatomyositis.[28]

Patients with paraneoplastic syndrome have decreased endurance, muscle weakness, pain, decreased joint motion, and problems with ambulation, self-care, sexual performance, and work-related activity. Treatment to increase joint motion with stretching exercise, to increase muscle strength with isometric exercise, to improve mobility with gait aides and bracing, and to improve ADL with assistive devices are all appropriate. The patient should be instructed in energy conservation, joint protection, and sexual and vocational counseling.

CARCINOMATOUS MYOPATHY

Carcinomatous myopathy may be seen with metastatic malignant disease. Histologically, there is widespread muscle necrosis and minimal or no inflammatory response. Clinically, there is proximal muscle weakness in this type of myopathy.[29] Because of the necrosis of muscle, it is thought that these patients would probably not respond well to an exercise program, but function should be maintained if possible. They should be given appropriate pain-relieving modalities and assistive and mobility devices to help with ADL and safe ambulation. The environment should be altered to help to ensure safety and easy access.

CARCINOMATOUS NEUROPATHY AND MYOPATHY

Simultaneous carcinomatous neuropathy and myopathy occur with metastatic disease and affect peripheral nerve and muscle due to either toxic or immunopathologic effects of the tumor. Diminished reflexes and diminished sensation ensue.[29] The rehabilitative treatment is similar to that recommended in the management of carcinomatous myopathy. However, distal weakness occurs in addition to the proximal weakness, and appropriate bracing to improve ankle dorsiflexion may be needed. If weakness is severe, an electric scooter may be needed. Several assistive devices to help with hand function are useful.

STEROID MYOPATHY

Steroid-induced muscle weakness is really a selective atrophy of type II fibers in proximal muscles. It tends not to affect neck flexor muscles. It may be superimposed on the weakness of carcinomatous myopathy or polymyositis- and dermatomyositis-associated myopathy and exacerbate it. It is caused by catabolic and anabolic effects of steroid on muscle. Amino acids leak into the circulation, and there is decreased incorporation of protein into muscle. The condition may be diminished by providing exercise to enhance protein metabolism by muscle.[30] Isometric exercise can be used to accomplish this goal. It may take up to 1 year after cessation of steroids for muscles weakened by steroid use to return to normal.[31]

BONE REPLACEMENT BY TUMOR

Bone can be invaded by tumor via direct extension, as is frequently seen in sarcoma; via embolization through the right side of the heart, the most frequent cause of distant metastasis; or via direct venous spread through Batson's plexus involving vertebral bodies and pelvis, the most frequent cause for metastatic bone disease in prostate cancer. Some tumors, such as leukemias, lymphomas, or myelomas, invade bone marrow.

Bony metastatic disease is most frequently associated with breast, lung, prostate, colon, or kidney tumors. It is important to note that the survival for patients with these tumors and bony metastases is years. Although any tumor can metastasize to bone, the most likely to spread are prostate, breast, lung, kidney, and thyroid.[32–35] The hematologic malignancies do frequently as well. Nearly 20% of tumors with distant spread will involve bone. Bony involvement is the third most frequent site for metastasis, with vertebral bodies, pelvis, femur, and ribs affected in order of frequency. Often, multiple sites are involved, of which 20% are in the upper extremities.[36]

Pain is the most frequent symptom associated with bony metastasis. This is characteristically dull, aching, and nocturnal. The spine is the most frequently involved area for metastatic spread, and the lumbar region is the most common site. When there is vertebral involvement, 50% of patients will have radicular symptoms. Cord compression, on the other hand, most frequently results from thoracic region involvement. Pain on weight bearing may be a sign of bony involvement or even a pathologic fracture. A bone scan is the simplest means of screening for bony tumor. Plain films offer definition of the local extent of the tumor, although computed tomography (CT) may be needed for better quantification of involvement.

PREVENTION AND MANAGEMENT OF PATHOLOGIC FRACTURES

Pathologic fractures can limit mobility in a marginally functioning patient and, in some cases, lead to significant morbidity and mortality. Hip fractures are particularly debilitating and often difficult to stabilize, and they may lead to a significant hemorrhage. Prevention of pathologic fracture is important. Fracture should be considered imminent when the size of a lytic lesion exceeds 60% of the total bone width (usually >2.5 cm in lower and >3.0 cm in upper extremities), if cortical involvement exceeds 50%, or if the axial extent of cortical destruction exceeds 13 mm in the femoral neck and 30 mm elsewhere.[37] These calculations are difficult to measure accurately, in part because local osteopenia is common and margins are often irregular and difficult to distinguish.

Pain with weight bearing suggests a need to reduce load on or immobilize the affected structure. A cane used in the hand opposite the affected lower extremity can theoretically remove approximately 50% of body weight from that extremity. Such attachments as a quadruped base (quad-cane) or a forearm support (forearm or Lofstrand crutch) may help to stabilize the cane, but they cannot overcome the simple physics of gravitation loading. Canes or a single crutch can be used for the patient who has pain with weight bearing, but they should not be used for the patient with a fracture or one that is imminent.

Bilateral support is essential for the patient in whom no weight bearing is required. For the more debilitated patient, a simple walker suffices. For the more active patient, axillary or forearm crutches may be used. Toe touch of the affected leg can usually be allowed but, in the patient who has difficulty coordinating the use of crutches or walker, total avoidance of weight bearing may be needed to avoid sudden weight bearing if the assistive device is not properly placed. Patients need to be evaluated for metastatic disease in the upper extremities. It is fairly possible to develop a pathologic fracture of an involved humerus if it is used as a weight bearing structure. The patient should be cautioned against torquing the affected extremity, because this can often lead to fracture, even without weight bearing.

After an affected extremity has been unweighted, options for stabilization can be considered. Radiation often can be used to treat lesions of the long bones. Irradiation does not directly repair damaged bone, and irradiated bone heals much more slowly than normal bone. For small lesions, irradiation, along with the use of a cane, may be all that is required. For larger lesions, surgical stabilization should be considered if possible. Intramedullary rods or methylmethacrylate can be used to increase strength of the invaded bone or, if used prophylactically, to stabilize a painful lesion and prevent fractures.[38] This gives the patient a more functional limb and allows increased mobility.

Destruction of the femoral head or acetabulum may be treated with hip joint arthroplasty, rendering ambulation a possibility while providing excellent palliation of pain. Fractures of the ischium may be painful during sitting and should be treated with cushions to reduce weight bearing over the fracture. Fractures of a single portion of the pelvic ring are generally not a problem. Multiple fractures, however, can interfere with ambulation and should be addressed appropriately. Fractures of the iliac wing may be painful during active hip flexion and abduction, due to the attachments of the iliacus and gluteal abductors, respectively. Assistive devices used to avoid activation of these muscles during ambulation can provide significant relief of pain.

When lower extremity and upper extremity are involved, use of gait aides may be contraindicated either because of pain or impending fracture. In this situation, a wheelchair may be needed until internal fixation can be performed. When upper extremity involvement is associated with pain but there is no immediate threat to bony integrity, a thermoplastic splint for forearm or a humeral cuff for lesions of the humerus may provide stability and symptom relief.

Ribs are also a common site of bony involvement and fracture. Generally, only a rib belt will be required. Pathologic fractures of non–weight-bearing bones can be managed with splinting or sling immobilization while irradiation is delivered. ROM or isometric exercises may be appropriate to maintain function. If a dominant upper extremity is involved, assistive devices and training in one-handed strategies by an OT can significantly improve function. Devices such as reachers and dressing aids can help the patient to avoid torquing the spine or hips if the risk of fracture is high.

In the patient who presents with neurologic deficits, the physician must always rule out spinal cord compression by tumor. Other causes of paraparesis in the cancer patient include peripheral neuropathy, lumbosacral plexitis, radiation myelitis, and pseudotumor, often from radiation fibrosis. Radiation-related paraparesis may not occur for some time after the completion of all treatment. We have seen patients with radiation myelitis presenting as long as 7 years after having been declared free of disease. Hyperreflexia may be masked by peripheral neuropathy or plexopathy related to chemotherapy or irradiation, and patients with extensive metastatic involvement of the vertebral column may even have little or no pain.

The prevention of serious spinal cord injury should be the primary goal of the cancer rehabilitation team in treating the patient with known vertebral destruction by primary or metastatic disease. Although radiation treatment may be used to control tumor growth and to relieve spinal cord compression, this does not address the issue of spinal stability.

Although no good models of vertebral collapse from tumor exist, it has been assumed that spinal stability in the cancer patient can be addressed in much the same way that it is in the patient with a traumatic injury of the spine.[39] The most widely accepted method of stability evaluation involves the concept of three columns.[40,41] This method considers the spine to be made up of three supporting columns—the anterior, middle, and posterior structures of the vertebrae—roughly divided into equal thirds. Any two of these supporting columns must be intact for the spine to be stable. For example, complete destruction of a vertebral body puts the spinal cord at risk for compression, because the posterior structures (facet joints) can easily sublux. A simple compression fracture, however, is usually stable because the posterior and middle columns are relatively intact. Of particular concern are lesions at the atlantoaxial and thoracolumbar junctions, due to the significant bending and torquing moments generated at these interfaces.

Whenever possible, an unstable lesion of the bony spine should be stabilized surgically, because virtually no brace can be completely effective in preventing subluxation. Irradiated bone heals slowly and often incompletely, and continued malignant destruction may sometimes occur. It is desirable from the rehabilitation standpoint to mobilize the patient as quickly as possible to prevent the complications associated with immobility. Even if there is extensive vertebral destruction, surgical stabilization can usually be accomplished by means of rods, strut grafts, and cement.[42,43] Occasionally, extensive multilevel involvement may render it impossible to find adequate healthy bone to which stabilizing hardware can be attached, or the patient's health may preclude any surgical option. In such cases, bracing may provide the only means of protecting the spinal canal.

If it becomes necessary to use a more "practical" cervical stabilization, orthosis selection should be based on the level of potential instability and the directions of motion that might lead to instability.[44] The Philadelphia collar, consisting of a foam collar with rigid supports, provides moderately successful stabilization of higher segments in flexion and extension but inadequate stabilization at lower levels and inadequate stabilization for side bending and rotation, and it is of limited usefulness as a spinal stabilization brace.

Two alternatives that provide excellent stabilization of lower segments in flexion and extension are the two-poster and sternal occipital mandibular immobilization (SOMI) braces (Fig. 57-1). The SOMI is particularly useful in managing debilitated patients, due to its open design and the ease with which it can be applied, because all components are attached from the front. It can be used with a light-weight chest piece, as supplied, or it can be bolted onto a lower spinal orthosis, making it useful in cases of multilevel instability (Fig. 57-2). An alternative cervical thoracic orthosis is the Yale brace, which essentially consists of a Philadelphia collar attached to a thoracic extension. With any of these orthoses, the patient must be informed that the brace is a compromise solution and that care is indicated, particularly with motions not well supported by the particular brace.

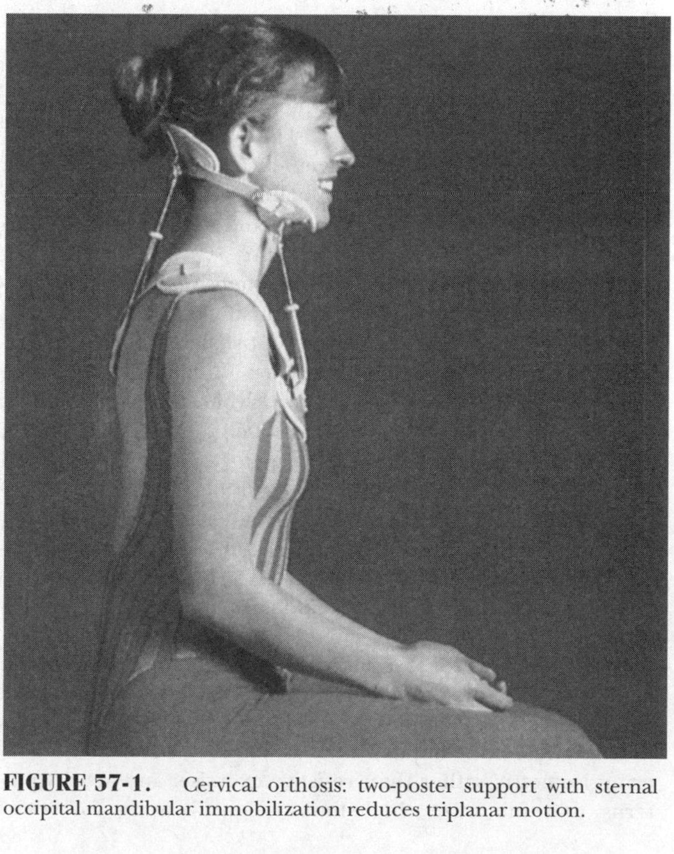

FIGURE 57-1. Cervical orthosis: two-poster support with sternal occipital mandibular immobilization reduces triplanar motion.

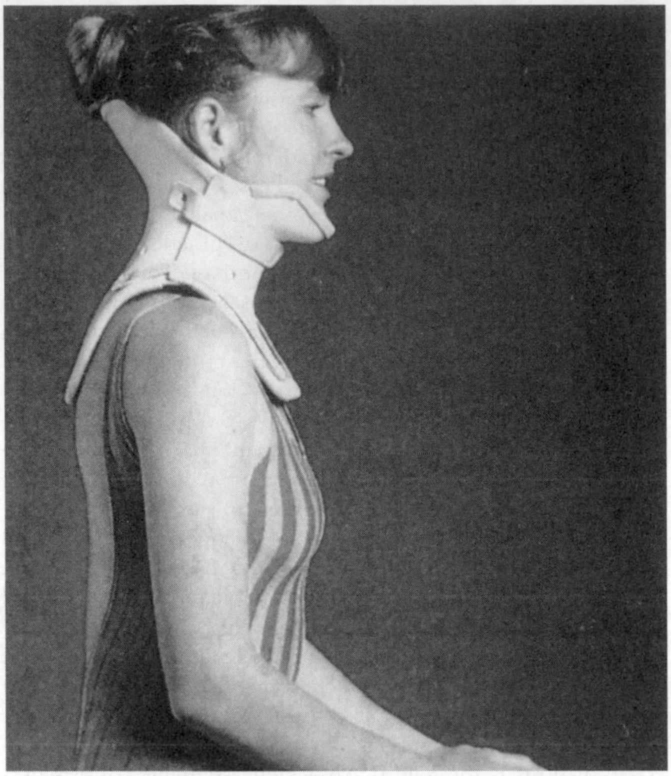

FIGURE 57-2. Sternal occipital mandibular immobilization orthosis with extended chest support reduces triplanar motion.

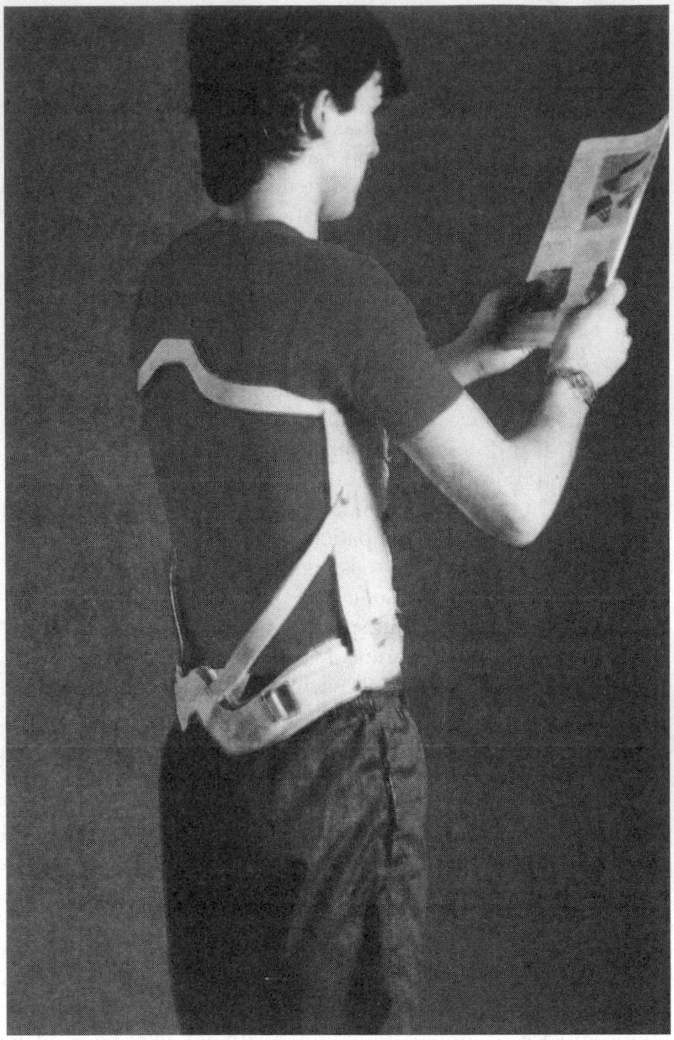

FIGURE 57-3. Thoracolumbar stabilization device (Taylor-Knight).

Stabilization of the thoracolumbar regions is generally achieved using two basic types of bracing. Metal braces, such as the Jewitt or the Taylor-Knight (Fig. 57-3) orthoses, can be fit to the patient rapidly, providing optimum limitation of flexion and extension. The custom-molded plastic thoracolumbosacral orthosis, or body jacket, additionally provides limitation in rotation as well. These braces are frequently poorly tolerated in the debilitated patient with atrophic skin. Elastic back braces and corsets, often used in the management of mechanical low back pain, do not provide adequate spinal stabilization, although rigid corsets may be worthy of consideration in the patient who absolutely cannot tolerate anything else.

High thoracic lesions and cases of extensive vertebral involvement may require the use of a combination orthosis. A cervical extension or SOMI brace can, for example, be attached to a body jacket (Fig. 57-4), providing restricted mobility of the entire spine. These braces should be worn whenever the patient is upright or travels in a motor vehicle. When the patient lies in bed without the brace, the head of the bed should not be elevated more than 30%. Patients should be cautioned against twisting or torquing their backs, because this may potentiate the injury. Cervical orthoses should be worn even when the patient is recumbent and should be removed only in a supervised setting.

The prescription of exercise and participation in vocational-avocation activity should be written by knowledgeable professionals. The goals for treatment should be limited to what the patient can do safely, and should promote independence and quality function at minimal risk. Exercise to promote fitness with minimal bony impact, such as aquatics; strengthening by using isometric rather than resistive exercise; and activity patterns that minimize single-limb weight bearing for lower extremities are recommended strategies. Education to help patients and caregivers to maximize safety is also important.

SPINAL CORD INJURY SYNDROMES AND REHABILITATION OF IMPAIRMENT

Spinal cord disorders in cancer patients may result from malignant invasion; bony compression or trauma; syrinx or hematoma formation; radiation myelitis; or vascular events. Radiation myelitis is directly related to radiation dose and often does not develop until years after the completion of therapy.[45] Spinal cord dysfunction has been associated with high-dose intrathecal chemotherapy.[46,47]

The degree of functional impairment in a spinal cord disorder is related to the level of the lesion and to its degree of completeness. The level of a lesion is, by American convention, the last fully functional spinal root level. For example, a C-5 (cervical root 5) quadriplegic has intact function of the biceps brachii (innervated primarily by C-5 and C-6), with intact sensation over the shoulders and lateral aspects of the arms. A C-5 quadriplegic is able to bring the hand to the mouth but will require assistance for most self-care. A level of C-4 is required for unassisted breathing. C-6 quadriplegics will

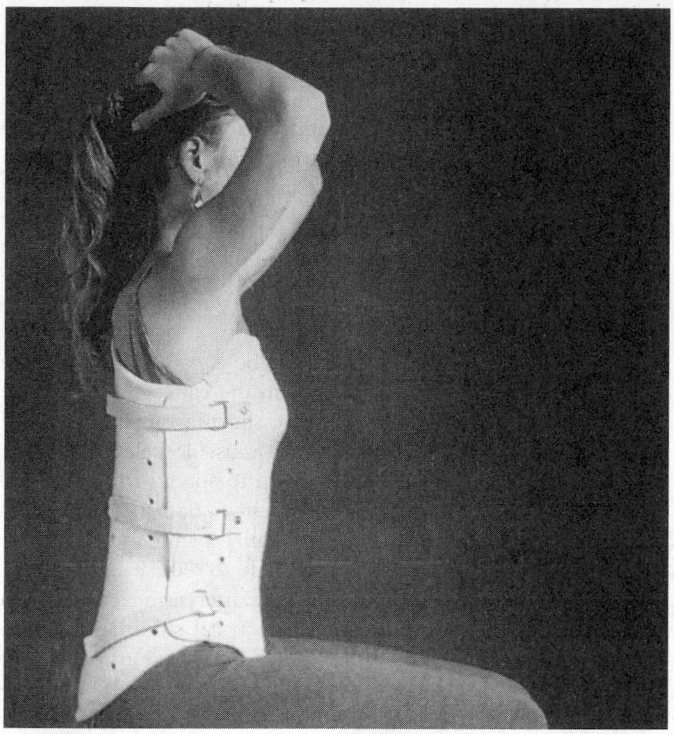

FIGURE 57-4. Body jacket for thoracic support and triplanar movement control.

have intact wrist extension, allowing some light grasp through the tenodesis effect. C-7 quadriplegics are able to extend the elbows, making it possible for them to lift themselves, performing their own weight shifts. C-8 and T-1 are required for intact hand function.

The remaining thoracic segments are of significance primarily in the motor control of trunk stability. In the lower spine, the degree of functional use of the legs is more vague, due to the extensive overlap of motor segments. Generally, hip and knee extensor strength of sufficient magnitude to overcome gravity (3/5) is essential for safe ambulation. Although long leg braces can be used for paraplegic ambulation, the level of energy required is usually beyond the capability of many healthy persons, let alone the patient debilitated by cancer. Short leg braces, or ankle-foot orthoses (AFOs) can be used effectively to compensate for the loss of ankle dorsiflexors and plantar flexors. In selected patients with intact hip musculature, AFOs that limit dorsiflexion can be used to create an extension moment at the knee, substituting for quadriceps function during the stance phase of gait.

Damage of the central portion of the spinal cord may occur, with the outer portions being spared. This may occur with intramedullary tumors, with syrinx formation, or in certain vascular events. The central cord syndrome is characterized by loss of upper extremity function, with relative sparing of function in the legs. If only one side of the spinal cord is involved, the Brown-Sequard syndrome results, in which motor function is affected on the ipsilateral side while most sensory function is affected on the contralateral side.

Because of the complexities involved with spinal cord dysfunction, rehabilitation should be provided by those familiar with management of spinal cord injury. Assisted mobility using manual or motorized wheelchairs or crutches or canes with braces will usually be required. Adaptive equipment and strategies for self-care may be needed in the cancer patient with spinal cord involvement.

Bowel and bladder dysfunction in this patient population is virtually universal, requiring particular attention. Even in the patient with apparent normal voiding, silent bladder and sphincter spasticity may lead to infection, bladder reflux, and significant morbidity. We have seen cases of hydronephrosis with almost complete destruction of the kidneys in asymptomatic persons. Foley catheters may be used for short-term management if there are other medical indications. Otherwise, intermittent catheterization done frequently enough to keep the bladder volume at less than 500 mL is the method of choice during the acute phase. A urologist should be consulted after the patient has stabilized. Regular use of laxatives as part of a bowel-training program is frequently required.

Autonomic dysreflexia or hyperreflexia is a true emergency in the spinal cord–impaired patient. When the spinal cord level is T-6 or above, uncontrolled vasoconstriction and severe hypertension may result. Paradoxically, the heart rate is often slowed, due to the intact vagus nerve. The first objective should be to lower the blood pressure as quickly as possible. Sitting the patient upright will help to reduce intracerebral pressure. A fast-acting agent, such as sublingual nifedipine, may be used initially, followed by a longer-acting agent, such as nitroprusside, if needed. After the blood pressure has been stabilized, the cause—usually a noxious stimulus—should be isolated and corrected. The most common cause is an overdistended bladder, and distended bowel and skin trauma are other possible explanations.

NEUROPATHIES AND PLEXOPATHIES

Peripheral nerve involvement is a common diagnostic dilemma in the cancer patient. Dysfunction of peripheral nerves usually results from the use of cisplatin or vincristine and irradiation.[48–50] Peripheral neuropathies and plexopathies can also be the result of direct tumor invasion or a paraneoplastic syndrome.

CHEMOTHERAPY-INDUCED NEUROPATHIES

Generally chemotherapy-related neuropathies tend to be distal and symmetric. Occasionally, initial symptoms are unilateral, mimicking a mononeuritis or invasive lesion. Vincristine and cisplatin are documented causes of autonomic neuropathies.[51,52] In some instances, this has been severe enough to mimic spinal cord involvement.[53] Cytarabine has caused brachial plexus neuropathy.[54] Suramin, largely an experimental drug, has caused a profound polyneuropathy, mimicking Guillain-Barré syndrome. Agents that are lipid-soluble or that have metabolites with a prolonged half-life may lead to a progressive neuropathy, even after discontinuance of the drug.[55]

Vincristine seems to induce distal axonal degeneration similar to that of other toxic neuropathies.[48] Because of this, the duration of the neuropathy tends to be prolonged because of the time needed for nerve fiber regeneration. Many patients receiving this agent develop sensory complaints of numbness and paresthesias. Some patients develop severe neuropathic pain. Often, the degree of motor neuropathy is significant, sometimes resulting in a virtual quadriparesis. Although it may take months after cessation of chemotherapy to recover function, recovery is usually complete. Neurotoxicity is one of the most common reasons for limiting the dosage of vincristine chemotherapy.

Neuropathies due to cisplatin generally tend to be less frequent and often milder. We have treated several patients who have developed a severe permanent neuropathy from the use of cisplatin. There does not seem to be any common factor that can be used to predict the development of lasting neuropathy. Rarely is an adjustment in cisplatin dosage indicated.[49]

BRACHIAL PLEXOPATHIES

Radiation-induced brachial plexopathy is an uncommon problem in the conservative management of breast cancer if supraclavicular and axillary lymph nodes are irradiated. It may be seen as a late effect of mantle irradiation for Hodgkin's disease. Onset of symptoms is usually delayed. In one study, symptoms began more than 1 year after therapy, and the overall prognosis for recovery was poor.[56]

Differentiation of radiation from neoplastic plexitis is essential. Severe pain has been documented in 80% of patients with infiltrating tumor, but only 19% of patients with radiation injury described this finding.[57] Horner's syndrome is more common in cases of tumor involvement, and lymphedema is a much more common concomitant finding in radiation injury. The distribution of involvement of the brachial plexus is an important diagnostic criterion, with 72% of patients with invasive tumor having involvement of the lower trunk and 78% of patients with radiation injury having involvement of the upper trunk.

Electrodiagnostically, myokymic discharges are virtually diagnostic of radiation plexitis, occurring in 63% of patients.[58] Other abnormalities are common in both types of injury, with nerve conduction studies being of limited usefulness.[59] Tumor detection by magnetic resonance imaging (MRI) provides definitive evidence of neoplastic involvement. Even without visible tumor during surgery, neoplastic disease has sometimes been found microscopically, and it may not be possible to rule out neoplastic plexopathy for many months after the onset of symptoms.[60,61]

LUMBOSACRAL PLEXOPATHY AND RADICULOPATHY

Involvement of the lumbosacral plexus is common in pelvic tumors due to direct invasion.[62] In a study of 11 patients with lumbosacral plexopathy, 6 had metastatic involvement, 2 had radiation-induced plexopathy, 1 had a primary tumor, and 2 had neuritis due to intraarterial chemotherapy.[63] Direct imaging of tumor with CT or MRI may be difficult after irradiation or surgery. We have seen a preponderance of delayed painful plexopathy in patients receiving intraoperative radiation. It is important to attempt to differentiate plexus lesions from those of the spinal cord, due to the difference in treatment, rehabilitation management, and prognosis.

Neuropathic pain is commonly seen with peripheral neuropathies. Loss of sensation may render the patient susceptible to skin injury. The patient with insensate skin should be cautioned about the avoidance of potential injuries from burns and sharp objects and about the need for daily skin inspection to avoid the development of infection. Loss of proprioceptive feedback, particularly in the patient with impaired vision, may interfere with simple fine-motor tasks and with ambulation. A cane can provide proprioceptive feedback to the upper extremities in the patient with impaired proprioception in the lower extremities. Motor impairment is treated similarly to other neurologic disorders, with bracing and adaptive devices as needed.

In addition to the use of narcotic agents, which has become the mainstay of palliative treatment in the cancer patient, the physical modalities of pain control may significantly help to alleviate suffering. More aggressive approaches, including nerve blocks and rhizotomies, have been used with limited success. Sympathetic nerve blocks and sympathectomies may be effective in patients with the reflex sympathetic dystrophy syndrome. Trigger point injections are also sometimes helpful in musculoskeletal pain disorders.

The use of physical modalities can be a particularly effective adjunct in the management of pain in the cancer patient. Heat modalities, including superficial heat, shortwave diathermy, and ultrasonography, may provide relief in musculoskeletal pain syndromes, but ultrasonography may help to spread lymphatic disease. Other heat modalities increase circulation to the affected area, questionably increasing the potential for metastatic spread. Therapeutic cold can also sometimes help to reduce pain.

Electrical stimulation has met with increasing criticism in the literature, but we have found electrical stimulation to be effective in reducing narcotics usage in a variety of cancer patients with a variety of pain syndromes. It seems to be particularly effective in the management of phantom limb pain and in treating radiculopathy and incisional pain. If effective, the patient can be provided with a pocket-sized transcutaneous electrical nerve stimulation (TENS) unit, which can be used as needed. Electrodes should be placed at the site of maximum pain or, in the case of referred pain, at the site of the lesion. A conventional high-frequency setting is usually most effective. Many TENS units are available at modest cost. Progressive muscle relaxation has also been reported to be useful.

LYMPHEDEMA AND DEEP VENOUS THROMBOSIS

The swollen extremity is often a diagnostic dilemma in the patient with a history of cancer. Because of the possibility of malignant compression or invasion of lymphatics or venous drainage, and because of the possibility of deep venous thrombosis, a swollen extremity should always be fully evaluated in the cancer patient or cancer survivor. Idiopathic lymphedema, rather than edema secondarily caused by infection or tumor, should be a diagnosis of exclusion. Tumor can usually be excluded by imaging studies, such as CT, MRI, or bone scan or, in extreme instances, by lymphangiogram.

Deep venous thrombosis can usually be ruled out using impedance plethysmography or ultrasonography.[64,65] If certainty is required, a venogram can be performed. Suspected pulmonary embolism can be evaluated with a ventilation-perfusion scan or, more definitively, by pulmonary angiography. The greatest risk of embolization is from proximal thromboses.

Lymphedema in the cancer patient is frequent, with lymph node involvement or after lymph node dissection. Late edema is usually related to radiotherapy and the gradual development of fibrous tissue and change in the protein content of the fluid. Edema in a nonirradiated extremity should always be thoroughly evaluated, and remediable causes, such as infection or cardiovascular causes, should be treated.

The simplest means of minimizing edema is to keep the affected extremity elevated as much as possible. Legs should be placed on an elevated foot support, preferably keeping the feet above the level of the heart. Arms should be rested on a high table surface. A sling may be of short-term benefit. Isometric exercises, by increasing muscle tone, may help to minimize edema.

The management of lymphedema varies from treatment center to treatment center and from country to country. Rehabilitative therapies have typically included education about limb position to minimize gravity, use of massage, exercise to enhance lymph flow and maintain mobility, and the use of pneumatic compression devices and compression garments to reduce lymphedema in the involved extremity. Because of a better understanding in the anatomy, physiology, and pathophysiology of the lymphatic system, a combination of techniques has evolved to manage lymphedema better.[66]

Manual lymph drainage (MLD)[67] is a specialized massage technique based on the concept of emptying the central regions first, to give the lymph from the periphery somewhere to go.[68,69] The lymph is moved proximally and, across lymphatic watersheds, into the nearest normally drained lymphotomes. The proximal region of the limb is always cleaned first, then the massage is extended distally; effleurage that starts at the distal end and attempts to push the lymph into the unemptied, proximal regions is ineffective.[70]

After MLD, some treatment centers will continue lymph drainage with the use of a sequential pneumatic compression device. Other centers will follow MLD immediately with compression bandaging, using the low-elastic Comprilan (Beiersdorf, Germany) applied over padding (Artiflex Soft, Beiersdorf, Germany) and an undergauze (Tricofix, Beiersdorf, Germany).[70] Once the compression bandages have been applied to the extremity, special exercises are performed to supplement the effects of the MLD.

The frequency and duration of the foregoing techniques vary from treatment center to treatment center. However, the greatest reduction in lymphedema usually occurs within the first week of treatment (when the treatment is provided by a highly trained and skilled PT). Just before discharge from the treatment program, the extremity is fitted with a compression garment to maintain the reduction in lymphedema. An example of a wrapped upper extremity in presented in Figure 57-5. The National Lymphedema Network located in San Francisco has a list of manual lymphatic drainage therapists and treatment centers throughout the United States.

BOWEL AND BLADDER DISORDERS

Bowel obstruction or ureteral or urethral compromise is usually the result of malignant invasion or spinal cord or nerve root compression. Constipation and urinary hesitancy are frequently related to the use of medication, particularly narcotics and drugs with anticholinergic properties. Input from the rehabilitation team is most often needed if there is neurologic dysfunction or in ostomy care.

MANAGEMENT OF BOWEL DYSFUNCTION

Disorders of fecal elimination are frequently the most significant complaint of the cancer patient. Constipation is extremely common and is best treated using dietary modifications and medication. Often, a high-fiber diet with copious fluid intake will be all that is required to ensure regularity. If fiber supplements are used, the patient should be cautioned about the absolute need for fluid intake, because bulk in the absence of fluid can lead to impaction. If necessary, stool softeners (e.g., docusate sodium, 50 to 200 mg/d) can be added to reduce straining. A stimulant medication (e.g., metoclopramide hydrochloride, 10 mg 30 minutes before meals and at bedtime) can be used for delayed gastric emptying.

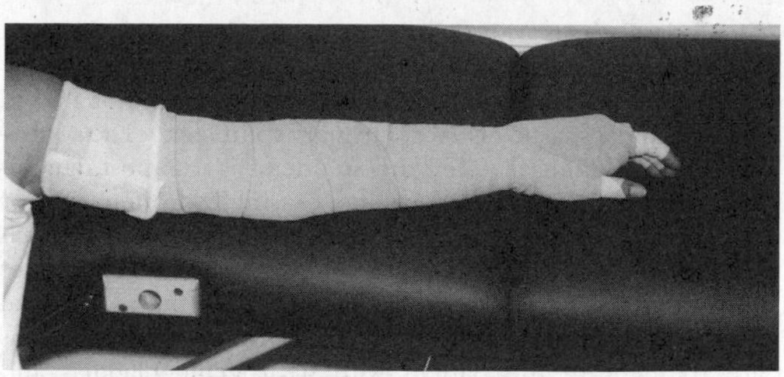

FIGURE 57-5. Wraps to reduce limb edema.

When spontaneous defecation does not occur, a stimulant agent may be required. A mild preparation with a well-controlled transit time, such as an over-the-counter senna preparation, is preferred. A standard dose of senna (e.g., Senokot, two tablets) at bedtime usually results in controlled defecation in the morning. Stronger agents, such as bisacodyl (5 to 15 mg) or magnesium hydroxide (milk of magnesia, 30 mL) may be used in more recalcitrant cases, although it should be kept in mind that magnesium is mildly nephrotoxic. Such cathartics as magnesium citrate should be used as a last resort and only if there is no suspicion of obstruction or impaction.

In the patient with neurogenic bowel dysfunction, stimulation from below may be required. Digital stimulation or, if needed, use of a glycerin or bisacodyl (10 mg) suppository should usually be sufficient to initiate evacuation. Rarely, an enema may be required. By instituting a regular bowel-training program in which full evacuation is achieved on a daily or every-other-day basis through the use of medications and rectal stimulation, it is usually possible to achieve continence.

Diarrhea in the cancer patient is usually the result of chemotherapy. Standard antidiarrheal preparations, narcotics, and anticholinergics may be used. If diarrhea occurs in the face of antibiotics, pseudomembranous colitis resulting from infection with *Clostridium difficile* should always be ruled out. Other bacterial or parasitic diarrhea should be treated with appropriate antibiotics, as determined by stool culture or smear. Narcotic antidiarrheal agents should be avoided in this case due to the potential for toxic megacolon development. Viral diarrhea should generally be allowed to run its course.

MANAGEMENT OF THE NEUROGENIC BLADDER

Proper evaluation and management of bladder dysfunction in cancer patients with neurologic abnormalities is essential to prevent significant morbidity. Although bladder dysfunction is often arbitrarily divided into disorders of incontinence or reduced bladder capacity and disorders of retention, this model is overly simplistic. Patients with spinal cord or brain stem involvement should always undergo formal evaluation of bladder function.

There may be various combinations of a spastic or flaccid bladder and a spastic or flaccid urinary sphincter.[71] The combination of a spastic bladder and sphincter is the most dangerous, because this can lead to reflux, causing hydronephrosis or upper tract infection or to autonomic hyperreflexia. Such medications as oxybutynin chloride, 5 mg two to four times daily, can be used to reduce bladder spasticity, but mechanical means of drainage may be needed.[72] Urinary tract infections are frequent in the patient with neurogenic bladder, and proper evaluation and treatment are mandatory.

In the acute phase of management, an indwelling catheter is usually sufficient if there are appropriate medical indications. Catheters should be removed as soon as the patient is stable, so as to minimize the risk of infection. In the patient who appears to be voiding normally, evaluation for possible retention should still be done. Postvoiding residual urine volumes as determined by catheterization or by ultrasonography should be less than 50 mL. If the patient does exhibit retention, intermittent catheterization should be instituted, taking care to catheterize frequently enough to keep bladder volumes at less than 500 mL. In the incontinent patient without retention, condom (Texas) catheters may be used for men. Collection devices for females are often less than satisfactory.

MANAGEMENT OF THE OSTOMY PATIENT

Cancer patients may have ostomies for a variety of reasons. Ureteral stints are often used in patients with ureteral obstruction, occasionally in combination with a temporary ostomy for kidney drainage. Patients with bladder carcinoma may have a ureteral diversion to an ileal loop, which is drained through an ostomy. Patients with bowel carcinoma or other types of bowel obstruction may need a temporary or permanent ostomy for fecal elimination. This may be required at any level of the small bowel or colon. Ileostomies, involving diversion of the terminal small bowel, are sometimes problematic because of the volume of fluid present in the fecal contents before entry into the colon. An ileal pouch is sometimes created surgically as a reservoir for urine or ileal fluid as a means of providing continence.

In cases of neck tumors or if there is impaired swallowing, a gastrostomy may be required for supplemental nutrition. This can often be placed by percutaneous endoscopic gastrostomy, eliminating the need for major surgery. Tracheostomies are often used in cases of head or neck tumors or if there is a need for prolonged access to the airway, as in the patient with severe cognitive impairment and uncontrolled tracheal secretions.

Ostomy training should be a regular part of the cancer patient's rehabilitation process.[73] Proper cleaning technique avoids the likelihood of infection. Proper attention to skin care should avoid maceration and breakdown. Occasionally, a bowel-training program can be instituted for colostomy patients, regularizing emptying and sometimes eliminating the need for an ostomy bag. A variety of ostomy collection systems are available, including one-piece collection bags, applied directly to the skin using an adhesive, and two-piece collection bags involving an occlusive seal that is applied to the skin and a separate detachable bag.[74] Collection bags may be closed and disposed of with each use or may be open, allowing for drainage and reuse. One- and two-piece barriers may be used to help patients to maintain continence. Support groups for ostomy patients are available in most areas, and a variety of patient information materials are available.[75–77]

PSYCHOSOCIAL ASPECTS OF CANCER REHABILITATION

Accommodating to change in daily performance, to loss of function, and to modifications in life style that accompany the diagnosis and treatment of cancer has relevance for all individuals. However, life management goals vary widely and may be influenced by each individual's values, stage in life and phase of disease, life experiences, and temperament. The challenge facing oncologists is identifying and addressing unique psychosocial reactions presented by the patient during all stages of oncologic management, including the terminal phase.

Table 57-8 summarizes some common emotional reactions to oncologic illness as they may be manifested during different stages of treatment. Also included are intervention approaches. Pivotal in medical and rehabilitation intervention is interdisciplinary management of these reactions to facilitate mastery of the long-term impact of cancer on function. With proper management, the likelihood of developing handicapping conditions and of impairing quality of life is decreased.

REHABILITATION AND MANAGEMENT OF SPECIFIC TUMORS

SARCOMA OF THE EXTREMITIES

Ablative extremity surgery (amputation), formerly the treatment of choice for local control of sarcomas, has been replaced by limb-sparing surgery in the majority of cases.[78,79] Since clinical trials indicate no benefit from amputation in overall survival rate in selected cases[80,81] and function and desirability favor limb preservation in many, limb-sparing surgery has become more prevalent.

Clinical trials have shown reduction of local tumor reoccurrence in soft tissue sarcomas (STS)[82–84] with preoperative and postoperative radiotherapy treatments and brachytherapy and of distal metastatic disease in osteosarcoma (OS)[85] with the use of preoperative and postoperative adjuvant chemotherapeutic regimens. Limb perfusion has reduced tumor size even when advanced, to permit limb-sparing surgery.[86] For those in whom there was still no option for limb-sparing surgery, a reduction in tumor size is often associated with palliation of pain and better cosmesis.

Tumor size, pathologic type, and adequacy of excision remain the main predictors of local control. Tumor location, involvement of neurologic tissue, and size often are the better predictors of function.

In recent years, the chance for better functional outcome in limb-spared patients has resulted from (1) refined surgical interventions (abandonment of origin-to-insertion whole-muscle group excision in favor of partial group excisions); (2) use of endoprostheses and bone allografts, muscle transfers, and sophisticated soft tissue reconstructive procedures; (3) refined radiotherapy

TABLE 57-8. Psychosocial Aspects of Cancer Rehabilitation

Psychosocial Aspect	*Diagnosis, Staging*	*E*	*I*	*L*	*T*	*Recommendations for Oncologic Management*	*Rehabilitation Intervention*
Denial	X				X	Show acceptance; allow denial system to operate	Expand self-protection strategies, build coping strategies
Anxiety, fear	X	X	X			Acknowledge control needs; foster realistic expectations; discuss genetic transmission	Teach relaxation and exercise, increase sense of control, use adaptive aids, orient to reality
Negative body image	X	X				Anticipate changes in body and image; recommend adapting fashion	Recommend prosthetic and cosmetic choices, suggest wig and stylish-adapted clothing
Grief, death and dying	X				X	Encourage self-expression; enable reconciliation to loss	Provide expressive groups, legacy building, gift giving, life review, supportive interaction
Depression, low self-esteem	X			X	X	Ensure safety; inspire hope; point out advances in medicine; acknowledge small gains	Develop support system; suggest lifestyle changes, foster motivation; structure time to include exercise, leisure education, and counseling
Frustration and anger	X	X	X	X	X	Acknowledge frustration and identify anger; offer possible solutions	Analyze tasks to allow enough time to complete, encourage expression of feelings; plan releases
Dependency		X				Encourage self-responsibility	Foster independence in tasks, increase task complexity
Resistance and maladaptation	X	X	X	X	X	Acknowledge resilient behaviors; anticipate changes in function	Provide challenges with unplanned activity; set realistic expectations, small goals; adapt self, environment, and tasks; clarify values and roles; foster community reintegration

E, early stage; I, intermediate stage; L, late stage; T, terminal stage.

procedures (abandonment of full-dose radiotherapy to the entire port in favor of advanced simulation techniques), which permit a cone-down high dose to the direct tumor site and lower doses to the rest of the port, with corrections also made to reduce dose and scatter to joints; and (4) the development of specific rehabilitation programs to follow up the limb-spared patient throughout the trajectory of the disease process.

In some patients, amputations are still needed. These tend to occur for large tumors involving other critical structures in which resection would result in poor functional outcome or poor local control. Often, these are high-level amputations. Amputation also occurs more often for hand and foot tumors where there is little leeway to obtain an adequate excision without severely compromising function. However, more sophisticated reconstructive procedures have recently been reported to salvage the hand and thumb.[87,88] Children younger than 13 years with OS are too young for limb-sparing procedures using endoprostheses. Other procedures may be used in some cases.

Functional deficits, impairments, and symptoms from limb-sparing surgery result from (1) the local procedure itself (depending on the extent of the resection and resection of adjacent structures, such as nerves and vessels); (2) adjuvant therapy (chemotherapy, radiotherapy, and limb perfusion); (3) the effects of local reoccurrence and distal metastasis; and (4) premorbid patient characteristics.

Specific impairments and symptoms include pain, edema, fatigue, reduced strength and joint motion, stress, and depression. Functional deficits occur in the areas of mobility; ADL; vocational, social, and sexual adjustment; and recreation and leisure.

Rehabilitation plays a major role in assessing the person's potential for limb sparing, predicting their functional outcome after the procedure, maximizing their function by treating their impairments and symptoms, and educating them in the proper care of their spared or amputated limb to prevent complications and encourage preservation and coping strategies related to impairment and handicap. Rehabilitation interventions should occur over the trajectory of the patient's life span as new problems emerge in different disease phases.

Role of Rehabilitation

Resection may involve partial muscle group removal, muscle transfer, and bony replacement by endoprosthesis or allograft (and less often, vessel and nerve removal). The surgeon predicts which structures will need to be removed for an adequate tumor excision. Based on the extent of the planned surgery, the physiatrist anticipates the level of function of the limb after surgery. Both surgeon and physiatrist discuss and concur on this prediction. A judgment is then made whether this would be acceptable function for the patient. A comparison of functional outcome resulting from amputation and limb sparing should be made before treatment selection. These discussions should be shared with affected patients before a treatment choice is selected, should be the best from such patients' perspective, and should be supportive of their needs.

For adequate function, the limb may need some permanent postoperative bracing or splinting. These are usually needed if there has been sacrifice of a key nerve or muscle. The patient should be informed preoperatively that these adjunctive devices may be necessary for independent functioning. Special age, wear, and fracture risk considerations take place if an endoprosthesis is used. In OS, usually a longer endoprosthesis must be placed, rendering the spared limb longer for patients aged 15 to 17 years. This compensates for growth arrest in the operative limb. A major growth plate may need to be stapled on the normal side in OS if the limb grows disproportionately and exceeds the affected side by more than 2 cm. A heel lift of up to 1 inch may be used if the endoprosthetic side is shorter than on the normal leg. Endoprosthetic loosening may occur, depending on the amount of wear and tear from activities, but endoprostheses can last up to 10 years. For long-term survivors, endoprosthetic replacement will be needed. There is generally a limit of two to three replacement reconstructions. Reconstructions are also necessary for prosthetic dislocation, bone fracture, and loosening. Removal of the prosthesis is often necessary for serious bony infection. Infections with some organisms (*Staphylococcus epidermidis*) have been successfully treated with 3 months of appropriate intravenous antibiotics.[89] Therefore, some patients who initially underwent limb-sparing procedures will need amputations later in their life. They need to be aware of the possibility of these problems preoperatively when choosing a limb-sparing surgery.

If the patient needs an amputation, the physiatrist should evaluate the patient preoperatively and recommend the most functional level. A very short above-knee amputation (AKA) can be fitted with a prosthesis and is much more functional and energy-efficient than a hip disarticulation. In some cases, a hip disarticulation can be converted to a short AKA by use of a custom-made short femoral endoprosthesis. A short below-elbow and below-knee amputation can be fitted appropriately with a prosthesis and is much more functional than its counterpart (above-elbow and AKA).

Treatment during Phases of Disease

INITIAL PHASE. Rehabilitation interventions begin preoperatively with instruction about crutch usage. The type of interventions and the rate at which rehabilitation progresses depend on a number of factors. Although general statements can be made about how a patient progresses, each resection is somewhat different, and the treatment plan and progression of treatment are individualized to each patient. Progression and intensity of rehabilitation are slower for bony reconstructive procedures.[90,91]

POSTSURGICAL PHASE. Postoperatively, the patient is reevaluated for level of pain, fatigue, stress, motivation, muscle strength, and joint motion. In general for STS patients, early treatment begins with correct positioning in bed to facilitate lymph drainage; a posterior splint or sling may be needed. Passive ROM by a PT or OT therapist is performed for joints distal to the resection and, in other joints, active motion is performed by the patient. On day 2, the patient is allowed to transfer out of bed with assistance and sit in a chair with proper limb positioning. For lower limb procedures, non–weight-bearing gait with crutches or a walker and posterior knee splint are initiated; if the upper extremity is the operative site, an appropriate sling or splint is used. The patient engages in active ROM of joints distal to the surgery. As drainage decreases and the drain is removed, gait progresses with toe touch and partial weight bearing. The joint near the surgical procedure receives active assistive ROM with the PT or OT therapist. Arc of motion is increased as the wound heals. Assessment of wound healing is made before ROM progression. When the staples are removed at around 14 days, the patient should be fully weight bearing and can come off crutches in a week.

Special procedures, such as the Tinkoff-Lindberg procedure for shoulder STS, require extensive soft tissue reconstruction and an endoprosthesis. The rehabilitation course is slower and similar to that of resections for proximal humeral OS tumors. The functional outcome is also the same.

Early rehabilitation for bony reconstruction is usually performed for OS but has a longer postoperative rehabilitation course, and the progression of treatment is highly dependent on the type and extent of the excision. Any complications that occur postoperatively alter the progression of rehabilitation. Two of the complications that occur are skin breakdown at the initial closure site and soft tissue or joint infection. The former often requires reoperation for closure or skin grafting (or both), and the latter requires intravenous antibiotic therapy and sometimes endoprosthesis removal. During these complications, rehabilitation is often put on hold and restarted when appropriate.

If no complications occur, patients with humeral excisions can be given passive hand ROM on day 2 and actively use their hand 2 weeks postoperatively. Passive ROM is performed on the elbow for 3 weeks postoperatively. Patients usually lack approximately 40 degrees of extension. Use of moist heat over the elbow followed by gentle stretching can be started at approximately 4 weeks after the reconstructive procedure involving the shoulder if the wound is sufficiently healed and can withstand the tension of biceps lengthening. The therapist performs progressive passive ROM of the shoulder beginning with 20 degrees flexion-extension, then adding abduction and internal-external rotation. Close contact with the surgeon is maintained in increasing the degree of ROM. Usually, passive ROM in abduction and internal-external ROM attained is approximately 60 degrees. Active ROM is not expected to be functional.

Patients with distal femoral endoprosthetic replacements generally wear a knee immobilizer for 3 weeks. The therapist performs passive ROM of distal joints. The therapist is allowed to perform limited-arc passive knee ROM of the involved joint between 2 to 3 weeks, carefully observing the wound closure for any signs of potential breakdown from increased tension with ROM. When the sutures are removed, active assistive ROM is performed, and the ROM arc is gradually increased. The patient should be able to perform some isometric exercise in the immobilizer on day 3 and begin active ROM at 1 month. Quadriceps strengthening to improve knee biomechanics is very important. Exercise intensity is advanced with addition of some isotonic light weight at 6 weeks. From a mobility point of view, patients walk with crutches and immobilizer and are non–weight bearing from days 4 to 10. Gradual weight bearing starts then with toe touching and progresses to tolerance, while monitoring pain and looking for development of any knee effusion. Usually, weight-bearing status is decreased if the latter occurs. By 2 to 3 months, when the quadriceps is sufficiently strengthened to support the knee and affected patients have no complications, they ambulate with a cane. Independent ambulation without a cane occurs anywhere from 3 to 4 months postoperatively.

Patients with proximal tibial resections have a slower course. One main reason for this is that the surgical procedure requires quadriceps reconstruction with a gastrocnemius flap and reattachment of the quadriceps mechanism to the metal endoprosthesis. Healing of the reconstruction takes longer. The limb is elevated for 10 days. Quadriceps isometrics are started on day 2. ROM and weight bearing are introduced at a slower pace. The patient wears a bivalved cast for a month. Knee ROM begins when the cast is removed. Active motion exercise starts when the patient is able to extend the knee. Often, the patient wears a long leg brace for an additional 2 months, which allows 30 degrees of flexion. Full weight bearing with a cane is not expected before 4 to 5 months. The quadriceps mechanism is initially weaker than with the distal femoral procedure, due to the quadriceps reconstruction. A more significant knee extension lag can occur. More intensive quadriceps strengthening is needed to help to reduce knee extension lag, allow for active knee extension, and ensure safe gait. Final functional outcomes are pain-free, independent ambulation without a cane and ADL around 6 to 8 months.

Early rehabilitation for amputees begins with fitting the residual limb with an immediate postoperative cast in the operating room. This is achieved for above-elbow amputation, below-elbow amputation, AKA, and below-knee amputation levels. The purpose is to shape the residual limb and to reduce pain and edema.

High-level amputees, or hemipelvectomies, may have considerable phantom pain because of surgical severance of large nerve trunks. Often, reduction of edema by elastic compression on manual drainage, use of TENS, and pharmacologic interventions help with pain reduction.

In most centers where limb-sparing surgeries are performed, the patient's function is evaluated at intervals to document clinical progress and to follow function in drug trials. Patients are followed up long term for 10 to 15 years and are often evaluated at 6-month intervals the first 3 to 5 years and yearly thereafter. If they are disease-free at 10 to 15 years, they are usually discharged.

Functional assessments include objective measures of strength (manual muscle test), ROM (goniometer), edema, and pain and fatigue by visual analog scales. A functional questionnaire may be used for determining level of participation in ADL and use of assistive devices and to identify psychosocial and vocational problems. A cancer-specific questionnaire is the Cancer Rehabilitation Evaluation Systems.[5] A combined physical evaluation and patient questionnaire for assessing function of OS patients is the Enneking or Musculoskeletal Tumor Society Rating Scale.[92] A recent questionnaire, the Toronto Extremity Salvage Score, was developed and validated for both STS and OS patients.[93] Patients with STS and OS may also be assessed from a biomechanical standpoint in motion analysis laboratories looking at velocity, stride length, and substitutive gait patterns.

Patients with STS who undergo wide local excision generally have satisfactory to excellent functional outcomes because one of the criteria for surgery is predicted satisfactory outcome. The specific outcome depends on the extent of the excision and adjacent structures and postoperative complications.[94,95]

Patients are generally independent either with or without assistive devices and braces. Some patients may need a change in vocational status. OS limb-spared patients generally have good to excellent function, as judged by the Enneking Assessment and Gait Analysis.[96] Some, however, fall into the poor to fair categories. Gait analysis reveals that such patients may have slower cadence and uneven stride lengths. They often use substitutive muscle strategies.[97] These vary widely. For instance, in the presence of a weak quadriceps, such patients strike their toe first on stance rather than heel strike. This creates an extension moment at the knee to help to stabilize it and, therefore, to improve gait safety. Limb-spared procedures require a reconstruction if there is dislocation, fracture at the bone cement interface, serious infection unresponsive to intravenous antibiotics, or worn-out components. Studies of these reconstructions are limited to case reports but indicate good to excellent function.[98]

Amputations are still necessary if limb salvage cannot be performed or if a former limb-sparing procedure cannot be done. Amputation levels for sarcoma (OS and STS) are performed at all levels, depending on tumor site and size. Skip lesions often occur in OS; thus, the amount of bone involved by the primary tumor in these lesions requires a higher amputation level for cure. In comparison to amputations for diabetes and vascular disease, which are usually midlevel below-knee amputations and AKAs, those for sarcomas tend to be high-level procedures (hemipelvectomy, hip disarticulation, high AKAs, short below-elbow amputations, and forequarters). Prosthetic fitting in these cases is more difficult. Achieved functional level and compliance with use of some prosthesis, as hemipelvectomies, is low, and energy requirements for use are higher. Forequarter prostheses are rarely functional and often not used.

In general, amputees are usually independent in mobility and ADL with or without crutches. Vocational status often needs to be changed. Phantom pain may interfere with function and needs to be treated.

The function of limb-spared patients versus amputees has been addressed. Some amputees may be more functional than limb-spared patients and vice versa. Since some prosthetic limbs are durable, participation in contact sports, running, high-impact dances, tennis, and golf are no problem. However, amputees with cosmetic limbs, humeral OS or lower limb sparing, should have more restriction in sport activities. Limited sport may be needed to preserve endoprostheses. However, an upper extremity Tinkoff-Lindberg procedure for humeral OS is much more functional than a forequarter amputation.

Pain. Management of pain postoperatively is essential. Pharmacologic management with narcotics is essential in the first postoperative week. Rehabilitation treatments begin with proper limb positioning to reduce edema and avoid contracture. Immobilization of operative sites using splints and use of TENS are common adjuncts. Acupuncture may also be useful to reduce pain.

Lymphedema. Edema can cause pain and interfere with function. Significant lymphedema commonly occurs with STS resections involving the adductor and hamstring, anterior compartment muscle groups, and breast sarcoma. This is controlled by proper positioning and the use of a compression garment. With these four excisions, edema is often chronic and needs to be treated long-term with combined modalities of massage, wrapping, and pumping. It can usually be well controlled or reduced. A new technique of nonelastic wrapping has proven very effective in management.[69]

Mobility. OS and STS limb-spared patients have short- and long-term mobility problems.

In the immediate postoperative phase, crutches and walkers are often needed. Often, patients will not need these devices at 6 months. Orthoses are needed after some soft tissue resections to replace lost function. The most common brace used is for knee control after excision of the quadriceps; for ankle control after gastrocnemius with peroneal nerve removal; and for wrist extension after radial nerve or forearm extensor removal. For knee control, an AFO with 5-degree plantar flexion is often used. This creates an extension movement to stabilize the knee. The peroneal nerve brace is a plastic AFO to correct equinovarus of the foot. A cock-up splint is used to maintain wrist extension or a dynamic outrigger brace is used to restore finger extension if the long extensors have been resected.

Below-knee and above-knee and above-elbow and below-elbow amputees are fitted with an immediate postoperative cast, after the suture line is closed, and a temporary pylon and foot are added at day 10 postoperatively for the below-knee and above-knee amputees. A permanent limb is ordered when the residual limb is well shaped and the patient does not have fluid and weight shifts from chemotherapy. If no chemotherapy is involved, a permanent prosthesis is made 6 weeks postoperatively. For chemotherapy patients, this may be delayed by 3 months.

Two main types of prostheses are used: endoskeletal and exoskeletal. Endoskeletal prostheses have an internal metal support system and an external molded, soft skin-color cover. They are more cosmetic and lighter in weight than exoskeletal. However, they will tear when subjected to contact sports or even walking in the woods. They are cosmetically more acceptable to many. Exoskeletal prosthesis have a hard durable shell and can be used for sports activities and are heavier.

New components using graphite for joint components have lessened the weight of prosthesis. The choice of the particular types of components, such as knees and ankles, and strength of cables for an upper extremity prosthesis depend on the activities in which the patient is engaged. Young amputees (common in the case of OS) prefer hydraulic knees that facilitate such activities as dancing and ankles that are flexible, which facilitate push-off in the gait cycle and render gait more propulsive. These are useful for sports activities.

Better form-fitting, more naturally aligned prosthetic sockets are routinely used. More sporty socket suspensions and prostheses are available, including swim legs and adaptations for skiing. Myoelectric upper extremity prostheses with switches are sometimes used but are very expensive. They are more cosmetic, but the hand component can lift only light objects.

Cosmesis. Cosmesis is very important to cancer patients. Wide local excision of STS often causes soft tissue deficits. Some of these can be ameliorated by soft, contoured fillers. Some examples of these are a buttock prosthesis for buttectomies, a gastrocnemius prosthesis, a shoulder prosthesis for forequarter amputations and after the Tinkoff-Lindberg procedure, and a foot prosthesis after partial-ray resection. Breast prostheses made of various materials (gels, fluff, etc.) are used for mastectomies secondary to sarcoma.

Fatigue. Fatigue results from inactivity, the disease itself, depression, and chemotherapy (Adriamycin). Exercise to increase strength and joint motion is an important component in facilitating and maintaining regain of function in limb-spared patients. Often, low-intensity, low-impact aerobic programs are prescribed. Frequently, particular muscles are targeted for exercise (e.g., quadriceps in distal femoral and proximal tibial limb-sparing procedures for OS and partial quadriceps removal for STS). General strengthening and ROM exercises are performed for uninvolved muscles. Isometrics and isotonic strengthening with weights to 2 pounds using a short lever arm are permitted in patients with endoprostheses. Isokinetic machine exercise is not permitted.

Maintaining at least critical joint motion for function is important. It is not necessary that the joint motion be completely normal for adequate function.

Vocational Activity. STS can occur in all age groups, but the median age tends to be midlife and later. This places people in that part of their lives when they are working and supporting families. As a result, some may need to change their vocation, though many remain in their jobs with reasonable accommodation. Some studies have shown individuals with STS often enter into retirement.[99]

OS occurs in children and young adults. Often, they are faced with career choices influenced by their level of physical as well as cognitive abilities. Career counseling is advised.

Recreational Activities. Recreational and social activities are important to cancer patients. Patients with wide local excision often can continue their premorbid recreational and social activities. With resections requiring bracing, some activities are not possible. Patients with STS and radiated bone and OS with endoprostheses must avoid contact sports and activities that cause torquing. In addition, impact activities (running, some dances) are not appropriate for limb-spared OS patients. These more aggressive activities can result in bony fracture, bone-prosthetic interface fracture, endoprosthetic dislocation, and early breakdown of prosthetic components.

Education of the patient about which activities are appropriate is important in preventing complications. Adaptive methods of participating in some sports are appropriate. For instance, modification of stance, position, and swing may reduce torque and allow some lower limb–spared patients to play golf. Doubles tennis played at less aggressive levels may also be appropriate. A young teen going to the prom can dance but needs to avoid torquing and high-impact dances.

LONG-TERM CARE PHASE. Limb-spared patients have had decreased morbidity, owing to appropriate adjunctive chemotherapeutic and radiotherapy regimens and defined and innovative surgical techniques. Limb-spared patients should be followed up from a rehabilitation standpoint to ensure that they are not developing any long-term radiotherapy problems (motion loss, radiculopathy, and cord syndromes) that would decrease function. Any new development of pain should signal local reoccurrence or fracture at the endoprosthetic junction. Amputees generally need new prostheses every 4 to 5 years, depending on level of use.

Special problem areas that arise in this treatment phase include adjustment to disability and vocational change and recreational, social, and schooling issues. The important goal is to maintain function.

METASTATIC DISEASE AND LOCAL RECURRENCE PHASE. When metastases occur with OS, they are most commonly to the lung or other bones. Often, it is a single metastasis or a few, possibly amenable to local resections. With STS, lung metastases occur. Patients may have multiple surgical procedures over time, usually a median sternotomy or thoracotomy with pleura and chest wall resections. A newer procedure allows for removal of lung metastases without major chest surgery. Chemotherapy is reintroduced after the local chest resection. These surgical treatment interventions often are associated with postoperative chest pain. The patients may become deconditioned and experience fatigue, anxiety, and weight loss during these treatment periods and may require rehabilitation interventions much as they did in the initial phase. Vocational and educational endeavors are disrupted. Rehabilitation strategies to relieve postoperative pain (TENS) and reduce fatigue (assistive devices, energy conservation techniques) and anxiety (stress management, relaxation techniques, and imagery) are helpful. Referral to a dietitian is made to support good nutrition.

When metastases return and are inoperable, experimental chemotherapy regimens are used. Often, these have low success rates and high toxicities. Likewise, local reoccurrence may happen, particularly with STS. These also require additional therapies. At this stage, emotional support, comfort, and education about problem solving to promote and preserve independence can be provided by the rehabilitation team.

MELANOMA

In advanced or recurrent melanoma, oncologists have reported the efficacy of isolated limb perfusion with various chemotherapeutic agents (e.g., melphalan) and biologic response modifiers (e.g., tumor necrosis factor and interferon) where mild to moderate limb toxicity has been reported.[100] Complications resulting from these procedures include transient peripheral neuropathy, edema, skin breakdown, and vascular compromise with tissue necrosis. As a result of these complications, rehabilitation of these patients is often protracted and requires careful daily monitoring of the skin for areas of pressure combined with an active program of exercises and progressive ambulation. Management of edema, using compression garments and inelastic wraps, may be achieved for symptom relief and control. Amputation rarely must be performed to treat complications of limb perfusion. Prosthetic fitting and training may be undertaken.

LUNG CANCER

Lung cancer patients may benefit from rehabilitation interventions addressing pain control, cardiopulmonary conditioning, and work and home modifications. Rehabilitation of the patient with lung cancer is generally divided into a preoperative or pretreatment phase and a postoperative phase. The pretreatment phase consists of a medical review of the chart to ascertain the stage and type of the tumor and whether metastases are present. The physician should review the planned medical treatment. In addition to assessment of current medical status in regard to cardiopulmonary function, tests should be performed for hemoglobin, hematocrit, and electrolyte levels. The current vocational status and family support situation should be assessed. A preoperative physical examination, with particular attention to chest wall expansion, musculoskeletal status, and cardiopulmonary status, is requisite. The patient is generally educated in proper coughing and breathing techniques (e.g., diaphragmatic, segmental). It should be explained to the patient that these exercises help air to enter the lungs better, increase the efficiency of the respiratory muscles, increase chest mobility, and decrease risk of pneumonia. Lower extremity exercises after surgery to prevent thrombophlebitis are also explained.

During the postoperative stage, the patient's pulmonary function and chest excursion are again assessed. Specific breathing exercises are started after the patient is extubated. Posture and lower extremity exercises are addressed. Chest wall pain is often relieved by use of a TENS unit. After pain is controlled and the patient is allowed to ambulate, some assessment of endurance should be made. Endurance exercises should be gradually introduced into the rehabilitation program.

In patients with metastatic disease of the brain, speech and language deficits should be included in a cognition, language, and swallowing evaluation. Depending on the location of the metastasis, there may also be focal motor and sensory deficits. Ambulatory aids, bracing or splinting, and occupational therapy intervention for assistive devices and safety equipment may be needed. Bone metastasis may need unweighting with crutches or a walker and spinal bracing and pain management.

Depending on the prognosis of patients, there should be discussions with them and their families about adjustment to whatever disabilities there may be. Careful assessment of whether such persons can continue working should be made.

CENTRAL NERVOUS SYSTEM NEOPLASMS

Brain damage may result from primary tumors of the brain, from metastatic disease, or from treatment of the cancer: surgery, radiation, or chemotherapy. The resultant symptoms, impairments, and disabilities may vary considerably but are similar to those that are seen in patients who have sustained a cerebrovascular accident or traumatic brain injury (TBI) affecting different parts of the brain. The crucial difference here is the potentially progressive or recurrent nature of the brain cancer and its uncertain prognosis. The greatest deficits are frequently seen immediately after surgery or during radiation and chemotherapy, after which extraordinary improvement may occur. Late brain injury from radiation with infarction or necrosis also may occur, but the subsequent disability has a less favorable prognosis for recovery.

Simple rehabilitation treatments can help the majority of patients, whereas those with more severe disease and deficits may require comprehensive inpatient rehabilitation, which should be provided when longer life expectancy allows. Structured, comprehensive cancer rehabilitation services have not been widely available, especially to patients with brain tumors. Nevertheless, there is good evidence that cancer patients can benefit significantly from rehabilitation intervention and that recurrent or metastatic tumors and ongoing aggressive tumor therapy should not preclude admission to a rehabilitation unit.[101]

Philip et al.[102] demonstrated that after definitive treatment of primary brain tumors in children, rehabilitation significantly improves outcome in self-care activities, transfers into and out of bed, and locomotion by a wheelchair or walking. Furthermore, preliminary evidence supports the efficacy of post–acute brain injury rehabilitation services for patients with primary malignant tumors, resulting in sustained increases in productivity.[103] Specific program interventions for these successful services include evaluation of cognitive, behavioral, affective, and social functioning; identification of impairments and their impact on patients' daily functioning; individualized therapies to improve functioning; and return to desired vocational status.

Rehabilitation intervention most commonly begins after removal of the brain tumor. When affected patients are medically stable, a referral to rehabilitation should be initiated so that they can be helped to sit up, get out of bed, and start an active restoration program that is tailored to their general condition. Recovery may be fairly rapid, initially due to control of edema. Hemiplegia or hemiparesis is a common sign of brain cancer and is often most profound just after the brain surgery. Some return of motor strength is common and may continue for several weeks or months. While muscles that are still paralyzed 4 to 8 weeks postoperatively generally remain so, functional improvement can still occur through routine daily activity as well as therapeutic exercise and use of appropriate assistive devices (orthoses or gait aids). Encouragement in the use of the affected limb is recommended, rather than learning to substitute for the affected side using one-sided activity. Data suggest that recovery of motor and language function can proceed over significant periods with proper encouragement and stimulation.

If patients are kept in bed, they should be placed on a special mattress designed to prevent pressure sores. To prevent capsular contractures of the shoulder, patients should lie with the affected arm abducted, externally rotated, and slightly elevated. The lower extremity should be positioned to minimize hip-knee flexion. Passive joint ROM exercises should be applied to the paralyzed extremities and active exercises to the unaffected parts twice a day.

Most patients are able to ambulate with assistive devices and training. Good sitting balance and standing balance are prerequisites for functional transfers and ambulation. Therapists use feedback mechanisms to correct patients' tendency to lean toward the affected side. For example, "handling" is a therapeutic technique designed to establish normal alignment, reduce or eliminate abnormal tone and movement, reeducate muscles in normal patterns in the trunk and limbs, and produce an active movement pattern in hemiplegic patients. "Inhibition" techniques are manual techniques and hand placements used to decrease or eliminate spasticity. Dynamic sitting balance is achieved through trunk exercises, use of mirrors, and verbal feedback regarding position. Potential ambulatory ability should be assessed by standing patients in the parallel bars. Patients should be taught bed-to-chair transfer activities as soon as sitting balance and weight shifting allow. Patients whose hip flexors and extensors remain weak will not ambulate independently because no satisfactory hip bracing is available. Weak knee extensors can be stabilized with a temporary knee-ankle-foot orthosis, which locks the knee in extension during weight bearing. Weak ankle dorsiflexors are often the last muscles to recover and can be stabilized with a plastic ankle-foot orthosis (AFO) to prevent toe dragging during the swing phase of gait. Elevation activities, such as climbing and descending stairs, ramps, or curbs, are started when a good gait pattern on level ground has been achieved. Patients with severe neurologic deficits may require a wheelchair, either for mobility at all times or only when ambulation endurance or safety is impaired.

The major goal in the rehabilitation of the patient with brain cancer is independence in ADL, which may be obtained through training, prescription of proper assistive devices (e.g., adaptive eating utensils, bathroom equipment, positioning and transferring equipment, and gait aids) and modification of the patient's home and work environment (Fig. 57-6).

Spasticity is a frequent impediment to mobility and performance of ADL. Factors that may aggravate spasticity, such as skin lesions, infections, and anxiety, need to be identified and treated. Thorough stretching of all joints should be performed daily. Medications, such as dantrolene, baclofen (starting at 5 mg three times daily and titrated until therapeutic dose is reached, usually 40 to 80 mg/d), and diazepam (2 to 10 mg three to four times daily), may be of some benefit but should be used sparingly because of their potential for producing somnolence. Selected nerve root blocks with dilute solutions of phenol or concentrated alcohol are usually effective in reducing spasticity. Botulinum toxin injections are also used, and proper dosage and administration site are essential for a favorable response. Surgical procedures for reducing spasticity in this population are rarely indicated.

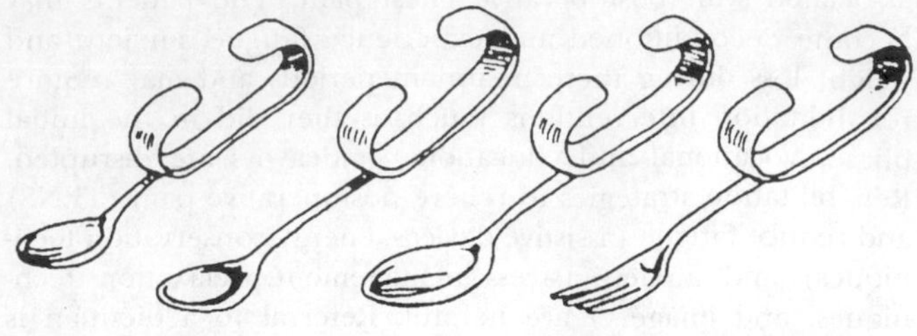

FIGURE 57-6. Adaptive eating utensils for patients with upper extremity spasticity or weakness.

Joint contractures may be caused by muscle imbalance, spasticity, poor nursing care, prolonged immobility, improper bed positioning, or an inadequate exercise program. Whatever the cause, the contractures may adversely affect the rehabilitation prognosis. For example, development of a frozen shoulder may render independent dressing impossible. Therefore, prevention of contractures by proper positioning and posture and joint ROM exercises is imperative, since treatment of contracture is relatively ineffective.

Cancer of the brain may cause pain in different parts of the body. Pain in the hemiplegic shoulder is common and may benefit from shoulder support by an arm sling or a lap board, administration of analgesics, application of heat or cold modalities, and gentle ROM and strengthening exercises. Complex regional pain syndrome of the shoulder (previously known as *shoulder-hand syndrome*) may also occur and requires similar treatment, but more effective relief may be obtained by prescribing oral steroids. Dysesthetic thalamic pain is notably refractory to treatment, though various centrally acting agents may be helpful.

Varying degrees of sensory loss are commonly seen in patients with brain cancer, either in the distribution of the cranial nerves or on one or both sides of the body. They may interfere with balance and mobility, since patients who cannot feel motion are unable to control it. Training with adaptive gait aids may help such patients to ambulate functionally again.

Vision deficits, such as double vision, homonymous hemianopsia, and anosognosia, may greatly interfere with function, especially in patients with a right brain lesion. Fortunately, specialized programs of cognitive remediation have been found to be effective with these patients.[104] Such programs include basic scanning training, somatosensory awareness and size estimation training, and complex visual perceptual training.

Aphasia, a disorder of both the expression and reception of propositional language secondary to cortical or subcortical disease, may be seen in patients with cancer in the left dominant hemisphere of the brain. Listening, speaking, reading, and writing are usually affected to varying degrees; thus, several types of aphasia are recognized. Expressive or nonfluent aphasia is caused by lesions in the Broca area of the brain. Reduced language production, vocabulary, and grammar are characteristic. The patient is well aware of these difficulties and becomes easily frustrated. Receptive or fluent aphasia is caused by lesions in the Wernicke area of the brain and results in difficulty in understanding language, both the patient's and that of others. Patients may be able to speak continuously at normal speed and with normal melody without giving any relevant information and be unaware of the errors. Speech therapy is indicated, whenever available, not only for psychological support but to stimulate patients to use their maximal speech ability and to adjust to new circumstances. It is also helpful to instruct affected families in proper communication with involved patients by such means as using proper sentences at a normal voice volume and using gestures and facial expressions while increasing respect, optimism, patience, and encouragement.

Dysarthria is a motor disturbance of speech characterized by weakness, slowness, or incoordination of the muscles that produce speech. Therefore, there is complete understanding of written or spoken language. The main problem is articulation, though speed, rhythm, sound, and intonation may also be impaired. Speech therapy emphasizes teaching the patient to use the remaining speech muscles more effectively or to bypass the effects of disturbed function.

Aprosopia is a communication disorder caused by lesions of the nondominant right hemisphere. It results in the inability to express and comprehend variations in pitch, rhythm, and stress, which give emotional meaning to speech. Affected patients may speak in a relatively flat voice and are often unable to recognize the emotional tones of speech, including the meaning of nonlanguage speech sounds, such as grunts or sighs. Therefore, the clinician and family should communicate with the patient strictly by words, because specific therapy does not exist. Fortunately, considerable improvement usually occurs over time.

Dysphagia, or impaired swallowing, is most commonly seen in lesions involving the brain stem. With severe involvement, the patient may be totally unable to swallow or, in milder cases, there may be difficulty only with the swallowing of liquids. Whatever the degree of severity, the patient is at risk for aspiration with resulting pneumonia, so suspicion of the condition with timely intervention is key to treatment. Serial radiographic swallowing studies are indicated for proper monitoring of the condition until it resolves or other and safer means of nutrition are provided. Speech therapy may institute a swallowing training program in which patients attempt to swallow food of different consistency using different techniques and positions. If indicated, a nasogastric tube can be used for several weeks while waiting for spontaneous recovery. A more persistent dysphagia may warrant a gastrostomy tube for prolonged feeding.

Neurobehavioral problems often have an underappreciated but large impact on the quality of life of patients with tumors and their families. Implementation of services directed toward these problems is only now receiving attention. The use of traditional cognitive and vocational rehabilitation for patients with brain tumors is complicated by the fact that existing programs are not entirely appropriate. The patterns and types of cognitive deficits experienced by these patients are different from those experienced by stroke or TBI patients. Anderson et al.[105] found that patients with brain tumors have milder cognitive deficits and greater variability in the nature and extent of their deficits, compared with people who have strokes that affect the same neuroanatomic site. Furthermore, the natural history of the disease process is different from that of cerebrovascular disease or TBI. The latter two are usually characterized by an acute onset and gradual recovery, while the onset of disease in brain tumors is relatively insidious. Although some recovery of function may be seen after surgery or other therapy, most patients experience a gradual deterioration of function as the tumor progresses.

The most common type of neurobehaviorally oriented program is the day treatment program, which emphasizes cognitive and vocational rehabilitation. Although these programs are frequently affiliated with an inpatient rehabilitation program, many are located in the community to provide better access to resources. The first step in cognitive and vocational rehabilitation is to identify realistic goals for the patient. Formal neuropsychological and vocational testing to identify preserved skills have been found to be useful. The major goal is to train patients to compensate for their neurobehavioral deficits at home and on the job. Memory, problem-solving skills, and social behavior are typical areas targeted for retraining. For example, patients with memory deficits may compensate by using tools, such as written reminders and alarm watches. Patients with behavioral problems should be taught to inhibit socially inappropriate remarks or to reduce frustration intolerance. Furthermore, patients and family members should be counseled about the need to select jobs that are less demanding although not as financially rewarding or prestigious.

In addition to providing rehabilitation to appropriate patients with brain cancer, patients' families should be offered education and emotional support. Families of such patients are often burdened by the patients' cognitive and behavioral changes in addition to the typical psychological problems of coping with cancer in a family member. Support groups for patients with brain cancer and their families may be of great benefit.

HEMATOPOIETIC TUMORS

Leukemias

Leukemia is the uncontrolled proliferation and incomplete maturation of leukocyte and lymphocyte precursors appearing in bone marrow and peripheral blood. Leukemia may occur in acute or chronic form. The acute leukemias include acute myelogenous leukemia (AML) and acute lymphoblastic leukemia (ALL). They are more common in childhood. Both leukemias are associated with anemia, fatigue, fever, bleeding gums, gastrointestinal tract or urinary tract symptoms, easy bruising, and pallor. Headache, mental changes, and cranial nerve palsy are common in ALL with CNS involvement. Joint pain is often seen with ALL but rarely in AML. The prognosis for AML, even with treatment, is poor. ALL responds much better to treatment, and complete remissions are often seen. Treatment of AML consists of cytarabine, daunorubicin, and amsacrine. The mainstay treatment in ALL consists of vincristine and prednisone.

Chronic myelogenous leukemia is not usually seen before 20 years of age, and chronic lymphocytic leukemia is generally seen after 50 years of age. Both present with abdominal discomfort, organ enlargement, malaise, and fatigue. Anemia, low platelet count, bruising, and cutaneous bleeding are seen with chronic myelogenous leukemia.

The rehabilitation team must address the effects of the leukemia itself and the side effects of medications and irradiation. A leukemia that does not respond completely to treatment has a course of remissions and exacerbations that seriously affects the ability to attend school or continue working. Long periods of rest may be needed during treatment or during times of low platelets. Generalized deconditioning and decreased muscle strength occur. Steroids contribute to decreased strength when they cause a myopathy. They may be associated with osteoporosis, compression fractures, and painful aseptic necrosis of bone. CNS leukemia is associated with altered cognition, cranial nerve abnormalities, and other neurologic deficits. Vincristine causes peripheral neuropathy. Hair loss occurs with some chemotherapeutic agents. Bone marrow transplantation requires a 6-week hospital stay, usually with confinement in a bone marrow hospital unit because of the necessary immunosuppression (e.g., leukocyte count <1000/mm^3).

Management of muscle weakness, decreased endurance, focal neurologic deficits, joint pain, cosmesis, and psychosocial and vocational problems are a challenge to rehabilitation specialists dealing with this group of patients. The type and intensity of exercises allowable depends mainly on the platelet count and hemoglobin level. Exercise should be nonresistive when the platelet count is less than 50,000/mm^3. No exercise is performed with counts below 20,000/mm^3.[106] Aerobic or endurance exercise is limited when hemoglobin measures less than 8 to 10 g/dL. Whenever exercise and activity are possible, they should be encouraged. Patients undergoing bone marrow transplantation are always placed on an exercise program to increase strength and endurance. Recent studies demonstrate the safety and efficacy of aerobic conditioning during bone marrow transplantation and during treatment with chemotherapy.[107–113] Exercise should be performed either 2 hours before or 2 hours after radiation is delivered, to avoid a radiation-enhancing effect that occurs during increased blood flow resulting from exercise. Those who are on high-dose steroid therapy and are particularly susceptible to steroid myopathy, osteoporosis, and aseptic necrosis. Their exercise program includes weight-bearing activities, upper extremity ROM, an isometric program, and back extension exercises. An aerobic program is introduced when platelet and hemoglobin levels permit. Exercise also seems to be effective for reducing symptoms of nausea and fatigue and for improving psychological well-being.[114]

Bracing and splinting are needed for neurologic deficits. A wig should be provided at initiation of treatment in anticipation of hair loss due to chemotherapy. Assessment of ADL and issuance of safety equipment and assistive devices may be needed. Energy conservation education is important. Assisting patients and their families in coping with acute and chronic problems is essential.

Lymphomas

Lymphomas constitute a group of malignant tumors that arise principally from lymph node cellular structures, other reticuloendothelial organs, and bone marrow. These tumors are classified as Hodgkin's disease and non-Hodgkin's lymphomas (NHLs). The type of cells and their growth pattern help to differentiate the types of lymphomas. Knowledge of the stage of the disease is important because medical and rehabilitation treatment regimens are oriented to the stage-specific problems and prognosis.

Treatment consists of combination chemotherapy and radiotherapy. Many multidrug regimens exist. Choice of an appropriate drug regimen depends on the stage of the disease. Most of the regimens include prednisone, and side effects of osteoporosis, compression fracture, myopathy, and aseptic necrosis may be seen in 10%.[114] Other drugs with potential side effects that need to be addressed by rehabilitation include doxorubicin, which produces decreased cardiac ejection fraction, and vincristine, which causes peripheral neuropathy. Combination regimens may result in hair loss, aspermia, and early menopause. Prolonged bed rest results in muscle weakness and decreased endurance. Treatment with radiotherapy can result in skin tightness, restricted joint motion, and aspermia.

The disease itself can be asymptomatic (subtype A) or symptomatic (subtype B). Systemic symptoms of fever, night sweats, weight loss, and decreased endurance are present with stage I through IVB disease.

Aggressive high-grade lymphomas, such as Burkitt's, have a high propensity for metastasis to the CNS (e.g., meningeal carcinomatosis), causing symptoms of headache, diplopia, cranial nerve palsy, and weakness. Spinal cord compression can occur if lymphoma involves the epidural space. CNS and spinal cord involvement can occur with NHL and Hodgkin's disease.

Other problems that arise with lymphomas include increased susceptibility to infection, pleural and pericardial effusion, and superior vena cava syndrome due to compression of the superior vena cava by enlarged lymph nodes.

Chemotherapy and irradiation regimens for NHL are chosen according to the grade and type of tumor. Vincristine, prednisone, and cyclophosphamide are commonly used in these regimens. (Side effects are similar to those described in Chapter 45.6 on Hodgkin's disease.)

As for patients with any type of cancer, it is important to know the type and stage of lymphoma, the treatment indicated, and side effects and the general prognosis when planning a rehabilitation regimen. In general, patients have to cope with disease-related problems and the effects of complex chemotherapeutic and radiotherapy regimens. Some patients may have an early complete cure and be left with no residual problems. Others may have had more advanced or more malignant disease with incomplete remissions or recurrences and disease- and treatment-related morbidity. In this latter group, vocational and school status should be assessed. All members of the rehabilitation team are involved in the management of these patients.

Neurologic involvement may require bracing, mobility aides, assistive devices, and speech and language evaluation. Unweighting lower extremity joints involved with aseptic necrosis is appropriate. Muscle weakness and deconditioning should be addressed with appropriate strengthening and endurance exercises. The same precautions about platelet and hemoglobin levels hold true for lymphomas and leukemias. Particular attention should be paid to unweighting bony lower extremity lesions if there is more than 50% cortical involvement. Appropriate spinal bracing for vertebral involvement should be addressed. Unstable lesions should be evaluated surgically. If the patient has advanced disease and surgery cannot be done, choice of a body jacket for thoracic and lumbar lesions and a four-poster brace for cervical lesions may need to be used to help prevent spinal cord compression. When treating patients in rehabilitation, any early signs of spinal cord compression, such as new weakness, sensory deficits, or reflex changes, should be reported to the primary physician, because radiotherapy may be effective in reducing the size of spinal metastasis and relieving spinal compression. Likewise, any signs of superior vena cava syndrome, such as increased dyspnea, facial edema, and dilated chest wall veins, should be reported, because radiation may palliate these symptoms.

CONCLUSION

The cancer population presents a significant challenge to health care professionals because management is complex and is unique to individual patients and their phase in life and stage of disease. A model for planning treatment for the entire life expectancy of these patients, which is likely to be measured in years, is that of managing a chronic illness. This chronic illness may also have acute phases. Treatment goals should always support those of the patients and promote, restore, or preserve functional activity that has value to patients in their unique social, vocational, and physical environment.

REFERENCES

1. Stolberg S. New cancer cases decreasing as deaths do, too. *New York Times,* March 13, 1998.
2. National Institutes of Health. *Cancer. rates and risks,* 4th ed. Bethesda, MD: National Institutes of Health, 1996:12.
3. Whelan TJ, ME, Willan AR, et al. The supportive care needs of newly diagnosed cancer patients attending a regional cancer center. *Cancer* 1997;80:1518.
4. Bergner M, et al. The sickness impact profile: development and final revision of a health status measure. *Med Care* 1981;19:787.
5. Ganz P. Long range effect of clinical trail interventions on quality of life. *Cancer* 1994;74[Suppl 9]:2620.
6. Osoba D. Lessons learned from mesuring health-related quality of life in oncology. *J Clin Oncol* 1994;12:608.
7. Karnofsky DA, Abelmann WH, Carver LF, Burchenal JH. *The use of nitrogen mustards in the palliative treatment of carcinoma,* vol 1. *Cancer* 1948;1:634.
8. Fawzy FI, Fawzy NW, Hyun CS, et al. Malignant melanoma: effects of an early structured psychiatric intervention, coping and affective state on recurrence and survival 6 years later. *Arch Gen Psych* 1993;50:681.
9. Given CW, Given BA, Stommel M. The impact of age, treatment and symptoms on the physical and mental health of cancer patients: a longitudinal perspective. *Cancer* 1994;74[Suppl 7]:2128.
10. Wilmore DW. Catabolic illness: strategies for enhancing recovery. *N Engl J Med* 1991;325(10):695.
11. Gross M, et al. Calcaneal bone density reduction in patients with restricted mobility. *Arch Phys Med Rehabil* 1987;68(3):158.
12. Stewart AF, et al. Calcium homeostasis in immobilization: an example of resorptive hypercalcemia. *N Engl J Med* 1982;306:1136.
13. Claus-Walker J, Halstead LS, Rodriguez GP, Henry YK. Spinal cord injury hypercalcemia: therapeutic profile. *Arch Phys Med Rehabil* 1982;63(3):108.
14. Akeson WH, Amiel D, Abel MF, Garfin SR, Woo SL. Effects of immobilization on joints. *Clin Orthop* 1987;(219):28.
15. Woo SL-Y, Gomez MA, Sites TJ, et al. The biomechanical and morphological changes in the medial collateral ligament of the rabbit after immobilization and remobilization. *J Bone Joint Surg Am* 1987;69(8):1200.
16. Mohr DN, Ryn JH, Litin SC, Rosenow EC 3rd. Recent advances in the management of venous thromboembolism. *Mayo Clin Proc* 1988;63:281.
17. Booth FW. Physiologic and biochemical effects of immobilization on muscle. *Clin Orthop* 1987;(219):15.
18. Häggmark TE, Eriksson E, Jansson E. Muscle fiber type changes in human skeletal muscle after injuries and immobilization. *Orthopedics* 1986;9(2):181.
19. O'Gorman P, McMillan DC, McArdle CS. Impact of weight loss, appetite and the inflammatory response on quality of life in GI cancer patients. *Nutr Cancer* 1998;32:76.
20. Ishihara K. Long term quality of life in patients after total gastrectomy. *Cancer Nurs* 1999;22:220.
21. Hautamaki RD, Souba WW . Principles and techniques of nutritional support in the cancer patient. In: Bland KI, Karakousis CP, Copeland EM, eds. Atlas of surgical oncology. Philadelphia: WB Saunders, 1995:740.
22. Moldawer LL, Copeland EM 3rd. Proinflammatory cytokines, nutritional support and the cachexia syndrome in interactions and therapeutic options. *Cancer* 1997;79:1828.
23. Lotze MT, Duncan MA, Gerber LH, et al. Early versus delayed shoulder motion following axillary dissection. *Ann Surg* 1981;193(325):288.
24. Sicard-Rosenbaum L, Lord D, Danoff JV, Thom AK, Eckhaus MA. Effects of continuous therapeutic ultrasound on growth and metastasis of subcutaneous murine tumors. *Phys Ther* 1995;75(25):3.
25. Dalakas M. Polymyositis dermatomyositis and inclusion body myositis. *N Engl J Med* 1991;325(25):1487.
26. Cairncross G. Effects of cancer on the nervous system. In: Wittes R, ed. *Manual of oncological therapeutics.* New York: JB Lippincott Co, 1991.
27. Lakhanpal S, Bunch TW, Strup IL, et al. Polymyositis-dermatomyositis and malignant lesions: Does an association exist? *Mayo Clin Proc* 1986;61:645.
28. Bohm A. Clinical presentation and diagnosis of polymyositis and dermatomyositis. In: Dalakas M, ed. *Polymyositis and dermatomyositis,* vol 28. London: Butterworth-Heinemann, 1987.
29. Rosenberg N, Carry M, Rengel S. Association of inflammatory myopathies with other connective tissue disorders and malignancies. In: Dalakas M, ed. *Polymyositis and dermatomyositis,* vol 28. London: Butterworth, 1987.
30. Dalakas, M. Treatment of polymyositis and dermatolyositis with corticosteroids. In: Dalakas M, ed. *Polymyositis and dermatomyositis,* vol 28. London: Butterworth, 1987.
31. David D, Greico H, Cushman P. Adrenal glucocorticoids after twenty years: a review of their clinically relevant consequences. *J Chron Dis* 1970;22:637.
32. Scher HI, Yagoda A. Bone metastases: pathogenesis, treatment, and rationale for use of resorption inhibitors. *Am J Med* 1987;82(2A):6.
33. Paterson AH. Bone metastases in breast cancer, prostate cancer and myeloma. *Bone* 1987;8[Suppl 1]:S17.
34. Nielsen OS, Munro AJ, Tannock IF. Bone mestatases: pathophysiology and management policy. *J Clin Oncol* 1991;9(3):509.
35. Tofe AJ, Francis MD, Harvey WJ. Correlation of neoplasms with incidence and localization of skeletal metastasis: an analysis of 355 diphosphonate bone scans. *J Nucl Med* 1975;16:986.
36. Tubiana-Hulin M. Incidence, prevalence, and distribution of bone metastasis. *Bone* 1991;12[Suppl 1]:9.
37. Menck H, Schulze S, Larsen E. Metastasis size in pathologic femoral fractures. *Acta Orthop Scand* 1988;59(2):151.
38. Galasko CSB. Skeletal metastases. *Clin Orthop* 1986;210:18.
39. Errico TJ, Kostuik JP. Diagnosis and treatment of metastatic disease of the spinal column: a review. *Contemp Orthop* 1986;13(5):15.
40. Denis F. Spinal instability as defined by the three-column spine concept in acute spinal trauma. *Clin Orhtop* 1984;(189):65.
41. Pal GP, Sherk HH. The vertical stability of the cervical spine. *Spine* 1988;13(5):447.
42. Önimus M, Schraub S, Bertin D, Basset JF, Guidet M. Surgical treatment of vertebral metastasis. *Spine* 1986;11(9):883.
43. Galasko CSB. Spinal instability secondary to metastatic cancer. *J Bone Joint Surg* 1991;73-B(1):104.
44. Johnson RO Jr, Hart DL, Callahan RA. Cervical orthoses: a guide to their selection and use. *Clin Orthop* 1981;154:34.
45. Sutherland IA, Myers SJ. Radiation myelopathy. *Arch Phys Med Rehabil* 1976;57:81.
46. Cooper PR, Maravilla KR, Sklar FH, Moody SF, Clark WK. Halo immobilization of cervical spine fractures. indications and results. *J Neurosurg* 1979;50(5):603.
47. Werner RA. Paraplegia and quadriplegia after intrathecal chemotherapy. *Arch Phys Med Rehabil* 1988;9(12):1054.
48. Ryan JR, Emami A. Vincristine neurotoxicity with residual equinocavus deformity in children with acute leukemia. *Cancer* 1983;51(3):423.
49. Loehrer PJ, Einhorn LH. Drugs five years later. Cisplatin. *Ann Intern Med* 1984;100(5):704.
50. Salner AL, Botnick LE, Herzog AG, et al. Reversible brachial plexopathy following primary radiation therapy for breast cancer. *Cancer Treat Rep* 1981;65(9):797.
51. Wheeler JS Jr, Siroky MB, Bell R, et al. Vincristine-induced bladder neuropathy. *J Urol* 1983;130(2):342.
52. Rosenfeld CS, Broder LE. Cisplatin-induced autonomic neuropathy. *Cancer Treat Rep* 1984;68(4):659.
53. Raphaelson MI Stevens JC, Newman RP. Vincristine neuropathy with bowel and bladder atony: mimicking spinal cord compression [Letter]. *Cancer Treat Rep* 1983;67(6):604.
54. Scherokman B, Filing-Katz MR, Tell D. Brachial plexus neuropathy following high-dose cytarabine in acute monoblastic leukemia. *Cancer Treat Rep* 1985;69(9):1005.
55. La Rocca RV, Meer J, Gilliatt RW, et al. Suramin-induced polyneuropathy. *Neurology* 1990;40(6):954.
56. Basso-Ricci S, della Costa C, Viganotti G, Ventafridda V, Zanolla R. Report on 42 cases of postirradiation lesions of the brachial plexus and their treatment. *Tumori* 1980;66(1):117.
57. Kori SH, Foley KM, Posner JB. Brachial plexus lesions in patients with cancer: 100 cases. *Neurology* 1981;31(1):45.
58. Harper CM Jr, Thomas JE, Cascino TL, Litchy WJ. Distinction between neoplastic and radiation-induced brachial plexopathy, with emphasis on the role of EMG. *Neurology* 1989;39:502.
59. Mondrup K, Olsen NK, Pfeiffer P, Rose C. Clinical and electrodiagnostic findings in breast cancer patients with radiation-induced brachial plexus neuropathy. *Acta Neurol Scand* 1990;81:153.
60. Barr LC, Kissin MW. Radiation-induced brachial plexus neuropathy following breast conservation and radical radiotherapy. *Br J Surg* 1987;74:855.
61. Hoang P, Ford DJ, Burke FDA. Post mastectomy pain after brachial plexus palsey: metastases or radiation neuritis. *J Hand Surg* 1986;11-B(3):441.
62. Jaeckle KA Young DF, Foley KM. The natural history of lumbosacral plexopathy in cancer. *Neurology* 1985;35(1):8.
63. Pettigrew LC, Glass JP, Maor M, Zornoza J. Diagnosis and treatment of lumbosacral plexopathies in patients with cancer. *Arch Neurol* 1984;41:1282.
64. Ricci MA. Deep venous thrombosis in orthopedic patients. Current techniques in precise diagnosis. *Orthop Rev* 1984;13(4):185.
65. Dauzat MM, Laroche JP Charras C, et al. Real-time B-mode ultrasonography for better specificity in the noninvasive diagnosis of deep venous thrombosis. *J Ultrasound Med* 1986;5(11):625.

66. Brennan MJ, Miller LT. Overview of treatment options and review of the current role and use of compression garments, intermittent pumps and exercise in the management of lymphedema. *Cancer* 1998;83:S2821.
67. Wittlinger H, Wittinger G, Harris RH, eds. *Textbook of Dr. Vodder's manual lymph drainage*, 5th ed, vol 1. Brussels: Haug International, 1992.
68. Foldi M. Treatment of lymphedema. *Lymphology* 1994;27:1.
69. Casley Smith J. Modern treatment of lymphoedema. *Mod Med Aust* 1992;35:70.
70. Habermann ET, Lopez RA. Metastatic disease of bone and treatment of pathological fractures. *Orthop Clin North Am* 1989;20(3):469.
71. Madersbacher H. The various types of neurogenic bladder dysfunction: an update of current therapeutic concepts. *Paraplegia* 1990;28:217.
72. Wyndaele JJ. Pharmacotherapy for urinary bladder dysfunction in spinal cord injury patients. *Paraplegia* 1990;28:146.
73. Broadwell D, Jackson BS. *Principles of ostomy care.* St Louis: Mosby, 1982.
74. ConvaTec. *A professionals guide for counseling ostomy patients.* Princeton: Squibb and Sons, 1989.
75. Broadwell D, Sorrells SL. *Ileostomy care*, vol 21. Plainfield, NJ: Patient Education Press, 1988.
76. Broadwell D, Broadhurst BB. *Colostomy care*, vol 26. Plainfield, NJ: Patient Education Press, 1989.
77. Broadwell D, Broadhurst BB, *Urinary diversion*, vol 24. Plainfield, NJ: Patient Education Press, 1989.
78. Brennan MF, Casper ES, Harrison LB. Sarcomas of soft tissue and bone. In: DeVita VT, Rosenberg SA, Hellman S, eds. *Cancer: principles and practice of oncology*, 5th ed. Philadelphia: Lippincott-Raven Publishers, 1997:1759.
79. Malawer MM, Link MP, Donaldson SS. Principles and techniques of limb-sparing surgery. In: DeVita VT, Rosenberg SA, Hellman S, eds. *Cancer: principles and practice of oncology*, 5th ed. Philadelphia: Lippincott-Raven Publishers, 1997:1800.
80. Rosenberg SA, Tepper J, Glatstein E, et al. The treatment of soft tissue sarcoma of the extremities: prospective randomized evaluations of 1) limb sparing surgery plus radiation therapy compared to amputation; 2) the role of adjuvant chemotherapy. *Ann Surg* 1982;196:305.
81. Simon MA, Aschliman MA, Thomas N, Mankin HJ. Limb salvage treatment versus amputation for osteogenic sarcoma of the distal end of the femur. *J Bone Joint Surg* 1986;68A:1331.
82. Yang JC, Chang AE, Baker AR, et al. Randomized prospective study of the benefit of adjuvant radiation in the treatment of soft tissue sarcomas of the extremity. *J Clin Oncol* 1998;16(1):197.
83. Brennan M. Long term results of a prospective randomized trial of adjuvant brachytherapy in soft tissue sarcoma. *J Clin Oncol* 1996;14(3):859.
84. Liu L, Glicksman AS. The role of radiation in the management of soft tissue sarcoma. *Med Health* 1997;80(1):32.
85. Link MP, Goorin AM, Horowitz M, et al. Adjuvant chemotherapy of high-grade osteosarcoma of the extremity: updated results of the Multi-Institutional Osteosarcoma Study. *Clin Orthop* 1991;270:8.
86. Eggermont AM, Schraffordt Koops H, Klausner JM, et al. Isolated limb perfusion with tumor necrosis factor and melphalan for limb salvage in 186 patients with locally advanced soft tissue sarcoma. The cumulative multicenter European experience. *Ann Surg* 1996;224(6):756.
87. Atiyeh BS, Zaatari AM. Fibrohistiocytic sarcoma of the thumb treated by wide resection and immediate free flap reconstruction. *Scand J Plast Reconstr Surg Hand Surg* 1996;30(1):75.
88. Bray PW, Bell RS, Bowen CV, et al. Limb salvage surgery and adjuvant radiotherapy for soft tissue sarcomas of the forearm and hand. *J Hand Surg* 1997;22A(3):495.
89. Malawer M. Personal communication of clinical experience with cases, 1999.
90. Lampert MH, Gahagen C. Rehabilitation of the sarcoma patient. In: MC, ed. *Physical therapy for the cancer patient.* New York: Churchill Livingstone, 1990:111.
91. Lampert MH, Gahagen C. Rehabilitation of patients with extremity sarcoma. In: Sugarbaker P, Malawar MM, eds. *Musculoskeletal surgery for cancer.* New York: Thieme Medical Publishers, 1992:55.
92. Enneking W. A system for the functional evaluation of the surgical management of musculoskeletal tumors. In: Enneking W, ed. *Limb-sparing surgery for musculoskeletal tumors.* New York: Churchill Livingstone, 1987:5.
93. Davis AM, Wright JG, Williams JI, et al. Development of a measure of function for patients with bone and soft tissue sarcoma. *Qual Life Res* 1996;55(5):508.
94. Robinson M. Post-treatment limb function in soft tissue sarcoma. *Cancer Treat Res* 1997;91:77.
95. Arzouman JM, Dudas S, Ferrans CE, et al. Quality of life in patients with sarcoma post-chemotherapy. *Oncol Nurs Forum* 1991;10(5):889.
96. Malawer M, Chow L, Seibel N, et al. Endoprosthetic (EP) survival and long-term functional and clinical outcome of 82 patients treated with limb sparing (LS) surgery with endoprosthetic replacement for high grade bone sarcomas. *Proc Annu Meet Ann Soc Clin Oncol* 1994;13:A1776.
97. Stanhope J, Hicks JE, Malawer MM, et al. Knee joint control mechanisms in the limb spared patient. *Arch Phys Med Rehabil* 1988;69(9):744.
98. Hicks J, Siegel K. Unpublished clinical data on gait analysis in limb-spared second endoprosthetic replacements. 1998
99. Lampert MH, Gerber LH, Glatstein E. Soft tissue sarcoma: functional outcome after wide local excision and radiation therapy. *Arch Phys Med Rehabil* 1984;65(8):477.
100. Schover LR, Schain WS, Montague DK. Sexual problems of patients with cancer. In: DeVita VT Jr, Hellman S, Rosenberg SA, eds, *Cancer: principles and practice of oncology.* Philadelphia: JB Lippincott Co, 1989:2206.
101. Marciniak C, Sliwa JA, Spill G, Heinemann AW, Semik PE. Functional outcome following rehabilitation of the cancer patient. *Arch Phys Med Rehabil* 1996;77:54.
102. Philip PA, Ayyanger R, Vanderbilt J, Gaebler-Spira DJ. Rehabilitation outcome in children after treatment of primary brain tumor. *Arch Phys Med Rehabil* 1994;75:36.
103. Sherer M, Meyers CA, Bergloff P. Efficacy of postacute brain injury rehabilitation for patients with primary malignant brain tumors. *Cancer* 1997;80:250.
104. Gordon WA, Hibbard MR, Egolko S, et al. Perceptual remediation in patients with right brain damage: a comprehensive program. *Arch Phys Med Rehabil* 1985;66:353.
105. Anderson SW, Damasio H, Tanel D. Neuropsychological impairments associated with lesions caused by tumor or stroke. *Arch Neurol* 1990;47:397.
106. Holtzman L, Chesney K. Rehabilitation of the leukemia/lymphoma patient. In: McGarvey C, ed. *Clinics in physical therapy: physical therapy for the cancer patient.* New York: Churchill Livingstone, 1990:85.
107. Dimeo F, Bertz H, Finke S, et al. An aerobic exercise program for patients with haematological malignancies after bone marrow transplantation. *Bone Marrow Transplant* 1996;18:1157.
108. Dimeo FC, Tilmann MH, Bertz H, et al. Aerobic exercise in the rehabilitation of cancer patients after high-dose chemotherapy and autologous peripheral stem cell transplantation. *Cancer* 1997;9:1117.
109. Dimeo F, Fetscher S, Lange W, Mertelsmann R, Keul J. Effects of aerobic exercise on the physical performance and incidence of treatment-related complications after high-dose chemotherapy. *Blood* 1997;90:3390.
110. Dimeo F, Rumberger BG, Keul J. Aerobic exercise as therapy for cancer fatigue. *Med Sci Sports Exerc* 1998;30(4):475.
111. MacVicar MG, Winningham ML, Nickel JL. Effects of aerobic interval training on cancer patients' functional capacity. *Nurs Res* 1989;38:348.
112. Winningham ML, MacVicar MG. The effect of aerobic exercise on patient reports of nausea. *Oncol Nurs Forum* 1988;15:447.
113. Dimeo FC, Stieglitz RD, Novelli-Fisher U, et al. Effects of physical activity on the fatigue and psychological status of cancer patients during chemotherapy. *Cancer* 1999;85:2273.
114. Proswitz LR, Lawson JP, Friedlander GE, et al. Avascular necrosis of bone in Hodgkin's disease patients treated with combined-modality therapy. *Cancer* 1981;47:2793.

M. Tish Knobf
Susan Anderson

CHAPTER 58

Advanced Practice Nurses and Physician Assistants in Oncology Care

The current health care environment has influenced the delivery of cancer care, with shifts in patient acuity levels, volume, and management of patients across care settings. In response to the dynamic health care changes and therapeutic advances in oncology over the past decade, a growing trend is evident to use advanced practice nurses (APNs) and midlevel practitioners [i.e., physician assistants (PAs)] in the effort to provide high-quality, cost-effective oncology care. This chapter describes the preparation and role implementation of the PA, defines the oncology APN, identifies the professional issues that influence regulations of practice, delineates the role components of the oncology APN, and identifies the benefits of a collaboration between physicians, APNs, and PAs in oncology practice.

PHYSICIAN ASSISTANTS

The first PA education program began at Duke in 1965. It was designed to train a general assistant, who could develop areas of expertise over time under the direct supervision of a physician, initially in the areas of primary care and general surgery. The American Academy of Physician Assistant estimates that there are 34,192 PAs practicing, predominantly in primary care (53%), family practice (40%), general surgery (19%), and emergency medicine (10%).[1] Currently, less than 6% of the PA population practices in one of the subspecialties of internal medicine, and only 1% work in adult or pediatric oncology.[2] PA practice includes history and physical examinations, diagnosis and management, prescription of controlled and noncontrolled medications in those states allowed by law,[3] screening procedures, ordering and interpreting laboratory and diagnostic tests, referrals and consultations, and counseling patients. Approximately one-half of the PAs in practice report performing invasive procedures, including bone marrows, lumbar punctures, and suturing and repair of lacerations.[1]

EDUCATION AND CERTIFICATION

There are 116 PA training programs in the United States, with 42% offering a master's degree. Among the PAs in practice, 64% hold bachelor degrees and 22% hold master's degrees.[1] Programs are divided into a didactic phase and a clinical phase. Postresidency programs at selected teaching hospitals offer advanced training in a specialty area.

Certification of PAs occurs at both national and state levels. National certification requires a certificate of completion from an accredited PA educational program and passing the Physician Assistant National Certification Examination, which is administered by the National Commission of National Certification of PAs. To maintain certification, PAs must fulfill annual continuing medical education requirements and must recertify every 6 years by written examination. Similar to initial certification, recertification focuses on primary care knowledge.

At the state level, 49 states plus the District of Columbia have licensing boards, which control prescriptive authority, reim-

TABLE 58-1. Recommended Course Content for a Master's Degree with a Specialty in Advanced Practice Oncology Nursing

Core Area	*Major Content Recommendations*
Clinical practice	Pathophysiology, cancer epidemiology, advanced health assessment, principles of disease treatment, principles of management across the continuum of care, pharmacology and therapeutics, clinical therapeutics, theories and models for clinical practice, ethical and legal aspects of oncology practice
Education	Teaching and learning theories, patient and family and community learning needs assessment, teaching objectives and strategies, development of educational programs
Consultation	Theories and practice, consultative roles, business and marketing strategies
Collaboration	Collaborative practice models, role delineation, negotiating skills, communication skills, team building, shared decision making
Systems	Organizational and change theories, health economics, delivery systems, health care reform, quality improvement, standards and policies, information systems
Role competency	Role theory, orientation, socialization, advanced practice nurse role, scope of practice, certification, licensure, professional and legal standards
Research and outcomes evaluation	Research process, skill in critique of research, scientific integrity, research utilization
Program development	Principles of program planning, program models, implementing and evaluating program outcomes, community assessment
Leadership	Group leadership skills, networking, mentoring, accountability and authority, support systems, development of standards and policies

(Adapted from ref. 5.)

bursement, and scope of practice. All states require physician collaboration in practice and for prescribing drugs.[3] Most states have legislation that mandates Medicaid and Medicare coverage for PAs, but few have statutes requiring reimbursement from private insurers.

FUTURE DIRECTIONS FOR PHYSICIAN ASSISTANTS

In 1998, the Department of Health and Human Services asked the American Association of Physician Assistant Programs to develop a 3-year strategic plan stimulated by the current environment of the medical profession and the proliferation of training programs for nonphysician clinicians.[4] Highlights of the plan include that education should continue to focus on primary care and allow for specialty developments over the course of one's career through continuing education requirements; competency should be promoted through continuing education programs and recertification examinations; PAs should continue to function in a delegated role under physician supervision, work with other health care disciplines to focus on underserved populations, enhance and empower patient populations through education, and attempt to provide cost-effective high-quality care.

ADVANCED PRACTICE IN ONCOLOGY NURSING

The oncology APN is defined as "a registered nurse, prepared with a minimum of a master's degree in nursing, who has acquired advanced, in depth knowledge and preceptored clinical experiences in oncology that enable her or him to exhibit a high degree of independent and collaborative judgment and clinical skill in providing nursing care to patients with cancer and their families."[5] In 2000, the Oncology Nursing Society includes nearly 5000 members who are prepared at the master's degree level or higher (World Wide Web site: http://www.ons.org). The acquired knowledge and clinical practice experience at the graduate level prepares the APN for expansion within areas of practice that overlap traditional medical practice and for integration of theory and research into practice.[6] Improved patient outcomes, cost-effective care, and improved quality of life for patients and family are well-documented advanced practice nursing outcomes.[7–9] Nursing, the core of advanced practice, is defined as assisting the individual in activities that contribute to health, recovery, or death[10] and the diagnosis and treatment of human responses to health and illness.[6] Collaborative practice between APNs and physicians results in better quality health care by combining the unique, documented contributions of the nursing discipline with the expert medical treatment of the illness.[11–13]

EDUCATIONAL PREPARATION OF ONCOLOGY ADVANCED PRACTICE NURSES

Understanding the educational preparation of APNs is critical to decision making for employment and role implementation. The current recommendation for a master's degree with a specialty in advanced practice oncology (Table 58-1), is designed for both the clinical nurse specialist (CNS) and nurse practitioner (NP), allowing for flexibility in emphasis of content for specific role preparation. Precepted clinical experiences in programs range from 600 to 800 hours.[14] These recommendations are consistent with national recommendations for advanced nursing practice education and should prepare nurses to practice across settings of care.[15–17]

The Oncology Nursing Society annually publishes a listing of master's programs in oncology nursing.[18] Common program characteristics of the schools that have provided information include four semesters of full-time study with greater than or equal to 600 clinical hours required. These programs include curriculum that prepare APNs as CNS, oncology NP, and acute care NP, and the majority provide a postmaster's option. The foundation for many of the oncology NP programs is the primary care adult NP curriculum, preparing students with a broad

TABLE 58-2. Certification for Advanced Practice Nurses Who Practice in Adult Oncology

Certification	*Master's Program*	*Certifying Body*	*Eligibility Criteria*
Adult nurse practitioner	Adult nurse practitioner; oncology nurse practitioner	American Nurses' Credentialing Center	Current RN license; master's level nurse practitioner or formal postmaster's program at graduate level
Adult nurse practitioner	Adult nurse practitioner; oncology nurse practitioner	American Academy of Nurse Practitioners	Current RN license; master's level nurse practitioner or formal postmaster's program at graduate level
Acute care nurse practitioner	Acute care nurse practitioner	American Nurses' Credentialing Center	Current RN license; master's level acute care nurse practitioner program or formal postmaster's program at graduate level
Clinical nurse specialist–medical surgical specialty	Clinical nurse specialist with or without oncology specialty	American Nurses' Credentialing Center	Current RN license; master's level nurse practitioner program or formal postmaster's program at graduate level
Advanced oncology certified nurse	Master's degree or higher in nursing, preferably with an oncology focus	Oncology Nursing Certification Corporation	Current RN license; master's degree or higher; greater than or equal to 30 months' RN experience within 5 years of application; greater than or equal to 2000 hours of oncology nursing practice within 5 years

RN, registered nurse.

base of knowledge about common clinical problems of midlife and older adults, such as hypertension, upper respiratory infections, arthritis, cardiac disease, and diabetes. The combination of primary care and oncology knowledge provides a strong foundation for assessment and management of patients with noncancer as well as cancer-related health problems.

REGULATING PRACTICE: CERTIFICATION, LICENSURE, AND PRESCRIPTIVE PRIVILEGES

Regulation of advanced practice nursing is the responsibility of state legislators and boards of nursing. There are four levels of regulation and it is important to know the individual state regulations as they affect implementation of the role and prescriptive authority.[19,20] The least restrictive is designation and recognition of the credentials of an APN, which in oncology is the CNS and the NP.[21] The second level of regulation is registration with the state board of nursing, and certification is the third level of regulation. Certification for advanced practice nursing is a process, usually a written examination, that a nongovernment organization uses to establish that a licensed registered nurse has mastered a certain body of knowledge and skills.[22,23] Certification is a voluntary professional activity but becomes mandatory for advanced practice licensure in most states.[20] The American Nurses Association has provided leadership for certification and established a credentialing center in 1993,[19] which offers advanced practice nursing certification (Table 58-2). Specialty organizations also offer certification. The Oncology Nursing Certification Corporation has objectively established criteria for delineating the role of advanced practice nursing in oncology.[24] Eligibility for the Advanced Oncology Certified Nurse certification is open to those not only with advanced clinical preparation but anyone with a master's degree or higher degree in administration, education, or research. Specialty certification is highly valued and recommended, but because Advanced Oncology Certified Nurse certification is *not* recognized by all states for licensure, many oncology APNs hold dual certification, one for licensure and one for specialty recognition (see Table 58-2).

Licensure is the fourth regulatory level that defines the scope of practice and qualifications, designed to protect public health, safety, and welfare and is associated with a high level of accountability.[19] Advanced Practice Registered Nurse (APRN) licensure is granted by a governmental agency at the state level, and Pearson[20] provides an annual review of the variations by each state on legal authority, reimbursement, prescriptive authority, scope of practice, and titling.

Reimbursement is provided by for-profit corporations and insurers, government [Medicare, Medicaid, Civilian Health and Medical Program of the Uniformed Services (CHAMPUS)], non-profit, and self-insured corporations.[23] Federal and state legislation dictate the level of reimbursement and the 1997 Balanced Budget Act provides direct reimbursement for NPs and CNSs across a variety of settings. NPs and CNSs are required to submit their own provider number in addition to the group practice number where applicable. Payments made to NPs and CNSs are "80% of the lesser of either the actual charge or 85% of the physician fee schedule amount."[25] The Health Care Financing Administration rules require a master's degree, state authority granted to practice as an NP or CNS, and certification by a nationally recognized certifying body (World Wide Web site http://www.nurse.org/acnp/medicare/hcfa9804.shtml). The educational requirement does not include a grandfather clause for NPs who were not prepared at the master's level and, thus, their services are not reimbursable under the current rules.

Prescriptive authority is part of state regulation and ranges from the APN as an independent prescriber to an interdependent relationship with a physician to the most restrictive, which only allows an APN to prescribe drugs from a list that has been preapproved by the state.[23] Prescriptive authority includes controlled substances, as allowed by the individual state law (Table 58-3). For those states that include prescriptive authority for controlled substances, the APN can apply to the Drug Enforcement Agency and obtain individual Drug Enforcement Agency authorization.

Credentialing is a general term that refers to validation of the educational preparation, licensure, credentials, certification, and advanced scope of nursing practice.[19] *Credentialing* is the

TABLE 58-3. Nurse Practitioner Prescriptive Authority by State[a]

State	*Independent of Physician Involvement*	*Requires Some Degree of Physician Involvement*	*Controlled Substance Prescriptive Authority*
Alabama			
Alaska	X		X
Arizona	X		X
Arkansas		X	X
California		X	X
Colorado		X	X
Connecticut		X	X
Delaware		X	X
District of Columbia	X		X
Florida		X	X
Georgia		X	X
Hawaii		X	
Idaho		X	X
Illinois		X	X
Indiana		X	X
Iowa		X	X
Kansas		X	X
Kentucky		X	
Louisiana		X	
Maine	X		X
Maryland		X	X
Massachusetts		X	X
Michigan		X	
Minnesota		X	X
Mississippi		X	X
Missouri		X	
Montana	X		X
Nebraska		X	X
New Hampshire	X		X
New Jersey		X	X
New Mexico	X		X
New York		X	X
Nevada		X	
North Carolina		X	X
North Dakota		X	X
Ohio		X	
Oklahoma		X	X
Oregon	X		X
Pennsylvania		X	
Rhode Island		X	X
South Carolina		X	X
South Dakota		X	
Tennessee		X	X
Texas		X	
Utah	X		X
Vermont		X	X
Virginia		X	X
Washington	X		X
West Virginia		X	X
Wisconsin	X		X
Wyoming		X	X

[a]May apply to other advanced practice nurses (clinical nurse specialist, certified nurse midwife, certified registered nurse anesthesist). Refer to ref. 20 for specific regulations and qualifications for prescriptive authority by state.

term often used by institutions for the process of evaluating and granting clinical practice privileges.[23]

ROLE IMPLEMENTATION OF ADVANCED PRACTICE NURSES

The APN implements the role as a direct caregiver, educator, consultant, administrator, and researcher. A role-delineation study[24] confirmed that these role components were relevant to both the CNS and NP APNs in oncology, with less than 10% of the items differentiating the roles. This study supports the standards of practice for advanced practice nursing in oncology,[5] supports identified competencies for role implementation,[17] and further validates the similar and overlapping role functions of the CNS and NP in clinical practice.[12,13,26,27]

Direct Care Provider

In provision of direct care to the patient, the roles of the CNS and NP are more blended than distinct, reflecting the similarity in advanced physical and psychosocial assessment and management.[13] The distinction between these APNs lies in the emphasis and time spent on specific role functions.[24,28] The NP direct care role is defined by comprehensive health assessment, diagnosis, health promotion, prescriptive authority, and management of acute and chronic problems.[6,12,20] Oncology NPs also perform procedures, write orders, prescribe chemotherapy, admit patients to the hospital, and write inpatient progress notes.[28] Some CNSs have adopted a practice model, in which the individual patient is the primary focus. In that model, the practice of the CNS and NP have little, if any, distinction. However, many CNSs continue a practice model, which was designed to promote improvement of nursing care by all nurses to a population of patients.[6] Thus, the direct hands-on care role for the oncology CNS refers to direct patient care but also to the supportive role for nursing staff related to assessment, clinical decision making, introducing new skills into practice, and interventions.[29] The reality of fewer professional registered nurses in hospitals, increased numbers of unlicensed personnel, continued specialization, and high patient acuity across settings of care have "recreated the scenario that first produced the need for specialized nurses earlier in the century."[30] In oncology, there is a real and persistent need to provide direction and consultation for direct patient care to less well-prepared nursing and nonnursing staff in order to deliver high-quality, safe, and competent nursing care.

Practice Setting

The changing nature of oncology practice creates continuous opportunities for diversity in role implementation across practice settings. The practice setting of the oncology APN is diverse, ranging from screening, detection, and genetic counseling programs to care of patients in the hospital, ambulatory clinics, private office practices, radiation therapy centers, home care, and hospice.[31] In the hospital, implementation of the role of the acute care NP with critically ill cancer patients is increasingly evident,[32–34] and a subacute NP role has been described for routine admissions of patients on a medical oncology service.[35] Consistent with changes in the health care environment, there has been a recognized shift of the oncology APN role to nontertiary settings, specifically home care,[8,36] palliative care,[37,38] ambulatory clinics and comprehensive cancer centers,[39–41] and radiation therapy.[42–44] Many APNs in clinics and private office settings have hospital privileges and provide care across settings.[28,39,45]

Educator

The APN's educator role addresses the learning needs of the patient and family, other nurses, disciplinary colleagues, and the community. Teaching the patient and family is a primary role of the NP and the CNS across all settings[46] and may include identification and use of appropriate culturally sensitive educational materials, development of practice standards for patient teaching, and evaluation of the effectiveness of educational interventions.

Another major responsibility of the oncology APN is to improve patient care through staff education.[47] In the current health care climate of high acuity and shortened stays in acute care settings and high volume and more complex care required for patients in ambulatory settings, informal on-site education for nurses by the APN for diagnostic, therapeutic, and ethical reasoning in clinical judgment provides a critical method to improve nursing care and patient outcomes.[46,48] Oncology APNs have made significant contributions to nursing education and clinical care through dissemination of clinical knowledge in specialty journals such as *Cancer Nursing, Oncology Nursing Forum, Clinical Journal of Oncology Nursing, Cancer Practice, Seminars in Oncology Nursing,* and oncology nursing texts.[49–63] Many of these texts serve as excellent on-site resources for clinical staff.

Consultant

Providing expert advice to nursing and professional colleagues on individual patient cases and on complex problems of a specific patient population is a well-established function of the oncology APN. Consultation can be informal (verbal) or formal (written) and can be initiated with APNs from within or outside of the oncology specialty or practice setting.[64] Symptom management, the need to acquire new skills, understanding and use of innovative technology, chemotherapy information for the non-oncology staff, and complex clinical problems are common examples for consulting with the oncology APN. In addition, the oncology APN provides important consultation in the development and revision of institutional policies, procedures, and clinical practice guidelines[32]; and professional consultation, such as educational programs and peer review for journal articles.

Clinical Leader

The clinical leader role should not be confused with institutional leadership activities of management.[32] The APN leadership is directed at the practice environment, patient outcomes, and improving nursing care. The APN functions as a change agent, the primary purpose of which is to effect change to maintain or improve the quality of care delivered. The oncology APN by virtue of specialty knowledge and change agent skills is uniquely qualified to assess the process of care delivery; evaluate the clinical, psychosocial, functional, fiscal, and patient satisfaction outcomes across the continuum of cancer care; determine what needs to be changed to achieve desired outcomes; and effectively implement change.[7] Creative change agency is needed to challenge the status quo, introduce new skills or technology, integrate research findings into practice, and adapt care delivery within and across settings to improve continuity.[65]

Researcher

Use of research in practice is dependent on the available body of research, dissemination of findings, and integration of the research findings by nurses in their clinical practice. Oncology nurses prepared at the doctoral level have made significant research contributions to the care of patients and families, with progression from earlier descriptive studies to intervention research. Symptom management is a major nursing focus[50] and a consistent research priority. In 1994, a metaanalysis was performed on 28 studies that addressed nausea and vomiting, pain, anxiety, alopecia, infection, chemotherapy side effects, shivering, radiodermatitis, anorexia, and mucositis.[66] Overall, interventions were successful in relieving symptoms and significant effectiveness was obtained for interventions used in the management of nausea and vomiting, pain, anxiety, alopecia, infection, and side effects of chemotherapy.[66] In that same year, a State of the Knowledge Conference on the symptom of fatigue summarized existing data.[67] That conference summary provided direction for future research, which has resulted in multiple publications from studies on measurement, prevalence, severity, perceived distress, and intervention effectiveness for the symptom of fatigue in cancer patients. These examples provide a small glimpse of the extent and scope of oncology nursing research that directly relates to practice.

RESEARCH UTILIZATION. Nursing is accountable to use research findings to support practice and maintain an evidence-based practice. As an example, Bookbinder and colleagues[68] spearheaded a research utilization project at Memorial Sloan-Kettering Cancer Center that was designed to improve quality patient care through integration of the Agency for Health Care Policy and Research Cancer Pain Management Clinical Practice Guideline into practice. APNs provided leadership for this project, which resulted in an organized clinical pain management program, pain management education programs, revision of assessment forms to include pain assessment and relief as the fifth vital sign, standards of care for professional and patient education and patient satisfaction, a systematic method to continually improve pain, and improved treatment outcomes. Collaboration of doctorally prepared clinical nurses and researchers with oncology APNs in clinical settings offers an opportunity to create environments that bridge the gap between practice and research, stimulate critical thinking among staff nurses, foster the value of research and application to practice, enhance practice-relevant nursing research, and ultimately, achieve the goal to improve patient care outcomes.[69,70]

NURSES' CONTRIBUTION TO THERAPEUTIC CLINICAL TRIAL RESEARCH. The growth in numbers of APNs over the next 10 years presents an opportunity to develop a unique role in clinical research.[4] Oncology nurses have traditionally played a major role in cancer clinical research by assuming the responsibility of safe study drug administration but also providing a full range of responsibilities related to research, including input into study design, feasibility assessments, and budgetary analysis; recruitment and education of patients; maintenance of regulatory documents; collection of data; and study summary and analysis.[71] The role and number of APNs currently working in clinical trial research is unknown. However, the depth of specialty knowledge, research preparation, and advanced clinical nursing skills of the oncology APN offer unique qualifications to meet the challenges of a research coordinator for clinical trials.[72] Additionally, the APN's autonomy as a direct care provider in toxicity assessment and in the management of complex cancer patients offers a model of care that combines resources to provide comprehensive care and maintain a high level of rigor in the research process. Few medical oncologists report any clinical research training, and many nurses involved in clinical trials do not have master's degrees. Thus, nursing has identified the need for advanced level knowledge and skill in this area and has implemented programs for master's degrees and postmaster's certificates in clinical trials management at Duke University, University of California in San Francisco, and Columbia University. The content includes protocol design, development strategies for drug development, principles of data management, and business practices for clinical research. Other schools such as Georgetown University have collaborated with pharmaceutical companies to offer continuing education programs in clinical research management. The courses at Georgetown include an explanation of the drug development process and preparation for advanced management of multisite trials.

Professional training in federal regulations governing clinical research, business aspects, and overall management roles are also addressed by the Cooperative Group Training Sessions, the Society of Research Nurses, the Association of Clinical Research Professionals (ACPR) and the Society of Clinical Research Professionals (SOCRA).

COLLABORATIVE PRACTICE

Collaborative practice among physicians and APNs or PAs is an appropriate model for oncology. The current health care environment and the increasing complexity of oncology have highlighted the need for professional interdependence and collaboration in order to provide safe care.[73,74] A multidisciplinary approach has been an established cornerstone of oncology practice, contributing to a more comprehensive plan of care and better overall patient outcomes. The PA and APN offer significant contributions to the delivery of high-quality comprehensive oncology care, although educational preparation and disciplinary practice focus differentiates their unique contributions. All APNs are prepared at the master's level and most within the specialty of oncology. Nursing is a distinct health profession and nurses practice under a professional nursing license. Primary care is the focus of the PA's educational preparation and PAs practice within the medical model in a delegated role under the supervision of a physician.[3] APNs may practice independently or collaboratively with physicians, as permitted by individual state law.[20] Collaborative practice between a physician and an APN represents a relationship in which both disciplines share knowledge and have diverse but complementary expertise and skills.[9] This type of interdisciplinary relationship between a physician and APN enhances communication and understanding, provides mutual support and results in an efficient approach to the delivery of comprehensive quality care, improved patient outcomes, and increased patient satisfaction.[38,43,45,75–77]

The current health care environment presents significant challenges to the delivery of high-quality patient-centered oncology care. Innovative collaborative models of care among providers can create environments that support the oncology health care team to achieve high-quality clinical outcomes, efficient use of resources, empowerment of the patient and family, and successful clinical research and maintain a state-of-the-art evidence-based practice.

Acknowledgments

For review of the manuscript: Mary Cooley, RN, PhD, NP; Janet van Cleve, RN, MSN, NP; Gail Melkus, RN, EdD; and Pamela Minarik, RN, MSN, CNS. Support for M. Tish Knobf: American Cancer Society Professor of Oncology Nursing.

REFERENCES

1. American Association of Physician Assistant (AAPA). *1998 Physician assistant census report.* 1998.
2. Hooker RS, Cawley JF. *Physician assistants in American medicine.* New York: Churchill Livingstone, 1997.
3. Cooper RA, Henderson T, Dietrich CL. Roles of nonphysician clinicians as autonomous providers of patient care. *JAMA* 1996;280:795.
4. Cooper RA, Laud P, Dietrich BS. Current and projected workforce of nonphysician clinicians. *JAMA* 1996;208:788.
5. Oncology Nursing Society. *Statement on the scope and standards of advanced practice in oncology nursing.* Pittsburgh, PA: Author, 1997.
6. American Nurses Association. *Nursing's social policy statement.* Washington, DC: Author, 1995.
7. Brooten D, Naylor MD. Nurses' effect on changing patient outcomes. *Image Journal Nursing Scholarship* 1995;27:95.
8. McCorkle R, Benoliel JQ, Donaldson G, et al. A randomized clinical trial of home nursing care for lung cancer patients. *Cancer* 1989;64:1375.
9. Freund CM, Fox JA. Research in support of nurse practitioners. In: Mezey MD, McGivern DO, eds. *Nurses, nurse practitioners.* New York: Springer, 1999:32.
10. Henderson V. *Nature of nursing.* New York: Macmillan, 1966.
11. Caitlin AJ, McAuliffe M. Proliferation of non-physician providers as reported in the Journal of the American Medical Association (JAMA), 1998. *Image Journal Nursing Scholarship* 1999;31:175.
12. Snyder M, Mirr MP. *Advanced practice nursing.* 2nd ed. New York: Springer, 1999.
13. Cooley M, Spatz DL, Yasko JM. Role implementation in cancer nursing. In: McCorkle R, Grant M, Frank-Stromberg M, Baird S, eds. *Cancer nursing: a comprehensive textbook.* 2nd ed. Philadelphia: WB Saunders, 1996:25.
14. Mezey MD, McGivern DO. *Nurses, nurse practitioners.* 3rd ed. New York: Springer, 1999.
15. American Association of Colleges of Nursing. *The essentials of master's education for advanced practice nursing.* Washington, DC: Author, 1997.
16. National Organization of Nurse Practitioner Faculties. *Advanced nursing practice: curriculum guidelines.* Washington, DC: Author, 1995.
17. American Cancer Society/Oncology Nursing Society. *The master's degree with a specialty in advanced practice oncology nursing, curriculum guide.* 3rd ed. American Cancer Society: 1994.
18. Brown J, Hinds P. Assessing master's programs in advanced practice oncology nursing. *Oncol Nurs Forum* 1999;26:1371.
19. Porcher FK. Licensure, certification and credentialing. In: Mezey MD, McGivern DO, eds. *Nurses, nurse practitioners.* 3rd ed. New York: Springer, 1999:422.
20. Pearson LJ. Annual update of how each state stands on legislative issues affecting advanced nursing practice. *Nurse Practitioner* 1999;24:16.
21. National Council of State Boards of Nursing. *National Council State Boards of Nursing position paper on the licensure of advanced nursing practice.* Chicago: Author, 1992.
22. Greco KE. Regulation of advanced nursing practice: part one—second licensure. *Oncol Nurs Forum* 1995;22(Suppl):35.
23. Lindeke L, Mirr MP. Professional issues: licensure and certification, prescriptive privileges and reimbursement. In: Snyder M, Mirr MP, eds. *Advanced practice nursing.* 2nd ed. New York: Springer, 1999:37.
24. McMillan SC, Huesinkveld KB, Spray JA, Murphy CM. Revising the blueprint for the AOCN examination using a role delineation study for advanced practice oncology nursing. *Oncol Nurs Forum* 1999;26:529.
25. American College of Nurse Practitioners. Medicare and Medicaid reimbursement for NPs. (http:/www.nurse.org/acnp/facts/reimbur.shtml), 1998.
26. Jacobs LA, Kreamer KM. The oncology clinical nurse specialist in a post-master's nurse practitioner program: a personal and professional journey. *Oncol Nurs Forum* 1997;24:1387.
27. Cobb MA. CNS role in women's health promotion and collaborative practice. *Clinical Nurse Specialist* 1998;12:112.
28. Kinney A, Hawkins R, Hudmon KS. A descriptive study of the role of the oncology nurse practitioner. *Oncol Nurs Forum* 1997;24:811.
29. Scott RA. A description of the roles, activities and skills of clinical nurse specialists in the United States. *Clinical Nurse Specialist* 1999;13:183.
30. McGivern DO, Mezey MD. Advanced practice nursing: preparation and clinical practice. In: Mezey MD, McGivern DO, eds. *Nurse, nurse practitioners.* 3rd ed. New York: Springer, 1999:3.
31. Galassi A. Role of the oncology advanced practice nurse. In: Groenwald S, Frogge M, Goodman M, Yarbro CH, eds. *Cancer nursing principles and practice.* 4th ed. Boston: Jones & Bartlett, 1997:1755.

32. Kaplow R. The role of the advanced practice nurse in the care of patients critically ill with cancer. *AACN Clinical Issues* 1996;7:120.
33. Daly BJ. *The acute care nurse practitioner.* New York: Springer, 1997.
34. Logan P. *Principles and practice of acute care nurse practitioner.* Stamford, CT: Appleton & Lange, 1999.
35. Suter S, Snow S. Integrating advanced practice nurses into in patient care. *Oncol Nurs Forum* 1999;26:975.
36. Haylock PJ. Home care for the person with cancer. *Home Healthcare Nurse* 1993;11:16.
37. Brant JM. The art of palliative care: living with hope, dying with dignity. *Oncol Nurs Forum* 1998;25:995.
38. Krammer LM, Muir JC, Gooding-Kellar N, Williams MB, vonGunten CF. Palliative care and oncology: opportunities for oncology nursing. *Oncology Nursing Updates* 1999;6:1.
39. Cooley ME, Lin EM, Hunter SW. The ambulatory oncology nurse's role. *Seminars Oncol Nurs* 1994;10:245.
40. Vooght S, Richardson A. A study to explore the role of a community oncology nurse specialist. *Eur J Cancer Care* 1996;5:217.
41. Poole K. The evolving role of the clinical nurse specialist within the comprehensive breast cancer centre. *J Clin Nurs* 1996;5:341.
42. Bodansky BE. The advanced practice nurse in radiation oncology. In: Dow KH, Bucholtz JD, Iwamoto R, Fieler V, Hilderley L, eds. *Nursing care in radiation oncology.* Philadelphia: WB Saunders, 1997:377.
43. Hilderley LJ. Nurse-physician collaborative practice: the clinical nurse specialist in radiation oncology private practice. *Oncol Nurs Forum* 1991;18:585.
44. Moore GJ. Collaborative role of a nurse practitioner in a university radiation oncology department. *Cancer Pract* 1996;4:285.
45. Mast ME. Nurse practitioners help to provide quality cost-effective care to patients with cancer. *ONS News* 1998;13:1.
46. Sparks RK. The APN as educator. In: Snyder M, Mirr MP, eds. *Advanced practice nursing.* New York: Springer, 1999;117.
47. Bakke SI. Implementing the staff educator component of the oncology clinical nurse specialist. *Oncol Nurs Forum* 1992;19:607.
48. Gordon M, Murphy CP, Candee D, Hiltunen E. Clinical judgement: an integrated model. *Adv Nurs Sci* 1994;16:55.
49. Groenwald S, Frogge MH, Goodman M, Yarbro CH. *Cancer nursing principles and practice.* 4th ed. Boston: Jones & Bartlett, 1997.
50. Yarbro CH, Frogge MH, Goodman M. *Cancer symptom management.* 2nd ed. Boston: Jones & Bartlett, 1999.
51. McCorkle R, Grant M, Frank-Stromberg M, Baird SB. *Cancer nursing: a comprehensive textbook.* 2nd ed. Philadelphia: WB Saunders, 1996.
52. Dow KH, Bucholtz KD, Iwamoto R, Fieler V, Hilderley L. *Nursing care in radiation oncology.* 2nd ed. Philadelphia: WB Saunders, 1997.
53. Dow KH. *Contemporary issues in breast cancer.* Boston: Jones & Bartlett, 1996.
54. Johnson BL, Gross J. *Handbook of oncology nursing,* 3rd ed. Boston: Jones & Bartlett, 1998.
55. Wilkes G, Barton Burke M, Ingwersen K. *2000 Oncology nursing drug handbook.* Boston: Jones & Bartlett, 1999.
56. Itano JK, Taoka KN. *Core curriculum for oncology nursing.* 3rd ed. Philadelphia: WB Saunders, 1998.
57. Rieger PT. *Clinical handbook for biotherapy.* Boston: Jones & Bartlett, 1999.
58. McGuire DB, Yarbro CH, Ferrell BR. *Cancer pain management.* 2nd ed. Boston: Jones & Bartlett, 1995.
59. Moore GJ. *Women and cancer: a gynecologic oncology nursing perspective.* Boston: Jones & Bartlett, 1997.
60. Varrichio C, Pierce M, Walker CL, Ades TB. *A cancer sourcebook for nurses.* 7th ed. Atlanta: American Cancer Society, 1997.
61. Shapiro TW, Davison DB, Rust DM. *A clinical guide to stem cell and bone marrow transplantation.* Boston: Jones & Bartlett, 1997.
62. King CR, Hinds PS. *Quality of life from nursing and patient perspectives.* Boston: Jones & Bartlett, 1998.
63. Winningham ML, Barton Burke M. *Fatigue in cancer.* Boston: Jones & Bartlett, 1999.
64. Moniken DR. Consultation in advanced practice nursing. In: Snyder M, Mirr MP, eds. *Advanced practice nursing.* 2nd ed. New York: Springer, 1999:149.
65. Hansen HE. The advanced practice nurse as a change agent. In: Snyder M, Mirr MP, eds. *Advanced practice nursing.* 2nd ed. New York: Springer, 1999:187.
66. Smith MS, Holcombe JK, Stullenbarger E. A meta-analysis of intervention effectiveness for symptom management in oncology nursing research. *Oncol Nurs Forum* 1994;21: 1201.
67. Winningham ML, Nail LN, Barton Burke M, et al. Fatigue and the cancer experience: the state of the knowledge. *Oncol Nurs Forum* 1994;21:23.
68. Bookbinder M, Goldstein ML, Derby S, et al. The research connection to quality care in the 21st century. *Oncology Nursing Updates* 1996;3:1.
69. Berger AM, Eilers JG, Heerman JA, et al. State-of-the-art patient care. The impact of doctorally prepared clinical nurses. *Clinical Nurse Specialist* 1999;13:259.
70. Goldberg NJ, Moch SD. An advanced practice nurse-nurse researcher collaborative model. *Clinical Nurse Specialist* 1998;12:251.
71. DiStasio SA, Hubbard SM. Principles of clinical research. In: Johnson BL, Gross J. *Handbook of oncology nursing.* 3rd ed. Boston: Jones & Bartlett, 1998:219.
72. Raybuck JA. The clinical nurse specialist as research coordinator in clinical drug trials. *Clinical Nurse Specialist* 1997;11:15.
73. Knox GE, et al. Downsizing, reengineering and patient safety: numbers, new-ness and resultant risk. *J Health Risk Manag* 1999;19:18.
74. Fischer DS, Alfano S, Knobf MT, Donovan C, Beaulieu N. Improving the cancer chemotherapy use process. *J Clin Oncol* 1996;14:3148.
75. Baggs JG, Schmitt MH. Collaboration between nurse and physicians. *Image Journal Nursing Scholarship* 1988;20:145.
76. Kavesh W. Physician and nurse practitioner relationships. In: Mezey MD, McGivern DO, eds. *Nurses, nurse practitioners.* 3rd ed. New York: Springer, 1999:186.
77. Neale J. Nurse practitioners and physicians: a collaborative practice. *Clinical Nurse Specialist* 1999;13:252.

Christopher Daugherty
Mark Siegler

CHAPTER 59

Ethical Issues in Oncology and Clinical Trials

This chapter begins with an overview of clinical medical ethics and the doctor–patient relationship (DPR) and then examines ethical issues, primarily in medical oncology, relating to both clinical care and clinical research. With regard to cancer clinical care, an effort has been made to cover those topics of greatest importance to the cancer physician: informed consent and decision making; prognosis determination and communication; and ethical issues in the care of patient with life-threatening and life-ending disease, including palliative care, advanced care planning, specific dilemmas related to providing end-of-life cancer care, and physician-assisted suicide (PAS). In examining cancer clinical research, the chapter focuses on specific ethical principles that ought to guide such research; the issues surrounding the concept and practice of informed consent for clinical trials; and the ethical issues and dilemmas associated with phase I, II, and III trials in oncology. Wherever possible, available empiric research is used in an attempt to address, and even resolve, the ethical issues and dilemmas that arise in cancer care and research settings.

ETHICAL ISSUES IN CANCER CLINICAL CARE

DOCTOR–PATIENT RELATIONSHIP AND CLINICAL MEDICAL ETHICS

To practice medicine competently and to provide high-quality care for cancer patients and others, physicians require both scientific and technical proficiency as well as a working knowledge of medical ethics.[1] This specialized knowledge and proficiency is used to assist patients, sometimes by curing or managing their illness and disease and sometimes by helping them overcome the fear, pain, and suffering that are often associated with illness. Competent physicians need not only practical and technical skills, but also the ability to manage such issues as informed consent, decision making, as well as end-of-life and palliative care. A working knowledge of practical ethics is not a substitute for the traditional standards of character and virtue expected of the good physician: competency, integrity, honesty, compassion, and respect for patients and colleagues. Since 1985, medical ethics has emerged as a new and useful component of medical practice and has assisted physicians and patients to reach ethically acceptable decisions. Clinical ethics focuses on how patients and physicians work within existing administrative, economic, and political structures to reach mutual agreement on clinical decisions that affect the patient.

The DPR is at the center of clinical medical ethics.[2] Most day-to-day ethical problems that arise in patient care present in the context of the DPR and most are resolved within this relationship. In the United States, the DPR has undergone two major changes in the past generation. Initially, in the 1970s and 1980s, the relationship began evolving from a paternalistic one, in which physicians made choices for patients based on physicians' values, to a more equal relationship of shared decision making, in which physicians advised patients, but patients ultimately made their own health care choices. Patient preferences are the ethical and legal nucleus of the DPR. In addition, respect for patients and their preferences is a clinical obligation because patients who reach a shared health care decision have greater trust and loyalty in the DPR, cooperate more fully to implement the shared decision, express greater satisfaction with their health care, and most important, have been shown to have better clinical outcomes in several chronic diseases.[3]

The second major change in the DPR has occurred more recently and relates to cost containment and managed care. To curtail health costs, private and government payers for health care have attempted to limit the freedom of decision making of both patients and physicians. Such actions have given rise to new and recurring ethical concerns within the DPR, as well as to potential repercussions[4] (e.g., the so-called patient bill of rights). Changes in the relationship between patients and physicians to a more equal relationship of shared decision making demand attention to ethical issues such as honest disclosure, effective communication, and informed consent.

Sound ethical analysis in clinical settings rests on a foundation of trust between the patient and physician, in other words, within the DPR. Crucial components in the analysis of any ethical issue include an understanding by both parties of the medical and scientific facts; the preferences, values, and goals of both patient and the physician; and the external constraints such as cost, limited resources, and legal duties that shape or restrict choices.[5] For instance, in the cancer setting, physicians have the excellent opportunity to cement trust and reduce the chances of conflict arising with respect to end-of-life care decisions by communicating clearly with patients about prognosis and treatment goals.

For a variety of reasons, ethical issues arise in oncology practice more frequently than in the past. Scientific advances and new technologies have raised unprecedented ethical problems: When should efforts to prolong life with ventilators or dialysis machines be stopped? To what populations of patients should potentially life-saving or life-prolonging (but highly toxic) therapies such as stem cell transplantation be applied? Changes in molecular medicine and genetics are generating new and different ethical problems in such traditional areas as informed consent and confidentiality: Who should have access to an individual's results of BRCA1 testing, and how should such information be used? Managed care has given rise to new ethical issues such as limitations on decision-making freedom for patients and physicians, and potential financial conflicts of interest associated with limiting the use of health resources.

Despite scientific developments of the past century, and despite the financial changes alluded to, the role of the medical profession in human societies has changed surprisingly little since the time of Hippocrates. In general, the DPR has also changed little and the encounter of healer and patient has remained the principal means by which medicine achieves its goals. Several reasons explain the extraordinary continuity over time of the DPR: (1) Medicine serves a universal and unchanging human need by responding to a patient's sense of illness or *disease*; (2) medicine has an unchanging central goal, which is to help patients; and (3) most medical help is delivered in the direct encounter of patient and physician (i.e., in the DPR). It is hardly surprising, therefore, that the DPR is the context in which the important ethical issues such as informed consent, decision making, prognosis communication, and the care of those with life-threatening and life-ending cancer diagnoses (e.g., advanced care planning, end-of-life care, and PAS) must be examined.

INFORMED CONSENT AND SHARED DECISION MAKING

The process by which physicians and patients make decisions together is often summarized in the phrase *informed consent.* This doctrine, which reflects respect for patients, is at the heart of the DPR and is based on the ethical principle of respect for individual autonomy, dignity, and self-determination.[6] Informed consent has three key components: disclosure, competency, and voluntariness.

Disclosure means that physicians tell patients about the medical diagnosis, prognosis, and risks and benefits associated with possible treatment options. Patients are entitled to enough information to permit them to ask reasonable questions about the diagnosis and the options that are available. *Competency* means that patients are able to understand relevant information, appreciate their own needs and values, manipulate information rationally, and communicate a treatment choice. *Voluntariness* means that a patient chooses freely, without coercion from the physician or anyone else.

Informed consent is not an event, nor does it refer to a patient's signature on a consent form. It is a process of continuous communication and dialogue between doctor and patient. In this process, physicians can help to empower patients to act in an autonomous manner by educating them about the nature of their medical problems and reasonable medical alternatives to resolve (or cope with) them. Patients are then in a position to choose treatment based on their own personal preferences, values, and goals. This subsequently enables them to directly exercise their autonomy or control over treatment decisions.[7–10]

From an ethical perspective, no cancer patient can make a truly informed decision about a particular plan of care until he or she has been made aware of, and understands, the potential alternatives. For cancer patients and others, either in clinical research or receiving clinical care, disclosure by the patient's health care provider of treatment alternatives is one of the central components of the informed consent process.[1,6,11] Such disclosure is essential if shared decision making is to occur.[6,7] Patient participation is also advocated because it has been linked to better health outcomes, including decreased anxiety, increased patient satisfaction, and improved compliance.[3,12–18] Moreover, many practitioners believe that improvement in overall quality of life can occur only when patients are fully informed of all reasonable alternatives and become equal partners in the decision-making process.[7,19]

Decision Making versus Information Seeking

The idea that treatment decision making and information seeking are distinctive and separate components of the medical encounter has become increasingly recognized within the doctor–patient communication literature.[14,20,21] Traditionally, the link between patients' desire for decision-making control has been assumed to be directly related to their information-seeking patterns.[18,22–24] It has also been assumed that patients are unable to achieve more involvement in treatment decision making because they have insufficient information.[22] Similarly, it has been expected that patients who want more control will also want more information about their treatment options.[22] Conversely, those who are information seekers are assumed to prefer involvement in decision making because of their proactive approach to maintaining their health. Increasingly, however, evidence suggests that, while patients generally express *preferences* for information about their illness and treatment,[11,18,22–25] they do not necessarily engage in information-*seeking* behaviors.[25] Further, their preferences for participating in treatment decision may vary and may not be linked to their wish for information.[21–26] In fact, several studies have shown no correlation between many cancer patients' information-seeking and decision-making preferences[11,24,26] or between information seeking and their level of participation in actual treatment decisions.[27] Many other variables seemingly unrelated to decision participation may also influence cancer patients' information-seeking patterns.[18,24,25,28]

PROGNOSIS DETERMINATION AND COMMUNICATION

Considering the life-threatening severity of their illness, it is not unreasonable to assume that prognostic information would play a pivotal role in shaping the overall medical decision-making process of cancer patients and lead to the most appropriate treatment decisions. In fact, from an ethical perspective, a discussion of prognosis should be an integral and necessary part of the communication and decision-making processes for cancer patients. This is the case, in part, because prognostic information has been shown to be significantly associated with cancer patients' treatment choices.[29] Nevertheless, several studies have suggested that advanced cancer patients have an inadequate understanding of their prognoses,[29–32] with patients generally overestimating the probability of their long-term survival. As well, many terminally ill cancer patients believe that the purpose of their treatment, even in the palliative care setting, is to cure them.[30,32,33] Despite this available empiric data, it should be recognized that this issue (i.e., awareness of prognosis) remains a difficult one to study because patient anxiety, fear, and the need to maintain hope in the face of a grave prognosis may affect advanced cancer patients' understanding of their prognoses. In addition, this research may be limited because, from a methodologic standpoint, these same emotions may affect their measured responses to queries about their awareness of when they believe they are going to die. Thus, these measured responses may not necessarily be an accurate reflection of cancer patients' true awareness of prognosis. Moreover, no studies have examined the effect of physician anxiety and physician desire to help patients maintain hope on actual communication of prognoses to cancer patients.

Physician Disclosure of Prognosis

Early research, some of which dates from the 1940s and 1950s, examining physician communication with cancer patients, clearly documented a great reluctance to disclose a cancer diagnosis and virtually no willingness to discuss prognosis.[34–39] Of those physicians surveyed in even the earliest of studies (most of whom did not disclose a cancer diagnosis), the majority said they would disclose the diagnosis if there was no other way to get the patient to comply with a needed diagnostic or therapeutic intervention.[34,35] Thus, it was not that cancer physicians did not wish to tell a *diagnosis*, but rather that they did not want to give a terminal *prognosis.* Interestingly, improvements in nonsurgical methods of evaluation (predominantly including radiologic, i.e., computed tomographic scans, and lesser invasive biopsy techniques) for confirming a cancer diagnosis have undoubtedly only resulted in the increasing need to better inform patients in order to obtain compliance for more complicated interventions. In addition, during the interval between these studies of the 1940s and 1950s and the late 1970s, when full disclosure of a cancer diagnosis had become the norm,[40] the perceived threat of a cancer diagnosis as a fatal disease has lessened. This is a result of multiple factors, including community and public health education efforts toward early cancer detection, and the U. S. government's declaration of the "War on Cancer," and the ever increasing range of treatment options now available (including many with high rates of success).[41]

Considering, and even in spite of, these events, it is still not difficult to imagine that physicians would remain reluctant to want to give a terminal prognosis. In fact, with regard to current practices toward disclosure of prognosis to cancer patients, the limited available empiric data document that physicians withhold information.[42,43] Physicians would appear to be reluctant to disclose grim prognostic information for the same ethical and psychological reasons they traditionally withheld a diagnosis.[39,44] Physicians may fear that the revelation of a grim prognosis would psychologically damage patients' hope to survive.[43–45] Physicians may also feel discomfort when placing odds on survival, recurrence, and cure. Thus, while the behavior of physicians has changed regarding disclosure of diagnosis, only limited information is available regarding whether they have changed in regard to practices of disclosure of prognosis.

While, from an ethical perspective, physicians have obligations to disclose a terminal prognosis, a question remains as to how such prognostic information ought to be provided.[10,46,47] Some cancer patients may better understand their prognosis when it is discussed through the use of numeric descriptors,[48] whereas others understand their prognoses when it is conveyed in qualitative descriptors.[49] Patients may also discern important information about their prognoses based on physicians' use of euphemisms, vague estimations, and nonverbal or nonlinguistic cues, for example, tone of voice, word choice, extent of eye contact, and so forth.[43] Further, situational factors, including the seriousness of the disease, patient characteristics, and seniority of the physician, have been shown to influence the extent to which physicians disclose prognostic information.[50] As mentioned, quantitative research has shown that patients generally have inaccurate estimates of their prognoses.[29–32] Most studies investigating how physicians foresee cancer patients' prognoses reveal that physicians themselves are often overly and incorrectly optimistic in their predictions of individual cancer patient survival.[51–58] Yet, how, and even whether, physicians' communication may contribute to patient misunderstanding remains unknown.

How oncologists make decisions about presenting prognostic information is undoubtedly a complex process, potentially influenced by multiple factors, including the patient's clinical condition and sociodemographics. As well, the physician's own sociocultural background may influence the depth and style of presenting prognostic information. In addition, the relationships between a particular oncologist and patient, the perceived patient desire for control over medical decisions, and a patient's information-seeking preferences may influence a physician's information-giving practices. An oncologist may provide more information about a patient's prognosis when a patient requests it, or may present little information based on their understanding of a patient's psychological state.

ETHICAL ISSUES IN THE CARE OF PATIENTS WITH LIFE-THREATENING AND LIFE-ENDING DISEASE

Oncologists deal almost exclusively with patients with serious and life-threatening diseases, many of whom are terminally ill.

It is therefore essential that oncologists have a working knowledge regarding the ethical issues related to palliative care, advanced care planning, the specific dilemmas present in end-of-life cancer care, and PAS.

Palliative Care

Oncologists must become experts in providing excellent palliative care, including both pain management and the relief of other symptoms such as nausea, dyspnea, and anxiety. Although palliative care has often come to be specifically emphasized in the setting of end-of-life care, oncologists must be equipped to provide excellent palliative care to all of their patients, not just to those who are terminally ill. For a complete discussion, see Chapters 56.1, 56.2, 56.3, 56.4, 56.5, 56.6, 56.7.

Advance Care Planning

ADVANCE CARE PLANNING FOR AWAKE PATIENTS WITH DECISION-MAKING CAPACITY. When oncologists and patients reach joint decisions about a plan for diagnosis and treatment, they are engaged in advance care planning. A fundamental ethical principle that underlies advance care planning is informed consent. Adult patients who have decision-making capacity, sometimes referred to by the legal term *competence*, have a right to make their own health care choices after being provided with appropriate information about the risks and benefits of reasonable alternative approaches. The principle of informed consent applies even to treatments that may be necessary to save a patient's life. Competent adult patients have the ethical and legal right to decline, or ask to have discontinued, treatments that may be life-saving, including intensive care unit care, life support measures such as dialysis and mechanical ventilation, and chemotherapy. Before accepting a patient's statement or decision, physicians must assess the following: (1) Has the patient been provided with adequate information to make life and death choices? (2) Does the patient understand the risks and benefits of the physician's recommendation and the alternatives? (3) Does the patient understand that the refusal of the proposed treatment will result in death? (4) Why is the patient making the choice against treatment? (5) Does the patient have adequate decision-making capacity to make a life and death choice?

None of these questions is easy to answer, but physicians nevertheless have a responsibility to make a good faith effort before acceding to a patient's wish to refuse life-sustaining treatment. Sometimes consultations with colleagues, including psychiatrists, may be necessary to resolve the question of decision-making capacity. In the end, however, the central principles of autonomy and patient rights mean that a competent patient may refuse life-sustaining treatment even if the physician believes such a refusal is a bad choice or is not consistent with the patient's prior wishes or is morally wrong.

ADVANCE CARE PLANNING FOR PATIENTS WHO LACK DECISION-MAKING CAPACITY. Decision making for unconscious patients, or for patients who are conscious but lack decision-making capacity, follows the same informed consent model as applies to competent adults. Essentially, incompetent patients are accorded the right to have their previous wishes made known and acted on by their physicians. Advance care planning is a process in which patients, their families, and their physicians plan in advance for treatment decisions, including decisions about life-sustaining treatment, that may have to made when the patient is no longer capable of participating in the decision. During the past 30 years, the traditional approach used for advance care planning in the United States has involved formal, written advance directives that indicate who should serve as the patient's proxy or surrogate and what end-of-life choices a patient would want if he or she were unable to participate in the decision. In our view, advance directives have not been a successful strategy for achieving patients' wishes and goals. There are many reasons to explain the failure of advance directives, but simply put, most people have not completed written advance directives and when they have, they are often overruled by a patient's family, ignored by physicians, or simply misunderstood.[59]

To achieve more successful advance care planning, written formal advance directives should not be exclusively relied on to make such extremely important decisions, but rather oncologists should commit themselves to the *process* of advance care planning. The process, rather than the simple *event* of signing a written advance directive form (sometimes months or years in advance of the need to make a decision), involves a series of conversations over time between the treating oncologist and the patient (and often the patient's family) in which the patient's goals and preferences are discussed and clarified. Such conversations should always be specific to the individual patient and to the actual clinical circumstances that are likely to be present at some near or distant future time when the patient may have lost decision-making capacity.

These conversations should determine two things: (1) Who would the patient want to serve as a proxy decision maker if the patient were unable to make decisions? (2) Based on the most likely future scenario for a particular patient, what choices would the patient want the surrogate to make (e.g., for aggressive or curative care, palliative care, or focusing more exclusively on end-of-life care). These conversations should be documented in the physician's notes and such conversations likely should occur on more than one occasion as the patient's clinical and life circumstances change. These are not easy conversations to have, and many physicians feel ill prepared to discuss these matters with their patients. This is an educational and behavorial failure. Physicians must learn how to conduct these important conversations. Good patient care requires that we advise and council our patients on what is possible and what is reasonable. The advance care planning process is an opportunity to do that.

Ethical Dilemmas in End-of-Life Cancer Care

As previously discussed, in the setting of cancer care in which prognosis is known to result in eventual death (i.e., advanced cancer) how and when such prognoses should be communicated remain matters of concern and controversy. In addition, several equally important concerns arise in the specific setting of advanced cancer regarding how and when palliative care may be implemented, as opposed to care that includes further attempts with anticancer agents. For advanced cancer patients who, by definition, have a life-ending diagnosis for which an anticancer standard of care has failed (or is unidentified), it remains unclear what factors influence their decisions to receive any particular form of care. For the more than 500,000 advanced cancer patients who die each year in the United States,[60] from both societal and medical perspectives, it is accepted that the ideal alternatives of care include receiving state-of-the-art palliative care, as available in hospice, and participation in clinical research involving an experimental agent (e.g., phase I trials). For reasons to be discussed, because of the complexities related to predicting time to death in those with advanced cancer, it may be difficult to know when referral to hospice might be appropriate or when it is still medically appropriate to continue attempts at anticancer therapy, including experimental agents.[51,61–64]

For advanced cancer patients to formally receive hospice care in the United States, through Medicare and insurance hospice benefits, they must be documented by their physician as having a prognosis of 6 months or less. Interestingly, for cancer patients participating in phase I trials of experimental agents, their median survival has been described as being almost identical to this prognostic milestone—6.5 months.[65] It is not clear which of these alternatives, experimental agents or hospice care, results in longer life or improved quality of life.[52,66–68] As well, there is limited data on the cost effectiveness of these alternatives.[69–72]

With regard to hospice care, as it is currently provided within third-party payer systems, it is clear that it remains greatly underused for advanced cancer patients. Only approximately 20% to 30% of cancer patients die each year while under hospice care. In addition, available Medicare data have shown that the median survival of cancer patients in hospice is only on the order of 2 to 3 weeks.[73] It has been argued that one of the obstacles to providing appropriate palliative care, as available in hospice, is a result of physician inaccuracy in predicting time to death.[52,73,74] While this undoubtedly plays some role in many physicians' hesitancy (and even unwillingness) to refer cancer patients to hospice, it does not provide a complete explanation for the apparent underuse of hospice services. Other reasons clearly exist for this hesitancy and unwillingness including perceived dilemmas related to physicians' desire to effectively communicate terminal prognoses to cancer patients and their families and still be able to facilitate the maintenance of hope; patients' and families' hesitancy or unwillingness to accept such prognoses; physician concerns regarding loss of control over their patients' medical care; and concerns about the methods by which the majority of hospice care is paid for in the United States, which may be insufficient to meet the needs of the dying.

Perceptions about damaging patient's and family's hope in the face of communicating a terminal prognosis remain a matter of concern among many clinicians. In fact, many clinicians believe that if they were to *effectively* communicate a terminal prognosis to a patient, they would essentially destroy the patient's hope.[44] Many physicians maintain that regardless of how sensitively or compassionately a terminal diagnosis is communicated, the ability of patients to sustain any meaningful hope is compromised. The effect of this physician belief clearly creates obstacles to quality end-of-life care and should not be underestimated.

In addition, for patients and families to accept referral to hospice, they presumably must (in some way) accept a terminal prognosis. This may not necessarily have to be the case, but patients or family members must sign consent forms for hospice care documenting that the terminal prognosis of the patient has been disclosed (even understood), and that they wish to receive no further treatment aimed at reversing their cancer. In addition, they must sign an advance directive stating that they wish no life-sustaining interventions be used in their care. Physicians often perceive that such disclosure of a terminal prognosis, and the requirements associated with signing such forms, may also severely damage a patient's and family members' hopes. As well, physicians may believe, with patients and family members often sharing this belief, that to agree to such care is to essentially give up. Patients are known to deny their terminal prognoses even in the face of explicit physician disclosure.[75] If this is the case, it obviously will be more difficult, perhaps even unethical, to refer such patients to hospice who willingly choose not to accept their terminal prognoses, as compared with those who have accepted their prognoses.

Some physicians and patients may also have fears or concerns regarding patient abandonment if and when they are referred to hospice. This may be the case in settings in which a cancer patient has been receiving significant amounts of anticancer therapy (e.g., chemotherapy) for several months or years before the recognition of a terminal prognosis. Now, with the introduction of the potential for hospice care, the care environment may be perceived as changing in dramatic ways. For example, such patients will no longer be receiving chemotherapy, or undergoing the pattern of physician and nursing visits as they had previously. This may be particularly true for those patients who have received their cancer care almost exclusively at hospitals or medical centers some distance from their homes or communities. Traditionally, when patients are referred to hospice in the United States, they typically undergo fewer (if any) physician office visits, receiving the vast majority of care in the home. Thus, patients may feel as though they are being abandoned by their physicians and health care providers. Some physicians may even perceive this threat of abandonment (real or otherwise) within patients or family members and, as a result, not pursue the option of hospice care.

Even further complicating matters, physicians may develop conflicts of interests when an appropriate time comes when adequate palliative care could be provided in hospice. These conflicts can relate to both financial and psychological issues. In a not uncommon example, consider a patient who is appropriate for referral to hospice yet a physician continues to make medical decisions that involve chemotherapy and receives reimbursement for such care. Here, a physician may have financial conflicts of interest and may be unwilling to refer to hospice for fear of lost income. Another more common (and perhaps more acceptable) example is physicians may perceive referral to hospice as implying loss of decision control and may be unwilling to refer because they have psychological needs to maintain decision control or maintain emotional attachments to their patients.

A final example of the dilemmas present in providing end-of-life care to advanced cancer patients relates to the Medicare and insurance benefits that exist to provide reimbursement for hospice care in the United States. In 2000, such care is paid for through a per diem benefit, with the Medicare per diem being approximately $120 a day (the actual rate depending on the region of the country in which the care is provided). A clear dilemma arises for some cancer patients, whose prognoses are undoubtedly terminal (i.e., consistent with less than 6 months of life) but who may have an otherwise excellent performance status and show evidence for continuing to benefit from rather expensive or aggressive palliative interventions. These might include such interventions as antibiotics, blood transfusions, and possibly even chemotherapy in some specific circumstances, for example, palliative chemotherapy for pancreatic carcinoma, indolent breast cancer, hormone-refractory prostate cancer, or those with hematologic malignancies. In these advanced cancer patient examples, such a per diem would not cover the costs of aggressive palliative care. As a result, physicians may not ever refer certain populations of patients to hospice. Or, they may perceive that hospices are not particularly interested in caring for such patients because of the high cost of such palliative interventions. Indeed, many hospices do have practical and appropriate concerns about cost containment. Thus, for a hospice that is attempting to maintain its solvency and continue to care for many terminally ill patients, many aggressive interventions may be financially prohibitive.

Some of the dilemmas present in providing end-of-life cancer care in the United States might be eliminated, or at least reduced in magnitude, by increasing or restructuring the Medicare hospice benefit.[76] As well, continuing medical education programs designed at improving communication techniques among oncologists may be effective in improving the ability of cancer physicians to communicate a terminal prognosis without the perceptions, real or otherwise, relating to the destruction of patient and family hope.[77] However, as long as perceptions and beliefs (appropriate or otherwise) exist among physicians, patients, and families that to accept (or disclose) a terminal cancer prognosis is equivalent to giving up hope,[78] there will likely always be hesitancy, resistance, and even unwillingness to accept end-of-life care as it has been traditionally provided.

Physician-Assisted Suicide

Oncologists must be informed about PAS so they are prepared to discuss this controversial issue if it is raised by patients or their families. Whenever PAS is raised in the clinical context, oncologists should be certain that the patient's pain is being controlled, that symptoms other than pain such as dyspnea, pruritus, and constipation are adequately managed, that advance care planning has been done, and that the patient is given the opportunity to maintain control over his or her situation (e.g., by being permitted to make medical choices).

RELEVANT DEFINITIONS AND DISTINCTIONS. PAS is defined as a physician prescribing a lethal dose of medication, and sometimes providing technical advice to a patient, who subsequently commits suicide without further assistance from the physician. The distinction between PAS and euthanasia is generally based on who administers the lethal dose: the patient (in PAS) or the physician (in euthanasia). PAS also differs from a competent adult patient's right to decline life-sustaining treatment in terms of the actual cause of death, the class of patients potentially affected by the practice, and the legality of the action. For example, PAS is currently illegal except in Oregon, whereas the right of patients to decline or forgo life support is clinically, ethically, and legally the standard of care throughout the United States.[1] The final distinction is the most subtle one (i.e., between PAS and aggressive pain management as occurs when a morphine drip is hung). Essentially, if the morphine drip is being used to palliate the patient's symptoms of pain, nausea, anxiety, and so forth, its use does not represent PAS, whereas if the morphine drip is being used deliberately to hasten the patient's death or kill the patient, it probably represents euthanasia rather than PAS.

ARGUMENTS FOR AND AGAINST PHYSICIAN-ASSISTED SUICIDE. The strongest arguments favoring PAS are claims based on autonomy and beneficence. The autonomy argument maintains that individuals have moral authority over their lives and should be permitted to control all aspects of life based on their own assessment of benefits and burdens, including the timing and means of their deaths. In this context, patients not only have a right to refuse treatment but also have a right to request PAS. Patients may exercise this choice if they are in pain, or are suffering, or perceive a loss of dignity, or indeed if they offer any reason, or none at all, for doing so.

The beneficence argument favoring PAS claims that the relief of pain and suffering is a central aspect of medical care and, therefore, PAS should be viewed as part of the continuum of care to relieve a patient's pain and suffering. Patients who have received appropriate pain management and adequate palliative care, but who continue to experience physical pain or unremitting suffering should be permitted to request PAS from compassionate physicians who are capable of providing the means to end the patient's life painlessly and efficiently.[79]

Both the autonomy and beneficent claims favoring PAS can be answered. The autonomy claim for PAS can be countered with the argument that no rights are absolute and the demand to be assisted by physicians to commit suicide must be balanced against the clinical, psychological, legal, and moral prohibitions against suicide and against assisting others to commit suicide. The central argument against the beneficence claim is that all physicians, especially oncologists who frequently care for patients who experience pain, must improve their ability to provide better pain management and comfort for patients, but this intervention does not have to include PAS.

Additional arguments against PAS are based on the following three risks of adverse consequences for individuals and for society:

- The risk that those requesting PAS are clinically depressed.
- The "slippery slope" risk that PAS may be performed in some patients who have not voluntarily requested it.
- The risk that PAS may harm the DPR by undermining trust between patients and physicians.

PHYSICIAN-ASSISTED SUICIDE AND DEPRESSION. Depression rather than physical pain is often associated with patient requests for PAS. Among cancer patients, depression is fairly common, probably two to four times more frequent than in the general population. Studies have found that 25% of cancer patients meet criteria for major or minor depression,[80] whereas another series reported that 25% of patients on palliative care services are depressed.[81] For these reasons, it is not surprising that suicide rates among cancer patients are substantially higher than those among the general public.[82] Most important, as in other populations, there is a high association between suicide and depression in cancer patients.[80,83–85] Among terminally ill patients with cancer, the disease often produces somatic symptoms of depression (insomnia, anorexia, fatigue) and makes it difficult to reach a diagnosis of depression. Furthermore, many physicians view depression following a diagnosis of cancer as *appropriate,* rather than as a symptom that needs treatment. Yet, depression among terminally ill patients can be treated with medications or with counseling. Despite the prevalence of potentially treatable mood disorders, data from the Netherlands suggest that only 3% of requests for PAS resulted in a psychiatric consultation.[80,87]

These data suggest that many depressed oncology patients who express an interest in PAS may have a reversible condition, depression, that often is not diagnosed and frequently is not treated. In addition, current safeguards in the Oregon PAS laws are inadequate and contain no mandatory requirement for a formal psychiatric evaluation of the patient, even in cases in which the diagnosis of depression is suspected.

PHYSICIAN-ASSISTED SUICIDE AND THE SLIPPERY SLOPE. One potential slippery slope concern is *encouraged* PAS, in which chronically ill or terminally ill patients may be encouraged or pressured by their families to choose PAS. In a benign variation of this approach, patients without direct coercion from their family may feel that the availability of the PAS option requires them to do the *noble* thing to prevent becoming a burden to their families.

Data on PAS and the slippery slope have come primarily from the experiences in the Netherlands. One of the most important findings to emerge from the empiric studies of Dutch practices regarding PAS and euthanasia concern the practice of voluntary euthanasia. A report commissioned by the Dutch government to empirically evaluate the practice of euthanasia reported that there were approximately 2300 cases of euthanasia per year (1.8% of all deaths) and 400 cases of PAS per year (0.3% of all deaths) in the Netherlands.[87] In addition, there were 1000 cases (0.8% of all deaths) in which patients received euthanasia either without explicitly requesting it or while deemed incompetent to make such a request.[88] In 56% of these cases, the patient was no longer competent when euthanasia was performed. Overall, 27% of Dutch physicians who were interviewed indicated that they had performed euthanasia at least once without an explicit voluntary request for euthanasia by the patient.

These data suggest that in the Netherlands a slippery slope has developed in which euthanasia has been extended from competent adults who voluntarily request it to incompetent patients (both adults and children) who have never made such a request. More recently, a group of Dutch physicians reported on the high complication rate (23%) associated with efforts to perform PAS in 114 cases.[89] In 21 of the 114 cases (18%), the physician decided to administer a lethal medication, which thus transformed the situation from PAS to actual direct euthanasia. This is another variation on the slippery slope that American physicians must be concerned with before PAS is legalized generally.[90]

Two studies of physicians in the state of Washington have been published to help characterize the current status of PAS in this country. In a 1994 study by Cohen and colleagues of 938 physicians (69% response rate),[91] although 54% thought that euthanasia should be legal in some situations, nearly one-half agreed with the statement that euthanasia is never ethically justified. Hematologists and oncologists were most likely to oppose PAS. Two years later, more research from Washington reporting on actual requests for PAS and physician responses was published.[92] The major finding of this 828 physician survey study was that 12% had received one or more explicit requests for PAS and 4% for euthanasia in the past year. The requests were generally from patients with cancer, neurologic disorders, and acquired immunodeficiency syndrome. Patients requests were most often based on concerns about loss of control, being a burden to others, and loss of dignity. Physicians in this study reported providing PAS in 24% of cases in which it had been requested and intended to provide PAS more often to patients with physical symptoms. The authors express concern that physicians did not consult their colleagues in many cases, raising questions about the appropriate regulatory framework to ensure quality in the evaluations of patient requests for physician-assisted death.

Further information regarding attitudes and practices regarding PAS in the United States is available form in an empiric, vignette-based study, by Emmanuel et al. The investigators examined the experiences of the public, cancer patients, and oncologists.[93] In the setting of unremitting pain, approximately two-thirds of cancer patients and the public found both euthanasia and PAS acceptable. They found it less acceptable in the setting of existential suffering, or in the setting in which there was the potential for a patient to be a "burden on the family" (vignette wording). Among patients actually experiencing pain, they were more likely to find euthanasia and PAS unacceptable. Among oncologists, more than one-half stated they had had a request for either euthanasia or PAS, and one in seven said they had performed either practice at least once. In a related set of data, nearly one-half of these oncologists could imagine a situation in which they would want PAS or euthanasia for themselves.[94] These oncologists were more than twice as likely to find euthanasia or PAS acceptable for their patients, as compared with oncologists who could not imagine a situation in which they would want PAS or euthanasia for themselves (86% vs. 42%, respectively). Many oncologists (42%) who would find PAS or euthanasia unacceptable for themselves still found these practices ethical for their patients.

These data can be viewed as concerning as they suggest that there is significant, although not majority support, for the use of PAS and euthanasia in at least some cancer care cases, and that as many as 15% of oncologists have carried out such practices at least once in their professional careers. Interestingly, in subsequent research, Emmanuel found that some oncologists suffered adverse consequences (emotional or psychological) from having performed PAS or euthanasia.[95] Further research is undoubtedly needed to better understand oncologists' attitudes to PAS and their perception of pain and suffering and their perceived obligations in helping cancer patient to end their lives.

Another data source that is being closely scrutinized for evidence of the slippery slope derives from the experience in the state of Oregon, which legalized PAS on October 27, 1997. During the first year of PAS activity, 23 persons requested lethal medications and 15 died after taking the medication.[96] Reports of the second-year experience indicate that 33 persons requested lethal medications and 26 died after taking the medication.[97] In both years, the median age of the patients was 69 to 71; the most common underlying diagnosis was cancer; and the most common reasons for PAS were not physical pain but rather "loss of autonomy due to illness, loss of control of bodily functions," and a wish to determine and control the manner of one's death. Based on the first two reports from Oregon, the use of PAS occurs infrequently and has generally involved patients who were well-insured, educated, and already in hospice programs. It is too soon to know whether vulnerable populations will also be recruited to participate in Oregon's PAS initiative.

THREAT TO PROFESSIONAL INTEGRITY AND TRUST BETWEEN PATIENT AND PHYSICIAN. Cancer patients often have a heightened sense of their own mortality and a need to trust a physician in a relationship that is based on honest communication but nurtures hope.[44] The conflation of the concept of healing with procedures designed to bring about the patient's death creates a serious threat to the integrity of the medical profession.[98] PAS and euthanasia distort the fundamental norms of medicine in at least three ways: (1) by diverting attention from the substantive issues of providing good care for dying patients; (2) by subverting the social role of the physician as healer; and (3) by often undermining the trust that patients place in their physicians. Many patients benefit from knowing that PAS is not an option that their physician would contemplate, and this reassurance strengthens the trust that cancer patients place in their doctors. Similarly, physicians efforts to prolong life and aggressively relieve pain and suffering are bolstered by the fundamental prohibition against actively ending the lives of their patients with PAS and euthanasia.

Based on our analysis of the scanty but worrying data on these practices (especially those available from the Netherlands), along with our view that PAS and euthanasia will ultimately weaken, not strengthen, the relationship of oncologists and patients and will attenuate the fundamental prohibition against killing in the medical context, we recommend that at this time oncologists resist appeals to participate in PAS and euthanasia.

ETHICAL ISSUES IN CANCER CLINICAL TRIALS

This section of the chapter examines the ethical issues associated with the clinical research of cancer. Following a brief overview of certain principles that guide the ethical conduct of clinical research, the chapter discusses the history and development of ethical guidelines and requirements regarding human experimentation. Further discussion and background pertaining to the concept and process of informed consent as it specifically relates to cancer patients and clinical research, including the use of consent forms for research, is also provided. The ethical aspects of clinical trials in oncology, including phase I, II, and III studies, are then examined. Wherever possible, empiric information is incorporated into these discussions from research on the informed consent and clinical trial process in cancer.

ETHICAL PRINCIPLES GUIDING CLINICAL RESEARCH

The main objective of clinical research in oncology is to improve medical care for future cancer patients. From both a societal and ethical perspective, this is viewed as a laudable and important goal. As such, no meaningful criticisms can truly be offered against the need and desire to better care for those with cancer. However, when one examines the methods by which this goal is pursued, problematic issues can be found. As is discussed, it is the process of using current patients as research subjects to achieve this goal in which true ethical dilemmas are created.

Whether in the context of clinical practice or clinical research, several specific principles guide the management of patients by physicians.[99,100] The first such principle worthy of mention in this context is, "One ought not to use others as means to an end." In the process of clinical research this general ethical principle is, in many ways, allowed to be violated. However, to allow violation of this principle, it is expected that no patient can participate as a research subject unless there is the potential for benefit. No doubt, in considering what is an acceptable degree of potential benefit, this safeguard is in place for a great proportion of clinical research. (Here, benefit is implied as it is traditionally measured in oncology, i.e., as a specific anticancer response or improvement in a patient–subject's symptoms.) However, as is discussed in the section regarding phase I trials (see Ethical Issues in Phase I Trials, later in this chapter), ethical dilemmas that challenge this safeguard are created in the early drug development process in which the potential for such benefit may be exceedingly small for involved cancer patients.

A second related ethical principle that must guide behavior in the research setting is, "One should not allow harm to come to others." Certainly, oversimplification or generalization of this principle would lead to the prohibition of specific patterns of behavior in the clinical (nonresearch) setting of cancer care, where the harm from toxicities is deemed acceptable because of the known benefits to be achieved. Thus, as with the first principle mentioned, the specific issue of harm cannot truly be weighed without consideration of the relative benefit that may be achieved for cancer patients. However, when cancer patients participate as research subjects in early clinical trials of anticancer agents, there is a greater relative potential for harm to come to patients as a result of the specific methodologies and research objectives employed in these trials. In addition to the recognition that benefit is not likely, there is even an expectation that harm will come. In fact, it may even be a goal of the study to produce harm. The safeguard that must be in place to allow violation of this principle is that the potential for harm to participating subjects must be warranted either as a result of the potential benefits to be achieved or (more commonly) that, given the circumstances of many advanced cancer patients participating in such trials, there are perceived to be no other available meaningful anticancer alternatives.

A third ethical principle that guides behavior in this context is, "One ought never to deceive others." Within clinical research, several safeguards are in place that are designed to prevent the deception of patients who become the subjects of research. The informed consent process itself, and other federal and institutional regulations, provide mechanisms in which oversight of both specific research protocols and the described methods of information provision are present to prevent any intentional deception of patients. More importantly, the conscientious communication efforts of participating physician–investigators are also relied on to prevent deception. However, in the setting of early trials of investigational agents, in which research subjects are most often those with far advanced disease, many have wondered about the potential vulnerability of these subjects and the potential for them to be unintentionally deceived. Indeed, the very fact that the agents under study in early drug trials have shown promise in preclinical models creates a variety of stated or unstated inducements that may play on some advanced cancer patients potentially overwhelming desire for therapeutic benefit and lead to a process akin to deception, albeit unintentional.

In a final principle worthy of mention, medical ethics itself teaches us that, "The interests of an individual physician's patient should be placed above the interests of others." One can easily argue that placing a cancer patient on a clinical trial involving a new investigational agent does not at all compromise their interest in receiving state-of-the-art care. However, one must keep in mind that the overall goal of clinical research (improving care for future patients) remains intact whenever a patient enters a clinical trial.

Thus, at the very least, other interests beyond the individual care of a patient are present when that patient enters a clinical trial. As is discussed, these potentially competing interests can lead to dilemmas. Further insight into these issues and dilemmas can be gained by specifically examining the early phases of cancer clinical research and the attendant informed consent process.

INFORMED CONSENT FOR CLINICAL RESEARCH

The concept of informed consent, which acknowledges the rights of patients to voluntarily participate in health care, applies both to clinical practice and clinical research.[6,101] Informed consent in clinical research is related to, but recognized as being more stringent than, informed consent outside the context of clinical trials.[102] This heightened consent standard exists for at least two reasons. First, from an ethical perspective, a patient considering clinical trial participation is always viewed as potentially vulnerable.[103] As a result of this potential vulnerability, he or she may have great difficulty in appreciating the differences between the therapeutic and research aspects of a given alternative of care or treatment. Without this distinction, patients cannot make uncoerced and autonomous health care decisions. Thus, the informed consent process, and the ethics of clinical research, require that such a clear distinction be made.[8,104] Second, the physician–investigator is seen as having an intrinsic conflict of interest in the role both as a physician for an individual patient and as a scientific investigator attempting to develop improved methods of medical care and treatment.[102,103,105] As previously mentioned, within the sole context of a therapeutic relationship, the physician places his or her patients' interests above all else.[1] However, within the context of clinical research, investigators have additional interests that may not be relative to their patients' interests.[105–110] From an ethical perspective, many concerns exist about the ability of clinical investigators to provide the requisite information to patients regarding participation in research in such a way that allows patients to recognize the distinction between research and therapy.[8,111–113]

A definition of informed consent for clinical research that encompasses all relevant aspects of the process remains somewhat elusive, with varying definitions having been described.[6,101–103] Generally, it is viewed as a process of communication between a patient–subject and a clinician–investigator regarding an investigational or experimental treatment. Within this communication process, several elements must be disclosed. These include the disclosure of the type of research to be performed, the risks and benefits of the treatment or research, the unproven nature of the research, the alternatives other than participation in the clinical trial, and finally, disclosure of the subject's freedom to withdraw or not to participate in the research without any detrimental effect on the patient's continued access to adequate health care. Separate from the issue of disclosure within this process is the issue of actual understanding on the part of the patient with regard to these disclosed elements. Whether the definition of informed consent should include an actual understanding of these elements, or how much of an understanding it should include, remain matters of controversy.[6,112,114] However, from an ethical standpoint it is accepted that the process of informed consent requires at least some attempt on the part of the clinician–investigator to help a patient understand those aspects of the consent process that have been disclosed so that the patient may autonomously and voluntarily decide to participate in research.[100,115] Other elements that have been described as important parts of the informed consent process include maintaining the confidentiality of a research subject's participation and, controversially, possible disclosure of potential conflicts of interest on the part of the clinician–investigator.

In an attempt to emphasize the importance of the distinctions between research and therapy, most ethical regulations governing clinical research have focused on the informed consent process as a means of protecting potentially vulnerable research subjects from physical and psychological harm.[102,103,113] These regulations have relied heavily on written informed consent documents to achieve full disclosure of the important elements of consent, including the risks of research participation, the nature of the research, and alternatives to research participation. Thus, informed consent is currently and most commonly viewed as a means of protection of a potentially vulnerable research subject from harm.[102,103] However, from their inception to the present day, many critics have recognized the imperfect nature of the methods used to regulate the informed consent process.[112,116–120] More recent empiric research on informed consent, a great proportion of which as been conducted in the cancer setting, may be helpful in attempting to objectively identify the current problems and deficiencies associated with written consent documents and their oversight. As reviewed elsewhere, several studies reported since 1980 have increasingly demonstrated that although regulations are being followed, informed consent documents have become increasingly unreadable, lengthy, and uninformative.[121–123] Indeed, they may actually be interfering with what might otherwise be an ethically appropriate informed consent process for patients, including not only those with cancer, but any patient considering therapeutic clinical trial participation.

Shaping of the Regulatory Process for Consent

Beginning in the 1960s, several events occurred that significantly changed the practice and process of informed consent in therapeutic research. One of the most important events, and clearly of greatest significance with regard to cancer and other related therapeutic research, was the publication of Henry Beecher's paper in the *New England Journal of Medicine* in 1966.[124] Beecher, a clinical investigator and anesthesiologist at Harvard, assembled 22 recent research reports that he pulled from the peer-reviewed medical literature that contained, in his view, clear violations of both patients' human rights and the recognized ethical principles of informed consent. Of note, several of the research reports that he described were specifically related to cancer clinical research. One such case was a published report regarding a young woman with metastatic melanoma. In this report, the investigators described excising one of the melanoma lesions from the patient and transplanting it onto the patient's mother. Subsequently, serum was withdrawn from the mother and given to the patient in hopes of producing an immune-mediated tumor response. The patient went on to die relatively quickly of widespread metastatic disease. Even more horrific, the mother subsequently died of metastatic melanoma approximately 1 year later. Another of Beecher's examples, although described without identifiers, clearly included the much publicized case of the Jewish Chronic Disease Hospital.[111] Researchers in this published study, in an attempt to gain information relevant to organ transplantation, injected malignant cells from cancer patients into elderly and debilitated noncancer patients at the hospital.

Beecher's cancer research examples, and the other reports described, put a great deal of the medical research process into the public spotlight. The subsequent outcry from the public and medical community led to regulations in the late 1960s and early 1970s that resulted in greatly increased scrutiny of government-sponsored clinical research.[102,111,125] Clinical researchers themselves undoubtedly became more sensitive to the issues regarding the use of patients, including those with cancer and others, as research subjects. Other events, including the disclosure to the public regarding the United States Public Health Service Syphilis Studies (also known as the Tuskegee Syphilis Study)[96,102,126] as well as the thalidomide experience and subsequent passage of the 1962 amendments to the Food, Drug, and Cosmetic Act,[127] also had a great effect on the regulatory requirements for informed consent in clinical research. All of these events eventually led to the creation of the National Commission for the protection of human subjects in biomedical and behavioral research. The resulting recommendations of the National Commission led to the now required and pervasive practice of formalized institutional review of clinical research protocols.[103]

Undoubtedly, the use of consent forms for clinical trials of new anticancer agents is one such setting in which these issues take on great significance, especially if we are to continue to recognize the value of patient–subject autonomy and the moral importance of the consent process as a mechanism of protection for potentially vulnerable patients attempting to make difficult decisions regarding their medical care. Separate from the content of the consent forms themselves, concerns also exist about the overall effect of the forms on different aspects of the consent process, including its outcome and the decision-making process of patients before the eventual decision to actually participate in a therapeutic clinical trial.

In the clinical trial setting, several studies have examined the potential effect of different information-provision methods on the informed consent process.[10,128–130] It is interesting to note that in a review by Edwards et al. of different methods of information provision in clinical trials across the entire spectrum of disease processes,[130] nearly 60% of these studies were conducted by cancer investigators and focused on clinical trials involving cancer patients as research subjects. In the review by Edwards et al., and as evidenced by the previously mentioned research, despite the format of presentation, information provision may have little effect on patient–subject understanding. Other significant research contributions within the cancer setting to the informed consent literature can be found elsewhere.[121,122,129]

In considering this available empiric data, one is certainly left to wonder about the utility and value of the current consent process for therapeutic clinical trials. Particular concerns develop when one recognizes that great emphasis continues to be placed on consent forms and their content. Such concerns become even more challenging in areas in which consent forms detail investigational therapies with relatively extreme toxicities, and in which the therapeutic goals of the alternatives to clinical trial participation may be quite different from the inherent or perceived goals of investigational therapy.

ETHICAL ISSUES IN PHASE I TRIALS

It is in the specific setting of cancer trials involving new agents (i.e., phase I trials) in which the general concerns about informed consent in therapeutic clinical trials become especially troubling and challenging.[103,131–133] This is because phase I trials typically involve patients with advanced, eventually life-ending disease in a research endeavor where the chance of meaningful objective therapeutic benefit has traditionally been described as being quite low, less than 5%.[134–137] As a result of the dose-escalation methods in these trials,[131] a more specific dilemma is the relative ratio of toxicity and benefit for patients who participate. Further complicating this is the need to adequately inform patients about these particular issues and then allow them to willingly and freely consent to participate in such studies. The complexities of the consent process for advanced cancer patients in phase I trials relate both to what degree such patients should be viewed as vulnerable, and to what extent a participating physician's own expectations and interests play a role in guiding patients to decide to participate. This unique form of therapeutic clinical research creates an intense environment of medical decision making in which arguably, many patients may not benefit from the traditional informed consent process.

If patients were to participate in phase I trials solely for altruistic reasons, in other words, to help forward cancer research and potentially help future cancer patients, phase I trials would probably carry less ethical conflict. As well, this would imply that the traditional informed consent process might more readily achieve the desired ideal outcome of understanding all elements of consent, including an understanding of the nature of phase I research and the alternatives to trial participation, as these less vulnerable patients would not necessarily be seeking benefit for themselves. However, the objective information available regarding the informed consent process for patients participating as research subjects in phase I trials tells us that altruism is not the primary motivating factor for patients participating in such clinical research. As reviewed in this section, the empiric studies examining the phase I consent process highlight the true ethical dilemmas associated with this early stage of clinical research.

In the first such study, Rodenhuis et al. evaluated the quality of informed consent among patients with advanced cancer who were offered participation in a phase I trial.[138] The majority of patients who gave their consent was motivated either by hope for improvement of their condition, pressure exerted by relatives and friends, or simply because they felt they had "no choice." Some patients did mention the desire to contribute to the progress of medicine. The investigators concluded that encouragement by relatives or friends appears to be a powerful force in motivating some patients to participate in phase I trials. In a similar but much smaller series of European advanced cancer patients, Willem and Sessa found corroborating results with regard to patient motivations for participation in such trials.[139]

Investigators at the University of Chicago conducted an in-depth survey study of 27 cancer patients who had given informed consent to participate in phase I trials at their institution.[33] Concurrently, the oncologists identified by the surveyed patients as responsible for their care and consent were surveyed as well. Eighty-five percent of patients decided to participate in a phase I trial for reasons of possible therapeutic benefit, 11% because of the advice or trust of physicians, and 4% because of family pressure. Ninety-three percent said they understood all (33%) or most (60%) of the information provided to them about the trial in which they had decided to participate. Only 33% were able to state the purpose of the trial in which they were participating, with patients able to state the purpose of phase I trials as dose-escalation or dose-finding studies being more educated ($P = .01$). The surveyed oncologists had wide ranging beliefs regarding expectations of possible benefits and toxicities for their patients participating in a phase I trial. The authors concluded that patients who participate in phase I trials are almost exclusively motivated by the hope of therapeutic benefit. Altruistic feelings, while perhaps present, appear to have a limited role in motivating patients to participate in these trials. Subsequent studies conducted by these investigators in a much larger series of subjects have found similar findings. In fact, in larger series of subjects, quantifiable survey data show that patients may even be less aware of the research purposes of phase I trials and are unable to recall whether alternatives to clinical trial participation, including palliative care or other nonexperimental therapies, were either discussed with or disclosed to them.[140] This is despite the fact that all surveyed patients had signed consent forms detailing the research purpose of phase I trials and the alternatives to trial participation.

Tomamichel and colleagues conducted an analysis of the communication process involved in informed consent for cancer patients agreeing to participate in phase I trials.[141] The authors concluded that the informed consent procedure was satisfactory from a quantitative point of view. Interestingly, they found that the most important items of information were acceptably communicated to patients. However, they also stated that greater attention should be paid to the indirect messages and implied criticism of patients to improve their participation in decision making. They also conclude that physicians should become more skillful in providing adequate information and to improve their methods of communication.

Yoder and colleagues conducted a prospective study involving entry and exit interviews of 37 advanced cancer patients participating in phase I trials.[142] The investigators found that patients expected slightly increased support from family members and received more support than expected. Perhaps not surprisingly, patients' expectations for tumor response and increased communication with their physician were not met. Their expectations were also not met with regard to improvement of symptoms such as fatigue, nausea and vomiting, and weight loss. They noted that one strong theme that emerged from the data was hope and optimism. They conclude that an issue that needs further exploration is the extent to which patients accurately understand information in the consent form and in the consent process itself. Their findings also support the importance of communication between the patient and family and all members of the health care team, and stress the importance of oncology nurses who may be able to mediate the flow of information between physicians and patients.

Research results providing a cross-cultural perspective are available as well. Japanese investigators, conducting a similar study, attempted to characterize the motivation, comprehension, and expectations of patients who had given informed consent to participate in phase I trials at the National Cancer Center in Japan.[143] Before receiving any investigational agents, 32 of 33 subjects were approached and completed a multiple choice questionnaire addressing these issues. When questioned regarding their expectations, more than one-half the subjects indicated that there might be personal benefit to themselves. As well, slightly more than one-third of the subjects (35%) believed that it was possible that their cancer could be cured, and 12 subjects fully expected to be cured as a result of participation in a phase I trial. The investigators found that older adults had slightly higher expectations of cure from participation in a phase I trial (although this did not reach statistical significance). With closed ended questioning, most patients appeared to comprehend the major features of a phase I trial, namely its investigational nature, the unknown effects of the agent investigated, and the unclear benefit to themselves. As well, nearly 60% of the patients anticipated they might suffer severe or life-threatening side effects from participation. As many as 43% of subjects were able to accurately indicate (again, in closed ended questioning) the research purpose of a phase I trial as a dose-determination study.

One disturbing finding from these studies is the potential discrepancies among what has been disclosed to patients, what they think they understand, and what they may actually understand. For example, the University of Chicago study found that 90% of patients stated they understood all or most of the information provided to them about the phase I trial in which they had agreed to participate.[33] However, only approximately one-third of the patients could state the purpose of a phase I trial, and an even smaller proportion of patients could state the research purpose of phase I trials in a much larger study.[140] This discrepancy likely results from several factors, including inadequate informed consent. It may also lie in the methodologic difficulties of determining what a patient actually understands in relation to the information they have been given.

The information gained from this research strongly supports the argument that the current process of obtaining informed consent for phase I trials may be inadequate to appropriately ensure that such advanced cancer patients understand both the nature of the research in which they are participating and the alternatives to trial participation. In addition, despite recognizing the existence of their potential vulnerability, we do not know how that vulnerability specifically affects an advanced cancer patient's ability to give what is otherwise perceived to be adequate informed consent. It is possible that several poorly understood and seldom studied factors play a vital role in shaping the informed consent process for potentially vulnerable advanced cancer patients considering participation in phase I trials. These likely include relatively subtle and less apparent factors as may exist in other health care decision-making environments for advanced cancer patients, for example, a patient's awareness of the certainty of his or her death[42,78,144] and the patient's cultural and ethnic background.[145] In addition, advanced cancer patients' religious or spiritual beliefs, their degree of hope and emotional well-being, and their attitudes toward medical decision making may likely influence the shape of the consent process in this setting. Further research will be required to better understand and delineate these issues and their importance on the informed consent process in this difficult and highly charged setting.

ETHICAL ISSUES IN PHASE II TRIALS

Some of the ethical issues related to phase II trials of new agents are similar to issues in phase I trials with regard to the participation of human subjects with otherwise incurable illnesses in biomedical research and the potential vulnerability of these patients in seeking therapy.[131–133] Although still troubling, issues in phase II trials can be viewed as potentially less complex for several reasons. In the phase II setting, there is less of the unknown for both oncologist–investigator and patient, as all agents studied in phase II trials have completed toxicity finding and dose-determination (phase I) studies. Thus, there may be greater attitudes of certainty with regard to expected toxicities. There may also be greater hope or expectations of benefit, in part because these agents are being administered at or near the maximum tolerated dose. Therefore, one unique issue in the phase II trial is the higher likelihood of toxicity developing for all patients in a trial, as they are being administered agents at relatively higher doses, as compared with patients in a prior phase I study investigating the same agents. The intentions and motivations of a participating oncologist, in the role of physician–healer or physician–investigator, are central issues in both phase I and II trials. Again, however, expectations or hope of benefit for their patients may be greater in the phase II setting. This may translate into greater therapeutic intent and subsequently be communicated to patients, resulting in greater expectations or hopes on their part as well.

Although these issues may be less complex and more easily examined in the phase II setting involving new agents, they are still troubling as there is an overall low probability of benefit with regard to tumor responses in these trials.[146] In fact, this concern may actually increase even as a phase II study is accruing patient–subjects. This relates to the accepted statistical requirements of phase II trials of new agents that are present to exclude, with an accepted amount of certainty or confidence, a low level of efficacy for a new agent.[147] Traditional stopping rules for many phase II trials would allow as many as 14 consecutive nonresponders to accrue to a trial before concluding that the agent lacks disease-specific efficacy. Yet, physician–investigators' attitudes and beliefs may change significantly with regard to an agent under study as response data accumulate that suggest a lack of efficacy, but the trial remains open in order to reach the statistically required accrual.

How should evolving data be handled during a phase II trial that suggests a lack of efficacy, but is not sufficiently substantiated from a statistical standpoint? In a study of even a small number of patients, if an agent is given to initial patient–subjects without apparent benefits or tumor responses, but not enough patients have been involved to satisfy statistical requirements, what information should be provided to prospective patient–subjects? For example, in a simple phase II single-agent study seeking to accrue 14 to 20 patients, if six evaluable patient–subjects have been administered the agent and are known to have not received any apparent benefits, what should the informed consent process consist of for prospective patient–subjects with regard to risks and benefits?

We know oncologists' attitudes, perceptions, and biases toward clinical trial chemotherapy may substantially affect clinical trial accrual.[148–150] These factors are likely to be important for phase II trial accrual. How oncologists, either as investigators or practitioners, interpret clinical trial data from ongoing trials could have a significant effect on their views toward continued accrual. How oncologists assimilate this information and communicate it to prospective cancer patient–subjects likely changes over the course of a trial. Yet, the consent forms for such trials are almost always static, potentially leading to subjects receiving conflicting information. As well, oncologists' enthusiasm or beliefs toward the potential efficacy of an agent may decline as information is acquired regarding nonresponders. What is troubling about this is that, quite often, accrual will continue unabated using the same consent process until the statistical requirements for accrual have been satisfied. This may well be justified in order to establish confidence regarding lack of efficacy of a new agent in a specific disease, but the potential dilemma remains and is no less troubling. Some might argue that as nonresponse information accumulates, such declining enthusiasm for a new agent should be allowed to affect accrual and should be uniformly communicated to prospective patient–subjects. However, traditionally, after the initiation of a phase II trial, subsequent patients are accrued with little formal response or toxicity information available to prospective subjects about prior evaluable patients in the trial. Interestingly, if such information could be fully and appropriately withheld from involved clinician–investigators, some of the described dilemmas in phase II trials might resolve themselves. As well, if one could guarantee an unprecedented quick rate of accrual of all the subjects necessary to meet the statistical requirements to a phase II trial, these dilemmas could potentially be less challenging. Practically speaking, these actions are not likely to be routinely achievable. Research on these issues in the phase II setting is needed.

ETHICAL ISSUES IN PHASE III TRIALS

Although ethical issues are present throughout all phases of clinical research, and early trials of new agents certainly present troubling dilemmas, it is randomized phase III trials that have undergone the most intense scrutiny. Indeed, much of this scrutiny has centered on the randomized trial process specifically in *cancer* clinical research. The overall informed consent process in phase III trials and, more specifically, how disclosure to potential subjects regarding the randomization process itself should be conducted, remain issues of controversy. An even more basic and primary ethical concern is the application of the phase III trial design itself, with much debate and controversy focused on when, rather than if, it is ethically appropriate to perform randomized comparative trials. Indeed, no ethical arguments have been made against the actual intended goals of phase III trials. Rather, it is phase III methodology, in which patient–subjects are randomly assigned to receive either an investigational therapy or a standard of care, that has caused concerns for some.[151–157] Such concerns deal with a perceived dilemma for the treating physician of a specific patient, and whether the physician's therapeutic responsibilities to that individual patient overwhelm any responsibilities to clinical research and the needs to improve medical care for future patients. Some have described this as a potential conflict that arises between the physician as investigator and the physician as healer for an individual patient.[110,155,156] Supporters of this view have argued that the responsibilities of the physician as healer carry far greater moral weight than those of the physician as investigator, to the extent that it becomes unethical to allow a random process to be the determining factor in what therapy a patient receives. Complicating this further is the fact that in the phase III setting the lines separating research from therapy are sometimes less clear.[8,104,153]

Much of the debate regarding ethical issues in phase III trials has centered around the issue of equipoise. As originally defined by Fried,[158] *equipoise* is viewed as a state of genuine uncertainty on the part of a clinical investigator or treating physician regarding the comparative merits of different treatments for a patient's specific disease process, such as cancer. Some have argued that equipoise must exist for an individual investigator or physician in regard to an individual patient, in order that he or she can ethically ask (or encourage) that patient to participate in an appropriately designed phase III trial. Others have argued that a broader definition of equipoise be accepted to justify randomized phase III trials; specifically, that clinical equipoise need not exist for an individual physician or investigator, but need only exist within a specified medical community.[159–161] In the cancer setting, clinicians, researchers, and ethicists have debated this issue of equipoise (whether it should be applied as an individual versus a community standard), and whether randomized studies are ethical at all.[155] The empiric research available from the cancer setting strongly suggests that the issue of equipoise remains quite unresolved for investigators, clinicians, and even patients.[162–169] The available evidence also suggests that many oncologists view the informed consent process requirements within randomized clinical trials as too cumbersome or potentially threatening to the patient, DPR, or both to the extent that they are a significant obstacle to patient accrual to phase III trials.[162,163,168]

Keeping this issue of equipoise in mind, and returning to the process of informed consent in phase III trials, Freedman has quite rationally argued that an individual physician or investigator is not the sole arbiter of appropriate or acceptable medical practice.[159] Rather, the medical community as a whole determines equipoise and, as long as equipoise truly exists, an individual physician can remain ethically and morally justified in consenting patients to participate in a phase III trial, even if the physician is not in equipoise. With regard to the informed consent process itself, Royall has extended this argument, noting that in situations involving an autonomous patient, the decision to participate in a randomized study does not rest with the physician but with the patient.[170] This is certainly the case as long as an adequate (perhaps ideal) process of informed consent can be carried out, including full disclosure of alternatives to randomized trial participation. Royall argues that what is needed for randomized trials to be justifiably conducted, beyond the presence of medical uncertainty (or equipoise) regarding particular therapies, is not physicians without preferences. Rather, it is patients who are informed of the uncertainty (i.e., the existence of perceived equipoise and are autonomously willing to consent to randomization). Thus, within the context of phase III trials, the informed consent process becomes one of utmost importance. In the cancer setting this may be especially true because of the life-threatening nature of these diseases and the relative toxicities of potential therapies contained within arms of many randomized trials.

Some efforts have been undertaken to examine different methods of obtaining consent for randomized trials and the effect of these methods on the quality of consent.[171–173] Many of these investigators have examined alternatives to the conventional methods of informed consent for phase III trials (i.e., in which subjects are first consented to the trial and then randomized to either standard or experimental treatment). The alternatives to this conventional method of consent and randomization include so-called preconsent randomization, where subjects are first randomized to one arm of the trial and then asked to consent to participation.

As reviewed by Altman and colleagues,[174] and originally proposed by Zelen,[175] these alternatives include single- and double-randomized consent designs. In the single-randomized consent design, eligible subjects are first randomized to one of the treatment arms under study in a trial before consent and without their knowledge. Subjects randomized to standard treatment are simply evaluated with routine follow-up and nothing is said to them about the trial or their participation (i.e., no formal consent is obtained from them). Subjects randomized to the experimental arm in such designs are consented to receive the investigational therapy. If these subjects refuse participation, they would then receive standard treatment and be followed similarly to those originally randomized to standard treatment. In the double-randomized consent design, all subjects are first randomized without their knowledge, then asked if they would consent to participate, receiving either the standard treatment or the experimental treatment to which they had already been randomized. Those refusing trial participation would then be offered treatment with the opposite arm to which they had been randomized (e.g., those refusing standard treatment would be treated with the experimental therapy).

Such designs were proposed in order to make the informed consent process less cumbersome and threatening for a participating physician–investigator. In fact, Zelen proposed such trial designs because of practical difficulties in getting physicians to participate in randomized trials, hoping to increase their willingness to participate.[175] The common theme of such designs is that patients are asked to consent to a specific treatment, rather than to participate in a randomized trial. Many statistical difficulties arise with such randomized consent designs, including an inability to blind subjects to the treatment. As well, such designs create both an underestimation and a dilution of possible differences in treatment effects, resulting in larger (and even unpredictable) accrual goals. Significant ethical issues also arise with such designs, including the fact that some subjects would be unaware that they are in a clinical trial. In addition, many subjects would likely receive biased information about the particular treatment to which they had already been prerandomized by the participating physician–investigator approaching them for inclusion in the trial.

Interestingly, even considering such criticisms, nearly a dozen cancer clinical trials have employed these or similar consent designs. As reviewed elsewhere,[174,175] many of these trials were in the cooperative group setting. Most of these trials had been originally initiated with conventional consent designs, but were then modified to include randomized consent designs in order to improve on slow patient accrual. Several of these trials increased their accrual rates substantially, some by a factor of three to six times the initial accrual rates.[176–178] Despite these improvements in accrual, these consent designs remain controversial. Gallo and colleagues examined the use of such trial designs, comparing different preconsent procedures for a hypothetical randomized trial among more than 2000 healthy subjects.[171] The investigators conclude that preconsent randomization methods are highly inefficient with regard to improving accrual, as subjects knowingly randomized to receive standard treatment would be likely to refuse clinical trial entry. In general, the ethical and statistical difficulties have prevented their implementation on a routine basis and they have not been recommended for such use.

CONCLUSIONS

If cancer physicians and investigators are to provide high-quality cancer care and conduct research according to the highest possible standards, they must maintain a heightened sensitivity to the ethical issues discussed. Certainly, continued study and debate regarding these complex issues is unquestionably needed if the dilemmas present in cancer care and research are to be addressed and, it is to be hoped, resolved. Considering their long-standing awareness, cancer physicians and investigators remain well qualified to continue to provide guidance in shaping this future study.

REFERENCES

1. Jonsen AR, Siegler M, Winslade WJ. *Clinical ethics.* 4th ed. New York: McGraw-Hill, 1998.
2. Siegler M, Pellegrino ED, Singer PA. Clinical medical ethics: the first decade. *J Clin Ethics* 1990;1:5.
3. Tarlov AL, Ware JE, Greenfield S, et al. The Medical Outcomes Study: an application of methods for monitoring the results of medical care. *JAMA* 1989;262:925.
4. Siegler M. Falling off the pedestal: what is happening to the traditional doctor-patient relationship? *Mayo Clin Proc* 1993;68:1.
5. Siegler M. The physician-patient accommodation: a central event in clinical medicine. *Arch Intern Med* 1982;142:1899.
6. Faden RR, Beauchamp TL, King NMP. *A history and theory of informed consent.* New York: Oxford University Press, 1986.
7. Vetch RM. Abandoning informed consent. *Hast Cent Rep* 1995;25:5.
8. Bok S. Shading the truth in seeking informed consent for research purposes. *Kennedy Institute of Ethics Journal* 1995;5:1.
9. Engelhardt HT. *The foundations of bioethics.* 2nd ed. New York: Oxford University Press, 1996.
10. Llewellyn-Thomas HA, McGreal J, Theil EC. Cancer patients' decision making and trial-entry preferences: the effects of "framing" information about short-term toxicity and long-term survival. *Med Decis Making* 1995;15:4.
11. Sutherland HJ, Llewellyn-Thomas HA, Lockwood GA, Tritchler DL, Till JE. Cancer patients: their desire for information and participation in treatment decisions. *J Royal Soc Med* 1989;82:260.
12. Margalith I, Shapiro A. Anxiety and patient participation in clinical decision-making: the case of patients with ureteral calculi. *Soc Sci Med* 1997;45:419.
13. Brockopp DY, Hayko D, Davenport W, Winscott C. Personal control and the needs for hope and information among adults diagnosed with cancer. *Cancer Nurs* 1989;12:112.
14. Charles C, Gafni A, Whelan T. Shared decision-making in the medical encounter: what does it mean? (or it takes at least two to tango). *Soc Sci Med* 1997;44:681.
15. Hall JA, Roter DL, Katz NR. Meta-analysis of correlates of provider behavior in medical encounters. *Med Care* 1988;26:657.
16. Pendleton DA, Bochner S. The communication of medical information in general practice consultations as a function of patients' social class. *Soc Sci Med* 1980;14A:669.
17. Waitzkin H, Stoeckle JD. The communication of information about illness: clinical, sociological, and methodological considerations. *Adv Psychosomat Med* 1972;8:180.
18. Cassileth BR, Zupkis RV, Sutton-Smith K, March V. Information and participation preferences among cancer patients. *Ann Intern Med* 1980;92:832.
19. Orona CJ, Koenig BA, Davis AJ. Cultural aspects of nondisclosure. *Camb Q Healthcare Ethics* 1994;3:338.
20. Ong LM, De Haes JCJM, Hoos AM, Lammes FB. Doctor-patient communication: a review of the literature. *Soc Sci Med* 1995;40:903.
21. Turner S, Maher EJ, Young T, Hudson GV. What are the information priorities for cancer patients involved in treatment decisions? An experienced surrogate study in Hodgkin's disease. *Br J Cancer* 1996;73:222.
22. Hack TF, Degner LF, Dyck DG. Relationship between preferences for decisional control and illness information among women with breast cancer: a quantitative and qualitative analysis. *Soc Sci Med* 1994;39:279.
23. Strull WM, Lo B, Charles G. Do patients want to participate in medical decision making? *JAMA* 1984;252:2990.
24. Blanchard CG, Labrecque MS, Ruckdeschel JC, Blanchard EB. Information and decision-making preferences of hospitalized adult cancer patients. *Soc Sci Med* 1988;27:1139.
25. Beisecker AE, Beisecker TD. Patient information-seeking behaviors when communicating with doctors. *Med Care* 1990;28:19.
26. Ende J, Kazis L, Ash A, Moskowitz MA. Measuring patients' desire for autonomy: decision making and information-seeking preferences among medical patients. *J Gen Intern Med* 1989;4:23.
27. Charles C, Redko C, Whelan T, Gafni A, Reyno L. Doing nothing is no choice: lay constructions of treatment decision-making among women with early-stage breast cancer. *Sociol Health Illness* 1998;20:71.
28. Turk-Charles S, Meyerowitz BE, Gatz M. Age differences in information seeking among cancer patients. *Intl J Aging Hum Dev* 1997;45:85.
29. Weeks JC, Cook F, O'Day SJ, et al. Relationship between cancer patients' predictions of prognosis and their treatment preferences. *JAMA* 1998;279:1709.
30. Eidinger RN, Schapira DV. Cancer patients' insight into their treatment, prognosis, and unconventional therapies. *Cancer* 1984;53:2736.
31. Mackillop WJ, Stewart WE, Ginsburg AD, Stewart SS. Cancer patients' perceptions of their disease and its treatment. *Br J Cancer* 1988;58:355.
32. Sulmassy DP, Terry PB, Weisman CS, et al. The accuracy of substituted judgments in patients with terminal diagnoses. *Ann Intern Med* 1998;128:621
33. Daugherty C, Ratain MJ, Grochowski E, et al. Perceptions of cancer patients and their physicians involved in phase I trials. *J Clin Oncol* 1995;13:1062.
34. Fitts WT, Ravdin IS. What Philadelphia physicians tell patients with cancer. *JAMA* 1953;153:901.
35. Oken D. What to tell cancer patients: a study of medical attitudes. *JAMA* 1961;175:1120.
36. Kelley WD, Friesen SR. Do cancer patients want to be told? *Surgery* 1950;27:822.
37. Koenig RR. Anticipating death from cancer: physician and patient attitudes. *Michigan Medicine* 1969;(Sept):899.
38. Gerle B, Lunden G, Sandlom P. The patient with inoperable cancer from the psychiatric and social standpoints. *Cancer* 1960;13:1206.
39. McIntosh J. Processes of communication, information seeking and control associated with cancer: a selective review of the literature. *Soc Sci Med* 1974;8:167.
40. Novack DH, Plumer R, Smith RL, et al. Changes in physicians' attitudes toward telling the cancer patient. *JAMA* 1979;241:897.
41. Patterson JT. *The dread disease: cancer and modern American culture.* Cambridge, MA: Harvard University Press, 1987.
42. Seale C. Communication and awareness about death: a study of a random sample of dying people. *Soc Sci Med* 1991;32:943.
43. Miyaji N. The power of compassion: truth-telling among American doctors in the care of dying patients. *Soc Sci Med* 1993;36:249.
44. Kodish E, Post SG. Oncology and hope. *J Clin Oncol* 1995;13:1817.
45. DelVecchio Good MJ, Good B, Schaffer C, et al. American oncology and the discourse on hope. *Cult Med Psychiatry* 1990;14:59.
46. Hux J, Naylor CD. Does the format of efficacy data determine patients' acceptance of treatment? *Med Decis Making* 1995;15:152.
47. Jacoby A, Baker G, Chadwick D, Johnson A. The impact of counseling with a practical statistical model on patients' decision-making about treatment for epilepsy: findings from a pilot study. *Epilepsy Res* 1993;16:207.
48. Siminoff LA, Fetting JH. Factors affecting treatment decisions for a life-threatening illness: the case of medical treatment of breast cancer. *Soc Sci Med* 1991;32:813.
49. Ravdin PM, Siminoff LA, Harvey JA. Survey of breast cancer patients concerning their knowledge and expectations of adjuvant therapy. *J Clin Oncol* 1998;16:515.
50. Amir M. Considerations guiding physicians when informing cancer patients. *Soc Sci Med* 1987;24:741.
51. Forster LE, Lynn J. Predicting life span for applicants to inpatient Hospice. *Arch Intern Med* 1988;148:2540.
52. Lamont EB, Christakis NA. Some elements of prognosis in terminal cancer. *Oncology* 1999;13:1165.
53. Evans C, McCarthy M. Prognostic uncertainty in terminal care: can the Karnofsky Index help? *Lancet* 1985;1:1204.
54. Heyse-Moore LH, Johnson-Bell VE. Can doctors accurately predict the life expectancy of patients with terminal cancer? *Palliat Med* 1987;1:165.
55. Maltoni M, Nanni O, Derni S, et al. Clinical prediction of survival is more accurate than the Karnofsky Performance Status in estimating life span of terminally ill cancer patients. *Eur J Cancer* 1994;30A:764.
56. Oxenham D, Cornbleet MA. Accuracy of prediction of survival by different professional groups in a hospice. *Palliat Med* 1998;12:117.
57. Parkes CM. Accuracy of predictions of survival in later stages of cancer. *BMJ* 1972;1:29.
58. Mackillop WJ, Quirt CF. Measuring the accuracy of prognostic judgments in oncology. *J Clin Epidemiol* 1997;50:21.
59. The SUPPORT Principal Investigators. A controlled trial to improve care for seriously ill hospitalized patients. The Study to Understand Prognoses and Preferences for Outcomes and Risks of Treatments (SUPPORT). *JAMA* 1995;274:1591.
60. Cancer statistics. *CA Cancer J Clin* 1998;48:6.
61. Parkes M. Accuracy of prediction of survival in later stages of cancer. *BMJ* 1972;2:29.
62. Yates JW, Chalmer B, McKegney FP. Evaluation of patients with advanced cancer using the Karnofsky Performance Status. *Cancer* 1980;45:2220.
63. Evans C, McCarthy M. Prognostic uncertainty in terminal care: can the Karnofsky Index help? *Lancet* 1985;1:1204.
64. Reuben DB, Mor V, Hiris J. Clinical symptoms and length of survival in patients with terminal cancer. *Arch Intern Med* 1988;148:1586.
65. Janisch L, Mick R, Schilsky RL, et al. Prognostic factors for survival in patients treated in phase I clinical trials. *Cancer* 1994;74:1965.
66. Barry ZS, Lynn J. Hospice medicine. *JAMA* 1993;270:221.
67. Levy MH. Living with cancer: hospice/palliative care. *J Natl Cancer Inst* 1993;85:1283.
68. Kinzbrunner BM. Hospice: what to do when anti-cancer therapy is no longer appropriate, effective, or desired. *Semin Oncol* 1994;21:792.
69. Bayer R, Callahan D, Fletcher J, et al. The care of the terminally ill: morality and economics. *N Engl J Med* 1983;309:1490.
70. Long SH, Gibbs JO, Crozier JP, et al. Medical expenditures of terminal cancer patients during the last year of life. *Inquiry* 1984;21:315.
71. Kedder D. The effects of hospice coverage on Medicare expenditures. *Health Services Research* 1992;27:195.
72. Emanuel EJ. Cost savings at the end of life. *JAMA* 1996;275:1901.
73. Christakis NA, Escarce JJ. Survival of Medicare patients after enrollment in hospice programs. *N Engl J Med* 1996;355:172.
74. Christakis N. *Death foretold: prophecy and progress in medical care.* Chicago: University of Chicago Press, 2000.
75. Daugherty CK, Hlubocky F, Ratain MJ, Banik DM. Assessing advanced cancer patients' awareness of prognosis: why simply asking may not be measuring. *Proc Am Soc Clin Oncol* 1999;18:417a.
76. Kinzbrunner BM. Ethical dilemmas in hospice and palliative care. *Support Care Cancer* 1995;3:28.

77. Fallowfield L, Lipkin M, Hall A. Teaching senior oncologists communication skills: results from a phase I of a comprehensive longitudinal program in the United Kingdom. *J Clin Oncol* 1998;16:1961.
78. Hinton J. How reliable are relatives' retrospective reports of terminal illness? Patients' and relatives' accounts compared. *Soc Sci Med* 1996;43:1229.
79. Quill TE, Cassel CK, Meier DE. Care of the hopelessly ill. Proposed clinical criteria for physician-assisted suicide. *N Engl J Med* 1992;327:1380.
80. Bukberg J, Penman D, Holland JC. Depression in hospitalized cancer patients. *Psychosom Med* 1984;46:199.
81. Chochinov HM, Wilson KG, Enns M, et al. Prevalence of depression in the terminally ill: effects of diagnostic criteria and symptom threshold judgments. *Am J Psychiatry* 1994;151:537.
82. Bolund C. Suicide and cancer: I. Demographical and suicidological description of suicides among cancer patients in Sweden. *J Psychosom Oncol* 1985;3:17.
83. Allebeck P, Bolund C, Ringback G. Increased suicide rate in cancer patients. A cohort study based on the Swedish Cancer-Environment Register. *J Clin Epidemiol* 1989;42:611.
84. Winokur G, Tsuang M. The Iowa 500: suicide in mania, depression, and schizophrenia. *Am J Psychiatry* 1975;132:650.
85. Barraclough B, Bunch J, Nelson B, et al. A hundred cases of suicide: clinical aspects. *Br J Psychiatry* 1974;125:355.
86. Groenewould JH, Van Der Maas J, Van Der Wal G, et al. Physician-assisted death in psychiatric practice in the Netherlands. *N Engl J Med* 1997;336:1795.
87. Van Der Maas PJ, Van Delden JJ, Pijnenborg L, et al. Euthanasia and other medical decisions concerning the end of life [see comments]. *Lancet* 1991;338:669.
88. Pijenborg L, van der Maas PJ, van Delden JJM, Looman CWN. Life terminating acts without explicit request of the patient. *Lancet* 1993;341:1196.
89. Groenewould JH, van der Heide A, Onwuteaka-Philipsen BN, et al. Clinical problems with performance of euthanasia and PAS in the Netherlands. *N Engl J Med* 2000;348:551.
90. Nuland SB. PAS and you in practice. *N Engl J Med* 2000;342:583.
91. Cohen JS, Fihn SD, Boyko EJ, et al. Attitudes toward assisted suicide and euthanasia among physicians in Washington state. *N Engl J Med* 1994;331:89.
92. Back AL, Wallace JI, Starks HE, et al. Physician-assisted suicide and euthanasia in Washington State. Patient requests and physician responses [see comments]. *JAMA* 1996;275:919.
93. Emanuel EJ, Fairclough DL, Daniels ER, et al. Euthanasia and physician-assisted suicide: attitudes and experiences of oncology patients, oncologists, and the public [see comments]. *Lancet* 1996;347:1805.
94. Howard OM, Fairclough DL, Daniels ER, et al. Physician desire for euthanasia and assisted suicide: would physicians practice what they preach? [see comments]. *J Clin Oncol* 1997;15:428.
95. Emanuel EJ, Daniels ER, Fairclough DL, et al. The practice of euthanasia and physician-assisted suicide in the United States: adherence to proposed safeguards and effects on physicians [see comments]. *JAMA* 1998;280:507.
96. Chiu AE, Hedberg K, Higgison GK, Fleming DW. Legalized physician-assisted suicide in Oregon—the first year's experience. *N Engl J Med* 2000;340:577.
97. Sullivan AD, Itedberg K, Fleming DW. Legalized physician-assisted suicide in Oregon—the second year. *N Engl J Med* 2000;342:598.
98. Gaylin W, Kass LR, Pellegrino ED, Siegler M. Doctors must not kill. *JAMA* 1988;259:2139.
99. Engelhardt HT. *The foundations of bioethics.* 2nd ed. New York: Oxford University Press, 1996:330.
100. *The final report of the president's advisory committee. The human radiation experiments.* New York: Oxford University Press, 1996.
101. Applebaum PS, Lindz CN, Meisel A. *Informed consent: legal theory and clinical practice.* New York: Oxford University Press, 1987.
102. Levine RJ. *Ethics and regulation of clinical research.* 2nd ed. Baltimore: Urban and Schwarzenburg, 1986.
103. National Commission for the Protection of Human Subjects of Biomedical and Behavioral Research. *Belmont Report; ethical principles and guidelines for the protection of human subjects of research.* Publication number (05) 78-0012. Washington, DC: USGPO, 1978.
104. Freedman B, Fuks A, Weijer C. Demarcating research in treatment: a systematic approach for the analysis of the ethics of clinical research. *Clin Res* 1992;40:655.
105. Pelligrino ED. Beneficence, scientific autonomy, and self-interest: ethical dilemmas in clinical research. *Cumb Q Health Ethics* 1992;1:361.
106. Schaffner KF. Ethical problems in clinical trials. *J Med Philos* 1986;11:297.
107. Markman M. The objective clinical scientist versus the advocate: a complex ethical and political dilemma facing cancer investigators and the public. *Cancer Invest* 1995;13:324.
108. Elks ML. Conflict of interest and the physician-researcher. *J Lab Clin Med* 1995;126:19.
109. Hammerschmidt DE. When commitments and interests conflict. *J Lab Clin Med* 1995;126:5.
110. Levine RJ. Clinical trials and physicians as double agents. *Yale J Biol Med* 1992;65:68.
111. Katz J. *Experimentation with human beings.* New York: Russell Sage Foundation, 1972.
112. Annas GJ. The changing landscape of human experimentation; Nuremberg, Helsinki, and beyond. *J Law Med* 1992;2:119.
113. The President's Commission for the Study of Ethical Problems in Medicine and Biomedical and Behavioral Research. *Implementing human research regulations: the adequacy and uniformity of federal rules and their implementation.* Washington, DC: USGPO, publication number 040-000-00471-8, 1983.
114. Engelhardt HT. *The foundations of bioethics.* 2nd ed. New York: Oxford University Press, 1996:330.
115. Jonas H. Philosophical reflections on experimenting with human subjects. In: Freund PA, ed. *Experimentation with human subjects.* New York: George Brazilier, 1969.
116. Epstein LC, Lasagna L. Obtaining informed consent, form or substance. *Arch Intern Med* 1969;123:682.
117. Gray BH, Cooke RA, Tannebaum AS. Research involving human subjects. The performance of institutional review boards is assessed in this empirical study. *Science* 1978;201:1094.
118. Hammerschmidt DE, Keanse MA. Institutional review board review lacks impact on the readability of consent forms for research. *Am J Med Sci* 1992;304:341.
119. Edgar H, Rothman DJ. The institutional review board and beyond: future challenges to the ethics of human experimentation. *J Milb Q* 1995;73:489.
120. Redshaw ME, Harris A, Baum JD. Research ethics committee audit: differences between committees. *J Med Ethics* 1996;22:78.
121. Kent G. Shared understandings for informed consent: the relevance of psychological research on the provision of information. *Soc Sci Med* 1996;43:1517.
122. Verheggen FWSM, van Wijmen FCB. Informed consent in clinical trials. *Health Policy* 1996;36:131.
123. Katz J. Human experimentation and human rights. *St. Louis University Law Journal* 1993;38:7.
124. Beecher HK. Ethics in clinical research. *N Engl J Med* 1966;274:1354.
125. Rothman DJ. Ethics and human experimentation: Henry Beecher revisited. *N Engl J Med* 1987;317:1195.
126. Jones JH. *Bad blood.* 2nd ed. New York: Free Press, 1993.
127. *The final report of the president's advisory committee. The human radiation experiments.* New York: Oxford University Press, 1996:98.
128. Simes RJ, Tattersal MHN, Coates AS, et al. Randomized comparison of procedures for obtaining informed consent in clinical trials of treatment for cancer. *BMJ* 1986;293:1065.
129. Daugherty CK. Impact of therapeutic research on informed consent and the ethics of clinical trials: a medical oncology perspective. *J Clin Oncol* 1999;17:1601.
130. Edwards SJL, Lilford RJ, Thornton J, et al. Informal consent for clinical trials: in search of the "best" method. *Soc Sci Med* 1998;47:1825.
131. Ratain MJ, Mick R, Schilsky R, Siegler M. Statistical and ethical issues in the design and conduct of phase I and II clinical trials of new anticancer agents. *J Natl Cancer Inst* 1993;85:1637.
132. Vanderpool HY. *The ethics of research involving human subjects. Facing the 21st Century.* Frederick, MD: University Publishing Group, 1996:306.
133. Freedman B. Cohort-specific consent: an honest approach to phase I cancer studies. *IRB Rev Human Subjects Res* 1990;12:5.
134. Von Hoff DD, Turner J. Response rates, duration of response, and dose response effect in phase I studies in antineoplastics. *Invest New Drugs* 1991;9:115.
135. Decoster G, Stein G, Holdener EE. Responses and toxic deaths in phase I clinical trials. *J Ann Oncol* 1990;2:175.
136. Estey E, Hoth D, Wittes R, et al. Therapeutic responses in phase I trials of antineoplastic agents. *Cancer Treat Rep* 1986;70:1105.
137. Smith TL, Lee JJ, Kantarjian HM, et al. Design and results of phase I cancer clinical trials: 3 year experience at MD Anderson Cancer Center. *J Clin Oncol* 1996;14:287.
138. Rodenhuis S, van-den Heuvel WJ, Annyas AA, et al. Patient motivation and informed consent in a phase I study of an anticancer agent. *Eur J Cancer Clin Oncol* 1984;20:457.
139. Willem Y, Sessa C. Informing patients about phase I trials—how should it be done? *Aeta Oncol* 1989;28:106.
140. Daugherty CK, Banik DM, Janisch L, Ratain MJ. Quantitative analysis of ethical issues in phase I trials: a survey interview study of 144 advanced cancer patients. *IRB Rev Hum Sub Res* 2000;22:6.
141. Tomamichel M, Sessa C, Herzig S, et al. Informed consent for phase I studies: evaluation of quantity and quality of information provided to patients. *Ann Oncol* 1995;6:321.
142. Yoder LH, O'Rourke TJ, Ethyre A, Spears DT. Expectations and experiences of patients with cancer participating in phase I clinical trials. *Oncol Nurs Forum* 1997;24:891.
143. Itoh K, Sasaki Y, Fuji H, et al. Patients in phase I trials of anti-cancer agents in Japan: motivation, comprehension and expectations. *Br J Cancer* 1997;76:107.
144. Mor V, Masterson-Allen S. A comparison of hospice vs conventional care of the terminally-ill cancer patients. *Oncology* 1990;4:85.
145. Trill MD, Holland J. Cross-cultural differences in the care of patients with cancer. A review. *Gen Hosp Psychiatry* 1993;15:21.
146. Marsoni S, Hoth D, Simon R, et al. Clinical drug development: an analysis of phase II trials. *Cancer Treat Rep* 1987;71:80.
147. Stores B, DeMetts D. Current phase I/II designs: are they adequate? *J Clin Res Drug Dev* 1987;1:121.
148. Rajagopal S, Goodman PJ, Tannock IF. Adjuvant chemotherapy for breast cancer: discordance between physicians' perception of benefit and the results of clinical trials. *J Clin Oncol* 1994;12:1296.
149. Belanger D, Moore M, Tannock I. How American oncologists treat breast cancer: an assessment of the influence of clinical trials. *J Clin Oncol* 1991;9:7.
150. Baar J, Tannock I. Analyzing the same data in two ways: a demonstration model to illustrate the reporting and misreporting of clinical trials. *J Clin Oncol* 1989;7:969.
151. Schafer A. The ethics of the randomized clinical trial. *N Engl J Med* 1982;307:719.
152. Gifford F. The conflict between randomized clinical trials and the therapeutic obligation. *J Med Philos* 1986;11:347.
153. Kodish E, Lantos JD, Siegler M. Ethical considerations in randomized controlled clinical trials. *Cancer* 1990;65(Suppl):2400.
154. Marquis D. Leaving therapy to chance: an impasse in the ethics of clinical trials. *Hast Cen Rep* 1983;13:40.
155. Hellman S, Hellman DS. Of mice but not men. Problems of the randomized clinical trial. *N Engl J Med* 1991;324:1585.
156. Markman M. Ethical difficulties with randomized clinical trials involving cancer patients: examples from the field of gynecologic oncology. *J Clin Ethics* 1992;3:193.
157. Emmanual EJ, Peterson WB. Ethics of randomized clinical trials. *J Clin Oncol* 1998;16:365.
158. Freid C. *Medical experimentation: personal integrity and social policy.* Amsterdam: North Holland Publishing, 1974.
159. Freedman B. Equipoise and the ethics of clinical research. *N Engl J Med* 1987;317:141.
160. Gifford F. Community equipoise and the ethics of randomized clinical trials. *Bioethics* 1995;9:127.

161. Freedman B. A response to a purported ethical difficulty with randomized clinical trials involving cancer patients. *J Clin Ethics* 1992;3:231.
162. Taylor KM, Margolese RG, Soskolne CL. Physicians' reasons for not entering eligible patients in a randomized clinical trial of surgery for breast cancer. *N Engl J Med* 1984;310:1363.
163. Taylor KM, Shapiro M, Soskolne CL, et al. Physician response to informed consent regulations for randomized clinical trials. *Cancer* 1987;60:1415.
164. Fetting JH, Simonoff LA, Piantodosi S, et al. The effects of patients' expectations of benefit with standard breast cancer adjuvant chemotherapy on participation in a randomized clinical trial: a clinical vignette study. *J Clin Oncol* 1990;8:1476.
165. Silverman WA, Altman DG. Patients' preferences and randomized trials. *Lancet* 1996;347:171.
166. Cassileth BR, Lusk ES, Hurwitz S, et al. Attitudes towards clinical trials among patients and the public. *JAMA* 1982;248:968.
167. Slevin MJ, Stubb L, Plant HJ, et al. Attitudes to chemotherapy: comparing views of patients with cancer with those of doctors, nurses, and the general public. *BMJ* 1990;300:1458.
168. Taylor KM, Feldstein ML, Skeel RT, et al. Fundamental dilemmas of the randomized clinical trial process: results of a survey of 1,737 Eastern Cooperative Oncology Group investigators. *J Clin Oncol* 1994;12:1796.
169. Lynoe N, Sandland M, Jacobson L. Cancer clinical research—some aspects on doctors' attitudes to informing participants. *Acta Oncol* 1996;35:749.
170. Royall RM. Ignorance and altruism. *J Clin Ethics* 1992;3:229.
171. Gallo C, Perrone F, Deplando S, Giust C. Informed versus randomized consent to clinical trials. *Lancet* 1995;346:1060.
172. Simel DL, Feussner JR. A randomized controlled trial comparing quantitative informed consent formats. *J Clin Epidemiol* 1991;44:771.
173. Baum M. New approach for recruitment into randomized controlled trials. *Lancet* 1993;341:812.
174. Altman DG, Whitehead J, Parman MK, et al. Randomized consent designs in cancer clinical trials. *Eur J Cancer* 1995;31A:1934.
175. Zelen M. Strategy and alternate randomized designs in cancer clinical trials. *Cancer Treat Rep* 1982;66:1095.
176. Riethmuller G, Schneider-Gadicke E, Schilmok G, et al. Randomized trial of monoclonal antibody for adjuvant therapy of resected Dukes' C colorectal carcinoma. *Lancet* 1994;343:1177.
177. Mansour EG, Gray R, Shatila AH, et al. Efficacy of adjuvant chemotherapy of high-risk node-negative breast cancer. *N Engl J Med* 1989;320:485.
178. Fisher B, Redmond C, Poisson R, et al. Eight-year results of a randomized clinical trial comparing total mastectomy and lumpectomy with or without irradiation in the treatment of breast cancer. *N Engl J Med* 1989;320:822.

Susan Molloy Hubbard

CHAPTER 60

Information Systems in Oncology

As the twentieth century slipped into history, there could be little doubt that we live in an age in which information technology will continue to catalyze dramatic changes in society that affect our daily lives, especially in the field of health care. The Internet has revolutionized telecommunications, enabling electronic devices with different operating systems and data formats to communicate with each other seamlessly and making the "Net" and the "Web" ubiquitous terms in our lives. Computing power continues to increase steadily as more powerful chips become available, and powerful hand-held computers with wireless access to the Internet are now available. Direct Internet connections, once only available in academic centers, are now readily available in the home, workplace, and a growing number of public settings, such as public libraries and shopping malls. Internet access is available through dial-up, cable, and wireless Internet service providers at a reasonable cost. The simplicity and accessibility of Internet access have now made the Web a primary mechanism for communicating health information. As a result, the Internet has rapidly become an extremely popular vehicle for information queries and research.

Effective communication is central to efficient, high-quality health care. Information empowers individuals, enabling them to make informed decisions. Changes in the accessibility of medical information and the way the public can acquire it are altering the field of health care and the relationship between health care professionals and patients. A federally funded science panel on interactive health communication has concluded that few other interventions have greater potential to improve health outcomes, decrease costs, and enhance consumer satisfaction than communication.[1] Data from CyberDialogue, a group that has followed Internet trends since 1993, reported that, in 1999, more than 69.3 million adult Americans (35% of the adult population) were actively online; more than 26.3 million (38%) searched the Internet to obtain health and medical information.[2] In 2000, more than 33.5 million adults are expected to use the Internet to search for health information.[3] Use of the Internet as a channel for communicating health and medical information will continue to increase as interactive health communication applications become more sophisticated and the cost of electronic devices and Internet access decreases. However, major gaps in knowledge exist about how consumers process and use health information; distinguish important from insignificant health risks; decide to modify risky behavior, such as smoking; resolve contradictory health messages; and make decisions about their health care options.[4]

Many of the health care applications currently in development are designed to support complex user interactions and sophisticated decision-making tools. Increasingly, applications feature multimedia assets that enable designers to communicate complex information on health to users in ways that can be tailored to the user's unique needs and perspectives. Applications are being designed for a variety of dissemination vehicles, including standalone systems; locally networked computers; and Internet access via personal computers, mobile wireless digital devices, kiosks, and Web television.

Innovative strategies to ensure that communication technologies fulfill the inherent promise they offer must take into consideration the "digital divide" that exists between those that can readily access computers and the Internet and those who cannot. This digital divide reflects the societal gap that exists between the "haves" and "have nots." Internet use by those who live in rural settings; blacks, Hispanics, and other central city minorities; and households headed by the poor, by females, and by the young (younger than 25 years of age) lags behind white users.[5] Efforts to address barriers to access for these disadvantaged populations deserve high priority by developers, because underserved and minority populations often carry a particularly heavy burden of one or more cancers. Studies have shown that patients in underserved populations do use computer-mediated advice services and rate them highly.[6,7]

The availability of accurate, credible information is essential for anyone making decisions about cancer care. Cancer patients, their families, and many of those who perceive themselves at risk of developing cancer face the arduous task of gathering and interpreting information they find or are given to make well-informed decisions about their care options. Cancer patients learn about their diagnosis and management options from many sources and, in today's health care environment, are more likely to ask health care providers sophisticated and pointed questions. When faced with the task of gathering cancer information either for oneself or for a family member, the Internet provides an instantaneous, inexpensive, and voluminous source of information. Valuable information resources are available on Web sites, e-mail services, news and usenet groups, and online discussion groups to anyone seeking information on cancer, whether the focus of the search is on treatment, prevention, screening, or support. An increasing number of cancer-oriented Web sites offer significant opportunities for individuals to profile themselves so that they can tailor information on the site to meet specific needs and preferences.

However, as Internet access and Web site development tools have become basic software for computer systems, anyone with a computer, an Internet connection, and the appropriate software can create a Web site, a fact with staggering implications for the amount and quality of medical information available to consumers. A search on the term "cancer" via any of the popular Web search engines retrieves more than 2,000 Web sites offering cancer information from one of the more than 20,000 health-related Web sites.[8] For patients and the lay public, the plethora of health information on the Internet often represents a mixed blessing. At present, the Internet is still an unregulated, uncensored medium. Information that is anecdotal, unreviewed, and undated can be found on many Web sites, e-mail services, and news and usenet groups. In an article on the accuracy of medical information on the Web, an oncologist searching the Web for information on Ewing's sarcoma found that 50% of the online material was irrelevant and 6% contained major errors. Inaccuracy of information is not the only cause for concern. Some health-oriented sites hawk health care products or refer users to e-commerce partners and then take a cut of the sales.[9,10] Some post information in an attempt to advance unproven approaches to disease management that are not medically or scientifically sound.

It can be difficult for a novice to determine whether the information is current, accurate, and complete unless the information provider clearly articulates the standards of quality that are being used for the inclusion of materials on the site and the criteria for linking to other Web sites. Users must prepare to take responsibility for making decisions about the value and applicability of the information, just as those using more traditional information sources do.

The National Cancer Institute (NCI) has always had a formal review process for the inclusion of content in its databases and information services.[11–15] It has established a formal process for ensuring that its Web site only provides hypertext links to Web sites that are accurate, useful, and current, and it provides information on how to evaluate electronic information (Table 60-1).[16,17] Other medical information providers have begun to rec-

TABLE 60-1. Cancer-Oriented Web Sites

Site	*URL*
Sites that address many topics	
American Cancer Society	http://www.cancer.org
CancerEducation.com	http://www.cancereducation.com
Cancer Care	http://www.cancercareinc.org
National Cancer Institute's (NCI) Cancer Information Service	http://cis.nci.nih.gov
CancerGuide: Steve Dunn's cancer information page	http://www.cancerguide.org/
CancerSource.com	http://www.cancersource.com
Cansearch	http://www.cansearch.org/canserch/canserch.htm
Healthfinder	http://www.healthfinder.gov
MEDLINE*plus*	http://www.nlm.nih.gov/medlineplus/cancers.html
OncoLink	http://oncolink.upenn.edu
Sustaining Oncology Studies Europe	http://sos.unige.it/soseuro.html
TeleSCAN Telematics Services in Cancer (European)	http://telescan.nki.nl
Cancer-specific Web sites	
Brain cancer	
American Brain Tumor Association	http://www.abta.org
National Brain Tumor Foundation	http://www.braintumor.org
Breast cancer	
Breast Cancer and Environmental Risk Factors Project	http://www.cfe.cornell.edu/bcerf
Breast Cancer Answers	http://www.medsch.wisc.edu/bca
Breast Cancer Awareness	http://www.tricaresw.af.mil/breastcd/index.html
Breast Cancer Online	http://www.bco.org
Community Breast Health Project	http://www-med.stanford.edu/CBHP/
ENCORE	http://www.ywca.org

(continued)

TABLE 60-1. (*Continued*)

Site	*URL*
Inflammatory Breast Cancer Research Foundation	http://www.ibcresearch.org
National Breast Cancer Coalition	http://www.natlbcc.org
Susan G. Komen Breast Cancer Foundation	http://www.breastcancerinfo.com
Y-ME National Breast Cancer Organization	http://www.y-me.org
Eye cancer	
The Eye Cancer Network	http://www.eyecancer.com
Genitourinary cancers	
American Foundation for Urologic Disease	http://www.afud.org
Kidney Cancer Association	http://www.nkca.org
Gynecologic cancers	
American College of Obstetricians and Gynecologists	http://www.acog.org
Center for Cervical Health	http://www.cervicalhealth.org
National Cervical Cancer Coalition	http://www.nccc-online.org
National Ovarian Cancer Coalition	http://www.ovarian.org
Ovarian Cancer National Alliance	http://www.ovariancancer.org
Head and neck cancers	
Support for People with Oral and Head and Neck Cancer, Inc.	http://www.spohnc.org
Leukemia	
Large Granular Lymphocyte Leukemia Registry	http://www.moffitt.usf.edu/lgl-leukemia
Leukemia Society of America	http://www.leukemia.org
Lung cancer	
Alliance for Lung Cancer Advocacy, Support, & Education	http://www.alcase.org
Lung Cancer Awareness Campaign	http://www.lungcancer.org/home.htm
Lymphomas	
Lymphoma Information Network	http://www.lymphomainfo.net
Lymphoma Research Foundation of America	http://www.lymphoma.org
Cure For Lymphoma Foundation (CFL)	http://www.cfl.org
Multiple myeloma	
International Myeloma Foundation	http://www.myeloma.org
Multiple Myeloma Research Foundation	http://www.multiplemyeloma.org
Pediatric cancers	
A Starting Point: Children's Brain & Spinal Cord Tumors	http://www.med.miami.edu/neurosurgery/start_intro.htm
Candlelighters Childhood Cancer Foundation	http://www.candlelighters.org
Children's Hospice International	http://www.chionline.org
National Childhood Cancer Foundation	http://www.nccf.org
Outlook: Life Beyond Childhood Cancer	http://www.outlook-life.org
Pediatric Oncology Group	http://www.pog.ufl.edu
The National Children's Cancer Society	http://www.children-cancer.com
Prostate cancer	
Prostate Cancer Answers	http://www.medsch.wisc.edu/pca
US TOO International, Inc.	http://www.ustoo.com
Skin cancer	
Melanoma Patients' Information Page	http://www.mpip.org
The Melanoma Education Fund	http://skincheck.com
Treatment-oriented Web sites	
Bone marrow transplantation sites	
BMT Support Online	http://www.bmtsupport.org
National Bone Marrow Transplant Link	http://comnet.org/nbmtlink
National Marrow Donor Program	http://www.marrow.org
Clinical guidelines for cancer treatment	
Agency for Health Care Policy and Research	http://www.ahcpr.gov
Cancer Care Ontario Practice Guidelines Initiative	http://hiru.mcmaster.ca/ccopgi
National Guideline Clearinghouse	http://www.guideline.gov
Treatment centers	
Current list of NCI's Cancer Center Web sites	http://www.nci.nih.gov/cancercenters/centerslist.html
HospitalWeb	http://neuro-www.mgh.harvard.edu/hospitalweb.shtml

(*continued*)

TABLE 60-1. (*Continued*)

Site	*URL*
Genetics	
Cancer Family Registries	http://www-dccps.ims.nci.nih.gov/EGRP/cfr.html
Cancer Genetics Network	http://www-dccps.ims.nci.nih.gov/CGN
Genomic and Genetic Data	http://www.nhgri.nih.gov/Data
Maize Genome Database	http://teosinte.agron.missouri.edu/top.htm
National Human Genome Research Institute	http://www.nhgri.nih.gov
Online Mendelian Inheritance in Man	http://www3.ncbi.nlm.nih.gov
The Genetics of Cancer	http://www.cancergenetics.org
The Genome Database at Johns Hopkins	http://gdbwww.gdb.org
Prevention	
American Institute for Cancer Research	http://www.aicr.org
Cancer Research Foundation of America	http://www.preventcancer.org
Harvard Center for Cancer Prevention	http://www.hsph.harvard.edu/cancer
NCI/Centers for Disease Control and Prevention (CDC) 5 A Day Online Tracking Chart	http://5aday.gov
Tobacco Related Disease Research Program	http://www.ucop.edu/srphome/trdrp/welcome.html
Testing for cancer	
Cancer Imaging Research	http://www.bccancer.bc.ca/research/imaging
Food and Drug Administration list of mammography screening facilities	http://www.fda.gov/cdrh/faclist.html
Coping with cancer	
CancerFatigue	http://www.cancerfatigue.org
Hospice Link	http://www.hospiceworld.org
Lymphatic Research Foundation	http://www.lymphaticresearch.org
National Hospice Organization	http://www.nho.org
National Lymphedema Network	http://www.lymphnet.org
Oral Complications	http://www.aerie.com/nohicweb/campaign
The Hospice Web	http://www.hospiceweb.com
The United Ostomy Association, Inc.	http://www.uoa.org
Washington-Alaska Cancer Pain Initiative	http://www.fhcrc.org/cipr/wacpi
Support and resources	
Association of Cancer Online Resources	http://www.acor.org/index.html
Helping Hand Resource Guide (Cancer Care, Inc.)	http://www.cancercareinc.org/hhrd/hhrd.htm
Cancer Hope Network	http://www.cancerhopenetwork.org
Cancer Supportive Care Programs	http://www.cancersupportivecare.com
Corporate Angel Network	http://www.corpangelnetwork.org
Gilda's Club, Inc.	http://www.gildasclub.org
NCI's Office of Cancer Survivorship	http://dccps.nci.nih.gov/ocs
National Coalition for Cancer Survivorship	http://www.cancsearch.org
Patient Advocate Foundation	http://www.patientadvocate.org
R. A. Bloch Cancer Foundation	http://www.blochcancer.org
Support for People with Oral and Head and Neck Cancer	http://www.spohnc.org
The National Children's Cancer Society	http://www.children-cancer.com
The Wellness Community	http://www.wellness-community.org
Vital Options & "The Group Room" Cancer Radio talk show	http://www.vitaloptions.org
Cancer literature	
American Association for Cancer Research	http://www.aacr.org
American Society of Clinical Oncology	http://www.asco.org
Cancer News on the Net	http://www.cancernews.com
Electronic Journal of Oncology	http://ejo.univ-lyon1.fr
Journal of the National Cancer Insitute (password required)	http://jnci.oupjournals.org
NCI Publications Locator	http://cancer.gov/publications
PubMed	http://www.ncbi.nlm.nih.gov/PubMed/fulltext.html
Sustaining Oncology Studies Europe Cancer-Related Publications On Line	http://sos.unige.it/soseuro/oncopubl/titles.html
Statistics	
American Cancer Society Statistics	http://www.cancer.org
CDC National Program of Cancer Registries	http://www.cdc.gov/nccdphp/dcpc/npcr/index.htm
Surveillance, Epidemiology and End Results	http://www-seer.ims.nci.nih.gov

(continued)

TABLE 60-1. (*Continued*)

Site	*URL*
Other resources	
Minority health	
Intercultural Cancer Council	http://icc.bcm.tmc.edu/home.htm
National Asian Women's Health Organization	http://www.nawho.org
Office of Minority Health Resource Center	http://www.omhrc.gov
Information in Spanish in addition to CancerNet	
Cancer Care	http://www.cancercareinc.org
NOAH: New York Online Access to Health	http://www.noah.cuny.edu
Y-ME National Breast Cancer Organization	http://www.y-me.org
Associations and societies	
American Association for Cancer Research	http://www.aacr.org
American Society for Clinical Oncology	http://www.asco.org
Association of Community Cancer Centers	http://www.accc-cancer.org
Oncology Nursing Society	http://www.ons.org
Society of Surgical Oncology (password required)	http://www.surgonc.org
Government	
Agency for Healthcare Research and Quality	http://www.ahcpr.gov
CDC	http://www.cdc.gov
ClinicalTrials.gov	http://www.clinicaltrials.gov
U.S. Food and Drug Administration	http://www.fda.gov/fdahomepage.html
Healthfinder	http://www.healthfinder.gov
National Cancer Institute	http://www.nci.nih.gov
National Center for Biotechnology Information	http://www.ncbi.nlm.nih.gov
National Center for Complementary & Alternative Medicine	http://nccam.nih.gov
National Institutes of Health	http://www.nih.gov
National Institute of Environmental Health Sciences	http://www.niehs.nih.gov
National Library of Medicine	http://www.ncbi.nlm.nih.gov
National Toxicology Program	http://ntp-server.niehs.nih.gov
National Women's Health Information Center	http://www.4women.gov
The White House	http://www.whitehouse.gov

ognize the need to take responsibility for ensuring that patients are not exposed to bogus and potentially harmful cancer information by using criteria for selecting information they disseminate.[18–24] To help users determine what Web sites are credible, the Health on the Net Foundation has established criteria for evaluating Web sites (Table 60-2).[25,26] The principles embodied in these criteria have been widely adopted by credible health-related Web sites.

As profiling of users becomes a more common feature of interactive health communication, understanding a site's position on the confidentiality of personal information is becoming increasingly important.[27] Users should determine what personally identifiable information is collected from them by the Web site; how the information will be used; with whom the information may be shared; what choices they have regarding

TABLE 60-2. Health on the Net Criteria for Site Evaluation

Criteria	*Description*
Authorship	Authors and contributors, their affiliations, and relevant credentials are provided. Medical and health professionals give medical and health advice.
Attribution	References and sources for content are clearly listed and relevant copyright information is noted. The site supports claims with clear references to scientific research results or published articles.
Disclosure	The site has a clear statement about the funding for the site. Web site "ownership" should be prominently and fully disclosed (e.g., sponsorship, advertising, underwriting).
Currency	Dates of posting and updates are indicated. The last update date is clearly displayed. The site's Web pages display the contact e-mail address of the webmaster or a link to it on all pages.
Linkage site	An accurate description of the link site's content, size, and location is provided. The site and site's linkages respect the legal requirements of medical information and privacy that apply. The information from other sources with a link is valid and regularly updated.
Other unique or innovative features	In addition, other variables that might be useful, such as interactive or tailored sites, surveys, and search options, might make it a user-friendly site.
Peer-reviewed process	Is there an editorial board or review process for the information included?

(Adapted from refs. 25 and 26.)

the collection, use, and distribution of the information; the kind of security procedures that are in place to protect the loss, misuse, or alteration of information; and how they can correct any inaccuracies in the information. TRUSTe is an independent, nonprofit initiative whose mission is to build trust and confidence in the Internet by promoting these principles of disclosure and informed consent. Many health-related sites explicitly state their privacy policy or display the TRUSTe mark.

NATIONAL CANCER INSTITUTE'S INFORMATION SERVICES

For more than two decades, the staff of NCI's International Cancer Information Center (ICIC) have striven to meet the challenge of assisting health professionals and the public to effectively use current medical knowledge by providing current, high-quality information through a variety of media. The primary information resources are Physician Data Query (PDQ), a comprehensive database of current, peer-reviewed syntheses of state-of-the-art information on cancer care (http://cancernet.nci.nih.gov/pdq.html), and CANCERLIT, a comprehensive source of bibliographic citations on published cancer research (http://cancernet.nci.nih.gov/cancerlit.html). These databases are distributed through a variety of media, including CancerFax, one of the first fully automated fax-back services; CancerMail, an automated e-mail service; and CancerNet (http://cancernet.nci.nih.gov), an Internet Web site that provides point and click access to NCI's information resources and has become a primary mechanism for disseminating PDQ and CANCERLIT information. These information resources undergo well-established peer-review processes that draw on a broad base of cancer experts to ensure that content is current and accurate. These systems are updated on a monthly basis, which ensures that users are provided with more current information than can be provided by most hard-copy publications.[9–14]

PHYSICIAN DATA QUERY

PDQ, the NCI's comprehensive cancer information database, first became available to health professionals in 1984.[9–12] It is unique in the fact that its content is developed based on systematic reviews of the medical literature and expert opinion. Five editorial boards synthesize information from the literature into concise, clear summaries that are updated on a regular basis.

PDQ consists of three main types of information: (1) literature-based, full-text summaries that reflect current, state-of-the-art information on the treatment of adult and pediatric malignancies, the prevention and screening of cancer, the supportive care for cancer and its complications, and cancer genetics; (2) summaries of clinical trials currently accruing patients and those that are closed or completed; and (3) directories of physicians who provide cancer care and listings of health professionals who provide services related to cancer genetic risk assessment, counseling, and testing.[13,14]

Cancer Information Summaries

TREATMENT OPTIONS. PDQ contains treatment information on all major types of cancer in children and adults, including autoimmune deficiency syndrome–related cancers (http://cancernet.nci.nih.gov/treatment.html). For each cancer, a detailed summary, designed to meet the information needs of health professionals, is provided that contains an overview, information on staging, and information on treatment options by important disease-specific parameters (e.g., stage, histology, anatomic location). Key citations to the literature are referenced to enable users to see the research data on which the texts of the PDQ summaries are based. Users can retrieve abstracts of these citations for review. Levels of evidence are provided for each summary (Table 60-3). A limited number of brief summaries on more rare cancers are also available. In addition, PDQ provides treatment summaries that contain similar information written in nontechnical language for patients and their families. All of the summaries are available in English and Spanish.

TABLE 60-3. Levels of Evidence for Therapeutic Benefit from Treatment Interventions

Rank	*Type of Evidence*
Strength of study design (ranked in descending order of strength)	
I.	Randomized controlled clinical trial(s)
i.	Double-blinded
ii.	Nonblinded (allocation schema or treatment delivery)
II.	Nonrandomized controlled clinical trial(s)
III.	Case series
i.	Population-based, consecutive series
ii.	Consecutive cases (not population-based)
iii.	Nonconsecutive cases
Strength of end points (ranked in descending order of strength)	
A.	Total mortality (or overall survival from a defined point in time)
B.	Cause-specific mortality (or cause-specific mortality from a defined point in time)
C.	Carefully assessed quality of life
D.	Indirect surrogates
i.	Disease-free survival
ii.	Progression-free survival
iii.	Tumor response rate

COPING WITH CANCER. PDQ contains summaries on issues that relate to coping with the management of side effects of cancer treatment, complications caused by cancer, and the psychosocial aspects of cancer and its treatment (http://cancernet.nci.nih.gov/coping.html).

SCREENING AND PREVENTION. The screening information in PDQ includes summaries on screening for breast, cervical, colorectal, endometrial, gastric, liver, lung, neuroblastoma, oral, ovarian, prostate, skin, and testicular cancers (http://cancernet.nci.nih.gov/testing.html). Each summary contains the available data concerning screening for that particular disease site, the levels of evidence for that summary, and the significance and evidence of benefit for the summary statement (Table 60-4). They include references to the current literature that support the information in the summary. In addition, PDQ contains a version of the summary on screening for breast cancer written for non–health professionals.

PDQ also contains summaries on the prevention of breast, cervical, colorectal, endometrial, gastric, lung, oral, ovarian,

TABLE 60-4. Levels of Evidence for Physician Data Query/CancerNet Screening Summaries

Evidence obtained from at least one randomized controlled trial
Evidence obtained from controlled trials without randomization
Evidence obtained from cohort or case-control analytic studies, preferably from more than one center or research group
Evidence obtained from multiple-time series, with or without intervention
Opinions of respected authorities based on clinical experience; reports of expert committees

prostate, and skin cancer (http://cancernet.nci.nih.gov/genetics_prevention.html). Similar in format to the PDQ information on screening, these summaries contain level(s) of evidence of the supporting research (Table 60-5).

CANCER GENETICS. An editorial board was established in 1998 to address issues that relate to the impact of research in cancer genetics on cancer prevention, screening, and treatment strategies (http://cancernet.nci.nih.gov/genetics_prevention.html). An overview of cancer genetics and the genetics of breast and ovarian cancer are currently available. Summaries on the genetics of colorectal and prostate cancer, the elements of cancer risk assessment and counseling, and the multiple endocrine neoplasia type 2 syndrome are in preparation.

COMPLEMENTARY AND ALTERNATIVE APPROACHES. In collaboration with the National Institutes of Health's National Center for Complementary and Alternative Medicine, ICIC staff are preparing evidence-based summaries on nontraditional approaches to cancer prevention, treatment, and symptom control. An advisory board composed of oncologists and representatives of the complementary and alternative medicine community review the summaries to ensure that they are accurate, informative, up to date, and well balanced. Summaries on cartilage and hydrazine sulfate are currently available, and summaries on Laetrile, antineoplastons, essaic, MTH-68 (Newcastle disease virus), 714-X, green and black tea, coenzyme Q10, mistletoe, IP-6 (inositol hexaphosphate), Cancell, and *Coriollus versicolorare* are in preparation (http://cancernet.nci.nih.gov/treatment.html).

Peer Review: The Process

The information in PDQ is reviewed by five core editorial boards, each handling one of the following topics: adult treatment, pediatric treatment, supportive care, screening and prevention, and cancer genetics. These core boards are comprised of more than 80 cancer specialists who meet regularly to review the current literature and to update PDQ summaries based on scientific data. Most (67%) are not government employees. Each core board is supplemented by an external advisory board that reviews summaries annually. More than 100 additional health professionals with expertise in cancer screening, prevention, treatment, genetics, coping, and complementary and alternative care serve on these advisory boards.

A process has been developed to assist board members to efficiently identify literature with important new data. Each month, more than 80 biomedical journals are screened by professionals who identify citations of potential relevance. The

TABLE 60-5. Levels of Evidence for Physician Data Query/CancerNet Prevention Summaries

Evidence obtained from at least one randomized controlled trial with
A cancer mortality end point
A cancer incidence end point
An accepted validated intermediate end point
Evidence obtained from controlled trials without randomization with
A cancer mortality end point
A cancer incidence end point
An accepted validated intermediate end point
Evidence obtained from cohort or case-control analytic studies, preferably from more than one center or research group with
A cancer mortality end point
A cancer incidence end point
An accepted validated intermediate end point
Evidence obtained from multiple-time series, with or without intervention, with
A cancer mortality end point
A cancer incidence end point
An accepted validated intermediate end point (e.g., large adenomatous polyps for colorectal prevention)
Ecologic studies (descriptive) (e.g., international patterns studies, migration studies) with
A cancer mortality end point
A cancer incidence end point
An accepted validated intermediate end point (e.g., large adenomatous polyps for colorectal prevention)
Opinions of respected authorities based on clinical experience, or reports of expert committees (e.g., any of the above study designs using nonvalidated surrogate end points)

investigators, including important, but unpublished, manuscripts that have been accepted for publication.

After the articles are screened, those considered the most relevant and significant are sent to appropriate board members for review. If the board members believe the data warrant a change in a state-of-the-art summary, the manuscript is put on the agenda of an upcoming board meeting. At the meeting, members discuss the positive and negative points of the research and make decisions about whether to modify summaries based on the data. Changes may involve the addition of a new management option, the deletion of one that is no longer supported by data, the integration of new data that lend additional support to existing options, or an interpretation of controversial data. Literature citations are provided for each option so that users can make their own assessment of the current literature. Users can link to these citations as well.

Use of Formal Evidence-Based Criteria in Physician Data Query/CancerNet

Editorial board members understand the volume of medical knowledge and the increased emphasis on physician accountability and cost-effective practice. In an attempt to assist health professionals to apply data from the medical literature in clinical practice, all of the editorial boards have moved from a consensus development approach to summary development to an evidence-based approach to evaluating the literature and summarizing it. The practice of developing evidence-based summaries of the existing literature enables the editorial boards to draw attention to significant gaps in medical evidence that are important to consider in making patient management decisions.[28,29] Pointing out these gaps is not only important for health professionals and patients in decision-making decisions; it also helps to define areas that are most in need of additional research.

Evidence-based criteria have been used exclusively by the screening and prevention board to develop and refine screening and prevention summaries since the board's inception. This approach has proven to be useful in the consideration of scientific data on cancer screening and prevention and has proven to be well suited to the presentation of controversial information. Evidence-based methodology allows editorial board members to summarize the information currently available on a particular topic and to indicate the strength of that evidence. Annotations on the strength of the evidence for a particular approach afford the user a good understanding of the intervention and the strength of the data supporting it (see Tables 60-3 to 60-5).

In therapeutic studies, a variety of end points may be measured and reported. These end points include total mortality (or survival from the initiation of therapy), cause-specific mortality, quality of life, or indirect surrogates of these three outcomes, such as disease-free survival, progression-free survival, or tumor response rate. End points may also be determined within study designs of varying strength, ranging from the gold standard (the randomized, double-blinded, controlled clinical trial) to case series experiences from nonconsecutive patients. The adult treatment editorial board uses a formal ranking system of levels of evidence to help the reader judge the strength of evidence linked to the reported results of a therapeutic strategy. For any given therapy, results can be ranked on each of the following two scales: (1) strength of the study design and (2) strength of the end points. Because studies or clinical experiences are ranked both by strength of design and importance of end points, a given study has a two-tiered ranking [e.g., I(ii)/A for a nonblinded randomized study showing a favorable outcome in overall survival, and III(iii)/D(iii) for a phase II trial of selected patients with response rate as the outcome]. Thus, the two rankings give an idea of the overall strength of evidence (see Table 60-3).

In addition, all recommendations try to take into account other issues that cannot be so easily quantified, such as toxicity, width of confidence intervals of observations, trial size, quality assurance in the trial, and cost. Depending on their perspectives, different expert panels, professional organizations, and individual physicians may use different cut points of overall strength of evidence in formulating therapeutic guidelines or in taking action.[30] Nevertheless, this ranking system does provide an ordinal categorization of strength of evidence as a starting point for discussions of study results, and the formal descriptions of the levels of evidence provide a uniform framework for the data. The editorial boards are currently integrating information on the levels of evidence into the summaries as they review and update summaries.

PDQ's state-of-the-art summaries are dynamic and can be updated as frequently as each month. On average in 1999, 15% of the summaries were revised each month. Approximately 90% of the changes were revisions of the summaries, and approximately 30% of the summaries underwent substantial revisions. All licensees are required to ensure that the information a user prints from PDQ is dated so that it is clear to the user when the information was retrieved from the database.

Physician Directory

The PDQ physician directory contains names, addresses, and telephone numbers for more than 25,000 physicians who devote a major portion of their practice to the treatment of cancer patients. Also included is information on medical specialties, oncologic subspecialty board certification, and organizational affiliations for each of these physicians. Physicians listed in the membership directories of major oncologic societies or organizations and clinical investigators who have protocols in PDQ or are members of NCI-sponsored clinical trials groups are also listed in this directory.

Organization Directory

The PDQ organization directory contains information on more than 3000 health care institutions that provide care for cancer patients, including NCI-designated comprehensive and clinical cancer centers, community clinical oncology programs, clinical trial groups, and members of the Association of Community Cancer Centers. Information on organizations is retrievable by any combination of name, city, state, country, or zip code. These directories are not yet available through CancerNet.

Cancer Genetics Services Directory

Cancer Genetics Services (http://cancernet.nci.nih.gov/genesrch.shtml) is a directory of approximately 300 health professionals of various disciplines, such as genetic counseling, oncology, nursing, psychology, social work, and clinical genetics, who provide services related to cancer genetics, including cancer risk assessment, genetic counseling, and genetic susceptibility testing. Each individual listed must be licensed, certified, or eligible for board certification in their profession; have specific training in cancer genetics; and be affiliated with an interdisciplinary team with substantial expertise in cancer genetics. They must also be members of one of the professional organizations listed on the application for inclusion in the directory (http://cancernet.nci.nih.gov/genetics/gc_application.html) and be willing to accept referrals.

Clinical Trials

PDQ and CancerNet contain more than 1700 summaries of clinical trials that are open or approved for patient accrual (http://cancernet.nci.nih.gov/trialsrch.shtml). Treatment, screening, prevention, and supportive care protocols supported by the NCI are listed in PDQ. Each can be retrieved by diagnosis, stage, treatment modality, phase of investigation, location, and drug name, or any combination of these and other parameters. Approximately 45% of the active trials in PDQ are not directly sponsored by NCI and are submitted voluntarily by the study chairperson; 10% are submitted by the pharmaceutical industry. Criteria for including voluntary submissions include whether the study design is reasonable, whether the trial is based on rational scientific information, whether the trial is likely to yield some useful information or is unduly risky to patients, and whether the entry criteria and statistical section are clear and complete. Trial summaries can be submitted to CancerNet online (http://cancernet.nci.nih.gov/protosub/protocol.html). CancerNet's trial summaries can also be found on ClinicalTrials.gov (http://www.clinicaltrials.gov), a

Web site developed by the National Library of Medicine to provide patients, family members, and members of the public information about clinical research studies currently under way for anyone with a life-threatening disease. Collaboration with U.S. Food and Drug Administration and other National Institutes of Health staff to encourage submissions from the pharmaceutical industry is ongoing.

A member of the clinical trials review editorial board reviews protocols voluntarily submitted by investigators who are not directly supported by the NCI before their inclusion. Phase II and III trials that have been submitted to the Food and Drug Administration under the investigational new drug application regulations do not require further editorial review. Foreign clinical trials are included after the review process of the sponsoring organization is approved by the PDQ editorial board. If the clinical trials editorial board finds a reason not to include a trial in PDQ and CancerNet, a letter containing the board's concern(s) is sent to the investigator, who is invited to respond by either modifying the protocol document according to the reviewers' comments or by clarifying the information in the protocol document. Once a response is received from the investigator, the protocol is re-reviewed by the clinical trials review board. More than 90% of the trials submitted for review are included.

An archival file of more than 10,800 closed protocols provides a rich source of data on previously completed clinical research, some of which is not published and is not available elsewhere. Whenever possible, ICIC staff link the protocol summaries to published reports on trial outcomes.

Since 1996, PDQ and CancerNet also has contained consumer-oriented summaries of active clinical trials. On CancerNet, the technical terms in each summary are hyperlinked to a glossary. The technical and consumer-oriented trial summaries are also linked to one another.

Since April 1998, NCI staff has provided additional contextual information on clinical trials on its cancerTrials Web site (http://cancertrials.nci.nih.gov). The site was established to raise awareness about clinical trials and to address some of the perceived barriers to participation. The information contained on cancerTrials falls into the following categories: a framework for understanding what clinical trials are and deciding about participation; information about clinical research grouped by type of cancer; information on how to find trials, which features a hyperlink to the CancerNet clinical trials search form (http://cancernet.nci.nih.gov/trialsrch.shtml); news and features highlighting topics under clinical investigation and trial results; and resources for researchers, such as a library of downloadable resources for clinical investigators that includes templates, guidelines, and policy documents. Information on specific cancers features hypertext links to the cancer information summaries in PDQ on CancerNet, as well as news about clinical trials.

CANCERLIT

CANCERLIT is a bibliographic archival database containing more than 1.5 million citations and abstracts of published research in cancer biology, etiology, screening, prevention, and treatment published from 1963 to the present from more than 4000 different sources. It is updated monthly and provides a comprehensive, up-to-date resource of cancer literature. Preformulated search "digests" for more than 90 clinical topics are also available (http://cancernet.nci.nih.gov/canlit/canlit.htm). The complete database can be searched on CancerNet (http://cancernet.nci.nih.gov/cancerlit.shtml).

Access to Physician Data Query, CancerNet, and CANCERLIT

The CancerNet Web site has become NCI's primary dissemination vehicle for PDQ and CANCERLIT data. At the end of 1999, monthly user statistics documented more than 9 million "hits" (2 million page views) in more than 400,000 user sessions per month. In addition to its own distribution outlet, staff manage a licensing program that allows for use of the databases by a variety of commercial and nonprofit distributors. Through a trademark license, these distributors deliver PDQ and CANCERLIT data to worldwide audiences through a variety of media. The mechanisms fall into two general categories: online time-sharing systems with dial-up or Internet access; and "local" implementations in which the database resides on a computer, CD-ROM, kiosk, or local area network. CANCERLIT is also available online through a variety of commercial database vendors as an online or CD-ROM product. The program began in 1982 with one agreement, has grown to 72 agreements (39 for PDQ, 15 for CANCERLIT, and 18 for CancerMail), and continues to grow. All new requests to license are reviewed and evaluated on the following criteria:

- Does the organization share NCI's goal of disseminating and sharing cancer information?
- What is the impact of the organization's efforts?
- Would licensing the information to the organization enable ICIC to reach a larger or new audience?
- Is the organization willing and able to update the information monthly and provide ICIC with user feedback and statistics?

Licensing efforts include partnerships with vendors that produce Web sites and public kiosks with credible health information, as well as those that are developing health information "portal" sites.

Toll-Free Search Services

One of the problems faced by those responsible for disseminating health care information is how to make it easily accessible to people without direct personal access to the technology. The Cancer Information Service (CIS) is an NCI-supported nationwide network of 14 regional offices located at 34 sites in the United States, Puerto Rico, and the U.S. Virgin Islands. Through its toll-free telephone service (1-800-4-CANCER) and Web site (http://cis.nci.nih.gov), certified information specialists trained by the NCI use a variety of printed and computer resources to provide accurate, up-to-date information on cancer. In 1999, the CIS responded to more than 890,000 calls from patients, family members, health professionals, and the general public. More than 300,000 inquiries came over the Internet, and 17% of callers reported that they obtained the toll-free number from the Internet. CIS staff conduct customized searches of PDQ and make more than 100,000 referrals to clinical trials from PDQ each year. Staff also interpret research findings; explain diagnostic and treatment information; inform callers about emerging areas of science, such as hereditary risk; clarify media stories about scientific discoveries; and provide smoking cessation counseling.

The CIS makes available nearly 600 publications and materials on a range of topics, including treatment information and research studies, specific types of cancer, community services, screening tests and examinations, adopting healthier behavior, coping with cancer, and cancer risk. The CIS offers printed and audio-visual materials that are easy to read and culturally appropriate; materials are also available in Spanish. A Web-based publication-ordering service is available (http://publications.nci.nih.gov).

Each year, the CIS Partnership Program assists 4500 organizations that serve minority and medically underserved populations within their communities. CIS staff provide partners with access to the latest, most accurate cancer information; assist with coalition building and networking; offer program planning, implementation, and evaluation assistance; provide media assistance; identify resource experts; and assist with training. Efforts involve breast and cervical cancer, tobacco education, science awareness, and overcoming barriers to clinical trial participation.

The CIS serves as a health communications laboratory through an NCI-funded research consortium. CIS staff are involved in studies that test and identify the most effective ways to communicate health information to help people adopt healthier behaviors. These studies have evaluated types of information messages provided, the manner in which they are delivered, how often messages should be communicated to affect health behaviors, and the value of tailoring messages to an individual's particular perspective.[31]

The CIS intends to apply the strengths of the telephone service to the Internet and plans to provide real-time interactions over the Web to position the CIS as the world's premier cancer information navigator. Under development is instant messaging, Web-based tailoring, Webcasting, an interactive voice response system for the publication ordering, and an interface with mobile wireless digital devices.

Physician Data Query/CANCERLIT Service Center

The PDQ/CANCERLIT Service Center provides customized searches from the NCI's PDQ database to health professionals, who can request and receive information through a toll-free telephone service, e-mail, or facsimile. The goal of the service center is to make the information from PDQ available to health professionals who do not have the time or resources to access electronic systems directly. The service center can be reached by calling toll-free 1-800-345-3300 (in the United States), Monday through Friday, 9 a.m. to 6 p.m. Eastern time. Alternatively, requests can be faxed to 1-800-380-1575 or sent via e-mail to pdqsearch@icicc.nci.nih.gov. More information on the search center can be found on the Web site.

PHYSICIAN DATA QUERY/CANCERNET REDESIGN

In mid-1990, ICIC staff recognized that the infrastructure supporting PDQ, CancerNet, CancerFax, and CancerMail was old and obsolete. The legacy system had become increasingly difficult to adapt for cutting edge information technology. It could only produce simple text (ASCII data) and could not support commonplace features, such as metatags, that make information easier to find on the Internet. Production processes were also hampered by a paper-based workflow/document management system used to identify, track, process, and update more than 480 peer-reviewed information summaries from more than 80 core editorial board members, many of whom receive materials for review every month.

In 1998, ICIC staff embarked on an initiative to restructure the infrastructure to take full advantage of advances in computing technology. A 2-day formal needs assessment was performed in February 1998 to identify functional requirements for the new system. This meeting provided an opportunity for more than 190 patients, advocates, clinical investigators, practicing oncologists, oncology nurses, librarians, health educators, social workers, and other health professionals, as well as experts in medical and consumer informatics and representatives from the pharmaceutical and insurance industries, to advise NCI on what should be included in the new system. Participants in the meeting provided specific input on the range of content, ease of navigation, user interface issues, use of current and emerging technologies, and barriers to access. Operational, marketing, and evaluation issues were also discussed. The recommendations were used to develop the specifications for a more robust and flexible system that could accommodate real-time updates and multimedia data and provide advanced concept search capabilities. Participants also directed NCI to develop evaluation strategies to ensure that user feedback is obtained on an ongoing basis and that enhancements are integrated and reevaluated in an iterative fashion.

Fundamental to the redesign initiative was the development of a flexible and scalable infrastructure to support a dynamic, broad-based, and modular information system. To meet this need, ICIC computer specialists developed a universal database (UDB) server that is both a repository and a powerful retrieval engine. It also contains pointers to data located in other databases and Web sites. The power of the UDB enabled ICIC staff to develop a flexible and scalable new user interface to CancerNet. The UDB allows users to search across different data types with a single query and obtain information on a specific topic from resources in Web sites and databases produced and maintained by other divisions, institutes, and organizations. The UDB links and organizes on the fly related documents for users to review, supports multiple dissemination media and delivery mechanisms, and can accommodate future delivery mechanisms with the addition of new access modules that will not require changing the system's infrastructure. Also under development is a new workflow/document management system that will enable ICIC staff to streamline the review and updating of peer-reviewed summaries and provide users with real-time updates to CancerNet as soon as quality control procedures are complete.

Additional research and development is under way and includes instant messaging; the development of a CancerFax system that does not require handsets on facsimile machines; CancerVoice, an automatic text-to-speech conversion and speech recognition system that will permit the physically challenged and those without access to computers, fax machines, or the Internet to access CancerNet information via the telephone; audio supplements that will enable CancerNet users to simultaneously see and hear information, a feature that will be beneficial for the elderly and vision-impaired; a Web-based protocol assembly application that will permit online clinical trial protocol submission, review, and updates; content enhancements that will provide information in additional levels of technical detail; intelligent software tools that will enable ICIC staff to customize output in response to user requests, download information to hand-held wireless communication devices, and dynamically link terms requiring explanation to the glossary; search wizards to help users find information; and improved indexing that will enhance search functionality. The UDB will enable ICIC staff to metatag each section of more than 480 PDQ information summaries as "independent" documents with unique identifiers, indexes, and links, so that it can compile responses on the fly that are precisely tailored to a user's requests. This feature will also enable ICIC staff to provide advocacy organizations serving highly focused audiences with information on specific cancers and import trial summaries from trusted partners for distribution, eliminating the need to duplicate their efforts.

Another core principle is that this new information infrastructure will be tightly integrated into the NCI clinical trials system, an apparatus that is undergoing change. Staff are working in other NCI offices to develop a comprehensive cancer informatics infrastructure that will support secure access to systems for electronic submission, review, manipulation, and updating of clinical trials data. The development of such resources will facilitate the rapid and efficient communication of information across systems and among the various components of the National Cancer Program.[32]

The NCI designated health communication as one of the extraordinary opportunities for investment in the bypass budget for 2001. ICIC staff are active participants in the development of a comprehensive strategy for funding research in cancer communications and developing strategies for improving access and use of cancer information regardless of race, ethnicity, health status, education, income, age, gender, or geographic area.[4]

Site Design

In a study of 15 large Web sites, users clicked away in frustration, complaining that they could not find the information they sought 58% of the time.[33] Despite attractive graphic identities and volumes of valuable content, these sites did not provide intuitive access to information because the information architecture did not assist users in finding information quickly and easily. Often, the site architecture is confusing because the developers did not obtain user input on the organization of information; hierarchy and layout of menus; ease of navigation; usability of search forms, site indexes, and instructions for users; and the overall graphic design of the system.

To ensure that the new CancerNet Web site would not fall prey to such problems, ICIC staff made use of emerging research on Web site usability engineering. The principles of usability engineering provide guidance on overall Web site design, navigation, and functionality. Usability engineering assists Web designers in achieving their objectives by requiring them to identify and focus on the goal of the Web site, the needs of the target audience, and the technical constraints that a typical user faces with regard to hardware, software, access, and experience *before* developing the Web site. It is a cost-effective technique that eliminates the need to build a site until key components of its functionality are evident from user input.

An integral part of the redesign was the prospective gathering of data on the information needs of the full spectrum of current and potential users. An online questionnaire provided input from more than 600 individuals; 37% were accessing the site for the first time, 23% were looking for information on a specific cancer, and 11% were seeking clinical trial information. After this stage, personal interviews were conducted with current and potential users to further define their information requirements. Based on this feedback, the first prototype was constructed and then subjected to iterative evaluations with current and potential users to see if their needs were being served by the prototype. Test participants representing the various target audiences were recruited to search for information in response to a series of specific questions. While attempting to find the information required to answer the questions, test participants were asked to "think out loud" so that their thought processes could be captured and recorded on videotape to identify flaws in terminology, layout of information, hierarchy, menu structure, and navigational elements. The process proved to be an effective method of validating the information architecture and drove the redesign process. For example, usability tests conclusively documented that there was no single preferred way to search for information. Therefore, the new site was designed to permit users to find information in multiple ways, with each path linking to the same page, so that a primary document exists in only one place on the Web site.

In November 1999, ICIC staff launched the first version of the redesigned CancerNet Web site. One of the things that ICIC staff were most proud of was the fact that the new site was built with user input at every stage of development. Major enhancements include a new user interface that makes site navigation easy; cancer-specific pages that provide ready access to all of the information on the site about that cancer (http://cancernet.nci.nih.gov/cancertypes.html); powerful new search capabilities (http://cancernet.nci.nih.gov/searchoptions.html); a network of hyperlinks between PDQ summaries, clinical trials, and CANCERLIT citations; a guide for first time visitors with hyperlinks to the information described (http://cancernet.nci.nih.gov/firsttime.html); a site map; a dictionary of more than 1200 medical terms; a greatly expanded list of hyperlinks to other cancer-related Web sites; and a publication locator that allows users to view and download NCI publications or order them by e-mail. Updates on new enhancements, content, search tools, and other changes are featured in a What's New area (http://cancernet.nci.nih.gov/whatsnew.html). This area also will be used to highlight feedback from users, enable them to automatically receive updates on enhancements to CancerNet, and sign up for the CancerNet listserv. Feedback from this area and iterative usability testing will continue to drive development and implementation activities.

Multiple approaches for increasing awareness about the new site are being used to heighten the visibility of CancerNet as a primary source for high-quality cancer information, including a robust system of metatags, an e-mail notification service for users, and reciprocal linking agreements with other Web sites. Licensing efforts include partnerships with vendors who produce kiosks and those developing health information "portal" sites. ICIC staff will also continue to work with public libraries to increase awareness and use. CancerNet information is featured in MEDLINE*plus*, the National Library of Medicine's health and medical information service for the public (http://www.nlm.nih.gov/medlineplus).

The "reinvention" of PDQ represents more than the mere updating of PDQ's content or the elaboration of new technologies. At a fundamental level, the redesign involves a complete rethinking of how technology products such as PDQ should be designed and maintained over time through a process of continuous refinement.[34,35] The phases of product conceptualization, development, testing, and dissemination are no longer thought of as being consecutive; rather, all of these phases overlap by design. Consumer input throughout product conceptualization helped to focus the developers. Continuous feedback from consumers during early stages of product development helped to inform and reshape the initial conceptualization, sometimes in dramatic departures from the site as originally conceived. Continued usability tests will provide additional input and result in further refinements and enhancements that are driven by continuous consumer review of blueprints and prototypes before new versions and major refinements are implemented and marketed.

CONCLUSION

The Internet will continue to revolutionize the way the world obtains and disseminates information, and rapidly advancing technology promises to continue to revolutionize the way that medicine is practiced. It is clear that computing and communication technologies have a major role to play in decision support in medicine. Medical students have access to huge collections of information and can participate in training sessions anywhere in the world. Collaborating physicians can share patient charts, laboratory results, and x-rays and other images without considering distance or time delays. However, legal considerations, such as malpractice liability, licensure, accreditation, and reimbursement for teleconsultation, remain to be addressed. With encryption authentication, some sites are already offering automated claims and payment services, and sensitive materials, such as digital medical records that contain digitized images and full-motion video clips, will cross the Internet, opening the doors for innovative patient evaluation and consultation, as well as remote assessment and monitoring of patients.

REFERENCES

1. U.S. Department of Health and Human Services, Science Panel on Interactive Communication and Health; Eng T, Gustafson D, eds. *Wired for health and well being: the emergence of interactive health communication.* Washington DC: U.S. Government Printing Office, 1999:1.
2. Cyber Dialogue. Internet Users, World Wide Web URL: http://www.cyberdialogue.com/resource/data/ic/index.html
3. Cyber Dialogue. Healthcare, World Wide Web URL: http://www.cyberdialogue.com/resource/data/cch/index.html
4. Cancer communications. In: *The Nation's investment in cancer research. A budget proposal for the year 2001.* NIH Publication No 99-4373, October 1999:69. World Wide Web URL: http://2001.cancer.gov.
5. McConnaughey JW, Lader W, Chin R, Everette D. Falling through the net II: new data on the digital divide. National Telecommunications and Information Administration. World Wide Web URL: http://www.ntia.doc.gov/ntiahome/net2/falling.html.
6. Gustafson DH, Hawkins RP, Boberg EW, et al. Impact of patient centered computer-based health information and support system. *Am J Prev Med* 1999;16:1.
7. Alemi F, Stephens R. Computer services to patients' homes through their telephones. Application to other disease management efforts. *Med Care* 1996;34[Suppl]:OS52.
8. Grimes B, Stuart PJ. Is the web bad for your health? *PC World* 2000;Feb:167.
9. Noble HB. E-MEDICINE—a special report: hailed as a surgeon general, Koop is faulted on web ethic. *New York Times* September 5, 1999.
10. Schwartz J. The fox in 'chick' Koop: the former surgeon general has gone public, and prospered in the process. *Washington Post* January 9, 2000.
11. Hubbard SM, Henney JE, DeVita VT. A computer data base for information on cancer treatment. *N Eng J of Med* 1987;316:315.
12. Hubbard SM, Shields V, Thurn A, DeVita VT. PDQ: access to cancer information: NCI's Physician's Data Query system. In: Dollinger M, Rosenbaum EH, Cable G, eds. *Everyone's guide to cancer therapy,* 3rd ed. Kansas City, MO: Andrews McMeel Publishing, 1997:302.
13. Hubbard SM. Access to cancer information, Part I. The Internet challenge. *Clin Oncol Alert* 1997;12:46.
14. Hubbard SM. Access to cancer information, Part II. The Internet challenge. *Clin Oncol Alert* 1997;12:54.
15. Hubbard SM, Thurn AL. PDQ: in information systems in oncology. In: DeVita VT, Hellman S, Rosenberg SA, eds. *Cancer: principles and practice of oncology,* 5th ed. Philadelphia: JB Lippincott Co, 1997:2983.
16. CancerNet, World Wide Web URL: http://cancernet.nci.nih.gov/pdq.html.
17. Robinson TN, Patrick K, Eng TR, Gustafson D: An evidence-based approach to interactive health communication: a challenge to medicine in the information age. *JAMA* 1998;280:1265.
18. CancerTrials, World Wide Web URL: http://cancertrials.nci.nih.gov/beyond/evaluating.html.
19. U.S. Department of Health and Human Services. Healthfinder, World Wide Web URL: http://www.healthfinder.gov/; selection criteria can be found at World Wide Web URL: http://www.healthfinder.gov/aboutus/selectionpolicy.htm.
20. Goldwein JW, Benjamin I. Internet-based medical information: time to take charge. *Ann Intern Med* 1995;123:152.
21. Larkin M. Internet accelerates spread of bogus cancer cure. *Lancet* 1999;353:331.
22. Sikorski R, Peters R. Oncology ASAP: where to find reliable cancer information on the Internet. *JAMA* 1997;277:1431.
23. Silberg W, Lundberg G, Musacchio R. Assessing, controlling, and assuring the quality of medical information on the Internet. *JAMA* 1997;277:1244.
24. Jadad A, Gagliardi A. Rating health information on the Internet: navigating to knowledge or to Babel. *JAMA* 1998;279:611.
25. Mayer D. Cancer patient empowerment. In: Hubbard S, Goodman M, Knobf T, eds. *Oncology nursing updates.* Cedar Knolls, NJ: Lippincott, Willliams & Wilkins Healthcare, 1999;6:1.
26. Health on the Net Foundation. *HON code of conduct for medical and health Web sites.* World Wide Web URL: http://www.hon.ch/HONcode/.
27. CancerNet. World Wide Web URL: http://cancernet.nci.nih.gov/aboutsite.html#privacy.
28. Hubbard SM, Thurn A. The National Cancer Institute's CancerNet: a reliable source of current cancer information on the Internet. *Health Care Internet* 1997;1:15.
29. Costa A, Hubbard S. Evidence-based medicine: a new challenge. *Eur J Cancer* 1997;33:987.
30. Cancer Care Ontario Practice Guidelines Initiative. World Wide Web URL: http://hiru.mcmaster.ca/ccopgi/.
31. Marcus AC, Morra ME, Bettinghaus E, et al. The Cancer Information Service Research Consortium: an emerging laboratory for cancer control research. *Prev Med* 1998;27[Suppl]:S3.
32. Informatics and information flow. In: *The nation's investment in cancer research. A budget proposal for the year 2001.* NIH Publication No 99-4373, October 1999:89. Also World Wide Web URL: http://2001.cancer.gov.
33. Spool J. *Web site usability: a designer's guide.* San Francisco: Morgan Kaufmann Publishers, 1999.
34. Iansiti M, McCormick A. Developing products on Internet time. *Harvard Business Review* September–October 1997:107 (reprint #975050).
35. Nielsen J. *Top ten mistakes of Web management.* Alert box for June 15, 1997; World Wide Web URL: http://www.useit.com/alertbox/9706b.htm.

Jeffrey D. White

CHAPTER 61

Complementary, Alternative, and Unproven Methods of Cancer Treatment

DEFINITIONS

Alternative medicine is a somewhat contentious but generally accepted term that refers to a diverse assortment of philosophies, theories, and diagnostic, preventive, and therapeutic practices not generally viewed as arising from or belonging to the modern Western biomedical paradigm. Many of these interventions are used around the world by indigenous peoples of non-Western cultures as their primary form of health care.[1] However, in most developed countries, these practices generally are used along with conventional Western medicine. Consequently, the terms *complementary medicine* and *integrative medicine* are used often to acknowledge the blending of these world views and therapeutic approaches. The term *complementary medicine* can be used also to refer to conventional modalities used in unconventional ways or to achieve unconventional end points (e.g., psychosocial support groups to prolong cancer patient survival).

In April 1995, the National Institutes of Health Office of Alternative Medicine established a Panel on Definition and Description, charging it "to establish a definition of the field of complementary and alternative medicine (CAM) for purposes of identification and research; and to identify factors critical to thorough and unbiased description of CAM systems and practices that would be applicable to both quantitative and qualitative research."[2] The panel defined CAM as follows:

> Complementary and alternative medicine (CAM) is a broad domain of healing resources that encompasses all health systems, modalities, and practices and their accompanying theories and beliefs, other than those intrinsic to the politically dominant health system of a particular society or culture in a given historical period. CAM includes all such practices and ideas self-defined by their users as preventing or treating illness or promoting health and well-being. Boundaries within CAM and between the CAM domain and the domain of the dominant system are not always sharp or fixed.

Other authors prefer to define complementary therapy separately, believing that it encompasses practices that can be integrated with conventional medicine, whereas so-called alternative medicines often are promoted as independent therapeutic approaches not amenable to combination with conventional therapy.[3,4] Many other terms have been used to define this subject: *unconventional, unproved, unorthodox, unsound, nontraditional, holistic,* and *non-Western.* Table 61-1 presents a partial list of CAM modalities used for the prevention or treatment of cancer, of cancer symptoms, or of conventional treatment side effects.

PHENOMENOLOGY OF COMPLEMENTARY AND ALTERNATIVE MEDICINE IN CANCER

CAM usage by cancer patients is very prevalent all over the world (Table 61-2). Recent surveys have reported CAM use by cancer populations in Austria,[5] Australia,[6] Finland,[7] Germany,[8,9] Italy,[10] the Netherlands,[11] Norway,[12–14] Taiwan,[15] the United Kingdom,[16] the United States,[17–23] and Canada.[24–28]

A systematic review of surveys of various cancer populations has given some validation to the general gestalt that the prevalence of CAM usage is increasing.[16] However, accurate assessment of trends in CAM usage by cancer patients is rendered difficult by the lack of consistency in the definition of CAM, by survey methodology, and by population demographics.

TABLE 61-1. Commonly Used Complementary and Alternative Medicine Modalities in Cancer

MEGAVITAMINS AND OTHER NUTRIENTS
Vitamin C[138]
CoQ10[139]
HERBAL PRODUCTS
Essiac
Hoxsey
Chapparal tea[140]
BIOELECTROMAGNETIC-BASED THERAPIES
Energy healing[141]
Therapeutic touch[142]
METABOLIC THERAPIES
Kelley therapy (and the Gonzalez variation)
Gerson
Revici therapy[143]
MANIPULATIVE AND BODY-BASED SYSTEMS
Reiki
MIND-BODY MEDICINE
Support group interventions
Relaxation therapy
Imagery
Hypnosis
UNCONVENTIONAL CHEMOTHERAPIES
Antineoplastons
Hydrazine sulfate
Laetrile
714-X[132,144]
UNCONVENTIONAL "IMMUNOMODULATIVE" THERAPIES
Immunoaugmentative therapy[145]
MGN-3[146]
β-D-glucans extracted from various mushrooms (e.g., *Coriolus versicolor*)[147]
OTHERS
Thymus therapy[148]

One study specifically attempted to gauge the change in prevalence of CAM use by cancer patients. Abu-Realh et al.[29] reviewed data from a subgroup of responders to the 1992 National Health Interview Survey to determine the growth in use of self-help therapies (e.g., relaxation exercises, imagery, humor, laughter, meditation, prayer, affirmations, self-hypnosis, and music, aroma, and color therapy) and psychosocial therapies (i.e., counseling and support groups). The authors compared the percentage of CAM users among individuals with diagnosed cancer prior to and after 1986 and found a 63% increase in use of those modalities (8.3% prior to 1986 vs. 13.6% after 1986).

The growth of general CAM usage in the United States has been investigated more thoroughly. Eisenberg et al.[30] reported results of a follow-up to their 1990 survey[31] of the American public for CAM use. The 1997 survey found that 42% of the interviewed participants had used at least one CAM modality in the last 12 months. Of the CAM users, 46% had at least one visit to an alternative medicine practitioner. These figures were significantly greater than the 34% overall CAM usage and the 36% of those visiting an alternative medicine practitioner reported in the 1990 survey. These surveys, and others from various countries, also found that CAM use was more prevalent among younger patients[5,26,28] and those with higher education[18,19,28] and higher income.[18,28]

The largest survey of CAM use by U.S. cancer patients was reported by the American Cancer Society in 1992.[32] Telephone interviews of approximately 36,000 households across the nation led to the identification of a group of 3272 living individuals who had had a cancer other than a nonmelanomatous skin cancer. Approximately two-thirds of these patients were interviewed, and information about the other one-third was obtained from family members. The authors found that 9% of cancer patients used CAM and that subpopulations of patients with certain tumor types had rates as high as 21% (e.g., brain cancer).

Ernst and Cassileth[16] performed a comprehensive review of surveys of cancer patients' use of CAM. Surveys of cancer patients in various settings have yielded rates ranging from 9% to 91%. Selected surveys are summarized in Table 61-2. The differences between the prevalence figures obtained likely are due to differences in the demographics of the populations, the definition of CAM, and the survey methodology.

Some recurring themes are seen across surveys. Most cancer patients who use CAM use more that one modality, often simultaneously.[18,19,33] Greater use has been noted among patients with advanced disease or a poor prognosis (or both).[9,11,32,34] Many studies have found that most users of CAM therapies for cancer judged them to be effective and were satisfied with their outcomes.[10,19,24,27]

Both similarities and some important differences are seen in the types of CAM modalities used by the general public, by individuals with a known noncancer illness, and by cancer patients. The most commonly used U.S. CAM modalities identified among patients with a variety of noncancer illnesses are chiropractic, relaxation, massage, herbal medicines, spiritual healing, and imagery.[30] Among U.S. and Canadian cancer patients, the modalities identified most frequently in the 1990s have been mind-body approaches (mediation, relaxation, hypnotherapy, visualization, and other imagery techniques); specialized diets and dietary supplements; herbal preparations; megavitamin therapy; and spirituality, prayer, and spiritual healing (see Table 61-2).

Two surveys reported the use of CAM approaches by pediatric cancer patients. Fernandez et al.[24] surveyed patients attending the only tertiary-care pediatric oncology center in British Columbia, Canada, and found that 42% of the patients in the study used a CAM modality, with herbal teas, plant extracts, relaxation therapy-imagery, and therapeutic vitamins being the most common. In a smaller study in the Netherlands,[11] 31% of the patients were using alternative treatments, with a greater rate of usage among the subgroup of relapsed patients (46%).

REASONS FOR CANCER PATIENT USE OF COMPLEMENTARY AND ALTERNATIVE MEDICINE MODALITIES

Many patients use CAM approaches to "boost" the immune system,[9,24] but many also choose them with hopes of slowing the progression of tumors or ultimately obtaining a cure.[21,26] Even

TABLE 61-2. Prevalence of Alternative Cancer Therapy Use Among Cancer Patients

Survey Source	*No. of Patients*	*Cancer Type*	*Location*	*Prevalence of CAM*[a]	*Most Frequently Used Modalities*[b]
UNITED STATES					
Adler et al., 1999[17]	86	Breast (adult)	San Francisco	72%	—
Burstein et al., 1999[18]	480	Breast (adult)	Massachusetts, United States	28%	Self-help groups, 44%; relaxation techniques, 44%; herbal medicines, 32%; megavitamins, 29%; imagery, 29%
Gotay et al., 1999[19]	343	Various types	Hawaii, United States	36%	Prayer, 50%; lifestyle changes, 38%; herbs, 33%; mind-body control, 20%
Sparber et al.[20]	100	Various types (adult)	NIH, United States	75%	Spirituality, 36%; relaxation, 26%; lifestyle, diet, 24%; high-dose vitamins–antioxidants, 22%
Vande Creek et al., 1999[21]	112	Breast (adult)	Midwestern United States	91%	Prayer, 76%; exercise, 38%; spiritual healing, 29%; megavitamins, 25%
Lerner et al., 1992[32]	3272	Various types (adult)	Continental United States	9%	"Mind" therapies, 49%; diets, 38%; drug or other methods, 33%
Goldstein et al., 1991[23]	40	Various types (adult)	New York	12.5%	Selenium, imagery
CANADA					
Nam et al., 1999[25]	232 (cancer patients); 36 (high-risk non-cancer)	Prostate	Toronto, Canada	33% of cancer patients; 33% of high-risk noncancer	Vitamin E, 65%; garlic, 49%; low-fat diet, 45%; saw palmetto, 40%
Verhoef et al., 1999[27]	167	Brain tumors	Alberta, Canada	24%	Herbal, 65%; mind-body, 33%; animal-vegetable-derived (e.g., shark cartilage, mushrooms), 25%; vitamins, 20%
Warrick et al., 1999[28]	200	Head and neck	Toronto, Canada	22.5%	Herbals, 50.5%; pharmacologic agents, 16.9%
Fernandez et al., 1998[24]	366	Various tumors (pediatric)	British Columbia, Canada	42%	Herbal teas, 61%; plant extracts, 56%; therapeutic vitamins, 55%; diet, 49%; Essiac tea, 46%
Oneschuk et al., 1998[26]	143	Various types	Alberta, Canada	37%	Herbs, 40%; vitamins, 33%
EUROPE					
Crocetti et al., 1998[10]	242	Breast	Italy	17%	Homeopathy, 24%; manual healing, 16%; herbs, 14%
Arkko et al., 1980[7]	151	Various types	Finland	45%	Herbal >70%; vitamin C, 10.3%
Jirillo et al., 1996[149]	450, 396	Solid tumors, unspecified	Argentina, Italy	17%, 19%	
Grothey et al., 1998[9]	103	Various types	Germany	45%	Vitamins, 50%; mistletoe, 45%
Risberg et al., 1995[34]	630	Various types	Norway	20%	Faith healing, herbs, vitamins, diets, and mistletoe
Grootenhuis et al., 1998[11]	84	Various types (pediatric)	Netherlands	31%	Cancer treatment based on autonomous medical concepts, 58%; physical and bioelectric methods, 35%; psychic and imagery healing, 23%
Mottonen et al., 1997[150]	15	ALL (pediatric)	—	40%	
Munstedt et al., 1996[75]	206	Gynecologic malignancies	Germany	38.3%	Mistletoe, 50%; trace minerals, 46%; megavitamins, 39%; enzymes, 22%
ASIA AND PACIFIC BASIN					
Liu et al., 1997[15]	100	Various tumors	Taiwan	64%	Traditional Chinese medicine, 100%
Sawyer et al., 1994[6]	100	Various tumor (pediatric)	Australia	46%	—

ALL, acute lymphocytic leukemia; CAM, complementary and alternative medicine; NIH, National Institutes of Health.
[a]Prevalence is of CAM use either since cancer diagnosis or specifically used for cancer prevention or treatment.
[b]Percentages are of the CAM user subpopulation.

in a study of patients referred to a pain and symptom management clinic, most CAM users had used the modalities for a potential anticancer effect.[26]

Some observers have suggested that disease recurrence or progression is the primary trigger for patients to seek CAM therapies.[35] However, for many patients, the initial diagnosis of cancer raises enough concerns to investigate alternative or complementary modalities.[18] For some patients, experimentation with CAM modalities may be due to fear of the uncertainty of response to conventional therapy; for others, this choice may be simply an attempt to participate in the healing process.[27]

Burstein et al.[18] reported that new use of CAM among a group of women with recently diagnosed early-stage breast cancer correlated with significantly more depression, less sexual satisfaction, greater fear of recurrence, and somatic symptoms. The problems of low sexual satisfaction and fear remained at the 12-month observation point, but the other areas improved and were not significantly different from those of nonusers. The authors suggested that initiation of CAM use should alert clinicians to inquire about anxiety, depression, or physical symptoms.

COMPLEMENTARY AND ALTERNATIVE MEDICINE THERAPIES

CAM therapies for cancer are legion, and many have multiple variations. In this section, some of the more prevalent therapies are described briefly, primarily from the standpoint of the published evidence. Other therapies are listed in Table 61-1 with references for those not discussed here. For most of these approaches, definitive clinical trials to assess their potential efficacy have not been performed. For many others, their use continues despite results of randomized controlled clinical trials indicating no efficacy.

ANTINEOPLASTONS

In the 1960s and 1970s, Dr. Stanislav Burzynski reported the identification of small peptide molecules in the blood and urine of normal humans, which he called *antineoplastons*.[36,37] Burzynski postulated that these compounds were components of a natural anticancer defense system or "chemo-surveillance system"[38] and named them for the original designation of the urine fractions from which they were extracted. Antineoplaston A10 is a 1:4 ratio of phenylacetylisoglutamine and phenylacetylglutamine, and AS2-1 is a 1:4 ratio of phenylacetylglutamine and phenylacetic acid.[39]

Burzynski reported his clinical experience with antineoplastons in cancer patients.[40–42] However, as pointed out in a comprehensive review of the subject,[43] the use of unconventional definitions of response and the confounding factors of concurrent conventional therapies hamper the interpretation of the results of these studies. One study by a Japanese group[44] evaluated the toxicity, and preliminarily evaluated the response rates, of patients with various tumors to AS2-1 and A10. Some of these patients received concurrent chemotherapy. The authors reported responses in 3 of 46 measurable tumors but gave insufficient information about the patients to assess the role of antineoplastons in these responses.

In 1991, the National Cancer Institute (NCI) reviewed a series of seven case reports of patients with brain tumors treated with antineoplastons. The reviewers found that presumptive evidence of antitumor activity was demonstrated, and phase II trials were initiated.

A trial of patients with recurrent high-grade glioma was designed and initiated with significant input from Burzynski.[39] Nine patients were treated with AS2-1 and A10 in the study before accrual was halted, owing to an inability to reach agreement with the supplier of the antineoplastons on protocol modifications designed to increase accrual. None of the six assessable patients manifested a radiographic remission, and all had progressive disease within less than 10 weeks of starting treatment. A recent study of continuous infusion of phenylacetate alone in patients with recurrent malignant gliomas has revealed low-level activity (3 partial responses of 40 patients).[45]

METABOLIC THERAPIES

Gerson Therapy

A therapy for cancer and other illnesses was developed empirically by Max B. Gerson, a German-born physician, and was administered in his sanitarium during the 1930s, 1940s, and 1950s until his death in 1959.[46,47] Gerson sought to "balance" potassium and sodium, as their "imbalance" was thought to support tumor growth. His therapy consisted of a low sodium, high potassium, lactovegetarian diet that emphasized fresh vegetables and fruit juices and vitamin supplements. Frequent enemas, including coffee enemas, and injections of a liver extract also were part of the regimen. Raw veal liver juice was discontinued in 1987, owing to contamination with *Campylobacter fetus*.

In 1977, the Gerson Institute was founded and based in Bonita, CA. The Institute oversees a clinic in Tijuana, Mexico [Centro Hospitalario Internacional del Pacifico, SA (CHIPSA)] where the Gerson therapy is offered along with other adjunctive measures.[48]

A retrospective study of 235 melanoma patients treated from 1975 to 1990 at the CHIPSA clinic has been published.[49] This report evaluated the 5-year survival rates of the 153 patients for which adequate staging information was available and compared them to historical controls. The authors reported 100% survival for stage I and stage II disease and a 71% survival for stage III disease, comparing favorably with the historical control. Other researchers have claimed that the Gerson regimen is useful to palliate pain and diminish the side effects of conventional irradiation and chemotherapy.[50]

Macrobiotic Diet

Apparently, the macrobiotic philosophy was developed by George Ohsawa (1893 to 1966) (also known as *Yukikazu Sakurazawa*), who first introduced his concepts to the United States in 1959. Subsequently, macrobiotic theories and practices were developed and promoted by Michio Kushi who, in 1978, founded the Kushi Institute. This establishment offers courses in physical and psychological health and in ecology, spiritual development, and world peace.

Originally, Ohsawa described 10 stages of diet designated −3 to +7. The +7 diet consisted of 100% cereals and was prescribed for short periods to patients with various illnesses, including cancer.[51] Reports of clinically significant vitamin and mineral deficiency states were reported with some versions of this diet.[52,53] However, the standard macrobiotic diet currently recommended by Kushi[54] is a better-balanced, high–complex carbohydrate, low-fat vegetarian diet that may include small amounts of seafood. Individuals consuming a macrobiotic diet have been found to have urinary levels of diphenolic phytoestrogens much higher than those of control groups of lacto-ovovegetarians or omnivores.[55]

Two unreported retrospective studies of survival of patients with pancreatic and prostate cancer and a series of case reports were reviewed by the Unconventional Cancer Therapies Panel of the Office of Technology Assessment.[51] Despite this, no consensus of compelling evidence for activity was obtained.

Kelley-Gonzalez Regimen

In the 1950s and 1960s, Dr. William D. Kelley,[57] a dentist from the Midwest, developed a theory of health and illness that classified people as metabolic types, with physiologies in which the activity either of the parasympathetic or of the sympathetic nervous system was dominant or the two were balanced.[56] He then prescribed diets ranging from purely vegetarian (for sympathetic types) to predominantly meat-containing (for parasympathetic types) to compensate for years of "wrong" diets that had resulted in illness. Kelley also believed that pancreatic proteolytic enzymes were secreted into the blood stream and acted as the body's first line of defense against malignancy.

The Kelley program for cancer treatment consists of six basic components: (1) the appropriate diet, (2) vitamin and mineral supplementation, (3) concentrates of raw beef organs and glands in pill form, (4) digestive aids, including pepsin, hydrochloric acid, bile, and various pancreatic enzymes, (5) frequent doses of proteolytic pancreatic enzymes between meals, and (6) a "detoxification" regimen that included frequent coffee enemas.[57]

Currently, variations of the Kelley regimen still are practiced by a few individuals in the United States. Dr. Nicholas Gonzalez has used this approach for several years and recently reported the results of a small prospective study in advanced pancreatic cancer patients.[58] Over the period of the study, 36 patients with pancreatic cancer were seen. Eleven of these patients were considered assessable, and the other 25 were deemed unassessable because they either did not start the regimen or stopped taking the therapy in less than 8 weeks (n = 13) or had one of six other exclusion criteria (n = 12). The patients had stage I to stage IV pancreatic cancer. All patients' tumors either were unresected or resected incompletely. The median survival was 17.0 months in the treatment group, compared to a literature control showing a 4- to 6-month median survival. A trial of this regimen versus gemcitabine in patients with advanced pancreatic cancer is under way at Columbia University.

BIOLOGICALLY BASED THERAPIES

Cartilage (Shark and Bovine)

Cartilage products of various sources long have been suspected of having anticancer activities and have been the subject of much lay literature. Frequently, shark cartilage is used by U.S. and Canadian cancer patients.[19,24] Estimates for 1992 maintained that more than 50,000 Americans used shark cartilage products.[59]

Some shark cartilage extracts and various isolated molecular species have *in vitro* antiangiogenesis and matrix metalloprotease inhibitor activity.[60–63] Evidence of oral bioavailability of the active components on a water-soluble shark cartilage extract has been demonstrated in a rat model.[64]

Reports of positive results from a Cuban trial of shark cartilage were aired on the television news magazine "60 Minutes" in 1994[65] but have not been followed by a published scientific article. Miller et al.[66] reported a phase I and II trial of a powdered shark cartilage product in which 60 patients with advanced, previously treated cancers were treated with 1 g/kg/d orally. The dose was increased to 1.3 g/kg if no response was seen after 6 weeks. No patient experienced a complete or partial remission, but 10 of 50 assessable patients had stable disease for at least 12 weeks. Another single-arm trial has been reported, but the results were confounded by the presence of concurrent conventional therapy.[67] Phase III trials of two oral shark cartilage products in advanced cancer patients are planned by the M.D. Anderson Community Clinical Oncology Program and the North Central Cancer Treatment Group.

Bovine cartilage has been administered either subcutaneously only[68] or both orally and subcutaneously.[69,70] Puccio et al.[70] reported 3 partial remissions in 22 metastatic renal carcinoma patients. Another study by Romano et al.[68] obtained one complete remission in nine patients with various types of tumors. The complete remission is reported to have been the resolution of lung metastases and a flank mass in a patient with metastatic renal cell carcinoma. This response had been continuous for 9 months when the trial was reported. The largest experience of human cancers treated with bovine cartilage was reported by Prudden.[69] He reported a 90% response rate (61% complete response) in 31 cases of a variety of malignancies.

Herbal Mixtures

ESSIAC. The Essiac herbal mixture has been used widely in Canada since the 1920s. The original recipe for this mixture is said to have been developed by an Ojibwa healer and was given to Rene Caisse (*Essiac* is *Caisse* spelled backward), a nurse working in Ontario, Canada, by a woman who believed herself to have been cured of breast cancer through its use.[71]

The original recipe contained four main herbs: burdock root (*Arctium lappa*) (also used in the Hoxsey treatment, discussed next in this chapter); Indian or turkey rhubarb (*Rheum palmatum*); sheep or sheepshead sorrel (*Rumex acetosella*); and the inner bark of slippery elm (*Ulmus fulva* or *Ulmus rubra*). Later, watercress (*Nasturtium officinale*), blessed thistle (*Cnicus benedictus* L.), red clover (*Trifolium pratense*), and kelp were added.[72] This mixture is manufactured by Essiac Products (New Brunswick, Canada) and is available directly from the manufacturer or, for Canadian patients, through the Emergency Drug Release Program of Health Canada.[73]

The individual herbal components of Essiac have been tested, and reports show varying activities despite the fact that certain purified chemical moieties from each of the herbs have reproducible antitumor activities.[72] To date, no published clinical trials have evaluated Essiac in cancer patients, but this product continues to be one of the CAM anticancer therapies used most commonly by American and Canadian cancer patients.[19,24]

HOXSEY TREATMENT. The Hoxsey therapy is composed of a variety of herbal preparations made famous by Harry Hoxsey beginning in the 1920s. After attaining a wide-ranging popularity in the United States, a series of violations of U.S. Food and Drug Administration regulations resulted in the closing of the U.S. clinics and the export of the treatment to a CHIPSA clinic in Tijuana, Mexico (see Gerson Therapy, earlier in this chapter).

The internal Hoxsey treatment is composed of licorice (*Glycyrrhiza glabra*), red clover (*Trifolium pratense*), burdock (*Arctium lappa*), stillingia root (*Stillingia sylvatica*), berberis root (*Berberis vulgaris*), poke root (*Phytolacca americana*), cascara (*Rhammus purshiana*), aromatic USP 14 (artificial flavor), prickly ash bark (*Zanthoxylum americanum*), and buckthorn bark (*Rhamnus frangula*).[74] The clinic treatment includes other dietary and hygiene manipulations. As with Essiac, some of the purified components of individual herbs within the mixture have reproducible anticancer activities, but the whole form of the herbs have yielded variable results. Neither clinical trials nor *in vitro* or animal model testing of the entire mixture has been reported. Series of case reports were submitted to the NCI in 1945 and 1950 but were judged to contain no evidence of anticancer activity.[74]

MISTLETOE. Mistletoe (*Viscum album* L.) is used extensively in Europe and is one of the CAM modalities used most frequently in Germany.[9,12,75] A semiparasitic plant member of the Loranthacea family, mistletoe draws water and minerals from host trees but produces carbohydrates by its own photosynthesis. Loranthacene species were proposed in 1916 to be useful in cancer by Rudolf Steiner, an Austrian who founded a system of health promotion called *anthroposophy*, attempting to link science and spirituality.

The active moieties in mistletoe are thought to be lectins (glycoproteins) and viscotoxins (proteins). The lectin component has been demonstrated to have immunostimulant activity *in vitro*. It induces macrophage production of tumor necrosis factor[76] and increases interleukin-1 and interleukin-6 production.[77] The viscotoxins have been shown to have direct cytotoxic activity against certain cancer cell lines.[78]

The currently available mistletoe products are Iscador, Helixor, Abnoba Viscum, Isorel, and Eurixor. They are whole or purified extracts, fermented or nonfermented. Iscador also has added metals (silver, copper, and mercury).

A large body of clinical literature (case reports, retrospective analysis, and a variety of clinical trials) deals with the commercially available mistletoe products. A few randomized, controlled cancer clinical trials of mistletoe have been reported from Europe. In the largest study, 677 women who had received radical or simple mastectomy for breast cancer were randomly assigned to Helixor (parenterally) with or without radiation therapy; to chemotherapy with cyclophosphamide, methotrexate, and fluorouracil with or without radiation therapy; or to no treatment.[79] A statistically significant survival advantage was identified for the Helixor arm as compared to no treatment, but no significant difference was found between the Helixor arm and the chemotherapy arm. Although side effects reportedly were not documented systematically, the primary adverse reactions associated with Helixor were said to be primarily inflammatory reactions at the injection site and occasional fevers.

In a study of patients with metastatic colorectal cancer, patients were randomly assigned to Helixor and fluorouracil and folinic acid (n = 20) versus fluorouracil and folinic acid (n = 20). Ten complete remissions were reported in the Helixor group, and six were reported in the control group. Median survival time was 14 months for controls and 26 months for the Helixor arm ($P = .06$). The difference in side effects between the two arms was small. Further randomized, multicenter clinical trials are under way.[80]

Other studies have investigated the immunomodulatory activity of mistletoe. A study of adjuvant therapy in glioma randomly assigned 35 patients either to receive subcutaneous injections of a standardized extract of mistletoe lectins for 3 months or to receive no therapy.[81] Increased lymphocyte numbers and activity were noted in the mistletoe lectin arm as was an improved quality of life determined by a standardized questionnaire.

SPES AND PC-SPES. SPES and PC-SPES are herbal mixtures developed by Dr. Sophie Chen, a researcher at New York Medical College, and distributed by BotanicLab in Brea, CA.[82] Reportedly, more than 2000 patients have used PC-SPES for the treatment of prostate cancer.[83]

SPES contains 14 herbs: *Agrimonia pilosa Ledeb*, *Cervus nippon Temminck*, Cheng-min chou, *Corydalis busbosa*, *Ganoderma lucidum*, *Panax ginseng* C.A. Meyer, glycyrrhiza, *Lycoris radiata*, Mou hui tou, *Phrola rotoundifolia L*, *Rabdosia rubescens*, *Stephania delavayi* Diels, *Stephania sinica* Diels, *Zanthozylum nitidum*. PC-SPES contains eight herbs: chrysanthemum, isatis, licorice, *Ganoderma lucidum*, *Panax pseudo-ginseng*, *Rabdosia rubescens*, saw palmetto, and *scutellaria* (skullcap).

Hsieh et al.[84] demonstrated the induction of apoptosis and down-regulation of bcl-6 in mutu I cells treated with ethanolic extracts of PC-SPES. Tumors induced in rats inoculated with a metastasizing prostate cancer cell line underwent apoptosis when the rats were fed rodent chow containing PC-SPES at levels of 0.05% and 0.045%. Neither obvious toxicity nor a significant difference in food intake was noted after 8 weeks. Dose-dependent inhibitory effects of dietary PC-SPES were observed on both tumor incidence and rate of tumor growth.[85]

A phase II study of PC-SPES has been performed at University of California, Los Angeles.[86] The results of the treatment of 34 patients (20 hormone-naïve, 14 androgen-independent) were reported. Prostatic-specific antigen (PSA) declined by more than 50% in 9 of 12 hormone-naïve patients and in 9 of 12 androgen-independent patients. Testosterone levels fell to anorchid levels by 1 month in 7 of 21 (33%). The toxicities noted were suggestive of estrogenic activity. Tender gynecomastia was seen in 71% of patients, and one patient had a thromboembolic event. Sixty percent of patients with previously normal testosterone levels lost libido and potency when present pretreatment.

Sixteen patients with advanced prostate cancer taking PC-SPES as a dietary supplement (2.7 g daily) were followed in another study.[82] At 3 months, 10 of 16 patients showed a decrease in PSA levels in excess of 50%. In a report of prostate cancer patients treated with PC-SPES, decreased serum testosterone levels were noted in six of six men, and drops in the PSA level were noted in eight of eight patients.[87]

HYDRAZINE (OR HYDRAZINIUM) SULFATE

Hydrazine is a chemical with a variety of uses and is an important intermediate in the synthesis of some pharmaceutical drugs, such as isoniazid, hydralazine, and procarbazine.[88] Gold[89] reported that the growth of Walker 256 tumor in mice was inhibited by hydrazine sulfate. Another study found that Morris hepatoma growth in rats was inhibited when the animals were fed hydrazinium sulfate, 15 mg/kg orally twice daily for 5 days.[90] However, this response was associated with reduction of body weight, anorexia, and decreased nitrogen metabolism and retention. An identical group that was fed parenterally sustained body weight but suffered stimulated tumor growth and symptoms of liver toxicity.

Hydrazine sulfate is also an inhibitor of phosphoenolpyruvate carboxykinase, a key enzyme in mammalian gluconeogenesis. This metabolic pathway has been recognized to play a role in cancer cachexia.[91] Gold[92] postulated that hydrazine sulfate interrupts host energy wasting by inhibiting the conversion of lactic acid to glucose in the liver. This process is also thought to decrease the glucose available to the tumor and therefore can lead to a slowing of tumor growth.

A report of a large patient experience (740 patients) from Russia calculated that 47% of the patients had symptomatic improvement.[93] They also reported some patients with objective responses (4% of lung cancer patients) or stable disease (22% of lung cancer patients).

Gold[94] studied 84 patients with various cancers and reported that 70% had symptomatic improvement (increased appetite, weight gain, decreased pain) and 17% had prolonged tumor stabilization or some degree of tumor regression. Three small single-arm trials by other investigators failed to substantiate these findings.[22,95,96]

There have been four randomized, controlled clinical trials of hydrazine sulfate in cancer patients that have yielded mixed results. The first study by Chelbowski et al.[97] had the most promising findings but did not show a significant difference in survival between the two arms until a subgroup analysis was done.

The NCI sponsored three follow-up clinical trials. Two trials studied lung cancer patients simultaneously treated with platinum-based chemotherapy regimens with hydrazine sulfate or placebo,[98,99] and a third study looked at hydrazine sulfate alone versus placebo alone in patients with advanced colorectal cancer.[100] None of these follow-up studies showed a statistically significant improvement in survival in the hydrazine sulfate arm, and the Cancer and Leukemia Group B study[98] showed a lesser quality of life in the hydrazine sulfate arm. All together, these three follow-up studies contained more than 600 patients.

There is still significant interest by the public in hydrazine sulfate and a feeling among some that the clinical trials were flawed and the results invalid. The General Accounting Office investigated the three NCI-supported randomized trials and found that they were accurate.[101]

LAETRILE

Laetrile is a mixture of amygdalin, a plant glycoside, and other compounds found in the pits of some fruits, raw nuts, and other plants.[102,103] Although frequently called *vitamin* B_{17} in the lay literature, amygdalin is not recognized as a vitamin by the Committee on Nomenclature of the American Institute of Nutrition. Laetrile has been given orally and intravenously, with different pharmacokinetics and toxicity profiles.

The NCI supported a trial at the Mayo Clinic using amygdalin and a "metabolic therapy" containing vitamins A, C, E, and B complex and pancreatic enzymes.[104] One hundred and seventy-nine patients with advanced cancer who had either failed attempts at prior standard therapy or for which no standard therapy with a curative potential was available were treated. Of the 175 assessable patients, only one met the criteria for a partial remission. There were no other responders, and all patients had progression by 7 months. The median survival from the start of therapy was 4.8 months.

Despite the fact that no new clinical trials have been reported, use of laetrile continues.[105] No further research appears to be under way.

SUPPORTIVE CARE (COMPLEMENTARY MEDICINE)

ACUPUNCTURE

Dundee et al.[106] found that acupuncture needling with 5 minutes of electrical stimulation at the P6 point (volar surface of the wrist) was effective in preventing chemotherapy-induced nausea and vomiting. Ten patients were studied in a randomized, crossover portion of the study in which patients received either P6 electroacupuncture or stimulation at a "dummy" point. The antiemetic effect lasted approximately 8 hours. After a systematic review of the literature, the NIH Consensus Development Panel on Acupuncture found sufficient evidence existed for efficacy in managing chemotherapy-induced nausea.[107]

Preliminary evidence suggests that acupuncture may also be effective in the treatment of vasomotor symptoms (i.e., hot flushes) in men receiving gonadotropin analogues for prostate cancer therapy. A pilot study used electroacupuncture to a fixed set of acupuncture points for 30 minutes, twice a week for 2 weeks followed by once a week for 10 weeks. The mean number of flushes per day for the six men who continued therapy for more than 2 weeks decreased from 7.9 during the week before therapy to 2.5 after 10 weeks.[108]

PAIN MANAGEMENT

A variety of CAM modalities have been used to aid in pain management. Reiki, an "energy healing system" based on Tibetan scriptures but developed in Japan, has been tested in at least one pilot study with reportedly positive effects.[109]

Use of relaxation, imagery, and cognitive-behavior training for the management of oral mucositis pain has been studied in a randomized, controlled trial.[110] Ninety-four patients at the Fred Hutchinson Cancer Research Center undergoing their first bone marrow transplant completed the study. Oral mucositis pain levels were evaluated in four groups of patients. The two groups receiving relaxation and imagery reported significantly lower pain levels as assessed by a visual analogue scale.

A randomized controlled trial of 96 women with newly diagnosed large or locally advanced breast cancer compared standard care versus standard plus relaxation training and imagery.[111] A significantly improved quality of life was seen in the group receiving relaxation and imaging. Other studies have used questionnaires designed to assess general patient comfort. One such randomized study by Kolcaba and Fox[112] demonstrated an improved level of comfort among the patients undergoing a guided imagery intervention.

SELF-HELP AND SUPPORT GROUPS AND HYPNOSIS

There appears to have been an increase in the number of cancer patients attending support groups.[29] Although patients are likely attending these groups mostly for psychosocial support, there is some evidence that these interventions may also be related to an increased survival for some groups.

Spiegel et al.[113] were the first to report evidence for a beneficial effect on survival of a support group intervention in a group of cancer patients. Eighty-six patients with metastatic breast cancer were randomly assigned to intervention (n = 50) or control group (n = 36). The intervention consisted of 1 year of weekly 90-minute support groups led by a therapist who had breast cancer in remission. The groups were structured to encourage discussion of how to cope with cancer and for patients to express their feelings about the illness and its effect on their lives. Also a self-hypnosis strategy was taught for pain control. The mean survival in control group was 18.9 months versus 36.6 months in the treatment group. Interestingly, a survival advantage was not seen until approximately 8 months after the completion of the group intervention (i.e., at 20 months from entry on study).

Spiegel and Spira[114] have written a manual explaining the details of their psychosocial intervention. Follow-up studies by Goodwin et al.[115] in Toronto, Canada, and Spiegel et al.[160] at the University of Rochester are under way.

Another study of a support group intervention with cognitive behavioral therapy in patients with metastatic breast cancer found no survival advantage for the treated group over a randomized control group.[116] Also a retrospective cohort study of a group of breast cancer patients with localized, regional, or distant disease found no advantage for the combination intervention of patient and family support groups with directed relaxation, imagery, and meditation.[117]

Fawzy et al.[118] reported the survival of surgically resected stage I melanoma patients randomly assigned to either six weekly 1.5-hour sessions of group support and education versus no intervention. An analysis of overall survival of the two groups, 6 years after the surgical excision of the melanoma, showed 10 of 34 dead in the control group and 3 of 34 in the treatment group. The difference was statistically significant.

COMPLEMENTARY AND ALTERNATIVE MEDICINE CANCER RESEARCH

Many medical and surgical oncologists as well as other health care practitioners and clinical and basic science researchers have recognized the need for good quality research into CAM modalities.[25,119] However, concerns have been raised about the use of different standards of evidence.[120]

Research programs are being established to focus on alternative medicine in cancer. The Osher Center for Integrative Medicine at the University of California at San Francisco has active protocols for patients with breast cancer and prostate cancer.[121] Memorial Sloan-Kettering Cancer Center (MSKCC) has recently added an Integrative Medicine Service, and the University of Texas-Houston has had a center supported by the National Center for Complementary and Alternative Medicine. The National Center for Complementary and Alternative Medicine (NCCAM) and the NCI plan to support other centers for basic and clinical research in CAM and cancer.

NATIONAL CANCER INSTITUTE OFFICE OF CANCER COMPLEMENTARY AND ALTERNATIVE MEDICINE AND THE BEST CASE SERIES PROGRAM

In 1998, the NCI established the Office of Cancer Complementary and Alternative Medicine to focus and extend the efforts of the Institute in the arena of CAM. This office seeks to promote and support research in the various disciplines and modalities associated with the field of CAM as they relate to the diagnosis, prevention, and treatment of cancer.

Since 1991, the NCI has had a process for the evaluation of data from alternative medicine practitioners of groups of patients with cancer treated with alternative medical approaches. This process, the Best Case Series Program, provides an independent review of the medical records and primary source materials (medical imaging and pathology) and an overall assessment of the evidence for a therapeutic effect.

In 1998, the NCCAM of the National Institutes of Health in collaboration with the NCI established a Cancer Advisory Panel for Complementary and Alternative Medicine that reviews evidence about CAM modalities and advises the director of the NCCAM about promising CAM approaches that warrant further research. The NCI works closely with this new body, and Best Case Series are now presented to this panel for their review and assessment.

EXAMPLES OF COMPLEMENTARY AND ALTERNATIVE MEDICINE TOPICS REQUIRING MORE RESEARCH

Controversy exists about the consequences of women with or at high risk for breast cancer using soy products or other plants containing phytoestrogens. Herbs such as dong quai (angelica sinensis), black cohosh, and ginseng as well as foods such as soy contain phytoestrogens. These estrogens bind both physiologic forms of the estrogen receptor, and some induce signs and symptoms of exogenous estrogen administration.[122] Some of these herbs are used by cancer patients to alleviate menopausal symptoms.[123] Further research is needed to assess the risk-benefit ratio of these various products. Similarly, with the recent growth of interest and use of the androgen dihydroepiandrosterone, which is available as a dietary supplement, research is needed about its potential effect on men with or at high risk for prostate cancer.

Another controversy rages over the potential risks and benefits of the use of antioxidants during chemotherapy or radiation therapy.[124,125] With preclinical evidence on both sides of the issue, definitive clinical trials are needed. The toxicity profiles of herbs and the mechanisms of herb-drug interactions are other areas in which further research would be immediately rewarding.

PRACTICAL ISSUES IN THE INTERFACE OF ONCOLOGY AND COMPLEMENTARY AND ALTERNATIVE MEDICINE

PHYSICIAN-PATIENT COMMUNICATION

Cases have been reported of patients with potentially very curable tumors who delayed or interrupted conventional treatment to pursue unsuccessful alternative approaches and subsequently died of advanced cancer.[126–128] Therefore, the physician's relationship with his or her patient and communication with patients about CAM are of primary importance.[129] Eisenberg[130] has described an approach for the physician to take in inquiring about and exploring a patient's use of CAM.

TABLE 61-3. Reported Toxicities or Drug Interactions of Herbs Used by Cancer Patients

Herb	*Reported Toxicity*
Chaparral (creosote bush, *Larrea tridentata*)	Hepatitis and hepatic failure[151]
Licorice (*Glycyrrhiza glabra*)	Pseudohyperaldosteronism (hypertension, and hypokalemia)[152,153]
Kombucha tea	Cardiac arrest[154]
Dong quai	Drug interaction with warfarin; increased INR[155]
Skullcap[a] (*Scutellaria lateriflora*)	Hepatoxicity[156]
PC-SPES (eight herbs; see text)	Estrogenic symptoms (breast tenderness, decreased libido, thrombosis)[87]

INR, international normalized ratio.
[a]Some herbal preparations purported to contain skullcap actually contain germander (*Teucrium canadense*), a known hepatotoxin. In one report of hepatotoxicity from an herbal product originally attributed to skullcap, germander had been substituted.[157]

TABLE 61-4. Potential and Documented Dietary Supplement–Drug Interactions

Herb	*Activity*	*Source*
Arnica	Contains coumarins; potential interaction with warfarin	158
Celery	Contains coumarins; potential interaction with warfarin	158
Chamomile	Contains coumarins; potential interaction with warfarin	158
Dan-shen	Increases the peak concentration of warfarin in rats	158
Dong quai	Drug interact with warfarin; increased INR	155
Fenugreek	Contains coumarins; potential interaction with warfarin	158
Feverfew	Inhibits platelet activity	158
Garlic	Decreases platelet aggregation; undocumented reports of increased INR in patients taking warfarin	158,159
Ginger	Potent inhibitor of thromboxane synthetase	158
Gingko	Reports of spontaneous hyphema, bilateral subdural hematomas; ginkgolide B, potent inhibitor of platelet-activating factor	158
Ginseng	Has antiplatelet component; can decrease INR in patients on coumadin	158

INR, international normalized ratio.

INTERACTIONS OF ALTERNATIVE MEDICINES WITH CONVENTIONAL MEDICINES

Oncologists often are not aware of their patients' use of CAM.[17,19,24,25,27] One study found that 29% of cancer patients reported taking an herbal supplement while they were receiving chemotherapy.[19] The potential for interactions of alternative medicines and conventional medicines is real. One group has reported that a mixture of naturopathic remedies used by a 7-year-old child reduced the bioavailability of oral mercaptopurine used as maintenance therapy for acute lymphoblastic leukemia.[131] Examples of other interactions are listed in Table 61-3. There are several herbs that theoretically could interact with anticoagulants or might be contraindicated in patients with thrombocytopenia. Some of these are listed in Table 61-4.

SOURCES OF INFORMATION FOR PATIENTS, PHYSICIANS, AND RESEARCHERS

A Canadian study of cancer patients attending an outpatient pain and symptom clinic found that the top two sources of information for CAM modalities that were used were health store staff and self-help literature followed by family members, friends, and herbalists.[26] Even in a setting with more cultural acceptance of specific CAM therapies (i.e., Taiwan), the majority of the patients make their decisions about the use of alternative approaches based on information obtained by word of mouth or through advertisement rather than through consulting with a licensed practitioner in alternative medicine or a conventional health care practitioner.[15]

The Office of Technology Assessment Report of the Unconventional Cancer Treatments Panel is a valuable source of background information about many CAM modalities still in use. This report may be downloaded from the Office of Technology Assessment Web site at http://www.ota.nap.edu/pdf/1990idx.html.

The American Cancer Society has summaries of various CAM modalities on its Web site at www.cancer.org. The NCCAM has a Web site at http://nccam.nih.gov that has links to useful information about CAM research.

The NCI's Cancer Information Service has summaries about CAM modalities available through its CancerNet Web site at www.cancernet.nci.nih.gov or via mail.

The Office of Cancer Complementary and Alternative Research of the NCI has a Web site (http://www.cancer.gov/cam) with information about CAM cancer research. The Task Force on Alternative Therapeutics of the Canadian Breast Cancer Research Initiative has produced several useful reviews of CAM modalities.[132–137]

REFERENCES

1. Bannerman RHO, Burton J, Ch'en W-C. *Traditional medicine and health care coverage: a reader for health administrators and practitioners.* Geneva: World Health Organization, 1983:342.
2. Panel on Definition and Description. Defining and describing complementary and alternative medicine. CAM Research Methodology Conference, April 1995. *Altern Ther* 1997;3:49.
3. Cassileth BR. "Complementary" or "alternative"? It makes a difference in cancer care. *Complement Ther Med* 1999;7:35.
4. Schimpff SC. Complementary medicine. *Curr Opin Oncol* 1997;9:327.
5. Rasky E, Stronegger WJ, Freidl W. [Use of unconventional therapies by cancer patients.] *Soz Praventivmed* 1999;44:22.
6. Sawyer MG, Gannoni AF, Toogood IR, Antoniou G, Rice M. The use of alternative therapies by children with cancer. *Med J Aust* 1994;160:320.
7. Arkko PJ, Arkko BL, Kari-Koskinen O, Taskinen PJ. A survey of unproven cancer remedies and their users in an outpatient clinic for cancer therapy in Finland. *Soc Sci Med [Med Psychol Med Sociol]* 1980;14A:511.
8. Kaiser G, Birkmann S, Buschel G, et al. [Unconventional, alternative therapy methods in oncology.] *Internist (Berl)* 1998;39:1159.
9. Grothey A, Duppe J, Hasenburg A, Voigtmann R. [Use of alternative medicine in oncology patients.] *Dtsch Med Wochenschr* 1998;123:923.
10. Crocetti E, Crotti N, Feltrin A, et al. The use of complementary therapies by breast cancer patients attending conventional treatment. *Eur J Cancer* 1998;34:324.
11. Grootenhuis MA, Last BF, de Graaf-Nijkerk JH, van der Wel M. Use of alternative treatment in pediatric oncology. *Cancer Nurs* 1998;21:282.
12. Risberg T, Wist E, Melsom H, Kaasa S. [Use of alternative medicine among Norwegian hospitalized cancer patients.] *Tidsskr Nor Laegeforen* 1997;117:2458.

13. Risberg T, Kaasa S, Wist E, Melsom H. Why are cancer patients using non-proven complementary therapies? A cross-sectional multicentre study in Norway. *Eur J Cancer* 1997;33:575.
14. Risberg T, Lund E, Wist E, Kaasa S, Wilsgaard T. Cancer patients use of nonproven therapy: a 5-year follow-up study. *J Clin Oncol* 1998;16:6.
15. Liu JM, Chu HC, Chin YH, et al. Cross sectional study of use of alternative medicines in Chinese cancer patients. *Jpn J Clin Oncol* 1997;27:37.
16. Ernst E, Cassileth BR. The prevalence of complementary/alternative medicine in cancer: a systematic review. *Cancer* 1998;83:777.
17. Adler SR, Fosket JR. Disclosing complementary and alternative medicine use in the medical encounter: a qualitative study in women with breast cancer. *J Fam Pract* 1999;48:453.
18. Burstein HJ, Gelber S, Guadagnoli E, Weeks JC. Use of alternative medicine by women with early-stage breast cancer. *N Engl J Med* 1999;340:1733.
19. Gotay CC, Hara W, Issell BF, Maskarinec G. Use of complementary and alternative medicine in Hawaii cancer patients. *Hawaii Med J* 1999;58:94.
20. Sparber A, Bauer L, Curt G, et al. Use of complementary medicine by adult patients participating in cancer clinical trials. *Oncol Nurs Forum* (in press).
21. VandeCreek L, Rogers E, Lester J. Use of alternative therapies among breast cancer outpatients compared with the general population. *Altern Ther Health Med* 1999;5:71.
22. Lerner HJ, Regelson W. Clinical trial of hydrazine sulfate in solid tumors. *Cancer Treat Rep* 1976;60:959.
23. Goldstein J, Chao C, Valentine E, Chabon B, Davis L. Use of unproven cancer treatment by patients in a radiation oncology department: a survey. *J Psychosoc Oncol* 1991;9:59.
24. Fernandez CV, Stutzer CA, MacWilliam L, Fryer C. Alternative and complementary therapy use in pediatric oncology patients in British Columbia: prevalence and reasons for use and nonuse. *J Clin Oncol* 1998;16:1279.
25. Nam RK, Fleshner N, Rakovitch E, et al. Prevalence and patterns of the use of complementary therapies among prostate cancer patients: an epidemiological analysis. *J Urol* 1999;161:1521.
26. Oneschuk D, Fennell L, Hanson J, Bruera E. The use of complementary medications by cancer patients attending an outpatient pain and symptom clinic. *J Palliat Care* 1998;14:21.
27. Verhoef MJ, Hagen N, Pelletier G, Forsyth P. Alternative therapy use in neurologic diseases: use in brain tumor patients. *Neurology* 1999;52:617.
28. Warrick PD, Irish JC, Morningstar M, et al. Use of alternative medicine among patients with head and neck cancer. *Arch Otolaryngol Head Neck Surg* 1999;125:573.
29. Abu-Realh MH, Magwood G, Narayan MC, Rupprecht C, Suraci M. The use of complementary therapies by cancer patients. *Nurs Conn* 1996;9:3.
30. Eisenberg DM, Davis RB, Ettner SL, et al. Trends in alternative medicine use in the United States 1990–1997: results of a follow-up national survey. *JAMA* 1998;280:1569.
31. Eisenberg DM, Kessler RC, Foster C, et al. Unconventional medicine in the United States. Prevalence costs and patterns of use. *N Engl J Med* 1993;328:246.
32. Lerner IJ, Kennedy BJ. The prevalence of questionable methods of cancer treatment in the United States. *CA Cancer J Clin* 1992;42:181.
33. Montbriand MJ. An overview of alternate therapies chosen by patients with cancer. *Oncol Nurs Forum* 1994;21:1547.
34. Risberg T, Lund E, Wist E, et al. The use of non-proven therapy among patients treated in Norwegian oncological departments. A cross-sectional national multicentre study. *Eur J Cancer* 1995;31A:1785.
35. Holland JC. Why patients seek unproven cancer remedies: a psychological perspective. *CA Cancer J Clin* 1982;32:10.
36. Burzynski SR. Antineoplastons: biochemical defense against cancer. *Physiol Chem Phys* 1976;8:275.
37. Burzynski SR. Antineoplastons: history of the research. *Drugs Exp Clin Res* 1986;12(Suppl 1):1.
38. Liau MC, Szopa M, Burzynski B, Burzynski SR. Chemo-surveillance: a novel concept of the natural defence mechanism against cancer. *Drugs Exp Clin Res* 1987;13(Suppl 1):71.
39. Buckner JC, Malkin MG, Reed E, et al. Phase II study of antineoplastons A10 (NSC 648539) and AS2-1 (NSC 620261) in patients with recurrent glioma. *Mayo Clin Proc* 1999;74:137.
40. Burzynski SR, Stolzmann Z, Szopa B, Stolzmann E, Kaltenberg OP. Antineoplaston A in cancer therapy. *Physiol Chem Phys* 1977;9:485.
41. Burzynski SR, Kubove E. Initial clinical study with antineoplaston A2 injections in cancer patients with five years' follow-up. *Drugs Exp Clin Res* 1987;13(Suppl 1):1.
42. Burzynski SR, Kubove E. Phase I clinical studies of antineoplaston A3 injections. *Drugs Exp Clin Res* 1987;13(Suppl 1):17.
43. U.S. Congress Office of Technology Assessment. Pharmacologic and biologic treatments. Unconventional cancer treatments. Washington, DC: U.S. Government Printing Office; 1990; OTA-H-405, 93.
44. Tsuda H, Iemura A, Sata M, et al. Inhibitory effect of antineoplaston A10 and AS2-1 on human hepatocellular carcinoma. *Kurume Med J* 1996;43:137.
45. Chang SM, Kuhn JG, Robins HI, et al. Phase II study of phenylacetate in patients with recurrent malignant glioma: a North American Brain Tumor Consortium report *J Clin Oncol* 1999;17:984.
46. Gerson M. Dietary considerations in malignant neoplastic disease. *Rev Gastroenterol* 1945;12:419.
47. Gerson M. *A cancer therapy: results of fifty cases.* San Diego: Gerson Institute, 1990.
48. U.S. Congress Office of Technology Assessment. Dietary treatments. Unconventional cancer treatments. Washington, DC: U.S. Government Printing Office; 1990; OTA-H-405, 44.
49. Hildenbrand GL, Hildenbrand LC, Bradford K, Cavin SW. Five-year survival rates of melanoma patients treated by diet therapy after the manner of Gerson: a retrospective review. *Altern Ther Health Med* 1995;1:29.
50. Lechner P, Kronberger I. Erfahrungen mit dem Einstaz. *Aktuel Ernahrungsmed* 1990;2:72.
51. U.S. Congress Office of Technology Assessment. Dietary treatments. Unconventional cancer treatments. Washington, DC: U.S. Government Printing Office; 1990; OTA-H-405, 58.
52. Sherlock P, Rothschild EO. Scurvy produced by a Zen macrobiotic diet. *JAMA* 1967;199:794.
53. Salmon P, Rees JR, Flanagan M, O'Moore R. Hypocalcaemia in a mother and rickets in an infant associated with a Zen macrobiotic diet. *Ir J Med Sci* 1981;150:192.
54. Kushi M, Denver J, Blauer S. *Macrobiotic way: the complete macrobiotic diet & exercise book,* 2nd ed. Garden City Park, NY: Avery Publishing Group, 1993.
55. Adlercreutz H, Fotsis T, Bannwart C, et al. Determination of urinary lignans and phytoestrogen metabolites potential antiestrogens and anticarcinogens in urine of women on various habitual diets. *J Steroid Biochem* 1986;25:791.
56. Gonzalez N. *One man alone: an investigation of nutrition, cancer and William Donald Kelly* [manuscript]. New York, 1987.
57. Kelley WD. *One answer to cancer,* 2nd ed. Mineral Wells, TX: Cancer Coalition, Inc.,1997:74.
58. Gonzalez NJ, Isaacs LL. Evaluation of pancreatic proteolytic enzyme treatment of adenocarcinoma of the pancreas with nutrition and detoxification support. *Nutr Cancer* 1999;33:117.
59. Workshop on Alternative Medicine. Pharmacological and biological treatments. In: Alternative medicine: expanding medical horizons. Washington, DC: U.S. Government Printing Office, 1992:162.
60. Beliveau R, Delbecchi L, Beaulieu E, Kachra Z. AE-941: a potent inhibitor of matrix metalloproteinase. *Proc Am Assoc Cancer Res* 1999;40:458.
61. Folkman J. The vascularization of tumors. *Sci Am* 1976;234:58.
62. Lee A, Langer R. Shark cartilage contains inhibitors of tumor angiogenesis. *Science* 1983;221:1185.
63. Oikawa T, Ashino-Fuse H, Shimamura M, Koide U, Iwaguchi T. A novel angiogenic inhibitor derived from Japanese shark cartilage: I. Extraction and estimation of inhibitory activities toward tumor and embryonic angiogenesis. *Cancer Lett* 1990;51:181.
64. Evans WK, Latreille J, Batist G, et al. Neovastat (AE-941) an inhibitor of angiogenesis: rationale for development in combination with induction chemotherapy/radiotherapy in patients with non-small-cell lung cancer (NSCLC). In: *European Cancer Conference in Oncology (ECCO-10).* Vienna, Austria, 1999.
65. Lane IW. Having my say. Shark cartilage therapy: a personal history of its development. *Altern Complement Ther* 1995;1:238.
66. Miller DR, Anderson GT, Stark JJ, Granick JL, Richardson D. Phase I/II trial of the safety and efficacy of shark cartilage in the treatment of advanced cancer. *J Clin Oncol* 1998;16:3649.
67. Milner M. Follow-up of cancer patients using shark cartilage. *Altern Complement Ther* 1996;2:99.
68. Romano CF, Lipton A, Harvey HA, et al. A phase II study of Catrix-S in solid tumors. *J Biol Response Mod* 1985;4:585.
69. Prudden JF. The treatment of human cancer with agents prepared from bovine cartilage. *J Biol Response Mod* 1985;4:551.
70. Puccio C, Mittelman A, Chun H, Baskind P, Ahmed T. Treatment of metastatic renal cell carcinoma with Catrix. *Proc Am Soc Clin Oncol* 1994;14:246(abst).
71. LeMoine L. Essiac: an historical perspective. *Can Oncol Nurs J* 1997;7:216.
72. U.S. Congress Office of Technology Assessment. Herbal treatments. Unconventional cancer treatments. Washington, DC: U.S. Government Printing Office 1990; OTA-H-405, 71.
73. Initiative CBCR Essiac: an information package. Toronto: CBCRI, 1996.
74. U.S. Congress Office of Technology Assessment. Herbal treatments. Unconventional cancer treatments. Washington, DC: U.S. Government Printing Office 1990; OTA-H-405, 75.
75. Munstedt K, Kirsch K, Milch W, Sachsse S, Vahrson H. Unconventional cancer therapy—survey of patients with gynaecological malignancy. *Arch Gynecol Obstet* 1996;258:81.
76. Mannel DN, Becker H, Gundt A, Kist A, Franz H. Induction of tumor necrosis factor expression by a lectin from *Viscum album. Cancer Immunol Immunother* 1991;33:177.
77. Bocci V. Mistletoe (*Viscum album*) lectins as cytokine inducers and immunoadjuvant in tumor therapy. A review. *J Biol Regul Homeost Agents* 1993;7:1.
78. Jung ML, Baudino S, Ribereau-Gayon G, Beck JP. Characterization of cytotoxic proteins from mistletoe (*Viscum album* L.). *Cancer Lett* 1990;51:103.
79. Gutsch J, Berger H, Scholz G, Denck H. Prospektive studie beim radikal operierten Mammakarzinom mit Polychemotherapie Helixor und unbehandelter Kontrolle. *Dtsch Zeitschrift Onkol* 1988;4:94.
80. Beuth J. Clinical relevance of immunoactive mistletoe lectin-I. *Anticancer Drugs* 1997;8(Suppl 1):S53.
81. Lenartz D, Stoffel B, Menzel J, Beuth J. Immunoprotective activity of the galactoside-specific lectin from mistletoe after tumor destructive therapy in glioma patients. *Anticancer Res* 1996;16:3799.
82. Tiwari RK, Geliebter J, Garikapaty VP, et al. Anti-tumor effects of PC-SPES, an herbal formulation in prostate cancer. *Int J Oncol* 1999;14:713.
83. Chen S. Personal communication,1999.
84. Hsieh TC, Ng C, Chang CC, et al. Induction of apoptosis and down-regulation of bcl-6 in mutu I cells treated with ethanolic extracts of the Chinese herbal supplement PC- SPES. *Int J Oncol* 1998;13:1199.
85. Mittelman A, Tiawari RK, Chen S, Geliebter J. Preclinical analysis of the in vivo and in vitro effects of PC-SPES on rat prostate cancer cells. *Proc ASCO* 1999;18:82a.
86. Kameda H, Small EJ, Reese DM, et al. A phase II study of PC-SPES, an herbal compound, for the treatment of advanced prostate cancer (PCa). *Proc ASCO* 1999;18:320a.
87. DiPaola RS, Zhang H, Lambert GH, et al. Clinical and biologic activity of an estrogenic herbal combination (PC- SPES) in prostate cancer. *N Engl J Med* 1998;339:785.
88. Schmidt EW. *Hydrazine and its derivatives: preparation properties applications.* New York: John Wiley & Sons, 1984:1059.
89. Gold J. Inhibition of Walker 256 intramuscular carcinoma in rats by administration of hydrazine sulfate. *Oncology* 1971;25:66.
90. Grubbs B, Rogers W, Cameron I. Total parenteral nutrition and inhibition of gluconeogenesis on tumor-host responses. *Oncology* 1979;36:216.
91. Keller U. Pathophysiology of cancer cachexia. *Support Care Cancer* 1993;1:290.

92. Gold J. Hydrazine sulfate: a current perspective. *Nutr Cancer* 1987;9:59.
93. Filov VA, Gershanovich ML, Danova LA, Ivin BA. Experience of the treatment with Sehydrin (Hydrazine Sulfate HS) in the advanced cancer patients. *Invest New Drugs* 1995;13:89.
94. Gold J. Use of hydrazine sulfate in terminal and preterminal cancer patients: results of investigational new drug (IND) study in 84 evaluable patients. *Oncology* 1975;32:1.
95. Ochoa M Jr, Wittes RE, Krakoff IH. Trial of hydrazine sulfate (NSC-150014) in patients with cancer. *Cancer Chemother Rep* 1975;59:1151.
96. Spremulli E, Wampler GL, Regelson W. Clinical study of hydrazine sulfate in advanced cancer patients. *Cancer Chemother Pharmacol* 1979;3:121.
97. Chlebowski RT, Bulcavage L, Grosvenor M, et al. Hydrazine sulfate influence on nutritional status and survival in non-small-cell lung cancer. *J Clin Oncol* 1990;8:9.
98. Kosty MP, Fleishman SB, Herndon JE 2nd, et al. Cisplatin, vinblastine, and hydrazine sulfate in advanced non-small-cell lung cancer: a randomized placebo-controlled, double-blind phase III study of the Cancer and Leukemia Group B. *J Clin Oncol* 1994;12:1113.
99. Loprinzi CL, Goldberg RM, Su JQ, et al. Placebo-controlled trial of hydrazine sulfate in patients with newly diagnosed non-small-cell lung cancer. *J Clin Oncol* 1994;12:1126.
100. Loprinzi CL, Kuross SA, O'Fallon JR, et al. Randomized placebo-controlled evaluation of hydrazine sulfate in patients with advanced colorectal cancer. *J Clin Oncol* 1994;12:1121.
101. Hydrazine sulfate trials were accurate GAO finds. *Cancer Lett* 1995;21:5.
102. Nout MJ, Tuncel G, Brimer L. Microbial degradation of amygdalin of bitter apricot seeds (*Prunus armeniaca*). *Int J Food Microbiol* 1995;24:407.
103. Tuncel G, Nout MJ, Brimer L, Goktan D. Toxicological, nutritional and microbiological evaluation of tempe fermentation with *Rhizopus oligosporus* of bitter and sweet apricot seeds. *Int J Food Microbiol* 1990;11:337.
104. Moertel CG, Fleming TR, Rubin J, et al. A clinical trial of amygdalin (Laetrile) in the treatment of human cancer. *N Engl J Med* 1982;306:201.
105. Diamond WJ, Cowden WL, Goldberg B. *An alternative medicine definitive guide to cancer.* Tiburon, CA: Futura Medicine Publishing Inc, 1997:1116.
106. Dundee JW, Ghaly RG, Fitzpatrick KT, Abram WP, Lynch GA. Acupuncture prophylaxis of cancer chemotherapy-induced sickness. *J R Soc Med 82:* 268-71 1989.
107. NIH Consensus Conference. Acupuncture. *JAMA* 1998;280:1518.
108. Hammar M, Frisk J, Grimas O, et al. Acupuncture treatment of vasomotor symptoms in men with prostatic carcinoma: a pilot study. *J Urol* 1999;161:853.
109. Olson K, Hanson J. Using Reiki to manage pain: a preliminary report. *Cancer Prev Control* 1997;1:108.
110. Syrjala KL, Donaldson GW, Davis MW, Kippes ME, Carr JE. Relaxation and imagery and cognitive-behavioral training reduce pain during cancer treatment: a controlled clinical trial. *Pain* 1995;63:189.
111. Walker LG, Walker MB, Ogston K, et al. Psychological clinical and pathological effects of relaxation training and guided imagery during primary chemotherapy. *Br J Cancer* 1999;80:262.
112. Kolcaba K, Fox C. The effects of guided imagery on comfort of women with early stage breast cancer undergoing radiation therapy. *Oncol Nurs Forum* 1999;26:67.
113. Spiegel D. Psychological support for women with metastatic carcinoma. *Psychosomatics* 1979;20:780.
114. Spiegel D, Spira J. *Supportive-expressive group therapy: a treatment manual of psychosocial intervention for women with recurrent breast cancer.* Stanford, CA: Psychosocial Treatment Laboratory, Stanford University School of Medicine, 1991.
115. Goodwin PJ, Leszcz M, Koopmans J, et al. Randomized trial of group psychosocial support in metastatic breast cancer: the BEST study. Breast-Expressive Supportive Therapy study. *Cancer Treat Rev* 1996;22(Suppl A):91.
116. Cunningham AJ, Edmonds CV, Jenkins GP, et al. A randomized controlled trial of the effects of group psychological therapy on survival in women with metastatic breast cancer. *Psychooncology* 1998;7:508.
117. Gellert GA, Maxwell RM, Siegel BS. Survival of breast cancer patients receiving adjunctive psychosocial support therapy: a 10-year follow-up study. *J Clin Oncol* 1993;11:66.
118. Fawzy FI, Fawzy NW, Hyun CS, et al. Malignant melanoma. Effects of an early structured psychiatric intervention, coping, and affective state on recurrence and survival 6 years later. *Arch Gen Psychiatry* 1993;50:681.
119. Herbert CP, Verhoef M, White M, O'Beirne M, Doll R. Complementary therapy and cancer: decision making by patients and their physicians setting a research agenda. *Patient Educ Counsel* 1999;38:87.
120. Tannock IF, Warr DG. Unconventional therapies for cancer: a refuge from the rules of evidence? [Editorial]. *Cmaj* 1998;159:801.
121. Study begins of Chinese medicine to ease chemotherapy side effects. *The Blue Sheet,* 1998;41:9.
122. Eagan CL, Elm ES, Teepe AG, Eagan PK. Medicinal botanicals: estrogenicity in rat uterus and liver. *Proc Am Assoc Cancer Res* 1997;38:293.
123. Boyle FM. Adverse interaction of herbal medicine with breast cancer treatment [Letter]. *Med J Aust* 1997;167:286.
124. Prasad KN, Kumar A, Kochupillai V, Cole WC. High doses of multiple antioxidant vitamins: essential ingredients in improving the efficacy of standard cancer therapy. *J Am Coll Nutr* 1999;18:13.
125. Labriola D, Livingston R. Possible interactions between dietary antioxidants and chemotherapy. *Oncology (Huntingt)* 1999;13:1003.
126. Jenkins CA, Scarfe A, Bruera E. Integration of palliative care with alternative medicine in patients who have refused curative cancer therapy: a report of two cases. *J Palliat Care* 1998;14:55.
127. Mehta P. Ineffectiveness of laetrile in the treatment of acute lymphoblastic leukemia. *Clin Pediatr (Phila)* 1980;19:363.
128. Coppes MJ, Anderson RA, Egeler RM, Wolff JE. Alternative therapies for the treatment of childhood cancer [Letter]. *N Engl J Med* 1998;339:846.
129. Risberg T, Bremnes RM, Wist E, Kaasa S, Jacobsen BK. Communicating with and treating cancer patients: how does the use of non-proven therapies and patients' feeling of mental distress influence the interaction between the patient and the hospital staff?*Eur J Cancer* 1997;33:883.
130. Eisenberg DM. Advising patients who seek alternative medical therapies. *Ann Intern Med* 1997;127:61.
131. Fernandez C, Pyesmany A, Stutzer C. Alternative therapies in childhood cancer [Letter]. *N Engl J Med* 1999;340:569.
132. Kaegi E. Unconventional therapies for cancer: IV. 714-X. Task Force on Alternative Therapeutic of the Canadian Breast Cancer Research Initiative. *Cmaj* 1998;158:1621.
133. Kaegi E. Unconventional therapies for cancer: V. Vitamins A, C and E. The Task Force on Alternative Therapies of the Canadian Breast Cancer Research Initiative. *Cmaj* 1998;158:1483.
134. Kaegi E. A patient's guide to choosing unconventional therapies. *Cmaj* 1998;158:1161.
135. Kaegi E. Unconventional therapies for cancer: III. Iscador. Task Force on Alternative Therapies of the Canadian Breast Cancer Research Initiative. *Cmaj* 1998;158:1157.
136. Kaegi E. Unconventional therapies for cancer: II. Green tea. The Task Force on Alternative Therapies of the Canadian Breast Cancer Research Initiative. *Cmaj* 1998;158:1033.
137. Kaegi E. Unconventional therapies for cancer: I. Essiac. The Task Force on Alternative Therapies of the Canadian Breast Cancer Research Initiative. *Cmaj* 1998;158:897.
138. U.S. Congress Office of Technology Assessment. Pharmacologic and biologic treatments. Unconventional cancer treatments. Washington, DC: U.S. Government Printing Office; 1990; OTA-H-405, 120.
139. Hodges S, Hertz N, Lockwood K, Lister R. CoQ10: could it have a role in cancer management? *Biofactors* 1999;9:365.
140. U.S. Congress Office of Technology Assessment. Herbal treatments. Unconventional cancer treatments. Washington, DC: U.S. Government Printing Office; 1990; OTA-H-405, 70.
141. Starn JR. Energy healing with women and children. *J Obstet Gynecol Neonatal Nurs* 1998;27:576.
142. Samarel N. Therapeutic touch dialogue and women's experiences in breast cancer surgery. *Holist Nurs Pract* 1997;12:62.
143. Cohen MA. Emanuel Revici M.D.: innovator in nontoxic cancer chemotherapy 1896–1997. *J Altern Complement Med* 1998;4:140.
144. Holzman D. Green tea, mistletoe, and more: Canadians test alternative cancer therapies. *J Natl Cancer Inst* 1997;89:683.
145. U.S. Congress Office of Technology Assessment. Immunoaugmentative therapy. Unconventional cancer treatments. Washington, DC: U.S. Government Printing Office; 1990; OTA-H-405, 129.
146. Ghoneum M. Enhancement of human natural killer cell activity by modified arabinoxylane from rice bran (MGN-3). *Int J Immunother* 1998;24:89.
147. Nakazato H, Koike A, Saji S, Ogawa N, Sakamoto J. Efficacy of immunochemotherapy as adjuvant treatment after curative resection of gastric cancer. Study Group of Immunochemotherapy with PSK for Gastric Cancer. *Lancet* 1994;343:1122.
148. Ernst E. Thymus therapy for cancer? A criteria-based systematic review. *Eur J Cancer* 1997;33:531.
149. Jirillo A, Lacava J, Leone BA, Lonardi F, Bonciarelli G. Survey on the use of questionable methods of cancer treatment. GOCS. Grupo Oncologico Cooperativo del Sur Republica Argentina. *Tumori* 1996;82:215.
150. Mottonen M, Uhari M. Use of micronutrients and alternative drugs by children with acute lymphoblastic leukemia. *Med Pediatr Oncol* 1997;28:205.
151. Gordon DW, Rosenthal G, Hart J, Sirota R, Baker AL. Chaparral ingestion. The broadening spectrum of liver injury caused by herbal medications. *JAMA* 1995;273:489.
152. Stormer FC, Reistad R, Alexander J. Glycyrrhizic acid in liquorice—evaluation of health hazard. *Food Chem Toxicol* 1993;31:303.
153. Farese RV Jr, Biglieri EG, Shackleton CH, Irony I, Gomez-Fontes R. Licorice-induced hypermineralocorticoidism. *N Engl J Med* 1991;325:1223.
154. Unexpected severe illness possibly associated with consumption of Kombucha tea—Iowa 1995. *MMWR* 1995;44:892.
155. Page RL 2nd, Lawrence JD. Potentiation of warfarin by dong quai. *Pharmacotherapy* 1999;19:870.
156. MacGregor FB, Abernethy VE, Dahabra S, Cobden I, Hayes PC. Hepatotoxicity of herbal remedies. *Br Med J* 1989;299:1156.
157. De Smet PA. Health risks of herbal remedies. *Drug Saf* 1995;13:81.
158. Miller LG. Herbal medicinals: selected clinical considerations focusing on known or potential drug-herb interactions. *Arch Intern Med* 1998;158:2200.
159. Reuter HD, Koch HP, Watson LD. Therapeutic effects and applications of garlic and its preparations. In: Koch HP, ed. *Garlic: the science and therapeutic application of* Allium sativum L. *and related species,* 2nd ed. Baltimore: Williams & Wilkins, 1996, 156.
160. Spiegel D, Morrow GR, Classen C, et al. Group psychotherapy for recently diagnosed breast cancer patients: a multicenter feasibility study. *Psychooncology* 1999;8:482.

PART 4

NEWER APPROACHES IN CANCER TREATMENT

CHAPTER 62

Genetic Therapy

SECTION 1 Gene Therapy

PATRICK HWU

Gene therapy can be defined as the introduction of new genetic material into cells for therapeutic intent. This encompasses a broad array of experimental cancer therapies, including immunization with cytokine or tumor antigen genes as well as the introduction of toxic genes directly into tumors (Table 62.1-1). Since the first gene transfer trial in 1989, a large number of cancer gene therapy clinical trials have been initiated (Table 62.1-2). Results of the first clinical trials have been published, and they highlight not only the potential promise of gene therapy but also the current limitations and areas where further efforts are needed. For example, because cancer is the result of mutation or loss of genetic material within cells, perhaps the most obvious approach to cancer gene therapy is the introduction of genes to correct these aberrations. Restoration of the normal p53 gene in human tumor cells deficient of this gene because of gene loss or mutation causes decreased tumorigenicity in nude mice.[1] However, current clinical efforts to apply this concept have been limited by the absence of technology that would allow efficient *in vivo* gene transfer into tumors. As vector technology improves, these approaches may become more feasible.

Many gene therapy protocols have used *ex vivo* gene transfer. This technique involves the removal of cells from an individual followed by gene transfer and growth in the laboratory before reinfusion into the patient.

Two requirements exist for successful genetic manipulation of a eukaryotic cell. First, a method must exist to provide successful gene insertion into the correct cell type with adequate efficiency for a particular therapeutic purpose. Some therapeutic approaches may require permanent gene transfer, whereas for others, transient activity may suffice. Second, the inserted gene must be adequately expressed by that cell. A high level of expression is required for some purposes, whereas a low level of gene expression is sufficient for others. Constitutive or regulated expression may be necessary, depending on the specific application.

METHODS OF GENE TRANSFER

Numerous techniques are available for gene transfer into mammalian cells (Table 62.1-3). The choice of a particular gene transfer technique depends on the biologic requirements of the specific therapeutic strategy. For example, to protect hematopoietic stem cells from the toxic effects of systemic chemotherapy, often given for several cycles, the multidrug resistance (MDR) gene must be stably integrated into stem cells, using gene transfer techniques that include retroviral vectors. However, to immunize patients against tumors, it is possible that only transient expression of antigen genes by viral vectors such as adenovirus will be sufficient.

Many techniques of gene transfer make use of viruses to introduce genetic material, because viruses in most cases can deliver genes to cells with higher efficiencies compared to nonviral methods.

RETROVIRAL VECTORS

Retroviruses are RNA viruses that are capable of stably integrating DNA within the host cell genome. The replication cycle of a retrovirus begins with viral attachment to a cell by a

TABLE 62.1-1. Cancer Gene Therapy Approaches

Strategies	*Examples of Potential Experimental Approaches*
Genetic modification of the immune response	
Active immunization	
Modification of tumor cells with genes that enhance tumor immunogenicity	Patient immunization with tumor cells modified by the introduction of cytokine genes (e.g., IL-2 or GM-CSF) or costimulatory molecules (e.g., B7-1). Gene transfer into tumor cells can be performed in the laboratory (*ex vivo*) or directly into the patient (*in vivo*).
Immunization with genes encoding tumor antigens	Patient immunization with genes encoding melanoma antigens recognized by T cells, such as MART-1. Immunization can be accomplished by direct injection of DNA or by injection of viral vectors encoding tumor antigens, such as vaccinia, fowlpox, or adenoviral or retroviral vectors. Immunization can be performed directly *in vivo* or by transduction of antigen-presenting cells (e.g., dendritic cells) with tumor antigen genes, followed by administration to the patient.
Genetic modification of immune effector cells	
Enhance survival of immune cells	Transduction of tumor-specific lymphocytes with the IL-2 gene to enhance their survival *in vivo.*
Increase tumor recognition	Use of novel receptor genes to allow lymphocytes to recognize new targets on tumor cells.
Increase antitumor efficacy of immune cells	Retroviral transduction of tumor infiltrating lymphocytes with the TNF gene in an attempt to deliver large quantities of TNF to the tumor site.
Decrease toxicity of effector cells	Treatment of BMT patients with donor T cells containing suicide gene to eliminate the cells before the development of graft-versus-host disease.
Modification of tumors with genes that have direct antitumor effects	
Tumor suppressor genes	Replace mutated or absent tumor suppressor genes to decrease tumor growth.
Antisense and ribozymes	Decrease expression of products of activated oncogenes.
Suicide genes	Kill tumor cells by introduction of genes that produce toxic products. Tumor-specific promoters or tumor-specific delivery can be used to decrease systemic toxicity.
Selective replication of virus in tumor	Use of E1B-defective adenovirus capable of replicating only in tumors lacking functional p53.
Introduction of genes into hematopoietic stem cells to decrease toxicity from chemotherapy	Transduce bone marrow cells with multidrug resistance gene to decrease hematopoietic toxicity from subsequent chemotherapy.
Antiangiogenic gene therapy	Express genes that have antiangiogenic properties or inhibit proangiogenic cytokines.

BMT, bone marrow transplantation; GM-CSF, granulocyte-macrophage colony-stimulating factor; IL-2, interleukin-2; TNF, tumor necrosis factor.

specific receptor (Fig. 62.1-1). The virus enters the cell, and the viral RNA is reverse transcribed to DNA by the virally encoded reverse transcriptase. The viral DNA is then transported to the nucleus, where it integrates into the host cell genome. The integrated viral DNA, termed the *provirus,* is transcribed, and then both spliced and unspliced transcripts are translated to form the viral proteins. Some of the unspliced transcripts are packaged, via a packaging signal sequence (ψ), into viral capsids. The mature viruses then bud from the host cell membrane.

Retroviral vectors for gene transfer have been constructed by substituting the gene of interest in place of the viral protein coding regions,[2,3] thus making these vectors replication incompetent (Fig. 62.1-2). These vectors are packaged into retroviral particles using helper, or packaging, cell lines that contain the structural viral protein genes in *trans* (i.e., from another site in the packaging cell genome). Because the retroviral vector contains the ψ sequences, it is packaged into the mature virus and is capable of infecting target cells, but it is incapable of replication because of the absence of the retroviral protein coding regions. The viral structural genes, provided in *trans*, are not packaged because of the absence of the ψ sequences (Fig. 62.1-3).

Retroviral vectors are one of the most common methods of gene transfer in currently approved gene therapy protocols. Their advantages include the ability to stably integrate into the host genome and the absence of viral protein expression. Current disadvantages of retroviral vectors include low titers, resulting in low levels of gene transfer efficiency, although new methods have been described to concentrate retroviral supernatants using ultracentrifugation.[4]

Retroviral packaging cells can use a variety of envelope genes from other viruses. Because the envelope protein is the primary determinant of the host range of the retrovirus, the particular envelope, or pseudotype, used can have a profound impact on transduction efficiencies.[5] Table 62.1-4 lists a num-

TABLE 62.1-2. Cancer Gene Therapy Clinical Trials Approved by the National Institutes of Health Recombinant Advisory Committee[a]

Approach	*Number of Trials* *In Vitro* Gene Transfer	*In Vivo* Gene Transfer	*Gene Transfer Method Used*	*Types of Cancers*	*Genes*
Immunotherapy approaches					
Tumor/fibroblast transduction to enhance tumor immunogenicity	50	41	Retrovirus, canarypox, liposomes, adenovirus, plasmid DNA, electroporation	Melanoma, renal, colon, breast, neuroblastoma, small cell, glioblastoma, lymphoma, head and neck, prostate, ovarian, sarcoma, NSCLC, angioendothelioma	GM-CSF, TNF-α, IL-2, HLA-B7, B7-1 (CD80), IL-4, IFN-γ, IL-12, IL-7, TGF-β antisense, CD40L, IFN-α, IFN-β
T cell/donor lymphocyte transduction	12	—	Retrovirus, electroporation	Melanoma, myeloma, ovarian, colon, CML, ALL, AML	TNF-α, HSV-TK, MOv-γ, CC49-ζ, αCEA-ζ, αCD20-ζ
Recombinant vaccines	5	27	DNA, adenovirus, canarypox, vaccinia, fowlpox, RNA/DC, adeno/DC, DNA/particle mediated	Melanoma, colorectal/GI/CEA+, breast, lung, prostate, non-Hodgkin's lymphoma, NSCLC, cervical	MART-1, GP100, GP100/GM-CSF, PSA, CEA, idiotypic DNA vaccine, MUC-1, MUC-1/IL-2, E6/E7, tyrosinase
Approaches that may result in direct antitumor effects					
Antisense	1	4	Retrovirus, liposomes	NSCLC, glioblastoma, breast, prostate, head and neck	Antisense to k-ras, c-fos, c-myc, IGF, EGFR
Tumor suppressor/oncogene regulation	—	29	Adenovirus, retrovirus, liposomes	NSCLC, colon, ovarian, head and neck, bladder, hepatocellular, HER-2+ tumors, breast, prostate, glioma	p53, retinoblastoma, BRCA-1, p16, E1A
Suicide gene	1	31	Retrovirus, adenovirus (replication defective and E1B-attenuated replication competent)	Brain tumors (glioblastoma, astrocytoma), leptomeningeal, mesothelioma, prostate, head and neck, ovarian, colorectal, liver metastases, NSCLC, melanoma, retinoblastoma	HSV-TK, cytosine deaminase
Chemoprotection approaches	10	—	Retrovirus	Ovarian, brain, breast, testicular, solid tumors, neuroblastoma, sarcoma	MDR-1, methylguanine DNA methyltransferase (mutant MGMT), DHFR
Other approaches	—	5	Adenovirus, HSV, replication-competent adenovirus (with PSA promoter elements)	Ovarian, glioblastoma, prostate	αerbB2 single-chain antibody

ALL, acute lymphoblastic leukemia; AML, acute myeloid leukemia; CEA, carcinoembryonic antigen; CML, chronic myeloid leukemia; DC, dendritic cell; DHFR, dihydrofolate reductase; EGFR, epidermal growth factor receptor; GI, gastrointestinal; GM-CSF, granulocyte-macrophage colony-stimulating factor; HSV-TK, herpes simplex virus/thymidine kinase; IFN, interferon; IGF, insulin-like growth factor; IL, interleukin; MDR-1, multidrug resistance-1; NSCLC, non–small cell lung carcinoma; PSA, prostate-specific antigen; TGF-β, transforming growth factor-β; TNF-α, tumor necrosis factor-α.
[a]Data as of November 19, 1999.

ber of envelope genes along with their relative host ranges. The development of packaging cell lines that use alternative envelope genes has resulted in significant advances in the ability to transduce primary lymphocytes. Retroviral vectors produced from the PG13 packaging cell line,[6] which uses the gibbon ape leukemia virus envelope (GALV), are capable of transducing B cells[7] and T cells[8] with significantly higher efficiencies compared with those derived from amphotropic packaging cell lines. In one study, transduction of primary T cells was 4- to 18-fold higher with PG13-packaged vectors compared with amphotropic PA317-packaged vectors.[8] This was found to correlate with an 8- to 19-fold higher expression of

TABLE 62.1-3. A Comparison of Gene Transfer Methods

	Gene Transfer Method						
Profile	Retrovirus[a]	Lentivirus	Adenovirus	Adenoassociated Virus	Vaccinia	Fowlpox	Nonviral
Efficiency of gene transfer	Moderate	Moderate	High	Moderate	High	High	Low
Stable versus transient	Stable	Stable	Transient	Stable	Transient	Transient	Transient
Gene expression	Variable[b]	Variable[b]	Variable[b]	Variable[b]	High	High	Variable[b]
Immunogenicity[c]	Low	Low	Moderate	Low	High	High	Low
In vitro toxicity	Low	Low	Low	Low	High	Low	Low
Titer	Low[d]	Low[d]	High	See comments	High	High	N/A
Comments	Requires replicating cells	Stable gene transfer to nondividing cells	New vector design should lead to decreased immunogenicity	High-titer preparations difficult to produce; production requires replication-competent adenovirus	Most infected cells die within 24 hours; replication competent	—	Easy to produce clinical-grade material; fewer safety issues compared with viral methods

N/A, not applicable.
[a]Murine leukemia virus–based vectors.
[b]Gene expression depends on specific promoter and cell type.
[c]Immunogenicity from expression of normal viral proteins.
[d]Can be concentrated to high titer with ultracentrifugation.

the GALV receptor (Pit-1) compared with the amphotropic receptor (Pit-2) in primary T cells, although other factors besides receptor expression have been found to play a role in transduction efficiency.[9] By combining the use of PG13-packaged vectors with a 1-hour centrifugation at 1000 *g*, Bunnell et al.[10] were able to obtain transduction efficiencies of primary T cells in the 40% range.

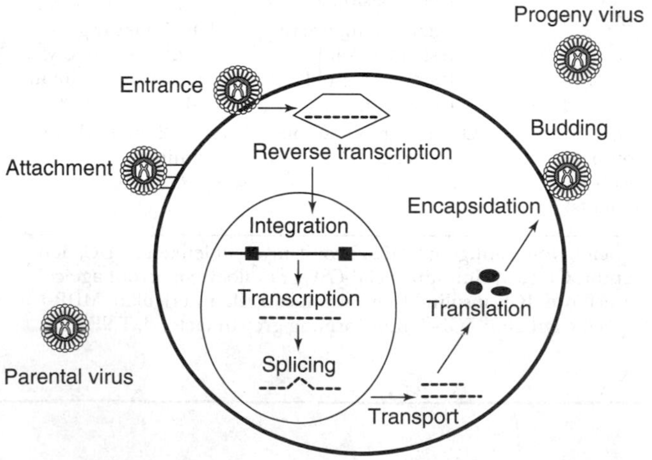

FIGURE 62.1-1. Retrovirus replication cycle. The retrovirus uses envelope glycoproteins to bind to specific receptors on the cell surface. Viral RNA then enters the cell and is reverse transcribed to DNA. The viral DNA is transported to the nucleus, where it integrates in the host chromosome and directs transcription of the provirus using the viral long terminal repeat. Viral transcripts are translated by the infected cell to form viral structural proteins. Some of the unspliced viral transcripts are packaged into the newly formed viral particles and are released by budding. (From ref. 243, with permission.)

The vesicular stomatitis virus (VSV) G glycoprotein can also be used to pseudotype retroviral vectors.[11] Unlike other envelope proteins, the VSV-G protein confers enhanced physical stability to retroviral particles, allowing concentration with ultracentrifugation to titers of 10^9 or higher. VSV-G pseudotyped retroviral vectors have a wide host range and have been used successfully to transduce primary T cells.[12,13]

In addition, future retroviral vectors may contain improved promoters for higher and regulatable levels of gene expression.

LENTIVIRAL VECTORS

Stable gene transfer using vectors based on murine retroviruses is only possible in dividing cells. Human immunodeficiency virus (HIV) can infect and integrate into the genome of nonproliferating cells because of proteins that mediate the active transport of the lentiviral preintegration complex through the nucleopore. These proteins—integrase, matrix, and *vpr*—interact with the nuclear import machinery to transport the HIV preintegration complex from the cytoplasm to the nucleus.

Naldini et al.[14] designed lentiviral vectors based on HIV that are capable of stably infecting nondividing cells. A packaging

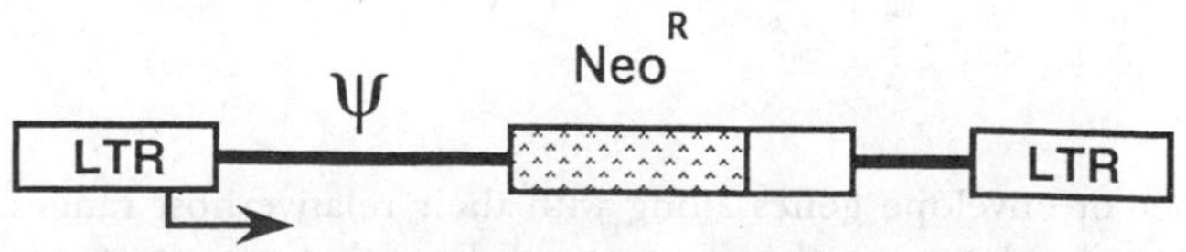

FIGURE 62.1-2. Schematic diagram of the LNL6 retroviral vector. The protein-coding regions of the virus have been removed and replaced with the gene for neomycin resistance (Neo[R]). The viral packaging site (ψ) has been left intact. The vector is a derivative of the Moloney murine leukemia virus.[244,245] LTR, long terminal repeats.

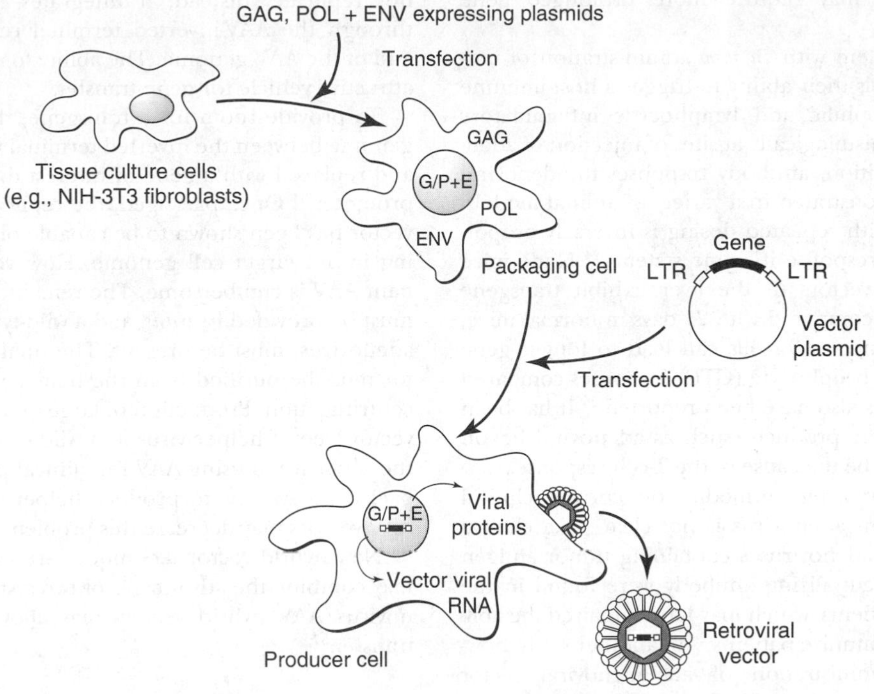

FIGURE 62.1-3. Production of retroviral vectors with packaging cells. The gene of interest is cloned into a retroviral vector (see Fig. 62.1-2), and then transfected into a helper cell line, which provides the retroviral structural genes in *trans*. The retroviral structural genes cannot be packaged because of the absence of a packaging sequence (ψ), whereas the retroviral vector can be packaged, thereby producing a replication-incompetent retrovirus. LTR, long terminal repeats. (From ref. 246, with permission.)

construct was used to express HIV proteins in *trans*. To avoid production of wild-type HIV, the construct is defective for the production of viral envelope and the accessory protein Vpu, and has deletions in the 5' signal sequence. To make defective lentiviral vectors, packaging cells are transiently transfected with the packaging construct, along with a separate plasmid encoding a heterologous envelope protein, such as VSV-G protein. A third plasmid, the transfer vector, encodes the gene of interest, along with the packaging signal and other *cis*-acting sequences of HIV required for packaging, reverse transcription, and integration.[14] Lentiviral vectors are currently being refined to enhance safety, transduction efficiency, and convenience.[15] HIV-based lentiviral vectors have been shown to be efficient vehicles of gene transfer into postmitotic cells, including brain, liver, muscle, CD34+ hematopoietic cells, and retina.[14,16–20] Current efforts are focused on the use of lentiviral vectors in the transduction of hematopoietic stem cells in an attempt to enhance long-term engraftment of gene-modified cells.[17,19]

TABLE 62.1-4. Envelopes Used for Retroviral Vectors

Envelope Source	*Host Range*
Ecotropic	Mouse, rat
Amphotropic	Human, mouse, rat, rabbit, cat, dog, monkey
Gibbon ape leukemia virus	Human, rat, rabbit, cat, dog, monkey (not mouse)
Vesicular stomatitis virus G protein	All

ADENOVIRAL VECTORS

The adenoviral genome is divided into four early gene regions, E1 to E4, which are expressed before viral DNA replication, and late genes, which primarily encode viral structural proteins. On infection, the E1 gene products are expressed first and are responsible for transcriptionally activating other genes that begin a cascade of events ultimately leading to viral replication. Removing the E1 region therefore results in an adenoviral particle that is replication deficient. These replication-deficient adenoviruses can be used for gene transfer by cloning the gene of interest into the deleted E1 region.[21] The recombinant adenovirus, however, must be produced using cell lines that provide the E1 products in *trans*, such as in 293 cells, which constitutively express Ad5 E1 genes.

Adenoviral gene transfer can be performed in many cells, both dividing and nondividing, with high efficiency, and it can result in high levels of gene expression. In addition, adenoviral vectors can be produced at high titers and are capable of infecting some tissues directly *in vivo*, such as pulmonary epithelial cells.[22] However, because adenoviral DNA exists episomally, with little or no incorporation into the host cell genome, expression of the transgene is transient, and it is lost as the infected cell divides. For some therapeutic strategies, this high-level transient expression may be adequate, whereas other treatment approaches may require more prolonged gene expression.

One potential problem with *in vivo* administration of current adenoviral vectors is their ability to trigger a host immune response. Both neutrophilic and lymphocytic inflammatory infiltrates can be seen histologically at sites of injection of adenoviral vectors.[23] In addition, antibody responses to adenoviral vectors have been demonstrated in a variety of animal models, and gene expression with repeated dosing is inversely proportional to the antibody response in some systems.[24] Nude mice expressing adenoviral vectors in the liver exhibit transgene expression for 60 days, compared with 21 days in normal mice, implying that the absence of T cells can lead to longer gene expression. Cytotoxic T lymphocyte (CTL) responses compared with adenoviral proteins also have been reported.[25] It has been postulated that late gene products, such as adenoviral hexon and fiber proteins, may be the cause of the T-cell response.

The effect of neutralizing antibodies on current clinical efforts with recombinant adenovirus is not clear. In a clinical trial with recombinant adenoviruses containing tumor antigen genes, high levels of neutralizing antibody were found in the pretreatment sera of patients, which may have impaired the ability of these viruses to immunize patients.[26] In another study, however, intratumoral administration of an adenoviral vector expressing β–galactosidase resulted in β-galactosidase–specific T helper, CTL, and antibody responses in three of four patients.[27]

New generations of adenoviral vectors are attempting to limit the antiviral immune response by eliminating much of the adenoviral genome. Besides reducing immunogenicity, this also allows an increased gene carrying capacity by the adenoviral vector. Packaging of these "gutless" adenoviral vectors requires helper virus or the expression of additional adenoviral genes by the helper cell lines. In addition, adenoviral vectors are being developed that may allow targeted, regulable gene expression.

Burcin and colleagues[28] have reported the construction of a recombinant adenovirus containing a tissue-specific, regulable target gene. The recombinant adenoviral vector lacked all viral coding sequences to avoid immunogenicity, and it contained a transgene that could be induced *in vivo* with the antiprogestin mifepristone. Tissue specificity was conferred by coupling the regulator cassette to the liver-specific transthyretin promoter region.[28] Inducible expression of the transgene was demonstrated *in vivo*, but the tissue specificity was not confirmed.

In an effort to confer targeting ability to adenoviral vectors, surface modification of the Ad fiber coat protein[29–31] or use of adenoviral/antibody complexes[32,33] has been attempted. Much work in vector development remains to be done for adenoviral vectors to be fully utilized in effective gene therapy strategies.

ADENOASSOCIATED VIRUS VECTORS

Adenoassociated virus (AAV), a member of the parvovirus family, can only replicate in the presence of a helper virus, such as adenovirus. The virus is nonenveloped and consists of a single-stranded linear DNA of 4.7 kilobases, which contains two major open reading frames. The left-hand open reading frame encodes the Rep proteins, which are responsible for AAV replication. The right-hand open reading frame encodes the Cap proteins, which form the structural proteins of the viral capsid. In the absence of a helper virus, such as adenovirus, AAV cannot replicate; instead, it integrates into the host genome through the AAV-inverted terminal repeats present on each end of the AAV genome. The ability to integrate makes AAV an attractive vehicle for gene transfer.

To provide room for a transgene, the majority of the AAV genome between the inverted terminal repeats can be removed and replaced with a gene of interest driven by an appropriate promoter.[34] Once packaged, the replication-incompetent AAV vector has been shown to be capable of infecting and integrating into a target cell genome. However, producing recombinant AAV is cumbersome. The remainder of the AAV genome must be provided in *trans*, and a wild-type helper virus, such as adenovirus, must be present. The final recombinant AAV vector must be purified from the helper virus by heat or density centrifugation. Production of large quantities of high-titer AAV vector free of helper virus and wild-type AAV has been one of the obstacles to using AAV for clinical purposes. However, new packaging systems to produce helper virus–free recombinant AAV vectors may decrease this problem.[35,36]

New hybrid vector techniques are under development that may combine the advantages of two systems. For example, adenovirus/AAV hybrid vectors may allow efficient, stable gene transfer.[37,38]

POX VECTORS

The poxviruses are a family of DNA viruses characterized by a large enveloped virion containing enzymes for messenger RNA (mRNA) synthesis, a genome composed of a single, linear, double-stranded DNA molecule of 130 to 300 kilobases, and the ability to replicate within the cytoplasm of the infected cell. The poxvirus genome encodes 150 to 200 genes, which can be divided into early and late genes. Early genes are expressed before viral DNA replication, and late genes are expressed after DNA replication.

Several properties of poxviruses make them attractive vectors for the introduction of foreign genes.[39–42] Because of the large size of the poxvirus genome, large amounts of foreign DNA can be incorporated without adversely effecting viral infectivity. Several silent or nonessential regions of the genome have been identified for the insertion of foreign DNA by homologous recombination. Plasmids that provide viral promoters and regions to facilitate homologous recombination into nonessential sites, such as the viral thymidine kinase (TK) region, have been constructed to produce recombinant vaccinia vectors. Multiple genes each can be inserted at a different site in the virus. Screening methods have been designed to isolate and expand recombinant clones containing the genes of interest.

A primary advantage of recombinant poxviruses is the large amount of gene expression that is possible because of the use of vaccinia transcription factors. Because gene expression is entirely cytoplasmic and does not rely on host-cell transcriptional machinery, it is not dependent on potential regulatory mechanisms of the host cell, and hence, large quantities of gene expression have been observed in a wide variety of cell types.

Disadvantages of poxviruses are the transient nature of gene expression and the cell lysis that results after infection. Some attenuated vaccinia strains[40] have been developed that result in delayed lysis of infected human target cells. Avipox viruses, such as fowlpox or canarypox, or swinepox viruses can infect human cells, but they do not result in cell lysis.[43] Another problem with recombinant poxviruses is that up to 200 viral gene products are expressed, many of which may be immunogenic or may adversely interact with the target cell or the gene product of interest.

NONVIRAL METHODS OF GENE TRANSFER

Cationic lipids, complexed to DNA, have been developed that are capable of mediating high gene transfer efficiencies *in vitro* for some cell types. Cationic lipids,[44] such as DOTMA (1,2-dioleyloxypropyl-3-trimethyl ammonium bromide), the prototype cationic lipid, along with a neutral lipid, such as DOPE (dioleoylphosphatidyletanolamine), can be complexed with DNA and added to cultured cells. New formulations of lipids are currently under development that may allow improved *in vitro* gene transfer as well as *in vivo* administration. Cationic lipid formulations have already been used to deliver genes to the lung *in vivo*,[45] as well as intratumorally.[46–48] Most recently, DNA-gelatin nanospheres have been used to allow the slow release of DNA *in vivo*. In a murine model, intramuscular injection of nanospheres containing the β-galactosidase marker gene led to higher expression levels than injection with naked DNA or DNA/lipid complexes.[49]

Physical methods of gene transfer include the "gene gun,"[50] which propels gold beads coated with DNA into cells. Although this method results in low transfection efficiencies, gene transfer to epithelial cells can be performed *in vivo*, giving it a potential role in immunization strategies.

The direct *in vivo* injection of DNA alone into selected tissues, such as muscle[51] and thyroid,[52] can result in gene transfer. This approach, termed *naked DNA*, has been used primarily for studies attempting to immunize against the products of the encoded genes.

Nonviral methods of gene delivery are more convenient and have obvious safety advantages over viral methods. However, the majority of current nonviral gene transfer methods result in transient gene expression, and the efficiency of gene transfer is lower compared with most viral methods.

GENE MARKING STUDIES

The first gene transfer study in humans in 1989 was designed to assess the safety and feasibility of gene transfer in humans, using a marker gene, neomycin phosphotransferase (Neo^R), an enzyme that inactivates neomycin and neomycin analogues.[53,54]

Subsequent goals of gene marking studies were to understand the biology of cancer and cancer treatments. For example, because a unique, foreign gene was introduced into cells, the fate of these cells could be followed *in vivo*. Adoptively transferred T cells could be followed for their survival *in vivo*, and patients receiving autologous bone marrow transplantations transduced with marker genes could be followed to see whether subsequent recurrences were in part due to viable tumor cells that were present in the transferred bone marrow.

T-CELL MARKING STUDIES

The first gene transfer study in humans was performed in 1989 in the Surgery Branch of the National Cancer Institute.[54] Tumor infiltrating lymphocytes (TILs) were genetically modified with a marker gene encoding Neo^R. The goals of the study were to evaluate the safety and feasibility of using gene-modified cells in humans. In addition, because a unique, foreign gene was placed into the TIL, survival and distribution studies of the infused cells could be done using polymerase chain reaction (PCR) assays on DNA from peripheral blood lymphocytes and tumor biopsies.

Because this was the first study of its kind, safety issues pertaining to the patients and the public were a major concern by regulatory agencies, such as the Recombinant DNA Advisory Committee (RAC). Consequently, many safety studies were required before approval of this and subsequent clinical trials. Ultimately, ten patients were treated, and no safety or toxicity problems were associated with the gene transfer. Using PCR analysis, TILs were found in tumor biopsies up to 64 days and in peripheral blood up to 189 days after infusion[54,55] (Fig. 62.1-4). Since this initial study, more than 300 human gene transfer and therapy studies have been approved by the RAC, and research in this field throughout the world has expanded tremendously.

T-cell marking studies have been performed using melanoma TILs,[56,57] renal TILs,[58] bone marrow stem cells,[59] and anti-HIV CTLs.[60] Using gene-marked Epstein-Barr virus (EBV)–specific CTLs in immunocompromised patients, Heslop et al.[61] found that EBV precursors could proliferate in response to *in vivo* or *ex vivo* viral challenge for as long as 18 months (Fig. 62.1-5).

Researchers at the University of Washington in Seattle have used Neo-marked, HIV-1, Gag-specific CD8+ CTL clones to treat HIV-infected individuals.[62] Using PCR amplification for the neo gene followed by *in situ* hybridization with fluorescein-labeled neo-specific oligonucleotides, the percentage of circulating transduced cells could be quantitated by flow cytometry. One day after cell infusion, 2.0% to 3.5% of CD8+ cells circulating in the periphery were neo-positive. The frequency of neo-modified CTL was found to correlate inversely with the percentage of HIV-infected cells in the peripheral blood after cell infusion. In addition, neo-positive CTLs were found to accumulate in lymph node biopsies obtained 4 days after cell infusion (2.2% to 7.9%), compared with the concurrent percentages of neo-positive CTLs circulating in the periphery (0.5% to 0.7%). Interestingly, neo-positive CTL aggregates were found in the parafollicular regions of the lymph node near cells that were productively infected with HIV. This finding illustrates the utility of cell marking to determine not only the overall traffic and survival of infused cells, but also their microanatomic localization.

HEMATOPOIETIC STEM CELL MARKING STUDIES

The ability to label stem cells with unique, integrated DNA sequences has enabled investigators to track stem cells and their differentiated progeny,[63] allowing such studies as, for example, the comparison of bone marrow stem cells with peripheral blood stem cells for their ability to reconstitute the host. In addition, because microscopic tumor deposits present within the marrow also are marked by retroviral vectors, attempts have been made to assess the source of disease recurrence after autologous bone marrow transplantation therapy in patients with acute myeloid leukemia and neuroblastoma. In one study, bone marrow was harvested during complete

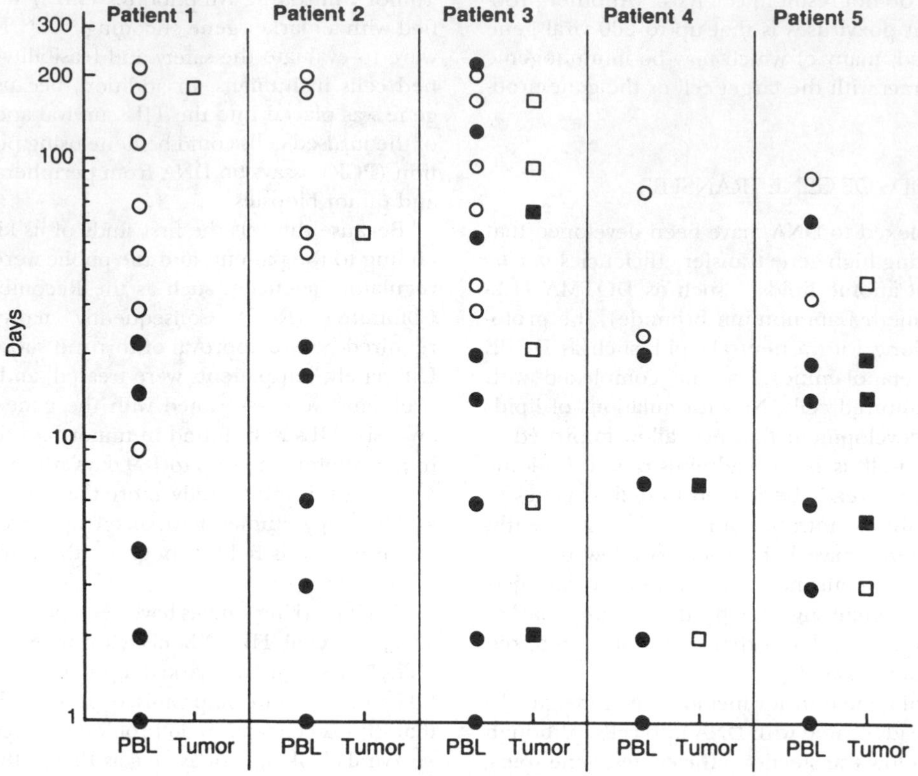

FIGURE 62.1-4. Results of polymerase chain reaction assays of peripheral blood lymphocytes (PBL, *circles*) and tumor-biopsy specimens (*squares*) obtained from patients at various intervals after the infusion of gene-transduced tumor-infiltrating lymphocytes. *Open symbols* denote negative results, and *solid symbols* indicate positive results. All results were corroborated in at least two separate Southern blot assays. The assays were performed and assessed in a blinded fashion. (From ref. 54, with permission.)

remission and retrovirally transduced with the Neo^R gene before reinfusion. Three of 12 acute myeloid leukemia patients have relapsed, and in two of these patients, tumor cells from the relapse contained the Neo^R gene. Of nine neuroblastoma patients studied, three have relapsed, and in all three cases, the Neo^R gene was found in the recurrent tumor cells.[63–66] Analysis of neuroblastoma DNA for discrete integration sites revealed that at least 200 malignant cells were introduced with the autologous marrow transplantation and contributed to the relapse.[66]

In a similar study using Neo^R transduced autologous CD34 cells in chronic myelogenous leukemia (CML) patients, two relapsing patients were studied, and both had leukemic cells that were positive for the Neo^R gene.[67] Thus, it is clear that remission marrow can contribute to disease relapse.

Using similar techniques, a variety of bone marrow purging regimens can be evaluated within the same patient to assess their success in eliminating tumor cells from the marrow.[68] This evaluation allows recurrent tumor cells to be analyzed genetically to determine if they had previously been exposed to a particular purging regimen.

Finally, gene transfer itself is being investigated as a purging technique, using antisense oligodeoxynucleotides against activated oncogenes as a means to eliminate tumor cells within the autologous marrow.[69–73]

GENETIC MODIFICATION OF THE IMMUNE RESPONSE

Several approaches have been proposed for cancer gene therapy (see Table 62.1-1). One strategy that has been pursued is an attempt to enhance the immune response against cancer using gene transfer techniques.

ACTIVE IMMUNIZATION

Much has been learned concerning the nature of the T-cell response to human cancers. Tumor antigens recognized by T cells have been cloned from melanoma cells.[74–81] These antigens have been shown to be nonmutated melanocyte differentiation antigens, nonmutated proteins expressed only in selected tissues such as testes, or mutated intracellular proteins. Despite the expression of known antigens on tumor cells, however, these tumors grow in their hosts, seemingly unopposed by any antitumor immune response. This lack of an adequate immune response could be due to a number of reasons, including deficient tumor antigen processing and presentation, lack of immune costimulation, production of inhibitory factors by the tumor cell, and insufficient helper activity from CD4 cells. In an attempt to bypass these potential deficiencies and stimulate a stronger antitumor response in the host, tumor

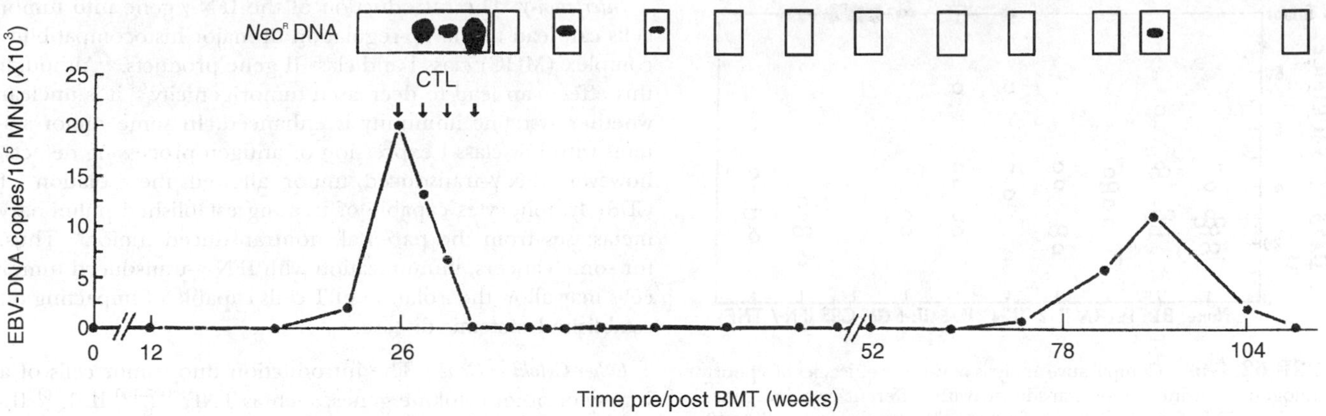

FIGURE 62.1-5. Recruitment of gene-marked, Epstein-Barr virus (*EBV*)-specific cytotoxic T lymphocyte (*CTL*) by antigenic stimulation *in vivo.* DNA was obtained from peripheral blood mononuclear cells (*MNC*) of a patient between 0 and 108 weeks after bone marrow transplantation (*BMT*), and it was divided into two portions. One was analyzed by polymerase chain reaction amplification using EBV-specific primers, whereas the second was amplified using neo-specific primers. The figure shows the relationship between levels of EBV-DNA and the presence of neomycin resistance (Neo[R])–marked, EBV-specific T cells. (From ref. 61, with permission.)

cells have been genetically modified with a variety of cytokine genes and costimulatory molecules, and these modified tumor cells have been used as antitumor vaccines.

Modification of Tumor Cells with Genes That Enhance Tumor Immunogenicity

CYTOKINE GENES. In contrast to the systemic administration of cytokines, which results in low concentrations *in vivo*, the introduction of genes encoding cytokines into tumor cells can result in the production of very high levels of cytokines in the tumor microenvironment. This approach is designed to more accurately mimic the paracrine nature by which cytokines normally interact to regulate immune responses. Tumors have been transduced with a variety of genes in an attempt to enhance immunogenicity.

Interleukin-2. In several murine models, tumors expressing the gene for interleukin-2 (IL-2) regress after an initial period of growth, leading to long-lasting protection from subsequent rechallenge.[82,83] In some cases, the immune response was shown to be dependent on CD8, but not CD4. This suggests that the IL-2 released by the tumor cells was bypassing the need for help from CD4 cells. In many studies, however, it was not clear whether systemic immunity was enhanced to levels greater than that which could be achieved using irradiated, nonmodified tumor cells.

In another study,[84] intraperitoneal, irradiated, IL-2–transduced murine bladder cancer cells were capable of treating 7-day parental tumors established by orthotopic implantation of tumor cells into the bladder wall. Irradiated nontransfected cells showed no antitumor response in these experiments.

Forty-five patients with renal cell cancer, melanoma, and sarcoma were treated with intratumoral injections of a DNA plasmid encoding human IL-2 complexed to the cationic lipids DMRIE/DOPE in a phase I/II study. Partial responses in uninjected tumors were observed in 2 of 14 patients with renal cell cancer and 1 of 16 patients with melanoma. On immunohistochemical evaluation of pre- and posttreatment biopsy specimens of injected tumors, an increase in IL-2 expression and CD8+ infiltration was observed in some patients.[46]

In another study, 23 patients with metastatic breast cancer and melanoma were treated with intratumoral injections of a recombinant adenovirus expressing IL-2. No clinical responses were seen, but IL-2 protein was detected by enzyme-linked immunoadsorbent assay in tumor at 48 hours but not at 7 days after injection. This finding demonstrated that some transgene expression could be detected, despite the presence of preexisting neutralizing antibodies against adenovirus.[85] Other trials have used autologous tumor or fibroblasts expressing IL-2 in melanoma[86] and colorectal cancer patients,[87] but no clinical responses have been reported.

Granulocyte-Macrophage Colony-Stimulating Factor. Granulocyte-macrophage colony-stimulating factor (GM-CSF) is a cytokine with the unique ability to stimulate the differentiation of hematopoietic progenitor cells into dendritic cells, a potent antigen-presenting cell. This property may allow increased presentation of tumor antigens on dendritic cells after immunization with tumors that express GM-CSF. In a comparative study,[88] mice were immunized with irradiated B16 melanoma cells that were transduced with either IL-2, IL-4, IL-5, IL-6, GM-CSF, interferon-γ (IFN-γ), tumor necrosis factor-α (TNF-α), intracellular adhesion molecule 1, or CD2. Only mice immunized with GM-CSF–transduced tumor cells were significantly protected against a subsequent tumor challenge (Fig. 62.1-6). IL-4– and IL-6–transduced tumor cells were minimally protective, but none of the other groups displayed a significant systemic antitumor response. GM-CSF–transduced B16 melanoma cells were also capable of significantly impacting on 3-day subcutaneous implants of a small inoculum of nontransduced B16 cells.[88] Immunization with GM-CSF–transduced tumor generated long-lasting systemic antitumor immunity that was dependent on both CD4+ and CD8+ T cells. Further studies have demonstrated that GM-CSF transduced tumor vaccines activate bone marrow–derived antigen-presenting cells to process and

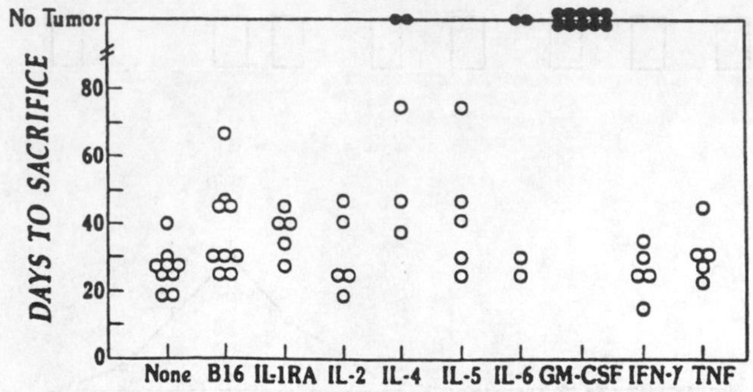

FIGURE 62.1-6. Comparative analysis of vaccine efficacies of a poorly immunogenic murine tumor transduced with different cytokine genes. Syngeneic C57BL/6 mice were vaccinated subcutaneously with 5×10^5 irradiated (3500 rad) B16 melanoma cells transduced with eight different cytokine genes using the MFG retroviral vector. Animals were challenged 14 days later with 1×10^6 live nontransduced B16 cells subcutaneously. (From ref. 88, with permission.) *Open circles,* animal succumbed to tumor challenge; *solid circles,* animal protected from tumor challenge. GM-CSF, granulocyte-macrophage colony-stimulating factor; IFN-γ, interferon-γ; IL, interleukin; TNF, tumor necrosis factor.

present tumor antigens to both CD4+ and CD8+ T cells.[89] Activated, tumor-specific CD4+ T cells were in turn shown to express both Th1 and Th2 cytokines that recruited other effector cells to the tumor, including eosinophils and macrophages. In addition, antitumor activity of GM-CSF–transduced vaccines were found to depend on the production of IFN-γ, IL-4, and IL-5.[90]

Three clinical studies have been reported that used GM-CSF–transduced tumors in renal cell cancer,[91] melanoma,[92] and prostate cancer.[93] In a phase I, randomized, double-blind dose-escalation study, patients with metastatic renal cell cancer were immunized with intradermal and subcutaneous injections of either nontransduced or GM-CSF–transduced autologous, irradiated renal cancer cells. Biopsy sites from patients receiving GM-CSF–transduced vaccines demonstrated infiltrates of macrophages, dendritic cells, eosinophils, neutrophils, and T cells consistent with preclinical studies. Delayed-type hypersensitivity responses using nontransduced autologous tumor cells revealed eosinophil infiltrates in only those patients who previously received GM-CSF–transduced vaccines. One partial response was seen out of nine patients treated with GM-CSF–transduced vaccines.[91]

In a phase I trial for patients with metastatic melanoma, 21 patients were immunized intradermally and subcutaneously with autologous melanoma cells transduced to express GM-CSF. Again, immunization sites were found to be infiltrated with T lymphocytes, dendritic cells, macrophages, and eosinophils in all 21 patients. Although only 1 of 21 patients had an objective partial response, 11 of 16 patients evaluated had T lymphocyte and plasma cell infiltrates in tumor biopsies after immunization.[92] In a phase I trial evaluating GM-CSF–transduced prostate cancer vaccination, delayed-type hypersensitivity reactions against nontransduced autologous tumor cells were positive in two of eight patients before vaccination and seven of eight patients after vaccination. However, no clinical responses were reported.[93]

Interferon-γ. The introduction of the IFN-γ gene into tumor cells can lead to the up-regulation of major histocompatibility complex (MHC) class I and class II gene products.[94] Although this effect can lead to decreased tumorigenicity,[95] it is unclear whether systemic immunity is enhanced. In some tumor systems with low class I expression or antigen processing defects, however, IFN-γ–transduced tumor allowed the isolation of CD8+ lymphocytes capable of treating established pulmonary metastases from the parental, nontransduced tumor.[96] Thus, for some cancers, immunization with IFN-γ–transduced tumor cells may allow the isolation of T cells capable of impacting on established, systemic disease.

Other Cytokine Genes. The introduction into tumor cells of a variety of other cytokine genes, such as TNF,[88,97–100] IL-1,[101] IL-4,[102–104] IL-6,[105–107] IL-7,[108–110] IL-13,[111] G-CSF,[112] MCP,[113,114] and RANTES,[115] can lead to decreased tumorigenicity. No evidence suggests, however, that these manipulations can increase systemic immunity above that which can be elicited from irradiated tumor cells.

Tahara et al.[116] introduced the IL-12 gene into murine MCA207 tumor cells (MCA207-IL-12), which resulted in decreased tumorigenicity. In addition, mice were injected with 3×10^5 MCA207 cells in the left flank on day 0, followed by treatment on day 3 with saline, MCA207-Neo^R, or MCA207-IL-12. Thirty-three percent of mice were free of tumor by day 21 when treated with MCA207-IL-12 tumor, compared to no animals free of tumor that were treated with saline or MCA207-Neo^R tumor.[116] However, it is not clear whether these effects were due to the paracrine secretion of IL-12 or to a systemic effect of secreted IL-12.

Although the transduction of tumor cells with a variety of cytokine genes can result in decreased tumorigenicity in murine models, few studies have demonstrated that this transduction leads to an enhanced immune response against the parental, nontransduced tumor compared to immunization with irradiated, nontransduced tumor cells. In one study, Hock et al.[117] demonstrated that tumor cells modified with different cytokine genes (IL-2, IL-4, IL-7, TNF, or IFN-γ) were only slightly superior to irradiated parental cells as immunogens. Moreover, parental cells admixed with the classical adjuvant *Cryptosporidium parvum* were found to be superior to the cytokine-modified tumors in their ability to immunize mice against the tumor.[117]

NONCYTOKINE GENES

B7-1 (CD80). The activation of T lymphocytes requires that they come in contact with a specific antigen and a costimulatory signal. One potential reason that some cancers develop and evade the immune system is that T lymphocytes are not adequately costimulated to become activated. The adhesion molecules B7-1 (CD80) and B7-2 (CD86) can bind to the CD28 receptor on T cells to provide costimulation.[118] Several groups have demonstrated that tumor cells transfected with B7-1 locally regress and lead to protection against subsequent tumor challenge with the parental tumor.[119–121] In one study,[122] regression of B7-transduced tumors was dependent on the intrinsic immunogenicity of the parental tumor.

Further studies are needed to assess the potency of B7 in the ability to stimulate an antitumor response.

HLA-B7. Several clinical trials based on murine models have been performed using intratumoral injection with plasmid DNA encoding HLA-B7 in HLA-B7–negative patients in the hopes of generating a stronger immune response against unmodified tumor cells.[123] Intratumoral injection of HLA-B7 plasmid DNA in a cationic lipid vector resulted in RNA or protein expression at the injection site in some patients,[47,48] but no tumor regression was seen in noninjected sites.

Immunization with Genes Encoding Tumor Antigens

RECOMBINANT VACCINES. Whole tumor cells have been used as immunogens because the specific antigens recognized by T cells have been largely unknown. However, the cloning of several melanoma antigens recognized by T cells[74–78] has opened new possibilities for active immunization strategies for cancer. Studies in murine models have demonstrated that antigens expressed at high levels in recombinant adenoviral, fowlpox, and vaccinia vector systems can induce a significant antitumor immune response against tumors bearing the same antigen.[124–127] Recombinant viral vaccines can result in the *in vivo* production of high quantities of heterologous proteins. However, expression of native viral proteins by these vectors can also result in a host immune response against the vector itself, thereby diminishing the effectiveness of repeated immunizations.

Immunization studies with "naked DNA" given intramuscularly, or DNA administered on gold beads using the "gene gun" technique, have resulted in significant antitumor effects. Because these methods do not use viral vectors, no irrelevant viral proteins are expressed, thus allowing repeated immunizations.

Current efforts are focused on enhancing immune responses through adjuvant exogenous cytokine administration or introduction of genes encoding cytokines or costimulatory molecules into the recombinant vectors.

DENDRITIC CELLS. Another strategy to actively immunize a patient against cancer is to use potent antigen-presenting cells, such as dendritic cells. These cells are capable of stimulating immune responses from quiescent lymphocytes. Dendritic cells pulsed with tumor peptide or protein antigens have been shown to have significant antitumor effects in murine models[128] and were reported to be effective in one study of patients with lymphomas. Nestle and colleagues[129] treated 16 metastatic melanoma patients with intranodal injections of dendritic cells pulsed with tumor lysates or peptides derived from known tumor antigens. Eleven of 16 patients demonstrated a positive delayed-type hypersensitivity reaction to peptide-pulsed dendritic cells, and clinical responses were observed in five patients.[129]

Although antitumor responses can be obtained in murine models by administering dendritic cells pulsed with peptide antigens or whole proteins, this approach limits immune responses to specific, defined MHC-binding epitopes within a given antigen or requires the production of recombinant proteins. For many tumor antigens, however, multiple epitopes have been described that bind to a variety of MHC molecules. One strategy that may enable the presentation of multiple, even undefined, epitopes within a given tumor antigen is the introduction of an antigen gene into the dendritic cell. This strategy may allow multiple epitopes to be presented in the context of both class I and class II molecules as well as the constitutive expression of these antigens in transduced dendritic cells. Several strategies have been proposed to genetically modify dendritic cells with tumor antigens. One is to transduce bone marrow cells and differentiate the cells *in vitro* into dendritic cells, using GM-CSF.[130–132] Another is the transient transfection of dendritic cells using cationic lipids,[133] gene gun, adenovirus,[134,135] or recombinant influenza virus.[136]

GENETIC MODIFICATION OF IMMUNE EFFECTOR CELLS

Several lines of evidence indicate that adoptively transferred T cells can be therapeutically effective. TILs have been shown to mediate significant responses in patients with melanoma, even in those who have not been successful with previous therapy with IL-2.[137] Adoptively transferred cytomegalovirus-specific T cells have been shown to prevent cytomegalovirus infections in patients after allogeneic bone marrow transplantation.[138] Infusion of donor T cells has been effective in treating the EBV-driven lymphoproliferative disease that sometimes complicates allogeneic bone marrow transplantation.[64] Patients with CML recurrence after allogeneic bone marrow transplantation can experience remission after transfer of donor T cells.[139] Several strategies for the genetic modification of transferred T cells attempt to increase their effectiveness.

Enhancing Survival of Immune Cells

For T cells to be functional against a tumor, they must survive *in vivo*, recognize the target, and then execute an adequate antitumor effector mechanism, either by direct cell lysis or release of cytokines that may attract and stimulate other immune cells. There are several ways to potentially enhance these steps. T cells grow in response to stimulation by various cytokines, such as IL-2. On adoptive transfer of TILs in murine models, the administration of systemic IL-2 potentiates the antitumor effect, presumably by maintaining growth and viability of the administered TILs.[140] By inserting the gene for IL-2, TILs may become able to stimulate themselves in an autocrine fashion, as demonstrated by Yamada et al.[141] and Karasuyama et al.[142] in CTL line and murine HT-2 T cells, respectively. Treisman et al.[143] demonstrated that a T-cell clone transduced with the IL-2 gene could grow in an IL-2–independent fashion while maintaining antigen specificity.[143] However, further work must be done to obtain sufficient IL-2 secretion in primary lymphocytes for this approach to be clinically useful. In addition, insertion of the gene encoding the IL-2 receptor, which is normally up-regulated by lymphocytes after antigen stimulation, may also be required to obtain a proliferative response to IL-2.

Increasing Tumor Recognition by Using Novel Receptor Genes

CHIMERIC ANTIBODY/T-CELL RECEPTOR GENES. Although adoptive immunotherapeutic strategies have been developed for some cancers, tumor-reactive T cells are difficult to isolate and expand from most types of cancer. A variety of monoclonal antibodies have been developed that bind to specific cancers. Although cancer therapy with antibodies has been largely disappointing, partially because of the lack of an adequate effec-

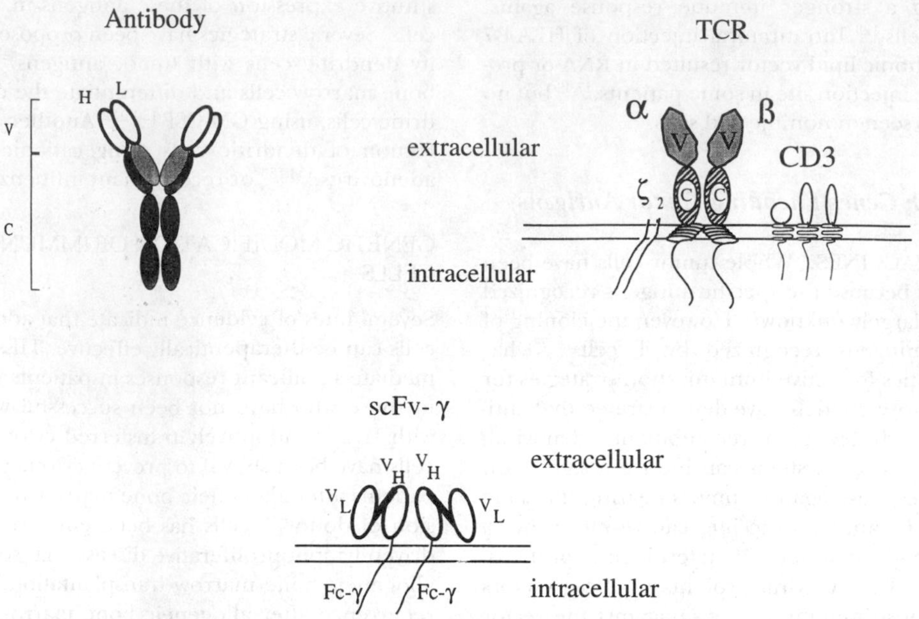

FIGURE 62.1-7. The chimeric immunoglobulin T-cell receptor (TCR) combines antibody-variable regions with T-cell signaling chains. In this diagram, a single-chain antibody variable (scFv) fragment derived from the variable regions of a monoclonal antibody is joined to the Fc receptor γ chain, which is related to the TCR-ζ chain and can mediate T-cell signal transduction.[149]

tor mechanism to destroy tumor cells on binding. By combining the antigen-recognition domains from antibodies with the intracellular, signaling chains of T cells, chimeric receptors can be generated that activate T cells based on antibody-like recognition (Fig. 62.1-7). This approach, which uses the antigen-binding capabilities of antibodies with the potent antitumor activity of T cells, would allow the production of specific T cells against any antigen for which a monoclonal antibody exists. This strategy could widely generalize the use of adoptive immunotherapy for cancer and infectious diseases.

The successful combination of antibody-variable regions with T-cell signaling chains has been established for several model antigens, such as phosphorylcholine, digoxin, and trinitrophenyl.[144–147] These initial approaches, however, required the use of two genes, because the antibody-variable region is encoded by a combination of light and heavy chains. This two-gene strategy, however, is impractical for use in clinical trials using primary T cells, because transduction efficiencies are relatively low for even one gene. Therefore, chimeric receptors encoded on a single gene[148,149] were designed by making use of single-chain antibody variable (scFv) regions in which the light- and heavy-chain variable regions are connected by a flexible linker.[150–152] These scFv fragments were joined to T-cell receptor (TCR) ζ or Fc receptor γ chains, both of which are closely related and have been demonstrated to be capable of mediating TCR signal transduction.[153–157]

Using this single-gene approach, receptors have been constructed using the mAb MOv18, which binds to a folate-binding protein overexpressed on most ovarian adenocarcinomas.[158,159] T cells retrovirally transduced with these receptor genes demonstrate specific cytokine secretion and cytolysis when cultured with human ovarian cancer cells. In addition, intravenously administered murine T cells transduced with this receptor could specifically treat experimental lung metastases from tumors that express the ovarian cancer antigen. Intraperitoneal administration of these T cells could also successfully treat human ovarian cancer cells growing intraperitoneally in nude mice.[160] These studies demonstrate that T cells can be manipulated genetically to recognize and destroy tumor cells based on antibody-type specificity.

Besides triggering direct T-cell activation with γ and ζ chains, antibody-variable regions can be coupled to other signaling chains, such as the intracellular portion of CD28, an important T-cell costimulatory receptor. This approach has been found to enhance T-cell survival and proliferation *in vitro*.[161]

Most recently, the transduction of hematopoietic stem cells with chimeric receptor genes has been under investigation, because this may not only provide a stable supply of redirected T cells, but also granulocytes, macrophages, and natural killer cells, all of which may have significant antitumor activity on expression of chimeric receptor genes. Mice that received MOv-g–transduced bone marrow cells exhibited significant antigen-specific antitumor activity *in vivo*.[162]

These strategies have the potential of widely generalizing the use of adoptive immunotherapy. scFv-γ and -ζ receptors have been constructed against breast cancer using an anti-HER2 mAb,[163] colon cancer using an anti-GA733 mAb,[164] and HIV using an anti-gp41 mAb.[165] This strategy could be applied to a wide range of cancer histologies or infectious diseases for which appropriate mAb exist.

NATIVE T-CELL RECEPTOR GENES. T-cell specificity can also be altered by the introduction of genes encoding native TCRs. The TCR consists of an α and β chain heterodimer that confers the ability to specifically recognize peptide/MHC complexes on antigen-presenting cells and target cells. TCRs derived from melanoma-specific CTLs have been identified, cloned, and characterized.[166] Clay et al.[167] transduced primary lymphocytes with a TCR gene specific for the MART-1 melanoma tumor rejection antigen. Because the TCR consists of two individual chains, a retroviral vector was constructed that uses internal ribosomal entry sites (IRES sequences) that allow the translation of multiple genes from a single transcript. Primary T cells transduced with this construct were capable of specifically recognizing tumor cells expressing the MART-1 melanoma tumor antigen in the context of HLA-A2. As more TCRs recognizing specific tumor antigens are characterized and cloned, this strategy may generalize the use of adoptive immunotherapy, circumventing the need to isolate T cells with specific reactivities from each individual patient.

Transduction of T Cells and Donor Lymphocytes with Suicide Genes

Adoptively transferred T cells have been safely administered to many patients for more than 10 years. In specific situations, however, the adoptively transferred cells may be toxic to the host, such as in the treatment of immunocompromised HIV patients. In the setting of allogeneic bone marrow transplantation for hematologic malignancies, donor lymphocyte infusions can be highly effective against tumor as well as EBV-induced lymphoma but may also incite graft-versus-host disease. In an attempt to increase the therapeutic index of adoptively transferred cells in these situations, "suicide" genes can be introduced into lymphocytes to specifically delete the transduced cells should they become toxic to patients *in vivo.* The gene for herpes TK (hTK) has been used for this purpose, because it specifically sensitizes cells to the antiviral agent ganciclovir.

In one study using hTK-transduced donor lymphocytes, three of eight patients receiving donor lymphocytes after allogeneic bone marrow transplantation for hematologic malignancies developed acute or chronic graft-versus-host disease. In these patients, ganciclovir administration significantly diminished the number of circulating hTK-transduced cells within 24 hours, resulting in complete or partial remissions of the disease[168] (Table 62.1-5).

In another study, anti-HIV CTLs were transduced with a fusion gene encoding hTK and the selectable marker hygromycin before administration in HIV-infected patients.[169] Because HIV patients are immunocompromised, the CTLs could be irradicated with ganciclovir should the transduced cells become toxic. However, initial results of the trial revealed that the patients were developing cellular immune responses against the hTK-hygromycin fusion protein, thus demonstrating that foreign genes, including selectable markers, can themselves become targets of the host immune response.

Increasing Antitumor Efficacy of Immune Cells

TNF has potent antitumor activity against large tumor burdens in some murine models.[170–172] However, humans can only tolerate 2% of the systemic TNF dose (by weight) required in mice, due to dose-limiting hypotension.[173–177] High doses of TNF, administered locally via direct tumor injection[178,179] or isolated limb perfusion,[180] can result in dramatic tumor regressions in some cancer patients. At the National Cancer Institute's Surgery Branch, regressions of liver metastases have been seen in patients treated with TNF administered as a component of an isolated hepatic perfusion.[181] Therefore, tumor regressions seem possible in patients when adequate local concentrations of TNF can be achieved. Because TILs have been demonstrated to accumulate at sites of tumor,[182–184] the transduction of TILs with the TNF gene may allow high concentrations of TNF to be delivered locally in the absence of systemic toxicity.[185]

Twelve patients have been treated with TNF-transduced TILs in a phase I trial using escalating doses of TILs and IL-2. No safety problems or toxicity have been detected. Replacement of the TNF transmembrane region with the signal peptide from interferon-γ, thus bypassing the transmembrane form,[186,187] resulted in a fivefold increase in TNF production.[185] Despite this improvement, however, primary lymphocytes transduced with the TNF gene probably do not produce high enough levels of TNF constitutively to be clinically effective. To optimize this treatment strategy, current efforts are directed toward identifying promoter/enhancer regions that direct higher levels of gene expression in primary lymphocytes.

MODIFICATION OF TUMORS WITH GENES THAT HAVE DIRECT ANTITUMOR EFFECTS

The gene therapies that have been discussed thus far have all focused on the stimulation of the immune system to react against tumor cells. Another approach to cancer gene therapy is to introduce genes into tumor cells that have direct antiproliferative or toxic effects on that cell. This approach, however, requires techniques to directly administer genes into tumor

TABLE 62.1-5. Effect of Ganciclovir Treatment on Elimination of Herpes Thymidine Kinase–Modified Donor Lymphocytes and on Graft-Versus-Host Disease (GVHD)

		Proportion of Transduced PBL (%)		*Clinical Out-*
Patient	*GVHD (Grade)*	Preganciclovir	24 Hr after Ganciclovir	*come of GVHD*
1	Acute skin (II/III)	13.4	$<10^{-4}$	CR
2	Acute liver (III)	2.0	$<10^{-4}$	CR
8	Chronic lung, skin, gastrointestinal tract	11.9	2.8	PR

CR, complete remission of GVHD; PBL, peripheral blood lymphocytes; PR, partial remission of GVHD.
(Adapted from ref. 168, with permission.)

cells *in vivo* with high efficiencies, which is not technically possible at this time. However, as vector development continues, the direct administration of genes into patients may play a more important role. Some preliminary studies have been initiated that use direct *in vivo* administration of genes into tumor cells.

TUMOR SUPPRESSOR GENES

Cancer can result from the abnormal expression of genes that control the cell cycle. Some genes, termed *tumor suppressor genes*, regulate cell growth, and their absence by mutation or deletion results in the malignant phenotype. One approach to treat tumors with deleted or mutated tumor suppressor genes is to replace these genes by *in vivo* gene transfer. Currently, gene transfer techniques do not exist that are capable of efficiently delivering these genes systemically to all tumor cells in the body, and significant technical improvements are required if this approach is to become practical.

Because of this limitation in systemic delivery, several groups have attempted local gene delivery of tumor suppressor genes.[188,189] Swisher and colleagues[190] treated 28 patients with non–small cell lung cancer with intratumoral administration of an adenovirus vector containing wild-type p53 complementary DNA. Reverse-transcriptase PCR analysis of posttreatment biopsies were positive for the presence of vector-specific p53 mRNA in 12 of 26 patients. Partial response of the injected lesion was observed in 2 of 25 evaluable patients (8%).[190] Because local therapy is of limited utility in the face of metastatic disease, these studies highlight the need for improved vectors that would allow efficient, systemic gene delivery.

ANTISENSE AND RIBOZYMES

Oncogenes are genes that cause uncontrolled cell growth when mutated or overexpressed, and neutralization of these genes can reverse the malignant phenotype. One approach to inactivate genes uses antisense oligodeoxynucleotides,[191,192] which are short sequences that are complementary to target RNA transcripts and can inhibit translation of the RNA into protein.

Oligonucleotides have been shown to enter cells by at least two pathways (i.e., endocytosis and pinocytosis), and significant activity of antisense constructs has been observed *in vitro* using tissue culture cell lines. *In vitro* growth suppression has been demonstrated using antisense oligonucleotides against BCL-2[193] in leukemia cells, BCR-ABL[194] in CML cells, MYC[195] in lymphoma cell lines, and MYB[196,197] in adenocarcinoma and leukemia cell lines.

Several studies have been performed in mice demonstrating *in vivo* efficacy of antisense oligonucleotides against tumors. Antisense inhibition of c-myb mRNA increased survival of scid mice bearing human K562 leukemia cells.[198] In another study, antisense against the p65 subunit of nuclear factor kB inhibited the growth of the murine fibrosarcoma K-BALB and the murine melanoma B16.[199]

Webb and colleagues[200] treated nine patients with non-Hodgkin's lymphoma with daily subcutaneous BCL-2 antisense oligonucleotide for 2 weeks. BCL-2 overexpression can promote tumorigenesis by causing resistance to programmed cell death (apoptosis). A complete response was observed in one of nine patients, with resolution of left axillary lymphadenopathy.[200]

A current limitation to this approach is the inability to successfully deliver antisense constructs to tumor cells *in vivo* with adequate efficiency. In addition, antisense studies must be interpreted carefully, because of the possibility of nonspecific effects. For example, because charged oligonucleotides are polyanions, they can bind nonspecifically to growth factors, such as basis fibroblast growth factor (bFGF).[201]

Another potential method to target activated oncogenes is through the use of ribozymes. These are RNA enzymes that catalyze endoribonucleolytic cleavage of RNA.[202] Several investigators have reported cleavage of the bcr-abl transcript, which is involved in the pathogenesis of chronic myelogenous leukemia, by specific hammerhead ribozymes. Anti-fos and anti-ras ribozymes also have been reported.[202] At the present time, however, no adequate *ex vivo* or *in vivo* systems can deliver ribozymes to target cells.

SUICIDE GENES

Because retroviral vectors integrate preferentially into dividing cells, replicating tumor cells might be targeted with relative specificity compared to normal tissues. To test this hypothesis, Culver et al.[203] implanted cell lines producing recombinant retrovirus containing the hTK gene into brain tumors in rats, then administered systemic ganciclovir therapy. Ganciclovir is a nucleotide analogue that is converted into a cytotoxic molecule by hTK, but it is a poor substrate for mammalian TK. Using this method, tumors regressed, and significant toxicity to surrounding normal tissues was not observed. Because the hTK gene can only be delivered locally *in vivo*, this treatment approach is limited to those cancers whose primary morbidity is due to local, unresectable disease. More than 30 clinical trials using suicide gene therapy have been approved by the RAC, including studies of patients with brain tumors, mesothelioma, prostate cancer, head and neck cancer, ovarian cancer, and colorectal cancer (see Table 62.1-2). These trials use retroviral and adenoviral gene transfer techniques to deliver the herpes simplex virus (HSV)-TK or cytosine deaminase suicide genes, which is followed by systemic therapy with ganciclovir (for HSV-TK) or 5-fluorocytosine (for cytosine deaminase).

Ram and colleagues[204] treated 15 patients with brain tumors, including malignant glioma ($n = 12$), metastatic melanoma ($n = 2$), and metastatic breast cancer ($n = 1$), with intratumoral implantation of up to 1×10^9 producer cells making retroviral vectors encoding HSV-TK, followed by systemic ganciclovir therapy for 14 days. *In situ* hybridization revealed that vector producer cells survived up to 7 days *in vivo* but were associated with only a low level of gene transfer to tumors. Five of the smaller tumors (1.4 ± 0.5 mL) showed evidence of antitumor activity, but larger tumors did not respond.

Several groups have reported the local administration of recombinant adenovirus containing HSV-TK,[205,206] but it is not clear whether these approaches have any advantages over other methods of local therapy. In addition, the tumor specificity of this approach is a potential problem, because, in contrast to retroviral vectors, no evidence indicates that adenovirus infects dividing tumor cells preferentially over nondividing normal tissue.

In an attempt to enhance the tissue specificity of suicide gene therapy, Pandha and colleagues[207] treated 12 breast cancer patients with intratumoral injections of a plasmid construct encoding the *Escherichia coli* cytosine deaminase suicide gene driven by the human erbB-2 promoter, followed by systemic prodrug administration. Significant levels of expression of the suicide gene were specifically restricted to erbB-2–positive tumor cells.[207]

A major limitation in the current application of *in vivo* gene therapy approaches for cancer, such as suicide gene strategies, is the absence of an adequate delivery system that could transfer the suicide gene to all cancer cells within a patient's body. Despite a potential "bystander effect," which may mediate the destruction of tumor cells surrounding those expressing the suicide gene, current gene transfer technology is too inefficient to allow the application of this strategy for the treatment of disseminated metastatic cancer. A second limitation to the use of suicide genes is that of specificity. For any cancer therapy to be effective, the toxicity for the tumor cells must be greater than for normal tissues. Retroviral vectors may theoretically be more selective for tumor cells than normal tissues, because retroviruses only infect proliferating cells. However, retroviruses are suboptimal for *in vivo* administration because of their low efficiency of transduction. Adenoviral vectors, on the other hand, show no selectivity towards tumor cells.

Enhanced tumor specificity might be accomplished by using tumor-specific promoter/enhancer regions to direct transcription of the suicide genes. For example, the α-fetoprotein promoter is primarily active in hepatoma cells,[208] whereas the tyrosinase promoter is specifically active in melanocytes and melanoma cells.[209] This approach also has been suggested to target tumor vasculature, using promoters that are relatively specific for endothelial cells, such as the E-selectin, vascular cell adhesion molecule, and CD31 promoters.[210] The use of tumor- or tumor-vasculature–specific promoters might decrease destruction of normal cells, because they would not express the suicide gene product. For these approaches, however, the fundamental problem of inadequate gene delivery still remains.

SELECTIVE REPLICATION OF VIRUS IN TUMORS

In vivo gene delivery to tumors using replication-defective viral systems are presently inadequate to obtain sufficient transduction efficiency. The design of a virus that could specifically replicate in and destroy tumor cells would be of obvious value. Some efforts[211] have used E1B-defective adenoviruses capable of specifically replicating and destroying tumor cells that lack p53 tumor suppressor function. The p53 protein is a transcription factor that acts as a potent tumor suppressor by its ability to induce cell-cycle arrest and apoptosis. Functional p53 is present in normal cells but is absent in more than 50% of the common solid tumors. Normally, on viral infection, p53 triggers early apoptosis of the cell, thereby limiting viral replication and spread. However, many viruses have evolved proteins, such as the adenoviral E1B 55-kD protein, that inhibit normal p53 function, thereby allowing maximal viral replication. E1B-defective adenoviruses, therefore, cannot fully replicate in normal tissues expressing p53, but they can replicate in tumor cells that lack functional p53.

Bischoff et al.[211] found that an E1B-deleted adenovirus (ONYX-015) could lyse p53-deficient human tumor cells but not cells with functional p53. Intratumoral injection of ONYX-015 caused regression of human cervical carcinomas grown in nude mice. Heise and colleagues[212] reported augmentation of antitumor effects of ONYX-015 by chemotherapy, as well as the efficacy of intravenously administered ONYX-015 in nude mice with subcutaneous human tumor xenografts.[213] Clinical trials are ongoing to test this approach in patients with head and neck cancer.

Studies have questioned whether the tumor specificity of ONYX-015 is strictly related to p53 expression by the tumor cells. Rothmann et al.[214] found that replication of ONYX-015 was independent of p53 status in tumor cells, and Hall and colleagues[215] reported that productive adenovirus infection was dependent on the p53 pathway. Therefore, much needs to be determined regarding the host range and mechanism of action of ONYX-015. In addition, the next generation of tumor-specific "smart viruses" must address enhanced specificity and systemic delivery of the virus, as well as methods to prevent humoral and cellular host immune responses against the virus.

INTRODUCTION OF GENES INTO HEMATOPOIETIC STEM CELLS TO DECREASE TOXICITY FROM CHEMOTHERAPY

Expression of the MDR gene decreases the toxicity from certain chemotherapy drugs, such as Taxol, Adriamycin, vincristine, and actinomycin D, by encoding for a transmembrane molecule that actively pumps these cytotoxic agents out of the cell.[216,217] Expression of the MDR gene in tumor cells is commonly associated with tumor resistance to these cytotoxic agents. Sorrentino et al.[218] transplanted MDR-transduced bone marrow cells into mice and substantially enriched for these cells after treatment with Taxol. Several clinical trials are now under way that attempt to genetically modify bone marrow cells with the MDR gene, then reinfuse them into the patient in an attempt to decrease hematopoietic toxicity from subsequent chemotherapy. However, clinical trials with patients receiving transduced bone marrow have shown that only a small percentage of hematopoietic cells are gene modified.[219,220] This limitation has been confirmed by several groups attempting to decrease chemotherapy toxicity with MDR-transduced hematopoietic progenitor cells. Cowan et al.[221] found low levels of short-term engraftment of MDR-transduced cells in three of four patients treated, and Hersdorffer and colleagues[222] had similar results in two of five patients. Hanania et al.[223] found that the method of transduction was important. They compared a 3-day transduction method on a stromal monolayer to a 4- to 6-hour transduction procedure in a culture bag. Three to 4 weeks after transplantation, none of ten patients receiving cells transduced with the supernatant method had MDR-positive cells, whereas five of eight patients receiving cells transduced with the stromal method had MDR-positive cells.[223] However, the percentage of positive cells was not quantified and was presumably low because of the requirement for sensitive PCR methods for detection.

Therefore, the success of this strategy may depend on whether the levels of gene transfer are sufficient to allow the administration of higher doses of chemotherapy. If this approach is to have a significant impact in cancer therapy, an effective chemotherapeutic regimen must exist that can eradicate tumor before the development of significant nonhematopoietic toxicities, such as liver failure.

ANTIANGIOGENIC GENE THERAPY

The discovery by Folkman[224] in the 1970s that tumors produce substances that stimulate the growth of their vasculature has led to intensive investigation into methods to inhibit tumor neovessel formation. Production of proangiogenic cytokines, including vascular endothelial growth factor (VEGF) and FGF, result in angiogenesis, which is required for tumor growth.[225] One gene therapy strategy, therefore, has focused on the inhibition of the production or function of proangiogenic cytokines. A second strategy involves the delivery of genes that encode inhibitors of angiogenesis.[226] A number of endogenous proteins have been described that are capable of inhibiting angiogenesis, and their expression *in vivo* may result in antitumor activity through interference with tumor blood supply.

GENES THAT INHIBIT PROANGIOGENIC CYTOKINES

VEGF is a proangiogenic cytokine that can bind to two high-affinity receptors (VEGFR-1/FLT-1 and VEGFR-2/KDR) expressed on vascular endothelial cells. An endogenous, alternatively spliced soluble form of FLT-1 (sFLT-1) has been identified[227] that is capable of inhibiting the effects of VEGF on vascular endothelial cells *in vitro*. Systemic administration of recombinant adenovirus expressing sFLT-1 resulted in tumor inhibition in mice with preexisting lung or liver metastases.[228] In another preclinical model using GS-9L gliosarcoma cells in rats, intracerebral or subcutaneous intratumoral injection of retrovirus-producing cells encoding a dominant-negative VEGFR-2 resulted in tumor inhibition that was associated with decreased vessel density within tumors.[229]

Antisense approaches also are being tested as a means to inhibit VEGF. Use of a recombinant adenovirus-encoding antisense VEGF for intratumoral injection of subcutaneous human gliomas in nude mice resulted in the inhibition of tumor growth.[230] The von Hippel-Lindau (VHL) gene[231] has been shown to down-regulate VEGF production by human renal cancer cells.[232] Therefore, gene therapy by introducing the VHL gene into tumors is a potential strategy to down-regulate VEGF expression *in vivo*. As with other approaches that depend on *in vivo* gene delivery into tumor cells, this approach is limited by the requirement for an efficient system that allows gene transfer to a majority of cancer cells *in vivo*.

Urokinase-type plasminogen activator (u-PA) is a FGF that can result in endothelial cell proliferation. Soluble N-terminal fragments of u-PA have been used to competitively inhibit the binding of endogenous u-PA with its receptor. Systemic administration of recombinant adenovirus encoding a competitor fragment of u-PA has been shown to inhibit liver metastases in an experimental model of human colon cancer in nude mice.[233]

Tie2 is an endothelium-specific receptor tyrosine kinase that plays an important role in angiogenesis of embryonic vasculature through the interaction with its ligand, angiopoietin 1.[234,235] Systemic administration of a recombinant adenovirus expressing a soluble Tie2 receptor (sTie2) capable of blocking Tie2 activation resulted in growth inhibition of subcutaneous murine mammary (4T1) and melanoma (B16F10.9) cells. In addition, the sTie2 recombinant adenovirus inhibited the development and neovascularization of pulmonary metastaes.[236]

GENES WITH ANTIANGIOGENIC PROPERTIES

A number of endogenous inhibitors of angiogenesis have been described. They include antiangiogenic proteolytic fragments, ILs, IFNs, thrombospondins, and tissue inhibitors of matrix metalloproteinases (TIMPs). Angiostatin is a 38-kD internal fragment of plasminogen, and endostatin is a 20-kD fragment derived from the C-terminal noncollagenous domain of the basement membrane constituent collagen XVIII.[237,238] Administration of angiostatin and endostatin can lead to tumor dormancy and regression in murine models.[237,238] However, these proteins have been difficult to produce in large quantities for clinical use because of instability. Because it may be necessary to administer antiangiogenic agents chronically to maintain long-term tumor suppression, other strategies besides administration of recombinant protein may be required for these approaches to be effective. Gene therapy using genes encoding these proteolytic fragments may be an attractive alternative to exogenous dosing.

Systemic administration of recombinant adenovirus expressing angiostatin resulted in dose-dependent inhibition of the establishment and growth of C6 rat gliomas in nude mice.[239] Using intravenous delivery of complexes of cationic liposomes and plasmid DNA-encoding angiostatin, Liu et al.[240] demonstrated reduced B16F10 melanoma metastases in a 7-day tumor model.

Feldman et al.[241] demonstrated inhibition of subcutaneous MC38 murine colon adenocarcinomas using intravenous administration of recombinant adenovirus expressing the endostatin gene. In this model, circulating levels of endostatin were as high as 2038 ng/mL in nude mice after injection of adenovirus.[241]

Preclinical gene therapy approaches have been investigated using genes encoding a number of other antiangiogenic agents, including IL-4, IL-10, IL-12, IFN-β, thrombospondin-1, TIMP-1, TIMP-2, and platelet factor-4. In addition, the combination of ionizing radiation and intratumoral administration of a recombinant adenovirus expressing TNF-α resulted in tumor suppression in a murine xenograft model mediated by the destruction of tumor microvasculature.[242]

REFERENCES

1. Cheng J, Yee JK, Yeargin J, Friedmann T, Haas M. Suppression of acute lymphoblastic leukemia by the human wild-type p53 gene. *Cancer Res* 1992;52:222.
2. Miller AD, Miller DG, Garcia JV, Lynch CM. Use of retroviral vectors for gene transfer and expression. *Methods Enzymol* 1993;217:581.
3. Danos O, Mulligan RC. Safe and efficient generation of recombinant retroviruses with amphotropic and ecotropic host ranges. *Proc Natl Acad Sci U S A* 1988;85:6460.
4. Burns JC, Friedmann T, Driever W, Burrascano M, Yee JK. Vesicular stomatitis virus G glycoprotein pseudotyped retroviral vectors: concentration to very high titer and efficient gene transfer into mammalian and nonmammalian cells [see comments]. *Proc Natl Acad Sci U S A* 1993;90:8033.
5. Miller AD. Cell-surface receptors for retroviruses and implications for gene transfer. *Proc Natl Acad Sci U S A* 1996;93:11407.
6. Miller AD, Garcia JV, von Suhr N, et al. Construction and properties of retrovirus packaging cells based on gibbon ape leukemia virus. *J Virol* 1991;65:2220.
7. Bauer TR Jr, Miller AD, Hickstein DD. Improved transfer of the leukocyte integrin CD18 subunit into hematopoietic cell lines by using retroviral vectors having a gibbon ape leukemia virus envelope. *Blood* 1995;86:2379.
8. Lam JS, Cowherd R, Rosenberg SA, Hwu P. Improved gene transfer into lymphocytes using retroviruses that express the gibbon ape leukemia virus envelope. *Hum Gene Ther* 1996;7:1415.

9. Uckert W, Willimsky G, Pedersen FS, Blankenstein T, Pedersen L. RNA levels of human retrovirus receptors Pit1 and Pit2 do not correlate with infectibility by three retroviral vector pseudotypes. *Hum Gene Ther* 1998;9:2619.
10. Bunnell BA, Muul LM, Donahue RE, Blaese RM, Morgan RA. High-efficiency retroviral-mediated gene transfer into human and nonhuman primate peripheral blood lymphocytes. *Proc Natl Acad Sci U S A* 1995;92:7739.
11. Yee JK, Friedmann T, Burns JC. Generation of high-titer pseudotyped retroviral vectors with very broad host range. *Methods Cell Biol* 1994;43[Pt A]:99.
12. Sharma S, Cantwell M, Kipps TJ, Friedmann T. Efficient infection of a human T-cell line and of human primary peripheral blood leukocytes with a pseudotyped retrovirus vector. *Proc Natl Acad Sci U S A* 1996;93:11842.
13. Gallardo HF. Recombinant retroviruses pseudotyped with the vesicular stomatitis virus G glycoprotein mediate both stable gene transfer and pseudotransduction in human peripheral blood lymphocytes. *Blood* 1997;90:952.
14. Naldini L, Blomer U, Gallay P, et al. *In vivo* gene delivery and stable transduction of nondividing cells by a lentiviral vector [see comments]. *Science* 1996;272:263.
15. Kafri T, van Praag H, Ouyang L, Gage FH, Verma IM. A packaging cell line for lentivirus vectors. *J Virol* 1999;73:576.
16. Naldini L, Blomer U, Gage F, Trono D, Verma I. Efficient transfer, integration, and sustained long-term expression of the transgene in adult rat brains injected with a lentiviral vector. *Proc Natl Acad Sci U S A* 1997;93:11382.
17. Case SS, Price MA, Jordan CT, et al. Stable transduction of quiescent CD34(+)CD38(−) human hematopoietic cells by HIV-1-based lentiviral vectors. *Proc Natl Acad Sci U S A* 1999;96:2988.
18. Kafri T, Blomer U, Peterson DA, Gage FH, Verma IM. Sustained expression of genes delivered directly into liver and muscle by lentiviral vectors. *Nat Genet* 1997;17:314.
19. Miyoshi H, Smith KA, Mosier DE, Verma IM, Torbett BE. Transduction of human CD34+ cells that mediate long-term engraftment of NOD/SCID mice by HIV vectors. *Science* 1999;283:682.
20. Miyoshi H, Takahashi M, Gage FH, Verma IM. Stable and efficient gene transfer into the retina using an HIV-based lentiviral vector. *Proc Natl Acad Sci U S A* 1997;94:10319.
21. Berkner KL. Expression of heterologous sequences in adenoviral vectors. *Curr Top Microbiol Immunol* 1992;158:39.
22. Rosenfeld MA, Yoshimura K, Trapnell BC, et al. *In vivo* transfer of the human cystic fibrosis transmembrane conductance regulator gene to the airway epithelium. *Cell* 1992;68:143.
23. Yei S, Mittereder N, Wert S, et al. *In vivo* evaluation of the safety of adenovirus-mediated transfer of the human cystic fibrosis transmembrane conductance regulator cDNA to the lung. *Hum Gene Ther* 1994;5:733.
24. Yei S, Mittereder N, Tank K, O'Sullivan C, Trapnell BC. Adenovirus-mediated gene transfer for cystic fibrosis: quantitative evaluation of repeated *in vivo* vector administration to the lung. *Gene Ther* 1994;1:192.
25. Yang Y, Nunes FA, Berencsi K, et al. Cellular immunity to viral antigens limits E1 deleted adenoviruses for gene therapy. *Proc Natl Acad Sci U S A* 1994;91:4407.
26. Rosenberg SA, Zhai Y, Yang JC, et al. Immunizing patients with metastatic melanoma using recombinant adenoviruses encoding MART-1 or gp100 melanoma antigens. *J Natl Cancer Inst* 1998;90:1894.
27. Gahery-Segard H, Molinier-Frenkel V, Le Boulaire C, et al. Phase I trial of recombinant adenovirus gene transfer in lung cancer. Longitudinal study of the immune responses to transgene and viral products. *J Clin Invest* 1997;100:2218.
28. Burcin MM, Schiedner G, Kochanek S, Tsai SY, O'Malley BW. Adenovirus-mediated regulable target gene expression *in vivo*. *Proc Natl Acad Sci U S A* 1999;96:355.
29. Wickham TJ, Tzeng E, Shears LL, et al. Increased *in vitro* and *in vivo* gene transfer by adenovirus vectors containing chimeric fiber proteins. *J Virol* 1997;71:8221.
30. Wickham TJ, Carrion ME, Kovesdi I. Targeting of adenovirus penton base to new receptors through replacement of its RGD motif with other receptor-specific peptide motifs. *Gene Ther* 1995;2:750.
31. Michael SI, Hong JS, Curiel DT, Engler JA. Addition of a short peptide ligand to the adenovirus fiber protein. *Gene Ther* 1995;2:660.
32. Wickham TJ, Segal DM, Roelvink PW, et al. Targeted adenovirus gene transfer to endothelial and smooth muscle cells by using bispecific antibodies. *J Virol* 1996;70:6831.
33. Douglas JT, Rogers BE, Rosenfeld ME, et al. Targeted gene delivery by tropism-modified adenoviral vectors. *Nat Biotechnol* 1996;14:1574.
34. Muzyczka N. Use of adeno-associated virus as a general transduction vector for mammalian cells. *Curr Top Microbiol Immunol* 1992;158:97.
35. Collaco RF, Cao X, Trempe JP. A helper virus-free packaging system for recombinant adeno-associated virus vectors. *Gene* 1999;238:397.
36. Inoue N, Russell DW. Packaging cells based on inducible gene amplification for the production of adeno-associated virus vectors. *J Virol* 1998;72:7024.
37. Lieber A, Steinwaerder DS, Carlson CA, Kay MA. Integrating adenovirus-adeno-associated virus hybrid vectors devoid of all viral genes. *J Virol* 1999;73:9314.
38. Recchia A, Parks RJ, Lamartina S, et al. Site-specific integration mediated by a hybrid adenovirus/adeno-associated virus vector. *Proc Natl Acad Sci U S A* 1999;96:2615.
39. Moss B. Vaccinia virus vectors. *Biotechnology* 1992;20:345.
40. Moss B. Poxvirus expression vectors. *Curr Top Microbiol Immunol* 1992;158:25.
41. Jenkins S, Gritz L, Fedor CH, et al. Formation of lentivirus particles by mammalian cells infected with recombinant fowlpox virus. *AIDS Res Hum Retroviruses* 1991;7:991.
42. Spehner D, Drillien R, Lecocq JP. Construction of fowlpox virus vectors with intergenic insertions: expression of the beta-galactosidase gene and the measles virus fusion gene. *J Virol* 1990;64:527.
43. Wild F, Giraudon P, Spehner D, Drillien R, Lecocq JP. Fowlpox virus recombinant encoding the measles virus fusion protein: protection of mice against fatal measles encephalitis. *Vaccine* 1990;8:441.
44. Felgner PL, Ringold GM. Cationic liposome-mediated transfection. *Nature* 1989;337:387.
45. Stribling R, Brunette E, Liggitt D, Gaensler K, Debs R. Aerosol gene delivery *in vivo*. *Proc Natl Acad Sci U S A* 1992;89:11277.
46. Galanis E, Hersh EM, Stopeck AT, et al. Immunotherapy of advanced malignancy by direct gene transfer of an interleukin-2 DNA/DMRIE/DOPE lipid complex: phase I/II experience. *J Clin Oncol* 1999;17:3313.
47. Stopeck AT, Hersh EM, Akporiaye ET, et al. Phase I study of direct gene transfer of an allogeneic histocompatibility antigen, HLA-B7, in patients with metastatic melanoma. *J Clin Oncol* 1997;15:341.
48. Nabel GJ, Gordon D, Bishop DK, et al. Immune response in human melanoma after transfer of an allogeneic class I major histocompatibility complex gene with DNA-liposome complexes. *Proc Natl Acad Sci U S A* 1996;93:15388.
49. Truong-Le VL, August JT, Leong KW. Controlled gene delivery by DNA-gelatin nanospheres. *Hum Gene Ther* 1998;9:1709.
50. Yang NS, Burkholder J, Roberts B, Martinell B, McCabe D. *In vivo* and *in vitro* gene transfer to mammalian somatic cells by particle bombardment. *Proc Natl Acad Sci U S A* 1990;87:9568.
51. Wolff JA, Malone RW, Williams P, et al. Direct gene transfer into mouse muscle *in vivo*. *Science* 1990;247:1465.
52. Sikes M, O'Malley BW, Finegold MJ, Ledley FD. *In vivo* gene transfer into rabbit thyroid follicular cells by direct DNA injection. *Hum Gene Ther* 1994;5:827.
53. Kasid A, Morecki S, Aebersold P, et al. Human gene transfer: characterization of human tumor-infiltrating lymphocytes as vehicles for retroviral-mediated gene transfer in man. *Proc Natl Acad Sci U S A* 1990;87:473.
54. Rosenberg SA, Aebersold P, Cornetta K, et al. Gene transfer into humans—immunotherapy of patients with advanced melanoma, using tumor-infiltrating lymphocytes modified by retroviral gene transduction. *N Engl J Med* 1990;323:570.
55. Rosenberg SA, Anderson WF, Blaese M, et al. The development of gene therapy for the treatment of cancer. *Ann Surg* 1993;218:455.
56. Favrot MC, Philip T. Treatment of patients with advanced cancer using tumor infiltrating lymphocytes transduced with the gene of resistance to neomycin. *Hum Gene Ther* 1992;3:533.
57. Lotze MT. The treatment of patients with melanoma using interleukin-2, interleukin-4 and tumor infiltrating lymphocytes. *Hum Gene Ther* 1992;3:167.
58. Miller AR, Skotzko MJ, Rhoades K, et al. Simultaneous use of two retroviral vectors in human gene marking trials: feasibility and potential applications. *Hum Gene Ther* 1992;3:619.
59. Brenner MK, Rill DR, Holladay MS, et al. Gene marking to determine whether autologous marrow infusion restores long-term haemopoiesis in cancer patients. *Lancet* 1993;342:1134.
60. Riddell SR, Greenberg PD, Overell RW, et al. Phase I study of cellular adoptive immunotherapy using genetically modified CD8+ HIV-specific T cells for HIV seropositive patients undergoing allogeneic bone marrow transplant. The Fred Hutchinson Cancer Research Center and the University of Washington School of Medicine, Department of Medicine, Division of Oncology. *Hum Gene Ther* 1992;3:319.
61. Heslop HE, Ng CY, Li C, et al. Long-term restoration of immunity against Epstein-Barr virus infection by adoptive transfer of gene-modified virus-specific T lymphocytes. *Nat Med* 1996;2:551.
62. Brodie SJ, Lewinsohn DA, Patterson BK, et al. *In vivo* migration and function of transferred HIV-1-specific cytotoxic T cells [see comments]. *Nat Med* 1999;5:34.
63. Brenner MK, Rill DR, Moen RC, et al. Gene marking and autologous bone marrow transplantation. *Ann N Y Acad Sci* 1994;716:204; discussion 214.
64. Brenner MK, Rill DR, Heslop HE, et al. Gene marking after bone marrow transplantation. *Eur J Cancer* 1994;30A:1171.
65. Brenner MK, Rill DR, Moen RC, et al. Gene-marking to trace origin of relapse after autologous bone-marrow transplantation. *Lancet* 1993;341:85.
66. Rill DR, Santana VM, Roberts WM, et al. Direct demonstration that autologous bone marrow transplantation for solid tumors can return a multiplicity of tumorigenic cells. *Blood* 1994;84:380.
67. Deisseroth AB, Zu Z, Claxton D, et al. Genetic marking shows that Ph+ cells present in autologous transplants of CML contribute to relapse after autologous bone marrow in CML. *Blood* 1994;83:3068.
68. Brenner M, Krance R, Heslop HE, et al. Assessment of the efficacy of purging by using gene marked autologous marrow transplantation for children with AML in first complete remission. *Hum Gene Ther* 1994;5:481.
69. Kirkland MA, O'Brien SG, McDonald C, et al. BCR-ABL antisense purging in chronic myeloid leukaemia [Letter]. *Lancet* 1993;342:614.
70. Gewirtz AM. Potential therapeutic applications of antisense oligodeoxynucleotides in the treatment of chronic myelogenous leukemia. *Leuk Lymphoma* 1993;11[Suppl 1]:131.
71. de Fabritiis P, Amadori S, Calabretta B, Mandelli F. Elimination of clonogenic Philadelphia-positive cells using BCR-ABL antisense oligodeoxynucleotides. *Bone Marrow Transplant* 1993;12:261.
72. Yuan T, Zhou YQ, Herst CV, et al. Molecular approaches to purging of chronic myelogenous leukemia marrow in autologous transplantation. *Prog Clin Biol Res* 1992;377:227.
73. Gewirtz AM. Bone marrow purging with antisense oligodeoxynucleotides. *Prog Clin Biol Res* 1992;377:215; discussion 225.
74. Kawakami Y, Eliyahu S, Sakaguchi K, et al. Identification of the immunodominant peptides of the MART-1 human melanoma antigen recognized by the majority of HLA-A2-restricted tumor infiltrating lymphocytes. *J Exp Med* 1994;180:347.
75. Kawakami Y, Eliyahu S, Delgado CH, et al. Cloning of the gene coding for a shared human melanoma antigen recognized by autologous T cells infiltrating into tumor. *Proc Natl Acad Sci U S A* 1994;91:3515.
76. Kawakami Y, Eliyahu S, Delgado CH, et al. Identification of a melanoma antigen recognized by tumor infiltrating lymphocytes associated with *in vivo* tumor rejection. *Proc Natl Acad Sci U S A* 1994;91:6458.

77. Van Der Bruggen P, Traversari C, Chomez P, et al. A gene encoding an antigen recognized by cytolytic T lymphocytes on a human melanoma. *Science* 1991;254:1643.
78. Brichard V, Van Pel A, Wölfel T, et al. The tyrosinase gene codes for an antigen recognized by autologous cytolytic T lymphocytes on HLA-A2 melanomas. *J Exp Med* 1993;178:489.
79. Wang RF, Robbins PF, Kawakami Y, Kang XQ, Rosenberg SA. Identification of a gene encoding a melanoma tumor antigen recognized by HLA-A31-restricted tumor-infiltrating lymphocytes [published erratum appears in *J Exp Med* 1995;181:1261]. *J Exp Med* 1995;181:799.
80. Robbins PF, el-Gamil M, Li YF, et al. Cloning of a new gene encoding an antigen recognized by melanoma-specific HLA-A24-restricted tumor-infiltrating lymphocytes. *J Immunol* 1995;154:5944.
81. Robbins PF, el-Gamil M, Kawakami Y, et al. Recognition of tyrosinase by tumor-infiltrating lymphocytes from a patient responding to immunotherapy [published erratum appears in *Cancer Res* 1994;54:3952]. *Cancer Res* 1994;54:3124.
82. Fearon E, Pardoll D, Itaya T, et al. Interleukin-2 production by tumor cells bypasses T helper function in the generation of an antitumor response. *Cell* 1990;60:397.
83. Gansbacher B, Zier K, Daniels B, et al. Interleukin 2 gene transfer into tumor cells abrogates tumorigenicity and induces protective immunity. *J Exp Med* 1990;172:1217.
84. Connor J, Bannerji R, Saito S, et al. Regression of bladder tumors in mice treated with interleukin 2 gene-modified tumor cells [published erratum appears in *J Exp Med* 1993;177:following 1831]. *J Exp Med* 1993;177:1127.
85. Stewart AK, Lassam NJ, Quirt IC, et al. Adenovector-mediated gene delivery of interleukin-2 in metastatic breast cancer and melanoma: results of a phase 1 clinical trial. *Gene Ther* 1999;6:350.
86. Palmer K, Moore J, Everard M, et al. Gene therapy with autologous, interleukin 2–secreting tumor cells in patients with malignant melanoma. *Hum Gene Ther* 1999;10:1261.
87. Sobol RE, Shawler DL, Carson C, et al. Interleukin 2 gene therapy of colorectal carcinoma with autologous irradiated tumor cells and genetically engineered fibroblasts: a phase I study. *Clin Cancer Res* 1999;5:2359.
88. Dranoff G, Jaffee E, Lazenby A, et al. Vaccination with irradiated tumor cells engineered to secrete murine granulocyte-macrophage colony-stimulating factor stimulates potent, specific, and long-lasting anti-tumor immunity. *Proc Natl Acad Sci U S A* 1993;90:3539.
89. Huang AY, Golumbek P, Ahmadzadeh M, et al. Role of bone marrow-derived cells in presenting MHC class I–restricted tumor antigens. *Science* 1994;264:961.
90. Hung K, Hayashi R, Lafond-Walker A, et al. The central role of CD4(+) T cells in the antitumor immune response. *J Exp Med* 1998;188:2357.
91. Simons JW, Jaffee EM, Weber CE, et al. Bioactivity of autologous irradiated renal cell carcinoma vaccines generated by *ex vivo* granulocyte-macrophage colony-stimulating factor gene transfer. *Cancer Res* 1997;57:1537.
92. Soiffer R, Lynch T, Mihm M, et al. Vaccination with irradiated autologous melanoma cells engineered to secrete human granulocyte-macrophage colony-stimulating factor generates potent antitumor immunity in patients with metastatic melanoma. *Proc Natl Acad Sci U S A* 1998;95:13141.
93. Simons JW, Mikhak B, Chang JF, et al. Induction of immunity to prostate cancer antigens: results of a clinical trial of vaccination with irradiated autologous prostate tumor cells engineered to secrete granulocyte-macrophage colony-stimulating factor using *ex vivo* gene transfer. *Cancer Res* 1999;59:5160.
94. Ogasawara M, Rosenberg SA. Enhanced expression of HLA molecules and stimulation of autologous human tumor infiltrating lymphocytes following transduction of melanoma cells with gamma-interferon genes. *Cancer Res* 1993;53:3561.
95. Watanabe Y, Kuribayashi K, Miyatake S, et al. Exogenous expression of mouse interferon gamma cDNA in mouse neuroblastoma C1300 cells results in reduced tumorigenicity by augmented anti-tumor immunity. *Proc Natl Acad Sci U S A* 1989;86:9456.
96. Restifo NP, Spiess PJ, Karp SE, Mule JJ, Rosenberg SA. A nonimmunogenic sarcoma transduced with the cDNA for interferon-gamma elicits CD8+ T cells against the wild-type tumor: correlation with antigen presentation capability. *J Exp Med* 1992;175:1423.
97. Asher AL, Mule JJ, Kasid A, et al. Murine tumor cells transduced with the gene for tumor necrosis factor-alpha. Evidence for paracrine immune effects of tumor necrosis factor against tumors. *J Immunol* 1991;146:3227.
98. Blankenstein T, Qin Z, Uberla K. Tumor suppression after tumor cell–targeted tumor necrosis factor alpha gene transfer. *J Exp Med* 1991;173:1047.
99. Teng MN, Park BH, Koeppen HKW. Long-term inhibition of tumor growth by tumor necrosis factor in the absence of cachexia or T-cell immunity. *Proc Natl Acad Sci U S A* 1991;88:3535.
100. Marincola FM, Ettinghausen SE, Cohen PA, et al. Treatment of established lung metastases with tumor-infiltrating lymphocytes derived from a poorly immunogenic tumor engineered to secrete hTNF-alpha. *J Immunol* 1994;152:3500.
101. Douvdevani A, Huleihel M, Zöller M, Segal S, Apte RN. Reduced tumorigenicity of fibrosarcomas which constitutively generate IL-1 alpha either spontaneously or following IL-1 alpha gene transfer. *Int J Cancer* 1992;51:822.
102. Tepper R, Pattengale P, Leder P. Murine interleukin-4 displays potent anti-tumor activity *in vivo*. *Cell* 1989;57:503.
103. Tepper RI, Coffman RL, Leder P. An eosinophil-dependent mechanism for the antitumor effect of interleukin-4. *Science* 1992;257:548.
104. Golumbek P, Lazenby A, Levitsky H, Jaffee E. Treatment of established renal cancer by tumor cells engineered to secrete interleukin-4. *Science* 1991;254:713.
105. Mullen CA, Coale MM, Levy AT, et al. Fibrosarcoma cells transduced with the IL-6 gene exhibited reduced tumorigenicity, increased immunogenicity, and decreased metastatic potential. *Cancer Res* 1992;52:6020.
106. Sun WH, Kreisle RA, Phillips AW, Ershler WB. *In vivo* and *in vitro* characteristics of interleukin 6-transfected B16 melanoma cells. *Cancer Res* 1992;52:5412.
107. Porgador A, Tzehoval E, Katz A, et al. Interleukin 6 gene transfection into Lewis lung carcinoma tumor cells suppresses the malignant phenotype and confers immunotherapeutic competence against parental metastatic cells. *Cancer Res* 1992;52:3679.
108. McBride WH, Thacker JD, Comora S, et al. Genetic modification of a murine fibrosarcoma to produce interleukin 7 stimulates host cell infiltration and tumor immunity. *Cancer Res* 1992;52:3931.
109. Hock H, Dorsch M, Diamantstein T, Blankenstein T. Interleukin 7 induces CD4+ T cell-dependent tumor rejection. *J Exp Med* 1991;174:1291.
110. Aoki T, Tashiro K, Miyatake S, et al. Expression of murine interleukin 7 in a murine glioma cell line results in reduced tumorigenicity *in vivo*. *Proc Natl Acad Sci U S A* 1992;89:3850.
111. Lebel-Binay S, Laguerre B, Quintin-Colonna F, et al. Experimental gene therapy of cancer using tumor cells engineered to secrete interleukin-13. *Eur J Immunol* 1995;25:2340.
112. Colombo MP, Ferrari G, Stoppacciaro A, et al. Granulocyte colony-stimulating factor gene transfer suppresses tumorigenicity of a murine adenocarcinoma *in vivo*. *J Exp Med* 1991;173:889.
113. Rollins BJ, Sunday ME. Suppression of tumor formation *in vivo* by expression of the JE gene in malignant cells. *Mol Cell Biol* 1991;11:3125.
114. Bottazzi B, Walter S, Govoni D, Colotta F, Mantovani A. Monocyte chemotactic cytokine gene transfer modulates macrophage infiltration, growth, and susceptibility to IL-2 therapy of a murine melanoma. *J Immunol* 1992;148:1280.
115. Mule JJ, Custer MC, Averbook B, et al. RANTES secretion by gene-modified tumor cells results in loss of tumorigenicity *in vivo*: role of immune cell subpopulations. *Hum Gene Ther* 1996;7:1545.
116. Tahara H, Zitvogel L, Storkus W, et al. Effective eradication of established murine tumors with IL-12 gene therapy using a polycistronic retroviral vector. *J Immunol* 1995;154:6466.
117. Hock H, Dorsch M, Kunzendorf U, et al. Vaccinations with tumor cells genetically engineered to produce different cytokines: effectivity not superior to a classical adjuvant. *Cancer Res* 1993;53:714.
118. Linsley PS, Clark EA, Ledbetter JA. T-cell antigen CD28 mediates adhesion with B cells by interacting with activation antigen B7/BB-1. *Proc Natl Acad Sci U S A* 1990;87:5031.
119. Chen L, Ashe S, Brady WA, et al. Costimulation of antitumor immunity by the B7 counterreceptor for the T lymphocyte molecules CD28 and CTLA-4. *Cell* 1992;71:1093.
120. Townsend SE, Allison JP. Tumor rejection after direct costimulation of CD8+ T cells by B7-transfected melanoma cells [see comments]. *Science* 1993;259:368.
121. Baskar S, Ostrand-Rosenberg S, Nabavi N, et al. Constitutive expression of B7 restores immunogenicity of tumor cells expressing truncated major histocompatibility complex class II molecules. *Proc Natl Acad Sci U S A* 1993;90:5687.
122. Chen L, McGowan P, Ashe S, et al. Tumor immunogenicity determines the effect of B7 costimulation on T cell-mediated tumor immunity. *J Exp Med* 1994;179:523.
123. Plautz GE, Yang ZY, Wu BY, et al. Immunotherapy of malignancy by *in vivo* gene transfer into tumors [see comments]. *Proc Natl Acad Sci U S A* 1993;90:4645.
124. Irvine KR, McCabe BJ, Rosenberg SA, Restifo NP. Synthetic oligonucleotide expressed by a recombinant vaccinia virus elicits therapeutic CTL. *J Immunol* 1995;154:4651.
125. Wang M, Bronte V, Chen PW, et al. Active immunotherapy of cancer with a nonreplicating recombinant fowlpox virus encoding a model tumor-associated antigen. *J Immunol* 1995;154:4685.
126. McCabe BJ, Irvine KR, Nishimura M, et al. Minimal determinant expressed by a recombinant vaccinia virus elicits therapeutic antitumor cytolytic T lymphocyte responses. *Cancer Res* 1995;55:1741.
127. Bronte V, Tsung K, Rao J, et al. IL-2 enhances the function of recombinant poxvirus-based vaccines in the treatment of established pulmonary metastases. *J Immunol* 1995;154:5282.
128. Celluzzi CM, Mayordomo JI, Storkus WJ, Lotze MT, Falo LD. Peptide-pulsed dendritic cells induce antigen-specific CTL-mediated protective immunity. *J Exp Med* 1996;183:283.
129. Nestle FO, Alijagic S, Gilliet M, et al. Vaccination of melanoma patients with peptide- or tumor lysate–pulsed dendritic cells. *Nat Med* 1998;4:328.
130. Inaba K, Inaba M, Romani N, et al. Generation of large numbers of dendritic cells from mouse bone marrow cultures supplemented with granulocyte/macrophage colony-stimulating factor. *J Exp Med* 1992;176:1693.
131. Specht J, Wang G, Do M, et al. Dendritic cells retrovirally transduced with a model antigen gene are therapeutically effective against established pulmonary metastases. *J Exp Med* 1997;186:1213.
132. Reeves ME, Royal RE, Lam JS, Rosenberg SA, Hwu P. Retroviral transduction of human dendritic cells with a tumor-associated antigen gene. *Cancer Res* 1996;56:5672.
133. Alijagic S, Moller P, Artuc M, et al. Dendritic cells generated from peripheral blood transfected with human tyrosinase induce specific T cell activation. *Eur J Immunol* 1995;25:3100.
134. Kaplan JM, Yu Q, Piraino ST, et al. Induction of antitumor immunity with dendritic cells transduced with adenovirus vector–encoding endogenous tumor-associated antigens. *J Immunol* 1999;163:699.
135. Song W, Kong HL, Carpenter H, et al. Dendritic cells genetically modified with an adenovirus vector encoding the cDNA for a model antigen induce protective and therapeutic antitumor immunity. *J Exp Med* 1997;186:1247.
136. Bhardwaj N, Bender A, Gonzalez N, et al. Influenza virus–infected dendritic cells stimulate strong proliferative and cytolytic responses from human CD8+ T cells. *J Clin Invest* 1994;94:797.
137. Rosenberg SA, Packard BS, Aebersold PM, et al. Use of tumor infiltrating lymphocytes and interleukin-2 in the immunotherapy of patients with metastatic melanoma. Preliminary report. *N Engl J Med* 1988;319:1676.
138. Walter EA, Greenberg PD, Gilbert MJ, et al. Reconstitution of cellular immunity against cytomegalovirus in recipients of allogeneic bone marrow by transfer of T-cell clones from the donor. *N Engl J Med* 1995;333:1038.
139. Drobyski WR, Keever CA, Roth MS, et al. Salvage immunotherapy using donor leukocyte infusions as treatment for relapsed chronic myelogenous leukemia after allogeneic bone marrow transplantation: efficacy and toxicity of a defined T-cell dose. *Blood* 1993;82:2310.

140. Shu S, Chou T, Rosenberg SA. *In vitro* sensitization and expansion with viable tumor cells and interleukin-2 in the generation of specific therapeutic effector cells. *J Immunol* 1986;136:3891.
141. Yamada G, Kitamura Y, Sonoda H, et al. Retroviral expression of the human IL-2 gene in a murine T cell line results in cell growth autonomy and tumorigenicity. *EMBO J* 1987;6:2705.
142. Karasuyama H, Tohyama N, Tada T. Autocrine growth and tumorigenicity of interleukin 2–dependent helper T cells transfected with IL-2 gene. *J Exp Med* 1989;169:13.
143. Treisman J, Hwu P, Minamoto S, et al. Interleukin-2-transduced lymphocytes grow in an autocrine fashion and remain responsive to antigen. *Blood* 1995;85:139.
144. Kuwana Y, Asakura Y, Utsunomiya N, et al. Expression of chimeric receptor composed of immunoglobulin-derived V regions and T-cell receptor–derived C regions. *Biochem Biophys Res Commun* 1987;149:960.
145. Gross G, Waks T, Eshhar Z. Expression of immunoglobulin–T-cell receptor chimeric molecules as functional receptors with antibody-type specificity. *Proc Natl Acad Sci U S A* 1989;86:10024.
146. Hwu P, Schwarz S, Custer M, et al. Use of soluble recombinant TNF receptor to improve detection of TNF secretion in cultures of tumor infiltrating lymphocytes. *J Immunol Methods* 1992;151:139.
147. Goverman J, Gomez SM, Segesman KD, et al. Chimeric immunoglobulin–T cell receptor proteins form functional receptors: implications for T cell receptor complex formation and activation. *Cell* 1990;60:929.
148. Eshhar Z, Waks T, Gross G, Schindler D. Specific activation and targeting of cytotoxic lymphocytes through chimeric single chains consisting of antibody-binding domains and the gamma or zeta subunits of the immunoglobulin and T-cell receptors. *Proc Natl Acad Sci U S A* 1993;90:720.
149. Hwu P, Shafer GE, Treisman J, et al. Lysis of ovarian cancer cells by human lymphocytes redirected with a chimeric gene composed of an antibody variable region and the Fc receptor gamma chain. *J Exp Med* 1993;178:361.
150. Huston JS, Levinson D, Mudgett-Hunter M, et al. Protein engineering of antibody binding sites: recovery of specific activity in an anti-digoxin single-chain Fv analogue produced in *Escherichia coli*. *Proc Natl Acad Sci U S A* 1988;85:5879.
151. Bird RE, Hardman KD, Jacobson JW, et al. Single-chain antigen-binding proteins. *Science* 1988;242:423.
152. Bird RE, Walker BW. Single chain antibody variable regions. *Trends Biotechnol* 1991;9:132.
153. Orloff D, Ra C, Frank SJ, Klausner RD, Kinet JP. Family of disulphide-linked dimers containing the zeta and eta chains of the T-cell receptor and the gamma chain of Fc receptors. *Nature* 1990;347:189.
154. Letourneur F, Klausner RD. T-cell and basophil activation through the cytoplasmic tail of T-cell-receptor zeta family proteins. *Proc Natl Acad Sci U S A* 1991;88:8905.
155. Romeo C, Amiot M, Seed B. Sequence requirements for induction of cytolysis by the T cell antigen/Fc receptor zeta chain. *Cell* 1992;68:889.
156. Romeo C, Seed B. Cellular immunity to HIV activated by CD4 fused to T cell or Fc receptor polypeptides. *Cell* 1991;64:1037.
157. Irving BA, Weiss A. The cytoplasmic domain of the T cell receptor zeta chain is sufficient to couple to receptor-associated signal transduction pathways. *Cell* 1991;64:891.
158. Coney LR, Tomassetti A, Carayannopoulos L, et al. Cloning of a tumor-associated antigen: MOv18 and MOv19 antibodies recognize a folate-binding protein. *Cancer Res* 1991;51:6125.
159. Miotti S, Canevari S, Ménard S, et al. Characterization of human ovarian carcinoma–associated antigens defined by novel monoclonal antibodies with tumor-restricted specificity. *Int J Cancer* 1987;39:297.
160. Hwu P, Yang JC, Cowherd R, et al. *In vivo* antitumor activity of T-cells redirected with chimeric antibody/T-cell receptor genes. *Cancer Res* 1995;55:3369.
161. Krause A. Antigen-dependent CD28 signaling selectively enhances survival and proliferation in genetically modified activated human primary T lymphocytes. *J Exp Med* 1998;188:619.
162. Wang G. A T cell-independent antitumor response in mice with bone marrow cells retrovirally transduced with an antibody/Fc-gamma chain chimeric receptor gene recognizing a human ovarian cancer antigen. *Nat Med* 1998;4:168.
163. Stancovski I, Schindler DG, Waks T, et al. Targeting of T lymphocytes to Neu/HER2-expressing cells using chimeric single chain Fv receptors. *J Immunol* 1993;151:6577.
164. Daly T, Royal RE, Kershaw MH, et al. Recognition of human colon cancer by T cells transduced with a chimeric receptor gene. *Cancer Gene Ther* 2000;7:284.
165. Finer MH, Dull TJ, Qin L, Farson D, Roberts MR. kat: a high-efficiency retroviral transduction system for primary human T lymphocytes. *Blood* 1994;83:43.
166. Cole DJ, Weil DP, Shilyansky J, et al. Characterization of the functional specificity of a cloned T-cell receptor heterodimer recognizing the MART-1 melanoma antigen. *Cancer Res* 1995;55:748.
167. Clay TM, Custer M, Sachs J, et al. Efficient transfer of a tumor antigen-reactive TCR to human peripheral blood lymphocytes confers anti-tumor reactivity. *J Immunol* 1999;163:507.
168. Bonini C, Ferrari G, Verzeletti S, et al. HSV-TK gene transfer into donor lymphocytes for control of allogeneic graft-versus-leukemia [see comments]. *Science* 1997;276:1719.
169. Riddell SR, Elliott M, Lewinsohn DA, et al. T-cell mediated rejection of gene-modified HIV-specific cytotoxic T lymphocytes in HIV-infected patients [see comments]. *Nat Med* 1996;2:216.
170. Haranaka K, Satomi N, Sakurai A. Antitumor activity of murine tumor necrosis factor (TNF) against transplanted murine tumors and heterotransplanted human tumors in nude mice. *Int J Cancer* 1984;34:263.
171. Creasey A, Reynolds MT, Laird W. Cures and partial regression of murine and human tumors by recombinant human tumor necrosis factor. *Cancer Res* 1986;46:5687.
172. Asher A, Mulé J, Reichert C, Shiloni E, Rosenberg SA. Studies on the anti-tumor efficacy of systemically administered recombinant tumor necrosis factor against several murine tumors *in vivo*. *J Immunol* 1987;138:963.
173. Feinberg B, Kurzrock R, Talpaz M, et al. A phase I trial of intravenously-administered recombinant tumor necrosis factor-alpha in cancer patients. *J Clin Oncol* 1988;6:1328.
174. Moritz T, Niederle N, Baumann J, et al. Phase I study of recombinant human tumor necrosis factor α in advanced malignant disease. *Cancer Immunol Immunother* 1989;29:144.
175. Rosenberg SA, Lotze M, Yang J, et al. Experience with the use of high-dose interleukin-2 in the treatment of 652 cancer patients. *Ann Surg* 1989;210:474.
176. Sherman M, Spriggs D, Arthur K, et al. Recombinant human tumor necrosis factor administered as a five-day continuous infusion in cancer patients: phase I toxicity and effects on lipid metabolism. *J Clin Oncol* 1988;6:344.
177. Spriggs D, Sherman M, Michie H, et al. Recombinant human tumor necrosis factor administered as a 24-hour intravenous infusion. A phase I and pharmacologic study. *J Natl Cancer Inst* 1988;80:1039.
178. Bartsch H, Pfizenmaier K, Schroeder M, Nagel G. Intralesional application of recombinant human tumor necrosis factor alpha induces local tumor regression in patients with advanced malignancies. *Eur J Cancer Clin Oncol* 1989;25:287.
179. Kahn JO, Kaplan LD, Volberding PA, et al. Intralesional recombinant tumor necrosis factor-alpha for AIDS-associated Kaposi's sarcoma: a randomized, double-blind trial. *J Acquir Immune Defic Syndr* 1989;2:217.
180. Lienard D, Ewalenko P, Delmotte J, Renard N, Lejeune F. High-dose recombinant tumor necrosis factor alpha in combination with interferon gamma and melphalan in isolation perfusion of the limbs for melanoma and sarcoma. *J Clin Oncol* 1992;10:52.
181. Fraker DL, Alexander HR. The use of tumour necrosis factor (TNF) in isolated perfusion: results and side effects. The NCI results. *Melanoma Res* 1994;4[Suppl 1]:27.
182. Fisher B, Packard B, Read E, et al. Tumor localization of adoptively transferred indium-111 labeled tumor infiltrating lymphocytes in patients with metastatic melanoma. *J Clin Oncol* 1989;7:250.
183. Griffith KD, Read EJ, Carrasquillo JA, et al. *In vivo* distribution of adoptively transferred indium-111 labeled tumor infiltrating lymphocytes and peripheral blood lymphocytes in patients with metastatic melanoma. *J Natl Cancer Inst* 1989;81:1709.
184. Pockaj BA, Sherry RM, Wei JP, et al. Localization of 111-indium-labelled tumor infiltrating lymphocytes to tumor in patients receiving adoptive immunotherapy. *Cancer* 1994;73:1731.
185. Hwu P, Yannelli J, Kriegler M, et al. Functional and molecular characterization of TIL transduced with the TNFα cDNA for the gene therapy of cancer in man. *J Immunol* 1993;150:4104.
186. Perez C, Albert I, DeFay K, et al. A nonsecretable cell surface mutant of tumor necrosis factor (TNF) kills by cell-to-cell contact. *Cell* 1990;63:251.
187. Kriegler M, Perez C, DeFay K, Albert I, Lu S. A novel form of TNF/cachectin is a cell surface cytotoxic transmembrane protein: ramifications for the complex physiology of TNF. *Cell* 1988;53:45.
188. Tait DL, Obermiller PS, Hatmaker AR, Redlin-Frazier S, Holt JT. Ovarian cancer BRCA1 gene therapy: phase I and II trial differences in immune response and vector stability. *Clin Cancer Res* 1999;5:1708.
189. Roth JA, Nguyen D, Lawrence DD, et al. Retrovirus-mediated wild-type p53 gene transfer to tumors of patients with lung cancer [see comments]. *Nat Med* 1996;2:985.
190. Swisher SG, Roth JA, Nemunaitis J, et al. Adenovirus-mediated p53 gene transfer in advanced non-small-cell lung cancer. *J Natl Cancer Inst* 1999;91:763.
191. Calabretta B. Inhibition of protooncogene expression by antisense oligodeoxynucleotides: biological and therapeutic implications. *Cancer Res* 1991;51:4505.
192. Mercola D, Cohen JS. Antisense approaches to cancer gene therapy. *Cancer Gene Ther* 1995;2:47.
193. Reed JC, Stein C, Subasinghe C, et al. Antisense-mediated inhibition of BCL2 protooncogene expression and leukemic cell growth and survival: comparisons of phosphodiester and phosphorothioate oligodeoxynucleotides. *Cancer Res* 1990;50:6565.
194. Szczylik C, Skorski T, Nicolaides NC, et al. Selective inhibition of leukemia cell proliferation by BCR-ABL antisense oligodeoxynucleotides. *Science* 1991;253:562.
195. McManaway ME, Neckers LM, Loke SL, et al. Tumour-specific inhibition of lymphoma growth by an antisense oligodeoxynucleotide. *Lancet* 1990;335:808.
196. Melani C, Rivoltini L, Parmiani G, Calabretta B, Colombo MP. Inhibition of proliferation by c-myb antisense oligodeoxynucleotides in colon adenocarcinoma cell lines that express c-myb. *Cancer Res* 1991;51:2897.
197. Anfossi G, Gewirtz AM, Calabretta B. An oligomer complementary to c-myb-encoded mRNA inhibits proliferation of human myeloid leukemia cell lines. *Proc Natl Acad Sci U S A* 1989;86:3379.
198. Ratajczak MZ, Kant JA, Luger SM, et al. *In vivo* treatment of human leukemia in a scid mouse model with c-myb antisense oligodeoxynucleotides. *Proc Natl Acad Sci U S A* 1992;89:11823.
199. Higgins KA, Perez JR, Coleman TA, et al. Antisense inhibition of the p65 subunit of NF-kappa B blocks tumorigenicity and causes tumor regression. *Proc Natl Acad Sci U S A* 1993;90:9901.
200. Webb A, Cunningham D, Cotter F, et al. BCL-2 antisense therapy in patients with non-Hodgkin lymphoma. *Lancet* 1997;349:1137.
201. Stein CA. Antisense oligodeoxynucleotides. In: DeVita VT, Hellman S, Rosenberg SA, eds. *Biologic therapy of cancer.* Philadelphia: JB Lippincott, 1995:759.
202. Poeschla E, Wong-Staal F. Antiviral and anticancer ribozymes. *Curr Opin Oncol* 1994;6:601.
203. Culver K, Ram Z, Wallbridge S, et al. *In vivo* gene transfer with retroviral vector-producer cells for treatment of experimental brain tumors. *Science* 1992;256:1550.
204. Ram Z, Culver KW, Oshiro EM, et al. Therapy of malignant brain tumors by intratumoral implantation of retroviral vector-producing cells [see comments]. *Nat Med* 1997;3:1354.
205. Herman JR, Adler HL, Aguilar-Cordova E, et al. *In situ* gene therapy for adenocarcinoma of the prostate: a phase I clinical trial. *Hum Gene Ther* 1999;10:1239.
206. Molnar-Kimber KL, Sterman DH, Chang M, et al. Impact of preexisting and induced humoral and cellular immune responses in an adenovirus-based gene therapy phase I clinical trial for localized mesothelioma. *Hum Gene Ther* 1998;9:2121.

207. Pandha HS, Martin LA, Rigg A, et al. Genetic prodrug activation therapy for breast cancer: a phase I clinical trial of erbB-2-directed suicide gene expression. *J Clin Oncol* 1999;17:2180.
208. Huber BE, Richards CA, Krenitsky TA. Retroviral-mediated gene therapy for the treatment of hepatocellular carcinoma: an innovative approach for cancer therapy. *Proc Natl Acad Sci U S A* 1991;88:8039.
209. Vile RG, Hart IR. *In vitro* and *in vivo* targeting of gene expression to melanoma cells. *Cancer Res* 1993;53:962.
210. Bicknell R. Vascular targeting and the inhibition of angiogenesis. *Ann Oncol* 1994;5[Suppl 4]:45.
211. Bischoff JR, Kirn DH, Williams A, et al. An adenovirus mutant that replicates selectively in p53-deficient human tumor cells [see comments]. *Science* 1996;274:373.
212. Heise C, Sampson-Johannes A, Williams A, et al. ONYX-015, an E1B gene–attenuated adenovirus, causes tumor-specific cytolysis and antitumoral efficacy that can be augmented by standard chemotherapeutic agents [see comments]. *Nat Med* 1997;3:639.
213. Heise CC, Williams AM, Xue S, Propst M, Kirn DH. Intravenous administration of ONYX-015, a selectively replicating adenovirus, induces antitumoral efficacy. *Cancer Res* 1999;59:2623.
214. Rothmann T, Hengstermann A, Whitaker NJ, Scheffner M, zur Hausen H. Replication of ONYX-015, a potential anticancer adenovirus, is independent of p53 status in tumor cells. *J Virol* 1998;72:9470.
215. Hall AR, Dix BR, O'Carroll SJ, Braithwaite AW. p53-dependent cell death/apoptosis is required for a productive adenovirus infection [see comments]. *Nat Med* 1998;4:1068.
216. Gottesman M. How cancer cells evade chemotherapy: sixteenth Richard and Hinda Rosenthal Foundation Award Lecture. *Cancer Res* 1993;53:747.
217. Kane S, Pastan I, Gottesman M. Genetic basis of multidrug resistance of tumor cells. *J Bioenerg Biomembr* 1990;22:593.
218. Sorrentino BP, Brandt SJ, Bodine D, et al. Selection of drug-resistant bone marrow cells *in vivo* after retroviral transfer of human MDR1. *Science* 1992;257:99.
219. Dunbar CE, Kohn DB, Schiffmann R, et al. Retroviral transfer of the glucocerebrosidase gene into CD34+ cells from patients with Gaucher disease: *in vivo* detection of transduced cells without myeloablation. *Hum Gene Ther* 1998;9:2629.
220. Dunbar CE, Young NS. Gene marking and gene therapy directed at primary hematopoietic cells. *Curr Opin Hematol* 1996;3:430.
221. Cowan KH, Moscow JA, Huang H, et al. Paclitaxel chemotherapy after autologous stem-cell transplantation and engraftment of hematopoietic cells transduced with a retrovirus containing the multidrug resistance complementary DNA (MDR1) in metastatic breast cancer patients [see comments]. *Clin Cancer Res* 1999;5:1619.
222. Hesdorffer C, Ayello J, Ward M, et al. Phase I trial of retroviral-mediated transfer of the human MDR1 gene as marrow chemoprotection in patients undergoing high-dose chemotherapy and autologous stem-cell transplantation. *J Clin Oncol* 1998;16:165.
223. Hanania EG, Giles RE, Kavanagh J, et al. Results of MDR-1 vector modification trial indicate that granulocyte/macrophage colony-forming unit cells do not contribute to post-transplant hematopoietic recovery following intensive systemic therapy [published erratum appears in *Proc Natl Acad Sci U S A* 1997;94:5495]. *Proc Natl Acad Sci U S A* 1996;93:15346.
224. Folkman J. Tumor angiogenesis: therapeutic implications. *N Engl J Med* 1971;285:1182.
225. Folkman J. What is the evidence that tumors are angiogenesis dependent? [Editorial]. *J Natl Cancer Inst* 1990;82:4.
226. Feldman AL, Libutti SK. Progress in antiangiogenic gene therapy of cancer. 2000 (*submitted*).
227. Kendall RL, Thomas KA. Inhibition of vascular endothelial cell growth factor activity by an endogenously encoded soluble receptor. *Proc Natl Acad Sci U S A* 1993;90:10705.
228. Kong HL, Hecht D, Song W, et al. Regional suppression of tumor growth by *in vivo* transfer of a cDNA encoding a secreted form of the extracellular domain of the flt-1 vascular endothelial growth factor receptor. *Hum Gene Ther* 1998;9:823.
229. Machein MR, Risau W, Plate KH. Antiangiogenic gene therapy in a rat glioma model using a dominant-negative vascular endothelial growth factor receptor 2. *Hum Gene Ther* 1999;10:1117.
230. Im SA, Gomez-Manzano C, Fueyo J, et al. Antiangiogenesis treatment for gliomas: transfer of antisense-vascular endothelial growth factor inhibits tumor growth *in vivo*. *Cancer Res* 1999;59:895.
231. Linehan WM, Lerman MI, Zbar B. Identification of the von Hippel-Lindau (VHL) gene. Its role in renal cancer. *JAMA* 1995;273:564.
232. Gnarra JR, Zhou S, Merrill MJ, et al. Post-transcriptional regulation of vascular endothelial growth factor mRNA by the product of the VHL tumor suppressor gene. *Proc Natl Acad Sci U S A* 1996;93:10589.
233. Li H, Lu H, Griscelli F, et al. Adenovirus-mediated delivery of a uPA/uPAR antagonist suppresses angiogenesis-dependent tumor growth and dissemination in mice. *Gene Ther* 1998;5:1105.
234. Suri C, Jones PF, Patan S, et al. Requisite role of angiopoietin-1, a ligand for the TIE2 receptor, during embryonic angiogenesis [see comments]. *Cell* 1996;87:1171.
235. Davis S, Aldrich TH, Jones PF, et al. Isolation of angiopoietin-1, a ligand for the TIE2 receptor, by secretion-trap expression cloning [see comments]. *Cell* 1996;87:1161.
236. Lin P, Buxton JA, Acheson A, et al. Antiangiogenic gene therapy targeting the endothelium-specific receptor tyrosine kinase Tie2. *Proc Natl Acad Sci U S A* 1998;95:8829.
237. O'Reilly MS, Boehm T, Shing Y, et al. Endostatin: an endogenous inhibitor of angiogenesis and tumor growth. *Cell* 1997;88:277.
238. O'Reilly MS, Holmgren L, Shing Y, et al. Angiostatin: a novel angiogenesis inhibitor that mediates the suppression of metastases by a Lewis lung carcinoma [see comments]. *Cell* 1994;79:315.
239. Griscelli F, Li H, Bennaceur-Griscelli A, et al. Angiostatin gene transfer: inhibition of tumor growth *in vivo* by blockage of endothelial cell proliferation associated with a mitosis arrest. *Proc Natl Acad Sci U S A* 1998;95:6367.
240. Liu Y, Thor A, Shtivelman E, et al. Systemic gene delivery expands the repertoire of effective antiangiogenic agents. *J Biol Chem* 1999;274:13338.
241. Feldman AL, Restifo NP, Alexander HR, et al. Antiangiogenic gene therapy of cancer utilizing a recombinant adenovirus to elevate systemic endostatin levels in mice. *Cancer Res* 2000;60:1503.
242. Staba MJ, Mauceri HJ, Kufe DW, Hallahan DE, Weichselbaum RR. Adenoviral TNF-alpha gene therapy and radiation damage tumor vasculature in a human malignant glioma xenograft. *Gene Ther* 1998;5:293.
243. Boris-Lawrie K, Temin HM. The retroviral vector: replication cycle and safety considerations for retrovirus-mediated gene therapy. *Ann N Y Acad Sci* 1994;716:59.
244. Miller AD, Rosman GJ. Improved retroviral vectors for gene transfer and expression. *Biotechniques* 1989;7:980.
245. Miller AD, Buttimore C. Redesign of retrovirus packaging cell lines to avoid recombination leading to helper virus production. *Mol Cell Biol* 1986;6:2895.
246. Eglitis MA, Anderson WF. Retroviral vectors for introduction of genes into mammalian cells. *Biotechniques* 1988;6:608.

ALBERT B. DEISSEROTH
AMANDA PSYRRI
DAVID J. AUSTIN

SECTION 2

Molecular Therapy

The modern age of chemotherapy has its origins in ancient civilizations thousands of years ago, when therapists went to the forests to dig up roots, to peel the bark from trees, and to pick the leaves and flowers from plants as the first step in drug development. Through the time-consuming process of trial and error, extracts of these natural substances were identified that conferred a beneficial effect on the natural history of life-threatening diseases, such as cancer. It was not until the middle of the twentieth century that sufficient quantities of the purified active ingredients of these plant extracts were available for clinical trials.

The structure of these plant alkaloids, which were complex polycyclic hydrocarbon molecules, barely soluble in aqueous solvents and associated with very significant toxicities for the central nervous system, the kidney, and the hematopoietic and the gastrointestinal tissues, posed challenges for the therapist. Despite these limitations, plant compounds, such as the epidophyllotoxins, the periwinkle alkaloids, the taxanes, and the camptothecins, have formed the basis of the most successful cancer treatment regimens of the first 30 years of chemotherapy.

Tremendous ingenuity has been displayed by pharmacologists and cancer treatment specialists, who have designed methods for limiting and circumventing the very significant toxicities of these compounds. Chemists working with synthetic organic compounds have continuously attempted to improve on the original natural products, which have spawned synthetic derivative compounds of the original natural products, such as vinorelbine tartrate, taxotere, and irinotecan, which are now displaying exciting patterns of activity in refractory epithelial neoplasms.

The next phase of the development of chemotherapy was the cloning of the genes for naturally occurring biologically active molecules, such as interferon, interleukin-2, and the growth factors. During the last decade of the twentieth century, the enormous power of structural biology and computational chemistry was used to design totally synthetic compounds, which have no relationship to natural products but have displayed exciting activity in disease states: the protease inhibitors for human immunodeficiency virus, the kinase inhibitors for chronic myelocytic leukemia (CML), and the low-molecular-weight chemical inhibitors for virally associated cancers.

Now, at the dawn of the twenty-first century, the power of protein structure analysis, computational chemistry, combinatorial chemistry, and the engineering of biopolymers are being combined to produce an entirely new generation of antineoplastic drugs that are already reaching the clinic.

STRATEGIES OF NEW DRUG DESIGN

TYPES OF TARGETS

The drugs discussed here are those that will be designed to modify the assembly of subunits in a multimeric protein or to alter the assembly of complexes of multiple proteins into a receptor or a multiprotein array that is promoting the formation of a transcription initiation complex or a replication initiation complex. Thus, the ideal types of protein domains as targets for inhibition by low-molecular-weight chemicals must be considered before proceeding to the design of an inhibitor.

ATTRIBUTES OF AN IDEAL TARGET PROTEIN FOR MOLECULAR THERAPY

The attributes of an ideal target protein are outlined in Table 62.2-1. The ideal target for molecular therapy is a protein the sequence of which is unique to the tumor cell and is one that confers a selective growth advantage to the tumor cells. In addition, it is important that the target sequence be present in the tumor cells of all patients with that type of cancer and that 100% of the tumor cells in every patient have the target sequence.

The ideal target is present in 100% of the cells of a tumor population, because the presence of this protein target confers on the cell in which it resides a selective advantage over cells that do not contain this change. This type of target has dual advantages: The inhibition of the function of this target protein will suppress the transformed phenotype and, at the very least, will halt the progression of the disease state. It may also induce cell death of the neoplastic cell.

Another attribute that is important for an ideal target is that it presents some feature unique to the regulatory environment of the tumor cell that is not shared by the normal noncancerous cell. This type of tumor-specific target enhances the probability that an inhibitor will be specifically toxic for the tumor cell and will not adversely affect the normal cells. Examples of targets that are totally unique for the tumor cell include viral oncoproteins (proteins that may not have a correlate in normal mammalian cells), a chimeric gene that produces proteins with protein junctional domains that are not present in normal cells, a mutant primary structure of a widely expressed protein, posttranslational modification of a protein that is unique to the tumor cell, and a protein that is either expressed inappropriately in a particular type of tissue or appears in an intracellular location that is unique to the tumor cell. Table 62.2-2 presents a list of examples of such target oncoproteins that exhibit one or more of these attributes.

In terms of the types of domains in the target protein that are more or less optimal for computational analysis and for interaction with low-molecular-weight chemical inhibitors of protein action, there is general consensus in the field that protein-protein contact regions are very poor regions for modulation by chemical inhibitors. The interactions that represent the contact points for proteins often are hydrophobic areas that are binding to one another through van Der Waals forces. Such forces are at any given point extremely weak in terms of affinity. Thus, the interposition of a chemical that blocks interaction at a single point in this broad surface has very little effect on the overall assembly of a protein.

TABLE 62.2-1. Ideal Attributes of a Target Protein Oncoprotein Domain for Molecular Therapy

STRUCTURE SPECIFICITY
Unique sequence by virtue of mutation, or chimeric junctional regions
Unique intracellular location
Unique pattern of expression
Origin from nonmammalian sources (DNA tumor virus oncoprotein)
PROTEIN DOMAIN
Receptors
Enzyme catalytic pocket
Crevices in DNA binding domains
Interdigitating subunits of a multimeric protein
G protein GTP domain
PREVALENCE IN TUMOR POPULATION
Confers selective advantage on tumor cell
Present in a significant percentage if not 100% of tumor cells
Tumor cell retains dependency on target protein

GTP, guanosine triphosphate.

TABLE 62.2-2. List of Candidate Target Oncoproteins

p210bcrabl
BCL-2
Mutant Myc
Mutant p53
Mutant p16, p27
Mutant RAS
Amplified or mutant growth factor receptor
Mutant p13 kinase
DNA tumor virus oncoproteins
EBNA I or LMP2 of Epstein-Barr virus
E6 and E7 of human papillomavirus

In contrast, receptors or pockets in which the catalytic site of an enzyme is located, or the crevice of a DNA binding domain, or a homodimerization domain that consists of interlocking invaginations, or stacking of flat aromatic amino acid side chains (e.g., tryptophans), which can bind to one another through sharing of electron orbitals, provide the structure within which a low-molecular-weight inhibitor can interact to disrupt a complex. Chemical inhibitors can act at multiple points with the local peptide domains to establish a very stable, high-affinity interaction that can have an impact on the entire protein.

Although receptors or enzyme pockets have a more stable conformation, all these regions of the protein are very mobile and are in continuous motion at the atomic level. Thus, interactions with low-molecular-weight chemical inhibitors may stabilize one of more of the conformations available to a protein domain. Low-molecular-weight chemicals that are designed to be inhibitors can stabilize a nonfunctional or inactive state of the protein. One example is the inactive state of a growth factor or an integrin receptor. Another example is the inactive state of the RAS proteins. A third example is a drug that can stabilize a conformal state of the protein, which limits access of a substrate, inhibits assembly of a multisubunit protein, or reduces the probability of assembly of a transcription initiation complex. Obviously, the more detailed the structural information, the more successful any design effort that is based on structure.

The alternative approach in developing drugs that stabilize one conformal state versus another is to select low-molecular-weight chemicals from a library of thousands of structural variants, each of which differs from the others by single atoms (i.e., two vs. one carbon atom in a side chain, etc.). Thus, the conformation of a chemical that best promotes the stabilization of an inactive conformal state of an enzyme or a receptor can be identified without any information about the structural details of the active and inactive states, merely by generating structural diversity, isolating relevant structures in a binding assay, and then assaying for loss of function of the protein molecules in the presence of that chemical. The same principle applies to the use of phage display libraries of random amino acid peptides. This requires the extra step of using computational and synthetic chemistry to create a chemical mimic of the peptide that produces the desired change in the protein. These two approaches can be combined by biasing the composition of the libraries on the basis of the structural information that exists about the target protein or the domain of the protein that is the contact point for the inhibitor.

Another issue is whether a domain that is in constant motion is a poor or good target as compared to a domain in which the order of the protein is so great as to reduce or restrict the excursions of the atoms and chemical functionalities. Accordingly, programs are available for simulating the possible trajectories of each atom in a biopolymer so that the dimensions of each state at very short expanses of time (nanoseconds) can be used to identify a useful target for engagement by a chemical inhibitor.

Thus, the true power of the use of structural data for drug design is revealed. Not only is there a possibility of identifying chemicals that could be selective for a particular primary amino acid sequence, but the possibility exists of identifying the chemical that is specific for the 1 in 1000 possible conformal states that can be engaged by a particular chemical structure for the purposes of stabilization or destabilization. The library approach exploits this vast expanse of possible targets by interrogating a large number of structural variants which can promote the conformal state of the target that is useful therapeutically.

APPROACHES TO DRUG DESIGN

STRUCTURE ANALYSIS OF TARGET

The recent example of the use of x-ray crystal structure of the human immunodeficiency virus protease for the development of successful drug treatment for the acquired immunodeficiency syndrome (AIDS) has led many researchers to apply this approach to the study of oncoproteins for drug development. The recent success in developing inhibitors of substrate-binding sites and cofactor-binding (adenosine triphosphate–binding) sites in the CML oncoprotein p210bcrabl led to the introduction into the clinic of a selective inhibitor of the p210bcrabl kinase in CML.[1] This new low-molecular-weight chemical inhibitor of CML was developed through the application of a structural model for the analysis of the cofactor-binding site of the p210bcrabl kinase oncoprotein of CML.[1]

MIMICS OF INHIBITORS OR SUBSTRATES

The application of analysis of substrates and mimics of ligands led to the RGD mimic inhibitors of integrin receptors that contribute to the ability of tumor cells to metastasize.[2] Mimics of guanosine triphosphate (GTP) are also being used to develop inhibitors of the membrane RAS signal transduction proteins.[3]

The development of chemical inhibitors of oncoproteins may start from computational analysis of the protein domain binding the cofactor or substrate, or it can start with the screening of combinatorial libraries of chemical mimics of a substrate or naturally occurring inhibitors of an oncoprotein. Alternatively, phage display libraries of random peptides can be used to collect all the peptide sequences that bind to an oncoprotein target.[4] Analysis of the peptide motifs that are associated with high-affinity binding to the target can then lead to the design of mimics of the peptide inhibitors of the oncoprotein.

Substrate Mimics for Tyrosine Kinase Inhibitors for Use in Chronic Myelocytic Leukemia

CML is an ideal disease for the development of molecular therapy, since there is a single genetic change that is absolutely essential for the development of the leukemia, which is present in 100% of the patients and is present in 100% of the cells of each patient.[5]

The first hint that inhibition of an oncoprotein would suppress the phenotype of a neoplastic disease came from the antisense oligonucleotide field.[6] Because CML is a disease of genetic instability and one in which the acquisition of sequential somatic mutations leads to evolution of the clinical phenotype of the disease, it was predicted that antisense oligonucleotides would have activity only in the very earliest stages of the disease process when the genetic complexity of the mutational change within the leukemic cells was lowest. Surprisingly, the anti-p210bcrabl antisense oligonucleotides were active in blast crisis cells both at the very end of the evolution of the disease process and at the very earliest stages of the disease process.[6] These findings now make sense in light of our understanding of the many actions of the p210bcrabl oncoprotein. Two of these pathways are activated within the CML cell. The first is the PI3 kinase/Alt kinase/BAD pathway that results in the release of BCL-2 in the leukemic cells, prolonging survival in the absence of growth factors and extracellular matrix apoptosis rescue ligands and conferring chemotherapy resistance on these cells.[7] The second results in increases in BCL-2 levels inside the CML cells through the GRB-2/RAS/RAF/BAD pathway. These two pathways are important, even at the blast crisis stage, in conferring resistance to chemotherapy on these cells.

The next stage in the evolution of molecular therapy for CML was the discovery that peptide ligands, which are parts of naturally occurring negative regulatory proteins for the abl kinase, could be used to suppress the transformed phenotype of CML cells.[8,9] This work led to the demonstration that expression vectors that carry inhibitory peptide transcription units directed to the ATP-binding sites of the tyrosine-specific protein kinases could also suppress the transformed phenotype of CML cells.[10]

It was a natural extension of these findings to proceed to an examination of chemical inhibitors of either the substrate-binding site or the cofactor-binding (ATP) site of the tyrosine-specific protein kinase oncoproteins in CML. A picture of the catalytic pocket of this oncoprotein is presented in Figure 62.2-1. The tryphostins were the class of compounds found that inhibit tyrosine-specific protein kinases by binding to the substrate-binding site of p210bcrabl.[11] These compounds were shown to decrease the *in vitro* proliferation of CML cells and to sensitize CML cells to the effects of chemotherapy. Interestingly, the tryphostins showed synergy when combined with cytokine therapy of chronic myelogenous leukemia cells.[11]

The next stage of development of chemical inhibitors was to engineer competitive inhibitors for the cofactor-binding (ATP) site of the tyrosine-specific protein kinase–binding site of p210bcrabl. This class of inhibitors is structurally distinct from the tryphostins. These compounds have been refined by Druker et al.,[12] who have introduced STI 571, a low-molecular-weight inhibitor of ATP binding, into the therapy of CML.

Druker et al.[12] have already shown that these compounds *in vitro* are remarkably selective for the abl kinase and are able to reduce the circulating level of the white blood cell count in chronic-phase CML. Although the evaluation of these compounds is still at its early stage, cytogenetic remissions have already been achieved in some chronic-phase patients. In addition, the level of circulating leukemic cells is reduced even in myeloid blast crisis patients. These compounds exhibit inhibitory activity for the abl kinase at micromolar concentrations and are remarkably specific for the abl kinase, showing cross-inhibitory activity only for the platelet-derived growth factor kinase. These compounds are already producing great interest on the part of therapists as a vindication of the use of structural analysis of biopolymers and computational chemistry. The duration of these remissions and the extent to which all chronic-phase patients will exhibit such remissions are the subject of current clinical trials.

Building on this advance, other workers are attempting produce low-molecular-weight inhibitors that are more selective and more effective than the compounds of Druker. At Yale, Austin has proposed (D. J. Austin, personal communication, 1998) that a chemical mimic of ATP can be constructed by attaching adenosine to a bicyclic scaffold molecule, which is a mimic of the triphosphate of ATP (Fig. 62.2-2).

The bicyclic scaffold molecule contains five ligands that can interact with local protein domains in the abl kinase pocket. As shown in Figure 62.2-2, these chemical functionalities can engage multiple local protein domains in the kinase pocket and can be projected into a spherical three-dimensional space through the use of the bicyclic scaffold. In the example pre-

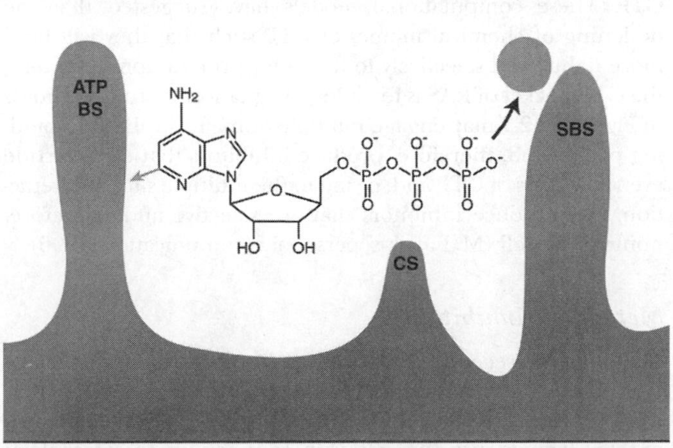

FIGURE 62.2-1. Adenosine triphosphate (ATP) kinase pocket of the p210bcrabl oncoprotein, in which the abl tyrosine-specific protein kinase catalytic site is depicted. This kinase pocket contains a substrate-binding site (SBS), a catalytic site (CS), and a cofactor-binding site (ATP BS). The ATP cofactor is shown donating its gamma high-energy phosphate to the substrate.

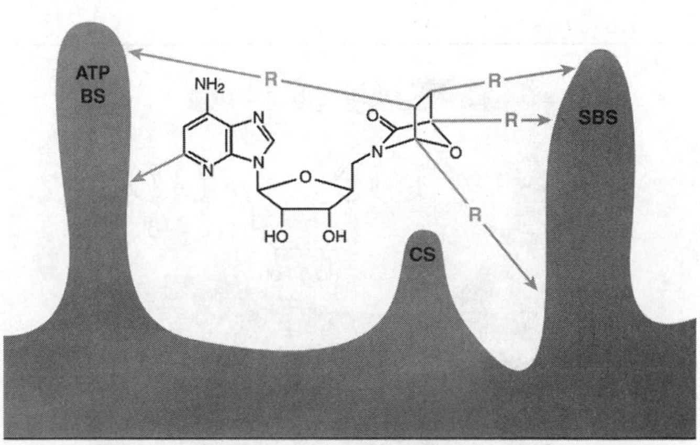

FIGURE 62.2-2. Adenosine-scaffold mimic in the adenosine triphosphate kinase pocket of the p210bcrabl oncoprotein. The interaction of the side chains of the adenosine scaffold with the local peptide domains of the kinase pocket is depicted. ATP BS, cofactor-binding site; CS, catalytic site; SBS, substrate-binding site.

sented in Figure 62.2-2, adenosine, the natural ligand for ATP to the cofactor kinase–binding site of abl, is attached to the scaffold, leaving four other positions where chemical functionalities can be attached.

Automated, convergent, synthetic, combinatorial chemical synthesis can be used to generate low-complexity libraries of compound, all of which have the scaffold and the adenosine but in which the structure of the other chemical functionalities can be varied automatically to generate diversity. Recombinant clones of the kinase pocket are used for screening the libraries for the high-affinity binders, which may identify molecules that display therapeutic activity that is greater than existing compounds.

RAS Oncoproteins (Farnesylation Inhibitors and G Pocket Inhibitors)

The RAS family of membrane-bound G proteins usually is activated in response to growth factor stimulation and trigger activation of at least two types of pathways within the cell: the MAP kinase pathway that ends in the nucleus at the level of transcription factor activation and the RAF/BAD pathway that results in the release of BCL-2 within the cell. In cancer, the acquisition of point mutations in RAS leads to continuous activation of these proteins, contributes to the dual phenotypes of chemotherapy resistance, and increases proliferation. This combination has the resultant effect of increasing the genetic instability of populations of cancer cells. These point mutations often are acquired as secondary mutations in a broad spectrum of epithelial neoplastic cells. In fact, very few neoplastic diseases exist in which RAS mutations do not occur. CML is an example of a disease in which the acquisition of RAS-activating point mutations is very rare, in part, perhaps, owing to the fact that the p210bcrabl kinase of CML results in activation of the RAS proteins.

The connections made by RAS, which are essential for it to be linked to its interacting pathways that link growth factor stimulation with gene expression of survival, depends on its localization to the plasma membrane. This localization depends on the action of a number of enzymes, which mediate

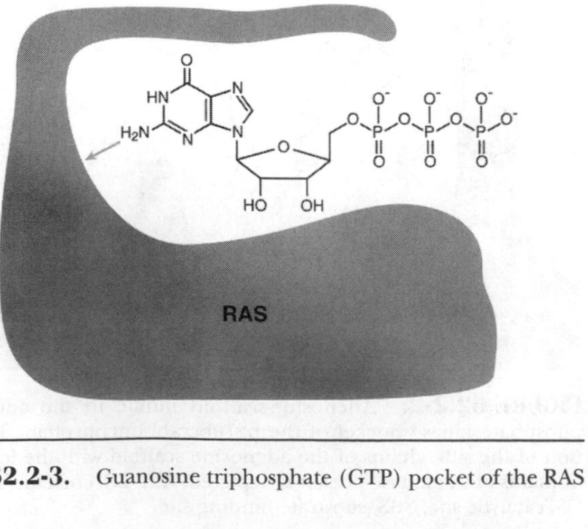

FIGURE 62.2-3. Guanosine triphosphate (GTP) pocket of the RAS G protein.

posttranslational modifications of the RAS protein.[14] Inhibitors of one of these posttranslational enzymes—protein farnesyltransferase—showed activity in animal models with respect to the suppression of human tumor xenografts. Interestingly, although the spectrum of clinical activity of the farnesylation inhibitors has been somewhat of a disappointment, the interesting surprise is that these agents appear to display activity even in tumor populations in which farnesylation of RAS is not playing a role in the natural history of the disease.[14]

Despite the initially disappointing spectrum of activity in trials of the farnesylation inhibitors, the inhibition of RAS activity is still an important goal. Every time a transdominant negative inhibitor of RAS activation has been tested in animal models or cell lines, a dramatic effect on the phenotype of the cancer cells has been observed in a spectrum of malignancies, including CML,[14] melanoma,[15] and gastrointestinal cancer.[17] Thus, many groups have been attempting to analyze the structure of RAS so as to design low-molecular inhibitors of RAS.

At the center of these new molecular approaches to the development of inhibitory agents for RAS is the GTP/GDP exchange role of RAS. As outlined previously, RAS acts as a molecular switch for cell growth. In its off state, p21RAS is bound to guanosine diphosphate (GDP), whereas on activation, GDP is exchanged for GTP (Fig. 62.2-3).

When GTP occupies the guanine nucleotide pocket of RAS, cell growth is promoted. In fact, many of the point mutations acquired in tumor cells by RAS prevent the hydrolysis of GTP. This maintains the activated state of RAS and prevents a return to its off state. The Karplus group at Harvard[17] has designed molecules that would recognize the dimensions and charge of the guanine nucleotide pocket of RAS in its activated state. Such molecules would bind to activated RAS, not to RAS proteins in their nonactivated state. This group is undertaking a computational analysis of the molecular switch regions of RAS (residues 30–38 and residues 60–75).

Karplus and his coworkers studied the bicyclic scaffold shown in Figure 62.2-2, now attached to a guanosine molecule (Fig. 62.2-4) and found that the guanosine scaffold was energetically a good mimic of the GTP and engaged the same amino acid side chains in the RAS guanine nucleotide–binding pocket as does GTP. These computational models have suggested that the designing of chemical mimics of GTP such that they will bind more tightly and selectively to the inner protein domains lining the GTP pocket of RAS is feasible. The guanosine scaffold shown in Figure 62.2-5 may engage multiple domains in the RAS-binding pocket and, therefore, produce inhibitors that can override even an excess of GTP and, owing to the multiple sites of interaction, can produce inhibitors that are selective and, therefore, nontoxic as well (M. Karplus, personal communication, 1996).

Metastasis Inhibitors

The integrin receptors constitute a complex class of surface cytoadhesion molecules that mediate apoptosis rescue signals from extracellular matrix proteins and stromal cells or supporting cell ligands into the cell, with connections to cytoskeletal structures and transcriptional regulation pathways within the cell.[18] The integrin receptors can exhibit changes in the number of receptors on the membrane and changes in the composition of the available subunits that contribute to the heterodimeric arrays of integrin receptors, and they can

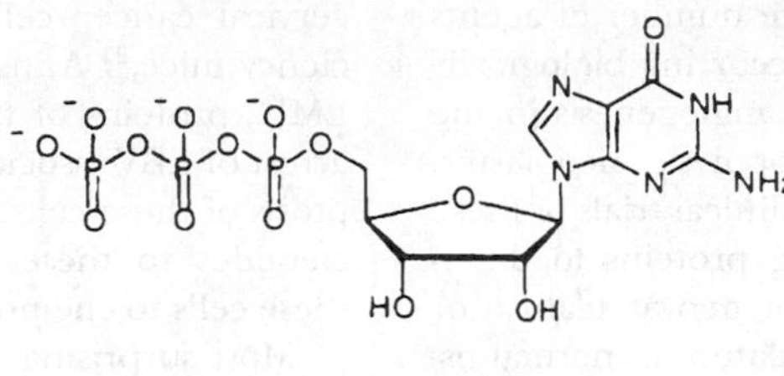

Guanosine triphosphate (GTP)

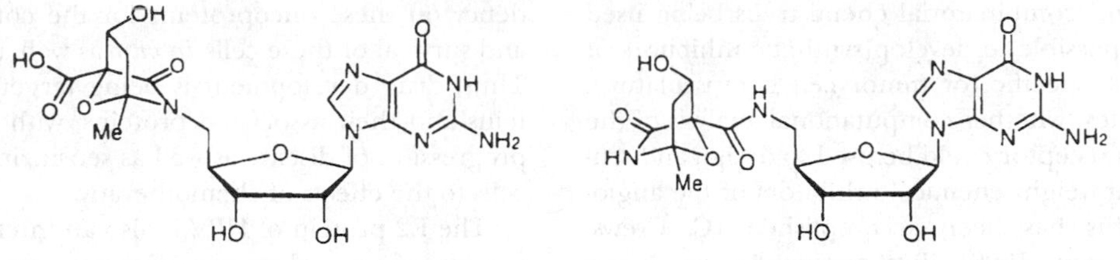

4 5

FIGURE 62.2-4. Austin bicyclic molecular scaffold as a mimic for the triphosphate domain of guanosine triphosphate (GTP). The natural cofactor of the abl kinase, GTP, is compared to the guanosine-scaffold mimic.

undergo changes in conformation, sometimes associated with posttranslational modification, which define differing states of functionality. Integrin receptors can also be activated to functionally active conformal states from signals arising from within the cell. Thus, the integrin receptors, which are apoptosis rescue signal transduction elements, can be activated from "inside out" and from "outside in."[18]

Several researchers have reported that the transfection of integrin expression vectors carrying specific integrin subunits, such as the β_3 integrin, can direct cells to metastasize to specific organs. Indeed, the $\alpha V\beta_3$ integrin receptor is commonly encountered in cancer cells that are metastatic and rapidly proliferating, whereas the $\alpha V\beta_5$ integrin receptor is often found in differentiating cells.

Extensive testing of the ligands and antibodies that can engage various integrin receptors have shown that the inhibitors of integrin receptors can be effective in suppressing particular patterns of metastatic spread in preclinical animal models. Some groups have used phage display libraries in which thousands of phage clones, each with a different peptide, are injected into the tail vein of a mouse. This is followed by analysis of the endothelial cells from the vessels of different tissues. These studies have shown that peptide sequences exist that are characteristic of the vessels of different tissues. This knowledge has led to the speculation that chemical mimics of trafficking molecules on the endothelial surface of different tissues could be used to prevent metastases to a particular target organ. An example would be the treatment of individuals with stage III colon cancer with chemical mimics of peptides, which would bind to the cytoadhesion molecules characteristic of vasculatures of hepatic tissues.

Several groups have reported the isolation of chemical mimics of the RGD peptide, which binds to the integrin receptor. The use of phage display peptide libraries led to the collection of peptide motifs, including RGD, that bind to integrin receptors. Now, combinatorial chemical libraries are being used to refine the structure of low-molecular chemical inhibitors of integrin receptors that appear to reduce the metastatic potential of a cell. These types of drugs should be highly exciting therapeutically when they are brought into the clinic.

LOW-MOLECULAR-WEIGHT INHIBITORS FOR THE ANGIOGENESIS RECEPTOR

One of the most exciting paradigm shifts has been the attempt to target drug development to normal tissues. Angiogenesis is a process that takes place during tumor growth. Now, inhibitors of this process are being tested in the therapy of solid tumor malignancies. This approach was stimulated by the correlation between the density of the neovasculature in histopathologic specimens and the aggressiveness of the natural history of the disease in a given patient. Also stimulating interest in this area was the demonstration in animal models that a number of naturally occurring modulators of angiogenesis also displayed activity in modulating the rate of tumor growth in animal mod-

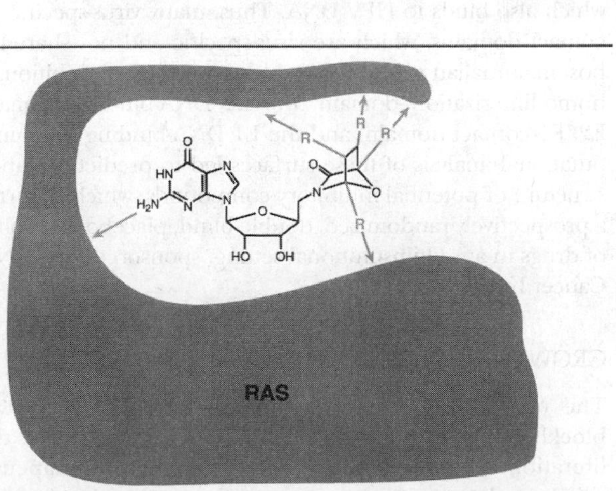

FIGURE 62.2-5. Guanosine-scaffold mimic in the guanosine triphosphate (GTP) pocket of the RAS G protein. The interaction of the side chains of the guanosine scaffold with the local peptide domains of the GTP pocket is depicted.

els. This has led to the isolation of a large number of agents (synthetic chemicals as well as naturally occurring biologically active proteins) that are known to affect angiogenesis in the treatment of solid tumors and hematopoietic neoplasms. There is immense interest in the current clinical trials of these natural products and naturally occurring proteins to determine whether they are selective for tumor neovasculature or whether they affect the formation of vasculature in normal tissues as well.

Computational and combinatorial chemistry is being used to test whether it is possible to develop synthetic inhibitors of angiogenesis that are specific for tumor cell neovasculature. The first step was to test whether computational analysis of the normal angiogenesis receptor could be used to design and synthesize low-molecular-weight chemical inhibitors of the angiogenesis receptor; this has been accomplished (C. Crews, personal communication, 1999). Two approaches are being used now to develop chemical therapy that is antiangiogenic. The first is to engineer low-molecular-weight inhibitors of the angiogenesis receptor. At Yale, Hu et al.[19] have taken a second approach: chimeric immunoconjugate molecules that are composed of an amino-terminal targeting domain that binds specifically to tumor endothelial cells, and a carboxyl-terminal end that carries the Fc fragment of IgG. The latter molecule is known to bind to natural killer cells. Hu et al.[19] have reported that the release of such chimeric immunoconjugate molecules into the systemic circulation of human tumor xenografts in nude mice results in regression of established tumor nodules. This reaction has been shown to depend on the binding of natural killer cells to the Fc fragment of the immunoconjugate molecules.

CHEMICAL INHIBITORS FOR ONCOPROTEINS OF DNA TUMOR VIRUSES

The oncoprotein products of DNA tumor viruses provide almost ideal targets for the development of low-molecular-weight chemical inhibitors for cancer treatment or prevention. As in many of the other targets we have discussed, the continued expression of these proteins is essential to the maintenance of the neoplastic phenotype. Moreover, since they are viral proteins, those proteins are unique targets that are not essential to the survival or proliferation of normal cells. Thus, drugs developed against these proteins may be highly selective for the tumor tissue and not toxic to the uninfected normal tissue.

The diseases associated with the DNA tumor viruses, human papilloma virus (HPV), and Epstein-Barr virus (EBV) are significant world health problems.[20] HPV-associated malignancies represent the second leading cause of cancer death in the world among women.[20] In addition, it is estimated that 40% of all AIDS patients alive today will eventually develop an EBV-associated non-Hodgkin's lymphoma.[21]

Again, the use of antisense oligonucleotides first showed convincingly that the continued expression of the protein products of the episomal DNA of these viruses was essential for the continued replication of tumor cell lines and growth of these cells in human tumor xenografts in severe combined immunodeficiency mice.[22] HPV E6/E7 antisense oligonucleotide transcription units were shown to suppress the growth of cervical cancer cell lines in severe combined immunodeficiency mice.[23] Antisense oligonucleotides to the EBNA I and LMP2 proteins of the EBV were shown to induce replication arrest of EBV-associated tumor cell lines and induction of apoptosis of these cells. Additionally, use of the antisense oligonucleotides to these unique targets produces sensitization of these cells to chemotherapy.

Most surprising is that cervical cancer cell lines harboring HPV-transforming proteins E6 and E7 still retained dependency on these oncoproteins for the continued proliferation and survival of these cells *in vitro* as well as in animal models.[24] Thus, drug development is being targeted to these two proteins and their associated proteins, with the aims of stopping progression of disease as well as sensitizing the cervical cancer cells to the effects of chemotherapy.

The E2 protein of HPV is also an interesting target for prevention of cervical cancer. Very commonly, the chronic infection of HPV in the cervical mucus, which is associated with dysplasia and chromosomal translocations, persists for years before the development of invasive cancer. In the United States, such dysplastic states of the cervical mucosa can be identified by repetitive Papanicolaou smear, and appropriate surgical action can be taken if the dysplasia is severe or persists. In contrast, in most areas of the world, the infrastructure necessary to screen women for HPV-associated dysplasia does not exist. Thus, the development of chemicals that will inhibit the formation of viral protein complexes necessary for the assembly of the replication initiation complex could be useful for the development of preventive therapy for cervical cancer.

Two of the viral proteins—E1, a helicase, and E2, a chaperone protein—are important for assembly of a functional replication initiation complex in HPV-infected cells. Once infected, the germinal epithelial cells of the cervical mucosa contain approximately 50 copies of HPV DNA per cell.[25] These copies of HPV are retained at a stable copy number because the replication of the HPV DNA episome is coupled to the replication of the host cells. This is probably owing to the need for host DNA polymerase for the replication of the HPV DNA.

E2 must form a homodimer before binding to the E2-binding sites in the HPV origin of replication. E2 also connects with E1, which also binds to HPV DNA. Thus, many virus-specific protein contact domains, which are virus-specific and not shared by the host mammalian cell, are available as targets for inhibition: the E2 homodimerization domain, the E2 DNA-binding domain, the E2/E1 contact domain, and the E1 DNA-binding domain. Computational analysis of these surfaces led to predictions about the structure of potential inhibitory compounds, which in turn led to a prospectively randomized, double-blind, placebo-controlled trial of drugs in a multiinstitutional setting, sponsored by the National Cancer Institute.

GROWTH FACTOR RECEPTOR INHIBITORS

The use of monoclonal antibodies has already shown that blocking of growth factor receptors can act to suppress the proliferation of tumor cells, enhance their chemotherapeutic sensitivity, and extend the duration of the progression-free interval in cancer patients. The Her2/neu receptor antibody Herceptin and the epidermal growth factor receptor (EGFR) inhibitory antibody C221 have been shown to sensitize tumor cells to

TABLE 62.2-3. Genetic Changes in Solid Tumor and Hematopoietic Neoplasms That Are Suitable Targets for Drug Development

Amplified growth factor receptors: Her2/Neu-R and EGFR in epithelial cancers
Point mutational change in RAS G proteins in gastrointestinal tract cancers
Amplification and translocation of MYC transcription factor lymphomas
MDM2 amplification in central nervous system tumors
Angiogenesis receptors and proteins
EWS protein in sarcomas
DNA tumor virus oncoproteins
Protein oncoprotein kinases

EGFR, epidermal growth factor receptor.

chemotherapy.[26] These clinical examples have shown that blocking of the appropriate domain on the growth factor receptor is sufficient to suppress the transformed phenotype of the cell.

Computational analysis of these two closely related receptors (EGFR and Her2/neu) is being directed to the development of low-molecular-weight chemical inhibitors of these receptors in such cancers as breast, gastric, and esophageal cancer, squamous cell carcinoma of the head and neck, and ovarian and lung cancer, which are associated with amplification of these receptors' genes.

SUMMARY AND FUTURE DIRECTIONS

In the twenty-first century, drug development will no longer depend on going to the forests to dig up roots, to pick flowers and leaves, or to strip the bark from the trees to discover new drugs for cancer treatment. It is now possible for a laboratory scientist to recapitulate in a few months what once required millions of years of evolution to produce. The ability to analyze protein structure, to decipher the dynamic array of conformal states of oncoproteins (both activating and inactive), and to characterize the genetic changes that may exert a dominant effect on the natural history of solid tumors and hematopoietic neoplasms (Table 62.2-3) has opened the door to selecting for drug development the best domains on target oncoproteins.

The availability of computational chemistry and the ability to generate diversity in chemical structure have enabled scientists to reach beyond the limits of available data about structure and activity relationships and to probe deeply in the unknown repository of untapped chemical structures for molecules that may exhibit favorable binding and specificity properties. It is apparent that the explosion of information about genetic changes in tumor cells will provide the necessary clues with which the chemist can direct structural diversification and screening to isolate newer and more effective compounds. Recent successes in the development of drugs for AIDS and CML on the basis of protein structure is a dramatic validation of this new approach to drug design. It is possible that this paradigm will be reiterated many times in the development of an entirely new generation of cancer treatment drugs based on inhibitors of receptors, transcription factors, adaptor molecules, viral and somatic cell oncoproteins, and apoptosis rescue proteins. The dividends for cancer patients and society may be substantial in terms of reducing the cost of therapy and enhancing its efficacy.

REFERENCES

1. Druker BJ, Lydon NB. Lessons learned from the development of an Abl tyrosine kinase inhibitor for chronic myelogenous leukemia. *J Clin Invest* 2000;105:3.
2. Wickham TJ, Mathias P, Cheresh DA, Memerow G. Integrins alpha$_v$ beta$_3$ and alpha$_v$ beta$_5$ promote adenovirus internalization but not virus attachment. *Cell* 1993;73:309.
3. Krengel U, Schlichting L, Scherer A, et al. Three-dimensional structures of H-ras p21 mutants: molecular basis for their inability to function as switch molecules. *Cell* 1990;62:539.
4. Sternberg N, Hoess RH. Display of peptides and proteins on the surface of bacteriophage lambda. *Proc Natl Acad Sci USA* 1995;92:1609.
5. Nowell PC, Hungerford DA. Chromosome studies on normal and leukemic human leukocytes. *J Natl Cancer Inst* 1960;25:85.
6. DeFabritiis P, Petti MC, Montefusco E, et al. Bcrabl antisense oligodeoxynucleotide in vitro purging and autologous bone marrow transplantation for patients with CML in advanced phase. *Blood* 1998;91:3156.
7. Skorski T, Palanisamy K, Nieborowska-Skorska M, et al. Phosphatidylinositol-3 kinase activity is regulated by BCR/ABL and is required for the growth of Philadelphia chromosome–positive cells. *J Natl Cancer Inst* 1995;86:726.
8. Knudsen ES, Buckmaster C, Chen TT, Feramisco JR, Wang JYJ. Inhibition of DNA synthesis by Rb: effects on G/S1 transition and S phase progression. *Growth Dev* 1998;12:2278.
9. Guo XYD, Cuillerot JM, Wang T, et al. Peptide containing the BCR oligomerization domain (AA 160) reverses the transformed phenotype of p210bcrabl positive 32D myeloid leukemia cells. *Oncogene* 1998;17:825.
10. Guo XYD, Balague C, Wang T, et al. The presence of the Rb c-box peptide in the cytoplasm inhibits p210bcrabl transforming function. *Oncogene* 1999;18:1589.
11. Anafi M, Gazit A, Zehavi A, et al. Tyrphostin-induced inhibition of p210bcrabl tyrosine kinase activity induces K562 to differentiate. *J Natl Cancer Inst* 1993;82:3524.
12. Druker B, Tamua S, Buchdunger E, et al. Effects of a selective inhibitor of the Abl tyrosine kinase on the growth of Bcr-Abl positive cells. *Nat Med* 1996;2:564.
13. Casey PJ, Seabra JC. Protein prenyltransferases. *J Biol Chem* 1996;271:5289.
14. Pendergast AM, Quilliam LA, Cripe LD, et al. Bcr-abl induced oncogenesis is mediated by direct interaction with the SH2 domain of the GRB-2 adaptor protein. *Cell* 1993;75:175.
15. Chin L, Tam A, Pumerante J, et al. Essential role for oncogenic ras in tumour maintenance. *Nature* 1999;400:468.
16. Breevik J, Meling GI, Spurkland A, et al. K-ras mutation in colorectal cancer: relations to patient age, sex, and tumor location. *Br J Cancer* 1994;69:367.
17. Caflisch A, Miranker A, Karplus M. Multiple copy simultaneous search and construction of ligands in binding sites: application to inhibitors of HIV-1 aspartic proteinase. *J Med Chem* 1993;36:2142.
18. Horwitz HF. Integrins and health. *Sci Am* 1997;276:68.
19. Hu Z, Sun Y, Garen A. Targeting tumor vasculature endothelial cells and tumor cells for immunotherapy of human melanoma in a mouse xenograft model. *Proc Natl Acad Sci USA* 1999;96:8161.
20. Parkin DM, Pisani P, Ferlay J. Estimates of the worldwide incidence of 25 major cancers in 1990. *Int J Cancer* 1990;80:827.
21. Pluda JM, Yarchoan R, Jaffe ES, et al. Development of non-Hodgkin's lymphoma in a cohort of patients with severe human immunodeficiency virus (HIV) infection on long-term antiretroviral therapy. *Ann Intern Med* 1990;113:276.
22. Roth G, Curiel T, Lacy J. Epstein-Barr viral nuclear antigen 1 antisense oligodeoxynucleotides inhibits proliferation of Epstein-Barr virus–immortalized B cells. *J Natl Cancer Inst* 1994;84:582.
23. Hu G, Liu W, Mendelsohn J, et al. High epidermal growth factor–receptor levels induced by the HPVE6/E7 proteins lead to unregulated growth in cervical carcinoma cells. *J Natl Cancer Inst* 1997;89:1271.
24. Hu G, Liu W, Hanania EG, et al. Suppression of tumorigenesis by transcription units expressing the antisense E6 and E7 messenger RNA (mRNA) for the transforming proteins of the human papilloma virus and the sense mRNA for the retinoblastoma gene in cervical carcinoma cells. *Cancer Gene Ther* 1995;2:19.
25. Schneider A, Oltersdorf T, Schneider V, et al. Distribution of human papillomavirus 16 genome in cervical neoplasia by molecular in situ hybridization of tissue sections. *Int J Cancer* 1987;39:717.
26. Pegram MD, Lipton A, Hayes DF, et al. Phase II study of receptor enhanced chemosensitivity using recombinant humanized anti-p185her2/neu monoclonal antibody plus cisplatin in patients with her2/neu-overexpressing metastatic breast cancer refractory to chemotherapy treatment. *J Clin Oncol* 1998;16:2659.

CHAPTER 63

Cancer Vaccines

SECTION 1 Preventive Cancer Vaccines

DOUGLAS R. LOWY
JOHN T. SCHILLER

The high rate of morbidity and mortality attributable to cancer has stimulated concerted efforts to prevent malignancies from developing. The recognition that environmental factors may account for the majority of cancers has encouraged researchers to identify the exogenous factors that trigger the carcinogenic process and to define their role in tumorigenesis. Infectious agents make up one important class of environmental factors implicated in tumor development.[1–3]

Although the oncogenic potential of some infectious agents, such as hepatitis B virus (HBV), was recognized more than two decades ago, many of the infectious agents now believed to be oncogenic were discovered after 1975 (Table 63.1-1).[2] These latter include the oncogenic papillomaviruses, hepatitis C virus, herpesvirus type 8, and *Helicobacter pylori.* It seems likely that further research will result in additional forms of cancer being attributed to infectious agents. The expanded list will arise via the demonstration that infectious agents already recognized as oncogenic may be causally involved with additional forms of cancer, by attributing these additional cancers to other infectious agents not yet recognized as oncogenic, or both.

Identification of an infectious agent in the etiology of a malignant process implies that timely interference with the infection could prevent the tumor from arising.[4,5] The development of effective vaccines against infectious carcinogenic agents represents a potentially powerful approach and is the main focus of this chapter. The prototype for this approach is the HBV vaccine, which can protect immunized individuals against both acute disease and the malignant consequences attributable to this virus.[6,7]

This chapter briefly considers how infectious oncogenic agents lead to cancer, discusses general issues related to developing vaccines against these agents, and presents individual sections devoted to the three agents that account for the most cancers worldwide. Vaccines against other infectious oncogenic agents are also in various stages of development.[8–10]

INFECTIOUS AGENTS AND CANCER

Reducing exposure to an identified carcinogen represents the principal approach to reducing the carcinogenic effects of many environmental carcinogens. For carcinogens such as cigarette smoke, entrenched human behavior and conflicting economic interests may present considerable obstacles to reducing or eliminating exposure. By contrast, a vaccine against an infectious carcinogen does not require modification of the behavior that leads to exposure because the vaccine attenuates the oncogenic activity of the infectious agent by reducing or preventing infection of target tissue.[4,5,11] Furthermore, the induction of *herd immunity* via the widespread use of an effective vaccine, offers the possibility of reducing the risk of nonimmunized individuals to exposure to the infectious agent. Vaccination also offers the long-term possibility of eliminating the agent from the environment.

Before considering vaccination itself, it is worthwhile reviewing some features of oncogenic infectious agents, as their characteristics may have implications for vaccine development,

TABLE 63.1-1. Oncogenic Infectious Agents

Agent	Tumor Types	Annual Cases Worldwide (Estimate)
BACTERIA		
Helicobacter pylori	Stomach cancer, gastric lymphoma	505,000
VIRUSES		
Human papillomavirus	Cervical, anal, vaginal, other cancers	447,000
Hepatitis B virus	Liver cancer	285,000
Hepatitis C virus	Liver cancer	113,000
Human immunodeficiency virus	Kaposi's sarcoma, non-Hodgkin's lymphoma	52,000
Human herpes type 8	Kaposi's sarcoma	44,000
Epstein-Barr virus	Lymphomas (Hodgkin's, non-Hodgkin's, Burkitt)	30,000
Human T-cell lymphotropic virus-1	Adult T-cell leukemia	3000
PARASITES		
Schistosomes	Bladder cancer	10,000
Liver flukes	Cholangiocarcinoma	800

(Adapted from ref. 2.)

testing, and implementation. Viruses, bacteria, and parasites have all been implicated in the pathogenesis of human cancer (see Table 63.1-1). Investigators at the International Agency for Research on Cancer estimated that in 1990 approximately 15% of cancers worldwide could be attributed to infectious agents (Table 63.1-2).[2] In the United States and other developed countries, a smaller proportion of cancers (approximately 9%) are associated with these agents, while they account for a higher proportion (approximately 20%) in developing countries.

Several factors probably account for these differences. Some of the infectious agents, such as parasites with oncogenic potential, are extremely uncommon in the United States, or the rate of infection may vary greatly, as with HBV.[12] For others, such as human papillomaviruses (HPV), infection in the United States is common, but Pap smear screening for premalignant lesions in the cervix leads to effective treatment before carcinomas develop.[13] In still other instances, strain differences or the interaction between the infectious agent and environmental, host factors, or both might help determine the rate of carcinogenic progression.[14]

The identified oncogenic infectious agents share at least four characteristics: the ability to establish chronic infection, the actual establishment of chronic infection in those individuals destined to develop malignancy attributable to the infection, an interval of many years between the initial infection and the development of malignancy, and a benign (i.e., nonmalignant) outcome for most infected individuals. These characteristics imply that cancer attributable to infectious agents develops only after prolonged infection and that a malignant outcome arises only after the development of infection-dependent changes in the host.

Consistent with current concepts of the multistep nature of carcinogenesis, the changes in the host probably involve genetic alterations in potential target cells, impairment of the immune system, or both. Since not all infectious agents that establish a chronic infection are carcinogenic, chronic infection with agents not implicated in carcinogenesis must be much less efficient in inducing the types of changes that lead to cancer than are those agents that are implicated in carcinogenesis.

Infection seems to induce tumors by three main mechanisms, either singly or in combination, depending on the agent.[5] In

TABLE 63.1-2. Cancers Attributable to Infection: Estimate of Worldwide Distribution According to Type (Annual Number of Cases in Thousands)[a]

Tumor Type	Developed Countries	Developing Countries	World	Percentage of Tumor Type Attributable to Infection
Stomach cancer	202	294	497	56
Cervical cancer	80	336	416	88
Liver cancer	47	352	399	81
Kaposi's sarcoma in acquired immunodeficiency syndrome	16	28	44	—
Vulva cancer	10	21	31	88
Hodgkin's disease	12	18	30	49
Bladder cancer	0	10	10	3
Non-Hodgkin's lymphoma in acquired immunodeficiency syndrome	4	4	9	—
Gastric lymphoma	3	5	8	76
Burkitt's lymphoma	0	8	8	81
Leukemias	1	2	3	—
Cholangiocarcinoma	0	1	1	—

[a]Figures in each column represent the estimated number of cases of that tumor type attributed to infection, except for the column on the right, which represents the percentage of all cancers of that type worldwide attributed to an infectious cause.
(Adapted from ref. 2.)

some instances, such as with the papillomaviruses, the agent infects the potential target cell population and induces a series of changes from within those cells that lead to cancer.[15] Some of the changes include alterations in the agent, so that only a subset of its genetic information is expressed. The viral genes that continue to be expressed contribute directly to the tumorigenic phenotype by, for example, inactivating the activity of tumor suppressor genes. Other genes from the virus are presumably silenced to lower the likelihood of the tumor cells being recognized and destroyed by the immune system.

In a second scenario, as occurs with *H pylori*, the infectious agent is present in the target tissue and induces cancer by local effects, usually chronic inflammation, but the agent remains outside the tumor cells.[16,17] By the time the tumor is capable of distant metastasis, if not sooner, its growth becomes independent of the infectious agent.

The third mechanism, which is more indirect, results in increased tumor risk secondary to suppression of the host immune system. This process has been identified in tumors that arise as a consequence of infection with the human immunodeficiency virus (HIV), which predisposes infected individuals to a variety of tumors.[18,19] As the immunosuppression associated with HIV renders patients much more susceptible to chronic infection with other agents, including some with oncogenic potential, many of the tumors result from the combined effects of coinfection with HIV and these other agents.

PROPHYLACTIC VERSUS THERAPEUTIC VACCINATION

Vaccination against an infectious oncogenic agent can be contemplated in three possible clinical settings: as a prophylactic vaccine to prevent infection or acute disease, as a therapeutic vaccine to treat an established infection before a malignancy has been induced, and as a therapeutic vaccine to treat the infection after the malignant tumor has developed, provided the growth, viability, or both growth and viability of the tumor still depend on the presence of the infectious agent. The use of vaccines in the treatment of cancer, which is the subject of intense investigation, is covered later in this chapter. This section examines the potential utility, complexity, and challenges for vaccines whose goals are to prevent established infection or to eradicate established infection before tumor development.

Ideally, a vaccine should be effective in both prevention and treatment. However, it has proven easier to develop prophylactic vaccines against infectious agents than therapeutic ones. Of the more than 20 approved vaccines in the United States, all are approved for prevention, rather than treatment, of established infection.[20]

The cellular and humoral arms of the immune system generally function together to interfere either with the initial phases of infection or the eradication of established infection. Antibodies capable of neutralizing the infectious agent appear to be the prime effectors in preventing infection, while CD8+ T cells appear to serve more critical roles in the resolution of established infection.[11,21,22] The success of prophylactic vaccines in inducing long-term protection against infection probably lies primarily in their ability to induce neutralizing antibodies, although other immune components probably also contribute to their overall effectiveness.

For infections that induce serious acute disease, such as polio, the main theoretical goal of vaccination is the prevention or modification of the acute disease. Since it is easier to reduce the incidence of acute disease by inducing widespread immunity with a prophylactic vaccine than by treating established infection, a prophylactic vaccine approach has an important theoretical advantage in this setting over a therapeutic one.

However, for cancer-causing microbes that induce benign primary infection, such as papillomaviruses, the long interval between infection and cancer, combined with the apparently necessary role played by the infectious agent during much of this period, provides a relatively long opportunity to identify and treat the infected population. Situations in which premalignant lesions attributable to the microbe are frequently identified, as in the case of Pap smear screening for cervical cancer, present an opportunity to intervene with a therapeutic vaccine.

The comparative ease with which prophylactic vaccines can be developed, relative to the continuing challenge posed by therapeutic vaccine development, makes prophylactic vaccination an important approach for cancer vaccines. Another advantage of prophylactic vaccines is that they do not depend on effective progress in identifying individuals with premalignant disease. Furthermore, worldwide public health vaccine efforts are designed primarily for the administration of prophylactic vaccines, and this vaccine approach has been extremely successful and highly cost-effective in combating many infectious disease. In addition, the primary disease induced by many oncogenic infectious agents can provide sufficient rationale for development of a prophylactic vaccine, in addition to the long-term prevention of cancer.

Numerous theoretical and practical concerns arise when considering development of a prophylactic vaccine against cancer. Safety is especially important for a vaccine whose primary goal is to prevent cancer, as many individuals will never be infected by the agent, the majority of infected individuals will never develop malignancy, and malignancy only develops many years after infection. In addition, it requires many years to determine whether a candidate prophylactic vaccine can prevent cancer. The minimum theoretical duration of efficacy trials whose end point was prevention of malignancy would be the length of the latent period between infection and malignancy. Thus, while vaccination against HBV was found more than 20 years ago to prevent primary infection, data showing this vaccination can actually reduce the frequency of hepatocellular carcinoma are only beginning to accumulate.[7]

Although cancer prevention might appear to be a necessary end point for establishing vaccine efficacy, there can be serious ethical obstacles to using this clinical end point. For those clinical situations in which the standard of care involves the treatment of premalignant lesions to prevent the development of malignancy, as with cervical abnormalities related to Pap smear screening, it may be unethical to delay treatment until cancer develops. In addition, once a vaccine has been shown to be effective in preventing infection, it might be considered unethical to withhold the vaccine from the control group, despite the possible ambiguities such vaccination might create for efforts to determine directly whether the vaccine could reduce cancer frequency.

The most critical information for vaccine development lies in determining which antigens can induce protective immunity. For HBV, many aspects of its immunology and its role in carcinogenesis remain incompletely understood, but identification of a *protective* viral antigen was able to lead to development of an effective vaccine.[6,12,23]

Many of the infectious agents with recognized oncogenic activity (see Table 63.1-1) induce nonmalignant diseases that carry significant morbidity and economic cost long before they cause cancer, although oncogenic HPV infection may be a notable exception. It may be more practical to use a nonmalignant end point in efforts to demonstrate efficacy, with the effect on cancer being determined, directly or indirectly, by follow-up studies. This was the approach taken with the hepatitis B vaccine, which has been approved for use in the United States because of its ability to prevent acute hepatitis. However, the presumption that the vaccine would prevent many liver cancers attributable to hepatitis B infection was also considered in recommending widespread use of the vaccine.

Some issues surrounding a therapeutic vaccine differ from those of a prophylactic one. As the individual is already infected, it is usually much easier to carry out therapeutic clinical trials that determine efficacy, compared with prophylactic trials. A therapeutic vaccine trial can limit its enrollment to infected individuals at a particular stage of disease, and the response to vaccine can be evaluated, usually within a short period, by suppression of infection and of the disease.

Another major theoretical advantage of an effective therapeutic vaccine is that it can have an effect on the incidence of malignant disease much sooner than a prophylactic vaccine. For cervical cancer, where the interval between HPV infection and cancer typically takes more than 20 years, it would take at least this length of time before a prophylactic vaccine, even if it were completely effective and were given to all at-risk individuals, would have any effect in the incidence of malignancy. By contrast, an effective therapeutic vaccine could reduce the incidence of cervical cancer after a much shorter interval. These considerations underscore the potential utility of determining whether successes with therapeutic vaccines in experimental animal systems, such as *H pylori*[17,24] and papillomaviruses,[25] can be achieved in people.

HEPATITIS B VIRUS

The identification of HBV in the 1960s led to epidemiologic studies that have clarified its worldwide role in hepatocellular cancer.[6,12,26,27] Although infection with this DNA virus can cause acute hepatitis, its most serious global consequences are chronic hepatitis, cirrhosis, and hepatocellular carcinoma, all of which are associated with chronic HBV infection. It is estimated that there are more than 1 million chronic HBV carriers in the United States and more than 300 million carriers throughout the world. The virus is believed to account for approximately 1 million deaths per year worldwide, approximately one-half of them secondary to hepatocellular carcinoma.

In highly endemic areas, the lifetime risk of exposure may exceed 50%, and most HBV infections occur perinatally or in early childhood. In areas of low endemicity, HBV transmission occurs mainly in adults, often via sexual exposure or parenteral exposure from infected shared needles used with illicit drugs. The risk of medical exposure to infected blood products has been greatly reduced by systematic screening of these materials for HBV.

The HBV carrier state, which is a measure of persistent infection, is a critical determinant of the long-term risk for hepatocellular carcinoma. HBV carrier rates vary dramatically in different populations, being less than 0.5% in the United States and many other countries with high standards of living, to rates of 10% to 20% in parts of Africa, Asia, and the South Pacific. The relative incidence of cancer attributable to HBV follows a similar geographic distribution, with many studies consistently showing chronic HBV infection is an important risk factor for hepatocellular carcinoma.

The frequency with which persistent HBV infection is established varies inversely with the age of exposure. The highest risk by far occurs during the perinatal period and the first year of life. More than 70% of neonates born to infected mothers become chronic carriers, compared with around 8% of those exposed at 3 years of age and an even lower proportion in immunocompetent adults.[26]

Conversely, HBV is much more likely to induce acute hepatitis in older age groups, while acute infection is usually asymptomatic when exposure occurs in the perinatal period. This difference occurs because the acute hepatic disease results from the immune response to infection, as HBV does not directly induce hepatocellular damage. Thus, the relative immunoincompetence of infants probably accounts for their lack of symptoms and for the high frequency with which the virus establishes persistent infection in this age group.

The precise role of the virus in the development of hepatocellular carcinoma has not been fully determined. Persistent infection appears to lead to cancer mainly as the result of chronic inflammation and repeated cellular regeneration, and some evidence implicates the viral X gene, which encodes a transcription factor, in this process.[28] Most cases of liver cancer associated with HBV infection arise after chronic hepatitis has lead to cirrhosis. Hepatocellular carcinoma may develop in as little as 5 to 10 years of infection, but it does not usually occur until an individual has been infected for at least 20 to 30 years. Ongoing infection continues to be a risk factor for carcinoma, with an estimated cumulative risk of 15% for an individual who has had persistent infection for 50 years.[12]

The rate of hepatocellular carcinoma attributable to HBV is at least three times higher in male than in female subjects, even when a similar proportion of male and female subjects are exposed to HBV. The difference is explained in part by the higher frequency with which the HBV carrier state is established in male subjects (close to 2:1) and the greater likelihood of female subjects to eliminate the carrier state.

The HBV vaccine is the prototype prophylactic vaccine against an oncogenic infectious agent.[6,12,29,30] A key to HBV vaccine development was the recognition that the neutralizing antibodies were directed against the hepatitis B surface antigen (HBsAg), and that there is only one HBV serotype. The HBsAg is expressed in relatively pure form as circulating enveloped virus-like particles (VLPs) in the blood of infected HBV carriers. The HBsAg particles do not carry the viral genome and are not infectious. It was possible to purify the particles, inactivate possibly contaminating infectious virus with formalin (which should also have inactivated other viruses), and to test the particles as a subunit vaccine in human clinical trials that were initiated in 1975.

The HBsAg vaccine was found to be well tolerated, to induce an immune response in almost all vaccinees, and to reduce the infection rate in adults by at least 95% and in neonates by at least 85%. The protection rates in neonates may be further increased by giving hepatitis B immune globulin in addition to the vaccine. The vaccine was licensed in the United States in 1981.

An analogous HBsAg particle vaccine has been produced in yeast by recombinant DNA technology, and it was licensed in the United States in 1986. The recombinant vaccine has replaced the blood-derived vaccine, although the immunogenic properties of the latter product are somewhat superior to the recombinant material. Efficacy trials have shown that the recombinant vaccine confers a similar rate of protection against HBV as the blood-derived vaccine.[12,29,30] In addition, the recombinant vaccine is less expensive to manufacture and does not have the theoretical concern of contaminating infectious material, although extensive analysis of the blood-derived vaccine recipients failed to document excess exposure to infectious agents.

The initial series of immunizations, with either vaccine preparation, confers protection against infection for at least several years. In instances in which breakthrough infection has occurred several years after immunization, it has not been associated with development of a chronic carrier state. Routine revaccination is not recommended at this time by vaccine advisory groups in the United States. Further studies, in progress, should determine whether this policy should remain in place or be modified.

The long interval between HBV infection and the development of hepatocellular carcinoma means that only limited data thus far indicate directly that vaccination can actually decrease the incidence of cancer attributable to HBV. Data from an HBV vaccination program in Taiwan, an area with high HBV endemicity where universal vaccination was instituted in 1984, do show such a reduction in children.[7] From 1990 through 1994, the incidence of cancer in children aged 6 to 14 was one-half the rate before implementing vaccination, and that for children aged 6 to 9 was only one-fourth the rate of the earlier period.

These results indicate that HBV vaccination can achieve the long-term goal of cancer reduction. However, such a reduction will occur only if the populations most at risk are given the vaccine in a timely manner. Even in such a setting, reduction in cancer among adults, in whom the incidence is greatest, would not be expected to be seen until these children achieve adulthood.

HUMAN PAPILLOMAVIRUS

Papillomaviruses are epitheliotropic agents that induce benign papillomas of the skin and mucous membranes.[31,32] In contrast to HBV, there are more than 100 HPV genotypes (types).[33] A subset of HPV types, which are almost always transmitted sexually, are the main cause of human cervical cancer. Infection with these HPV types is a strong risk factor for cervical cancer, and HPV DNA from one or more of these types is found in virtually all cervical tumors.[31,34–36] The virus encodes oncoproteins that appear to be required both for the induction and the maintenance of the cancer.[32]

HPV infection has also been linked to the majority of anal cancers, in which the molecular pathogenesis seems to be similar to that of the cervix, as well as to other anogenital malignancies and to tumors of the upper aerodigestive tract.[37,38] The precise relationship between HPV infection and the development of some of these cancers is not as firmly established as that with cervical cancer.

As with HBV, cancer attributable to HPV develops only after many years of persistent HPV infection and is an infrequent outcome of infection. Cervical HPV infection is remarkably common, with sensitive polymerase chain reaction assays indicating prevalence rates of 20% to 40% among young sexually active women. Most infections are self-limited, and clinical cures are associated with resistance to reinfection. The antigenic divergence between HPV types is such that protection appears to be largely type specific.

The HPVs associated with cervical and anal cancer are usually designated high-risk types, as contrasted with the low-risk types, which also participate in anogenital infection but are almost never found in cervical or anal cancers.[15,32] Although there are several high-risk HPV types, HPV-16 is the most common type, being present in more than one-half of cervical cancers worldwide. The viral E6 and E7 genes are preferentially retained and expressed in the tumors, where they inactivate the p53 and Rb tumor suppressor proteins, respectively.

In principle, cervical cancer is already a largely preventable disease. In countries in which Pap smear screening reaches most women, the incidence of cervical cancer has decreased markedly. In the United States, for example, the rate of cervical cancer has decreased several-fold since the 1950s, from more than 50 in 100,000 to less than 10 in 100,000. This decrease in cancer rates is even more impressive because it has occurred during a period in which increased sexual promiscuity has been associated with an increased frequency of genital HPV infection.

However, the cost of Pap smear screening and follow-up is high (estimated to be more than $5 billion annually in the United States), and Pap smear screening is not routinely available in many less well-developed countries. This situation has made cervical cancer the leading cancer among women in many developing countries, and it remains the third most common female cancer worldwide.[39]

Establishing the etiologic link between HPV infection and cervical cancer (and other tumors) has focused interest on developing an HPV vaccine.[35,40,41] The main goal would be to protect against cervical cancer, which accounts for approximately 75% of the cancers worldwide attributable to HPV infection (see Table 63.1-1).[2] Since cervical cancer is especially prevalent in developing countries, such a vaccine would potentially have its greatest public health effect in these populations. However, in the United States, an effective HPV vaccine might further reduce the current incidence of cervical cancer by reaching populations that currently do not receive adequate Pap screening. In addition, by decreasing the frequency of genital HPV infection, a vaccine could decrease the anxiety and morbidity associated with cervical dysplasia and its treatment and reduce the social stigma associated with genital HPV infection. If widely used, a vaccine might reduce the frequency and overall cost of cervical cancer screening. The overall effectiveness of a vaccine, even for prevention of cervical cancer, would be greater if it were given to male subjects as well as to female subjects.

As papillomaviruses contain oncogenes, and a prophylactic vaccine would be directed toward healthy young individuals, efforts to develop a prophylactic vaccine have emphasized a subunit approach, analogous to that used for HBV.[40–42] Indeed, constitutive high-level expression of the L1 major structural viral protein, even in nonmammalian cells, will lead to its efficient self-assembly into VLPs that resemble authentic viral capsids structurally and antigenically. Preparative amounts of VLPs can be synthesized in insect cells or yeast. Such VLPs are suitable immunogens that, as is true of authentic virions, possess the immunodominant conformational epitopes capable of raising high titer neutralizing antibodies.

Since papillomaviruses are species specific, animal papillomavirus models have been used preclinically to evaluate VLPs as a candidate subunit prophylactic vaccine.[40–42] Excellent results (90% to 100% protection, even without adjuvant, against high-dose virus challenge) have been obtained with systemic immunization in three models, one cutaneous and two oral mucosal. The neutralizing antibodies appear to be largely responsible for the protection, which can last at least 1 year. Excellent protection has also been reported in the cutaneous animal model when a vaccinia vector was used to express L1 or when the L1 gene was injected as naked DNA. However, administration of protein seems more likely to be readily accepted by regulatory authorities in developed countries.

Alternative approaches are also being considered.[40–42] These include mucosal immunization via purified VLPs or via nonpathogenic enteric bacteria or the use of nonstructural viral proteins either alone or as incorporated into VLPs. Nonstructural viral proteins have been shown to prevent and, in some cases treat, animal papillomavirus infection,[25,43] in addition to working in tumorigenic models with cells that express a papillomavirus protein.[42] The utility of a vaccine that might treat established infection, especially if it were also effective prophylactically, makes it highly worthwhile to pursue the development of therapeutic HPV vaccines.

HPV-11 and HPV-16 L1 VLPs have been tested in early safety and immunogenicity trials of intramuscular injection of healthy human volunteers.[44,45] The vaccines were well tolerated and induced serum antibody titers, with or without adjuvant, comparable with the protective levels induced in animals. Large-scale efficacy trials will be needed to determine if this approach, which is not specifically directed toward the mucosal immune system, will confer protection against cervical HPV infection.

As noted in the Prophylactic versus Therapeutic Vaccination section, it would take many years to establish unequivocally if a vaccine actually had an effect on cervical cancer, since cervical HPV infection usually precedes the development of malignancy by more than 20 years. In addition, ethical considerations would argue against allowing cervical lesions arising in women in a vaccine study population to progress to malignancy. However, since infection with high-risk HPV is highly associated with the development of Pap smear cytologic abnormalities, which in turn place women at increased risk of progression,[34] it is likely that surrogate intermediate end points of infection will be used to determine vaccine efficacy in prospective trials.

If prophylactic vaccination with VLPs proves efficacious, the type specificity of neutralizing antibodies makes it likely that protection will also be type specific. Since multiple HPV types are found in cervical cancer, the type-specific nature of the immune protection implies that a polyvalent vaccine would be required to inhibit the majority of cervical cancers. For example, a vaccine that contained VLPs against HPV-16, 18, 31, and 45, might theoretically prevent close to 80% of cervical cancers.

Helicobacter pylori

H pylori, which was discovered in 1982, induces chronic gastric infection of almost one-half the world population. Infection with *H pylori* is associated with a variable proportion of several disorders, including duodenal ulcer, gastric ulcer, carcinoma of the gastric antrum and fundus, which is the second most common cancer worldwide, and gastric mucosa-associated lymphoid tissue lymphomas.[2,16,24,46]

H pylori is usually acquired in childhood. It disproportionately affects people of lower socioeconomic status, and the majority of adults from developing countries are infected. The bacterium is found less frequently among individuals in developed countries such as the United States, and the low rate of infection in children from developed countries suggests the proportion in adults will continue to fall.[24]

Most *H pylori* infections are asymptomatic and have a benign outcome. When infection does lead to stomach cancer, it usually takes decades.[46] In this process, bacterially induced chronic gastritis is believed to progress to atrophic gastritis and metaplasia, and then to cancer. The bacterium appears to be required only until atrophic gastritis develops, at which stage it frequently can no longer be cultured from the stomach. Experimental *H pylori* infection of Mongolian gerbils can induce these sequential pathologic changes, including gastric adenocarcinoma.[47]

Gastric mucosa-associated lymphoid tissue lymphoma is much less common than gastric carcinoma and has a distinct pathogenesis.[16] This B-cell lymphoma arises from *H pylori*–dependent chronic stimulation of the Peyer's patches in the gastric mucosa. Localized mucosa-associated lymphoid tissue tumors often remain dependent on continued stimulation by bacterial antigens, and eradication of the bacteria with antibiotic treatment may frequently be associated with lymphoma regression at this stage. However, the growth of more invasive tumors, which may become widely disseminated, is usually autonomous, and these tumors typically do not respond to antibacterial therapy.

Several bacterial virulence factors account for the ability of *H pylori* to colonize and persist in the gastric mucosa.[17,24] Although different isolates of *H pylori* are closely related antigenically, type I isolates, which are associated with carcinoma, contain a cassette of genes that are designated a pathogenicity-associated island called *cag*.

In principle, *H pylori* infection can be eradicated by combined treatment with several antimicrobial agents plus proton pump inhibitors. However, the high cost and the emergence of antibiotic resistance make this approach poorly suited for bacterial eradication from whole populations. These limitations have fostered efforts to develop *H pylori* vaccines.[17,24] Encouraging preclinical studies have been obtained with a variety of animal models. Mucosal immunization with bacterial lysates, purified bacterial antigens, or with attenuated salmonellae encoding *H pylori* antigen can all prevent experimental infection. Some of these vaccines have also been used successfully to eradicate established infection in the animal models. It remains to be determined which of these approaches will prove efficacious in human vaccine trials. The most desirable outcome would be a cost-effective vaccine that could eradicate established infection while also protecting against new infections. Such a vaccine would have the long-term benefits of a purely prophylactic vaccine while reducing the incidence of gastric cancer after a much shorter interval.

REFERENCES

1. Ames BN, Gold LS. The prevention of cancer. *Drug Metab Rev* 1998;30:201.
2. Pisani P, Parkin DM, Munoz N, Ferlay J. Cancer and infection: estimates of the attributable fraction in 1990. *Cancer Epidemiol Biomarkers Prev* 1997;6:387.
3. Tominaga S. Major avoidable risk factors of cancer. *Cancer Lett* 1999;143(Suppl 1):S19.

4. Hilleman MR. Overview of viruses, cancer, and vaccines in concept and in reality. *Recent Results Cancer Res* 1998;154:345.
5. Persing DH, Prendergast FG. Infection, immunity, and cancer. *Arch Pathol Lab Med* 1999;123:1015.
6. Blumberg BS. Hepatitis B virus, the vaccine, and the control of primary cancer of the liver. *Proc Natl Acad Sci U S A* 1997;94:7121.
7. Chang MH, Chen CJ, Lai MS, et al. Universal hepatitis B vaccination in Taiwan and the incidence of hepatocellular carcinoma in children. Taiwan Childhood Hepatoma Study Group [see comments]. *N Engl J Med* 1997;336:1855.
8. Abrignani S, Houghton M, Hsu HH. Perspectives for a vaccine against hepatitis C virus. *J Hepatol* 1999;31:259.
9. Cohen J. The scientific challenge of hepatitis C [see comments]. *Science* 1999;285:26.
10. Khanna R, Moss DJ, Burrows SR. Vaccine strategies against Epstein-Barr virus-associated diseases: lessons from studies on cytotoxic T-cell-mediated immune regulation. *Immunol Rev* 1999;170:49.
11. Murphy BR, Chanock RM. Immunization against virus disease. In: Fields BN, Knipe DM, Howley PM, eds. *Fields Virology*. Philadelphia: Lippincott–Raven, 1996:467.
12. Hollinger FB. Hepatitis B virus. In: Fields BN, Knipe DM, Howley PM, eds. *Fields Virology*. Philadelphia: Lippincott–Raven, 1996:2739.
13. Rinas AC. The gynecological Pap test. *Clin Lab Sci* 1999;12:239.
14. Maeda S, Ogura K, Yoshida H, et al. Major virulence factors, VacA and CagA, are commonly positive in *Helicobacter pylori* isolates in Japan. *Gut* 1998;42:338.
15. Lazo PA. The molecular genetics of cervical carcinoma. *Br J Cancer* 1999;80:2008.
16. Isaacson PG. Gastric MALT lymphoma: from concept to cure. *Ann Oncol* 1999;10:637.
17. Vyas SP, Sihorkar V. Exploring novel vaccines against *Helicobacter pylori*: protective and therapeutic immunization. *J Clin Pharm Ther* 1999;24:259.
18. Blattner WA. Human retroviruses: their role in cancer. *Proc Assoc Am Physicians* 1999;111:563.
19. Weiss RA. Viruses, cancer and AIDS. *FEMS Immunol Med Microbiol* 1999;26:227.
20. Katz SL. Future vaccines and a global perspective. *Lancet* 1997;350:1767.
21. Ahmed R, Gray D. Immunological memory and protective immunity: understanding their relation. *Science* 1996;272:54.
22. Zajac AJ, Murali-Krishna K, Blattman JN, Ahmed R. Therapeutic vaccination against chronic viral infection: the importance of cooperation between CD4+ and CD8+ T cells. *Curr Opin Immunol* 1998;10:444.
23. Lee WM. Hepatitis B virus infection [see comments]. *N Engl J Med* 1997;337:1733.
24. Covacci A, Telford JL, Del Giudice G, Parsonnet J, Rappuoli R. *Helicobacter pylori* virulence and genetic geography. *Science* 1999;284:1328.
25. Selvakumar R, Borenstein LA, Lin YL, Ahmed R, Wettstein FO. Immunization with nonstructural proteins E1 and E2 of cottontail rabbit papillomavirus stimulates regression of virus-induced papillomas. *J Virol* 1995;69:602.
26. Beasley RP, Hwang LY. Overview on the epidemiology of hepatocellular carcinoma. In: Hollinger FB, Lemon SM, Margolis HS, eds. *Viral hepatitis and liver disease*. Baltimore: Williams & Wilkins, 1991:532.
27. IARC. Hepatitis viruses. Monographs on the evaluation of carcinogenic risks to humans. Lyon: *IARC Monographs*, Vol. 59, 1994.
28. Chen PJ, Chen DS. Hepatitis B virus infection and hepatocellular carcinoma: molecular genetics and clinical perspectives. *Semin Liver Dis* 1999;19:253.
29. Lemon SM, Thomas DL. Vaccines to prevent viral hepatitis. *N Engl J Med* 1997;336:196.
30. Mahoney FJ. Update on diagnosis, management, and prevention of hepatitis B virus infection. *Clin Microbiol Rev* 1999;12:351.
31. IARC. Human papillomaviruses. IARC Monographs on the evaluation of carcinogenic risks to humans. Lyon: *IARC Monagraphs*, Vol. 64, 1995.
32. Shah KV, Howley PM. Papillomaviruses. In: Fields BN, Knipe DM, Howley PM, eds. *Fields virology*. Philadelphia: Lippincott–Raven, 1996:2077.
33. De Villiers EM. Papillomavirus and HPV typing. *Clin Dermatol* 1997;15:199.
34. Schiffman MH. New epidemiology of human papillomavirus infection and cervical neoplasia [editorial; comment]. *J Natl Cancer Inst* 1995;87:1345.
35. Munoz N, Bosch FX. The causal link between HPV and cervical cancer and its implications for prevention of cervical cancer. *Bull Pan Am Health Organ* 1996;30:362.
36. Walboomers JM, Jacobs MV, Manos MM, et al. Human papillomavirus is a necessary cause of invasive cervical cancer worldwide. *J Pathol* 1999;189:12.
37. Melbye M, Frisch M. The role of human papillomaviruses in anogenital cancers. *Semin Cancer Biol* 1998;8:307.
38. Frisch M, Biggar RJ. Aetiological parallel between tonsillar and anogenital squamous-cell carcinomas. *Lancet* 1999;354:1442.
39. Parkin DM, Pisani P, Ferlay J. Estimates of the worldwide incidence of 25 major cancers in 1990. *Int J Cancer* 1999;80:827.
40. Hines JF, Ghim SJ, Jenson AB. Prospects for human papillomavirus vaccine development: emerging HPV vaccines. *Curr Opin Obstet Gynecol* 1998;10:15.
41. Lowy DR, Schiller JT. Papillomaviruses: prophylactic vaccine prospects. *Biochim Biophys Acta* 1999;1423:M1.
42. Tindle RW. Immunomanipulative strategies for the control of human papillomavirus associated cervical disease. *Immunol Res* 1997;16:387.
43. Han R, Cladel NM, Reed CA, Peng X, Christensen ND. Protection of rabbits from viral challenge by gene gun-based intracutaneous vaccination with a combination of cottontail rabbit papillomavirus E1, E2, E6, and E7 genes. *J Virol* 1999;73:7039.
44. Reichman R, Balsley J, Carlin D, et al. Evaluation of the safety and immunogenicity of a recombinant HPV-11 L1 virus like particle vaccine in healthy adult volunteers. *(Submitted).*
45. Harro CD, Pang Y-YS, Rodan RBS, et al. A safety and immunogenicity trial of a candidate HPV16 virus-like particle vaccine. *(Submitted).*
46. Asaka M, Kudo M, Kato M, Sugiyama T, Takeda H. Review article: long-term *Helicobacter pylori* infection—from gastritis to gastric cancer. *Ailment Pharmacol Ther* 1998; 12(Suppl 1):9.
47. Watanabe T, Tada M, Nagai H, Sasaki S, Nakao M. *Helicobacter pylori* infection induces gastric cancer in mongolian gerbils [see comments]. *Gastroenterology* 1998;115:642.

SECTION 2

NICHOLAS P. RESTIFO
MARIO SZNOL
WILLEM W. OVERWIJK

Therapeutic Cancer Vaccines

The term *vaccine* originally referred to use of live cowpox virus inoculated in the skin as prophylaxis against smallpox, and hence is derived from the Latin *vacca*, which means cow. This meaning was extended to include the use of live, attenuated, or killed microbes or derivatives of microbes given by virtually any route to prevent the development of an infectious disease. The most recent incarnations of this term include the use of any antigen or fragment of an antigen, or any collection of antigens used alone, or together with an adjuvant, to modulate an immune response.

Vaccines are traditionally thought of as *preventing* infectious diseases, but they may have new uses in the *treatment* of malignancies. In the case of cancer, it is now clear that the immune system can recognize and destroy even large quantities of established tumor. Evidence for this immune-mediated destruction comes primarily from clinical trials using interleukin-2 (IL-2), which is now approved by the U.S. Food and Drug Administration for treatment for melanoma and renal cell carcinoma.[1] Although data are limited, experimental therapeutic vaccines have also been demonstrated to cause regression of cancer in a small percentage of patients.[2–4]

The goal of designing vaccines to prevent cancer may be appealing, but a variety of practical and theoretical problems arise in creating a prophylactic vaccine. Predicting which patients will develop cancer remains difficult, although assessment of risk becomes more accurate with the expansion in knowledge of genetic and environmental factors that contribute to carcinogenesis. There are also theoretical reasons why prophylactic vaccination against defined antigens may not be feasible. For example, the difficulty in predicting which of myriad mutations may occur in any one of a large number of genes makes vaccination against mutated tumor antigens unlikely to be successful. Similarly, vaccination against self-antigens may be subject to chronic immunologic tolerization, or may produce untoward side effects resulting from the destruction of normal tissues that express the same antigen.

The only truly preventive cancer vaccines that are under serious consideration are vaccines designed to prevent infectious diseases linked to the development of cancer.[5] For example, vaccines that prevent human papillomavirus or hepatitis B virus infections should also prevent cervical cancer and liver cancer, respectively. However, most cancers affecting individu-

TABLE 63.2-1. Candidate Vaccines for the Treatment of Established Cancer

WHOLE TUMOR CELL VACCINES MODIFIED *IN VIVO* OR *EX VIVO*
Admixture with adjuvant (chemical, bacterial, or viral)
Physical alteration (gamma irradiation)
Gene modification (with interleukin-2, tumor necrosis factor-α, interferon-γ, granulocyte-macrophage colony-stimulating factor, B7-1/B7-2)
TUMOR-DERIVED HEAT SHOCK PROTEINS
RECOMBINANT AND SYNTHETIC VACCINES
Peptides and proteins (given with adjuvants such as IFA)
Plasmid DNA (intramuscular injection, gene gun)
Self-replicating DNA or RNA (intramuscular injection, gene gun)
Recombinant viruses (fowlpox, vaccinia, adenovirus)
Recombinant bacteria (bacillus Calmette-Guérin, *Listeria, Salmonella*)
DENDRITIC CELL–BASED VACCINES
Pulsed with recombinant or protein or tumor cell lysate
Pulsed with synthetic or tumor-derived peptides
Transfected with recombinant or tumor-derived DNA or RNA
Infected with recombinant viruses or bacteria
Fused to whole tumor cells

IFA; incomplete Freund's adjuvant.

als in developed countries have not been associated with viruses. Thus, prophylactic vaccines for cancer are likely to be the exception rather than the rule. Most research in the field of cancer vaccines is devoted to vaccines designed to activate the immune system to destroy established cancer cells.

The notion that cancer cells could be recognized by the immune system has been the subject of scientific investigation for over 100 years. The nineteenth-century physician William Coley attempted to treat tumor-bearing patients by injecting fluid cultures of living *Streptococcus erysipelas* and reported an apparent decrease in tumor burden in some of his patients.[6] Since then, results from experiments first done by Gross, then by Prehn and Main, and finally expanded on by Klein and colleagues, indicated that mice could be immunized against subsequent challenge with methylcholanthrene-induced sarcomas.[7,8] Advances in molecular biology and immunology have since led to the identification of prospective tumor antigens and improved methods of immunization. Clinical studies of human immunotherapies and work done in experimental animal tumor systems have been mutually enhancing efforts. A number of broad categories of anticancer vaccine approaches have emerged from this research (Table 63.2-1).

IMMUNE MECHANISMS UNDERLYING VACCINE FUNCTION

CRITICAL ROLE OF T CELLS IN THE ANTITUMOR IMMUNE RESPONSE

The principle that T cells were critically important in the immune response against cancer was derived originally in mice with methylcholanthrene-induced tumors.[9–13] In both animal tumors and some human malignancies, T cells that accumulate within the mass of a tumor have been shown to specifically recognize autologous tumor cells *in vitro*, and to proliferate and specifically secrete cytokines, such as IL-2, interferon-γ (IFN-γ), granulocyte-macrophage colony-stimulating factor (GM-CSF), and tumor necrosis factor-α (TNF-α), in response to stimulation with autologous tumor cells.[14–16] The adoptive transfer of these antitumor T cells can treat substantial tumor burdens in both humans and mice.[17,18] Furthermore, the antitumor activity observed with systemic administration of the T-cell growth factor IL-2 in animal models, and perhaps also in patients, appears to be mediated in large part by tumor antigen-specific T lymphocytes.[19,20]

Several mouse studies have suggested that tumor rejection is largely dependent on CD8+, cytolytic T cells, with little if any role for CD4+ T cells.[21] In addition, adoptive transfer of pure populations of CD8+ T lymphocytes was shown to mediate tumor regression in mice.[22–24] Thus, many efforts to develop therapeutic anticancer vaccines have focused on CD8+ T lymphocytes, and the molecular targets of these cells have been identified in human and mouse systems.[25,26]

Compared with the comprehensive studies using CD8+ T cells in tumor models, relatively little is known about how CD4+ T cells influence antitumor immunity. Early work demonstrated that disseminated murine leukemia could be eradicated by a combination of cyclophosphamide and adoptive transfer of CD4+ T cells.[27,28]

We now understand some aspects of how CD4+ T lymphocytes help initiate and maintain the antitumor immune response.[29,30] CD4+ T cells regulate antigen-specific immune responses by regulating the functions of other components of the immune system, including B lymphocytes and CD8+ T lymphocytes. In the B16 murine melanoma system, CD4+ T cells appear crucial for the induction of both antitumor and autoimmunity that is mediated by B lymphocytes, as well as eosinophils and macrophages.[31–37]

Activated CD4+ T cells express CD40 ligand (gp39), which can engage the CD40 receptor on antigen-presenting cells (APCs) such as dendritic cells (DCs). These DCs can secrete proinflammatory cytokines such as IL-12, which in turn trigger the activation of CD8+ T cells and their production of IFN-γ and IL-2, resulting in the attraction of a host of other immune cells to the site.[38,39]

One potentially important experimental thrust in the use of adoptively transferred T cells may be the intentional addition of helper CD4+ T cells to adoptively transferred CD8+ T cells. Walter and colleagues found that the cytotoxic activity of adoptively transferred cytomegalovirus-specific CD8+ T-cell clones declined in patients deficient in cytomegalovirus-specific helper CD4+ T cells.[40]

Perhaps the most dramatic examples of the power of CD4+ T cells in the immune response to self proteins can be found in murine models of autoimmune diseases such as experimental allergic encephalomyelitis, systemic lupus erythematosus, and diabetes. In these models, disease can often be transferred to naive mice with purified, self-reactive CD4+ splenocytes or specific CD4+ T lymphocyte clones.[41,42] These studies suggest that the full activation of autoreactive CD4+ T cells may be a key element missing from many current clinical cancer vaccine trials. Attempts to identify the molecular targets of antitumor CD4+ T cells have already been successful.[43–48] Thus, current work focuses on efforts to harness the potential capabilities of tumor-specific CD4+ T cells.

TABLE 63.2-2. Examples of Defined Tumor-Associated Antigens in Cancer Vaccine Clinical Trials

CANCER TESTES ANTIGENS
MAGE-1 (melanoma, breast, lung, and others)
MAGE-3 (melanoma, breast, lung, and others)
NY-ESO-1 (melanoma, breast, lung, and others)
LAGE-1/CAMEL (melanoma, breast, lung, and others)
MELANOCYTE-DIFFERENTIATION ANTIGENS
MART-1/MelanA
gp100/pmel-17
Tyrosinase
Tyrosinase-related protein-1 (gp75)
Tyrosinase-related protein-2
NORMAL SELF-PROTEINS
Carcinoembryonic antigen (gastrointestinal malignancies, other adenocarcinomas)
Prostate-specific antigen
Prostate-specific membrane antigen
Human chorionic gonadotropin-β (adenocarcinomas)
Melanocyte-stimulating hormone receptor (melanoma)
HER-2/neu (breast, ovarian, others)
CA125 (ovarian)
GA733 (colon)
Gp72 (colon)
Proteinase-3 (myeloid leukemia)
MUC-1 core protein (breast, other adenocarcinomas)
VIRAL PROTEINS ASSOCIATED WITH MALIGNANCY
Human papillomavirus-16 E6 (cervical carcinoma)
Human papillomavirus-16 E7 (cervical carcinoma)
MUTATIONS, CHROMOSOMAL TRANSLOCATIONS, AND TUMOR-UNIQUE PROTEINS
Mutated ras (many tumors)
Mutated p53 (many tumors)
Pax3-fkhr translocation (alveolar rhabdomyosarcoma)
Ews-fli-1 translocation (Ewing's sarcoma)
Mutated von Hippel-Lindau (renal cell carcinoma)
Lymphoma idiotypes
Myeloma idiotypes
GANGLIOSIDE OR CARBOHYDRATE ANTIGENS
Fucosyl-GM1 (neural crest derivatives, melanoma, small cell lung)
GM2 (neural crest derivatives, melanoma, small cell lung)
GD2 (neural crest derivatives, melanoma, small cell lung)
GD3 (neural crest derivatives, melanoma, small cell lung)
Sialyl-Tn epitope of mucins (breast, colon, ovarian)
Globo H hexasaccharide (prostate)

TUMOR-ASSOCIATED ANTIGENS

Now that many tumor antigens have been identified (Table 63.2-2), how does one go about choosing an antigen appropriate for use in the design of a cancer vaccine? Some workers have picked target antigens because they are frequently mutated in tumors, as in the case of p53[49] or ras,[50,51] are at the site of joining of a translocation such as bcr-abl,[52] or are aberrantly glycosylated and thus the subject of recognition by antibodies as is the case for MUC-1.[53,54]

It is clear that not every peptide that can be generated from a protein will be presented in a major histocompatibility complex (MHC) class I–restricted fashion. The chances that any given peptide will be presented on the tumor cell surface are in the range of 1%, although this number is approximate. Because not every MHC-binding tumor-derived peptide will be naturally presented on the tumor cell surface, it is possible to induce a cytotoxic T lymphocyte (CTL) that can kill peptide-pulsed targets but not actual tumors.[56]

Identifying Tumor Antigens Recognized by T Lymphocytes

Because of the difficulty in predicting what peptides from a given potential antigen will be present on the cell surface, one of the most successful approaches to identifying tumor-associated antigens suitable for the development of cancer vaccines starts with the antitumor immune response. In many cases, the antitumor T cells were derived from cultures of tumor-infiltrating lymphocyte. Our own group [the Surgery Branch of the National Cancer Institute (NCI)] has focused on the T-cell reactivities that were associated with objective regressions of metastatic melanoma lesions after their adoptive transfer.[57] cDNA libraries of expressed melanoma genes were screened by transfecting these genes, along with the gene for the restricting MHC molecule, into an antigen-negative cell line that was then admixed with T lymphocytes that have antitumor activity. If the T cells recognize the transfected cell line, they lyse it and release cytokines such as GM-CSF, TNF-α, and IFN-γ, any of which can be measured.[2,14] This process of cloning genes encoding tumor antigens is under constant improvement and has become considerably faster and more streamlined.[58]

Targeting Self-Antigens

The identification of self-antigens as potential targets in the immunotherapy of cancer has been an important factor driving interest in cancer vaccine development. Many of the tumor antigens that have been identified, in the case of melanoma, are tissue differentiation antigens in melanocytes and include gp100,[59–65] MART-1/MelanA,[66–70] tyrosinase,[61,71–74] and tyrosinase-related protein-1/gp75[75] and tyrosinase-related protein-2.[76–78] Interestingly, these antigens are involved in the synthesis of melanin that gives both melanocytes and deposits of melanoma tumor their dark pigment. CEA expressed in gastrointestinal and some other malignancies, and prostate-specific antigen (PSA), are other examples of differentiation antigens that have relatively restricted expression in normal tissues and could be targeted by cancer vaccines.[79]

A second group of self-antigens are expressed by a diversity of tumor histologies but are not expressed by normal tissues other than testis. Cloned in large part by Dr. Thierry Boon and his colleagues, these antigens are encoded by genes with family names like MAGE, BAGE, GAGE, RAGE, LAGE, and CAMEL.[80–82] NY-ESO-1 also falls into this group and is expressed in a significant proportion of human melanoma cells as well as tumors arising from breast, ovary, bladder, prostate, and liver.[83–88]

The fact that differentiation antigens are nonmutated in most tumors has two important implications. First, expression of these antigens would be expected in subsets of patients with a defined tumor histology, thus an *off-the-shelf* vaccine strategy targeting these antigens is possible (a strategy that targets a mutated antigen may have to be individualized for every mutation). Second, the nonmutated nature of these antigens suggests that immunotherapies that target these antigens could elicit autoreactivity. One consequence of this autoreactivity may be vitiligo, the patchy and permanent loss of pigment from the skin and hair thought to result from the autoimmune destruction of pigment cells.[31] Vitiligo has been correlated with objective shrinkage of deposits of metastatic melanoma in patients receiving high-dose IL-2, a cytokine known to activate and expand T lymphocytes.[89] This correlation is among the strongest evidence that the antitumor effects of IL-2 are mediated by antigen-specific immune responses and supports the notion that targeting immune responses to recognize self-antigens expressed by tumor can lead to tumor regression.

Are Mutated Tumor Antigens Better Targets for Immune Recognition?

Besides shared antigens, human tumors also express mutated antigens that can be processed and presented for recognition by T cells. Neoantigens produced as a result of mutation often are found to originate in ubiquitously expressed proteins. Examples include epitopes from β-catenin,[90] CDK4,[91] MUM1,[92] FLICE (caspase 8),[93] HLA-A2,[94] and a mutant gene from a bladder carcinoma that is recorded in databases under the name KIAA0205, whose function is unknown.[93,95] Interestingly, some of these antigens are also oncogenic, including the mutations described for β-catenin and CDK4.[90,91]

Mutated antigens may not lend themselves easily to off-the-shelf vaccines consisting of purely recombinant and synthetic components, because each neoantigen for each patient must be checked for sequence and that sequence must be verified to be present on the surface of a tumor cell. Some workers have asserted that mutated tumor antigens are superior targets for vaccine design because immune cells will not be tolerized to these antigens.[96] However, work has shown that even the most immunogenic *foreign* antigen, such as the hemagglutinin antigen from the influenza A virus, can be tolerizing when expressed peripherally (i.e., outside the thymus) either in normal cells[97] or tumor cells.[98] Thus, mutated or otherwise foreign antigens may also induce peripheral tolerance when expressed by tumor cells.

ROLE OF DENDRITIC CELLS IN VACCINE FUNCTION

It is likely that DCs are a key mediator of vaccine function.[99–101] DCs activate T-cell responses by capturing, processing, and presenting antigens in the context of MHC molecules to T lymphocytes. In addition, DCs express the costimulatory molecules B7-1 (CD80) and B7-2 (CD86), which provide a second signal on interaction with their receptors on the surface of T cells known as CD28 and CTLA-4.[102,103] Engagement of CD28 is associated with proliferation and differentiation whereas CTLA-4 may trigger functional unresponsiveness.[104,105] Blocking CTLA-4 engagement has been reported to enhance immune responses to tumor cells.[106] Activating T cells by DC is thus accomplished by presenting antigen/MHC complexes in the context of a variety of other activating signals.[107]

DCs can undergo maturation or *super activation* through the activity of GM-CSF and TNF-α and other macrophage-derived cytokines, greatly enhancing their ability to activate naive T cells. In addition, CD40 and its ligand have been shown to be important in B-cell activation, in the production of type 1 cytokines by T-helper cells, and in the generation of cytotoxic T-cell memory responses. We and others have found that the addition of CD40L trimer to DNA vaccination can significantly increase antitumor efficacy.[108] Another molecule called FLT3 ligand can induce the apparent growth and differentiation of functional DC and has been reported to have antitumor effects,[109,110] and its effect on the function of recombinant and synthetic anticancer vaccines is the subject of a great deal of investigation in experimental mouse models.

ROLE OF ANTIBODIES IN IMMUNE-MEDIATED ANTITUMOR RESPONSES

Much of the experimental data generated with cancer vaccines in animal models suggests that immune-mediated antitumor activity is attributable to T cells. Nevertheless, adoptive transfer of antibodies directed against surface tumor antigens can cause regression of cancer in animal models, and vaccine-induced antibody responses have been demonstrated to reject a tumor challenge and to cause regression of small-volume established cancer.[111] Antibodies mediate antitumor effects by complement-dependent lysis or by antibody-dependent cellular cytotoxicity. In addition, antibodies directed against growth factor receptors or other cell surface molecules have demonstrated antitumor activity in animal models and in human clinical trials, by mechanisms that appear to involve blocking or stimulating a cell signal. For example, trastuzumab (Herceptin) is a humanized monoclonal antibody that blocks the function of the HER-2/neu protooncogene, which is overexpressed in 25% to 30% of breast cancers, and causes objective tumor responses in approximately 15% of breast cancer patients with metastatic disease. It also significantly enhances the therapeutic effect of paclitaxel in these patients. Although the mechanism of action is thought to involve the inhibition of stimulatory signals provided by multiple neuregulins and epidermal growth factor–like molecules,[112–116] there is some evidence that the therapeutic effect may also have an immunologic component through direct killing of antibody-coated tumor cells by natural killer cells.[117]

Antibody responses are generally directed toward cell surface components of tumor cells. Similar to T-cell responses, several factors may influence the antitumor activity of an antibody response, including the density of the target on the cell surface; the type of target; the type of antibody response; the affinity of the antibody for its target; the magnitude of the response (titer); the amount of circulating antigen; the presence of antigen on normal cells; and perhaps the availability at the tumor site of effector immune cells bearing the appropriate Fc receptors. Entry of antibodies into tumors can be limited by physiologic barriers, for example, by high tumor pressure, and the presence of complement inhibitors has been documented on various tumor cell lines,[118,119] perhaps limiting the activity of antibodies that require complement activation for antitumor activity.

MONITORING OF CANCER VACCINE TRIALS

A major challenge for cancer vaccine trials is determination of efficacy, as measured by immune response and patient benefit. Techniques for measuring antibody response have become relatively well established, although it is important to verify that the antibody responses actually recognize tumor cells bearing the antigen, and that affinity, titer, and biologic activity are sufficiently high to expect antitumor activity *in vivo*.

T-cell responses can be measured through a biologic assay, for example, a skin test of delayed-type hypersensitivity (DTH), by assessment of number and function of antigen-specific T cells in peripheral blood, and by assessment of histologic changes and antigen-specific T-cell number and function within the tumor. DTH is commonly used to measure responses to autologous and allogeneic cell vaccines. Application of appropriate controls for DTH testing is often difficult, and it is often not possible to be certain that a positive reaction truly indicates response to a relevant tumor antigen and not, for example, serum or other components of the tumoral growth medium.

Detection of antigen-specific T cells in blood or tumor can be accomplished by a physical characteristic (presence of a particular T-cell receptor) or function (production of cytokine in response to the binding of a peptide-MHC complex with the T-cell receptor). If the peptide to which the immune response is directed is known, peptide-MHC complexes can be joined to form a tetramer, which can be used to detect T cells bearing the appropriate T-cell receptor in a flow cytometer.[120] By this technique, the number of peptide-specific T cells in a bulk population can be enumerated, and after sorting, the functional capacity of the T cells can be characterized.[121,122] The tetramer technique is promising but is still limited by the sensitivity of the flow cytometer.

Perhaps the most sensitive techniques for assessing a T-cell response to immunization are based on detecting a particular function of a T cell when exposed to its antigen, most commonly secretion of cytokines, cytotoxicity toward antigen pulsed cells, tumor expressing the antigen, or all these. Ultimately, it is important to demonstrate induction of immune responses that recognizes tumor cells and not just antigen presented by a target cell, since efficacy is based on the immune response recognizing naturally processed and presented antigen. If immunization results in an increased frequency of T cells against the immunizing antigen, posttreatment bulk cultures of T cells exposed to the appropriate target should produce greater amounts of cytokines than pretreatment bulk cultures. Indeed, the latter has been shown after immunization with various peptides including MART-1 and modified gp100 melanoma peptides, although the posttreatment cultures still require some expansion of precursors *in vitro* before measuring cytokine release.[123] Limiting dilution assays allow a more accurate enumeration of T-cell precursors that are ultimately detected based on function such as cytokine release or cytotoxicity.[2]

The enzyme-linked immunosorbent assay–spot (ELISPOT) technique involves plating T cells with targets and fixed antibodies to a particular cytokine. The plate is developed by a second antibody to the cytokine, so that a spot appears wherever a T cell has recognized a target and has been stimulated to produce the indicator cytokine. By counting the number of spots and dividing by the number of T cells plated, an estimate of the frequency of antigen-specific T cells can be made. The ELISPOT technique also has sensitivity limitations, but may become a useful tool in monitoring of some cancer vaccine trials.[124]

The Surgery Branch of the NCI has explored the use of quantitative reverse transcriptase polymerase chain reaction techniques to detect evidence of immunization to a peptide vaccine directly from peripheral blood and from tumor. The technique involves measurement of mRNA message for a particular cytokine normalized to a standard curve. Measurements can be made on fine-needle aspirates of tumor. Since the mechanism of vaccine antitumor response likely involves infiltration of tumor by T cells, and activity is dependent on cytokine production by the infiltrating T cells, an efficient measure of vaccine biologic activity is an increase in mRNA for a particular cytokine at the tumor site.[125]

ANTICANCER VACCINE APPROACHES DERIVED FROM AUTOLOGOUS AND ALLOGENEIC TUMOR CELLS

Many cancer vaccines in current development use autologous or allogeneic tumor cells as the source of antigen for immunizing patients. Autologous tumor cell vaccines must be prepared individually for each patient, but offer the potential to immunize against antigens generated by patient- and tumor-specific gene mutations. Allogeneic tumor cells provide a more reliable and uniform source of antigen for preparation of vaccines, but target only antigens that are shared between the cell lines in the vaccine and the patient's tumor.

Final preparations of autologous or allogeneic tumor cell vaccines contain either whole cells, lysates, or extracts from the cells. Some attempts have been made to immunize with live autologous cancer cells, but to avoid the concern that live cells might implant or metastasize, whole tumor cells are irradiated or otherwise killed before reinjection. To ensure adequate presentation of antigens to the immune system, adjuvants such as bacille Calmette-Guérin (BCG),[126,127] *Corynebacterium parvum*,[128,129] DETOX, and alum must be added to the cells or cell extracts. Attempts to increase immunogenicity have also included the infection of allogeneic tumor cells with vaccinia virus,[130,131] vesicular stomatitis virus,[132] as well as other viruses to create *oncolysates* that contain both viral and tumor antigens. The strong foreign viral antigens serve as an immunologic adjuvant that enhances immune responses to the tumor antigens.

A significant body of work in experimental animals has shown that transfection of genes into tumor cells is capable of increasing their immunogenicity.[133–135] Based on these results, patients have been treated with tumor cells genetically modified *ex vivo* or *in vivo* to express several different classes of genes, including cytokines, T-cell costimulatory molecules, or foreign genes encoding allogeneic or xenogeneic MHC class I molecules. The substantial work with gene-modified tumor cells is described in greater detail in Chapter 62.1.

More recent efforts to improve the immunogenicity of autologous and allogeneic cancer cell vaccines have involved the direct transfer to, or expression of, potential antigens in host APC. Methods under investigation in animal models, and either ongoing or planned for clinical trials, include expressing whole tumor cell RNA in host APC,[136] pulsing APC with peptides extracted by acid elution from the surface of tumor cells,[137,138] and creating DC–tumor cell fusions.[139,140]

An alternative to the use of whole tumor cells in vaccines has been to enrich the relevant and immune-activating components of tumor cells while excluding the irrelevant and immune-suppressing substances that may be present. Partially purified fractions of allogeneic tumor cell lines, in this instance shed tumor antigens into the culture media, have been shown to yield preparations that are capable of stimulating immune responses in experimental murine models.[141] This method of preparing a tumor vaccine has been extended into the clinic,[142,143] in combination with adjuvants such as alum[144] or DETOX.[145] Srivastava and colleagues have shown that heat shock proteins carry antigenic peptide determinants of cellular proteins, including tumor antigens, to the MHC molecules in the endoplasmic reticulum.[146,147] When isolated from tumor cells and administered as a vaccine, the heat shock proteins can apparently gain access to both the class I and class II antigen-processing pathways of certain APCs, including macrophages, and can induce both tumor-antigen specific helper and cytotoxic T-lymphocyte responses.[147] The heat shock protein preparations have generated protective and therapeutic antitumor activity in animal models, and on this basis, have entered clinical trials.[148–152]

CLINICAL EXPERIENCE

Some of the vaccines that have progressed to randomized trials are listed in Table 63.2-3. Most of the clinical experience has been in patients with melanoma. A large number of clinical trials have been conducted including vaccinia-induced lysates of allogeneic melanoma cell lines[131]; shed antigens from cultures of allogeneic melanoma cell lines (admixed with alum)[142,143]; Melacine, lysates from two allogeneic melanoma cell lines (administered with DETOX)[145,153]; CancerVax, a combination of three allogeneic melanoma cell lines (with BCG as adjuvant)[154,155]; and autologous melanoma cells chemically modified with dinitrophenyl (DNP).[156–158] For several of the vaccines, including Melacine, CancerVax, and the DNP-modified autologous melanoma cells, low rates of objective responses were observed in patients with metastatic disease, although usually not in patients with large tumor burdens or visceral involvement. A striking observation in trials of the DNP-modified autologous melanoma cells was the induction of inflammation and lymphocytic infiltrates in distant metastatic lesions. For all the vaccines, single-arm studies suggested that the vaccine improved disease-free survival of stage III patients (in general, patients following resection of their primary or regional nodes, or both, and at high risk for recurrence), and for some of the vaccines improved survival was also suggested for patients with metastatic disease. Comparisons were made with historical controls, or within the study, immune responders were compared with patients who had poor or no immunologic response to the vaccine.

Based on these data, several of the vaccines were tested or are currently in phase III randomized trials (see Table 63.2-3). The vaccinia melanoma oncolysate showed no benefit for patients with stage III disease in one trial, although another larger study of a vaccinia melanoma oncolysate is pending analysis. Melacine, a vaccine composed of lysates from two allogeneic melanoma cells lines admixed with DETOX, did not improve survival of patients with metastatic melanoma compared with chemotherapy. Two randomized trials of an autologous colon cancer vaccine admixed with BCG adjuvant involving stage II/III patients have been published.[159] One of the studies indicated an improvement in disease-free survival for stage II patients only. The difference in outcome between the two trials was attributed to improved quality control in vaccine preparation and administration of an additional dose

TABLE 63.2-3. Moderate and Large Randomized Trials of Cancer Vaccines

Vaccine	*Adjuvant*	*Disease/Stage*	*Total No. of Patients*	*Results*	*References*
Melanoma vaccinia oncolysate	NA	Stage III (1–5 lymph nodes)	250, 217 evaluable	No survival improvement compared with control (live vaccinia virus); at 5 y, 48% alive	263
Melanoma vaccinia oncolysate	NA	Stages IIB and III	700	Pending	Hersey et al. (personal communication, 2000)
Melanoma cell-line lysate (Melacine)	DETOX, low-dose cyclophosphamide	Metastatic	140	No survival improvement compared with chemotherapy	264
Melanoma cell-line lysate (Melacine)	DETOX	Stage IIA (1.5–4.0 mm primary)	689, 590 evaluable	Pending analysis February 2000, no effect on disease-free survival in eligible patients	Sondak et al. (meeting presentation, February 2000)
GM2 ganglioside	Bacille Calmette-Guérin, low-dose cyclophosphamide	Melanoma stage III	122	Trend toward improved disease-free and overall survival; disease-free survival 50% at 4 y versus 30% in controls	265
GM2 ganglioside, conjugated to KLH	QS-21	Melanoma stage IIB, III	880	Pending, control arm is interferon-α_{2b}	Kirkwood et al. (personal communication, 2000)
Autologous colon cancer cells	Bacille Calmette-Guérin	Stage II, III	412, 303 evaluable	No survival improvement compared with controls	266
Autologous colon cancer cells	Bacille Calmette-Guérin	Stage II, III	254	Improvement in disease-free interval, benefit in stage II patients only	159

for late boosting of the immune response in the positive trial. Additional studies may be required to assess the true efficacy of the vaccine when administered optimally.

Various autologous tumor cell vaccine approaches have been explored in patients with advanced renal cell cancer. Among 20 evaluable patients immunized with autologous tumor cells and a bacterial (*Corynebacterium parvum*) adjuvant, one complete and four partial responses were observed, all in lung metastases.[160] Positive DTH responses to the autologous tumor cells correlated with response and survival.[161] Kugler et al. reported on 17 metastatic renal cell cancer patients immunized with a vaccine composed of autologous tumor cells fused to allogeneic monocyte-derived DCs.[140] Theoretically, the tumor self-MHC molecules are presenting unique cancer antigens to the host immune system, and the allogeneic DC fusion partner is providing the necessary costimulation to T cells to ensure optimal activation. Four complete and two partial responses were observed. Regression was noted primarily in metastases of lung, bone, lymph node, and local recurrences and appeared durable in some patients, although median follow-up was only 13 months at the time of the report. DTH responses to autologous tumor developed in 11 of the 17 patients, which included all the objective antitumor responses.

The clinical experience obtained with tumor cells modified with genes encoding cytokines or other immune-stimulatory molecules is covered in Chapter 62.1. Whether gene modification of tumor cells enhances their immunogenicity and therapeutic outcome in comparison with a simple admixture of tumor cells with nonspecific adjuvants remains a subject of debate and further study in preclinical models and clinical trials. Nevertheless, a large number of clinical trials involving gene-modified tumor cells have been initiated. An occasional antitumor response has been reported, but in general the vaccines have had minimal activity against advanced disease. Of note, in a trial of GM-CSF–transfected autologous melanoma cells, the vaccine appeared to induce T-cell infiltrates in distant metastatic lesions, similar to results reported for the DNP-modified autologous tumor cell vaccine. Despite the biologic activity, systemic antitumor response as measured by standard criteria was observed in only a few patients.[162]

APPROACHES USING RECOMBINANT AND SYNTHETIC ANTICANCER VACCINES

Because cancer cells are notoriously poor immunogens, workers in a number of laboratories have attempted to isolate tumor antigens and present them to the immune system in more immunogenic formulations. This has led to the development of recombinant and synthetic cancer vaccines, which are predicated on the identification of tumor-associated antigens.

Among the most effective immunization strategies for defined antigens in animal models has been to insert the gene for the antigen in recombinant vectors. A partial list of recombinant viral immunogens includes vaccinia, fowlpox, canarypox, adenovirus, influenza, polio, and sindbis.[163] Recombinant organisms include *Listeria*, *Salmonella*, and BCG.[164,165] In addition, *naked* nucleic acid–based vectors include the administration of DNA by intramuscular or intradermal injection or by *gene gun* and most recently, the administration of *self-replicating* nucleic acid-based immunogens.[166,167]

RECOMBINANT VIRUS–BASED VACCINES

Recombinant virus–based cancer vaccines are created by inserting genes encoding tumor antigens into the viral genome. The safety of these recombinant viruses can be ensured in a number of ways. Some of the recombinant vaccines are composed of viruses incapable of replicating in mammalian cells because of their host range (e.g., the avian poxviruses),[168] whereas others are highly attenuated (such as certain influenza A viruses[169] or the Wyeth and MVA strains of vaccinia virus[170]), and still others are made safe by the removal of viral genes that are critical to viral replication and virulence (such as adenoviruses).[171]

Vaccines based on live, attenuated, or killed viruses can be highly effective in preventing human viral diseases such as polio, smallpox, and even influenza A. However, recombinant viruses encoding tumor antigens have an important shortcoming: The only component of the immune response that can be tumor specific is the response elicited by the expression of the transgene(s) encoding the tumor antigen(s). Although viral elements might help boost immune reactivity through their activity as helper epitopes, they will not contribute any specificity of immune reactivity for tumors, with the exception of recombinant virus-based immunogens used to vaccinate against a virally induced cancer (e.g., the use of recombinant human papillomavirus to treat cervical cancer).

Problem of Preexisting Immunity to Viral Immunogens

Although viral vaccines are potent inducers of antitumor immunity in animal models, the obstacle of preexisting immunity remains an important problem in the translation of these strategies to the clinic. We have learned in the conduct of our own clinical trials that humans have high neutralizing titers to recombinant viral vaccines based on adenoviruses, likely due to the ubiquitous presence of adenovirus in the environment of the upper respiratory systems.[172–175]

Vaccinia virus was widely used in the campaign to eradicate smallpox.[176] Thus, anyone born in the United States before approximately 1970 (the majority of patients who currently have cancer) have already been immunized to vaccinia.[177] Elsewhere in the world, immunization with vaccinia was continued well after the early 1970s.[178] Indeed, most patients appear to be able to rapidly clear these viruses, making it difficult or impossible to effectively use cancer vaccines based on these viruses. One way of circumventing the problem of preexisting immunity is the use of viruses whose natural hosts are nonmammalian, such as the avian poxviruses.[168]

Clinical Experience

Viruses engineered to express some tumor antigens induce potent immune responses in murine models, which serve as the basis for initiating human clinical studies. However, the animal models may overestimate the efficacy of the recombinant viral vaccines in clinical trials. In addition to the problem of preexisting immunity to several of the viral vectors, patients also are likely to have preexisting immunologic tolerance to the tumor antigen, which is often a self-antigen in the human trials. The results of clinical studies to date seem to bear out these concerns (Table 63.2-4). Limited data from a trial of vaccinia-CEA, and separately ALVAC-CEA, the latter a nonreplicating poxvirus in

TABLE 63.2-4. Clinical Trials Using Vaccines Based on Recombinant Viruses[a]

Antigen	*Method of Gene Delivery*	*Route of Administration, Dose Range*	*Patient Population (Disease and Stage)*	*No. of Patients*	*Clinical Responses*	*Immunologic Effects*	*Comments*	*References*
MART-1	Adenovirus	Subcutaneous or IM, 10^7 to 10^{11}	Metastatic melanoma	36	CR 31+ mo without IL-2, 2 CR+ 2 PR with IL-2	5 of 23 HLA-A201 patients developed increased CTL activity to MART-1 :27–35 peptide	Most patients had substantial preexisting titers against adenovirus	172
MART-1	Vaccinia	Scarification, IM, 10^7 to 5×10^8	Metastatic melanoma	6	Pending	Pending	Overall response rate identical to IL-2 alone	
MART-1	Fowlpox	IM, 10^7 to 5×10^9	Metastatic melanoma	17	Pending	Pending		
gp100	Adenovirus	IM	Metastatic melanoma	18	1 CR with IL-2	No reactivity to three different HLA-A2 restricted gp100 peptides (n = 16)	Most patients had substantial preexisting titers against adenovirus	172
gp100	Vaccinia	Scarification, IM, 10^7 to 10^9	Metastatic melanoma	47	Pending	Pending	Overall response rate identical to IL-2 alone	Surgery Branch, NCI
gp100	Fowlpox	IM, 10^7 to 5×10^9	Metastatic melanoma	15	Pending	Pending		Surgery Branch, NCI, in progress
gp100	DNA plasmid	0.1–1 mg, divided over two sites, IM or intradermal	Metastatic melanoma	23	Pending	Pending		Surgery Branch, NCI
CEA	Vaccinia	Scarification, monthly × 3, 2×10^5 to 10^7	CEA + metastatic malignancy	17 + 26	None	Postvaccination weak CTL responses to a CEA HLA-A2 restricted peptide in some patients	Two separate trials	179,267
CEA	Vaccinia	Monthly × 2, Intradermal vs. subcutaneous jet device, 10^7 to 10^8	CEA+ metastatic malignancy	20	None	No T-cell proliferative or antibody responses to CEA protein	Both ID and SQ routes effective for immune responses to vaccinia antigens	180
CEA	ALVAC	IM monthly × 3, 2.5×10^5 to 2.5×10^7	CEA+ metastatic malignancy, no evidence of disease patients eligible	20	None	Two- to tenfold increase in precursor CTL to CAP-1 (an HLA-A2 CEA peptide) in HLA-A2+ patients	Highest CTL frequency 1 of 37,434 postimmunization	268,269
CEA and B7.1	ALVAC	Intradermal, q2wk × 4, and IM monthly, 4.5×10^6 to 4.5×10^8	CEA + metastatic malignancy	39 + 18	None	Too early	Two different trials	Lee et al., Von Mehren et al.
PSA	Vaccinia	Intradermal, monthly × 3, 2.65×10^6 to 2.65×10^8	PSA + prostate cancer	23	4 of 23 progression-free at 14–24+ mo	Pending		Eder et al.
HPV-16 and HPV-18 E6 and E7	Vaccinia	Scarification, once, 2×10^6	HPV16+ postsurgery/radiation or recurrent cervical cancer	8	No objective regression	3 of 8 Ab response to HPV-18 E7		270

CEA, carcinoembryonic antigen; CR, complete response; CTL, cytologic T lymphocyte; HPV, human papillomavirus; IL, interleukin; NCI, National Cancer Institute; PR, partial response; PSA, prostate-specific antigen.

[a]Trials of prime boost with vaccinia-CEA + ALVAC-CEA, vaccinia-PSA + fowlpox-PSA, and vaccinia-tyrosinase + fowlpox-tyrosinase are in progress.

humans, suggest that weak cellular responses to CEA can be induced *in vivo*, as measured by T-cell responses to an HLA-A201 restricted peptide from CEA.[179] Antibody responses to the CEA protein were not detected in a separate study.[180] The Surgery Branch, NCI, has conducted clinical trials of adenovirus, vaccinia, and fowlpox separately carrying the MART-1 and gp100 melanoma genes[172] (S. A. Rosenburg, personal communication, 2000). One patient treated with the adenovirus-MART-1 vector experienced a durable complete regression, but otherwise, no clinical responses were observed with any of the vaccines used alone in patients with metastatic melanoma. Furthermore, the viral vaccines were not able to elicit immune responses to the viral-encoded tumor antigens, as measured against known HLA-A201 restricted peptide epitopes of the antigen. Because of the methodologies used to detect immune responses in the latter trials, it is not possible to exclude weak immune responses to known or unknown epitopes of the tumor antigens. Clinical trials of recombinant vaccinia and fowlpox vectors containing PSA and MUC-1 are in progress. Preliminary results of the vaccinia-PSA trial, in patients with rising PSA levels postsurgery, suggest that some patients may remain progression-free for an extended period, although actual benefit from the vaccine must be proven in randomized trials.

Table 63.2-4 demonstrates that trials of recombinant viral vaccines have employed different routes of administration including scarification (multiple punctures of the vaccine solution into the skin), intradermal, subcutaneous, and intramuscular injection. Some patients also received the nonreplicating fowlpox-gp100 vaccine intravenously (S. A. Rosenberg et al., personal communication, 2000). A large range of doses has been explored in the phase I trials. Immunizations were repeated monthly in most trials for a maximum of three to four doses. Using immune responses to the viral vector antigens as a guide, no route of administration has proven to be superior, and a relationship between dose and immune response has not been established, although higher doses are predicted to be more effective for the nonreplicating vectors. Exploration of schedule issues (e.g., a longer interval between doses) has been difficult in the selected patient populations with progressing metastatic disease. For the vaccinia vectors, a *take* (formation of an inflammatory response and a bleb at the injection site) has occurred in most patients receiving the vaccine by scarification or intradermal injection despite preexisting immunity to vaccinia. However, second and third doses of vaccinia are usually not associated with a significant local reaction, suggesting that the vaccinia is cleared too quickly to allow boosting of immune responses to the encoded tumor antigen.

In order to improve the effects of these vectors, current studies are combining different viral vectors that are non–cross-reactive in patients, or viral vectors combined with the corresponding peptide epitopes of the antigen gene, administered sequentially. These heterologous boost strategies were superior to repeated immunizations with single vectors in animal models.[181,182] Examples of ongoing trials include sequential immunizations with vaccinia-CEA and ALVAC-CEA in patients with CEA-expressing malignancies, and vaccinia-tyrosinase sequenced with fowlpox-tyrosinase in metastatic melanoma patients. Investigators are also combining genes for T-cell costimulatory signals with the antigen gene within a single viral vector, or combining viral vectors that respectively express the antigen gene and genes for cytokines or one or more T-cell costimulatory signals. Clinical trials of vaccinia containing genes for both CEA and B7-1 (CD80) have been initiated, but results are pending. Several of the recombinant viral vaccines encoding tumor antigens have also been administered in combination with systemic or local administration of GM-CSF, and with systemic IL-2. The Surgery Branch, NCI, administered high-dose IL-2 following immunization with adenovirus, fowlpox, and vaccinia vectors containing either the MART-1 or gp100 genes in patients with metastatic melanoma[172] (S. A. Rosenberg, personal communication, 2000). Although some clinical response were observed, the response rates did not appear higher than expected with IL-2 alone, and no enhancement of immunologic responses to the tumor antigens was observed. Results of studies employing lower doses of IL-2 with other recombinant viral vaccines have not been completed.

RECOMBINANT VACCINES BASED ON NAKED NUCLEIC ACID

Reports dating from the early 1990s indicated the surprising finding that the intramuscular injection of *naked* plasmid DNA (i.e., DNA without a viral coat) could result in an immune response.[183] Like viral vaccines, the activity of DNA vaccines appears to be mediated through DCs and other *professional* APCs.[100]

In the case of gene-gun delivery, nucleic acid is precipitated onto an inert particle (generally gold beads) and forced into the cells with a helium blast. Transfected cells then express the antigen encoded on the plasmid, resulting in an immune response. Like live or attenuated viruses, DNA vaccines effectively engage both MHC I and MHC II pathways, allowing for the induction of CD8+ and CD4+ T cells.

DNA-based vaccines are relatively safe and easy to engineer and produce. In animal models, they are generally not as potent as recombinant viruses at eliciting immune responses capable of destroying tumors. Important innovations in the design of DNA vaccines include promoter optimization, enhancement of polyadenylation sequences, the removal of 5' and 3' untranslated regions from the inserted gene, and the use of intronic sequences to improve nuclear export.

Clinical trials using naked DNA vaccines encoding tumor antigens have begun. One of the first of these trials was launched at the Surgery Branch, NCI. It uses a plasmid encoding a modified form of the human gp100 melanoma antigen first alone then in combination with IL-2, previously shown in murine studies to enhance vaccination with plasmid.[166] Preliminary results indicate no clear signs of immunization and no objective tumor regressions.

One promising new approach to the development of nucleic acid vaccines may be strategies designed to make them self-replicating. Self-replication can be accomplished by using a gene encoding an RNA replicase polyprotein derived from alphaviruses, a family of viruses that includes Semliki Forest virus, Sindbis virus, and the Venezuelan encephalitis virus. A gene encoding a tumor antigen can be added to such a construct under the control of a viral promoter. Such constructs can elicit antigen-specific antibody and CD8+ T-cell responses at doses as low as 0.1 μg.[166]

PEPTIDE VACCINES

Table 63.2-5 describes the clinical results of selected trials conducted with peptide vaccines. Peptides have been derived from various antigens, including melanoma antigens MART-1, gp100, tyrosinase, and tyrosinase-related protein-1; cancer tes-

TABLE 63.2-5. Clinical Trials Using Vaccines Based on Synthetic Peptides or Purified Proteins

Peptide Antigen/Human Leukocyte Antigen Restriction	*Adjuvant*	*Route of Administration*	*Dose Range*	*Patient Population*	*No. of Patients*	*Clinical Results*	*Immunologic Results*	*Reference*
MART-1:27-35–A201	Montanide ISA 51	SQ, q3wk	0.1–10.0 mg	Metastatic melanoma	23 (18 analyzed)	None	15 of 18 had new or increased CTL reactivity toward peptide	123
gp100:209-217-A201	Montanide ISA 51	SQ, q3wk	1 mg	Metastatic melanoma	9	1 PR , 4 mo duration	2 of 8 developed CTL reactivity to peptide	2
gp100:209-217 (210M)-A201	Montanide ISA 51	SQ, q3wk	1 mg	Metastatic melanoma	11	3 mixed responses	10 of 11 developed CTL reactivity to native peptide, 4 of 5 to HLA-A2 matched melanoma	2
gp100:154-162-A201	Montanide ISA 51	SQ, q3wk	1–10 mg	Metastatic melanoma	10 (7 analyzed)	None	No CTL reactivity	274
gp100:280-288	Montanide ISA 51	SQ, q3wk	1–10 mg	Metastatic melanoma	9 (6 analyzed)	None	3 of 6 developed CTL response to immunizing peptide	274
gp100, MART-1, and tyrosinase HLA-A201 restricted melanoma peptides/ Montanide ISA 51 adjuvant	Montanide ISA 51	SQ, q3wk	1–10 mg	Metastatic melanoma, HLA-A201+, stage IV with no evidence of disease	Ongoing	Ongoing	Ongoing	ECOG trial, 212,363
Mage3-A1	None	Monthly × 3	100 µg	Metastatic melanoma	39 (25 evaluable)	3 CR, 4 other with tumor regression, all but 1 cutaneous	No CTL response	184
Mage3-A1	Pan-DR helper peptide + Montanide ISA 51	SQ, q4wk × 4	0.1 to 2.0 mg	Resected stage III/IV melanoma	18	NA	No CTL response to MAGE3+, HLA-A1 tumor, 5 of 14 and 2 of 8 with lytic and cytokine response to peptide-pulsed targets	275
HER-2/ neu:369-377-A201	Montanide ISA 51	SQ, q3wk	1 mg	HLA-A2 Her2+ expressing metastatic cancer	4	None	CTL to peptide-pulsed target but not to her2+ tumor	56
HER-2/neu peptides (six 15–18 aa peptides)	Granulocyte-macrophage colony-stimulating factor, 125 µg	Intradermal, monthly × 6	500 µg/ peptide, 3 peptides per patient	Stage IV breast and ovarian, no evidence of disease or minimal residual disease	Full study report pending	NA	6 of 8 developed proliferative responses to the protein; evidence of epitope spreading; and + DTH to immunizing peptides	188
MUC-1 105-mer (5 tandem repeats)	BCG	SQ, q3wk × 3	100 µg	Adenocarcinoma	63	NA	3 of 63 DTH+ to peptide, T-cell infiltrate in biopsy of DTH test site despite no reaction in 44 of 55	189
MUC-1 mannan fusion protein	None	SQ, weekly × 4, q2 wk × 4	10–500 µg	Metastatic breast, colon, stomach, and rectal cancers	25	NA	High-titer anti-MUC-1 Ab in 13 of 25, T-cell proliferative and cytotoxic responses in 4 of 15 and 2 of 10	190
β-Human chorionic gonadotropin, carboxy-terminal oligopeptide, CTP37	Conjugated to diphtheria toxoid, combined with CRL1005, 3–75 mg	IM, q4wk × 4	1 mg	Metastatic pancreas, lung, or colon	21	2 patients had liver lesions regress	Low-level Ab and T-cell proliferative responses to human chorionic gonadotropin in some patients	191
13-Mer mutant ras peptides, codon 12 mutations	DETOX	SQ, monthly × 3	0.1–5.0 mg	Advanced cancer containing ras mutations at codon 12	10	None	3 of 10 CD4+ or CD8+ response, tumor recognition documented in 1	276

(continued)

TABLE 63.2-5. *(Continued)*

Peptide Antigen/Human Leukocyte Antigen Restriction	*Adjuvant*	*Route of Administration*	*Dose Range*	*Patient Population*	*No. of Patients*	*Clinical Results*	*Immunologic Results*	*Reference*
HPV-16 E7, 2 HLA-A201 peptides, and 1 helper peptide	Montanide ISA 51	SQ	0.1–1.0 mg	Advanced cervical cancer	19	None	NA	187
Lipidated HPV-16 E7 peptide (86–83) linked to helper peptide PADRE	None	SQ, q3wk × 4	0.1–2.0 mg	HLA-A201 advanced cervical cancer	12	None	3 of 7 induction of peptide-specific CTL	186

CR, complete response; CTL, cytologic T lymphocyte; DTH, delayed-type hypersensitivity; HPV, human papillomavirus; PR, partial response.

tes antigen MAGE-3; PSA and prostate-specific membrane antigen; CEA; the mucin MUC-1; the hormone human chorionic gonadotropin-α; the oncogene HER-2/neu; mutated ras and p53; and human papillomavirus E6 and E7 proteins. Several conclusions can be drawn from the series of studies conducted with MHC class I (HLA-A201 in most trials) restricted peptides derived from the melanoma antigens. In those trials, doses of 1 mg administered in an emulsion with a type of incomplete Freund's adjuvant were adequate to induce immune responses, and within the range of doses studied (100 μg to 10 mg), the immune response did not appear to be dose related. While scheduling was not examined in detail, the studies revealed that administration of the vaccine every 3 to 4 weeks was effective in inducing immune responses. Cytotoxic T-cell responses to the peptide and to HLA-A201+, antigen-positive tumor cells could be detected by several techniques, and the strength of the immune response was dependent on the peptide. The ability to induce detectable T-cell responses to peptides in patients, using current immune monitoring techniques, was found to be dependent on coadministration of an adjuvant (S. A. Rosenberg et al., personal communication, 2000).

Occasional mixed and true objective antitumor responses have been observed in a small minority of patients receiving melanoma peptide vaccines. However, no correlation has been made between detection of immune response and clinical outcome in these trials. In a study of an HLA-A1 restricted peptide from the cancer testis antigen MAGE-3, administered without an adjuvant to 39 patients with metastatic melanoma, three complete responses and four other patients with objective regression were reported, despite the inability to detect immune responses to the peptide.[184]

A substantial experience has been developed in studies of a synthetic peptide immunogen corresponding to an epitope from the gp100 melanoma antigen. The epitope, consisting of amino acids 209 to 217 and restricted by HLA-A*0201, was identified by determining reactivities of tumor-infiltrating lymphocytes from patients with metastatic melanoma. When the second amino acid from the amino terminus was modified from a threonine to a methionine to create a peptide called g209-2M, binding to the HLA-A*0201 molecule could be increased ninefold compared with the native peptide in an *in vitro* competitive binding assay.[185] *In vivo*, 91% of patients vaccinated with this peptide were successfully immunized on the basis of immunologic assays in peripheral blood, a substantial improvement over the immunization rate observed with the native peptide. CD8+ T-cell responses to the modified peptide recognized the native peptide as well as tumor cells expressing the gp100 protein. Despite the increased immunogenicity of the peptide in patients, antitumor responses were not observed. Clinical trials of immunization with a combination of several HLA-A201 restricted peptides from different melanoma antigens including gp100, MART-1, and tyrosinase have been initiated, but preliminary results do not indicate a marked improvement in activity against metastatic disease (S. A. Rosenberg et al., personal communication, 2000). However, a randomized trial of immunization with the combined g209-2M, MART-1, and tyrosinase peptides in HLA-A201 stage IV melanoma patients who have had resection of all metastatic disease, compared with placebo, is ongoing, and is designed to test whether immunization against these antigens will have greater effect in patients with minimal tumor burdens.

The clinical experience with other peptides selected to induce only CD8+ lymphocyte responses remains limited. Results of studies involving peptide-pulsed DCs are discussed in the section on DC tumor vaccines [see Vaccination Using Host Antigen-Presenting Cells (Dendritic Cell Vaccines), later in this chapter]. HLA-A201 restricted peptides from the E7 human papillomavirus-16 have been administered in adjuvant or attached to a lipidated peptide designed to elicit broad nonspecific T-cell helper responses.[186,187] Human papillomavirus-16 E7 peptide-specific T-cell responses were observed in several patients without evidence of antitumor activity. A small experience with an HLA-A201 restricted peptide from the her2 protein illustrates an important principle in selection of peptides for clinical trials. The her2 peptide was shown to bind to HLA-A201 *in vitro*, and CTL raised to the peptide and some tumor-infiltrating lymphocyte preparations could kill peptide-pulsed target cells. On this basis, a clinical trial was initiated administering the peptide in Montanide ISA 51 similar to the melanoma trials.[56] While the HER-2/neu peptide could be demonstrated to induce peptide-specific T-cell responses in patients, the CTL did not recognize HER-2/neu+ HLA-A201+

tumors, suggesting that the peptide is not naturally processed and presented on HLA-A201 molecules sufficiently by most tumor cells to allow T-cell activation. Therefore, it is possible to generate potent T-cell responses to various MHC class I binding peptides in patients, but these immune responses do not necessarily recognize tumor, and therefore would not be expected to have antitumor effects.

Various peptides of longer length, usually greater than 10 to 12 amino acids, have also been studied in clinical trials. Longer peptides are most often intended to induce CD4+ T-helper cell responses, although long peptides are capable of inducing CD8+ lymphocyte responses if they are trimmed or processed *in vivo* to a peptide of correct length that can bind to the patient's class I MHC molecules. Disis et al. demonstrated that immunization with peptides 15 to 18 amino acids in length and selected from the HER-2/neu protein could induce T-cell proliferative responses to the her2 protein in six of eight patients with HER-2/neu+ tumors.[188] Demonstration of responses to the protein, rather than just the peptide itself, suggests that the immune responses are relevant and could recognize antigen presented by tumor cells or picked up by host APC. The investigators also reported evidence of epitope spreading, manifest as the induction of proliferative responses to her2 peptide epitopes not in the vaccine. Clinical antitumor responses could not be assessed as most patients had minimal or no disease at the start of vaccination. Immunization with a 105 aa *peptide* composed of five tandem repeats derived from MUC-1 did not produce antitumor activity among 63 patients with advanced adenocarcinomas, although T-cell infiltrates were observed in the peptide delayed-type hypersensitivity skin test sites of 44 of 55 patients.[189] Immunization of 25 metastatic adenocarcinoma patients with a MUC-1 mannan fusion protein produced high antibody titers in 13, but T-cell responses were limited.[190] Low-level antibody and T-cell proliferative responses, as well as regression of liver lesions in two patients, were reported among 21 patients immunized against a carboxy-terminal peptide of human chorionic gonadotropin-β, conjugated to diphtheria toxoid.[191] The results have been extended to a randomized controlled trial in advanced colon cancer.

Cytokines have been administered together with peptide vaccines to enhance presentation, for example, by recruiting and activating host APC, or to affect the developing T-cell response by directly interacting with the T cells. When the T-cell growth and differentiation cytokine IL-2 was added to the g209-2M melanoma peptide treatment regimen, 13 of 31 patients (42%) had objective clinical responses and four additional patients had mixed or minor responses (Table 63.2-5).[2] These results are significantly different from results obtained in clinical trials using high-dose IL-2 alone, in which objective response rates are in the range of 15%, and a randomized trial comparing IL-2 plus peptide with IL-2 alone is due to start in 2000. Of note, high-dose IL-2 diminished the CTL response to peptide as measured in peripheral blood. Coadministration of IL-12 or GM-CSF with the g209-2M peptide in adjuvant also diminished CTL reactivity to the peptide, and among the 14 patients treated with peptide and IL-12 and 13 treated with peptide and GM-CSF, there were no objective antitumor responses.[192] GM-CSF has been an effective adjuvant in studies of the her2 peptides, which were not admixed with a nonspecific adjuvant.[188] The cytokine flt3, which increases the number of circulating and tissue APC, has generated substantial interest and is being administered before peptide vaccination in a number of clinical studies, although results are not yet available.

Future directions in the development of synthetic peptide vaccines may include the use of modified peptides embedded into microspheres or coated onto microbeads, a maneuver that can target antigen for uptake and MHC class I restricted presentation by professional APCs.[193,194] Other novel strategies developed in experimental animal systems use toxin-linked peptides[195,196] and peptides linked to endoplasmic reticulum insertion signal sequences covalently attached to the amino terminus of a peptide immunogen.[197]

VACCINATION USING PURIFIED OR SYNTHETIC DEFINED PROTEINS

In relative terms, only a few vaccines are in development that are composed of synthetic or purified proteins. Proteins provide the opportunity for immunization against multiple epitopes, and also have the potential for inducing both CD4+ and CD8+ T-cell responses. However, for some self-antigens, immunization with proteins may be limited by tolerance to its dominant epitopes. Animal models have shown that immunization with xenogeneic proteins may be superior to the syngeneic self-protein, due to amino acid differences that induce helper CD4+ T-cell responses, and the chance occurrence that the xenogeneic protein will contain a peptide epitope just different enough from the native epitope to be highly immunogenic, but still induce T-cell responses to the native epitope.[198,199] An alternative to immunization with a purified or recombinant protein is to insert the gene into a viral vector, which theoretically enters the cytoplasmic compartment of an APC to produce large amounts of the protein for processing and antigen presentation.

Clinical experience with vaccines containing defined proteins is limited, with the exception of idiotype lymphoma vaccines (see Vaccination Using Idiotypes or Antiidiotypes, later in this chapter). Results of trials of liposome-encapsulated PSA protein vaccines have been presented in abstract form.

VACCINATION USING HOST ANTIGEN-PRESENTING CELLS (DENDRITIC CELL VACCINES)

In order to improve the immunogenicity of antigens, investigators have increasingly adopted the approach of placing the antigen directly into host APCs, which when fully differentiated present surface molecules and produce cytokines that result in optimal activation of T cells. Interpretation of the many clinical trials is confounded by the different approaches to generating APC *in vivo* and *in vitro*; by the different types and functions of APC; by difficulty in fully defining the characteristics of APC that result in optimal antigen presentation; by the many different approaches to place antigen into or onto APC; and by the variety in dose, route of administration, and use of concurrent cytokines in the clinical studies. Few if any studies have compared APC-based vaccines with other immunization approaches, for example, peptide pulsed on APC to peptide in adjuvant. A representative sample of tumor vaccines employing host APC is presented in Table 63.2-6. APC used to deliver antigens derived from autologous tumor cells, for example, tumor cell-DC fusions, is discussed earlier (see Anticancer Vaccine Approaches Derived from Autologous and Allogeneic Tumor Cells, earlier in this chapter).

TABLE 63.2-6. Clinical Trials Using Vaccines Based on Antigen-Presenting Cells

Antigen-Presenting Cell Type	*Dose Range of Antigen-Presenting Cells*	*Route of Administration*	*Antigen(s)*	*Patient Population (Disease/Stage)*	*No. of Patients*	*Clinical Results*	*Immunologic Results*	*References*
PBMC	N/A	IV	Individually determined peptides spanning ras and p53 mutations	Solid tumors	33, 26 with evident disease	No responses	Immune responses to immunizing peptide in at least 1 assay in >50%	Carbone et al. (personal communication, 2000)
PBMC cultures in IL-4 + GM-CSF	6–20 × 10^7	IV	gp100:209–217 (210M), MART-1 peptides	Metastatic melanoma	10	No responses	1 of 5 tested had increase in pCTL to gp100 peptide	Marincola et al., 2000, submitted
PBMC cultures in IL-4 + GM-CSF	10^6	Direct injection into lymph nodes, qwk × 4, week 6, then monthly	Tumor lysate, or A2-restricted Mart-1 and gp100 peptides (check), or A1-restricted MAGE-1 and MAGE-3 peptides	Metastatic melanoma	16	2 CR, 3 PR	DTH to DC pulsed with peptides or tumor lysate increased postimmunization in 15 of 16, 5 >10 mm	3
PBMC cultures in IL-4 + GM-CSF + monocyte-conditioned media	6–12 × 10^6	Every 14 × 5; first 3 given ID and SQ, last 2 given IV	MAGE3-A1 peptide (HLA-A1 restricted)	HLA-A1+, MAGE3+ metastatic melanoma	13 (11 received all five vaccines)	None, but 6 of 11 had mixed response	8 of 11 had increase in pCTL to MAGE-3A1 peptide	271
PBMC cultures in IL-4 + GM-CSF	10^7 to 10^8	IV, and IV + ID, weekly × 4 or q2wk × 4	CAP1 (CEA HLA-A201 peptide)	HLA-A2+, CEA+ metastatic cancer	21 (19)	1 MR	DTH to CEA peptide not observed in most patients	272
DC isolated by gradients from monocyte and lymphocyte-depleted PBMC	2–32 × 10^6	IV, monthly × 3, boost at 5–6 mo; idiotype protein SQ on day 16 of each cycle	Lymphoma idiotypes	Follicular lymphoma	4 (16 total in 1999 abstract)	1 CR, 1 MR	4 of 4 proliferative T-cell responses to idiotype protein (8 of 16 cellular response, no humoral response)	202
PBMC cultures in IL-4 + GM-CSF		IV, q6wk × 6	2 HLA-A2 peptides from prostate-specific membrane antigen	Advanced hormone-refractory, and presumed local recurrence with rising PSA	33 advanced, 37 locally recurrent	6 PR, 2 CR in advanced, 1 CR and 10 PR in locally recurrent	No consistent peptide-specific responses, no correlation to clinical outcome	200,273
APC8015, dendritic cells obtained by density centrifugation, matured by culture with Ag for 40 hr	0.2 to 1.2 × 10^9	IV, q4wk × 3	Recombinant prostatic acid phosphatase fused to GM-CSF	Advanced prostate cancer	28	2 of 22 had PSA decrease >50%	Consistent T-cell proliferative response to PAP in all patients, Ab response in <20%	320
Allogeneic PBMC cultures in IL-4 + GM-CSF + tumor necrosis factor	5 × 10^7	SQ near inguinal lymph node, q6wk × 2, then q3mo	Fusion of DC with equal number of autologous tumor cells	Metastatic renal cell cancer	17	4 CR, 2 PR	11 of 17 + DTH to autologous tumor cells postvaccine	140

CEA, carcinoembryonic antigen; CR, complete response; DC, dendritic cells; DTH, delayed-type hypersensitivity; GM-CSF, granulocyte-macrophage colony-stimulating factor; IL, interleukin; N/A, not applicable; PBMC, peripheral blood mononuclear cells; PR, partial response; PSA, prostate-specific antigen.

The majority of clinical studies have produced APC by *ex vivo* culture of nonadherent peripheral blood mononuclear cells (PBMC) in the presence of the cytokines IL-4 and GM-CSF (monocyte-derived APC). After several days of culture, the APC are incubated with the antigen, and then administered to the patient. In some cases an additional signal to mature APC is provided before the final harvest for injection, for example, addition of TNF or monocyte-conditioned media. Some clinical studies use as the APC preparation all PBMC obtained from a pheresis with minimal *ex vivo* manipulation, or apply centrifugation and elutriation techniques to isolate circulating APC from blood, which are then directly cultured *in vitro* with antigen only. The optimal route of administration for APC has not been determined, but clinical protocols have employed intravenous, intradermal, subcutaneous, and intralymphatic routes, as well as direct injection into lymph nodes.

Preliminary data from immunization with monocyte-derived APC pulsed with melanoma peptides suggest that the approach is less effective than administering peptide in adjuvant for generating CTL responses in peripheral blood (F. M. Marincola, personal communication, 2000). Nevertheless, some antitumor responses have been observed in the clinical trials. Nestle et al. reported two complete and three partial responses among 16 melanoma patients treated with melanoma peptides or tumor lysates pulsed onto monocyte-derived APC and injected directly into lymph nodes.[3] Immune response was assessed by delayed-type hypersensitivity reactions to APC alone versus APC plus antigen, and 15 of the 16 patients appeared to have increased delayed-type hypersensitivity responses to the antigen-pulsed APC.

Declines in the PSA levels of prostate cancer patients have been observed following administration of APC-based vaccines. Approximately 25% of 70 patients, including 33 with hormone-refractory disease, were reported to achieve complete or partial responses when treated with monocyte-derived APC pulsed with two HLA-A2 restricted peptides from prostate-specific membrane antigen.[200]

VACCINATION USING IDIOTYPES OR ANTIIDIOTYPES

The antigen-binding region of an antibody (the idiotype), which is formed from recombination of genes within the B cells, can theoretically be processed by the B cells to peptides that bind self-MHC molecules and are presented on the surface of the cell, thus forming a unique antigen that can be recognized by T cells. Antigen-binding regions of antibodies can also be recognized by other antibodies; therefore, it is possible to raise antibodies to the idiotype present on the surface of malignant B cells. The specific antibody idiotype to be used in a vaccine must be prepared individually from each patient using hybridoma or recombinant DNA techniques, processes that can take several weeks to months to generate a clinical product. Nevertheless, a substantial clinical experience is now available with these unique lymphoma idiotype vaccines.[201–203] Optimal induction of immune responses requires conjugation of the idiotype protein to KLH and administration with a strong nonspecific adjuvant. The Stanford group demonstrated induction of antibody responses to the idiotype in 20 of 41 immunized patients with follicular lymphoma.[202] Fifteen of the immune responders were among the 20 patients who were in complete remission at the beginning of vaccine treatment. There was a marked increase in progression-free survival and overall survival in immune responders versus nonresponders. Two of 21 patients had regression of residual disease with the vaccine treatment. A similar vaccine was studied at the NCI in follicular lymphoma patients in their first complete remission.[203] T-cell responses, including proliferation to the idiotype and cytotoxicity toward autologous tumor, were reported in 19 of the 20 patients, and antibody responses to the idiotype in 15 of 20. Eight of 11 patients with detectable bcl-2 translocations in peripheral blood following chemotherapy developed molecular complete remissions with vaccination. Furthermore, 18 of 20 patients were relapse-free from 28+ to 53+ months from initiation of initial chemotherapy. Although the results of the two series are promising, the data must be interpreted with caution since the beneficial clinical effects are occurring primarily in complete remission patients whose natural history of disease is already quite favorable. A phase III randomized trial of the lymphoma idiotype vaccine is expected to begin in 2000.

The antibodies directed to the antigen-binding regions of other antibodies carry within their own antigen-binding region a physical resemblance to the original antigen. For example, if CEA is the intended tumor antigen, an antibody is first raised to CEA. That antibody (termed Ab1) is itself used as an immunogen in mice to raise a second group of antibodies (Ab2), some of which recognize the CEA-binding site of the Ab1. The antigen-binding site of Ab2 physically resembles CEA, and when used to immunize animals or patients, can generate antibodies (Ab3) that recognize CEA. The Ab2 is capable of generating more potent immune responses to the original antigen than the antigen itself in some circumstances, since the antigenic epitope is being presented outside of immune-tolerizing influences.

Clinical results of representative antiidiotype vaccines are presented in Table 63.2-7.[156,204–211] The antiidiotype antibodies are most often of murine origin and are administered together with a nonspecific immunologic adjuvant. Several antiidiotypes have been developed to immunize against melanoma cell surface antigens. An antiidiotype developed to mimic the melanoma high-molecular-weight antigen generated antibody responses that recognized melanoma cells expressing the antigen and was also associated with regression of metastatic disease in 3 of 52 patients.[212] Only a subset of the 52 patients received the antiidiotype conjugated to KLH and administered with BCG, which appeared to be necessary to induce the antimelanoma antibodies. An antiidiotype mimicking the ganglioside GD2 produced antibody responses to GD2 in 40 of 47 patients and was associated with one complete response and 12 patients who had stable disease for greater than 14 months.[213] Another antiidiotype mimicking the ganglioside GD3 has been examined in patients with melanoma and small cell lung cancer.[214,215] Approximately one-third of the patients receiving the GD3 antiidiotype developed antibodies to GD3, some despite having completed intensive chemotherapy. In the 15 patients with small cell lung cancer who were immunized while in partial or complete remission from chemotherapy, disease-free survival appeared to be prolonged compared with historical controls. The latter results formed the basis for an ongoing randomized phase III trial in the same patient population.

Antiidiotypes mimicking colorectal cancer antigens are also in clinical trials. A polyclonal goat antiidiotype mimicking the 17-1A antigen was the subject of a small randomized trial in advanced colon cancer, and despite inducing antibodies to 17-1A

TABLE 63.2-7. Clinical Trials Using Vaccines Based on Idiotypes and Antiidiotypes

Antigen	*Adjuvant*	*Route of Administration, Dose Range*	*Patient Population*	*No. of Patients*	*Clinical Results*	*Immunologic Results*	*Reference*
Lymphoma idiotypes	Conjugated to KLH, granulocyte-macrophage colony-stimulating factor, 100 or 500 μg/m² SQ d × 4	Subcutaneous, monthly × 4	Follicular lymphoma > 6 mo in complete remission post first chemotherapy regimen	20	18 of 20 without relapse 28+ to 53+ mo, 8 of 11 molecular remission	CD4+ and CD8+ responses to autologous tumor in 19 of 20, antibody responses to idiotype in 15 of 20	203
Lymphoma idiotypes	Conjugated to KLH (0.5 mg), in threonyl-muramyl dipeptide	0.5 mg protein plus adjuvant, subcutaneous, weeks 0, 2, 6, 10, 20	Follicular lymphoma, following first or second chemotherapy remission	41 (21 CR, 20 residual disease)	Progression-free survival and survival greater in immune responders compared with nonresponders, 2 patients developed CR	Anti-ID Ab responses in 20 of 41, 15 of immune responders in CR group, cytotoxic T lymphocyte responses also observed	202,201
GD3 antiidiotype (BEC2)	BCG	ID q2wk × 5, BEC2, 2.5 mg/dose	Small cell lung cancer, PR or CR postchemotherapy	15	Median survival 20.5+ months, long-term disease-free survival greater than historical control	5 of 13 detectable anti-GD3 IgG	277
GD2 antiidiotype	QS-21, 100 μg	SQ, qw × 4, then monthly, 1–8 mg	Metastatic melanoma	47	1 CR 24+ mo, 12 SD 14+ to 37+ mo, median survival >16+ mo	40 of 47 developed antibody to GD2	211,213
High-molecular-weight melanoma-associated antigen, antiidiotypes	None, CTX, KLH/BCG, or CTX/KLH/BCG	2 mg SQ days 0, 7, 28, 35, and when titers fell to <1:8	Metastatic melanoma	58, 52 evaluable	3 objective responses, correlation of antibody response to high-molecular-weight melanoma-associated antigen with survival	18 of 52 Ab response to melanoma cells, all but 1 in patients receiving KLH/BCG adjuvant	212
CEA antiidiotype	Alum or QS-21	ID, q2wk × 4, then monthly, 2 mg	CEA+, colon cancer, completely resected Duke's B, C, D, or Duke's D minimal residual disease, 14 received concurrent chemotherapy	32	8 of 9 with residual disease progressed, 18 of 23 with no evidence of disease, progression-free, including 8 of 9 Duke's D (no evidence of disease)	32 of 32 developed Ab responses to CEA, 80% T-cell proliferative responses to a CEA peptide	217
17-1A goat antiidiotype	Alum	4 mg SQ weekly × 4, boost q6wk	Metastatic colon	42 (21 nonspecific goat polyclonal Ab as control)	No survival difference from control, no clinical responses	12 of 21 Ab response to 17-1A	216
791Tgp72 (CD55) antiidiotype	Alum, also KLH + Freund's	5–100 μg	Adjuvant and metastatic colon	13 metastatic, 35 adjuvant	No clinical responses, effect on survival suggested	Dependent on dose and adjuvant; Ab and cellular responses to Ag+ tumor cells	278,279

BCG, bacille Calmette-Guérin; CEA, carcinoembryonic antigen; CR, complete response; CTX, cyclophosphamide; PR, partial response.

in 12 of the 21 patients in the treatment arm, no survival benefit was observed compared with the control (immunization with nonspecific goat polyclonal antibody).[216] An antiidiotype mimicking CEA was reported to induce high titer anti-CEA antibodies in all 32 immunized patients.[217] Furthermore, because the antiidiotype contained sequences that were similar to the protein sequence of CEA, some patients developed CD4+ T-cell proliferative responses to CEA. No antitumor responses were observed, but 18 of 23 patients with no evidence of disease, including eight of nine with completely resected metastatic disease, were progression free at the time of the publication. Combination with 5-fluorouracil–containing regimens did not appear to reduce the immunogenicity of the antiidiotype, and a phase III trial in the adjuvant setting is planned.

VACCINES USING CARBOHYDRATE AND GANGLIOSIDE CELL SURFACE ANTIGENS

Certain tumors, particularly melanoma and small cell lung cancer, are known to express gangliosides that can be recognized by antibodies. Induction of antibody responses against the ganglioside antigens can have therapeutic value in animal models, particularly in micrometastatic settings. A vaccine composed of purified GM2 combined with BCG was administered subcutaneously in a randomized controlled trial in patients with stage IIb/III melanoma. Patients received low-dose cyclophosphamide before immunization. The GM2/BCG vaccine was shown to induce low to moderate titers of IgM anti-GM2 antibodies in the majority of patients, and produced a trend toward improved disease-free survival.[218] When patients with preexisting anti-GM2 responses, which are associated with a better prognosis, were excluded from the analysis of both arms, the differences between arms became statistically significant. Pilot studies of GM2 conjugated to the protein KLH and admixed with QS-21 produced higher titers of IgM antibodies to GM2 compared with the GM2/BCG vaccine, and also high titers of IgG antibodies to GM2, although the IgG anti-GM2 antibodies did not appear recognize cell surface GM2 in the majority of patients.[219,220] Among the patients who develop IgM anti-GM2 antibodies, only approximately 40% to 50% have antibody responses that are cytotoxic for GM2-expressing melanoma cells. A phase III trial of the GM2-KLH/QS-21 vaccine compared with high-dose IFN for patients with stage IIb/III melanoma completed accrual in 1999 and is awaiting analysis.

A vaccine containing both GM2 and GD2 gangliosides has been developed and appears to induce IgM and IgG antibody responses to both gangliosides.[221] Another ganglioside, Fucosyl-GM1, which is expressed on small cell lung cancer, has been conjugated to KLH and administered with QS-21 to ten patients with small cell lung cancer in partial or complete remission following chemotherapy.[215] The vaccine induced cytotoxic antibody responses in the majority of patients.

STn is a carbohydrate antigen from the MUC-1 glycoprotein, expressed on various adenocarcinomas including breast, ovarian, and colon cancer.[53,222,223] The carbohydrate epitopes are revealed due to abnormal glycosylation patterns in tumors. A synthetic STn was conjugated to KLH and administered with the DETOX adjuvant in several trials involving patients with metastatic breast, ovarian, and colon cancer. High-titer IgG responses to natural mucin STn epitopes were demonstrated, and a correlation was found between survival and development of IgM (colon cancer) or IgG (breast cancer) titers above the median.[224–226] Of note, there was no correlation in these same studies between survival and anti-KLH antibody responses. The STn-KLH/QS-21 vaccine is the subject of a large randomized phase III trial in metastatic breast cancer patients who are stable or have a partial or complete response after initial chemotherapy.

ENHANCING VACCINE-INDUCED IMMUNE RESPONSES

OPTIMIZING DOSE, BOOSTING, AND ROUTE OF THE IMMUNIZATION

There are a bewildering number of choices that the immunotherapist must make when designing an anticancer vaccine, including choice of antigen, immunogen, and adjuvant. In addition, it becomes important to consider the appropriate dose, route of administration, and the length of intervals between boosting. The answers to these questions require an understanding of the immunophysiology of vaccination *in vivo. In vitro* work with human cells is of limited benefit, while work in human subjects must necessarily be limited in its scope. Thus, in practice, questions regarding dose, route, and boosting are generally addressed in mouse models.

Based on the idea that more antigen is better, most viral and DNA vaccines are geared toward maximum expression and use the strongest available promoters. In our own preclinical trials using immunogens based on vaccinia viruses, as well as DNA given by blasts with the gene gun, efficacy improves as the dose of immunogen increases.[166,227]

It has long been known that boosting an immune response can increase its intensity. When primary and booster immunization using a single vector (i.e., homologous boosting) is compared with a regimen that uses two different vectors (i.e., heterologous boosting), the heterologous boosting generally resulted in significantly more potent antigen-specific cytotoxic T-lymphocyte responses.[181,182] This is likely due to absence of a neutralizing antivector immune response during the booster immunization.

The route of immunization can determine its efficacy; for example, administration of a synthetic peptide by the intraperitoneal route can lead to tolerization, whereas administration of the same peptide immunogen subcutaneously leads to activation.[228] For poxviral vectors, the intravenous route of immunization is optimal in mice.[229] For any given immunogen, we surmise that the optimal route of immunization is likely to be dictated by the route that leads to the presence of the antigen on the maximal number of activated DCs, perhaps with the least amount of antigen presentation by normal, potentially tolerizing cells.

CYTOKINES, CHEMOKINES, AND COSTIMULATORY MOLECULES AS MOLECULARLY DEFINED ADJUVANTS

From the vaccinologist's point of view, cytokines, chemokines, and costimulatory molecules can be used as molecularly defined adjuvants, significantly improving vaccine-induced immune responses. They can be administered systemically as protein or through insertion of their genes into recombinant vaccines.[166,230–232] We have found that gene gun delivery of a model antigen was protective by itself, but was only therapeutic

TABLE 63.2-8. Potential Impediments to Immunization against Tumor Antigens and Development of Effective Antitumor Immune Responses

DEFECTS IN CANCER CELLS PREVENTING RECOGNITION OR RESPONSE
Loss of antigen expression[258,280,281]
Loss or mutation of restricting major histocompatibility complex molecule[282–285]
Loss of interferon-γ signaling pathway[286]
POSSIBLE MECHANISMS OF ACTIVE SUPPRESSION OF ANTIGEN PRESENTATION OR T-CELL FUNCTION
Tumor cell expression of certain major histocompatibility complex class I molecules that bind to natural killer receptor on CTL and block CTL activity[287]
Tumor cell expression of *fas* ligand or other death receptor ligands that bind to receptors on T cells and cause T-cell apoptosis (alone or in combination with tumor growth factor-β expression)[252,254,288]
Induction or presence of granulocyte-macrophage regulatory cells that induce T-cell apoptosis by contact[289,290]
Tumor-related alterations in T-cell signaling[291–294]
Expression of immunosuppressive cytokines, blocking maturation and function of professional antigen-presenting cells (interleukin-10, VEGF)[295–299]
During the growth of tumor, tumor antigen is presented by immature or dysfunctional antigen-presenting cells leading to tolerance/anergy[98] or immune deviation (ineffective immune responses)[300–302] toward the tumor antigens
OBSTACLES TO GENERATING EFFECTIVE IMMUNE RESPONSES BASED ON LIMITATIONS TO SELF-REACTIVITY
Preexisting central or peripheral tolerance to proposed tumor antigen (self-antigen)[198,199,303–307] and inability of tumor antigen to induce T cells with high avidity for the tumor[308–310]
Induction or presence of suppressor T cells preventing antitumor immune response[311–313]
Tumor antigen-specific CTL encounter natural antagonist peptides *in vivo* that inhibit function[314]
Lack of CD4+ help to initiate memory responses, sustain CTL, or produce cytokines and recruit other cellular effectors to tumor site[37]
OBSTACLES TO MAINTAINING AND AMPLIFYING ANTITUMOR IMMUNE RESPONSES LOCALLY
Tumor vasculature lacks adhesion molecules necessary for penetration of T cells, or T cells lack necessary adhesion molecules[315]
Lack of costimulation at tumor site to support effector activity[316,317]
Inability of tumor to sustain active antitumor immune response[318,319]

CTL, cytotoxic T lymphocyte.

when delivered with IL-2, IL-6, IL-7, or especially IL-12.[166] Other useful cytokine adjuvants include GM-CSF, a cytokine thought to play an important role in the recruitment and maturation of DCs.[162,233,234] Studies using vaccinia virus-based immunogens have revealed that IL-2 and IL-12[166,230,231] are extremely potent in their ability to increase the efficacy of cancer vaccines. In addition, the costimulatory molecules B7-1, B7-2, and CD40L have a beneficial effect on vaccination.[108,231,232,235] Less studied as vaccine adjuvants, chemokines induce the activation and directional migration in a variety of immune cells.[236–239] They are produced locally in the tissues, often as a result of the presence of pathogens, and act on leukocytes through a family of at least a dozen receptors.

Importantly, not all of the findings in murine models were confirmed in human clinical trials. When patients with metastatic melanoma were immunized with a modified immunodominant peptide derived from gp100, no increase in efficacy as measured by objective clinical response was observed using GM-CSF or IL-12.[2,192] Only IL-2 was found to have a beneficial effect as an adjuvant for peptide immunization.[2]

Bacterial DNA sequences called *immunostimulatory sequences* have been reported to be potent adjuvants. Nonmethylated, palindromic DNA sequences containing CpG-oligodinucleotides can activate an innate immune response by activating monocytes, natural killer cells, DCs, and B cells in an antigen-independent manner.[240] Thus, the use of large amounts of plasmid for immunization may not only overcome the low transfection efficiency *in vivo*, but may also serve as an adjuvant, driving a Th1 response.[241]

FUTURE CHALLENGES: TUMOR ESCAPE FROM IMMUNE RECOGNITION

Every cancer that kills a person is a cancer that has not been destroyed by the immune system, and many mechanisms have been hypothesized for this apparent lack of immunogenicity (Table 63.2-8).

LACK OF INFLAMMATION

One mechanism that may explain why patients with cancer usually do not reject their tumors involves the lack of inflammation at the tumor site. There are important differences between the site of a tumor deposit and a site of infection. Tumors produce few, if any, immunologic danger signals to stimulate the immune response.[242,243] In contrast, at a site of infection, the innate immune response is triggered because of tissue destruction. Inflammatory cells, such as monocytes, macrophages, and DCs, are activated as a result of this tissue destruction, and by components of the infectious agents themselves, such as lipopolysaccharide, nonmethylated CpG sequences, and double-stranded RNA, each of which are components of invading microbes that are not shared by either normal host cells or growing cancer cells. In the absence of these danger signals, the immune system may not become fully activated.[107,244]

INDUCTION OF TOLERANCE BY TUMOR CELLS

Despite cancer cells' expression of clearly immunogenic molecules, the host usually does not mount an effective immune response to these antigens. One reason could be the lack of expression of costimulatory molecules necessary for efficient T-cell activation by tumor cells. In the absence of costimulation, T cells tend to become anergic, a process thought to protect against autoimmune disease. The costimulatory molecules CD80 (B7-1) and CD80 (B7-2) are expressed on professional APC and on a variety of other tissues after exposure to inflammatory cytokines.[245] Transfection of tumor cells with both B7 isoforms has been used successfully to trigger their immune-mediated rejection of experimental mouse tumors, which have some inherent immunogenicity.[246] However, this strategy is insufficient for nonimmunogenic tumors, a category into which most, if not all, human tumors would likely fall.[247]

A number of groups have conducted experiments in which highly immunogenic foreign antigens, such as the hemagglutinin protein from influenza,[98] the β-galactosidase enzyme from *Escherichia coli*,[168] and the ovalbumin protein from chicken are expressed in tumor cells.[248] The results are fairly uniform: Tumors tend to grow progressively, retaining their lethality despite the expression of a foreign and highly immunogenic protein by the tumor cell.

Alternative immune mechanisms designated *tolerance* and *ignorance* have been used to explain why the immune system fails to recognize tumors expressing even these normally highly immunogenic antigens. Tolerance generally refers to the lack of a destructive immune reaction to a given antigen. In the tumor context, we might distinguish an active state of tolerance, in which the immune system undergoes a functional and phenotypic change after encounter with antigen, from ignorance, a passive process in which immune cells do not have any contact with the antigen that alters their phenotype or function.[249,250] Both mechanisms likely play a role in the immune system's unresponsiveness to tumor cells.

PRODUCTION OF IMMUNOSUPPRESSIVE FACTORS

Tumor cells may ectopically employ normal immunosuppressive mechanisms, such as the production of transforming growth factor-β, normally produced by certain immune and other somatic cells, but potentially antiproliferative for CTL, natural killer, and lymphokine-activated killer cells.[251] Another example, IL-10, produced by activated T cells, B cells, monocytes, and keratinocytes may be produced by certain solid tumors and may interfere with macrophage-mediated antigen presentation and other immune functions.[251]

It has been reported that expression of Fas ligand (FasL/CD95L) by melanoma cells was responsible for their escape from immune recognition.[252] Because FasL was reportedly expressed in areas of immune privilege such as the eye and testis, it was reasoned that expression of FasL by melanoma cells indicated that the tumor bed was also an "immune privileged" site. In our own study, however, we found no FasL expressed by a panel of 26 human melanoma lines we tested.[253–255] Thus, our data do not support a role for FasL expression in the escape of melanoma cells from immune destruction.

TUMOR AS A MOVING TARGET

Tumor cells can be a *moving target* when it comes to immune recognition. The field of chemotherapy has produced a number of well-known examples of tumor escape from treatment including the induction of the expression of the multidrug resistance (MDR) gene. As recombinant and synthetic vaccines become more effective, the selective pressure on the loss of particular target antigens may increase. Indeed, there is some evidence that tumor cells may preferentially loose the gp100 tumor antigen as a result of treatment with the gp100 209 to 217 (2M) peptide plus IL-2.[256,257]

Tumors have unstable genomes that lead them to be heterogenous for the expression of tumor-associated antigens. Further, their unstable genomes may enable them to escape immune recognition because they loose or mutate key elements of the antigen processing machinery such as the TAP [transporter associated with antigen processing] transporters, β_2-microglobulin, or the MHC class I α chain molecules.[258–262] Other mechanisms underlying the poor immunogenicity of tumors includes the down-regulation of two IFN-γ–inducible proteasomal components called LMP2 and LMP7 in certain human tumors.[258] The proteasome is a large multicatalytic complex involved in the degradation of many of the peptides that later find their way into the MHC class I pathway.

CONCLUSION

The field of cancer vaccines has been greatly advanced by a wave of technological innovation as well as a deeper understanding of the immunologic response to both cancer cells and potential vaccines. Vaccines using whole tumor cells have been optimized by transfection or addition of costimulatory molecules, cytokines, and chemokines. In addition, target antigens that can mediate tumor cell recognition by immune cells have been cloned and are currently used in a variety of vaccine approaches. The antigens that are most practical for application in vaccines are the self-antigens shared among cancer patients. Encoded in recombinant viruses and bacteria, naked nucleic acids, or delivered as minimal peptide epitopes, these antigens can induce immune responses that can destroy established tumors in animal models and in some instances even in cancer patients. The great genomic plasticity and poor inherent immunogenicity of tumor cells make them difficult targets for complete eradication by the immune system. Yet our growing understanding of the important roles of CD4+ and CD8+ T cells and APC, as well as the importance of dosing and the frequency and route of vaccine administration, will further improve on these initial attempts at therapeutic cancer vaccines.

REFERENCES

1. Rosenberg SA. Keynote address: perspectives on the use of interleukin-2 in cancer treatment. *Cancer J Sci Am* 1997;3(Suppl 1):S2.
2. Rosenberg SA, Yang JC, Schwartzentruber DJ, et al. Immunologic and therapeutic evaluation of a synthetic peptide vaccine for the treatment of patients with metastatic melanoma. *Nat Med* 1998;4:321.
3. Nestle FO, Alijagic S, Gilliet M, et al. Vaccination of melanoma patients with peptide- or tumor lysate-pulsed dendritic cells. *Nat Med* 1998;4:328.
4. Jaeger E, Bernhard H, Romero P, et al. Generation of cytotoxic T-cell responses with synthetic melanoma- associated peptides in vivo: implications for tumor vaccines with melanoma-associated antigens. *Int J Cancer* 1996;66:162.
5. Lowy DR, Schiller JT. Papillomaviruses and cervical cancer: pathogenesis and vaccine development. *J Natl Cancer Inst Monogr* 1998;23:27.

6. Oettgen HF. The history of cancer immunotherapy. In: DeVita VT Jr, Hellmann S, Rosenberg S, eds. *Biologic therapy of cancer.* Philadelphia: Lippincott, 1991:87.
7. Prehn RT, Main JM. Immunity to methylcholanthrene-induced sarcomas. *J Natl Cancer Inst* 1957;18:769.
8. Klein G, Sjogren HO, Klein E, Hellstrom KE. Demonstration of resistance against methylcholanthrene-induced sarcomas in the primary autochthonous host. *Cancer Res* 1960;20:1561.
9. Greenberg PD. Adoptive T cell therapy of tumors: mechanisms operative in the recognition and elimination of tumor cells. *Adv Immunol* 1991;49:281.
10. Schreiber H, Ward PL, Rowley DA, Stauss HJ. Unique tumor-specific antigens. *Annu Rev Immunol* 1988;6:465.
11. Greenberg PD, Cheever MA, Fefer A. H-2 restriction of adoptive immunotherapy of advanced tumors. *J Immunol* 1981;126:2100.
12. Rosenberg SA, Spiess P, Lafreniere R. A new approach to the adoptive immunotherapy of cancer with tumor-infiltrating lymphocytes. *Science* 1986;233:1318.
13. Shimizu K, Shen FW. Role of different T cells sets in the rejection of syngeneic chemically induced tumors. *J Immunol* 1979;122:1162.
14. Hom SS, Schwartzentruber DJ, Rosenberg SA, Topalian SL. Specific release of cytokines by lymphocytes infiltrating human melanomas in response to shared melanoma antigens. *J Immunother* 1993;13:18.
15. Topalian SL, Solomon D, Rosenberg SA. Tumor-specific cytolysis by lymphocytes infiltrating human melanomas. *J Immunol* 1989;142:3714.
16. Itoh K, Platsoucas CD, Balch CM. Autologous tumor-specific cytotoxic T lymphocytes in the infiltrate of human metastatic melanomas. Activation by interleukin 2 and autologous tumor cells, and involvement of the T cell receptor. *J Exp Med* 1988;168:1419.
17. Rosenberg SA, Packard BS, Aebersold PM, et al. Use of tumor-infiltrating lymphocytes and interleukin-2 in the immunotherapy of patients with metastatic melanoma. A preliminary report [see comments]. *N Engl J Med* 1988;319:1676.
18. Rosenberg SA, Yannelli JR, Yang JC, et al. Treatment of patients with metastatic melanoma with autologous tumor-infiltrating lymphocytes and interleukin 2. *J Natl Cancer Inst* 1994;86:1159.
19. Mule JJ, Yang JC, Afreniere RL, Shu SY, Rosenberg SA. Identification of cellular mechanisms operational in vivo during the regression of established pulmonary metastases by the systemic administration of high-dose recombinant interleukin 2. *J Immunol* 1987; 139:285.
20. Rosenberg SA. Immunotherapy of cancer using interleukin 2: current status and future prospects [see comments]. *Immunol Today* 1988;9:58.
21. Prehn RT. Relationship of tumor immunogenicity to concentration of the oncogen. *J Natl Cancer Inst* 1975;55:189.
22. Barth RJJ, Bock SN, Mule JJ, Rosenberg SA. Unique murine tumor-associated antigens identified by tumor infiltrating lymphocytes. *J Immunol* 1990;144:1531.
23. Melief CJ, Kast WM. T-cell immunotherapy of tumors by adoptive transfer of cytotoxic T lymphocytes and by vaccination with minimal essential epitopes. *Immunol Rev* 1995;145:167.
24. Yee C, Riddell SR, Greenberg PD. Prospects for adoptive T cell therapy. *Curr Opin Immunol* 1997;9:702.
25. De Smet C, Lurquin C, De Plaen E, et al. Genes coding for melanoma antigens recognised by cytolytic T lymphocytes. *Eye* 1997;11(Pt 2):243.
26. Restifo NP, Rosenberg SA. Developing recombinant and synthetic vaccines for the treatment of melanoma. *Curr Opin Oncol* 1999;11:50.
27. Greenberg PD, Cheever MA, Fefer A. Eradication of disseminated murine leukemia by chemoimmunotherapy with cyclophosphamide and adoptively transferred immune syngeneic Lyt-1+2- lymphocytes. *J Exp Med* 1981;154:952.
28. Greenberg PD, Kern DE, Cheever MA. Therapy of disseminated murine leukemia with cyclophosphamide and immune Lyt-1+,2- T cells. Tumor eradication does not require participation of cytotoxic T cells. *J Exp Med* 1985;161:1122.
29. Toes RE, Ossendorp F, Offringa R, Melief CJ. CD4 T cells and their role in antitumor immune responses. *J Exp Med* 1999;189:753.
30. Ossendorp F, Mengede E, Camps M, Filius R, Melief CJ. Specific T helper cell requirement for optimal induction of cytotoxic T lymphocytes against major histocompatibility complex class II negative tumors. *J Exp Med* 1998;187:693.
31. Overwijk WW, Lee DS, Surman DR, et al. Vaccination with a recombinant vaccinia virus encoding a "self" antigen induces autoimmune vitiligo and tumor cell destruction in mice: Requirement for CD4(+) T lymphocytes. *Proc Natl Acad Sci U S A* 1999;96:2982.
32. Pardoll DM. Inducing autoimmune disease to treat cancer. *Proc Natl Acad Sci U S A* 1999;96:5340.
33. Weber LW, Bowne WB, Wolchok JD, et al. Tumor immunity and autoimmunity induced by immunization with homologous DNA. *J Clin Invest* 1998;102:1258.
34. Clynes R, Takechi Y, Moroi Y, Houghton A, Ravetch JV. Fc receptors are required in passive and active immunity to melanoma. *Proc Natl Acad Sci U S A* 1998;95:652.
35. Hara I, Takechi Y, Houghton AN. Implicating a role for immune recognition of self in tumor rejection: passive immunization against the brown locus protein. *J Exp Med* 1995;182:1609.
36. Hirschowitz EA, Leonard S, Song W, et al. Adenovirus- mediated expression of melanoma antigen gp75 as immunotherapy for metastatic melanoma. *Gene Ther* 1998;5:975.
37. Hung K, Hayashi R, Lafond-Walker A, et al. The central role of CD4(+) T cells in the antitumor immune response. *J Exp Med* 1998;188:2357.
38. Ridge JP, Di Rosa F, Matzinger P. A conditioned dendritic cell can be a temporal bridge between a CD4+ T- helper and a T-killer cell. *Nature* 1998;393:474.
39. Schoenberger SP, Toes RE, van der Voort EI, Offringa R, Melief CJ. T-cell help for cytotoxic T lymphocytes is mediated by CD40-CD40L interactions. *Nature* 1998;393:480.
40. Walter EA, Greenberg PD, Gilbert MJ, et al. Reconstitution of cellular immunity against cytomegalovirus in recipients of allogeneic bone marrow by transfer of T-cell clones from the donor [see comments]. *N Engl J Med* 1995;333:1038.
41. McDevitt HO. The role of MHC class II molecules in susceptibility and resistance to autoimmunity. *Curr Opin Immunol* 1998;10:677.
42. Goodnow CC. Balancing immunity, autoimmunity, and self-tolerance. *Ann N Y Acad Sci* 1997;815:55.
43. Wang RF, Wang X, Atwood AC, Topalian SL, Rosenberg SA. Cloning genes encoding MHC class II-restricted antigens: mutated CDC27 as a tumor antigen. *Science* 1999;284:1351.
44. Wang RF, Wang X, Rosenberg SA. Identification of a novel major histocompatibility complex class II- restricted tumor antigen resulting from a chromosomal rearrangement recognized by CD4(+) T cells. *J Exp Med* 1999;189:1659.
45. Topalian SL, Gonzales MI, Parkhurst M, et al. Melanoma- specific CD4+ T cells recognize nonmutated HLA-DR-restricted tyrosinase epitopes. *J Exp Med* 1996;183:1965.
46. Pieper R, Christian RE, Gonzales MI, et al. Biochemical identification of a mutated human melanoma antigen recognized by CD4(+) T Cells. *J Exp Med* 1999;189:757.
47. Chaux P, Vantomme V, Stroobant V, et al. Identification of MAGE-3 epitopes presented by HLA-DR molecules to CD4(+) T lymphocytes. *J Exp Med* 1999;189:767.
48. Manici S, Sturniolo T, Imro MA, et al. Melanoma cells present a MAGE-3 epitope to CD4(+) cytotoxic T cells in association with histocompatibility leukocyte antigen DR11. *J Exp Med* 1999;189:871.
49. Yanuck M, Carbone DP, Pendleton CD, et al. A mutant p53 tumor suppressor protein is a target for peptide-induced CD8+ cytotoxic T-cells. *Cancer Res* 1993;53:3257.
50. Bristol JA, Schlom J, Abrams SI. Persistence, immune specificity, and functional ability of murine mutant ras epitope-specific CD4(+) and CD8(+) T lymphocytes following in vivo adoptive transfer. *Cell Immunol* 1999;194:78.
51. Abrams SI, Hand PH, Tsang KY, Schlom J. Mutant ras epitopes as targets for cancer vaccines. *Semin Oncol* 1996;23:118.
52. Chen W, Qin H, Reese VA, Cheever MA. CTLs specific for bcr-abl joining region segment peptides fail to lyse leukemia cells expressing p210 bcr-abl protein. *J Immunother* 1998;21:257.
53. Hiltbold EM, Ciborowski P, Finn OJ. Naturally processed class II epitope from the tumor antigen MUC1 primes human CD4+ T cells. *Cancer Res* 1998;58:5066.
54. Magarian-Blander J, Ciborowski P, Hsia S, Watkins SC, Finn OJ. Intercellular and intracellular events following the MHC-unrestricted TCR recognition of a tumor-specific peptide epitope on the epithelial antigen MUC1. *J Immunol* 1998;160:3111.
55. Kass E, Schlom J, Thompson J, et al. Induction of protective host immunity to carcinoembryonic antigen (CEA), a self-antigen in CEA transgenic mice, by immunizing with a recombinant vaccinia-CEA virus. *Cancer Res* 1999;59:676.
56. Zaks TZ, Rosenberg SA. Immunization with a peptide epitope (p369-377) from HER- 2/neu leads to peptide-specific cytotoxic T lymphocytes that fail to recognize HER- 2/neu+ tumors. *Cancer Res* 1998;58:4902.
57. Rosenberg SA. A new era for cancer immunotherapy based on the genes that encode cancer antigens. *Immunity* 1999;10:281.
58. Wang RF, Wang X, Johnston SL, et al. Development of a retrovirus-based complementary DNA expression system for the cloning of tumor antigens. *Cancer Res* 1998;58:3519.
59. Kawakami Y, Eliyahu S, Delgado CH, et al. Identification of a human melanoma antigen recognized by tumor- infiltrating lymphocytes associated with in vivo tumor rejection. *Proc Natl Acad Sci U S A* 1994;91:6458.
60. Kawakami Y, Eliyahu S, Jennings C, et al. Recognition of multiple epitopes in the human melanoma antigen gp100 by tumor-infiltrating T lymphocytes associated with in vivo tumor regression. *J Immunol* 1995;154:3961.
61. Kawakami Y, Robbins PF, Wang X, et al. Identification of new melanoma epitopes on melanosomal proteins recognized by tumor infiltrating T lymphocytes restricted by HLA-A1, -A2, and -A3 alleles. *J Immunol* 1998;161:6985.
62. Bakker AB, Schreurs MW, de Boer AJ, et al. Melanocyte lineage-specific antigen gp100 is recognized by melanoma- derived tumor-infiltrating lymphocytes. *J Exp Med* 1994;179:1005.
63. Skipper J, Kittlesen DJ, Hendrickson RC, et al. Shared epitopes for HLA-A3 restricted melanoma reactive human CTL include a naturally processed epitope from Pmel-17/gp100. *J Immunol* 1996;157:5027.
64. Cox A, Skipper J, Cehn Y, et al. Identification of a peptide recognized by five melanoma-specific human cytotoxic T cell lines. *Science* 1994;264:716.
65. Robbins PF, El-Gamil M, Li YF, et al. The intronic region of an incompletely spliced gp100 gene transcript encodes an epitope recognized by melanoma-reactive tumor-infiltrating lymphocytes. *J Immunol* 1997;159:303.
66. Kawakami Y, Eliyahu S, Delgado CH, et al. Cloning of the gene coding for a shared human melanoma antigen recognized by autologous T cells infiltrating into tumor. *Proc Natl Acad Sci U S A* 1994;91:3515.
67. Kawakami Y, Eliyahu S, Sakaguchi K, et al. Identification of the immunodominant peptides of the MART-1 human melanoma antigen recognized by the majority of HLA-A2-restricted tumor infiltrating lymphocytes. *J Exp Med* 1994;180:347.
68. Schneider J, Brichard VG, Boon T, Buschenfelde K, Wolfel T. Overlapping peptides of melanocyte differentiation antigen MELAN-A/MART-1 recognized by autologous cytolytic T lymphocytes in association with HLA-B45.1 and HLA-A2.1. *Int J Cancer* 1998;75:451.
69. Valmori D, Gervois N, Rimoldi D, et al. Diversity of the fine specificity displayed by HLA-A*0201-restricted CTL specific for the immunodominant Melan-A/MART-1 antigenic peptide. *J Immunol* 1998;161:6956.
70. Romero P, Gervois N, Schneider J, et al. Cytolytic T lymphocyte recognition of the immunodominant HLA-A*0201-restricted Melan-A/MART-1 antigenic peptide in melanoma. *J Immunol* 1997;159:2366.
71. Wolfel T, van Pel A, Brichard VG, et al. Two tyrosinase nonapeptides recognized on HLA-A2 melanomas by autologous cytolytic T lymphocytes. *Eur J Immunol* 1994;24:759.
72. Kittlesen DJ, Thompson LW, Gulden PH, et al. Human melanoma patients recognize and HLA-A1-restricted CTL epitope from tyrosinase containing two cysteine residues: implications for vaccine development. *J Immunol* 1998;160:2099.
73. Brichard VG, Herman J, van Pel A, et al. A tyrosinase nonapeptide presented by HLA-B44 is recognized on a human melanoma by autologous cytolytic T lymphocytes. *Eur J Immunol* 1996;26:224.
74. Kang X-Q, Kawakami Y, Sakaguchi K, et al. Identification of a tyrosinase epitope recognized by HLA-A24 restricted tumor-infiltrating lymphocytes. *J Immunol* 1995;155:1343.
75. Wang RF, Parkhurst MR, Kawakami Y, Robbins PF, Rosenberg SA. Utilization of an alternative open reading frame of a normal gene in generating a novel human cancer antigen. *J Exp Med* 1996;183:1131.

76. Wang RF, Appella E, Kawakami Y, Kang X, Rosenberg SA. Identification of TRP-2 as a human tumor antigen recognized by cytotoxic T lymphocytes. *J Exp Med* 1996;184:2207.
77. Wang RF, Johnston SL, Southwood S, Sette A, Rosenberg SA. Recognition of an antigenic peptide derived from tyrosinase-related protein-2 by CTL in the context of HLA-A31 and -A33. *J Immunol* 1998;160:890.
78. Parkhurst MR, Fitzgerald EB, Southwood S, et al. Identification of a shared HLA-A*0201-restricted T-cell epitope from the melanoma antigen tyrosinase-related protein 2 (TRP2). *Cancer Res* 1998;58:4895.
79. Gilboa E. The makings of a tumor rejection antigen. *Immunity* 1999;11:263.
80. De Plaen E, De Backer O, Arnaud D, et al. A new family of mouse genes homologous to the human MAGE genes. *Genomics* 1999;55:176.
81. van Baren N, Chambost H, Ferrant A, et al. PRAME, a gene encoding an antigen recognized on a human melanoma by cytolytic T cells, is expressed in acute leukaemia cells. *Br J Haematol* 1998;102:1376.
82. Lethe B, Lucas S, Michaux L, et al. LAGE-1, a new gene with tumor specificity. *Int J Cancer* 1998;76:903.
83. Jager E, Chen YT, Drijfhout JW, et al. Simultaneous humoral and cellular immune response against cancer-testis antigen NY-ESO-1: definition of human histocompatibility leukocyte antigen (HLA)-A2-binding peptide epitopes. *J Exp Med* 1998;187:265.
84. Stockert E, Jager E, Chen YT, et al. A survey of the humoral immune response of cancer patients to a panel of human tumor antigens. *J Exp Med* 1998;187:1349.
85. Chen YT, Scanlan MJ, Sahin U, et al. A testicular antigen aberrantly expressed in human cancers detected by autologous antibody screening. *Proc Natl Acad Sci U S A* 1997;94:1914.
86. Boon T, Old LJ. Cancer tumor antigens. *Curr Opin Immunol* 1997;9:681.
87. Wang RF, Johnston SL, Zeng G, et al. A breast and melanoma-shared tumor antigen: T cell responses to antigenic peptides translated from different open reading frames. *J Immunol* 1998;161:3598.
88. Aarnoudse CA, van den Doel PB, Heemskerk B, Schrier PI. Interleukin-2-induced, melanoma-specific T cells recognize CAMEL, an unexpected translation product of LAGE-1. *Int J Cancer* 1999;82:442.
89. Rosenberg SA, White DE. Vitiligo in patients with melanoma: normal tissue antigens can be targets for cancer immunotherapy. *J Immunother Emphasis Tumor Immunol* 1996;19:81.
90. Robbins PF, El-Gamil M, Li YF, et al. A mutated beta- catenin gene encodes a melanoma-specific antigen recognized by tumor infiltrating lymphocytes. *J Exp Med* 1996;183:1185.
91. Wolfel T, Hauer M, Schneider J, et al. A p16INK4a-insensitive CDK4 mutant targeted by cytolytic T lymphocytes in a human melanoma. *Science* 1995;269:1281.
92. Coulie PG, Lehmann F, Lethe B, et al. A mutated intron sequence codes for an antigenic peptide recognized by cytolytic T lymphocytes on a human melanoma. *Proc Natl Acad Sci U S A* 1995;92:7976.
93. Mandruzzato S, Brasseur F, Andry G, Boon T, van der Bruggen P. A CASP-8 mutation recognized by cytolytic T lymphocytes on a human head and neck carcinoma. *J Exp Med* 1997;186:785.
94. Brandle D, Brasseur F, Weynants P, Boon T, van den Eynde B. A mutated HLA-A2 molecule recognized by autologous cytotoxic T lymphocytes on a human renal cell carcinoma. *J Exp Med* 1996;183:2501.
95. Gueguen M, Patard JJ, Gaugler B, et al. An antigen recognized by autologous CTLs on a human bladder carcinoma. *J Immunol* 1998;160:6188.
96. Blachere NE, Srivastava PK. Heat shock protein-based cancer vaccines and related thoughts on immunogenicity of human tumors. *Semin Cancer Biol* 1995;6:349.
97. Lo D, Freedman J, Hesse S, et al. Peripheral tolerance to an islet cell-specific hemagglutinin transgene affects both CD4+ and CD8+ T cells. *Eur J Immunol* 1992;22:1013.
98. Staveley-O'Carroll K, Sotomayor E, Montgomery J, et al. Induction of antigen-specific T cell anergy: an early event in the course of tumor progression. *Proc Natl Acad Sci U S A* 1998;95:1178.
99. Bronte V, Carroll MW, Goletz TJ, et al. Antigen expression by dendritic cells correlates with the therapeutic effectiveness of a model recombinant poxvirus tumor vaccine. *Proc Natl Acad Sci U S A* 1997;94:3183.
100. Porgador A, Irvine KR, Iwasaki A, et al. Predominant role for directly transfected dendritic cells in antigen presentation to CD8+ T cells after gene gun immunization. *J Exp Med* 1998;188:1075.
101. Banchereau J, Steinman RM. Dendritic cells and the control of immunity. *Nature* 1998;392:245.
102. Bluestone JA. Cell fate in the immune system: decisions, decisions, decisions. *Immunol Rev* 1998;165:5.
103. Schwartz RH. T cell clonal anergy. *Curr Opin Immunol* 1997;9:351.
104. Van Parijs L, Abbas AK. Homeostasis and self-tolerance in the immune system: turning lymphocytes off. *Science* 1998;280:243.
105. Walunas TL, Bluestone JA. CTLA-4 regulates tolerance induction and T cell differentiation in vivo. *J Immunol* 1998;160:3855.
106. Leach DR, Krummel MF, Allison JP. Enhancement of antitumor immunity by CTLA-4 blockade. *Science* 1996;271:1734.
107. Gallucci S, Lolkema M, Matzinger P. Natural adjuvants: endogenous activators of dendritic cells. *Nat Med* 1999;5:1249.
108. Gurunathan S, Irvine KR, Wu CY, et al. CD40 ligand/trimer DNA enhances both humoral and cellular immune responses and induces protective immunity to infectious and tumor challenge. *J Immunol* 1998;161:4563.
109. Esche C, Subbotin VM, Maliszewski C, Lotze MT, Shurin MR. FLT3 ligand administration inhibits tumor growth in murine melanoma and lymphoma. *Cancer Res* 1998;58:380.
110. Shurin MR, Pandharipande PP, Zorina TD, et al. FLT3 ligand induces the generation of functionally active dendritic cells in mice. *Cell Immunol* 1997;179:174.
111. Zhang H, Zhang S, Cheung NK, Ragupathi G, Livingston PO. Antibodies against GD2 ganglioside can eradicate syngeneic cancer micrometastases. *Cancer Res* 1998;58:2844.
112. Klapper LN, Glathe S, Vaisman N, et al. The ErbB- 2/HER2 oncoprotein of human carcinomas may function solely as a shared coreceptor for multiple stroma-derived growth factors. *Proc Natl Acad Sci U S A* 1999;96:4995.
113. Pegram MD, Lipton A, Hayes DF, et al. Phase II study of receptor-enhanced chemosensitivity using recombinant humanized anti-p185HER2/neu monoclonal antibody plus cisplatin in patients with HER2/neu-overexpressing metastatic breast cancer refractory to chemotherapy treatment. *J Clin Oncol* 1998;16:2659.
114. Pekarek LA, Starr BA, Toledano AY, Schreiber H. Inhibition of tumor growth by elimination of granulocytes. *J Exp Med* 1995;181:435.
115. Baselga J, Norton L, Albanell J, Kim YM, Mendelsohn J. Recombinant humanized anti-HER2 antibody (Herceptin) enhances the antitumor activity of paclitaxel and doxorubicin against HER2/neu overexpressing human breast cancer xenografts. *Cancer Res* 1998;58:2825.
116. Baselga J, Tripathy D, Mendelsohn J, et al. Phase II study of weekly intravenous recombinant humanized anti-p185HER2 monoclonal antibody in patients with HER2/neu-overexpressing metastatic breast cancer. *J Clin Oncol* 1996;14:737.
117. Cooley S, Burns LJ, Repka T, Miller JS. Natural killer cell cytotoxicity of breast cancer targets is enhanced by two distinct mechanisms of antibody-dependent cellular cytotoxicity against LFA-3 and HER2/neu. *Exp Hematol* 1999;27:1533.
118. Thorsteinsson L, O'Dowd GM, Harrington PM, Johnson PM. The complement regulatory proteins CD46 and CD59, but not CD55, are highly expressed by glandular epithelium of human breast and colorectal tumour tissues. *APMIS* 1998;106:869.
119. Schmitt CA, Schwaeble W, Wittig BM, Meyer ZBK, Dippold WG. Expression and regulation by interferon-gamma of the membrane-bound complement regulators CD46 (MCP), CD55 (DAF) and CD59 in gastrointestinal tumours. *Eur J Cancer* 1999;35:117.
120. Altman JD, Moss PH, Goulder PR, et al. Phenotypic analysis of antigen-specific T lymphocytes. *Science* 1996;274:94.
121. Lee PP, Yee C, Savage PA, et al. Characterization of circulating T cells specific for tumor-associated antigens in melanoma patients. *Nat Med* 1999;5:677.
122. Lee KH, Wang E, Nielsen MB, et al. Increased vaccine-specific T cell frequency after peptide-based vaccination correlates with increased susceptibility to in vitro stimulation but does not lead to tumor regression. *J Immunol* 1999;163:6292.
123. Cormier JN, Salgaller ML, Prevette T, et al. Enhancement of cellular immunity in melanoma patients immunized with a peptide from MART-1/Melan A. *Cancer J Sci Am* 1997;3:37.
124. Pass HA, Schwarz SL, Wunderlich JR, Rosenberg SA. Immunization of patients with melanoma peptide vaccines: immunologic assessment using the ELISPOT assay. *Cancer J Sci Am* 1998;4:316.
125. Kammula US, Lee KH, Riker AI, et al. Functional analysis of antigen-specific T lymphocytes by serial measurement of gene expression in peripheral blood mononuclear cells and tumor specimens. *J Immunol* 1999;163:6867.
126. Key ME, Hanna MGJ. Mechanism of action of BCG-tumor cell vaccines in the generation of systemic tumor immunity. I. Synergism between BCG and line 10 tumor cells in the induction of an inflammatory response. *J Natl Cancer Inst* 1981;67:853.
127. Key ME, Hanna MGJ. Mechanism of action of BCG-tumor cell vaccines in the generation of systemic tumor immunity. II. Influence of the local inflammatory response on immune reactivity. *J Natl Cancer Inst* 1981;67:863.
128. Likhite VV, Halpern BN. Lasting rejection of mammary adenocarcinoma cell tumors in DBA-2 mice with intratumor injection of killed *Corynebacterium parvum*. *Cancer Res* 1974;34:341.
129. Halpern BN, Biozzi G, Stiffel C, Mouton D. Inhibition of tumour growth by administration of killed *Corynebacterium parvum*. *Nature* 1966;212:853.
130. Bash JA. Active specific immunotherapy of murine colon adenocarcinoma with recombinant vaccinia/interleukin-2-infected tumor cell vaccines. *Ann NY Acad Sci* 1993;690:331.
131. Arroyo PJ, Bash JA, Wallack MK. Active specific immunotherapy with vaccinia colon oncolysate enhances the immunomodulatory and antitumor effects of interleukin-2 and interferon alpha in a murine hepatic metastasis model. *Cancer Immunol Immunother* 1990;31:305.
132. Livingston PO, Albino AP, Chung TJ, et al. Serological response of melanoma patients to vaccines prepared from VSV lysates of autologous and allogeneic cultured melanoma cells. *Cancer* 1985;55:713.
133. Colombo MP, Forni G. Cytokine gene transfer in tumor inhibition and tumor therapy: where are we now? *Immunol Today* 1994;15:48.
134. Colombo MP, Rodolfo M. Tumor cells engineered to produce cytokines or cofactors as cellular vaccines: do animal studies really support clinical trials? *Cancer Immunol Immunother* 1995;41:265.
135. Pardoll DM. Paracrine cytokine adjuvants in cancer immunotherapy. *Annu Rev Immunol* 1995;13:399.
136. Ashley DM, Faiola B, Nair S, et al. Bone marrow-generated dendritic cells pulsed with tumor extracts or tumor RNA induce antitumor immunity against central nervous system tumors. *J Exp Med* 1997;186:1177.
137. Celluzzi CM, Mayordomo JI, Storkus WJ, Lotze MT, Falo LDJ. Peptide-pulsed dendritic cells induce antigen-specific CTL-mediated protective tumor immunity. *J Exp Med* 1996;183:283.
138. Zitvogel L, Mayordomo JI, Tjandrawan T, et al. Therapy of murine tumors with tumor peptide-pulsed dendritic cells: dependence on T cells, B7 costimulation, and T helper cell 1-associated cytokines. *J Exp Med* 1996;183:87.
139. Gong J, Chen D, Kashiwaba M, Kufe D. Induction of antitumor activity by immunization with fusions of dendritic and carcinoma cells. *Nat Med* 1997;3:558.
140. Kugler A, Stuhler G, Walden P, et al. Regression of human metastatic renal cell carcinoma after vaccination with tumor cell-dendritic cell hybrids. *Nat Med* 2000;6:332.
141. Johnston D, el Rouby S, Bystryn JC. Identification of melanoma cell surface antigens immunogenic in mice. *Cancer Biother* 1994;9:29.
142. Bystryn JC. Immunogenicity and clinical activity of a polyvalent melanoma antigen vaccine prepared from shed antigens. *Ann NY Acad Sci* 1993;690:190.

143. Bystryn JC, Henn M, Li J, Shroba S. Identification of immunogenic human melanoma antigens in a polyvalent melanoma vaccine. *Cancer Res* 1992;52:5948.
144. Bystryn JC, Oratz R, Roses D, et al. Relationship between immune response to melanoma vaccine immunization and clinical outcome in stage II malignant melanoma. *Cancer* 1992;69:1157.
145. Schultz N, Oratz R, Chen D, et al. Effect of DETOX as an adjuvant for melanoma vaccine. *Vaccine* 1995;13:503.
146. Blachere NE, Li Z, Chandawarkar RY, et al. Heat shock protein-peptide complexes, reconstituted in vitro, elicit peptide-specific cytotoxic T lymphocyte response and tumor immunity. *J Exp Med* 1997;186:1315.
147. Suto R, Srivastava PK. A mechanism for the specific immunogenicity of heat shock protein-chaperoned peptides. *Science* 1995;269:1585.
148. Srivastava PK, Udono H. Heat shock protein-peptide complexes in cancer immunotherapy. *Curr Opin Immunol* 1994;6:728.
149. Udono H, Srivastava PK. Comparison of tumor-specific immunogenicities of stress-induced proteins gp96, hsp90, and hsp70. *J Immunol* 1994;152:5398.
150. Udono H, Levey DL, Srivastava PK. Cellular requirements for tumor-specific immunity elicited by heat shock proteins: tumor rejection antigen gp96 primes CD8+ T cells in vivo. *Proc Natl Acad Sci U S A* 1994;91:3077.
151. Heike M, Blachere NE, Wolfel T, et al. Membranes activate tumor- and virus-specific precursor cytotoxic T lymphocytes in vivo and stimulate tumor-specific T lymphocytes in vitro: implications for vaccination. *J Immunother Emphasis Tumor Immunol* 1994;15:165.
152. Tamura Y, Peng P, Liu K, Daou M, Srivastava PK. Immunotherapy of tumors with autologous tumor-derived heat shock protein preparations [published erratum appears in *Science* 1999;283(5405):preceding 1119]. *Science* 1997;278:117.
153. Elliott GT, McLeod RA, Perez J, Von Eschen KB. Interim results of a phase II multicenter clinical trial evaluating the activity of a therapeutic allogeneic melanoma vaccine (theraccine) in the treatment of disseminated malignant melanoma. *Semin Surg Oncol* 1993;9:264.
154. Stover CK, de la Cruz VF, Fuerst TR, et al. New use of BCG for recombinant vaccines. *Nature* 1991;351:456.
155. Berd D, Maguire HCJ, McCue P, Mastrangelo MJ. Treatment of metastatic melanoma with an autologous tumor-cell vaccine: clinical and immunologic results in 64 patients. *J Clin Oncol* 1990;8:1858.
156. Sensi M, Farina C, Maccalli C, et al. Clonal expansion of T lymphocytes in human melanoma metastases after treatment with a hapten-modified autologous tumor vaccine. *J Clin Invest* 1997;99:710.
157. Berd D, Murphy G, Maguire HCJ, Mastrangelo MJ. Immunization with haptenized, autologous tumor cells induces inflammation of human melanoma metastases. *Cancer Res* 1991;51:2731.
158. Berd D, Maguire HCJ, Schuchter LM, et al. Autologous hapten-modified melanoma vaccine as postsurgical adjuvant treatment after resection of nodal metastases. *J Clin Oncol* 1997;15:2359.
159. Vermorken JB, Claessen AM, van Tinteren H, et al. Active specific immunotherapy for stage II and stage III human colon cancer: a randomised trial. *Lancet* 1999;353:345.
160. Sahasrabudhe DM, deKernion JB, Pontes JE, et al. Specific immunotherapy with suppressor function inhibition for metastatic renal cell carcinoma. *J Biol Response Mod* 1986;5:581.
161. McCune CS, O'Donnell RW, Marquis DM, Sahasrabudhe DM. Renal cell carcinoma treated by vaccines for active specific immunotherapy: correlation of survival with skin testing by autologous tumor cells. *Cancer Immunol Immunother* 1990;32:62.
162. Simons JW, Jaffee EM, Weber CE, et al. Bioactivity of autologous irradiated renal cell carcinoma vaccines generated by ex vivo granulocyte-macrophage colony-stimulating factor gene transfer. *Cancer Res* 1997;57:1537.
163. Restifo NP. The new vaccines: building viruses that elicit antitumor immunity. *Curr Opin Immunol* 1996;8:658.
164. Paterson Y. Rational approaches to immune regulation. *Immunol Res* 1998;17:191.
165. Paterson Y, Ikonomidis G. Recombinant *Listeria monocytogenes* cancer vaccines. *Curr Opin Immunol* 1996;8:664.
166. Ying H, Zaks TZ, Wang RF, et al. Cancer therapy using a self-replicating RNA vaccine. *Nat Med* 1999;5:823.
167. Polo JM, Dubensky TWJ. DNA vaccines with a kick. *Nat Biotechnol* 1998;16:517.
168. Wang M, Bronte V, Chen PW, et al. Active immunotherapy of cancer with a nonreplicating recombinant fowlpox virus encoding a model tumor-associated antigen. *J Immunol* 1995;154:4685.
169. Restifo NP, Surman DR, Zheng H, et al. Transfectant influenza A viruses are effective recombinant immunogens in the treatment of experimental cancer. *Virology* 1998;249:89.
170. Carroll MW, Overwijk WW, Chamberlain RS, et al. Highly attenuated modified vaccinia virus Ankara (MVA) as an effective recombinant vector: a murine tumor model. *Vaccine* 1997;15:387.
171. Chen PW, Wang M, Bronte V, et al. Therapeutic antitumor response after immunization with a recombinant adenovirus encoding a model tumor-associated antigen. *J Immunol* 1996;156:224.
172. Rosenberg SA, Zhai Y, Yang JC, et al. Immunizing patients with metastatic melanoma using recombinant adenoviruses encoding MART-1 or gp100 melanoma antigens. *J Natl Cancer Inst* 1998;90:1894.
173. Gurwith MJ, Horwith GS, Impellizzeri CA, et al. Current use and future directions of adenovirus vaccine. *Semin Respir Infect* 1989;4:299.
174. Wood DJ. Adenovirus gastroenteritis. *BMJ (Clin Res Ed)* 1988;296:229.
175. Zahradnik JM. Adenovirus pneumonia. *Semin Respir Infect* 1987;2:104.
176. Wehrle PF. A reality in our time—certification of the global eradication of smallpox. *J Infect Dis* 1980;142:636.
177. Gregorio L. The smallpox legacy: a history of pediatric immunizations. *Pharos* 1996;59:7.
178. Fenner F. Risks and benefits of vaccinia vaccine use in the worldwide smallpox eradication campaign. *Res Virol* 1989;140:465.
179. Tsang KY, Zaremba S, Nieroda CA, et al. Generation of human cytotoxic T cells specific for human carcinoembryonic antigen epitopes from patients immunized with recombinant vaccinia-CEA vaccine. *J Natl Cancer Inst* 1995;87:982.
180. Conry RM, Khazaeli MB, Saleh MN, et al. Phase I trial of a recombinant vaccinia virus encoding carcinoembryonic antigen in metastatic adenocarcinoma: comparison of intradermal versus subcutaneous administration. *Clin Cancer Res* 1999;5:2330.
181. Irvine KR, Chamberlain RS, Shulman EP, et al. Enhancing efficacy of recombinant anticancer vaccines with prime/boost regimens that use two different vectors. *J Natl Cancer Inst* 1997;89:1595.
182. Hodge JW, McLaughlin JP, Kantor JA, Schlom J. Diversified prime and boost protocols using recombinant vaccinia virus and recombinant non-replicating avian pox virus to enhance T-cell immunity and antitumor responses. *Vaccine* 1997;15:759.
183. Liu MA. Vaccine developments. *Nat Med* 1998;4:515.
184. Marchand M, van Baren N, Weynants P, et al. Tumor regressions observed in patients with metastatic melanoma treated with an antigenic peptide encoded by gene MAGE-3 and presented by HLA-A1. *Int J Cancer* 1999;80:219.
185. Parkhurst MR, Salgaller ML, Southwood S, et al. Improved induction of melanoma-reactive CTL with peptides from the melanoma antigen gp100 modified at HLA-A*0201-binding residues. *J Immunol* 1996;157:2539.
186. Steller MA, Gurski KJ, Murakami M, et al. Cell-mediated immunological responses in cervical and vaginal cancer patients immunized with a lipidated epitope of human papillomavirus type 16 E7. *Clin Cancer Res* 1998;4:2103.
187. van Driel WJ, Ressing ME, Kenter GG, et al. Vaccination with HPV16 peptides of patients with advanced cervical carcinoma: clinical evaluation of a phase I-II trial. *Eur J Cancer* 1999;35:946.
188. Disis ML, Grabstein KH, Sleath PR, Cheever MA. Generation of immunity to the HER-2/neu oncogenic protein in patients with breast and ovarian cancer using a peptide-based vaccine. *Clin Cancer Res* 1999;5:1289.
189. Goydos JS, Elder E, Whiteside TL, Finn OJ, Lotze MT. A phase I trial of a synthetic mucin peptide vaccine. Induction of specific immune reactivity in patients with adenocarcinoma. *J Surg Res* 1996;63:298.
190. Karanikas V, Hwang LA, Pearson J, et al. Antibody and T cell responses of patients with adenocarcinoma immunized with mannan-MUC1 fusion protein. *J Clin Invest* 1997;100:2783.
191. Triozzi PL, Stevens VC, Aldrich W, et al. Effects of a beta-human chorionic gonadotropin subunit immunogen administered in aqueous solution with a novel nonionic block copolymer adjuvant in patients with advanced cancer. *Clin Cancer Res* 1997;3:2355.
192. Rosenberg SA, Yang JC, Schwartzentruber DJ, et al. Impact of cytokine administration on the generation of antitumor reactivity in patients with metastatic melanoma receiving a peptide vaccine. *J Immunol* 1999;163:1690.
193. Falo LDJ, Kovacsovics-Bankowski M, Thompson K, Rock KL. Targeting antigen into the phagocytic pathway in vivo induces protective tumour immunity. *Nat Med* 1995;1:649.
194. Kovacsovics-Bankowski M, Rock KL. A phagosome-to-cytosol pathway for exogenous antigens presented on MHC class I molecules. *Science* 1995;267:243.
195. Goletz TJ, Klimpel KR, Arora N, et al. Targeting HIV proteins to the major histocompatibility complex class I processing pathway with a novel gp120-anthrax toxin fusion protein. *Proc Natl Acad Sci U S A* 1997;94:12059.
196. Goletz TJ, Klimpel KR, Leppla SH, Keith JM, Berzofsky JA. Delivery of antigens to the MHC class I pathway using bacterial toxins. *Hum Immunol* 1997;54:129.
197. Minev B, McFarland BJ, Spiess PJ, Rosenberg SA, Restifo NP. Insertion signal sequence fused to a minimal peptide elicits specific CD8+ T cell responses and prolongs survival of thymoma-bearing mice. *Cancer Res* 1994;54:4155.
198. Naftzger C, Takechi Y, Kohda H, et al. Immune response to a differentiation antigen induced by altered antigen: a study of tumor rejection and autoimmunity. *Proc Natl Acad Sci U S A* 1996;93:14809.
199. Overwijk WW, Tsung A, Irvine KR, et al. gp100/pmel 17 is a murine tumor rejection antigen: induction of "self"-reactive, tumoricidal T cells using high-affinity, altered peptide ligand. *J Exp Med* 1998;188:277.
200. Murphy GP, Tjoa BA, Simmons SJ, et al. Phase II prostate cancer vaccine trial: report of a study involving 37 patients with disease recurrence following primary treatment. *Prostate* 1999;39:54.
201. Nelson EL, Li X, Hsu FJ, et al. Tumor-specific, cytotoxic T-lymphocyte response after idiotype vaccination for B-cell, non-Hodgkin's lymphoma. *Blood* 1996;88:580.
202. Hsu FJ, Caspar CB, Czerwinski D, et al. Tumor- specific idiotype vaccines in the treatment of patients with B-cell lymphoma—long-term results of a clinical trial. *Blood* 1997;89:3129.
203. Bendandi M, Gocke CD, Kobrin CB, et al. Complete molecular remissions induced by patient-specific vaccination plus granulocyte-monocyte colony-stimulating factor against lymphoma [see comments]. *Nat Med* 1999;5:1171.
204. Singhai R, Levy JG. Isolation of a T-cell clone that reacts with both antigen and anti-idiotype: evidence for anti-idiotype as internal image for antigen at the T-cell level. *Proc Natl Acad Sci U S A* 1987;84:3836.
205. Somasundaram R, Zaloudik J, Jacob L, et al. Induction of antigen-specific T and B cell immunity in colon carcinoma patients by anti-idiotypic antibody. *J Immunol* 1995;155:3253.
206. Herlyn D, Benden A, Kane M, et al. Anti-idiotype cancer vaccines: pre-clinical and clinical studies. *In Vivo* 1991;5:615.
207. Ferrone S. Anti-idiotypes in melanoma. *Hybridoma* 1993;12:509.
208. Foon KA, Chakraborty M, John WJ, et al. Immune response to the carcinoembryonic antigen in patients treated with an anti-idiotype antibody vaccine. *J Clin Invest* 1995;96:334.

209. Levitsky HI, Montgomery J, Ahmadzadeh M, et al. Immunization with granulocyte-macrophage colony-stimulating factor-transduced, but not B7-1-transduced, lymphoma cells primes idiotype-specific T cells and generates potent systemic antitumor immunity. *J Immunol* 1996;156:3858.
210. Foon KA, Bhattacharya-Chatterjee M. Idiotype vaccines in the clinic. *Nat Med* 1998;4:870.
211. Foon KA, Sen G, Hutchins L, et al. Antibody responses in melanoma patients immunized with an anti-idiotype antibody mimicking disialoganglioside GD2. *Clin Cancer Res* 1998;4:1117.
212. Mittelman A, Chen GZ, Wong GY, et al. Human high molecular weight-melanoma associated antigen mimicry by mouse anti-idiotypic monoclonal antibody MK2-23: modulation of the immunogenicity in patients with malignant melanoma. *Clin Cancer Res* 1995;1:705.
213. Foon KA, Lutzky J, Baral RN, et al. Clinical and immune responses in advanced melanoma patients immunized with an anti-idiotype antibody mimicking disialoganglioside GD2. *J Clin Oncol* 2000;18:376.
214. McCaffery M, Yao TJ, Williams L, et al. Immunization of melanoma patients with BEC2 anti-idiotypic monoclonal antibody that mimics GD3 ganglioside: enhanced immunogenicity when combined with adjuvant. *Clin Cancer Res* 1996;2:679.
215. Dickler MN, Ragupathi G, Liu NX, et al. Immunogenicity of a fucosyl-GM1-keyhole limpet hemocyanin conjugate vaccine in patients with small cell lung cancer. *Clin Cancer Res* 1999;5:2773.
216. Samonigg H, Wilders-Truschnig M, Kuss I, et al. A double-blind randomized-phase II trial comparing immunization with antiidiotype goat antibody vaccine SCV 106 versus unspecific goat antibodies in patients with metastatic colorectal cancer. *J Immunother* 1999;22:481.
217. Foon KA, John WJ, Chakraborty M, et al. Clinical and immune responses in resected colon cancer patients treated with anti-idiotype monoclonal antibody vaccine that mimics the carcinoembryonic antigen. *J Clin Oncol* 1999;17:2889.
218. Livingston PO, Adluri S, Helling F, et al. Phase 1 trial of immunological adjuvant QS-21 with a GM2 ganglioside-keyhole limpet haemocyanin conjugate vaccine in patients with malignant melanoma. *Vaccine* 1994;12:1275.
219. Helling F, Zhang S, Shang A, et al. GM2-KLH conjugate vaccine: increased immunogenicity in melanoma patients after administration with immunological adjuvant QS-21. *Cancer Res* 1995;55:2783.
220. Kitamura K, Livingston PO, Fortunato SR, et al. Serological response patterns of melanoma patients immunized with a GM2 ganglioside conjugate vaccine. *Proc Natl Acad Sci U S A* 1995;92:2805.
221. Takahashi T, Johnson TD, Nishinaka Y, Morton DL, Irie RF. IgM anti-ganglioside antibodies induced by melanoma cell vaccine correlate with survival of melanoma patients. *J Invest Dermatol* 1999;112:205.
222. Jerome KR, Barnd DL, Bendt KM, et al. Cytotoxic T-lymphocytes derived from patients with breast adenocarcinoma recognize an epitope present on the protein core of a mucin molecule preferentially expressed by malignant cells. *Cancer Res* 1991;51:2908.
223. Taylor-Papadimitriou J, Finn OJ. Biology, biochemistry and immunology of carcinoma-associated mucins. *Immunol Today* 1997;18:105.
224. von Mensdorff-Pouilly S, Gourevitch MM, Kenemans P, et al. Humoral immune response to polymorphic epithelial mucin (MUC-1) in patients with benign and malignant breast tumours. *Eur J Cancer* 1996;32A:1325.
225. Reddish MA, MacLean GD, Poppema S, Berg A, Longenecker BM. Pre-immunotherapy serum CA27.29 (MUC-1) mucin level and CD69+ lymphocytes correlate with effects of Theratope sialyl-Tn-KLH cancer vaccine in active specific immunotherapy. *Cancer Immunol Immunother* 1996;42:303.
226. Kotera Y, Fontenot JD, Pecher G, Metzgar RS, Finn OJ. Humoral immunity against a tandem repeat epitope of human mucin MUC-1 in sera from breast, pancreatic, and colon cancer patients. *Cancer Res* 1994;54:2856.
227. Restifo NP, Bacik I, Irvine KR, et al. Antigen processing in vivo and the elicitation of primary CTL responses. *J Immunol* 1995;154:4414.
228. Aichele P, Brduscha-Riem K, Zinkernagel RM, Hengartner H, Pircher H. T cell priming versus T cell tolerance induced by synthetic peptides. *J Exp Med* 1995;182:261.
229. Irvine KR, Chamberlain RS, Shulman EP, Rosenberg SA, Restifo NP. Route of immunization and the therapeutic impact of recombinant anticancer vaccines. *J Natl Cancer Inst* 1997;89:390.
230. Bronte V, Tsung K, Rao JB, et al. IL-2 enhances the function of recombinant poxvirus-based vaccines in the treatment of established pulmonary metastases. *J Immunol* 1995;154:5282.
231. Rao JB, Chamberlain RS, Bronte V, et al. IL-12 is an effective adjuvant to recombinant vaccinia virus-based tumor vaccines: enhancement by simultaneous B7-1 expression. *J Immunol* 1996;156:3357.
232. Carroll MW, Overwijk WW, Surman DR, et al. Construction and characterization of a triple-recombinant vaccinia virus encoding B7-1, interleukin 12, and a model tumor antigen. *J Natl Cancer Inst* 1998;90:1881.
233. Dranoff G, Jaffee E, Lazenby A, et al. Vaccination with irradiated tumor cells engineered to secrete murine granulocyte-macrophage colony-stimulating factor stimulates potent, specific, and long-lasting anti-tumor immunity. *Proc Natl Acad Sci U S A* 1993;90:3539.
234. Witmer-Pack MD, Olivier W, Valinsky J, Schuler G, Steinman RM. Granulocyte/macrophage colony-stimulating factor is essential for the viability and function of cultured murine epidermal Langerhans cells. *J Exp Med* 1987;166:1484.
235. Chamberlain RS, Carroll MW, Bronte V, et al. Costimulation enhances the active immunotherapy effect of recombinant anticancer vaccines. *Cancer Res* 1996;56:2832.
236. Mantovani A. The chemokine system: redundancy for robust outputs. *Immunol Today* 1999;20:254.
237. Sallusto F, Lanzavecchia A. Mobilizing dendritic cells for tolerance, priming, and chronic inflammation. *J Exp Med* 1999;189:611.
238. Ward SG, Bacon K, Westwick J. Chemokines and T lymphocytes: more than an attraction. *Immunity* 1998;9:1.
239. Baggiolini M. Chemokines and leukocyte traffic. *Nature* 1998;392:565.
240. Krieg AM, Yi AK, Schorr J, Davis HL. The role of CpG dinucleotides in DNA vaccines. *Trends Microbiol* 1998;6:23.
241. Brazolot MC, Weeratna R, Krieg AM, Siegrist CA, Davis HL. CpG DNA can induce strong Th1 humoral and cell-mediated immune responses against hepatitis B surface antigen in young mice. *Proc Natl Acad Sci U S A* 1998;95:15553.
242. Fuchs EJ, Matzinger P. Is cancer dangerous to the immune system? *Semin Immunol* 1996;8:271.
243. Matzinger P. An innate sense of danger. *Semin Immunol* 1998;10:399.
244. Matzinger P. Tolerance, danger, and the extended family. *Annu Rev Immunol* 1994;12:991.
245. Liebowitz DN, Lee KP, June CH. Costimulatory approaches to adoptive immunotherapy. *Curr Opin Oncol* 1998;10:533.
246. La Motte RN, Sharpe AH, Bluestone JA, Mokyr MB. Importance of B7-1-expressing host antigen-presenting cells for the eradication of B7-2 transfected P815 tumor cells. *J Immunol* 1998;161:6552.
247. Chen L, McGowan P, Ashe S, et al. Tumor immunogenicity determines the effect of B7 costimulation on T cell-mediated tumor immunity. *J Exp Med* 1994;179:523.
248. McCabe BJ, Irvine KR, Nishimura MI, et al. Minimal determinant expressed by a recombinant vaccinia virus elicits therapeutic antitumor cytolytic T lymphocyte responses. *Cancer Res* 1995;55:1741.
249. Ochsenbein AF, Klenerman P, Karrer U, et al. Immune surveillance against a solid tumor fails because of immunological ignorance. *Proc Natl Acad Sci U S A* 1999;96:2233.
250. Chen L. Immunological ignorance of silent antigens as an explanation of tumor evasion. *Immunol Today* 1998;19:27.
251. Stearns ME, Garcia FU, Fudge K, Rhim J, Wang M. Role of interleukin 10 and transforming growth factor beta1 in the angiogenesis and metastasis of human prostate primary tumor lines from orthotopic implants in severe combined immunodeficiency mice. *Clin Cancer Res* 1999;5:711.
252. Hahne M, Rimoldi D, Schroter M, et al. Melanoma cell expression of Fas(Apo-1/CD95) ligand: implications for tumor immune escape. *Science* 1996;274:1363.
253. Chappell DB, Restifo NP. T cell-tumor cell: a fatal interaction? *Cancer Immunol Immunother* 1998;47:65.
254. Chappell DB. Human melanoma cells do not express Fas (Apo-1/CD95) ligand. *Cancer Res* 1999;59:59.
255. Zaks TZ, Chappell DB, Rosenberg SA, Restifo NP. Fas-mediated suicide of tumor- reactive T cells following activation by specific tumor: selective rescue by caspase inhibition. *J Immunol* 1999;162:3273.
256. Riker A, Cormier J, Panelli M, et al. Immune selection after antigen-specific immunotherapy of melanoma. *Surgery* 1999;126:112.
257. Cormier JN, Abati A, Fetsch P, et al. Comparative analysis of the in vivo expression of tyrosinase, MART-1/Melan-A, and gp100 in metastatic melanoma lesions: implications for immunotherapy. *J Immunother* 1998;21:27.
258. Restifo NP, Esquivel F, Kawakami Y, et al. Identification of human cancers deficient in antigen processing. *J Exp Med* 1993;177:265.
259. Restifo NP, Kawakami Y, Marincola F, et al. Molecular mechanisms used by tumors to escape immune recognition: immunogenetherapy and the cell biology of major histocompatibility complex class I. *J Immunother* 1993;14:182.
260. Restifo NP, Marincola FM, Kawakami Y, et al. Loss of functional beta 2-microglobulin in metastatic melanomas from five patients receiving immunotherapy. *J Natl Cancer Inst* 1996;88:100.
261. Marincola FM, Shamamian P, Simonis TB, et al. Locus-specific analysis of human leukocyte antigen class I expression in melanoma cell lines. *J Immunother Emphasis Tumor Immunol* 1994;16:13.
262. Cormier JN, Panelli MC, Hackett JA, et al. Natural variation of the expression of HLA and endogenous antigen modulates CTL recognition in an in vitro melanoma model. *Int J Cancer* 1999;80:781.
263. Wallack MK, Sivanandham M, Balch CM, et al. Surgical adjuvant active specific immunotherapy for patients with stage III melanoma: the final analysis of data from a phase III, randomized, double-blind, multicenter vaccinia melanoma oncolysate trial. *J Am Coll Surg* 1998;187:69.
264. Mitchell MS. Perspective on allogeneic melanoma lysates in active specific immunotherapy. *Semin Oncol* 1998;25:623.
265. Livingston PO, Wong GY, Adluri S, et al. Improved survival in stage III melanoma patients with GM2 antibodies: a randomized trial of adjuvant vaccination with GM2 ganglioside. *J Clin Oncol* 1994;12:1036.
266. Harris JE, Ryan L, Hoover HCJ, et al. Adjuvant active specific immunotherapy for stage II and III colon cancer with an autologous tumor cell vaccine: Eastern Cooperative Oncology Group Study E5283. *J Clin Oncol* 2000;18:148.
267. McAneny D, Ryan CA, Beazley RM, Kaufman HL. Results of a phase I trial of a recombinant vaccinia virus that expresses carcinoembryonic antigen in patients with advanced colorectal cancer. *Ann Surg Oncol* 1996;3:495.
268. Zhu MZ, Marshall J, Cole D, Schlom J, Tsang KY. Specific cytolytic T-cell responses to human CEA from patients immunized with recombinant avipox-CEA vaccine. *Clin Cancer Res* 2000;6:24.
269. Marshall JL, Hawkins MJ, Tsang KY, et al. Phase I study in cancer patients of a replication-defective avipox recombinant vaccine that expresses human carcinoembryonic antigen. *J Clin Oncol* 1999;17:332.
270. Borysiewicz LK, Fiander A, Nimako M, et al. A recombinant vaccinia virus encoding human papillomavirus types 16 and 18, E6 and E7 proteins as immunotherapy for cervical cancer [see comments]. *Lancet* 1996;347:1523.
271. Thurner B, Haendle I, Roder C, et al. Vaccination with mage-3A1 peptide-pulsed mature, monocyte-derived dendritic cells expands specific cytotoxic T cells and induces regression of some metastases in advanced stage IV melanoma. *J Exp Med* 1999;190:1669.
272. Morse MA, Deng Y, Coleman D, et al. A phase I study of active immunotherapy with carcinoembryonic antigen peptide (CAP-1)-pulsed, autologous human cultured dendritic

cells in patients with metastatic malignancies expressing carcinoembryonic antigen. *Clin Cancer Res* 1999;5:1331.
273. Murphy GP, Tjoa BA, Simmons SJ, et al. Infusion of dendritic cells pulsed with HLA-A2-specific prostate-specific membrane antigen peptides: a phase II prostate cancer vaccine trial involving patients with hormone-refractory metastatic disease. *Prostate* 1999;38:73.
274. Salgaller ML, Marincola FM, Cormier JN, Rosenberg SA. Immunization against epitopes in the human melanoma antigen gp100 following patient immunization with synthetic peptides. *Cancer Res* 1996;56:4749.
275. Weber JS, Hua FL, Spears L, et al. A phase I trial of an HLA-A1 restricted MAGE-3 epitope peptide with incomplete Freund's adjuvant in patients with resected high-risk melanoma. *J Immunother* 1999;22:431.
276. Khleif SN, Abrams SI, Hamilton JM, et al. A phase I vaccine trial with peptides reflecting ras oncogene mutations of solid tumors. *J Immunother* 1999;22:155.
277. Grant SC, Kris MG, Houghton AN, Chapman PB. Long survival of patients with small cell lung cancer after adjuvant treatment with the anti-idiotypic antibody BEC2 plus Bacillus Calmette- Guérin. *Clin Cancer Res* 1999;5:1319.
278. Durrant LG, Maxwell-Armstrong C, Buckley D, et al. A neoadjuvant clinical trial in colorectal cancer patients of the human anti-idiotypic antibody 105AD7, which mimics CD55 [In Process Citation]. *Clin Cancer Res* 2000;6:422.
279. Durrant LG, Doran M, Austin EB, Robins RA. Induction of cellular immune responses by a murine monoclonal anti-idiotypic antibody recognizing the 791Tgp72 antigen expressed on colorectal, gastric and ovarian human tumours. *Int J Cancer* 1995;61:62.
280. Cormier JN, Hijazi YM, Abati A, et al. Heterogeneous expression of melanoma-associated antigens and HLA-A2 in metastatic melanoma in vivo. *Int J Cancer* 1998;75:517.
281. Sanda MG, Restifo NP, Walsh JC, et al. Molecular characterization of defective antigen processing in human prostate cancer. *J Natl Cancer Inst* 1995;87:280.
282. Jager E, Ringhoffer M, Altmannsberger M, et al. Immunoselection in vivo: independent loss of MHC class I and melanocyte differentiation antigen expression in metastatic melanoma. *Int J Cancer* 1997;71:142.
283. Kageshita T, Wang Z, Calorini L, et al. Selective loss of human leukocyte class I allospecificities and staining of melanoma cells by monoclonal antibodies recognizing monomorphic determinants of class I human leukocyte antigens. *Cancer Res* 1993;53:3349.
284. Cabrera T, Collado A, Fernandez MA, et al. High frequency of altered HLA class I phenotypes in invasive colorectal carcinomas. *Tissue Antigens* 1998;52:114.
285. Cabrera T, Angustias FM, Sierra A, et al. High frequency of altered HLA class I phenotypes in invasive breast carcinomas. *Hum Immunol* 1996;50:127.
286. Kaplan DH, Shankaran V, Dighe AS, et al. Demonstration of an interferon gamma-dependent tumor surveillance system in immunocompetent mice. *Proc Natl Acad Sci U S A* 1998;95:7556.
287. Ikeda H, Lethe B, Lehmann F, et al. Characterization of an antigen that is recognized on a melanoma showing partial HLA loss by CTL expressing an NK inhibitory receptor. *Immunity* 1997;6:199.
288. Chen JJ, Sun Y, Nabel GJ. Regulation of the proinflammatory effects of Fas ligand (CD95L). *Science* 1998;282:1714.
289. Bronte V, Wang M, Overwijk WW, et al. Apoptotic death of CD8+ T lymphocytes after immunization: induction of a suppressive population of Mac-1+/Gr-1+ cells. *J Immunol* 1998;161:5313.
290. Watson GA, Lopez DM. Aberrant antigen presentation by macrophages from tumor-bearing mice is involved in the down-regulation of their T cell responses. *J Immunol* 1995;155:3124.
291. Correa MR, Ochoa AC, Ghosh P, et al. Sequential development of structural and functional alterations in T cells from tumor-bearing mice. *J Immunol* 1997;158:5292.
292. Zea AH, Curti BD, Longo DL, et al. Alterations in T cell receptor and signal transduction molecules in melanoma patients. *Clin Cancer Res* 1995;1:1327.
293. Mizoguchi H, O'Shea JJ, Longo DL, et al. Alterations in signal transduction molecules in T lymphocytes from tumor-bearing mice. *Science* 1992;258:1795.
294. Ling W, Rayman P, Uzzo R, et al. Impaired activation of NFkappaB in T cells from a subset of renal cell carcinoma patients is mediated by inhibition of phosphorylation and degradation of the inhibitor, IkappaBalpha. *Blood* 1998;92:1334.
295. Ishida T, Oyama T, Carbone DP, Gabrilovich DI. Defective function of Langerhans cells in tumor-bearing animals is the result of defective maturation from hemopoietic progenitors. *J Immunol* 1998;161:4842.
296. Gabrilovich D, Ishida T, Oyama T, et al. Vascular endothelial growth factor inhibits the development of dendritic cells and dramatically affects the differentiation of multiple hematopoietic lineages in vivo. *Blood* 1998;92:4150.
297. Steinbrink K, Jonuleit H, Muller G, et al. Interleukin-10-treated human dendritic cells induce a melanoma-antigen- specific anergy in CD8(+) T cells resulting in a failure to lyse tumor cells. *Blood* 1999;93:1634.
298. Mule JJ, Schwarz SL, Roberts AB, Sporn MB, Rosenberg SA. Transforming growth factor-beta inhibits the in vitro generation of lymphokine-activated killer cells and cytotoxic T cells. *Cancer Immunol Immunother* 1988;26:95.
299. Torre-Amione G, Beauchamp RD, Koeppen H, et al. A highly immunogenic tumor transfected with a murine transforming growth factor type beta 1 cDNA escapes immune surveillance. *Proc Natl Acad Sci U S A* 1990;87:1486.
300. Hu HM, Urba WJ, Fox BA. Gene-modified tumor vaccine with therapeutic potential shifts tumor-specific T cell response from a type 2 to a type 1 cytokine profile. *J Immunol* 1998;161:3033.
301. D'Orazio TJ, Niederkorn JY. A novel role for TGF-beta and IL-10 in the induction of immune privilege. *J Immunol* 1998;160:2089.
302. Sarzotti M, Robbins DS, Hoffman PM. Induction of protective CTL responses in newborn mice by a murine retrovirus. *Science* 1996;271:1726.
303. Shimizu Y, Guidotti LG, Fowler P, Chisari FV. Dendritic cell immunization breaks cytotoxic T lymphocyte tolerance in hepatitis B virus transgenic mice. *J Immunol* 1998;161:4520.
304. Rowse GJ, Tempero RM, VanLith ML, Hollingsworth MA, Gendler SJ. Tolerance and immunity to MUC1 in a human MUC1 transgenic murine model. *Cancer Res* 1998;58:315.
305. Clarke P, Mann J, Simpson JF, Rickard-Dickson K, Primus FJ. Mice transgenic for human carcinoembryonic antigen as a model for immunotherapy. *Cancer Res* 1998;58:1469.
306. Wei C, Willis RA, Tilton BR, et al. Tissue-specific expression of the human prostate-specific antigen gene in transgenic mice: implications for tolerance and immunotherapy. *Proc Natl Acad Sci U S A* 1997;94:6369.
307. Fong L, Ruegg CL, Brockstedt D, Engleman EG, Laus R. Induction of tissue-specific autoimmune prostatitis with prostatic acid phosphatase immunization: implications for immunotherapy of prostate cancer. *J Immunol* 1997;159:3113.
308. Alexander-Miller MA, Leggatt GR, Berzofsky JA. Selective expansion of high- or low-avidity cytotoxic T lymphocytes and efficacy for adoptive immunotherapy. *Proc Natl Acad Sci U S A* 1996;93:4102.
309. Morgan DJ, Kreuwel HT, Fleck S, et al. Activation of low avidity CTL specific for a self epitope results in tumor rejection but not autoimmunity. *J Immunol* 1998;160:643.
310. Targoni OS, Lehmann PV. Endogenous myelin basic protein inactivates the high avidity T cell repertoire. *J Exp Med* 1998;187:2055.
311. Suri-Payer E, Amar AZ, Thornton AM, Shevach EM. CD4+CD25+ T cells inhibit both the induction and effector function of autoreactive T cells and represent a unique lineage of immunoregulatory cells. *J Immunol* 1998;160:1212.
312. Thornton AM, Shevach EM. CD4+CD25+ immunoregulatory T cells suppress polyclonal T cell activation in vitro by inhibiting interleukin 2 production. *J Exp Med* 1998;188:287.
313. Marelli-Berg FM, Weetman A, Frasca L, et al. Antigen presentation by epithelial cells induces anergic immunoregulatory CD45RO+ T cells and deletion of CD45RA+ T cells. *J Immunol* 1997;159:5853.
314. Loftus DJ, Squarcina P, Nielsen MB, et al. Peptides derived from self-proteins as partial agonists and antagonists of human CD8+ T-cell clones reactive to melanoma/melanocyte epitope MART1(27-35). *Cancer Res* 1998;58:2433.
315. Ganss R, Hanahan D. Tumor microenvironment can restrict the effectiveness of activated antitumor lymphocytes. *Cancer Res* 1998;58:4673.
316. Wick M, Dubey P, Koeppen H, et al. Antigenic cancer cells grow progressively in immune hosts without evidence for T cell exhaustion or systemic anergy. *J Exp Med* 1997;186:229.
317. Allison J, Stephens LA, Kay TW, et al. The threshold for autoimmune T cell killing is influenced by B7-1. *Eur J Immunol* 1998;28:949.
318. Speiser DE, Miranda R, Zakarian A, et al. Self antigens expressed by solid tumors do not efficiently stimulate naive or activated T cells: implications for immunotherapy. *J Exp Med* 1997;186:645.
319. Prevost-Blondel A, Zimmermann C, Stemmer C, et al. Tumor-infiltrating lymphocytes exhibiting high ex vivo cytolytic activity fail to prevent murine melanoma tumor growth in vivo. *J Immunol* 1998;161:2187.
320. Burch PA, Breen JK, Buckner JC, et al. Priming tissue-specific cellular immunity in a Phase I trial of autologous dendritic cells for prostate cancer. *Clin Cancer Res* 2000;6:2175.

Nick Bryan
Steven K. Libutti

CHAPTER 64

Image-Guided Surgery

With the introduction of the x-ray at the turn of the twentieth century heralding the advent of modern medical imaging, the surgeon's eye has been supplemented with indirect imaging data that better defines local disease. Conventional x-ray techniques have been supplemented, or even supplanted, by radiographic contrast agents, nuclear imaging techniques, ultrasound (US), computed tomography (CT), and magnetic resonance (MR) imaging. There is no reason to believe that even more powerful imaging techniques will not follow. These increasingly sophisticated imaging techniques have steadily improved the identification of local disease, and this development, in combination with concomitant improvements in surgical techniques, has resulted in dramatic improvements in surgical outcomes. Newer imaging techniques now allow disease that cannot easily be visualized with the naked eye to be "seen." Furthermore, the diseased tissue can be better visualized in relationship to adjacent normal tissue, allowing for more precise anatomic treatment. In contemporary practice, fewer and fewer diseases are treated on the basis of direct observation alone. Such is the heritage of twentieth-century medicine.

Until relatively recently, however, the surgeon was still personally responsible for transferring the imaging data to the patient. That is, the surgeon usually reviewed the various imaging studies before surgery and then mentally, but indirectly, incorporated this information into the actual surgical procedure. The future of image-guided surgery (IGS) rests with the development of techniques that allow the operator to more directly incorporate the images into delivery of the therapy. The goal is to enable more precise and less invasive access to a tumor and to monitor its resection, ablation, or other form of local therapy.

MEDICAL IMAGING TECHNIQUES

Any type of image (medical or other) has two intrinsic properties: spatial and signal.[1] The former defines the location and geometric features of a structure or lesion. The latter, generally reflected by gray tone or color, is important for lesion detection and the definition of tissue type. Spatial features of an image include the number of dimensions represented and the resolution. Most medical images are either two-dimensional (2D) projections, such as with a chest film, or three-dimensional (3D), such as with thin section CT or MR. Obviously, 3D images provide more data for guiding a therapeutic device (including a scalpel) into a 3D object (a patient). High spatial resolution, although generally desirable, is often impractical, being associated with longer examination times or poorer image quality. There is also no reason to have higher resolution images than is necessary to detect a lesion or guide therapy. In general, "high-resolution" medical images have 0.5 to 1.0 mm^3 resolution. The biophysical interactions of the imaging technique and the tissues of the body determine the "signal" properties of medical images. Different imaging techniques report different features of tissues. The following are general characteristics of current medical imaging techniques.[2]

X-RAY IMAGES

The measurements of x-ray emitted by a point source and transmitted through the human body depends on the integral of the electron density along rays projected through the body, which is a function of the mean atomic number of the tissue. These measurements of "radiodensity" have traditionally been made on films or by image intensifiers, both of which are devices that create analog images that can then be digitized. Digital images are required for most IGS applications. More recently, x-ray–sensitive solid state detector systems in linear or planar arrays are being used to directly generate digital x-ray images.[3] The spatial resolution of most 2D x-ray images is less than 0.5 mm. Conventional x-ray images are used primarily to image bony structures, but also to image the distribution and temporal evolution of contrast agents such as iodine in soft tissues (e.g., blood vessels). Soft tissue contrast is very poor on conventional x-ray studies.

Rotation of the x-ray source and detector around the longitudinal axis of a patient produces projections that can be used for tomographic reconstruction of slices, with typical series of parallel 1- to 10-mm thick sections of 512×512 pixels, each 0.25 to 1.0 mm^2 in size. Because this reconstruction process provides a correct approximation of tissue densities and not integrals of tissue densities as in x-ray projections, CT images accurately differentiate bony and soft tissues. Since the advent of CT in the 1970s, the technology has rapidly evolved. Now a common technique, the spiral CT uses a continuous rotation of the x-ray source and a 2D-detector array synchronized with a linear continuous motion of the patient.[4] This technique provides individual slices in approximately 1 second. On the horizon is the use of planar detectors for real 3D volumetric acquisitions instead of reconstruction of 3D images from 2D sections. These x-ray volume imagers will become increasingly important for IGS.

MAGNETIC RESONANCE IMAGING

MR imaging (MRI) provides information about molecular properties of tissues.[5] A body first is set into an intense constant magnetic field (ranging from 0.1 T to a few Teslas). MRI studies the way tissues behave when they are submitted to a weak, transient perturbation of this strong magnetic field. Radiofrequency (RF) pulses induce spinning motions of nuclei that come back to an equilibrium. Using a select sequence of perturbations, information is provided about the concentration (often called *density*) of atoms (mainly hydrogen in H_2O) and about their physicochemical environment. Several components of the received signals, which relate to intrinsic MR parameters (proton density, relaxation times $T1$ and $T2$) are used to create images. Although each of these MR tissue parameters reflects a unique aspect of the biophysical milieu of tissue water, they remain poorly understood from a biologic perspective. However, they have been empirically shown to provide great contrast between different types of normal and abnormal tissues, including benign and malignant neoplasms. MRI is a true 3D-imaging technique, because the application of magnetic field gradients can define any point of the volume studied. Whereas most standard devices provide series of parallel sections in sagittal, coronal, or axial planes, it is possible to obtain homogeneous 3D volumes of $256 \times 256 \times 256$ voxels having a spatial resolution of 1 mm^3. A valuable modification of MRI is MR angiography, which produces clear images of blood vessels noninvasively.[6]

MR spectroscopy allows for metabolic studies of complex biologic systems: Spectra in the frequency domain correspond to the composition of molecules of a region.[7] Clinical applications of MR spectroscopy are increasing, with protons being the main nuclei that are observed. Chemical shift imaging techniques (multivoxel spectroscopy) have been developed,[8] but more work still is necessary before these will be ready for routine clinical use. Miniaturization of RF coils for ultra-high-resolution imaging of small regions is another interesting trend in MRI research, which may be important for IGS applications.[9]

ULTRASOUND

US is a relatively inexpensive, portable, real-time imaging system with a typical spatial resolution of 1 mm.[10] These features make US a major imaging tool for IGS. After the emission of an US wave from a piezoelectric element, the sound signal reflected by the discontinuities of acoustic impedances of tissues is analyzed. Time of flight measurements of the reflected echoes gives spatial information of acoustical interfaces. Acoustic impedances of tissues are primarily related to physical features rather than to their biologic properties. Selection of US frequency depends on a trade-off of resolution versus attenuation. High-resolution, 12-MHz US images of the thyroid gland have 0.5 mm^3 resolution, but the depth of view is only a few centimeters. Mechanically or electronically moving the direction of US allows one to obtain a 2D or 3D image. Images may be corrupted by a rather strong texture noise and by distortions due to such things as bone and air.

The analysis of blood velocities is achievable through the use of Doppler US probes, some of which have been miniaturized and mounted at the tip of a needle. Newer US imaging modalities include color and power Doppler sonography, which produce 2D or 3D color images of blood velocities superimposed on a standard grayscale US image.[11]

NUCLEAR MEDICINE

In contrast to the imaging techniques already described, which are primarily dependent on physical, morphologic properties of tissue, nuclear imaging is usually directly dependent on biochemical or physiologic properties. In nuclear medicine imaging, or scintigraphy, a source of photons (gamma) or positrons (beta) is attached to a specific radiopharmaceutical and injected into the body. External detectors observe the emission of such radioactive elements. A typical image corresponds to an orthogonal projection of the density of radioactive elements, which is related to the metabolism of the radiopharmaceutical in the studied region.[12] Rotation of the gamma camera around the patient provides a set of projections that is fed onto tomographic algorithms similar to those used for x-ray CT. The result is a 3D volume of data—tomoscintigraphy, or single photon emission CT (SPECT).[13] A more complex strategy studies the emission of positrons (negative electrons). Each emitted positron collides with an electron of the environment and gives rise to two high-energy photons that go in opposite directions. A ring of detectors set around the patient detects these two photons at very near instants. Thus, the associated events lie on a straight line between these two corresponding detectors. The intersection of such lines gives rise to a 3D region of emission from which a 3D image can be reconstructed. Such is the technique of positron emission tomography (PET).[14] Both SPECT and PET have relatively poor spatial resolution when compared with CT or MRI (typically a set of 64^3 or 128^3 voxels, each 2 to 10 mm^3, is obtained), but these methods provide functional information that is not available with other techniques.

IMAGE GUIDANCE

These various modalities provide images of anatomic or pathologic structures that can form the basis for surgical planning and subsequent image guidance of a procedure. In contrast to traditional surgery that depends heavily on physician inferences and qualitative decisions based on human perception of these images (and other data), IGS depends on quantitative decisions (e.g., direction and depth of a needle) based on digital image data processed by computers that are directly linked to surgical devices. The engineering requirements of such a system are extraordinarily demanding; system fidelity and reliability must be superb. Even with the most sophisticated system, however, the physician operator remains the critical unit.

Generally, five important elements make up IGS: (1) high-quality digital images, (2) advanced computer image processing that includes tissue classification or segmentation algorithms and 2D and 3D visualization tools, (3) a computer modeling system for simulation, (4) a registration system that links the medical images with the real patient, and (5) digital interfaces to therapeutic devices.[15]

DATA ACQUISITION

In most cases, image information is provided by preoperative or intraoperative studies. Medical *a priori* knowledge (e.g., an anatomic atlas) as well as video images or different types of signals (e.g., Doppler, electrophysiology) can also be used.

IMAGE PROCESSING

The "raw" image data must be processed to allow the surgeon to intuitively perceive the pertinent image information and relate it to the planned surgical procedure. Often, this process requires that images be reformatted into 3D or pseudo-3D images and that key structures or tissues be identified, either implicitly or explicitly. The former step requires state of the art computer visualization tools, whereas the latter step requires accurate tissue classification or segmentation algorithms. Although current segmentation techniques can quickly and accurately classify spatially well-defined and high-contrast tissues, such as bone on x-ray CT, much more work is necessary for the accurate segmentation of subtle soft tissue differences, such as those related to infiltrating neoplasms.

REGISTRATION

The problem of matching all of the image data available for a patient into a unique coordinate system is commonly referred to as *registration.* Registration is a crucial technology in IGS for three reasons. First, the coregistration of medical data allows the surgeon to plan an operation using all of the available information. Second, registration of preoperative and postoperative data is crucial for individual patient follow-up and statistical analysis of results. Third, registration of preoperative and intraoperative data provides the crucial step required to relate the "virtual patient" created from the medical images to the actual patient on the operating table. Ideally, all patient data should be correlated with the physical space of the real surgery and made available to the surgeon. A variety of registration techniques have been developed, some of which use external markers or fiducials placed on the patient, whereas other methods use intrinsic anatomic structures to register images and physical spaces.[16] This latter capability is important because it is more direct, logistically easier, and potentially more robust. Although accurate rigid registration is now routinely performed, a continuing challenge is still the elastic registration of nonrigid tissues—for instance, tracking deformations due to surgery, respiration, and temporal changes of structures.

SURGICAL PLANNING

A 3D model of the patient and pathology is created into which all the relevant image data has been incorporated. The operator (surgeon or physician) can then manipulate the model in a virtual reality mode. This permits the surgeon to define the surgical strategy, which can then be simulated and modified.

PERFORMING THE SURGERY

Different types of guiding systems can be used to execute the surgical plan. Passive systems enable the surgeon to compare the actual intervention with the planned one. This is the case with systems such as the ISG Wand (ISG Technologies, Mississauga, Ontario, Canada),[17] in which previously obtained images have been registered to the patient using a computer system with a digital articulated arm. Surgical instruments are then attached to the articulated arm and manipulated by the surgeon who can observe the tool in real, patient space as well as on the workstation in image, or virtual, space. Semiactive systems enable the physical guiding of the instrument that is still controlled by the operator, which is the case, for example, with the stereotactic neurosurgical system described by Lavallee and Troccaz.[16] Finally, active systems execute part of the intervention. Kelly[18] developed a system in which a laser is used for brain microsurgery. The laser is directed toward a tumor that has been localized by MRI. The laser is digitally manipulated until a synthesized image built from MRI data can be superimposed on an intraoperative video image.

The use of active robots, perhaps the ultimate IGS, remains rare and experimental. However, there are some potential advantages to the use of robots in surgery, including (1) repeatable tool position and trajectory; (2) steady motion; (3) ability to react rapidly to changes in force level; (4) remote operation; and (5) ability to remain poised in a fixed position.[19] Because of such attributes, the use of robots could lead to more effective treatment. In the case of contagious diseases, reducing human contact might lower the risk of infection. In other cases, robots might reduce risks to the patient by offering the potential of less invasive surgery.

However, a number of points should be considered before a suitably autonomous device is implemented, not least of which is the role of "expert systems" for high-level system control. It is not reasonable that a robot system should operate without continuous backup from a surgeon who is in a position to define and check the step-by-step progress of the task and to override the system in case of unforeseen difficulties. The robotic device would be driven to an acceptable start under position control by the surgeon and, on instruction, would perform the defined task, prompted by the surgeon at each stage. The system would be required to react to given situations in real time by comparison of actual behavior with sophisticated reference models, few of which exist.

SPECIFIC APPLICATIONS OF IMAGE-GUIDED SURGERY

A variety of imaging techniques have become an integral part of the surgeon's approach to managing tumors, both benign and malignant. Many can be used for both preoperative and intraoperative localization. Several surgical specialties have incorporated IGS into their approach to patient management.

NEUROSURGERY

IGS has its origins in the development of techniques for stereotactic brain biopsy.[20–23] These early studies used CT to localize lesions in the brain through coordinates provided by a device fixed to the patient's skull. In one study, RF ablation was applied to a deep brain lesion with symptomatic relief for the patient.[20] This may represent one of the earliest applications of IGS.

The techniques and equipment used for image-guided neurosurgery have evolved substantially since the late 1970s. Improvements in biopsy techniques paved the way for therapeutic interventions using a variety of ablative procedures, culminating in dedicated operating suites with real-time imaging from CT and MRI.[24] The success of these techniques is predicated on their ability to allow surgeons to perform their procedures more safely and efficiently.[25] The approach to lesions that are located deep in the brain presents challenges that help to illustrate where image guidance may prove its utility.

Microsurgery of deep brain lesions is often complicated by the close proximity of major vessels, eloquent brain, and the need to work in a confined space where standard microscopic visualization may be limited. By combining images from CT, MRI, and digital angiography, a 3D rendering of the surgical field has been successfully applied to guide microsurgical resections of deep-seated cerebral lesions.[26] The information obtained allows the surgeon to visualize the relationship between the lesion and cerebral vessels as well as brain structures of high functional significance. 3D rendering allows the surgeon to overlay the position of surgical instruments and to predict and simulate the trajectory of the approach.[26]

Similar guidance systems have been used to allow for the ablation of brain tumors using heat generated by RF devices. In this setting, the accurate position of the RF ablation probe is critical to minimizing the potential for collateral thermal injury of adjacent structures. In a study of 12 patients (14 lesions treated) with primary or metastatic brain tumors, an MR-guided stereotactic RF procedure was evaluated.[27] Using MRI, the stereotactic coordinates of the tumor and the angle of the RF ablation probe were calculated. Once the probe was properly positioned, the tissue was heated to the target temperature, and full ablation of the tumor was confirmed by real-time MRI. All procedures were performed in awake patients, and patients were followed for up to 10 months. MRI was successful in demonstrating well-defined lesions in all cases, documenting accurate placement of the RF probe. Characteristic changes in the appearance of the lesions during treatment on T2-weighted images allowed for confirmation of focal energy delivery during the procedure.[27]

In addition to providing for accurate localization and real-time anatomic feedback, newer computer-guided imaging systems also have been designed to give functional information during the surgical procedure. Using real-time MR images in conjunction with superimposed functional data from somatosensory evoked potentials derived from dipole tracings, investigators have been able to localize the central sulcus in 12 patients with intracranial disorders.[28] In six of the patients, 3D computer graphics were reconstructed from MRIs, which allowed for the visualization of lesions deep in the brain. The 3D functional images were then superimposed on the anatomic images. This technique allowed the surgeons to see the 3D relationship between the lesion and the functional sensorimotor cortex. This type of data can potentially allow for greater preservation of normal brain function during surgery.

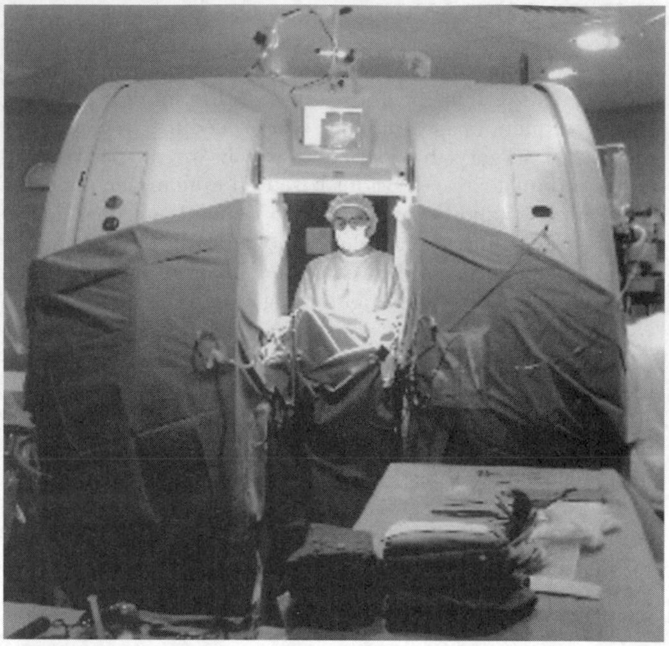

FIGURE 64-1. Open magnetic resonance imaging for image-guided surgery as implemented at the Brigham and Women's Hospital, Boston.

A significant advance for intraoperative IGS has been the open-bore MR unit (Fig. 64-1). This is an open MR device, which allows for optimal vertical access of the surgeon and assistant to the patient. Using such a system, surgeons at the Brigham and Women's Hospital in Boston published their experience with 110 cases, which included 47 biopsies, six catheter placements, four cyst drainage procedures, 47 craniotomies for resection, three spinal cases, and three laser tumor ablations.[29] This intraoperative MR surgery unit was especially useful in guiding biopsies and resections near cysts, ventricles, and critical vascular structures. Standard approaches using prior image data with framed and frameless techniques would be inadequate to show anatomic changes during the procedure. The acquisition of real-time images of the biopsy needle within the lesion were found to be very useful. The information obtained from this system allowed for more complete resection of infiltrative tumors. Image fusion of SPECT and neurofunctional data into the imaging space enabled the surgeons to better visualize tumor invasion or neural function with real-time imaging during resection.[29]

The true test of whether image-guided techniques are of benefit in neurosurgery is whether an impact on outcome is the result. Studies focusing on outcome analysis are beginning to emerge.[30–33] Early data indicate that the addition of image-guided techniques can reduce operative time, patient morbidity, and the need for repeat procedures. Further prospective studies of cost analysis are necessary to definitively demonstrate these benefits.

HEAD AND NECK SURGERY

Because of anatomic similarities, IGS techniques developed for neurosurgery have found several applications in the management of patients with both benign and malignant tumors of the head and neck. For patients with skull base tumors, an intraoperative guidance system has been used to provide nearly instantaneous CT and MRI images with computer reconstruction to the surgeons. The ISG viewing wand can correlate any point within the operative field to its corresponding locus on the reformatted images.[34–36] The use of this wand in 14 patients with skull base, cerebellopontine angle, or temporal bone lesions has allowed for minimally invasive incisions, intraoperative navigation, and identification of important anatomic structures. This precision allowed for a greater margin of safety and a more precise assessment of the extent of lesion resection.[34]

Endoscopic techniques have revolutionized the approach to nasal and sinus surgery. A computer-assisted surgery system has been applied to help in intraoperative localization during endoscopic surgery of the paranasal sinus region.[37] This system allows for the continuous orientation of the scope by using a 3D reconstruction of the preoperative CT scan with superimposed positioning of the endoscope. By using a dual display on the endoscopic monitor, the surgeon can see the video-endoscopic picture and the information from the localizer simultaneously. This allows for positional adjustments of the scope without the need for the surgeon to look away from his or her operative field. This system also has been used for complex skull base and head and neck resections.[38]

3D intraoperative navigational systems have been used to assist in craniofacial procedures ranging from corrections of craniofacial asymmetry to tumor resections. A study of 17 patients undergoing craniofacial procedures demonstrated the utility of the ISG navigation system in precisely orienting the surgeon to his exact location throughout the procedure.[39] The system was particularly useful in defining intraorbital anatomy, in determining ocular globe position, and in delineating tumor margins. No additional operative time or adverse events were attributed to the use of the system.

The development of virtual endoscopy is another useful application of real-time imaging. A virtual otoscope has been designed that provides a precise view of the structures of the inner ear.[40] The precision of the images derived from this device may replace the more invasive endoscopes in current use.

SURGICAL ONCOLOGY

The application of IGS to the management of malignancies of soft tissues in the abdominal cavity has required imagination as well as modifications of the approaches used in neurosurgery. Unlike the brain, which is fixed in its position, the abdominal contents, such as small bowel, are more fluid and present certain difficulties in making use of imaging techniques for "target" acquisition. The liver, however, represents a relatively fixed anatomic structure for which image-guided therapies have been used.

A variety of ablation techniques have been applied to the treatment of liver tumors in situations in which surgical resection may not be appropriate. These techniques, such as RF ablation, cryotherapy, and interstitial laser thermoablation are discussed in greater detail elsewhere in this text. These techniques share in common the need to not only localize the target lesion, but also to monitor the effects of the therapy during the time it is being applied.

Several imaging modalities, including US, CT, and MRI, have been used to accurately position the ablation probes into the lesion and to monitor the effects of the therapy. Using an Nd-YAG (neodymium:yttrium-aluminum garnet) laser system and real-time MRI, a group of 12 patients had a total of 27 lesions in the liver treated under local or general anesthesia.[41] An MR colorization sequence was used to monitor changes in the tissue temperature during therapy. The patients tolerated the procedure well, with 8 of the 12 being discharged home on the day after the procedure. Thermal zones of ablation up to 5 cm were achieved with two patients with 3-cm lesions, achieving complete ablation with a single procedure. Seven of the patients required multiple procedures to successfully ablate their lesions. Similar procedures also have been performed laparoscopically.[42]

Using intraoperative US and a laparoscopic approach, RF ablation has been applied to the treatment of liver metastases from neuroendocrine tumors.[43] In six patients (13 lesions treated) no intraoperative complications were reported. US was used successfully to position the thermal ablation probe and to monitor the treatment effect in the operating room to determine when an adequate zone of necrosis was achieved. US is able to detect the "outgassing," which occurs as the tissue is heated and gas is released into the surrounding parenchyma.

A trial at the National Cancer Institute is currently under way to evaluate US, CT, and MRI to determine the best modality for positioning the probes and monitoring the effects of RF ablation in the liver. Figure 64-2 demonstrates a real-time CT image of a lesion in the liver before and after RF ablation. Patients are imaged with dynamic enhanced MRI preoperatively and in follow-up as a means of following response.

Nuclear imaging has been applied to the preoperative and intraoperative detection of malignancy in the abdominal cavity. This approach has been most extensively evaluated with respect to colon and rectal cancer. Two strategies have been pursued, one using anti-carcinoembryonic antigen (CEA) antibody immunoscintigraphy and the other using PET and the radiopharmaceutical [^{18}F]fluorodeoxyglucose (FDG).

Radioimmunoguided surgery (RIGS) has relied on the ability of radiolabeled monoclonal antibodies or antibody fragments to bind specifically to markers expressed on tumor tissue. The sensitivity and specificity of these antibodies is based to a large degree on the tumor marker itself and how restricted its expression is to neoplastic tissue. CEA has been extensively studied as a target for this approach.[44–52]

Radioimmunoguided surgery using an intraoperative probe to detect radioactivity has been evaluated as an adjunct to second-look laparotomy in the evaluation of colorectal cancer patients with rising serum CEA levels.[44] Sixteen asymptomatic patients with a history of colorectal cancer surgery and a rising serum CEA level underwent second-look surgery using the RIGS approach. Patients received the anti–tumor-associated glycoprotein iodine 125–labeled monoclonal antibody (MoAb) B72.3 preoperatively. RIGS exploration was combined with a standard

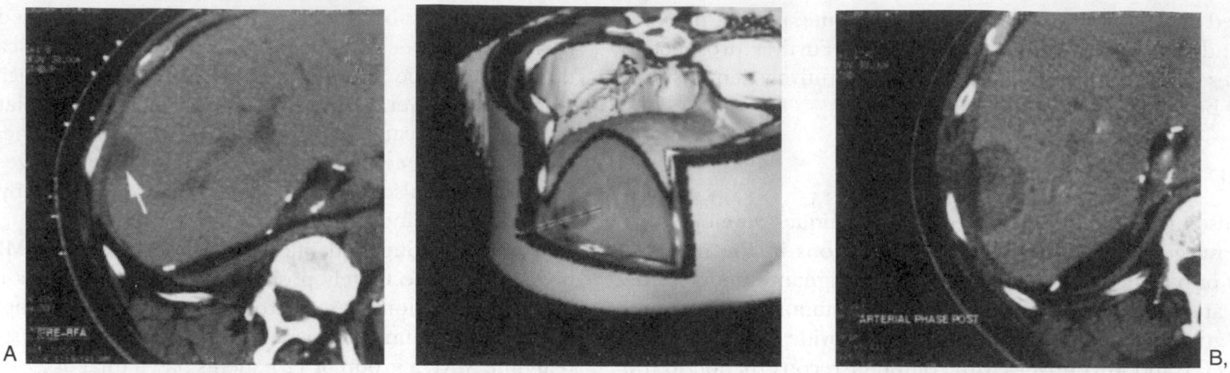

FIGURE 64-2. A tumor (*arrow*) located in the right lobe of the liver in a patient with metastatic adrenal cancer as seen on computed tomographic (CT) scan. Panel **A** shows the lesion before radiofrequency (RF) ablation on a noncontrast scan. Panel **B** shows a three-dimensional rendering of the lesion, illustrating the path of the needle. This image was obtained while the patient was on the table, as a means of directing the therapy. Panel **C** demonstrates the lesion post–RF ablation on an arterial phase postcontrast CT scan. Note that the lesion appears larger than at preablation. This is because of the 1-cm zone of necrosis achieved around the lesion.

exploratory laparotomy. Recurrent disease was observed in 14 of the 16 patients as the result of this combined exploration. Standard exploration alone demonstrated recurrent disease in 9 of 16 patients (56.2%). In five patients (31.2%), RIGS detected disease that would otherwise have been overlooked. The additional RIGS-detected tumor sites were resectable for cure. In this study, RIGS improved the results of colorectal cancer, CEA-guided, second-look procedures in asymptomatic patients by recruiting one-third of patients to curative resections.[44]

Preoperative SPECT imaging studies can be obtained using a gamma camera in addition to the use of the intraoperative probe. This combined approach was used in a study evaluating *in vivo* posttargeting of tumor by means of anti-CEA monoclonal antibodies and the avidin-biotin three-step system.[52] Six patients with primary or recurrent rectal cancer were preoperatively injected with 1 mg of FO23C5 (anti-CEA) and/or B72.3 anti–tumor-associated glycoprotein (TAG-72) biotinylated monoclonal antibody. At 24 hours after injection, 1 mg of avidin was administered and, after a further 24 hours, biotin-labeled indium 111 was also injected. Eight tumor sites were localized in the six patients. Four of the eight lesions were identified preoperatively by the gamma camera; and six intraoperatively using a nuclear probe. An advantage of this method was the ability to perform preoperative scintigraphy and intraoperative radioimmunodetection with a single radioactive compound injection of biotin labeled with ^{111}In within a few days before surgery.[52]

Radioguided surgery using antibody-directed immunoscintigraphy relies on the ability of the antibody to bind efficiently to the target tissue and to be imaged above background. It also requires multiple antibodies to be derived against a number of tumor markers, depending on the histology of the target lesion. Many of these limitations could be overcome by using a more universal reagent that would be taken up by tumor tissue selectively, regardless of the tumor histology and independent of the need for antibody-antigen interactions. The radiopharmaceutical FDG has many of these properties.

Several studies have shown that malignant lesions demonstrate elevated glycolysis when compared to normal tissues.[53,54] By using the radiolabeled glucose analog FDG, investigators have documented increased uptake of FDG in cancer tissues.[55,56] PET scanning with FDG has been used to image a variety of malignant neoplasms, including breast cancer, head and neck tumors, lung cancer, lymphoma, melanoma, ovarian tumors, bone cancers, and colorectal carcinomas.

The mechanism whereby FDG is selectively accumulated in neoplastic tissue is based primarily on increased uptake of FDG and conversion to FDG-6-phosphate. The inability of cells to further metabolize FDG-6-phosphate causes the molecule to be trapped in the cells, facilitating accurate imaging. Figure 64-3 shows a representative PET image using FDG. The intensity in this image is proportional to the amount of FDG that has entered the cells, begun the first steps of the metabolic conversion of sugar to energy, and then been trapped. The reasons why so many tumors avidly accumulate glucose are only partly understood. The energy needs of rapidly dividing cells obviously plays a role.

Currently, a study is under way at the National Cancer Institute evaluating the use of FDG-PET scanning and anti-CEA antibody immunoscintigraphy in the preoperative and intraoperative detection of recurrent colon and rectal cancers. Patients are recruited based on a rising serum CEA value in the absence of imageable disease, or with a single site of otherwise resectable disease. Patients are explored, and in some cases, a probe designed to detect FDG is used intraoperatively. This study is ongoing and is designed to evaluate the sensitivity, specificity, and predictive value of these scans as well as second-look laparotomy for the detection of recurrent tumor.

IGS has made possible a more minimally invasive approach to the diagnosis and management of breast lesions. The use of mammography and breast US has resulted in successful localization of lesions. Percutaneous core sampling of lesions, guided by specialized, computerized, stereotactic radiographic equipment is less painful and can be done under local anesthesia.[57,58] Tissue cores obtained are adequate to make the diagnosis in most cases.

Using an open MRI scanner, excisional biopsies of breast lesions have been successfully performed.[59] Intraoperative real-time scanning assisted in determining adequacy of resection margin and in positioning and minimizing the size of the incision. In a study of women undergoing excision of benign lesions, the MR demonstrated that all lesions were adequately excised with pathologic confirmation of clean margins.[59]

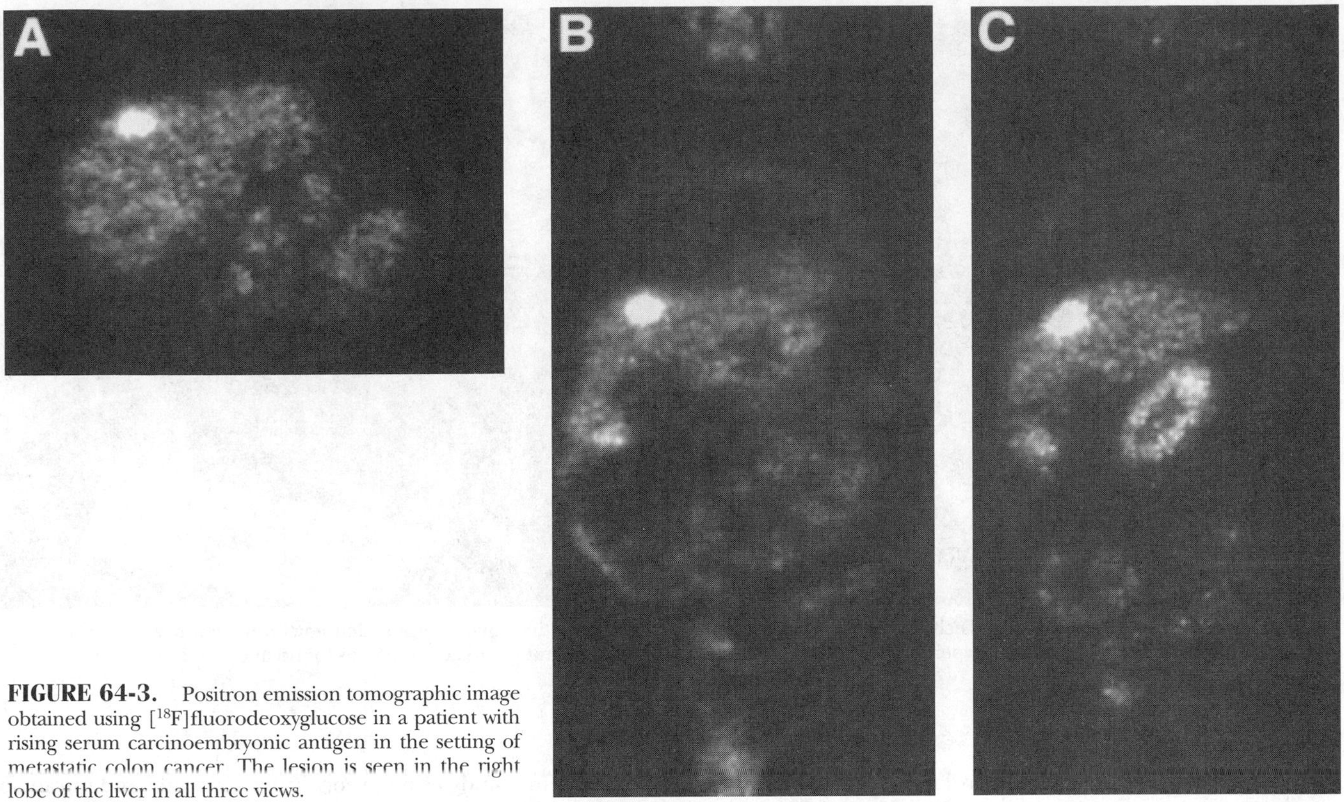

FIGURE 64-3. Positron emission tomographic image obtained using [^{18}F]fluorodeoxyglucose in a patient with rising serum carcinoembryonic antigen in the setting of metastatic colon cancer. The lesion is seen in the right lobe of the liver in all three views.

During an exploratory laparotomy, the surgeon is limited in the examination of the hollow viscera by the inability to adequately assess the mucosal surfaces. Although intraoperative endoscopy can be performed, this procedure is often difficult logistically and complicates the exploration because of the need to insufflate gas into the bowel. Furthermore, the small bowel is virtually inaccessible. Virtual endoscopy may help to overcome these limitations.

Virtual colonoscopy, for example, is a method of colon examination in which computer-aided 3D visualization of spiral CT simulates fiberoptic colonoscopy. In one study, a colon phantom containing spheres of various sizes was used to determine the influence of CT acquisition parameters on lesion detectability and sizing.[60] Results demonstrated that detection of beads of 4 mm or more was 100%. Detection decreased to 78% to 94% for 2.5 mm beads. The authors concluded that CT scanning at 5 mm collimation and up to pitch 2 is adequate for detection of high-contrast lesions as small as 4 mm in their model. As the imaging algorithms are improved, virtual colonoscopy may be used as a screening modality both preoperatively and intraoperatively in a CT-equipped operating suite.

Virtual endoscopic techniques also have been applied to the examination of the biliary and pancreatic ducts. MR cholangiography is a noninvasive technique that allows one to image the biliary system without the need for a contrast agent. Depending on the MR sequence chosen and the image processing, the ductal anatomy can be highlighted as a light or dark image.[61] Because this is an MRI-based approach, there is no radiation exposure. Images can be rendered in three dimensions to give an accurate representation of the ductal anatomy. Studies have demonstrated that the image quality compares favorably to endoscopic retrograde cholangiopancreatography of pancreatic (duct).[61]

A similar approach has been used to image the pancreatic duct in patients with mucin-producing pancreatic tumors. In a group of 13 patients with a total of 18 lesions, a computer-based virtual endoscopy system was used to render 3D reconstructions of the pancreatic ductal anatomy.[62] The virtual pancreatoscopy was successful in demonstrating the surfaces of the bile and pancreatic duct and could distinguish cystic from solid tumors. The surfaces of the malignant mucin-producing tumors were shown to be more irregular than those of the benign lesions. The data were useful for surgical planning with regard to extent of resection.

ENDOCRINE SURGERY

Nuclear imaging, making use of radioisotopes that target specific tissue types, has made significant contributions to IGS, allowing for more minimally invasive procedures. The application of technetium Tc 99m sestamibi scanning to the preoperative and intraoperative localization of parathyroid adenomas has improved detection and allowed for less morbid surgical procedures. For the majority of patients, routine preoperative imaging may not be necessary.[63] In experienced hands, 95% of patients with primary hyperparathyroidism (HPT) are cured after a careful bilateral neck exploration.[64]

Imaging becomes critical for those patients who have persistent or recurrent HPT. In this patient population, reexploration is complicated by scarring, which not only makes it difficult to identify the parathyroid glands, but also increases the risk of injury to the recurrent laryngeal nerves.[65,66] Furthermore, in patients who are not cured at the first operation, it is

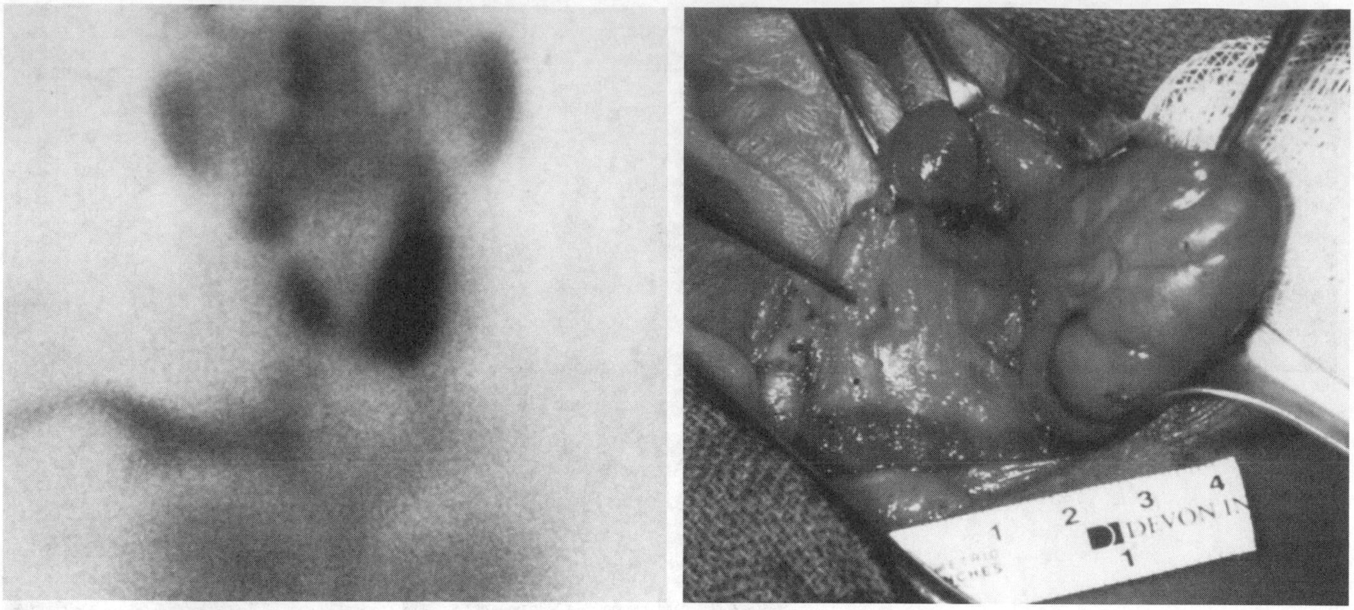

A B

FIGURE 64-4. **A:** Technetium Tc 99m sestamibi scan demonstrating a parathyroid adenoma on the left in a patient with primary hyperparathyroidism. **B:** A large left inferior parathyroid adenoma was found at operation.

possible that the abnormal parathyroid gland is located in an ectopic site, such as the pharynx or mediastinum.[67–70]

Compared to other noninvasive imaging studies, such as CT, US, and MRI, the sestamibi scan has been shown to be superior, with a positive predictive value as high as 90%.[65,71] Sestamibi scans can localize the parathyroid adenoma to the correct side of the neck and to the position within the neck relative to other structures (Fig. 64-4). The accuracy of sestamibi has led to the introduction of a minimally invasive approach to parathyroid surgery.

The standard approach of bilateral neck exploration for the patient with primary hyperparathyroidism has been questioned. In a retrospective study, a group of 68 patients was reviewed with respect to localization studies and the need for bilateral neck exploration.[72] Forty-four patients were treated with localization study–aided unilateral neck exploration, whereas 24 patients were treated with the standard bilateral approach without localization studies. In 15 patients, the preoperative localization study was a sestamibi scan, which correctly localized the adenoma in all cases. All 15 patients with unilateral neck exploration guided by sestamibi results were cured, as were all 24 patients who underwent a bilateral neck exploration. Based on their results, the authors recommend a preoperative sestamibi scan for patients with primary hyperparathyroidism who have not undergone previous neck exploration, followed by a unilateral approach if the scan demonstrates a single lesion. They suggest that the second gland on the explored side be identified and biopsied. They conclude that bilateral exploration should be reserved for patients with multiple glands seen on sestamibi, or an abnormal biopsy of the second gland. This approach has been further supported by the use of an intraoperative probe for the detection of sestamibi during the procedure.[73,74]

However, caution should still be exercised in pursuing less than a bilateral neck exploration at the time of primary surgery for HPT. In a study using preoperative sestamibi and intraoperative measurements of parathyroid hormone levels, a success rate of unilateral exploration of 67% at 3 months was reported.[75] Failed unilateral exploration was due to multigland disease (31%), erroneous localization (31%), slow metabolism of parathyroid hormone (13%), and need for improved exposure (25%). The authors suggest that, at best, the success rate of unilateral exploration using intraoperative parathyroid hormone measurements can be expected to be 85%.[75] Although these strategies are a good example of how image guidance can change surgical management, the ultimate utility of this approach compared with standard bilateral neck exploration with a historical success rate of 95% awaits more definitive prospective studies.

CONCLUSIONS

The ultimate goal of any medical therapy is obvious: precisely define the site and nature of disease and deliver the most effective therapy to the diseased tissue while doing no harm to normal tissue. Two main therapeutic approaches have been followed: systemic (generally medicinal) and surgical. The fundamental basis of surgery, for cancer or any other disease, is the concept of "local treatment of local disease." This presumes that the disease, or a major component of the disease to be treated, is (1) confined to a local region, (2) can be accurately defined, (3) is accessible, and (4) can be treated locally by resection or other ablative techniques.

Simplistically, this means that the surgeon is directly responsible for targeting the therapy. Systemic therapy, on the other hand, is based on the assumption that the therapy (i.e., antibiotic or chemotherapy) will self-target the disease, which can be local or disseminated. Given these precepts, *IGS* is a redundant term. Some type of "imaging" of the local disease must guide surgery and other forms of local therapy. Traditionally, the imaging has been performed by the surgeon's naked eye, supplemented by other, cruder sensory facilities, such as palpation. As advanced imaging techniques and technology become available, the surgeon will be able to expand the repertoire of available information and deliver local therapy in a more precise fashion.

REFERENCES

1. Taylor RH, Lavallee S, Burdea GC, eds. *Computer-integrated surgery: technology and clinical applications.* Boston: MIT Press, 1996.
2. Webb S. *The physics of medical imaging.* Medical Science Series. Bristol, UK: IOP Publishing, 1988.
3. Chotas HG, Dobbins JT III, Ravin CE. Principles of digital radiography with large-area, electronically readable detectors: a review of the basics. *Radiology* 1999;210:595.
4. Kalender WA, Polacin G, Baert AL. Current status and new perspective in spiral CT. Advances in CT: Second European Scientific User Conference. Berlin: Springer-Verlag, 1992:85.
5. Wehrli FW, McGowan JC. The basis of MR contrast. In: Atlas SW, ed. *Magnetic resonance imaging of the brain and spine.* Philadelphia: Lippincott–Raven, 1996:29.
6. Perl J, Turski PA, Masaryk TJ. MR angiography: techniques and clinical applications. In: Atlas SW, ed. *Magnetic resonance imaging of the brain and spine.* Philadelphia: Lippincott–Raven, 1996:1547.
7. Lenkinski RE, Schnall MD. MR spectroscopy and the biochemical basis of neurologic disease. In: Atlas SW, ed. *Magnetic resonance imaging of the brain and spine.* Philadelphia: Lippincott–Raven, 1996:1619.
8. Barker PB, Soher BJ, Blackband SJ, et al. Quantitation of proton NMR spectra of the human brain using tissue water as an internal concentration reference. *NMR Biomed* 1993;6:89.
9. Peck TL, Lavalle L, Magin RL, et al. RF microcoils patterned using microlithographic techniques for use as microsensors in NMR. *IEEE Engineering in Medicine and Biology Society Proceedings* 1993:174.
10. Hottier F, Billion AC. 3-D echography: status and perspective. In: Hohne KH, ed. *3D Imaging in Medicine,* vol F60. Berlin: Springer-Verlag, 1990:21.
11. Curry TS, Dowdy JE, Murry RC. *Christensen's introduction to the physics of diagnostic radiology.* Philadelphia: Lea & Febiger, 1984.
12. Mazziotta JC, Gilman S. *Clinical brain imaging: principles and applications.* Philadelphia: FA Davis Co, 1992.
13. Lassen NA, Holm S. Single photon emission computed tomography (SPECT). In: Mazziotta JC, Gilman S, eds. *Clinical brain imaging: principles and applications.* Philadelphia: FA Davis Co, 1992:108.
14. Frost JJ, Wagner HN. *Quantitative imaging: neuroreceptors, neurotransmitters, and enzymes.* New York: Raven Press, 1990.
15. Kikinis R, Gleason PL. Surgical planning using computer-assisted three-dimensional reconstructions. In: Taylor RH, Lavallee S, Burdea GC, eds. *Computer-integrated surgery.* Boston: MIT Press, 1996:147.
16. Lavallee S, Troccaz J. Image guided operating robot: a clinical application in stereotactic neurosurgery. In: Taylor RH, Lavallee S, Burdea GC, eds. *Computer-integrated surgery.* Boston: MIT Press, 1996:343.
17. Zinreich SJ, Tebo SA, Long DM, et al. Frameless stereotaxic integration of CT imaging data: accuracy and initial applications. *Radiology* 1993;188:735.
18. Kelley PJ. Technical approaches to identification and stereotactic reduction of tumor burden. In: Walker MD, Thomas DGT, eds. *Biology of brain tumor.* The Hague, The Netherlands: Martinus Nijhoff, 1986:237.
19. Khodabandehloo K, Brett PN. Special-purpose actuators and architectures for surgery robots. In: Taylor RH, Lavallee S, Burdea GC, eds. *Computer-integrated surgery.* Boston: MIT Press, 1996:263.
20. Gleason CA, Wise BL, Feinstein B. Stereotactic localization (with computerized tomographic scanning), biopsy, and radiofrequency treatment of deep brain lesions. *Neurosurgery* 1978;2:217.
21. Penn RD, Whisler WW, Smith CA, Yasnoff WA. Stereotactic surgery with image processing of computerized tomographic scans. *Neurosurgery* 1978;3:157.
22. Boethius J, Collins VP, Edner G, Lewander R, Zajicek J. Stereotactic biopsies and computer tomography in gliomas. *Acta Neurochir (Wien)* 1978;40:223.
23. Lewander R, Bergstrom M, Boethius J, et al. Stereotactic computer tomography for biopsy of gliomas. *Acta Radiol Diagn (Stockh)* 1978;19:867.
24. Lunsford LD, Coffey RJ, Cojocaru T, Leksell D. Image-guided stereotactic surgery: a 10-year evolutionary experience. *Stereotact Funct Neurosurg* 1990;55:375.
25. Wadley J, Kitchen N, Thomas D. Image-guided neurosurgery. *Hosp Med* 1999;60:34.
26. Giorgi C, Casolino DS, Ongania E, et al. Guided microsurgery by computer-assisted three-dimensional analysis of neuroanatomical data stereotactically acquired. *Stereotact Funct Neurosurg* 1990;55:482.
27. Anzai Y, Lufkin R, DeSalles A, et al. Preliminary experience with MR-guided thermal ablation of brain tumors. *AJNR Am J Neuroradiol* 1995;16:39; discussion, 49.
28. Hayashi N, Endo S, Kurimoto M, et al. Functional image-guided neurosurgical simulation system using computerized three-dimensional graphics and dipole tracing. *Neurosurgery* 1995;37:694.
29. Alexander E III, Moriarty TM, Kikinis R, Black P, Jolesz FM. The present and future role of intraoperative MRI in neurosurgical procedures. *Stereotact Funct Neurosurg* 1997;68:10.
30. Alberti O, Dorward NL, Kitchen ND, Thomas DG. Neuronavigation—impact on operating time. *Stereotact Funct Neurosurg* 1997;68:44.
31. Barnett GH. The role of image-guided technology in the surgical planning and resection of gliomas. *J Neurooncol* 1999;42:247.
32. Samii M, Brinker T, Samii A. Image-guided neurosurgery—state of the art and outlook. *Wien Klin Wochenschr* 1999;111:618.
33. Jolesz FA, Kettenbach J, Grundfest WS. Cost-effectiveness of image-guided surgery. *Acad Radiol* 1998;5[Suppl 2]:S428.
34. Carney AS, Patel N, Baldwin DL, Coakham HB, Sandeman DR. Intra-operative image guidance in otolaryngology—the use of the ISG viewing wand. *J Laryngol Otol* 1996; 110:322.
35. McDermott MW, Gutin PH. Image-guided surgery for skull base neoplasms using the ISG viewing wand. Anatomic and technical considerations. *Neurosurg Clin North Am* 1996;7:285.
36. Freysinger W, Gunkel AR, Thumfart WF. Image-guided endoscopic ENT surgery. *Eur Arch Otorhinolaryngol* 1997;254:343.
37. Kruckels G, Korves B, Klimek L, Mosges R. Endoscopic surgery of the rhinobasis with a computer-assisted localizer. *Surg Endosc* 1996;10:453.
38. Vannier MW, Marsh JL. Three-dimensional imaging, surgical planning, and image-guided therapy. *Radiol Clin North Am* 1996;34:545.
39. Demianczuk AN, Antonyshyn OM. Application of a three-dimensional intraoperative navigational system in craniofacial surgery. *J Craniofac Surg* 1997;8:290.
40. Frankenthaler RP, Moharir V, Kikinis R, et al. Virtual otoscopy. *Otolaryngol Clin North Am* 1998;31:383.
41. de Jode MG, Lamb GM, Thomas HC, Taylor-Robinson SD, Gedroyc WM. MRI guidance of infra-red laser liver tumour ablations, utilising an open MRI configuration system: technique and early progress. *J Hepatol* 1999;31:347.
42. Germer CT, Albrecht D, Roggan A, Buhr HJ. Technology for *in situ* ablation by laparoscopic and image-guided interstitial laser hyperthermia. *Semin Laparosc Surg* 1998; 5:195.
43. Siperstein AE, Rogers SJ, Hansen PD, Gitomirsky A. Laparoscopic thermal ablation of hepatic neuroendocrine tumor metastases. *Surgery* 1997;122:1147; discussion, 1154.
44. Bertoglio S, Benevento A, Percivale P, et al. Radioimmunoguided surgery benefits in carcinoembryonic antigen-directed second-look surgery in the asymptomatic patient after curative resection of colorectal cancer. *Semin Surg Oncol* 1998;15:263.
45. Bertoglio S, Percivale P, Schenone F, et al. Role of tumor-associated antigen expression in radioimmunoguided surgery for colorectal and breast cancer. *Semin Surg Oncol* 1998;15:249.
46. Bonjer HJ, Bruining HA, Pols HA, et al. Intraoperative nuclear guidance in benign hyperparathyroidism and parathyroid cancer. *Eur J Nucl Med* 1997;24:246.
47. Buchegger F, Mach JP, Pelegrin A, et al. Radiolabeled chimeric anti-CEA monoclonal antibody compared with the original mouse monoclonal antibody for surgically treated colorectal carcinoma. *J Nucl Med* 1995;36:420.
48. Buchegger F, Gillet M, Doenz F, et al. Biodistribution of anti-CEA F(ab')2 fragments after intra-arterial and intravenous injection in patients with liver metastases due to colorectal carcinoma. *Nucl Med Commun* 1996;17:500.
49. Chetanneau A, Barbet J, Peltier P, et al. Pretargeted imaging of colorectal cancer recurrences using an 111In-labelled bivalent hapten and a bispecific antibody conjugate. *Nucl Med Commun* 1994;15:972.
50. de Nardi P, Stella M, Magnani P, et al. Combination of monoclonal antibodies for radioimmunoguided surgery. *Int J Colorectal Dis* 1997;12:24.
51. Di Carlo V, Stella M, De Nardi P, Fazio F. Radioimmunoguided surgery: clinical experience with different monoclonal antibodies and methods. *Tumori* 1995;81:98.
52. Di Carlo V, De Nardi P, Stella M, Magnani P, Fazio F. Preoperative and intraoperative radioimmunodetection of cancer pretargeted by biotinylated monoclonal antibodies. *Semin Surg Oncol* 1998;15:235.
53. Conti PS, Lilien DL, Hawley K, et al. PET and [18F]-FDG in oncology: a clinical update. *Nucl Med Biol* 1996;23:717.
54. DiChiro G. Positron emission tomography using [18F]fluorodeoxyglucose in brain tumors: a powerful diagnostic and prognostic tool. *Invest Radiol* 1986;22:360.
55. Valk PE, Abella-Columna E, Haseman MK, et al. Whole-body PET imaging with [18F] flourodeoxglucose in management of recurrent colorectal cancer. *Arch Surg* 1999;134(5):503–511.
56. Ito K, Kato T, Tadokoro M, et al. Recurrent rectal cancer and scar: differentiation with PET and MR imaging. *Radiology* 1992;182:549.
57. Burns RP. Image-guided breast biopsy. *Am J Surg* 1997;173:9; discussion, 12.
58. Graves TA, Bland KI. Surgery for early and minimally invasive breast cancer. *Curr Opin Oncol* 1996;8:468.
59. Gould SW, Lamb G, Lomax D, Gedroyc W, Darzi A. Interventional MR-guided excisional biopsy of breast lesions. *J Magn Reson Imaging* 1998;8:26.
60. Beaulieu CF, Napel S, Daniel BL, et al. Detection of colonic polyps in a phantom model: implications for virtual colonoscopy data acquisition. *J Comput Assist Tomogr* 1998;22:656.
61. Meakem TJ III, Schnall MD. Magnetic resonance cholangiography. *Gastroenterol Clin North Am* 1995;24:221.
62. Nakagohri T, Jolesz FA, Okuda S, et al. Virtual pancreatoscopy of mucin-producing pancreatic tumors. *Comput Aided Surg* 1998;3:264.
63. Allerheiligen DA, Schoeber J, Houston RE, Mohl VK, Wildman KM. Hyperparathyroidism [published erratum appears in *Am Fam Physician* 1998;58:52]. *Am Fam Physician* 1998;57:1795, 1807.
64. Mundschenk J, Klose S, Lorenz K, Dralle H, Lehnert H. Diagnostic strategies and surgical procedures in persistent or recurrent primary hyperparathyroidism. *Exp Clin Endocrinol Diabetes* 1999;107:331.
65. Jaskowiak N, Norton JA, Alexander HR, et al. A prospective trial evaluating a standard approach to reoperation for missed parathyroid adenoma. *Ann Surg* 1996;224:308; discussion 320.
66. Thompson GB, Grant CS, Perrier ND, et al. Reoperative parathyroid surgery in the era of

sestamibi scanning and intraoperative parathyroid hormone monitoring. *Arch Surg* 1999;134:699; discussion, 704.

67. Doppman JL, Skarulis MC, Chen CC, et al. Parathyroid adenomas in the aortopulmonary window [see comments]. *Radiology* 1996;201:456.
68. Doppman JL, Shawker TH, Fraker DL, et al. Parathyroid adenoma within the vagus nerve. *AJR Am J Roentgenol* 1994;163:943.
69. Buell JF, Fraker DL, Doppman JL, et al. High cervical intravagal hypercellular parathyroid gland as the etiology of severe persistent primary hyperparathyroidism. *Am Surg* 1995;61:943.
70. Billingsley KG, Fraker DL, Doppman JL, et al. Localization and operative management of undescended parathyroid adenomas in patients with persistent primary hyperparathyroidism. *Surgery* 1994;116:982; discussion, 989.
71. George EF, Komisar A, Scharf SC, Ferracci A, Blaugrund S. Diagnostic value of the preoperative sestamibi scan in intraoperative localization of parathyroid adenomas: a case study. *Laryngoscope* 1998;108:627.
72. Kountakis SE, Maillard AJ. Parathyroid adenomas: is bilateral neck exploration necessary? *Am J Otolaryngol* 1999;20:396.
73. Singer JA, Sardi A, Conaway G, Spiegler EJ. Minimally invasive parathyroidectomy utilizing a gamma detecting probe intraoperatively. *Md Med J* 1999;48:55.
74. Costello D, Norman J. Minimally invasive radioguided parathyroidectomy. *Surg Oncol Clin North Am* 1999;8:555.
75. Moore FD Jr, Mannting F, Tanasijevic M. Intrinsic limitations to unilateral parathyroid exploration. *Ann Surg* 1999;230:382; discussion, 388.

Ira J. Spiro Anthony Lomax
Alfred R. Smith Jay S. Loeffler

CHAPTER 65

Proton Beam Radiation Therapy

There is a growing interest in developing techniques that produce extremely conformal x-ray dose distributions. Several means of reducing treatment volumes are under active development and clinical testing. These new techniques include three-dimensional treatment planning, stereotactic patient positioning, and conformal delivery technology, such as intensity-modulated radiation therapy. The results of these efforts support the concept that higher doses of radiation can be delivered with equal or reduced normal tissue complications. The ability to deliver higher doses of radiation using proton radiation therapy should lead to improved local control and survival rates.

PHYSICAL ASPECTS OF PROTONS

Protons have comparable biologic effects in tissue relative to high-energy x-rays used in conventional radiation therapy. Evidence of this comes from the fact that the relative biologic effectiveness (RBE) of protons is approximately 1.1. The RBE of a proton beam is the ratio of the dose required to produce a specified effect using a reference radiation, usually cobalt 60 photons, to the proton dose required to produce the same effect. Most recent studies have reported RBE values for clinical protons in the range of 1.0 to 1.25.[1–3] Therefore, the advantage of proton radiation therapy is because of the superiority of the physical dose distributions compared with those for conventional therapy beams, rather than a biologic advantage.

A proton loses its energy in tissue through coulombic interactions with electrons, although a small fraction of energy is transferred through nuclear collisions. The energy loss per unit path length is relatively small and constant until near the end of the proton range, where the residual energy is lost over a short distance, resulting in a steep rise in the absorbed dose (energy absorbed per unit mass). This portion of the particle track, where energy is rapidly lost over a short distance, is known as the *Bragg peak* (see the curve labeled "Unmodulated Proton Beam" in Fig. 65-1). In physical terms, the magnitude of the transfer of energy to tissue per unit path length traversed by the protons is inversely proportional to the square of the proton velocity. The initial low-dose region in the depth-dose curve, before the Bragg peak, is referred to as the *plateau of the dose distribution* and is 30% to 40% of the maximum dose.

The Bragg peak is too narrow to treat any but the smallest of targets. For irradiation of larger targets, the beam energy is modulated to widen the Bragg peak, which is accomplished by superimposing several beams of closely spaced energies (ranges) to create a region of uniform dose over the depth of the target; these extended regions of uniform dose are called *spread-out Bragg peaks.* This is illustrated in Figure 65-1. For comparison, Figure 65-1 also shows the depth-dose curve for a 10-MV x-ray beam, an energy commonly used to treat deep-seated tumors. Note that the x-ray beam dose rises to a maximum value at relatively shallow depths, then falls off exponentially as depth increases. This fundamental difference in energy loss in tissue leads to superior dose distributions with protons.

The physical superiority of proton dose distributions is illustrated for the treatment of a paranasal sinus cancer (Fig. 65-2) and a large Ewing's sarcoma of the pelvis (Fig. 65-3). In this comparison, intensity-modulated x-ray therapy and intensity-modulated proton therapy are used. Both x-ray and proton treatment plans of the paranasal sinus make use of multiple beam portals and identical constraints. The two treatment plans are designed to provide equal doses of 76 Gy to the target volume. The differences in the two plans are shown in the lower

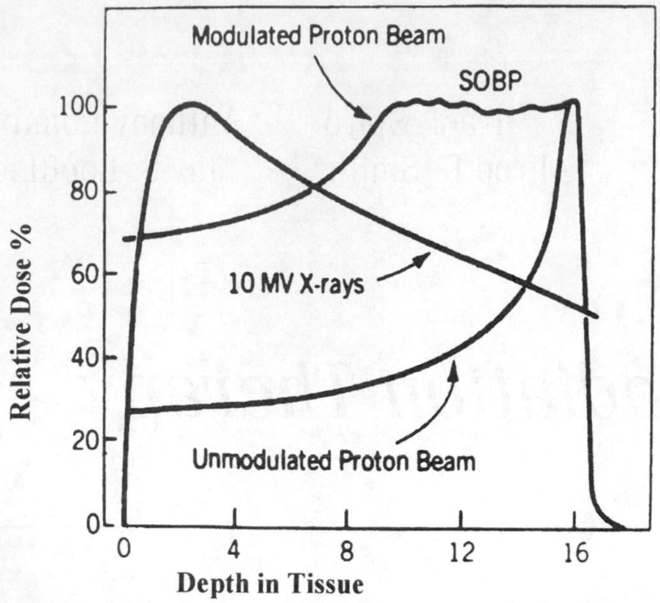

FIGURE 65-1. Depth dose curves (relative percent dose vs. depth in tissue) for an unmodulated proton beam (Bragg peak), a modulated proton peak (spread-out Bragg peak; SOBP), and 10-MV x-rays.

panels of Figure 65-2. This illustration reveals that x-rays deliver an additional 5 to 15 Gy throughout the brain. In the region of the right eye, which is magnified, the x-ray plan delivers up to 40 Gy more than the proton plan. The constraint on the right eye retina was 50 Gy. Had this been reduced, the x-ray dose would have been lower in this region, but at the expense of increased dose elsewhere or greater dose inhomogeneity in the target. This comparison illustrates that protons can be made to stop sharply beyond a target volume, sparing a critical structure distal to the target.

The second example is a Ewing's sarcoma of the ilium in an 18-year-old man as shown in the transverse computed tomography images in Figure 65-3. The x-ray plan delivers greater dose to the anterior small bowel and midline structures, such as the bladder, prostate, and large bowel. This plan also dispels the commonly held misconception that protons only offer significant advantages over x-rays for small treatment volumes. The effects of excess dose outside of the target volume are not well understood, although late effects of radiation do not occur in unirradiated tissues. Such excess radiation may also be important in the acute tolerance to treatment as well as the tolerance to combined treatment with chemotherapy and radiation. These two examples illustrate the superiority of protons in treating both small and large targets.

PROTON BEAM RADIATION TREATMENT: HISTORICAL NOTE

In 1946, Robert Wilson proposed that proton beams would provide superior dose distributions and should be considered for clinical radiation treatment. Initial efforts were directed at intracranial targets and used single-dose protocols. The first treatments using proton or helium ion beams were at the University of California at Berkeley (1955), University of Uppsala, Sweden (1957), Massachusetts General Hospital (MGH; 1961), Physics Research Institute, Dubna, Russia (1964), and the Institute for Experimental and Theoretical Physics, Moscow (1969). As of 1999, approximately 24,500 patients have received part or all of their radiation treatment by proton beams (for a historical review, see ref. 4). Today 19 proton treatment centers are established worldwide. Only one prospective randomized trial reporting on the efficacy of proton beam radiation therapy versus photon therapy has been published.[5]

The proton treatment program at MGH began in 1961. It was led by the neurosurgical group of W. Sweet and R. Kjellberg using the 160-MeV cyclotron in the department of physics at Harvard University. Their targets were principally pituitary adenomas, arteriovenous malformations, and other benign intracranial neoplasms and were treated by single-dose protocol. In January 1974, the MGH department of radiation oncology began a program of fractionated proton treatment. This clinical research program represents an active collaboration between the Harvard Cyclotron Laboratory (HCL), the Massachusetts Eye and Ear Infirmary, the Harvard Medical School, and MGH.

CLINICAL RESULTS

PROSTATE CARCINOMA

Investigators at MGH completed a phase III trial comparing 67.2 Gy of photons versus 75.6 Cobolt Grey Equivalent (CGE) using a conformal perineal proton boost.[5] From 1982 through 1992, 202 patients with T3–T4 prostate cancer received 50.4 Gy by four-field photons. Patients then received either 25.2 CGE with conformal protons or a 16.8 Gy photon boost. No differences were found in overall survival, total recurrence-free survival, or local recurrence-free survival in the two groups. The local recurrence-free survival rate at 7 years for patients with poorly differentiated (Gleason 9 and 10) tumors was 85% on the proton arm and 37% on the photon arm. Grade 1 and 2 rectal bleeding was higher in the proton arm (32% vs. 12%), as was urethral stricture (19% vs. 8%). In conclusion, dose escalation to 75.6 CGE by conformal proton boost led to increased late radiation sequelae, but not to increased total survival in any subgroup. However, there was an improved local recurrence-free survival in patients with poorly differentiated tumors.

Based on the results of this trial, the Proton Radiation Oncology Group (PROG) 95-09 was initiated. Participants in the trial were MGH and Loma Linda University (LLU) Medical Center. PROG 95-09 is a randomized phase III trial using conformal photons with proton boost in early-stage prostate cancer. The study was proposed because long-term follow-up of T1–T2 irradiated patients demonstrated biochemical disease-free survival rates of 50%, 35%, and 20% for well, moderate, and poorly differentiated tumors, respectively. This study randomized patients to two different proton boost dose levels, with patients receiving a total dose of either 79.2 Gy or 70.2 Gy. Patients deemed to be a low risk for local failure (prostate-specific antigen less than 4 ng/ml) and patients with high risk for distant disease (prostate-specific antigen greater than 15 ng/ml and/or positive lymph nodes) are not likely to benefit from this dose escalation and thus were excluded. This randomized trial was designed to

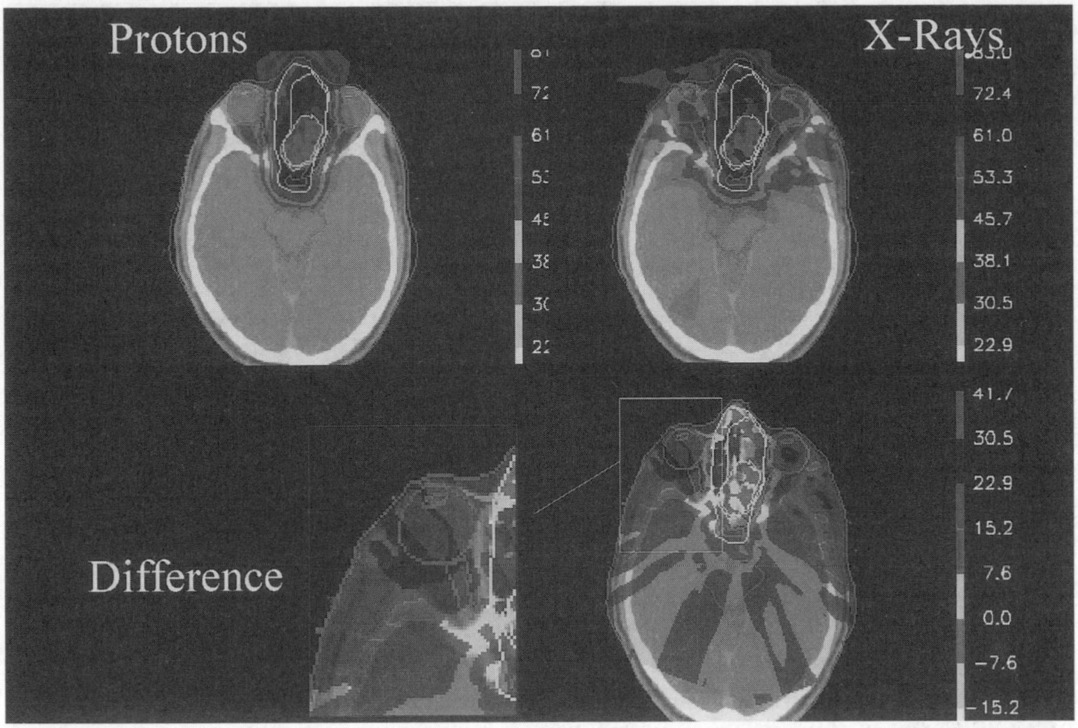

FIGURE 65-2. Paranasal sinus tumor treated with intensity-modulated proton therapy (upper left) and intensity modulated x ray therapy (upper right). The difference in the two plans is shown in the lower right panel and magnified in the lower left panel. Note the additional 5 to 15 Gy that the brain receives and the increased dose to the right eye. The plans were developed by one of the authors (A. L.) at the Paul Scherrer Institute in Villigen, Switzerland. (See Color Fig. 65-2 in the CD-ROM and on the Web at www.LWWoncology.com.)

detect a 20% increase in freedom from local failure and biochemical relapse at 5 years. With 390 patients entered, this trial is now closed and is awaiting analysis.

The results of the LLU experience in early-stage prostate cancer have been published.[6] Three hundred and nineteen men with T1–T2b tumors were treated with 74 to 75 CGE protons, or combined protons and x-rays. The overall 5-year biochemical disease-free survival rate was 88%. No severe treatment-related morbidity was observed.

UVEAL MELANOMA

As of October 1998, a total of 2586 patients have been treated for uveal melanoma at MGH with protons in collaboration with the Massachusetts Eye and Ear Infirmary.[7] Patients were treated with 70 CGE in five fractions over 7 to 9 days. The 5-year actuarial local control rate is 96% for all sites within the globe, with an 80% survival. The probability of eye retention at 5 years was estimated to be 90% for the entire group and 97%, 93%, and 78% for patients with small, intermediate, and large tumors, respectively. Independent risk factors for enucleation were involvement of the ciliary body, tumor height more than 8 mm, and distance between the posterior tumor edge and the fovea. These results compare favorably with local control rates of 89% reported with protons in Nice, France.[8]

Because some patients have experienced deteriorating vision after doses of 70 CGE, a randomized trial compared 50 and 70 CGE for small- and intermediate-size lesions located within 6 mm of the optic disc or macula. This dose-reduction study was completed in June 1994 with accrual of 188 patients. Interim analysis based on patients followed through September 1997 (median follow-up 60 months) suggested no reduction in either local control or survival rate. No marked improvement in visual outcome or complications has been observed. However, visual field analysis does show a smaller mean defect in the patients randomized to 50 CGE.[7]

A study has been completed comparing iodine 125 plaques to helium ions by the group at University of California, San Francisco (UCSF) and Lawrence Berkeley Laboratories (LBL).[9] Patients with melanomas less than 10 mm in height and less than 15 mm in diameter were randomized by the UCSF/LBL group to receive either 70 CGE in five treatments with helium ions, or 70 Gy to the tumor apex with ^{125}Iodine plaque brachytherapy. Local control was 100% in those patients treated with helium ions compared with 87% in those patients treated with ^{125}I plaques.

SARCOMAS OF THE SKULL BASE AND CERVICAL SPINE

Treatment of patients with a sarcoma of the skull base is challenging because of the large number of critical structures penetrating the skull base and the proximity of these tumors to the brain stem and optic pathways. These factors have limited the success of conventional photon radiation therapy and surgery. The results of the MGH series has been analyzed.[10] One hundred and sixty-nine patients with chordoma and 165 patients with chondrosarcoma were treated with protons between 1975 and 1998. The 5-year actuarial local control rates for skull-base chondrosarcomas was 98% and was 73% for chordoma patients. For cervical spine patients, local

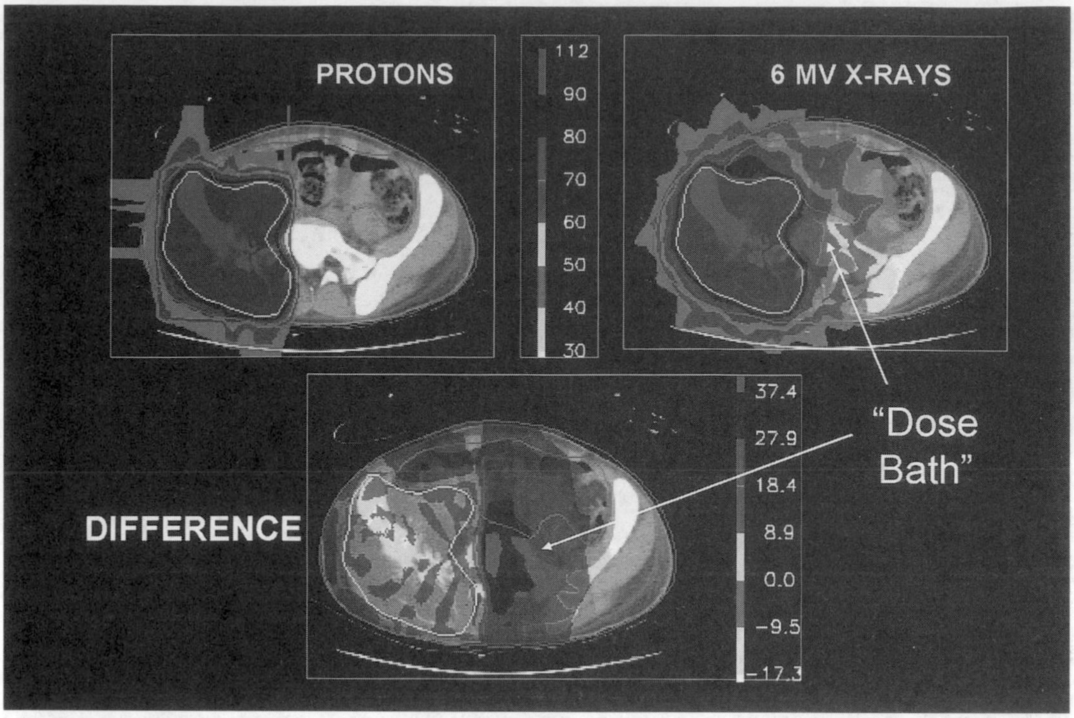

FIGURE 65-3. Ewing's sarcoma of the right pelvis treated with intensity-modulated proton therapy (upper left) and intensity-modulated x-ray therapy (upper right). The lower panel shows the difference in the two plans. Note the additional 8 to 28 Gy that the small bowel, midline structures, and contralateral sacrum receive. The plans were developed by one of the authors (A. L.) at the Paul Scherrer Institute in Villigen, Switzerland. (See Color Fig. 65-3 in the CD-ROM and on the Web at www.LWWoncology.com.)

control rates were 54% and 48% for chondrosarcoma and chordoma patients, respectively. The LLU proton experience for skull-base tumors showed 5-year actuarial local control rates of 75% for chondrosarcoma and 59% for chordoma.[11] The MGH results compare favorably with the experience (median dose 50 Gy) from Princess Margaret Hospital in Toronto of 55%.[12]

OPTIC PATHWAY GLIOMA

Seven patients with optic pathway glioma were treated at LLU between 1992 and 1997.[13] Tumor volumes ranged from 3.9 cm^3 to 127 cm^3. At a median follow-up of 37 months, all patients were locally controlled. A reduction in tumor volume was seen in three patients, and tumor volumes remained stable in four patients. Visual acuity remained stable in patients who presented with useful vision. Proton radiation therapy was shown to reduce the dose to the contralateral optic nerve by 47%, compared with three-dimensional photon techniques.

ASTROCYTOMA

Between 1993 and 1998, 48 patients were treated for nonresectable grade II and III intracranial tumors at the Center for Proton Therapy in d'Orsay, France.[14] Mean tumor doses ranged from 63 to 67 Gy at 1.8 Gy per fraction. With a median follow-up of 18 months, local control was 97% (33 of 34 cases) and 43% (6 of 14 cases) for nonparenchymal and parenchymal lesions, respectively.

Twenty-three patients with the diagnosis of glioblastoma multiforme were treated to 90 CGE with twice-daily protons.[15] Median survival time was 20 months from the date of surgery and 18.6 months from the start of radiation treatment. Actuarial survival at 2 and 3 years was 34% and 18%, respectively. Sixteen of the 23 patients were judged to have had tumor progression. Of these 16, 15 had progression in tissues that received 60 to 70 CGE (or less). In only one patient was there evidence of failure within the 90-CGE volume. All patients developed new areas of gadolinium enhancement during the follow-up period. Pathologic material was examined in 15 patients. Radiation necrosis only was demonstrated in seven patients. The survival rate for this group of 23 patients is comparable to that of the best brachytherapy or radiosurgery series. However, a trend towards larger and less accessible tumors was seen in this patient population. This regimen has achieved an apparent high frequency of tumor eradication in the 90-CGE volume, although toxicity has been significant.

BENIGN MENINGIOMA

Between 1981 and 1996, 46 patients with incompletely resected or recurrent benign meningioma were treated at the HCL with a combined proton-photon technique. The median dose to the tumor volume was 59.0 CGE. Overall survival at 5 and 10 years was 93% and 77%, respectively, and recurrence-free survival at 5 and 10 years was 100% and 88%. Three patients developed local tumor recurrence at 61, 95, and 125 months, although no patient died from recurrent disease. Complications have included focal brain stem necrosis in two patients and grade 3 memory loss in another patient. In four patients who developed ophthalmologic toxicity, the maximum dose to the optic structures was 58.4, 59.2, 59.3, and 63.0 CGE. Unilateral sensineural hearing loss developed in two patients and endocrinopathy in 11 patients.

Nineteen patients with inextirpable skull-base meningiomas were treated at the Svedberg Laboratory in Uppsala, Sweden, with 24 Gy in four fractions. With a minimum follow-up time of 36 months, no patients have experienced disease progression.[16]

PARANASAL SINUS CARCINOMA

Between 1991 and 1996, 32 patients with carcinomas of the paranasal sinuses were treated on an accelerated-dose proton-photon protocol.[17] The stage distribution was T3 in two cases and T4 in 30 cases, and all were N0 and M0. Four patients had had a gross total resection, whereas the others had had only a biopsy (7) or subtotal resection (19). The median observation period was 2.7 years. Actuarial disease-specific survival at 3 years was 62%. Ten deaths—three with intercurrent disease and seven with metastatic tumor—have been reported. Three patients developed local failure. The 3-year actuarial local control rate was 89%. Late toxicity has included temporal lobe necrosis in three patients, although all have regressed with steroid treatment. Three patients have required surgical soft tissue repair. These local-control results appear to constitute a substantial gain over conventional surgery and photon treatment techniques.

HEPATOCELLULAR CARCINOMA

Investigators at Tsukuba University, Japan, have reported impressive long-term control and survival results in patients with primary hepatocellular carcinoma treated with proton radiation therapy.[18] The dose per fraction was 4 Gy and the mean total dose was 72 Gy. The 7-year local control and survival results in this series of 122 patients were reported as 94% and 27%. Proton therapy did not cause clinically symptomatic changes in liver function.[19] The only notable change observed was a transient increase in liver transaminases.

LUNG CARCINOMA

Between 1994 and 1998, 37 patients with medically inoperable stage I–IIIa lung cancer were treated at LLU with conformal photons and protons.[20] Patients received either photons and protons or protons alone to 73.8 CGE over 5 weeks. Patients with poor lung function received 51 CGE in ten fractions over 2 weeks to the gross tumor volume. With a median follow-up time of 14 months, disease-free survival at 2 years was 63% for all patients and 86% for stage I patients.

PROTON RADIOSURGERY

Between 1961 and 1993, 2987 patients were treated with single-fraction proton therapy (proton radiosurgery). This effort was led by the late Dr. Raymond Kjellberg, a neurosurgeon at MGH. The majority of patients were treated for inoperable arteriovenous malformations and pituitary adenomas.[21] Beginning in 1991, a second proton radiosurgery technique was developed using a patient positioning system capable of stereotactic alignment for radiosurgery (STAR).[22] This system was developed because of the inherent restrictions of the fixed horizontal beam at the HCL. The STAR unit was based on target coordinates obtained directly from computed tomography, magnetic resonance imaging, or angiography. Early results with arteriovenous malformations, acoustic neuromas, and brain metastases are comparable with those produced by other stereotactic technologies (Gamma Knife, linear accelerator, Elecktra Corporation, Stockholm, Sweden).

DESIGN OF CLINICAL TRIALS USING PROTON BEAMS

The fixed horizontal, 160-MeV HCL proton beam, with an effective treatment depth of 15.9 cm, constrained the number of sites that could effectively be treated. For this reason, past efforts have focused on intracranial targets, skull-base tumors, head and neck tumors, eye tumors, and prostatic carcinoma. The Northeast Proton Therapy Center (NPTC) at MGH will have a more energetic beam (220 MeV) capable of treating to depths of 32 cm, a gantry-based delivery system, and state-of-the-art patient positioners. These improvements will increase the numbers of patients that can be treated and will facilitate treatment at a number of new sites, including lung, rectum, and liver. In addition, a major effort will be placed on developing protocols for the treatment of pediatric malignancies.

Several examples of the potential advantages of the NPTC proton beam have been documented. Medulloblastoma is a pediatric malignancy that occurs in the posterior fossa and can spread through the cerebrospinal fluid to seed in the cranial cavity and the spinal axis, requiring radiation treatment to the cranial contents as well as the spinal axis. As a result, these patients frequently experience hearing, neurologic, neuropsychological, endocrine, musculoskeletal, cardiac, and fertility deficits because of the combined chemotherapy and radiation treatment. Figure 65-4 illustrates the dramatic reduction in the volume of normal tissue irradiated in the thorax (heart, lung, and esophagus) seen with protons. In addition, similar reductions would be seen in the abdomen (stomach, small bowel, pancreas, and liver) and pelvis (ovaries, bladder, and bowel). Also, not illustrated here, the dose to the middle ear can be reduced by 50% using photon techniques. Another example for which protons would reduce treatment-related morbidity is the treatment of rectal carcinoma. Current treatment of patients with stage II and III rectal carcinoma includes surgical resection, pelvic radiation, and infusional 5-fluorouracil. Significant treatment-related morbidity results from this regimen because of the irradiation of large volumes of normal bowel and bladder with conventional photon radiation techniques. Proton beam treatment allows for irradiation of the target lymph nodes with minimal dose to the small bowel and the bladder (Fig. 65-5).

The reduction in normal tissue irradiation with protons has significant implications for combined radiation and chemotherapy protocols. Even when modest doses of radiation are prescribed, as in the case of rectal carcinoma, proton radiation should improve tolerance to the combined regimen. This should result in fewer dose-limiting toxicities and improved treatment intensity and

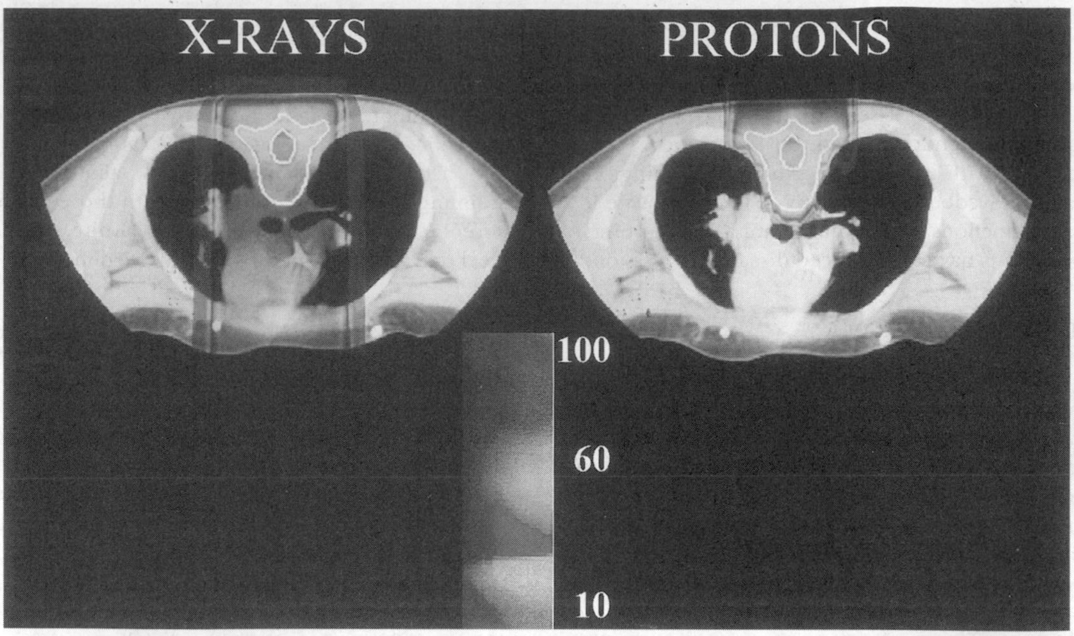

FIGURE 65-4. Comparison of x-ray and proton single posterior portals for craniospinal irradiation in medulloblastoma. The x-ray plan results in exit irradiation of the heart, lung, carina, esophagus (not visualized), and anterior soft tissues. (See Color Fig. 65-4 in the CD-ROM and on the Web at www.LWWoncology.com.)

treatment compliance, which may allow for higher chemotherapy doses and, ultimately, lead to higher cancer control rates.

CONCLUSIONS AND FUTURE DIRECTIONS

The history of radiation oncology has demonstrated that major improvements in local control have occurred because of improvements in dose distributions. Proton radiation therapy represents one of the most precise and sophisticated treatment delivery systems in radiation oncology. Proton therapy will also make use of some of the same improvements that have developed in conformal x-ray therapy (intensity modulation, rotational delivery, multileaf collimation, stereotactic localization) to further improve the dose distribution of protons. Such improvements will allow for continued escalation in tumor doses while minimizing dose to normal, nontarget tissues. With the installation of a high-energy (220 MeV) hospital-based proton therapy facility at the NPTC at MGH and the existing facility at LLU Medical Center, the technology exists for continuing clinical research in proton radiation therapy. Efforts for the first decade of the twenty-first century will include: (1) comparing intensity-modulated x-ray therapy and intensity-modulated proton therapy, (2) assessing the gains in treatment intensity in combined modality therapy with protons, and (3) assessing the impact of proton therapy on improving cure rates in pediatric cancer and reducing late effects.

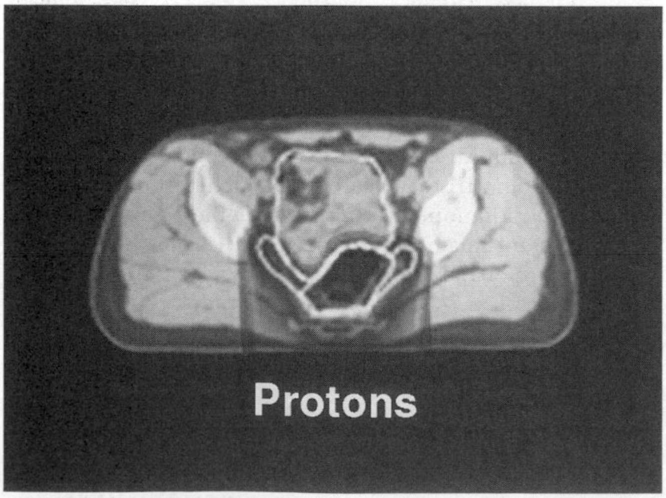

FIGURE 65-5. Posterior proton portal for the treatment of rectal carcinoma. The tumor bed and internal iliac lymph nodes are targeted, whereas the small bowel and anterior soft tissues are not treated. (See Color Fig. 65-5 in the CD-ROM and on the Web at www.LWWoncology.com.)

REFERENCES

1. Tepper J, Verhey L, Goitein M, Suit HD, Koehler AM. *In vivo* determinations of RBE in a high energy modulated proton beam using normal tissue reactions and fractionated dose schedules. *Int J Radiat Oncol Biol Phys* 1977;2:1115.
2. Urano M, Verhey LJ, Goitein M, et al. Relative biological effectiveness of modulated proton beams in various murine tissues. *Int J Radiat Oncol Biol Phys* 1984;10:509.
3. Gerweck LE, Kozin SV. Relative biological effectiveness of proton beams in clinical therapy [Review]. *Radiother Oncol* 1999;50:135.
4. Raju MR. Proton radiobiology, radiosurgery and radiotherapy [Review]. *Int J Radiat Oncol Biol Phys* 1995;67:237.
5. Shipley WU, Verhey LJ, Munzenrider JE, et al. Advanced prostate cancer: the results of a randomized comparative trial of high dose irradiation boosting with conformal protons compared with conventional dose irradiation using photons alone [see comments]. *Int J Radiat Oncol Biol Phys* 1995;32:3.
6. Slater JD, Rossi CJJ, Yonemoto LT, et al. Conformal proton therapy for early-stage prostate cancer. *Urology* 1999;53:978.
7. Munzenrider JE. Proton therapy for uveal melanomas and other eye lesions. *Strahlentherapie und Onkologie* 1999;175[Suppl 2]:68.
8. Courdi A, Caujolle JP, Grange JD, et al. Results of proton therapy of uveal melanomas treated in Nice. *Int J Radiat Oncol Biol Phys* 1999;45:5.
9. Char DH, Quivey JM, Castro JR, Kroll S, Phillips T. Helium ions versus iodine 125 brachytherapy in the management of uveal melanoma. A prospective, randomized, dynamically balanced trial. *Ophthalmology* 1993;100:1547.
10. Munzenrider JE, Liebsch NJ. Proton therapy for tumors of the skull base [Review]. *Strahlentherapie und Onkologie* 1999;175[Suppl 2]:57.

11. Hug EB, Loredo LN, Slater JD, et al. Proton radiation therapy for chordomas and chondrosarcomas of the skull base. *J Neurosurg* 1999;91:432.
12. Catton C, O'Sullivan B, Bell R, et al. Chordoma: long-term follow-up after radical photon irradiation. *Radiother Oncol* 1996;41:67.
13. Fuss M, Hug E, Schaefer RA, et al. Proton Radiation Therapy (PRT) for pediatric optic pathway gliomas: comparison with 3D planned conventional photons and a standard photon technique. *Int J Radiat Oncol Biol Phys* 1999;45:1117.
14. Habrand JL, Haie-Meder C, Rey A, et al. [Radiotherapy using a combination of photons and protons for locally aggressive intracranial tumors. Preliminary results of protocol CPO 94-C1]. *Cancer Radiother* 1999;3:480.
15. Fitzek MM, Thornton AF, Rabinov JD, et al. Accelerated fractionated proton/photon irradiation to 90 cobalt gray equivalent for glioblastoma multiforme: results of a phase II prospective trial. *J Neurosurg* 1999;91:251.
16. Gudjonsson O, Blomquist E, Nyberg G, et al. Stereotactic irradiation of skull base meningiomas with high energy protons. *Acta Neurochir* (Wien) 1999;141:933.
17. Thornton AF, Fitzek MM, Varvarres M, et al. Accelerated, hyperfractionated proton/photon irradiation for advanced paranasal sinus cancer: results of a prospective phase I-II study. *Int J Radiat Oncol Biol Phys* 1998;42:222(abst).
18. Matsuzaki Y, Osuga T, Chiba T, et al. New, effective treatment using proton irradiation for unresectable hepatocellular carcinoma. *Intern Med* 1995;34:302.
19. Tsuji H, Okumura T, Maruhashi A, et al. [Dose-volume histogram analysis of patients with hepatocellular carcinoma regarding changes in liver function after proton therapy] [Japanese]. *Nippon Igaku Hoshasen Gakkai Zasshi* 1995;55:322.
20. Bush DA, Slater JD, Bonnet R, et al. Proton-beam radiotherapy for early-stage lung cancer. *Chest* 1999;116:1313.
21. Amin-Hanjani S, Ogilvy CS, Candia GJ, Lyons S, Chapman PH. Stereotactic radiosurgery for cavernous malformations: Kjellberg's experience with proton beam therapy in 98 cases at the Harvard cyclotron [see comments]. *Neurosurgery* 1998;42:1229.
22. Harsh G, Loeffler JS, Thornton A, et al. Stereotactic proton radiosurgery. *Neurosurg Clin North Am* 1999;10:243.

INDEX

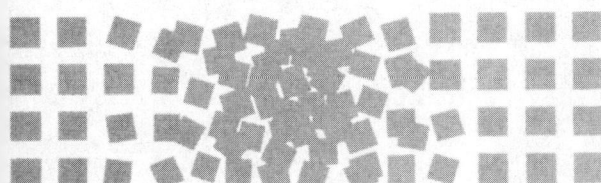

Index

Page numbers followed by *f* indicate figures; those followed by *t* indicate tables.

B

F

H

L

M

O

S

V

W

X

Y

Z